HURST'S
THE HEART

NOTICE

NINTH EDITION

HURST'S
THE HEART
ARTERIES AND VEINS

Editors

R. WAYNE ALEXANDER, M.D., Ph.D.

R. Bruce Logue Professor of Medicine
Director, Division of Cardiology
Department of Medicine
Emory University School of Medicine
Chief of Cardiology, Emory Hospital and Emory Clinic
Atlanta, Georgia

ROBERT C. SCHLANT, M.D.

Professor of Medicine (Cardiology)
Emory University School of Medicine
Chief of Cardiology, Grady Memorial Hospital
Atlanta, Georgia

VALENTIN FUSTER, M.D., Ph.D.

Director, Cardiovascular Institute
Richard Gorlin, M.D. / Heart Research Foundation
Professor of Cardiology
Dean for Academic Affairs
Vice Chairman, Department of Medicine
The Mount Sinai Medical Center
New York, New York

Associate Editors

ROBERT A. O'ROURKE, M.D.

Charles Conrad Brown Distinguished Professor
   in Cardiovascular Disease
University of Texas Health Science Center at San Antonio
San Antonio, Texas

ROBERT ROBERTS, M.D.

Don W. Chapman Professor of Medicine and Chief
   of Cardiology
Professor of Cell Biology
Director, Bugher Foundation Center for Molecular Biology
Baylor College of Medicine
Houston, Texas

EDMUND H. SONNENBLICK, M.D.

Edmond J. Safra Distinguished University Professor
   of Medicine
Chief Emeritus, Division of Cardiology
The Albert Einstein College of Medicine
Bronx, New York

McGRAW-HILL
Health Professions Division

New York St. Louis San Francisco Auckland Bogotá Caracas Lisbon London Madrid
Mexico City Milan Montreal New Delhi San Juan Singapore Sydney Tokyo Toronto

McGraw-Hill

A Division of The McGraw·Hill Companies

Hurst's THE HEART
Ninth Edition

Copyright © 1998, 1994, 1990, 1986, 1982, 1978, 1974, 1970, 1966 by *The McGraw-Hill Companies, Inc.* All rights reserved. Printed in the United States of America. Except as permitted under the United States Copyright Act of 1976, no part of this publication may be reproduced or distributed in any form or by any means, or stored in a data base or retrieval system, without the prior written permission of the publisher.

1234567890 DOWDOW 9987

ISBN 0-07-057717-X (Single vol. ed.)
      0-07-912951-X (2-vol. set ed.)
      0-07-057718-8 (Vol. 1)
      0-07-057719-6 (Vol. 2)

FOREIGN LANGUAGE EDITION
Italian (Eighth Edition)—McGraw-Hill Libri Italia srl © 1995

This book was set in Times Roman by Monotype Composition Company, Inc.
The editors were Joseph Hefta and Muza Navrozov.
The production supervisor was Helene G. Landers.
The text and cover were designed by Marsha Cohen / Parallelogram Graphics.
The index was prepared by Barbara Littlewood.
R. R. Donnelley and Sons Company was printer and binder.

This book is printed on acid-free paper.

Cover illustration reproduced with permission from S. B. King and J. S. Douglas, "Coronary Arteriography and Angioplasty," copyright © 1985, McGraw-Hill, N.Y. Illustration by Michael Budowick, Medical Artist, Emory University School of Medicine, Office of Medical Illustration.

Library of Congress Cataloging-in-Publication Data

Hurst's the heart, arteries and veins / editors, R. Wayne Alexander,
  Robert C. Schlant, Valentin Fuster ; associate editors, Robert
  A. O'Rourke, Robert Roberts, Edmund H. Sonnenblick. — 9th ed.
    p.   cm.
  Rev. ed. of: The heart, arteries, and veins. 8th ed. © 1994.
  Includes bibliographical references and index.
  ISBN 0-07-912951-X (2 vol. set ed.). — ISBN 0-07-057719-6 (v. 2).
— ISBN 0-07-057718-8 (v. 1). — ISBN 0-07-057717-X (1 vol. ed.)
    1. Cardiovascular system—Diseases. 2. Cardiology.
I. Alexander, R. Wayne. II. Schlant, Robert C., date.
III. Fuster, Valentin. IV. Title: Heart, arteries and veins.
[DNLM: 1. Cardiovascular Diseases. WG 100 H9662 1998]
RC667.H88   1998
616.1—DC21 :
DNLM/DLC
for Library of Congress

To

Jane, Kate, Melissa, and David (R.W.A.)
Mia and Stephanie (R.C.S.)
Maria, Silvia, and Pablo (V.F.)
Suzann, Michael, Kevin, Sean, Katie, and Ryan (R.A.O.)
Donna, Brandon, and Allison (R.R.)
and
Linda, Emily and Charlotte (E.H.S.).

CONTENTS

CONTRIBUTORS*

Masood Akhtar, M.D. [29]

Professor of Medicine
Chief, Cardiovascular Disease Section
University of Wisconsin Medical School
Milwaukee Clinical Campus
Milwaukee, Wisconsin

James K. Alexander, M.D. [93]

Professor of Medicine (Cardiology)
Baylor College of Medicine
Houston, Texas

R. Wayne Alexander, M.D., Ph.D.
  [4, 44, 45, 47]

R. Bruce Logue Professor of Medicine
Director, Division of Cardiology
Department of Medicine
Emory University School of Medicine
Chief of Cardiology, Emory Hospital and Emory Clinic
Atlanta, Georgia

Joseph S. Alpert, M.D. [60]

Robert S. and Irene P. Flinn Chair of Medicine
Head, Department of Medicine
University of Arizona College of Medicine
Tucson, Arizona

W. Banks Anderson, Jr., M.D. [11]

Professor of Ophthalmology
Duke University Eye Center
Durham, North Carolina

Robert J. Bache, M.D. [43]

Professor of Medicine
Department of Medicine
Division of Cardiology
University of Minnesota School of Medicine
Minneapolis, Minnesota

Arthur C. Beall, Jr., M.D. [98]

Professor of Surgery
Baylor College of Medicine
Houston, Texas

Gerald J. Berry, M.D. [25]

Associate Professor of Pathology
Director of Cardiac Pathology
Stanford University School of Medicine
Stanford, California

Margaret E. Billingham, M.B., B.S.,
  F.R.C. Path. [25]

Professor of Pathology Emerita
Stanford University School of Medicine
Stanford, California

Daniel G. Blanchard, M.D. [14]

Associate Professor of Medicine
University of California at San Diego School of Medicine
Director, Noninvasive Cardiac Laboratories
University of California at San Diego Medical Center
San Diego, California

Teresa J. Bohlmeyer, M.D. [73]

Assistant Professor of Medicine
University of Colorado Health Sciences Center
Denver, Colorado
Staff Pathologist, Sterling Regional Medical Center
Sterling, Colorado

Harisios Boudoulas, M.D. [35]

Professor of Medicine and Pharmacy
Division of Cardiology
The Ohio State University Medical Center
Director, Overstreet Teaching and Research Laboratory
Division of Cardiology
The Ohio State University College of Medicine
Columbus, Ohio

Michael R. Bristow, M.D., Ph.D. [73]

Professor of Medicine
Head, Division of Cardiology
University of Colorado Health Sciences Center
Denver, Colorado

*Numbers in brackets refer to chapters written or cowritten by the contributor.

Bruce H. Brundage, M.D. [18]

Professor of Medicine and Radiological Sciences
UCLA School of Medicine
Chief, Division of Cardiology
Harbor-UCLA Medical Center
Scientific Director, Saint John's Cardiovascular
   Research Center
Torrance, California

Peter M. Buttrick, M.D. [95]

Professor of Medicine and Physiology
Chief of the Section of Cardiology
University of Illinois at Chicago
Chicago, Illinois

Louis R. Caplan, M.D. [99]

Professor and Chairman
Department of Neurology
Tufts University School of Medicine
Professor of Medicine
Tufts University School of Medicine
Neurologist-in-Chief, New England Medical Center
Boston, Massachusetts

Agustin Castellanos, M.D. [12, 27, 34]

Professor of Medicine
Director, Clinical Electrophysiology
University of Miami School of Medicine
Miami, Florida

Nisha Chibber Chandra, M.D. [37]

Professor of Medicine
Johns Hopkins University School of Medicine
Director, Coronary Intensive Care Unit
Johns Hopkins Bayview Medical Center
Baltimore, Maryland

Melvin D. Cheitlin, M.D. [79]

Professor of Medicine Emeritus
University of California, San Francisco
Former Chief of Cardiology, San Francisco
   General Hospital
San Francisco, California

James T. T. Chen, M.D. [13]

Professor of Radiology
Department of Radiology
Duke University Medical Center
Durham, North Carolina

Michael B. Clark, M.D. [104]

Associate Medical Director
Metropolitan Life Insurance Company
New York, New York

Stephen D. Clements, Jr., M.D. [51]

Professor of Medicine (Cardiology)
Emory University School of Medicine
Atlanta, Georgia

Denton A. Cooley, M.D. [86]

Clinical Professor of Surgery
University of Texas Medical School
Surgeon-in-Chief, Texas Heart Institute
President, Texas Heart Institute
Houston, Texas

Ralph B. D'Agostino, Sr., Ph.D. [1]

Professor of Mathematics/Statistics and Public Health
Director, Statistics and Consulting Unit
Co-Director, Biostatistics Graduate Program
Boston University
Boston, Massachusetts

James Eugene Dalen, M.D., M.P.H. [60]

Vice President for Health Sciences
Dean, College of Medicine,
University of Arizona College of Medicine
Tucson, Arizona

Michael J. Davies, M.D., F.R.C.P., F.R.C.Path. [40]

British Heart Foundation Professor of Cardiovascular
   Pathology
St. George's Hospital Medical School
University of London
London, England

John E. Deanfield, M.B., B.Ch., F.R.C.P. [71]

Professor of Cardiology
University of London
Consultant Cardiologist, Great Ormond Street Hospital
   for Children
London, England

Michael E. DeBakey, M.D. [98]

Chancellor Emeritus, Baylor College of Medicine
Olga Keith Wiess Professor of Surgery and Distinguished
   Service Professor
Baylor College of Medicine
Director, The DeBakey Heart Center
Houston, Texas

Anthony N. DeMaria, M.D. [14]

Professor of Medicine and Chief
Division of Cardiology
University of California, San Diego
San Diego, California

Regis A. DeSilva, M.D., M.B. [32]

Assistant Professor of Medicine
Harvard Medical School
Physician, Cardiology Division
Beth Israel Deaconess Medical Center
Boston, Massachusetts

Thomas F. Dodson, M.D. [101]

Associate Professor of Surgery
Program Director and Vice Chairman for Education
Department of Surgery
Emory University School of Medicine
Atlanta, Georgia

Gerald W. Dorn II, M.D. [6]

Associate Professor of Medicine and Pharmacology
    and Biophysics
University of Cincinnati Medical Center
Director, VA Cardiac Catheterization Laboratory
Cincinnati, Ohio

John S. Douglas, Jr., M.D. [16, 48]

Associate Professor of Medicine (Cardiology)
Emory University School of Medicine
Co-Director, Cardiac Catheterization Laboratory
Emory University Hospital
Atlanta, Georgia

David T. Durack, M.B., D.Phil. [82]

Worldwide Medical Director
Becton Dickinson Microbiology Systems
Baltimore, Maryland
Consulting Professor of Medicine
Duke University Medical Center
Durham, North Carolina

Victor J. Dzau, M.D. [9]

Hersey Professor of the Theory and Practice of Medicine
Harvard Medical School
Chairman, Department of Medicine
Director of Research and Physician-in-Chief
Brigham and Women's Hospital
Boston, Massachusetts

Kim A. Eagle, M.D. [83]

Professor of Internal Medicine
Senior Associate Chair
Department of Internal Medicine
Chief of Clinical Cardiology
Division of Cardiology
Co-Director, Heart Care Program
University of Michigan
Ann Arbor, Michigan

Jesse E. Edwards, M.D. [66]

Professor of Pathology
University of Minnesota
Minneapolis, Minnesota
Senior Consultant
Registry of Cardiovascular Disease of United Hospital
St. Paul, Minnesota

Robert L. Eisner, Ph.D. [17]

Associate Professor of Radiology
Emory University School of Medicine
Co-Director, Nuclear Cardiology
Crawford Long Hospital of Emory University
Atlanta, Georgia

Robert S. Eliot, M.D.† [89]

Clinical Professor of Medicine (Cardiology)
University of Nebraska College of Medicine
Omaha, Nebraska
Director, Institute of Stress Medicine
Jackson Hole, Wyoming

Erica Diana Engelstein, M.D. [36]

Assistant Professor of Medicine
Indiana University School of Medicine
Director of Electrophysiology Services
Richard L. Roudebush VA Medical Center
Indianapolis, Indiana

Maurice Enriquez-Sarano, M.D. [64]

Associate Professor of Medicine
Consultant, Cardiovascular Diseases and Internal Medicine
Mayo Medical School
Rochester, Minnesota

Stephen M. Factor, M.D. [43]

Professor of Pathology and Medicine (Cardiology)
Director of Pathology
Jacobi Medical Center
Albert Einstein College of Medicine
Bronx, New York

Alfred P. Fishman, M.D. [59]

William Maul Measey Professor of Medicine
University of Pennsylvania School of Medicine
Chairman, Department of Rehabilitation Medicine
University of Pennsylvania Medical Center
Philadelphia, Pennsylvania

†Deceased May 1996.

Gerald F. Fletcher, M.D. [15]

Professor of Medicine
Mayo Medical School
Senior Associate Consultant
Mayo Clinic
Jacksonville, Florida

Robert E. Foster, M.D. [19]

Cardiologist, Birmingham Heart Clinic
Birmingham, Alabama

Robert H. Franch, M.D. [16]

Professor of Medicine (Cardiology)
Emory University School of Medicine
Atlanta, Georgia

O. Howard Frazier, M.D. [86]

Chief, Cardiopulmonary Transplantation
Director, Surgical Research
Texas Heart Institute
Professor of Surgery and Director, Division
    of Thoracic Surgery
University of Texas Medical School at Houston
Clinical Professor
Department of Surgery, Baylor College of Medicine
Clinical Associate Professor of Surgery
Department of Thoracic Surgery
University of Texas M. D. Anderson Cancer Center
Houston, Texas

Michael D. Freed, M.D. [70]

Associate Professor of Pediatrics
Harvard Medical School
Senior Associate in Cardiology and Chief
    of Cardiology Services
Children's Hospital
Boston, Massachusetts

William T. Friedewald, M.D. [104]

Clinical Professor of Medicine and of Public Health
    (Epidemiology)
College of Physicians and Surgeons
    of Columbia University
Senior Vice-President and Chief Medical Advisor
Metropolitan Life Insurance Co.
New York, New York

Gottlieb C. Friesinger II, M.D. [38]

Betty and Jack Bailey Professor of Cardiology
Vanderbilt University School of Medicine
Nashville, Tennesee

William H. Frishman, M.D. [23, 54]

Professor and Associate Chairman
Albert Einstein College of Medicine/Montefiore
    Medical Center
Bronx, New York

Edward D. Frohlich, M.D. [56]

Vice President for Academic Affairs
Alton Ochsner Medical Foundation
Professor, Department of Medicine
    and Department of Physiology
Louisiana State University
Clinical Professor of Medicine and Adjunct Professor
    of Pharmacology
Tulane University
New Orleans, Louisiana

Robert L. Frye, M.D. [64]

Professor of Medicine
Rose M. and Maurice Eisenberg Professor of Medicine
Mayo Medical School
Chair, Department of Medicine
Mayo Clinic
Rochester, Minnesota

Valentin Fuster, M.D., Ph.D. [52]

Director, Cardiovascular Institute
Richard Gorlin, M.D. / Heart Research Foundation
Professor of Cardiology
Dean for Academic Affairs
Vice Chairman, Department of Medicine
The Mount Sinai Medical Center
New York, New York

Bernard J. Gersh, M.B., Ch.B., D.Phil., F.R.C.P. [71]

Professor of Medicine
Chief, Division of Cardiology
W. Proctor Harvey Teaching Professor of Cardiology
Georgetown University Medical Center
Washington, D.C.

Ray W. Gifford, Jr., M.D., M.S. [58]

Professor of Internal Medicine
The Ohio State University College of Medicine
Columbus, Ohio
Consultant, Department of Nephrology/Hypertension
Acting Chairman of the Office of Regional Health Affairs
    and Physician Outreach
Cleveland Clinic Foundation
Cleveland, Ohio

Edward M. Gilbert, M.D. [73]

Associate Professor of Medicine
Division of Cardiology
Director, Heart Failure Treatment Program
University of Utah School of Medicine
Salt Lake City, Utah

Emilio B. Gonzalez, M.D. [85]
Associate Professor of Medicine
Division of Rheumatology
Department of Medicine
Emory University School of Medicine
Chief, Rheumatology Service
Grady Memorial Hospital
Atlanta, Georgia

Antonio M. Gotto, Jr., M.D., D.Phil. [53]
The Stephen and Suzanne Weiss Dean
Medical College Provost for Medical Affairs
Cornell University
New York, New York

Kathy K. Griendling, Ph.D. [4, 44]
Associate Professor of Medicine
Department of Medicine
Division of Cardiology
Emory University School of Medicine
Atlanta, Georgia

Robert F. Grover, M.D., Ph.D. [88]
Professor Emeritus of Medicine
University of Colorado School of Medicine
Denver, Colorado

Scott M. Grundy, M.D., Ph.D. [53]
Professor of Internal Medicine
Director, Center for Human Nutrition
Chairman, Department of Clinical Nutrition
University of Texas Southwestern Medical Center at Dallas
Dallas, Texas

Gary L. Grunkemeier, Ph.D. [67]
Director, Medical Data Research Center
Providence Health System
Portland, Oregon

Robert J. Hall, M.D. [86]
Clinical Professor, Department of Medicine
Baylor College of Medicine
Clinical Professor of Medicine, The University of Texas
    Medical School at Houston
Director, Cardiology Education
St. Luke's Episcopal Hospital/Texas Heart Institute
Houston, Texas

W. Dallas Hall, M.D. [57]
Professor of Medicine
Director, Division of Hypertension
Emory University School of Medicine
Atlanta, Georgia

Carl C. Hug, Jr., M.D., Ph.D. [51]
Professor of Anesthesiology and Pharmacology
Emory University School of Medicine
Director, Cardiothoracic Anesthesiology
The Emory Clinic
Atlanta, Georgia

Sharon A. Hunt, M.D. [25]
Professor, Cardiovascular Medicine
Director, Post Heart Transplant Program
Stanford University School of Medicine
Stanford, California

J. Willis Hurst, M.D. [38]
Consultant to the Division of Cardiology
Emory University School of Medicine
Former Chairman (1957–1986)
Department of Medicine
Emory University School of Medicine
Atlanta, Georgia

Jeffrey M. Isner, M.D. [102]
Professor of Medicine and Pathology
Tufts University School of Medicine
Chief, Cardiovascular Research
St. Elizabeth's Medical Center of Boston
Boston, Massachusetts

Peter H. Jones, M.D. [53]
Associate Professor of Medicine
Section of Atherosclerosis and Lipid Research
Department of Medicine
Baylor College of Medicine
Houston, Texas

John W. Joyce, M.D. [100]
Professor Emeritus of Medicine
Mayo Medical School
Mayo Foundation
Rochester, Minnesota

William B. Kannel, M.D., M.P.H. [1]
Professor of Medicine and Public Health
Boston University School of Medicine
Boston, Massachusetts
Framingham Heart Study
Framingham, Massachusetts

Edward L. Kaplan, M.D. [62]
Professor, Department of Pediatrics
University of Minnesota Medical School
Professor, Division of Epidemiology
School of Public Health
University of Minnesota
Minneapolis, Minnesota

Joel A. Kaplan, M.D. [84]

Horace W. Goldsmith Professor of Anesthesiology
The Mount Sinai School of Medicine
New York, New York

Robert B. Karp, M.D. [66]

Professor of Surgery
Chief, Cardiac Surgery
Pritzker School of Medicine
The University of Chicago
Chicago, Illinois

Arnold M. Katz, M.D., D.Med. (Hon.) [3, 21]

Professor of Medicine
Division Chief Emeritus
University of Connecticut Health Center
Farmington, Connecticut

Nevin M. Katz, M.D. [66]

Professor of Surgery
Chief of Adult Cardiac Surgery
Georgetown University Medical Center
Washington, D.C.

Bradley B. Keller, M.D. [8]

Associate Professor of Pediatrics
Department of Pediatrics
University of Rochester School of Medicine and Dentistry
Rochester, New York

Kenneth M. Kessler, M.D. [12, 27]

Professor of Medicine
Associate Director, Division of Cardiology
University of Miami School of Medicine
Chief, Cardiology Section
Department of Veterans Affairs Medical Center
Miami, Florida

Spencer B. King III, M.D. [16, 48]

Professor of Medicine (Cardiology)
Emory University School of Medicine
Co-Director, Cardiac Catheterization Laboratories
Director, Interventional Cardiology
Emory University Hospital
Atlanta, Georgia

Juha P. Kokko, M.D., Ph.D. [24]

Asa G. Candler Professor of Medicine
Chairman, Department of Medicine
Emory University School of Medicine
Atlanta, Georgia

Naresh Kumar, M.D., M.R.C.P., F.R.C.P. [89]

Chief of Internal Medicine
Whitby General Hospital
Medical Director, Whitby Cardiovascular Institute
    and Cardiac Rehabilitation
Whitby, Canada
Medical Director, Institute of Stress Medicine, Canada
Associate Director, Institute of Stress Medicine
Jackson Hole, Wyoming

Joel Kupersmith, M.D. [103]

Dean of the School of Medicine
Texas Tech University Health Sciences Center
School of Medicine
Lubbock, Texas

Thierry H. LeJemtel, M.D. [23]

Professor of Medicine
Albert Einstein College of Medicine
Bronx, New York

Richard P. Lewis, M.D. [35]

Professor of Internal Medicine
The Ohio State University College of Medicine
Columbus, Ohio

Joseph Lindsay, Jr., M.D. [98]

Professor of Medicine
The George Washington University School
    of Health Care Sciences
Director, Division of Cardiology
Washington Hospital Center
Washington, D.C.

Floyd D. Loop, M.D. [50]

Chief Executive Officer
The Cleveland Clinic Foundation
Cleveland, Ohio

Bernard Lown, M.D. [32]

Professor of Cardiology Emeritus
Harvard School of Public Health
Senior Physician
Brigham and Women's Hospital
Boston, Massachusetts

Douglas D. Mair, M.D. [71]

Professor of Pediatrics and Associate Professor of Medicine
Mayo Medical School
Rochester, Minnesota

Michael J. Mann, M.D. [9]
Instructor of Medicine
Harvard Medical School
Brigham and Women's Hospital
Boston, Massachusetts

Frank I. Marcus, M.D. [97]
Distinguished Professor of Medicine
Director, Arrhythmia Service
University of Arizona College of Medicine
Tucson, Arizona

Roger R. Markwald, Ph.D. [8]
Professor and Chairman
Department of Cell Biology and Anatomy
Professor, Department of Pediatrics
Director, Cardiovascular Developmental Biology Center
Medical University of South Carolina College of Medicine
Charleston, South Carolina

Barry J. Maron, M.D. [74]
Director, Cardiovascular Research Division
Minneapolis Heart Institute Foundation
Minneapolis, Minnesota

David J. Maron, M.D. [41]
Assistant Professor of Medicine
Director, Preventive Cardiology
Vanderbilt University School of Medicine
Nashville, Tennessee

Jay W. Mason, M.D. [72]
Chief, Division of Cardiology
Professor of Medicine
University of Utah School of Medicine
Salt Lake City, Utah

Hugh A. McAllister, Jr., M.D. [86]
Clinical Professor of Pathology
Baylor College of Medicine and University of Texas
    Medical School, Houston
Chief, Department of Pathology
St. Luke's Episcopal Hospital and Texas Heart Institute
Houston, Texas

John H. McAnulty, M.D. [68, 92]
Professor of Medicine and Head
Division of Cardiology
Oregon Health Sciences University
Portland, Oregon

James Metcalfe, M.D. [92]
Professor of Medicine
Oregon Health Sciences University
Associate Chief of Staff for Extended Care
Portland Veterans Affairs Medical Center
Portland, Oregon

William E. Mitch, M.D. [94]
Garland Herndon Professor of Medicine
Director, Renal Division
Department of Medicine
Emory University School of Medicine
Atlanta, Georgia

Raul D. Mitrani, M.D. [34]
Assistant Professor of Medicine
University of Miami School of Medicine
Director, Arrhythmia and Pacemaker Center
Miami, Florida

Hugo M. Morales-Ballejo, M.D. [89]
Director of Medical Affairs
Boehringer Mannheim Therapeutics
Gaithersburg, Maryland

Douglas C. Morris, M.D. [51]
J. Willis Hurst Professor of Medicine (Cardiology)
Emory University School of Medicine
Director, The Emory Heart Center
Director, Carlyle Fraser Heart Center
Crawford Long Memorial Hospital of Emory University
Director of Clinical Cardiology Services
The Emory Clinic, Emory University Hospital, and
    Crawford Long Memorial Hospital of Emory University
Atlanta, Georgia

Derek D. Muehrcke, M.D. [50]
Smithwick Cardiovascular Group
Jacksonville, Florida

Robert J. Myerburg, M.D. [12, 27, 34]
Professor of Medicine and Physiology
Director, Division of Cardiology
University of Miami School of Medicine
Jackson Memorial Medical Center
Miami, Florida

Steven D. Nelson, M.D. [35]
Associate Professor of Medicine
The Ohio State University College of Medicine
Director, Cardiac Electrophysiology Laboratory
Director, Arrhythmia Monitoring Services
Columbus, Ohio

John H. Newman, M.D. [61]
Elsa S. Hanigan Chair in Pulmonary Medicine
Professor of Medicine
Vanderbilt University School of Medicine
Chief, Medical Service
Nashville Veterans Affairs Medical Center
Nashville, Tennessee

Steven E. Nissen, M.D. [49]

Professor of Medicine
The Ohio State University College of Medicine
Vice Chairman, Department of Cardiology
Director, Clinical Cardiology
Cleveland Clinic Foundation
Cleveland, Ohio

R. Joe Noble, M.D. [28]

Northside Cardiology
Clinical Professor of Medicine
Indiana University School of Medicine
Indianapolis, Indiana

Paul E. Nolan, Jr., Pharm.D. [97]

Associate Professor, College of Pharmacy
Associate Clinical Scientist, University Heart Center
Cardiovascular Clinical Pharmacist
University of Arizona Medical Center
Tucson, Arizona

Peter A. O'Callaghan, M.B., B.A.O., B.Ch. [33]

Clinical Assistant in Medicine
Massachusetts General Hospital
Instructor in Medicine
Harvard Medical School
Boston, Massachusetts

John B. O'Connell, M.D. [76]

Professor and Chairman
Department of Internal Medicine
Wayne State University School of Medicine
Physician-in-Chief
Detroit Medical Center
Detroit, Michigan

Robert A. O'Rourke, M.D. [10, 65, 66]

Charles Conrad Brown Distinguished Professor
  in Cardiovascular Disease
University of Texas Health Science Center at San Antonio
San Antonio, Texas

Lionel H. Opie, M.D., Ph.D. [91]

Professor of Medicine
University of Cape Town
Director, Hypertension Clinic and Cape Heart Centre
Groote Schuur Hospital
Cape Town, South Africa

Stephen O. Pastan, M.D. [94]

Assistant Professor of Medicine
Emory University School of Medicine
Medical Director
Gambro Peachtree Dialysis Center
Atlanta, Georgia

Randolph E. Patterson, M.D. [17]

Professor of Medicine (Cardiology)
Emory University School of Medicine
Director of Cardiovascular Imaging
Emory Heart Center
Director of Nuclear Cardiology
Carlyle Fraser Heart Center
Crawford Long Hospital of Emory University
Medical Director, Atlanta Life Tech
Atlanta, Georgia

Thomas A. Pearson, M.D., M.P.H., Ph.D. [41]

Albert B. Kaiser Professor and Chair
Department of Community and Preventive Medicine
University of Rochester School of Medicine
Rochester, New York

Claude A. Piantadosi, M.D. [88]

Professor of Medicine
Assistant Professor of Anesthesiology
Director, F.G. Hall Center for Hypobaric
  and Hyperbaric Medicine
Duke University Medical Center
Durham, North Carolina

William H. Plauth, Jr., M.D. [70]

Emory-Egleston Children's Heart Center
Professor of Pediatrics
Emory University School of Medicine
Atlanta, Georgia

Gerald M. Pohost, M.D. [19]

Professor of Medi cine
Professor of Radiology
Mary Gertrude Waters Professor
  in Cardiovascular Medicine
University of Alabama at Birmingham School of Medicine
Director, Center for NMR Research and Development
Birmingham, Alabama

Craig M. Pratt, M.D. [47]

Professor of Medicine
Section of Cardiology, Department of Internal Medicine
Baylor College of Medicine
Director, Clinical Cardiology Research
Baylor College of Medicine and Affiliated Hospitals
Director, Coronary Care Unit, The Methodist Hospital
Houston, Texas

Charles E. Rackley, M.D. [66]

Professor of Medicine
Georgetown University School of Medicine
Director of Lipid Disorder Center
Georgetown University Medical Center
Washington, D.C.

Shahbudin H. Rahimtoola, M.B., F.R.C.P., [63, 64, 67, 68]

Distinguished Professor
George C. Griffith Professor of Cardiology
Chairman, Griffith Center
Professor of Medicine
University of Southern California
Los Angeles, California

B. Ashok Raj, M.D. [90]

Associate Professor of Psychiatry
Department of Psychiatry
Director, Division of Geriatric Psychiatry
University of South Florida College of Medicine
Tampa, Florida

Richard N. Re, M.D. [56]

Vice-President and Director
Division of Research
Alton Ochsner Medical Foundation
New Orleans, Louisiana

John T. Reeves, M.D. [88]

Professor Emeritus of Medicine and Pediatrics
University of Colorado Health Sciences Center
Denver, Colorado

Timothy J. Regan, M.D. [77]

Professor of Medicine
University of Medicine and Dentistry of New Jersey
New Jersey Medical School
Newark, New Jersey

David L. Reich, M.D. [84]

Associate Professor of Anesthesiology
Co-Director of Cardiac Anesthesia
The Mount Sinai Medical Center
New York, New York

Dale G. Renlund, M.D. [76]

Professor of Medicine
Department of Internal Medicine
Division of Cardiology
University of Utah School of Medicine
Medical Director
Utah Transplantation Affiliated Hospitals (UTAH) Cardiac
   Transplant Program
Salt Lake City, Utah

Paul M. Ridker, M.D., M.P.H. [41]

Associate Professor of Medicine
Harvard Medical School
Associate Physician
Brigham and Women's Hospital
Division of Cardiovascular Disease
   and Division of Preventive Medicine
Boston, Massachusetts

Robert Roberts, M.D. [7, 47, 69]

Don W. Chapman Professor of Medicine and Chief of
   Cardiology
Professor of Cell Biology
Director, Bugher Foundation Center for Molecular Biology
Baylor College of Medicine
Houston, Texas

William C. Roberts, M.D. [85]

Executive Director
Baylor Cardiovascular Institute
Dean, A. Webb Roberts Center for Continuing Education
Baylor University Medical Center
Dallas, Texas

Thom W. Rooke, M.D. [100]

Associate Professor of Medicine
Director, Gonda Vascular Center
Mayo Medical Center
Rochester, Minnesota

Kenneth Rosenfield, M.D. [102]

Assistant Professor of Medicine
Tufts University School of Medicine
Boston, Massachusetts

John Ross, Jr., M.D. [22]

Professor of Medicine
Co-Director for Scientific Affairs
Division of Cardiology
University of California San Diego School of Medicine
La Jolla, California

Joseph C. Ross, M.D. [61]

Professor of Medicine
Associate Vice Chancellor for Health Affairs
Vanderbilt University, School of Medicine
Nashville, Tennessee

Russell Ross, Ph.D. [39]

Professor, Department of Pathology
Adjunct Professor
Department of Biochemistry
Director, Center for Vascular Biology
University of Washington School of Medicine
Seattle, Washington

Loring B. Rowell, Ph.D. [88]

Professor Emeritus of Physiology and Biophysics
   and Medicine (Cardiology)
University of Washington School of Medicine
Seattle, Washington

Jeremy N. Ruskin, M.D. [33]
Associate Professor of Medicine
Harvard Medical School
Director, Cardiac Arrhythmia Service
Massachusetts General Hospital
Boston, Massachusetts

Elliot L. Sagall, M.D. [105]
Assistant Clinical Professor of Medicine
Harvard Medical School
Boston, Massachusetts
Founder and First President
The American Society of Law, Medicine and Ethics
Chestnut Hill, Massachusetts

Rosemarie Salerni, M.D. [10]
Associate Professor of Medicine
University of Pittsburgh School of Medicine
Pittsburgh, Pennsylvania

Herbert A. Saltzman, M.D. [88]
Professor of Medicine
Duke University School of Medicine
Durham, North Carolina

Stephen F. Schaal, M.D. [35]
Professor of Medicine
The Ohio State University College of Medicine
Columbus, Ohio

Hartzell V. Schaff, M.D. [64]
Stuart W. Harrington Professor of Surgery
Mayo Medical School
Consultant, Thoracic and Cardiovascular Surgery
Mayo Clinic
Rochester, Minnesota

Robert M. Schainfeld, D.O. [102]
Assistant Professor of Medicine
Director, Noninvasive Vascular Laboratory
St. Elizabeth's Medical Center
Tufts University School of Medicine
Boston, Massachusetts

Melvin M. Scheinman, M.D. [31]
Professor of Medicine
University of California San Francisco
    School of Medicine
San Francisco, California

Heinrich R. Schelbert, M.D., Ph.D. [20]
Professor of Pharmacology and Radiological Sciences
Chief of Service, Nuclear Medicine
Vice Chairman, Department of Molecular
    and Medical Pharmacology
UCLA School of Medicine
Los Angeles, California

James Scheuer, M.D. [95]
Baumritter Professor and Chairman
Department of Medicine
Albert Einstein College of Medicine
Bronx, New York

Robert C. Schlant, M.D. [2, 3, 10, 15, 21, 45, 80, 83, 85]
Professor of Medicine (Cardiology)
Emory University School of Medicine
Chief of Cardiology, Grady Memorial Hospital
Atlanta, Georgia

John S. Schroeder, M.D. [25]
Professor of Medicine
Cardiovascular Medicine Division
Chief, Cardiovascular Medicine Clinic
Stanford University School of Medicine
Stanford, California

Steven P. Schulman, M.D. [96]
Associate Professor of Medicine
Johns Hopkins University School of Medicine
Director, Coronary Care Unit
Johns Hopkins Hospital
Baltimore, Maryland

Robert J. Schwartz, Ph.D. [7]
Professor of Cell Biology
Baylor College of Medicine
Houston, Texas

Ralph Shabetai, M.D. [75, 81]
Professor of Medicine, University of California, San Diego
    School of Medicine
Chief, Cardiology Section
San Diego Veterans Affairs Medical Center
San Diego, California

James A. Shaver, M.D. [10]
Professor of Medicine
University of Pittsburgh School of Medicine
Pittsburgh, Pennsylvania

David V. Sheehan, M.D., M.B.A. [90]
Professor of Psychiatry
Director, Office of Research
Department of Psychiatry
University of South Florida College of Medicine
Tampa, Florida

Halit Silbershatz, Ph.D. [1]
Research Associate
College of Arts and Sciences
Department of Mathematics
Boston University
Boston, Massachusetts

Mark E. Silverman, M.D. [10]

Professor of Medicine (Cardiology)
Emory University School of Medicine
Chief of Cardiology
Piedmont Hospital
Atlanta, Georgia

Andrew L. Smith, M.D. [80]

Assistant Professor of Medicine (Cardiology)
Medical Director
Heart Failure and Cardiac Transplantation
Emory University School of Medicine
Atlanta, Georgia

Robert B. Smith III, M.D. [101]

John E. Skandalakis Professor of Surgery
Head, General Vascular Surgery
Emory University School of Medicine
Medical Director and Associate Chief of Surgery
Emory University Hospital
Atlanta, Georgia

Edmund H. Sonnenblick, M.D. [3, 21, 23, 54, 78]

Edmond J. Safra Distinguished University Professor of Medicine
Chief Emeritus, Division of Cardiology
The Albert Einstein College of Medicine
Bronx, New York

Albert Starr, M.D. [67]

Director, The Heart Institute at St. Vincent Hospital
Professor of Surgery
Oregon Health Sciences University
Consultant in Thoracic Surgery
Portland Veterans Affairs Medical Center
Portland, Oregon

Gary L. Stiles, M.D. [5]

Professor of Medicine and Pharmacology
Chief, Division of Cardiology
Vice Chair, Department of Medicine
Medical Director
Duke University Health System Network Development
Duke University Medical Center
Durham, North Carolina

Panagiotis N. Symbas, M.D. [87]

Professor of Cardiothoracic Surgery
Emory University School of Medicine
Director, Cardiothoracic Surgery
Grady Memorial Hospital
Atlanta, Georgia

Pierre Théroux, M.D. [46]

Professor of Medicine
University of Montreal
Chief, Coronary Care Unit
Montreal Heart Institute
Montreal, Quebec, Canada

Thomas J. Thom, B.A. [1]

Statistician, Epidemiology and Biometry Program
Division of Epidemiology and Clinical Applications
National Heart, Lung, and Blood Institute
National Institutes of Health
Bethesda, Maryland

Jeffrey A. Towbin, M.D. [69]

Associate Professor
Departments of Pediatrics (Cardiology) and Molecular and Human Genetics
Director, Phoebe Willingham Muzzy Pediatric Molecular Cardiology Laboratory
Medical Director, Pediatric Cardiac Transplant Service
Baylor College of Medicine and Texas Children's Hospital
Houston, Texas

E. Murat Tuzcu, M.D. [49]

Associate Professor of Medicine
The Ohio State University, Columbus, Ohio
Director, Intravascular Ultrasound Laboratory
Interventional Cardiologist
Department of Cardiology
The Cleveland Clinic Foundation
Cleveland, Ohio

Kent Ueland, M.D. [92]

Professor Emeritus
Department of Gynecology and Obstetrics
Stanford University School of Medicine
Stanford, California

Marc Verstraete, M.D., Ph.D., F.R.C.P. [52]

Professor of Medicine
University of Leuven
Center for Molecular and Vascular Biology
Leuven, Belgium

Heiko E. von der Leyen, M.D. [9]

Assistant Professor
Division of Cardiology
Department of Medicine,
Hannover Medical School
Hannover, Germany

Albert L. Waldo, M.D. [26]

The Walter H. Pritchard Professor of Cardiology
Professor of Medicine and Professor
   of Biomedical Engineering
Case Western Reserve University School of Medicine
Director, Clinical Cardiac Electrophysiology Program
University Hospitals of Cleveland
Cleveland, Ohio

Bruce F. Waller, M.D. [2, 42]

Clinical Professor of Medicine and Pathology
Indiana University School of Medicine
Director, Cardiovascular Pathology Registry
St. Vincent Hospital
Cardiologist, Nasser Smith Pinkerton Cardiology
Indiana Heart Institute
Indianapolis, Indiana

Richard A. Walsh, M.D. [6]

Mabel S. Stonehill Professor of Medicine
University of Cincinnati College of Medicine
Director, Division of Cardiology and Cardiovascular Center
Cincinnati, Ohio

Carole A. Warnes, M.D., M.R.C.P. [71]

Associate Professor of Medicine
Mayo Medical School
Consultant, Division of Cardiovascular Diseases
   and Internal Medicine
Consultant, Section of Pediatric Cardiology
Director, Adult Congenital Heart Disease Clinic
Rochester, Minnesota

David Waters, M.D. [46]

Professor of Medicine
University of Connecticut School of Medicine
Director of Cardiology, Hartford Hospital
Hartford, Connecticut
Director of Cardiology, University of Connecticut
   Health Center
Farmington, Connecticut

Myron L. Weisfeldt, M.D. [37, 96]

Samuel Bard Professor of Medicine
Columbia University College of Physicians and Surgeons
Chairman, Department of Medicine
Director, Medical Service
Head, Cardiovascular Center
Columbia Presbyterian Medical Center
New York, New York

Nanette Kass Wenger, M.D. [55]

Professor of Medicine (Cardiology)
Emory University School of Medicine
Director, Cardiac Clinics, Grady Memorial Hospital
Consultant, Emory Heart Center
Atlanta, Georgia

Byron R. Williams, Jr., M.D. [17]

Chief of Cardiology
Crawford Long Memorial Hospital of Emory University
Associate Professor of Medicine
Emory University School of Medicine
Atlanta, Georgia

Andrew L. Wit, Ph.D. [26]

Professor of Pharmacology
College of Physicians and Surgeons
Columbia University
New York, New York

Raymond L. Woosley, M.D., Ph.D. [30]

Professor of Pharmacology and Medicine
Chairman, Department of Pharmacology
Co-Director, The Cardiovascular Institute
Georgetown University School of Medicine
Washington, D.C.

Douglas P. Zipes, M.D. [28, 36]

Distinguished Professor of Medicine, Pharmacology,
   and Toxicology
Director, Division of Cardiology and the Krannert Institute
   of Cardiology
Indiana University School of Medicine
Indianapolis, Indiana

Joel Zonszein, M.D. [78]

Associate Professor of Medicine
Albert Einstein College of Medicine
Director, Clinical Diabetes Center
The Jack D. Weiler Hospital of the Albert Einstein College
   of Medicine, Division of Montefiore Medical Center
Bronx, New York

PREFACE

In this ninth edition of *Hurst's **The Heart,*** we continue the tradition of previous editions in providing the reader with a practical approach to the treatment of patients with cardiovascular disease that is based both on the latest evidence available from clinical trials and observational studies and on the underlying scientific principles. The ninth edition has been reorganized extensively, and the number of chapters has been decreased by about thirty percent in order to facilitate the comprehensive treatment of each subject in a well-integrated fashion while reducing duplication. The increasing importance of molecular biology and genetics in the understanding and treatment of cardiovascular disease is reflected in the expansion of the chapter on genetic diseases and in the inclusion of a chapter on gene therapy. On the other hand, the underlying objective of providing guidance in the handling of common problems such as the management of the postoperative patient who has had cardiac surgery is manifest in a new chapter on this subject. Specific therapeutic recommendations generally take into account the most current clinical guidelines for management of a given problem as well as providing the underlying scientific rationale and deviations that might be considered by experienced clinicians.

We thank our authors for their superb contributions and our students, residents, and fellows for their curiosity and challenging questions, which provide a source of continued stimulation.

We thank J. Willis Hurst, M.D., editor of the first seven editions, for his continued enthusiastic support.

We give special thanks and appreciation to Marty Wonsiewicz and Joe Hefta and their colleagues at McGraw-Hill, particularly Lucinda Bauer, Marsha Cohen, Rose Derario, Daniel J. Green, Robert Laffler, Helene Landers, Elissa Lavacca, Muza Navrozov, Eileen Scott, and Heidi Thaens, each of whom gave wise advice and made great personal sacrifice to ensure the accurate and timely birth of this edition.

This edition would not have been possible without the many extensive contributions and personal sacrifices of many individuals, particularly Kate W. Harris, Nell McDonald, Shirley Ballou, William Payne, Lynda Mathews, Barbara Merchant-Bailey, Carolyn Morris, Jackie Cosgrove, Nathalie Harden, Debora Weaver, Joanne Cioffi, and Eddie Jackson. Their extra efforts and those of many others have made this edition possible.

Finally, we wish to acknowledge the support of our families and the many sacrifices they have made to make this volume possible. Our wives remain our greatest support and strength: Jane W. Alexander, Maria Ellingsen-Schlant, Maria Fuster, Suzann O'Rourke, Donna Roberts, and Linda Sonnenblick.

HURST'S
THE HEART

BASIC FOUNDATIONS OF CARDIOLOGY

1

INCIDENCE, PREVALENCE, AND MORTALITY OF CARDIOVASCULAR DISEASES IN THE UNITED STATES

Thomas J. Thom / William B. Kannel / Halit Silbershatz / Ralph B. D'Agostino, Sr.

Life expectancy in the United States is now at its highest. Accounting for most of the improvement over the past 30 years has been the 53 percent decline in the age-corrected death rate for cardiovascular diseases between 1964 and 1994. This indicates the extent to which these leading causes of death are subject to preventive and therapeutic measures. These diseases, however, still account for 42 percent of all deaths and are leading causes of morbidity and health care utilization. Control of these diseases should focus on prevention because of its inherent benefits, apparent role in the mortality reductions, and potential benefits given the presence of modifiable risk factors in millions of Americans.

CARDIOVASCULAR DISEASES

Major Cause of Morbidity and Mortality

The most common cardiovascular diseases are hypertension and heart disease, but the basis for most cardiovascular diseases is atherosclerosis, which is almost universally present in U.S. adults and is manifest clinically as *coronary heart disease* (CHD), cerebrovascular disease (stroke), or peripheral arterial disease. The likelihood of developing one of these diseases is high, and they affect the health of tens of millions of Americans. In 1993, these diseases accounted for $126 billion in health care expenditures in the United States— 2 percent of the gross domestic product (Fig. 1-1).[1,2] These diseases also account for an estimated $84 billion in lost productivity due to illness and premature mortality.[2] These expenditures and indirect costs are by far the largest for any diagnostic group.[3]

During the past 30 years there have been major reductions in mortality rates for the various forms of cardiovascular disease (Fig. 1-2). Cardiovascular diseases, however, continue to be the most common serious threat to life and health. One in every three men in the United States can expect to develop some major cardiovascular disease before reaching age 60; the odds for women are 1 in 10.[4] CHD is the major cause of death beginning around age 40 in men and 65 in women.[5] An estimated 8 percent of the U.S. population, 20 million persons, have some form of heart disease.[6] About 50 million, 20 percent of the total population and one-fourth of the adult population, have hypertension, defined as a systolic blood pressure of ≥140 mmHg, a diastolic blood pressure of ≥90 mmHg, or normal blood pressure levels maintained by use of antihypertensive medication.[2,7] One-fourth of persons with heart disease and 36 percent of those with stroke are

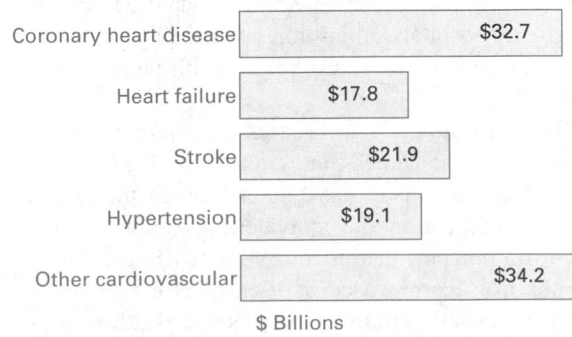

	$ Billions
Coronary heart disease	$32.7
Heart failure	$17.8
Stroke	$21.9
Hypertension	$19.1
Other cardiovascular	$34.2

FIGURE 1-1

Health expenditures for cardiovascular diseases, United States, 1993 (includes expenditures for hospital, home, and nursing home care; physician and other professionals; and drugs). (From National Heart, Lung, and Blood Institute.[2])

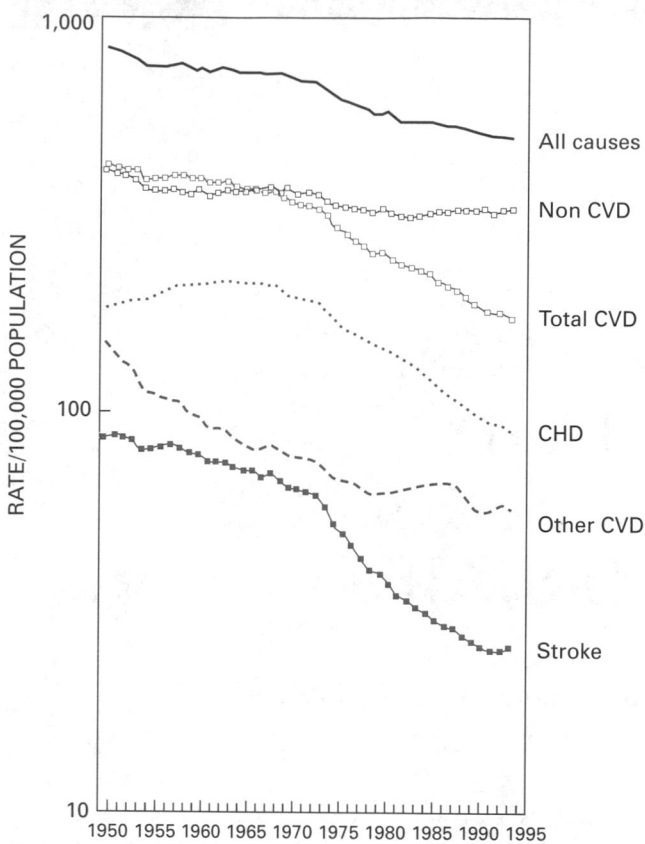

FIGURE 1-2

Age-adjusted death rates for selected causes of death; United States, 1950–1994. CVD = cardiovascular disease; CHD = coronary heart disease. (From *Vital Statistics of the United States,* National Center for Health Statistics.)

limited in their usual activity by the condition.[8] Heart disease and hypertension, respectively, are the third and fourth most common chronic condition causing limitation of activity.[2] A large proportion of individuals with hypertension are under 65 years of age, and 40 percent of persons with heart disease are under that age.[6] The prevalence and mortality from the cardiovascular diseases increase with decreasing levels of family income and education.[6,9] In 1990 to 1992 in the United States, heart disease and hypertension accounted for an estimated 542 million days of restricted activity and 206 million bed days.[8] In 1994, there were an estimated 37 million days in short-stay hospitals, 54 million visits to physicians' offices, and 503,000 patients receiving home health care for the cardiovascular diseases.[10–12]

In 1994, cardiovascular diseases accounted for 42 percent of all deaths in the United States, a total of 955,000.[3] Largely because there are many more older women than older men in the U.S. population, the equivalent percentage is higher in women (45 percent) than men (39 percent), and the number of deaths from cardiovascular diseases is greater in women than men.[5] Of all cardiovascular disease deaths, 36 percent occurred "prematurely," i.e., before 75 years of age, the approximate average life expectancy in 1994.[13] Atherosclerosis, when manifested as CHD, cerebrovascular disease, or peripheral arterial disease, accounted for 72 percent of all deaths

from the cardiovascular diseases in 1994.[3] Heart disease was the leading cause of death, followed by cancer and then cerebrovascular diseases.[1] This is true for the white, black, and Asian U.S. population. In American Indians and in Hispanic Americans, heart disease is the leading cause of death, and stroke ranks sixth highest. Age-adjusted death rates for cardiovascular disease in 1993 were highest in black males, next highest in white males, then followed by black females and were lowest in white females.

Unfortunately, national incidence and case fatality data for the cardiovascular diseases do not exist. Data from the Framingham (Massachusetts) Heart Study, which began in 1948, provide reliable estimates for 40 years of follow-up of a defined population sample of 5209 men and women aged 35 to 94. The average annual rates of first major cardiovascular events rose from 5 per 1000 men at ages 35 to 44 years to 73 per 1000 at ages 85 to 94 (Table 1-1). For women, comparable rates are achieved 10 years later in life, with the gap closing with advancing age. CHD is the predominant cardiovascular event, comprising more than one-half of all such events in men and in women under age 75 (Table 1-2). The proportions of cardiovascular events due to CHD decline with age, as the proportions due to stroke and congestive heart failure (CHF) increase with age. Under age 75, there is a higher proportion of cardiovascular events due to CHD in men than women, and a higher proportion due to congestive heart failure in women than men (Tables 1-1 and 1-2).

Secular Trends

The trend in mortality from total cardiovascular disease has been downward since about 1940, with long-term declines for the three subgroups—rheumatic, cerebrovascular, and hypertensive diseases—and a decline for CHD since the mid-1960s.[2] The coronary decline antedates effective antithrombolytic and antihypertensive treatment. Prior to 1940, cardiovascular mortality increased and became the predominant cause of death because of control of infectious and parasitic diseases and an epidemic increase in fatal coronary attacks. Cardiovascular mortality declined just under 1 percent per year in the 1950s and 1960s. The decline became more precipitous in the 1970s, with the rate falling 3 percent per year since then. For CHD, there has been more than a 58 percent decline in the age-adjusted death rate between the peak of mortality in 1963 and 1994; the current decline is about 2 to 3 percent per year. For stroke, the rate of decline was 4 to 6 percent per year in the 1970s and early 1980s, but the decline slowed and has been less than 1 percent per year since 1990.

The decline in cardiovascular mortality, including the steep rise and fall in CHD mortality, indicates that the major force of mortality is controllable. Whether attributable more to beneficial changes in disease-promoting lifestyle or to better medical care of those already afflicted, it is clear that cardiovascular disease in most patients is not an inevitable burden of aging or genetic makeup. Although the causes of the decline in cardiovascular mortality are uncertain, the decline has been substantial, sustained, and real. The decline has coincided with increased efforts to achieve healthier living habits and with improvements in the ambient burden of cardiovascular risk factors.

Unfortunately, there are very few statistics on trends in morbidity, particularly incidence. Some, but not all, studies suggest that there have been declines in incidence and case fatality of CHD and stroke.[14-18] This is important because reduction in mortality without a decline in the incidence rate would indicate better medical care was responsible, whereas a reduction in both incidence and mortality suggests environmental influences and/or preventive measures have improved. If reduction in mortality continues, the size of the elderly population will continue to increase over and above the increase related to demographic effects.

Risk Factors

Observational studies in populations such as those observed in the Framingham Study have documented factors that increase the risk of cardiovascular diseases.[19] These include atherogenic attributes, living habits that promote them, indicators of unstable lesions, and signs of compromised circulation. Risk factors can be classified into the lipids, metabolic factors, hemostatic factors, blood pressure, and lifestyle factors. Some are modifiable. They promote cardiovascular disease in both sexes at all ages, but with different strengths. Diabetes and high-density lipoprotein (HDL) cholesterol operate with greater power in women. Cigarette smoking is particularly influential in men, is noncumulative, and loses some of its adverse impact shortly after quitting. Fibrinogen levels, leukocyte count, homocystinemia, and Lp(a) lipoprotein are more recent additions to major risk factors for cardiovascular disease. Some risk factors, such as blood lipids, impaired glucose tolerance, uric acid, and fibrinogen, have smaller risk ratios in advanced age, but this lower relative risk is offset by a high absolute risk. In fact, the major risk factors remain relevant in the elderly. Obesity or weight gain promotes or aggravates all the atherogenic risk factors, and physical indo-

lence worsens some of them and predisposes to cardiovascular events at all ages. Systolic blood pressure and isolated systolic hypertension are major risk factors at all ages in both sexes. The ratio of total to HDL cholesterol is used by many as a convenient lipid risk factor profile (see also Chap. 53).

Beyond age 65, women become nearly as vulnerable to cardiovascular mortality as men.[5] The predisposing modifiable risk factors for CHD, stroke, peripheral arterial disease, and cardiac failure are similar in the young and old in men and women.[19] An attenuated risk ratio for some risk factors at advanced age is offset by a greater incidence of cardiovascular disease, consequently, the attributable risk and the potential benefit of treatment rise with age. In old age, average atherogenic total and low-density lipoprotein cholesterol are considerably higher in women than men. Cardiovascular risk profiles comprising the major risk factors predict CHD as efficiently in the elderly as in the young. This, and the fact that the decline in cardiovascular mortality has included the elderly, suggests the potential for intervention.

TABLE 1-1

INCIDENCE OF MAJOR CARDIOVASCULAR EVENTS: FRAMINGHAM STUDY, 40-YEAR FOLLOW-UP[a]

Age	Cardiovascular Disease (All Types)		Coronary Heart Disease		Stroke and TIA		Congestive Heart Failure		Peripheral Arterial Disease	
	Men	Women	Men	Women	Men	Women	Men	Women	Men	Women
35–44	5	2	5	1	b	b	b	b	b	b
45–54	15	7	11	4	2	1	2	1	2	1
55–64	28	16	21	11	5	3	5	3	5	3
65–74	39	24	26	14	10	8	9	6	7	4
74–84	59	40	33	19	21	14	19	13	6	4
85–94	73	58	31	22	9	26	28	25	4	1
35–64[c]	18	10	14	6	3	2	3	2	3	2
65–94[c]	44	29	28	16	13	11	12	9	7	4

[a] Average annual incidence per 1000 persons free of specified disease.
[b] Results are omitted when fewer than five individuals experience an event.
[c] Age-adjusted rates.
Note: TIA = Transient ischemic attack.
Source: The Framingham Study.

TABLE 1-2

PERCENTAGE OF FIRST CARDIOVASCULAR EVENTS BY TYPE OF EVENT: FRAMINGHAM STUDY, 40-YEAR FOLLOW-UP

Age	Cardiovascular Disease (All Types) n		Coronary Heart Disease, %		Stroke and TIA, %		Congestive Heart Failure, %		Peripheral Arterial Disease, %	
	Men	Women	Men	Women	Men	Women	Men	Women	Men	Women
35–54	264	139	77.3	58.3	8.7	18.7	6.8	13.7	7.2	8.6
55–64	435	347	70.1	62.8	11.0	12.7	6.4	11.0	12.2	13.3
65–74	365	362	62.2	56.4	19.2	23.8	6.8	9.4	11.8	10.5
75–94	182	275	54.4	44.7	25.3	33.8	12.1	15.3	5.1	6.9

Source: The Framingham Study.

Evidence from the Framingham Study suggests that the presence of certain risk factors in women can eliminate their advantage in cardiovascular risk over that in men. These are as follows:

Age: The male-female gap in incidence closes with advancing age.

Menopause: Risk escalates two- to threefold, with more infarction and sudden death.

High total/HDL cholesterol ratio of 7.5 or greater: This eliminates the female advantage.

Diabetes: Twice the impact on risk in women, virtually canceling the female advantage.

Electrocardiographic evidence of left ventricular hypertrophy: Greater impact on risk in women.

High triglyceride/HDL ratio: Correlates with dyslipidemic hypertension.

Ingrained in the American lifestyle are major modifiable risk factors, including cigarette smoking, elevated lipid levels, hypertension, and overweight. Contributing to this last factor is the sedentary lifestyle of many Americans. These risk factors contribute powerfully to cardiovascular disease and are highly prevalent in the population. Trends in their prevalence and differences in their impact on the various atherosclerotic sequelae are noteworthy. Despite 30 years of decline in the percent of persons who smoke cigarettes, in 1994 one-fourth of adults, 46 million, still smoked.[1] Despite declining trends in mean total serum cholesterol, an estimated 52 percent of American adults (97 million) have blood cholesterol levels ≥200 mg/dL, and of these, 38 million have levels ≥240 mg/dL.[20] Fifty million Americans have hypertension.[1,2,7] Fortunately, treatment and control of this condition have improved considerably.[21] Not improving, however, is obesity. One-third of adults (62 million) are overweight, defined as a *body mass index >27.7 kg/m² in men and >27.2 kg/m² in women.*[1,20] An estimated 7.8 million persons are at increased risk of cardiovascular disease because they have diabetes.[6] Another highly prevalent risk factor is sedentary lifestyle. It plays a role in the prevalence of overweight and hypertension and, thus, cardiovascular disease. There also are persons under 18 years of age who have one or more modifiable risk factors.[1,20]

No individual risk factor is essential or sufficient in the causation of cardiovascular disease; causation is multifactorial. Indeed, the risk posed by one factor may be influenced by presence of another. Thus, multivariate risk factor assessment gives the most useful measure of the joint effect of the risk factors.[19] Multivariate analyses help provide better understanding of the pathogenesis of the disease and guidelines for prevention. Based on the absolute, relative, and attributable risks imposed by the various risk factors, the older concepts of *normal* have evolved to optimal values associated with long-term freedom from disease. As a consequence, acceptable blood pressures, blood glucose levels, and lipid values have been revised downward[19] (see also Chap. 41).

CORONARY HEART DISEASE

Coronary heart disease (CHD) kills and disables people in their most productive years and in 1993 accounted for $33 billion in medical care costs and $38 billion in indirect economic costs.[2] Each year there are more hospitalizations for CHD than for any broad diagnostic group with the exceptions of births, all respiratory diseases, all digestive diseases, and all injuries.[10] CHD is the leading cause of premature, permanent disability in the U.S. labor force, accounting for 19 percent of disability allowances by the Social Security Administration.[22]

Prevalence

In the United States, an estimated 13.7 million have CHD, about one-half of whom have acute myocardial infarction and half have angina pectoris.[20] For men, prevalence of CHD is 7 percent at ages 40 to 49 years, 13 percent at 50 to 59 years, 16 percent at 60 to 69 years, and 22 percent at ages 70 to 79 years (Fig. 1-3). For women, the corresponding estimates by age are 5, 8, 11, and 14 percent, substantially lower than in men.

Incidence

In the United States, coronary heart disease causes about 800,000 new heart attacks each year and 450,000 recurrent attacks.[2] The incidence in women lags behind men by 10 years for total CHD and by 20 years for more serious clinical manifestations such as myocardial infarction and sudden death (Tables 1-1 and 1-3). Male predominance is least striking for uncomplicated angina pectoris. The first coronary presentation for women is more likely to be angina, whereas in men it is more likely to be myocardial infarction (Table 1-4). In men, more angina occurs after infarction than before. Only 20 percent of coronary attacks are preceded by long-standing angina; the percentage is lower if the infarction is silent or unrecognized. In the premenopausal female, serious manifestations of CHD such as infarction or sudden death are relatively rare. The incidence and severity of CHD increase with age in both sexes. There seems to be a more precipitous increase for women after menopause, with CHD rates in postmenopausal women two to three times those of women the same age who remain premenopausal.[23] This applies whether the menopause is natural or surgical and, in the latter case, whether or not the ovaries are removed. The sex ratio in incidence narrows progressively with advancing age.

Unrecognized myocardial infarctions are common in the Framingham Study, numbering at least one in four infarctions (Fig. 1-4). Half of the unrecognized infarctions are silent, and the rest are atypical so that neither the patient nor the physician entertains the possibility. More than half of these persons eventually develop some overt clinical manifestations of CHD and hence come under medical care. Angina is less frequent in individuals with unrecognized infarction than in those with recognized symptomatic myocardial infarction, either before or after the infarction occurs. Despite the apparent mild nature of unrecognized infarction, the risk of subsequent mortality is nearly the same as in patients with recognized infarction. Diabetic men and hypertensive persons of both sexes are particularly susceptible to silent or unrecognized infarctions.

Prognosis

In patients who survive the acute stage of a myocardial infarction, the morbidity and mortality range from 1.4 to 10 times that of the general population, depending on the person's sex and clinical outcome (Table 1-5). The rates of occurrence of reinfarction, sudden death, angina pectoris, cardiac failure, and stroke are all substantial. The relative and absolute risks of these events are as great in women as in men. Within 6 years following a recognized myocardial infarction, 21 percent of men and 33 percent of women have a recurrent infarction, and 29 percent of men and 15 percent of women develop angina. About 21 percent of men and 30 percent of women are disabled with cardiac failure; 9 percent of men and 13 percent of women will have a stroke. Sudden death will be experienced by 7 percent. The prognosis is nearly as bad, sometimes worse, following an unrecognized infarction (Table 1-5). Although about two-thirds of patients with myocardial infarction do not make a complete recovery, 88 percent under age 65 are able to return to their usual occupations[24] (see also Chap. 38).

Mortality

Coronary heart disease is the leading cause of death in adults in the United States, accounting for almost one-fourth of the deaths in persons over age 35.[13] In 1994, there were 487,000 coronary deaths. Mortality from this disease increases with age, but CHD is also a prominent cause of death in adults at the peak of their productive lives. It is either the leading cause or one of the leading causes of death in men and women and in every racial

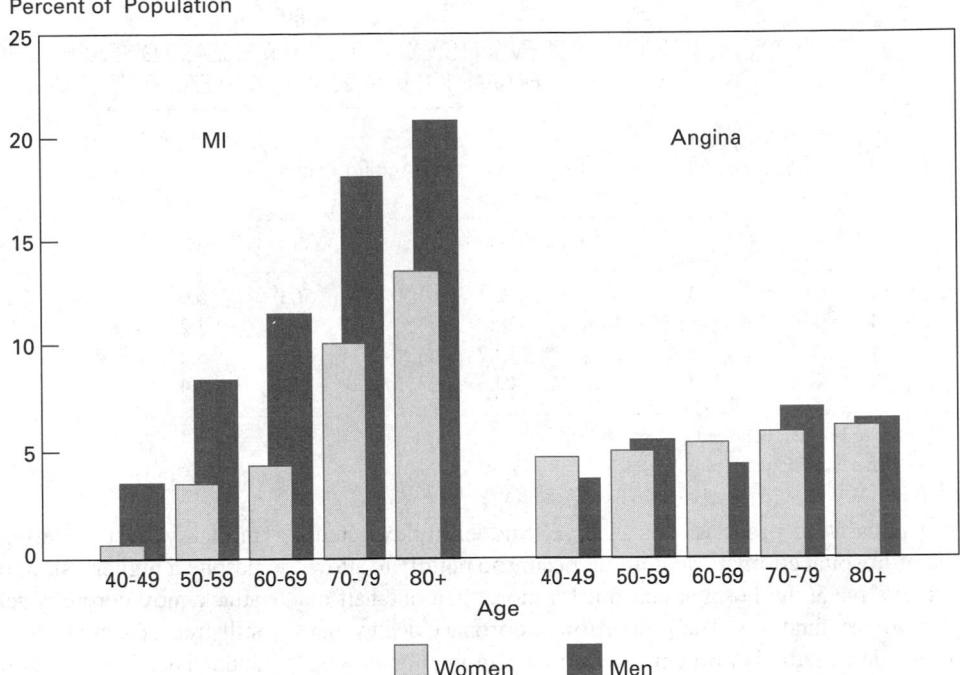

Percent of Population

FIGURE 1-3
Prevalence of myocardial infarction and angina pectoris by age and sex, United States, 1988–1991 (self-reported myocardial infarction and Rose angina from health interviews). MI = myocardial infarction. (From the National Health and Nutrition Examination Survey, 1988–1991, National Center for Health Statistics.)

or ethnic group.[2] The death rate is three times higher in men than in women at ages 25 to 34, but this ratio declines to 1.6 by ages 75 to 84. The coronary death rate is twice as high in blacks than in whites at ages 25 to 34, and that difference disappears by age 75. CHD mortality is not as high among the Hispanic population as it is among blacks and whites.

In a substantial number of CHD deaths, the progression from inapparent clinical disease to death is swift. Much of the premature mortality from CHD comes with little warning

TABLE 1-3

INCIDENCE OF SPECIFIED CLINICAL MANIFESTATIONS OF CORONARY HEART DISEASE: FRAMINGHAM STUDY, 40-YEAR FOLLOW-UP[a]

Age, years	Angina Pectoris		Myocardial Infarction		Sudden Death	
	Men	Women	Men	Women	Men	Women
35–44	2	<1	3	b	b	b
45–54	5	2	5	1	1	b
55–64	10	7	10	3	2	1
65–74	9	7	15	6	3	1
75–84	6	7	20	9	7	3
85–94	b	b	23	14	b	5
35–64[c]	6	4	7	2	1	<1
65–94[c]	9	7	16	7	1	2

[a] Average annual incidence rate per 1000 persons free of coronary heart disease.
[b] Results are omitted when fewer than five individuals experienced event.
[c] Age-adjusted rates.
Source: The Framingham Study.

TABLE 1-4

PERCENTAGE OF FIRST EVENTS OF CORONARY HEART DISEASE (CHD) BY TYPE OF EVENT:
FRAMINGHAM STUDY, 40-YEAR FOLLOW-UP

Age	Coronary Heart Disease (All Types) n		Myocardial Infarction[a], %		Angina Pectoris, %		Coronary Insufficiency, %		Sudden Death from CHD, %		Non-Sudden Death from CHD, %	
	Men	Women	Men	Women	Men	Women	Men	Women	Men	Women	Men	Women
35–54	212	84	49.5	32.1	30.7	56.0	6.6	4.8	9.4	4.8	3.8	2.4
55–64	340	245	47.4	28.2	37.9	57.1	3.2	6.1	8.8	5.7	2.6	2.9
65–74	277	242	56.7	39.7	26.0	46.3	3.2	4.5	10.8	7.0	3.2	2.5
75–94	124	152	61.3	49.3	15.3	27.6	2.4	4.6	16.9	14.5	4.0	2.0

[a] Recognized or unrecognized.

Source: The Framingham Study.

in a population prone to this disease. Sudden, unexpected, out-of-hospital coronary deaths that occur too rapidly to allow arrival alive at the hospital account for more than one-half of all coronary fatalities. The proportion of coronary deaths that are sudden deaths is lower in women than in men and lower in elderly men than in the young (Fig. 1-5). The percentage of sudden coronary deaths that occur without prior CHD, however, is much greater in women than in men (Fig. 1-6). In 57 percent of men and 64 percent of women who died suddenly, there was no prior evidence of overt coronary disease (see also Chap. 36).

In persons under age 65, about 80 percent of coronary mortality occurs during the initial coronary attack.[4] Thus, despite a higher risk of death in patients with a prior coronary attack, most coronary deaths arise from the population who are still free of symptomatic CHD. After myocardial infarction, sudden death occurs at four to six times the rate in the general population. Hence, primary prevention ultimately appears to offer more to society than secondary prevention. The first year following a recognized myocardial infarction is especially dangerous, with 24 percent of men and 42 percent of women succumbing (Fig. 1-7). Long-term survival following unrecognized myocardial infarction is only slightly better than for recognized infarctions, and survival is better for women than for men (Table 1-6). In men under age 65 with uncomplicated angina pectoris, the survival picture is nearly the same as it is for recognized myocardial infarction and is much worse than the survival in women (see also Chap. 38).

HYPERTENSION

Hypertension is the most prevalent cardiovascular disease in the United States and it is one of the most powerful contributors to cardiovascular morbidity and mortality. It is the most important factor contributing to the 500,000 cases of stroke that occur each year in the United States and is a major factor in the estimated 1.5 million annual heart attacks.[20] In 1994, only 4 percent of the cardiovascular disease deaths[13] were attributed to hypertensive disease as the underlying cause. On the other hand, it is the main contributor to the 154,000

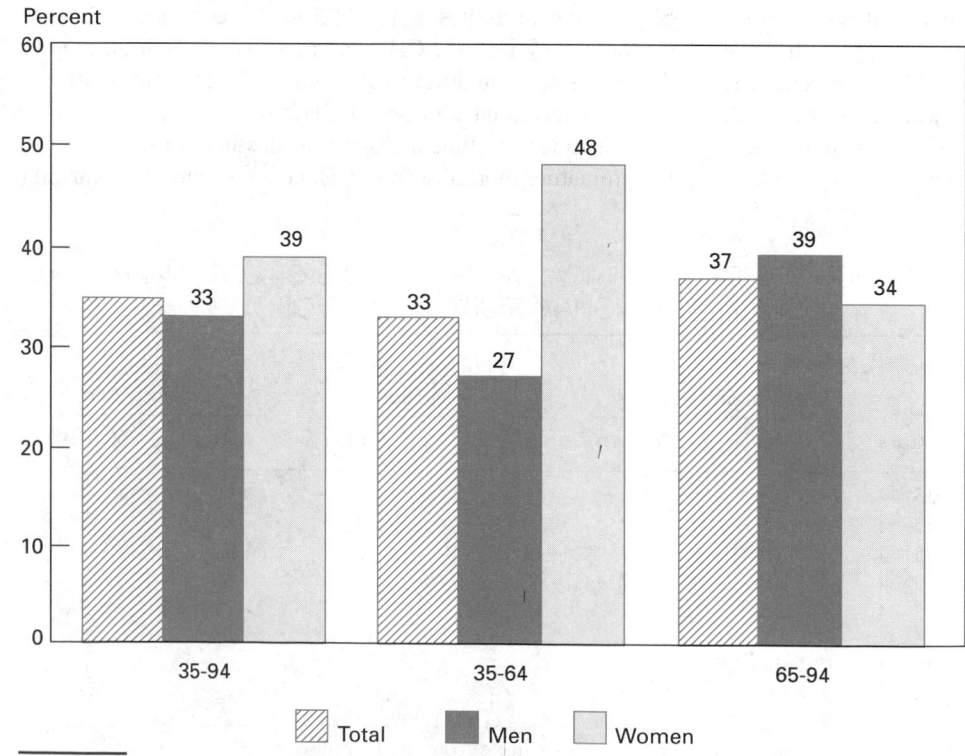

FIGURE 1-4

Percent of myocardial infarctions that are unrecognized: Framingham study, 40-year follow-up. (From the Framingham Study.)

deaths from stroke, 45,000 deaths from cardiac failure, many of the 487,000 deaths from CHD, and many of the 22,000 deaths from kidney disease that occurred in 1994.[2,13] In 1993, an estimated $19 billion in national medical care expenditures were attributed to hypertension, apart from its role in coronary, cerebrovascular, and kidney diseases and cardiac failure.[2]

Prevalence

Data from the National Health and Nutrition Examination Survey for 1988 to 1991 indicate a hypertension prevalence of 24 percent for persons 18 years of age and over in the United States.[7] For that estimate, the definition of hypertension is that either the patient's blood pressure is ≥140/90 mmHg or the patient is on antihypertensive medication. When these data are extrapolated to 1993 for all ages, the prevalence is about 50 million—one-fifth of the total population or just over one-fourth of the adult population.[2]

The percent prevalence increases with age and is highest among blacks and the elderly (Fig. 1-8). Isolated systolic hypertension is a common and distinctly hazardous condition in the elderly. There is recent evidence from the Systemic Hypertension in the Elderly Program (SHEP) that treatment of this form of hypertension in the elderly is distinctly efficacious, not only against stroke but also against coronary disease.[25] This benefit accrued despite the use of a diuretic (chlorthalidone). The benefit in spite of diuretic use may derive from the lower impact of side effects on lipids and glucose tolerance in the elderly or from the lower dose of diuretics used in this trial than in former trials. Persons with hypertension face serious excess risks of cardiovas-

TABLE 1-5

SIX-YEAR PROGNOSIS FOLLOWING MYOCARDIAL INFARCTION: FRAMINGHAM STUDY, 40-YEAR FOLLOW-UP[a]

	Men		Women	
	Percent	Risk Ratio[b]	Percent	Risk Ratio[b]
RECOGNIZED				
Death	40	2.7	49	4.2
Sudden death	7	4.0	7	5.1
Myocardial infarction	21	2.6	33	9.0
Angina pectoris	29	4.4	15	2.5
Cardiac failure	21	5.2	30	10.1
Stroke/TIA	9	2.7	13	3.7
UNRECOGNIZED				
Death	47	2.5	36	2.5
Sudden death	5	1.7	2	2.1
Myocardial infarction	16	1.7	18	3.6
Angina pectoris	10	1.4	18	3.4
Cardiac failure	24	5.2	22	6.5
Stroke/TIA	14	3.8	7	1.5

[a] Surviving 30 days.
[b] Standardized morbidity and mortality ratios (times 0.01).
Note: TIA = transient ischemic attack.
Source: The Framingham Study.

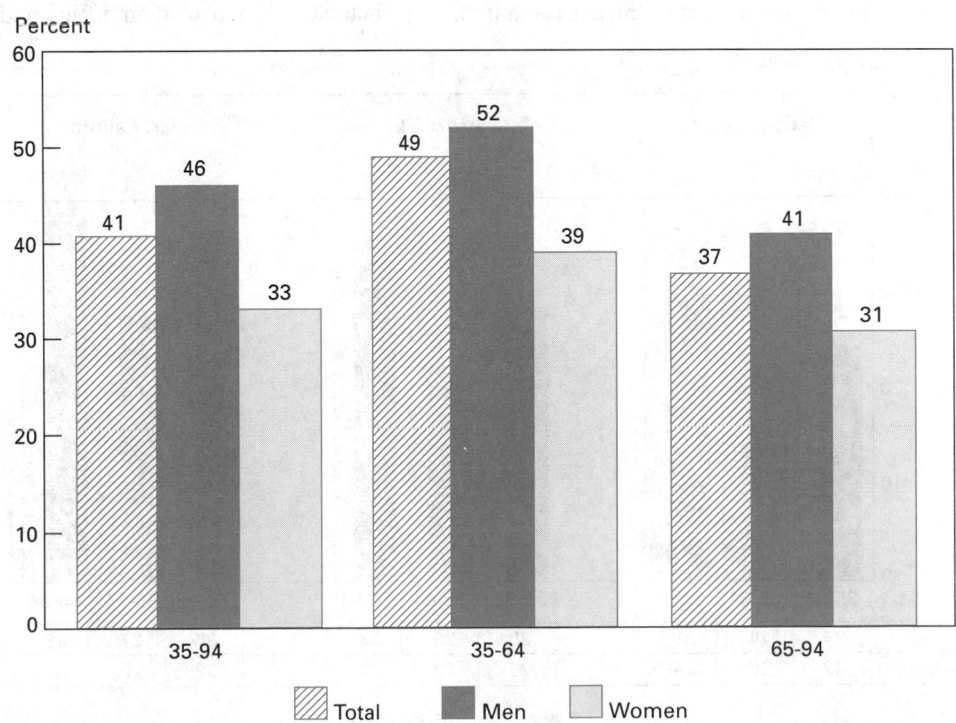

FIGURE 1-5

Percent of coronary heart disease deaths as sudden deaths: Framingham study, 40-year follow-up. (From the Framingham Study.)

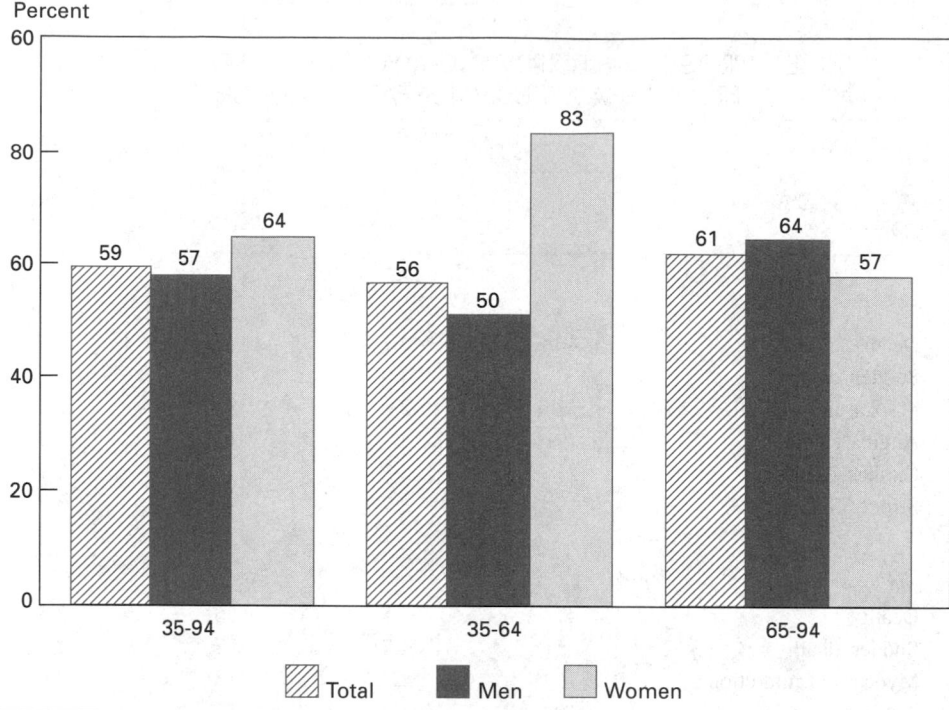

FIGURE 1-6

Percent of sudden deaths without prior coronary heart disease: Framingham Study 40-year follow-up. (From the Framingham Study.)

to hypertension comes from this blood pressure range. *The risks of cardiovascular sequelae are proportional to the blood pressure level at any age and in both sexes and are the same whether the elevation is systolic or diastolic.* Approximately one-half of the persons who suffer a first heart attack and two-thirds who suffer a first stroke have blood pressures >160/95 mmHg.

Although there is a rise in blood pressure with age in most affluent populations in both sexes, this is not universal and it does not imply that blood pressure must inevitably rise with age or that in those whose pressures do rise it reflects a normal aging process. In the United States, there is about a 20-mmHg systolic and 10-mmHg diastolic rise in mean pressures from age 30 to age 64. Systolic pressures continue to rise in women in their eighties and in men into their seventies. Diastolic pressures level off earlier, and in men decline beyond age 55. The pressures start lower in young adult women and rise more steeply in middle age (50 and over), and they equal those of men in their fifties and then progressively exceed those of men in later life; this crossover is observed for both systolic and diastolic pressures. In some populations in the world, blood pressure does not rise with age.

For the following discussion, *hypertension* means that a patient has blood pressure ≥160/95 mmHg or is on antihypertensive medication; *under control* means that a patient is on antihypertensive medication and has blood pressure <160/95 mmHg. Between the periods 1960 to 1962 and 1988 to 1991, there have been large improvements in the percentage of hypertensive patients who (1) are aware of their hypertension (from 53 to 89 percent), (2) are on antihypertensive medication (from 35 to 79 percent), and (3) are under control (from 16 to 64 percent).[21]

Although an improving trend is also seen at the 140/90+ mmHg level of control, using that

cular sequelae, and since much of this excess risk is attributable to mild hypertension, there is need for intervention through preventive lifestyle modification, if not through drug treatment. Because of the higher prevalence of milder hypertension, almost 60 percent of the excess mortality attributable

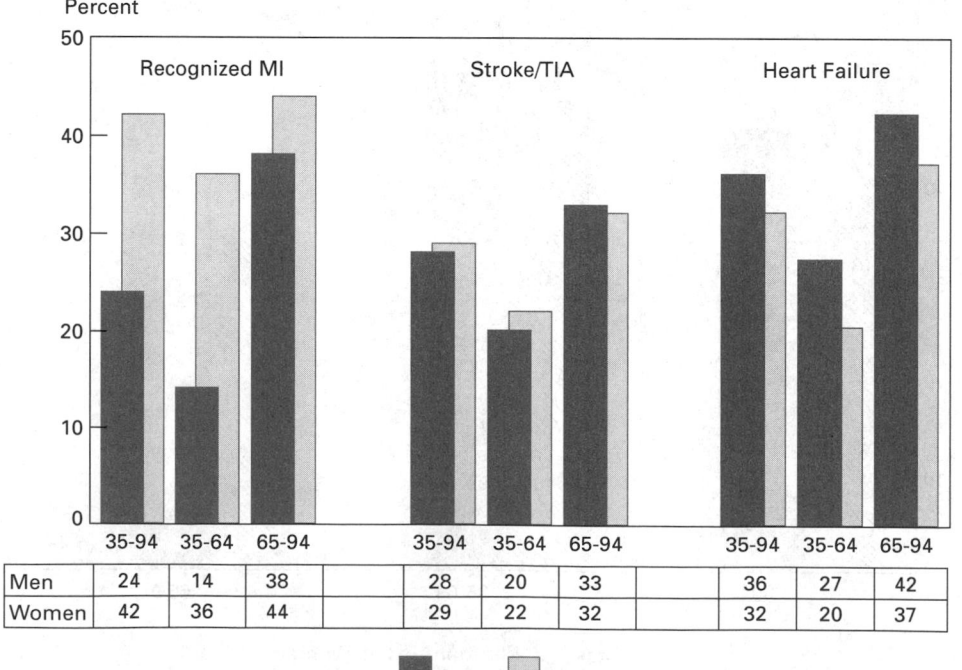

	35-94	35-64	65-94		35-94	35-64	65-94		35-94	35-64	65-94
Men	24	14	38		28	20	33		36	27	42
Women	42	36	44		29	22	32		32	20	37

FIGURE 1-7

Percent of deaths within one year following initial cardiovascular event: Framingham study, 40-year follow-up. (From the Framingham Study.)

TABLE 1-6

DEATHS PER 100 PERSONS AT RISK BY TIME INTERVAL FOLLOWING INITIAL CARDIOVASCULAR EVENT
AND SURVIVAL FOR 30 DAYS: FRAMINGHAM STUDY, 40-YEAR FOLLOW-UP

Age	Angina Pectoris Uncomplicated		Recognized Myocardial Infarction		Unrecognized Myocardial Infarction		Stroke/Transient Ischemic Attacks		Intermittent Claudication		Congestive Heart Failure	
	Men	Women	Men	Women	Men	Women	Men	Women	Men	Women	Men	Women
					AGES 35–64 YEARS							
1–2	2	1	5	12	4	2	9	11	1	1	23	12
2–4	6	3	10	15	9	7	15	16	2	1	37	20
4–8	14	10	20	29	25	19	26	22	12	9	54	32
8–12	31	21	39	46	48	34	45	42	31	23	77	59
12–16	50	34	53	63	70	46	64	57	56	44	86	71
16–20	65	47	66	81	81	55	76	67	69	66	91	81
					AGES 65–94 YEARS							
1–2	1	3	12	19	9	7	16	15	1	1	29	23
2–4	8	6	19	23	17	20	24	23	3	2	45	34
4–8	17	20	39	48	38	45	38	32	15	9	65	51
8–12	41	36	64	68	63	62	63	59	44	30	87	80
12–16	69	52	82	81	81	74	79	75	71	60	95	90
16–20	87	72	92	91	90	87	89	89	89	80	99	93

Source: The Framingham Study.

definition, 45 percent still do not have medication prescribed for their hypertension.

Incidence

Longitudinal observation of blood pressures as people age reveals a different pattern than cross-sectional data. The reason for this difference is obscure. Diastolic pressures are essentially parallel in both sexes, with women's pressures consistently below those of men. In women, systolic pressures are initially lower than in men but subsequently rise more steeply. They converge at age 60 with those of men but never exceed them. With advancing age in both genders, a progressive and disproportionate rise in systolic pressure is presumed to result from loss of arterial elasticity. Blacks have higher blood pressures than whites in most western cultures.

Determinants

While genetic susceptibility plays a large role in hypertension,

this may be only permissive, requiring one or more environmental cofactors such as salt intake, alcohol, or weight gain to bring on hypertension. Of all the identifiable determinants of hypertension, weight gain and adiposity, particularly abdominal in distribution, seem to be predominant. New under-

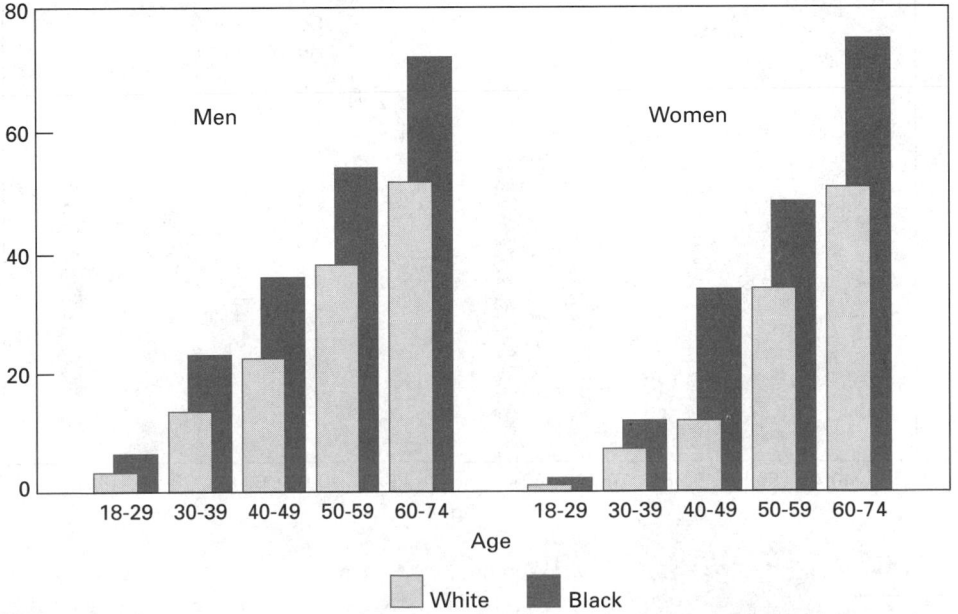

FIGURE 1-8

Prevalence of hypertension by age, race, and sex; United States, 1988–1991 (hypertension: 140/90 + or on antihypertensive medication). (From the National Health and Nutrition Examination Survey, National Center for Health Statistics.

lying causes of hypertension are discovered every decade, but the causes of the vast majority of cases remain undetermined. Of the identifiable causes, chronic renal diseases, renovascular disease, and hypertension induced by oral contraceptives head the list. Routine search for underlying causes not suggested by signs or symptoms is usually unrewarding and often counterproductive. Recent research suggests that insulin resistance occurring in association with obesity may play a fundamental role[26] (see also Chaps. 41 and 56).

STROKE

Prevalence

Two percent of the U.S. adult population, 3.9 million, have cerebrovascular disease (stroke).[2] More than 1 million of these individuals are limited in their usual activity.[8] The prevalence rises from 16 per 1000 men at 40 to 49 years to 121 per 1000 for men ages 75 and over and from 5 to 128 per 1000 in the respective age groups in women (Fig. 1-9). In the Framingham Study, the most common variety of stroke is atherothrombotic brain infarction, which accounts for 64 percent of all strokes (excluding transient ischemic attacks).[27] Next most common are cerebral embolus, subarachnoid hemorrhage, and intracerebral hemorrhage. Intracerebral hemorrhage has apparently declined most in recent years (see also Chap. 99).

Incidence

In the Framingham Study, the chance of having a stroke before age 70 was 1 in 20 for both sexes.[27] The incidence rates vary depending on (1) the age of the patients studied, (2) whether the sample is derived from the general population or from some select subgroup such as hospitalized patients, and (3) whether or not recurrent strokes are included. Thirty-one percent of stroke survivors needed assistance in self-care, 20 percent required help in ambulation, and 71 percent had an impaired vocational capacity when examined an average of 7 years after their stroke.[28]

Cerebrovascular disease is not a necessary consequence of aging. Modifiable contributing factors offer the possibility of prevention by identifying stroke candidates for corrective measures. Stroke prevention requires early treatment of persons with hypertension, cardiac disorders, and transient cerebral ischemic attacks.

Mortality

Cerebrovascular disease, the third leading cause of death, was responsible for 207,000 deaths in 1974, but by 1994 the number had declined to 154,000.[2,13] This decline is remarkable because the population of older persons increased substantially during that time. The age-adjusted death rate declined by 55 percent over this period, although the rate of decline diminished, and in the past few years there has been a slight increase. The rate of decline in mortality for stroke accelerated from a 1 percent per year decline in the 1940s and 1950s and a 2 percent per year decline in the 1960s to a 6 percent per year decline in the 1970s. From 1985 to 1990, the decline slowed to 3 percent per year before a possible upturn. This disease still accounts for 1 of every 15 deaths, and 44,000 of them occur in individuals less than 75 years of age. Under age 65, the mortality rate is three times greater in the black than in the white population, largely as a result of the higher prevalence and increased severity of hypertension in that population. The proportion of strokes that result in death within 1 year is about 29 percent, less if the stroke occurs before age 65 (Fig. 1-7). The long-term survivorship is worse in men than in women; more than one-half of men with stroke die within 8 years (Table 1-6) (see also Chap. 99).

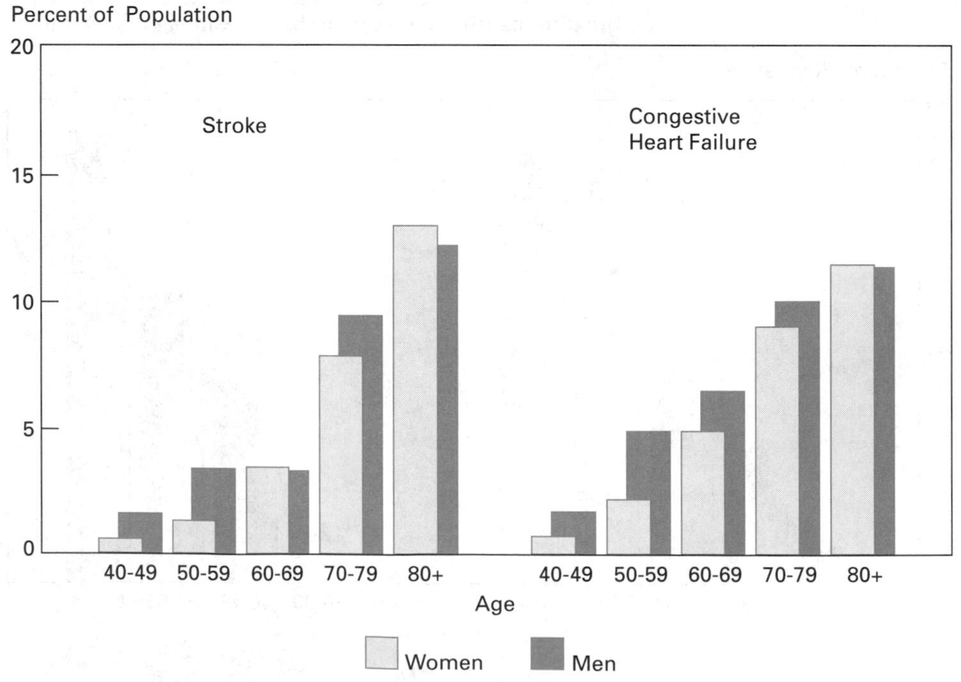

HEART FAILURE

Heart failure is the end stage of cardiac disease after the myocardium has used all its reserve and compensatory mechanisms. Once overt signs appear, half of

FIGURE 1-9

Prevalence of stroke and congestive heart failure by age and sex; United States, 1988–1991 (self-reported stroke and congestive heart failure from health interviews). (From the National Health and Nutrition Examination Survey, National Center for Health Statistics.)

the patients die within 5 years despite medical management.[29] Heart failure is most often a consequence of hypertension, CHD, valve deformity, diabetes, or cardiomyopathy.[30] The various etiologies tend to coexist. CHD, frequently accompanied by hypertension, is responsible in more than 50 percent of cases and has been increasing in prevalence among new cases of heart failure.[31] Isolated hypertension and valvular diseases are diminishing determinants. The risk of cardiac failure is increased two- to sixfold with CHD, angina conferring half the risk compared to myocardial infarct. The dominant cause is hypertension, which precedes failure in 75 percent of cases.

An estimated 4.8 million Americans have CHF.[20] The prevalence increases with age to exceed 10 percent after age 60 (Fig. 1-9). Each year there are an estimated 400,000 new cases.[2] In 1993, there were 45,000 deaths nominally classified to heart failure as the underlying cause and about another 200,000 where heart failure was listed on the death certificates as the leading "diagnostic related group" in hospitalized patients over 65 years of age.[32] The death rate increased in most years between 1968 and 1993. The rate of hospitalizations for heart failure increased three to four times between 1970 and 1994 in patients aged 45 to 64 and 65 and over.[2] In 1994, heart failure was the first-listed discharge diagnosis in 887,000 hospital discharges and a secondary diagnosis in another 1.8 million discharges.[10] One in five of all discharges of patients aged 65 and over had heart failure as a primary or secondary diagnosis. The percentage of CHF patients who died in hospitals, however, decreased from 11.3 percent in 1981 to 6.1 percent in 1993.[2] Visits to physicians' offices for CHF increased from 1.7 million in 1980 to 2.9 million in 1993.[2] The prevalence is similar in men and women, but it is higher in blacks than whites. It increased substantially as measured in national surveys in 1976 to 1980 and 1988 to 1991[2] (see also Chaps. 23 and 41).

Based on the Framingham Study, heart failure is equally frequent in men and women, and the annual occurrence approaches 10 per 1000 population after 65 years of age (Table 1-1). Survival following the diagnosis of heart failure is worse in men than women, but even in women fewer than 20 percent survive much longer than 8 to 12 years (Table 1-6). The prognosis is not much better than for most forms of cancer. The 1-year fatality rate for heart failure is high, with one in five dying. Sudden death is a common mode of exitus, occurring at six to nine times the general population rate. With an increasing geriatric population, heart failure is a formidable problem.

There is little indication that the declines in death rates from heart disease in general and from CHD in particular in the United States have been accompanied by an improvement in the incidence of heart failure.[32,33] This cannot be readily explained. Some postulate that improved survival of patients with angina, myocardial infarction, and hypertensive heart disease may result in an increased prevalence of chronic heart disease and ultimately heart failure.[32] Data from the Framingham Study indicate very little improvement to date in the ominous outlook following the onset of CHF. The median

survival of 652 incident cases of CHF was only 1.7 years in men and 3.2 years in women,[31,32] and the overall survival rates at 5 years were only 25 percent for men and 38 percent for women. The mortality increased with age in both sexes. If one adjusts for age, no significant changes in the prognosis of CHF are evident over the past four decades despite improvements in treatment. Thus, CHF remains a highly lethal condition with a better prognosis in women and younger patients. Advances in treatment of hypertension, myocardial ischemia, and valvular heart disease have not resulted in dramatic improvements in survival once heart failure ensues.

Despite the availability of potent glycosides, diuretics, and antihypertensive agents, heart failure continues at a high incidence. There is evidence that treatment of hypertension and left ventricular systolic dysfunction can decrease the incidence of clinical cardiac failure and that use of angiotensin-converting enzyme inhibitors or vasodilators can prolong survival after onset.[31,34] If preventive programs are to be developed, identification of factors that predispose and influence the course of the disease is essential.

IDIOPATHIC CARDIOMYOPATHY

Reliable estimates of the prevalence and incidence of idiopathic dilated (congestive) and hypertrophic cardiomyopathies are unavailable because of their comparatively uncommon occurrence in the general population. The National Center for Health Statistics data from 1993 assigned 26,214 deaths to cardiomyopathy.[35] Hypertrophic cardiomyopathy accounted for only 1 percent of deaths. Alcoholic heart muscle disease (cardiomyopathy) appears to account for 8 percent of deaths due to cardiomyopathy. This condition appears to be 2.5 times as frequent in blacks as in whites.

In 1994, cardiomyopathy was responsible for 37,000 hospitalizations and 270,000 days of hospital care in the United States.[10] Mortality was highest in older persons, men, and blacks. Death rates rose sharply between 1970 and 1993, but for reasons that are unclear. This apparent increase could be an artifact of changes in diagnostic criteria and death certification practices[35] (see also Chaps. 72 and 73).

ARRHYTHMIAS

Arrhythmias can be a manifestation of many cardiac diseases; they are a major cause of morbidity in heart failure and rheumatic heart disease and are a contributor to half of the mortality from CHD. Many such victims die suddenly, without warning. Together with heart failure, arrhythmias are often the final common pathways of heart disease.

Although true frequency of arrhythmias is not known, in 1994 there were an estimated 614,000 hospital discharges with arrhythmias listed first on the hospital record and an additional 3 million with arrhythmia as a secondary diagnosis.[10] In 1993, there were an estimated 3.6 million visits to physicians' offices for arrhythmias, larger than the number due to stroke. It is not known how many deaths are directly attributed to arrhythmias each year because it is the immediate cause, not the underlying cause, of much cardiac mortality.

The Framingham Study reported incidence rates for atrial fibrillation. In that population the chance of developing this condition was about 2 percent within 20 years.[36] About 70 percent of the cases evolved following development of overt cardiovascular disease. Heart failure and valvular heart disease were the most powerful precursors, with the relative risks as much as fivefold.[37] Hypertensive cardiovascular disease was the most common prior cardiovascular disease, largely because of its great frequency in the general population. On the other hand, neither hypertension alone nor CHD was a significant precursor. Among the risk factors, only diabetes and left ventricular hypertrophy on electrocardiogram were significantly or substantially related to the occurrence of atrial fibrillation. Cardiovascular mortality was doubled by the development of atrial fibrillation (see Chap. 27).

RHEUMATIC FEVER AND RHEUMATIC HEART DISEASE

Rheumatic fever is the chief cause of serious valvular heart disease. Acute rheumatic fever and subsequent rheumatic heart disease remain important cardiovascular problems in the tropical and subtropical developing countries in South America, Africa, the Middle East, and Asia,[38] where they occur with a frequency seen in the United States and Europe a century ago. Although preventable, rheumatic fever occurs more frequently because of overcrowding, the deceptive self-limited nature of symptoms in streptococcal pharyngitis, and the mild and often clinically inapparent nature of streptococcal infections. The availability of penicillin to treat these infections, living conditions that are less crowded than formerly, and evolution of different strains of streptococcus have made rheumatic fever uncommon in the United States, although the incidence remains high in subgroups such as blacks, Puerto Ricans, Mexican Americans, and American Indians[39] (see Chap. 62). Because this disease has not been eradicated in this country, there is need to define its incidence and prevalence more accurately as well as those of the infective endocarditis that may follow in order to pinpoint those at risk (see also Chap. 82).

The estimated prevalence in 1994 of active rheumatic fever and chronic rheumatic heart disease in the United States was 1.4 million persons—5 per 1000 persons of all ages.[20] About 15 percent of these persons are limited in activity because of the resulting chronic carditis.[8] There is no good recent estimate of annual incidence. The occurrence tends to be concentrated in the lower socioeconomic subgroups. Rheumatic fever is rare before age 3, occurring most frequently between 5 and 15 years of age, when streptococcal infections are most frequent. During epidemics of streptococcal pharyngitis, the rheumatic fever attack rate may be 3 percent, whereas in endemic situations it is usually only 0.3 percent (see also Chap. 62).

With the decline in rheumatic fever in the United States, its clinical manifestations have also moderated so that carditis is detected in fewer than 20 percent of acutely affected patients.[39] The annual mortality has declined to fewer than 6000 deaths per year, which reflects a 91 percent decline in the age-adjusted death rate from 1950 to 1993. Because the cardiac sequelae of rheumatic fever are still seen in adults and adequate treatment can reduce attacks by 90 percent, rheumatic fever and rheumatic heart disease remain the two most preventable serious cardiovascular disorders. It seems clear that at least part of the decline in rheumatic fever was due to prompt antistreptococcal treatment by physicians. The decline in rheumatic fever, however, appears to have antedated the advent of antistreptococcal agents. We are currently unable to explain the reasons for the decline in rheumatic fever definitely, possibly because we do not fully understand its etiologic factors (see Chap. 62).

In developing countries, rheumatic fever is the most frequent cause of heart disease in the 5- to 13-year-old group, causing 25 to 40 percent of all cardiovascular diseases and 33 to 50 percent of all hospital admissions.[38]

OTHER VALVULAR DISEASE

In the two decades since mitral valve prolapse was described, the syndrome has changed from being a curiosity to being the most frequently diagnosed valvular deformity. The exact prevalence is not clear. It appears to occur in about 6 to 10 percent of presumably normal young women[40] and is reported in about 4 percent of healthy young men.[41] Although the condition may become manifest at any age, it is reported most frequently in young women aged 14 to 30, where it may reach a prevalence exceeding 10 percent. Echocardiographic studies indicate that it may be even more common, with 10 to 15 percent of the population possibly afflicted; however, many allegedly diagnosed by echocardiography exhibit neither clinical nor angiographic evidence of the syndrome. The fact that 6 to 10 percent of asymptomatic young women may have this syndrome is *prima facie* evidence that it is generally a benign condition. The natural history is not well established. Few cases progress to a severe form, and the risk of sudden death appears to be much less than originally thought. The major importance may be the threat of endocarditis, which must be rare, and arrhythmias, which may be common (see Chap. 65).

CONGENITAL HEART DISEASE

The 1990 to 1992 National Health Interview Survey in the United States estimated that 960,000 persons reported being told they have congenital heart disease.[20] The prevalence of congenital heart disease at birth as determined during the infant's brief stay in the hospital is likely to be underestimated, and recognition of specific lesions may be inaccurate.[42] Most data are deficient for congenital heart disease diagnosed after the first week of life. Prevalence data based on autopsy findings are unreliable because they reflect a fraction of the deaths and relate only to fatal lesions. Most information comes from retrospective studies based extensively on referral practices.

Structural abnormalities of the heart or intrathoracic great vessels seem to affect 8 to 10 of every 1000 infants born alive in the United States. If bicuspid aortic valves and mitral valve prolapse manifested later in life are included, the rate may well exceed 1 percent of live births. About 1 newborn per 1000 live births has a cardiac birth defect that cannot be managed medically or surgically. Most infants who previously would have died now survive to adult life because of improved treatment, but 5 to 6 of these infants per 1000 live births require frequent medical or surgical attention shortly after birth or later in childhood.

Except for the recent unexplained twofold increase in ventricular septal defects and the threefold increase in patent ductus arteriosus, the incidence of most congenital heart diseases has remained stable. Rubella vaccine has reduced rubella-caused congenital heart disease, and congenital heart defects associated with Down's syndrome are less common because older women are having fewer babies. Pregnancies may be terminated if prenatal screening reveals Down's syndrome. Preventive strategies are impeded by lack of knowledge of the cause of most congenital heart disease, although it is known that alcohol, trimethadione, and lithium can cause cardiac defects. The majority of congenital heart disease may involve complex genetic-environmental interactions that remain to be elucidated (see Chaps. 69 and 70).

About 73 of each 1000 live births in the United States are premature, with the infants weighing less than 2500 g.[43] Almost half of premature infants weighing less than 1750 g will maintain patency of their ductus arteriosus, possibly because their immature lungs do not properly metabolize prostaglandins that cause the ductus to remain open.[44] The growing number of teratogens identified appears to account for only 5 percent of all human malformations, and single mutant genes are said to be responsible for only 3 percent of cases.

In all evaluations of mortality from congenital heart disease, death in infancy predominates at 1.3 to 2.8 per 1000 live births. Later mortality is more speculative, about 0.4 per 1000 live births over the subsequent 3 years. About 25 percent of infants with congenital heart disease have a malformation incompatible with life beyond the first year; possibly half of these can be treated surgically to improve the quality of life, if not to produce a cure. About 2.5 per 1000 live-born infants require specialized services for diagnosis and treatment of congenital heart disease shortly after birth, and another 2.5 per 1000 will need these resources later in childhood.

With the exception of mitral valve prolapse and bicuspid aortic valve in older patients, ventricular septal defect is the most common variety, accounting for 30 percent of congenital heart disease. Some 75 percent of congenital heart disease in infants and children is encompassed by seven defects: ventricular septal defect, pulmonary stenosis, patent ductus arterio-

sus, tetralogy of Fallot, aortic stenosis, coarctation of the aorta, and transposition of the great arteries. There is an excess of birth defects in blacks. The rate among siblings is 17 per 1000 compared to 2.6 per 1000 in the general population (see Chap. 70).

PULMONARY THROMBOEMBOLISM

More than 95 percent of pulmonary emboli arise from deep venous thrombi in the legs (above the knee); the remainder arise from the right cardiac chambers or other veins. The majority of deaths occur suddenly and can be avoided only by prophylaxis. Patients who survive to reach the hospital for medical treatment generally have a good outlook, with little morbidity and resolution of the emboli.

Estimates of mortality from pulmonary embolism vary widely, depending on the source and accuracy of the data. Pulmonary emboli are probably directly responsible for 50,000 deaths annually in the United States. If untreated, recurrent episodes are frequent and more than 25 percent will be fatal. More than 60 percent of fatalities occur within 1 h of onset; hence, pulmonary embolism is likely to be confused with sudden coronary death. It is estimated that pulmonary embolism is grossly underdiagnosed, since only 10 to 30 percent of autopsied cases with evidence of embolism had an antemortem diagnosis.[45]

Among the white U.S. population, the age-adjusted death rate for pulmonary embolism decreased 12 percent in men and 20 percent in women between 1970 and 1978.[46] Despite protocol changes that increased the number of diagnoses coded and the introduction of prospective payment and diagnosis-related groups from 1983 to 1985, no increases in rates were noted from 1979 to 1985. The rate of hospital discharges with the diagnosis of pulmonary embolism declined 15 to 45 percent, particularly in younger age groups, between 1979 and 1985. Death rates and hospital rates for pulmonary embolism increase with age and are higher in men than in women and in blacks than in whites.[5] It was listed on 101,000 hospital records in 1994.[10] The incidence is even more uncertain. Only 10 percent of cases occur in normal persons without predisposing factors such as chronic cardiopulmonary and malignant disease, estrogen therapy, orthopedic trauma, immobilization, operative procedures, obesity, pregnancy, or blood dyscrasias. The elderly are more vulnerable.

Postoperative pulmonary emboli alone produce 4000 to 8000 deaths annually.[47] It is a major cause of death post partum and in patients hospitalized for orthopedic conditions. Evidence from Britain suggests that the annual mortality from pulmonary embolism has been increasing for several decades despite anticoagulant drugs. More than 5 million persons over age 45 undergo major surgery each year in the United States; 1 or 2 of each 1000 will die postoperatively from pulmonary embolism. The recent advent of low-dose heparin prophylaxis may substantially reduce this risk (see Chap. 60).

PREVENTIVE IMPLICATIONS

Examination of the incidence, prevalence, mortality, and natural history of cardiovascular disease suggests the need for a preventive approach. Further innovations in diagnosis and treatment for cardiovascular disease will undoubtedly improve the outlook of patients surviving the initial attack, but this can have only a limited impact because of the high initial mortality. When the heart or brain is infarcted, no therapy can be expected to restore full function. If the initial presentation is sudden death, therapy is unavailing. A preventive approach involving correction of predisposing factors in advance of the overt clinical expression of the disease can be expected to have a greater impact.

CHD often strikes without warning: One in five coronary attacks presents as sudden death, and two-thirds of the deaths occur in the community too precipitously to be brought under medical attention.

While some strokes may give warning by transient ischemic attacks, most do not. Even when they do, intervention at that stage does not necessarily avoid a permanently damaging stroke or prolong life.

Heart valves damaged by rheumatic heart disease and infective endocarditis can be surgically repaired or replaced by prosthetic appliances; this approach often requires potentially dangerous anticoagulants to prevent emboli, and valve failure and hemolysis are distressingly common. Although such patients live longer, more comfortable lives than formerly, their survival does not approach that of patients with rheumatic fever who have been kept from progressing to severe valve damage by antibiotic prophylaxis against recurrent disease.

Hypertension that progresses to target organ involvement is less manageable than if vigorously treated prior to such manifestations. The first sign of target organ involvement is often a stroke, myocardial infarction, or sudden death. Half such events occur before evidence of organ involvement is discovered on routine biennial examination. In some respects, the occurrence of symptoms may be more properly regarded as a medical failure rather than as the initial indication for treatment (see Chap. 58).

A major impact on cardiovascular morbidity and mortality should derive from the practice of preventive medicine, from public health measures to alter lifestyle to one more favorable to cardiovascular health, and from health education to inform people of what they must do to protect their cardiovascular health.[48,49] Recent expansion and improvements in these measures have occurred, conceivably contributing significantly to the 43 percent decline in cardiovascular mortality during the past two decades, which is responsible for 90 percent of the decline in overall mortality.[3]

REFERENCES

1. National Center for Health Statistics. *Health, United States, 1995.* DHHS pub no (PHS) 96-1232. US Government Printing Office; 1996.

2. National Heart, Lung, and Blood Institute: *Morbidity and Mortality Chartbook on Cardiovascular, Lung, and Blood Diseases/1996.* US Dept of Health and Human Services; 1996.

3. National Heart, Lung, and Blood Institute. *NHLBI Fact Book, Fiscal Year 1995.* US Dept of Health and Human Services, National Institutes of Health; March 1996.

4. Gordon T, Kannel WB: Premature mortality from coronary heart disease: The Framingham Study. *JAMA* 1971; 215:1617–1625.

5. National Center for Health Statistics: *Vital Statistics of the United States, 1993,* vol II, *Mortality,* pt A. DHHS pub no (PHS) 97-1101. US Government Printing Office (in press).

6. National Center for Health Statistics, Adams PF, Marano MA. Current estimates from the National Health Interview Survey, United States, 1994. *Vital and Health Statistics.* DHHS pub no (PHS) 96-1521. US Government Printing Office; 1995.

7. Burt VL, Whelton P, Roccella EJ, Brown C, Cutler JA, Higgins M, et. al. Prevalence of hypertension in the US adult population: Results from the third National Health and Nutrition Examination Survey, 1988–1991. *Hypertension* 1995; 25:3:305–313.

8. National Center for Health Statistics, Collins JG. Prevalence of selected chronic conditions, United States, 1990–92. *Vital and Health Statistics,* 10 (194). DHHS pub no (PHS) 97-1522. US Government Printing Office; 1997.

9. Rogot E, Sorlie PD, Johnson NJ, Schmitt C. Second data book; a study of 1.3 million persons: By demographic, social, and economic factors: 1979–1985 follow-up: US National Longitudinal Mortality Study. US Dept of Health and Human Services, National Institutes of Health pub no 92-3297; 1992.

10. National Center for Health Statistics, Graves EJ. Detailed diagnoses and procedures, National Hospital Discharge Survey, 1994. *Vital and Health Statistics,* ser 13, no. 127. DHHS pub no (PHS) 97-1788. US Government Printing Office; 1997.

11. National Center for Health Statistics, Schappert SM. National ambulatory medical care survey: 1994 summary. *Advance Data from Vital and Health Statistics.* No. 273, DHHS pub no (PHS) 96-1250. US Government Printing Office; 1996.

12. National Center for Health Statistics, Strahan GW. An overview of home health and hospice care patients: 1994 National Home and Hospice Care Survey. *Advance Data from Vital and Health Statistics.* No. 274, DHHS pub no (PHS) 96-1250. US Government Printing Office; 1996.

13. National Center for Health Statistics. Annual summary of births, marriages, divorces, and deaths; United States, 1994. *Monthly Vital Statist Rep:* vol 43, no 13, October 23, 1995.

14. Higgins MW, Luepker RV, eds. *Trends in Coronary Heart Disease Mortality: The Influence of Medical Care.* New York: Oxford University Press; 1988.

15. Higgins MW, Luepker RV. Trends and determinants of coronary heart disease mortality: International comparisons. *Int J Epidemiol* 1989; 18(suppl 1):S1–S2.

16. Sytkowski PA, Kannel WB, D'Agostino RB. Changes in risk factors and the decline in mortality from cardiovascular disease: The Framingham Study. *N Engl J Med* 1990; 322:1635–1641.

17. D'Agostino RB, Kannel WB, Belanger AJ, Sytkowski PA. Trends in CHD and risk factors at age 55–64 in the Framingham Study. *Int J Epidemiol* 1989; 18(3, suppl 1):567–572.

18. Burke GL, Sprafka JM, Folsom AR, Luepker RV, Norsted SW, Blackburn H. Trends in CHD mortality, morbidity and risk factor levels from 1960 to 1986: The Minnesota Heart Survey. *Int J Epidemiol* 1989; 18(3, suppl 1):573–581.

19. Kannel WB, Wilson PWF. An update on coronary risk factors. *Med Clin North Am* 1995; 79:5:951–971.

20. American Heart Association. *Heart and Stroke Facts: 1995 Statistical Supplement.* American Heart Association; 1994. Dallas, TX 75231-4596.

21. Burt VL, Cutler JA, Higgins M, Horan MJ, Labarthe D, Whelton P, et al. Trends in the prevalence, awareness, treatment, and control of hypertension in the adult US population: Data from the health examination surveys, 1960 to1991. *Hypertension* 1995; 26:60–69.

22. US Dept of Health and Human Services, Social Security Administration. *Characteristics of Social Security Disability Insurance Beneficiaries.* SSA pub no 13-11947, 1982.

23. Gordon T, Kannel WB, Hjortland MC, McNamara PM. Menopause and coronary heart disease. *Ann Intern Med* 1978; 89:157–161.

24. Kannel WB: *The Natural History of Myocardial Infarction: The Framingham Study.* Leiden: Leiden University Press; 1973.

25. SHEP Cooperative Working Group. Prevention of stroke by antihypertensive drug treatment in older persons with isolated systolic hypertension: Final results of the Systolic Hypertension in the Elderly Program (SHEP). *JAMA* 1991; 265:3255–3264.

26. Reaven GM, Hoffman BB. A role for insulin, the aetiology and causes of hypertension? *Lancet* 1987; 2:435–437.

27. Gresham GE, Fitzpatrick TE, Wolf PA, McNamara PM, Kannel WB, Dawber TR. Residual disability in survivors of stroke: The Framingham Study. *N Engl J Med* 1975; 293:954–956.

28. Kannel WB, Wolf PA, Dawber TR. An evaluation of the epidemiology of atherothrombotic brain infarction. *Milbank Q* 1975; 53:405–448.

29. Kannel WB, Belanger AJ. Epidemiology of heart failure. *Am Heart J* 1991; 121(3, pt 1):951–957.

30. Kannel WB, Ho K, Thom T. Changing epidemiological features of cardiac failure. *Br Heart J* 1994; 72:S3–S9.

31. Ho KKL, Anderson KM, Kannel WB, Grossman W, Levy D. Survival after the onset of congestive heart failure in Framingham Heart Study subjects. *Circulation* 1993; 88:1:107–115.

32. Gillum RF. Epidemiology of heart failure in the United States. *Am Heart J* 1993; 126:1042–1047.

33. Gillum RF, Folson AR, Blackburn H. The decline in coronary heart disease mortality: Old questions and new facts. *Am J Med* 1984; 76:1055–1065.

34. Ho KKL, Pinsky JL, Kannel WB, Levy D. The epidemiology of heart failure: The Framingham Study. *J Am Coll Cardiol* 1993; 22:4:6A–13A.

35. Gillum RF. Idiopathic cardiomyopathy in the United States, 1970–1982. *Am Heart J* 1986; 111:752–755.

36. Kannel WB, Abbott RD, Savage DD, McNamara PM. Epidemiologic features of chronic atrial fibrillation: The Framingham Study. *N Engl J Med* 1982; 306:1018–1022.

37. Benjamin EJ, Levy D, Vaziri SM, D'Agostino RB, Belanger AJ, Wolf PA. Independent risk factors for atrial fibrillation in a population-based cohort: The Framingham Heart Study. *JAMA* 1994; 271:11:840–844.

38. Gillum RF. Trends in acute rheumatic fever and chronic rheumatic heart disease: A national perspective. *Am Heart J* 1986; 111:430–432.

39. Persellin RH. Acute rheumatic fever: Changing manifestations. *Ann Intern Med* 1978; 89:1002–1004.

40. Procacci PM, Savran SV, Schreiter SL, Bryson AL. Prevalence of clinical mitral valve prolapse in 1969 young women. *N Engl J Med* 1976; 294:1086–1088.

41. Sbarbaro JA, Mehlman DJ, Wu L, Brooks HL. A prospective study of mitral valvular prolapse in young men. *Chest* 1979; 75:555–559.

42. Gillum RF. Epidemiology of congenital heart disease in the United States. *Am Heart J* 1994; 127:919–927.

43. National Center for Health Statistics. Advance report of final natality statistics, 1994. *Monthly Vital Statistics Rep:* vol 44, no 11, June 24, 1996.

44. Michaelson M. *Report on a Study of Congenital Cardiovascular Malformations—Etiology, Incidence, Natural History and Organization of Diagnostic and Therapeutic Services.* World Health Organization, Regional Office for Europe, 1979.

45. Moser KM: Pulmonary thromboembolism. In: Isselbacher KJ, Braunwald E, Wilson JD, Martin JB, Fauci AS, Kasper DL, eds. *Harrison's Principles of Internal Medicine,* 13th ed. New York: McGraw-Hill; 1994:1214–1220.

46. Gillum RF. Pulmonary embolism and thrombophlebitis in the United States, 1970–1985. *Am Heart J* 1987; 114:1262–1266.

47. Clagett GP, Anderson FA Jr, Levine MN, Heit J, Levine M, Wheeler HB. Prevention of venous thromboembolism. *Chest* 1995; 108(suppl):3125–3345.

48. Havlik RJ, Feinleib M, eds. *Proceedings of the Conference on Decline of Coronary Heart Disease Mortality.* Washington, DC; National Institutes of Health: 1979.

49. Thom TJ, Kannel WB. Factors in the decline of coronary disease mortality. In: Connor WE, Bristow JD, eds. *Coronary Heart Disease: Prevention, Complications, and Treatment.* Philadelphia: Lippincott; 1985:5–20.

2

ANATOMY OF THE HEART

Bruce F. Waller / Robert C. Schlant

GROSS ANATOMY OF THE HEART AND BLOOD VESSELS

Andreas Vesalius (1514–1564) is considered the "father" of modern anatomy. Since his day, however, new observations have been made that provide an important framework for understanding cardiac physiology and pathophysiology, examining the patient, and interpreting noninvasive and invasive tests of the heart.[1–14]

The heart is situated in the middle mediastinum with its "long axis" oriented from the right shoulder to the left upper abdominal quadrant. The heart has a base, which is formed by the atria and great arteries, and an apex, which is formed by the junction of the ventricles and ventricular septum.

The sternum and costal cartilages of the third, fourth, and fifth ribs overlie the heart anteriorly. About two-thirds of the heart is left of the midline. The heart rests upon the diaphragm and is tilted forward and to the left so that the apex is anterior to the rest of the heart. The normal apex impulse can be palpated in the fourth or fifth intercostal space near the midclavicular line. The weight and size of the heart vary considerably depending on age, sex, body length, epicardial fat, and general nutrition. The average human adult heart averages approximately 325 ± 75 g in men and 275 ± 75 g in women.[10]

The borders of the normal cardiac silhouette in a frontal view are formed by the following structures (Fig. 2-1): The top of the cardiac silhouette is formed by the transverse and ascending aorta. The upper right margin is delineated by the superior vena cava. The right atrium provides the remaining right lateral cardiac border. Most of the inferior border is composed of right ventricle. The apex and the lower left lateral cardiac border consist of the left ventricle. The left atrial

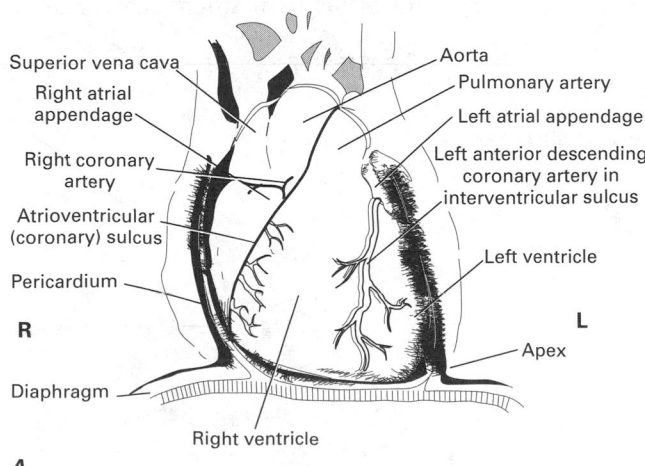

Superior vena cava
Right atrial appendage
Right coronary artery
Atrioventricular (coronary) sulcus
Pericardium
R
Diaphragm
Right ventricle

Aorta
Pulmonary artery
Left atrial appendage
Left anterior descending coronary artery in interventricular sulcus
Left ventricle
L
Apex

A

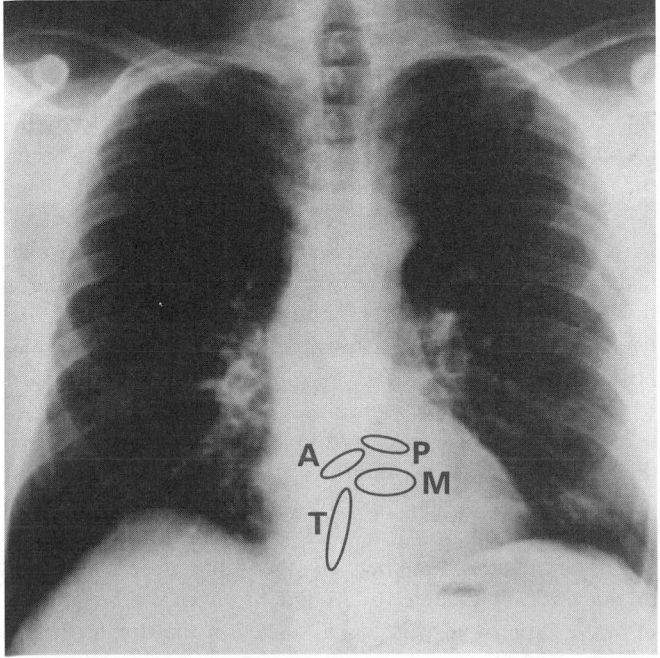

B

FIGURE 2-1

A. Diagram showing the normal relations of the pericardium, great vessels, ventricles, and atria as viewed in the frontal position. R = right; L = left. *B.* Frontal (AP) roentgenogram of the heart. The components that form the cardiac silhouette can be readily identified from *A.* A = aortic valve ring; P = pulmonary valve ring; M = mitral valve ring; T = tricuspid valve ring. (Diagram by McClaren Johnson, Jr., M.D.)

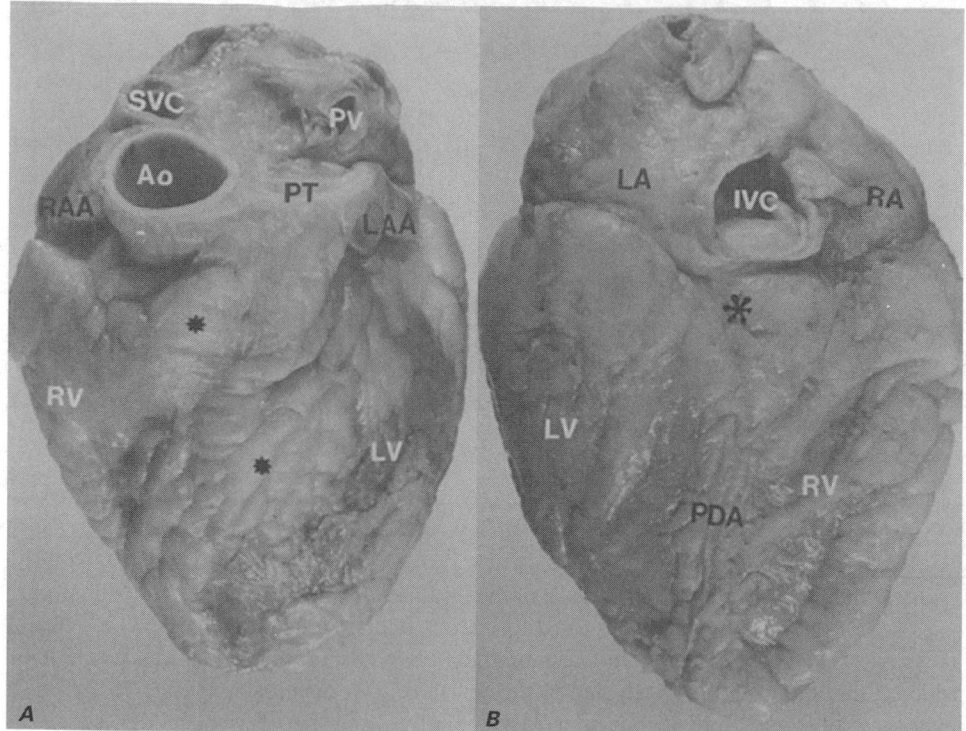

FIGURE 2-2

External views of the heart. *A.* Anterior surface showing epicardial fat, *, which obscures the interventricular sulci containing the left anterior descending artery. Ao = aorta; LAA = left atrial appendage; LV = left ventricle; PT = pulmonary trunk; PV = pulmonary vein; RAA = right atrial appendage; RV = right ventricle; SVC = superior vena cava. *B.* Posterior surface of heart showing location of posterior descending artery (PDA), crux of the heart, *, and inferior vena cava (IVC). LA = left atrium; RA = right atrium.

The posterior interventricular sulcus is the pathway for the posterior descending coronary artery, which is usually the terminal branch of the right coronary artery or, less frequently, of the left circumflex artery (Fig. 2-2). The two atria may be delineated externally by a groove on the posterior surface between the right pulmonary veins and the venae cavae.

The *crux* of the heart is the area on the posterior basal surface where the coronary sulcus meets the posterior interventricular sulcus (Fig. 2-2). Internally at this junction, the atrial septum joins the ventricular septum. The coronary artery that crosses this area makes a sharp inward turn at the crux and provides a small artery to the nearby AV node. The area of the heart below the crux is referred to as the diaphragmatic, or inferior, surface of the heart. A transverse section through the heart is extremely helpful in demonstrating the relations of the cardiac chambers (Figs. 2-3 to 2-5). The ventricular and atrial septa are aligned obliquely 45° to the left of the midline, with the planes of the septa directed approximately from right scapula to left nipple.[7] The entire right side of the heart is to the right of this plane, placing most of the right atrium anterior to the

appendage perches atop the left ventricle and to the side of the pulmonary artery, interjecting its auricle on the cardiac border between the left ventricle and pulmonary outflow tract. The pulmonary outflow area forms the rest of the upper left border.

External Features

The atria are separated from the ventricles externally by the coronary sulcus [atrioventricular (AV) sulcus], which circles the heart between the atria and ventricles (Figs. 2-1 and 2-2). The right coronary artery, after leaving the aorta, travels in this sulcus between the right atrium and right ventricle until it descends on the posterior surface of the heart. Similarly, the left circumflex artery is found in the coronary sulcus between the left atrium and left ventricle until the artery ramifies posteriorly.

Externally, the two ventricles are delineated by interventricular sulci, which descend from the coronary sulcus toward the apex. Epicardial fat often obscures these landmarks (Fig. 2-2). The anterior interventricular sulcus contains the left anterior descending coronary artery and courses over the muscular ventricular septum between the right and left ventricles to the apex. It then turns around the apex and continues in the posterior interventricular sulcus on the diaphragmatic surface of the heart.

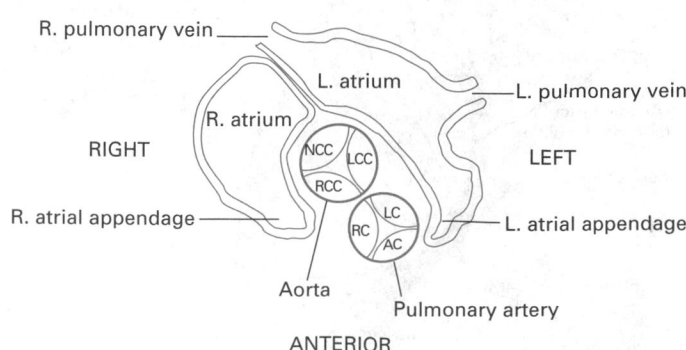

FIGURE 2-3

Schematic transverse section through the heart at approximately the level of the second intercostal space. The relation between the left and right atria and the interatrial septum is illustrated. The relative positions of the aortic and pulmonary valves and their cusps are shown. AC = anterior cusp; RC = right cusp; LC = left cusp of the pulmonary valve; LCC = left coronary cusp; RCC = right coronary cusp; NCC = noncoronary cusp of the aortic valve.

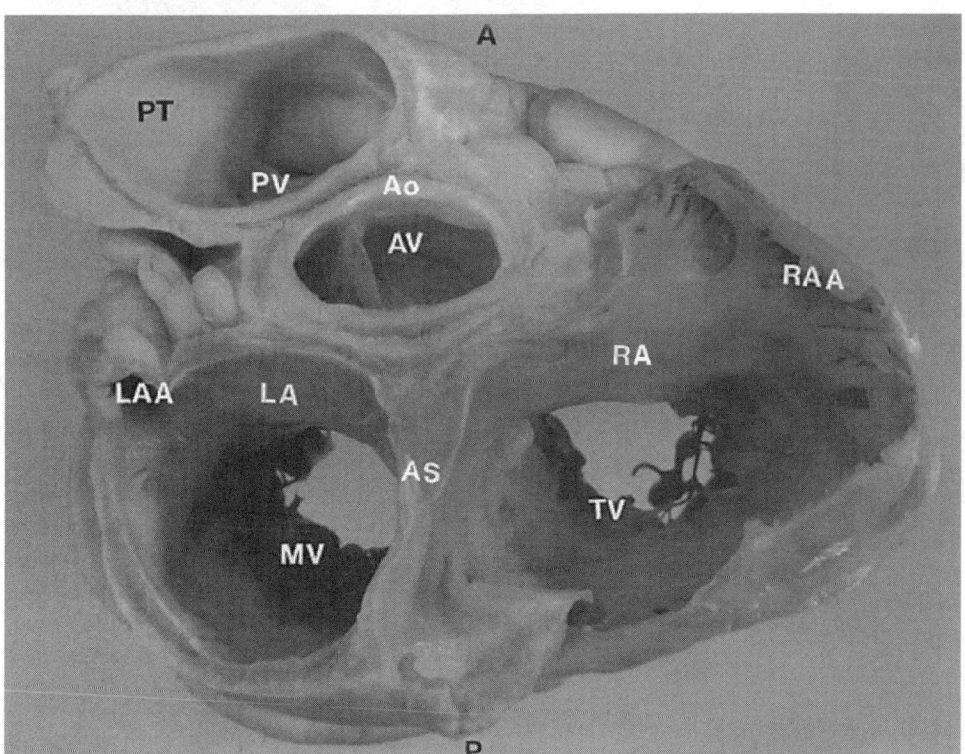

FIGURE 2-4

Transverse section through base of heart
showing relationship of various chambers
and great vessels. A = anterior; Ao =
aorta; AS = atrial septum; AV = aortic
valve; LA = left atrium; LAA = left
atrial appendage; MV = mitral valve;
RA = right atrium; RAA = right atrial
appendage; P = posterior; PT = pulmonary trunk; PV = pulmonic valve;
TV = tricuspid valve. [From Waller BF,
et al. Tomographic views of normal and
abnormal hearts: The anatomic basis for
various cardiac imaging techniques. *Clin
Cardiol* 1990; 13:802(pt I), 877(pt II).
Reproduced with permission from the
publisher and authors.]

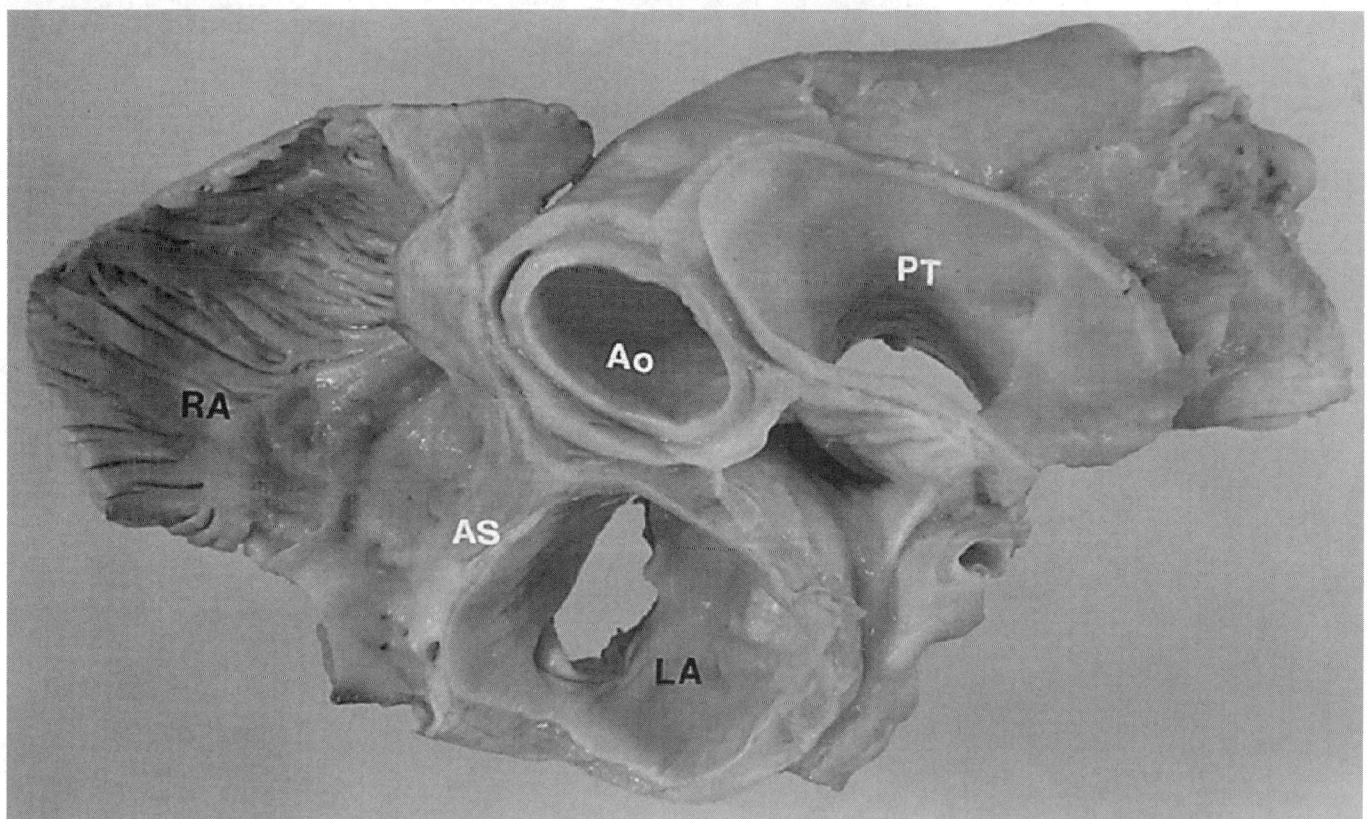

FIGURE 2-5

Basal view of heart showing relationship of great vessels and atria. The
left atrium (LA) has a smooth endocardium while the right atrium (RA) is
trabeculated. The aorta (Ao) is posterior to the pulmonary trunk (PT) but
anterior to the atrial septum (AS). [From Waller BF, et al. Tomographic
views of normal and abnormal hearts: The anatomic basis for various cardiac
imaging techniques. *Clin Cardiol* 1990; 13:802(pt I), 877(pt II). Reproduced
with permission from the publisher and authors.]

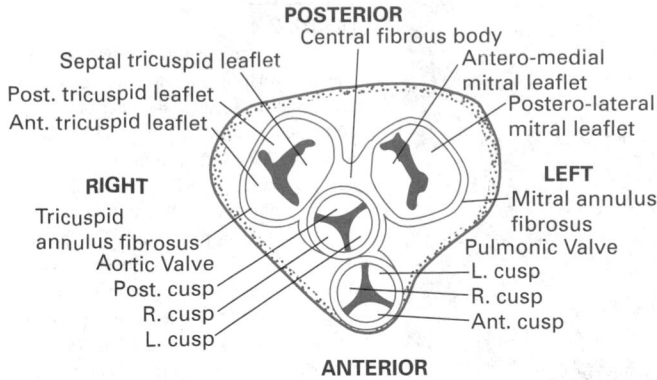

POSTERIOR
Central fibrous body

Septal tricuspid leaflet
Post. tricuspid leaflet
Ant. tricuspid leaflet

Antero-medial
mitral leaflet
Postero-lateral
mitral leaflet

RIGHT
Tricuspid
annulus fibrosus
Aortic Valve
Post. cusp
R. cusp
L. cusp

LEFT
Mitral annulus
fibrosus
Pulmonic Valve
L. cusp
R. cusp
Ant. cusp

ANTERIOR

FIGURE 2-6

Schematic anterosuperior view of the heart with the atria removed. The components of the fibrous skeleton and the orientation of the leaflets of each valve are shown.

left atrium and most of the right ventricle anterior to the left ventricle.

Fibrous Skeleton

A fibrous tissue framework affords a firm anchor for the attachments of the atrial and ventricular musculature as well as the valvular tissue (Figs. 2-6 and 2-7). At the center of the heart, the central fibrous body (right fibrous trigone) fuses together the medial aspect of the mitral and tricuspid valves and the aortic root. The left fibrous trigone is formed by compact bundles of connective tissue that course from the central fibrous body to the left, posterior inferiorly and anteriorly. Continuations of fibroelastic tissue from the central fibrous body (right fibrous trigone) and the left fibrous trigone partially encircle the mitral and tricuspid valves. These rings of tissue are the mitral and tricuspid annuli, which serve as attachments for the mitral and tricuspid valves as well as for the atrial and ventricular muscle. In general, the fibrous skeleton is less well developed around the tricuspid valve. A triple scalloped line of heavy collagenous tissue extends

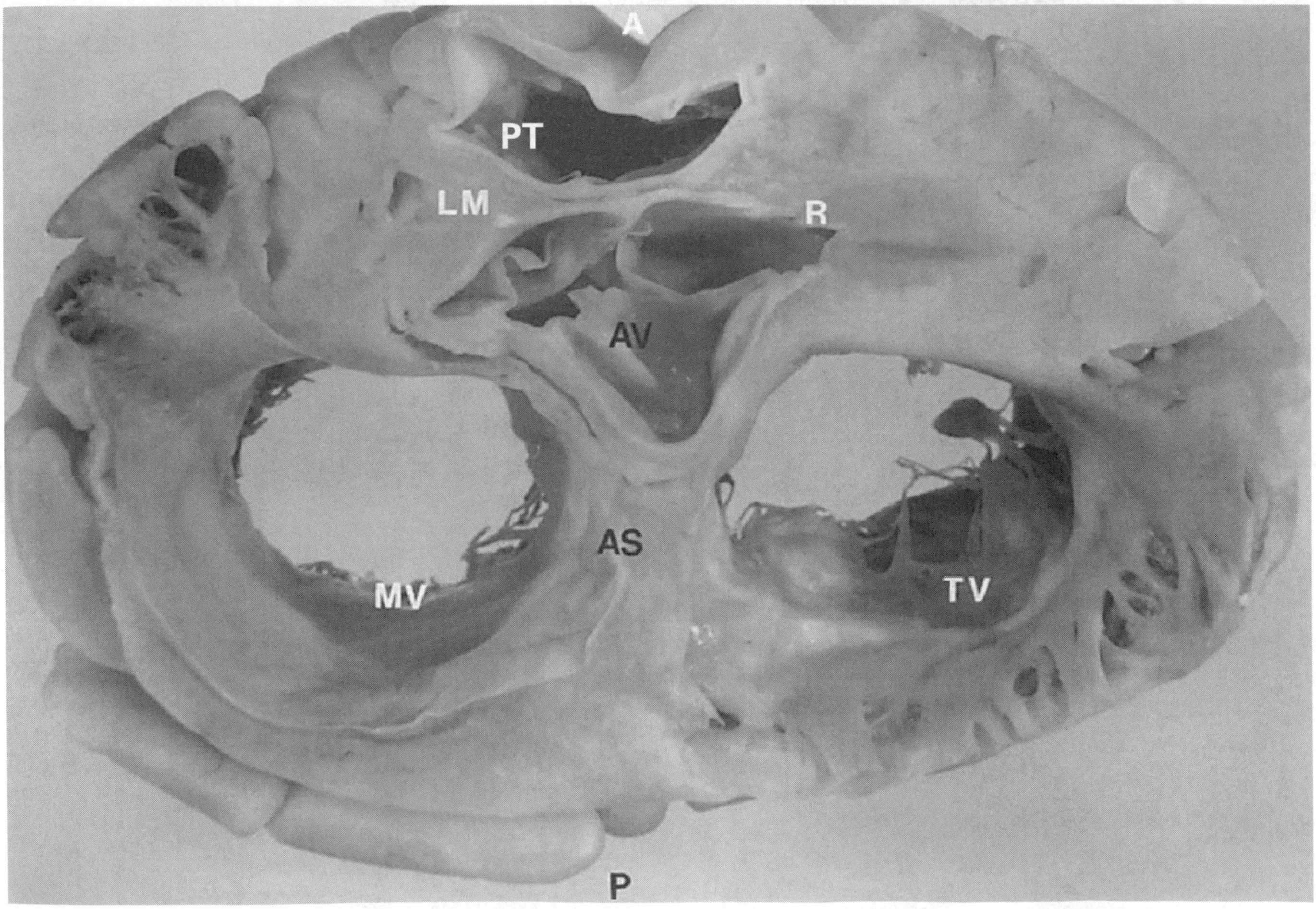

FIGURE 2-7

Cross-sectional view of heart showing aortic valve (AV), pulmonary trunk (PT), origin of the right (R) and left main (LM) coronary arteries, tricuspid (TV) and mitral (MV) valves, and atrial septum (AS). A = anterior; P = posterior. [From Waller BF, et al. Tomographic views of normal and abnormal hearts: The anatomic basis for various cardiac imaging techniques. *Clin Cardiol* 1990; 13:802(pt I), 877(pt II). Reproduced with permission from the publisher and authors.]

anteriorly from the left and right fibrous trigones to provide a three-pointed, crownlike skeletal support for the aortic root and cusps. A substantial ligament of tissue, the conus ligament, passes from the right side of the aortic root to a similar arrangement of scalloped tissue that surrounds the pulmonic root.

An important extension of the fibrous skeleton, the membranous ventricular septum, extends inferiorly and anteriorly from the central fibrous body (right fibrous trigone).[7,9,15] This membranous septum is located at the summit of the muscular ventricular septum, where it provides support for the right coronary and noncoronary aortic cusps (Fig. 2-8). A portion of the membranous ventricular septum extends slightly above the tricuspid valve, forming a small portion of the medial wall of the right atrium.[16] The bundle of His penetrates the central fibrous body and travels along the inferior margin of the membranous portion of the ventricular septum.[17] At the crest of the muscular septum, above the level of junction of the right coronary and posterior (noncoronary) aortic cusps, the His bundle separates into a left bundle branch and a right bundle branch. The left bundle subsequently subdivides into multiple branches that fan out as they spread to the left ventricle.

Cardiac Chambers

RIGHT ATRIUM

Venous blood returns to the heart via the superior and inferior venae cavae into the right atrium, where it is stored during right ventricular systole. During ventricular diastole, blood flows from the right atrium into the right ventricle (Figs. 2-1, 2-2, 2-4, 2-7, and 2-9 to 2-11). The right atrium forms the right lateral cardiac border and is above, behind, and to the right of the right ventricle (Figs. 2-4 and 2-7). Most of the right atrium is to the right and anterior to the left atrium (Figs. 2-4 and 2-7). Anteromedially, the right atrial appendage protrudes from the right atrium and overlaps the aortic root (Figs. 2-1 and 2-2). On the posterior external surface of the right atrium a ridge, the sulcus terminalis (or terminal groove), extends vertically from the superior to the inferior vena cava. This corresponds to an internal muscular bundle, the crista

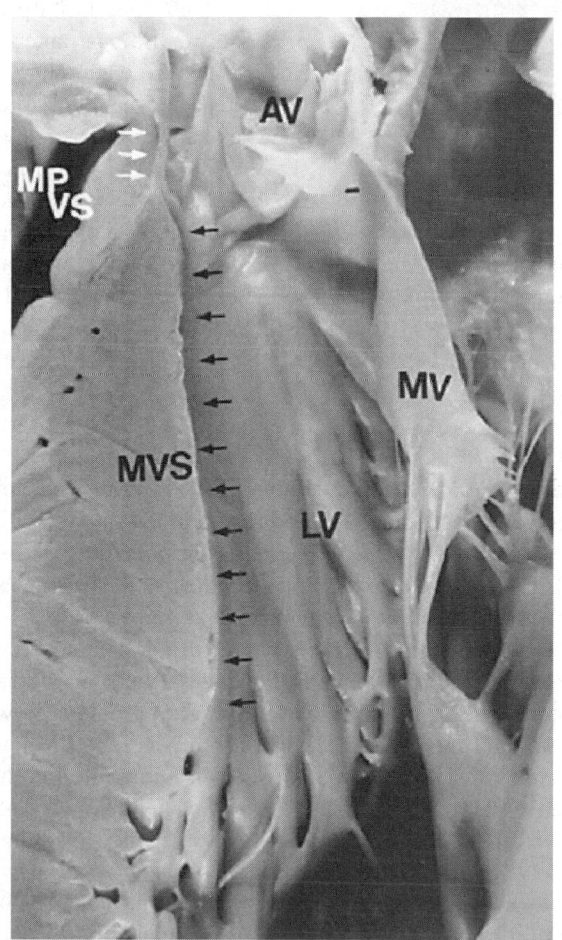

FIGURE 2-8
Specimen showing the muscular ventricular septum (MVS) (*black arrows*) and membranous portion of the ventricular septum (MPVS) (*white arrows*). LV = left ventricle; MV = mitral valve.

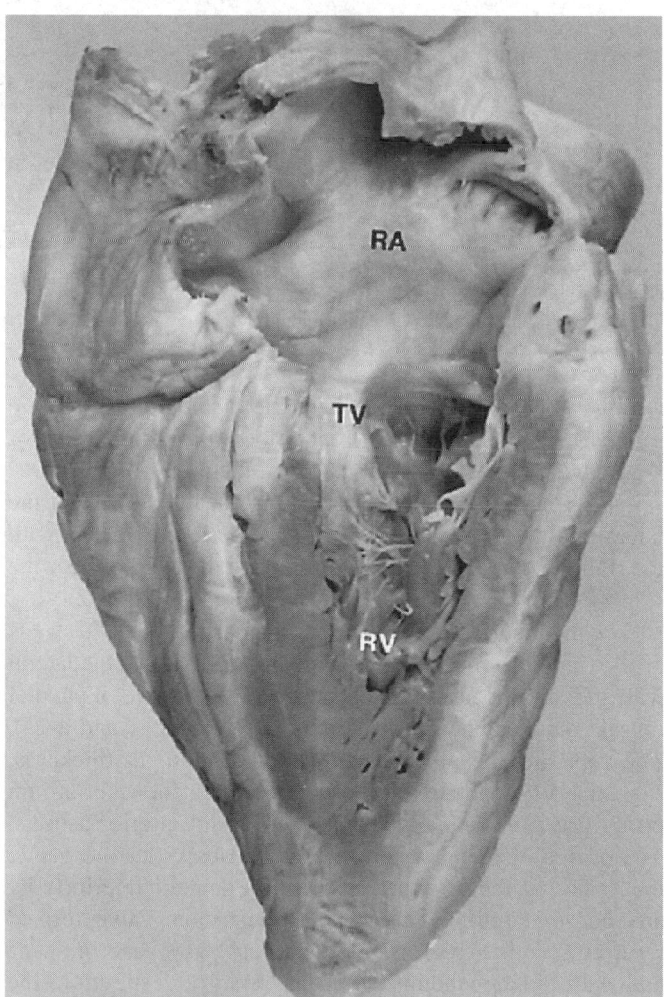

FIGURE 2-9
Long-axis view of right side of heart showing right ventricle (RV), right atrium (RA), and tricuspid valve (TV). The RV walls are heavily trabeculated. [From Waller BF, et al. Tomographic views of normal and abnormal hearts: The anatomic basis for various cardiac imaging techniques. *Clin Cardiol* 1990; 13:802(pt I), 877(pt II). Reproduced with permission from the publisher and authors.]

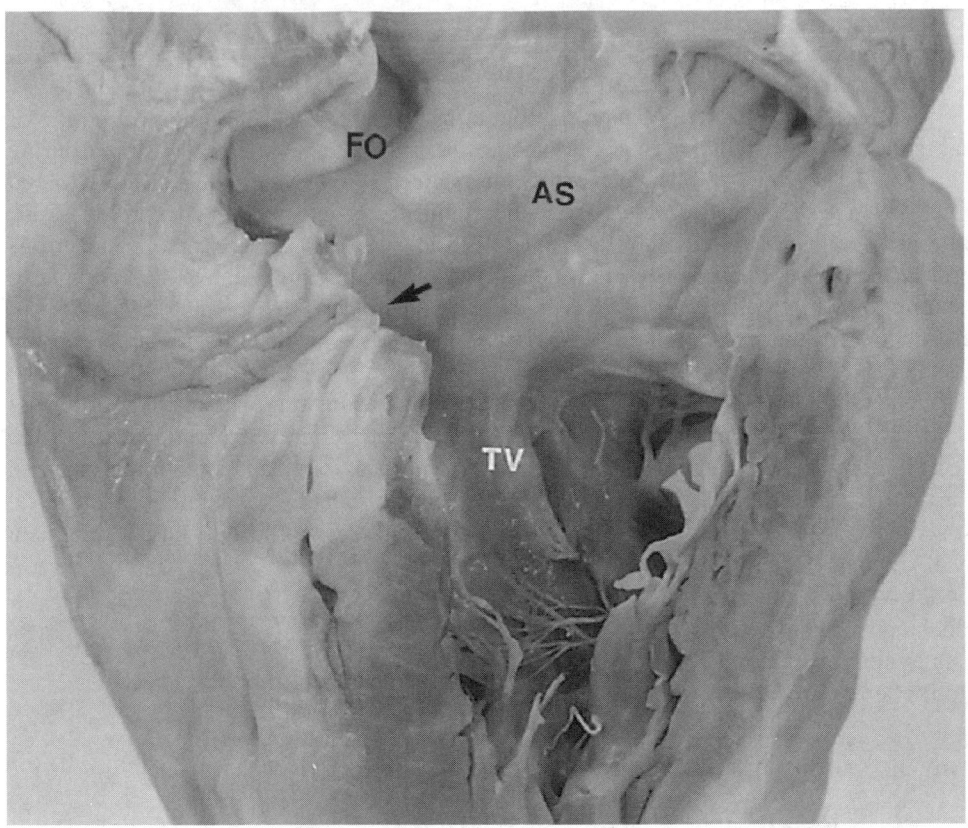

FIGURE 2-10

Close-up of right atrium showing atrial septum (AS), foramen ovale (FO), entrance to orifice of coronary sinus (*arrow*), and tricuspid valve (TV).

the aortic root lean against the medial right atrium, forming a normal slight bulge known as the *torus aorticus*, which is a useful landmark during transseptal catheterization of the left side of the heart. The proximal right coronary artery is in the immediate vicinity as it enters the coronary sulcus. The proximity of the aortic root to the right atrium permits an aneurysm of the sinus of Valsalva to rupture into the right atrium.

The atrial septum (Figs. 2-3, 2-4, 2-7, and 2-9 to 2-11) is found in the posteroinferior portion of the medial wall of the right atrium and extends obliquely forward from right to left.[18] Near the center of the atrial septum there is a shallow depression, the fossa ovalis, which often has a prominent fold, or limbus, anteriorly. The ostium of the coronary sinus is located between the inferior vena cava and the tricuspid valve (Figs. 2-9 to 2-11). The orifice of the coronary sinus is guarded by a rudimentary flap of tissue, the Thebesian valve. The AV node is located in the lower atrial septum, anterior and medial to the coronary sinus, just above the septal leaflet of the tricuspid valve. The sinus and AV nodes, as well as the entire conducting pathways, are not grossly visible.

terminalis, which runs along the edge of the entrance to the right atrial appendage to the front of the orifice of the superior vena cava and then to the right side of the inferior vena cava[7] (Figs. 2-9 to 2-11). The sinus node is usually located at the lateral margin of the junction of the superior vena cava with the right atrium and the atrial appendage, beneath or near the sulcus terminalis (terminal groove) (Figs. 2-1 and 2-2).

The inner surface of the posterior and medial (septal) walls of the right atrium is smooth, while the surfaces of the lateral wall and of the right atrial appendage are composed of parallel muscle bundles, the pectinate muscles[7] (Figs. 2-7 and 2-11). The right atrial wall measures almost 2 mm in thickness. The superior and inferior venae cavae enter the right atrium posteriorly and medially at its superior and inferior aspects. The orifice of the superior vena cava usually has no valve; the orifice of the inferior vena cava is flanked anteriorly by an inconstant, rudimentary valve, the eustachian valve, formed by a crescentic fold. The caval orifices may vary in shape and diameter depending upon the phase of respiration, the cardiac cycle, and the contraction or relaxation of surrounding muscular bands. The variation in the orifice may play some role in promoting venous return or preventing atrial reflux.

The medial wall of the right atrium includes the atrial septum and is also important because of its proximity to several structures[7] (Figs. 2-7 and 2-9 to 2-11). Anteriorly, the posterior (noncoronary) cusp and the right coronary cusp of

RIGHT VENTRICLE

The right ventricle receives venous blood from the right atrium during ventricular diastole and propels blood into the pulmonary circulation during ventricular systole (Figs. 2-9 to 2-14). The right ventricle is normally the most anterior cardiac chamber, lying directly beneath the sternum (Figs. 2-1 and 2-2). Enlargement or hyperactivity of the right ventricle may often be detected by palpation of the sternum or the lower left sternal border. The right ventricle is partially below, in front of, and medial to the right atrium but anterior and to the right of the left ventricle. Most of the entire inferior border of the frontal roentgenogram view of the heart consists of the right ventricle (Fig. 2-1). The striking difference in configuration between the two ventricles is illustrated by a transverse section (Figs. 2-12 and 2-13). The left ventricular chamber is an ellipsoidal sphere surrounded by relatively thick (8 to 15 mm at autopsy) musculature, well suited to ejecting blood against the high resistance of the systemic vessels. The right ventricle, which normally contracts against very low resistance, has a crescent-shaped chamber and a thin outer wall,

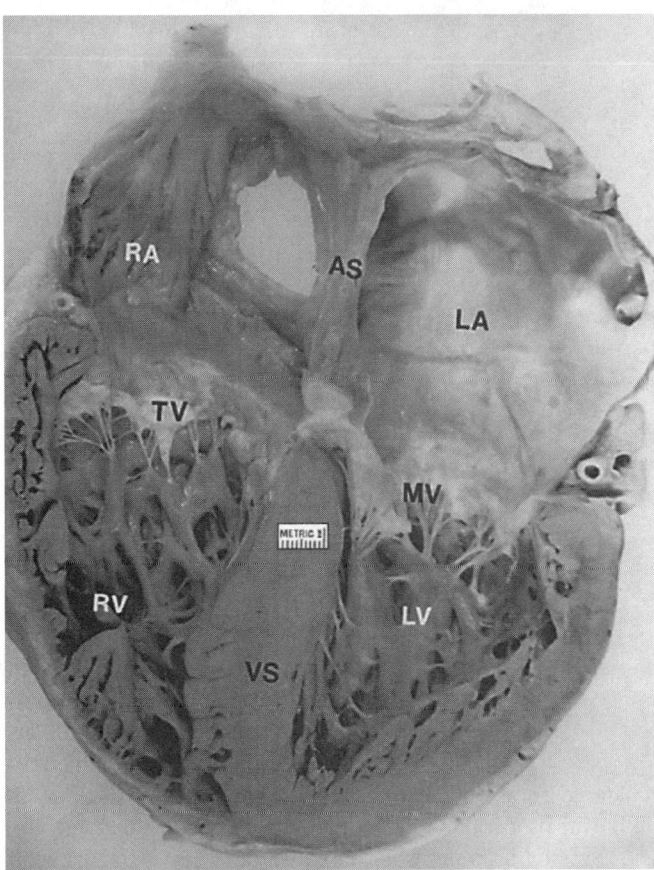

FIGURE 2-11

Four-chamber view of heart showing morphologic differences between the four chambers. The right atrium (RA) is more trabeculated than the left (LA), and the right ventricle (RV) is more heavily and coarsely trabeculated compared to the left ventricle (LV). AS = atrial septum; MV = mitral valve; TV = tricuspid valve; VS = ventricular septum. [From Waller BF, et al. Tomographic views of normal and abnormal hearts: The anatomic basis for various cardiac imaging techniques. *Clin Cardiol* 1990; 13:802(pt I), 877(pt II). Reproduced with permission from the publisher and authors.]

The inflow tract, consisting of the tricuspid valve and the trabecular muscles of the anterior and inferior walls, directs entering blood anteriorly, inferiorly, and to the left at an angle of 60° to the outflow tract[20] (Fig. 2-9). The smooth-walled outflow tract, also referred to as the *infundibulum*, forms the superior portion of the right ventricle. It is separated from the inflow tract by a thick muscle, the crista supraventricularis, which arches from the anterolateral wall over the anterior leaflet of the tricuspid valve to the septal (medial) wall, where it joins other constrictor bands of muscle that encircle the outflow tract[14,21] (Figs. 2-9 and 2-14). Blood entering the infundibulum is ejected superiorly and posteriorly into the pulmonary trunk.

LEFT ATRIUM

The left atrium receives blood from the pulmonary veins and serves as the reservoir during left ventricular systole and as a conduit during left ventricular filling. In addition, left atrial contraction provides a significant increment of blood to the left ventricle, stretching the ventricle and priming it for ventricular ejection. This is sometimes referred to as the "atrial kick," or atrial component of ventricular filling (see Chap. 3).

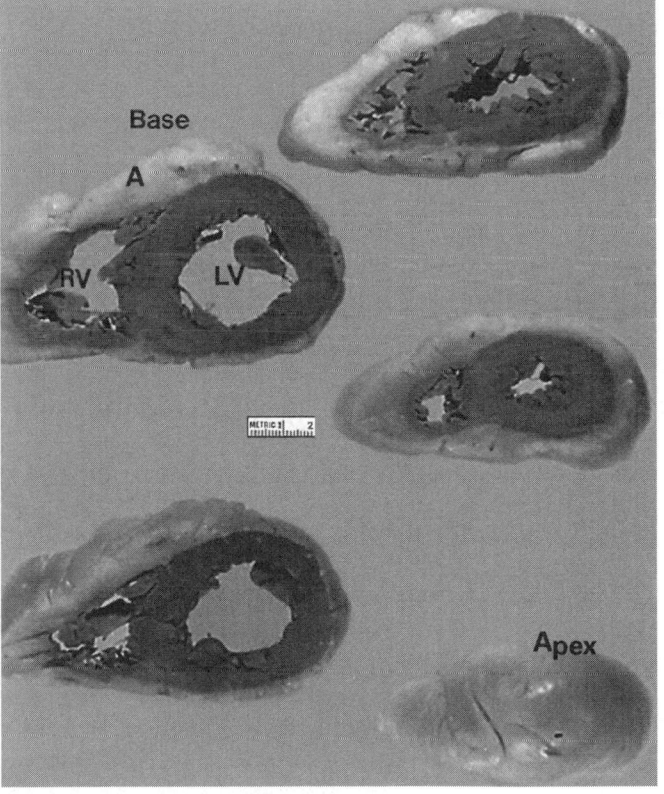

FIGURE 2-12

Family of ventricular slices from base to apex. A = anterior; LV = left ventricle; RV = right ventricle; P = posterior; VS = ventricular septum. The LV cavity is more "circular" shaped compared to the more "triangular" shaped RV cavity. [From Waller BF, et al. Tomographic views of normal and abnormal hearts: The anatomic basis for various cardiac imaging techniques. *Clin Cardiol* 1990; 13:802(pt I), 877(pt II). Reproduced with permission from the publisher and authors.]

measuring 4 to 5 mm in thickness.[19] The anterior right ventricular wall curves over the ventricular septum, which normally bulges into the right ventricular cavity. Although the ventricular septum forms the medial wall of both ventricles, it seems to contribute predominantly to left ventricle function in normal subjects. The anterior and inferior walls of the right ventricular cavity are lined by muscle bundles, the trabeculae carneae, which often form ridges along the inner surface of the wall or cross from one wall to the other (Figs. 2-9 to 2-14). A rather constant muscle, the moderator band, crosses from the lower ventricular septum to the anterior wall, where it joins the anterior papillary muscle (Figs. 2-9 to 2-11). The right bundle branch, after traveling through the muscular ventricular septum, courses through the moderator muscle to the endocardium of the right ventricle.

Functionally, the right ventricle can be partitioned into an inflow tract, an outflow tract, and an apical trabecular component (body). The trabecular muscles in the apex of the right ventricle are much coarser than those in the left ventricle.

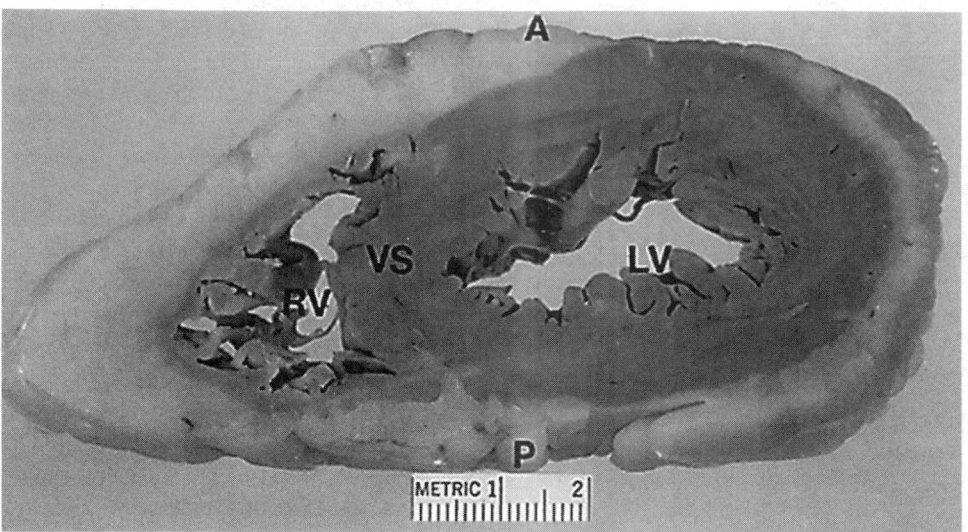

FIGURE 2-13

Close-up of ventricular slice seen in Fig. 2-12. This view corresponds to the short-axis echocardiographic views of the ventricular cavities. A = anterior; LV = left ventricle; RV = right ventricle; VS = ventricular septum. [From Waller BF, et al. Tomographic views of normal and abnormal hearts: The anatomic basis for various cardiac imaging techniques. *Clin Cardiol* 1990; 13:802(pt I), 877(pt II). Reproduced with permission from the publisher and authors.]

The left atrium is located superiorly, in the midline, and posterior to the other cardiac chambers (Figs. 2-3, 2-4, 2-7, 2-11, and 2-15). As a consequence of this posterior position, the left atrium is not normally seen in the frontal roentgenogram. The esophagus abuts directly on its posterior surface, while the aortic root impinges on its anterior wall. The right

atrium is located to the right and anterior (Fig. 2-3). The left ventricle is to the left, anterior, and inferior. The posterior position of the left atrium makes it impossible to palpate externally unless it is massively dilated. With severe mitral regurgitation, however, expansion of the left atrium from the regurgitation and the ejection recoil of the anteriorly located ventricles may force the heart anteriorly, producing a late systolic sternal lift. The left atrium usually enlarges posteriorly and laterally in mitral stenosis or regurgitation, occasionally even reaching the right or left lateral chest wall.

The wall of the left atrium is 3 mm thick, slightly thicker than that of the right atrium. Two pulmonary veins enter posterolaterally on each side, conveying oxygenated blood from the lungs. Though there are no true valves at the junction of the pulmonary veins and the left atrium, "sleeves" of atrial muscle extend from the left atrial wall around the pulmonary veins for 1 or 2 cm and may exert a partial sphincter-like influence, tending to lessen reflux during atrial systole or mitral regurgitation (Figs. 2-11 and 2-15).

The endocardium of the left atrium is smooth and slightly opaque (Figs. 2-11 and 2-15). Pectinate muscles are present only in the left atrial appendage, which projects from the anterolateral left atrium, alongside the pulmonary artery. The atrial septum is smooth but may contain a central shallow area, corresponding to the fossa ovalis (Figs. 2-11 and 2-15).

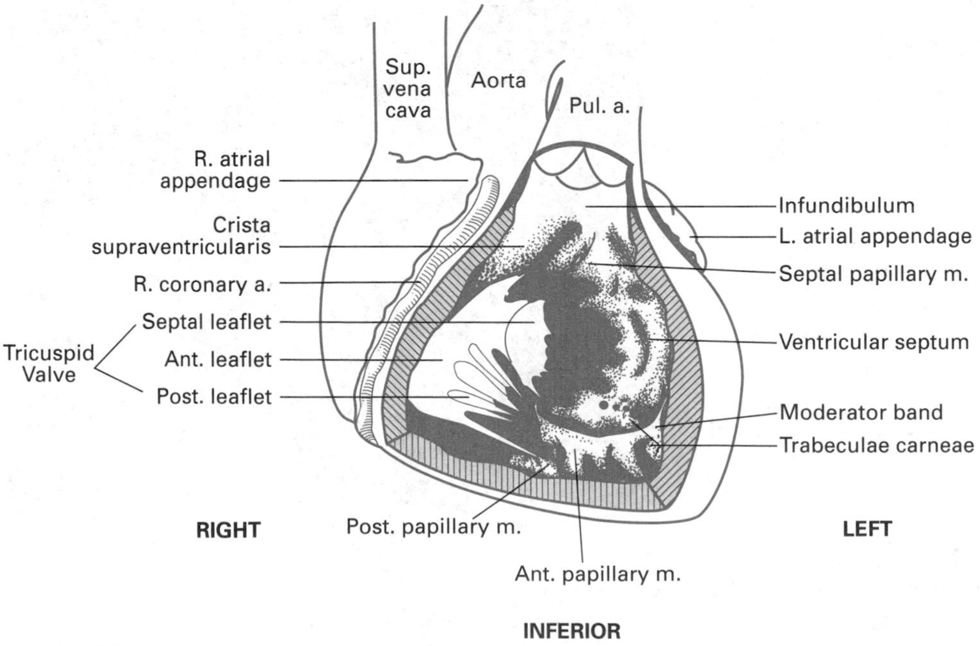

LEFT VENTRICLE

The left ventricle receives blood from the left atrium during ventricular diastole and ejects blood into the systemic arterial circulation during ventricular systole (Figs. 2-11 to 2-13 and 2-15). The left ventricle is roughly bullet-shaped, with the blunt tip directed anteriorly, inferiorly, and to the left, where it contributes, with the lower ventricular septum, to the apex of the heart.[22]

Sup. vena cava

Aorta

Pul. a.

R. atrial appendage

Crista supraventricularis

R. coronary a.

Tricuspid Valve
Septal leaflet
Ant. leaflet
Post. leaflet

Infundibulum

L. atrial appendage

Septal papillary m.

Ventricular septum

Moderator band

Trabeculae carneae

RIGHT

Post. papillary m.

Ant. papillary m.

LEFT

INFERIOR

FIGURE 2-14

Schematic representation of a frontal view of the heart. The anterior right ventricular wall has been removed to demonstrate the orientation of the tricuspid leaflets and the papillary muscles. The anterior papillary muscle is sectioned. The trabeculated inflow portion of the right ventricle is contrasted with the smooth infundibular (outflow) area.

Although the left ventricle forms the lower left lateral cardiac border in the frontal roentgenogram, the major portion of its external surface is posterolateral (Fig. 2-1). The left ventricle is posterior and to the left of the right ventricle and inferior, anterior, and to the left of the left atrium. The left ventricular chamber is approximately an ellipsoidal sphere, surrounded by thick muscular walls measuring 8 to 15 mm, or approximately two to three times the thickness of the right ventricular wall. The tip of the left ventricular apex is often thin, sometimes measuring 2 mm or less. The medial wall of the left ventricle is the ventricular septum, which is shared with the right ventricle (Figs. 2-2, 2-11 to 2-13, and 2-15). The septum, which is roughly triangular in shape, with the base of the triangle at the level of the aortic cusps, is entirely muscular except for the small membranous septum, located superiorly just below the right coronary and the posterior coronary cusps (Figs. 2-8, 2-11, and 2-15). The upper third of the septum is smooth endocardium. The remaining two-thirds of the septum and the remaining ventricular walls are ridged by interlacing muscles, the trabeculae carneae. The ventricular wall exclusive of the septum is often referred to as the free wall of the left ventricle.

The anteromedial leaflet of the mitral valve, which is the larger and more mobile of the two mitral leaflets, extends from the top of the posteromedial septum across the ventricular cavity to the anterolateral ventricular wall and separates the left ventricular cavity into an inflow and an outflow tract (Figs. 2-15 and 2-16). The funnel-shaped inflow tract, which is formed by the mitral annulus and by both mitral leaflets and their chordae tendineae, directs the entering atrial blood inferiorly, anteriorly, and to the left (Figs. 2-15 and 2-16). The outflow tract, surrounded by the inferior surface of the anteromedial mitral leaflet, the ventricular septum, and the left ventricular free wall, orients the blood flow from left ventricular apex to the right and superiorly at an angle of 90° to the inflow tract.[7] With the onset of ventricular systole, both mitral leaflets are propelled together and upward, converting the entire left ventricle into an expulsion chamber. The apical portion of the left ventricle is characterized by fine trabeculations.

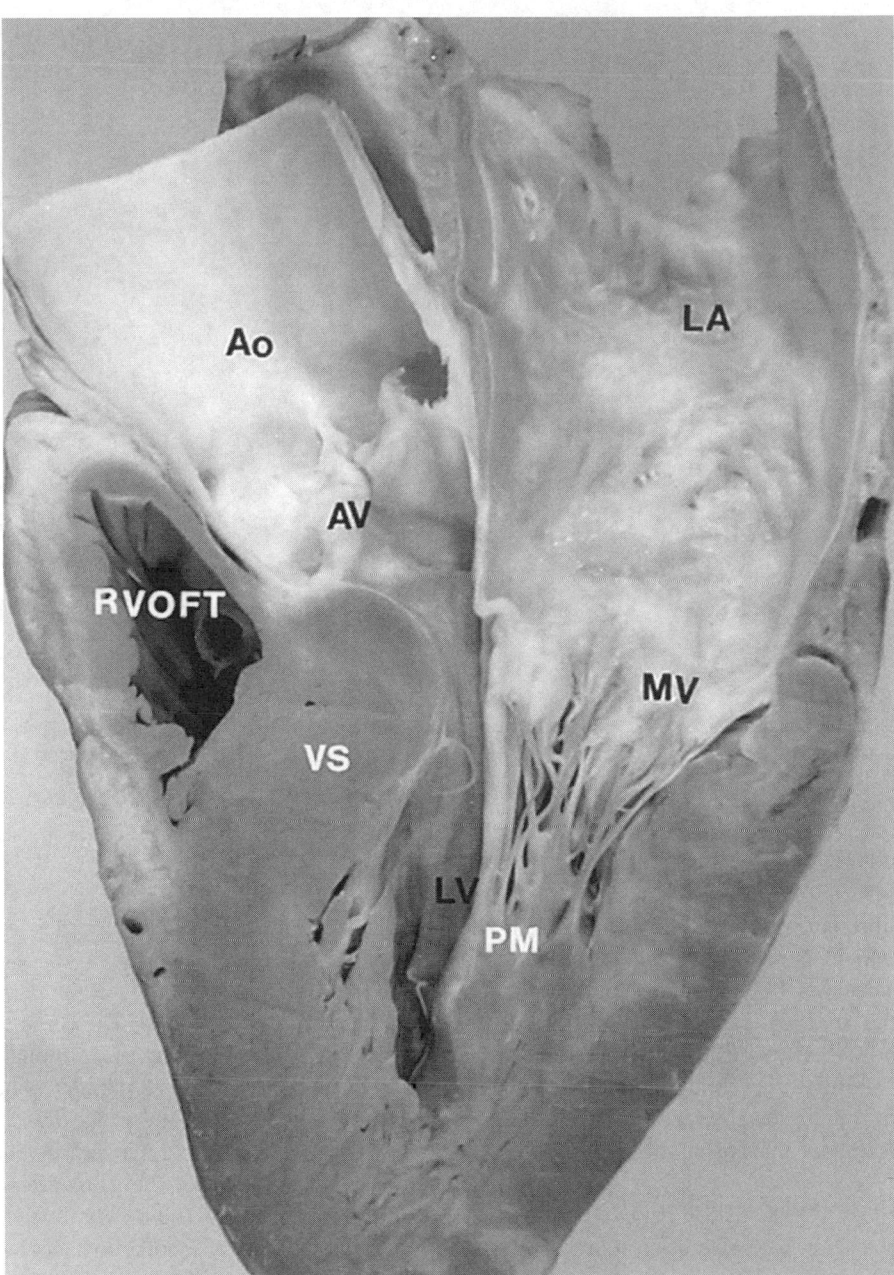

FIGURE 2-15

Long-axis view of left side of heart showing aorta (Ao), left atrium (LA), left ventricle (LV), mitral valve (MV), papillary muscle (PM) of mitral valve, aortic valve (AV), and right ventricular outflow tract (RVOFT). [From Waller BF, et al. Tomographic views of normal and abnormal hearts: The anatomic basis for various cardiac imaging techniques. *Clin Cardiol* 1990; 13:802(pt I), 877(pt II). Reproduced with permission from the publisher and authors.]

Cardiac Valves

The heart contains four cardiac valves: two semilunar and two atrioventricular.[23] The two semilunar valves, aortic and pulmonic, guard the outlet orifice of their respective left and right ventricles. The two AV valves, mitral and tricuspid, guard the inlet orifice of their respective left and right ventricles. The four cardiac valves are surrounded by fibrous tissue forming partial or complete "rings" (valve annulus). These

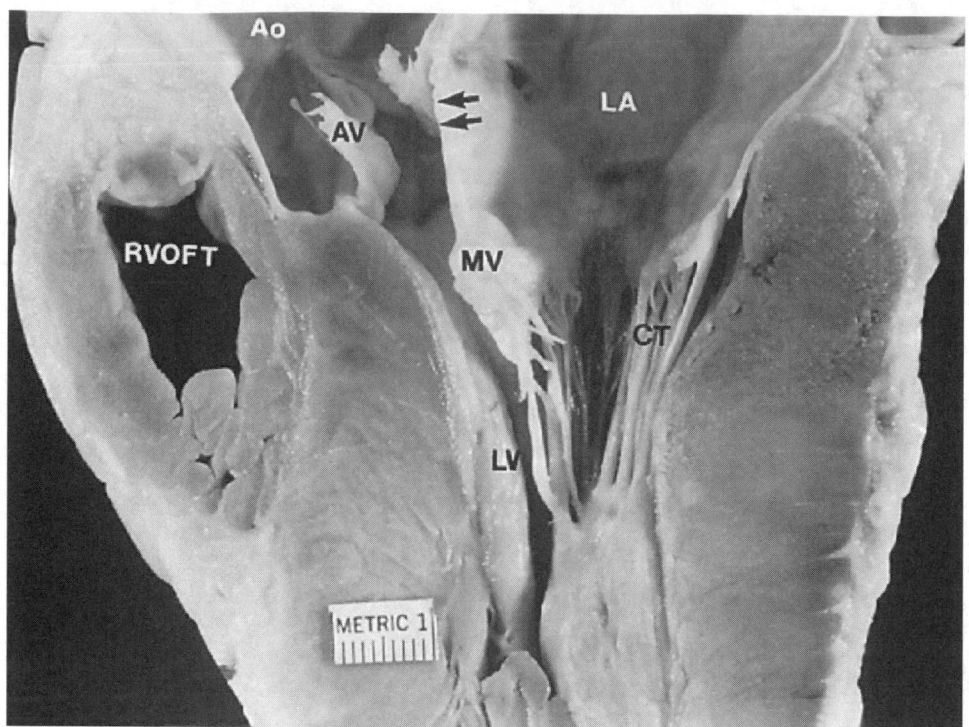

FIGURE 2-16

Long-axis view of left ventricle showing continuity of aortic (AV) and mitral (MV) valves (arrows) and chordae tendineae (CT) of MV. Ao = aorta; LA = left atrium; LV = left ventricle; RVOFT = right ventricular outflow tract.

SEMILUNAR VALVES

The semilunar aortic and pulmonary valves are similar in configuration except that the aortic cusps are slightly thicker.[23,28–30] They are situated at the summit of the outflow tract of their corresponding ventricle, the pulmonary valve being anterior, superior, and slightly to the left of the aortic valve (Figs. 2-4, 2-6 to 2-8, and 2-14 to 2-19). Each valve is composed of the three fibrous cusps. The pulmonary valve differs from the aortic valve by having no discrete annulus or fibrous ring. The U-shaped convex lower edges of each cusp are attached to and suspended from the root of the aorta or pulmonary artery, with the upper, free valve edges projecting into the lumen. The cusps circle the inside of the vessel root.[31]

Each semilunar valve consists of three equal-sized or nearly equal-sized semicircular cusps. Each cusp is attached by its semicircular border to the wall of the aorta or pulmonary trunk. The small space between attachments of adjacent cusps is called a *commissure*. Each semilunar valve has three commissures. The three commissures lie equally spaced around the aorta or pulmonary trunk, and the circumference connecting these points has been termed the *sinotubular junction*, which may also be described as the portion of the great vessel separating the sinuses of Valsalva from the adjacent tubular portion of the great artery. In the aorta a distinctive circumferential "hump" or line marks this junction, originally described by Leonardo da Vinci as the "supraaortic ridge." Each of the ventricular surfaces of the semilunar cusps has a small nodule [much more prominent on the aortic valve (*noduli Arantii*)] in the center of the free edge marking the contact sites of closure (Figs. 2-18, 2-19, and 2-23).

Behind each cusp the vessel wall bulges outward, forming a pouchlike dilatation known as the *sinus of Valsalva*. The free edge of each cusp is concave, with a nodular interruption at the center of the cusp, the nodulus Arantii. The portion of the cusp adjacent to the rim is not as thick and may normally contain small perforations. During ventricular systole, the cusps are passively thrust upward away from the center of the aortic lumen. During ventricular diastole, the cusps fall passively into the lumen of the vessel as they support the column of blood above. The noduli Arantii meet in the center and contribute to the support of the leaflets. The geometry of the cusps and the strong fibrous tissue support provide excellent approximations of the cusps and prevent regurgitation of blood.

fibrous rings join to form the fibrous skeleton of the heart, to which also is attached the atrial and ventricular myocardium. The area between the septal leaflet of the tricuspid valve, the anterior leaflet of the mitral valve, and the posterior or noncoronary cusp of the aortic valve forms one part of the central fibrous body. The remaining portion is made up of fibrous tissue connecting the left aortic cusp and the anterior leaflet of the mitral valve.[23]

HISTOLOGIC STRUCTURE

Each cardiac valve has a central collagenous core, the *fibrosa*, which is continuous with the collagen of the cardiac skeleton and of the chordae tendineae. Both sides of the fibrosa are covered by loose fibroelastic tissue, usually containing mucopolysaccharides, and the entire valve is covered by endothelium. The endothelium and connective tissue of the AV valves are continuous with the atrial and ventricular endocardium, and those of the semilunar valves are continuous with the aortic and pulmonary intima. Gross and Kugel[24] have proposed that the loose connective tissue on the atrial aspect of the AV valves be termed the *atrialis*, that on the ventricular surface of all four valves the *ventricularis*, and that on the aortic or pulmonary side of the semilunar valves the *arterialis*. Smooth and striated cardiac muscle may extend onto the proximal one-third of the atrialis in the AV valves and often contains blood vessels. The distal two-thirds of the normal AV valve and all the semilunar valves are avascular.[23–27]

FIGURE 2-17
Short-axis view of three-cuspid aortic valve (AV) and pulmonary trunk (PT). LM = left main coronary ostium; R = right coronary ostium. [From Waller BF, et al. Tomographic views of normal and abnormal hearts: The anatomic basis for various cardiac imaging techniques. *Clin Cardiol* 1990; 13:802(pt I), 877(pt II). Reproduced with permission from the publisher and authors.]

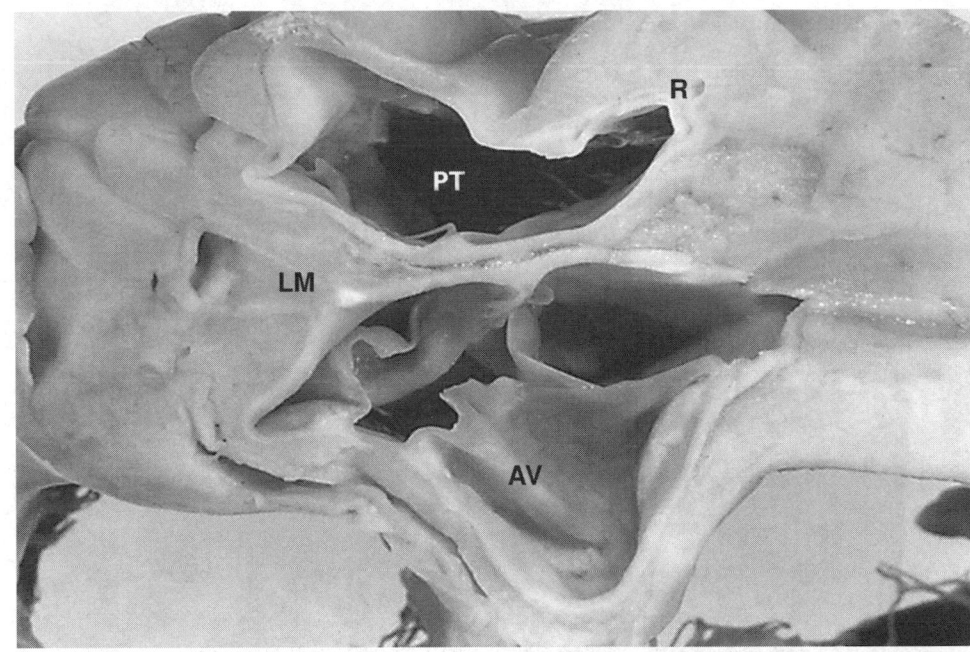

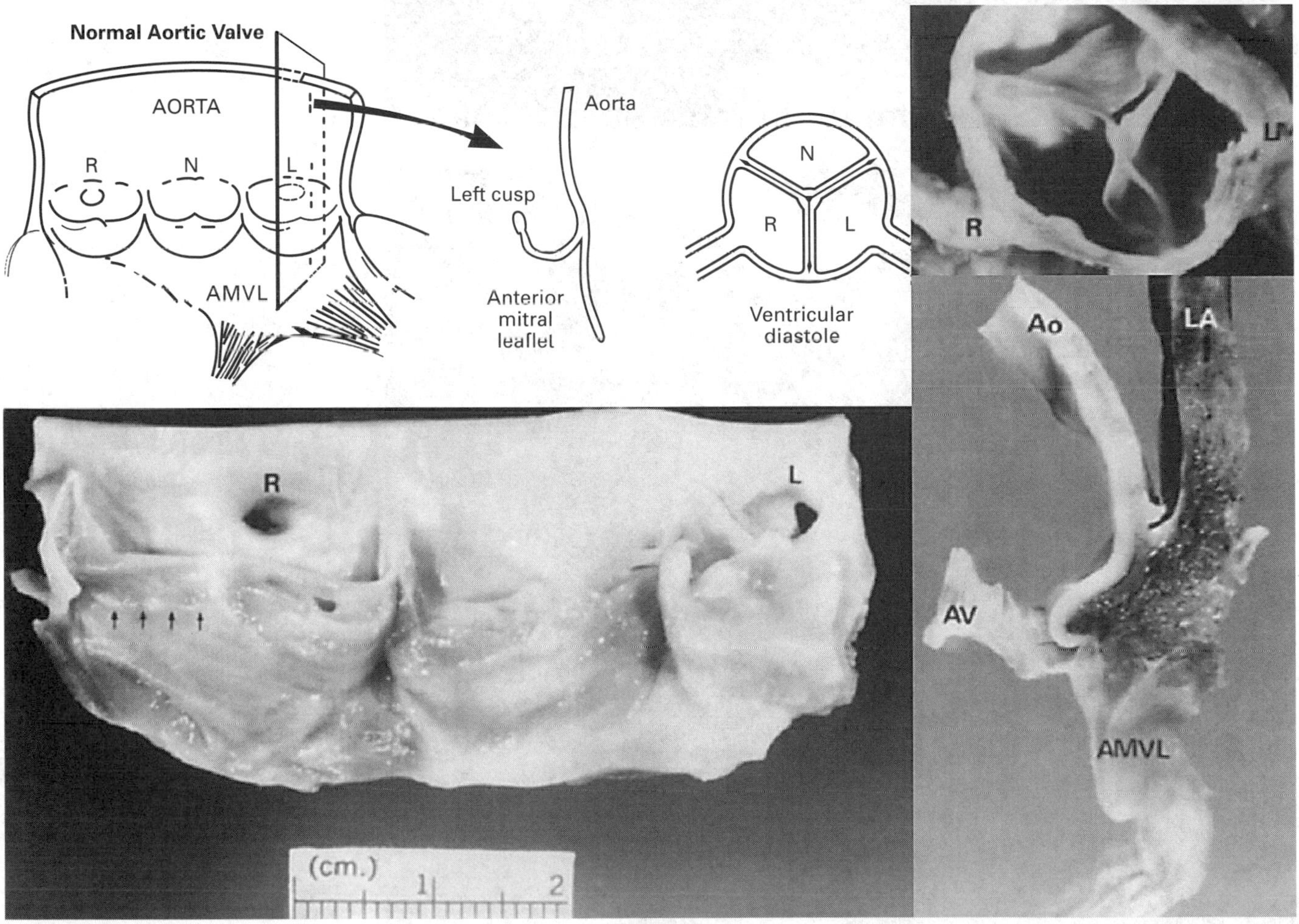

FIGURE 2-18
Morphology of the normal aortic valve. AMVL = anterior mitral valve leaflet; Ao = aorta; AV = aortic valve; LM = left main; N = noncoronary cusp; LA = left atrium; R = right; RC = right coronary artery. Arrows point to line of closure. Portion of aortic cusp above the line of closure is called the *lunula.* (From Waller BF. Morphologic aspects of valvular heart disease: Part I. *Curr Probl Cardiol* 1985; 9:13. Reproduced with permission from the publisher and author.)

Normal Pulmonic Valve

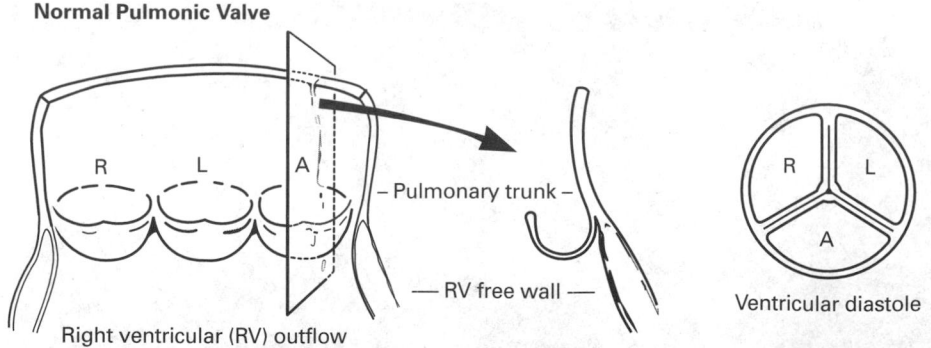

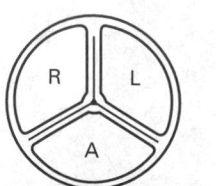

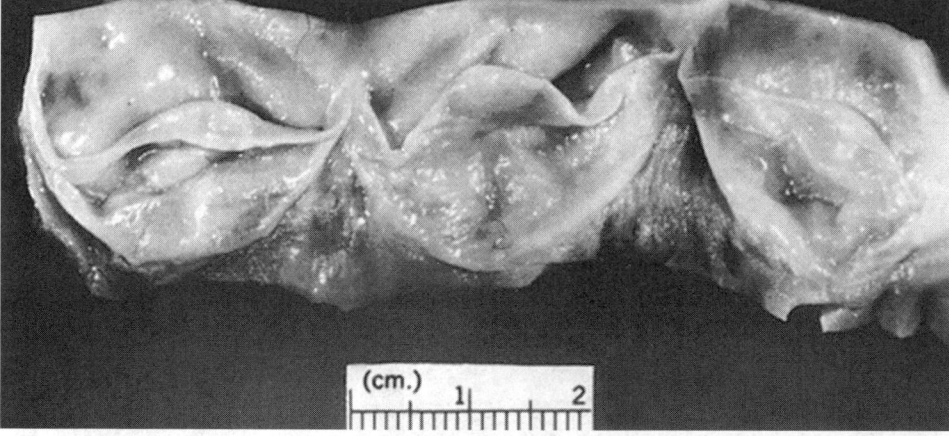

FIGURE 2-19
Morphology of the normal pulmonic valve. A = anterior; L = left; R = right. (From Waller BF. Morphologic aspects of valvular heart disease: Part I. *Curr Probl Cardiol* 1985; 9:13. Reproduced with permission from the publisher and author.)

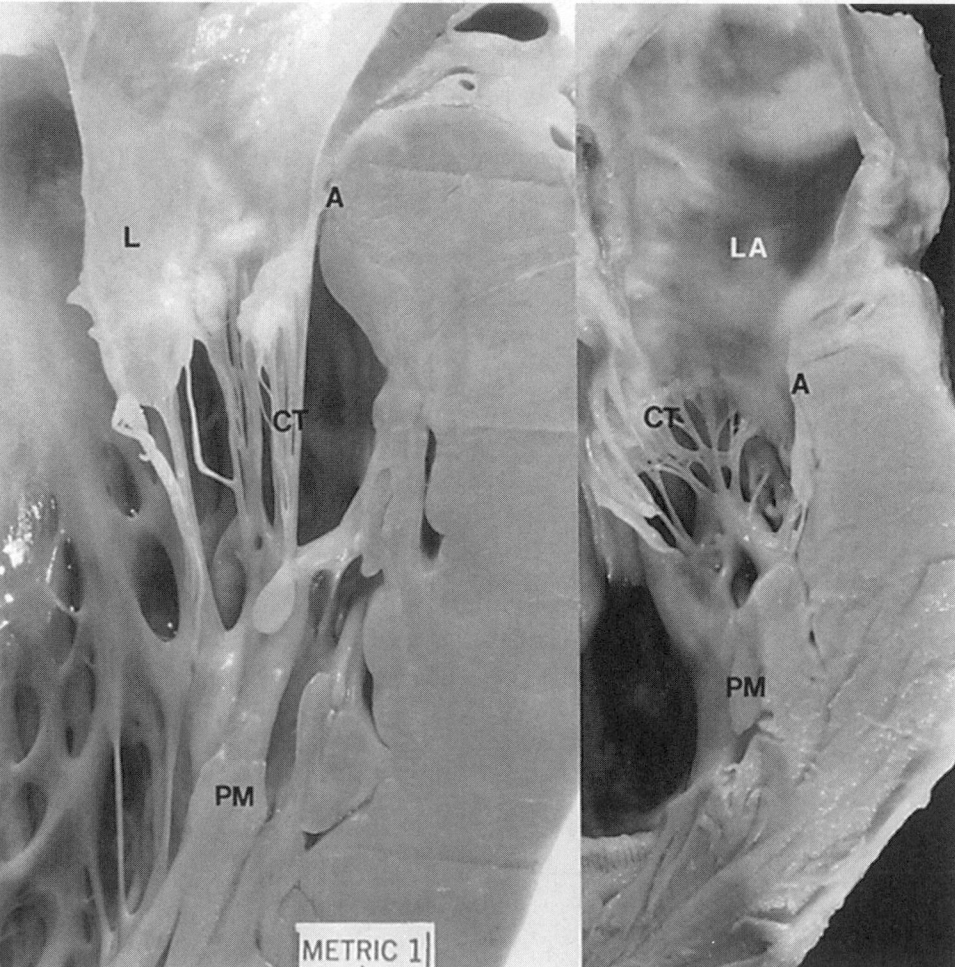

FIGURE 2-20
Mitral valve apparatus. *Left:* Chordae tendineae (CT); leaflet (L); annulus (A); papillary muscle (PM). *Right:* Left atrium (LA). Note the interchordal connections and chordal connections from both anterior and posterior mitral leaflets to the posteromedial papillary muscle (*right*). [From Waller BF, et al. Tomographic views of normal and abnormal hearts: The anatomic basis for various cardiac imaging techniques. *Clin Cardiol* 1990; 13:802(pt I), 877(pt II). Reproduced with permission from the publisher and authors.]

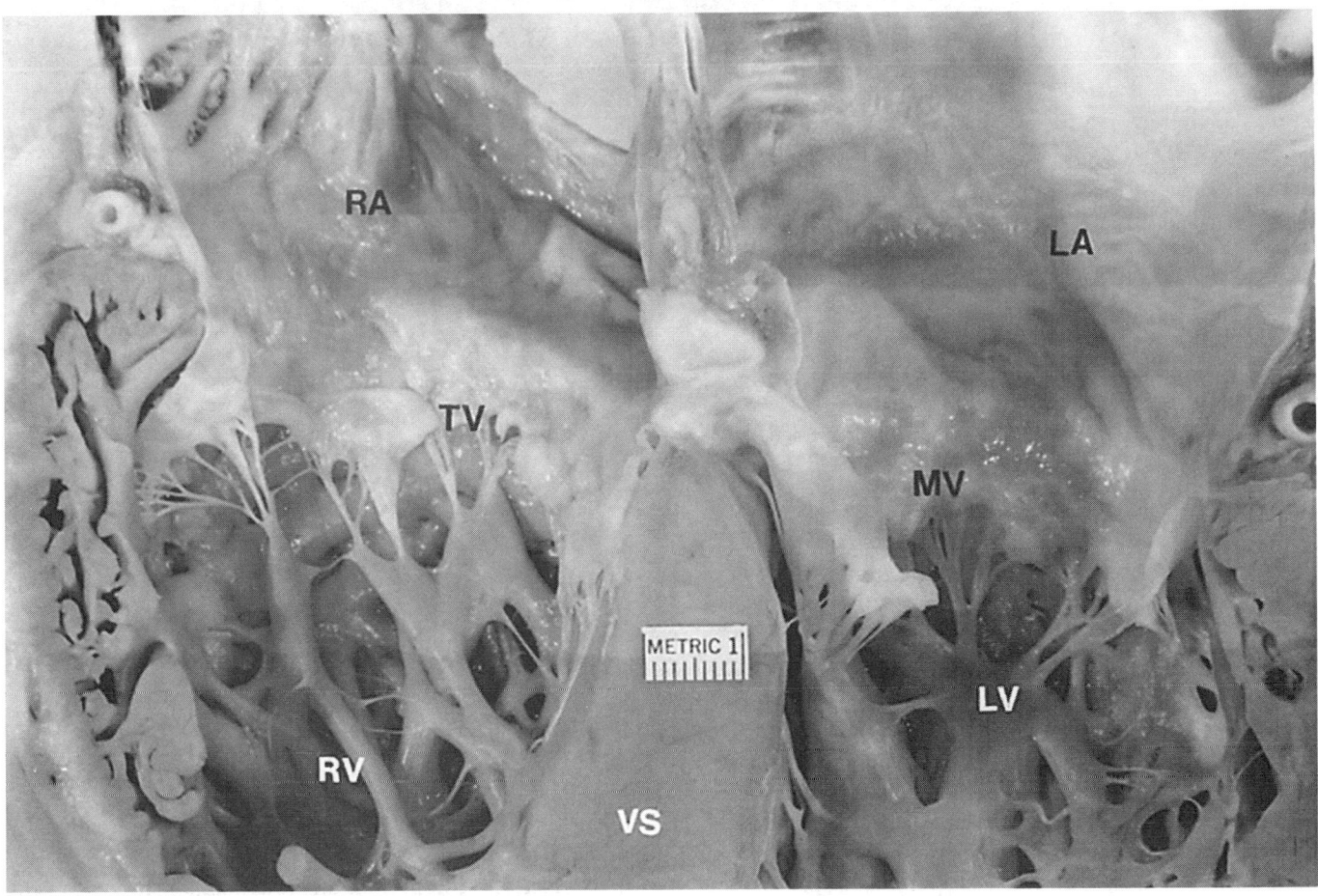

FIGURE 2-21

Four-chamber view showing mitral (MV) and tricuspid (TV) valves. The annulus of the tricuspid valve is more spiral than the annulus of the mitral valve. LA = left atrium; LV = left ventricle; RA = right atrium; RV = right ventricle; VS = ventricular septum. [From Waller BF, et al. Tomogra-phic views of normal and abnormal hearts: The anatomic basis for various cardiac imaging techniques. *Clin Cardiol* 1990; 13:802(pt I), 877(pt II). Reproduced with permission from the publisher and authors.]

The anatomy of the two AV valves is considerably more complex than the anatomy of the semilunar valves (Figs. 2-6, 2-7, 2-9, 2-11, 2-15, and 2-20 to 2-23). Both AV valves consist of leaflets (two mitral and three tricuspid), chordae tendineae, papillary muscles (two or three, respectively), and valve annuli. The leaflets are demarcated by commissures located along the valve annular attachment. The anterior leaflet of each of the AV valves is the largest and is roughly semicircular in shape. The posterior mitral leaflet and the posterior and septal tricuspid leaflets have shorter annulus-to-free-edge distances but longer basal attachments compared to the respective anterior leaflet. Complex chordal structures arise from papillary muscles or directly from ventricular myocardium and insert onto the free edge and several millimeters from the margin on the ventricular surface. The annular structure of the mitral valve primarily surrounds the posterior leaflet, while the anterior leaflet does not have a true annulus but is continuous with the wall of ascending aorta, aortic valve, and membranous ventricular septum. The annulus of the tricuspid is nearly circumferential, is larger than the mitral annulus, and lies at a lower level (i.e., it is more apical) than the mitral annulus. On the atrial surface of the AV valves, 0.5 to 1.0 cm from the free edge, is a line of nodular thickening (more prominent on the mitral valve), marking the contact points of closure.[23]

SPECIFIC VALVE STRUCTURE

Aortic Valve

General The normal tricuspid aortic valve (Figs. 2-17 and 2-18) is a symmetric structure in which the orifice of the fully opened valve is central and the cusps are easily mobile and retract to the aortic commissures. When the valve is closed, all three cusps meet and overlap equally. The circumferential distances between each of the three commissures and the depth of the aortic valve sinus (from sinotubular junction to base of sinus) in a normally formed valve are similar (Fig. 2-18). Each of the ventricular surfaces of the aortic cusps has a small nodule in the center of the free edge that marks the closure contact site. A small rim of valve tissue above this nodule, known as the *lunula*, overlaps the neighboring cusp and serves as a supporting strut. Fenestrations of the lunula are quite common but are of no functional consequence. Fenestrations of the aortic valve lunula increase with age.[30]

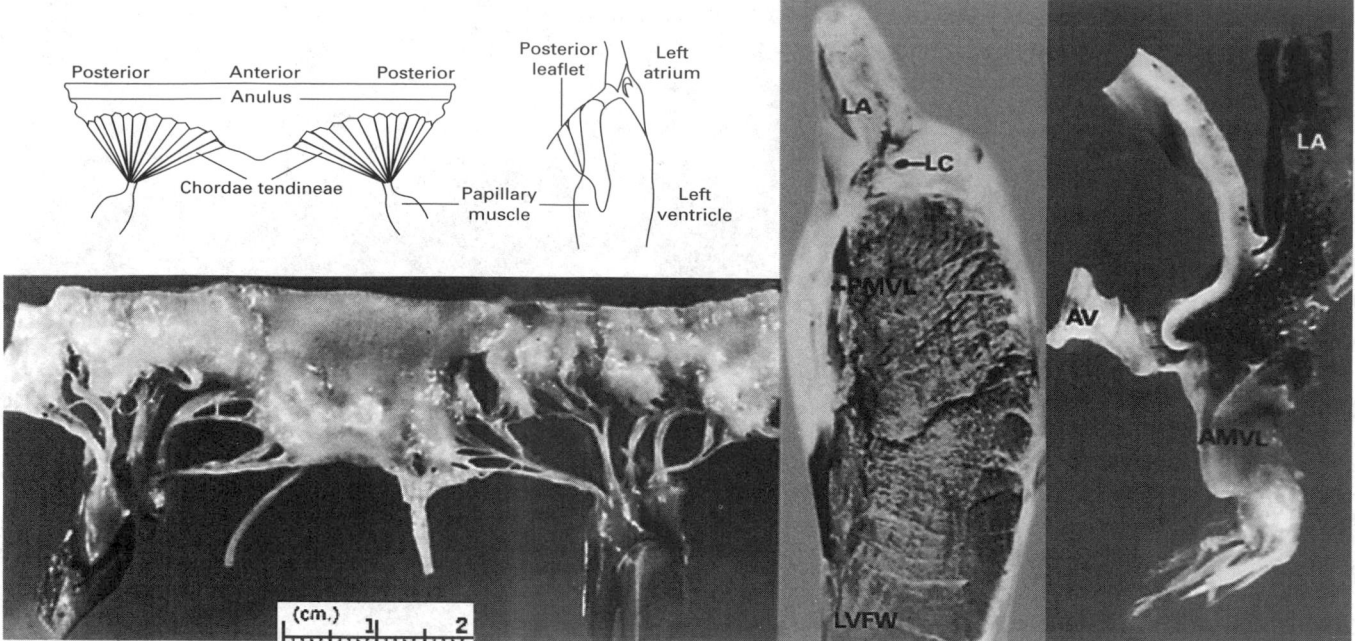

FIGURE 2-22

Morphology of the normal mitral valve. AMVL = anterior mitral valve leaflet; AV = aortic valve; LA = left atrium; LC = left circumflex coronary artery; LVFW = left ventricular free wall; PMVL = posterior mitral valve leaflet. (From Waller BF. Morphologic aspects of valvular heart disease: Part I. *Curr Probl Cardiol* 1985; 9:13. Reproduced with permission from the publisher and author.)

The sinotubular junction, the aortic sinuses of Valsalva, the valve cusps and commissures, and the junction of the aortic valve with the ventricular septum and anterior mitral valve leaflet make up the aortic valve complex. The narrowest circumference is at the lowermost portion of this complex, the junction with the ventricular septum. This circumference (diameter), referred to as the *aortic ring*, is measured by surgeons to determine the size of an aortic prosthetic valve. Pathologists at necropsy, on the other hand, measure the circumference (8 to 10 cm) at the sinotubular junction, which more closely corresponds to the measurements made by the echocardiographers during life.

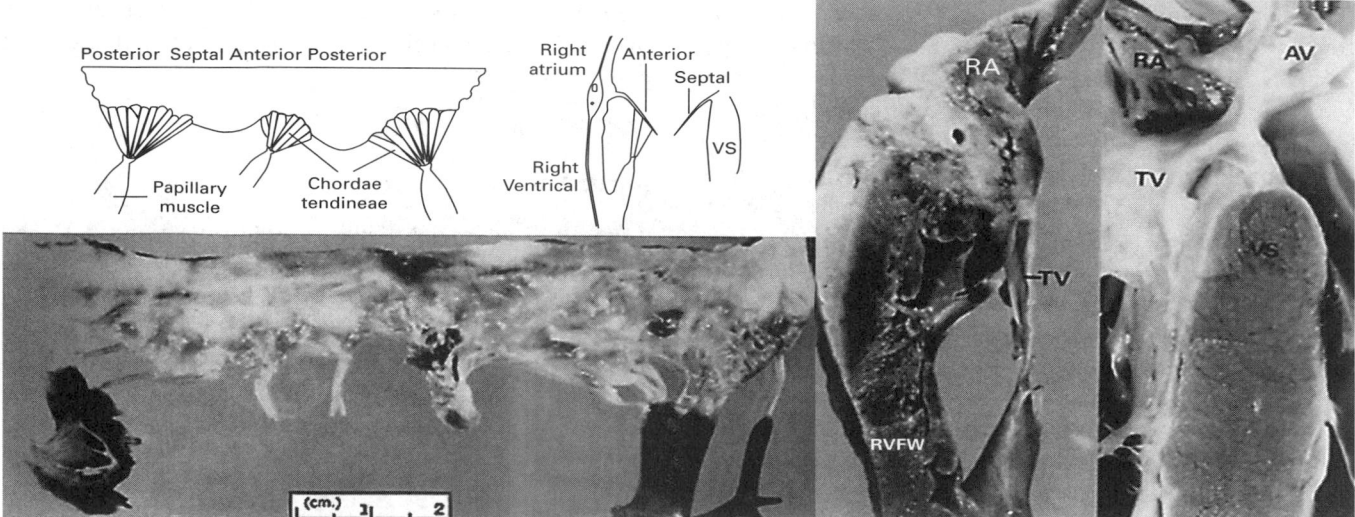

FIGURE 2-23

Morphology of the normal tricuspid valve. AV = aortic valve; RA = right atrium; RVFW = right ventricular free wall; TV = tricuspid valve; VS = ventricular septum. (From Waller BF. Morphologic aspects of valvular heart disease: Part I. *Curr Probl Cardiol* 1985; 9:13. Reproduced with permission from the publisher and author.)

The three aortic valve cusps have been termed the left, right, and noncoronary (posterior) cusps, with each of the left and right sinuses of Valsalva giving rise to the left and right main epicardial coronary artery, respectively. Knowledge of the adjacent anatomic structures or chambers of the aortic valve is important in determining potential sites of left-to-right shunting. Rupture of the right and noncoronary sinuses of Valsalva may communicate with right-sided chambers (right ventricular outflow tract, right atrium), while rupture of the left sinus of Valsalva generally communicates with left-sided chambers (left atrium or left ventricular outflow tract). Portions of the left and noncoronary cusps are continuous with the anterior leaflet of the mitral valve.

Anatomic Variations   The normal tricuspid aortic valve is a symmetric structure composed of three equal-sized cusps. Detailed measurements of commissural diameters and cuspal depth show that some tricuspid aortic valves have marked variation in these measurements.[31,32] The circumference between one set of commissures may be longer or shorter than in the remaining two sets of commissures, one sinus of Valsalva may be deeper or shallower than the remaining two sinuses, or the combination of these variables may occur in the same aortic valve. These variations in cusp size result in asymmetric lines of closure and may result in accelerated "wear and tear" (aging) of the valve structure. These congenitally malformed tricuspid valves may be the basis for some of the isolated aortic valve stenoses seen in patients over 65 years of age[31,32] (see also Chap. 63).

Age-Related Changes   The normal cuspal markings become more prominent with age. The central cuspal nodules thicken and enlarge and the bases of the sinuses of Valsalva typically contain calcific deposits. The body of the aortic valve cusps also thickens, while the cusp lunula often thins and develops fenestrations. Commissures characteristically remain open with normal aging, and the sinuses of Valsalva dilate.[33]

Pulmonic Valve

General   Like the aortic valve, the normal tricuspid aortic valve is a symmetric structure (Figs. 2-7 and 2-19) in which the orifice of the fully opened valve is central and the cusps are easily mobile and retract to the pulmonary trunk attachments. The circumferential distances between each of the three commissures and the depth of the pulmonary valve sinus in a normally formed valve are similar. With the exception of adjacent anatomic connections and coronary ostia, the normal pulmonic and aortic valves are identical in design. The lines of cusp apposition and the central nodules are less prominent in pulmonic valves than in aortic valves, as might be expected from the lower right-sided ventricular pressures. With age, fenestrations of the cusp lunulae appear but, as in the aortic valve, have no apparent functional significance. The three pulmonic valve cusps are named in relation to the aortic cusps—right, left, and anterior. The pulmonic valve annulus is about 1.5 cm above the level of the aortic valve annulus, but its circumference is similar (7 to 9 cm). The pulmonic valve is discontinuous with the tricuspid valve because of muscular structures of the right ventricular outflow tract.

Anatomic Variations   As with the aortic valve, detailed measurements of commissural diameters and cuspal depth reveal variations. The long-term functional significance of these congenitally abnormal tricuspid pulmonic valves with asymmetric closure lines differs from that of the aortic valve in that acquired "senile" (old age) pulmonic stenosis does not occur. This difference presumably is due to the difference in right- and left-sided ventricular systolic pressures.

Age-Related Changes   With increasing age, the pulmonic valve cusps thicken slightly, but far less than the aortic valve leaflets. Calcific deposits in the base of the pulmonic sinuses were not observed in 40 hearts from patients aged 90 to 103 years.[33]

Mitral Valve

General   The mitral valve is much more complex than the semilunar valves. The mitral valve consists of six major anatomic components[34] (Figs. 2-6, 2-7, 2-15, 2-16, and 2-20 to 2-22): posterior left atrial wall, annulus, leaflets, chordae tendineae, papillary muscles, and left ventricular free wall. Alterations of one, more than one, or all of these components can cause mitral valve dysfunction. The mitral valve annulus forms a major part of the basal attachment of the posterior leaflet. This bundle of fibrous tissue separates left ventricular from left atrial myocardium and is located posterior to the posterior mitral leaflet. The anterior leaflet does not have a true annulus but is continuous with the wall of ascending aorta, aortic valve, and membranous ventricular septum. The valve measurement used by surgeons ("mitral ring") or that obtained by pathologists at autopsy is not really a measurement of the mitral annulus but of the mitral valve circumference. The circumference of the normal mitral valve ranges from 8 to 10.5 cm (mean, 9.4 cm).[34–36]

Unlike the other three cardiac valves, each of which has three leaflets or cusps, the mitral valve consists of only two leaflets. The anterior leaflet has a much longer width from the base to the margin of closure (2.3 cm) than the posterior leaflet (1.2 cm),[37] but the circumference (6 cm) of the posterior leaflet (annular attachment) is about twice that of the anterior leaflet (3 cm). Whereas the base-to-margin widths and circumferences of each mitral leaflet are different, the surface area of each leaflet is similar.[34,35] The total surface area of both leaflets is about 2½ times that of the orifice area calculated using the mitral valve circumference.[38] The leaflets are connected to each other at junctions called *commissures*. In distinction to the semilunar commissures, which represent "spaces" between cusps, the commissures of the AV valves are "junctions" of continuous leaflet tissue.

The chordae tendineae of the mitral valve consist of primary, secondary, and tertiary chordae[34] that subdivide as they extend from papillary muscles to leaflets (Figs. 2-20 to 2-22). Some chordae tendineae from each papillary muscle attach to both anterior and posterior mitral leaflets. The spaces between the multiple chordal subdivisions function as secondary orifices between the left atrium and left ventricle.[34] The two left ventricular papillary muscles are termed *anterolateral* and *posteromedial*. The anterolateral papillary muscle is usually larger than the posteromedial. The major blood supply of the anterolateral muscle is the left anterior descending coronary artery, while the right coronary artery supplies the posteromedial muscle.[39] The left circumflex artery supplies blood to both papillary muscles. The apices of papillary muscles appear to be sensitive indicators of myocardial hypoxia, since blood supply to the papillary muscle must travel the full thickness of the left ventricular free wall and then retrogradely up the longer axis of the papillary muscle body.[40]

Anatomic Variations The posterior leaflet of the mitral valve shows considerable variation in its subdivision into one to three scallops—lateral, middle, and medial.[37] Virtually all posterior leaflets (96 percent) are triscalloped, with the middle scallop being the largest. The width of the middle scallop is about 1.3 cm, compared to about 1.0 cm for the lateral and medial scallops.[37] Variation in number, width, and circumference of the posterior leaflet scallops, however, constitutes the major anatomic variation of the mitral valve. Rare congenital variations of mitral leaflets and chordae include abnormal supernumerary orifices of the mitral valve (bridging leaflet tissue or actual duplication) and aberrant chordae tendineae from atrial septum to mitral valve leaflets.[41] Some hearts have "muscular chords," representing direct insertion of papillary muscles into leaflet edges.[36]

Age-Related Changes Expected age-related changes of the mitral valve include focal areas of leaflet fibrous thickening, lipid deposits over the ventricular surface of the anterior mitral leaflet, progressive prominence of the lines of closure, and calcification of the mitral valve annulus.[33] Since the size of the left ventricular cavity decreases with increasing age, the mitral valve annulus also decreases with age.[40] This latter change promotes further leaflet contact and increases leaflet fibrous changes. This change in the ventricular cavity also creates disproportion in the ventriculoleaflet area, as a result of which the segments of normal leaflet may prolapse into the left atrium.[33]

Tricuspid Valve

General The tricuspid valve, like the mitral valve, is a complex structure made up of six major anatomic components: right atrial wall, annulus, three leaflets, chordae tendineae, papillary muscles, and right ventricular free wall. The three leaflets are termed *anterior*, *posterior*, and *septal* (Figs. 2-6, 2-7, 2-9 to 2-11, 2-14, and 2-23). The anterior leaflet is usually

the largest, with a width of 2.2 cm. The septal and posterior leaflets measure about 1.5 and 2.0 cm in width, respectively.[42] The tricuspid annulus is a nearly circular fibrous structure, much less prominent than the mitral valve annulus but slightly larger in circumference (10 to 12.5 cm). The posterior leaflet makes up the largest portion of the annulus (7.5 cm), followed by the anterior (3.7 cm) and septal (3.6 cm) leaflets. The septal leaflet has a characteristic fold or indentation where its annulus passes from the posterior ventricular free wall to the membranous septum (Fig. 2-23). The chordae tendineae of the tricuspid valve are made up of five types: fan-shaped, rough-zone, basal, free-edge, and deep[42] (Fig. 2-23). Of these, the free-edge and deep chordae are unique to the tricuspid valve.[42] The chordae arise from a single large anterior papillary muscle, double or multiple septal papillary muscles, and several small posterior papillary muscles. The papillary muscles are attached to the corresponding walls of the right ventricle.

Anatomic Variations The posterior leaflet of the tricuspid valve shows considerable variation in its subdivisions into one to three scallops. The scallops are produced by small clefts marked by fan-shaped chordae. Rare congenital anomalies of the tricuspid valve include supernumerary orifices created by bridging leaflet tissue or actual valve duplication.[43,44]

Age-Related Changes With increasing age, the margins of closure of the tricuspid valve leaflet become more prominent, and the leaflet acquires focal areas of fibrous thickening. Leaflet or annular calcification is rarely seen unless there is an abnormal calcium balance[45] or the patient has inborn metabolic abnormalities.[36]

Papillary Muscles

The papillary muscles of both ventricles are located below the commissures of the AV valves.[46] These muscles project from the trabeculae carneae and may be single or bifid, or they may occasionally occur as a row of muscles arising from the ventricular wall. In the left ventricle the two groups of papillary muscles, located below the anterolateral and posteromedial commissures, arise from the junction of the apical and middle thirds of the ventricular wall (Figs. 2-8 to 2-11, 2-15, 2-16, 2-20, 2-21, and 2-24). In the right ventricle there are usually three papillary muscles (Figs. 2-10 and 2-11). The largest is the anterior papillary muscle, which is found below the commissure between the anterior and posterior leaflets, originating from the moderator band as well as from the anterolateral ventricular wall. The posterior papillary muscle lies beneath the junction of the posterior and septal leaflets. A small septal papillary muscle, originating from the wall of the infundibulum, tethers the anterior and septal leaflets high against the infundibular wall. At times this muscle is virtually absent, and the chordae tendineae arise from a small tendinous connection to the infundibulum. The septal leaflet of the tricuspid valve usually has extensive attachments to the ventricular septum. The papillary muscles, because of their relatively parallel alignment to the ventricular wall and their chordal attachments to two adjacent valve leaflets, pull the leaflets of the mitral valve and tricuspid valve together and downward at the onset of isovolumic ventricular contraction.

Chordae Tendineae

Strong cords of fibrous tissue, the chordae tendineae,[47] spring from the tip of each papillary muscle (Figs. 2-8, 2-11, 2-15, 2-16, 2-20, and 2-21). They often subdivide and interconnect before they attach to the two leaflets directly above. The chordae may attach directly into a fibrous band running along the free edge of the valves or they may become incorporated into the ventricular surface of the leaflet a few millimeters back from the edge. Additional chordae run directly from the ventricular wall into the undersurface of the posterolateral leaflet of the left ventricle and the septal and posterior leaflets of the right ventricle. The chordae tendineae, by their attachments to most of the free valvular border and their numerous cross connections, allow the valve leaflets to balloon upward and against each other and evenly distribute the forces of ventricular systole. Dysfunction or rupture of a papillary muscle or rupture of a chorda tendinea may undermine the support of one or more valve leaflets, producing regurgitation.

Endocardium

Endocardium endothelium appears to share many if not all of the functions of vascular endothelium, described below. A newly found agent from endocardial endothelial cells that prolongs myocardial contraction has been provisionally referred to as *endocardin*. The prolongation of contraction by endocardin can be overridden by stimulation of endothelium-derived relaxing factor (EDRF), which shortens the duration of contraction (see Chaps. 3, 4, 21, and 44).

Pericardium

The heart is enclosed by the pericardium,[48,49] the two surfaces of which can be visualized by considering the heart as a fist that is plunged into a large balloon or serous pericardium (Figs. 2-1 and 2-25). The surface of the balloon in intimate contact with the fist is analogous to the visceral pericardium or epicardium. This surface encases the heart, extending several centimeters onto each of the great vessels. It is then reflected back, as is the outer surface of the balloon, to form the parietal

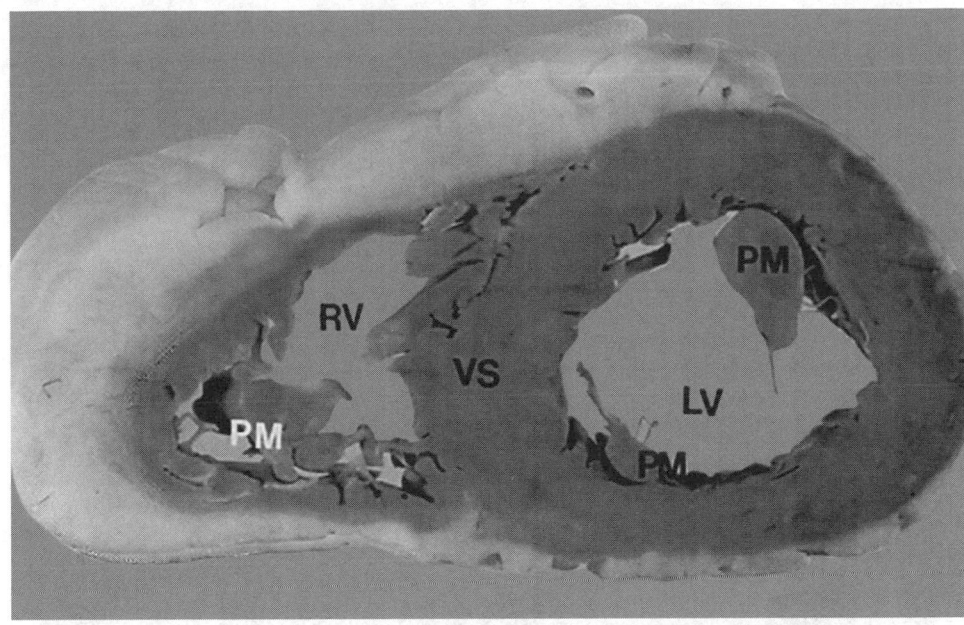

FIGURE 2-24

Short-axis view of ventricles showing papillary muscles (PM) of mitral valve (PM black) and tricuspid valve (PM white). LV = left ventricle; RV = right ventricle; VS = ventricular septum.

pericardium, which is fused to the fibrous pericardium to form the fibrous layer. The two pericardial surfaces are lined by smooth, glistening serous tissue and are separated by a thin layer of lubricating fluid, which allows the heart to move freely within the parietal pericardium. The parietal pericardium is attached by ligaments to the manubrium, the xiphoid process, the vertebral column, and the diaphragm. There is normally about 10 to 50 mL of thin, clear pericardial fluid, which moistens the contracting surfaces of the visceral and parietal pericardium. Four recesses are frequently present in images or examination of the pericardial space: the superior sinus, the transverse sinus, the postcaval recess, and the oblique sinus.[49]

TOMOGRAPHIC VIEWS OF NORMAL HEART: ANATOMIC BASIS FOR VARIOUS CARDIAC IMAGING TECHNIQUES

During the last several years, dramatic developments have taken place in the diagnosis of cardiovascular disorders in the area of cardiac imaging techniques.[13,14] From a previous era of imaging by silhouettes (chest roentgenography, fluoroscopy, angiocardiography), we have emerged into an era of imaging by tomographic scanning [echocardiography, radionuclide tomography, computed tomography (CT), magnetic resonance imaging (MRI)]. An understanding of tomographic anatomy is the foundation for proper use and interpretation of these new imaging modalities.

Position of Heart and Tomographic Axis

New tomographic imaging techniques result in various depictions of the heart that have similarities and differences. The

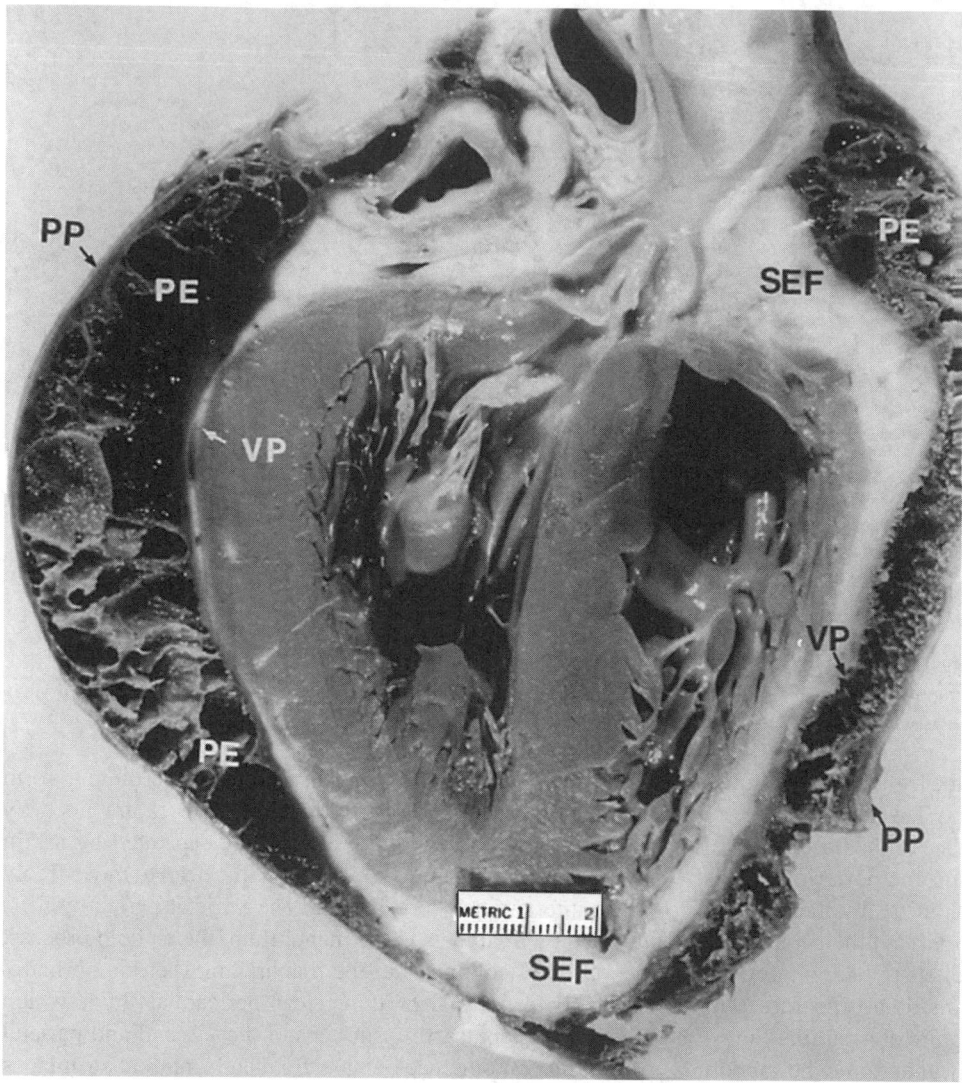

FIGURE 2-25

Fibrous pericardial effusion (PE) helps to delineate the two normal layers of the pericardial sac: visceral pericardium (VP) and parietal pericardium (PP). Subepicardial fat (SEF) is located just beneath the visceral layer of pericardium.

chamber, the left atrium is a midline posterior chamber, the right ventricle is an anterior chamber, and the left ventricle is a posterior chamber. Sectioning the heart in tomographic planes using the thorax as the axis of reference necessarily results in "distortions" of cardiac cavities, valve structures, and thickness of chamber walls. Oblique sectioning of the cavities and chamber walls may not provide precise anatomic correlates but produces truncated or inflated measurements. Technical changes in CT and MRI presently under development will permit tomographic cardiac sectioning using the heart as the axis of reference. In contrast to imaging modalities using the thorax as the axis of sectioning, echocardiography uses the heart.

Thus, precise anatomic correlates can be made in terms of measurements of wall thickness and chamber sizes. Debate among pathologists and anatomists concerning the "proper anatomic orientation" and "display" of tomographic cardiac images[50–53] centers around the principle of reference axis. Arguments that depiction of the heart in an echocardiographic four-chamber view ("valentine shape") is "unconventional" and "nonanatomic" are based upon tomographic imaging that uses the body as the reference axis. When one uses the heart as the reference axis, however, the echocardiographic four-chamber view is quite conventional and anatomic.[4,13,14]

major similarity in the techniques is the planar method of cardiac sectioning. The major difference in these various tomographic techniques is the axis of sectioning relative to the position of the heart in the thorax. Two-dimensional echocardiographic imaging, transthoracic or transesophageal, cuts the heart in transverse and longitudinal planes perpendicular and parallel to the heart itself (Figs. 2-26 to 2-28). The heart serves as the axis of tomographic sectioning. The cavities and chamber walls are sectioned perpendicular and/or parallel to their respective axis. In contrast, CT and MRI cut the thorax in transverse and longitudinal planes. The body serves as the axis of tomographic sectioning. The heart sits in an oblique position relative to the thorax: the atria are located posteriorly and only slightly superiorly; the cardiac apex is directed leftward, anteriorly, and somewhat inferiorly; and the atrial and ventricular septae and AV valves are directed anteriorly and somewhat inferiorly. Thus, the right atrium is a right lateral

Preparation of Necropsy Heart and Methods of Cutting to Display Tomographic Anatomy

At necropsy, planar sectioning of the heart requires formalin fixation with or without perfusion for 12 to 24 h before cutting. If pressure fixation is not available, gentle "stuffing" of the atria with paper towels can help distend these chambers. The paper towels should not be placed through the AV valves, as this will abnormally distort the valve leaflets. Adult as well as infant hearts can be sectioned in tomographic planes if they are prepared by the methods described above. Actual tomographic cutting of the heart can be done with the use of

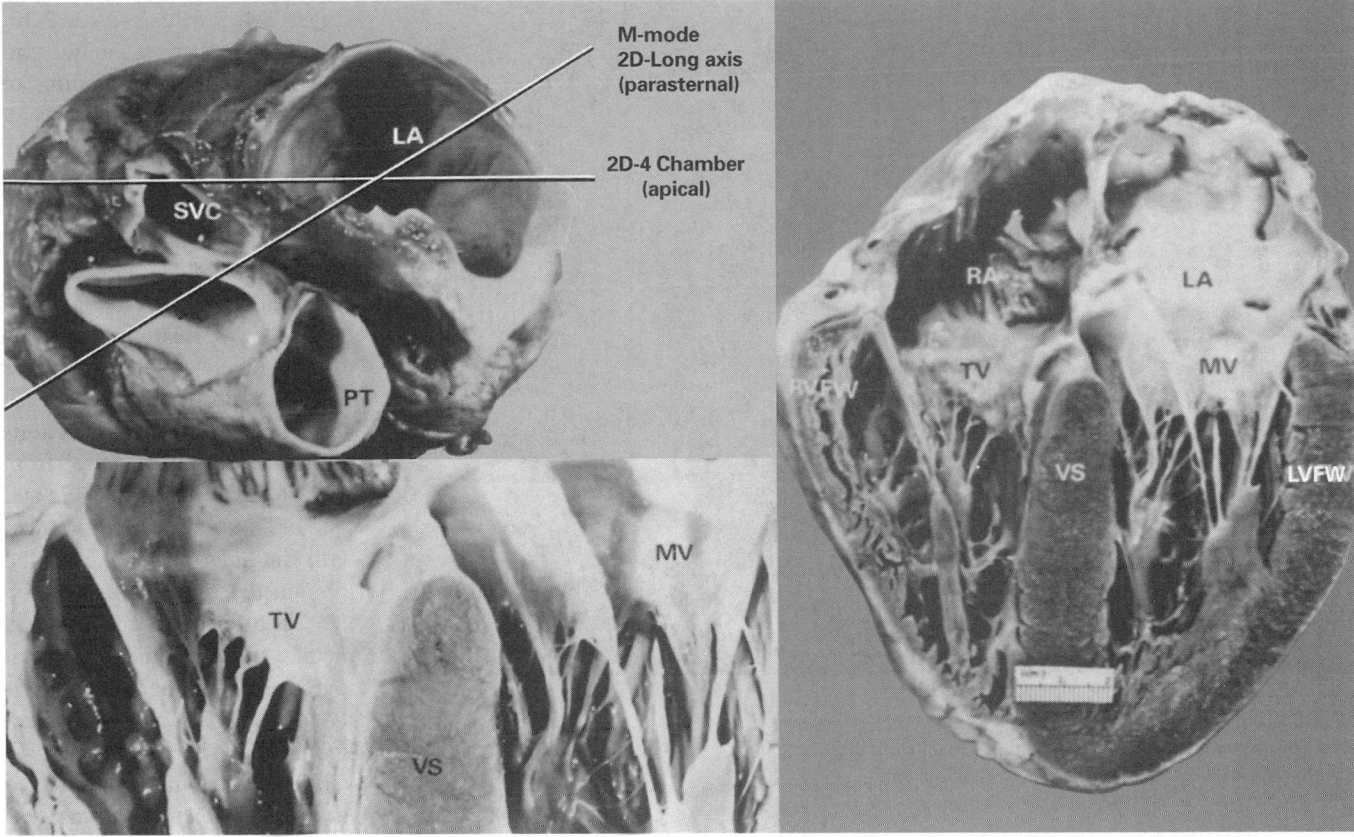

FIGURE 2-26

Composite showing method of cutting a heart and resultant tomographic views. *Upper left.* Basal view of heart showing planes of base-apex sectioning in order to obtain two-dimensional long-axis and two-dimensional, four-chamber echocardiographic views. The parasternal long-axis view is also used to correlate images obtained from M-mode echocardiography. *Lower left.* Close-up of four-chamber view showing atrioventricular valves [tricuspid (TV), mitral valve (MV)]. The annulus of the TV is located more apically than the MV annulus. VS = ventricular septum. *Right.* Four-chamber view of heart. LA = left atrium; LVFW = left ventricular free wall; RA = right atrium; RVFW = right ventricular free wall. (From Waller BF. Morphologic aspects of valvular heart disease: Part I. *Curr Probl Cardiol* 1985; 9:13. Reproduced with permission from the publisher and author.)

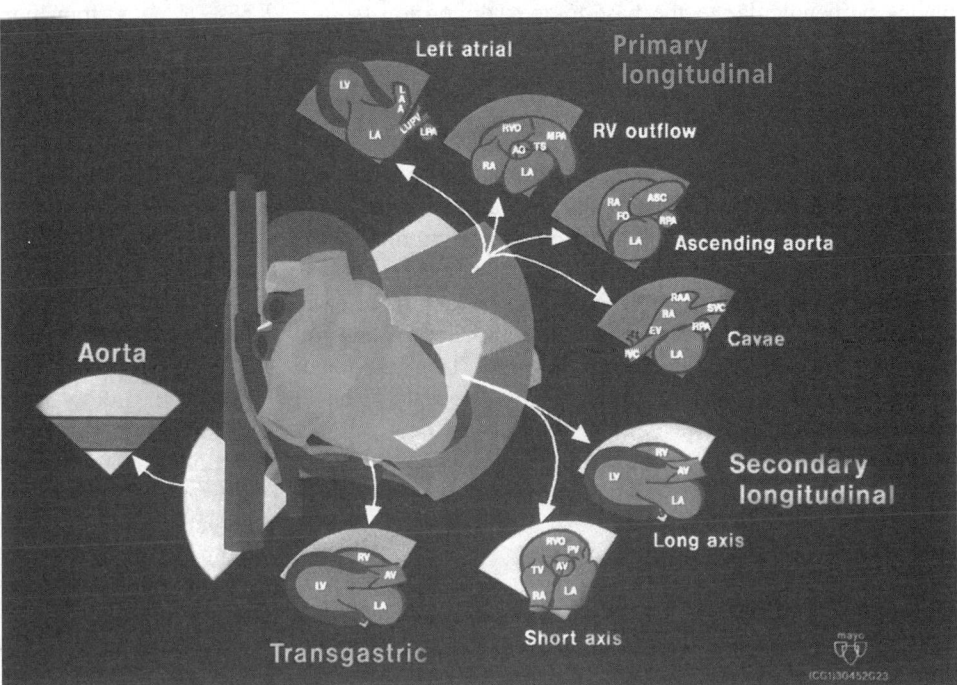

FIGURE 2-27

Schematic depiction of various views of the heart obtained in the horizontal plane by transesophageal echocardiography. (From Khandheria K, Oh J,[53] with permission).

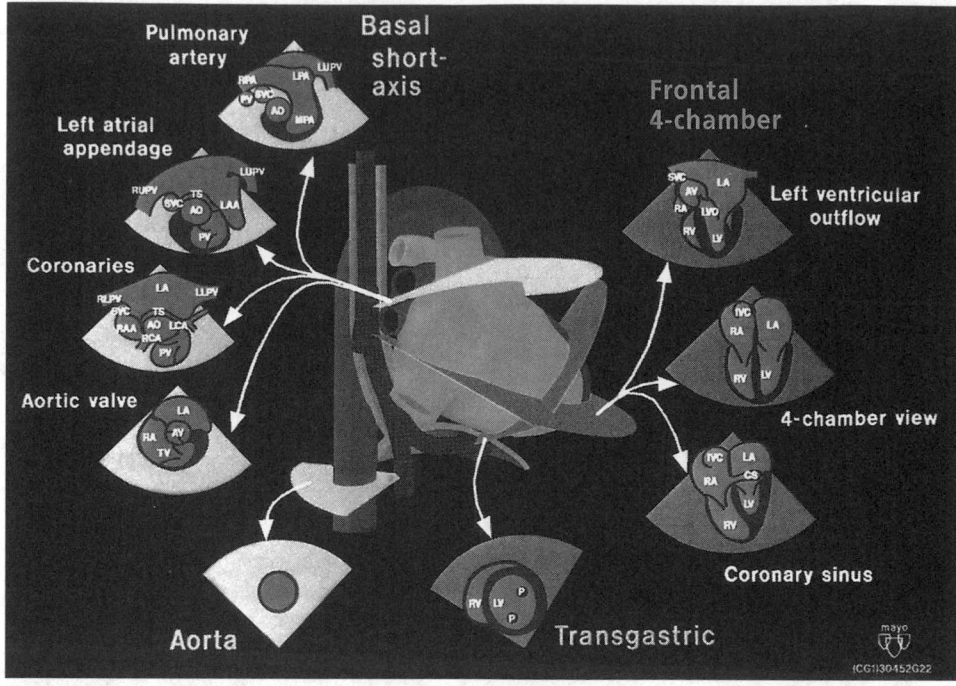

FIGURE 2-28
Schematic depiction of various views of the heart obtained in the longitudinal plane by transesophageal echocardiography. (From Khandheria K, Oh J,[53] with permission).

a large 30- to 40-cm knife, which allows smooth, straight sectioning. Sectioning the heart in tomographic planes without formalin fixation will result in irregular, rough cavity walls and distortions in the cardiac chambers.

Clinically, multiple cuts in different planes are obtained in each patient. Anatomically, multiple cuts in different planes are more difficult to achieve but can be obtained with the use of cyanoacrylate glue. The formalin-fixed heart can be cut in planes perpendicular to the base-to-apex dimension (short-axis view) or parallel to it (long-axis, two-chamber, four-chamber views) or cut in planes parallel to the thorax (transverse, frontal, parasagittal views) (Figs. 2-4, 2-5, 2-7, 2-9 to 2-12, and 2-29 to 2-33). The short-axis, two-chamber, and four-chamber planes and the transverse, frontal, and parasagittal planes are orthogonal sets of images but use the heart or body, respectively, as the reference axis for sectioning.

A particular method of cutting a heart should be chosen so as to demonstrate the specific disease or lack of disease in each heart. Each necropsy specimen is different, and no "standard" or "universal" cut can be used. The traditional "flow of blood" method of cutting a heart appears to have lost its clinical relevance with respect to the new cardiac imaging techniques. This method is particularly poor for demonstrating myocardial or valvular anatomy or heart disease.

The Heart as the Reference Axis

SHORT-AXIS METHOD
The short-axis method of sectioning the heart also has been referred to as the "bread loaf" or "ventricular slice" method

(Figs. 2-4, 2-5, 2-7, 2-12, 2-13, and 2-33). The technique involves transverse sectioning of the right and left ventricles at about 1-cm intervals from apex to base perpendicular to the axis of the atrial and ventricular septum. Near the base of the heart (about the level of chordae tendineae–papillary muscle junction), the transverse sections may skip to the level of the semilunar valves and atria (Figs. 2-12, 2-13, and 2-33). The resulting sections produce a "family of slices" from apex to base (Figs. 2-12 and 2-13). These slices are oriented with the anterior surface on the top and the posterior surface on the bottom. The short-axis method allows clinical morphologic correlation of wall and cavity dimensions and cross-sectional analysis of the cardiac valves. It is the method of choice in cases of atherosclerotic coronary heart disease, in which recent and remote myocardial infarcts are likely; in cases of neoplastic infiltration, in which metastatic implants are possible; and in cases of aortic and mitral valve disease, in which assessment of valve structure and value function (stenotic, purely regurgitant) is necessary. This method of sectioning the heart also allows classification of myocardial infarcts into location and size: anterior, posterior, septal, and/or lateral; basal, midventricular, apical, or base to apex; transmural or nontransmural (subendocardial, subepicardial). Another use of the short-axis view of the aortic valve and adjacent anatomic structures is recognition of the right and left main coronary arteries (Figs. 2-4, 2-5, and 2-7). The bifurcation of the left main into left anterior descending and left circumflex arteries and proximal portions of these main arteries can often be identified with two-dimensional (2D) echocardiography. Anomalous origin of the right and left coronary ostia can also occasionally be recognized.

TWO-CHAMBER METHOD
The two-chamber method involves sectioning the heart through the inflow tract of the left ventricle and a portion of the outflow track of the left ventricle. The plane of left ventricular sectioning is through the left ventricle and left atrium in an anteroposterior fashion and extending from base to apex. The two-chamber left ventricular plane discloses views of left atrium, anterior (septal), and posterior (mural) portions of the mitral valve leaflets, left ventricular cavity, and the anterior, apical, and posterior walls of the left ventricle. This view is currently used in assessment of the left ventricle in patients with atherosclerotic coronary heart disease. It provides another

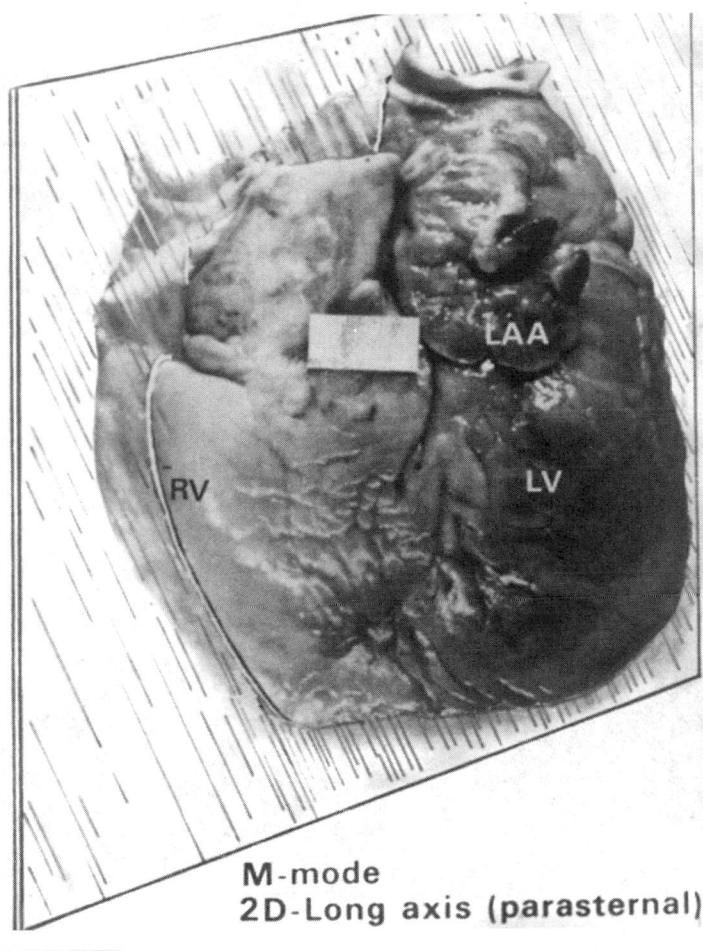

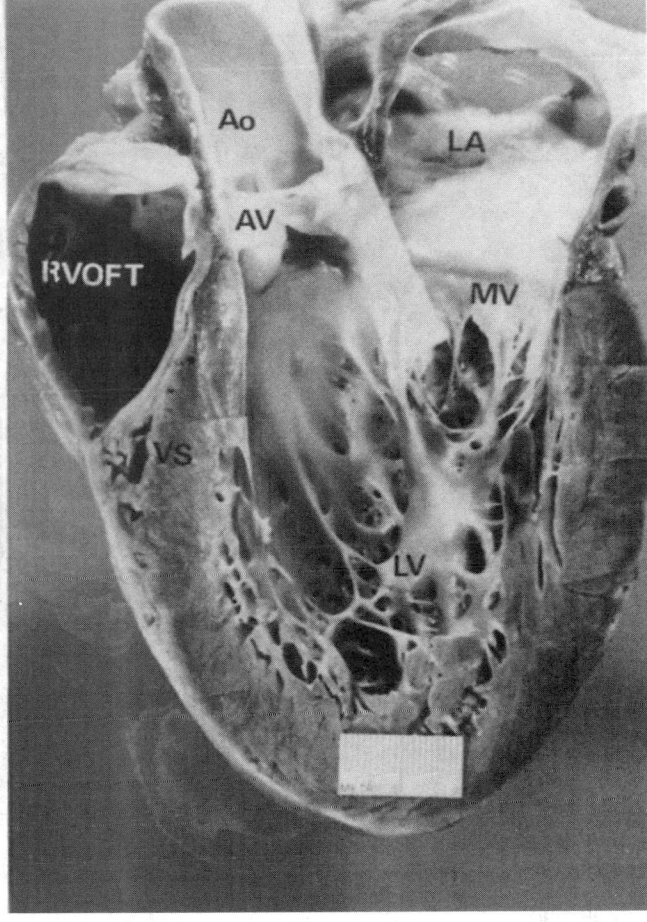

FIGURE 2-29

Tomographic sectioning of the heart from base to apex along the planar lines shown in Fig. 2-2 produces views that correlate with echocardiographic parasternal long-axis images. Ao = aorta; AV = aortic valve; LA – left atrium; LAA – left atrial appendage, LV = left ventricle; MV = mitral valve; RV – right ventricle; RVOFT = right ventricular outflow tract; VS = ventricular septum. (From Waller BF. Morphologic aspects of valvular heart disease. Part I. *Curr Probl Cardiol* 1985; 9:13 Reproduced with permission from the publisher and author.)

plane of sectioning for classification of left ventricular damage. A parallel cut on the right side of the heart discloses a similar view of the right ventricular inflow (right atrium, tricuspid valve, right ventricular body) but also discloses a portion of the right ventricular outflow tract. Although this particular tomographic view has been used less commonly in echocardiography, it would appear to be ideal in assessing right ventricular wall damage, intracavitary masses, and right ventricular outflow tract obstruction.

FOUR-CHAMBER METHOD

The four-chamber method involves sectioning the heart from base to apex in a right-to-left plane along the acute margins of right and left ventricles and corresponding walls of the atria (Figs. 2-11, 2-21, and 2-26). In the bisected specimen, portions of the tricuspid valve (posterior and septal leaflet), mitral valve (primarily posterior leaflet), AV valve annuli, chordae tendineae, papillary muscles, and each of the four cardiac chambers are visualized. In this view, it is readily apparent that the tricuspid valve annulus is located more api-

cally than the mitral valve annulus. This anatomic finding is useful in identification of the right ventricle in complex congenital heart disease. Once the ventricle is identified, the AV valve follows concordantly. The corollary is also true in that if the AV valve can be morphologically identified, the ventricle follows concordantly (i.e., recognition of the tricuspid valve as the most apical AV valve also identifies the morphologic right ventricle). The four-chamber view is useful in cardiomyopathies for measurement of all four chambers and wall thickness and for identification of cavitary thrombus or tumor.

LONG-AXIS METHOD

The long-axis method of cutting or imaging the heart produces a unique left ventricular inflow/outflow tract view (Figs. 2-9, 2-10, 2-15, 2-16, 2-27, 2-30, and 2-34). The left ventricular long-axis view is obtained by sectioning the heart in an antero-lateral plane from base to apex. In this longitudinal plane, evaluation of the aortic and mitral valves, proximal portion of the ascending aorta (sinus portion and proximal tubular

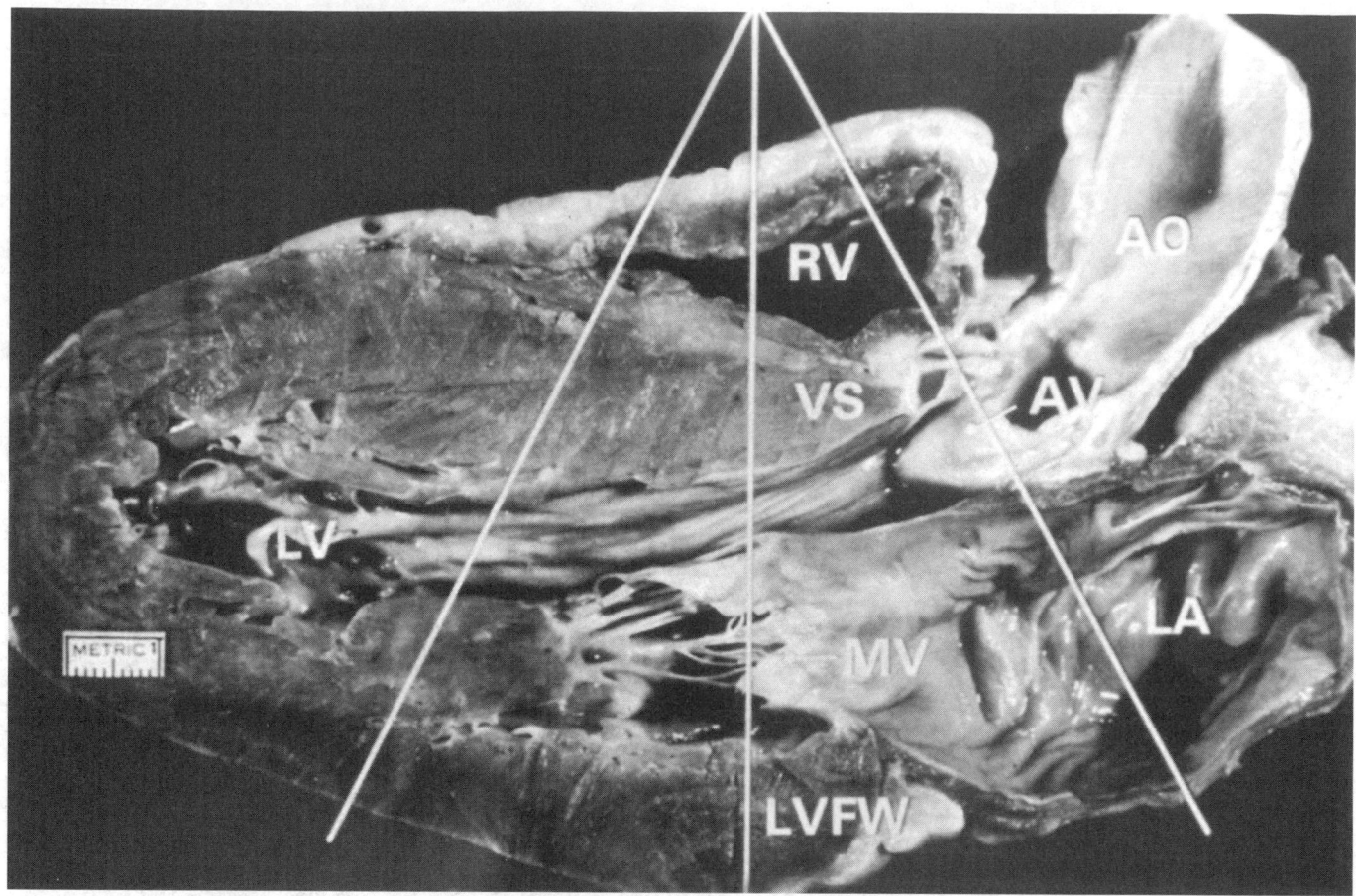

FIGURE 2-30

M-mode echocardiographic view showing "ice-pick" views of selected areas of the heart. One view displays the right ventricle (RV), aortic valve (AV), portions of aorta (AO), and left atrium (LA). Another more apical view shows the RV, ventricular septum (VS), left ventricular cavity (LV), and left ventricular free wall (LVFW). MV = mitral valve. [From Waller BF, et al. Tomographic views of normal and abnormal hearts: The anatomic basis for various cardiac imaging techniques. *Clin Cardiol* 1990; 13:802(pt I), 877(pt II). Reproduced with permission from the publisher and authors.]

portion), left ventricular outflow, left ventricular and atrial walls, and chamber is possible. Also, a portion of right ventricular outflow tract just apical to the pulmonic valve is viewed on the left ventricular long-axis plane. The right-sided parallel longitudinal section views the right atrium, tricuspid valve, and body of the right ventricle.

The left ventricular long-axis view is one of the "standard" 2D echocardiographic views of the heart and thus is used for coronary, valvular, and myocardial heart disease. The long-axis left ventricular section also corresponds to the traditional M-mode echocardiographic image, with "ice pick" views of the aorta and left atrium, left ventricular outflow tract and mitral valve, and proximal portion of the ventricular septum, left ventricular cavity, and left ventricular free wall. Anatomically, the left ventricular free wall imaged in this plane represents the lateral left ventricular free wall.

The Body (Thorax) as the Reference Axis

Tomographic sections of the heart obtained by use of the body as the reference axis result in cardiac images that differ from those described earlier. Three standard anatomic planes are generally used in CT and MRI: transverse (horizontal), frontal (coronal), and parasagittal (paramedian) (Fig. 2-35). Corresponding anatomic cardiac sections produced by these tomographic planes have been well illustrated in several anatomic atlases.[54–57]

TRANSVERSE (HORIZONTAL) METHOD

Transverse tomographic planes of the thorax produce sections of the heart with truncated or expanded views of chambers and walls because of the oblique position of the heart within the thorax (Fig. 2-35). Some of the transverse views appear similar to the echocardiographic short-axis views. Transverse sectioning at the level of the great vessels provides an anatomic display of the pulmonary trunk and its bifurcation into the right and left main pulmonary arteries and an adjacent cross section of the ascending aorta. Transverse sections taken of the heart "from the head to the feet" produce a family of oblique cross sections. One horizontal view produces a foreshortened four-chamber view that, when viewed from the left, appears as a two-chamber echocardiographic cut, and,

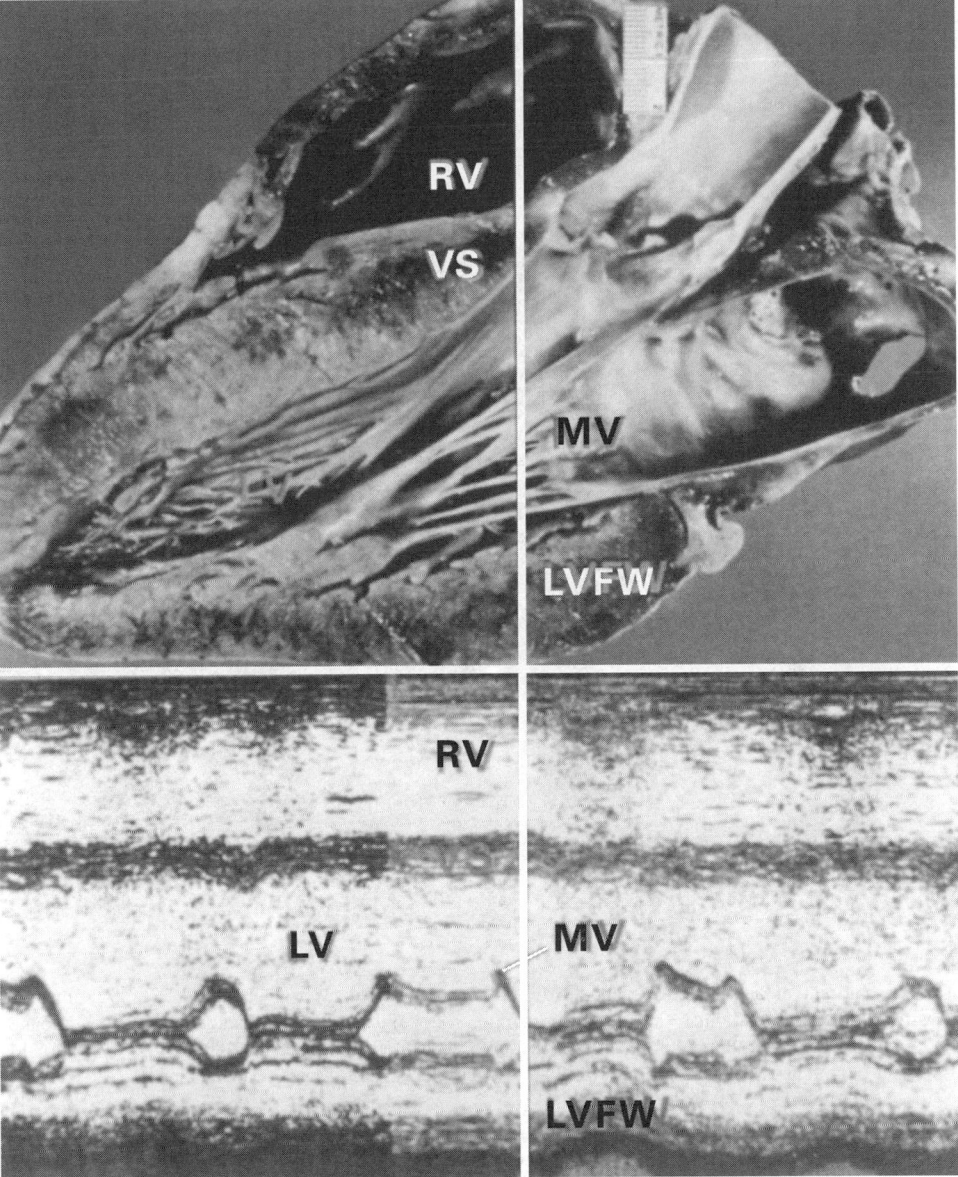

FIGURE 2-31
Parasternal long-axis view of heart with correlating M-mode echocardiogram. The ice-pick view through the midportion of the heart shows the right ventricle (RV) outflow tract, the ventricular septum (VS), left ventricular (LV) cavity, mitral valve (MV), and left ventricular free wall (LVFW). Systolic measurements on M-mode echocardiogram correspond to measurements on the formalin-fixed heart. [From Waller BF, et al. Tomographic views of normal and abnormal hearts: The anatomic basis for various cardiac imaging techniques. *Clin Cardiol* 1990; 13:802(pt I), 877(pt II). Reproduced with permission from the publisher and authors.]

when viewed from the right, appears as a truncated view of right ventricular inflow and an inflated view of the right atrium. Horizontal planes are useful in the evaluation of patients with coronary and pericardial heart disease and in those with diseases of the great vessels (dissection, aneurysm, mediastinal masses).

FRONTAL (CORONAL) METHOD
Frontal tomographic planes of the body (thorax) produce the least familiar cardiac images compared with echocardiographic images. Sectioning the thorax from the anterior to the posterior (sternum to spine) results in cardiac sections that, at any one time, contain portions of left and right ventricles, aorta and pulmonary trunks, and left and right atria. These cardiac sections also cut the heart obliquely, preventing adequate assessment of chamber size and wall thickness or thinness. This method provides excellent views of the right ventricular out-

flow tract, pulmonary trunk, and pulmonary trunk bifurcation that are not available in the previously described tomographic cardiac sections. Also, the frontal plane is useful in evaluation of the aortopulmonary window and the vena cava.

PARASAGITTAL (PARAMEDIAN) METHOD
Parasagittal tomographic planes of the body (thorax) produce another set of generally unfamiliar views of the heart. Planes of sectioning cut the heart in right-to-left fashion from shoulder to shoulder. Thus, the right-sided structures (venae cavae, right atrium, right ventricle) are viewed last. Some sections resemble the echocardiographic two-chamber views of the right and left sides. This method also cuts chambers and vessels in an oblique fashion that precludes adequate assessment of chamber size and wall thickness in most images. This method is excellent in anatomic evaluation of the aortic aneurysm, dissection, and coarctation.

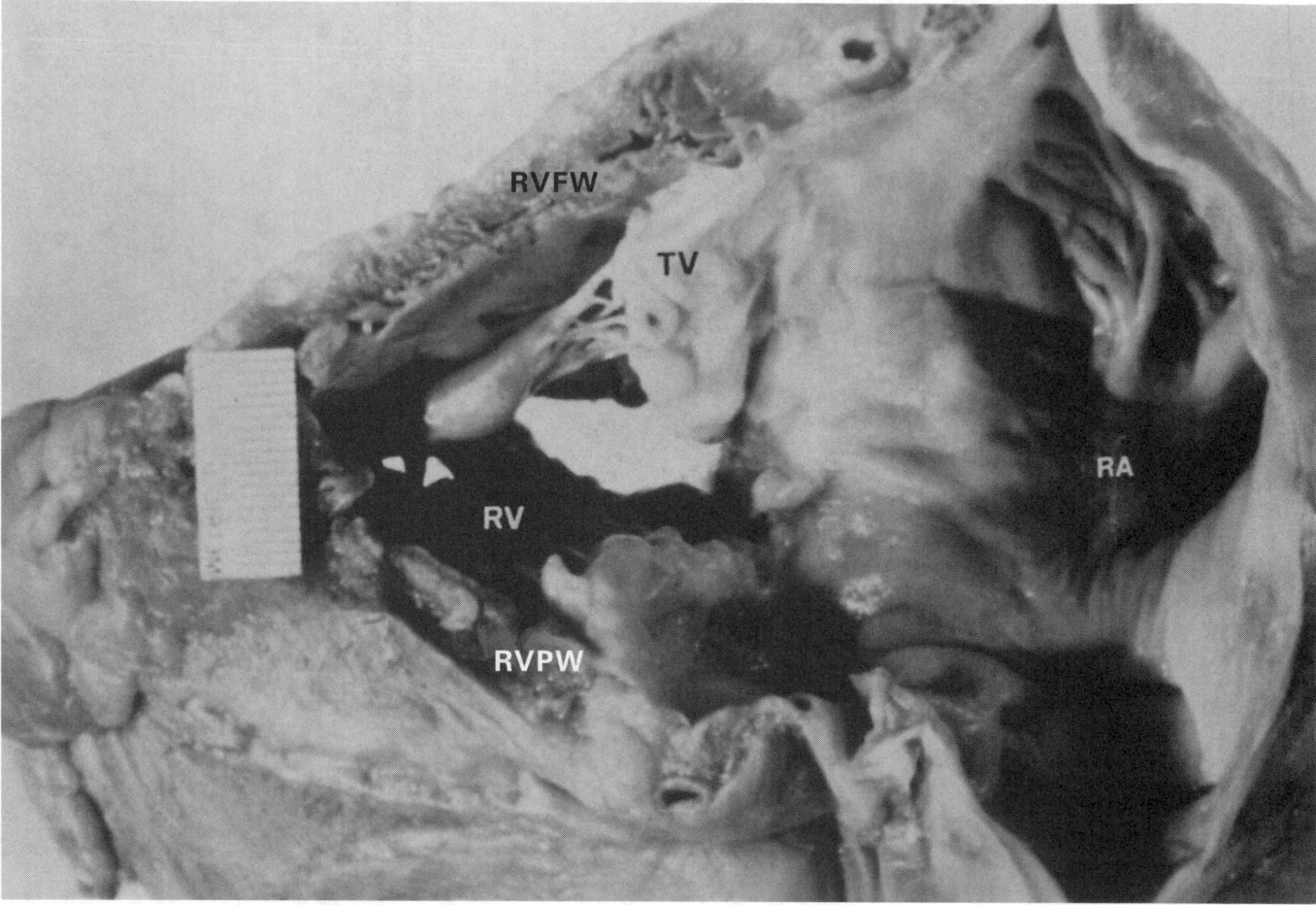

FIGURE 2-32

Tomographic cut of heart through right-sided structures as viewed by a parasternal long-axis, two-dimensional echocardiogram. RA = right atrium; RV = right ventricle; RVFW = right ventricular free wall (anterior); RVPW = right ventricular posterior wall; TV = tricuspid valve. [From Waller BF, et al. Tomographic views of normal and abnormal hearts: The anatomic basis for various cardiac imaging techniques. *Clin Cardiol* 1990; 13:802(pt I), 877(pt II). Reproduced with permission from the publisher and authors.]

In addition to conventional transverse, coronal, and sagittal imaging, oblique imaging planes are possible with MRI.[58–60] Oblique planes permit cuts of the heart along its long and short axes. The resultant cuts are analogous to the angiographic right and left anterior oblique views.

The newer cardiac imaging modalities (MRI, cine CT, positron emission tomography) provide not only depiction of cardiac anatomy with the limitations mentioned above but also an excellent technique for characterization of myocardial tissue. Distinctions between ischemic and scarred myocardium, tumor and fat infiltration, and intracavitary tumor versus thrombus are useful morphologic data that cannot be assessed using present echocardiographic modalities[59–61] (see Chap. 14).

Scintigraphic Thallium Imaging

Scintigraphic thallium testing is a popular technique used in conjunction with exercise testing. Present methods of sec-

tioning the heart produce images that closely resemble 2D echocardiographic views yet are variants of the oblique and sagittal planes. The similarity of these images to that of the echocardiographic views results from using the heart primarily as the axis for imaging (see Chap. 17).

Three- and Four-Dimensional Cardiac Reconstruction

IMAGING

Several echocardiographic, CT, and MRI techniques have been developed that permit reconstruction of the entire heart or specific portions of its anatomy: coronary arteries, valves, and chambers (Figs. 2-36 to 2-41). The development of three-dimensional (3D) echocardiography has been facilitated by advances in techniques for image acquisition, digital data processing, storage, and display.[62–79] Dynamic 3D imaging [also known as four-dimensional (4D) imaging] uses the traditional three physical dimensions of *length*, *width*, *depth* and

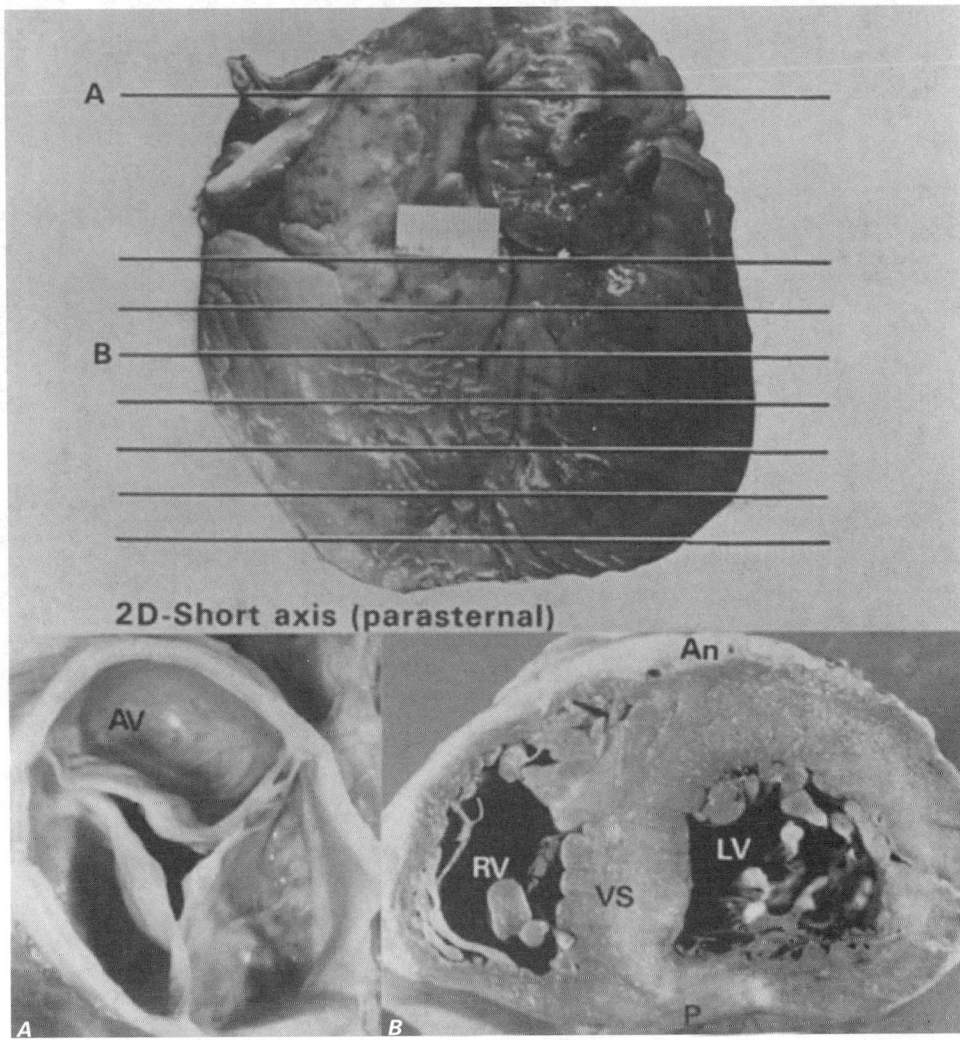

2D-Short axis (parasternal)

FIGURE 2-33
Tomographic sectioning of the heart in a "breadloaf" fashion produces a series of short-axis views of the left ventricle (LV) from apex to base. This "family of ventricular slices" is seen in Fig. 2-12. A very basal view of the heart (line A) produces a view of the aortic valve (AV)(A). Line B corresponds to a basal view of the ventricles (B) showing right ventricle (RV) and LV, anterior (An) and posterior (P) surfaces of the heart, and the ventricular septum (VS).

adds the dimension of *time* to import the cinematic perception of motion.[61] The internal structure(s) of a 3D object can be displayed by "opening and flattening" the object. This image of surface features resembles a topographic map.[62] This display is similar to views at necropsy when the internal structures of chambers or opened blood vessels are examined. Additional specialized 3D displays such as volume displays,[62,69,70,72,73] flow displays, function displays, and small-parts displays permit assessment of volumes,[1,8–12,15] distribution of blood flow,[62,66–68,78] contraction patterns,[1,14] and such structures as atrial or ventricular septae[79] and valves, respectively.[62] Electronic dissection and tissue characterization are also feasible.

The heart can also be reconstructed by CT using ultrafast (or cine) CT and scanning electron beam technology (Figs. 2-42 and 2-43).[67,80–83] Data processing advances now permit reconstruction of cardiac cavities and 3D anatomy of the major coronary arteries.[84] MRI using MBEST and FLASH techniques also is capable of reconstruction of cardiac chambers, walls, valves, and coronary arteries (Figs. 2-44 to 2-47).[85,86]

INNERVATION OF THE HEART

Although the sinus or SA (sinoatrial) node, AV (atrioventricular) node, and specialized conduction system of the heart possess the inherent ability for spontaneous, rhythmic initiation of the cardiac excitation impulse, the autonomic nervous system also influences the rate of spread of the excitation impulse, the depolarization and repolarization of the myocardium, and the contractility of both the atria and the ventricles.

The parasympathetic innervation of the heart originates in the medulla and passes through the right and left vagus nerves (Fig. 2-48). Two sets of cardiac nerves arise from each vagus nerve: the superior (superior and inferior cervical) cardiac nerves, which arise from the vagi in the neck, and the inferior (thoracic) cardiac nerves, which arise from either the vagus nerves or the recurrent branches of the vagi. The sympathetic innervation of the heart passes from the spinal cord to the upper four or five thoracic ganglia. Some fibers from the upper thoracic ganglia pass up the cervical sympathetic to the

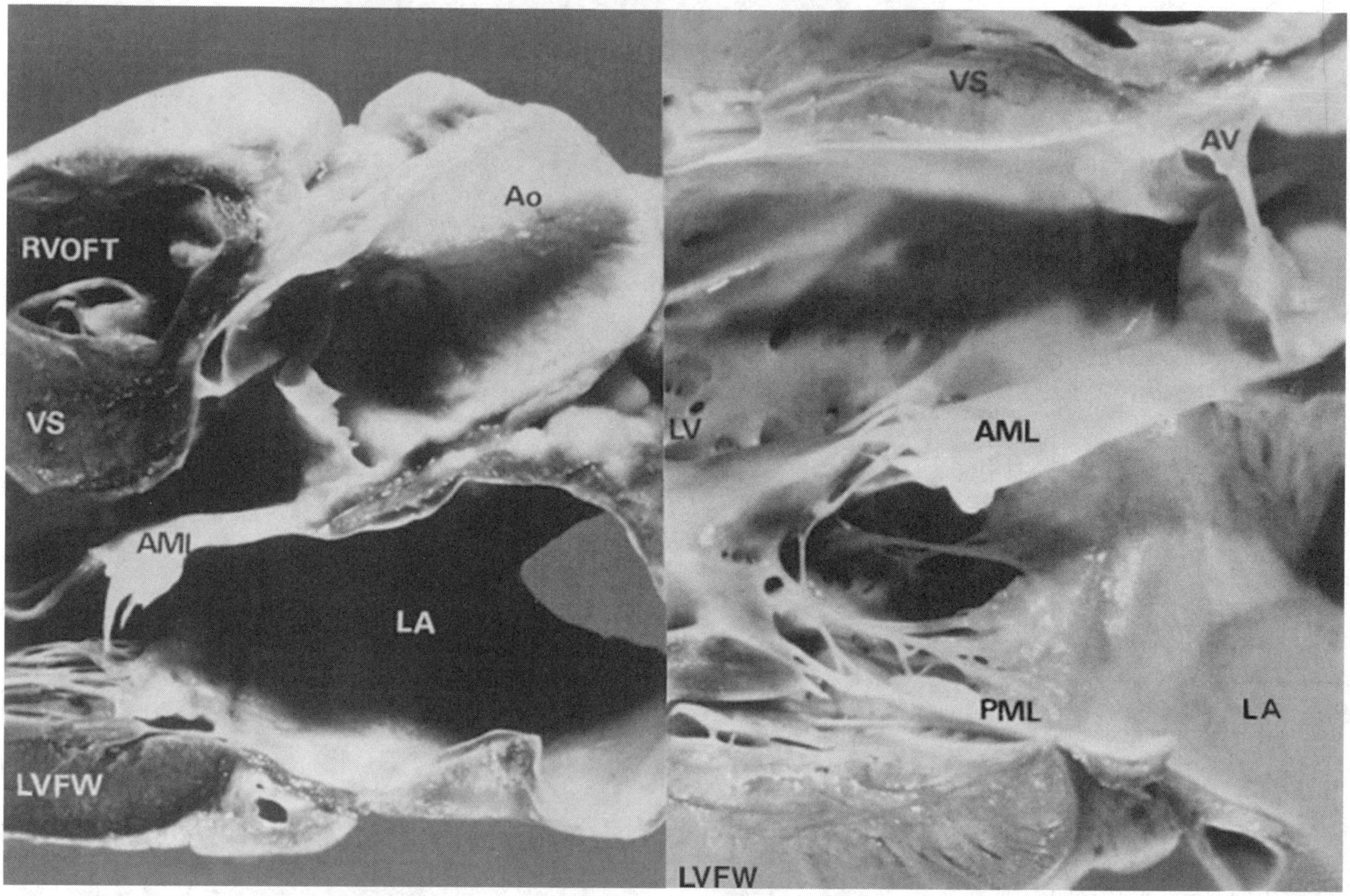

FIGURE 2-34

Parasternal long-axis view of the heart as viewed on a two-dimensional echocardiogram. *Left:* This view provides anatomic information about the basal ventricular septum (VS), left ventricular (LV) cavity, and aortic (AV) and mitral (MV) valves. AML = anterior mitral leaflet; Ao = aorta; LA = left atrium; LVFW = left ventricular free wall; RVOFT = right ventricular outflow tract. *Right:* Close-up view of LV outflow tract showing fibrous continuity of AV and AML. PML = posterior mitral leaflet. (From Waller BF. Morphologic aspects of valvular heart disease: Part I. *Curr Probl Cardiol* 1985; 9:13. Reproduced with permission from the publisher and author.)

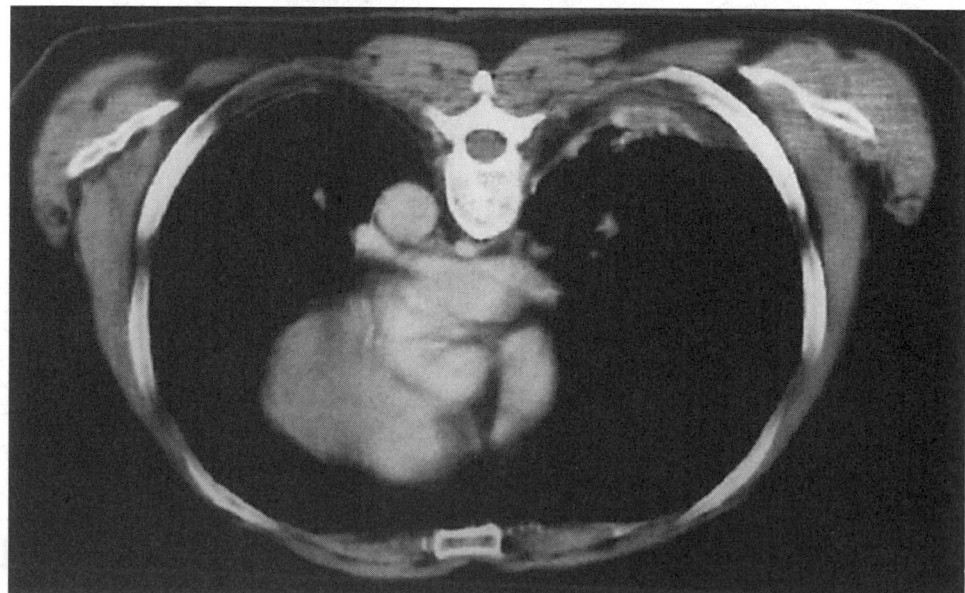

FIGURE 2-35

Transverse section of the heart from a CT scan. The perpendicular cut of the thorax creates oblique cuts of the heart. [From Waller BF, et al. Tomographic views of normal and abnormal hearts: The anatomic basis for various cardiac imaging techniques. *Clin Cardiol* 1990; 13:802(pt I), 877(pt II). Reproduced with permission of the publisher and authors.]

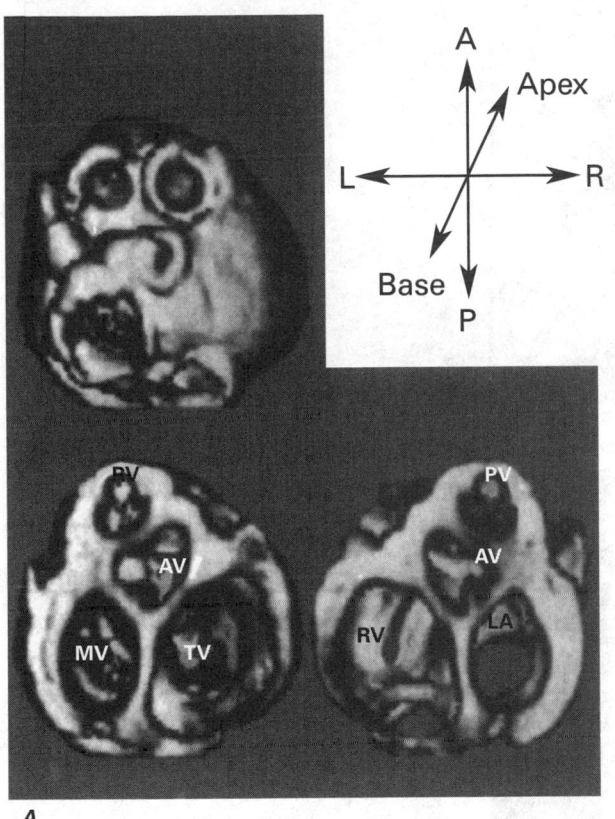

A

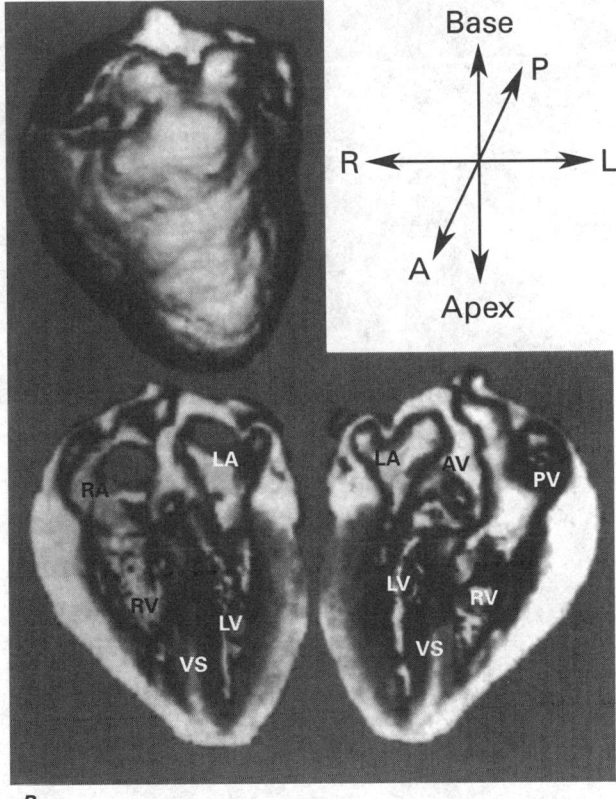

B

FIGURE 2-36

Volume-rendered image of in vitro human heart. *A*. Short-axis view. *B*. Two-chamber long axis. A = anterior; AV = aortic valve; L = left; LA = left atrium; LV = left ventricle; MV = mitral valve; P = posterior; PV = pulmonary valve; R = right; RA = right atrium; RV = right ventricle; TV = tricuspid valve; VS = ventricular septum. (From Belohlavek et al.,[62] with permission.)

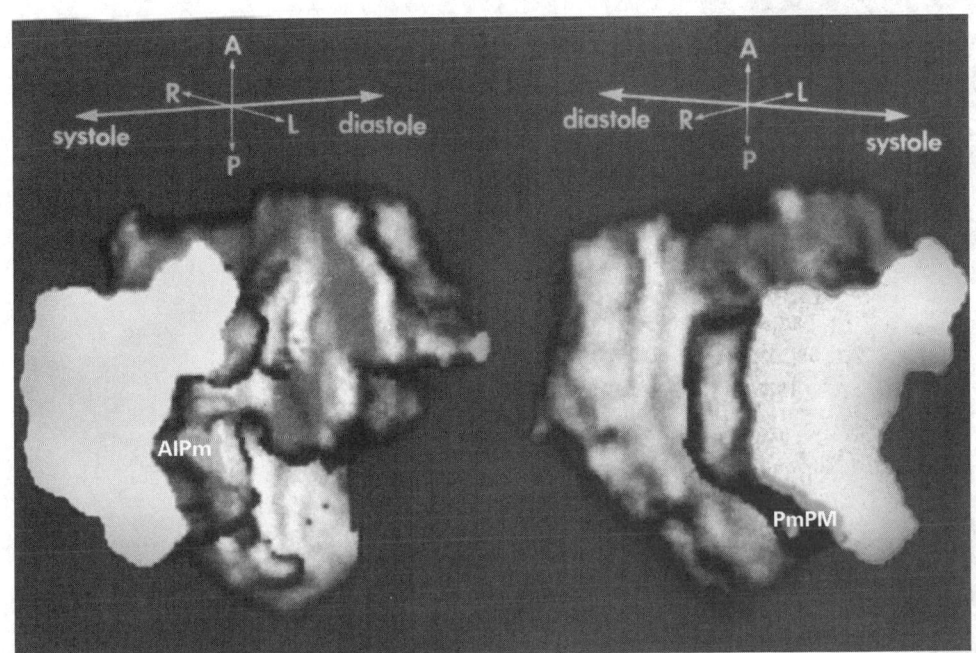

FIGURE 2-37

Function display of cross section of left ventricle. Time series of 15 cross-section images of left ventricle at level of papillary muscles was used to create a cast that demonstrated regional left ventricular contractile function. *Left:* Lateral left ventricular cavity. Anterolateral papillary = muscle (AIPm). *Right:* Septal left ventricular cavity. Smaller indentation from posteromedial papillary muscle (PmPM) is evident. Undulations of contours of the "tube" in this type of display represent cardiac cycle–dependent regional contraction and relaxation. A = anterior; L = left; P = posterior; R = right. (From Belohlavek et al.,[62] with permission.)

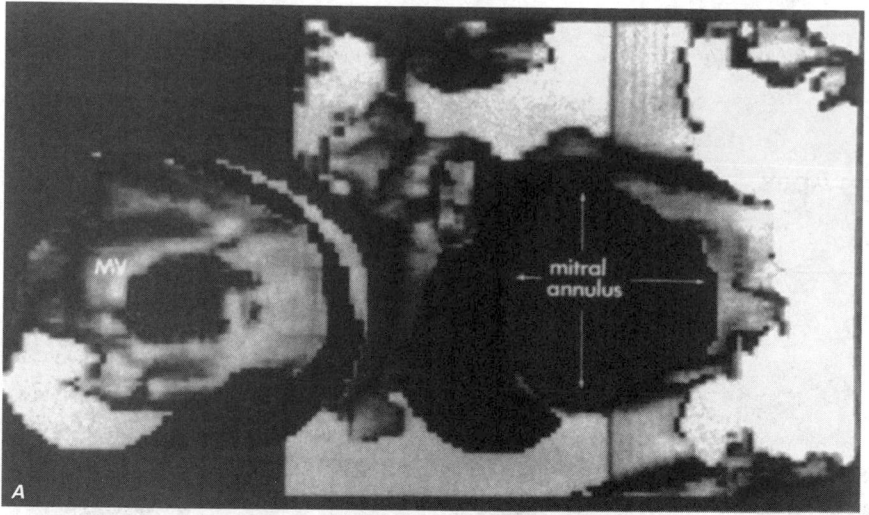

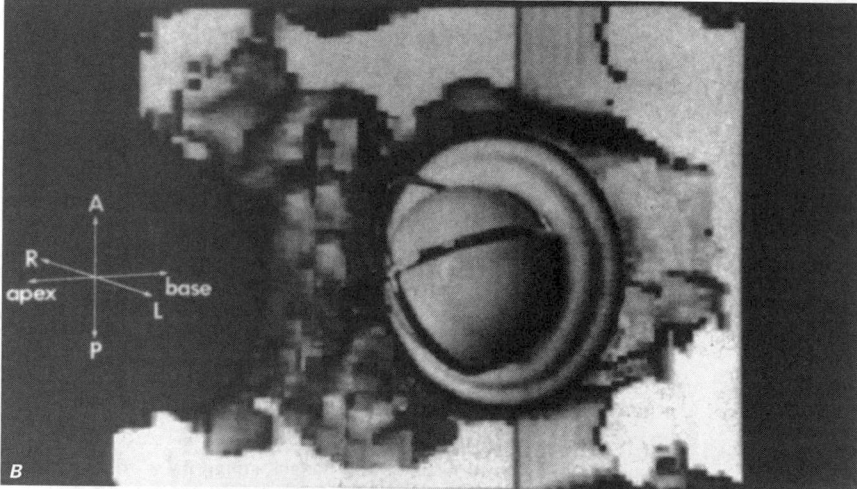

FIGURE 2-38

Electronic dissection. *A.* Three-dimensional computer rendition of stenotic mitral valve (MV) has been electronically removed from mitral annulus. *B.* Potential of three-dimensional electronic surgical procedure is illustrated by electronic positioning of a sized valvular prosthesis into mitral valve annulus to simulate surgical replacement. A = anterior; L = left; P = posterior; R = right. (From Belohlavek et al.,[62] with permission.)

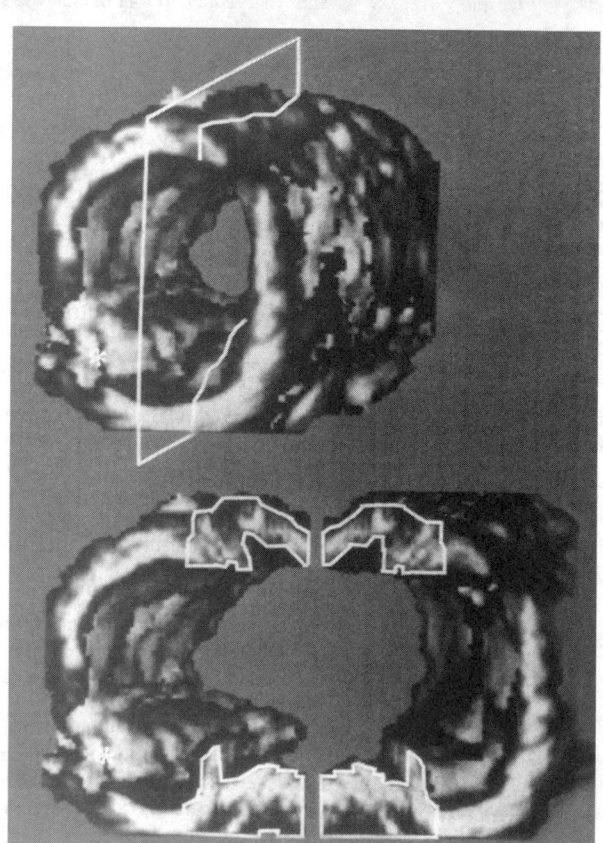

FIGURE 2-39

Intravascular 3D imaging: volume-rendered images from an in vitro pullback scan. *Top:* Three-dimensional view of intact arterial segment. *Bottom:* Same segment electronically bisected along its longitudinal axis. Note intraluminal debris and brightness of calcified arterial wall. (From Belohlavek et al.,[62] with permission.)

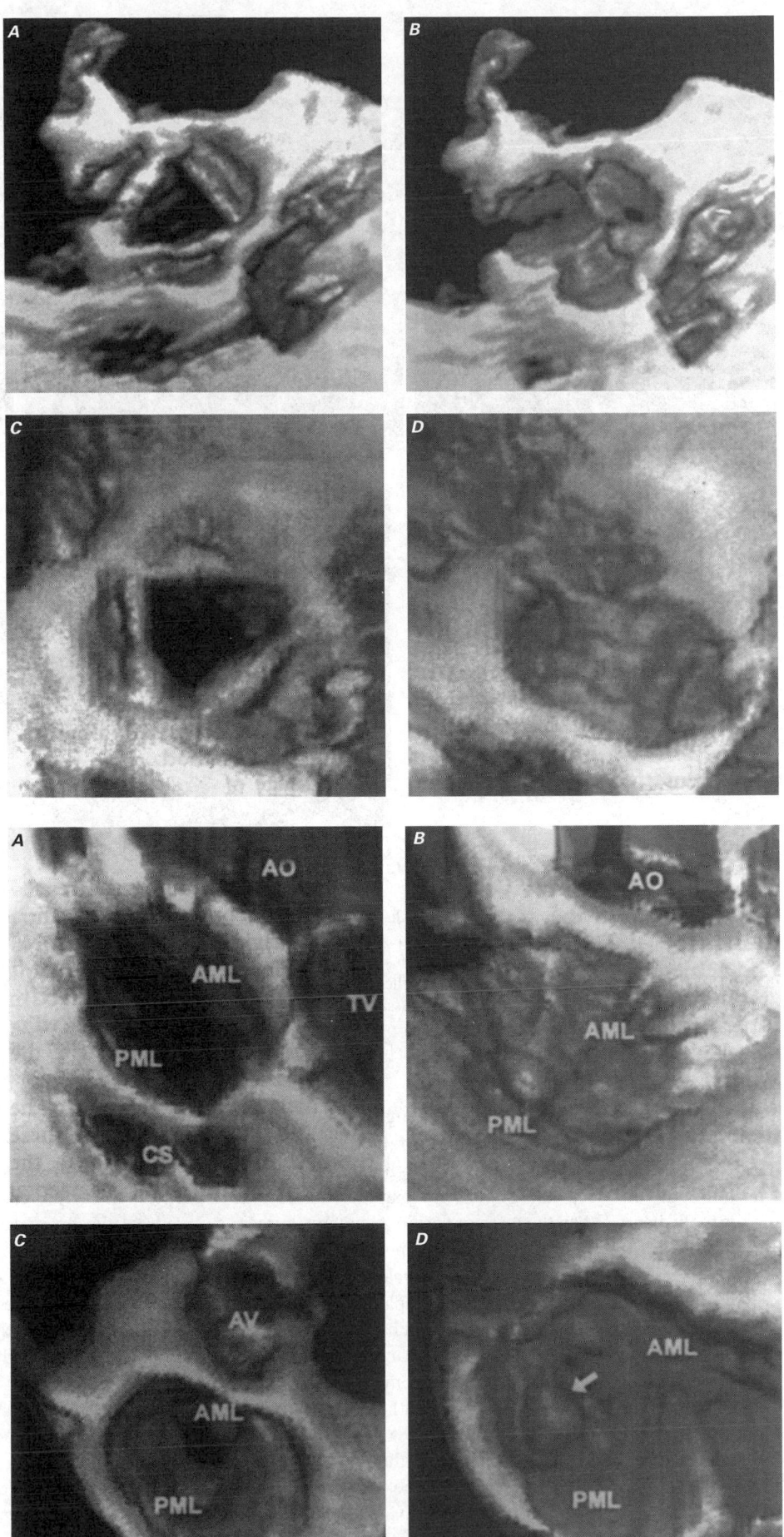

FIGURE 2-40
Normal aortic valve. Three-dimensional reconstruction from transesophageal (*A* and *B*) and precordial (*C* and *D*) acquisition. View of the valve from above shows the open leaflets in systole (*A* and *C*) and its typical arrangement in diastole (*B* and *D*). (From Salustri,[72] with permission.)

FIGURE 2-41
3D reconstruction of the mitral valve. (*A* and *B*. Prerecorded acquisition. *C* and *D*. Transesophageal acquisition.) An unroofed view of the left atrium shows a normal valve in diastole (*A*) and in systole (*B*). *C*. The orifice of a stenotic mitral valve in diastole. *D*. A prolapse of the lateral scallop of the posterior leaflet is clearly seen in systole (*arrow*). AO = aorta; AV = aortic valve; AML = anterior mitral leaflet; CS = coronary sinus; PML = posterior mitral leaflet; TV = tricuspid valve. (From Salustri,[72] with permission.)

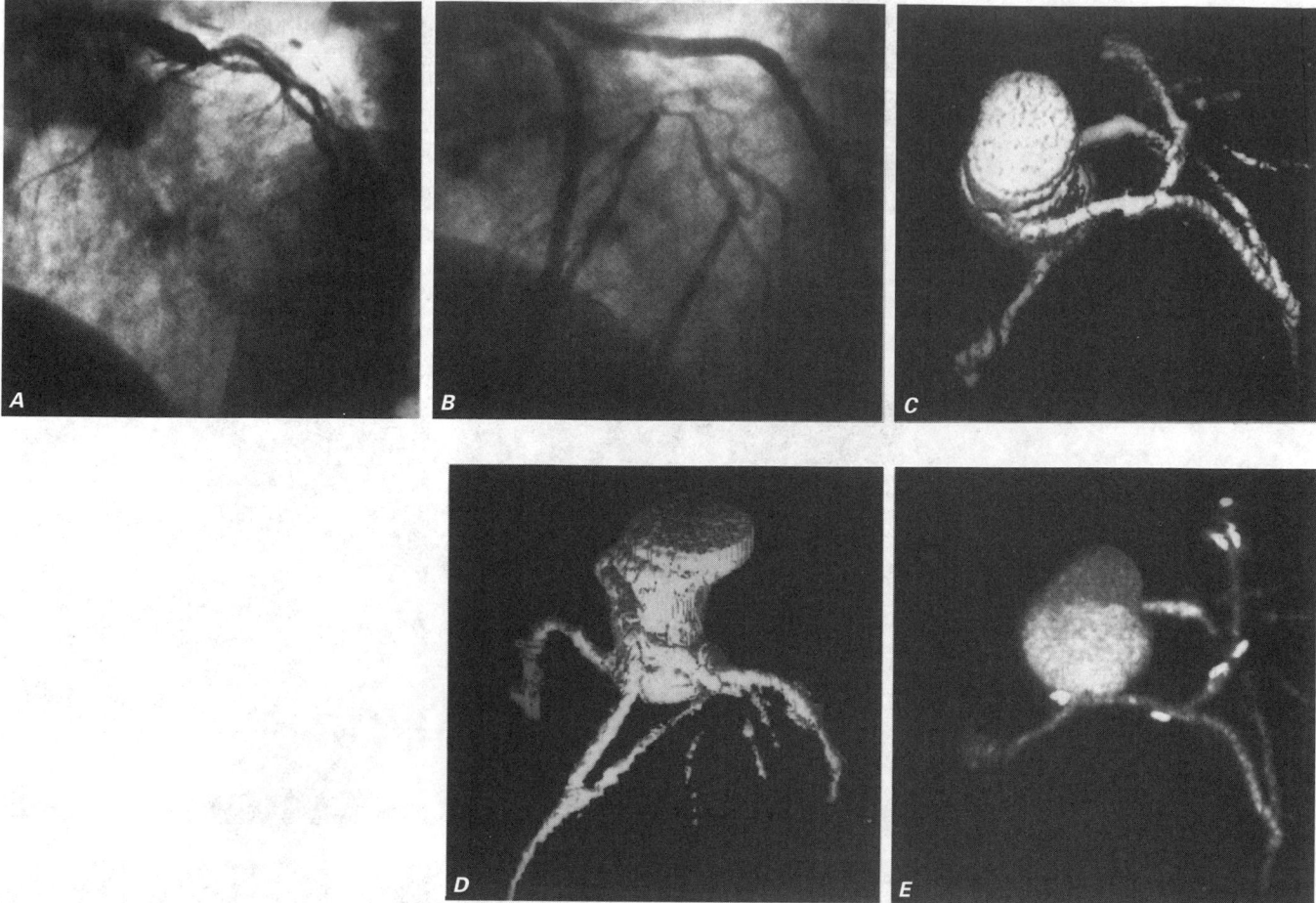

FIGURE 2-42

CT imaging of coronary arteries. Coronary artery disease in a 51-year-old man with completely intact aortocoronary bypass grafts to LADA and LCXA. *A* and *B*. Coronary angiograms demonstrate an occlusion near the origin of the LADA. The vessel distal to the occlusion is filled through the bypass graft. *C* and *D*. Corresponding 3D electron-beam CT surface reconstructions (shaded-surface display) of the inner vessel lumina demonstrate intact bypass grafts to LADA and LCXA with retrograde filling of the LADA by means of the bypass graft (owing to proximal occlusion). No major stenoses seen in the RCA. *E*. Electron-beam CT maximum-intensity projection with view identical to that in (*C*) demonstrates flow of contrast agent in the vein grafts and RCA and retrograde flow in the LADA (owing to proximal occlusion). Metal clips can be seen along the vein grafts. (From Moshage et al.,[80] with permission.)

superior, middle, or inferior cervical ganglia. The superior (cervical), middle (cervical), and inferior (cervical) cardiac nerves originate from their respective ganglia and pass downward through the deep and superficial parts of the cardiac plexus to the heart. When the inferior cervical and first thoracic ganglia are fused, the resulting ganglion is known as the *stellate ganglion*. Additional cardiac branches arise from the upper four or five thoracic ganglia and pass to the cardiac plexuses, which surround the root and arch of the aorta near the tracheal bifurcation. The cardiac and coronary plexuses are formed by cardiac branches from both the sympathetic and parasympathetic systems. Both sympathetic and parasympathetic fibers influence the SA node, the AV node, and both the atrial and ventricular myocardium, although vagal fibers to the ventricles are rather sparse. Sympathetic fibers are dense to the epicardial coronary arteries and veins and are moderate to intramural vessels. Sympathetic stimulation to the heart is largely mediated by the release of norepinephrine. Cardiac parasympathetic impulses are transmitted by acetylcholine.

Afferent impulses from chemoreceptors and mechanoreceptors in the pericardium, connective tissue, adventitia, and walls of the heart pass by peripheral sensory axons through sympathetic plexuses and through the lower two cervical and upper four thoracic sympathetic ganglia to thoracic dorsal ganglia, where the cell bodies of the neurons are located. The impulses are carried by the central axon of this neuron through the dorsal roots to the posterior gray column of the spinal cord, where the fibers synapse with the second-order neuron. From this neuron, fibers cross the median plane, ascend in the ventral spinothalamic tract, and terminate in the posteroventral nucleus of the thalamus. Some afferent vagal ganglia have been found in the left coronary artery system. Impulses passing through these neurons and ganglia are thought to be important in the Bezold-Jarisch reflex.[87–89]

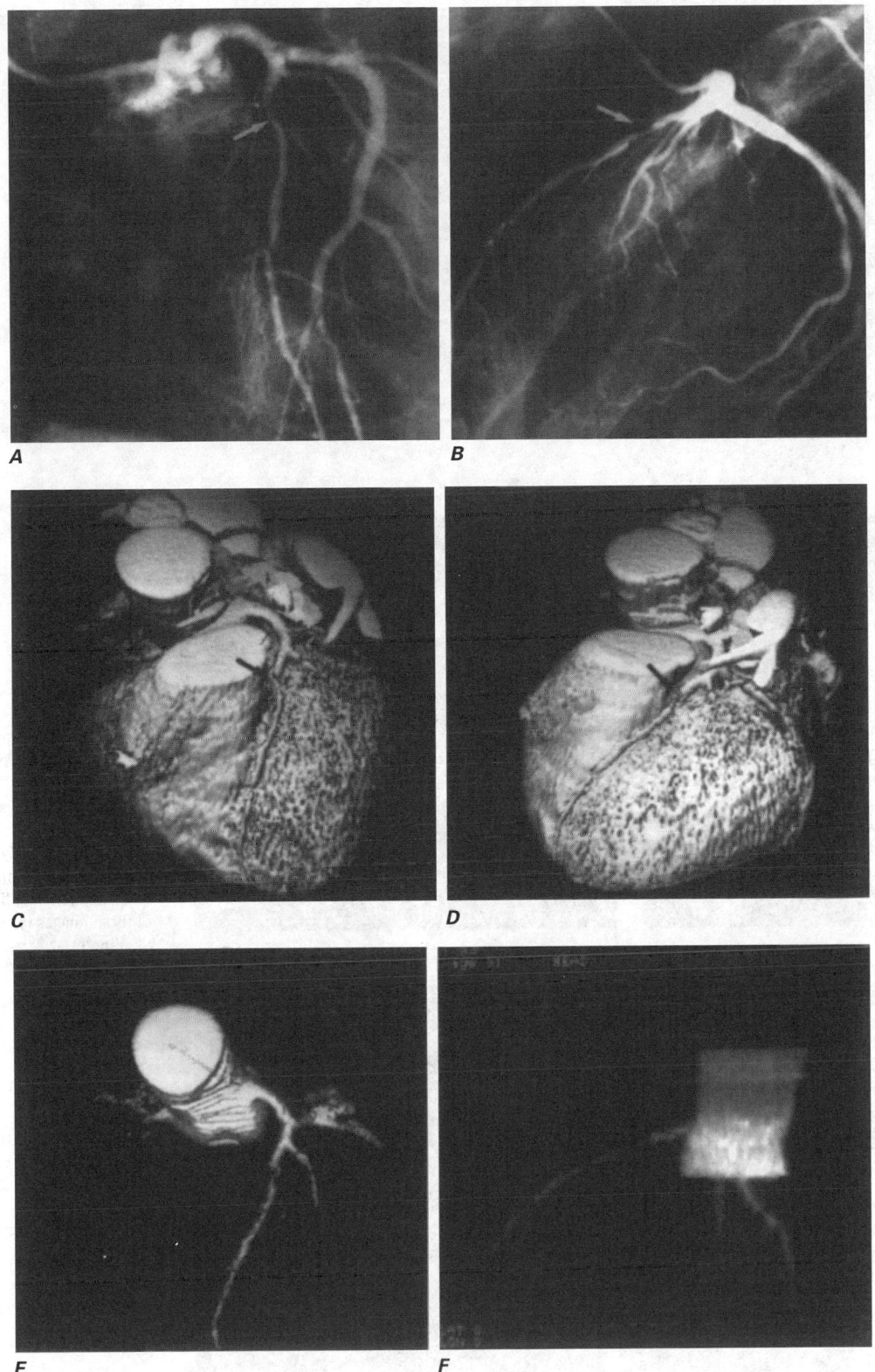

FIGURE 2-43

CT imaging of coronary arteries. *A* and *B*. Coronary artery disease in a 58-year-old man with a high-grade stenosis of the proximal LADA. Coronary angiograms demonstrate the stenosis (*arrow*) after the origin of the first diagonal branch. *C* and *D*. Electron-beam CT three-dimensional surface reconstructions (shaded-surface display). *E*. Manually edited image shows isolated LADA and stenosis. *F*. Maximum-intensity projection reconstruction of electron-beam CT data demonstrates calcifications just proximal to the stenosis. No relevant calcifications in the stenotic segment, which has a reduced vessel lumen, are shown. (From Moshage et al.,[80] with permission.)

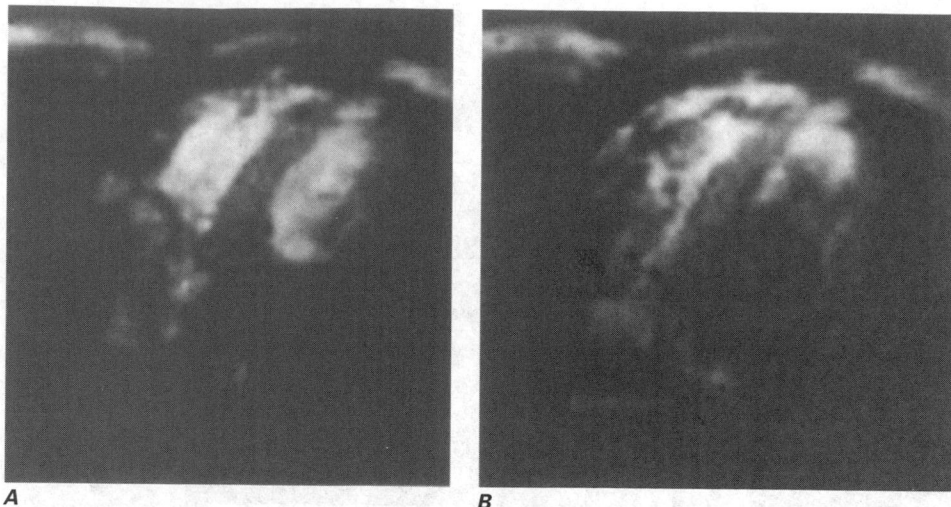

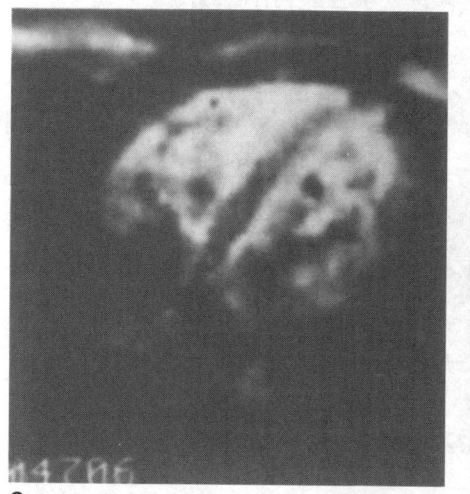

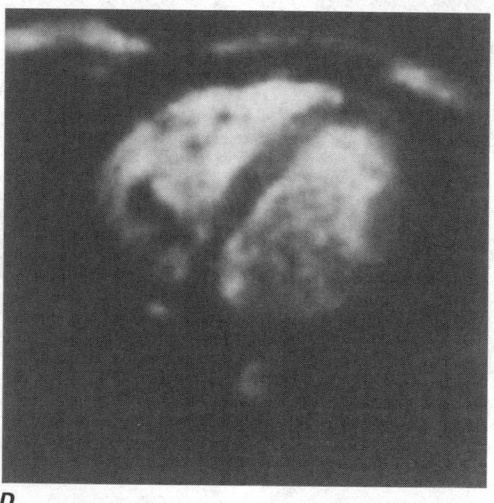

FIGURE 2-44

Planar MR imaging. Snapshot images through the heart obtained with use of a surface coil. *A.* Transection obtained during systole shows left ventricular myocardial wall thickening. *B.* Rapid ventricular filling in early diastole. *C* and *D.* Transections obtained during diastole show thinner wall. The spatial resolution of these images is less than 2 mm. (From Stehling et al.,[85] with permission.)

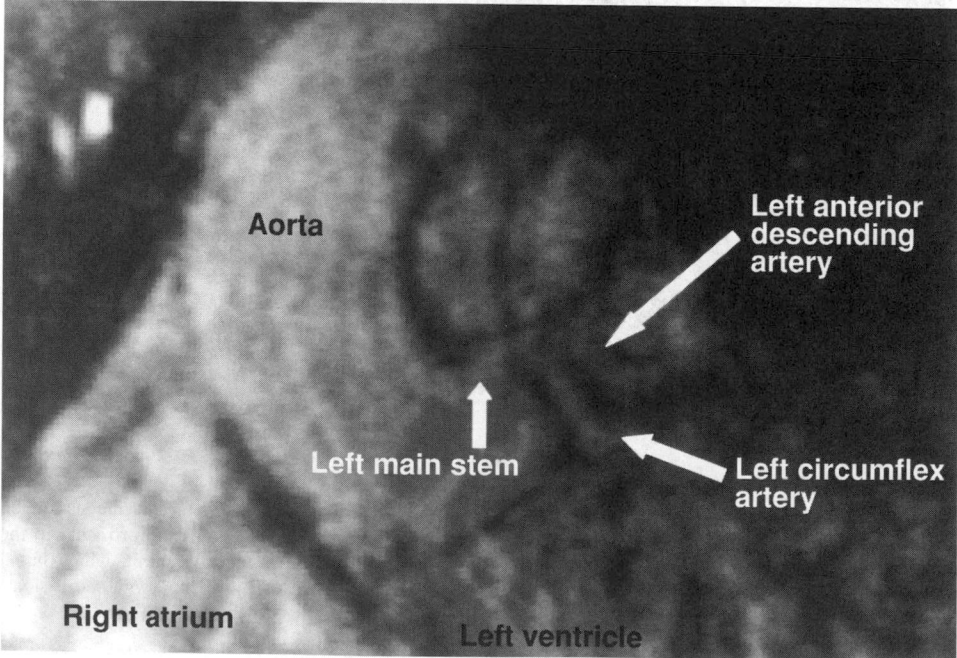

FIGURE 2-45

MRI of coronary arteries. Fast gradient-echo technique. Coronal images of the coronary sinuses showing the left main stem, left anterior descending, and left circumflex arteries. (From Pennell et al.,[86] with permission.)

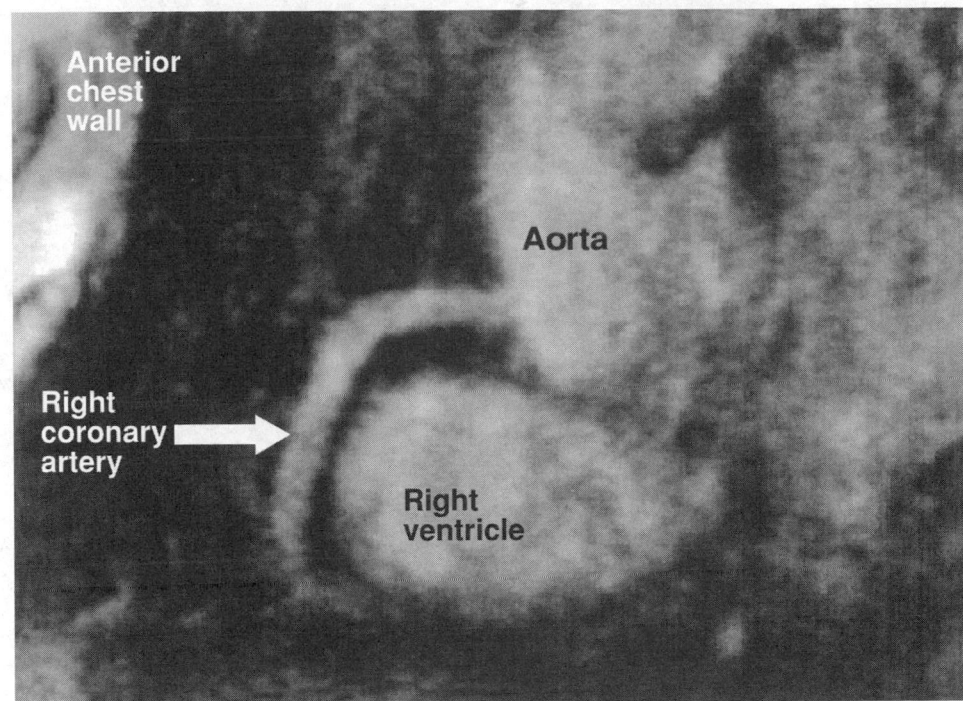

FIGURE 2-46
MRI of coronary arteries. Fast gradient-echo technique. Longitudinal image of the right coronary artery in an oblique sagittal plane. (From Pennell et al.,[86] with permission.)

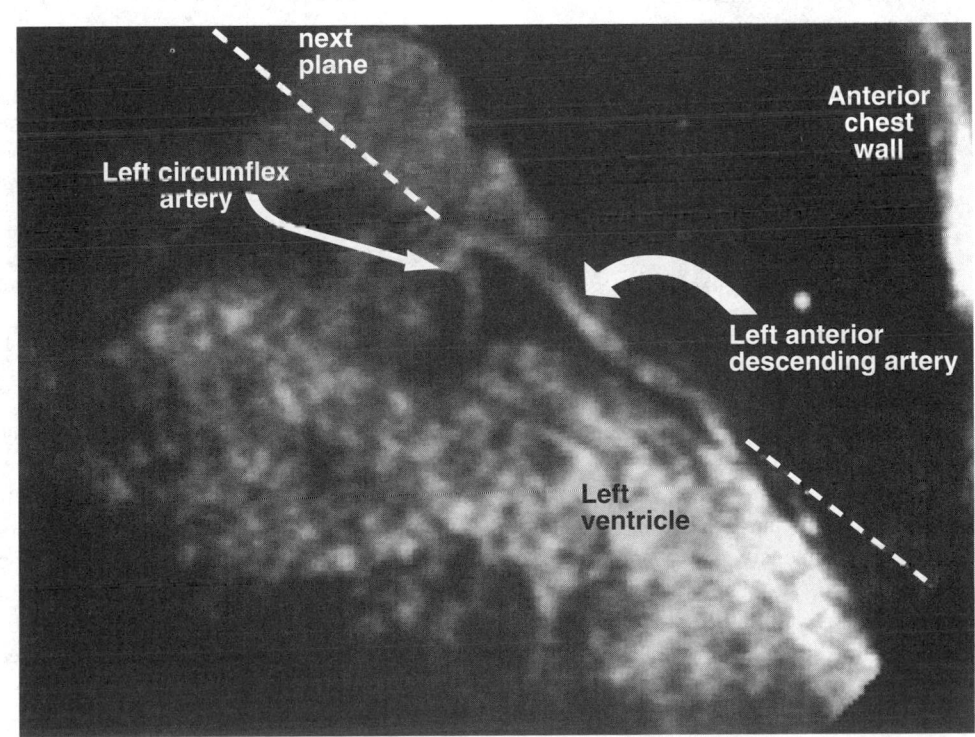

FIGURE 2-47
Longitudinal MRI image (fast gradient-echo technique) of the proximal left anterior descending artery in an oblique sagittal plane. This includes the origin of the left circumflex artery. (From Pennell et al.,[86] with permission.)

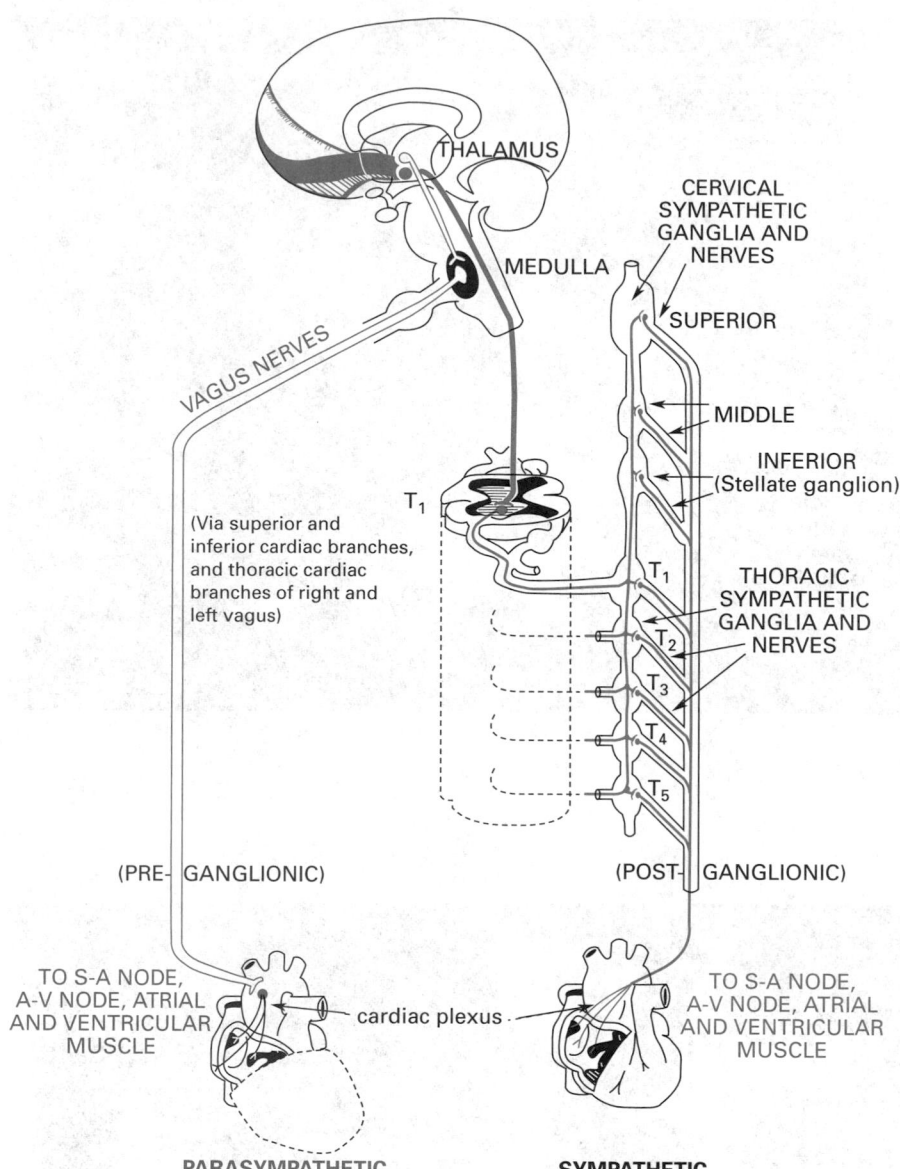

THALAMUS

MEDULLA

CERVICAL
SYMPATHETIC
GANGLIA AND
NERVES

SUPERIOR

VAGUS NERVES

MIDDLE

INFERIOR
(Stellate ganglion)

T_1

(Via superior and
inferior cardiac branches,
and thoracic cardiac
branches of right and
left vagus)

T_1

T_2

T_3

T_4

T_5

THORACIC
SYMPATHETIC
GANGLIA AND
NERVES

(PRE- GANGLIONIC)

(POST- GANGLIONIC)

TO S-A NODE,
A-V NODE, ATRIAL
AND VENTRICULAR
MUSCLE

cardiac plexus

TO S-A NODE,
A-V NODE, ATRIAL
AND VENTRICULAR
MUSCLE

PARASYMPATHETIC

SYMPATHETIC

FIGURE 2-48
A simplified, diagrammatic representation of the
efferent autonomic innervation of the heart. The
parasympathetic and sympathetic nerves to the
heart, many of which closely accompany each
other in and through the various cardiac and coronary plexuses, have been separated for illustrative
purposes. See text for details. (Diagram by
McClaren Johnson, Jr., M.D.)

LYMPHATIC SYSTEM OF THE HEART

The lymphatic drainage of the heart flows from subendocardial
vessels to an extensive capillary plexus lying throughout the
subepicardium.[90,91] These capillaries converge in collecting
lymphatic channels that run alongside the coronary vessels:
a posterior interventricular trunk paralleling the posterior descending coronary artery up to the crux of the heart and then
circling around to the right from posterior to anterior in the
right coronary sulcus; an anterior interventricular trunk ascending from the apex to the base next to the left anterior
descending coronary artery; and an obtuse marginal trunk
running alongside the left circumflex artery (Fig. 2-49).

The two major left ventricular channels—the anterior interventricular trunk and the obtuse marginal trunk—join near
the base of the pulmonary artery to form the left coronary
channel. More often, the right coronary channel unites with
the left coronary channel to become a main supracardiac
channel, the principal cardiac lymphatic, which passes upward
beneath the left atrial appendage, behind the pulmonary artery,
to enter a pretracheal node between the arch of the aorta and
the pulmonary artery. From there the right lymphatic duct
runs cephalad in the mediastinum to drain into the junction
of the internal jugular and right subclavian veins.

EPICARDIAL CORONARY ARTERIES

The epicardial coronary artery system[92] consists of the left
and right coronary arteries, which normally arise from ostia
located in the left and right sinuses of Valsalva, respectively

(Figs. 2-50 and 2-51). In about 50 percent of humans a "third coronary artery" ("conus artery") arises from a separate ostium in the right sinus. Additional smaller ostia may be found in the right sinus, which give rise to multiple right ventricular branches. Up to five separate coronary ostia have been described (Figs. 2-52 and 2-53).[93]

The left main (LM) coronary artery ranges in length from 1 to 25 mm before bifurcating into the left anterior descending (LAD) and left circumflex (LC) branches.[94] The LAD coronary artery measures from 10 to 13 cm in length, whereas the usual nondominant LC artery measures about 6 to 8 cm in length. The dominant right coronary artery (RCA) is about 12 to 14 cm in length before giving rise to the posterior descending artery (PDA). The luminal diameters of the major coronary arteries in adults range as follows: LM, 2.0 to 5.5 mm (mean 4 mm); LAD, 2.0 to 5.0 mm (mean 3.6 mm); LC, 1.5 to 5.5 mm (mean 3.0 mm); and RCA, 1.5 to 5.5 mm (mean 3.2 mm).[94] Although the LAD and LC arteries generally taper in diameter as each extends from the left main bifurcation, the RCA maintains a fairly constant diameter until just before the origin of its posterior descending branch. The subepicardial coronary arteries run on the surface of the heart embedded in various amounts of subepicardial fat. Portions of the epicardial coronary arteries may dip into the myocardium ("mural artery" or "tunneled artery") and be covered for a variable length (1 to several millimeters)[21] by ventricular muscle ("myocardial bridge") (Figs. 2-54 and 2-55). Tunneled epicardial coronary arteries probably represent a normal variant, being recognized in up to 86 percent of vessels[95,96] (see also Chap. 16).

Branches of the Major Epicardial Arteries

The branches (Fig. 2-51) of the LAD artery, in their usual order of origin, are the first diagonal, the first septal perforator, the right ventricular (not always seen in normal hearts), other septal perforators, and other diagonal branches. There may be two to six diagonal arteries, including the first diagonal, which may originate separately from the LM trunk. These diagonal branches course laterally over the free wall of

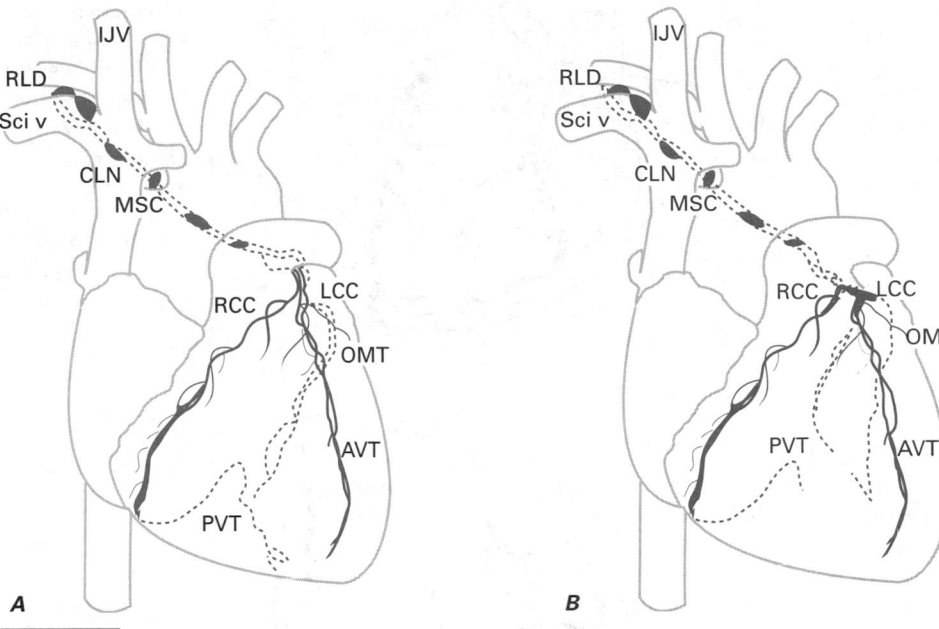

A   **B**

FIGURE 2-49

Diagrams of two different anatomic patterns (*A* and *B*) of lymphatic drainage channels of the heart. PVT = posterior interventricular trunk; RCC = right coronary channel; LCC = left coronary channel; AVT = anterior interventricular trunk; OMT = obtuse marginal trunk; MSC = main supracardiac channel; CLN = cardiac lymph node; RLD = right lymphatic duct; Sci v = right subclavian vein; IJV = internal jugular vein. (From Feola M, Merklin R, Cho S, et al. The terminal pathway of the lymphatic system of the human heart. *Ann Thorac Surg* 1977; 22:531. Reproduced with permission from the publisher and authors.)

the left ventricle in the angle between the LAD and the LC. There are also three to five septal branches, which leave the LAD artery at a right angle and plunge deeply into the ventricular septum (Fig. 2-51).

The branches of the LC are variable but may include the sinus node artery (40 to 50 percent), the left atrial circumflex branch, the anterolateral marginal, the distal circumflex, one or more posterolateral marginals, and the PDA (10 to 15 percent). The anterolateral marginal, which is usually the largest branch, is directed along the anterolateral wall toward the apex.

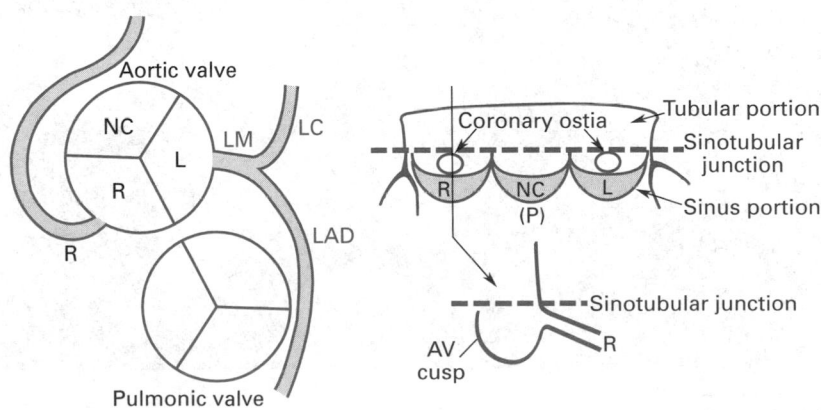

FIGURE 2-50

Diagram showing normal aortic origin and initial distribution of four major coronary arteries: left anterior descending (LAD), left circumflex (LC), left main (LM), and right (R). AV = aortic valve; NC = noncoronary; P = posterior.

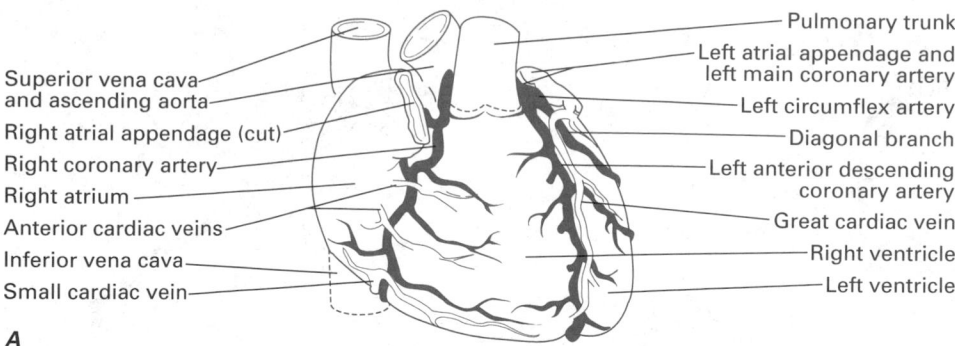

A

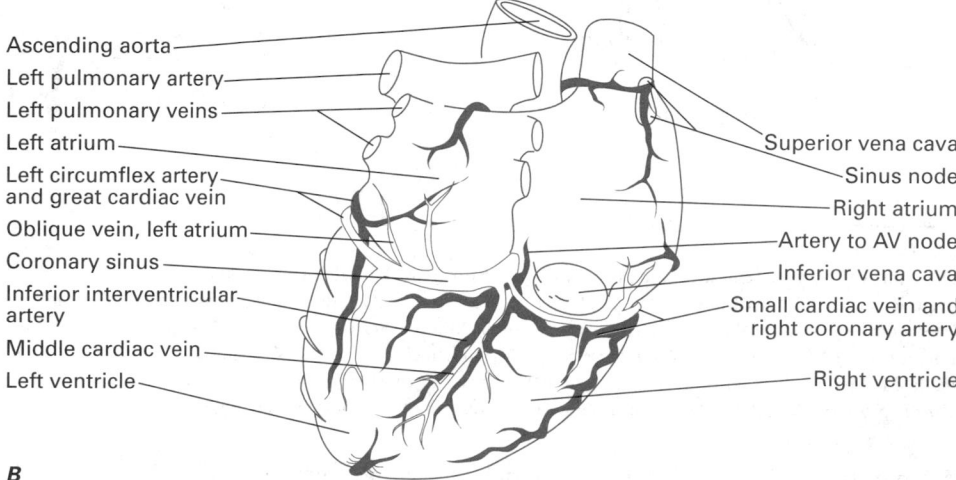

B

FIGURE 2-51

Diagram illustrating the principal arteries and veins on (*A*) the anterior surface of the heart and (*B*) the posterior and inferior surfaces of the heart. Part of the right atrial appendage has been resected to show the proximal right coronary artery. In *B* the heart is shown more vertically oriented to expose the inferior surface. (From Walmsley R, Watson H. *Clinical Anatomy of the Heart.* New York: Churchill Livingstone; 1978. Reproduced with permission from the publisher and authors.)

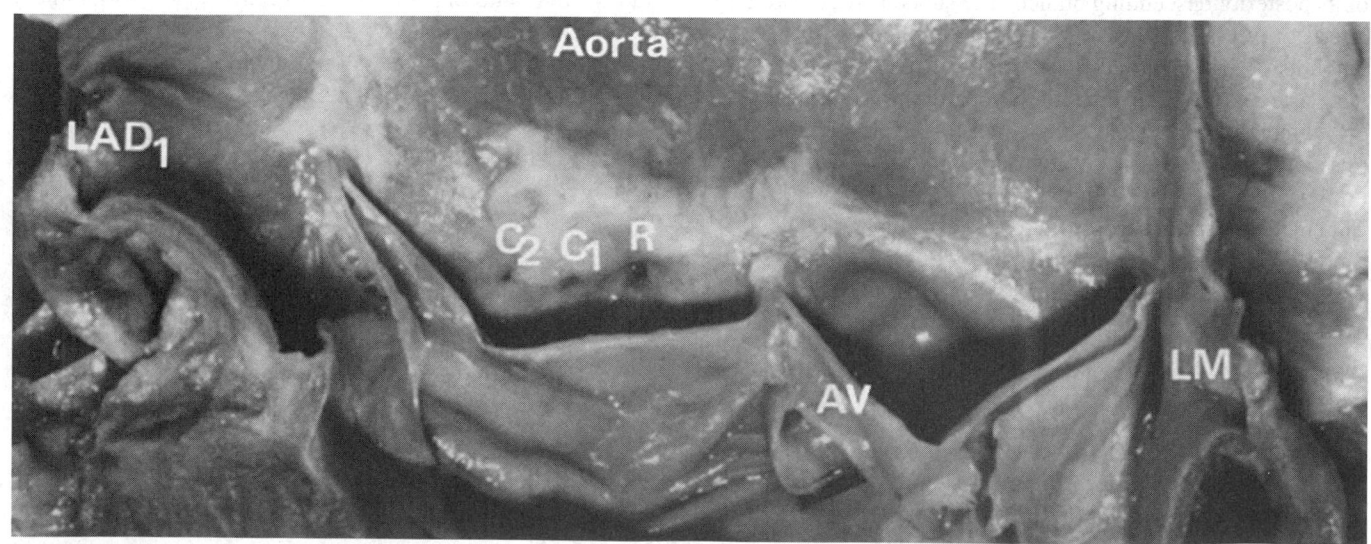

FIGURE 2-52

Photograph of ascending aorta showing five separate coronary ostia: duplicate left anterior descending (LAD$_1$), duplicate conal arteries (C$_1$, C$_2$), left main (LM), and right (R). AV = aortic valve. (From Waller BF. Five coronary ostia: Duplicate left anterior descending and right conus coronary arteries. *Am J Cardiol* 1983; 52:137. Reproduced with permission from the publisher and author.)

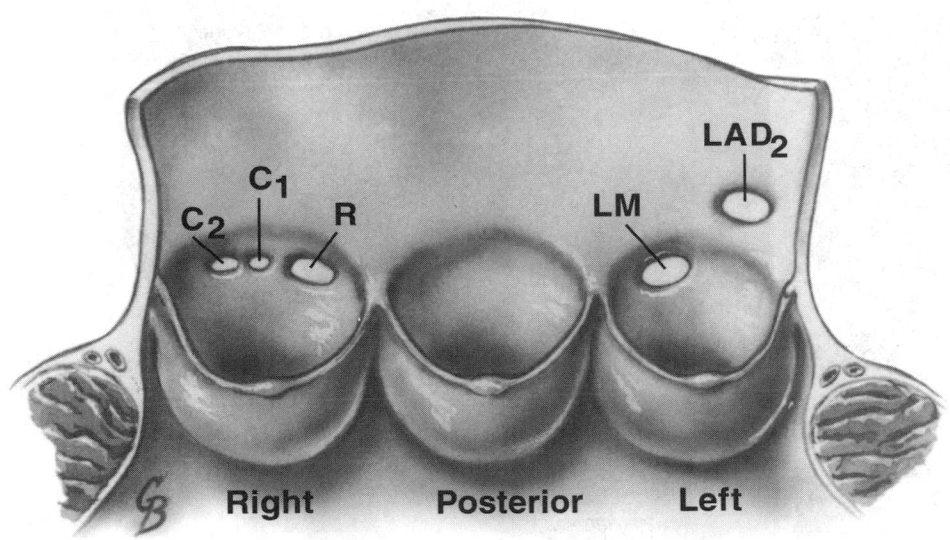

FIGURE 2-53

Diagram showing origin of the left main (LM) and right (R) coronary arteries and accessory conal branches (C_1, C_2) and a duplicate left anterior descending artery (LAD_2).

Coronary Artery Distribution and Myocardial Supply

In the current era of reperfusion therapy for evolving acute myocardial infarction, it has become popular to refer to the "infarct-related artery" of the "ventricular myocardium at risk." These phrases indicate that there is a well-established relation between a given epicardial coronary artery and its myocardial supply. Although general statements can be made about the coronary distribution, the amount of myocardium supplied by a vessel is variable and is affected by collateral vessels, congenital variations, and other factors. Figure 2-56 shows a scheme whereby certain areas on various views of the 2D echocardiogram can provide a reasonable prediction of the coronary artery perfusion pattern. Generally, the basal half of the ventricular septum and the anterior left ventricular free wall are perfused by the LAD coronary artery. A dominant right coronary artery perfuses anterior, lateral, and posterior right ventricular myocardium. The posterior coronary artery (most commonly arising from the RCA) supplies blood to the

The branches of the RCA include the conus artery (which may originate from a separate ostia in the right coronary sinus in 40 to 50 percent of hearts) to the right ventricular outflow area, the artery to the sinus node (50 to 60 percent), several anterior right ventricular branches, right atrial branches, the acute marginal branch, the artery to the AV node and proximal bundle branches, the PDA, and terminal branches to the left ventricle and left atrium. When the sinus node artery originates from the RCA, it runs along the anterior right atrium to the superior vena cava, which it encircles in a clockwise or counterclockwise direction before it penetrates the sinus node.[97] In 40 to 50 percent of hearts, the sinus node artery originates from the proximal LC and crosses behind the aorta and in front of the left atrium to reach the superior vena cava.

Coronary Ostia

The left and right coronary ostia arise normally within a sinus of Valsalva or at the junction of the sinus and tubular portions of the aorta (sinotubular junction) (Figs. 2-50 and 2-52). This ostial location allows maximal coronary filling during ventricular diastole. Occasionally, the right or left coronary ostium arises 1 cm or more above the sinotubular junction. This ostial dislocation has been termed a *high-takeoff coronary artery*. The record position for such a coronary artery is 2.5 cm above the sinotubular junction.[98] In addition to the normal variants of a separate conus ostium or several right ventricular branch ostia, certain congenital coronary artery anomalies give rise to a reduced number (single coronary artery), increased number (separate origin of the LAD, LC, or both) (Figs. 2-50, 2-52, and 2-53), or altered shapes (acute-angle takeoff, slitlike) of the coronary ostia (see Chap. 70).

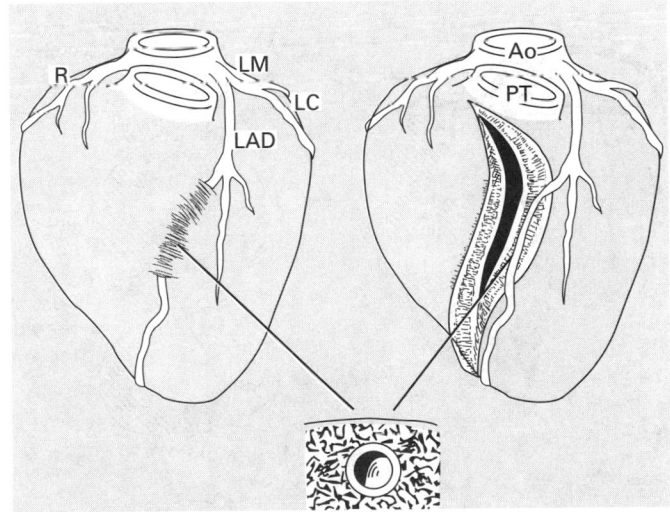

FIGURE 2-54

Diagram and photomicrograph showing tunneled epicardial coronary artery. *Left:* Middle portion of left anterior descending coronary artery (LAD) lies within ventricular myocardium. Ao = aorta; LC = left circumflex; LM = left main; PT = pulmonary trunk; R = right. (×100) (From Waller BF. Anatomy, histology, and pathology of the major epicardial coronary arteries relevant to echocardiographic imaging techniques. *J Am Soc Echocardiogr* 1989; 2:232. Reproduced with permission from the publisher and author.)

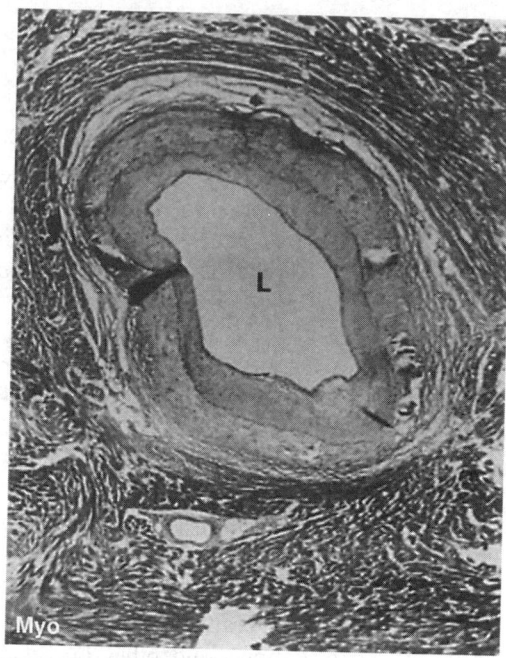

FIGURE 2-55

Tunneled left anterior descending coronary artery. The artery is surrounded by myocardium (Myo). L = lumen. (From Waller BF. Anatomy, histology, and pathology of the major epicardial coronary arteries relevant to echocardiographic imaging techniques. *J Am Soc Echocardiogr* 1989; 2:232. Reproduced with permission from the publisher and author.)

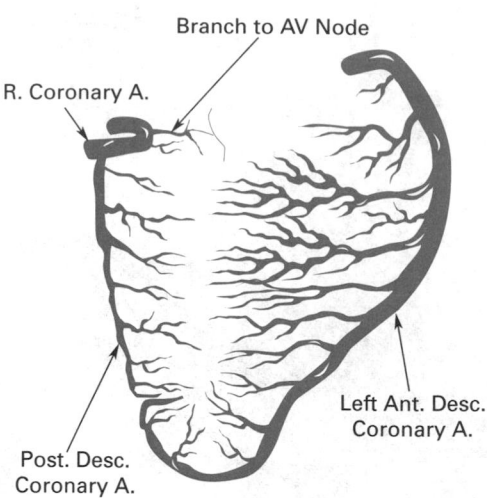

FIGURE 2-57

Drawing illustrating the normal blood supply of the human ventricular septum. (From James TN, Burch GE. Blood supply of the human interventricular septum. *Circulation* 1958; 17:391. Reproduced with permission from the American Heart Association and the authors.)

posterior quarter of the ventricular septum and posterior left ventricular free wall. The LC coronary artery usually perfuses the lateral wall of the left ventricle (defined as that portion of ventricular myocardium located between anterolateral and posteromedial papillary muscles).

Unappreciated areas of coronary perfusion include the basal ventricular septum and left ventricular apex. The basalmost portion of the ventricular septum is usually perfused by branches of the PDA (Figs. 2-56 and 2-57). The apical third of the posterior left ventricle may be predominantly perfused by the LAD artery as it wraps around the cardiac apex for variable lengths along the posterior left ventricle. At present it is believed that the LAD artery and its branches nourish the apical wall of the left ventricle, most of the right and left bundle branches, and the anterolateral papillary muscle of the left ventricle. When the PDA is provided by the circumflex artery, the entire ventricular septum is vascularized by the left coronary system.[99] The LAD artery can also provide collateral circulation to the anterior right ventricle via the circle of Vieussens, to the posterior ventricular septum by the septal perforators,

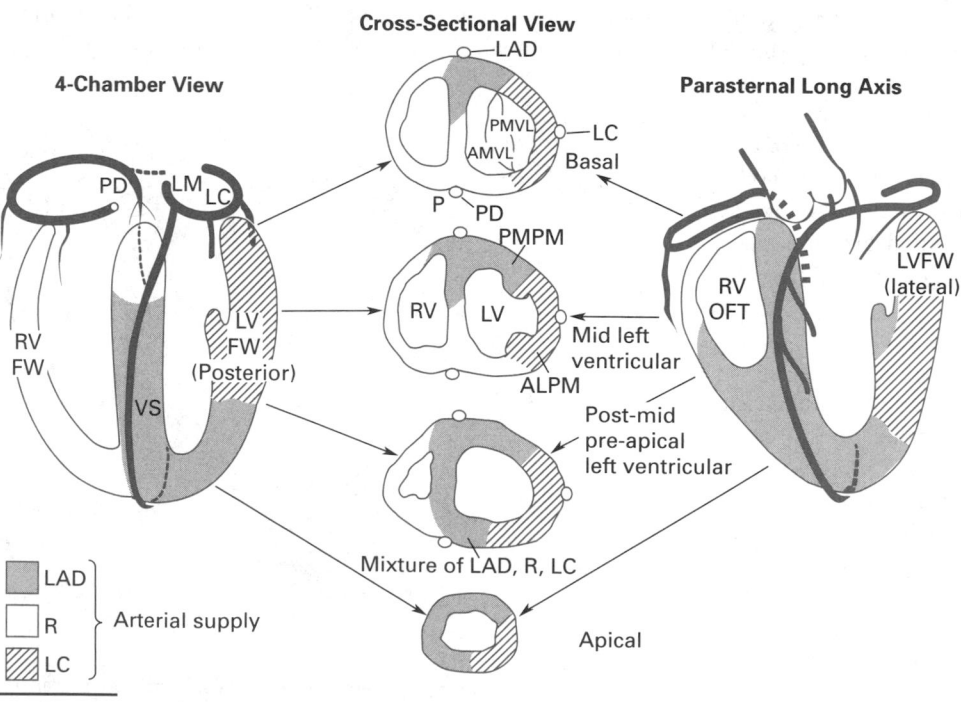

FIGURE 2-56

Diagram showing myocardial perfusion patterns of major epicardial coronary arteries as viewed from three tomographic cuts: four-chamber view, cross-sectional view, and parasternal long axis. A = anterior; ALPM = anterolateral papillary muscle; LC = left circumflex; LAD = left anterior descending; LM = left main; LV = left ventricle; LVFW = left ventricular free wall; P = posterior; PMPM = posteromedial papillary muscle; RV = right ventricle; RVFW = right ventricular free wall; RVOFT = right ventricular outflow tract. (Modified from Feigenbaum H. *Echocardiography*. Philadelphia: Lea & Febiger; 1986:262.)

and to the PDA from the distal LAD artery or a diagonal branch.

Kogel's artery[100] arises from the proximal RCA or LC or, rarely, the LM; it courses posteriorly into the lower portion of the atrial septum and anastomoses with the AV node artery.

Histologic Features of the Normal Coronary Artery

The basic organization of the coronary arterial wall is similar to all arteries in that three concentric layers can be distinguished (Figs. 2-58 and 2-59): an inner (luminal) layer, the intima (tunica intima, intimal layer); a medial layer; and an outer (external) layer, the adventitia (tunica adventitia, adventitial layer).

The intima consists of a lining layer of endothelial cells, a subendothelial layer containing connective tissue, and smooth muscle cells. The endothelium provides a smooth luminal lining and a selective diffusion barrier between the blood and the other wall layers. The endothelial cells are oriented longitudinally relative to the artery and are attached by occluding junctions and gap (communicating) junctions. Until recently, the endothelium was considered a simple, passive barrier modulating diffusion. In contrast, it is now known that endothelial cells have a number of metabolic and endocrine functions that play a critical role both normally and in various disease states. EDRF, which is now thought to be nitric oxide produced from L-arginine, stimulates guanylate cyclase to produce vasodilating cyclic guanosine monophosphate. EDRF is an important modulator of subadjacent vascular smooth muscle tone and of the vascular response to a number of vasoactive hormones (such as adenosine, acetylcholine, serotonin, and bradykinin) in both conduit and resistance vessels. The release of EDRF under the stimulus of increased shear stress plays an important role in the production of vasodilatation in some vascular beds during conditions of increased flow (see also Chaps. 3, 4, and 44). Some of the many other functions of the arterial endothelial cell include production of endothelin, a potent vasoconstrictor peptide; an antithrombotic agent (prostacyclin, PGI_2); a prothrombotic agent (factor VIII or von Willebrand's factor); a fibrinolytic agent (tissue plasminogen activator); an inflammatory mediator (interleukin-1); and important growth factors, including PDGF and fibroblast growth factor. It contains receptors for low-density lipoprotein, thrombin, and factor X.[101] The intimal layer is also the site of many of the pathologic changes seen in elastic arteries, such as atherosclerosis. The intimal layer is separated from the medial layer by the internal elastic membrane (internal elastic lamina, elastica interna), which is a fenestrated sheet of elastic tissue (Figs. 2-58 and 2-59). The internal elastic membrane may be fragmented, duplicated, or focally lost with advancing age or intimal disease (see Chap. 40).

The media consists of multiple layers of smooth muscle cells and connective tissue (elastic fibers, collagen, proteoglycans). The amount of elastic tissue is less and the number of smooth muscle cells greater in the epicardial coronary arteries compared with other elastic vessels.[94] The media consists of up to 40 layers of circumferentially or helically oriented smooth muscles. The normal media ranges in thickness from 125 to 350 μm (average, 200 μm).[102] Medial thicknesses underlying diseased intima (atherosclerotic plaque) are considerably thinner, ranging from 16 to 190 μm (mean 80 μm).[102] The smooth muscle cells are embedded in a glycoprotein mix that stains heavily with the periodic acid–Schiff (PAS)–positive reaction. Collagen and elastic fibers are also present in this layer. The medial layer is separated from the adventitial layer by the external elastic membrane (external elastic lamina, elastica externa). The external elastic membrane is composed of interrupted layers of elastin and is considerably thinner than the internal elastic membrane. Closely adherent to the outer border of the external elastic membrane are unmyelinated nerve axons. The neural stimulation of the medial smooth muscles apparently results from diffusion of the neurotransmitter through the fenestrations of the external elastic membrane.[103] The resulting depolarization of the smooth muscle cells is propagated throughout the media by low-resistance gap junctions or nexuses.[103]

The adventitial layer consists of fibrous tissue (collagen, elastic fibers) surrounded by vasa vasorum, nerves, and lymphatic vessels. Surrounding bundles of collagen are oriented primarily longitudinally.

The orientation of the collagen and the relatively "loose" consistency of the adventitia permit continual changes in the coronary diameter.[103] The thickness of the adventitia ranges from 300 to 500 μm.

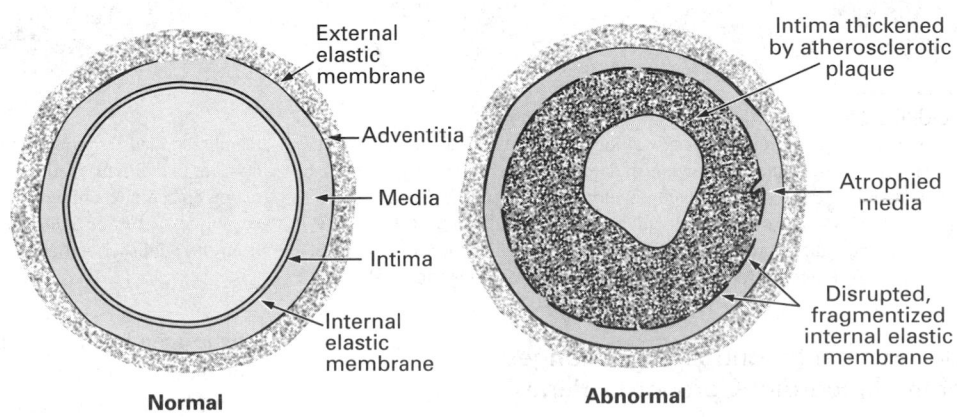

Normal **Abnormal**

FIGURE 2-58

Diagram showing histologic structure of normal and diseased epicardial coronary artery. (From Waller BF. Anatomy, histology, and pathology of the major epicardial coronary arteries relevant to echocardiographic imaging techniques. *J Am Soc Echocardiogr* 1989; 2:232. Reproduced with permission from the publisher and author.)

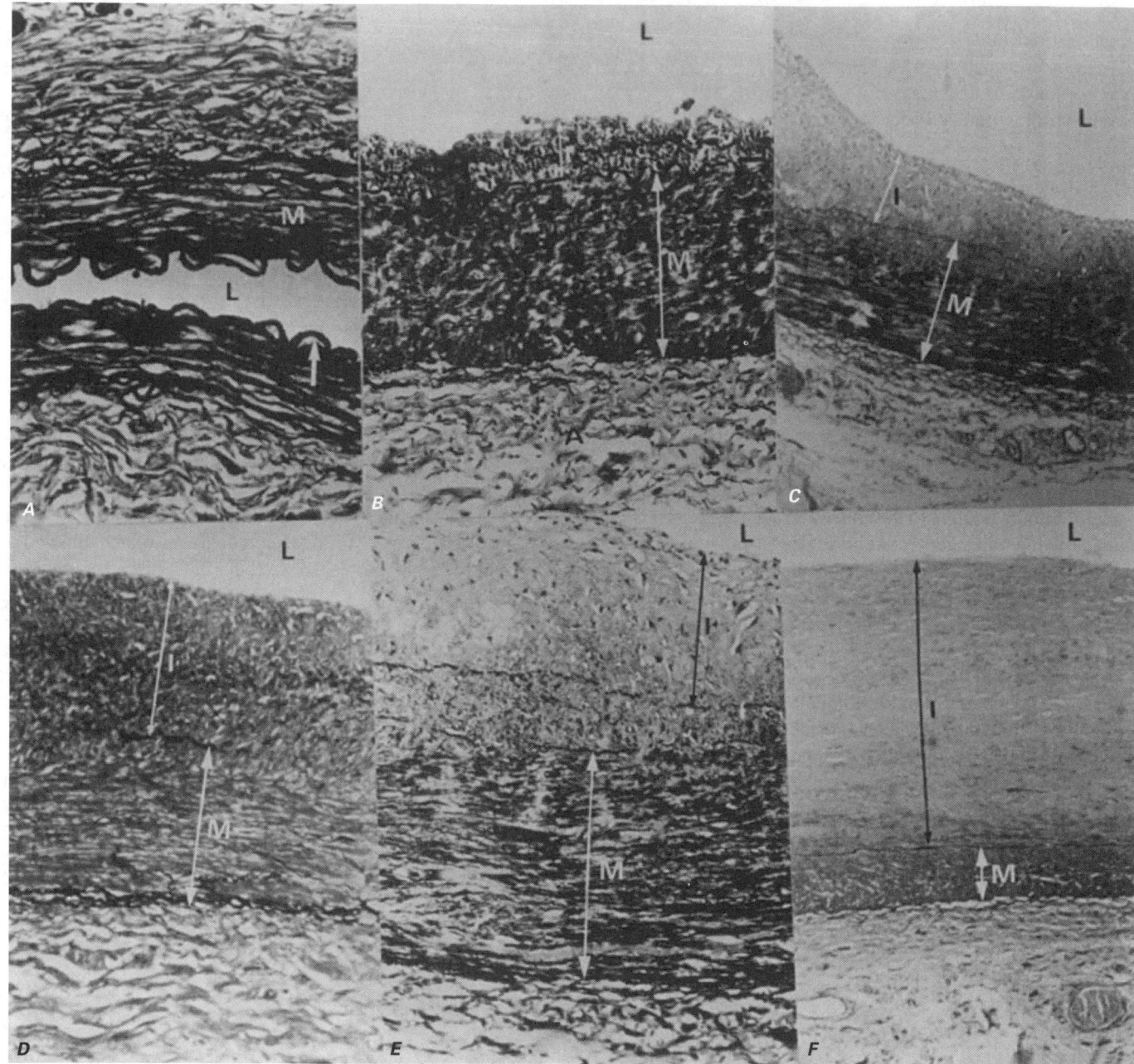

FIGURE 2-59

Composite of histologic sections of wall of various epicardial coronary arteries. *A.* One-day-old artery showing underdeveloped intima, wavy internal elastic membrane (*arrow*), and well-developed media (M). *B.* Teenage coronary artery showing further development of intima and media. *C* through *F.* Diseased epicardial coronary arteries showing varying degrees of intimal thickening by atherosclerotic plaque, fragmented or disrupted internal elastic membrane, and thinning of media. A = adventitia; L = coronary lumen; I = intima. (From Waller BF. Anatomy, histology, and pathology of the major epicardial coronary arteries relevant to echocardiographic imaging techniques. *J Am Soc Echocardiogr* 1989; 2:232. Reproduced with permission from the publisher and author.)

Developmental and Aging Changes of the Epicardial Coronary Arteries

The epicardial coronary arteries normally undergo significant changes between the fetal state and old age (Fig. 2-60).[104,105] In fetal coronary arteries the intima is not well developed, consisting of a thin layer of elongated endothelial cells in close contact with the internal elastic membrane. The internal elastic membrane appears as a continuous tube (Fig. 2-60). The media in fetal coronary arteries is well developed, consisting of a layer of circular smooth muscle cells and fine elastic fibers (Fig. 2-60). The adventitia is less well developed and consists of a thin layer of connective tissue.[104] Changes in various layers begin after birth and consist of splitting and fragmenting of the internal elastic membrane, proliferation of fibroblasts, and an increase in ground substance in the

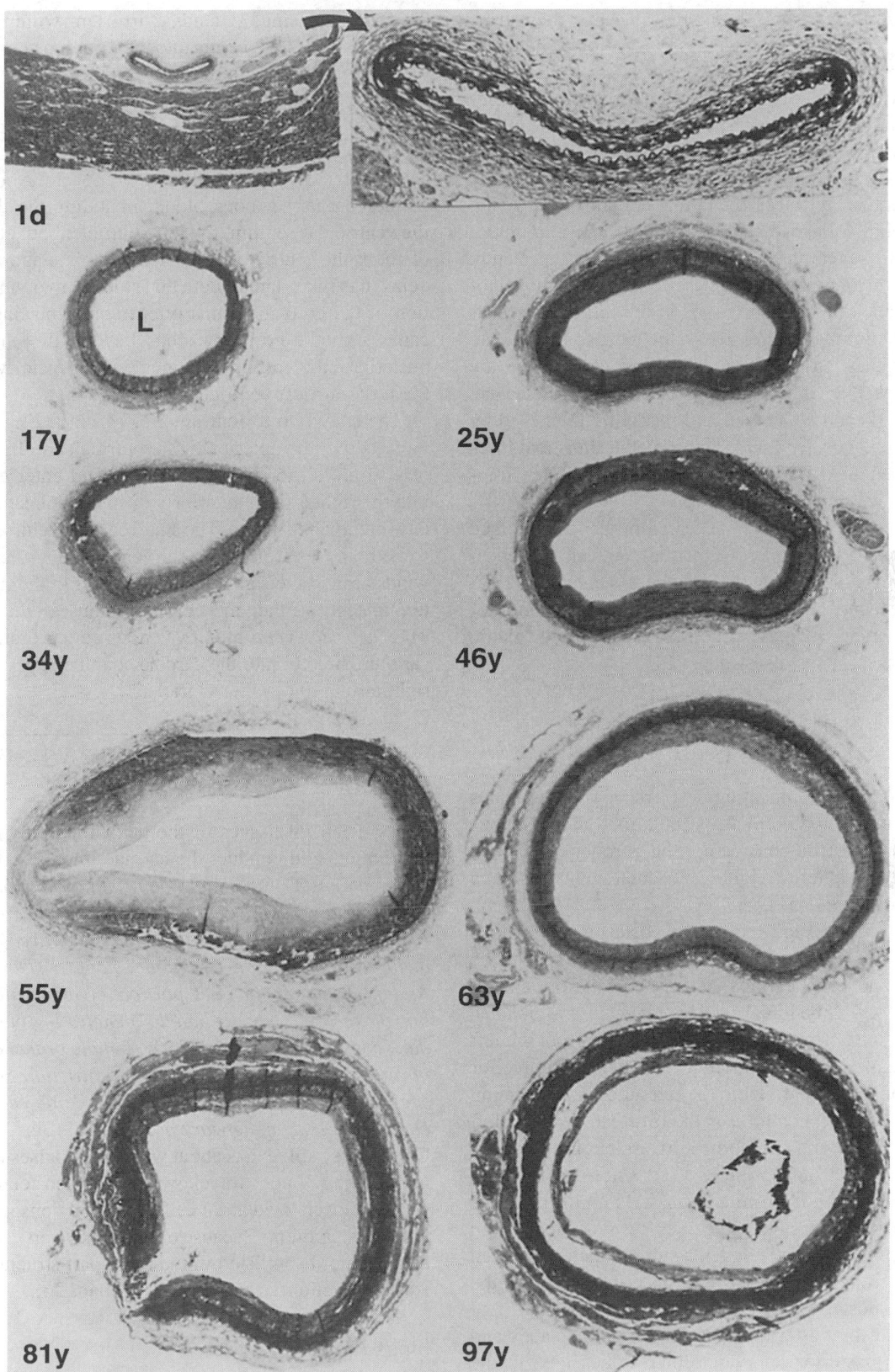

FIGURE 2-60

Photomicrographs of left anterior descending coronary artery from nine patients spanning nine decades of life. All arteries except top right are photographed at same magnification (×10). Top right is higher magnification (×40) of artery in top left. With advancing age, luminal diameter and cross-sectional area increase, intima thickens, and media thins. All arteries are from patients dying of noncardiac disease. D = day; y = year. (From Waller BF. Anatomy, histology, and pathology of the major epicardial coronary arteries relevant to echocardiographic imaging techniques. *J Am Soc Echocardiogr* 1989; 2:232. Reproduced with permission from the publisher and author.)

subendothelium. The medial smooth muscles alter their shape and position, presumably as a result of a reaction to hemodynamic changes after birth.[104] In the next several months, smooth muscles appear between the split internal elastic membrane and form the "musculoelastic layer" between the intima and media. Intimal "cushions" of fibroblasts and elastic fibers occur focally along the intima. The external elastic membrane forms by 6 months. By 1 year, the intima contains a collection of subendothelial collagen and elastic fibers and a musculoelastic layer that eventually is incorporated into the mature media. In normal human coronary arteries, the amount of smooth muscle and fibroelastic tissue in the intima is a function of age. The intima progressively thickens, so that by late adolescence it is as thick as the media; after adolescence, the intima becomes thicker than the media.[105] In middle age, the intima may become diseased and markedly thickened by atherosclerotic plaque. The underlying media thins and loses smooth muscle cells. The internal elastic membrane fragments, duplicates, or disappears focally.

Degenerative changes such as calcium deposition take place in the intima (atherosclerotic plaque), but calcific deposits rarely involve the media (Monckeberg's medial sclerosis).[106] In old age, the coronary arteries become tortuous, the luminal diameter increases, the media thins, and calcific deposits increase[107] (see also Chap. 40).

THE CORONARY VEINS

An extensive intercommunicating network of veins provides venous drainage for the coronary circulation. Three venous drainage systems can be considered: the coronary sinus and its tributaries, the anterior right ventricular veins, and the *Thebesian veins* (Fig. 2-51).[108]

The coronary sinus, located in the posterior AV groove near the crux of the heart, receives venous blood from the great, middle, and small cardiac veins, the posterior veins of the left ventricle, and the left atrial *oblique vein (of Marshall)*. The coronary sinus predominantly drains blood from the left ventricle. The anterior interventricular vein lies in the anterior interventricular sulcus, parallel to the left anterior descending coronary artery. It ascends to near the bifurcation of the left main coronary artery and then turns leftward to circle posteriorly under the left atrium in the left AV sulcus, where it is referred to as the *great cardiac vein*. Along its posterior course, the great cardiac vein receives venous blood from large marginal and posterior left ventricular branches and then becomes the coronary sinus near the posterior margin of the left atrium. The posterior interventricular vein (*middle cardiac vein*) arises near the posterior aspect of the cardiac apex and ascends in the posterior interventricular sulcus next to the posterior descending coronary artery and drains either into the right atrium directly or into the coronary sinus just before it empties into the right atrium. The oblique vein of Marshall runs along the posterior left atrium and joins the great cardiac vein at the point where the latter becomes the coronary sinus.

The coronary sinus extends 2 to 3 cm within the posterior AV groove before it opens into the inferoposteromedial aspect of the right atrium, between the orifice of the inferior vena cava and the septal tricuspid leaflet. A crescent-shaped, rudimentary valve, the *Thebesian valve*, can be seen at its entrance. The total distance from the bifurcation of the left coronary artery to the Thebesian valve is about 9 cm. About 85 percent of the coronary venous blood, including the drainage from the ventricular septum, the left ventricle, both atria, and some of the right ventricle, is carried by this elaborate system of veins. It is important to note that studies involving catheterization of the coronary sinus often require placing the tip of a catheter in the coronary sinus beyond the entrance of the posterior interventricular vein and other major veins draining the posterior left ventricle.

There are two to four anterior cardiac veins that originate in and drain the anterior right ventricular wall, travel superiorly to cross the right AV sulcus, and enter either directly into the right atrium anteriorly or into a collecting vein at the base of the right atrium. The small cardiac vein, which receives some branches from the right ventricle and the right atrium, winds around the right side of the heart in the AV sulcus and terminates in either the coronary sinus or the right atrium. The *Thebesian veins* are tiny venous outlets draining the myocardium directly into the cardiac chambers, primarily into the right atrium and right ventricle.

THE CONDUCTION SYSTEM OF THE HEART

The specialized tissues of the heart (neuromyocardial cells) that initiate and conduct the cardiac impulse consist of three major parts: (1) the *sinus node (sinuatrial node, sinoatrial node, SA node, sinoauricular node, pacemaker, node of Keith-Flack)*; (2) the *atrioventricular junctional area*, including the *atrioventricular node (AV node, node of Tawara, node of Aschoff-Tawara, compact portion of atrioventricular junctional area)* and the *His bundle (penetrating bundle, AV bundle, common bundle)*; and (3) the *bundle branches (branching portion of AV bundle, bifurcation, ventricular conduction tissue)* and *terminal Purkinje fibers (Purkinje cells, peripheral conduction system, network of Purkinje)* (Figs. 2-61 to 2-76). Controversy still exists about whether impulses from the sinus node to the AV node travel over specialized conducting "pathways" ("specialized atrial cells") or over nonspecialized plain atrial myocardium. Because of this controversy, the internodal area has not been listed in the three-part structure of specialized conduction tissues (see also Chap. 26).

Sinus Node

The sinus node, first reported by Keith and Flack in 1907,[109–111] is an oval-shaped, elongated mass (spindle-shaped) measuring about 10 to 20 mm long and up to 5 mm thick. The "head" of the node extends toward the interatrial groove, while its "tail" extends toward the orifice of the

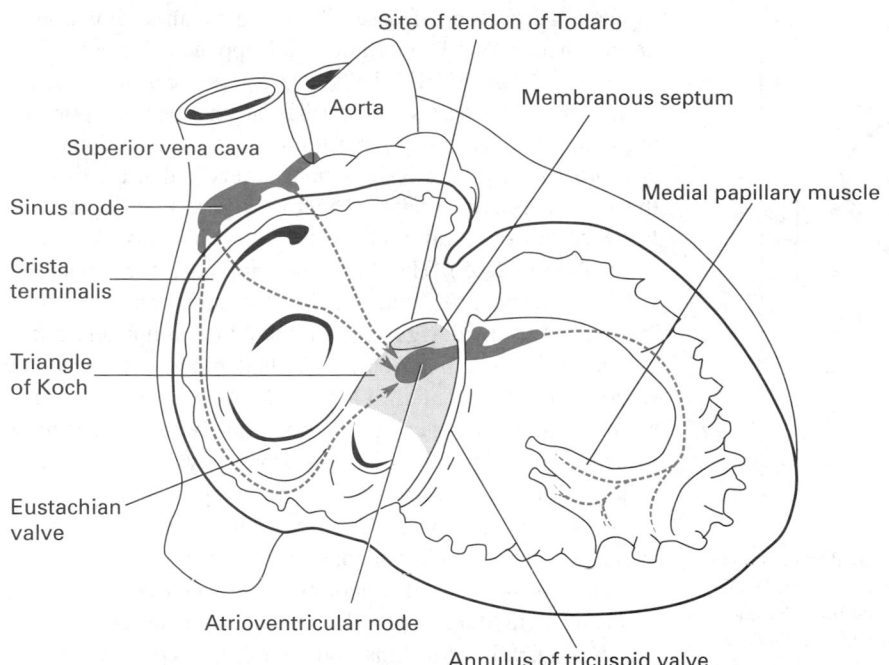

FIGURE 2-61
Diagram showing the anatomic landmarks of the cardiac conduction system.

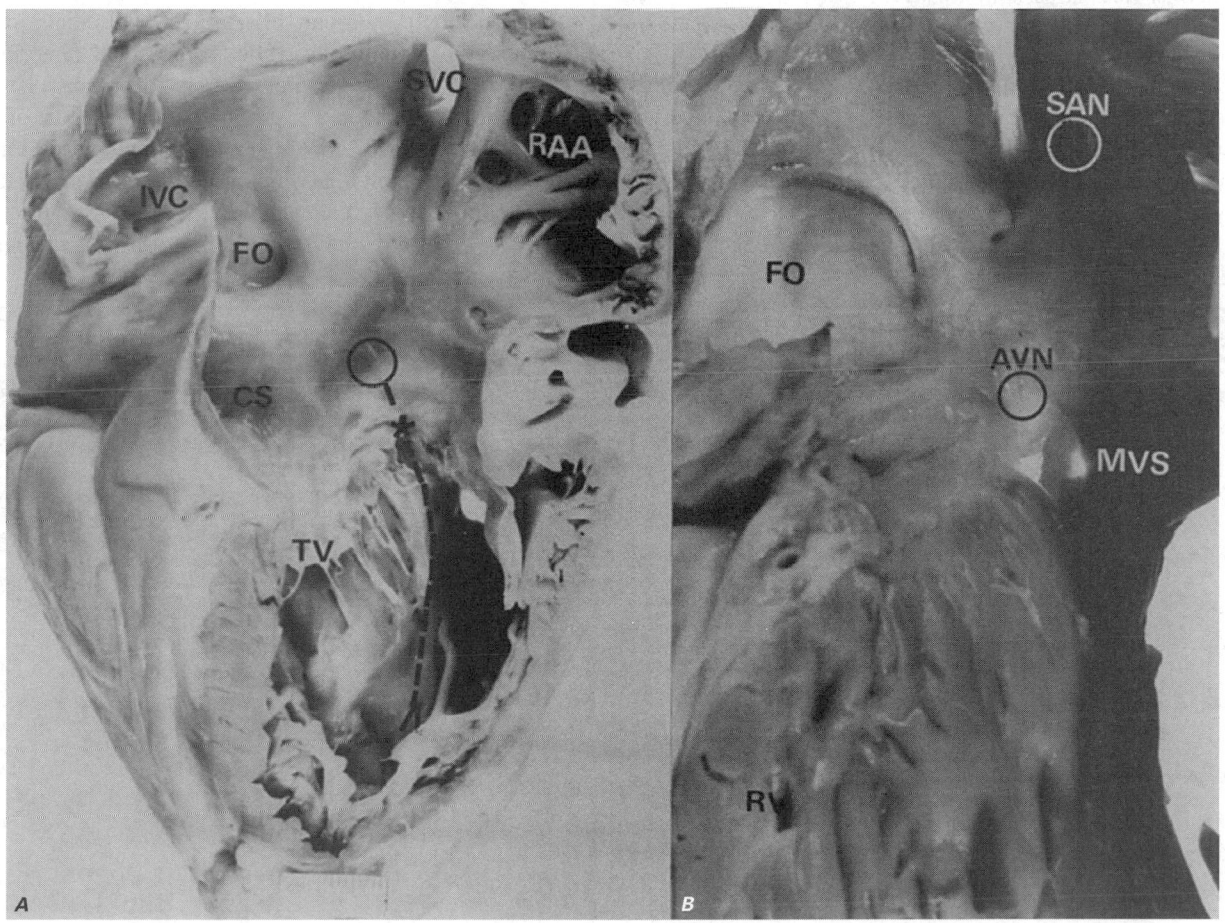

FIGURE 2-62
Photographs of heart showing anatomic landmarks of the cardiac conduction system. *A.* Tomographic cut of the right side of the heart showing the location of the atrioventricular node (circle) and right bundle branch (* – – –). CS = coronary sinus; FO = fossa ovale; IVC = inferior vena cava; RAA = right atrial appendage; SVC = superior vena cava; TV = tricuspid valve. *B.* Close-up of annulus of tricuspid valve showing approximate location of sinoatrial node (SAN) and atrioventricular node (AVN, circle). MVS = membranous ventricular septum; RV = right ventricle.

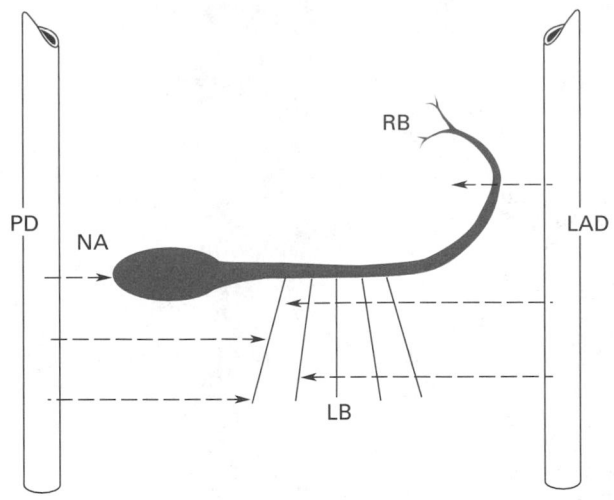

FIGURE 2-63

Diagram showing arterial blood supply of the cardiac conduction system. The nodal artery (NA) arises from the posterior descending artery (PD). The bulk of the arterial blood supply to right and left bundle branches comes from the left anterior descending artery (LAD). (From Davies MJ. *Pathology of Conducting Tissue of the Heart.* London: Butterworth; 1979. Reproduced with permission from the publisher and author.)

inferior vena cava (Figs. 2-61 and 2-62). In most hearts its location is in the subepicardial region (less than 1 mm from the epicardial surface) at the lateral junction of the superior vena cava and right atrium (Fig. 2-62A and B). In a serial reconstruction analysis by Anderson et al.,[112] the human sinus node was most commonly found in the lateral location, but

in about 10 percent of cases it was found in a "horseshoe" arrangement around the right atrial appendage crest as described by Blair and Davies.[113] The superficial layer of the node is surrounded by subepicardial fat, and the inner portions anastomose with atrial myocardium. Supplying the sinus node is a prominent artery ("sinus node artery") that arises from the right coronary artery in 55 to 60 percent of cases and from the left circumflex coronary artery in 40 to 45 percent (Figs. 2-63 to 2-65). The artery may approach the sinus node from a clockwise or counterclockwise direction around the superior vena caval–right atrial junction or completely encircle the atriocaval junction.[114] A dual blood supply to the sinus node is present in 11 percent of individuals.[115] The relationship of the artery to the node has been thought to be fairly constant, provoking concepts of a physiologic relationship between arterial pulsation, arterial diameter, and sinus node discharge rate in a feedback control system ("servomechanism").[116] On the other hand, variation in arterial disposition suggests an inconsistent relationship between the artery and node and casts doubt upon the servomechanism concept.[112]

Histologically, the sinus node is easily recognized at low magnifications (Figs. 2-66 to 2-68). Specific cell types in the sinus node include nodal cells, transitional cells, and atrial muscle cells. Nodal cells (P cells) are small (3 to 10 μm), ovoid, pale-staining, and poorly striated compared with the general myocardial cells.[117] Although the nuclei are of normal size, the nodal cells contain fewer mitochondria compared with contractile cells. The nodal cells are grouped together in interconnecting fascicles placed in a background of fibrous matrix.[118] The interweaving fascicles of nodal cells surround

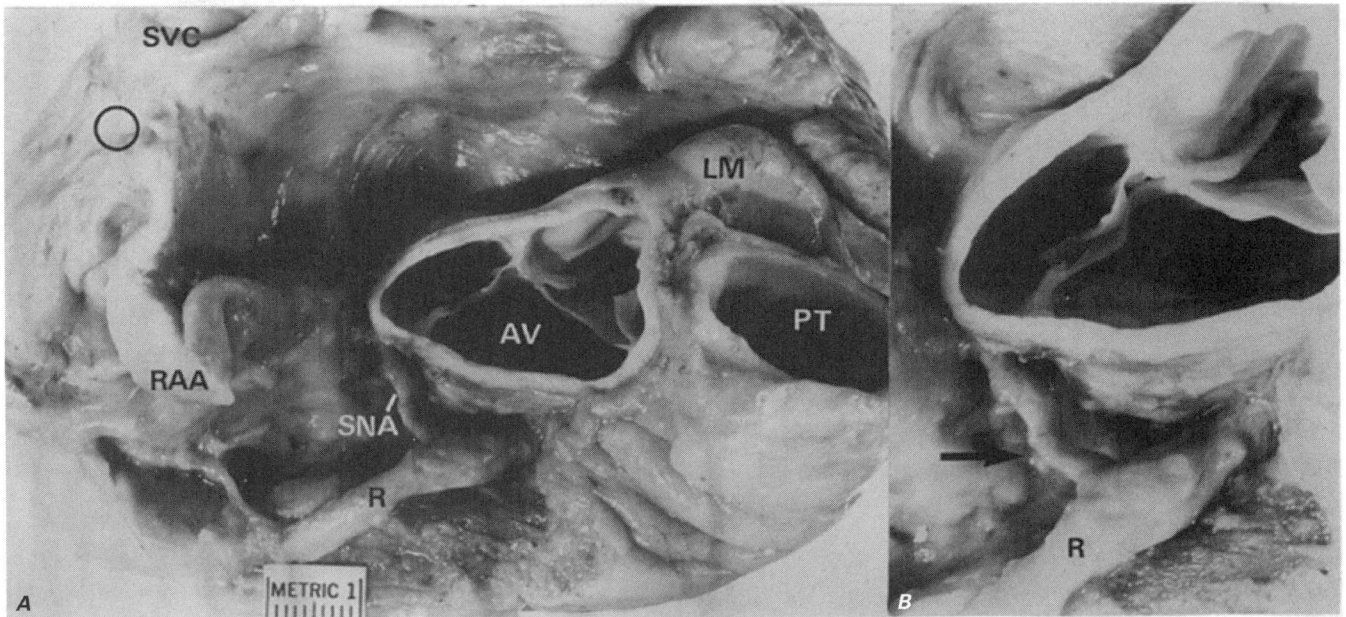

FIGURE 2-64

Photographs of heart showing origin of the sinus nodal artery (SNA). *A.* Sinus nodal artery arising as early branch of the right (R) coronary artery. Dark circle indicates approximate location of the sinus node (SN). PT =

pulmonary trunk, RAA = right atrial appendage, SVC = superior vena cava. *B.* Close-up of right coronary artery.

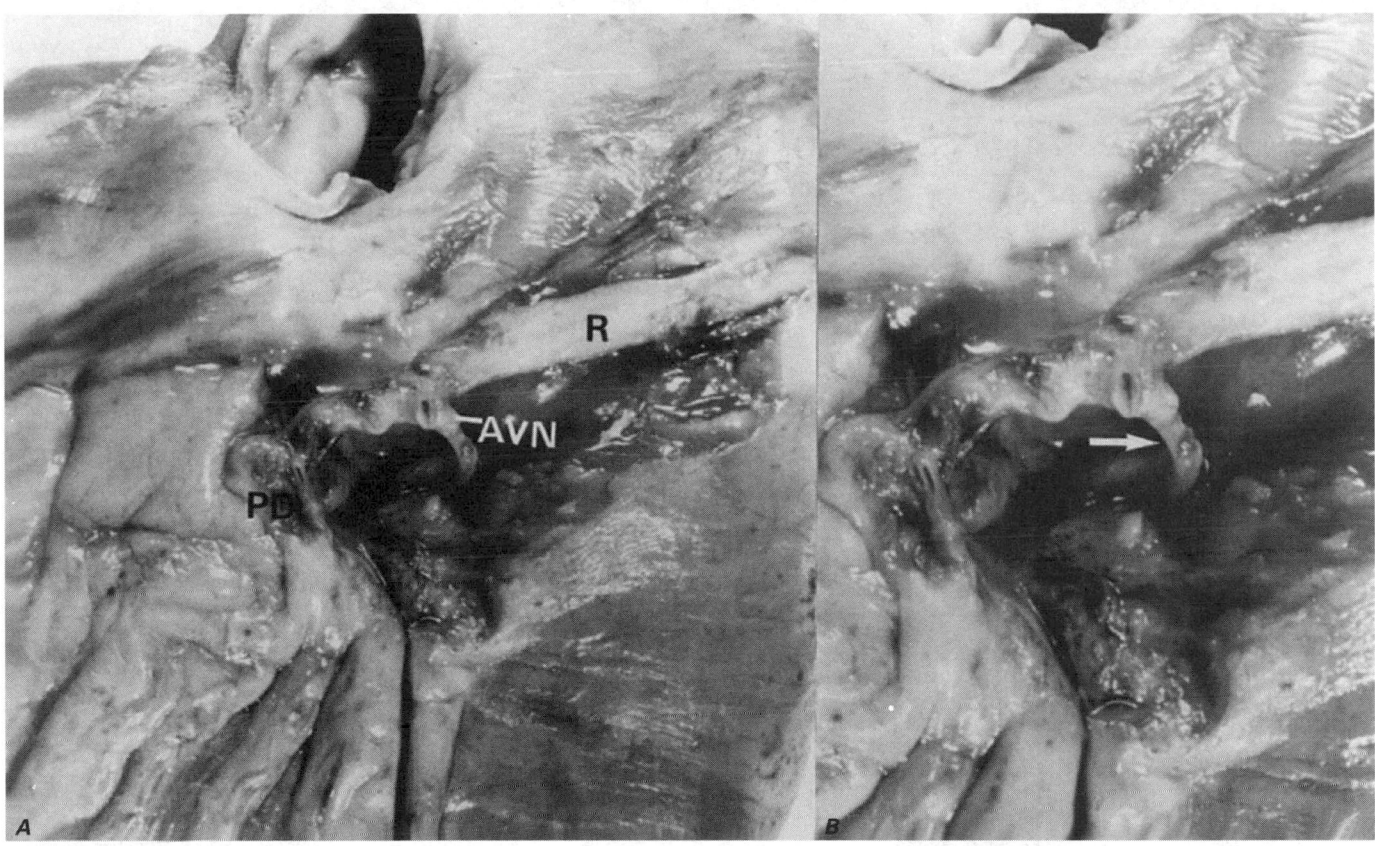

FIGURE 2-65

Photographs of posterior surface of the heart at the crux showing the origin of the atrioventricular nodal (AVN) artery from the right (R) coronary artery.

A. The AVN artery arises near the origin of the posterior descending (PD) coronary artery. *B.* Close-up of origin of AVN artery (*arrow*).

the sinus nodal artery (body of node). Although contact between nodal cells was thought to occur by opposing cell membranes (a factor possibly correlating with the slow conduction within the sinus node), more recent studies suggest the presence and role of nexus connections.[119,120] Nodal cells are thought to be the source of normal impulse formation in the sinus node.[121–123] Transitional cells (T cells) are elongated cells with characteristics intermediate between the packed nodal cells and the individual atrial myocardial cells.[118] The T cells are located at the margins of the node, where the nodal cells become contiguous with atrial myocardium. T cells near nodal cells have simple intercellular connections, while more fully developed intercalated disks exist in T cells near atrial myocardium.[92] In some areas, discrete fibrous septae form junctions that separate the node from atrial myocardium; in other areas, projections of transitional cells ("tongues") extend for short distances into the working atrial myocardium[118] (Fig. 2-67). Since nodal cells make contact with each other or with T cells, the T cells may provide a "functional pathway" for distribution of the sinus impulses formed in the nodal cells to the rest of the atrial myocardium.[123] The third type of cell present in the sinus node is the working atrial myocardial cell. These cells also extend as projections or tongues into the nodal boundaries. James[123] has described large, clear ("Purkinje") cells at the margins of the sinus node, whereas Becker and colleagues[124] have not found these cells in infant hearts.

There are marked differences between the histology of the sinus node in an infant and that in an adult.[98] In the infant sinus node, the nodal cells predominate relative to the fibrous matrix. In contrast, in the adult sinus node, the fibrous tissue is predominant, with the nodal cells scattered within the connective tissue.[98] Part of the increase in fibrosis is likely to be related to an imbalance between proliferating fibrous tissue and more static nodal cells.[118] Surrounding fat also increases with advancing age.[125]

Internal Atrial Myocardium

As noted, the method of travel of the sinus impulse to the AV node remains controversial.[111,126–136] Investigators agree that the electrophysiologic properties of a certain population of atrial cells differ from those of other atrial cells. The controversy revolves around whether or not the population of atrial cells with "specialized" action potentials is involved in the orderly transmission of the sinus impulse within the atrium and whether or not these "specialized" cells can be distinguished

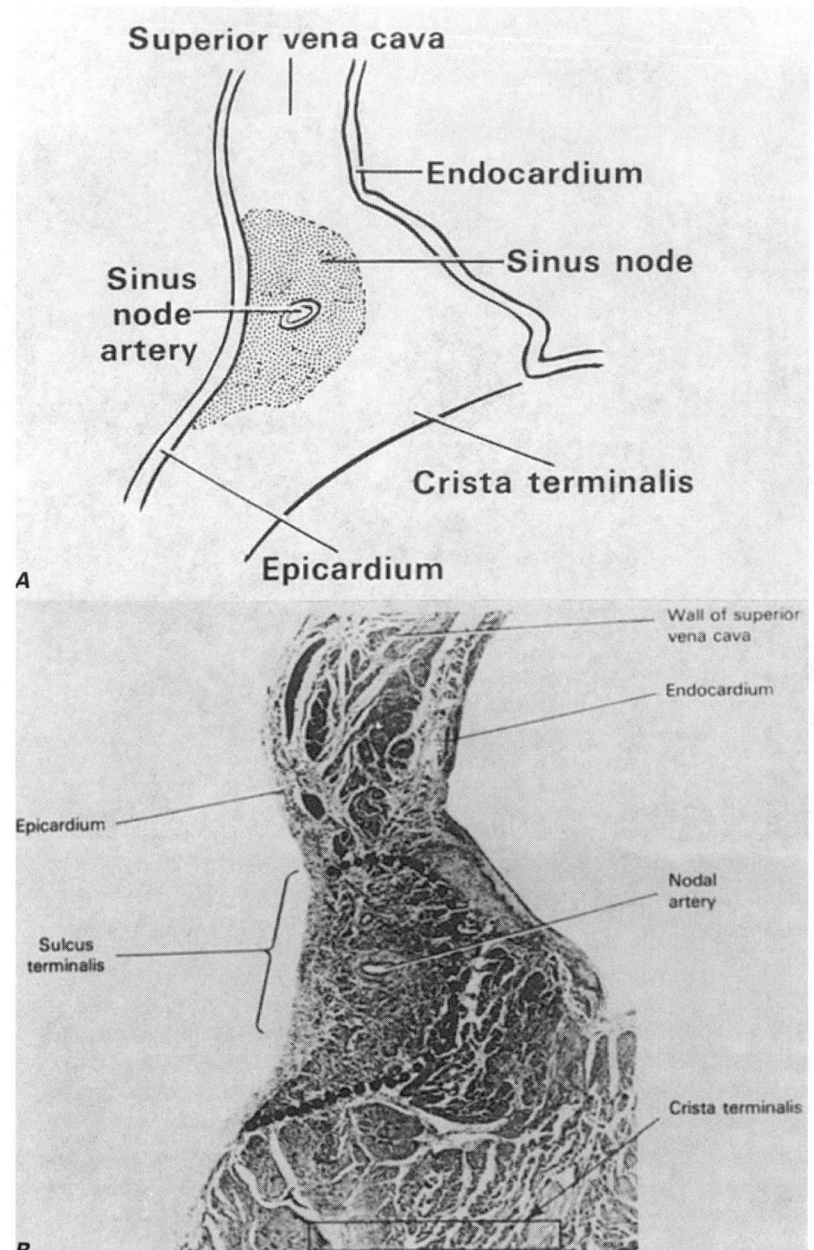

FIGURE 2-66

Diagram (*A*) and photomicrograph (*B*) of sinus node. (*B.* from Davies MJ, et al. *The Conduction System of the Heart.* London: Butterworth; 1983. Reproduced with permission from the publisher and authors.)

histologically from "working" atrial myocardium.[91] James[131] and James and Sherf[137] have reviewed the original studies of Bachman,[138] Wenckebach,[139] and Thorel[126] and have supported the concept of three specific internodal tracts between sinus and atrioventricular nodes: anterior internodal tract (*Bachmann-James'*), middle internodal tract (*Wenckebach's*), and posterior internodal tract (*Thorel's*). All three tracts anastomose with each other above the AV node. In these bundles are transitional cells and common atrial myocardial cells. Purkinje cells have been reported near the proximal and distal course of these fascicles,[140] whereas in the middle course, common atrial myocardial cells are prevalent, making it difficult and uncertain to follow the fascicles anatomically. In contrast to the concept of specialized atrial "tracts," Janse and

Anderson[136] favor the preferential transmission of the sinus node impulse by the shortest routes between the nodes over the thickest bundles of working atrial myocardium. These investigators also question the presence of Purkinje-like cells in the internodal atrial myocardium. Thus, the issue of atrial conduction pathways (or tracts) has not been settled,[141] but presently the evidence does not strongly support the presence of specialized internodal tracts resembling the discrete histologically identifiable bundle branches in the ventricles.[142] Preferential internodal conduction in some parts of the atrium compared to other parts probably does exist and may be due to atrial myocardial fiber orientation, size, geometry, or other factors rather than specialized tracts located between the nodes.[112,118,119]

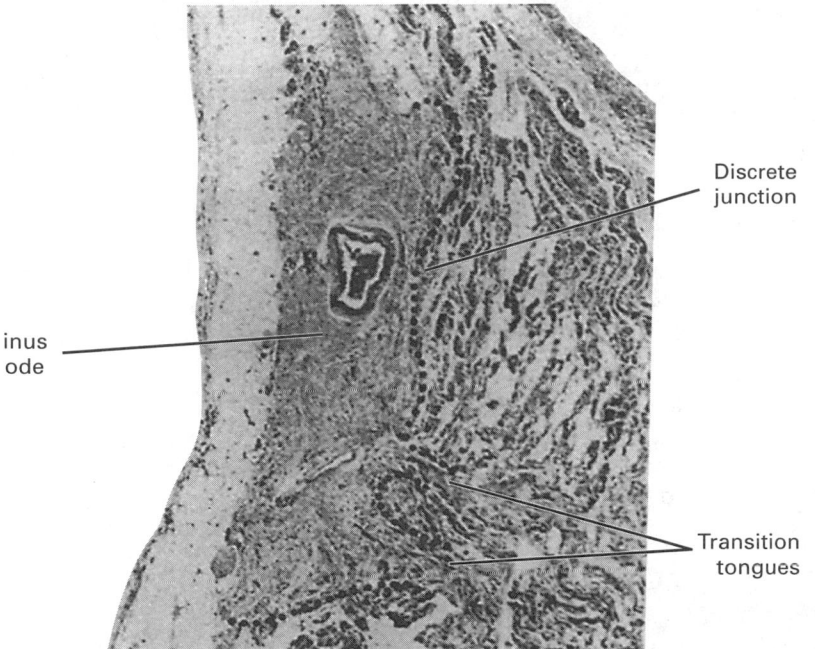

inus
ode

Discrete
junction

Transition
tongues

FIGURE 2-67
Photomicrographs of section of sinus node showing junction
of sinus node and atrial myocardium and area of transitional
cells. (From Davies MJ, et al. *The Conduction System of
the Heart.* London: Butterworth; 1983. Reproduced with
permission from the publisher and authors.)

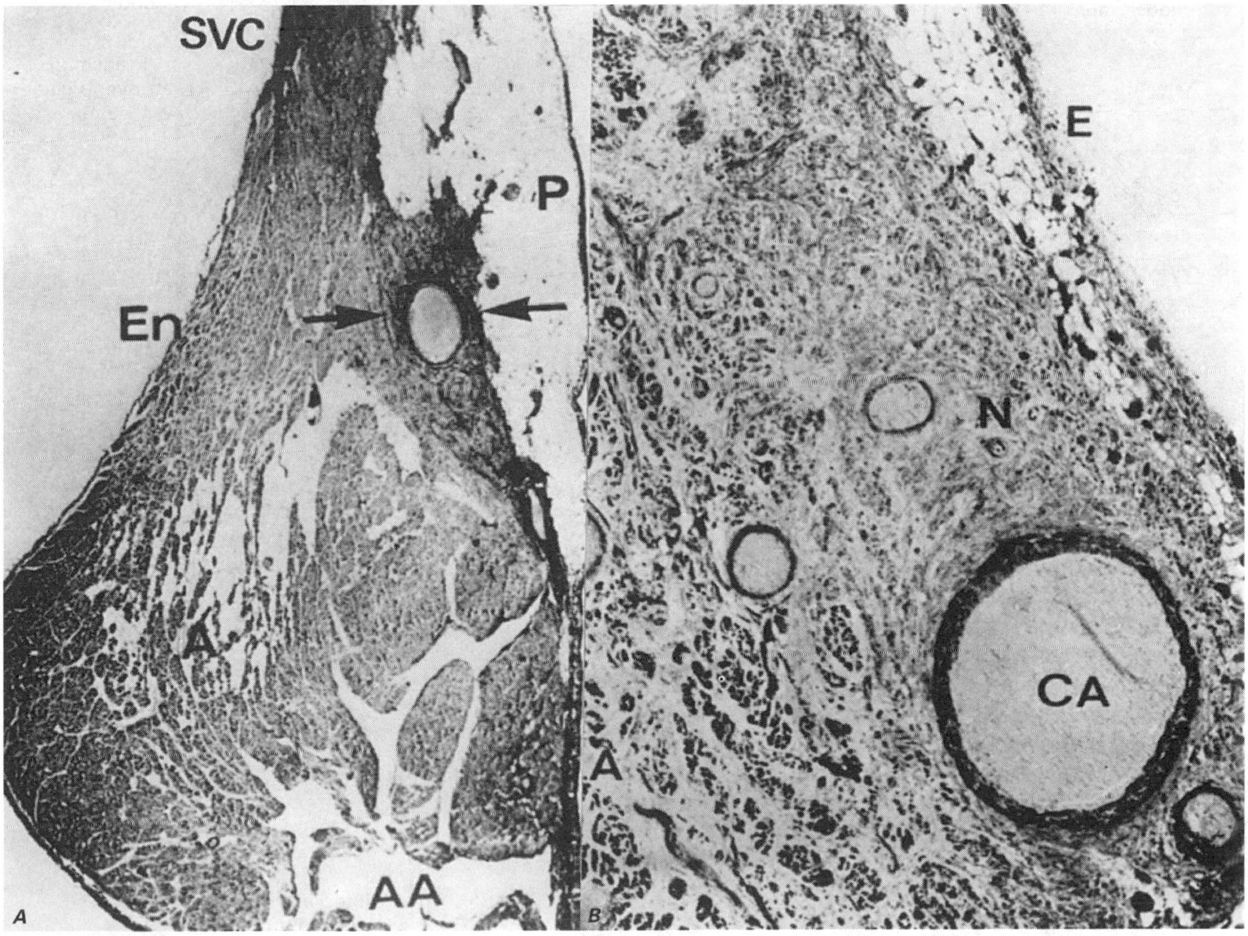

SVC

P

E

En

N

CA

A

A

AA

A

B

FIGURE 2-68
Photomicrographs of the sinus node. *A.* Sinus node (*arrows*) is identified by
a central artery located just beneath the epicardial surface. A = right atrium;
AA = atrial appendage; En = endocardium; SVC = superior vena cava.
B. Close-up of sinus node (N) showing a matrix of collagen and muscle
fibers. A = atrium; CA = central artery; E = endocardium. (From Davies
MJ. *Pathology of Conducting Tissue of the Heart.* London: Butterworth;
1979. Reproduced with permission from the publisher and author.)

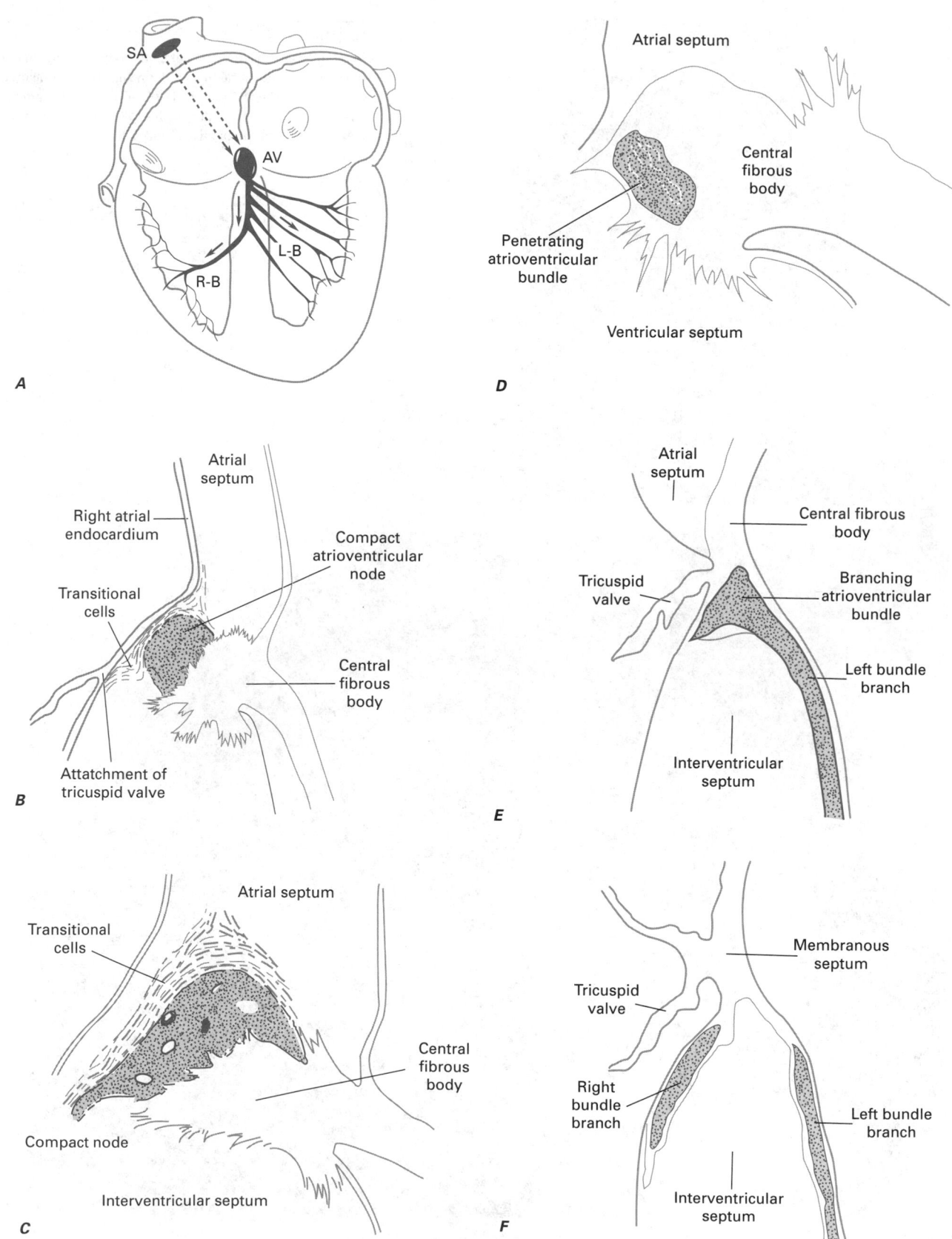

FIGURE 2-69

Diagrammatic composite showing the anatomy of the atrioventricular junctional area from the proximal area of atrioventricular node (*B* and *C*) to the penetrating bundle (*D*), branching atrioventricular bundle (*E*), to the distal area of the right (R) and left (L) bundle (B) branches (*F*). AV = atrioventricular node; SA = sinus node.

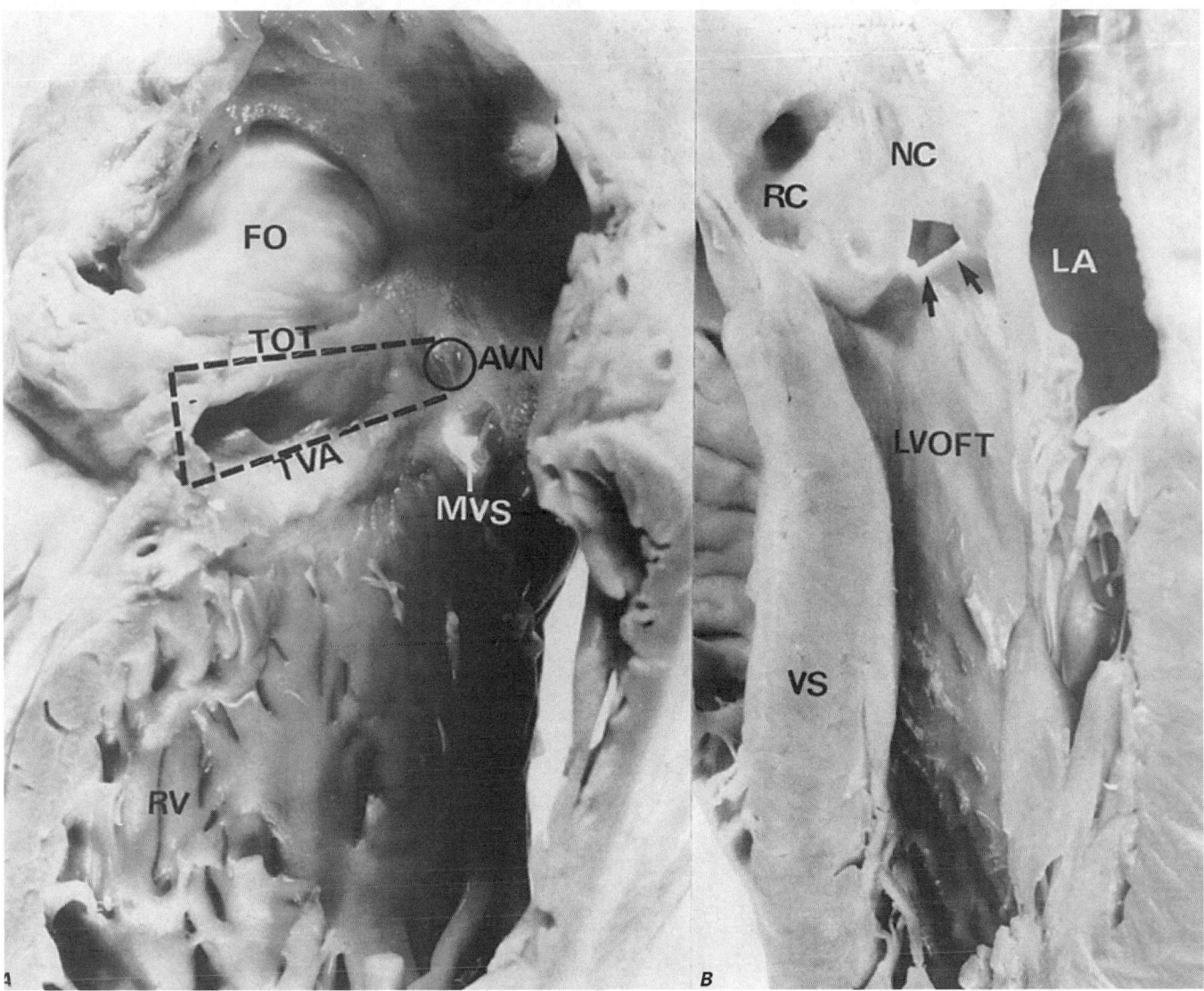

FIGURE 2-70

Photomicrographs of the heart showing anatomic landmarks of the atrioventricular node (AVN). *A.* Triangle of Koch (*dashed lines*) showing location of AVN. The membranous ventricular septum (MVS) has been excised. CS = coronary sinus; FO = fossa ovale; RV = right ventricle; TOT = tendon of Todaro; TVA = tricuspid valve annulus. *B.* View of left ventricular outflow tract (LVOFT) showing location of excised MVS (*arrows*) beneath the noncoronary (NC) cusp of aortic valve. LA = left atrium; RC = right coronary cusp; VS = ventricular septum.

Interatrial Conduction

Bachmann's bundle appears to conduct the cardiac impulse preferentially from the right to the left atrium. This large muscle bundle (see earlier) begins along the anterior margin of the sinus node and travels posteriorly around the aorta to the left atrium. James[123] indicates that the middle and posterior internodal tracts may also extend fibers from the right atrium to the left atrium.

Atrioventricular Junctional Area

The normal AV junctional area can be divided into three distinct regions: *transitional cell zone*[143] ("*nodal approaches*"[144]), *atrioventricular node* (*compact portion, Taw-* *ara's node*[145]), and *penetrating portion of the AV bundle* (*His bundle, common bundle*) (Figs. 2-61 to 2-63). Some authors[118] include the *branching AV bundle* (*bundle branches*) as the fourth region.

Transitional-Cell Zone (Nodal Approaches)

The connections by which the myocardium of the right atrium anastomoses with the AV node can be regarded as a "transitional" area between working and specialized cardiac muscle or as an "outer layer" of the AV node (Figs. 2-69 and 2-70). This outer zone concept was originally described by Tawara[143] in 1906 and recently reemphasized by Anderson and colleagues.[145] Rossi[146] indicates that the transitional zone

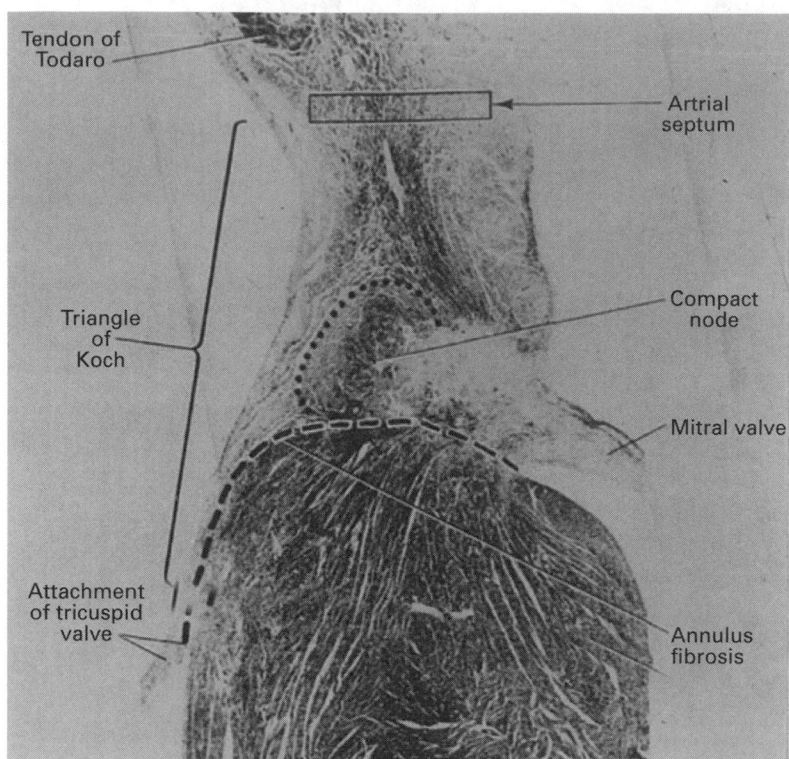

FIGURE 2-71

Photomicrograph showing the boundaries of the triangle of Koch and location of the atrioventricular node (compact node). (From Davies MJ, et al. *The Conduction System of the Heart.* London: Butterworth; 1983. Reproduced with permission from the publisher and authors.)

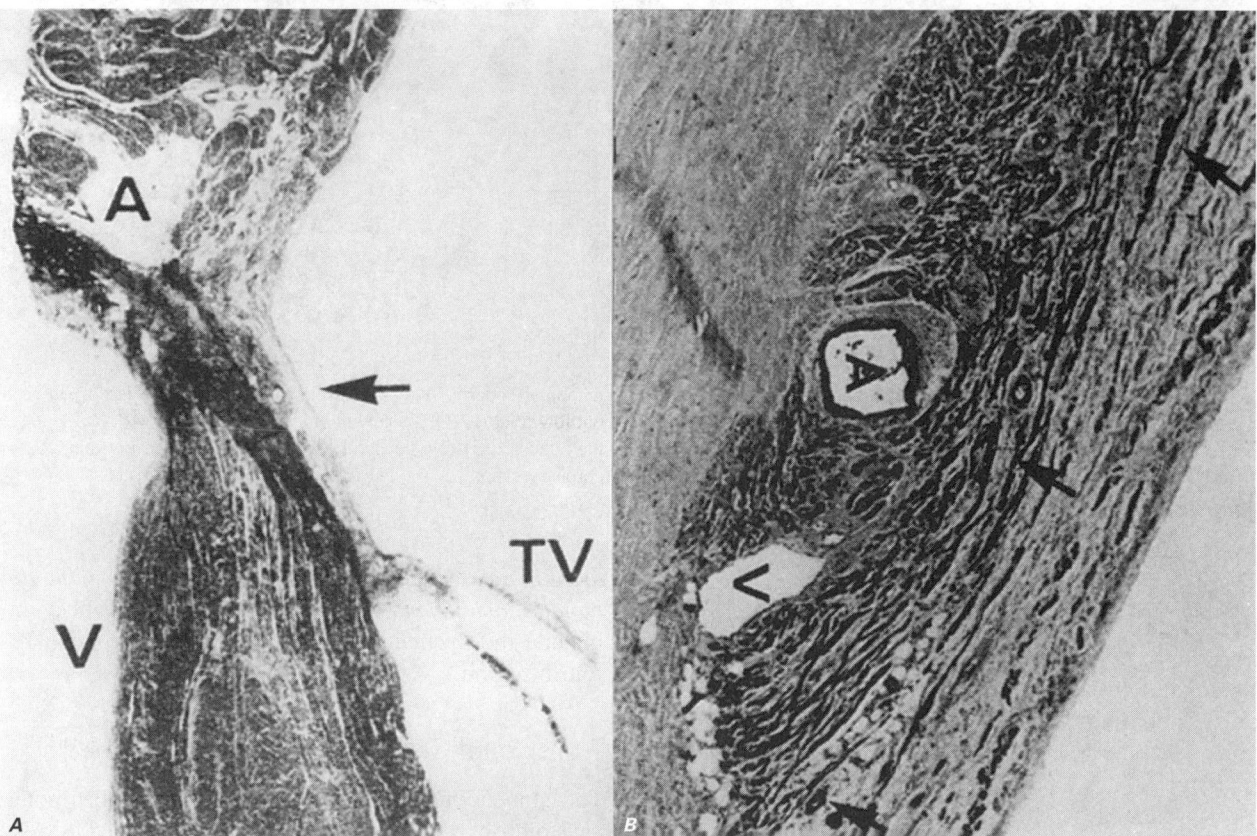

FIGURE 2-72

Photomicrographs of normal atrioventricular node (AVN). *A.* The AVN (*arrow*) is adjacent to the central fibrous body (CFB) and lies beneath the right atrial endocardium just above the insertion of the tricuspid valve (TV). V = left ventricle. *B.* Close-up of AVN (*arrows*) showing artery (A) and vein (V). (From Davies MJ. *Pathology of Conducting Tissue of the Heart.* London: Butterworth; 1979. Reproduced with permission from the publisher and author.)

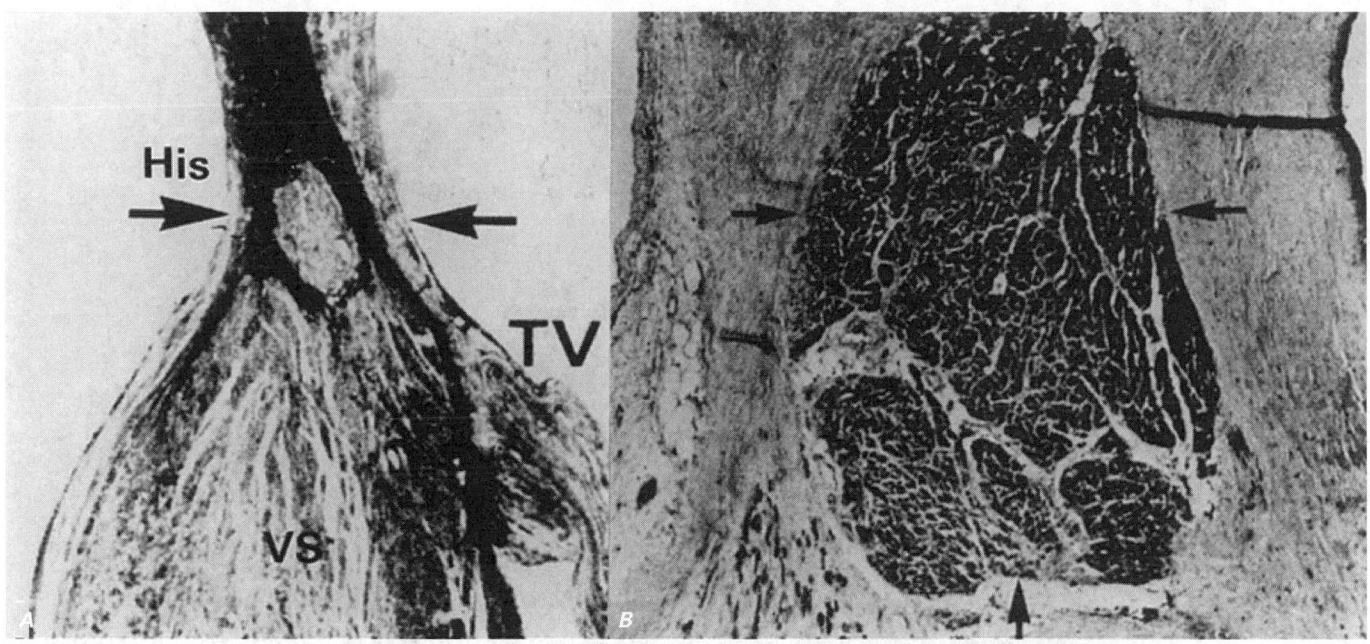

FIGURE 2-73

Photomicrographs of normal main bundle of His. *A.* Emerging from the central fibrous body is the main bundle of His (*arrow*). TV = tricuspid valve; VS = ventricular septum. *B.* Close-up of normal main bundle of His.

(From Davies MJ. *Pathology of Conducting Tissue of the Heart.* London: Butterworth; 1979. Reproduced with permission from the publisher and author.)

is not a definite layer external to the compact AV node but is made up of thin separate fascicles. These junctional bundles have been subdivided into three main groups: anterior (superior), middle, and posterior (inferior).[131,147] James[110] described some fibers passing from the posterior internodal tract to the distal portion of the AV node (His bundle), which may provide an anatomic substrate for a bypass tract. Other

investigators have been unable to confirm these findings, and the functional significance of these fibers has not been demonstrated.

Atrioventricular Node

The compact portion of the AV junction (AV node) seems to occupy a position in the middle of the heart but actually

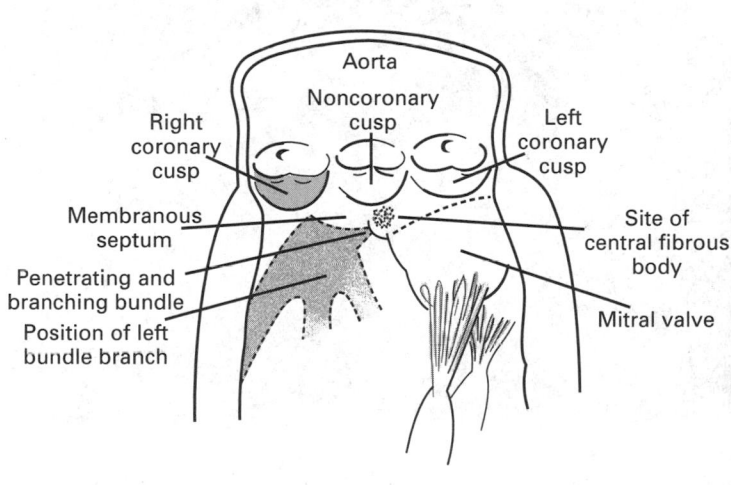

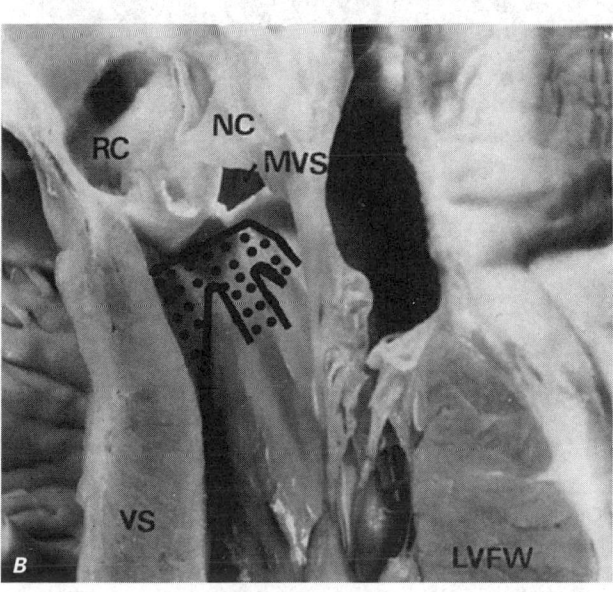

FIGURE 2-74

Anatomy of the left side of the heart showing landmarks of the conduction system. *A.* Diagram of conduction system. *B.* Photograph of heart showing excised membranous ventricular septum and location of left bundle branch.

NC = noncoronary cusp; RC = right cusp of aortic valve; LVFW = left ventricular free wall; VS = ventricular septum.

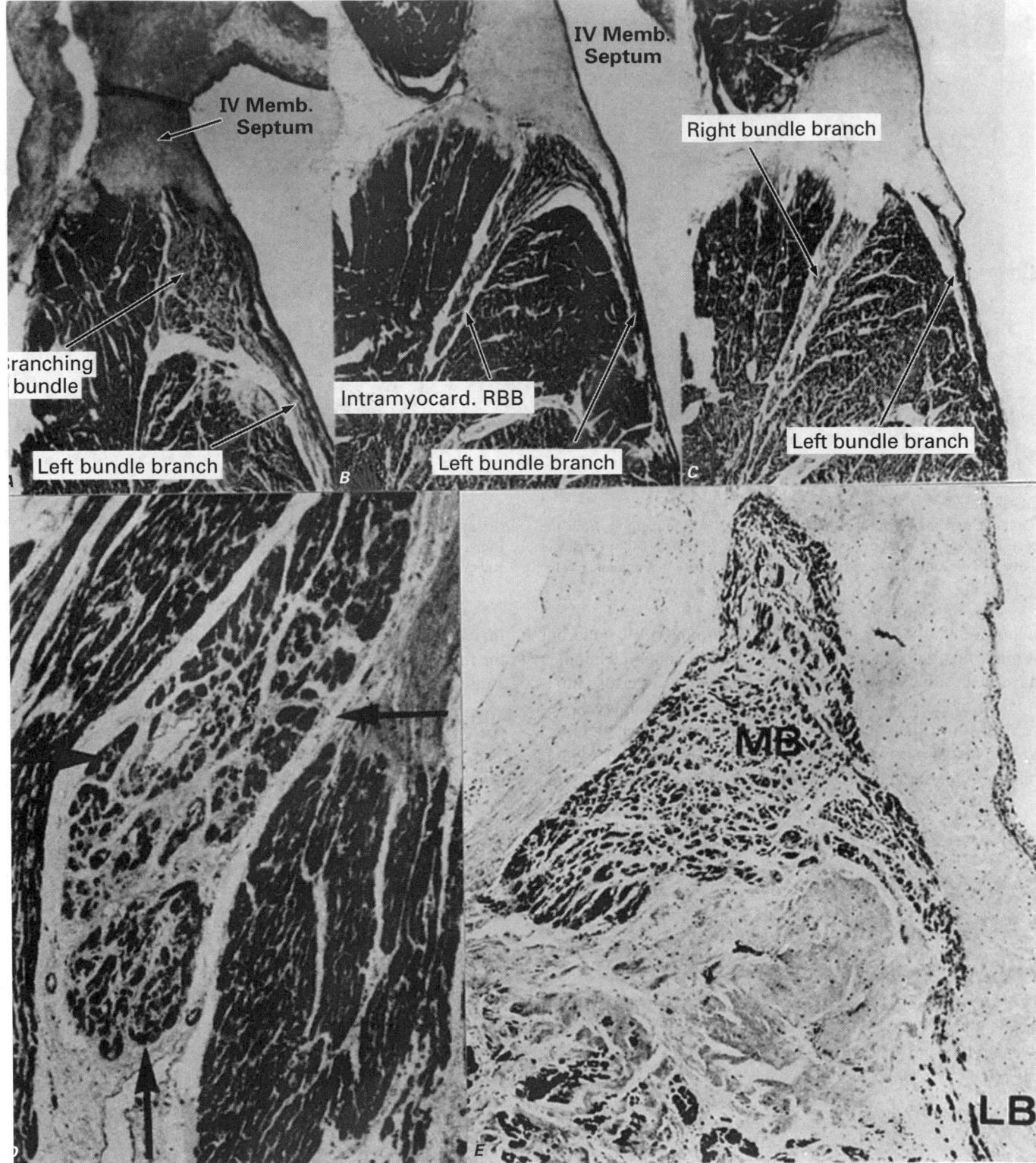

FIGURE 2-75

Photomicrographs of normal branching atrioventricular bundle and right (R) and left (L) bundle branches (BB). *A* through *C.* Series showing origin of branching bundle. *D* through *E.* Close-ups showing origin of left bundle (LB) from main bundle (MB). (*A* through *C.* From Davies MJ, et al. *The Conduction System of the Heart.* London: Butterworth; 1983. *D* and *E.* From Davies MJ. *Pathology of Conducting Tissue of the Heart.* London: Butterworth; 1979. Reproduced with permission from the publisher and authors.)

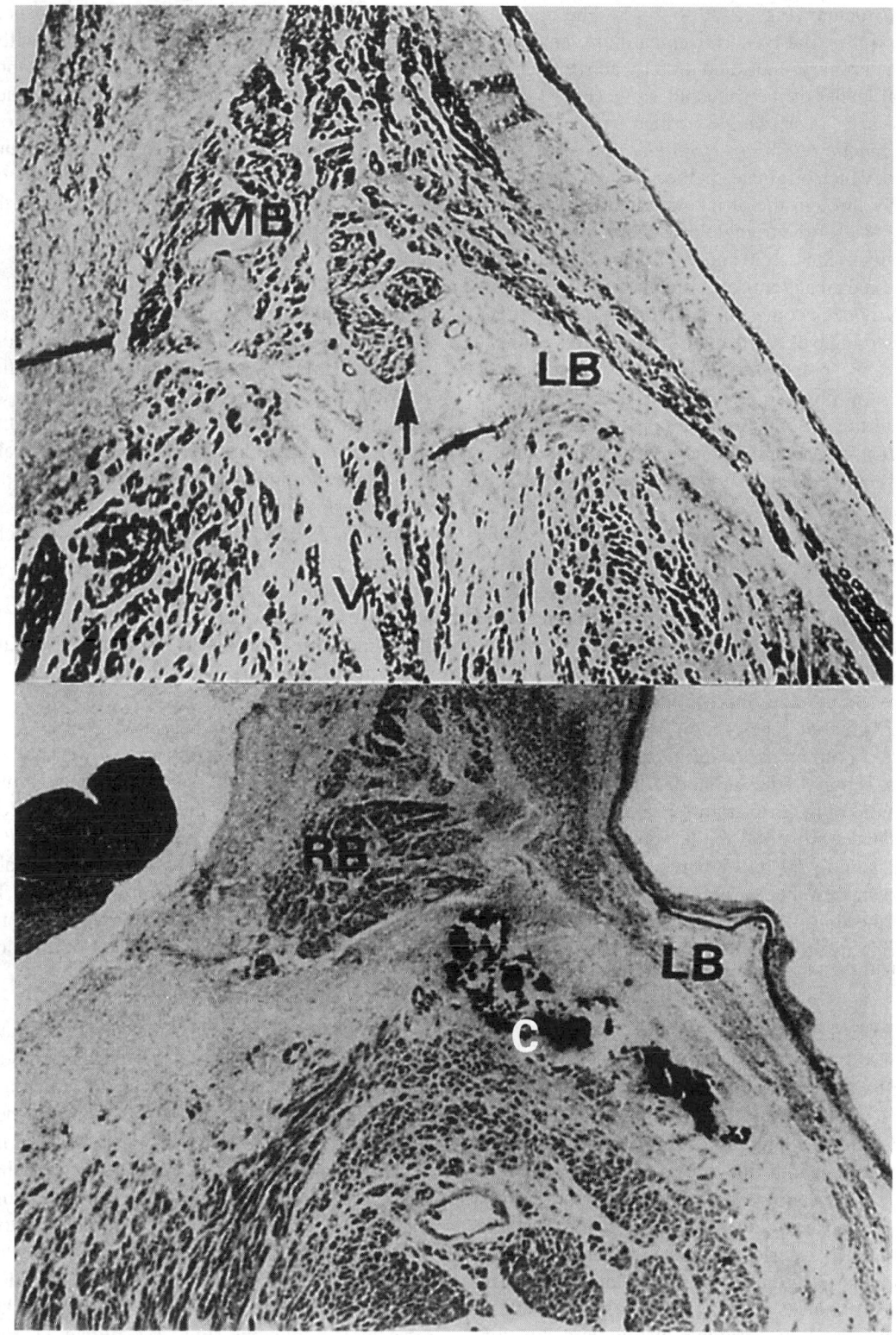

FIGURE 2-76

Variants of normal main bundle and branching bundles. *Top:* Close-up of main bundle (MB) and origin of left bundle (LB). A muscle strand (*arrow*) leaves the main bundle to enter the upper ventricular septum (V) bypassing the bundle branches. *Bottom:* Normal origin of left bundle (LB) showing calcium (C) as aging change in the crest of ventricular septum. RB = right bundle. (From Davies MJ. *Pathology of Conducting Tissue of the Heart.* London: Butterworth; 1979. Reproduced with permission from the publisher and author.)

is an epicardial structure (Figs. 2-70 to 2-72). The node lies just beneath the right atrial posterior epicardium, anterior to the ostium of the coronary sinus, and directly above the insertion of the septal leaflet of the tricuspid valve (Fig. 2-72). It is located at the apex of a triangle formed by the tricuspid annulus and the *tendon of Todaro* (*triangle of Koch*).[128] The tendon of Todaro, which originates in the central fibrous body, passes posteriorly through the atrial septum with the eustachian valve. The base of the triangle of Koch[128] is the ostium of the coronary sinus (Figs. 2-70 and 2-71). The atrial component of the junctional area is entirely contained in this triangle. The compact AV node becomes the penetrating bundle of His at the apex of the triangle of Koch and passes into the ventricular tissues below the point of attachment of the tendon of Todaro to the central fibrous body. Within the ventricles, the gross landmark of the AV junctional area is the membranous septum (Fig. 2-70). The branching and nonbranching bundles are located between the membranous and the muscular ventricular septum.

In the adult human, the AV node is a compact ovoid structure measuring about 1 by 3 by 5 mm. Histologically, the AV node is composed of a thick mesh of tiny pale cells, which anastomose with one another by short pluridirectional projections of their cytoplasm ("star cells").[126] These cells are interwoven with collagen and elastic fibers. At the electron microscopic level, James and Sherf[137] examined two human hearts and described four types of AV nodal cells: P cells, transitional cells, common myocardial cells, and Purkinje cells. The arterial supply to the AV node ("AV nodal artery") is a branch from the right coronary artery in 85 to 90 percent of human hearts and a branch of the left circumflex coronary artery in the remaining 10 to 15 percent[8] (Figs. 2-63 and 2-65). The innervation of the AV junction, though less prominent than that of the sinus node, is richly supplied by adrenergic and cholinergic fibers, with regional differences relevant to function.[128,149]

THE BUNDLE OF HIS (PENETRATING PORTION OF THE AV BUNDLE)

The penetrating bundle (*His bundle*) is a continuation of the distal part of the AV node without any definite histocytological boundary (Fig. 2-73). The bundle of His is a cordal structure measuring 20 mm in length and up to 2 mm in diameter. Conventionally, the beginning of the common bundle is at a point where the specialized myocardial cells lose their network arrangement and form parallel strands just before entering into the membranous septum.[126] These changes are quite variable, but the differences in structure may be quite abrupt and distinct enough to allow a reliable histologic distinction. Proximal cells of the penetrating portion are heterogeneous, resembling those of the compact node, whereas the distal cells of the common bundle are similar to cells in the proximal bundle branches. In general, the Hisian fibers have larger diameters and more parallel arrangement compared to the nodal structures.

The course of the common bundle has been subdivided

anatomically into three portions: (1) nonpenetrating (proximal, distal to AV node), (2) penetrating (within the fibrous tissue of the central body and membranous septum, "tunneled segment"), and (3) branching (bifurcation at the crest of muscular ventricular septum).[126] The names "proximal," "middle," and "distal" tract of the AV common bundle have also been applied to these subdivisions. "Upper connections"[126] sometimes connect the common bundle with the crest of the ventricular septum (Fig. 2-76). These fibers were first described by Mahaim[150] in 1927 and are termed either *Mahaim fibers* or *paraspecific fibers*. These "bypass" fibers can be separated into "nodoventricular" and "fasciculoventricular" fibers and have been implicated as a substrate for preexcitation in adult hearts. These fibers may connect the node to the ventricular septum or connect various portions of the penetrating bundle to the septal crest. The presence of these fibers as islands of conduction tissue within the central fibrous body has also been implicated in sudden infant death syndrome[151] and as a possible cause for circus-rhythm circuits[152] (see Chap. 26). Arterial branches from both the left anterior and posterior descending coronary arteries supply the upper muscular ventricular septum, making this portion of the conduction system less subject to ischemic damage.[121] Nerve trunks are found along blood vessels, and small strands of beaded nerve fibers lie inside and near the bundle.[151]

BIFURCATION AND BUNDLE BRANCHES

Anatomically, the bifurcation is the lowest part of the common bundle (Figs. 2-69 and 2-74 to 2-76). The bifurcation begins on the left side at about the point where the common bundle emerges from the central fibrous body, while the right bundle divides at a more anterior point in the distal membranous septum.[126] Variations in the bifurcation site have potential clinicopathologic correlates, including right- or left-sided His bundle bifurcation[154] and intraseptal bifurcation.[126]

BUNDLE BRANCHES

The bundle branches begin at the crest of the muscular ventricular septum immediately distal to the membranous septum, with fibers of the left bundle branch forming a cascade down the left ventricular septal surface beneath the noncoronary aortic cusp (Figs. 2-69, 2-74, and 2-75). The morphology of the left bundle branch has been a subject of debate. The initial left bundle fibers separate from the branching bundle as a continuous "fan" of cells along the left ventricular septum. The disagreement concerns the fashion in which the fan of cells divides as it passes into the left ventricle. Tawara[146] showed that the left bundle radiates in a fanlike fashion with three major divisions (Fig. 2-77, Plate 1). Rosenbaum and colleagues[155] have postulated that the left bundle has a bifascicular structure. More recent reconstruction studies have indicated a trifascicular division of the left bundle.[154,156] Al-

FIGURE 2-77
See color Plate 1.

though the anatomy may not conform to a bifascicular system on the left (thin anterosuperior and thick posteroinferior), the concept of a trifascicular bundle branch system (right, bifascicular left) remains useful to clinicians.[119]

The right bundle branch is the direct continuation of the penetrating bundle positioned along the right side of the ventricular septum (Figs. 2-69 and 2-74). The right bundle becomes a subendocardial structure in the middle and lower thirds of the ventricular septum and can be seen grossly. In some hearts, the right bundle branch forms an obtuse angle with the His bundle.[154] It remains unbranched to the apex of the right ventricle.

The cells of the bundle branches are traditionally described as *Purkinje cells* (large and vacuolated). As in the His bundle, the proximal portions of the bundle branches have longitudinal strands of Purkinje-like cells. These cells have loosely arrayed mitochondria with few myofibrils. While the Purkinje fibers also exhibit side-to-side connections, the major intercellular connections are end to end through intercalated disks that may facilitate rapid longitudinal conduction[121,157] (see Chap. 26).

The left bundle branch receives blood from both the LAD and posterior descending (right) coronary arteries (Figs. 2-63 to 2-65). The anterior and middle radiations of the left bundle branch are supplied mainly through septal perforations of the LAD coronary artery. The right bundle branch is supplied from both right and left anterior descending coronary arterial systems.[158]

Terminal Purkinje Fibers

These fibers connect with the ends of the bundle branches to form interweaving networks on the endocardial surface of both ventricles. Practically, however, it is very difficult to trace the distal connections of the bundle branch system in humans. Purkinje fibers tend to be concentrated at papillary muscle tips rather than at the base of the ventricles. These fibers, which penetrate the subendocardium and myocardium at varying distances (species-dependent), appear to be more resistant to ischemia than common myocardial fibers.[124]

ULTRASTRUCTURE OF THE MYOCARDIUM

The functions of the heart may be classified into the following three types: electrical, mechanical, and endocrine. Many myocardial cells are specialized for one of these functions. The myocardial cells concerned primarily with mechanical shortening are similar, although there are some differences between atrial and ventricular myocardium.[159] Several different types of cells have electrical or endocrine activity as a major function, and the structure of such cells is significantly different from that of contractile, or "working," myocardial cells.[110,117,131–160]

Some special cells of the heart are particularly developed for the generation and very rapid conduction of an electrical impulse to the working cells.[131] Four types of cells are generally recognized in this system of impulse formation and rapid conduction: P cells, transitional cells, ameboid cells, and Purkinje cells. The P cells are numerous in the sinus node and are also present in the AV node and internodal pathways.[137] Transitional cells are found predominantly in the sinus node, the AV node, internodal pathways, and for considerable distances the atrial tissue adjacent to both nodes. Ameboid cells are found primarily in the eustachian ridge area. Purkinje cells are found at the margins of the sinus node; in the internodal pathways, which also contain intermingled transitional cells and ordinary working myocardial cells; adjacent to the AV node; and in the His bundle and its branches. The His bundle consists primarily of Purkinje cells, while the bundle branches consist of Purkinje cells intermingled with ordinary working cells.

The P cells are so named[90,161] because of their pale appearance on microscopy and their resemblance to primitive myocardial cells and because they are thought to be the site of origin of the pacemaker impulse. They are usually ovoid or rounded, in contrast to the usual elongated shape of other myocardial cells. They measure 5 to 10 μm in greatest diameter and are the smallest type of myocardial cell.

Transitional cells are a heterogeneous group of cells that include all cells with a microscopic appearance intermediate between the P cells and the more complex working myocardial cells. They are more elongated than P cells but shorter and narrower than working myocardial cells.

Ameboid cells have been described[161,162] in electron micrographs from the eustachian ridge. They may be elongated, triangular, oval, or nongeometric in shape. They have multilobular nuclei and pseudopodic prolongations that fill the spaces between neighboring cells and are often filled with a heavy concentration of electron-opaque granules that tend to give the cells a dark appearance. They have many mitochondria and myofibrils. Although the exact function of the ameboid cells is unknown, they may act as an auxiliary pacemaker or may be a source of atrial natriuretic factor.

Purkinje cells are identified primarily on the basis of their ultrastructure. They tend to be both broader and shorter than working myocardial cells and measure from 10 to 30 μm in cross section and 20 to 50 μm in length. Contractile or "working" myocardial cells are similar, whether they are from atrial or ventricular myocardium. They are characterized by hundreds of myofibrils in a special arrangement. Working myocardial cells are arranged longitudinally in series, with multiple cells forming a "fiber." Multiple fibers are generally arranged in parallel. Although cardiac muscle fibers have many lateral and end-to-side connections, the contractile cells are not a true anatomic syncytium. Intercalated disks at the terminal margins and junctions of contractile cells form a specialized transversely oriented cell boundary.[164] The myofibrils of working myocardial cells insert in the region of the intercalated disk. Contractile cells have many mitochondria and a nucleus, which tends to be centrally located and slightly elongated. These myocardial cells are about 10 to 20 μm in diameter and 50 to 100 μm in length.

Contractile cells contain an intricate sarcotubular system of tubules, vesicles, and cisternae.[165,166] One component of this system consists of the periodic invagination of the sarcolemma by transversely oriented tubules known as the T system. Focal dilatations of the T-system tubules are seen in the area of the Z band, forming a cistern-like structure, the intermediary vesicle.[167] A second component of the sarcotubular system is the series of interconnecting longitudinal tubules that tend to be oriented parallel to the myofibrils, which they surround. Near the Z band, these tubules have local dilatations, lateral sacs, or terminal cisternae, which, together with the intermediary vesicle, form a triad. A triad consists

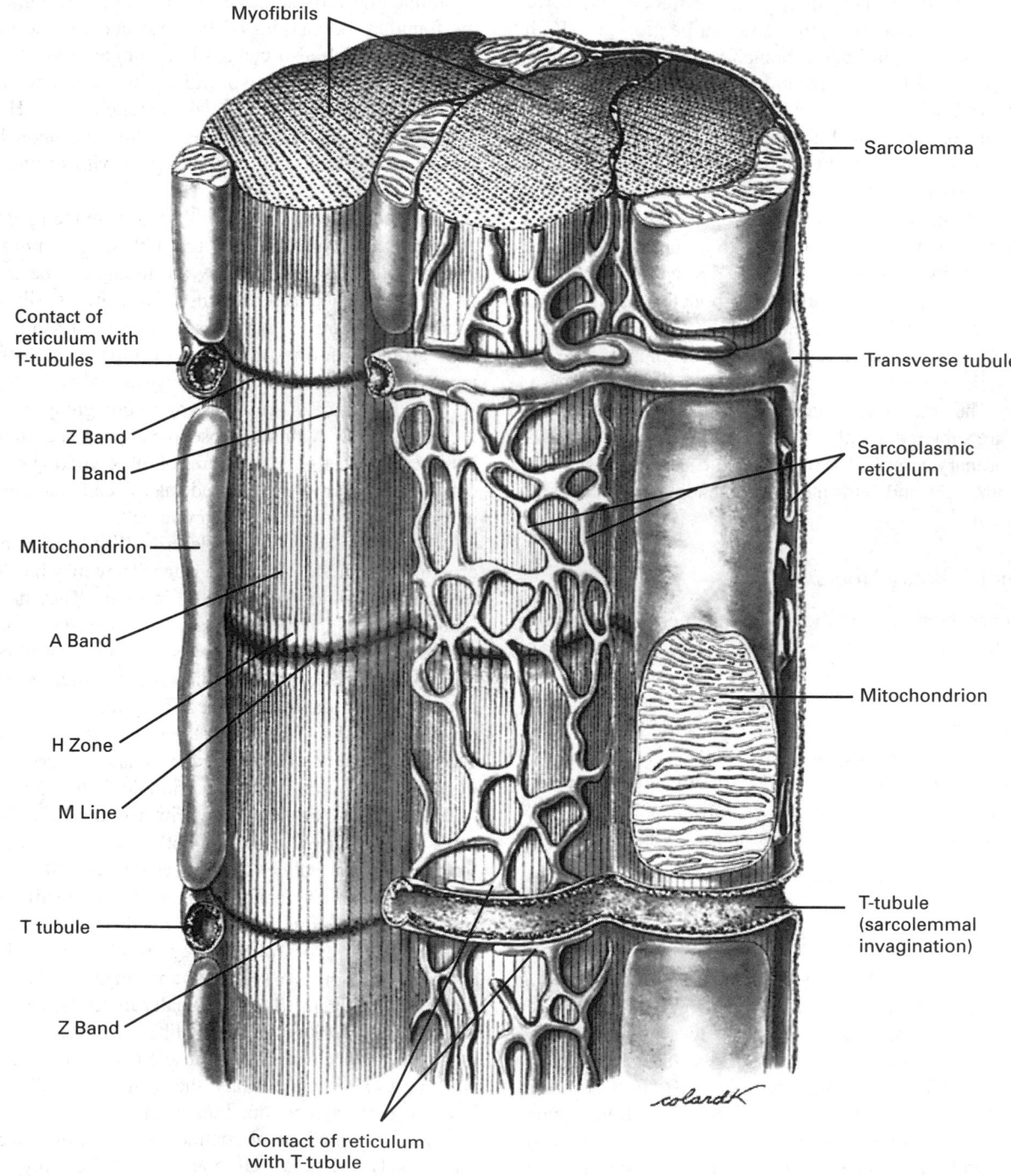

FIGURE 2-78

Schematic representation of myocardium. One sarcomere extends from one Z band to the other. Mitochondria, sarcoplasmic reticulum, and T tubules are also shown. (From Bloom W, Fawcett DW. *Textbook of Histology.* Philadelphia: Saunders; 1969, and Fawcett DW, McNutt NC. Ultrastructure of the myocardium: I. Ventricular papillary muscle. *J Cell Biol* 1969; 22:1. Copyright and permission of the Rockefeller University Press. Modified and reproduced with permission from the publishers and authors.)

of an intermediary vesicle from the T system and two lateral sacs from the longitudinal system. Although the three components of the triad are very close to each other, they probably are not in direct communication. The term *subsarcolemma cisternae* describes both the central (T system) and peripheral (sarcolemma) sites of proximity (see Chap. 3).

Transverse tubules are arranged perpendicular to the long axis of the cell but branch longitudinally and can directly connect with other transverse tubules.[168,169] In contrast, the internal longitudinal system (or sarcoplasmic reticulum) is a plexiform labyrinth of vesicles and tubules, some of which may also be transversely oriented.[170]

The sarcotubular system plays an important role in both electrical impulse conduction[171] and electromechanical coupling.[167] The impulse spreads rapidly on the surface of cells and down the transverse tubules; it stimulates the lateral sacs or vesicles and the entire sarcoplasmic reticulum to release large amounts of calcium around the contractile elements of the cell and initiate myocardial contraction.[172,173]

The myofibrils form longitudinally oriented strands of interdigitating myosin and actin filaments, which are the contractile elements of working, contractile myocardial cells (Figs. 2-78 and 2-79). The repeating morphologic and functional unit of contractile cells, the *sarcomere*, produces a regular band pattern of dark and light areas. The length of each sarcomere varies from 1.5 to 2.2 μm.[171] The dark Z bands, where the intercalated disks are located, provide a boundary at the ends of the sarcomere to which the actin filaments are attached. These thin filaments of actin and some tropomyosin B project into the center of the sarcomere, where they interdigitate with the thick myosin filaments, which lie in the central part of the sarcomere. The thick filaments of myosin measure 1.5 μm in length and have small excrescences produced by cross bridges.[174] On microscopy, the dark and light zones of the sarcomere are produced by the periodic, interdigitating relations between the thin actin and the thick myosin filaments (Figs. 2-78 and 2-79). When the myofibrils are moderately stretched, the following pattern is seen: The I band consists

of thin actin filaments attached to each side of the dark Z band. The A band is the wide dark area between two peripherally located I bands. The H zone is a lighter band of thick myosin filaments in the center of the A band. Crossing the center of the H zone is a thin dark line, the M line, consisting of the knoblike excrescences of the myosin filaments. The portions of the A band that extend in either direction from the H zone to each adjacent I band are darker than the H zone because they contain both thin actin and thick myosin filaments.

The appearance of a transverse section of myofibril depends upon the level of the sarcomere at which the cut is made. The H zone and M line area contain only thick myosin filaments arranged in a hexagonal pattern; the I band contains only evenly spaced thin actin filaments except in the H zone; the A band shows the thick myosin and thin actin filaments arranged in a hexagonal pattern with six thin actin filaments surrounding each thick myosin filament. Each working myocardial cell contains hundreds of parallel myofibrils with rows

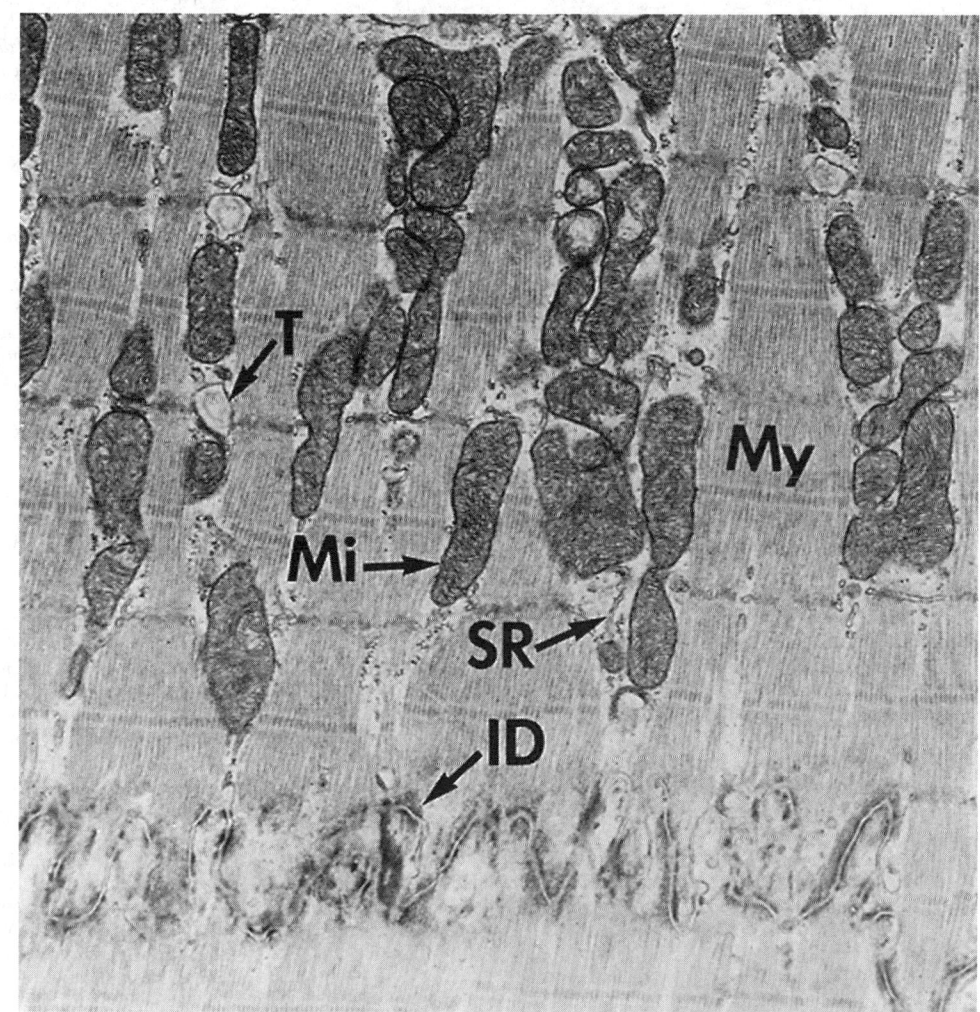

FIGURE 2-79
Electron micrograph of human myocardium, longitudinal section. Cytoplasm is packed with a regular array of myofibrils (My), showing the distinct banding pattern. Mitochondria (Mi) and elements of the sarcoplasmic reticulum (SR) and the T-tubule system (T) are arranged around the myofibrils. Portions of two cells are shown joined end to end at the intercalated disk (ID). (Courtesy of Claudia R. Adkison, Ph.D.)

of mitochondria between them (Figs. 2-78 and 2-79). The alignment of Z bands, I bands, and A bands of adjacent myofibrils is responsible for the typical cross striations seen on light microscopy.

Many studies have supported the application of Huxley and Hanson's "sliding filament hypothesis"[175-177] to both skeletal and myocardial muscle. In their theory, linkages between the actin and myosin pull or propel the actin filaments toward the center of the sarcomere. The two sets of filaments slide past each other, causing the muscle fiber to shorten. The myosin component for the linkage is heavy (H) meromyosin,[176] which combines with actin and also contains the adenosine triphosphatase (ATPase) necessary to split the ATP to provide the energy for contraction. When a myocardial cell is activated, the concentration of free intracellular Ca^{2+} combines with troponin and releases the actinmyosin inhibition, thereby permitting the actin and myosin fibers to slide and the muscle fiber to shorten. The mitochondria of working myocardial cells (Figs. 2-78 and 2-79) are cylindrically shaped and measure 2 by 0.5 μm. They have many infoldings, or cristae, which project inward from the membrane. Mitochondria are very numerous and make up 25 to 50 percent of the total mass of myocardium[171] (see also Chap. 3).

REFERENCES

1. Anderson RH, Wilcox BR, Becker AE. Anatomy of the normal heart. In: Hurst JW, ed. *Atlas of the Heart.* New York: McGraw-Hill and Gower; 1988:1–10.
2. Burton AC. The importance of the shape and size of the heart. *Am Heart J* 1957; 52:801–810.
3. Zimmerman J. The functional and surgical anatomy of the heart. *Ann R Coll Surg Engl* 1966; 39:328–366.
4. Waller BF. Anatomic basis for newer imaging techniques. *Am J Cardiac Imag* 1987; 1:311–322.
5. Davies MJ, Pomerance A, Lamb D. Techniques in examination and anatomy of the heart. In: Pomerance A, Davies MJ, eds. *The Pathology of the Heart.* Oxford: Blackwell; 1975:1–10.
6. McAlpine WA. *Heart and Coronary Arteries.* New York: Springer-Verlag; 1975:1–50.
7. Walmsley R, Watson H. *Clinical Anatomy of the Heart.* New York: Churchill Livingstone; 1978:1–22.
8. Nazarian GK, Julsrud PR, Ehman RL, Edwards WD. Correlation between magnetic resonance imaging of the heart and cardiac anatomy. *Mayo Clin Proc* 1987; 62:573–583.
9. Wilcox BR, Anderson RH. *Surgical Anatomy of the Heart.* New York: Raven Press; 1985:1–96.
10. Edwards WD. Applied anatomy of the heart. In: Brandenburg RO, Fuster V, Giuliani ER, et al, eds. *Cardiology: Fundamentals and Practice.* Chicago: Year Book; 1987:27–112.
11. Scholz DG, Kitzman DW, Hagan PT, Ilstrup DM, Edwards WD. Age-related changes in normal human hearts during the first 10 decades of life: Part I. (Growth). A quantitative anatomic study of 200 specimens from subjects from birth to 19 years old. *Mayo Clin Proc* 1988; 63:126–136.
12. Anderson RH, Becker AE. *Cardiac Anatomy.* London: Gower; 1980:1–30.
13. Waller BF, Taliercio CP, Slack JD, Orr CM, Howard J, Smith ML. Tomographic views of normal and abnormal hearts: The anatomic basis for various cardiac imaging techniques. Part I. *Clin Cardiol* 1990; 13:802–812.
14. Waller BF, Taliercio CP, Slack JD, Orr CM, Howard J, Smith ML. Tomographic views of normal and abnormal hearts: The anatomic basis for various cardiac imaging techniques. Part II. *Clin Cardiol* 1990; 13:877–882.
15. Lev M, Bharati S. The fibrous skeleton of the heart. In: Hurst JW, ed. *Update* IV: *The Heart.* New York: McGraw-Hill; 1982:7–12.
16. Rosenquist GC, Sweeney LJ. The membranous ventricular septum in the normal heart. *Johns Hopkins Med J* 1972; 135:9–16.
17. Titus JL. Normal anatomy of the human cardiac conduction system. *Mayo Clin Proc* 1973; 28:22–30.
18. Sweeney LF, Rosenquist GC. The normal anatomy of the atrial septum in the human heart. *Am Heart J* 1979; 98:192–199.
19. Prakash R. Determination of right ventricular wall thickness in systole and diastole: Echocardiographic and necropsy correlation in 32 patients. *Br Heart J* 1978; 20:1257–1261.
20. Grant RP, Downey FM, MacMahon H. The architecture of the right ventricular outflow tract in the normal heart and in the presence of ventricular septal defects. *Circulation* 1961; 22:223–235.
21. James TN. Anatomy of the crista supraventricularis: Its importance for understanding right ventricular function, right ventricular infarction and related conditions. *J Am Coll Cardiol* 1985; 6:1083–1095.
22. Kennedy JW, Baxley WA, Figley MM, Dodge HT, Blackmon JR. Quantitative angiocardiography: I. The normal left ventricle in man. *Circulation* 1966; 32:272–278.
23. Waller BF. Morphologic aspects of valvular heart disease: Part I. *Curr Probl Cardiol* 1985; 9:13–26.
24. Gross L, Kugel MA. Topographical anatomy and histology of the valves in the human heart. *Am J Pathol* 1931; 7:225–276.
25. Clark JA. An x-ray microscopic study of the blood supply to the valves of the human heart. *Br Heart J* 1965; 27:220–223.
26. Duran CMG, Gunning AJ. The vascularization of the heart valves: A comparative study. *Cardiovasc Res* 1968; 3:290–296.
27. Montiel MM. Muscular apparatus of the mitral valve in man and its involvement in left-sided cardiac hypertrophy. *Am J Cardiol* 1970; 26:321–322.
28. Zimmerman J. The functional and surgical anatomy of the aortic valve. *Isr J Med Sci* 1969; 5:862–868.
29. Merklin RJ. Position and orientation of the heart valves. *Am J Anat* 1969; 125:375–380.
30. Davies MJ. *Pathology of Cardiac Valves.* London: Butterworth; 1980.
31. Vollebergh FEMG, Becker AE. Minor congenital variations of cusp size in tricuspid aortic valves: Possible link with isolated aortic stenosis. *Br Heart J* 1977; 39:1006–1011.
32. Roberts WC. The structure of the aortic valve in clinically isolated aortic stenosis—An autopsy study of 162 patients over 15 years of age. *Circulation* 1970; 22:91–97.
33. Waller BF, Roberts WC. Cardiovascular disease in the very elderly: Analysis of 40 necropsy patients aged 90 years and over. *Am J Cardiol* 1983; 51:203–221.
34. Perloff JK, Roberts WC. The mitral apparatus: Functional anatomy of mitral regurgitation. *Circulation* 1972; 26:227–239.
35. Waller BF, Morrow AG, Maron BJ, DelNegro AA, Kent KM, McGrath FJ, et al. Etiology of clinically isolated, severe, chronic, pure mitral regurgitation: Analysis of 97 patients over 30 years of age having mitral valve replacement. *Am Heart J* 1982; 102:276–288.
36. Roberts WC. Morphologic features of the normal and abnormal mitral valve. *Am J Cardiol* 1983; 51:1005–1028.
37. Ranganathan N, Lam JHC, Wigle ED, Silver MD. Morphology of the human mitral valve: II. The valve leaflets. *Circulation* 1970; 21:259–267.
38. Brock RC. The surgical and pathologic anatomy of the mitral valve. *Br Heart J* 1952; 12:289–513.
39. Estes EH Jr, Dalton FM, Entman ML. The anatomy and blood supply of the papillary muscles of the left ventricle. *Am Heart J* 1966; 71:356–362.
40. Roberts WC, Perloff JK. Mitral valve disease: A clinicopathologic survey of the conditions causing the mitral valve to function abnormally. *Ann Intern Med* 1972; 77:939–975.
41. Edwards BS, Edwards WD, Bambara JF, Van der Bel-Kahn J, Bove KE, Edwards JE. Anomalies of the left atrium and mitral valve: Cords, flaps and duplication of valves. *Arch Pathol Lab Med* 1983; 107:29–33.
42. Silver MD, Lam JHC, Ranganathan N, Wigle ED. Morphology of human tricuspid valve. *Circulation* 1971; 23:333–338.
43. Cascos AS, Rabago P, Sokolowski M. Duplication of the tricuspid valve. *Br Heart J* 1967; 29:923–926.
44. Elfenbein B, Paplanus SH. Duplication of the mitral and tricuspid valves. *Arch Pathol* 1968; 85:675–680.
45. Roberts WC, Waller BF. Effect of chronic hypercalcemia on the heart: An analysis of 18 necropsy patients. *Am J Cardiol* 1981; 71:371–382.

46. Estes EH Jr, Dalton FM, Entman ML, Dixon HB II, Hackel DB. The anatomy and blood supply of the papillary muscles of the left ventricle. *Am Heart J* 1966; 71:356–362.

47. Lam JHC, Ranganathan N, Wigle ED, Silver MD. Morphology of the human mitral valve: I. Chordae tendineae. *Circulation* 1970; 21:229–258.

48. Holt JP. The normal pericardium. *Am J Cardiol* 1970; 26:255–265.

49. Choe YH, Im J-G, Park JH, Ho MC, Kim CW. The anatomy of the pericardial space: A study in cadavers and patients. *Am J Radiol* 1987; 129:693–698.

50. Edwards WD, Tajik AJ, Seward JB. Standardized nomenclature and anatomic bases for regional tomographic analysis of the heart. *Mayo Clin Proc* 1981; 56:279–297.

51. Silverman NH, Hunter S, Anderson RH, Ho SY, Davies MJ, Sutherland GR. Anatomic basis for cross-sectional echocardiography. *Br Heart J* 1983; 50:221–231.

52. Edwards WD. Anatomic basis for tomographic analyses of the heart at autopsy. In: Waller BF, ed. *Cardiac Morphology.* Philadelphia: Davis; 1982:285–506.

53. Khandheria K, Oh J. Transesophageal echocardiography: State of the art and future directions. *Am J Cardiol* 1992; 69:61H–75H.

54. Carter BL, Morehead J, Wolpert SM, Hammerschlag SB, Griffiths HJ, Kahn PC. *Cross-Sectional Anatomy, Computed Tomography and Ultrasound Correlation.* New York: Appleton-Century-Crofts; 1977:1–60.

55. Bo WJ, Mechan I, Krueger WA. *Basic Atlas of Cross-Sectional Anatomy.* Philadelphia: Saunders; 1980:1–28.

56. Gambarelli J, Guerinel G, Chevrot L, Matteri M. *Computerized Axial Tomography. An Anatomic Atlas of Serial Sections of the Human Body.* Berlin: Springer-Verlag; 1977:1–21.

57. Han MC, Kim CW. *Sectional Human Anatomy: Transverse, Sagittal and Coronal Sections Correlated with Computed Tomography and Magnetic Resonance Imaging.* Seoul: Ilchokok; 1985:1–20.

58. Nazarian GK, Julsrud PR, Ehman RL, Edwards WD. Correlation between magnetic resonance imaging of the heart and cardiac anatomy. *Mayo Clin Proc* 1987; 62:573–583.

59. Higgins CB. New horizons in cardiac imaging. *Radiology* 1985; 156:577–588.

60. Higgins CB. Overview of MR of the heart—1986. *Am J Radiol* 1986; 126:907–912.

61. Higgins CB, Carlsson E, Lipton MJ. *CT of the Heart and Great Vessels.* Mount Kisco, NY: Futura; 1983:1–28.

62. Belohlavek M, Foley DA, Gerber TC, Kinter TM, Greenleaf JF, Seward JB. Three- and four-dimensional cardiovascular ultrasound imaging: A new era for echocardiography. *Mayo Clin Proc* 1993; 68:221–230.

63. Silberbach M, Sahn DJ. Three-dimensional echocardiographic reconstruction: From "ice pick" to virtual reality. *Mayo Clin Proc* 1993; 68:311–312.

64. Raqueno R, Ghosh A, Nanda NC, Schott J, Moos S. Four-dimensional reconstruction of 2-dimensional echocardiographic images. *Echocardiography* 1989; 6:323–337.

65. Ofili EO, Nanda NC. Three-dimensional and four-dimensional echocardiography. *Ultrasound Med Biol* 1992; 20:669–675.

66. Speidel CM, Walkup RK, Abendschein DR, Kenzora JL, Vannier MW. Coronary artery mapping: A method for three-dimensional reconstruction of epicardial anatomy. *Am J Digital Imag* 1995; 8:22–35.

67. Di Mario C, von Birgelen C, Prati F, Soni B, Li W, Bruining N, et al. Three-dimensional reconstruction of cross sectional intracoronary ultrasound: Clinical or research tool? *Br Heart J* 1995; 73:26–32.

68. von Birgelen C, Erbel R, Di Mario C, Li W, Prati F, Ge J, et al. Three-dimensional reconstruction of coronary arteries with intravascular ultrasound. *Herz* 1995; 20:277–289.

69. Ritman RL. Rationale for, and recent progress in, 3-D reconstruction of the heart and lungs. *Comput Med Imag Graphics* 1993; 17:263–271.

70. Gerber TC, Belohlavek M, Greenleaf JF, Foley DA, Seward JB. Dynamic spatial reconstruction of cardiovascular ultrasound images: Four-dimensional ultrasound imaging. *Am J Cardiac Imag* 1992; 8:199–205.

71. Levine RA, Weyman AE, Handschumacher MD. Three-dimensional echocardiography: Techniques and applications. *Am J Cardiol* 1992; 69:121H–130H.

72. Salustri A, Roelandt J. Three-dimensional reconstruction of the heart with rotational acquisition: Methods and clinical applications. *Br Heart J* 1995; 73:10–15.

73. Martin RW, Bashein G, Nessly ML, Sheehan FH. Methodology for three-dimensional reconstruction of the left ventricle from transesophageal echocardiogram. *Ultrasound Med Biol* 1993; 19:27–38.

74. Salustri A, Roelandt JR. Ultrasonic three-dimensional reconstruction of the heart. *Ultrasound Med Biol* 1995; 21:281–293.

75. Aakhus S, Maehle J, Bjoernstad K. A new method for echocardiographic computerized three-dimensional reconstruction of left ventricular endocardial surface: In vitro accuracy and clinical repeatability of volumes. *J Am Soc Echocardiogr* 1992; 7:571–581.

76. Handschumacher MD, Lethor JP, Siu SC, Mele D, Rivera JM, Picard MH, et al. A new integrated system for three-dimensional echocardiographic reconstruction: Development and validation for ventricular volume with application in human subjects. *J Am Coll Cardiol* 1993; 21:723–753.

77. Levine RA, Weyman AE, Handschumacher MD. Three-dimensional echocardiography: Techniques and applications. *Am J Cardiol* 1992; 69:121H–132H.

78. Halmann M, Sideman S, Lessick J, Beyar R. Relating coronary perfusion to myocardial function using three-dimensional reconstruction of heart and coronary arteries. *Med Biol Eng Comput* 1992; 32:S122–S150.

79. Belohlavek M, Foley DA, Gerber TC, Greenleaf JF, Seward JB. Three-dimensional ultrasound imaging of the atrial septum: Normal and pathologic anatomy. *J Am Coll Cardiol* 1993; 22:1673–1678.

80. Moshage WE, Achenbach S, Seese B, Bachmann K, Kirchgeorg M. Coronary artery stenoses: Three dimensional imaging with electrocardiographically triggered, contrast agent-enhanced, electron-beam CT. *Radiology* 1995; 196:707–712.

81. Demaria R, Godlewski G, DeGuilhermier P, Tang J, Seguin J, Chaptal PA. Static morphometric bases for CT identification and evaluation of the outflow chamber of the left ventricle: Preliminary study in formalin-fixed heart. *Surg Radiol Anat* 1993; 15:125–150.

82. Rumberger JA, Bell MR. Measurement of myocardial perfusion and cardiac output using intravenous injection methods by ultrafast (cine) computed tomography. *Invest Radiol* 1992; 27:S20–S26.

83. Taratorin AM, Sideman S. 3D functional mapping of the left ventricular dynamics. *Comput Med Imag Graphics* 1995; 19:113–129.

84. Thomas PJ, McCollough CH, Ritman EL. An electron-beam CT approach for transvenous coronary arteriography. *J Comput Assist Tomogr* 1995; 19:383–389.

85. Stehling MJ, Howseman AM, Ordidge RJ, Chapman B, Turner R, Coxon R, et al. Whole body echo-planar MR imaging at 0.5 T1. *Radiology* 1989; 170:257–263.

86. Pennell DJ, Keegan J, Firmin DN, Gatehouse PD, Underwood SR, Longmore DB. Magnetic resonance imaging of coronary arteries: Technique and preliminary results. *Br Heart J* 1993; 70:315–326.

87. Mitchell GAG. *Cardiovascular Innervation.* Baltimore: Williams & Wilkins; 1956.

88. Janes RD, Brandys JC, Hopkins DA, Johnstone DE, Murphy DA, Armour JA. Anatomy of human extrinsic cardiac nerves and ganglia. *Am J Cardiol* 1986; 57:299–309.

89. Randall WC, ed. *Nervous Control of Cardiovascular Function.* New York: Oxford University Press; 1982.

90. Feola M, Merrlin R, Cho S, Brockman SK. The terminal pathway of the lymphatic system of the human heart. *Ann Thorac Surg* 1977; 22:531–536.

91. Miller AJ. *Lymphatics of the Heart.* New York: Raven Press; 1982.

92. Waller BF. Anatomy, histology, and pathology of the major epicardial coronary arteries relevant to echocardiographic imaging techniques. *J Am Soc Echocardiogr* 1989; 2:232–252.

93. Waller BF. Five coronary ostia: Duplicate left anterior descending and right conus coronary arteries. *Am J Cardiol* 1983; 52:126–137.

94. Baroldi G. Diseases of the coronary arteries. In: Silver MD, ed. *Cardiovascular Pathology, I.* New York: Churchill Livingstone; 1983:317–391.

95. Schulte MA, Waller BF, Hull MT, Pless JE. Origin of the left anterior descending coronary artery from the right aortic sinus with intramyocardial tunneling to the left side of the heart via the ventricular septum: A case against clinical and morphologic significance of myocardial bridging. *Am Heart J* 1985; 110:299–501.

96. Polacek P. Relation of myocardial bridges and loops on the coronary arteries to coronary occlusions. *Am Heart J* 1961; 61:22–52.

97. Anderson KR, Ho SY, Anderson RH. Location and vascular supply of sinus node in human heart. *Br Heart J* 1979; 21:28–32.

98. Spring DJ, Thomsen JH. Severe atherosclerosis in the "single coronary artery." Report of a previously undescribed pattern. *Am J Cardiol* 1973; 31:662–665.

99. James TN, Burch GE. Blood supply of the human interventricular septum. *Circulation* 1958; 17:391–396.

100. Kugel MA. Anatomical studies on the coronary arteries and their branches: I. Arteria anastomotica auricularis magna. *Am Heart J* 1927; 3:260–270.

101. Benditt EP, Schwartz SM. Blood vessels. In: Rubin E, Farber JL, eds. *Pathology.* Philadelphia: Lippincott; 1988:252–265.

102. Waller BF. The eccentric coronary atherosclerotic plaque: Morphologic observations and clinical relevance. *Clin Cardiol* 1989; 12:12–20.

103. Fawcett DW. Blood and lymph vascular systems. In: Fawcett DW, ed. *A Textbook of Histology.* Philadelphia: Saunders; 1986:367–381.

104. Neufeld HN, Schneeweiss A. *Coronary Artery Disease in Infants and Children.* Philadelphia: Lea & Febiger, 1983:1–22.

105. Vlodaver Z, Edwards JE. Pathology of coronary atherosclerosis. *Prog Cardiovasc Dis* 1971; 12:256–272.

106. Monckeberg JG. Uber die reine Mediaverkalkung der Extremitatenarterien und ihr Vorhalten zur Arterioskierwose. *Virchows Archiv [A]* 1903; 171:12–30.

107. Waller BF, Morgan R. The very elderly heart. *Cardiovasc Clin* 1987; 18:361–370.

108. James TN. *Anatomy of the Coronary Arteries.* New York: Hoeber Medical Division, Harper & Row; 1961:1–77.

109. Keith A, Flack M. The form and nature of the muscular connections between the primary division of the vertebrate heart. *J Anat Physiol* 1907; 21:172–182.

110. James TN. Anatomy of the human sinus node. *Anat Rec* 1961; 121:109–139.

111. Lev M, Bharati S. Anatomy of the conduction system in normal and congenitally abnormal hearts. In: Roberts NK, Gelband H, eds. *Cardiac Arrhythmias in the Neonate, Infant and Child.* New York: Appleton-Century-Crofts; 1977:29–53.

112. Anderson KR, Ho SY, Anderson RH. The location and vascular supply of the sinus node in the human heart. *Br Heart J* 1979; 21:28–32.

113. Blair DM, Davies F. Observations on the conducting system of the heart. *J Anat* 1935; 69:303–325.

114. James TN. *Anatomy of the Coronary Arteries.* New York: Harper & Row; 1961:1–50.

115. Vieweg WVR, Alpert JS, Hagan AD. Origin of the sinoatrial node and atrioventricular node arteries in right, mixed and left inferior emphasis systems. *Cathet Cardiovasc Diagn* 1975; 1:361–373.

116. James TN. The sinus node as a servomechanism. *Circ Res* 1973; 32:307–313.

117. James TN, Sherf L, Fine G, Morales AR. Comparative ultrastructure of the sinus node in man and dog. *Circulation* 1966; 32:139–163.

118. Davies MJ, Anderson RH, Becker AE. *The Conduction System of the Heart.* London: Butterworth; 1983:1–200.

119. Zipes DP. Genesis of cardiac arrhythmias: Electrophysiological consideration. In: Braunwald E, ed. *Heart Disease: A Textbook of Cardiovascular Medicine,* 2d ed. Philadelphia: Saunders; 1982:581–620.

120. Masson-Pevel M, Bleeker WK, Gas D. The plasma membrane of leading pacemaker cells in the rabbit sinus node: A qualitative and quantitative ultrastructural analysis. *Circ Res* 1979; 25:621–629.

121. Trautwein W, Uchizono K. Electron microscopic and electrophysiologic study of the pacemaker in the sinoatrial node of the rabbit heart. *Z Zellforsch Mikrosk Anat* 1963; 61:96–101.

122. Bleeker WK, Mackaay AJ, Masson-Pevet M, Bowman LN, Becker AE. Functional and morphological organization of the rabbit sinus node. *Circ Res* 1980; 26:11–21.

123. James TN. Anatomy of the conduction system of the heart. In: Hurst JW, Logue RB, Rackley CE, Schlant RC, Sonnenblick EH, Wallace AG, et al, eds. *The Heart,* 5th ed. New York: McGraw-Hill; 1982:26–56.

124. Becker AE, Bowman LN, Janse MJ, Anderson RH. Functional anatomy of the cardiac conduction system. In: Harrison DC, ed. *Cardiac Arrhythmias: A Decade of Progress.* Boston: Hall; 1981:3–24.

125. Lev M. Aging changes in the human sinoatrial node. *J Gerontol* 1952; 9:1–10.

126. Thorel C. Verlaufige Mitteilung uber eine besondere Muskelverbindung Zwischen der Cava Superior und dem Hisschen Bundel. *Munch Med Wochenschr* 1909; 56:2159–2163.

127. Condorelli L. Uber die Bahnen der Reizleitung von Keith-Flackschen Knoten zeiden Vorhofen. *Z Gesam Exp Med* 1929; 68:293–297.

128. Franco PM. Recherches sur les faisceaux de connexion auriculaires dans les condition normales et pathologues. *Arch Mal Coeur* 1951; 22:287–292.

129. Osawa M. Histologic study on the conducting systems in the atrial portion of the dog's heart: 3. Specific pathways conducting between the sinus node and the Tawara node. *Jpn Circ J* 1959; 23:1012–1019.

130. Robb JS, Petri R. Expansions of the atrio-ventricular system in the atria. In: Paes de Carvalho A, de Mello WC, Hoffman BF, eds. *The Specialized Tissues of the Heart.* Amsterdam: Elsevier; 1961:1–21.

131. James TN. The connecting pathways between the sinus node and the A-V node and between the right and left atrium in the human heart. *Am Heart J* 1963; 66:498–508.

132. Meredith J, Titus JL. The anatomical atrial connections between sinus and AV node. *Circulation* 1968; 37:566–579.

133. Spach MS, King TD, Barr RC, Boaz DE, Marrow MN, Giddens SH. Electrical potential distribution surrounding the atria during depolarization and repolarization in the dog. *Circ Res* 1969; 22:857–873.

134. Truex RC. The sinoatrial node and its connections with the atrial tissues. In: Wellens HJJ, Lie KI, Janse MJ, eds. *The Conduction Systems of the Heart—Structure, Function and Clinical Implications.* Philadelphia: Lea & Febiger; 1976:209–215.

135. Lev M, Bharati S. Lesions of the conduction system, and their functional significance. *Pathol Annu* 1972; 9:157–207.

136. Janse MJ, Anderson RH. Specialized internodal atrial pathways—Fact or fiction. *Eur J Cardiol* 1982; 2:117–136.

137. James TN, Sherf L. Specialized tissue and preferential conduction in the atria of the heart. *Am J Cardiol* 1971; 28:212–227.

138. Bachman G. The interauricular time interval. *Am J Physiol* 1916; 21:309–320.

139. Wenckebach KF. Beitrangae zur Kenntnis der menschlichen Herztatigkeit. *Arch Anat Physiol* 1908; 3:53–58.

140. Isa L, Matturri L, Rossi L. Contributo isto-citologico al riconoscimento delle connessioni internodali atriali. *G Ital Cardiol* 1976; 2:1022–1025.

141. Hoffman BF. Fine structure of the internodal pathways. *Am J Cardiol* 1979; 22:385–386.

142. Becker AE, Bouman LN, Janse MK, Anderson RH. Functional anatomy of the cardiac conduction system. In Harrison DC, ed. *Cardiac Arrhythmias: A Decade of Progress.* Boston: Hall; 1981:1–18.

143. Tawara S. *Das Reizleitungssystem des Saugetierkerzens.* Jena: Gustav Fischer, 1906.

144. Hecht HH, Kossmann CE, Childers RW, Langendorf R, Ler M, Rosen KM, et al. Atrioventricular and intraventricular conduction: Revised nomenclature and concepts. *Am J Cardiol* 1973; 31:222–232.

145. Anderson RH, Becker AE, Brechenmacher C, Davies MJ, Rossi L. The human atrioventricular junctional area: A morphological study of the AV node and bundle. *Eur J Cardiol* 1975; 3:11–25.

146. Rossi L. *Histopathology of Cardiac Arrhythmias,* 2d ed. Milan: Casa Editrice Ambrosiana; 1979:1–75.

147. Becker AE, Anderson RH. Morphology of the human atrioventricular junctional area. In: Wellens JHH, Lie KI, Janse MJ, eds. *The Conduction System of the Heart—Structure, Function and Clinical Implications.* New York: Lea & Febiger; 1976:263–271.

148. Thaemert JC. Atrioventricular node innervation in ultrastructural three dimensions. *Am J Anat* 1970; 128:229–239.

149. Thaemert JC. Fine structure of the atrioventricular node in ultrastructural three dimensions. *Am J Anat* 1973; 136:23–65.

150. Mahaim I. Kent's fiber in the A-V paraspecific conduction through the upper connection of the bundle of His—Tawara. *Am Heart J* 1927; 33:651–653.

151. James TN. Sudden death in babies: New observations in the heart. *Am J Cardiol* 1968; 22:279–282.

152. James TN, Marshall ML. De Subitaneis Mortibus 18: Persistent fetal dispersion of the atrioventricular node and His bundle within the central fibrous body. *Circulation* 1976; 53:1026–1032.

153. Rossi L. *Sistema di Conduzione e Nervi nel Aiore dell'Uomo.* Milano: Casa Editrice Ambrosiana; 1952:1–66.

154. Massing GK, James TN. Anatomical configuration of the His bundle and bundle branches in the human heart. *Circulation* 1976; 53:609–621.

155. Rosenbaum MB, Elizari MV, Lazzari JO. *The Hemiblocks.* Tampa, FL: Tampa Tracings; 1970.

156. Demoulin JC, Kulbertus HE. Histopathological examination of concept of left hemiblock. *Br Heart J* 1972; 32:807–812.

157. Weidmann S. The diffusion of radiopotassium across intercalated disks of mammalian cardiac muscle. *J Physiol* 1966; 187:323–328.

158. Davies MJ. *Pathology of Conducting Tissue of the Heart.* London: Butterworth; 1971:1–29.

159. Anderson RH, Becker AE, Tranum-Jensen J, Janse MJ. Anatomic-electrophysiological correlations in the conduction system—A review. *Br Heart J* 1981; 25:67–82.

160. Sommer JR, Jennings RB. Ultrastructure of cardiac muscle. In: Fozzard HA, Haber E, Jennings RD, et al, eds. *The Heart and Cardiovascular System: Scientific Foundations.* New York: Raven Press; 1986:61–75.

161. James TN, Sherf L. Ultrastructure of the human atrioventricular node. *Circulation* 1968; 37:1029–1070.

162. Sherf L, James TN. Fine structure of cells and their histological organization within internodal pathways of the heart: Clinical and electrocardiographic implications. *Am J Cardiol* 1979; 22:325–369.

163. Sherf L, James TN. Functional anatomy and ultrastructure of the internodal pathways. In: Little RC, ed. *Physiology of Atrial Pacemakers and Conductive Tissues.* New York: Futura; 1980:67–72.

164. Sjostrand FS, Andersson-Cedergran E. Intercalated discs of heart muscle. In: Bourne GH, ed. *The Structure and Function of Muscle.* New York: Academic Press; 1960:221–229.

165. Porter KR, Palade GE. Studies on the endoplastic reticulum: III. Its form and distribution in striated muscle cells. *J Biophys Biochem Cytol* 1957; 3:269–276.

166. Hoffman BF. Physiology of atrioventricular transmission. *Circulation* 1961; 22:506–517.

167. Essner E, Novikoff AB, Quintana N. Nucleoside phosphatase activities in rat cardiac muscle. *J Cell Biol* 1965; 25:201–215.

168. Fawcess DW, McNutt NS. The ultrastructure of the cat myocardium: I. Ventricular papillary muscle. *J Cell Biol* 1969; 22:1–25.

169. Forssmann WG, Giardier L. A study of the T system in rat heart. *J Cell Biol* 1970; 22:1–19.

170. Sommer JR, Johnson EA. A comparative study of Purkinje fibers and ventricular fibers. *J Cell Biol* 1968; 36:297–526.

171. Huxley AF, Taylor RE. Local activation of striated muscle fibers. *J Physiol* 1958; 122:221–226.

172. Huxley AF. The links between excitation and contraction. *Proc R Soc Lond Ser B* 1962; 160:286–288.

173. Braunwald E, Ross J Jr, Sonnenblick EH. Mechanisms of contraction of the normal and failing heart. *N Engl J Med* 1967; 277:792–800.

174. Hasselbach W. ATP driven active transport of Ca in the membranes of the sarcoplasmic reticulum. *Proc R Soc Lond Ser B* 1962; 160:501–502.

175. Huxley HE, Hanson J. Changes in the cross-striations of muscle during contraction and stretch and their structural interpretation. *Nature* 1952; 173:973–976.

176. Huxley HE. Structural arrangement and the contraction mechanism in striated muscle. *Proc R Soc Lond Ser B* 1962; 160:222–228.

177. Huxley HE. Structural evidence concerning mechanism of contraction in striated muscle. In: Paul WM, Kay CM, Monckton G, eds. *Muscles.* Toronto: Pergamon, 1965:3–18.

3

NORMAL PHYSIOLOGY OF THE CARDIOVASCULAR SYSTEM

Robert C. Schlant / Edmund H. Sonnenblick / Arnold M. Katz

The cardiovascular system has the following three basic functions: (1) to transport oxygen and other nutrients to the cells of the body, (2) to remove metabolic waste products from the cells, and (3) to carry substances such as hormones from one part of the body to another. In addition, the heart and blood vessels themselves have important neurohumoral functions.

With every beat, the performance of the heart may be considered the net result of the following four major determinants: *preload*, *afterload*, *contractility* (the inotropic state), and *distensibility* (the lusitropic state). The heart rate then determines the performance of the heart relative to time. Cardiac performance is further influenced by many factors, including the synchrony of ventricular contraction, atrial function, neural control, drugs, hormones and metabolic products, and pericardial properties. This chapter reviews myocardial excitation-contraction coupling, the fundamentals of muscle mechanics, the major factors influencing cardiac performance, the major mechanisms of cardiac reserve, the coronary circulation, the response to exercise, and the cardiac cycle. Detailed discussions are found in the general reference sources.[1-18] The evaluation of cardiac and myocardial function is further discussed in Chap. 22, and the pathophysiology of heart failure in Chap. 21.

MYOCARDIAL EXCITATION-CONTRACTION COUPLING

The action potential generated along the surface of the myocyte initiates the contractile process in heart muscle. The calcium ion (Ca^{2+})[11,14,19-29] plays a central role in excitation-contraction coupling, as noted in classic studies of Ringer.[30] Ca^{2+} has several roles in excitation-contraction coupling. Because it is a cation, Ca^{2+} serves as a charge carrier that carries an inward (depolarizing) current across the plasma membrane that contributes to the plateau of the cardiac action potential. This Ca^{2+} also serves as a "trigger" that releases a much larger amount of this cation from internal stores in the sarcoplasmic reticulum (SR). Ca^{2+} binds to and activates the cardiac contractile apparatus and by an indirect signal transduction system that mediated by calmodulin initiates smooth muscle contraction. Variations in the amounts of activator Ca^{2+} play a major role in the regulation of myocardial contractility and vascular tone. Ca^{2+} binds to other intracellular proteins and so regulates a number of cellular processes, including protein synthesis.

With the initiation of the action potential in ventricular myocardium (Fig. 3-1), opening of sodium channels initiates a very rapid influx of Na^+ (or change in Na^+ *conductance*), which produces the rapid electrical spike and overshoot during phase zero of the action potential[31,32] (see Chap. 26). During the plateau phase of the action potential (phase 2), there is a slow inward flux of Ca^{2+} through calcium channels in the myocardial cell membrane, or sarcolemma, into the intracellular fluid (sarcoplasm, or cytosol).[33,34] Some extracellular Ca^{2+} ions may be temporarily bound to special sites on the sarcolemmal surface for one or more beats prior to being transported into the sarcoplasm by subsequent action potentials.[7,23] The action potential also spreads from the myocardial cell membrane down the extensive *transverse tubular (t) system*, which consists of sarcolemma invaginations, especially near the Z bands, that are in direct continuity with the extracellular or interstitial space (see Chap. 2 for anatomic details). During the passage of the action potential, the t system allows for the rapid activation of the entire myocyte. The action potential descends the t system near the Z bands into *triadic junctions*, in which a single t-system tubule is in extremely close proximity to, but not in open communication with, two terminal *cisternae*, or extensions (lateral sacs), of the SR, which contain the calcium-release channels of the SR. The latter, often called ryanodine receptors,[34] are opened by the

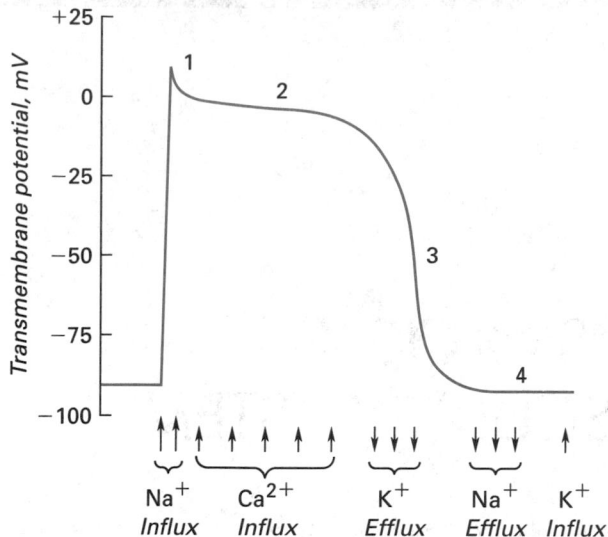

FIGURE 3-1

Schematic action potential of human ventricular myocardium together with probable electrolyte movements. The initial phase 0 spike and overshoot is related to a sudden influx of Na^+. This is followed by a slower, maintained influx of Ca^{2+} during the plateau phase 2. The phase of Ca^{2+} efflux is not well defined for human ventricular myocardium, but presumably it occurs during phase 4.

Ca^{2+} that enters through voltage-gated L-type calcium channels in the sarcolemma. Because the small Ca^{2+} influx releases much more Ca^{2+} for activating contraction, this process is termed *calcium-induced calcium release.*

The SR is an extensive system of intracellular tubules more or less floating in the sarcoplasm and surrounding the myofibrils. It has many branches near the transverse tubules and the surface membranes (sarcolemma) and invests every myofibril in the cell. While the SR is present in all mammalian cardiac cells, the t system is usually present where the cells are relatively large and serves to extend the surface membrane deep into the fiber. In small atrial fibers and cells of the conduction system, the t system is generally absent.

The mechanism by which the action potential depolarization "signal" is transferred from the sarcolemma and the t system to the intracellular sarcoplasmic reticulum occurs when the relatively small initial transsarcolemmal calcium flux releases large amounts of Ca^{2+} from the SR into the sarcoplasm (Fig. 3-2). This Ca^{2+} binds to troponin C, which is one of four regulatory proteins (tropomyosin-troponin) in the thin filament that normally inhibit actin from interacting with myosin in the thick filament (see below). When Ca^{2+} is bound to troponin C, this inhibition is removed and sites of actin can now interact with myosin, permitting the sarcomere to contract (Fig. 3-3). Ca^{2+} is released from the terminal cisternae (or vesicles or lateral sacs) of the SR through channels that, because they bind to the plant alkaloid ryanodine, are called *ryanodine receptors* (Fig. 3-4). The heart's mitochondria may serve as a buffer under conditions of high cellular Ca^{2+} load.[35,36] Additional Ca^{2+} enters through Ca^{2+} channels during the later portion of the plateau phase of the

action potential, and a small amount of Ca^{2+} enters by the Na^+/Ca^{2+} exchanger. Neither appears to contribute to the continued calcium-triggered calcium release, which is initiated by Ca^{2+} entry via L-type calcium channels. Instead, this late-entering Ca^{2+} is stored in the SR to provide Ca^{2+} for subsequent contractions.[11,21,22,24–29,33,37]

The increase in sarcoplasmic "free," or "activating," Ca^{2+} allows this cation to bind to the troponin C component of the troponin-tropomyosin complex, which is located along the thin actin filaments. In the absence of Ca^{2+}, troponin and tropomyosin, which are found with actin in the thin filament, prevent actin from interacting with myosin. There are three proteins in the troponin complex: troponin C, which binds Ca^{2+}; troponin I, which interacts with tropomyosin so as to keep actin from associating with myosin; and troponin T, which attaches these units to tropomyosin. Once Ca^{2+} binds to troponin C, a conformational change occurs in these regulatory proteins that allows the formation of cross-bridges between myosin and actin, resulting in contraction.[11,14,21,22,24–29,33,38] This allows adenosine triphosphatase (ATPase) enzyme sites on myosin cross-bridges to interact with actin. The result is transduction of energy in myosin-bound adenosine triphosphate (ATP) and magnesium, which allows cross-bridge motion and myocardial contraction to occur through the sliding filament mechanism. An increase in the free Ca^{2+} concentration from 5×10^{-7} to 6×10^{-6} M results in the production of approximately 90 percent of the maximum force. The increased sarcoplasmic Ca^{2+} also stimulates myocardial energy production by activating glycogen phosphorylase, which results in increased glycogenolysis; phosphofructokinase, which increases glycolysis; and pyruvate dehydrogenase, which stimulates the citric acid cycle. The energy for myocardial contraction is obtained when ATP is split by the ATPase site on the myosin cross-bridges during their interactions with actin.

Relaxation occurs when the rise in cytosolic Ca^{2+} increases the uptake of Ca^{2+} into the SR, thereby causing Ca^{2+} to dissociate from troponin C.[28,39–44] The Ca^{2+} taken up by the calcium pump (SERCA), located mainly along the longitudinal tubules of the SR, diffuses back to the terminal cisternae within the SR. A smaller amount of Ca^{2+} is pumped back into the interstitial space by a plasma membrane calcium pump (PMCA).[42–46] Relaxation is regulated by another protein, phospholamban, which, when phosphorylated, increases the rate of Ca^{2+} uptake by sensitizing the SR ATPase to Ca^{2+}.[47] This phosphorylation is initiated by activation of the β_1 receptors on the cardiac cell surface membrane, which not only increases Ca^{2+} entry into the myocardium, thus increasing force development, but also increases relaxation rates by phosphorylating phospholamban. Phosphorylation of troponin I, which reduces the Ca^{2+} affinity of troponin C, also facilitates relaxation.

The primary transport system for the efflux of Ca^{2+} from myocardial cells appears to be the Na^+/Ca^{2+} exchanger, in which one calcium ion leaves the cell in exchange for three sodium ions, which are subsequently pumped out of the cell

FIGURE 3-2

Two Ca^{2+} cycles regulate excitation-contraction coupling and relaxation in the adult mammalian heart. Key structures are diagrammed in *A*. The major Ca^{2+} fluxes are shown in *B*, where the thickness of each arrow indicates the magnitude of the Ca^{2+} flux and the direction of each arrow describes the "energetics" of the Ca^{2+} fluxes: *downward arrows* describe passive Ca^{2+} fluxes and *upward arrows* described energy-dependent Ca^{2+} transport.

In the extracellular cycle, Ca^{2+} enters the cell from the extracellular fluid via plasma membrane Ca^{2+} channels A. In the adult heart, most of this Ca^{2+} triggers Ca^{2+} release from the sarcoplasmic reticulum; a small portion directly activates the contractile proteins (A_1). Ca^{2+} is transported uphill, out of the cytosol into the extracellular fluid by two plasma membrane systems: the Na^+/Ca^{2+} exchanger (B_1), and the plasma membrane Ca^{2+} pump (B_2). In the intracellular Ca^{2+} cycle, this ion is released into the cytosol from the subsarcolemmal cisternae of the sarcoplasmic reticulum during activation (C), and pumped back into the sarcotubular network of the sarcoplasmic reticulum during relaxation (D). Ca^{2+} diffuses within the sarcoplasmic reticulum in a third Ca^{2+} flux (G), returning to the subsarcolemmal cisternae where it is stored in complex with calsequestrin and other Ca^{2+}-binding proteins. Binding, (E), and dissociation, (F), of Ca^{2+} with the high-affinity Ca^{2+}-binding sites of troponin C allow changes in cytosolic Ca^{2+} to regulate the contractile process. Movements of Ca^{2+} into and out of mitochondria (H) can buffer cytosolic Ca^{2+} concentration when there is an abnormal Ca^{2+} overload. (Modified from Katz.[12] Reproduced with permission of the publisher and author.)

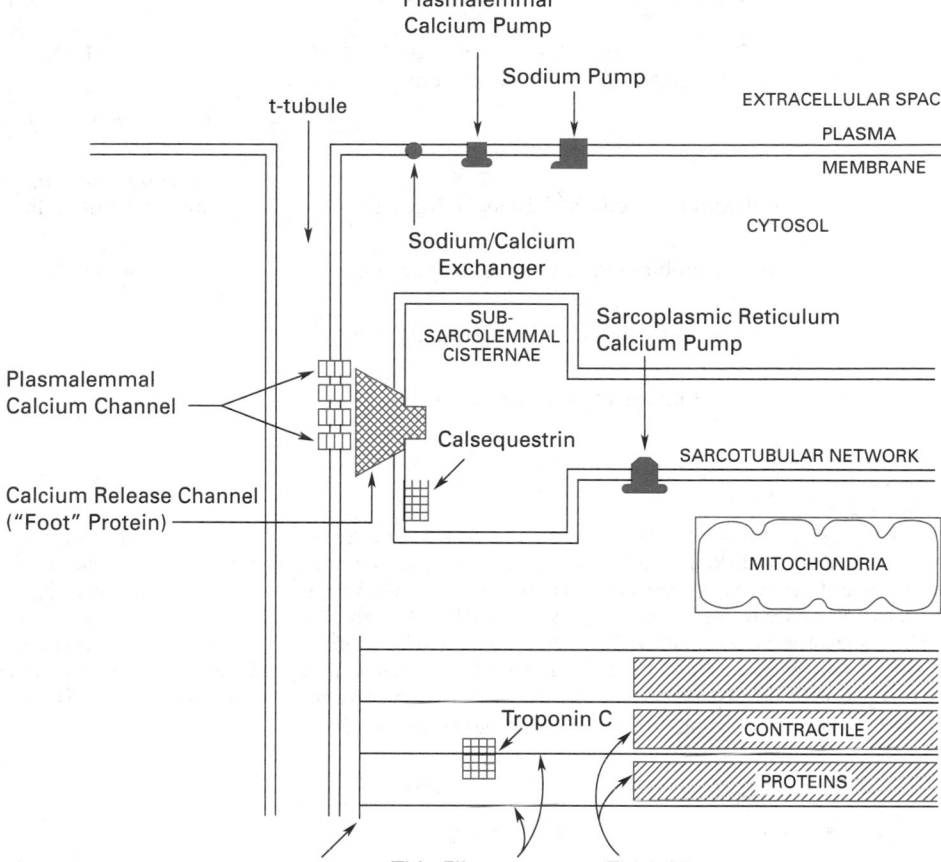

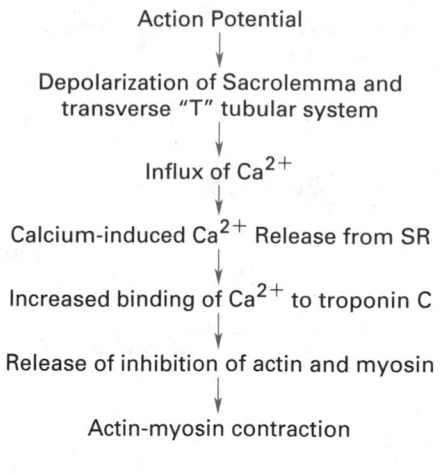

Action Potential
↓
Depolarization of Sacrolemma and
transverse "T" tubular system
↓
Influx of Ca^{2+}
↓
Calcium-induced Ca^{2+} Release from SR
↓
Increased binding of Ca^{2+} to troponin C
↓
Release of inhibition of actin and myosin
↓
Actin-myosin contraction

A

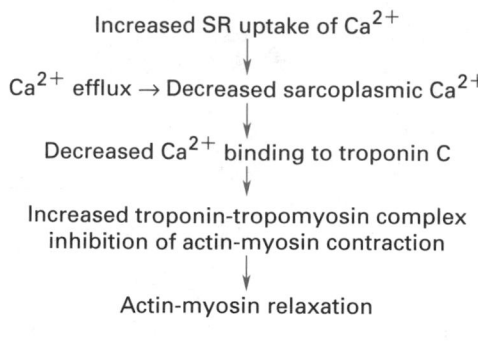

Increased SR uptake of Ca^{2+}
↓
Ca^{2+} efflux → Decreased sarcoplasmic Ca^{2+}
↓
Decreased Ca^{2+} binding to troponin C
↓
Increased troponin-tropomyosin complex
inhibition of actin-myosin contraction
↓
Actin-myosin relaxation

B

FIGURE 3-3

Schematic diagram of the events that produce (*A*) myocardial excitation-contraction coupling and (*B*) myocardial relaxation. With depolarization of the cardiac cell membranes [sarcolemma and transverse (T) system], the inward current carried by Na^+ channels opens L-type Ca^{2+} channels. The initial transsarcolemmal influx of Ca^{2+} triggers the release of Ca^{2+} from the sarcoplasmic reticulum (SR). The Ca^{2+} in higher concentration then binds to troponin C; this produces conformational changes in the thin filament that exposes active sites on actin, allowing the interaction of actin and myosin

to produce contraction. Relaxation is initiated when the calcium pump of the sarcoplasmic reticulum (SERCA), which is activated by the rise in cytosolic Ca^{2+} concentration, pumps Ca^{2+} back into the sarcoplasmic reticulum. This lowers cytosolic Ca^{2+} concentration and dissociates Ca^{2+} from troponin C, which initiates conformational changes in the thin filament that again inhibit actin-myosin interactions, causing relaxation. During relaxation, Ca^{2+} is also pumped back to the extracellular space by a plasma membrane calcium pump (PMCA).

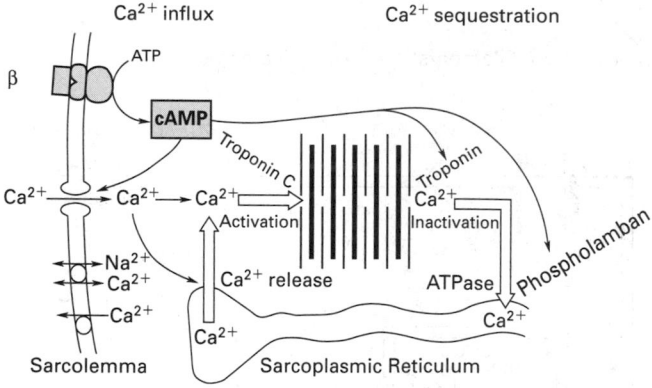

FIGURE 3-4

Effect of Ca^{2+} cycling on activation and inactivation of contractile proteins. Calcium influx across the sarcolemma initiates Ca^{2+} release from sarcoplasmic reticulum stores. Binding of this Ca^{2+} to troponin C allows interactions between the myofibrillar proteins actin and myosin, to utilize the chemical energy of ATP to effect cellular contraction. Intracellular Ca^{2+} concentration is then lowered by rapid sequestration of Ca^{2+} into the sarcoplasmic reticulum by the calcium pump, also called "sarco-endoplasmic reticulum calcium ATPase" (SERCA). The decrease in intracellular Ca^{2+} concentration removes this activator from the regulatory proteins of the thin filament. This dissociates actin and the myosin cross-bridges, with resultant cellular relaxation. Stimulation of sarcolemmal β-adrenergic receptors increases the intracellular concentration of cyclic AMP (cAMP), which augments contractility by increasing Ca^{2+} entry through plasma membrane calcium channels and also facilitates relaxation by phosphorylation of troponin I (which reduces its Ca^{2+} affinity) and of phospholamban (which stimulates the calcium pump of the sarcoplasmic reticulum.) (Adapted from Bonow RO, Udelson JE. Left ventricular diastolic dysfunction as a cause of congestive heart failure: Mechanisms and management. *Ann Intern Med* 1992; 117:502–510. Reproduced with permission from the publisher and authors.)

by Na^+, K^+-ATPase in exchange for two potassium ions.[10,12–15]

The velocity and the amount of tension developed by the actin-myosin myofilaments are directly related to the amount of Ca^{2+} available to induce contraction. It should also be noted that the Ca^{2+} that enters the cells via the plasma membrane calcium channels indirectly modulates myocardial contractility in subsequent beats by contributing to the stores of intracellular calcium. When the heart rate is abruptly increased, there is an associated progressive increase in contractile force, known as the *Bowditch, staircase,* or *treppe phenomenon.* A similar inotropic effect is also seen when the amount of Ca^{2+} available for activation is increased. Many drugs (such as digitalis,[26,47–51] sympathomimetic amines,[37,51–55] and phosphodiesterase inhibitors), as well as conditions such as an increase in heart rate,[56–59] paired pacing,[60] or postextrasystolic potentiation,[61] ultimately have their influence on myocardial contractility through their effect upon available intracellular Ca^{2+}.[11,24,26,52,62,63] The negative inotropic effect of acidosis upon myocardial contractility may also be related to a decrease in the Ca^{2+} sensitivity of the troponin complex and the quantity of Ca^{2+} released from the sarcoplasmic reticulum.[12,64] An increase in the intracellular Na^+ concentration decreases the influx of Na^+ via the bidirectional Na^+/Ca^{2+} exchange system and thereby decreases the efflux of Ca^{2+}. The net result is an increase in intracellular Ca^{2+} and in contractility.[11,24,26,65] Figure 3-5 diagrammatically illustrates the major components that regulate calcium homeostasis in myocardial membranes and that directly influence myocardial contractility by their influence upon intracel-

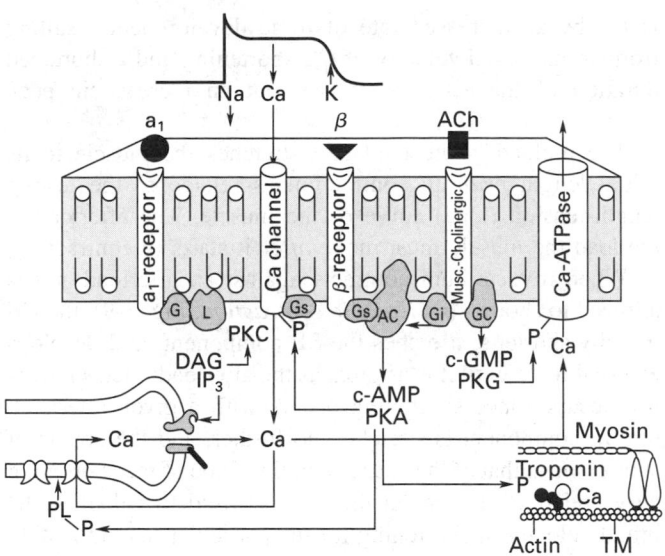

FIGURE 3-5

Schematic representation of adrenergic and cholinergic modulation of myocardial calcium. Alpha- and β-adrenergic receptor stimulation act synergistically to increase cytosolic calcium by both increased calcium entry and calcium release from the sarcoplasmic reticulum. Conversely, cholinergic stimulation can both directly (increase calcium extrusion) and indirectly (oppose action of adrenergic stimulation) decrease cytosolic calcium. Heterotrimeric G proteins, both inhibitory and stimulatory, act as signal transducers between activation of receptors and cytoplasmic changes leading to cellular response. AC, adenylate cyclase; ACh, acetylcholine; DAG, diacylglycerol; GC, guanylate cyclase; G_s, stimulatory G protein; G_i, inhibitory G protein; IP_3, inositol trisphosphate; L, membrane-bound phospholipase; PKC, protein kinase C; PKA, cAMP-dependent protein kinase, protein kinase A; PKG, cGMP-dependent protein kinase, protein kinase G; PL, phospholamban; TM, tropomyosin. (From Billman GE. Cellular mechanisms for ventricular fibrillation. *News Physiol Sci* 1992; 7:254–258. Reproduced with permission from the publisher and author.)

lular Ca^{2+}. It is also clear that at shorter sarcomere lengths, the Ca^{2+} sensitivity of troponin is reduced, which decreases force development at short sarcomere length.

Digitalis, which binds to and inhibits the plasma membrane Na^+-K^+-ATPase and thereby inhibits the active extrusion of sodium that enters with each systole in exchange for potassium, produces much of its effect by increasing intracellular Na^+, which, by inhibiting Ca^{2+} efflux through the Na^+/Ca^{2+} exchanger, results in an increased concentration of intracellular activator Ca^{2+} [26,43,50,51] (see Chap. 23). Other conditions that increase intracellular Na^+ may also increase myocardial contractility. [26,65] Significant abnormalities in the many calcium fluxes shown in Fig. 3-4 are present in the myocardium of patients with heart failure (see Chap. 21).

FUNDAMENTAL MYOCARDIAL MUSCLE MECHANICS

The contraction of heart muscle is regulated by five distinct, although interrelated, factors:

1. The *preload* (Starling's law of the heart), which is the passive load that establishes the initial muscle length of the cardiac fibers prior to contraction. Preload is described by the resting length-tension curve in isolated muscle. In the intact heart, this comprises the diastolic pressure-volume curve.

2. The *afterload*, which is the sum of all the loads against which the myocardial fibers must shorten during systole, including the aortic impedance, the arterial resistance, the peripheral vascular resistance, the intraventricular pressure, acting through the Laplace relationship, and the mass of blood in the aorta and great arteries, as well as the viscosity of the blood.

3. The *contractility*, or *inotropic state*, of the heart, which is reflected in the speed and shortening capacity of the myocardium at a given instantaneous load.

4. *Diastolic compliance (distensibility)*, or *lusitropic state*, of the heart, which describes the ability of the heart to fill at any given diastolic pressure.

5. The *heart rate*, or frequency of contraction.

These five factors are interrelated in the intact organism and are not independent. As will be described, fiber length appears to influence primarily the number of active force-generating sites in the myocardium that are activated by a given amount of Ca^{2+}, which decreases as sarcomere length is decreased. In contrast, a change in the contractile state (or contractility) is related to a qualitative change in the force generated by the sites, that is, a change in their activations, with or without a change in their number, that is independent of changes in sarcomere length. [66–70] Before discussing these mechanisms, however, a brief review of fundamental myocardial mechanics as described by force-velocity-length relationships is appropriate. [71] More detailed discussions are presented in specialized reviews. [10,71–93]

Hill[94,95] suggested a model for muscular contraction that has been exceedingly useful for understanding myocardial mechanics and predicting their changes under a number of different circumstances. In this model (Fig. 3-6), muscle contraction behaves as if there were a *contractile element* (CE), which is capable of developing force and of shortening; a

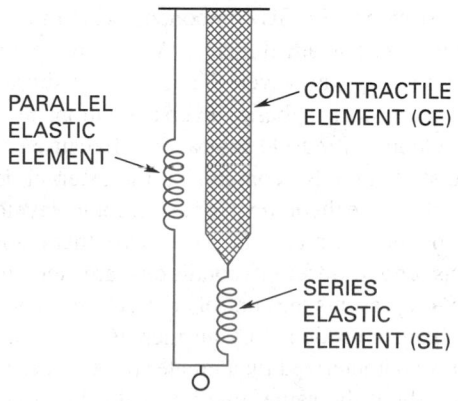

FIGURE 3-6

Hill's three-component model for muscle. See the text for details. (From Sonnenblick.[77] Reproduced with permission from the publisher and author.)

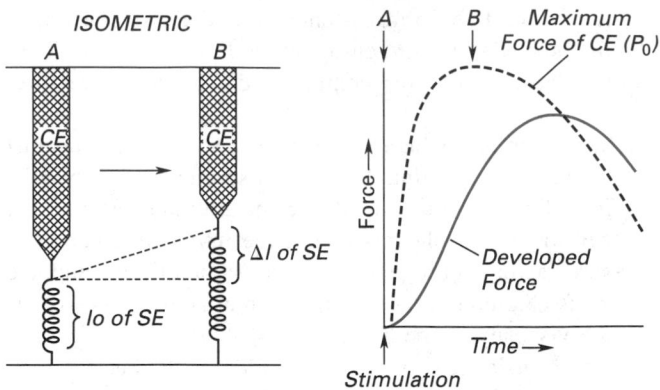

FIGURE 3-7

Schematic model of an isometric contraction of a strip of heart muscle. *Left:* The muscle model with a contractile element (CE) and a series elastic component (SE). The initial length of the SE (l_0) increases by Δl between A and B. *Right:* The time course of development of external force together with the hypothetical instantaneous force of CE that it might develop if no SE attachments were present. Point A, the initial resting state; Point B, some time during active activation. See the text for details. (From Sonnenblick.[77] Reproduced with permission from the publisher and author.)

series elastic (SE) *component*, which is passively stretched by shortening the CE; and a *parallel elastic component*, which supports resting tension but plays little role during contraction. The model does not denote specific anatomic sites of the components or, indeed, their arrangement. Rather, it describes how force and shortening are transferred from contractile sites to the external world, and anatomic reality is not implied. As such, it is a useful "working" model for understanding how isometric and isotonic contractions are related. In isolated muscle preparations, this SE component is created by damaged elastic ends of the muscle; in the intact heart, the SE component includes valves and elastic structures. For these reasons, when compared to skeletal muscle, the functional SE component of heart muscle is four to five times as compliant.

After stimulation of a strip of heart muscle that is not allowed to shorten (*isometric contraction*, Fig. 3-7), the CE is activated rapidly by the amount of Ca^{2+} available and begins to shorten at its maximal velocity (V_{max}). As the CE shortens, it stretches the SE component, which transmits the force to the external attachments. As the force in the SE component develops, however, the velocity of shortening declines in accord with a basic inverse relationship between force and velocity of muscle contraction. Because of the time required to stretch the SE component, the external developed force lags behind the theoretical force CE could develop (P_0) if no SE component were present. Three hypothetical isometric contractions under different conditions are shown in Fig. 3-8. Curve A represents the control contraction; curve B represents the changes produced by an increase in initial muscle length and is characterized by a greater peak force, P_0, which occurs after about the same time interval following stimulation; and curve C represents an increased frequency of contraction from curve B, illustrating the increased contractility mani-

fested by an increased rate of force development resulting from an increased velocity of CE shortening and a shortened duration of the active state, without an increase in peak force.

The preload is the load that stretches the muscle to its initial length *prior* to contraction as related to the resting length-tension (load) curve of the muscle. The afterload is the load the muscle must move *after* it starts to contract.

When myocardium contracts against an afterload and is allowed to shorten (an *isotonic contraction*, Fig. 3-9), the CE initially shortens, stretches the SE component, and develops external force until it is as great as the afterload; then shortening occurs. Once shortening occurs with a given afterload, the SE component is stretched no further, and the course of shortening is that of the CE. The initial slope of the shortening curve relative to time on the right is used to calculate the initial velocity of shortening for the particular load (P). With progressively increasing afterload, the time interval from stimulus to the onset of shortening is prolonged, but the time to maximal shortening is essentially unchanged (Fig. 3-10). In addition, the initial velocity of isotonic shortening for each load decreases with increasing loads. This basic curvilinear relationship is further illustrated in Figs. 3-11 and 3-12, in which the force-velocity relationships of isolated papillary muscles are plotted to illustrate the basic principle of a decrease in the initial velocity of shortening with increasing loads. As shown in Fig. 3-11, extrapolation of the curve to zero load yields the theoretical maximal velocity (V_{max}) of shortening of the CEs in the unloaded muscle. V_{max} in turn is altered by factors that modify the activation of the muscle but not by a change in initial muscle length within physiologic resting lengths.[2,71] Thus, it forms one index of the contractility of the myocardial fibers being examined.

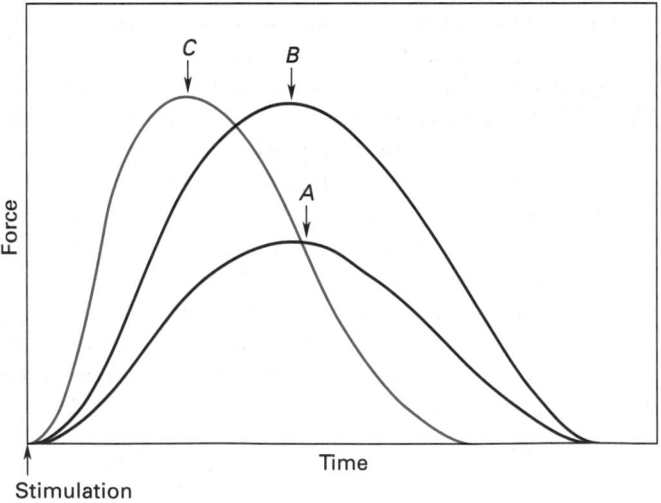

FIGURE 3-8

Hypothetical isometric force developed by three hypothetical contractions. A. Control. B. Increased initial muscle length. C. The muscle in curve B contracting more frequently. See the text for details. (From Sonnenblick.[77] Reproduced with permission from the publisher and author.)

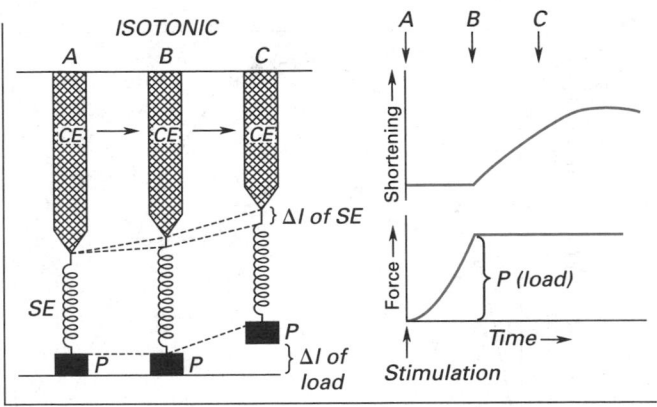

FIGURE 3-9

An afterloaded isotonic contraction of myocardium. On the left is the muscle model attached to a load P, which is supported when the muscle is at rest (A). This type of load P that is encountered by the CE only when the CE attempts to shorten is the afterload, whereas the small load used to stretch the system to its initial length is the preload. With stimulation of the system, the CE begins to shorten at maximum speed V_{max}. During the isometric portion of the contraction, between A and B, the CE shortens, the SE matches the load P, and the load starts to move. Once the load begins to move to point B, the SE remains constant in length, and shortening of the system reflects shortening of the CE alone. The curves on the right reflect force and shortening as functions of time after stimulation. The tangent to the slope of the curve of initial shortening is used to obtain the initial velocity of isotonic shortening for a given load. After plotting the initial velocity of shortening for different loads, one may extrapolate the curve to zero load to obtain the theoretic intrinsic or maximal velocity V_{max}. See Fig. 3-11. (From Sonnenblick.[77] Reproduced with permission from the publisher and author.)

PRELOAD IN THE INTACT HEART: THE FRANK-STRAUB-WIGGERS-STARLING PRINCIPLE

In 1871, Bowditch[96] showed that if the condition of the heart muscle remains unaltered, contractions remain equal in strength, regardless of the strength of stimuli applied. This *all-or-nothing law of the heart* implied that cardiac muscle either does not contract at all or responds to the fullest extent, but that the magnitude of the all-or-none response is determined by the inherent "condition" of the muscle, what we now term its *contractility*, or *relative degree of activation*. In 1884, Howell and Donaldson[97] showed that the heart itself has intrinsic mechanisms by which its output is adjusted to the venous input, in that increasing the venous return increased cardiac output and stroke as well as right atrial pressure. In 1895, Frank[98] correlated the reactions of cardiac muscle with the responses of skeletal muscle. Force of contraction, as previously shown by Fick,[99] von Kries,[100] and Blix,[101] was related to the initial length and resting tension. Frank studied the frog atria and ventricles and showed that, within limits, stepwise increases in diastolic volume and pressure just before contraction—the presystolic or end-diastolic volume and pressure—determine the magnitude of the all-or-none response.

In 1914, Wiggers[102] demonstrated that the reactions established by Frank for the frog's ventricle also apply to the

naturally beating right ventricle of dogs. He concluded that the rate of isometric pressure rise and the peak systolic pressure are determined by changes in the initial tension, as long as marked changes in inherent contractility are not simultaneously produced by experimental procedures. Also in 1914, Straub[103] and Starling and associates[104,105] independently reported their studies of the effect of changes in initial tension and length on the response of isolated hearts. The general principle of these studies is often referred to as the *Frank-Starling law of the heart*.[106]

In 1951, Wiggers[107] pointed out that, although there is a general impression that the often-reproduced representation of the law by Starling and associates was based on data from their own experiments, the published curves were reproductions of graphs previously published by Blix and by Frank. Although it is not certain whether the responsiveness of the heart is fundamentally related to changes in presystolic pressure (initial tension) or to changes in volume (initial length), fiber length and resting tension are interrelated.

Wiggers[107] also emphasized the importance of other factors affecting the responsiveness of the myocardium and stressed that the statement of the law of the heart, in which the energy of contraction is a function of the length of the muscle fiber, should be modified by the phrase "under equivalent states of responsiveness," or what today one would call contractility.[108] Sarnoff and Berglund[109,110] demonstrated this principle as a "family of curves" relating stroke work to

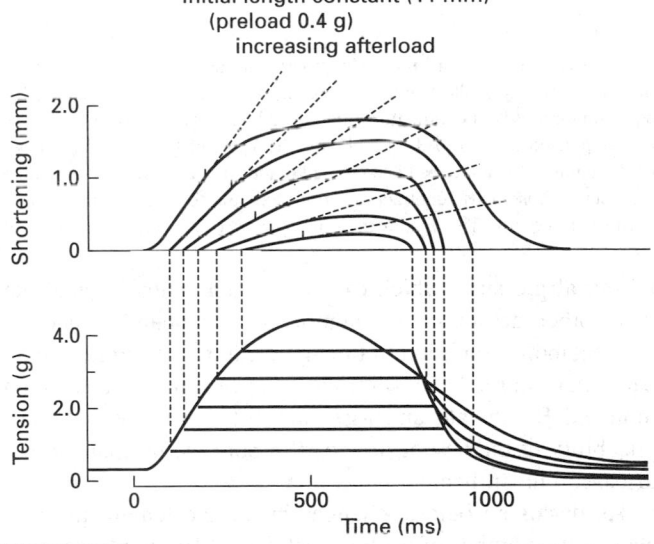

FIGURE 3-10

A series of superimposed tracings made from isolated papillary muscle that was arranged in such a manner that both initial isometric contraction and subsequent isotonic shortening are possible. *Below:* Serial isometric contraction at increasing afterloads (*horizontal lines*). *Above:* Successive isotonic shortening corresponding to the increasing afterloads in the lower tracing (*dashed lines*). The dashed lines on the upper tracing represent the initial velocity of shortening. As the afterload increases, the initial velocity of shortening decreases and the extent of shortening decreases, but the isometric relaxation phase increases. (From Sonnenblick.[77] Reproduced with permission from the publisher and author.)

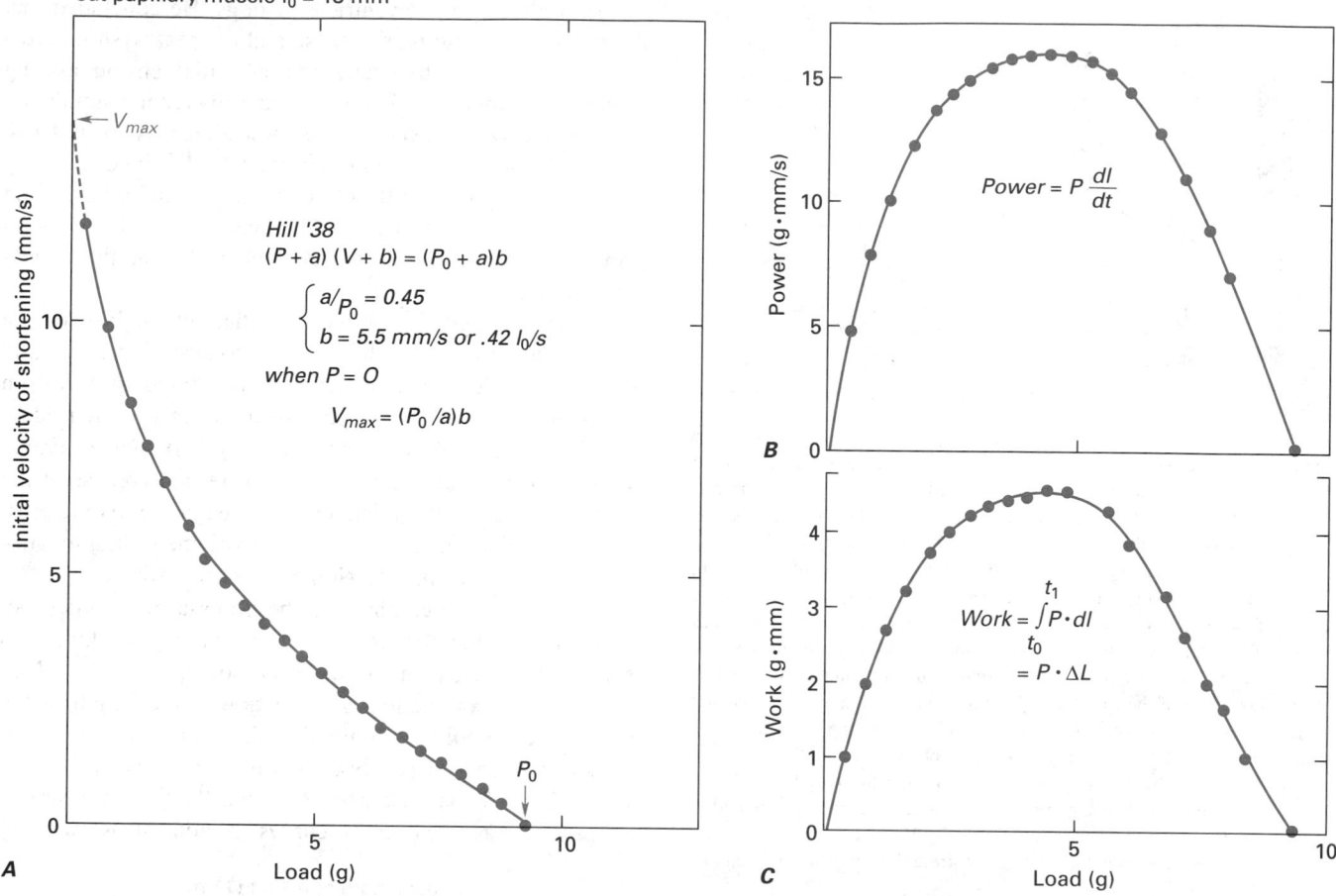

Cat papillary muscle l_0 = 13 mm

V_{max}

Initial velocity of shortening (mm/s)

Hill '38
$(P + a)(V + b) = (P_0 + a)b$
$\begin{cases} a/P_0 = 0.45 \\ b = 5.5 \text{ mm/s or } .42 \, l_0/s \end{cases}$
when $P = O$
$V_{max} = (P_0/a)b$

P_0

A   Load (g)

$Power = P\dfrac{dl}{dt}$

Power (g·mm/s)

B

$Work = \int_{t_0}^{t_1} P \cdot dl$
$= P \cdot \Delta L$

Work (g·mm)

C   Load (g)

FIGURE 3-11

A. Force-velocity relationships of a papillary muscle, illustrating the decreasing initial velocity of shortening with increasing loads. The insert gives Hill's equation for muscular contraction with the derived constants. When the curve is extrapolated to zero load, one obtains the V_{max}, or the intrinsic velocity of shortening. When the load is increased to the point at which no shortening can occur (an isometric contraction), the maximum force is manifest (P_0 or intrinsic force). *B.* The load versus the power (force versus velocity of shortening). *C.* The load versus work (force or load versus displacement). Note that peak power and work are obtained at loads approximately 50 percent of the maximal force of contraction P_0 obtained during isometric conditions. Instantaneous force-velocity of shortening is measured at a constant time after stimulation by quick-release techniques. (From Sonnenblick.[77] Reproduced with permission from the publisher and author.)

left atrial pressure, which exists for each ventricle, and that many other factors, such as humoral agents, neural influences, and metabolic condition of the myocardium, determine which particular "curve" the ventricle is operating on at a given moment. Braunwald and associates[2,111,112] showed the applicability of the law of the heart in both the normal and the diseased human heart.

As discussed below, changes in muscle length not only change the number of bridges that can be formed to develop force but also affect the amount of force produced by the same amount of Ca^{2+} activation.[66-69,72] Thus, although V_{max} is not altered by changing muscle length, the sensitivity of the contractile system to Ca^{2+} is length-dependent. In this sense, muscle length (preload) and contractility (inotropism) are interrelated.

Although pressure and volume (initial fiber length) are related, the relationship may be altered under certain circumstances. *Distensibility*, or *compliance*, is the ratio of change in ventricular volume to change in ventricular diastolic pressure ($\Delta V/\Delta P$), while ventricular *stiffness* is the reciprocal, or the change in pressure for a given change in volume ($\Delta P/\Delta V$).[93,113-121] Steady-state compliance determined just before systolic contraction comprises only part of the determinants of ventricular filling. Early ventricular filling following closure of the aortic valves depends on rapidity of the ventricular relaxation, with *elastic recoil* creating a gradient of rapid early ventricular filling. This active elastic recoil depends on a small end-systolic volume and helps early filling, especially during tachycardia. Late filling depends on passive diastolic compliance as well as completed ventricular relaxation. Defining changes in compliance is especially complex in certain pathologic conditions. For example, with chronic volume overloads, eccentric hypertrophy moves the curve relating diastolic volume to pressure to the right so there is greater volume for any given filling pressure and a greater volume at zero filling pressure (V_0). Nevertheless, at larger volumes, very small changes in volume may produce large diastolic pressure changes that are consistent with increased wall stiff-

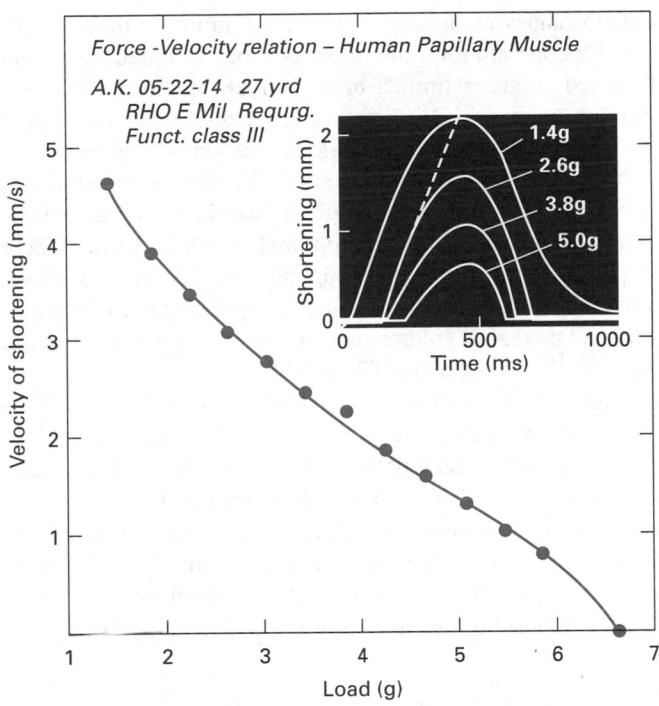

FIGURE 3-12

Relationship between the initial velocity of isotonic shortening and afterload of a human papillary muscle stimulated at a rate of 12 stimuli per minute. The preload was 1.4 g, with a muscle length of 15 mm. Note the significant decrease in initial velocity as the load increases. The insert shows four recordings with different afterloads; the decrease in rate of shortening with increasing afterload is apparent from the altered slopes of the length-time curves (From Sonnenblick et al.[74] Reproduced with permission from The American Society for Clinical Investigation and the author.)

ness. Thus, the curve is changed with increased compliance at small volumes but with reduced compliance at large volumes. Such alterations reflect ventricular wall remodeling due to the volume overload (see Chap. 21).

Most of the recognized changes in static ventricular compliance occur chronically. Conditions that may change ventricular compliance include ventricular distension, resulting in increased compliance; ventricular hypertrophy, resulting in reduced compliance; fibrosis; infiltrative diseases; pericardial tamponade or constriction; lymphatic obstruction; engorgement of the coronary circulation; ventricular septal hypertrophy; or disease or dilatation of the contralateral ventricle (decreased compliance). Aging is also associated with an increase in ventricular stiffness or decreased compliance, reflecting age-dependent myocyte loss, fibrosis, and reactive hypertrophy.[122,123] Except in response to hypoxia, ischemia, acidosis, afterload, or tachycardia, significant acute changes in the pressure-volume relationship or in the relaxation and distensibility of ventricles probably do not occur, nor do many inotropic agents produce significant acute changes.[113,120,124] On the other hand, the rate of ventricular relaxation can be increased by late systolic loading or catecholamines.[125–127] There is some evidence that some calcium channel blockers and other agents may favorably influence early relaxation and distensibility, particularly in the hypertrophied heart.[128–130]

Marked tachycardia and asynchrony also influence relaxation and ventricular filling[131,132] (see also Chap. 21).

Ventricular distensibility is often significantly influenced by filling of the opposite ventricle, especially when filling pressures are acutely elevated with an intact pericardium.[133–139] Thus, the pressure-volume relationships of one ventricle can be immediately influenced by acute changes in the filling of the contralateral ventricle. At cardiac catheterization, it is possible to obtain reasonable estimations of ventricular end-diastolic volumes (EDV) and end-systolic volumes and very accurate measurements of end-diastolic pressure (EDP). As discussed in Chap. 21, the ventricular EDP may be elevated either by an altered compliance due to myocardial hypoxia, fibrosis, infiltrative processes, pericardial tamponade or constriction, or failure or by ventricular hypertrophy itself.[2,113–117,121,140,141] The term *lusitropy* is used to refer to the diastolic properties of myocardium and cardiac chambers.[142]

The Frank-Starling law of the heart is one of the major mechanisms by which the normal right and left ventricles maintain equal minute outputs even though their stroke outputs may vary considerably during normal respiration. Thus, if the right ventricle temporarily pumps more blood into the pulmonary circulation than the left ventricle pumps into the systemic circulation, the proper balance between the two pumps is soon achieved, since the venous return to the left atrium and ventricle causes the left ventricular end-diastolic fiber length to be greater, increasing left ventricular stroke output. In addition, a decreased left ventricular stroke output would eventually lead to decreased return of blood to the right atrium and ventricle, producing a decrease in right ventricular stroke output. By this mechanism the two ventricles, which function as two pumps in series, are able to balance their outputs and prevent pulmonary edema despite marked variations in stroke volumes (SV).

A left ventricular "function curve" is shown in Fig. 3-13, in which left ventricular SV is plotted as a function of left ventricular EDP. The initial ventricular function curves[109] utilized stroke work (stroke volume × blood pressure); however, SV and derived stroke work are greatly dependent on the blood pressure, and thus the use of SV is more appropriate. Because end-diastolic fiber length and intraventricular pressure are normally related to each other, it is common in clinical situations to measure left ventricular EDP, since fiber length is difficult to determine in patients. In Fig. 3-13, curve A represents a hypothetical normal left ventricular function curve. Curve B represents a "shift to the left" of the function curve of the same ventricle under the influence of sympathetic stimulation or the infusion of epinephrine, norepinephrine, or other catecholamines. Curve C represents a "shift to the right" of curve A, such as might occur with myocardial depression from hypoxia, cardiodepressant drugs, or myocardial "failure." Note that under normal conditions (curve A), very slight changes in fiber length, which can be produced by small changes in filling pressure, are associated with significant increases in SV. As mentioned above, this is one of the major

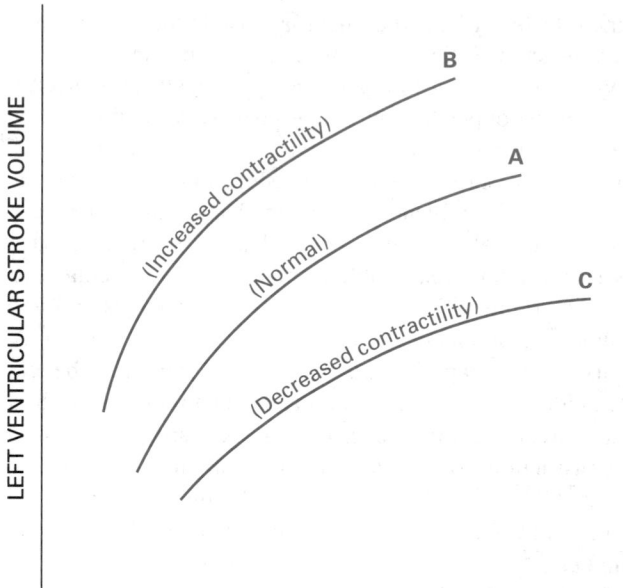

FIGURE 3-13

Relationship between left ventricular end-diastolic pressure and left ventricular stroke volume. A: The normal function. B: The shift to the left of the original curve associated with increased contractility, such as might result from sympathetic stimulation of the ventricle or the infusion of epinephrine or norepinephrine. C: A shift to the right of the original curve associated with decreased contractility, such as might result from ventricular failure from ischemia or myocardial depressant drugs. A ventricle functioning on a curve C might be restored to a curve A by the action of digitalis or inotropic drugs, such as norepinephrine or epinephrine. Similar but not identical curves are obtained when left ventricular stroke volume or cardiac output is plotted against left ventricular end-diastolic pressure or left atrial mean pressure. Function curves such as these may be obtained from both ventricles and both atria.

mechanisms by which the two ventricles have balanced outputs over any period of time, even though their stroke outputs may vary considerably from beat to beat, particularly during the respiratory cycle. Cardiac output is increased by an increase in preload (i.e., the Frank-Starling relationship) in many conditions, including those associated with an increase in venous return and a decrease in peripheral vascular resistance, such as exercise, anemia, fever, pregnancy, or other forms of peripheral arteriovenous fistulas. Changes in external pressure on the body, such as those encountered in immersion of the lower body in water, are associated with increased preload and increased intrathoracic blood volume.

Sympathetic stimulation increases cardiac output not only by producing an increase in heart rate but also by increasing the contractile force of both the atria and the ventricles, with a resultant increase in SV for any extent of filling. The increase in ventricular contractile force produced by sympathetic stimulation may be depicted graphically as a "shift to the left" of the ventricular function curve. Thus, sympathetic impulses can produce an increase in ventricular SV without the necessity of a change in end-diastolic fiber length or pressure. While there is good evidence that the normal heart utilizes alterations in preload (or the Starling law of the heart) during normal resting

circumstances or during exercise, the failing, dilated heart, which is operating on the upper portions of a depressed and flattened curve, is limited in the amount it can increase SV through increased filling pressure. At this point, the failing ventricle is operating at a higher portion of the pressure-volume curve where any increase in filling pressure produces only a very small increase in diastolic volume and the sarcomeres in the wall are at their optimal length (2.2 μm). There is probably no true descending limb for a function curve, although changes in afterload reflecting the Laplace relationship and increased volume may produce an apparent descending limb[143–146] (see also Chap. 21).

Figure 3-14 illustrates the interrelationships between ventricular EDV, EDP, and stroke work. As indicated in Fig. 3-14*A*, the relationship between SV and EDV is nearly linear. On the other hand, the relationship between EDP and EDV (Fig. 3-14*B*) is curvilinear, with a finite volume at zero pressure and a rather sharp increase in pressure above a certain volume. Figure 3-14*C* illustrates the resultant familiar curvilinear relationship between ventricular EDP and SV.

Ultrastructural Basis of Starling's Law

The length-tension relationship of a papillary muscle is shown in Fig. 3-15. The length of a myocardial sarcomere at which maximal force develops is approximately 2.2 μm after fixation, at which length the thin actin and thick myosin myofilaments are optimally overlapped to provide the greatest number of force-generating sites.[2,70,76,147–157] When the sarcomere is stretched beyond about 2.2 μm, the myocardium becomes very stiff and resting tensions rise greatly while developed tension starts to decline. In addition, actual damage to the myocardial cells and sarcomeres occurs when the fibers are excessively stretched.[145] In skeletal muscle, the actin and myosin myofilaments are completely disengaged at a length of 3.65 μm, and developed tension drops to zero. These long sarcomeres are seen only in skeletal fibers. Cardiac sarcomeres and cells are too stiff to become overstretched, so that longer sarcomere lengths at which force falls with increasing length are not seen physiologically. At sarcomere lengths less than 2.2 μm, the actin myofilaments first pass into the center of the sarcomere, and at 2.0 μm, they bypass one another and developed tension decreases. The cause for the decreasing force with decreasing length may be multifactorial. Of major importance is a decrease in Ca^{2+} sensitivity of sarcomeres as they become shorter. Interference of their filaments creating internal restoring forces may also play a role at shortened lengths.[69,158] As the papillary muscle in Fig. 3-15 is increasingly stretched, the resting tension increases, at first slowly and then more markedly. The stiffness of myocardial muscle can be defined as the slope of the curve relating the change in resting tension to the change in length. Relative to skeletal muscle, cardiac muscle is very stiff, with resting tension rising exponentially. If there is no resting tension, diastolic sarcomere length is about 1.95 μm. As sarcomeres reach 2.2 μm, resting tension is very great. Compressive forces occur in systole at shorter lengths, i.e., less than 1.95 μm, and this creates elastic recoil on relaxation.

A sarcomere length (after fixation) of 2.2 μm, which produces peak active tension (L_{max}), occurs in normal dogs at about the upper limit of normal left ventricular filling pressure (10 to 12 mmHg). At normal filling pressures, the sarcomere length in the midwall of the left ventricle varies from about 2.07 μm at end-diastole to 1.8 μm at end-systole.[150,151] Theoretically, the normal ventricle may have an ejection fraction (EF) of 55 percent with a shortening of individual sarcomere length of only 13 percent.[106,107] Endocardial sarcomeres

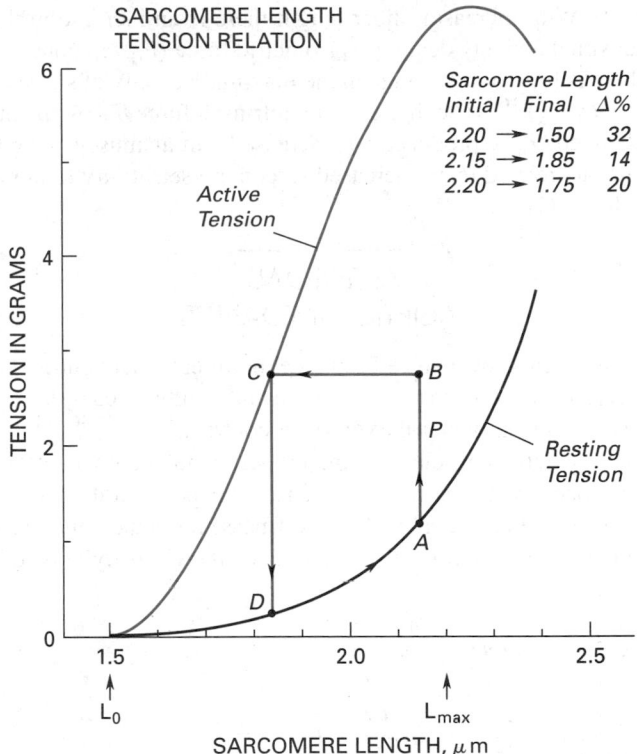

FIGURE 3-15

Relationship among papillary sarcomere length, resting tension, and developed or active tension. Note that active tension increases up to a sarcomere length of 2.2 μm (L_{max}) and then decreases. The resting tension increases markedly above a sarcomere length of 2.0 to 2.2 μm, which corresponds to an end-diastolic pressure of about 10 to 12 mmHg. The course of a normal contraction is shown in *ABCD*. Contraction starts at point *A* and develops a force equal to an imposed load *P*, reaching point *B*. The fiber then shortens until the active tension curve is reached at *C*, when relaxation occurs and returns the course to *D* at the end of systole. Normally, the ventricle functions on the ascending limb of the active tension curve at length below L_{max}, where greatest active tension develops, with sarcomere lengths between 1.8 and 2.2 μm. The descending limb of the length–active tension curve occurs at sarcomere lengths greater than L_{max}. There is normally moderate heterogeneity of sarcomere lengths in the heart, sarcomeres in the subendocardial layers tending to be longer and to shorten more than sarcomeres from the midwall or epicardium. In patients with marked ventricular dilatation, most of the dilatation is due to rearrangement and plastic "slippage" of the muscle fibers and myofibrils together with an increase in length of fibers due to synthesis of sarcomeres in series rather than to stretching of individual sarcomeres. (From Sonnenblick et al.[147] Reproduced with permission from the American Heart Association and the authors.)

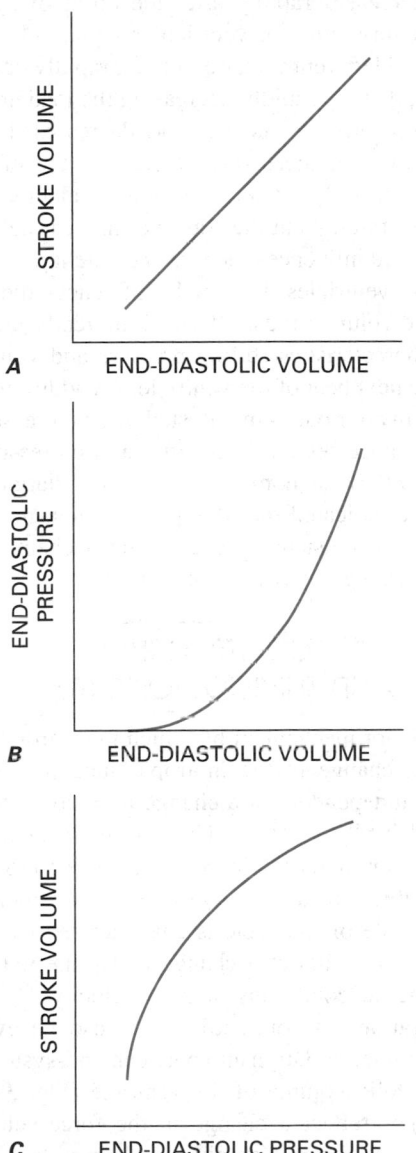

FIGURE 3-14

Illustration of the approximate interrelationships among stroke work, ventricular end-diastolic volume, and end-diastolic pressure. *A*. The relationship between stroke volume and end-diastolic volume is nearly linear. *B*. The relationship between end-diastolic pressure and end-diastolic volume is curvilinear, with a definite volume at zero pressure and a rather sharp increase in pressure above a certain volume. *C*. The familiar curvilinear relationship between stroke volume and ventricular end-diastolic pressure, similar to that shown in Fig. 3-13.

must, of course, shorten more than epicardial sarcomeres. Theoretically, 50 percent of the normal SV can be accounted for by the piston-like effect produced by about 25 to 35 percent ventricular wall thickening[159]; thus, the ejection of blood from the ventricles results from the generation of intraventricular pressure that is produced by both shortening and thickening of individual myocardial sarcomeres.

Influences of Fiber Length on Force-Velocity Relationships

The influence of increased initial fiber length on the force-velocity relationships of a papillary muscle is shown in Fig.

3-16. With increasing fiber length there is an increase in the maximal actively developed isometric force (P_0). In contrast, there is little or no change in the maximal velocity of shortening (V_{max}).[160] The increase in intrinsic force P_0 with unchanged V_{max} produced by increased initial muscle length appears related to an increased sarcomere sensitivity to intracellular Ca^{2+}.[66-68]

AFTERLOAD: AORTIC IMPEDANCE

It has been known since Frank's experiments that ventricular ejection and performance are significantly influenced by the resistance against which the ventricles contract.[104,107,146,161-168] For the left ventricle, the major peripheral components of afterload are the aortic impedance, the peripheral vascular resistance, the arterial wall (or stiffness) resistance, the mass of the column of blood in the aorta, and the viscosity of blood.

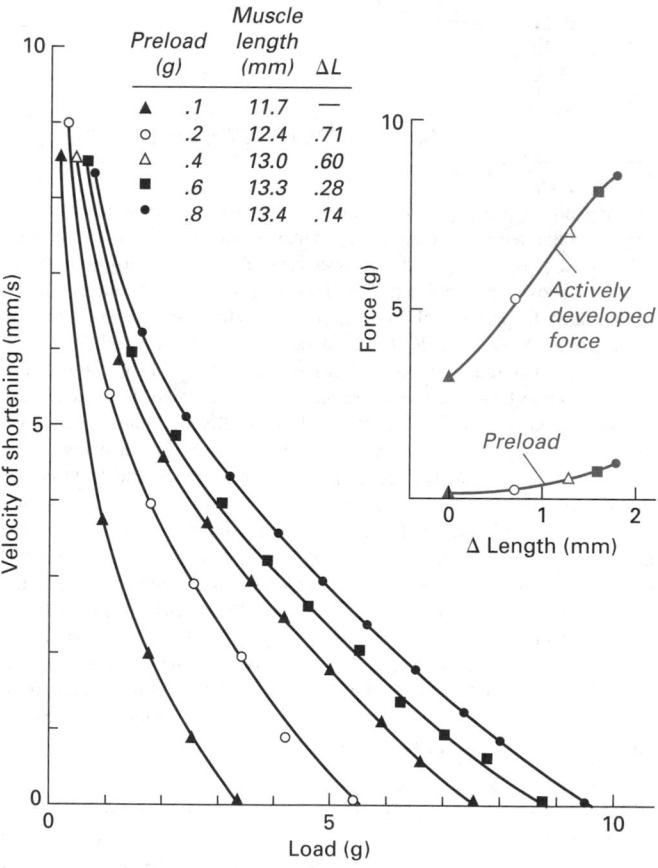

FIGURE 3-16
The effects of increasing initial muscle length on the force-velocity relationship. The initial velocity of shortening is plotted against preload, increases in which increase the initial length. In the insert, the maximal force developed is plotted against the change in muscle length. It is apparent that an increased muscle length produces little or no increase in V_{max}, the velocity of shortening at zero load obtained by extrapolation, but increases the actively developed maximal force P_0, which is produced under isometric conditions when the load is increased so much that no shortening can occur. (From Sonnenblick.[160] Reproduced with permission from the American Physiological Society and the author.)

The corresponding factors for the right ventricle are the main pulmonary artery impedance, the pulmonary vascular resistance, the mass of blood in the pulmonary circulation, and the viscosity of blood. In addition to these peripheral factors, the preload, or EDV, of each ventricle is a major determinant of ventricular afterload. Thus, the amount of blood in the ventricle at end-diastole directly determines the radius of the ventricle at the onset of systole and thereby (by the Laplace relationship) the amount of myocardial wall tension generated during the onset of the next ventricular contraction.

In conditions in which the volume of blood in the left ventricle decreases rapidly after the onset of systole (such as mitral regurgitation or ventricular septal defect), the total impedance to left ventricular emptying rapidly decreases during systole, thereby rapidly decreasing the load upon the ventricle significantly.[166] As the load decreases, the speed of muscle shortening increases. In general, the effects of afterload continuously influence the force-velocity-length-time relationships throughout the course of myocardial shortening. Since afterload influences the rate and extent of systolic emptying of the ventricles, it directly influences the ventricular end-systolic volume; thus, afterload indirectly influences the diastolic characteristics (filling pressure and volume or preload) of the next beat of the ventricle. An additional influence of changes in afterload is manifested by an increase in ventricular performance several beats after aortic pressure is raised (the *Anrep effect*, or homeometric autoregulation).[169] Some studies have indicated that this phenomenon may be due to recovery from transient subendocardial ischemia caused by the sudden change in arterial pressure.[170]

CONTRACTILITY AND THE INOTROPIC STATE

The third major mechanism by which myocardial function is altered is a change in the inotropic state (contractility) of the muscle independent of a change in preload (fiber length) or afterload.[2,16,68-91,171-179] The biochemical events that are responsible for increases in contractility, or inotropism, remain the subject of active investigation. An increase in the contractile state of a muscle is characterized by an increase in V_{max} with or without a change in P_0, the maximal force under isometric conditions at zero velocity[180] (Fig. 3-16). Acute alterations in contractility can also be evaluated by shifts in the linear relationship between end-systolic pressure and end-systolic volume of the ventricle (Fig. 3-12). All of these changes reflect a change in the force-velocity-length relationships of the myocardium and thus the ventricle, as noted below (see also Chap. 22).[71,181-187]

The change in contractility associated with an increase in heart rate occurring in both atrial and ventricular muscle is shown by the *force-frequency relationship;* it is also termed the *Bowditch effect,* or *treppe.*[57-59,74,76,79,178,179] In many conditions associated with an increase in heart rate, there is associated increased sympathetic stimulation of the myocardium, which activates adenylate cyclase, resulting in increased production of cyclic adenosine 3′,5′-monophosphate (cAMP, or second messenger), which causes an increased influx of Ca^{2+} through L-type calcium channels and an increase in myocardial contractility.

An increase in heart rate increases the contractile state, as shown by an increase in the velocity of shortening at any level of tension and by changes in location of V_{max}, obtained by extrapolating to zero load, without a change in P_0. An increase in heart rate also increases the rate of relaxation, or negative dP/dt.[188] Strophanthidin and norepinephrine both produce a significant shift to the right in the force-velocity curves and an increase in both V_{max} and P_0 in association with a decrease in the time from stimulation to peak shortening.[75] Increased contractility can also be characterized by a shift in the developed pressure (or developed tension) relative to filling pressure (or resting tension) as seen in Fig. 3-12. This dynamic relation can thus be portrayed by pressure-volume loops, which express force and shortening but not speed. Ventricular function curves (Fig. 3-13) express the same type of information but tend to be a less sensitive indicator of changes in the contractile state of isolated myocardium than a force-velocity curve.[79] The increased contractility produced by an increase in heart rate (the force-frequency relationship, or the Bowditch phenomenon)[56–59,78,178,179,188] affects pri-

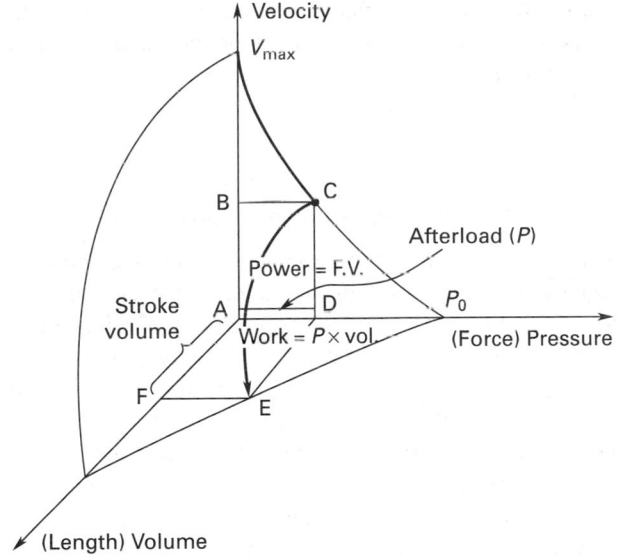

FIGURE 3-17

Force-velocity-length (force-velocity-volume) diagram of the intact ventricle. The force is the equivalent of load, which is the sum of preload (end-diastolic pressure) and afterload (aortic pressure). The length axis is derived from intraventricular volume. The superimposed dark line portrays the course of a single contraction. Starting at A, with activation, the contractile element (CE) velocity rises toward V_{max}. With CE shortening, force is built up and velocity of shortening decreases to C. This represents the isometric (isovolumic) phase of contraction. At C, the force equals the load, and shortening begins from C to E. During muscle shortening between C and E, velocity of shortening changes as a function of the decrease in muscle length that ensues. The rectangle on the force-velocity (vertical) plane represents calculated power ($ABCD$); the rectangle on the base represents work for a load P ($ADEF$). (From Sonnenblick.[77] Reproduced with permission from the publisher and author.)

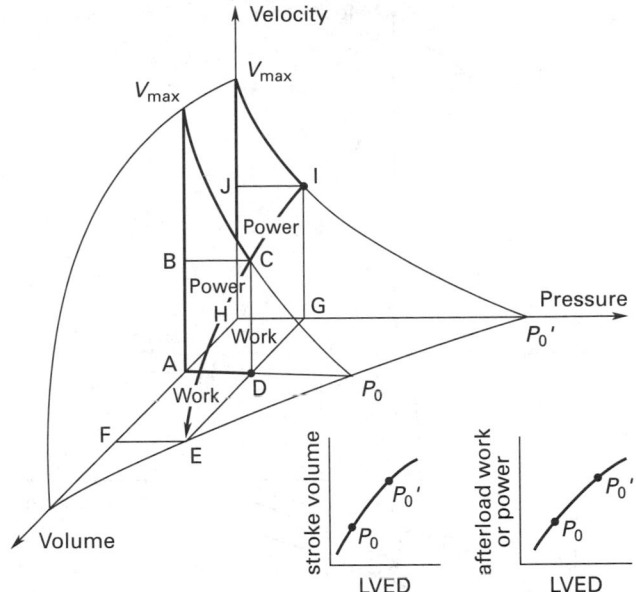

FIGURE 3-18

The effect of increasing preload (left ventricular end-diastolic pressure) on the force-velocity-volume relationship. Blood pressure remains the same. Maximum isometric force increases from P_0 to P_0'; work increases from $ADEF$ to $HGEF$, while power increases from $ABCD$ to $HGIJ$. This increase in the end-diastolic volume of the ventricle does not represent a change in the contractile state of the myocardium, since V_{max} is not changed. The insert in the lower right shows the predicted relations of stroke volume, stroke work, and stroke power to left ventricular end-diastolic pressure (LVED), reflecting changes in work and power areas from the three-dimensional diagram. (From Sonnenblick.[77] Reproduced with permission from the publisher and author.)

marily the speed of contraction and is thus more readily shown by force-velocity curves than by ventricular function curves. On the other hand, the increased contractility produced by large amounts of norepinephrine or by large increases in heart rate may be apparent in both types of curves.

The complex interrelationships among *force*, *velocity*, and *length* of both isolated myocardium and intact ventricles is best represented by a three-dimensional graph.[2,71,77,171,172] Figure 3-17 is a diagram of such a graph for a ventricle with the superimposed course of a single contraction; Fig. 3-18 illustrates the effect of increasing preload or initial muscle length; Fig. 3-19 illustrates the effects of an increased contractile state. This indicates that when contractility is augmented, the myocardium shortens faster at any given muscle length for any given load and also shortens further or generates more force. It should be noted that myocardial contractility at any moment can be well defined by the *surface* of the curved surface relating force, velocity, and length.[71]

When sympathetic stimulation causes the heart to beat with increased contractility and at a faster rate, not only is the contraction more forceful and faster, but the relaxation and elastic recoil of the ventricular musculature ("diastolic suction") are also more rapid.[188–194] Both the more forceful contraction and the more vigorous relaxation tend to increase the SV of the next beat, since the diastolic filling period is

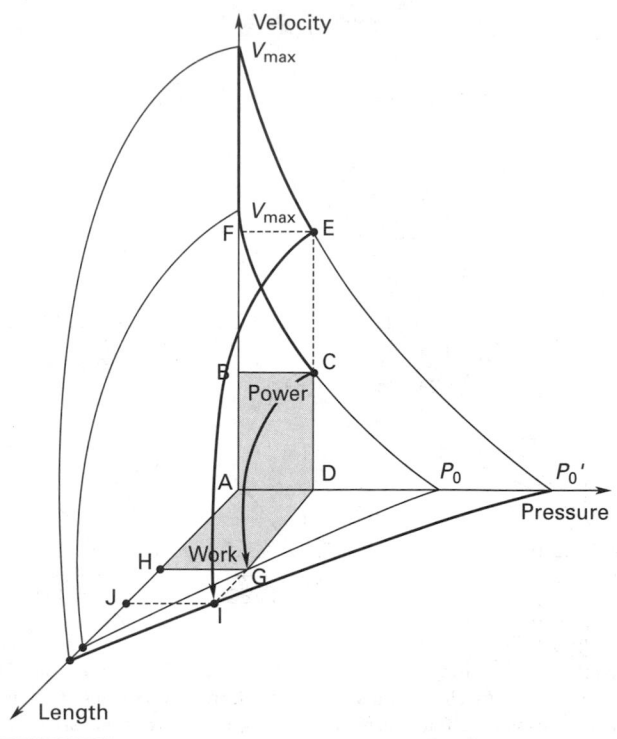

FIGURE 3-19

The effect of increasing the contractile state on the force-velocity-volume relation of the ventricle. Both V_{max} and P_0 are augmented, while the load (pressure) has been kept constant. Work and power are augmented. (From Sonnenblick.[77] Reproduced with permission from the publisher and author.)

longer than it would otherwise be and since, with the more rapid elastic recoil, the ventricular pressure is lower earlier and more rapidly, and possibly absolutely. The increased emptying produced by increased contractility also means that the fiber length will be less at the beginning of the next diastole. This shorter length tends to increase the distensibility of the ventricle, augment rapid early filling, and allow greater filling at a lower filling pressure.

DIASTOLIC COMPLIANCE (DISTENSIBILITY) AND THE LUSITROPIC STATE

The lusitropic state of the heart, which describes its ability to fill at any given diastolic pressure, is influenced not only by the passive viscoelastic properties of the heart's walls but also by dynamic interactions between the cardiac contractile proteins. The most important physiologic determinant of the ability of the ventricle to fill is β-adrenergic stimulation, which both desensitizes the contractile proteins to Ca^{2+} and increases the Ca^{2+} sensitivity of the calcium pump of the sarcoplasmic reticulum.[195,196] Together, these changes accelerate relaxation and, by reducing any Ca^{2+}-dependent tension that persists throughout diastole, can increase filling at any level of diastolic pressure. Energy starvation, as seen in the ischemic and failing heart, is probably the most important pathologic cause of a change in lusitropic state and plays an important role in the reduced diastolic compliance following myocardial infarction[197,198] (see Chap. 47). Other more slowly evolving

causes of loss of normal diastolic compliance include alterations in the extracellular matrix (e.g., fibrosis), abnormal geometry (e.g., hypertrophy), and pericardial constriction or tamponade.[142]

HEART RATE

The fifth major determinant of cardiac function is the heart rate, or the frequency of cardiac contraction. This is probably the major mechanism by which most individuals increase their cardiac output during periods of modest increased demand or exercise. An increase in heart rate may also increase myocardial contractility and relaxation and improve diastolic performance; the systolic force-interval relationship is known as *treppe*, the *staircase phenomenon*, or the *Bowditch effect*.[56–59,78,79,178,179,188] This effect is much more apparent in an anesthetized animal or depressed heart than in the intact, conscious state.[2,178,179,199] Even in the intact individual, however, the duration of each systole decreases as the heart rate increases, within limits. The rate of relaxation also increases with an increase in heart rate. Nevertheless, since there are more systoles per minute, the total time per minute spent in systole increases. Presumably, the increase in heart rate results in the release of more Ca^{2+} from the stores within the myocardial cell, thus enhancing myofibrillar contraction. The "recuperative effect of a long pause" upon the strength of contraction is known as the *Woodworth phenomenon*, or as the negative, or reverse, staircase phenomenon.[200,201]

MOLECULAR BASIS FOR EXCITATION-CONTRACTION COUPLING AND RELAXATION

The pumping action of the heart depends on interactions between the contractile proteins that transform chemical energy, derived from hydrolysis of the high-energy phosphate bonds of ATP, into mechanical work.[2,7,12–15] Activation of the contractile proteins is initiated by a signaling process, called *excitation-contraction coupling*, that begins when the action potential depolarizes the cell and ends when ionized calcium (Ca^{2+}) appears within the cytosol and binds to the Ca^{2+} receptor of the contractile apparatus. The Ca^{2+} fluxes into the cytosol that initiate systole are passive ("downhill") processes in which Ca^{2+} passes through open ion channels, while diastole depends on the active ("uphill") Ca^{2+} transport out of the cytosol by ion exchangers and ion pumps. These Ca^{2+} fluxes determine not only the onset and end of systole but also the intensity of the contractile process (inotropy) and the speed and completeness of relaxation (lusitropy) (Fig. 3-2).

Two key membrane structures, the plasma membrane and the sarcoplasmic reticulum, regulate contraction and relaxation in the adult human heart (Fig. 3-20). The plasma membrane is divided structurally into the sarcolemma, which surrounds the cell to separate the cytosol from the extracellular space, and the transverse tubular (t) system that penetrates deep into the cell. The t tubules, whose lumens open to the extracellular space, transmit the action potential into the cell interior, thereby facilitating the activation of the center of the muscle cell. Composite structures, called *dyads*, are formed by the membranes of the sarcolemma, or t system, and those of the SR (Fig. 3-20). The dyads contain the membrane proteins that couple membrane depolarization during the action potential to the release of activator Ca^{2+} during excitation-contraction coupling.

The SR, an intracellular membrane system that takes up, stores, and releases Ca^{2+}, is divided into two regions. The first is the *subsarcolemmal cisternae*, dilated extensions of the SR, which contain binding proteins that store Ca^{2+} within the cell and Ca^{2+}

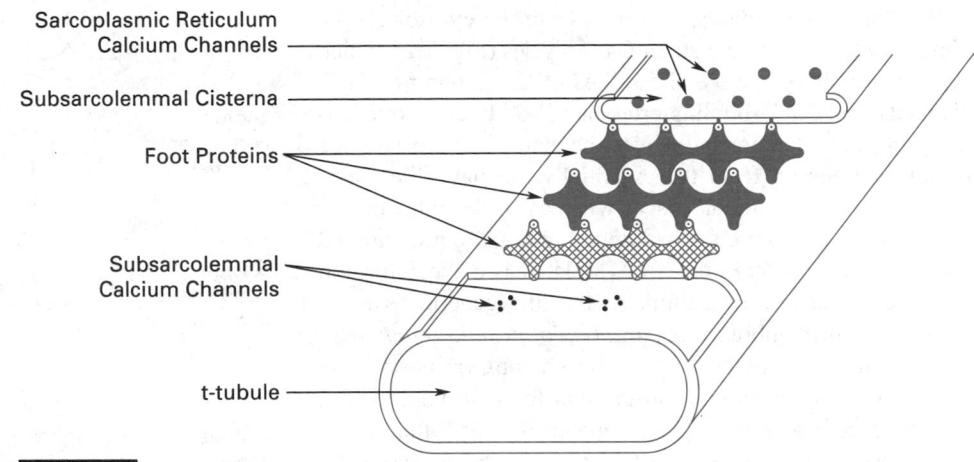

FIGURE 3-20
Schematic diagram of a dyad showing the Ca^{2+}-release channels (foot proteins) of the sarcoplasmic reticulum through which this cation leaves the subsarcolemmal cisternae of the sarcoplasmic reticulum. The Ca^{2+}-release channels, which are tetrameric structures that surround a central channel, are in close approximation to the plasma membrane Ca^{2+} channels. (From Katz.[12] Reproduced with permission from the publisher and author.)

channels that release this activator cation into the cytosol.[202] The second is the more extensive *sarcotubular network*, which surrounds the contractile proteins and contains a densely packed array of Ca^{2+}-pump ATPase proteins that transport Ca^{2+} out of the cytosol into the lumen of the SR to relax the heart.

As noted previously, excitation-contraction coupling begins when an inward Na^+ current depolarizes the plasma membrane and ends when Ca^{2+} is released from the intracellular stores for binding to troponin C. Relaxation, which involves much more than simply the reversal of the processes involved in excitation-contraction coupling, is brought about by entirely different structures. Major structures and their function in excitation-contraction coupling and relaxation are listed in Table 3-1 and depicted in Fig. 3-2.

Energy is needed for both contraction and relaxation, although this energy is used in different ways and by different structures in the two processes. During systole, chemical energy of ATP is released by the contractile proteins to effect muscle shortening and tension development, whereas during diastole, ATP is hydrolyzed by the ion pumps that remove activator Ca^{2+} from the cytosol. The latter is an active process because extracellular Ca^{2+} and the Ca^{2+} concentra-

tion in the SR are very high, about 1 mM, whereas the Ca^{2+} concentration needed to saturate troponin is 100-fold less ($\sim$10 μM). As both are much higher than the cytosolic Ca^{2+} concentration in the resting heart, Ca^{2+} fluxes that activate contraction are downhill, whereas those involved in relaxation are uphill and require the expenditure of energy.

TABLE 3-1

STRUCTURE-FUNCTION RELATIONSHIPS IN EXCITATION-CONTRACTION (E-C) COUPLING OF WORKING CARDIAC MYOCYTES

Structure	Role in E-C Coupling	Role in Relaxation
PLASMA MEMBRANE		
Sarcolemma		
Na^+ channel	Action potential upstroke	
Ca^{2+} channel	Action potential plateau	
	Ca^{2+}-triggered Ca^{2+} release	
Ca^{2+} pump (PMCA)		Ca^{2+} removal
Na^+/Ca^{2+} exchanger	Ca^{2+} entry (minor)	Ca^{2+} removal
Na^+ pump		Repolarization
		Na^+ gradient
Transverse tubule		
Na^+ channel	Action potential propagation	
Ca^{2+} channel	Ca^{2+}-triggered Ca^{2+} release	
SARCOPLASMIC RETICULUM		
Subsarcolemmal cisternae		
Ca^{2+}-release channel	Ca^{2+} release	
Sarcotubular network		
Ca^{2+} pump (SERCA)		Ca^{2+} removal
MYOFILAMENTS		
Actin and myosin	Contraction	
Troponin C	Ca^{2+} receptor	
Other proteins	Allosteric regulation	

Source: Adapted from Katz.[12] Reproduced with permission of the publisher and author.

The entry and removal of Ca^{2+} from the cytosol can be viewed in terms of two distinct Ca^{2+} cycles (Fig. 3-2), which involve members of several families of Ca^{2+} pumps, Ca^{2+} channels, and Ca^{2+}-binding proteins.[203,204] In the extracellular cycle, Ca^{2+} enters and leaves the cytosol by crossing the plasma membrane from the essentially inexhaustible Ca^{2+} store in the extracellular space, whereas in the intracellular Ca^{2+} cycle, this activator is pumped into and out of limited stores contained within the SR. The latter is a specialization of the endoplasmic reticulum, so that the generic term for these internal membranes is *sarco(endo)plasmic reticulum.*

The source of activator Ca^{2+} differs among various muscle types. In vascular smooth muscle and the embryonic heart, excitation-contraction coupling depends on Ca^{2+} that enters the cytosol from the extracellular space (the extracellular Ca^{2+} cycle), whereas the more specialized myocytes of skeletal muscle and the adult heart derive most of their activator Ca^{2+} from intracellular stores in the sarcoplasmic reticulum (the intracellular Ca^{2+} cycle). Both Ca^{2+} cycles are regulated by membrane proteins that are imbedded in a Ca^{2+}-impermeable phospholipid bilayer. These proteins include the Ca^{2+} pumps and exchangers that actively transport this cation uphill, back into the extracellular space and the lumen of the SR. The plasma membrane Ca^{2+} channels (extracellular Ca^{2+} cycle) and the SR Ca^{2+}-release channels (intracellular Ca^{2+} cycle) differ structurally, which reflects the fact that they are members of two distinct protein families. The ATP-dependent Ca^{2+} pumps in the plasma membrane and SR are members of a single family of "P-type" ion pumps that also includes the Na^+,K^+-ATPase. The Na^+/Ca^{2+} exchanger, which couples the downhill flux of Na^+ across the plasma membrane into the cell to the active transport of Ca^{2+} out of the cytosol, belongs to a different family of membrane proteins.

In skeletal muscle, the functional link between plasma membrane depolarization (the action potential) and the opening of intracellular Ca^{2+}-release channels is provided by a mechanical coupling that allows plasma membrane depolarization to remove a "plug" formed by part of an L-type plasma membrane Ca^{2+} channel that occludes the intracellular Ca^{2+}-release channel in the resting muscle.[204] In the heart, a different L-type plasma membrane Ca^{2+} channel couples membrane depolarization to Ca^{2+} release from the cardiac SR by a very different mechanism, in this case by opening to cause a localized increase in cytosolic Ca^{2+} concentration, called a *Ca^{2+} spark.*[205] This localized area of high Ca^{2+} concentration opens adjacent intracellular Ca^{2+}-release channels to cause a much greater Ca^{2+} release from the SR by a process often referred to as *Ca^{2+}-induced Ca^{2+} release.*[206,207]

The plasma membrane contains channels, named for the ions that they carry (Table 3-1); they are complex proteins made up of as many five subunits, called α_1, α_2, β, γ, and δ.[208–212] Most important are large proteins (called α or α_1 subunits in different channels) that make up and surround the channel pore (Fig. 3-21) and that determine ion specificity and contain the activation and inactivation gates that respond

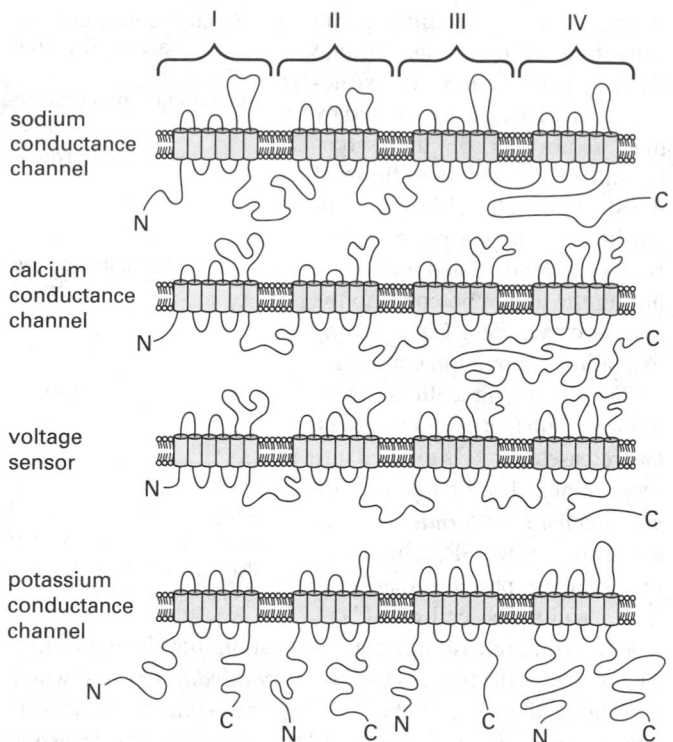

FIGURE 3-21
Four members of the family of ion channel proteins. The major subunits of the Ca^{2+} and Na^+ channels are tetramers made up of four covalently linked domains that are numbered I to IV. The voltage sensor that initiates contraction in depolarized mammalian skeletal muscle is a specialized Ca^{2+} channel that lacks a portion of the C-terminal amino acid sequence. K^+ channels also contain four domains, but unlike Ca^{2+} and Na^+ channels, these domains are not covalently linked. (From Katz.[12] Reproduced with permission from the publisher and author.)

to changes in membrane voltage by opening, closing, and inactivating the channels. The α and α_1 subunits of plasma membrane channels are tetramers made up of four domains, each of which contains six α-helical transmembrane segments (Fig. 3-22). The S_4 α-helical transmembrane segment, which is rich in charged amino acids, represents the "voltage sensor" that responds to membrane depolarization, generally by opening the channel; as described above, one exception is the Ca^{2+}-channel protein in skeletal muscle, where depolarization causes a conformational change. The "pore" region of the channel is made up of the S_5 and S_5 α-helical transmembrane segments and intervening sequence of amino acids, while many channels are inactivated by movements of the peptide chain that links domains III and IV.

In most plasma membrane Na^+ and Ca^{2+} channels, the four domains of the α and α_1 subunits are linked covalently to make up a single, large membrane protein (Fig. 3-21). The four domains in most potassium (K^+) channels, however, are members of a large family of proteins that are not linked covalently to each other, an arrangement that allows these domains to exchange amongst each other so as to generate a large and highly variable number of channel subtypes. This complexity is increased by interactions of these K^+ channel

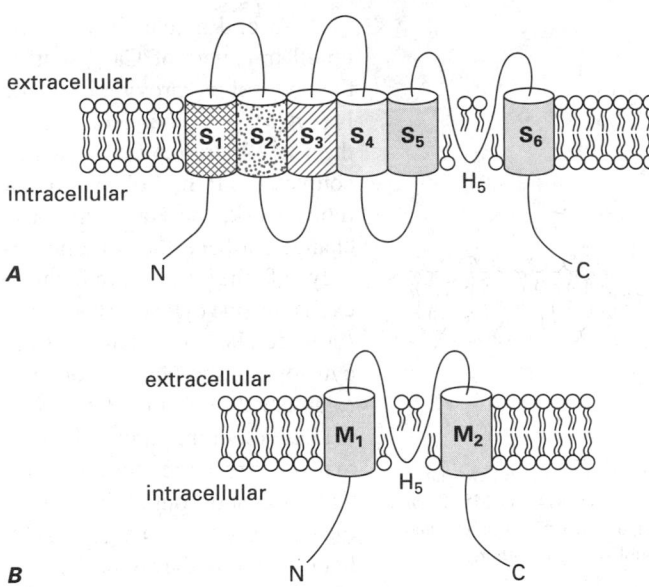

FIGURE 3-22

An ion channel domain. The ion channels depicted are tetramers made up of four domains, each of which contains six α-helical transmembrane segments. Known ion channel domains are believed to have evolved from a common ancestral protein. The S_4 segment, which is rich in positively charged amino acids, is believed to open the channel in response to membrane depolarization. The transmembrane segments S_5 and S_6, along with the intervening peptide chain that dips into the hydrophobic core of the membrane bilayer, probably surround the pore through which ions cross the lipid barrier in the core of the membrane bilayer. (From Katz.[12] Reproduced with permission from the publisher and author.)

subunits with other, smaller, peptides that consist of only a portion of the ancestral channel domain.[213–215] The major subunit of the L-type plasma membrane Ca^{2+} channels, called α_1, like that of the Na^+ channel, contains four covalently linked domains,[216–222] which illustrates the high degree of structural homology among these channels.

There are also several classes of the plasma membrane Ca^{2+} channels. In the heart, the most important members of this family are the L-type Ca^{2+} channels, which bind the familiar classes of Ca^{2+} channel blockers (*dihydropyridines* such as nifedipine, *phenylalkylamines* such as verapamil, and *benzothiazepines* such as diltiazem). These are sometimes called *dihydropyridine receptors* because of their high-affinity binding to this class of Ca^{2+} channel blockers. The T-type Ca^{2+} channels, a recently characterized class of plasma membrane Ca^{2+} channels, are involved in smooth muscle contraction and the sinoatrial (SA) node pacemaker but appear not to be important in excitation-contraction coupling.[34,204]

Intracellular Ca^{2+}-release channels (Fig. 3-23), whose structure differs considerably from that of the Ca^{2+} channels in the plasma membrane, are members of another family that includes at least two classes of related proteins.[212,223–226] The larger are the *ryanodine receptors*, found in the subsarcolemmal cisternae where they project into the space between the SR and plasma membrane or t tubule. This allows them to open in response to Ca^{2+} sparks, thereby mediating the step in excitation-contraction coupling where plasma membrane

depolarization initiates Ca^{2+} release from the SR. The role of the smaller *InsP₃ receptors*, which bind to and are activated by inositol triphosphate (InsP₃), in the heart is less clear (see below). Both the ryanodine and InsP₃ receptors are tetrameric structures, each subunit of which includes a large cytosolic domain and four α-helical transmembrane segments (Fig. 3-21). Although the InsP₃ receptors are only about half the size of the ryanodine receptors, there is considerable homology between these two classes of intracellular Ca^{2+}-release channel. For example, their three-dimensional structures are quite similar in that the four subunits are believed to surround a central pore through which activator Ca^{2+} is released when the channel is opened.

The explosive contractile responses of cardiac and skeletal muscle occur when the opening of high-conductance ryanodine-receptor Ca^{2+} channels releases large amounts of Ca^{2+} from the interior of the SR. The InsP₃ receptors, whose single-channel conductance is less than that of the larger ryanodine receptors,[225] are the predominant Ca^{2+} channels that initiate the much slower contractile responses in smooth muscle.[226] Because InsP₃ is generated by signal transduction systems that are activated by such chemical mediators as α-adrenergic agonists and angiotensin II, this process is called *pharmacomechanical coupling*. The function of the small numbers of InsP₃-regulated Ca^{2+} channels found in the heart is not clearly understood. Evidence that they release only a small amount of Ca^{2+} at a slow rate indicates that they are unable to participate in the beat-to-beat Ca^{2+} cycles that trigger excitation-contraction coupling. Instead, the InsP₃-regulated Ca^{2+} channels in the heart may regulate diastolic tension, and because the InsP₃-gated Ca^{2+} channels often participate in signal transduction systems other than those that activate muscle contraction, these channels may play a role in regulating cell growth, differentiation, and perhaps programmed cell death (apoptosis).[204]

The Ca^{2+}-pump ATPases are members of a family of closely related proteins that contain membrane-spanning α-helices and a large "head" that projects into the cytosol (Fig. 3-24). All couple hydrolysis of the high-energy phosphate bond of ATP to the uphill transport of Ca^{2+} out of the

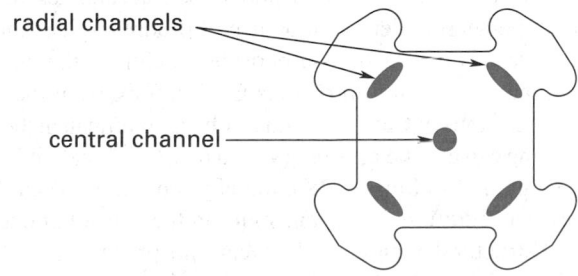

FIGURE 3-23

Schematic representation of the Ca^{2+}-release channel (foot protein) of the subsarcolemmal cisternae based on negative staining data showing fourfold symmetry. The central channel, which is surrounded by the four subunits of the protein, has been suggested to connect to four radial channels that lie in the foot (see Fig. 3-21) seen on the cytoplasmic surface of this membrane. (From Katz.[12] Reproduced with permission from the publisher and author.)

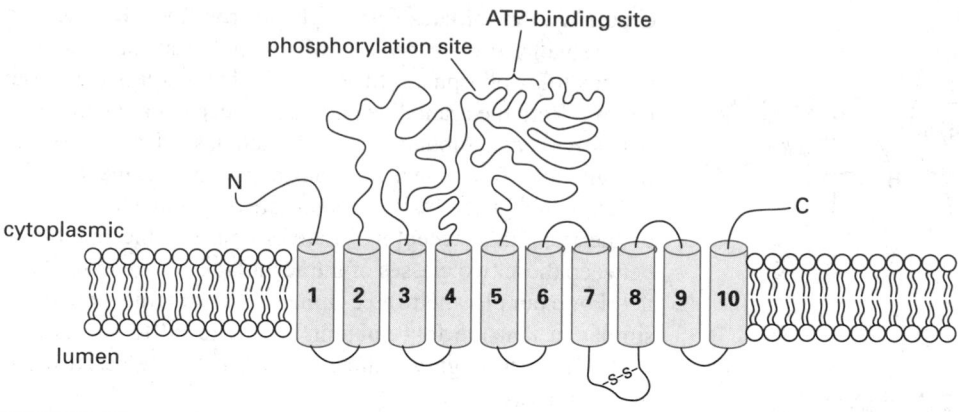

FIGURE 3-24

Depiction of the Ca^{2+}-pump ATPase showing 10 membrane-spanning segments (M1 to M10) and two large cytoplasmic loops. The ATP-binding site is found on the large cytoplasmic loop between M4 and M5. Polar amino acids in the membrane-spanning loops M4, M5, M6, and M8 may participate in Ca^{2+} binding and transfer across the bilayer. (From Katz.[12] Reproduced with permission from the publisher and author.)

cytosol.[43,227] Members of this family of proteins, which are found in the endoplasmic reticulum of noncontractile cells and SR of muscle cells, are called *SERCA* [sarco(endo)plasmic reticulum Ca^{2+}-ATPase], while the plasma membrane Ca^{2+} pump is referred to as *PMCA* (plasma membrane Ca^{2+} ATPase). The plasma membrane Ca^{2+}-pump ATPase molecule is larger than that of the SR, and both share a similar reaction mechanism that allows the energy released by ATP hydrolysis to pump Ca^{2+} out of the cytosol; however, they are regulated differently.

The SR Ca^{2+} pump is stimulated when cAMP promotes a phosphorylation reaction that transfers a phosphate group to phospholamban, an inhibitory membrane protein distinct from the Ca^{2+}-pump ATPase. When phosphorylated, phospholamban accelerates Ca^{2+} uptake from the cytosol[228,229] (see above). The larger plasma membrane Ca^{2+}-pump ATPase, on the other hand, is stimulated when the Ca^{2+}-calmodulin complex binds to an inhibitory site located on the C-terminal domain of the molecule.[43] This binding site is not found in the homologous SR protein but, like phospholamban, regulates Ca^{2+} transport out of the cytosol. Cyclic AMP–activated phosphorylation of phospholamban accelerates relaxation of the heart under the influence of β-adrenergic stimulation, whereas Ca^{2+}-activated phosphorylation of the plasma membrane Ca^{2+} pump promotes Ca^{2+} efflux from the cell under conditions of Ca^{2+} overload. [Phospholamban in the SR membrane can also be phosphorylated by a Ca^{2+}-calmodulin-dependent protein kinase (PK), thereby providing the cardiac myocyte an additional mechanism to rid the cytosol of excess Ca^{2+}.] Structural homologies between phospholamban and the inhibitory site on the plasma membrane Ca^{2+} pump suggest that these are related gene products, except that a separate gene for the analogous peptide chain in the SR Ca^{2+} pump encodes a distinct protein (phospholamban) that participates in β-adrenergic signaling, whereas the homologous C-terminal peptide chain of the ancestral Ca^{2+} pump remains attached to the ion pump where it stimulates the Ca^{2+} pump in response to a rise in cytosolic Ca^{2+}.

A second mechanism for the uphill transport of Ca^{2+} out of the cytosol is provided by the Na^+/Ca^{2+} exchanger. Unlike the Ca^{2+}-pump ATPase, which couples ATP hydrolysis to osmotic work, the Na^+/Ca^{2+} exchanger utilizes the osmotic energy of the Na^+ gradient to exchange one cytosolic Ca^{2+} ion for three Na^+ ions that enter the cytosol. As the Na^+ gradient is established by the Na^+,K^+-ATPase (sodium pump), the ultimate energy source for the uphill Ca^{2+} transport out of the cell via the Na^+/Ca^{2+} exchanger is ATP hydrolyzed by the sodium pump. The overall structure of the Na^+/Ca^{2+} exchanger differs markedly from that of the Ca^{2+}-pump ATPases. The ion exchanger is a larger membrane protein that contains twelve α-helical transmembrane segments.[230] Although the Na^+/Ca^{2+} exchanger contains a high-affinity cytosolic Ca^{2+}-binding site, the amino acid sequence of this Ca^{2+}-binding site does not show homologies to the cytosolic Ca^{2+}-binding proteins.[231]

Because the Na^+/Ca^{2+} exchanger moves three positively charged Na^+ ions across the membrane in exchange for one Ca^{2+} ion, it generates an electric current. This current, however, is small and of little importance in generating the normal action potential. Under conditions of Ca^{2+} overload, however, the exchanger can generate currents that depolarize the cell membrane, generally at the end of the action potential where these so-called transient depolarizations can be arrhythmogenic (see Chap. 26). In addition to its normally small effect on membrane potential, the charge movement associated with Na^+/Ca^{2+} exchange extensions influences ion exchange. The negative intracellular potential of the resting cell tends to "pull" Na^+ into the cell, so that during diastole the exchanger favors Ca^{2+} efflux. Reversal of membrane potential during systole, when the cell interior becomes positively charged, has the opposite effect to promote Ca^{2+} influx.

Although some of the Ca^{2+} stored in the SR is in a free, ionized form, most appears to be associated with Ca^{2+}-binding proteins within this intracellular membrane system.[227] Most important of the latter is *calsequestrin*, a 45-kDa protein that traps calcium within this membrane system. Other calcium-binding proteins found in smaller amounts include the 44-kDa protein *calreticulin* and a 170-kDa *histidine-rich calcium-binding protein*.

Mitochondria, of course, serve primarily to regenerate ATP, but they can also take up Ca^{2+}. The Ca^{2+} affinity of the mitochondrial Ca^{2+} pump is low, however, and mitochondrial Ca^{2+} transport at physiologic cytosolic Ca^{2+} concentrations is very slow.[232] Although these energy-producing structures do not normally play a role in the calcium fluxes involved in excitation-contraction coupling, the mitochondria can "buffer" cytosolic Ca^{2+} and so protect the myocardium from the detrimental effects of Ca^{2+} overload when abnormally large amounts of this ion gain access to the cytosol in pathologic states such as myocardial ischemia.

OTHER FACTORS INFLUENCING VENTRICULAR FUNCTION AND CONTRACTILITY

Sequence of Ventricular Contraction

Since the ventricular myocardial fibers contract sequentially, the strength of contraction of the later-contracting myocardial fibers theoretically is influenced by the strength, the rate, and the sequence of contraction of the fibers that contract earlier and that stretch the later-contracting fibers.[233–235] This phenomenon has been referred to as *idioventricular kick*,[236] in analogy with the increased ventricular filling and performance, the *atrial kick*, produced by atrial systole. An abnormal sequence of ventricular contraction or *dyssynergy* is also mechanically less efficient and relatively wasteful of energy, particularly if there are areas of akinesis or dyskinesis (see Chap. 43).

Ventricular Suction

Ventricular filling is enhanced by any increases in the pressure difference between the atrium and ventricle, whether produced by increased atrial pressure or by lower ventricular diastolic pressure. The latter phenomenon, which can be produced by increased elastic recoil and ventricular relaxation, is referred to as *diastolic suction*. One form is present normally during early diastole, immediately following opening of the atrioventricular (AV) valve, and its extent is inversely related to ventricular volume. During this earliest phase of rapid ventricular filling, the pressure in the ventricle *decreases* despite a rapid simultaneous increase in ventricular volume. Other forms of diastolic suction have been reviewed by Brecher,[237] although the physiologic significance of the phenomenon is still uncertain. This phenomenon enhances filling of the ventricle in early diastole, especially when the end-systolic volume is small.[193,238] Such a mechanism would be of special value during exercise, when tachycardia may limit the time for filling. Significantly, increases in contractility not only increase the rate of pressure change during systole (dP/dt) but also increase the rate of relaxation, reflected as negative dP/dt.[188,194] In the failing ventricle, where ventricular volume is large, diastolic suction is much less, and higher mean atrial pressures are needed to fill the ventricle.

Atrial Function

The atria have two main functions: a transport, or pump, function and a reservoir function to contain blood available for rapid ventricular filling.[239–244] Like the ventricles, the atria respond to an increase in fiber length by an increased force of contraction. Increased atrial contractility characterized by a shift to the left of atrial function curves (or a shift to the right of their force-velocity curves) may be produced by increased sympathetic stimulation, by inotropic agents such as digitalis or catecholamines, or by decreased vagal stimulation. Each of these causes the atrium to pump a greater amount of blood forward into the ventricle, with a resultant increase in ventricular end-diastolic fiber length and EDP (the *atrial kick*), thereby causing the ventricle to increase its force of contraction. When the atrial transport function is lost (e.g., by atrial fibrillation) in a person with an otherwise normal heart, the normal circulatory reserve mechanisms are able to maintain the cardiac output at rest within normal limits, although the response of the cardiac output to strenuous exercise is usually diminished. In a patient with ventricular disease, however, where compliance of the ventricle may be reduced and thus produce diastolic dysfunction, the mean diastolic pressure may be elevated and result in pulmonary congestion, and even the resting cardiac output may be diminished significantly by this form of *atrial failure* (see Chap. 21).

The atria and ventricles also produce atrial natriuretic peptides (ANPs) and brain natriuretic peptides (BNPs) that have natriuretic and diuretic actions and relax intestinal smooth muscle.[245–255] Some ANPs and BNPs also relax vascular muscle. It is probable that atrial distention triggers the release of ANP, leading to diuresis and natriuresis. ANPs also inhibit the production of aldosterone.[256] The importance of ANPs (or *atrial natriuretic factor*) and BNPs in normal homeostasis, congestive heart failure, or essential hypertension remains under active investigation.

Nervous Control[13,54,257–263]

The nerve endings of sympathetic fibers, which lie between the myocardial fibers, synthesize norepinephrine and store it in granules. Both atria and ventricles contain β_1 and β_2 receptors, with the atria usually having somewhat more. Other studies have indicated that β_2 receptors are located especially in vascular smooth muscle or in the SA and AV nodes.[264] On stimulation, sympathetic fibers cause the local release of norepinephrine, which binds to β receptors on the fiber surface. In reaction mediated by G proteins, this activates the enzyme adenyl cyclase, which catalyzes the conversion of ATP to cAMP.[265] Cyclic AMP activates cAMP-dependent protein kinases (PK A) that phosphorylate L-type calcium channels, increasing myocellular Ca^{2+} entry and myocardial contractility (inotropic effect)[54,55,195,196] (Fig. 3-5). At the same time, PK A phosphorylates two proteins, phospholamban, which causes the SR to take up Ca^{2+} more rapidly, and troponin I, which desensitizes the myofilaments to Ca^{2+}. Both reactions enhance relaxation (lusitropic effect). Once nerve stimulation stops, the same nerve endings take up and store norepinephrine for reutilization. A small amount of the norepinephrine is also metabolized locally. Sympathetic nerve fibers reach the entire atria and ventricles, as well as the sinus or SA and AV nodes, while vagal fibers, which cause the local release of acetylcholine, influence the atrial musculature and SA and AV nodes predominantly. Some vagal innervation, however, has also been shown to reach the ventricles, and vagal stimulation can decrease ventricular contractility modestly.[266] Further, vagal stimulation reduces the extent of the inotropic response produced by the sympathetic stimulation.[266] In general, sympathetic stimulation increases atrial and ventricular contractility, promotes relaxation, increases heart rate, and speeds the spread of excitation through the AV node and, very slightly, through the ventricles. The coronary vessels and heart muscle may also produce neuropeptides that can influence coronary vascular resistance and myocardial contractility.[267,268]

Vagal stimulation generally exerts effects opposite to those of sympathetic stimulation on the sinus node of the atria. At any given instant, the effect of the nervous system on the heart is the net balance of these two opposing controls, which usually vary reciprocally. It is probable that the vagal parasympathetic stimulation, which is generally inhibitory, normally predominates in the conscious state and maintains the usual resting heart rate of about 65 to 75 beats per minute. The resting bradycardia of exercise training is due predominantly to a slowing of the intrinsic rate of the sinus node pacemaker due to enhanced vagal activity in association with a decrease in the adrenergic influence.[269] Neural reflexes, particularly from stretch receptors in the carotid sinus and aorta, form a major extrinsic control mechanism that influences myocardial performance directly and indirectly.[258–261] When carotid sinus stretch decreases, as with arterial hypotension, a reflex venoconstriction is produced by the sympathetic nervous system that increases venous return and thereby increases ventricular end-diastolic fiber length. Simultaneously, carotid sinus hypotension produces reflex arterial vasoconstriction, increasing peripheral vascular resistance and aortic impedance. In addition, carotid sinus hypotension elicits reflexes that increase atrial and ventricular contractility. Stimulation of the carotid sinus nerve, such as might occur with carotid sinus hypertension, produces opposite effects.

Cardiac Renin-Angiotensin System

There is good evidence of a cardiac renin-angiotensin system that produces active peptides with physiologic effects. All of the components of such a system, [renin, angiotensinogen, angiotensin-converting enzyme (ACE), as well as the products angiotensin I and angiotensin II] have been localized in the myocardium.[270–274] In addition, angiotensin II receptors are found on cardiac fibroblasts and myocytes. This has led to the autocrine-paracrine theory, which suggests that local release of angiotensin II may mediate local responses such as cellular hypertrophy.[275] This system may also play an important role in responses to stress and in the presence of heart failure.[276]

Drugs and Hormones

Myocardial contractility is increased by an enhanced availability of Ca^{2+} ions inside the cell.[11,24–28] Increased Ca^{2+} bath-

ing the heart produces this action. Some of the major mechanisms that regulate myocardial cellular Ca^{2+} homeostasis are illustrated in Fig. 3-5. Catecholamines, including norepinephrine, epinephrine, and isoproterenol, act on β-adrenergic receptors on the myocardial cells, which activate a G protein as the signal transducer to activate adenylyl cyclase, increasing the production of cAMP, which in turn activates PK A that phosphorylates L-type calcium channels, resulting in increased intracellular Ca^{2+}.[277] As noted previously, PK A also enhances relaxation. These actions together result in a stronger but shorter contraction. Digitalis glycosides enhance contractility by inhibiting the Na^+,K^+-ATPase in the cell surface membrane, thereby leaving larger amounts of Na^+ within the cell, decreasing the Na^+/Ca^{2+} exchange and resulting in an increased concentration of Ca^{2+} within the fiber (Fig. 3-5)[50,51] (see also Chaps. 21 and 23). Contractility is also increased to some degree by glucorticoids, aldactone, angiotensin II, serotonin,[278] and glucagon.[279]

The physiologic role of other substances such as prostaglandins,[280] secretin,[281] neurotensin, endogenous opiates, and enkephalins and nucleotide and polypeptide systems such as kinekard, vasoactive intestinal polypeptide, and neuropeptide Y[267,282–284] in the regulation of myocardial contractility is unclear. Vascular endothelial cells release substances that may affect myocardial contractility, such as *endothelin*, which is also a potent vasoconstrictor.[285–295] Endocardial cells also appear to affect contractility.[296–300] Overall, these effects, when demonstrated, are relatively small and their relative importance is unclear (see below). The actions of thyroxine on myocardial contractile functions are complex, but in general its effects are to increase rates of contraction and relaxation (see Chap. 78).

Myocardial contractility is decreased by hypoxia and ischemia and by many drugs, including barbiturates, quinidine, procainamide, disopyramide, lidocaine, most beta blockers, and calcium channel blockers (Chap. 54). Acidosis also depresses myocardial contractility, particularly if the sympathoadrenal system function is impaired.[301] Morphine produces a very mild negative inotropic effect upon isolated myocardial strips, but in the conscious dog it can produce a β-adrenergic-mediated increase in myocardial contractility and α-adrenergic-mediated coronary vasoconstriction.[302]

A number of neuropeptides have been shown to have significant effects on myocardial contractility and coronary vascular resistance.[267,282–284] Some of these occur in significant amounts in the heart and may play important roles in the normal regulation of myocardial contractility and coronary blood flow.

Anesthesia

General anesthesia from halothane or pentobarbital may depress myocardial contractility significantly. In addition, the reflex control mechanisms influencing heart rate may be significantly altered by anesthesia. For example, in the conscious state, the reflex bradycardia of acute hypertension is caused mainly by withdrawal of sympathetic stimulation, while under anesthesia, it is caused almost entirely by parasympathetic restraint.[199] In the intact conscious animal, the force-frequency relationship (the Bowditch phenomenon) appears to influence myocardial contractility relatively little, whereas an increase in heart rate causes a much larger increase in contractility if the level of contractility is first depressed by generalized anesthesia.[199] Similarly, in anesthetized animals, the increase in heart rate produced by acute volume loading and presumed stimulation of low-pressure receptors in the atria (the *Bainbridge reflex*) is erratic; on the other hand, the reflex is consistently found in conscious animals and can be blocked by the combination of atropine and propranolol.[303] In contrast, the Anrep effect, or the positive inotropic effect of an acute increase in afterload, has been demonstrated in the anesthetized animal but is difficult to demonstrate in the conscious subject with a low spontaneous heart rate.[199]

Postextrasystolic Potentiation

When an extraventricular depolarization is imposed or occurs spontaneously between normal beats, the subsequent normal beat is potentiated. The extent of *postextrasystolic potentiation* is generally related to the closeness of the extra beat to the previous normal beat. The mechanism of this type of postextrasystolic potentiation is probably related to increased availability of calcium ions near the contractile sites of the actin and myosin myofilaments. Advantage has even been taken clinically of this phenomenon by placing an electrically induced extra beat close to the spontaneous beat and continuing it.[304–306] The clinical use of "paired electrical stimulation," which markedly increases myocardial contractility, is limited by the danger of inducing ventricular fibrillation.

MECHANISMS OF CARDIAC RESERVE

Normal homeostatic mechanisms regulate cardiac output to meet metabolic demands of the body, which can increase cardiac output five- to sixfold during exercise. It is not possible to separate sharply those mechanisms by which the cardiovascular system is normally controlled from those mechanisms of cardiac reserve (Table 3-2) that the heart may utilize to meet increased demands to maintain cardiac function in the presence of disease of the heart or circulatory system. Many of these homeostatic and regulatory mechanisms act synergistically in the intact organism; others, such as the sympathetic and parasympathetic nervous control of the heart, are in a state of constantly varying balance. Although the relative contributions of each mechanism in the experimental animal can be separated and quantified, in humans this is generally not possible. Indeed, the demonstration of mechanisms during physiologic experiments indicates only potential mechanisms of reserve or control, not what actually happens in the intact organism. Furthermore, since most of the mechanisms are interrelated and affect one another, the contribution of one mechanism depends on, and changes with, the contribution of

TABLE 3-2

MECHANISMS OF CARDIAC RESERVE

Increased heart rate
Increased stroke volume
Increased oxygen extraction
Redistribution of blood flow
Anaerobic metabolism
Cardiac dilatation
Cardiac hypertrophy

the other mechanisms. In the following discussion, some of these mechanisms will be considered from the standpoint of their use as forms of cardiac reserve, although many of the same mechanisms are utilized in the normal circulatory regulation (see also Chaps. 21 and 22).

The two basic mechanisms of cardiac reserve by which the heart or any other pulsatile pump can increase its output in the face of increased demand (or attempt to maintain output in the presence of myocardial disease) are (1) change in rate, and (2) change in stroke volume.

Heart Rate

A change in pulse rate is one of the simplest and most effective ways of increasing cardiac output in response to an increase in venous return. In individuals who are not trained athletes, under conditions of moderately increased demands, an increase in cardiac output occurs primarily by an increase in heart rate mediated by decreased parasympathetic (vagal) tone. An increase in heart rate by itself may mediate an increase in cardiac output about four- to fivefold in highly trained athletes. Above certain limits, however, cardiac output may actually begin to fall as heart rate rises. This rate is about 170 to 180 beats per minute for most normal young individuals but may be 200 to 220 in trained athletes or only 120 to 140 in older, untrained persons or in patients with heart disease. The decrease in cardiac output above a certain rate is due largely to the shortening of the time of diastole per minute, limiting the time for both adequate filling of the ventricles and coronary blood flow, which occurs primarily during diastole in the left ventricle.

Although an increase in heart rate may produce a modest increase in myocardial contractility and a shortening in the absolute duration of each systole,[56–59,76–78,178,179,186] negative inotropic effects of tachycardia can become apparent above a certain rate.[59] The shape of the curve relating heart rate to contractility varies according to species and the conditions under which it is studied. Most changes in pulse rate during normal activities are effected by decrease in vagal inhibition and by the addition of sympathetic stimulation of the sinus node of the heart during more vigorous stress.[237–261]

Stroke Volume

In a normal individual in the recumbent position, the ratio of left ventricular SV to EDV, termed the ejection fraction (EF), is about 60 to 75 percent and tends to be linear. Since the curve relating EDV to filling pressure is curvilinear, when EDP is substituted for EDV, the curve relating SV to filling pressure is curved and, due to the exponential rise in filling pressure relative to volume, tends to flatten at high filling pressures (Fig. 3-15).[71] Increased contractility may increase the EF and the SV with a decreased end-systolic volume, with the EDV either decreasing or remaining the same. An increased SV can also be produced either by a primary increase in venous return, which utilizes preload reserve and increases the end-diastolic fiber length of the atria and ventricles, or by a decrease in afterload, which permits enhanced emptying of the ventricle.[168] In the early stages of heart failure, since there is often an increase in EDV and fiber length, which tends to maintain the SV, the EF is decreased. Indeed, a decrease in EF is a hallmark of ventricular failure. Since SV is load-dependent, the EF may be increased when impedance of ventricular emptying is reduced (e.g., mitral regurgitation) or reduced when impedance is high (e.g., aortic stenosis) (see Chaps. 21 and 22).

Increased Oxygen Extraction

When the tissue requirements for oxygen increase or the supply of blood decreases, the tissues may, up to a point, extract more oxygen from the volume of blood passing through the tissue. The diffusion of oxygen into myocardial cells is facilitated by myoglobin, which has oxygen dissociation characteristics favorable to the diffusion of oxygen into the cells.[307] Increased oxygen extraction is a major reserve mechanism utilized by the tissues of the body acutely during extreme exertion or chronically when the cardiac output is diminished. This reserve mechanism is of less value to the myocardium, which even normally extracts about 75 percent of its arterial oxygen content.

Redistribution of Blood Flow

The redistribution of cardiac output is a major mechanism of reserve for the body under conditions of increased demand, as during exercise or under conditions of diminished cardiac output.[13,17,18,273,289,291,294,308–311] The general result is to maintain blood flow to the brain, the heart, and the tissues acutely requiring blood flow while sacrificing blood flow to tissues and organs not being utilized or less essential to immediate survival. The mechanisms by which this redistribution occurs are complex. Although the following explanation is oversimplified, redistribution may be considered the integrated response of two mechanisms: (1) a local autoregulation of the metabolically active tissue or organ, by which local changes in P_{O_2}, P_{CO_2}, pH, K^+ concentration, and other metabolic products and mechanical shear stress affect the endothelium of local blood vessels, reducing small vessel resistance and increasing blood flow (see below); and (2) an integrated response of the central nervous system, mediated by the sympathetic and parasympathetic nervous systems, producing vasodilation of the active or exercising organ and vasoconstric-

tion of many other tissues and organs. In addition, there often appears to be a venoconstriction mediated by the sympathetic nervous system, which increases venous return to the heart and performs a type of internal transfusion or shifting of blood from the large venous reservoirs to the heart, arterial system, and active organs.

Anaerobic Metabolism

Many tissues, particularly skeletal muscle, utilize anaerobic metabolism as a reserve mechanism, although the value of this mechanism for the myocardium is also quite limited. In a normal individual during moderate exercise, anaerobic metabolism may account for about 5 percent of the energy utilized; patients with heart failure may obtain 30 percent of their immediate total energy requirements by anaerobic metabolism during exercise.

Dilatation and Hypertrophy

Dilatation and hypertrophy are forms of compensatory reserve, in that, at least in the early stages of a response to overload, they tend to normalize wall stress.[312–314] Neither, however, represents perfect compensation. The maladaptive effects of dilatation are readily understood as arising from consequences of the law of Laplace, because augmented cavity dimensions increase wall stress, a major determinant of cardiac energy demands. Hypertrophy also has important maladaptive consequences that appear to reflect abnormalities that accompany the hypertrophic response itself.[315,316]

REGULATION OF REGIONAL BLOOD FLOW

The amount of blood flowing to an individual organ of the body is determined by the difference between the arterial and venous pressures in the vessels supplying the organ and by the vascular resistance of the organ. Although the arterial and venous pressures change in situations such as exercise, eating, or emotional stress, most of the alterations in the distribution of blood flow are the consequence of changes in vascular resistance of the organ.[5,13,17,273,289,291,294,308–311,317–323] The major mechanisms by which decreases in organ vascular resistance are effected are an increase in caliber of the vessels and an opening of new vascular channels. Since most of the vascular resistance appears to be located at the level of the small arteries and arterioles, it is probable that most of the regulation occurs by changes in caliber of these vessels, although changes in the capillaries and veins may at times play an important role. In a consideration of the local control of blood flow, several fundamental relationships and definitions should first be introduced.

The *resistance* to blood flow through a given portion of the circulation is usually expressed by the ratio of the mean pressure difference between two points in the vascular system to the mean amount of blood passing from one point to the other. It is usually calculated using mean pressures and flows, although most vascular flow is pulsatile. If it were possible to measure instantaneous pressure differences and flows accurately, it would be theoretically more proper to calculate vascular *impedance*, which is the ratio of pulsatile pressure to pulsatile flow and which varies with the frequency of the pulse. Vascular resistance may be expressed in various units: by *peripheral resistance units* (PRU), or pressure gradient (mmHg) per unit blood flow (mL/s); by Aperia's formula, to give results in absolute or metric (cgs, or centimeter-gram-second) units by multiplying PRU units by a conversion factor of 1332 to express resistance in terms of dynes · second per centimeter^5; or by the ratio of pressure gradient (mmHg) to blood flow (L/min) to give *R units*. R units may be converted approximately to dynes · second per centimeter^5 by multiplying by 80.

Minor changes in calculated resistance are usually of no significance, not only because of possible errors in pressure or flow measurements but also because changes in apparent resistance may result from the distending effect of inflow or exit pressures. Since resistance is the slope of the relationship of pressure to flow and this relationship is curvilinear, resistance can change merely by changing either pressure or blood flow. Moreover, if both are changing, the change in resistance is difficult or impossible to evaluate. In addition, alterations in the distending force may mask changes in the vascular bed. Because of such considerations and the nonlinear relationship between pressure and flow in most vascular beds, changes in calculated resistance cannot be equated simply with vasoconstriction or vasodilatation. This is particularly true if there are changes in both pressure and flow.

The relationship of the various factors affecting the resistance to fluid flow in rigid tubing is expressed by *Poiseuille's equation:*

$$\text{Fluid flow} = \frac{\pi(\text{pressure difference})(\text{radius})^4}{8(\text{vessel length})(\text{fluid viscosity})}$$

Since the experiments from which the equation was derived were performed in straight, rigid tubes with steady, streamlined flow of an ideal, viscous fluid, the relationship cannot be directly applied to the vascular system, in which the vessels are neither straight nor rigid, the blood is not a simple viscous fluid, and the flow is not always streamlined. Nevertheless, the predominant influence on flow of the radius of the vessel, which is raised to the *fourth* power in the above equation, is apparent. Of the other factors, changes in vessel length are thought to be ordinarily relatively unimportant; however, changes in viscosity related to changes in hematocrit, temperature, and serum protein levels are often of marked significance, particularly in small blood vessels. It should also be noted that in most vascular beds, most of the blood vessels are connected in parallel rather than in series. The total resistance of vessels connected in parallel is calculated by adding the *conductance* of each individual vessel (1/R, the reciprocal of the individual resistance) to obtain the total conductance of all the vessels (Fig. 3-25). Because of these relationships for vessels in parallel and in accordance with Poiseuille's law,

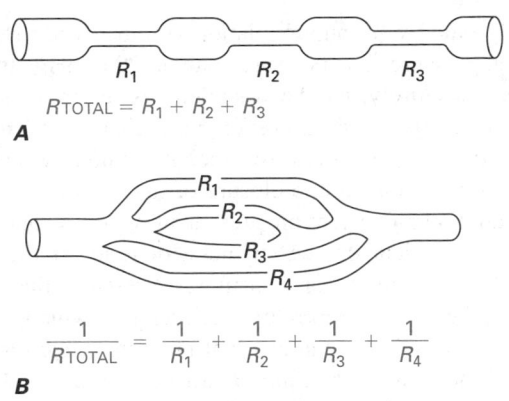

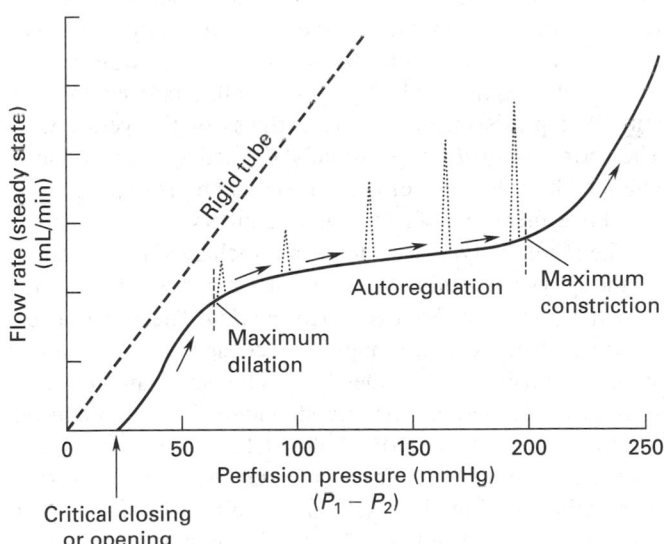

FIGURE 3-25

Comparison of the calculation of vascular resistance of vessels in series (*A*) and in parallel (*B*). In most vascular beds, most of the blood vessels of the same size are connected in parallel.

the resistance of four small tubes in parallel is four times as great as that of a single large tube of equal total cross-sectional area. Actually, it requires 16 small tubes with four times the total cross-sectional area to have a resistance as low as a single wide tube or vessel.

Since all normal blood vessels are distensible at least to some extent, it follows that increasing the *intraluminal pressure* will increase the *transmural pressure* on the vessel wall and increase the diameter and radius of the vessel. This effect is seen in Fig. 3-26, which illustrates the pressure-flow curve of an isolated peripheral vascular bed. Flow is maintained

FIGURE 3-26

Effect of perfusion pressure on flow rate in a rigid tube perfused with a Newtonian fluid (---) and in a vascular bed (muscle) perfused with blood (—). Note the autoregulation of steady-state blood flow within certain limits of perfusion pressure in the circulation through muscle. The dotted lines represent the immediate increase in blood flow, which declines to the steady level when vascular smooth muscle reacts to stretch and washout of vasodilator metabolites. (Figure modified by Dr. Badeer from Badeer HS. *Cardiovascular Physiology: A Synopsis.* Basel: Karger; 1984:146. Reproduced with permission from the publisher and author.)

relatively equally by autoregulation within a wide range of perfusion pressure. The pressure at about 20 mmHg, at which flow ceases entirely, has been sometimes referred to as the *critical closure pressure;* however, it is perhaps better referred to as the *critical flow pressure,* since it is unlikely that there is often complete anatomic closure of the vessels.

The amount of distention present in an individual blood vessel is dependent on the stiffness, or tone, of the vessel and on the distending, or transmural, pressure, that is, the difference between the intraluminal pressure, which tends to expand the vessel, and the external pressure, which tends to compress the vessel. The *tone,* or stiffness, of a blood vessel is determined by the geometry of the vessel and by the mechanical properties of the vessel wall. *Myogenic tone* refers to the contraction of vascular smooth muscle in response to stretch.[18,324–327] Such tone, which may be either maintained or rhythmic, is important in the local autoregulation of blood flow.

Important relationships between the distending pressure and the tension in the wall of a blood vessel are expressed in the following form of the *law of Laplace:*

$$\text{Wall tension} = \text{distending pressure} \times \frac{\text{vessel radius}}{2 \times \text{wall thickness}}$$

From this equation it is apparent that the tension in the wall of a blood vessel tending to expand it is greater either if the radius of the vessel is greater or if the blood vessel wall is thinner. Thus, veins with greater radii and thinner walls than their arterial counterparts have a greater wall tension than their arterial counterparts *at the same pressure.* As noted previously, the same considerations hold for the heart. The degree of stretching of the vessel wall produced by wall tension depends on the elastic stiffness of the vessel wall. The term *distensibility* is usually defined by the pressure-volume characteristics of a given vessel and is dependent on the above-mentioned factors, among others.

The regulation of vascular stiffness achieved by alterations in the physicochemical-mechanical properties of vascular smooth muscle is referred to as *vasomotion.* The major factors by which changes in vasomotion and changes in vessel caliber are accomplished are (1) metabolic, chemical, and hormonal substances carried in the blood and/or locally produced; (2) pressure (wall stretch); (3) flow (shear stress)[328,329]; and (4) the activity of fibers from the autonomic nervous system innervating the blood vessels and locally releasing norepinephrine or acetylcholine. The relative importance of these mechanisms varies markedly from one vascular bed to another and in different sizes of vessels in the same bed.[329] The relative importance is also significantly different at rest and during activity of the organ.

Most systemic arteries, and probably veins, respond to hypoxia and/or an increase in P_{CO_2} with vasodilatation.[305–308] The vasodilatation produced by hypoxia in many vascular beds is significantly augmented by an increase in K^+ concentration. Many substances are important in the local control of vasomotion, including endothelium-derived relaxing factor (EDRF), which is thought to be nitric oxide[322,330]; endothelin, a very potent vasoconstricting substance released by the endothelium[285–295,331]; prostaglandins[310,332]; lactic acid; histamine; neuropeptides and other vasoactive peptides; and unknown "metabolic products." The cerebral vessels are particularly sensitive to P_{CO_2}, whereas the coronary vessels respond strikingly to changes in P_{O_2},[308,321,333–337] although qualitatively similar changes are found in most other systemic vessels. It is probable that the myocardial vasodilatation produced by hypoxia is ordinarily mediated by the metabolite adenosine rather than by a direct effect of lowered P_{O_2}, unless the hypoxia is extreme.[6,13,18,273,290,322,327,338] Local prostaglandins and neuropeptides released in the heart may also be important (see below).[267,281,332,333] In most organs, the effects of P_{O_2}, P_{CO_2}, K^+, prostaglandins, and metabolic products work synergistically with the autonomic nervous system to regulate regional blood flow.[326] In contrast to systemic vessels, the pulmonary vessels seem to respond in the opposite manner to changes in P_{CO_2}, pH, and P_{O_2}. Thus, alveolar hypoxia results in regional vasoconstriction of the pulmonary arterioles, which tends to decrease perfusion of poorly ventilated areas and to help maintain normal O_2 saturation of arterial blood. In addition to their regional effects, P_{O_2} and P_{CO_2} in the mixed venous blood returned to the heart appear to be involved in the control of the total output of the heart through poorly understood mechanisms.

Endothelial Control of Blood Vessels

The endothelium plays a very active role in the modulation of arteriolar and arterial tone.[268,273,287–295,330,337–341] EDRF, one form of which is nitric oxide (NO) produced from L-arginine, stimulates guanylate cyclase to produce cyclic guanosine monophosphate (cGMP), which produces relaxation of vascular smooth muscle by decreasing cytosolic free Ca^{2+}.[330,342] EDRF is an important modulator of the local vascular response to vasoactive substances such as acetylcholine, ATP, adenosine diphosphate (ADP), adenosine monophosphate (AMP), substance P, histamine, serotonin, and bradykinin. In most vascular beds, the release of EDRF is stimulated by an increase in shear stress associated with an increase in the velocity of flow and thereby plays an important role in vasodilatation (Fig. 3-27).[289–291,294,322,328,329,337–348] EDRF may also help modulate the response to changes in oxygen tension.[287,294,330,340,343–345,349–351] Metabolic dilatation of distal arterioles can result in dilatation of upstream arterioles by both flow-dependent and myogenic mechanisms and can result in decreased vascular resistance and improved oxygen delivery (Fig. 3-28). The endothelium is often functionally impaired in atherosclerosis[287,291,294,340,344,345,350–358] (see Chaps. 4 and 44).

The endothelium also forms prostacyclin (PGI_2) from arachidonic acid. PGI_2 inhibits platelet adherence to the endothelium[359] and also produces relaxation of vascular smooth muscle. Nitrates, sodium nitroprusside, adenosine, hydrogen ions,

CO_2, and K^+ act directly on vascular smooth muscle cells, and their actions are not endothelium-mediated.

The endothelium can also release vasoconstricting substances. One of these is *endothelin*, which produces very strong vascular smooth muscle vasoconstriction by acting on an endothelin receptor to stimulate Ca^{2+} entry through the Ca^{2+} channel[286] and to stimulate the formation of $InsP_3$,[285–288, 292, 293, 295, 331, 360] which increases cytosolic calcium in vascular smooth muscle by stimulating the release of Ca^{2+} from intracellular sources. Many substances cause endothelin to be released, including vasopressor hormones, such as angiotensin II, epinephrine, and arginine vasopressin; coagulation products, such as thrombin; cytokines, such as interleukin 1; oxygen free radicals; and substances derived from aggregating platelets, such as transforming growth factor β.[295,351] Endothelium can also synthesize endothelial-derived contracting factors, which are not endothelin.

Plasma endothelin-1 concentration is increased in patients with unstable angina, acute myocardial infarction, heart failure, or renal insufficiency and in some patients with systemic arterial hypertension (see Chaps. 4 and 44). Impaired endothelial function in advanced heart failure leads to decreased vasodilatation of the vasculature in exercising skeletal muscles and to decreased capacity for exercise. The same deadaptation occurs with inactivity of muscle and is restored over time with muscle use (exercise). (See Chaps. 4 and 44 for more detailed discussions of endothelial function.)

Neural Control of Blood Vessels

Three main types of nerve fibers are important in the control of blood vessels: (1) sympathetic vasoconstrictor fibers, (2) sympathetic vasodilator fibers, and (3) parasympathetic vasodilator fibers.[3,13,18,260,261,309,317,318,361]

Sympathetic vasoconstrictor fibers are found in both arteries and veins throughout the body but not in capillaries. These fibers appear to effect vasoconstriction by the release of norepinephrine at the nerve fiber endings, which acts on α_1-adrenergic receptors in vascular smooth muscle. Vasodilatation may be produced by inhibition of the discharge rate of these nerve fibers. These fibers are important in responding to local or regional stimuli of many types. During exercise, they also produce arterial vasoconstriction in nonworking muscles and venous vasoconstriction of capacitance vessels, thereby helping to restrict blood flow to those areas and to

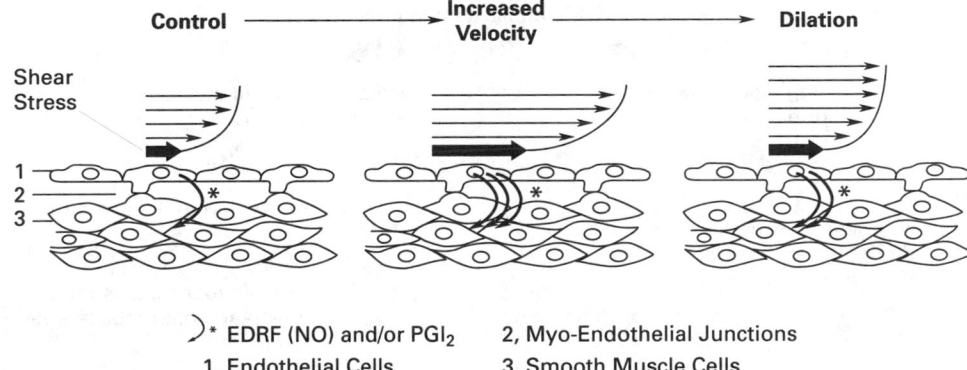

FIGURE 3-27

Schematic diagram of current concept of flow-induced dilation showing changes that occur during a period of increased blood flow velocity. Under control conditions (*left*), there is a continuous release of endothelium-derived relaxing factor (EDRF) and/or prostacyclin (PGI_2). When blood velocity increases (*middle*), rise in shear stress of the bloodstream acting on the endothelial layer of the blood vessel causes greater release of EDRF and/or PGI_2, as well as possibly vasodilator signals through the myoendothelial junctions, leading to vessel dilation (*right*) and partial return of shear stress toward control state. NO, nitric oxide. (From Smiesko V, Johnson PC. The arterial lumen is controlled by flow-related shear stress. *News Physiol Sci* 1993; 8:34–38. Reproduced with permission from the publisher and authors.)

maintain blood flow to either vital beds or exercising muscle. In addition, these fibers are the major pathways for reflex changes in peripheral resistance secondary to changes in carotid sinus and aortic stretch receptors, as well as reflex changes from the carotid body chemoreceptors and from stretch receptors in the low-pressure areas of the intrathoracic vascular bed.[260] They are thought to be the principal mechanism by which impulses from the cortical and subcortical areas of the brain influence total and regional peripheral resistance. The effect of these nerve fibers on the coronary and cerebral blood vessels is ordinarily very slight, being overshadowed by the influence of P_{O_2} and P_{CO_2}, although the adrenergic vasoconstriction may limit the concomitant metabolic vasodilatation and may help maintain blood flow to the inner layer of the left ventricle during tachycardia.[308–311,362,363] The influence of sympathetic stimulation[361] and coronary reflexes is further considered in Chap. 43.

Sympathetic vasodilator fibers appear to be of importance in skeletal muscles, although it is possible that some cutaneous blood vessels and coronary vessels also receive this type of fiber. Probably these fibers are not normally active tonically and are not influenced significantly by the carotid sinus or aortic arch stretch receptors, but they may be important in increasing blood flow to active muscles during the initiation of exercise. The effector agent at the nerve fiber ending is thought to be acetylcholine.

Parasympathetic vasodilator fibers are restricted to the tongue and salivary glands and to the sacral area, particularly the erectile vessels of the genital organs. In the sacral area they subserve local regulation of blood flow through the release of acetylcholine. Parasympathetic stimulation of the salivary glands releases *kallikrein*, which acts on kininogen, a plasma α_2 globulin synthesized in the liver, to form lysyl-bradykinin, which is converted by an aminopeptidase to *bradykinin*, a sub-

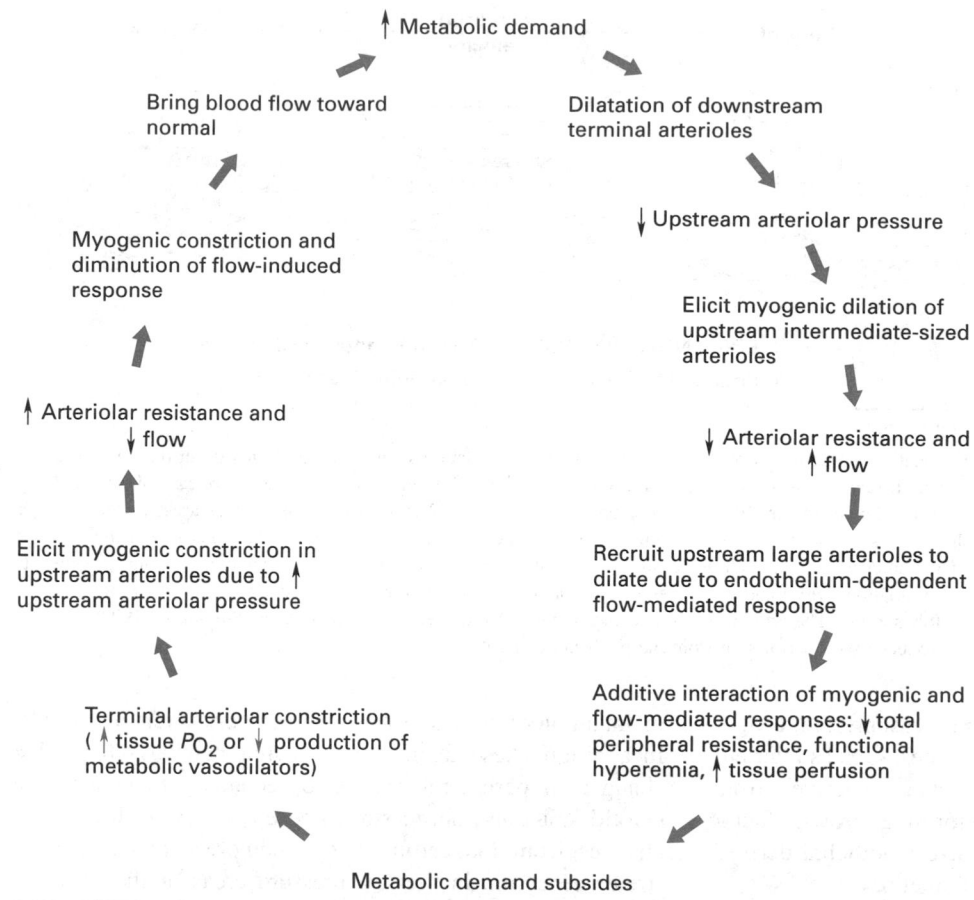

FIGURE 3-28

Integrative role of metabolic, myogenic, and flow-mediated regulation of coronary arteriolar tone during functional hyperemia. Note that metabolic dilatation of small arterioles can result in dilatation of upstream arterioles by flow-dependent and myogenic mechanisms that lessen overall vascular resistance and improve tissue oxygenation. (From Kuo L, Davis MJ, Chilian WM. Endothelial modulation of arteriolar tone. *News Physiol Sci* 1992; 7:5–9. Reproduced with permission from the publisher and authors.)

stance with powerful vasodilating properties. This is the same enzyme that converts inactive angiotensin I to the active angiotensin II. The sweat glands of the skin, innervated by sympathetic cholinergic fibers, may also liberate a kallikrein, and a kallikrein precursor in plasma may be activated by certain physical and chemical factors. In addition, the release of kallikrein and the formation of kinins may contribute to the hypotension associated with endotoxin and anaphylactic shock, the dumping syndrome, and carcinoid syndrome.[364–366]

In general, vasoconstriction occurs as the result of increased activity of the sympathetic nervous system, which causes the local release of norepinephrine at the nerve fiber endings in blood vessels, whereas vasodilatation is produced by the inhibition of sympathetic vasoconstrictor impulses and/or by endothelial and metabolic vasoactive products and local environmental conditions (P_{O_2}, P_{CO_2}, pH, K^+, etc.; Fig. 3-29). Localized vasodilatation may also be produced in exercising muscle by sympathetic vasodilator fibers and in the sacral area and salivary glands by parasympathetic fibers. In some areas, vasodilatation may be produced by the formation of neuropeptides and other polypeptides under autonomic nervous system

influence.[273,282,284,364–366] Prostaglandins are also very important in local circulatory control.

The anatomic pathways by which the central nervous system helps to control cardiovascular function are still poorly defined. The mechanisms by which the nervous system is able to integrate impulses from all levels—the cortex and limbic system, reticular system, diencephalon, mesencephalon, medulla oblongata, and spinal cord—and to synthesize these impulses in order to provide the organism with responses varying from the massive sympathetic discharge associated with shock to very discrete vasomotor changes are also not well delineated. Three major pools of spontaneously active neurons appear important in control of both the heart and the peripheral blood vessels: the *cardiovascular excitatory center* (pressor area), located in the rostrolateral portion of the medulla; the *cardiovascular inhibitory center* (depressor area), located in the mediocaudal portion of the medulla; and the *dorsal motor nucleus of the vagus nerve*, which exerts a cardiac inhibitory influence.[3] It is also apparent that impulses from high levels at times bypass lower integrative areas. There is also little information regarding the mechanisms of conditioning involving the autonomic nervous system.

MYOCARDIAL OXYGEN CONSUMPTION

The hemodynamic determinant of myocardial oxygen consumption ($M\dot{V}_{O_2}$) was related in 1907 by Barcroft and Dixon to external work, or the product of aortic pressure and flow.[367] In 1912, Rohde concluded that ventricular pressure and heart rate together determined myocardial oxygen consumption,[368] and in 1915 Evans and Matsuoka[369] reported a "relation between the tension set up on contraction and the metabolism of the contractile tissue." They noted that volume work was performed with less oxygen consumed than was an equal amount of pressure work and noted that the tension in the wall of the heart "varies roughly as the endocardiac pressure and as the square of the radius of the heart cavities," the nowfamiliar Laplace relationship. Subsequently, many studies have confirmed the importance of active intramyocardial tension or wall stress developed by the ventricle, or a related variable, as a major determinant of myocardial oxygen consumption.[370] Related variables have been correlated with $M\dot{V}_{O_2}$, including the product of pressure and heart rate, the product of integrated ventricular pressure and heart rate (the "tension-time index"),[371] developed wall tension, and contractile element work. Clearly, *wall tension* and *heart rate* are the major determinants of myocardial oxygen consumption. The inotropic state (contractility, or the velocity of contraction) is another major determinant of myocardial oxygen consumption.[370–373]

The results of several earlier studies relating $M\dot{V}_{O_2}$ to ventricular end-diastolic fiber length or diastolic volume were probably related to changes in developed tension or velocity of contraction. Similarly, the net effect on myocardial oxygen consumption of various positive inotropic interventions, such as sympathetic nerve stimulation or excitement, paired electrical stimulation, or the infusion of digitalis glycosides, catecholamines, or calcium, depends to a large degree on the relative effects on the tension developed and on the contractile state.[370] Most of the increase in myocardial oxygen uptake produced by catecholamines is related to the hemodynamic alterations they induce, although large doses can increase oxygen uptake in the nonbeating heart by a small amount. The effect of digitalis and other positive inotropic agents on $M\dot{V}_{O_2}$ depends on its relative effects on the contractile state of the heart, which it increases, causing $M\dot{V}_{O_2}$ to increase, and upon ventricular wall tension, which can decrease $M\dot{V}_{O_2}$ significantly if the heart radius decreases sufficiently.[370,373]

As shown in Table 3-3, the seven determinants of myocardial oxygen consumption can be classified as four major determinants and three minor determinants. The oxygen cost of electrical activation is probably less than 1 percent of the total $M\dot{V}_{O_2}$, and the costs for contractile-state activation and deactivation and for the maintenance of the active state are also small.[370,372] Clinically, relative myocardial oxygen requirements can be estimated by determining the product of systolic blood pressure and heart rate, the *tension-time index*,[373] or *pressure-time per minute*.[374] One may also factor the product of pressure and heart rate by the total duration of systole per minute.

Coronary flow and pressure affect oxygen consumption in the nonworking heart but have variable effects in the beating heart.[375] Alcohol stimulates the myocardial uptake of oxygen, whereas hypothermia markedly decreases oxygen consumption.

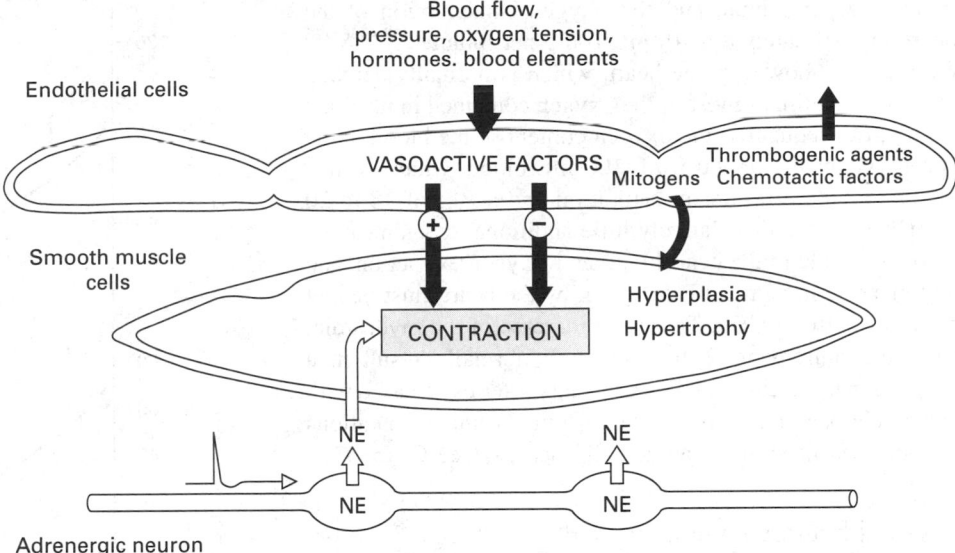

FIGURE 3-29

Schematic representing regulatory systems responsible for control of peripheral vascular tone. Adrenergic neurons, through release of norepinephrine (NE), regulate adjustments in tone relative to the activity of cardiopulmonary, baro-, and chemoreceptors. In response to changes in blood flow, oxygen tension, circulating levels of hormones, and substances released from blood elements (aggregating platelets and activated macrophages), the endothelium releases vasoactive substances that can either contract or relax the smooth muscle. Some vasoactive factors can also be mitogenic and inhibit platelet and macrophage adhesion or aggregation. (From Miller VM. Interactions between neural and endothelial mechanisms in control of vascular tone. *News Physiol Sci* 1991; 6:60–63. Reproduced with permission from the publisher and author.)

CORONARY CIRCULATION

The normal coronary circulation is able to provide oxygen to the heart under a wide range of conditions and is able to increase its flow five to six times the value at rest.[290,322,327,333–336,340,363,376–382] *Coronary vascular reserve* is the capacity of the coronary circulation to provide additional oxygenated blood to the myocardium. At rest, the coronary blood flow (CBF) is approximately 70 to 90

TABLE 3-3

DETERMINANTS OF MYOCARDIAL OXYGEN CONSUMPTION

Major determinants
    Myocardial mass
    Intramyocardial tension or wall stress
      (pressure × volume)
    Inotropic state (contractility)
    Heart rate
Minor determinants
    External work (load × shortening)
    Basal oxygen requirements
    Activation energy

mL/100 g per minute and the oxygen consumption of the heart approximately 8 to 10 mL/100 g per minute.[333–336,376] Even at rest, however, the heart, which is normally aerobic, extracts and utilizes most of the oxygen contained in its blood supply. Consequently, the oxygen content of the blood in the coronary sinus is about 5 mL/100 mL blood, which corresponds to about 30 percent saturation and a P_{O_2} of 18 to 20 mmHg. As a result, relatively little additional oxygen can be made available to the heart by greater oxygen extraction, and any increase in demand for oxygen by the heart must be met by an increase in CBF. Thus, any increase in the myocardial oxygen requirement (Table 3-3) will normally result in a proportional increase in CBF. Coronary arteries diseased with atherosclerosis may fail to dilate normally under conditions of increased need and may actually narrow (see Chap. 43).

Physical Factors Influencing CBF

The arterial pressure gradient (aortic–left ventricular diastolic pressure) and the time spent in diastole are the major determinants of CBF. Excessively elevated diastolic pressure, however, does not result in unneeded perfusion because of autoregulation.[383] On the other hand, when the perfusion pressure is very low, the coronary circulation is maximally dilated, and CBF is linearly related to the perfusion pressure. In general, CBF is maintained throughout a fairly wide range of perfusion pressure by autoregulation via myogenic changes in coronary artery tone.[324,325,327,367] CBF may be decreased by factors decreasing effective coronary perfusion pressure, such as congenital anomalies of the coronary arteries or obstruction of a coronary artery by atherosclerosis, thrombosis, or vasoconstriction. In general, it is necessary to decrease the lumen, or cross-sectional area, of an epicardial coronary vessel by at least two-thirds to cause a significant decrease in resting coronary flow. CBF also varies with the length and character of the obstruction, and lesser degrees of obstruction can cause a significant obstruction under conditions that increase the need for coronary blood flow (see also Chap. 43).

During ventricular systole, the left ventricular intramyocardial pressure exceeds left ventricular cavitary pressure or aortic systolic pressure, and the penetrating coronary vessels in the wall of the left ventricle are markedly compressed, or "throttled," preventing forward blood flow and even producing retrograde flow.[384] In addition to the physical systolic compression of the vessels, CBF is impeded by increased shear produced by twisting of the coronary vessels during systole.[385] Thus, the left ventricule receives the majority of its CBF during diastole, while the right ventricle receives flow more nearly equally during both systole and diastole (Fig. 3-30). In patients with coronary artery disease or even with marked left ventricular hypertrophy, tachycardia predisposes to myocardial ischemia, not only by the direct increase in oxygen consumption but also by significantly limiting the amount of time occupied by diastole. Indeed, in the markedly hypertrophied left ventricle, coronary reserve is significantly reduced, although resting flow corrected for mass may be normal. Furthermore, as noted

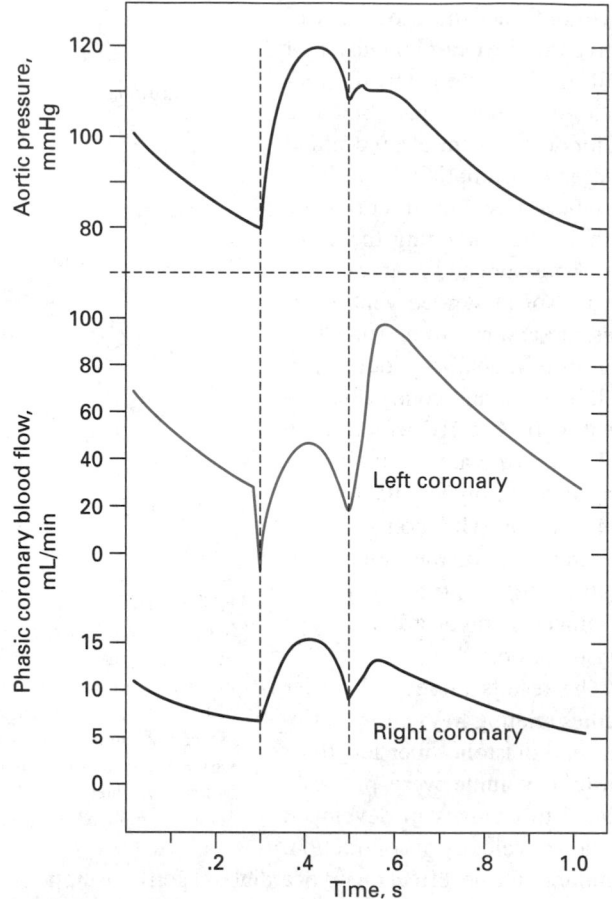

FIGURE 3-30

Comparison of phasic coronary blood flow in the left and right coronary arteries. Note the marked decrease in flow in the left coronary artery during left ventricular ejection. The decrease in blood flow to the left ventricle begins with the onset of left ventricular systole, shortly before the beginning of ejection of blood from the left ventricle, which is indicated by the first vertical line. (From Berne and Levy.[13] Reproduced with permission from the publisher and authors.)

above, coronary vascular resistance may actually increase during conditions of stress, such as exercise, in patients with coronary atherosclerosis (see Chap. 43).

Tissue pressure and especially left ventricular diastolic pressure also influence and can decrease CBF, especially to the subendocardium of a "failing" left ventricle and particularly if arterial hypotension is also present. An elevation of outlet pressure in the coronary sinus or right atrium can also offer some impediment to coronary perfusion, although this is seldom a significant factor in the absence of severe coronary artery disease. Blood viscosity is an additional factor that may contribute to a limitation of CBF, particularly in the presence of coronary artery disease.

A myogenic mechanism, or *Bayliss phenomenon*, also contributes to the autoregulation of CBF.[324,325,327,367] Additional physical factors affecting the adequacy of CBF include the total myocardial mass and the diffusion distance of oxygen from coronary capillaries to the center of hypertrophied myocardial cells.

Metabolic Factors Influencing CBF

CBF normally increases linearly with increased myocardial oxygen requirements, and most of the increase in CBF is by coronary vasodilatation secondary to metabolic autoregulation (Table 3-3). Several mediators or metabolic vasodilators are responsible for the metabolic autoregulation of the coronary circulation. Adenosine, which is formed when large amounts of AMP are broken down and which has strong coronary vasodilating properties, has most of the criteria for the physiologic regulation of CBF and may play a major role in the metabolic control of coronary resistance.[327,333–337,378,379,385–388] Other potential mediators include other nucleotides, prostaglandins, carbon dioxide, EDRF, and pH concentration.[273,290,291,327,338,339] It is unlikely that K^+, Ca^{2+}, or osmolality function as mediators in the normal control of coronary circulation.[333–337,378,379] The oxygen tension appears to influence coronary resistance secondarily by influencing the release of other mediators rather than by a direct influence on the coronary vessels. Changes in pH and P_{CO_2} also have a slight effect on myocardial oxygenation by producing changes in the oxygen-hemoglobin dissociation curve. Locally derived angiotensin II may help modulate CBF, as well as inotropy and chronotropy.[270–272,274] The endothelium of the coronary circulation plays an important role in modulating coronary tone through the release of dilating factors such as EDRF,[268] now generally believed to be nitric oxide, and constricting substances such as endothelin (see Chaps. 4 and 44).

Although many prostaglandins can produce coronary vasodilatation, at present they are not thought to play a major role in the normal control of coronary resistance. Some studies, however, have suggested that thromboxane A_2, an extremely strong coronary vasoconstrictor, may be important in producing coronary spasm.[378,379,388–392] Serotonin and vasopressin also produce coronary vasoconstriction. Local atherosclerosis may also potentiate the vasoconstrictor effects of alpha agonists,[393] norepinephrine, serotonin,[394–396] or histamine.[397] Such potentiation could cause coronary spasm. Focal loss of coronary vessel wall endothelium or endothelial function results in loss of the EDRF mechanism for dilatation. In this circumstance, acetylcholine produces paradoxical vasoconstriction in diseased coronary vessels[350–358,398] (see Chaps. 44 and 45).

Humoral Factors Influencing CBF

Catecholamines such as norepinephrine and epinephrine stimulate α receptors in the coronary vessels and produce direct coronary vasoconstriction, but indirectly they produce coronary vasodilatation and an increase in CBF due to the marked increase in myocardial contractility and thus increased myocardial oxygen consumption.[273,399] The effects of dopamine on the coronary circulation vary markedly with the dose administered, but in general it produces mild coronary vasodilatation. Isoproterenol stimulates β-adrenergic vasodilator receptors and produces an increase in coronary venous oxygen saturation in normal animals.[400]

Angiotensin II produces coronary vasoconstriction, although this effect is partially obscured by its other effects that increase myocardial oxygen consumption by increases in systemic pressure and left ventricular wall stress, heart rate, and myocardial contractility. It may also release prostaglandins E_2 and F, which produce coronary vasodilatation.[401,402]

High concentrations of vasopressin produce direct coronary vasoconstriction.[403–405] Coronary vascular tone is probably not significantly affected by changes in concentration of Na^+, K^+, Ca^{2+}, or Mg^{2+}, although studies have suggested that Ca^{2+} produces mild vasoconstriction; Mg^{2+} produces vasodilatation; Na^+ produces no effect; and K^+ produces a biphasic response, with small doses producing vasodilatation and large doses vasoconstriction.

Thyroid hormone produces coronary vasodilatation secondary to its effects on heart rate and myocardial contractility to increase myocardial oxygen consumption.[406,407] Adrenal steroids affect CBF and resistance secondarily by their tendency to produce systemic hypertension and left ventricular hypertrophy. Glucagon produces coronary vasodilatation that is secondary to an increase in heart rate and contractility. Beriberi is associated with increased CBF and decreased myocardial oxygen extraction,[408] perhaps as part of generalized arterial vasodilatation.

Adenosine and acetylcholine both produce marked coronary vasodilatation in normal vessels. As noted above, in patients with coronary atherosclerosis and endothelial dysfunction, acetylcholine may produce paradoxic coronary artery vasoconstriction[350–358,398] (see also Chaps. 44 and 45). Histamine produces coronary vasodilatation, both directly and indirectly, by its positive inotropic and chronotropic effects.[333] Serotonin also produces direct and, to a lesser degree, indirect coronary vasodilatation.

Polypeptides are also possibly important in the regulation of CBF.[333–337,364,385,386] Bradykinin increases CBF, possibly by the actions of prostaglandins.[409,410] Substance P produces moderate endothelium-dependent coronary vasodilatation, but its role in the normal regulation of CBF is unknown.[327,411–413] Vasoactive intestinal polypeptide appears to produce both direct coronary vasodilatation (strong endothelium-dependent, weaker endothelium-independent) and indirect vasodilatation due to its positive inotropic effects.[284,413–416] Neuropeptide tyrosine Y, which is very widespread, coexists with norepinephrine in the peripheral nervous system, including nerves to coronary blood vessels. Neuropeptide tyrosine Y may play a role in some instances of coronary spasm.[267,327,414] Calcitonin gene–related peptide produces endothelium-dependent coronary vasodilatation. Its importance in the control of CBF in normal individuals or patients with disease is unknown.[327]

Many prostaglandins produce coronary vasodilatation, especially PGI_2, which is synthesized by endothelial cells and which also inhibits platelet aggregation.[273,417] Thromboxane A_2 is a very strong coronary vasoconstrictor released from platelets that may be important in producing episodic, vasospastic, clinically significant decreases in coronary blood flow[366,388] (see Chap. 46).

Neural Factors Influencing CBF

SYMPATHETIC NERVES

As described in Chap. 2, sympathetic nerves to the heart and coronary vessels arise from the three cervical and the first four thoracic sympathetic ganglia.[262] Sympathetic adrenergic fibers extensively innervate both the epicardial and the intramural arteries and veins. Large coronary vessels appear to have both α and β_2 receptors, while small vessels have predominantly β_2 receptors. The coronary vessels do not appear to have either β_1-adrenergic receptors, which appear to be limited to the myocardium, or sympathetic cholinergic fibers.[418]

Stimulation of cardiac sympathetic nerves produces a direct vasoconstriction of the coronary arteries. This vasoconstriction, however, is normally overwhelmed by vasodilatation secondary to the increase in myocardial metabolism produced by the sympathetic stimulation of heart rate and myocardial contractility.[262,263] Coronary vascular β-adrenergic receptors are not thought to contribute to the response to nerve stimulation.

PARASYMPATHETIC NERVES

Experimentally, stimulation of the vagus nerves produces some direct coronary vasodilatation that is mediated by the release of acetylcholine and can be blocked by atropine.[419] In the intact organism, however, vagal stimulation produces bradycardia and may decrease myocardial contractility, both of which decrease myocardial oxygen requirements and result in secondary coronary vasoconstriction. Acetylcholine inhibits adenylate cyclase by a guanine inhibitory protein and decreases myocardial cAMP but augments cGMP, both of which decrease myocardial contractility[262] (see Fig. 21-15). Since vagal fiber innervation of ventricular myocardium is relatively small, however, the effect on function is minor.

Coronary Reflexes

Although coronary vascular resistance is determined primarily by metabolic autoregulation, it is also modulated by the sympathetic nervous system in response to changes in arterial pressure that are sensed by baroreceptors in the carotid sinus.[3,5,162,257–260] Carotid chemoreceptors, which may be initiated by acidosis, hypoxemia, or hypercapnia, can also influence coronary resistance by a predominant vasodilator effect mediated by the vagi and perhaps by a lesser vasoconstrictor effect mediated by the sympathetic nerves and only apparent if the vagal reflex is blocked.[258,260,333,336] There is no convincing evidence, however, of a coronary-to-coronary reflex except following the intracoronary administration of veratridine, which is known to elicit the *Bezold-Jarisch reflex*, a coronary-to-periphery reflex producing hypotension and bradycardia.[263,376] There is evidence that reflex vasodilatation

of some peripheral vascular beds as well as changes in heart rate and contractility may occur in some patients following coronary occlusion.[263,420] On the other hand, there is little substantial evidence of reflex vasoconstriction of coronary vessels from peripheral phenomena such as gastritis or cholecystitis. There is good evidence for a pulmonary inflation reflex that produces coronary vasodilatation in part mediated by a withdrawal of sympathetic tone.[421] The role of cardiac mechanoreceptors in the regulation of CBF is uncertain.[263,422]

Coronary Collateral Circulation

The stimuli and mechanisms for the development of coronary collateral circulation are not precisely known.[423–426] Hypoxia appears to play a major role. It has been postulated that hypoxia releases vasodilator metabolites that dilate preexisting microscopic collateral vessels without a smooth muscle component, increasing their pressure and tangential wall stress and damaging the vessel walls. This initial damage is then followed by reparative processes and the development of large-lumen, thick-walled collateral vessels with smooth muscle responsive to constrictive and dilating influences.[263,423–426] Fibroblast-stimulating factor increases coronary collateral flow into acutely ischemic areas and reduces resultant infarct size.[427] In human beings, the presence of coronary collateral circulation usually signifies the presence of significant coronary artery disease.[423–426] Once formed by hypoxia, collateral circulation may persist, although it may not be evident when primary flow sources are adequate.

Distribution of CBF

Current evidence indicates that the blood flow to the left ventricle is closely related to its oxygen demands. In experimental animals, this is also true within the left ventricle, where the left ventricular subendocardium at rest consumes 10 to 30 percent more oxygen per gram than the subepicardium and has a proportionately higher blood flow.[380,428–430] During tachycardia or other conditions that increase myocardial oxygen requirements and CBF of the experimental animal, however, CBF is more nearly equal in different layers of left ventricular myocardium. Estimates of CBF distribution in normal human beings, however, have suggested a fairly homogeneous distribution of coronary flow in the layers of the left ventricle at rest.[431] Most studies have indicated that the left ventricular subendocardium, which possesses a very dense vasculature, has a higher systolic intramyocardial pressure, calculated wall stress, and oxygen consumption than the subepicardium.[428,432] CBF to the left ventricular subendocardium is especially likely to be compromised by tachycardia, hypertrophy, an aged ventricle, or elevation of left ventricular diastolic pressure. The latter may be seen chronically in patients with hypertension, aortic stenosis, or hypertrophic cardiomyopathy[433] and may produce chronic diastolic dysfunction (see Chaps. 21 and 23). It may occur acutely secondary to myocardial ischemia with angina pectoris or myocardial infarction. In this situation, it may produce acute or even "flash" pulmonary edema.[434,435]

THE CARDIAC CYCLE

The successive mechanical events of the cardiac cycle may be described by a modification (Fig. 3-31, Plate 2) of Wiggers' classic diagram, which divided the cardiac cycle into two *periods*, systole and diastole, and subdivided these periods into *phases* of cardiac activity.[436–438] In the following discussion, the cardiac cycle is divided according to events on the left side of the heart. Corresponding periods and phases may also be described for events on the right side of the heart, with some differences (see below). The echocardiogram is very useful for estimating changes in ventricular volume and for timing valvular events.[439,440]

The first phase of ventricular systole is *isovolumic (isovolumetric* or *isochoric) contraction*. This phase begins with the first detectable rise in left ventricular pressure after the *z point* (see below); it is associated with the initial, mitral component (MC) of the first heart sound and the beginning of the isovolumic contraction (IC) wave of the apex cardiogram. The end of the isovolumic contraction phase and the beginning of the succeeding *rapid ventricular ejection* phase are indicated by the opening of the aortic valve (AO), a rise in aortic pressure, a decrease in ventricular volume, and the peak of the ejection E wave of the apex cardiogram. The onset and termination of the next phase of *reduced ventricular ejection* are less well defined; however, the slope of the aortic pressure pulse can be used to distinguish the phases of reduced and rapid ejection. *Rapid ejection* occurs when aortic pressure is rising, which means that blood is flowing into the aorta from the left ventricle more rapidly than it is leaving to perfuse the tissue, whereas *reduced ejection* represents that phase of the cardiac cycle before aortic valve closure, during which blood flows out of the aorta more rapidly than it enters. The phase of reduced ejection lasts until the end of actual ventricular ejection and the beginning of diastole, which occurs just before the recording of the *incisura* (notch) on the aortic pressure tracing. The very brief initial phase of diastole preceding the incisura is referred to as *protodiastole* and represents the time required for the reversal of flow in the aorta to close the aortic valve, which is responsible for the incisura of the aortic pressure tracing.

The beginning of the next phase of *isovolumic relaxation* of the left ventricle is signified by the closure of the aortic valve, as indicated by the aortic component (AC) of the second heart sound and by an inward isovolumic relaxation (IR) wave of the apex cardiogram. Isovolumic relaxation lasts until the left ventricular pressure falls below the left atrial pressure when the mitral valve opens and blood begins to flow from the atrium into the ventricle. Usually, the left ventricular pressure falls below the left atrial pressure tracing slightly *after* the peak of the left atrial *v* wave, since there is a slight fall in left atrial pressure caused by a decrease in the upward

bulging of the AV valve structures during ventricular isovolumic relaxation. In a sense, this is the opposite of the mechanism thought to produce the *c* wave in the atria during early ventricular systole. Both isovolumic relaxation and the following phase of rapid ventricular filling are produced by elastic recoil and active relaxation of the ventricular myocardium.

The end of the isovolumic relaxation phase and the beginning of the *rapid ventricular filling phase* are indicated by an increase in ventricular volume and by the O point of the apex cardiogram, which coincides with the opening of the mitral valve (MO). If the mitral leaflets are fused in a pliable valve, the opening of the valve may be audible as an "opening snap" (OS). This rapid ventricular filling phase is associated with a continuation of the decrease in atrial pressure (the *y descent*) begun during isovolumic relaxation, a rapid increase in ventricular volume, and an outward rapid-filling wave (RFW) in the apex cardiogram.

The end of the rapid ventricular filling phase and the beginning of the *slow ventricular filling phase* (sometimes called *diastasis*) are evidenced by a change in the slope of the ventricular volume curve, which indicates a change in the rate of ventricular filling. At times, rapid ventricular filling is associated with low-frequency vibrations or a sound, termed the S_3 or *ventricular gallop,* which occurs very shortly before the nadir of the *y* descent of the atrial pressure tracing. On the apex cardiogram, the end of the rapid ventricular filling phase (and the identification of S_3) is indicated at the moment when an abrupt change in slope occurs at the transition from the RFW to the slow-filling wave (SFW). This may be associated with a brief outward pulsation which is referred to as an *F wave,* or *peak,* on the apex cardiogram; frequently an S_3 is both visible and palpable (see Chap. 10).

During the phase of slow ventricular filling, or diastasis, the pressures in the left atrium and left ventricle slowly increase as the ventricle is passively filled until the next atrial systole produces the *a wave* in the left atrial pressure tracing. At times, an *h wave* is present in late diastasis prior to the *a* wave. Atrial contraction and the increased ventricular filling produced by atrial contraction (or "atrial kick") are reflected in an increase in ventricular pressure, an increase in ventricular volume, and an outward *a* wave of the apex cardiogram. Toward the peak or the second half of the atrial *a* wave, there may be a sound (S_4), particularly if there is a vigorous atrial contraction and relaxation. After the *a* wave of atrial contraction and relaxation, there is a very brief period or point (*z* point) when the atrial and ventricular pressures are essentially equal in normal individuals. The next cardiac cycle begins when the next ventricular contraction causes a definite sharp rise in pressure from the *z* point.

As one would expect from the location of the sinus node, contraction of the right atrium and opening of the tricuspid valve occur slightly before the corresponding events on the left side of the heart (Fig. 3-31, Plate 2; Fig. 3-32, Plate 3).

FIGURE 3-31
See color Plate 2.

FIGURE 3-32
See color Plate 3.

On the other hand, excitation and contraction of the left ventricle begin prior to contraction of the right ventricle, although the beginning of ejection of blood into the pulmonary artery slightly precedes ejection into the aorta, since the pressure in the right ventricle does not have to increase to such a high level before ejection begins (Fig. 3-31, Plate 2). Right ventricular ejection lasts beyond left ventricular ejection, producing the normal interval between the aortic component of the second heart sound (A_2) and the pulmonic component of the second heart sound (P_2). The shorter duration of left ventricular ejection is related to the greater contractile force of the left ventricle and to differences in the aorta and the pulmonary artery impedance and compression-chamber (*Windkessel*) characteristics.

During the brief phase of left ventricular isovolumic systole, the central aortic pressure pulse may show a slight positive wave that is produced by slight bulging of the aortic valve due to the rapidly increasing left ventricular pressure. During left ventricular ejection, the left ventricular pressure exceeds aortic pressure only during the early part of ejection and actually is slightly less than aortic pressure during most of systole.[441] It should also be noted that, although the components of the first and second heart sounds are referred to by the name of the valve commonly associated with the production of that sound (M_1, T_1, A_2, P_2), the sounds are not produced by the actual closure or striking together of the valve leaflets. *The sounds are more properly considered to be produced by the sudden acceleration and deceleration of blood, with tensing of the entire valve structures and vibrations of all cardiac structures. Actually, there is evidence that the AV valves and the aortic valve may be closed physiologically at a slightly different time than when these sounds occur.*[442–448] In most clinical situations, the two components of the first heart sound, the mitral (M_1) and the tricuspid (T_1) component, are produced by sudden acceleration-deceleration of blood, the valves, and cardiac structures in association with abrupt closure of the mitral and tricuspid valves, respectively. It is useful to consider the heart sounds as similar to the booming of a drum, where the ventricular walls are analogous to the drumhead, and the forces that cause the ventricle to vibrate (relaxation and valve closure) are the drumstick. This helps to understand the difference between a "physiological third sound" and a "diastolic gallop," both of which occur at the same time and so represent S_3 (Fig. 3-31, Plate 2). In the case of a physiologic third sound, common in healthy young people, the causes are rapid relaxation of a normal ventricle and closure of a pliable valve, which are analogous to a sharp tap from the drumstick. In contrast, the diastolic gallop heard in the failing heart, where both flow and valve closure are often slowed, occurs when ventricular wall tension is abnormally high, which is analogous to a taut drumhead.

While ventricular pressure is traditionally expressed in relation to time (Fig. 3-31, Plate 2), pressure can also be expressed in relation to ventricular volume in pressure-volume loops of individual heartbeats (see Fig. 22-5). Such loops are very useful in the evaluation of systolic and diastolic ventricular function and of myocardial contractility.[403] The slope of the line connecting the points at the end of systole (point *C* in Fig. 22-5) on different pressure-volume loops is called the *end-systolic elastance* (Ees), reflecting the shortening capacity of the ventricle (i.e., the end-systolic length-tension curve). As such, it has been used as one index of contractility[183–187,449] (see Chap. 22).

THE ARTERIAL PULSE

The arterial pressure pulse is produced by the ejection of blood from the left ventricle into the aorta and great vessels at a rate faster than its runoff into the peripheral circulation. In human beings, an average left ventricular stroke volume of 60 to 100 mL is ejected in about 0.25 s; and, of this volume, approximately two-thirds is ejected during the rapid-ejection phase. Although the peak rate of ejection of blood occurs prior to the peak pressure in the left ventricle or aorta, the pressure continues to rise in the aorta as long as blood is ejected into the aorta faster than it runs off into the peripheral arteries. Sometimes there is a slight notch in the central arterial pulse wave during or toward the end of the rapid-ejection phase. This is referred to as the *anacrotic notch*, or *shoulder*, and is accentuated in valvular aortic stenosis. At the end of ventricular ejection (and after the very brief phase of protodiastole), the aortic valve closes. In central aortic pressure tracings, this event is reflected by a sharp downward deflection, or *incisura*, on the descending limb of the pressure tracing and a gradual fall during diastole. At times, left ventricular isovolumic contraction causes a slight positive deflection in central arterial tracings just before the onset of the main arterial pulse wave.

As the arterial pressure pulse wave passes to the periphery, there are significant changes in its form (Fig. 10-38).[450] As the pulse moves away from the heart, the initial upstroke of the pulse becomes steeper, there is normally no anacrotic pause on the ascending limb, and the systolic maximum becomes peaked and increased in magnitude. The *dicrotic notch*, or *halt*, which corresponds to the incisura recorded more centrally, tends to occur later and lower and to be smoother in contour than the incisura. The positive wave that follows the dicrotic notch is referred to as the *dicrotic wave;* in many peripheral arteries this is normally more prominent than the slight upward deflection recorded centrally following the incisura. Although the systolic pressure may increase as the wave moves to the periphery, the diastolic and mean arterial pressures decrease slightly. The major factors responsible for these changes in the arterial pulse contour are (1) distortion of the components of the pulse waves as they travel peripherally, (2) different rates of transmission of various components of the pulse wave, (3) amplification or distortion of different components of the pulse by *standing waves* or *reflected waves,* (4) differences in elastic behavior and in caliber of the arteries, and (5) conversion of some kinetic energy to hydrostatic energy. Further details of the arterial pulse are discussed in Chap. 10.

THE VENOUS PULSE

The form of the venous pressure pulse[240,451] is determined by the rate of return of the blood from the peripheral tissues into the venous segment, the pressure-volume characteristics of the segment of the vein, the nature of the resistance to flow or distensibility offered by the right atrium and ventricle during the different phases of the cardiac cycle, and, to a slight degree, the tissues overlying the veins at the point of observation. Although the venous pressure pulse wave travels peripherally away from the heart, there is at the same time a venous flow of blood in the opposite direction toward the heart.

The a wave of the venous pressure pulse is related to contraction of the right atrium and is followed by the z point immediately preceding ventricular systole. In the jugular venous pulse, the c wave as usually recorded is predominantly produced by the systolic impulse in the adjacent carotid artery, with some contribution produced by right ventricular contraction and upward bulging of the tricuspid valve. In the early part of ventricular systole and following the brief c wave, there is a rapid inflow of blood to the right atrium, produced in part by descent of the tricuspid valve ring, which produces the normal negative venous wave during ventricular systole, the negative x wave, or x *descent* (or systolic collapse). The x descent is also produced by recoil of the right ventricle caused by the ejection of blood from both ventricles and by the decrease in the intrapericardial pressure during ejection, which reduces the pressure in both atria. As the venous inflow continues into the atria after the x descent, the pressure in the atria and in the veins builds up, producing the v wave during approximately the second half of ventricular systole. The peak of the right atrial v wave occurs shortly before or simultaneously with opening of the tricuspid valve and the beginning of the phase of right rapid ventricular filling. During early ventricular diastole, the rapid flow of blood from the great veins and right atrium into the right ventricle produces the negative y descent (or diastolic collapse) of the peripheral venous pulse wave. When recorded externally, the venous pulse wave is somewhat damped, and even when recorded directly, the waves are usually less steep in rise and descent than the corresponding waves of the atria. In part this is due to the damping effect of the large veins, which can accommodate markedly increased volumes of blood without a marked change in pressure.

Clinically, venous pulse waves are particularly difficult to evaluate in the presence of tachycardia, obesity, or shock or during the administration of drugs that produce venoconstriction. Further details of the venous pulse are discussed in Chap. 10.

NORMAL PRESSURE AND FLOW RATES IN THE CARDIOVASCULAR SYSTEM[452–454]

In general, the pressure in the systemic arteries is about five to six times greater than in the pulmonary arteries, although the amount of blood flowing in each unit is essentially the same. The left ventricular output may be slightly greater than the right ventricular output, due to the small amount of bronchial artery flow that returns via the pulmonary veins and the drainage of a few thebesian veins into the left atrium and ventricle. In order to compare measurements between individuals of different sizes, measurements of flow and resistance are often expressed in terms of square meters of body surface area; that is, instead of comparing cardiac output in absolute number of liters per minute, the output of the heart is expressed as the *cardiac index*, or liters per minute per square meter of body surface area. There is still a need for additional data to establish the limits of "normal" for vascular pressures, flow, and resistance for normal individuals of all ages under conditions of rest, exercise, or emotional stress. Furthermore, some of the slight differences in normal values reported from different laboratories are related to the use of different methods of measurement or different baselines for measurement of pressure. Table 3-4 lists the mean and range of hemodynamic measurements for normal resting adults, and Table 3-5 gives the distribution of systemic blood flow and oxygen consumption in a hypothetical 70-kg normal resting male.

RESPONSE TO EXERCISE[2,5,76,455–467]

The mechanisms utilized to increase the cardiac output during dynamic exercise vary, depending on the age, condition, posture, and athletic training of the person (see also Chap. 95). In particular, the relative contribution of heart rate and SV has been the subject of considerable interest. In general, pulse rate may increase threefold (or even fivefold in some highly trained athletes), whereas SV increases considerably less.[468] With extreme increases in heart rate, SV may even decline slightly. Most "normal" but untrained individuals in the supine position increase their cardiac output during mild to moderate dynamic exercise predominantly by an increase in pulse rate rather than by an increase in SV. With the increase in ventricular contractility, EDV tends to decrease with an increase in EF. With more extreme exercise, SV increases about 10 to 15 percent in the supine position and by 30 to 100 percent in the upright position, despite a considerably shortened systolic ejection period. In individuals who are accustomed to physical exertion, there is an earlier and more marked increase in SV in both positions, and SV often doubles during extreme upright exercise. The increase in EF during supine exercise is often associated with an increase in EDV in untrained subjects but with a decrease in end-systolic volume in well-trained individuals.[469] During upright exercise in some normal subjects, the increase in EF is associated with an increase in EDV.[470] The EF may decrease rather than increase during upright exercise in some apparently normal individuals over 65 years of age[471] (see also Chap. 95).

Dynamic exercise results in increased sympathetic adrenergic nervous activity to the resistance vessels of the kidney and splanchnic area and to the uninvolved muscles, while

TABLE 3-4

HEMODYNAMIC VALUES OF NORMAL RECUMBENT ADULTS

Measurement	Mean	Range
Cardiac index, liters/min per m^2	3.4	2.8–4.2
Stroke index, mL/beat	47	30–65
Arteriovenous oxygen difference, mL		
per liter of blood	38	30–48
Arterial saturation, %	98	94–100
Pressure,^{a} mmHg		
Brachial artery		
Systolic	130	90–140
Diastolic	70	60–90
Mean	85	70–105
Left ventricle		
Systolic	130	90–140
End-diastolic	7	4–12
Left atrium		
Maximum	13	6–20
Minimum	3	−2–+9
Mean	7	4–12
Pulmonary artery wedge (PC)		
Maximum	16	9–23
Minimum	6	1–12
Mean	9	6–15
Pulmonary artery		
Systolic	24	15–28
Diastolic	10	5–16
Mean	16	10–22
Right ventricle		
Systolic	24	15–28
End-diastolic	4	0–8
Right atrium		
Maximum	7	2–14
Minimum	2	−2–+6
Mean	4	−1–+8
Venae cavae		
Maximum	7	2–14
Minimum	5	0–8
Mean	6	1–10
End-diastolic volume		
Left ventricular, mL/m^2	70	50–90
Resistance, dyn·s/cm^5		
Total systemic	1150	900–1400
Systemic arteriolar	850	600–900
Total pulmonary	200	150–250
Pulmonary arteriolar	70	45–120

^{a} Baseline for pressure measurements one-half of anteroposterior chest diameter. 1 mmHg = 133.332 Pascal (Pa) = 0.133 kPa.

total arterial resistance normally decreases considerably during exercise.

An increase in cardiac output is further moderated by an increase in venous return produced by the combination of vasodilatation of the exercising muscles and the increased mechanical activity of the skeletal muscles, which rhythmically compress the peripheral veins, and by the rhythmic increase and decrease of the pressure in the peritoneal and thoracic cavities. The latter is sometimes referred to as the *abdominothoracic pump.* Exercise also produces a decrease in the volume of blood in venous reservoirs, especially the splanchnic blood volume. The result of these shifts makes more blood available to the heart, arterial vessels, and exercising muscles. On the other hand, during prolonged exercise, plasma volume may decrease significantly, with a resultant increase in hematocrit.[472,473] An increase in venous return to the atria may also produce an increase in heart rate by the *Bainbridge reflex;* this is more apparent in patients with a low resting heart rate or with hypervolemia in association with hemodilution. Isometric exercises of relatively mild degree may produce significant increases in blood pressure and pulse rate,[474–479] factors of considerable importance in patients with coronary artery disease (see Chaps. 43 and 45).

During exercise, there is a significant redistribution of the elevated cardiac output. During mild-to-moderate dynamic exercise, CBF and blood flow to the active skeletal muscles increase and cerebral flow is maintained, whereas renal and splanchnic flows diminish. During more severe exercise, these changes are exaggerated, and flow to the resting skeletal muscles may decrease. During maximal exercise, cerebral flow may also decrease, in association with hyperventilation and respiratory alkalosis. Skin blood flow may decrease initially during exercise, but it increases with continued exercise and contributes to the elimination of body

increasing blood flow to the exercising muscles by sympathetic vasodilatation and by locally mediated vasodilatation resulting from increased metabolic activity. The increase in sympathetic nervous system activity is roughly proportional to the intensity of exercise. The arterial systolic blood pressure often increases by 40 to 60 mmHg during moderate or severe exercise, although the mean arterial blood pressure increases much less. The diastolic pressure changes variably. Calculated

TABLE 3-5

DISTRIBUTION OF SYSTEMIC BLOOD FLOW AND OXYGEN CONSUMPTION IN A NORMAL SUBJECT[a] AT REST IN A COMFORTABLE ENVIRONMENT

Circulation	Blood Flow, mL/min	Percentage of Total Flow	AV[b] O_2 Difference, mL/dL	O_2 Consumption, mL/min	Percentage of Total Consumption
Splanchnic	1400	24	4.1	58	25
Renal	1100	19	1.3	16	7
Cerebral	750	13	6.3	46	20
Coronary	250	4	11.4	27	11
Skeletal muscle	1200	21	8.0	70	30
Skin	500	9	1.0	5	2
Other organs	600	10	3.0	12	5
Total	5800	100	4.0	234	100

[a] Weight, 70 kg; surface area, 1.7 m^2.
[b] AV = arteriovenous.
Source: Wade and Bishop.[454] Reproduced with permission from the publisher and authors.

heat. Exercise at high altitude imposes special problems, including sustained stimulation of the sympathetic nervous system[480] (see also Chap. 88).

In general, there is evidence of a generalized sympathetic discharge during exercise that in active muscles is overridden by local endothelial control, vasodilator metabolites, and changes in P_{O_2}, P_{CO_2}, pH, and K^+. In exercising skeletal muscles, there may be increased activity of sympathetic vasodilator fibers in addition to decreased vasoconstrictor activity. Venoconstriction during exercise tends to shift blood toward the central circulation and to the active skeletal muscles. Similar venoconstriction may occur in response to cold, emotion, hyperventilation, or norepinephrine. The plasma levels of both norepinephrine and epinephrine increase during dynamic exercise, but the level of norepinephrine is increased much less during isometric exercise.

REFERENCES

1. Hamilton WF, Dow P, eds. *Handbook of Physiology*, sec 2: *Circulation*, vols 1–3. Bethesda, MD: American Physiological Society; 1962–1965.
2. Braunwald E, Ross J Jr, Sonnenblick EH. *Mechanisms of Contraction of the Normal and Failing Heart*, 2d ed. Boston: Little, Brown; 1976.
3. Berne RM, ed. *Handbook of Physiology*, sec 2: *The Cardiovascular System*, vol 1: *The Heart*. Bethesda, MD: American Physiological Society; 1979.
4. Braunwald E, Ross J Jr. Control of cardiac performance. In: Berne RM, ed. *Handbook of Physiology*, sec 2: *The Cardiovascular System*, vol 1: *The Heart*. Bethesda, MD: American Physiological Society; 1979:533–580.
5. Shepherd JT, Abboud FM, eds. *Handbook of Physiology*, sec 2: *The Cardiovascular System*, vol III: *Peripheral Circulation and Organ Blood Flow*, parts 1 and 2. Bethesda, MD: American Physiological Society; 1983.
6. Renkin EM, Michel CC, eds. *Handbook of Physiology*, sec 2: *The Cardiovascular System*, vol IV: *Microcirculation*, part 1. Bethesda, MD: American Physiological Society; 1984:1–626.
7. Langer GA, ed. *Calcium and the Heart*. New York: Raven; 1990:1–387.
8. Chien S, ed. *Molecular Biology of the Cardiovascular System*. Philadelphia: Lea & Febiger; 1990:1–262.
9. Zucker IH, Gilmore JP, eds. *Reflex Control of the Circulation*. Boca Raton, FL: CRC Press; 1991:1–1053.
10. Opie LH. *The Heart: Physiology, Metabolism, Pharmacology, and Therapy*. Orlando, FL: Grune & Stratton; 1984.
11. Fozzard HA, Haber E, Jennings RB, Katz AM, Morgan HE, eds. *The Heart and Cardiovascular System: Scientific Foundations*, 2d ed. New York: Raven; 1991:1–2193.
12. Katz AM. *Physiology of the Heart*, 2d ed. New York: Raven; 1992.
13. Berne RM, Levy MD. *Cardiovascular Physiology*, 7th ed. St. Louis: Mosby Year Book; 1997:1–298.
14. Bers DM. *Excitation-Contraction Coupling and Cardiac Contractile Force*. Dordrecht, The Netherlands: Kluwer; 1991.
15. Rüegg C. *Calcium in Muscle Contraction. Cellular and Molecular Physiology*, 2d ed. Berlin: Springer; 1992.
16. Roberts R, ed. *Molecular Basis of Cardiology*. Oxford: Blackwell; 1993.
17. Spooner PM, Brown AM, eds. *Ion Channels in the Cardiovascular System. Function and Dysfunction*. Armonk, NY: Futura; 1994.
18. Loscalzo J, Creager MA, Dzau VJ, eds. *Vascular Medicine*. Boston: Little, Brown; 1992:1–1211.
19. Langer GA. Calcium at the sarcolemma. *J Mol Cell Cardiol* 1984; 16:147–153.
20. McDonald TF. Excitation-contraction coupling: Relationship of the slow inward current to contraction. In: Sperelakis N, ed. *The Physiology and Pathophysiology of the Heart*. Boston: Martinus Nijhoff; 1984:187–198.
21. Fabiato A, Baumgarten CM. Methods for detecting calcium release from the sarcoplasmic reticulum of skinned cardiac cells and the relationships between calculated transsarcolemmal calcium movements and calcium release. In: Sperelakis N, ed. *The Physiology and Pathophysiology of the Heart*. Boston: Martinus Nijhoff; 1984:215–254.
22. Tada M, Shigekawa M, Nimura Y. Uptake of calcium by the sarcoplasmic reticulum and its regulation and functional consequences. In: Sperelakis N, ed. *The Physiology and Pathophysiology of the Heart*. Boston: Martinus Nijhoff; 1984:255–277.
23. Pierce GN, Rich TL, Langer GA. Trans-sarcolemmal Ca^{2+} movements associated with contraction of the rabbit right ventricular wall. *Circ Res* 1987; 61:805–814.
24. Katz AM. Regulation of cardiac muscle contractility. *J Gen Physiol* 1967; 50:185–196.
25. Ebashi S. Excitation-contraction and the mechanism of muscle contraction. *Annu Rev Physiol* 1991; 53:1–16.
26. Sheu S-S, Blaustein MP. Sodium/calcium exchange and control of cell calcium and contractility in cardiac and vascular smooth muscles. In: Fozzard HA, Haber E, Jennings RB, Katz AM, Morgan HE, eds. *The Heart and Cardiovascular System*, 2d ed. New York: Raven; 1991:903–943.

27. Gibbons WR, Zygmunt AC. Excitation-contraction coupling in the heart. In: Fozzard HA, Haber E, Jennings RB, Katz AM, Morgan HE, eds. *The Heart and Cardiovascular System*, 2d ed. New York: Raven; 1991:1249–1279.

28. Callewaert G. Excitation-contraction coupling in mammalian cardiac cells. *Cardiovasc Res* 1992; 26:923–932.

29. Langer GA. Calcium and the heart: Exchange at the tissue, cell, and organelle levels. *FASEB J* 1992; 6:893–902.

30. Ringer S. A further contribution regarding the influence of the different constituents of the blood on the contraction of the heart. *J Physiol (Lond)* 1885; 4:29–42.

31. Coraboeuf E. Ionic basis of electrical activity in cardiac tissue. In: Levy MN, Vassale M, eds. *Excitation and Neural Control of the Heart*. Baltimore: Williams & Wilkins; 1982:1–35.

32. Fozzard HA, Hauck DA. Sodium channels. In: Fozzard HA, Haber E, Jennings RB, Katz AM, Morgan HE, eds. *The Heart and Cardiovascular System*, 2d ed. New York: Raven; 1991:1091–1119.

33. Philipson KD, Bers DM, Nashimoto AY, Langer GA. Binding of Ca^{2+} and N^+ to sarcolemmal membranes: Relating to control of myocardial contractility. *Am J Physiol* 1980; 238:H373–H378.

34. Fleischer S, Inui M. Biochemistry and biophysics of excitation-contraction coupling. *Annu Rev Biophys Chem* 1989; 18:333–364.

35. Lehninger AL. Ca^{2+} transport by mitochondria and its possible role in the cardiac contraction-relaxation cycle. *Circ Res* 1974; 35(suppl 3):83–90.

36. Carafoli E, Tiozzo R, Lugli G, Crovetti F, Kratzing C. The release of calcium from heart mitochondria by sodium. *J Mol Cell Cardiol* 1974; 6:361–371.

37. Sperelakis N. Regulation of calcium slow channels of cardiac muscle by cyclic nucleotides and phosphorylation. *J Mol Cell Cardiol* 1988; 20(suppl II):75–105.

38. Winegrad S. Regulation of cardiac contractile proteins. *Circ Res* 1984; 55:565–574.

39. Carafoli E. The homeostasis of calcium in heart cells. *J Mol Cell Cardiol* 1985; 17:203–212.

40. Carafoli E. The intracellular homeostasis of calcium: An overview. *Ann NY Acad Sci* 1988; 551:147–157.

41. Lepeuch CJ, Demaille JG. Covalent regulation of the cardiac sarcoplasmic reticulum calcium pump. Review article. *Cell Calcium* 1989; 10:397–400.

42. Schatzmann HJ. The calcium pump at the surface membrane and at the sarcoplasmic reticulum. *Annu Rev Physiol* 1989; 51:473–485.

43. Carafoli E. Calcium pump of the plasma membrane. *Physiol Rev* 1991; 71:129–153.

44. Missiaen L, Waytack F, Raeymaekers L, Demedt H, Droogmans G, Declerck I, et al. Ca^{2+} extrusion across plasma membrane and Ca^{2+} uptake by intracellular stores. *Pharmacol Ther* 1991; 50:191–232.

45. Caroni P, Carafoli E. The Ca^{++}-pumping ATPase of heart sarcolemma. *J Biol Chem* 1981; 256:3263–3270.

46. Siri FM, Kruoger J, Nordin C, Ming Z, Aronson RS. Depressed intracellular calcium transients and contractions in myocytes from hypertrophied and failing guinea pig hearts. *Am J Physiol* 1991; 26:H514–H540.

47. Hicks MJ, Shigekawa M, Katz AM. Mechanism by which cyclic adenosine 3′:5′-monophosphate-dependent protein kinase stimulates calcium transport in cardiac sarcoplasmic reticulum. *Circ Res* 1979; 44:384–391.

48. Barry WH, Biedert S, Miura DS, Smith TW. Changes in cellular Na, K, and Ca contents, monovalent cation transport rate, and contractile state during washout of cardiac glycosides from cultured chick heart cells. *Circ Res* 1981; 49:141–149.

49. Mullins LJ. The role of Na-Ca exchange in heart. In: Sperelakis N, ed. *The Physiology and Pathophysiology of the Heart*. Boston: Martinus Nijhoff; 1984:199–214.

50. Eisner DA, Smith TW. The Na-K pump and its effectors in cardiac muscle. In: Fozzard HA, Haber E, Jennings RB, Katz AM, Morgan HE, eds. *The Heart and Cardiovascular System*, 2d ed. New York: Raven; 1991:863–902.

51. Smith TW. Digitalis: Mechanisms of action and clinical use. *N Engl J Med* 1988; 318:358–365.

52. Sperelakis N. Cyclic AMP and phosphorylation in regulation of Ca^{++} influx into myocardial cells and blockade by calcium antagonist drugs. *Am Heart J* 1984; 107:347–357.

53. Colucci WS, Wright RF, Braunwald E. New positive inotropic agents in the treatment of congestive heart failure. *N Engl J Med* 1986; 314:290, 349–358.

54. Vatner SA. Sympathetic mechanisms regulating myocardial contractility in conscious animals. In: Fozzard HA, Haber E, Jennings RB, Katz AM, Morgan HE, eds. *The Heart and Cardiovascular System*, 2d ed. New York: Raven; 1991:1709–1728.

55. Williamson JR, Monck JR. Second messengers of inositol lipid metabolism and Ca^{2+} signaling. In: Fozzard HA, Haber E, Jennings RB, Katz AM, Morgan HE, eds. *The Heart and Cardiovascular System*, 2d ed. New York: Raven; 1991:1729–1744.

56. Koch-Weser J, Blinks JR. The influence of the interval between beats on myocardial contractility. *Pharmacol Rev* 1963; 15:601–652.

57. Covell JW, Ross J Jr, Taylor R, Sonnenblick EH, Braunwald E. Effects of increasing frequency of contraction on the force-velocity relation of left ventricle. *Cardiovasc Res* 1967; 1:2–8.

58. Arentzen CE, Rankin JS, Anderson PAW, Freezor MD, Anderson RW. Force-frequency characteristics of the left ventricle in the conscious dog. *Circ Res* 1978; 42:64–71.

59. Johnson EA. Force-interval relationship of cardiac muscle. In: Berne RM, ed. *Handbook of Physiology*, sec 2: *The Cardiovascular System*, vol 1: *The Heart*. Bethesda, MD: American Physiological Society; 1979:475–496.

60. Braunwald E, Sonnenblick EH, Frommer PL, Ross J Jr. Paired electrical stimulation of the heart: Physiologic observations and clinical implications. *Adv Intern Med* 1967; 13:61–96.

61. Hoffman BF, Bindler E, Suckling EE. Postextrasystolic potentiation of contraction in cardiac muscle. *Am J Physiol* 1956; 185:95–102.

62. Braunwald E. Mechanisms of action of calcium channel blocking agents. *N Engl J Med* 307:1618–1627.

63. Watanabe AM, Lindemann JP. Mechanisms of adrenergic and cholinergic regulation of myocardial contractility. In: Sperelakis N, ed. *Physiology and Pathophysiology of the Heart*. Boston: Martinus Nijhoff; 1984:377–404.

64. Fabiato A, Fabiato F. Effects of pH on the myofilaments and sarcoplasmic reticulum of skinned cells from cardiac and skeletal muscles. *J Physiol* 1978; 276:233–255.

65. Eisner DA, Lederer WJ, Vaughan-Jones RD. The quantitative relationship between twitch tension and intracellular sodium activity in sheep cardiac Purkinje fibers. *J Physiol (Lond)* 1984; 355:251–266.

66. Allen DG, Kentish JG. The cellular basis of the length-tension relation in cardiac muscle. *J Mol Cell Cardiol* 1985; 17:821–840.

67. Hoh JFY, Rossmanith GH, Kwan LJ, Hamilton AM. Adrenaline increases the rate of cycling of crossbridges in rat cardiac muscle as measured by pseudo-random binary noise–modulated perturbation analysis. *Circ Res* 1988; 62:452–461.

68. Lakatta EG. Starling's law of the heart is explained by an intimate interaction of muscle length and myofilament calcium interaction. *J Am Coll Cardiol* 1987; 10:1157–1164.

69. Babu A, Sonnenblick EH, Gulati J. Molecular basis for the influence of muscle length on myocardial performance. *Science* 1988; 240:74–76.

70. Lakatta EG. Length modulation of muscle performance: Frank-Starling law of the heart. In: Fozzard HA, Haber E, Jennings RB, Katz AM, Morgan HE, eds. *The Heart and Cardiovascular System*, 2d ed. New York: Raven; 1991:1325–1351.

71. Brutsaert DL, Sonnenblick EH. Cardiac muscle mechanics in the evaluation of myocardial contractility and pump function: Problems, concepts and directions. *Prog Cardiovasc Dis* 1973; 16:337–361.

72. Sonnenblick EH. Implications of muscle mechanics in the heart. *Fed Proc* 1962; 21:975–990.

73. Sonnenblick EH. Instantaneous force-velocity-length determinants in the contraction of heart muscle. *Circ Res* 1965; 16:441.

74. Sonnenblick EH, Braunwald E, Morrow AG. The contractile properties of human heart muscle: Studies on myocardial mechanics of surgically excised papillary muscles. *J Clin Invest* 1965; 44:966–977.

75. Glick G, Sonnenblick EH, Braunwald E. Myocardial force-velocity relations studied in intact unanesthetized man. *J Clin Invest* 1965; 44:978–988.

76. Sonnenblick EH, Braunwald E, Williams JF Jr, Glick G. Effects of exercise on myocardial force-velocity relations in intact unanesthetized man: Relative roles of changes in heart rate, sympathetic activity, and ventricular dimensions. *J Clin Invest* 1965; 44:2051–2062.

77. Sonnenblick EH. The mechanics of myocardial contraction. In: Briller SA, Conn HL Jr, eds. *The Myocardial Cell: Structure, Function and Modification by Cardiac Drugs*. Philadelphia: University of Pennsylvania Press; 1966:173–250.

78. Sonnenblick EH, Morrow AG, Williams JF Jr. Effects of heart rate on the dynamics of force development in the intact human ventricle. *Circulation* 1966; 33:945–951.

79. Covell JW, Ross J Jr, Sonnenblick EH, Braunwald E. Comparison of the force-velocity relation and the ventricular function curve as measures of the contractile state of the intact heart. *Circ Res* 1966; 19:364–372.

80. Braunwald E, Sonnenblick EH, Ross J Jr, Gault JH. Insights into cardiovascular physiology derived from muscle mechanics. *Am J Cardiol* 1967; 20:705–711.

81. Pool PE, Sonnenblick EH. Mechanochemistry of heart muscle: I. The isometric contraction. *J Gen Physiol* 1967; 50:951–965.

82. Gault JH, Ross J Jr, Braunwald E. Contractile state of the left ventricle in man: Instantaneous tension-velocity-length relations in patients with and without disease of the left ventricular myocardium. *Circ Res* 1968; 22:451–463.

83. Pool PE, Chandler BM, Seagren SC, Sonnenblick EH. Mechanochemistry of cardiac muscle: II. The isotonic contraction. *Circ Res* 1968; 22:465–472.

84. Barns JW, Covell JW, Ross J Jr. The mechanics of isotonic left ventricular contractions. *Am J Physiol* 1973; 224:725–732.

85. Langer GE, Brady AJ. *The Mammalian Myocardium*. New York: John Wiley; 1974.

86. Mahler F, Ross J Jr, O'Rourke RA, Covell JW. Effects of changes in preload, afterload and inotropic state on ejection and isovolumic phase measures of contractility in the conscious dog. *Am J Cardiol* 1975; 35:626–634.

87. Skelton CL, Sonnenblick EH. Physiology of cardiac muscle. In: Levine JH, ed. *Clinical Cardiovascular Physiology*. New York: Grune & Stratton; 1976:57–120.

88. Jewell BR. A reexamination of the influence of muscle length on myocardial performance. *Circ Res* 1977; 40:221–230.

89. Alpert NR, Hamrell BB, Mulieri LA. Heart muscle mechanics. *Annu Rev Physiol* 1979; 41:521–537.

90. Brady AJ. Mechanical properties of cardiac fibers. In: Berne RM, ed. *Handbook of Physiology*, sec 2: *The Cardiovascular System*, vol 1: *The Heart*. Bethesda, MD: American Physiological Society; 1979:461–474.

91. Strobeck JE, Sonnenblick EH. Myocardial contractile properties and ventricular performance. In: Fozzard HA, Haber E, Jennings RB, Katz AM, Morgan HE, eds. *The Heart and Cardiovascular System: Scientific Foundations*. New York: Raven; 1986:31–49.

92. Shroff SG, Janick JS, Weber KT. Mechanical and energetic behavior of the intact left ventricle. In: Fozzard HA, Haber E, Jennings RB, Katz AM, Morgan HE, eds. *The Heart and Cardiovascular System*, 2d ed. New York: Raven; 1991:129–150.

93. Grossman W, Lorell BH, eds. *Diastolic Relaxation of the Heart: Basic Research and Current Applications for Clinical Cardiology*. Boston: Martinus Nijhoff; 1988:1–310.

94. Hill AV. The heat of shortening and the dynamic constants of muscle. *Proc R Soc Lond B* 1938; 126:136–195.

95. Hill AV. *First and Last Experiments in Muscle Mechanics*. Cambridge: Cambridge University Press; 1970:141.

96. Bowditch HP. Ueber die Eigenthumlichkeiten der Reizbarkeit, welche die Muskelfasern des Herzens zeigen. *Verh K Sachs Ges Wochenshr, Leipzig Math Phys Cl* 1871; 23:652.

97. Howell WH, Donaldson F Jr. Experiments upon the heart of the dog with reference to maximum volume of blood sent out by left ventricle in a single beat. *Philos Trans R Soc Lond B* 1884; 175:139.

98. Frank O. Zur Dynamik des Herzmuskels. *Z Biol* 1895; 32:370; Chapman CB, Wasserman E (trans). *Am Heart J* 1958; 58:282–317, 467–478.

99. Fick A. *Mechanische Arbeit und Warmeentwickelung bei der Muskeltatigheit*. Leipzig: FA Brockhaus; 1882.

100. von Kries J. Untersuchungen zur Mechanik der quergestreiften Muskels. *Arch Physiol Leipzig* 1885; 67:348–374.

101. Blix M. Die Lange und die Spannung des Muskels. *Skand Arch Physiol* 1895; 5:173.

102. Wiggers CJ. Some factors controlling the shape of the pressure curve in the right ventricle. *Am J Physiol* 1914; 33:382–396.

103. Straub H. I. Dynamik des Saugetierherzens; II. Mitteilung Dynamik des Rechten Herzens. *Dtsch Arch Klin Med* 1914; 115:531–595, 116:409–436.

104. Patterson SW, Starling EH. On the mechanical factors which determine the output of the ventricles. *J Physiol* 1914; 48:357–379.

105. Patterson SW, Piper H, Starling EH. The regulation of the heart beat. *J Physiol* 1914; 48:465–513.

106. Starling EH. *The Linacre Lecture on the Law of the Heart*. London: Longman, Green; 1918.

107. Wiggers CJ. Determinants of cardiac performance. *Circulation* 1951; 4:485–495.

108. Strobeck JE, Krueger J, Sonnenblick EH. Load and time considerations in the force-length relations of cardiac muscle. *Fed Proc* 1980; 39:175–182.

109. Sarnoff SJ, Berglund E. Ventricular function: I. Starling's law of the heart studied by means of simultaneous right and left ventricular function curves in the dog. *Circulation* 1954; 9:706–718.

110. Sarnoff SJ. Myocardial contractility as described by ventricular function curves: Observations on Starling's law of the heart. *Physiol Rev* 1955; 35:107–122.

111. Braunwald E, Ross J Jr. Applicability of Starling's law of the heart to man. In: Evans JR, guest ed. Symposium: Structure and function of heart muscle. *Circ Res* 1964; 15(suppl 2):169–178.

112. Braunwald E. The control of ventricular function in man. *Br Heart J* 1965; 27:1–16.

113. Levine HJ. Compliance of the left ventricle. *Circulation* 1972; 46:423–426.

114. Gaasch WH, Cole JS, Quinones MA, Alexander JK. Dynamic determinants of left ventricular diastolic pressure-volume relations in man. *Circulation* 1975; 51:317–323.

115. Mirsky I. Assessment of passive elastic stiffness of cardiac muscle: Mathematical concepts, physiologic and clinical considerations, directions for future research. *Prog Cardiovasc Dis* 1976; 18:277–308.

116. Grossman W, McLaurin LP. Diastolic properties of the left ventricle. *Ann Intern Med* 1976; 84:316–326.

117. Gaasch WH, Levine HJ, Quinones MA, Alexander JK. Left ventricular compliance: Mechanisms and clinical implications. *Am J Cardiol* 1976; 38:645–653.

118. Nayler WG, Williams A. Relaxation in heart muscle: Some morphological and biochemical considerations. *Eur J Cardiol* 1978; 7(suppl):35–50.

119. Mirsky I. Elastic properties of the myocardium: A quantitative approach with physiological and clinical applications. In: Berne RM, ed. *Handbook of Physiology*, sec 2: *The Cardiovascular System*, vol 1: *The Heart*. Bethesda, MD: American Physiological Society; 1979; 497–531.

120. Smith V-E, Zile MR. Relaxation and diastolic properties of the heart. In: Fozzard HA, Haber E, Jennings RB, Katz AM, Morgan HE, eds. *The Heart and Cardiovascular System*, 2d ed. New York: Raven, 1991:1353–1367.

121. Grossman W, Lorell BH, eds. *Diastolic Relaxation of the Heart: Basic Research and Current Applications for Clinical Cardiology*. Boston: Martinus Nijhoff; 1988.

122. Weisfeldt ML, Loeven WA, Shock NW. Resting and active mechanical properties of trabeculae carneae from aged male rats. *Am J Physiol* 1971; 220:1921–1927.

123. Olivetti G, Melissari M, Capasso JM, Anversa P. Cardiomyopathy of the aging human heart: Myocyte loss and reactive cellular hypertrophy. *Circ Res* 1991; 68:1560–1568.

124. Nakamura Y, Wiegner AW, Bing OHL. Measurement of relaxation in isolated rat ventricular myocardium during hypoxia and reoxygenation. *Cardiovasc Res* 1986; 20:690–697.

125. Blaustein AS, Gaasch WH. Myocardial relaxation: VI. Effects of adrenergic tone and asynchrony on LV relaxation rate. *Am J Physiol* 1983; 244:H417–H422.

126. Hori M, Inoue M, Kitakaze M, Tsujioka K, Ishida Y, Fukunami M. Loading sequence is a major determinant of afterload-dependent relaxation in intact canine heart. *Am J Physiol* 1985; 249:H747–H754.

127. Gaasch WH, Ariel Y, McMahon TA. Dynamics of left ventricular diastolic filling (abstr). *J Am Coll Cardiol* 1986; 7:243A.

128. Hanrath P, Mathey DG, Kremer P, Sonntag F, Bleifeld W. Effect of verapamil on left ventricular isovolumic relaxation time and regional left ventricular filling in hypertrophic cardiomyopathy. *Am J Cardiol* 1980; 45:1258–1264.

129. Lorell BH, Paulus WJ, Grossman W. Modification of abnormal left ventricular diastolic properties by nifedipine in patients with hypertrophic cardiomyopathy. *Circulation* 1982; 65:499–507.

130. Suwa M, Hirota Y, Kawamura K. Improvement in left ventricular diastolic function during intravenous and oral diltiazem therapy in

patients with hypertrophic cardiomyopathy: An echocardiographic study. *Am J Cardiol* 1984; 54:1047–1053.

131. Bahler RC, Martin P. Effects of loading conditions and inotropic state on rapid filling phase of left ventricle. *Am J Physiol* 1985; 248:H523–H533.

132. Heyndrickx GR, Vantrimpont PJ, Rousseau MF, Pouleur H. Effects of asynchrony on myocardial relaxation at rest and during exercise in conscious dogs. *Am J Physiol* 1988:254 (*Heart Circ Physiol* 23):H817–H822.

133. Taylor RR, Covell JW, Sonnenblick EH, Ross J Jr. The independence of ventricular distensibility in the filling of the opposite ventricle. *Am J Physiol* 1967; 213:711–718.

134. Bemis CE, Serur JR, Borkenhagen D, Sonnenblick EH, Urschel CW. Influence of right ventricular filling pressure on left ventricular pressure and dimension. *Circ Res* 1974; 34:498–504.

135. Shirato K, Shabetai R, Bhargava V, Franklin D, Ross J Jr. Alteration of the left ventricular diastolic pressure–segment length relation produced by the pericardium: Effects of cardiac distention and afterload reduction in conscious dogs. *Circulation* 1978; 57:1191–1198.

136. LeWinter MM, Pavelec R. Influence of the pericardium on left ventricular end-diastolic pressure-segment relations during early and late stages of experimental chronic volume overload in dogs. *Circ Res* 1981; 50:501–509.

137. Bhargava V, Shabetai R, Ross J Jr, Pavelec RS, Mason PA. Influence of the pericardium on left ventricular diastolic pressure-volume curves in dogs with sustained volume overload. *Am Heart J* 1983; 105:995–1001.

138. Hess OM, Bhargava V, Ross J Jr, Shabetai R. The role of the pericardium in interactions between the cardiac chambers. *Am Heart J* 1983; 106:1377–1383.

139. Little WC, Badke FR, O'Rourke RA. Effect of right ventricular pressure on the end-diastolic left ventricular pressure-volume relationship before and after chronic right ventricular pressure overload in dogs without pericardia. *Circ Res* 1984; 54:719–730.

140. Braunwald E, Ross J Jr. The ventricular end-diastolic pressure: Appraisal of its value in the recognition of ventricular failure in man. *Am J Med* 1963; 34:147–150.

141. DiDonna G, LeWinter M, Johnson A, Peterson K. Effects of left ventricular hypertrophy on diastolic wall stiffness. *Circulation* 1974; 50(suppl 3):45–49.

142. Smith VE, Katz AM. Inotropic and lusitropic abnormalities in the genesis of heart failure. *Eur Heart J* 1983; 4(suppl A):7–17.

143. Katz AM. The descending limb of the Starling curve and the failing heart. *Circulation* 1965; 32:871–875.

144. Monroe RG, Gamble WJ, LaFarge CG, Kumar AE, Manasek FJ. Left ventricular performance at high end-diastolic pressure in isolated perfused dog hearts. *Circ Res* 1970; 26:85–99.

145. Ross J Jr, Sonnenblick EH, Taylor RR, Spotnitz HM, Spiro D. Diastolic geometry and sarcomere lengths in the chronically dilated canine left ventricle. *Circ Res* 1971; 28:49–61.

146. MacGregor DC, Covell JW, Mahler F, Dilley RB, Ross J Jr. Relations between afterload, stroke volume, and the descending limb of Starling's curve. *Am J Physiol* 1974; 227:884–890.

147. Sonnenblick EH, Spotnitz HM, Spiro D. Role of the sarcomere in ventricular function and the mechanism of heart failure. *Circ Res* 1964; 15(suppl 2):70–80.

148. Spiro D, Sonnenblick EH. The structural basis of the contractile process in heart muscle under physiological and pathological conditions. *Prog Cardiovasc Dis* 1965; 7:295–335.

149. Spiro D. The fine structure and contractile mechanism of heart muscle. In: Briller SA, Conn HL Jr, eds. *The Myocardial Cell: Structure, Function, and Modification by Cardiac Drugs*. Philadelphia: University of Pennsylvania Press; 1966:13.

150. Ross J Jr, Sonnenblick EH, Covell JW, Kaiser G, Spiro D. Architecture of the heart in systole and diastole: Technique for rapid fixation and analysis of left ventricular geometry. *Circ Res* 1967; 21:409–421.

151. Sonnenblick EH, Ross J Jr, Covell JW, Spotnitz HM, Spiro D. The ultrastructure of the heart in systole and diastole: Changes in sarcomere length. *Circ Res* 1967; 21:423–431.

152. Sonnenblick EH, Ross J Jr. Some ultrastructural considerations in myocardial failure: Sarcomere overextension and length dispersion. In: Tanz RD, Kavaler F, Roberts J, eds. *Factors Influencing Myocardial Contractility*. New York: Academic; 1967:43–48.

153. Leyton RA, Sonnenblick EH. The sarcomere as the basis of Starling's law of the heart in the left and right ventricles. In: Bajusz E, Jasmin G, eds. *Methods and Achievements in Experimental Pathology*, vol 5. Basel: Karger; 1971:22–59.

154. Yoran C, Covell JW, Ross J Jr. Structural basis for the ascending limb of left ventricular function. *Circ Res* 1973; 32:297–303.

155. Sonnenblick EH, Skelton CL. Reconsideration of the ultrastructural basis of cardiac length-tension relations. *Circ Res* 1974; 35:517–526.

156. Skelton CL, Sponitz WW, Feldman D, Serur JR, Mirsky I, Sonnenblick EH. Ultrastructural and functional correlates of acute cardiac distension (abstr). *Clin Res* 1974; 22:304a.

157. Sommer JR, Jennings RB. Ultrastructure of cardiac muscle. In: Fozzard HA, Haber E, Jennings RB, Katz AM, Morgan HE, eds. *The Heart and Cardiovascular System*, 2d ed. New York: Raven; 1991:3–50.

158. Allen DG, Kurihara S. Calcium transients at different muscle length in rat ventricular muscle. *J Physiol (Lond)* 1979; 292:68p–69p.

159. Dodge HT, Frimer M, Stewart DK. Functional evaluation of the hypertrophied heart in man. *Circ Res* 1974; 35(suppl 2):122–127.

160. Sonnenblick EH. Series elastic and contractile elements in heart muscle: Changes in muscle length. *Am J Physiol* 1964; 207:1330–1338.

161. Imperial ES, Levy MN, Zieske HJ Jr. Outflow resistance as an independent determinant of cardiac performance. *Circ Res* 1961; 9:1145–1155.

162. Sarnoff SJ, Mitchell JH. The control of the function of the heart. In: Hamilton WF, Dow P, eds. *Handbook of Physiology*, sec 2: *Circulation*, vol 1. Bethesda, MD: American Physiological Society; 1962:489.

163. Sonnenblick EH, Downing SE. Afterload as a primary determinant of ventricular performance. *Am J Physiol* 1963; 204:604–610.

164. Levine HJ, Forward SA, McIntyre KM, Schechter E. Effect of afterload on force-velocity relations and contractile element work in the intact dog heart. *Circ Res* 1966; 18:729–744.

165. Evans GL, Smulyan H, Eich RH. Role of peripheral resistance in the control of cardiac output. *Am J Cardiol* 1967; 20:216–221.

166. Urschel CW, Covell JW, Sonnenblick EH, Ross J Jr, Braunwald E. Myocardial mechanics in aortic and mitral valvular regurgitation: The concept of instantaneous impedance as a determinant of the performance of the heart. *J Clin Invest* 1968; 47:867–883.

167. Milnor WR. Arterial impedance as ventricular afterload. *Circ Res* 1975; 36:565–570.

168. Ross J Jr. Mechanisms of cardiac contraction. What roles for preload, afterload and inotropic state in heart failure? *Eur Heart J* 1983; 4(suppl A):19–28.

169. Von Anrep G. On the part played by suprarenals in the normal vascular reactions of the body. *J Physiol* 1912; 45:307–317.

170. Vatner SF, Monroe RG, McRitchie RJ. Effects of anesthesia, tachycardia and autonomic blockade on Anrep effect in intact dogs. *Am J Physiol* 1974; 226:1450–1456.

171. Brutsaert DL, Sonnenblick EH. Force-velocity-length-time relations of the contractile elements in heart muscle of the cat. *Circ Res* 1969; 24:137–149.

172. Brutsaert DL, Claes VA, Sonnenblick EH. Effects of abrupt load alterations on force-velocity-length and time relations during isotonic contractions of heart muscle: Load clamping. *J Physiol* 1971; 216:319–330.

173. Noble MIM. Problems concerning the application of concepts of muscle mechanics to the determination of the contractile state of the heart. *Circulation* 1972; 45:252–255.

174. Peterson KL, Skloven D, Ludbrook P, Uther JB, Ross J Jr. Comparison of isovolumic and ejection phase indices of myocardial performance in man. *Circulation* 1974; 49:1088–1101.

175. Brady AJ. Mechanics of the myocardium. In: Langer GA, Brady AJ, eds. *The Mammalian Myocardium*. New York: John Wiley; 1974:163–192.

176. Sonnenblick EH, Strobeck JE. Derived indices of ventricular and myocardial function. *N Engl J Med* 1977; 296:978–982.

177. Brady N. Contractile and mechanical properties of the myocardium. In: Sperelakis N, ed. *The Physiology and Pathophysiology of the Heart*. Boston: Martinus Nijhoff; 1984:279–299.

178. Higgins CB, Vatner SF, Franklin D, Braunwald E. Extent of regulation of the heart's contractile state in the conscious dog by alteration in the frequency of contraction. *J Clin Invest* 1973; 52:1187–1194.

179. Mahler F, Yoran C, Ross J Jr. Inotropic effect of tachycardia and poststimulation potentiation in the conscious dog. *Am J Physiol* 1974; 227:569–575.

180. Abbott BC, Mommaerts WFHM. A study of inotropic mechanisms in the papillary muscle preparation. *J Gen Physiol* 1959; 42:533–551.

181. Tanz RD, Kavaler F, Roberts J, eds. *Factors Influencing Myocardial Contractility.* New York: Academic; 1967.

182. Mehmel HC, Stocking B, Ruffmann K, von-Olshausen K, Schuler G, Kubler W. The linearity of the end-systolic pressure-volume relationship in man and its sensitivity for assessment of left ventricular function. *Circulation* 1981; 63:1216–1222.

183. Sagawa K. The end systolic pressure-volume relation of the ventricle: Definition, modifications and clinical use. *Circulation* 1981; 63:1223–1227.

184. McKay RG, Aroesty JM, Heller GV, Royal H, Parker JA, Silverman KJ, et al. Left ventricular pressure-volume diagrams and end-systolic pressure-volume relations in human beings. *J Am Coll Cardiol* 1984; 3:301–312.

185. Maughan WL, Sunagawa K, Burkhoff D, Sagawak K. Effect of arterial impedance changes on end-systolic pressure-volume relation. *Circ Res* 1984; 54:595–602.

186. Kaseda S, Tomoike H, Ogaa I, Ogata I, Nakamura M. End-systolic pressure-volume, pressure-length, and stress-strain relations in canine hearts. *Am J Physiol* 1985; 18:H648–H654.

187. Lee J, Tajimi T, Widmann TF, Lee JD, Tajimi T, Widmann TF, et al. Application of end-systolic pressure-volume and pressure-wall thickness relations in conscious dogs. *J Am Coll Cardiol* 1987; 98:136–146.

188. Freeman GL, Little WC, O'Rourke RA. Influence of heart rate on left ventricular performance in conscious dogs. *Circ Res* 1987; 61:455–464.

189. Parmley WW, Sonnenblick EH. Relation between mechanics of contraction and relaxation in mammalian cardiac muscle. *Am J Physiol* 1969; 216:1084–1091.

190. Cohn PF, Liedtke AJ, Serur J, Sonnenblick EH, Urschel CW. Maximal rate of pressure fall (negative *dp/dt*) during ventricular relaxation. *Cardiovasc Res* 1972; 6:263–267.

191. Weisfeldt ML, Scully HE, Frederiksen J, Rubenstein JJ, Pohost GM, Beierholm E, et al. Hemodynamic determinants of maximum negative *dp/dt* and the periods of diastole. *Am J Physiol* 1974; 227:613–621.

192. Strobeck JE, Bahler AS, Sonnenblick EH. Isotonic relaxation in cardiac muscle. *Am J Physiol* 1975; 229:646–651.

193. Brutsaert DL, Rademakers FE, Sys SU, Gillebert TC, Housmans PR. Analysis of relaxation in the evaluation of ventricular function of the heart. *Prog Cardiovasc Dis* 1985; 28:143–163.

194. Chemla D, Lecarpentier Y, Martin JL, Clerque R, Antonetti A, Hatt P. Relationship between inotropy and relaxation in rat myocardium. *Am J Physiol* 1986; 250:H1008–H1016.

195. Katz AM. Cyclic AMP effects on the myocardium. A man who blows hot and cold with one breath. *J Am Coll Cardiol* 1983; 2:143–149.

196. Katz AM. Interplay between inotropic and lusitropic effects of cyclic adenosine monophosphate on the myocardial cell. *Circulation* 1990; 82(suppl I):1-7-1–11.

197. Kass DA, Midei M, Brinker J, Maughan WL. Influence of coronary occlusion during PTCA on end-systolic and end-diastolic pressure volume relations in humans. *Circulation* 1990; 81:447–460.

198. Monomura SI, Ferguson JJ, Miller MJ, Parker JA, Grossman W. Regional myocardial blood flow and left ventricular diastolic properties in pacing-induced ischemia. *J Am Coll Cardiol* 1991; 17:781–789.

199. Vatner SF, Braunwald E. Cardiovascular control mechanisms in the conscious state. *N Engl J Med* 1975; 293:970–976.

200. Woodworth RS. Maximal contraction, staircase contraction, refractory period, and compensatory pause of the heart. *Am J Physiol* 1902; 8:213–249.

201. Hajdu S. Mechanism of the Woodworth staircase phenomenon in heart and skeletal muscle. *Am J Physiol* 1969; 216:206–214.

202. Page E. Cardiac gap junctions. In: Fozzard H, Haber E, Katz AM, Jennings R, Morgan HE, eds. *The Heart and Cardiovascular System,* 2d ed. New York: Raven; 1991; 1003–1047.

203. Clapham DE. Calcium signalling. *Cell* 1995; 80:259–268.

204. Katz AM. Calcium channel diversity in the cardiovascular system. *J Am Coll Cardiol* 1996; 28:522–528.

205. Cheng H, Lederer WJ, Cannell MB. Calcium sparks: Elementary events underlying excitation-contraction coupling in heart muscle. *Science* 1993; 262:740–743.

206. Fabiato A. Calcium-induced release of calcium from the cardiac sarcoplasmic reticulum. *Am J Physiol* 1983; 245:C1–C14.

207. Wier WG, Egan TM, López JR, Balke CW. Local control of excitation-contraction coupling in rat heart cells. *J Physiol (Lond).* 1994; 474:463–471.

208. Caterall WA. Structure and function of voltage-sensitive ion channels. *Science* 1988; 242:50–61.

209. Hille B. *Ionic Channels of Excitable Membranes.* Sunderland, MA: Sinauer; 1992.

210. Catterall WA. Cellular and molecular biology of voltage-gated sodium channels. *Physiol Rev* 1992; 72(suppl):S15–S48.

211. Jan LY, Jan YN. Tracing the roots of ion channels. *Cell* 1992; 69:715–718.

212. Katz AM. Cardiac ion channels. *N Engl J Med* 1993; 328:1244–1251.

213. Ho K, Nichols CG, Lederer WJ, Lytton J, Vassilev PM, Kabazirska MV, et al. Cloning and expression of an inwardly rectifying ATP-regulated potassium channel. *Nature* 1993; 362:127–133.

214. Kubo Y, Baldwin TJ, Jan YN, Jan LY. Primary structure and functional expression of a mouse inward rectifier potassium channel. *Nature* 1993; 362:127–133.

215. Attali B. A new wave for heart rhythms. *Nature* 1997; 384:24–25.

216. Tsien RW, Tsein RY. Calcium channels, stores, and oscillations. *Annu Rev Cell Biol* 1990; 6:715–760.

217. Hoffman F, Biel M, Bosse E, Flockerzi V, Ruth P, Welling A. Functional expression of cardiac and smooth muscle calcium channels. In: Spooner PM, Brown AM, Catterall WA, Kaczorowski GJ, Strauss HC, eds. *Ion Channels in the Cardiovascular System: Function and Dysfunction.* Armonk, NY: Futura; 1994:369–381.

218. McDonald TF, Pelzer S, Trautwein W, Pelzer D. Regulation and modulation of calcium channels in cardiac, skeletal, and smooth muscle cells. *Physiol Rev* 1994; 72:365–507.

219. Melzer W, Hermann-Frank A, Lüttgau HC. The role of Ca^{2+} ions in excitation-contraction coupling of skeletal muscle fibres. *Biochem Biophys Acta* 1995; 1241:59–116.

220. Bean BP. Classes of calcium channels in vertebrate cells. *Ann Rev Physiol* 1989; 51:367–384.

221. Vassort G, Alvarez J. Cardiac T-type calcium current. Pharmacology and roles in cardiac tissues. *J Cardiovasc Electrophysiol* 1994; 5:376–393.

222. Sperelakis N. Properties of calcium channels in cardiac and vascular smooth muscle. *Mol Cell Pharmacol* 1990; 99:97–109.

223. Henzi V, MacDermott AB. Characteristics and function of Ca^{2+}- and inositol 1,4,5-trisphosphate-releasable stores of Ca^{2+} in neurons. *Neuroscience* 1992; 46:251–273.

224. Berridge M. Inositol trisphosphate and calcium signalling. *Nature* 1993; 361:315–325.

225. Ehrlich BE, Watras J. Inositol 1,4,5-triphosphate activates a channel from smooth muscle sarcoplasmic reticulum *Nature* 1988; 336:583–586.

226. Somlyo AP, Somlyo AV. Smooth muscle structure and function. In: Fozzard H, Haber E, Katz AM, Jennings R, Morgan HE, eds. *The Heart and Cardiovascular System,* 2d ed. New York: Raven; 1991:1295–1324.

227. Lytton J, MacLennan DH. Sarcoplasmic reticulum. In: Fozzard H, Haber E, Katz AM, Jennings R, Morgan HE, eds. *The Heart and Circulation,* 2d ed. New York: Raven; 1991:1203–1222.

228. Tada M, Katz AM. Phosphorylation of the sarcoplasmic reticulum and sarcolemma. *Annu Rev Physiol* 1982; 44:401–423.

229. Kim HW, Steenaart NAE, Ferguson DG, Kranias EG. Functional reconstitution of the cardiac sarcoplasmic reticulum Ca^{2+}-ATPase with phospholamban in phospholipid vesicles. *J Biol Chem* 1990; 265:1702–1709.

230. Nicoll DA, Longoni S, Philipson KD. Molecular cloning and functional expression of the cardiac sarcolemmal Na^{+}-Ca^{2+} exchanger. *Science* 1990; 250:469–471.

231. Levitsky DO, Nicoll DA, Philipson KD. Identification of the high affinity Ca^{2+}-binding domain of the cardiac Na^{+}-Ca^{2+} exchanger. *J Biol Chem* 1994; 269:22847–22852.

232. Ebashi S, Kitazawa T, Kodama K, Van Eerd P-C. Calcium ion in cardiac contractility. In: Kobayashi T, Sano T, Dhalla NS, eds. *Recent Advances in Studies on Cardiac Structure and Metabolism,* vol. II, *Heart Function and Metabolism.* Baltimore, MD: University Park Press; 1978:93–101.

233. Hawthorne EW. Instantaneous dimensional changes of the left ventricle in dogs. *Circ Res* 1961; 9:110–119.

234. Schlant RC, Dixon F, Elson SH, Rawls WJ, Williamson FR Jr. Modification of the law of the heart: Influence of early contracting areas (abstr). *Circulation* 1964; 30(suppl 3):153.

235. Schlant RC, Rawls WJ, Dixon F, Elson S. An additional determinant of ventricular performance (abstr). *Clin Res* 1965; 13:62.

236. Schlant RC. Idoventricular kick (abstr). *Circulation* 1966; 34(suppl 3):209.

237. Brecher GA. Experimental evidence of ventricular diastolic suction. *Circ Res* 1956; 4:513–518.

238. Sonnenblick EH. The structural basis and importance of restoring forces and elastic recoil for the filling of the heart. *Eur Heart J* 1980; 1(suppl A):107–110.

239. Mitchell JH, Gilmore JP, Sarnoff SJ. The transport function of the atrium: Factors influencing the relation between mean left atrial pressure and left ventricular end diastolic pressure. *Am J Cardiol* 1962; 9:237–247.

240. Brecher GA, Galletti PM. Functional anatomy of cardiac pumping. In: Hamilton WF, Dow P, eds. *Handbook of Physiology*, sec 2: *Circulation*, vol 2. Bethesda, MD: American Physiological Society; 1963:759–798.

241. Braunwald E. Hemodynamic significance of atrial systole. *Am J Med* 1964; 37:778–779.

242. Burchell HB. A clinical appraisal of atrial transport function. *Lancet* 1964; 1:775–779.

243. Williams JF Jr, Sonnenblick EH, Braunwald E. Determinants of atrial contractile force in the intact heart. *Am J Physiol* 1965; 209:1061–1068.

244. Mitchell JH, Gupta DN, Payne RM. Influence of atrial systole on effective ventricular stroke volume. *Circ Res* 1965; 17:11–18.

245. Dietz JR. Release of natriuretic factor from rat heart-lung preparations by atrial distention. *Am J Physiol* 1984; 247:R1093–R1096.

246. Debold AJ. Atrial natriuretic factor: A hormone produced by the heart. *Science* 1985; 230:767–770.

247. Yamaji T, Ishibashi M, Takaka F. Atrial natriuretic factor in human blood. *J Clin Invest* 1985; 76:1705–1709.

248. Tikkanen I, Fyhrquist F, Metsarinne K, Leidenius R. Plasma atrial natriuretic peptide in cardiac disease and during infusion in healthy volunteers. *Lancet* 1985; 2:66–69.

249. Espiner EA, Crozier IG, Nicholls MG, Cuneo R, Yondle TG, Ikram H. Cardiac secretion of atrial natriuretic peptide. *Lancet* 1985; 2:398–399.

250. Ballermann BJ, Brenner BM. Role of atrial peptides in body fluid homeostasis. *Circ Res* 1986; 58:619–630.

251. Raine AE, Erne P, Burgisser E, Muller FB, Bolli P, Burkart F, et al. Atrial natriuretic peptide and atrial pressure in patients with congestive heart failure. *N Engl J Med* 1986; 315:533–537.

252. Mulrow PJ, Schrier R, eds. *Atrial Hormones and Other Natriuretic Factors*. Bethesda, MD: American Physiological Society; 1987:1–178.

253. Genest J, Cantin M. Atrial natriuretic factor. *Circulation* 1987; 75(suppl 1):118–124.

254. Wildey GM, Misono KS, Graham RM. Atrial natriuretic factor: Biosynthesis and mechanisms of action. In: Fozzard HA, Haber E, Jennings RB, Katz AM, Morgan HE, eds. *The Heart and Cardiovascular System*, 2d ed. New York: Raven; 1991:1777–1796.

255. Marcus LS, Hart D, Packer M, Yushak M, Medina IV, Danziger RS, et al. Hemodynamic and renal excretory effects of human brain natriuretic peptide infusion in patients with congestive heart failure. A double-blind, placebo-controlled, randomized crossover trial. *Circulation* 1996; 94:3184–3189.

256. Atarashi K, Mulrow PJ, Franco-Saenz R, Snajdar R, Rapp J. Inhibition of aldosterone production by an atrial extract. *Science* 1984; 224:992–994.

257. Levy MN, Martin PJ. Neural control of the heart. In: Berne RM, ed. *Handbook of Physiology*, sec 2: *The Cardiovascular System*, vol 1: *The Heart*. Bethesda, MD: American Physiological Society; 1979:581–620.

258. Brown AM. Cardiac reflexes. In: Berne RM, ed. *Handbook of Physiology*, sec 2: *The Cardiovascular System*, vol 1: *The Heart*. Bethesda, MD: American Physiological Society; 1979:677–689.

259. Korner PI. Central nervous control of autonomic cardiovascular function. In: Berne RM, ed. *Handbook of Physiology*, sec 2: *The Cardiovascular System*, vol 1: *The Heart*. Bethesda, MD: American Physiological Society; 1979:691–739.

260. Mancia G, Mark AL. Arterial baroreceptors in humans. In: Shepherd JT, Abboud FM, eds. *Handbook of Physiology*, sec 2: *The Cardiovascular System*, vol III: *Peripheral Circulation and Organ Blood Flow*, part 2. Bethesda, MD: American Physiological Society; 1983:755–793.

261. Randall WC, ed. *Nervous Control of Cardiovascular Function*. New York: Oxford University Press; 1984.

262. Armour JA. Anatomy and function of the intrathoracic neurons regulating the mammalian heart. In: Fozzard HA, Haber E, Jennings RB, Katz AM, Morgan HE, eds. *The Heart and Cardiovascular System*, 2d ed. New York: Raven; 1991:1–37.

263. Hainsworth R. Reflexes from the heart. *Physiol Rev* 1991; 71:617–658.

264. Susanni EE, Vatner DE, Homcy CJ. The beta-adrenergic receptor/adenylyl cyclase system. In: Fozzard HA, Haber E, Jennings RB, Katz AM, Morgan HE, eds. *The Heart and Cardiovascular System*, 2d ed. New York: Raven; 1991:1685–1708.

265. Sutherland EW. On the biological role of cyclic AMP. *JAMA* 1970; 214:1281–1288.

266. DeGeest H, Levy MN, Zieske H, Lipman RI. Depression of ventricular contractility by stimulation of the vagus nerves. *Circ Res* 1965; 17:222–235.

267. Franco-Cerecada A, Lundberg JM, Dahlof C. Neuropeptide Y and sympathetic control of heart contractility and coronary vascular tone. *Acta Physiol Scand* 1985; 124:361–365.

268. Bassenge E, Busse R. Endothelial modulation of coronary tone. *Prog Cardiovasc Dis* 1988; 30:349–380.

269. Badeer HS. Resting bradycardia of exercise training: A concept based on currently available data. In: Roy PE, Rona G, eds. *The Metabolism of Contraction*, vol 10: *Recent Advances in Studies on Cardiac Structure and Metabolism*. Baltimore: University Park Press; 1975:553–560.

270. Dzau VJ, Re RN. Evidence for the existence of renin in the heart. *Circulation* 1987; 75:1134–1136.

271. Dzau VJ. Cardiac renin-angiotensin system: Molecular and functional aspects. *Am J Med* 1988; 84:22–27.

272. Lindpainter K, Ganten D. The cardiac renin-angiotensin system: An appraisal of present experimental and clinical evidence. *Circ Res* 1991; 68:905–921.

273. O'Rourke ST, Vanhoutte PM. Vascular pharmacology. In: Loscalzo J, Creager MA, Dzau VJ, eds. *Vascular Medicine: A Textbook of Vascular Biology and Diseases*. Boston: Little, Brown; 1992:133–155.

274. Dostal DE, Baker KM. Evidence for a role of an intracardiac renin-angiotensin system in normal and failing hearts. *Trends Cardiovasc Med* 1993; 3:67–74.

275. Sadoshima J, Malhotra R, Izumo S. The role of the cardiac renin-angiotensin system in load-induced cardiac hypertrophy. *J Cardiac Failure* 1996; 2(suppl 4):S1–S6.

276. Dzau VJ. Tissue renin-angiotensin system in myocardial hypertrophy and failure. *Arch Intern Med* 1993; 153:937–942.

277. Holmer SR, Homey CJ. G proteins in the heart: A redundant and diverse transmembrane signaling network. *Circulation* 1991; 84:1891–1902.

278. Saman S, Thandroyen F, Opie LH. Serotonin and the heart: Effects of ketanserin on myocardial function, heart rate, and arrhythmias. *J Cardiovasc Pharmacol* 1985; 7(suppl 7):S70–S75.

279. Zaritsky AL, Horowitz M, Chernow B. Glucagon antagonism of calcium channel blocker-induced myocardial dysfunction. *Crit Care Med* 1988; 16:246–251.

280. Dzau VJ, Packer M, Lilly LS, Swartz SL, Hollenberg NK, Williams GH. Prostaglandins in severe congestive heart failure: Relation to activation of the renin-angiotensin system and hyponatremia. *N Engl J Med* 1984; 310:347–352.

281. Gunnes P, Reikeras O. Distribution of the increased cardiac output secondary to the vasodilating and inotropic effects of secretin. *Scand J Clin Lab Invest* 1987; 47:383–388.

282. Gu J, Adrian TE, Tatemoto K, Polak JM, Allen JM, Bloom SR. Neuropeptide tyrosine (NPY): A major cardiac neuropeptide. *Lancet* 1983; 1:1008–1010.

283. Su C. Extracellular functions of nucleotides in heart and blood vessels. *Annu Rev Physiol* 1985; 47:665–676.

284. Franco-Cereceda A, Bengtsson L, Lundberg JM. Inotropic effects of calcitonin gene–related peptide, vasoactive intestinal polypeptide and somatostatin on the human right atrium in vitro. *Eur J Pharmacol* 1987; 134:69–76.

285. Marsden PA, Danthuluri NR, Brenner BM, Ballermann BJ, Brock TA. Endothelin action on vascular smooth muscle involves inositol triphosphate and calcium mobilization. *Biochem Biophys Res Commun* 1988; 158:86–93.

286. Goto K, Kasuya Y, Matsuki N, Takuwa Y, Kurihara H, Ishikawa T, et al. Endothelin activates the dihydropyridine-sensitive, voltage-dependent Ca^{2+} channel in vascular smooth muscle. *Proc Natl Acad Sci U S A* 1989; 86:3915–3918.

287. Lüscher TF, Yang Z, Diederich D, Bühler FR. Endothelium-derived vasoactive substances: Potential role in hypertension, atherosclerosis, and vascular occlusion. *J Cardiovasc Pharmacol* 1989; 14:563–569.

288. Vane JR, Botting R, Masaki T, eds. Endothelin. *J Cardiovasc Pharmacol* 1989; 13(suppl):S1–S231.

289. Vanhoutte PM. Endothelium and control of vascular function. *Hypertension* 1989; 13:658–667.

290. Bassenge E, Heusch G. Endothelial and neuro-humoral control of coronary blood flow in health and disease. *Rev Physiol Biochem Pharmacol* 1990; 116:77–165.

291. Vane JR, Änggärd EE, Botting RM. Regulatory functions of the vascular endothelium. *N Engl J Med* 1990; 323:27–36.

292. Masaki T, Kimura S, Yanagisawa M, Goto K. Molecular and cellular mechanisms of endothelin regulation: Implications for vascular function. *Circulation* 1991; 84:1457–1468.

293. Rubany GM, Botelho LHP. Endothelins. *FASEB J* 1991; 5:2713–2720.

294. Lerman A, Burnett JC Jr. Intact and altered endothelium in regulation of vasomotion. *Circulation* 1992; 86(suppl III):III12–III19.

295. Lüscher TF, Boulanger CM, Dohi Y, Yang Z. Endothelium-derived contracting factors. *Hypertension* 1992; 19:117–130.

296. Brutsaert DL. Role of endocardium in cardiac overloading and failure. *Eur Heart J* 1991; 11(suppl G):G8–G16.

297. Brutsaert DL, Andries LJ. The endocardial endothelium. *Am J Physiol* 1992; 263(*Heart Circ Physiol* 32):H985–H1002.

298. Brutsaert DL, DeKeulenaar GW, Fransen P, Mohan P, Kaluza GL, Andries LJ, et al. The cardiac endothelium: Functional morphology, development, and physiology. *Prog Cardiovasc Dis* 1966; 39:239–262.

299. Shah AM, Grocott-Mason RM, Pepper CB, Mebazaa A, Henderson AH, Lewis MJ, et al. The cardiac endothelium: Cardioactive mediators. *Prog Cardiovasc Dis* 1996; 39:263–284.

300. Henderson AH, Lewis MJ, Shah AM, Smith JA. Endothelium, endocardium, and cardiac contraction. *Cardiovasc Res* 1992; 26:305–308.

301. Rocamora JM, Downing SE. Preservation of ventricular function by adrenergic influences during metabolic acidosis in the cat. *Circ Res* 1969; 24:373–381.

302. Vatner SF, Marsh JD, Swain JD. Effects of morphine on coronary and left ventricular dynamics in conscious dogs. *J Clin Invest* 1975; 55:207–217.

303. Horwitz LD, Bishop VS. Effect of acute volume loading on heart rate in the conscious dog. *Circ Res* 1972; 30:316–332.

304. Frommer PL, Robinson BF, Braunwald E. Paired electrical stimulation: A comparison of the effects on performance of the failing and nonfailing heart. *Am J Cardiol* 1966; 18:738–774.

305. Cranefield PF, Hoffman BF. The physiologic basis and clinical implications of paired pulse stimulation of the heart. *Dis Chest* 1966; 49:561–567.

306. Braunwald E, Sonnenblick EH, Frommer PL, Ross J Jr. Paired electrical stimulation of the heart: Physiologic observations and clinical implications. *Adv Intern Med* 1967; 13:61–96.

307. Wittenberg JB. Myoglobulin-facilitated oxygen diffusion: Role of myoglobin in oxygen entry into muscle. *Physiol Rev* 1970; 50:559–636.

308. Korner PI. Control of blood flow to special vascular areas: Brain, kidney, muscle, skin, liver, and intestine. In: Guyton AC, Jones CE, eds. *Cardiovascular Physiology*, ser I. vol 1. Baltimore: University Park Press; 1974:123–162.

309. Zelis R, ed. *The Peripheral Circulations*. New York: Grune & Stratton; 1975.

310. Messina EJ, Weiner R, Kaley G. Prostaglandins and local circulatory control. *Fed Proc* 1976; 35:2367–2375.

311. Abboud FM, Schmid PG, Heistad DD, Mark AL. Regulation of peripheral and coronary circulation. In: Levine HJ, ed. *Clinical Cardiovascular Physiology*. New York: Grune & Stratton; 1976:143–205.

312. Sandler H, Dodge HT. Left ventricular tension and stress in man. *Circ Res* 1963; 13:91–104.

313. Hood WP Jr, Rackley CE, Rolett EL. Wall stress in the normal and hypertrophied human left ventricle. *Am J Cardiol* 1968; 22:5550–5558.

314. Grossman W, Jones D, McLaurin LP. Wall stress and patterns of hypertrophy in the human left ventricle. *J Clin Invest* 1975; 56:56–64.

315. Katz AM. Cardiomyopathy of overload. A major determinant of prognosis in congestive heart failure. *N Engl J Med* 1990; 322:100–110.

316. Katz AM. Cardiomyopathy of overload. An unnatural growth response in the hypertrophied heart. *Ann Intern Med* 1994; 121:363–371.

317. Shepherd JT, Vanhoutte PM. *Veins and Their Control*. Philadelphia: Saunders; 1975:269.

318. Abboud FM, Schmid PG, Heistad DD, Mark AL, Barnes RW. The venous system. In: Levine HJ, ed. *Clinical Cardiovascular Physiology*. New York: Grune & Stratton; 1976:207–257.

319. Dobrin PB. Vascular mechanics. In: Shepherd JT, Abboud FM, eds. *Handbook of Physiology*, sec 2: *The Cardiovascular System*, vol III: *Peripheral Circulation and Organ Blood Flow*, part 2. Bethesda, MD: American Physiological Society; 1983:65–102.

320. Zweifach BW, Lipocosky HH. Pressure-flow relations in blood and lymph microcirculation. In: Renkin EM, Michel CC, eds. *Handbook of Physiology*, sec 2: *The Cardiovascular System*, vol III: *Microcirculation*, part 1. Bethesda, MD: American Physiological Society; 1984:251–307.

321. Rose CP, Goresky CA. Interactions between capillary exchange, cellular entry, and metabolic sequestration processes in the heart. In: Renkin EM, Michel CC, eds. *Handbook of Physiology*, sec 2: *The Cardiovascular System*, vol III: *Microcirculation*, part 1. Bethesda, MD: American Physiological Society; 1984:781–798.

322. Parent R, Paré R, Lavallée M. Contribution of nitric oxide to dilation of resistance coronary vessels. *Am J Physiol* 1992; 262(*Heart Circ Physiol* 31):H10–H16.

323. Stamler JS, Loh E, Roddy M-A, Currie KE, Creager MA. Nitric oxide regulates basal systemic and pulmonary vascular resistance in healthy humans. *Circulation* 1994; 89:2035–2040.

324. Bevan JA. Vascular myogenic or stretch-dependent tone. *J Cardiovasc Pharmacol* 1985; 7(suppl 3):S129–S136.

325. Nichols WW, O'Rourke MF. *McDonald's Blood Flow in Arteries*, 3d ed. Philadelphia: Lea & Febiger; 1990:1–456.

326. Davis MJ. Myogenic response gradient in an arteriolar network. In: Mulvany MJ, Aalkjaer C, Heagerty AM, Nyborg NCB, Strandgaard S, eds. *Resistance Arteries: Structure and Function*. Amsterdam: Elsevier; 1991:51–55.

327. Olsson RA, Bunger R, Spaan JAE. Coronary circulation. In: Fozzard HA, Haber E, Jennings RB, Katz AM, Morgan HE, eds. *The Heart and Cardiovascular System*, 2d ed. New York: Raven; 1991:1393–1425.

328. Smiesko V, Lang DJ, Johnson PC. Dilator response of rat mesenteric arcading arterioles to increased blood flow velocity. *Am J Physiol* 1989; 257(*Heart Circ Physiol* 26):H1958–H1965.

329. Kuo L, Davis MJ, Chilian WM. Endothelium-dependent, flow-induced dilation of isolated coronary arterioles. *Am J Physiol* 1990; 259(*Heart Circ Physiol* 28):H1063–H1070.

330. Moncada S, Palmer RM, Higgs EA. Nitric oxide: Physiology, pathophysiology, and pharmacology. *Pharmacol Rev* 1991; 43:109–142.

331. Simonson MS, Dunn MJ. Endothelin. Pathways of transmembrane signaling. *Hypertension* 1990; 15(suppl I):I5–I12.

332. Needleman P. The synthesis and function of prostaglandins in the heart. *Fed Proc* 1976; 35:2376–2381.

333. Marcus ML. *The Coronary Circulation in Health and Disease*. New York: McGraw-Hill; 1983.

334. Feigl EO. Coronary physiology. *Physiol Rev* 1983; 63:1–2095.

335. Olsson RA, Bunger R, Spaan JAE. Coronary circulation. In: Fozzard HA, Haber E, Jennings RB, Katz AM, Morgan HE, eds. *The Heart and Cardiovascular System*, 2d ed. New York: Raven; 1991:1393–1425.

336. Spaan JAE, Bruschke AVG, Gittenberger-DeGroot AC, eds. *Coronary Circulation*. Dordrecht: Martinus Nijhoff; 1987.

337. Busse R, Trogisch G, Bassenge E. The role of endothelium in the control of vascular tone. *Basic Res Cardiol* 1985; 80:475–490.

338. Vanhoutte PM, Miller VM, Houston DS. Modulation of vascular smooth muscle contraction by the endothelium. *Annu Rev Physiol* 1986; 48:307–320.

339. Vanhoutte PM. Endothelium-dependent contractions in arteries and veins. *Blood Vessels* 1987; 24:141–144.

340. Bassenge E, Busse R. Endothelial modulation of coronary tone. *Prog Cardiovasc Dis* 1988; 30:349–380.

341. Inoue T, Tomoike H, Hisano K, Nakamara M. Endothelium determines flow-dependent dilation of the epicardial coronary artery in dogs. *J Am Coll Cardiol* 1988; 11:187–191.

342. Murad F. Signal transduction using nitric oxide and cyclic guanosine monophosphate. *JAMA* 1996; 276:1189–1192.

343. Rubanyi GM, Romero JC, Vanhoutte PM. Flow-induced release of endothelium-derived relaxing factor. *Am J Physiol* 1986; 250:H1145–H1149.

344. Vanhoutte PM, Shimokawa H. Endothelium-derived relaxing factor and coronary vasospasm. *Circulation* 1989; 80:1–8.

345. Henderson AH. Endothelium in control. *Br Heart J* 1991; 65:116–125.

346. Holtz J, Forstermann U, Pohl U, Giesler M, Bassonge E. Flow-dependent, endothelium-mediated dilatation of epicardial coronary arteries in conscious dogs: Effects of cyclooxygenase inhibition. *J Cardiovasc Pharmacol* 1984; 6:1161–1169.

347. Pohl U, Holtz J, Busse R, Bassenge E. Crucial role of endothelium in vasodilator response to increased flow in vivo. *Hypertension* 1986; 8:37–44.

348. Kuo L, Davis MJ, Chilian WM. Endothelium-dependent flow-induced dilation of isolated coronary arterioles. *Am J Physiol* 1990; 259:H1063–H1070.

349. Dewey JG, Vanhoutte PM. Anoxia and endothelium-dependent reactivity in canine femoral artery. *J Physiol (Lond)* 1983; 335:65–74.

350. Yasue H, Horio Y, Nakamura N, Fujii H, Imoto N, Sonoda R, et al. Induction of coronary artery spasm by acetylcholine in patients with variant angina: Possible role of the parasympathetic nerve system in the pathogenesis of coronary artery spasm. *Circulation* 1986; 74:955–963.

351. Vanhoutte PM, Mombouli J-V. Vascular endothelium: Vasoactive mediators. *Prog Cardiovasc Dis* 1996; 39:229–238.

352. Okumura K, Yasue H, Horio Y, Takaoka K, Matsuyama K, Fujii H, et al. Multivessel coronary spasm in patients with variant angina: A study with intracoronary injection of acetylcholine. *Circulation* 1988; 77:535–542.

353. Ludmer PL, Selwyn AP, Shook TL, Wayne R, Mudge GH, Alexander RW, et al. Paradoxical vasoconstriction induced by acetylcholine in atherosclerotic coronary arteries. *N Engl J Med* 1986; 315:1046–1051.

354. Yamamoto H, Bossaller C, Cartwright J Jr, Henry PD. Videomicroscopic demonstration of defective cholinergic arteriolar vasodilatation in atherosclerotic rabbit. *J Clin Invest* 1988; 81:1752–1758.

355. Cox DA, Vita JA, Treasure CB, Fish RD, Alexander RW, Ganz P, et al. Atherosclerosis impairs flow-mediated dilation of coronary arteries in humans. *Circulation* 1989; 80:458–465.

356. Yasue H, Matsuyama K, Matsuyama K, Okumura K, Morikami Y, Ogawa H. Responses of angiographically normal human coronary arteries to intracoronary injection of acetylcholine by age and segment: Possible role of early coronary atherosclerosis. *Circulation* 1990; 81:482–490.

357. Marshall JJ, Kontos HA. Endothelium-derived relaxing factors: A perspective from in vivo data. *Hypertension* 1990; 16:371–386.

358. Flavahan NA. Atherosclerosis or lipoprotein-induced endothelial dysfunction: Potential mechanisms underlying reduction in EDRF/nitric oxide activity. *Circulation* 1992; 85:1927–1938.

359. Ware JA, Heistad DD. Platelet-endothelium interactions. *N Engl J Med* 1993; 328:628–635.

360. Rubanyi GM, Vanhoutte PM. Hypoxia releases a vasoconstrictor substance from the canine vascular endothelium. *J Physiol (Lond)* 1985; 364:45–56.

361. Di Carli MF, Tobes MC, Mangner T, Levine AB, Muzik O, Chakroborty P, et al. Effects of cardiac sympathetic innervation on coronary blood flow. *N Engl J Med* 1997; 336:1208–1215.

362. Feigl EO. The paradox of adrenergic coronary vasoconstriction. *Circulation* 76:737–745.

363. Gutterman DG, Brody MJ, Marcus ML. Neural regulation of coronary blood flow. In: Fozzard HA, Haber E, Jennings RB, Katz AM, Morgan HE, eds. *The Heart and Cardiovascular System*, 2d ed. New York: Raven; 1991:695–736.

364. Sander GE, Huggins CG. Vasoactive peptides. *Annu Rev Pharmacol* 1972; 12:227–264.

365. Oates JA, Fitzgerald GA, Branch RA, Jackson EK, Knapp HR, Roberts LJ. Clinical implications of prostaglandins and thromboxane A2 formation. *N Engl J Med* 1988; 319:689–698.

366. Zusman RM. Eicosanoids: Prostaglandins, thromboxane, and prostacyclin. In: Fozzard HA, Haber E, Jennings RB, Katz AM, Morgan HE, eds. *The Heart and Cardiovascular System*, 2d ed. New York: Raven; 1991:1797–1815.

367. Barcroft J, Dixon WE. The gaseous metabolism of the mammalian heart. *J Physiol* 1907; 35:182–204.

368. Rohde E. Uber den Einfluss der mechanischen Bedingungen auf die Tatigkeit und den Sauerstoffverbrauch des Warmbluterherzens. *Arch Exp Pathol Pharmakol* 1912; 68:401–420.

369. Evans CL, Matsuoka Y. The effect of various mechanical conditions on the gaseous metabolism and efficiency of the mammalian heart. *J Physiol* 1915; 49:378–405.

370. Sonnenblick EH, Skelton CL. Oxygen consumption of the heart: Physiological principles and clinical implications. *Mod Concepts Cardiovasc Dis* 1971; 40:9–16.

371. Sarnoff SJ, Braunwald E, Welch GH, Case RB, Stainsby WN, Macruz R. Hemodynamic determinants of oxygen consumption of the heart with special reference to the tension-time index. *Am J Physiol* 1958; 192:148.

372. Sonnenblick EH, Ross J Jr, Covell JW, Kaiser GA, Braunwald E. Velocity of contraction as a determinant of myocardial oxygen consumption. *Am J Physiol* 1965; 209:919–927.

373. Covell JW, Braunwald E, Ross J Jr, Sonnenblick EH. Studies on digitalis: XVI. Effects on myocardial oxygen consumption. *J Clin Invest* 1966; 45:1535–1542.

374. Neill WA, Levine HJ, Wagman RJ, Gorlin R. Left ventricular oxygen utilization in intact dogs: Effect of systemic hemodynamic factors. *Circ Res* 1963; 12:163–169.

375. Gregg DE. Effect of coronary perfusion pressure or coronary flow on oxygen usage of the myocardium. *Circ Res* 1963; 13:497–500.

376. Berne RM, Rubio R. Coronary circulation. In: Berne RM, ed. *Handbook of Physiology*, sec 2: *The Cardiovascular System*, vol 1: *The Heart.* Bethesda, MD: American Physiological Society; 1979:873.

377. Rose CP, Goresky CA. Interactions between capillary exchange, cellular entry, and metabolic sequestration processes in the heart. In: Renkin EM, Michel CC, eds. *Handbook of Physiology*, sec 2: *The Cardiovascular System*, vol IV: *Microcirculation*, part 2. Bethesda, MD: American Physiological Society; 1984:781–798.

378. Dole WP. Autoregulation of the coronary circulation. *Prog Cardiovasc Dis* 1987; 29:293–323.

379. Olsson RA, Bunger R. Metabolic control of coronary blood flow. *Prog Cardiovasc Dis* 1987; 29:369–387.

380. Hoffman JI. Transmural myocardial perfusion. *Prog Cardiovasc Dis* 1987; 29:429–464.

381. McHale PA, Dube GP, Greenfield JC Jr. Evidence for myogenic vasomotor activity in the coronary circulation. *Prog Cardiovasc Dis* 1987; 30:139–146.

382. Young MA, Knight DR, Vatner SF. Autonomic control of large coronary arteries and resistance vessels. *Prog Cardiovasc Dis* 1987; 30:211–234.

383. Hanley FL, Messina LM, Grattan MT, Hoffman IE. The effect of coronary inflow pressure on coronary vascular resistance in the isolated dog heart. *Circ Res* 1984; 54:760–772.

384. Wiggers CJ. The interplay of coronary vascular resistance and myocardial compression in regulating coronary flow. *Circ Res* 1954; 2:271–214.

385. Bache RJ, Dymek DJ. Local and regional regulation of coronary vascular tone. *Prog Cardiovasc Dis* 1981; 24:191–212.

386. Belardinelli L, Linden J, Berne RM. The cardiac effects of adenosine. *Prog Cardiovasc Dis* 1989; 32:73–97.

387. Mubagwa K, Mullane K, Flameng W. Role of adenosine in the heart and circulation. *Cardiovasc Res* 1996; 32:797–813.

388. Conti CR, ed. *Coronary Artery Spasm: Pathophysiology, Diagnosis and Treatment.* New York: Marcel Dekker; 1986:1–347.

389. Folts JD, Crowell EB Jr, Rowe GG. Platelet aggregation in partially obstructed vessels and its elimination with aspirin. *Circulation* 1976; 54:365–370.

390. Kuzuya T, Tada M, Inoue M, Kodama K, Takeda H, Mishima M, et al. Increased levels of thromboxane A2 in peripheral and coronary circulation in patients with angina pectoris (abstr). *Am J Cardiol* 1980; 45:454.

391. Robertson RM, Robertson D, Roberts LJ, Maas RL, Fitzgerald GA, Friesinger GC, et al. Thromboxane A2 in vasotonic angina pectoris. *N Engl J Med* 1981; 304:998–1000.

392. Esumi K, Tada M, Kuzuya T, Ohmori M, Matsuda H, Inoue M, et al. Thromboxane A2 and prostaglandin I$_2$ in canine circulation during transient myocardial ischemia (abstr). *Circulation* 1981; 64(suppl 4):266.

393. Yokoyama M, Goldman M, Henry PD. Supersensitivity of atherosclerotic arteries to ergonovine is partially mediated by a serotonergic mechanism (abstr). *Circulation* 1979; 60(suppl 2):100.

394. Heistad DD, Armstrong ML, Marcus ML, Marcus ML, Piegors DJ, Mark AL. Augmented responses to vasoconstrictor stimuli in hypercholesterolemic and atherosclerotic monkeys. *Circ Res* 1984; 54:711–718.

395. Mudge GH Jr, Goldberg S, Gunther S, Mann T, Grossman W. Comparison of metabolic and vasoconstrictor stimuli on coronary vascular resistance in man. *Circulation* 1979; 59:544–550.

396. Johannsen UJ, Mark AL, Marcus ML, Armstrong ML. Effects of dietary hyperlipoproteinemia on coronary vascular responsiveness in vivo (abstr). *Circulation* 1980; 64(suppl 4):267.

397. Shimokawa H, Tomoike H, Nabeyama S, Yamamoto H, Araki H, Nakamura M, et al. Coronary artery spasm induced in atherosclerotic miniature swine. *Science* 1983; 221:560–562.

398. Harrison DG, Minor RL, Guerra R, Quillen JE, Selke FW. Endothelial dysfunction in atherosclerosis. In: Rubanyi GM, ed. *Cardiovascular Significance of Endothelium-Derived Vasoactive Factors.* Mt Kisco, NY: Futura; 1991:263–280.

399. Vatner SF, Higgins CB, Braunwald E. Effects of norepinephrine on coronary circulation and left ventricular dynamics in the conscious dog. *Circ Res* 1974; 34:812–823.

400. Krasnow N, Rolett EL, Yurchak PM, Hood WB, Gorlin R. Isoproterenol and cardiovascular performance. *Am J Med* 1964; 37:514–525.

401. Dusting GJ, Moncada S, Vane JR. Prostaglandins, their intermediates and precursors: Cardiovascular actions and regulatory roles in normal and abnormal circulatory systems. *Prog Cardiovasc Dis* 1979; 21:405–430.

402. Gunther S, Cannon PJ. Modulation of angiotensin II coronary vasoconstriction by cardiac prostaglandin synthesis. *Am J Physiol* 1980; 238:H895–H901.

403. Nakano J. Cardiovascular actions of vasopressin. *Jpn Circ J* 1973; 37:363–381.

404. Nakano J. Cardiovascular responses to neurohypophysial hormones. In: Greep RO, Astwood EB, eds. *Handbook of Physiology*, sec 7: *Endocrinology*, vol 4. Bethesda, MD: American Physiological Society; 1974:395–442.

405. Khayyal MA, Eng C, Franzen D, Breall JA, Kirk ES. Effects of vasopressin on the coronary circulation reserve and regulation during ischemia. *Am J Physiol* 1985; 248:H516–H522.

406. Buccino RA, Spann JF Jr, Pool PE, Sonnenblick EH, Braunwald E. Influence of thyroid state on the intrinsic contractile properties and energy stores of the myocardium. *J Clin Invest* 1967; 46:1669–1682.

407. Skelton CL, Sonnenblick EH. Cardiovascular system. In: Werner SC, Ingbar SH, eds. *Hyperthyroidism.* New York: Harper & Row; 1978:688–697.

408. Hackel DB, Kleinerman J. Effects of thiamin deficiency on myocardial metabolism in intact dogs. *Am Heart J* 1953; 46:1.

409. Needleman P, Marshall GR, Sobel BE. Hormone interactions in the isolated rabbit heart: Synthesis and coronary vasomotor effects of prostaglandins, angiotensin, and bradykinin. *Circ Res* 1975; 37:802–808.

410. Regoli D, Barabe J, Therialult B. Does indomethacin antagonize the effects of peptides and other agents on the coronary circulation of rabbit isolated hearts? *Can J Physiol Pharmacol* 1977; 55:307–310.

411. Losay J, Mroz EA, Treagear GW, Leeman SE, Gamble WJ. Action of substance P on the coronary blood flow in the isolated dog heart. In: von Euler US, Pernow B, eds. *Substance P.* New York: Raven; 1976.

412. Carretero OA, Scicli AG. The kallikrein-kinin system. In: Fozzard HA, Haber E, Jennings RB, Katz AM, Morgan HE, eds. *The Heart and Cardiovascular System*, 2d ed. New York: Raven; 1991:1851–1874.

413. Brum JM, Bove AA, Vanhoutte PM. Participation of the endothelium in the vasodilator effects of vasoactive intestinal peptide and substance P in the coronary arteries (abstr). *Circulation* 1985; 72(suppl III):III-83.

414. Said SI. VIP: Overview. In: Bloom SR, ed. *Gut Hormones.* Edinburgh: Churchill Livingstone; 1978:465–469.

415. Rudehill A, Solleri A, Franco-Cereceda A, Lundberg JM. Neuropeptide Y (NPY) and the pig heart: Release and constrictor effects. *Peptides* 1987; 7:821–826.

416. DeNeef P, Robberecht P, Chatelain P, Waelbroeck M, Christophe J. The in vitro chronotropic and inotropic effects of vasoactive intestinal peptide (VIP) on the atria and ventricular papillary muscle from *Cyanomologus* monkey heart. *Regul Pept* 1984; 8:237–244.

417. Needleman P, Kaley S. Cardiac and coronary prostaglandin synthesis and function. *N Engl J Med* 1978; 298:1122–1128.

418. Stiles GL, Lefkowitz RJ. Cardiac adrenergic receptors. *Annu Rev Med* 1984; 35:149–164.

419. Feigl EO. Parasympathetic control of coronary blood flow in dogs. *Circ Res* 1969; 25:509–519.

420. Hanley HG, Costin JC, Skinner NS Jr. Differential reflex adjustments in cutaneous and muscle vascular beds during experimental coronary artery occlusion. *Am J Cardiol* 1971; 27:513–521.

421. Vatner SF, McRitchie RJ. Interaction of the chemoreflex and the pulmonary inflation reflex in the regulation of coronary circulation in conscious dogs. *Circ Res* 1975; 37:664–673.

422. Shepherd JT. Cardiac mechanoreceptors. In: Fozzard HA, Haber E, Jennings RB, Katz AM, Morgan HE, eds. *The Heart and Cardiovascular System*, 2d ed. New York: Raven; 1991:1481–1504.

423. Schaper W. Collateral circulation. In: Schaper W, ed. *The Paraphysiology of Myocardial Perfusion.* Amsterdam: Elsevier/North-Holland; 1979:1–276.

424. Schaper W, Bernotat-Danielowski S, Nienaber C, Schaper J. Collateral circulation. In: Fozzard HA, Haber E, Jennings RB, Katz AM, Morgan HE, eds. *The Heart and Cardiovascular System*, 2d ed. New York: Raven; 1991:1427–1464.

425. Schaper W. *Collateral Circulation: Heart, Brain, Kidney, Limbs.* Norwell, MA: Kluwer Academic; 1993.

426. Gregg DE, Patterson RE. Functional importance of the coronary collaterals. *N Engl J Med* 1980; 303:1404–1406.

427. Yanagisawa-Miwa A, Uchida Y, Nakamuru F, Tomara T, Kido H, Kamijo T, et al. Salvage of infarcted myocardium by angiogenic action of basic fibroblast growth factor. *Science* 1992; 25:1401–1403.

428. Hoffman JIE, Buckberg GD. Transmural variations in myocardial perfusion. In: Yu PN, Goodwin JF, eds. *Progress in Cardiology.* Philadelphia: Lea & Febiger; 1976:37–89.

429. Hoffman JIE. Determinants and prediction of transmural myocardial perfusion. *Circulation* 1978; 58:381–391.

430. Wangler RD, Peters KG, Marcus ML, Tomanek RJ. Effects of duration and severity of arterial hypertension on cardiac hypertrophy and coronary vasodilator reserve. *Circ Res* 1982; 51:10–18.

431. Schelbert HR, Phelps ME, Hoffman EJ, Huang SC, Selin CE, Kuhl DE. Regional myocardial perfusion assessed with N-13 labeled ammonia and positron emission computerized axial tomography. *Am J Cardiol* 1979; 43:209–218.

432. Hoffman JIE. The effect of intramyocardial forces on the distribution of intramyocardial blood flow. *J Biomed Eng* 1979; 1:33–40.

433. Bache R. Effects of hypertrophy on the coronary circulation. *Prog Cardiovasc Dis* 1988; 30:403–440.

434. Lee FA, Cabin HS, Francis CK. The syndrome of flash pulmonary edema: Clinical definition and angiographic findings (abstr). *J Am Coll Cardiol* 1988; 11(suppl A):151A.

435. Schlant RC. "Flash" pulmonary edema. *Am Coll Cardiol Curr J Rev* 1992; 1:74–75.

436. Wiggers CJ. Studies on the consecutive phases of the cardiac cycle: I. The duration of the consecutive phases of the cardiac cycle and the criteria for their precise determination. *Am J Physiol* 1921; 56:415–438.

437. Wiggers CJ. Studies on the consecutive phases of the cardiac cycle: II. The laws governing the relative durations of ventricular systole and diastole. *Am J Physiol* 1921; 56:439–459.

438. Schlant RC. Events during cardiac cycle. In: Altman PL, Dittmer DS, eds. *Respiration and Circulation*, 2d ed. Bethesda, MD: Federation of American Society for Experimental Biological Proceedings; 1973:304.

439. Laniado S, Yellin E, Kotler M, Levy L, Stadler J, Terdiman R. A study of the dynamic relations between the mitral valve echogram and phasic mitral flow. *Circulation* 1975; 51:104–113.

440. Laniado S, Yellin E, Terdiman R, Meytes I, Stadler J. Hemodynamic correlates of the normal aortic valve echogram: A study of sound, flow, and motion. *Circulation* 1976; 54:729–737.

441. Spencer MP, Greiss FC. Dynamics of ventricular ejection. *Circ Res* 1962; 10:274–279.

442. Grant C, Greene DG, Bunnell IL. The valve-closing function of the right atrium: A study of pressures and atrial sounds in patients with heart block. *Am J Med* 1963; 34:325–328.

443. MacCanon DM, Arevalo F, Meyer EC. Direct detection and timing of aortic valve closure. *Circ Res* 1964; 14:387–391.

444. Piemme TE, Barnett GO, Dexter L. Relationship of heart sounds to acceleration of blood flow. *Circ Res* 1966; 18:303–315.

445. Delman AJ. Hemodynamic correlations of cardiovascular sounds. *Annu Rev Med* 1967; 18:139–158.

446. Craige E, Fortuin NJ. Genesis of heart sounds and murmurs as demon-

strated by echocardiography. In: Joyner CR, ed. *Ultrasound in the Diagnosis of Cardiovascular-Pulmonary Disease.* Chicago: Year Book Medical; 1974:119–132.

447. Waider W, Craige E. First heart sound and ejection sounds: Echocardiographic and phonocardiographic correlation with valvular events. *Am J Cardiol* 1975; 35:346–356.

448. Chandraratna PAN, Lopez JM, Cohen LS. Echocardiographic observations on the mechanism of production of the second heart sound. *Circulation* 1975; 51:292–296.

449. Sagawa K, Maughan L, Suga H, Sunagawa K. *Cardiac Contraction and the Pressure-Volume Relationship.* New York: Oxford University Press; 1988:1–480.

450. Marshall HW, Helmholz HF, Wood EH. Physiologic consequences of congenital heart disease. In: Hamilton WF, Dow P, eds. *Handbook of Physiology,* sec 2: *Circulation,* vol 1. Bethesda, MD: American Physiological Society; 1962:417–487.

451. Mackay IFS. The true venous pulse wave, central and peripheral. *Am Heart J* 1967; 74:48–57.

452. Barratt-Boyes BG, Wood EH. Cardiac output and related measurements and pressure values in the right heart and associated vessels, together with an analysis of the hemodynamic response to the inhalation of high oxygen mixtures in healthy subjects. *J Lab Clin Med* 1958; 51:72–90.

453. Braunwald E, Brockenbrough EC, Fraham CJ, Ross J Jr. Left atrial and left ventricular pressures in subjects without cardiovascular disease. *Circulation* 1961; 24:267–269.

454. Wade OL, Bishop JM. *Cardiac Output and Regional Blood Flow.* Oxford: Blackwell Scientific; 1962.

455. Dexter L, Whittenberger JL, Haynes FW, Goodale WT, Gorlin R, Sawyer CG. Effect of exercise on circulatory dynamics of normal individuals. *J Appl Physiol* 1951; 3:439–453.

456. Barratt-Boyes BG, Wood EH. Hemodynamic response of healthy subjects to exercise in the supine position while breathing oxygen. *J Appl Physiol* 1957; 11:129–135.

457. Wang Y, Marshall RJ, Shepherd JT. The effect of changes in posture and of graded exercise on stroke volume in man. *J Clin Invest* 1960; 39:1051–1061.

458. Epstein SE, Beiser GD, Stampfer M. Characterization of the circulatory response to maximal upright exercise in normal subjects and patients with heart disease. *Circulation* 1967; 35:1049.

459. Braunwald E, Sonnenblick EH, Ross J Jr, Glick G, Epstein SE. An analysis of the cardiac response to exercise. *Circ Res* 1967; 20(suppl 1):1–58.

460. Chapman CB, ed. Physiology of muscular exercise. *Circ Res* 1967; 20(suppl 1):I-1–I-226.

461. Bevegard BS, Shepherd JT. Regulation of the circulation during exercise in man. *Physiol Rev* 1967; 47:178–213.

462. Smith EE, Guyton AC, Manning RD, White RJ. Integrated mechanisms of cardiovascular response and control during exercise in the normal human. *Prog Cardiovasc Dis* 1976; 18:421–444.

463. Astrand PO, Rodahl K. *Textbook of Work Physiology: Physiological Bases of Exercises,* 3d ed. New York: McGraw-Hill; 1986.

464. Scheuer J, Tipton CM. Cardiovascular adaptations of physical training. *Annu Rev Physiol* 1977; 39:221–251.

465. Blomqvist CG, Saltin B. Cardiovascular adaptations to physical training. *Annu Rev Physiol* 1983; 45:169–189.

466. Brengelmann GL. Circulatory adjustments to exercise and heat stress. *Annu Rev Physiol* 1983; 45:191–212.

467. Schlant RC. Physiology of exercise. In: Fletcher GF, ed. *Exercise in the Practice of Medicine,* 2d ed. Mount Kisco, NY: Futura; 1988:1–47.

468. Upton MT, Rerych SK, Roeback JR Jr, Newman GE, Douglas JM Jr, Wallace AG, et al. Effect of brief and prolonged exercise on left ventricular function. *Am J Cardiol* 1980; 45:1154–1160.

469. Bar-Shlomo B-Z, Druck MN, Morch JE, Jablonsky G, Hilton JO, Feiglin DH, et al. Left ventricular function in trained and untrained healthy subjects. *Circulation* 1982; 65:484–488.

470. Kelbaek H, Gjorup T, Christensen WJ, Vestergaard B, Godtredsen J. Cardiac function and plasma catecholamines during upright exercise in healthy young subjects. *Int J Cardiol* 1986; 10:223–235.

471. Port S, Cobb FR, Coleman RE, Jones RH. Effect of age on the response of the left ventricular ejection fraction to exercise. *N Engl J Med* 1980; 303:1133–1137.

472. Astrand PO, Saltin B. Plasma and red cell volume after prolonged severe exercise. *J Appl Physiol* 1964; 19:819–832.

473. Lundvall J, Mellander S, Westling H, White T. Fluid transfer between blood and tissues during exercise. *Acta Physiol Scand* 1972; 85:258–269.

474. Lind AR, McNicol GW. Circulatory responses to sustained hand-grip contractions performed during other exercise, both rhythmic and static. *J Physiol* 1967; 192:595–607.

475. Lind AR, McNicol GW. Cardiovascular responses to holding and carrying weights by hand and by shoulder harness. *J Appl Physiol* 1968; 25:261–267.

476. Nutter DO, Schlant RC, Hurst JW. Isometric exercise and the cardiovascular system. *Mod Concepts Cardiovasc Dis* 1972; 41:11–15.

477. Fisher ML, Nutter DO, Jacobs W, Schlant RC. Haemodynamic responses to isometric exercise (handgrip) in patients with heart disease. *Br Heart J* 1973; 35:422–432.

478. Martin CE, Shaver JA, Leon DF, Thompson ME, Reddy PS, Leonard JJ. Autonomic mechanism in hemodynamic responses to isometric exercise. *J Clin Invest* 1974; 54:104–115.

479. McCloskey DI, Streatfield KA. Muscular reflex stimuli to the cardiovascular system during isometric contractions of muscle groups of different mass. *J Physiol* 1975; 250:431–441.

480. Grover RF, Weil JV, Reeves JT. Cardiovascular adaptation to exercise at high altitude. *Exercise Sports Sci Rev* 1986; 14:269–302.

4

CELLULAR BIOLOGY
OF BLOOD VESSELS

Kathy K. Griendling / R. Wayne Alexander

Knowledge of the biology of the vascular wall is essential to understanding the pathophysiology of atherosclerosis, vasospasm, and hypertension, as well as the rationale behind the development and application of new therapeutic strategies for vascular disease. As the major strategy for treating vascular disease shifts from treating secondary manifestations to treating the primary dysfunction, understanding the biologic basis of disease becomes of central importance. It is likely that much cardiovascular disease reflects *dysfunctional endothelium*. This chapter is designed to give an introduction to vascular biology with emphasis on the function of the endothelium.

STRUCTURE
OF THE VESSEL WALL

Arteries consist of three layers: the innermost *intima*, the *media*, and the outermost *adventitia*. The intima is composed of a single layer of endothelial cells embedded in an extracellular matrix. The media is separated from the intima by the internal elastic lamina and consists of smooth muscle cells, elastic laminae, bundles of collagen fibers, and elastic fibrils, all embedded in an extracellular matrix. The adventitia is the most variable layer, containing dense fibroelastic tissue, nutrient vessels, and nerves.

The actual composition of each of these layers varies with the type of blood vessel. Large, conduit arteries are typically referred to as *elastic arteries* because of their high ratio of elastic laminae to smooth muscle cells. Muscular arteries are generally smaller and have a prevalence of smooth muscle cells, while arterioles consist of only one to two layers of smooth muscle cells. The smallest vessels are the capillaries, made up of a single layer of endothelial cells that are occasionally apposed to pericytes—smooth muscle-like cells that serve a contractile function. The venous system has a similar architecture to that of the arterial system, the main difference being the orientation of the smooth muscle cells within the wall.

Physiologically, the two most important cell types in the vascular system are the *endothelial cell* and the vascular *smooth muscle cell*. The endothelial cell is generally oriented with the direction of blood flow parallel to the main axis of the vessel. Endothelial cells are held together by junctional complexes that regulate permeability and control cell-to-cell communication. The smooth muscle cell is a spindle-shaped cell the orientation of which varies with the type of artery, but it is generally helical in large, elastic arteries and concentric in muscular arteries. Vascular smooth muscle cells contain three types of filaments: *thick* (myosin), *thin* (actin), and *intermediate*. The proteins that form these filaments undergo phosphorylation upon exposure to certain vasoactive agonists, thus altering their orientation and interactions and supporting force development (see below). In normal arteries, the smooth muscle cells are primarily in the "contractile" phenotype described above. Under conditions where smooth muscle cells are proliferating, however—such as atherosclerotic plaques, intimal hyperplasia as a result of angioplasty, or placement in culture—these cells "modulate" morphologically and biochemically to a growth mode and lose their differential contractile features.

PHYSIOLOGY
OF THE ENDOTHELIAL CELL

Normal endothelial cell function is crucial to homeostasis in the vascular system. As mentioned above, diseases such as atherosclerosis ultimately are manifestations of endothelial dysfunction. The endothelium has three major functions: as a metabolically active, secretory tissue; as an anticoagulant, antithrombotic surface; and as a barrier to indiscriminant passage of blood constituents into the arterial wall. The implications of these physiologic properties for vascular biology will be considered separately. In this subsection we discuss the processing of various substances by the endothelium.

Endothelial Cell Metabolism and Secretion of Vasoactive Factors

As discussed in more detail below, endothelial cells secrete vasoactive substances that play a major role in the control of vascular tone. These molecules include *prostacyclin, endothelial-derived relaxing factor* (EDRF), and *endothelial-derived hyperpolarizing factor* (EDHF), which serve as vasodilators,[1–3] as well as endothelin[4] and *endothelial-derived contracting factor* (EDCF), which act as vasoconstrictors.

Endothelial cells also manufacture and secrete substances such as factor VIII antigen, von Willebrand's factor, and plasminogen activator, which are involved in the coagulation/fibrinolytic pathways. Structural components of the extracellular matrix synthesized by these cells include *collagen, elastin, glycosaminoglycans,* and *fibronectin.*[5,6] The composition of the extracellular matrix is dynamically modulated by *matrix metalloproteinases,* enzymes that degrade matrix proteins and participate in its remodeling. These enzymes are secreted by both endothelial and smooth muscle cells.[7,8] In addition, endothelial cells synthesize and secrete heparans and growth factors that regulate smooth muscle cell proliferation.[9–12] Finally, endothelial cells are able to clear and metabolically alter blood-borne and locally produced substances including plasma lipids and lipoproteins,[13] adenine nucleotides and nucleosides,[14] serotonin, catecholamines, bradykinin, and angiotensin I.[15]

Endothelial cells are involved in the metabolism of plasma lipids in several ways. Lipoprotein lipase, an enzyme that hydrolyzes triglycerides into constituent fatty acids, is bound to the endothelial cell surface by heparan sulfates.[16] The interaction of this enzyme with chylomicrons or very low density lipoprotein (VLDL) particles results in the release of free fatty acids, which can then cross the subendothelial space to the underlying smooth muscle or inflammatory cells in atherosclerosis. In addition, endothelial cells possess receptors for low-density lipoprotein (LDL),[17] which regulate the transport and modification of LDL. Normally, LDL receptors are downregulated because receptor processing is inhibited in the nongrowing monolayer.[17] There are, however, two other pathways for uptake of LDL. First, LDL can be transported across the endothelium by an unknown, active, receptor-independent mechanism.[18] Second, modified, or oxidized LDL can be taken up by "scavenger" LDL receptors,[19] the expression of which is unaffected by the growth state of the endothelial cells. These cells also have the capacity to modify LDL,[20] thus enhancing its uptake and ultimately leading to an increase in cholesterol esters in the vessel wall and, importantly, facilitating LDL uptake by inflammatory cells in disease.

The Endothelial Cell and Thrombosis

Quiescent endothelial cells normally present an antithrombotic surface that resists platelet adhesion and does not activate coagulation. (For a more detailed discussion of thrombosis, see Chap. 52.) The continuity of the endothelium is essential to this function, and nonthrombogenicity has been attributed in part to the negative charge on the surface of these cells.[21] Endothelial cells are, however, capable of synthesizing and secreting prothrombotic factors, especially when stimulated with cytokines or other inflammatory agents. The endothelium thus represents a functional antithrombotic-thrombolytic/thrombotic balance (Fig. 4-1). Potent anticoagulants elaborated by the endothelium include prostacyclin, which inhibits platelet aggregation,[22] heparin-like molecules,[23] and thrombomodulin, which activates protein C.[24] In addition, antithrombin III binds to the surface-bound heparin-like molecules and serves as a clearance (via internalization) molecule for thrombin, as well as a thrombin inhibitor.[25] These cells also produce tissue plasminogen activator (tPA) and plasminogen activator inhibitor I (PAI-I), and can bind plasminogen on their surface via fibronectin and thrombospondin.[26] The relative amounts of tPA and PAI-I can be up- or downregulated, respectively, by thrombin and other vasoactive substances to control clot lysis.

As mentioned above, under conditions of injury or inflammation, the endothelium may become prothrombotic (Fig. 4-2). On stimulation with inflammatory cytokines, endothelial cells increase the surface expression of tissue factor[27] and leukocyte adhesion molecules[28] and decrease the expression of thrombomodulin.[27] Thrombin itself stimulates further production of von Willebrand's factor,[29] which, along with thrombospondin and fibronectin, participates in the thrombotic response. Furthermore, endothelial cells can bind factor IX,[30] which, when tissue factor is expressed, can be activated by tissue factor-VIIa complex, leading to activation of factor X in the presence of factor VIII. Activated factor X (Xa) can then promote assembly of the prothrombinase complex. Thus, under inflammatory conditions, endothelial cells can amplify the prothrombotic response. All of the factors controlling the expression of pro- and antithrombotic/fibrinolytic molecules

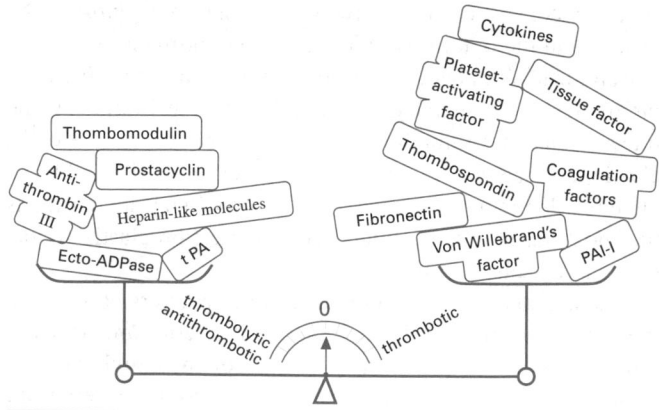

FIGURE 4-1

Hemostatic/thrombotic balance in endothelial cells. Endothelial cells express and secrete both prothrombotic and antithrombotic/thrombolytic molecules. Under normal conditions, endothelial cells present an antithrombotic surface. Upon stimulation with cytokines or other inflammatory agents, they synthesize and secrete prothrombotic factors. The hemostatic status of the endothelium is thus highly dependent upon the balance between these two opposing classes of compounds. tPA = tissue plasminogen activator; PAI-I = plasminogen activator inhibitor I. (Courtesy of Bernard Lassègue, Ph.D.)

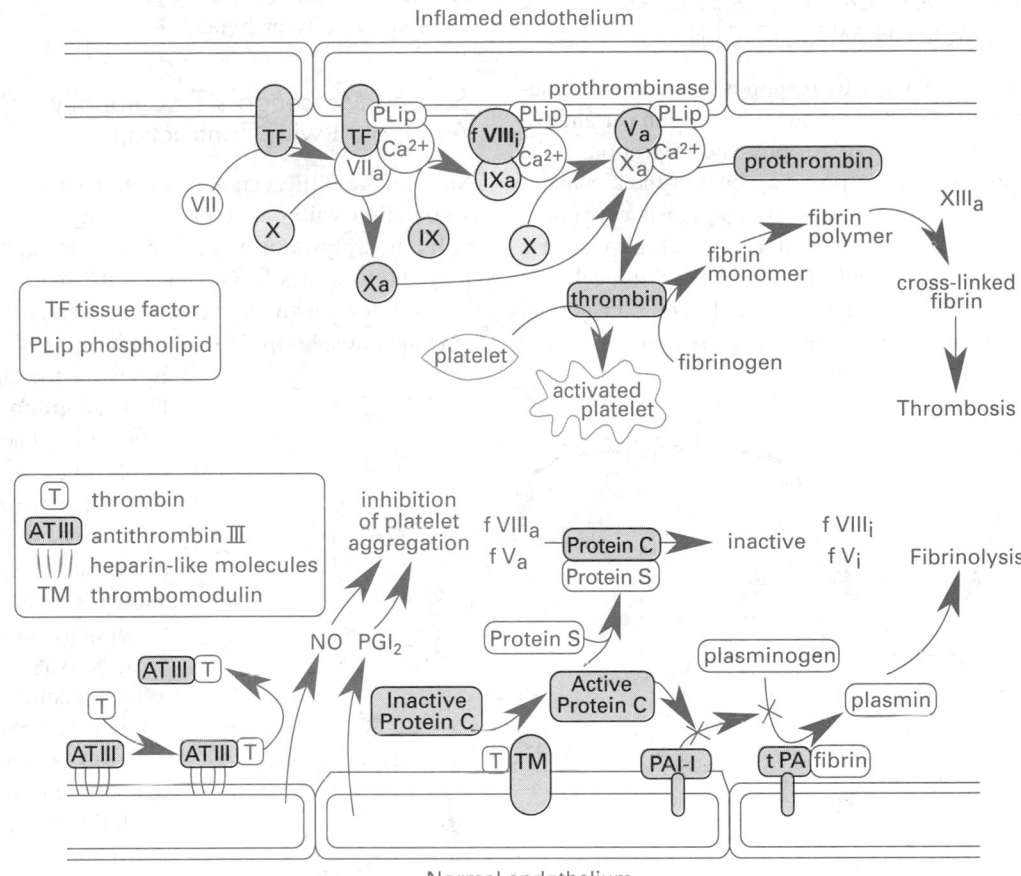

FIGURE 4-2

Pathways of thrombosis and thrombolysis. Under normal conditions, the endothelium is antithrombotic. Antithrombin III (ATIII) binds thrombin and serves to clear thrombin from the circulation. Prostacyclin (PGI$_2$) inhibits platelet aggregation, and thrombomodulin (TM) activates protein C, which inhibits plasminogen activator inhibitor I (PAI-I) and interacts with protein S to inactivate activated factors V and VIII, thus limiting thrombosis. Since PAI-I inhibits the tissue plasminogen activator (tPA)-catalyzed conversion of plasminogen to plasmin, PAI-I inhibition leads to accumulation of plasmin and fibrinolysis. Upon stimulation with inflammatory cytokines, there is increased expression of tissue factor on the endothelial cell surface. Tissue factor participates in the activation of factor X, which, in turn, promotes assembly of the prothrombinase complex, producing thrombin. Under these conditions, endothelial cells thus amplify the thrombotic response. (Courtesy of Bernard Lassègue, Ph.D.)

are not known, but it is clear that the endothelium functions as a major regulator of hemostasis.

Barrier Function and Endothelial Cell Permeability

There are three routes by which the endothelium selectively regulates the influx of plasma macromolecules into the arterial wall: intercellular tight junctions, vesicles and/or transendothelial channels, and the lipid phase of the endothelial membrane. These pathways enable the intact endothelium to serve as a barrier, preventing or impeding highly mitogenic, thrombotic, or vasoactive substances from coming into direct contact with the underlying vascular smooth muscle. Each route has both active and passive components, and the extent to which they are utilized depends to a certain degree on the location of the endothelial cells. Thus, capillaries and postcapillary venules respond to vasoactive agents, some of which (histamine, prostaglandins) are secreted by the endothelial cell it-self, with increased flux through tight junctions.[31] The tight junctions found in arteries tend to be the most occlusive but may also be influenced by hypertension[32] and various agonists. Vesicular transport is mainly utilized by the cell to transfer water-soluble macromolecules from the luminal surface to the abluminal surface, but the permanence of such structures and whether they form transendothelial channels are matters of debate. Lipid-phase transport has been proposed as a mechanism whereby lipid-soluble molecules (e.g., free fatty acids) could be transferred to the abluminal surface of the endothelial cell.[33] These molecules could enter the outer leaflet of the membrane from the circulation and diffuse along the lipid bilayer to be released or bind to extracellular matrix components in the subintimal area. Thus, the endothelium has both passive and active roles in the control of vascular permeability by acting as a physical permeability barrier and by modulating the expression of cell-surface and secreted agonists and molecules that are capable of altering permeability.

PHYSIOLOGY OF THE VASCULAR SMOOTH MUSCLE CELL

The smooth muscle cell normally responds to hormonal stimulation with contraction or relaxation. However, in certain disease states, growth and/or hypertrophy and migration to the intima are the predominant responses. Some of the biochemical signals generated by these vasoactive agonists are similar for both types of responses, with the final physiologic response dictated by the phenotype and environment of the cell and the exact biochemical pathways activated. Thus, in normal arteries, growth factors can act as vasoconstrictors,[34] while in modulated smooth muscle cells, vasoconstrictors can stimulate hypertrophy or hyperplasia.[35]

Second Messengers Traditionally Associated with Contraction

Some of the earliest signals generated within the cell following stimulation with calcium-mobilizing vasoactive agonists involve hydrolysis of a specific class of membrane lipids, the phosphoinositides[36]. There are three major inositol phospholipids in the plasma membrane that serve as substrates for the enzyme phospholipase C. Phospholipase C cleaves phospholipids to liberate the water-soluble head group and the lipophilic molecule diacylglycerol (Fig. 4-3). The water-soluble head group that is most important for signal generation is inositol trisphosphate (IP$_3$), which has been shown to release Ca^{2+} from intracellular stores.[37] Ca^{2+}, in turn, activates a cascade of enzymes leading to contraction or growth (see below). Diacylglycerol is a potent activator of protein kinase C, a Ca^{2+}- and phospholipid-dependent enzyme that phosphorylates numerous cellular proteins.[38] Diacylglycerol can be further metabolized to phosphatidic acid or to glycerol, fatty acids, and, ultimately, eicosanoids and leukotrienes, which may themselves modulate tone. Additionally, vasoconstrictor agents cause a sustained intracellular alkalinization[39] and an influx of extracellular Ca^{2+},[40] both of which serve to sustain and enhance vasoconstriction.

Biochemical Signals Traditionally Associated with Proliferation

Classical growth factors, such as platelet-derived growth factor (PDGF), activate many of the same signaling pathways as do vasoconstrictors: phosphoinositide hydrolysis, Ca^{2+} mobilization and influx, Na$^+$/H$^+$ exchange, and intracellular alkalinization. Vasoactive agonists and growth factors also stimulate phosphorylation of numerous proteins on tyrosine, a

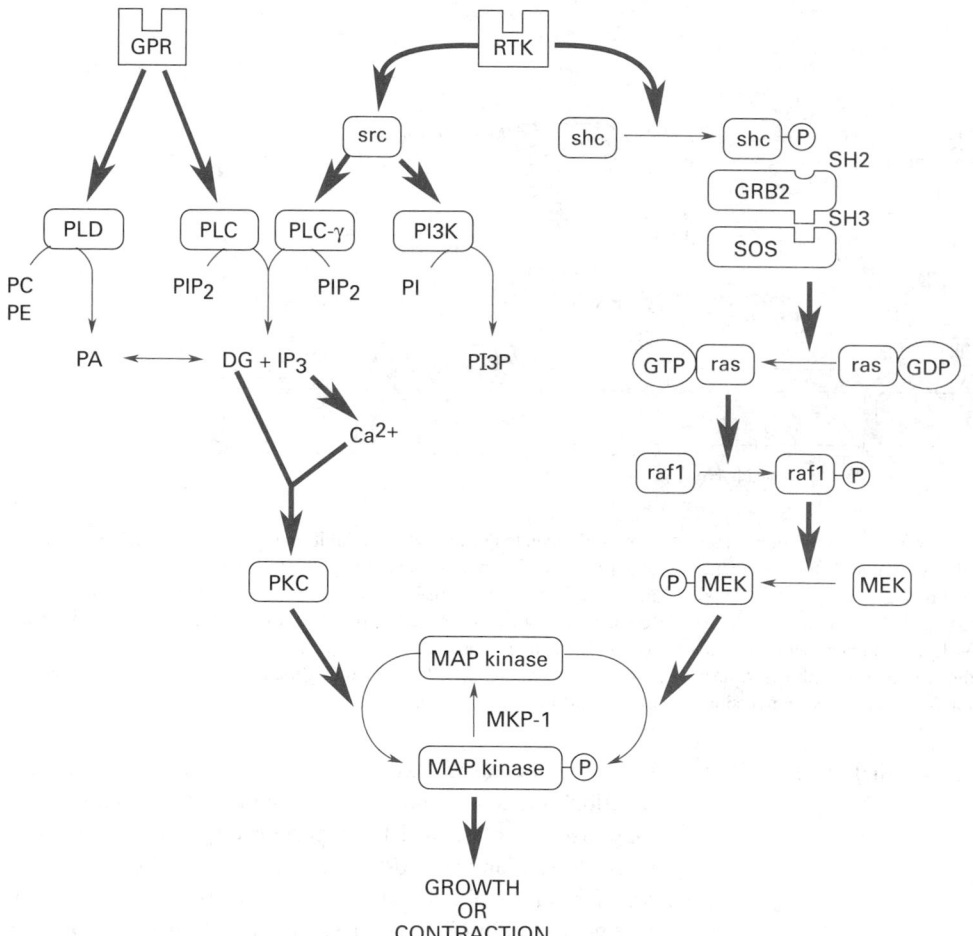

FIGURE 4-3

Signaling pathways in vascular smooth muscle. Vasoconstrictor agonists interact with specific G protein coupled receptors (GPR) on vascular smooth muscle. These receptors are linked to a G protein, which then couples to one or more phospholipase Cs (PLC) or phospholipase D (PLD). PLC cleaves the inositol phospholipids to yield diacylglycerol (DG) and inositol phosphates, in particular, inositol trisphosphate (IP$_3$). IP$_3$ releases calcium from intracellular stores, and, along with DG, activates the Ca^{2+}- and phospholipid-dependent enzyme protein kinase C (PKC). PLD cleaves phosphatidylcholine (PC) to release phosphatidic acid (PA) and choline. DG and PA can be interconverted; in vascular smooth muscle, PLD-mediated PC hydrolysis is probably the main source of DG. PKC is involved in activation of the mitogen activated protein (MAP) kinase cascade. Growth factors activate receptor tyrosine kinases (RTK), which activate src and subsequently PLC-γ, initiating IP$_3$ release and PKC activation. Involved in this coupling is phosphatidylinositol 3-kinase (PI3K). RTKs also phosphorylate and form a signaling complex with adapter proteins such as shc, which bind grb-2 and sos and ultimately mediate the conversion of ras to its active form. Ras phosphorylates raf1, which in turn phosphorylates MEK, leading to activation of the MAP kinase cascade. PI = phosphatidylinositol; PI3P = phosphatidylinositol 3-phosphate; PIP$_2$ = phosphatidylinositol 4,5-bisphosphate. (Courtesy of Bernard Lassègue, Ph.D.)

signaling pathway that is essential for growth. The importance of tyrosine phosphorylation in mediating the growth response is shown by the observation that mutant PDGF receptors, which lack the normal, intrinsic tyrosine kinase domain, are incapable of mediating proliferation in response to PDGF.[41] In addition, tyrosine kinase inhibitors have been shown to inhibit growth.[42] There is also increasing evidence that tyrosine phosphatases are able to counteract the mitogenic effects of growth factors by inhibiting tyrosine phosphorylation of specific substrates.[43]

A complex of substrates is postulated to become associated with activated growth factor receptor complexes and subsequently to activate a cascade of intracellular events leading to the final cellular response (Fig. 4-3).[44] This complex is proposed to be composed of phospholipase C-γ and phosphatidylinositol-3-kinase. Upon addition of PDGF to various cell types, the receptor dimerizes and auto-tyrosine phosphorylates, and each of the above proteins is phosphorylated on tyrosine, presumably leading, either directly or indirectly via association with the activated receptor to their activation. In addition, adapter proteins such as Shc and Grb2 link these receptors to ras, a ubiquitous GTPase that initiates a kinase cascade that includes mitogen-activated protein kinase (MAP kinase) and ultimately leads to growth. Recent evidence suggests that many of these proteins are also activated by seven transmembrane–spanning hormone receptors[45]—an observation that may partially explain the growth-promoting properties of some vasoconstrictor hormones such as angiotensin II.

An additional pathway that is activated under some conditions by growth factors and vasoactive agonists is phospholipase D–mediated hydrolysis of plasma membrane phosphatidylcholine.[46] In this reaction, phosphatidic acid and choline are released. This pathway is receiving increasing attention because phosphatidic acid may have a role in mediating the growth response[47] and phospholipase D activation seems to be required for the proliferative response.[48]

Contraction Cascade

Contractions induced by various vasoactive hormones differ not only in magnitude and time course but also between vessels. In general, there is an initial, rapid component of force generation and a more sustained phase of contraction. Some agonists, such as angiotensin II, induce only a transient constriction of many vessels, while others, including norepinephrine and vasopressin, nearly always cause a sustained contraction. The initial phase of force development shown to depend on the formation of actin-myosin cross bridges, but the mechanisms underlying the sustained phase of contraction are less clear.

Phasic contraction of smooth muscle is proposed to be regulated by a sliding-filament mechanism similar to that seen in skeletal muscle. Force generation is accomplished by attachment of the myosin heads (or cross bridges) to actin filaments. This attachment catalyzes adenosine triphosphate (ATP) hydrolysis to generate tension and occurs in a cyclic

manner for the duration of the stimulus. Smooth muscle has a relatively greater content of actin and a lower content of myosin than does skeletal muscle, and in contrast to skeletal muscle, the major site of calcium regulation of smooth muscle actomyosin is on the myosin molecule. Smooth muscle myosin consists of two large subunits, each with molecular mass of 200 kDa, and two small subunits of 20 and 16 to 17 kDa, known as the myosin light chains. Force generation in smooth muscle is regulated by phosphorylation/dephosphorylation of the 20-kDa protein (Fig. 4-4). Once phosphorylation occurs, actin-activated Mg^{2+}-ATPase activity is stimulated, resulting in cross-bridge cycling. Myosin light chain phosphorylation is mediated by an enzyme known as myosin light chain kinase (MLCK). This protein associates with calmodulin, a calcium-binding protein required for activation of numerous cytoplasmic enzymes. Thus, when Ca^{2+} increases within the cell in response to hormonal stimulation, it binds to calmodulin, which, in turn, associates with MLCK, converting it from an inactive to an active form. MLCK then phosphorylates the myosin light chain, permitting actin activation of the Mg^{2+}-ATPase and resulting in cross-bridge formation. When the intracellular Ca^{2+} concentration drops below about 100 nM, Ca^{2+} dissociates from calmodulin, calmodulin detaches from MLCK, and MLCK becomes inactive. Myosin light chain phosphatase activity then predominates, myosin is dephosphorylated, and cross-bridge cycling ceases. However, during sustained contraction, the intracellular Ca^{2+} concentration is low and energy consumption is reduced, suggesting the development of a latch bridge or of a low cycling state.[49] Alternatively, the sensitivity of the contractile apparatus to

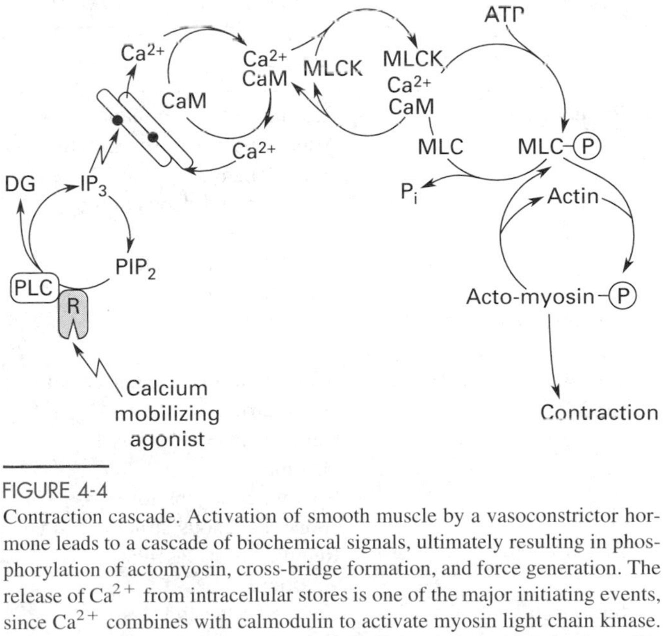

FIGURE 4-4

Contraction cascade. Activation of smooth muscle by a vasoconstrictor hormone leads to a cascade of biochemical signals, ultimately resulting in phosphorylation of actomyosin, cross-bridge formation, and force generation. The release of Ca^{2+} from intracellular stores is one of the major initiating events, since Ca^{2+} combines with calmodulin to activate myosin light chain kinase. This enzyme phosphorylates the myosin light chain, which is then able to interact with actin. R = receptor; PLC = phospholipase C; DG = diacylglycerol; PIP_2 = phosphatidylinositol 4,5-bisphosphate; IP_3 = inositol trisphosphate; CaM = calmodulin; MLCK = myosin light chain kinase; MLC = myosin light chain; P = phosphate. (Courtesy of Bernard Lassègue, Ph.D.)

Ca^{2+} may be increased, a response posited to be regulated by protein kinase C.[50]

Growth

Vascular smooth muscle cell growth takes two forms: hypertrophy and hyperplasia. In general, hypertrophy appears to occur in response to long-term stimulation with vasoconstrictor-type agents, while hyperplasia occurs in response to the classical growth factors. Hypertrophy is characterized by an increase in smooth muscle cell mass due to increased protein synthesis and has been shown to occur in response to angiotensin II[51] and thrombin,[52] as well as in large vessels during hypertension. Hyperplasia is characterized by cell replication, and is stimulated by growth factors such as PDGF and fibroblast growth factor (FGF)[53–55] following vascular injury.

THE EXTRACELLULAR MATRIX

The extracellular matrix is a major component of the vessel wall. It is the medium through which nutrients are transported, a repository for products secreted by the cells of the vascular wall, the site of accumulation of cell debris, and a substrate for migration and proliferation of endothelial cells, monocytes, and vascular smooth muscle cells. The matrix consists of several proteins that have distinct functions in maintaining the integrity of the wall (Table 4-1).

TABLE 4-1
COMPONENTS OF THE EXTRACELLULAR MATRIX

Matrix Component	Function
Proteoglycans	Resistance to deformation
	Arterial permeability, filtration, ion exchange
	Transport and deposition of plasma elements
	Regulation of cellular metabolism
Collagens (types I and III)	Mechanical strength
Collagens (types IV, V, and VI)	Attachment of vascular cells to the matrix
	Components of the basal lamina
	Linking collagens to noncollagenous structures
Elastin	Regulation of vascular elasticity
Fibronectin	Cell-cell adhesion
	Cell-substrate adhesion
	Cell motility
	Specific binding of collagen, heparin
Laminin	Attachment of endothelial cells to type IV collagen

Extracellular matrix degradation and reformation is an integral part of vascular remodeling. For example, one of the earliest events in angiogenesis is degradation of the extracellular matrix to permit tube (capillary) formation. Microvascular and venous endothelial cells have been shown to synthesize both matrix metalloproteinases (MMPs), enzymes that selectively digest the individual components of the matrix, and tissue inhibitors of metalloproteinases (TIMPs).[7] Smooth muscle cells also synthesize matrix metalloproteinases.[8]

MMPs belong to three main groups: the type IV collagenases (also called gelatinases), the stromelysins, and interstitial collagenase. The characteristics of these proteins are described in Table 4-2. MMPs are produced as inactive zymogens which can be activated by plasmin.[8] The activity of MMPs is also regulated by cytokines at transcriptional and post-translational levels, as well as by the relative levels of tissue inhibitors of metalloproteinases. MMP-2 is usually found complexed with its specific inhibitor, TIMP-2.

In venous or microvascular endothelial cells, MMP-1 (interstitial collagenase), MMP-2 (72 kDa-gelatinase) and TIMP-1 and -2 are constitutively expressed. Although MMP-3 is only weakly expressed, it can be induced synergistically by incubation of the cells with the cytokine TNF-α with the tumor promoter PMA.[7] This treatment also induces MMP-9 expression. Since MMP-2 and TIMP-2 are unaffected by TNF-α, cytokine activation of endothelial cells can change the complement of metalloproteinases produced. In vascular smooth muscle cells, MMP-2 is constitutively expressed, while MMP-1, MMP-9 (92-kDa gelatinase) and MMP-3 (stromelysin) are induced by cytokines such as interleukin 1 (IL-1) and TNF-α.[8] Cytokines are also able to activate MMP-2 zymogen.[56] Thus, cytokine stimulation increases the range of active metalloproteinases secreted by smooth muscle cells to encompass proteases capable of degrading all the major matrix components. In contrast, although TIMP-1 and TIMP-2 are constitutively expressed by vascular smooth muscle, their expression is unaffected by cytokines.[8] *The net effect of cytokines on the vascular wall may be to tip the balance between the production of MMPs and TIMPs in favor of extracellular matrix degradation and remodeling.*

ENDOTHELIAL CELL–VASCULAR SMOOTH MUSCLE INTERACTIONS

Endothelial Control of Vascular Tone

The endothelium serves a dual function in the control of vascular tone (Fig. 4-5). It secretes relaxing factors such as nitric oxide and adenosine and constricting factors such as the endothelins. Vessel tone is thus dependent on the balance between these factors as well as upon the ability of the smooth muscle cell to respond to them. The most important regulatory molecules are discussed separately.

ENDOTHELIUM-DERIVED RELAXING FACTOR/NITRIC OXIDE
An endothelium-derived relaxing factor (EDRF) was first described by Furchgott and Zawadzki,[2] who observed that aortic

TABLE 4-2

MATRIX METALLOPROTEINASES AND INHIBITORS

Class	Nomenclature	Molecular Weight[a]	Vascular Cell Type	Expression
Interstitial collagenase	MMP-1	~45	VSMC, EC, microvascular EC	Inducible by PDGF, PMA, IL-1, vEGF
Type IV collagenase	MMP-9, gelatinase B, type V gelatinase	92	VSMC, EC	Inducible by IL-1α, PMA; inhibited by retinoic acid
	MMP-2, gelatinase A, type IV gelatinase	72	VSMC, wounded EC, microvascular EC	Constitutive, ↑ by TNF-α, IL-1α (VSMC); ↑↓ by retinoic acid (EC)
Stromelysin	MMP-3	50	VSMC, EC, microvascular EC	Inducible by IL-1 (VSMC); TNF-α, PMA (EC)
TIMP-1	inhibits MMPs	30	VSMC, EC, microvascular EC	Constitutive
TIMP-2	inhibits MMP-2	~20	VSMC, EC, microvascular EC	Constitutive, ↑ by retinoic acid (EC)

[a] The molecular weight of MMP-1 and MMP-3 depends on the species.

rings dilated in response to acetylcholine only when the rings maintained an intact endothelium. The predominant form of EDRF, derived from L-arginine by the action of the enzyme nitric oxide synthase, is nitric oxide (NO), or a closely related nitroso compound.[55] This conclusion is based on the observation that both EDRF and NO activate guanylate cyclase, are inhibited by oxygen free radicals, methylene blue, and heme-containing proteins; and have a mechanism of action that is independent of prostaglandins generated by the cyclooxygenase pathway.[57] Like EDRF, NO is highly unstable and is rapidly oxidized to form nitrite and nitrate.

Many factors have been shown to regulate the release of EDRF/NO[58] by increasing intracellular Ca^{2+}. These include hormones such as acetylcholine, norepinephrine, bradykinin, thrombin, ATP, and vasopressin; the platelet-derived factors, serotonin and histamine; fatty acids; ionophores; and physical forces. NO easily crosses the smooth muscle cell membrane and binds to the heme moiety of the soluble guanylate cyclase, thereby enhancing the formation of the cyclic guanosine monophosphate (GMP). Cyclic GMP, in turn reduces intracellular Ca^{2+} concentrations, leading to dephosphorylation of the myosin light chain and relaxation.[59] It should be noted that the drug nitroglycerin exerts its vasodilator effects by being converted to NO, thus substituting for a natural product. Deficiency in release of active NO is an important contributing factor leading to vasospasm (see Chap. 44).

NO is produced by the action of the enzyme NO synthase, which oxidizes the guanidino nitrogens of L-arginine to form citrulline and NO. This enzyme has been cloned from brain (bNOS, type I),[60] macrophages (iNOS, for inducible NOS, type II),[61] and endothelial cell (eNOS, type III).[62] The three isoforms of NOS share important consensus sequences for nicotinamide-adenine dinucleotide phosphate (NADPH), flavin adenine dinucleotide (FAD) and flavin mononucleotide (FMN) cofactor binding sites as well as a Ca^{2+}-calmodulin binding site. Although expression of the endothelial enzyme was originally thought to be constitutive, it has recently been shown that

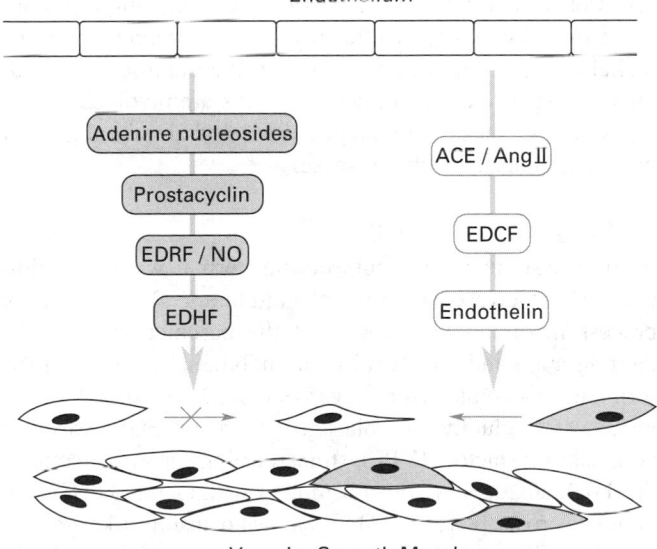

Endothelium

Adenine nucleosides
Prostacyclin
EDRF / NO
EDHF

ACE / Ang II
EDCF
Endothelin

Vascular Smooth Muscle

FIGURE 4-5
Endothelial control of vascular tone. Endothelial cells synthesize and secrete both vasodilator substances (*colored boxes*) and vasoconstrictor compounds (*white boxes*). Vessel tone is dependent on the balance between these factors as well as on the ability of the smooth muscle cells to respond to them. EDRF = endothelial-derived relaxing factor; NO = nitric oxide; EDHF = endothelial-derived hyperpolarizing factor; ACE = angiotensin-converting enzyme; AngII = angiotensin II; EDCF = endothelium-derived contracting factor. (Courtesy of Bernard Lassègue, Ph.D.)

fluid shear stress is a potent regulator of eNOS.[62] The cytokine TNF-α is also a powerful modulator of eNOS mRNA expression, decreasing eNOS levels several-fold in 24 h.[62] Endothelial NOS expression is also regulated by the growth state of the cell: NOS levels are much lower in growth-arrested than in proliferating cells.[63] Although the NO produced during the proliferative phase has no apparent effect on endothelial growth,[63] it may serve an important role during regrowth of the endothelium after vascular injury and in inhibiting smooth muscle cell proliferation[64] and platelet aggregation.[65]

PROSTACYCLIN

Prostacyclin, or PGI$_2$, is a prostanoid derived from the action of cyclooxygenase on arachidonic acid. It is released by the endothelium and relaxes vascular smooth muscle by increasing its intracellular content of cyclic adenosine monophosphate (AMP).[66] Prostacyclin is also platelet-suppressant and antithrombotic, and it reduces the release of growth factors from endothelial cells and macrophages.[22] Among the agonists that stimulate prostacyclin synthesis are bradykinin (one of the most potent), substance P, PDGF and epidermal growth factor (EGF), and adenine nucleotides,[22] while aspirin has been shown to inhibit it transiently. Therapeutically, the debate about the appropriate dose of aspirin in ischemic coronary syndrome revolves around finding a dose that will inhibit platelet function without inhibiting endothelial PGI$_2$ synthesis.

ADENOSINE AND RELATED COMPOUNDS

Both adenine nucleosides (adenosine) and nucleotides (adenosine diphosphate, or ADP, and ATP) are released by the endothelium in response to such stimuli as thrombin[67] and flow.[68] Adenine nucleosides bind to P1 purinergic receptors that activate cyclic AMP, leading to relaxation, while adenine nucleotides stimulate P2 receptors that are coupled to phosphoinositide hydrolysis. Stimulation of P2 receptors in endothelial cells results in an increase in intracellular Ca^{2+} and release of EDRF/prostacyclin,[69] while P2 receptors on vascular smooth muscle mediate contraction.[70] Thus, depending on the relative amounts of adenosine, ATP, and ADP in the vessel wall and the presence of a functional endothelium, these compounds can have a net dilatory or constrictor effect on vascular smooth muscle. Additionally, the endothelium possesses an extracellular ectonucleotidase enzymatic system that mediates the conversion of ATP or ADP to adenosine, thereby regulating the local levels of these compounds.[14] These systems are important in determining the vascular response to ADP released from platelets at the site of thrombus formation.

ENDOTHELIN

The endothelins are a family of closely related peptides made and secreted by endothelial cells in some but not all vascular beds. There are three endothelins (endothelin-1, -2, and -3), all of which are 18 amino acid peptides. Endothelins are initially synthesized as preproendothelin, released in precursor form, and activated by endothelin-converting enzyme. The vascular effects of endothelin are mediated by endothelin receptors, of which subtypes have been identified (ET-A, -B, and -C). The receptors have differing specificity for the individual endothelin peptides and activate somewhat different signaling pathways.

Endothelins have numerous effects on the vascular wall.[71] First and foremost, endothelin-1 is the most potent endogenous vasoconstrictor ever identified. The slow, sustained contraction appears to be the result of activation of the phosphoinositide/protein kinase C signaling pathway as well as of opening voltage-dependent L-type calcium channels.[72] Endothelin is also a potent growth factor for smooth muscle. In endothelial cells, endothelin is linked to nitric oxide and/or prostacyclin release, which can cause a transient vasodilation.[71] Endothelin has also been shown to act as a chemoattractant for monocytes[73] and to play a role in nitroglycerin tolerance.[74]

ANGIOTENSIN-CONVERTING ENZYME

Endothelial cells synthesize and express on their surface angiotensin-converting enzyme (ACE),[75] the protein that converts angiotensin I to the potent vasoconstrictor angiotensin II and that degrades and inactivates bradykinin. ACE associated with the endothelial cell membrane serves to modify both locally produced or circulating angiotensin I and bradykinin and hence contributes importantly to the regulation of vasomotor tone.

Endothelial Control of Vascular Growth

As with vascular tone, the endothelium also exerts a dual effect on vascular growth (Fig. 4-6). Both growth-promoting and growth-inhibitory factors are made and secreted by endothelial cells, making them pivotal in the control of smooth muscle responsiveness. Endothelial cells are involved in two types of vascular growth: angiogenesis and abnormal growth of smooth muscle during disease.

ANGIOGENESIS

Angiogenesis in vivo occurs during normal wound healing and during the vascularization of solid tumors. It is a complex process involving degradation of the basement membrane, the migration and proliferation of endothelial cells, and tube formation. Several factors have been shown to stimulate angiogenesis, including fibroblast growth factor (FGF), vascular permeability factor (VPF), transforming growth factor-α (TGF-α), angiogenin, transforming growth factor-β (TGF-β), tumor necrosis factor-α (TNF-α),[76] and insulin-like growth factor I (IGF-I).[77] Their properties are summarized in Table 4-3. Some of these factors stimulate angiogenesis by inducing endothelial cell migration and proliferation (FGF, VPF); others appear to do so by stimulating endothelial cell differentiation (TGF-β, TNF-α) or by activating a secondary cell type to produce angiogenic factors (angiogenin, TGF-β, TNF-α). Angiogenesis may be negatively regulated by both naturally occurring and synthetic compounds. It can be inhibited by

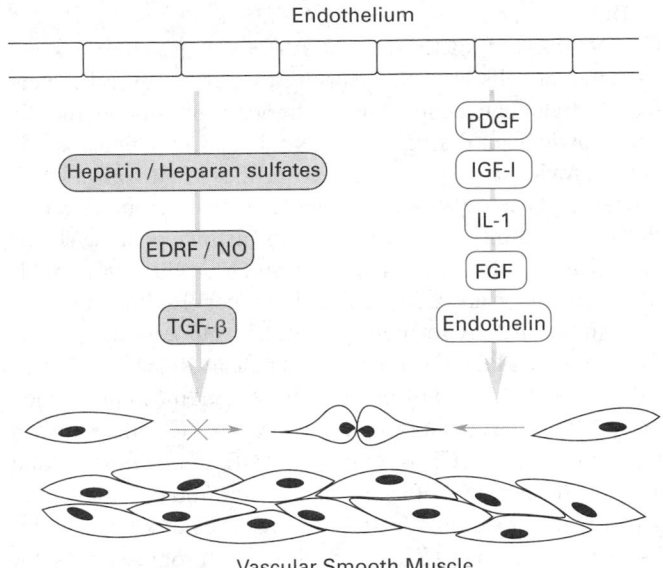

Endothelium

Vascular Smooth Muscle

FIGURE 4-6

Endothelial control of vascular growth. As with vasoactive substances, endothelial cells make and secrete both growth-promoting (*white boxes*) and growth-inhibitory (*colored boxes*) compounds. Under normal conditions, the net effect of the endothelium is growth-inhibitory. EDRF = endothelial-derived relaxing factor; NO = nitric oxide; TGF-β = transforming growth factor β; PDGF = platelet-derived growth factor; IGF-I = insulin-like growth factor 1; IL-1 = interleukin 1; FGF = fibroblast growth factor. (Courtesy of Bernard Lassègue, Ph.D.)

the combination of heparin and cortisone,[78] thrombospondin, platelet factor IV, and γ-interferon. Many of these agents bind to heparin, suggesting that they exert their growth-inhibitory effects by blocking the action of heparin-binding growth factors, such as FGF. It is likely that the control of angiogenesis rests on the maintenance of a balance between the stimulatory and inhibitory factors, the regulation of which is not yet fully understood.

ENDOTHELIUM-DERIVED INHIBITORS OF SMOOTH MUSCLE CELL GROWTH

Normally, smooth muscle cells are relatively refractory to growth stimuli and are maintained in a quiescent, differentiated state. It has been proposed, based on at least two lines of evidence, that the endothelium is important in maintaining this smooth muscle phenotype. First, removal of the endothelium experimentally allows initiation of the mitogenic response, and second, regrowth of normal endothelium inhibits further proliferation.[79] One mechanism by which such a tonic inhibitory influence on smooth muscle cell growth could be effected is the secretion by endothelial cells of specific inhibitors of cell proliferation. Alternatively, the endothelium could be an effective barrier limiting access of blood-borne growth factors to vascular smooth muscle. Attention so far has focused on heparin and other glycosaminoglycans (including heparan sulfate) as possible candidates for endothelial-derived growth

TABLE 4-3

ANGIOGENIC STIMULATORS AND INHIBITORS

	Angiogenesis	Origin	Release	Endothelial Cell Proliferation	Endothelial Cell Chemotaxis	Tubule Formation
FGF	+	Endothelial cells	Cell lysis	+ +	+ (EC)	+
VPF	+	Follicular cells, (neuroblastoma glioma)	Secreted	+ +		
TGF-α	+	Transformed fibroblasts, macrophages (adenocarcinoma cells)	Secreted	+ +		
Angiogenin	+	Lymphocytes, Liver	Secreted	0	−	
TGF-β	+	Endothelial cells	Secreted	−	− (EC) + (monocytes)	+
TNF-α	+	Activated macrophage tumor cells	Secreted	−	+	+
Angiostatic Steroids	−	Synthetic		−	−	
Thrombospondin	−	Platelets	Secreted		−	
Platelet Factor IV	−	Platelets	Secreted		−	
γ-interferon	−	Activated T cells, macrophages	Secreted		−	

inhibitory factors. Heparin inhibits vascular smooth muscle cell (VSMC) mitogenesis and migration in vivo and in vitro and reduces neointimal proliferation if administered during the first 3 days after vascular injury.[80] However, the inhibition is not complete, and it seems likely that other endothelial cell factors may be involved. Another possibility is NO, which is usually associated with vascular relaxation. NO is released tonically from the endothelium of large arteries, which have a relatively minor role in the control of vascular resistance, suggesting that it may have additional functions in these vessels, such as being anti-inflammatory and anti-thrombotic (see Chap. 44). Studies on cultured VSMC have shown that pharmacologic agents such as sodium nitroprusside and 8-bromo-cyclic GMP, which mimic the effect of NO on vascular smooth muscle G kinase, can inhibit mitogenesis.[64] This raises the possibility that NO may have an important role in maintaining the normal artery in a state refractory to mitogens. Finally, endothelial cells have been shown to make and secrete TGF-β,[11] which is subsequently activated by smooth muscle cells. This growth factor inhibits smooth muscle growth directly[81] and also alters PDGF secretion[82] as well as extracellular matrix composition. The extracellular matrix may have a very important influence on smooth muscle proliferation.

The response of vascular smooth muscle cells to growth factors depends on the balance of the hormonal and environmental influences to which the cells are subjected. For example, intact arteries are relatively unresponsive to FGF, only showing a proliferative response when the endothelium has been damaged or removed.[54] This raises the possibility that the cellular mechanism of action of factors secreted by the endothelial cells is to induce a protein or factor in smooth muscle cells that makes them refractory to mitogenic stimulation. One candidate for such a protein is a *tyrosine phosphatase*. As noted above, most growth factors activate a cascade of tyrosine kinases as an initial step in the mitogenic stimulus. The level of tyrosine in cellular proteins is also controlled by tyrosine phosphatases, enzymes that remove phosphates from tyrosine residues. Thus, in cells with very active tyrosine phosphatases, tyrosine kinases may be unable to induce a sustained phosphorylation of proteins on tyrosine, theoretically inhibiting the growth response. Evidence for such a mechanism of growth control is only now becoming available with the recent isolation and cloning of membrane-spanning and cytosolic tyrosine phosphatases.[83] Somatostatins act as growth inhibitors in neoplastic cells through activation of a tyrosine phosphatase.[43] Furthermore, angiopeptin, a somatostatin analog, has been shown to inhibit neointimal proliferation after ballon injury,[84] suggesting that activators of tyrosine phosphatases may be important in growth control. TGF-β, one of the major growth inhibitors produced by endothelial cells, has also been proposed to stimulate tyrosine phosphatase activity.[85] These observations raise the possibility that one of the mechanisms by which endothelial cells help to maintain smooth muscle quiescence is by the induction of tyrosine phosphatase activity in the smooth muscle cells.

ENDOTHELIUM-DERIVED STIMULATORS OF SMOOTH MUSCLE CELL GROWTH

Endothelial cells have the capacity to secrete several factors that are thought to be involved in the abnormal smooth muscle cell growth seen during atherogenesis and hypertension. As noted previously, the best studied of these factors is PDGF, so named because it was originally isolated from platelets. PDGF is a dimer composed of two distinct peptide chains (designated A and B chains), and can be produced as an AB heterodimer, or an AA or BB homodimer. Endothelial cells contain the mRNA for both peptides,[82] although the precise form in which PDGF is secreted is unclear. Release of PDGF from the endothelium is regulated by second messengers such as cAMP and activators of protein kinase C; other growth factors including TGF-β, FGF, and TNF; circulating factors; and locally produced factors such as thrombin.[82] A second growth factor made and secreted by endothelial cells is insulin-like growth factor I (IGF-I).[12] IGF-I is a progression factor that facilitates movement of cells through the cell cycle but by itself is not a particularly strong mitogen. In vitro, it enhances the mitogenic effect of PDGF on smooth muscle.[86] IGF-I production by endothelium has been shown to be regulated by PDGF and hydrostatic pressure. It has recently been shown to be a major player in vascular hypertrophy and hyperplasia.[87]

Other factors made by the endothelium that are able to alter smooth muscle proliferation include interleukin 1 (IL-1), FGF, and endothelin. IL-1 is an inflammatory cytokine that has numerous vascular effects in addition to mitogenesis, including the stimulation of procoagulant activity,[88] induction of leukocyte adhesiveness (see below), and inhibition of contraction.[89] IL-1 regulates its own expression[90]; in addition, its production is regulated by TNF-α,[76] lipopolysaccharide, and γ-interferon.[90] As noted above, basic FGF has been detected in endothelial cells[16] and acts as a potent smooth muscle mitogen, particularly after denuding injury.[54] FGF does not contain the signal peptide that usually provides a mechanism for transporting proteins out of cells and thus is thought not to be secreted by endothelial cells. It is, however, present and stored in the subendothelial matrix and may be released on cell lysis or death.[91] FGF released from vascular smooth muscle cells may be particularly important in the growth response induced by injury to the arterial wall after balloon angioplasty. FGF bound to the matrix can be released by heparin and proteinases,[92] suggesting that the matrix may serve as a store for rapidly mobilizing this growth factor. Finally, the vasoconstrictor endothelin has also been shown under certain circumstances to act as a smooth muscle mitogen,[93] possibly by increasing PDGF–A chain secretion in the smooth muscle cells themselves.

ENDOTHELIAL CELL–LEUKOCYTE INTERACTIONS

Endothelial cells have been shown to participate actively in the development of inflammatory reactions. They are central to the recruitment of leukocytes to sites of inflammation by secreting *chemotactic molecules* and expressing *adhesion molecules* that interact with surface proteins on leukocytes.

Inflammatory cytokines increase synthesis of vasodilators by the endothelium, which causes increased blood flow to the injured area. Histamine, which is released at the site of vascular inflammation, also contracts endothelial cells in certain areas, thus increasing permeability.[94] Cytokines stimulate endothelial secretion of leukocyte chemoattractant proteins (IL-8) and monocyte chemotactic protein (MCP-1), and expression of adhesion molecules such as intercellular adhesion molecules-1 and -2 (ICAM-1 and ICAM-2), endothelial leukocyte adhesion molecule-1 (ELAM-1 or E-selectin), vascular cell adhesion molecule-1 (VCAM-1), and GMP-140 which are important regulators of leukocyte accumulation on the vascular surface.[95] ELAM-1 and GMP-140 bind resting but not activated, neutrophils; VCAM-1 binds to the VLA-4 antigen on monocytes and T lymphocytes; and ICAM-1 and -2 bind to the LFA-1 integrin receptor on B lymphocytes.[95] The expression of these molecules appears to be differentially regulated by cytokines, thrombin, and histamine,[95] so that their surface expression determines the type of leukocytes attached to the endothelial monolayer. It has been suggested that the sequential accumulation of different leukocyte classes at sites of inflammation can be explained by the differential induction of these endothelial cell adhesion molecules.[96] Leukocyte adhesion molecules and chemoattractant proteins are also likely to be important in atherogenesis (see below).

ENDOTHELIAL RESPONSES TO HEMODYNAMIC INFLUENCES

In addition to being influenced by the interaction of circulating blood cells, vascular smooth muscle cells, and matrix, the endothelium responds to the physical forces of pressure, stretch, and shear stress imposed by the hemodynamics of the circulation. Flow-mediated, endothelium-dependent vasodilation has been described in many vascular beds,[97] and shear stress has been proposed to play a role in controlling endothelial cell proliferation.[98] Elevated pressure, stretch of the vessel wall, and shear stress have all been shown independently to affect endothelial cell morphology and/or function. Pressure alone appears to have a role in the generalized hypertrophy of the vessel wall that occurs during hypertension. Studies in cultured cells have shown that stretching of endothelial cells leads to changes in cell shape and intracellular signal generation, with an increase in calcium concentration and proliferation.[98] Shear stress has numerous effects on endothelial cells. Initially, it was found that exposure of endothelial cell monolayers to elevated shear stresses in vitro caused them to align in the direction of flow. This reorientation was accompanied by changes in the cytoskeleton of the cells, including reorganization and alignment of the actin filaments and microtubules (Fig. 4-7). Similar mechanisms presumably also account for the orientation of endothelial cells parallel to the longitudinal axis in areas of laminar flow in the arterial system. The function of endothelial cells is also altered by shear stress: a K^+ current is activated; secretion of vasoactive and growth factors, including NO, endothelin, prostacyclin, and bFGF is increased; tissue factor expression is increased; uptake of LDL is elevated; and tissue plasminogen activator secretion is increased.[98]

The importance of these observations lies in the variation in hemodynamic forces throughout the circulation. High pressure, such as that which occurs in hypertension, causes changes in the morphology and function of the vessel wall.[99] In addition, the areas of the vasculature exposed to low shear stress (branch points and curvatures) exhibit a predilection to the formation of atherosclerotic lesions.[100] *It is thus clear that the hemodynamic environment of the endothelium and underlying smooth muscle is a potentially powerful regulator of vascular function.*

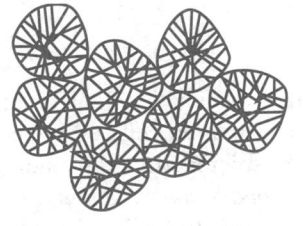 Shear Stress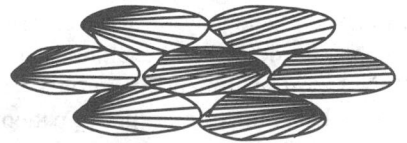

K+ current
NO release
endothelin release
prostacyclin release
SOD expression
LDL uptake
tPA secretion
fos, jun expression
growth factor expression
tissue factor expression

FIGURE 4-7
Effect of shear stress on endothelial cells. In endothelial cells grown in static conditions, actin filaments (indicated by lines inside the cell) assume a random orientation. Upon exposure to shear stress, these filaments align and the listed cellular functions are stimulated. (Courtesy of Barbara Merchant-Bailey).

The mechanism(s) by which the endothelial cell can sense and transduce mechanical signals is unknown. Possibilities include a surface mechanoreceptor, a flow-sensitive ion channel, changes in cytoskeletal stress due to deformation, and flow-dependent gradients of bioactive substances along the surface of the cell.

ENDOTHELIAL DYSFUNCTION AND VASCULAR SMOOTH MUSCLE ABNORMALITIES

In general, the normal endothelium is in an inhibitory mode—inhibiting contraction, thrombosis, white cell adhesion, and vascular smooth muscle growth (Figs. 4-1, 4-5, and 4-6). *Endothelial dysfunction* is one of the important concepts that has developed in vascular biology over the last decade. Implicit in the term is the recognition that the fundamental or normal functions of the endothelium are not fixed, but are regulatable. Thus, the endothelium in a given area may lose its vasodiolator predominance, become prothrombotic or less thrombolytic, begin to support leukocyte adherence (which may be a normal response in the inflammatory process), or stimulate rather than inhibit smooth muscle migration and proliferation. *It is likely that endothelial dysfunction accounts ultimately for a large portion of all cardiovascular disease.*

Atherosclerosis

Atherosclerosis is the prototypical disease characterized by endothelial dysfunction. Many of its cardinal features are directly explainable in this context. Thus, mononuclear and lymphocytic infiltration, hypercontractility, LDL modification, smooth muscle cell growth, and intimal migration are likely related to abnormalities of the endothelium induced by hyperlipidemia, hypertension, smoking, and unknown hereditary factors. The pathogenesis of atherosclerosis viewed as a disease of endothelial dysfunction is depicted in Fig. 4-8. (For a more detailed discussion, see Chap. 44).

Clinically, endothelial dysfunction in atherosclerosis has primarily been defined by impairment of endothelium-dependent relaxation.[101] This defect, which likely contributes to the vasospastic tendency of diseased arteries, appears to be attributable to defective generation or delivery of active EDRF/NO.[102] Impairment of coronary endothelium-dependent vasodilator function occurs in patients with risk factors such as hypercholesterolemia prior to angiographically demonstrable coronary disease.[103] In hypercholesterolemic animals, Minor et al.[102] have found marked decreases in EDRF activity accompanied by increases in the release of NO metabolites. This apparent paradox is likely explained by the fact that the enhanced NO produced by the hypercholesterolemic endothelium is rapidly degraded to inactive metabolites of NO. Since the vasodilator defect in these animals could be corrected both in vivo and in vitro by administration of polyethylene glycol-linked superoxide dismutase (PEG-SOD),[104] an enzyme that inactivates intracellular superoxide radicals, it is probable that excessive oxygen free radicals produced by the endothelium as a consequence of the oxidative metabolic stress induced by hypercholesterolemia degrade NO and account for the decreased vasodilator activity.

A second manifestation of a dysfunctional endothelium that is apparent very early after initiation of cholesterol feeding in animals is the recruitment of monocytes and macrophages into the vessel wall.[105] This recruitment is likely the result of induction of VCAM-1 expression[106] as well as of secretion of MCP-1.[107] The molecular linkage between hyperlipidemia and MCP-1/adhesion molecule expression is unknown but may reflect in part the metabolic (oxidative) stress imposed by this change in milieu. Inflammatory cytokines are also important mediators of adhesion molecule expression, and their production by the endothelium and inflammatory cells in the vessel wall may also contribute to adhesion molecule expression in both the early and late stages of the disease.

The intimal proliferation observed in atherosclerotic lesion formation results from migration and hyperplasia of vascular smooth muscle cells[108] and accumulation of extracellular matrix. Proliferation has been attributed to growth factors such as PDGF, FGF, and IGF-I. Since these growth factors can be produced by the endothelium in vitro, it is very likely that the dysfunctional endothelium in atherosclerosis also produces growth factors while shifting from a growth-inhibitory to a growth-promoting mode. Furthermore, there is evidence that products of oxidative metabolism may also release growth factors and activate matrix metalloproteinases,[109] thus contributing to intimal lesion formation on multiple levels.

The recent rapid advance in our understanding of vessel wall biology provides insight into the biological mechanisms responsible for the pathogenesis of atherosclerosis. *There is now a basis for developing a unifying concept of the disease that revolves around endothelial dysfunction mediated by changes in oxidative metabolism.* Oxidative modification of LDL thus assumes a central role in atherogenesis (Fig. 4-8). The role of oxidized LDL is discussed more completely in Chap. 39, and the relationship of the cell biology of atherosclerosis to coronary ischemic syndrome is discussed in Chap. 44.

Vasospasm

When the endothelium becomes dysfunctional, as in atherosclerosis, the underlying smooth muscle cells often become hyperreactive to certain vasoconstrictor stimuli, including serotonin and ergonovine.[110] *Coronary spasm leading to myocardial infarction is one of the most clinically relevant problems arising from this phenomenon.* Proposed mechanisms to account for this vasoconstrictor abnormality, which can result in total occlusion, include supersensitivity of the smooth muscle cells themselves to constrictor stimuli and loss of endothelium-dependent relaxing mechanisms. The increased tendency toward thrombus formation is due to a loss of the normal anticoagulant function of the endothelium. This latter event would also promote the release of thrombus-related factors (serotonin, thromboxane A2, ADP, thrombin, PDGF) in the vicinity of the smooth muscle cells, any of which can cause vasoconstriction in the absence of a functional endothelium.[111]

Hypertension

Hypertension is characterized by dysfunction of both endothelium and vascular smooth muscle. *In chronic hypertension, endothelium-dependent relaxations are impaired in both conduit and resistance arteries.* Relaxations to some platelet factors are also altered but have been found to be augmented or diminished, depending on the hypertensive model studied.[112]

Furthermore, the endothelium-dependent constrictor activity is increased in some models of hypertension.[112] These alterations in endothelial function would tend to increase the tone of hypertensive vessels. The mechanism responsible for this effect is not entirely clear. Data from experimental animals makes it seem likely that the alterations in endothelium-dependent responses in hypertension result from a combination of altered endothelial and vascular smooth muscle cell function.

Hypertension is also characterized by an increase in vessel wall mass. In the aortas of spontaneously hypertensive and

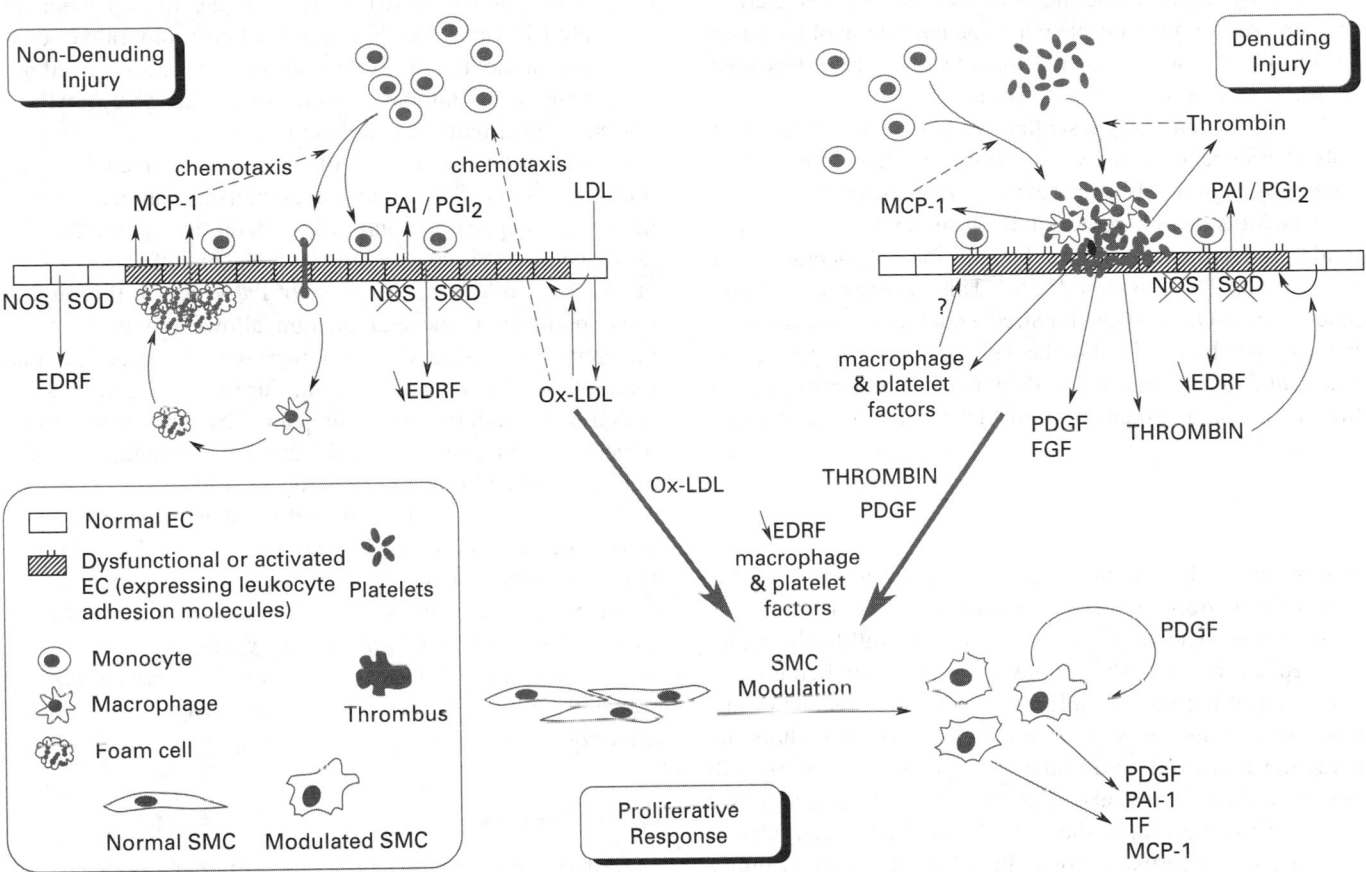

FIGURE 4-8

Theoretical initiating events in vascular lesion formation. *Nondenuding injury*: LDL enters the subendothelial space where it is converted to oxidized LDL (ox-LDL), which induces monocyte chemoattraction and endothelial dysfunction. Dysfunctional endothelial cells (EC) express cell adhesion molecules (ICAM, ELAM, and VCAM) leading to increased monocyte adhesion and movement into the vessel wall. Monocytes in the vessel wall differentiate into macrophages, take up lipids, and remain locally as foam cells, subsequently evolving into fatty streaks. The foam cells in the fatty streak and the overlying endothelium express monocyte chemotactic protein-1 (MCP-1), resulting in further enhanced monocyte chemoattraction and adhesion. Dysfunctional EC may synthesize less nitric oxide synthase (NOS) or superoxide dismutase (SOD, an enzyme that metabolizes oxygen radicals that have been shown to inactivate NO). This decreases endothelial-derived relaxing factor (EDRF) release/activity. The loss of EDRF together with the direct effects of ox-LDL, or growth factors secreted by the foam cells or endothelium, act on the quiescent contractile smooth muscle cells in the vessel wall, giving rise to the proliferative phenotype, with division and migration into the intima. *Denuding injury*: Loss of endothelium leads to platelet deposition, tissue factor-mediated activation of extrinsic coagulation to generate thrombin, cleavage of fibrinogen to fibrin, and the formation of thrombus. Thrombin gives rise to endothelial expression of adhesion molecules and consequent monocyte attachment, together with secretion of platelet granular constituents. Monocytes enter the thrombus and differentiate into phagocytic macrophages, expressing tissue factor and MCP-1. This leads to further monocyte chemoattraction into the vessel wall. Smooth muscle cell proliferation is produced by (1) thrombin generation at the site of denuding injury; (2) platelet-derived growth factor (PDGF) or other growth factors released from platelets in the thrombus; (3) factors secreted by the macrophages ingesting the thrombus; and (4) the loss of EDRF activity caused by endothelial dysfunction. *Proliferative response*: modulated smooth muscle cells (SMCs) proliferate and synthesize factors that promote plaque development. SMCs synthesize (1) PDGF and other growth factors, which cause self-perpetuating autocrine or paracrine stimulation of SMC proliferation; (2) tissue factor (TF) and plasminogen activator inhibitor 1 (PAI-I), which act locally to produce thrombin or inhibit fibrinolysis of the fibrin network used to facilitate cell migration; and (3) MCP-1, which increases monocyte chemoattraction into the lesion, thereby leading to lesion development. (We thank Drs. Laurence Harker, Josiah Wilcox, and Bernard Lassègue for their creative and intellectual development of this figure.)

Goldblatt hypertensive rats, this increase can be attributed to an increase in the size of the existing smooth muscle cells.[113,114] Hypertrophy is accompanied by an increase in ploidy; that is, an increased DNA content per cell.[113,114] In contrast, resistance vessels from these same animals appear to increase their mass by hyperplasia of the smooth muscle cells.[115] The stimuli responsible for these changes in the hypertensive vascular wall are unknown. Vascular remodeling appears to have two stages: (1) an initial, reversible, intense vasoconstriction mediated by neural or endogenous signals, followed by (2) a remodeling of the vessel wall characterized by increased smooth muscle mass and narrowing of the vessel lumen. There is some evidence that this response is dependent on the presence of the endothelium.[99]

Recent evidence suggests that oxidative stress may be involved in some forms of hypertension, especially those characterized by high levels of circulating angiotensin II. In animal models, infusion of angiotensin II causes an increase in superoxide production by the vascular nicotinamide adenine dinucleotide (NADH) oxidase.[116,117] This superoxide not only inactivates NO, causing impaired endothelial relaxation,[117] but also may be involved in the development of hypertension, since infusion of superoxide dismutase significantly impairs the ability of angiotensin II to chronically increase blood pressure.[116]

Restenosis

Restenosis is the development of a neointima that occurs following angioplasty, often leading to reocclusion of the initial lesion. The response of the arterial wall to the injury induced by angioplasty (removal of the endothelium and stretching of the vessel wall) involves several distinct events (Fig. 4-8). Removal of the endothelium not only alters the paracrine hormonal environment in which vascular smooth muscle cells exist but also exposes a thrombogenic surface to which platelets and other circulating factors can adhere, resulting in the formation of a thrombus. In addition, injury to the underlying smooth muscle may release factors such as FGF, which have mitogenic effects on the remaining smooth muscle cells. Finally, infiltration and subsequent activation of macrophages into the denuded vessel wall bring an additional set of hormonal influences to bear on the vascular smooth muscle. The pathophysiologic consequences of these complex events include migration and proliferation of smooth muscle cells into the intimal area, resulting in the formation of a neointima over a period of weeks to months.

Balloon injury has been extensively studied in several animal models, including pig, rabbit, rat, and baboon. In the rat carotid artery, the events following injury can be divided into three stages: initial (injury to 48 h), migratory (3 to 7 days), and proliferative (7 days to 3 to 4 weeks). During the initial response to injury, growth-related genes in the smooth muscle cells are induced, including c-fos, PDGF-A, PDGF-β receptor,[118] and MCP-1.[119] It also appears that deep injury to smooth muscle cells results in an outpouring of FGF, a potent smooth muscle mitogen.[91] This initial response does not appear to be dependent on platelet factors but does appear to be directly related to the removal of the endothelium.[79] During the migratory phase, a large increase of thymidine incorporation in the vessel wall occurs, accompanied by further increases in the mRNA encoding IGF-I[120] and the PDGF-β receptor.[118] This phase of the response can be modulated by platelet factors and inhibited by the endothelium.[79] Finally, the proliferative phase is characterized by marked intimal thickening, with a decreased percentage of thymidine-labeled cells. Some of the increased area is due to deposition of extracellular matrix, and the majority of the proliferative activity occurs at the luminal surface of the vessel. This proliferative phase seems ultimately to be inhibited by regrowth of normally functioning endothelium.

Thus, during the process of restenosis after angioplasty, both the loss of endothelium and the transformation of smooth muscle cells appear to contribute to neointimal formation. At least two lines of evidence implicate the endothelium as having a crucial role in the response of the vessel wall to injury. First, removal of the endothelium allows initiation of the mitogenic response, and second, regrowth of normal endothelium inhibits further proliferation. Furthermore, gentle denudation with a nylon loop, accompanied by rapid regeneration of endothelium, results in significantly less neointimal proliferation.[121] In addition, proliferating smooth muscle cells have characteristics distinct from the differentiated smooth muscle cells in the medial layer. Their cytoskeleton is similar to that found in cultured cells. It seems likely, therefore, that *two of the most important causes of restenosis are the loss of endothelium-derived growth inhibitory factors, and the transformation of smooth muscle cells into a phenotype able to respond to platelet- and endothelium-derived factors with proliferation.*

Gene Therapy

One of the most interesting and potentially promising new approaches to development of treatments for restenosis and abnormal vascular growth in atherosclerosis is gene therapy. Gene therapy can be defined as the introduction of genetically engineered genes into the somatic cells of patients to correct inherited or acquired disorders through the induction of in vivo synthesis of the missing or defective gene product (see Chap. 9). Gene therapy applied to cardiovascular pathology is still in its early stages, but several approaches have been successfully used in animal models of vascular disease. In some instances autologous endothelial or smooth muscle cells have been removed and cultured, transfected in vitro, and reintroduced into a denuded artery by means of a double balloon catheter.[122] A second method that has been tested involves direct genetic modification of vascular cells in vivo using adenoviral or retroviral vectors or DNA liposomes. Examples of successful transfer in model systems include adenosine deaminase,[122] tPA,[123] vascular endothelial growth factor,[124] TIMP-1,[125] and class I major histocompatibility complex (MHC).[126] These methods have been used experimentally to investigate mechanisms of intimal proliferation,[125,126] angiogenesis,[124] and smooth muscle cell hypertrophy[127] as well as to improve stent function by local delivery of thrombolytic molecules.[123] Gene transfer thus holds promise as a potential treatment for diverse vascular diseases.

REFERENCES

1. Moncada S, Vane JR. Arachidonic acid metabolites and the interaction between platelets and blood vessel walls. *N Engl J Med* 1979; 300:1142–1147.

2. Furchgott RF, Zawadski JV. The obligatory role of endothelial cells in the relaxation of arterial smooth muscle by acetylcholine. *Nature* 1980; 228:373–376.

3. Taylor SG, Weston AH. Endothelium-derived hyperpolarizing factor: A new endogenous inhibitor from the vascular endothelium. *Trends Pharmacol Sci* 1988; 9:272–274.

4. Yanagisawa Y, Kurihara H, Kimura S, Tomobe Y, Kobayashi M, Mitsui Y, et al. A novel potent vasoconstrictor peptide produced by vascular endothelial cells. *Nature* 1988; 332:411–415.

5. Stenmark KR, Orton EC, Reeves JT, Voelkel NF, Crouch EC, Parks WC, et al. Vascular remodeling in neonatal pulmonary hypertension. *Chest* 1988; 93:127S–133S.

6. Sato T, Arai K, Ishiharajima S, Asano G. Role of glycosaminoglycan and fibronectin in endothelial cell growth. *Exp Mol Pathol* 1987; 47:202–210.

7. Hanemaaijer R, Koolwijk P, le Clercq L, de Vree WJ, van Hinsbergh VW. Regulation of matrix metalloproteinase expression in human vein and microvascular endothelial cells: Effects of tumor necrosis factor alpha, interleukin 1 and phorbol ester. *Biochem J* 1993; 296:803–809.

8. Galis ZS, Muszynski M, Sukhova GK, Simon-Morrissey E, Unemori EN, Lark MW, et al. Cytokine-stimulated human vascular smooth muscle cells synthesize a complement of enzymes required for extracellular matrix digestion. *Circ Res* 1994; 75:181–189.

9. Castellot JJ Jr, Addonizio ML, Rosenberg R, Karnovsky MJ. Cultured endothelial cells produce a heparin-like inhibitor of smooth muscle cell growth. *J Cell Biol* 1981; 90:372–379.

10. Zerwes HG, Risau W. Polarized secretion of a platelet-derived growth factor–like chemotactic factor by endothelial cells in vitro. *J Cell Biol* 1987; 105:2037–2041.

11. Hannan RL, Kourembanas S, Flanders KC, Rogel SJ, Roberts AB, Faller DV, et al. Endothelial cells synthesize basic fibroblast growth factor and transforming growth factor beta. *Growth Factors* 1988; 1:7–17.

12. Delafontaine P, Bernstein KE, Alexander RW. Insulin-like growth factor I gene expression in vascular cells. *Hypertension* 1991; 17:693–699.

13. Wang-Iverson P, DeRosa PM, Brown WV. Plasma lipoprotein interaction with endothelial cells. In: Ryan U (ed). *Endothelial Cells*. Boca Raton, FL: CRC Press; 1988.

14. Gordon EL, Pearson JD, Slakey LL. The hydrolysis of extracellular adenine nucleotides by cultured endothelial cells from pig aorta. *J Biol Chem* 1986; 33:15496–15504.

15. Cary DA, Mendelsohn FA. Effect of forskolin, isoproterenol and IBMX on angiotensin converting enzyme and cyclic AMP production by cultured bovine endothelial cells. *Mol Cell Endocrinol* 1987; 53:103–109.

16. Shimada K, Gill PJ, Silbert JE, Douglas WHJ, Fanburg BL. Involvement of cell surface heparan sulfate in the binding of LDL to cultured bovine endothelial cells. *J Clin Invest* 1981; 68:995–1002.

17. Vlodavsky I, Fielding PE, Johnson LK, Gospodarowicz D. Inhibition of low density lipoprotein uptake in confluent endothelial cell monolayers correlates with a restricted surface receptor redistribution. *J Cell Physiol* 1979; 100:481–495.

18. Hashida R, Anamizu C, Kimura J, Ohkuma S, Yoshida Y, Takano T. Transcellular transport of lipoprotein through arterial endothelial cells in monolayer culture. *Cell Struct Funct* 1986; 11:31–42.

19. Baker DP, van Lenten BJ, Fogelman AM, Edwards PA, Kean C, Berliner JA. LDL, scavenger and beta-VLDL receptors on aortic endothelial cells. *Arteriosclerosis* 1984; 4:357–364.

20. Morel DW, DiCorleto PE, Chisolm GM. Endothelial and smooth muscle cells alter low density lipoprotein in vitro by free radical oxidation. *Arteriosclerosis* 1984; 4:357–364.

21. Danon D, Skutelsky E. Endothelial surface charge and its possible relationship to thrombogenesis. *Ann NY Acad Sci* 1976; 275:47–63.

22. Gryglewski RJ, Botting RM, Vane JR. Mediators produced by the endothelial cell. *Hypertension* 1988; 12:530–548.

23. Rosenberg RD, Rosenberg JS. Natural anticoagulant mechanisms. *J Clin Invest* 1984; 74:1–6.

24. Esmon CT, Owen WG. Identification of an endothelial cofactor for thrombin-catalyzed activation of protein C. *Proc Natl Acad Sci USA* 1981; 78:2249–2252.

25. van Iwaarden F, Acton DS, Sixma JJ, Meijers, JCM, de Groot PG, Bouma BN. Internalization of antithrombin III by cultured human endothelial cells and its subcellular localization. *J Lab Clin Med* 1989; 113:717–726.

26. Podor TJ, Curriden SA, Loskutoff DJ. The fibrinolytic system of endothelial cells. In: Ryan US (ed). *Endothelial Cells*. Boca Raton, FL: CRC Press; 1988.

27. Schorer AE, Moldow CF. Production of tissue factor. In: Ryan US (ed). *Endothelial Cells*. Boca Raton, FL: CRC Press; 1988.

28. Whelan J, Ghersa P, Hooft-an-Huijsduijnen R, Gray J, Chandra G, Talabot F. An NF kappa B-like factor is essential but not sufficient for cytokine induction of endothelial leukocyte adhesion molecule 1 (ELAM-1) gene transcription. *Nucleic Acids Res* 1991; 19:2645–2653.

29. Sporn LA, Marder VJ, Wagner DD. Von Willebrand factor released from Weibel-Palade bodies binds more avidly to extracellular matrix than that secreted constitutively. *Blood* 1987; 69:1531–1534.

30. Stern DM, Nawroth PP. Modulation of endothelial cell coagulant properties. In: Ryan US (ed). *Endothelial Cells*. Boca Raton, FL: CRC Press; 1988.

31. Svensjo E, Grega GJ. Evidence for endothelial cell-mediated regulation of macromolecular permeability by post-capillary venules. *Fed Proc* 1986; 45:89–95.

32. Huttner I, Boutet M, Rona G, More RH. Studies on protein passage through arterial endothelium: III. Effect of blood pressure levels on the passage of fine structural protein tracers through rat arterial endothelium. *Lab Invest* 1973; 29:536–546.

33. Scow RO, Blanchette-Mackie EJ, Smith LC. Role of capillary endothelium in the clearance of chylomicrons: A model for lipid transport from blood by lateral diffusion in cell membranes. *Circ Res* 1976; 39:149–162.

34. Berk BC, Alexander RW, Brock TA, Gimbrone MA Jr, Webb RC. Vasoconstriction: A new activity for platelet-derived growth factor. *Science* 1986; 232:87–90.

35. Owens GK. Control of hypertrophic vs. hyperplastic growth of vascular smooth muscle cells. *Am J Physiol* 1989; 257:H1755–H1765.

36. Berridge MJ, Irvine RF. Inositol trisphosphate, a novel second messenger in cellular signal transduction. *Nature* 1984; 312:315–321.

37. Yamamoto H, van Breeman C. Inositol 1,4,5-trisphosphate releases calcium from skinned cultured smooth muscle cells. *Biochem Biophys Res Commun* 1985; 130:270–274.

38. Nishizuka Y. The role of protein kinase C in cell surface signal transduction and tumour promotion. *Nature* 1984; 308:693–698.

39. Berk BC, Aronow MS, Brock TA, Cragoe EJ, Gimbrone MAJ, Alexander RW. Angiotensin II-stimulated Na+/H+ exchange in cultured vascular smooth muscle cells: Evidence for protein kinase C-dependent and -independent pathways. *J Biol Chem* 1987; 262:5057–5064.

40. Brock TA, Alexander RW, Ekstein LS, Atkinson WJ, Gimbrone MAJ. Angiotensin increases cytosolic free calcium in cultured vascular smooth muscle cells. *Hypertension* 1985; 7:I-105–I-109.

41. Williams LT. Signal transduction by the platelet-derived growth factor receptor. *Science* 1989; 243:1564–1570.

42. Clegg KB, Sambhi MP. Inhibition of epidermal growth factor–mediated DNA synthesis by a specific tyrosine kinase inhibitor in vascular smooth muscle cells of the spontaneously hypertensive rat. *J Hypertens* 1989; 7:S144–S145.

43. Liebow C, Reilly C, Serrano M, Schally AV. Somatostatin analogues inhibit growth of pancreatic cancer by stimulating tyrosine phosphatase. *Proc Natl Acad Sci USA* 1989; 86:2003–2007.

44. Ullrich A, Schlessinger J. Signal transduction by receptors with tyrosine kinase activity. *Cell* 1990; 81:203–212.

45. Bourne HR. Team blue sees red. *Nature* 1995; 376:727–729.

46. Lassègue B, Alexander RW, Clark M, Griendling KK. Angiotensin II-

induced phosphatidylcholine hydrolysis in cultured vascular smooth-muscle cells: Regulation and localization. *Biochem J* 1991; 276:19–25.

47. Moolenaar WH, Kruijer W, Tilly BC, Verlaan I, Bierman AJ, de Laat SW. Growth factor-like action of phosphatidic acid. *Nature* 1986; 323:171–173.

48. Kondo T, Inui H, Konishi F, Inagami T. Phospholipase D mimics platelet-derived growth factor as a competence factor in vascular smooth muscle cells. *J Biol Chem* 1992; 267:23609–23616.

49. Dillon PF, Aksoy MO, Driska SP, Murphy RA. Myosin phosphorylation and the cross-bridge cycle in arterial smooth muscle. *Science* 1981; 211:495–497.

50. Morgan KG. Role of calcium ion in maintenance of vascular smooth muscle tone. *Am J Cardiol* 1987; 59:24A–28A.

51. Berk BC, Vekshtein V, Gordon HM, Tsuda T. Angiotensin II-stimulated protein synthesis in cultured vascular smooth muscle cells. *Hypertension* 1989; 13:305–314.

52. Berk BC, Taubman MB, Griendling KK, Cragoe EJ Jr, Fenton JW II, Brock TA. Thrombin-stimulated events in cultured vascular smooth muscle cells. *Biochem J* 1991; 274:799–805.

53. Golden MA, Au YPT, Kirkman TR, Wilcox JN, Raines EW, Ross R, et al. Platelet-derived growth factor activity and mRNA expression in healing vascular grafts in baboons. *J Clin Invest* 1991; 87:406–414.

54. Lindner V, Lappi DA, Baird A, Majack RA, Reidy MA. Role of basic fibroblast growth factor in vascular lesion formation. *Circ Res* 1991; 68:106–113.

55. Myers PR, Minor RL, Guerra R, Jr, Bates JN, Harrison DG. The vasorelaxant properties of the endothelium derived relaxing factor more closely resemble S-nitrosocysteine than nitric oxide. *Nature* 1990; 345:161–163.

56. Sato H, Takino T, Okada Y, Cao J, Shinagawa A, Yamamoto E, et al. A matrix metalloproteinase expressed on the surface of invasive tumor cells. *Nature* 1994; 370:61–65.

57. Ignarro LJ. Endothelium-derived nitric oxide: Actions and properties. *FASEB J* 1989; 3:31–36.

58. Furchgott RF, Vanhoutte PM. Endothelium-derived relaxing and contracting factors. *FASEB J* 1989; 3:2007–2018.

59. Rapoport RM, Draznin MB, Murad F. Endothelium-dependent relaxation in rat aorta may be mediated through cyclic GMP-dependent protein phosphorylation. *Nature* 1983; 306:174–176.

60. Bredt DS, Hwang PM, Glatt CE, Lowenstein C, Reed RR, Snyder SH. Cloned and expressed nitric oxide synthase structurally resembles cytochrome P-450 reductase. *Nature* 1991; 351:714–718.

61. Lyons CR, Orloff GJ, Cunningham JM. Molecular cloning and functional expression of an inducible nitric oxide synthase from a murine macrophage cell line. *J Biol Chem* 1992; 267:6370–6374.

62. Nishida K, Harrison DG, Navas JP, Fisher AA, Dockery SP, Uematsu M, et al. Molecular cloning and characterization of the constitutive bovine aortic endothelial nitric oxide synthase. *J Clin Invest* 1992; 90:2092–2096.

63. Arnal J-F, Yamin J, Dockery S, Harrison DG. Regulation of endothelial nitric oxide synthase mRNA, protein, and activity during cell growth. *Am J Physiol* 1994; 267:C1381–C1388.

64. Garg UC, Hassid A, Nitric oxide generating vasodilators and 8-bromo cyclic GMP inhibit mitogenesis and proliferation of cultured rat vascular smooth muscle cells. *J Clin Invest* 1989; 83:1774–1777.

65. Radomski MW, Palmer RMJ, Moncada S. Endogenous nitric oxide inhibits human platelet adhesion to vascular endothelium. *Lancet* 1987; 2:1057–1058.

66. Ito, T, Ogawa, K, Enomoto I, Hashimoto H, Kai I, Satake T. Comparison of the effects of PGI₂ and PGE₁ on coronary and systemic hemodynamics and coronary arterial cyclic nucleotide level in dogs. *Adv Prostaglandin Thromboxane Leukot Res* 1980; 7:641–646.

67. Carwile LE, Ager A, Gordon JL. Effects of neutrophil elastase and other proteases on porcine aortic endothelial prostaglandin I2 production, adenine nucleotide release, and responses to vasoactive agents. *J Clin Invest* 1984; 74:1003–1010.

68. Milner P, Bodin P, Loesch A, Burnstock G. Rapid release of endothelin and ATP from isolated aortic endothelial cells exposed to increased flow. *Biochem Biophys Res Commun* 1990; 170:649–656.

69. Pearson JD, Slakey LL, Gordon JL. Stimulation of prostaglandin production through purinoceptors on cultured porcine endothelial cells. *Biochem J* 1983; 214:273–276.

70. O'Connor SE, Wood BE, Leff P. Characterization of P2x-receptors in rabbit isolated ear artery. *Br J Pharmacol* 1990; 101:640–644.

71. Luscher TF, Wenzel RR. Endothelin and endothelin antagonists: Pharmacology and clinical implications. *Agents Actions Suppl* 1995; 45:237–253.

72. Simonson MS, Dunn MJ. Cellular signaling by peptides of the endothelin gene family. *FASEB J* 1990; 4:2989–3000.

73. Achmad TH, Rao GS. Chemotaxis of human blood monocytes toward endothelin-1 and the influence of calcium channel blockers. *Biochem Biophys Res Commun* 1992; 189:994–1000.

74. Münzel T, Giaid A, Kurz S, Stewart DJ, Harrison DG. Evidence for a role of endothelin 1 and protein kinase C in nitroglycerin tolerance. *Proc Natl Acad Sci USA* 1995; 92:5244–5248.

75. Gumkowski F, Kaminska F, Kaminiski M, Morrissey LW, Auerbach R. Heterogeneity of mouse vascular endothelium: In vitro studies of lymphatic, large blood vessel and microvascular endothelial cells. *Blood Vessels* 1987; 24:11–23.

76. Klagsbrun M, D'Amore PA. Regulators of angiogenesis. *Annu Rev Physiol* 1991; 53:217–239.

77. Hansson HA, Brandsten C, Lossing C, Petruson K. Transient expression of insulin-like growth factor I immunoreactivity by vascular cells during angiogenesis. *Exp Mol Pathol* 1989; 50:125–138.

78. Folkman J, Langer R, Linhardt RJ, Haudenschild C, Taylor S. Angiogenesis inhibition and tumor regression caused by heparin or a heparin fragment in the presence of cortisone. *Science* 1983; 221:719–725.

79. Clowes AW, Clowes MM, Fingerle J, Reidy MA. Regulation of smooth muscle cell growth in injured artery. *J Cardiovasc Pharmacol* 1989; 14:S12–S15.

80. Clowes AW, Clowes MM. Kinetics of cellular proliferation after arterial injury: IV. Heparin inhibits rat smooth muscle mitogenesis and migration. *Circ Res* 1986; 58:839–845.

81. Owens GK, Geisterfer AA, Yang YW, Komoriya A. Transforming growth factor-beta-induced growth inhibition and cellular hypertrophy in cultured vascular smooth muscle cells. *J Cell Biol* 1988; 107:771–780.

82. Kavanaugh WM, Harsh GR IV, Starksen NF, Rocco CM, Williams LT. Transcriptional regulation of the A and B chain genes of PDGF in microvascular endothelial cells. *J Biol Chem* 1988; 263:8470–8472.

83. Hunter T. Protein-tyrosine phosphatases: The other side of the coin. *Cell* 1989; 58:1013–1016.

84. Conte JV, Foegh ML, Calcagno D, Wallace RB, Ramwell PW. Peptide inhibition of myointimal proliferation following angioplasty in rabbits. *Trans Proc* 1989; 21:3686–3688.

85. Gruppuso PA, Mikumo R, Brautigan DL, Braun L. Growth arrest induced by transforming growth factor beta 1 is accompanied by protein phosphatase activation in human keratinocytes. *J Biol Chem* 1991; 266:3444–3448.

86. Clemmons DR. Exposure to platelet-derived growth factors modulate the porcine aortic smooth muscle cell response to somatomedin-C. *Endocrinology* 1985; 117:77–83.

87. Delafontaine P. Insulin-like growth factor I and its binding proteins in the cardiovascular system. *Cardiovasc Res* 1995; 30:825–834.

88. Bevilaqua MP, Gimbrone MA, Jr. Modulation of endothelial cell procoagulant and fibrinolytic activities by inflammatory mediators. In: Ryan US (ed). *Endothelial Cells*. Boca Raton, FL: CRC Press; 1988.

89. Beasley D, Cohen RA, Levinsky NG. Interleukin 1 inhibits contraction of vascular smooth muscle. *J Clin Invest* 1989; 83:331–335.

90. Schindler R, Ghezzi P, Dinarello CA. IL-1 induces IL-1 IV: IFN-gamma suppresses IL-1 but not lipopolysaccharide-induced transcription of IL-1. *J Immunol* 1990; 144:2216–2222.

91. Lindner V, Reidy MA. Proliferation of smooth muscle cells after vascular injury is inhibited by an antibody against basic fibroblast growth factor. *Proc Natl Acad Sci USA* 1991; 88:3739–3743.

92. Bashkin P, Doctrow S, Klagsbrun M, Svahn CM, Folkman J, Vlodavsky I. Basic fibroblast growth factor binds to subendothelial extracellular matrix and is released by heparinase and heparin-like molecules. *Biochemistry* 1989; 28:1737–1743.

93. Hirata Y, Takagi Y, Fukuda Y, Marumo F. Endothelin is a potent mitogen for rat vascular smooth muscle cells. *Atherosclerosis* 1989; 78:225–228.

94. Majno G, Shea SM, Leventhal M. Endothelial contraction induced by histamine-type mediators: An electron microscopic study. *J Cell Biol* 1969; 42:647–672.

95. Pober JS, Cotran RS. What can be learned from the expression of endothelial adhesion molecules in tissues? *Lab Invest* 1991; 64:301–305.

96. Pober JS, Cotran RS. The role of endothelial cells in inflammation. *Transplantation* 1990; 50:537–544.

97. Marshall JJ, Kontos HA. Endothelium-derived relaxing factors: A perspective from in vivo data. *Hypertension* 1990; 16:371–386.

98. Nerem RM, Girard PR. Hemodynamic influences on vascular endothelial biology. *Toxicol Pathol* 1990; 18:572–582.

99. Schwartz SM, Majesky MW, Dilley RJ. Vascular remodeling in hypertension and atherosclerosis. In: Laragh JH, Brenner BM (eds). *Hypertension: Pathophysiology, Diagnosis and Management*. New York: Raven Press; 1990.

100. Asakura T, Karino T. Flow patterns and spatial distribution of atherosclerotic lesions in human coronary arteries. *Circ Res* 1990; 66:1045–1066.

101. Freiman PC, Mitchell GG, Heistad DD, Armstrong ML, Harrison DG. Atherosclerosis impairs endothelium-dependent vascular relaxation to acetylcholine and thrombin in primates. *Circ Res* 1986; 58:783–789.

102. Minor RL, Myers PR, Guerra R, Bates JN, Harrison DG. Diet-induced atherosclerosis increases the release of nitrogen oxides from rabbit aorta. *J Clin Invest* 1990; 86:2109–2116.

103. McLenachan JM, Williams JK, Fish RD, Ganz P, Selwyn AP. Loss of flow-mediated endothelium-dependent dilation occurs early in the development of atherosclerosis. *Circulation* 1991; 84:1273–1278.

104. Mügge A, Elwell JH, Peterson TE, Hofmeyer TG, Heistad DD, Harrison DG. Chronic treatment with polyethylene-glycolated superoxide dismutase partially restores endothelium-dependent vascular relaxations in cholesterol-fed rabbits. *Circ Res* 1991; 69:1293–1300.

105. Hansson GK, Seifert PS, Olsson G, Bondjers G. Immunohistochemical detection of macrophages and T lymphocytes in atherosclerotic lesions of cholesterol-fed rabbits. *Arterioscler Thromb* 1991; 1:745–750.

106. Cybulsky MI, Gimbrone MAJ. Endothelial expression of a mononuclear leukocyte adhesion molecule during atherogenesis. *Science* 1991; 251:788–791.

107. Wang JM, Sica A, Peri G, Walter S, Padura IM, Libby P, et al. Expression of monocyte chemotactic protein and interleukin-8 by cytokine-activated human vascular smooth muscle cells. *Arterioscler Thromb* 1991; 11:1166–1174.

108. Ross R. The pathogenesis of atherosclerosis—an update. *N Engl J Med* 1986; 14:488–500.

109. Rajagopalan S, Meng XP, Ramasamy S, Harrison DG, Galis ZS. Reactive oxygen species produced by macrophage-derived foam cells regulate the activity of vascular matrix metalloproteinases in vitro. *J Clin Invest* 1996; 98:2572–2579.

110. Vita JA, Treasure CB, Nabel EG, McLenachan JM, Fish RD, Yeung AC, et al. Coronary vasomotor response to acetylcholine relates to risk factors for coronary artery disease. *Circulation* 1990; 81:491–497.

111. Rubanyi GM. Endothelium-derived relaxing and contracting factors. *J Cell Biochem* 1991; 46:27–36.

112. Luscher TF, Vanhoutte PM. Endothelium-dependent contractions to acetylcholine in the aorta of the spontaneously hypertensive rat. *Hypertension* 1986; 8:344–348.

113. Owens GK, Schwartz SM. Alterations in vascular smooth muscle mass in the spontaneously hypertensive rat: Role in cellular hypertrophy, hyperploidy and hyperplasia. *Circ Res* 1982; 51:280–289.

114. Owens GK, Schwartz SM. Vascular smooth muscle cell hypertrophy and hyperploidy in the Goldblatt hypertensive rat. *Circ Res* 1983; 53:491–501.

115. Halpern W, Warshaw DM, Mulvany MJ. Mechanical and morphological properties of arterial resistance vessels in young and old spontaneously hypertensive rats. *Circ Res* 1979; 45:250–259.

116. Fukui T, Ishizaka N, Rajagopalan S, Bech Laursen J, Capers Q IV, Taylor WR, et al. p22phox mRNA expression and NADPH oxidase activity are increased in aortas from hypertensive rats. *Circ Res* 1996; 80:45–51.

117. Rajagopalan S, Kurz S, Münzel T, Tarpey M, Freeman BA, Griendling KK, et al. Angiotensin II mediated hypertension in the rat increases vascular superoxide production via membrane NADH/NADPH oxidase activation: contribution to alterations of vasomotor tone. *J Clin Invest* 1996; 97:1916–1923.

118. Majesky MW, Reidy MA, Bowen-Pope DF, Hart CE, Wilcox JN, Schwartz SM. PDGF ligand and receptor gene expression during repair of arterial injury. *J Cell Biol* 1990; 111:2149–2158.

119. Taubman MB, Rollins BJ, Poon M, Marmur J, Green RS, Berk BC, et al. JE mRNA accumulates rapidly in aortic injury and in platelet-derived growth factor-stimulated vascular smooth muscle cells. *Circ Res* 1992; 70:314–325.

120. Cercek B, Fishbein MC, Forrester JS, Helfant RH, Fagin JA. Induction of insulin-like growth factor I messenger RNA in rat aorta after balloon denudation. *Circ Res* 1990; 66:1755–1760.

121. Fingerle J, Au YP, Clowes AW, Reidy MA. Intimal lesion formation in rat carotid arteries after endothelial denudation in absence of medial injury. *Atherosclerosis* 1990; 10:1082–1087.

122. Lynch CM, Clowes MM, Osborne WRA, Clowes AW, Miller AD. Long-term expression of human adenosine deaminase in vascular smooth muscle cells of rats: A model for gene therapy. *Proc Natl Acad Sci USA* 1992; 89:1138–1142.

123. Dichek DA, Neville RF, Zwiebel JA, Freeman SM, Leon MB, Anderson WF. Seeding of intravascular stents with genetically engineered endothelial cells. *Circulation* 1989; 80:1347–1353.

124. Takeshita S, Tsurumi Y, Couffinahl T, Asahara T, Bauters C, Symes J, et al. Gene transfer of naked DNA encoding for three isoforms of vascular endothelial growth factor stimulates collateral development in vivo. *Lab Invest* 1996; 75:487–501.

125. Forough R, Koyama N, Hasenstab D, Lea H, Clowes M, Nikkari ST, et al. Overexpression of tissue inhibitor of matrix metalloproteinase-1 inhibits vascular smooth muscle cell functions in vitro and in vivo. *Circ Res* 1996; 79:812–820.

126. Nabel EG. Direct gene transfer into the arterial wall. *J Vasc Surg* 1992; 15:931–932.

127. Morishita R, Gibbons GH, Ellison KE, Lee W, Zhang L, Yu H, et al. Evidence for direct local effect of angiotensin in vascular hypertrophy: In vivo gene transfer of angiotensin converting enzyme. *J Clin Invest* 1994; 94:978–984.

STRUCTURE AND FUNCTIONING OF CARDIOVASCULAR MEMBRANES, CHANNELS, AND RECEPTORS

Gary L. Stiles

The concepts and techniques that have accrued from the development of modern cellular and molecular biology have revolutionized how we think about cell growth, function, development, and signaling. The great unknowns about how receptors signal, how ion channels gate ions, and how the two systems interact are rapidly becoming unraveled. In order to understand these concepts and their implications for clinical medicine and the development of new therapeutic approaches, it is required that at least a cursory knowledge of cell membranes be understood.

MEMBRANE STRUCTURE

Every living cell must have the ability to maintain a controlled intracellular environment. In order to accomplish this, a variety of substances such as ions, water, and proteins must be transported into or out of the cell as needed. In addition, cells must be responsive to environmental perturbations such as hormones, drugs, or other molecules, even when these factors do not physically enter the cell. The structural entity that allows this to be accomplished is the plasma membrane. The plasma membrane effectively gives structure to the cells while selectively insulating the extracellular from the intracellular world. Although the plasma membrane can be thought of as a simple cellular envelope, it is anything but simple and inert.[1–4] The membrane is, in fact, a highly organized structure composed of lipids, proteins, and carbohydrates dynamically interacting and largely associated through noncovalent bonds. The general structure for a membrane is shown in Fig. 5-1; there is a lipid bilayer in which the charged portions of the lipids face the extracellular and intracellular spaces while hydrophobic (nonpolar) fatty acyl chains interact with each other.

As can be seen in Fig. 5-1, there is not only a very heterogeneous population of substances that constitute the membrane, but these molecules are arranged in an asymmetric distribution with certain substituents having a predilection for the extracellular surface (glycoproteins), whereas others are more frequently encountered on the cytoplasmic surface (phosphatidylserine).

Approximately 50 percent of the mass of the plasma membrane is lipid. The phospholipids, the major type of lipid, have a polar head group and two hydrophobic hydrocarbon tails. Phospholipids themselves are a mixture of different compounds that vary in the length of the hydrocarbon tails, the

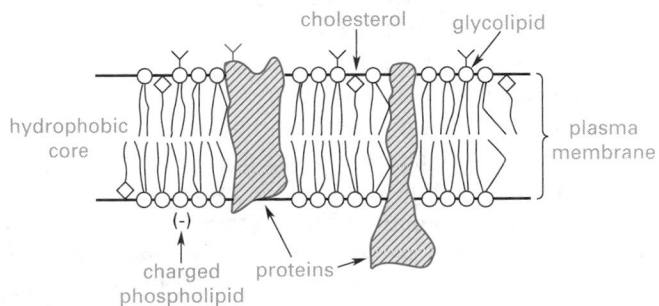

Extracellular Space

FIGURE 5-1

Schematic representation of plasma membrane. The polar head groups represented by small circles are arranged at the extracellular and intracellular surfaces. The lipid (fatty acid) chains face each other to form the hydrophobic core. The unsaturated fatty acid chains (contain double bonds) are represented by the "kinked" tails. The large proteins shown represent transmembrane proteins embedded in the lipid matrix. One of the proteins and several of the lipids (glycolipids) are represented as containing a carbohydrate substituent (Y). The charged phospholipids are shown on the intracellular surface.

degree of double-bond saturation in the tail, and the type of substituents in the polar head groups. Of particular importance in the functioning of the membrane is the degree of saturation or unsaturation in the fatty acid tails of the phospholipids. When the fatty acid chains are unsaturated, i.e., have double bonds between carbon atoms, the chain is kinked (as depicted in Fig. 5-1) and, hence, cannot be packed as tightly together, which leads to a greater mobility or fluidity within the membranes. Theoretically at least, there may be an association between the diet content of saturated versus unsaturated fats and the composition of plasma membrane. This possibility could ultimately provide a link between diet and how cells function and respond to stimuli. This may directly affect how the proteins can move or function within the lipid bilayer.[1–3]

Cholesterol is another major constituent of the membrane and tends to promote membrane rigidity rather than fluidity.[1,2,4] Cholesterol, which is a rigid heterocyclic compound, aligns itself in the membrane with its hydroxyl group near the polar head groups of the phospholipid and its hydrophobic tail interacting with the fatty acid tails within the lipid bilayer. Cholesterol's rigidity decreases the ability of fatty acid tails to move and thereby promotes membrane rigidity.

Glycolipids make up the last large class of lipids that comprise the lipid bilayer. These lipids contain carbohydrates in the form of oligosaccharides. The oligosaccharides are a very heterogeneous group of compounds, ranging from a single sugar substituent to very complex gangliosides that contain multiple sugar residues terminating in sialic acid, giving them an overall negative charge. As mentioned earlier, glycolipids are found only on the extracellular face where their glycan components are exposed to the extracellular environment. The function of this class of molecules remains speculative but may relate to cell-cell interaction or may act as specific cell-surface receptors.

The very nature of lipid molecules makes them form bilayers spontaneously when exposed to a water environment. The association of lipids occurs when the hydrophobic tails associate to exclude water, thus aligning the charged head groups towards the water and the tails towards a core. This hydrophobic core acts as an effective insulation preventing the passage of charged molecules. For example, a sodium (Na^+) ion is 10 billion times less likely to cross a lipid bilayer than is a water molecule. If the structure of the plasma membrane contained only lipids as described, it would be an effective barrier, although it would, by and large, not allow for the transport of substances into or out of the cell nor for the transduction of transmembrane signals.

To accomplish these specific functions, the lipid bilayer acts as a matrix to support proteins in the appropriate conformation to allow them to carry out their appointed tasks. Although there is the general scheme described above for the types of lipids found in plasma membranes, there is great diversity and disparity from cell to cell among the types of proteins embedded in the plasma membrane. There are, however, two general classes of proteins. The first consists of integral membrane proteins that either pass through the lipid bilayer directly (transmembrane protein) or are attached via a lipid side chain interaction to the lipid bilayer. These proteins do not readily dissociate from the plasma membrane and can be released only through disruption of the membrane structure by detergents or organic solvents. The other class comprises proteins (peripheral or loosely associated) that do penetrate the lipid bilayer but are more closely associated with integral membrane proteins by noncovalent associations and can be dissociated from the membrane without physically disrupting the membrane bilayer.

For the purposes of this chapter, the integral membrane proteins are most important. This class of proteins is the major constituent of both membrane-bound receptors and ion channels. These integral membrane proteins can pass through the membrane once or multiple times. Proteins that span an odd number of times will have their N- and C-terminals on opposite sides of the lipid bilayer, while proteins that span an even number of times will have their C- and N-terminals on the same side.

Since these proteins must interact with the relatively aqueous (hydrophilic) cytosolic and extracellular spaces as well as with the hydrophobic lipid bilayer, most proteins contain stretches of hydrophilic amino acids interspersed with hydrophobic domains. The hydrophobic domains are incorporated into the lipid bilayer so that the nonpolar regions of the amino acids interact with the fatty acid chains while the polar peptide bonds and polar side chains are grouped to shield themselves from the fatty acids. As we shall see, when the proteins span the lipid bilayer multiple times, the transmembrane segments can arrange themselves in a bundle to create a hydrophilic core, pore, or channel and a hydrophobic perimeter to interact with the fatty acid chains. This pore can be utilized as a site for interaction of ligands, hormones, or drugs to interact with the protein (receptor) or as a hydrated channel through which ions or other small molecules can pass into or out of the cell. As might be imagined, the orientation of the protein in the membrane is critical to its function. A significant proportion of integral membrane proteins has posttranslational modifications including glycosylation (addition of sugars) or fatty acid acylation. The carbohydrate chains are always on the extracellular face of the cell, while the lipid modifications can be attached to either face of the membrane. In some cases, these modifications are absolutely required for function of the protein; in other cases, the alterations have no apparent effect.

Membranes, as mentioned earlier, display a property known as fluidity, which permits proteins and lipids to have mobility in the lipid bilayer. This property allows distinct proteins to come together and interact to produce a functional coupling (lateral diffusion), e.g., receptors and guanine nucleotide binding proteins (G proteins) or the clustering of low-density lipoprotein receptors. The lipid bilayer cannot, however, be viewed as an unstructured liquid through which proteins float at random. Membranes, in fact, have discrete structural domains in which certain ion channels or enzymes are confined to specific areas and are not free to diffuse around the cell.[1]

ION CHANNELS

Few fields in science have witnessed a more rapid expansion in knowledge than that of ion channel structure and function. Ion channels function primarily to regulate the flow of ions across the cell membrane and thereby modulate the electrical potential of the cell.[5] It has long been recognized that channel proteins must in some way form a regulatable water-filled pore through which select ions can pass. Under the appropriate conditions, a single channel can maintain a high degree of specificity towards a single type of ion yet allow more than a million of these ions to pass per second. Ion channels can be thought of as a passive conduit through which ions move down a concentration gradient. That is to say, energy in the form of adenosine triphosphate (ATP) is not expended during the ion movement. This is in contrast to an energy-dependent ion pump, which can move ions against a concentration gradient.[1]

Channels must inherently have the ability to open and close in response to the cells' need or appropriate stimuli. If the channel were to remain open, an ionic equilibrium would quickly be reached between the outside and inside of the cells and no ionic gradient or electrical potential across the membrane would be maintained. This would lead to cellular dysfunction and/or death.

The "gating" function of ion channels is intrinsic to the protein structure of the channel and can be regulated by several distinct signaling processes, including mechanical stimulation of the channel such as stretch (mechanically gated channel), voltage changes across the membrane (voltage-gated channels), or the binding of hormones or drugs (ligand-gated channels).[6–13] This last class of channels can be regulated via external neurotransmitters such as acetylcholine, epinephrine, or adenosine.[7,10–13] These substances may interact directly with the channel protein (acetylcholine) or through distinct receptors, such as the β-adrenergic receptor (epinephrine) or A$_1$ adenosine receptor (adenosine), which in turn activate specific G proteins. The G proteins can then modulate channel activity either through direct intramembrane interactions or indirectly via a second messenger system, such as cyclic adenosine monophosphate (cAMP) or cyclic guanosine monophosphate (cGMP).[7,10–13] These channel subtypes should not be taken to be mutually exclusive since a voltage-sensitive channel may also have its function modulated by receptor-mediated G protein interactions.

The fact that external stimuli can regulate channel pore opening and closing immediately begins to provide insight into the protein architecture of the channel. First, the protein must span the membrane to allow a pore to form. Next, the pore must have inherent properties that allow only specific ions to enter and traverse the pore. Third, the pore must have the ability to close and open (gate). Finally, the channel protein must have regulatory regions through which the appropriate signals can be imparted to the channel, such as sites for G protein interaction, sites that sense changes in voltage, or sites

for covalent modifications such as phosphorylation (see Fig. 5-2 for schematic representation).

In addition to classification of channels by regulatory mechanisms, categorization is frequently made by their ion selectivity and whether they promote outward or inward currents. For example, in the outward-current channel class, the K$^+$-selective channels are by far the most important and the most abundant of the different subtypes. This class of channels acts to hyperpolarize the cell and, therefore, is frequently responsible for repolarizing cells after the action potential, created largely by the Na$^+$ channel (inward current), has depolarized the cell. As mentioned previously, the K$^+$ movement is down its concentration gradient, and hence K$^+$ moves outward. K$^+$ channels are highly regulated in the heart.[5,10] Acetylcholine, acting through muscarinic receptors, and adenosine, acting via A$_1$ adenosine receptors, activate a pertussis toxin–sensitive G protein that subsequently activates a K$^+$ channel to promote hyperpolarization of the cell.[5,10] The effect of hyperpolarization on pacemaker and conducting system cells would be to decrease spontaneous depolarization and hence to decrease chronotropy and slow conduction. This response is consistent with the known effects of adenosine, for example, to slow heart rate and atrioventricular nodal conduction.[14] In extracardiac tissues such as neurons, muscarinic receptors, acting through pertussis toxin–insensitive G proteins, can inhibit K$^+$ channels (M currents) through mechanisms distinct from those described above.[10] In addition, there are several other types of K$^+$ channels in the heart, including the ATP depletion–dependent K$^+$ channel, the Na$^+$-dependent K$^+$ channels, and the delayed rectifying K$^+$ channels.[5] The term *rectifying channels* refers to channels that have a net current, usually in the outward direction, and that rectify or counteract the depolarized state. A delayed rectifying channel simply opens late in the depolarization

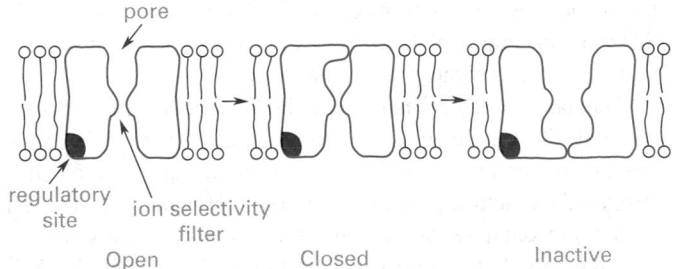

Extracellular Space

Intracellular Space

FIGURE 5-2

Schematic representation of a generic ion channel in lipid bilayer. The major functional features of an ion channel are depicted. These include a central pore, or "channel," through which ions can pass. A selectivity filter permits only a specific ion to pass. The regulatory site represents a domain on the protein responsible for regulating the function (ability of ions to pass) of the channel. This could range from a phosphorylation site, an actual hormone binding site, or the site for interaction with G proteins. Three discrete states of the channel are shown—open, closed, or inactive. See description in text.

process. This latter group of channels functions primarily during the most depolarized states of the cell. In the heart, cAMP will increase the outward current, thereby accelerating repolarization and shortening the action potential. There are a variety of additional outward rectifying K^+ channels that are modulated by time (A current channels) or Ca^{2+}—the Ca^{2+}-activated outward rectifying K^+ channels. The great diversity of K^+ channels makes a detailed description of each type impossible in this chapter, and the reader is referred to the references.[5,6,8,15–17]

There are two main types of inward channels that promote depolarization of the cell: the Na^+ and Ca^{2+} channels. The Ca^{2+} channels are primarily responsible for increasing intracellular Ca^{2+} leading to contraction of muscle.[5,6,18] The three major classes of voltage-dependent Ca^{2+} channels have been designated L type, N type, and T type.[5] The channels can be differentiated by their sensitivity to the dihydropyridine class of Ca^{2+} channel blockers, by the membrane potential at which they are activated and inactivated, and by their gating and permeation characteristics. These channels are positively and negatively regulated by G protein–coupled receptors. For example, in the heart β-adrenergic receptors acting via the G_s protein promote the opening of Ca^{2+} channels. This effect can be mediated by two distinct pathways. The first is mediated by an enhanced level of intracellular cAMP, which activates protein kinase A leading to phosphorylation of the Ca^{2+} channels.[7,10]

The second involves the direct activation of the channel by activated G_s protein independent of cAMP. A number of receptors are capable of inhibiting the activity of Ca^{2+} channels via distinct mechanisms. Certain muscarinic (M_2) receptors and A_1 adenosine receptors inhibit Ca^{2+} currents by suppressing cAMP levels following activation of inhibitory G_i proteins. In contrast, atrial natriuretic factor acting via its receptor can activate cGMP, leading to an enhancement of a cyclic nucleotide phosphodiesterase that degrades cAMP.[5] This produces the same effect functionally as that mediated by the A_1 adenosine receptor described above but by a distinctly different mechanism. Receptors that activate protein kinase C may also inactivate Ca^{2+} channels.

The last class of channels to be described are the Na^+ channels. These channels are largely responsible for the rapid inward movement of Na^+ ions that results in the rapid upstroke of the action potential. The Na^+ channel will be used as a representative of the larger class of voltage-sensitive ion channels that undergo inactivation and that includes K^+ channels (A channel) and dihydropyridine-sensitive Ca^{2+} channels, since they all share structural and functional homologies.[6,18,19] The voltage-gated Na^+ channels are largely responsible for generating the action potential so critical in cardiac muscle and conducting tissue.[20] The action potential is a rapid, transient self-propagating electrical current that traverses the membrane. The cell normally has a potential difference across the membrane of ~ -80 to -100 mV. A depolarization of the membrane, i.e., a shift in the membrane potential to a less negative value, leads to the opening of

voltage-gated Na^+ channels and an influx of Na^+ (down its concentration gradient) into the cell. This leads to a further depolarization that permits additional Na^+ to enter. This positive-feedback loop enhances the propagation of the depolarization wave. There must, however, be a mechanism to terminate this process, since the cell obviously does not find itself in a situation where all Na^+ channels are open and no Na^+ gradient exists. The process that protects the cell against this possibility is called the *inactivation state* of the channel. This state of the channel is distinctly different from simple channel closure (Fig. 5-2). When "inactivated" the channel cannot reopen until the local membrane potential has returned to its resting negative value and the channel protein reassumes its closed configuration. The exact mechanism(s) responsible for this inactivation state and the process returning the protein to its closed state remain largely unknown.

Molecular studies undertaken in the past few years have revealed strong structural similarities among Na^+, K^+, and Ca^{2+} channels.[6,18,19] These channels may be a single subunit protein complex or may contain multiple subunits.[6,18,19] There are, however, homologous motifs within the primary subunit of each channel. For example, each channel has multiple membrane-spanning hydrophobic domains, including a so-called S4 sequence in which positively charged basic amino acid residues, such as arginines, are located every third amino acid within the transmembrane domain. This specialized sequence may function as the voltage sensor.[6,18,19] In addition, there are multiple hydrophilic regions that traverse the membrane to form the aqueous pore through which the ions pass. The gating function is envisioned as a twisting or "screwlike" motion of the helices upward in the membrane, resulting in the opening of the channel.[15,16]

Multiple Na^+ channels have now been cloned and/or purified.[6,21–23] Purification studies indicate that there is one large subunit (of over 1800 amino acids) and several smaller subunits.[6,19] The large subunit by itself can form functional Na^+ channels with many but not all of the properties expected of the native Na^+ channel. Within the large subunit there are multiple repeats of similar sequences[6]; that is to say, the large protein is composed of four homologous domains linearly arranged in series. Within each of these domains lie multiple stretches of hydrophobic amino acids that likely represent the transmembrane-spanning regions and a single S4 sequence described above (see Fig. 5-3A).

In contrast to the Na^+ channel, the K^+ channel is much simpler and contains only one of the basic repeat units contained in the Na^+ channel (Fig. 5-3B). Multiple K^+ channels have been cloned, and all have the basic single subunit motif but differ in their N- and C-terminals.[6,8] This suggests that the common, or shared, portions of these channels are responsible for the ion pore, the ion selectivity, and the voltage sensitivity mechanisms, whereas the two ends may function to impart specific regulatory functions.

The Ca^{2+} channels are known to be multimeric, having both large and small subunits. The large α_1 subunit has many of the structural features of the Na^+ channel, as shown in

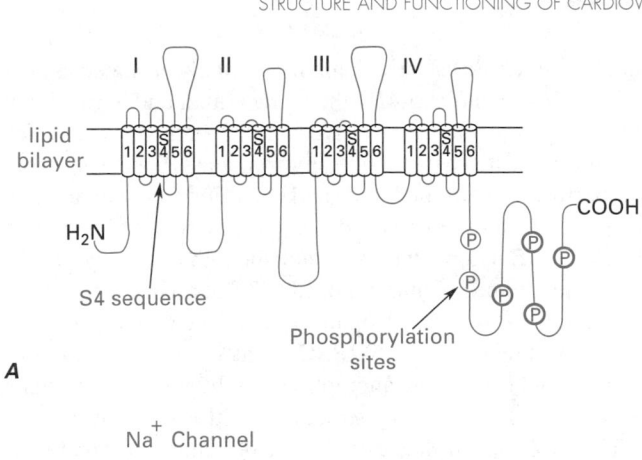

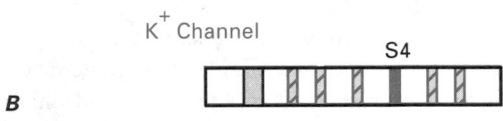

FIGURE 5-3

Structural characteristics of sodium channels. *A.* Schematic representation of Na$^+$ channel protein/membrane architecture. The large protein traverses the membrane multiple times with both the N- and C-terminals on the intracellular side of the membrane. The transmembrane regions are grouped into four motifs, each containing six transmembrane spans. Within each motif there is a specific span termed the *S4 region*, which likely contains the voltage sensing region. Phosphorylation sites shown on the carboxyl tail help to regulate channel function. *B.* Comparison of a schematic representation of the Na$^+$ channel with its four motifs with that of a K$^+$ channel in which a single similar motif comprises the channel pore.

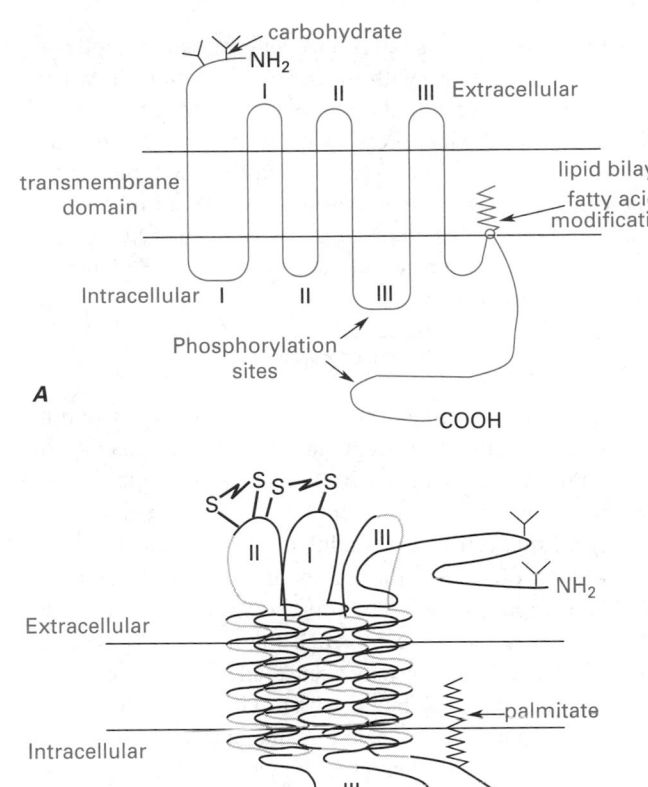

FIGURE 5-4

Receptor structure. *A.* Planar model of a prototypic G protein–coupled receptor and its arrangement in the lipid bilayer. These receptors have their N-terminal on the extracellular surface. Most receptors have carbohydrate modifications on the extracellular surface either on the N-terminal (as shown) or on the second extracellular loop. Sites for protein phosphorylation exist on the third intracellular loop and/or the C-terminal. Phosphorylation of these sites likely results in less efficient coupling of the receptor to the effector system. Some receptors have lipid modifications that attach the protein to the lipid bilayer. *B.* Model of receptor with the transmembrane domains bundled together to form a ligand pocket. Disulfide bonds (both intraloop and interloop) are shown and are known to be important in maintaining the receptors' three-dimensional architecture necessary for appropriate ligand binding.

Fig. 5-4*A*, in that it has four homologous domains that contain multiple membrane-spanning regions and a single S4 sequence.[18,19,24]

The insight derived from these molecular studies when combined with modern genetics has made a tremendous impact on our understanding of ion channels at the protein and cellular levels. This work now has consequences at the clinical level. An example is the long QT syndrome. This is an inherited cardiac disorder that causes an increased risk of sudden death from ventricular arrhythmias[25–30] (see Chaps. 27 and 36). In the affected individuals, there is an abnormality in repolarization of cardiac tissue demonstrated by a prolonged QT interval on the electrocardiogram.[25] Recent studies document that long QT syndrome results from abnormalities (mutations) in genes that encode ion channels. Three separate genes have been identified: *SCN*5A is located on chromosome 3, *HERG* is on chromosome 7, and *KVLQT* is on chromosome 11.[25–30] *SCN*5A encodes the cardiac Na$^+$ channel described above. The abnormality (mutation) in this case causes an enhanced function of the channel rather than a loss-of-function problem. The inactivation gate of the abnormal ion channel is rendered unstable, allowing it to open and close rather than to keep the channel closed, which leads to a prolonged action potential.[25–27]

The *HERG* gene codes for the α subunit of a delayed rectifying K$^+$ channel. Activation of the normal *HERG* K$^+$ channel leads to a termination of the cardiac action potential. Mutations in *HERG* lead to a loss of function of the channel, which results in a prolonged action potential.[25–28,30] The exact nature of the *KVLQT*1 gene is not known, but the predicted amino acid sequence would suggest that it codes for a new type of K$^+$ channel.[25,26,29]

The common feature of all these gene mutations is that they prolong action potential duration by some mechanism. The insight gained from these studies into the mechanisms involved has already provided a rationale for therapies. For example, in the gain-of-function mutations in the Na$^+$ channel (*SCN*5A), in which case the channel remains active for too long a period of time, the use of medications to block Na$^+$

channel function appears to produce a beneficial effect[26] (see Chap. 27). For patients with the *HERG* mutation, in whom the K^+ channel does not allow enough K^+ ions to flow out of the cell, a paradoxical property of the channel can be used to create a potential therapy. Even though the K^+ moves out of the cell (down its concentration gradient), an increase in extracellular K^+ does increase the overall activity of the channel. Therefore, dietary supplementation with K^+ may be used to treat this disorder.[26]

RECEPTORS

Cell-surface (transmembrane) receptors function to permit extracellular substances to regulate intracellular function or metabolism without necessarily having to enter the cell. A number of different types of receptors can initiate a transmembrane signal that ultimately modulates cellular function. We shall focus here only on the largest group—the G protein–coupled receptors that utilize G proteins to act as the intermediary between a given receptor and the actual inhibition or activation of an effector system, such as adenylyl cyclase.[31–33] The other classes of receptors, which will not be discussed, include those that have intrinsic tyrosine kinase activity, such as the receptor for epidermal growth factor or insulin[34]; those that transport the ligand itself into the cell, such as those for the low-density lipoprotein[35]; or the ion channels that themselves contain the receptor for their own ligand, such as the nicotinic acetylcholine receptor.[7]

Receptor Structure

As alluded to in the previous section, there is a close functional association between ion channels and membrane receptors. In addition, there are structural similarities between the G protein–coupled receptors and ion channels. The past 10 years have witnessed the purification and cloning of a large number of these G protein–coupled receptors, which have provided an abundance of information about their structure, function, and regulation.[32,36] The G protein–coupled receptors are part of an ever-growing, large gene family that binds such diverse agonists (ligands) as adenosine, catecholamines, "light," odorants, acetylcholine, prostaglandins, angiotensin, vasoactive intestinal protein, and histamine.[31–33,36,37] The receptors for all of these endogenous substances are integral membrane proteins that contain seven transmembrane domains that likely associate to form a "bundle" with a central "pocket"—much like that described for ion channels (see Figs. 5-3A, 5-4A). Instead of forming an aqueous pore, however, the pocket forms the binding site for the ligand. Just as the ion pore has a selectivity filter that permits only selective ions to pass through it, the pocket determines the ligand specificity for each receptor. In addition, each receptor contains an extracellular N-terminal tail and three extracellular loops connecting the transmembrane domains. There are three intracellular loops and an intracellular carboxyl tail (see Fig. 5-4A).

All these receptors are single subunit proteins, and each of the seven transmembrane domains contains 20 to 28 hydro-

phobic amino acids. These domains are likely arranged as an α helix as shown in Fig. 5-4B. The extracellular and intracellular loops largely contain more hydrophilic amino acids, which can interact with the aqueous environment. Pioneering work was performed with rhodopsin and bacteriorhodopsin (a member of the G protein–coupled receptors) and high-resolution electron diffraction studies established the validity of the seven-membrane-spanning motif.[37,38] This work has permitted models for other G protein–coupled receptors to be proposed, as shown in Fig. 5-4B. Currently, many laboratories throughout the world are attempting to validate and understand the secondary and tertiary structures of these receptors.

The functions of the extracellular domains are largely unknown, although it is clear that the N-terminal tail or extracellular loop II is the site for glycosylation.[39] The role of glycosylation in the functioning of the receptor remains unclear.[39] The extracellular loops I and II contain cysteine residues that likely form disulfide bonds, which are important in stabilizing the ligand binding pocket.[39,40]

As mentioned above, the transmembrane domains contain the ligand binding site and determine the pharmacologic specificity of the receptors. At present, the exact regions (and amino acids) of the domains responsible for the ligand binding site for agonists and antagonists are largely unknown. For further details see Refs. 32 and 41 to 43.

The cytoplasmic regions, particularly loop III and the carboxyl tail, are important for receptor coupling to its G protein and contain sites for posttranslational modifications such as phosphorylation, which are important for regulation of receptor function.[39] The function of cytoplasmic loops I and II remains largely unknown.

Receptor Coupling

G protein–coupled receptors functionally interact with a wide variety of G proteins, which are heterotrimeric protein complexes consisting of α, β, and γ subunits.[44,45] The α subunits are likewise an ever-expanding superfamily of proteins that currently has more than 12 members, some of which are listed in Table 5-1. The more common α subunits are α_s, which is responsible for activating adenylyl cyclase; α_i (three subtypes known), which inhibit adenylyl cyclase; α_0 (two types), which likely regulate Ca^{2+} channels and phospholipase C; and α_z, which may activate phospholipase C.

All the α subunits are capable of coupling to receptors and are multifunctional proteins of molecular mass ~40 kDa. Within the α subunit resides a specific domain that allows it to interact with its attendant receptor, a site for interacting with the appropriate effector system, and a region that binds guanosine triphosphate (GTP) and then has the ability to hydrolyze GTP to guanosine diphosphate (GDP) (GTPase activity).[46]

A full understanding of receptor-mediated transmembrane signaling requires insight into how the three known components of a prototypic stimulatory adenylyl cyclase system interact.[31,32,39] For this system, the β-adrenergic receptor (βAR), the stimulatory G_s protein, and the enzyme adenylyl cyclase are the three protein components. The βAR acts as the recognition unit for a hormone—epinephrine (see Fig. 5-5). When an agonist such as epinephrine binds to the receptor in its appropriate pocket, it induces a conformational change in the receptor that allows it to interact functionally with its G protein, G_s, which, basally is in its heterotrimeric state—$\alpha\beta\gamma$. In the basal state, GDP (inactive guanine nucleotide) is bound to the α subunit. Under the influence of the agonist, an agonist-specific, high-affinity receptor–G protein complex forms and the G protein is induced to undergo a conformational change that promotes the exchange of GTP (active guanine nucleotide) for GDP. The binding of GTP likely results in the dissociation of the receptor from the G protein as well as the dissociation of the α-GTP from the $\beta\gamma$ subunit. These reactions are all known to require the presence of Mg^{2+}. The activated α-GTP is then able to interact functionally with the catalytic unit of adenylyl cyclase, thereby activating it to convert ATP to cAMP.

The mechanism responsible for terminating this process is the hydrolysis of GTP to GDP + Pi (orthophosphate). This GTPase activity resides within the α subunit itself.[39,44] When the GTP is hydrolyzed to GDP, α-GDP is no longer able to activate adenylyl cyclase and the α subunit reassociates with $\beta\gamma$, allowing the complex to recycle back to interact with the receptor if an agonist is present to start the process again. If no agonist is present, then the α-GDP($\beta\gamma$) remains in its basal state.

An analogous process is likely responsible for G protein–mediated activation of ion channels; phospholipases C, D, and A; and the cGMP-phosphodiesterase. The exact mechanism by which the A_1 adenosine or the α_2-adrenergic receptors act to suppress cAMP is still debated, but most investigators believe that activation of the G_i protein by these prototypical inhibitory receptors is analogous to that described above. Following the dissociation of α_i-GTP from $\beta\gamma$, however, the mechanism for inhibition of adenylyl cyclase becomes less clear. The most likely scenario is that following the release of $\beta\gamma$, the $\beta\gamma$ may (by the process of mass action) promote the reassociation of α_s with $\beta\gamma$, thereby inactivating α_s. Thus, G_i appears to inactivate G_s rather than directly inhibiting the catalytic unit. The other potential mechanism would be that activated

TABLE 5-1

GUANINE NUCLEOTIDE BINDING PROTEINS (G PROTEINS)

G Proteins	α Subunits (Types)	Location	Effector	Response
G_s FAMILY				
G_s	4 splice variants	Ubiquitous	Adenylyl cyclase	+
			Ca^{2+} channel	+
G_{olf}	1	Olfactory epithelium	Adenylyl cyclase	+
G_i FAMILY				
Transducin	2	Rods/cones	cGMP PDE	+
G_{i1}	1	Neurons	??	+
G_{i2}	1	Ubiquitous	Adenylyl cyclase	−
G_{i3}	1	Nonneuronal	??	
G_0	2	Neuronal endocrine	Ca^{2+} channels	−
G_z	1	Neuronal platelet	??	
G_q FAMILY				
G_q	1	Ubiquitous	Phospholipase C-β	+
G_{11}	1	Nonhematopoietic	Phospholipase C-β	+
G_{14}	1	Diverse	Phospholipase C-β	+
$G_{15,16}$	1	Hematopoietic	Phospholipase C-β	+
G_{12} FAMILY				
G_{12}	1	Ubiquitous	??	
G_{13}	1	Ubiquitous	??	

Abbreviation: PDE = phosphodiesterase.

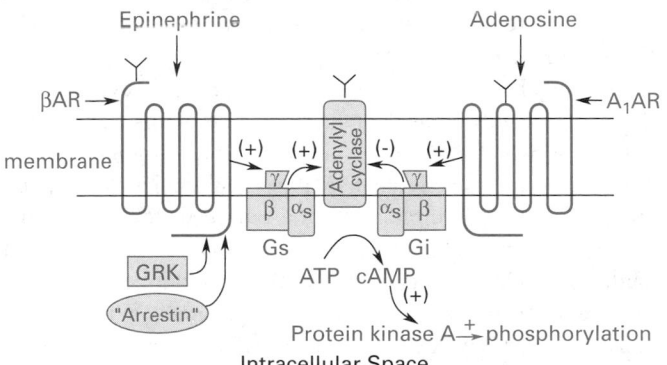

FIGURE 5-5

Typical hormone-sensitive adenylyl cyclase system. The β-adrenergic receptor (βAR) is a typical stimulating receptor that interacts with the stimulatory G protein (G_s) shown in its heterotrimeric form with the α, β, γ subunits. The enzyme adenylyl cyclase is shown as a transmembrane protein (actually has multiple transmembrane domains) with a carbohydrate chain (γ) shown on its extracellular surface. The A_1 adenosine receptor (A_1AR) is a typical inhibitory receptor that interacts with the inhibitory guanine nucleotide binding protein (G_i) to inhibit the enzyme adenylyl cyclase. Each receptor contains a carbohydrate chain (γ). GRK refers to the G protein–coupled receptor kinase, which, upon agonist activation of a receptor, leads to receptor phosphorylation with subsequent binding of an "arrestin" molecule (see text for full description).

α_i GTP directly inhibits the catalytic unit itself.[25,39] In the final analysis, both mechanisms may be operative but under different conditions.

Receptor Function

The original concept of transmembrane signaling put forward by Robison et al. in 1967 was that a hormone activated a specific receptor that, in turn, directly activated an effector.[47] This model was constructed based on what was known about multisubunit enzymes. As the complexity of the signaling systems in terms of components, cofactors, and component interactions became apparent, more diverse pathways and interactions had to be expected and explained.

Traditionally, for example, receptor classes were defined by their relative affinities for specific agonists and antagonists. Thus, a distinct pharmacologic potency series defined a given receptor type or class. Evidence slowly accumulated that there appeared to be pharmacologic variations within receptor classes, leading to the concept of receptor subtypes. With the recent application of the techniques of molecular biology to the field of receptor classification, we are only now beginning to appreciate the great diversity nature has to offer. For illustrative purposes, we can again use adrenergic receptors as a model. Ahlquist, in 1948, first demonstrated that catecholamines exerted their effects through two different receptors based on a pharmacologic profile.[48] He termed these *alpha* and *beta receptors*. With the advent of radioligand binding studies and the synthesis of new ligands, it became clear that each of these types could be subdivided into β_1- and β_2- and α_1- and α_2-adrenergic receptor subtypes by pharmacologic criteria. Now with molecular cloning techniques, it is clear that there is a β_3 receptor, found predominantly in fat tissues, and that there are at least three subtypes of each of the α_1- and α_2-adrenergic receptors.

Not only has the number of known receptor subtypes grown dramatically but so has the number of G proteins and effector systems to which each receptor may couple. Dogma has been that βARs always activate cAMP as their mechanism for cell signaling, and, by implication, the only effector system that the G_s protein could activate was adenylyl cyclase. Recent studies now clearly document that β-adrenergic receptors acting via G_s can directly open Ca^{2+} channels without first activating adenylyl cyclase and cAMP.[10] Similarly, the A_1 adenosine receptor, which was thought to produce its effect only via inhibition of adenylyl cyclase, is now known to open K^+ channels also.[10] Whether there are separate and distinct G_i-like proteins that mediate these two effects remains unproven. To further complicate matters, a single receptor subtype may well be capable of activating several different G proteins.[10]

As is evident from this brief discussion, our ability to find and study the components of the signaling apparatus has far outstripped our ability to define how each component interacts to maintain selectivity and specificity in a physiologically relevant manner. Much additional work will be necessary to define the processes (pathways) involved between receptor activation and physiologic responses more accurately.

Receptor Regulation

G protein–coupled receptors have long been recognized to be dynamic entities capable of being regulated by pathophysiologic processes.[31,39,49–55] This regulation is now known to occur at multiple levels, i.e., transcriptional, translational, and posttranslational. In addition, it is clear that activation of certain G protein–coupled receptors can lead to alterations in the quantity and functionality of G proteins.[52–54] These multiple levels of regulation make possible a very fine "tuning" mechanism for controlling the transmembrane signal transduction process for either an enhancement or a diminution of receptor signaling. It has been demonstrated during the past decade that each of the components of hormone-sensitive adenylyl cyclase systems can be modified either quantitatively, functionally, or both in a variety of model systems. Table 5-2 lists the known or possible modes of regulation. Obviously, not all of these changes occur in any one cell system or for any pathophysiologic perturbation.

There are now a large number of conditions known to modulate receptor signaling, including agonist-induced desensitization, antagonist-induced sensitization, changes in steroid and thyroid hormone levels, cAMP changes, congestive heart failure, diabetes, and ischemia.[31,49,51] One of the physiologically and therapeutically important modes of regulation is the phenomenon of agonist-induced desensitization. *Desensitization* refers to the attenuation of responsiveness to an agonist in its continued presence—a phenomenon well appreciated in clinical medicine. At least two major mechanisms are responsible for agonist-mediated desensitization, including regulation of receptor number on the cell surface and the ability of these receptors to interact with the appropriate G proteins to transmit a signal. These two final pathways for regulation can result from changes occurring at many different levels. In the βAR system, at least three different processes are involved with desensitization. The first is uncoupling of the receptor from its G_s protein, which is rapid (seconds to minutes).

TABLE 5-2

MODES OF RECEPTOR SIGNALING REGULATION

Changes in receptor number
   Increase or decrease in transcriptional rate (mRNA)
   Alteration in translatability or stability of mRNA
   Alteration in protein half-life or stability
   Removal of receptor from membrane
Covalent alterations of receptor
   Phosphorylation
   Fatty acid acylation
Alterations in receptor–G protein coupling
Changes in G protein quantity and/or functionality
? Alterations in G protein–effector interaction
? Alterations in effector unit quantity or functionality

Second is sequestration of the receptor away from its normal cell-surface membrane domain to a less accessible compartment. Finally, there is downregulation, wherein there is an absolute decrease in the total cellular receptor population. Agonist-specific or homologous desensitization is usually defined as a decrease in adenylyl cyclase responsiveness to a single agonist after chronic exposure to that agonist. In contrast, heterologous desensitization occurs when the responsiveness of a number of receptor-mediated agonists or nonreceptor activators of adenylyl cyclase, such as guanine nucleotides or sodium fluoride, are decreased after an exposure to a single agonist.[39,55] These two processes may not be mutually exclusive, however, and heterologous desensitization may occur in addition to homologous desensitization, particularly if agonist exposure is prolonged.[39,55] Recent evidence links the phosphorylation of the receptor with the rapid uncoupling of the receptor from the effector units.

A major step forward in elucidating potential mechanisms involved in homologous desensitization was the discovery and characterization of a new receptor-specific kinase by Benovic et al.[56] This kinase has been called the β-adrenergic receptor kinase (βARK), although it is now known that it can phosphorylate other integral membrane receptors. This kinase is different and distinct from other kinases, such as the cAMP-dependent protein kinase or protein kinase C. This kinase is now known to be a member of a family of kinases known as G protein–receptor kinases (GRK)s.[57] At least six different kinases have thus far been identified and characterized.[57] The original βARK, which was βARK I, is now known as GRK2. The structure and functions of this family of kinases have recently been reviewed.[57] The most interesting property of the GRKs is that they preferentially phosphorylate the agonist-occupied receptor rather than an antagonist-occupied or unoccupied receptor. This preferential phosphorylation raises the prospect that in vivo phosphorylation of the agonist-occupied receptor may play a direct role in the desensitization process. There is compelling evidence that this may be the case. First, the phosphorylated receptor under the appropriate in vitro conditions displays an 80 percent decrease in its ability to interact with G_s (uncoupled). Second, the time course for phosphorylation of the βAR in intact cells parallels the time course of desensitization. Third, GRKs display wide tissue distribution. Finally, the sequestration of phosphorylated receptors into the cell is subsequently associated with their dephosphorylation and recycling back to the cell membrane.

Homologous desensitization is not thought to be a cAMP-mediated event, i.e., elevated concentrations of cAMP without receptor activation and consequent increased protein kinase A activity do not mimic catecholamine-induced desensitization. In contrast, heterologous desensitization may involve multiple pathways that include both receptor protein changes as well as alterations in the other components of the adenylyl cyclase system. This form of desensitization usually results from a prolonged exposure to agonists and proceeds at a slower rate than does homologous desensitization. In contrast, heterologous desensitization can be induced directly by increases in cAMP concentrations in some systems.[55] Thus, administration of stable analogues of cAMP to cells can totally mimic the phenomenon of catecholamine-induced desensitization in some model systems. This suggests that activation of protein kinase A may be a mediator of some forms of desensitization.

The mechanism(s) responsible for sequestration of the receptor is much less clear and may not involve phosphorylation. The sequestration does appear to be agonist-dependent and may involve a specific conformation of the receptor, which initiates the translocation process. Where this sequestered region is and how the receptor stays there are also unknown.

Downregulation, as mentioned above, refers to the state wherein there is an actual decrease in the total cellular pool of receptors associated with a decreased agonist responsiveness. This downregulation appears to be a much slower process than uncoupling and sequestration. There is at present an incomplete understanding of how downregulation occurs. When the quantity of any protein changes, there are always at least two possible mechanisms involved including altered synthesis, altered degradation, or both. In the case of G protein–coupled receptors, both possibilities appear to be implicated. Evidence has recently been put forth to suggest that there is enhanced proteolysis of the receptor during desensitization.[39] In addition, altered synthesis of new messenger RNA (mRNA) involving regulation of transcription likewise has been documented.[45] The cloning of the genes for G protein receptors has now permitted the evaluation of receptor regulation at the DNA/RNA levels.[51]

Several groups have now documented that prolonged exposure of cells to β-adrenergic agonists, cAMP analogues, or forskolin (a diterpine that activates adenylyl cyclase) all produce a downregulation of βARs, which is accompanied by a significant decrease in βAR mRNA levels.[51] The above agents increase cAMP and hence activate protein kinase A. A logical assumption, therefore, is that the protein kinase A activation must be involved in this pathway. The pathway leading to decreased transcription, however, is likely independent of the well-known cAMP-regulating motif (CRE) found in many promoter-enhancer regions of genes that act to increase transcription.[51] A mechanism for decreasing the quantity of mRNA is that of decreasing messenger stability and hence decreasing its half-life. A decreased half-life results in less time available for the mRNA to be translated. Evidence for just such a mechanism has now been described for the βAR. When a smooth muscle cell line was treated with agonist, the half-life of the βAR mRNA was significantly decreased. Although the mechanism responsible for the change in stability is not known, the 3'-untranslated region of the β_2AR mRNA contains sequences that have been found in other mRNAs that are short lived and highly regulated.[51]

Although agonist-induced receptor regulation has been highlighted here, for completeness the effect of endocrine modulation on receptor regulation should be briefly mentioned. Hormones, such as cortisol and thyroid hormone, have long been recognized to modulate receptor responsiveness.[31]

The glucocorticoids increase βAR number and ephinephrine responsiveness in many cells. In addition, cotreatment of cells with glucocorticoids and catecholamines leads to a diminished desensitization, compared to treatment with catecholamines alone.[51] This suggests that glucocorticoids might act by enhancing receptor synthesis or preventing downregulation. Recent studies have documented that glucocorticoids can directly increase the rate of β_2AR gene transcription and that a rapid elevation of mRNA precedes an increase in the number of βARs found at the cell surface.[51] Glucocorticoids are known to promote increases in gene transcription via a specific DNA motif in the 5′ enhancer/promoter region, which has been termed a *glucocorticoid response element* (GRE). This enhancer is a 15-bp element that binds a specific glucocorticoid/protein complex.[51] A similar GRE has been identified in the β_2AR gene and may explain the effect of glucocorticoid responsiveness of the βAR.[51]

G PROTEIN REGULATION

Not only are receptors capable of being regulated but so, too, are G proteins. This regulation of G proteins by G protein–coupled receptor activation remains enigmatic, compared to what is known concerning receptor regulation. The earliest pathophysiologic condition known to modulate G protein quantity was probably altered thyroid hormone levels.[31] The most common scenario is that hyperthyroidism is associated with an increased quantity of G_s, while hypothyroidism is associated with a decrease in G_s.[31] This is, however, not found in all cell types studied. Chronic activation of G protein receptors has been associated with modulation of G proteins.[53,54] An excellent example of this is the activation of the A_1 adenosine receptor in adipocytes. In an in vivo rat model, following long-term activation of the A_1 adenosine receptor by agonists, there is a decrease in the ability of adenosine to mediate inhibition of adenylyl cyclase. This desensitization occurs concomitantly with a sensitization to the effects of agonists that stimulate adenylyl cyclase.[53,54] These changes are associated with a decreased quantity of the G_i proteins and an increased quantity of the G_s proteins.[53,54] These changes occur with no alteration in the quantity of the mRNAs for these proteins.[54] The mechanisms involved remain speculative. The changes in the G proteins may well explain the phenotypic changes seen in the cellular responsiveness that is seen following desensitization in this system.[53,54] Similar changes in G proteins have now been described for a variety of receptor systems.[58]

RECEPTOR SIGNALING IN THE HEART

The heart has been the focus of a large number of studies relating pathophysiologic conditions to modification of G protein–coupled receptor-initiated transmembrane signaling. The reasons for this expansive body of work are intuitively obvious

given the dramatic impact of heart disease on human morbidity and mortality. As described above, much has been learned concerning how regulation of receptors comes about in model systems, but detailed understanding of receptor systems in the heart has lagged behind. There are several reasons for the disparity in knowledge. First, there were no continuous cell lines of myocardial cells. Second, the number of receptors in myocardial cells is typically much lower (by a factor of 10 to 100) than found in many other cells and tissues. Third, myocardial membranes are labile and sensitive to proteinases, which renders them unresponsive to agonist-mediated effector activation as assessed by in vitro studies. Even with these difficulties, many pathophysiologic conditions have been shown to modulate receptors, G proteins, and responsiveness of adenylyl cyclase systems.[59,60] If we have learned anything about these systems, it has been that regulation is complex and multifactorial. Simply to quantitate receptors or G proteins is not sufficient, and detailed studies of each of the components and their interactions must be undertaken if we are to have any hope of comprehending how a complex organ such as the heart is regulated. Even when much information is available, it is still not always clear whether the changes seen are cause or effect. An example of this is what occurs during congestive heart failure (CHF) in the human heart. Many studies have documented that a number of alterations occur in the adenylyl cyclase system of the heart in CHF.[59,60] These include a decreased cAMP responsiveness to catecholamines, decreases in βAR number, an uncoupling of βARs from G_s, and an increased quantity of the inhibitory G protein, G_i.

All of these changes could help explain the decreased contractile responsiveness to catecholamines in CHF. The finding that hearts from such patients and animals are less responsive to the inotropic effects of catecholamines and that βARs are decreased in number has lead to the development of new animal models for studying the processes involved and to attempts to create potential therapeutic strategies. The approach has been to use transgenic technology to create animals (usually mice) in which gene(s) that code for various components of the signaling pathway can be introduced in a mouse germ line to overexpress a normal or abnormal form of a receptor, G protein, or enzyme in a tissue-specific manner.

For example, when human β_2ARs are overexpressed in the hearts of a transgenic mouse line, a number of fascinating changes occur in mouse heart function.[61] First, the mice express 50 to 150 times the normal βAR density. Second, this is associated with resting tachycardia (450 versus 350 beats per minute) compared to control. Third, contractility is maximal even without stimulation by catecholamines. Finally, the mice appear to be healthy and have not developed congestive heart failure or had premature death. These types of approaches highlight the potential use of gene therapy, i.e., introduction of additional receptors into the heart as a means to enhance cardiac function in disease states.

Equally interesting was the creation of transgenic mice that express excess GRKs or dominant negative GRKs (which block the function of endogenous GRKs) to assess their effect on cardiac function. It was found that animals overexpressing GRK2 demonstrated an attenuated inotropic response to catecholamines similar to the response seen in CHF. Conversely, animals overexpressing a GRK2 inhibitor displayed enhanced cardiac contractility in vivo, both with and without catecholamines.[62] These new approaches should provide many new insights into the pathophysiology of cardiac diseases and even raise the specter of gene therapy.

SUMMARY

This chapter has highlighted some of the recent advances in the areas of cell membrane structure, ion channels, and G protein–coupled receptors. A major aim has been to illustrate that these topics are not in any way distinct or separate but rather are intimately related structurally, functionally, and in how they are regulated. As our knowledge of these membrane components is increased, we shall be able to understand cardiac pathophysiology better and hence develop rational therapeutic and preventive modalities to decrease the morbidity and mortality associated with heart disease.

REFERENCES

1. Alberts B, Bray D, Lewis J, Raff M, Roberts K, Watson JD, eds. *Molecular Biology of the Cell*, 3d ed. New York: Garland; 1994.
2. Vouce DE, Vouce JE, eds. *Biochemistry of Lipids and Membranes*. Menlo Park, CA: Benjamin/Cummings; 1985.
3. Benga G, Tager JM. *Biomembranes: Basic and Medical Research*. New York: Springer-Verlag; 1988.
4. Jain M, Wagner R. *Introduction to Biological Membranes*. New York: Wiley; 1980.
5. Lewis DL, Lechleiter JD, Kim D, Nanavati C, Clapham DE. Intracellular regulation of ion channels in cell membranes. *Mayo Clin Proc* 1990; 65:1127–1143.
6. Catterall WA. Structure and function of voltage-gated ion channels. *Annu Rev Biochem* 1995; 64:493–531.
7. Wickman K, Clapham DE. Ion channel regulation by G proteins. *Physiol Rev* 1995; 75:865–885.
8. Rehm H, Tempel BL. Voltage-gated K$^+$ channels of the mammalian brain. *FASEB J* 1991; 5:164–170.
9. Sather WA, Yang J, Tsien RW. Structural basis of ion channel permeation and selectivity. *Curr Opin Neurobiol* 1994; 4:313–323.
10. Brown AM, Birnbaumer L. Ionic channels and their regulation by G protein subunits. *Annu Rev Physiol* 1990; 52:197–213.
11. Numa S. A molecular view of neurotransmitter receptors and ionic channels. *Harvey Lect* 1989; 83:121–165.
12. Green WN, Millar NS. Ion-channel assembly. *Trends Neurosci* 1995; 18:280–287.
13. Birnbaumer L, Codina J, Yatani A, Mattera R, Graf R, Olate J, et al. Molecular basis of regulation of ionic channels by G proteins. *Recent Prog Horm Res* 1989; 45:121–208.
14. Belardinelli L, Linden J, Berne RM. The cardiac effects of adenosine. *Prog Cardiovasc Dis* 1989; 32:73–97.
15. Guy HR, Conti F. Pursuing the structure and function of voltage-gated channels. *Trends Neurosci* 1990; 13:201–206.
16. Montal M. Molecular anatomy and molecular design of channel proteins. *FASEB J* 1990; 4:2623–2635.
17. Agnew WS. A Rosetta stone for K channels. *Nature* 1988; 331:114–115.
18. Catterall WA. Excitation-contraction coupling in vertebrate skeletal muscle: A tale of two calcium channels. *Cell* 1991; 64:871–874.
19. Catterall WA. Structure and function of voltage-sensitive ion channels. *Science* 1988; 242:50–61.
20. Hille B. *Ionic Channels of Excitable Membranes*. Sunderland, MA: Sinauer; 1984.
21. Loughney K, Kreser R, Ganetzley B. Molecular analysis of the paralocus, a sodium channel in *Drosophila*. *Cell* 1989; 58:1143–1154.
22. Kayano T, Noda M, Flockerzi V, Takahashi H, Numa S. Primary structure of rat brain sodium channel III deduced from the cDNA sequence. *FEBS Lett* 1988; 228:187–194.
23. Noda M, Ikeda T, Suzaki H, Takeshima H, Takahashi T, Kuno M, et al. Expression of functional sodium channels from cloned cDNA. *Nature* 1986; 322:826–828.
24. Froehner SC. New insights into the molecular structure of the dihydropyridine-sensitive calcium channel. *Trends Neurosci* 1988; 11:90–92.
25. Roden DM, George AL Jr, Bennett PB. Recent advances in understanding the molecular mechanisms of the long QT syndrome. *J Cardiovasc Electrophysiol* 1995; 6:1023–1031.
26. Keating MT, Sanguinetti MC. Molecular genetic insights into cardiovascular disease. *Science* 1996; 272:681–685.
27. Schwartz PJ, Priori SG, Locati EH, Napolitano C, Cantú F, Towbin JA, et al. Long QT syndrome patients with mutations of the SCN5A and HERG genes have differential responses to Na$^+$ channel blockade and to increases in heart rate: Implications for gene-specific therapy. *Circulation* 1995; 92:3381–3386.
28. Sanguinetti MC, Jiang C, Curran ME, Keating MT. A mechanistic link between an inherited and an acquired cardiac arrhythmia: HERG encodes the I$_{Kr}$ potassium channel. *Cell* 1995; 81:299–307.
29. Wang Q, Curran ME, Splawski I, Burn TC, Millholland JM, VanRaay TJ, et al. Positional cloning of a novel potassium channel gene: KVLQT1 mutations cause cardiac arrhythmias. *Nat Genet* 1996; 12:17–23.
30. Curran ME, Splawski I, Timothy KW, Vincent GM, Green ED, Keating MT. A molecular basis for cardiac arrhythmia: HERG mutations cause long QT syndrome. *Cell* 1995; 80:795–803.
31. Barnes PJ. Beta-adrenergic receptors and their regulation. *Am J Respir Crit Care Med* 1995; 152:838–860.
32. Strade CD, Fong TM, Tota MR, Underwood D. Structure and function of G protein–coupled receptors. *Annu Rev Biochem* 1994; 63:101–132.
33. Caron MG. The guanine nucleotide regulatory protein-coupled receptors for nucleosides, nucleotides, amino acids and amine neurotransmitters. *Cell Biol* 1989; 1:159–166.
34. Carpenter G, Cohen S. Epidermal growth factor. *J Biol Chem* 1990; 265:7709–7712.
35. Brown MS, Goldstein JL. Lipoprotein receptors: Therapeutic implication. *J Hypertens Suppl* 1990; 8:533–535.
36. Dohlman HG, Caron MG, Lefkowitz RJ. A family of receptors coupled to guanine nucleotide regulatory proteins. *Biochemistry* 1987; 26:2657–2664.
37. Nathans J, Thomas D, Hogness DS. Molecular genetics of human color vision. The genes encoding blue, green, and red pigments. *Science* 1986; 232:193–202.
38. Henderson R, Unwin PNT. Three-dimensional model of purple membrane obtained by electron microscopy. *Nature* 1975; 257:28–32.
39. Raymond JR, Hnatowich M, Lefkowitz RJ, Caron MG. Adrenergic receptors: Models for regulation of signal transduction processes. *Hypertension* 1990; 15:119–131.
40. Dohlman HG, Caron MG, DeBlasi A, Frielle T, Lefkowitz RJ. A role of extracellular disulfide bonded cysteines in the ligand binding function of the β$_2$-adrenergic receptor. *Biochemistry* 1990; 29:2335–2342.
41. Lefkowitz RJ, Caron MG. Adrenergic receptors: Models for receptors coupled to guanine nucleotide regulatory proteins. *J Biol Chem* 1988; 263:4993–4996.
42. Strader CD, Sigal IS, Dixon RAF. Structural basis of β-adrenergic receptor function. *FASEB J* 1989; 3:1825–1832.
43. Hibert MF, Trumpp-Kallmeyer S, Bruinvels A, Hoflack J. Three-dimensional models of neurotransmitter G-binding protein-coupled receptors. *Mol Pharmacol* 1991; 40:8–15.
44. Gilman AG. G proteins: Transducers of receptor-generated signals. *Annu Rev Biochem* 1987; 56:615–649.
45. Nürnberg B, Gudermann T, Schultz G. Receptors and G proteins as primary components of transmembrane signal transduction. Part 2. G proteins: Structure and function. *J Mol Med* 1995; 73:123–132.
46. Birnbaumer L. Transduction of receptor signal into modulation of effector activity by G proteins: The first 20 years or so.... *FASEB J* 1990; 4:3068–3078.
47. Robison GA, Butcher RW, Sutherland EW. Adenyl cyclase as an adrenergic receptor. *Ann NY Acad Sci* 1967; 139:703–723.
48. Ahlquist RP. A study of the adrenotropic receptors. *Am J Physiol* 1948; 153:585–600.

49. Stiles GL. Adenosine receptors and beyond: Molecular mechanisms of physiological regulation. *Clin Res* 1990; 38:10–18.

50. Sibley DR, Benovic JL, Caron MG, Lefkowitz RJ. Regulation of transmembrane signaling by receptor phosphorylation. *Cell* 1987; 48:913–922.

51. Collins S, Caron MG, Lefkowitz RJ. Regulation of adrenergic receptor responsiveness through modulation of receptor gene expression. *Annu Rev Physiol* 1991; 53:497–508.

52. Ramkumar V, Bumgarner JR, Jacobson KA, Stiles GL. Multiple components of the A_1 adenosine receptor–adenylate cyclase system are regulated in rat cerebral cortex by chronic caffeine ingestion. *J Clin Invest* 1988; 82:242–247.

53. Parsons WJ, Stiles GL. Heterologous desensitization of the inhibitory A_1 adenosine receptor–adenylate cyclase system in rat adipocytes: Regulation of both N_s and N_i. *J Biol Chem* 1987; 262:841–847.

54. Longabaugh JP, Didsbury J, Spiegel A, Stiles GL. Modification of the rat adipocyte A_1 adenosine receptor–adenylate cyclase system during chronic exposure to an A_1 adenosine receptor agonist: Alterations in the quantity of $G_{s\alpha}$ and $G_{i\alpha}$ are not associated with changes in their mRNAs. *Mol Pharmacol* 1989; 36:681–688.

55. Hausdorff WP, Caron MG, Lefkowitz RJ. Turning off the signal: Desensitization of β-adrenergic receptor function. *FASEB J* 1990; 4:2881–2889.

56. Benovic JL, DeBlasi A, Stone WC, Caron MG, Lefkowitz RJ. β-Adrenergic receptor kinase: Primary structure delineates a multigene family. *Science* 1989; 246:235–240.

57. Premont RT, Inglese J, Lefkowitz RJ. Protein kinases that phosphorylate activated G protein–coupled receptors. *FASEB J* 1995; 9:175–182.

58. Rich KA, Codina J, Floyd G, Sekura R, Hildebrandt JD, Iyengar R. Glucagon-induced heterologous desensitization of the MDCK cell adenylyl cyclase: Increases in the apparent levels of the inhibitory regulator (N_i). *J Biol Chem* 1984; 259:7893–7901.

59. Stiles GL, Lefkowitz RJ. Cardiac adrenergic receptors. *Annu Rev Med* 1984; 35:149–164.

60. Stiles GL. Adrenergic receptor responsiveness and congestive heart failure. *Am J Cardiol* 1991; 67:13C–17C.

61. Milano CA, Allen LF, Rockman HA, Dolber PC, McMinn TR, Chien KR, et al. Enhanced myocardial function in transgenic mice overexpressing the β2-adrenergic receptor. *Science* 1994; 264:582–586.

62. Koch WJ, Rockman HA, Samama P, Hamilton R, Bond RA, Milano CA, et al. Cardiac function in mice overexpressing the β-adrenergic receptor kinase or a βARK inhibitor. *Science* 1995; 268:1350–1353.

6

GROWTH AND HYPERTROPHY OF THE HEART AND BLOOD VESSELS

Richard A. Walsh / Gerald W. Dorn II

Growth of the heart and blood vessels is a dynamic process that occurs during embryogenesis, postnatal development, maturity, and senescence and in response to changing environmental and pathologic conditions. Cardiovascular growth occurs at the cellular level as a consequence of the interplay between *hyperplasia* (increase in cell number) and *hypertrophy* (increase in cell size) or a combination of both processes. The relative importance of each of these two mechanisms depends upon the cell type, developmental stage, and the nature of the growth stimulus. These two forms of cell growth are variably modulated by *apoptosis*, or programmed cell death.[1,2] This phenomenon is of importance in the determination of heart shape during cardiogenesis and may contribute to altered cardiac chamber and vascular geometry in response to pathologic stimuli. Physiologic and pathologic cardiovascular growth are generally mediated by developmental programs, mechanical deformation, and injury in various combinations. Physical forces stimulate a repertoire of biochemical signals that alter the cardiovascular phenotype. The application of molecular and cell biology (see Chap. 7) to this problem is rapidly defining the precise factors responsible for mechanotransduction-induced growth in the cardiovascular system.

CARDIAC GROWTH AND HYPERTROPHY

Cardiac hypertrophy is a process wherein there is an increase in chamber mass produced largely by an increase in the size of terminally differentiated cardiomyocytes. Although cardiomyocytes comprise only one-third of the total cell number, they are responsible in aggregate for over 70 percent of cardiac volume. Cardiac hypertrophy may be reasonably categorized as either physiologic or pathologic (Fig. 6-1).

Physiologic Hypertrophy

Physiologic hypertrophy includes cardiogenesis during embryonic development, postnatal cardiac growth, a modest additional increase in heart size that evolves during senescence, and the increase in heart size that occurs during physical conditioning in athletes. The earliest stage of cardiac growth *in utero* depends on a genetically determined developmental program since it can occur in the absence of contractile activity. Subsequently, mechanical forces become increasingly important in the development of the normal cardiac phenotype. Throughout the embryonic period and for a few weeks after birth, cardiac growth occurs as a consequence of hyperplasia and hypertrophy of myocytes. Classically, adult myocytes have been described as terminally differentiated, that is, incapable of reentering the cell cycle (see Chap. 7). This issue is currently undergoing reexamination. It is critical to make a distinction between DNA synthesis and cell division. In the adult cardiomyocyte, DNA synthesis may clearly result in either multinucleation or polyploidy (an increase in the DNA content of a single nucleus). By contrast, there is little evidence that cardiomyocytes are capable of division under normal conditions after the early postnatal period.[3,4] The capacity to reactivate hyperplasia in the terminally differentiated cardiomyocyte is an area of intense research interest, with potentially important therapeutic implications in the hypertrophied and failing heart.[5]

From birth to maturation the mammalian heart undergoes a sixfold increase in mass. The normal heart/body weight ratio is species-specific. The largest hearts relative to body size occur in animals with survival requirements that depend on sustained exercise rather than on burst activity.[6] In humans, intense, prolonged exercise training can produce an increase in cardiac mass. Isotonic exercise such as running produces *eccentric hypertrophy*, characterized by a normal ratio of wall thickness to dimension, whereas isometric exercise such as weight lifting stimulates *concentric hypertrophy*, associated with an increased ratio of wall thickness to dimension.[7] Senescent animals and humans free of organic heart disease develop mild concentric left ventricular hypertrophy as a consequence of age-related decreases in the distensibility of the peripheral vasculature.[8] The molecular biochemical and physiologic changes associated with physiologic hypertrophy differ both qualitatively and quantitatively from those that occur during pathologic hypertrophy.

Pathologic Hypertrophy

Pathologic hypertrophy is an important adaptive response to abnormal global or regional increases in cardiac work. Initially, the increase in cardiac mass serves to normalize wall stress and permit normal cardiovascular function at rest and during exercise in *compensated hypertrophy*. If the stimulus for pathologic hypertrophy is sufficiently intense or prolonged, *decompensated hypertrophy* and heart failure ensue. Pathologic hypertrophy may be caused by pressure overloading such as systemic or pulmonary arterial hypertension, left ventricular outflow obstruction, or aortic coarctation. Pressure overloading produces an increase in systolic wall stress and results in concentric ventricular hypertrophy. Volume overloading, such as occurs in mitral or aortic regurgitation or as a result of arteriovenous fistulae, also produces pathologic hypertrophy. These conditions induce an increase in either diastolic wall stress (mitral regurgitation) or both systolic and diastolic wall stress (aortic regurgitation and arteriovenous fistulae) and result in eccentric left ventricular hypertrophy. Regional hypertrophy that occurs in viable myocardium adjacent to and remote from an area of infarction has the characteristics of eccentric hypertrophy. An exception to the principle that pathologic hypertrophy occurs as a result of excessive increases in external work is hypertrophic cardiomyopathy. In the familial autosomal dominant form, point mutations of the sarcomeric proteins, in particular the β-myosin heavy chain, produce massive asymmetric or concentric hypertrophy in the absence of augmented peripheral hemodynamic requirements[9,10] (see also Chaps. 69 and 74). It is possible that the massive myofibrillar disarray that characterizes this genetic form of hypertrophy increases internal cardiac work, which in turn increases cardiac mass.

Mechanisms for the Development of Cardiac Hypertrophy

STIMULI AND SIGNAL TRANSDUCTION PATHWAYS

Dynamic or static stretch of neonatal or adult cardiomyocytes, papillary muscle, isolated heart, or intact hearts appears to be necessary and sufficient to produce increased cardiac protein synthesis and resultant hypertrophy.[11] The process by which stimuli in the physical domain activate intracellular growth-signaling pathways is known as *mechanotransduction*.[12] There is evidence that this process may be accomplished in the cardiomyocyte by stretch-activated sarcolemmal ion channels, G protein–coupled receptors, Na^+/H^+ antiporters, tyrosine kinase–containing receptors, and/or an extracellular matrix–integrin linked pathway. These cell-surface mechanotransducers then activate cytosolic signal transduction pathways that initiate gene transcription and translation of increased quantities of protein (Fig. 6-2). Important signal transduction pathways that are clearly activated by mechanical deformation include protein kinase C (PKC) and cyclic adenosine monophosphate (cAMP)-dependent protein kinase.[13] In particular, stretch of neonatal cultured cardiomyocytes produces G protein–mediated activation of membrane-bound phospholipase C, which in turn hydrolyzes phosphatidylinositol bisphosphate (PIP_2) to inositol trisphosphate (IP_3) and diacylglycerol (DAG). Diacylglycerol then activates PKC.[14,15] Phosphorylation of downstream cytosolic and nuclear proteins by PKC is known to be of critical importance for growth in a number of cell types, while inositol triphosphate is an important modulator of cytosolic calcium homeostasis by the interaction with its receptor on the sarcoplasmic reticulum. Angiotensin II receptor coupling appears to play a critical role in the activation of phospholipase C[16,17]; however, α_1-adrenergic and endothelin receptor stimulation can also activate this pathway, with resultant

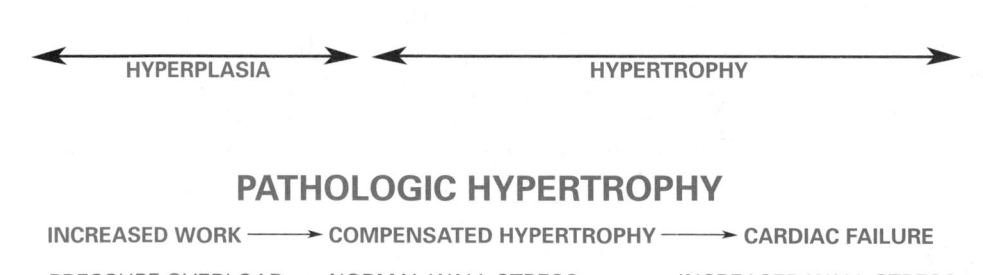

PHYSIOLOGIC HYPERTROPHY
(DEVELOPMENT, CONSTITUTIVE, EXERCISE)

CARDIOGENESIS ⟶ POSTNATAL GROWTH ⟶ MATURITY ⟶ SENESCENCE

⟵————— HYPERPLASIA —————⟶ ⟵————————— HYPERTROPHY —————————⟶

PATHOLOGIC HYPERTROPHY

INCREASED WORK ⟶ COMPENSATED HYPERTROPHY ⟶ CARDIAC FAILURE

PRESSURE OVERLOAD / NORMAL WALL STRESS / INCREASED WALL STRESS
VOLUME OVERLOAD / NL OR ABNL LV FUNCTION / ABNL LV FUNCTION
BOTH OR OTHER / NORMAL MYOCYTE FUNCTION / ABNL MYOCYTE FUNCTION

⟵————————————— HYPERTROPHY —————————————⟶

⟵——— ?HYPERPLASIA ———⟶
?APOPTOSIS

FIGURE 6-1

Relative roles of cardiomyocyte hypertrophy hyperplasia and apoptosis in physiologic and pathologic cardiac hypertrophy, along with the functional differences between compensated hypertrophy and heart failure.

hypertrophy in the neonatal cardiomyocyte.[18,19] In transgenic mice, α_1 receptor overexpression produces increased heart weight.[20] In addition to mechanotransduction by G protein–coupled receptor agonists, there is evidence that stimulation of tyrosine-kinase receptors can elicit a hyperplastic or hypertrophic response in neonatal cardiomyocytes.[21] Both acidic and basic fibroblast growth factors (FGF), which act as ligands for tyrosine-kinase receptors, can induce myocyte growth.[22] Acidic FGF produces a hyperplastic response, whereas basic FGF stimulates an increase in protein synthesis with resultant hypertrophy.[23] In contrast to its role in vascular smooth muscle growth, transforming growth factor β (TGFβ) does not induce a growth response under these conditions.[24] Whether or not and to what extent various G protein–coupled and tyrosine kinase–coupled receptor ligands can induce hypertrophy in the terminally differentiated adult cardiomyocyte is unclear at this time. The role of mechanotransduction-stimulated activation of cAMP-dependent protein kinases in the heart is more controversial, although overexpression of β_2-adrenergic receptor was reported in one study to produce cardiomyocyte hypertrophy in transgenic mice.[25]

Current information suggests that mechanotransduction and a number of interrelated autocrine, paracrine, and endocrine effects of hormones and growth factors mediate cardiac hypertrophy (Fig. 6-2). The resultant activation of multiple signal transduction pathways, which have demonstrable cross talk and considerable redundancy, provides a powerful mechanism by which the heart can respond to changing chronic hemodynamic requirements. A point of downstream convergence of multiple signal transduction pathways in the heart and noncardiac systems appears to be the phosphorylation of *m*itogen-*a*ctivated *p*rotein *k*inase [MAPK, also known as *e*xtracellular *s*ignal *r*egulated *k*inase (ERK)]. Mammalian MAPKs are serine-threonine protein kinases that are activated by signal transduction pathways coupled to both phosphatidylinositol hydrolysis/

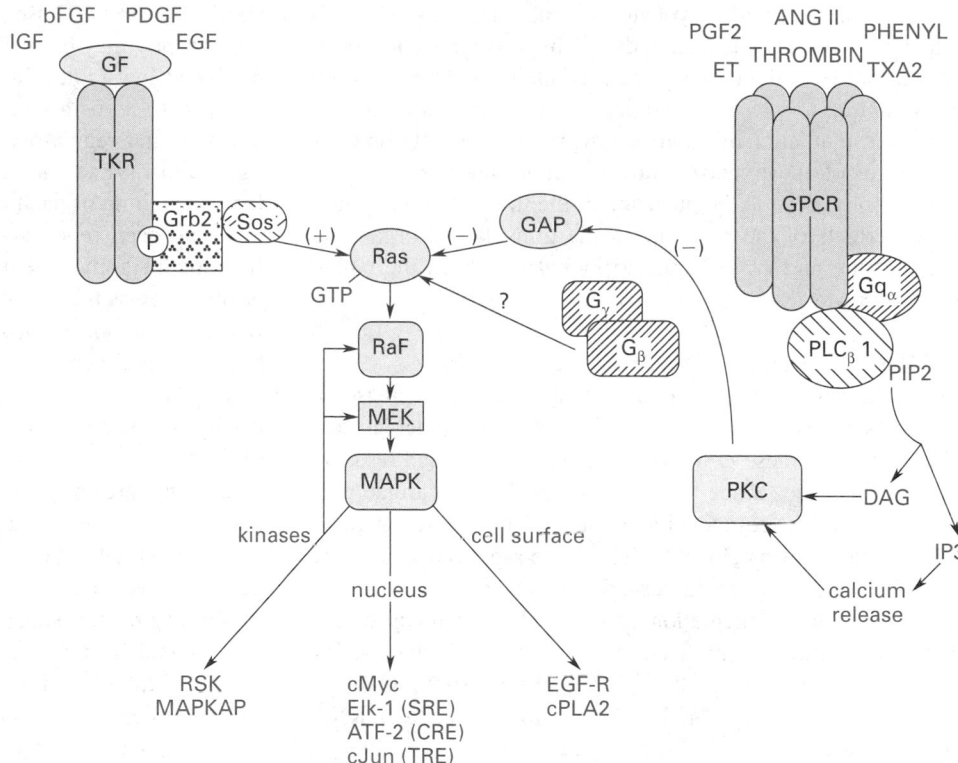

FIGURE 6-2

Simplified model for growth factor (GF) and G protein–coupled receptor (GPCR) stimulation of myocardial and vascular signal transduction pathways that stimulate mitogen-activated protein kinase (MAPK). Insulin-like growth factor (IGF), basic fibroblast growth factor (bFGF), platelet-derived growth factor (PDGF), or epidermal growth factor (EGF) interacts with its membrane tyrosine-kinase receptors (TKR), which, by autotyrosine phosphorylation (P), activate Ras by the facilitator proteins growth factor receptor–bound protein (Grb2) and sone of sevenless (SOS).

In contrast, angiotensin II (Ang II), prostaglandin $F_2\alpha$ (PGF$_2$), endothelin (ET), thrombin, thromboxane A$_2$ (TXA2), or phenylephrine (Phenyl) binding to their GPCR activates phospholipase C$_\beta$1 (PLC$_\beta$1) via the dissociated α subunit of a GTP-binding protein of the Gq class (Gqα). PLC$_\beta$1 catalyzes the hydrolysis of phosphatidylinositol biphosphate (PIP2) into diacylglycerol (DAG), which activates protein kinase C (PKC), and inositol triphosphate (IP$_3$), which stimulates the release of calcium from intracellular stores. PKC activated by calcium and DAG phosphorylates and inactivates Ras-associated GTPase-activating protein (GAP), thereby disinhibiting Ras. Ras may also be activated by dissociated β and γ subunits of Gq heterotrimers (Gβ and Gγ). Activated GTP-bound Ras initiates a cascade of phosphorylation events that in turn activate Raf, MAPK/ERK-activating kinase (MEK), and MAPK. Activated MAPK has numerous targets including Raf and MEK, thus forming a positive-feedback signal in the tyrosine-kinase and protein kinase C cascades; the kinases ribosomal S-6 kinase (RSK) and MAPK-activated protein (MAPKAP); nuclear factors such as c-*myc*; Elk-1, which binds to the serum response element (SRE); ATF-2, which binds to the cAMP response element (CRE); and c-*jun*, which binds to the 12-0-tetradecanoyl-phorbol-13-acetate response element (TRE). MAPK also targets cell-surface proteins such as EGF receptors (EGF-R) and cytosolic phospholipase A$_2$ (cPLA$_2$). The ultimate consequence of MAPK activation is transcriptional and translational regulation.

PKC activation and receptor protein tyrosine kinases (Fig. 6-2). Of particular importance to cardiac hypertrophy is the observation that important transcription factors (c-*jun*, c-*myc*, p62^{TCF}) are known substrates of MAPK. Recently, transfection of an antisense nucleotide to MAPK was shown to prevent hypertrophy in cardiomyocytes.[26]

Thyroid hormone is generally considered an endocrine mediator of cardiac hypertrophy. Administration of excess thyroid hormone to small and large experimental animals produces increased heart weight that is associated with transcriptionally mediated alterations in the myosin heavy chains (MHC), calcium-cycling proteins, and other functional constituents of the cardiomyocyte in small animals and primates.[27] Thyroid hormone–induced hypertrophy appears to be an indirect effect of the T_3-mediated increased oxygen consumption and resultant augmented cardiac work. Heterotopic transplantation of a nonworking rat heart into the abdominal aorta of the hyperthyroid animal is unassociated with hypertrophy, despite the presence of the transcriptionally mediated effects of the hormone in the transplanted organ and hypertrophy and typical transcriptional events in the native working heart.[28,29]

PROTEIN CONTENT AND ISOFORM DIVERSITY

The hallmark of cardiac hypertrophy is a net increase in protein synthesis above protein degradation. Under normal circumstances, these two processes are matched and result in nitrogen balance. Since the average half-life of cardiac proteins is 5 days, the composition of the adult heart is regenerated approximately every 3 weeks. The more rapid rate of cardiac growth in response to increased hemodynamic load could result from an augmentation in either the efficiency or the capacity of protein synthesis or a combination of the two.[30,31] Efficiency of protein synthesis is usually measured as moles of amino acid incorporated per milligram of cellular RNA per hour; capacity is assessed by determining the number of milligrams of RNA per gram of tissue. Experiments in a variety of systems indicate that the critical determinant for cardiac hypertrophy is an increased capacity for protein synthesis, which is mediated by augmented ribosomal content. Protein degradation appears to be modestly increased in cardiac hypertrophy and may play a critical role in the variably altered geometry of the ventricles in response to pressure or volume overloading, hypertrophy, regression, and atrophy.[32,33] The mechanisms for protein degradation in the heart involve the activation of both lysosomal and cytosolic proteases. Posttranslational processes are increasingly being recognized as important factors in the production of the cardiac phenotype in cardiac hypertrophy and failure.[27,34]

In addition to increased total protein content, cardiac hypertrophy is characterized by alterations in the relative abundance and isoform composition of the cardiomyocyte contractile, regulatory, and calcium-cycling proteins and other subcellular constituents. These processes provide an additional degree of plasticity for the heart to adapt to changing functional requirements. It is clear that there is considerable species specificity in the capacity for isoform switching. In small mammals with rapid heart rates, imposition of a pressure overload produces a transcriptionally mediated shift from the α- to the β-MHC and from cardiac to skeletal α-actin.[35–37] α-Myosin has a three- to sevenfold greater ATPase activity than β-myosin. The greater abundance of β-MHC in response to pressure overload in small animals increases the efficiency of force development by producing the same absolute muscle tension at a slower rate.[38] Despite identical cardiac muscle mechanics in response to hypertrophy, large animals with slower heart rates and humans possess β-MHC almost exclusively throughout embryogenesis and postnatal development.[39] It is possible that, in higher mammalian species, al-

tered myosin ATPase in response to pressure overload hypertrophy may be mediated in part by a posttranslationally produced low-molecular-weight variant of the β-MHC.[34] In addition to myosin and actin, cardiac isoforms exist for the essential and regulatory light chains, troponin (I, C, and T), tropomyosin, and the sarcolemmal Na^+, K^+-ATPase. Isoform switching of each of the components of the cardiomyocyte has been reported in hypertrophy and failure, but the functional significance has been unclear. The ability to ablate or overexpress these isoforms in genetically engineered mice will unambiguously determine their role in the normal and hypertrophied heart.

In addition to altered isoform composition, cardiac hypertrophy is associated with changes in the relative abundance of the various structural and functional proteins. All forms of cardiac hypertrophy are associated with increased collagen deposition in the extracellular matrix, which contributes to the observed alterations in passive chamber or muscle properties.[40–42] Pressure overload, but not volume overload, hypertrophy has been associated with changes in the levels of the cytoskeletal proteins titin, desmin, and tubulin.[43] Depolymerization of tubulin with colchicine reversed abnormalities in cardiac function in feline right ventricular hypertrophy[44] but not in guinea pig left ventricular hypertrophy.[43]

Calcium cycling in the heart is accomplished by voltage-dependent entry of calcium through the dihydropyridine-sensitive l-channel (Fig. 6-3). Calcium interacts with the ryanidine receptor on the surface of the sarcoplasmic reticulum, further augmenting cytosolic calcium concentration.[45] After binding to troponin C to trigger actin-myosin cross-bridge formation and cycling, calcium is resequestered into the sarcoplasmic reticulum by an ATPase the action of which is inhibited by the phosphoprotein phospholamban. Phosphorylation of phospholamban by CAMP-dependent protein kinases and calcium calmodulin–dependent kinases relieves the inhibition and results in improved contraction and relaxation. Decompensated pressure overload hypertrophy is associated with decreases in the sarcoplasmic reticulum ATPase and variable alterations in phospholamban.[45] Isolated changes in the stoichiometry between the sarcoplasmic reticulum ATPase and its inhibitor, phospholamban, have been demonstrated to have functional signficance in genetically engineered mice. Targeted ablation of phospholamban enhanced cardiac inotropic and lusitropic function,[46] whereas cardiac-specific overexpression produced the opposite result.[47] These findings strongly implicate changes in the relative abundance of the calcium-cycling proteins in the altered cardiac function observed in the hypertrophied and failing heart. The *cis* and *trans* acting factors, which are responsible for alterations in the calcium-cycling proteins in hypertrophy and failure, are poorly understood.

CARDIAC FUNCTION OF THE HYPERTROPHIED HEART

The phenotypic consequences of the increased cardiac mass and altered protein abundance and composition of the hypertrophied heart are considerable and depend upon the model utilized; animal species; and the nature, intensity, and duration of the hypertrophic stimulus. Taken together, available clinical and animal studies suggest that functional alterations evolve along a continuum from normal chamber and myocyte function to abnormal chamber and normal myocyte function to abnormalities of both chamber and myocyte function (Fig. 6-1).

Electrical Properties

The most typical electrical abnormality of the hypertrophied heart is prolongation of the duration of the action potential.[48] Recent studies using single-cell voltage clamp technique have begun to elucidate the ionic mechanisms responsible for this phenomenon. In mild hypertrophy, increases in calcium and calcium-activated currents (including the Na^+/Ca^{2+} exchanger) appear to be important.

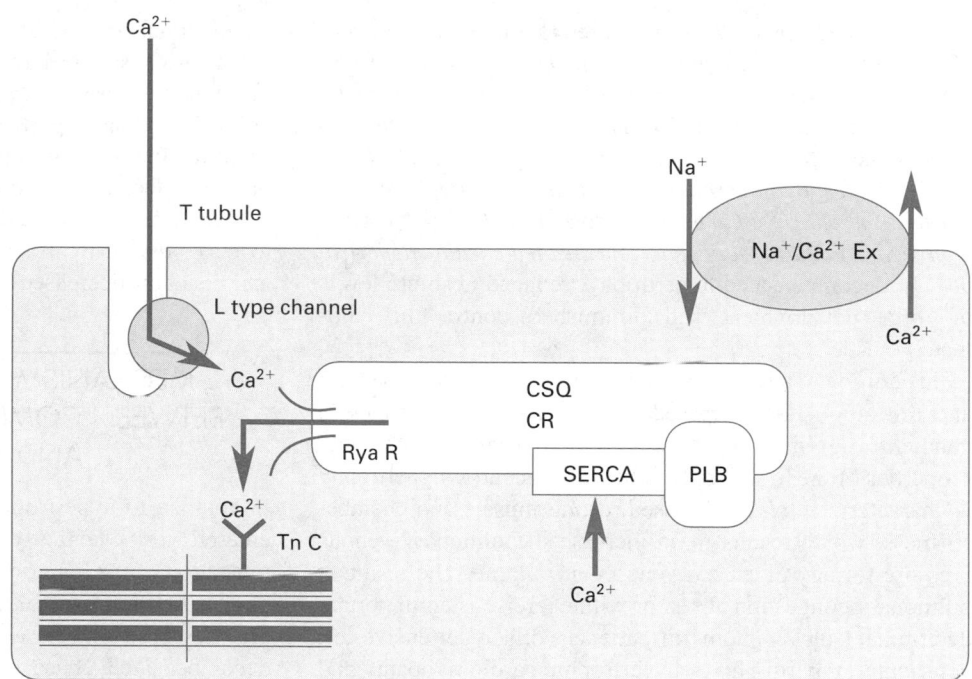

FIGURE 6-3

Schematic diagram of a cardiomyocyte that demonstrates excitation-contraction relaxation coupling by calcium. Calcium (Ca^{2+}) enters the cytosol via the voltage sensitive *l* channel. Ca^{2+} then interacts with the ryanodine receptor (RYAR), which triggers augmented calcium release from the sarcoplasmic reticulum (SR). Calcium is transiently bound to troponin C (TNC), which activates actin myosin cross-bridge development and shortening. Calcium is then released and resequestered in the SR by an ATPase (SERCA), which is inhibited by phospholamban (PLB) in its dephosphorylated state. Calsequestrin (CSQ) and calreticulum (CR) are calcium-binding storage proteins in the luminal SR.

In severe hypertrophy and failure, calcium current density is reduced, inward rectifier current density is reduced, and transient outward current density is also diminished. In severe hypertrophy, prolongation of the action potential is also determined importantly by a reduction in the potassium currents I_{K1} and I_{to}. The relations between these changes in membrane current properties of hypertrophied hearts and altered mechanical behavior at the myocyte and whole-heart level are not clearly understood at present.

Hypertrophied myocardium is more likely to precipitate arrhythmias than normal tissue. The mechanisms for arrhythmogenesis are multifactorial and are operant at the tissue and cardiomyocyte levels. Increased dispersion of refractoriness and slowed conduction results from myocyte loss and fibrosis. Prolongation of the duration of the action potential increases the likelihood of early after-depolarizations, which may result in triggered arrhythmias. Reduced coronary artery flow reserve and accelerated atherosclerosis of epicardial coronary vessels predispose toward ischemia-induced arrhythmias.[49] In concert, these mechanisms contribute to the fact that cardiac hypertrophy was the most powerful predictor of cardiovascular mortality in the Framingham Study (see Chap. 1).

Mechanical Properties

Mechanical function of the hypertrophied heart has been studied at the isolated myocyte, muscle, and chamber levels and in the intact circulation.[50-52] The results of these studies have revealed variable alterations in rate and extent of contraction and relaxation, in the amount of force development, and in resting muscle and chamber properties. In the intact circulation, altered systolic and diastolic function is a composite result of subcellular changes in the myocyte, changes in the extracellular matrix, altered chamber geometry and mass, altered ventricular-vascular coupling, and the modulatory effects of neural and hormonal influences.

The earliest changes in mechanical performance observed in isometrically contracting papillary muscles extracted from hypertrophied hearts consist of a prolongation of time to peak tension and relaxation, despite normal peak twitch tension normalized for cross-sectional area of the muscle.[53] Afterloaded isotonically shortening papillary muscle preparations from hypertrophied hearts of a variety of animal species typically reveal a decrease in the force-velocity relationship and a depression of V_{max} (the extrapolated maximal unloaded shortening velocity).[54] V_{max} has been directly related to the calcium-activated myosin ATPase activity. Both myosin and myofibrillar ATPase activity are typically depressed in hypertrophied myocardium. In small rodents, this is due to the transcriptionally mediated switch from α- to β-MHC. In higher mammals and humans, the decreased myosin ATPase activity of the hypertrophied heart may be due to alterations in the troponin isoform composition[55] or the posttranslational generation of a lower molecular variant of the β-MHC, as noted above.[34]

The dissociation between depressed rate-dependent indices of contraction and relaxation and normal maximal force development and extent of shortening in early cardiac hypertrophy has also been demonstrated in isolated cardiomyocytes and in the intact circulation of the nonhuman primate.[50,52] *These results suggest that the rate of cross-bridge cycling is reduced but that the effective number of active cross-bridges per unit of myocardium is preserved in compensated cardiac hypertrophy.* In decompensated hypertrophy, reduced absolute levels of force development and diminished contractility ultimately ensue.

In addition to alterations in excitation-contraction coupling and relaxation, the increased cardiac mass and changes in geometry significantly affect passive muscle and chamber properties of the hypertrophied heart. Concentric hypertrophy is characterized by an increased resting muscle and chamber stiffness, which results in an increase in pulmonary venous pressure for any given left ventricular volume. The resultant pulmonary congestion at rest or with exercise is an important determinant of symptoms in patients with hypertensive left ventricular hypertrophy or hypertrophic cardiomyopathy and normal or elevated ejection fraction. Pure volume overload hypertrophy, as occurs with mitral regurgitation, is typically associated with no change or a decrease in passive muscle or chamber stiffness. As a result, patients with chronic volume overload may remain asymptomatic for long periods despite appreciable increases in regurgitant fraction (see also Chap. 21).

Coronary Circulation

Clinicians have long recognized that myocardial blood flow may be abnormal in the hypertrophied heart since such patients may have exertional angina, resting or exercise-induced electrocardiographic or perfusion abnormalities, or pathologic evidence of subendocardial fibrosis, despite the presence of angiographically normal epicardial coronary arteries.

Morphologic studies of hypertrophied hearts from experimental animals and patients with pressure overload hypertrophy demonstrate that the ratio of capillaries to myocytes remains unchanged.[56] Since myocyte cross-sectional area increases, there is a resultant increase in nutrient diffusion distance in the hypertrophied heart. This anatomic change results in a reduced vasodilatory reserve in response to various stimuli in experimental and clinical studies.[57] Myocardial blood flow and oxygen consumption per unit myocardium are normal in compensated pressure overload–left ventricular hypertrophy, where wall stress has been normalized by an increase in wall thickness. The impairment in vasodilatory reserve produces evidence of ischemia during increased myocardial oxygen demand. In right ventricular pressure overload hypertrophy, differences in perfusion between the ventricles result in increased right ventricular blood flow per unit myocardial mass at rest and no increase in minimum coronary resistance of hypertrophied right ventricular myocardium.[58]

Fewer data are available regarding changes in the coronary circulation in experimental or clinical volume overload hypertrophy. Most studies have reported normal resting flow values per unit myocardial mass. In contrast to pressure overload, volume overload hypertrophy has been associated with normal or mildly increased minimum coronary resistance and normal or mildly decreased coronary reserve.[59] The coronary circulatory abnormalities associated with cardiac hypertrophy appear to be reversible with removal of the hypertrophic stimulus and resultant decreased chamber mass.[60]

MECHANISMS FOR THE TRANSITION BETWEEN COMPENSATED HYPERTROPHY AND HEART FAILURE

In contrast to hypertrophied skeletal muscle, chronically increased work eventually results in depressed contractility and relaxation of the hypertrophied heart. Compensated hypertrophy, which is characterized by abnormal chamber function but preserved muscle and myocyte function, evolves into a decompensated phase characterized by abnormal chamber, muscle, and myocyte function (Fig. 6-1). Attempts to elucidate the underlying mechanisms for this transition have involved multidisciplinary studies of clinical end-stage heart failure, longitudinal studies in experimental animals, and characterization of cardiovascular function in genetically engineered mice where attempts are made to mimic human disease[61] (Fig. 6-4).

Current information suggests that decompensated hypertrophy may result from a number of mechanisms that are both intrinsic and extrinsic to the cardiomyocyte. These include necrosis; apoptosis[62,63]; inadequate growth secondary to altered signal transduction pathways; alterations in cardiomyocyte contractile, regulatory, calcium-cycling, and structural proteins; alterations in the extracellular matrix, and remodeling (Fig. 6-4). Because of the complex combinatorial alterations that occur in human heart failure and conventional animal models of hypertrophy, studies in genetically engineered mice in which a protein of interest is either overexpressed or ablated using homologous recombination hold particular promise in determining the relative importance of various candidate genes. For example, mice bearing the mutation in the β-MHC that occurs in familial cardiomyopathy have many features of the human disease.[64] Overexpression of the α subunit of the G protein that couples to the β-adrenergic receptor has produced dilated fibrotic hearts with altered cardiovascular function.[65] Overexpression or ablation of genes involved in cardiomyocyte calcium-cycling proteins has been associated with altered heart function and abnormal calcium kinetics. It is of interest that, with few exceptions,[66] the resultant cardiac phenotype has failed to reproduce completely human decompensated hypertrophy and failure. This observation further supports the multifactorial nature of the condition.

A common and prominent feature of many experimental and clinical studies of decompensated hypertrophy and failure is a derangement of cardiomyocyte calcium homeostasis (Fig. 6-3). Studies of human cardiomyocytes extracted from the hearts of patients with end-stage heart failure have revealed elevated diastolic calcium levels with either no change or a reduction in the amplitude of the calcium transient.[67–70] Longitudinal studies of hypertrophy in experimental animals have revealed depression of steady-state mRNA levels[71] and sarcoplasmic reticulum ATPase and phospholamban proteins[51] in decompensated, but not compensated, pressure overload hypertrophy. These changes were associated with distinctive contractile depression of isovolumically contracting heart function and increases in the EC_{50} and decreases in the V_{max} for sarcoplasmic reticular membrane uptake of calcium.[51] Transgenic overexpression of the sarcoplasmic reticulum ATPase inhibitor phospholamban depressed cardiomyocyte function and calcium kinetics,[47] whereas targeted ablation of the phosphoprotein produced the opposite result.[46] Whether altered levels of the calcium-cycling proteins occur by transcriptional, translational, or posttranslational levels is currently unknown (see also Chap. 21).

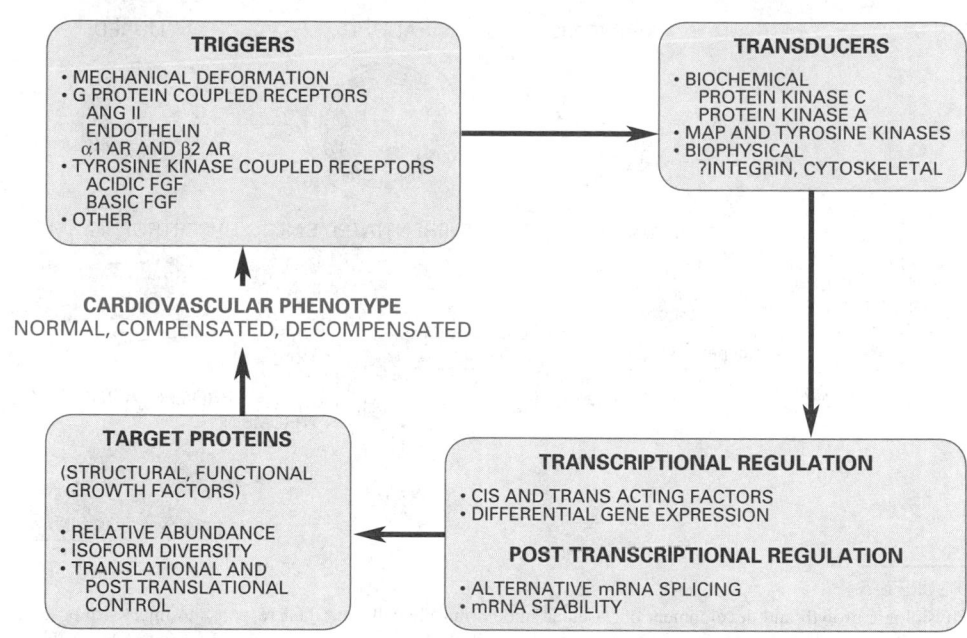

FIGURE 6-4

Schematic diagram of the mechanisms responsible for the development of the anatomic and functional cardiac phenotypes in physiologic and pathologic hypertrophy. Abnormalities at one or multiple levels in this putative closed-loop system may be responsible for the transition between compensated and decompensated hypertrophy.

VASCULAR SMOOTH MUSCLE GROWTH

The vasculature is a complex organ with several functional roles: containing and directing blood elements, regulating local tissue flow and systemic perfusion pressure via altered vascular tone, adapting to increased perfusion pressure, and repair of vascular injury via vascular growth. Thus, the vasculature must autonomously regulate its structure in order to carry out its various functions. The effector cell for vasoconstriction and growth of preexisting vessels is the smooth muscle cell.

Embryonic Vascular Smooth Muscle Development

During embryonic development, the first recognizable blood vessels arise from coalescence of isolated angioblasts into tubular structures composed of a single layer of endothelial cells.[72] Because of the role of endothelial cells in defining the organization of the early vascular tree, it is thought that the endothelium may organize and recruit vascular smooth muscle cells from the surrounding local mesenchyme. Thus, a primordial organ is invaded by endothelial vascular cords, and the primordium itself contributes the vascular smooth muscle layers to the developing blood vessels (Fig. 6-5).

Within the embryonic vasculature, smooth muscle cells secrete extracellular matrix proteins that, together with the smooth muscle cells per se, endothelial cells, and fibroblasts, form the structure of the vascular wall. Embryonic vascular smooth muscle cells actively proliferate, migrate, secrete extracellular matrix, and exhibit an immature pattern of gene expression.[73] By birth, however, the vasculature is essentially completely organized, and mature vascular smooth muscle cells are quiescent and do not proliferate or develop contractile fibers under normal conditions.[74]

Vascular Smooth Muscle Hypertrophy and Hyperplasia

In normal adult arteries, the muscular wall, or media, consists of quiescent vascular smooth muscle cells that constrict when exposed to vasopressive agonists but are unresponsive to growth factors.[74,75] Unlike skeletal and cardiac muscle cells, quiescent smooth muscle cells can reenter the cell cycle and exhibit different growth responses depending upon intrinsic capacity and the extrinsic stimulus. In certain disease entities where vascular smooth muscle cells are exposed to increased hemodynamic load, arterial injury, or other physiologic stresses, they display one of two distinct growth responses. In the large blood vessels of *chronic* hypertensive animals and patients, smooth muscle cell growth is primarily due to hypertrophy, with little or no hyperplasia.[76,77] In contrast, after induction of severe *acute* experimental hypertension, aortic and carotid vascular smooth muscle cells undergo a

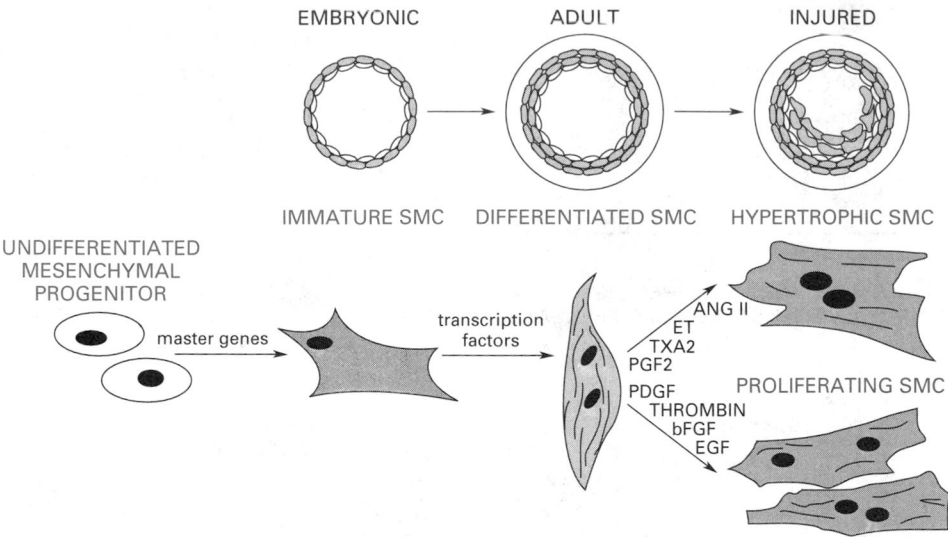

EMBRYONIC   ADULT   INJURED

IMMATURE SMC   DIFFERENTIATED SMC   HYPERTROPHIC SMC

UNDIFFERENTIATED MESENCHYMAL PROGENITOR

master genes — transcription factors

ANG II
ET
TXA2
PGF2
PDGF
THROMBIN
bFGF
EGF

PROLIFERATING SMC

FIGURE 6-5

Physiologic growth and development of vascular smooth muscle cells and their response to injury. Embryonic endothelial vascular tubes acquire immature smooth muscle cell layers from the surrounding mesenchyme. Fully differentiated adult smooth muscle cells are quiescent and express contractile elements. In response to injury, however, vascular smooth muscle cells de-differentiate, reenter the cell cycle, and undergo either hypertrophy or hyperplasia as dictated by the particular growth stimulus.

more classic migratory and proliferative response.[78] It has also been noted that a mixed cellular growth response can occur under certain circumstances. For instance, the increase in mesenteric medial thickness observed in spontaneously hypertensive rats is the result of smooth muscle hyperplasia. As these rats age, however, there is only a small increase in aortic smooth muscle cell number compared with Wistar-Kyoto controls of the same age, with hypertrophy accounting for most of the increase in medial thickness.[79]

Based on the pathologic states in which they occur, vascular hypertrophy and hyperplasia probably have distinct physiologic roles. Proliferation of vascular smooth muscle cells (medial hyperplasia) is not only observed in intermediate arteries during acute severe hypertension but also after balloon injury in animals and in human coronary arteries that restenose after balloon angioplasty. Thus, hyperplasia tends to occur after vessel injury or inflammation and may represent an exuberant attempt to repair damaged arterial walls. In contrast, the smooth muscle hypertrophy observed in large vessels in animals and patients with chronic hypertension may be an adaptive response that, because of additional force-developing capacity and normalized vessel wall stress, confers upon blood vessels a heightened capacity to withstand increased luminal pressures. This augmented capacity for vasoconstriction has the potential to lead to an amplified response to contractile agonists, thereby paradoxically exaggerating or perpetuating hypertension.

Clinical conditions associated not with increased hemodynamic load, but with abnormal hypertrophic or hyperplastic growth of vascular smooth muscle cells play a major pathophysiologic role and include coronary restenosis following balloon angioplasty or atherectomy, pulmonary hypertension,

and the accelerated coronary atherosclerosis that follows orthotopic heart transplantation.[75,80–82] The histologic, functional, and morphologic changes of vascular smooth muscle cells that transition from a normal quiescent/contractile state to a proliferative state are, to a large degree, recapitulated in tissue culture. Normal quiescent smooth muscle cells are characterized immunohistologically by high-level expression of α smooth muscle actin and the SM_1 and SM_2 isoforms of vascular MHC[83,84] and by low-level expression of platelet-derived growth factor (PDGF) AA (see below). During in vitro tissue culture, however, passaged cells express relatively less α actin and myosin but more fibronectin, collagen α_2 (type I), collagen α_1 (type III), thrombospondin, and PDGF AA. The many common features of both cultured and hyperplastic vascular smooth muscle cells resulting from vascular balloon injury support the utilization of tissue-cultured vascular smooth muscle cells as a model system for identification of the stimuli for and mechanisms of vascular smooth muscle growth. Such tissue culture studies have established three major classes of growth stimuli for vascular smooth muscle cells: peptide growth factors, vasoconstricting growth promoters, and mechanical deformation.

Vascular Smooth Muscle Growth Factors

The first class of proliferative agents, peptide growth factors, is typified by PDGF, a dimeric protein derived in large part from platelet α granules but also secreted from vascular smooth muscle and other cells.[85] PDGF binds to and activates two subtypes of membrane receptors (α and β) that possess intrinsic tyrosine-kinase activity and that activate the cascade of tyrosine phosphorylation reactions described in Fig. 6-2. PDGF exists as A or B peptide chains, which can form either homo- or heterodimers. PDGF BB is secreted by platelets, binds preferentially to PDGFβ-type receptors, and is the more mitogenic of the two PDGF homodimers.[86] Heterodimeric PDGF AB is intermediate in mitogenic potency between BB and AA. PDGF AA is secreted from vascular smooth muscle cells in response to growth stimuli and may serve as an autocrine enhancer of vascular smooth muscle growth.[85,87] Other peptide growth factors, such as FGF, epidermal growth factor (EGF), and vascular endothelial growth factor (VEGF), stimulate vascular smooth muscle hyperplasia in like manner by activating their individual tyrosine kinase–coupled receptors.[88]

The second class of growth stimuli, vasoconstricting growth promoters, is typified by angiotensin II and also includes thrombin, thromboxane, prostaglandins, serotonin, and endothelin.[89–91] In general, vasoconstrictors are less potent growth factors than the peptide growth factors described above and their major role in vivo is likely to be enhancement of other stimulators of vascular smooth muscle cell growth. A common feature of the vasoconstricting growth promoters is that they all activate transmembrane receptors coupled, via guanosine triphosphate (GTP)-binding proteins of the Gq class, to activation of phospholipase C. The precise cellular events that transduce Gq/phospholipase C–stimulated vascular smooth muscle growth are not yet completely defined. It is clear, however, that the proliferative tyrosine-kinase cascade is also activated to some degree by each of these agents, possibly via PKC-mediated inhibition of Ras-GTPase or Gβ/γ-mediated activation of tyrosine kinases via stimulation of a calcium/calmodulin-dependent kinase[92,93] (see Fig. 6-2).

An interesting feature of the vasoconstricting growth promoters is that they are incomplete mitogens. As described in detail for angiotensin II and thromboxane A_2,[94,95] stimulation of quiescent vascular smooth muscle cells with these agonists (in the absence of exogenous peptide growth factors) results generally in cellular hypertrophy defined by increased amino acid incorporation, protein content, and cell size without cell proliferation. The lack of a full mitogenic response to vasoconstrictors may reflect activation of only selective components of the tyrosine-kinase cascade[96] or, as described below, by increased expression of endogenous growth inhibitors.[91,97]

Angiotensin II is not only the prototypical vasoconstricting vascular smooth muscle growth promoter but is arguably also the most important because the vascular wall possesses a local renin-angiotensin system that may be activated by injury. Both angiotensinogen and angiotensin-converting enzyme have been detected in the vascular wall, and expression of both enzymes is increased in the neointima of balloon-injured arteries.[98,99] Furthermore, neointimal cells express angiotensin II receptors. Finally, prolonged infusion of angiotensin has been shown to stimulate medial and neointimal vascular smooth muscle cell growth,[100] thus demonstrating in vivo relevance of angiotensin II as a vascular growth promoter.

Recent studies have established that mechanical deformation, or "stretch," is a proliferative stimulus for vascular smooth muscle cells.[101,102] It appears that autocrine production of PDGF may play a role in stretch-induced vascular growth[103] in a manner analogous to the autocrine role proposed for growth factors in angiotensin II, thrombin, and thromboxane-stimulated vascular hypertrophy.[89–91] Clearly, mechanical deformation can activate vascular smooth muscle tyrosine kinases via some mechanism, either directly or indirectly by the actions of endogenously produced growth promoters.[102] *Therefore, the three classes of vascular smooth muscle growth stimuli each appear to activate tyrosine kinases as a common signal transduction pathway to stimulate cellular growth.*

Growth Signaling in Vascular Smooth Muscle Cells

There is an ongoing explosion of information regarding receptor-mediated growth signaling in vascular smooth muscle cells. Peptide growth factors, vasoconstricting growth promoters, and mechanical deformation each activate protein tyrosine kinases in vascular smooth muscle cells with convergent phosphorylation and activation of MAPK.[96,102,104–106] Thus, MAPK represents a common signaling molecule that integrates signals from multiple divergent physical and chemical stimuli in order to transduce a growth response. MAPK is activated by both threonine and tyrosine phosphorylation[107] and has numerous downstream targets, as depicted in Fig. 6-2. MAPK substrates can be divided into three classes—protein kinases, nuclear factors, and cytosolic proteins. The number of different proliferative stimuli that activate MAPK and the number of different MAPK substrates make this enzyme a "funnel" through which growth signaling is processed in multiple cell types.

Peptide growth factors and vasoconstricting growth promoters interact at different subclasses of receptors and therefore activate MAPK via different mechanisms.[108] In both cases, the MAPK ERK1 and ERK2 are activated by threonine/tyrosine phosphorylation by *MAPK/ERK-activating kinase* (MEK) which, in turn, is activated when phosphorylated by c-Raf, itself activated by the GTP-binding protein Ras. The events transducing peptide growth factor activation of Ras, Raf, MEK, and MAPK have been elucidated.[109,110] Activated growth factor receptors that possess intrinsic tyrosine kinase activity undergo autophosphorylation. Tyrosine phosphorylation permits binding of growth factor receptor–bound (Grb)-2 protein at an Src homology 2 domain, and Grb-2 recruits the Ras activator Sos (son of sevenless) to form a receptor-Grb 2–Sos complex. Sos promotes GTP binding to Ras, thus activating it and the entire tyrosine-kinase cascade (Fig. 6-2).

The pathway leading from Gq-coupled vasoconstrictor receptors to Ras activation is not as clear but appears to involve PKC activation, with phosphorylation of Ras–GTPase-activating protein, thus inhibiting hydrolysis of Ras-bound GTP. In this manner PKC activates Ras by maintaining it in the GTP-bound form. Additional tyrosine kinases that are sensitive to calcium/calmodulin may also play a role in transducing Gq or G_i protein–coupled receptor activation of Ras via dissociated Gβ/γ subunits.[92,93]

Endogenous Growth Modifiers in Vascular Smooth Muscle Growth

It has been observed that the most probable functional role of vasoconstricting growth promoters is synergistic enhancement of peptide growth factor effects. Yet the two events cannot be separated, because synthesis of endogenous growth factors is an intrinsic regulatory mechanism for modifying vascular smooth muscle growth stimulated by vasoconstricting agents or mechanical injury. When specific growth factors are assayed after balloon injury, basic FGF protein and PDGF

A-chain (but not PDGF B-chain) mRNA increase.[111–113] The beneficial effects of antibodies against PDGF or basic FGF, which reduce intimal thickening after balloon injury in rats,[111,113,114] support an important functional role for autocrine growth factors in vascular smooth muscle proliferation after intimal disruption. Furthermore, the relative abundance of endogenous growth inhibitors and growth promoters appears to be a critical determinant of whether agonist-stimulated growth will be hypertrophic or hyperplastic (Fig. 6-5).

TRANSFORMING GROWTH FACTOR β_1

One cellular mechanism that appears to determine the nature of vascular smooth muscle growth (hypertrophy or hyperplasia) is expression of endogenous transforming growth factor β_1 (TGFβ_1).[97] TGFβ_1 is a multifunctional growth modulator originally described as a tumorigenic factor that stimulated anchorage-independent growth of certain mesenchymal cell lines. TGFβ_1 is synthesized as an inactive polypeptide and undergoes proteolysis to form an active 25-kDa homodimer.[115] It is released by platelets but is also synthesized by vascular smooth muscle cells,[97] and both TGFβ_1 mRNA and protein are increased in the neointima of balloon-injured vessels.[116] Infusion of TGFβ_1 after balloon injury increases [^{3}H]thymidine labeling of neointimal smooth muscle cells, and TGFβ_1 overexpression in porcine arteries increases the synthesis of extracellular matrix protein.[116,117] These in vivo data strongly suggest that TGFβ_1 is an important factor that influences smooth muscle cell growth after vascular injury.

In vitro studies have shown that TGFβ_1 has a bimodal effect on cultured vascular smooth muscle cells. Lower concentrations stimulate growth or augment the growth response to other growth factors. At higher concentrations, however, TGFβ_1 inhibits cell proliferation. A possible explanation for the opposing effects of TGFβ_1 is that lower concentrations increase autocrine PDGF A-chain synthesis, which stimulates growth, but that higher concentrations diminish PDGFα-receptor expression, thus interrupting the autocrine effects of PDGF A.[118] It should be noted that the effects of TGFβ_1 on autocrine PDGF production only partially explain its growth-stimulating activity, as TGFβ_1 can be mitogenic in 3T3 cells derived from PDGFα-receptor knockout mice.[119]

Another well-described action of TGFβ_1 on vascular smooth muscle cells is interruption of the cell growth cycle. Topical application of TGFβ_1 causes cell cycle arrest in late G_1 phase (see Chap. 7). The transition from G_1 to S phase is regulated by cyclin E activation of cyclin-dependent kinase 2, and TGFβ_1 causes the release of p29^{Kip1}, a protein inhibitor of cyclin E–dependent cyclin-dependent kinase 2 activity,[120] thereby preventing cell cycle progression into S phase.

The growth-inhibitory effects of TGFβ_1 play an important role in regulating vasoconstrictor-stimulated vascular smooth muscle hypertrophy. As described by Gibbons et al.,[97] upregulation of endogenous TGFβ_1 expression after angiotensin II or thromboxane stimulation prevents cell proliferation and DNA synthesis. Inhibition of TGFβ_1 with neutralizing antibodies or antisense oligodeoxynucleotides permits completion of the full cell growth cycle. These studies suggest that endogenous expression of TGFβ_1 is a key regulatory event that determines whether vascular smooth muscle growth will be hypertrophic or hyperplastic.

BASIC FIBROBLAST GROWTH FACTOR AND VASCULAR SMOOTH MUSCLE GROWTH

While TGFβ_1 is a key endogenous negative regulator of vascular smooth muscle growth, basic FGF is an important endogenous activator of growth in cells stimulated with thrombin, thromboxane, or angiotensin II.[89–91] Basic FGF is a multifunctional protein initially recognized for its angiogenic properties but that is now known to also affect mitogenicity, invasiveness, and migration of a variety of cell types. At the tissue level, basic FGF induces angiogenesis in vivo and in vitro,[121,122] promotes collateral vessel development in ischemic myocardium,[123,124] stimulates endothelial and vascular smooth muscle migration and proliferation in injured arteries,[125,126] and may contribute to tumor expansion.[122] Basic FGF is generally thought to transduce at least some of these effects via interactions with membrane receptors coupled to tyrosine phosphorylation reactions.[88] The biological importance of basic FGF on abnormal neointima formation after endovascular injury has been experimentally demonstrated through the use of neutralizing antibodies or heparin to inhibit basic FGF.[111,114,125,126] In tissue culture, quiescent vascular smooth muscle cells exposed to angiotensin II, thrombin, or thromboxane increase expression of basic FGF; and inhibition of basic FGF, using antisense oligonucleotides or neutralizing antibodies, attenuates agonist-stimulated growth.[89–91] Increased endogenous basic FGF, while necessary for angiotensin II– or thromboxane-stimulated vascular smooth muscle hypertrophy, is not sufficient without simultaneous activation of PKC.[127] This may explain the lack of a vascular phenotype in transgenic mice overexpressing human basic FGF.[128]

The isolation and complete structural characterization of human, bovine, and rat basic FGF cDNAs and the human basic FGF gene demonstrated that basic FGF represents multiple, closely related proteins ranging in molecular mass from 23 to 18 kDa.[129] The variations in protein size result from N-terminal extensions that are produced by alternate CUG translation start sites located 5′ of the more typical AUG start site. Interestingly, the N-terminal extensions encode nuclear targeting sequences that result in higher-molecular-weight basic FGFs being preferentially localized in cell nuclei.[130] In contrast, low-molecular-mass (18 kDa) basic FGF is equally distributed throughout the cell. Although all basic FGF isoforms appear to have identical effects when applied to cells from the outside, the nuclear localization of endogenous higher-molecular-weight forms suggests that they may play unique roles in cell growth or development.

All basic FGF isoforms lack signal sequences and are therefore not "secreted" proteins in the classic sense. Nevertheless, basic FGF is exported from cells, and the biological effects of endogenously derived basic FGF can be partially inhibited by neutralizing antibodies. Postulated physiologically relevant mechanisms for basic FGF release include cell death or damage and exocytosis (independent of the endoplasmic reticulum–golgi pathway). Although vascular smooth muscle and other tissues produce basic FGF, its effects clearly arise in part from extracellular actions (which are inhibited by antibodies and can downregulate membrane basic FGF receptors).[111,114,125] The fact that basic FGF is not found in tissue culture medium suggests that (18 kDa) basic FGF is released from cells but remains associated with the cell membranes, perhaps by binding to heparan sulfate proteoglycans. Heparan sulfate–bound basic FGF can be released by the actions of glycosylphosphatidylinositol-specific phospholipases C and D and thus be free to interact with membrane receptors.[131,132] It has been suggested that exportation of basic FGF is regulated and, in turn, can modulate tissue phenotype and function.[122]

TRANSFECTION STUDIES OF BASIC FGF ISOFORMS

It has been difficult to design experimental systems in which to address questions regarding the physiologic significance of higher-molecular-weight/nuclear targeted basic FGF isoforms relative to low-molecular-weight, nontargeted basic FGF. One approach has been to use transfected cell systems to endogenously overexpress individual basic FGF isoforms. This has been accomplished by constructing expression vectors in which the complete basic FGF cDNA has been altered to permit expression of only distinct basic FGFs. Mutation of one or more upstream CTG codons to CTT eliminates synthesis of the corresponding nuclear-targeted higher-molecular-weight basic FGF. In contrast, mutation of the initiator ATG prevents synthesis of the low-molecular-weight, nontargeted basic FGF. Higher-molecular-weight basic FGFs expressed in Cos-7 cells using these types of constructs localize to the nucleus, whereas low-molecular-weight basic FGF is found in the cytoplasm and cell surface.[133] Furthermore, these types of studies demonstrate that 18-kDa basic FGF is formed de novo and is not simply a degradation product of high-molecular-weight basic FGF. Finally, only the 18-kDa nontargeted basic FGF appears to be exported to the surface of the cell.[133] The differences in localization and export of basic FGF isoforms suggest that there are either unknown functions of higher-molecular-weight forms, or that some of the autocrine functions currently ascribed to exported (18 kDa) basic FGF are actually the intracrine consequences of nuclear-targeted basic FGF. This notion has been examined in transfection studies using NIH 3T3 fibroblasts. A specific functional role for higher-molecular-weight basic FGFs was suggested because low-level overexpression of high-molecular-weight basic FGFs inhibited cell growth and stimulated formation of multinuclear cells. In contrast, low-level overexpression of 18-kDa basic FGF failed to produce these changes. High-level expression of both high- and low-molecular-weight basic FGF, however, transformed the fibroblasts and caused tumor formation.[134] In separate but similar studies, NIH 3T3 cells transfected with low-molecular-weight basic FGF (in the presence or absence of high-molecular-weight basic FGFs) exhibited enhanced migration and decreased basic FGF receptor number. Cells transfected with high-molecular-weight basic FGF encoding cDNA did not show altered migration but instead demonstrated an ability to grow to high density in low serum or in the presence of a cotransfected dominant negative mutant basic FGF receptor.[135] Different functions of high- and low-molecular-weight basic FGF isoforms have also been compellingly demonstrated by Couderec et al.,[136] who overexpressed high- or low-molecular-weight basic FGFs in bovine aortic endothelial cells (using recombinant retroviral infection) and found that expression of 18-kDa basic FGF resulted in cellular transformation, whereas expression of higher-molecular-weight CUG-initiated forms caused cell immortalization. Taken together, these studies suggest that low-molecular-weight secreted basic FGF interacts with basic FGF membrane receptors to stimulate cell migration and proliferation, whereas intracellular high-molecular-weight basic FGF can enhance cell growth independent of the cell surface receptor.

REFERENCES

1. Vaux DL, Strasser A. The molecular biology of apoptosis. *Proc Natl Acad Sci USA* 1996; 93:2239–2244.
2. Thompson CB. Apoptosis in the pathogenesis and treatment of disease. *Science* 1995; 267:1456–1462.
3. Peter M, Herskowitz I. Joining the complex: Cyclin-dependent kinase inhibitory proteins and the cell cycle. *Cell* 1994; 79:181–184.
4. Dorée M, Galas S. The cyclin-dependent protein kinases and the control of cell division. *FASEB J* 1994; 8:1114–1121.
5. Field LJ. Atrial natriuretic factor-SV40 T antigen transgenes produce tumors and cardiac arrhythmias in mice. *Science* 1988; 239:1029–1033.
6. Clark AJ. General physiology of hearts of cold-blooded vertebrates. In: Barcroft J, Saunders JT, eds. *Comparative Physiology of the Heart.* New York: MacMillan; 1927:22 151.
7. Ford LE. Heart size. *Circ Res* 1976; 39:297–303.
8. Walsh RA. Cardiovascular effects of the aging process. *Am J Med* 1987; 82:34–40.
9. Watkins H, Rosenzweig A, Hwang DS, Levi T, McKenna W, Seidman CE, et al. Characteristics and prognostic implications of myosin missense mutations in familial hypertrophic cardiomyopathy. *N Engl J Med* 1992; 326:1108–1114.
10. Marian AJ, Roberts R. Recent advances in the molecular genetics of hypertrophic cardiomyopathy. *Circulation* 1995; 92:1336–1347.
11. Cooper G IV. Cardiocyte adaptation to chronically altered load. *Annu Rev Physiol* 1987; 49:501–518.
12. Watson PA. Mechanical activation of signaling pathways in the cardiovascular system. *Trends Cardiovasc Med* 1996; 6:73–79.
13. Sugden PH, Bogoyevitch MA. Intracellular signalling through protein kinases in the heart. *Cardiovasc Res* 1995; 30:478–492.
14. Komuro I, Katoh Y, Kaida T, Shibazaki Y, Kurabayashi M, Hoh E, et al. Mechanical loading stimulates cell hypertrophy and specific gene expression in cultured rat cardiac myocytes. *J Biol Chem* 1991; 266:1265–1268.
15. Sadoshima J, Jahn L, Takahashi T, Kulik TJ, Izumo S. Molecular characterization of the stretch-induced adaptation of cultured cardiac cells. *J Biol Chem* 1992; 267:10551–10560.
16. Sadoshima J, Xu Y, Slayter HS, Izumo S. Autocrine release of angiotensin II mediates stretch-induced hypertrophy of cardiac myocytes *in vitro*. *Cell* 1993; 75:977–984.
17. Yamazaki T, Komuro I, Kudoh S, Zou Y, Shiojima I, Mizuno T, et al. Angiotensin II partly mediates mechanical stress-induced cardiac hypertrophy. *Circ Res* 1995; 77:258–265.
18. Knowlton KU, Michel MC, Itani M, Shubeita HE, Ishihara K, Brown JH, et al. The α_{1A}-adrenergic receptor subtype mediates biochemical, molecular, and morphologic features of cultured myocardial cell hypertrophy. *J Biol Chem* 1993; 268:15374–15380.

19. Bogoyevitch MA, Glennon PE, Andersson MB, Clerk A, Lazou A, Marshall CJ, et al. Endothelin-1 and fibroblast growth factors stimulate the mitogen-activated protein kinase signaling cascade in cardiac myocytes. *J Biol Chem* 1994; 269:1110–1119.

20. Milano CA, Dolber PC, Rockman HA, Bond RA, Venable ME, Allen LF, et al. Myocardial expression of a constitutively active α_{1B}-adrenergic receptor in transgenic mice induces cardiac hypertrophy. *Proc Natl Acad Sci USA* 1994; 91:10109–10113.

21. Sadoshima J, Izumo S. Mechanical stretch rapidly activates multiple signal transduction pathways in cardiac myocytes: Potential involvement of an autocrine/paracrine mechanism. *EMBO J* 1993; 12:1681–1692.

22. Cummins P. Fibroblast and transforming growth factor expression in the cardiac myocyte. *Cardiovasc Res* 1993; 27:1150–1154.

23. Parker TG, Packer SE, Schneider MD. Peptide growth factors can provoke "fetal" contractile protein gene expression in rat cardiac myocytes. *J Clin Invest* 1990; 85:507–514.

24. Roberts AB, Roche NS, Winokur TS, Burmester JK, Sporn MB. Role of transforming growth factor-β in maintenance of function of cultured neonatal cardiac myocytes. *J Clin Invest* 1992; 90:2056–2062.

25. Milano CA, Allen LF, Rockman HA, Dolber PC, McMinn TR, Chien KR, et al. Enhanced myocardial function in transgenic mice overexpressing the β_2-adrenergic receptor. *Science* 1994; 264:582–586.

26. Glennon PE, Kaddoura S, Sale EM, Sale GJ, Fuller SJ, Sugden PH. Depletion of mitogen-activated protein kinase using an antisense oligodeoxynucleotide approach downregulates the phenylephrine-induced hypertrophic response in rat cardiac myocytes. *Circ Res* 1996; 78:954–961.

27. Khoury SF, Hoit BD, Dave V, Pawloski-Dahm CM, Shao Y, Gabel M, et al. Effects of thyroid hormone on left ventricular performance and regulation of contractile and Ca^{2+}-cycling proteins in the baboon: Implications for the force-frequency and relaxation-frequency relationships. *Circ Res* 1996; 79:727–735.

28. Klemperer JD, Ojamaa K, Klein I. Thyroid hormone therapy in cardiovascular disease. *Prog Cardiovasc Dis* 1996; 38:329–336.

29. Klein I, Hong C. Effects of thyroid hormone on cardiac size and myosin content of the heterotopically transplanted rat heart. *J Clin Invest* 1986; 77:1694–1698.

30. Morgan HE, Gordon EE, Kira Y, Chua BHL, Russo LA, Peterson CJ, et al. Biochemical mechanisms of cardiac hypertrophy. *Annu Rev Physiol* 1987; 49:533–543.

31. Hannan RD, Luyken J, Rothblum LI. Regulation of ribosomal DNA transcription during contraction-induced hypertrophy of neonatal cardiomyocytes. *J Biol Chem* 1996; 271:3213–3220.

32. Samarel AM. Hemodynamic overload and the regulation of myofibrillar protein degradation. *Circulation* 1993; 87:1418–1420.

33. Samarel AM, Parmacek MS, Magid NM, Decker RS, Lesch M. Protein synthesis and degradation during starvation-induced cardiac atrophy in rabbits. *Circ Res* 1987; 60:933–941.

34. Henkel RD, VandeBerg JL, Shade RE, Leger JJ, Walsh RA. Cardiac beta myosin heavy chain diversity in normal and chronically hypertensive baboons. *J Clin Invest* 1989; 83:1487–1493.

35. Morkin E. Regulation of myosin heavy chain genes in the heart. *Circulation* 1993; 87:1451–1460.

36. Walsh RA, Henkel R, Robbins J. Cardiac myosin heavy- and light-chain gene expression in hypertrophy and heart failure. *Heart Failure* 1990/91; 6:238–243.

37. Boheler KR, Chassagne C, Martin X, Wisnewsky C, Schwartz K. Cardiac expressions of α- and β-myosin heavy chains and sarcomeric α-actins are regulated through transcriptional mechanisms. *J Biol Chem* 1992; 267:12979–12985.

38. Cooper G IV. Load and length regulation of cardiac energetics. *Annu Rev Physiol* 1990; 52:505–522.

39. Hixson JE, Henkel RD, Britten ML, Vernier DT, deLemos RA, VandeBerg JL, et al. α-Myosin heavy chain cDNA structure and gene expression in adult, fetal, and premature baboon myocardium. *J Mol Cell Cardiol* 1989; 21:1073–1086.

40. Weber KT, Brilla CG. Pathological hypertrophy and cardiac interstitium. *Circulation* 1991; 83:1849–1865.

41. Borg TK, Rubin K, Carver W, Samarel A, Terracio L. The cell biology of the cardiac interstitium. *Trends Cardiovasc Med* 1996; 6:65–70.

42. Prockop DJ, Kivirikko KI. Collagens: Molecular biology, diseases, and potentials for therapy. *Annu Rev Biochem* 1995; 64:403–434.

43. Collins JF, Pawloski-Dahm C, Davis MG, Ball N, Dorn GW II, Walsh RA. The role of the cytoskeleton in left ventricular pressure overload hypertrophy and failure. *J Mol Cell Cardiol* 1996; 28:1435–1443.

44. Tsutsui H, Kshihara K, Cooper G. Cytoskeletal role in the contractile dysfunction of hypertrophied myocardium. *Science* 1993; 260:682–687.

45. Arai M, Matsui H, Periasamy M. Sarcoplasmic reticulum gene expression in cardiac hypertrophy and heart failure. *Circ Res* 1994; 74:555–564.

46. Luo W, Grupp IL, Harrer J, Ponniah S, Grupp G, Duffy JJ, et al. Targeted ablation of the phospholamban gene is associated with markedly enhanced myocardial contractility and loss of β-agonist stimulation. *Circ Res* 1994; 75:401–409.

47. Kadambi VJ, Ponniah S, Harrer JM, Hoit BD, Dorn GW II, Walsh RA, et al. Cardiac-specific overexpression of phospholamban alters calcium kinetics and resultant cardiomyocyte mechanics in transgenic mice. *J Clin Invest* 1996; 97:533–539.

48. Hart G. Cellular electrophysiology in cardiac hypertrophy and failure. *Cardiovasc Res* 1994; 28:933–946.

49. Pye MP, Cobbe SM. Mechanisms of ventricular arrhythmias in cardiac failure and hypertrophy. *Cardiovasc Res* 1992; 26:740–750.

50. Dorn GW II, Robbins J, Ball N, Walsh RA. Myosin heavy chain regulation and myocyte contractile depression after LV hypertrophy in aortic-banded mice. *Am J Physiol* 1994; 267:H400–H405.

51. Kiss E, Ball NA, Kranias EG, Walsh RA. Differential changes in cardiac phospholamban and sarcoplasmic reticular Ca^{2+}-ATPase protein levels: Effects on Ca^{2+} transport and mechanics in compensated pressure-overload hypertrophy and congestive heart failure. *Circ Res* 1995; 77:759–764.

52. Hoit BD, Shao Y, Gabel M, Walsh RA. Disparate effects of early pressure overload hypertrophy on velocity-dependent and force-dependent indices of ventricular performance in the conscious baboon. *Circulation* 1995; 91:1213–1220.

53. Cooper G IV, Tomanek RJ, Ehrhardt JC, Marcus ML. Chronic progressive pressure overload of the rat right ventricle. *Circ Res* 1981; 48:488–497.

54. Bing OHL, Matsushita S, Fanburg BL, Levine HJ. Mechanical properties of rat cardiac muscle during experimental hypertrophy. *Circ Res* 1971; 28:234–245.

55. Anderson PAW, Greig A, Mark TM, Malouf NN, Oakeley AE, Ungerleider RM, et al. Molecular basis of human cardiac troponin T isoforms expressed in the developing, adult, and failing heart. *Circ Res* 1995; 76:681–686.

56. Bache RJ. Effects of hypertrophy on the coronary circulation. *Prog Cardiovasc Dis* 1988; 31:403–440.

57. Breisch EA, White FC, Bloor CM. Myocardial characteristics of pressure overload hypertrophy. A structural and functional study. *Lab Invest* 1984; 51:333–342.

58. Murray PA, Vatner SF. Reduction of maximal coronary vasodilator capacity in conscious dogs with severe right ventricular hypertrophy. *Circ Res* 1981; 48:25–33.

59. Hultgren PB, Bove AA. Myocardial blood flow and mechanics in volume overload-induced left ventricular hypertrophy in dogs. *Cardiovasc Res* 1981; 15:522–528.

60. Isoyama S, Ito N, Kuroha M, Takishima T. Complete reversibility of physiological coronary vascular abnormalities in hypertrophied hearts produced by pressure overload in the rat. *J Clin Invest* 1989; 84:288–294.

61. Wagoner LE, Walsh RA. The cellular pathophysiology of progression to heart failure. *Curr Opin Cardiol* 1996; 11:237–244.

62. Teiger E, Dam TV, Richard L, Wisnewsky C, Tea BS, Gaboury L, et al. Apoptosis in pressure overload-induced heart hypertrophy in the rat. *J Clin Invest* 1996; 97:2891–2897.

63. Cheng W, Li B, Kajstura J, Li P, Wolin MS, Sonnenblick EH, et al. Stretch-induced programmed myocyte cell death. *J Clin Invest* 1995; 96:2247–2259.

64. Geisterfer-Lowrance AAT, Christe M, Conner DA, Ingwall JS, Schoen FJ, Seidman CE, et al. A mouse model of familial hypertrophic cardiomyopathy. *Science* 1996; 272:731–734.

65. Iwase M, Bishop SP, Uechi M, Vatner DE, Shannon RP, Kudej RK, et al. Adverse effects of chronic endogenous sympathetic drive induced by cardiac $G_{s\alpha}$ overexpression. *Circ Res* 1996; 78:517–524.

66. Edwards JG, Lyons GE, Micales BK, Malhotra A, Factor S, Leinwand LA. Cardiomyopathy in transgenic *myf5* mice. *Circ Res* 1996; 78:379–387.

67. D'Agnolo A, Luciani GB, Mazzucco A, Gallucci V, Salviati G. Contractile properties and Ca^{2+} release activity of the sarcoplasmic reticulum in dilated cardiomyopathy. *Circulation* 1992; 85:518–525.

68. Schwinger RHG, Böhm M, Schmidt U, Karczewski P, Bavendick U, Flesch M, et al. Unchanged protein levels of SERCA II and phospholamban but reduced Ca^{2+} uptake and Ca^{2+}-ATPase activity of cardiac sarcoplasmic reticulum from dilated cardiomyopathy patients compared with patients with nonfailing hearts. *Circulation* 1995; 92:3220–3228.

69. Meyer M, Schillinger W, Pieske B, Holubarsch C, Heilmann C, Posival H, et al. Alterations of sarcoplasmic reticulum proteins in failing human dilated cardiomyopathy. *Circulation* 1995; 92:778–784.

70. Hasenfuss G, Reinecke H, Studer R, Meyer M, Pieske B, Holtz J, et al. Relation between myocardial function and expression of sarcoplasmic reticulum Ca^{2+}-ATPase in failing and nonfailing human myocardium. *Circ Res* 1994; 75:434–442.

71. Feldman AM, Weinberg EO, Ray PE, Lorell BH. Selective changes in cardiac gene expression during compensated hypertrophy and the transition to cardiac decompensation in rats with chronic aortic banding. *Circ Res* 1993; 73:184–192.

72. Poole TJ, Coffin JD. Vasculogenesis and angiogenesis: Two distinct morphogenetic mechanisms establish embryonic vascular pattern. *J Exp Zool* 1989; 251:224–231.

73. Katoh Y, Periasamy M. Growth and differentiation of smooth muscle cells during vascular development. *Trends Cardiovasc Med* 1996; 6:100–106.

74. Gordon D, Reidy MA, Benditt EP, Schwartz SM. Cell proliferation in human coronary arteries. *Proc Natl Acad Sci USA* 1990; 87:4600–4604.

75. Schwartz S, Ross R. Cellular proliferation in atherosclerosis and hypertension. *Prog Cardiovasc Dis* 1984; 26:355–372.

76. Owens G, Schwartz S. Alterations in vascular smooth muscle mass in the spontaneously hypertensive rat: Role of cellular hypertrophy, hyperploidy, and hyperplasia. *Circ Res* 1982; 51:280–289.

77. Schwartz S, Campbell GR, Campbell JH. Replication of smooth muscle cells in vascular disease. *Circ Res* 1986; 58:427–444.

78. Owens G, Reidy M. Hyperplastic growth response of vascular smooth muscle cells following induction of acute hypertension in rat by aortic coarctation. *Circ Res* 1985; 57:695–705.

79. Owens, GK. Influence of blood pressure on development of aortic medial smooth muscle hypertrophy in spontaneously hypertensive rats. *Hypertension* 1987; 9:178–187.

80. Johnson DE, Hinohara T, Selmon MR, Braden LJ, Simpson JB. Primary peripheral arterial stenoses and restenoses excised by transluminal atherectomy: A histopathologic study. *J Am Coll Cardiol* 1990; 425:419–425.

81. Haworth SG. Primary pulmonary hypertension. *Br Heart J* 1983; 49:517–521.

82. Johnson DE, Alderman EL, Schroeder JS, Gao S-Z, Hunt S, DeCampli WM, et al. Transplant coronary artery disease: Histopathologic correlations with angiographic morphology. *J Am Coll Cardiol* 1991; 17:449–457.

83. Nagai R, Larson DT, Periasamy M. Characterization of a mammalian smooth muscle myosin heavy chain cDNA clone and its expression in various smooth muscle types. *Proc Natl Acad Sci USA* 1988; 85:1047–1051.

84. Nagai R, Kuro OM, Babij P, Periasamy M. Identification of two types of smooth muscle myosin heavy chain isoforms by cDNA cloning and immunoblot analysis. *J Biol Chem* 1989; 264:9734–9737.

85. Naftilan AJ, Pratt RE, Dzau VJ. Induction of platelet-derived growth factor A-chain and c-*myc* gene expressions by angiotensin II in cultured rat vascular smooth muscle cells. *J Clin Invest* 1989; 83:1419–1424.

86. Inui H, Kitami Y, Tani M, Kondo T, Inagami T. Differences in signal transduction between platelet-derived growth factor (PDGF) α and β receptors in vascular smooth muscle cells. *J Biol Chem* 1994; 269(48):30546–30552.

87. Negoro N, Kanayama Y, Haraguchi M, Umetani N, Nishimura M, Konishi Y, et al. Blood pressure regulates platelet-derived growth factor A-chain gene expression in vascular smooth muscle cells in vivo. *J Clin Invest* 1995; 95:1140–1150.

88. Heldin C-H. Dimerization of cell surface receptors in signal transduction. *Cell* 1995; 80:213–223.

89. Ali S, Davis MG, Becker MW, Dorn GW II. Thromboxane A_2 stimulates vascular smooth muscle hypertrophy by upregulating the synthesis and release of endogenous basic fibroblast growth factor. *J Biol Chem* 1993; 268:17397–17403.

90. Weiss RH, Maduri M. The mitogenic effect of thrombin in vascular smooth muscle cells is largely due to basic fibroblast growth factor. *J Biol Chem* 1993; 268:5724–5727.

91. Itoh H, Mukoyama M, Pratt RE, Gibbons GH, Dzau VJ. Multiple autocrine growth factors modulate vascular smooth muscle cell growth response to angiotensin II. *J Clin Invest* 1993; 91:2268–2274.

92. Eguchi S, Matsumoto T, Motley ED, Utsunomiya H, Inagami T. Identification of an essential signaling cascade for mitogen-activated protein kinase activation by angiotensin II in cultured rat vascular smooth muscle cells. *J Biol Chem* 1996; 271:14169–14175.

93. van Biesen T, Hawes BE, Luttrell DK, Krueger KM, Touhara K, Porfiri E, et al. Receptor-tyrosine-kinase- and Gβ/γ-mediated MAPkinase activation by a common signaling pathway. *Nature* 1995; 376:781–784.

94. Berk BC, Vekshtein V, Gordon HM, Tsuda T. Angiotensin II–stimulated protein synthesis in cultured vascular smooth muscle cells. *Hypertension* 1988; 13:305–314.

95. Dorn GW II, Becker MW, Davis MG. Dissociation of the contractile and hypertrophic effects of vasoconstrictor prostanoids in vascular smooth muscle. *J Biol Chem* 1992; 267:24897–24905.

96. Ali S, Dorn GW II. Patterns of tyrosine phosphorylation differ in vascular hypertrophy and hyperplasia. *Am J Physiol* 1994; 36:C1674–C1681.

97. Gibbons GH, Pratt RE, Dzau VJ. Vascular smooth muscle cell hypertrophy vs. hyperplasia: Autocrine transforming growth factor-β_1 expression determines growth response to angiotensin II. *J Clin Invest* 1992; 90:456–461.

98. Naftilan AJ, Zuo WM, Inglefinger J, Ryan TJ Jr, Pratt RE, Dzau VJ. Localization and differential regulation of angiotensinogen mRNA expression in the vessel wall. *J Clin Invest* 1991; 87:1300–1311.

99. Dzau VJ, Gibbons GH, Pratt RE. Molecular mechanisms of vascular renin-angiotensin system in myointimal hyperplasia. *Hypertension* 1991; 18:II-100–II-105.

100. Daemen MJAP, Lombardi DM, Bosman FT, Schwartz SM. Angiotensin II induces smooth muscle cell proliferation in the normal and injured rat arterial wall. *Circ Res* 1991; 68:450–456.

101. Sudhir K, Wilson E, Chatterjee K, Ives HE. Mechanical strain and collagen potentiate mitogenic activity of angiotensin II in rat vascular smooth muscle cells. *J Clin Invest* 1993; 92:3003–3007.

102. Davis MG, Ali S, Leikauf GD, Dorn GW II. Tyrosine kinase inhibition prevents deformation-stimulated vascular smooth muscle growth. *Hypertension* 1994; 24:706–713.

103. Wilson E, Mai Q, Sudhir K, Weiss RH, Ives HE. Mechanical strain induces growth of vascular smooth muscle cells via autocrine action of PDGF. *J Cell Biol* 1993; 123:741–747.

104. Force T, Kyriakis JM, Avruch J, Bonventre JV. Endothelin, vasopressin, and angiotensin II enhance tyrosine phosphorylation by protein kinase C–dependent and –independent pathways in glomerular mesangial cells. *J Biol Chem* 1991; 266:6650–6656.

105. Weiss RH, Nuccitelli R. Inhibition of tyrosine phosphorylation prevents thrombin-induced mitogenesis, but not intracellular free calcium release, in vascular smooth muscle cells. *J Biol Chem* 1992; 267:5608–5613.

106. Vallius M, Kazlauskas A. Phospholipase C-γ1 and phosphatidylinositol 3 kinase are the downstream mediators of the PDGF receptor's mitogenic signal. *Cell* 1993; 73:321–334.

107. Anderson NG, Maller JL, Tonks NK, Sturgill TW. Requirement for integration of signals from two distinct phosphorylation pathways for activation of MAP kinase. *Nature* 1990; 343:651–653.

108. Linseman DA, Benjamin CW, Jones DA. Convergence of angiotensin II and platelet-derived growth factor receptor signaling cascades in vascular smooth muscle cells. *J Biol Chem* 1995; 270:12563–12568.

109. Blenis J. Signal transduction via the MAP kinases: Proceed at your own RSK. *Proc Natl Acad Sci USA* 1993; 90:5889–5892.

110. Davis RJ. The mitogen-activated protein kinase signal transduction pathway. *J Biol Chem* 1993; 268:14553–14556.

111. Lindner V, Reidy MA. Proliferation of smooth muscle cells after vascular injury is inhibited by an antibody against basic fibroblast growth factor. *Proc Natl Acad Sci USA* 1991; 88:3739–3743.

112. Majesky MW, Daemen MJAP, Schwartz SM. α_1-Adrenergic stimulation of platelet-derived growth factor α-chain gene expression in rat aorta. *J Biol Chem* 1990; 265:1082–1088.

113. Ferns GAA, Raines EW, Sprugel KH, Motani AS, Reidy MA, Ross R. Inhibition of neointimal smooth muscle accumulation after angioplasty by an antibody to PDGF. *Science* 1991; 253:1129–1133.

114. Galloway AC. Suppression of neointimal lesions after vascular injury: A role for polyclonal anti-basic fibroblast growth factor antibody. *Surgery* 1994; 116:456–462.

115. Derynck R, Jarrett JA, Chen EY, Eaton DH, Bell JR, Assoian RK, et al. Human transforming growth factor-β complementary DNA sequence and expression in normal and transformed cells. *Nature* 1985; 316:701–705.

116. Majesky MW, Lindner V, Twardzik DR, Schwartz SM, Reidy MA. Production of transforming growth factor β₁ during repair of arterial injury. *J Clin Invest* 1991; 88:904–910.

117. Nabel EG, Shum L, Pompili VJ, Yang Z-Y, San H, Shu HB, et al. Direct transfer of transforming growth factor β₁ gene into arteries stimulates fibrocellular hyperplasia. *Proc Natl Acad Sci USA* 1993; 90:10759–10763.

118. Stouffer GA, Owens GK. TGF-β promotes proliferation of cultured SMC via both PDGF-AA-dependent and PDGF-AA-independent mechanisms. *J Clin Invest* 1994; 93:2048–2055.

119. Seifert RA, Coats SA, Raines EW, Ross R, Bowen-Pope DF. Platelet-derived growth factor (PDGF) receptor α-subunit mutant and reconstituted cell lines demonstrate that transforming growth factor-β can be mitogenic through PDGF A-chain-dependent and -independent pathways. *J Biol Chem* 1994; 269:13951–13955.

120. Koff A, Ohtsuki M, Polyak K, Roberts JM, Massague J. Negative regulation of G1 in mammalian cells: Inhibition of cyclin E-dependent kinase by TGF-β. *Science* 1993; 260:536–539.

121. Montesano R, Vassalli J-D, Baird A, Guillemin R, Orci L. Basic fibroblast growth factor induces angiogenesis *in vitro*. *Proc Natl Acad Sci USA* 1986; 83:7297–7301.

122. Kandel J, Bossy-Wetzel E, Radvanyi F, Klagsbrun M, Folkman J, Hanahan D. Neovascularization is associated with a switch to the export of bFGF in the multistep development of fibrosarcoma. *Cell* 1991; 66:1095–1104.

123. Yanagisawa-Miwa A, Uchida Y, Nakamura F, Tomaru T, Kido H, Kamijo T, et al. Salvage of infarcted myocardium by angiogenic action of basic fibroblast growth factor. *Science* 1992; 257:1401–1403.

124. Unger EF, Banai S, Shou M, Lazarous DF, Jaklitsch MT, Scheinowitz M, et al. Basic fibroblast growth factor enhances myocardial collateral flow in a canine model. *Am J Physiol* 1994; 266:H1588–H1595.

125. Lindner V, Olson NE, Clowes AW, Reidy MA. Inhibition of smooth muscle cell proliferation in injured rat arteries. Interaction of heparin with basic fibroblast growth factor. *J Clin Invest* 1992; 90:2044–2049.

126. Lindner V, Majack RA, Reidy MA. Basic fibroblast growth factor stimulates endothelial regrowth and proliferation in denuded arteries. *J Clin Invest* 1990; 85:2004–2008.

127. Ali S, Becker MW, Davis MG, Dorn GW II. Dissociation of vasoconstrictor-stimulated basic fibroblast growth factor expression from hypertrophic growth in cultured vascular smooth muscle cells: Relevant roles of protein kinase C. *Circ Res* 1994; 75:836–843.

128. Coffin JD, Florkiewicz RF, Neuman J, Hopkins TM, Dorn GW II, Lightfoot P, et al. Abnormal bone growth and selective translational regulation in basic fibroblast growth factor (FGF-2) transgenic mice. *J Cell Biol* 1995; 6:1861–1873.

129. Florkiewicz RZ, Sommer A. Human basic fibroblast growth factor gene encodes four polypeptides: Three initiate translation from non-AUG codons. *Proc Natl Acad Sci USA* 1989; 86:3978–3981.

130. Bugler B, Amalric F, Prats H. Alternative initiation of translation determines cytoplasmic or nuclear localization of basic fibroblast growth factor. *Mol Cell Biol* 1991; 11:573–577.

131. Bashkin P, Neufeld G, Gitay-Goren H, Vlodavsky I. Release of cell surface–associated basic fibroblast growth factor by glycosylphosphatidylinositol-specific phospholipase C. *J Cell Physiol* 1992; 151:126–137.

132. Brunner G, Metz CN, Nguyen H, Gabrilove J, Patel SR, Davitz MA, et al. An endogenous glycosylphosphatidylinositol-specific phospholipase D releases basic fibroblast growth factor–heparan sulfate proteoglycan complexes from human bone marrow cultures. *Blood* 1994; 83(8):2115–2125.

133. Florkiewicz RZ, Shibata F, Barankiewicz T, Baird A, Gonzalez A-M, Florkiewicz E, et al. Basic fibroblast growth factor gene expression. *Ann NY Acad Sci* 1991; 638:109–126.

134. Quarto N, Talarico D, Florkiewicz R, Rifkin DB. Selective expression of high-molecular-weight basic fibroblast growth factor confers a unique phenotype to NIH 3T3 cells. *Cell Reg* 1991; 2:699–708.

135. Bikfalvi A, Klein S, Pintucci G, Quarto N, Mignatti P, Rifkin DB. Differential modulation of cell phenotype by different molecular weight forms of basic fibroblast growth factor: Possible intracellular signaling by the high-molecular-weight forms. *J Cell Biol* 1995; 129:233–243.

136. Couderec B, Prats H, Bayard F, Amalric F. Potential oncogenic effects of basic fibroblast growth factor require cooperation between CUG and AUG-initiated forms. *Cell Reg* 1991; 2:709–718.

7

PRINCIPLES OF MOLECULAR BIOLOGY AND CARDIAC DEVELOPMENT

Robert Roberts / Robert J. Schwartz

The application of the techniques of recombinant DNA to cardiovascular disorders appears to be both essential and ideally suited to overcome several of the major obstacles to immediate and future progress.[1–3] The heart exhibits three characteristic adaptive responses to changes in its environment: The constitutive adaptive mechanism—namely, myofibril stretch that regulates cardiac output on a beat-to-beat basis (Starling's Law)[4]; modulation of excitation contraction coupling through intramyofibril calcium leading to increased heart rate and force of contraction; and the long-term adaptation of compensatory growth (see Chap. 6). The first two adaptations have been characterized extensively in this century through the development, refinement, and application of hemodynamic techniques. To understand the long-term adaptive mechanism of cardiac growth will require an elucidation of the molecular genetic basis of this response and ultimately of cardiac differentiation and development, particularly if one desires to modulate growth therapeutically. Similarly, elimination of restenosis after angioplasty will probably require disruption of the smooth-muscle proliferative response.[5–7] To unravel the molecular basis of hereditary cardiac disorders, including the cardiomyopathies, will definitely require molecular genetics[8,9] (see Chap. 69).

Analogously, genetically engineered drugs such as tissue plasminogen activator required recombinant DNA techniques,[10] which initiated a paradigmatic shift in the therapy of myocardial infarction resulting in an acute mortality of only 6 percent; this was quickly followed by recombinant hirudin, superoxide dismutase, urokinase, prourokinase, and multiple mutant forms of tissue plasminogen activator.[11]

HISTORICAL PERSPECTIVE OF MOLECULAR BIOLOGY

In 1953, Watson and Crick[12,13] proposed the double-helix model for DNA structure based on the results of x-ray defrac-tion by Franklin, Wilkins, and others.[14,15] The implications of DNA being a double helix were evident; namely, that one strand could serve as a template for the synthesis of another strand, thus providing the means whereby genetic information could be perpetuated from parent to offspring. In 1957, Schekman et al.[16] described DNA polymerase, the enzyme necessary for the synthesis of DNA that was essential to recombinant DNA technology. Marmor and colleagues[17] showed that the double helix of DNA could be separated by high temperatures[18] into its separate strands (denatured) and that decreasing the temperature resulted in the strands reannealing, or hybridizing, thus returning to their previous double stranded nature. This specific hybridization, or "base-pairing" of complementary nucleotide strands, provides both the rationale and the practical basis for much of recombinant DNA technology. Crick had suggested correctly that the genetic code would be written in codons of three nucleotides for each amino acid.[13] The specific combination of three nucleotides that code for each amino acid was unraveled by Nirenberg, Khorana, and colleagues.[19,20] Several other necessary components were discovered subsequently including the enzyme DNA ligase, which joins DNA fragments together.[21] All of this information was known in the 1960s, as was the complete DNA code, mRNA, and the cytoplasmic ribosomal RNA for protein synthesis; but recombinant technology was not yet born and, in fact, for the next few years did not appear promising.

Many important discoveries, including those from the 1950s, played a role in recombinant technology, but four that really brought it to fruition and made possible modern molecular biology occurred between the years of 1970 and 1977. A major obstacle to the manipulation of DNA was its large size with no means to cut it into smaller pieces of known specific size. This obstacle was overcome by the discovery of restriction endonucleases, which made it possible to cut DNA into smaller pieces in a predictable fashion.[22,23] These endonucleases, more commonly referred to as *restriction en-*

zymes, recognize specific sequences of DNA consisting of anywhere from four to eight nucleotides and specifically cut the DNA molecules at their recognition sites, making it possible to utilize and manipulate DNA fragments in a variety of procedures and reactions. In 1972, the enzyme reverse transcriptase was discovered by Baltimore and by Temin and Mizutani simultaneously,[24,25] making it possible to translate messenger RNA (mRNA) into its complementary DNA (cDNA). Shortly after, the group at Stanford[26] cloned the first molecule, and recombinant DNA techniques were born, as was modern molecular biology. Modern molecular biology rapidly accelerated into reality, and development has continued to accelerate. In 1977, Sanger and Coulson[27] and Maxam and Gilbert[28] developed techniques for the rapid sequencing of DNA. In addition to these four developments, the recent development of polymerase chain reaction (PCR), a technique that can be used to amplify rapidly small amounts of DNA or RNA several millionfold, is having a revolutionary effect on the application of these techniques in medicine and other fields.

NUCLEIC ACIDS

The Essentials of Nucleic Acids

The human genome is known to contain about 3 billion base pairs (bp), which contain information that would more than fill a 500,000-page textbook. The DNA is contained in 46 chromosomes consisting of 44 autosomal and two sex chromosomes, but each chromosome is one continuous DNA molecule around which is wrapped several proteins. The smallest chromosome, twenty-one, has more than 50 million bp, while chromosome one, the largest has over 250 million bp. There is enough DNA to form several hundred thousand genes; however, it is estimated that only about 67,000 genes encode for a human being. This would indicate that less than 5 percent of DNA is used to code for protein. The remainder of the DNA is used to provide spacing, structure, regulatory information, and other as-yet-unknown functions.

DNA consists of four building blocks referred to as *nucleotides,* or merely as bases. A nucleotide consists of a nitrogenous base, a 5-carbon sugar, deoxyribose, and a phosphate group (Fig. 7-1). There are two purine bases (adenine and guanine) and two pyrimidine bases (cytosine and thymine) (Fig. 7-2). The triphosphate molecule is bonded to the 5′ carbon of the sugar, and the base is bonded to the 1′ carbon of the sugar. Each DNA molecule consists of millions of nucleotides joined together in a linear fashion through the phosphate group, which forms a bond with the hydroxyl group of the 3′ carbon of the next sugar. The water-soluble phosphate groups form the backbone and face outward. Attached to the inner side of the sugar is the hydrophobic base, shielded from the aqueous environment. The molecule forms a right-sided spiral coil with a turn every 10 nucleotides (3.4 nM), referred to as a right-sided α-helix, and pairs with its complementary strand to form the so-called double helix (Fig. 7-3). The center of the molecule consists of the bases, which face inward and

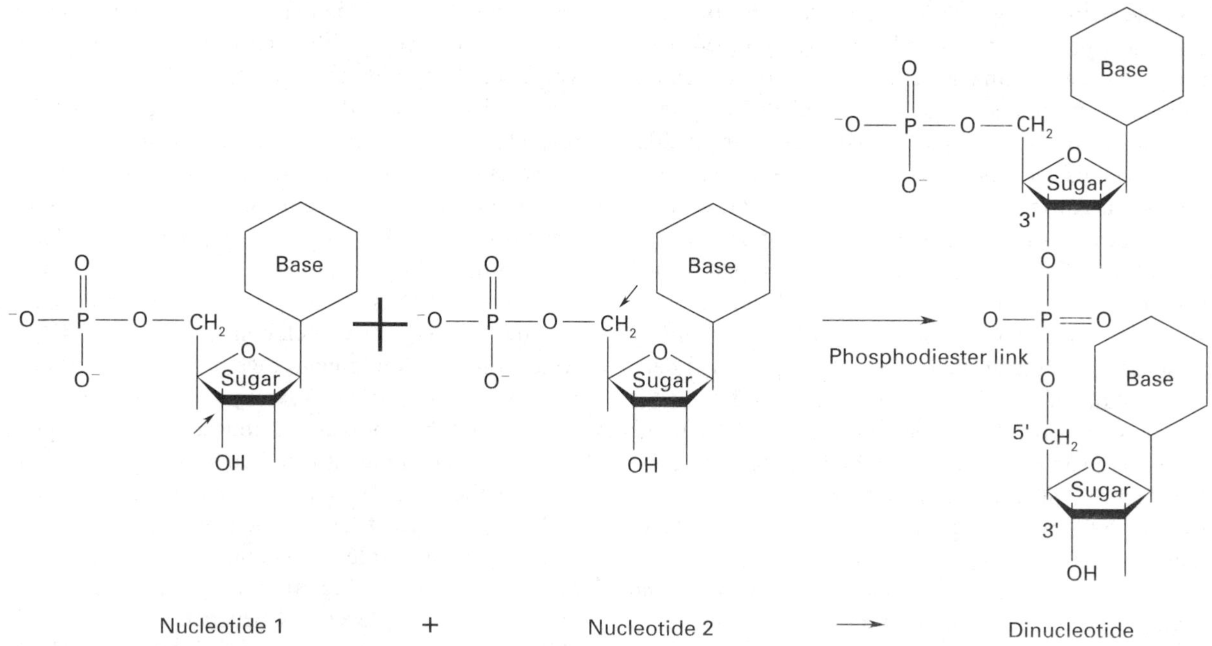

Nucleotide 1   +   Nucleotide 2   ⟶   Dinucleotide

FIGURE 7-1

Formation of polynucleotides from nucleotide precursors. Nucleotides are joined together by a phosphodiester linkage to form a nucleic acid. Arrows indicate the carbon atoms of deoxyribose that are joined by phosphodiester bonds to form polynucleotides. Note that the bases are attached to 1′ carbon position of the sugar molecule and face the interior of the molecule. The backbone is formed by the sugar linked by phosphate groups binding to 5′ and 3′ carbons of the sugar. (From Mares A Jr. et al. Molecular biology for the cardiologist. *Curr Probl Cardiol* 1992; 17:9–72. Reproduced with permission from the publisher and authors.)

Purine bases

Adenine
(A)

Guanine
(G)

Pyrimidine bases

Cytosine
(C)

Thymine
(T)

FIGURE 7-2

The common purine and pyrimidine bases found in DNA. Uracil is substituted for thymine in RNA. (From Mares A Jr. et al. Molecular biology for the cardiologist. *Curr Probl Cardiol* 1992; 17:9–72. Reproduced with permission from the publisher and authors.)

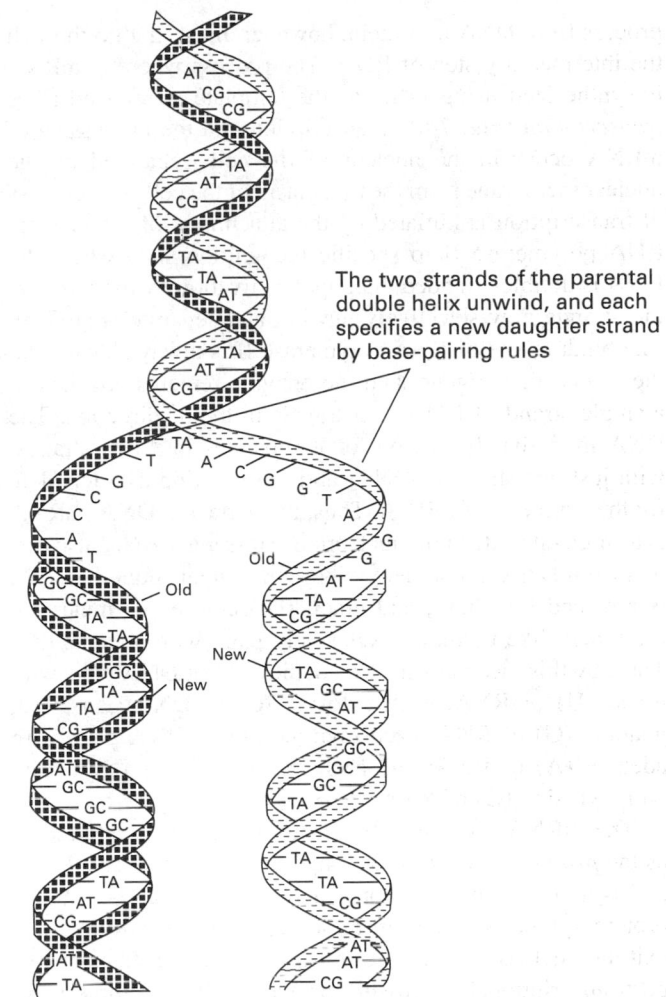

The two strands of the parental double helix unwind, and each specifies a new daughter strand by base-pairing rules

FIGURE 7-3

DNA replication conserves the nucleotide sequence. DNA is a double-stranded helical molecule bound together by the nucleotide bases contained on each individual strand. During cell division, two identical copies of the original parental strand are made by unwinding the DNA and then synthesizing a complementary second strand to make two identical new daughter strands.

are opposite to each other. This arrangement provides for the hydrogen bonding between the bases that keeps the two strands together. The hydrogen bonds are perpendicular to the helical axis. The directionality of the strands is referred to as 5′ to 3′ or 3′ to 5′, which refers to the position of the carbons in the sugar. The end of the molecule with a phosphate or hydroxyl group on the 5′ carbon is termed the *5′ end,* whereas the end with a free terminal 3′ carbon is referred to as the *3′ end.* It is important to distinguish the two ends, since DNA replication always proceeds from the 5′ to the 3′ end. There seem to be no constraints on which bases can be adjacent to each other; however, the hydrogen binding between the bases of the two chains is highly specific, as adenine (A) always pairs with thymine (T), and guanine (G) always pairs with cytosine (C). The sugars and the phosphate groups are always the same, whereas the sequence of the bases determines the nature of the hereditary information to be passed on to the progeny. The specificity of this "base pairing" is the basis of the ability of DNA to replicate itself and pass on the genotype characteristics; it also forms the basis for the specificity of essentially all of the procedures used in recombinant DNA technology. During the process of DNA replication, the strands separate and new strands form complementary to the original strands, resulting in two additional identical molecules.

Transcription

The central dogma of molecular biology is that DNA produces RNA, which in turn produces a polypeptide, the latter being the molecules that make up the proteins that provide the cell

structure and perform the functions of the cell (Fig. 7-4). The genetic information inherited by each individual is encoded by the sequence of the bases of the DNA (the *genotype*), which is translated into proteins and provides the observable characteristics of the individual (the *phenotype*). This overall

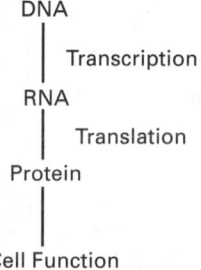

DNA
| Transcription
RNA
| Translation
Protein
|
Cell Function

FIGURE 7-4
Central dogma of molecular biology.

process from DNA to protein, however, must first go through the intermediary step of RNA. The process whereby mRNA is synthesized using DNA as the template is referred to as *transcription* (Fig. 7-5). Transcription and the processing of mRNA occur in the nucleus of the cell, separated by the nuclear membrane from the cytoplasm of the cell. The process of transcription is initiated by the attachment of the enzyme RNA polymerase II to specific recognition sites where the DNA is double-stranded, but, upon activation by the enzyme, the strands now selectively unwind and separate (Fig. 7-6). The binding site of RNA polymerase II is always located on the 5′ end of the gene, and the enzyme remains attached to a single strand of DNA as it travels in the 3′ direction. The DNA immediately in front of it separates into two strands, with just one strand of DNA (antisense) acting as a template for the synthesis of mRNA. Thus, in contrast to DNA, mRNA is a single-stranded polynucleotide. Messenger RNA also differs from DNA in that deoxyribose, the sugar found in DNA, is replaced by ribose, and uracil (U) replaces thymine (T); the uracil, like thymine, exclusively pairs with adenine (A). Thus, by this mechanism each adenine (A) of DNA pairs with uracil (U) of RNA; each cytosine (C) of DNA pairs with guanine (G) of RNA; each thymine (T) of DNA pairs with adenine (A) of RNA; and each guanine (G) of DNA pairs with cytosine (C) of RNA.

The mRNA, as transcribed from the DNA, is referred to as the *primary transcript,* or sometimes as immature mRNA, and is a complementary copy of the DNA (Fig. 7-7). Since protein synthesis occurs in the cytoplasm, the mRNA must exit the nucleus, but prior to transport it undergoes extensive posttranscriptional processing primarily through three main events: (1) Addition of a methylated guanosine (7-methylguanosine residue) to the 5′ end, referred to as a cap, which is important for the initiation of translation; (2) addition of a long tail of repeated adenine nucleotides, called the poly (A) tail, to the 3′ region of the mRNA, essential for stability of

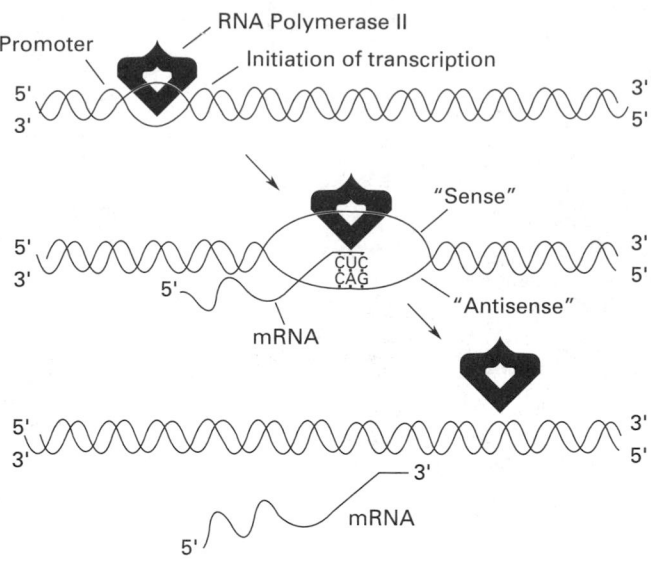

FIGURE 7-6

Illustration of how RNA polymerase II interacts with DNA and the promoter to generate a single-stranded mRNA. RNA polymerase II attaches to the initiation site promoted by the 5′ promoter sequence. mRNA is synthesized in the 5′ to 3′ direction from just one stand, the antisense strand. The specificity of base pairing between mRNA and the antisense strand provides for a mRNA with sequences complementary to that of the antisense and identical to that of the sense strands.

the message in the cytoplasm; and (3) the primary transcript, which contains introns and exons, undergoes a specific splicing process whereby the introns are removed and the exons are properly respliced together prior to exit from the nucleus as mature mRNA. The process of splicing is, in part, performed by molecules referred to as *small nuclear ribonucleoproteins,* which consist of RNA molecules tightly associated with a group of about 10 different proteins. Exons survive the mRNA processing and exit the nucleus (hence the name) as part of the mature mRNA. The mRNA consist of three

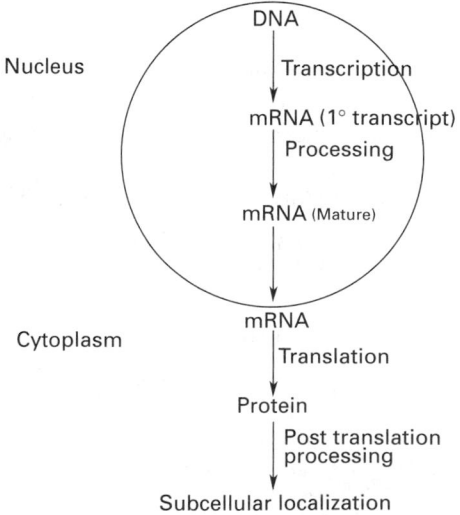

FIGURE 7-5

Schematic localization of the processes of transcription and translation.

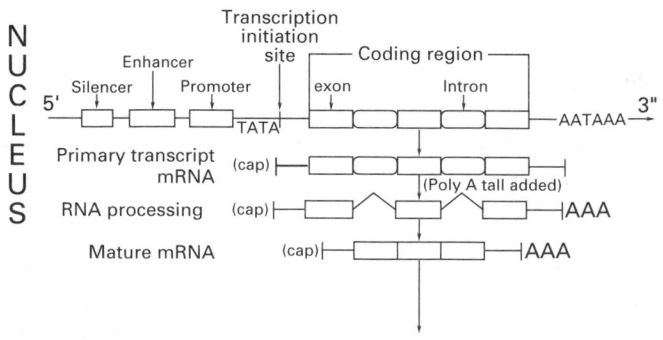

FIGURE 7-7

Transcription. Transcription occurs in the nucleus, producing mRNA that is processed into mature mRNA and transported to the cytoplasm. In the cytoplasm, translation occurs with the mRNA coding for specific amino acids, which are linked together to form a polypeptide and ultimately to form a mature protein. (From Mares A Jr. et al. Molecular biology for the cardiologist. *Curr Probl Cardiol* 1992; 17:9–72. Reproduced with permission from the publisher and authors.)

distinct regions. The exons of the 5′ end are not translated into protein but signal the beginning of mRNA translation and contain sequences that direct the mRNA to the ribosome in the cytoplasm for protein synthesis. The exons in the second region, referred to as the *coding region,* contain the information that determines the amino acid sequence of the protein. The exons of the 3′ end do not code for protein but for signals that terminate translation and direct the addition of the poly (A) tail. Introns are portions of the gene included in the primary mRNA transcript but are spliced out of the mature mRNA. The process of splicing out of introns and the rejoining of exons is an important means of introducing genetic diversity, since one mRNA may provide several different mRNAs that code for different polypeptides; this will be discussed further under gene regulation. The primary transcript undergoes extensive shortening such that the mature mRNA often represents only 10 percent of the primary transcript. The mature mRNA exits the nucleus through nuclear pores, enters the cytoplasm, and attaches to a ribosome to initiate protein synthesis.

Translation

The final process whereby the nucleic acids of the mRNA code for a specific polypeptide is referred to as *translation.* This process is the most complex of the various processes that occur in the flow from genomic DNA (gene) to the mature protein. The alphabet of the DNA or its single-stranded complementary mRNA is that of the four nucleotides (bases), while that of the protein is the 20 amino acids. Crick in 1961,[12] while trying to determine the code for translation from DNA to protein, showed that the genetic code was written in triplets of bases, with each amino acid being encoded by three bp, referred to as a *codon,* and specific amino acids determined by the sequence of the codon. The mRNA codons dictate which amino acids are to be selected, and the order of the codons dictates the sequence of the amino acids in the protein. Determination of the codons for each amino acid was completed in 1966. There are four different nucleotides to form the triplets; thus, the number of combinations (4^3) is 64, but there are only 20 amino acids. There is considerable redundancy, referred to as *degeneracy,* which results in most of the amino acids having more than one codon. In addition to codons for each amino acid, there is also the codon AUG, which is the start codon that

initiates protein synthesis and also codes for methionine. To stop translation, there are three codons, UAA, UAG, and UGA, which signal the end of a particular polypeptide. Translation into protein requires two other RNA species, ribosomal RNA (rRNA) and transfer RNA (tRNA). The mRNA, after exiting the nucleus, recognizes the ribosome, which is the site of protein synthesis. The ribosome moves along an mRNA molecule, translating each of its codons in a 5′ to 3′ direction to assemble the polypeptide from its amino (N-terminal) to its carboxy (C-terminal) ends (Fig. 7-8).

The mRNA does not interact directly with amino acids but rather through adaptor molecules—tRNA—to which amino acids are covalently joined by a highly specific enzyme (amino acid tRNA synthetase) utilizing ATP. There is at least one tRNA species corresponding to each of the 20 naturally occurring amino acids. The aminoacyl tRNA synthetase performs a special function of activating the amino acids and assuring that each amino acid is joined to its tRNA and to no other. The structure of tRNA is now known in great detail, and its specificity is attributed to the sequence of three nucleotides complementary to the codon exposed at one end of the folded tRNA molecule which, on the tRNA, is referred to as the *anticodon.* The amino acid receptor site is exposed at the other end. Amino acids are thus specified at two recognition steps: one in which a specific enzyme joins the amino acid to a specific tRNA and the other in which the tRNA, serving

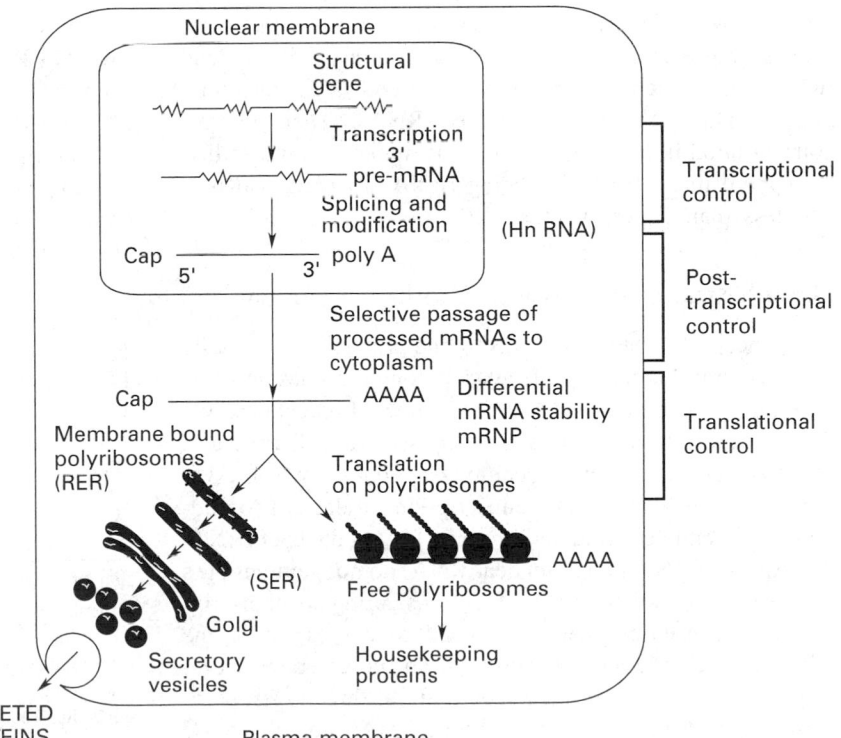

FIGURE 7-8

A summary of the multiple steps involved in gene expression from the genomic DNA to the protein, showing how the protein destined for secretion follows a systematic path different from those destined to remain in the cytoplasm. (From Nucleic acids and protein biosynthesis. In: Campbell PN, Smith AD, eds. *Biochemistry Illustrated,* 2d ed. New York: Churchill Livingstone; 1988:111. Reproduced with permission from the publisher.)

as an adaptor molecule, joins the amino acid to the ribosomal-mRNA complex through a codon-anticodon specific-base-pairing interaction between the mRNA and the tRNA. Once the process of protein synthesis is initiated, the ribosome moves along the mRNA, joining the amino acids via peptide bonds in the sequence specified by the mRNA to form the mature polypeptide. The process of protein synthesis from this complex of mRNA and ribosome involves over 100 enzymes. The steps involved consist of initiation, elongation, and termination of the polypeptide, with each process having its own enzymes.

The mature polypeptide consists of amino acids joined together by peptide bonds; however, the mature protein often consists of multiple covalently bound polypeptides, and many undergo other modifications referred to as *posttranslational changes*. Encoded in the polypeptide are other features that have been determined by the mRNA; namely, leader sequences that will direct the protein to either intracellular membranes, the plasma membrane, or to organelles, such as the mitochondria. There is also considerable proteolytic activity following entry of the molecule into its organelle, or membrane, as the leader sequences are removed. There are also the processes whereby disulfhydryl bonds are formed or glycosylation occurs (in the Golgi apparatus) (Fig. 7-8). The mRNAs generally are not long-lived due to their rapid degradation by RNAses and so may last from only a few minutes to many hours. A single mRNA may code for only a few copies of the polypeptide or several thousand. The average estimate is 1400. In contrast, rRNAs and tRNAs are much less rapidly degraded and, therefore, have acquired the name "stable" RNAs. Their relative concentration in the cell, in large part, reflects their stability, with more than 80 percent being rRNA, 15 percent tRNA, and less than 5 percent mRNA.

Gene Structure, Expression, and Its Regulation

The concept that one gene leads to one protein remains basic to the central dogma of molecular biology but does, in some cases, need to be modified slightly in view of recent observations. In the classic sense, a gene consists of a discrete unit of DNA that encodes for a specific *polypeptide*. Two observations must be noted. First, transcription produces two endpoints—ribonucleic acid and protein. The products of rRNA, tRNA, and snRNA (small nuclear RNA) do not get translated into protein but rather perform functions during posttranscription and translation that are pivotal to expression of the mRNA, which does code for protein. The polymerases necessary for transcription of these genes are of three types, polymerase I for rRNA, polymerase II for mRNA, and polymerase III for tRNA and some other smaller nuclear RNAs. Second, in part because of snRNA and certain proteins, alternative splicing of the exons in the primary mRNA can lead to different mature mRNAs, with each coding for a slightly different polypeptide. The forms, however, are generally isoforms of the same protein, such as multiple forms of tropomyosin from the same gene. The class of genes that encode for proteins

do so only through mRNA. The following discussion will address the regulation of those genes that encode for proteins.

The anatomy of a protein-coding gene is composed of introns and exons. The average exon is about 300 bp, while introns are much larger and are spliced out of the mature mRNA and thus do not code for protein. A typical mRNA has three regions: the 5' untranslated region that contains the *cis*-acting sequences that regulate translation; the central portion, referred to as the *coding region*, which codes for protein; and the 3' untranslated end, which also has regulatory sequences and coding signals for stability of the mature mRNA. The first nucleotide to be transcribed is given the $+1$ number, and everything 5' to it is referred to as upstream or proximal and is numbered with the first base pair as -1, etc. The initiation site for transcription is always upstream from the 5' end of the translated region. The 5' regulatory untranslated region has variable sequences, but there are several consistent sequences present in the same position in most human genes. Polymerase II has no affinity for DNA and can only bind after several transcription factors (TF) have bound. The site of transcription and its direction are determined by the TATA box, which has a consensus sequence of TATAA(T)AA(T) and is found at -25 to -30 bp upstream from the start site. A large complex of TF (more than 25 proteins) bind to the TATA box in preparation for RNA polymerase II binding and transcription. Collectively they are referred to as TFII (transcription factors for polymerase II), with letters designating the different factors. TFIID binds first, then TFIIB followed by RNA polymerase II followed by several TFII factors such as E, F, G, H, and J. TFIIH has kinase activity and phosphorylates RNA polymerase II, which now, independent of transcription factors, can initiate transcription. Also in many human genes located at about -200 bp upstream is the GGG CG box to which SP1 binds; it is felt to be a regulatory of "housekeeping" genes (see below; Fig. 7-9).

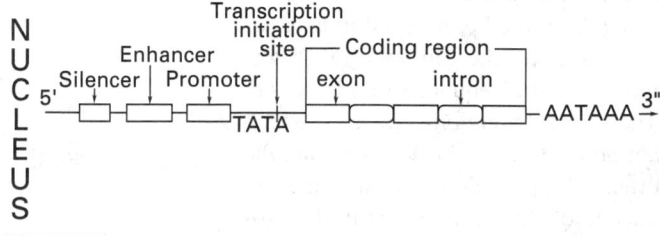

FIGURE 7-9

Structure of a gene. These small functional units within the nucleus contain the coding information for the synthesis of a polypeptide and on its 5' end have regulatory sequences that include silencers, enhancers, and promoters. The coding region consisting of exons (code for protein) as well as intervening noncoding sequences (introns) is followed by a 3' non-coding region that is translated into the mRNA. The 3' end appears important for exit of the mRNA from the nucleus and its stability in the cytoplasm but does not code for protein. The TATA is the initiation site for polymerase and is present in most eukaryotes at about 10 to 30 bp 5' from the start codon (TAC) of the coding region. The AATAA will become the recognition site on the mRNA to which attaches an enzyme that cleaves the 3' region and replaces the distal portion with a poly A tail. (From Mares A Jr. et al. Molecular biology for the cardiologist. *Curr Probl Cardiol* 1992; 17:9–72. Reproduced with permission from the publisher and authors.)

Gene expression refers to all of the processes required to go from DNA to protein, from the initial unfolding of the nuclear chromatin in preparation for transcription until the mature protein emerges following completion of posttranslational changes. Regulation of this process occurs at all levels in response to signals both from within the cell and from the environment. The latter mechanism is of particular interest as it represents one of the major areas of research in molecular biology and cardiology and is also an area that has great potential for therapeutic intervention. The cell maintains its integrity and responds to external stimuli through signals that activate receptors (generally in the cell membrane). These in turn use signaling proteins to transfer the message to the cytoplasm or nucleus, which in some way modifies gene expression. Delineation of the receptor, the signaling proteins, and where and how gene expression is altered is of prime importance.

The most fundamental level of gene regulation involves cell differentiation (discussed below). The body contains at least 200 different types of cells that have been programmed by their genes to perform highly specialized functions. All cells have the same DNA and the same genes, but only those genes that are expressed determine the cell's phenotype. Cardiac myocytes, for example, are characterized by a set of proteins that specialize in contractile activity, while hepatocytes specialize in the synthesis and catabolism of proteins. Selective gene expression is the basis of cell differentiation. Cell growth and replication occur in what is termed the undifferentiated cell but, through complex mechanisms, give rise to cells that cease to replicate and are programmed to take on specialized functions (cell differentiation). In the process of cell differentiation, genes—particularly those concerned with cell proliferation and undifferentiated functions—are downregulated, while those genes coding for the proteins that perform the specialized functions are upregulated. Once cells are differentiated, however, protein synthesis remains a dynamic process to maintain cell integrity. Most of gene regulation is concerned with the maintenance of cellular integrity, and the genes responsible for this basal function are referred to as *housekeeping genes*. Housekeeping genes are constitutively regulated, as opposed to genes responsible for cell differentiation and growth that are developmentally regulated. It is estimated that organs utilize about 10,000 genes (constitutive) to maintain their integrity, with one exception—the brain, which is estimated to utilize around 20,000 genes. Regulation may be classified under the following headings: pretranscription, transcription, posttranscription, translation, and posttranslation.[29]

Pretranscriptional regulation refers to the decompaction of the DNA and exposure of the region about to undergo transcription. The total DNA of a single cell would measure about 1 m in length, yet in the nucleus it is markedly compacted and is folded around specific proteins, the dominant class being histone. The coiling of the DNA appears to be in domains that can be exposed when transcription is activated. It is also at this level that methylation plays a role, in that heavily methylated genes tend not to be transcribed, while other areas sensitive to digestion by the enzyme DNase appear to be very active in transcription. The precise mechanisms involved with chromatin conformational changes or exposure of the gene for transcription are, at present, relatively unknown. There is evidence, however, that methylation is involved in regulating cell differentiation.

The role of transcriptional control is a major rate-limiting step to gene expression. While transcription is catalyzed by the enzyme RNA polymerase II, the enzyme by itself cannot initiate transcription and acts only with the help of additional TFs. In addition to the promoter sequences previously described (TATA box and CG box), several DNA sequences in conjunction with their DNA binding proteins act as either promoters, enhancers, or silencers of transcription and will be subsequently defined (Fig. 7-9). The 5' upstream region immediately adjacent to the transcription initiation site, and including the area that binds RNA polymerase II, is referred to as the *promoter region*. This region contains sequences that are specific binding sites for proteins—TFs, also referred to as *transacting factors*. The protein binding sites are often referred to as *cis*-acting sequences since they are on the same DNA molecule on which they act. The TFs (also referred to as DNA-binding proteins) are also called transacting factors (acting at a distance) since they are encoded by genes that may even be on another chromosome. The average promoter binding site consists of several hundred bp grouped into motifs of 4 to 10 bp.[30] It is hypothesized that all of the motifs have to be bound by TFs of the appropriate nature and in the appropriate sequence for transcription to occur.

The promoter sequences and their corresponding DNA-binding proteins may act ubiquitously or may be tissue specific. Promoters often increase transcription of a class of genes rather than a single gene. Another type of DNA sequence that increases transcription is referred to as an *enhancer* (Fig. 7-9). These differ from promoter sequences in that they may be upstream or downstream from the coding region and be separated by as much as hundreds of thousands of bp and are effective whether in the 5' to 3' or 3' to 5' direction. An extreme example is the DNA sequence that enhances expression of the gene for hemoglobin that is located more than 1 million bp from the transcription initiation site. These enhancers, like promoters, consist of several small motifs of 4 to 10 bp and, when bound by their corresponding DNA-binding proteins (TFs), have a positive influence on gene transcription. Another regulatory DNA sequence that is similar to enhancers in size and location but exerts a negative influence on transcription is referred to as a *silencer* or *repressor*. It is believed that enhancer and silencer sequences, when bound by TFs, communicate with promoters by DNA looping that is induced by the binding. This DNA binding that brings the enhancer, silencer, and promoter in close proximity is the mechanism responsible for the action-at-a-distance phenomenon seen in human gene regulation.

The genes that encode proteins regulating cardiac growth are many: growth factors, growth factor receptors, intracellular signaling proteins that relay growth signals from the extracellular milieu, and, ultimately, the TFs that regulate RNA polymerase and selectively induce or downregulate gene expression.[31] There are at least 10 motifs of DNA-binding proteins (TFs) (Fig. 7-10), including the zinc fingers, leucine zippers, helix-loop-helix (HLH), MADS domain, and the helix-turn-helix proteins. The zinc-finger type is utilized by developmental genes, called GATA factors, and the receptors for circulating hormones, including the glucocorticoids, progesterones, androgens, mineralocorticoids, estrogen, thyroxine, vitamin D_3, and retinoic acid. These hormones, which are lipophilic, penetrate the cell membrane and activate an intracellular receptor or nuclear receptor, which, in turn, activates gene expression through the zinc-finger transcription proteins. Many of the growth-related signaling proteins, such as *c-fos, jun-B,* and *c-jun,* dimerize through leucine zippers prior to binding to DNA. For example, *c-fos* dimerizes with *c-jun* and subsequently binds to DNA.[32] TFs such as the myo-D family genes, which are the master genes for inducing differentiation of skeletal muscle, contain an HLH motif. The MADS domain–containing proteins include myocyte enhancer factor 2 (MEF2) and the serum response factor (SRF). The helix-turn-helix proteins include homeodomain-containing proteins, which are important in the development of prokaryotes and eukaryotes.

Another level at which gene expression may be regulated is that of mRNA processing, whereby the introns are removed and the exons spliced together to provide the mature mRNA. In the majority of instances, each exon present in the gene is incorporated into a mature mRNA via ligation of consecutive pairs of exons with removal of all introns. This constitutive splicing process produces a single gene product from each transcriptional unit, even when the coding sequence is split into many separated exons. In other instances, however, nonconsecutive exons are joined in the processing of some gene transcripts, and this alternative pattern of primary mRNA splicing can exclude individual exons from mature mRNA in some transcripts and include them in others. The use of such differential splicing patterns creates mRNAs that generate a variety of proteins from a single gene. Differential splicing is particularly prevalent in genes of muscles and has been shown to occur in three of the eight major sarcomeric proteins studied thus far—myosin heavy chains (MHC), tropomyosin, and troponin T (skeletal and cardiac).

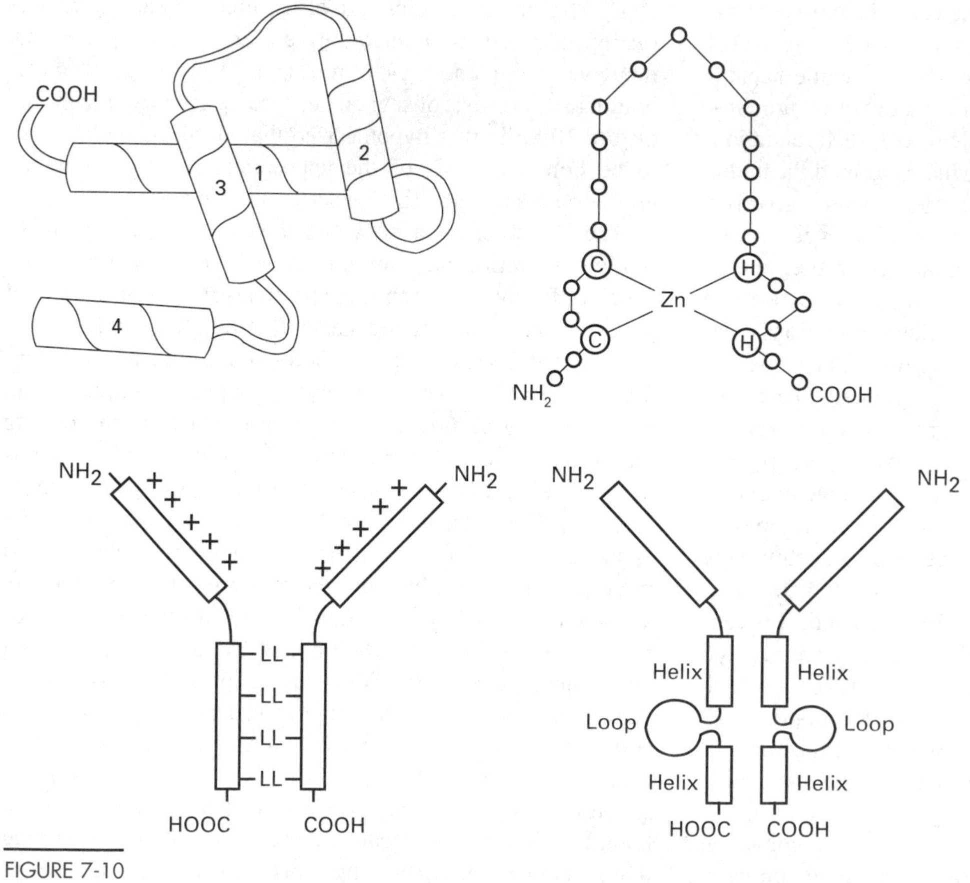

The 3′ non-protein-coding region of the mature mRNA contains the poly (A) tail that is essential for message stability. It is believed that protein synthesis is, in part, regulated on the basis of alterations in message stability. The precise mechanism whereby an mRNA is induced to remain stable and encode for several thousand polypeptides as opposed to being extremely unstable and encoding for only a few molecules is not well understood. Nevertheless, it is likely to be an important step in regulating the response to cytoplasmic signals that require rapid synthesis of a particular polypeptide. Synthesis of a polypeptide initiated via transcription is estimated to take several minutes, while synthesis of a protein initiated through translation requires only seconds. Regulation of gene expression also occurs at the translational and posttranslational levels. Proteins are often translated as precursors, which must undergo proteolytic cleavage. Others must undergo cleavage of leader sequences attached to direct them to their particular subcellular compartment. Other posttranslational modifications

FIGURE 7-10

Type of transcription factors that effect gene activation. Schematic representation of the shape of four types of protein transcription factors that bond to DNA and influence gene activation. Helix-turn-helix is a protein with two α-helices separated by a β-turn. Leucine zippers are protein dimers with entering leucine amino acids. Zinc fingers have a peptide loop connected at the base by a zinc ion tetrahedran between cysteine and/or histidine in amino acids. The helix-loop-helix consists of α-helix but utilizes leucine zippers and has a loop between the α-helices. The darkened areas are believed to be the regions of the protein that interact with the DNA to modulate transcription.

include protein glycosylation, or the addition of polysaccharides and lipids, and the formation of disulfide bonds. Finally, polypeptides often require polymerization into complex tertiary structures to form the mature proteins.

Modern Molecular Biology and the Basis for Recombinant DNA Technology

Modern molecular biology, initiated in the 1970s,[28,33] was in part due to four pivotal discoveries or inventions: restriction enzymes, reverse transcription, cloning, and DNA sequencing. Since DNA consists simply of four nucleotides joined together, it is a monotonous, repetitive molecule that, at first glance, offers no landmarks for recognizing that a particular segment of DNA codes for a particular mRNA. The discovery of the restriction endonucleases provided the genetic scalpel to cut DNA into smaller pieces of predictable size, which could be utilized in a variety of procedures. The unique feature of these enzymes is that each recognizes a specific sequence of DNA of 4 to 8 bp and cleaves the molecule at that particular site. Thus, one knows precisely where the enzyme cuts and, using a variety of different enzymes, one can identify the site and number of recognition sites for each enzyme in a fragment of DNA of interest and develop what is referred to as *restriction map*. These enzymes also made it possible to cut DNA from different sources in a predictable manner in preparation for ligating them together into a recombinant molecule. Restriction endonucleases have now been obtained from over 400 strains of bacteria that recognize more than 100 different cleavage sites. A restriction endonuclease is named after the bacterium from which it is isolated, taking the first letter of the genus of the bacterium, the first two letters of the species, and the first letter of the strain. An example of this would be an enzyme from *Haemophilus influenza* referred to as Hind-III. The III simply refers to the third restriction endonuclease enzyme isolated from that particular species of bacteria. Thus, the availability of restriction endonucleases made it possible to digest DNA into smaller molecules that could be manipulated and utilized in a variety of reactions and to develop a restriction map and chimeric DNA molecules, the latter being the essence of recombinant DNA technology.

The discovery that retroviruses contain an enzyme that catalyzes the formation of DNA from RNA, referred to as *reverse transcriptase*, revolutionized molecular biology. The resulting so-called complementary DNA (cDNA) (represented by the appropriate complementary bases for the mRNA except, of course, with thymine replacing uracil) will then bind to the nucleotide sequences from which the particular mRNA was originally derived (Fig. 7-11). Messenger RNA, as discussed previously, codes for a specific polypeptide and was derived from a discrete, specific unit of DNA referred to as a gene. Reverse transcriptase reverses this process so that the cDNA generated from the mRNA-coding part of the gene can be used as a gene to express the protein. The process whereby cDNA is reinserted into the genome of a vector (virus or

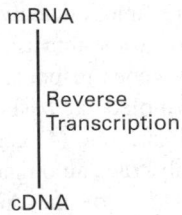

mRNA

Reverse
Transcription

cDNA

FIGURE 7-11

Generation of a complementary DNA (cDNA). Taking advantage of the enzyme, reverse transcriptase, mRNA is converted to DNA, referred to as complementary DNA, or cDNA. The DNA is single-stranded and complementary to the sequence of RNA, except thymine now replaces uracil. Utilizing DNA polymerase, one can then make the single-stranded DNA into double-stranded cDNA. The cDNA can be used as a probe to identify specific sequences or genes of the genomic DNA or it can be inserted into vectors to be cloned or expressed in a variety of hosts.

plasmid) and subsequently replicated in an appropriate host, such as a bacterium, made possible the first cloning of the gene. Radioactive labeling of a cDNA as a probe or indicator molecule provides an extraordinarily powerful tool for developing known chromosomal landmarks and for isolating and identifying particular genes. The labeled cDNA, referred to as a *probe,* is a routine, essential tool used to identify and isolate DNA or RNA fragments of interest.

Development of rapid-sequencing techniques made it possible to sequence several thousand bases per day. It is expected that a by-product of the Human Genome Project will be technology to sequence up to 100,000 bases per day.

Two features essential to all techniques of recombinant DNA technology need to be highlighted: First, the property of DNA to denature and anneal, or hybridize. The double-stranded DNA held together by hydrogen bonding of the corresponding complementary bases will, upon exposure to high temperatures (95°C), separate into two strands, but, under appropriate conditions (55°C), the complementary strands will again anneal precisely as originally and the DNA will return to its normal double-stranded state. The process of separating into separate strands is referred to as *denaturation* and the recombining process as *annealment* or *hybridization,* with the latter term preferred if the two DNA fragments are from different sources. Second, the strands come together identically to the parent molecule because of complementary base-pairing, whereby A must bind to T and C to G.

Unique Features of Recombinant DNA Technology

The techniques routinely used in molecular biology consist of electrophoresis, Southern and Northern blotting, DNA cloning, PCR, electrophoretic mobility shift assay, and the development of gene libraries. Techniques related to vessel-wall biology and gene transfer are discussed in Chap. 9. The techniques of recombinant DNA are unique and are not limited by some of the restrictions imposed on other scientific techniques.[3] Some of these are the ability to do the following:

(1) perform the structure-function analysis of a selected molecule or a portion thereof in the intact living cell or organism; (2) isolate and identify genes responsible for hereditary diseases; (3) unravel the molecular basis for the regulation of growth, including the heart; and (4) generate large quantities of protein present in only trace amounts that would not otherwise be available, and provide the opportunity to engineer proteins genetically for maximum benefit with the fewest side effects.

Isolation of DNA

Since the DNA of all human tissues is the same, practically any tissue can be utilized to obtain a DNA sample. It requires only a microgram for most procedures. In humans, lymphocytes are commonly used since they are very accessible and the DNA can be easily extracted. Lymphocytes are also used because they can be transformed by Epstein-Barr virus into an immortal cell line that can provide a continuous, renewable source of DNA. A blood sample of 10 to 15 mL of whole blood would typically yield about 50 to 100 μg of genomic DNA. If one's interest is restricted to DNA that is expressed, then one would isolate mRNA and using it as a template employ reverse transcriptase to derive its cDNA. cDNA molecules represent the expressed form of a gene and, thus, can be used as probes to select the specific genome DNA segments from which the mRNA was transcribed. Myocardial biopsies provide adequate tissue for most DNA or RNA analysis.

Digestion and Electrophoretic Separation of DNA

One of the important physical properties of the DNA molecule is that each individual nucleotide possesses a net negative charge resulting from the phosphate group. Thus, fragments of different sizes exposed to an electric field tend to migrate toward the positive electrode at differential rates depending on their size, with small fragments migrating faster than larger ones. This process of separation based on electric charge is called *electrophoresis*.[34] The DNA sample, after being digested into fragments of different size by a restriction endonuclease, is added to a gel matrix such as agarose or acrylamide. After electrophoresis, the pattern of the DNA can be visualized under an ultraviolet lamp after staining with a fluorescent dye such as ethidium bromide[35] (Fig 7-12). Agarose gel electrophoresis will separate fragments from 1000 to 60,000 bp (60 kb) in size, and polyacrylamide gels effectively separate fragments smaller than 1000 bp (1 kb). Until recently, resolution of large fragments was not possible, but the recent development of pulsed-field gel electrophoresis (PFGE) has made possible the separation of DNA fragments even up to 2000 kb. In this technique the electric field is alternated in different directions, forcing the molecules of DNA to reorient between each pulse of electric current. Thus, this technique is particularly suitable for isolating and characterizing large segments of DNA, such as to identify a known gene.

As noted previously, prior to electrophoresis, the DNA had to be digested with one of the restriction endonucleases. The size of the fragments resulting from digestion will depend on the type of restriction endonuclease used as to whether they recognize a 4-, 5-, 6-, or 8-bp sequence. Enzymes recognizing a 4-bp sequence will cut the DNA into much smaller fragments than one that recognizes an 8-bp sequence.

Development of a DNA Probe

A nucleic acid probe is a fragment of nucleic acid to which has been attached a label such as a radioisotope or a fluorescent compound, making it possible to detect and recognize the desired fragment easily among other complex native DNA molecules. The fragment labeled is usually cDNA or

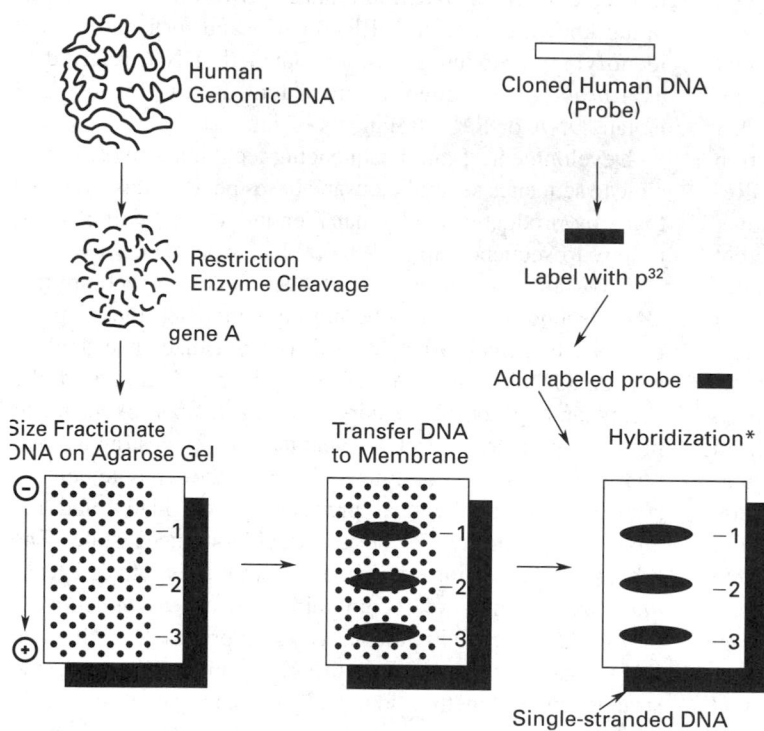

FIGURE 7-12
Southern blotting technique. The DNA is cleaved with an appropriately selected restriction endonuclease. The digested fragments are separated by electrophoresis on agarose gel, and the fragments of gene A are located at positions 1, 2, and 3 but cannot be seen against the background of many other randomly occurring DNA fragments. The DNA is denatured and transferred to a membrane in an identical pattern to what it was on the agarose gel. It is difficult to manipulate anything on a soft gel or to remove it. Once transferred to the membrane (filter), a solid support system, the DNA is much easier to handle. A DNA probe (cDNA) that has been labeled with ^{32}P is hybridized to its complementary DNA and visualized after exposure of the nylon membrane to an autoradiograph. The transfer of the DNA from the gel to the membrane developed by Southern was a major innovation illustrated in the next figure. (From Mares A Jr. et al. Molecular biology for the cardiologist. *Curr Probl Cardiol* 1992; 17:9–72. Reproduced with permission from the publisher and authors.)

a synthetic oligonucleotide, although it could be RNA. It is now possible to synthesize DNA fragments of up to 30 to 40 bp, referred to as *oligonucleotides,* that, with an attached label, can be used as probes to identify DNA in the human genome or mRNA in the cytoplasm. This takes advantage of the fact that at high temperatures the double-stranded DNA probe and the native DNA will separate into separate strands. On recombining at random, the labeled DNA probe will bind not only to its original complementary strand but also equally well to that of the native DNA that is complementary to the probe, and thus provide a means of isolating a fragment of native genomic DNA. A probe is necessary in most recombinant DNA procedures to detect the molecule of interest following electrophoresis.

Southern, Northern, and Western Blotting

The procedure to separate and detect specific DNA fragments, which is now referred to as *Southern blotting,* is named after E. M. Southern, who developed it in 1975.[36] Genomic DNA is isolated and digested, and electrophoresis is performed on a gel as described previously. Following separation, DNA fragments are denatured chemically into single-strand fragments. It is very difficult to handle gels, and even more impractical to store them. Southern developed a technique whereby these separated single-strand fragments on gel can be transferred by capillary action to a solid support medium (nylon or nitrocellulose membrane) and permanently fixed by heating. The pattern on the membrane reflects identically the pattern induced by electrophoresis on the gel. The process used to produce a Southern blot is illustrated schematically in Fig. 7-12. The nylon membrane and its attached single-strand DNA fragments are then incubated with a radioactively labeled complementary probe. The hybridized radioactive, double-strand product, upon exposure to x-ray film (autoradiography), will exhibit the pattern of the radiolabeled DNA fragments (Fig. 7-13). In summary, Southern blotting is the electrophoretic separation of DNA, followed by its transfer to a nylon membrane for subsequent identification by radioactive hybridization. The autoradiogram is called *Southern blot.* The same approach for detecting mRNA is referred to as *Northern blotting.* This procedure can also be used for detection of proteins, in which case it is referred to as *Western blotting* (Table 7-1). The only significant difference in detecting protein versus nucleic acid by this procedure is the probe, which

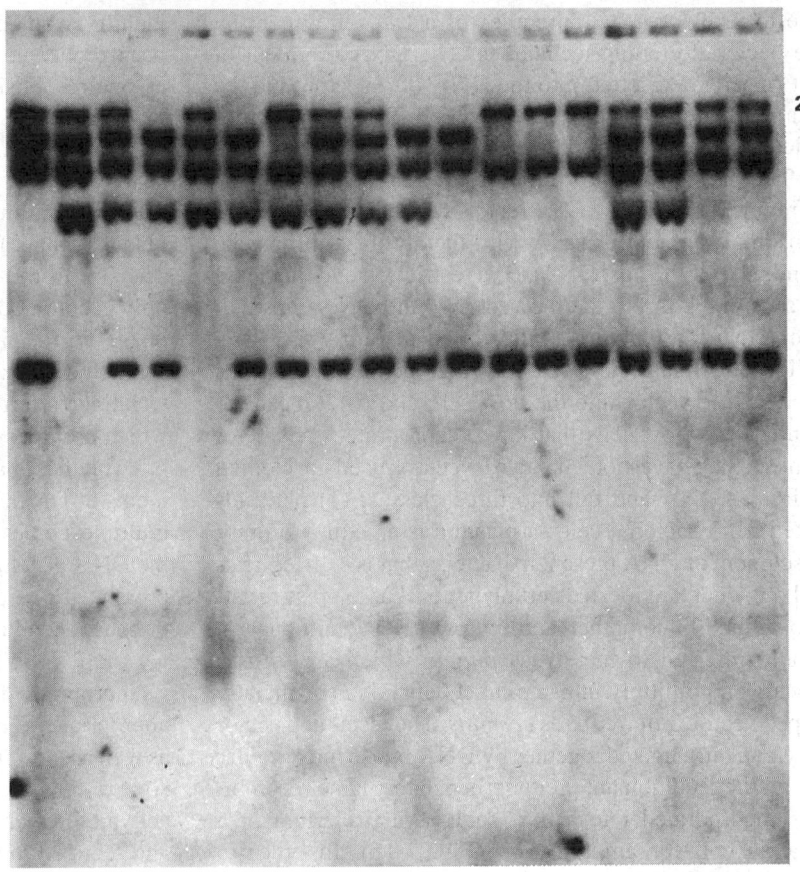

FIGURE 7-13

A typical Southern blot with distinct bands. Each vertical lane consists of DNA from a separate individual. All of the individual DNAs were digested with the same restriction endonuclease. Following separation on electrophoresis and transfer to a nylon membrane, hybridization was performed with the selected radioactive probe and thus only those fragments complementary to the probe are visualized. This is an analysis of a family with hypertrophic cardiomyopathy, and the different patterns reflect restriction fragment length polymorphisms (RFLP) characteristic of the marker locus which is linked to the disease locus. (From Mares A Jr. et al. Molecular biology for the cardiologist. *Curr Probl Cardiol* 1992; 17:9–72. Reproduced with permission from the publisher and authors.)

is an antibody rather than an oligonucleotide or cDNA. However, as in Southern and Northern blotting, the probe may be labeled with a radioactive isotope, a fluorescent tag, or some visual colorimetric substance.

Cloning of a Gene

DNA cloning is a technique used to produce large quantities of a specific DNA fragment of interest.[37] It is generally quite

TABLE 7-1

SEPARATION AND IDENTIFICATION OF MOLECULAR SPECIES

Procedures	Molecule	Labeled Probe
Southern blotting	DNA	DNA or cDNA
Northern blotting	RNA	DNA or cDNA
Western blotting	Protein	Antibody

feasible to produce a billion copies of a DNA fragment by routine bacterial cloning techniques. The DNA fragment of interest (insert) is inserted into the DNA of a vector, and the vector amplified in an appropriate host cell. The host provides amplification of the DNA of both the vector and the foreign insert. The prerequisites for cloning are (1) isolation of the DNA fragment of interest; (2) a vector, which is often an extra chromosomal segment of DNA with the ability to propagate independently of the host DNA; (3) a restriction endonuclease to digest both the insert and the vector so the DNA ends will be compatible for ligation, as illustrated in Fig. 7-14; (4) a DNA ligase to ligate the insert into the vector; (5) a means to introduce the vector into the host cell; and (6) a means to differentiate the host cells that have incorporated the vector from those that have not. Standard vectors used in cloning have circular DNA and fall into three classes: (1) plasmids harvested from bacterial cells; a plasmid is an extra chromosomal segment of DNA present in bacteria that is self-replicating and on which are located certain genes that express resistance to ampicillin or other antibiotics; (2) bacteriophages, commonly referred to merely as *phage,* which are viruses that invade and multiply in bacterial cells; and (3) artificially developed vectors referred to as *cosmids.* The insert and vector are enzymatically ligated together by DNA ligase into circular DNA, and the recombinant product (hence the name recombinant) is incorporated into a host such as a bacterium or a mammalian cell for amplification (Fig. 7-15). In order to

identify whether or not the particular DNA of interest has been replicated in the host, a so-called selection gene, such as one responsible for ampicillin resistance, is incorporated into the vector. The bacteria are grown in media containing ampicillin, so only those that have the resistance gene will survive. Since the resistance gene is attached to the DNA fragment of interest, it indicates that colonies (bacteria) or plaques (phage) that survive must contain the gene of interest. The size of the insert is a limitation in cloning. Plasmids can only accommodate inserts of up to approximately 15,000 bp, phage up to 25,000 bp, and cosmids up to 45,000 bp. This limitation in size has been overcome by the development of a technique referred to as yeast artificial chromosome (YAC),[38] which provides for DNA inserts of up to 100,000 to 2 million bp. This has markedly accelerated the cloning of large fragments of DNA. Cloning, as discussed, is performed to obtain multiple copies of DNA, and, unless specifically designed, the DNA is neither transcribed into mRNA nor translated into protein. If one desires to express a particular DNA fragment or gene, one must then use what is referred to as an *expression vector.* It is imperative to provide a promoter element that is appropriate for the host, and the gene must contain the appropriate 5′ untranslated region for binding to the ribosome as well as the appropriate 3′ region for stability of the message. An example would be the expression of tissue plasminogen activator in mammalian cells, whereby the protein is expressed and secreted to be harvested and commercially processed for use as a thrombolytic agent.

Development of Gene Libraries

Gene libraries are usually referred to as either genomic or cDNA. A genomic library refers to one made from nuclear DNA. A library is really a collection of DNA fragments that have been cloned in an appropriate vector and grown in a particular host, usually bacteria. A major difference between a genomic and a cDNA library is that a *genomic library* contains DNA fragments composed of introns, exons, and large intragenic sequences, whereas the *cDNA library* is made from mRNA that represents genes expressed in that organ and does not have introns or intragenic sequences. The cDNA library contains genes specifically expressed in that tissue only. In contrast, a genomic library, whether made from the heart or another tissue, will have the same genes. To make a human genomic library one must first isolate the whole genome of a cell, cut it into fragments with a restriction enzyme, and insert the fragments into a vector replicated in an appropriate host, usually bacteria.[39] To increase the odds that enough fragments are cloned to represent the whole genome, certain calculations are necessary. It is assumed that the recognition site for a particular restriction enzyme occurs at random. The restriction enzyme EcoR₁ has a 6-bp recognition site, and the average size of each fragment produced will be $4^6 = 4096$ bp. In contrast, if the recognition site involves 4 bp, each fragment would be $4^4 = 256$ bp. Using the 6-bp cutter for the human genome of 3 billion bp, dividing by 4096

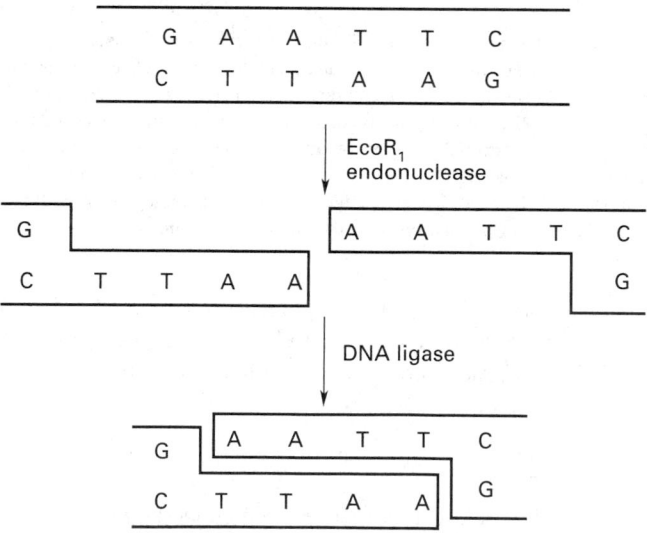

FIGURE 7-14

Restriction endonucleases recognize specific sequences and cut in a specific manner. The sequences recognized may be anywhere from 3 to 8 bp and may cut to give a blunt end or a staggered end (ECoR₁). Enzymes that provide staggered ends (cohesive or sticky ends) have unpaired bases, which are easy to ligate together since they are complementary to each other, as shown in this illustration. This feature is exploited in cloning or in the formation of any recombinant DNA molecule. For cloning purposes, the fragment of DNA to be inserted is digested with the same restriction enzyme as is used to digest the DNA of the vector into which it will be inserted. Thus, the sticky ends of the DNA insert and the vector will be complementary and easy to ligate together in the presence of the enzyme DNA ligase, as illustrated in Fig. 7-15.

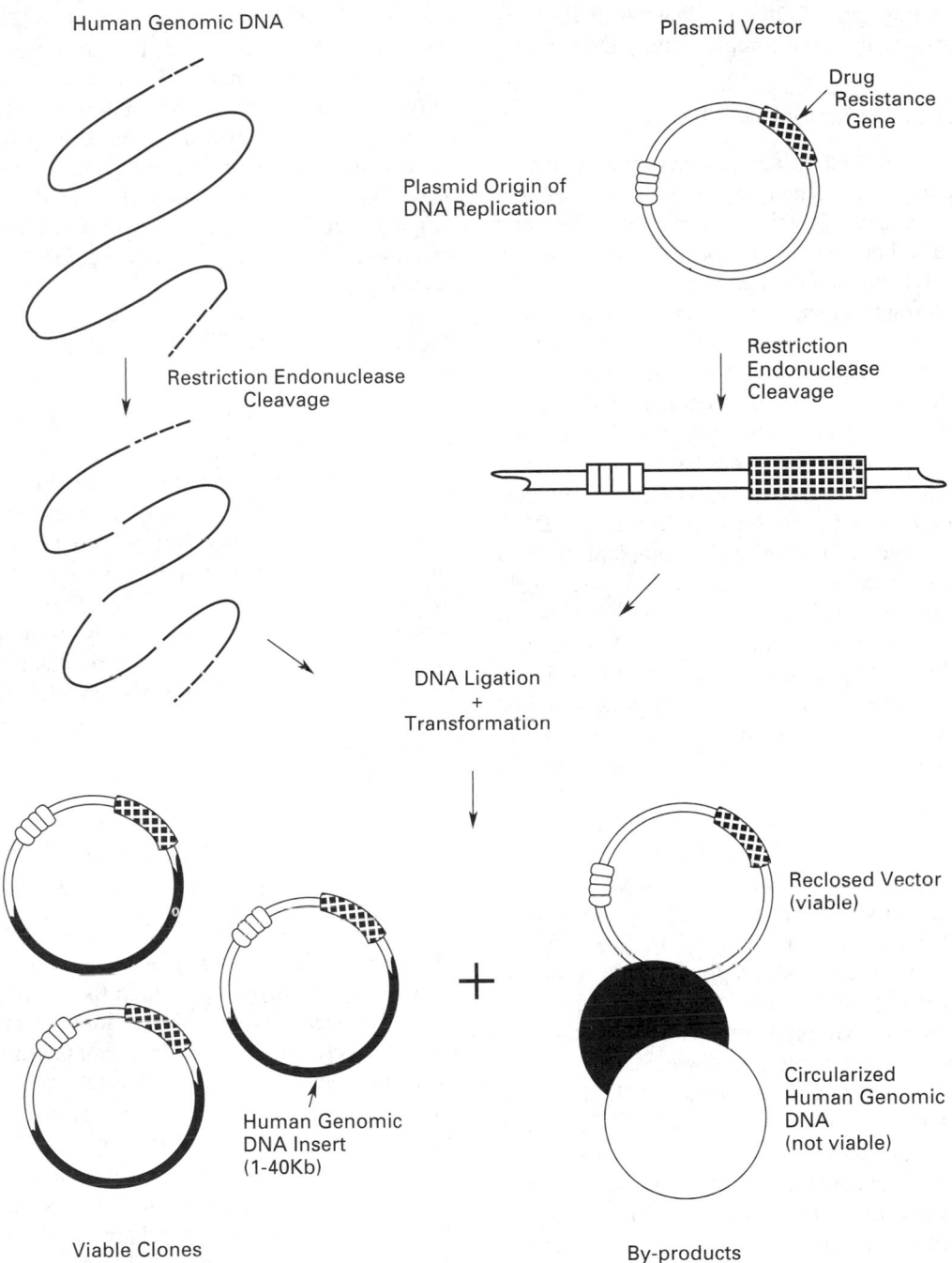

FIGURE 7-15

DNA cloning. The basic objective of cloning is to provide multiple copies of a DNA fragment of interest. The fundamental principles for in vitro cloning of specific DNA fragments are: (1) the human genome DNA of interest is isolated after digestion by a restriction endonuclease, which is often referred to as the DNA insert; (2) a DNA vector is selected (shown on the right); the vector is a plasmid that has circular DNA and contains the necessary replication site and the reporter gene (drug resistance) to subsequently recognize which host has the insert; the vector and the DNA fragment to be inserted are digested with the same restriction endonuclease so that the ends are complementary for ligation; (3) DNA ligase ligates compatible insert and vector ends together; and (4) host cells are transformed by incorporating vectors containing insert fragments and are identified by characteristics encoded by resident genes on the vector. Some of the clones will be viable and others not. (From Mares A Jr. et al. Molecular biology for the cardiologist. *Curr Probl Cardiol* 1992; 17:9–72. Reproduced with permission from the publisher and authors.)

will produce roughly 750,000 fragments, requiring 750,000 colonies or clones. The recognition sites are not evenly or randomly distributed, however, and so some fragments are larger, others smaller; to be certain, at least 1 million colonies would be required. Other factors must also be considered, such as the choice of vector with respect to the insert size. The part of the library utilized can be replaced by regrowing it and thus is a permanent, renewable source of DNA. cDNA libraries of the whole heart and specific structures of the heart, such as the Purkinje system, are now available. To isolate a particular gene or fragment of DNA or cDNA from a library generally requires a radioactive complementary DNA probe.

Polymerase Chain Reaction

The PCR has revolutionized the application of the techniques of molecular biology. This technique was not developed until 1985,[40,41] but its impact already has been felt throughout medicine and biotechnology. This procedure, conveniently and without the tedium of cloning, can provide 1 million copies of a DNA fragment in 3 to 4 h and a billion copies within 24 h. PCR simply and ingeniously takes advantage of the natural DNA replication process. The sequence of the two ends of the DNA fragment desired to be amplified must be known, but short sequences of 15 to 30 bp are adequate, and fragments in between these sequences as large as 20 kb can be amplified. The sequence is used to make two oligonucleotides, referred to as *primers,* with one for each end of the DNA fragment. The sequence of one primer is complementary to the sense direction, and the sequence of the other is made complementary to the antisense direction. The primers are used to prime the synthesis of complementary DNA strands and are designed so that the DNA between the primers is the fragment of interest to be amplified. If mRNA is to be amplified, it is first converted to a cDNA using the enzyme reverse transcriptase. The primers (oligonucleotides) and the necessary bases are added in excess, together with the enzyme Taq DNA polymerase (to catalyze DNA synthesis) and a sample containing the DNA to be amplified. There are three steps to each cycle: Initially, one must denature the DNA (separate the primers and the native DNA) into separate strands, which is done by increasing the temperature to 95°C. The temperature is then decreased to 50°C so the primers and the native DNA will reanneal to their complementary base sequences. The native DNA strands will bind not only to each other but also to the primers. The temperature is now increased to 65°C for synthesis of the new DNA fragments. Synthesis in the presence of Taq1 polymerase is initiated at the 5′ end, and further nucleotides are added in the 5′ to 3′ direction to provide the desired double-stranded DNA fragment. Taq1 DNA polymerase, isolated from *thermus aquaticus,* is thermostable, which is of tremendous advantage in performing the PCR reaction. Since the high temperatures of up to 95°C do not destroy this polymerase, it negates the need to add DNA polymerase between each cycle. Furthermore, since Taq polymerase has an optimal activity temperature of around 70°C, one can significantly accelerate DNA synthesis. The cycle is then repeated; after about 30 cycles over 3 h, one should have about a million copies.

There are many clinical applications for PCR. To make a diagnosis of viral myocarditis, for example, one can use PCR to amplify from a myocardial biopsy any specific viral RNA or DNA for which primers can be made. The sensitivity of most conventional techniques is inadequate to detect molecules unless present in 50,000 to 100,000 copies per cell. In contrast, only one copy of RNA or DNA is needed for detection by PCR, and in 3 to 4 h up to 1 million copies can be generated, which is adequate abundance for detection by most conventional techniques. PCR offers exquisite diagnostic sensitivity and specificity for determining the etiology of cardiac disorders such as myocarditis and, in patients undergoing cardiac transplantation, for detecting infection or immunologic rejection. Another application of PCR is to detect and amplify mutations associated with hereditary disorders. One can also sequence DNA directly from PCR without the need for cloning.

Electrophoretic Mobility-Shift Assay (Band-Shift Assay)

This technique is used routinely to study transcriptional factors. On gel electrophoresis, DNA exhibits a certain migratory pattern due to the large fragments moving more slowly, and these show up as the stained bands closer to the negative electrode. If a transcription factor is bound to its DNA-binding site, migration is slowed and the decreased mobility will be detected as a shift in the migrating band through the gel—hence the name. Using an antibody to the protein one can also study the protein specifically. It was this technique that identified a unique family of DNA- and RNA-binding proteins that are specific for the triplet repeat, CTG (or CUG), and these proteins may play a role in the pathogenesis of myotonic dystrophy.[42]

MOLECULAR BASIS OF CARDIAC CONTRACTION

Cardiac myocytes are large cells of up to 120 μm in length.[43] They are joined together in a syncytium. The sarcolemma surrounding the myocyte through the intercalated disk joins to adjacent cells and invaginates into the myofibril through the T-tubules. Cardiac muscle is composed of fibers, which in turn are composed of myofibrils. The myofibril has a periodicity imparted to it by the sarcomere, which is the working unit of contraction. The sarcomeres are joined in series with each other via the Z-lines. The sarcomere is composed of myosin and actin, primarily the thick and thin filaments, respectively. There are four regulatory proteins attached to the actin filament—tropomyosin and troponins C, T, and I—and two myosin light chain molecules attached to the MHC. The sarcomeres comprise about 50 percent of the mass of the cardiac myocyte and, depending on the state of contraction, vary from 1.6 to 2.2 μm in length as shown in Fig. 7-16.

The Contractile Proteins

The proposed mechanism[44] whereby the actin filaments slide over the myosin filaments and induce shortening or contraction is illustrated in Fig. 7-17. Cardiac contraction and relaxation are regulated in part by calcium. Calcium released from sarcoplasmic reticulum (SR) induces contraction by releasing calcium and relaxation by sequestering it in SR. Hydrolysis of ATP at a rate of one molecule per myosin head is required

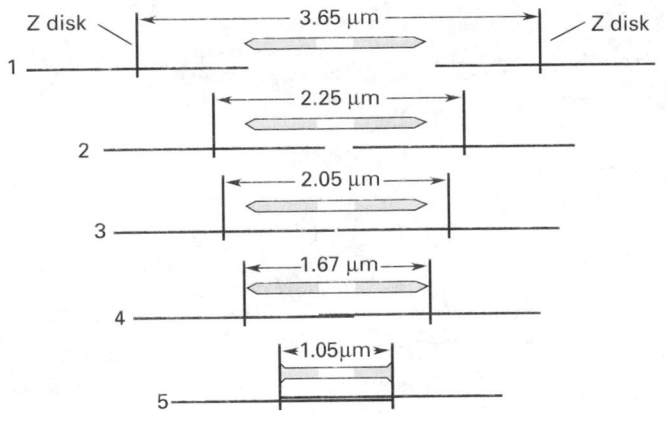

FIGURE 7-16

Relationship of sarcomere length and tension generated during isometric contraction of striated muscle. Maximum tension is generated at sarcomere lengths that allow maximum interaction of myosin heads and actin filaments (positions 2 and 3). If the sarcomere length is too short (positions 4 and 5), actin filaments overlap one another and prevent optimum interaction with myosin heads (From Darnell J et al., eds. *Molecular Cell Biology*. New York: Freeman; 1990. Reproduced with permission from the publisher.)

for each cycle, as the actin filament moves a distance of about 7 nm. In the relaxed state, myosin is prohibited from binding to actin by the presence of tropomyosin and troponin, which block the binding site for myosin. Myosin has minimal ATPase activity in the absence of actin; nevertheless, it does induce some hydrolysis of ATP to ADP and P_i. Systolic contraction is induced by calcium, which, upon release from SR, binds to troponin C to induce a slight movement of tropomyosin that exposes the binding site on actin for myosin. The resulting binding of actin to myosin increases the ATPase activity of myosin by about 200-fold, which hydrolyzes the ATP to ADP. The ADP is released from the head of the myosin, which further enhances the binding of the myosin to

actin. The head of the myosin, which is oriented at a 90° angle to the actin, flexes to a 45° angle and in so doing moves the actin filaments closer together. Subsequently, the calcium is again sequestered by SR, and ATP binds to the myosin head, which inhibits binding to the actin, relaxes the sarcomere, and reinitiates diastole (Fig. 7-18). Using high intensity x-ray from a synchrotron, it has been possible to follow the changes in muscle diffraction patterns during muscle contractions. The increase in cytosolic calcium and tropomyosin movement occurs 17 ms after a muscle is stimulated. The myosin head attaches to actin after about 25 ms, and the tension is generated after about 40 ms (see also Chap. 6).

THE CYTOSKELETAL PROTEINS

Cytoskeleton refers to the fibrous proteins that are present in the cytoplasm. The cytoskeletal fibers give the cell strength and rigidity and control movement within the cell. For example, the microtubules provide the tracks along which vesicles are transported by tubulin-binding molecules. These cytoskeletal proteins form three major classes, subdivided according to their size into microfilaments,[45] microtubules,[46] and intermediate filaments.[47] The microfilaments are polymers of the protein subunit actin; the microtubules are polymers of the subunits of α and β tubulin and the intermediate filaments of five different rod-shaped protein subunits. The polymerization and depolymerization of these fibers are closely regulated by the cell.

Microfilaments

In addition to the organized actin of the sarcomere, actin filaments are distributed throughout the cytoplasm of essentially all cells and serve to anchor many proteins crucial to

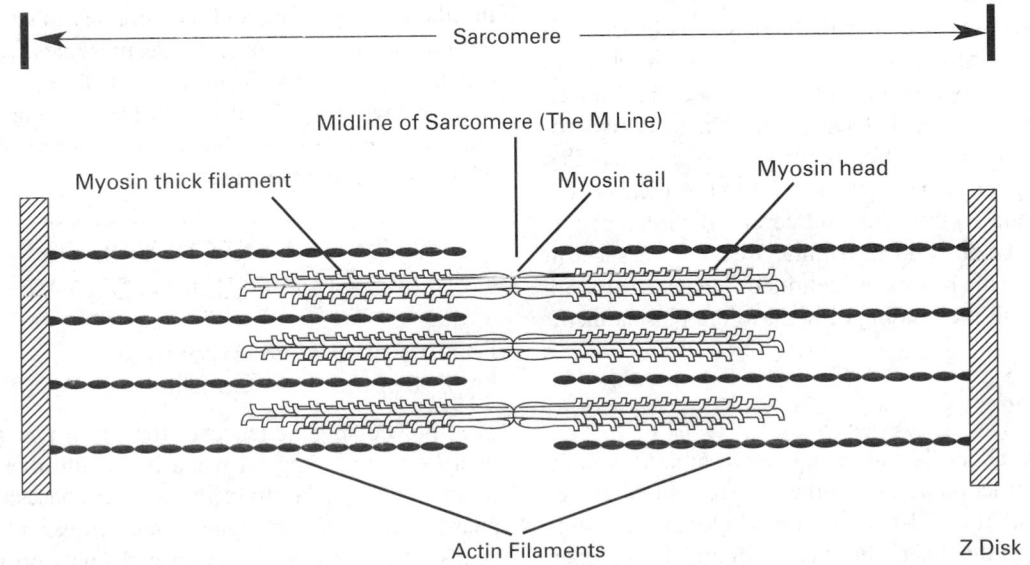

FIGURE 7-17

Sarcomere ultrastructure.

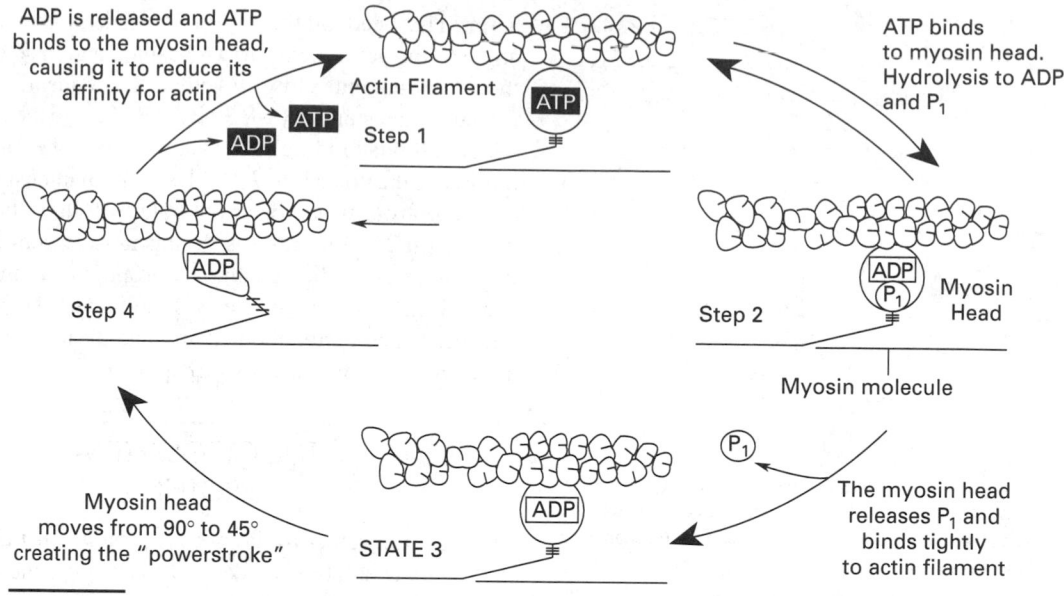

FIGURE 7-18

Molecular basis of myocardial contraction. (Adapted from Alberts B et al., eds. *Molecular Biology of the Cell*, 2d ed. New York: Garland; 1991:621. Reproduced with permission from the publisher and authors.)

cell survival. In addition, actin is associated with several other proteins that enable the actin filaments to perform their specific functions. The full normal function of actin and its associated proteins and their alteration during pathologic states are not known. In the growth response of cardiac hypertrophy or the healing and remodeling following myocardial infarction, it is possible that these proteins play pivotal roles. *Titan*, which binds myosin to the Z-line, is essential to the velocity and force developed by myosin-actin interaction, as is *nebulin*, which attaches actin to the Z-line. Abnormalities related to these proteins, both acquired and inherited, are beginning to emerge. *Dystrophin* is the protein encoded by the gene responsible for Duchenne's muscular dystrophy and is known to be a subsarcolemmal protein with the function of anchoring actin to the plasma membrane. Elucidation of the mechanism by which defective dystrophin induces the well-recognized cardiomyopathy associated with Duchenne's muscular dystrophy should provide information applicable to many cardiac disorders.[48,49] *Spectrin* has several isoforms critical to the cytoskeleton of the erythrocyte, and certain inherited abnormalities are known to induce anemia. Recently, a spectrin isoform specific to the heart was identified[50] that also appears to be involved with the binding of actin to the plasma membrane.

Microtubules

Microtubules are about 24 nm in diameter and vary widely in length from a fraction of a micrometer to tens of micrometers. The microtubule wall is made up of globular subunits about 4 to 5 nm in diameter, and these subunits are arranged in 13 longitudinal rows encircling the hollow-appearing center. This basic design is present in practically all microtubules.

Colchicine, which inhibits microtubule assembly, does so by binding to the tubulin. Microtubules are involved in movement and organization of cell organelles.

Intermediate Filaments

In contrast to actin and tubulin, which are widely distributed among cell types, the rather insoluble intermediate filaments are tissue- and cell-specific. Actin and tubulin are globular, and the polymers they form are rather like beads on a string. In contrast, intermediate filament subunit proteins are extended molecules that form ropelike polymers. The intermediate filament proteins include desmin, vimentin, neurofilaments, glial fibrillary acid protein, and the keratins. In cardiac myocytes, desmin filaments connect the desmosomes from one muscle cell to the other and form the scaffold for both the Z-disk and the myofibrils. The desmin filament plays a role in the transmission of the stress and strain of the contractile force between cardiac myocytes.

MOLECULAR BASIS FOR CELLULAR GROWTH

Patterns of Growth (Hyperplasic, Hypertrophic, and Constitutive)

The molecular genetic basis for growth is somewhat distinct,[51,52] depending on when in the life of the organism it occurs, and may be divided into four phases: the embryonic phase in utero of development and cellular differentiation (to be discussed later), the rapid-growth phase prior to and during puberty, the normal constitutive maintenance growth throughout life, and compensatory growth in response to stimuli such as exercise or injury. Growth may be associated with an increase in the number of cells (*hyperplasia*) or just an increase in their size (*hypertrophy*), or it may be just replacement of proteins as they are catabolized, with no change in the number of cells or their size or function (*constitutive growth*). During early development in the fetal and embryonic stages, practically all cells proliferate as well as increase in size and are said to be in cell cycle (Fig. 7-19). Throughout this process, certain cells drop out of cell cycle, cease proliferating, and undergo the process of differentiation. At birth or within weeks thereafter, certain cells of organs such as the heart and brain lose their ability to proliferate, and growth is restricted to constitutive growth or hypertrophy. Some cells undergo programmed cell death, called *apoptosis*. Many of the genes responsible for embryonic development subsequently downregulate after birth. Conversely, genes that code for proteins serving specialized functions in the differentiated cell are inhibited in the proliferating, undifferentiated cell and are expressed only upon differentiation. For example, the muscle cell, upon differentiation, downregulates the gene that encodes for BB creatine kinase and upregulates the gene for MM creatine kinase. Similarly, upregulation occurs for the genes that encode for myosin, actin, and other sarcomeric proteins essential to the contractile performance of the cell. It is estimated that the human body has a total of 10^{14} cells, but only 200 to 250 different types are defined by their specific function. The specialized functions of a cell are determined by the repertoire of genes expressed in that particular cell.

In the adult heart, most of normal growth is constitutive. It is estimated that most of the proteins of the heart are replaced every 5 days, except collagen, which replaces itself every 120 days; however, with hypertrophy, the half-life of collagen is only 17 days. It is estimated that all human functions are determined by about 67,000 genes, and about 10,000 genes (proteins) are required to maintain basal cellular integrity of a particular organ, except the brain, which requires about 20,000 genes. Thus, maintaining normal cellular homeostasis is a dynamic growth process. For example, in every second of a human being's life, more than a million trillion hemoglobin molecules are synthesized.

Growth Factors and Receptors Underlying the Growth Response

Normal and pathologic growth is initiated by multiple factors.[53] Several of the circulating hormones, such as growth hormone, thyroxine, mineralocorticoids, glucocorticoids, and angiotensin II, act as growth factors. Growth factors[54] such as transforming growth factor β and the fibroblastic growth factors are produced locally, released into the immediate environment, and mediate their effect on growth through what are termed paracrine or autocrine mechanisms. *Paracrine* refers to a growth factor that is secreted and affects the growth of adjacent cells. *Autocrine* refers to a growth factor that binds to the receptors of the same cell from which it was produced and secreted. *Intracrine* refers to a growth factor that induces growth in the same cell from which it was produced without being secreted. An external stimulus that influences growth is detected by a receptor, which usually sits on the cell's surface as an intramembrane receptor, and is relayed through several signaling or transducing proteins to the nucleus of the cell where the ultimate effector molecule is a TF (Table 7-2). The effector molecule may also affect growth through regulation of translation. The latter, however, usually more transient, while a sustained change in growth is almost always mediated through transcription. The signaling proteins involve kinases and phosphatases, which, through phosphorylation, transfer ATP to amplify the signal and, by dephosphorylation, decrease it or in some way alter it (Fig. 7-20). Regulation of protein synthesis may also result from altered stability of mRNA. The growth response to circulating hormones or locally produced growth factors occurs several hours after the initial stimulation and is more likely to occur if two or more growth factors have been activated (see also Chap. 6). In

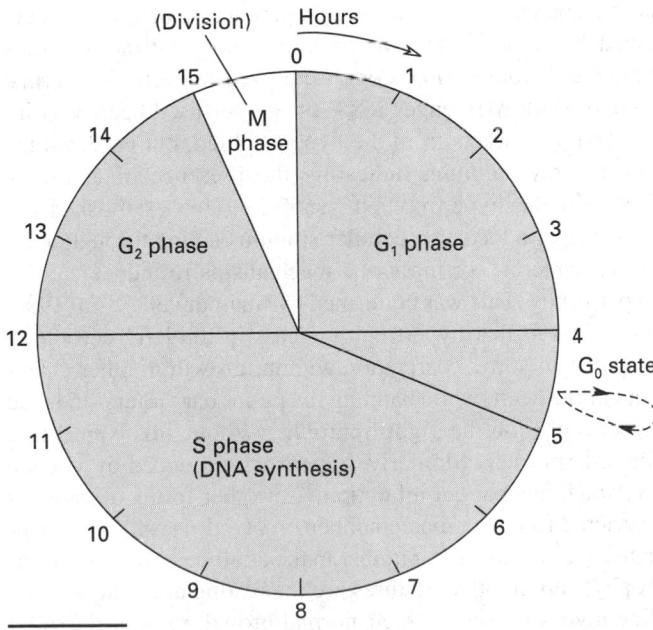

FIGURE 7-19
The cell cycle in a mammalian cell having a generation time of 16 h. The three phases spanning the first 15 h or so—the G_1 (first gap) phase, the S (synthetic) phase, and the G_2 (second gap) phase—make up the interphase, during which DNA and other cellular macromolecules are synthesized. The remaining hour is the M (mitotic) phase, during which the cell actually divides.

TABLE 7-2

CASCADE FOR RELAYING GROWTH SIGNALS

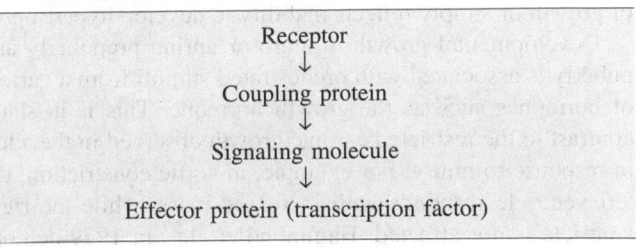

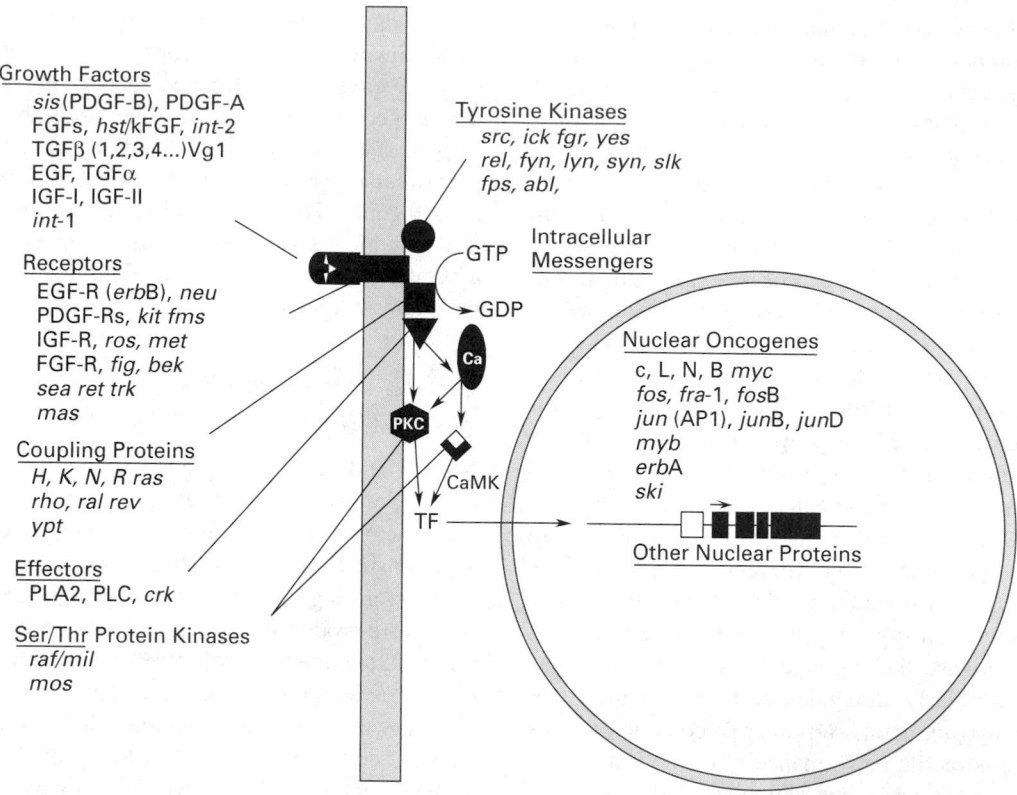

FIGURE 7-20

Illustration of many proteins with varied functions for which oncogenes are known to encode. It is clear from this diagram that oncogenes encode proteins that function as growth factors, receptors, coupling proteins, signaling proteins, and transcription factors.

the case of the heart, a common signal is increased intraventricular pressure, which results in compensatory hypertrophy (Chap. 6).

THE CARDIAC GROWTH RESPONSE

The growth response of the myocardium to injury, whether it be myocardial infarction, hypertension, or valvular disease, is a major determinant of morbidity and mortality. Growth is the major long-term adaptive mechanism of the heart (see also Chap. 6). The response of the heart to physiologic or pathologic stimuli is limited to hypertrophy, dilatation, or their combination. The clinical and pathologic features associated with cardiac hypertrophy have been described extensively.[55] Meerson[56] put forward the concept that early compensatory growth is beneficial, while subsequent growth may become pathologic and contribute to increased mortality. It remains to be determined whether cardiac dilatation is a form of growth or simply reflects inability to develop hypertrophy.

Developmental growth in utero or during prepuberty and puberty is associated with orchestrated stimuli from a variety of hormones such as the growth hormone. This is in sharp contrast to the restricted cardiac growth observed in the adult in response to injury. For example, in aortic constriction, the left ventricle responds with increased mass, while the right ventricle is not affected. Hammond et al.[57] in 1979 demon-

strated that the growth stimulus was indeed localized to the affected organ. Left ventricular hypertrophy was induced by aortic coarctation in the dog. Supernatants of the homogenized, hypertrophied left ventricle from dogs with aortic coarctation and from normal dogs were used to perfuse a normal canine heart. Messenger RNA of the perfused heart was increased by extracts from the hypertrophied, but not from the normal, myocardium, indicating the presence of a growth factor in the hypertrophied ventricle. This established the presence of a localized cellular stimulus acting through autocrine, paracrine, or intracrine mechanisms to induce cardiac hypertrophy. This was confirmed by Imamura et al.[58] in 1990; they showed that hypertrophy occurs in the left ventricle in response to aortic coarctation without growth in other chambers of the heart, while banding the pulmonary artery–induced hypertrophy of the right ventricle without involvement of the left ventricle. Similarly, hypertrophy induced by volume overload, myocardial infarction,[59] or other forms of injury is restricted to the cardiac chamber involved. Despite the myocytes not increasing in number in the adult heart during hypertrophy, certain other features are interesting and unique. Cardiac myocytes, during their normal growth response, exhibit DNA synthesis (multiple nuclei)[60] and the reexpression of several fetal proteins otherwise expressed only in the embryonic cells.[61] The rational basis for the reexpression of fetal protein is not obvious. The response has been referred to as adaptive, maladaptive, or part of a triggered program response.[29] The atrial natriuretic factor gene is expressed in the atria and ventricles in the embryonic state but not in the normal adult ventricle; however, it is reexpressed in the ventricle during hypertrophy.[62,63] Calcium ATPase, an enzyme essential to cardiac contractility, is decreased in the hypertrophied human ventricle.[64] It is well documented in the developing mammalian heart in utero that the initial actin gene expressed is that of smooth muscle type, followed by that of skeletal and finally cardiac muscle.[65] The functional significance, if any, of the reexpression of fetal genes when the cardiac growth program is turned on in the adult heart is unknown. It is possible that the growth response can be activated only through expression of a family of genes. The master gene controlling expression of such a family could be triggered by a growth factor stimulated by pressure overload; this could result in a cascade of genes expressed, most of which are incidental rather than adaptive or maladaptive. For example, in skeletal muscle there is a master gene, myo-D,[66,67] that triggers the differentiation of the skeletal muscle. When this occurs, a cascade of genes are downregulated and another cascade of genes upregulated. Myo-D is not expressed in cardiac muscle, and no such triggering factor has been found for cardiac myocyte differentiation (discussed below).

DIFFERENTIATION AND DEVELOPMENT OF THE HEART

Congenital cardiovascular malformations are a major cause of morbidity and mortality. The fifth ranking cause of premature mortality in the United States is congenital cardiovascular anomalies and malformations. Heart development begins in the human embryo at day 18 and is completed by day 56. This is an exceptionally critical period in development since the heart is very sensitive to teratogenic agents, and, in many cases, this is too soon for the mother to know she is pregnant. Heart defects are some of the most frequent of all major birth defects, occurring at a frequency of approximately 8 per 1000 births. The study of heart formation is, therefore, important for the understanding of these defects. A postulated outline of the hierarchy of the known genes in the development of the heart is illustrated in Fig. 7-21 and will be discussed in detail throughout this section.

Formation of the Heart Tube

In vertebrates, the heart is the first organ to form from paired regions of anterior lateral mesoderm called the cardiogenic plate, which lies on the floor of the pericardial cavity. These cells become committed to a cardiac fate in response to inductive signals emanating from underlying anterior pharyngeal endoderm, and they form a true epithelium with the ability to form both the endocardial (inner endothelial cell lining) and myocardial (outer heart muscle) cell lineages[68] (see Chap. 8).

On the nineteenth day, the parallel cardiac primordia fuse at the midline to form the primitive heart tube. Just prior to

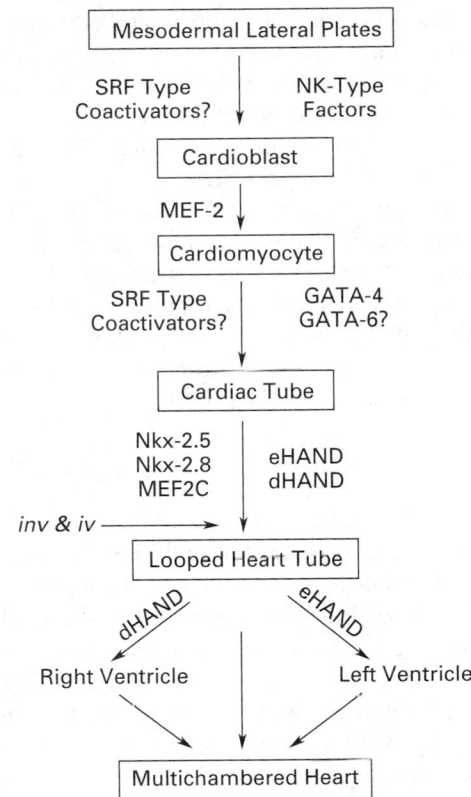

FIGURE 7-21

A lateral plate of mesoderm on each side of the midline forms the progenitor for development of the heart and portions of the great vessels. The homeobox genes, such as Nkx, have yet to be elucidated but, in combination with multiple other genes such as the serum response factor (SRF), are responsible for activating commitment of these undifferentiated cells to cardioblast. Myocyte enhancer factor (MEF) has a binding site in practically all muscle genes and is essential to the development of cardiac myocytes. The genes responsible for the fusion of the two lateral mesodermal plates into a single tube remain unknown, but experiments show that GATA-4 is necessary, along with SRF and many other genes yet to be identified. The cardiac tube that forms a loop to the right requires Nkx genes and the eHAND and dHAND as well as *inv* (inversion of embryonic turning) and *iv* genes. The dHAND gene is responsible for formation of the right ventricle and the eHAND for the left ventricle. (Courtesy of Drs. Eric Olson, Michael D. Schneider, and Robert J. Schwartz.)

the process described as *cardiac looping,* the heart consists of four regions aligned in series as follows: (1) The aortic sac, which will become part of the aorta and pulmonary trunk; (2) the bulbus cordis, consisting of three regions; the dilated end will form the right ventricle, the conus-bridging region will form the outflow tracts of the two ventricles, and the tapered end the truncus arteriosus; (3) the primitive ventricle, which will ultimately form the left ventricle; and (4) the atrium, which will form the atria. The sinus venosus and sinous horns do not fuse. This straight heart tube contains an outer myocardium and an inner endocardium separated by extracellular matrix known as *cardiac jelly.* Atrial and ventricular chambers appear following morphogenesis of the looped heart. Atrial and ventricular cardiac myocytes proceed to express different subgroups of cardiac muscle genes that bestow the contractile and electrophysiologic properties particular to each chamber. Early commitment and later diversification of cardiogenic precursors to atrial and ventricular phenotypes appear to originate from separate lineages, which have been shown to occur before looping by stage HH3 in chicken embryos.[69] These lineages differentiate according to their positions along the anteroposterior axis of the embryo such that the heart tube can be divided into segments that give rise to the atrium, left ventricle, right ventricle, and the ventricular outflow tract (conotruncus). The heart tube achieves anterior-to-posterior polarity during or shortly after commitment to the cardiac lineage by specifying positional information by as-yet-unknown developmental mechanism(s).

Molecular Factors Involved in Cardiogenesis

Defining the molecular basis underlying the establishment and maintenance of cardiac muscle differentiation presents a fundamental challenge in developmental biology and molecular genetics. Despite the shared expression of numerous contractile protein genes by striated muscles, common to cardiac and skeletal types, there is little information including whether the *cis*-acting elements and *trans*-acting factors (defined earlier) governing skeletal muscle cells are similar to or different from those operating in cardiac muscle cells.

Myo-D Myogenic Basic Helix-Loop-Helix Factor Determines Skeletal Muscle

It has been shown that myo-D expressed in myoblasts[67] is sufficient to convert a variety of mesodermal and nonmesodermal cell types to stable myoblasts and active muscle-specific gene expression. Using myo-D as a probe, several additional regulatory factors that specify skeletal muscle cell lineage in fibroblasts have been identified: myogenin,[70,71] Myf5,[72] MRF4-herculin, and Myf6.[73–75] These factors share extensive homology within a basic region and an HLH motif that mediate DNA-binding and dimerization, respectively.[76] HLH proteins share the ability to recognize the DNA consensus sequence CANNTG, known as an *E-box*, first identified with the immunoglobulin enhancer[76] and subsequently found in regulatory regions of most muscle-specific genes. Thus, the regulatory paradigm for skeletal muscle differentiation is centered upon the βHLH myogenic regulatory factors, but neither myo-D, myogenin, Myf5, MRF-4, or Myf6 are expressed in the heart.[77] However, the E-box is present in most, if not all, skeletal and cardiac muscle genes.

It is unknown whether a corresponding "determination" gene controls the onset of cardiac muscle development. Several factors under study that could regulate cardiac gene expression will be discussed.

Drosophila Tinman Is Required for Insect Heart Development

Homeotic genes are genes that determine a change in structure and have in common a domain that codes for 60 amino acids.

Genes with this sequence, referred to as *homeobox* (Hox) *genes,* are generally upregulated during early differentiation, and appear in a time-dependent sequence. Homeobox genes have been studied extensively in *Drosophila*, where they are involved in commitment of cells to specific developmental pathways and play an important role in pattern formation.[78] Recently, the NK homeobox family of genes (NK-1/S59, NK-2/vnd, NK-3/bagpipe, and NK-4/msh-2/tinman and H6) was identified.[79] Nkx-2 factors are DNA-binding proteins (transcriptional factors) capable of activating transcription; their 60-amino-acid homeodomain comprises three helices, in which helix II and helix III form a helix-turn-helix motif.[80] Helix III fits across the AT-rich major groove of the DNA binding site. Nkx-2.5 has been shown to bind to novel NKE sites,[81] certain serum response elements of the cardiac α-actin promoter[82] and the NKE sites in the cardiac atrial natriuretic factor promoter.[83] Gajewski et al.[84] showed that two NKE promoter sites direct *Drosophila* MEF2 (dMEF2) expression in response to *tinman*. Mutations in the *tinman* gene result in loss of heart formation in the *Drosophila* embryo.[85] In addition, *tinman* is known to regulate NK-3/bagpipe expression in the visceral mesoderm[86] and the expression of dMEF2.[84] These observations suggest that *tinman* may be involved in cardiac mesoderm patterning and make it a likely marker for cardiac mesoderm induction.

Tinman and Other Related NK-2 Genes Are Required for Normal Heart Morphogenesis

Homeobox genes of the NK class may also function in early cardiac development in vertebrates. The murine NK-2 homeobox gene, Nkx-2.5/Csx, is expressed in early cardiac progenitor cells, prior to cardiogenic differentiation, and continues through adulthood.[87,88] Superimposed upon the appearance of Nkx-2.5 in cardiac progenitor cells is the sequential expression of the cell type–restricted cardiac α-actin and MHC genes.[87] The Nkx-2.5 factors identified in other vertebrates such as zebrafish,[89] *Xenopus*,[90] and chickens[91] were highly related in sequence and expression pattern to the mouse gene and to cardiac development (Fig. 7-22).

The similarity in expression patterns between Nkx-2.5, XNkx-2.5, ceh-22, *tinman,* and *bagpipe* suggested that the function of these genes might be conserved. Another member of the Nkx-2 family, Nkx-2.8, recently isolated from avian species, is closely related to *Xenopus*, chicken, and zebrafish Nkx-2.5 homeoboxes and is expressed in the developing embryo in the lateral plate mesoderm and underlying pharyngeal endoderm.[92] An attractive hypothesis is that these homeodomain factors function in phylogenetically conserved myogenic pathways occurring in muscle types that do not utilize the myo-D family. Whether the vertebrate Nkx-2.5 or other Nkx-2-related genes expressed in the early heart play a role in heart specification or whether they are downstream regulators

FIGURE 7-22
See color Plate 4.

of cardiac gene expression remains to be determined. In fact, recent homologous recombination knockouts of the endogenous murine Nkx-2.5 gene caused embryonic lethality.[69]

The partially overlapping expression pattern of Hox genes in embryos has led to the concept of a "Hox code."[93] The term *Hox code* means that a particular combination of Hox genes is functionally active in a region and thereby specifies the developmental fate of this region. The existence of eight Nkx-2 family members, their overlapping DNA binding specificities, and, most importantly, their partially overlapping patterns of expression raise the possibility of an "Nkx code."[92]

Overexpression of Nkx-2.5 in zebrafish embryo results in an enlarged heart.[89] Thus, inactivation of the Nkx genes by homologous recombination and overexpression as transgenes offer promise to address the functional significance of the expression domains and thus also of the Nkx code.

SRF and MEF2, MADS Box Factors Involved with Cardiogenesis

Serum response factor was generally presumed to be an ubiquitous and constitutive TF[94] but was recently shown to be highly expressed in the embryonic heart.[95] SRF represents an ancient DNA-binding protein, whose relatives shared a highly conserved DNA-binding/dimerization domain of 90 amino acids, termed the *MADS box*. SRF-related proteins capable of binding to sites found in the regulatory regions of both non-muscle- and muscle-specific genes also belong to the MADS box family of TFs.[96]

SRF-related proteins are capable of binding MEF2 sites, CTA(A/T)4TAG, which can be found in the regulatory regions of both non-muscle- and muscle-specific genes.[97,98] Like SRF, MEF2 factors contain a MADS box and an adjacent MEF2 box. Expression and mutagenesis studies in *Drosophila* have shown that MEF2 proteins are necessary for myogenic differentiation during development[99,100] and are activated by *tinman*.[84]

In the mouse embryo, MEF2 genes are highly expressed in the early heart and skeletal muscle progenitor cells prior to the induction of cardiac and skeletal muscle structural genes, implicating MEF2 as key regulator of cardiac and skeletal muscle differentiation programs.[101] Four MEF2 genes have been isolated in vertebrate species and are referred to as MEF2A-MEF2D.[102,103] The four MEF2 gene products are highly homologous in the MADS box domain but divergent in the carboxy termini, arising from alternative splicing mechanisms. MEF2C shows a tissue-restricted expression pattern being expressed exclusively in skeletal muscle, brain, and spleen and is induced by myogenin in fibroblasts during myogenic differentiation in tissue cultures.[104]

Transactivation of the Cardiac α-Actin Gene by Nkx-2.5 and SRF

Gilman and coworkers[105,106] showed that human SRF interacts with a novel human homeodomain protein, Phox, which shows similarity to the homeodomains of two murine Pax genes. The highest similarity is to a partial murine cDNA termed S8[107] and to MHox, a novel homeodomain protein expressed in mesoderm.[108] Phox interacts with SRF to enhance the exchange of SRF with its binding site in the *c-fos* gene. Recently, it was shown that Nkx-2.5 transactivates the cardiac α-actin gene by binding to SRF, but only after SRF has bound to DNA.[109]

The Role of The GATA Family in Cardiogenesis

The GATA family of proteins has been subdivided, with GATA-1/2/3 being linked to hematopoiesis and GATA-4/5/6 thought to be involved with cardiac, gut, and blood vessel formation. Each of the six GATA proteins contains a highly specific DNA-binding domain, consisting of two C4 zinc fingers that bind to the DNA sequence element (A/T)GATA(A/G) and that may be able to interchange with each other. GATA-4 has been found to be expressed in a developmentally and lineage-specific pattern within cardiac mesoderm and gut epithelium.[110–112] Experiments have shown that GATA-4 regulates expression of cardiac-specific genes, such as cardiac troponin C[113] and α MHC.[114] Mice without the GATA-4 gene display a severe defect in formation of the cardiac tube. Several studies have demonstrated that the GATA-4 transcription factor plays an important role in regulating cardiac-specified genes and appears to be downstream to the Nkx-2.5 gene.

Cardiogenesis, an Nkx-2-Dependent Paradigm

An attractive hypothesis from the analysis of these NK-2 homologues is that these homeodomain factors function in phylogenetically conserved pathways in muscle cell types that do not utilize the myo-D family. Expression of Nkx-2.5 in fibroblasts demonstrated that downstream targets such as the cardiac α-actin gene were not directly activated by Nkx-2.5 alone but required the collaboration of additional factors, such as SRF.[82,109] Whether the vertebrate Nkx-2.5 or other Nkx-2-related genes with SRF are sufficient to play the primary role in heart specification and serve as regulators of other downstream cardiac genes remains to be determined. It is reasonable to postulate that the vertebrate MEF2C genes and the GATA-4 factor are high in the hierarchical order of regulatory factors that in combination with Nkx-2.5 and SRF specify the cardiac cell lineage.

Role for Bone Morphogenic Proteins in Initiating Early Myocardial Cell Differentiation

One type of signaling molecule responsible for cardiogenic commitment was recently identified to be composed of the bone morphogenic proteins (BMPs), which are members of the transforming growth factor β family of signaling molecules. BMP-2 and -4 appear to be capable of inducing the cardiac regulatory factors Nkx-2.5 and GATA-4 when ectopically applied to regions of chick embryos that are not usually specified to become heart tissue.[91] In mice with the BMP-4 gene eliminated (knock-out mice), there was little or no mesoderm differentiation. Some of the mice deficient for

BMP-2 gene that lacked Nkx-2.5 expression also failed to enter early heart development.[115] Thus, BMPs appear to have an early influence on cardiogenesis and Nkx-2.5 expression.

Left-Right Looping of the Cardiac Tube

The first grossly asymmetric feature to develop is the heart tube, which forms from the fusion of cardiac primordia at the midline. Subsequently, the initially symmetric heart acquires a dextral loop. The tubular heart initiates rhythmic contractions at about day 23 in humans and then undergoes rightward looping. The molecular mechanisms underlying left-right axial patterning in vertebrate embryos are not well understood.

There is a genetic basis for left-right asymmetry, as several types of unlinked mutations affecting left-right laterality exist in mice and humans. For example, in the offspring of *iv* mice (lacking the *iv* gene), 50 percent have situs inversus.[116] The *iv* gene has been mapped to chromosome 12 but has not been identified. The *inv* (inversion of embryonic turning) gene mapped to chromosome 4 causes complete reversal of left-right symmetry and cardiac looping.[117] Recently, a yeast artificial chromosome containing a portion of chromosome 4 was found to cure the *inv* mutation, and it is likely that identification of the *inv* gene will be forthcoming (Overbeek PA, personal communication).

Cardiac Chamber Specification

dHAND and eHAND are two βHLH proteins that share high homology in their βHLH regions and are expressed in the developing heart and neural crest. In the mouse, HAND expression coincides with that of other cardiac transcription factors. dHAND expressed in the endocardium is maintained throughout the straight heart tube but is restricted to the conotruncus and future right ventricle as the heart tube forms a loop. eHAND expressed in the myocardium becomes rapidly restricted to the conotruncus and left ventricle.[118] Expression of dHAND and eHAND precedes separation of the two ventricles, representing early chamber specification. It is of interest that Nkx-2.8 has an expression pattern that overlaps eHAND, being restricted to the rostral and caudal regions of the heart tube following looping and expressed in the endoderm of the pharyngeal arches. The recent deletion of dHAND by gene targeting showed that dHAND expression is necessary for the formation of the right ventricle.[118,119] Thus, it appears that dHAND specifies the right ventricle and eHAND the left ventricle. Expression of cardiac-specified genes, αMHC, MLC2A, MLC2V, ANF, and Nkx-2.5, were unaffected by elimination of the dHAND gene. GATA-4 in the myocardium was downregulated by dHAND-deficient hearts and appears to be a downstream target of dHAND.

FUTURE DEVELOPMENT

Three important branches of research are proceeding in parallel, namely, sequencing of the human genome (the Human Genome Project), developmental biology, and identification of genes responsible for disease; together, these will provide an avalanche of information with respect to the regulation of cardiac growth. Identification of genes responsible for inherited cardiac disease and congenital abnormalities and determination of gene function from transgenic and knockout mice will give rise to new dimensions with respect to diagnosis, prevention, and treatment.

REFERENCES

1. Roberts R. Impact for molecular biology in cardiology. *Am J Physiol* 1991; 261:8–14.
2. Roberts R. Integrated program for the training of cardiovascular fellows in molecular biology. In: Albertini A, Lenfant C, Paoletti R, eds. *Biotechnology in Clinical Medicine.* New York: Raven; 1987:99–104.
3. Katz AM. Molecular biology in cardiology, a paradigmatic shift. *J Mol Cell Cardiol* 1988; 20:355–366.
4. Patterson SW, Piper H, Starling EH. The regulation of the heart beat. *J Physiol* 1914; 48:465.
5. Haudenschild CC, Grunwald J. Proliferative heterogeneity of vascular smooth muscle cells and its alteration by injury. *Exp Cell Res* 1985; 157:364–370.
6. Grunwald J, Haudenschild CC. Intimal injury in vivo activates vascular smooth muscle cell migration and explant outgrowth in vitro. *Arteriosclerosis* 1984; 4:183–188.
7. Califf RM, Ohman EM, Frid DJ, Forti DF, Mark DB, Hlatky MA, et al. Restenosis: The clinical issues. In: Anonymous. *Textbook of Interventional Cardiology.* Philadelphia: Saunders; 1990:363–394.
8. Jarcho JA, McKenna W, Pare JAP, Solomon SD, Holcombe RF, Dickie S, et al. Mapping a gene for familial hypertrophic cardiomyopathy to chromosome 14q1. *N Engl J Med* 1989; 321:1372–1378.
9. Hejtmancik JF, Brink PA, Towbin J, Hill R, Brink L, Tapscott T, et al. Localization of the gene for familial hypertrophic cardiomyopathy to chromosome 14q1 in a diverse U.S. population. *Circulation* 1991; 83:1592–1597.
10. Pennica D, Holmes WE, Kohr WJ, Harkins RN, Vehar GA, Ward CA, et al. Cloning and expression of human tissue-type plasminogen activator cDNA in *E. coli. Nature* 1983; 301:214–221.
11. Smalling RW, Bode C, Kalbfleisch J, Sen S, Limbourg P, Forycki F, et al. More rapid, complete, and stable coronary thrombolysis with bolus administration of reteplase compared with alteplase infusion in acute myocardial infarction. *Circulation* 1995; 91:2725–2732.
12. Watson JD, Crick FHC. Molecular structure of nucleic acids: A structure for deoxyribose nucleic acid. *Nature* 1953; 171:737–738.
13. Watson JD, Crick FHC. Genetic implications of the structure of deoxyribonucleic acid. *Nature* 1953; 171:964–967.
14. Franklin RE, Gosling RG. Molecular configuration in sodium thymonucleate. *Nature* 1953; 171:740–741.
15. Wilkins MHF, Stokes AR, Wilson HR. Molecular structure of deoxypentose nucleic acids. *Nature* 1953; 171:738–740.
16. Schekman R, Weiner A, Kornberg A. Multienzyme systems of DNA replication. *Science* 1956; 186:987–993.
17. Marmor J, Lane L. Strand separation and specific recombination of deoxyribonucleic acids: Biologic studies. *Proc Natl Acad Sci USA* 1960; 46:453–461.
18. Doty P, Marmor J, Eigner J, Schildkraut C. Strand separation and specific recombination in deoxyribonucleic acids: Physical chemical studies. *Proc Natl Acad Sci USA* 1960; 46:461–476.
19. Leder P, Nirenberg M. RNA codewords and protein synthesis. II. Nucleotide sequence of a valine RNA codeword. *Proc Natl Acad Sci USA* 1964 52:420–427.
20. Nishimura S, Jones DS, Khorana HG. The in vitro synthesis of a co-polypeptide containing two amino acids in alternative sequence dependent upon a DNA-like polymer containing two nucleotides in alternating sequence. *J Mol Biol* 1981; 146:1–21.
21. Olivera BM, Hall ZW, Lehman IR. Enzymatic joining of polynucleotides. V. A DNA adenylate intermediate in the polynucleotide joining reaction. *Proc Natl Acad Sci USA* 1968; 61:237–244.

22. Smith HO, Wilcox KW. A restriction enzyme from *Hemophilias influenzae*. I. Purification and general properties. *J Mol Biol* 1970; 51:379–391.

23. Kelly TJ Jr, Smith HO. A restriction enzyme from *Hemophilias influenzae*. II. Base sequence of the recognition site. *J Mol Biol* 1970; 51:393–409.

24. Baltimore D. Viral RNA-dependent DNA polymerase. *Nature* 1970; 226:1209–1211.

25. Temin HM, Mizutani S. RNA-dependent DNA polymerase in virions of Rous sarcoma virus. *Nature* 1970; 226:1211–1213.

26. Cohen S, Chang A, Boyer H, Helling R. Construction of biological functional bacterial plasmids in vitro. *Proc Natl Acad Sci USA* 1973; 70:3240–3244.

27. Sanger F, Coulson AR. A rapid method for determining sequences in DNA by primed synthesis and DNA polymerase. *J Mol Biol* 1975; 94:444–448.

28. Maxam AM, Gilbert W. A new method of sequencing DNA. *Proc Natl Acad Sci USA* 1977; 74:560–564.

29. Roberts R. Modern molecular biology: Historical perspective and future potential. In: Roberts R, ed. *Molecular Basis of Cardiology*. Hamden, CT: Blackwell Scientific; 1992:1–15.

30. Knight SL. Molecular zippers in gene regulation. *Sci Am* 1991; 264:54–64.

31. Schneider MD, Roberts R, Parker TG. Modulation of cardiac genes by mechanical stress. The oncogene signalling hypothesis. *Mol Biol Med* 1991; 8:167–183.

32. Falvey E, Schibler U. How are the genes regulators regulated? *FASEB J* 1991; 5:309–314.

33. Anonymous. *Molecular Biology; A Selection of Papers*. San Diego: Academic Press; 1989.

34. Aaij C, Borst P. The gel electrophoresis of DNA. *Biochim Biophys Acta* 1972; 269:192–200.

35. Sharp PA, Sugden B, Sambrook J. Detection of two restriction endonuclease activities in *Haemophilus parainfluenzae* using analytical agarose-ethidium bromide electrophoresis. *Biochemistry* 1973; 12:3055–3062.

36. Southern EM. Detection of specific sequences among DNA fragments separated by gel electrophoresis. *J Mol Biol* 1975; 98:503–517.

37. Sambrook J, Fritsch EF, Maniatis T. Analysis and cloning of eucaryotic genomic DNA. In: Anonymous. *Molecular Cloning, A Laboratory Manual*. New York: Cold Spring Harbor Laboratory; 1989:9.14–9.23.

38. Schwarz DC, Cantro CR. Separation of yeast chromosome-sized DNAs by pulsed field gradient gel electrophoresis. *Nucleic Acids Res* 1984; 37:67.

39. Hunt T, Kozak M, Lindahl T, Varmus HE. The molecular organization of cells. In: Alberts B, Bray D, Lewis J, Raff M, Roberts K, Watson JD, eds. *Molecular Biology of the Cell*. New York; Garland; 1989:201–274.

40. Saiki RK, Scharf S, Faloona F, Mullis KB, Horn GT, Erlich HA, et al. Enzymatic amplification of beta-globin genomic sequences and restriction site analysis for diagnosis of sickle cell anemia. *Science* 1985; 230:1350–1354.

41. Saiki RK, Gelfand DH, Stoffel S, Scharf SJ, Higuchi R, Horn GT, et al. Primer-directed enzymatic amplification of DNA with a thermostable DNA polymerase. *Science* 1988; 239:487–491.

42. Timchenko LT, Timchenko NA, Caskey CT, Roberts R. Novel proteins with binding specificity for DNA CTG repeats and RNA CUG repeats: Implications for myotonic dystrophy. *Hum Mol Genet* 1996; 5:115–121.

43. Darnell J, Lodish H, Baltimore D. Actin, myosin, and intermediate filaments: Cell movements and cell shape. In: Darnell J. Lodish H, Baltimore D, eds. *Molecular Cell Biology*. New York: Freeman; 1990:859–903.

44. Cooke R. The mechanism of muscle contraction. *CRC Crit Rev Biochem* 1986; 21:53–118.

45. Pollard TD, Cooper JA. Actin and actin-binding proteins. A critical evaluation of mechanisms and functions. *Annu Rev Biochem* 1986; 55:987–1035.

46. Darnell J, Lodish H, Baltimore D. Microtubules and cellular movements. In: Darnell J, Lodish H, Baltimore D, eds. *Molecular Cell Biology*. New York: Freeman; 1990:815–858.

47. Steinert PM, Roop DR. Molecular and cellular biology of intermediate filaments. *Annu Rev Biochem* 1988; 57:593–626.

48. Bies RD, Friedman DL, Roberts R, Perryman MB, Caskey CT. Expression and localization of dystrophin in human cardiac purkinje fibers. *Circulation* 1992; 86:147–153.

49. Bies RD, Phelps SF, Cortez MD, Roberts R, Caskey CT, Chamberlain JS. Human and murine dystrophin mRNA transcripts are differentially expressed during skeletal muscle, heart and brain development. *Nucleic Acids Res* 1992; 20:1725–1731.

50. Vybiral T, Williams JK, Winkelman JC, Roberts R, Joe EH, Casey DL, et al. Human cardiac and skeletal muscle spectrins: Differential expression and localization. *Cell Motil Cytoskeleton* 1992; 21:291–304.

51. Olson EN. Molecular pathways controlling heart development. *Science* 1996; 272:671–676.

52. Borg TK, Nakagawa M, Carver W, Terracio L. Overview: Extracellular matrix, receptors, and heart developments. In: Clark EB, Markwald RR, Takao A, eds. *Developmental Mechanisms of Heart Disease*. Armonk, NY: Futura; 1995:175–184.

53. Rayter SI, Iwata KK, Michitsch RW, Sorvillo JM, Valenzuela DM, Foulkes JG. Biochemical functions of oncogenes. In: Glover DM, Hames BD, eds. *Oncogenes*. New York: IRL Press; 1989:113–189.

54. Robert AR, Sporn MB. The transforming growth factor-β. In: Sporn MB, Roberts AR, eds. *Peptide Growth Factors and Their Receptors. Handbook of Experimental Pharmacology*. Heidelberg: Springer-Verlag; 1990:419–472.

55. Roberts R, Towbin J, Parker TG, Bies RD, eds. *A Primer of Molecular Biology*. New York: Elsevier; 1992.

56. Meerson FZ, ed. *The Failing Heart: Adaptations and Maladaptations*. New York: Raven; 1983.

57. Hammond GL, Wieben E, Markert CL. Molecular signals for initiating protein synthesis in organ hypertrophy. *Proc Natl Acad Sci USA* 1979; 76:2455–2459.

58. Imamura SI, Matsuoka R, Hiratsuka E, Kimura M, Nishikawa T, Takao A. Local response to cardiac overload on myosin heavy chain gene expression and isozyme transition. *Circ Res* 1990; 66:1067–1073.

59. Rubin SA, Correa M, Rabines A, Fishbein MC. Beta blockade alters myosin heavy chain gene expression after rat infarction (abstr). *Circulation* 1989; 80:II-458.

60. Clubb JR, Bishop FJ, Bishop SP. Formation of binucleated myocardial cells in the neonatal rat: An index for growth hypertrophy. *Lab Invest* 1984; 40:571–577.

61. Parker TG, Packer SE, Schneider MD. Peptide growth factors can provoke "fetal" contractile protein gene expression in rat cardiac myocytes. *J Clin Invest* 1990; 85:507–514.

62. Seidman CE, Wong DW, Jarcho JA, Bloch JD, Seidman JG. Cis-acting sequences that modulate atrial natriuretic factor gene expression. *Proc Natl Acad Sci USA* 1988; 85:4104–4108.

63. Schwarz F, Faure A, Katus H, Von Olshausen K, Hofmann M, Schuler G, et al. Intracoronary thrombolysis in acute myocardial infarction: An attempt to quantitate its effect by comparison of enzymatic estimate of myocardial necrosis with left ventricular ejection fraction. *Am J Cardiol* 1983; 51:1573–1578.

64. Mercadier JJ, Lompre AM, Duc P, Boheler KR, Fraysse JB, Wisnewsky C, et al. Altered sacroplasmic reticulum Ca^{2+}-ATPase gene expression in the human ventricle uring end-stage heart failure. *J Clin Invest* 1990; 8:305–309.

65. Ruzicka DL, Schwartz RJ. Sequential activation of a α-actin gene transcripts mark the onset of cardiomyocyte differentiation. *J Cell Biol* 1988; 107:2575–2586.

66. Olson EN. MyoD family: A paradigm for development? *Genes Dev* 1990; 4:1454–1461.

67. Davis RL, Weintraub H, Lassar AB. Expression of a single transfected cDNA converts fibroblasts to myoblasts. *Cell* 1987; 51:987–1000.

68. DeHaan RL. Organogenesis. In: DeHaan RL, Ursprung H, eds. New York: Holt, Rinehart, and Winston; 1965:377–420.

69. Lyons I, Parsons LM, Hartley L, Li R, Andrews JE, Robb L, et al. Myogenic and morphogenic defects in the heart tubes of murine embryos lacking the homeobox gene Nkx2-5. *Genes Dev* 1995; 9:1654–1666.

70. Edmondson DG, Olson EN. A gene with homology to the myc similarity region of MyoD1 is expressed during myogenesis and is sufficient to activate the muscle differentiation program. *Genes Dev* 1989; 3:628–640.

71. Wright WE, Sassoon DA, Lin VK. Myogenin, a factor regulating myogenesis, has a domain homologous to Myo D. *Cell* 1989; 56:607–617.

72. Braun T, Buschhausen-Denker G, Bober E, Tannich E, Arnold HH. A novel human muscle factor related to but distinct from MyoD1

induces myogenic conversion in 10T1/2 fibroblasts. *EMBO J* 1989; 8:701–709.

73. Rhodes SJ, Konieczny SF. Identification of MRF4: A new member of the muscle regulatory factor gene family. *Genes Dev* 1989; 3:2050–2061.

74. Miner JH, Wold B. Herculin, a fourth member of the MyoD family of myogenic regulatory genes. *Proc Natl Acad Sci USA* 1990; 87:1089–1093.

75. Braun T, Bober E. Winter B, Rosenthal N, Arnold HH. Myf-6, a new member of the human gene family of myogenic determination factors: Evidence for a gene cluster on chromosome 12. *EMBO J* 1990; 9:821–831.

76. Murre C, McCaw PS, Baltimore D. A new DNA binding and dimerization motif in immunoglobulin enhancer binding, daughterless, MyoD, and myc proteins. *Cell* 1989; 56:777–783.

77. Sasson D, Lyons G, Wright WE, Lin V, Lassar A, Weintraub H, et al. Expression of two myogenic regulatory factors myogenin and MyoD1 during mouse embryogenesis. *Nature* 1989; 41:303–307.

78. Harvey RP. NK-2 homeobox genes and heart development. *Dev Biol* 1996; 178:203–216.

79. Kim Y, Nirenberg M. *Drosophila* NK-homeobox genes. *Proc Natl Acad Sci USA* 1989; 86:7716–7720.

80. Scott MP, Tamkun JW, Hertzell GW III. The structure and function of the homeodomain. *Biochim Biophys Acta* 1989; 989:25–48.

81. Chen CY, Schwartz RJ. Identification of novel DNA binding targets and regulatory domains of a murine *tinman* homeodomain factor, Nkx-2.5. *J Biol Chem* 1995; 270:15628–15633.

82. Chen CY, Croissant J, Majesky M, Topouzis S, McQuinn T, Frankovsky MJ, et al. Activation of the cardiac α-actin promoter depends upon serum response factor, *tinman* homologue, Nkx-2.5, and intact serum response elements. *Dev Genet* 1996; 19:119–130.

83. Durocher D, Chen CY, Ardati A, Schwartz RJ, Nemer M. The atrial natriuretic factor promoter is a downstream target for Nkx-2.5 in the myocardium. *Mol Cell Biol* 1996; 16:4648–4655.

84. Gajewski K, Kim Y, Lee YM, Olson EN, Schultz RA. D-mef2 is a target for *tinman* activation during *Drosophila* heart development. *EMBO J* 1997. (In Press)

85. Bodmer R. The gene *tinman* is required for specification of the heart and visceral muscles in *Drosophila*. *Development* 1993; 118:719–729.

86. Azpiazu N, Frasch H. *Tinman* and bagpipe: Two homeo box genes that determine cell fates in the dorsal mesoderm of *Drosophila*. *Genes Dev* 1993; 7:1325–1340.

87. Lints TJ, Parsons LM, Hartley L, Lyons I, Harvey RP: Nkx-2.5: A novel murine homeobox gene expressed in early heart progenitor cells and their myogenic descendants. *Development* 1993; 119:419–431.

88. Komuro I, Izumo S. Csx: A murine homeobox-containing gene specifically expressed in the developing heart. *Proc Natl Acad Sci USA* 1993; 90:8145–8149.

89. Chen JN, Fishman MC. Zebrafish tinman homolog demarcates the heart field and initiates myocardial differentiation. *Development* 1996; 122:3809–3816.

90. Tonissen KF, Drysdale TA, Lints TJ, Havey RP, Krieg PA. XNkx-2.5, a *Xenopus* gene related to Nkx-2.5 and *tinman*: Evidence for a conserved role in cardiac development. *Dev Biol* 1994; 162:325–328.

91. Schultheiss TM, Xydas S, Lassar AB. Induction of avian cardiac myogenesis by anterior endoderm. *Development* 1995; 121:4203–4214.

92. Reecy JM, Yamada M, Cummings K, Sosic D, Chen CY, Eichele G, et al. Chicken Nkx-2.8: A novel homeobox gene expressed in early heart progenitor cells and pharyngeal pouch-2 and -3 endoderm. *Dev Biol* 1997. (In Press)

93. Kessel M, Gruss P. Homeotic transformations of murine vertebrae and concomitant alteration of Hox codes induced by retinoic acid. *Proc Natl Acad Sci USA* 1989; 67:89–104.

94. Teisman R. Identification of a protein-binding site that mediates transcription response of the *c-fos* gene to serum factors. *Cell* 1986; 46:567–574.

95. Croissant JD, Kim JH, Eichele G, Goering L, Lough J, Prywes R, et al. Avian serum response factor expression restricted primarily to muscle cell lineages is required for α-actin gene transcription. *Dev Biol* 1996; 177:250–264.

96. Dalton S, Treisman R. Characterization of SAP-1, a protein recruited by serum response factor to the *c-fos* serum response element. *Cell* 1992; 68:597–612.

97. Pollock R, Treisman R. Human SRF-related proteins: DNA-binding properties and potential regulatory targets. *Genes Dev* 1991; 5:2327–2341.

98. Gossett LA, Kelvin DJ, Sternberg EA, Olson EN. A new myocyte-specific enhancer-binding factor that recognizes a conserved element associated with multiple muscle-specific genes. *Mol Cell Biol* 1989; 9:5022–5033.

99. Bour BA, O'Brien MA, Lockwood ML, Goldstein ES, Bodmor R, Taghert PH, et al. *Drosophila* MEF2, a transcription factor is essential for myogenesis. *Genes Dev* 1995; 9:730–741.

100. Lilly B, Zhao B, Ranganayakulu G, Paterson BM, Schulz RA, Olson EN. Requirement of MADS domain transcription factor D-MEF2 for muscle formation in *Drosophila*. *Science* 1995; 267:688–693.

101. Edmondson DG, Lyons GE, Martin JF, Olson EN. *Mef-2* gene expression marks the cardiac and skeletal muscle lineages during mouse myogenesis. *Genes Dev* 1994; 120:1251–1263.

102. Yu Y, Reitbart RE, Smoot LB, Lee Y, Mahdavi V, Nadal-Ginard B. Human myocyte-specific enhancer factor 2 comprises a group of tissue-restricted MADS box transcription factors. *Genes Dev* 1992; 1783–1798.

103. Breitbart RE, Liang C, Smott LB, Laheru DA, Mahdavi V, Nadal-Ginard B. A fourth human MEF-2 transcription factor, hMEF-2d, is an early marker of the myogenic lineage. *Development* 1993; 118:1095–1106.

104. Martin JF, Miano JM, Hustad CM, Copeland NG, Jemkins NA, Olson EN. A Mef2 gene that generates a muscle-specific isoform via alternative mRNA splicing. *Mol Cell Biol* 1994; 14:1647–1656.

105. Grueneberg DA, Natesan S, Alexandre C, Gilman MZ. Human and *Drosophila* homeodomain proteins that enhance the DNA-binding activity of serum response factor. *Science* 1992; 257:1089–1095.

106. Grueneberg DA, Simon KJ, Brennan K, Gilman M. Sequence-specific targeting of nuclear signal transduction pathways by homeodomain proteins. *Mol Cell Biol* 1995; 15:3318–3326.

107. Opsltsein D, Vogels JE, Robert B, Kalkhoven E, Zwartkruis LL, Destree OH, et al. The mouse homeobox gene, S8, is expressed during embryogenesis predominantly in mesenchyme. *Mech Dev* 1991; 34:29–42.

108. Cserjesi P, Lilly B, Bryson L, Want Y, Sasson DA, Olson EN. MHox: A mesodermally-restricted homeodomain protein that binds an essential site in the muscle creatine kinase enhancer. *Development* 1992; 115:1087–1101.

109. Chen CY, Schwartz RJ. Recruitment of the *tinman* homolog Nkx-2.5 by serum response factor activates cardiac α-actin gene transcription. *Mol Cell Biol* 1996; 16:6372–6384.

110. Merika M, Orkin SH. DNA binding specificity of the GATA family transcription factors. *Mol Cell Biol* 1993; 13:3999–4010.

111. Laverriere AC, MacNeill C, Mueller C, Poelmann RE, Burch JBE, Evans T. GATA4/5/6 a subfamily of three transcription factors transcribed in developing heart and gut. *J Biol Chem* 1994; 269:23177–23184.

112. Morrisey EE, Ip HH, Lu MM, Parmaceh MS. GATA-6: A zinc finger transcription factor that is expressed in multiple cell lineages derived from lateral mesoderm. *Dev Biol* 1996; 177:309–322.

113. Ip HS, Wilson DB, Heikinheimo M, Tang Z, Ting CN, Simon MC, et al. The GATA-4 transcription factor transactivates the cardiac muscle specific troponin C promoter-enhancer in nonmuscle cells. *Mol Cell Biol* 1994; 14:7515–7526.

114. Mokentin JD, Lin Q, Duncan S, Olson EN. Requirement of the transcription factor GATA4 for heart tube formation and ventral morphogenesis. *Genes Dev* 1997; 11:1061–1072.

115. Zhang HB, Bradley A. Mice deficient for BMP2 are nonviable and have defects in amnion/chorion and cardiac development. *Development* 1996; 122:2977–2986.

116. Layton WM. Random determination of developmental process: Reversal of normal visceral asymmetry in the mouse. *J Hered* 1976; 67:336–338.

117. Yokoyama T, Copeland NG, Jenkins NA, Montgomery CA, Elder FFB, Overbeek PA. Reversal of left-right assymmetry: A situs inversus mutation. *Science* 1993; 260:679–682.

118. Srivastava D, Thomas T, Lin Q, Brown D, Olson EN. Regulation of cardiac mesodermal and neural crest development by the bHLH transcription factor, dHAND. *Nat Genet* 1997. (In Press)

119. Lin Q, Schwarz J, Bucana C, Olson EN. Control of mouse cardiac morphogenesis and myogenesis by transcription factor MEF2C. *Science* 1997; 276:1404–1407.

120. Lazzaro D, Price M, DeFelice M, DiLauro R. The transcription factor TTF-1 is expressed at the onset of thyroid and lung morphogenesis and in restricted regions of the foetal brain. *Development* 1991; 113:1093–1104.

121. Evans SM, Yan W, Murillo MP, Ponce J, Papalopulu N. *Tinman*, a *Drosophila* homeobox gene required for heart and visceral mesoderm specification, may be represented by a family of genes in vertebrates: XNkx-2.3, a second vertebrate homologue of *tinman*. *Development* 1995; 121:3889–3899.

122. Buchberger A, Pabst I, Brand T, Seidl K, Arnold H. Chick NKx-2.3 represents a novel family member of vertebrate homologues to the *Drosophila* homeobox gene *tinman:* Differential expression of cNKx-2.3 and cNKx-2.5 during heart and gut development. *Mech Dev* 1996; 56:151–163.

123. Lee KH, Xu Q, Breitbart RE. A new *tinman*-related gene, Nkx2.7, anticipates the expression of Nkx2.5 and Nkx2.3 in zebrafish heart and pharyngeal endoderm. *Dev Biol* 1996; 180:722–731.

8

EMBRYOLOGY OF THE HEART

Bradley B. Keller / Roger R. Markwald

The wide spectrum of congenital cardiovascular anomalies found from the prenatal period into adulthood has challenged clinicians and scientists for centuries.[1,2] Equally daunting historically have been the complex and varied descriptions of cardiac embryology and the pathogenesis of congenital cardiovascular malformations.[3-6] Fortunately, scientific advances—including the availability of cell-specific immunohistochemistry, rapid advances in molecular biological techniques, expansion of investigations into integrated embryonic cardiovascular physiology, and, finally, dramatic improvements in the three-dimensional imaging of embryonic cardiovascular anatomy—make the specific determination of pathogenesis for most cardiovascular anomalies a realistic goal over the next decade (Fig. 8-1).[7-11]

As with all complex subjects, cardiovascular structural maturation must be defined in a stepwise fashion. This chapter is organized in part in relation to the temporal maturation of the heart and vasculature and in part in relation to the sequence of important events that occur at specific regions of the developing heart and vasculature over time. The information presented in this chapter is focused on human development, though cardiovascular embryology is now under investigation in a wide range of mammalian and nonmammalian species.

DEVELOPMENT OF THE HEART TUBE

Embryo Patterning

The morphogenesis of the heart begins with the initial patterning that determines the three axes of the embryo: anterior-posterior, dorsal-ventral, and left-right. These axes are imprinted onto the cellular program as cell populations expand to form the embryo and extraembryonic tissues. Structural asymmetry is apparent at the blastodisk stage, when the primitive streak defines the anterior-posterior axis and the dorsal-ventral axis is defined by the position of the yolk sac. Specific genes have been identified that alter axis determination in a range of species, including the mouse.[12,13]

The process of mesoderm formation is integral to the organization of the primary axis of the embryo and the differentiation of right and left sides. At the blastodisk stage of development, there are two primitive germ layers, endoderm and ectoderm. Mesoderm is formed as ectodermal cells migrate through the primitive streak coursing adjacent to Hensen's node. Hensen's node contains retinoic acid and serves as an embryonic organizer, conferring positional information on the mesodermal cells.[14] At this critical phase in cell determination, exogenous retinoic acid is extremely teratogenic. Interestingly, retinoic acid has a gradient-like effect on determination of the heart tube, with the greatest effect at the arterial pole and least effect at the venous pole.[15] Following migration, this crescent of mesodermal cells forms the precardiac region from which heart and great vessels precursor cells originate.

Correct laterality is fundamental to the developing embryo and situs solitus has the lowest risk of congenital cardiovascular malformations.[16] There is a progressive increase in the rate of defects in situs inversus totalis, bilateral left-sidedness, and bilateral right-sidedness; bilateral same-sidedness is consistently associated with congenital heart defects in humans. There are several theories regarding the determination of laterality; however, the important point is that laterality may be altered by a single gene mutation, with life-threatening consequences.[17,18]

Following determination of the embryo axes, subpopulations of cells are programmed in a segmental body plan. Much of our understanding of the body plan comes from developmental studies of *Drosophila*, an insect with a head, thorax, and abdomen.[19] In mammals, maternal gene products control the cell through the first two cell cycles; then control switches to the embryonic genome. These patterning genes are arranged along the vertical axis of the neural crest, which is relevant to the spectrum of conotruncal defects that are a consequence of abnormal neural crest cell migration.[20] Recent

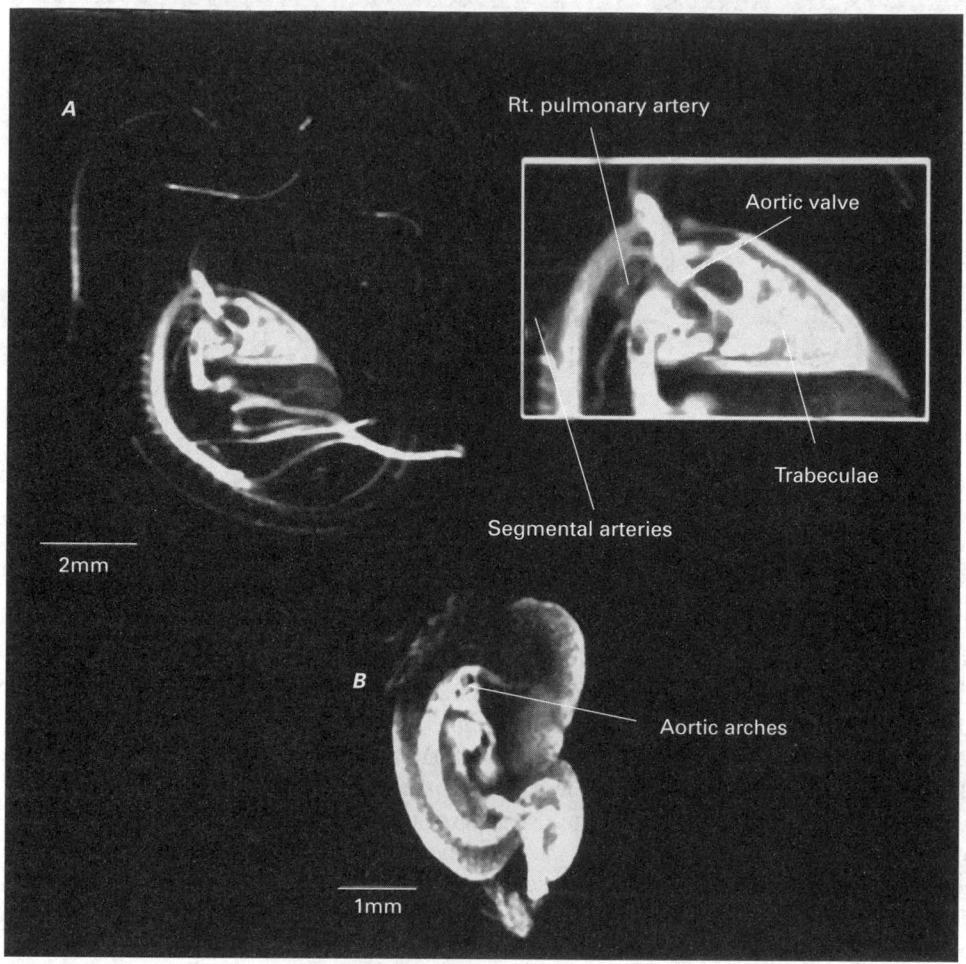

FIGURE 8-1

Magnetic resonance microscopy of mouse embryos at embryonic days 12.5 (*A*) and 9.5 (*B*). These embryos were perfused with BSA-DTPA-Gd, an MR contrast agent to enhance the signal from cardiovascular structures. These volume-rendered images, based on three-dimensional T1-weighed scans, demonstrate the cardiac chambers, cardiac valves, aortic arches, intersegmental vessels, cranial vasculature, and hepatic vasculature. Scale bars are marked as 1 or 2 mm. (Data courtesy of Brad Smith, the NIH National Research Resource Center for In Vivo Microscopy, Duke University.)

cellular protease, and morphogenetic signals from the transforming growth factor beta (TGF-β) and fibroblast growth factor 2 (FGF-2) growth and differentiation factors.[24–27] The genetic events that mediate the transformation of stem cell to cardiac myocyte are now becoming clear. In skeletal muscle, differentiation is mediated by a group of proteins including MYO D and helix-loop-helix proteins that bind to E-box regions. Specific muscle gene induction within the myocyte is also likely related to unique transcription factors for skeletal, cardiac, and smooth muscle.[28,29]

In the human embryo, the heart begins to contract at day 17 as the machinery of contraction and relaxation becomes functional. These functional units include the sarcomere, composed of the contractile elements; the mitochondria, containing the enzymes for energy production and modulation; and the sarcolemma, the cell envelope with specialized components of the t-tubular system linked to the sarcoplasmic reticulum. In the mature myocardium, sarcomeres are organized parallel to the lines of peak systolic stress. In the embryonic myocyte, myofibrils initially appear disarrayed and become aligned as development proceeds.[30] Despite this disordered appearance, the contraction pattern of the early embryonic heart is isotropic.[31]

The temporal and spatial expression of contractile proteins in the developing heart is under intense investigation. At the pre–cardiac tube stage, smooth muscle alpha actin is the only isoform present. With formation of the cardiac tube, there is progressive expression of the cardiac form of sarcomeric actin with the onset of cardiac pumping. The alpha smooth muscle actin may act as a scaffolding during assembly of the sarcomere.[32,33]

Mitochondria multiply concurrently with the myofibrils in the differentiating myocyte. In the mature heart, mitochondrial enzymes are the major source of the high-energy phosphate necessary for contraction and likely begin this function during embryonic development. In the chick, the mitochondria account for about 10 percent of the myocyte volume.[30] In the rat embryo, the total volume increases from 22 to 34 percent

molecular studies have also confirmed the segmental patterning of the cardiac tube, linking gene products with morphologic boundaries between the atria, ventricle, and outflow tract in chick, mouse, and human hearts.[21]

Myocyte Determination, Migration, and Differentiation

There is intense interest in the origin and signals that transform precardiac mesoderm into myocardium. The primordial myocytes arise in the splanchnic fold of the lateral mesothelium. Retrovirus labeling studies define at least two populations of myocyte progenitors in the ventricle and show that these myocytes migrate in response to a variety of factors. Clusters of cells within the tubular heart form units that coalesce to segments of the cardiac wall.[22,23] The regulation of myocyte migration and further differentiation is complex and likely involves cell adhesion molecules including *N*-cadherin, extra-

between days 6 and 10, and the mitochondria also change morphologically with development, becoming larger with more cristae and denser matrix.[34] The myocyte mitochondrial volume fraction correlates directly with heart rate and oxygen consumption among animals.[35]

Maturation of the sarcoplasmic reticulum (SR) and apparatus for excitation-contraction coupling occurs coincident with the structural morphogenesis of the embryonic heart. The sarcolemma contains ion pumps, channels, and exchangers that maintain chemical and charge differences between extracellular and intracellular spaces.[36] During maturation of the heart, the resting potential increases (becomes more negative) in both birds and mammals.[37,38] Ca^{2+} influx through Ca^{2+} channels may play a relatively important role in transsarcolemmal Ca^{2+} influx in the immature heart. However, peak Ca^{2+} current density is actually decreased as compared to that measured in mature cells.[39,40] Although Ca^{2+} influx by way of the Na^+-Ca^{2+} exchanger is less important for excitation-contraction coupling in mature myocardium, Na^+-Ca^{2+} exchange may play an important role in myocytes from relatively immature rabbit hearts.

Relaxation, an active process by which the myocardium returns to steady state after contraction, depends on rapid removal of Ca^{2+} from troponin C. This is mediated primarily by active transport of Ca^{2+} back into the SR. The SR Ca^{2+} pump ATPase (SERCA2a) usually couples hydrolysis of ATP to active Ca^{2+} transport. The rate of SR Ca^{2+} uptake correlates well with the observed rate of myocardial relaxation. Regulation of SR Ca^{2+} pump activity is mediated by the intrinsic SR protein, phospholamban. Ca^{2+} is also removed from the myofilaments by extrusion across the cell membrane. In the steady state, the amount of Ca^{2+} removed from the myocyte equals the amount entering through the Ca^{2+} channels.[41]

Neural Crest Cell Migration

The neural crest is another major cell mass contributing to the morphogenesis of the heart. The neural crest arises from the dorsal margin of the neural tube prior to fusion and migrates ventrally to form the autonomic ganglia, melanocyte, and Schwann cells. The crest cells move in waves through the branchial arches during the first 4 weeks of human development. The eventual fate of the neural crest cells is likely determined long before the initial phenotypic expression of a heart tube by activation of the cellular gradients of *Hox* genes and other morphoregulating factors.[42,43] The cranial neural crest region

defines a developmental field that includes the heart, hindbrain, face, and branchial arch derivatives.

Experimental disruption of cranial neural crest produces a spectrum of abnormalities. In a series of elegant ablation and chick quail chimera studies, Kirby and colleagues defined the range of cardiac neural crest that is integral to the septation of the conotruncal region of the heart and branchial arch derivatives, including facial abnormalities, thymus, parathyroid, and autonomic derivatives.[42] These neural crest cells are site-specific and carry information for formation of structures appropriate to their origin rather than being defined at the destination of migration.

Hox gene abnormalities are associated with defects in the derivatives of cranial neural crest. A transgenic murine model of *Hox* 1.1 overexpression has neural crest ectomesenchymal tissue abnormalities including cleft palate, nonfused pinnae, and open eyes. *Hox* 1.5–deficient mice have features of DiGeorge syndrome.[43] In humans, DiGeorge syndrome and velocardiofacial syndrome are associated with chromosomal abnormalities, teratogens, and deletions in the long arm of chromosome 22 DiGeorge.[44–47] In addition, retinoic acid is a potent teratogen in humans and produces a syndrome involving all the derivatives of the cranial neural crest.[48]

Formation of the Heart Tube

Formation of the cardiac tube is a complex morphogenetic event. Myocyte commitment occurs in the early blastula stage followed by clonal expansion in the bilateral heart forming regions located in the lateral splanchnic folds (Fig. 8-2). The bilateral heart tubes each contain an inner layer of endoderm, a middle layer of cardiac jelly, and an outer layer of myocardium. At the cephalic end of the embryo (on each side of the

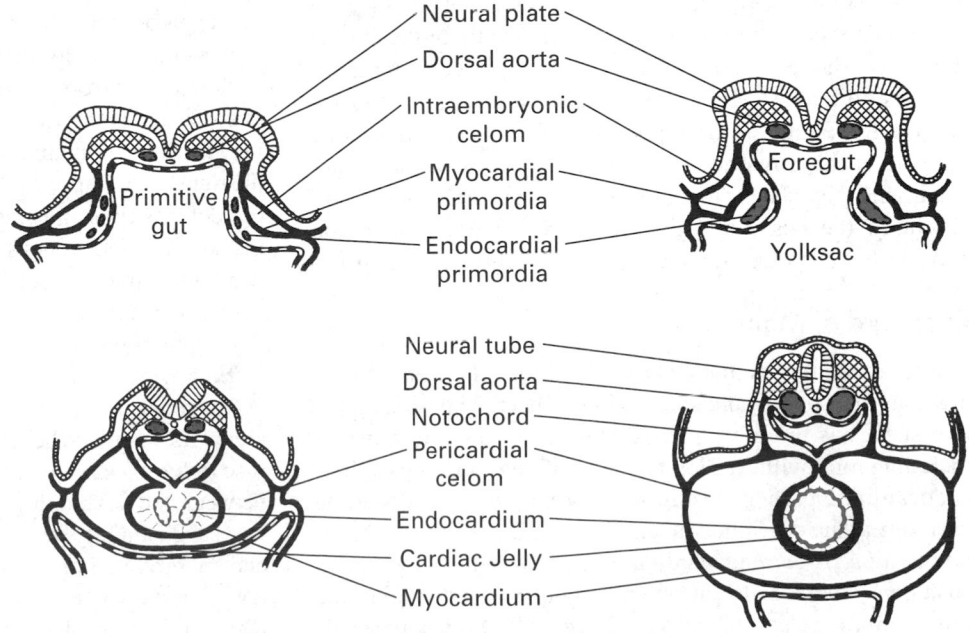

FIGURE 8-2

Schematic transverse section through embryos of different ages showing the formation of the midline heart tube.

midsagittal plane), myocytes within a section of each heart tube acquire contractile elements, and the position of the heart tubes shifts first to be parallel and close to each other within the cephalic part of the developing body cavity (intraembryonic coelom), ventral to the foregut, followed by fusion of the heart tubes in the ventral midline to form the embryonic ventricle and bulbus cordis.[4,5,49–51]

Cardiac Jelly

Between the myocardium and endocardium is an acellular mass of extracellular matrix called *cardiac jelly*. Cardiac jelly forms prior to cardiac tube fusion and is closely associated with the primordial myocytes.[52] At the pretubular heart stages, the extracellular matrix contains collagen types I and IV, fibronectin, and laminin. The primordial endothelial cells destined to form the endocardium interact and migrate through this matrix during the establishment of the primitive bilateral heart tubes. Radioactive labeling demonstrates that proteins produced in the myocardium flow toward the endocardium and are incorporated into the basal lamina.[53] The cardiac jelly has a variety of functions related to hemodynamic performance, cardiac looping, and cell migration in cardiac septation and formation of the endocardial cushion valves at the atrioventricular (AV) junction and outflow tract of the heart.

The protein composition in cardiac jelly modulates differentiation of the endothelium. Recent information explains the role of genes from the TGF-β family of peptide growth factors as regulators of morphogenesis.[54] TGF-β_2 proteins are in the extracellular matrix and an integral component to the morphogenetic changes at the AV cushion level, acting through second messengers like protein kinase C.[55] In addition, fibronectin likely serves to set up migratory pathways in the cardiac jelly. These protein strands are arranged radially in the cushion, presumably along the lines of stress. The fibronectin strands may also serve as a template for the fibrous skeleton of the AV valve leaflets.[56–58] The extracellular matrix proteins stimulate cellular dedifferentiation of the endocardium in these regions, prompting endothelial cells to migrate into the cushion matrix. Laminin and type IV collagen are stabilizing signals or markers, since these compounds are absent in the cushion regions but present adjacent to the endocardial cells that maintain a typical epithelial integrity.

Endocardial Maturation

The endothelial cells that make up the lining of the embryonic heart are initially arranged as a single sheet. This squamous-like sheet has the morphologic features of an active tissue, including microvilli, ruffles, and intercellular openings.[59] The endocardium participates in the formation of endocardial cushions at the AV junction and in the outflow tract.[60] Dedifferentiation of the endocardium occurs over the endocardial cushions, where cells round up, produce pseudopodia, and migrate into the cardiac jelly.[61] These cells eventually make up a portion of the fibrous skeleton of the cardiac valves. Chemical signals from the endocardium to the myocardium

regulate the cardiac jelly extracellular matrix. In addition, hemodynamic alterations can influence the orientation of endocardial cells on the endocardial cushions[62] and the loci of dead and dying cells in the chick embryo heart.[63] This interaction is likely similar to the relationship between the endothelium and smooth muscle of the mature vascular bed.[64] Finally, expansion of the endocardium is critical to the process of ventricular trabeculation, as discussed below.

Looping

Following complete fusion of the heart tube, the embryo is about 2 mm long and 23 days old. From the dilated cephalic, extrapericardial portion of the bulboventricular tube—the aortic sac—originates the first pair of aortic arches and later also the second, third, fourth, and sixth arches (the fifth pair of aortic arches does not normally develop in mammals or is very rudimentary). The caudal part of the bulboventricular tube expands to form the early embryonic ventricle. It receives the paired confluence of veins that lie extrapericardially, caudal to the embryonic ventricles, embedded in mesenchyme.

The growing bulboventricular tube bends to the right and anteriorly into a compound sigmoid structure: the bulboventricular loop (Fig. 8-3). The deepening concavity on the left side of the bulboventricular loop is referred to as the *bulboventricular groove* or *sulcus*. Internally, the bulboventricular sulcus corresponds to a fold, the bulboventricular fold. At this stage the descending limb of the loop is called the embryonic ventricle and the ascending limb, the bulbus cordis. The AV junction, which at first lies in the midline, is displaced laterally to the left. The embryonic ventricle is thus positioned in the left side of the pericardial cavity, and the right side of this cavity is now occupied by the rapidly enlarging bulbus cordis.

Cardiac looping appears to be due to a fundamental property of the myocardium[65–68] rather than being a passive phenomenon brought about by flexure of the rapidly lengthening bulboventricular loop within the space available in the coelomic (pleuropericardial) cavity, as was thought previously.[69,70] At least three different biomechanical mechanisms may act in combination to generate the characteristic bend to the right of the cardiac tube: locally constrained growth, active cell deformation, and prestressed dorsal mesocardium.[71] Since the arterial and venous poles of the heart tube are fixed, bending of the tube imparts to it a certain amount of torsion that may be responsible partly for the spiral orientation of the developing outlet septum.

Following looping of the primitive heart tube, subsequent events relate primarily to the development of sequential events along its length. The originally paired venous confluences fuse to form a large common atrium and endocardial cushions between the developing atrium and ventricle are shifted leftward and cranially, remaining relatively narrow. The ventricle and the proximal one-third of the bulbus cordis expand, while the junction between them, the primary interventricular foramen (also referred to as the bulboventricular foramen), remains narrow and comes to lie approximately in the midsagittal plane[70] (Figs. 8-4 and 8-5).

ANOMALIES

Ventricular Inversion with Transposition of the Great Arteries

If the cardiac loop forms to the left and anterior, rather than to the right and anterior, then all structures derived from the bulboventricular loop—i.e., the AV valves, the ventricles, and the arterial roots—will develop in an inverted position. Since the sinus venosus, the atria, and the truncoaortic sac lie extrapericardially, these parts of the heart remain normally located. The aorticopulmonary septum also develops in a normal fashion, but since partitioning of the inverted truncus arteriosus takes place in mirror image, the end result is transposition of the great arteries with the aorta arising anteriorly from a left-sided, morphologically right (systemic) ventricle and the pulmonary trunk arising posteriorly from a right-sided, morphologically left (venous) ventricle—hence the term *corrected transposition* commonly used for this anomaly.

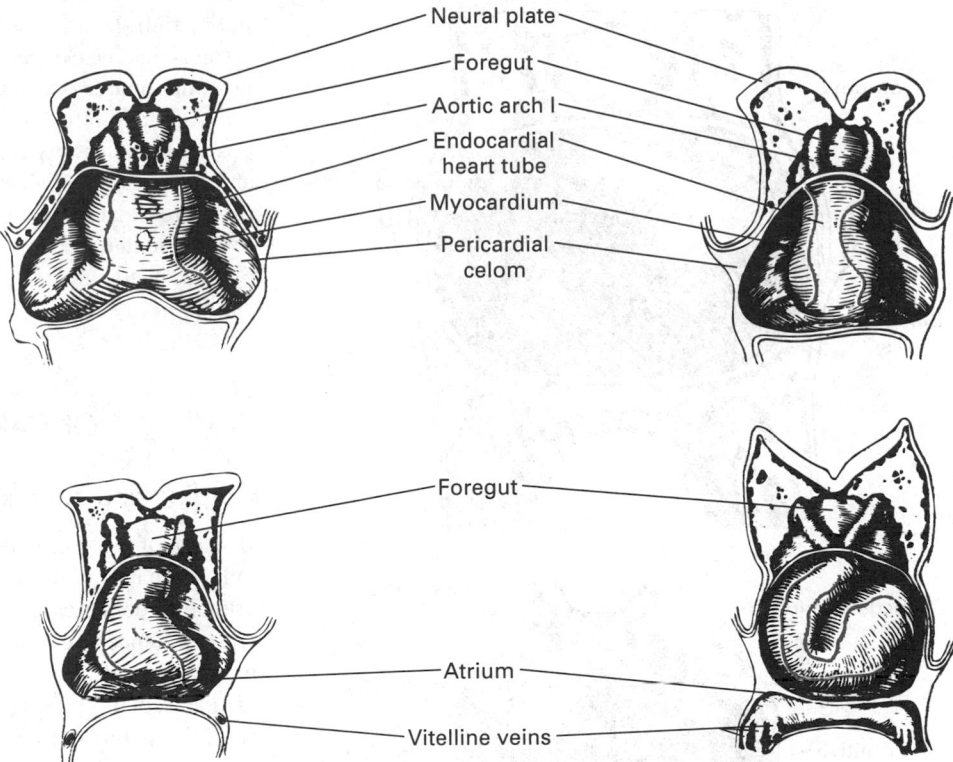

FIGURE 8-3
Schematic ventral dissections of human embryos of different ages showing formation of the heart loop. (Adapted from Davis CL. Development of the human heart from its first appearance to the state found in embryos of 20 paired somites. *Contrib Embryol* 1927; 19:245. Reproduced with permission from the Carnegie Institution of Washington.)

Double-Outlet Right Ventricle

This anomaly appears to be due to lack of medial shift of the conus cordis, which retains its original embryologic relationships with the right ventricle only. The bulboventricular fold is retained and separates the two arterial ostia from the AV ostia (aortic-mitral valve discontinuity). This anomaly can be produced experimentally following a wide range of hemodynamic, metabolic, and genetic insults, suggesting that the phenotype of double-outlet right ventricle may be a final common expression of a range of primary abnormalities.[72]

Myocardial Trabeculation

The processes of primary myocardial trabeculation, expansion of secondary and tertiary myocardial trabeculae, and myocardial compaction are critical to the structural maturation of the ventricular chambers. This process results in the transformation of the smooth-walled endocardial lining into complex three-dimensional structure of the right and left ventricular myocardium. Rapid cell division and interposition of endothelial cells along the right and left ventrolateral borders of the endocardial tube is associated with a rapid resorption of cardiac jelly, resulting in myocardial ridges and trabeculae lined with single layers of endocardial cells.[73] The initial number and orientation of the myocardial ridges differs between species.[74] In general, myocardial trabeculation begins at the ventricular outer curvature (future apex) and then extends proximally and distally. The intersection between the outer, compact myocardium and the base of the trabeculae is likely a site of peak wall stress, and myocyte division is most active at this site (Fig. 8-5).[75,76] Retroviral marker studies have also shown that ventricular myocardial growth is associated with a transmural distribution of clonally related myocardial cells extending from the epicardium to the endocardium.[27] Of note, these cells reside in muscle bundles that are oriented at an angle to the longitudinal axis of the heart, consistent with the adult myocardial architecture that results in efficient twist and contraction.[27] However, the mechanisms that regulate clonal myocardial expansion and compaction remain undefined.

With the onset of myocardial trabeculation, diverticula first appear as two sharply defined areas along the right and left ventrolateral borders of the endocardial tube.[77] These diverticula develop initially at the expense of the cardiac jelly and later also penetrate the myocardium as the latter increases in thickness, producing a spongy mass of trabeculae.[73] The filling capacity of the heart is increased by the added intertrabecular spaces. The trabeculating embryonic heart can be now divided into primitive right and left ventricles, as there are distinct morphologic differences between the trabecular architecture of the developing ventricular chambers. The devel-

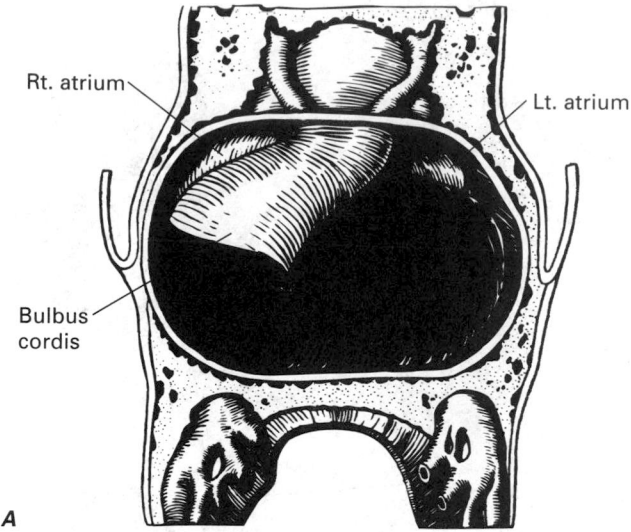

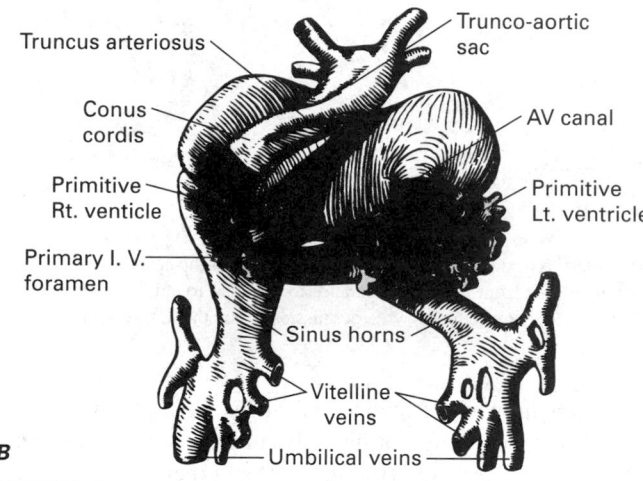

FIGURE 8-4

Twenty-somite human embryo, ovulation age about 25 days. *A.* Ventral dissection. *B.* Reconstruction of cardiac lumen. (Adapted from an original painting by Netter FH. In: Netter FH, ed. *The CIBA Collection of Medical Illustrations.* Summit, NJ: CIBA Pharmaceutical Company; 1969:112. Copyright by CIBA Pharmaceutical Company, Division of CIBA-GEIGY Corporation. Reproduced with permission from the publisher.)

oping left ventricle is trabecular over the majority of its greater curvature, while the developing right ventricle has a significant portion that is smooth-walled.[78] At this stage of development, the embryo is approximately 3 mm long and has an ovulation age of about 25 days.[49] Because of future developments, it is helpful to distinguish three sections in developing right ventricle and common outflow tract: the bulbus cordis, of which the proximal one-third includes the trabeculated portion of the primitive right ventricle; the conus cordis, representing the smooth-walled middle one-third, from which the outflow portions of both ventricles will be derived; and the truncus arteriosus, which is the terminal one-third which, after partitioning, develops into the aortic and pulmonary roots. The later two-thirds are occasionally referred to as the *conotruncus.*

The rapid growth and expansion of the primitive atria cause the conotruncal section of the bulbus cordis to shift from its initial right-lateral position to a more medial location. The result is that the truncus arteriosus comes to lie in a midsagittal position, in a depression of the atrial roof between the primitive right and left atria; the conus cordis assumes an oblique position and lies between the roof of the primitive left ventricle and the anteromedial wall of the right atrium. In an embryo of approximately 4 to 5 mm in crown-rump (CR) length (ovulation age of approximately 27 days), the external shape of the heart already suggests its future four-chambered condition.

MECHANISMS OF CARDIAC SEPTATION

Cardiac and Extracardiac Orientation

Because of rapid growth and the progressive curvature of the longitudinal axis of the embryo during organogenesis, it is critical to define cardiac morphogenesis, including septation, with reference to extracardiac markers that relate to the longitudinal axis of the embryo.[79] In the following discussion on cardiac septation, therefore, the diaphragm (septum transversum) is assumed to maintain an approximately horizontal position as in the mature heart. The terms *anterior, posterior, superior,* and *inferior* are employed accordingly. Although the formation of the various cardiac septa occurs almost simultaneously, it is necessary, for clarity, to consider their development individually.

Mechanisms of Cardiac Septation

There are two basic methods by which a septum can be formed in a hollow organ such as the heart.[78,80] First, differential growth may occur between a relatively slow-growing "passive" segment of the circumference versus a rapidly growing region (Fig. 8-6*A* and *B*). The portions of the walls of the expanded regions on either side of the narrow intervening segment come to face each other, appose, and fuse. However, expansive growth takes place mainly in one direction, resulting in the formation of a septum with an eccentrically placed communication between the two adjoining chambers. A septum formed in this fashion can never be complete: there is always an opening in it somewhere. A second mechanism of septation is seen in portions of the heart that possess a well-developed layer of cardiac mesenchyme (endocardial cushion tissue) between the myocardium and the endocardium (e.g., the AV canal, the conus cordis, and the truncus arteriosus). Local elaborations of such cardiac mesenchyme form two apposing masses of tissue that grow toward each other and fuse. This active fusion process may include the participation of cells of extracardiac origin, as with neural crest cell involvement in outlet septation.[42] Because of their appearance, these masses of mesenchymal tissue are called *cushions* (Fig. 8-6*C*). Occasionally a septum in its initial phases of development is formed passively but is completed by actively growing cushion tissue present along its free edge (Fig. 8-6*D*).

Partitioning of the embryonic heart is accomplished by the formation of seven basic septa. Of these, three are formed passively (septum secundum of the atrium, muscular portion of the ventricular septum, and aorticopulmonary septum) and three are formed actively (septum of the AV canal, conal septum, and truncal septum). One, the atrial septum primum, starts out as a passively formed septum, but it is completed by actively growing tissue along its border.

The Ventricles

In an embryo of about 5 mm in CR length, the AV canal communicates exclusively with the primitive left ventricle, and blood reaches the primitive right ventricle only by way of the primary interventricular foramen. Until the completion of ventricular septation, the primary interventricular foramen is bordered by the developing muscular interventricular septum inferiorly and anteriorly and by the bulbo-(cono-)ventricular fold superiorly and posteriorly (Fig. 8-7A). The interventricular septum and the conoventricular fold are continuous with each other anterosuperiorly.

The ventricles enlarge by centrifugal growth of the myocardium. The trabecular myocardium progresses from primary to secondary to tertiary trabeculations, while the compact outer myocardial layer remains relatively thin.[81] Coalescence of the secondary trabeculations into larger tertiary trabeculations occurs following septation, coincident with formation of the AV valve leaflets.[82] The trabeculae positioned at the border between the developing left and right ventricles coalesce to form the major portion of the muscular ventricular septum.[82] On the right side, a large trabecula, the trabecula septomarginalis,[83] appears early (in embryos of about 9 mm in CR length) and runs from the anteroinferior border of the primary interventricular foramen toward the apex (Fig. 8-7B).

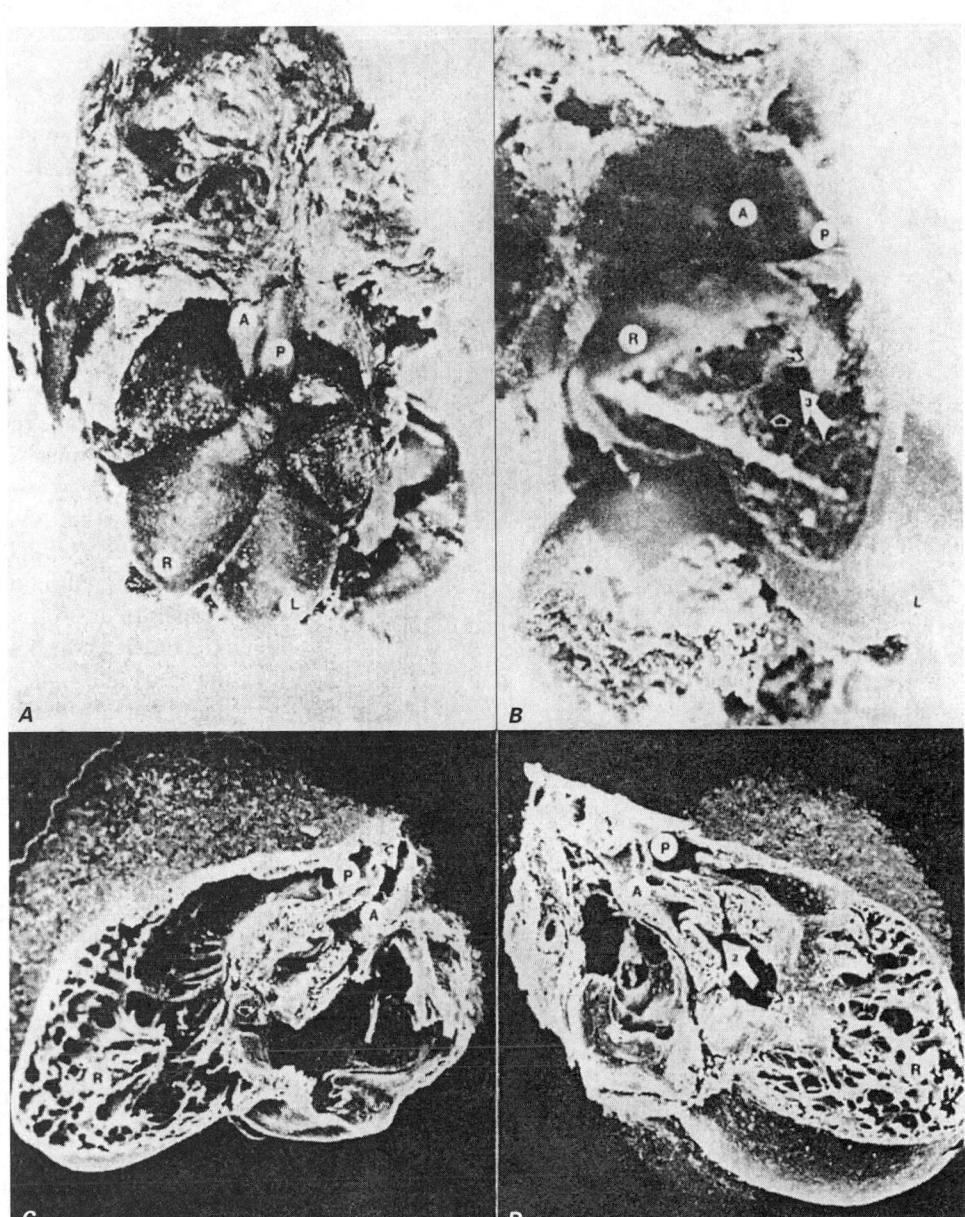

FIGURE 8-5
Human embryo heart, stage XIX, 45 days of gestation. *A.* Frontal view, ×25. *B.* Microdissected right ventricle, ×25; small arrow indicates fusion line of conal cushions. The arrowhead is situated on the fused AV cushions. The large arrow indicates the axis of the foramen interventriculae tertium. *C.* Right (parietal) half of the right ventricle, ×44; arrowhead labels the superior lateral AV cushion. *D.* Left (septal) half of the right ventricle, ×44; large arrow is within the foramen interventriculae secundum, directed toward the left ventricular outflow tract, and the small arrow is positioned in the foramen interventricular tertium. (From Pexieder T, Janecek P. Organogenesis of the human embryonic and early fetal heart as studied by microdissection and SEM. In: Nora JJ, Takao A, eds. *Congenital Heart Disease: Causes and Processes.* Mt Kisco, NY: Futura; 1984:401–421. Reproduced with permission from the publisher.)

ANOMALIES

Muscular Ventricular Septal Defect
Failure of compaction and fusion of the trabecular portion of the ventricular septum results in the most common congenital cardiovascular anomaly, the isolated muscular ventricular septal defect.

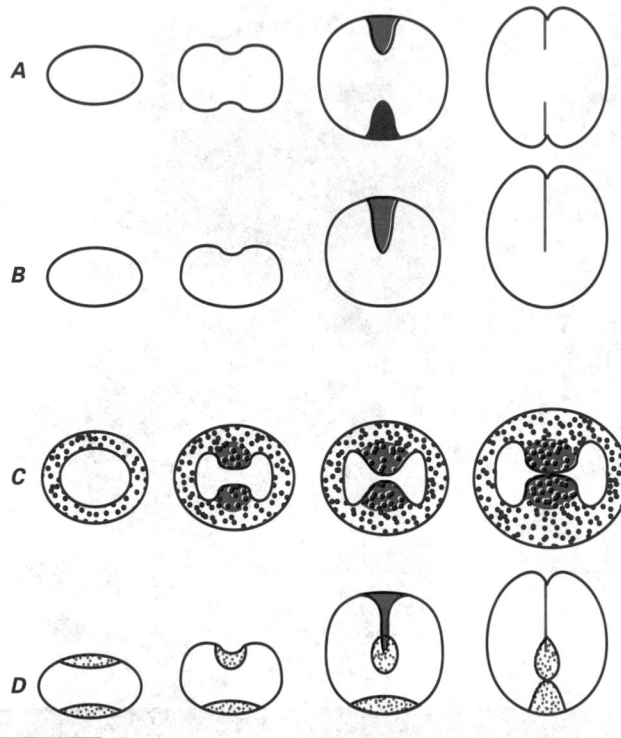

FIGURE 8-6

Mechanism of cardiac septation. *A* and *B*. Passively formed septum. *C*. Actively formed septum. *D*. Combination of *B* and *C*. [From Van Mierop LHS. Morphological development of the heart. In: Berne RM, ed. *Handbook of Physiology:* Sec 2. *The Cardiovascular System.* Vol 1: *The Heart.* Bethesda, MD: American Physiological Society; 1979:11. Reproduced with permission from the American Physiological Society.]

The Atrioventricular Canal

Division of the AV canal into right- and left-sided orifices occurs as the result of fusion of the superior and inferior AV endocardial cushions, which are first evident in the 6-mm CR-length human embryo (Fig. 8-7). First, the AV canal expands rightward while the conotruncus shifts medially. At 6 mm, this shift has not been completed and the AV canal gives access to the primitive left ventricle only and is separated from the conus cordis by the bulboventricular fold. With further development, the central portion of this fold recedes, and blood can now enter the primitive right ventricle directly from the right-sided atrium (Fig. 8-7). In 9-mm CR-length embryos, the left-sided portion of the fold terminates almost midway along the base of the superior endocardial cushion and is less prominent (Fig. 8-7B), while the right-sided portion becomes part of the parietal band. In older embryos, both the medial shift of the conotruncus and the effacement of the central part of the bulboventricular fold continue until the plane of the primary interventricular foramen is repositioned to left from an original vertical position, providing direct access from the primitive left ventricle to the posteromedial portion of the conus cordis and the aorta. Rather than closing, the primary interventricular foramen enlarges, resulting in the aortic infundibulum in the mature heart.[83]

ANOMALIES

Single Ventricle, Left Ventricular Type with Rudimentary Outflow Chamber, or Double-Inlet Left Ventricle

If the early embryonic AV canal fails to shift medially, retains its far leftward position, and divides into right and left AV ostia, then both of these ostia continue to empty into the primitive left ventricle. The proximal one-third of the bulbus (primitive right ventricle) thus does not receive the right AV ostium, its inflow portion will not develop, and as a result, it remains small. The communication between the large ventricular chamber and the rudimentary outflow chamber represents the persistent primary interventricular foramen of the young embryo heart.

Meanwhile, the AV canal has enlarged to the right while the growing endocardial cushions project into the lumen (Fig. 8-7B). Smaller cushions appear on the lateral borders of the AV canal. In the 10-mm CR-length embryo, the major cushions reach each other and fuse, resulting in a complete division of the canal into right and left AV orifices. At the same time the cushions also bend, and after fusion they form an arch that is concavely directed anteriorly and toward the left ventricle[70]; its convexity is directed anteriorly and toward the atria (Figs. 8-7C and 8-8). The free margin of the atrial septum primum fuses with the convex atrial side of the fused endocardial cushions (Fig. 8-8C). The left limb of the fused AV cushion eventually becomes incorporated into the anterior cusp of the mitral valve. The right half of the fused endocardial cushions comes to lie within the ventricles in a sagittal orientation somewhat to the right of the muscular interventricular septum. Thus the communication remaining between right and left ventricles, the secondary interventricular foramen, is bordered by the muscular ventricular septum inferiorly and anteriorly, the right extremity of the fused endocardial cushions posteriorly, and the conal septum superiorly (Fig. 8-8C). The plane of the secondary interventricular foramen, therefore, inclines somewhat to the right; that of the primary interventricular foramen, as we have seen, has come to deviate to the left. Both interventricular foramens share the top of the muscular septum as part of their inferior borders.

ANOMALIES

Partial and Complete Atrioventricular Canal Defect

The several forms of persistent AV canal are due to various degrees of failure of fusion of the superior and inferior AV canal cushions. Total lack of fusion results in a single AV ostium, i.e., the complete form of the anomaly. Since the arch or bay normally formed after the fusion of the endocardial cushions fails to develop, the lower border of the atrial septum cannot fuse with the endocardial cushions. The result is a low-lying, large interatrial communication, and the AV part of the cardiac septum is absent. The upper part of the ventricular septum remains deficient to a greater or lesser degree, and

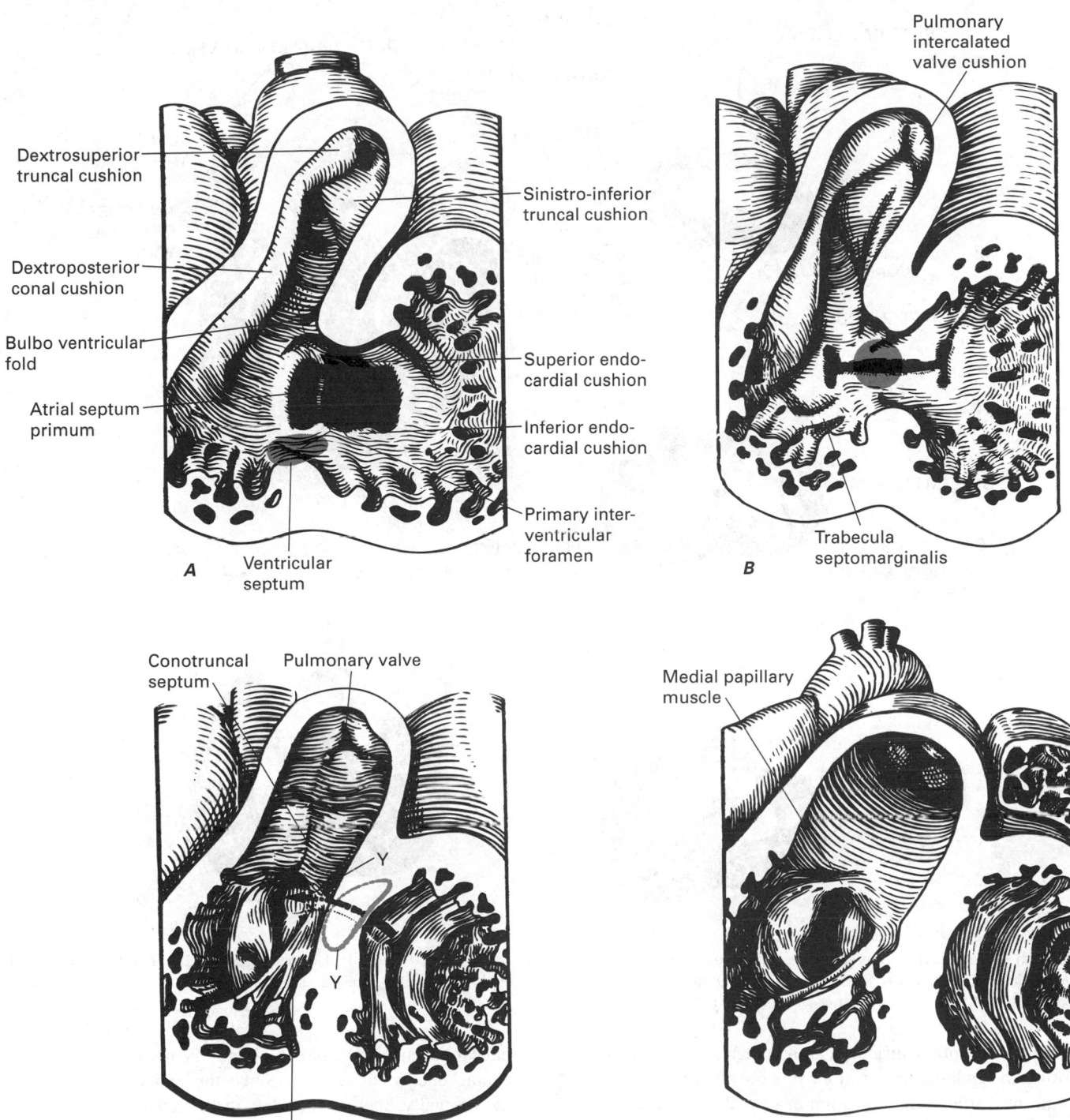

Dextrosuperior truncal cushion

Dextroposterior conal cushion

Bulbo ventricular fold

Atrial septum primum

Sinistro-inferior truncal cushion

Superior endo-cardial cushion

Inferior endo-cardial cushion

Primary inter-ventricular foramen

Ventricular septum

A

Pulmonary intercalated valve cushion

Trabecula septomarginalis

B

Conotruncal septum

Pulmonary valve

Y

Y

Trabecula septomarginalis

C

Medial papillary muscle

D

FIGURE 8-7

Schematic frontal section through the heart of embryos: 6.5 mm CR length (*A*); 9 mm CR length (*B*); 16 mm CR length (*C*); and 40 mm CR length (*D*). X = primary interventricular foramen; Y = secondary interventricular foramen. (Redrawn from Van Mierop LHS, Alley RD, Kausel HW, et al. The anatomy and embryology of endocardial cushion defects. *J Thorac Cardiovasc Surg* 1962; 43:71. Reproduced with permission from the publisher and author.)

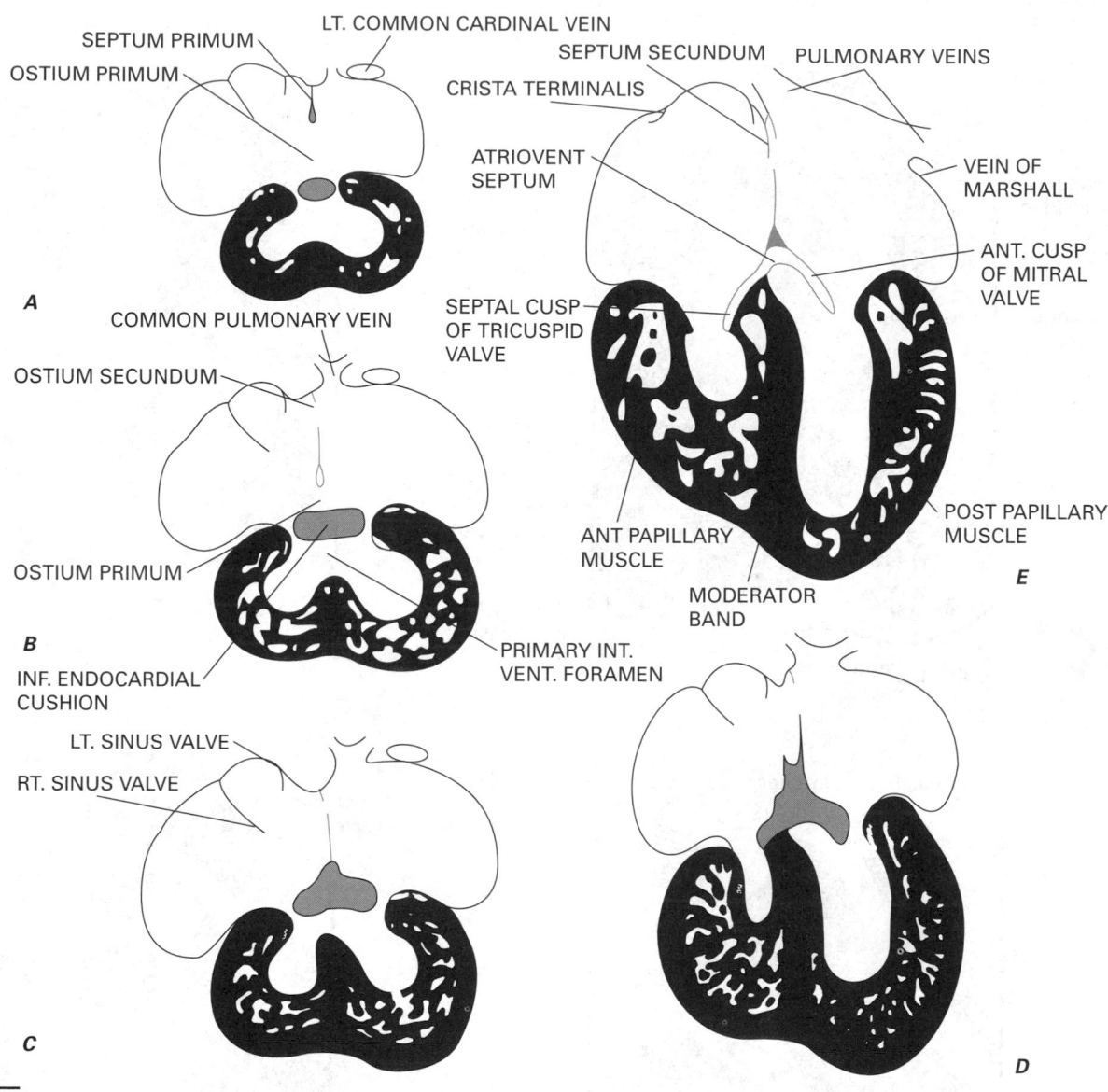

FIGURE 8-8
Diagram showing sections through heart in embryos of 6 mm (*A*), 9 mm (*B*), 12 mm (*C*), 17 mm (*D*), and 40 mm (*E*). [From Van Mierop LHS. Embryology of the atrioventricular canal region. In: Feldt RH, ed. *Atrioven-* *tricular Canal Defects.* Philadelphia: Saunders; 1976:6. Reproduced with permission from the publisher and author.]

there is an interventricular communication. In the partial forms, the endocardial cushions fuse only centrally. The result is an interatrial communication or so-called ostium primum–type atrial septal defect. The upper part of the muscular ventricular septum remains deficient, but this area of the ventricular septum is closed by fibrous tissue. Because the left side of the endocardial cushions does not fuse, the anterior or aortic cusp of the mitral valve is cleft. AV septal defects are frequently associated with trisomy 21 in humans and trisomy 16 in mice.[72] Genetic markers in patients without trisomy 21 are also under investigation.

Ventricular Septal Defect

Some forms of perimembranous ventricular septal defect may be due to failure of fusion of the right extremity of the fused

endocardial cushions, upper border of the muscular ventricular septum, and conal septum. Since the endocardial cushions fuse normally, there is no cleft in the anterior mitral valve cusp, nor is there an interatrial communication.

The Truncus Arteriosus

Septation of the conotruncal area of the bulbus cordis begins in embryos of about 6 mm in CR length with the appearance of two opposing truncal cushions (Fig. 8-8). One of these is located along the dextrosuperior truncal endocardium (dextrosuperior truncal cushion), the other on the sinistroinferior wall (sinistroinferior truncal cushion). Coincident with the expansion of the conotruncus, the cushions rapidly enlarge and fuse to form the truncal septum, thus dividing the truncus into aortic and pulmonary channels. The truncus is the first part of the heart to septate (at the 7-mm CR-length stage). Proximally, the truncal cushions merge with the superior aspects of the conal cushions, which are the comparable mesenchymal masses within the conus cordis. Distally, the undivided portion of the truncus and the aortic sac enlarge to form the truncoaortic sac. Simultaneously, the origin and course of the sixth arches shift leftward, aligning with right ventricular outflow, and the origin and course of the fourth aortic arches shift rightward, aligning with left ventricular outflow. At the same time, the dorsal wall of the truncoaortic sac invaginates between the origins of the fourth and sixth arches to form a vertical septum, the aorticopulmonary septum, which approaches and then fuses with the truncal septum.[70,72,78,83,84]

ANOMALIES

Persistent Truncus Arteriosus

If the truncal cushions remain hypoplastic and fail to fuse, partitioning of the truncus arteriosus does not take place. If, in addition to the hypoplastic truncal cushions, both intercalated valve cushions persist, the result is a quadricuspid truncal valve. Usually, fusion occurs between adjacent valve anlagen, resulting in an apparently tricuspid truncal valve with one larger cusp containing a fused raphe. In the great majority of cases, the aorticopulmonary septum does develop, and a short common pulmonary trunk arises from the persistent trunk. The ductus arteriosus is almost always absent except when associated with interruption of the aortic arch. In experimental models, persistent truncus arteriosus can be produced following selected ablation of neural crest tissue, as mentioned above.[42]

Aorticopulmonary Septal Defect

This anomaly may be due to malalignment and/or failure of fusion between the distal truncal septum and the aorticopulmonary septum. Both arterial valves are present, but there is a communication of varying size between the ascending aorta and the pulmonary trunk.

The Conus Cordis

The conal cushions make their appearance at about the same time as the truncal cushions (Fig. 8-8). One is located on the dextrodorsal wall, the other on the sinistroventral wall of the conus cordis. On the right side, the dorsal conal cushion becomes continuous with the superior truncal cushion; on the left, the ventral conal cushion becomes continuous with the inferior truncal cushion. Fusion of the conal cushion begins proximally and then progresses rapidly, completing the partition of the conal septum by the 14- to 15-mm CR-length stage. Conal septation reduces and then closes the small secondary interventricular foramen, which was bordered by the conal septum, the top of the muscular ventricular septum, and the right extremities of the fused endocardial cushions. The portion of the endocardial cushion arch between the junction with septum primum and the ventricular septum becomes the AV portion of the membranous septum (Fig. 8-8).

ANOMALIES

Ventricular Septal Defect, Eisenmenger Type

A large basilar septal defect, dextroposition of the aortic valve, and a hypoplastic or absent infundibular septum are likely due to hypoplasia or absence of the conal cushions.

Ventricular Septal Defect, Supracristal Type

The supracristal type of ventricular septal defect is likely due to either simple failure of truncal and conal septal fusion or to septal malalignment, which prevents fusion.

Tetralogy of Fallot

The primary anomaly in tetralogy of Fallot is likely an anterior displacement to a varying degree of the conal septum, which leads to unequal partitioning of the conus and reduction of the right ventricular infundibulum. A large basilar ventricular septal defect and dextroposition of the aortic valve result from failure of the displaced conal septum to participate in closure of the interventricular foramen. Pulmonary vascular hypoplasia is likely a secondary result of diminished forward blood flow.

The Sinus Venosus

In the 4-mm human embryo, the sinus venosus consists of a central, transverse portion of the sinus venosus, and the right and left sinus horns (Figs. 8-4 and 8-9). The sinus venosus receives three pairs of veins: the omphalomesenteric (vitelline), umbilical (allantoic), and common cardinal veins. The proximal portions of the umbilical veins soon disappear. As a result of the increased blood flow associated with the right and left systemic veins, the right sinus horn and proximal cardinal and vitelline veins attain a vertical position, increase in size, and form the smooth-walled, intercaval part of the atrium. The transverse portion and proximal left sinus horn become the coronary sinus. Rightward infolding of the cardiac wall at the sinoatrial junction forms the right sinus valve (Figs. 8-4 and 8-8), while a leftward, smaller fold appears somewhat later on at the sinoatrial junction. Thus, the vertical sinoatrial orifice is flanked on each side by a valvelike structure in the 4- to 6-mm human embryo (Fig. 8-8). Superiorly, the sinus valves join to form the septum spurium. The sinus valves, particularly the right sinus valve, are relatively large in the 16-mm embryo, but they then disappear almost completely. The left sinus valve fuses with the atrial septum, and the inferior part of the right sinus valve divides into a larger inferior vena caval (eustachian) valve and a smaller coronary sinus (thebesian) valve.

ANOMALIES

Cor Triatriatum Dexter

Complete persistence of the right sinus valve of the embryonic heart produces a septum in the right atrium separating the intercaval part of the right atrium from the atrial body. The remaining opening may be quite small and restrictive.

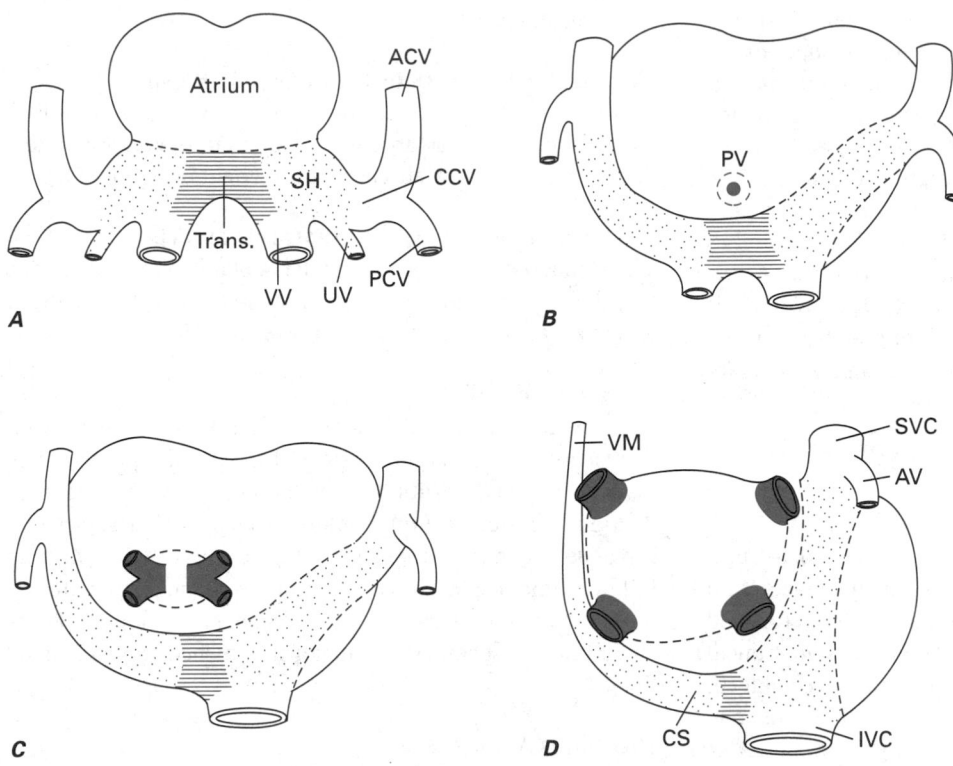

FIGURE 8-9

Diagrammatic posterior views of the atria and sinus venosus in embryos: 3-mm CR length (*A*), 5-mm CR length (*B*), 12-mm CR length (*C*), and newborn (*D*). A(C)CV = anterior (common) cardinal vein; AV = azygos vein; CS = coronary sinus; IVC = inferior vena cava; PCV = posterior cardinal vein; PV = pulmonary vein; SH = sinus horn; UV = umbilical vein; VM = vein of Marshall; VV = vitelline vein. (From Van Mierop LHS, Wiglesworth FW. Isomerism of the cardiac atria in the asplenia syndrome. *Lab Invest* 1962; 11:1303. Copyright by U.S. and Canadian Academy of Pathology.)

ovale is the opening bordered by the free edge of the septum secundum. After fusion of the septum primum and the septum secundum, the foramen ovale becomes the fossa ovalis. The limbus fossa ovalis is a remnant of the free edge of the septum secundum.

Until recently the embryonic pulmonary vein (Figs. 8-8 and 8-9) was thought to develop as an outgrowth of the posterior left atrial wall leftward of the septum primum and then to fuse with the splanchnic venous plexus in the region of the developing lung buds.[86] However, in the alligator, the common pulmonary vein initially enters the sinus venosus and is then assigned to the left atrium during the process of atrial septation.[87] The pulmonary vein then expands to form the larger, smooth part of the adult left atrium, including the orifice for each of the mature pulmonary veins. Of note, the trabeculated left atrial appendage is the remnant of the original embryonic left atrium.

Persistent Left Superior Vena Cava

Persistence of the left common cardinal vein and left sinus horn results in a left superior vena cava draining into the coronary sinus.

The Atria, Atrial Septum, and Pulmonary Veins

Rapid enlargement of the atrial and ventricular chambers occurs shortly after cardiac looping. A depression is formed in the roof of the common atrium underneath the midline truncus arteriosus, resulting internally in a sickle-shaped crest. This is the first indication of the septum primum, which is directed toward the AV canal; the ostium primum is formed by the inferior rim between the developing right and left atria (Fig. 8-8). Closure of the ostium primum occurs through the extension and fusion of the superior and inferior endocardial cushions, which occurs by the 10- to 11-mm CR-length stage. Perforations then appear in the septum primum, and these coalesce to form the ostium secundum, ensuring continued communication between the right- and left-sided atria. The posterosuperior portion of the septum secundum is formed by an infolding of the atrial wall between the left sinus valve and septum. The anteroinferior part of the septum secundum is derived from the expanding sinus vestibuli.[85] The foramen

ANOMALIES

Atrial Septal Defect at the Fossa Ovalis

This defect, often referred to as a *secundum-type* atrial septal defect, is due to overresorption of septum primum, producing a very large ostium secundum. Frequently, the atrial defect is further enlarged by a hypoplastic septum secundum. Total absence of both septum primum and septum secundum (common atrium) is rare and almost always associated with a form of persistent AV canal.

Anomalous Pulmonary Venous Connection

The total form of anomalous pulmonary venous connection is presumably due either to lack of development or to a premature involution of the common pulmonary vein. A number of types of pulmonary venous to systemic venous connections occur, depending on which of the early embryonic channels connecting the pulmonary venous bed to the systemic venous circulation remains patent. Partial anomalous pulmonary venous return is due to retention of a connection between part of the pulmonary venous system with the systemic venous circulation.

Cor Triatriatum Sinister

If incorporation of the common pulmonary vein into the left atrium does not take place and the common pulmonary venous ostium remains narrow, the result is a septum-like structure that divides the left atrium into two components: one receives the pulmonary veins and the other gives access to the mitral valve and left atrial appendage.

DEVELOPMENT OF THE HEART VALVES

The Atrioventricular Valves

Beginning with the tubular heart, the primitive endocardial cushions function as thick valves to facilitate forward blood flow. However, the thin, mature AV valve cusps, chordae, and papillary muscles are derived predominantly by delamination of the muscular ventricular wall.[88] All AV valve cusps are therefore initially thick and fleshy; only later in development are they transformed into thin, fibrous cusps.[77]

ANOMALIES

Tricuspid Valve Atresia, Mitral Valve Atresia

Tricuspid and mitral valve atresias are anomalies that are probably due to premature fusion of endocardial cushion tissue that borders the AV canal during or shortly after partitioning of the AV canal.

Ebstein's Anomaly of the Tricuspid Valve

Ebstein's anomaly of the tricuspid valve is likely due to an abnormality in the process of myocardial delamination required for AV valve and chordal formation.

The Arterial Valves

The primordia of the semilunar valves become visible as small tubercles on the distal extensions of each truncal cushion after truncal partitioning in the 9-mm embryo. One of each pair is assigned to pulmonary and aortic channels, respectively. On the walls of both aortic and pulmonary channels, opposite the fused truncus cushions, a third small cushion appears.[84] These two intercalated valve cushions form the third member of each arterial valve primordium (Figs. 8-7 and 8-10). Both the aortic and pulmonary roots, consisting of the sinuses of Valsalva and the semilunar valves, are likely derived from the truncus arteriosus and the truncal and intercalated valve cushions.

ANOMALIES

Bicuspid Arterial Valves

A bicuspid aortic or pulmonary valve is due to a failure of development of an intercalated valve cushion, resulting in a valve with two equal sized cusps, neither containing a raphe,

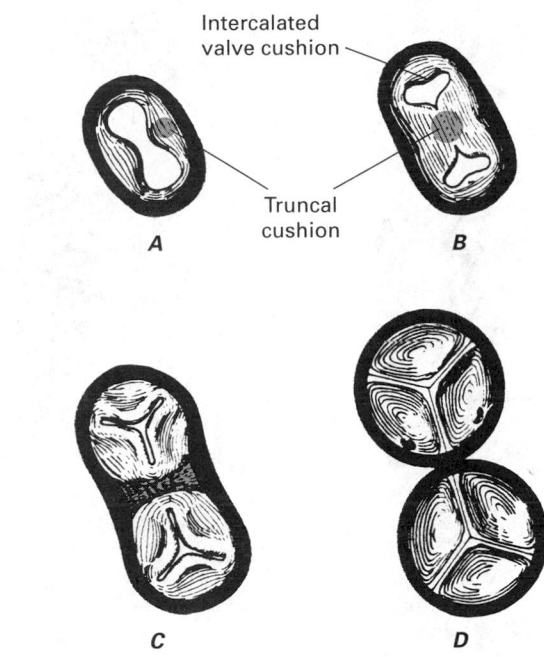

FIGURE 8-10
Diagram showing the development of the arterial valves.

or to fusion of adjacent valve anlagen, in which case the cusps are generally unequal in size with the larger containing a raphe of varying length.

Arterial Valve Stenosis or Atresia

Fusion of two or all three of the arterial valve anlagen likely results in stenosis or atresia of the valve.

Absent Arterial Valves

Failure of the arterial valve anlagen to develop likely explains the rare occurrence of absence of the pulmonary or aortic valve.

DEVELOPMENT OF THE AORTIC ARCH

Aortic arch development involves the sequential development and then involution of six arch pairs. The first pair of arches in the 3-mm CR-length embryo is large when the second pair is just forming (Fig. 8-11A). Caudally, the dorsal aortas fuse to form a single vessel, and then vessel fusion progresses cranially. In a 4-mm CR-length embryo, the first and second arches have largely disappeared (Fig. 8-11B). The third aortic arch is well developed, and the fourth and sixth arches are being formed as ventral and dorsal sprouts of the aortic sac and dorsal aorta, respectively. The ventral portion of the sixth arch already has as its major branch the primitive pulmonary artery, even though the arch itself has not yet been completed. Of note, in mammals the fifth aortic arch is rudimentary. By the 10-mm CR-length stage, the first two aortic arches have regressed and the third, fourth, and sixth are present; the

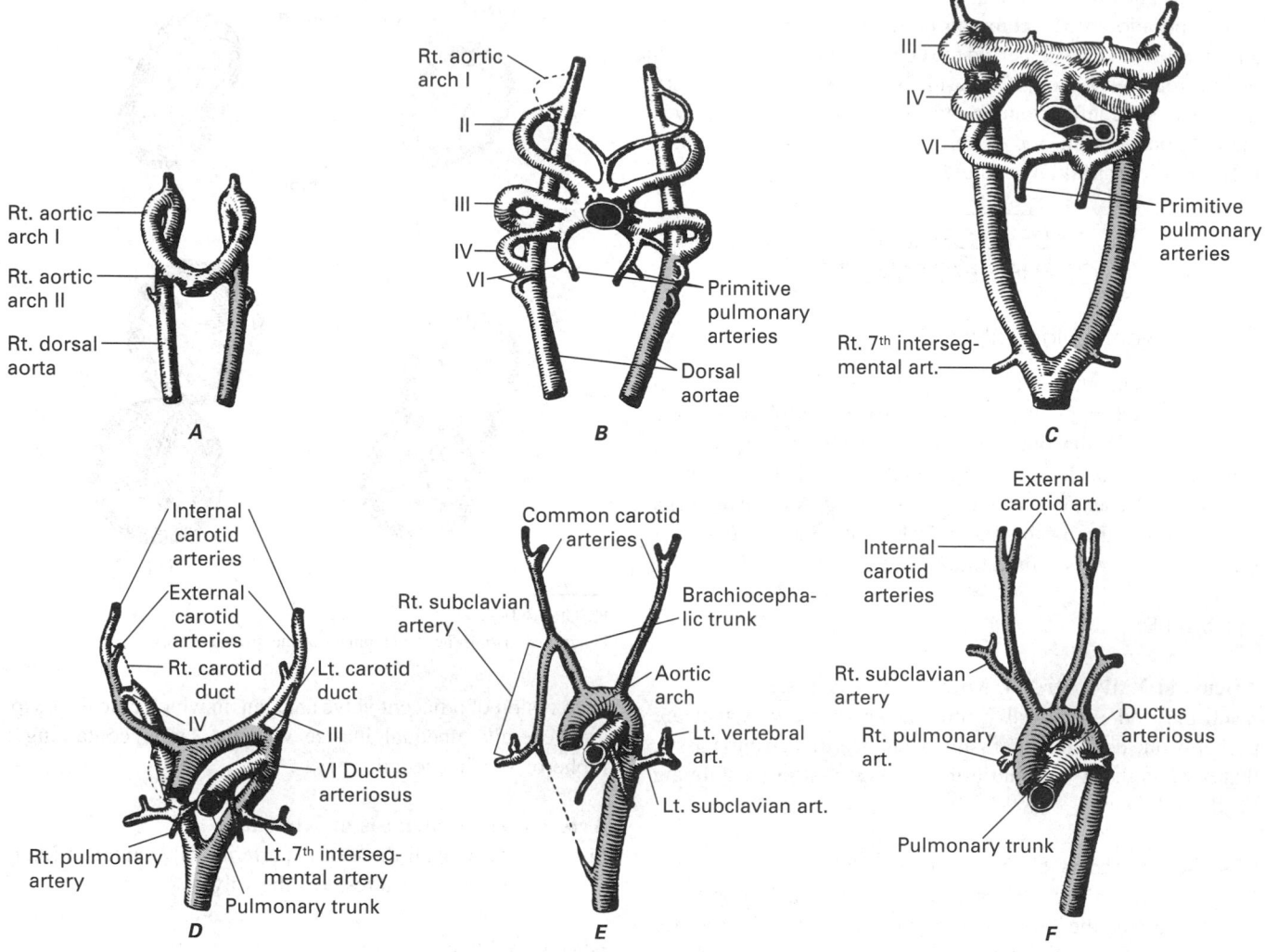

FIGURE 8-11
Development of the aortic arch system in embryos of 3 mm (*A*), 4 mm (*B*), 10 mm (*C*), 14 mm (*D*), and 17 mm (*E*) and in a neonate (*F*). (After Congdon ED. Transformation of the aortic arch system during the development of the human embryo. *Contrib Embryol* 1922; 14:47, with permission.)

truncoaortic sac has been divided by the formation of the aorticopulmonary septum so that the sixth arches are now continuous with the pulmonary trunk (Fig. 8-11*C*). Of note, the seventh cervical intersegmental arteries arise from the dorsal aorta near the midline and form the subclavian arteries. In a 14-mm CR-length embryo, the dorsal aortas between the third and fourth arches have disappeared and the third arches begin to elongate (Fig. 8-11*D*). At this point, the dorsal portion of the right sixth arch has disappeared, though the left sixth arch persists as the ductus arteriosus. The aortic sac has been broadened to contribute to the brachiocephalic trunk on the right and part of the definitive aortic arch up to the origin of the left third arch (common carotid artery). Finally, by the 17-mm CR-length stage, the right dorsal aorta has become atrophic between its junction with the left dorsal aorta, and the origin of the right seventh intersegmental artery has become attenuated and later disappears (Fig. 8-11*E*). The remaining components of the right dorsal aorta and right fourth aortic arch form the proximal subclavian artery. After birth, the distal part of the left sixth aortic arch, the ductus arteriosus, normally also involutes to form the ligamentum arteriosum. Thus, most aortic arch anomalies are secondary to abnormal retention or disappearance of various embryonic segments.

ANOMALIES

Patent Ductus Arteriosus

Persistence of the ductus arteriosus postnatally frequently occurs in premature infants due to delayed ductal involution. However, persistence of a large ductus arteriosus also occurs in isolation and in association with a variety of congenital cardiovascular malformations.

Double Aortic Arch

Double aortic arch is the result of persistence and continued patency of the segment of the right dorsal aorta between the origin of the right seventh intersegmental artery and its junction with the left dorsal aorta.

Right Aortic Arch

In the right aortic arch anomaly, the right rather than the left dorsal aorta is maintained in its entirety. The branching pattern of the aortic arch, therefore, will be the mirror image of normal, with the brachiocephalic (innominate) artery arising as the first vessel on the left rather than the right side.

Anomalous Subclavian Artery

The subclavian artery can arise from the aortic arch distal to the left subclavian artery if the right dorsal aorta between the origin of the right seventh intersegmental artery and the junction with the left dorsal aorta is maintained to form the proximal portion of the right subclavian artery.

Interrupted Aortic Arch

Interrupted aortic arch anomaly type B results from the disappearance of the left fourth aortic arch (type A is a form of coarctation of the aorta). The ascending aorta terminates as the brachiocephalic and left common carotid arteries and is isolated from the descending aorta, which is perfused by the pulmonary trunk by way of a patent ductus arteriosus.

Absent Left Pulmonary Artery

The left pulmonary artery is almost always absent in that it arises from a left-sided ductus arteriosus (or ligamentum arteriosum). This anomaly is the result of disappearance of the proximal left sixth arch. If, in this anomaly, the aortic arch is on the left side, the ductus arteriosus that feeds the intrapulmonary part of the left pulmonary artery arises from the usual position on the underside of the arch. If the aortic arch is on the right, the ductus arteriosus usually arises from the brachiocephalic trunk, with the left common carotid and left subclavian arteries as a trifurcation or, rarely, from a diverticulum of the descending aorta. Usually the left subclavian artery in such cases also arises from the diverticulum.

CORONARY ARTERY DEVELOPMENT

Endothelial Cell Origin

Coronary vascular endothelial maturation closely parallels the development of the embryonic epicardium.[89] The first coronary endothelial cells migrate from the region of the developing liver and first contact the sinus venosus. Vascular precursor cells and small vessels then invade the sinus venosus wall, ventricular and atrial myocardium, and mesenchymal border of the aortic annulus.[89] Initially, multiple connections between the coronary vascular plexus and the aortic myocardium are present; however only two connections persist. Of note, coronary endothelial cells do not participate in the formation of the intramyocardial vascular network. In addition, it is interesting to note that the heart begins to pump blood before perfusion of the coronary vasculature occurs, consistent with the hypothesis that the early trabecular myocardium is metabolically supplied by local diffusion of nutrients.

Origin of Vascular Smooth Muscle Cells

Antibodies to smooth muscle alpha actin document that the maturation of coronary smooth muscle precedes the maturation of the outflow vessels.[90] Of note, the orderly development of the coronary arterial branching pattern and elastic lamina is dependent upon the presence of neural crest. Following experimental neural crest ablation in the chick embryo, persistent truncus arteriosus associated with a single origin of the coronary arterial tree occurs.[90] The distribution and symmetry of the coronary vasculature is distinctly abnormal following injury to the neural crest. In addition, the elastic lamina and collagen organization of the great vessels is markedly abnormal following neural crest ablation, as has been noted in some congenital cardiovascular anomalies.[91]

Vasculogenesis and Adaption

It is important to note that the maturation of the coronary vasculature, as with the systemic vasculature, represents both angiogenesis (sprouting of existing vessels) and vasculogenesis (fusion of precursor cells).[92] Following increased ventricular pressure loading in the chick embryo, myocardial vasculogenesis increases to match increased ventricular mass.[93] This finding is consistent with the investigation of children with pressure-overload left ventricular hypertrophy, where capillary density remains unchanged.[94]

ANOMALIES

Anomalous Origin of the Left Coronary Artery

Occasionally, the left coronary artery is found to arise from the pulmonary artery and, rarely, from other aortic arch vessels. The developing coronary vessels perforate the aortic annulus in association with specific immunohistochemical markers, so it is likely that anomalies occur when this patterning event is altered.

Abnormal Origin and Course of Coronary Arteries

Numerous variations in the architecture and course of the coronary arteries occur in association with structural cardiovascular malformations. For example, an anomalous origin of the left anterior descending coronary artery from the right coronary artery occurs in association with tetralogy of Fallot. Unfortunately, the mechanisms for these associations have not yet been defined.

Coronary Arterial Fistulas

Coronary arterial fistulas occasionally occur in isolation and also in association with pulmonary valve atresia with intact ventricular septum. The mechanisms responsible for these anomalies are also unknown.

CONDUCTION SYSTEM DEVELOPMENT

Recently there has been a renewed interest in investigating the immunohistochemical maturation of the cardiac conduction system.[95,96] Unfortunately, a detailed discussion of the competing theories regarding the origin and maturation of the specialized conduction system are beyond the scope of this chapter.

CARDIOVASCULAR INNERVATION

Despite numerous descriptive studies regarding the location of cardiac ganglia, little is known regarding the immunohistochemical cues required for the patterning of myocardial innervation. Neural crest cell migration is critical for this process, as neural crest cells serve as precursors for the cardiac nerves and ganglia.[42] Cardiac ganglia and nerves are present in the human embryo at 7 weeks' gestation.[97] The density of cardiac innervation exhibits a gradient of decreasing density from the atrium to the ventricle. It is interesting to note that functional adrenergic receptors are present on the embryonic heart prior to histologic evidence of autonomic nerves.[98] The differential appearance and distribution of peptide-containing nerves indicates that there is a maturational order to the autonomic and sensory components of the developing human heart.[97]

FUNCTIONAL MATURATION OF THE EMBRYONIC HEART

Obviously, cardiovascular morphogenesis is directly influenced by the dynamic mechanical environment of the pulsatile embryonic heart. Unfortunately, an overview of functional maturation, while critical, is beyond the scope and space of this chapter. The reader is therefore referred to several recent reviews of embryonic functional maturation in vertebrate and invertebrate species.[99,100]

REFERENCES

1. Von Haller A. *Sur la Formation du Coeur dans le Poulet.* Lausanne: 1758.
2. Neill CA, Clark EB. Tetralogy of Fallot: The first 300 years. *Texas Heart Inst J* 1994; 21:272–279.
3. Anderson RH. Simplifying the understanding of congenital malformations of the heart. *Int J Cardiol* 1991; 32:131–142.
4. Van Mierop LHS. Morphological development of the heart. In: Berne RM, ed. *Handbook of Physiology.* Vol I, Sec 2. Bethesda, MD: American Physiological Society; 1979:1–28.
5. Clark EB, Van Mierop LHS. Cardiac development. In: Adams FH, Emmanoulides GC, Riemenschneider TA, eds. *Heart Disease in Infants, Children, and Adolescents.* 4th ed. Baltimore: Williams & Wilkins; 1989:1–22.
6. Wenick ACG. Embryology of the heart. In: Anderson RH, Macartney FJ, Shinebourne EA, Tynan M, eds. *Paediatric Cardiology.* Vol. 1. New York: Churchill Livingstone; 1987:83–107.
7. Ferrens VJ, Rosenquist GC, Weinstein C. *Cardiac Morphogenesis.* New York: Elsevier; 1985.
8. Nora JJ, Takao A. *Congenital Heart Disease: Causes and Processes.* Mt Kisco, NY: Futura; 1984.
9. Clark EB, Takao A. *Developmental Cardiology: Morphogenesis and Function.* Mt Kisco, NY: Futura; 1990.
10. Bockman DE, Kirby ML. *Embryonic Origins of Defective Heart Development.* New York: New York Academy of Sciences; 1990.
11. Clark EB, Markwald RR, Takao A. *Developmental Mechanisms of Heart Disease.* Mt Kisco, NY: Futura; 1995.
12. Brueckner M, D'Eustachio P, Horwich AL. Linkage mapping of a mouse gene, iv, that controls left-right asymmetry of the heart and viscera. *Proc Natl Acad Sci USA* 1989; 86:5035–5038.
13. Yokoyama T, Copeland NG, Jenkins NA, Montgomery CA, Elder FFB, Overbeek PA. Reversal of left-right asymmetry: A situs inversus mutation. *Science* 1993; 260:679–682.
14. Osmond MK, Butler AJ, Voon FCT, Bellairs R. The effects of retinoic acid on heart formation in the early chick embryo. *Development* 1991; 113:1405–1417.
15. Chen Y, Solursh M. Comparison of Hensen's node and retinoic acid in secondary axis induction in the early chick embryo. *Dev Dyn* 1992; 195:142–151.
16. Morgan MJ. The asymmetrical genetic determination of laterality: Flatfish, frogs and human handedness. In: *Biological Asymmetry and Handedness. CIBA Found Symp* 1991; 162:234–250.
17. Brown NA, Wolpert L. The development of handedness in left/right asymmetry. *Development* 1990; 109:1–9.
18. Layton WM Jr. The biology of asymmetry and the development of the cardiac loop. In: Ferrans VJ, Rosenquist GC, Weinstein C, eds. *Cardiac Morphogenesis.* New York: Elsevier; 1985:134–140.
19. Akam M, Dawson I, Tear G. Homeotic genes and the control of segment diversity. *Development* 1988; 104:123–168.
20. Hunt P, Krumlauf R. HOX codes and positional specification invertebrate embryonic axes. *Annu Rev Cell Biol* 1992; 8:227–256.
21. Lamers WH, Wessels A, Verbeek FJ, Moorman AFM, Viragh S, Wenink ACG, et al. New findings concerning ventricular septation in the human heart: Implications for maldevelopment. *Circulation* 1992; 86:1194–1205.
22. Mikawa T, Borisov A, Brown AM, Fischman DA. Clonal analysis of cardiac morphogenesis in the chicken embryo using a replication-defective retrovirus: I. Formation of the ventricular myocardium. *Dev Dyn* 1992; 193:11–23.
23. Mikawa T, Cohen-Gould L, Fischman DA. Clonal analysis of cardiac morphogenesis in the chicken embryo using a replication-defective retrovirus: III. Polyclonal origin of adjacent ventricular myocytes. *Dev Dyn* 1992; 195:133–141.
24. Linask KK. N-Cadherin localization in early heart development and polar expression of Na^+, K^+-ATPase, and integrin during pericardial coelom formation and epithelialization of the differentiating myocardium. *Dev Biol* 1992; 151:213–224.
25. Parlow MH, Bolender DL, Kokan-Moore NP, Lough J. Localization of bFGF-like proteins as punctate inclusions in the preseptation myocardium of the chicken embryo. *Dev Biol* 1991; 146:139–147.
26. Lyons KM, Jones CM, Hogan BL. The TGF-beta-related *DVR* gene family in mammalian development. *CIBA Found Symp* 1992; 165:219–230.
27. Sugi Y, Sasse J, Lough J. Inhibition of precardiac mesoderm cell proliferation by antisense oligodeoxynucleotide complementary to fibroblast growth factor-2 (FGF-2). *Dev Biol* 1993; 157:28–37.
28. Yu Y-T, Breitbart RE, Smoot LB, Lee Y, Mahdavi V, Nadal-Ginard B. Human myocyte-specific enhancer factor 2 comprises a group of tissue restricted MADS box transcription factors. *Genes Dev* 1992; 6:1783–1798.
29. Chien KR, Zhu H, Knowlton KU, Miller-Hance W, van-Bilsen M, O'Brien TX, et al. Transcriptional regulation during cardiac growth and development. *Annu Rev Physiol* 1993; 55:77–95.
30. Clark EB, Hu N, Dummett JL, Vandekieft GK, Olson C, Tomanek R. Ventricular function and morphology in the chick embryo stage 18 to 29. *Am J Physiol* 1986; 250:H407–H413.
31. Taber LA, Keller BB, Clark EB. Cardiac mechanics in the stage 16 chick embryo. *J Biomech Eng* 1992; 114:427–434.
32. Ruzicka DL, Schwartz RJ. Sequential activation of alpha actin genes during avian cardiogenesis: Vascular smooth muscle alpha actin gene transcripts mark the onset of cardiomyocyte differentiation. *J Cell Biol* 1988; 107:2575–2586.
33. Sugi Y, Lough J. Onset of expression and regional deposition of alpha-smooth and sarcomeric actin during avian heart development. *Dev Dyn* 1992; 193:116–124.
34. Sordahl LA, Crow CA, Draft GH, Schwartz A. Some ultrastructural and biochemical aspects of heart mitochondria associated with development. *J Mol Cell Cardiol* 1972; 4:1–10.
35. Barth E, Stammler G, Speiser B, Schaper J. Ultrastructural quantitation of mitochondria and myofilaments in cardiac muscle from 10 different animal species including man. *J Mol Cell Cardiol* 1992; 24:669–681.

36. Mahony L. Cardiac Membrane Structure and Function. In: Burggren WW and Keller BB, eds. *Development of Cardiovascular Systems: Molecules to Organisms*. New York: Cambridge University Press; 1997:18–26.

37. Bernard C. Establishment of ionic permeabilities of the myocardial membrane during embryonic development of the rat. In: Lieberman M and Sano T, eds. *Development and Physiological Correlates of Cardiac Muscle*. New York: Raven Press; 1975:169–184.

38. Rosen MR, Danilo P Jr. Developmental electrophysiology of the heart. In: Polin RA, Fox WW, eds. *Fetal and Neonatal Physiology*. Philadelphia: Saunders; 1992:656–665.

39. Osaka T, Joyner RW. Developmental changes in calcium currents of rabbit ventricular cells. *Circ Res* 1991; 68:788–796.

40. Wetzel GT, Chen F, Klitzner TS. Ca²⁺ channel kinetics in acute isolated fetal, neonatal and adult rabbit cardiac myocytes. *Circ Res* 1993; 72:1065–1074.

41. Bridge JHB, Smolley JR, Spitzer KW. The relationship between charge movements associated I_{Ca} and $I_{Na\text{-}Ca}$ in cardiac myocytes. *Science* 1990; 248:376–378.

42. Kirby ML, Waldo KL. Role of neural crest in congenital heart disease. *Circulation* 1990; 82:332–340.

43. Chisaka O, Capecchi MR. Regionally restricted developmental defects resulting from targeted disruption of the mouse homeobox gene *Hox-1.5*. *Nature* 1991; 350:473–474.

44. Lammer EJ, Opitz JM. The DiGeorge anomaly as a developmental field defect. *Am J Med* (genet suppl) 1986; 2:113–127.

45. Wilson DI, Cross IE, Goodship JA, Coolthard S, Carey AM, Scambler PJ, et al. DiGeorge syndrome with isolated aortic coarctation and isolated ventricular septal defect in three sibs with a 22q11 deletion of maternal origin. *Br Heart J* 1991; 66:308–312.

46. Scambler PJ, Kelly D, Lindsay E, et al. Velo-cardio-facial syndrome associated with chromosome 22 deletions encompassing the DiGeorge locus. *Lancet* 1992; 339:1138–1139.

47. Driscoll DA, Budarf ML, Emanuel BS. A genetic etiology for DiGeorge syndrome: Consistent deletions and microdeletions of 22q11. *Am J Hum Genet* 1992; 50:924–933.

48. Lammer EJ, Chen DT, Hoar R, et al. Retinoic acid embryopathy. *N Engl J Med* 1985; 313:837–841.

49. Davis CL. Description of a human embryo having 20 paired somites. *Contrib Embryol* 1923; 15:1–52.

50. Davis CL. The cardiac jelly of the chick embryo. *Anat Rec* 1924; 27:201–202.

51. Van Mierop LHS. Embryology of the heart. In: Netter FH, ed. *The CIBA Collection of Medical Illustrations*. Vol 5, pt 1. Summit, NJ: CIBA Pharmaceutical Co; 1969:112–130.

52. Drake CJ, Davis LA, Walters L, Little CD. Avian vasculogenesis and the distribution of collagens I, IV, laminin and fibronectin in the heart primordia. *J Exp Zool* 1990; 255:309–322.

53. Markwald RR, Mjaatvedt CH, Krug EL. Induction of endocardial cushion tissue formation by adheron-like molecular complexes derived from the myocardial basement membrane. In: Clark EB, Takao A. *Developmental Cardiology: Morphogenesis and Function*. Mt Kisco, NY: Futura, 1990:191–204.

54. Lyons KM, Jones CM, Hogan BLM. The TGF-β-related DVR gene family in mammalian development. In: *Postimplantation Development in the Mouse*. *CIBA Found Symp* 1992; 165:219–234.

55. Runyan RB, Potts JD, Sharma RV, Loeber CP, Chiang JJ, Bhalla RC. Signal transduction of a tissue interaction during embryonic heart development. *Cell Reg* 1990; 1:301–313.

56. Chin C, Gandour-Edwards R, Oltjen S, Choy M. Fate of the atrioventricular endocardial cushions in the developing chick heart. *Pediatr Res* 1992; 32:390–393.

57. Garcia-Martinez V, Sanchez-Quintana D, Hurle JM. Histogenesis of the semilunar valves: An immunohistochemical analysis of tenascin and type-I collagen distribution in developing chick heart valves. *Cell Tissue Res* 1990; 259:299–304.

58. Potts JD, Vincent EB, Runyan RB, Weeks DL. Sense and antisense TGF beta 3 mRNA levels correlate with cardiac valve induction. *Dev Dyn* 1992; 193:340–345.

59. Pexieder T. Prenatal development of the endocardium: A review. *SEM* 1981; 2:223–253.

60. Noden DM. Origins and patterning of avian outflow tract endocardium. *Development* 1991; 111:867–876.

61. Markwald RR, Mjaatvedt CH, Krug EL, Sinning AR. Inductive interac-

tion in heart development: Role of cardiac adherons in cushion tissue formation. In: Bockman DE, Kirby ML, eds. *Embryonic Origins of Defective Heart Development*. *Ann NY Acad Sci* 1990; 588:13–25.

62. Icardo JM, Hurle JM, Ojeda JL. Endocardial cell polarity during the looping of the heart in the chick embryo. *Dev Biol* 1982; 90:203–209.

63. Pexieder T. Cell death in the morphogenesis and teratogenesis of the heart. *Adv Anat Embryol Cell Biol* 1975; 51:1–100.

64. Dzau VJ, Krieger JE. Molecular biology of hypertension. In: Roberts R, ed. *Molecular Basis of Cardiology*. Boston: Blackwell; 1993:325–354.

65. Castro-Quezada A, Nadal-Ginard B, de la Cruz MV. Experimental study of the formation of the bulboventricular loop in the chick. *J Embryol Exp Morphol* 1972; 27:623–637.

66. Manasek FJ, Burnside MB, Waterman RE. Myocardial cell shape change as a mechanism of embryonic heart looping. *Dev Biol* 1972; 29:349–371.

67. Stalsberg H. Origin of heart asymmetry: Right and left contributions to the early chick embryo heart. *Dev Biol* 1969; 19:109–127.

68. Stalsberg H. Mechanism of dextral looping of the embryonic heart. *Am J Cardiol* 1970; 25:265–271.

69. Patten BM. The formation of the cardiac loop in the chick. *Am J Anat* 1922; 30:373–397.

70. Van Mierop LHS, Alley RD, Kausel HW, Stranahan A. Pathogenesis of transposition complexes: I. Embryology of the ventricles and great arteries. *Am J Cardiol* 1963; 12:216–225.

71. Taber LA, Lin IE, Clark EB. Mechanics of cardiac looping. *Dev Dyn* 1995; 203:42–50.

72. Gittenberger-de Groot A. Principles of abnormal cardiac development. In: Burggren WW, Keller BB, eds. *Development of Cardiovascular Systems: Molecules to Organisms*. New York: Cambridge University Press; 1997:259–267.

73. Icardo JM, Fernandez-Teran A. Morphologic study of ventricular trabeculation in the embryonic chick heart. *Acta Anat* 1987; 130:264–274.

74. Pexieder T, Christen Y, Vuillemin M, Patterson DR. Comparative morphometric analysis of cardiac organogenesis in chick, mouse, and dog embryos. In: Nora JJ, Takao A, eds. *Congenital Heart Disease: Causes and Processes*. Mt Kisco, NY: Futura; 1984:423–438.

75. Taber LA, Hu N, Pexieder T, Clark EB, Keller BB. Residual strain in the ventricle of the stage 16–24 chick embryo. *Circ Res* 1993; 72:455–462.

76. Thompson RP, Lindroth JR, Wong YMM. Regional differences in DNA-synthetic activity in the preseptation myocardium of the chick. In: Clark EB, Takao A, eds. *Developmental Cardiology: Morphogenesis and Function*. Mt Kisco NY: Futura; 1990:219–234.

77. Streeter GL. Developmental horizons in human embryos: Description of age groups XI, 13–20 somites, and age group XII, 21–29 somites. *Contrib Embryol* 1942; 30:211–246.

78. Van Mierop LHS, Alley RD, Kausel HW, Stranahan A. The anatomy and embryology of endocardial cushion defects. *J Thorac Cardiovasc Surg* 1962; 43:71–83.

79. Pexieder T, Christen Y. Quantitative analysis of the shape development in the chick embryo heart. In: Pexieder T, ed. *Mechanisms of Cardiac Morphogenesis and Teratogenesis*. New York: Raven Press; 1981:49–67.

80. Pexieder T. Development of the outflow tract of the embryonic heart. In: Rosenquist GC, Bergsma D, eds. *Morphogenesis and Malformation of the Cardiovascular System: Birth Defects*. Original Article Series: Vol XIV, No 7. New York: Liss, 1978:29–68.

81. Pexieder T, Janecek P. Organogenesis of the human embryonic and early fetal heart as studied by microdissection and SEM. In: Nora JJ, Takao A, eds. *Congenital Heart Disease: Causes and Processes*. Mt. Kisco, NY: Futura; 1984:401–402.

82. Streeter GL. Developmental horizons in human embryos: Description of age groups XV, XVI, XVII, XVIII, being the third issue of a survey of the Carnegie Collection. *Contrib Embryol* 1948; 32:133–204.

83. Grant RP. Embryology of ventricular flow pathways in man. *Circulation* 1962; 25:756–779.

84. Pexieder T. Conotruncus and its septation at the advent of the molecular biology era. In: Clark EB, Markwald RR, Takao A, eds. *Developmental Mechanisms of Heart Disease*. Mt Kisco, NY: Futura; 1995:227–247.

85. Asami I, Koizumi K. Development of the atrial septal complex in the human heart: Contribution of the spina vestibuli. In: Clark EB, Markwald RR, Takao A, eds. *Developmental Mechanisms of Heart Disease*. Mt Kisco, NY: Futura; 1995:255–260.

86. Neill CA. Development of the pulmonary veins. *Pediatrics* 1956; 18:880–887.

87. Kutsche LM, Van Mierop LHS. Development of the pulmonary vein in the American alligator (*Alligator mississippiensis*). *Anat Rec* 1988; 222:170–176.

88. Dor X, Corone P. Embryologie cardiaque: Malformations (I). In: *Embryologie Cardiaque—Editions Techniques* Paris: *Encyclopedie Medico-Chirurgicale.* 1992:1–20.

89. Poelman RE, Gittenberger-de Groot AC, Metlink MMT, Bokenkamp R, Hogers B. Development of the cardiac coronary vascular endothelium, studied with antiendothelial antibodies, in chicken-quail chimeras. *Circ Res* 1993; 73:559–568.

90. Hood LC, Rosenquist TH. Coronary artery development in the chick: Origin and deployment of smooth muscle cells, and the effects of neural crest ablation. *Anat Rec* 1992; 234:291–300.

91. Rosenquist TH, Modis L. Spatial disorder of collagens in the great vessels, associated with congenital heart defects. *Anat Rec* 1991; 229:116–124.

92. Risau W. Vasculogenesis, angiogenesis and endothelial cell differentiation during embryonic development. In: Feinberg RN, Sherer GK, Auerbach R, eds: *The Development of the Vascular System.* Basel: Karger; 1991; 14:58–68.

93. Rakusan K, Flanagan MF, Geva T, Southern J, Van Praagh R. Morphometry of human coronary capillaries during normal growth and the effect of age in left ventricular pressure-overload hypertrophy. *Circulation* 1992; 86:38–46.

94. Tomanek RJ, Phan BP, Hu N, Clark EB. Myocardial vascularization is accelerated in chick embryos with increased afterload and ventricular mass (abstr). *FASEB J* 1996; 10:A579.

95. Anderson RH, Becker AE, Wenink ACG. The development of the conducting tissues. In: Roberts EA, ed. *Cardiac Arrhythmias in the Neonate, Infant and Child.* New York: Appleton-Century-Crofts; 1978.

96. Wessels A, Vermeulen JLM, Verbeek FJ, Viragh S, Kalman F, Lamers WH, et al. Spatial distribution of "tissue-specific" antigens in the developing human heart and skeletal muscle: III. An immunohistochemical analysis of the distribution of the neural tissue antigen G1N2 in the embryonic heart: Implications for the development of the atrioventricular conduction system. *Anat Rec* 1992; 231:97–111.

97. Gordon L, Polak JM, Moscoso GJ, Smith A, Kuhn DM, Wharton J. Development of the peptidergic innervation of human heart. *J Anat* 1993; 183:131–140.

98. St Petery LB, Van Mierop LHS. Evidence for the presence of adrenergic receptors in 3-day-old chick embryo. *Am J Physiol* 1977; 232:H250–H254.

99. Keller BB. Functional maturation and coupling of the embryonic cardiovascular system. In: Clark EB, Markwald RR, Takao A, eds: *Developmental Mechanisms of Heart Disease,* Mt Kisco, NY: Futura; 1995:367–386.

100. Keller BB. Embryonic cardiovascular function, coupling, and maturation: A species view. In: Burggren W, Keller BB, eds. *Development of Cardiovascular Systems: Molecules to Organisms.* New York: Cambridge University Press, 1997:65–87.

9

GENE THERAPY OF CARDIOVASCULAR DISORDERS

Heiko E. von der Leyen / Michael J. Mann / Victor J. Dzau

Several pivotal events in (molecular) biology and biochemistry as well as in medicine made possible the new concept of *gene transfer* as a therapeutic tool to treat diseases. The importance of deoxyribonucleic acid (DNA) as a carrier of genetic information was first discovered by F. Griffith,[1] an English microbiologist. He found that live, nonpathogenic bacteria (*Diplococcus pneumoniae*) that were mixed with heat-inactivated pathogenic bacteria were partly transformed into pathogenic bacteria when injected into living animals. Thus, Griffith described a heat resistant "genetic" substance that could transform nonpathogenic bacteria into pathogenic ones. The molecular principle behind Griffith's observation was determined in 1944, when three physicians at the Rockefeller Institute showed that the factor that transformed the pneumococcus to a virulent state was DNA.[2] A decade later, Watson and Crick revealed the molecular structure of DNA, and, for the first time, presented a hypothesis for genetic replication.[3,4] By the mid- to late 1960s, it was discovered that, in the course of transforming a cell from the normal to the neoplastic phenotype, the papovaviruses SV40 and polyoma integrated their genetic information or specific transforming regions covalently, stably, and heritably into the genomes of target cells.[5] These experiments showed, for the first time, that an efficient genetic transformation of a cell by exogenous genetic information is possible,[6] and it was suggested that SV40 could be developed as a transducing vector to introduce exogenous DNA into mammalian cells.[7] Thus, before the beginning of the era of recombinant DNA, viruses were used to transfer genes into cells. Even an experimental clinical application was performed—unsuccessfully.[8] In 1972, Friedmann and Roblin,[9] stimulated by the advent of recombinant DNA techniques,[10,11] first suggested that tumor viruses can be modified to carry (recombinant) genetic information to complement genetic defects and correct disease phenotypes. This concept was supported by Berg and colleagues,[12] who prepared a recombinant SV40 vector that indeed was able to transfer foreign DNA sequences efficiently into mammalian cells. In 1979, the same group showed that even total cellular DNA could be introduced into mammalian cells efficiently and functionally.[13]

The use of recombinant DNA has altered both the way scientific questions are formulated and the way solutions are sought. The isolation of genes and their introduction in cells and experimental animals is now standard practice in research laboratories.[14] The identification of genes involved in cardiovascular disease created the possibility of targeting genes as a potential approach to treat such disease. For establishing the concept of *cardiovascular gene therapy*, it was essential to create the "molecular" approach to cardiovascular disease. This approach includes (1) the elucidation of pathobiological processes, especially at the cellular and molecular level, using Northern blot reverse transcription polymerase chain reaction (RT-PCR), in situ hybridization, etc. (see Chap. 7); (2) in vivo gene manipulation and development of animal models of diseases using gene transfer, antisense oligonucleotide application, or transgenic animals; and (3) the development of novel therapeutic strategies such as gene replacement, gene correction, or gene augmentation.

GENE TRANSFER TECHNIQUES AND THEIR APPLICATION IN VASCULAR DISEASE

Genetic material can be delivered to the vasculature either by a direct in vivo, vector-based gene transfer or by an ex vivo, indirect cell-based gene transfer. Ex vivo gene transfer approaches require individualized recipient-related cell harvest, preparation of transduced cells, and reimplantation of genetically engineered cell material.[15] In contrast, the direct in vivo gene transfer approach circumvents these problems and is theoretically easier to handle. The success of this approach, however, depends on the development of efficient gene transfer methods. Currently, several transduction systems have been employed (Table 9-1). In this chapter, we focus on gene transfer methods currently applied to the cardiovascular system.

Virus-Mediated Gene Transfer

RETROVIRUS-MEDIATED GENE TRANSFER

Retroviral expression vectors, which are constructed by incorporating exogenous cDNA into their genomes, can deliver the inserted gene into actively dividing cells.[16] A retroviral vector is constructed in several steps.[17] First, the structural genes required for viral replication are deleted to render the vector nonreplicating. After insertion of the exogenous gene of interest into the viral backbone, the recombinant retrovirus contains the exogenous gene, regulatory sequences, and packaging signals but lacks the actual structural genes required to produce a complete virion. It requires a helper cell to produce infectious viral particles.[18] Nabel et al.[19,20] first demonstrated the feasibility of transfecting blood vessels with foreign DNA in vivo by transfecting pig iliofemoral arteries with a recombinant amphotropic retroviral vector containing a the β-galactosidase gene. Several cell types in the vessel wall were transduced, including endothelial and vascular smooth muscle cells. Using a β-galactosidase retroviral vector to modify endothelial cells, Wilson et al.[15] demonstrated β-galactosidase expression up to 5 weeks after transfection in prosthetic vascular grafts seeded with the genetically transformed cells. Other studies could show only low transfection efficiency when retroviral vectors were used.[21,22] Possible explanations for inefficient retrovirus-mediated gene transfer include the requirement of actively dividing cells for integration and expression of the viral genome,[23] the moderately high titers of infectious virions that must be propagated,[24] and rapid inactivation by complement-mediated processes.[25–27] Since the retroviral vectors stably integrate into chromosomal DNA of the transfected cell, the potentially stable gene expression may result in insertional mutagenesis.[16,28]

ADENOVIRUS-MEDIATED GENE TRANSFER

Adenovirus vectors are widely used for cardiovascular gene transfer. Adenoviruses can transfect nondividing cells and generally do not integrate into the host genome. Two different methods using adenoviral gene transfer are currently under investigation: (1) a replication-deficient adenoviral vector with features similar to those described for the retroviral approach and (2) coupling of adenoviral coat to transferrin-polylysine/DNA complexes. For the first approach, adenoviral vectors commonly used are based on serotype 5, with the majority of E1a and E1b deleted to provide a replication-deficient vector. The E3 region can be deleted to provide space for inserting plasmid DNA of up to 7.5 kb.[29,30] Usually, an expression cassette containing essential viral elements, a promoter, and the exogenous gene are inserted in the E1 position. The vectors are propagated in a helper cell line that expresses E1 protein for the production of the replication-deficient (E1⁻) virus in high titers for in vivo delivery. Adenovirus vectors enter mammalian cells by receptor-mediated endocytosis and $\alpha_2\beta_3$ integrins.[31] Aortic smooth muscle cells[32] and cardiac myocytes[33] were successfully transfected using replication-defective adenovirus carrying the β-galactosidase or chloramphenicol acetyltransferase reporter gene, respectively. In vivo transfection by adenoviral vectors was demonstrated in vascular tissue by direct infusion into vessels,[32,34–36] in myocardial tissue by direct injection into the myocardium,[33,37] and in the circulation after adenoviral infection of skeletal muscle.[38] Limitations of the current vector (first generation) include transient gene expression, inflammatory reactions in organs expressing the transgene,[39–41] and viral antigen-induced immunity.[42]

An alternative, adenovirus-mediated gene transfer approach consists of an adenovirus-augmented, receptor-mediated gene delivery system developed by coupling inactivated adenovirus to DNA polylysine complexes.[43] Using the endosome-disruptive activity of inactivated adenovirus particles and poly-L-lysine, gene constructs (up to 48 kb) have been transfected with high efficiency in vitro[44] and in vivo to autologous rabbit jugular vein grafts.[45] Complexing unmodified plasmid DNA with replication-deficient adenovirus via cationic lipids enhanced gene transfer both in vitro and in vivo.[46]

Adeno-associated virus (AAV) is a dependent human parvovirus that is not able to replicate unless a helper virus, such as adenovirus or herpesvirus, is also present.[47] AAV vectors preferentially transduce cells in S phase.[48] Interestingly, transduction efficiency of fibroblasts by AAV vectors was increased by prior exposure to DNA synthesis inhibitors or topoisomerase inhibitors.[49] Among the favorable properties of AAV vectors as gene transfer agents are a lack of known human pathogenicity, a wide range of target cell lines that can be infected, and the ability of the virus to establish a latent infection by integration into the genome of the cell.[50]

TABLE 9-1

EXPERIMENTAL GENE TRANSFER METHODS

Virus-mediated
  Retrovirus
  Adenovirus
  Adenoviral coat/transferrin polylysine
  Adeno-associated virus
Lipid-mediated
  Liposomes
  Cationic lipids (Lipofectin)
Fusigenic liposome-mediated
  Sendai virus (HVJ) liposomes
Other methods
  "Naked" DNA
  Microinjection
  Microparticle bombardment
  Myoblast implantation

Early applications of AAV vectors to human gene therapy have included phenotypic correction of Fanconi anemia in human hematopoietic cells[51] and stable in vivo expression of the cystic fibrosis transmembrane conductance regulator in airway epithelial cells.[52] The potential use of AAV vectors for vascular gene transfer remains to be determined.

Lipid-Mediated Gene Transfer

The encapsulation of DNA in artificial lipid membranes (liposomes) can facilitate its uptake and cellular transport. Cationic liposomes have been used extensively during the last 5 years for cellular delivery of DNA[53,54] and antisense oligonucleotides.[55,56] The activity of cationic liposomes is postulated to be mediated by (1) spontaneous capture of the negatively charged polynucleotides with cationic lipids by a condensation reaction, (2) increased cellular uptake due to interaction of positively charged complexes with negatively charged biological membranes, and (3) membrane fusion (or transient membrane destabilization) with the plasmalemma or the endosome to achieve delivery into the cytoplasm while avoiding degradation in the lysosomal compartment.[57,58] Recent data indicate that movement of DNA from the cytoplasm to the nucleus and successful dissociation of DNA from the lipid complex appear to be important variables for lipid-mediated gene transfer.[59] Expression of recombinant genes after cationic lipid–mediated gene transfer has been demonstrated in vivo in several animal models.[20,21,60–62] Gene expression after liposome-mediated arterial gene transfer may be augmented in the presence of ongoing proliferation (e.g., intimal proliferation after balloon injury).[63]

Fusigenic Liposome–Mediated Gene Transfer

This method utilizes a combination of fusigenic proteins of the Sendai virus (hemagglutinating virus of Japan, or HVJ) in conjunction with neutral liposomes. HVJ is an RNA virus and belongs to the paramyxovirus family, which has HN and F glycoproteins on its envelope.[64] HN binds with glycol-type sialic acid and degrades the receptor by its own neuraminidase activity. F glycoprotein is cleaved to generate a hydrophobic fusion peptide by proteases, and the activated F protein can interact directly with the cellular lipid bilayer and induces fusion. A nuclear protein (high-mobility group 1 [HMG-1]) that binds DNA enhances the integration of transfected DNA into the nucleus.[65,66] HVJ liposomes consist of neutral liposomes complexed with ultraviolet (UV) light–inactivated HVJ virus. An interesting feature of the HVJ liposome–mediated gene transfer method is that after fusion of the liposome complex with the cell membrane, the DNA is directly released into the cytosol without undergoing endocytosis, thereby reducing lysosomal destruction of the DNA construct and facilitating the nuclear uptake.[67] HVJ liposome–mediated in vivo gene transfer of an SV40 large T-antigen cDNA expression vector in rat carotid arteries yielded up to 30 percent SV40 T-antigen–positive cells within the vascular wall without ap-

parent toxic effects.[68] HVJ liposome methods have been successfully employed for gene transfer in vivo to many tissues, including liver,[66] kidney,[69,70] and vascular wall.[71,72]

Other in Vivo Gene Transfer Methods

Microinjection has been used successfully to introduce purified recombinant proteins, neutralizing antibodies, and competitor oligonucleotides into cells.[73,74] By applying direct gene injection to the heart muscle, the expression of a reporter gene was demonstrated for up to 4 weeks after the initial injection.[75] Furthermore, expression of injected genes can be targeted to specific cell types in vivo (e.g., cardiac muscle cells) and can be modulated by the hormonal status of the animal.[76]

Ex Vivo Gene Transfer

As mentioned above, ex vivo gene transfer methods utilize the transfer of recombinant genes into the vessel wall by reimplanting cells that have been genetically modified to express new genetic material. Nabel et al.[19] first demonstrated a cell-based vascular gene transfer technique. By reimplanting endothelial cells transfected ex vivo with a retroviral β-galactosidase vector on the surface of balloon-injured porcine iliofemoral arteries, genetically modified cells could be detected up to 2 to 4 weeks following reimplantation. Conte et al.[77] reported a high degree of variation in the persistence of seeded endothelial cells transfected with a recombinant β-galactosidase containing retroviral vector. In addition to endothelial cells, ex vivo–transfected smooth muscle cells have been introduced in the vasculature.[78] Lynch et al.[79] reported the seeding of smooth muscle cells transfected with adenosine deaminase gene into endothelium-denuded blood vessels. Another application of ex vivo gene transfer is the engineering of vascular grafts seeded with endothelial cells previously transfected in a culture dish.[15,80] Dichek and colleagues[81,82] focused on the development of a stent coated with genetically modified endothelial cells for the prevention of restenosis. They were able to detect small quantities of tissue-type plasminogen activator (t-PA) from stents seeded with genetically modified endothelial cells containing recombinant t-PA. Gene targeting and gene transfer studies of the plasminogen/plasmin system with implications in thrombosis, hemostasis, neointima formation, and atherosclerosis are discussed elsewhere.[83,84] Seeding of vascular grafts with soluble vascular cell adhesion molecule (sVCAM) (see Chap. 4) using adenoviral ex vivo gene transfer was reported by Chen et al.[85] The potential of this approach to prevent or slow progression of vein graft disease is not yet determined.

Implantation of genetically modified myoblasts or fibroblasts to skeletal muscle is an attractive gene transfer method, because the gene product can be delivered systemically. Indeed, several investigators have reported successful gene delivery using these approaches.[86–88] In a mouse model, myoblasts were transplanted and supported sustained delivery of functionally active erythropoietin to correct anemia associated

TABLE 9-2

CURRENT STRATEGIES FOR LOCAL GENETIC
ENGINEERING IN VASCULAR DISEASE

Oligonucleotide	Plasmid DNA
Intracellular effects	Intracellular effects
Antisense: inhibition of translation	Cytostatic
Decoy: inhibition of transcription	Cytotoxic
	Extracellular effects
	Paracrine

with renal failure.[89] The myoblast method could potentially provide an approach for the delivery of insulin (diabetes), atrial natriuretic peptide (hypertension or heart failure), or apolipoprotein AI (atherosclerosis).

GENE TRANSFER AND VASCULAR DISEASE

Most studies dealing with genetic engineering in vascular disease have focused on the delivery of genetic material locally to the site of disease using oligonucleotides or plasmid DNA (Table 9-2). The development of catheter-based drug delivery systems that permit exposure times necessary for efficient gene transfer and that simultaneously permit maintenance of tissue perfusion will be necessary to elucidate the full potential of in vivo gene transfer.[90] As described in the following sections, current in vivo models for studying gene expression are mainly focused on iliac and carotid arteries or, in a few examples, on coronary arteries. In extending the range of vascular gene delivery, recent reports described adenovirus-mediated gene transfer in vivo to cerebral blood vessels[91] and pulmonary arteries.[92]

Genetic Engineering Using Synthetic Oligonucleotides

ANTISENSE OLIGONUCLEOTIDES
Antisense oligonucleotides can be employed as therapeutic agents that exert their molecular actions during different steps of DNA-RNA processing, either at the translational or at the transcriptional level—e.g., uncoiling of DNA, transcription of DNA, export of RNA, DNA splicing, RNA stability, or RNA translation. *Oligonucleotides are most widely applied to inhibit gene expression as inhibitors of ribosomal translation, with the complementary or "antisense" base sequence targeted to a specific "sense" sequence in the mRNA.*[93,94] Interestingly, antisense mRNAs occur naturally as a cellular regulatory mechanism.[95,96] Mechanisms of antisense inhibition include interference with ribosome binding and processing of mRNA, interference with mRNA conformation or mRNA splicing, and RNase-H activation of mRNA digestion.[94,97] Antisense inhibition is usually targeted at the 5′ initiation codon. An antisense oligonucleotide generally consists of 15 to 20 bases, since it should be complementary to only one unique target sequence in the genome.[98] Three features of nucleic acids are relevant for the use of antisense oligonucleotides as pharmacologic agents:[99] (1) coding properties for gene transfer or gene therapy; (2) binding and recognition properties of antisense-, antigene-, or sense-directed oligonucleotides leading to inhibition or modulation of expression, targeting mRNA, double-stranded DNA with formation of a triple helix, and nucleic acid–binding proteins; and (3) catalytic properties of ribozymes against sequence-specific sites on mRNA. Instability of oligonucleotides has been a significant problem in their experimental use. By chemically modifying the phosphate backbone of the oligonucleotide (phosphorothioate or phosphoroamidate bonding), the stability of oligonucleotides against nucleolytic phosphodiesterases could be improved.[94,100,101] Under some conditions, phosphorothioate analogs can exert non-sequence-specific antiviral activity.[102] Antisense oligonucleotides can exhibit sequence-specific effects in mimicking bacterial DNA and triggering rather than inhibiting a specific immune response.[103] Furthermore, a stretch of four contiguous guanosine (4G) residues, which is present in antisense c-myb and c-myc oligonucleotides that were used in previous studies,[104–106] may have nonspecific though antiproliferative effects.[107–109] The uptake of modified oligonucleotides can be enhanced by complexing the oligonucleotide with cationic liposomes[56,110] or fusigenic liposomes (HVJ liposomes).[71,72] In the area of vascular gene therapy, several groups have investigated the effects of antisense oligonucleotides on intimal hyperplasia after balloon injury (Table 9-3).

TRANSCRIPTIONAL FACTOR DECOY
Synthetic double-stranded oligonucleotides functioning as transcriptional factor "decoys" can block the binding of nuclear factors to promoter regions of targeted genes, resulting in the inhibition of gene transactivation.[111,112] This "decoy"

TABLE 9-3

APPLICATION OF ANTISENSE OLIGONUCLEOTIDES
IN VASCULAR DISEASE

Target of Antisense Oligonucleotide	Definition of Target Protein	Reference
c-*myb*	DNA-binding nuclear protein	105
cdc2/PCNA	Cell cycle–regulatory proteins	65, 110, 116
c-*myc*	DNA-binding nuclear protein	98, 100, 104
PCNA	Cell cycle–regulatory protein	114
Angiotensinogen	Angiotensin I precursor	112, 140, 146

strategy may be useful for treating a wide range of human diseases (Fig. 9-1). Recently, our group showed that a single administration of an E2F decoy (containing the E2F cis element) that binds the transcription factor E2F inhibits smooth muscle cell hyperplasia in a rat carotid balloon injury model.[113] The binding of E2F prevents it from transactivating the gene expression of cell-cycle regulatory proteins such as PCNA, c-myc, and cdk2, thereby inhibiting vascular smooth muscle cell proliferation and subsequent neointima formation in vivo.

Experimental Applications of Antisense Oligonucleotides

INTIMAL HYPERPLASIA

Simons et al.[105] first reported that the administration of antisense oligonucleotides against *c-myb* applied by pluronic gel to the adventitial layer of rat carotid arteries inhibited neointimal hyperplasia in response to balloon injury. Data from our laboratory demonstrated that a single HVJ liposome–mediated administration of antisense oligonucleotides against proliferating cell nuclear antigen (PCNA) and cdc2 kinase inhibited neointimal lesion formation after balloon injury at least up to

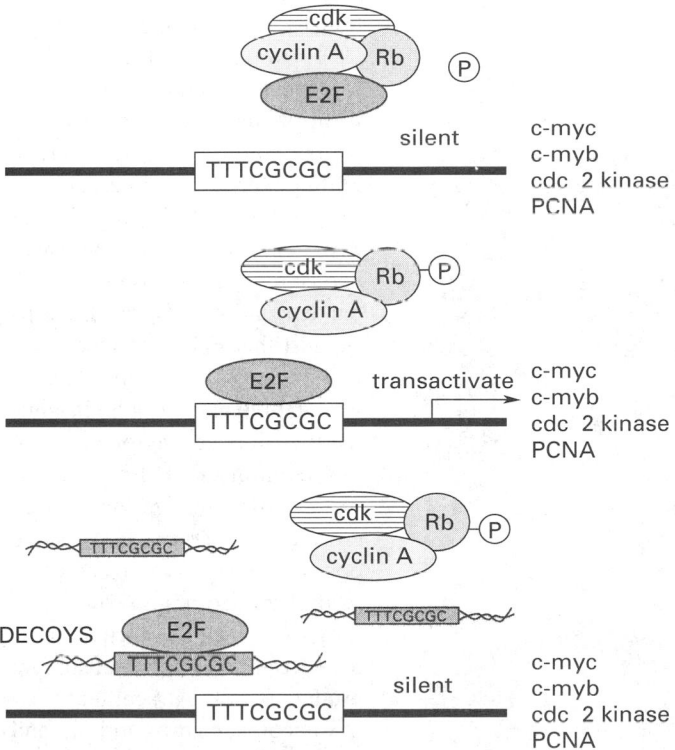

FIGURE 9-1

Principal of E2F "decoy" strategy. TTTCGCGC is the consensus sequence for the E2F binding site. In the quiescent cell state, the transcription factor E2F is complexed with Rb (retinoblastoma gene product), cyclin A, and the cyclin dependent kinase cdk2 (*top*). Phosphorylation of Rb releases free E2F, which binds to cis elements of the cell cycle–regulatory genes, resulting in the transactivation of these genes (*middle*). The E2F decoy cis-element double stranded oligonucleotide binds to free E2F, preventing E2F-mediated transactivation of cell cycle–regulatory genes (*bottom*). (From Morishita et al.,[113] with permission.)

8 weeks after transfection.[71] The combination of antisense cdc2 kinase and cdk2 kinase oligonucleotides also resulted in almost complete inhibition of neointima formation.[72] Bennett et al.[104] showed an inhibition of vascular smooth muscle cell proliferation by administration of c-myc antisense oligonucleotides to the adventitial surface of injured carotid arteries in a pluronic gel solution. Two other studies reported inhibition of neointima formation after application of antisense oligonucleotides. Delivery of antisense PCNA oligonucleotides by pluronic gel (in a rat carotid model) and of antisense c-myc oligonucleotides by direct application through a porous balloon (in a porcine coronary artery model) resulted in significant inhibition of neointimal hyperplasia.[106,114]

VEIN GRAFT DISEASE

Autologous vein grafts remain the most commonly used conduits for surgical revascularization of the heart and lower extremities. Given the failure of traditional therapies at improving long-term vein graft function,[115] gene therapy offers a new opportunity for reducing the morbidity and increased costs associated with the current limitations on functional graft survival. The vein graft offers an unusual opportunity for combining intact tissue in vivo gene transfer techniques with the increased safety of an ex vivo application of the transfection medium. Manipulation of transfection conditions, including increased exposure time and controlling components of the transfection medium, can also be more easily achieved. Some researchers have begun to explore the possibility of ex vivo viral-mediated gene transfer in autologous vein grafts. Chen et al.[85] demonstrated the expression of the marker gene β-galactosidase along the luminal surface and in the adventitia of porcine vein grafts infected with a replication-deficient adenoviral vector at the time of surgery. In this same study, short-term expression of soluble VCAM-1 (sVCAM-1) was documented after transfection of vein grafts. Kupfer et al.[45] explored the use of a novel adenovirus-based transfection system (adenoviral particles, plasmid DNA, and biotin/streptavidin transferrin/polylysine complexes) to deliver the gene for β-galactosidase to the walls of rabbit vein grafts. β-galactosidase expression was again greatest on the luminal surfaces of the grafts at 3 and 7 days after surgery, although the presence of transfected cells in the medial and adventitial layers was also reported.

We hypothesized that we could, through genetic engineering, alter the ability of the grafts to mount a hyperplastic response to acute injury while leaving intact their ability to respond to chronic hemodynamic stress via a hypertrophic response, such as that seen in arteries exposed to hypertension. We therefore used HVJ liposomes to deliver a combination of antisense oligonucleotides (ODN) to cdc2/PCNA to rabbit veins at the time of grafting into the carotid artery and observed a greater than 90 percent inhibition of increased smooth muscle cell (SMC) proliferation during the first postoperative week.[116] This blockade of cell cycle progression resulted in a near complete inhibition of neointimal hyperplasia. Instead, the vein graft wall was shifted to an adaptive process of medial hypertrophy. Having redirected the genetically engineered grafts away from neointimal hyperplasia and toward medial hypertrophy as an adaptation to the arterial environment, we then tested the susceptibility of these antisense ODN–treated grafts to accelerated atherogenesis. Control ODN–treated and untreated grafts placed in cholesterol-fed rabbits developed significant foam-cell lesions and plaque within 6 weeks after surgery. Antisense ODN–treated grafts that had remained free of neointima formation, however, resisted macrophage invasion and the development of macroscopic plaque (Fig. 9-2). We have subsequently found that this inhibition of cell cycle progression is likely to have profound effects on the phenotypes of the vascular cells undergoing remodeling after vein grafting and that these changes are likely to affect the proatherogenic environment of the normal graft wall. For example, the endothelium of antisense ODN–treated grafts retained more of its capacity to produce nitric oxide and resist monocyte adhesion in comparison to untreated or control ODN–treated grafts.[117]

GENE TRANSFER AND THE STUDY OF VASCULAR REMODELING

Molecular cardiovascular research has resulted in significant gains in the knowledge of disease processes at cellular as well as molecular levels and has led to the characterization of locally expressed genes in diseased blood vessels that have been postulated to play autocrine and/or paracrine roles in vascular pathophysiology. Table 9-4 summarizes recent studies in which local overexpression of a specific gene (gene construct) was used to investigate genes putatively involved in vascular diseases.

Using a retrovirus-mediated transfection method, Nabel et al.[61] overexpressed an expression vector encoding a secreted form of fibroblast growth factor 1 (FGF-1) in porcine arteries. FGF-1 expression was associated with intimal thickening of the transfected vessels together with neocapillary formation in the expanded intima. These findings suggest that FGF-1 induces intimal hyperplasia in the arterial wall in vivo and, through its ability to stimulate angiogenesis in the neointima, FGF-1 could stimulate neovascularization of atherosclerotic plaques. In the same porcine model, the overexpression of transforming growth factor β_1 (TGF-β_1) in normal arteries resulted in substantial production of extracellular matrix accompanied by intimal and medial hyperplasia.[120] These findings showed that TGF-β_1 differentially modulates extracellular matrix production and cellular proliferation in the arterial wall and could play a reparative role in response to arterial injury. The increased production of extracellular matrix that accompanied the

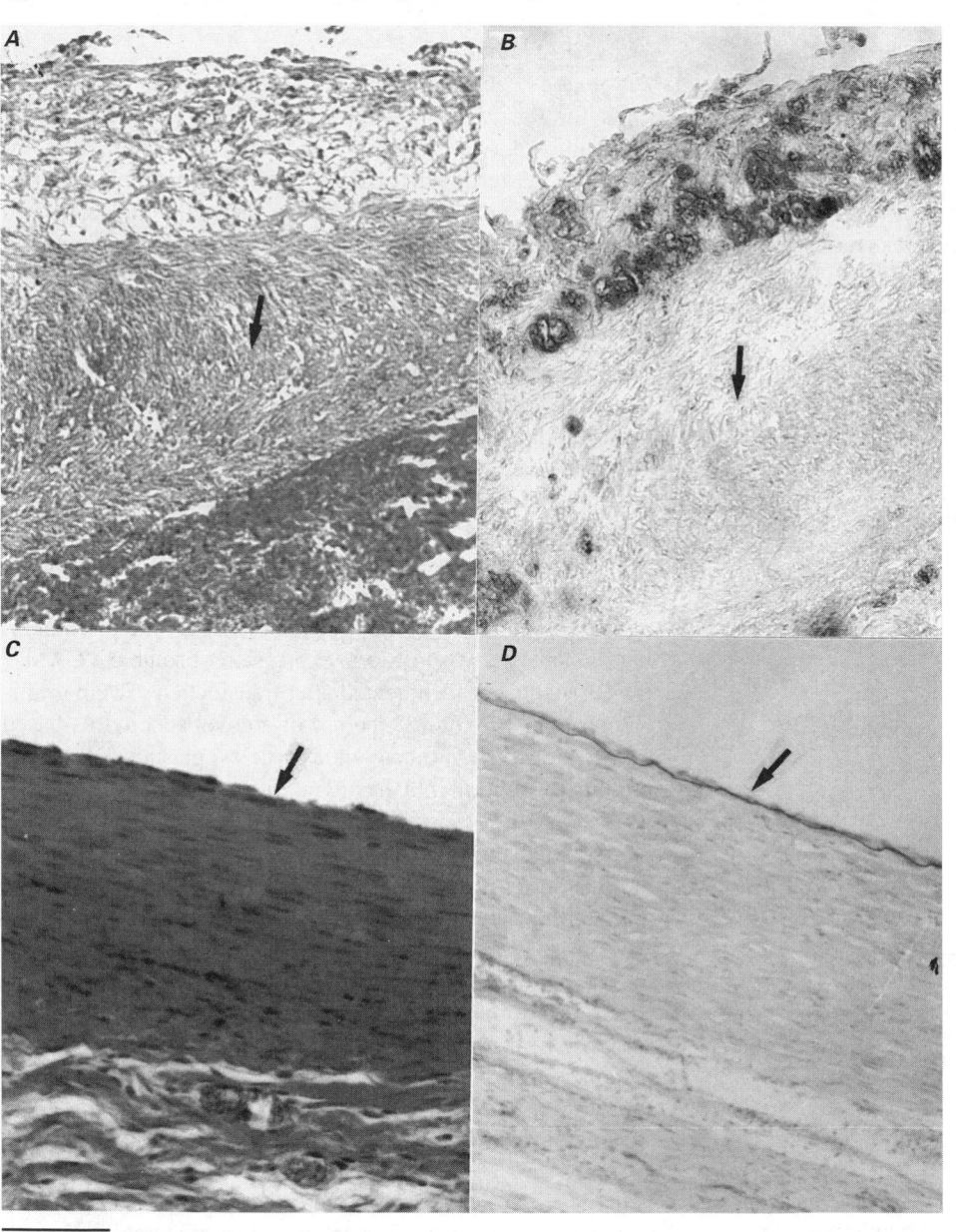

FIGURE 9-2
Control oligonucleotide-treated (*A* and *B*) and antisense oligonucleotide (against cdc2 kinase/PCNA)-treated vein grafts (*C* and *D*) in hypercholesterolemic rabbits, 6 weeks after surgery (×70). Sections of 5 μm were stained with hematoxylin/van Gieson (*A* and *C*) and a monoclonal antibody against rabbit macrophages (*B* and *D*). Arrows indicate the location of the internal elastic lamina. (From Mann et al.,[116] with permission.)

intimal and medial hyperplasia was not observed following expression of other growth factor genes in the vessel wall, including genes for platelet-derived growth factor (PDGF-BB)[60,121] or the secreted form of FGF-1.[61] Porcine arteries transfected with human PDGF-BB demonstrated intimal hyperplasia with increased numbers of intimal SMC. An increased deposition of procollagen, however, as seen in TGF-β_1–transfected vessels, was not observed. By stimulating the formation of extracellular matrix, it is possible that TGF-β_1 could help to promote healing following vascular injury

TABLE 9-4

OVEREXPRESSION OF GROWTH MEDIATING FACTORS
BY GENE TRANSFER FOR THE STUDY OF VASCULAR REMODELING

Transfected DNA	Remodeling Effect	Reference
Fibroblast growth factor (FGF-1)	Neointima formation Angiogenesis	61
Transforming growth factor (TGF-β_1)	Cellular proliferation Extracellular matrix formation	120
Platelet-derived growth factor (PDGF-BB)	Intimal hyperplasia	60, 121
Angiotensin converting enzyme (ACE)	Medial hypertrophy	123
Angiotensin II type 2 (AT2) receptor	Antiproliferative counteracting AT1 receptor	124
Nitric oxide synthase (ecNOS)	Inhibition of neointima formation	127

limiting the extensive cellular intimal hyperplasia observed with PDGF-BB.[120]

The pathogenesis of vascular diseases such as hypertension involves a process of vascular remodeling associated with increased vascular hypertrophy and the activation of the local angiotensin system.[118,119,122] Angiotensin II has been shown to stimulate the growth and proliferation of vascular smooth muscle as well as collagen biosynthesis in vitro. Its in vivo role has been inferred from experiments using angiotensin converting enzyme (ACE) inhibitors. Since these drugs produce hemodynamic effects, a direct role of local angiotensin in vascular remodeling has not been proved. To study the local effects of an autocrine/paracrine factor like angiotensin, Morishita et al.[123] overexpressed ACE within the vascular wall by using fusigenic liposomes (HVJ liposomes) as the delivery vehicle. Immunohistochemistry localized immunoreactive ACE activity in the medial vascular SMC as well as in the intimal endothelial cells. The increase in vascular ACE activity was associated with increased DNA synthesis and vascular protein content via the local production and action of vascular angiotensin II without changes in systemic blood pressure. Parallel to these biochemical changes, morphometric analysis documented a medial thickening of the ACE-transfected vessel segments, with unchanged luminal diameters implicating a medial wall hypertrophy via local autocrine/paracrine angiotensin II production. Indeed, the vascular hypertrophic response to local ACE overexpression was inhibited by the angiotensin antagonist Dup 753. In a subsequent study, Nakajima et al.[124] demonstrated by overexpression of the type 2 angiotensin II (AT2) receptor in balloon-injured rat carotid arteries that the AT2 receptor exerts an antiproliferative effect, counteracting the growth action of AT1 receptors. These experiments demonstrated that gene transfer techniques provide the unique opportunity to selectively investigate the role of autocrine-paracrine factors and their receptors, respectively, in vascular remodeling independent of systemic factors or hemodynamic stimuli.

Injury to the endothelium plays an essential role in the pathogenesis of vasculoproliferative disorders,[125] and endothelium-derived relaxing factor/nitric oxide has an important regulatory function in maintaining vascular homeostasis.[126] As described below in detail, transfection of the cDNA-encoding endothelial cell nitric oxide synthase (ecNOS) in injured carotid arteries inhibited neointimal hyperplasia after balloon injury, demonstrating an important role for vascular-derived nitric oxide in modulating vascular remodeling.[127]

THERAPEUTIC APPLICATIONS OF GENE TRANSFER IN CARDIOVASCULAR DISEASES

Neointimal Hyperplasia and Restenosis

Besides using synthetic oligonucleotides for inhibiting specific mRNA processing, gene constructs (plasmid DNA) can be delivered into the vessel wall for therapeutic purposes. Table 9-5 lists recent approaches using in vivo transfer of plasmid DNA to treat neointimal hyperplasia after vascular injury. We recently reported the construction of an expression vector containing the *ec-NOS* cDNA driven by a β-actin promoter and cytomegalovirus (CMV) enhancer.[127] To assess the biological response to transfection of the *ec-NOS* gene on vascular lesion formation in vivo, we chose the well-characterized rat carotid artery balloon injury model, in which no significant regrowth of endothelium is observed within 2 to 3 weeks after injury. Four complementary experimental methods were used to verify successful in vivo *ec-NOS* gene transfer into the vessel wall: (1) transgene protein expression was documented by Western blot; (2) localization of enzyme expression in the vessel wall was verified by in situ histochemical staining using the NADPH-diaphorase assay; (3) enzymatic activity of the transgene product was confirmed by measurement of increased generation of nitric oxide from transfected vessel segments using chemiluminescence methods; and (4) biological effectiveness of the transgene product

TABLE 9-5

PLASMID DNA TRANSFER AND THERAPEUTIC EFFECTS IN BLOOD VESSELS

Transfected DNA	Therapeutic Effect	Reference
Nitric oxide synthase (*ec-NOS*)	Inhibition of neointima formation Improvement of vascular reactivity	127
Herpes simplex virus thymidine kinase (HSV *tk*)	Inhibition of neointima formation	128, 147
Constitutive active form of retinoblastoma (Rb) gene product	Inhibition of neointima formation	129
Vascular endothelial growth factor (VEGF)	Angiogenesis	133
ras transdominate negative mutants	Inhibition of neointima formation	131
p21	Inhibition of neointima formation	130

was assessed by changes in vascular reactivity induced by the increased local generation of nitric oxide, thereby potentially counterbalancing vasospasm induced by vascular injury. Thus, in vivo transfection of *ec-NOS* in balloon-injured rat carotid arteries not only restored production of nitric oxide within the vessel wall but also significantly improved the vasomotor reactivity of the vessel. Furthermore, *ec-NOS* transgene expression resulted in a 70 percent inhibition of neointima formation after balloon injury (Fig. 9-3). This study

documented the therapeutic effects utilizing direct in vivo gene transfer of a cDNA encoding a functional enzyme. Although the rat carotid model may not be a good model of human disease, this study provides direct evidence that endothelium-derived nitric oxide is an important local inhibitor of neointimal hyperplasia in vivo. Since the regulation of vascular growth and migration in vivo involves a delicate balance of stimulatory versus inhibitory factors, the loss of endothelial-derived nitric oxide may play a fundamental role in the pathogenesis of vasculoproliferative diseases, including atherosclerosis. The overexpression of *ec-NOS* may be useful for gene therapy of neointimal hyperplasia and associated local vasospasm after vascular injury.

Another therapeutic approach using gene transfer was reported recently using an adenoviral vector–mediated transfer of the herpesvirus thymidine kinase (HSV *tk*).[128] After introduction of the vector into injured porcine arteries and vascular smooth muscle cells, respectively, the *tk* gene rendered the SMC sensitive to the nucleoside analog ganciclovir given immediately after balloon injury. After one course of ganciclovir treatment, intimal hyperplasia decreased by about 50 percent. Chang et al[129] showed that localized arterial infection with a replication-defective adenovirus encoding a nonphosphorylatable, constitutively active form of the retinoblastoma gene product at the time of balloon angioplasty significantly reduced SMC proliferation and neointima formation in both the rat carotid and porcine femoral artery models of restenosis. Similar results were obtained by adenovirus-mediated overexpression of human *p21* in vivo.[130] Ras proteins are key transducers of mitogenic signals from membrane to nucleus in many cell types. The local delivery of DNA vectors expressing ras transdominant negative mutants, which interfere with ras function, reduced neointimal lesion formation in a rat carotid artery balloon injury model.[131]

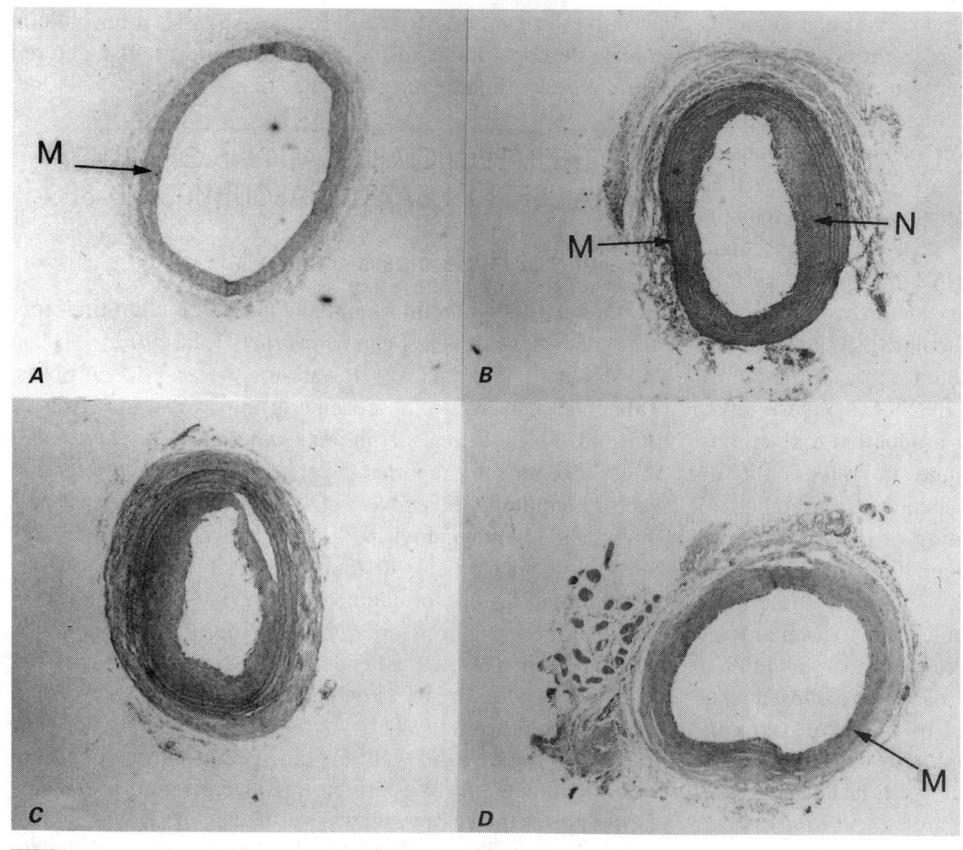

FIGURE 9-3
Inhibition of neointimal hyperplasia by in vivo gene transfer of endothelial cell-nitric oxide synthase (ecNOS) in balloon-injured rat carotid arteries. *A*. Normal artery. *B*. Injured, untransfected artery. *C*. Injured, control vector–transfected artery. *D*. Injured, *ec-NOS*-transfected. M = media; N = neointima. (From von der Leyen et al.,[127] with permission.)

Angiogenesis

Angiogenic growth factors may be useful to expedite and/or augment collateral artery development in animal models of myocardial and hindlimb ischemia (see Chap. 102). Enhanced angiogenesis was demonstrated in a model of rabbit ischemic hindlimb following hydrogel polymer-mediated gene transfer of vascular endothelial growth factor (VEGF),[132] and improvement of resting and maximum flow was achieved that was comparable to a single administration of VEGF protein.[133] Recently, a Phase I study was initiated to study the effect of arterial gene transfer of VEGF using a hydrogel polymer–coated angioplasty balloon in patients with peripheral artery disease.[134]

MYOCARDIAL GENE TRANSFER

Direct injection of DNA into myocardial tissue has been shown to be effective in local delivery of a transgene to the heart. Lin et al.[75] first reported in vivo expression of bacterial β-galactosidase in cardiac myocytes for at least 4 weeks after direct injection into the left ventricle. Direct injections of α-major histocompatibility complex (*MHC*) gene and the reporter gene luciferase under the control of an *MHC* promoter also resulted in the regulated expression of these genes.[76] Subsequent studies also showed increased gene expression after myocardial injection of adenoviral vectors.[33,37] Using cationic lipids of HVJ liposome–mediated gene transfer, detectable expression of reporter genes was reported after direct coronary injection.[21,34,135]

Healing and remodeling of the ventricle after myocardial infarction remain as important clinical problems. Some candidate genes (e.g., transforming growth factor β [TGF-β_1] and myogenin) may enhance the healing and recovery of myocytes after injury associated with infarction. The induction of neovascularization or angiogenesis in ischemic myocardium after coronary artery occlusion using gene transfer may salvage myocardium at risk by enhancing blood supply to the ischemic areas. Indeed, intracardiac myoblast grafts stably transfected with an inducible TGF-β_1 construct that were transplanted into mice hearts were accompanied by increased DNA synthesis in vascular endothelial cells, consistent with a sustained angiogenic response.[136] The success of intracardiac grafting with genetically modified cardiomyocytes depends on the ability of grafts to couple with host myocytes. Soonpaa et al.[137] demonstrated that fetal cardiomyocytes isolated from transgenic mice carrying a fusion protein of the cardiac α-*MHC* promoter with a β-galactosidase reporter gene were connected to the host myocardium by nascent intercalated disks formed after grafting. Chronic heart failure is accompanied by a reduction in the number of myocardial β-adrenergic receptors and in inotropic responsiveness. Cardiac-specific overexpression of the β_2-adrenergic receptor in a transgenic animal model with subsequent increased myocardial function suggests a potential gene therapy approach to heart failure.[138]

HEPATIC GENE TRANSFER AND CARDIOVASCULAR DISEASE

Perhaps the most dramatic effect of hepatic gene transfer has been achieved in the development of therapy of familial hypercholesterolemia, an inherited disease in humans caused by deficiency of LDL receptors. Infusion of an LDL receptor gene–protein complex into the portal vein of the Watanabe heritable hyperlipidemic rabbit, which has a similar receptor deficiency, resulted in hepatocyte-specific gene transfer and a temporary amelioration of hypercholesterolemia.[139] Using an ex vivo approach the introduction of hepatocytes transformed by a retroviral LDL receptor (LDLR) vector resulted in a long-term improvement of hypercholesterolemia in LDLR-deficient rabbits.[140] Treatment of hypercholesterolemia in *apoE*-deficient mice by adenovirus-mediated gene transfer of human *apoE3* cDNA resulted in a shift in the plasma lipoprotein distribution from primarily VLDL and LDL in the control mice to predominantly HDL in transfected mice.[141] Furthermore, in normal mice, adenovirus-mediated transfer of a gene encoding apoA-I produced transient, physiologically relevant elevations of HDL cholesterol comparable to those in animals transgenic for a copy of the *apoA-I* gene.[142] Thus, the liver is thought to be a highly desirable target for gene therapy of inheritable metabolic disorders affecting the cardiovascular system.

CURRENT STATUS OF GENE THERAPY IN HUMAN TRIALS

The first clinical trial with a marker gene in an approved protocol began on March 22, 1989. The first federally approved human gene therapy protocol began on September 14, 1990, for patients with adenosine deaminase (ADA) deficiency. Since then, successful human gene transfer has been demonstrated in 28 ex vivo and 10 in vivo studies.[143] In the cardiopulmonary field, two studies [ex vivo: LDL receptor to hepatocytes; in vivo: cystic fibrosis transmembrane conductance regulator (CFTR) to nasal epithelium] have been reported in which transfer of genetic material has evoked a biological response that is relevant to the underlying disease, hypercholesterolemia and cystic fibrosis, respectively.[144,145] As mentioned earlier, a clinical Phase I trial investigating the effect of intravascular delivery of VEGF-plasmid DNA is currently being performed.[134] The objectives of current human gene therapy trials are, in general, the evaluation of (1) in vivo efficacy of gene transfer methods, (2) safety of gene transfer methods, and (3) possible therapeutic efficacy.

REFERENCES

1. Griffith F. The significance of pneumococcal types. *J Hyg* 1928; 27:113–159.
2. Avery OT, MacLeod CM, MacCarty M. Studies on the chemical nature of the substance inducing transformation of pneumococcal types. *J Exp Med* 1944; 36:137–158.
3. Watson JD, Crick FHC. Molecular structure of nucleic acids: A structure for deoxyribose nucleic acid. *Nature* 1953; 171:737–738.

4. Watson JD, Crick FHC. Genetical implications of the structure of deoxyribonucleic acid. *Nature* 1953; 171:964–967.

5. Sambrook J, Westphal H, Srivansan PR, Dulbecco R. The integrated state of viral DNA in SV40-transformed cells. *Proc Natl Acad Sci USA* 1968; 59:1288–1293.

6. Rogers S, Pfuderer P. Use of viruses as carriers of added genetic information. *Nature* 1968; 219:749–751.

7. Subramani S, Southern PJ. Analysis of gene expression using simian virus 40 vectors. *Anal Biochem* 1983; 135:1–15.

8. Rogers S, Lowenthal A, Terheggen HG, Colombo JP. Induction of arginase activity with the Shope papilloma virus in tissue culture cells from an argininemic patient. *J Exp Med* 1973; 137:1091–1096.

9. Friedmann T, Roblin R. Gene therapy for human genetic disease? *Science* 1972; 175:949–955.

10. Cohen S, Chang H, Boyer H, Helling R. Construction of biologically functional bacterial plasmids in vitro. *Proc Natl Acad Sci USA* 1973; 70:3240–3244.

11. Berg P. Dissections and reconstructions of genes and chromosomes. *Science* 1981; 213:296–303.

12. Jackson DA, Symons RH, Berg P. Biochemical method for inserting new genetic information into DNA of simian virus 40: Circular SV40 DNA molecules containing lambda phage genes and the galactose operon of *Escherichia coli*. *Proc Natl Acad Sci USA* 1972; 69:2904–2909.

13. Mulligan RC, Howard BH, Berg P. Synthesis of rabbit beta-globin in cultured monkey kidney cells following infection with a SV40 beta-globin recombinant genome. *Nature* 1979; 277:108–114.

14. Berg P, Singer MF. The recombinant DNA controversy: Twenty years later. *Proc Natl Acad Sci USA* 1995; 92:9011–9013.

15. Wilson JM, Birinyi LK, Salomon RN, Libby P, Callow AD, Mulligan RC. Implantation of vascular grafts lined with genetically modified endothelial cells. *Science* 1989; 244:1344–1346.

16. Cone RD, Mulligan RC. High-efficiency gene transfer into mammalian cells: Generation of helper-free recombinant retrovirus with broad mammalian host range. *Proc Natl Acad Sci USA* 1984; 81:6349–6353.

17. Danos O, Mulligan RC. Expression of retroviral trans-acting functions from complementary crippled genomes: A system for helper free packaging of retroviral vectors. *J Cell Biochem* 1988; 12:172–178.

18. Boris-Lawrie K, Temin HM. The retroviral vector: Replication cycle and safety considerations for retrovirus-mediated gene therapy. *Ann NY Acad Sci* 1994; 716:59–70.

19. Nabel EG, Plautz G, Boyce FM, Stanley JC, Nabel GJ. Recombinant gene expression in vivo within endothelial cells of the arterial wall. *Science* 1989; 244:1342–1344.

20. Nabel EG, Plautz G, Nabel GJ. Site-specific gene expression in vivo by direct gene transfer into the arterial wall. *Science* 1990; 249:1285–1288.

21. Lim CS, Chapman GD, Gammon RS, Muhlestein JB, Bauman RP, Stack RS, et al. Direct in vivo gene transfer into the coronary artery and peripheral vasculature in the intact dog. *Circulation* 1991; 83:2007–2011.

22. Flugelman MY, Jaklitsch MT, Newman KD, Casscells W, Bratthauer GL, Dichek DA. Low level in vivo gene transfer into the arterial wall through a perforated balloon catheter. *Circulation* 1992; 85:1110–1117.

23. Miller DG, Adam MA, Miller AD. Gene transfer by retrovirus vectors occurs only in cells that are actively replicating at the time of transfection. *Mol Cell Biol* 1990; 10:4239–4242.

24. Friedmann T, Yee JK. Pseudotyped retroviral vectors for studies of human gene therapy. *Nature Med* 1995; 1:275–277.

25. Cooper NR, Jensen FC, Welsh RM, Oldstone MBA. Lysis of RNA tumor viruses by human serum: Direct antibody-independent triggering of the classical complement pathway. *J Exp Med* 1976; 144:970–984.

26. Cornetta K, Moen RC, Culver K, Morgan RA, McLachlin JR, Sturm S, et al. Amphotropic murine leukemia retrovirus is not an acute pathogen for primates. *Hum Gene Ther* 1990; 1:15–30.

27. Takeuchi Y, Cosset FLC, Lachmann PJ, Okada H, Weiss RA, Collins MKL. Type C retrovirus inactivation by human complement is determined by both the viral genome and the producer cell. *J Virol* 1994; 68:8001–8007.

28. Donahue RE, Kessler SW, Bodine D, McDonagh K, Dunbar C, Goodman S, et al. Helper virus induced T cell lymphoma in nonhuman primates after retroviral mediated gene transfer. *J Exp Med* 1992; 176:1125–1135.

29. Berkner KL. Expression of heterologous sequences in adenoviral vectors. *Curr Top Microbiol Immunol* 1992; 158:39–66.

30. Brody SL, Crystal RG. Adenovirus-mediated in vivo gene transfer. *Ann NY Acad Sci* 1994; 716:90–101.

31. Wickman TJ, Mathias P, Cheresh DA, Nemerow GR. Integrins $\alpha v \beta 3$ and $\alpha v \beta 5$ promote adenovirus internalization but not virus attachment. *Cell* 1983; 73:309–319.

32. Guzman RJ, Lemarchand P, Crystal RG, Epstein SE, Finkel T. Efficient and selective adenovirus-mediated gene transfer into vascular neointima. *Circulation* 1993; 2838–2848.

33. Kass-Eisler A, Falck-Pedersen E, Alvira M, Rivera J, Buttrick PM, Wittenberg BA, et al. Quantitative determination of adenovirus-mediated gene delivery to rat cardiac myocytes in vitro and in vivo. *Proc Natl Acad Sci USA* 1993; 90:11498–11502.

34. Barr J, Kalynych AM, Tripathy SK, Kozarsky K, Wilson JM, Leiden JM. Efficient catheter-mediated gene transfer into the heart using replication-defective adenovirus. *Gene Ther* 1994; 1:51–58.

35. Lemarchand P, Jones M, Yamada I, Crystal RG. In vivo gene transfer and expression in normal uninjured blood vessels using replication-deficient recombinant adenovirus vectors. *Circ Res* 1993; 72:1132–1138.

36. Losordo DW, Pickering JG, Takeshita S, Leclerc G, Gal D, Weir L, et al. Use of the rabbit ear artery to serially assess foreign secretion after site-specific arterial gene transfer in vivo. *Circulation* 1994; 89:785–792.

37. Guzman RJ, Lemarchand P, Crystal RG, Epstein SE, Finkel T. Efficient gene transfer into myocardium by direct injection of adenovirus vectors. *Circ Res* 1993; 73:1202–1207.

38. Tripathy SK, Goldwasser E, Lu MM, Barr E, Leiden JM. Stable delivery of physiological levels of recombinant erythropoietin to the systemic circulation by intramuscular injection of replication-defective adenovirus. *Proc Natl Acad Sci USA* 1994; 91:11557–11561.

39. Engelhardt JF, Simon RH, Yang Y, Zepeda M, Weber-Pendleton S, Grossman M, et al. Adenovirus-mediated transfer of CFTR gene to lung of nonhuman primates: Biological efficacy study. *Hum Gene Ther* 1993; 4:759–769.

40. Gerard RD, Herz J. Adenovirus-mediated low density lipoprotein receptor gene transfer accelerates cholesterol clearance in normal mice. *Proc Natl Acad Sci USA* 1993; 90:2812–2816.

41. Simon RH, Engelhardt JF, Yang Y, Zepeda M, Weber-Pendleton S, Grossman M, et al. Adenovirus-mediated gene transfer of CFTR gene to lung of nonhuman primates: Toxicity study. *Hum Gene Ther* 1993; 4:771–780.

42. Quantin B, Perricaudet LD, Tajbakhsh S, Mandel JL. Adenovirus as an expression vector in muscle cells in vivo. *Proc Natl Acad Sci USA* 1992; 89:2581–2584.

43. Wagner E, Zatloukal K, Cotten M, Kirlappos H, Mechtler K, Curiel DT, et al. Coupling of adenovirus to transferrin-polylysine/DNA complexes greatly enhances receptor-mediated gene delivery and expression of transfected genes. *Proc Natl Acad Sci USA* 1992; 89:6099–6103.

44. Cotten M, Wagner E, Zatloukal K, Phillips S, Curiel DT, Birnstiel ML. High-efficiency receptor-mediated delivery of small and large (48 kilobase) gene constructs using the endosome-disruption activity of defective or chemically inactivated adenovirus particles. *Proc Natl Acad Sci USA* 1992; 89:6094–6098.

45. Kupfer JM, Ruan XM, Liu G, Matloff J, Forrester J, Chaux A. High-efficiency gene transfer to autologous rabbit jugular vein grafts using adenovirus-transferrin/polylysine-DNA complexes. *Hum Gene Ther* 1994; 5:1437–1443.

46. Raja-Walia R, Webber J, Naftilan J, Chapman GD, Naftilan AJ. Enhancement of liposome-mediated gene transfer into vascular tissue by replication deficient adenovirus. *Gene Ther* 1995; 2:521–530.

47. Muzyczka N. Use of adeno-associated virus as a general transduction vector for mammalian cells. *Curr Top Microbiol Immunol* 1992; 158:97–129.

48. Russell DW, Miller DA, Alexander IE. Adeno-associated virus vectors preferentially transduce cells in S phase. *Proc Natl Acad Sci USA* 1994; 91:8915–8919.

49. Russel DW, Alexander IE, Miller DA. DNA synthesis and topoisomerase inhibitors increase transduction by adeno-associated virus vectors. *Proc Natl Acad Sci USA* 1995; 92:5719–5723.

50. Linden RM, Ward P, Giraud C, Winocour E, Berns KI. Site-specific integration by adeno-associated virus. *Proc Natl Acad Sci USA* 1996; 93:11288–11294.

51. Walsh CE, Nienhuis AW, Samulski RJ, Brown MG, Miller JL, Young NS, et al. Phenotypic correction of Fanconi anemia in human hematopoietic cells with a recombinant adeno-associated virus vector. *J Clin Invest* 1994; 94:1440–1448.

52. Flotte TR, Afione SA, Conrad C, McGrath SA, Solow R, Oka H, et al. Stable in vivo expression of the cystic fibrosis transmembrane conductance regulator with an adeno-associated virus vector. *Proc Natl Acad Sci USA* 1993; 90:10613–10617.

53. Felgner PL, Gader TR, Holm M, Roman R, Chan HW, Wenz M, et al. Lipofectin: A highly efficient, lipid mediated DNA-transfection procedure. *Proc Natl Acad Sci USA* 1987; 84:7413–7417.

54. Felgner PL, Rhodes G. Gene therapeutics. *Nature* 1991; 349:351–352.

55. Chiang MY, Chan H, Zounes MA, Freier SM, Lima WF, Bennett CF. Antisense oligonucleotides inhibit intercellular adhesion molecule 1 expression by two distinct mechanisms. *J Biol Chem* 1991; 266:18162–18171.

56. Bennett CF, Chiang MY, Chan H, Shoemaker JE, Mirabelli CK. Cationic lipids improve antisense oligonucleotide uptake and prevent degradation in cultured cells and in human serum. *Mol Pharmacol* 1992; 41:1023–1033.

57. Düzgünes N, Goldstein JA, Friend DS, Felgner PL. Fusion of liposomes containing a novel cationic lipid, *N*-[2,3-(Dioleyloxy)propyl]-*N,N,N*-trimethylammonium: Induction by multivalent anions and asymmetric fusion with acidic phospholipid vesicles. *Biochemistry* 1989; 28:9179–9184.

58. Felgner JH, Kumar R, Sridhar CN, Wheeler CJ, Tsai YJ, Border R, et al. Enhanced gene delivery and mechanism studies with a novel series of cationic lipid formulations. *J Biol Chem* 1994; 269:2550–2561.

59. Zabner J, Fasbender AJ, Moninger T, Poellinger KA, Welsh MJ. Cellular and molecular barriers to gene transfer by a cationic lipid. *J Biol Chem* 1995; 270:18997–19007.

60. Nabel EG, Yang Z, Liptay S, San H, Gordon D, Haudenschild CC, et al. Recombinant platelet-derived growth factor B gene expression in porcine arteries induces intimal hyperplasia in vivo. *J Clin Invest* 1993; 91:1822–1829.

61. Nabel EG, Yang Z, Plautz G, Forough R, Zhan X, Haudenschild C, et al. Recombinant fibroblast growth factor-1 promotes intimal hyperplasia and angiogenesis in arteries in vivo. *Nature* 1993; 362:844–846.

62. Leclerc G, Gal D, Takeshita S, Nikol S, Weir L, Isner JM. Percutaneous arterial gene transfer in a rabbit model: Efficiency in normal and balloon dilated atherosclerotic arteries. *J Clin Invest* 1992; 90:936–944. .

63. Takeshita S, Gal D, Leclerc G, Pickering JG, Riessen R, Weir L, et al. Increased gene expression after liposome-mediated arterial gene transfer associated with intimal smooth muscle cell proliferation. *J Clin Invest* 1994; 93:652–661.

64. Okada Y. Sendai virus-induced cell fusion. *Methods Enzymol* 1993; 221:18–41.

65. Kaneda Y, Morishita R, Tomita N. Increased expression of DNA cointroduced with nuclear protein in adult rat liver. *J Mol Med* 1995; 73:289–297.

66. Kaneda Y, Iwai K, Uchida T. Increased expression of DNA cointroduced with nuclear protein in adult rat liver. *Science* 1989; 243:375–378.

67. Okada Y, Koseki I, Kim J, Hashimotot T, Kanno Y, Matsui Y. Modification of cell membranes with viral envelopes during fusion of cells with HVJ (Sendai virus). *Exp Cell Res* 1975; 93:368–378.

68. Morishita R, Gibbons GH, Kaneda Y, Ogihara T, Dzau VJ. Novel and effective gene transfer technique for study of vascular renin angiotensin system. *J Clin Invest* 1993; 91:2580–2585.

69. Tomita N, Higaki J, Morishita R, Kato K, Mikami H, Kaneda Y, et al. Direct in vivo gene introduction into rat kidney. *Biochem Biophys Res Commun* 1992; 186:129–134.

70. Isaka Y, Fujiwara Y, Ueda N, Kaneda Y, Kamada T, Imai E. Glomerulosclerosis induced by in vivo transfection of transforming growth factor-β or platelet-derived growth factor gene into the rat kidney. *J Clin Invest* 1993; 92:2597–2601.

71. Morishita R, Gibbons GH, Ellison KE, Nakajima M, Zhang L, Kaneda Y, et al. Single intraluminal delivery of antisense cdc2 kinase and proliferating-cell nuclear antigen oligonucleotides results in chronic inhibition of neointimal hyperplasia. *Proc Natl Acad Sci USA* 1993; 90:8474–8478.

72. Morishita R, Gibbons GH, Ellison KE, Nakajima M, von der Leyen H, Zhang L, et al. Intimal hyperplasia after vascular injury is inhibited by antisense cdk 2 kinase oligonucleotides. *J Clin Invest* 1994; 93:1458–1464.

73. Capecchi M. High efficiency transformation by direct microinjection of DNA into mammalian cells. *Cell* 1980; 22:479–488.

74. Adams BA, Tanabe T, Mikami A, Numa S, Beam KC. Intramembrane charged movement restored in dysgenic skeletal muscle by injection of dihydropyridine receptor cDNAs. *Nature* 1990; 345:569–572.

75. Lin H, Parmacek MS, Morle G, Bolling S, Leiden JM. Expression of recombinant gene in myocardium in vivo after direct injection of DNA. *Circulation* 1990; 82:2217–2221.

76. Kitsis RN, Buttrick PM, McNally EM, Kaplan ML, Leinwand LA. Hormonal modulation of a gene injected into rat heart in vivo. *Proc Natl Acad Sci USA* 1991; 88:4138–4142.

77. Conte MS, Birinyi LK, Miyata T, Fallon JT, Gold HK, Whittemore AD, et al. Efficient repopulation of denuded rabbit arteries with autologous genetically modified endothelial cells. *Circulation* 1994; 89:2161–2169.

78. Plautz G, Nabel EG, Nabel GJ. Introduction of vascular smooth muscle cells expressing recombinant genes in vivo. *Circulation* 1991; 83:578–583.

79. Lynch CM, Clowes MM, Osborne RA, Clowes AW, Miller AD. Long-term expression of human adenosine deaminase in vascular smooth muscle cells of rats: A model for gene therapy. *Proc Natl Acad Sci USA* 1992; 89:1138–1142.

80. Dichek DA, Neville RF, Zwiebel JA, Freeman SM, Leon MB, Anderson WF. Seeding of intravascular stents with genetically engineered endothelial cells. *Circulation* 1989; 80:1347–1353.

81. Dichek DA, Nussbaum O, Degen SJF, Anderson WF. Enhancement of the fibrinolytic activity of sheep endothelial cells by retroviral vector-mediated gene transfer. *Blood* 1991; 77:533–541.

82. Dichek DA, Anderson J, Kelly AB, Hanson SR, Harker LA. Enhanced in vivo antithrombotic effects of endothelial cells expressing recombinant plasminogen activators transduced with retroviral vectors. *Circulation* 1996; 93:301–309.

83. Carmeliet P, Collebn D. Gene targeting and gene transfer studies of the plasminogen/plasmin system: Implications in thrombosis, hemostasis, neointima formation, and atherosclerosis. *FASEB J* 1995; 9:934–938.

84. Flugelman MY. Inhibition of intravascular thrombosis and vascular smooth muscle cell proliferation by gene therapy. *Thromb Hemost* 1995; 74:406–410.

85. Chen S, Wilson JM, Muller DWM. Adenovirus-mediated gene transfer of soluble vascular cell adhesion molecule to porcine interposition vein grafts. *Circulation* 1994; 89:1922–1928.

86. Yao SN, Smith KJ, Kurachi K. Primary myoblast-mediated gene transfer: Persistent expression of human factor IX in mice. *Gene Ther* 1994; 1:99–107.

87. Barr E, Leiden JM. Systemic delivery of recombinant proteins by genetically modified myoblasts. *Science* 1991; 254:1507–1509.

88. Dhawan J, Pan LC, Pavlath GK, Travis MA, Lanctot AM, Blau HM. Systemic delivery of human growth hormone by injection of genetically engineered myoblasts. *Science* 1991; 254:1509–1512.

89. Hamamori Y, Samal B, Tian J, Kedes L. Myoblast transfer of human erythropoietin gene in a mouse model of renal failure. *J Clin Invest* 1995; 95:1808–1813.

90. Riessen R, Isner JM. Prospects for site-specific delivery of pharmacologic and molecular therapies. *J Am Coll Cardiol* 1994; 23:1234–1244.

91. Ooboshi H, Welsh MJ, Rios CD, Davidson BL, Heistad DD. Adenovirus-mediated gene transfer in vivo to cerebral blood vessels and perivascular tissue. *Circ Res* 1995; 77:7–13.

92. Schachtner SK, Rome JJ, Hoyt RF, Newman KD, Virmani R, Dichek DA. In vivo adenovirus-mediated gene transfer via the pulmonary artery of rats. *Circ Res* 1995; 76:701–709.

93. Zamecnik PC, Stephenson ML. Inhibition of Rous sarcoma virus replication and cell transformation by a specific oligodeoxynucleotide. *Proc Natl Acad Sci USA* 1978; 75:280–284.

94. Cohen JS. Oligonucleotide therapeutics. *Trends Biotechnol* 1992; 10:87–91.

95. Inouye M. Antisense RNA: Its functions and applications in gene regulation—Review. *Gene* 1988; 72:25–34.

96. Krystal GW, Armstrong BC, Battey JF. N-myc mRNA forms an RNA-RNA duplex with endogenous antisense transcripts. *Mol Cell Biol* 1990; 10:4180–4191.

97. Colman A. Antisense strategies in cell and developmental biology. *J Cell Sci* 1990; 97:399–409.

98. Stein CA, Cheng YC. Antisense oligonucleotides as therapeutic agents—Is the bullet really magical? *Science* 1993; 261:1004–1012.

99. Bricca G. Sense, antisense, nonsense: Where's the right way? *J Mol Med* 1995; 73:417–419.

100. Uhlmann E, Peyman A. Antisense oligonucleotides: A new therapeutic principle. *Chem Rev* 1990; 90:544–552.

101. Crooke ST. Progress toward oligonucleotide therapeutics: Pharmacodynamic properties. *FASEB J* 1993; 7:533–539.

102. Matsukura M, Shinozuka K, Zon G, Mitsuya H, Reitz M, Cohen JS, et al. Phosphorothioate analogs of oligodeoxynucleotides: Inhibitors of replication and cytopathic effects of human immunodeficiency virus. *Proc Natl Acad Sci USA* 1987; 84:7706–7710.

103. Krieg AM, Yi A, Matson S, Waldschmidt T, Bishop GA, Teasdale R, et al. CpG motifs in bacterial DNA trigger direct B-cell activation. *Nature* 1995; 374:546–549.

104. Bennett MR, Anglin S, McEwan JR, Jagoe R, Newby AC, Evan GI. Inhibition of vascular smooth muscle cell proliferation in vitro and in vivo by C-*myc* antisense oligonucleotides. *J Clin Invest* 1994; 93:820–828.

105. Simons M, Edelman ER, DeKeyser JL, Langer R, Rosenberg RD. Antisense c-*myb* oligonucleotides inhibit intimal arterial smooth muscle cell accumulation in vivo. *Nature* 1992; 359:67–70.

106. Shi Y, Fard A, Galeo A, Hutchinson HG, Vermani P, Dodge GR, et al. Transcatheter delivery of c-myc antisense oligomers reduces neointimal formation in a porcine model of coronary artery balloon injury. *Circulation* 1994; 90:944–951.

107. Yaswen P, Stampfer MR, Ghosh K, Cohen JS. Effects of sequence of thioated oligonucleotides on cultured human mammary epithelial cells. *Antisense Res Dev* 1993; 3:67–77.

108. Villa AE, Guzman LA, Poptic EJ, Labhasetwar V, D'Souza S, Farrell CL, et al. Effects of antisense c-*myb* oligonucleotides on vascular smooth muscle cell proliferation and response to vessel wall injury. *Circ Res* 1995; 76:505–513.

109. Burgess TL, Fisher EF, Ross SL, Bready JV, Qian Y, Bayewitch LA, et al. The antiproliferative activity of c-myb and c-myc antisense oligonucleotides in smooth muscle cells is caused by a nonantisense mechanism. *Proc Natl Acad Sci USA* 1995; 92:4051–4055.

110. Loke S, Stein C, Zhang X, Avigan M, Cohen JLN. Delivery of c-myc antisense phosphorothioate oligodeoxynucleotides to haemopoietic cells in culture by liposome fusion: Specific reduction in c-myc protein expression correlates with inhibition of cell growth and DNA synthesis. *Curr Top Microbiol Immunol* 1988; 14:282–289.

111. Bielinska A, Schivdasani RA, Zhang L, Nabel GJ. Regulation of gene expression with double-stranded phosphothioate oligonucleotides. *Science* 1990; 250:997–1000.

112. Sullenger BA, Gallardo HF, Ungers GE, Gilboa E. Overexpression of TAR sequences renders cells resistant to human immunodeficiency virus replication. *Cell* 1990; 63:601–608.

113. Morishita R, Gibbons GH, Horiuchi M, Ellison KE, Nakajima M, Zhang L, et al. A novel molecular strategy using cis element "decoy" of E2F binding site inhibits smooth muscle proliferation in vivo. *Proc Natl Acad Sci USA* 1995; 92:5855–5859.

114. Simons M, Edelman ER, Rosenberg RD. Antisense proliferating cell nuclear antigen oligonucleotides inhibit intimal hyperplasia in a rat carotid artery injury model. *J Clin Invest* 1994; 93:2351–2356.

115. Cox JL, Chiasson DA, Gotlieb AI. Stranger in a strange land: The pathogenesis of saphenous vein graft stenosis with emphasis on structural and functional differences between veins and arteries. *Prog Cardiovasc Dis* 1991; 34:45–68.

116. Mann MJ, Gibbons GH, Kernoff RS, Diet FD, Tsao PS, Cooke JP, et al. Genetic engineering of vein grafts resistant to atherosclerosis. *Proc Natl Acad Sci USA* 1995; 92:4502–4506.

117. Mann MJ, Gibbons GH, Tsao PS, von der Leyen HE, Cooke JP, Buitrago R, et al. Cell cycle inhibition leads to preservation of endothelial function in genetically engineered vein grafts. *J Clin Invest* 1997; 99:1295–1301.

118. Wielbo D, Sernia C, Gyurko R, Phillips MI. Antisense inhibition of hypertension in the spontaneously hypertensive rat. *Hypertension* 1995; 25:314–319.

119. Tomita N, Higaki J, Kaneda Y, Yu H, Morishita R, Mikami H, et al. Hypertensive rats produced by in vivo introduction of the human renin gene. *Circ Res* 1993; 73:898–905.

120. Nabel EG, Shum L, Pompili VJ, Yang Z, San H, Shu HB, et al. Direct transfer of transforming growth factor β1 gene into arteries stimulates fibrocellular hyperplasia. *Proc Natl Acad Sci USA* 1993; 90:10579–10763.

121. Pompili VJ, Gordon D, San H, Yang Z, Muller DW, Nabel GJ, et al. Expression and function of a recombinant PDGF B gene in porcine arteries. *Arterioscl Thromb Vasc Biol* 1995; 15:2254–2264.

122. Dzau VJ. The role of mechanical and humoral factors in growth regulation of vascular smooth muscle and cardiac myocytes. *Curr Opin Nephrol Hypertens* 1993; 2:27–32.

123. Morishita R, Gibbons GH, Ellison KE, Lee W, Zhang L, Yu H, et al. Evidence for direct local effect of angiotensin in vascular hypertrophy: In vivo gene transfer of angiotensin converting enzyme. *J Clin Invest* 1994; 94:978–984.

124. Nakajima M, Hutchinson HG, Fujinaga M, Hayashida W, Morishita R, Zhang L, et al. The angiotensin II type 2 (AT2) receptor antagonizes the growth effects of the AT1 receptor: Gain-of-function study using gene transfer. *Proc Natl Acad Sci USA* 1995; 92:10663–10667.

125. Ross R. The pathogenesis of atherosclerosis: A perspective for the 1990s. *Nature* 1993; 362:801–809.

126. Vane JR, Änggård EE, Botting RM. Regulatory functions of the endothelium. *N Engl J Med* 1990; 323:27–36.

127. von der Leyen HE, Gibbons GH, Morishita R, Lewis NP, Zhang L, Nakajima M, et al. Gene therapy inhibiting neointimal vascular lesion: In vivo gene transfer of endothelial-cell nitric oxide synthase gene. *Proc Natl Acad Sci USA* 1995; 92:1137–1141.

128. Ohno T, Gordon D, San H, Pompili VJ, Imperiale MJ, Nabel GJ, et al. Gene therapy for vascular smooth muscle cell proliferation after arterial injury. *Science* 1994; 265:781–784.

129. Chang MW, Barr E, Seltzer J, Jiang Y, Nabel GJ, Nabel EG, et al. Cytostatic gene therapy for vascular proliferative disorders with a constitutively active form of the retinoblastoma gene product. *Science* 1995; 267:518–522.

130. Chang MW, Barr E, Lu MM, Barton K, Leiden JM. Adenovirus-mediated over-expression of the cyclin/cyclin-dependent kinase inhibitor, p21 inhibits vascular smooth muscle cell proliferation and neointima formation in the rat carotid artery model of balloon angioplasty. *J Clin Invest* 1995; 96:2260–2268.

131. Indolfi C, Avvedimento EV, Rapacciuolo A, Lorenzo ED, Esposito G, Stabile E, et al. Inhibition of cellular *ras* prevents smooth muscle cell proliferation after vascular injury in vivo. *Nature Med* 1995; 1:541–545.

132. Takeshita S, Zheng LP, Asahara T, Riessen R, Brogi E, Ferrara N, et al. In vivo evidence of enhanced angiogenesis following direct arterial gene transfer of the plasmid encoding vascular endothelial growth factor (abstr). *Circulation* 1993; 88:I-476.

133. Takeshita S, Bauters C, Asahara T, Zheng L, Rossow ST, Keamey M, et al. Physiologic assessment of angiogenesis by arterial gene therapy with vascular endothelial growth factor (abstr). *Circulation* 1994; 90:I-90.

134. Isner JM, Walsh K, Symes J, Pieczek A, Takeshita S, Lowry J, et al. Arterial gene therapy for therapeutic angiogenesis in patients with peripheral artery disease. *Circulation* 1995; 91:2687–2692.

135. Sawa Y, Suzuki K, Bai HZ, Shirakura R, Morishita R, Kaneda Y, et al. Efficiency of in vivo gene transfection into transplanted rat heart by coronary infusion of HVJ liposome. *Circulation* 1995; 92(suppl): II-479–II-482.

136. Koh GY, Kim S, Klug MG, Park K, Soonpaa MH, Field LJ. Targeted expression of transforming growth factor-β1 in intracardiac grafts promotes vascular endothelial cell DNA synthesis. *J Clin Invest* 1995; 95:114–121.

137. Soonpaa MH, Koh GY, Klug MG, Field LJ. Formation of nascent intercalated disks between grafted fetal cardiomyocytes and host myocardium. *Science* 1994; 264:98–101.

138. Milano CA, Allen LF, Rockman HA, Dolber PC, McMinn TR, Chien KR, et al. Enhanced myocardial function in transgenic mice overexpressing the β2-adrenergic receptor. *Science* 1994; 264:582–586.

139. Wilson JM, Grossman M, Cabrera JA, Wu CH, Wu GY. A novel mechanism for achieving transgene persistence in vivo after somatic gene transfer into hepatocytes. *J Biol Chem* 1992; 267:11483–11489.

140. Chowdhury JR, Grossman M, Gupta S, Chowdhury NR, Baker JR, Wilson JM. Long-term improvement of hypercholesterolemia after ex vivo gene therapy in LDLR-deficient rabbits. *Science* 1991; 254:1802–1805.

141. Stevenson SC, Marshall-Neff J, Teng B, Lee CB, Roy S, McClelland A. Phenotypic correction of hypercholesterolemia in apoE-deficient mice by adenovirus-mediated in vivo gene transfer. *Arterioscler Thromb Vasc Biol* 1995; 15:479–484.

142. Kopfler WP, Willard M, Betz T, Willard JE, Gerard RD, Meidell RS. Adenovirus-mediated transfer of a gene encoding human apolipoprotein A-I into normal mice increases circulating high-density lipoprotein cholesterol. *Circulation* 1994; 90:1319–1327.

143. Crystal RG. Transfer of genes to humans: Early lessons and obstacles to success. *Science* 1995; 270:404–410.

144. Crystal RG, McElvaney NG, Rosenfeld MA, Chu CS, Mastrangeli A, Hay JG, et al. Administration of an adenovirus containing the human CFTR cDNA to the respiratory tract of individuals with cystic fibrosis. *Nature Genet* 1994; 8:42–51.

145. Grossman M, Rader DJ, Muller DWM, Kolansky DM, Kozarsky K, Clark III BJ, et al. A pilot study of ex vivo gene therapy for homozygous familial hypercholesterolemia. *Nature Med* 1995; 1:1148–1154.

146. Tomita N, Morishita R, Higaki J, Aoki M, Nakamura Y, Mikami H, et al. Transient decrease in high blood pressure by in vivo transfer of antisense oligonucleotides against rat angiotensinogen. *Hypertension* 1995; 26:131–136.

147. Guzman RJ, Hirschowitz EA, Brody SL, Crystal RG, Epstein SE, Finkel T. In vivo suppression of injury-induced vascular smooth muscle cell accumulation using adenovirus-mediated transfer of the herpes simplex virus thymidine kinase gene. *Proc Natl Acad Sci USA* 1994; 91:10732–10736.

GENERAL EVALUATION OF THE PATIENT

10

THE HISTORY, PHYSICAL EXAMINATION, AND CARDIAC AUSCULTATION

Robert A. O'Rourke / James A. Shaver / Rosemarie Salerni / Mark E. Silverman / Robert C. Schlant

In evaluating patients with definite or suspected heart disease, important information can be obtained from the history, physical examination, chest roentgenogram, electrocardiogram, and other routine laboratory tests. This data base provides the necessary background for making an accurate diagnosis and appropriate decisions concerning therapy in many patients. In other patients, more information is necessary and additional, more technical, noninvasive cardiac tests such as echocardiography or radionuclide studies are needed. In certain patients, the general assessment indicates the need for cardiac catheterization and contrast angiography, with or without additional noninvasive cardiac testing. For example, the proper approach to specific patients with symptomatic coronary artery disease may include both coronary arteriography and cardiac catheterization (anatomy and hemodynamics) as well as myocardial perfusion imaging with thallium or technetium sestamibi (extent of inducible ischemia).

Not all patients need every test, and the skillful use of low technology including the history and general examination may preclude the need for additional studies or may be important in determining which of a wide variety of available sophisticated tests should be chosen for a particular patient. This chapter is divided into three sections. The first section concerns the proper application of the *history* and its use to delineate the differential diagnosis in patients who present with certain common cardiovascular symptoms. The second section details the essential components of the *physical examination* and their usefulness in establishing a likely diagnosis when specific abnormal findings are detected. Finally, the third section focuses on cardiac auscultation.

THE HISTORY

ELEMENTS OF ACCURATE HISTORY TAKING

A carefully obtained history is the cornerstone in the assessment of a patient with known or suspected cardiac disease.[1,2] A deliberate, compassionate interview forms the basis for a patient-physician relationship that will continue for days, months, or years to come. Unfortunately, the interview may result in adversary roles for the physician and the patient if the interviewer appears hurried, demands exact answers, and shows impatience; demonstrates contempt when the answers are not known; insists on exploring areas that are uncomfortable to the patient; fails to establish eye contact; accepts multiple interruptions during the interview; seems to treat dreaded diseases casually; gives nonverbal signs of personal unhappiness; and appears to be unsympathetic.[2] When the medical interview is unsatisfactory because of poor communication and lack of rapport, the medical information obtained will often be inaccurate.[2] Also, important facts that are not revealed during a meticulous initial history usually are not detected later, as workup progresses and the patient and physician become focused on high-technology studies and more aggressive therapeutic interventions.[1]

The patient's chief complaint, which requires further elaboration and investigation, may not identify the patient's most serious problem. The interviewer must not fail to define symptoms other than the patient's chief complaint.[2] Rather than focusing entirely on the patient's present illness as related to the chief complaint, the interviewer should note all existing symptoms and establish a present illness for each of these.[2]

A medical questionnaire given to the patient well in advance of the interview is useful. The patient can then record important data more accurately because of the time available for reflection and the checking of details.[2] Any abnormalities indicated on the questionnaire must be defined more completely during the interview, and related areas should be discussed.[2]

A proper interpretation of the past history (see below) is important, and the physician may erroneously accept a past event as a fact when the evidence is not well established or only hearsay in nature. Information obtained from family members about the patient's symptoms and his or her response to the illness is extremely important and a doctor-family relationship as well as a doctor-patient relationship should be established.[2]

Importantly, serious heart disease can occur in patients with mild or no symptoms. Also, knowing the sensitivity, specificity, and predictive value of an answer to a question and of the presence or absence of a physical sign provides the physician with a better perspective. The physician must determine whether or not the history obtained suffices to support a decision-making process about the patient.[2] While many patients with severe heart disease have no symptoms, others have many symptoms associated with minor or no disease. Some patients deny the presence of symptoms because they cannot accept the reality of the situation, while others may purposefully withhold information because they might lose their jobs if the truth were revealed.[2] Still other patients may overstate their symptoms for personal gain. Elderly patients, sedentary patients, and patients whose physical activity is limited by another illness may have no symptoms because they do not exert sufficient physical effort to produce them.[2]

Past and Family History

The past history may provide important clues to the presence of cardiovascular disease. A definite history of rheumatic fever may be useful in defining the cause of a heart murmur, whereas a negative history of rheumatic fever does not exclude it.[2] A history of hypertension in a family member increases the likelihood that the patient has essential hypertension.[2] Previous trauma may be the cause of constrictive pericarditis, a thoracic aortic aneurysm, an arteriovenous fistula, and other types of cardiac lesions. A detailed history of the use of medications, addicting drugs, and alcohol, each of which may cause heart disease, is essential. A past history of pulmonary embolism, thrombophlebitis, or systemic embolism should be ascertained.

A history of dental work, some other diagnostic or therapeutic procedure, or recent infection suggests the possibility of infective endocarditis in a patient with valvular heart disease.

Patients commonly give the history of having had a "heart attack," which, in fact, may have been an episode of unstable angina, heart failure, or arrhythmia. The "heart attack" history often becomes "myocardial infarction" in the patient's medical record unless more information about the episode is obtained or documentation of the event is reviewed.[1] Many patients are referred who have had several catheterizations, angioplasties, and one or more bypass operations in addition to multiple noninvasive tests. A thorough and often time-consuming review of records from the other institutions, operative notes, catheterization films, and noninvasive studies will often provide an accurate assessment of the patient's current status without the unnecessary repetition of expensive and potentially risky procedures.[1]

Past and present therapeutic regimens must be reviewed carefully. Various treatment programs may have been inappropriate or suboptimal. The drugs currently used for the treatment of cardiovascular diseases have a larger number of potential side effects that can result in both cardiovascular and noncardiovascular symptoms (see Chap. 91).

Multiple risk factors for developing coronary heart disease have been identified, including age, male sex, hypertension, hypercholesterolemia, low HDL cholesterol, cigarette smoking, diabetes, and a family history of premature atherosclerosis (see Chap. 41). The presence or absence of risk factors can increase or decrease the statistical likelihood that an individual patient has coronary heart disease.

Patients should be questioned about previous health evaluations. In addition to being examined at the time of routine physicals or in association with other medical treatment, patients have often been examined for the military service, for athletics, or for insurance and they may have been told of a heart murmur or hypertension on those occasions.[1] Rejection by the military or an insurance company is often due to a cardiovascular abnormality. Many patients have not seen a physician in the recent past or ever had a careful examination of the cardiovascular system.

The increasing hemodynamic burden of pregnancy may cause an otherwise marginally compensated cardiac patient to become symptomatic. Specific inquiry should be made about heart failure, edema, dyspnea, or requirement for prolonged periods of bed rest during pregnancy.[1] Many normal women have had a murmur detected during pregnancy (Chap. 92). The history of illicit parenteral drug use should raise the suspicion of infective endocarditis, especially in a febrile patient (Chap. 82). Cocaine can cause coronary artery vasospasm and also raise myocardial oxygen demand by increasing heart rate and blood pressure. Angina, myocardial infarction, and sudden cardiac death have been well documented after cocaine use (see Chap. 80).

A history of moderate to excessive alcohol consumption (Chap. 77), an enlarged heart on prior chest roentgenogram, periods of rapid weight gain or loss, and history of other illnesses may provide important information, as may questions concerning prior diagnoses made by the patient or by medical personnel.[1]

A family history of congenital heart disease indicates a higher risk of a congenital heart lesion (Chap. 70). The patient's mother may give a history of rubella during the first few months of pregnancy; this increases the likelihood that the patient has patent ductus arteriosus, pulmonary valve stenosis, coarctation of the pulmonary arteries, or atrial septal defect.

Although most of the common cardiovascular diseases are sporadic, there are several examples in which genetic transmission can occur (Chap. 69). These include mitral valve prolapse and the hypertrophic or dilated cardiomyopathies. Other genetically determined disorders include some of the inborn errors of metabolism, muscular dystrophies, Ehlers-Danlos syndrome, Marfan's syndrome, and the long Q-T syndromes with or without deafness (Chap. 69).

SYMPTOMS ASSOCIATED WITH CARDIOVASCULAR DISEASE

Chest Pain

Chest pain or chest discomfort is the foremost manifestation of myocardial ischemia and results from a disparity between myocardial oxygen demand and coronary blood flow in patients with coronary artery disease.[3] The most common causes of myocardial ischemia are coronary atherosclerosis, coronary vasoconstriction, and coronary artery thrombosis, the latter occurring particularly in patients with acute coronary syndromes such as acute myocardial infarction and unstable angina (Chaps. 46 and 47). It is now recognized that an increase in myocardial oxygen demand (MV_{O_2}) or demand ischemia, a decrease in or inadequate blood flow (supply ischemia), or their combination may be responsible for anginal chest pain.

The mechanism responsible for cardiac pain is not clearly understood.[4] Nonmedullated small sympathetic nerve fibers that parallel the coronary arteries are thought to provide the afferent sensory pathway for angina; these enter the spinal cord in the C8-T4 segments.[5] Impulses are transmitted to corresponding spinal ganglia and then through the spinal cord to the thalamus and cerebral cortex. Angina pectoris, like other pain of visceral origin, is often poorly localized and is commonly referred to the corresponding segmental dermatomes.

The differential diagnosis of chest pain is extensive.[6] In addition to angina pectoris and myocardial infarction, other cardiovascular diseases, gastrointestinal diseases, psychogenic disease, neuromuscular disease, and diseases of the pulmonary system must be considered (Tables 10-1 and 45-4). An accurate interpretation of the etiology of chest discomfort and its significance in individual patients is critically dependent on a carefully taken history. Important clinically relevant information may be missed if the overenthusiastic use of noninvasive or invasive diagnostic methods replaces rather than augments direct physician-patient communication (see Chap. 45).

TABLE 10-1
DIFFERENTIAL DIAGNOSIS OF CHEST PAIN

1. Angina pectoris/myocardial infarction
2. Other cardiovascular causes
   a. Likely ischemic in origin
      (1) Aortic stenosis
      (2) Hypertrophic cardiomyopathy
      (3) Severe systemic hypertension
      (4) Severe right ventricular hypertension
      (5) Aortic regurgitation
      (6) Severe anemia/hypoxia
   b. Nonischemic in origin
      (1) Aortic dissection
      (2) Pericarditis
      (3) Mitral valve prolapse
3. Gastrointestinal
   a. Esophageal spasm
   b. Esophageal reflux
   c. Esophageal rupture
   d. Peptic ulcer disease
4. Psychogenic
   a. Anxiety
   b. Depression
   c. Cardiac psychosis
   d. Self-gain
5. Neuromusculoskeletal
   a. Thoracic outlet syndrome
   b. Degenerative joint disease of cervical/thoracic spine
   c. Costochondritis (Tietze's syndrome)
   d. Herpes zoster
   e. Chest wall pain and tenderness
6. Pulmonary
   a. Pulmonary embolus with or without pulmonary infarction
   b. Pneumothorax
   c. Pneumonia with pleural involvement
7. Pleurisy

The original subjective description of angina pectoris by William Heberden[7] of his own chest pain in the late eighteenth century has not been surpassed. He wrote the following:

> **But there is a disorder of the breast marked with strong and peculiar symptoms, considerable for the kind of danger belonging to it and not extremely rare, which deserves to be mentioned more at length. The seat of it and sense of strangling and anxiety with which it is attended make it not improperly called angina pectoris. They who are afflicted with it are seized while they are walking (more especially if it be up a hill and soon after eating) with a painful and most disagreeable sensation in the breast, which seems as if would extinguish life if it were to increase or to continue; but the moment they stand still, all this uneasiness vanishes.**

Angina pectoris is defined as chest pain or discomfort of cardiac origin that usually results from a temporary imbalance between myocardial oxygen supply and myocardial oxygen demand. It may occur only with exertion or spontaneously at rest; various subtypes are defined in Chap. 45. The *quality* of the chest discomfort is usually described as "tightness," "pressure," "burning," "heavy," "aching," "strangling," or "compression." Usually the patient is able to describe a deep rather than a superficial origin of the pain. Since the qualitative description of the pain is greatly influenced by the patient's intelligence, education, and social/cultural background, a definition of other characteristics of the chest discomfort is often extremely important in evaluating the symptoms appropriately. The most important of these characteristics are the *precipitating factors* for the onset of pain, its *mode of onset* and *duration*, its *pattern of disappearance*, and its *location*. Classically, the discomfort is induced by exercise, emotion, eating, or cold weather. A recognizable pattern of reproducibility of chest pain by certain activities is an important characteristic of angina, and the patient should be questioned specifically along these lines. Often, patients develop pain with exertion after meals, and there is a greater tendency for arm work, which involves a greater element of isometric exercise than isotonic leg exercise, to produce distress.[8–11] Chest pain occurring only after exercise has been concluded or at the end of the day is rarely due to myocardial ischemia. Occasionally, angina will dissipate despite continued exercise (the walk-through phenomenon) or will not occur when a second exercise effort is undertaken that previously produced chest discomfort (warm-up phenomenon). Both circumstances may be attributed to the opening of functioning coronary arterial collaterals during the initial myocardial ischemia. Pain is more likely to occur when the patient is outdoors, especially when the temperature is extremely high or low and when the patient is walking uphill against the wind. Angina commonly occurs after the patient has eaten a heavy meal or when the patient is excited, angry, or tense. Cold showers increase blood pressure and heart rate, while hot showers cause an augmented cardiac output in response to vasodilation.[8–11] Either may precipitate angina after exercise. The chest pain during any type of activity is often made worse by the use of tobacco. All of the hemodynamic changes resulting from the use of nicotine increase the myocardial oxygen demand.[12]

Angina pectoris characteristically has a crescendo *pattern at onset* and "builds up." Pains, often described as "shooting" or "stabbing" that reach their maximum intensity virtually instantaneously are often not angina but are of musculoskeletal or neural origin. Angina is usually relieved within 5 to 15 min by rest, with or without the use of vasodilator drugs such as nitroglycerin, although nitroglycerin characteristically hastens relief. Failure to obtain relief with rest or nitroglycerin suggests another cause of pain or actual impending myocardial infarction. The reproducible relief of chest pain in an appropriate time frame (within 10 min) can be strong evidence favoring ischemia. A trial of nitroglycerin can be a useful diagnostic strategy. Patients with angina pectoris are usually classified functionally from class I to class IV (Table 10-2), depending on the amount of activity necessary to induce chest pain.[13]

TABLE 10-2

CANADIAN CARDIOVASCULAR SOCIETY FUNCTIONAL CLASSIFICATION OF ANGINA PECTORIS

I.	Ordinary physical activity, such as walking and climbing stairs, does not cause angina. Angina results from strenuous or rapid or prolonged exertion at work or recreation.
II.	Slight limitation of ordinary activity. Walking or climbing stairs rapidly, walking uphill, walking or stair climbing after meals, in cold, in wind, or when under emotional stress, or only during the few hours after awakening. Walking more than two blocks on the level and climbing more than one flight or ordinary stairs at a normal pace and under normal conditions.
III.	Marked limitations of ordinary physical activity. Walking one to two blocks on the level and climbing more than one flight under normal conditions.
IV.	Inability to carry on any physical activity without discomfort—anginal syndrome may be present at rest.

Source: Modified from Campeau L. Letter to the editor. *Circulation* 1976; 54:522. Reproduced with permission from the American Heart Association, Inc., and the author.

Localizing the *site* of chest discomfort provides additional information in determining its cause. Anginal pain is ordinarily retrosternal or felt slightly to left of the midline, beside or partly under the sternum. It is rarely isolated to the cardiac apex in the inframammary region. The chest pain of myocardial ischemia tends to *radiate* bilaterally across the chest into the arms (left more than right), and into the neck and lower jaw. Occasionally radiation to the back or occiput is noted. In the arms, the pain passes down the ulnar and volar surface to the wrist and then only into the ulnar fingers, rarely into the thumb or down the outer (extensor) surface of the arm, which have a different dermatome pattern.[5–11] Pain may occasionally be felt only in the arm or may start in the arm and radiate to the chest. Attention to the gestures that the patient utilizes in characterizing and localizing the site of pain may be useful in determining its etiology. One or two clenched fists held by the patient over the sternal area (Levine's sign) is much more indicative of ischemic pain than is a finger pointed to a small, circumscribed area in the left inframammary region.[5–11] The latter more likely represents chest pain of psychogenic origin.

As indicated above, the *duration* of chest pain may also be a useful differentiating feature. Angina pectoris rarely lasts less than 1 min or more than 15 min in the absence of myocardial infarction or persistent arrhythmias. Most patients with angina report prompt *relief* in less than 5 min after cessation of activity or with the use of sublingual nitroglycerin. Delayed relief of chest pain by sublingual nitroglycerin may be ascribed to a placebo effect. Since nitrates are generalized relaxants of smooth muscle, pain due to diffuse esophageal spasm or biliary colic may also be relieved by these same agents. Carotid sinus massage by the physician frequently will relieve anginal chest pain because of the reflex production of a relative bradycardia and a decrease in systolic blood pressure, thus reducing myocardial oxygen demand.[14] Carotid sinus massage should be performed only in the absence of extracranial occlusive cerebrovascular disease as manifest by carotid bruits or decreased carotid arterial pulsations and with careful auscultatory monitoring of the heart rate. The Valsalva maneuver may also relieve anginal pain by decreasing myocardial wall tension as a result of the reduced venous return and left ventricular volume accompanying the increase in intrathoracic pressure. *Associated symptoms*—such as nausea, vomiting, faintness, fatigue, or diaphoresis—often accompany severe episodes of myocardial ischemia both in men and in women.[15] Severe myocardial ischemia often produces severe dyspnea due to a marked increase in left ventricular diastolic filling pressure, sometimes producing an "angina equivalent" in the absence of chest discomfort.

Linked angina is a term applied to genuine episodes of angina in patients with established coronary artery disease caused by gastrointestinal factors not related to an increase in cardiac work.[16] Episodes are typically induced by stooping or occur after eating; they can be mimicked by esophageal acid stimulation, which can reduce coronary blood flow.[16]

No consideration of myocardial ischemia as a likely cause of chest discomfort is complete without carefully considering the chest pain in the context of known risk factors for coronary artery disease (see above).

Angina pectoris should be considered as a symptom and not as a specific disease. Coronary arteriographic studies have demonstrated that more than 90 percent of patients with chest pain precipitated by exercise and relieved by rest have angiographic evidence of significant coronary disease.[5–11] However, other diseases may be associated with classic angina pectoris (see below).

Several reports have described certain patients with typical exertional chest discomfort and arteriographically normal coronary arteries.[17–21] These patients are more likely to be females, have fewer coronary risk factors, have variable responses to various antianginal agents, and, less commonly, have more relief of pain by sublingual nitroglycerin than patients with occlusive coronary artery disease. Although the underlying cause of this condition remains unsettled, the life expectancy of these patients appears no different from that of an age- and sex-matched population without chest discomfort.

There is some evidence that abnormal function of small coronary arteries may cause limited coronary flow responses to stress or pharmacologic vasodilators in a subset of patients with anginal chest pain despite angiographically normal coronary arteries (*microvascular angina*).[22–29] In the past, investigators arguing for or against the existence of this syndrome have often used the term *syndrome X* to describe their patient cohort.[30–31] Syndrome X appears to include a heterogenous group of patients with a wide spectrum of chest pain and a variety of vascular and smooth muscle hypersensitive constrictor responses. Multiple research studies continue in an effort to explain syndrome X.[32–40] It should be distinguished from the metabolic syndrome X of insulin resistance (glucose intolerance), hypertension, and upper body obesity (see Chap. 45).

Some patients with coronary artery disease experience angina at rest as a complication or an isolated clinical manifestation of ischemic heart disease.[8–11] Myocardial ischemic pain at rest more likely results from an acute reduction in myocardial oxygen supply than from an increase in myocardial oxygen demand. Possible causative factors include isolated coronary artery spasm or embolism, coronary artery spasm superimposed on coronary atherosclerosis, and coronary thrombosis with spontaneous thrombolysis.[41–44] In patients with progressive coronary atherosclerosis, however, ischemic rest pain may also result from intermittent arrhythmias that increase myocardial oxygen demand or decrease diastolic coronary blood flow, or from labile hypertension with its increased wall stress. Chest pain at rest may occur only as nocturnal angina. In addition to the above mechanisms, nocturnal angina, also known as *angina decubitus*, may be produced by the increase in wall stress and, thus, $M\dot{V}_{O_2}$ secondary to redistribution of the intravascular blood volume in the recumbent position. The relative hypercapnia and acidosis that occur during sleep may also contribute to nocturnal angina. This condition has also been accompanied by concomitant rapid eye movement sleep patterns on the electroencephalogram, which may result from augmented sympathetic discharge increasing $M\dot{V}_{O_2}$ or causing coronary constriction[8–11] (Chaps. 45 and 46).

Despite the more malignant natural history observed in many patients with rest angina, particularly in those with coincident ST-T wave changes, the predictive value of the history alone is not as accurate as with exertional angina. The quality of pain is usually similar to that of exertional angina, but the discomfort may be more severe and its duration longer. In addition, angina at rest is commonly associated with nausea, vomiting, and diaphoresis. The onset of shortness of breath during or after the beginning of chest discomfort suggests that the pain is due to extensive myocardial ischemia and usually results from an acute elevation of left ventricular filling pressure secondary to the development of a large, transiently ischemic myocardial segment. Such patients are commonly found to have multivessel occlusive coronary artery disease on arteriography.

Chest pain or discomfort resulting from *myocardial infarction* is qualitatively similar to angina at rest. The differentiation between the pain resulting from ischemia and that due to myocardial necrosis is usually impossible to ascertain from the history alone.[8–11] Pain associated with transmural Q-wave infarction is usually more severe and longer lasting than anginal pain and is often associated with nausea, vomiting, and diaphoresis. In addition, myocardial infarction is frequently accompanied by symptoms of sustained left ventricular dysfunction (dyspnea, orthopnea) and evidence of autonomic nervous system hyperactivity (tachycardia, diaphoresis, bradycardia).[8–11] Painless or atypical presentations of myocardial infarction, however, occur in up to 30 percent of patients, particularly in diabetic patients and the elderly. Thus, determination of serial serum enzymes and isoenzymes, providing evidence of myocardial necrosis, and serial electrocardiograms (ECGs), indicating myocardial injury, are necessary to establish the diagnosis in most patients (see Chap. 47).

There are two groups of *cardiovascular diseases causing chest pain that is not due to coronary atherosclerosis* (Table 10-1). The first group consists of cardiac diseases causing myocardial ischemia–related angina in the absence of coronary artery disease; ischemia is due to hemodynamic changes associated with an inadequate myocardial oxygen supply in relation to a normal or increased myocardial oxygen demand. Among these are *aortic valve stenosis* (Chap. 63), *hypertrophic cardiomyopathy* (Chap. 74), and *systemic arterial hypertension* (Chap. 56), in which left ventricular systolic pressure and left ventricular wall tension are greatly increased or left ventricular hypertrophy is present.[8–11,45–47] Chest pain due to myocardial ischemia can also occur with severe aortic regurgitation (Chap. 63). The large ventricular volume load and increased ventricular dimensions result in increased myocardial oxygen demand, and the reduced diastolic perfusion pressure of the coronary arteries results in a relatively inadequate coronary blood flow. Occasionally, very severe anemia or hypoxia may also produce myocardial ischemia by an inadequate oxygen blood supply even in the absence of associated coronary artery disease as well as increases in angina in the presence of obstructive coronary disease.[48] In addition, severe right ventricular systolic hypertension, as often occurs with pulmonic stenosis or pulmonary hypertension, may cause exertional angina, presumably on the basis of right ventricular subendocardial ischemia.[49]

A second group of cardiac diseases causing chest pain that is not usually due to myocardial ischemia includes *pericarditis* (Chap. 81), *aortic dissection* (Chap. 98), and *mitral valve prolapse* (Chap. 65). Pericarditis is a relatively common cause of chest pain.[50,51] The chest pain of pericarditis is most often sharp and penetrating in quality, and patients often obtain relief by sitting up and bending forward (Chap. 81). The cardinal diagnostic feature of pericardial pain is its frequent worsening by changes in body position, during deep inspiration, and occasionally upon swallowing. The chest discomfort may radiate to the shoulders, upper back, and neck because of irritation of the diaphragmatic pleura, which is innervated through the phrenic nerve by fibers originating in cervical sympathetic ganglia C3 to C5. Therefore, the chest discomfort associated with pericarditis is due predominantly to parietal pleural irritation. Occasionally, the pain of acute benign, presumptive viral pericarditis may mimic that observed in acute myocardial infarction. Importantly, the most common cause of pericarditis in middle-aged or older people is acute myocardial infarction. The pericarditis usually occurs several days after the myocardial necrosis and must be distinguished from recurrent infarction or ischemia. Pericarditis may also be a cause of chest pain after cardiac surgery and may be a complication of aortic dissection, with leakage into the pericardium.

Aortic dissection (Chap. 98) may be misdiagnosed on initial presentation as an acute myocardial infarction; indeed, myocardial infarction is a recognized complication of aortic dissection. The pain with dissection, however, is usually of sudden onset as compared to the pain of myocardial ischemia, which builds in intensity with time.[52] Patients frequently characterize the pain as excruciating, the most severe discomfort that they have ever experienced, and as having a tearing quality, commonly localized to the interscapular area. The discomfort may radiate widely into the neck, back, abdomen, flanks, and legs and may migrate, depending on the location and progression of the aortic dissection and the amount of arterial luminal compression. Neurologic symptoms and signs may occur when dissection involves the cerebral arteries. With the exception of patients with Marfan's syndrome (Chap. 85) or idiopathic cystic medial necrosis, most patients with aortic dissection have a history of long-standing systemic arterial hypertension or evidence of it on physical examination.

Psychogenic chest discomfort is a common type of recurrent chest pain that may be difficult to separate from angina pectoris, particularly when it occurs in patients with multiple risk factors for coronary artery disease or in otherwise asymptomatic patients with well-documented coronary artery disease. The most common psychogenic cause of chest discomfort is anxiety[53,54] (see also Chap. 89). Psychogenic chest pain is often described as sharp or stabbing, is commonly localized to the left inframammary area, and is usually sharply circumscribed. Terms such as *stabbing* or *lightning-like* may be used to describe extremely short (less than 1 min) episodes of pain. At times, the pain may persist for many hours or several days, in contrast to the pain of myocardial ischemia. Patients often note psychogenic pain at rest. Also, nonvocal communication, such as a flat or worried facial expression, retarded motor activity, and hand wringing may indicate underlying depression. Observation of the patient during pain that occurs spontaneously or during exercise testing often provides insight into a potential psychogenic etiology. Patients with anxiety often have multiple complaints such as breathlessness, giddiness, and palpitation. Associated symptoms, such as air hunger, circumoral paresthesias, globus hystericus, and multiple somatic complaints may suggest a neurasthenic personality or hyperventilation syndrome.

Pain originating in the gastrointestinal tract, particularly that of esophageal origin, is commonly confused with ischemic chest pain.[55] Diffuse esophageal spasm, a neuromuscular motor disorder of the esophagus characterized by chest pain, is the extracardiac condition most frequently confused with angina pectoris.[56–62] Esphageal spasm may occur at any age but is more common in individuals in the fifth decade. The pain is usually retrosternal; may be burning, squeezing, or aching in quality; and often radiates to the back, arms, and jaw. It usually begins during or after a meal and can last minutes or hours. In some patients, the pain may be precipitated or exacerbated by exercise, and relief may be obtained with nitroglycerin, which also relaxes esophageal smooth muscle. A useful feature in the differentiation of diffuse esophageal spasm from ischemic chest discomfort is its frequent association with pain as a result of swallowing, dysphagia, and the regurgitation of gastric contents. Episodes of pain are frequently precipitated either by extremely hot or cold drinks, or an emotional upset. The diagnosis of diffuse esophageal spasm is based on the history, the exclusion of cardiac and musculoskeletal causes of chest pain, and the demonstration of abnormal esophageal motility on cineesophagograms or by esophageal manometry.[56–62]

Reflux esophagitis results from mucosal irritation produced by failure of the lower esophageal sphincter to prevent regurgitation of highly acidic gastric contents into the distal esophagus.[62–67] The pain is usually epigastric or retrosternal, burning in quality, and frequently precipitated by the recumbent position or by bending over. "Heartburn" and regurgitation often occur after meals or ingestion of coffee or after postural changes. Patients are often awakened by chest discomfort due to acid reflux occurring in the recumbent position. Many of these patients are obese and report relief of discomfort from food, antacids, or elevation of the head of the bed. Dysphagia may result from stricture formation secondary to long-standing esophageal reflux. An upper gastrointestinal series may demonstrate hiatal hernia, but this does not establish the diagnosis of esophagitis or esophageal reflux. Esophagoscopy and esophageal biopsy may demonstrate mucosal lesions and are useful for assessing the severity of inflammation and for excluding malignancy. Sphincter incompetence may be documented by the use of esophageal manometry.[56] Esophageal acid perfusion testing (Berstein test) will often provoke the patient's characteristic symptoms, and distal esophgeal pH monitoring will detect gastroesophageal reflux.

Acute esophageal rupture, a serious and often rapidly lethal event, causes severe retrosternal pain secondary to the chemical mediastinitis produced by acidic gastric contents.[8–11,55] Spontaneous rupture usually results from a prolonged bout of vomiting or retching after a heavy meal. Rupture is a recognized iatrogenic complication of esophageal instrumentation. The pain varies in location depending on the rupture's site and position. The diagnosis is based on symptoms and signs of mediastinal air following vomiting or esophageal instrumentation.

Although peptic ulcer disease and biliary colic are less commonly confused with chest pain of cardiac origin, myocardial ischemic pain may occasionally be described as burning in character and located near the epigastrium.

Diseases involving the neuromuscular-skeletal systems may cause pain affecting dermatome patterns similar to those occurring with angina pectoris.[8–11] The thoracic outlet syndromes, in which various neural and vascular structures are compressed, may produce symptoms that are sometimes confused with cardiac chest pain. Although compression of the neurovascular bundle by a cervical rib or the scalenus anterior muscle may cause discomfort radiating to the head and neck, the shoulder region, or the axilla, most patients experience pain in the upper extremity resulting from somatic nerve compression, usually in the distribution of the ulnar nerve.[8–11]

The presence of associated paresthesias, the presence of pain unrelated to physical exercise, the worsening of discomfort, and its aggravation by certain body positions are useful differentiating characteristics. The diagnosis of thoracic outlet syndrome can be confirmed in many patients by careful physical and neurologic examination.

Tietze's syndrome, or idiopathic costochondritis, is an occasional cause of anterior chest wall pain that is aggravated by movement and deep breathing.[68] The reproduction of the chest pain syndrome by direct pressure over the involved costochondral junction or the relief of pain after local infiltration with lidocaine is a helpful diagnostic maneuver.[69] Degenerative arthritis of the cervical and thoracic vertebrae may cause bandlike pain confined to the chest, neck, or back that often radiates to the arms.[70] Radiologic evidence of degenerative changes involving the cervical and thoracic vertebrae is often found in asymptomatic elderly patients. The production or exacerbation of pain by various postures, movement, sneezing, or coughing is more useful in the diagnosis of chest discomfort due to vertebral disease.[8–11]

The *preeruptive stage of herpes zoster* may be characterized by bandlike chest pain over one or more dermatomes. The advanced age of the patient, additional symptoms of malaise, headache and fever, the presence of hyperesthesia of the involved area on physical examination, and the eventual eruption of typical lesions 4 or 5 days after the onset of symptoms will result in the correct diagnosis. Chest wall pain and tenderness may occur for unknown reasons.[71] The discomfort may be reproduced by pressure over the painful area and by movements of the thorax such as bending, twisting, or turning. The variable duration of the pain and the absence of relief by nitroglycerin distinguish it from angina.

The syndrome of acute massive *pulmonary embolism* with its associated acute pulmonary hypertension and low cardiac output may occasionally simulate acute myocardial infarction, since myocardial ischemia may be present in both conditions.[72] The quality of chest pain may be identical to that observed in patients with nonradiating ischemic chest pain or may be pleuritic, as described below. The associated signs of severe dyspnea, tachypnea, and intense cyanosis, accompanied by profound anxiety and agitation, however, favor the diagnosis of pulmonary embolism[8–11] (Chap. 60). The clinical setting may suggest the diagnosis because of the known increased likelihood of pulmonary embolism in the postpartum or postoperative state, during long trips, in patients with congestive heart failure and peripheral edema, and in those with deep vein thrombophlebitis.[8–11] Measurements of arterial blood gases, abnormal pulmonary perfusion-ventilation scans and, if needed, pulmonary arteriography will establish the correct diagnosis.[8–11]

Other pulmonary conditions associated with chest discomfort, such as pneumothorax, are rarely confused with ischemic chest pain because of additional characteristic clinical features. Spontaneous pneumothorax usually occurs in otherwise healthy males in the third and fourth decades. The clinical presentation is usually characterized by the abrupt onset of agonizing unilateral pleuritic chest pain associated with severe shortness of breath. The plain or expiratory chest film provides the definitive diagnosis. Chest pain associated with pneumonias of various etiologies, as well as pulmonary infarctions as a consequence of pulmonary embolus, may result from pleural irritation. The discomfort is sharp, varies acutely with breathing, and is frequently accompanied by a reduced inspiratory effort. Associated signs of pulmonary parenchymal infection or infarction usually indicate the underlying diagnosis.

Extrathoracic Pain

Intermittent claudication of the *lower extremities* due to peripheral atherosclerosis (Chap. 100) may present as discomfort during exercise in the arch of the foot, calf of the leg, thighs, hips, or gluteal region.[73] Acute arterial occlusion in the lower extremities due to systemic embolism may cause the sensation of hypoesthesia.[2] Intermittent claudication of the upper extremities or masseter muscles is usually due to nonatherosclerotic causes of arterial disease, such as arteritis.[2] The pain of Raynaud's disease may be noted in the fingers after exposure to cold, with pallor of the fingers prior to the sensation of pain.[74] Pain and swelling of lower extremities may be caused by thrombophlebitis[75] (see Chap. 100).

Head pain secondary to myocardial ischemia may be felt in the jaw, hard palate, cheek, and sometimes deep in the ear canals. The pain of temporal arteritis, commonly localized to the temporal area, is often associated with abnormal vision and polymalagia rheumatica.[76] Migraine headache, frequently accompanied by nausea, scotoma, and intolerance to light, is vascular in origin and may be incapacitating.[2] A severe headache may be present in patients with uncontrolled hypertension (Chap. 56).

Pain in the abdomen, often localized to the midabdomen and lower portion of the back, may be produced by an expanding or rupturing atherosclerotic abdominal aneurysm. Abdominal angina due to vascular disease of the mesenteric arteries is discussed in Chap. 98. The liver is often painful and tender in severe right heart failure, with worsening of the pain during activity.[2]

Various types of *joint pain* may be associated with heart disease. Rheumatic fever, rheumatoid arthritis, lupus erythematosus, psoriatic arthritis, ankylosing spondylitis, gonococcal arthritis, Reiter's syndrome, and Lyme disease may be associated with valvular, myocardial, or pericardial disease.[2]

RESPIRATORY
SYMPTOMS

Dyspnea is defined as difficult or labored respiration or the unpleasant awareness of one's respiration. It has many causes. A clue to the etiology is obtained from the factors that precipitate or relieve it.[1] Chronic dyspnea can be caused by heart failure, pulmonary disease, anxiety, obesity, poor physical fitness, pleural effusions, and asthma.[2] Acute dyspnea may occur with acute pulmonary edema, hyperventilation, pneu-

mothorax, pulmonary embolism, pneumonia, and airway obstruction.[2]

Dyspnea on effort, a frequent symptom, is usually due to congestive heart failure, chronic pulmonary disease, or physical deconditioning (Chap. 23). The amount of activity necessary to produce dyspnea needs definition. A recent or dramatic increase in the dyspnea is more likely to be due to the development of heart failure than to lung disease. When heart and lung disease coexist, however, the determination of the relative contribution of pulmonary and cardiac dysfunction to dyspnea can be very difficult.

Cheyne-Stokes respiration is a form of periodic breathing characterized by cycles beginning with shallow respirations that increase in rate and depth to significant hyperpnea, followed by decreasing rate and depth of respiration, then a period of apnea that may last 15 s or longer.[1] This form of respiration occurs in advanced congestive heart failure and in some forms of central nervous system disease. Cheyne-Stokes respiration often occurs during sleep without the patient's awareness and is often reported by others.

Orthopnea results from an increase in hydrostatic pressure in the lungs that occurs with assumption of the supine position. It consists of cough and dyspnea in some patients with left ventricular failure or mitral valve disease and necessitates the use of two or more pillows on lying down. The patient with severe obstructive lung disease, especially acute asthma, also cannot lie flat comfortably.

Paroxysmal nocturnal dyspnea (PND) is the occurrence of dyspnea during sleep, commonly 2 to 3 h after going to bed, that is relieved by assuming the upright position. Dyspnea usually does not recur after the patient goes back to sleep. Episodes can be mild, or they can be severe with wheezing, coughing, gasping, and apprehension.[1] Some episodes will progress to pulmonary edema. The probable mechanism for this relatively specific symptom of left heart failure is the increase in central blood volume in the supine position.

A drying, nonproductive *cough*, occurring with effort or at rest, may be related to the pulmonary congestion associated with heart failure (Chap. 23). Although dyspnea is usually present, cough may dominate the clinical picture. The cough that accompanies acute pulmonary edema is often associated with frothy, pink-tinged sputum, whereas the sputum associated with chronic bronchitis is usually white and mucoid.[2] The sputum associated with pneumonia is often thick and yellow, and that due to pulmonary infarction may be bloody, as may the sputum associated with cancer of the lung or bronchiolectasis. Cough also may be caused by angiotension converting enzyme inhibitors, which are often prescribed for heart failure or hypertension.

Recurrent coughing due to heart failure is often thought to be due to bronchitis, and patients with chronic bronchitis may cough more when heart failure ensues.[2] Patients with a high pulmonary blood flow due to congenital left-to-right shunts are subject to pulmonary infection. Patients with a high pulmonary venous pressure are more vulnerable to the development of pulmonary edema when they have viral pneumonitis than are patients with normal pulmonary venous pressure. This particularly applies to patients with mitral stenosis.

Hemoptysis occurs in many cardiac disorders. Posterior epistaxis due to systemic hypertension may cause blood-streaked sputum; patients on anticoagulants may have epistaxis that mimics hemoptysis. Epistaxis, however, is usually easily differentiated from bloody sputum. Bright red pulmonary venous blood from rupture of submucosal pulmonary venules may be expectorated by patients with pulmonary venous hypertension due to mitral stenosis or severe left ventricular failure.[2] Darker blood or clots often occur with pulmonary emboli. Pink, frothy sputum may be produced during acute pulmonary edema. Blood-streaked sputum is a feature of the "winter bronchitis" of mitral stenosis.[2] Massive hemoptysis with exsanguination or death from asphyxiation can follow rupture of an aortic aneurysm or one of the cardiac chambers into the bronchial tree.[2] Rupture of a pulmonary artery by the balloon of an indwelling pulmonary artery catheter can cause abrupt, severe hemoptysis in hospitalized patients.

Wheezing associated with dyspnea may be due to lung or heart disease. If the symptoms have developed recently in an adult over the age of 40, other clues indicating heart disease should be sought. Wheezing due to heart disease is termed *cardiac asthma*.

EDEMA
AND ASCITES

Edema is a common symptom or finding in patients with right or left heart failure. Fluid retention in heart failure results from increased venous pressure and abnormal activity of salt-retaining hormones (Chap. 21). In an average-size person, 5–10 lb of excess fluid are required for edema to become apparent; a history of recent weight gain will often correlate with a deterioration in clinical status.[1] The amount of weight loss in response to treatment for heart failure in the past will relate to the severity of the problem. Minor degrees of edema are evident only after a period of dependency of the legs and will decrease after rest. Presacral edema may be most obvious when the patient has been at bed rest. Although edema of cardiac origin may progress to anasarca, cardiac edema rarely involves the face or upper extremities. Edema mainly affecting the face and arms is more likely to be due to venous or lymphatic obstruction by clot or neoplasm.[1] Facial edema is a feature of the nephrotic syndrome, angioneurotic edema, and glomerulonephritis. Swelling or "puffiness" of hands and fingers is not usually a symptom of cardiac disease. Persistent edema in the legs from which veins were harvested at the time of bypass surgery is common. Other causes of edema—such as varicosities, obesity, tight girdle, renal insufficiency, or cirrhosis with hypoproteinemia—must be considered.[1] A patient with chronic congestive heart failure may detect edema of the ankles and lower legs during the day and note that it diminishes during the night. It is important to ascertain whether edema of the extremities preceded or followed dyspnea on effort. The calcium antagonists, such as nifedipine, may produce bilateral edema of the lower legs.

Patients will be aware of *ascites* because of increased abdominal girth. Previously comfortable trousers or skirts may no longer fit. Bending at the waist is uncomfortable with ill-defined abdominal fullness. Patients with severe edema due to congestive heart failure may develop ascites; however, ascites is particularly common in patients with constrictive pericardial disease, sometimes occurring before peripheral edema becomes obvious (Chap. 81). Ascitic fluid is formed when elevated venous pressure leads to transudation of fluids from the serosal surfaces. Other causes of ascites—such as cirrhosis, nephrosis, and tumor—must be excluded.[1]

FATIGUE
AND WEAKNESS

Fatigue and *weakness* may be due to many causes and therefore are not specific symptoms for heart disease. The most common cause of these symptoms is anxiety and depression. Anemia, thyrotoxicosis, and other chronic disease states may be associated with fatigue and weakness.

When a patient with heart disease is volume overloaded or when there is pulmonary congestion due to heart disease, the patient is likely to complain of dyspnea. With vigorous diuretic therapy, this complaint may be replaced by symptoms of fatigue and weakness,[2] probably related to inadequate cardiac output (Chap. 21). The heart fails in its prime objective of nourishing all the tissues and organs of the body, including the skeletal muscles. As congestive heart failure worsens, fatigue may replace dyspnea as the major symptom. Beta blockers used to treat angina or hypertension will commonly cause fatigue and lethargy. Hypotension or hypokalemia caused by diuretics can cause fatigue and weakness, as can relative hypovolemia due to the use of angiotensin converting enzyme inhibitors.

Severe fatigue related to effort may result from transient global myocardial ischemia in patients with extensive coronary artery disease. Dyspnea and hypotension may also occur at the same time as the severe fatigue as "angina equivalents."[2]

PALPITATION

Most normal individuals are intermittently aware of their heart action, particularly at the time of physical and emotional stress. When the heart action is more vigorous than usual or its perception is unpleasant, the term *palpitation* is appropriate.[1] The patient may complain of a "pounding," "stopping," "jumping," or "racing" in the chest. Palpitation is frequently a benign symptom without any serious cardiac disease present; at other times it may indicate a potentially life-threatening condition. Simple premature beats may be perceived as a floating or flopping sensation in the chest due to the more forceful beat that occurs after the pause following the premature beat. Sometimes a transient feeling of fullness in the neck (due to cannon *a* waves) is perceived with premature beats. Certain patients perceive almost every premature beat, while others are totally unaware of frequent or advanced arrhythmias. A report of skips or irregularity during uninterrupted sinus rhythm is not uncommon. Generally, thin, tense individuals are likely to be more aware of their cardiac activity than others. Individuals with and without arrhythmias are often aware of their cardiac activity when they first lie down on their sides to sleep, especially if they lie on their left sides.[1]

Rapid heart action of a paroxysmal tachycardia usually begins and terminates suddenly and causes a pounding sensation in the chest.[1] Patients will often indicate whether the tachycardia is regular or irregular and may be able to tap out the rate and rhythm of the episode (Chap. 27). Chest pressure suggesting angina may occur with an episode of tachycardia even in young, healthy patients without coronary heart disease. Patients with coronary disease, however, often develop severe angina with a sustained arrhythmia because of increased myocardial oxygen demand. Depending on the rate and mechanism of the arrhythmia, faintness and syncope may be described during questioning. Nevertheless, sustained ventricular tachycardia can occur in the setting of serious underlying cardiac disease without a significant compromise in hemodynamics (Chap. 27). Syncope due to tachyarrhythmias may occur without the patient being aware of palpitations.

SYNCOPE

Cardiac *syncope* (fainting) (Chap. 35) is defined as the transient loss of consciousness due to inadequate cerebral blood flow secondary to an abrupt decrease in cardiac output. *Near syncope* refers to the clinical situation in which the patient feels dizzy and weak and tends to lose postural tone but does not lose consciousness. In assessing the patient with syncope, one determines if there were precipitating factors, premonitory symptoms, injury with the episode, seizure activity or incontinence, or a postictal state.[1] Injury during an episode suggests a sudden profound loss of body tone and increases the likelihood of the more serious causes. Brief, unsustained seizure activity can occur with syncope due to a cardiac arrhythmia.

The patient may be incontinent during cardiogenic syncope, but an aura, sustained tonic-chronic movements, tongue biting, and confusion or drowsiness after the event are more characteristic of syncope due to central nervous system disease.[1] In contrast, return of consciousness to the alert state is prompt after the reversal of the arrhythmia causing cardiac syncope.[1] The common faint (*vasovagal syncope*) results from bradycardia and hypotension caused by excessive vagal discharge. It is often associated with some precipitating event such as a "heavy" meal in a warm room and has brief premonitory signs and symptoms such as nausea, yawning, diaphoresis, and sometimes the feeling of decreased hearing or vision.[1] There is frequently sufficient warning that the patient does not fall abruptly. The results of head-up tilt-table testing indicate a vasovagal mechanism in some patients with syncope who do not have premonitory symptoms (Chap. 35). Following a

fainting episode, the patient may be pale and diaphoretic and have a slow heart rate. Syncope occurring in the setting of any gastrointestinal symptoms is likely to be vagal in origin. A history of similar episodes during the preceding several years is common in patients with vagal syncope.

A hypersensitive carotid sinus can cause syncope. A history of episodes during an activity such as shaving, wearing of a tight collar, or extreme turning of the head may occur but is unusual even when a sensitive carotid sinus is shown to be the cause of syncope. Syncope following urination (micturition syncope) may occur at the time of rapid decompression of a distended bladder, which typically occurs after a period of sleep. Paroxysms of coughing, usually in patients with underlying pulmonary disease, can result in syncope. Very fast or slow arrhythmias may decrease the cardiac output enough to cause alterations in consciousness, ranging from abrupt profound syncope to mild light-headedness. Stokes-Adams syncope is caused by intermittent complete heart block, sinus arrest, or ventricular tachyarrhythmias[77] (Chap. 35). It is characterized by abrupt loss of consciousness without warning, a variable period of unconsciousness (seconds to minutes), and then a rapid return of normal mental status without amnesia or postictal state.

In the presence of several left ventricular outflow obstruction (aortic stenosis or hypertrophic cardiomyopathy), loss of consciousness with effort may occur. Syncope can be due either to the heart's inability to increase its output in response to the peripheral vasodilatation that occurs during exercise, or to a tachyarrhythmia. Intermittent obstruction of a cardiac valve by a intracavitary tumor or thrombus is a rare cause of syncope which occasionally may be precipitated when the patient changes position.

Many normal subjects experience transient light-headness with rapid changes in position. This is more common in older patients, since the ability of the peripheral vasculature to respond is attenuated with aging (see Chap. 96). Postural hypotension is a well-defined cause of fainting or dizziness that usually occurs when the individual is upright and often just after rising from a supine or sitting position. Possible causes include peripheral neuropathy, autonomic dysfunction, volume depletion, or drug side effects.[1]

OTHER CEREBRAL SYMPTOMS

Patients with decreased cardiac output secondary to heart failure may become mentally confused and disoriented. Such symptoms may also be due to hypoxia, to drugs that are invariably prescribed for such patients, and to renal or hepatic failure.[2] A completed stroke may be caused by a lacunar infarct, cerebral hemorrhage, cerebral arterial thrombosis, or a cerebral embolus (Chap. 99). A transient cerebral ischemic attack is commonly due to an embolus. The embolus may originate in an atheromatous ulcer in the carotid artery system or the aortic arch; be related to infective endocarditis, a recent myocardial infarction, atrial fibrillation, or clots on a prosthetic valve; or originate in the leg veins and pass through a patent foramen ovale to the brain (Chap. 99).

The patient with cardiogenic shock or with a severe tachyarrhythmia who also has considerable intracranial or extracranial vascular disease may develop such severe cerebral hypoxia that coma occurs. Hypoxic encephalopathy may follow cardiac resuscitation and occasionally occurs after cardiopulmonary bypass for cardiac surgery. A cerebral abscess may occur in patients with congenital heart disease and a right-to-left shunt.[2]

FEVER, CHILLS, AND SWEATS

Patients with rheumatic fever usually do not have chills. Chills are common in patients with bacterial endocarditis. Symptoms of *fever, chills, or sweats* in any patient with a heart murmur should lead one to suspect infective endocarditis (Chap. 82). A history of valvular heart disease is not a prerequisite for a diagnosis of endocarditis, since previously normal valves become infected. A history of recent dental work, genitourinary surgery, or illicit drug use increases the suspicion of infective endocarditis. Fever may accompany pericarditis. Myalgia, chills, and fever may on rare occasions be related to myocardial infarction, presumably because of some form of immunologic response to the necrotic myocardial tissue. An intracardiac tumor (myxoma) may produce systemic symptoms in the absence of infection. Low-grade fever in a patient with heart failure may be a sign of pulmonary emboli.[2] A profuse "cold sweat" mediated by sympathetic discharge often accompanies early stages of acute myocardial infarction. Excessive sweating may occur in patients with severe aortic regurgitation. Diaphoresis is often a sign of congestive heart failure in infants.

HOARSENESS

Although usually unrelated to cardiovascular disease, *hoarseness* can occur in patients with an aortic aneurysm that involves the left recurrent laryngeal nerve. Mitral stenosis may occasionally produce hoarseness due to the pressure of a large pulmonary artery on the recurrent laryngeal nerve. Pericardial effusion may be related to myxedema, which may be associated with a coarse, low-pitched voice. Hoarseness and loss of voice may occur following the use of an endotracheal tube during cardiac surgery.

INDIGESTION, HICCUPS, AND DYSPHAGIA

Many patients with angina pectoris due to coronary artery disease erroneously attribute their symptoms to *indigestion* or heartburn. Also, patients with heartburn, esophageal reflux, and esophageal spasm may believe they have angina pectoris. *Hiccups* may occasionally occur in patients with myocardial infarction and are common during the postoperative period after cardiac surgery. *Dysphagia* may occur in patients with progressive systemic sclerosis, an aortic arch anomaly, or an extremely large left atrium.

GASTROINTESTINAL SYMPTOMS

Anorexia, nausea, and vomiting may occur as a result of digitalis excess.[1] Hepatomegaly associated with tricuspid valve disease or severe right heart failure may cause right-upper-quadrant epigastric pain and fullness as well as anorexia. Abdominal pain due to visceral ischemia or infarction may occur in a patient who has had a period of very low cardiac output.[1] The pain of some gastrointestinal diseases may be referred or extend to the chest or back and lead to confusion with myocardial ischemia.

ABNORMAL SKIN COLOR

Although *cyanosis* is a sign rather than a symptom, patients or family members may describe cyanosis during the history. Cyanosis is a bluish color of the skin or mucous membranes caused by excess amounts of reduced hemoglobin. About 4 g of reduced hemoglobin is required for cyanosis to be apparent (Chap. 70). Severely anemic patients will not exhibit cyanosis. A distribution of cyanosis involving the mucous membranes as well as the periphery (central cyanosis) is caused by the admixture of venous blood at the level of the heart or great vessels. A patient or a family member may detect that the cyanosis is more intense in the feet than in the hands. This differential cyanosis suggests a right-to-left shunt through a patent ductus arteriosus in a patient with Eisenmenger physiology (Chap. 70). Peripheral cyanosis does not involve the mucous membranes but is the result of slow peripheral flow with accumulation of excess reduced hemoglobin in the setting of circulatory failure, shock, or peripheral vasospasm.[1]

Jaundice may be detected by a patient or by a member of the family. As a rule, hepatic congestion due to heart failure will not produce jaundice. When jaundice does occur in a patient with heart failure, it is appropriate to consider pulmonary infarction in addition to hepatic congestion or cirrhosis of the liver. Hemolysis of red blood cells may occur in patients with prosthetic valves and can produce jaundice.[2]

A history of *flush* of face and trunk, sometimes accentuated by alcohol, should lead one to search for the other signs and symptoms of carcinoid heart disease.[2] Cardiomyopathies due to hemochromatosis should be considered in the patient with diabetes whose skin color has changed from normal to bronze.[2] A slatelike color of the skin, hands, and nose may develop in patients who take amiodarone.

EMBOLIZATION

The entry of a blood clot, vegetation, or tumor fragment from the heart into the systemic circulation results in arterial embolus. Clots may occur in the left atrium behind a stenotic mitral valve, within a ventricular aneurysm, or in the left ventricle of a patient with cardiomyopathy. While many emboli originate in the heart, arteriosclerotic material in the ascending and descending aorta often embolizes to the periphery.[1] Many emboli are asymptomatic. Symptoms of a stroke occur with emboli to the cerebral vessels. Myocardial infarction can result from an embolus to a coronary artery. Hematuria, flank pain, and hypertension can result from embolization to a renal artery. The abrupt development of a cold, painful extremity follows embolic obstruction of an arm or leg artery.[1] Emboli from the vegetations of acute endocarditis may produce characteristic areas of vascular necrosis in the fingers or toes (Chap. 82). Severe atherosclerosis in the abdominal aorta and iliac vessels can be responsible for showers of peripheral emboli with multiple small, reddish-blue lesions on the lower extremities sometimes causing small areas of gangrene. An embolic event may be the presenting manifestation of previously unrecognized cardiac disease.

INSOMNIA

The most common causes of *insomnia* are mental conflict, emotional disturbances, and depression. Heart failure, however, may also cause insomnia. The patient with Cheyne-Stokes (see above) respiration may sleep during the apneic phase and wake during the hyperpneic phase of the condition. Occasionally, patients with pulmonary congestion due to heart failure have insomnia before they develop nocturnal dyspnea.

CLASSIFICATION OF CARDIAC DISABILITY

Several classifications have been proposed and used for many years for the systematic and reproducible grading of disability due to cardiac disease. Although the complete New York Heart Association method of classifying cardiac diagnoses, originally proposed many years ago, is not widely used now, the portion of the classification that concerns functional capacities[78] is still commonly used (Table 10-3). Although the Canadian Cardiovascular Society's grading system for angina (Table 10-2) is more widely utilized for patients with chest pain, both classifications continue to be used in the medical literature and in clinical practice, particularly as criteria for the inclusion of heart patients in multicenter clinical trials.

THE PHYSICAL EXAMINATION

Important information concerning the patient with definite or suspected heart disease is often obtained by a careful and

TABLE 10-3

THE OLD NEW YORK HEART ASSOCIATION FUNCTIONAL CLASSIFICATION

Class 1	No symptoms with ordinary physical activity.
Class 2	Symptoms with ordinary activity. Slight limitation of activity.
Class 3	Symptoms with less than ordinary activity. Marked limitation of activity.
Class 4	Symptoms with any physical activity or even at rest.

Source: The Criteria Committee of the New York Heart Association. *Diseases of the Heart and Blood Vessels: Nomenclature and Criteria for Diagnosis of the Heart and Great Vessels.* 6th ed. New York: New York Heart Association/Little Brown; 1964. Reproduced with permission from the New York Heart Association, Inc., and the publisher.

deliberate physical examination, which includes a general inspection of the patient, an indirect measurement of the arterial blood pressure in both arms and one or more lower extremities, an examination of central and peripheral arterial pulses, an evaluation of the jugular venous pressure and pulsations, palpation of the precordium, and cardiac auscultation. Based on the results of this rather inexpensive evaluation, a definite diagnosis is often made and selected noninvasive and invasive testing is ordered when appropriate.

GENERAL INSPECTION OF THE PATIENT

The art of bedside medicine, as practiced by William Osler[79] and other great clinicians, begins with a careful head-to-toe appraisal of the patient. This visual approach is of great advantage in seeking clues to the etiology of cardiovascular disease, as shown in the following section. Since this discussion is organized according to the specific type of heart involvement, diseases that cause several problems are mentioned more than once. Each disorder is italicized, and its major manifestations are described the first time it is named.

SYNDROMES ASSOCIATED WITH CONGENITAL HEART DISEASE

Congenital heart disease syndromes may be classified into heritable disorders, connective tissue disorders, inborn areas of metabolism, chromosomal abnormalities, sporadic disorders, and teratogenic disorders (see also Chaps. 69, 70, and 85). Occasionally, a particular syndrome falls into more than one category. In the first category, the *Ellis-van Creveld syndrome*, a common disorder in the Amish population, is a heritable form of dwarfism characterized by short extremities, polydactyly, dysplastic teeth and nails, and multiple frenula binding the upper eyelid to the alveolar ridge (Fig. 10-1).

Over half of the patients have heart disease, usually a large atrial septal defect or a single atrium.[80] The *thrombocytopenia–absent radius (TAR) syndrome* includes bilateral radial aplasia with a persistent thumb and thrombocytopenia and may be associated with an ostium secundum atrial septal defect and/or tetralogy of Fallot. The *Holt-Oram syndrome*, an autosomal dominant trait, combines an atrial septal defect or other congenital heart disease with a thumb (Fig. 10-2)[81] that may be absent, hypoplastic, bifid, triphalangeal, or unusually long. *Tabatzniks syndrome* (heart-hand syndrome type II) is characterized by hypoplastic deltoids, skeletal anomalies of the forearm, bradydactyly, and atrial fibrillation. In the *Laurence-Moon-Bardet-Biedl syndrome*, mental retardation, polydactyly, obesity, retinitis pigmentosa, and hypogonadism occur with a variety of congenital heart diseases.[82]

Arteriovenous fistulas involving the lung, liver, and mucous membranes are associated with multiple telangiectasia in patients with the hereditary hemorrhagic telangiectasis (*Osler-Weber-Rendu syndrome*).[83] *Cornelia de Lange's syndrome* is characterized by bushy, confluent eyebrows, downward-

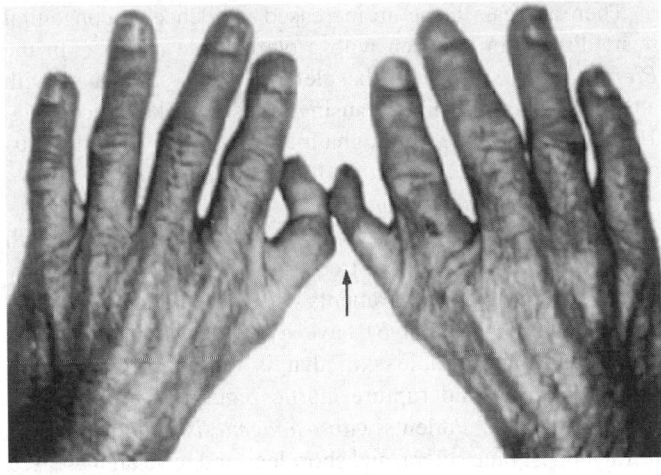

FIGURE 10-2

Holt-Oram syndrome: fingerized thumb (*arrow*) associated with an atrial septal defect.

slanting eyes, a small mandible, low-set ears, hirsutism, long eyelashes, a broad, flat, upturned nose, severe growth and mental retardation, and a peculiar "chicken-wing" extremity with a single thumblike digit (Fig. 10-3). A ventricular septal defect, patent ductus arteriosus, pulmonic stenosis, anomalous venous return, or atrial septal defect may be present.

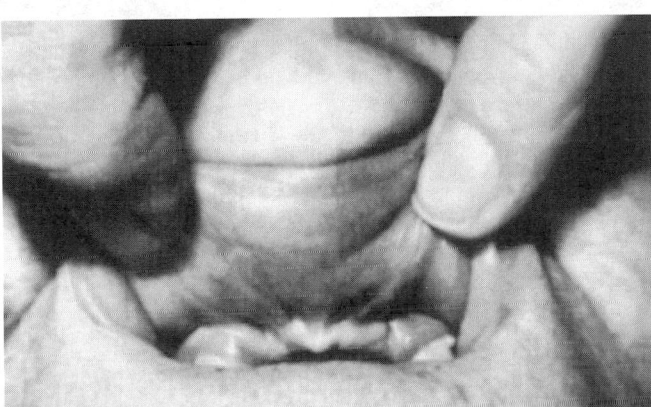

A

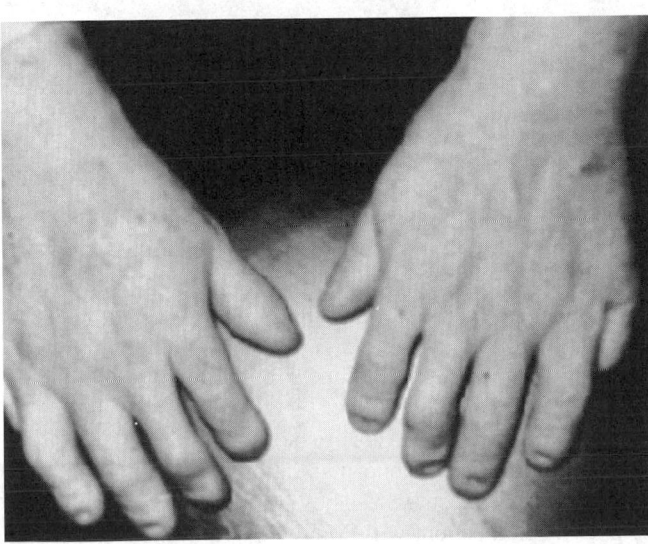

B

FIGURE 10-1

Ellis-van Creveld syndrome. *A*. Typical "lip tie" due to multiple frenulum. *B*. Polydactyly. This patient has a large septal defect.

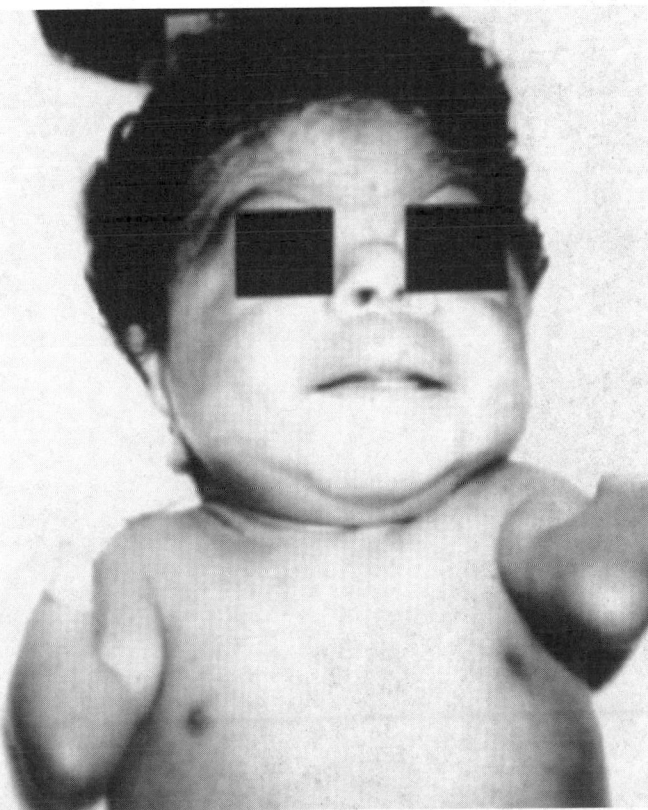

FIGURE 10-3

Cornelia de Lange's syndrome: low hairline, hirsutism, bushy brows, phocomelia, and a single thumblike digit. May be associated with ventricular septal defect.

There appears to be an increased incidence of congenital heart disease in children with a cleft palate or lip.[84] In the *Pierre Robin syndrome*, the cleft palate is associated with a hypoplastic mandible causing a "shrewlike" face (Fig. 10-4). A cleft palate, micrognathia, low-set ears, and truncus arteriosus may be present in the familial *third and fourth pharyngeal pouch syndromes.*

Cutis laxis is a generalized disruption of elastic fibers with diminished skin resilience, frequent hernias, and pulmonary artery branch stenosis.[85] Patients with the *Ehlers-Danlos syndrome* (Fig. 10-5*A* and *B*) have hyperextensible joints and hyperelastic and friable skin that is often associated with arterial dilation and rupture, aortic regurgitation, or mitral valve prolapse.[86] Patients with *osteogenesis imperfecta* have brittle bones, blue sclera, and short legs and have an increased incidence of aortic and mitral regurgitation.[87] Patients with *pseudoxanthoma elasticum* (see also Chap. 85), who have degeneration of dermal elastic fibers and retinal angioid streaks, can develop aortic regurgitation and coronary artery disease (Fig. 10-6).

Marfan's syndrome, an autosomal dominant trait, is suggested by skeletal features such as increased height, long

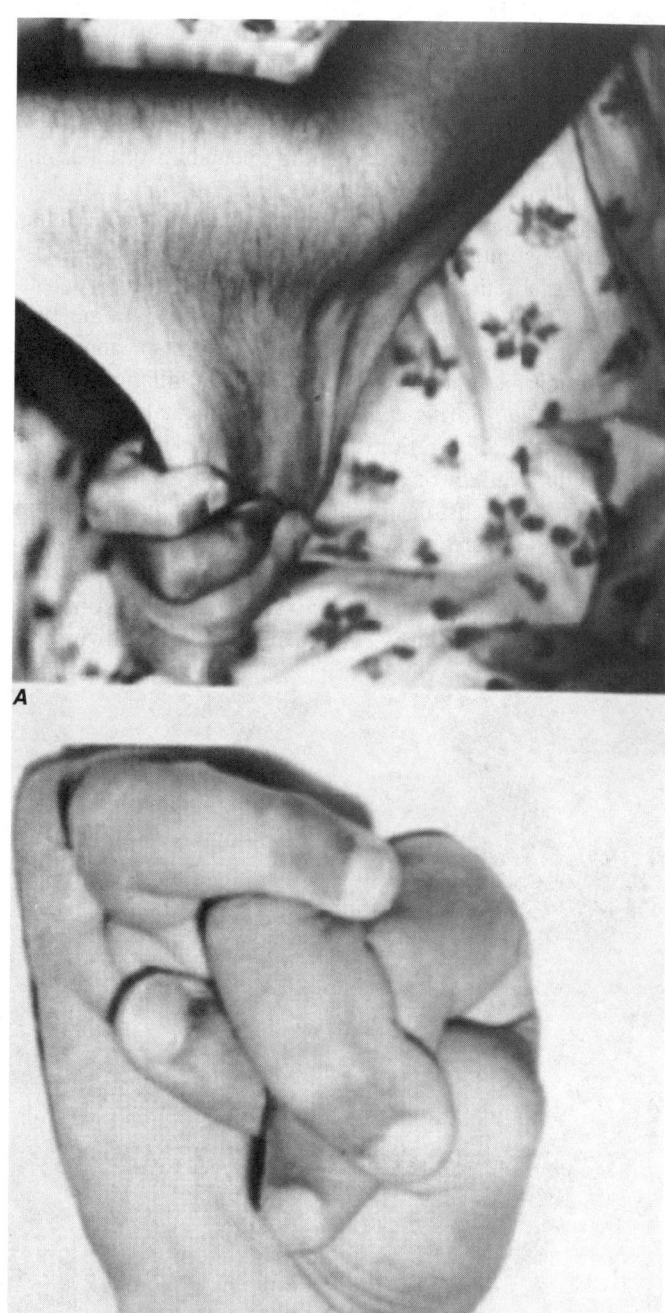

A

B

FIGURE 10-5

Ehlers-Danlos syndrome. *A.* Hyperextensible skin. *B.* Lax joints. Redundant chordae tendineae and arterial rupture may occur.

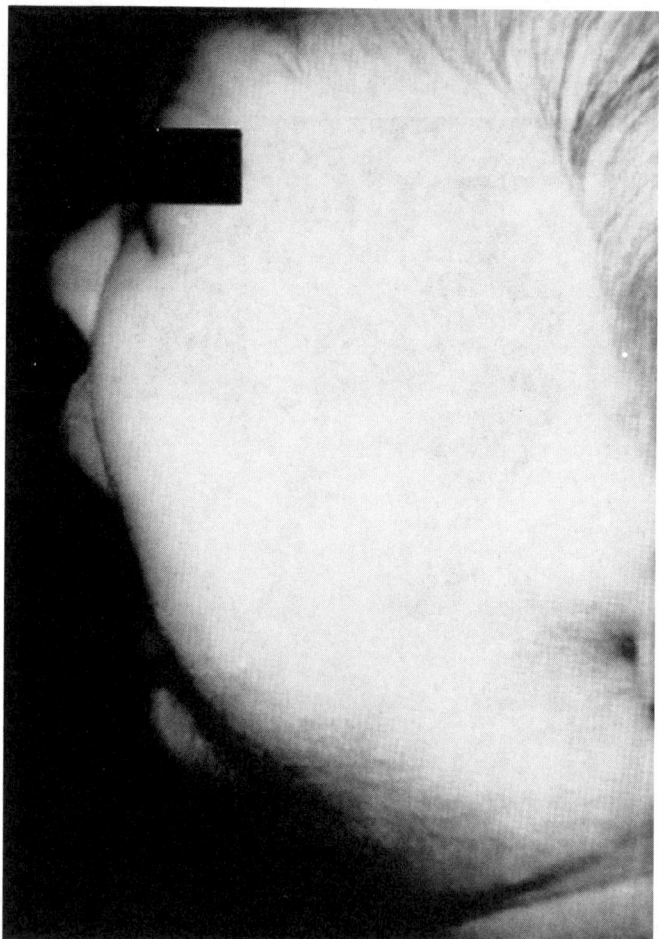

FIGURE 10-4

Pierre Robin syndrome: hypoplastic mandible associated with a ventricular septal defect.

fingers, narrow palms, lax joints, kyphoscoliosis, pectus excavatum or carinatum, an elongated face, high-arched palate, and flat feet (Fig. 10-7*A–C*).[88] The legs are disproportionally long, resulting in an abnormal ratio of the upper-to-lower segments of at most 0.85. The arm span many exceed the height. When a patient with Marfan's syndrome clenches the hand around a flexed thumb, the thumb protrudes past the ulnar side of the hand. Such a patient can also easily encircle the wrist by grasping it with the fifth finger and thumb of the other hand (Fig. 10-7*B*). Other signs include bilateral

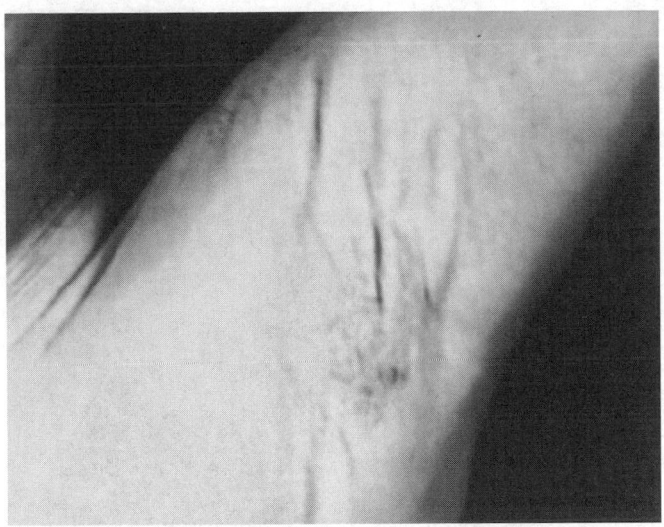

FIGURE 10-6
Pseudoxanthoma elasticum: grooved skin in a typical location. Arterial calcification may occur.

subluxation of the lens, severe myopia, and blue sclera (Fig. 10-7*D*). Subcutaneous tissue is sparse. Valvular disease is common; patients with Marfan's syndrome may have mitral valve prolapse, minimal to severe mitral regurgitation, a dilated and often calcified mitral annulus, and eventual chordal rupture. Aortic regurgitation is a consequence of a dilated aortic root, prolapse of the aortic cusps, or aortic dissection (see also Chap. 85).

Aortic regurgitation has also been described in patients with inborn errors of metabolism including *Morquio's syndrome* (mucopolysaccharidosis IV) and *Scheie's syndrome* (mucopolysaccharidosis V).[89] Patients with Morquio's syndrome are identified by their short stature, short neck, barrel chest, broad mouth, short nose, widely spaced teeth, and cloudy cornea. In Scheie's syndrome, growth retardation, sternal protrusion, facial abnormalities, and cloudy cornea are present. In *Fabry's disease*, angiokeratomas identified as purplish, pinpoint skin lesions occur on the lips, underarm, buttocks, scrotum, and penis (Fig. 10-8). Conduction defects, cardiomyopathy, ischemic heart disease and conduction defects beginning in the third decade are associated with this sex-linked recessive disorder, in which there is a genetic deficiency of the enzyme α-galactosidase A.[90]

Many chromosomal abnormalities have been associated with congenital heart disease. The well-recognized characteristics of *Down's syndrome* (trisomy 21) include a small head, shallow orbits, epicanthal folds, low-set ears, widely spaced eyes (hypertelorism), Brushfield's white spots of the iris, protruding tongue, transverse palmar creases, and mental retardation (Chap. 69). Congenital heart disease occurs in 40 to 60 percent of patients; a ventricular septal defect or endocardial cushion defect are the most frequent.[91] Less commonly, tetralogy of Fallot, secundum atrial septal defect, patent ductus arteriosus, and other abnormalities are present.[92,93]

Klinefelter's syndrome is characterized by gynecomastia, small testicles, a eunuchoid appearance, tall stature, and long extremities. Associated atrial septal defects have been described.[92]

Patients with abnormalities involving chromosomes 1, 9, 11, and 22 often have congenital heart disease.[93] The findings with *chromosome 1 abnormalities* include a peaked nose, micrognathia, and long, tapering fingers. Children with *chromosome 9 abnormalities* have a prominent forehead, hypertension, anteverted nostrils, long upper lip, a short neck, mental retardation, and external ear malformations. A child with a *chromosome 11 abnormality* shares similar features plus retraction of the lower lip. Psychomotor retardation, coloboma, hypertelorism (widely spread eyes), downward slanting of the eyes, and preauricular tags or fistulas are clues to a *chromosome 22 defect*.

Congenital heart disease, primarily patent ductus arteriosus, has been associated with the 49 *XXXXY syndrome*. This unusual disorder should be suspected when a child has psychomotor retardation, hypoplastic genitals, prognathism, clinodactyly (inward curving of the fifth finger), and radioulnar synostoses.

Congenital heart disease of varied types is common in *trisomy 13* and *trisomy 18 syndromes*.[94] In *trisomy 13 syndrome*, the child has a cleft palate and lip; the ocular tissue and the nose may be missing. Polydactyly in combination with retroflexible thumbs, transverse creases, hyperconvex narrow nails, and flexion of the fingers and hands are characteristic of this syndrome. The features of the *trisomy 18 syndrome* are a small, triangular mouth with receding chin, small mandible, webbed neck, and tightly clenched fists with the index finger overlapping the third finger and the fifth finger over the fourth (Fig. 10-9).

Low hairline, low-set ears, deafness, small jaw, and short, webbed neck are physical findings common to both *Turner's syndrome* and the *Klippel-Feil syndrome*. Turner's syndrome also includes short stature, broad chest with widely spaced nipples, epicanthal folds, widely spaced eyes, pigmented moles, ptosis, clinodactyly, and a shortened fifth finger (Fig. 10-10).[95] Coarctation of the aorta, aortic stenosis, and hypertrophic cardiomyopathy are the usual cardiovascular considerations. The Klippel-Feil syndrome may cause facial asymmetry, cleft palate, torticollis, scoliosis, deafness, strabismus, and hydrocephaly. Ventricular septal defect is the most common associated cardiac disorder.[96]

There are many sporadic disorders associated with congenital heart disease. An imperforate anus may be associated with a cardiovascular malformation.[97] This may occur as an isolated finding or as a component of the *VATER association*,[98] the *asplenia syndrome*,[99] the *CHARGE syndrome*[100] (coloboma, heart disease, atresia choanae, retarded growth, genital hypoplasia, ear anomalies), or *cat's-eye pupil*[101] (a fissure of the iris and choroid associated with a cardiac defect). The VATER association includes vertebral defect, tracheoesophageal fistula, and radial and renal dysplasia. A ventricular defect occurs in 80 percent of these patients. The asplenia

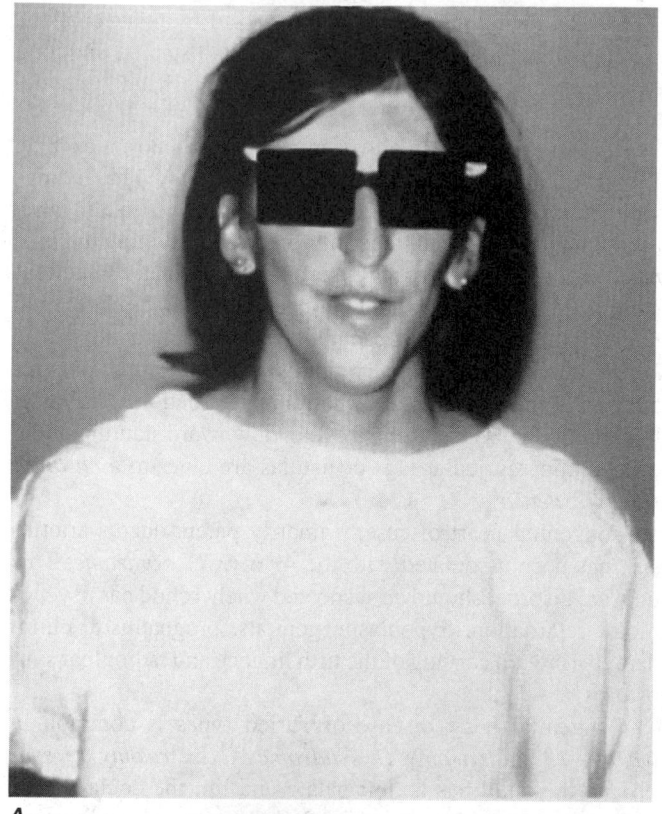

A

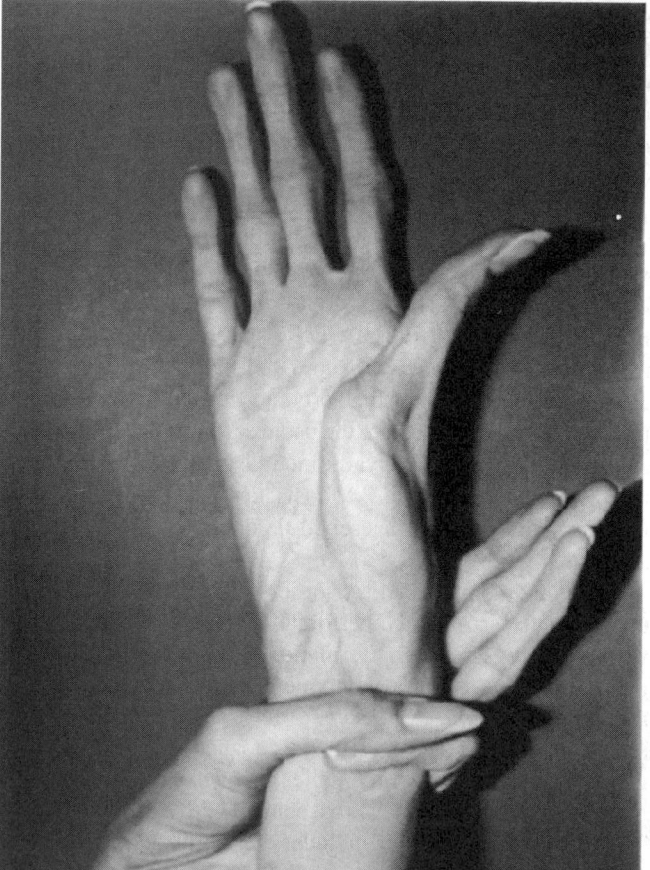

B

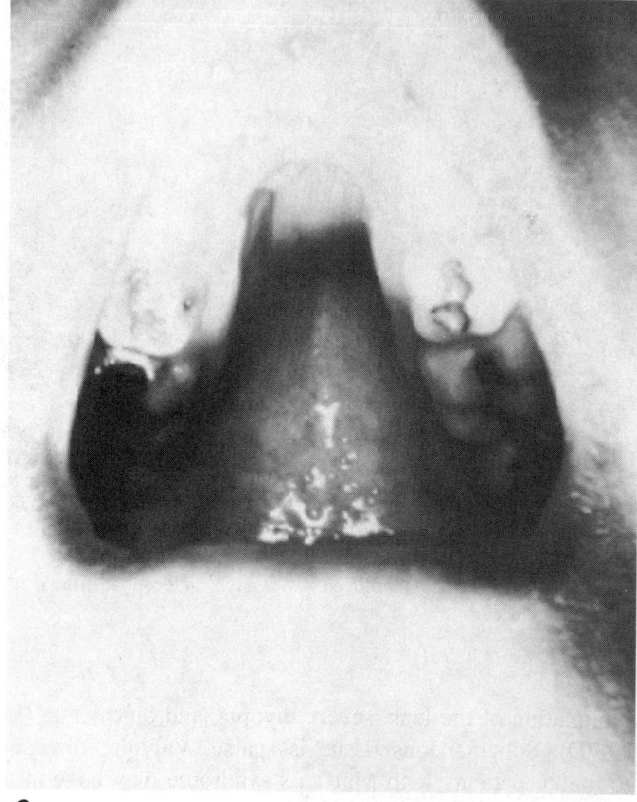

C

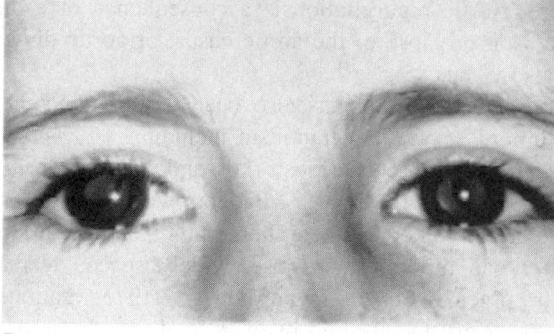

D

FIGURE 10-7

Marfan's syndrome. *A*. Long, narrow face. *B*. Arachnodactyly and positive wrist sign. *C*. High-arched palate. *D*. Ectopia lentis associated with aortic aneurysm and severe aortic regurgitation in a teenage girl.

syndrome is associated with a high incidence of complex congenital heart disease. Cardiovascular malformations are found in 15 to 25 percent of newborns with omphalocele.[102]

Teratogenic effects resulting in congenital heart disease may be alcohol-induced, the result of rubella during pregnancy, or induced by phenytoin, thalidomide, or lithium.[103]

From 30 to 40 percent of children born to alcoholic mothers are affected with the *fetal alcohol syndrome*.[104] These children have an undeveloped-appearing central face because of maxillary hypoplasia, a small and upturned nose, an indistinct or smooth philtrum, micrognathia, and a thin upper lip and vermilion (Fig. 10-11). Atrial and ventricular septal defects are most common, but many other cardiac defects can also be

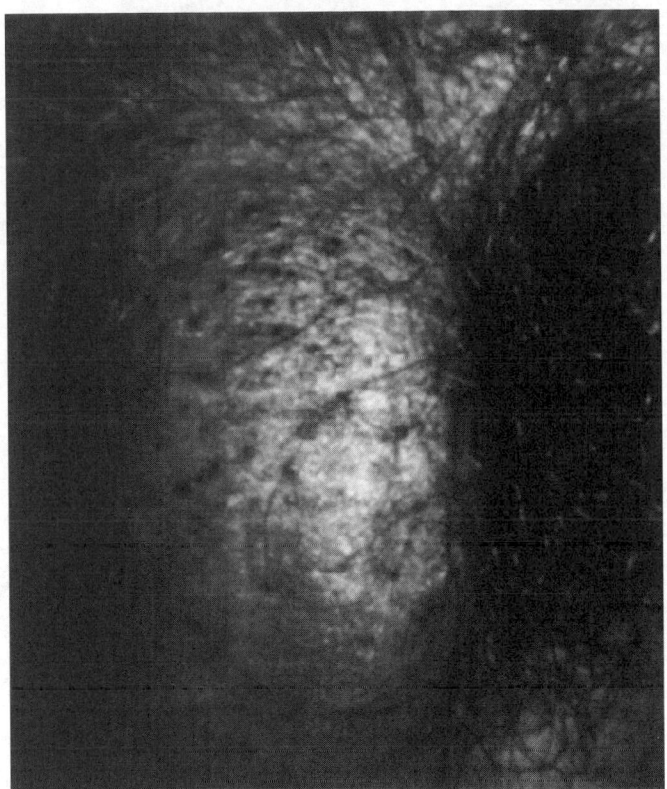

FIGURE 10-8
Fabry's disease: dark red angiokeratomas on the penis may be linked with coronary artery disease.

found. The teratogenic effects of the *rubella syndrome* include cataracts, deafness, and microcephaly. The most frequent congenital cardiac disorders are patent ductus arteriosus, pulmonic valvular and/or arterial stenosis, and atrial septal defect.[105]

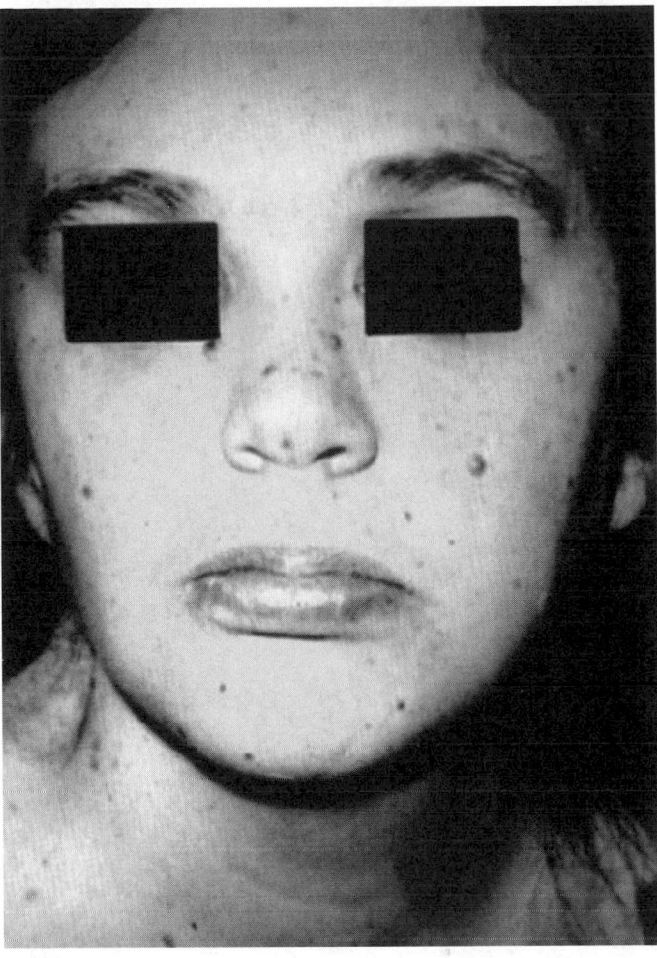

FIGURE 10-10
Turner's syndrome: epicanthal folds, pigmented moles, hypertelorism, and scars on the neck where webs have been removed may be associated with coarctation of the aorta.

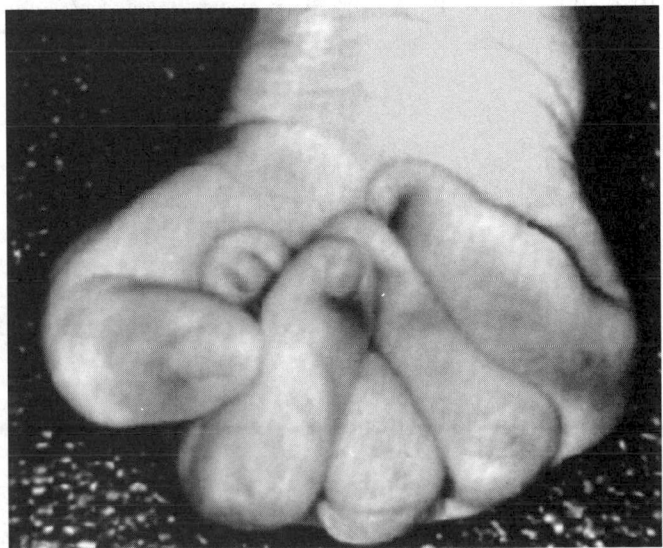

FIGURE 10-9
Trisomy 18 syndrome: tightly clenched fist with overlapping index and fifth fingers. A ventricular septal defect was present.

Important clues to the diagnosis of underlying congenital heart disease may be obtained from careful observation of the thorax and extremities. Bilateral prominence of the anterior chest with bulging of the upper two-thirds of the sternum is commonly present in children with a large ventricular septal defect. A unilateral bulge at the fourth and fifth intercostal spaces at the lower left sternal border often is found in adults with ventricular septal defects. A bulge in the area of the second and third intercostal spaces at the left sternal border may result from an underlying atrial septal defect. Scoliosis is commonly present in cyanotic congenital heart disease. Underdeveloped musculature of the lower extremities compared with the upper extremities occurs with coarctation of the aorta. Clubbing of the digits and cyanosis of the skin or nails suggest congenital heart disease with right-to-left shunting of blood (Fig. 10-12, Plate 5).

Differential cyanosis often provides a clue to exact pathological anatomy.[106] Cyanosis and clubbing of the toes associated with pink fingernails of the right hand and minimal cyanosis and clubbing of the left hand are due to pulmonary

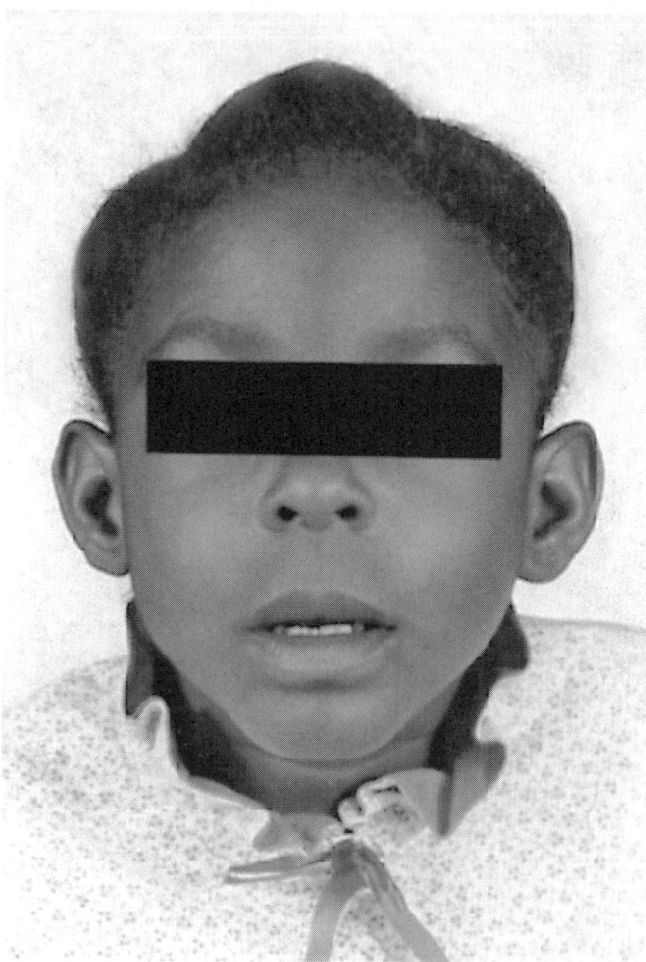

FIGURE 10-11
Fetal alcohol syndrome: midface hypoplasia, absent philtrum, and microcephaly associated with a ventricular septal defect.

hypertension with normally related great vessels and a reversed shunt, with the patent ductus arteriosus bringing unoxygenated blood to the left arm and lower extremities (Fig. 10-13, Plate 6). The same pattern results from interruption of the aortic arch and a patent ductus arteriosus delivering desaturated blood to the legs. If the right subclavian artery arises proximal to the aortic obstruction, the right hand may be pink and the left hand cyanotic. When an anomalous right subclavian artery originates from the descending aorta, however, both hands are cyanotic. Cyanosis of the fingers greater than that in the toes suggests complete transposition of the great vessels with preductal coarctation or complete interrup-

FIGURE 10-12
See color Plate 5.

FIGURE 10-13
See color Plate 6.

FIGURE 10-14
See color Plate 7.

FIGURE 10-15
See color Plate 8.

FIGURE 10-16
See color Plate 9.

tion of the aortic arch, pulmonary hypertension, and a reverse shunt through a patent ductus arteriosus delivering oxygenated blood to the lower extremities (Fig. 10-14, Plate 7). In this anomaly, the presence of aortic coarctation can be distinguished from complete interruption of the aortic arch. Slightly less cyanosis of the left arm when compared with the right arm favors aortic coarctation; while intense symmetric cyanosis of both arms is seen with complete aortic interruption. Red fingertips ("tuft erythema") may signify a small, intermittent right-to-left shunt with only slight reduction in arterial oxygen saturation (Fig. 10-15, Plate 8).

Anotia (congenital absence of the pinna) and facial paralysis may be signs of an underlying ventricular septal defect and pulmonic stenosis.[107] The presence of any congenital somatic abnormality should always prompt a search for congenital heart disease. Extracardiac anomalies were found in 25 percent of infants seen during the first year for significant cardiac disease in one study.[108] The defects were commonly found in the musculoskeletal system and were associated with specific syndromes.

DISORDERS AFFECTING THE VALVES

The cutaneous lesions of *infective endocarditis* (Chap. 82) include Osler's nodes, Janeway lesions, clubbing of the fingers (Fig. 10-16, Plate 9), splinter hemorrhages of the nails, and petechiae.[109,110] *Osler's nodes* are reddish-purple, tender nodules typically found in the distal pad of the finger or toe (Fig. 10-17; Fig. 10-18, Plate 10). By contrast, *Janeway lesions*

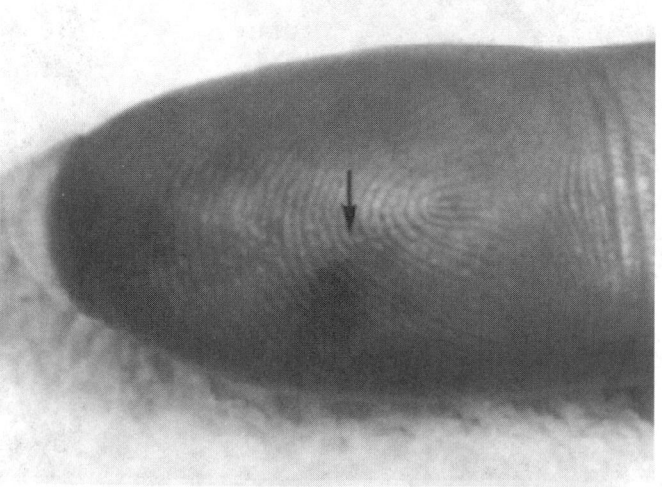

FIGURE 10-17
Bacterial endocarditis: valvular infection associated with a tender, purplish nodule (Osler's node) in the finger pad (*arrow*).

FIGURE 10-18
See color Plate 10.

are hemorrhagic but nontender and involve the palms or soles. Splinter hemorrhages are linear and black and affect the distal third of the fingernail. They are also present in many unrelated diseases and may result from trauma in otherwise healthy people.

Certain features suggest primary valvular heart disease (Chaps. 63, 64, 66). Pulmonic stenosis may be part of Noonan's syndrome, Turner's syndrome (previously discussed), Rubinstein-Taybi syndrome, rubella syndrome (see above), the multiple lentigines syndrome, pulmonary valve dysplasia, or Watson's syndrome. In *Noonan's syndrome*,[111] the characteristic findings include ptosis, low-set ears, downward-slanting eyes, webbed neck, hypertelorism, low posterior hairline, short stature, mental retardation, and normal chromosomes (Fig. 10-19). Broad toes and thumbs, a slanting forehead, a thin, beaked nose, and large, low-set ears are seen in *Rubinstein-Taybi* syndrome (Fig. 10-20).[112] Café au lait spots and mental retardation are linked to pulmonic valve stenosis in *Watson's syndrome.*

The *multiple lentigines syndrome* is identified by the presence of multiple tan-to-brown macules varying in size from pinpoint to 5 cm in diameter (Fig. 10-21). These cutaneous lesions may affect the entire body but are most heavily concentrated on the neck and upper thorax. Other findings in this syndrome include hearing loss, short stature, hypertelorism, ptosis, prognathism, pectus excavatum or carinatum, kyphoscoliosis, café au lait spots, and other skeletal defects.[113]

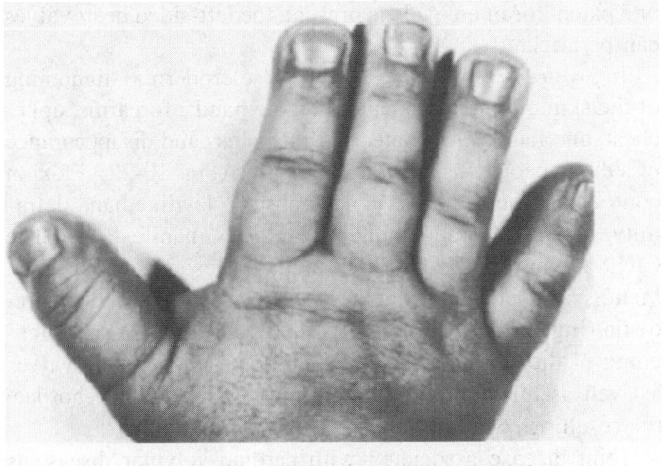
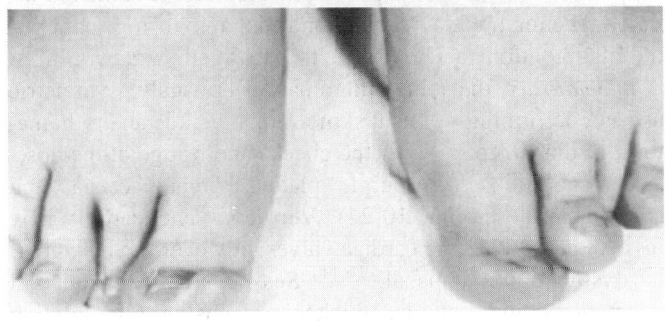

FIGURE 10-20
Rubinstein-Taybi syndrome may be associated with a variety of congenital heart defects. (From Silverman ME, Hurst JW. The hand and heart. *Am J Cardiol* 1968; 22:718. Reproduced with permission from the publisher and authors.)

The *carcinoid syndrome* may present as intense flushing of the face; a chronic cyanotic hue and telangiectasia may be present. Stenosis and/or regurgitation of the tricuspid and/or pulmonic valves often result when hepatic metastases are present.[114] When a patent ductus arteriosus, lung metastases,

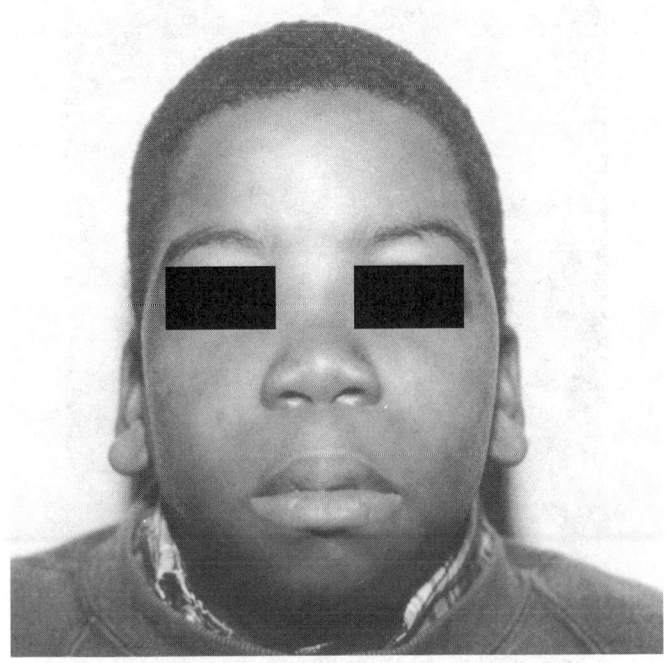

FIGURE 10-19
Noonan's syndrome: ptosis, hypertelorism, and low-set ears associated with valvular pulmonic stenosis.

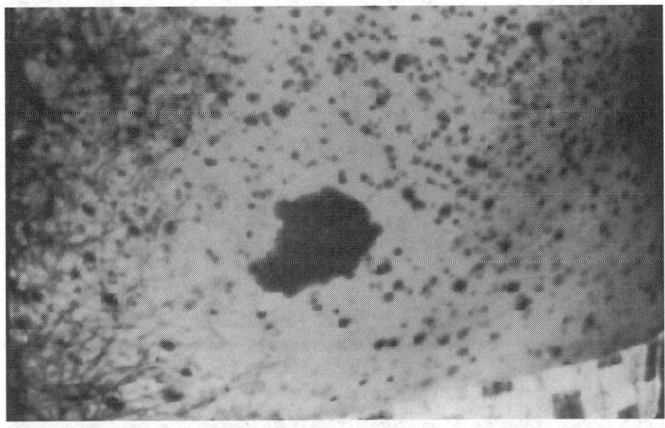

FIGURE 10-21
Multiple lentigines syndrome: dark brown macular lesions of the abdomen associated with hypertrophic subaortic stenosis. (From Silverman ME. Visual clues to diagnosis. *Primary Cardiology*, October 1986. Reproduced with permission from the publisher and author.)

or a patent foramen ovale is present, the left-sided heart valves can be affected.

In *progressive systemic sclerosis* (scleroderma), tightening of the skin on the fingers and then the hands, forearms, upper chest, and face is associated with hair loss and disappearance of subcutaneous tissue and skin creases (Fig. 10-22). Flexion contractures on the fingers may cause a clawlike hand deformity. Raynaud's phenomenon is an early manifestation. The CREST syndrome (calcinosis, Raynaud's esophageal involvement, sclerodactyly, and telangiectasia) is a variant of scleredema (Fig. 10-23). Although valvular changes include thickening of the edges of the mitral, aortic, and tricuspid valves as well as thickening and shortening of the mitral chordae, the resulting valve disease is rarely significant.[115]

Joint disease associated with cardiac valvular disease is frequent with systemic lupus erythematosus, rheumatoid arthritis, rheumatic fever, polychondritis, ankylosing spondylitis, alkaptonuria, and Whipple's disease. In *systemic lupus erythematosus*, the joint inflammation is usually symmetric and nondeforming. Typical skin lesions include an erythematous, scaling eruption over the cheeks and bridge of the nose, circumscribed reddish-purple plaques, telangiectasia, and patchy hair loss (Fig. 10-24). Verrucous endocarditis may involve any of the four cardiac valves; however, severe valvular dysfunction is unusual.[116,117] Sessile, small, nonbacterial vegetations and valvular thickening causing regurgitation rather than stenosis may be more common in patients with antiphospholipid antibodies[118] (see also Chap. 85).

In patients with *rheumatoid arthritis*, the metacarpophalangeal joints, proximal interphalangeal joints, wrists, metatarsophalangeal joints, shoulders, knees, ankles, and elbows are

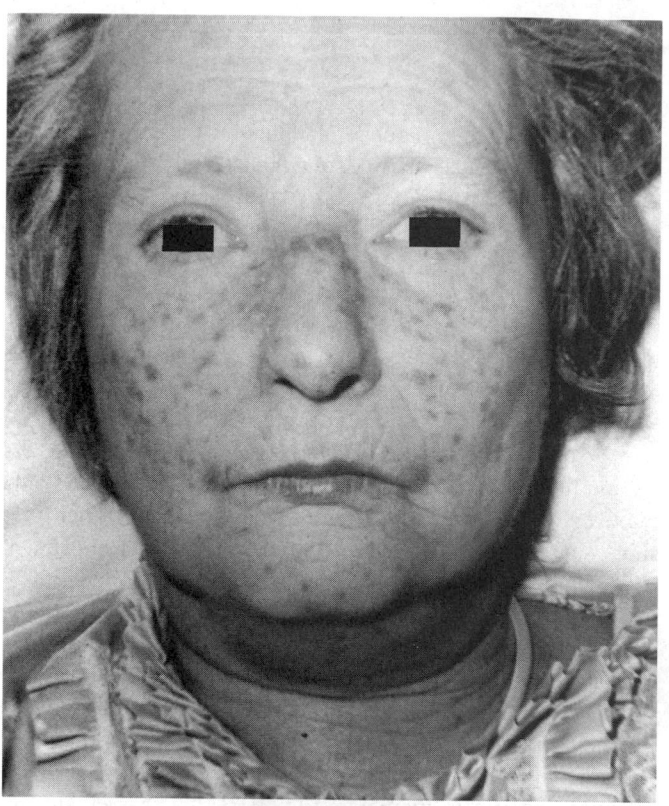

FIGURE 10-23
CREST syndrome: Telangiectasia of the face in a patient with Raynaud's phenomenon and sclerodactyly.

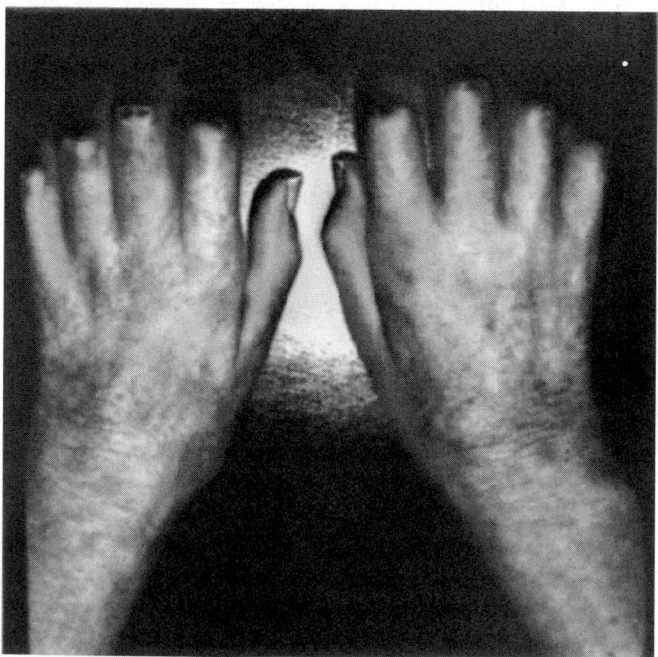

FIGURE 10-22
Scleroderma: clawlike hand deformity and shiny, tight skin may be linked with myocardial fibrosis.

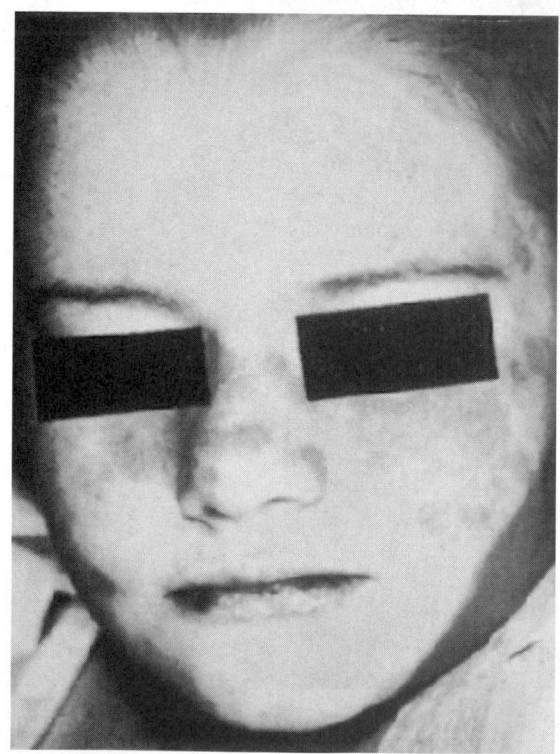

FIGURE 10-24
Systemic lupus erythematosus: butterfly rash associated with pericardial, myocardial, and endocardial disease.

involved with inflammation and subsequent destruction. Advanced disease results in ulnar deviation of the fingers, flexion of the distal interphalangeal joints with hyperextension of the proximal interphalangeal joints, producing a "swan-neck" deformity, and a Z-shaped configuration of the thumb. Subluxation of the metacarpophalangeal joints with interosseal muscle wasting and thickening of the wrists are common. Granulomatous aortic or mitral valve disease with regurgitation is most common in patients who are seropositive and have subcutaneous nodules or classic rheumatoid deformities.[119] *Rheumatic fever*, often with cardiac involvement, should be suspected in patients with erythema marginatum, urticaria, and migratory polyarthritis involving the large joints (see Chap. 62). Subcutaneous nodules are less frequently found. Marked ulnar deviation at the metacarpophalangeal joints, suggesting rheumatoid arthritis, can be due to repeated attacks of rheumatic fever and is known as *Jaccoud's or postrheumatic fever arthritis*. In contrast to rheumatoid arthritis, the fingers can be moved freely into a correct alignment and x-rays of the hands are normal.

Polychondritis causes an inflammatory destruction of the cartilage of the face, resulting in a saddle-shaped collapse of the nose or a cauliflower ear. Aortic regurgitation, aortic aneurysm, and rarely aortic root dissection are associated (Fig. 10-25).[120]

Chronic synovitis involving the fibrocartilaginous joints of the spine occurs in patients with *ankylosing spondylitis*. The disease may be confined to a sacroiliac area or spread slowly upward. The patient with advanced disease is bent forward, is unable to stand upright, and must walk with a stiff and halting gait (Fig. 10-26). Aortic regurgitation, due to thickening and shortening of the aortic cusps from perivascular inflammation and fibrosis, occurs in up to 10 percent of patients.[121] Mitral regurgitation and complete heart block may also occur. *Cogan's syndrome*, consisting of ophthalmic inflammation and audiovestibular symptoms, is another cause of vasculitis involving the aortic root and leading to aortic regurgitation and coronary disease.[122]

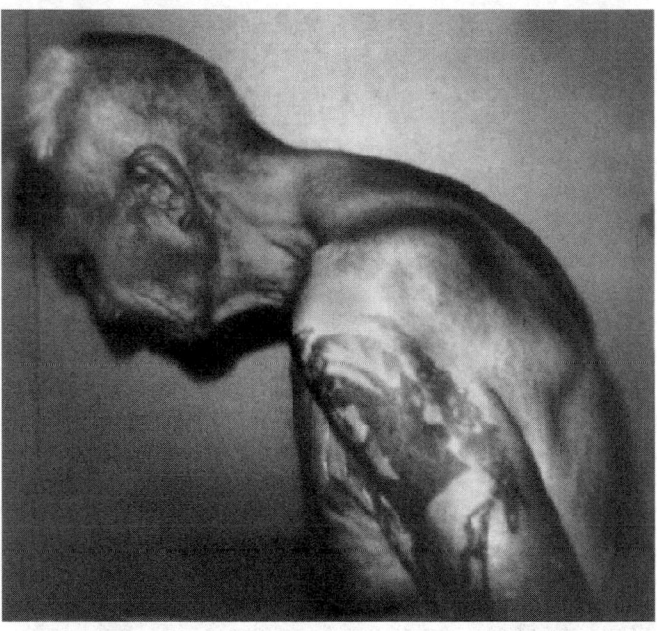

Whipple's disease is suggested by the combination of polyarthritis, abdominal pain, and diarrhea. Aortic and mitral regurgitation and endocarditis are known complications.[123] Aortic or mitral valvular disease may also be due to an accumulation of homogentisic acid in *alkaptonuria*. Blue-black, stiff pinnae and joints are important clues to this inherited disorder of tyrosine metabolism.

External signs of mitral valve prolapse (see also Chap. 65) include a straight thoracic spine, pectus excavatum, scoliosis, hypomastia, joint laxity, and various neuromuscular disorders. Systolic and rarely diastolic murmurs have been described with chest wall deformities due to *straight-back syndrome* and *pectus excavatum*, which may impinge on or displace the heart.

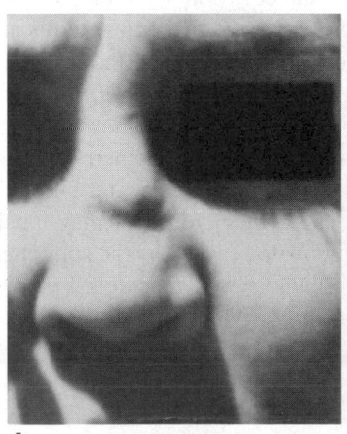 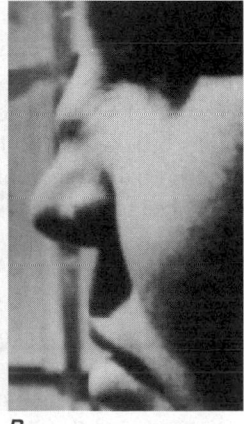

FIGURE 10-25
Polychondritis. *A, B*. Destruction of cartilage of nose, producing a "saddle nose" in association with aortic regurgitation. (Courtesy of Dr. Warren Sarrell, Anniston, AL.)

DISORDERS ASSOCIATED WITH CARDIOMYOPATHY

Hypertrophic cardiomyopathy (Chap. 74) has been associated with Friedreich's ataxia, Turner's syndrome, Noonan's syndrome, Fabry's disease, neurofibromatosis, and the multiple lentigines syndrome. *Friedreich's ataxia* is a spinocerebellar degenerative disorder that results in a broad-based, lurching gait, impaired vibration, position, and joint sense, and incoordination. Kyphoscoliosis and pes cavus (high instep, retraction of the toes at the metatarsal-phalangeal joints, and hammer toes) are two important physical signs (Fig. 10-27). Concentric and asymmetric left ventricular hypertrophy that may evolve into a dilated cardiomyopathy have each been described.[124]

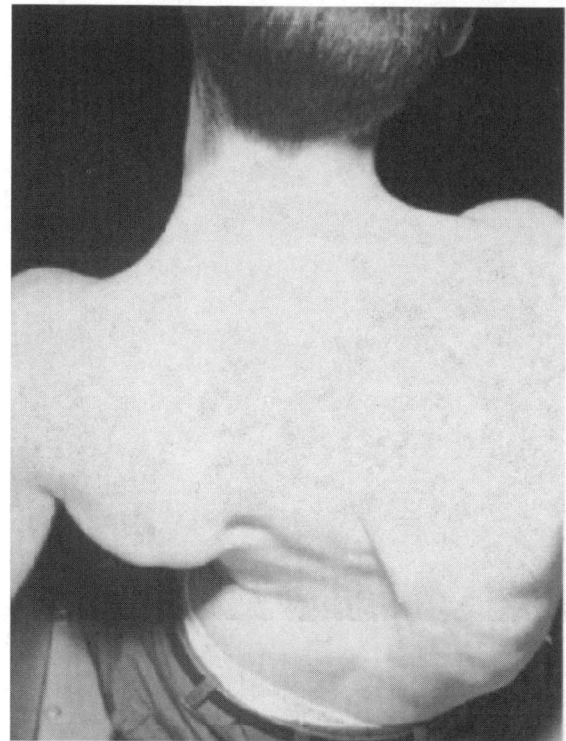

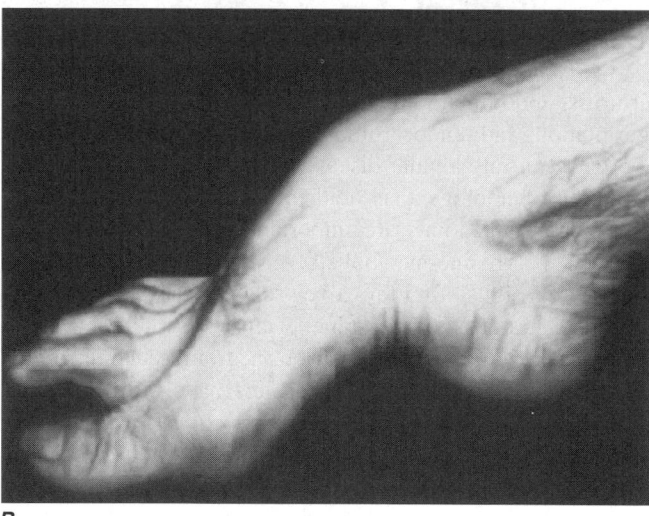

FIGURE 10-27
Friedreich's ataxia (photographs from different patients). *A.* Kyphoscoliosis. *B.* Pes cavus. Myocardial fibrosis and hypertrophy are often present. (From Silverman ME. Visual clues to diagnosis. *Primary Cardiology*, June 1987. Reproduced with permission from the publisher and authors.)

Myocardial hypertrophy may be secondary to extreme *obesity* or *acromegaly*. With acromegaly, the broad forehead, thickened skin, and enlarged nose, lip, and tongue produce coarsened facial features (Fig. 10-28), while elongation of the mandible leads to prognathism and overbite. The large, sausage-shaped fingers and spadelike configuration of the hands are typical.[125]

Cor pulmonale and right ventricular hypertrophy may be secondary to pulmonary hypertension caused by *kyphoscolio-*

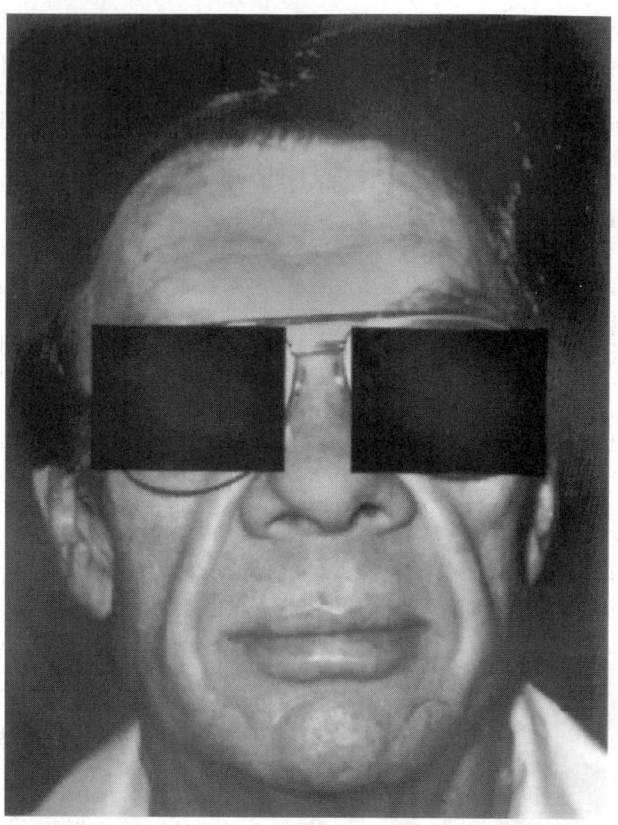

FIGURE 10-28
Acromegaly: coarse facial features, folds of skin, and prognathism are associated with myocardial hypertrophy and fibrosis. (From Silverman ME. Visual clues to diagnosis. *Primary Cardiology*, February 1987. Reproduced with permission from the publisher, author, and patient.)

sis, restrictive lung disease, progressive systemic sclerosis, *upper airway blockade* by enlarged tonsils[126] and adenoids, or the *sleep apnea syndrome* associated with extreme obesity.[127]

Myocarditis (Chap. 76) occurs with systemic lupus erythematosus, rheumatic fever, Reiter's syndrome,[128] Kawasaki's disease,[129] Lyme arthritis,[130] and occasionally Whipple's disease. *Reiter's syndrome* is characterized by conjunctivitis and hyperkeratotic coalescing lesions encrusted on the soles and palms, associated with arthritis and urethritis. *Kawasaki's disease* begins with fever, nonexudative conjunctivitis, dry, fissured lips, cervical adenopathy, and a strawberry tongue. Later, the palms and soles become indurated and purplish-red and then peel. A widespread erythematous rash may appear and then desquamate. *Lyme arthritis*, caused by the spirochete *Borrelia burgdorferi*, begins with a red macule or papule, then develops into an expanding erythematous rash with a bright red border known as erythema migrans (Fig. 10-29). The center of the rash may clear, indurate, blister, or become necrotis. Multiple annular lesions may develop.

Diseases that cause myocardial fibrosis include dermatomyositis, Duchenne's and Becker's muscular dystrophy, myotonic muscular dystrophy, Kearns-Sayres syndrome, Friedreich's ataxia, sarcoidosis, and progressive systemic sclerosis (see also Chaps. 69 and 85). With *dermatomyositis*, an erythe-

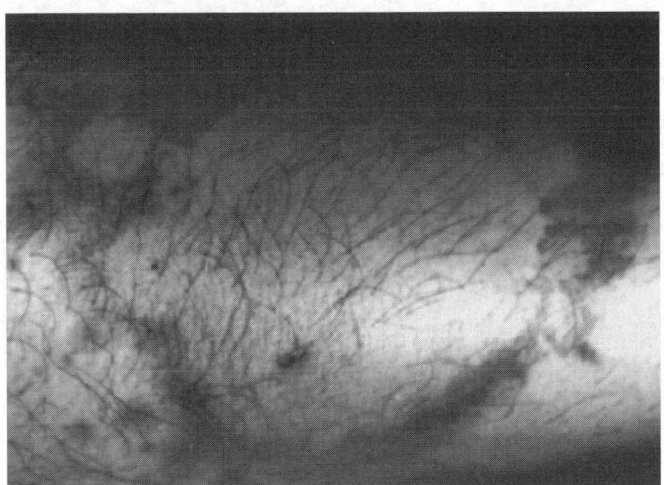

FIGURE 10-29

Lyme arthritis: annular expanding rash with a clear central area may be associated with pericarditis and AV block. (From Silverman ME. Visual clues to diagnosis. *Primary Cardiology*, December 1986. Reproduced with permission from the publisher and author.)

matous eruption and periorbital heliotrophic discoloration affects the face (Fig. 10-30, Plate 11) and a scaly, erythematous rash may cover the knuckles, sparing the interphalangeal region.[131] A waddling gait and pseudohypertrophic calves are characteristic of Duchenne's muscular dystrophy. The electrocardiogram ECG is commonly consistent with fibrosis of the posterior left ventricle.[132] In *myotonic dystrophy* drooping eyelids, cataracts, a receding hairline, and a masklike expression are present.[133] The *Kearns-Sayre syndrome* is a form of ocular muscular dystrophy in which external ophthalmoplegia, ptosis, and retinitis pigmentosa occur.[134] The skin manifestations of *sarcoidosis* include erythema nodosum, lupus pernio (a red or violet plaque with a predilection for the nose, cheeks, eyelids, and ears), and waxy translucent papules found on the cheeks, periorbital area, ears, nasolabial folds, and elsewhere.[135] Uveitis, bilateral parotid and lacrymal gland enlargement, and arthritis are other signs (see also Chap. 69).

Isolated noncompaction of the left ventricular myocardium is characterized by numerous, prominent ventricular trabeculations, deep intertrabecular recesses, arrhythmias, and a distinctive facial dysmorphism.

Infiltrative diseases of the myocardium include Wilson's disease, Cori's disease, Fabry's disease, hemochromatosis, amyloidosis, glycogen storage disease, and sarcoidosis (see also Chap. 75). Wilson's disease is an autosomal recessive disorder in which copper accumulates in tissues, including the myocardium.[136] Arrhythmias, autonomic dysfunction, and cardiomyopathy have been reported. Kayser-Fleischer rings, usually golden-brown in color and circling the edge of the cornea, provide a major clue to the correct diagnosis. *Cori's disease* (type III glycogenosis) is suspected when a patient has xanthomas and a yellowish skin. In *hemochromatosis*,

FIGURE 10-30
See color Plate 11.

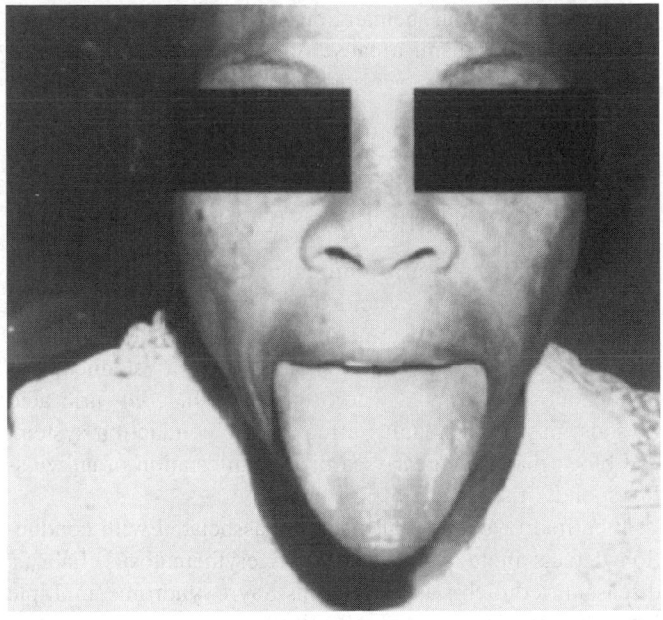

FIGURE 10-31

Amyloidosis: enlarged tongue may be a sign of an infiltrative cardiomyopathy. (From Silverman ME. Visual clues to diagnosis. *Primary Cardiology*, November 1987. Reproduced with permission from the publisher, author, and patient.)

the skin has a bronze or slate-gray coloration; myocardial infiltration with iron deposits often causes a dilated or rarely a restrictive cardiomyopathy associated with arrhythmias and heart failure[137] Macroglossia and waxy nodules of the skin and eyelids, which may hemorrhage when pinched, are clues to the diagnosis of *amyloidosis* (Fig. 10-31).[138] (see also Chap. 75). Glycogen storage disease and myxedema can also enlarge the tongue.

DISORDERS ASSOCIATED WITH PERICARDIAL DISEASE

Pericarditis may be a result of Reiter's syndrome, Whipple's disease, Kawasaki's disease, systemic lupus erythematosus, rheumatoid arthritis,[139] rheumatic fever, sarcoidosis, scleroderma, dermatomyositis, hemochromatosis, Behçet's disease, Degos' disease, uremia, mulibrey nanism, polychondritis, hypothyroidism, or metastatic disease among others (see also Chap. 81). The components of *Behçet's disease* include erythema nodosum, superficial phlebitis, oral and genital ulcers, and iritis.[140] Patients with *Degos' disease* (malignant atrophic papulosis) present with painless, oval cutaneous lesions that have a white center and surrounding erythema. In this rapidly fatal disease, occlusive fibrosis of small- and medium-size arteries produces pleuritis and pericarditis. In far-advanced renal disease, urochrome pigmentation of the skin and uremic frost are cutaneous manifestations. The term *mulibrey nanism* describes a syndrome involving muscle, liver, brain, and eyes.[141] These patients have a triangular face, bulging forehead, low nasal bridge, growth retardation, pigmentary changes in the fundus, hemangiomas, and constrictive pericarditis. Hypothyroidism, a cause of often massive pericardial effusions, thickens the face and causes dry hair, puffy eyelids, and an enlarged tongue.

DISORDERS CAUSING CONDUCTION SYSTEM DISEASE

Acquired causes of atrioventricular (AV) block or bundle branch block include sarcoidosis,[135] rheumatic fever, gout, Reiter's syndrome,[142] dermatomyositis, amyloidosis, Kawasaki's disease,[143] ankylosing spondylitis,[129] systemic lupus erythematosus,[117] and Lyme arthritis.[130] In *gout*, uric acid crystals may form nodules affecting the conduction system. AV block may be an early cardiac manifestation of ankylosing spondylitis.

Inherited or congenital disorders associated with conduction defects include systemic lupus erythematosus, Fabry's disease, Friedreich's ataxia, Kearns-Sayre syndrome, multiple lentigines syndrome, muscular dystrophy, myotonic dystrophy, tuberous sclerosis, and Refsum's disease. Maternal lupus is an important cause of congenital complete AV block in the newborn.[116] In *Refsum's disease*, a lipidosis and genetically determined neuropathy characterized by high levels of phytanic acid, cerebellar ataxia, night blindness, deafness, ichthyosis, cataracts, and polyneuropathy have been associated with myocardial disease and conduction abnormalities.

Syndactyly (webbing of the hands or feet) has been found with a long QT interval—a syndrome with a high risk of sudden death.[144]

DISORDERS AFFECTING THE VASCULAR SYSTEM

Aortic aneurysms and dissection (Chap. 98) are frequent cardiovascular complications of the Marfan and Ehlers-Danlos syndromes.[86,88,144] Aneurysms of other vessels and arterial rupture may also occur. A progressive looseness of skin, producing pendulous folds and droopy eyelids, can be due to *cutis laxa*, a generalized destruction of elastic tissue that can cause dilatation of the aorta or pulmonary artery and aortic rupture.[85]

Coronary artery stenosis from atherosclerosis can be associated with hyperlipidemia,[145] cerebrotendinous xanthomatoses, Werner's syndrome, uremia, progeria, acromegaly, and diabetes mellitus. *Hyperlipidemia* may be suspected when xanthomas or arcus senilis are present. Xanthelasma usually involve the upper eyelid. When they occur before age 50, there is a strong association with familial hypercholesterolemia and premature coronary artery disease. Eruptive xanthomata are recognized as papules with yellow centers surrounded by an erythematous halo. They often appear with a sudden outbreak of discrete 1- to 4-cm lesions on the buttocks, back, thighs, and exterior surfaces of the knees and elbows. They indicate a very high level of triglycerides and are associated with hyperlipidemia, diabetes mellitus, pancreatitis, myxedema,

and the nephrotic syndrome. Tendon xanthomata are firm, painless nodules that thicken the exterior tendons of the hand, the Achilles tendons, and sometimes the tendons of the knees and elbows (Fig. 10-32). *Cerebrotendinous xanthomatosis* is a rare disorder in which tendon xanthomas, cataracts, dementia, ataxia, neuropathy, and accelerated atherosclerosis are present. Tuberous xanthomata are yellow to deep-orange papules erupting over the elbows, knees, buttocks, and heels. They may coalesce or be pedunculated and are a manifestation of hyperlipidemia, myxedema, and liver disease. Large, orange, lobulated tonsils are a finding in *Tangier disease*, in which there is deficiency of high-density lipoprotein.

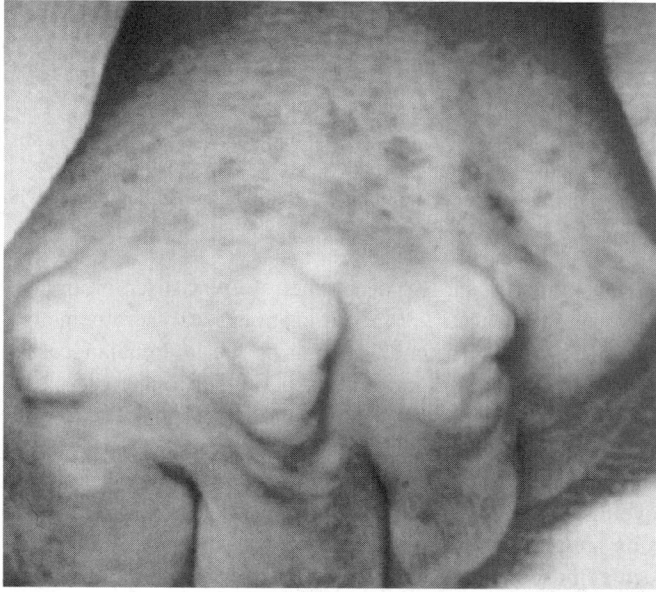

A

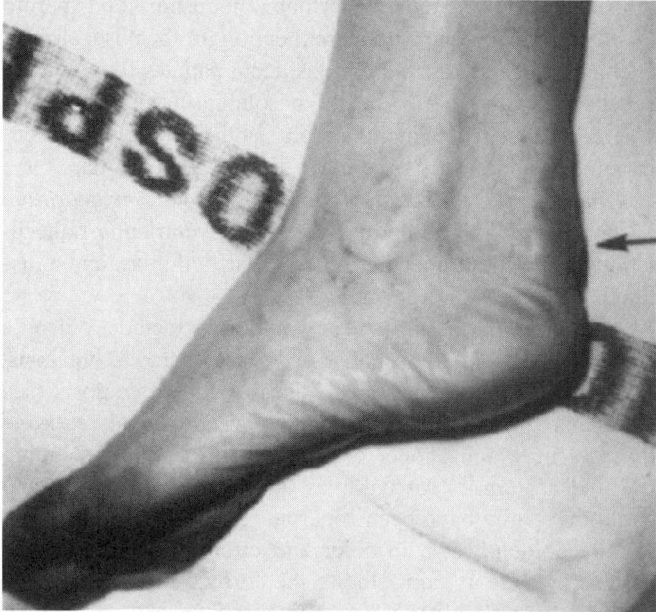

B

FIGURE 10-32

Hyperlipidemia: xanthomata associated with coronary artery disease. *A.* On the extensor tendons of the hand. *B.* On the Achilles tendon (*arrow*).

In *Werner's syndrome*, the skin is tightly stretched over the underlying bones.[146] There is marked loss of subcutaneous tissue, and ulcerations occur over the legs. Severe coronary atherosclerosis often results in myocardial infarction at an early age. Physical findings in diabetes mellitus may include tight skin and *necrobiosis diabeticorum*, an atrophy of the skin of the lower extremities characterized by ovoid plaques with central telangectasia and a violet, undurated perimeter. *Progeria* is a rare disorder in which the face is small and prematurely aged, the eyes bulge, and the nose is beaked. Severe atherosclerosis with early myocardial infarction is a common cause of death in early life.[147] A diagonal earlobe crease and short tufts of ear-canal hair have been curiously associated with coronary artherosclerosis.[148] There is a modest correlation between male-pattern baldness involving the vertex of the scalp in men under 55 years of age and an increased risk of myocardial infarction.[149] Patients resemble those with Marfan's syndrome because they have long extremities, pectus carinatum, and kyphoscoliosis. Pseudoxanthoma elasticum has been associated with fibrosis of coronary artery and calcification of peripheral arteries[150] (Chap. 85). A glycosphingolipid is deposited in the arterial endothelium of patients with Fabry's disease and may result in angina pectoris or myocardial infarction. Patients with Hurler's syndrome have mental retardation; a large, boat-shaped head; a broad nose; large lips; small, widely spaced teeth; and a large, protuberant tongue. Glycosaminoglycan deposition in the coronary arteries is present.[151] Myocardial fibrosis due to repeated coronary small-vessel spasm has been postulated to be a result of progressive systemic sclerosis.[115]

Vasculitis may be due to systemic lupus erythematosus, rheumatoid arthritis, Behçet's disease,[140] Kawasaki's disease,[179] and polyarteritis. Cutaneous infarction, nodules, petechiae, livedo reticularis, gangrenous digits, myocardial infarction, heart failure, and hypertension may be due to polyarteritis[152] (see also Chap. 85).

Arteriovenous shunts may be found in extensive skin disease, hereditary hemorrhagic telangiectasia (HHT), and the Klippel-Trenaunay-Weber syndrome. *Kaposi's sarcoma* or *exfoliative dermatitis* due to psoriasis may divert the blood supply through shunts in the skin to produce high-output cardiac failure. Clues to underlying *arteriovenous fistula* as a cause of high-output failure include a barely discernible scar from a knife wound or a surgical incision. Telangiectasia of the fingertips, face, palate, lips, and tongue as well as pulmonary and hepatic arteriovenous fistulas are components of *hereditary hemorrhagic telangiectasia*.[83] The triad of anomalies that *Klippel-Trenaunay-Weber syndrome* comprises are vascular nevus, large varices, and bony or soft-tissue hypertrophy.[153] Marked enlargement of a limb(s) and facial hemihypertrophy are features of this disorder, in which part or all of the deep venous system is absent and arteriovenous malformation is often present. Hemangiomas of the skin may also indicate multinodular hemangiomatosis of the liver, a cause of high-output heart failure in infancy (Fig. 10-33).

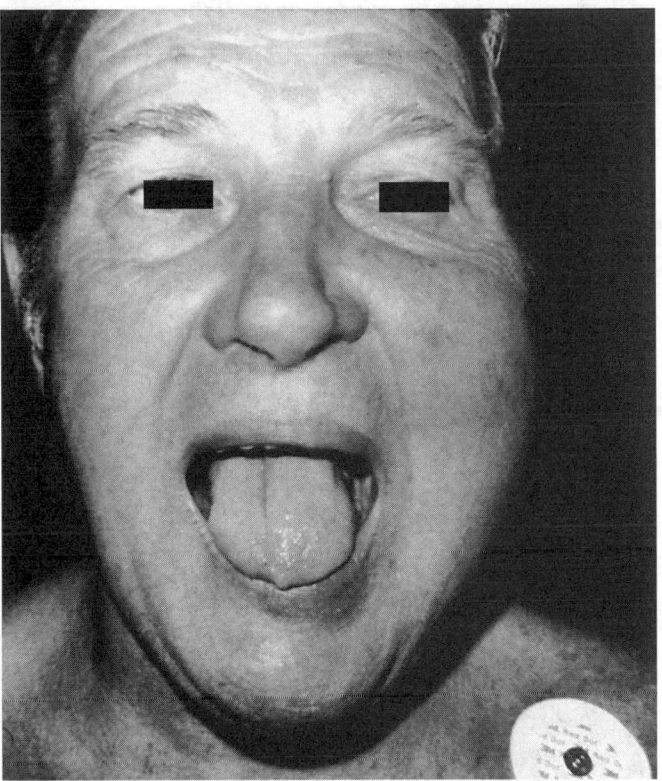

FIGURE 10-33
Klippel-Trenaunay syndrome: hypertrophy of left side of face and tongue in patient with port-wine stains, gigantism of digits, and varicose veins.

Stenosis of large arteries may occur with supravalvular aortic stenosis, rubella syndrome, Turner's syndrome, and neurofibromatosis. The face of a child with supravalvular aortic stenosis (Williams syndrome) is almost diagnostic (Fig. 10-34). The head is small, with an elflike appearance; the cheeks are full and baggy, and the mouth is large.[154] Thick lips and peg-shaped, widely spaced teeth are typical findings. The forehead is prominent and broad. Mental retardation is often present. The supravalvular aortic stenosis may be a localized ridge or a diffuse narrowing of the aorta beginning just above the sinuses of Valsalva. Pulmonic artery branch stenosis is frequently present. Coarctation of the aorta is a common cardiac lesion in Turner's syndrome,[95] and neurofibromatosis has been associated with renal artery stenosis.

Facial swelling and jugular venous distention may be early signs of *superior vena caval obstruction* from clot or tumor.

MISCELLANEOUS DISORDERS

Multiple lentigines, cutaneous myxomas, myxoid fibroadenomas of the breast, and various endocrine abnormalities are features of a recently described inherited disorder in which single or multiple cardiac myxoma occur.[155]

Telangiectasia of the tongue and lips or under the fingernails may be associated with a pulmonary arteriovenous fistula (Figs. 10-35 and 10-36, Plates 12 and 13).

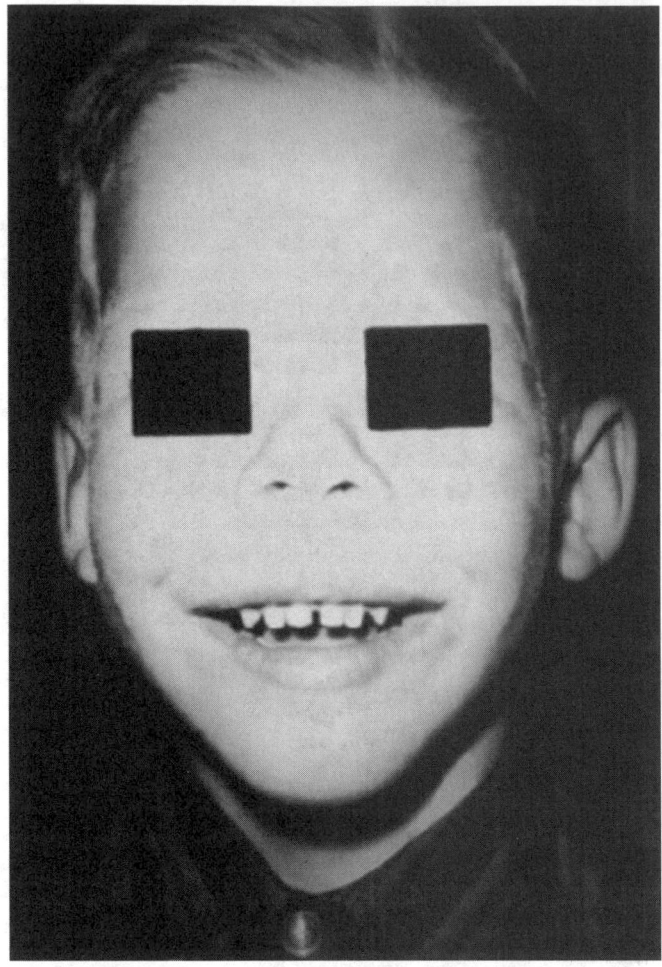

FIGURE 10-34
Supravalvular aortic stenosis: turned-up nose, broad cheeks, large mouth with peg-shaped teeth, and large ears.

A susceptibility to atrial fibrillation and atrial flutter has been documented in patients who have *facioscapulohumeral muscular dystrophy*.[156] Sinus node dysfunction, elbow contractures, and humeroperoneal weakness are manifestations of *Emery-Dreifuss muscular dystrophy*.[157]

Single or multiple rhabdomyomas may develop within the myocardium and cause heart failure, valvular obstruction, or arrhythmias in patients with tuberous sclerosis (Fig. 10-37, Plate 14).[158] The diagnosis is suggested by the presence of yellow-brown angiofibromas ("adenoma sebaceum") on the face, subungual fibromas around the fingernail, café au lait spots, and subcutaneous nodules.

FIGURE 10-35
See color Plate 12.

FIGURE 10-36
See color Plate 13.

FIGURE 10-37
See color Plate 14.

MEASUREMENT OF ARTERIAL BLOOD PRESSURE

The use of a pneumatic cuff for the noninvasive assessment of the arterial blood pressure is the most commonly used method for determining the status of the circulation and the interaction between the heart and arterial system. Blood pressure deviations from normal often provide important diagnostic information in patients with a variety of cardiac and noncardiac diseases.

Physical Determinants of the Arterial Pressure

The arterial blood pressure, a measure of lateral force per unit area of vascular wall, is quantitated as millimeters of mercury or dynes per square centimeter. The factors responsible for the peak systolic blood pressure include the volume and velocity of left ventricular ejection, the peripheral arteriolar resistance, the distensibility of the arterial wall, the viscosity of the blood, and the end-diastolic volume in the arterial system.[159] The subsequent diminution in pressure during diastole is, in turn, determined by blood viscosity, arterial distensibility, peripheral resistance to flow, and length of the cardiac cycle.[159] Important physical factors affecting arterial distensibility include (1) the elastic modulus of the arterial wall, the ratio of stress (force acting to deform the wall) to strain (the proportional deformation produced), and (2) the geometry of the arterial wall, i.e., the internal radius (r) and wall thickness (h), which govern wall tension (T) according to the modified Laplace equation $T = Pr/h$, where P is intravascular pressure. A decrease in elasticity or an increase in radius results in diminished distensibility and a greater rise in pressure per unit volume of blood.[160]

The mean arterial pressure is the product of the cardiac output and the total peripheral resistance, the latter often being increased by many mechanisms, including alpha-adrenergic stimulation, the renin-angiotensin system, or other circulating hormonal or humoral factors.[161]

Methods for Measuring the Arterial Pressure

DIRECT METHODS

In 1733, Stephen Hales recorded the arterial pressures in animals by cannulation and use of a blood-filled glass column.[162] Current techniques for the direct and continuous measurement of arterial pressure utilize the electromanometer, a transducer that converts mechanical energy into an electric signal suitable for amplification, display, and recording. The artery is cannulated with a saline-filled catheter or needle that mechanically couples the circulation to the arterial manometer. Pressures are recorded using atmospheric pressure as the "zero" reference level, and intravascular pressures are further referenced to the level of the heart by addition or subtraction of a gravitation factor. The gravitation factor is expressed by the formula pgh, where p is the density of blood (in grams per milliliter), g is the acceleration due to gravity

(980 cm/s^2), and h is the transducer height (centimeter) above or below the horizontal plane of the heart.

The strain-gauge manometer is commonly used for the precise and accurate measurement of the arterial pressure. However, error may originate in the catheter or coupling system, in which the properties of inertia, friction, and elasticity interact to produce damping of the frequency response. Systems may be overdamped or underdamped, both of which can result in signal distortion. Nevertheless, the appropriate combination of an inelastic cardiac catheter and connecting tube filled with bubble-free fluid produces "critical" damping in which the system response is constant to some desirable frequency level and adequate for the clinical recording of intravascular pressures.[159]

Measurement errors also occur when an end-hole catheter is positioned axial to flow in a vessel and may become especially important during high arterial flow, when kinetic energy may exceed 10 percent of the total fluid energy. The use of a side-hole catheter positioned in a large, patent artery allows measurement of the true arterial pressure. Also, pressure transients due to catheter whip can falsely elevate the measured arterial pressure.[159]

Miniature, self-flushing strain-gauge manometers attached directly to an intravascular catheter or needle eliminate many of the problems related to transducer mounting and flushing and overdamping by connective tubing. The most satisfactory method for reducing measurement errors, however, is the use of intravascular electromanometers mounted on cardiac catheters or surgically implanted in the vascular wall.

INDIRECT METHODS

The invention of the pneumatic cuff manometer (Riva-Rocci, 1896) and the subsequent discovery and use of the arterial sounds (Korotkoff, 1905) permitted indirect measurement of the arterial pressure. The most commonly used noninvasive method is based on the auscultatory detection of low-pitched Korotkoff sounds over a peripheral artery at a point distal to cuff compression of the artery. McCutcheon and Rushmer[163] described two major components of these sounds: the initial transient (k_i) and the compression murmur (k_c), which coincide with the opening tap and rumble sounds of Rodbard.[164] The initial sound k_i occurs when cuff pressure reaches arterial pressure and likely results from abrupt arterial opening and vascular distension. The intensity of this initial sound depends on the slope of the pressure pulse and the level of the distal arterial pressure at the time of arterial opening, the sound being louder with vasodilatation and high-velocity flow and softer with arterial constriction or circulatory collapse. The initial transient is probably caused by oscillation of the arterial walls as the occluded segment is suddenly opened by systolic pressure, and the compression murmur is caused by a turbulent jet of flow distal to the partially compressed segment.

The Korotkoff sounds have been divided into five phases occurring in sequence as the occluding pressure declines. Phase I consists of clear tapping sounds (k_i) that occur when the cuff pressure has fallen to the arterial peak systolic level.

These sounds are initially soft and gradually become louder as cuff pressure falls. Phase II consists of k_i sounds followed by swishing sounds or murmurs (k_c). Phase III is an augmentation of phase II sounds as an increased volume of blood passes through the partially compressed artery. Phase IV is signaled by the abrupt, distinct muffling of the sounds, resulting in a blowing quality that slowly diminishes in intensity. It is due to diminution and loss of component k_i as cuff pressure approaches arterial diastolic levels and reduction in component k_c as the flow period lengthens and velocity decreases. Phase V, complete cessation of sound, occurs when the artery is no longer compressed to an extent that produces turbulent flow. The cuff pressure at which sound disappears may be extremely low or nonexistent when high-flow velocities (e.g., from exercise, anemia, fever) exist in the circulation. This indirect method slightly underestimates the true arterial pressure.

Proper technique is important for obtaining accurate measurements of blood pressure by the indirect method. The inflatable rubber bag within the compression cuff should have a width that is 20 percent greater than the limb diameter and a length adequate to encompass two-thirds the limb. The cuff should be applied snugly, with the inflatable bag positioned over the artery, at the level of the heart. Before auscultation, the cuff is quickly inflated to a pressure 20 mmHg above the systolic, as indicated by obliteration of the radial pulse. The stethoscope is then applied lightly but firmly over the artery and auscultatory pressure is determined by noting the onset (peak systole) and behavior of the Korotkoff sounds as the cuff is deflated at a rate of about 3 mmHg per second. When the sounds disappear, the bag should be rapidly decompressed and 1 or 2 min allowed to pass before repeat determinations are made. When possible, the blood pressure should be taken with the subject upright as well as supine. Determination of the blood pressure in both arms is recommended, especially in the elderly. An American Heart Association report[165] recommends that the systolic pressure be recorded as the point at which the first tapping sounds occur for two consecutive beats (phase I) and that the diastolic pressure in adults be recorded as the point at which sounds become inaudible. In children and in adults with a hyperkinetic circulation, the diastolic pressure should be recorded as the point at which muffling of the sounds occurs (onset of phase IV). The arterial pressures at both the onset of muffling (phase IV) and the disappearance of sound (phase V) should be recorded. The mean blood pressure can be estimated by the addition of one-third the pulse pressure (systolic pressure minus diastolic pressure) to the diastolic pressure.

Patients with atrial fibrillation may have a significant beat-to-beat variation in their arterial pressure. Accordingly, the indirect blood pressure should be measured several times and the average noted.

This indirect method provides several potential sources of error due to improper equipment, inaccurate detection of the Korotkoff sounds, and observer techniques.[159] For example, a cuff with a smaller than the recommended width may result in falsely elevated arterial pressure measurements. The standard pneumatic cuff may often be unsatisfactory for pressure measurement in the arms or in the legs of very obese subjects.[166] The arterial pressure may be underestimated if the cuff is deflated too rapidly, particularly when bradycardia or an irregular rhythm is present or if inadequate inflation does not result in complete arterial occlusion. When the cuff is deflated too slowly or is immediately reinflated for multiple pressure determinations, the resultant venous congestion may artificially elevate the diastolic pressure and falsely decrease the systolic pressure by decreasing the intensity of phase I or phase II sounds to an inaudible level. An erroneously low systolic pressure may also result from the failure to detect the presence of an auscultatory gap—a silent interval occasionally present just below the systolic pressure level.[159]

Studies correlating direct and indirect blood pressure measurements have been characterized by considerable variability between individual subjects but in general have shown a good correlation between indirect and direct measurements of blood pressure in the arm.[166] The observed trend has been for the indirect method to underestimate systolic pressure by several millimeters of mercury, to overestimate diastolic pressure by several millimeters of mercury when phase IV is used as an end point, and to slightly underestimate diastolic pressure in normal individuals when phase V is taken as the end point.

Home blood pressure recordings using manual or automatic inflation, and deflation of the cuff and detection of Korotkoff sounds by a microphone, stethoscope, or ultrasonic transducer are being used with increasing frequency for the ambulatory assessment of patients with hypertension.[167–169] Ambulatory blood pressure devices are not available that meet the standards for automated devices of the Association for the Advancement of Medical Instrumentation.[170–172]

More recently, arterial tonometry has been used as a completely noninvasive method for monitoring the arterial pressure. This probe, with a micromanometer in its tip, operates on the principle of a piezo-resistive transducer of cantilever construction.[173–176]

NORMAL ARTERIAL PRESSURE

Normal pressures have been defined on the basis of values included within two standard deviations of the mean of pressures obtained in a large population of apparently healthy individuals. The normal blood pressure range varies with age, sex, and socioracial grouping.[177] In the United States, the pressure increases rapidly during the first few days of life and then increases gradually, with a slightly greater increment in systolic than in diastolic values, throughout life. The pressure tends to be higher in Western, industrialized societies than in Asian, African, and technically undeveloped societies.

With increasing age beyond maturity and into senescence, the aorta undergoes progressive dilation and elongation, with increasing stiffness of its walls.[178,179] As a result of this diminished vascular distensibility, there is an increase in systolic arterial pressure with less change in diastolic pressure.[180]

The normal blood pressure limits for adults (below 40 years of age and of mixed sex and race) living in the United States are approximately 100 to 140 mmHg systolic and 60 to 90 mmHg diastolic. In an individual subject, however, baseline pressures above or below these levels do not define a pathologic state, since the physiologic range of normal for an individual may overlap with the statistical range of abnormality.[159] The systolic arterial pressure rises slowly and progressively in most Americans between ages 20 and 60 and more rapidly later, increasing by about 20 mmHg between ages 60 and 80.[181] Diastolic pressure usually rises very little after age 45.[182]

In mildly to moderately hypertensive persons, the blood pressure "casually" recorded by a physician is significantly higher than the average value of a series of intermittent, indirect determinations or continuous direct recordings made during normal activity.[182] To estimate basal blood pressure, measurements have been obtained during sleep, when the subject first awakens in the morning while still recumbent, or after several hours of reclining.

Many factors contribute to variations in an individual's blood pressure during daily activities. These include (1) body posture; (2) state of muscular, cerebral, or gastrointestinal activity; (3) emotional or painful stimuli; (4) environmental factors such as temperature and noise level; and (5) the use of tobacco, coffee, alcohol, and other drugs with direct or neurally mediated vasomotor properties.[159,183] Twenty-four-hour pressures, obtained from normal and hypertensive subjects with an automatic recorder, have shown considerable variability with activity and emotional stimuli.[184,185] The average diurnal pattern of blood pressure consists of an increase throughout the day and early evening and a significant, rapid decline to a low point during the early, deep stage of sleep.

With normal respiration, the peak systolic blood pressure is greater during expiration than during inspiration by as much as 10 mmHg. An augmentation of this difference occurs in patients with pericardial tamponade (pulsus paradoxus; see Chap. 81) and during hyperventilation.

Isotonic exercise in both the supine and upright positions produces a moderate increase in blood pressure (systolic pressure greater than mean greater than diastolic pressure). Sustained isometric muscular contractions produce an abrupt increase in systolic, mean, and diastolic blood pressure that is dependent on the strength of the contraction.[186]

ABNORMAL ARTERIAL PRESSURE

Increased Pulse Pressure

An increase in arterial pulse pressure is commonly observed during routine blood pressure recordings. This usually results from an increase in stroke volume and ejection velocity, often associated with a decrease in peripheral resistance. Fever, anemia, hot weather, exercise, pregnancy, hyperthyroidism, or arteriovenous fistulas may produce this change. Several cardiac diseases, such as aortic regurgitation, patent ductus arteriosus, or truncus arteriosus, can also result in a widened pulse pressure. An increased pulse pressure due to a large stroke volume may occur with complete heart block or marked sinus bradycardia.[159]

Atherosclerosis of the large arteries often reduces arterial compliance and results in an elevated systolic pressure with a normal or even decreased stroke volume. The systolic hypertension of the elderly does not necessarily represent a change in arteriolar resistance. Efforts to lower this type of systolic pressure elevation are often appropriate but can result in diminished peripheral perfusion (see Chap. 58). The increased pulse pressure associated with systemic arteriovenous fistulas is less common; a relative tachycardia may be the only clinical clue. Compression of a systemic arteriovenous fistula can produce a prompt slowing of the heart rate (Branham's sign).

Reduced Pulse Pressure

A narrow pulse pressure is uncommon in normal subjects but may result from an increased peripheral resistance (increased circulating catecholamines in heart failure), decreased stroke volume (severe aortic stenosis), and/or markedly decreased intravascular volume (diabetic ketoacidosis).[159]

Unequal Pulse Pressures

The diagnostic importance of blood pressure differences between right and left arms has been enhanced in recent years by the recognition of supravalvular aortic stenosis[187] in children and the subclavian steal syndrome in adults. Most patients with the former have greater than 20 mmHg higher blood pressure in the right arm. The subclavian steal syndrome, often accompanied by symptoms of cerebrovascular insufficiency, usually results in a pronounced lowering or absence of brachial artery pressure in the ipsilateral extremity.[159]

A progressive increase in systolic pressure normally occurs as the point of measurement is moved peripherally from the central aorta, and the increment in systolic pressure is equivalent in the large arteries of the upper arm and the thigh. Direct recordings of femoral and brachial arterial pressures (systolic, diastolic, and mean) in adults[188] and children[189] and indirect measurement of popliteal and brachial pressures using appropriate pressure cuffs[190] have demonstrated that mean pressures are equal at these sites. A difference in arm and leg pressures may occur because of coarctation of the aorta or acquired disease such as aortic dissection, aortic arch syndrome, or the subclavian steal syndrome.[159]

Pulsus Alternans

Pulsus alternans may be detected by palpating a peripheral artery. The femoral artery is probably best for this purpose. One must, of course, be certain the heart rhythm is normal. The sphygmomanometer can be used to measure accurately the beat-to-beat variation in pressure that characterizes pulsus alternans.

Pulsus alternans, which is discussed at greater length later in this chapter, occurs in patients with severe heart disease who exhibit impaired left ventricular contraction. It can also occur for a few beats following supraventricular tachycardia

in normal persons or when the respiratory rate is half the pulse rate. This may be apparent when pulsus paradoxus is present in patients with cardiac tamponade.

Pulsus Paradoxus

A normal person may exhibit a 10- to 12-mmHg drop in systolic pressure during normal inspiration. A fall in pressure greater than this amount may be identified in patients with acute cardiac tamponade, constrictive pericarditis, severe obstructive lung disease, and restrictive cardiomyopathy.

Pulsus paradoxus is best detected by inflating the blood pressure cuff above systolic pressure and then slowly releasing it. As the cuff pressure is gradually reduced, the blood pressure sounds become audible during expiration. The difference in pressure between the first audible sound heard on expiration and the pressure level at which the sounds are heard during all phases of respiration gives a measurement of magnitude of pulsus paradoxus.

The mechanism of pulsus paradoxus is discussed in Chap. 81.

THE ARTERIAL PULSE

Palpation of the arterial pulse is a basic and important element of the physical examination.[191–193] Any discussion of the arterial pulse must include recent advances in measurement of arterial hemodynamics, assessment of the arterial wave contour, and frequency analysis of the pressure pulse.[192–202]

Physical Determinants of the Arterial Pulse

GENESIS OF THE ARTERIAL PULSE

Pressure and blood flow measurements in the ascending aorta result from the interaction between the heart and arterial system. When left ventricular pressure exceeds the aortic pressure it becomes the driving force for the movement of blood into the ascending aorta.[200,201] This driving force is dependent on the intrinsic contractility of ventricle muscle, the size and shape of the left ventricle, and the heart rate. It is opposed by several forces that impede the development of flow and are interrelated in a complex manner. Three major determinants of arterial impedance include (1) resistance, (2) inertia, and (3) compliance. Resistance is related to blood viscosity and the geometry of the vasculature; it opposes flow and is unaffected by changes in heart rate. Inertia, which is related to the mass of the column of blood, opposes the rate of change of arterial blood flow (i.e., acceleration) and is heart rate–dependent. Compliance is related to the distensibility of the vascular walls, opposes changes in arterial blood volume, and is also heart rate–dependent. The heart rate dependency of inertia and compliance introduces phase shifts between instantaneous pressure and flow in a pulsatile system.[200] Inertia and compliance are important determinants of the character of ventricular ejection, especially in early systole, when flows and pressures are changing rapidly.

The arterial pulse wave begins with aortic valve opening and the onset of left ventricular ejection. Aortic pressure rises rapidly in early systole since the left ventricular stroke volume enters the aorta faster than it flows to distal sites. The rapid-rising portion of the arterial pressure curve is often termed the *anacrotic limb* (from the Greek, meaning "upbeat"). In experimental animals and in humans, peak proximal aortic flow velocity occurs slightly earlier than peak pressure.[195] After its peak, aortic pressure declines as ventricular ejection slows and peripheral blood flow continues. During isovolumic relaxation, a transient reversal of flow from the central arteries toward the ventricle just prior to aortic valve closure is associated with an incisura on the descending limb of the aortic pressure pulse. The subsequent smaller, secondary positive wave has been attributed to the elastic recoil of the aorta and aortic valve but is partially due to reflected waves from more distal arteries. Subsequently, aortic pressure decreases again as further "runoff" in the peripheral circulation occurs in diastole (see also Chap. 3).

The proximal aortic pulse pressure is directly proportional to the ratio of stroke volume to arterial distensibility, but multiple factors influence this complex relationship.[202] Arterial distensibility diminishes as the distending arterial pressure increases. Accordingly, the pulse pressure for a constant stroke volume will be larger if the mean blood pressure is elevated. In addition, arterial distensibility varies inversely with the rate of rise of intraluminal pressure. When the systolic ejection rate increases, the stiffer arterial wall results in a greater pulse pressure. Finally, the arterial pulse pressure is modified by reflected pressure waves and by the rate of blood flow from arterioles to veins.

CONTOUR OF THE ARTERIAL PULSE

Pulsatile changes in arterial diameter are virtually identical to the pressure pulse, with minor differences explained in terms of nonlinear elasticity and viscosity of the arterial wall. In 1939, Hamilton and Dow defined the pressure wave contour in different arteries in terms of wave reflection between the aortic valve and peripheral sites.[203] In their explanation, the arterial pulse bounded back and forth between the aortic valve and peripheral reflecting sites, setting up a system of "standing waves" in the aorta. The standing-wave hypothesis is not completely accurate, however, since some attenuation to the wave in travel occurs and there is incomplete reflection of the wave.[204]

More precise information about the arterial pulse has been obtained from quantitative studies in which a regularly repeated pressure of flow wave is considered as a series of harmonics.[194,205] Each harmonic component has a definite modulus (amplitude) and a definite phase (delay) from a set point of reference. Given the modulus and phase of the different harmonics of the pulse, the original wave can be resynthesized, and corresponding components of waves recorded simultaneously can be compared. By measuring and correlating mean values of the waves, one can calculate vascular resistance and interpret the resistance properties of vessels down-stream. The corresponding frequency components of pressure and flow can be compared in order to determine vascular impedance, the relation of pressure to flow at frequencies that are multiples of the heart rate.[194]

Usually, there is a linear relation between pressure and flow at the same point in an artery and between pressure and pressure at different points in the arterial system. From impedance curves, it is possible to identify the factors responsible for the relation between the pulsatile pressure and flow.[195,196,201,206] Furthermore, the coefficient of reflection in peripheral vessels can be calculated from the relation of resistance to the minimal and subsequent values of impedance modulus. The peripheral arterial pressure wave recorded is the summation of the incident (initial) and the reflected waves. The systemic circulation has been represented by a simple asymmetric T-tube model that emphasizes the importance of wave reflection at two arteriolar reflecting sites in the upper and lower parts of the body.[194,197] An important patient study indicates major reflection sites at the aortic level of the renal arteries and at a point distal to the terminal abdominal aorta bifurcation.[198]

PERIPHERAL TRANSMISSION OF THE ARTERIAL PULSE

As the normal aortic pulse wave is transmitted peripherally, significant changes in its contour occur due to (1) distortion and damping of pulse wave components; (2) different rates of transmission of various components; (3) distortion or exaggeration by reflected, resonant, or standing waves; (4) conversion of kinetic energy into hydrostatic or potential energy; (5) differences in distensibility and caliber of the arteries; and (6) changes in the vessel wall due to age and/or disease.[207]

The arterial pressure pulse enters the proximal aorta and travels distally at a velocity many times faster than maximum blood flow. The pressure wave is accompanied by a traveling wave distending the arterial wall, the pulse wave velocity increasing as arterial wall distensibility diminishes.[202] This normally occurs distally, as the arteries branch into smaller channels and their walls become stiffer. With increasing age or with systemic hypertension, however, arterial wall distensibility diminishes and pulse wave velocity is correspondingly greater.[194,208–212]

The pulse wave arrives progressively later at more peripheral sites when timed from the QRS complex on the ECG. Representative time delays from the central aorta are as follows: carotid, 30 ms; brachial, 60 ms; radial, 80 ms; and femoral, 75 ms.

The arterial pulse wave undergoes a progressive change in shape during its transmission distally (Figs. 10-38 and 3-27). The pulse pressure and systolic amplitude increase, and the ascending limb of the pulse wave becomes steeper. The incisura of the central aorta pulse is gradually replaced by a smoother, somewhat later, dicrotic notch that occurs at lower pressure levels. The dicrotic notch and the following positive secondary or dicrotic wave probably result from the summation of the forward pulse wave and reflected waves from the peripheral vessels (see also Chap. 3).

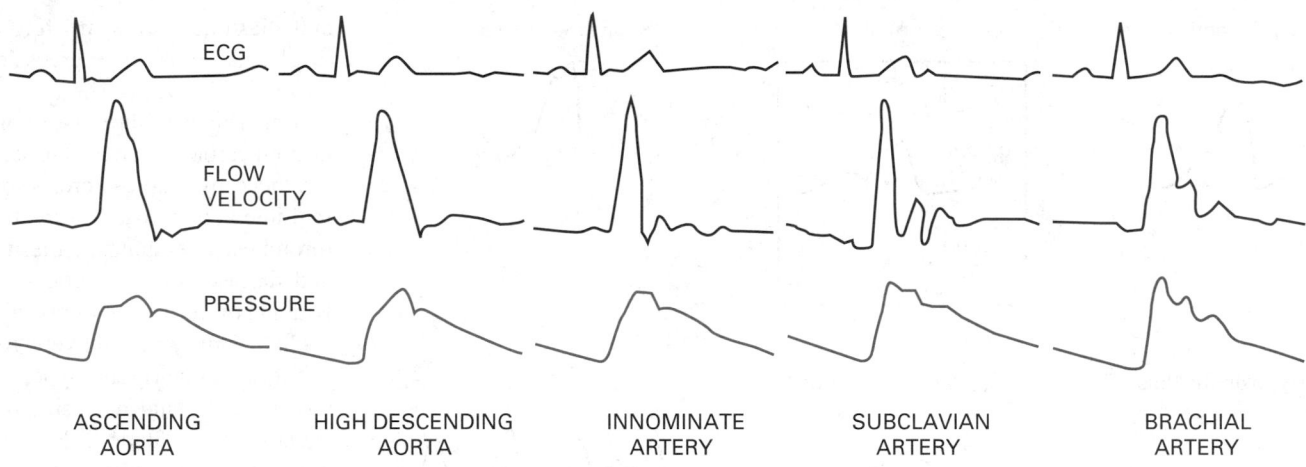

ECG

FLOW VELOCITY

PRESSURE

| ASCENDING AORTA | HIGH DESCENDING AORTA | INNOMINATE ARTERY | SUBCLAVIAN ARTERY | BRACHIAL ARTERY |

FIGURE 10-38

Simultaneous recording of ECG, catheter-tip flow velocity, and micromanometer pressure in a normal subject as the catheter is moved distally from the ascending aorta. (From Stein JH, ed. *Internal Medicine*, 2d ed. Boston: Little Brown; 1987:315. Used with permission from the publisher and author.)

Examination of the Arterial Pulse

All major arterial pulses should be examined bilaterally both for patency and for waveform characteristics. The thickness and hardness of the arterial walls often can be assessed by "rolling" the vessel against underlying tissue. A pulse in the foot should not be considered absent unless examined with the foot in the dependent position. Otherwise, the arterial pulses usually are examined with the patient supine and with the trunk of the body slightly elevated.

The examiner uses tactile receptors in the tips of the fingers to sense movement of the arterial wall associated with the pressure pulse as it passes the site of palpation. Measurements in the proximal aorta show cyclic movement in both diameter and length proportional to the pulse pressure.[213] In more peripheral arteries with connective tissue attachments, however, the detectable movement is small and variable, with radial expansion by only about 2 percent of the end-diastolic cross-sectional area.[214]

The usual technique for palpating the arterial pulse is to press with the examining fingers until the maximum pulse is sensed. The pulse is felt as changing displacement superimposed on the "baseline" displacement produced by compressing the artery. The examiner should apply varying degrees of pressure while concentrating on the separate phases of the pulse wave. This method, referred to as *trisection*, is useful for assessing the upstroke, systolic peak, and diastolic slope of the arterial pulse.[207] Controversy exists as to how many fingers should be used to palpate the pulse; the examiner should use whichever method he or she prefers, being careful not to perceive the examiner's fingertip pulse as well.

Palpation of the carotid artery is preferred for assessing cardiac performance, since the carotid pulse corresponds more closely to the central aortic pressure. In certain cardiac diseases (e.g., aortic regurgitation), however, the abnormalities detected in the carotid pulse are accentuated in the more peripheral pulses. For determining the cardiac rate and rhythm, the radial pulse most often is used; but if it is irregular, cardiac auscultation often provides more reliable information. To evaluate the integrity of the peripheral arterial blood supply and to localize any lesions that exist, the arterial pulses in all four extremities should be examined and compared (Chap. 100).

Inspection of the carotid arterial and jugular venous pulsations should be performed at the same time. The carotid pulse is usually best examined with the sternocleidomastoid muscles relaxed and with the head rotated slightly toward the examiner. The carotid pulse may be timed from the first heart sound, which is heard slightly before the pulsation. The carotid pulse should be palpated in the lower half of the patient's neck in order to avoid carotid sinus compression. Occasionally, it is useful to palpate two arteries simultaneously (e.g., radial and femoral) to detect an apparent pulse wave delay, such as occurs in patients with coarctation of the aorta.

The examination of arterial pulses in the abdomen and upper and lower extremities should be performed carefully in all patients and compared using a scale such as the following: 0 = complete absence of pulsation; 1+ = small or reduced pulsation; 2+ = normal or average pulsation; and 3+ = large or bounding pulsation. Furthermore, auscultation over the major arteries should be performed, since an audible bruit may be a clue to partial occlusion or may (e.g., carotid) indicate transmission of a cardiac murmur.

NORMAL ARTERIAL PULSE

The normal carotid pulse has a smooth, rapid upstroke or ascending limb to a smooth, dome-shaped summit (Fig. 10-39). Then a downstroke occurs that is somewhat less rapid than the upstroke. The dicrotic notch and secondary diastolic wave usually are not felt but may be palpable in some normal individuals, particularly during fever, exercise, or excitement. The dicrotic notch usually occurs about 300 ms after the onset of the pulse wave when corrected for heart rate.

In arteries distal to the carotid, the pulse wave arrives later and has a steep initial wave that rises to a high peak pressure,

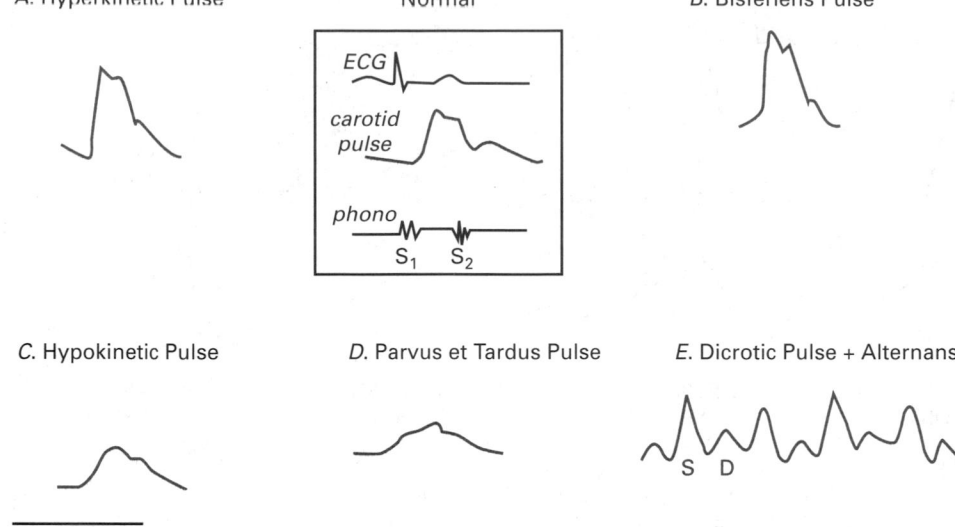

A. Hyperkinetic Pulse   Normal   *B.* Bisferiens Pulse

ECG

carotid
pulse

phono
S₁   S₂

C. Hypokinetic Pulse   *D.* Parvus et Tardus Pulse   *E.* Dicrotic Pulse + Alternans

S   D

FIGURE 10-39

Schematic representation of the normal carotid arterial pulse, five types of abnormal pulses, and pulsus alternans. ECG = electrocardiogram; phono = phonocardiogram; S₁, S₂ = first and second heart sounds; S = systole; D = diastole.

whereas the diastolic pressure and the mean pressure are slightly lower. The systolic upstroke time (onset of pulse wave to its peak) tends to be shorter but the apparent left ventricular ejection time (onset of pulse wave to incisura) longer in more peripheral arterial pulses. In the brachial artery, the heart rate–corrected systolic upstroke time averages 120 ms (range, 90 to 160 ms) and the systolic ejection time about 320 ms (range, 280 to 360 ms).

Graphic recordings of the arterial pulses frequently show two positive deflections during systole; the first shoulder being referred to as the *percussion wave* and the second as the *tidal wave*. In the normal proximal aortic pulse, the percussion wave is due to arrival of the impulse generated by left ventricular ejection, the tidal wave may represent its echo from the upper part of the body, and the dicrotic or diastolic wave is a reflection from the lower part of the body.[194] The contour of the distal pulses can be explained in similar terms, with altered time relations between incident and reflected waves at different distances from peripheral reflecting sites.

With aging, there is a relative increase in the second (tidal) systolic wave and the height of the incisura relative to the first systolic wave.[181,196,206,210,215] The systolic upstroke time is longer, and the amplitude and duration of the diastolic wave tend to be less prominent.

ABNORMAL ARTERIAL PULSES

In hypertension and arteriosclerosis, the pressure pulse amplitude is increased, the tidal wave is prominent, and the diastolic wave is absent. All features of the pulse can be explained by increased wave velocity.[181,196] Reflected waves return to the proximal aorta during late systole, augmenting the tidal wave and increasing systolic pressure.[181] With systemic hypotension, the pulse wave velocity is decreased and the later tidal

and diastolic waves are further displaced from the percussion wave.

Impairment of the pulse of one or both carotid arteries is usually produced by atherosclerosis, but multiple other causes include thrombosis, embolus, arteritis, and diseases of the aortic arch. Kinking of the carotid or brachiocephalic artery is relatively frequent, particularly in hypertensive patients, and may simulate aneurysmal dilatation. Femoral pulses may be diminished in the child or young adult as a result of coarctation of the aorta. In most adults, however, the diminution of the femoral pulsation is caused by atherosclerosis of the abdominal aorta, aortic bifurcation, or ileofemoral arteries (Chap. 100).

Hyperkinetic Arterial Pulse

Large, bounding arterial pulses usually indicate the rapid ejection of an increased volume of blood from the left ventricle (Fig. 10-39A). Commonly, the arterial pulse pressure is increased and the peripheral arterial resistance diminished. The hyperdynamic arterial pulse is sometimes referred to in terms that describe a particular component of the pulse wave. Thus, the "water-hammer pulse," named after a Victorian toy, refers to an extremely rapid, forceful ascending limb of the arterial pulse wave.[216] By contrast, "collapsing pulse" refers to a quick, marked decrease in the arterial pulse wave following its peak. Hyperkinetic pulses often are more prominent in the brachial, radial, or femoral arteries than in the carotid artery. The term *Quincke pulse* refers to visible small pulsations in the nail bed of patients with hyperdynamic arterial pulses from any cause, including aortic regurgitation.

Hyperkinetic arterial pulses occur in normal subjects with a hyperkinetic circulation (e.g., exercise, fever), patient with cardiovascular diseases associated with increased stroke volume, and subjects with marked bradycardia and an extremely large stroke volume (e.g., athletes). A hyperdynamic arterial pulse also occurs in patients with an abnormally rapid runoff of blood from the arterial system (e.g., patent ductus arteriosus, arteriovenous fistulas). Patients on chronic hemodialysis often have hyperdynamic pulses produced by the combination of a surgical arteriovenous fistula, anemia, and hypertension.

In aortic regurgitation, the rapid-rising, bounding arterial pulse results from increases in both stroke volume and the rate of left ventricular ejection. The early systolic flow often produces palpable vibrations manifest as a thrill on the steep ascending limb. Later in systole, the rate of ventricular ejection and the arterial pulse wave decrease sharply, often resulting in systolic collapse.[201]

Bisferiens Arterial Pulse

The *bisferiens* (from the Latin, meaning "twice beating") pulse has a waveform characterized by two positive waves during systole (Fig. 10-39*B*). The pulse wave upstroke rises rapidly and forcefully, producing the first systolic peak (*percussion wave*). A brief decline in pressure is followed by a smaller and somewhat slower-rising positive pulse wave (*tidal wave*). Abnormalities of left ventricular ejection and reflected waves from peripheral arteries contribute to the prominence of the second systolic wave in the bisferiens pulse. The bisferiens pulse, usually felt in the carotid artery, is sometimes more easily palpable in a brachial or radial artery. A bisferiens pulse often occurs in patients with pure aortic regurgitation and in patients with combined aortic stenosis and severe aortic regurgitation.[217–220] It can also occur in other conditions associated with the rapid ejection of an increased stroke volume from the left ventricle (e.g., exercise, fever, patent ductus arteriosus).

The bisferiens pulse often is present in patients with hypertrophic cardiomyopathy, many of whom have a pressure gradient in the left ventricular outflow tract.[221] In this syndrome, the midsystolic negative wave usually coincides with a marked decrease in the rate of left ventricular ejection. The second systolic wave, or tidal wave, most likely is produced by reflected waves from the periphery. The bisferiens pulse may be elicited by maneuvers that decrease the left ventricular size or increase its contractility. The most characteristic aspect of the arterial pulse in hypertrophic cardiomyopathy is its rapid rate of rise. A physical finding nearly specific for hypertrophic cardiomyopathy is a much smaller arterial pressure pulse in the cardiac cycle following a premature ventricular beat (Chap. 74).

Hypokinetic Arterial Pulse

A small, weak arterial pulse is frequently present in patients with a diminished stroke volume (Fig. 10-39*C*). Usually, the decreased stroke output is associated with decreased rate and duration of left ventricular ejection, and there is a narrow arterial pulse pressure despite an increased arterial resistance. Common causes include hypovolemia, left ventricular failure, and mitral or aortic valve stenosis.

Parvus et Tardus Pulse

Patients with moderate or severe valvular aortic stenosis often have an arterial pulse that is small and has a delayed systolic peak.[222–225] Occasionally, there may be a detectable shoulder on the upstroke of the carotid pulse, referred to as *anacrotic* (Fig. 10-39*D*).[226] Palpable coarse vibrations are often present as a systolic thrill over the slowly rising carotid pulse. The *parvus et tardus* pulse is much easier to detect in the carotid arteries than in more distal arteries.

Most middle-aged patients with uncomplicated severe aortic stenosis have a parvus et tardus pulse, but this pulse may also occur in relatively mild stenosis. Conversely, an apparently normal arterial pulse is not unusual in elderly patients with severe aortic stenosis who have decreased distensibility of the large arteries, which also alters the character of the arterial pulse.[182,227] Severe left ventricular failure often results in a small, weak pulse which may be difficult to distinguish from that of aortic stenosis.

Dicrotic Arterial Pulse

The *dicrotic* (from the Greek *dikrotos*, meaning "double beating") pulse is a twice-peaked pulse with one peak in systole and the second in diastole, the latter due to an accentuated and palpable dicrotic wave that follows the second heart sound (Fig. 10-39*E*).[228] It is usually felt best in the carotids, although it may also be palpated over more peripheral arteries. Major abnormalities include a short systolic ejection phase, a low dicrotic notch, a large diastolic wave, a narrow pulse pressure, a diminished rate of rise of the pulse, and the lack of distinct percussion and tidal waves. The dicrotic pulse is most common in young or middle-aged patients with impaired left ventricular performance. It is usually associated with a low cardiac output, markedly diminished stroke volume, elevated left ventricular end-diastolic pressure, and high systemic arterial resistance. In general, the dicrotic wave becomes less prominent with age, hypertension, generalized atherosclerosis, and diabetes. Rarely, the dicrotic wave can be palpated in young, febrile patients in whom none of the other abnormal features of the dicrotic pulse are present.

Pulsus Alternans

In pulsus alternans, beats occur at regular intervals with a regular alternation of the systolic height of the pressure pulses (Fig. 10-39*E*).[229,230] Rarely, pulsus alternans is so marked that the weaker pulses are not felt at all. When pulsus alternans is noticed first after a premature beat, the extent of the difference in systolic pressure in alternating beats may decline for several cycles until the pulse amplitude is again constant. The initiation of postpremature ventricular beat pulsus alternans is probably related to the increased duration of left ventricular filling after the premature beat, resulting in a greater end-diastolic volume and hence increased contractile force due to the Frank-Starling mechanism.[231]

Sustained pulsus alternans (see also Chap. 21) is seen in severe depression of left ventricular performance with an alteration in aortic flow, systolic left ventricular pressure, aortic systolic pressure, left ventricular *dP/dt*, and left ventricular end-diastolic pressure. Sustained pulsus alternans likely is due to alteration of the contractile state of at least part of the myocardium, which may be caused by the failure of electromechanical coupling in some cells during the weaker contraction.[232] A subsequent stronger contraction would then represent contraction of all cells, some of which were potentiated.[233]

Pulsus alternans may be better appreciated when palpating a distal artery, which normally has a slightly wider pulse pressure than the carotid artery. It is often brought out or accentuated when the patient assumes the upright position, thus decreasing venous return. The patient's respiration should be held since the small changes in arterial pressure caused by normal respiration may obscure the recognition of pulsus alternans. Pulsus alternans can be confirmed by using a sphygmomanometer and is usually associated with a left ventricular third heart sound.

Pulsus Paradoxus

A paradoxical pulse (Chap. 81) is defined as a marked decrease in the pulse amplitude during normal quiet inspiration or a decrease in the systolic arterial pressure by more than 10 mmHg. The normal small decline in systolic blood pressure probably is produced predominantly by relative pooling of blood in the pulmonary vessels during inspiration and may also reflect the delayed transmission through the lungs of the preceding expiratory fall in venous pressure and right ventricular cardiac output.[207]

In patients with cardiac tamponade, fluid accumulation in the pericardium increases intrapericardial pressure, and the heart's filling capacity is reduced. During inspiration, the expected augmentation of venous return to the right side of the heart occurs despite the elevated intrapericardial pressure.[234] The diminished thoracic pressure also causes a pooling of blood in the pulmonary veins and capillaries and diminishes pulmonary venous return to the left atrium. Since the high intrapericardial pressure limits flow to the heart and the total cardiac filling capacity is limited, the increase in right-sided heart volume with inspiration causes an obligatory decrease in left-sided heart filling. This, along with the pooling of blood in the pulmonary bed, produces a decline in left ventricular stroke volume and systolic blood pressure during inspiration.[235] Pulsus paradoxus is common with cardiac tamponade but infrequent with constrictive pericarditis (see also Chap. 81). Different hemodynamic mechanisms contribute to the production of a paradoxical pulse in certain patients with superior vena cava obstruction, asthma, or obstructive airway disease, in some patients with pulmonary embolism or shock, or postthoracotomy.[207]

The extent of pulsus paradoxicus can be quantitated by cuff sphygmomanometry as the pressure difference between the first discernible Korotkoff sound on expiration and the pressure level at which Korotkoff sounds are audible during all phases of respiration.

EFFECTS OF ARRHYTHMIAS ON THE ARTERIAL PULSE

Premature Ventricular Depolarizations

A premature ventricular depolarization may be associated with no pulse, a small-amplitude pulse, or a normal arterial pulse, depending on timing and whether or not the left ventricular pressure generated is able to open the aortic valve.[236] The arterial pulse following a premature beat usually is greatly enhanced because of decreased aortic impedance, increased left ventricular filling, and augmented left ventricular contractility. At times, premature ventricular beats are so common

as to produce an irregularly irregular pulse. Then the presence of cannon *a* waves in the jugular venous pulse should alert one to the correct diagnosis.

Tachyarrhythmias

The ECG is usually needed for the definitive diagnosis of any abnormality of heart rate or rhythm. On the other hand, careful observation of the arterial and jugular venous pulses frequently leads to the correct diagnosis. Simultaneous cardiac auscultation is also frequently helpful.

Most tachycardias associated with a regular pulse are of supraventricular origin. In sinus tachycardia, the arterial pulse will gradually slow with carotid sinus pressure and then again gradually increase. Paroxysmal atrial tachycardia has an "all-or-none" response. In patients with atrial flutter, carotid sinus pressure will increase the block at the AV junction, the pulse rate slowing and subsequently returning to its original rate in a "jerky" fashion.

In patients with ventricular tachycardia and AV dissociation, the variation in the atrial-ventricular sequence of contraction and resulting variation in pulse amplitude may often be detected by palpation.[237]

An irregularly irregular pulse with a varying pulse pressure is usually the result of atrial fibrillation; however, multifocal atrial tachycardia is also a common cause of this finding in patients with severe chronic obstructive lung disease (see also Chap. 27).

Bradyarrhythmias

An unusually slow heart rate frequently is associated with a decrease in the rate of rise and amplitude of the arterial pressure pulse. Complete heart block is often readily diagnosed by the variability in the arterial pulse amplitude, the changing intensity of the first heart sound, and intermittent cannon *a* waves in the jugular venous pulse, all due to the time-dependent variable contribution of atrial contraction to ventricular filling.

VENOUS PULSE

An accurate assessment of the venous pulse is an integral part of the physical examination since it provides information concerning both the mean right atrial pressure and the hemodynamic events in the right atrium.[193] Factors influencing the right atrial and central venous pressure (CVP) include the total blood volume, the distribution of blood volume, and the strength of right atrial contraction.

Venous blood returning from the systemic capillaries is nonpulsatile. Changes in volume flow created by skeletal muscles and respiratory pump are nonsynchronous with the pulsatile activity of the heart. Changes in flow and pressure caused by right atrial and ventricular filling, however, produce pulsations in the central veins that are transmitted toward the peripheral veins, opposite to the direction of blood flow. With the possible exception of the *c* wave, which is the combined result of carotid arterial impact and an upward movement of the tricuspid valve, the pulsations observed in the neck are produced by right atrial and ventricular activity.[238]

EXAMINATION OF THE JUGULAR VENOUS PULSE

The two main objectives of the bedside examination of the neck veins are the estimation of the CVP and the inspection of the waveform. Usually, the right internal jugular vein is superior for both purposes. In most normal subjects, the maximum pulsation of the internal jugular vein is observed when the trunk is inclined by less than 30°. In patients with an elevated venous pressure, it may be necessary to elevate the trunk further, sometimes to as much as 90°.[239] When the neck muscles are relaxed, shining a beam of light tangently across the skin overlying the internal jugular vein often exposes its pulsations. Simultaneous palpation of the left carotid artery aids the examiner in deciding which pulsations are venous.

Measurements of Venous Pressure

The difference between venous distension and venous pressure elevation must be considered. Veins may be markedly dilated with minimal increase in pressure or may not be visibly distended despite a very high venous pressure. Venous pressure may be estimated by examining the veins on the dorsum of the hand. With the patient sitting or lying at a 30° elevation or greater, the arm is slowly and passively raised from a dependent position. When the venous pressure is normal, the veins collapse when the dorsum of the hand reaches the level of the sternal angle of Louis. Unfortunately, local venous obstruction or augmented peripheral venous constriction may diminish the accuracy of estimating CVP by this method.

The external or internal jugular veins may also be used to estimate venous pressure.[240] Because of its more direct route to the right atrium, the internal jugular vein is superior for the estimation of venous pressure and assessment of the venous waveform. The patient is examined at the optimum degree of trunk elevation for visualization of venous pulsations. The vertical distance from the top of the oscillating venous column to the level of the sternal angle is generally less than 3 cm. Greatly elevated venous pressure may be missed by failing to elevate adequately the

patient's head. It may be necessary to actually have the patient sit upright. If the "pulsating meniscus" is very high, pulsations may not be apparent in the lower neck. When venous engorgement is marked, the patient's earlobe may pulsate and even the veins on the top of the head may be distended.

In patients suspected of right ventricular failure but having normal resting venous pressure, the abdominojugular (also known as hepatojugular) test is useful.[241] With the patient breathing normally, firm pressure is applied with the palm of the hand to the upper right quadrant of the abdomen for 10 or more seconds. The patient should be instructed to continue to breathe normally during the test. In most subjects the jugular venous pressure is not altered significantly. In some normal patients there is a transient increase in jugular venous pressure with a *rapid return* to or near baseline in less than 10 s. The dysfunctioning right ventricle, however, is unable to accept the increment in blood volume due to enhanced venous return without a marked increase in its filling pressure, which is transmitted to the neck veins. In patients with right ventricular failure, which often results from left-sided heart failure, the venous pressure either rises rapidly and then partially declines slowly during continued abdominal compression or remains elevated by 4 cm of blood or more until the abdominal pressure is released (Fig. 10-40).[242] Ducas et al. also studied the abdominojugular test and confirmed its clinical value.[243]

Analysis of Venous Waveforms

Again, the patient's trunk should be inclined to whatever elevation is necessary to reveal the top of the oscillating

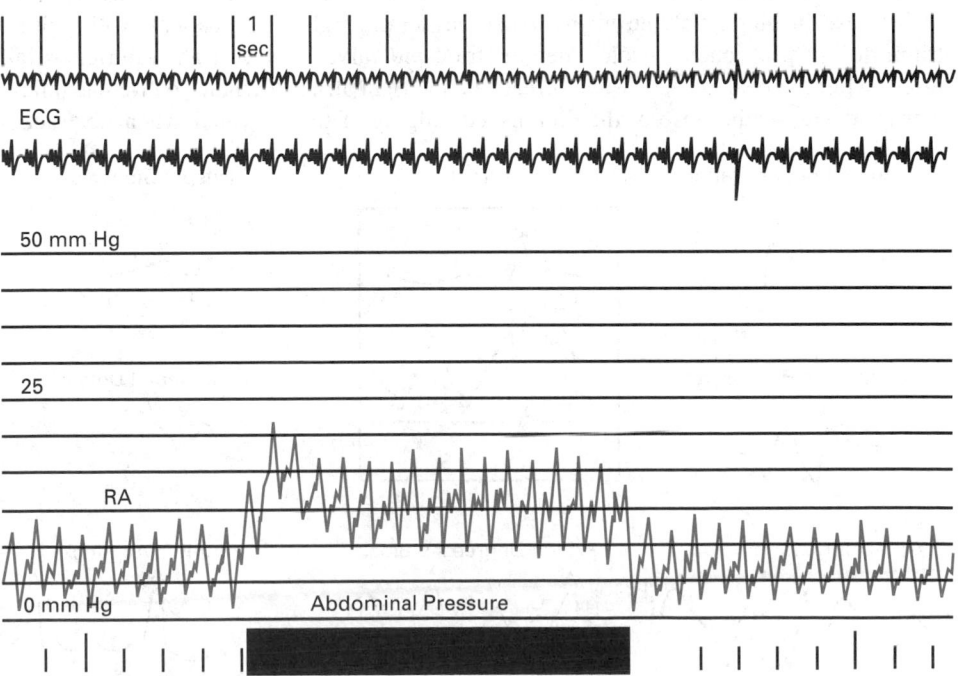

FIGURE 10-40
Elevation in right atrial (RA) pressure observed during abdominal pressure in patient with mild congestive heart failure. (From Ewy GA. The abdominojugular test: Technique and hemodynamic correlates. *Ann Intern Med* 1989; 109:456. Used with permission from the publisher and author.)

venous column.[192,244] Slow, deep inspiration will increase the amplitude of the presystolic *a* wave while decreasing the mean right atrial pressure. This is a useful technique for identifying the site at which the pulsations will be best visualized. Simultaneous palpation of the left carotid artery and cardiac auscultation aid the examiner in relating the venous pulsations to the timing of the cardiac cycle.

NORMAL VENOUS PULSE

The normal jugular venous pulse (JVP) reflects phasic pressure changes in the right atrium and consists of three positive waves and two negatives troughs (Fig. 10-31). It is useful to refer to the events of the cardiac cycle (Fig. 3-31, Plate 2). The positive presystolic *a* wave is produced by right atrial contraction and is the dominant wave in the JVP, particularly during inspiration.

During atrial relaxation, the venous pulse descends from their summit of the *a* wave. Depending on the PR interval, this descent may continue until a plateau (*z* point) is reached just prior to right ventricular systole. More often, the descent is interrupted by a second positive venous wave, the *c* wave, which is produced by bulging of the tricuspid valve into the right atrium during right ventricular isovolumic systole and by the impact of the carotid artery adjacent to the jugular vein.[245] Following the summit of the *c* wave, the JVP contour declines, forming the normal negative systolic wave, the *x* wave. The *x* descent is due to a combination of atrial relaxation, the downward displacement of the tricuspid valve during right ventricular systole, and the ejection of blood from both ventricles (see also Chap. 3).

The positive, later systolic *v* wave in the JVP results from the increase in blood volume in the venae cavae and right atrium during ventricular systole when the tricuspid valve is closed. After the peak of the *v* wave is reached, the right atrial pressure decreases because of the diminished bulging of the tricuspid valve into the right atrium and the decline in right ventricular pressure that follow tricuspid valve opening. In the JVP the latter occurs at the peak of the *v* wave. Following the summit of the *v* wave, there is a negative descending limb, referred to as the *y* descent or diastolic collapse, which is due to the tricuspid valve opening and the rapid inflow of blood into the right ventricle. The initial *y* descent corresponds to the right ventricular rapid-filling phase. The trough of the *y* wave occurs in early diastole and is followed by the ascending limb of the *y* wave, which is produced by the continued diastolic inflow of blood into the right side of the heart. The velocity of this ascending pressure curve depends on the rate of venous return and the distensibility of the chambers of the right side of the heart. When diastole is long, the ascending limb of the *y* wave is often followed by a small, brief, positive wave, the *h* wave, which occurs just prior to the next *a* wave. At times, there is a plateau phase rather than a distinct *h* wave. With increasing heart rate, the *y* trough and *y* ascent are followed immediately by the next *a* wave (see also Fig. 3-31, Plate 2).

Usually, there are three visible major positive waves (*a,c,v*) and two negative waves (*x,y*) when the pulse rate is below 90 beats per minute and the PR interval is normal. With faster heart rates, there is often fusion of some of the pulse waves, and an accurate analysis of the waveform is more difficult.

ABNORMAL VENOUS PULSE

Elevated Venous Pressure

The most common cause of an elevated jugular venous pressure is an increased right ventricular pressure such as occurs in patients with pulmonic stenosis, pulmonary hypertension, or right ventricular failure secondary to left heart failure or right ventricular infarction. The venous pressure also is elevated when obstruction to right ventricular inflow occurs, as with tricuspid stenosis or right atrial myxoma, or when constrictive pericardial disease impedes right ventricular inflow. It may also result from vena cava obstruction and, at times, an increased blood volume. Patients with obstructive pulmonary disease may have an elevated venous pressure only during expiration.

Küssmaul's Sign

Normally during inspiration there is an increase in the *a* wave of the JVP but a decrease in the mean jugular venous pressure as a result of the increased filling of the right-sided chambers associated with the decrease in intrathoracic pressure. *Küssmaul's sign*

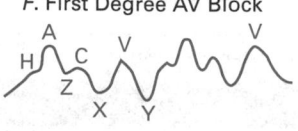

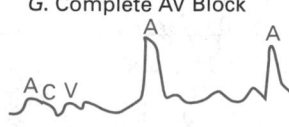

FIGURE 10-41

Schematic representation of the normal jugular venous pulse (JVP), four types of abnormal JVPs, and the JVPs in three arrhythmias. See text for definition of H, A, Z, C, X, V, and Y.

denotes an inspiratory increase in the venous pressure, which may occur in patients with severe constrictive pericarditis when the heart is unable to accept the increase in right ventricular volume without a marked increase in the filling pressure.[229] Although Küssmaul's sign was first described in patients with constrictive pericarditis, its most common cause is severe right-sided heart failure, regardless of etiology. The presence of Küssmaul's sign is also useful in the diagnosis of right ventricular infarction[246] (Chap. 81).

Abnormalities of the *a* Wave

The *a* wave in the JVP is absent when there is no effective atrial contraction, such as in atrial fibrillation (Fig. 10-41*E*). In certain other conditions, the *a* wave may not be apparent. In sinus tachycardia the *a* wave may fuse with the preceding *v* weave, particularly if the PR interval is prolonged. In some patients with sinus tachycardia, the jugular *a* wave may occur during the *v* or *y* descent and may be small or absent. In the presence of first-degree AV block, a discrete *a* wave with ascending and descending limbs is often completed prior to the first heart sound and the *ac* interval is prolonged (Fig. 10-41*F*).

Large *a* waves are of considerable diagnostic value (Fig. 10-41*B*). When giant *a* waves are present with each beat, the right atrium is contracting against an increased resistance. This may result from obstruction at the tricuspid valve (tricuspid stenosis or atresia, right atrial myxoma) or conditions associated with increased resistance to right ventricular filling.[247] A giant *a* wave is more likely to occur in patients with pulmonic stenosis or pulmonary hypertension in whom both the atrial and ventricular septa are intact.

Cannon *a* waves occur when the right atrium contracts while the tricuspid valve is closed during right ventricular systole.[238] Cannon waves may occur either regularly or irregularly and are most common in the presence of arrhythmias (Fig. 10-41*G*).

Abnormalities of the *x* Wave

The most important alteration of the normally negative systolic collapse (*x* wave) of the JVP is its obliteration or even replacement by a positive wave. This is usually due to tricuspid regurgitation.[248,249] Although atrial relaxation may contribute to the normal *x* descent, the development of atrial fibrillation does not obliterate the *x* wave except in the presence of tricuspid regurgitation. Accordingly, the occurrence of a positive wave in the JVP during ventricular systole is strong evidence of tricuspid regurgitation (Figs. 10-41*A* and 10-42). Mild tricuspid regurgitation lessens and shortens the downward *x* wave as the regurgitation of blood into the right atrium produces a positive wave that diminishes the usual systolic fall in venous pressure. In some patients with moderate tricuspid regurgitation, there is a fairly distinct positive wave during ventricular systole between the *c* and *v* waves. This abnormal systolic waveform is usually referred to as a *v* or *cv* wave, although it has also been referred to as an *r* (regurgitant) or an *s* (systolic) wave.

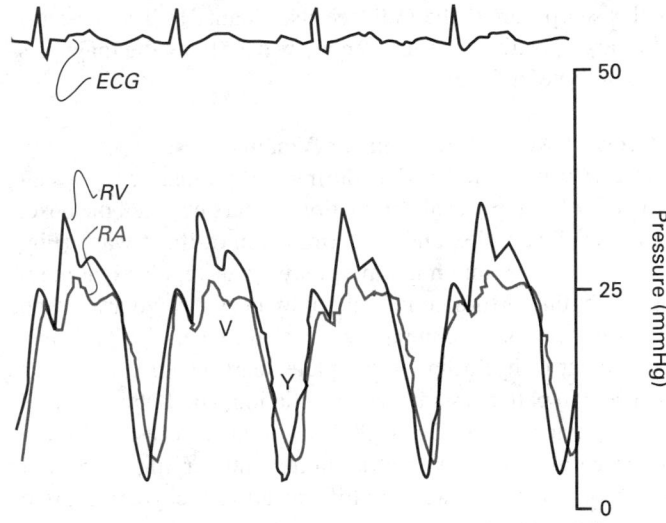

FIGURE 10-42

Right ventricular (RV) and right atrial (RA) pressure curves and simultaneous ECG from a patient with severe tricuspid regurgitation. Note ventricularization of the RA pressure curve.

In patients with constrictive pericarditis, the *x* descent wave during systole is often more prominent than the early diastolic *y* wave (Fig. 10-41*C*) (see Chap. 81).

Abnormalities of the *v* Wave

The positive, late systolic *v* wave results from the increasing right atrial blood volume during ventricular systole when the tricuspid valve normally is closed. With mild tricuspid regurgitation, the *v* wave and the obliteration of the *x* descent result in a single, large positive systolic wave (ventricularization) (Figs. 10-41*A* and 10-42).

Normally in the JVP the *v* wave is lower in amplitude than the *a* wave. In patients with an atrial septal defect, however, the *a* and *v* waves are often equal in the right atrium and the JVP (Fig. 10-41*D*).[250] In patients with constrictive pericarditis and sinus rhythm, the right atrial *a* and *v* waves may also be equal, but the venous pressure is increased, which is unusual with isolated atrial septal defect. In patients with constrictive pericarditis who are in atrial fibrillation, the *cv* wave is prominent and the *y* descent rapid.

Abnormalities of the *y* Trough

The *y* descent, or diastolic collapse, is produced mainly by the tricuspid valve opening and the rapid inflow of blood into the right ventricle. A rapid, deep *y* descent in early diastole occurs with severe tricuspid regurgitation (Fig. 10-41*A*). A venous pulse characterized by a sharp *y* descent, a deep *y* trough, and a rapid ascent to the baseline is seen in patients with constrictive pericarditis or with severe right-sided heart failure. A slow *y* descent in the JVP suggests an obstruction to right ventricular filling and may be the only abnormal finding in patients with tricuspid stenosis or right atrial myxoma (Fig. 10-41*B*).[251] In both constrictive pericarditis and severe right-sided heart failure, the venous pressure is elevated with a sharp *y* dip in the JVP (see also Chap. 81). The presence of a large positive systolic venous wave favors the diagnosis of severe heart failure.

Effects of Arrhythmias on the Venous Pulse

Large *a* waves in the JVP during arrhythmias are present when the *P* wave (atrial contraction) occurs between the onset of the QRS complex and the termination of the *T* wave (Fig. 10-41*G*). Such cannon *a* waves may occur regularly in junctional rhythm. More commonly, they occur irregularly when AV dissociation accompanies premature ventricular beats, ventricular tachycardia, or complete heart block. The *a* wave is absent in patients with atrial fibrillation, and flutter *a* waves at a regular rate of 250 to 300 per minute occasionally are observed in patients with atrial flutter and varying degrees of AV block. Patients with multifocal atrial tachycardia often have prominent and somewhat variable *a* waves in the JVP. In these patients, many of whom have pulmonary hypertension secondary to lung disease, the *a* waves are often very large.

INSPECTION AND PALPATION OF THE PRECORDIUM

Inspection and palpation of the cardiac pulsations of the anterior chest have been practiced by physicians since ancient times and have a solid scientific basis.[252–254] The results of precordial inspection and palpation have been correlated with noninvasive studies, hemodynamic data, and surgical and autopsy studies[253,254] and remain an important part of the cardiovascular examination.[255–259] Their usefulness depends on an understanding of cardiovascular physiology, the proficiency of the examiner and his or her ability to integrate findings with history, the information obtained by other portions of the physical examination, the ECG, the chest roentgenogram, and other diagnostic tests.[254]

Precordial Pulsations Due to the Heartbeat

Precordial pulsations, reflecting underlying movement of the heart and great vessels, occur principally in seven areas of the anterior chest[253,254] (Fig. 10-43):

1. The sternoclavicular area
2. The aortic area
3. The pulmonic area
4. The right ventricular (left parasternal) area
5. The apical (left ventricular) area
6. The epigastric area
7. Ectopic (variable-location) areas

While the cardiac apex is usually produced by the left ventricle, it is sometimes produced by an enlarged right ventricle that displaces the left ventricle laterally and posteriorly.[253] Occasionally, the cardiac position is abnormal due to dextroposition, dextroversion, dextrocardia, or other changes in intrathoracic structures. Although the cardiac apex impulse is commonly referred to as the *point of maximal impulse* (PMI),

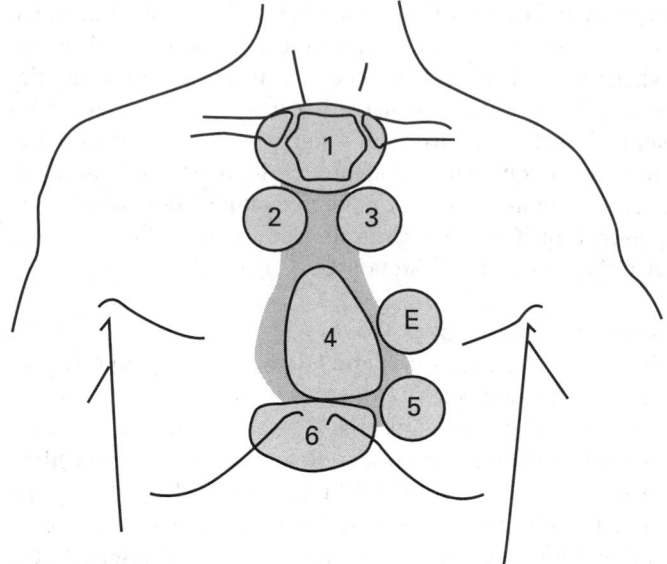

FIGURE 10-43
Seven areas to be examined for abnormal cardiovascular pulsations by inspection and palpation. (From Schlant RC, Hurst JW. *Examination of the Precordium: Inspection and Palpation.* New York: American Heart Association; 1990:1–28. Used with permission from the publisher and authors.)

the two terms are not necessarily synonymous, since the maximal precordial pulsation may be produced by an enlarged or hypertrophied right ventricle, a dilated aorta or pulmonary artery, or a left ventricular wall-motion abnormality. Therefore, precordial pulsations should be described by their location, timing, contour, and duration.[253,254,258]

INSPECTION OF THE PRECORDIUM

The examiner should first inspect the thorax from the foot of the bed with the subject supine, the legs horizontal, and the head and trunk elevated to approximately 30°.[253] The patient may have a barrel-shaped chest with an increased anteroposterior diameter, a straight-back syndrome, pectus excavatum, pectus carinatum, kyphoscoliosis, or ankylosing spondylitis. Each may produce or be associated with cardiac abnormalities. Asymmetry of the thorax due to convex bulging of the precordium suggests the presence of heart disease since childhood. Exaggerated movements of the cardiac apex can often be detected from this observation point.

Next, the examiner should move to the patient's right side and observe the patient's chest tangentially rather than from above. A light beam directed across the precordium may enhance subtle findings.[253,254] Precordial movements can frequently be more easily recognized if the tip of an applicator stick, tongue blade, or light pencil is held against the impulse as a fulcrum. Motion of the underlying chest wall is transmitted to the free end of the instrument and exaggerated, making the movements more obvious.[253,254]

In patients with an abnormally prominent apical impulse and in some thin, normal individuals, the apical impulse or apex beat can be seen. The presystolic apical motion associated with the atrial contribution to ventricular filling (a fourth heart sound) may sometimes be visualized, as may the diastolic waveform due to rapid ventricular filling a third heart sound. A late systolic bulge either at the apex or in an ectopic area, usually located either medial and superior or lateral to the apical impulse, may be observed in patients with a large dyskinetic ventricular aneurysm.[254] When precordial pulsations are exaggerated, they become visible as well as palpable. In general, however, outward movements are best discerned by palpation, whereas inward movements are usually more easily seen than felt.[253,254]

PALPATION OF THE PRECORDIUM

With Tietze's syndrome, pain, sometimes with swelling and tenderness, may affect the costochondral, chondrosternal, or xiphosternal joints and may be reproduced by touching. Palpation may also reveal tender superficial veins on the anterior chest (Mondor's disease), a rare etiology of chest discomfort.[254] Collateral vessels in the posterior intercostal spaces may be palpable in patients with aortic coarctation.[254]

Palpation of the precordium is also best performed from the right side, with the patient supine and the upper trunk elevated 30°. Palpation with the right hand usually provides more information. Patients with suspected cardiovascular disease should also be examined in the left lateral decubitus position, rotated 45 to 90°.[254,255,260] In this position, the normal left ventricular impulse may be displaced several centimeters leftward and may appear more prominent and sustained. The size of the apex impulse rather than its distance from the midsternal or midclavicular line determines its normality.[260] Often, the apex impulse and other palpable events such as a left ventricular rapid filling wave (S_3) or presystolic *a* wave (S_4) may be felt only in this position.[254–260]

The location and size of the cardiac apex impulse should be defined, its contour characterized, and any abnormal precordial pulsations identified.[261] The palm of the hand, ventral surface of the proximal metacarpals, and fingers should all be used for the optimal appreciation of specific movements.[262] The fingers appear to be particularly insensitive to movements of relatively large amplitude and very low frequency.[262] This is consistent with the clinical observation that an examiner's hand can occasionally be visualized to move up and down with precordial motion, although the same movements are imperceptible by palpation alone.[253] By contrast, higher-frequency events, such as the vibrations associated with abnormally loud aortic or pulmonic components of the second heart sound, are easily palpable, even though the amplitude of their movement is not readily visible.[253]

The pads of the fingers are most useful for detecting left ventricular and normal right ventricular motion, while the palm and proximal metacarpals are usually best used for palpating larger, low-frequency movements such as the parasternal systolic lift of right ventricular hypertrophy.[253] Varying pressure with the hand is often quite useful. High-frequency movements such as ejection sounds, valve closure sounds, and mitral opening snaps are more easily detected with the hand held firmly against the chest, while low-frequency movements such as ventricular diastolic filling events are best recognized with light pressure with the fingertips.

Thrills are palpable vibrations from murmurs or bruits ordinarily associated with grade 4/6 murmurs or louder (discussed later in this chapter). The location of a thrill often helps identify its origin. Thrills are most easily palpated with the fingertips or with firm pressure, using either the palm of the hand or proximal metacarpals. Sometimes thrills are felt better during a held-end expiration with moderate pressure applied from the right hand on top of the left hand, which is placed on the chest.[254] Occasionally, palpable murmurs are more readily detected with the right palm placed over the anterior chest and the left hand supporting the posterior thorax with equal force.[254]

To detect abnormal right ventricular motion, the heel of the hand should be placed over the lower half of the sternum with the patient's breath held at end-expiration.[253] The parasternal lift due to right ventricular hypertrophy is often better visualized than actually felt. In patients with chronic obstructive pulmonary disease, subxyphoid and epigastric palpation with the patient's breath held at end-inspiration is useful for assessing right ventricular motion.[254]

As indicated above, proper patient positioning is important. The location of the apex impulse is usually described in terms of its distance from the midsternal or midclavicular line and the intercostal space in which it is located. Although heart size is commonly estimated based on the size and location of the apex impulse with the patient supine, this is not always a reliable indicator of left ventricular end-diastolic volume.[260–262] The apex impulse is often faint or not palpable with the patient supine because of the distance of the ventricular apex from the chest wall. Palpation of the cardiac apex with the patient in the left lateral position, however, permits optimal assessment of the size (diameter) and contour of the systolic outward movement at the apex; diastolic movements are also best appreciated with the patient in this position.[260–263] Since the apex impulse may shift several centimeters laterally when the patient rotates to the left lateral position, however, the location of the apex impulse may be incorrect in this position. Palpation with simultaneous cardiac auscultation often is useful for identifying the systolic or diastolic timing of precordial pulsations. Simultaneous palpation of the apical impulse and carotid pulse may be helpful in assessing the severity of aortic stenosis. An appreciable lag time between the onset of the apex impulse and carotid pulse usually indicates severe aortic stenosis[264] (see also Chap. 63).

PHYSIOLOGY OF PRECORDIAL MOTION

Although only the apical impulse is palpable normally, a brief right ventricular systolic motion can be felt at the left sternal edge in asthenic individuals. With the onset of isovolmic left ventricular contraction, there is anterior movement of the left ventricle toward the chest wall (Fig. 10-44).[196] Counterclockwise rotation of the left ventricle along its longitudinal axis occurs as the cardiac apex moves anteriorly and makes contact with the chest wall in early systole.[264–268] The maximal out-

Graphic Representation
(palpable features in heavy line)

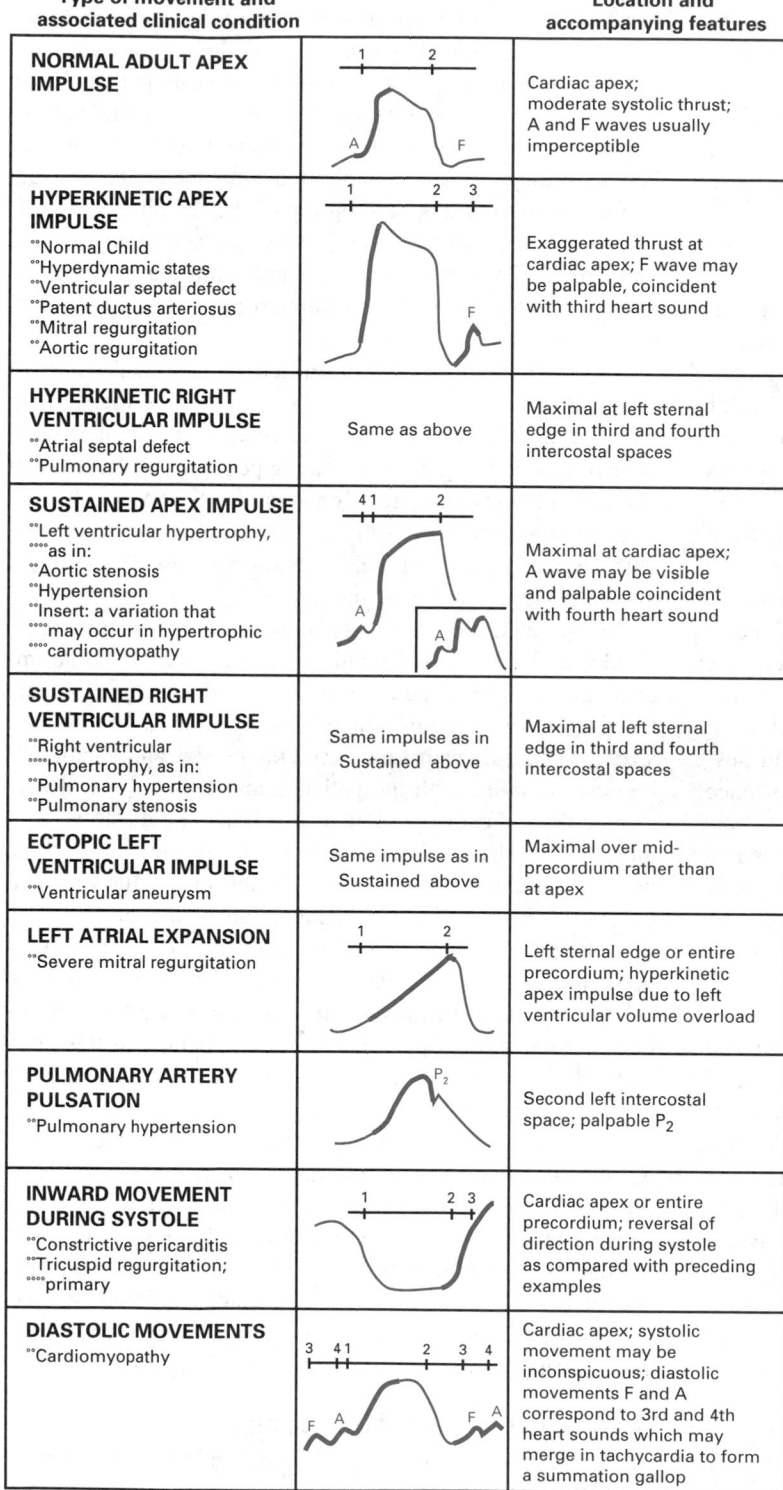

Type of movement and associated clinical condition	Graphic Representation	Location and accompanying features
NORMAL ADULT APEX IMPULSE		Cardiac apex; moderate systolic thrust; A and F waves usually imperceptible
HYPERKINETIC APEX IMPULSE °°Normal Child °°Hyperdynamic states °°Ventricular septal defect °°Patent ductus arteriosus °°Mitral regurgitation °°Aortic regurgitation		Exaggerated thrust at cardiac apex; F wave may be palpable, coincident with third heart sound
HYPERKINETIC RIGHT VENTRICULAR IMPULSE °°Atrial septal defect °°Pulmonary regurgitation	Same as above	Maximal at left sternal edge in third and fourth intercostal spaces
SUSTAINED APEX IMPULSE °°Left ventricular hypertrophy, °°°°as in: °°Aortic stenosis °°Hypertension °°Insert: a variation that °°°°°may occur in hypertrophic °°°°°cardiomyopathy		Maximal at cardiac apex; A wave may be visible and palpable coincident with fourth heart sound
SUSTAINED RIGHT VENTRICULAR IMPULSE °°Right ventricular °°°°hypertrophy, as in: °°Pulmonary hypertension °°Pulmonary stenosis	Same impulse as in Sustained above	Maximal at left sternal edge in third and fourth intercostal spaces
ECTOPIC LEFT VENTRICULAR IMPULSE °°Ventricular aneurysm	Same impulse as in Sustained above	Maximal over mid-precordium rather than at apex
LEFT ATRIAL EXPANSION °°Severe mitral regurgitation		Left sternal edge or entire precordium; hyperkinetic apex impulse due to left ventricular volume overload
PULMONARY ARTERY PULSATION °°Pulmonary hypertension		Second left intercostal space; palpable P_2
INWARD MOVEMENT DURING SYSTOLE °°Constrictive pericarditis °°Tricuspid regurgitation; °°°°°primary		Cardiac apex or entire precordium; reversal of direction during systole as compared with preceding examples
DIASTOLIC MOVEMENTS °°Cardiomyopathy		Cardiac apex; systolic movement may be inconspicuous; diastolic movements F and A correspond to 3rd and 4th heart sounds which may merge in tachycardia to form a summation gallop

FIGURE 10-44

Graphic representation of apical movements in health and disease. Heavy line indicates palpable features. P_2, pulmonary component of second heart sound; A, atrial wave, corresponding to a fourth heart sound (S_4) or atrial gallop; F, filling wave, corresponding to third heart sound (S_3) or ventricular gallop. (From Willis P IV. Inspection and palpation of the precordium. In: Hurst JW, ed. *The Heart*, 7th ed. New York: McGraw-Hill; 1990:164. Reproduced with permission.)

ward movement occurs coincident with or just after aortic valve opening. After rapid early ejection, the left ventricle moves away from the chest wall and the apex retracts during latter systole and returns to baseline well before the second heart sound.[253] The outward apex movement in early systole normally is palpable, but the later systolic inward movement is only visible (Fig. 10-44). Palpable movements of the apex in diastole result from left ventricular filling. The early diastolic outward movement due to rapid ventricular filling (*F* wave), which corresponds to the normal S_3, is occasionally palpable in normal children and young adults (Fig. 10-44). Later diastolic filling due to left atrial contraction (*A* wave) is not normally palpable. Precordial motion is modified by age, chest wall thickness, lung disease, and pleural or pericardial effusion.[196]

Area 1: Sternoclavicular Area Pulsations

The sternoclavicular area (Fig. 10-43) includes the right and left sternoclavicular joints, the manubrium, and the upper sternum. Usually, no pulsation is noted in this area. A slight, brief systolic pulsation of a sternoclavicular joint or the manubrium may be due to aortic regurgitation. Abnormal pulsations and movements in the sternoclavicular area are commonly produced by enlargement, dilatation, or diseases of the aorta, particularly aortic dissection, atherosclerotic aneurysm, or syphilitic aneurysm.[254] An abnormal pulsation of a sternoclavicular joint in patients with chest pain may be an early clue to diagnosis of aortic dissection.[269,270] A slight pulsation in the right sternoclavicular area may suggest a right-sided aortic arch in patients with cyanotic heart disease, particularly tetralogy of Fallot.[271] A kinked, tortuous right carotid artery or dilation and tortuosity of other brachiocephalic vessels may produce visible and palpable pulsations in the suprasternal notch or the supraclavicular areas.[254]

Area 2: Aortic Area Pulsations

Vibrations of the aortic component (A_2) of the second heart sound may be palpated when they are accentuated, as in arterial hypertension. With valvular aortic stenosis, a systolic thrill is present frequently in the second and less commonly in the first and third right intercostal spaces near the sternum (Fig. 10-43). It often radiates upward toward the right side of the neck and to the suprasternal notch and right supraclavicular area. Less frequently, the thrill is palpable at the second or third left interspace next to the sternum or at the apex. A systolic thrill in the aortic area and in the right carotid artery can also occur in patients with severe aortic regurgitation without stenosis. Abnormal systolic pulsations in the aortic area may be due to dilation of the ascending aorta due to aneurysm and/or chronic aortic regurgitation.

Area 3: Pulmonic Area Pulsations

Vibrations associated with a loud pulmonic component (Fig. 10-43) of S_2 are often palpable in patients with pulmonary hypertension from any cause. During simultaneous palpation of the carotid pulse, a palpable P_2 or A_2 coincides with the early downslope of the carotid pulse. A systolic thrill in the second and third left intercostal space near the sternum often occurs with pulmonic valve stenosis. The thrill often radiates toward the left side of the neck, in contrast to the thrill with aortic stenosis, which radiates upward and to the right.

Pulsations of a dilated pulmonary artery may be seen or felt in the second or third left intercostal space near the sternum.[272] In normal infants and children or anxious adults with thin chest walls, a slight, brief, early systolic pulsation may be present in this area. This pulsation is accentuated by conditions that cause an increased cardiac output (e.g., fever, pregnancy). Idiopathic dilatation of the pulmonary artery may also cause a palpable systolic impulse in the same area.[254]

The common causes of an accentuated and sustained systolic pulsation in the pulmonary artery area are pulmonary hypertension, increased pulmonary blood flow, or their combination. In general, pulmonary hypertension causes a relatively slow, sustained, and forceful pulmonary artery pulsation, while a large pulmonary blood flow (e.g., atrial septal defect) produces an extremely active, more vigorous, but less sustained pulsation. Valvular pulmonary stenosis with poststenotic dilation of the pulmonary artery may be associated with a palpable, sustained pulsation in this area, often with a slow rise of the initial phase.[254]

Area 4: Left Parasternal–Right Ventricular or Tricuspid Area Pulsations

A systolic thrill in the third, fourth, or fifth intercostal space in the parasternal area to the left of the sternum (Fig. 10-43) is characteristic of ventricular septal defect, although tricuspid regurgitation can also produce a thrill here.

Normally the lower left parasternal region retracts very slightly during systole, and right ventricular activity is not palpable. Slight, gentle outward pulsations of the lower sternum and left parasternal area may be recorded in normal children and young adults, in thin adults with a small anterior-posterior thoracic diameter, or in patients with pectus excavatum. Sometimes, these pulsations can be palpated in the subxiphoid area, and are increased by hyperdynamic cardiac function.[254]

Abnormal pulsations of the sternal and left parasternal areas are most commonly due to right ventricular hypertrophy or dilation. The pulsation associated with right ventricular hypertension is usually more sustained throughout systole and tends to rise more gradually than the pulsation produced by

a right ventricular volume load, which usually is more vigorous but often briefer.[273]

A predominant right ventricular pressure load occurs with pulmonic stenosis and pulmonary hypertension due to left ventricular failure, mitral valve disease, a left-to-right shunt, or pulmonary vascular disease. The sustained anterior precordial pulsation associated with isolated valvular pulmonic stenosis may not occur with tetralogy of Fallot because the thick right ventricle is not excessively dilated.[254] Atrial septal defect and ventricular septal defect are two congenital lesions frequently associated with a right ventricular volume load.[274]

Moderate or severe mitral regurgitation may produce an abnormal late systolic anterior left parasternal pulsation even in the absence of pulmonary hypertension.[275–277] This precordial lift is brisk, and its greatest force coincides with the accentuated *V* wave in the left atrial pressure wave. It likely is due to the large volume of blood regurgitated into the expanding left atrium, which is located centrally behind the right ventricle and anterior to the spine. While expansion of the left atrium may contribute somewhat to the anterior motion of the heart, it is likely that most of the anterior motion and force is the result of a jet or squid effect.

Conditions associated with a decrease in right ventricular compliance, such as right ventricular hypertrophy secondary to pulmonary hypertension, may be associated with a palpable "right-sided" S_4 in this area or, occasionally, in the epigastric area. Although a palpable S_3 in this area may reflect a large right ventricular volume load, it usually indicates right ventricular dysfunction or failure. Right ventricular S_3 and S_4 vibrations may be augmented during inspiration and may be attenuated or even disappear during expiration (see later in this chapter).

Area 5: Apical Area Pulsations

As mentioned above, the apex impulse (Fig. 10-43) is not synonymous with maximum impulse or PMI. The location, size, and character (duration, contour or shape, amplitude, and apparent force) of the apex impulse should be determined.[254] The examiner should focus on one phase of the cardiac cycle at a time and correlate the findings with other cardiovascular events.

The normal apex (apical) impulse usually is located within 10 cm of the sternal midline, at or within the left midclavicular line in the fifth intercostal space when the patient is supine. It may be located lateral to the midclavicular line when associated with a high diaphragm, pregnancy, marked pectus excavatum, or other conditions that displace a normal heart to the left. The normal apex impulse is less than 3 cm in diameter and in most instances is considerably smaller.[260] The early systolic outward movement of the apical area (Fig. 10-44) begins at about the same time as that of the S_1, just before the upstroke of the carotid pulse. Peak outward motion normally occurs with or just after blood is ejected into the aorta; then the apex normally moves inward. The outward movement of the apical impulse is normally not excessively forceful and is felt only during the first third of systole.

The apex impulse may be hyperkinetic or hyperdynamic with increased amplitude in normal individuals who have a thin chest wall, a flat chest, or a depressed sternum. Lying on the left side may cause a normal apical impulse to move laterally and to have increased amplitude and duration[254,260]; however, it should still not exceed a diameter of greater than 3 cm.[203] A hyperdynamic apex impulse may also be found in anxious children, in patients with high cardiac output states, and in patients with a mild to moderate left ventricular volume load from mitral or aortic regurgitation.[254] The apex impulse is more sustained when mitral or aortic regurgitation is more severe or when left ventricular systolic function is decreased.[278,279] In general, a greatly sustained apex impulse indicates either marked left ventricular hypertrophy or depressed left ventricular systolic function, while left ventricular dilation displaces the apex impulse laterally and inferiorly[254] (Fig. 10-44).

Concentric left ventricular hypertrophy without an increase in left ventricular cavity size may occur in systemic hypertension, valvular aortic stenosis, and hypertrophic cardiomyopathy. Characteristically, the apex impulse is not displaced but is both abnormally forceful and sustained.[280,281] An S_4 vibration may be palpable or visible or both.

Severe left ventricular dilation—whether due to volume load or ventricular failure—may displace the apex impulse laterally and inferiorly and cause a marked increase in size. The duration of the apex impulse is more sustained in patients with left ventricular systolic dysfunction, particularly when associated with marked left ventricular dilation.

Important information about relative amounts of ventricular hypertrophy and dilatation often can be obtained from the apex impulse. Thus, in valvular aortic stenosis, with marked concentric left ventricular hypertrophy but little or no dilation, the apex impulse characteristically is small, forceful, and sustained but not displaced.[282] A presystolic S_4 is often palpable at the apex. By contrast, in severe aortic regurgitation with marked dilation of the left ventricle plus considerable eccentric hypertrophy, there is a diffuse apex impulse with increased force, duration, and amplitude, and it is displaced laterally and inferiorly.[254]

In some patients with acute myocardial infarction, a sustained apex impulse may simulate that due to left ventricular hypertrophy.[283–285] Those developing mitral regurgitation secondary to myocardial infarction (papillary muscle dysfunction) may manifest left ventricular dilation and hypertrophy by a displaced and sustained, forceful, large apex impulse.[254] A late systolic bulge at the cardiac apex may be due to a functional left ventricular aneurysm, occasionally resulting in a bifid apex impulse. In other patients, a late systolic bulge may be palpable in an ectopic area between the apex impulse and the left parasternal area.[254]

A bifid apex impulse during systole may also be due to marked left ventricular dilation and hypertrophy in patients with both aortic stenosis and regurgitation or in patients with hypertrophic cardiomyopathy.[286] Infrequently, a faint systolic notch or vibration is palpable in the apex impulse of patients

with mitral valve prolapse at the moment of a nonejection midsystolic click. Systolic retraction of the apical impulse usually indicates either constrictive pericarditis or severe tricuspid regurgitation with marked right ventricular dilation (Fig. 10-44).[287] An apical systolic thrill most commonly is produced by mitral regurgitation and often is diffuse, whereas a diastolic thrill is usually produced by mitral stenosis and is localized to a small, discrete area.

DIASTOLIC EVENTS: PALPABLE THIRD AND FOURTH HEART SOUNDS

During early diastole, brief outward chest wall movement corresponding to a left ventricular rapid filling or a third heart sound (S_3) may occasionally be seen or felt, even if not audible with a stethoscope (Fig. 10-44). In children and young adults, the presence of an early diastolic ventricular filling sound (S_3) and movement is usually normal. On the other hand, the presence of such a movement or sound in a sedentary adult or a patient with heart disease usually indicates an elevated left ventricular diastolic pressure and volume, and likely ventricular decompensation, often with a decreased ejection fraction. Patients with acute myocardial infarction or transient myocardial ischemia during angina pectoris frequently develop a transient palpable and audible ventricular filling S_3, which reflects the acutely decreased ventricular compliance. A palpable ventricular rapid filling wave (S_3) may be present in patients with left ventricular failure from any cause; however, hemodynamic systolic ventricular failure is often not always present when a ventricular filling wave or sound occurs in the presence of volume loading and dilation of the left ventricle, as with mitral regurgitation or aortic regurgitation.

The presystolic left atrial contribution to the apical impulse (referred to as the atrial impulse or *a* wave) may be detected during late diastole, just prior to S_1 (Fig. 10-44). Usually a palpable atrial impulse coincides with an audible fourth heart sound and is associated with an increased left ventricular end-diastolic pressure and decreased compliance. In general, an S_4 is not normally palpable but may be felt at the apex with its associated S_4 in some normal adults if the PR interval is long and circulation is hyperdynamic.[254] In some patients with ischemic heart disease, a palpable apical S_4 may develop or become more prominent during an episode of angina pectoris or even during exertion without chest pain.[288] A palpable presystolic impulse, S_4, or both occur frequently in patients with acute myocardial infarction, and these are also frequently is present in other conditions producing a decrease in left ventricular compliance and increased end-diastolic pressure.

In a patient with mitral valve disease, the presence of a palpable left-sided atrial impulse or S_4, a palpable left-sided ventricular filling sound or S_3, or an abnormally sustained apical impulse is evidence against the diagnosis of isolated important mitral stenosis and suggests the presence of coincident left ventricular disease.

A double, or bifid, apical impulse may be present in various circumstances, most commonly in the combination of an outward movement during ventricular systole and a second outward pulsation during diastole.[254] The diastolic impulse may occur either in early diastole (S_3) or in late diastole or presystole (S_4).

A bifid apical impulse with two systolic impulses may be present in patients with hypertrophic obstructive cardiomyopathy, complete left bundle branch block, or myocardial infarction. If these patients also develop a palpable impulse during either early (S_3) or late (S_4) diastole, a triple or trifid apical impulse may occur.[254] When such patients develop both a palpable S_3 and a palpable S_4, it is occasionally possible to see and feel a quadruple apical impulse.

Area 6: Epigastric Area Pulsations

Some normal and many hyperkinetic individuals have visible or palpable pulsations of the aorta in the epigastric area (Fig. 10-43). Abnormally large pulsations of the aorta may be due to an aortic aneurysm or aortic regurgitation. Hepatic movements may be identified in the epigastric area, particularly in patients with tricuspid regurgitation, tricuspid stenosis, or marked right ventricular dilatation, hypertrophy, and hyperactivity.

In some patients with pulmonary hypertension due to chronic lung disease, the detection of right ventricular hypertrophy by precordial palpation is difficult because the shape of the chest often conceals the enlarged right ventricle. To detect abnormal right ventricular pulsations in patients with emphysema, the palm of the right hand should be placed on the epigastric area and moved cephalad while gently sliding the fingers under the rib cage.[254] Aortic pulsations can be detected by the palmar surface of the fingers, and pulsations due to right ventricular hypertrophy can be felt in the fingertips.

Area 7: Ectopic Area Pulsations

Occasionally, cardiac pulsations are encountered in areas other than those previously described; that is, between the pulmonary and apical areas (Fig. 10-43). Ischemic heart disease is the most common cause of an ectopic systolic pulsation, which may occur transiently during an episode of angina pectoris. A similar paradoxical systolic outward movement may be detected after acute myocardial infarction and may persist; more commonly, it disappears within a few weeks. A persistent paradoxical ectopic pulsation may also be found in patients who develop a ventricular aneurysm after myocardial infarction.

Ectopic pulsations on the anterior chest wall can also be found in patients with cardiomyopathies of varying etiologies. In patients with severe mitral regurgitation and a giant left atrium that extends to the right, an ectopic systolic pulsation of the atrium may occasionally be felt in the right anterior or lateral chest or in the left axilla.[254]

PERCUSSION VERSUS INSPECTION AND PALPATION OF THE PRECORDIUM

When performed by a skilled examiner, percussion of the heart can provide an estimate of cardiac size and shape. Percussion of the heart only gives information about the location of the borders of cardiac dullness, while precordial inspection and palpation provide both information about the location of the outer limits of cardiac pulsations and a determination of the size and character of the pulsations. Although percussion has been used in the diagnosis of pericardial effusion, it has limited value when the results are objectively correlated with the diagnosis as determined by more sensitive and specific noninvasive and invasive testing.

PHYSICAL EXAMINATION OF THE CHEST, ABDOMEN, AND EXTREMITIES

Physical examination of the lungs is a painless, noninvasive technique, requiring only a stethoscope.[289,290] An abnormal examination often indicates the need for a chest roentgenogram. Wheezing and a pleural friction rub are detected only by the clinical evaluation. The pleural friction rub may be a clue to the diagnosis of pulmonary infarction. Pleural fluid due to heart failure is usually located in the right pleural space. When pleural fluid is localized predominately to the left, a cause other than or in addition to heart failure, such as pulmonary infarction, should be considered.[290]

A pneumothorax may develop as a consequence of spontaneous mediastinal emphysema or may be iatrogenic, due to procedures.[290] Hyperresonance and diminished breath sounds may be due to pulmonary emphysema. Signs of pulmonary consolidation may be due to pneumonia or pulmonary infarction. Wheezing and rales may be due to bronchial disease. Heart failure may be associated with rales in the lung bases, wheezing, and pleural fluid. Importantly, heart failure frequently is *not* associated with rales, since interstitial pulmonary edema usually does *not* produce rales.[290]

The diameter of the *abdominal* aorta should be determined in every patient (see also Chap. 98).[290] An abdominal aortic aneurysm may be missed if the examiner fails to assess the area above the umbilicus.

Specific abnormalities of the abdomen may be secondary to heart disease. A large, tender liver is common in patients with heart failure or constrictive pericarditis. Systolic hepatic pulsations are frequent in patients with tricuspid regurgitation. A palpable spleen is a common but late sign in patients with severe heart failure and is also often present in patients with infective endocarditis.

Although hepatic cirrhosis is the most common cause of ascites, the latter may occur with heart failure alone, although it is less common with the use of diuretic therapy. Severe tricuspid regurgitation, as caused by infective endocarditis in drug addicts, may produce prominent systolic pulsation of the internal jugular veins in the neck; a large, moving, and pulsating liver; and ascites. Constrictive pericarditis should be considered when the ascites is out of proportion to peripheral edema. In many such patients, the heart is normal in size or only slightly enlarged, a pericardial "knock" is heard, and there is a rapid x and/or y descent in the internal jugular vein pulsation.[290] Restrictive cardiomyopathy can mimic constrictive pericarditis, but the heart is usually moderately large in patients with restrictive cardiomyopathy. When there is an arteriovenous fistula in the abdomen, a continuous murmur may be heard over the abdomen. Fistulas due to trauma and surgery may occur.

A systolic bruit may be heard over the kidney areas and may signify renal artery stenosis, particularly in patients with systemic hypertension. A systolic bruit often is auscultated over the abdominal aorta, but its presence does not indicate the severity of disease of the aorta.[290]

Examination of the upper and lower *extremities* may provide important diagnostic information (see also Chap. 100). The clinical detection of arterial disease and thrombophlebitis is important.[2] Atherosclerosis of the peripheral arteries may produce intermittent claudication of the buttock, calf, thigh, or foot, with severe disease resulting in tissue damage of the toes. Peripheral atherosclerosis is an important risk factor for ischemic heart disease, and its presence increases the likelihood of coronary atherosclerosis. Thrombophlebitis often causes pain in the calf or thigh or edema, and its presence should raise the consideration of pulmonary emboli as well. Edema is a late sign of heart failure, and its predictive value as a diagnostic sign is poor. It frequently involves the right leg prior to the left. Considerable heart failure and a resulting weight gain may be present without edema being present. Edema of the lower extremities may be secondary to local factors such as varicose veins or thrombophlebitis or the removal of veins at coronary artery bypass surgery. Under such circumstances, the edema often occurs in only one leg.

Edema may result from restrictive garments, and venous stasis often is secondary to a long trip in a car or airplane.[290] Edema may be due to salt and water retention in patients with primary renal disease. In the differential diagnosis of edema, local factors should be considered first. If local factors can be excluded, the cause of the salt and water retention should be determined with an assessment for evidence of primary renal disease. Rarely, peripheral edema can be an early sign of lymphatic obstruction produced by metastatic disease in the pelvis or abdomen.

Since the invention of the stethoscope by Laennec in 1826,[291] cardiac auscultation has played a key role in the evaluation of the patient with cardiovascular disease. New diagnostic techniques developed in recent years have led to a better understanding of the relationship between intracardiac pressure, flow, and valve motion and the resultant sound phenomena on the other. The analysis of heart sounds and murmurs by phonocardiography together with informa-

tion obtained by cardiac catheterization, angiography, echocardiography, and cardiac surgery have made cardiac auscultation a precise discipline based on firm physiologic principles.[292]

CARDIAC AUSCULTATION

THE STETHOSCOPE

The physician must choose a stethoscope that fits the ears comfortably with the right angulation, has as short a segment of flexible tubing as possible, and is equipped with a diaphragm and a bell. Selection of the proper earpieces for comfort and the best transmission of sound is based on individual preference and is best evaluated by trial and error. A snug, comfortable fit depends on the size of the earpieces as well as the angle at which they enter the ear canal; the angulation of the rigid metal tubing must therefore be chosen to suit the comfort of the individual. The rubber tubing should be as short as feasible; experience indicates that tubing about 12 in. (30 cm) long is the best compromise. Rapaport and Sprague[293] have shown that thick-walled tubing about ⅛ in. (3 mm) in diameter is best suited to transmit sounds and murmurs.

The human ear is most sensitive to auditory vibrations that occur in the frequency range between 1000 and 4000 to 5000 Hz; the sensitivity falls off sharply when the frequency of vibration is below 1000 Hz. This is particularly true of low-frequency sounds, which must be of considerably greater amplitude to reach the threshold of audibility than sounds of higher frequency. Most cardiovascular sounds and murmurs of diagnostic importance are between 30 and 1000 Hz, thereby placing the auscultator at considerable disadvantage.[294] Therefore, a stethoscope requires both a diaphragm and a bell and each must be applied to the chest wall with optimal pressure. The diaphragm, which is fairly rigid, brings out the high frequencies and attenuates the lows. When the diaphragm is used to accentuate high-pitched sounds, it should be pressed very firmly against the skin. This technique will make a high-frequency murmur, such as the faint diastolic blowing murmur of aortic valve regurgitation, audible along the left sternal border when it would otherwise be missed. The bell tends to accentuate the low-frequency sounds and to filter out the high-pitched tones. Often, low-frequency sounds are more easily appreciated by palpation than by auscultation; in these situations, the stethoscope should be placed very lightly on the skin, with just enough pressure to seal the edge at the point of maximal impulse. With very light pressure of the bell, the low-pitched sounds are accentuated; however, with firm pressure of the bell against the skin, the skin itself becomes a relatively tight diaphragm and the low-frequency sounds are suppressed. Although this technique can be very helpful, the stethoscope should always be equipped with a valve system that permits one to switch from the diaphragm to the bell with ease.

EXAMINATION OF THE PATIENT

The examination should take place in a quiet room that is well lighted and comfortably heated. The patient should be properly gowned, with adequate exposure to the waist. The examining table should be large enough that the patient can be instructed to lie flat, sit up, or roll to one side with complete ease. Usually, the physician will examine from the right side, and it is equally important that the physician be comfortable.

Prior to auscultation, the clinician should take advantage of the information obtained from the history as well as from the examination of the arterial, venous, and cardiac pulsations. When abnormalities are found, their auscultatory counterparts should be diligently pursued. For example, prominent a waves in the jugular venous pulse should alert the clinician to search carefully for a low-pitched, right-sided fourth heart sound (S_4) or the subtle presystolic murmur of tricuspid stenosis, while large v waves that augment with inspiration should suggest tricuspid regurgitation. The presence of pulsus alternans should always demand a careful search for third and fourth heart sounds (S_3, S_4) as well as for the presence of functional mitral or tricuspid regurgitation, often present in severe cardiac decompensation. A rapid, jerky rise of the carotid pulse may be the clue to the diagnosis of hypertrophic cardiomyopathy, which can be confirmed by manipulating the systolic murmur with maneuvers that change the pre- and afterloading conditions of the heart. Since every patient cannot be examined in every position or with complete evaluation by physiologic or pharmacologic interventions, the extent of the examination must be dictated by the patient's overall clinical presentation.

There are four primary areas of cardiac auscultation: (1) the primary and secondary aortic areas in the second right interspace and the third left interspace adjacent to the sternum, respectively; (2) the pulmonary area in the second left interspace; (3) the tricuspid area in the fourth and fifth interspaces adjacent to the left sternal border; and (4) the mitral area at the cardiac apex. This does not mean to imply that auscultatory events arising from each valve are heard only in their respective areas. The murmur of aortic stenosis in the elderly is often heard best (and at times only) at the apex, whereas the murmur of a flail posterior mitral leaflet may radiate to the base and simulate the murmur of aortic stenosis. Ejection sounds arising from the stenotic aortic valve are usually most prominent at the apex, while the opening snap of mitral stenosis is heard best midway between the tricuspid and mitral areas. The murmur of tricuspid regurgitation may be appreciated best at the classical mitral area if the right ventricle occupies the apex. Furthermore, cardiac auscultation should not be restricted to just these four areas. For example,

the murmur of aortic regurgitation secondary to abnormalities of the aortic root may be heard best to the right of the sternum, while the murmur of tricuspid regurgitation in the emphysematous patient with pulmonary hypertension may be best heard in the epigastrium. The continuous murmur of a patent ductus arteriosus is heard just below the left clavicle, while the murmur of large bronchial collaterals may be most prominent in the posterior thorax. Again, the overall clinical presentation will guide one to the appropriate area to auscultate.

During auscultation, one listens both specifically and selectively for heart sounds and then for murmurs, first during systole and then during diastole. As described by Levine and Harvey,[295] the physician should adopt a systematic way of listening: starting at the apex, then moving to the lower left sternal border, and progressing along the sternal border to the base of the heart. The patient should be lying on his or her back, and each area should be surveyed with both chest pieces. In each area examined, the physician listens specifically for the first heart sound (S_1), noting its intensity, constancy, presence of splitting, and variation with respiration. This is followed by selective listening to the second heart sound (S_2), noting the same characteristics. Then extra sounds are searched for and carefully listened to, first in systole, then in diastole, with mental notations as to their time of appearance, pitch, and other characteristics that may identify them as gallop sounds, ejection sounds, or valve opening sounds. Whether the examination is initiated at the base by listening to S_2 or at the apex listening to S_1 depends on the physician's preference. Of greater importance is that the examination be performed in a methodical, systematic way, with the physician listening intently for one event at a time. Attention is then first turned to systole and then to diastole for the presence of murmurs. After this general survey, the physician listens selectively for certain sounds and murmurs. With the bell applied lightly to the skin at the apex, the patient is instructed to roll onto the left side and the clinician selectively "tunes in" to diastole and the low-frequency range. This allows the physician to determine the presence or absence of diastolic filling sounds or diastolic rumbles arising from the atrioventricular valves. The examination is continued with the patient in the sitting position. While the patient leans slightly forward during quiet respiration, the clinician can optimally appreciate splitting of S_2. With the patient's breath held in deep expiration, the physician examines the aortic and pulmonic areas with the diaphragm firmly pressed against the chest wall, selectively "tuning in" to the high-frequency range in an effort to hear the faint blowing diastolic murmur of aortic regurgitation or, if the clinical situation warrants, the presence of a pericardial friction rub. Sounds and murmurs such as these are discovered only when they are searched out carefully with intent listening and concentration.

Auscultation of the heart should be considered a dynamic exercise. In addition to being auscultated in the left lateral ducubitus position, the patient should, when possible, also be examined[296] while standing, squatting, and during the Valsalva maneuver and following its release. This type of dynamic examination changes the pre- and afterloading conditions of the heart and may yield diagnostic information because of the typical response of heart sounds and murmurs to these maneuvers.

Once the attentive physician has heard an unusual sound or murmur, it will never be forgotten. An analogy can be made with the distinctiveness of the sounds emanating from a violin versus those from the piccolo. Once heard and defined, they will never be confused. Likewise, the whooping murmur of a prolapsed mitral valve, once heard, will never be confused with the rough systolic ejection murmur of aortic stenosis; nor will the high-frequency opening snap of a mobile mitral valve be confused with a loud summation gallop. Often, the experienced clinician can arrive at a definitive diagnosis by careful attention to the very specific characteristics of certain heart sounds and murmurs.

PHONOCARDIOGRAPHY

Modern phonocardiography is a graphic representation of the cardiovascular examination[296] and is used to demonstrate what we see, feel, and hear at the bedside. Although inferior to the actual cardiac examination at the bedside, it can complement the written word. It includes the recording not only of the auscultatory events of the precordium but also the of the carotid, venous, and apical precordial pulsations simultaneously with the ECG. This technique may enhance the accuracy of the cardiac examination because it allows precise timing of cardiac auscultatory events as well as accurate and quantitative reproduction of physiologic events of the cardiac cycle. It is an excellent teaching aid, particularly in terms of training the clinician's ear to the timing of closely sequenced sounds. On the other hand, many high-frequency events—such as the soft murmur of aortic regurgitation—are almost impossible to record. In that situation, the "tuned-in" ear is far superior. When phonocardiography is combined with echocardiography (phonoechocardiography), instantaneous valvular and ventricular wall motion can be correlated with sound and pressure events, further enhancing its diagnostic and teaching value.

HEART SOUNDS

Heart sounds are of two types: high-frequency transients associated with the abrupt terminal checking of valves that are closing or opening, and low-frequency sounds related to early and late diastolic filling events of the ventricles. Sounds related to closing and opening of the atrioventricular valves include mitral and tricuspid closing sounds (M_1, T_1), nonejection sounds, and the opening snaps; sounds related to closing and opening of the semilunar valves include aortic and pulmonic closure sounds (A_2, P_2) and early valvular ejection sounds or clicks. Low-frequency sounds include the physiologic heart sound (S_3) and the pathologic S_3 gallop associated with early ventricular filling events and the presystolic atrial S_4 gallop associated with late diastolic events resulting from

the atrial contribution to ventricular filling. With tachycardia, these sounds may fuse, producing a summation gallop.

In recent years, sophisticated studies using phonoechocardiography, high-fidelity micromanometry, instantaneous flow and flow velocity measurements, and high-speed cineangiography have given us better understanding of the sound, pressure, flow, and motion correlates of these heart sounds.[297–299] These approaches are emphasized in subsequent sections to provide a better understanding of both the mechanisms of production and the clinical relevance of these sounds in health and disease.

THE FIRST HEART SOUND

The first heart sound (S_1) as recorded by high-resolution phonocardiography consists of four sequential components: (1) small, low-frequency vibrations, usually inaudible, that coincide with the beginning of left ventricular contraction and felt to be muscular in origin; (2) a large, high-frequency vibration, easily audible, related to mitral valve closure (M_1); (3) a second high-frequency component, following closely, related to tricuspid valve closure (T_1); and (4) small, low-frequency vibrations that coincide with accelerated flow of blood into the great vessel (Fig. 10-45). The two major components normally audible at the left lower sternal border are the louder M_1 followed by T_1. They are separated by only 20 to 30 ms and at the apex in the normal subject and only as a single sound (M_1) is usually appreciated. Although some controversy still exists regarding the genesis of these two major components, several hemodynamic and phonoechocardiographic studies have supported the original observations of Dock[300] and Leatham[301] regarding the role played by the atrioventricular valves in generating these sounds.

Echocardiographic Correlates and Splitting of S_1

The first high-frequency component of S_1 coincides with the complete coaptation of the anterior and posterior leaflets of the mitral valve.[302–309] This sound is not due to the clapping together of the two delicate leaflets but rather to the sudden deceleration of blood setting the entire cardiohemic system into vibration when the elastic limits of the closed, tensed valves are met.[310] It is unlikely that complete coaptation of the complex valve leaflets and final tensing are simultaneous; presumably it is the latter event that is associated with vibrations perceived as M_1. For practical purposes, however, the resolution of M-mode echocardiography is inadequate to distinguish between these two events, and M_1 and the C point of the mitral valve echocardiogram are considered to be coincident.[309] Similar echocardiographic correlates are more difficult to demonstrate for T_1 in the normal subject because it is often impossible to clearly identify the onset of T_1, since two components of S_1 are often synchronous or narrowly split (Fig. 10-45). When T_1 is more widely separated from M_1, however, identical echocardiographic correlates have been demonstrated in patients with wide splitting of S_1 due to Ebstein's anomaly of the tricuspid valve.[297,311] This exaggerated T_1, or "sail sound," and its wide separation from M_1 has been a helpful sign in the diagnosis of this entity.[311] Wide splitting of S_1 with normal sequencing (M_1, T_1) is also present in right bundle branch block of the proximal type as well as in left ventricular pacing, ectopic beats, and idioventricular rhythms originating from the left ventricle due to a delayed contraction of the right ventricle.[312] In a similar manner, pacing from the right ventricle and ectopic beats and idioventricular rhythms originating from the right ventricle will produce reversed splitting of S_1 (T_1, M_1) due to delay in left ventricular contraction. Reversed splitting of S_1 may also be present in patients with hemodynamically significant obstruction of the mitral valve, as mitral valve closure is delayed due to the increased left atrial pressure, which must be overcome by the rising left ventricular pressure before closure can occur.[313] Similar delay in M_1 may also be found in mitral obstruction secondary to left atrial myxoma.

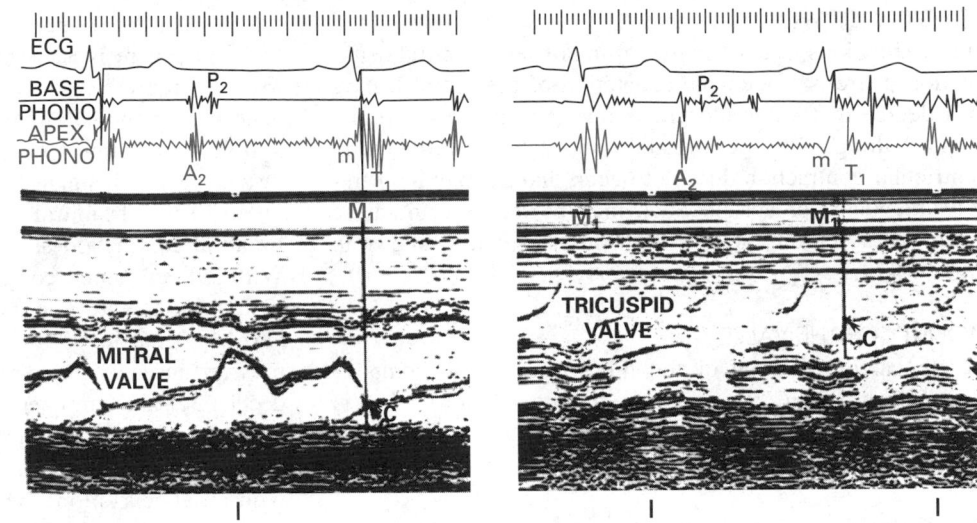

FIGURE 10-45

The apex phonocardiogram is recorded with the mitral valve echocardiogram (*left panel*) and tricuspid valve echocardiogram (*right panel*) in a normal subject. The mitral (M_1) and tricuspid (T_1) components of the first heart sound are coincident with the closure point (C) of the mitral and tricuspid valves, respectively. A small, low-frequency vibration (m) is seen prior to M_1, and a few low-frequency vibrations follow T_1 in early systole.

Hemodynamic Correlates of S_1

In Fig. 10-46, the sound and pressure correlates of M_1 are shown. The first high-frequency component of M_1 coincides with the downstroke of the left atrial *c* wave and is delayed from the left ventricular–left atrial pressure crossover by 30 ms. Similar delays in M_1 following atrioventricular pressure crossover have been reported by other investigators.[314,315] In the past, these findings have caused considerable confusion regarding the origin of both M_1 and T_1, as it was assumed that these sounds occurred at atrioventricular pressure crossover. However, the elegant studies of Laniado et al.,[303] who recorded both valve motion and phasic flow across the mitral valve simultaneously, resolved this issue. This study established that forward flow continued for a short period following left ventricular–left atrial pressure crossover due to the inertia of mitral flow, with M_1 occurring 20 to 40 ms later, coincidentally with cessation of mitral flow and closure of the valve. An even greater delay between the occurrence of T_1 and right ventricular-right atrial pressure crossover has been shown by Mills and associates,[316] and the micromanometer study of O'Toole and associates[316] has shown that T_1 also coincides with the downstroke of the right atrial *c* wave. These hemodynamic data, together with the echocardiographic correlates of M_1 and T_1, confirm the prime role played by the arterioventricular valves in the genesis of S_1.

Intensity of S_1

The primary factors determining intensity of S_1 are (1) integrity of valve closure, (2) mobility of the valve, (3) velocity of valve closure, (4) status of ventricular contraction, (5) transmission characteristics of the thoracic cavity and thorax, and (6) physical characteristics of the vibrating structures.

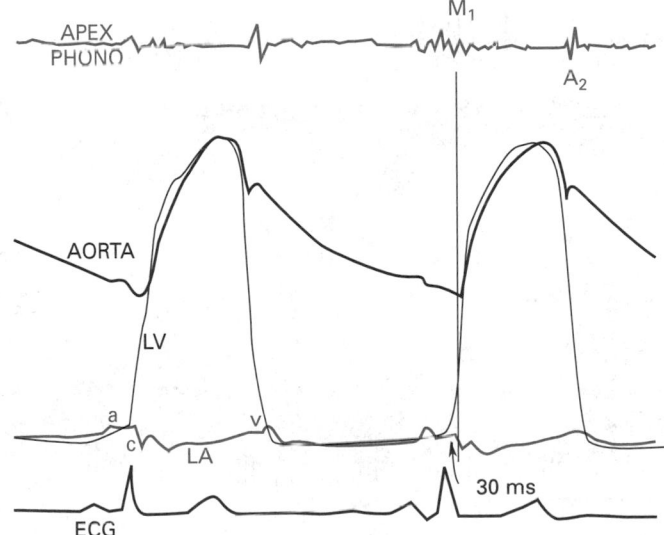

FIGURE 10-46

The apex phonocardiogram is displayed simultaneously with the cardiac cycle, as recorded by high-fidelity catheter-tipped micromanometers in the central aorta, left ventricle (LV), and left atrium (LA). The first high-frequency component of M_1 is coincident with the downstroke of the left atrial *c* wave and is separated from left ventricular–left atrial pressure crossover by an interval of 30 ms. [From Shaver JA et al. Normal and abnormal heart sounds in cardiac diagnosis. Part I: systolic sounds. *Curr Probl Cardiol* 1985; 10(3):10. Reproduced with permission from the publisher and authors.]

INTEGRITY OF VALVE CLOSURE

In rare situations, usually in the setting of severe mitral regurgitation, there is inadequate coaptation of the mitral leaflets to a degree that valve closure is not effective. As a result, abrupt halting of the retrograde blood column during early ventricular contraction does not occur, and S_1 may be markedly attenuated or absent. Such may be the case in severe mitral regurgitation due to a flail mitral leaflet, as shown in Fig. 10-47.

MOBILITY OF THE VALVE

Severe calcific fixation of the mitral valve with complete immobilization will cause a markedly attenuated M_1. This is most commonly seen in the setting of long-standing mitral stenosis, as shown in Fig. 10-48.

VELOCITY OF VALVE CLOSURE

The velocity of valve closure is the most important factor affecting the intensity of S_1 and is determined by the timing of mitral valve closure in relation to the left ventricular pressure rise in early systole.[302,305,309,317–319] The relative timing of left atrial and left ventricular systole may vary this relationship, as shown in Fig. 10-49, in an anesthetized dog preparation using the technique of sequential atrioventricular pacing.[317] As the PR interval progressively decreased from 130 to 30 ms, there is a progressive increase in the intensity of M_1 and progressive delay in M_1 relative to the onset of left ventricular contraction. When left atrial and left ventricular systole occur almost simultaneously at a PR interval of 10 ms, however, S_1 again becomes soft. At short PR intervals (30 to 70 ms), the mitral valve leaflets are maximally separated by atrial contraction at the onset of left ventricular systole. With left ventricular contraction, the mitral valve closes at a high velocity with a large excursion. This results in a loud, late M_1 occurring on a steeper part of the left ventricular pressure curve when the retrograde blood column is suddenly decelerated at the moment the elastic limits of the mitral valve are met. At longer PR intervals, there is less separation of the mitral valve leaflets, which have already begun to close with atrial relaxation. When left ventricular systole begins, there is less excursion of the mitral valve until tensing occurs, and S_1 occurs earlier relative to the onset of left ventricular contraction at a lower left ventricular pressure. Thus, less force is applied to the mitral valve, its closing velocity is decreased, and less energy is generated when a column of retrograde blood is abruptly halted, resulting in a softer M_1. Although simultaneous motion of the mitral valve is not shown in Fig. 10-49, subsequent investigations using cineradiography and echocardiographic techniques to visualize the mitral valve during variations of the PR interval have further confirmed the relationship between the rate of mitral valve closure and the intensity of M_1.[305,315,320]

The clinical finding of marked variation in the intensity of S_1 in a patient with a slow heart rate will often alert the clinician at the bedside to the diagnosis of complete heart block with atrioventricular (AV) dissociation. Other conditions in which there are beat-to-beat variations in the intensity of S_1 include Mobitz type I heart block and ventricular tachycardia with AV dissociation. Variations in the intensity of S_1 also occur with atrial fibrillation with both normal and stenotic atrioventricular valves. The loud S_1 occurs at short RR intervals, while a softer S_1 occurs at longer RR intervals when the valve leaflets have partially closed.[321] Mills and Craige[309] have shown an excellent correlation ($R = .90$) between the terminal closing rate of the anterior mitral leaflet and amplitude of

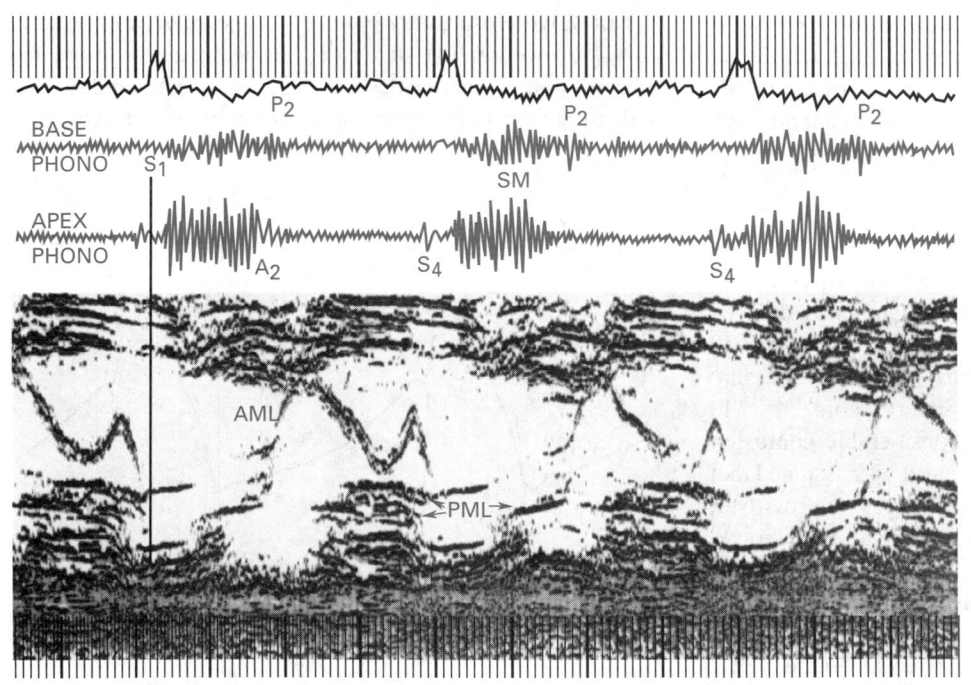

FIGURE 10-47

Base and apex phonocardiograms are recorded simultaneously with the mitral valve echocardiogram in a 62-year-old man who developed acute mitral regurgitation secondary to rupture of the chordae tendinae of a myxomatous valve. During diastole, multiple echoes arise from the flail posterior mitral leaflet (PML), and during early ventricular systole, effective mitral valve closure does not occur, resulting in an inaudible low-frequency vibration on the apex phonocardiogram. During systole, there is separation of the anterior (AML) and posterior mitral leaflets, resulting in severe mitral regurgitation. The murmur has a crescendo-decrescendo contour simulating the murmur of aortic stenosis ending prior to A_1. Wide physiologic splitting of S_1 is present. The prominent S4 present on the apex phonocardiogram was associated with an apical presystolic impulse. [From Shaver JA. The physical examination in cardiac diagnosis. *Cardiol Consult* 1985; 6(3):3. Reproduced with permission from the publisher and author.]

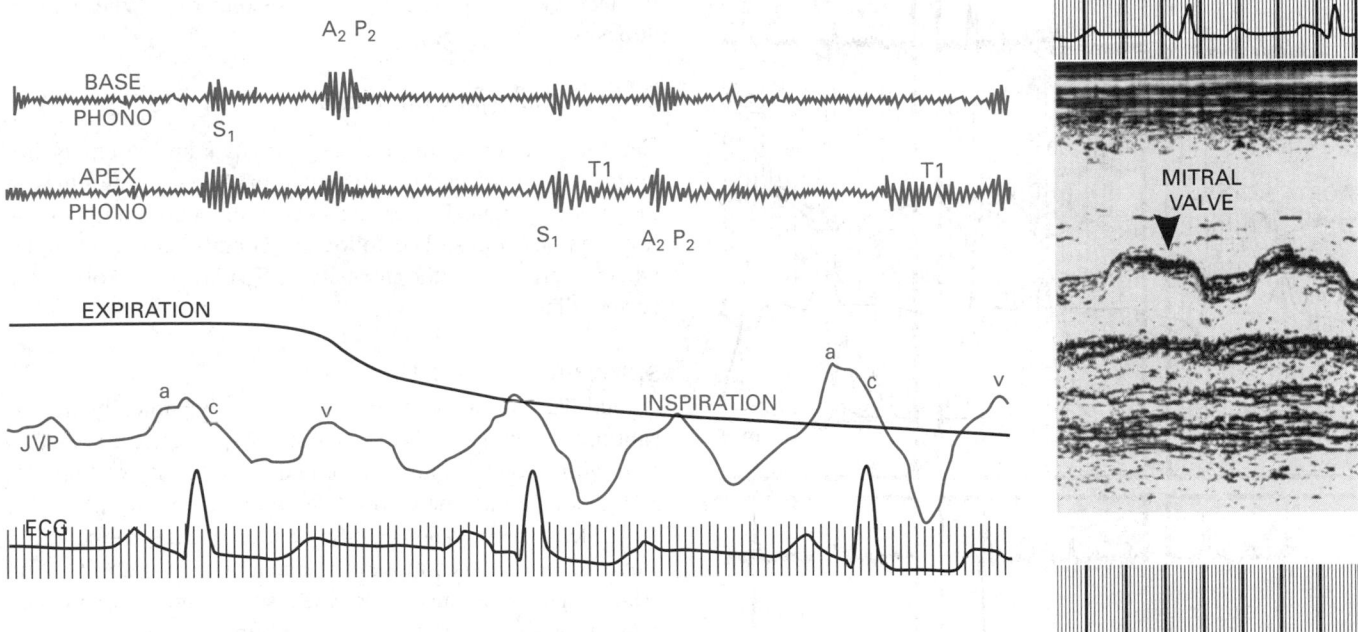

FIGURE 10-48

Left panel: Base and apex phonocardiograms are recorded simultaneously with the jugular venous pulse (JVP) and ECG in a patient with calcific fixation of a severely stenotic mitral valve (*right panel*). S_1 is soft, and there is no evidence of an opening snap during early diastole or a diastolic rumble. Note that with inspiration, a functional tricuspid regurgitation murmur develops in the apex phonocardiogram, and the *a* wave on the JVP becomes more prominent. Cardiac catheterization confirmed severe mitral stenosis and pulmonary hypertension. [From Shaver JA. Current uses of phonocardiography in clinical practice. In: Rapaport E, ed. *Cardiology Update—Reviews for Physicians*. New York: Elsevier; 1981; 362. Reproduced originally in part (left panel) with permission of the publisher and authors; and from Shaver JA et al. Normal and abnormal heart sounds in cardiac diagnosis: Part I. Systolic sounds. *Curr Probl Cardiol* 1985; 10(3):20. Reproduced with permission from the publisher and authors.]

M_1 in patients with atrial fibrillation without mitral obstruction.

The position of the mitral valve at the onset of ventricular systole may be altered not only by the relative timing of atrial and ventricular systole but also by altering the rate of left ventricular filling during atrial systole. Leonard and associates[322] have shown that the timing and intensity of both S_1 and S_4 in hypertensive patients can be influenced by variations in venous return (Fig. 10-39). It is suggested that the mitral leaflets have a greater separation when venous return is decreased to the noncompliant hypertensive left ventricle because there is more effective atrial volume transport into a relatively underfilled ventricle. As shown in the right panel of Fig. 10-50, this results in a softer S_4 that migrates toward an increased S_1. When venous return is increased (center panel), the atrial contribution of ventricular filling is now operating on the steeper portion of the left ventricular pressure volume curve. The S_4 becomes louder and earlier, and S_1 is decreased in amplitude due to partial atriogenic closure of the mitral valve. This is the most likely explanation of a soft S_1 frequently noted in hypertensive patients with normal PR intervals.

STATUS OF VENTRICULAR CONTRACTION

The status of ventricular contractility is also an independent factor determining the amplitude of S_1.[317,318,320,323] In nor-mal subjects, both exercise and catecholamine infusion have been shown to increase the amplitude of S_1, while administration of beta-blocking agents decreases it.[318,324] In both situations, the prime factor in altering the intensity of S_1 is the rate of pressure development in the ventricle. This increased rate of pressure development partially explains why S_1 is increased in patients with anemia, arteriovenous fistulas, pregnancy, anxiety, and fever.[318,320] It is also likely that these high-output states, often associated with tachycardia, result in wider separation of the AV valves at the onset of ventricular systole due to high flow through a shortened diastolic period. Similarly, the loud T_1 in an atrial septal defect is due to high flow through the tricuspid valve, secondary to the left-to-right shunt at the atrial level. A decrease in the intensity of S_1 associated with a decrease in the rate of left ventricular pressure development may be found in myxedema, cardiomyopathy, and acute myocardial infarction.[325,326] Beat-to-beat variation in the intensity of S_1 (auscultatory alternans) has also been found in patients with pulsus alternans, in whom beat-to-beat alteration in the rate of left ventricular pressure development occurs.[327]

TRANSMISSION CHARACTERISTICS OF THE THORACIC CAVITY AND CHEST WALL

The degree of attenuation of heart sounds generated by the vibrating cardiohemic system is a function of both sound

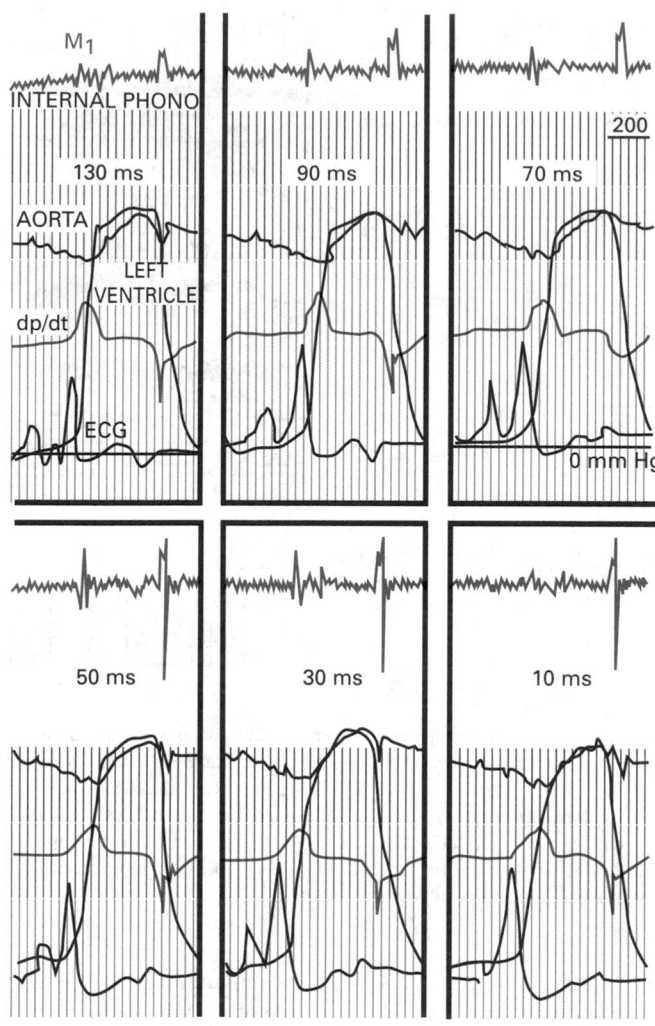

FIGURE 10-49

The effect of changing the PR interval on left ventricular sound and pressure events, as recorded by high-fidelity catheter-tipped micromanometers in an anesthetized dog preparation. The M_1 amplitude is markedly increased at the shorter PR intervals, while the maximum *dP/dt* is decreased. At the 10-ms PR interval, the M_1 amplitude is again decreased. Note that as the PR interval shortens, both M_1 and the notch on the *dP/dt* tracing occur later in systole and a plateau develops preceding the notch. (From Stept ME et al. Effect of altering P-R interval on the amplitude of the first heart sound in the anesthetized dog. *Circ Res* 1969; 25:259. Reproduced with permission from the American Heart Association, Inc, and the authors.)

frequency and the distance of the heart from the chest wall. The higher-frequency heart sounds are attenuated to a greater extent than are lower frequency sounds.[328] Conditions such as obesity, emphysema, or large pleural or pericardial effusions will decrease the intensity of all auscultatory events, while a thin body habitus would tend to increase the intensity.

PHYSICAL CHARACTERISTICS OF THE VIBRATING STRUCTURES

Alterations in the physical characteristics of the vibrating structures may also vary the intensity of S_1. Both myocardial infarction and ischemia induced by pacing have been shown

to decrease the intensity of S_1 secondary to these alterations.[329,330]

S_1 in Pathologic Conditions

Careful attention to the intensity of S_1 is an extremely important aspect of cardiac auscultation, often giving clues to the proper diagnosis and the degree of abnormality of the involved structures. The following conditions are examples where alterations in the intensity of S_1 play a key role in the correct diagnosis.

S_1 IN MITRAL STENOSIS

A loud, late M_1 is the hallmark of hemodynamically significant mitral stenosis.[318,331–333] When M_1 is loud, it is associated with a loud opening snap, and the intensity of both M_1 and the opening snap correlate with valve motility (Fig. 10-51, left panel). When calcific fixation of the stenotic mitral valve occurs, M_1 is soft and the opening snap is absent (Fig. 10-48). The relationship between sound and pressure and echocardiographic mitral valve motion is shown in Fig. 10-52. Significant scarring of the mitral valve is evident as a result of the rheumatic process. The increased left atrial pressure delays the time of pressure crossover between the left atrium and the left ventricle. As a result, M_1 occurs later and at a much higher than normal left ventricular pressure, at a time when there is a more rapid rate of development of left ventricular pressure. The presystolic gradient between the left atrium and left ventricle prevents preclosure of the mitral valve leaflets. As a result, the closure of the leaflet begins from a domed position within the left ventricular cavity and takes place over a much greater distance than normal following the onset of left ventricular contraction. Both of these factors increase the velocity of mitral valve closure and the momentum of blood directed toward the mitral valve leaflets, resulting in a loud M_1 when the elastic limits of the stenotic mitral valve are met. A similar mechanism is responsible for the booming S_1 with aftervibrations in left atrial myxoma (Fig. 10-51, center panel).[334,335]

S_1 IN MITRAL VALVE PROLAPSE

Tei and colleagues[336] have reported a loud M_1 heard over the apex in patients with nonrheumatic mitral regurgitation; this is indicative of holosystolic mitral valve prolapse (Fig. 10-51, right panel). Patients with the more common middle to late systolic prolapse have a normal S_1, while a soft or absent S_1 may indicate a flail mitral leaflet (Fig. 10-47). The increased amplitude of leaflet excursion with prolapse beyond the line of closure explains the loud M_1 associated with holosystolic prolapse. An alternate explanation may be a summation of a normal M_1 and an early nonejection click of valvular prolapse.

S_1 AND LEFT BUNDLE BRANCH BLOCK

In left bundle branch block (LBBB), M_1 is decreased in intensity and is frequently delayed, at times resulting in reversal of sequence of S_1 (Fig. 10-53).[318,337–339] The reason for the delay and the decreased intensity of M_1 in this condition is multi-factional, with different mechanisms operative in different patients, depending on the degree of completeness of the LBBB, the site of block (proximal versus peripheral), and especially the status of left ventricular function.[340–342] The primary factors involved are (1) delay in onset of left ventricular contraction, (2) degree of left ventricular dysfunction, (3) presence of concomitant first-degree heart block, and (4) presence of a noncompliant left ventricle facilitating atriogenic preclosure of the mitral valve. It is likely that more than one factor is operative in most patients with LBBB, with one or two factors predominating.

S_1 IN ACUTE AORTIC REGURGITATION

One of the important auscultatory findings in acute aortic regurgitation is attenuation or absence of M_1, as shown in Fig. 10-54.[318,320,343,344] Severe regurgitation into a left ventricle that has not had time to adapt to the acute volume overload causes a marked increase in the left ventricular end-diastolic pressure, resulting in premature closure of the normal mitral valve in middiastole. With the onset of left ventricular systole, minimal mitral valve excursion occurs, causing a marked reduction in the intensity of M_1.

SYSTOLIC EJECTION SOUNDS

Ejection sounds are early systolic ejection events that can originate from either the left or the right side of the heart. These sounds may be classified as valvular, arising from deformed aortic or pulmonic valves, or as vascular, or root events caused by the rapid, forceful ejection of blood into the great vessels. The presence or absence of valvular ejection sounds is of great benefit in defining the level of right or left ventricular outflow tract obstruction while root ejection sounds give insight into abnormalities of the great vessels with or without systemic or pulmonary hypertension.

Aortic Valvular Ejection Sounds

Aortic valvular ejection sounds are found in nonstenotic congenital bicuspid valves and in the entire spectrum of mild to

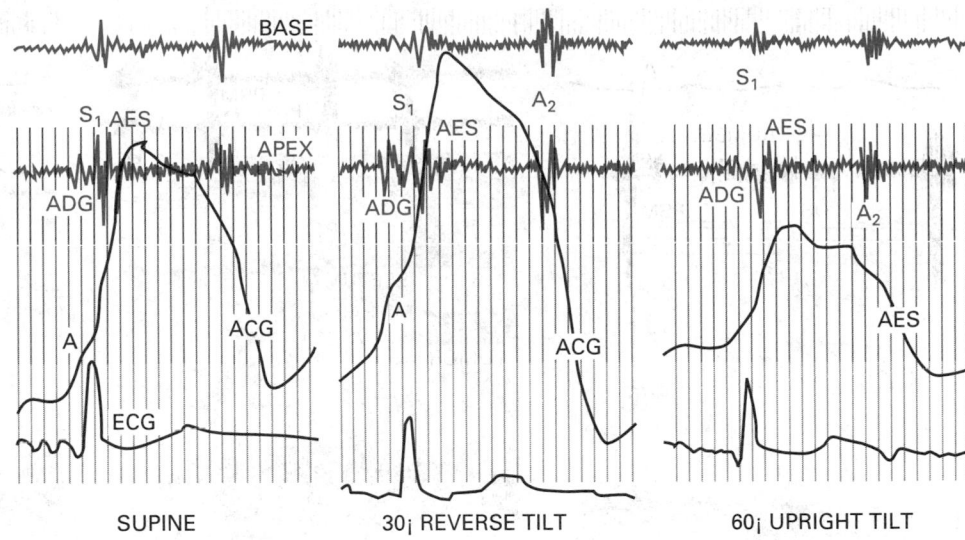

FIGURE 10-50

Base and apex phonocardiograms are recorded simultaneously with the apex cardiogram (ACG) and ECG in a 52-year-old man experiencing significant systemic hypertension. In all three postures, an atrial diastolic gallop (ADG) precedes the mitral component of S_1. In turn, M_1 is followed by a prominent second component that is most likely an aortic root ejection sound in this clinical setting. In the supine position, S_1 is of moderate intensity. During a 30° reverse tilt with increased venous return, there is significant increase in the amplitude of the ADG as well as prominence of the a wave on the ACG. The ADG is also further separated from the mitral component of S_1, which is slightly softer. In contrast, with 60° of upright tilt and a decrease in venous return, there is a significant decrease in the intensity of the ADG and loss of the a wave on the ACG. Note also the migration of the ADG toward S_1, which has increased significantly in intensity. With these postural changes, there is no significant change in the intensity of the aortic ejection sound (AES), which is well recorded at the apex and at the base. These simple maneuvers at the bedside can be particularly helpful in distinguishing an ADG-S_1 sequence versus a split S_1. (From Shaver JA et al. Ejection sounds of left-sided origin. In: Leon DF, Shaver DF, eds. *Physiologic Principles of Heart Sounds and Murmurs*. Monograph 46. Dallas: American Heart Association, 1975:31. Reproduced with permission from the publisher and authors.)

severe stenosis of the aortic valve. This sound introduces the typical ejection murmur of aortic stenosis, is widely transmitted, and is often heard best at the apex. As shown in the left panel of Fig. 10-55, the aortic valvular ejection sound is delayed 20 to 40 ms after the onset of pressure rise in the central aorta and is coincident with the sharp anacrotic notch on the upstroke of the aortic pressure curve. The sound is coincident with the maximal excursion of the domed valve when its elastic limits are met.[345–348] The abrupt deceleration of the oncoming column of blood sets the entire cardiohemic system into vibration, the lower-frequency components being recorded as the anacrotic notch and the high-frequency components representing the valvular ejection sound. Inherent in this mechanism of sound production is the ability of the deformed valve to move. With severe calcific fixation of the valve, no excursion or piston-like ascent of the deformed valve is possible; therefore, no sudden tensing of the valve leaflets or abrupt deceleration of the column of blood occurs. As shown in the right panel of Fig. 10-55, neither an anacrotic notch on the upstroke of the aortic pressure nor a valvular ejection sound is recorded in this situation. Sound and motion correlates identical to those demonstrated by cineangiography have been found with phonoechocardiography, clearly showing the onset of the ejection sound to be coincident with the maximal opening of the valve (Fig. 10-56).[306–349] The

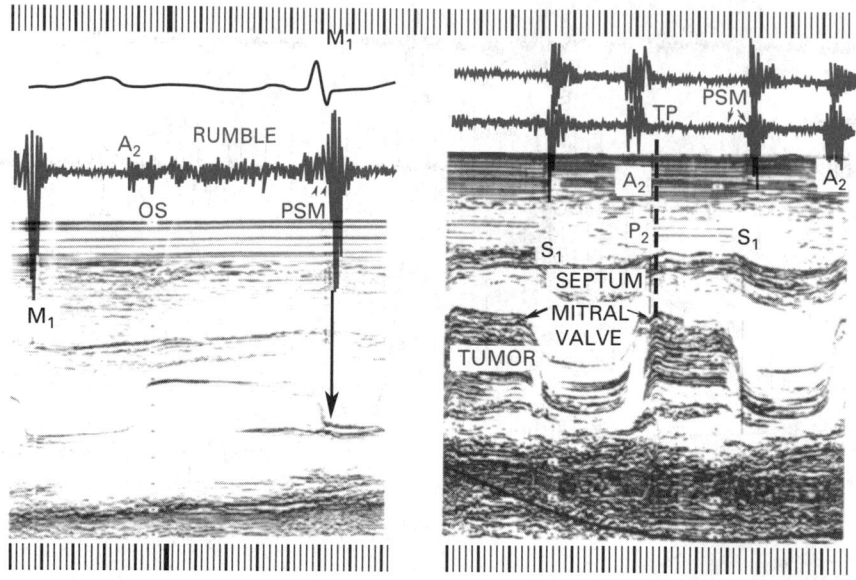

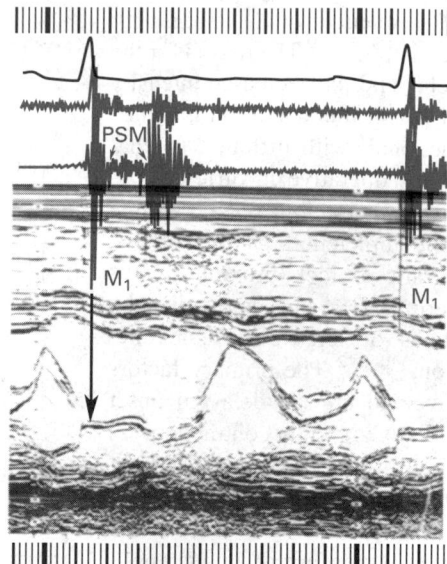

FIGURE 10-51

Simultaneous phonocardiograms are recorded with the mitral valve echocardiograms in three patients: mitral stenosis (*left panel*), left atrial myxoma (*center panel*), and prolapse of the mitral valve (*right panel*). In each condition, a loud M_1 is present and coincident with the closing point of the mitral valve echocardiogram. Common to each condition is wide separation of the mitral leaflets at the onset of left ventricular systole, with high-velocity closure occurring over a large excursion. In the left panel, a mobile stenotic valve is demonstrated, and a loud opening snap is coincident with the E point. In the center panel, an early diastolic tumor plop (TP) is coincident with the maximal excursion of the tumor during its rapid descent into the ventricle. Note the presystolic crescendo murmur (PSM) occurring during the rapid closure of the mitral valve in both mitral stenosis and left atrial myxoma. In the right panel, a pansystolic murmur (PSM) with late systolic accentuation is secondary to the prolapse of the mitral valve with late systolic hammocking. [From Shaver JA. Current uses of phonocardiography in clinical practice. In Rapaport E, ed. *Cardiology Update—Reviews for Physicians*. New York: Elsevier; 1981:370. Reproduced in part (center panel) with permission from the publisher and author. Copyright 1981 by Elsevier Science Publishing Co, Inc.]

intensity of the ejection sound correlates directly with the mobility of the valve, but there is no correlation between intensity and the severity of the obstruction. In mobile, nonstenotic bicuspid valves, the ejection sound is not only loud but also widely separated from S_1 due to the prolonged excursion of the mobile valve (Fig. 10-57, left panel).[350] The presence of an aortic valvular ejection sound is a valuable physical finding at the bedside; it not only defines the left ventricular outflow obstruction at the valvular level but also gives insight into the mobility of the valve (Fig. 10-56).

Pulmonary Valvular Ejection Sounds

Pulmonary valvular ejection sounds have identical sound and pressure correlates as aortic valvular ejection sounds.[351] Echocardiographic correlations have also shown that the onset of the pulmonary ejection sound occurs at the maximal excursion of the stenotic pulmonary valve.[306,349] In contrast to the aortic valvular ejection sounds and to most right-sided auscultatory events, the pulmonic sound or ejection click decreases in intensity or disappears with inspiration in mild to moderate pulmonic stenosis. The hemodynamic mechanism responsible for this phenomenon[351-353] is shown in Fig. 10-58. Phonoechocardiographic studies by Weyman and associates[354] and Mills and Craige[309] have documented this dynamic movement of the pulmonary valve with respiration. In very mild valvular

pulmonic stenosis, respiratory variation may be absent.[351] In very severe valvular obstruction, a vigorous atrial contraction can completely preopen the pulmonic valve in diastole, causing a crisp preejection sound.[355,356] In this situation, right ventricular pressure at the time of the atrial kick can actually exceed pulmonary artery end-diastolic pressure.[351] As the severity of the pulmonic stenosis increases, both the excursion of the deformed valve and the right ventricular isovolumic contraction time decrease. The net effect of both of these events is migration of the pulmonary ejection sound toward S_1.

Aortic Vascular Ejection Sounds

Ejection sounds originating from the aortic root are common in systemic arterial hypertension in the setting of a tortuous sclerotic aortic root, a tight, noncompliant arterial tree, and forceful left ventricular ejection. They are coincident with the upstroke of the high-fidelity central aortic pressure and have been interpreted as an exaggeration of the ejection component of the normal S_1.[345,346] Echocardiographic correlations by Mills and associates,[349] however, have shown that this sound occurs at the moment of complete opening of the aortic valve and always on the pressure upstroke of the high-fidelity aortic pressure curve. These observations have led them to conclude that this sound probably originates from the valve leaflets. At present, these minor discrepancies regarding the exact

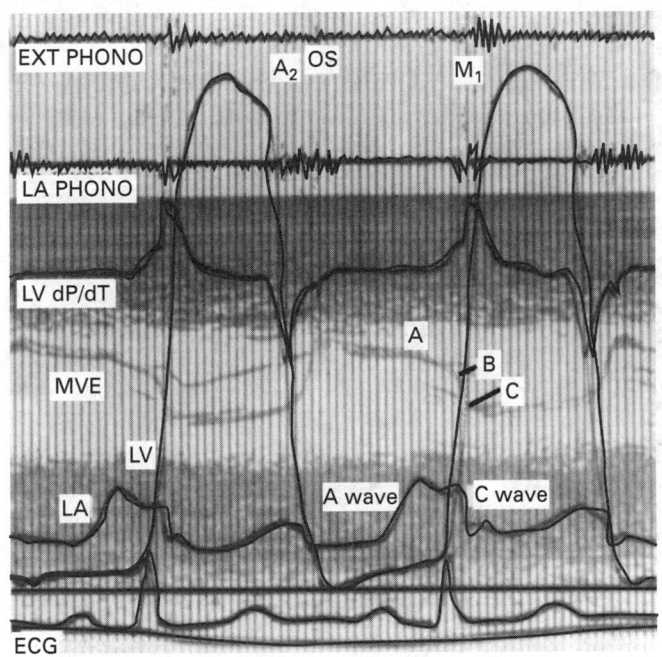

FIGURE 10-52

External sound, equisensitive left ventricular and left atrial pressures (catheter-tipped micromanometer), left ventricular *dP/dt*, and left atrial sound are recorded simultaneously with the mitral valve echocardiogram in a patient with hemodynamically significant mitral stenosis. A significant presystolic gradient is present due to atrial contraction, and the onset of the rapid closure of the mitral valve (B) is delayed until the left ventricular pressure exceeds left atrial pressure. This occurs 40 ms after the beginning of the left ventricular pressure rise at a time when left ventricular *dP/dt* is much higher than normal. Following left atrial-left ventricular pressure crossover, there is rapid ventriculogenic closure of the mitral valve (B-C), resulting in a very loud M_1 coincident with the C point of the mitral valve echocardiogram. Its separation from A_2 is determined by both the level of the left atrial pressure and the rate of left ventricular pressure decline. [From Shaver JA et al. Normal and abnormal heart sounds in cardiac diagnosis: Part I. Systolic sounds. *Curr Probl Cardiol* 1985; 10(3):21. Reproduced with permission from the publisher and the authors.]

mechanisms of production of this sound have not been resolved.

In contrast to the ejection sound of the stenotic aortic valve, these root sounds tend to be poorly transmitted from the aortic area and are not heard well at the apex. It may be difficult or impossible to differentiate this sound from the tricuspid component of a widely split S_1, which is best heard at the fourth left parasternal area and often increases with inspiration. The bedside decision as to whether this is T_1 or an ejection sound will often be dictated by the clinical situation. In either condition, it should be emphasized that the benign S_1 ejection sound or M_1-T_1 complex is frequently misinterpreted as a pathologic S_4-S_1 sequence. Factors that favor the presence of an S_4-S_1 complex are an associated palpable presystolic apical impulse, optimal audibility of the S_4 with the stethoscope bell applied lightly at the apex, and a change in the intensity of the S_4 with maneuvers that vary venous return (Fig. 10-50).

Pulmonary Vascular Ejection Sounds

Vascular or root ejection sounds may also arise from the pulmonary artery, and the common denominator is dilation of the pulmonary artery.[351] This dilation can be idiopathic or secondary to severe pulmonary hypertension. Although Leatham and Vogelpoel[357] have stated that this sound is louder during expiration, there is no consensus on this point. Unlike splitting of S_1, which is heard best at the mitral or tricuspid area, this sound is louder in the second and third left intercostal spaces.

Echocardiographic correlates of the pulmonary root ejection sound show it to be coincident with complete opening of the pulmonary valve, occurring during the upstroke of the high-fidelity pulmonary artery pressure recording.[349,358] This has led to the conclusion that these vascular ejection sounds may originate from semilunar valve cusps that have undergone changes in structure in response to increased pressure.[309] Other investigators have found that the pulmonary root ejection sounds in the setting of pulmonary hypertension coincide with the upstroke of the high-fidelity pulmonary artery pressure tracing, while in both idiopathic dilation of the pulmonary artery and atrial septal defect, this sound occurs during the upstroke of the pulmonary pressure tracing.[351] In each of these conditions, it has been suggested that this sound is related to sudden checking of the rapidly accelerating blood column by the "tight" or "loose" pulmonary artery when its elastic limits are met. At the present time, it is not possible to state with certainty whether the coincidence of this sound with the maximal opening of the pulmonary valve as found by some investigators is cause and effect or a chance relationship.

NONEJECTION SOUNDS

The midsystolic click due to prolapse of the mitral or tricuspid valve is the most frequent cause of systolic nonejection sounds and is often associated with a systolic regurgitant murmur. Such sounds were first described in 1887 and termed systolic gallop.[359] Although originally thought to be extracardiac in origin,[360] confirmation of their valvular origin has been shown by angiographic[361,362] intracardiac phonocardiographic[363,364] and echocardiographic studies.[365–367] As originally proposed by Reid[368] the cause of this sound is due to tensing of the AV valves during systole. As with other high-frequency cardiac sounds, it is produced by vibrations of the entire cardiohemic system when the elastic limits of the prolapsed valve are suddenly reached.

The presence of a nonejection click on physical examination is sufficient to make the diagnosis of mitral valve prolapse (MVP). The sound has a sharp, high-frequency clicking quality and, although often confined to the apex, can be transmitted widely on the precordium. It may be an isolated finding occur-

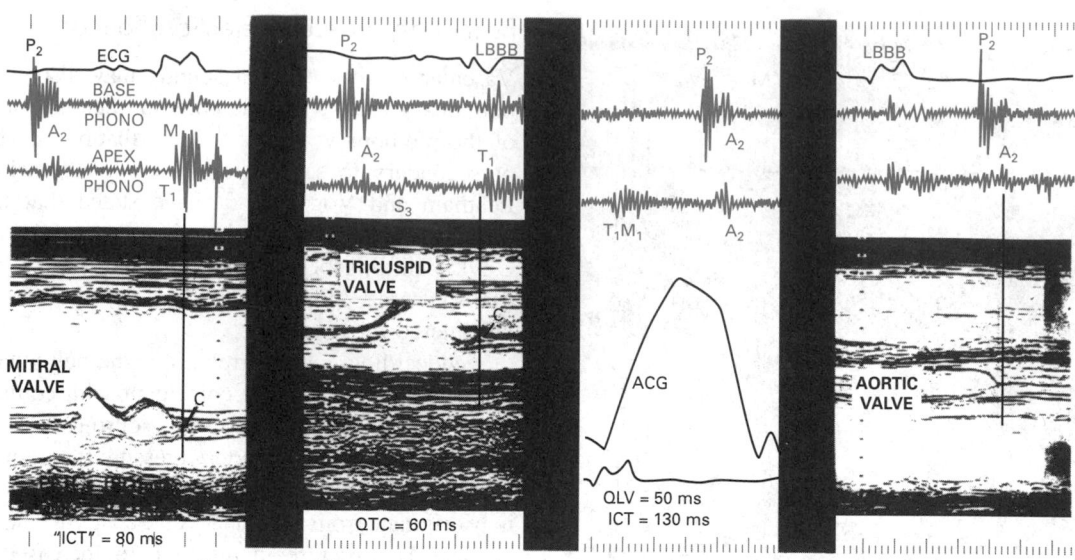

FIGURE 10-53

Base and apex phonocardiograms are recorded simultaneously with the mitral and tricuspid valve echocardiogram, the apex cardiogram (ACG), and the aortic valve echocardiogram in a patient with LBBB and significant left ventricular dysfunction. A markedly delayed M_1 is coincident with complete coaptation of the anterior and posterior leaflets of the mitral valve. The sequence of S_1 is reversed. The mitral valve echocardiogram shows significant atriogenic preclosure of the anterior and posterior leaflets, which is followed by slow ventriculogenic closure of the valve, resulting in a soft M_1. In the next panel, T_1 is clearly shown to be coincident with the final closure point

of the tricuspid valve and precedes M_1. Reversed splitting of S_2 is present and is confirmed by simultaneous recording of the aortic valve echocardiogram in the far right panel. In this patient with LBBB, the electromechanical interval (Q—left ventricular) was within normal limits, and the reversed splitting of S_1 and S_2 was due to severe left ventricular dysfunction with marked prolongation of isovolumic contraction time. (From Shaver JA et al. Effects of left bundle branch block on the events of the cardiac cycle. *Acta Cardiol* 1988; 43:461–462. Reproduced with permission from the publisher and the authors.)

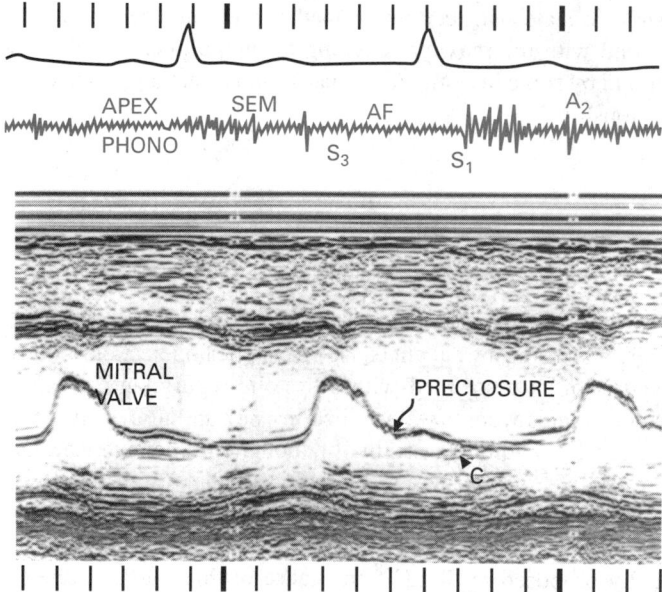

FIGURE 10-54

The apex phonocardiogram is recorded simultaneously with the mitral valve echocardiogram in a patient with acute aortic regurgitation. There is middiastolic preclosure of the mitral valve, and a very soft S_1 is recorded coincident with the terminal closing motion of the mitral valve following the onset of ventricular systole. A systolic ejection murmur (SEM) is present during systole, and an Austin Flint murmur (AF) is introduced by an S_3 gallop during early diastole. Note the absence of the presystolic component of the Austin Flint murmur. [From Shaver JA et al. Normal and abnormal heart sounds in cardiac diagnosis: Part I. Systolic sounds. *Curr Probl Cardiol* 1985; 10(3):25. Reproduced with permission from the publisher and the authors.]

ring most often in middle to late systole or there may be multiple clicks, presumably as a result of different areas of the large, redundant, scalloped mitral leaflets prolapsing at different times (Fig. 10-59). Numerous echocardiographic studies have shown the presence of the characteristic mid- to late-systolic prolapse as well as holosystolic prolapse in patients with clicks. All of these patterns may be seen in the presence of an isolated systolic click, click and late systolic murmur, or a late systolic murmur alone. The click usually occurs at the time of maximum prolapse; the lack of exact correlation of maximal valvular prolapse and the auscultatory findings is the result of the M-mode echocardiographic technique, which allows visualization of only a small portion of the valve.

A feature of MVP is the variability of the auscultatory findings from examination to examination and even from beat to beat (Fig. 10-60). The timing of the click, or click and the late systolic murmur, vary considerably with changes in posture (Fig. 10-61).[369] In the upright posture, the heart becomes smaller due to decreased venous return and the click moves earlier in systole. Angiographic studies have confirmed an earlier and greater degree of prolapse in the upright posture compared to the supine position.[370] Squatting, which causes an immediate increase in venous return and afterload, increases left ventricular volume, resulting in later prolapse and movement of the click toward S_2. At the bedside, these simple maneuvers are helpful in differentiating the nonejection click from early ejection sounds, a split S_2, or an S_3.

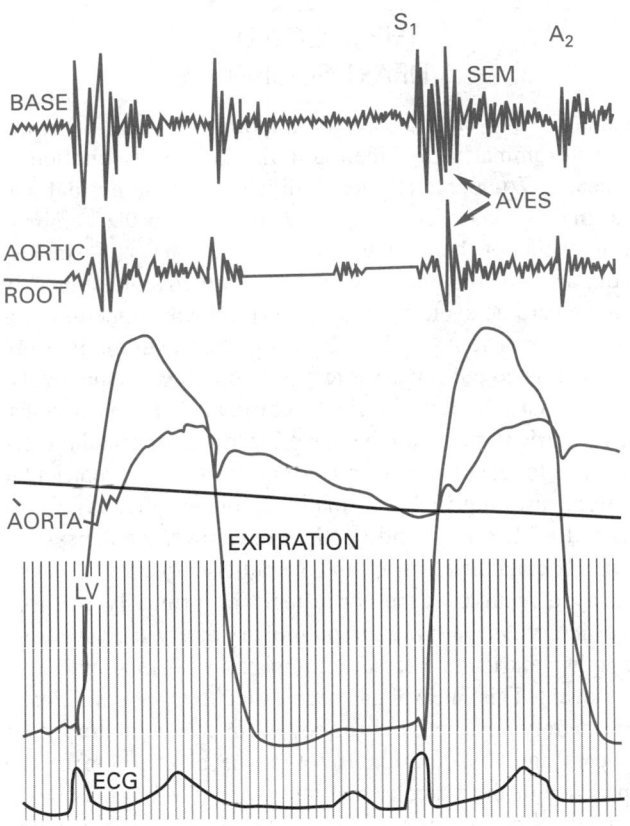

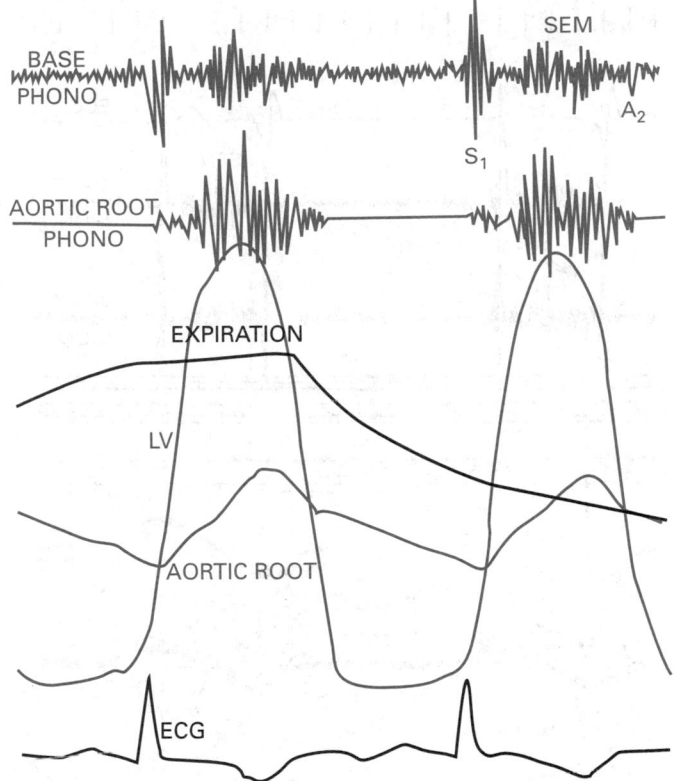

FIGURE 10-55

Base and aortic root phonocardiograms are recorded simultaneously with high-fidelity catheter-tipped micromanometers in the central aorta and left ventricle in a 23-year-old man with mild valvular aortic stenosis (*left panel*) and in an elderly patient with severe calcification of the aortic valve (*right panel*). In valvular aortic stenosis, the murmur is introduced by a loud aortic valvular ejection sound (AVES). The peak gradient across the aortic valve was less than 30 mmHg, and the systolic ejection murmur ends well before the prominent aortic closure sound. With calcific fixation of the aortic valve, a valvular ejection sound is not recorded on either the base or the aortic root phonocardiogram, nor is an anacrotic notch present on the upstroke of the central aortic pressure trace. Note also that the aortic closure sound is barely recordable at the base. [From Shaver JA. Innocent murmurs. *Hosp Med*, April 1978:25. © 1978. Reproduced from *Hospital Medicine* in part (*left panel*) with permission of Hospital Publications, Inc, and the author; and from Shaver JA, et al. Ejection sounds of left-sided origin. In: Leon DF, Shaver JA, eds. *Physiologic Principles of Heart Sounds and Murmurs*. Monograph 46. Dallas: American Heart Association; 1975:33. Reproduced in part (*right panel*) with permission from the publisher and the authors.]

Other physiologic and pharmacologic maneuvers that vary the loading conditions of the heart also cause changes in the timing of the auscultatory event. Phonoechocardiographic correlations during the inhalation of amyl nitrite have confirmed the cause-and-effect relationship between the echocardiographically demonstrated prolapse and the timing of the click.[367] Mathey and associates[371] have demonstrated that echocardiographically determined left ventricular diameter was relatively constant at the time of the click during supine, upright, and amyl nitrite conditions, indicating that a critical size was necessary for prolapse to occur. Increased contractility or velocity of shortening will also affect the click timing, as the critical size will be reached earlier in systole. The documentation of this consistent relationship of left ventricular size to the timing of the click is in keeping with what is thought to be the cause of mitral valve prolapse—that is, valvuloventricular disproportion or a valve too big for the ventricle.[372] In general, maneuvers that decrease left ventricular volume—such as sitting, standing,

or strain of the Valsalva maneuver as well as amyl nitrite administration—cause the click to move closer to S_1. Maneuvers that increase left ventricular volume (squatting, vasopressor infusion, and the supine position) move the click toward S_2. If the diastolic left ventricular volume is large enough that the critical prolapse size does not occur in systole, the click will be absent. Conversely, if the diastolic volume is too small, the click will fuse with S_1 (see also Chap. 65).

Although the most common cause of nonejection clicks is prolapse of the AV valves, systolic sounds have been reported in patients with left-sided pneumothorax, adhesive pericarditis, atrial myxomas, left ventricular aneurysm, aneurysm of the membranous ventricular septum associated with a ventricular septal defect, and incompetent heterograft valves.[373–376] The presence of these conditions can usually be recognized by the clinical setting and by the absence of the typical changes in the timing of the click associated with physiologic and pharmacologic maneuvers.

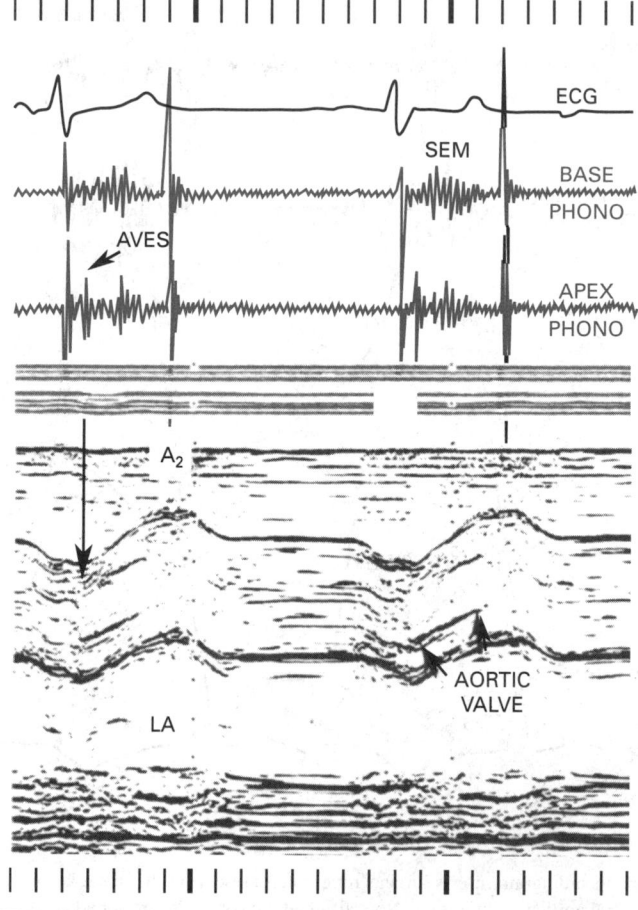

FIGURE 10-56

Base and apex phonocardiograms are recorded simultaneously with the aortic valve echocardiogram in a young man with valvular aortic stenosis. A prominent aortic valvular ejection sound (AVES) is recorded at the apex and is coincident with the maximal excursion of the aortic valve in early systole. It is followed by a crescendo-decrescendo systolic ejection murmur (SEM) that ends well before a loud A_2.

THE SECOND HEART SOUND

Leatham[377] has emphasized the importance of the S_2 in the cardiac examination by labeling it the "key to auscultation of the heart." To appreciate the significance of the normal and abnormal S_2, knowledge of its relationship to the hemodynamic events of the cardiac cycle is essential.[378–380] In Fig. 10-62, the two components of S_2 are recorded simultaneously with the cardiac cycle by high-fidelity catheter-tipped micromanometers. The A_2 and P_2 are coincident with the incisura of the aorta and pulmonary artery pressure trace, respectively, and terminate the left and right ventricular ejection periods. Right ventricular ejection begins prior to left ventricular ejection, has a longer duration, and terminates after left ventricular ejection, resulting in P_2 normally occurring after A_2 (Figs. 3-31 and 3-32; Plates 2 and 3). Right and left ventricular systole are nearly equal in duration, and the pulmonary artery incisura is delayed relative to the aortic incisura, primarily due to a larger interval separating the pulmonary artery incisura from the right ventricular pressure compared with the same left-sided event. This interval has been called the "hangout" interval, a purely descriptive term coined in our laboratory over 15 years ago. Its duration is felt to be a reflection of the impedance of the vascular bed into which the blood is being received.[381–383] Normally, it is less than 15 ms in the systemic circulation and only slightly prolongs the left ventricular ejection time. In the low-resistance, high-capacitance pulmonary bed, however, this interval is normally much greater than on the left, varying between 43 and 86 ms, and therefore contributes significantly to the duration of right ventricular ejection.[381] Awareness of this interval is essential for proper understanding of normal physiologic splitting and for the abnormal splitting seen in conditions where significant alterations in pulmonary vascular impedance have occurred.

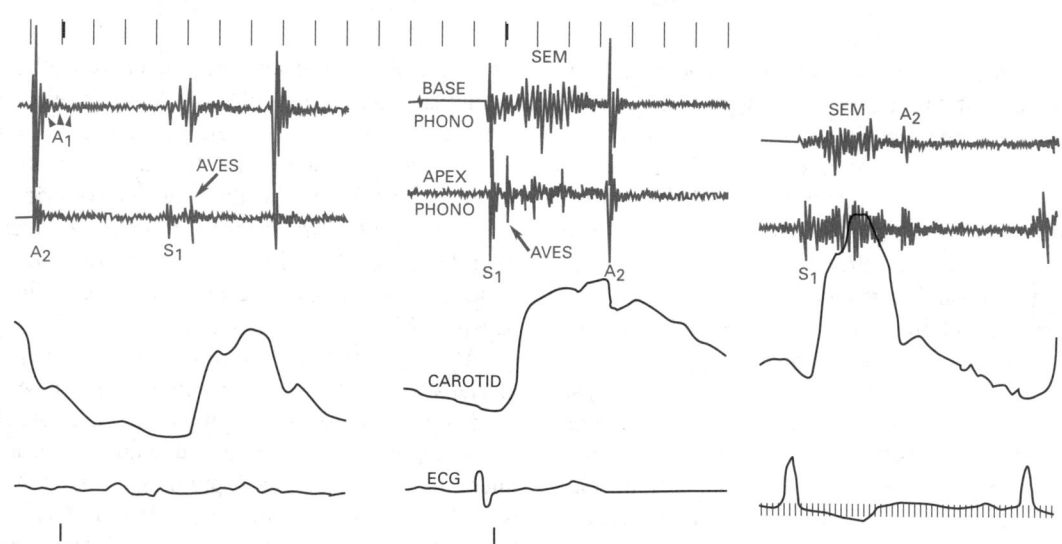

FIGURE 10-57

A prominent aortic valvular ejection sound (AVES) of a congenital nonstenotic and stenotic bicuspid aortic valve is shown on the left and center panels, respectively. On the right panel there is no evidence of a valvular ejection sound in a patient with severe fixed orifice subaortic stenosis. The valvular ejection sound of the nonstenotic bicuspid valve is widely separated from S_1 and unassociated with a subsequent murmur. The ejection sound of the stenotic bicuspid valve introduces the typical crescendo-decrescendo murmur of valvular aortic stenosis. In both conditions, A_1 is well preserved.

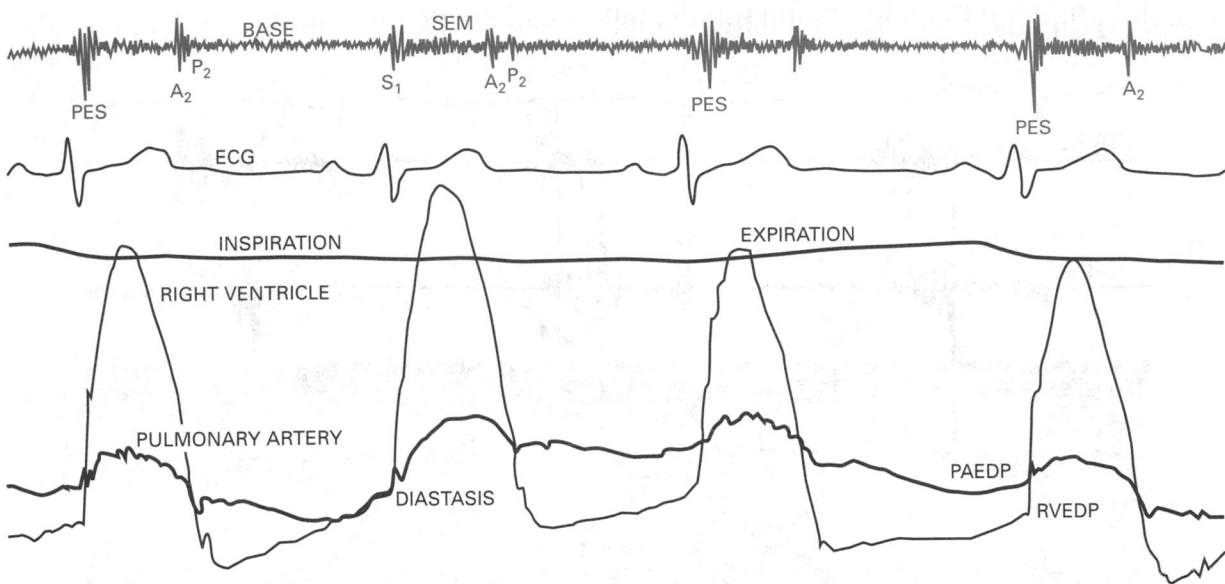

FIGURE 10-58

Simultaneous right ventricular and pulmonary artery pressures are recorded with the phonocardiogram showing the mechanism of the attenuation of the pulmonary valvular ejection sound (PES) during respiration in a patient with mild valvular pulmonic stenosis. In the second complex, the valvular ejection sound has disappeared and there is complete equalization of the diastolic pressure in the right ventricle and pulmonary artery. With equalization of pressure, there is preopening of the deformed stenotic valve, and with the onset of right ventricular systole, no further excursion of the domed valve is possible, and the ejection sound is absent. During expiration, the pulmonary artery diastolic pressure is significantly higher than the right ventricular end-diastolic pressure, and the prominent ejection sound is again recorded. Considerable variation of the ejection sound occurs during various phases of respiration and is caused by varying degrees of preopening of the valve. Note the tendency for the ejection sound to occur later during the expiratory phase. (From Reddy PS et al. Cardiac systolic murmurs: Pathophysiology and differential diagnosis. *Prog Cardiovasc Dis* 1974; 14:14. Reproduced in part with permission from the publisher and the authors.)

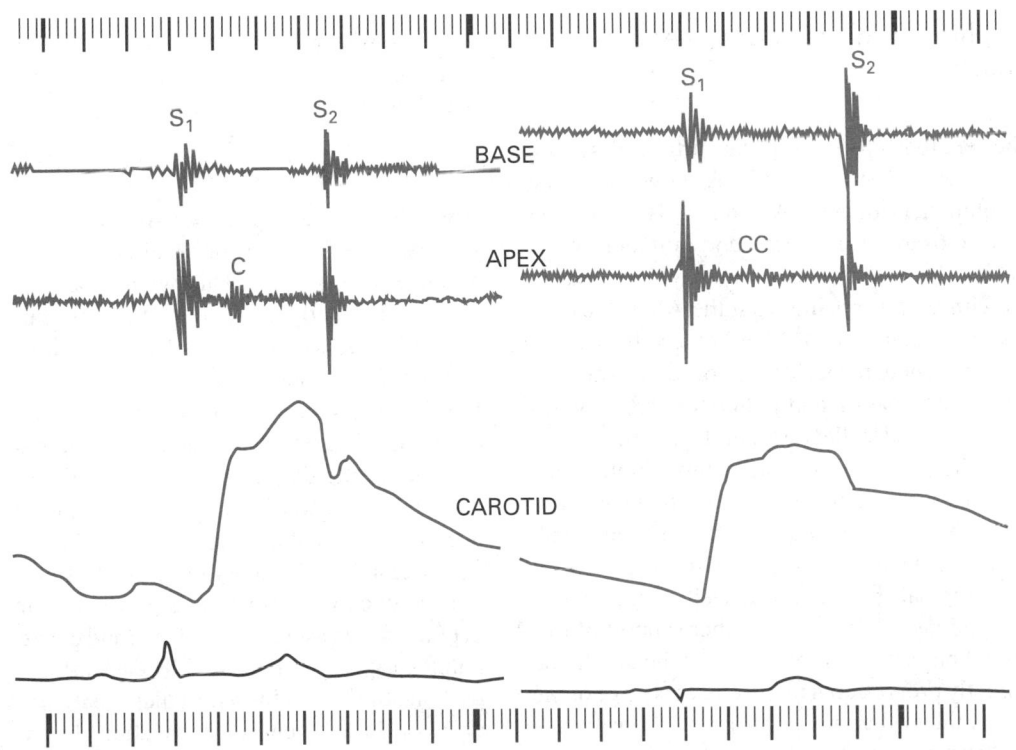

FIGURE 10-59

Base and apex phonocardiograms in two patients with nonejection clicks. The apex phonocardiogram shows an isolated systolic click (*left*). In the right panel are two close clicks 40 ms apart. On examination, multiple clicks may sound like a scratchy murmur rather than individual clicks. [From Shaver JA et al. Normal and abnormal heart sounds in cardiac diagnosis: Part I. Systolic sounds. *Curr Probl Cardiol* 1985; 10(3):38. Reproduced with permission from the publisher and the authors.]

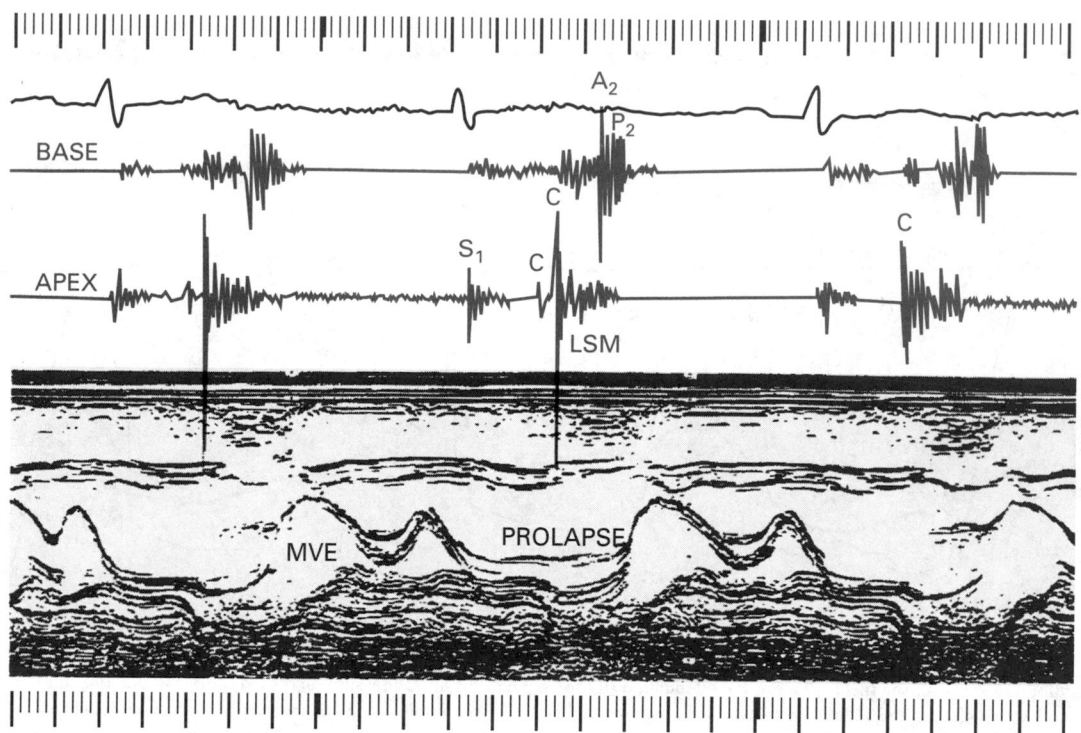

FIGURE 10-60

Simultaneously recorded base and apex phonocardiograms and mitral valve echocardiogram (MVE) demonstrating the frequent association of a late systolic murmur with a prominent late systolic click. Although the murmur is well transmitted to the base, the click transmits poorly. In the first two complexes, an additional softer click precedes the click murmur complex. The last complex shows only a single click, demonstrating the variability of the auscultatory findings even at rest. The large click occurs at maximal prolapse and the smaller click occurs near the onset of echocardiographic prolapse.

Echocardiographic Correlations and Mechanisms of Sound Production

In Fig. 10-63, the relationship between the aortic and pulmonary valve echocardiogram and A_2 and P_2 is shown. The first high-frequency component of both A_2 and P_2 is coincident with completion of closure of the aortic and pulmonic valve leaflets. Identical correlations have been found by other investigators.[384,385] As with sounds arising from the AV valves, A_2 and P_2 are not due to the clapping together of the valve leaflets but are produced by the sudden deceleration of retrograde flow of the blood column in the aorta and pulmonary artery when the elastic limits of the tensed leaflets are met. This abrupt deceleration of flow sets the cardiohemic system into vibration; the lower-frequency vibrations are recorded as in the incisura of the great vessels, while the higher-frequency components result in A_2 and P_2. This mechanism of sound production is consistent with Rushmer's[310] original observations as well as with several subsequent investigations.[381,386,387] In further support of this theory are additional observations showing that the amplitude of A_2 and P_2 is directly proportional to the rate of change of the diastolic pressure gradient that develops across the valves— that is, the driving force accelerating the blood mass retrograde into the base of the great vessels.[386,388] This pressure gradient is the result of both the level of the diastolic pressure in the great vessel and the rate of pressure decline in the ventricle

and is consistent with the well-known clinical observation of increased intensity of A_2 and P_2 in systemic and pulmonary hypertension.

Normal Physiologic Splitting

Normally during expiration, A_2 and P_2 are separated by an interval of less than 30 ms and are heard by the clinician as a single sound.[389,390] During inspiration, both components become distinctly audible as the splitting interval widens, primarily due to a delayed P_2,[301,391] although an earlier A_2 contributes to a lesser degree (Fig. 10-64).[391–397] The traditional explanation of normal splitting was that the delayed P_2 during inspiration was secondary to increased venous return, prolonging the duration of right ventricular systole, while a concomitant decrease in venous return to the left heart shortened left ventricular systole.[398–400] More recent studies have shown that the delayed P_2 and early A_2 associated with inspiration are due to a complex interplay between dynamic changes in pulmonary vascular impedance and changes in systemic and pulmonary venous return.[397] The net effect of these changes is prolongation of right ventricular ejection and a concomitant decrease in left ventricular ejection that results in widening of the splitting interval during inspiration.

On auscultation, splitting of S_2 is usually best heard at the second or third left intercostal space; the normal P_2 is softer than A_2 and is rarely audible at the apex.[396] When P_2 is

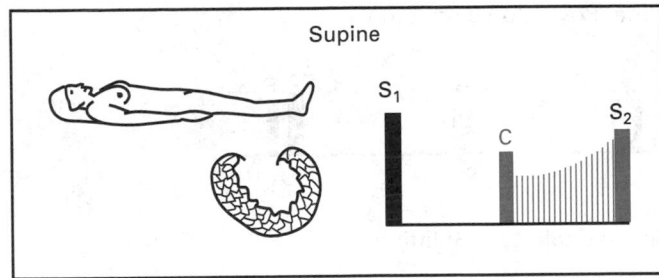

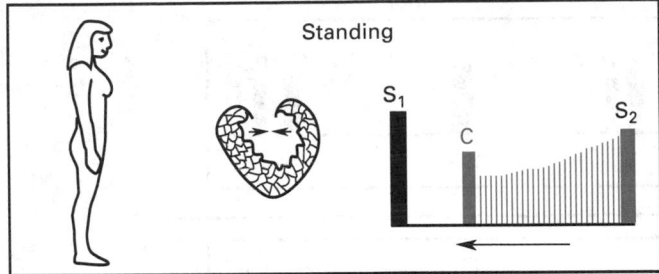

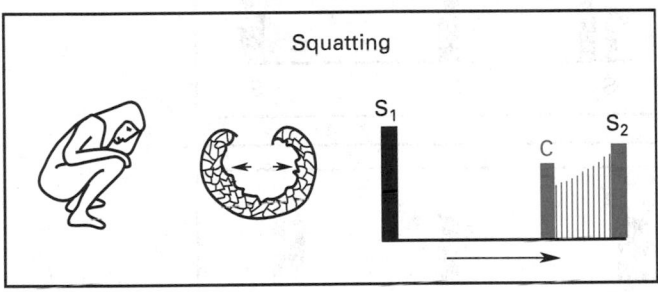

FIGURE 10-61

A midsystolic nonejection sound (C) occurs in mitral valve prolapse and is followed by a late systolic murmur that crescendo to S_1. With the assumption of the upright posture, venous return decreases, the heart becomes smaller, the C moves closer to S_1, and the mitral regurgitant murmur has an earlier onset. With prompt squatting, both venous return and afterload increase, the heart becomes larger, the C moves toward S_2, and the duration of the murmur shortens. (From Shaver JA et al. *Examination of the Heart: Part IV. Auscultation*. Dallas: American Heart Association; 1990:13. Reproduced with permission from the publisher and the authors.)

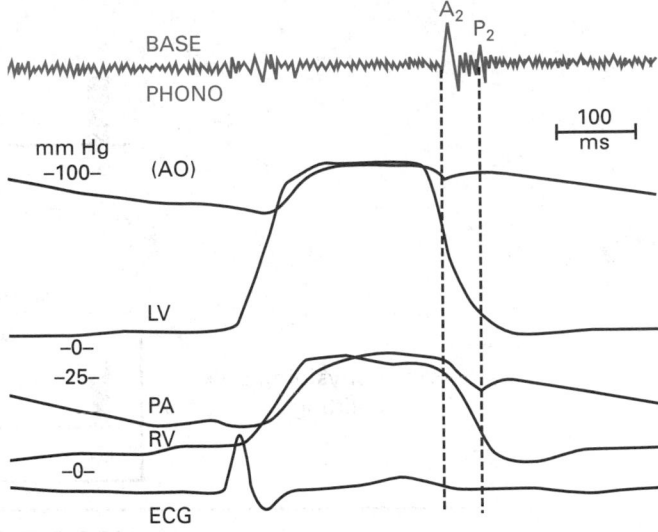

FIGURE 10-62

The cardiac cycle recorded by high-fidelity catheter-tipped micromanometers. The aortic (A_2) and pulmonic (P_2) closure sounds are coincident with the incisurae of their respective arterial traces. Although the left and right ventricular mechanical systoles are nearly equal in duration, the right ventricular (RV) systolic ejection period terminates after left ventricular (LV) ejection because of an increased right-sided "hangout" interval. (From Shaver JA et al. The second heart sound: Newer concepts: Part 1. Normal and wide physiological splitting. *Mod Concepts Cardiovasc Dis* 197; 46:7. Reproduced with permission from the American Heart Association, Inc, and the authors.)

heard at the apex, either significant pulmonary hypertension is present or the apex is occupied by the right ventricle—a situation commonly seen in normotensive atrial septal defect. The absolute value of inspiratory splitting varies with age and the depth of respiration. In younger subjects, maximal splitting during inspiration averages 40 to 50 ms; with age, this value decreases such that a single S_2 during both phases of respiration may be normal in subjects older than 40 years.[396,401–403]

Abnormal Splitting

All conditions in which abnormal splitting of S_2 exist can be identified at the bedside by the presence of audible expiratory splitting (more than 30 ms)—that is, the ability to hear two distinct sounds during expiration (Fig. 10-64).[378,401] This finding must be present when the patient is auscultated in both the supine and upright positions, as some normal subjects have audible expiratory splitting in the recumbent position

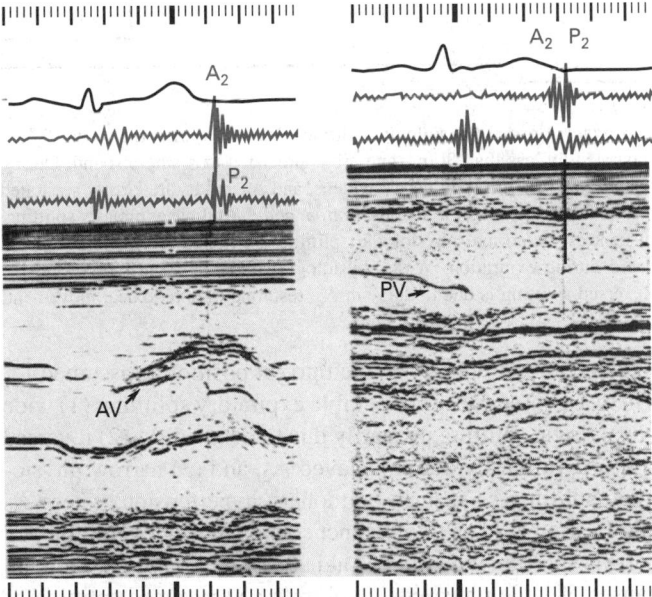

FIGURE 10-63

Left panel: The base and apex phonocardiograms are recorded simultaneously with the aortic valve echocardiogram. The first high-frequency component of A_2 is coincident with the completion of closure of the aortic valve. *Right panel*: Base and apex phonocardiograms are recorded with the pulmonary valve echocardiogram. The first high-frequency component of P_1 is coincident with the completion of closure of the pulmonic valve. [From Shaver JA et al. Normal and abnormal heart sounds in cardiac diagnosis: Part I. Systolic sounds. *Curr Probl Cardiol* 1985: 10(3):43. Reproduced with permission from the publisher and the authors.]

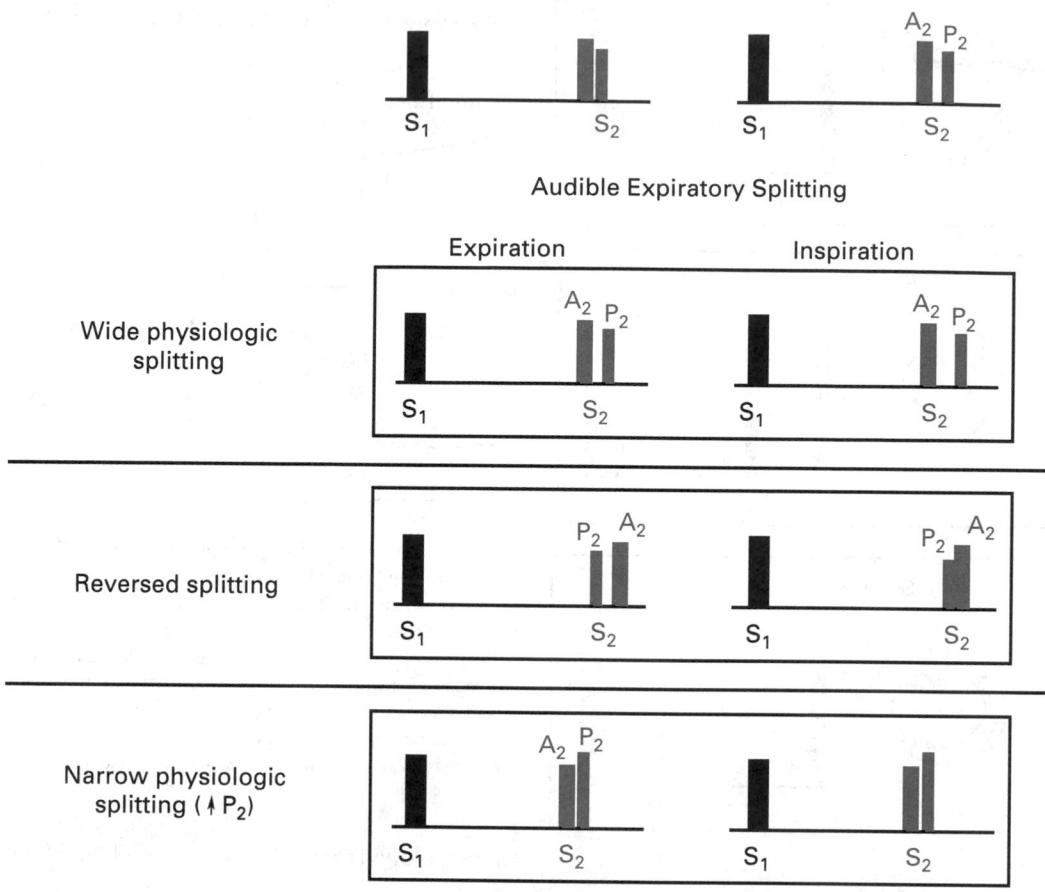

FIGURE 10-64

Top panel: Normal physiologic splitting. During expiration, A_2 and P_2 are separated by less than 30 ms and are appreciated as a single sound. During inspiration, the splitting interval widens, and A_2 and P_2 are clearly separated into two distinctly audible sounds. *Bottom panel*: Audible expiratory splitting. In contrast to normal physiologic splitting, two distinct sounds are easily heard during expiration. Wide physiologic splitting is due to delay in P_2. Reversed splitting is due to delay in A_2, resulting in paradoxical movement; that is, with inspiration, P_2 moves toward A_2, and the splitting interval narrows. Narrow physiologic splitting is seen in pulmonary hypertension, and both A_2 and P_2 are heard during expiration at a narrow splitting interval due to an increased intensity and high-frequency composition of P_2. (From Shaver JA et al. *Examination of the Heart: Part IV. Auscultation.* Dallas: American Heart Association; 1990:17. Reproduced with permission from the publisher and the authors.)

that becomes single when the upright position is assumed.[110] There are three causes of audible expiratory splitting: (1) wide physiologic splitting primarily due to delayed P_2, (2) reversed splitting primarily due to delayed A_2, and (3) narrow physiologic splitting as seen in pulmonary hypertension, where A_2 and P_2 are heard as two distinct sounds during expiration at a narrow splitting interval. In Tables 10-4 and 10-5, the common causes of wide physiologic splitting and reversed splitting of S_2 are classified according to the abnormality of the cardiac cycle responsible for the altered timing of A_2 and P_2. In each table, the cardiac cycle has been divided into three phases (Fig. 10-62): (1) the electromechanical couple interval, the time from the onset of the Q wave to the rise of ventricular pressure; (2) ventricular mechanical systole, the sum of the isovolumic contraction time plus the ejection period minus the "hangout" interval (abnormalities of this interval exclude those conditions in which prolongation of the hangout interval is primarily responsible for the increased ejection time); and (3) hangout or impedance interval, the time between the incisura of the arterial trace and the ventricular pressure at the same level as the incisura (includes all conditions in which prolongation of this interval is primarily responsible for the increased ejection time).

WIDE PHYSIOLOGIC SPLITTING OF S_2

An example of wide physiologic splitting of S_2 due to delayed electrical activation of the right ventricle secondary to right bundle branch block is shown in Fig. 10-65. In Figs. 10-66 and 10-67, prolongation of right ventricular mechanical systole secondary to severe pulmonary hypertension and pulmonic stenosis is responsible for the delayed P_2. In Fig. 10-68, the classic wide, fixed splitting of S_2 found in atrial septal defect is demonstrated. A composite in Fig. 10-69 documents the role played by decreased impedance of the pulmonary vascular

TABLE 10-4

WIDE PHYSIOLOGIC SPLITTING OF THE SECOND HEART SOUND

Delayed pulmonic closure
  Delayed electrical activation of the right ventricle
    Complete RBBB (proximal type)[312]
    Left ventricular paced beats[312]
    Left ventricular ectopic beats[312]
  Prolonged right ventricular mechanical systole
    Acute massive pulmonary embolus[404,405]
    Pulmonary hypertension with right heart failure[406,407]
    Pulmonic stenosis with intact septum (moderate to severe)[355,408]
  Decreased impedance of the pulmonary vascular bed (increased "hangout")
    Normotensive atrial septal defect[378,409]
    Idiopathic dilation of the pulmonary artery[378,381]
    Pulmonic stenosis (mild)[378,381]
    Atrial septal defect, postoperative (70%)[29,389]
    Unexplained AES in the normal[410]
Early aortic closure
  Shortened left ventricular mechanical systole (LVET)
    Mitral regurgitation[378,389,391]
    Ventricular septal defect[389]

Abbreviations: RBBB = right bundle branch block; AES = audible expiratory splitting; LVET = left ventricular ejection time.

Source: From Shaver JA et al. The second heart sound; Newer concepts. Part 1: Normal and wide physiological splitting. *Mod Concepts Cardiovasc Dis* 1977; 46:9. Reproduced with permission from the American Heart Association, Inc., and the authors

TABLE 10-5

REVERSED SPLITTING OF THE SECOND HEART SOUND

Delayed aortic closure
  Delayed electrical activation of the left ventricle
    Complete LBBB[a] (proximal type)[340,412,413]
    Right ventricular paced beat[312]
    Right ventricular ectopic beats[312]
  Prolonged left ventricular mechanical systole
    Complete LBBB (peripheral type)[340,401,412,413]
    Left ventricular outflow tract obstruction[380,412,414,415]
    Hypertensive cardiovascular disease[417]
    Arteriosclerotic heart disease
      Chronic ischemic heart disease[418,420]
      Angina pectoris[418–420]
  Decreased impedance of the systemic vascular bed (increased "hangout")
    Poststenotic dilation of the aorta secondary to aortic stenosis or regurgitation[412,415,416]
    Patent ductus arteriosus[412,421]
Early pulmonic closure
  Early electrical activation of the right ventricle
    Wolff-Parkinson-White syndrome, type B[422,423]

[a] LBBB = left bundle branch block.

Source: From Shaver JA et al: The second heart sound: Newer concepts. Part 2: Paradoxical splitting and narrow physiological splitting. *Mod Concepts Cardiovasc Dis* 1977; 46:13. Reproduced with permission from the American Heart Association, Inc., and the authors.

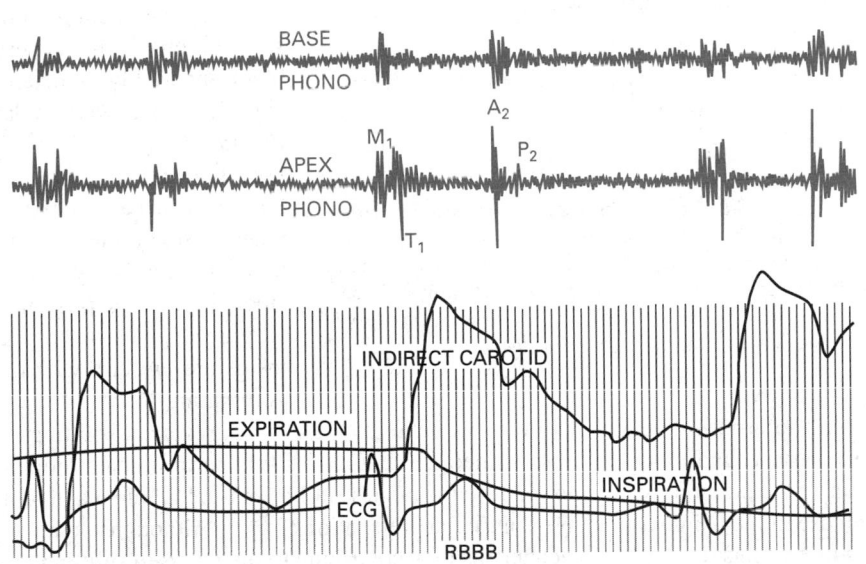
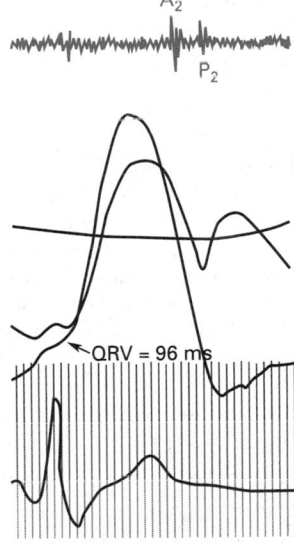

FIGURE 10-65

Left panel: Wide physiologic splitting of S_2 is seen in a patient with complete right bundle branch block. Audible expiratory splitting that widens normally with inspiration is present. Note also the wide splitting of the first heart sound into its mitral (M_1) and tricuspid (T_1) components, as recorded at the apex. *Right panel*: The base phonocardiogram is recorded simultaneously with high-fidelity catheters in the right ventricle and pulmonary artery during cardiac catheterization. There is marked prolongation of the Q to the onset of the right ventricular pressure rise of 96 ms, resulting in wide physiologic splitting of S_2. The delayed P_2 is secondary to the delayed activation of the right ventricle. [From Shaver JA. Current uses of phonocardiography in clinical practice. In: Rapaport E, ed. *Cardiology Update—Reviews for Physicians*. New York: Elsevier; 1981:337. Reproduced originally in part (*left panel*) with permission from the publisher and author; and from Shaver JA et al. Normal and abnormal heart sounds in cardiac diagnosis: Part I. Systolic sounds. *Curr Probl Cardiol* 1985; 10(3):48. Reproduced in total with permission from the publisher and authors.]

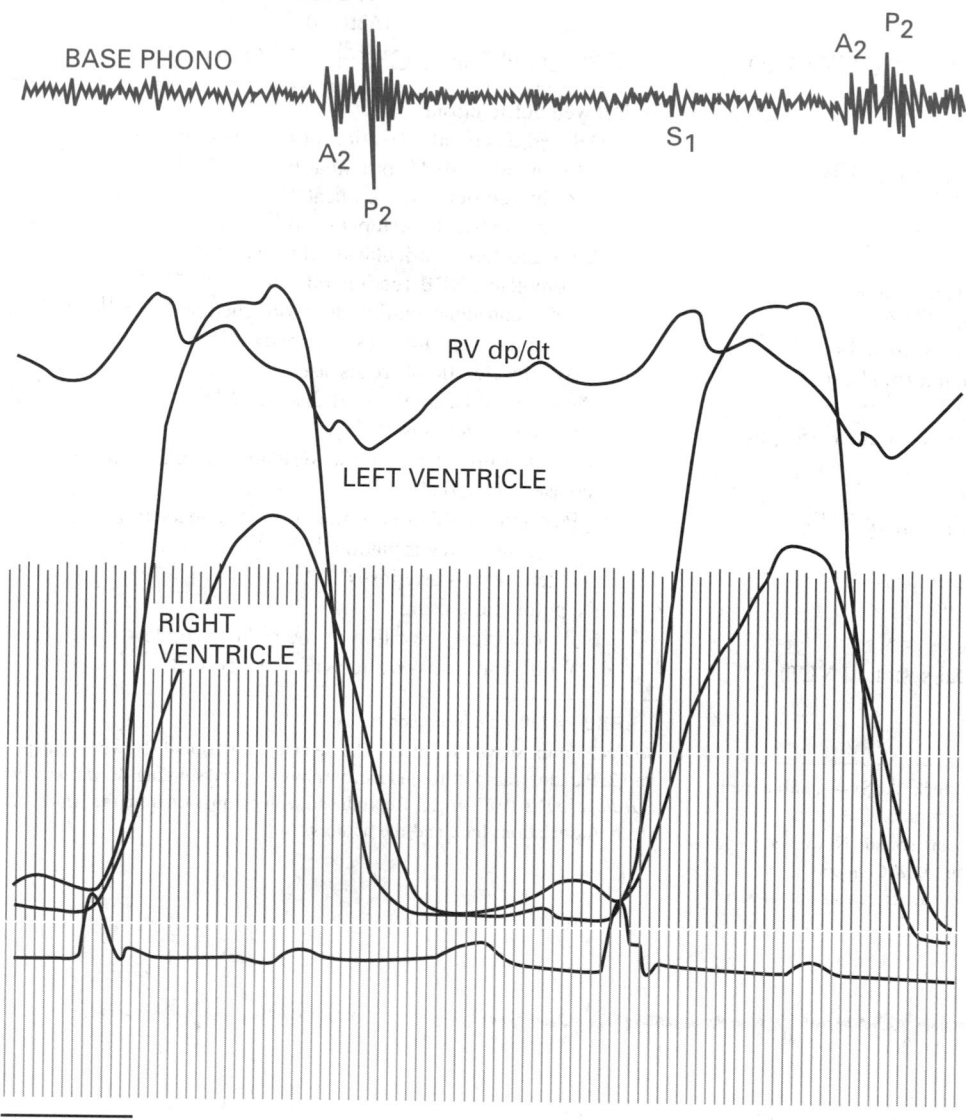

FIGURE 10-66

Simultaneous high-fidelity left and right ventricular pressures are recorded with the base phonocardiogram in a 35-year-old chronic drug abuser with severe pulmonary hypertension. Wide, fixed splitting of S_2 is recorded, and the intensity of P_2 is greater than that of A_2. Significant prolongation of right ventricular systole is responsible for the delay in P_2, due primarily to prolongation of the right ventricular isovolumic contraction time. [From Shaver JA et al. Normal and abnormal heart sounds in cardiac diagnosis: Part I. Systolic sounds. *Curr Probl Cardiol* 1985; 10(3):50. Reproduced in total with permission from the publisher and authors.]

with P_2 preceding A_2. At the bedside, this abnormality is recognized by paradoxical movement of A_2 and P_2 with respiration.[411] During inspiration, P_2 moves toward A_2 and the splitting interval narrows, whereas during expiration the two components separate, and audible expiratory splitting is present (Fig. 10-64). The presence of paradoxical splitting of S_2 almost always indicates significant underlying cardiovascular disease.

Both right ventricular ectopic and paced beats produce a delay in the onset of left ventricular contraction, resulting in reversed splitting of S_2.[312] The mechanism responsible is a delayed activation of the left ventricle, prolonging the Q to left ventricular pressure rise interval. The most common cause of reversed splitting is complete LBBB, which can be due either to delayed activation of the left ventricle, as seen in isolated proximal block (Fig. 10-70), or to prolonged mechanical systole (primarily isovolumic contraction time), as seen in proximal or peripheral block invariably associated with significant left ventricular dysfunction (Fig. 10-53).[339–341] Delay often exists in the onset of left ventricular pressure rise when isovolumic contraction time is markedly prolonged, since in most cases of LBBB varying degrees of both mechanisms are present, with one predominating.[412,413]

bed in the audible expiratory splitting found in atrial septal defect, idiopathic dilation of the pulmonary artery, and mild pulmonic stenosis with aneurysmal dilation of the pulmonary artery. In each case, there is a marked increase in the hangout interval as measured by high-fidelity pressure tracings. In Fig. 10-47, wide physiologic splitting secondary to a decreased left ventricular ejection time is shown in a patient with acute mitral regurgitation. For a more detailed analysis of each of the conditions producing wide physiologic splitting of S_2, the reader is referred to the references listed in Table 10-4.

REVERSED SPLITTING OF S_2

Almost all cases of reversed splitting of S_2 are due to a delay in A_2. As a result, the sequence of closure sounds is reversed,

In the left panel of Fig. 10-71, reversed splitting of S_2 is demonstrated in a patient with hypertrophic cardiomyopathy and is due to the large systolic pressure gradient and prolonged left ventricular relaxation.[380,414] Although both of these mechanisms may contribute to the reversed splitting observed in patients with valvular aortic stenosis, an additional mechanism is shown in the right panel of Fig. 10-71, where an exaggerated hangout interval of 30 ms is present and is primarily responsible for the delayed A_2.[415,416]

In hypertensive cardiovascular disease, splitting is usually physiologic with the intensity of A_2 increased; however, rare instances of reversed splitting do occur. The elevation of blood pressure produced by intravenous administration of methoxamine has been shown to produce reversed splitting

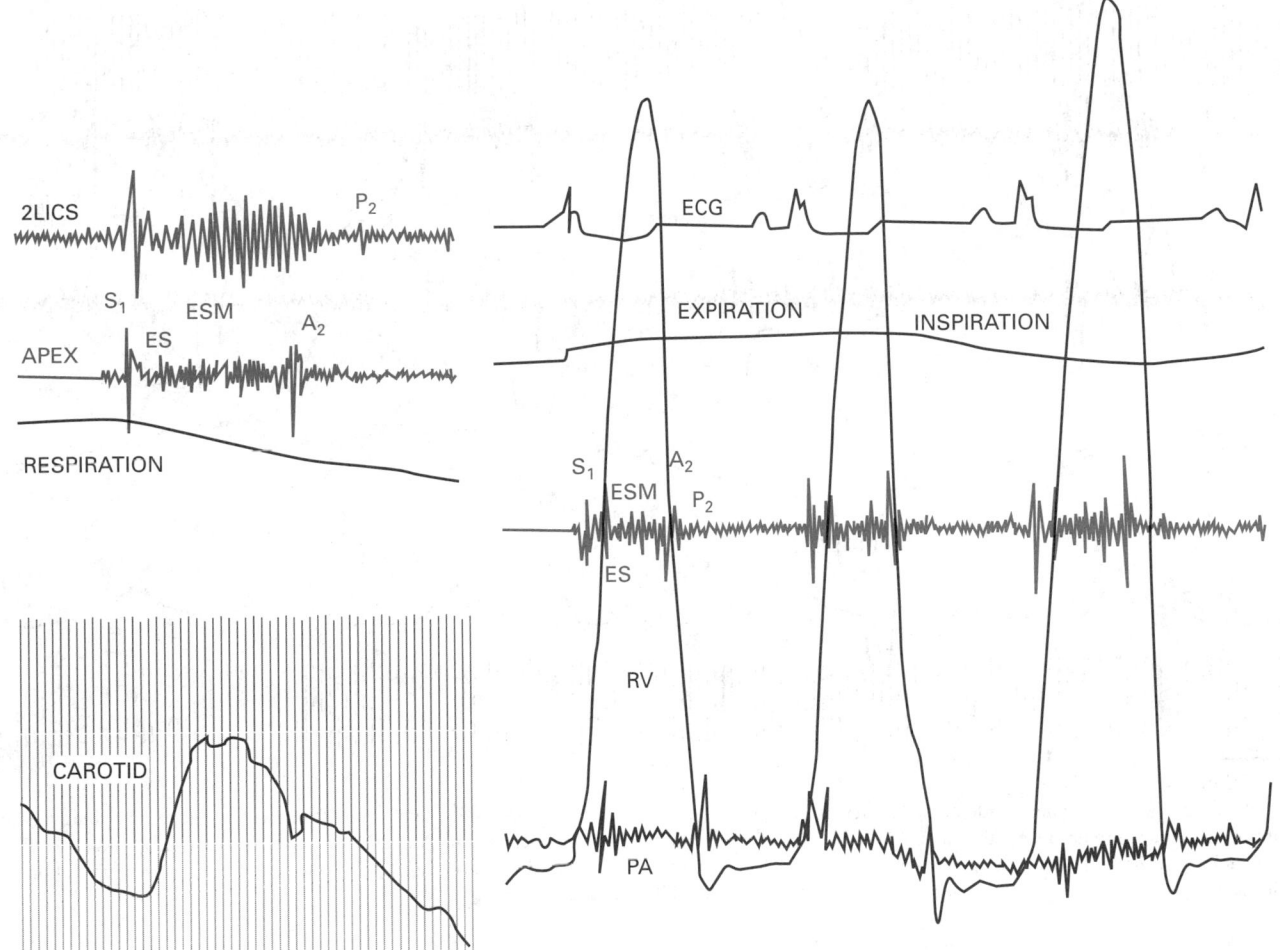

FIGURE 10-67

Left panel: The phonocardiogram of a patient with severe valvular pulmonic stenosis as recorded at the second left intercostal space (2LICS) and the apex. The long ejection murmur (ESM) has late systolic peaking and spills through A_2. There is a marked delay in P_2, which is very small in amplitude. *Right panel*: At cardiac catheterization, the markedly delayed P_2 is shown to be secondary to a very large systolic pressure gradient, and its decreased intensity is due to the low pulmonary artery pressure at the time of valve closure. The late peaking of the ejection murmur correlates with the maximal pressure gradient between the right ventricle and the pulmonary artery. (From Curtiss EI et al. First and second heart sound. In: Horwitz LD, ed. *Signs and Symptoms in Cardiology*. Philadelphia: Lippincott; 1985:200. Reproduced with permission from the publisher and authors.)

in a normal subject due to prolongation of both left ventricular ejection time and the isovolumic contraction time in the face of an increased afterload.[417]

Reversed splitting of S_2 has also been reported in ischemic heart disease and during episodes of angina pectoris.[418,419] The latter is extremely uncommon and has rarely been documented by phonocardiography. It is most likely due to a prolonged isovolumic contraction time of the ischemic left ventricle, although during angina it may also be due to an increase in systemic arterial pressure or transient LBBB.[420]

Decreased impedance in the systemic vascular bed can also contribute to the delayed A_2 seen in poststenotic dilation of the aorta, as shown in the right panel of Fig. 10-71. It also plays a role in the reversed splitting occasionally seen in both chronic aortic regurgitation and patent ductus arteriosus.[412,421] Reversed splitting of S_2 has also been reported in some cases of type B Wolff-Parkinson-White syndrome, where early activation of the right ventricle through an accessory pathway has caused P_2 to occur prematurely.[422,423]

NARROW PHYSIOLOGIC SPLITTING

Narrow physiologic splitting of S_2 is a common finding in severe pulmonary hypertension, as shown in Fig. 10-64.[406,424] In contrast to the normal situation, where only a single sound is heard during expiration, both A_2 and P_2 are easily heard, even though the splitting interval is less than 30 ms because of the increased intensity and high-frequency composition of P_2. Narrow splitting, although common in severe pulmonary hypertension, is not always the case, as shown in Fig. 10-66, where wide splitting with an increased amplitude of P_2 is present. Shapiro and associates[407] suggested that a wide split in pulmonary hypertension may indicate a more severely compromised ventricle than a normal split. Similar observations have also been made by Perloff,[406] who states that wide, persistent splitting becomes a useful sign of abnormal right ventricular performance in patients with primary pulmonary hypertension. In order to reconcile these different responses in S_2 when pulmonary hypertension develops, it is essential to appreciate that normally the duration of right and left ven-

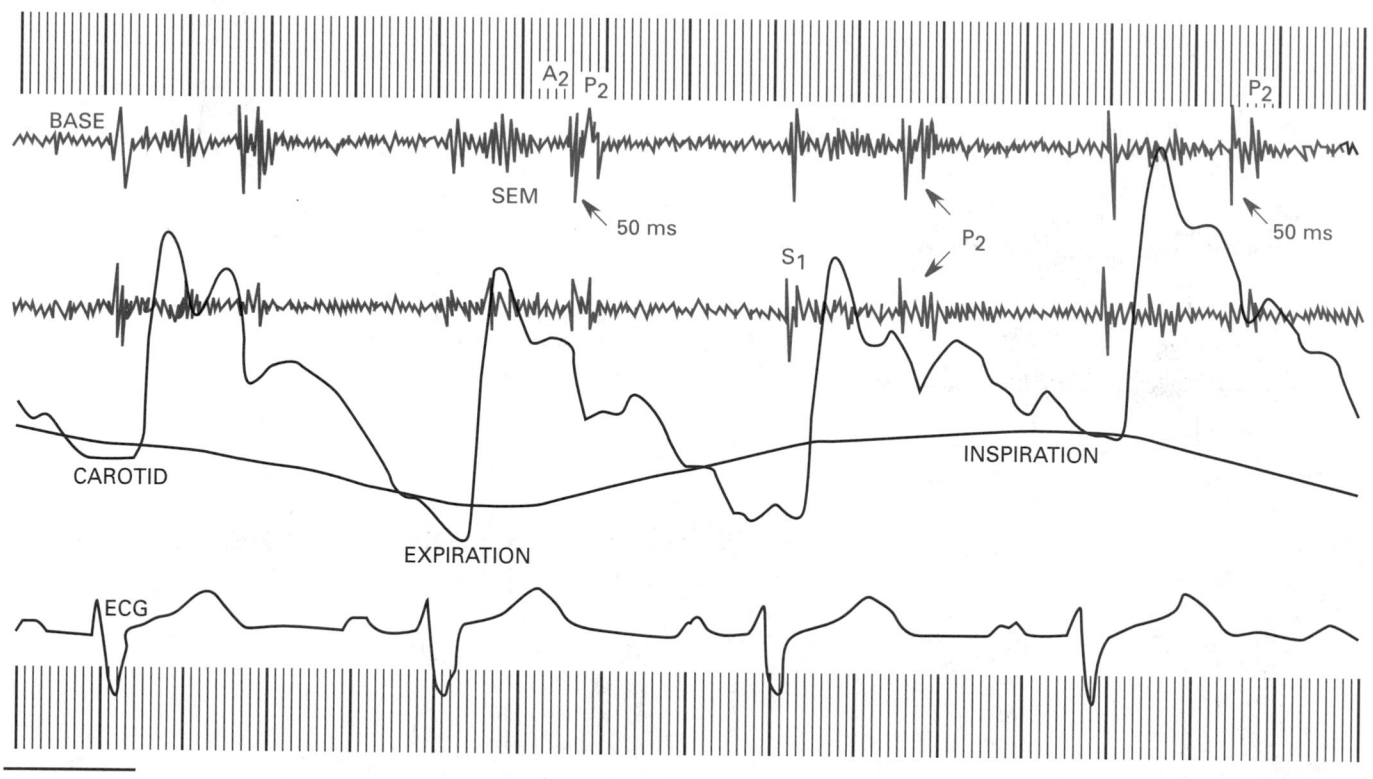

FIGURE 10-68

Simultaneous base and apex phonocardiograms are recorded together with the carotid pulse during quiet respiration in a young woman with a large atrial septal defect. Wide, fixed splitting of S_2 is present, and P_2 is easily recorded at the apex. A prominent systolic ejection murmur (SEM) is recorded at the base and is due to the large stroke volume across the right ventricular outflow tract. (From JA Shaver: Innocent murmurs. *Hosp Med,* April 1978, p. 15. © 1978. Reproduced with permission of Hospital Publications, Inc., and the author.)

tricular systole is nearly equal and that a potential interval (the normally wide right-sided hangout interval) can be encroached upon as the pulmonary hypertension progressively decreases the capacitance and increases the resistance of the pulmonary vascular bed (Fig. 10-62).[379–382,412–425] In Fig. 10-72, the sound and pressure correlates of two patients with severe pulmonary hypertension are shown, one having narrow splitting of S_2 and the other having wide splitting of S_2. Common to both patients is marked narrowing of the normally wide right-sided hangout interval. In the center panel, the duration of right and left ventricular mechanical systole is nearly equal at the time of the pulmonary artery incisura, and the splitting interval is narrow. In contrast, the right panel shows that there has been a marked prolongation of right ventricular mechanical systole in the face of chronic pressure overload, and the net effect is a delayed P_2 resulting in wide splitting of S_2. Thus, a spectrum of the width of splitting may be seen in pulmonary hypertension, depending on the degree of selective prolongation of right ventricular systole, always in the setting of a narrow hangout interval. Furthermore, it is clear that varying degrees of splitting may be seen in the same patient during different stages of the disease process producing the pulmonary hypertension. Similar hemodynamic correlates have been found in patients having hyperkinetic pulmonary hypertension secondary to large atrial septal defects.[382,409] Fixed splitting of S_2 has occasionally been documented in

severe right ventricular failure secondary to pulmonary hypertension. This has usually been attributed to the inability of the compromised right ventricle to accept the augmented venous return associated with inspiration. Curtiss and associates[397] have shown that another factor—the altered pulmonary vascular impedance associated with severe pulmonary hypertension—may also play an important role in the diminished inspiratory split observed in such cases.

Single S_2

All conditions listed in Table 10-5 that delay A_2 may produce a single S_2 when the splitting interval becomes less than 30 ms. Also, conditions in which one component of S_2 is either absent or inaudible will produce a single S_2 (for example, truncus arteriosus, severe tetralogy of Fallot, severe semilunar valve stenosis, pulmonary atresia, and most cases of tricuspid atresia). In Eisenmenger's ventricular septal defect, the duration of right and left ventricular systole is necessarily equal and a loud, single S_2 is appreciated because A_2 and P_2 occur simultaneously. The most common cause of an apparently single S_2 is the inability to hear the fainter of the two components of the sound (usually P_2) because of emphysema, obesity, or respiratory noise. Another common cause of single S_2 is seen in individuals over age 50. Although this has been attributed to a delayed A_2,[403,421] a decreased inspiratory delay

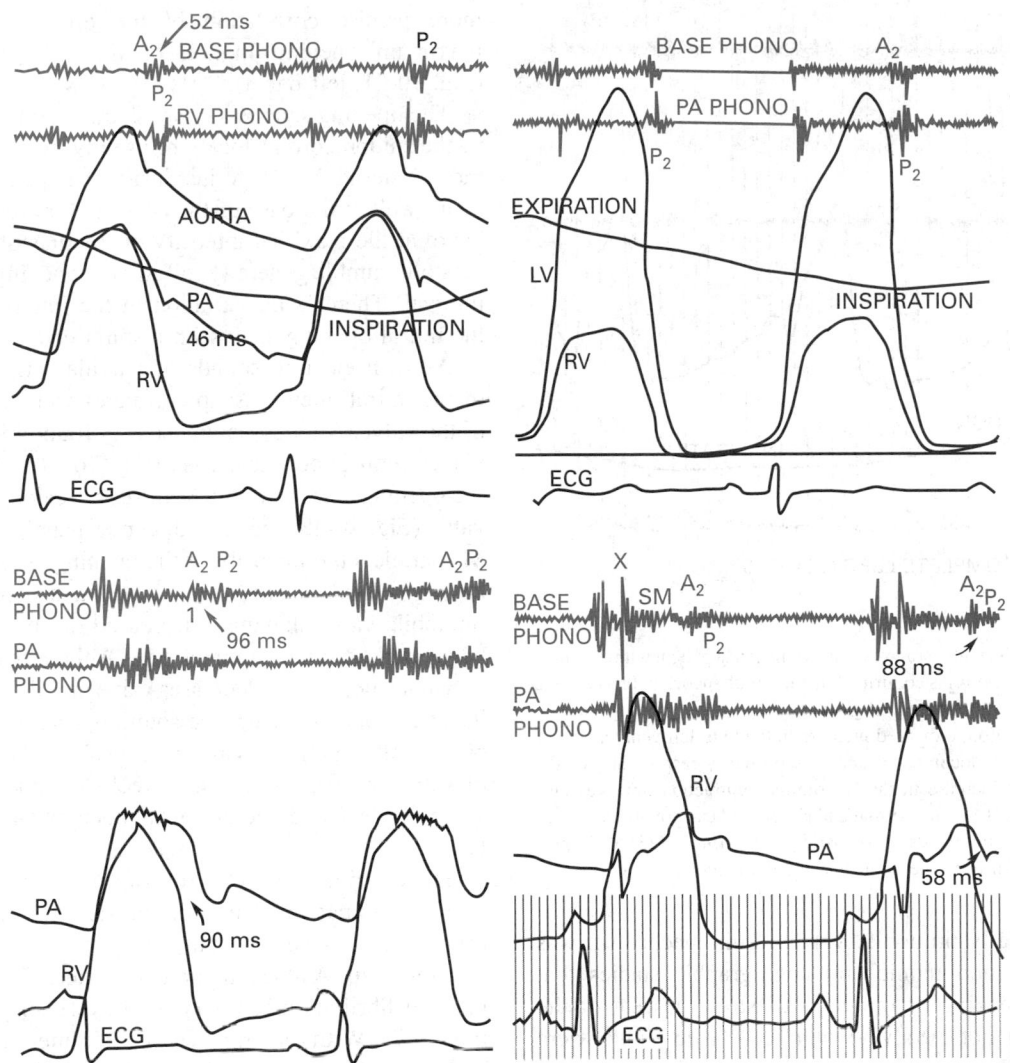

FIGURE 10-69

Upper left panel: Sound and pressure correlates of S_2 in a 45-year-old woman with a normotensive atrial septal defect (shunt 2:1). Wide, fixed splitting of S_2 is demonstrated; P_2 and A_2 are coincident with their respective incisurae, and the duration of the hangout interval is nearly equal to the A_2-P_2 interval. *Upper right panel*: Simultaneous right and left ventricular pressures clearly show that the duration of right and left ventricular systole is equal. *Lower left panel*: Sound and pressure correlates of a patient with idiopathic dilation of the pulmonary artery. P_2 is coincident with the incisura of the pulmonary artery and separated from the right ventricular pressure tracing by a hangout interval of 90 ms (almost identical to the splitting interval). *Lower right panel*: Similar sound and pressure correlates in a patient with mild valvular pulmonic stenosis and aneurysmal dilation of the pulmonary artery. Most of the delay in P_2 is due to a wide hangout interval of 56 ms. In each patient all pressures are recorded by catheter-tipped micromanometers. [From Shaver JA et al. Second heart sound: The role of altered greater and lesser circulation. In: Leon DF, Shaver JA, eds. *Physiologic Principles of Heart Sounds and Murmurs*. Monograph 46. New York: American Heart Association; 1975:63. Reproduced originally in part (*top panel*) with permission from the publisher and the authors; and from Shaver JA. The second heart sound: Hemodynamic determinants. *Acta Cardiol* 1985; 40:12. Reproduced in total with permission from the publisher and authors.]

in P_2 has also been reported.[402] This latter finding has been shown to be due to a decreased right-sided hangout interval, most likely related to aging changes in the pulmonary vascular bed.[390]

OPENING SNAPS

Opening of the normal atrioventricular valve is almost always a silent event. With thickening and deformity of the leaflets, usually rheumatic in origin, however, a sound is generated in early diastole in a manner analogous to ejection sounds arising from deformed semilunar valves. The term *opening snap* was first used by Thayer[426] in 1908 to describe the high-frequency early diastolic sound in mitral stenosis. Margolies and Wolferth[427] provided the first extensive description of the sound and its timing and proposed that the mechanism of production was a sudden stopping of the opening movement of the valve. They also recognized that the sound had been absent in those patients who, on autopsy, had markedly thick-

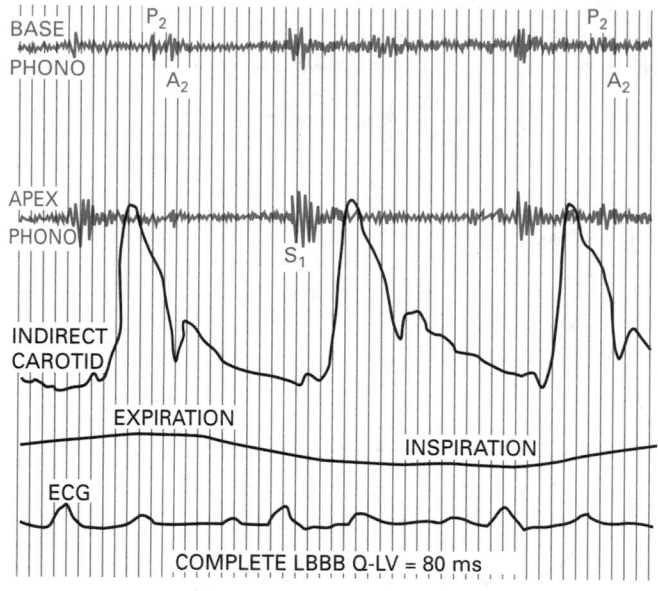

FIGURE 10-70

Reversed splitting of S_2 with paradoxical movement in a patient with complete left bundle branch block. A_2 is confirmed by the simultaneous indirect carotic pulse, and with inspiration there is slight narrowing of the splitting interval. At cardiac catheterization, a marked increase in the Q to left ventricular rise interval of 80 ms was documented and was primarily responsible for the delayed A_2. A slight increase in the isovolumic contraction time was also present. [From Shaver JA et al. Normal and abnormal heart sounds in cardiac diagnosis: Part I. Systolic sounds. *Curr Probl Cardiol* 1985; 10(3):56. Reproduced with permission from the publisher and the authors.]

ened and essentially immobile valves. This mechanism was confirmed by hemodynamic and angiographic studies that show sudden checking of the early diastolic descent of the funnel-shaped stenotic valve when its elastic limits were met.[332,428,429] Phonoechocardiography has given an even

more precise correlation of the opening snap with the maximum opening motion of the anterior mitral leaflet (Fig. 10-51, left panel).[340,430]

The opening snap is a crisp, sharp sound that can be heard in the midprecordial location, usually best in the area from the left sternal border to just inside the apex. It may often be heard well at the base of the heart and is frequently not well heard at the maximal intensity of the diastolic murmur. The diastolic rumble generally follows the opening snap by a short interval. There is no variation in the intensity or timing of the mitral opening snap with respiration.

As with ejection sounds of valvular origin, the intensity of the mitral opening snap correlates well with the mobility of the valve. A loud opening snap is found in mobile stenotic valves with good excursions (Fig. 10-51, left panel), while the opening snap is absent with severe calcific fixation of the valve (Fig. 10-48; Fig. 10-73, center panel). The intensity of M_1 parallels the intensity of the opening snap; mobile valves having a loud opening snap have an accentuated M_1, and immobile valves having a decreased or absent opening snap have marked attenuation of M_1. Although the presence of valvular calcification decreases valve mobility and the audibility of the opening snap, the sound is actually found in 50 to 60 percent of patients with calcific valves. The mere presence of valvular calcium does not preclude some mobility of the valve leaflets and therefore an opening snap (Fig. 10-73, left panel).

The opening snap (OS) follows A_2 by an interval of 0.03 to 0.15 s. In patients with mild mitral stenosis, the interval is usually long, whereas with more severe stenosis, the A_2-opening snap (A_2-OS) interval is shorter. The A_2-OS interval in atrial fibrillation can vary with cycle length, as shown in Fig. 10-74. With a short preceding RR interval, the left atrium has not had time to empty, the left atrial pressure remains

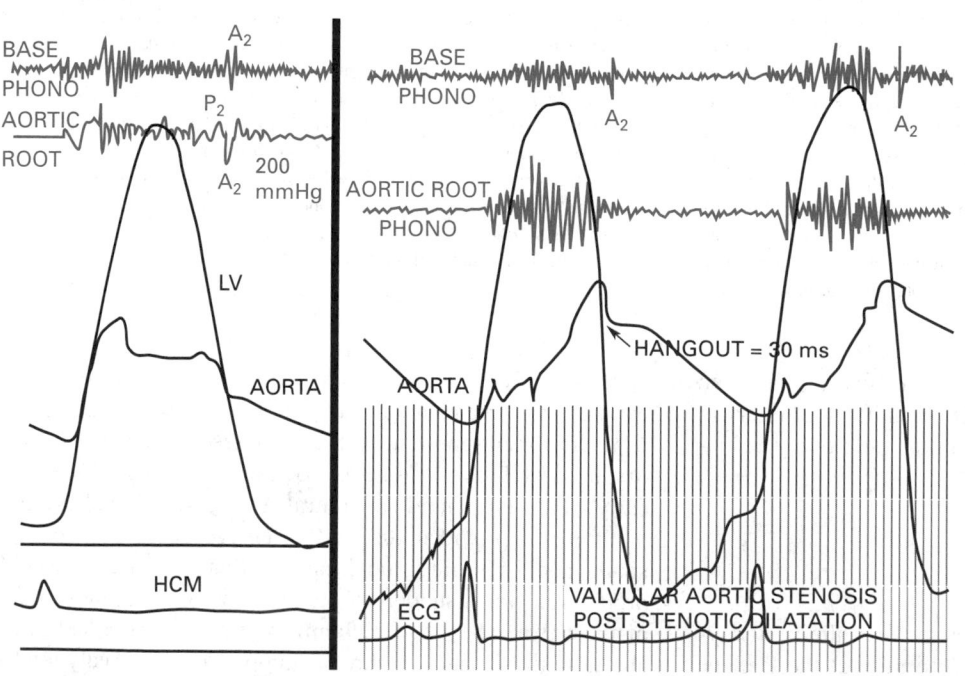

FIGURE 10-71

Left panel: External sound and aortic root sound are recorded simultaneously with pressures in the left ventricle and central aorta (catheter-tipped micromanometers) in a patient with hypertrophic cardiomyopathy. Reversed splitting of S_2 is present, and the delayed A_2 is due to the large systolic pressure gradient and the prolonged left ventricular relaxation. *Right panel*: Catheter-tipped micromanometers are recording pressures in the left ventricle and central aorta in a patient with valvular aortic stenosis having marked poststenotic dilation of the aorta; A_2 is coincident with the central aortic incisura and separated from the left ventricular pressure by a wide hangout interval of 30 ms. This interval is nearly twice as long as the normal left ventricular hangout interval, as shown in Figs. 10-46 and 10-62. (From Shaver JA. The second heart sound: Hemodynamic determinants. *Acta Cardiol* 1985; 40:7. Reproduced with permission from the publisher and the author.)

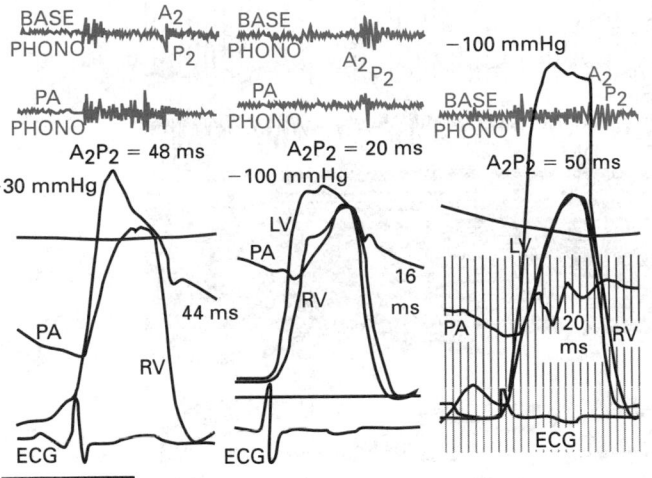

FIGURE 10-72

The sound and pressure correlates of S_2 in a 17-year-old patient with normal pulmonary artery pressure (*left panel*) are contrasted with the sound and pressure correlates of two patients having severe pulmonary hypertension. The center panel shows narrow splitting of S_2 on the external phonocardiogram, while in the right panel there is wide splitting of S_2. There is a marked reduction in the hangout interval in both patients with severe pulmonary hypertension compared to the patient with normal pulmonary artery pressure. In the center panel, the duration of left and right ventricular systole is nearly equal, and narrow splitting of S_2 results. In the right panel, significant prolongation of right ventricular mechanical systole beyond left ventricular systole delays P_2, producing wide splitting of S_2. (From Shaver JA. Clinical implications of the hangout interval. *Int J Cardiol* 1984; 5:396. Reproduced with permission from the publisher and the author.)

high, and the A_2-OS interval is short. With a longer preceding RR interval, the left atrial pressure falls, and the A_2-OS interval widens.

There have been a number of attempts to use the A_2-OS interval to predict the level of the left atrial pressure and severity of mitral stenosis.[431–433] The hemodynamics responsible for the timing of the opening snap are shown in Fig. 10-52. The opening snap occurs at the maximal mitral valve opening shortly after left ventricular–left atrial pressure crossovers. Factors that influence the timing of the opening snap relative to A_2 are (1) the rate of left ventricular pressure decline, (2) the level of the left ventricular pressure at the time of A_2, and (3) the level of the left atrial pressure. Increasing severity of mitral stenosis is usually accompanied by an increasing left atrial pressure and therefore a shortening of the A_2-OS interval. Because this interval is multifactorially determined, there is an imperfect correlation between the A_2-OS interval and the mitral valve area.[434,435] Tricuspid valve stenosis can also produce an opening snap.[436–438] This sound is frequently not detected because the findings of coexisting mitral stenosis, which is almost invariably present, overshadow those of tricuspid stenosis. The maximum intensity of the tricuspid opening snap tends to be found closer to the left sternal border and, unlike the mitral snap, the intensity of the tricuspid snap increases with inspiration. When present, it generally follows the mitral opening snap.[437] An early diastolic sound can also be caused by a right or left atrial

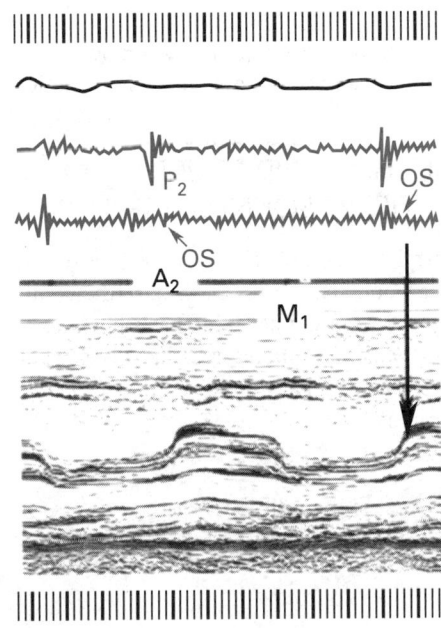
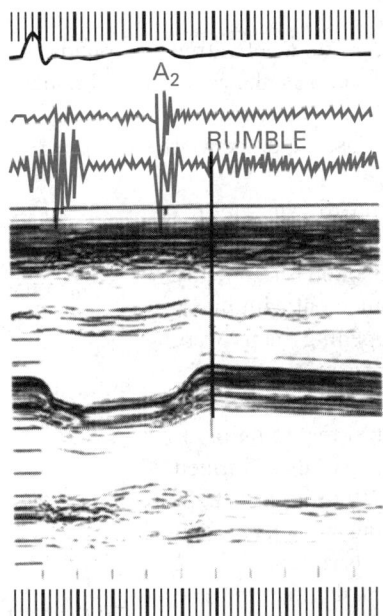
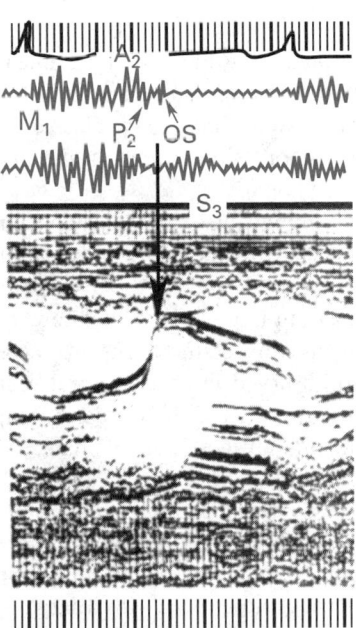

FIGURE 10-73

Base and apex phonocardiograms are recorded simultaneously with the mitral valve echocardiogram in three patients with chronic rheumatic mitral valve disease. In the left panel, a soft opening snap is coincident with the maximal opening of a thickened, relatively immobile stenotic mitral valve. In the center panel, calcific fixation of a severely stenotic mitral valve is present, and an opening snap is absent. Note that the onset of the diastolic rumble begins after the maximal anterior excursion of the heavily calcified valve. In the right panel, an opening snap occurs at the maximal opening of the nonstenotic rheumatic valve. A holosystolic murmur of mitral regurgitation is present, and no gradient was found across the mitral valve at cardiac catheterization. A loud S_2 gallop follows the opening snap and occurs during the early E-F slope of the rheumatic mitral valve.

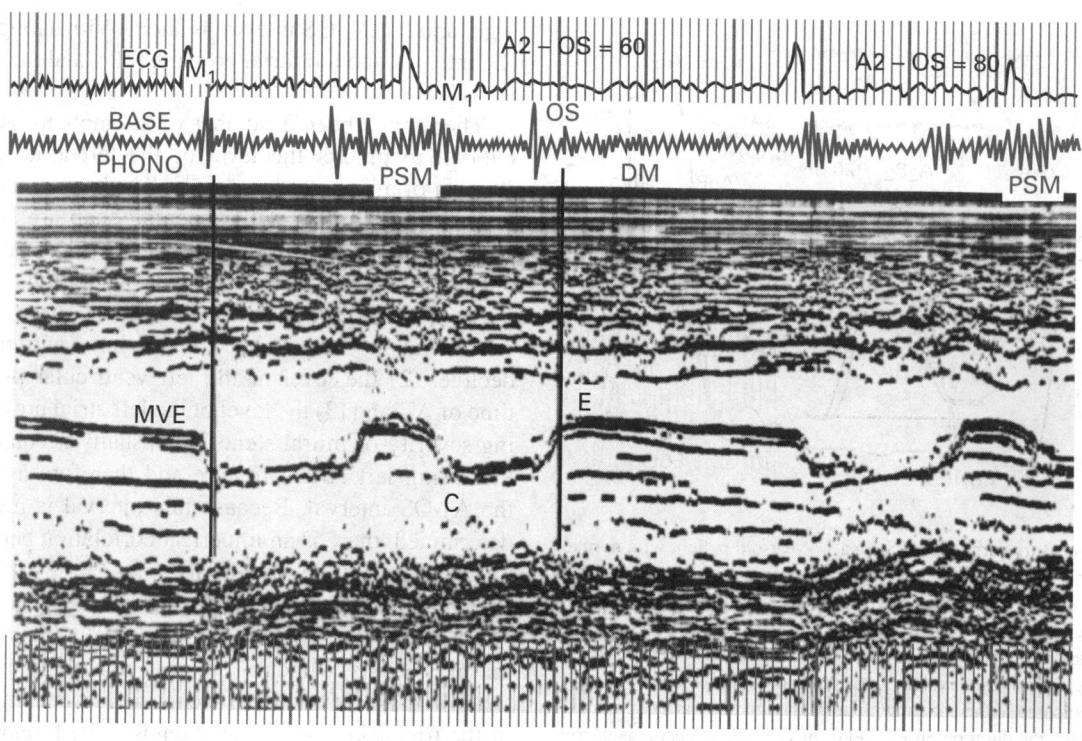

FIGURE 10-74

The base phonocardiogram is recorded with the mitral valve echocardiogram in a patient having mitral stenosis with atrial fibrillation and varying RR cycles. Following a short diastolic filling period, the A_2-OS interval in complex 2 is 60 ms. After a longer diastolic filling period, the A_2-OS interval in complex 3 is lengthened to 80 ms because of the decrease in left atrial pressure. The crescendo presystolic murmur (PMS) preceding complex 2 is caused by ventriculogenic closure of the stenotric mitral valve shortly after it has opened. The PSM is absent in complex 3 following a longer diastolic filling period. DM = diastolic murmur; E = maximal point of mitral valve opening. [From Reddy PS, et al. Normal and abnormal heart sounds in cardiac diagnosis: Part 2. Diastolic sounds. *Curr Probl Cardiol* 1985; 10(3):12. Reproduced with permission from the publisher and the authors.]

myxoma.[334] Although the clinical findings of a left atrial myxoma may be similar to those of mitral stenosis, the echocardiographic picture is classic (Fig. 10-51, center panel). The tumor "plop" occurs at the maximal diastolic descent of the myxoma.

Although an opening snap is rarely heard with normal valves, it may be heard in situations where high flow exists across the AV valves.[439] An early diastolic sound is frequently present in large atrial septal defects[440] coincident with maximal opening of the tricuspid valve.[441] Opening snaps were also observed in severe mitral regurgitation in reports prior to the routine use of echocardiography.[442,443] It may well be that some of these patients had severe mitral regurgitation of rheumatic origin with typical diastolic doming of the deformed valves, as seen with mitral stenosis (Fig. 10-73, right panel). Other conditions in which functional opening snaps have been found include large ventricular septal defects, thyrotoxicosis, and tricuspid atresia with a large atrial septal defect.[439] The opening snap must be differentiated from other early diastolic sounds such as the S_3, the pulmonary component of a widely split S_2, and a pericardial knock. At the bedside, differentiation of an opening snap from P_2 is made by noting that the maximal intensity is near the apex rather than at the pulmonary area and that there is lack of movement with respiration. During continuous respiration, it is often possible to appreciate three sounds on inspiration, occurring in rapid sequence in the pulmonary area, and only two components on expiration.

THE THIRD AND FOURTH HEART SOUNDS

The third and fourth heart sounds (S_3, S_4) are low frequency events related to early and late diastolic filling of the ventricles (Fig. 10-75). When they are heard in disease states, they are called *gallop sounds*, and their presence gives valuable information to the clinician regarding the status of ventricular function and compliance.

THE THIRD HEART SOUND

Physiologic S_3

The physiologic S_3 is a benign finding commonly heard in children, adolescents, and young adults,[444,445] but it is rarely present in the adult after age 40 and, when present, is often associated with a thin, asthenic body habitus.[446] This is a low-frequency sound that follows A_2 by 120 to 200 ms and occurs during the rapid filling wave of the apexcardiogram

Diastolic Filling Sounds

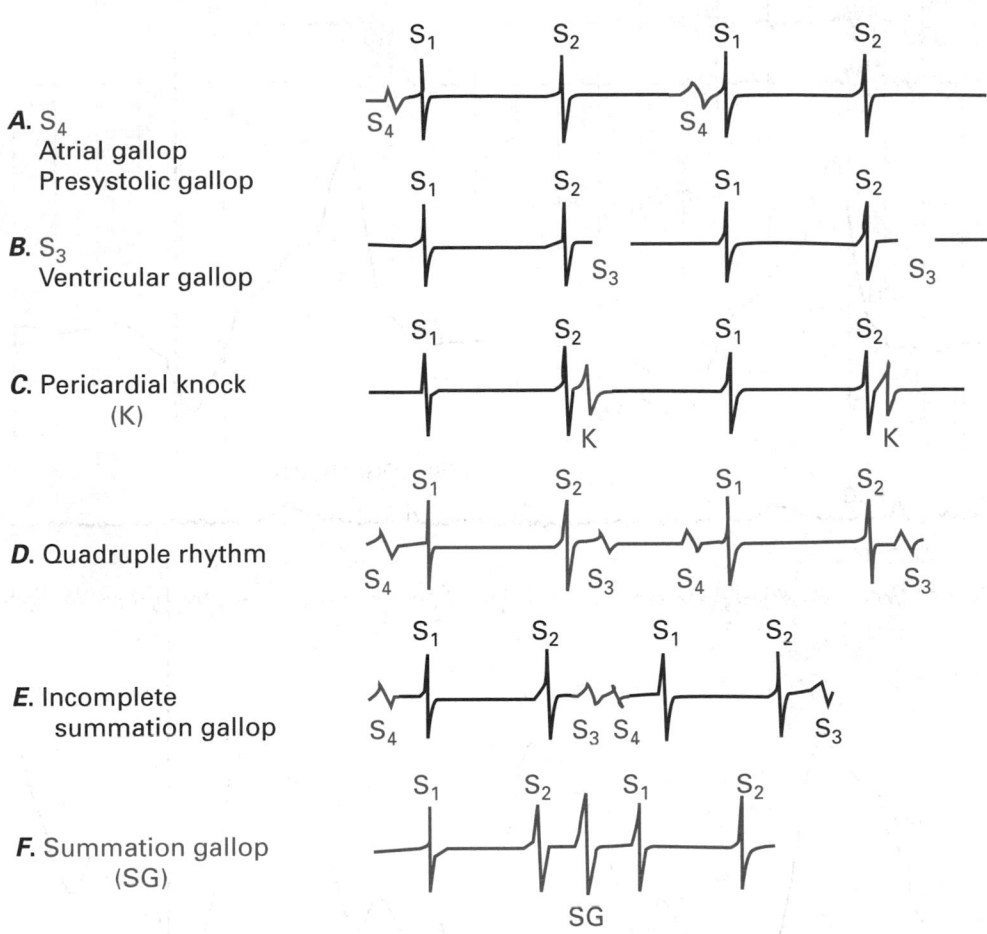

FIGURE 10-75

A. The S_4 occurs in presystole and is frequently called an *atrial*, or *presystolic, gallop. B.* The S_3 occurs during the rapid phase of ventricular filling. It is a normal finding and is commonly heard in children and young adults, disappearing with increasing age. When it is heard in the patient with cardiac disease, it is called a *pathologic* S_3, or *ventricular, gallop* and usually indicates ventricular dysfunction or AV valvular incompetence. *C.* In constrictive pericarditis, a sound in early diastole, the pericardial knock (K), is heard earlier and is louder and higher-pitched than the usual pathologic S_3.

D. A quadruple rhythm results if both S_4 and S_3 are present. *E.* At faster heart rates, the S_3 and S_4 occur in rapid succession and may give the illusion of a middiastolic rumble. *F.* When the heart rate is sufficiently fast, the two rapid phases of ventricular filling reinforce each other, and a loud summation gallop (SG) may appear; this sound may be louder than either the S_3 or S_4 alone. (From Shaver JA et al. *Examination of the Heart*: Part IV. *Auscultation*. Dallas: American Heart Association; 1990:27. Reproduced with permission from the publisher and the authors.)

(Fig. 10-76, top panel).[448] It is best heard at the apex in the left lateral position with the stethoscope bell pressed lightly against the skin and differentiated from the pathologic S_3 primarily by the "company it keeps."[449,450]

Pathologic S_3

Most agree that the pathologic S_3 is an exaggeration of the physiologic S_3, with a common mechanism of production.[310,451,452] The exact genesis of the S_3 remains controversial. Three major mechanisms of production have been proposed: the valvular theory, the ventricular theory, and the impact theory. Recent phonoechocardiographic studies have clearly shown that the valvular theory implicating diastolic tensing of the AV valves at the termination of rapid ventricular

filling is no longer tenable.[450,452,453] The most popular theory has indicated that these sounds have their origins within the left or right ventricle or their walls.[454–468] The dynamic interplay between the force of delivery of blood into the ventricle on one hand and the ability of the ventricle to accept this flow on the other hand is thought to be the important factor in the genesis of this sound. When there is appropriate interaction between these factors, the S_3 occurs when the ventricle suddenly reaches its elastic limits and abruptly decelerates the onrushing column of blood, thereby setting the entire cardiohemic system into vibration. In keeping with this theory, an S_3 may be produced by excessive rapid filling into a ventricle with normal or increased compliance, as with high-output states and mitral regurgitation, or by a normal or less than normal rate of filling into a ventricle with decreased compli-

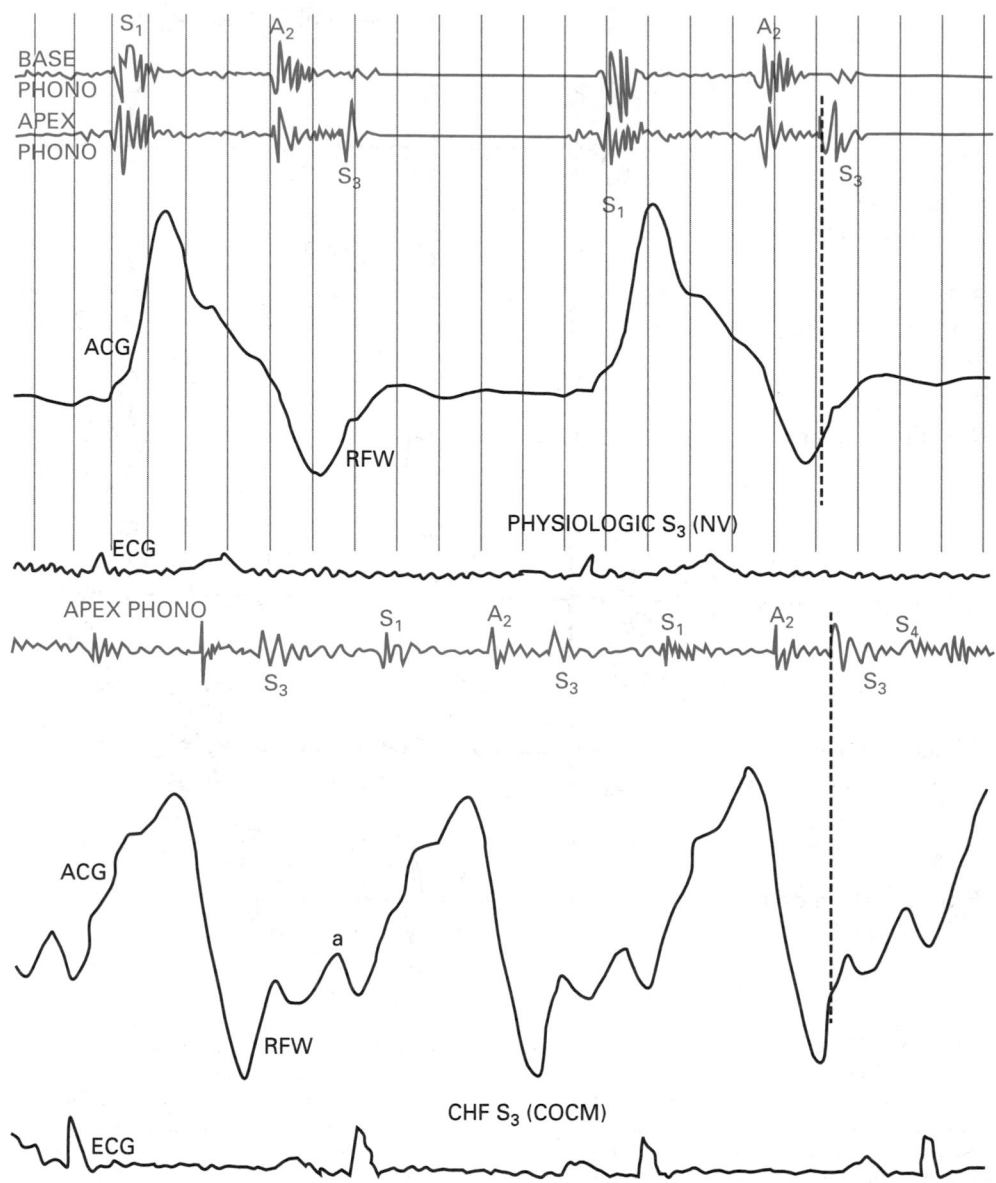

FIGURE 10-76

Top panel: A physiologic S_3 (normal variant) recorded in a 24-year-old woman without evidence of cardiovascular disease. The onset of the S_3 occurs during the rapid filling wave (RFW) of the ACG between the O and F points. The remainder of the cardiovascular examination was entirely within normal limits. *Bottom panel*: A very prominent S_3 gallop is recorded in a patient with severe congestive cardiomyopathy (COCM). On physical examination, there was a small-volume carotid pulse and marked engorgement of the neck veins with elevated venous pressure. The ACG shows a very prominent presystolic pulsation (*a*) and extremely rapid filling wave is present. The onset of the S_3 occurs during the RFW of the ACG. The first heart sound is soft. [From Shaver JA et al. Early diastolic events associated with the physiologic and pathologic S_3. *J Cardiog* 1984; 14(suppl 5):30. Reproduced with permission from the publisher and the authors.]

ance, as in patients with hypertrophic cardiomyopathy. Likewise, decreased rates of filling into overfilled ventricles with large end-systolic volumes, as seen in patients with poor left ventricular function and congestive heart failure, will produce this sound.[469,470]

Although this mechanism is likely responsible for the sound recorded within the ventricular cavity and on its epicardial surface, Reddy and associates[298,470–473] have reported convincing data that the sound heard with the stethoscope can be due to the dynamic impact of the heart with the chest wall.

Using equisensitive high-fidelity transducers with identical electronic filters, they recorded external and left ventricular sound and pressure simultaneously and consistently found that the S_3 within the left ventricle was softer or absent as compared to the external sound.[470] Furthermore, when both sounds were present, they often occurred at different times, clearly indicating that the external S_3 was not due to passive transmission of a sound originating from the left ventricle through the intervening structures to the chest wall. The force of the impact and resultant intensity of S_3 are dependent primarily on the size of the heart, the motion of the heart within the thorax, and the chest wall configuration. This theory explains the S_3 present in hyperdynamic states as well as those with an increased end-systolic volume secondary to left ventricular dysfunction. In the latter, the space between the enlarged heart and lateral chest wall is diminished, thereby facilitating a more forceful impact in early diastole. This results in an exaggerated rapid filling wave on the apexcardiogram and the prominent S_3 pathognomonic of congestive failure (Fig. 10-76, lower panel). Table 10-6 tabulates the major factors responsible for the production of the S_3 as recorded within the left ventricle and on the chest wall. In most disease states, it is likely that a complex interplay between these factors is responsible for the genesis of this sound, with impact of the heart on the chest wall playing the primary role in the production of this sound as recorded and auscultated at the chest wall.

A convenient classification of physiologic and pathologic states with an S_3 is presented in Table 10-7. Both the intensity and timing of the pathologic S_3 associated with left ventricular dysfunction are related to the patient's volume status. With diuresis, the S_3 may decrease in intensity or disappear and it tends to move away from A_2. Careful attention to these subtle changes in the S_3 is a simple and accurate way to follow the response to therapy in patients with congestive heart failure. A loud, persistent S_3 with cardiomyopathy or acute myocardial infarction is an ominous sign associated with high mortality, while prompt subsidence with therapy suggests a more favorable outlook.[457,474] Often, the pathologic S_3 is quite faint and easily overlooked; it may require intense listening in a quiet room with the bell of the stethoscope pressed lightly on the skin in the left lateral position. Very often, an abnormal S_3 is heard only intermittently rather than with each beat. Maneuvers that increase venous return (e.g., passive leg raising) are helpful in increasing the intensity of the S_3. Conversely,

TABLE 10-6
HEMODYNAMIC DETERMINANTS OF THE S_1

Ability of the ventricle to accept flow during the rapid
  phase of diastolic filling
    Rate of relaxation of the ventricle
    End-systolic or residual volume of the ventricle
    Compliance of the relaxed ventricle
    Nonobstructed atrioventricular valve
Atrial pressure head
    Atrial blood volume
    Atrial compliance
Dynamic impact of the heart with the chest wall
    Architecture of the thorax
    Cardiac size
    Cardiac motion within the thorax
    Phase of respiration
    Position of the patient

Source: From Shaver JA et al. Early diastolic events associated with the physiologic and pathologic S_3. *Am J Cardiol* 1984; 14(suppl 5):45. Reproduced with permission from the publisher and authors.

TABLE 10-7
THIRD HEART SOUND (S_3), VENTRICULAR DIASTOLIC GALLOP, PROTODIASTOLIC GALLOP, AND PERICARDIAL KNOCK

Physiological S_3—children and young adults
  Decreased prevalence with increasing age
Pathologic S_3
  Ventricular dysfunction—poor systolic function, in-
    creased end-diastolic and end-systolic
      volume, decreased ejection fraction, and high filling
        pressures
    Idiopathic dilated cardiomyopathy
    Ischemic heart disease
    Valvular heart disease
    Congenital heart disease
    Systemic and pulmonary hypertension
  Excessively rapid early diastolic ventricular filling
    Hyperkinetic states
      Anemia
      Thyrotoxicosis
      Arteriovenous fistula
    Atrioventricular valve incompetence
    Left-to-right shunts
  Restrictive myocardial or pericardial disease
    Constrictive pericarditis (pericardial knock)
    Restrictive cardiomyopathy
    Hypertrophic cardiomyopathy?

decreased venous return, as with the upright posture or tourniquets about the extremities, will decrease the intensity.[475] Left ventricular third heart sounds are heard best at the apex, while right ventricular third heart sounds are heard at the lower left sternal edge and may increase in intensity with inspiration.

In chronic aortic regurgitation, even though end-diastolic volume is increased, end-systolic volume may not be increased until left ventricular dysfunction develops. As left ventricular dysfunction develops, the ejection fraction decreases, resulting in an increased end-systolic volume, and a pathologic S_3 appears in these patients.[476] An S_3 is very common in acute aortic regurgitation and is usually followed by the middiastolic component of the Austin Flint rumble (Fig. 10-54).[434]

A pathologic S_3 resulting from excessive early diastolic filling is common in hyperkinetic states and AV valve regurgitation (Fig. 10-73, right panel) and often initiates a short flow rumble. It is often present in large left-to-right shunts due to high flow across the mitral valve with ventricular septal defect or patent ductus arteriosus and with high flow across the tricuspid valve with atrial septal defect. The presence of this sound in these conditions does not imply congestive heart failure, and such patients may maintain normal myocardial contractility for years after the S_3 is detected.[477] Pathologic third heart sounds are heard is both restrictive and hypertrophic cardiomyopathy. At times, they occur somewhat earlier after A_2 and may have durations that simulate a short diastolic rumble. In constrictive pericarditis, an early prominent sound of a somewhat higher frequency is heard—the pericardial

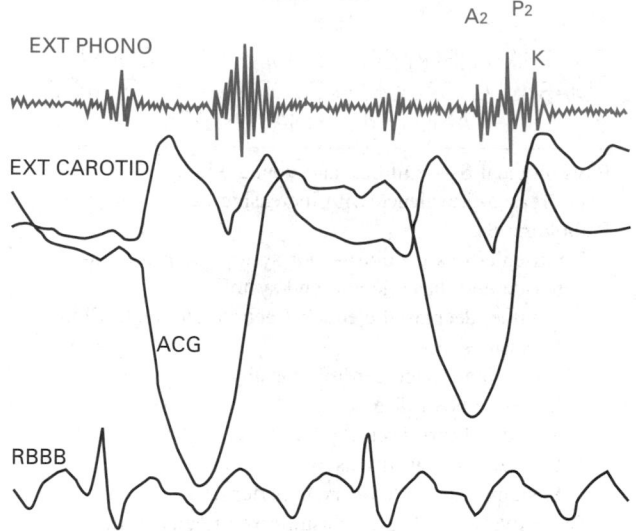

FIGURE 10-77

The ACG, external phonocardiogram, and external carotid pressure are recorded in a patient with chronic constrictive pericarditis, atrial flutter, and right bundle branch block (RBBB). Note the wide splitting of S2 and the presence of a pericardial diastolic knock (K). The ACG shows systolic retraction and a prominent diastolic wave that peaks at the time of occurrence of the knock. (From Reddy PS. Hemodynamics of constrictive pericarditis. In: Reddy PS, et al, eds. *Pericardial Disease*. New York: Raven Press; 1982:291. Reproduced in part with permission from the publisher and the authors.)

knock. The evidence to date points to the simultaneous occurrence of the pericardial knock and the termination of rapid filling of the ventricles.[478] Whether this relationship is causal or coincidental is unclear. The apex cardiac pulsation may show systolic retraction followed by an exaggerated diastolic impulse. As shown in Fig. 10-77, this results in an apexcardiogram that is a mirror image of the normal, with the knock occurring at the peak of the diastolic impulse, consistent with the impact theory of Reddy.[298] The pericardial knock usually increases in intensity with inspiration and occurs near the nadir of the y descent of the jugular venous pulse (Fig. 10-78). Atrial fibrillation is commonly present in severe constrictive pericarditis, and at times the loud early knock may be confused with the opening snap of mitral stenosis. Careful attention to the classic contour of the jugular venous pulse in this condition will usually allow the correct diagnosis at the bedside (see also Chap. 81).

THE FOURTH HEART SOUND

Precordial vibrations resulting from atrial contraction are normally neither palpable nor audible. Under pathologic conditions, forceful atrial contraction generates a low-frequency sound (S_4) just prior to S_1 (also termed the *atrial diastolic*

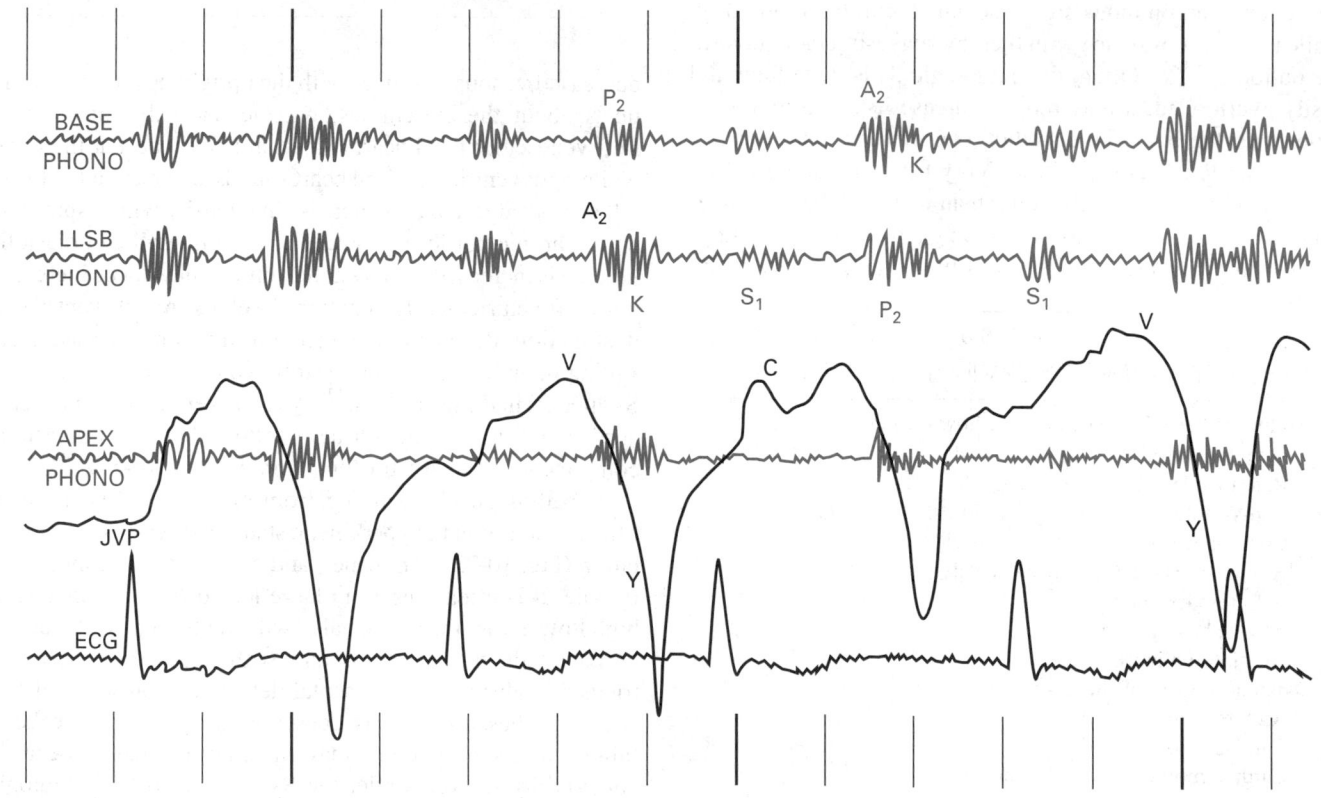

FIGURE 10-78

Phonocardiograms at the base, left sternal border, and apex are recorded with the jugular venous pulse in a patient with constrictive pericarditis and chronic atrial fibrillation. Wide splitting of S_2 is present and a relatively high frequency sound, the pericardial knock (K), occurs near the nadir of the y descent of the jugular venous pulse (JVP). Note the increase in the intensity of the knock associated with the more prominent y descent during inspiration on the first complex.

gallop or the *presystolic gallop*). Atrial contraction must be present for production of an S_4. It is absent in atrial fibrillation and in other rhythms in which atrial contraction does not precede ventricular contraction. The S_4 follows the onset of the P wave of the ECG by approximately 70 ms. Audibility of the S_4 depends not only on its intensity and frequency but also on its separation from S_1. The degree of this separation is determined primarily by the PR interval, but it is also somewhat influenced by the P-S_4 and the Q-S_1 intervals.[298,451] A loud S_1 may also mask the audibility of a preceding softer S_4. The S_4 is best heard at the apex impulse with the patient turned in the left lateral position. It varies considerably with respiration, usually being heard best during expiration. Both the intensity and timing of the S_4 are closely related to the end-diastolic volume of the ventricle. Maneuvers that increase venous return increase the audibility by increasing the intensity of the sound and by causing it to occur earlier, thereby separating it further from S_1 (Fig. 10-50).[322] Decreased venous return does the opposite. Audible fourth heart sounds are usually accompanied by a palpable presystolic apical impulse in the absence of obesity, emphysema, etc.; but occasionally palpable presystolic impulses are not audible. The S_4 generated by a forceful right atrial contraction is usually heard best at the lower left sternal border. Unlike the left-sided S_4, it tends to be accentuated with inspiration (Fig. 10-79). It is also accompanied by prominent *a* waves in the jugular venous pulse and is occasionally audible over the right jugular vein.[479]

As with the S_3, both the ventricular origin of the S_4 sound due to the abrupt deceleration of the atrial contribution to late diastolic filling[461] and the impact theory[298] have been proposed. It is likely that the former is responsible for the sounds recorded within the ventricular cavities or on their epicardial surfaces, while the latter mechanism is responsible for the S_4 auscultated at the chest wall.

Regardless of the exact mechanism of production, the presence of an S_4, particularly when associated with a palpable presystolic apical impulse, is an abnormal finding. Although considered to be a normal finding in older subjects by some investigators,[480] others feel strongly that a definite S_4 in a middle-aged or older person is unlikely to be a normal

event.[479,481] The study of Reddy and associates[446] has shed light on this controversy, showing that the absolute intensity of S_4 does not decrease with age, as does the absolute intensity of S_1, resulting in a relative increase in the intensity of S_4 compared to S_1. This relative change in intensity may well explain the increased frequency of recordable and audible fourth heart sounds in older subjects. Conditions such as obesity, emphysema, or barrel-chest deformity may hinder the clinical detection of both an S_4 and an apical presystolic impulse.

The common pathologic conditions in which S_4 is heard are listed in Table 10-8. A forceful atrial contraction into a hypertrophied noncompliant ventricle almost always produces an early and easily audible and recordable S_4. The severe left ventricular hypertrophy present in systemic hypertension, severe valvular aortic stenosis, and hypertrophic cardiomyopathy is responsible for the loud S_4 recorded in Figs. 10-48, 10-80, and 10-81. In each case, the S_4 is associated with a prominent apical presystolic impulse and is widely separated from S_1. Although Goldblatt et al.[482] have reported that an S_4 in patients with aortic stenosis correlates with a peak systolic gradient of 70 mmHg or more and a left ventricular end-diastolic pressure of 13 mmHg or greater, Caulfield and associ-

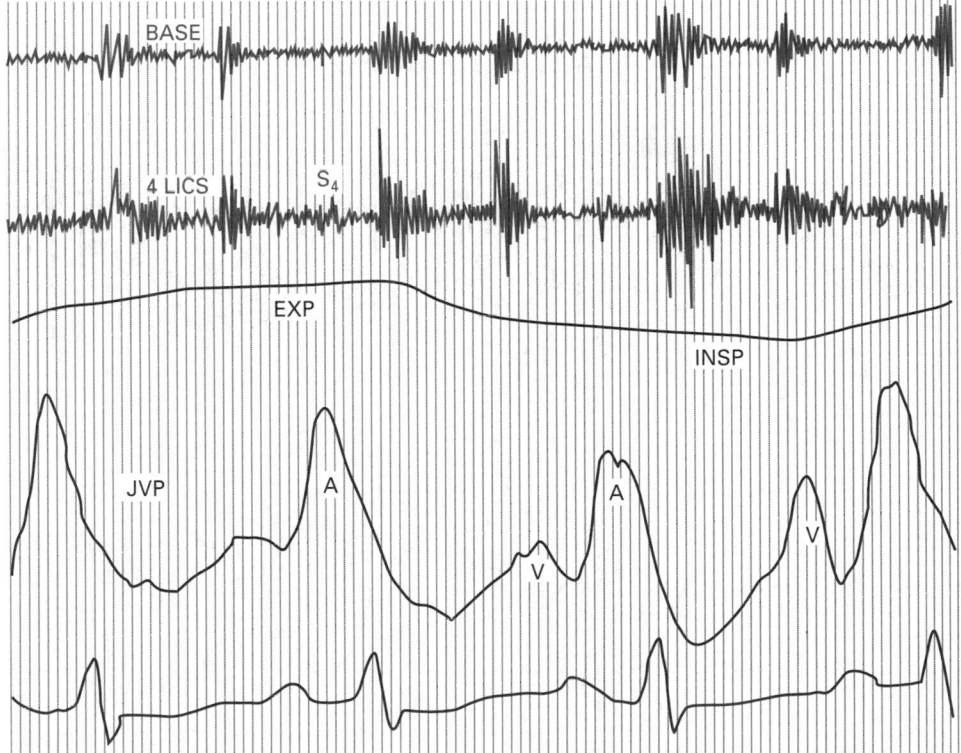

FIGURE 10-79

The external phonocardiogram and jugular venous pulse (JVP) tracing are recorded in a patient with severe pulmonary hypertension. The increased force of right atrial contraction is evident from the prominent *a* wave in the JVP. The S_4 is recorded in the fourth left intercostal space (4LICS) along the lower left sternal border. Note the increased amplitude of the S_4 with inspiration. (From Shaver JA. Current uses of phonocardiography in clinical practice. In: Rapaport E, ed. *Cardiology Update*. New York: Elsevier; 1981:352. Reproduced with permission from the publisher and the author. Copyright 1981 by Elsevier Publishing Co., Inc.)

TABLE 10-8

FOURTH HEART SOUND (S$_4$), ATRIAL DIASTOLIC
GALLOP, AND PRESYSTOLIC GALLOP

Physiologic—recordable, rarely audible
Pathologic
   Decreased ventricular compliance
      Ventricular hypertrophy
         Left or right ventricular outflow obstruction
         Systemic or pulmonary hypertension
         Hypertrophic cardiomyopathy
      Ischemic heart disease
         Angina pectoris
         Acute myocardial infarction
         Old myocardial infarction
         Ventricular aneurysm
      Idiopathic dilated cardiomyopathy
   Excessively rapid late diastolic filling secondary to
      Vigorous atrial systole
      Hyperkinetic states
         Anemia
         Thyrotoxicosis
      Arteriovenous fistula
      Acute atrioventricular valve incompetence
   Arrhythmias
      Heart block

ates[483] have modified this observation, concluding that an S$_4$ is good evidence of significant aortic stenosis only in patients under age 40.

An audible S$_4$ with a palpable presystolic impulse is common in patients with ischemic heart disease during an acute episode of angina and in the early phases of transmural myocardial infarction. Its prevalence is also increased with prior myocardial infarction; however, audible fourth heart sounds in patients with ischemic heart disease without prior infarction or hypertension are uncommon.[298] In patients with left ventricular aneurysm or idiopathic or ischemic cardiomyopathy, abnormal fourth heart sounds are commonly present and often associated with an S$_3$, producing a quadruple rhythm. If tachycardia is present or if the PR interval is prolonged, S$_3$ and S$_4$ may fuse, giving rise to a loud summation gallop (Fig. 10-75).

Quadruple rhythms are common in hyperkinetic states where the S$_3$ is due to excessively rapid early diastolic filling and the S$_4$ results from a forceful atrial contraction into a volume-loaded ventricle. With varying degrees of tachycardia, incomplete summation may occur, simulating a diastolic rumble, or complete fusion may occur, generating a loud summation gallop (Fig. 10-75). In acute incompetence of the AV valve, vigorous atrial contraction into an acutely volume-loaded ventricle can produce an S$_4$ associated with a presystolic apical impulse (Fig. 10-47).[484] At times it may be diffi-

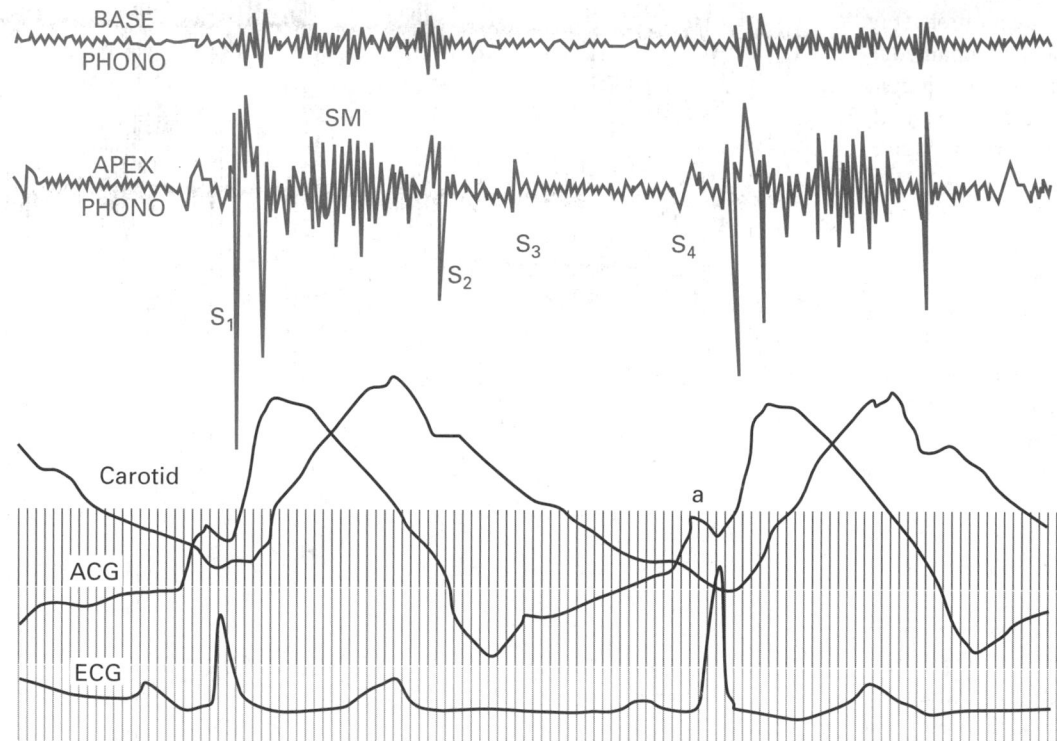

FIGURE 10-80

Atrial diastolic (ADG) and ventricular diastolic (VDG) gallops are recorded in an adult with severe calcific aortic stenosis. The ADG is associated with a prominent presystolic apical impulse (*a*) and the VDG occurs during the rapid filling wave of the ACG. The carotid pulse has a very slow rate of rise and a markedly prolonged left ventricular ejection time. The classic diamond-shaped systolic ejection murmur (SM) is present at the base and apex. Note the higher-frequency composition of the SM at the apex but preservation of the crescendo-decrescendo pattern. (From Shaver JA. Current uses of phonocardiography in clinical practice. In: Rapaport E, ed. *Cardiology Update—Reviews for Physicians*. New York: Elsevier; 1981:356. Reproduced with permission from the publisher and author. Copyright 1981 by Elsevier Publishing Co., Inc.)

cult to appreciate because of the masking effect of the loud systolic murmur. This contrasts with most patients with chronic mitral regurgitation, who do not have an S_4 but frequently have an S_3 (see also Chap. 80).

Presystolic and isolated diastolic fourth heart sounds as well as summation gallops may be heard with varying degrees of heart block. First-degree heart block facilitates audibility of the S_4 because it further separates S_4 from S_1. In 2:1 heart block, an isolated S_4 may be heard in diastole and also a presystolic S_4 may be audible because of the increase in diastolic volume. In complete heart block, S_4 may be heard randomly throughout diastole, and when it occurs simultaneously with rapid early ventricular filling, a loud summation gallop may occur (Fig. 10-82). Fourth heart sounds have also been reported in ventricular systole when atrial contraction occurred during systole in a patient with heart block. The occurrence of an S_4 when the mitral valve is closed excludes its ventricular origin due to either a pressure or volume change and is in keeping with the impact theory of S_4 sound production.[298]

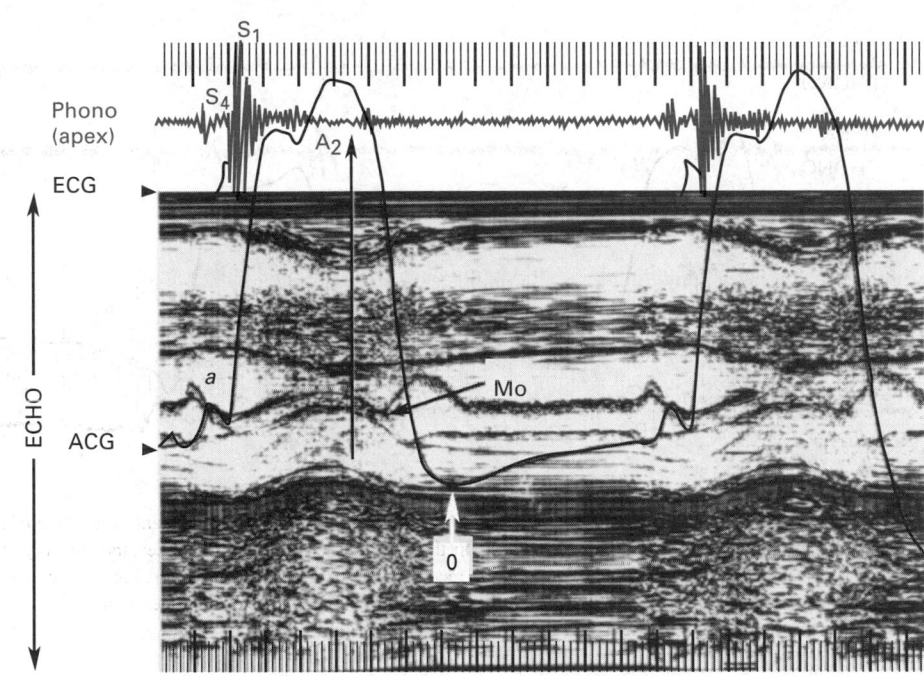

FIGURE 10-81

The apex phonocardiogram is recorded simultaneously with the ACG and mitral valve echocardiogram. A prominent S_4 is widely separated from S_1 and is coincident with the rapid upstroke of the *a* wave on the ACG. Asymmetric septal hypertrophy is present, and the left ventricular cavity is small. At cardiac catheterization, no gradient was found across the left ventricular outflow tract. [From Alvares RF et al. Isovolumic relaxation period in hypertrophic cardiomyopathy. *J Am Coll Cardiol* 1984; 3(1):75. Reproduced with permission from the American College of Cardiology and the authors.]

PROSTHETIC VALVE SOUNDS

The sounds produced by prosthetic valves are varied, depending on the type of valve, its position, and whether or not it is functioning normally. Mechanical valves produce opening and closing clicks that are easily audible and in many patients can be heard even without a stethoscope. Ball-in-cage valves such as the Starr-Edwards produce the loudest and most distinctive opening and closing clicks in any position as long as there is normal valve and ventricular function (Fig. 10-83).[485,486] In the aortic position, a crisp opening click occurs 0.06 to 0.07 s after S_1 and is coincident with maximal ball excursion as demonstrated by echocardiography.[487] The metallic ball of the Starr-Edwards valve also produces multiple early systolic clicks when the freely moving ball bounces against the cage during early systolic ejection.[486,488] These clicks occur during the harsh systolic ejection murmur. Absence or decrease in intensity of these clicks can occur with valve obstruction or left ventricular dysfunction. A decrease in the intensity of the opening and closing clicks, which normally have an intensity ratio of more than 0.5, and the absence of the opening click are also indications of valve malfunction.[486,487]

In the mitral position, a prominent opening click occurs

0.05 to 0.15 s after A_2.[489] Narrowing of this interval indicates an elevation of left atrial pressure, which may be due to either valvular obstruction or regurgitation. Interference with ball motion can also produce prolongation or significant beat-to-beat variation of this interval. A closing click is also prominent. Just as is seen with the normal S_1, there is variability in the intensity of the closing click, with the changing RR intervals of atrial fibrillation being louder with short RR intervals and softer with long. A decreased intensity with first-degree AV block also occurs due to partial atriogenic closure of the valve, thus reducing the ball excursion and therefore the click intensity. Although a decreased intensity of the valve clicks occurs with valve malfunction, the presence of normal ball motion on an echocardiogram suggests that a nonvalvular cause such as severe left ventricular dysfunction is responsible for the decreased intensity.[485]

The auscultatory findings of disk valve prostheses vary, depending upon the type of disk valve. Central occluder valves such as the Beall valve, which was used predominantly in the mitral and tricuspid positions, produce distinct, audible opening and closing sounds.[486,487] The more commonly used tilting-disk valves do not ordinarily produce audible opening sounds in either the aortic or mitral position, although a soft opening sound can usually be demonstrated by phonocardiography (Fig. 10-84). Phonoechocardiography has shown that these sounds occur at the onset rather than at the maximal opening of the disk.[486,490] In the mitral position, the A_2-OS

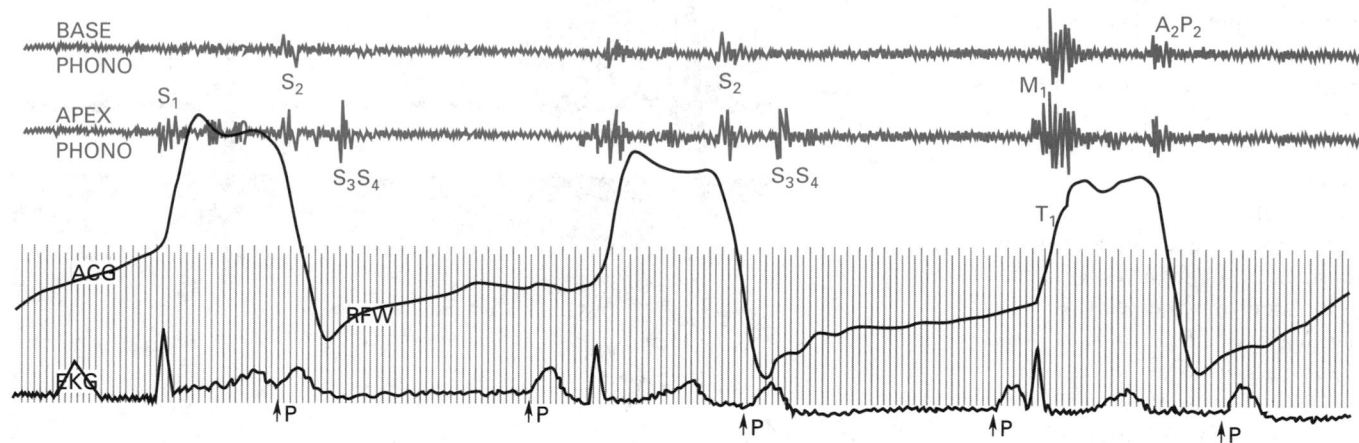

FIGURE 10-82

Base and apex phonocardiograms are recorded with the ACG in a patient having complete heart block with AV dissociation. In the first and second complexes a prominent summation gallop (S_3S_4) is recorded due to atrial contraction occurring during the rapid filling phase of the left ventricle. In the third complex, atrial contraction occurs later, and only minimal vibrations are present at the time of the rapid filling wave of the ACG. In the first two complexes, the intensity of S_1 is soft, while in the third complex in the setting of a short PR interval, there is a marked increase in the mitral and tricuspic components of S_1.

interval is 0.05 and 0.09 s; abbreviation of this interval occurs with valvular regurgitation or obstruction, both of which elevate the left atrial pressure. The aortic opening click usually follows S_1 by 0.04 s. The closing sounds of disk valves are distinct and easily heard in both aortic and mitral positions.

Left ventricular dysfunction, first-degree AV block, or other arrhythmia that causes the disk to move to a partially closed position prior to the onset of ventricular contraction will result in a softer sound. This finding must be distinguished from malfunction caused by either fibrosis or thrombus disturbing

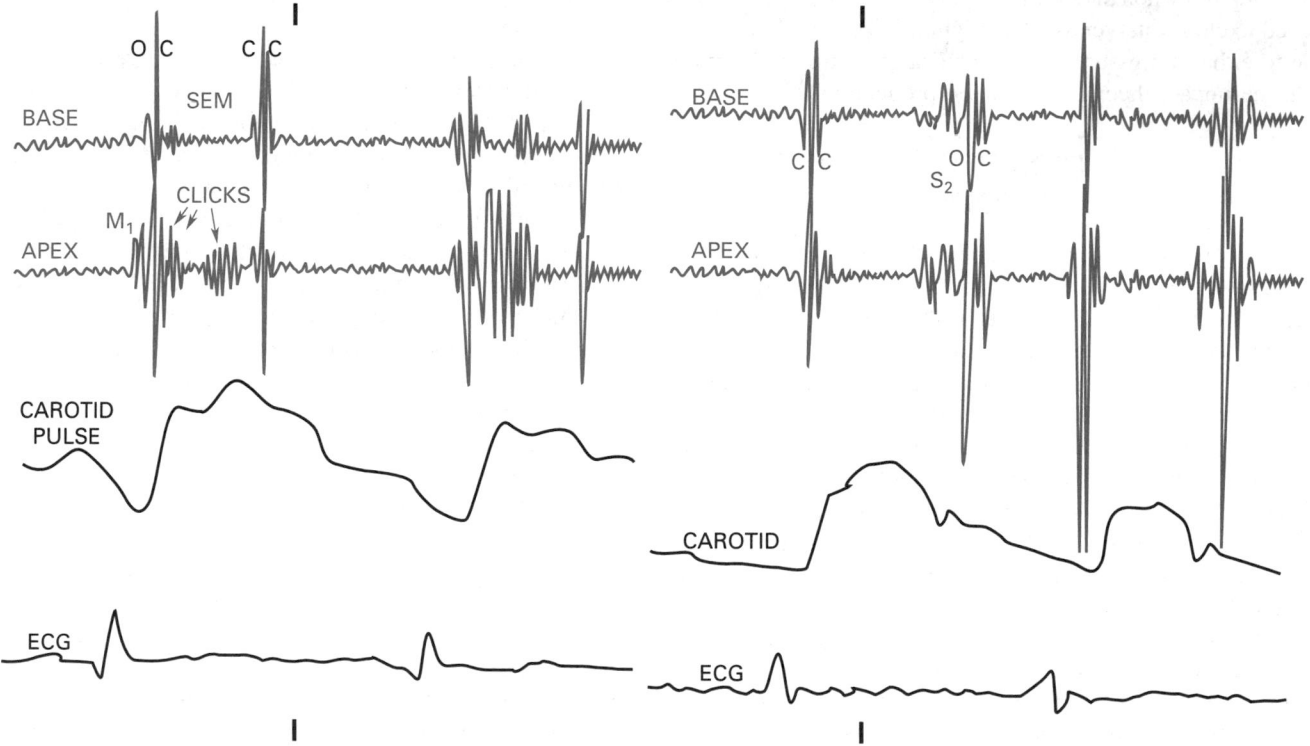

FIGURE 10-83

Left panel: Phonocardiogram of a patient with a Starr-Edwards aortic valve. A loud aortic closing click (CC) is present. A slightly softer aortic opening click (OC) follows a much softer S_1 ($S_1 - OC = 55$ ms). A harsh ejection murmur with overlying systolic clicks is recorded (*arrows*). *Right panel*: Phonocardiogram of a patient with a Starr-Edwards mitral valve. There is a very loud mitral closing click (CC). A prominent opening click (OC) occurs 65 ms after aortic closure (A_2). A softer sound follows the OC and is due to the ball bouncing against the cage.

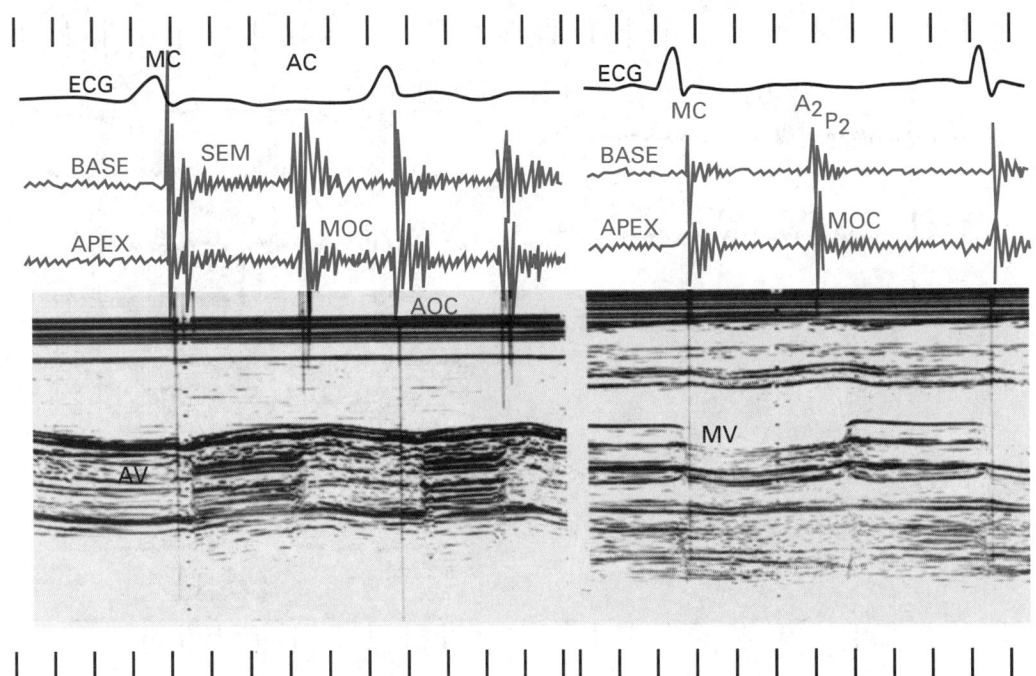

FIGURE 10-84

Left panel: Phonoechocardiogram of a patient with tilting-disk (Bjork-Shiley) aortic and mitral valves. There is a prominent mitral closing (MC) and opening click (MOC) (A₂ − MOC = 55 to 110 ms). The click interval varies with the RR cycle length. Unlike the case with most tilting-disk valves, a prominent aortic opening click (AOC) was audible and is recorded. The

aortic closing clock (AD) is also loud. *Right panel*: Phonocardiogram of a patient with tilting-disk (Hall-Kaster) mitral valve showing the more usual auscultatory findings of a loud closure sound (MC) and a very soft opening sound that was not audible. (A₂ − MOC = 65 ms). The OC occurs at the onset of disk motion.

the disk motion. Auscultation of the bileaflet St. Jude valve is similar to that of the tilting-disk valve.[491]

The sounds produced by tissue prosthetic valves are more like normal heart sounds than the sounds from a mechanical valve (Fig. 10-85).[186,487] In the aortic position, an opening sound is usually not audible. In the mitral position, an opening sound is audible in about 50 percent of patients at an interval of 0.07 to 0.11 s after A₂.

EXTRACARDIAC SOUNDS

Pacemaker Sounds

High-frequency sounds of brief duration are occasionally present in patients with transvenous pacemakers located in the right ventricular apex. They are extracardiac in origin, occurring nearly synchronously (within 6 to 10 ms) with the pacemaker spike, and are due to stimulation of intercostal nerves adjacent to endocardial electrodes.[492] This stimulus results in contraction of the intercostal muscles, and frequently twitching of the muscle can be observed. The presence of these sounds should always suggest possible myocardial perforation by the endocardial lead, although this is not always present. Stimulation of the pectoral muscles as well as diaphragmatic stimulation has also been reported to produce

these extracardiac sounds. They have also been observed in patients having transthoracically placed epicardial leads.

Pericardial Friction Rub

Inflammation of the pericardial sac with or without fluid may cause a pericardial friction rub. These friction sounds are very high-pitched, leathery, and scratchy in nature. They seem close to the ear and are ausculted best with the patient leaning forward or in the knee-chest position, holding his or her breath after forced expiration. The pericardial rub may have three components during the intervals of the cardiac cycle when the heart has the greatest excursions within the pericardial sac—at the time of atrial systole, at the time of ventricular contraction, and during rapid early diastolic filling. The usual friction rub occurs during the first two intervals, although three-component rubs may be heard. Triple-component friction rubs are common in uremic pericarditis, particularly when the underlying cardiac disease is hypertension. In this situation, the heart is hyperkinetic due to both pressure and volume overload as well as to the anemia associated with renal failure. Pericardial friction rubs are very common in the acute phase of transmural myocardial infarction, although they often last for only a few hours. There is a common misconception that friction rubs are not heard when there is a large amount of fluid in the pericardial sac; this is not the case, because usually some portions of the visceral and parietal pericardial surfaces

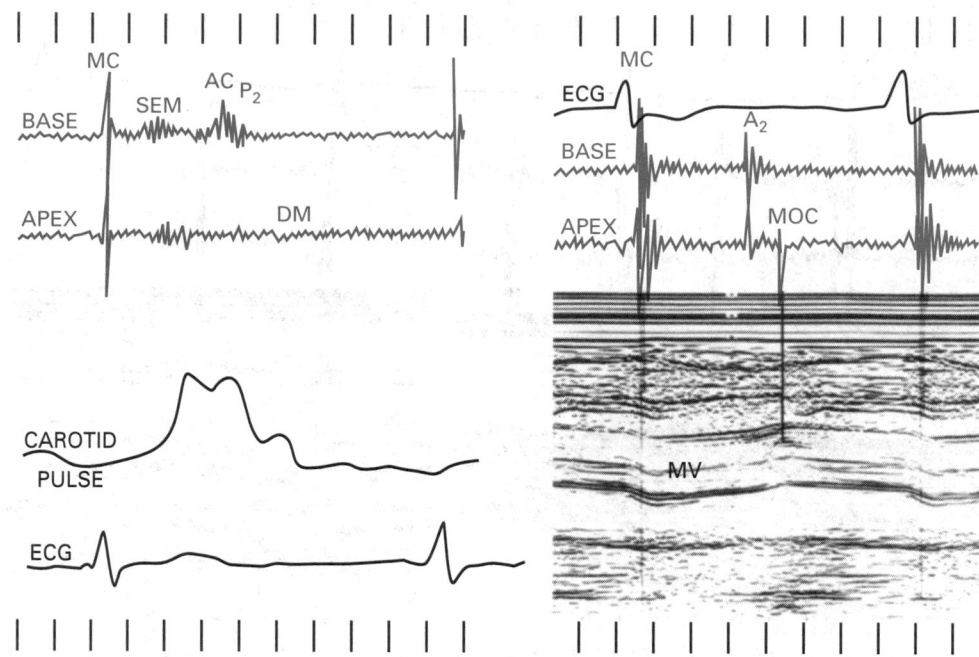

FIGURE 10-85

Left panel: Phonocardiogram of a patient with heterograft aortic and mitral valves. There is no distinct aortic or mitral opening click. Closing clicks of both valves are prominent. (AD = aortic closure; MC = mitral closure). There is a mitral middiastolic rumble at the apex (DM) and a systolic ejection murmur (SEM); both are frequently found with heterograft valves.

Right panel: Phonoechocardiogram of a patient with the more typical auscultatory findings of a heterograft mitral valve. There is a prominent mitral closing sound (MC). A softer but still audible mitral opening sound (MOC) occurs just after maximum excursion of the valve leaflets. A₂ − MOC = 90 ms. No diastolic rumble was recorded.

are in contact in spite of the large amount of fluid[292] (see also Chap. 81).

Occasionally, certain midsystolic (ejection) murmurs have a scratchy character and may be misinterpreted as friction rubs. This is particularly true of the short, scratchy pulmonic ejection murmur heard in hyperthyroidism (Means-Lerman sign).[493] Such scratchy sounds should not be considered to be a friction rub unless both systolic and diastolic components are heard.

Mediastinal Crunch: Hamman's Sign

When air is present in the mediastinum, a series of scratchy sounds (Hamman's sign[494]) may occur, related indirectly to both heartbeat and respiratory excursion. These sounds occur most frequently during ventricular systole and in a random fashion. The diagnosis of mediastinal emphysema may be confirmed by crepitation in the neck secondary to subcutaneous air. Often, the patient is aware of the sound and may volunteer what position or phase of respiration will accentuate it. These crunching sounds due to air in the mediastinum are common following cardiac surgery.

HEART
MURMURS

A cardiac murmur is defined as a relatively prolonged series of auditory vibrations of varying intensity (loudness), frequency

(pitch), quality, configuration, and duration.[495] Although the exact physical principles that govern the production of murmurs have been debated for years, most authorities now agree that turbulence is the prime factor responsible for most murmurs.[310,496] Turbulence arises when blood velocity becomes critically high due to high flow, flow through an irregular or narrow area, or a combination of both. Leatham has attributed the production of murmurs to three main factors[497]: (1) high flow rate through normal or abnormal orifices, (2) forward flow through a constricted or irregular orifice or into a dilated vessel or chamber, and (3) backward or regurgitant flow through an incompetent valve, septal defect, or patent ductus arteriosus. Frequently, a combination of these factors is operative.

While the intensity of a systolic murmur is not always proportional to the hemodynamic disturbance, grading the loudness of a murmur from 1 to 6 as described by Freeman and Levine[498] is generally utilized. A grade 1 murmur is so faint that it can be heard only with special effort. A grade 2 murmur is faint but can be easily heard. A grade 3 murmur is moderately loud; a grade 4 murmur is very loud; and a grade 5 murmur is extremely loud and can be heard if only the edge of the stethoscope is in contact with the skin but cannot be heard if the stethoscope is removed from the skin. A grade 6 murmur is exceptionally loud and can be heard with the stethoscope just removed from contact with the chest. Experience has shown that systolic murmurs of grade 3 or more in intensity are usually hemodynamically significant.

Systolic thrills are usually associated with murmurs of grade 4 or louder. As pointed out by Leatham, the intensity of the murmur varies directly with the velocity of blood flow across the area of murmur production. The velocity, in turn, is directly related to the pressure head that drives the blood across the murmur-producing area. For example, high velocity of flow through a small ventricular septal defect produces a loud murmur, whereas a large flow at low velocity through an atrial septal defect produces no murmur. The intensity of a murmur as asculted at the chest wall is also determined by the transmission characteristics of the tissues intervening between the source of the murmur and the stethoscope. Obesity, emphysema, and the presence of significant pericardial or pleural effusion will decrease the intensity of a murmur, while a thin, asthenic body habitus will often accentuate it.

McKusick[499] has shown that the frequency of a murmur bears a direct relationship to the velocity of blood flow, as does the intensity of the murmur. The low-velocity flow resulting from a small pressure head across a stenotic mitral valve produces a low-pitched rumbling murmur, while the large diastolic pressure gradient across an incompetent aortic valve causes a high-pitched murmur. A recent study has further demonstrated that the dominant frequencies contained in heart murmurs due to stenotic lesions are directly related to the instantaneous jet velocities distal to the associated obstruction.[500] Occasionally, the frequency composition of the same systolic murmur may vary, depending on the area asculted. For example, the systolic murmur of aortic stenosis frequently sounds higher-pitched at the apex than at the base.[501] Some murmurs—such as the "cooing dove" regurgitant murmur of a ruptured or retroverted aortic cusp,[502] the systolic "whoop" or "honk" of mitral valve prolapse,[503] or the high-pitched systolic murmur of a degenerated bioprosthetic valve[504]—have a very distinctive musical quality. Recent data support the theory that such musical murmurs result from a uniform periodic vibration of a cardiac structure such as a valve leaflet or chordae tendineae that begins to resonate in response to turbulent energy.[504–506]

In addition to the intensity and frequency of murmurs, their timing should also be described. There is seldom any difficulty distinguishing between systole and diastole, since systole is considerably shorter at normal heart rates. At rapid heart rates, however, the durations of these two intervals approach each other. Under such circumstances, the examiner can usually time the murmur by simultaneous palpation of the lower right carotid artery or can rely on the fact that the second heart sound (S_2) is usually the louder sound at the base. Once S_2 is identified, murmurs can be properly located in the cardiac cycle as systolic or diastolic. If the murmur in question is at the apex, the proper timing can be ensured by the "inching" technique popularized by Harvey and Levine.[295] This consists of slowly moving the stethoscope down from the base to the apex while repeatedly fixing the cardiac cycle in mind, using S_2 as a reference point. With sinus tachycardia, carotid sinus pressure may temporarily slow the rate and make it possible to differentiate systole from diastole. If extra systoles are

occurring and one listens carefully to identify the beat that follows a compensatory pause, the first subsequent sound will be the first heart sound (S_1). Continuous murmurs are heard throughout the cardiac cycle in systole and diastole and usually have their peak intensity around S_2.

The location and radiation of a murmur is multifactorially determined by its site of origin, intensity, and direction of blood flow as well as by the physical characteristics of the chest.[507] The duration and time intensity contour (murmur "envelope") of a specific murmur is intimately related to the instantaneous pattern of blood flow velocity causing the murmur.

SYSTOLIC MURMURS

Systolic murmurs may be classified into two basic categories—ejection murmurs and regurgitant murmurs (Fig. 10-86). This simple classification, popularized by Leatham,[497] is attractive because it has a physiologic as well as a descriptive basis. Systolic "ejection" murmurs are due to forward

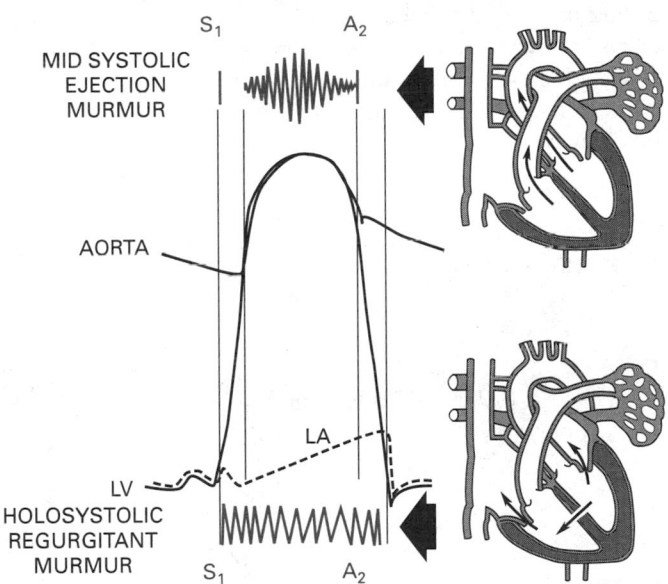

FIGURE 10-86

Midsystolic ejection murmurs are caused by forward flow across the left or right ventricular outflow tract, whereas pansystolic regurgitant murmurs are caused by retrograde flow from a high-pressure cardiac chamber to a low-pressure one. *Left panel*: diagrammatic representation of the midsystolic ejection murmur and the pansystolic regurgitant murmur, as related to left ventricular (LV), aortic, and left atrial (LA) pressures. The systolic ejection murmur occurs during the period of LV ejection; the onset of the murmur is separated from S_1 by the period of isovolumic contraction and the crescendo-decrescendo murmur terminates before A_2. The pansystolic regurgitant murmur begins with, or may replace, S_1, and the murmur continues up to and through A_2 as left ventricular pressure exceeds left atrial pressure during the period of isovolumic relaxation. The murmur has a plateau configuration and varies little with respiration. *Right panel*: flow diagram. (Left panel reproduced from Reddy PS, Shaver JA, Leonard JJ. Cardiac systolic murmurs: Pathophysiology and differential diagnosis. *Prog Cardiovasc Dis* 1971; 14:19. Entire figure reproduced with permission from Shaver JA. Systolic murmurs. *Heart Dis Stroke* 1993; 2:10.)

flow across the left or right ventricular outflow tract, while systolic "regurgitant" murmurs are due to retrograde flow from a high-pressure cardiac chamber to a low-pressure chamber.[508]

Systolic Ejection Murmurs

The systolic "ejection" murmur begins shortly after the pressure in the left or right ventricle exceeds the aortic or pulmonic diastolic pressure sufficiently to open the aortic or pulmonic valve. As a result, there is a delay between the S_1, which occurs shortly after AV pressure crossover, and the beginning of the murmur (Fig. 10-86). The murmur then waxes and wanes in a crescendo-decrescendo fashion often described as "diamond-shaped" or "spindle-shaped" in configuration. The murmur ends before the semilunar valve closure of the side from which it originates. The contour of the time-intensity pattern or "envelope" of the murmur corresponds to the contour of the flow velocity, and the murmur is heard when the sound produced during the peak turbulence exceeds the audible threshold.[509] Thus, not only is the overall intensity of the murmur proportional to the rate of ventricular ejection, but also its shape depends on the instantaneous flow velocity during the period of ejection. As can be seen in Fig. 10-87, during normal left ventricular ejection, a disproportionately large volume flow occurs in early systole. If velocity of flow exceeds the murmur threshold, a short midsystolic or "ejection" murmur results, and its envelope corresponds to the

flow velocity pattern. If the stroke volume of the ventricle is increased, this pattern of ejection persists in an exaggerated fashion; the resultant murmur has a tendency to peak early in systole and fade out about halfway through the ejection phase. Such murmurs have been referred to as "kite-shaped," and are common in high-output states or conditions such as aortic regurgitation or heart block, where stroke volume is high.

The flow characteristics of normal right ventricular ejection are somewhat different. Early ejection rates are not nearly as high and the flow curve peaks somewhat later, having a more rounded contour.[510] This flow pattern may well explain some of the long systolic ejection murmurs heard in atrial septal defects and the straight-back syndrome, where only minimal gradients are found across the right ventricular outflow tract.[511] With true valvular obstruction, rapid early ejection is no longer possible; the aortic flow velocity patterns becomes rounded, resulting in the more symmetric murmur of aortic stenosis. In such cases, the instantaneous flow pattern is determined by the instantaneous pressure head with the resultant high correlation between the contour of the pressure gradient and the murmur envelope (Fig. 10-88). If left or right ventricular obstruction is severe, systole is prolonged and closure sound of the semilunar valve is delayed. The murmur, however, always stops before the closure sound of the side from which it originates, although it may envelop the closure sound of the opposite side of the circulation. Because of the high correlation between the shape of the murmur and its underlying flow velocity characteristics, careful attention must be given during auscultation to the shape and duration of the murmur as well as to its intensity.

The intensity of ejection murmurs closely parallels changes in cardiac output. Any condition that increases forward flow—such as exercise, anxiety, fever, or increased stroke volume associated with the long diastolic filling period after a premature beat—increases the intensity of the murmur. Likewise, conditions that decrease cardiac output—congestive heart failure, beta blockade, or other negative inotropic agents—will decrease the intensity of the ejection murmur. This intimate relationship to flow, particularly with beat-to-beat variations, will usually allow the clinician to differentiate a systolic ejection murmur from a systolic regurgitant murmur. Furthermore, the definitive diagnosis

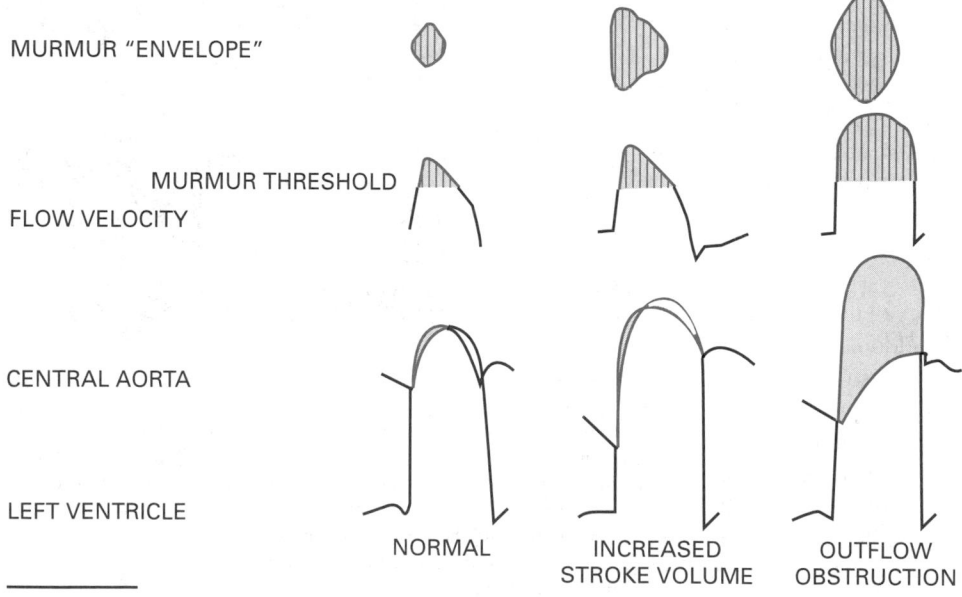

MURMUR "ENVELOPE"

MURMUR THRESHOLD
FLOW VELOCITY

CENTRAL AORTA

LEFT VENTRICLE

NORMAL   INCREASED   OUTFLOW
                STROKE VOLUME   OBSTRUCTION

FIGURE 10-87

The simultaneous time-intensity course of the murmur "envelope," aortic flow velocity, and left ventricular (LV) and central aortic pressure. During normal LV ejection (*left panel*), peak flow velocity is early, with two-thirds of the ventricular volume ejected during the first half of systole. The murmur threshold may be exceeded during the early peak flow and the corresponding murmur envelope inscribed. The center panel shows exaggeration of the normal pattern of LV ejection with a high stroke volume, as in high-output states. With critical aortic stenosis (*right panel*), rapid early ejection is no longer possible; the flow velocity is increased and the contour becomes rounded and prolonged, producing the typical diamond-shaped murmur of aortic stenosis. (Modified from Reddy PS et al. Cardiac systolic murmurs: Pathophysiology and differential diagnosis. *Prog Cardiovasc Dis* 1971; 14:4. Reproduced with permission from the publisher and the authors.)

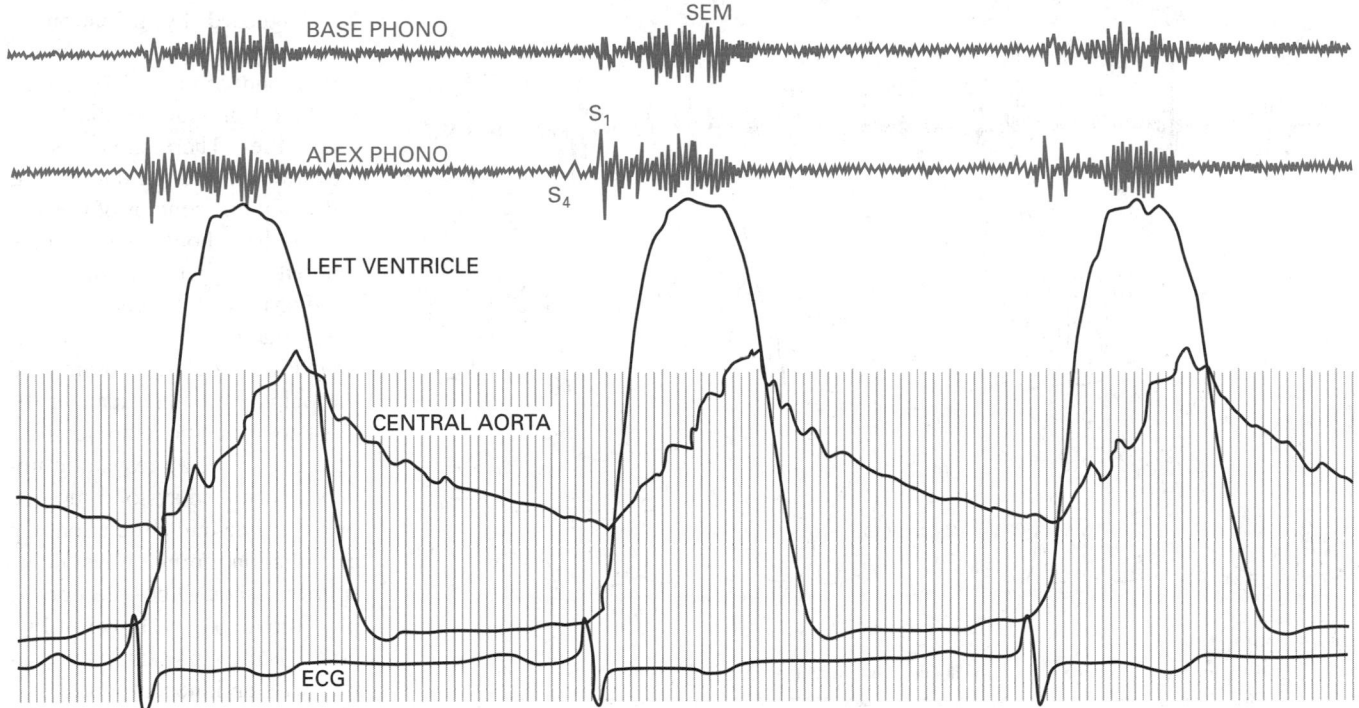

FIGURE 10-88

Base and apex phonocardiograms are recorded simultaneously with left ventricular (LV) and central aortic pressures in a patient with severe calcific aortic stenosis. A valvular ejection sound is absent, and A_2 is not recorded. The murmur is crescendo-decrescendo, and its contour correlates well with the instantaneous pressure gradient. Note that the murmur has a much higher frequency content on the apex phonocardiogram. A soft S_4 gallop is also recorded at the apex.

of the systolic murmur can often be made during auscultation by careful attention to the response of the murmur to various bedside maneuvers that alter the flow and loading conditions of the heart.[512] These maneuvers include respiration, the strain and release phases of the Valsalva maneuver, standing, squatting, passive leg elevation, isometric hand-grip exercise, inhalation of amyl nitrite, and transient arterial occlusion.

INNOCENT MURMURS

Innocent murmurs are always systolic ejection in nature and occur without evidence of physiologic or structural abnormalities in the cardiovascular system when peak flow velocity in early systole exceeds the murmur threshold.[513] These murmurs are almost always less than grade 3 in intensity and vary considerably from examination to examination and with body position and level of physical activity. They are not associated with a thrill or with radiation to the carotid arteries or axillae. They may arise from flow across either the normal left or right ventricular outflow tract and always end well before semilunar valve closure.

Innocent murmurs are found in approximately 30 to 50 percent of all children. In young children, especially ages 3 to 8, the vibratory systolic (Still's) murmur is common (Fig. 10-89). It has a very distinctive quality described as "groaning," "croaking," "buzzing," or "twanging." It is heard best along the left sternal border at the third or fourth interspace

and disappears by puberty. Considerable controversy exists as to the origin of the vibratory systolic murmur. Some have suggested that left ventricular bands, which cross the left ventricular outflow tract, could be responsible for the production of turbulence resulting in the vibratory murmur. They found left ventricular bands of this type in 76 percent of patients with the Still's murmur.[515] This finding was not confirmed in another study using Doppler and two-dimensional echocardiography,[516] and it was suggested that the origin of the Still's murmur was related to the finding of a small ascending aortic diameter associated with a concomitant high aortic blood flow velocity. Similar findings were recently reported by Van Oort et al.[517] Regardless of the exact cause, most authorities agree that this murmur originates from flow in the left ventricular outflow tract.

Innocent systolic ejection murmurs have also been attributed to flow in the normal right ventricular outflow tract and have been termed *innocent pulmonic systolic murmurs* because the site of their maximal intensity is ausculted best in the pulmonary area at the second left interspace with radiation along the left sternal border. These are low to medium in pitch, with a blowing quality, and are common in children, adolescents, and young adults. Stein et al.,[518] who used high-fidelity catheter-tipped micromanometers to record intracardiac sound and pressure in the aorta and pulmonary artery in adults with normal valves, invariably recorded the ejection murmur in the region of the aortic valve. They concluded that

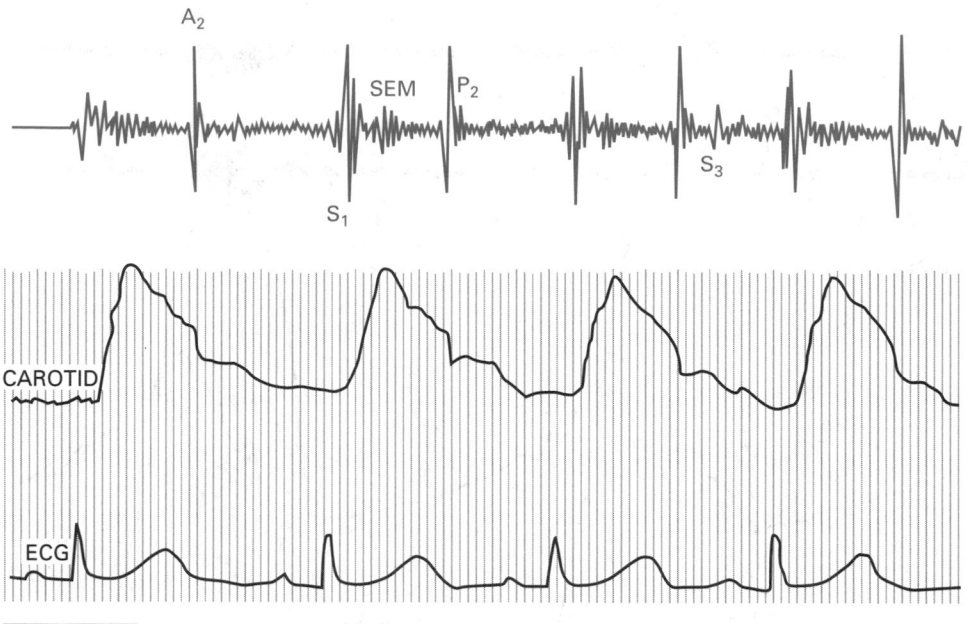

FIGURE 10-89

Typical Still's murmur as recorded in a 4-year-old boy. Note the vibratory quality of the systolic ejection murmur (SEM). The murmur begins well after S_1, peaks before midsystole, and ends well before A_2. A physiologic third heart sound (S_3) is present, and the carotic arterial pressure tracing is normal. (From Shaver JA. Innocent murmurs. *Hosp Med*, April 1978, p 15. © 1978. Reproduced with permission from Hospital Publications, Inc., and the author.)

these murmurs, in spite of their precordial location, were aortic in origin.

In adults over age 50, innocent murmurs due to flow in the left ventricular outflow tract are often heard and may be of a higher frequency, with a musical quality, and frequently loudest at the apex. They may be associated with a tortuous, dilated sclerotic aortic root, often in the setting of systolic hypertension. Mild sclerosis of the aortic valve may also be present.

The preceding descriptive breakdown of innocent murmurs is based primarily on age, precordial location, and distinctive acoustic qualities. Since all of these murmurs are equally innocent and because there is considerable overlap among them in respect to origin, transmission, and frequency composition, they are best characterized as systolic ejection murmurs without associated abnormalities of the cardiovascular system. Since both innocent and pathologic ejection murmurs have the same mechanism of production, it is not the nature of the murmur itself that allows differential diagnosis but rather the associated cardiac findings. Thus, it is "the company the murmur keeps" that affords the differential diagnosis of the pathologic systolic ejection murmur from the innocent murmur (Fig. 10-90).[519]

For a murmur to be considered innocent, the examination of the cardiovascular system must disclose no abnormalities. Blood pressure and contour of the carotid, femoral, and brachial arteries should always be evaluated carefully. For example, a seemingly innocent murmur in the setting of hypertension, particularly in a younger patient, should always suggest the diagnosis of coarctation of the aorta, which can readily

be diagnosed by palpation of weak or nearly absent femoral pulses and confirmed by taking the blood pressure in the lower extremities. There should be no elevation of the jugular venous pulse, and the contour of the jugular pulse should be normal, without exaggeration of either the *a* or *v* wave. Evidence of cardiac enlargement on physical examination should be absent, and the palpation of the apex in the left lateral position should show no evidence of a presystolic impulse, sustained systolic motion, or hyperdynamic circulation. On auscultation, normal physiologic splitting should be present. A physiologic S_3, as shown in Fig. 10-89, is often present in association with an innocent murmur in children and young adults but should not be heard after age 30. An S_4 is rarely heard in normal children and adults (younger than 50 years) and should always be considered to be abnormal when associated with a presystolic impulse. Systolic ejection sounds of valvular origin as well as midsystolic nonejection sounds should be absent, as they point to minor abnormalities of the semilunar and AV valves, respectively (Fig. 10-90). The remainder of the physical examination should show no evidence of a cardiac cause of pulmonary or systemic congestion. In almost all patients with innocent murmurs, the ECG and the cardiac silhouette on chest x-ray should be normal.

The supraclavicular arterial murmur or bruit is a common finding in normal individuals, particularly children and adolescents.[520] These murmurs are maximal in intensity above the clavicles and tend to be louder on the right, although they are often heard bilaterally. The bruit begins shortly after S_1, is diamond-shaped, and is of brief duration, usually occupying less than half of systole. Although the exact mechanism of production is unknown, it is related to peak flow velocity near the origin of the normal subclavian, innominate, or carotid artery. When particularly prominent, this murmur may transmit to the basal region of the heart and simulate a systolic ejection murmur. However, unlike the cardiac ejection murmur, the supraclavicular murmur is always louder above the clavicles than below them. Complete compression of the subclavian artery may cause the murmur to disappear completely, while partial compression may occasionally intensify it. Hyperextension of the shoulders is a simple bedside maneuver that may decrease the intensity of the murmur and cause it to disappear completely.[521] In the adult, the supraclavicular murmur must be distinguished from the murmur of true organic carotid obstruction, this latter murmur being longer, often extending through S_2, and frequently associated with a history suggestive of transient ischemic attacks.

FUNCTIONAL SYSTOLIC EJECTION MURMURS

Systolic ejection murmurs produced by high cardiac output states are functional and flow-related but are excluded from the category of innocent murmurs because of their associated altered physiologic state.[513] These include the cardiac murmurs of thyrotoxicosis, pregnancy, anemia, fever, exercise, and peripheral arteriovenous fistula, which are best interpreted in light of the total presentation of the patient (Fig. 10-90).[522] Although these murmurs are often grade 3 and occasionally grade 4 in intensity, they always end well before S_2 and are only rarely confused with obstruction of the left or right ventricular outflow tract. The large stroke volume associated with high-degree heart block often produces a functional systolic murmur; when found in the setting of complete heart block, beat-to-beat variations in the intensity of the murmur are present due to the random contribution of atrial systole to left ventricular filling.

The functional systolic murmur in patients with a hemodynamically significant atrial septal defect is due to the increased flow in the right ventricular outflow tract secondary to the left-to-right shunt at the atrial level. It is easily diagnosed at the bedside "by the company it keeps" (Fig. 10-68). The hallmark of this condition is wide, fixed splitting of S_2.[440] When the shunt is large (more than 2.5:1), a hyperdynamic parasternal impulse is usually present, and a diastolic flow rumble is often heard in the tricuspid area. In addition, the tricuspid closure is loud, and prominent a and v waves are seen in the jugular venous pulse. An important condition to be differentiated from an atrial septal defect is narrowing of the anterior-posterior diameter of the bony thorax. Prominent systolic murmurs—often grade 3 or 4—are heard in patients having the "straight-back" syndrome and/or pectus excavatum.[523] Audible expiratory splitting is frequently present and, coupled with a prominent pulmonary artery on the chest x-ray (secondary to the narrow anterior-posterior diameter), can lead to additional unnecessary procedures to rule out an atrial septal defect. Careful attention at the bedside to the physical examination of the spine, thoracic cage, and sternum should be part of the routine evaluation of any patient with a murmur. Often, confirmation of the thoracic abnormality with a lateral chest film is all that is necessary for definitive evaluation. Similar systolic murmurs from the right ventricular outflow tract are also present in patients having significant left-to-right shunting at the ventricular level. In this situation, one may be able to hear both the holosystolic murmur of the

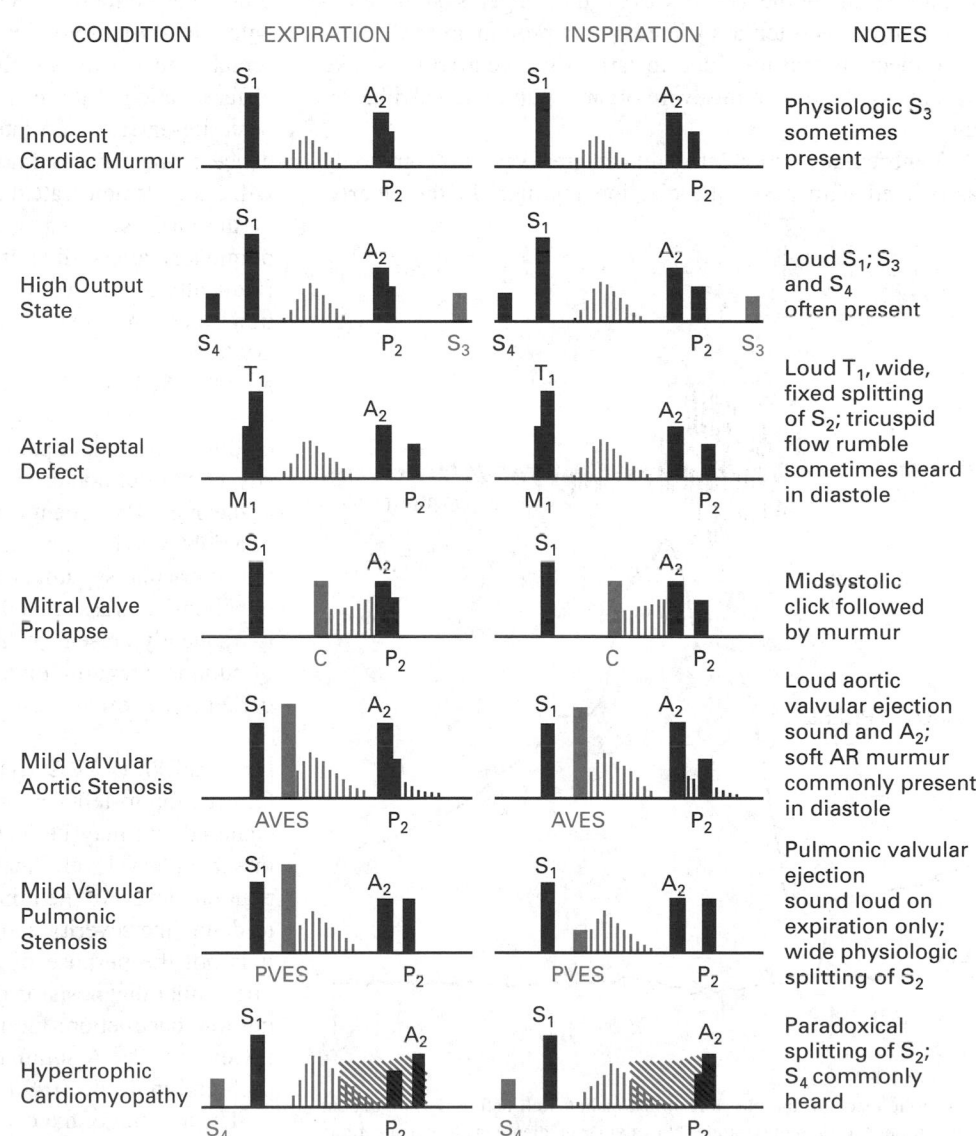

FIGURE 10-90

The differential diagnosis of the innocent murmur versus the pathologic systolic murmur is made by the "company the murmur keeps." The innocent murmur must be found in the setting of an otherwise normal cardiovascular examination. C = midsystolic nonejection sound; AVES = aortic valvular ejection sound; PVES = pulmonary valvular ejection sound; AR = aortic regurgitation. (From Shaver JA et al. *Examination of the Heart: Part IV. Auscultation*. Dallas: American Heart Association; 1990:40. Reproduced with permission from the publisher and the authors.)

ventricular septal defect along the left sternal border and the spindle-shaped systolic murmur loudest at the base.

Prominent systolic ejection murmurs are the rule in patients with significant aortic regurgitation secondary to the large forward stroke volume (Fig. 10-91). Although no significant left ventricular outflow gradient is found in these patients, the intensity of such murmurs may be grade 4 or 5, and occasionally they are associated with a thrill. They always end well before aortic closure and are clearly separated from the early regurgitant murmur. Such a murmur is rarely confused with significant valvular obstruction because of the peripheral findings of wide-open aortic regurgitation. When true valvular obstruction is present (mixed stenosis and regurgitation of the aortic valve), the longer systolic ejection murmur is often associated with a prominent thrill. Systolic ejection murmurs due to large right ventricular stroke volume are also seen in severe organic pulmonic valvular regurgitation.

Ventricular ejection into a dilated great vessel is commonly associated with a systolic ejection murmur. In the elderly,

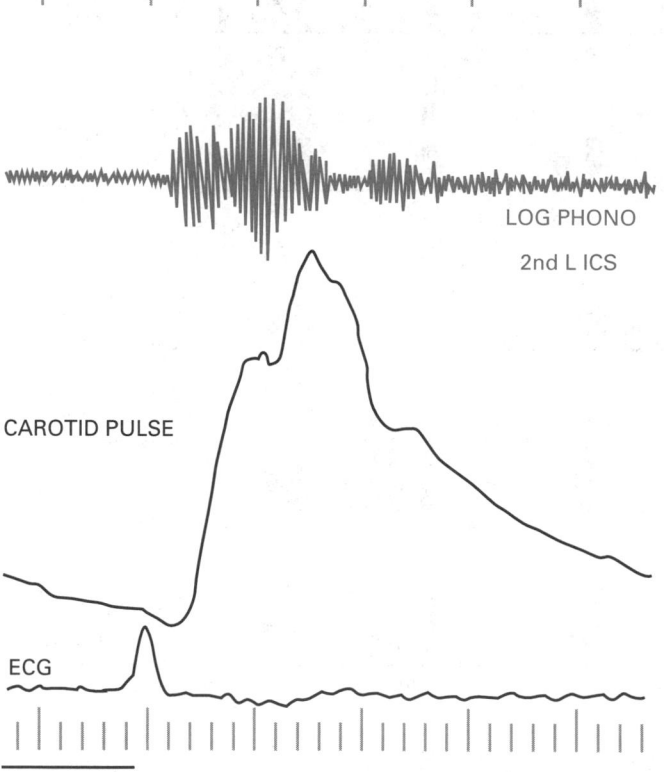

FIGURE 10-91

A systolic ejection murmur is recorded ending well before S_2 in a patient with chronic aortic regurgitation. No valvular gradient was found at cardiac catheterization. The carotid pulse is rapid-rising and has a wide pulse pressure. A long decrescendo–early diastolic murmur is recorded throughout diastole. On physical examination, a systolic thrill was associated with a grade 5 systolic murmur. (From Shaver JA. Current uses of phonocardiography in clinical practice. In: Rapaport E, ed. *Cardiology Update: Reviews for Physicians.* New York: Elsevier; 1981:363. Reproduced with permission from the publisher and the author. Copyright 1981 by Elsevier Science Publishing Co., Inc.)

such murmurs are due to ejection into a dilated, sclerotic aorta and are often best appreciated at the apex. Frequently, degenerative changes of mild sclerosis of the aortic valve are also present, and the clinician is faced with a difficult decision as to whether or not true obstruction exists. The presence of significant calcification on fluoroscopic examination favors true obstruction and can be confirmed when a significant gradient is demonstrated by Doppler studies. A systolic ejection murmur due to right ventricular ejection into a massively dilated pulmonary artery is frequently present in idiopathic dilation of the pulmonary artery (Fig. 10-69),[357] which is often confused with an atrial septal defect due to the wide auditory expiratory splitting present in this condition. The prominent pulmonary ejection sound may also be confused with a loud tricuspid closure sound of a patient with an atrial septal defect. Careful clinical examination may not allow differentiation of these two conditions; however, the standard posterior-anterior and lateral chest x-ray will not show evidence of increased pulmonary flow, and the echocardiogram will easily demonstrate the large hyperdynamic right ventricle of the atrial septal defect, which is not seen with isolated pulmonary artery dilation. Short systolic ejection murmurs, frequently associated with a prominent late pulmonary ejection sound, are also seen in dilated pulmonary arteries secondary to severe pulmonary hypertension of any cause.[357] They are identified by "the company they keep." Physical findings of severe pulmonary hypertension are always present, including a prominent parasternal impulse and increased intensity of the pulmonic component of S_2, which is well heard at the apex. Prominent *a* waves in the neck and the presence of a right-sided S_4 that increases with inspiration are present if the ventricular septum is intact (Fig. 10-79). If the pulmonary hypertension is associated with intracardiac shunting, cyanosis is frequently present. A high-pitched, early diastolic murmur of pulmonic regurgitation secondary to severe pulmonary hypertension is often present.

LEFT VENTRICULAR OUTFLOW TRACT MURMURS

Obstruction to left ventricular outflow may be congenital or acquired and may be located at the valvular, supravalvular, or subvalvular level. Stenosis is occasionally present at more than one level. In the clinical evaluation, one should attempt to define the severity and the level of obstruction. However, it is not the purpose of this chapter to give an exhaustive differential diagnosis of the various forms of left ventricular outflow obstruction; the reader is referred to three excellent reviews.[524–526] A summary of this differential diagnosis can be found in Table 10-9 (see also Chap. 63).

The murmur of fixed stenosis of the left ventricular outflow tract, regardless of the site, is crescendo-decrescendo, and its contour closely parallels the instantaneous pressure gradient (Fig. 10-88). A long as cardiac output is maintained, there is an excellent correlation between the intensity and length of the murmur with severity of obstruction, as shown in Figs. 10-55 and 10-88. Although there is a tendency toward late peaking of the murmur with increasing severity of the obstruc-

TABLE 10-9

DIFFERENTIAL DIAGNOSIS OF LEFT VENTRICULAR OUTFLOW OBSTRUCTION

Parameter	Congenital Aortic Stenosis			Acquired Aortic Stenosis	Hypertrophic "Obstructive" Cardiomyopathy
	Valvular	Subvalvular	Supravalvular		
Physical appearance	Normal	Normal	Characteristic facies	Normal	Normal
Arterial pulse	Slow rise, sustained peak	Slow rise, sustained peak	Right brachial and carotid > left	Slow rise, sustained peak	Brisk rise, unsustained double peak
S_4 presystolic impulse	Yes	Yes	Yes	Yes	Yes
Left ventricular systolic impulse	Sustained, single	Sustained, single	Sustained, single	Sustained, single	Sustained, may be double
Aortic ejection sound	Typical ↓ with calcif.	Rare	Rare	Common ↓ with calcif.	Rare exception
Midsystolic ejection murmur; maximal site	First or second right interspace	First or second right interspace	First right interspace and over right carotid	First or second right interspace; apex in elderly	Apex, lower left sternal edge
Second sound splitting	Usually normal or single	Usually normal or single	Usually normal or single	Usually single or reversed	Usually reversed or single
Intensity of aortic closure	Normal or increased or ↓ with calcif.	Normal or decreased	Normal or decreased	Decreased or absent with calcif.	Normal
Murmur of aortic regurgitation	Common	Common	Uncommon	Common	Rare exception

a Calcif. = calcification.

Source: Modified from Reddy PS, et al. Cardiac systolic murmurs: Pathophysiology and differential diagnosis.
Prog Cardiovasc Dis 1971; 14:6. Reproduced with permission from the publisher and authors.

tion, this delayed peaking has not been found to correlate as well with the severity of valvular obstruction in aortic stenosis as it has in pulmonic stenosis.[527] The murmur of significant fixed left ventricular outflow tract obstruction is usually best heard in the second right and second and third left interspaces near the sternum. It radiates widely into the neck and along the great vessels. With radiation to the apex, particularly in the elderly patient, the high-frequency components of the murmur predominate and the apical murmur has a high pitch and often a musical quality (Figs. 10-80 and 10-88).[501] This characteristic change in the pitch between the proximal and distal radiation of the murmur is a repeated source of confusion on auscultation. There is an almost overpowering urge to call it a separate murmur of mitral regurgitation; however, observations repeatedly demonstrate that this murmur, regardless of its timbre or harmonics, retains a spindle-shaped configuration whenever it is heard or recorded. Of help in confirming the ejection nature of such a high-pitched murmur is the relationship between the intensity of the systolic murmur and the length of preceding diastole as described by Henke and associates.[528] They noted that the murmur of aortic steno-

sis varied directly with the length of the preceding diastole; the longer the preceding ventricular filling period, the louder the systolic murmur (Fig. 10-92). In contrast, the apical murmur of mitral regurgitation is associated with little or no variation in intensity with varying cycle lengths. This observation is useful in patients with atrial fibrillation or frequent premature contractions and helps to identify whether an apical murmur is due to radiation of an ejection murmur or is an additional regurgitant murmur of mitral regurgitation. Beat-to-beat variations in the intensity of the murmur of aortic stenosis have been noted in both pulsus alternans[529] and AV dissociation,[530] again demonstrating the intimate relationship between beat-to-beat changes in stroke volume and the intensity of the systolic ejection murmur.

A loud early systolic valvular ejection sound or click is the hallmark of congenital valvular aortic stenosis, and its presence defines the obstruction at the valvular level (Fig. 10-56).[531] As discussed earlier in this chapter, its intensity correlates well with the motility of the valve, and there is little correlation with the severity of the obstruction. As shown in Fig. 10-55, it disappears when the valve becomes immobile

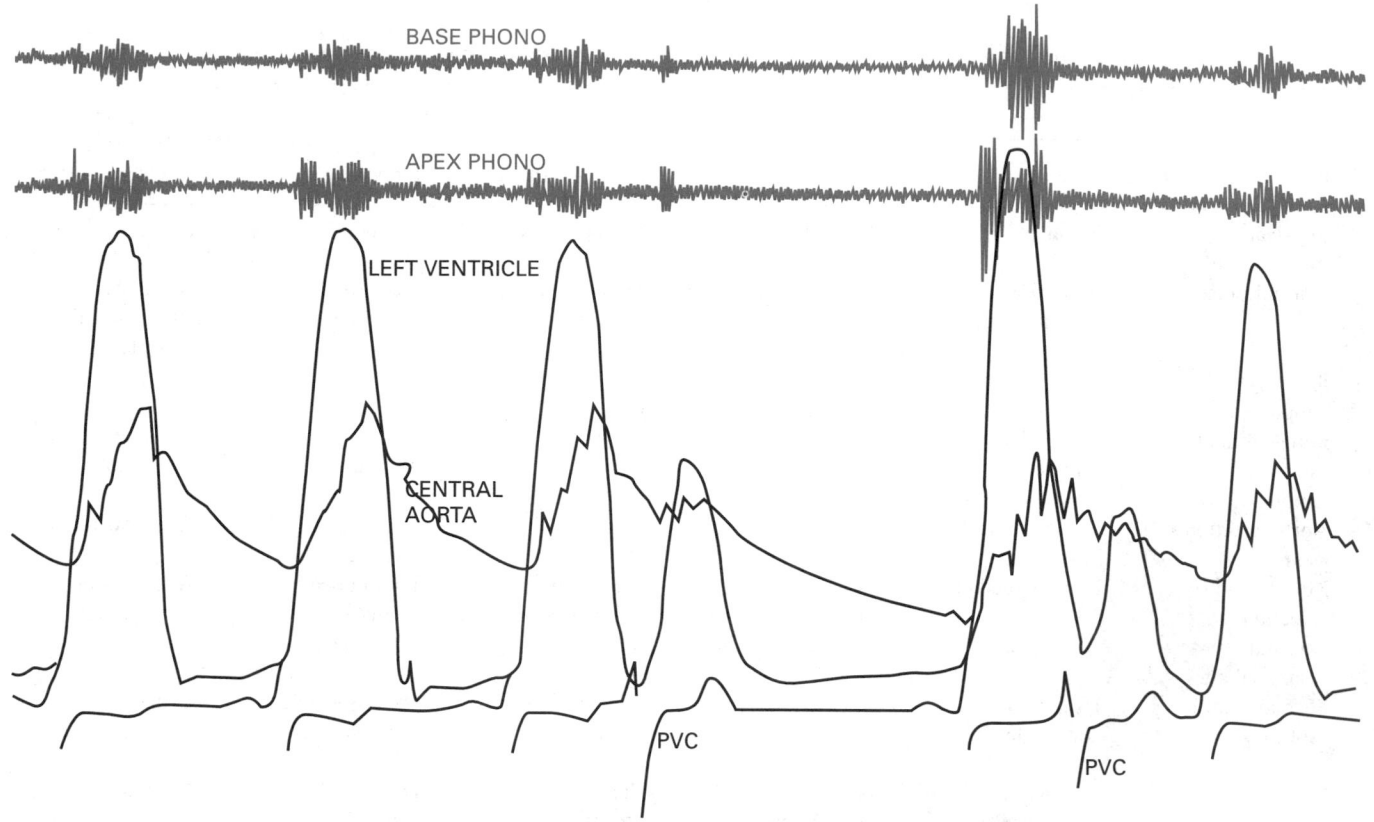

FIGURE 10-92

Effect of the long diastolic filling period following a premature ventricular contraction (PVC) on the intensity of the systolic ejection murmur (SEM) in the same patient as in Fig. 10-88. There is a marked increase in the intensity of the aortic stenosis murmur recorded at the base and at the apex. In spite of the higher-frequency content of the apical murmur, this response clearly identifies this murmur as ejection in nature. (From Paley H. Left ventricular outflow tract obstruction: Heart sounds and murmurs. In Leon DF, Shaver JA, eds. *Physiologic Principles of Heart Sounds and Murmurs*. Monograph 46. Dallas: American Heart Association; 1975:112. Reproduced with permission from the publisher and the author.)

due to calcific fixation and is absent in fixed subaortic stenosis (Fig. 10-58). With progressive increase in the severity of the outflow obstruction, the duration of left ventricular ejection is prolonged,[532,533] resulting in narrow, single, or reversed splitting of S_2. Reversed splitting of S_2 in aortic stenosis in the absence of LBBB is always associated with severe obstruction (see also Chap. 63).

Regardless of the site of obstruction, significant stenosis always results in left ventricular hypertrophy, with a decreased diastolic compliance. Clinically, this is manifest as a presystolic apical pulsation on palpation and as an S_4 on auscultation (Fig. 10-80). In patients above age 12, the S_4 is generally associated with a left ventricular diastolic pressure above 11 mmHg and a left atrial a-wave peak of about 13 mmHg.[482] The relationship between the severity of obstruction and the presence of S_4 gallops is indirect, reflecting hypertrophy and decreased compliance of the left ventricle rather than obstruction per se.

Because of the frequent coexistence of hypertensive or arteriosclerotic heart disease in the elderly patient with calcific aortic stenosis, the presence of an S_4 is nonspecific and correlates poorly with the severity of obstruction.[483] The S_3 gallops may also be heard in left ventricular outflow tract obstruction, particularly when decompensation occurs (Fig. 10-80).

The diagnosis of hemodynamically significant aortic stenosis in the elderly presents a particularly difficult problem.[534] The murmur is often of low intensity due to the decreased cardiac output and poor left ventricular function. An ejection sound or click is rarely present, due to calcific fixation of the valve leaflets, and S_2 is of low amplitude. The murmur is often loudest at the apex, has a high-frequency content, and may be difficult to define as ejection in nature because S_1 and A_2 may be poorly heard and therefore lost as landmarks defining the onset and end of mechanical systole. In most patients with severe aortic stenosis, no A_2 is heard and the systolic murmur obliterates P_2. In the elderly the rate of rise of the carotid pulse may be nearly normal due to the hard, sclerotic vessels even with severe obstruction. As shown in Fig. 10-92, the response of the murmur following a premature ventricular contraction (PVC) may be very helpful in confirming the ejection nature of the murmur. Differentiation from the benign murmur of mild aortic sclerosis may be difficult and often necessitates confirmation of obstruction and its quantitation by echo-Doppler examination[535] (see also Chaps. 14 and 63).

RIGHT VENTRICULAR OUTFLOW TRACT OBSTRUCTION

Obstructions to right ventricular outflow are congenital anomalies and may be at the level of the valve, infundibulum, and proximal or distal branches of the pulmonary artery. Isolated infundibular pulmonic stenosis with an intact septum is rare and is usually associated with a large ventricular septal defect (tetralogy of Fallot). When the ventricular septum is intact, there is an excellent correlation between both the intensity and duration of the murmur and the severity of obstruction.[355,536] In Fig. 10-93, the auscultatory findings of progressively more severe valvular pulmonic stenosis with intact ventricular septum are contrasted with those found in tetralogy of Fallot with progressively more severe right ventricular outflow obstruction.[537,538] As with valvular aortic stenosis, an early systolic ejection sound defines the level of obstruction at the valve. In mild to moderate valvular obstruction, the intensity of this sound is markedly attenuated or may disappear with inspiration (Fig. 10-58).[353] In more severe valvular obstruction, this sound may fuse with S_1 or may actually present

as a presystolic click when the pressure generated by a forceful right atrial contraction exceeds right ventricular end-diastolic pressure, causing doming of the stenotic valve in late diastole. Although obstruction to right ventricular outflow in tetralogy of Fallot is usually at the infundibular level, valvular stenosis may also be present. In this setting a pulmonary valvular ejection sound introduces a systolic murmur, and little variation in the intensity of the ejection sound is found with respiration.[539]

The classic late peaking of the systolic ejection murmur of severe pulmonic stenosis with intact ventricular septum is demonstrated in Fig. 10-67. Note that the late vibrations of the murmur completely envelop A_2, while P_2 is markedly delayed and decreases in intensity secondary to the low pulmonary artery closing pressure. In moderate to severe valvular pulmonic stenosis, an excellent correlation has been found between the A_2-P_2 interval and the right ventricular peak pressure.[355] When the ventricular septum is intact in severe right ventricular outflow obstruction, prominent a waves are present in the jugular venous pulse, in association with a right-sided S_4 that may increase with inspiration. Neither of these findings is present in uncomplicated tetralogy of Fallot. Occasionally, in very severe pulmonic stenosis, a low-pitched, presystolic murmur may be present due to forward flow across the stenotic valve that has been prematurely opened by forceful right atrial contraction in late diastole.[355] Such patients are often cyanotic due to right-to-left shunting through a patent foramen ovale.

In isolated infundibular obstruction, a pulmonic ejection sound is usually not encountered[540] and the pulmonic closure (P_2) is usually not audible except in the mildest cases. The site of maximal intensity of the murmur is of little help in differentiating the site of obstruction. Both valvular pulmonic stenosis and isolated infundibular pulmonic stenosis with intact septum can be differentiated from tetralogy of Fallot by noting the marked intensification of the ejection murmur after the inhalation of amyl nitrite. In contrast, the murmur of tetralogy of Fallot shortens and decreases in intensity.[541]

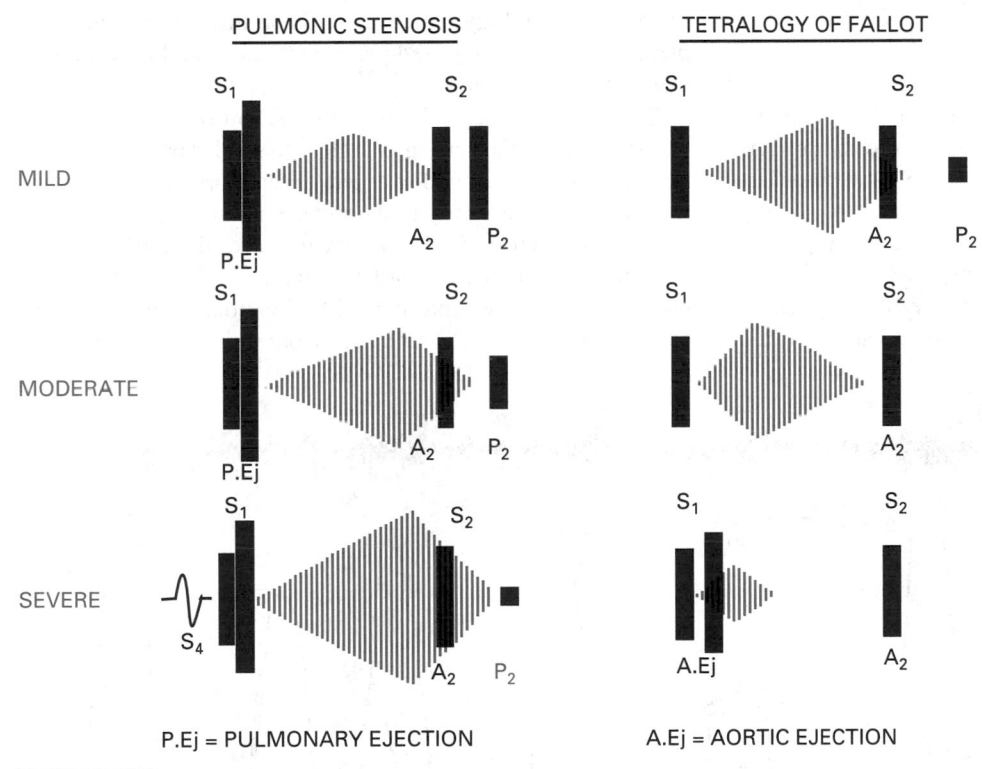

PULMONIC STENOSIS **TETRALOGY OF FALLOT**

MILD

MODERATE

SEVERE

P.Ej = PULMONARY EJECTION   A.Ej = AORTIC EJECTION

FIGURE 10-93

In valvular pulmonic stenosis with intact ventricular septum, right ventricular systolic ejection becomes progressively longer with increasing obstruction to flow. As a result, the murmur becomes louder and longer, enveloping the aortic closure sound. At the same time, pulmonic closure occurs later; splitting becomes wider but is more difficult to appreciate because the aortic closure sound is lost in the murmur; and the pulmonic closure sound becomes progressively softer due to the low pulmonary artery pressure. With increasing severity of pulmonic stenosis, the pulmonary ejection sound may fuse with S_1. In severe obstruction with concentric hypertrophy and decreased right ventricular compliance, an S_4 appears. In tetralogy of Fallot, with increasing obstruction at the infundibular area, more and more right ventricular blood is shunted across a silent ventricular septal defect with less flow across the obstructed right ventricular outflow tract. With increasing obstruction, the murmur becomes shorter, earlier, and fainter. The pulmonic closure sound is absent in severe tetralogy of Fallot. The dilated aorta receives almost all of the cardiac output from both ventricular chambers, and there is an aortic ejection sound (Aej). (From Leonard J et al: *Examination of the Heart* series: Part four. *Ausculatation.* Dallas: American Heart Association; 1974:45. Reproduced with permission from the publisher and authors.)

In branch stenosis of the pulmonary artery, there is a systolic murmur of varying intensity at the upper left sternal border that is widely transmitted to the right chest, back, and both axillae. The murmur is usually less harsh and of higher pitch than the murmur of valvular stenosis. With more peripheral branch stenosis, systolic ejection murmurs or even continuous murmurs may be heard over the lung fields. The wide radiation of this murmur is particularly helpful in alerting the clinician to this type of right-sided obstruction.

Systolic Regurgitant Murmurs

Systolic regurgitant murmurs are produced by retrograde flow from a chamber of high pressure to a chamber of lower pressure.[492,542] The classic examples of such murmurs are the holosystolic (pansystolic) murmur of mitral regurgitation, tricuspid regurgitation, and ventricular septal defect. Since there is usually a high-pressure differential between the two chambers throughout systole, the murmurs are holosystolic in duration, high-pitched and blowing in quality, and plateau-like in configuration.

HOLOSYSTOLIC REGURGITANT MURMURS

The murmur of chronic mitral regurgitation is the prototype of the holosystolic regurgitant murmur, as shown in Figs. 10-86 and 10-94. It begins with or replaces S_1 and continues throughout systole in a plateaulike fashion beyond A_2, finally terminating when the left ventricular pressure drops to the level of the left atrial pressure during isovolumic relaxation.[443,543,544] In contrast to the systolic ejection murmur, there is little variation in its intensity with varying cycle

lengths (Fig. 10-94).[545] It is heard best at the apex and radiates well into the axilla; only the loudest murmurs are associated with a thrill at the apex. There is little variation in its intensity with respiration, and it is frequently accompanied by a loud diastolic filling sound followed by a short rumble.[546] In this situation, the loud S_3 is not a manifestation of congestive failure but a reflection of hemodynamically significant mitral regurgitation. Likewise, the short rumble does not mean concomitant obstruction at the mitral valve but rather is secondary to extremely rapid early diastolic filling. As shown in Fig. 10-95, the intensity of the murmur is directly related to the pressure gradient between the left ventricle and the left atrium. With amyl nitrite, there is a dramatic decrease in the left ventricular–left atrial gradient and in the intensity of the murmur. The opposite response is seen with vasoconstrictive agents that increase the left ventricular–left atrial pressure gradient.

The diagnosis of hemodynamically significant mitral regurgitation is established by the presence of the holosystolic regurgitant murmur and loud S_3 associated with a short flow rumble. The etiology, however, is determined by the clinical presentation and associated physical findings and is best confirmed by echocardiography.[547]

The classic holosystolic (pansystolic) murmur of tricuspid regurgitation in the setting of right ventricular pressure overload is best heard at the lower left sternal border.[292] At times it may be heard laterally to the midclavicular line, indicating that the right ventricle occupies the region of the cardiac apex. Although occasionally heard this far laterally, the murmur does not radiate well into the axillary region. Furthermore, it can generally be differentiated from mitral regurgitation

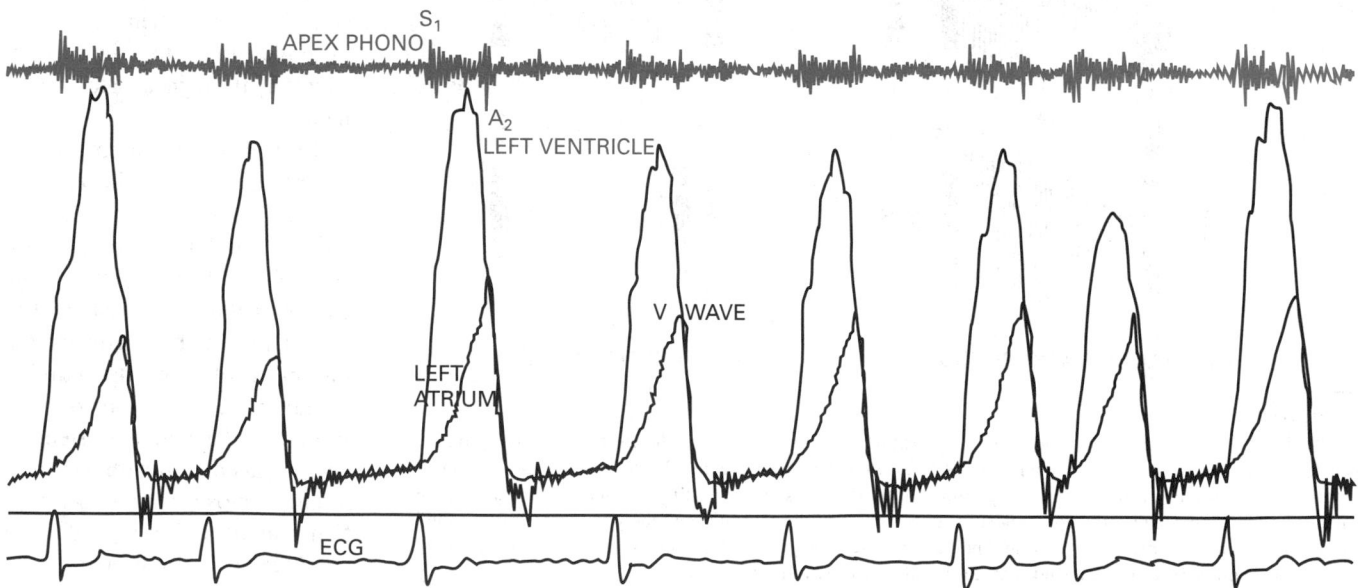

FIGURE 10-94

The apex phonocardiogram is recorded simultaneously with the left ventricular (LV) and left atrial (LA) pressures in a patient with chronic mitral regurgitation. The murmur is plateaulike in character, spilling through A_2 and having minimal variation in intensity with the varying cycle lengths of atrial fibrillation. This is in marked contrast to the post-PVC response of valvular aortic

stenosis as shown in Fig. 10-92. (From Paley H. Left ventricular outflow tract obstruction: Heart sounds and murmurs. In: Leon DF, Shaver JA, eds. *Physiologic Principles of Heart Sounds and Murmurs.* Monograph 46. Dallas: American Heart Association; 1975:112. Reproduced with permission from the publisher and the authors.)

because its intensity is usually strongly influenced by respiration.[548,549] As shown in Fig. 10-96, during continuous and accentuated respiration, the murmur increases in intensity with inspiration due to the increased venous return and right ventricular filling associated with inspiration.[550] The inspiratory increase in loudness of right-sided auscultatory events is known as Carvallo's sign. Careful inspection of the jugular venous pulse while auscultating the murmur will be of further help in defining its tricuspid origin, showing a prominent v wave with a rapid y descent that augments during inspiration. In severe right ventricular failure, this respiratory variation may be absent, but it may reappear as the state of compensation improves. With severe tricuspid regurgitation, a short flow rumble introduced by an S_3 can be present, just as with mitral regurgitation, and both will increase with inspiration.[550]

The holosystolic murmur of ventricular septal defect (VSD) is heard best just off the sternal border in the fourth, fifth, and sixth intercostal spaces and is usually accompanied by a forceful thrill.[551,552] The murmur does not radiate to the axilla as with mitral regurgitation and does not have the respiratory variation characteristic of tricuspid regurgitation. Wide physiologic splitting with an easily heard P_2 is usually present when the left-to-right shunt is hemodynamically significant. When the shunt is large, there is a left ventricular S_3 followed by a short flow rumble. The regurgitant murmur is due to high-velocity flow from the high-pressure left ventricle to the lower pressure right ventricle, and its intensity correlates poorly with the degree of left-to-right shunting. For example, a grade 5 murmur may be associated with a very high velocity flow through a small hemodynamically insignificant muscular VSD (Roger).[553] On the other hand, an equally loud murmur associated with a thrill may be present with a larger defect having massive left-to-right shunting. When the defect is very large and the right and left ventricular pressures are equal, however, no murmur may be produced across the defect; instead, the short pulmonary ejection murmur of severe pulmonary hypertension is present (Eisenmenger's VSD).[554] As shown in Fig. 10-97, the murmur of ventricular septal defect is very sensitive to vasoactive agents that alter vascular impedance, and a marked decrease in both the left ventricular–right ventricular pressure gradient and the intensity of the murmur is seen following the administration of amyl nitrite.

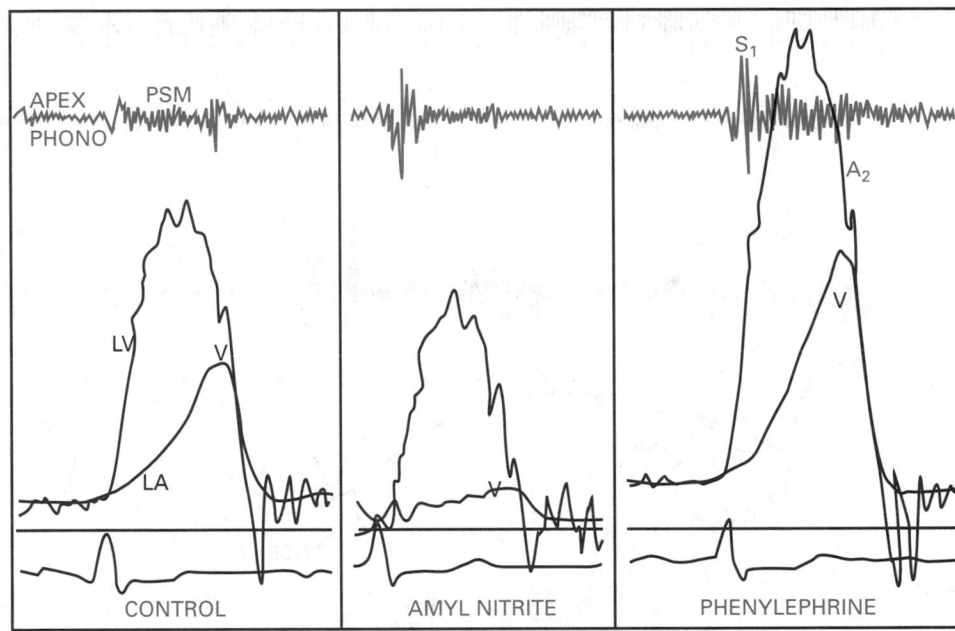

FIGURE 10-95

Simultaneous apex phonocardiogram. Left atrial (LA) and left ventricular (LV) pressures are recorded during the control state, the inhalation of amyl nitrite, and phenylephrine infusion in a patient with long-standing mitral regurgitation. During control observation, a significant LV-LA pressure gradient was associated with a pansystolic murmur (PSM) recorded at the apex. After inhalation of amyl nitrite, the peak LV pressure, the height of the v wave, and the LV-LA pressure gradient are decreased. Associated with this is a marked diminution in the intensity of the pansystolic murmur. In contrast, after the infusion of phenylephrine, all three pressure parameters as well as the intensity of the murmur are increased. [From Shaver J. The physical examination in cardiac diagnosis. *Cardiol Consult* 1985; 6(3):8. Reproduced with permission from the publisher and the author.]

EARLY SYSTOLIC REGURGITANT MURMURS

Rarely, a regurgitant murmur confined to early systole is seen in the presence of a small ventricular septal defect. This murmur begins in the usual manner at the onset of ventricular systole and stops suddenly in early or midsystole.[555,556] The sudden cessation of the murmur is due to the fact that as ejection continues and ventricular size decreases, the small defect is sealed shut as the ventricular septum thickens during systole and the flow ceases. This murmur is important because it is characteristic of the type of ventricular septal defect that may disappear with age.

In contrast to the holosystolic murmur of chronic mitral regurgitation, acute severe mitral regurgitation may present as an early systolic spindle-shaped murmur.[557–559] Common conditions producing acute mitral regurgitation include spontaneous rupture of the chordae tendineae of a myxomatous valve, acute or subacute bacterial endocarditis of the mitral valve, papillary muscle rupture or dysfunction secondary to acute myocardial infarction, and disruption of the mitral apparatus due to chest trauma.[560–563] In each of these conditions, large-volume flow regurgitates into a relatively normal left atrium that has not had the time to make the adaptive changes in compliance seen in chronic longstanding mitral regurgitation. As a result, an extremely high v wave is generated in the left atrium.

This high v wave abolishes the left ventricular–left atrial

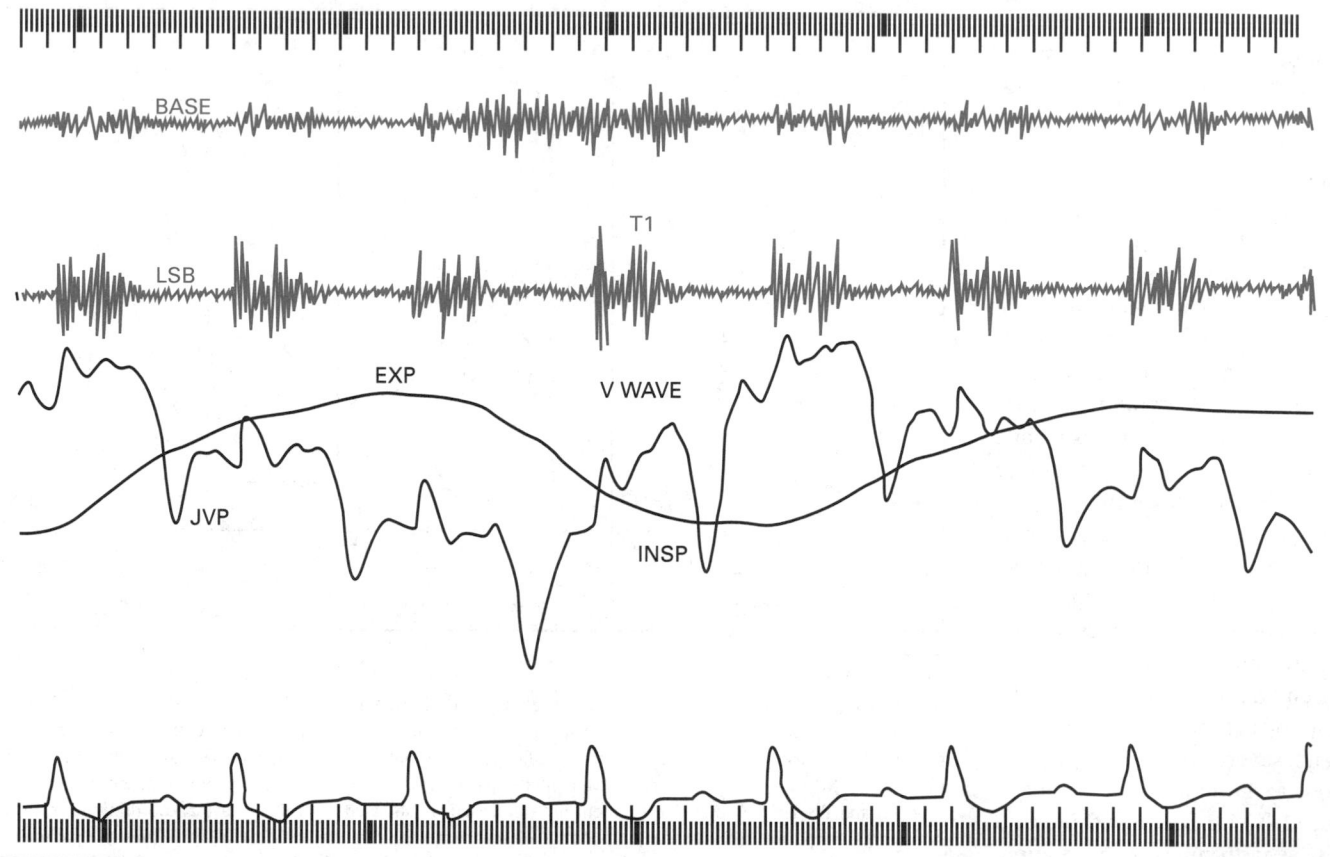

FIGURE 10-96

Phonocardiograms at the base and left sternal border (LSB) are recorded with the jugular venous pulse during exaggerated respiration in a patient with cor pulmonale. Augmentation of the pansystolic murmur at the left sternal border confirms its tricuspid origin. The jugular venous pulse shows prominent *v* waves having an increased pulse pressure and *y* descent during inspiration, characteristic of tricuspid regurgitation. (From Salerni R et al. Noninvasive graphic evaluation: Phonocardiography and echocardiography. In: Frankl WS, Brest AN, eds. *Cardiovascular Clinics: Valvular Heart Disease—Comprehensive Evaluation and Management.* Philadelphia: Davis; 1986:201. Reproduced with permission from the publisher and the authors.)

gradient during the latter part of systole, resulting in termination of retrograde flow and abbreviation of the systolic murmur. As shown in Fig. 10-47, in a patient with acute mitral regurgitation secondary to spontaneous rupture of the chordae tendineae of a myxomatous valve, the murmur ends before A_2. Audible expiratory splitting with an accentuated P_2 is present at the base, and a loud S_4 is recorded at the apex. The presence of the S_4 associated with a prominent presystolic impulse on palpation is an important clue that indicates the acute nature of the mitral regurgitation and is rarely present in mitral regurgitation of a chronic nature.[484] The systolic murmur of acute mitral regurgitation, which can mimic "ejection" murmurs, may have classic radiation to the axilla and back, especially if it is due to prolapse of the anterior leaflet of the valve with flow directed over the posterior leaflet. When the murmur is loud, it may be conducted to the top of the head and to the sacrum along the spinal column. Occasionally, the murmur is conducted to the base of the heart and great vessels, simulating aortic stenosis.[564] The quick-rising carotid pulse with rapid fall-off as well as the wide physiologic splitting of the second heart sound help differentiation from aortic stenosis.[565]

The systolic murmur of organic tricuspid regurgitation is often unimpressive and presents as an early systolic murmur ending well before A_2, even in the presence of severe regurgitation.[566] In this condition, the right ventricular pressure is nearly normal, and massive regurgitation may be present with only a small pressure differential between the right ventricle and the right atrium (Fig. 10-98). The small pressure head results in a low-velocity flow, minimal turbulence, and a soft, abbreviated murmur. Occasionally, only minimal early systolic vibrations are heard, as demonstrated in Fig. 10-98. In most patients, large *v* waves are readily apparent in the jugular venous pulse. The murmur retains the characteristic inspiratory augmentation seen in right-sided regurgitant murmurs and is frequently associated with an S_4 that increases in intensity with inspiration. A right-sided S_4 together with a prominent diastolic tricuspid flow rumble are the rule when the tricuspid regurgitation is acute, as in endocarditis of the tricuspid valve. After total excision of the tricuspid valve for infective endocarditis related to intravenous drug abuse, the systolic murmur is often very unimpressive or may be completely absent. Giant *v* waves in the neck are easily visible, however, and palpable venous thrills and a murmur at the

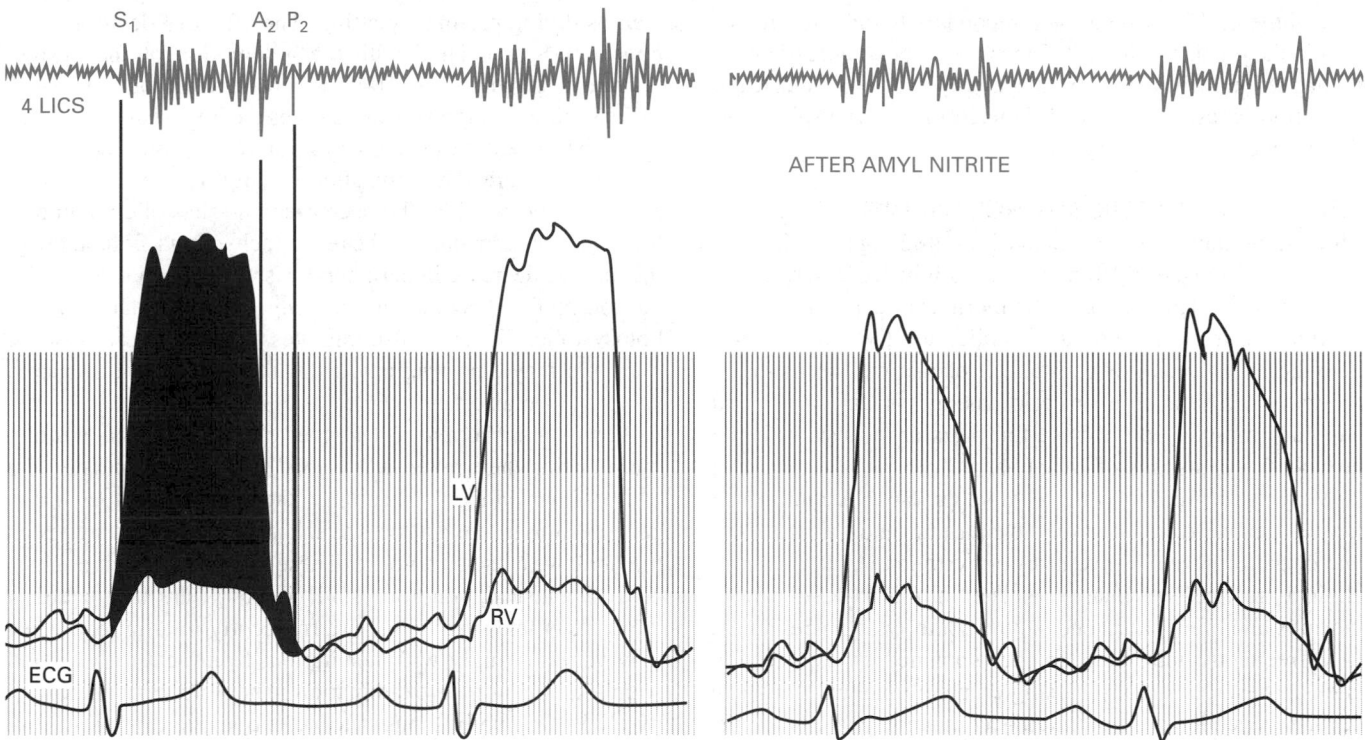

FIGURE 10-97

Right (RV) and left ventricular (LV) pressures are recorded with the phonocardiogram at rest and following inhalation of amyl nitrite in a 26-year-old woman with a ventricular septal defect without pulmonary hypertension. The pansystolic murmur extends through A₂, corresponding to the LV-RV pressure gradient. Following inhalation of amyl nitrite, there is a marked decrease in the LV-RV pressure gradient and a concomitant decrease in the intensity of the murmur. (From Reddy PS et al. Cardiac systolic murmurs: Pathophysiology and differential diagnosis. *Prog Cardiovasc Dis* 1971; 14:21. Reproduced with permission from the publisher and the authors.)

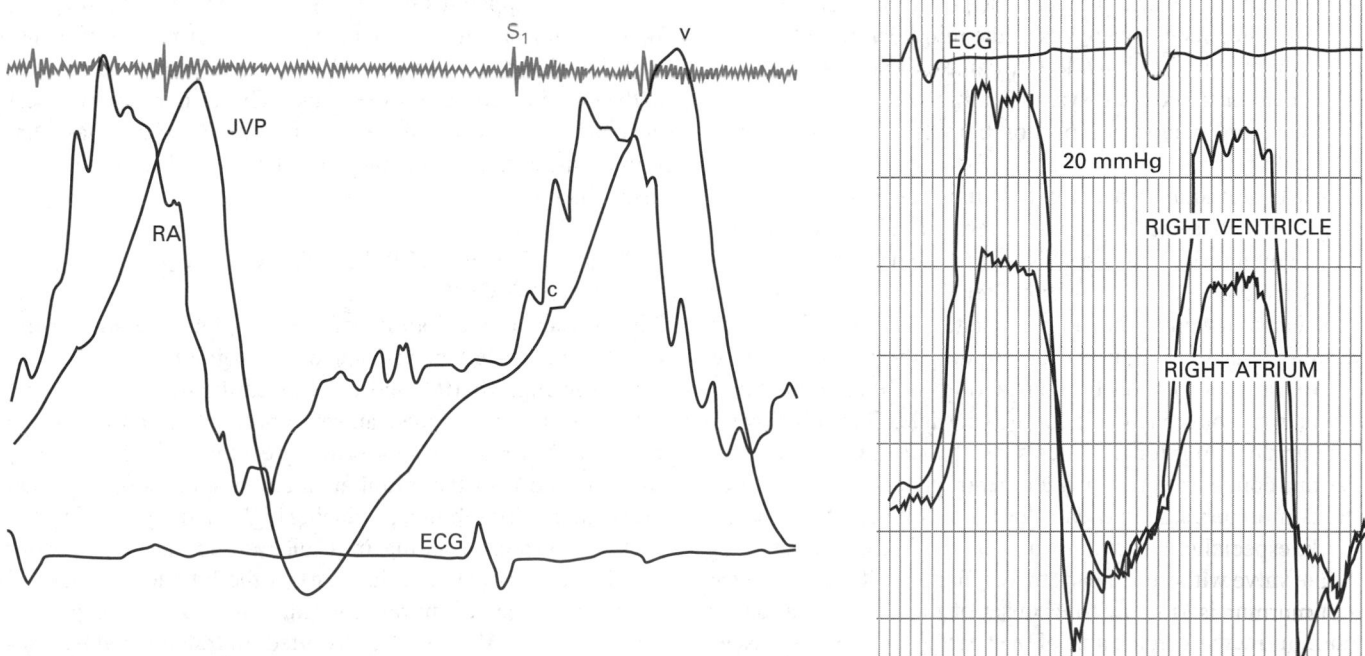

FIGURE 10-98

The phonocardiogram is recorded simultaneously with the jugular venous pulse and right atrial pressure in a patient with severe organic tricuspid regurgitation. Only minimal early systolic vibration is recorded on the phonocardiogram, and a huge CV wave is present on the jugular venous pulse. In the right panel, simultaneous right ventricular and right atrial pressures are shown, demonstrating ventricularization of the right atrial pressure. There is a minimal pressure gradient across the tricuspid valve, resulting in low-velocity retrograde flow and absence of a significant murmur.

base of the neck may be present secondary to rapid retrograde flow in the jugular system.[567] Other causes of organic tricuspid regurgitation include carcinoid heart disease, right ventricular infarction, chest trauma, and damage of the tricuspid valve during open heart surgery.

MID- AND LATE-SYSTOLIC REGURGITANT MURMURS

Midsystolic murmurs can occur with mitral regurgitation due to papillary muscle dysfunction, as originally described by Burch et al.[568] The timing of the murmur of papillary muscle dysfunction may also be late systolic, and the murmur may be either intermittent or constant. It occurs with ischemia or infarction of either the posterior medial or anterior lateral papillary muscle. Often these murmurs are transient, being provoked by episodes of ischemia.

Varying degrees of mitral valve prolapse are the most frequent cause of a late-systolic murmur, and this entity is one of the most common causes of systolic murmurs seen in clinical practice (see Chap. 65). The murmur is best heard at the apex and often has a tendency to a late systolic crescendo. It is frequently introduced or accompanied by nonejection clicks. These clicks may be single or multiple, and they can occur independently without an accompanying systolic murmur (Fig. 10-59). A shown in Fig. 10-60, the click occurs near the time of maximal prolapse in midsystole, and the late-systolic murmur continues up to and through A_2 due to prolapse of the posterior leaflet during the remainder of systole. In the past, the late-systolic murmurs and mid- and late-systolic clicks were considered to be innocent and thought to be extracardiac in origin—that is, pleural or pericardial.[569,570] Subsequent studies with intracardiac phonocardiography have localized these acoustic events to the mitral valve and subvalvular structures,[363,364] while left ventricular cineangiograms have demonstrated late-systolic mitral regurgitation with billowing or prolapse of one or both leaflets into the left atrium.[361,362,571]

The timing and intensity of these murmurs vary with physiologic and pharmacologic maneuvers that alter the end-diastolic volume of the heart (Fig. 10-61). These murmurs are also sensitive to conditions that alter the peripheral vascular impedance as well as the inotropic state of the heart.[372] These variations in the timing and duration of the murmur can be most easily understood by considering MVP as a condition in which the valve is too big for the ventricle. This valvuloventricular disproportion manifests itself at a given geometric size and configuration during left ventricular contraction. Situations that decrease the end-diastolic volume of the heart, decrease peripheral vascular impedance, or increase the inotropic state allow the heart to reach this critical geometry sooner, resulting in an earlier onset of the click and a longer murmur. Increase in the size of the heart and peripheral vascular impedance and a decrease in the inotropic state will result in the opposite changes, with the click moving toward S_2 and the murmur becoming shorter. These dynamic changes can best be appreciated at the bedside by examining the patient in the supine, left lateral, sitting, and standing positions as

well as during prompt squatting. The effect of decreased venous return associated with the assumption of the upright posture is shown in Fig. 10-99 in a patient without a murmur in the supine position and emphasizes the importance of examining the patient suspected of mitral valve prolapse in more than one posture. The inhalation of amyl nitrite is also very helpful at the bedside; the decreased end-diastolic volume of the ventricle secondary to the reflex tachycardia, coupled with the marked decrease in peripheral vascular impedance, causes the murmur to become earlier, longer, louder, and at times holosystolic. The click also migrates toward S_1. Late systolic murmurs may also originate from prolapse of the tricuspid valve[550] (see also Chap. 66).

Levine and Harvey[295] described a musical, apical systolic murmur that they called a "whoop" because it simulated the "whoop" of whooping cough. Rackley and associates[572] called a similar sound a "precordial honk" because it suggested the honking noise of a goose. These murmurs are loud, high-pitched, musical, sonorous, and vibratory; are best heard at the apex in late systole and are frequently intermittent. They may vary strikingly with respiration, from beat to beat, and from examination to examination. They are often preceded by clicks originally thought to be extracardiac in origin but confirmed by intracardiac phonocardiography to originate in the mitral valve.[364] They are associated with ballooning of the mitral valve or mitral regurgitation (or both),[503] and their unusual quality is secondary to the high-frequency vibrations of the mitral apparatus. The systolic whoop or honk together with late systolic murmurs, with or without associated clicks, are part of a continuum representing abnormalities of the mitral valve apparatus of varying etiologies. Similar honking noises, with or without clicks, may arise from the tricuspid valve and have also been produced by transvenous pacemaker catheters situated across the valve. These murmurs are best auscultated at the fourth left intercostal space and have the typical inspiratory augmentation of tricuspid murmurs (see also Chap. 66).

MURMUR OF HYPERTROPHIC "OBSTRUCTIVE" CARDIOMYOPATHY

The classic cardiac findings of hypertrophic cardiomyopathy (HCM) with a left ventricular outflow gradient are demonstrated in Fig. 10-100, and the echocardiogram on the right gives insight into the mechanism of production of the systolic murmur. Most authorities now agree that systolic anterior motion (SAM) of the mitral apparatus impinges on the massively thickened septum, producing high-velocity flow in mid- and late systole, resulting in a midsystolic ejection murmur usually with its maximal intensity at the left sternal edge.[573] Varying degrees of mitral regurgitation may also be present during systole due to the distorted mitral apparatus. Frequently, on auscultation, the skilled clinician has difficulty deciding whether the systolic murmur found in HCM is ejection or regurgitant in nature.[574] The explanation for this confusion is readily understood by analysis of the intracardiac sound and pressure recordings shown in Fig. 10-101. A typical

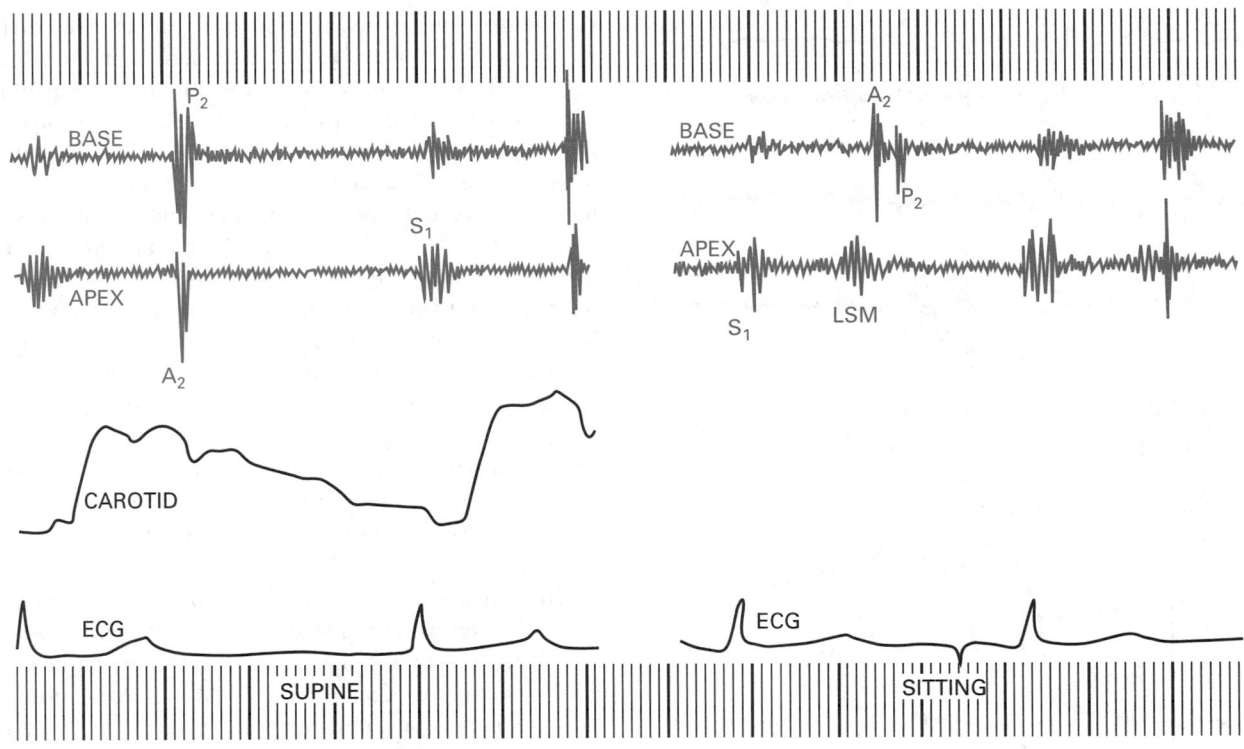

FIGURE 10-99

Base and apex phonocardiograms are recorded in the supine and sitting positions in a patient with late mitral valve prolapse. Note the absence of a late systolic murmur in the supine position. When the patient assumes the sitting posture, a late systolic murmur is produced secondary to the decreased venous return. A nonejection click is not present in this patient. (From Brandenburg RO et al, eds. *Cardiology: Fundamentals and Practice*. Chicago: Year Book; 1987:256. Reproduced with permission from the publisher and the authors.)

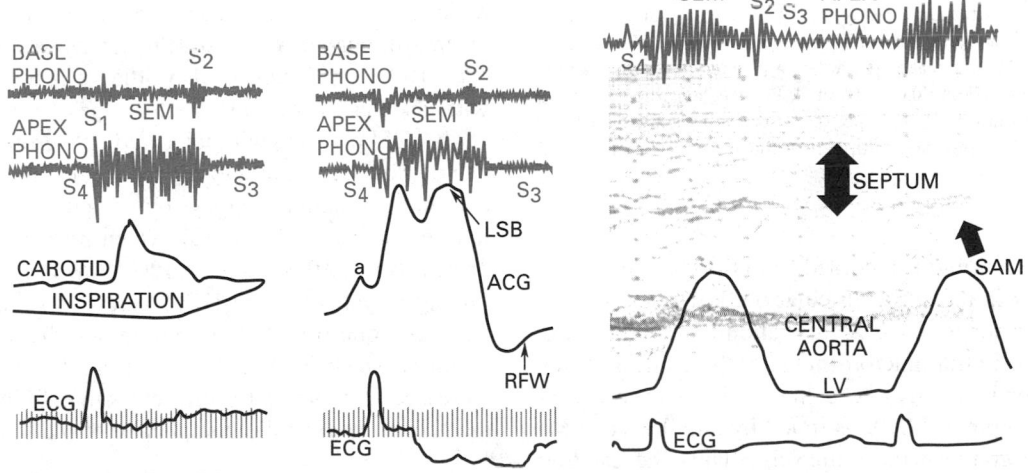

FIGURE 10-100

Simultaneous base and apex phonocardiograms are recorded with the carotid pulse and ACG in the left and center panels, respectively, in a 54-year-old man with hypertrophic cardiomyopathy. The carotid pulse rises rapidly and has a late systolic plateau and a prolonged ejection period. Prominent S_4 and S_1 are demonstrated and are associated with the a wave and the rapid filling wave (RFW), respectively, of the ACG. Note the late systolic bulge (LSB) on the ACG. S_2 is single. A loud, grade 5 systolic ejection murmur is present and is of greatest intensity at the apex. In the right panel, the apical systolic murmur is recorded together with the M-mode echocardiogram. Simultaneous high-fidelity left ventricular and central aortic pressures are recorded by catheter-tipped micromanometers. Marked thickening of the interventricular septum and SAM of the mitral valve are present on the echocardiogram. A large systolic pressure gradient is demonstrated beginning shortly after the onset of the SAM. (From Shaver JA et al. Phonoechocardiography and intracardiac phonocardiography in hypertrophic cardiomyopathy. *Postgrad Med J* 1986; 62:538. Reproduced with permission from the publisher and the authors.)

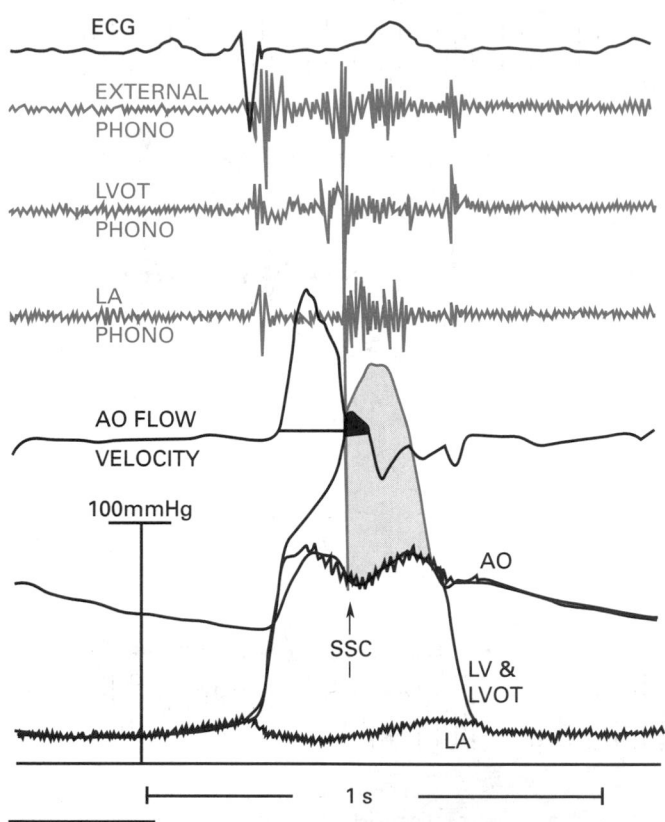

FIGURE 10-101

Catheter-tipped micromanometer pressures are recorded from the left atrium, left ventricle, left ventricular outflow tract (LVOT), and aorta, together with external and intracardiac sound recorded from micromanometers in the left atrium and LVOT in a patient with hypertrophic cardiomyopathy. Aortic flow velocity is recorded by a flow probe in the central aorta. The vertical line denotes the time of SAM-septal contact (SSC) as determined by simultaneous M-mode echocardiography of the mitral valve. Note that the majority of aortic flow occurs before SSC. A systolic ejection murmur is recorded from the LVOT, and a late systolic mitral regurgitant murmur is recorded from the left atrium. The external phonocardiogram represents the summation of these two murmurs. (From Shaver JA et al. Phonoechocardiography and intracardiac phonocardiography in hypertrophic cardiomyopathy. *Postgrad Med J* 1986; 62:539. Reproduced with permission from the publisher and the authors.)

systolic ejection murmur is recorded from the catheter-tipped micromanometer in the left ventricular outflow tract, while a late systolic murmur of mitral regurgitation is recorded from the transseptal left atrial micromanometer. The onset of this latter murmur begins shortly after contact of the anterior mitral leaflet with the septum (SSC), as timed by simultaneous M-mode echocardiography of the mitral valve. Thus, the resulting external murmur recorded by the precordial phonocardiogram is the summation of the murmurs as transmitted to the chest wall.[352,575,576]

In patients with dynamic left ventricular outflow gradients, the intensity of both the systolic ejection murmur and the mitral regurgitant murmur varies directly with the magnitude of the pressure gradient.[573,574,577] Thus, physiologic maneuvers and pharmacologic interventions that increase the pres-

sure gradient will increase the intensity of the precordial murmur, and vice versa. Decreases in left ventricular preload and afterload or increases in left ventricular contractility are associated with increases in the pressure gradient and the intensity of the murmur, while increases in left ventricular preload and afterload or decreases in left ventricular contractility will decrease the pressure gradient and the intensity of the murmur.[352,573,577–579] For example, the upright posture and the strain phase of the Valsalva maneuver decrease venous return and left ventricular preload, and the murmur increases in intensity. Upon reclining or with prompt squatting, augmented venous return increases left ventricular preload and the murmur decreases in intensity. Vasoactive drugs such as amyl nitrite decrease blood pressure, and a marked increase in the intensity of the murmur occurs; whereas vasoconstrictive drugs such as phenylephrine increase the afterload, and the murmur is decreased or abolished (Fig. 10-102)[578] (see also Chap. 74).

These responses to vasoactive drugs should be compared to the diametrically opposite responses shown in Fig. 10-95 in a patient with a holosystolic murmur of chronic mitral regurgitation. In patients with HCM, inotropic drugs such as digitalis and catecholamines increase the intensity of the murmur, while beta blockade usually decreases it. The responses to these interventions are relatively specific for HCM, although occasionally patients with mitral valve prolapse (MVP) behave similarly.[576] The clinical setting of MVP is usually easily differentiated from HCM; when this is not possible, echocardiography provides the definitive diagnosis.

In the absence of a left ventricular outflow gradient at rest or with provocation, the murmur of HCM is less impressive. Although a short ejection murmur is usually recorded due to rapid early left ventricular ejection, it is often softer and extends through less of systole than when a gradient is present (Fig. 10-81).[580] There is also little variation in the intensity with changes in preload, afterload, or contractility.

In HCM with and without a gradient across the left ventricular outflow tract, massive left ventricular hypertrophy is present, and a prominent presystolic impulse associated with a left ventricular S_4 is the rule when normal sinus rhythm is present (Figs. 10-81 and 10-100). An S_3 is also a common finding in patients with HCM, and occasionally there is an early diastolic rumble that may mimic the diastolic murmur of mitral stenosis. Such rumbles are felt to be due to the increased impedance to left ventricular filling secondary to the decreased diastolic compliance of the left ventricle.[574]

DIASTOLIC MURMURS

Diastolic murmurs have two basic mechanisms of production. Diastolic filling murmurs or rumbles are due to forward flow across an AV valve, while diastolic regurgitant murmurs are due to retrograde flow across an incompetent semilunar valve[581,582] (Fig. 10-103).

Diastolic Filling Murmurs (Rumbles)

Diastolic rumbles are caused by forward flow across the AV valves and are delayed from their respective semilunar closure sound by the isovolumic relaxation period. Only following this period, when the atrial pressure exceeds the declining ventricular pressure, do the AV valves open and filling begins. Since there are two phases of rapid ventricular filling—early diastole and presystole—these murmurs have a tendency to be most prominent during these two filling periods.[292] Because the velocity of flow is relatively low, these murmurs have a low-frequency content and are rumbling in character.

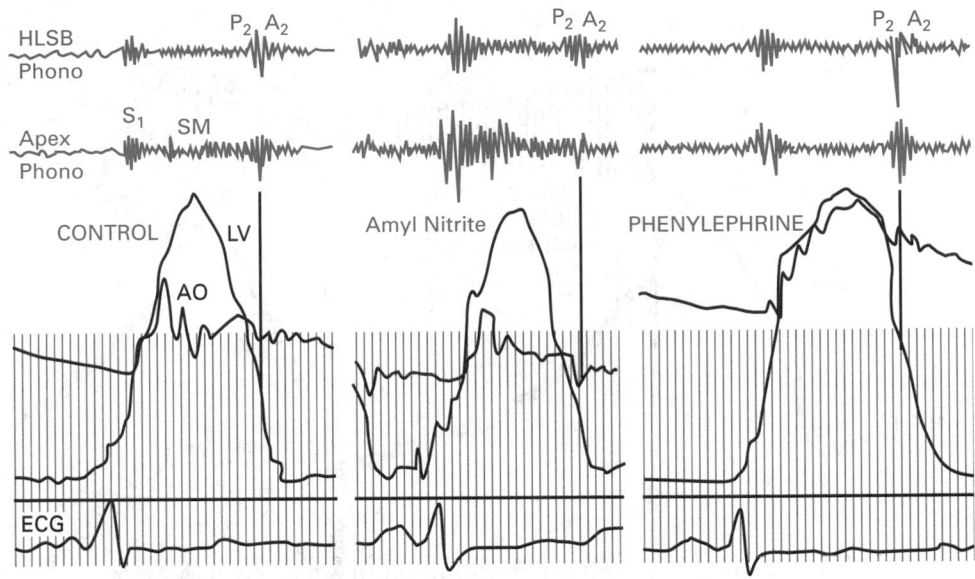

FIGURE 10-102

Simultaneous high left sternal border (HLSB) and apex phonocardiograms are recorded with left ventricular (LV) and central aortic pressure in the control state, following inhalation of amyl nitrite and the intravenous administration of phenylephrine in an 18-year-old woman with hypertrophic cardiomyopathy. In the control state, a large LV-aortic pressure gradient is present, and the duration of LV ejection is markedly prolonged, resulting in reversed splitting of S_2. A grade 3 systolic ejection murmur is recorded by the apex phonocardiogram during the pressure gradient. Following the administration of amyl nitrite, there is an increase in the LV-aortic pressure gradient and a marked increase in the intensity of the systolic murmur as recorded at the apex. Note that on the base phonocardiogram, reversed splitting of S_2 persists, with an even greater delay in A_2. Following administration of phenylephrine, there is complete obliteration of the LV-aortic pressure gradient and almost total disappearance of the apical murmur. The contour of the central aortic pressure is normalized, and physiologic splitting of S_2 is now present. As compared with the control state, the inhalation of amyl nitrite and the infusion of phenylephrine result in no significant change in peak LV pressure; the increased gradient during inhalation of amyl nitrite was secondary to a decrease in aortic pressure. Contrast these responses to the administration of amyl nitrite and phenylephrine with those shown in Fig. 10-84—a patient with chronic mitral regurgitation. (From Reddy PS et al. cardiac systolic murmurs: Pathophysiology and differential diagnosis. *Prog Cardiovasc Dis* 1971; 14:31. Reproduced in part with permission from the publisher and the authors.)

DIASTOLIC RUMBLES DUE TO OBSTRUCTION OF THE ATRIOVENTRICULAR VALVE

The murmur of mitral stenosis is heard best at the apex in the left lateral position, and its duration correlates well with the duration of the mitral diastolic gradient. Its intensity is related to the severity of the obstruction and to the flow across the valve.[583] As a result, there is poor correlation between the intensity of the murmur and the severity of the obstruction; for example, high flow across a mild obstruction may produce a loud rumble, while low flow across a severely stenotic valve may produce a very soft murmur or may be silent.[584] When the stenotic mitral valve is mobile, the murmur is introduced by a prominent opening snap (OS) (Fig. 10-51, left panel). The duration of the interval between A_2 and the opening snap correlates well with the level of left atrial pressure; the shorter the A_2-OS interval, the higher the left atrial pressure, and vice versa.[431,435,438] The S_1 is also loud when the stenotic valve is mobile and is usually preceded by a crescendo murmur. Although originally attributed to increased flow secondary to left atrial systole, phonoechocardiographic studies by Criley et al.[589] have suggested that this short "presystolic" murmur is actually due to high-velocity antegrade flow through a progressively narrowing mitral orifice during very early (isovolumic) ventricular systole (Fig. 10-51, left panel). This mechanism may also be responsible for the brief crescendo presystolic murmur observed in patients with mitral stenosis in atrial fibrillation following a short cycle length (Fig.

10-75).[586] The exact physical principles causing the production of this crescendo murmur are still in question, as a study by Hada and associates[587] has not confirmed high-velocity flow by Doppler echocardiography during the rapid closing motion of the stenotic mitral valve. Regardless of the exact mechanism, these sounds are dependent on the presence of antegrade mitral flow at the time of very early ventricular contraction.[588]

Although the intensity of the diastolic rumble in mitral stenosis correlates poorly with the severity of obstruction, there is an excellent correlation of severity with the duration of the murmur. When sinus tachycardia or rapid atrial fibrillation is present, a rumble starting with an opening snap and continuing to S_1 may not be meaningful because of the short diastolic time. Carotid sinus pressure may be very helpful in temporarily slowing the heart rate, thereby allowing the clinician to uncover the potential length of the rumble.

Obstruction of the mitral orifice can also be produced by a left atrial tumor. The diastolic murmur may be very similar to that produced by mitral stenosis, as shown in Fig. 10-51, center panel.[334] A loud tumor "plop" is present instead of the

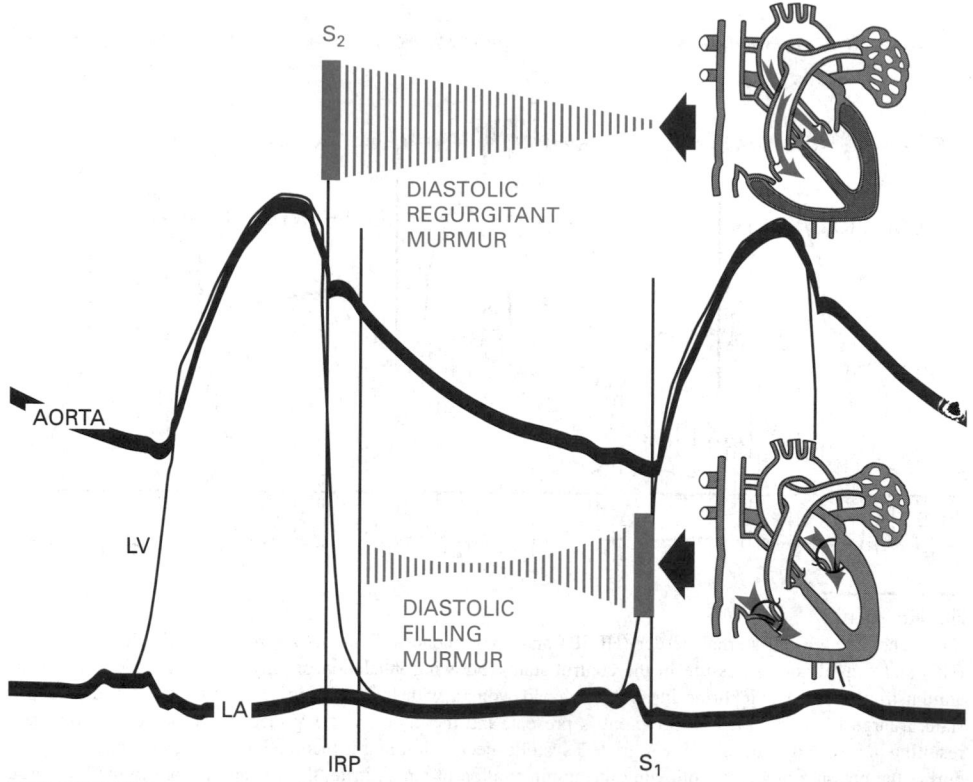

FIGURE 10-103

Diastolic filling murmurs or rumbles are caused by forward flow across the atrioventricular valves, whereas diastolic regurgitant murmurs are caused by retrograde flow across incompetent semilunar valves. *Left panel*: diagrammatic representation of the diastolic filling murmur and the diastolic regurgitant murmur as related to left ventricular (LV), aortic, and left atrial (LA) pressures. The diastolic filling murmur occurs during the diastolic filling period and is separated from S_2 by the isovolumic relaxation period. The rumbling murmur is most prominent during rapid, early ventricular filling and presystole, terminating with S_1. The diastolic regurgitant murmur begins immediately after S_2 and continues in a decrescendo fashion up to S_1, closely paralleling the aortic left ventricular diastolic pressure gradient. *Right panel*: flow diagram. (From Shaver JA. Diastolic murmurs. *Heart Dis Stroke* 1993; 1:98–103. Reproduced with permission from the American Heart Association.)

opening snap, and the presystolic crescendo murmur occurs as the protruding tumor mass returns rapidly through the mitral orifice into the left atrium during early ventricular systole. A systolic murmur of mitral regurgitation may also be present, and both murmurs may vary from examination to examination and with changes in body position.

The murmur of tricuspid stenosis is usually heard in the xiphoid area just off the sternal border. Since right atrial systole occurs earlier than left, the diastolic murmur of tricuspid stenosis may have a crescendo-decrescendo configuration (Fig. 10-104).[589] Even when the PR interval is normal, the presystolic accentuation of the diastolic rumble may terminate before S_1. Since tricuspid stenosis almost always occurs in the presence of mitral stenosis, this diastolic diamond-shaped murmur, which augments during inspiration, and the presence of large *a* waves in the jugular venous pulse are clues to this additional diagnosis.[590] When atrial fibrillation is present, the murmur is in middiastole and has the typical inspiratory augmentation. It is often very difficult to appreciate and must be carefully sought out, however, since both the presystolic murmur and large *a* waves alerting the clinician to this diag-

nosis are absent.[591] A tricuspid opening snap, which usually follows the mitral opening snap, may also be present and may initiate the murmur.[438]

DIASTOLIC RUMBLES DUE TO HIGH FLOW ACROSS THE ATRIOVENTRICULAR VALVES

High-velocity flow across the normal or insufficient AV valve may result in short middiastolic rumbles often accompanied by an S_3 and should not be confused with murmurs produced by true obstruction of the AV valves. Such rumbles are common in both ventricular septal defect and patent ductus arteriosus due to the large flow across the mitral valve secondary to the left-to-right shunt.[592,593] Likewise, the left-to-right shunt in a large atrial septal defect often produces a tricuspid rumble.[440] Similar low-pitched rumbling murmurs may also be present in hyperkinetic states. Common to all these conditions is high-volume flow during the latter phase of the rapid filling period. Phonoechocardiography has shown that these murmurs occur during the rapid closing motion of the mitral valve, suggesting a functional "obstruction" during the period of rapid early diastolic filling.[594] Identical phonoechocardiographic correlates have also been shown with mitral and tricuspid regurgitation, where early diastolic filling is also extremely rapid. With tricuspid regurgitation, the early rumble will increase with inspiration, typical of right-sided murmurs across the tricuspid valve. During rapid atrial fibrillation, ventriculogenic closure of the normal mitral valve during the rapid filling phase of a short cardiac cycle may cause a "presystolic" murmur by a similar mechanism (Fig. 10-105).

Mitral valvulitis during an episode of acute rheumatic fever may cause a short diastolic rumble, the Carey Coombs murmur.[595] This rumble, especially in children or in the presence of fever and anemia, may be introduced by an S_3 rather than by an opening snap. This combination of an S_3 with a short rumble indicates that there is not enough obstruction to the valve to alter the characteristics of rapid early ventricular filling.

The Austin Flint murmur, as originally described by Flint in 1862,[596] consisted of an apical presystolic murmur observed in two patients with considerable aortic regurgitation

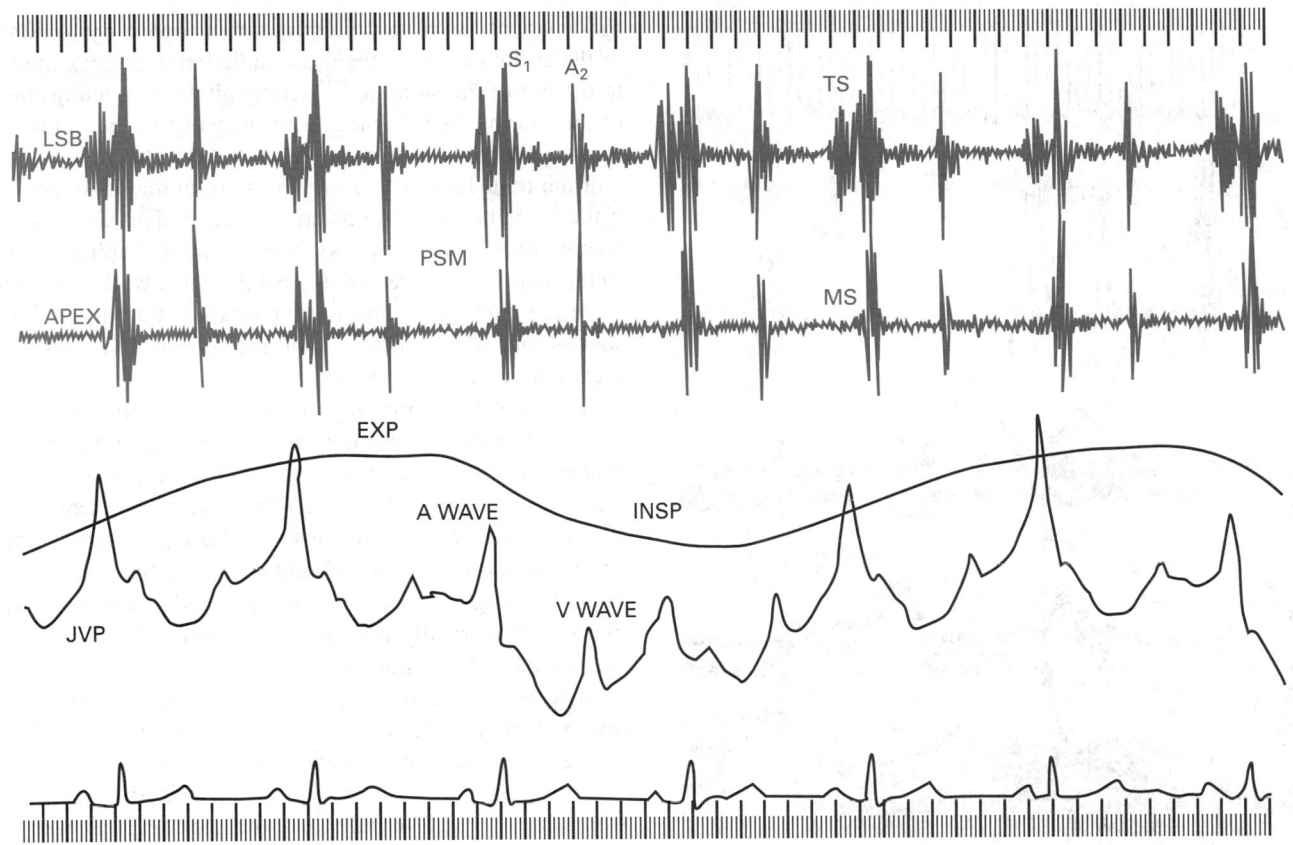

FIGURE 10-104

Phonocardiograms at the left sternal border (LSB) and apex are recorded together with the jugular venous pulse in a patient originally thought to have only mitral stenosis. The jugular venous pulse shows prominent *a* waves and the phonocardiogram at the LSB clearly shows inspiratory augmentation of a diamond-shaped presystolic murmur (TS) of tricuspid stenosis, in contrast to the apical mitral stenosis murmur (MS) that begins later and crescendos to S_1. (From Salerni R et al. Noninvasive graphic evaluation: Phonocardiography and echocardiography. In: Frankl WS, Brest AN, eds. *Cardiovascular Clinics: Valvular Heart Disease—Comprehensive Evaluation and Management*. Philadelphia: Davis, 1986:199. Reproduced with permission from the publisher and the authors.)

and no evidence of mitral stenosis at autopsy. Since its original description, the timing of this murmur has been extended to include a middiastolic component (Fig. 10-106). It is heard best at the apex and has many of the qualities of the murmur of mitral stenosis. It is introduced by an S_3 rather than by an opening snap, however, and S_1 is of normal or decreased amplitude.[597] Maneuvers or pharmacologic agents that increase the degree of aortic regurgitation, such as hand grip or vasoconstricting drugs, will increase the intensity of the rumble, while vasodilating agents such as amyl nitrite will decrease its intensity. In most cases of severe aortic regurgitation, particularly when the regurgitation is acute, the presystolic component of the Austin Flint murmur is lost (Fig. 10-54). In this situation, there is marked elevation of the left ventricular end-diastolic pressure (LVEDP), and the reverse pressure gradient between the left ventricle and left atrium causes premature closure of the mitral valve.

A complete understanding of the origin of this murmur is still forthcoming, but most investigators agree that it is not secondary to late diastolic mitral regurgitation or isolated vibrations of the mitral leaflets. Elegant phonoechocardiographic studies have shown that the murmur is associated with the rapid closing motion of the mitral valve leaflets during middiastole and presystole, presumably due to antegrade flow across a closing orifice in a manner similar to the flow rumble of AV valvular regurgitation and high-output states.[598,599] Austin Flint murmurs have been observed in the absence of rapid closing of the mitral valve, however, and Reddy et al.[600] have suggested that incomplete valve opening rather than excessively rapid closure rates may be the essential requirement for producing the increased mitral flow velocity. One echo-Doppler study has suggested that patients with an Austin Flint murmur usually have an aortic regurgitant jet aimed directly at the mitral valve, causing deformity and shuddering of the valve, in contrast to patients with equally severe regurgitation in whom the murmur is absent.[601] A combination of these factors is most likely responsible for the turbulence that occurs across the mitral valve when the regurgitant jet collides with the antegrade flow through the mitral orifice and with the mitral leaflets. Right-sided Austin Flint murmurs of similar quality have been reported in association with severe pulmonic regurgitation associated with pulmonary hypertension.[602] These murmurs have not been reported in organic pulmonic regurgitation with normal pulmonary artery pressures.

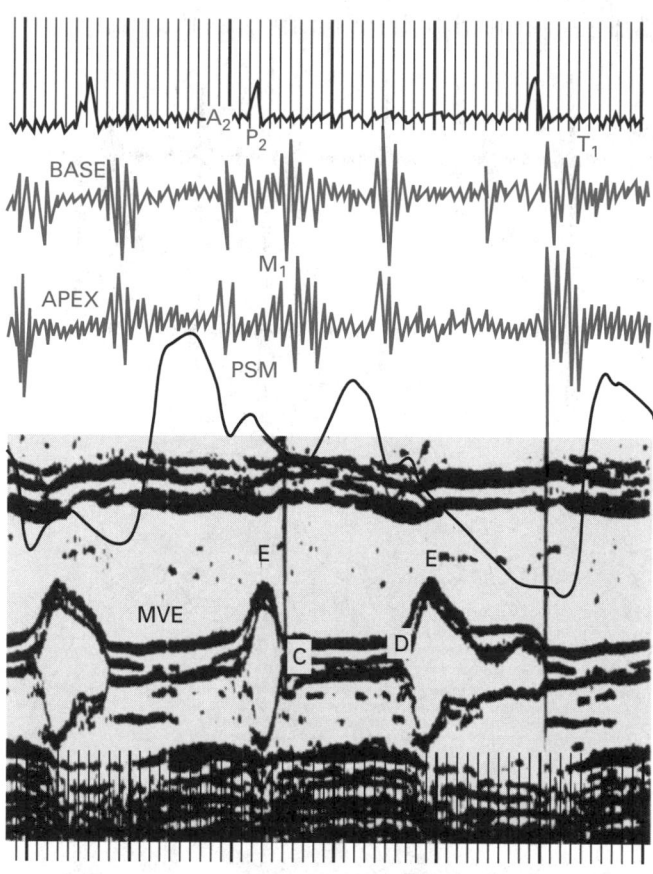

FIGURE 10-105

Phonoechocardiogram showing the mechanism of the presystolic murmur (PSM) in rapid atrial fibrillation without obstruction at the mitral valve. A rapidly closing normal mitral valve causes a crescendo murmur in complex 2. This finding is not present at longer cycle lengths. (From Salerni R et al. Noninvasive graphic evaluation: Phonocardiography and echocardiography. In: Frankl WS, Brest AN, eds. *Cardiovascular Clinics: Valvular Heart Disease—Comprehensive Evaluation and Management.* Philadelphia: Davis; 1986:178. Reproduced with permission from the publisher and the authors.)

Diastolic Regurgitant Murmurs

HOLODIASTOLIC AORTIC REGURGITANT MURMURS

The early diastolic murmur of aortic regurgitation is blowing and high-pitched in character and if often more difficult to record than to hear because of its high-frequency content. Since isovolumic relaxation of the left ventricle is very rapid, a large gradient quickly develops between the aortic and left ventricular diastolic pressures, and the murmur builds up to maximum intensity almost immediately after A_2. As diastole progresses, the gradient between the two chambers slowly falls, and the murmur envelope closely parallels the pressure drop in a decrescendo fashion up to S_1 (Figs. 10-91 and 10-106). When the aortic regurgitation is valvular in origin, the murmur is usually best heard at the third and fourth left parasternal areas. The finding that the murmur is heard best to the right of the sternum should alert the clinician to an aortic root etiology of the regurgitation.[603] It should be pointed out that this finding is helpful only if present, as

most patients with aortic regurgitation secondary to dilation of the aortic root have the usual radiation with peak intensity to the left of the sternum.[604] Although the frequency content of the murmur is in a range advantageous to the human ear, the amplitude of the vibrations may be quite small and the murmur quite faint. Therefore, the murmur may be overlooked if the examiner does not listen with the patient sitting up and leaning forward and does not listen with the diaphragm of the stethoscope firmly pressed against the chest wall. In addition, since the pitch of the murmur approaches that of respiratory sounds, one should listen while the patient holds his or her breath after deep expiration.

The degree of aortic regurgitation is directly proportional to the pressure head driving the flow in a retrograde fashion. Maneuvers or pharmacologic agents that increase or decrease the diastolic aortic–left ventricular pressure gradient will increase or decrease the intensity of the regurgitant murmur. Prompt squatting will often bring out a very faint aortic regurgitant blowing murmur at the bedside, and inhalation of amyl nitrite will markedly decrease its intensity. It should be remembered that the murmur of mild aortic regurgitation often disappears during the latter stages of pregnancy due to the low peripheral vascular resistance. As shown in Fig. 10-91, pure aortic regurgitation without associated valvular stenosis may present with a prominent systolic ejection murmur as well as an Austin Flint rumble at the apex (Fig. 10-106). The carotid pulse is rapid-rising and has a large volume. The A_2 is often diminished or even absent when the regurgitation is valvular in origin, due to inadequate coaptation and checking of the retrograde blood column by the deformed leaflets.[605]

The etiology of the aortic regurgitation usually cannot be determined by the quality of the murmur. An exception to this rule is the presence of a "cooing dove" or musical diastolic murmur, which usually denotes a rupture or retroversion of an aortic cusp. Such ruptures occur secondary to trauma, bacterial endocarditis, and occasionally in the presence of arteriosclerotic involvement of the aortic valve.[502] Retroversion and subsequent rupture of the aortic valve with a musical murmur is also a complication of syphilitic aortic regurgitation[606] (see also Chap. 63).

ABBREVIATED AORTIC DIASTOLIC REGURGITANT MURMUR

The murmur of very mild aortic regurgitation may be abbreviated and may end by middiastole. This is particularly true of the functional aortic regurgitant murmur of systemic arterial hypertension. As the volume of blood in the aorta decreases during diastole, the aortic ring becomes smaller and coupled with the decreasing aortic-left ventricular diastolic gradient, retrograde flow ceases, and the murmur disappears.

The murmur of aortic regurgitation may also be abbreviated if the aortic regurgitation is acute.[343] Acute regurgitation of blood into a ventricle that has not had time to adapt to a large-volume load results in marked elevation of the LVEDP and equilibration of the aortic and left ventricular diastolic pressures. With this, retrograde flow ceases and the murmur disappears in the latter part of diastole, as demonstrated in

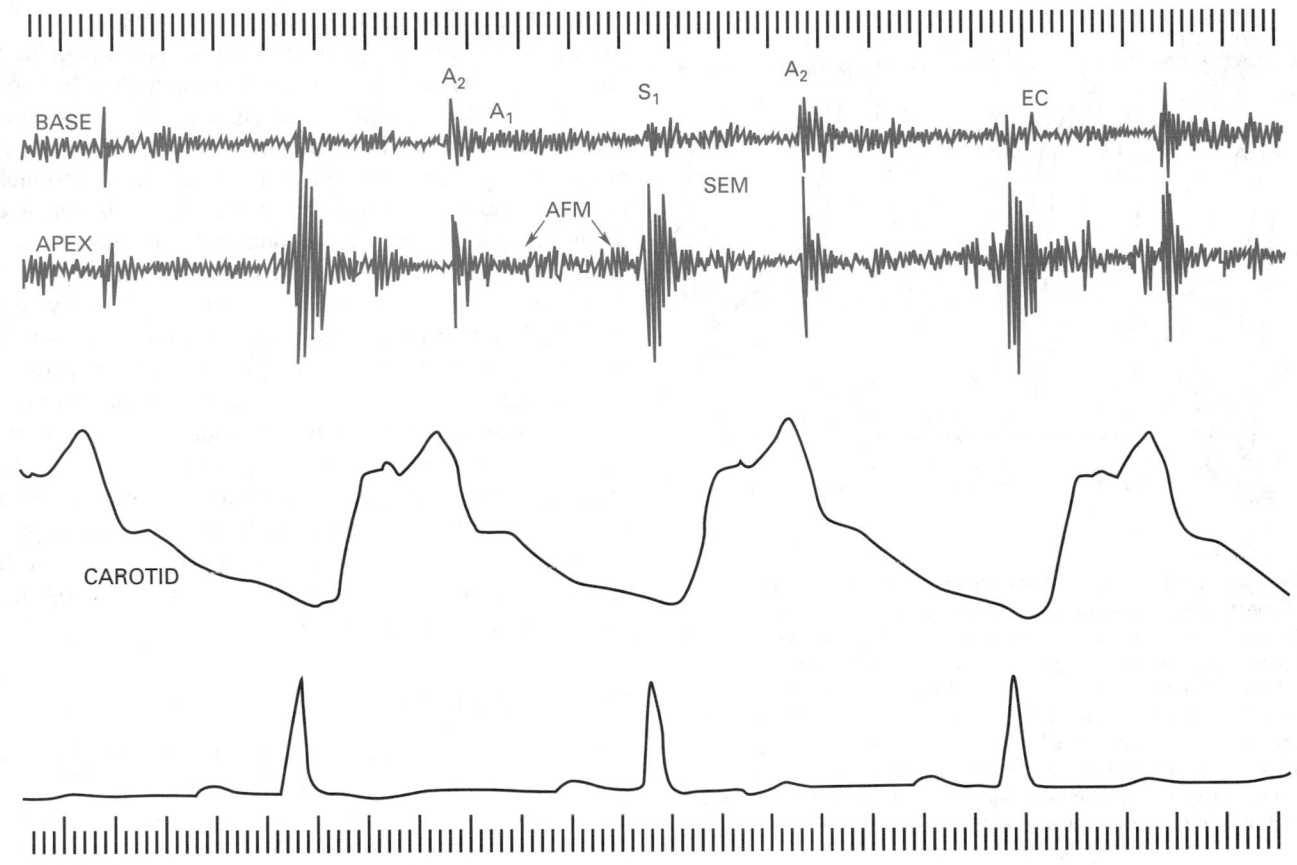

FIGURE 10-106

The early diastolic and presystolic component of the Austin Flint murmur (AFM) is recorded in a 26-year-old man with chronic aortic regurgitation. S_1 and S_2 are normal. A soft ejection click (EC) introduces a systolic ejection murmur (SEM), the latter being due to the increased forward stroke volume. The early diastolic murmur at the base (AI) begins with A_2 and extends through most of diastole. The carotid pulse is full, with a wide pulse pressure.

(From Salerni R et al. Noninvasive graphic evaluation: Phonocardiography and echocardiography. In: Frankl WS, Brest AN, eds. *Cardiovascular Clinics: Valvular Heart Disease—Comprehensive Evaluation and Management*. Philadelphia: Davis; 1986:193. Reproduced with permission from the publisher and the authors.)

Fig. 10-107. In the syndrome of acute aortic regurgitation, there may be preclosure of the mitral valve, resulting in a soft or absent S_1 as well as absence of the presystolic component of the Austin Flint murmur (Fig. 10-54). The auscultatory findings of acute versus chronic aortic regurgitation are contrasted in Fig. 10-108. Common causes of acute aortic regurgitation include aortic valve endocarditis, trauma, acute aortic dissection, and dehiscence of an aortic valve prosthesis (see also Chap. 63).

HOLODIASTOLIC PULMONIC REGURGITANT MURMUR

Pulmonic regurgitation is most commonly found in the setting of severe pulmonary hypertension and dilation of the pulmonary artery with inadequate coaptation of the leaflets of the pulmonic valve. The functional murmur of pulmonic regurgitation (Graham Steell murmur)[607] is similar in both frequency and contour to that of aortic regurgitation because the hemodynamics responsible for their production are identical. These murmurs cannot be differentiated by either their quality or location on the chest wall. Thus, the differential diagnosis is made by the "company the murmur keeps," and when associ-

ated with the peripheral signs of hemodynamically significant aortic regurgitation or with the findings of severe pulmonary hypertension, there is rarely a problem. However, when rheumatic mitral stenosis is the primary lesion, the semilunar regurgitant murmur may be secondary either to associated rheumatic aortic regurgitation or to the Graham Steell murmur if the pulmonary hypertension is severe. Careful investigation of the semilunar blowing murmur in the setting of mitral stenosis has shown that it is almost always due to aortic regurgitation, even when significant pulmonary hypertension is present.[608] More common causes of the Graham Steell murmur of functional pulmonary regurgitation are primary pulmonary hypertension and Eisenmenger's syndrome.

Early diastolic murmurs are occasionally heard in end-stage renal failure, particularly when there is concurrent anemia, hypertension, and fluid overload. Doppler echocardiography demonstrated that these murmurs are usually pulmonic in origin.[609] They are often transient in nature and are related to fluid overload. Such murmurs are diminished by extracellular fluid removal and reflect correctable pulmonary hypertension.[609]

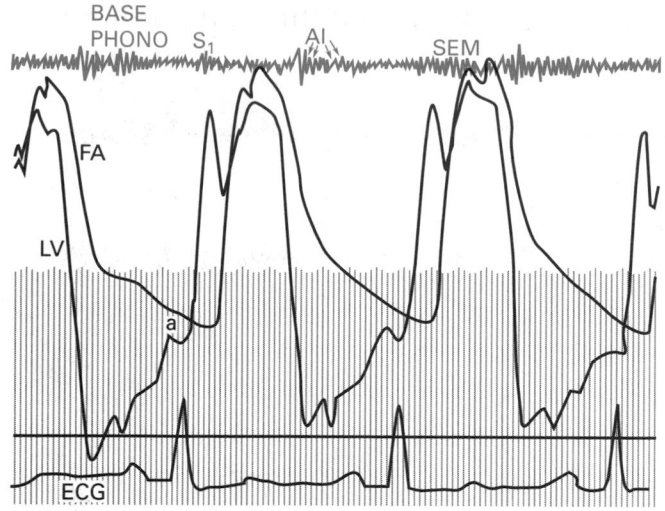

FIGURE 10-107

The base phonocardiogram is recorded simultaneously with the left ventricular and femoral artery pressures in a patient with acute aortic regurgitation, producing a number of atypical auscultatory findings as compared with chronic compensated aortic regurgitation. There is marked elevation of the LVEDP to 32 mmHg, with equilibration of the aortic and LVEDPs. With this equilibration of pressures, there is abbreviation of the aortic regurgitation murmur with a silent gap before S_1. The decreased intensity of S_1 is due to partial preclosure of the mitral valve secondary to the elevated LVEDP owing to regurgitant flow into a noncompliant left ventricle. (From Shaver JA. Current uses of phonocardiography in clinical practice. In Rapaport E, ed. *Cardiology Update—Reviews for Physicians.* New York: Elsevier; 1981:338. Reproduced with permission from the publisher and the author. Copyright 1981 by Elsevier Science Publishing Co., Inc.)

DELAYED PULMONIC REGURGITANT MURMUR

The murmur of organic pulmonary regurgitation is quite different in quality and duration as compared to either aortic regurgitation or the Graham Steell murmur of pulmonary hypertension.[610] As shown in Fig. 10-109, the murmur is delayed from P_2 by a short interval and then builds up quickly to a crescendo followed by a decrescendo that ends well before S_1. In organic pulmonic regurgitation, the pulmonary artery pressure may be normal, and the diastolic gradient between the pulmonary artery and right ventricle may be very small, resulting in low-velocity retrograde flow and a lower-pitched murmur. The murmur is heard only during the period of maximal gradient in early and middiastole, as the pulmonary artery pressure begins to equilibrate with the right ventricular end-diastolic pressure in the latter part of diastole. This type of murmur may be congenital or acquired, as with pulmonary valve endocarditis, carcinoid syndrome, or surgical procedures on the pulmonic valve. It is often associated with a prominent systolic ejection murmur secondary to the large right ventricular stroke volume.

Continuous Murmurs

A continuous murmur is defined as one that begins in systole and extends through S_2 into part or all of diastole.[495] It need not occupy the entire cardiac cycle; therefore, a systolic murmur that extends into diastole without stopping at S_2 is considered to be continuous even if it fades completely before the subsequent S_1. A physiologic classification of continuous murmurs as described by Myers[611] is detailed in Table 10-10.

CONTINUOUS MURMURS DUE TO RAPID BLOOD FLOW

High-velocity blood flow through veins and arteries may cause a continuous murmur. The cervical venous hum is a continuous murmur with diastolic accentuation and is easily heard in almost all children.[612] This murmur can also be heard in healthy adults and is present in nearly all women in the later stages of pregnancy. High cardiac output states such as thyrotoxicosis and anemia are also associated with easily heard venous hums. This murmur is usually poorly heard in the supine position, and its presence in this position in an adult strongly suggests a hyperdynamic circulatory state. Peak intensity is in the supraclavicular fossa just lateral to the sternocleidomastoid muscle, and it is usually more prominent on the right side. When the murmur

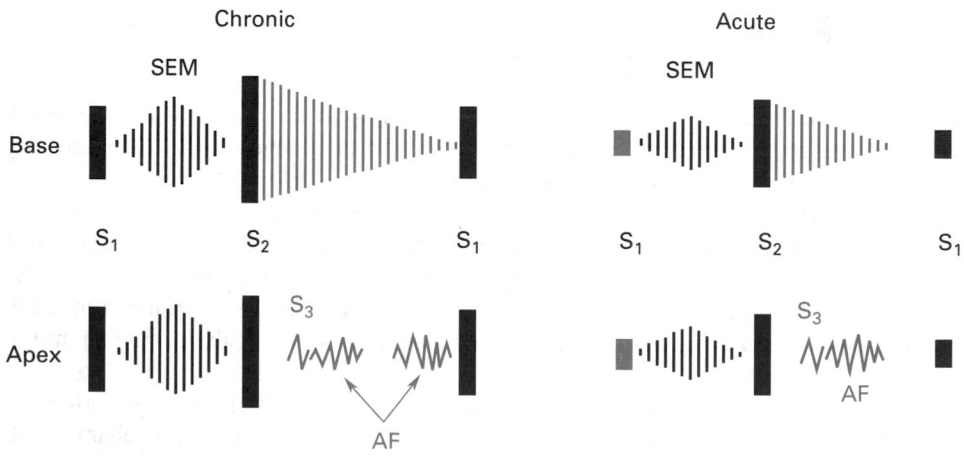

FIGURE 10-108

Diagram contrasting the auscultatory findings in chronic and acute aortic regurgitation. In chronic aortic regurgitation, a prominent systolic ejection murmur (SEM), resulting from the large forward stroke volume, is heard at the base, apex, and ends well before S_2. The aortic diastolic regurgitant murmur begins with S_2 and continues in a decrescendo fashion, terminating before S_1. At the apex, the early diastolic component of the Austin Flint murmur (AF) is introduced by a prominent S_3. A presystolic component of the AF is also heard. In acute aortic regurgitation, there is a significant decrease in the intensity of the SEM compared with chronic aortic regurgitation because of the decreased forward stroke volume. S_1 is markedly decreased in intensity because of preclosure of the mitral valve, and at the apex the presystolic component of the AF murmur is absent. The early diastolic murmur at the base ends well before S_1 because of the equilibration of the left ventricular and aortic end-diastolic pressure. Significant tachycardia is usually present. (From Shaver JA. Diastolic murmurs. *Heart Dis Stroke* 1993; 1:98–103. Reproduced with permission from the American Heart Association.)

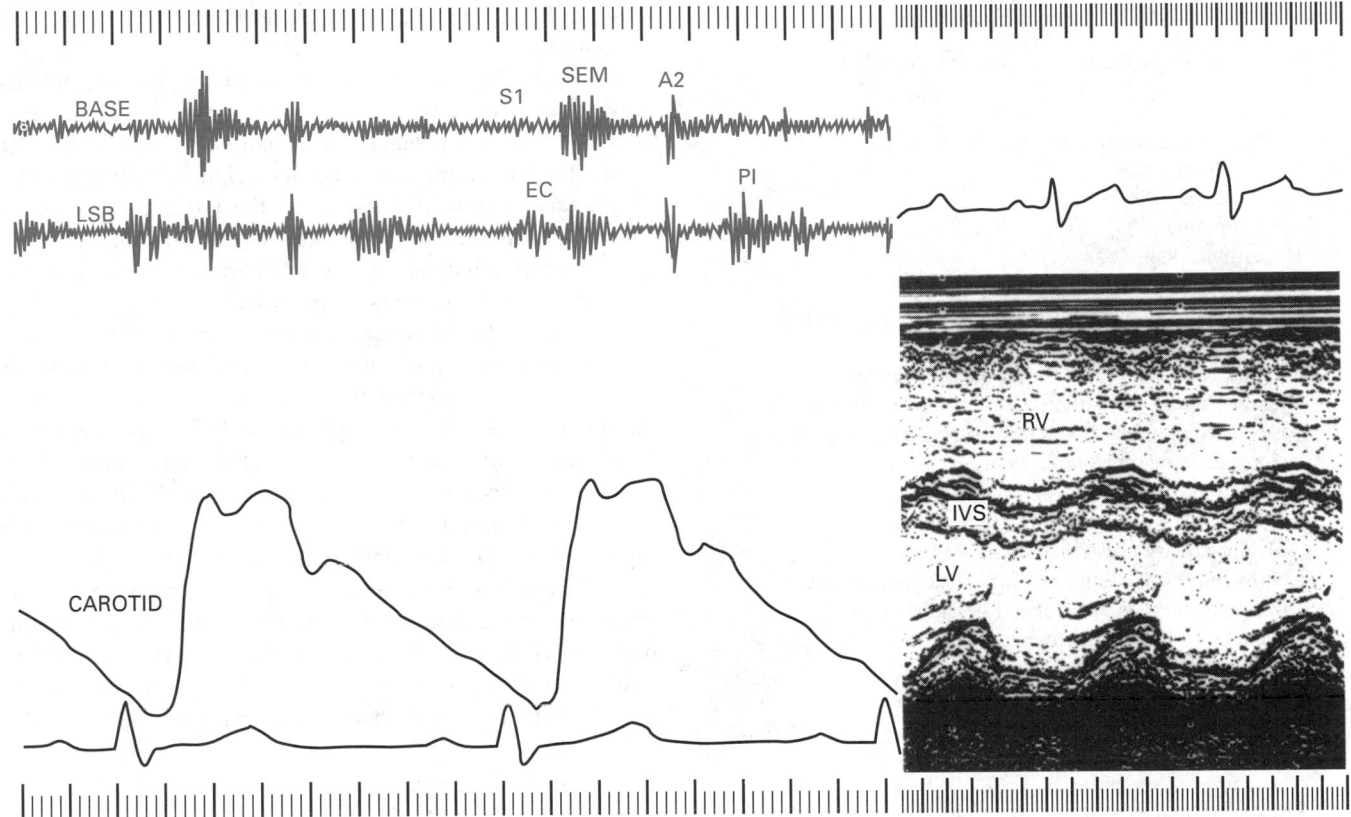

FIGURE 10-109

Phonocardiogram and echocardiogram of a 32-year-old man with organic pulmonic regurgitation. At the left sternal border (LSB), a middiastolic diamond-shaped murmur (PI) that is delayed from the soft P_2 is typical of organic pulmonic regurgitation. A prominent systolic ejection murmur is present due to the increased stroke volume across the right ventricular outflow tract. The echocardiogram shows a dilated right ventricle (RV) and a paradoxical septal motion of right ventricular volume overload. (From Salerni R et al. Noninvasive graphic evaluation: Phonocardiography and echocardiography. In: Frankl WS, Brest AN, eds. *Cardiovascular Clinics: Valvular Heart Disease—Comprehensive Evaluation and Management.* Philadelphia: Davis; 1986:206. Reproduced with permission from the publisher and the authors.)

is loud, it may radiate below the clavicles and occasionally can be confused with the continuous murmur of patent ductus arteriosus. This error should never be made, however, because the cervical venous hum can easily be terminated by digital compression of the jugular venous pulse.

The mammary souffle is another example of a continuous murmur occurring in 10 to 15 percent of pregnant women during the second and third trimesters and in the early postpartum period, particularly in lactating women, and is heard between the second and sixth anterior intercostal spaces.[613] This murmur may be obliterated by firm pressure on the stethoscope or by digital pressure applied just lateral to the site of auscultation and should therefore not be confused with the continuous murmur of patent ductus arteriosus or with arteriovenous fistula.[592] The mammary souffle disappears after termination of lactation. Other causes of continuous murmurs due to rapid blood flow through arterial or venous channels are outlined in Table 10-10.

CONTINUOUS MURMURS DUE TO HIGH-TO-LOW–PRESSURE SHUNTS

A group of congenital cardiovascular anomalies has shunting from the high-pressure systemic (aortic) circulation to the low-pressure pulmonary arterial circulation, resulting in a large gradient between the two systems throughout the cardiac cycle. The murmur of patent ductus arteriosus is the classic example of this type of anomaly (Fig. 10-110). It is heard best in the left infraclavicular area and the second left intercostal space. The peak intensity of the murmur is at the time of S_2, after which it gradually wanes until it terminates before S_1.[318] The length of the murmur is determined by the difference in the vascular resistance between the greater and lesser circulation.[406] As the pulmonary vascular resistance increases, the diastolic pressure in the pulmonary artery approaches and finally reaches systemic levels, diminishing and finally abolishing diastolic flow and the diastolic portion of the murmur. With equilibration of aortic and pulmonary artery pressure, systolic flow across the shunt diminishes and finally disappears, leaving the ductus silent [Eisenmenger's patent ductus arteriosus (PDA)]. Surgically produced aortopulmonary connections (Blalock, Waterston, or Pott's shunts) as well as the murmur of aortic pulmonary window have identical qualities, and the effect of pulmonary hypertension on their length is analogous. It is important to distinguish these types of continuous murmurs from to-and-fro murmurs. The latter is a combination of the systolic ejection murmur and a semilunar

TABLE 10-10

PHYSIOLOGIC CLASSIFICATION OF CONTINUOUS MURMURS

Continuous murmurs due to rapid blood flow
  Venous hum
  Mammary souffle
  Hemiangioma
  Hyperthyroidism
  Acute alcoholic hepatitis
  Hyperemia of neoplasm (hepatoma renal cell carcinoma, Paget's disease)
Continuous murmurs due to high-to-low pressure shunts
  Systemic artery to pulmonary artery (patent ductus arteriosus, aortopulmonary window, truncus arteriosus, pulmonary atresia, anomalous left coronary, bronchiectasis, sequestration of the lung)
  Systemic artery to right heart (ruptured sinus of Valsalva, coronary artery fistula)
  Left-to-right atrial shunting (Lutembacher's syndrome, mitral atresia plus atrial septal defect)
  Venovenous shunts (anomalous pulmonary veins, portosystemic shunts)
  Arteriovenous fistula (systemic or pulmonic)
Continuous murmurs secondary to localized arterial obstruction
  Coarctation of the aorta
  Branch pulmonary stenosis
  Carotid occlusion
  Celiac mesenteric occlusion
  Renal occlusion
  Femoral occlusion
  Coronary occlusion

Source: From Myers JD. The mechanisms and significances of continuous murmurs. In: Leon DF, Shaver JA (eds). *Physiologic Principles of Heart Sounds and Murmurs*. Monograph 46. New York: American Heart Association; 1975:202. Reproduced with permission from the American Heart Association, Inc., and author.

diastolic murmur. The classic example of a to-and-fro murmur is the murmur of aortic stenosis and regurgitation. The continuous murmur builds to a crescendo around S_2, whereas the to-and-fro murmur has two components. The midsystolic ejection component decrescendos and may disappear as it approaches S_2, leaving a silent period before the onset of the regurgitant murmur (Fig. 10-91). Truncus arteriosus is a rare congenital anomaly and probably produces a continuous murmur only if there is coexisting pulmonary artery stenosis. In the presence of severe right ventricular outflow obstruction, bronchial collateral arteries can enlarge their normal precapillary anastomoses with pulmonary arteries, and the resultant aortic pulmonary fistula can produce a continuous murmur. This murmur can be heard in the same location as the patent ductus but radiates widely, especially over the posterior thorax. Large bronchial collateral arteries producing such continuous murmurs are more common with pulmonary atresia but also occur with tetralogy of Fallot.[616] Bronchial artery–pulmonary artery collaterals sufficient to produce continuous murmurs are also found in far advanced bronchiectasis[617] and sequestration of the lung.

An anomalous left coronary artery arising from the pulmonary artery may cause a continuous murmur when the left-to-right shunt flow is large; it is usually best heard at the left sternal border. In this condition, the origin of the right coronary artery is from the aorta, and the left-to-right shunt is from the high-pressure right coronary arterial bed through large arterial collaterals to the left coronary system, which empties into the low-pressure pulmonary artery.

Sinus of Valsalva aneurysms may cause continuous murmurs when they rupture into the right heart. In almost all cases, rupture occurs from the right and noncoronary sinuses into the right atrium or the right ventricle.[618] The murmur is heard maximally at the lower sternal border or xiphoid over the area corresponding to the fistulous tract.[581] Diastolic accentuation of this murmur is an important sign to differentiate ruptured sinus from patent ductus arteriosus or AV fistula. Systolic suppression of the murmur is due to both mechanical narrowing of the fistulous tract during systole as well as the probable Venturi effect created by the rapid ejection of blood past the aortic origin of the fistula.[581] The continuous murmur may be very loud and occasionally can be heard from the foot of the bed.

Coronary artery fistulas usually empty into the right atrium or ventricle and cause a continuous murmur that is best heard to either the left or the right of the lower sternal area. Since the majority of coronary flow occurs during diastole, the diastolic component of the murmur is louder. When the coronary artery fistula empties into a high-pressure right ventricle, only a diastolic murmur may be heard because the pressure gradient across the shunt is reduced during systole. Left-to-right shunting through an uncomplicated atrial septal defect produces no murmur audible on the chest wall because of the minimal pressure gradient and absence of turbulence. When mitral valve obstruction is present, as with Lutembacher's syndrome or mitral atresia, however, there can be a high-pressure gradient between the left and right atria across a small defect, and a continuous murmur may be present.[619] This murmur increases in intensity with inspiration and decreases with the Valsalva maneuver. Occasionally, a small atrial septal defect is produced following transseptal catheterization or balloon valvuloplasty for mitral stenosis, and a continuous murmur is produced due to high-velocity flow resulting from the large pressure gradient from left to right atrium. This is especially likely to occur if the mitral obstruction is not adequately relieved by the balloon valvuloplasty.

Total anomalous pulmonary venous drainage into a systemic vein may produce a continuous venous hum usually heard in the pulmonary area or the left infraclavicular area.[620] Frequently, a constriction at the junction of the anomalous venous conduit and the innominate vein or superior vena cava may cause augmentation of the murmur.

Arteriovenous fistulas between peripheral vessels produce a classic continuous murmur with systolic accentuation caused by shunting of a large volume of blood at rapid flow rates

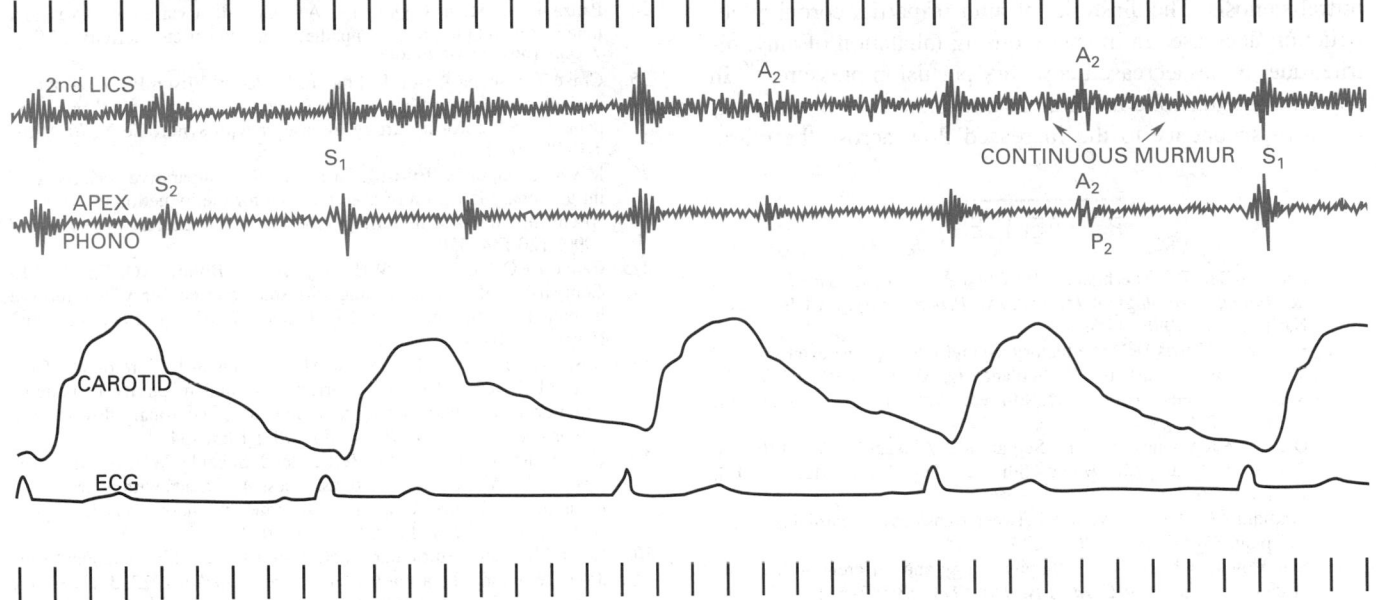

FIGURE 10-110

The classic contour of a continuous murmur of a large patent ductus arteriosus (PDA) as recorded at the second intercostal space. The murmur begins in systole, peaks at S_2, and continues in a decrescendo manner during diastolic runoff. The carotic pulse in prominent, with a prolonged left ventricular ejection time. (From Shaver JA. Current uses of phonocardiography in clinical practice. In Rapaport E, ed. *Cardiology Update—Reviews for Physicians*. New York: Elsevier; 1981:366. Reproduced with permission from the publisher and the author. Copyright 1981 by Elsevier Science Publishing Co., Inc.)

from a high-pressure artery into a low-pressure vein. These murmurs are best heard at the site of the fistula. Local compression of the veins may decrease the intensity of the murmur by raising venous pressure and reducing the arteriovenous pressure gradient. Complete obliteration of the fistula will terminate the murmur, and if the shunt is of considerable magnitude, a baroreceptor-mediated reflex bradycardia may occur (Branham's sign). Likewise, a reflex tachycardia will occur upon release of the obstruction. Pulmonary arteriovenous fistulas usually produce only a systolic murmur because the peripheral vascular resistance of the normal lung is very low, and the normally small diastolic pressure gradient from pulmonary artery to pulmonary vein is not significantly increased by the presence of the fistula.[611]

CONTINUOUS MURMUR SECONDARY TO LOCALIZED ARTERIAL OBSTRUCTION

Localized stenosis of systemic or pulmonary arteries may produce a continuous murmur or bruit if the obstruction is critical and adequate collateral flow is not available.[621] Most partially obstructed arteries have only systolic murmurs that are delayed relative to cardiac systole, depending upon the transit time of pulsatile flow from the heart to the site of obstruction. Edholm and associates[622] have shown that a considerable systolic pressure gradient exists across partial arterial obstructions, but there is usually no diastolic gradient. This lack of diastolic gradient was explained by the fact that the collateral arteries around the obstruction deliver adequate flow such that the diastolic pressure on either side of the localized obstruction is essentially equal. Thus, a localized,

partial arterial obstruction characteristically produces only a systolic murmur or bruit. If adequate collateral flow is not present, however, a diastolic and a systolic pressure gradient can be produced, together with a continuous murmur with systolic accentuation. Depending on the degree of inadequacy of collaterals, the murmur is truly continuous when collateral circulation is essentially nonexistent or it extends only partially through diastole when collateral flow is somewhat compromised. Such is the case in severe coarctation of the aorta, where, in addition to the systolic and/or continuous murmurs heard over the thorax and produced by rapid blood flow through the tortuous intercostal collaterals, a continuous murmur may be produced at the site of the coarctation.[623] This latter murmur is best heard over the back midline between the scapulae.

Continuous murmurs may also arise from branch pulmonary stenosis or partial obstruction of a major pulmonary artery occluded by a massive pulmonary embolus. Other common locations of continuous murmurs secondary to localized arterial obstructions are listed in Table 10-10. Common to all these murmurs is critical narrowing of the vessel with inadequate collateral flow, such that a continuous pressure gradient is produced throughout the cardiac cycle. Murmurs produced by obstruction of major coronary arteries are rarely loud enough to be transmitted to the chest wall. When audible, they produce only diastolic murmurs, even with inadequate collateral circulation.[624,625] This is because most coronary flow normally occurs during diastole due to the high wall tension in the left ventricle during systole. Inhalation of amyl nitrite is helpful in differentiating this murmur from that of mitral stenosis. The diastolic murmur of partial coronary obstruction decreases in intensity during inhalation of amyl nitrite, due to the decreased coronary perfusion pressure.[626] In contrast, the diastolic murmur of mitral stenosis increases in intensity secondary to the increased flow across the mitral valve.

REFERENCES

1. Vanden Belt RJ. The history. In: Chizner M, ed. *Classic Teachings in Clinical Cardiology: A Tribute to W. Proctor Harvey.* Cedar Grove, NJ: Laennec; 1996:41–54.
2. Hurst JW, Morris DC. The history: Symptoms and past events related to cardiovascular disease. In: Schlant RC, Alexander RW, O'Rourke RA, et al., eds. *The Heart,* 8th ed. New York: McGraw-Hill; 1994:205–216.
3. O'Rourke RA. Chest pain. In: Schlant RC, Alexander RW, O'Rourke RA, et al., eds. *The Heart,* 8th ed. New York: McGraw-Hill; 1994:459–467.
4. Malliani AM. The elusive link between transient myocardial ischemia and pain. *Circulation* 1986; 73:201–204.
5. Sampson JJ, Cheitlin M. Pathophysiology and differential diagnosis of cardiac pain. *Prog Cardiovasc Dis* 1971; 13:507–531.
6. O'Rourke RA. Diagnostic approach to the patient with chest pain compatible with definite or suspected angina pectoris. In: Sobel BE, ed. *Medical Management of Heart Disease.* New York: Marcel Dekker; 1996:4–22.
7. Heberden W: Some accounts of a disorder of the breast. *Med Trans* 1772; 2:59.
8. Murray DR, O'Rourke RA, Walling AD, Walsh RA: History and physical examination in myocardial ischemia and acute myocardial infarction. In Francis G, Alpert J, eds. *Coronary Care,* 2d ed. Boston: Little Brown; 1995:73–95.
9. Levine HJ. Difficult problems in the diagnosis of chest pain. *Am Heart J* 1980; 100:108–118.
10. Dell'Italia LJ. Chest pain. In: Stein JH, ed. *Internal Medicine,* 4th ed. Boston: Little, Brown, 1994:86–91.
11. Christie LG Jr, Conti CR. Systemic approach to evaluation of angina-like chest pain: Pathophysiology and clinical testing with emphasis on objective documentation of myocardial ischemia. *Am Heart J* 1981; 102:897–912.
12. Oram S, Souton E. Tobacco angina. *Q J Med* 1963; 32:115–120.
13. Campeau L. Letter to the editor. *Circulation* 1976; 54:522.
14. Levine SA. Carotid sinus massage: A new diagnostic test for angina pectoris. *JAMA* 1962; 182:1332–1356.
15. Douglas PS, Ginsberg GS. The evaluation of chest pain in women. *N Engl J Med* 1996; 334:1311–1315.
16. Chauhan A, Mullins PA, Taylor G, Petch MC, Schofield PM. Cardio-esophageal reflex: A mechanism for "linked angina" in patients with angiographically proven coronary artery disease. *J Am Coll Cardiol* 1996; 27:1621–1628.
17. Epstein SE, Talbot TL. Dynamic coronary tone in precipitation, exacerbation and relief of angina pectoris. *Am J Cardiol* 1981; 48:797–803.
18. Proudfit WL, Shrey ED, Sones FM Jr. Selective cine coronary arteriography: Correlation with clinical findings in 1000 patients. *Circulation* 1996; 33:901–910.
19. Ockene IS, Shay MJ, Alpert JS, Weiner BH, Dalen JE. Unexplained chest pain in patients with normal coronary arteriograms. *N Engl J Med* 1980; 303:1249–1258.
20. Braschke AVG, Proudfit WL, Sones FM. Clinical course of patients with normal coronary arteriograms and chest pain resembling angina pectoris. *Am J Cardiol* 1971; 28:25–32.
21. Waxler EB, Kimbiris D, Driefus LS. The fate of women with normal coronary arteriograms and chest pain resembling angina pectoris. *Am J Cardiol* 1971; 28:25–32.
22. Cannon RO III: Microvascular angina: Cardiovascular investigations regarding pathophysiology and management. *Med Clin North Am* 1991; 75:1097–1118.
23. Cannon RO III, Cattau EL Jr, Yakshe PN, Maher K, Schenke WH, Benjamin SB, et al. Coronary flow reserve, esophageal motility, and chest pain in patients with angiographically normal coronary arteries. *Am J Med* 1990; 88:217–222.
24. Panza JA, Epstein S, Quyyumi AA. Circadian variation in vascular tone and its relation to α-sympathetic vasoconstrictor activity. *N Engl J Med* 1991; 325:986–990.
25. Crake T, Canepa-Anson R, Shapiro L, Poole-Wilson PA. Continuous recording of coronary sinus oxygen saturation during atrial pacing in patients with coronary artery disease or with syndrome X. *Br Heart J* 1988; 59:31–38.
26. Miwa K, Fujita M, Ejiri M, Sasayama S. Comparative sensitivity of intracoronary injection of acetylcholine for the induction of coronary spasm in patients with various types of angina pectoris. *Am Heart J* 1990; 120:544–550.
27. Cannon RO III, Schenk WH, Quyyumi A, Bonow RO, Epstein SE. Comparison of exercise testing with studies of coronary flow reserve in patients with microvascular angina. *Circulation* 1991; 83(suppl III):III-77–III-81.
28. Kaski JC, Tousoulis D, Galassi AR, McFadden E, Pereira WI, Crea P, et al. Epicardial coronary artery tone and reactivity in patients with normal coronary arteriograms and reduced coronary flow reserve (syndrome X). *J Am Coll Cardiol* 1991; 18:50–54.
29. Cannon RO III, Peden DB, Berkebile C, Schenke WH, Kaliner MA, Epstein SE. Airway hyperresponsiveness in patients with microvascular angina: Evidence for a diffuse disorder of smooth muscle responsiveness. *Circulation* 1990; 82:2011–2017.
30. Kemp HG. Left ventricular function in patients with the anginal syndrome and normal coronary arteries. *Am J Cardiol* 1973; 32:375–376.
31. Abrogast R, Bourassa MG. Myocardial function during atrial pacing in patients with angina pectoris and normal coronary arteriograms. *Am J Cardiol* 1973; 32:257–263.
32. Attilio M. Syndrome X: Still an appropriate name. *J Am Coll Cardiol* 1991; 17:1471–1472.
33. Levy RD, Cunningham D, Shapiro LM, Wright C, Mockus L, Fox KM. Diurnal variation in left ventricular function: A study of patients with myocardial ischaemia, syndrome X, and of normal controls. *Br Heart J* 1987; 57:148–153.
34. Turiel M, Galassi AR, Glazier JJ, Kaski JC, Maseri A. Pain threshold and tolerance in women with syndrome X and women with stable angina pectoris. *Am J Cardiol* 1987; 60:503–507.
35. Spinelli L, Ferro G, Genovese A, Ginquegrana G, Spadafora M, Condorelli M. Exercise-induced impairment of diastolic time in patients with X syndrome. *Am Heart J* 1990; 119:829–833.
36. Kern MJ. Extracting the coronary artery from syndrome X: Is epicardial vasomotion physiologic in patients with normal coronary arteriograms and reduced coronary flow reserve? *J Am Coll Cardiol* 1991; 18:55–56.
37. Opherk DO, Schuler G, Wetterauer K, Mathey J, Schwarz F, Kubler W. Four-year follow-up study in patients with angina pectoris and normal coronary arteriograms ("syndrome X"). *Circulation* 1989; 80:1610–1616.
38. Galassi AR, Kaski JC, Pupita G, Margarita V, Crea F, Maseri A. Lack of evidence for alpha-adrenergic receptor-mediated mechanisms in the genesis of ischemia in syndrome X. *Am J Cardiol* 1989; 64:264–269.
39. Epstein SE, Cannon RO III, Bonow RO. Exercise testing in patients with microvascular angina. *Circulation* 1991; 83(suppl III):III-73–III-76.
40. Cannon RO III, Quyyumi AA, Schenke WH, Fananapazir L, Tucker EE, Gaughan AM, et al. Abnormal cardiac sensitivity in patients with chest pain and normal coronary arteries. *J Am Coll Cardiol* 1990; 16:1359–1366.
41. Maseri A, ed. *Ischemic Heart Disease.* New York: Churchill Livingstone, 1995:1–713.
42. Hillis DL, Braunwald E. Medical progress: Coronary-artery spasm. *N Engl J Med* 1978; 229:695–702.
43. Prinzmetal M, et al. Angina pectoris: 1. A variant form of angina pectoris. *Am J Med* 1959; 26:375–388.
44. Herrick JB. Clinical features of sudden obstruction of the coronary arteries. *JAMA* 1912; 59:2015–2020.
45. Wood P. Aortic stenosis. *Am J Cardiol* 1958; 1:553–571.
46. Pasternac A, Noble J, Streulens Y, Elie R, Herschke C, Bourassa MG. Pathophysiology of the chest pain in patients with cardiomyopathies and normal coronary arteries. *Circulation* 1982; 65:778–789.
47. Ouzts HG, Turner JL, Douglas JS Jr, Hurst JW. Prolonged chest pain suggesting myocardial infarction in patients with hypertrophic cardiomyopathy. In: Hurst JW, ed. *The Heart, Update III.* New York: McGraw-Hill; 1980:139–146.
48. Pickering GW, Wayne EJ. Observations on angina pectoris and intermittence claudication in anemia. *Clin Sci* 1933; 1:305–309.

49. Ross RS, Babe BM. Right ventricular hypertension as a cause of angina. *Circulation* 1960; 22:801–802.

50. Barnes AR, Burchell HB. Acute pericarditis simulating myocardial infarction. *Am Heart J* 1942; 23:247–268.

51. Spodick DH. Pitfalls in the recognition of pericarditis. In: Hurst JW, ed. *Clinical Essays on the Heart, V.* New York: McGraw-Hill; 1985:95–111.

52. Eagle KA, DeSanctis RW. Dissecting aortic aneurysm. *Curr Probl Cardiol* 1989; 14:227–228.

53. Cohen ME. White PD, Johnson RE. Neurocirculatory asthenia, anxiety necrosis or the effect syndrome. *Arch Intern Med* 1948; 81:260–281.

54. Katon W, Hall ML, Russo J, Cormier L, Hollifield M, Vitaliano PP. Chest pain: Relationship of psychiatric illness to coronary arteriographic results. *Am J Med* 1988; 84:1–9.

55. Mellow MH. A gastroenterologist's view of chest pain. *Curr Probl Cardiol* 1983; 9:1–36.

56. Cassella RR, Ellis FH, Brown AL. Diffuse spasm of the esophagus: Fine structure of esophageal smooth muscle and nerve. *JAMA* 1965; 191:379–382.

57. Castell DO: The spectrum of esophageal motility disorders. *Gastroenterology* 1979; 76:639–640.

58. Brand DL, Martin D, Pope CE. Esophageal manometrics in patients with angina-like chest pain. *Dig Dis Sci* 1977; 22:300–304.

59. Gillis M, Nicks R, Skyring A. Clinical, manometric and pathogenic studies in diffuse esophageal spasm. *Br Heart J* 1967; 2:537.

60. Creamer B, Denoghue FE, Code CF. Pattern of esophageal motility in diffuse spasm. *Gastroenterology* 1958; 34:782–796.

61. Ferguson SC, Hodges K, Hersh T, Jinch H. Esophageal manometry in patients with chest pain and normal arteriograms. *Am J Gastroenterol* 1981; 75:124–129.

62. Rose S, Achkar E, Easley KA. Follow-up of patients with noncardiac chest pain. Value of esophageal testing. *Dig Dis Sci* 1994; 39:2063–2068.

63. Richter JE, Castell DO. Gastroesophageal reflux: Pathogenesis, diagnosis and therapy. *Ann Intern Med* 1982; 97:93–103.

64. Johnson LF, DeMeeter TR. Twenty-four hours pH monitoring of the distal esophagus: A quantitative measure of gastrointestinal reflux. *Am J Gastroenterol* 1974; 62:325–332.

65. Bernstein LM, Grain RC, Pacini R. Differentiation of esophageal pain from angina pectoris: Role of esophageal acid perfusion test. *Medicine* 1962; 41:145–162.

66. Beng LJ, Hookin LA, Marguies S, Donner MW, Cauthorne RJ, Hendrix TR. A comparison of clinical measurements of gastroesophageal reflux. *Gastroenterology* 1972; 62:1–5.

67. Atkinson M. Monitoring esophageal pH. *Gut* 1987; 28:509–514.

68. Tietze A. Uber eine eigenartige Haufung on Fallen mit Dystrophie der Ripenknorpel. *Berl Klin Wehr* 1921; 58:829.

69. Wolf E, Stern S: Costosternal syndrome: Its frequency and importance in differential diagnosis of coronary heart disease. *Arch Intern Med* 1976; 136:1289–1291.

70. Gunther L, Sampson JJ. The radicular syndrome in hypertrophic osteoarthritis of the spine: Root pain and its differentiation from the heart pain. *JAMA* 1929; 93:514–519.

71. Epstein SE, Gerber LN, Boren JS. Chest wall syndrome: A common cause of unexpected pain. *JAMA* 1979; 241:2793–2797.

72. Bettmann MA, Salzman EW. Current concepts in the diagnosis of pulmonary embolism. *Mod Conc Cardiovasc Dis* 1984; 53:1–6.

73. De Weese JA. Pedal pulse disappearing with exercise. *N Engl J Med* 1960; 262:1214–1217.

74. De Takas G, Fowler EF. Raynaud's phenomenon. *JAMA* 1962; 179:99–106.

75. Haeger K. Problems of acute deep-vein thrombosis: The interpretation of signs and symptoms. *Angiology* 1969; 20:219–223.

76. Gonzalez EB, Varner WT, Lisse JR, et al. Giant-cell arteritis in the southern United States: An 11-year retrospective study from the Texas Gulf coast. *Arch Intern Med* 1989; 149:1561–1565.

77. Kapoor W, Karpf M, Wieand S, Peterson JR, Levey GS. A perspective evaluation and follow-up of patients with syncope. *N Engl J Med* 1983; 309:197–204.

78. The Criteria Committee of the New York Heart Association. *Diseases of the Heart and Blood Vessels: Nomenclature and Criteria for Diagnosis of the Heart and Great Vessels*, 6th ed. New York: New York Heart Association/Little Brown; 1964.

79. Bean WB. *Sir William Osler: Aphorisms.* Springfield, IL: Charles C Thomas; 1968.

80. McKusick VA, Egeland JA, Eldridge R, Krusem DE. Dwarfism in the Amith. I. The Ellis–van Creveld syndrome. *Bull Johns Hopkins Hosp* 1964; 115:306–330.

81. Basson CT, Solomon SD, Weissman B, MacRae CA, Poznanski AK, Prieto F, et al. Genetic heterogeneity of heart-hand syndromes. *Circulation* 1995; 91:1326–1329.

82. Green JS, Parfrey PS, Harnett JD, Farid NR, Cramer BC, Johnson G, et al. The cardinal manifestations of Bardet-Biedl syndrome, a form of Laurence-Moon-Biedl syndrome. *N Engl J Med* 1989; 321:1002–1009.

83. Guttmacher AE, Marchuk DA, White RI Jr. Hereditary hemorrhagic telangiectasia. *N Engl J Med* 1995; 333:918–926.

84. Shah CV, Pruyansky S, Harris WS. Cardiac malformations with facial clefts. *Am J Dis Child* 1970; 119:238–244.

85. Beighton P. The dominant and recessive forms of cutis laxa. *J Med Genet* 1972; 9:916–925.

86. Takahashi T, Koide T, Yamaguchi H, Nakamura N, Ohshima Y, Suzuki J, et al. Ehlers-Danlos syndrome with aortic regurgitation, dilation of the sinuses of Valsalva, and abnormal dermal collagen fibrils. *Am Heart J* 1992; 123:1709–1712.

87. Hortop J, Tsipouras P, Hanley JA, Maron BJ, Shapiro JR. Cardiovascular involvement in osteogenesis imperfecta. *Circulation* 1986; 73:54–61.

88. Marsalese DL, Moodie DS, Vacante M, Lytle BW, Gill CC, Sterba R, et al. Marfan's syndrome: Natural history and long-term follow-up of cardiovascular involvement. *J Am Coll Cardiol* 1989; 14:422–428.

89. Schieken RM, Kerber RE, Iowasecu VV, Zellinger H. Cardiac manifestations of the mucopolysaccharidoses. *Circulation* 1975; 52:700–705.

90. Fisher EA, Desnick RJ, Gordon RE, Eng CM, Griepp R, Goldman ME. Fabry disease: An unusual cause of severe coronary disease in a young man. *Ann Intern Med* 1992; 117:221–223.

91. Tandon R, Edwards JE. Cardiac malformations associated with Down's syndrome. *Circulation* 1973; 47:1349–1355.

92. Rosenthal A. Cardiovascular malformations in Klinefelter's syndrome: Report of three cases. *J Pediatr* 1972; 80:471–473.

93. Lewandowski RC Jr, Yunis J. New chromosomal syndromes. *Am J Dis Child* 1975; 129:515–529.

94. Musewe NN, Alexander DJ, Teshima I, Smallhorn JF, Freedom RM. Echocardiographic evaluation of the spectrum of cardiac anomalies associated with trisomy 13 and trisomy 18. *J Am Coll Cardiol* 1990; 15:673–677.

95. Subramaniam PN. Turner's syndrome and cardiovascular anomalies. *Am J Med Sci* 1989; 297:260–262.

96. Helmi C, Pruzansky S. Craniofacial and extracranial malformations in the Klippel-Feil syndrome. *Cleft Palate J* 1980; 17:65–88.

97. Greenwood RD, Rosenthal A, Nadas AS. Cardiovascular malformations associated with imperforate anus. *J Pediatr* 1975; 86:576–579.

98. Quan L, Smith DW. The VATER association. *J Pediatr* 1973; 82:104–107.

99. Freedom RM. The asplenia syndrome: A review of significant extracardiac structural abnormalities in 29 necropsied patients. *J Pediatr* 1972; 81:1130–1133.

100. Cyran SE, Martinez R, Daniels S, Dignan P, Kaplan S. Spectrum of congenital heart disease in CHARGE association. *J Pediatr* 1987; 110:576–578.

101. Ho CK, Kaufman RL, Podos SM. Ocular colobomata, cardiac defect, and other anomalies. *J Med Genet* 1975; 12:289–293.

102. Greenwood RD, Rosenthal A, Nadas AS. Cardiovascular malformations associated with omphalocele. *J Pediatr* 1974; 85:818–821.

103. Nora JI, Nora AH. Maternal transmission of congenital heart diseases: New recurrence risk figures and the questions of cytoplasmic inheritance and vulnerability to teratogens. *Am J Cardiol* 1987; 59:459–463.

104. Sandor GGS, Smith DF, McLeod PM. Cardiac malformations in the fetal alcohol syndrome. *J Pediatr* 1981; 98:771–773.

105. Rowe RD. Maternal rubella and pulmonary artery stenosis. *J Pediatr* 1963; 32:180–185.

106. Aziz K, Sanyal SK, Goldblatt E. Reversed differential cyanosis. *Br Heart J* 1968; 30:288–290.

107. Pearl W. Syndrome of anotia, facial paralysis, and congenital heart disease. *J Pediatr* 1984; 105:441–442.

108. Jaigesimi P, Antia AV. Extracardiac defects in children with congenital heart disease. *Br Heart J* 1979; 42:475–479.

109. Hermans PE: The clinical manifestations of infective endocarditis. *Mayo Clin Proc* 1982; 57:15–21.

110. Proudfit WL. Skin signs of infective endocarditis. *Am Heart J* 1983; 106:1451–1453.

111. Burch M, Sharland M, Shinebourne E, Smith G, Patton M, McKenna W. Cardiologic abnormalities in Noonan syndrome: Phenotypic diagnosis and echocardiographic assessment of 118 patients. *J Am Coll Cardiol* 1993; 22:1189–1192.

112. Gellis SS, Feingold M. Rubinstein-Taybi syndrome. *Am J Dis Child* 1971; 121:327–328.

113. St. John Sutton MG, Tajik AJ, Giuliana ER, Gordon H, Daniel WP. Hypertrophic obstruction cardiomyopathy and lentiginosis: A little known neural ectodermal syndrome. *Am J Cardiol* 1981; 47:214–217.

114. Pellikka PA, Tajik AJ, Khandheria BK, Seward JB, Callahan JA, Pitot HC, et al. Carcinoid heart disease: Clinical and echocardiographic spectrum in 74 patients. *Circulation* 1993; 87:1188–1196.

115. Goldman AP, Kotler MN. Heart disease in scleroderma. *Am Heart J* 1985; 110:1043–1046.

116. Waltuck J, Buyon JP. Autoantibody-associated congenital heart block: Outcome in mothers and children. *Ann Intern Med* 1994; 120:544–551.

117. Boumpas DT, Austin HA III, Fessler BJ, Balow JE, Kippel JH, Lockshin MD. Systemic lupus erythematosus: Emerging concepts: Part 1. renal, neuropsychiatric, cardiovascular, pulmonary and hematologic disease. *Ann Intern Med* 1995; 122:940–950.

118. Hojnik M, George J, Ziporen L, Shoenfeld Y. Heart valve involvement (Libman-Sacks endocarditis) in the antiphospholipid syndrome. *Circulation* 1996; 93:1579–1587.

119. Nomier AM, Turner RA, Watts LE. Cardiac involvement in rheumatoid arthritis. *Arthritis Rheum* 1979; 22:561–564.

120. Bowness P, Hawley JC, Morris T, Dearden A, Walport MJ. Complete heart block and severe aortic incompetence in relapsing polychondritis. *Arthritis Rheum* 1991; 34:97–100.

121. Bergfeldt L, Edhag O, Rajs J. HLA-B27-associated heart disease. *Am J Med* 1984; 77:961–967.

122. Livingston JZ, Casale AS, Hutchins GM, Shapiro EP. Coronary involvement in Cogan's syndrome. *Am Heart J* 1992; 123:528–530.

123. McAllister HA, Fenogho JJ. Cardiac involvement in Whipple's disease. *Circulation* 1975; 52:152–156.

124. Casazza F, Morpurgo M. The varying evolution of Friedreich's ataxia cardiomyopathy. *Am J Cardiol* 1996; 77:895–898.

125. Lie JT, Grossman SJ. Pathology of the heart in acromegaly: Anatomic findings in 27 autopsied patients. *Am Heart J* 1980; 100:41–52.

126. Sofer S, Weinhouse E, Tal A, Wanderman KL, Margulis G, Leiberman A. Cor pulmonale due to adenoidal or tonsillar hypertrophy or both in children. *Chest* 1988; 93:119–127.

127. Parish JM, Shepard JW. Cardiovascular effects of sleep disorders. *Chest* 1990; 97:1220–1225.

128. Collins P. Aortic incompetence and active myocarditis in Reiter's disease. *Br J Vener Dis* 1972; 48:300–303.

129. Dajani AS, Taubert KA, Gerber MA, Shulman ST, Ferrieri P, Freed M, et al. Diagnosis and therapy of Kawasaki disease in children. *Circulation* 1993; 87:1776–1780.

130. Cox J, Krajden M. Cardiovascular manifestations of Lyme disease. *Am Heart J* 1991; 122:1449–1455.

131. Stern R, Goldbold JH, Chess O, Kagen LJ. ECG abnormalities in polymyositis. *Arch Intern Med* 1984; 144:2185–2189.

132. Perloff JK. Cardiac rhythm and conduction in Duchenne's muscular dystrophy: A prospective study of 20 patients. *J Am Coll Cardiol* 1984; 3:1263–1268.

133. Badano L, Autore C, Fragola PV, Picelli A, Antonini G, Vichi R, et al. Left ventricular myocardial function in myotonic dystrophy. *Am J Cardiol* 1993; 71:987–991.

134. Kenny D, Wetherbee J. Kearns-Sayre syndrome in the elderly: Mitochondrial myopathy with advanced heart block. *Am Heart J* 1990; 120:440–443.

135. Shammas RL, Movahed A. Sarcoidosis of the heart. *Clin Cardiol* 1993; 16:462–472.

136. Kuan P. Cardiac Wilson's disease. *Chest* 1987; 91:579–583.

137. Olson LJ, Edwards WD, McCall JT, Ilstrup DM, Gersh BJ. Cardiac iron deposition in idiopathic hemochromatosis: Histologic and analytic assessment of 14 hearts from autopsy. *J Am Coll Cardiol* 1987; 10:1239–1243.

138. Kyle RA. Amyloidosis. *Circulation* 1995; 91:1269–1271.

139. Hara KS, Ballard DJ, Ilstrup DM, Connolly DC, Vollertsen RS. Rheumatoid pericarditis: Clinical features and survival. *Medicine* 1990; 69:81–91.

140. Di Eusanio G, Mazzola A, Gregorini R, Esposito G, DiNardo W, DiManici G, et al. Left ventricular aneurysm secondary to Behçet's disease. *Ann Thorac Surg* 1991; 51:131–135.

141. Turiteri L, Perheentupa J, Rapola J. The cardiopathy of mulibrey nanism: A new inherited syndrome. *Chest* 1974; 65:628–631.

142. Deer T, Rosencrance JG, Chillag SA. Cardiac conduction manifestations of Reiter's syndrome. *South Med J* 1991; 84:799–800.

143. Bergfeldt L, Edhag O, Vedin L, Vallin H. Anklosing spondylitis: An important cause of severe disturbances of the cardiac conduction system. *Am J Med* 1982; 73:187–191.

144. Marks ML, Trippel DL, Keating MT. Long QT syndrome associated with syndactyly identified in females. *Am J Cardiol* 1995; 76:744–745.

145. Sprecher DL, Schaefer EJ, Kent KM, Gregg RE, Zech LA, Hoeg JM. Cardiovascular features of homozygous familial hypercholesterolemia: Analysis of 16 patients. *Am J Cardiol* 1984; 54:20–30.

146. Cohen JI, Arnett EN, Kolodny AL, Roberts WC. Cardiovascular features of the Werner syndrome. *Am J Cardiol* 1987; 59:493–495.

147. Dyck JD, David TE, Burke B, Webb GD, Henderson MA, Fowler RS. Management of coronary artery disease in Hutchinson-Gilford syndrome. *J Pediatr* 1987; 111:407–410.

148. Elliott WJ, Powell LH. Diagonal earlobe creases and prognosis in patients with suspected coronary artery disease. *Am J Med* 1996; 100:205–211.

149. Lesko SM, Rosenberg L, Shapiro S. A case-control study of baldness in relation to myocardial infarction in men. *JAMA* 1993; 269:998–1003.

150. Bowen J, Boudoulas H, Wooley CF. Cardiovascular disease of connective tissue origin. *Am J Med* 1987; 82:481–488.

151. Braunlin EA, Hunter DW, Krivit W, Burke BA, Hesslein PS, Porter PT, et al. Evaluation of coronary artery disease in the Hurler syndrome by angiography. *Am J Cardiol* 1992; 69:1487–1489.

152. Przybojewski JZ. Polyarteritis nodosa in the adult: Report of a case with repeated myocardial infarction and a review of cardiac involvement. *S Afr Med J* 1981; 60:512–518.

153. You CK, Rees J, Gillis DA, Steeves J. Klippel-Trenaunay syndrome: A review. *Can J Surg* 1983; 26:399–403.

154. Pagon RA, Bennett FC, LaVeek B, Stewart KB, Johnson J. Williams syndrome. *J Pediatr* 1987; 80:85–91.

155. Carney JA, Kruska LS, Beauchamp CD, Gordon H. Dominant inheritance of the complex of myxomas, spotty pigmentation, and endocrine overactivity. *Mayo Clin Proc* 1986; 61:165–172.

156. Stevenson WG, Perloff JK, Weiss JN, Anderson TL. Facioscapulohumeral muscular dystrophy: Evidence for selective, genetic electrophysiologic cardiac involvement. *J Am Coll Cardiol* 1990; 15:292–299.

157. Hopkins LC, Jackson JA, Elsas LJ. Emery-Dreifuss humero-peroneal muscular dystrophy: An X-linked myopathy with unusual contractures and bradycardia. *Ann Neurol* 1981; 10:230–237.

158. Gibbs JL. The heart and tuberous sclerosis. *Br Heart J* 1985; 54:596–599.

159. Nutter DO. Measurements of the systolic blood pressure. In: Hurst JW, ed. *The Heart*, 5th ed. New York: McGraw-Hill; 1982.

160. Asmar R, Benetos A, London G, Hugue C, Weiss Y, Topouchian J, et al. Aortic distensibility in normotensive, untreated and treated hypertensive patients. *Blood Pressure* 1995; 4:48–54.

161. Frohlich ED. Hypertension in the elderly. *Curr Probl Cardiol* 1988; 13:313–367.

162. Hales S. *Statistical Essays: Containing Haema-staticks; or, an Account of Some Hydraulick and Hydrostatical Experiments Made on the Blood and Blood-Vessels of Animals.* London: Innys W, Manby R; 1733.

163. McCutcheon EP, Rushmer RF. Korotkov sounds: An experimental critique. *Circ Res* 1967; 20:149–161.

164. Rodbard S. The components of the Korotkov sounds. *Am Heart J* 1967; 74:278–282.

165. Kirkendall WM, Feinleib M, Freis ED, Mark AL. AHA committee report: Recommendations of human blood pressure determination by sphygmomanometers. *Circulation* 1980; 62:1146A–1155A.

166. Neilsen PR, Janniche H. The accuracy of auscultatory measurement of arm blood pressure in very obese subjects. *Acta Med Scand* 1974; 196:403–409.

167. Hla KM, Feussner JR. Screening for pseudohypertension: A quantitative non-invasive approach. *Arch Intern Med* 1988; 148:673–676.

168. Krakoff LR, Eison H, Phillips RH, Leiman SJ, Lev S. Effect of ambulatory blood pressure monitoring on the diagnosis and cost of treatment for mild hypertension. *Am Heart J* 1988; 116:1152–1154.

169. Zachariah PK, Sheps SG, Ilstrup DM, Long CR, Bailey KR, Wiltgen CM. Blood pressure load: A better determinant of hypertension. *Mayo Clin Proc* 1988; 63:1085–1091.

170. Littler WA, Komsuoglar B. Which is the most accurate method of measuring blood pressure? *Am Heart J* 1989; 117:723–728.

171. Evans CE, Haynes RB, Goldsmith CH, Hewson SA. Home blood pressure-measuring devices: A comparative study of accuracy. *J Hypertens* 1989; 7:133–142.

172. White SB, Berson AS, Robbins C, Jamieson MJ, Prisant LM, Roccella E, et al. National standard for measurement of resting and ambulatory blood pressure with automated sphygmamomanometers. *Hypertension* 1993; 21:504–509.

173. Kelly RP, Haywood C, Ganis J, Avolio A, O'Rourke M. Noninvasive registration of the arterial pressure waveform using high-fidelity applanation tonometry. *J Vasc Med Biol* 1989; 1:142–149.

174. Sato T, Nishinaga M, Kawamoto A, Ozawa T, Takatsuji H. Accuracy of a continuous blood pressure monitor based on arterial tonometry. *Hypertension* 1993; 21(6 pt 1):866–874.

175. Lal SK, Henderson RJ, Cejnar M, Hart MG, Hunyor SN. Physiological influences on continuous finger and simultaneous intra-arterial blood pressure. *Hypertension* 1995; 26:307–314.

176. Asmar R, Benetos A, Topouchian J, Laurent P, Pannier B, Brisac AM, et al. Assessment of arterial distensibility by automatic pulse wave velocity measurement: Validation and clinical application studies. *Hypertension* 1995; 26:485–490.

177. Frohlich ED, Gifford RW, Hall WD. Hypertensive cardiovascular disease. In: 18th Bethesda Conference Report: Cardiovascular disease in the elderly. *J Am Coll Cardiol* 1987; 10(suppl A):57A–59A.

178. LaKatta ED, Mitchell JH, Pomerance A, Rowe GG. Human aging: Changes in structure and function. In: 18th Bethesda Conference Report: Cardiovascular disease in the elderly. *J Am Coll Cardiol* 1987; 10(suppl A):42A–47A.

179. Cohn JN, Finkelstein SM. Abnormalities of vascular compliance in hypertension, aging and heart failure. *J Hypertens* 1992; 10:S61–S64.

180. O'Rourke MF: *Arterial Function in Health and Disease.* New York: Churchill Livingstone, 1982.

181. Wei Y, Gersh BJ. Heart disease in the elderly. *Curr Probl Cardiol* 1987; 12:1–65.

182. Kaplan NM. *Clinical Hypertension*, 5th ed. Baltimore: Williams & Wilkins; 1990.

183. Safar ME, Frohlich ED. The arterial system in hypertension: A prospective view. *Hypertension* 1995; 26:10–14.

184. Littler WA, Honour AJ, Pugsley DJ, Sleight PL. Continuous recording of direct arterial pressure in unrestricted patients. *Circulation* 1975; 51:1101–1106.

185. Richardson DW, Honour AJ, Fenton DW, Scott FH, Pickering GW. Variation in arterial pressure throughout the day and night. *Clin Sci* 1964; 26:445–460.

186. Donald KW, Lind AR, McNicol GW, Humphreys PW, Taylor SH, Staunton HP. Cardiovascular response to sustained contractions. *Circ Res* 1967; 20(suppl 1):15–30.

187. Wooley CF, Hosier DM, Booth RW, Molnar W, Sirak HD, Ryan JM. Supravalvular aortic stenosis. *Am J Med* 1961; 31:717–725.

188. Pascarelli EF, Bertrand CA. Comparison of blood pressure in the arms and legs. *N Engl J Med* 1964; 270:693–698.

189. Park MK, Guntheroth WG. Direct blood pressure measurements in brachial and femoral arteries in children. *Circulation* 1979; 42:231–237.

190. Felix WR, Hochbert HM, George MED, Schmalzback EL, Vaserberg R. Ultrasound measurement of arm and leg blood pressure. *JAMA* 1973; 226:1096–1099.

191. Crawford MH. Inspection and palpation of venous and arterial pulses: In: *Examination of the Heart*: Part 2. New York: American Heart Association; 1990.

192. O'Rourke MF, Kelly R, Avolio A. *The Arterial Pulse*. Philadelphia: Lea & Febiger; 1992.

193. Ewy GA. Venous and arterial pulsations: Bedside insights into hemodynamics. In: Chizner M, ed. *Classic Teachings in Clinical Cardiology. A Tribute to W Proctor Harvey*. Cedar Grove, NJ: Laennec, 1996:65–84.

194. O'Rourke MF. The arterial pulse in health and disease. *Am Heart J* 1971; 82:687–702.

195. Murgo JP, Westerhof N, Giolma JP, Altobelli SA. Aortic input impedance in normal man: Relationship to pressure wave shapes. *Circulation* 1980; 62:105–116.

196. O'Rourke MF. Pressure and flow waves in systemic arteries and the anatomic design of the arterial system. *J Appl Physiol* 1967; 23:139–149.

197. O'Rourke MF, Auido AP. Pulsatile flow and pressures in human systemic arteries: Studies in man and in a multibranched model of the human systemic arterial tree. *Circ Res* 1980; 46:363–372.

198. Murgo JP, Westerhof N, Giolma JO, Altobelli SA. Effects of exercise on aortic impedance and pressure wave shapes in normal man. *Circ Res* 1981; 48:334–343.

199. Latham RD, Westerhof N, Sipkema P, Rubal BJ, Reuderick P, Murgo JP. Regional wave travel and reflections along the human aorta: A study with six simultaneous micromanometer pressures. *Circulation* 1985; 72:1257–1269.

200. Murgo JP, Altobelli SA, Dorethy JF. Normal ventricular ejection dynamics in man during rest and exercise. *AHA Monogr* 1975; 46:92.

201. Westerhof N, Murgo JP, Sipkema P. Arterial impedance. In: Hwang NHC, Gross DR, Patel DJ, eds. *Quantitative Cardiovascular Studies*. Baltimore: University Park Press; 1979:111–150.

202. Marx HJ, Yu PN. Clinical examination of the arterial pulse. *Prog Cardiovasc Dis* 1967; 10:207–235.

203. Hamilton WF, Dow P. An experimental study of the standing waves in the pulse propagated through the aorta. *Am J Physiol* 1939; 125:48.

204. McDonald DA, Taylor MG. The hydrodynamics of the arterial circulation. *Prog Biophys* 1959; 9:105–173.

205. McDonald DA. The relation of pulsatile pressure to flow in arteries. *J Physiol* 1955; 127:533–552.

206. O'Rourke MF, Taylor MG. Input impedance of the systemic circulation. *Circ Res* 1967; 20:365–380.

207. Schlant RC, Felner MJ. The arterial pulse—Clinical manifestations. *Curr Prob Cardiol* 1977; 2:1–50.

208. O'Rourke MF, Blazek JV, Morreels CL, Korveta LJ. Pressure wave transmission along the human aorta. *Circ Res* 1968; 23:567–579.

209. Freis ED, Heath WC, Luchsinger PC, Snell RE. Changes in the carotid pulse which occurs with age and hypertension. *Am Heart J* 1966; 72:757–765.

210. Benetos A, Laurent S, Hoeks AP, Boutouyrie PH, Safar ME. Arterial alterations with aging and high blood pressure: A noninvasive study of carotid and femoral arteries. *Arterioscler Thromb* 1993; 13:90–97.

211. Armentano R, Megnien JL, Simon A, Bellenfant F, Barra J, Levenson J. Effects of hypertension on viscoelasticity of carotid and femoral arteries in humans. *Hypertension* 1995; 26:48–54.

212. Safar ME, Frohlich ED. The arterial system in hypoertension: A prospective view. *Hypertension* 1995; 26:10–14.

213. Patel DJ, Greenfield JC, Dry DL: In vivo pressure length-radius relationships of certain blood vessels in man and dog. In: Attinger EO, ed. *Pulsatile Blood Flow*. New York: McGraw-Hill; 1964: chap 17.

214. Stead EA, Greenfield JC. Pressures and pulses. *Physiol Phys* 1964; 2:1–6.

215. Freis ED, Kyle MC. Computer analysis of carotid and brachial pulse waves: Effects of age in normal subjects. *Am J Cardiol* 1968; 22:691–695.

216. Corrigan DJ. On permanent patency of the mouth of the aorta, or inadequacy of the aorta valves. *Edinburgh Med Surg* 1832; 37:225–245.

217. Clarke JM. On the pulsus bisferiens of aortic regurgitation. *Lancet* 1894; 2:1529–1541.

218. Broadbent W. Pulsus bisferiens. *Br Med J* 1899; 1:75–77.

219. Fleming PR. The mechanism of the pulsus bisferiens. *Br Heart J* 1951; 19:519–524.

220. Ikram H, Nixon PGF, Fox JA. The hemodynamic implications of the bisferiens pulse. *Br Heart J* 1964; 26:452–459.

221. Wigle ED. The arterial pressure pulse in muscular subaortic stenosis. *Br Heart J* 1963; 25:97–105.

222. Steell G. The pulse in aortic stenosis. *Lancet* 1894; 2:1206–1217.

223. Feil HS, Katz LN. The transformation of the central into the peripheral pulse in patients with aortic stenosis. *Am Heart J* 1926; 2:12–17.

224. Deane CR, Needleman L. The cause of pulsus tardus in arterial stenosis. *Radiology* 1995; 194:28–30.

225. Bude RO, Rubin JM, Platt JF, Fechner KP, Adler RS. Pulsus tardus: Its cause and potential limitations in detection of aortic stenosis. *Radiology* 1994; 190:779–784.

226. Dow P. The development of the anacrotic and tardus pulse of aortic stenosis. *Am J Physiol* 1940; 131:432.

227. Rahimtoola SH, Cheitlin MD, Hutter AM. Valvular and congenital heart disease. In: 18th Bethesda Conference Report: Cardiovascular disease in the elderly. *J Am Coll Cardiol* 1987; 10(suppl A):60–62.

228. Ewy GA, Rios JC, Marcus FI: The dicrotic arterial pulse. *Circulation* 1969; 39:655–661.

229. White PD. Alternation of the pulse: A common clinical condition. *Am J Med Sci* 1915; 150:82–96.

230. Cohn KE, Sandler H, Hancock EW. Mechanisms of pulsus alternans. *Circulation* 1967; 36:372–380.

231. Mitchell JH, Sarnoff SJ, Sonnenblock EH. The dynamics of pulsus alternans: Alternating end-diastolic fiber length as a causative factor. *J Clin Invest* 1963; 42:55–63.

232. Pace JB, Priola DV, Randall WC. Alternatives in cardiac synchrony and contractility during induced pulsus alternans. *Physiologist* 1966; 9:259.

233. Freeman GL, Widman LE, Campbell JM, Colston JT. An evaluation of the onset of pulsus alternans in closed-chest dogs. *Am J Physiol* 1992; 262:H278–H284.

234. Shabetai R, Fowler NO, Fenton JC, Masangkay M. Pulsus paradoxus. *J Clin Invest* 1965; 44:1882–1898.

235. Shabetai R, Fowler NO, Guntheroth WG. The hemodynamics of cardiac tamponade and constrictive pericarditis. *Am J Cardiol* 1970; 26:480–498.

236. Otsuji Y, Toda H, Kisanuki A, Kuroiwa R, Murayama T, Matsushita R, et al. Influence of left ventricular filling profile during preceding control beats on pulse pressure during ventricular premature contractions. *Eur Heart J* 1994; 15:462–467.

237. Garratt CJ, Griffith MJ, Young G, Curzen N, Brecker S, Rickards AF, et al. Value of physical signs in the diagnosis of ventricular tachycardia. *Circulation* 1994; 90:3103–3107.

238. Hurst JW, Schlant RC. Examination of the veins and their pulsation. In: Hurst JW, ed. *The Heart*, 4th ed. New York: McGraw-Hill; 1978; 15:193–201.

239. Fowler NO, Marshall WJ. Cardiac diagnosis from examination of arteries and veins. *Circulation* 1964; 30:272–283.

240. Ewy GA, Marcus FI. Bedside estimation of the venous pressure. *Heart Bull* 1968; 17:41.

241. Ewy GA. The abdominojugular test: Technique and hemodynamic correlates. *Ann Intern Med* 1989; 108:456–460.

242. Kussmaul A: Uber schwielige Mediastino-pericarditis und Den Parodoxen Pulse. *Berl Klin Wochenschr* 1873; 10:433.

243. Ducas J, Magder S, McGregor M. Validity of the hepatojugular reflux as a clinical test for congestive heart failure. *Am J Cardiol* 1983; 52:1299–1303.

244. Fowler NO. Inspection and palpation of venous and arterial pulses: In: *Examination of the Heart*. New York: American Heart Association; 1972:1–41.

245. Wood P. *Diseases of the Heart and Circulation*, 2d ed. Philadelphia: Lippincott; 1957.

246. Dell'Italia L, Starling MR, O'Rourke RA. Physical examination for exclusion of hemodynamically important right ventricular infarction. *Ann Intern Med* 1983; 99:608–612.

247. Stonjic BB, Brecker SJ, Xiao HB, Gibson DG. Jugular venous "a" wave in pulmonary hypertension: New insights from a Doppler echocardiographic study. *Br Heart J* 1992; 68:187–191.

248. Messer AL, Hurst JW, Rappaport MB, Sprague HB. A study of the venous pulse in tricuspid valve disease. *Circulation* 1950; 1:388–393.

249. Meuller O, Shillingford J. Tricuspid incompetence. *Br Heart J* 1954; 16:195–207.

250. Dexter L. Atrial septal defect. *Br Heart J* 1956; 18:209–225.

251. Perloff JK, Harvey WP. Clinical recognition of tricuspid stenosis. *Circulation* 1960; 22:346–364.

252. Corvisart JN. *An Essay on the Organic Diseases and Lesions of the Heart and Great Vessels*. Translated from the French, with notes, by Jacob Gates. New York: Hafner; 1962.

253. Willis PW IV. Inspection and palpation of the precordium. In: Hurst JW ed. *The Heart*, 7th ed. New York: McGraw-Hill; 1990:163–169.

254. Schlant RC, Hurst JW. *Examination of the Precordium: Inspection and Palpation*. New York: American Heart Association; 1990:1–28.

255. Stapleton JF, Groves BM. Precordial palpation. *Am Heart J* 1971; 82:409–427.

256. Basta LL, Bettinger JJ. The cardiac impulse: A new look at an old art. *Am Heart J* 1979; 97:96–111.

257. Perloff JK. The physiologic mechanisms of cardiac and vascular physical signs. *J Am Coll Cardiol* 1983; 1:184–198.

258. Abrams J. Precordial motion in health and disease. *Mod Concepts Cardiovasc Dis* 1980; 49:55–60.

259. Abrams J. Precordial palpation: Let your fingers do the walking. In: Chizner M, ed. *Classic Teachings in Clinical Cardiology: A tribute to W. Proctor Harvey*. Cedar Grove, NJ: Laennec; 1996:85–103.

260. Eilen SD, Crawford MH, O'Rourke RA. Accuracy of precordial palpation for detecting increased left ventricular volume. *Ann Intern Med* 1983; 99:628–630.

261. Smith D, Craige E. Enhancement of tactile perception as employed in palpation. *Circulation* 1980; 62:1114–1118.

262. Corn RD, Cole JS. The cardiac apex impulse. *Ann Intern Med* 1971; 75:185.

263. Bethell HJN, Nixon PGF. Examination of the heart in supine and left lateral positions. *Br Heart J* 1973; 35:902–907.

264. Chun PKC, Dunn BE. Clinical care of severe aortic stenosis. *Arch Intern Med* 1982; 142:2284–2288.

265. Deliyannis A, Gillam PMS, Mounsey JPD, Steiner RE. The cardiac impulse and the motion of the heart. *Br Heart J* 1964; 26:396–411.

266. McDonald IG. The shape and movements of the human left ventricle during systole. *Am J Cardiol* 1970; 26:221–230.

267. Sutton GC, Prewitt TA, Craige E. Relationship between quantitated precordial movement and left ventricular function. *Circulation* 1970; 41:179–190.

268. Abrams J. *Essentials of Cardiac Physical Diagnosis*. Philadelphia: Lea & Febiger, 1987.

269. Logue RB, Sikes C. A new sign in dissecting aneurysm of aorta: Pulsation of a sternoclavicular joint. *JAMA* 1952; 148:1209–1212.

270. Lindsey J Jr, Hurst JW. Clinical features and prognosis in dissecting aneurysm of the aorta: A re-appraisal. *Circulation* 1967; 35:880–888.

271. Perloff JK. The movements of the heart—Observation, palpation, and percussion. In: *Physical Examination of the Heart and Circulation*. Philadelphia, Saunders, 1982; 130–170.

272. Burstin L. Determination of pressure in the pulmonary artery by external graphic recordings. *Br Heart J* 1967; 29:396–404.

273. Eddleman EE Jr, Thomas HD. The recognition and differentiation of right ventricular pressure and flow loads: A correlative study of kinetocardiograms, electrocardiograms, fluoroscopy, and cardiac catheterization data in patients with mitral stenosis, septal defect, pulmonic stenosis and isolated pulmonary hypertension. *Am J Cardiol* 1959; 4:652–661.

274. Nagle RE, Tamara FA. Left parasternal impulse in pulmonary stenosis and atrial septal defect. *Br Heart J* 1967; 29:735–741.

275. Ronon JA Jr, Steelman RB, DeLeon AC Jr, Waters TJ, Perloff JK, Harvey WP. The clinical diagnosis of acute severe mitral insufficiency. *Am J Cardiol* 1971; 27:284–290.

276. Sutton GC, Craige E, Grizzle JE. Quantitation of precordial movement: II. Mitral regurgitation. *Circulation* 1967; 35:483–491.

277. Basta LL, Wolfston P, Eckberg DL, Abboud FM. The value of left parasternal impulse recordings in the assessment of mitral regurgitation. *Circulation* 1973; 48:1055–1065.

278. Eddleman EE Jr. Kinetocardiographic findings in aortic insufficiency. *Am Heart J* 1957; 53:530–541.

279. Abrams J. Precardial palpation. In: Horwitz LD, Graves BM, eds. *Signs and Symptoms in Cardiology*. Philadelphia: Lippincott; 1985:156–177.

280. Nagle RE, Boicourt OW, Gillam PM, Mounsey JP. Cardiac impulse in hypertrophic obstructive cardiomyopathy. *Br Heart J* 1966; 28:419–425.

281. Rios JC, Massumi RA. Correlation between the apex cardiogram and left ventricular pressure. *Am J Cardiol* 1965; 15:647–655.

282. Tafur E, Cohen LS, Levine HD. The apex cardiogram in left ventricular outflow tract obstruction. *Circulation* 1964; 30:392–399.

283. Harvey WP. Some pertinent physical findings in the clinical evaluation of acute myocardial infarction. *Circulation* 1969; 39/40(suppl IV):IV-175–IV-181.

284. Heikkila J, Luomanmaki K, Pyroala K. Serial observations on left ventricular dysfunction in acute myocardial infarction: 1. Gallop sounds, ventricular asynergy, and radiological signs. *Acta Med Scand* 1971; 190:89–104.

285. Lane FJ, Carroll JM, Levine HD, Gorlin R. The apexcardiogram in myocardial asynergy. *Circulation* 1968; 37:890–899.

286. Shah PM. Newer concepts in hypertrophic obstruction cardiomyopathy: II. *JAMA* 1979; 242:1771–1776.

287. Boicourt OW, Nagle RE, Mounsey JP. The clinical significance of systolic retraction of the apical impulse. *Br Heart J* 1965; 27:379–391.

288. Eddlemand EE Jr, Harrison TR. The kinetocardiogram in patients with ischemic heart disease. *Prog Cardiovasc Dis* 1963; 6:189–211.

289. Walker HK, Hall WD, Hurst JW. *Clinical Methods: The History, Physical, and Laboratory Examination*, 2d ed. Boston: Butterworths; 1980:200, 628–648, 726, 740–775.

290. Hurst JW, Robinson PH. Physical examination of the chest, abdomen and extremities. In: Hurst JW, et al (eds). *The Heart*, 7th ed. New York: McGraw-Hill, 1990:242–243.

291. Lannec RTH. *Traite de l'auscultation mediate*, 2d ed. Paris: Brosson et Chaude; 1826.

292. Shaver JA, Leonard JJ, Leon DF. *Examination of the Heart*: Part 4. *Auscultation of the Heart*. Dallas: American Heart Association; 1990.

293. Rapaport MB, Sprague HB. The effects of tubing bore on stethoscope efficiency. *Am Heart J* 1951; 42:605–609.

294. Butterworth JS, Chassin MR, McGrath R, et al. *Cardiac Auscultation*. New York: Grune & Stratton; 1960.

295. Levine SA, Harvey SP. *Clinical Auscultation of the Heart*, 2d ed. Philadelphia: Saunders; 1959.

296. Shaver JA. Current uses of phonocardiography in clinical practice. In: Rapaport E, ed. *Cardiology Update—Reviews for Physicians*. New York: Elsevier; 1981:327–378.

297. Shaver JA, Salerni R, Reddy PS. Normal and abnormal heart sounds in cardiac diagnosis: Part I. Systolic sounds. *Curr Probl Cardiol*, March 1985; 10:1–68.

298. Reddy PS, Salerni R, Shaver JA. Normal and abnormal heart sounds in cardiac diagnosis: Part II. Diastolic sounds. *Curr Probl Cardiol*, April 1985; 10:1–55.

299. Shaver JA. Cardiac auscultation: A cost-effective diagnostic skill. *Curr Probl Cardiol* 1995; 20:443–530.

300. Dock W. Mode of production of the first heart sound. *Arch Intern Med* 1933; 51:737–746.

301. Leatham A. Splitting of the first and second heart sounds. *Lancet* 1954; 267:607–614.

302. Mills PG, Chamusco RF, Moos S, Craige E. Echophonocardiographic studies of the contribution of the atrioventricular valves to the first heart sound. *Circulation* 1976; 54:944–951.

303. Laniado S, Yellin EL, Miller H, Frater WM. Temporal relation of the first heart sound to closure of the mitral valve. *Circulation* 1973; 47:1006–1014.

304. Shah PM, Kramer DH, Gramiak R. Influence of the timing of atrial systole on mitral valve closure and on the first heart sound in man. *Am J Cardiol* 1970; 26:231–237.

305. Burggraf GW, Craige E. The first heart sound in complete heart block: Phono-echocardiographic correlations. *Circulation* 1974; 50:17–24.

306. Waider W, Craige E. First heart sound and ejection sounds: Echocardiographic and phonocardiographic correlation with valvular events. *Am J Cardiol* 1975; 35:346–356.

307. Criley JM, Chambers RD, Blaufuss AH, Friedman NJ. Mitral stenosis: Mechanico-acoustical events. In: Leon DF, Shaver JA, eds. *Physiologic Principles of Heart Sounds and Murmurs*. Monograph 46. New York: American Heart Association, 1975:149–159.

308. Brooks N, Leech G, Leatham A. Factors responsible for normal splitting of first heart sound: High-speed echophonocardiographic study of valve movement. *Br Heart J* 1979; 42:695–702.

309. Mills P, Craige E. Echophonocardiography. *Prog Cardiovasc Dis* 1978; 20:337.

310. Rushmer RF: *Cardiovascular Dynamics*, 3d ed. Philadelphia: Saunders; 1970:305.

311. Milner S, Meyer RA, Venables AW, Korfhagen J, Kaplan S. Mitral and tricuspid valve closure in congenital heart disease. *Circulation* 1976; 53:513–518.

312. Haber E, Leatham A. Splitting of heart sounds from ventricular asynchrony in bundle-branch block, ventricular ectopic beats, and artificial pacing. *Br Heart J* 1965; 27:691–696.

313. Hultgren HN, Leo TF. The tricuspid component of the first heart sound in mitral stenosis. *Circulation* 1958; 18:1012–1016.

314. DiBartolo G, Nunez-Dey D, Muiesan G, et al. Hemodynamic correlates of the first heart sound. *Am J Physiol* 1961; 201:888–892.

315. Wexler LF, Pohost GM, Rubenstein JJ, O'Keefe DD, Vezeridis MP, Daggett WM. The relationship of the first heart sound to mitral valve closure in dogs. *Circulation* 1982; 66:235–243.

316. O'Toole JD, Reddy PS, Curtiss EI, Griff FW, Shaver JA. The contribution of tricuspid valve closure to the first heart sound: An intracardiac micromanometer study. *Circulation* 1976; 53:752–758.

317. Stept ME, Heid CE, Shaver JA, Leon DF, Leonard JJ. Effect of altering P-R interval on the amplitude of the first heart sound in the anesthetized dog. *Circ Res* 1969; 25:255–263.

318. Thompson ME, Shaver JA, Leon DF, Reddy PS, Leonard JJ. Pathodynamics of first heart sound. In: Leon DF, Shaver JA, eds. *Physiologic Principles of Heart Sounds and Murmurs*. Monograph 46. New York: American Heart Association; 1975:8–18.

319. Leech G, Brooks N, Green-Wilkinson A, Leatham A. Mechanisms of influence of P-R interval on loudness of first heart sound. *Br Heart J* 1980; 43:138–142.

320. Shah PM: Hemodynamic determinants of the first heart sound. In: Leon DF, Shaver JA, eds. *Physiologic Principles of Heart Sounds and Murmurs*. Monograph 46. New York: American Heart Association; 1975:2–7.

321. Rytand DA. The variable loudness of the first heart sound in auricular fibrillation. *Am Heart J* 1949; 37:187–204.

322. Leonard JJ, Weissler AM, Warren JV. Observations on the mechanism of atrial gallop rhythm. *Circulation* 1958; 17:1007–1012.

323. Sakamoto T, Kusukawa R, MacCanon DM, Luisada AA. Hemodynamic determinants of the amplitude of the first heart sound. *Circ Res* 1965; 16:45–57.

324. Hume L, Reuben SR. The effects of exercise on the amplitude of the first heart sound in normal subjects. *Am Heart J* 1978; 95:4–11.

325. Delman AJ. Hemodynamic correlates of cardiovascular sounds. *Annu Rev Med* 1967; 18:139–158.

326. Stein PD, Sabbah HN, Barr I. Intensity of heart sounds in the evaluation of patients following myocardial infarction. *Chest* 1979; 75:679–684.

327. Sakamoto T, Kusukawa R, MacCanon DM, Luisada AA. First heart sound amplitude in experimentally induced alternans. *Dis Chest* 1966; 50:470–475.

328. Ravin A. *Auscultation of the Heart*, 2d ed. Chicago: Yearbook, 1967.

329. Adolph RJ, Stephens JF, Tanaka K. The clinical value of frequency analysis of the first heart sound in myocardial infarction. *Circulation* 1970; 41:1003–1014.

330. Clarke WB, Austin SM, Shah PM, Griffen PM, Dove JT, McCullough J, et al. Spectral energy of the first heart sound in acute myocardial ischemia. *Circulation* 1978; 57:593–598.

331. Wooley CF, Klassen KP, Leighton RF, Goodwin MS, Ryan JM. Left atrial and left ventricular sound and pressure in mitral stenosis. *Circulation* 1968; 38:295–307.

332. Thompson ME, Shaver JA, Heidenreich FP, Leon DF, Leonard JJ. Sound, pressure and motion correlates in mitral stenosis. *Am J Med* 1970; 49:436–450.

333. Salerni R, Reddy PS, Sherman ME, O'Toole JD, Leon DF, Shaver JA. Pressure and sound correlates of the mitral valve echocardiogram in mitral stenosis. *Circulation* 1978; 58:119–125.

334. Nasser WK, Davis RH, Dillon JC, Tavel ME, Helmen CH, Feigenbaum H, et al. Atrial myxoma: II. Phonocardiographic, echocardiographic, hemodynamic and angiographic features in nine cases. *Am Heart J* 1972; 83:810–824.

335. Gershlick AH, Leech G, Mills PG, Leatham A. The loud first heart sound in left atrial myxoma. *Br Heart J* 1984; 52:403–407.

336. Tei C, Shah PM, Cherian G, Wong M, Ormiston JA. The correlates of an abnormal first heart sound in mitral valve prolapse syndromes. *N Engl J Med* 1982; 307:334–339.

337. Burggraf GW. The first heart sound in left bundle branch block: An echophonocardiographic study. *Circulation* 1981; 63:429–435.

338. Hultgren HN, Craige E, Nakamura T, Fujii J, Bilisoly J. Left bundle branch block and mechanical events of the cardiac cycle. *Am J Cardiol* 1983; 52:755–762.

339. Grines CL, Bashore TM, Boudoulas H, Olson S, Shafer P, Wooley CF. Functional abnormalities in isolated left bundle branch block: The effect of interventricular asynchrony. *Circulation* 1989; 79:845–853.

340. Baragan J, Fernandez-Caamano F, Sozutek Y, Coblence B, Lenegre J. Chronic left complete bundle-branch block: Phonocardiographic and mechanocardiographic study of 30 cases. *Br Heart J* 1968; 30:196–202.

341. Shaver JA, Rahko PS, Grines CL, Boudoulas H, Wooley CF. Effect of left bundle branch block on the events of the cardiac cycle. *Acta Cardiol* 1988; 4:459–467.

342. Rahko PS, Shaver JA, Salerni R. Reversed closure sequence of the mitral and tricuspid valves in congestive heart failure. *J Am Coll Cardiol* 1993; 21:1114–1123.

343. Reddy PS, Leon DF, Krishnaswami V, O'Toole JD, Salerni R, Shaver JA. Syndrome of acute regurgitation. In: Leon DF, Shaver JA, eds. *Physiologic Principles of Heart Sounds and Murmurs*. Monograph 46. New York: American Heart Association; 1975:166–174.

344. Meadows WR, VanPraagh S, Indreika M, Sharp JT. Premature mitral valve closure: A hemodynamic explanation for absence of the first sound in aortic insufficiency. *Circulation* 1963; 28:251–258.

345. Whittaker AV, Shaver JA, Gray S III, Leonard JJ. Sound-pressure correlates of the aortic ejection sound: An intracardiac sound study. *Circulation* 1969; 39:475–484.

346. Shaver JA, Griff FW, Leonard JJ. Ejection sounds of left-sided origin. In Leon DF, Shaver JA (eds): *Physiologic Principles of Heart Sounds and Murmurs*. Monograph 46. New York: American Heart Association; 1975:27–34.

347. Ross RS, Criley JM, Cineangiocardiographic studies of the origin of cardiovascular physical signs. *Circulation* 1964; 30:255–261.

348. Epstein EJ, Criley JM, Raftery EB, Humphries JO, Ross R. Cineradiographic studies of the early systolic click in aortic valve stenosis. *Circulation* 1965; 31:842–853.

349. Mills PG, Brodie B, McLaurin L, Schall S, Craige E. Echocardiographic and hemodynamic relationships of ejection sounds. *Circulation* 1977; 56:430–436.

350. Leech G, Mills P, Leatham A. The diagnosis of a non-stenotic bicuspid aortic valve. *Br Heart J* 1978; 40:941–950.

351. Martin CE, Shaver JA, O'Toole JD, Leon DF, Reddy PS. Ejection sounds of right-sided origin. In Leon DF, Shaver JA, eds. *Physiological Principles of Heart Sounds and Murmurs*. Monograph 46. New York: American Heart Association; 1975:35–44.

352. Reddy PS, Shaver JA, Leonard JJ. Cardiac systolic murmurs: Pathophysiology and differential diagnosis. *Prog Cardiovasc Dis* 1971; 14:1–37.

353. Hultgren HN, Reeve R, Cohn K, McLeod R. The ejection click of valvular pulmonic stenosis. *Circulation* 1969; 40:631–639.

354. Weyman AE, Dillon JC, Feigenbaum H, Chang S. Echocardiographic patterns of pulmonary valve motion in valvular pulmonary stenosis. *Am J Cardiol* 1974; 34:644–651.

355. Leatham A, Weitzman D. Auscultatory and phonocardiographic signs of pulmonary stenosis. *Br Heart J* 1957; 19:303–317.

356. Flanigan WH, Shah PM. Echocardiographic correlate of presystolic pulmonary ejection sound in congenital valvular pulmonic stenosis. *Am Heart J* 1977; 94:633–636.

357. Leatham A, Vogelpoel L. The early systolic sound in dilatation of the pulmonary artery. *Br Heart J* 1954; 16:21–33.

358. Sakamoto T, Matsuhisa M, Hayashi T, Ichiyasu H. Echocardiogram and phonocardiogram related to the movement of the pulmonary valve. *Jpn Heart J* 1975; 16:107–117.

359. Cuffer B. Nouvelle recherches sur le bruit galop. *Arch Gen Med* 1887; 1:131, 301.

360. Gallavardin L. Nouvelle observation avec autopsie d'un pseudodevoublement mitral. *Prat Med Fra* 1932; 13:19.

361. Barlow JB, Pocock WA, Marchand P, Denny M. The significance of late systolic murmurs. *Am Heart J* 1963; 66:443–452.

362. Criley JM, Lewis KB, Humphries JO, Ross RS. Prolapse of the mitral valve: Clinical and cine-angiocardiographic findings. *Br Heart J* 1966; 28:488–496.

363. Ronan JA, Perloff JK, Harvey WP. Systolic clicks and the late systolic murmur. *Am Heart J* 1965; 70:319–325.

364. Leon DF, Leonard JJ, Kroetz FW, Page WL, Shaver JA, Lancaster JF. Late systolic murmurs, clicks, and whoops arising from the mitral valve. *Am Heart J* 1966; 72:325–336.

365. Kerber RE, Isaeff DM, Hancock EW. Echocardiographic patterns in patients with the syndrome of systolic click and late systolic murmur. *N Engl J Med* 1971; 284:691–693.

366. Popp RL, Brown OR, Silverman JF, Harrison D. Echocardiographic abnormalities in the mitral valve prolapse syndrome. *Circulation* 1974; 49:428–433.

367. Winkle RA, Goodman DJ, Popp RL. Simultaneous echocardiographic phonocardiographic recordings at rest and during amyl nitrite administration in patients with mitral valve prolapse. *Circulation* 1975; 51:522–529.

368. Reid JVO. Mid-systolic clicks. *S Afr Med J* 1961; 35:353–355.

369. Fontana ME, Pence HL, Leighton RF, Wooley CF. The varying clinical spectrum of the systolic click-late systolic murmur syndrome: A postural auscultatory phenomenon. *Circulation* 1970; 41:807–816.

370. Fontana ME, Wooley CF, Leighton RF, Lewis R. Postural changes in left ventricular and mitral valvular dynamics in the systolic click-late systolic murmur syndrome. *Circulation* 1975; 51:165–173.

371. Mathey DG, Decoodt PR, Allen HN, Swan HJC. The determinants of onset of mitral valve prolapse in the systolic click-late systolic murmur syndrome. *Circulation* 1976; 53:872–878.

372. Fontana ME, Kissel GL, Criley JM. Functional anatomy of mitral valve prolapse. In: Leon DF, Shaver JA, eds. *Physiological Principles of Heart Sounds and Murmurs*. Monograph 46. New York: American Heart Association; 1975:126–132.

373. Roelandt J, Willems J, van der Hauwaert LG, deGeest H. Clicks and sounds (whoops) in left-sided pneumothorax: Clinical and phonocardiographic study. *Dis Chest* 1969; 56:31–36.

374. Martin CE, Hufnagel CA, deLeon AC Jr. Calcified atrial myxoma: Diagnostic significance of the "systolic tumor sound" in a case presenting as tricuspid insufficiency. *Am Heart J* 1969; 78:245–250.

375. Pickering D, Keith JD. Systolic clicks with ventricular septal defects: A sign of aneurysm of ventricular septum? *Br Heart J* 1971; 33:538–539.

376. Killebrew E, Cohn K. Observations on murmurs originating from incompetent heterograft mitral valves. *Am Heart J* 1971; 81:490–493.

377. Leatham A. The second heart sound, key to auscultation of the heart. *Acta Cardiol* 1964; 19:395–416.

378. Shaver JA, O'Toole JD. The second heart sound: Newer concepts. Part I: Normal and wide physiologic splitting. *Mod Concepts Cardiovasc Dis* 1977; 46:7–12.

379. Shaver JA. Clinical implications of the hangout interval. *Int J Cardiol* 1984; 5:391–398.

380. Shaver JA. The second heart sound: Hemodynamic determinants. *Acta Cardiol* 1985; 40:7–18.

381. Shaver JA, Nadolny RA, O'Toole JD, Thompson ME, Reddy PS, Leon DF, et al. Sound pressure correlates of the second heart sound: An intracardiac sound study. *Circulation* 1974; 49:316–325.

382. Shaver JA, O'Toole JD, Curtiss EI, Thompson ME, Reddy PS, Leon DF. Second heart sound: Role of altered greater and lesser circulation. In: Leon DF, Shaver JA, eds. *Physiologic Principles of Heart Sounds and Murmurs*. Monograph 46. New York: American Heart Association; 1975:58–67.

383. Curtiss EI, Reddy PS, O'Toole JD, Shaver JA. Alterations of right ventricular systolic time intervals by chronic pressure and volume overloading. *Circulation* 1976; 53:997–1003.

384. Craige E. Echocardiography in studies of the genesis of heart sounds and murmurs. In: Yu P, ed. *Progress in Cardiology*, Philadelphia: Lea & Febiger; 1975:1–21.

385. Hirschfeld S, Liebman J, Borkat G, Bormuth C. Intracardiac pressure-sound correlates of echocardiographic aortic valve closure. *Circulation* 1977; 55:602–604.

386. Kusukawa R, Bruch DW, Sakamoto T, MacCanon DM, Luisada AA. Hemodynamic determinants of the amplitude of the second heart sound. *J Appl Physiol* 1966; 21:938–946.

387. Brough RD, Talley RC. Temporal relation of the second heart sound to aortic flow in various conditions. *Am J Cardiol* 1972; 30:237–241.

388. Stein PD, Sabbah HN, Anbe DT, Khaja F. Hemodynamic and anatomic determinants of relative differences in amplitude of the aortic and pulmonary components of the second heart sound. *Am J Cardiol* 1978; 42:539–544.

389. Adolph RJ. Second heart sound: Role of altered electromechanical events. In: Leon DF, Shaver JA, eds. *Physiologic Principles of Heart Sounds and Murmurs*. Monograph 46. New York: American Heart Association; 1975:45–57.

390. Curtiss EI, Shaver JA, Reddy PS, O'Toole JD. Newer concepts in physiologic splitting of the second heart sound. In: Leon DF, Shaver JA, eds. *Physiologic Principles of Heart Sounds and Murmurs*. Monograph 46. New York: American Heart Association; 1975:68–73.

391. Leatham A, Towers M. Splitting of the second heart sound in health. In: Proceedings of the Thirtieth Annual General Meeting of the British Cardiac Society, Glasgow, May 10, 1951. *Br Heart J* 1951; 13:575.

392. Boyer SH, Chisholm AW. Physiologic splitting of the second heart sound. *Circulation* 1958; 18:1010–1011.

393. Shafter HA. Splitting of the second heart sound. *Am J Cardiol* 1960; 6:1013–1022.

394. Castle RF, Jones KL. Mechanism of respiratory variations in splitting of the second heart sound. *Circulation* 1961; 24:180–184.

395. Aygen MM, Braunwald E. Splitting of the second heart sound in normal subjects and in patients with congenital heart disease. *Circulation* 1962; 25:328–345.

396. Harris A, Sutton G. Second heart sound in normal subjects. *Br Heart J* 1968; 30:739–742.

397. Curtiss EI, Matthews RG, Shaver JA. Mechanism of normal splitting of the second heart sound. *Circulation* 1975; 51:157–164.

398. Shuler RH, Ensor C, Gunning RE, Moss WG, Johnson V. The differential effects of respiration on the left and right ventricles. *Am J Physiol* 1942; 137:620–627.

399. Lauson HD, Bloomfield RA, Cournand A. Influence of the respiration on the circulation in man: With special reference to pressures in the right auricle, right ventricle, femoral artery and peripheral veins. *Am J Med* 1946; 1:315–335.

400. Brecher GA, Hubay CA. Pulmonary blood flow and venous return during spontaneous respiration. *Circ Res* 1955; 3:210–214.

401. Adolph RJ, Fowler NO. The second heart sound: A screening test for heart disease. *Mod Concepts Cardiovasc Dis* 1970; 39:91–96.

402. Shah PM, Slodki SJ. The Q-II interval: A study of the second heart sound in normal adults and in systemic hypertension. *Circulation* 1964; 29:551–561.

403. Slodki SJ, Hussain AT, Luisada AA. The Q-II interval: III. A study of the second heart sound in old age. *J Am Geriatr Soc* 1969; 17:673–679.

404. Logue RB, Cobbs BW, Dorney ER. The second heart sound in pulmonary embolism and pulmonary hypertension. *Trans Am Clin Climatol Assoc* 1966; 78:38–50.

405. Susmano A, Kefer J, Kumar LV. Abnormal pulmonic sound during acute massive pulmonary embolism. *Chest* 1978; 74:45–49.

406. Perloff JK. Auscultatory and phonocardiographic manifestations of pulmonary hypertension. *Prog Cardiovasc Dis* 1967; 9:303–338.

407. Shapiro S, Clark TJH, Goodwin JF. Delayed closure of the pulmonary valve in obliterative pulmonary hypertension. *Lancet* 1965; 2:1207–1211.

408. Vogelpoel L, Schrire V. Auscultatory and phonocardiographic assessment of pulmonary stenosis with intact ventricular septum. *Circulation* 1960; 22:55–72.

409. O'Toole JD, Reddy PS, Curtiss EI, Shaver JA. The mechanisms of splitting of the second heart sound in atrial septal defect. *Circulation* 1977; 56:1047–1053.

410. Ehlers KH, Engle MA, Farnsworth PB, Levin AR. Wide splitting of the second heart sound without demonstrable heart disease. *Am J Cardiol* 1969; 23:690–696.

411. Gray IR. Paradoxical splitting of the second heart sound. *Br Heart J* 1956; 18:21–28.

412. Shaver JA, O'Toole JD. The second heart sound: Newer concepts. Part 2: Paradoxical splitting and narrow physiological splitting. *Mod Concepts Cardiovasc Dis* 1977; 46:13–16.

413. Luisada AA, Kumar S, Pouget MJ. On the causes of the changes of the second heart sound in left bundle branch block. *Jpn Heart J* 1972; 13:281–294.

414. Alvares RF, Shaver JA, Gamble WH, Goodwin JF. The isovolumic relaxation period in hypertrophic cardiomyopathy. *J Am Coll Cardiol* 1984; 3:71–81.

415. Gamble WH, Shaver JA, Alvares RF, Salerni R, Reddy PS. A critical appraisal of diastolic time intervals as a measure of relaxation in left ventricular hypertrophy. *Circulation* 1983; 68:76–87.

416. Kumar S, Luisada AA. Mechanism of changes in the second heart sound in aortic stenosis. *Am J Cardiol* 1971; 28:162–167.

417. Shaver JA, Kroetz FW, Leonard JJ, Paley HW. Effect of steady-state increases in systemic arterial pressure on the duration of left ventricular ejection time. *J Clin Invest* 1968; 47:217–230.

418. Agnew T, Bucher H, McDonald L, Seymour J. Delayed closure of the aortic valve in ischaemic heart disease. *Br Heart J* 1967; 29:775–777.

419. Yurchak PM, Gorlin R. Paradoxical splitting of the second heart sound in coronary heart disease. *N Engl J Med* 1963; 269:741–743.

420. Martin CE, Shaver JA, Leonard JJ. Physical signs, apexcardiography, phonocardiography, and systolic time intervals in angina pectoris. *Circulation* 1972; 46:1098–1114.

421. Luisada AA. The second heart sound in normal and abnormal conditions. *Am J Cardiol* 1971; 28:150–161.

422. Zuberbuhler JR, Bauersfeld SR. Paradoxical splitting of the second heart sound in the Wolff-Parkinson-White syndrome. *Am Heart J* 1965; 70:595–602.

423. Ito M, Fujino T, Kanaya S, Imanishi S, Mashiba H. Phono-, echo-, and electrocardiographic correlation in the Wolff-Parkinson-White syndrome, with special reference to the split pattern of second heart sound. *Jpn Heart J* 1977; 18:329–339.

424. Wood P. Pulmonary hypertension. *Br Med Bull* 1952; 8:348–353.

425. Dell'Italia LJ, Walsh RA. Acute determinants of the hangout interval in the pulmonary circulation. *Am Heart J* 1988; 16:1289–1297.

426. Thayer WS. The early diastolic heart sound. *Trans Assoc Am Phys* 1908; 13:326–357.

427. Margolies A, Wolferth CC. The opening snap (claquement d'ouverture de la mitrale) in mitral stenosis: Its characteristics, mechanism of production and diagnostic importance. *Am Heart J* 1932; 7:443–470.

428. Ross RS, Criley JM, Morgan RH. Cineangiography in mitral valve disease. *Trans Assoc Am Phys* 1961; 74:271–279.

429. McCall BW, Price JL. Movement of the mitral cusps in relation to the first heart sound and opening snap in patients with mitral stenosis. *Br Heart J* 1967; 29:417–421.

430. Friedman NJ. Echocardiographic studies of mitral valve motion: Genesis of the opening snap in mitral stenosis. *Am Heart J* 1970; 80:177–187.

431. Wells B. The assessment of mitral stenosis by phonocardiography. *Br Heart J* 1954; 16:261–266.

432. Oriol A, Palmer WH, Nakhjavan F, McGregor M. Prediction of left atrial pressure from the second sound-opening snap interval. *Am J Cardiol* 1965; 16:184–188.

433. Bayer O, Loogen F, Wolter HH. The mitral opening snap in the quantitative diagnosis of mitral stenosis. *Am Heart J* 1956; 51:234–245.

434. Rackley CE, Craig RJ, McIntosh HD, Orgain E. Phonocardiographic discrepancies in the assessment of mitral stenosis. *Arch Intern Med* 1968; 121:50–53.

435. Rahko PS, Shaver JA, Salerni R, Gamble WH, Reddy PS. Echophonocardiographic estimates of pulmonary artery wedge pressure in mitral stenosis. *Am J Cardiol* 1985; 55:462–469.

436. Bousvaros GA, Stubington D. Some auscultatory and phonocardiographic features of tricuspid stenosis. *Circulation* 1964; 29:26–33.

437. Luisada AA, Slodke SJ, Krol B. Double (mitral and tricuspid) opening snap in patients with valvular lesions. *Am J Cardiol* 1965; 16:800–806.

438. Tavel ME. Opening snaps: Mitral and tricuspid. In: Leon DF, Shaver JA, eds. *Physiologic Principles of Heart Sounds and Murmurs*. Monograph 46. New York: American Heart Association; 175:85–91.

439. Millward DK, McLaurin LP, Craige E. Echocardiographic studies to explain opening snaps in presence of nonstenotic mitral valves. *Am J Cardiol* 1973; 31:64–70.

440. Leatham A, Gray I. Auscultatory and phonocardiographic signs of atrial septal defect. *Br Heart J* 1956; 18:193–208.

441. Tavel ME, Baugh D, Fisch C, Feigenbaum H. Opening snap of the tricuspid valve in atrial septal defect. *Am Heart J* 1970; 80:550–555.

442. Nixon PGF, Wooler GH, Radigan LR. The opening snap in mitral incompetence. *Br Heart J* 1960; 22:395–402.

443. Perloff JK, Harvey WP. Auscultatory and phonocardiographic manifestations of pure mitral regurgitation. *Prog Cardiovasc Dis* 1962; 5:172–194.

444. Sloan AW, Campbell FW, Henderson AS. Incidence of the physiological third heart sound. *Br Med J* 1952; 2:853–855.

445. Harvey WP, Stapleton J. Clinical aspects of gallop rhythm with particular reference to diastolic gallops. *Circulation* 1958; 18:1017–1024.

446. Reddy PS, Haidet K, Meno F. Relation of intensity of cardiac sounds to age. *Am J Cardiol* 1985; 55:1383–1388.

447. Kupari M, Koskinen P, Virolainen J, Hekali P, Keto P. Prevalence and predictors of audible physiological third heart sound in a population sample aged 36 to 37 years. *Circulation* 1994; 89:1189–1195.

448. Tavel ME, Campbell RW, Feigenbaum H, Steinmetz EF. The apex cardiogram and its relationship to haemodynamic events with the left heart. *Br Heart J* 1965; 27:829–839.

449. Craige E. Gallop rhythm. *Prog Cardiovasc Dis* 1967; 10:246–260.

450. Shaver JA, Reddy PS, Alvares FR. Early diastolic events associated with the physiologic and pathologic S3. *J Cardiol* 1984; 14(suppl V):30–46.

451. Warren JV, Leonard JJ, Weissler AM. Gallop rhythm. *Ann Intern Med* 1958; 48:580–596.

452. Nixon PGF. The genesis of the third heard sound. *Am Heart J* 1963; 65:712–714.

453. Dock W, Grandell F, Taubman F. The physiologic third heart sound: Its mechanism and relation to protodiastolic gallop. *Am Heart J* 1955; 50:449–464.

454. Shah PM, Jackson D. Third heart sound and summation gallop. In: Leon DF, Shaver JA, eds. *Physiologic Principles of Heart Sounds and Murmurs*. Monograph 46. New York: American Heart Association; 1975:79–84.

455. Sakamoto T, Ichiyasu H, Hayashi T, Kawarantani H, Amano K, Hada Y. Genesis of the third heart sound: Phonoechocardiographic studies. *Jpn Heart J* 1976; 17:150–162.

456. Kuo PT, Schnabel TG Jr, Blakemore WS, Whereat A. Diastolic gallop sounds: The mechanism of production. *J Clin Invest* 1957; 36:1035–1042.

457. Shah PM, Gramiak R, Kramer DH, Yu P. Determinants of atrial (S4) and ventricular (S3) gallop sounds in primary myocardial disease. *N Engl J Med* 1968; 278:753–758.

458. Potain C. Du bruit de galop. *Gars d'Hop* 1880; 53:529.

459. Ozawa Y, Smith D, Craige E. Origin of the third heart sound: I. Studies in dogs. *Circulation* 1983; 67:393–398.

460. Ozawa Y, Smith D, Craige E. Origin of the third heart sound: II. Studies in human subjects. *Circulation* 1983; 67:399–404.

461. VandeWerf F, Minten J, Carmeliet P, DeGeest H, Kesteloot H. The genesis of the third and fourth heart sounds: A pressure-flow study in dogs. *J Clin Invest* 1984; 73:1400–1407.

462. VandeWerf F, Boel A, Geboers J, Minten J, Willems J, DeGeest H, et al. Diastolic properties of the left ventricle in normal adults and in patients with third heart sounds. *Circulation* 1984; 69:1070–1078.

463. VandeWerf F, Geboers J, Kesteloot H, DeGeest H, Barrios L. The mechanism of disappearance of the physiologic third heart sound with age. *Circulation* 1986; 73:877–884.

464. Wilken MK, Meyers DG, Laski PA, Yi FP, Starke H. Mechanism of disappearance of S3 with maturation. *Am J Cardiol* 1989; 64:1394–1396.

465. Vancheri F, Gibson D. Relation of third and fourth heart sounds to blood velocity during left ventricular filling. *Br Heart J* 1989; 61:144–148.

466. Lavine SJ, Arends D. Diastolic filling correlates of the third heart sound. *Am J Noninvas Cardiol* 1989; 3:51–57.

467. Pozzoli M, Febo O, Tramarin R, Pinna G, Cobelli F, Specchia G. Pulsed Doppler evaluation of left ventricular filling in subjects with pathologic and physiologic third heart sound. *Eur Heart J* 1990; 11:550–508.

468. Glower DD, Murrah RL, Olsen CO, Davis JW, Rankin JS: Mechanical correlates of the third heart sound. *J Am Coll Cardiol* 1992; 19:450–457.

469. Porter CM, Baxley WA, Eddleman EE Jr, Frimer M, Rackley CE. Left ventricular dimensions and dynamics of filling in patients with gallop heart sounds. *Am J Med* 1971; 50:721–727.

470. Reddy PS, Meno F, Curtiss EI, O'Toole JD. The genesis of gallop sounds: Investigation by quantitative phono- and apexcardiography. *Circulation* 1981; 63:922–933.

471. Gamble WH, Reddy PS: Preservation of the third heart sound in mitral stenosis. *N Engl J Med* 1983; 308:498–502.

472. Aubert AE, Denys BG, Meno F, Reddy PS: Investigation of genesis of gallop sounds in dogs by quantitative phonocardiography and digital frequency analysis. *Circulation* 1985; 71:987–993.

473. Shaver JA, Reddy PS, Alvares RF, Salerni R. Genesis of the physiologic third heart sound. *Am J Noninvas Cardiol* 1987; 1:39–55.

474. Riley C, Russell R, Rackley C. Left ventricular gallop sound and acute myocardial infarction. *Am Heart J* 1973; 86:598–602.

475. Leonard J, Weissler A, Warren J. Modification of ventricular gallop rhythm induced by pooling of blood in the extremities. *Br Heart J* 1958; 20:502–506.

476. Abdulla AM, Frank MJ, Erdin RA Jr, Canedo M. Clinical significance and hemodynamic correlates of the third heart sound gallop in aortic regurgitation. *Circulation* 1981; 64:464–471.

477. Stapleton JF. Third and fourth heart sounds. In: Horwitz LD, Groves BM, eds. *Signs and Symptoms in Cardiology*. Philadelphia: Lippincott; 1985:214–226.

478. Tyberg TI, Goodyer AVN, Langou RA. Genesis of pericardial knock in constrictive pericarditis. *Am J Cardiol* 1980; 46:570–575.

479. Fowler NO, Adolph RJ. Fourth sound gallop or split first sound? *Am J Cardiol* 1972; 30:441–444.

480. Spodick DH, Quary-Pigotti VM. Fourth heart sound as a normal finding in older persons. *N Engl J Med* 1973; 288:140–141.

481. Tavel ME. The fourth heart sound: A premature requiem? *Circulation* 1974; 49:4–6.

482. Goldblatt A, Aygen MM, Braunwald E. Hemodynamic-phonocardiographic correlations of the fourth heart sound in aortic stenosis. *Circulation* 1962; 26:92–98.

483. Caulfield WH, deLeon AC, Perloff JK, Steelman RB. The clinical significance of the fourth heart sound in aortic stenosis. *Am J Cardiol* 1971; 28:179–182.

484. Cohen LS, Mason DT, Braunwald E. Significance of an atrial gallop sound in mitral regurgitation. *Circulation* 1967; 35:112–118.

485. Kotler MN, Segal BL, Parry WR. Echocardiographic and phonocardiographic evaluation of prosthetic heart valves. *Cardiovasc Clin* 1978; 9:187–207.

486. Smith ND, Raizada V, Abrams J: Auscultation of the normally functioning prosthetic valve. *Ann Intern Med* 1981; 95:594–598.

487. Kotler MN, Mintz GS, Panidis I, Morganroth J, Segal BL, Ross J. Noninvasive evaluation of normal and abnormal prosthetic valve function. *J Am Coll Cardiol* 1983; 1:151–173.

488. Simon EB, Kotler MN, Segal BL, Parry W. Clinical significance of multiple systolic clicks from Starr-Edwards prosthetic aortic valves. *Br Heart J* 1977; 39:645–650.

489. Hultgren HN, Hubis H. A phonocardiographic study of patients with the Starr-Edwards mitral valve prosthesis. *Am Heart J* 1965; 69:306–319.

490. Gibson TC, Starek PJK, Moos S, Craige E. Echocardiographic and phonocardiographic characteristics of the Lillehei-Kaster mitral valve prosthesis. *Circulation* 1974; 49:434–440.

491. DePace NL, Kotler MN, Mintz GS, Lichtenberg R, Coel IP, Segal BL. Echocardiographic and phonocardiographic assessment of the St. Jude cardiac valve prosthesis. *Chest* 1981; 80:272–277.

492. Harris A. Pacemaker "heart sound." *Br Heart J* 1967; 29:608–615.

493. Lerman J, Means JH, Cardiovascular symptomatology in exophthalmic goiter. *Am Heart J* 1932; 8:55–65.

494. Hamman L. Spontaneous mediastinal emphysema. *Bull Johns Hopkins Hosp* 1939; 64:1–21.

495. Soffer A, Feinstein A, Luisada AA, Perloff JK, Rosner S, Schlant R, et al. Glossary of cardiologic terms related to physical diagnosis and history. *Am J Cardiol* 1967; 20:285–286.

496. Stein PD. *A Physical and Physiologic Basis for the Interpretation of Cardiac Auscultation: Evaluations Based Primarily on the Second Sound and Ejection Murmurs*. Mt. Kisco, NY: Futura; 1981.

497. Leatham A. Systolic murmurs. *Circulation* 1958; 17:601–611.

498. Freeman AR, Levine SA. Clinical significance of systolic murmurs: Study of 1000 consecutive "non-cardiac" cases. *Ann Intern Med* 1933; 6:1371–1385.

499. McKusick VA. *Cardiovascular Sound in Health and Disease*. Baltimore: Williams & Wilkins, 1958.

500. Donnerstein RL. Continuous spectral analysis of heart murmurs for evaluating stenotic cardiac lesions. *Am J Cardiol* 1989; 64:625–630.

501. Gallavardin L, Ravault P. Le souffle du retrecissement aortique puet changer de timbre et devenir musical dans sa propagation apexienne. *Lyon Med* 1925; 135:523–529.

502. Gelfand D, Bellet S. The musical murmur of aortic insufficiency: Clinical manifestations; Based on a study of 18 cases. *Am J Med Sci* 1951; 221:644–654.

503. Behar VS, Whalen RE, McIntosh HD. The ballooning mitral valve in patients with the "precordial honk" or "whoop." *Am J Cardiol* 1967; 20:789–795.

504. Sabbah HN, Magilligan DJ, Lakier JB, Stein PD. Hemodynamic determinants of the frequency and amplitude of a musical murmur produced by a regurgitant mitral bioprosthetic valve. *Am J Cardiol* 1982; 50:53–58.

505. Stein PD, Sabbah HN, Lakier JB. Origin and clinical relevance of musical murmurs. *Int J Cardiol* 1983; 4:103.

506. Pennestri F, Boccardi L, Minardi G, DiSegni M, Pucci E, Biasucci LM, et al. Doppler study of precordial musical murmurs. *Am J Cardiol* 1989; 63:1390–1394.

507. Rushmer RF, Morgan CL. Meaning of murmurs. *Am J Cardiol* 1968; 21:722–730.

508. Shaver JA. Systolic murmurs. *Heart dis Stroke* 1993; 2:9–17.

509. Spencer MP, Greiss FC. Dynamics of ventricular ejection. *Circ Res* 1962; 10:274–279.

510. Franklin DL, VanCitters RL, Rushmer RF. Balance between right and left ventricular output. *Circ Res* 1962; 10:17–26.

511. Murgo JP, Altobelli SA, Dorethy JF, Logsdon JR, McGranahan GM. Normal ventricular ejection dynamics in man during rest and exercise. In: Leon DF, Shaver JA, eds. *Physiologic Principles of Heart Sounds and Murmurs*. Monograph 46. New York: American Heart Association; 1975:92–101.

512. Lembo NJ, Dell'Italia LJ, Crawford MH, O'Rourke RA. Bed side diagnosis of systolic murmurs. *N Engl J Med* 1988; 318:1572–1578.

513. Tavel ME. Innocent murmurs. In: Leon DF, Shaver JA, eds. *Physiologic Principles of Heart Sounds and Murmurs*. Monograph 46. New York: American Heart Association; 1975:102–106.

514. Still GF. *Common Disorders and Diseases of Childhood*. London: Frowde; 1909.

515. Darazs B, Hesdorfer CS, Butterworth AM, Ziady F. The possible

etiology of the vibratory systolic murmur. *Clin Cardiol* 1987; 10:341–346.

516. Schwartz ML, Goldberg SJ, Wilson N, Allen HD, Mark GR. Relation of Still's murmur, small aortic diameter and high aortic velocity. *Am J Cardiol* 1986; 57:1344–1348.

517. Van Oort A, Hopman J, De Boo T, Van Der Werf T, Rohmer J, Daniels O. The vibratory innocent heart murmur in schoolchildren: A case-control Doppler echocardiographic study. *Pediatr Cardiol* 1994; 15:275–181.

518. Stein PD, Sabbah HN. Aortic origin of innocent murmurs. *Am J Cardiol* 1977; 39:665–671.

519. Shaver JA. Innocent murmurs. *Hosp Med*, April 1978; 8–35.

520. Fowler NO, Marshall WJ. The supraclavicular arterial bruit. *Am Heart J* 1965; 69:410–418.

521. Nelson WP, Hall RJ. The innocent supraclavicular arterial bruit—Utility of shoulder maneuvers in its recognition. *N Engl J Med* 1968; 278:778.

522. Leonard JJ, Renfro NL, deGroot WJ, Page WL. The auscultatory diagnosis of the hyperkinetic state. In: Segal BL, ed. *The Theory and Practice of Auscultation*. Philadelphia: Davis; 1964:180–190.

523. deLeon AC Jr. "Straight back" syndrome. In: Leon DF, Shaver JA, eds. *Physiologic Principles of Heart Sounds and Murmurs*. Monograph 46. New York: American Heart Association; 1975:197–208.

524. Perloff JK. Clinical recognition of aortic stenosis: The physical signs and differential diagnosis of the various forms of obstruction to left ventricular outflow. *Prog Cardiovasc Dis* 1968; 10:323–352.

525. Vogel JH, Blount SG. Clinical evaluation in localizing levels of obstruction to outflow from left ventricle. *Am J Cardiol* 1965; 15:782–792.

526. Paley HW. Left ventricular outflow tract obstruction: Heart sounds and murmurs. In: Leon DF, Shaver JA, eds. *Physiologic Principles of Heart Sounds and Murmurs*. Monograph 46. New York: American Heart Association; 1975:107–121.

527. Gamboa R, Hugenholtz PG, Nadas AS. Accuracy of the phonocardiogram in assessing severity of aortic and pulmonic stenosis. *Circulation* 1964; 30:35–46.

528. Henke RP, March HW, Hultgren HN. An aid to identification of the murmur of aortic stenosis. *Am Heart J* 1960; 60:354–363.

529. Tavel ME, Nasser WK. Murmur alternans in aortic stenosis. *Chest* 1970; 57:176–179.

530. Kroetz FW, Leonard JJ, Shaver JA, Leon DF, Lancaster JF, Beamer VL. The effect of atrial contraction on left ventricular performance in valvular aortic stenosis. *Circulation* 1967; 35:852–867.

531. Hancock EW. Differentiation of valvular and supravalvular stenosis. *Guys Hosp Rep* 1961; 110:1–30.

532. Bonner AJ, Sacks HN, Tavel ME. Assessing the severity of aortic stenosis by phonocardiography and external carotid pulse recordings. *Circulation* 1973; 48:247–252.

533. Kligfield P, Okin P. Effect of ventricular function on left ventricular ejection time in aortic stenosis. *Br Heart J* 1979; 42:438–441.

534. Thompson ME, Shaver JA. Aortic stenosis in the elderly. *Geriatrics* 1983; 38:50–65.

535. Aronow WS, Kronzon I. Correlation of prevalence and severity of valvular aortic stenosis determined by continuous-wave Doppler echocardiography with physical signs of aortic stenosis in patients aged 62 to 100 years with aortic systolic ejection murmurs. *Am J Cardiol* 1987; 60:399–401.

536. Vogelpoel L, Schrire V. Auscultatory and phonocardiographic assessment of pulmonary stenosis with intact ventricular septum. *Circulation* 1960; 22:55–72.

537. Vogelpoel L, Schrire V. Auscultatory and phonocardiographic assessment of Fallot's tetralogy. *Circulation* 1960; 22:73–89.

538. Zuberbuhler JR, Lenox CC, Neches WH, Park SC, Shaver JA. Auscultatory spectrum of the tetralogy of Fallot. In: Leon DF, Shaver JA, eds. *Physiologic Principles of Heart Sounds and Murmurs*. Monograph 46. New York: American Heart Association; 1975:187–192.

539. Martin CE, Reddy PS, Leon DF, Shaver JA. Genesis, frequency and diagnostic significance of the ejection sound in adults with tetralogy of Fallot. *Br Heart J* 1973; 35:402–412.

540. Mills P, Wolfe C, Redwood D, Leech G, Craige E, Leatham A. Noninvasive diagnosis of subpulmonary outflow tract obstruction. *Br Heart J* 1980; 43:276–283.

541. Vogelpoel L, Schrire V, Nellen M, Swanepoel A. The value of amyl nitrite in the differentiation of Fallot's tetralogy and pulmonary stenosis with intact ventricular septum. *Am Heart J* 1959; 57:803–819.

542. Leatham A. Auscultation of the heart. *Lancet* 1958; 2:757–765.

543. O'Rourke RA, Crawford MH. Mitral valve regurgitation. *Curr Probl Cardiol* 1984; 9:1–52.

544. Brigden W, Leatham A. Mitral incompetence. *Br Heart J* 1953; 15:55–73.

545. Karliner JS, O'Rourke RA, Kearney DJ, Shabetai R. Hemodynamic explanation of why the murmur of mitral regurgitation is independent of cycle length. *Br Heart J* 1973; 35:397–401.

546. Nixon PGF. The third heart sound in mitral regurgitation. *Br Heart J* 1961; 23:677–689.

547. Burgess J, Clark R, Kamigaki M, Cohen K. Echocardiographic findings in different types of mitral regurgitation. *Circulation* 1973; 48:97–106.

548. Rivero Carvallo JM, Signo para el diagnostico de las insuficiencias tricuspideas. *Arch Inst Cardiol Mex* 1946; 16:531–540.

549. Leon DF, Leonard JJ, Lancaster JF, Kroetz FW, Shaver JA. Effect of respiration on pansystolic regurgitant murmurs as studied by biatrial intracardiac phonocardiography. *Am J Med* 1965; 39:429–441.

550. Wooley CF. The spectrum of tricuspid regurgitation. In: Leon DF, Shaver JA, eds, *Physiologic Principles of Heart Sounds and Murmurs*. Monograph 46. New York: American Heart Association; 1975:139–148.

551. Leatham A, Segal BL. Auscultatory and phonocardiographic findings in ventricular septal defect with left-to-right shunt. *Circulation* 1962; 25:318–327.

552. Craige E. Phonocardiography in interventricular septal defects. *Am Heart J* 1960; 60:51–60.

553. Roger H. Recherches cliniques sur la communication congénitale des deux coeurs par inocclusion du septum interventriculaire. *Bull Acad Med (Paris)* 1879; 8:1074–1094.

554. Wood P. The Eisenmenger syndrome or pulmonary hypertension with reversed central shunt. *Br Med J* September 1958; 701–709.

555. Vogelpoel L, Schrire V, Beck W, Nellen M, Swanepoel A. Atypical systolic murmur of minute ventricular septal defect and its recognition by amyl nitrite and phenylephrine. *Am Heart J* 1961; 62:101–118.

556. Leatham A. The spectrum of ventricular septal defect. In: Leon DF, Shaver JA, eds. *Physiologic Principles of Heart Sounds and Murmurs*. Monograph 46. New York: American Heart Association; 1975:135–138.

557. Leonard JJ, Shaver JA. Acute mitral insufficiency. *Hosp Pract*, May 1985; 75–96.

558. Sutton GC, Craige E. Clinical signs of severe acute mitral regurgitation. *Am J Cardiol* 1967; 20:141–144.

559. Ronan JA Jr, Steelman RB, DeLeon AC, Waters TJ, Perloff JK, Harvey WP. The clinical diagnosis of acute severe mitral insufficiency. *Am J Cardiol* 1971; 27:284–290.

560. Roberts WC, Braunwald E, Morrow AG. Acute severe mitral regurgitation secondary to ruptured chordae tendineae. *Circulation* 1966; 33:58–70.

561. Morrow AG, Cohen LS, Roberts WC, Braunwald NS, Braunwald E. Severe mitral regurgitation following acute myocardial infarction and ruptured papillary muscle. *Circulation* 1968; 37–38(suppl 2):124–132.

562. Perloff JW, Roberts WC. The mitral apparatus: Functional anatomy of mitral regurgitation. *Circulation* 1972; 46:227–239.

563. DePace NL, Nestico PF, Morganroth J. Acute severe mitral regurgitation: Pathophysiology, clinical recognition, and management. *Am J Med* 1985; 78:293–306.

564. Shapiro HA, Weiss DR. Mitral insufficiency due to ruptured chordae tendineae. *N Engl J Med* 1959; 261:272–276.

565. Braunwald E. Mitral regurgitation. *N Engl J Med* 1969; 281:425–433.

566. Rios JC, Massumi RA, Breesmen WT, Sarin RK. Auscultatory features of acute tricuspid regurgitation. *Am J Cardiol* 1969; 23:4–11.

567. Amidi M, Irwin JM, Salerni R, Lavine SJ, Zuberbuhler JR, Shaver JA, et al. Venous systolic thrill and murmur in the neck: A consequence of severe tricuspid insufficiency. *J Am Coll Cardiol* 1986; 7:942–945.

568. Burch GE, DePasquale NP, Phillips HJ. Clinical manifestations of papillary muscle dysfunction. *Arch Intern Med* 1963; 112:158–163.

569. Humphries JO, McKusick VA. The differentiation of organic and innocent "systolic murmurs." *Prog Cardiovasc Dis* 1962; 5:152–171.

570. Reid JA, Humphries JO. Systolic clicks (so-called systolic gallops): A study of their clinical significance. *Bull Johns Hopkins Hosp* 1955; 97:177–181.

571. Barlow JB, Bosman CK, Pocock WA, Marchand P. Late systolic murmurs and non-ejection ("mid-late") systolic clicks. *Br Heart J* 1968; 30:203–217.

572. Rackley CE, Whalen RE, Floyd WL, Orgain ES, McIntosh HD. The precordial honk. *Am J Cardiol* 1966; 17:509–515.
573. Wigle ED, Sasson Z, Henderson MA, Ruddy TD, Fulop J, Rakowski H, et al. Hypertrophic cardiomyopathy: The importance of the site and the extent of hypertrophy. A review. *Prog Cardiovasc Dis* 1985; 28:1–83.
574. Shaver JA, Alvares RF, Reddy PS, Salerni R. Phonoechocardiography and intracardiac phonocardiography in hypertrophic cardiomyopathy. *Postgrad Med J* 1986; 62:537–543.
575. Murgo JP, Miller JW. Hemodynamic, angiographic and echocardiographic evidence against impeded ejection in hypertrophic cardiomyopathy. In: Goodwin JF, ed. *Heart Muscle Disease.* Lancaster, England: MTP Press; 1985:187–211.
576. Criley M, Siegel RJ. Has "obstructive" hindered our understanding of hypertrophic cardiomyopathy? *Circulation* 1985; 72:1148–1154.
577. Shah PM. Controversies in hypertrophic cardiomyopathy. *Curr Probl Cardiol* 1986; 11:563–613.
578. Braunwald E, Lambrew CT, Rockoff SD, Ross J, Morrow A. Idiopathic hypertrophic subaortic stenosis: I. A description of the disease based upon an analysis of 64 patients. *Circulation* 1964; 30(suppl 4):3–119.
579. Shaver JA, Salerni R, Curtiss EI, Follansbee WP. A clinical presentation and noninvasive evaluation of the patient with hypertrophic cardiomyopathy. In Shaver JA, Brest AN, eds. *Cardiomyopathies: Clinical Presentation, Differential Diagnosis, and Management. Cardiovascular Clinics.* Philadelphia: Davis, 1988:149–192.
580. Murgo JP, Alter BR, Dorethy JF, Altobelli SA, McGranahan GM. Dynamics of left ventricular ejection in obstructive and nonobstructive hypertrophic cardiomyopathy. *J Clin Invest* 1980; 66:1369–1382.
581. Craige E, Millward DK. Diastolic and continuous murmurs. *Prog Cardiovasc Dis* 1971; 14:38–56.
582. Shaver JA. Diastolic murmurs. *Heart Dis Stroke* 1993; 2:98–103.
583. Wood P. An appreciation of mitral stenosis. *Br Med J* 1954; 1:1051–1063.
584. Ueda H, Sakamoto T, Kawai N, Watanabe H, Uozumi Z, Okada R, et al. "Silent" mitral stenosis: Pathoanatomical basis of the absence of diastolic rumble. *Jpn Heart J* 1985; 6:206–219.
585. Criley JM, Chambers RD, Blaufuss AH, Friedman NJ. Mitral stenosis: Mechanico-acoustical events. In: Leon DF, Shaver JA, eds. *Physiologic Principles of Heart Sounds and Murmurs.* Monograph 46. New York: American Heart Association; 1975:149–159.
586. Criley JM, Hermer AJ. The crescendo presystolic murmur of mitral stenosis with atrial fibrillation. *N Engl J Med* 1971; 285:1284–1287.
587. Hada Y, Amano K, Yamaguchi T, Takenaka K, Takahashi H, Takikawa R, et al. Noninvasive study of the presystolic component of the first heart sound in mitral stenosis. *J Am Coll Cardiol* 1986; 7:43–50.
588. Tavel ME. Presystolic murmur of mitral stenosis revisited. *J Am Coll Cardiol* 1986; 7:51–52.
589. Wooley CF, Fontana ME, Kilman JW, Ryan JM. Tricuspid sounds: Atrial systolic murmur, tricuspid opening snap, and right atrial pressure pulse. *Am J Med* 1985; 78:375–384.
590. Killip T III, Lukas DS. Tricuspid stenosis: Clinical features in 12 cases. *Am J Med* 1958; 24:836–452.
591. Sanders CA, Hawthorne JW, DeSanctis RW, Austen G. Tricuspid stenosis: A difficult diagnosis in the presence of atrial fibrillation. *Circulation* 1966; 33:26–33.
592. Craige E. Phonocardiography in interventricular septal defects. *Am Heart J* 1960; 60:51–60.
593. Ravin A, Darley W. Apical diastolic murmurs in PDA. *Ann Intern Med* 1950; 33:903–914.
594. Fortuin NJ, Craige E. Echocardiographic studies of genesis of mitral diastolic murmurs. *Br Heart J* 1973; 35:75–81.
595. Coombs CF. *Rheumatic Heart Disease.* New York, William Wood, 1924:190.
596. Flint A. On cardiac murmurs. *Am J Med Sci* 1862; 44:29–54.
597. Segal JP, Harvey WP, Corrado MA. The Austin Flint murmur: Its differentiation from the murmur of rheumatic mitral stenosis. *Circulation* 1958; 18:1025–1033.
598. Fortuin NJ, Craige E. On the mechanism of the Austin Flint murmur. *Circulation* 1972; 45:558–570.
599. Craige E. The Austin Flint murmur. In: Leon DF, Shaver JA, eds. *Physiologic Principles of Heart Sounds and Murmurs.* Monograph 46. New York: American Heart Association; 1970:160–165.
600. Reddy PS, Curtiss EI, Salerni R, O'Toole JD, Griff FW, Leon DF, et al. Sound pressure correlates of the Austin Flint murmur: An intracardiac sound study. *Circulation* 1976; 53:210–217.
601. Rahko PS. Doppler and echocardiographic characteristics of patients having an Austin Flint murmur. *Circulation* 1991; 83:1940–1950.
602. Green EW, Agruss NS, Adolph RJ. Right-sided Austin Flint murmur. *Am J Cardiol* 1973; 32:370–374.
603. Harvey WP, Corrado MA, Perloff JK. "Right-sided" murmurs of aortic insufficiency. *Am J Med Sci* 1963; 245:533–543.
604. Sakamoto T, Kawai N, Uozumi Z, Yamada T, Inove K, Change SY, et al. The point of maximum intensity of aortic diastolic regurgitant murmur. *Jpn Heart J* 1968; 9:117–133.
605. Sabbah HN, Khaja F, Anbe DT, Stein PD. The aortic closure sound in pure aortic insufficiency. *Circulation* 1977; 56:859–863.
606. Stembridge VA, Hejtmancik MR, Herrmann GR. Unusual musical murmurs of anterior cusp aortic regurgitation: Report of 10 cases. *Am Heart J* 1954; 48:163–172.
607. Steell G. The murmur of high pressure in the pulmonary artery. *Med Chron* 1888; 9:182–188.
608. Runco V, Molnar W, Meckstroth CV, Ryan JM. The Graham Steell murmur versus aortic regurgitation in rheumatic heart disease. *Am J Med* 1961; 31:71–80.
609. Perez JE, Smith CA, Meltzer VN. Pulmonic valve insufficiency: A common cause of transient diastolic murmurs in renal failure. *Ann Intern Med* 1985; 103:497–502.
610. Runco V, Levin HS. The spectrum of pulmonic regurgitation. In: Leon DF, Shaver JA. eds. *Physiologic Principles of Heart Sounds and Murmurs.* Monograph 46. New York: American Heart Association; 1975:175–182.
611. Myers JD. The mechanisms and significances of continuous murmurs. In: Leon DF, Shaver JA, eds. *Physiologic Principles of Heart Sounds and Murmurs.* Monograph 46. New York: American Heart Association; 1975:201–208.
612. Fowler NO, Gause R. The cervical venous hum. *Am Heart J* 1964; 67:135–136.
613. Tabatznik B, Randall TW, Hersch C. The mammary souffle of pregnancy and lactation. *Circulation* 1960; 22:1069–1073.
614. Hurst JW, Staton J, Hubbard D. Precordial murmurs during pregnancy and lactation. *N Engl J Med* 1958; 259:515–517.
615. Gibson GA. Lecture on patent ductus arteriosus. *Edinburgh Med J* 1900; 8:1–10.
616. Ongley PA, Rahimtoola SH, Kincaid OW, Kirklin JW. Continuous murmurs in tetralogy of Fallot and pulmonary atresia with ventricular septal defect. *Am J Cardiol* 1966; 18:821–826.
617. Victor S, Lakshmikanthan C, Shankar G, Parameswaran PG, Sreenivasan H, Sadasivan CS. Continuous murmur as sequel of augmented collateral circulation in suppurative lung disease: Report of 3 cases. *Chest* 1972; 62:504–505.
618. Minkoff SM, Fort ML, Sharp JT. Rupture of an aneurysm of the sinus of Valsalva into the right atrium. *Am J Cardiol* 1967; 19:278–284.
619. Ross J Jr, Braunwald E, Mason DT, Braunwald NS, Morrow AG. Interatrial communication and left atrial hypertension: A cause of continuous murmur. *Circulation* 1963; 28:853–860.
620. Keith JD, Rowe RD, Vlad P, O'Hanley JH. Complete anomalous pulmonary venous drainage. *Am J Med* 1954; 16:23–38.
621. Myers JD, Murdaugh HV Jr, McIntosh HD, Blaisdell RK. Observations on continuous murmurs over partially obstructed arteries. *Arch Intern Med* 1956; 97:726–737.
622. Edholm OG, Howarth S, Sharpey-Schafer EP. Resting blood flow and blood pressure in limbs with arterial obstruction. *Clin Sci* 1951; 10:361–367.
623. Spencer MP, Johnston FR, Meredith JH. Origin and interpretation of murmurs in coarctation of aorta. *Am Heart J* 1958; 56:722–736.
624. Dock W, Zoneraich S. Diastolic murmur arising in stenosed coronary artery. *Am J Med* 1967; 42:617–619.
625. Sangster JF, Oakley CM. Diastolic murmur of coronary artery stenosis. *Br Heart J* 1973; 35:840–844.
626. Cheng TO. Diastolic murmur caused by coronary artery stenosis. *Ann Intern Med* 1970; 72:543–546.

11

EXAMINATION OF THE RETINA

W. Banks Anderson, Jr.

Inspection of the smaller vessels of the body is possible in only three areas: the retina, the conjunctiva, and the nail beds. The ophthalmoscope has made the retina by far the easiest and most rewarding of these observation sites. Viewing this two-dimensional vascular display is generally much easier, especially in the aged, if the pupils are dilated. One drop of tropicamide 1% ophthalmic solution (Mydriacyl) will dilate the pupils in 15 or 20 min. Pulse and blood pressure determinations should be made prior to the instillation of such rapidly acting mydriatics, as both may increase after absorption of the drops. Although complications of mydriasis are rare, the pupils are best left undilated in patients in whom the iris seems closely apposed to the cornea and in those with a history of closed-angle glaucoma. Examination of the retina should proceed methodically. Best pupillary dilatation is maintained if the optic disk is observed first. Look for evidence of edema and blurred margins and for cupping with sharp contours. Rule out neovascularization or the pallor of optic atrophy. Next, scan along the superior temporal arcade, inspecting the arteries carefully for embolic plaques at each bifurcation. Note the arteriovenous crossings for evidence of obscuration of the vein and for pronounced nicking and banking of the vessels. The lower arcade and the nasal vessels may be inspected next. Avoid the macular area until all else has been viewed, as the pupil constricts most intensely when this area is illuminated. To find diabetic microaneurysms early, look just temporal to the fovea, along the horizontal raphe. To discover cotton-wool infarcts, look circularly around the disk two disk diameters out. With such a plan in mind, the retina can be efficiently searched for evidence of cardiovascular disease (see Table 11-1).

An appreciation of the pathophysiological variations in retinal architecture is essential for recognizing its disease processes. The following sections describe morphologic changes helpful in assessing the cardiac patient.

TABLE 11-1
RETINAL TOPOGRAPHY

Finding	Most Common Location
Arteriovenous crossings	Upper temporal quadrant
Cotton-wool spots	Around optic disk
Hard exudates	Between disk and fovea
Microaneurysms	Temporal to fovea
Emboli	Arterial bifurcations
Diabetic new vessels	Nerve head and arcades

CHANGES IN RETINAL VESSEL CALIBER

Changes in caliber along the course of a single artery or vein are of much greater significance than are estimates of arteriovenous ratios or absolute vascular diameter. Estimates of the degree of tortuosity or straightening are also generally valueless except in the situation where the veins are large, dark, and tortuous. This constellation of findings implies outflow obstruction, arterial inflow obstruction, hypoxia, or all three.[1] Such dark and dilated veins may occur in patients with large right-to-left shunts, in the leukemias, and in hyperviscosity syndromes.

Autonomic innervation of the retinal vessels does not exist.[2] Nevertheless, the retinal vessels may change in caliber both acutely and chronically. Autoregulation of the retinal vessels does occur, and oxygen is the most active vasomotor substance. With hyperoxia, there is rapid constriction of both the arteries and veins, while in hypoxia, vasodilatation occurs.[3] Elevated carbon dioxide tension is also a retinal vasodilator.[4] Striking clinical examples of these combined effects are the vasodilatation (darkening of the blood column) and retinal and disk edema seen in patients with marked pulmonary insufficiency and right-sided cardiac failure[5] and in children with cyanotic congenital heart disease.[6] At the opposite extreme, the marked vasoconstrictor effect of oxygen may produce retinal vasoobliteration in immature infants, with resulting retinopathy of prematurity.

Estimates of arteriovenous ratios are of little clinical utility.[7] Of much greater significance are variations in the caliber of a single vessel. These changes may take the form of focal narrowing, sometimes called *beading* or *spasm*. Beading is produced by an abnormal constriction that may be contiguous with an abnormally dilated segment. Usually seen in the venous system where there is venous outflow obstruction, such beading is particularly common in diabetic retinopathy. Beading of the arteries is not generally associated with systemic disease but is seen in congenital conditions such as von Hippel's angiomatosis, Coats' disease, and Leber's miliary aneurysms.

Segmental narrowing or spasm of the retinal vessels has been much described in the older literature. Most descriptions of rapid waves of "spasm" were probably observations of patients with moving fibrin or platelet emboli. Narrowing of the retinal vessels has been observed in response to injections of norepinephrine and angiotensin.[8] Autoregulatory narrowing of the retinal vessels is a response to hypertension and upon occasion may be focal. This narrowing is chronic, and "spasm" is not an apt description.

THICKENING OF THE VASCULAR WALL

Normally only the blood column is visible when the retinal vessels are viewed. When changes in the walls do occur, they are most visible along the sides of the vessels, since in this location the tangential line of sight presents a greater thickness to the viewer. Vessels at the disk often appear sheathed. This normal variant may be associated with a veil of tissue in front of the disk (Bergmeister's papilla). More peripheral retinal vessels become sheathed or cuffed in response to intraocular inflammation, vasculitis, or multiple sclerosis. Fatty exudate (hard exudate) may collect along venous walls (never arteries), particularly in diabetic exudative retinopathy. These deposits are not intrinsic to the wall itself. After venous obstructive disease of some duration, a white, uniform line may develop along either side of the retinal veins in the involved area. Ballantyne[9] terms this *halo sheathing*, and Kennedy and Wise[10] have found it to consist of increased collagen deposition in the vessel wall.

ARTERIOSCLEROSIS

Should the retinal arterial circulation be considered arterial or arteriolar? If vessel size is the criterion, then *arteriolar* might be proper. Nevertheless, Hogan and Feeney[11] have demonstrated smooth muscle cells several layers thick in the media of the retinal arterial vessels both posteriorly and in the periphery. We therefore use the terms *arteriosclerosis* and *artery* without respect to the size of the vessels. In arteriosclerosis, the medial smooth muscle (which may hypertrophy in chronic hypertension) becomes hyalinized with the deposition of collagen. As the wall thickens, the vessel takes on a burnished coppery luster; with further thickening, this may transmute to silver. Obscuration of the venous blood column at arterial crossings is early evidence of this process. Even when the artery walls become so thick as to resemble "silver wires," flow can ordinarily still be demonstrated by fluorescein angiography. The intensity of the light reflex from these older vessels is increased, although the width of the vascular light reflex itself does not appear to be related to age or blood pressure.[12]

ARTERIOVENOUS COMPRESSION

Arteriovenous compression, or "nicking," has as its histologic basis the sharing by the artery and vein of a common adventitial sheath at their crossings. Arteriosclerotic thickening impedes venous outflow at these locations, with venous tortuosity, engorgement, and darkening of the blood column distal to the compression. Where the vein dives beneath the thick artery wall, sometimes "banking" to intersect at right angles, its blood column is obscured and it appears nicked.

ATHEROSCLEROSIS

Atherosclerosis, or fatty infiltration of the intima, was once thought not to occur in the retina. Clinicopathologic confirmation of retinal atherosclerosis has been obtained.[13] Retinal atheromata have a predilection for the bifurcations and bends within the first two branches of the central retinal artery, appearing as segments of irregular yellowish sheathing and having the crystalline knobbiness of a salted pretzel stick. On occasion the thickening may progress to the point where no blood column is visible, although total obstruction is rare.

COTTON-WOOL SPOTS

Cotton-wool spots are generally a sign of serious systemic disease. They may be seen in patients with severe hypertension, blood dyscrasias, collagen diseases, or hemorrhagic shock. Cotton-wool spots are also frequently seen in patients with acquired immunodeficiency syndrome (AIDS).[14] They are almost invariably found within three disk diameters of the optic disk and have a feathery, woolly character because of their anterior involvement of the nerve fiber layer (Fig. 11-1, Plate 15). Cotton-wool "exudates" are not exudates but consist of a cluster of cell-like swollen ends of fragmented axons (cytoid bodies) in an area of edematous retina. They

FIGURE 11-1
See color Plate 15.

are evanescent and will often disappear within a few weeks, leaving behind no observable trace of their presence. Ischemia is almost certainly the cause of these spots, which may occur secondary to occlusion of peripapillary capillaries, occlusion of a small artery, or hypoxia. The presence of these cotton-wool spots is usually indicative of serious systemic disease.

HARD EXUDATES

Hard exudates are most probably edema residues. They occur in situations where the vessels become leaky, and as the more watery component of the extravasation is resorbed, the lipid residue forms hard, yellow, waxy deposits. They may surround the leaking vessel in a circinate ring or may accumulate in the macula, radiating from the fovea in the spokes of a macular "star" (Fig. 11-2, Plate 16). Histologically found deep in the retina, these exudates will disappear in some months if the source of the leakage is eliminated. These exudates indicate a loss of vascular wall integrity and are associated with hypertension, diabetes, venous outflow obstruction, and retinal angiomas. They are not ischemic in origin but indicate chronic fluid extravasation and retinal edema.

MICROANEURYSMS

Microaneurysms are not unique to diabetes but occur in many disease states, including retinal venous obstructive disease, sickle cell disease, the dysproteinemias, Behçet's disease, sarcoidosis, and other forms of uveitis. A common factor in all these conditions seems to be the presence of both retinal hypoxia and viable capillary endothelial cells. Microaneurysms are outpouchings in capillary walls that range in size from 20 to 100 μm. They are commonly found adjacent to zones of capillary obliteration or "dropout," and it has been suggested that they represent abortive attempts at revascularization of a compromised capillary bed (Fig. 11-3, Plate 17). Their etiology is, however, still unknown.

NEOVASCULARIZATION

Neovascularization also occurs in conditions where microaneurysms are found. The new vessels generally originate from capillaries or from the venous side of the circulation and are associated with greater or lesser degrees of fibrosis. In all cases, however, the new vessels are incorporated in an associated fibrous membrane (Fig. 11-4, Plate 18; and Fig. 11-5).

FIGURE 11-2
See color Plate 16.

FIGURE 11-3
See color Plate 17.

FIGURE 11-4
See color Plate 18.

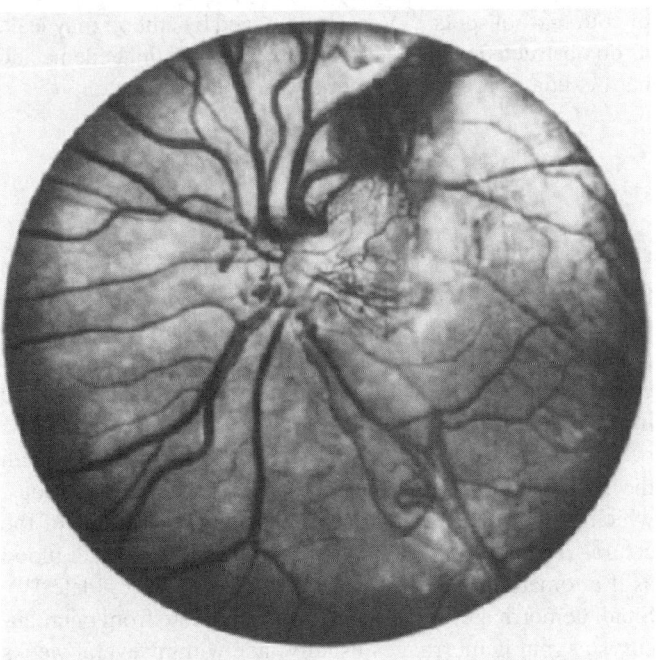

FIGURE 11-5
Proliferative diabetic retinopathy, left eye. There is extensive neovascularization of the disk with an associated small intravitreal hemorrhage that obscures the upper temporal vessels. Along the inferior temporal arcade is another area of neovascularization. These new vessels are incorporated in fibrous membranes that may tent up the vessels and cause traction detachments of the retina, as at the lower right edge of the photograph.

Some of the channels appear to function as shunts and, in cases of venous outflow obstruction, may serve to bypass the obstructed site. Other neovascular channels branch in a fanlike fashion toward an avascular zone or forward into the vitreous cavity, proliferating along a posterior hyaloid membrane. Such a *rete mirabile* does not appear to have any shunting function and is more suggestive of an attempt at revascularization of an unperfused tissue. Clinically the likelihood of blinding vitreous hemorrhage is greatly increased in the presence of such neovascularization.[15]

RETINAL VESSEL LEAKAGE

Normally the retinal vessels are permeable only to quite small molecules. This blood-retina barrier is analogous to the blood-brain barrier and is facilitated by the overlapping of the endothelial cells and the tight endothelial cell junctions in retinal vessels. Enclosed within the basement membrane of the capillary is an intramural pericyte whose investment may contribute to the relative impermeability of these vessels.

The sodium fluorescein molecule normally does not traverse this vascular barrier, and by fluorescein angiography, abnormal sites of leakage can be conveniently defined. With this technique, neovascular channels are found to leak profusely, as do microaneurysms. In severe hypertension, small areas of leakage may be seen along tiny arteries in the vicinity of cotton-wool spots.[16] Vessels damaged by emboli may leak, as do obstructed veins or inflamed vessels. Retinal edema and hard exudates are the consequences of this leakage.

RETINAL HEMORRHAGE

Hemorrhage into the retina indicates further breakdown in the integrity of the vascular wall. When the hemorrhage occurs in the inner retina, as in hypertension, it assumes a feathery flame shape as it is molded and dispersed by the nerve fibers coursing toward the disk. Deeper hemorrhages, such as those in diabetics, take on a more rounded dot or blot shape. Diabetic neovascularization may result in large hemorrhages beneath the retinal internal limiting membrane or into the vitreous, which obscures the underlying retina. In obstructions of the central retinal vein, the fundus may be splattered with blood as if a tomato had ruptured on the disk (Fig. 11-6, Plate 19). Small hemorrhages are difficult to differentiate from microaneurysms, but hemorrhages usually fade within several weeks while microaneurysms may persist for months to years.

Hemorrhage may occur beneath the retina and usually originates not from the retinal vessels but from proliferation of a choroidal neovascular membrane growing through Bruch's membrane. These hemorrhages commonly occur beneath the macula and may destroy central vision. They have the appearance of a gray-black mass with a red fringe and have been mistaken for malignant melanomas of the choroid.

VASCULAR OCCLUSION

When the central artery or one of its branches is occluded, the nonperfused retinal area becomes cloudy in a matter of minutes. At the fovea, where the retina is one cell layer thick and nourished by the choroid, the normal color and transparency persist. By contrast with the surrounding pallor, the fovea then has a cherry-red appearance (Fig. 11-7, Plate 20). Occlusion at the capillary level is identified by the surrounding microaneurysms or adjacent cotton-wool spots. With fluorescein angiography, such areas can be directly identified by their lack of perfusion.

Occlusion of the central retinal vein results in retinal edema and the "squashed tomato" hemorrhages noted above. Occlusions of branches of the central vein produce edema and hemorrhage in the drained area (Fig. 11-6, Plate 19). These branch vein occlusions always occur at arteriovenous crossings. Examination of the retina of the opposite eye of such patients will generally reveal significant arteriovenous com-

pression. As collateral drainage channels develop (Fig. 11-8, Plate 21), the edema and hemorrhagic retinopathy subside, leaving white-walled veins, neovascularization, and microaneurysms in the affected area. Hemorrhage into the vitreous may occur as a late complication from the neovascularization. There is a very high incidence of diabetes and hypertension in patients with venous obstructive disease,[17] and retinal and systemic arteriosclerosis is usually present.

OPTIC DISK EDEMA

Increased intracranial pressure, retinal venous outflow obstruction, inflammation, and ischemia are the four major causes of optic disk edema. The term *papilledema* is reserved by ophthalmologists and neurologists for the form of disk edema that is the result of increased intracranial pressure. It therefore has an etiologic connotation and is not used generally to mean optic disk edema. Patients with papilledema see well, while other forms of disk edema are associated with poor vision. *Papillitis* is the term applied to inflammatory disk edema. Patients with anterior ischemic optic neuropathy commonly have a pale, edematous disk with an altitudinal field effect. When this is associated with elevations of the sedimentation rate, such patients should be suspected of having giant-cell arteritis (temporal arteritis). If this diagnosis can be established, steroid therapy is indicated to prevent loss of vision in the opposite eye.

RETINAL DYSTROPHY

In the equatorial periphery can be seen the irregular pigment clumps typical of retinitis pigmentosa, or "night blindness." Such pigment spicules in association with bilateral palsies of ocular movement occur in Kearns-Sayre syndrome. Affected patients develop progressive atrioventricular block, which in turn may cause sudden death. The syndrome is the result of mutated mitochondrial deoxyribonucleic acid (DNA).[18]

OPTIC ATROPHY

In eyes with retinal dystrophy or with the resolution of disk edema in papillitis or ischemic optic neuropathy, the disk will become flat and pale. Both pallor and impaired visual function are necessary for the diagnosis of optic atrophy, since both the color and vascularity of the disk are highly variable. If the disk is atrophic and cupped with a shift of the vessels to the nasal side, glaucoma should be suspected. Optic atrophy without cupping may indicate intracranial tumor and should be investigated. It is unlikely that tumor has caused the atrophy if vision was once poor and has returned to near normal

FIGURE 11-6
See color Plate 19.

FIGURE 11-7
See color Plate 20.

FIGURE 11-8
See color Plate 21.

TABLE 11-2
EMBOLI OF CARDIOVASCULAR SIGNIFICANCE

Type	Appearance	Significance
Platelet	Dull pink to gray often with associated fibrin	Downstream vegetations, mural thrombi
Hollenhorst plaque	Glistening yellow-orange plaques at bifurcations	Downstream atheroma (containing cholesterol)
Calcium plaque	Glistening white plaques	Calcific aortic stenosis
Roth spot	Hemorrhage with gray-white center (Plate 23, 12-5)	Blood dyscrasia or septic embolus as in subacute bacterial endocarditis (SBE)
Fat embolus	Fuzzy-bordered gray-white spot without hemorrhage	Severe trauma with long-bone fractures; prognosis grave
Myxoma	Disk edema, retinal edema in arterial supply zone	Life-threatening atrial myxoma

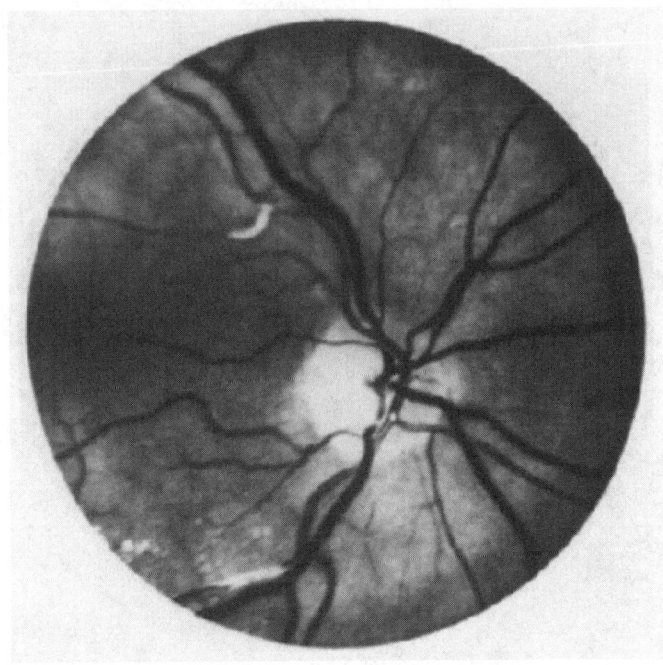

FIGURE 11-9
Retinal emboli often lodge at bifurcations, as in this patient with carotid atherosclerosis. Note that the embolic material often seems larger than the containing vessel, as in the embolus at the lower left edge of the photograph. Emboli may damage the vessel wall and cause leakage, as can be seen by the exudate deposited about the inferior embolus. Hollenhorst cholesterol plaques rarely obstruct arterial flow completely, and this patient maintained vision.

levels. This is the situation often observed in patients with demyelinating disease.

EMBOLISM

Embolism from the heart and great vessels occurs more commonly than is generally appreciated. A sudden increase in tinnitus in one ear, a fleeting woozy sensation, a scintillating scotoma, and a transient monocular visual loss all may be symptoms of embolic ischemia. This clinical suspicion may be confirmed by ophthalmoscopy. Table 11-2 lists the characteristics of retinal emboli of cardiovascular significance. Of these, platelet emboli are at once the most common and the most evanescent. Within minutes after vision has returned, platelet emboli have usually broken into fragments too small to be identified ophthalmoscopically. Most other emboli persist for days or years and are more lasting evidence of an embolic episode. Hollenhorst cholesterol plaques may be identified at the same bifurcations for months to years after the embolic shower. Platelet emboli, Hollenhorst plaques (Fig. 11-7, Plate 20; and Fig. 11-9), and calcium emboli (Fig. 11-10, Plate 22) are usually seen along the course of a retinal artery. Roth spots (Fig. 11-11, Plate 23) and fat emboli may not appear to be intravascular and may not be associated with a vessel that is ophthalmoscopically visible (see Table 11-2).

Inspection of the retina may identify emboli that were deposited during cardiac catheterization or surgery. Valvular surgery is an especially likely source. In one series of 81 such patients, 12 percent were noted to have postoperative signs of retinal emboli.[19] Embolic central retinal artery occlusion has been reported during cardiac catheterization.[20]

DISEASES

The eye is a major target for two extremely common diseases of cardiovascular significance: diabetes and hypertension. Blindness from the former now ranks as the second leading cause of acquired adult blindness in the United States, and these diabetic changes are commonly paralleled by severe renal and cardiac vasculopathy.

Diabetes Mellitus

The average diabetic develops ophthalmoscopically visible retinal changes after 16 years of the disease. Focal loss of a portion of the capillary bed is followed by microaneurysm formation and vascular dilatation around the borders of the area of capillary dropout (Fig. 11-3, Plate 17). Vascular leakage occurs with dot and blot hemorrhages and deposits of

FIGURE 11-10
See color Plate 22.

FIGURE 11-11
See color Plate 23.

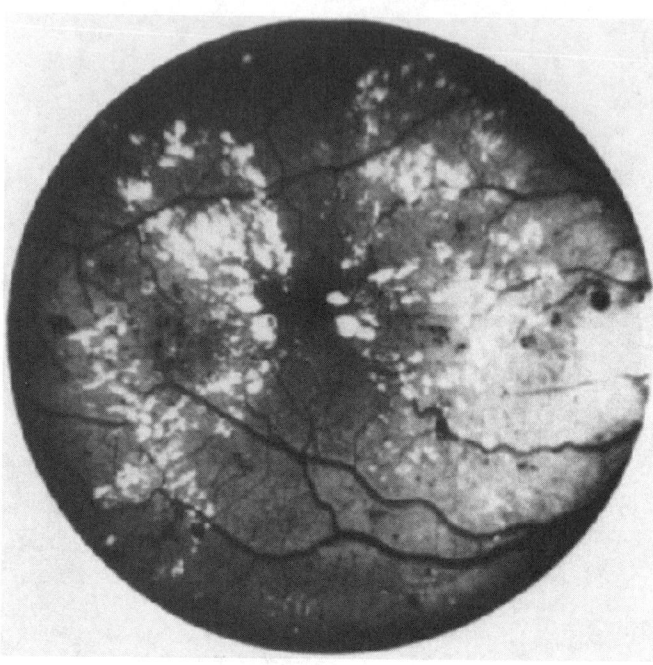

FIGURE 11-12
Exudative diabetic retinopathy, right eye, illustrating microaneurysms, dot-and-blot hemorrhages, and venous engorgement with extensive deposits of hard, yellow exudate.

hard exudate (Fig. 11-12). New blood vessels develop along the vascular arcades and at the optic nerve head (Fig. 11-4, Plate 18; and Fig. 11-5). The proliferation of new blood vessels with their associated membranes often results in blinding hemorrhage into the vitreous cavity and tractional detachment of the retina.

The clinician must recognize early proliferative diabetic retinopathy, for not only are these changes associated with renal and cardiac disease but immediate laser photocoagulation of the retina may be sight-saving.[21] Control of the commonly associated hypertension is also of great importance, as elevations of systemic blood pressure compound the difficulty in controlling retinal vascular leakage. Even the presence of "high-normal" blood pressure has been correlated with diabetic retinopathy,[22] although a cause-and-effect relationship has not been established (see also Chap. 78).

Systemic Arterial Hypertension

When the systemic blood pressure rises, the retinal circulation becomes especially vulnerable, since its capillary pressure floor is determined by the intraocular pressure (about 16 mmHg) and not by the jugular or cavernous sinus pressure. The intraocular pressure does not increase in hypertension, and increases in systemic blood pressure would be directly reflected in increased retinal capillary perfusion pressure were it not for the homeostatic responses of the retinal vasculature.

Vasoconstriction of the arterial tree and thickening of the arterial vessel walls with consequent reduction in lumen diameter are homeostatic responses to hypertension. Arteriosclerotic narrowing of the vessels acts to insulate the capillary bed from the elevated pressure of the arterial supply. These arteriosclerotic changes are visible as narrowing, increases in central light reflexes, and copper and silver "wiring" of the arteries (Fig. 11-13, Plate 24). If, however, increases in the systemic blood pressure are either very marked or very rapid, these homeostatic mechanisms are overwhelmed. The resulting decompensation of the capillary bed results in accumulations of fluid in the retina and optic nerve head. The aqueous portion of the fluid is more rapidly cleared than the lipid component, which accumulates as hard exudate. Radial arrangement of such exudate deposits in the macula produces a "star" (Fig. 11-2, Plate 16). Hemorrhage may occur in the inner retinal layers in a characteristic flame pattern, and focal ischemia in the nerve fiber layer may result in cotton-wool microinfarcts. In severe hypertensive decompensation, the optic nerve head becomes swollen and edematous (Fig. 11-2, Plate 16). In older classifications,[23,24] patients with disk edema would be assigned to the grade IV category of hypertensive retinopathy. Patients with eclampsia or pheochromocytoma may have such marked and rapid elevations of capillary pressure that edema fluid floats the retina off the choroid, producing an exudative (nonrhegmatogenous) detachment of the retina and visual loss. Such retinal signs of capillary bed decompensation are usually paralleled by severe renal vasculopathy, and therapeutic efforts are indicated immediately. The likelihood that the patient suffers from a nonessential variety of hypertension is also markedly increased, especially if the patient is Caucasian.[25] It is clinically useful, therefore, to categorize hypertensive patients as to whether or not their retinal circulation is compensated or has decompensated with observable edema, cotton-wool spots, flame hemorrhages, or swelling of the optic disk.

FIGURE 11-13
See color Plate 24.

REFERENCES

1. Wise GN, Dollery CT, Henkind P. *The Retinal Circulation.* New York: Harper & Row; 1971:220–221.
2. Laties AM. Central retinal artery innervation: Absence of adrenergic innervation to the intraocular branches. *Arch Ophthalmol* 1967; 77:405–409.
3. Cusick PL, Benson OO, Boothby WM. Effect of anoxia and of high concentrations of oxygen on the retinal vessels. *Mayo Clin Proc* 1940; 15:500–502.
4. Frayser R, Hickam JB. Retinal vascular response to breathing increased carbon dioxide and oxygen concentrations. *Invest Ophthalmol* 1964; 3:427–431.
5. Stevens PM, Austen F, Knowles JH. Prognostic significance of papilledema in course of respiratory insufficiency. *JAMA* 1963; 183:161–164.
6. Petersen RA, Rosenthal A. Retinopathy and papilledema in cyanotic congenital heart disease. *Pediatrics* 1972; 49:243–249.
7. Stokoe NL, Turner RW. Normal retinal vascular pattern: Arteriovenous ratio as a measure of arterial caliber. *Br J Ophthalmol* 1966; 50:21–40.
8. Dollery CT, Hill DW, Hodge JV. The response of normal retinal blood vessels to angiotensin and noradrenaline. *J Physiol* 1963; 165:500–507.
9. Ballantyne AJ. The state of the retina in diabetes mellitus. *Trans Ophthalmol Soc UK* 1966; 66:503–543.

10. Kennedy JE, Wise GN. Retinochoroidal vascular anastomosis in uveitis. *Am J Ophthalmol* 1971; 71:1221–1225.

11. Hogan MJ, Feeney L. The ultrastructure of the retinal blood vessels. *J Ultrastruct Res* 1963; 9:10–28.

12. Brinchmann-Hansen O, Myhre K, Sandvik L. The light reflex in retinal vessels and its relations to age and systemic blood pressure. *Acta Ophthalmol* 1987; 65:206–212.

13. Brownstein S, Font RL, Alper MG. Atheromatous plaques of the retinal blood vessels: Histologic confirmation of ophthalmoscopically visible lesions. *Arch Ophthalmol* 1973; 90:49–52.

14. Rosenberg PR, Uliss AE, Friedland GH, Harris CA, Small CB, Klein RS. Acquired immunodeficiency syndrome—Ophthalmic manifestations in ambulatory patients. *Ophthalmology* 1983; 90:874–878.

15. The Diabetic Retinopathy Study Research Group. Four risk factors for severe visual loss in diabetic retinopathy: The third report from the diabetic retinopathy study. *Arch Ophthalmol* 1979; 97:654–655.

16. Hodge VJ, Dollery CT. Retinal soft exudates: A clinical study by color and fluorescence photography. *Q J Med* 1964; 33:117–131.

17. Quinlan PM, Elman MJ, Bhatt AK, Mardesich P, Enger C. The natural course of central retinal vein occlusion. *Am J Ophthalmol* 1990; 110:118–123.

18. Moraes CT, DiMauro S, Zeviani M, Lombes A, Shanske S, Miranda AF, et al. Mitochondrial DNA deletions in progressive external ophthalmoplegia and Kearns-Sayre syndrome. *N Engl J Med* 1989; 320:1293–1299.

19. Pe'er J, Milgalter E, Matmoros N, Silberman S, Vidaurri L. Retinal emboli after open heart surgery (letter). *Arch Ophthalmol* 1989; 107:317.

20. Stefansson E, Coin T, Lewis WR, Belkin RN, Behar VS, Morris JJ, et al. Central retinal artery occlusion during cardiac catheterization. *Am J Ophthalmol* 1985; 99:586–589.

21. The Diabetic Retinopathy Study Research Group. Photocoagulation treatment in proliferative diabetic retinopathy: The second report of diabetic retinopathy study findings. *Ophthalmology* 1978; 85:82–106.

22. Chase PH, Garg SK, Jackson WE, Thomas MA, Harris S, Marshall G, Crews MJ. Blood pressure and retinopathy in type I diabetes. *Ophthalmology* 1990; 97:155–159.

23. Scheie HG. Evaluation of ophthalmoscopic changes of hypertension and arteriolar sclerosis. *Arch Ophthalmol* 1953; 49:117–138.

24. Keith NM, Wagener HP, Barker NW. Some different types of essential hypertension: Their course and prognosis. *Am J Med Sci* 1939; 197:332–343.

25. Davis BA, Crook JE, Vestal RE, Oates JA. Prevalence of renovascular hypertension in patients with grade III or IV hypertensive retinopathy. *N Engl J Med* 1979; 301:1273–1276.

CHAPTER

12

THE RESTING ELECTROCARDIOGRAM

Agustin Castellanos / Kenneth M. Kessler / Robert J. Myerburg

What is commonly called an *electrocardiogram* (ECG) is the graph obtained when the electrical potentials of an electrical field originating in the heart are recorded at the body surface.[1–3] Emphasis should be placed on the fact that only potential differences in the field are registered, since the ECG does not record *directly* the electrical activity of the heart itself. Classically, there are two major subdivisions of clinical electrocardiography[4]: (1) the analysis of arrhythmias (see Chap. 27) and (2) the study of the resting 12- (and occasionally more) lead ECG, which is discussed in this chapter. Although the ECG provides very useful clinical information, it affords only an approximation of the voltage produced by the source. Unfortunately, the ECG has not been able to achieve major *new* insights into its own basic theoretical limitations, which some have considered as the solutions of the "forward" problem and the "inverse" problem of electrocardiography.[1,2] Whereas the former seeks the description of a specific ECG pattern in response to a specific local or regional intracardiac change in electrical activity, the inverse problem seeks to predict the behavior of the cardiac generator from potentials recorded at the body surface.[1,2] Despite these limitations, the ECG has many uses: it may serve as an independent marker of myocardial disease; it may reflect anatomic, hemodynamical, molecular, ionic, or drug-induced abnormalities of the heart; and it may provide information that is essential for the proper diagnosis and therapy of many cardiac problems[4] (see also Chap. 27). In fact, it is the most commonly used laboratory procedure for the diagnosis of heart disease. Underreading or misreading due to insufficient knowledge of pathologic conditions, overreading due to inability to recognize technical errors, and—most important—failure to correlate ECG findings with the clinical findings may result in iatrogenic heart disease. Every physician interpreting ECGs as well as those learning ECG interpretation should read the *Guidelines for Electrocardiography of the American College of Cardiology, American Heart Association Task Force.*[4]

VENTRICULAR DEPOLARIZATION AND REPOLARIZATION

Fluxes of ions across the cell membrane cause the differences in voltage between resting and activated myocardial cells. To understand the electrical forces produced by the heart as a whole at the body surface, it has been conventional to first discuss the electrical properties of a hypothetical muscle strip from the free wall of the left ventricle extending from endocardium to epicardium.[5–7] In the resting or polarized state, the charges are at rest. A unipolar electrode facing the epicardial side of the strip, such as V_6, registers an isoelectric line.[5–13] If activation of this relatively large muscle strip starts in the endocardial side, it initiates the process called *depolarization.*[5–13] The *sequence* of this process is thus from endocardium to epicardium. Depolarization has been described as a moving wave *with the positive charges in front of* the negative charges. The previously mentioned lead V_6 overlying the epicardium of the left ventricle (LV) will record a positivity because it consistently faces positive charges throughout the entire depolarization sequence.[5–13] On the other hand, the *sequence* of ventricular repolarization is from epicardium to endocardium.[5–13] The *negative charges*, however, travel *in front*, since repolarization tends to reestablish the resting, polarized state of the previously depolarized cells. Consequently, V_6 will record a positive deflection (T wave) because it constantly faces positive charges throughout the entire repolarization sequence. The earlier epicardial onset of repolarization has been attributed to the shorter duration of repolarization that epicardial cells have in comparison to endocardial cells. Thus, repolarization finishes at the epicardium while it still has not been completed at the endocardium. Hence, the *sequence* of repolarization is, as previously noted, from epicardium to endocardium. In contrast, in isolated (small) muscle strips the *sequence* of repolarization is from endocardium to epicardium (see "Ventricular Gradient," below).

ELECTROCARDIOGRAPHIC LEADS

To record an ECG, an electric circuit between the heart and the electrocardiograph must be completed.[11] For this purpose, electrodes are placed on different parts of the body surface and are connected to the instrument by means of cables.[11] Thus, the whole system consists of an instrument, electrodes, cables, and leads.

Bipolar Standard Leads

An ECG lead can be defined as a pair of terminals with designated polarity, each of which is connected either directly or through passive-active network to recording electrodes. In 1913, Einthoven et al.[3] developed a method of studying the electrical activity of the heart by representing it graphically in a two-dimensional geometric figure—namely, an equilateral triangle. While this is not strictly (mathematically) true, it has provided the clinician with a practical concept with which to work. None of the many objections held against the theory has done away with it.[9,13] Einthoven's hypothesis is founded upon several simplifying assumptions[3–13]: (1) The body is a homogeneous volume conductor. Although the conductivity of the various tissues is not the same, the differences are not great and the body can be considered as a homogeneous volume conductor. (2) The sum of all the electric forces, or the mean of all the forces generated during the cardiac cycle, can be considered as originating in a dipole located in the electrical center of the heart. (3) Electrodes placed on the right arm (RA), left arm (LA), and left leg (LL) are used to pick up the potential variations on these extremities. Standard (bipolar) leads (I, II, and III) are obtained by recording, respectively, the potential differences between LA and RA, LL and RA, and LL and LA. These leads record potential variations in the frontal plane only. (4) Attachment between these limb electrodes, on the forearms and limbs, corresponds to a position in the root of the corresponding limb. For example, an electrode in the right forearm records the electrical activity that reaches the right shoulder. It should be pointed out that when the electrodes are placed proximally to the roots of the extremities, they lose their relatively "far" distance from the heart. Hence, Einthoven's equilateral theory does not hold. The latter explains why limb leads placed proximally to the roots of the extremities, like some used for coronary care unit and ambulatory electrocardiographic (Holter) monitoring or during exercise testing, by being only "equivalent" to the corresponding bipolar leads, are in some cases markedly different from the "true" standard bipolar leads.

Wilson Central Terminal

The sum of the potentials from RA, LA, and LL is equal to zero throughout the cardiac cycles with respect to any point at the body surface.[3,5,6,13] Lead wires attached to electrodes on each limb are connected together, through 5000-ohm resis-

tors, at a point. When this common point—Wilson's central terminal—is attached to the negative pole of the ECG machine and an "exploring" electrode is connected to the positive pole, the potential variations recorded will be those of the latter only. A lead taken by this method is called a *unipolar* lead. Actually, the electrical potential of the central terminal is not truly zero because the right arm, left arm, and left leg are not equidistant from each other and from the heart; the body tissues vary in resistance; and the heart and the extremities do not lie in exactly the same plane in the body. The potential of the central terminal has been said to average around 0.3 mV.[9]

Unipolar Extremity Leads

Unipolar extremity leads were initially recorded by a system in which the central terminal of Wilson constituted the indifferent electrode and the exploring electrode was one of the three of the limb electrodes. A lead is called *indifferent* if it approximates, for arbitrary sources in the heart, the potential existing at an infinite distance from these sources.[13] Such leads were known as V_R, V_L, and V_F. At present, unipolar extremity leads are obtained by disconnecting the input to the central terminal of Wilson from the extremity being explored. This results in a $1\frac{1}{2}$ increase in their voltage. These *augmented* (a) extremity leads are the ones currently used for clinical electrocardiography and are labeled aV_R, aV_L, and aV_F.[5,9,13]

Unipolar Precordial Leads

The unipolar precordial ECG is obtained by placing the exploring electrode (connected to the positive pole of the ECG machine) on the classical six locations of the anterior and left portions of the chest.[5,6,13] The central terminal is used as the indifferent electrode. Unipolar leads made by this method are prefixed by the letter V (which stands for *voltage*), followed by subscript numbers 1 through 6, which indicate the corresponding chest sites. Precordial leads yield a positive deflection when facing positive charges and a negative deflection when facing negative charges.[5,13] They do this according to what Wilson called the *solid angle concept*.[5,13] A solid angle is merely an imaginary cone extending from the site in the chest throughout the heart. The precordial electrode is at its apex, and its base is at the opposite epicardial surface.[13] This concept is important in order to understand precordial lead morphologies. For example, a lead displaying an old (Q-wave) infarction may show changes consistent with a new infarction. This occurs because the solid angle subtended by the corresponding lead explores more than the region generating the old scar. Precordial leads record the electrical activity from the regions of the heart over which they are placed as well as from distant regions.[5] Thus, if V_2 is placed over (thereby facing) the right ventricle, part of the initial positive ventricular deflection reflects right ventricular activation, with the corresponding electrical forces moving toward the electrode.[13] Most portions of the terminal S wave represent activation of muscle other than the right ventricle (septum and free left ventricular wall), reflecting electric forces moving away from the electrode.[13] Lead V_2 is a right ventricular lead only because the electrode faces the right ventricle, not because it records only the electrical activity of the right ventricle. For practical purposes, the peak of the r (or R) wave in this and all other precordial leads gives a rough estimate of the moment of arrival of excitation (*intrinsicoid* deflection) at the muscle underneath the electrode.[13] This, however, encompasses a considerable amount of muscle fibers (given by the solid-angle concept); in fact, the amount is greater than if the electrode is placed directly on the epicardial surface.[13] In the latter situation, the amount of arrival of excitation at the electrode affects a lesser number of fibers and is thus given by the *intrinsic* deflection.[13]

NORMAL ACTIVATION OF THE HEART: VENTRICULAR DEPOLARIZATION

After emerging from the sinus node, the cardiac impulse propagates throughout the atria in its journey toward the atrioventricular (AV) node. The normal P wave (due to activation of the myocardium of both atria) is a consequence of but does not directly represent sinus node activity. During sinus rhythm, the right atrium is activated before the left atrium.[6] This explains why high-fidelity recordings of the P waves of some normal persons show a small notch at the top. The latter simply reflects the normal asynchrony existing between the atria.[6] Because of the anatomic position of the sinus node, the sequence of atrial depolarization occurs in an inferior, leftward, and somewhat posterior direction. The normal P waves are always positive in leads I, II, aV_F, and V_3 to V_6 and negative in lead aV_R. According to the anatomic position of the heart, the P wave may be diphasic in V_1 and aV_L or negative in the latter lead. Atrial repolarization, also called T_a, is directly opposite in polarity to the P wave.[6,11] It is usually not seen because it coincides with the PR segment (not to be confused with the PR interval) and QRS complex. Since the cardiac impulse reaches the AV node before the end of atrial depolarization, arrival of excitation at the AV node occurs at an undetermined moment (which can be roughly estimated by catheter recordings) within but before the end of the P wave. Activation of the ordinary ventricular muscle (onset of the QRS complex) starts as soon as the impulse emerging from the most distal ramifications of the bundle branches depolarizes a sufficiently large number of cells.[6,7,11] Therefore, the PR interval (used to estimate AV conduction time) includes conduction through the "true" AV structures (AV node, His bundle, bundle branches, and main divisions of the left bundle branch) as well as through those parts of the atria located between sinus and AV nodes.[8] The onset of ventricular depolarization (given by the beginning of the normal q wave) reflects activation of the left side of the interventricular septum. This has been attributed to the fact that the left bundle system is shorter than the right bundle branch.[8,15] In addition, the large fanlike distribution of the ramifications of the fascicles of the left bundle branch on the left septal surface pro-

duces activation of a greater number of ordinary muscle cells per unit of time.[8,15] For this reason, the normal initial depolarization is oriented from left to right, therefore explaining the small q wave in lead V_6 and the small r wave in V_1. After the cardiac impulse descending through the right bundle branch reaches the right septal surface, the interventricular septum is activated in both directions. Septal activation is therefore encompassed within or neutralized by free wall activation. The most distal ramifications of both bundle branches (Purkinje fibers) form networks within the subendocardial regions of both ventricular walls. The latter are activated as soon as the multiple ramifications emerge from the Purkinje fibers.[15] The greater mass of the left ventricular (LV) free wall explains why LV free wall events overpower those of the interventricular septum and right ventricular free wall.

ELECTRICAL AXIS

The electrical axis (EA) may be defined as a vector originating in the center of Einthoven's equilateral triangle.[3,13] A *vector* is a mathematical value expressed as an arrow that has magnitude, sense, and direction. On the other hand, scalar values have only magnitude. Moreover, *vector* is a term for *force*, and since all electrocardiography deals with electrical forces, all electrocardiography can be considered vectorial. In practice, however, the term vectorial is used in referring to forces represented by arrows and loops rather than by complexes and waves. When applied to the EA, the vector that represents it also gives the direction of the activation process as projected in the plane of the limb leads. Its length represents the manifest potential of the dipole in the center of the triangle. These general considerations apply either to the instantaneous EA (the vector indicating the direction of the impulse at the instant at which it is determined) as well as the mean EA (which is the resultant of all instantaneous electrical axes). Although the term *EA* can be used in reference to any of the major components of the ECG (P, T, or QRS), it is generally applied to the QRS. There are many methods for determining the mean EA. The one recommended by electrocardiographers of the classical school consists of calculating the net areas enclosed by the QRS complex in leads I, II, and III.[3,6,7,12,13] The net area is the absolute sum of the positive and negative areas of the QRS complex in the corresponding lead. One of the drawbacks of this method is that the absolute values of the net area cannot be determined *accurately* by inspection. Since the absolute magnitude of the EA is not of fundamental clinical importance, it has been recommended that arbitrary units be used. When this is done, the results can be counterchecked by using Einthoven's law. For example, if, in a given case, lead I is $+4$ units, lead II is $+2$ units, and lead III is -2 units, the calculation is accurate, since the sum of leads I and III ($+4$ plus -2) must always equal lead II ($+2$). After having determined the net area, the results are plotted on the sides of the triangle, and perpendiculars are dropped from two or all three leads. The perpendiculars will meet at a point away from the center of the triangle. A line drawn from the latter to the former defines the mean EA. A simpler though less precise method of calculating the quadrant (or parts of a quadrant) in which the EA is located consists of using the maximal QRS deflection in leads I and aV_F and, when necessary, lead II. This method is inexact from the mathematical viewpoint but has the value of simplicity.[15,16]

Ventricular Repolarization

Although the depolarization process in the free LV wall has been extensively studied, less known is how repolarization spreads throughout the interventricular septum and both ventricles.[12,13] This is probably related to the fact that in these structures repolarization is not a propagated process in the sense that depolarization is. It is for this reason that it is slower (takes longer time) and has a smaller voltage than depolarization. Moreover, it does not follow the same pathways.[12]

VENTRICULAR GRADIENT

The relationship between the EA of the QRS complex and the T wave was referred to by Wilson as the *ventricular gradient*.[17] In contrast to what occurs in an epicardial-to-endocardial muscle strip (as previously mentioned), in the isolated muscle strip the *sequence* of ventricular depolarization occurs in the same direction as that of repolarization.[12] Although the QRS and T deflections have opposite polarity, the algebraic sum of QRS and T *areas* is zero. In the human heart, however, not only is the sequence different, but the pathways of ventricular depolarization and repolarization are not exactly the same.[12] Thus, the algebraic sum of QRS and T *areas* is no longer zero. Therefore, a gradient is said to exist. The ventricular gradient can be calculated by determining the electrical axis of the QRS and T (using *areas*) and then obtaining the resultant by the parallelogram method. Wilson considered that the ventricular gradient could be useful in differentiating between T-wave inversion of various causes (*primary changes*) and the obligatory *secondary T-wave*

changes resulting from abnormalities in depolarization, such as bundle branch block, ventricular hypertrophy, ventricular pacing, and preexcitation syndromes.[12,13,17] In practice, calculation of the ventricular gradient is difficult and time consuming, since it must be determined by areas and not maximal amplitude.

Apparent Challenges to the Concept of the Ventricular Gradient

Rosenbaum et al. studied the prolonged depolarization occurring during long periods of ventricular stimulation and found two types of altered ventricular repolarization.[18] One, corresponding to Wilson's classical theory, was transient and proportional in magnitude to the QRS complex but of opposite polarity. The other, concealed by (and during) the former, required a longer time (even days) to reach maximal effect as well as to disappear, becoming apparent *only when* normal activation recurred. The latter type was attributed to modulated electronic interactions occurring during cardiac activation in such a way that repolarization was accelerated at ventricular sites where depolarization begins and delayed in areas where depolarization terminates. T-wave changes appearing after prolonged depolarization was no longer present showed accumulation and (fading) memory that persisted for variable time (see "Secondary ST-T–Wave Changes," below).[18] The term *memory* refers to the capacity of the myocardial cells to "remember" the previously concealed repolarization changes even after the causative effects had ceased to exist.[18] These abnormalities are primary according to Wilson's classical schema.

ABNORMAL ST-SEGMENT CHANGES

In orthodox ECG language, *injury* implies *abnormal* ST-segment changes, *necrosis* implies *abnormal* Q waves, and *ischemia* implies *symmetric* T-wave inversion (or elevation).[5–7,9–13,16] Following conventional ECG theory, several authors consider that ECG "injury" occurs because the affected cells are unable to maintain their normal polarization during diastole.[5–7,12,16,19] Various hypotheses have been postulated to explain how this diastolic hypopolarization or generalized diastolic depolarization is manifest as abnormal ST-segment shifts in the surface ECG (Fig. 12-1).[20–22] One hypothesis is based on the existence of a diastolic current of "injury." During the control (diastolic) period, both membrane resting potential and surface ECG baseline are at their normal level. At the onset of injury, the resting intracellular

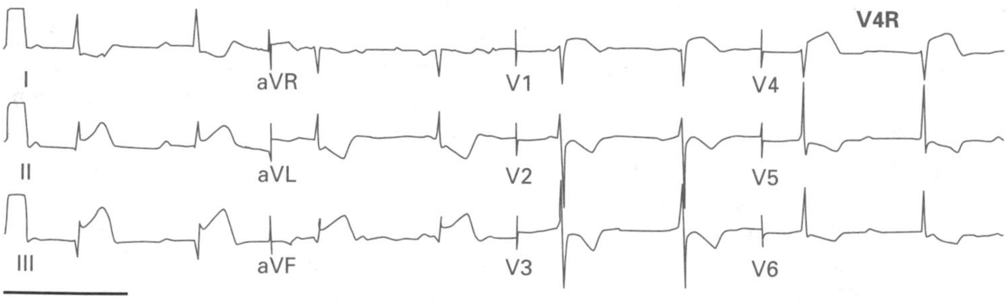

FIGURE 12-1

Acute inferior (diaphragmatic) myocardial infarction showing "indicative" ST-segment elevation in leads reflecting the inferior wall (II, III, and aV_F). Reciprocal changes are seen in the diametrically opposed leads (I and aV_L) located in the same (frontal) plane. V_4R showed evidence of right ventricular myocardial infarction. There was complete AV block with an AV junctional rhythm. QRS duration: 0.10 s.

potential decreases (for example, from -90 to -70 mV) and the ECG baseline shifts below its preinjury level. Because the injured cells leak negative ions, their *exterior* becomes relatively negative (or less positive) than that of the normal cells. Thus, a "current of injury" flows between the negative ("injured") zone and the positive (normal) region.[10] This produces a negative displacement of the surface ECG *baseline* in the leads facing the injured region. In the surface ECG, depolarization (by virtue of the electrical negativization of the nonaffected area) practically reduces the potential difference between noninjured and injured regions. Therefore, the ST segment remains at the preinjury level, which is relatively *elevated* in reference to the injury baseline. Consequently, the ST segment appears to be abnormally displaced above the latter. Note that the apparent presence of a systolic current of injury actually reflects disappearance of the diastolic current of injury. Finally, after the end of repolarization, the current of injury between injured and noninjured regions is reestablished and the ECG baseline is again depressed (as it was immediately before depolarization). Since the precise moment at which injury starts is not recorded in the surface ECG, the baseline that is almost invariably recorded is the postinjury baseline, which has been placed at an apparently adequate position by the recording instrument or by the ECG technician.[10] It also has been shown that the abnormal ST-segment elevation in leads facing the affected zone does not merely represent the (passive) return of the baseline to its preinjury level but reflects a true, active, positive displacement.[10,20–23] Thus, when depolarization of both normal and injured regions has occurred, the surface of the normal cells will (because of their greater initial polarization) be able to accumulate more negative ions. Hence, the normal regions become more negative than the injured regions, which are relatively more positive. In consequence, the ST segment becomes actively elevated above and beyond the preinjured baseline because of the relative potential difference existing at the end of depolarization. Most likely, injury reflects both disappearance of diastolic baseline shifts plus active ST elevation.[10,22] According to the current-of-injury theory, this process results in ST-segment elevation when the injured muscle is located between normal muscle and the corresponding unipolar electrode. On the other hand, ST-segment depression occurs when normal muscle is located between the injured tissue and the corresponding electrode (Fig. 12-1).[10,12] The mechanism of abnormal ST segment elevation in anatomically defined ventricular aneurysms has not been fully established. Some authors consider

that it results from the earlier repolarization of a ring of persistently viable (but nevertheless affected) tissue surrounding the aneurysm.[10] For other investigators, chronic ST-segment elevation reflects functional (echocardiographic) dyskinesia, thus not necessarily being due to a pathologic ventricular aneurysm.[8,23–25] Coronary artery disease is the most frequent cause of abnormal ST-segment elevation. The latter, when generalized, can also be due to epicardial injury due to pericarditis. Pericarditis should be differentiated from the benign "early repolarization" pattern, a normal variant.[26,27] In its classical form, there is J-point elevation (of no more than 3 mm) with an upwardly concave ST segment. R waves may be tall and at times have a distinct notch and slur on the downstroke (Fig. 12-2). ST-segment elevation is more frequent in chest leads but can occur in leads I and II. These dynamic ECG changes may be affected by exercise and hyperventilation. Isoproterenol reduces while propranolol increases ST-segment elevation.[28,29] Although the mechanism of early repolarization has not been fully elucidated, it has been related to enhanced activity of the right sympathetic nerves.[28] A high-takeoff ST segment of either the coved or saddleback type localized to the right chest leads, associated with right bundle branch block and sudden cardiac death, is known as the *Brugrada syndrome*.[30] Finally, advanced hyperkalemia can also produce ST-segment elevation in the right chest leads.

ABNORMAL Q WAVES

Abnormal Q waves appearing several hours after total occlusion of a coronary artery result from the necrosis secondary to the decreased blood supply. The number of affected cells

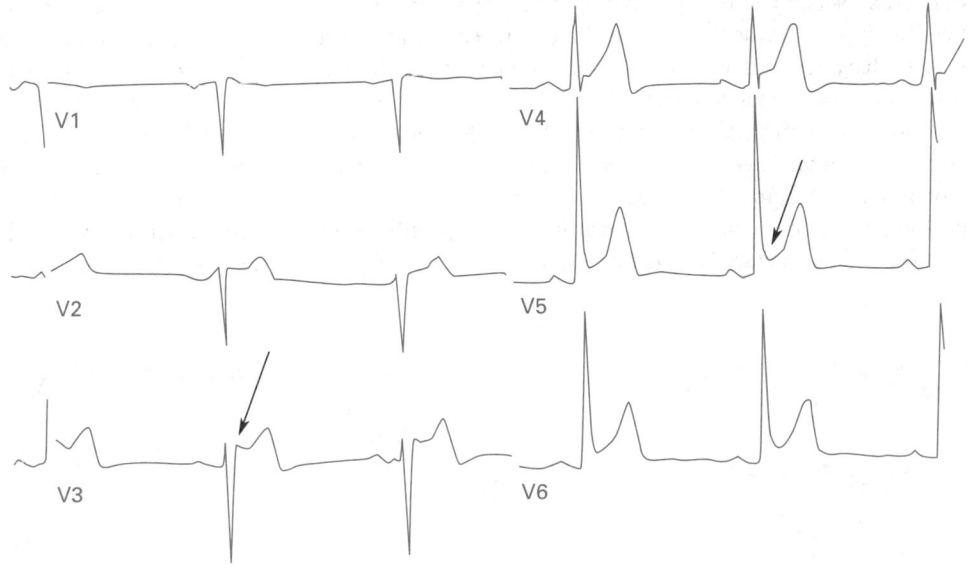

FIGURE 12-2

Early repolarization. This normal variant is characterized by narrow QRS complexes with J point and ST-segment elevation in the chest leads. Left chest leads often show tall R waves with a distinct notch or slur in their downstroke (*arrow* in V₅), while the right chest leads may display ST segments having a "saddleback" or "humpback" shape (*arrow* in V₃).

must be large enough to produce changes reflected at the body surface. In general, the depth of the Q wave is proportional to wall thickness involved.[7] Thus, in leads I and V_4 to V_6, a QS complex reflects transmural necrosis. The duration of the Q wave is proportional to the extent of the area of necrosis parallel to the epicardial surface.[7] If the latter starts in the subendocardium and extends toward (but not quite reaches) the epicardium, the corresponding leads will record QR or Qr complexes depending on the amount of living tissue located between dead tissue and the recording electrode. Therefore, abnormal Q waves may occur in infarctions that are not completely transmural.[7] In the course of the clinical entity known as acute *myocardial* infarction (MI), persisting Q waves are usually but not invariably due to anatomic (lack of blood flow-related) necrosis. Abnormal Q waves can also occur transiently in unstable angina, Prinzmetal's angina, coronary artery spasm, and exercise-induced ischemia. This has been attributed to an intensity of cellular affectation ("injury") severe enough to produce a significant degree of hypopolarization (to around -60 mV). Because the cells become electrically unexcitable (even though they are not, anatomically, irreversibly necrotic),[7,8,15,16] abnormal Q waves occur. Spontaneous recanalization of an occluded vessel, spontaneous reversion of the ischemia, or spasm and interventions (pharmacologic or mechanical) that improve cellular metabolism and oxygenation can restore the normal polarization. If these cells become again excitable, the abnormal Q waves may disappear or vanish.[16,31] Ischemic necrosis takes some hours to appear.[5] This contrasts with the accelerated occurrence of abnormal Q waves in the majority of patients with Q-wave MI after successful thrombolysis or following coronary artery angioplasty performed early in the course of the process. The genesis of these Q waves is not well understood.[31] Some authors consider them an expression of the acceleration of necrosis secondary to explosive cell swelling in already irreversibly injured tissue.[31] Because some of these Q waves also tend to disappear quickly, other authors consider that they reflect factors other than myocardial necrosis, such as reversal of regional metabolic abnormalities or transient interstitial ischemia or hemorrhage.[32] Q waves that persist for more than 1 day may result from other causes than necrosis. Profound and prolonged ischemia can cause myocardial stunning with reversible functional, metabolic, ultrastructural, and electrophysio-

logic abnormalities.[33] Thus, transient Q waves may be the ECG counterpart (electrical stunning) of the corresponding mechanical stunning.[31–34] It is possible for myocardial stunning to lag behind electrical recovery.[31] *Myocardial stunning* should be differentiated from *myocardial hibernation*. The latter is a term used in reference to chronic, not transient mechanical dysfunction of an ischemic area.[35,36] Although the ECG counterpart of this type of mechanical dysfunction requires further studies, it is conceivable that (in some cases) the disappearance of chronic Q waves after coronary artery bypass surgery with improvement of wall motion abnormalities indicates that these Q waves were due not to cellular death but to cellular hibernation.[35,36] (see also Chaps. 43 to 45). Finally, abnormal Q waves need not be the end result of coronary artery disease, since they may be seen after primary (due to infections or drugs) cellular necrosis and in other pathologic processes such as myocardial infiltration and certain types of interventricular septal (and LV) hypertrophy, Wolff-Parkinson-White syndrome, and muscular dystrophies.[37]

ISCHEMIC T-WAVE CHANGES

Symmetric T waves, upright or inverted, characteristic of ECG "ischemia" have been considered to reflect a type or degree of cellular affection resulting only in action potentials of increased duration.[7,10,16] Because the QT interval recorded at the body surface can be considered as the sum of all action potentials (that is, of the QT intervals of individual cells), any process (such as ECG ischemia) that increases the duration of action potentials will cause prolongation of ventricular depolarization and QT interval. In subendocardial ischemia, the increased duration of the action potentials occurs in a group of cells where it was already longer than in the epicardium. Because this is an exaggeration of normality, repolarization (though taking a longer time than usual) still spreads from epicardium to endocardium.[7,10] In consequence, the QT interval is prolonged and the T wave appears symmetrically positive. On the other hand, the increase in the duration of action potentials that occurs in epicardial ischemia results not only in delayed repolarization (QT prolongation) but also in a change in the sequence of repolarization, which now starts at the endocardium repolarized earlier and then spreads toward the epicardium with the negative charges in front. The latter produces the characteristic symmetric T-wave inversion,[7,10] which does not always reflect "physiologic" ischemia (due to decreased blood supply), since they can also be seen in evolving pericarditis, myocardial contusion, increased intracranial pressure (Fig. 12-3), and in the right chest leads of young patients (persistent juvenile pattern).[5,37]

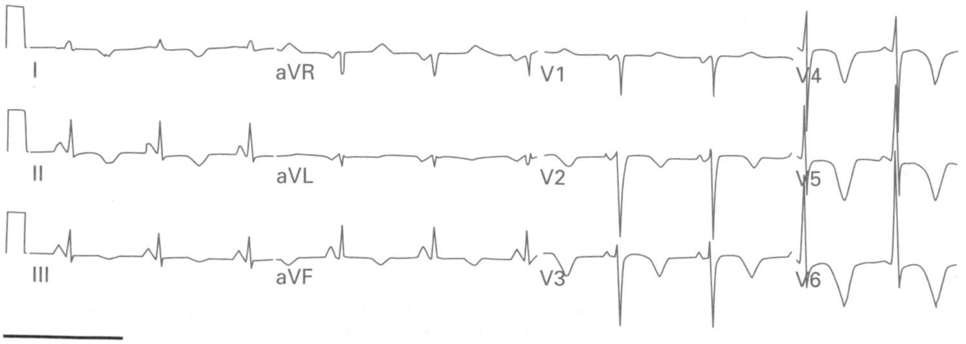

FIGURE 12-3

Electrocardiographic ischemia. Symmetric T-wave inversion is more evident in left chest leads. The uncorrected and corrected QT intervals were prolonged (0.52 and 0.54 s, respectively).

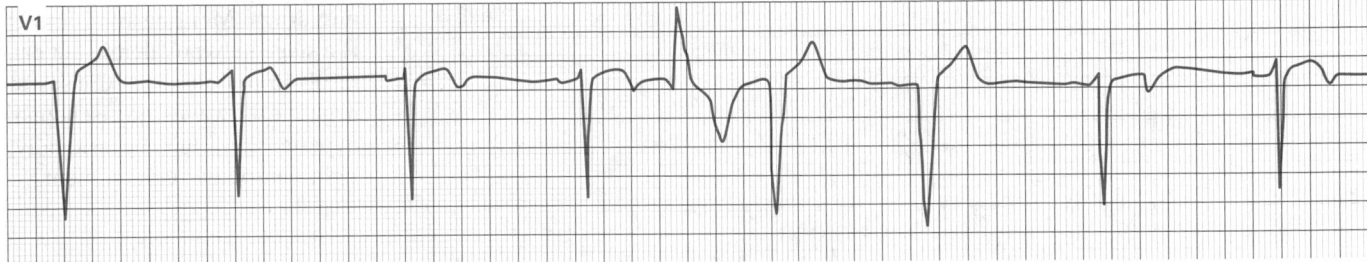

FIGURE 12-4
Tachycardia-dependent complete left bundle branch block. Negative, non-ischemic T waves were manifest (when the left bundle branch block disappears) in leads showing a predominant negative (S-waves) deflection. The patient had "primary" conduction system disease with no other evidence of organic heart disease. These changes have been attributed to accumulation and cardiac memory.[18]

SECONDARY ST-T–WAVE CHANGES

Alterations in the sequence of (and sometimes delay in) ventricular depolarization—as occurs with bundle branch blocks, ventricular pacing, ectopic ventricular impulse formation, pre-excitation syndromes, and ventricular hypertrophy—result in a change in the sequence of ventricular repolarization. The latter causes nonischemic T-wave inversions (secondary T-wave changes) in leads showing predominantly positive QRS deflections.[6,10,12,17] As mentioned in the section on ventricular gradient, disappearance of these alterations of ventricular depolarization may be followed by narrow QRS complexes with negative T waves.[18] An example (attributed to electrotonic modulation, memory, and accumulation) is shown in (Fig. 12-4). In intermittent chronic "complete" left bundle branch block (LBBB), when the ventricular complexes become narrow, inverted T waves appear in leads (such as V_1 and V_2) where the S wave predominates (Fig. 12-4). That changes in the ventricular activation sequence can produce primary but nonischemic T-wave changes capable of persisting long after cessation of the triggering factors has important clinical implications in intermittent bundle branch block (BBB), preexcitation syndromes, and posttachycardia syndrome and in patients with implanted pacemakers.[18] Finally, marked ST-segment changes may occur during rapid supraventricular tachycardias in young patients without metabolic evidence of (physiologic) ischemia.[38]

NONSPECIFIC ST-SEGMENT–T-WAVE CHANGES

ST-segment and T-wave changes will be considered together because of their often coexistence. While nonspecific (or rather nondiagnostic) ST-segment–T wave changes are the most commonly diagnosed ECG abnormalities, they have not been adequately categorized and represent different findings for various interpreters.[39] In their classical paper, Friedberg and Zager considered depth of ST-segment depression and T-wave inversion as well as their contour (Fig. 12-5).[40] When analyzed without clinical information, this diagnosis was made in 40 percent of 410 abnormal ECGs. But the number was reduced to 10 percent when clinical data became available. In absence of structural heart disease, these changes can be due to a variety of physiologic (hyperventilation, anxiety, body position, food, neurogenic influences, and temperature), pharmacologic (antiarrhythmic and psychotropic drugs, digoxin) and extracardiac (electrolyte abnormalities, upper gastrointestinal processes, allergic reactions, etc.) factors.[39]

U WAVE

Several hypotheses have been advanced to explain its genesis. Foremost among them is their relationship to late repolariza-

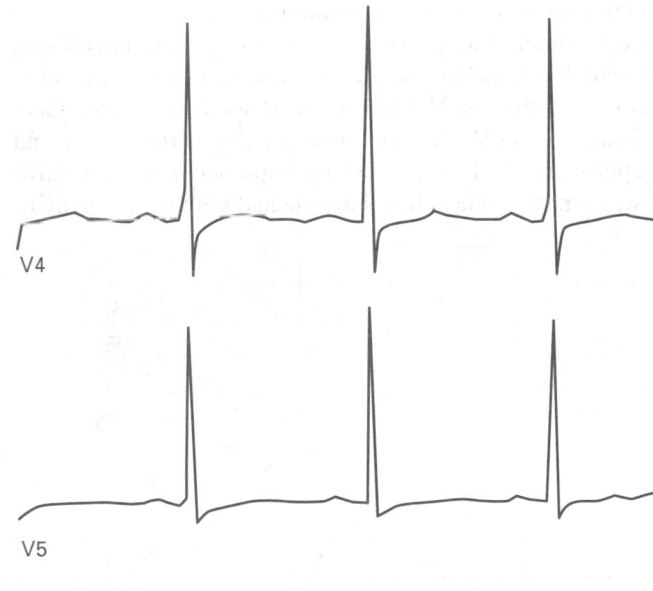

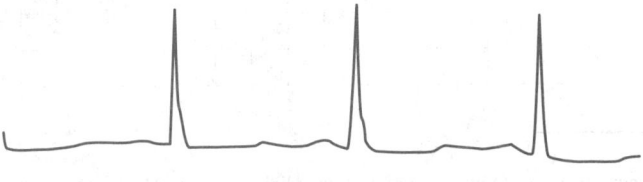

FIGURE 12-5
Nonspecific (nondiagnostic) ST-segment–T wave changes, the most common abnormalities in ECG interpretation.

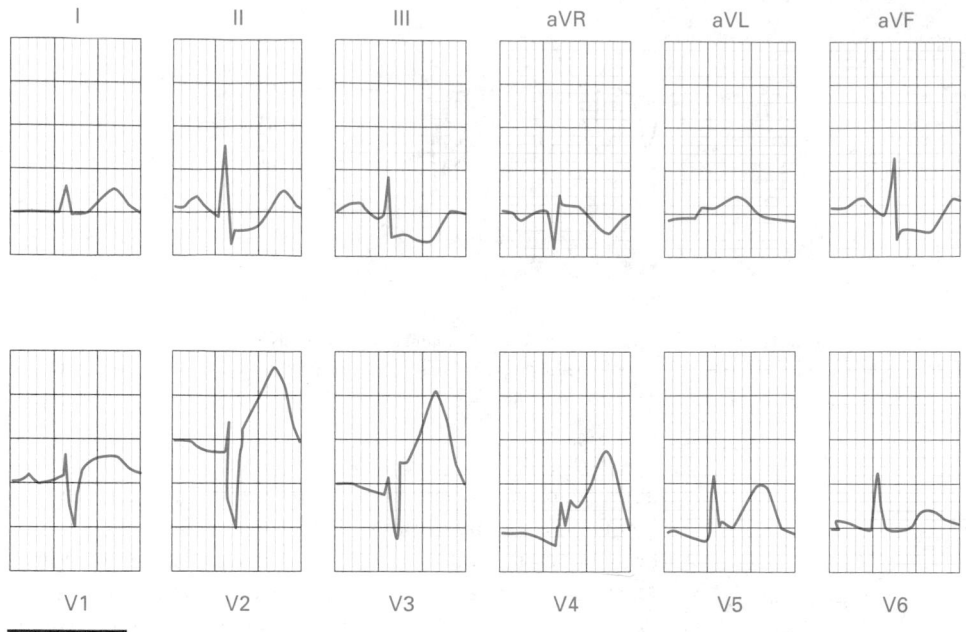

FIGURE 12-6

Acute extensive anterior wall myocardial infarction showing abnormal ST-segment changes and hyperacute T waves.

mic drugs. Merging of T and U is a stage in hypokalemia but can result from quinidine. Causes of negative U waves are ischemia, hypertension, and, occasionally, right ventricular enlargement.

ACUTE MI

Myocardial infarctions are no longer classified as transmural and subendocardial but rather as Q-wave and non–q wave.[42–45] In the thrombolytic era the prevalence of the latter seems to be greater than that of the former (see Chap. 47) presumably because of a reduction infarct size.[42–44] The prethrombolytic "classical" evolution of acute MI has been transformed by pharmacologic therapy and interventional techniques.[44,45] The suc-

tion of the Purkinje system. A criticism of this hypothesis is that the conducting system does not have sufficient mass to generate a large deflection at the body surface. The recent identification of another population of (M) cells in the deep subepicardium may provide the necessary mass to produce, not only U waves but also the J (or Osborn) wave characteristics of hypothermia.[41] The normal U wave, most prominent in leads V_2 and V_3, has the same polarity as the T wave and is approximately 10 percent of its amplitude. A large positive U wave may be due to hypokalemia and multiple antiarrhyth-

cession of events in the course of a Q-wave MI is from hyperacute positive T waves (on occasion) to ST-segment elevation to abnormal Q waves to T-wave inversion (Figs. 12-1, 12-6, and 12-7).[44,45] Commonly two or more of these findings appear together, depending on the timing of the first recorded static ECG. Acceleration of these phases can occur with effective reperfusion. The time course of ST-segment elevation is a good predictor of reperfusion. Because prethrombolytic 12-lead ECG studies on ST-segment evolutions were based on static recordings obtained at fixed time intervals, it became clear that frequent monitoring was essential to adequately record the dynamics of ST-segment trends (Fig. 12-8). Sensitivity increases as frequency of monitoring increases.[46,47] Continuous monitoring is thus essential to evaluate occurrence of reperfusion. Resolution of ST-segment elevation has been defined as a progressive decrease within 40 min to less than 50 percent of its maximally elevated value.[46,47] It has been suggested that in patients treated with thrombolytics, the dichotomization for Q- and non–Q wave MI should be made by the predischarge rather than the 24-h ECG due to possible crossover from one group to another.[48]

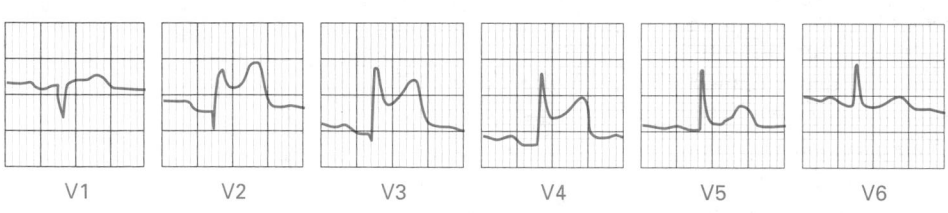

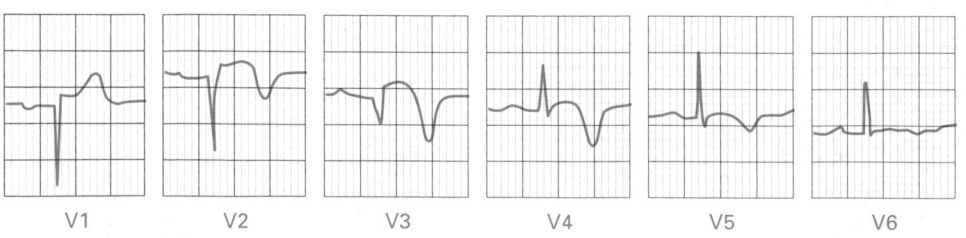

FIGURE 12-7

Acute extensive Q-wave anterior myocardial infarction. The top row shows abnormal ST-segment elevation at the moment of appearance of (small) q waves in V_1, V_2, and V_3. In the bottom row Q waves are deeper, ST segments are less elevated, and ischemic T waves can be clearly seen.

LOCATION OF THE SITE OF ACUTE MI

Table 12-1 shows the ECG location of MI according to a slight modification of the latest edition of the *Nomenclature and Criteria* of the Criteria Committee of the New York Heart Association.[49] In addition, it depicts other processes which may also result in false patterns of MI.

RECIPROCAL ST-SEGMENT CHANGES

In an inferior MI with abnormal ST-segment elevation limited to this wall, the reciprocal ST-segment changes will occur in diametrically opposed leads located in the *same* plane. For example, "indicative" ST elevation in leads III and aV_F, which record the electrical activity of the inferior (posteroinferior, or diaphragmatic) wall, yields "reciprocal" ST-segment depression in leads I and aV_L because they face the superior (anterolateral) wall (Fig. 12-1).[11,50,51] ST-segment depression in lead V_2 may reflect injury in the anterior subendocardial wall as well as injury in the posterobasal (or true posterior) wall.[10] The ECG by itself cannot distinguish with absolute certainty between these two possibilities.[10] The differential diagnosis can perhaps be made best by performing cardiac catheterization or radionuclear studies in the acute phase of the MI, when the ST changes are still present. Another way is by analyzing ST-segment changes occurring during percutaneous transluminal coronary angioplasty in patients with proven single-vessel disease.[52] This has shown that reciprocal ST-segment depression in leads V_2 and V_3 can occur during balloon occlusions of either dominant right or dominant left coronary arteries.[53]

RIGHT VENTRICULAR MI

According to Braat et al.,[54] an ST-segment elevation of at least 1 mm in lead V_4R in patients with *acute inferior MI* had a sensitivity of 100 percent, a specificity of 87 percent, and a predictive accuracy of 92 percent for the diagnosis of right ventricular infarction in patients with ST-segment elevation in leads II, III, and aV_F (Fig. 12-1). These changes disappeared within 10 to 18 h after the onset of chest pain in 50 percent of their patients and after 72 h in the remaining patients.[54] In addition to V_4R, ST-segment elevation can be seen in leads V_5 and V_6R and in some cases (with decreasing amplitude) in V_1, V_2, and even V_3. It is possible for ST-segment depression in V_5 and V_6 to be reciprocal to right ventricular involvement (Fig. 12-1) (see also Chap. 47).

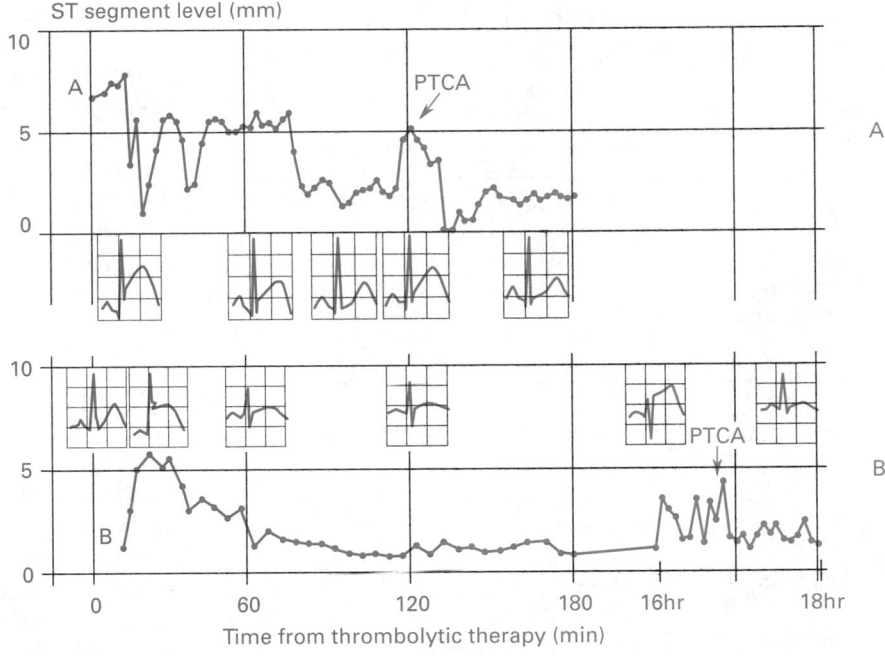

FIGURE 12-8

Assessment of thrombolytic therapy in patients with acute myocardial infarction by ST-segment monitoring. Plots of ST segment levels versus time from initiation of therapy in two selected patients with angiographic reocclusion. Patient A showed wide ST-segment shifts in the first 40 min, angiographic and electrocardiographic reperfusion at 90 min, and reocclusion at 120 min that required percutaneous coronary angioplasty (PTCA). Patient B had successful thrombolysis with 60 min of initiation of therapy; at 16 h, ST-segment elevation recurred and PTCA was performed.

ATRIAL MI

Atrial infarction has been related to extensive ventricular MI.[55] In histopathologic studies, important atheromatotic obstructions of the proximal portions of the right, left anterior descending, and circumflex coronary arteries are found.[55] Atrial infarction is suspected (but not proved) when an atrial arrhythmia develops in a patient with a large ventricular MI. Changes in morphology of the sinus P waves are also seen, but this finding is also nonspecific.[11,55] Other abnormalities, perhaps more diagnostic, are widespread PR-segment changes in the presence of an atrial reciprocal depression in the right chest leads or elevation in lead I with reciprocal depression in lead III.[11,56]

PERICARDITIS

The ECG pattern of acute (generalized) pericarditis not due to MI is produced by the associated epicardial epimyocarditis, which, in turn, results in diffuse epicardial "injury."[6] The ST segments can be elevated in all leads except aV_R and, rarely, in

TABLE 12-1

ELECTROCARDIOGRAPHIC LOCATION OF INFARCTION SITES

Site	Leads	False Patterns
Inferior (diaphragmatic)	II, III, aV_F	WPW (PSAP), IHSS, PE
Inferolateral	II, III, aV_F, V_4–V_6	WPW (PSAP)
"True" posterior (posterobasal)	V_1^a	RVH, "atypical" incomplete RBBB, LFWAP
Inferoposterior	II, III, aV_F, V_1^a	WPW (left PSAP), HCM
Anteroseptal	V_1, V_2, V_3	LVH, chronic lung disease, LBBB, chest electrode misplacement
Anterolateral	I, II, aV_L, V_4–V_6	HCM, ventricular septal defect
Extensive anterior	I, aV_L, V_1–V_6	
High anterolateral	I, aV_L	
Anterior (apical)	V_2–V_4	
Posterolateral	V_4–V_6, V_1^a	WPW (LFWAP)
Right ventricular	V_4R with V_4R–V_6R or V_1-V_3	ASMI

^{a} Tall R wave, "reciprocal" to changes in "indicative" back lead.

Abbreviations: ASMI = anteroseptal myocardial infarction; HCM = hypertrophic cardiomyopathy; LBBB = left bundle branch block; LFWAP = left free-wall accessory pathway; LVH = left ventricular hypertrophy; PE = pulmonary emphysema; PSAP = posteroseptal accessory pathway; WPW = Wolff-Parkinson-White syndrome.

V_1 (Fig. 12-9). Symmetric T-wave inversion (due to epicardial "ischemia") usually develops after the ST segments have returned to the baseline (but can appear during the injury stage).[6] Neither reciprocal ST-segment changes nor abnormal Q waves are seen. In most cases of acute pericarditis, the PR segment is depressed at some time (Fig. 12-9). Average ECG resolution occurs in about 2 weeks.[11] The ECG pattern of acute pericarditis has to be differentiated from the normal variant, referred to as "early repolarization" (Fig. 12-2).

FASCICULAR BLOCKS

Generalities

A brief review of how our current knowledge regarding the fascicular blocks was obtained is appropriate. There are several ways of proving that a given QRS pattern is due to a specific type of conduction abnormality.[15,51,57] First is extrapolation from animal experiments.[5,58–63] Second is ECG-pathologic correlation.[64–73] Third is the analysis of QRS changes produced by the inadvertent section of the conduction fascicles during open heart surgery or catheter-induced trauma.[74] Fourth is the comparison of tracings obtained before, during, or after the appearance or disappearance of conduction disturbances that are either persistent or intermittent. Under such circumstances, the QRS changes produced by fascicular block occur side by side with the control morphologies.[15,57,75,76] The various criteria proposed for diagnosis of fascicular blocks, though empirical, have been accepted in the need to interpret clinical ECGs. In reality, the sensitivity and specificity of these criteria require independent confirmation.[57,77] One can speculate that the latter may be provided by newer methods of intraoperative and body-surface mapping and refinements in the technique of phase imaging, since few centers are currently performing histopathologic studies of the distal intraventricular conduction system.

Left Anterior Fascicular Block

In left anterior fascicular block (LAFB), the posteroinferior regions of the LV endocardium are activated abnormally before the anterosuperior LV area.[8,15] After emerging from the posteroinferior division of the left bundle branch, the impulse first propagates in an inferior, rightward, and usually anterior direction for a short period of time. This orientation is responsible for the small

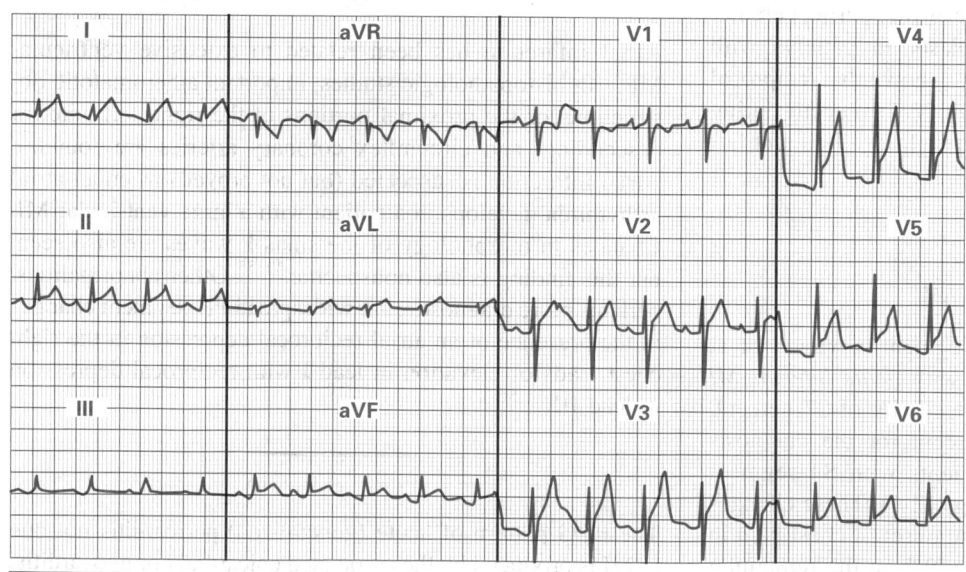

FIGURE 12-9

Acute nonspecific pericarditis showing ST-segment elevation in all leads except aV_R and V_1.

q waves in leads I and aV_L and for the r waves in leads II, III, and aV_F (Fig. 12-10). Occasionally, small q waves are not present in leads I and aV_L.[15] In the absence of MI, these initial QRS abnormalities have been attributed to "anatomic clockwise rotation of the heart" or to coexisting septal fibrosis or to incomplete LBBB.[15] In pure LAFB, the general direction of the activation process (which determines the direction of the EA) occurs in a superior and leftward direction. Consequently, from the ECG viewpoint, the fascicles of the left branch behave more as if they were "superior" and "inferior" rather than "anterior" and "posterior" (Figs. 12-10 and 12-11). Accordingly, the most significant abnormalities produced by LAFB—in the absence of complete right bundle branch block (RBBB)—occur in the standard and unipolar extremity leads rather than in the precordial leads[15] (Figs. 12-10 and 12-11). S waves are frequently recorded V_5 and V_6 because the depolarization wave first moves toward them and later, because of their relatively low position, away in a more superior direction. The degree of left axis deviation required for the diagnosis of complete LAFB has been a subject of debate and speculation.[8] It has been stated that if the EA lies between -30 and $-60°$, LAFB is probably present; if the EA is between -60 and $-90°$, it is almost certainly present.[8] In our opinion, a cutoff of $-45°$ is a valid compromise. The analysis of QRS changes produced by atrial extrasystoles with aberration has shown that conduction delays through the left anterior fascicle can occur with a lesser degree of left axis deviation. Incom-

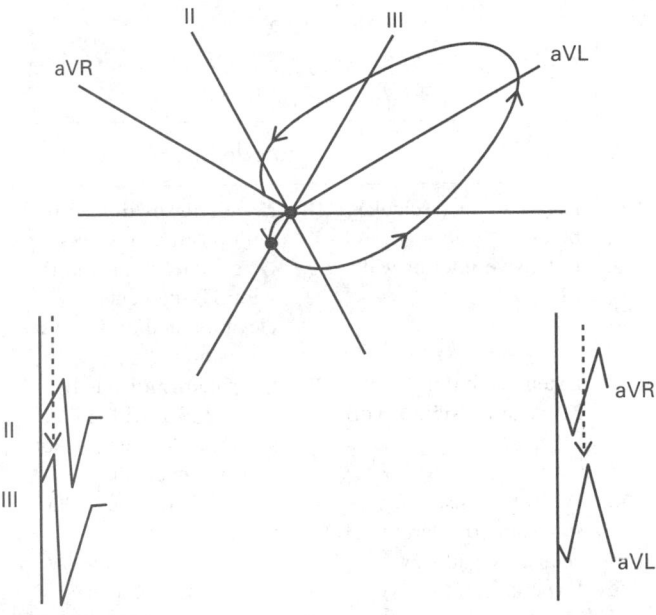

FIGURE 12-11

Derivation of ECG leads from a frontal plane QRS loop showing LAFB. Due to the counterclockwise rotation of the left superior loop, the peak of the R in aV_L preceded the peak of this deflection in aV_R (*lower right*). Furthermore, because the initial portion of the loop was inscribed on the positive half of the axis of lead III before it was inscribed in the positive half of the axis of lead II, the peak of the R in the former lead occurred before that in the latter lead. (From Castellanos A, Pina L, Zaman L, et al. Recent advances in the diagnosis of fascicular blocks. *Cardiol Clin* 1987; 5:469–488. Reproduced with permission from the publisher and the authors.)

plete LAFB, however, can be diagnosed in these dynamic situations only when the original (control) location of the EA is known. It should be remembered that LAFB is but one of the causes of left (superior and leftward) axis deviation (Table 12-2). Criteria for the diagnosis of pure LAFB are presented in (Table 12-3)[77–81]; illustrative examples are shown in Figs. 12-10, 12-11, and 12-12. When LAFB coexists with certain congenital types of right ventricular enlargement and extensive anterolateral MI, the EA can be shifted to the "undeterminate" (right superior) quadrant (Fig. 12-12). Thus, the constant feature of the axis deviation produced by LAFB is its superior orientation, not its superior and leftward orientation (abnormal left axis deviation).[57] Because of the multiple interconnections between the fascicles of the left bundle branch system, the appearance of LAFB does not increase QRS duration by more than 0.025 s.[8] Therefore, an LAFB pattern with prolonged QRS duration generally indicates the presence of additional conduction disturbances such as RBBB (Fig. 12-13, top), MI, or nonspecific intraventricular conduction delays due to diffuse fibrosis. Masquerading RBBB is said to be present when (with classical findings in lead V_1) lead I shows what seems to be an LBBB due to the absence of q and s waves (Fig. 12-13, bottom). This pattern has been attributed to a terminal delay perpendicular to lead I associated with diffuse intramyocardial fibrosis.[44]

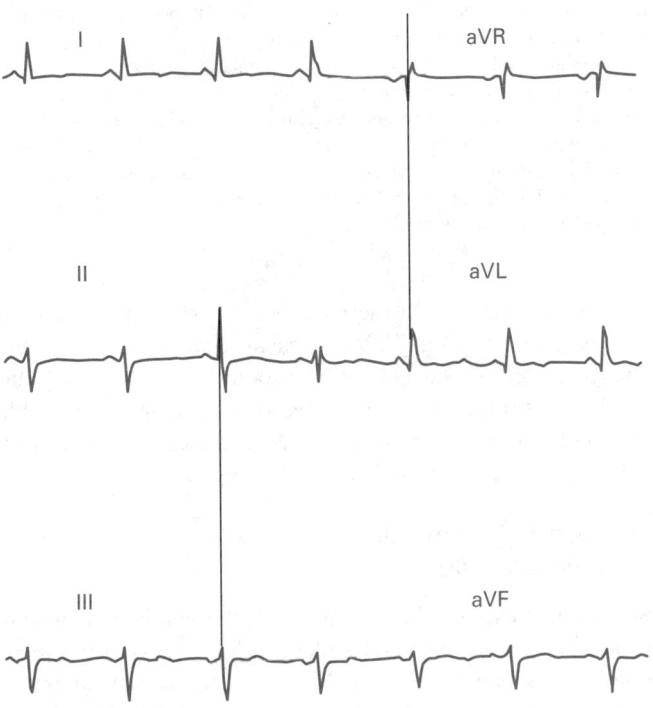

FIGURE 12-10

Left anterior fascicular block (LAFB) in a patient with primary conduction system disease. QRS duration: 0.10 s. At normal paper speeds (25 mm/s) the relationship between the peaks of the R waves (*vertical lines*) in simultaneously recorded leads II and III and aV_L and aV_R cannot be determined with the desired accuracy (see Fig. 12-11).

TABLE 12-2

CAUSES OF ABNORMAL (−30° TO −90°) LEFT AXIS DEVIATION

Cause	Characteristic Features
1. Left anterior fascicular block	1. rS complexes in lead II with positive T waves
2. Extensive inferior wall MI	2. Qr complexes in lead II with ST-segment elevation and/or T-wave inversion
3. Extensive inferior wall MI with possible LAFB	3. QS pattern in leads II, III, and aV_F with ST-segment elevation and/or T-wave inversion
4. Wolff-Parkinson-White syndrome (posteroseptal accessory pathway)	4. Short PR interval; delta wave
5. Hyperkalemia	5. Wide QRS complexes; peaked T waves
6. Pulmonary emphysema	6. Low voltage; peaked P waves
7. Right ventricular apical pacing	7. Pacemaker spikes; predominantly negative ventricular deflections in V_1
8. Middle cardiac vein pacing	8. Pacemaker spikes; predominantly positive QRS deflections in V_1
9. Left coronary arteriography	9. Knowledge that dye was injected in left coronary artery

Source: From Castellanos and Myerburg,[15] with permission.

Left Anterior Fascicular Block Coexisting with MI

The ECG changes imposed by MIs of different locations on the LAFB are shown in (Fig. 12-14). An inferior wall MI can be masked by an LAFB if the infarction does not involve the areas first depolarized by the impulse emergency from the

TABLE 12-3

CRITERIA FOR DIAGNOSIS OF PURE LEFT ANTERIOR FASCICULAR BLOCK

1. Abnormal left axis deviation (usually between −45° and −60°)
2. rS complexes in leads II, III, and aV_F and qR complexes in leads I and aV_L
3. Delayed intrinsicoid deflection in leads I and aV_L
4. Peak of r wave in lead III occurring earlier than peak of r wave in lead II
5. Peak of R wave in lead aV_L occurring earlier than peak of R wave in aV_R

Source: From Castellanos et al.[57] and Milliken,[77] with permission.

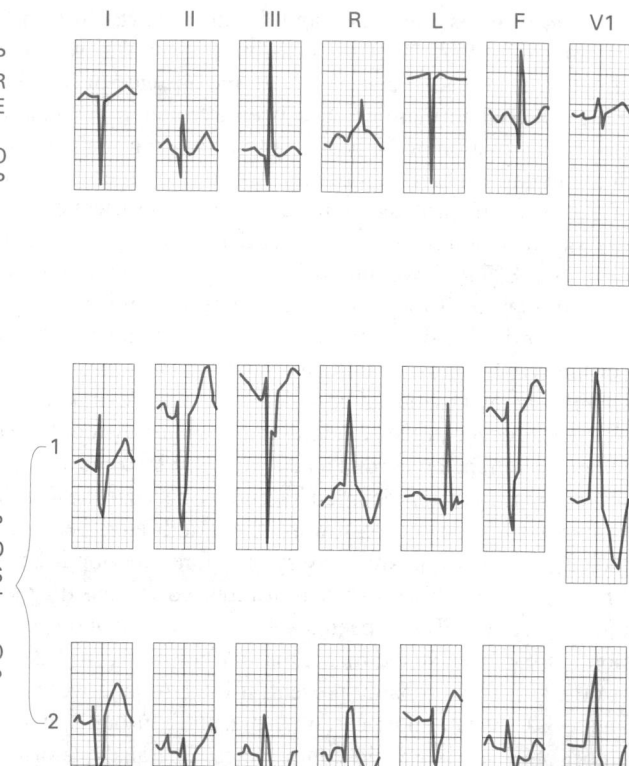

FIGURE 12-12

Transient postsurgical LAFB with right (not left) *superior* electrical axis (and an R wave in the left arm lead) coexisting with persistent RBBB in a patient with tetralogy of Fallot (*middle tracing*). The top (control) tracing shows right axis deviation due to right ventricular hypertrophy with narrow QRS complexes. In the bottom tracing, recorded after disappearance of LAFB, right axis deviation due to right ventricular hypertrophy coexists with the persistent RBBB. The left arm lead now shows an S wave. (From Castellanos A, Pina L, Zaman L, et al. Recent advances in the diagnosis of fascicular blocks. *Cardiol Clin* 1987; 5:469–488. Reproduced with permission from the publisher and the authors.)

unaffected fascicle.[8] In these cases an r (slurred or not) can be seen as leads III and aV_F. It has also been stated that the change in left septal activation produced by the fascicular block may produce small r waves in V_1, V_2, and V_3 capable of modifying the characteristics QS complexes produced by anteroseptal MI in these leads.[8]

Nonspecific Intraventricular Conduction Delays

Several names have been applied to the conduction disturbances occurring in the left-sided Purkinje-myocardial junctions, left septal surface, or free wall of the left ventricle: arborization block, diffuse (nonspecific) intraventricular block, peri-infarction block, parietal block, focal block, and so on.[8,81–88] These conduction disturbances have different electrogenetic mechanisms. Thus, the cellular "affectation" due to acute injury resulting from coronary artery disease, hyperkalemia, drugs, and intracoronary injections of contrast material occurs within (inside) the affected regions.[5,15,88]

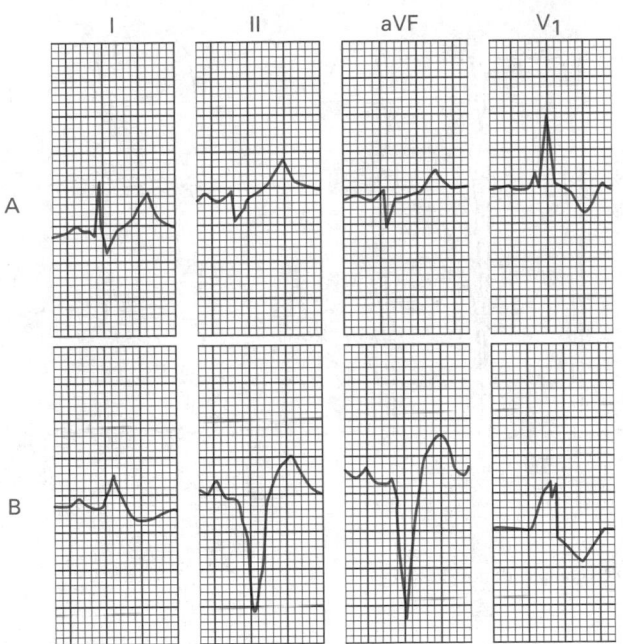

FIGURE 12-13
Left anterior fascicular block with wide QRS complexes. Whereas panel *A* shows LAFB with RBBB, these conduction disturbances coexist with diffuse septal and inferoposterior fibrosis in panel *B*. Consequently, the expected small q wave and the wide s wave in lead I are not present. This pattern has been called "masquerading" BBB, since the standard leads suggest LBBB while the chest leads are diagnostic of RBBB.

Blocks occurring in subacute or chronic MI after the appearance of abnormal Q waves (peri-infarction block) (Fig. 12-15), as well as those occurring in the presence of diffuse myocardial fibrosis (Fig. 12-16), are due to the circuitous and irregular activation of living cells surrounding areas of fibrotic tissue (Fig. 12-16).[5,81-88]

Left Posterior Fascicular Block

In pure left posterior fascicular block (LPFB), the impulse emerges from the unblocked anterosuperior division, producing small q waves in leads II, III, and aV$_F$.[8,15] Thereafter, the impulse moves through the electrically predominant left ventricle in an inferior and rightward direction, thus explaining the S waves in leads I and aV$_L$ as well as the R waves in leads II, III, and aV$_F$.[8,15] Radiologic studies of the human heart in situ have shown that the paraseptal regions of the posteroinferior (diaphragmatic) surface of the anatomic *left* ventricle are spatially located more to the *right* than certain (anterior) portions of the anatomic right ventricle.[15] Since the portions of the left ventricle that are

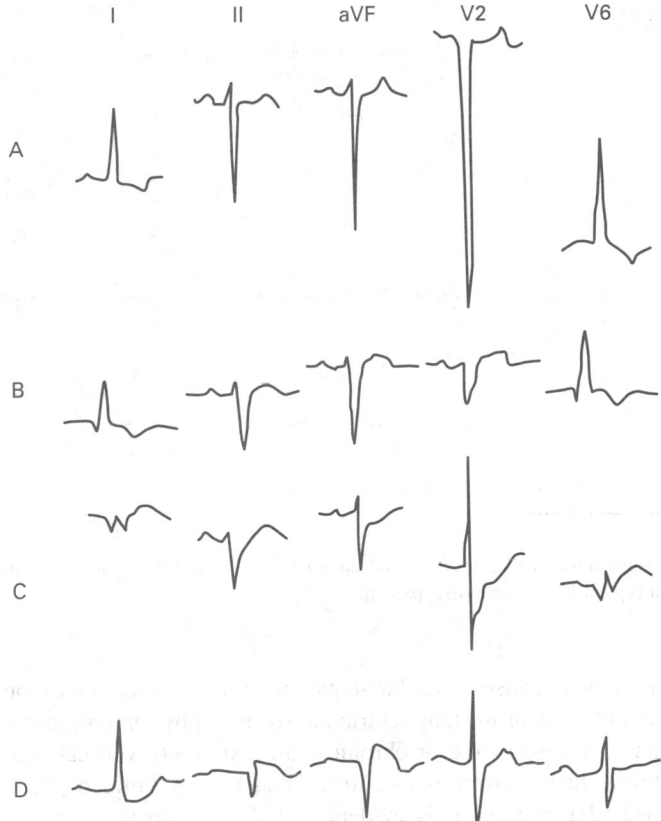

FIGURE 12-14
Diagnosis of LAFB associated with MI. Diagnostic feature given in parentheses. *A.* Left anterior fascicular block and anteroseptal MI (Qr or QS complex in right chest leads). *B.* Left anterior fascicular block and anterolateral MI (abnormal Q wave in leads I and V$_6$). *C.* Left anterior fascicular block and anterolateral MI with electrical axis in right superior quadrant (Q wave in leads I and V$_6$). *D.* Left anterior fascicular block and inferior wall MI (Qr or QS complexes and elevation of J point and ST segments in leads II and III).

spatially located to the right are less than those located superiorly, the degree of right axis deviation produced by pure LPFB is of lesser magnitude than that of left axis deviation produced by LAFB.[15] The hallmark of LPFB is, therefore, an "inferior" axis shift as much as "right" axis deviation (Figs. 12-17 to

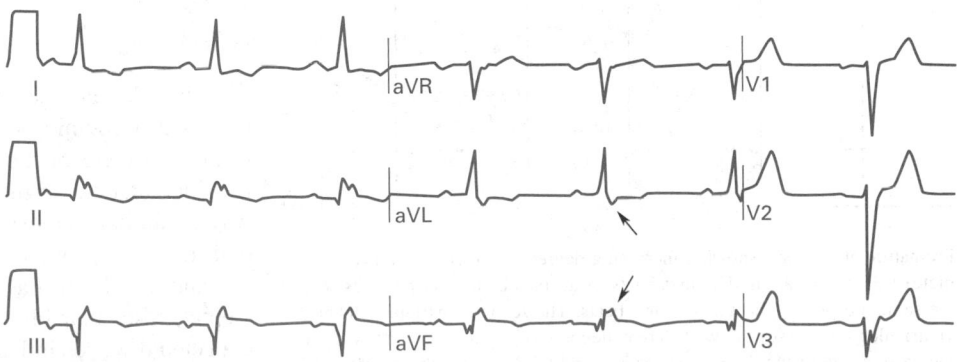

FIGURE 12-15
Type of nonspecific intraventricular conduction delay known as peri-infarction block. The patient had an evolving inferior wall myocardial infarction. The wide (0.14 s) ventricular complexes show a predominantly terminal delay (*arrows*) and notching (more evident in the inferior leads) without a typical LBBB or RBBB morphology.

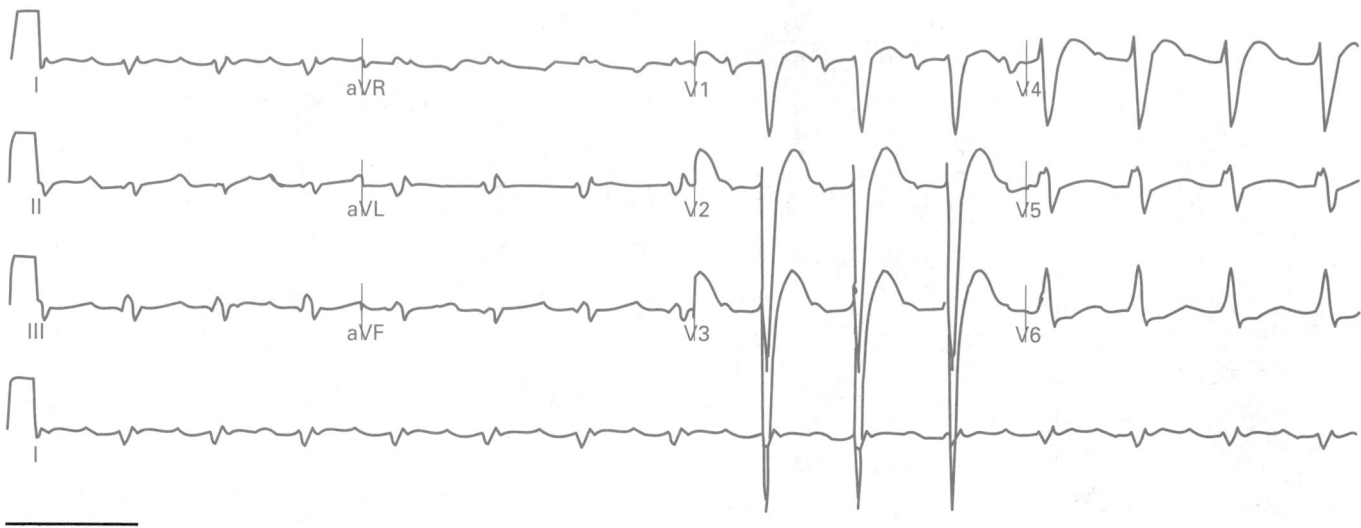

FIGURE 12-16
Nonspecific intraventricular conduction delay characterized by very wide (0.17 s) QRS complexes not showing a typical RBBB or LBBB pattern.

12-19). Because a similar sequence of ventricular activation can also occur in right ventricular hypertrophy, pleuropulmonary disease (acute or chronic), and extremely vertical anatomic heart positions due to a slender body build or chest wall deformities, it is evident that the diagnosis of "pure" LPFB cannot be made from ECG alone. Additional clinical, radiologic, or pathologic information is required for this purpose.[8,15,57,70] The changes imposed in LPFB by MIs of different locations are depicted in Figs. 12-18 and 12-19.

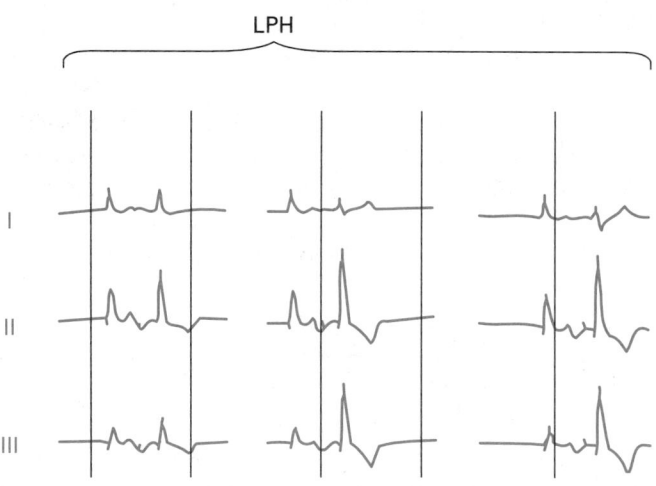

FIGURE 12-17
Premature atrial beats showing increasing degrees of (incomplete and complete) LPFB aberration. The first beats in all panels are escape beats with the same morphology as that of sinus beats. The second, aberrantly induced ventricular complexes show different degrees of right axis shift with an increase in size of the R waves in leads II and III. Note that the fundamental characteristic of LPFB was not right axis deviation (beyond +90°) but an inferior axis shift. (From Castellanos and Myerburg.[15] Reproduced with permission from the publisher and the authors.)

Left Fascicular Blocks Produced by Intra-His Bundle Lesions

Rosenbaum and coworkers[74] attributed surgically induced LAFB (coexisting with RBBB) to a lesion of the "pseudobifurcating" part of the His bundle. The production of LBBB and LPFB by catheters located in the right-sided cavities, however, cannot be explained by assuming direct affectation of these left-sided structures.[89,90] Nevertheless, they have been reported and attributed to the His bundle trauma produced by Swan-Ganz catheters.[89,90] In fact, certain clinical and experimental studies have shown that some BBB patterns could be normalized by distal His bundle pacing.[91–94] Longitudinal dissociation of conduction within a usually diseased His bundle should be present for this to occur. There is, however, disagreement as to the mechanism involved, especially in regard to the predestination of fibers (within the His bundle) to specific right- or left-sided structures and to the role played by the transverse fibers connecting the various longitudinal strands.[90–94]

Left-Middle (Septal) Fascicular Blocks

This disorder has been anatomically demonstrated and associated with ischemic heart disease and fibrosis of the middle (septal) fascicle of the left branch.[95,96] While some authors consider that the right precordial leads show prominent R waves (similar to those found in true posterior, basal myocardial infarction), others have described Q waves in leads V_1, V_2, and V_3.[95,96] It has also been considered that left-middle (septal) fascicular blocks are manifest by the absence of the expected q waves in leads V_5 and V_6 in electrocardiographic intermediate or horizontal hearts. Such a diversity of diagnostic criteria shows that there are marked discrepancies regarding the ECG characteristics of this conduction disturbance.

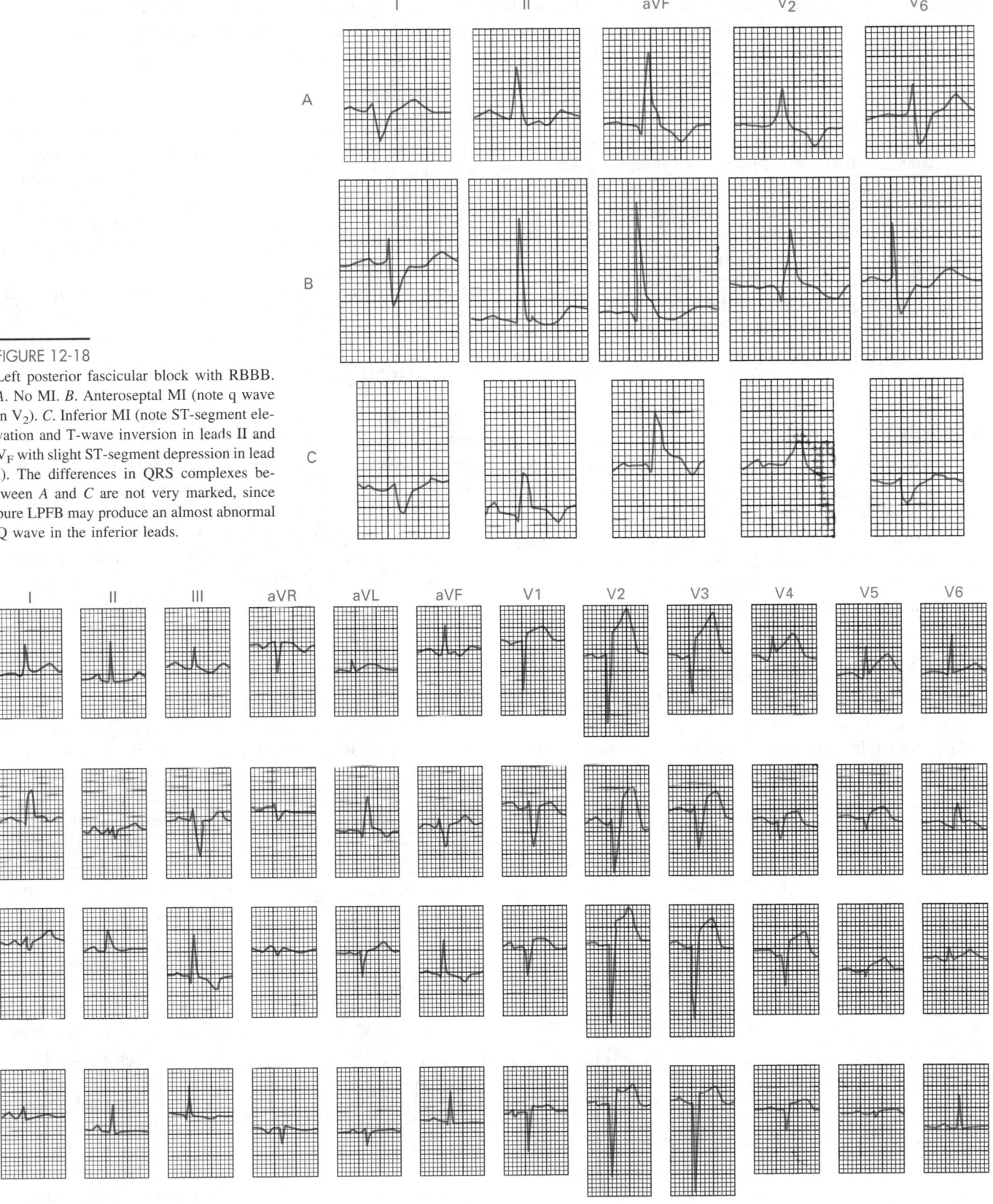

FIGURE 12-18

Left posterior fascicular block with RBBB. *A.* No MI. *B.* Anteroseptal MI (note q wave in V_2). *C.* Inferior MI (note ST-segment elevation and T-wave inversion in leads II and V_F with slight ST-segment depression in lead I). The differences in QRS complexes between *A* and *C* are not very marked, since pure LPFB may produce an almost abnormal Q wave in the inferior leads.

FIGURE 12-19

Pure (without RBBB) LPFB (*third row*) and LAFB (*second row*) occurring during acute anterior wall MI. Pre- and postfascicular block QRS morphologies are shown in the top and bottom rows, respectively.

Recently, Dhala et al. described "unmasking" of the trifascicular conduction system by catheter ablation of the right bundle branch with a diseased left intraventricular conduction system.[97] Ablation-induced damage to "predestined" fibers in diseased His bundle, however, cannot be totally excluded.

Complete RBBB

A "complete" BBB pattern (with QRS duration greater than 0.11 s) does not necessarily reflect the existence of a total conduction block in the right branch. This pattern only indicates that the entire or major parts of both ventricles are activated by the impulse emerging from the left branch.[15,98–100] Thus, a significant degree of conduction delay ("high-grade" or "incomplete" RBBB) can produce a similar pattern. In pure complete RBBB, the EA should not be deviated *abnormally* either to the left or to the right. These axis deviations reflect coexisting fascicular block or right ventricular (RV) hypertrophy.

Incomplete RBBB Pattern

For many years what has been proved with endocardial (catheter) and epicardial mapping has been recognized—namely, that incomplete RBBB "patterns" can be produced by various mechanisms[98–110]: (1) different degrees of conduction delays through the main trunk of the right bundle branch; (2) an increased conduction time through an elongated right bundle branch that is stretched because of a concomitant enlargement of the right septal surface; (3) a diffused Purkinje-myocardial delay due to RV stretch or dilatation; (4) surgical trauma or disease-related interruption of the major ramifications of the right bundle branch ("distal" RBBB); or (5) congenital variations of the distribution of the major distal ramifications resulting in a slight delay in activation of the crista supraventricularis.[6] In arrhythmogenic RV dysplasia, the S wave in V_1 is followed by a sharp, wide, positive deflection (epsilon wave) attributed to delayed ventricular activation (postexcitation) in some RV myocardial fibers.[39]

Concealed RBBB

A conduction delay in the main trunk of the right bundle branch or in its major ramification may be concealed (not manifest in the surface ECG) when there are coexisting (and of greater degree) conduction disturbances in the main left bundle branch, the anterosuperior division of the left bundle branch, and/or the free left ventricular wall.[15] An RBBB can also be concealed in some patients with Wolff-Parkinson-White syndrome if the ventricular insertion of the accessory pathway causes preexcitation of the right ventricular regions that would be activated late because of the RBBB.[111]

Complete LBBB

This conduction disturbance is characterized by wide (greater than 0.11 s) QRS complexes. The diagnostic criterion consist of prolongation of the QRS complexes (over 0.11 s) with neither a q nor an S wave in leads I and aV_L and in the *properly placed* V_6. A wide R wave with a notch on its top ("plateau") is seen in these leads. Apparently, the EA of most *uncomplicated* complete LBBB blocks is usually not located beyond $-30°$.[15,16] Complete LBBB with abnormal left axis deviation indicates a great degree of left Purkinje and myocardial disease.

Complete LBBB with Acute MI

The classical pattern of LBBB may not be modified by a small area of myocardial necrosis. This explains why thrombolytics may be given if clinical findings characteristic of MI occur in patients with an LBBB pattern. Recent studies, however, have shown that occlusions of a coronary artery by either an angioplasty balloon or (a presumably large) MI can produce ST segment changes as in absence of the conduction disturbance.[112] Recently, Sgarbossa has suggested that ST elevation ≥ 1 mm concordant with QRS polarity has a high specificity and sensitivity. ST elevation ≥ 5 mm discordant with QRS-polarity ST-segment depression ≥ 1 mm in V_1, V_2, and V_3, and (sudden) positive T waves in V_5 and V_5 have a high specificity but a low sensitivity.[112] The latter can occur transiently during acute ischemia (pseudonormalization) without myocardial necrosis or be persistently present in cases where its significance is unclear.

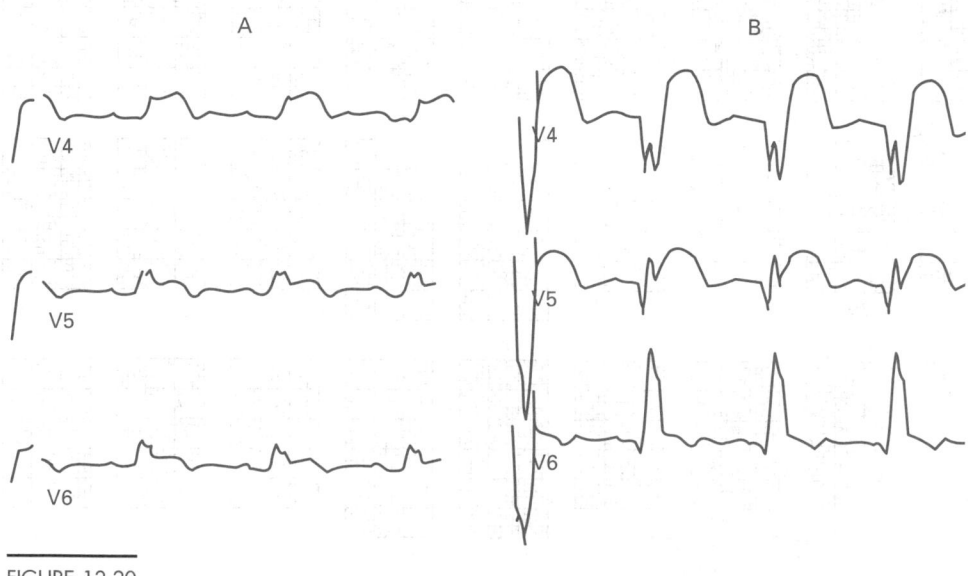

A   B

FIGURE 12-20

Morphologic characteristics of complete LBBB complicated by acute anterior MI. *A* shows abnormal ST-segment elevation without q waves (QRS duration: 0.14 s). In *B*, obtained from another patient, abnormal ST-segment elevation persisted after the appearance of abnormal Q waves (QRS duration: 0.15 s).

Examples of LBBB complicated by acute anterior and inferior MI are shown in Figs. 12-20 and 12-21. Sgarbossa et al. have suggested that the criteria mentioned above can also be applied to diagnose acute MI in patients with pacemakers.[112]

Complete LBBB with Old MI

Normally, in complete LBBB, the impulse emerges from the right bundle branch and propagates inferiorly, to the left and slightly anteriorly. This orientation of the initial forces tends to abolish previously present inferiorly and laterally located abnormal Q waves characteristic of inferior and lateral wall MIs.[15,113–115] If the infarction is anteroseptal, however, the impulse cannot propagate toward the left. Instead, the initial vectors point toward the free wall of the RV because now the RV free wall forces are not neutralized by the normally preponderant septal and/or initial left ventricular free wall forces. Thus, a small q wave will be recorded in leads (I, V_5, and V_6), where it is not normally present in complete LBBB (Fig. 12-22A). For a recent review of this subject, see Ref. 112. Similar findings can be seen in paced beats when in lead I, the spike is followed by a well-defined q wave (Fig. 12-22B). Several studies reported that Q waves in lead I or in two or more lateral leads (I, aV_L or V_5 and V_6) have high specificity but moderate sensitivity.[112] The sign of Cabrera and Friedland (late notching of S waves in V_3–V_5) has been found to have high-to-moderate specificity and moderate-to-low sensitivity.[116] Notching of the upstroke of the R wave in I, aV_L, V_5, and V_6 (sign of Chapman) has a sensitivity of 21 percent and a specificity of 82 percent).[116]

Complete LBBB with Left Ventricular Hypertrophy

This is discussed under "Left Ventricular Hypertrophy," below.

Incomplete LBBB Pattern

An incomplete LBBB pattern can be diagnosed in leads I and in an appropriately placed V_6 showing an R wave not preceded by a q wave.[6] Lead V_1 shows rS or QS complexes, and lead V_2 shows rS complexes. Although QRS duration usually ranges between 0.08 and 0.11 s, this *pattern* can be observed with QRS durations of 0.12 and 0.13 s.

Wide QRS Complexes in Patients with Manifest Preexcitation Syndromes

The characteristic pattern of manifest Wolff-Parkinson-White

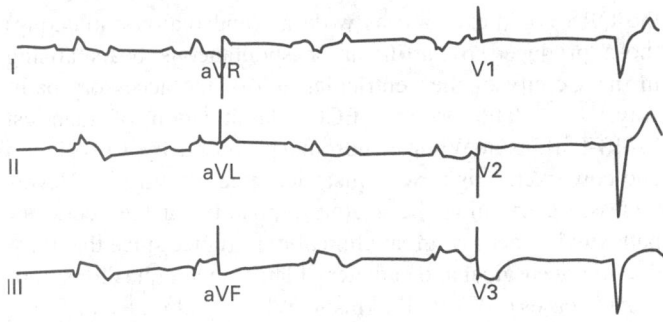

FIGURE 12-21

Morphologic features of complete LBBB complicated by acute inferior MI. There is abnormal ST-segment elevation in leads II, III, and aV_F. QRS duration: 0.14 s. Atrioventricular block is also present.

syndrome during sinus rhythm is well known.[116] The ventricular complex is a fusion beat resulting from ventricular activation by two wave fronts.[116–126] The degree of preexcitation (amount of muscle activated through the accessory pathway) is variable and depends on many factors. Foremost among these are the distance between the sinus node and atrial insertion of accessory pathway and, more important, the differences in conduction time through the normal pathway and accessory pathway. Other things being equal, a patient with rapid (enhanced) AV nodal conduction will have a smaller delta wave than a patient with slow conduction through the AV node. Moreover, if there is total block at the AV node or His-Purkinje system, the impulse will be conducted exclusively via the accessory pathway bundle.[120–122] Consequently, the QRS complexes are different from fusion beats, though the direction of the delta wave remains the same. Moreover,

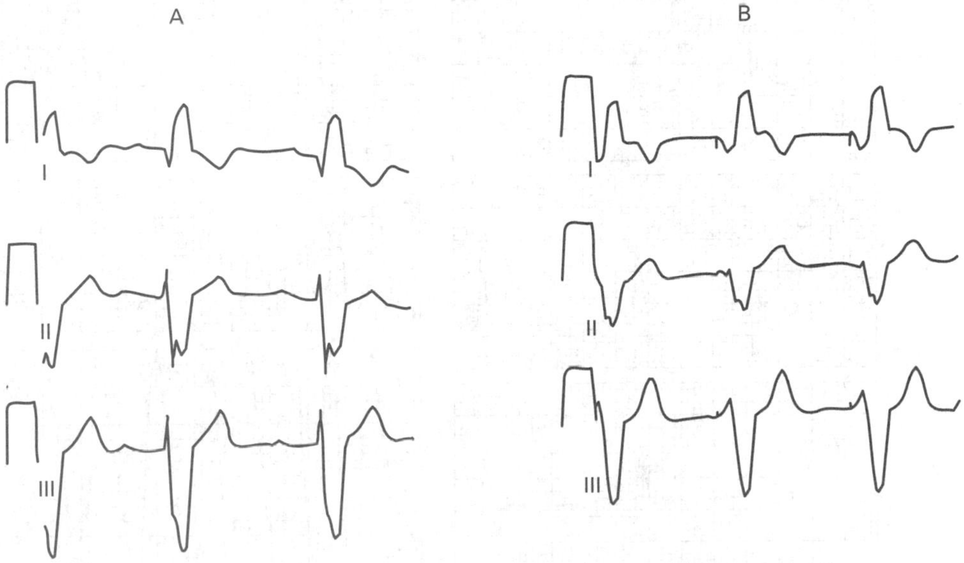

FIGURE 12-22

A. Complete LBBB with old anterior MI. Abnormal Q waves are present in lead I. QRS duration: 0.18 s. *B.* Pacing-induced complete LBBB pattern in a patient with old anterior MI. There are abnormal Q waves in lead I after spikes. QRS duration: 0:20 s. Note resemblance between natural and artificial (electrically induced) QRS patterns.

the QRS complexes are as wide as (and really stimulating) those produced by artificial or spontaneous beats arising in the vicinity of the ventricular end of the accessory pathway.[117–124] The original ECG classification of manifest Wolff-Parkinson-White syndrome proposed by Rosenbaum and coworkers[99] is now of historical interest only.[118] Nevertheless, determining the anatomic position of the accessory pathway has been of great clinical importance since the introduction of surgical and catheter-ablative techniques for symptomatic cases of Wolff-Parkinson-White syndrome (see Chap. 31). Currently there are two noninvasive electrical methods available for the anatomic localization of accessory pathways—namely, body-surface potential mapping and analysis of the 12-lead ECG.

Milstein and coworkers[125] analyzed the direction of the delta wave and divided the mitral and tricuspid ring areas where the pathways are located into various segments. These investigators considered that only four segments were necessary. This appeared logical, for at the time that this method was proposed, most ablations were performed surgically.[125,126] Left free wall accessory pathways are characterized by negative, isoelectric, and even positive delta waves in one of leads I, aV_L, V_5, or V_6. Lead V_1 shows R or Rs complexes (Fig. 12-23). During sinus rhythm, the electrical axis may be normal; but when atrial fibrillation develops and exclusive accessory pathway conduction occurs, the EA is deviated to the right and inferiorly (Fig. 12-23). Posteroseptal accessory pathways show negative delta waves in leads III, and aV_F and R waves in V_2. An Rs (or RS) wave in V_1 suggests a left posteroseptal pathway; a QS complex in the

same lead may correspond to a right posteroseptal pathway (Fig. 12-24). Right free wall accessory pathways display an LBBB pattern, defined, for lead I and rS complexes in leads V_1 and V_2 with an electrical axis ranging between +30 and −60° (Fig. 12-25). The most rare right anteroseptal accessory pathways show an LBBB pattern (as defined) with an electrical axis ranging between +30 and +120° (Fig. 12-26). A q wave may be present in lead aV_L but *not* in leads I or V_6. Mixed patterns resulted from the existence of two separate accessory pathways.

Since accessory pathways can traverse almost any part of the atrioventricular annulus, this classification is insufficient when catheter ablation is contemplated. Multiple algorithms have been proposed. Since the most useful are complex, electrocardiographers find them difficult to memorize. They are also not completely satisfactory, since smaller degrees of preexcitation seem to limit diagnostic accuracy and the polarity delta waves [positive, biphasic (+ − or − +), negative, and isoelectric] have to be properly categorized. Figure 12-27 illustrates a useful algorithm to predict accessory pathway location from the 12-lead ECG.[127]

Nodoventricular (Mahaim) Fibers

As a rule, the so-called classical pattern appears only during atrial pacing.[126,127] According to data from intraoperative mapping, what had usually been considered to be Mahaim fiber conduction in most instances represents anterograde propagation through a slowly conducting right free wall accessory pathway.[128]

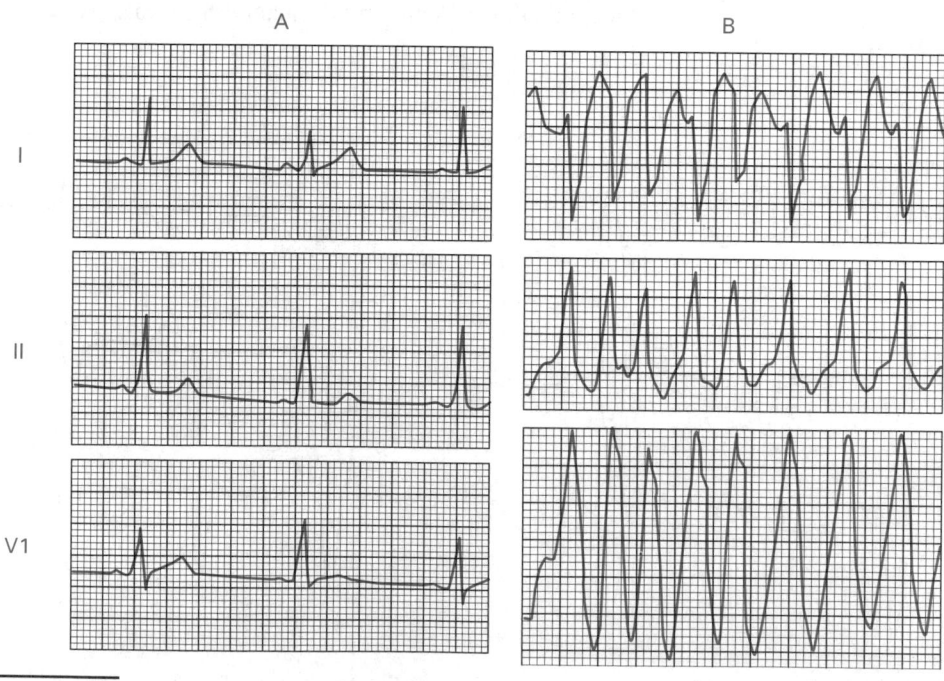

FIGURE 12-23
Wolff-Parkinson-White syndrome in a patient with left free wall accessory pathway. *A.* Sinus rhythm with fusion beats showing different degrees of preexcitation. *B.* Maximal preexcitation during atrial fibrillation. Note marked change in QRS duration and electrical axis.

Wide QRS Complexes Produced by Ventricular Pacing from Different Sites

In determining the location of the stimulating electrodes, one should take special care not to consider that the distortion produced by large unipolar spikes constitutes parts of the pacing-induced QRS complexes. It is best *not* to describe the electrically produced ventricular beats as having an RBBB or LBBB morphology, since what is relevant is the polarity of the *properly positioned* V_1 and V_2 electrodes and the direction of the EA (Fig. 12-28).[129,130] For example, endocardial or epicardial stimulation of the *anteriorly* located RV at any site [apical (inferior), or mid/outflow tract (superior)] yields predominantly negative deflections in the right chest leads

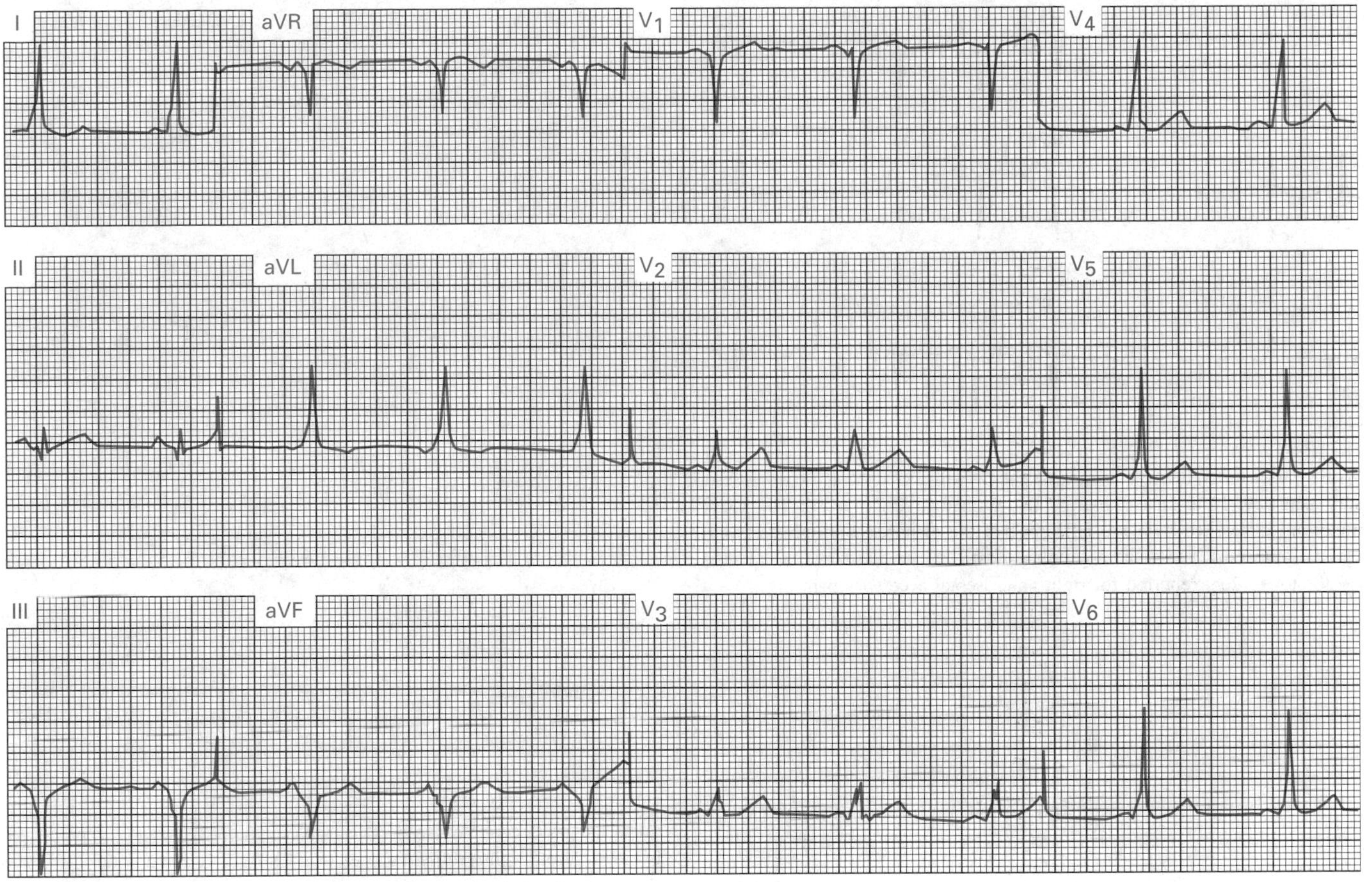

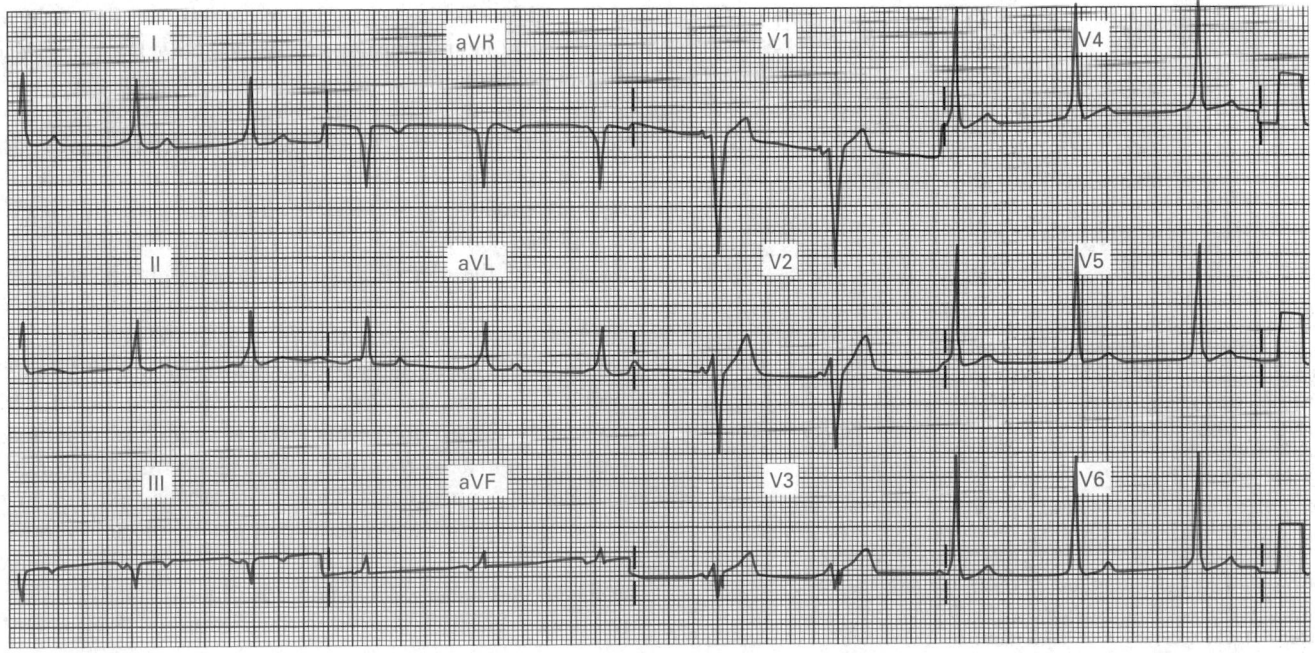

FIGURE 12-24
Wolff-Parkinson-White syndrome in a patient having a (most likely right) posteroseptal accessory pathway. Note short PR intervals with negative delta waves in III and aV$_F$. (False pattern of inferior MI.) Lead V$_2$ shows all positive QRS complexes.

FIGURE 12-25
Wolff-Parkinson-White syndrome in a patient with right free wall accessory pathway. Note LBBB "pattern" characterized for diagnostic (of accessory pathway location) purposes by a QRS deflection greater than 0.09 s in lead I with rS complexes in leads V$_1$ and V$_2$. The electrical axis is approximately +15°.

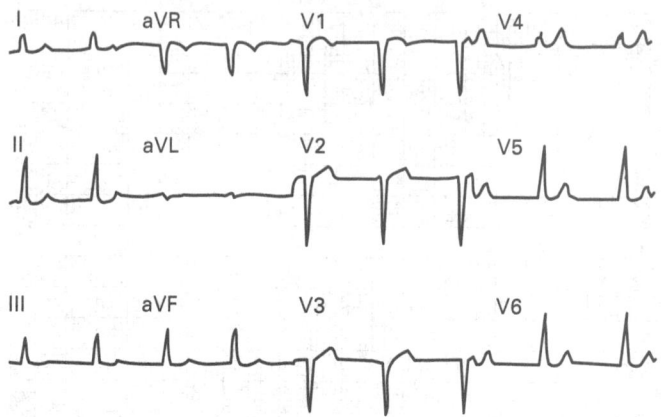

FIGURE 12-26

Wolff-Parkinson-White syndrome in a patient with a right anteroseptal accessory pathway. Note LBBB pattern (as defined in Fig. 12-25). The most important difference with the latter is that the electrical axis points more vertically, toward +60°, thereby being located within the range of the axis (+30° to +120°) reported for right anteroseptal accessory pathways.

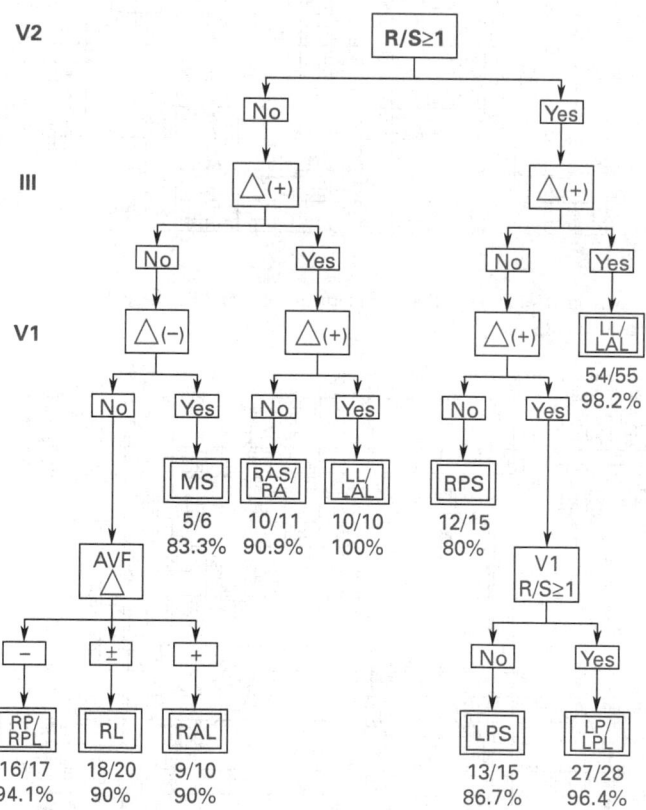

FIGURE 12-27

Useful algorithm to predict accessory pathway location from the 12-lead ECG. Step 1 = analysis of R/S ratio in V₂. Step 2 = existence of positive (+) delta wave in lead III (initial 40 ms). Step 3 = existence of positive or negative (−) delta wave in V₁ (initial 60 ms). Step 4 = delta-wave polarity in a V$_F$ (initial 40 ms) or analysis of R/S ratio in V₁ (± = biphasic or isoelectric). The accuracy of the algorithm for each location in 187 prospective patients is also shown at the bottom. LAL = left anterolateral; LL = left lateral; LP = left posterior; LPL = left posterolateral; LPS = left posteroseptal; MS = midseptal; RA = right anterior; RAL = right anterolateral; RAS = right anteroseptal; RL = right lateral; RP = right posterior; RPL = right posterolateral; RPS = right posteroseptal. (From Chiang et al.[127] Reproduced with permission from the publishers and the authors.)

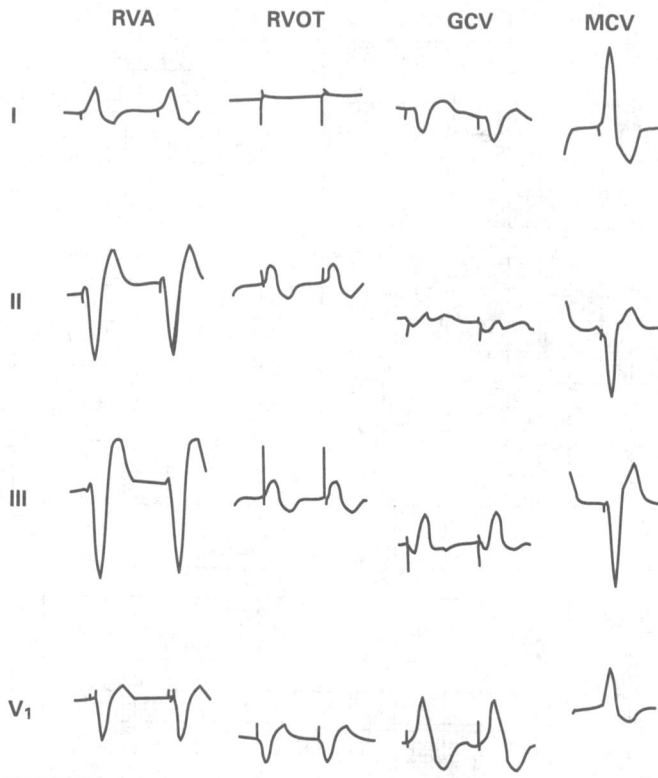

FIGURE 12-28

QRS changes (location of the electrical axis and polarity of lead V₁) produced by pacing from right ventricular apex (RVA), right ventricular outflow tract (RVOT), great cardiac vein (GCV), and middle cardiac vein (MCV).

due to the *posterior* spread of activation (first and second vertical rows in Fig. 12-26). The reverse (positive deflections in V₁ and V₂) occurs when the epicardial stimulation of the superior and lateral portions of the posterior LV by catheter electrodes in the distal coronary sinus or great and middle cardiac veins (or by implanted electrodes in the nearby muscle) results in *anteriorly* oriented forces (third and fourth vertical rows in Fig. 12-26). Right ventricular apical pacing may produce positive deflections in V₁ if this lead is (mis)placed above its usual level. On the other hand, *superior* deviation of the electrical axis indicates only that a spatial *inferior* ventricular site has been stimulated, regardless of whether this site is the apical portion of the RV or the inferior part of the LV, the latter being paced through the middle cardiac vein (first and fourth vertical rows in Fig. 12-26). Conversely, an *inferior* vertical axis is simply a consequence of pacing from a *superior* site, which can be the endocardium of the right ventricular outflow tract or the epicardium of the posterosuperior and lateral portions of the left ventricle (second and third vertical rows in Fig. 12-26). The changes produced on the basic ECG patterns of paced beats produced by MI were briefly discussed in the section of LBBB and MI.

Left Atrial Hypertrophy

Munuswamy et al.,[131] using M-mode echocardiography as the gold standard, evaluated the specificity and sensitivity of the most important clues for determining left atrial hypertrophy. These included (1) P-wave duration greater than 0.11 s and notched P wave with an interpeak interval in excess of 0.04 s and (2) negative phase of P in V_1 longer than 0.04 s and greater than 1 mm in lead V_1. There are, however, problems in applying these criteria in a given ECG. For example, according to Josephson,[132] the mechanism of prolonged duration of the P wave and of (posteriorly directed) terminal forces is delayed left atrial activation, not left atrial enlargement. In fact, most criteria mentioned above also apply for intraatrial block. Moreover, the previously mentioned findings in lead V_1[132] may reflect improper (high) placement of this lead, a common error made by ECG technicians. Generally, if the previously mentioned findings are found in patients with LV enlargement or mitral stenosis, left atrial hypertrophy is most likely present; but in their absence, such findings most likely indicate an intraatrial conduction defect. In any case, the ECG pattern of left atrial hypertrophy results from a hypertrophy-induced intraatrial conduction delay.

LEFT VENTRICULAR HYPERTROPHY

As emphasized by Surawicz, since the advent of other noninvasive techniques, there has been a changing role for the ECG in the diagnosis of ventricular hypertrophy.[133] Necropsy studies have demonstrated the superiority of echocardiography (see Chap. 14) in respect to electrocardiography to detect LV hypertrophy (LVH).[133] Echocardiography is also a better method for the serial follow-up of changes during progression or regression of LVH. Multiple criteria have been proposed to diagnose LVH using necropsy or echocardiography information (Tables 12-4 and 12-5).[44,134–137] Of these, the Sokolow-Lyon criterion ($SV_1 + RV_{5–6} \geq 35$ mm) is the most specific (>95 percent), but it is not very sensitive (around 45 percent) (Table 12-4). The Romhilt-Estes score has a specificity of 90 percent and a sensitivity of 60 percent in studies

TABLE 12-4

ELECTROCARDIOGRAPHIC CRITERIA FOR LEFT VENTRICULAR ENLARGEMENT

Voltage Criteria	Sensitivity, %	Specificity, %	Accuracy, %
RI + S_{III} > 25 mm	10.6	100	55
RV_L > 7.5 mm	22.5	96.5	59.5
RV_L > 11 mm	10.6	100	55
RV_F > 20 mm	1.3	99.5	50
$SV_1 + RV_{5–6}$ > 35 mm (Sokolow-Lyon)	55.6	89.5	73
In V_1–V_6, the tallest S + the tallest R > 45 mm	45	93	69
$RV_{5–6}$ > 26 mm	25	98	62
Romhilt-Estes score	See Table 12-5		

Source: From Bayes de Luna,[44] with permission.

TABLE 12-5

POINT SCORE SYSTEM OF ROMHILT AND ESTES FOR DIAGNOSIS OF LEFT VENTRICULAR HYPERTROPHY

1. Amplitude, 3 points
   Any of the following:
   a. Largest R or S wave in the limb leads $\geq$ 20 mm
   b. S wave in V_1 or V_2 $\geq$ 30 mm
   c. R wave in V_5 or V_6 $\geq$ 30 mm
2. ST-T-segment changes (typical pattern of left ventricular strain with the ST-T-segment vector shifted in direction opposite to the mean QRS vector)
   Without digitalis, 3 points
   With digitalis, 1 point
3. Left atrial involvement, 3 points
   Terminal negativity of the P wave in V_1 is 1 mm or more in depth with a duration of 0.04 s or more
4. Left axis deviation: $-30°$ or more, 2 points
5. QRS duration $\geq$ 0.09 s, 1 point
6. Intrinsicoid deflection in V_5, V_6 = 0.05 s, 1 point

Note: Sensitivity, 54%; specificity, 97%.
Sources: From Bayes de Luna[44] and Romhilt and Estes,[137] with permission.

correlated with echocardiography. The following are some of the other criteria[44]: The Casale (modified Cornell) criterion ($Ra_{VL} + SV_3 > 28$ mm in men and >20 in women) is somewhat more sensitive, but less specific than the Sokolow-Lyon criterion.[138] The Talbot criterion[139] (R $\geq$ 16 mm in aV_L) is very specific (>90 percent), even in the presence of myocardial infarction and ventricular block, but not very sensitive. The Koito and Spodick criterion[140] ($RV_6 > RV_5$) claims a specificity of 100 percent and a sensitivity of more than 50 percent. According to Hernandez Padial, a total 12-lead QRS voltage >120 mm is a good ECG criterion of LVH in systemic hypertension and is better than those most frequently used.[141] With echocardiography as the gold standard, several authors postulated ECG criteria for diagnosis of LVH in the presence of complete LBBB and LAFB (Tables 12-6 and 12-7).[142,143] The high sensitivity and specificity reported by Gertsch et al.[143] for diagnosis of LVH and LAFB have not been corroborated in preliminary studies performed in our department (unpublished observation; nevertheless indicated in Table 12-7).

PROCESSES PRODUCING OR LEADING TO RVH AND ENLARGEMENT

Right ventricular hypertrophy (RVH) is manifest in the ECG only when the RV forces predominate over those of the LV. Since the latter has, roughly, three times more mass than the former, the RV may double in size (when the LV is normal) or triple its weight (when there is significant LVH) and still not result in the necessary requirements to pull the electrical forces anteriorly and to the right. For these reasons, RVH cannot be recognized easily in adult patients. Despite these limitations, the ECG manifestations of RVH or enlargement can be subdivided into the following main types[1,133]: (1)

TABLE 12-6

CRITERIA FOR DIAGNOSIS OF LEFT VENTRICULAR
HYPERTROPHY IN PRESENCE OF COMPLETE
LEFT BUNDLE BRANCH BLOCK

1. $RaV_L \geq 11$ mm
2. Electrical axis $\leq 40°$ (or $S_2 > R_1$)
3. $SV_1 + RV_5$ or $RV_6 \geq 40$ mm
4. $SV_2 \geq 30$ and $SV_3 \geq 25$ mm

SENSITIVITY (%)	SPECIFICITY (%)
24	100
39	100
58	97
75	90

Note: Left ventricular hypertrophy diagnosed by echocardiography when left ventricular mass is ≥ 115 g/m^2.
Source: From Kafka et al.,[142] with permission.

the posterior and rightward displacement of the QRS forces associated with low voltage, as seen in patients with pulmonary emphysema (Fig. 12-29); (2) the incomplete RBBB pattern *with right axis deviation* occurring in patients with chronic lung disease and **some** congenital cardiac malformation resulting in volume overloading of the right ventricle (Fig. 12-30); (3) the true posterior wall myocardial infarction pattern with normal to low voltage of the R wave in V_1 of mitral stenosis (Fig. 12-31); (4) and the classical RVH and strain pattern seen in young patients with congenital heart disease (producing pressure overloading) or in adult patients with high-pressure ("primary") pulmonary hypertension (Fig. 12-32).[133] False patterns of RVH may occur in patients with

TABLE 12-7

CRITERIA FOR DIAGNOSIS OF LEFT VENTRICULAR HYPERTROPHY
IN PRESENCE OF LEFT ANTERIOR FASCICULAR BLOCK[a]

Study	ECG Criteria	Sensitivity, %	Specificity, %	Positive Predictive Value, %	Negative Predictive Value, %
Bozzi and Figini	$SV_1 + (RV_5 + SV_5) \geq 25$ mm	69	92	90	73
Milliken	$RaV_L \geq 13$ mm	35	92	82	56
Milliken	$SIII \geq 15$ mm	38	87	77	57
Gertsch et al.	$SIII$ + maximal sum of R + S in any single precordial lead	96	87	89	95
Reevaluated Gertsch criteria[b]		80	55	78	58

[a] Left ventricular hypertrophy diagnosed by echocardiography when left ventricular mass is ≥ 124 g/m^2.
Unpublished observations performed in our department; see text.
Source: From Gertsch et al.,[143] with permission.

true posterior (basal) MI, complete RBBB with LPFB and Wolff-Parkinson-White syndrome resulting from AV conduction through the left free wall, or posteroseptal accessory pathways.

ELECTROLYTE IMBALANCES

Because multiple factors can affect ventricular repolarization in diseased hearts, the finding characteristic of a specific electrolyte abnormality may be modified and even mimicked by various pathologic processes and the effects of certain drugs. In practice, the major problem with the ECG diagnosis of electrolyte imbalance is not the negative ECG with abnormal serum values but the production of similar changes by other conditions in patients with normal serum values.[144]

Hyperkalemia

The initial effect of acute hyperkalemia is the appearance of peaked T waves with a narrow base (Fig. 12-33, left). The diagnosis of hyperkalemia is almost certain when the duration of the base is 0.20 s or less (with rates between 60 and 110/min).[144] As the degree of hyperkalemia increases, the QRS complex widens (Fig. 12-34), with the electrical axis usually being deviated abnormally to the left and only rarely to the right. In addition, the PR interval prolongs, and the P wave flattens until it disappears.[144] If the condition is untreated, death ensues either because of ventricular standstill or coarse slow ventricular fibrillation. Death can also result if wide QRS complexes occurring at fast rates are diagnosed as ventricular tachycardia and the patient is treated with antiarrhythmic drugs. On the other hand, class IA, IC, and III drugs as well as large doses of tricyclic antidepressants (especially when ingested for suicidal purposes) can also produce marked QRS widening. These processes, however, do not coexist with narrow-based, peaked T waves. Rarely, hyperkalemia produces (in the absence of coronary artery disease) a degree of ST-segment elevation in the right chest leads capable of suggesting anteroseptal myocardial injury (Fig. 12-34). These constitute the "dialyzable currents of injury in potassium intoxication" reported by Levine et al.[145]

Hypokalemia

The abnormal and delayed repolarization that occurs in hypokalemia is best expressed as QU rather than QT prolongation, since at times it can be difficult

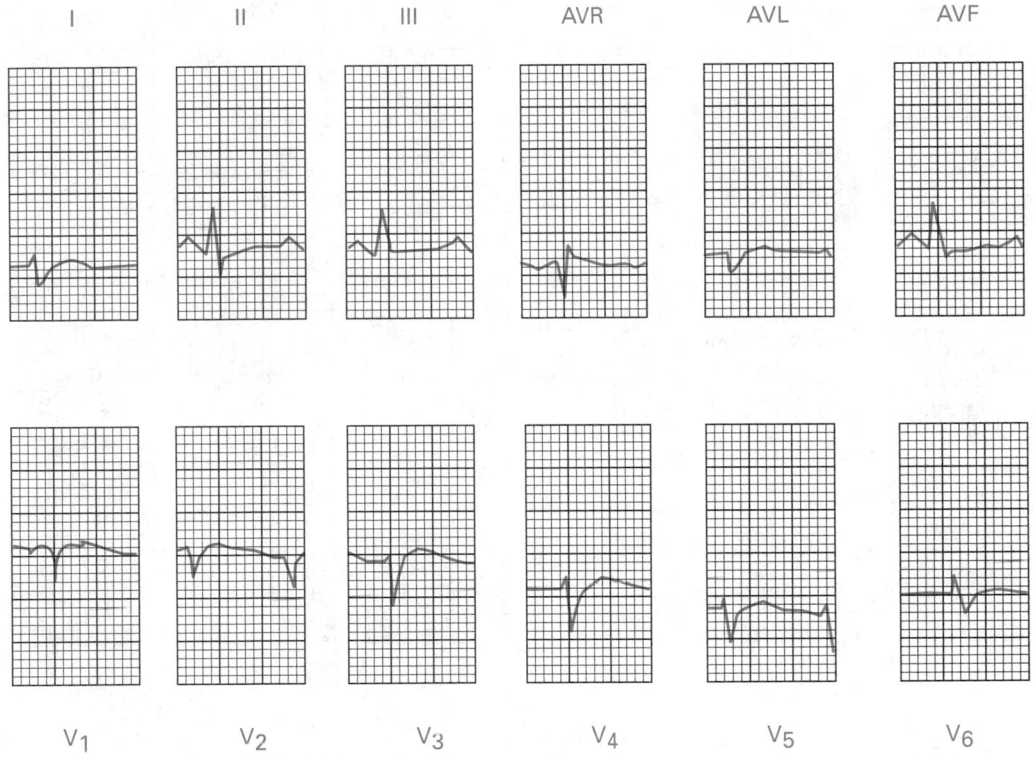

FIGURE 12-29

Electrocardiogram taken on a patient with pulmonary emphysema, showing slight right axis deviation with small rS complexes in lead I, and electrically vertical heart position, overall tendency to low voltage, and rS complexes in all chest leads. (From Lemberg and Castellanos.[169] Reproduced with permission from the publisher and the authors.)

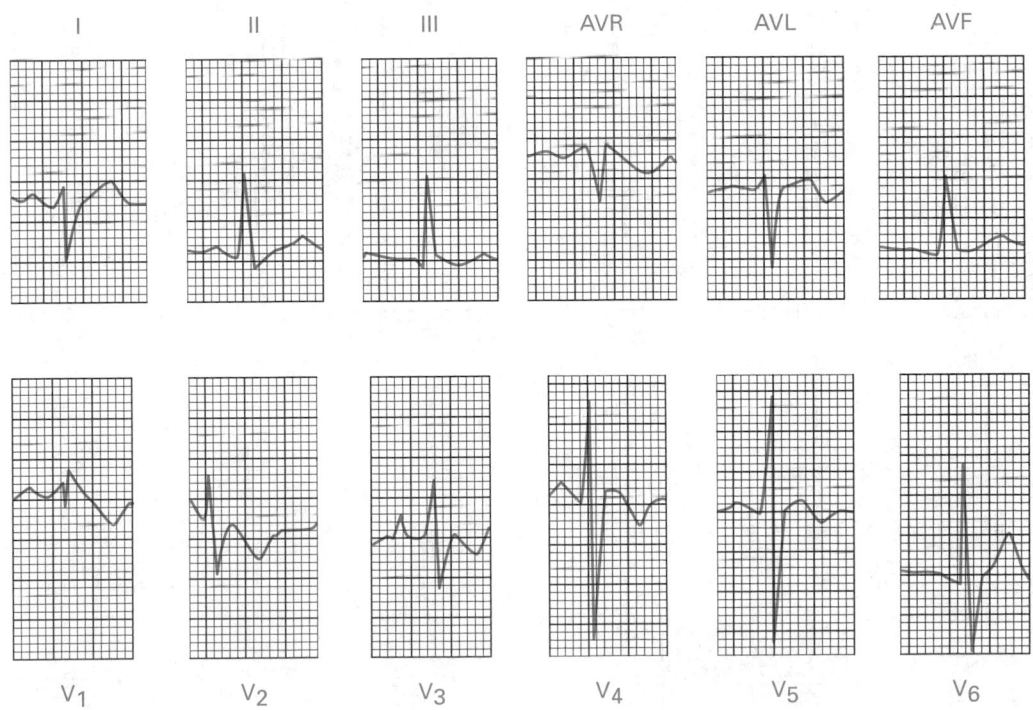

FIGURE 12-30

Electrocardiogram from a patient with right ventricular enlargement (volume overload in type) due to a small atrial septal defect (ostium secundum). Right axis deviation was associated with an incomplete RBBB pattern (rsR′ complexes in lead V₁). (From Lemberg and Castellanos.[169] Reproduced with permission from the publisher and the authors.)

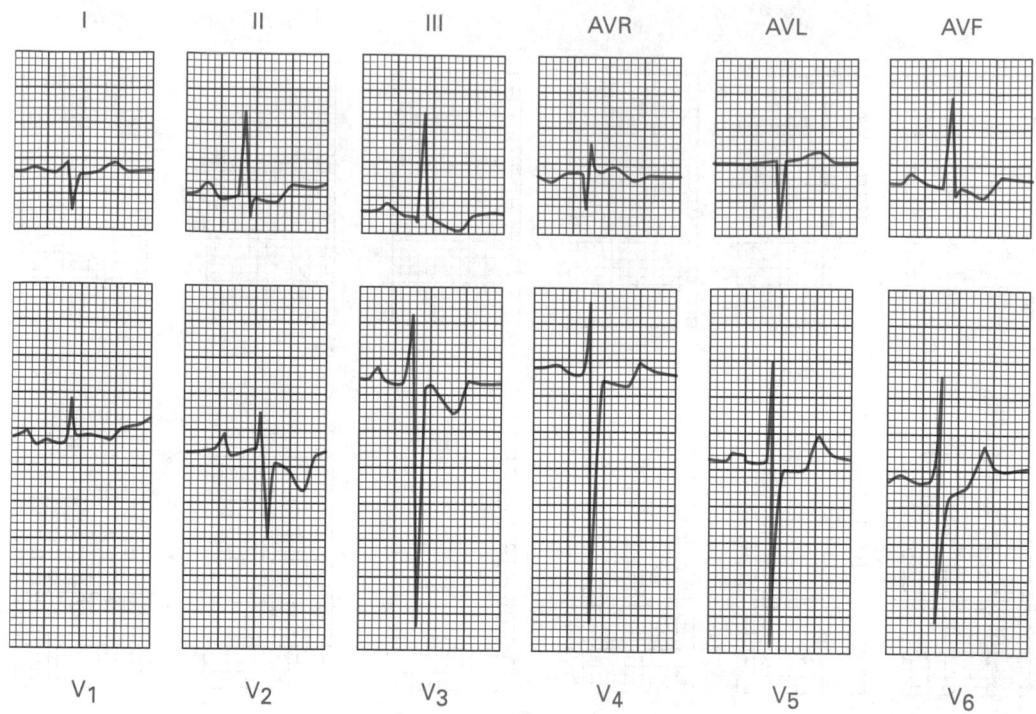

FIGURE 12-31

Electrocardiogram from a patient with right ventricular hypertrophy due to pure mitral stenosis showing P "mitrale," right axis deviation, an all-positive deflection (R wave of only approximately 5 mm) in V_1, and rS complexes from V_2 to V_6. (From Lemberg and Castellanos.[169] Reproduced with permission from the publisher and the authors.)

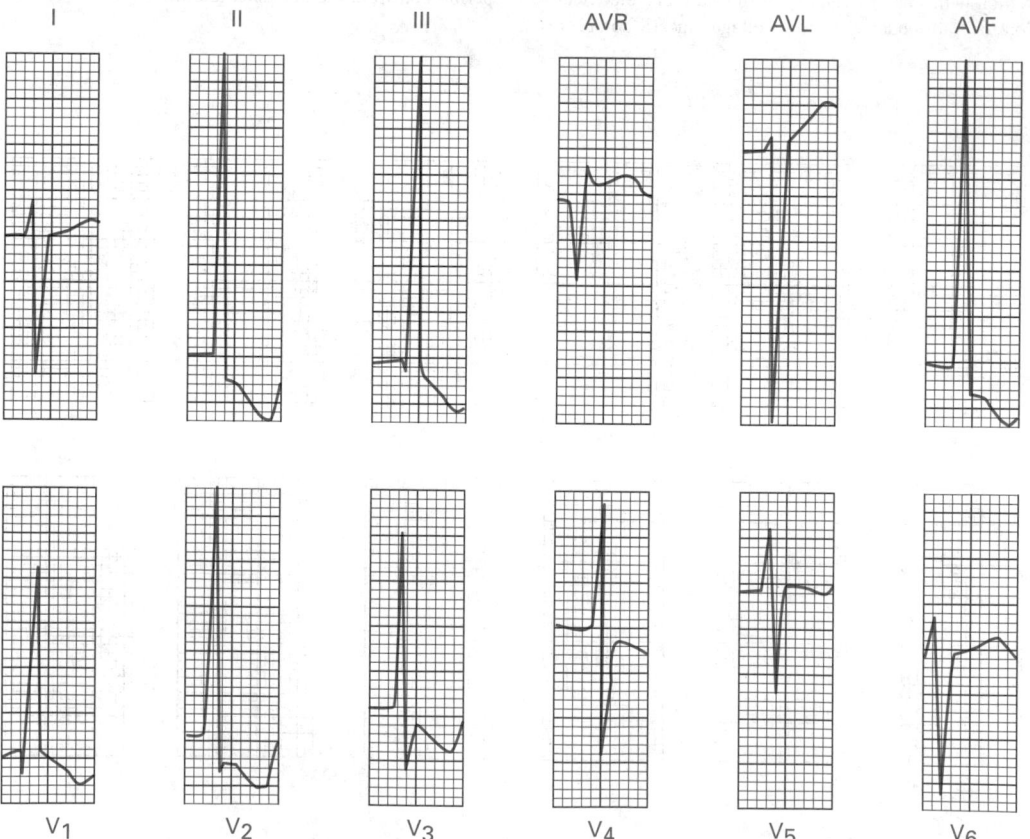

FIGURE 12-32

Electrocardiogram from a 17-year old patient who had right ventricular enlargement (pressure overloading in type) due to severe pulmonic stenosis. Note extreme right axis deviation, overall high voltage, and qR complexes in lead V_1 without an incomplete RBBB pattern. (From Lemberg and Castellanos.[169] Reproduced with permission from the publisher and the authors.)

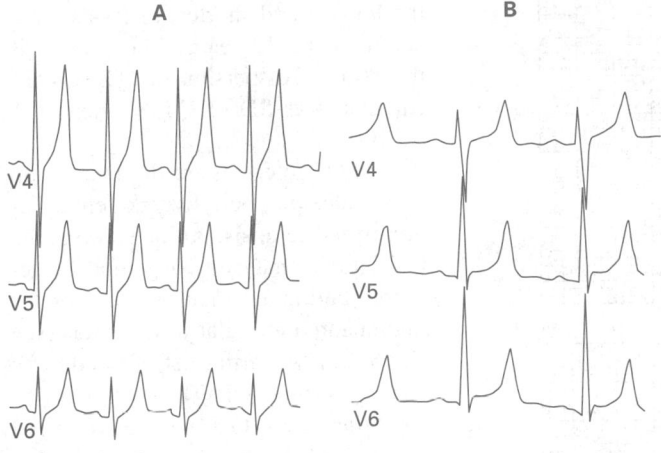

FIGURE 12-33

Electrocardiographic manifestations of early hyperkalemia. The unprolonged QRS complex is followed by a peaked T wave having a very narrow base. Uncorrected and corrected QT intervals of 0.32 and 0.44 s, respectively (*A*). Hyperkalemia with hypocalcemia characterized by prolongation of the QT interval at the expense of the ST segment preceding the narrow-based T wave. Uncorrected and corrected QT intervals of 0.52 and 0.53 s, respectively (*B*).

to differentiate between notching of the T wave and T- and U-wave fusion.[144] As the serum potassium falls, the ST segment becomes progressively more depressed and there is a gradual blending of the T wave into what appears to be a tall U wave (Fig. 12-35, top). An ECG pattern similar to that of hypokalemia can be produced by some antiarrhythmic drugs, especially quinidine. In any case, when repolarization is greatly prolonged, ventricular arrhythmias, including the so-called torsades de pointes, can occur.

Hypomagnesemia

Hypomagnesemia does not produce QU prolongation unless the coexisting hypokalemia (with which it is almost invariably associated) is severe.[144] Long-standing and very marked magnesium deficiency lowers the amplitude of the T wave and depresses the ST segment.[144] It may be difficult to differentiate between the changes produced by magnesium from those produced by potassium. For this reason it has been stated that hypomagnesia does not cause any changes in the ECG.[39]

Hypermagnesemia

Similarly, in clinical tracings the effects of hypermagnesemia on the ECG are difficult to identify because the changes are dominated by calcium.[146] According to some authors, administration

of intravenous magnesium to patients with normal ECGs may shorten the QT interval.[39] Other authors found no effects on ventricular refractoriness that are reflected by changes in the QT interval.[147] Intravenous magnesium given to patients with torsades de pointes controls the arrhythmia in a high percentage of patients without changing the prolonged QT interval significantly.[148] The calcium-blocking activity of magnesium was suggested to be one of the mechanisms responsible for this antiarrhythmic activity.[146]

Hypercalcemia

During sinus rhythm with normal rates, the QT interval is short (Fig. 12-35, bottom). In some cases the Q-to-apex of T intervals is also short. If factors known to modify the QT interval are not present, it has been said that a reasonably accepted correlation exists between the duration of the interval and serum calcium levels.[144] Occasionally, the ST segment disappears and the T waves may become inverted in left and right chest leads. Digitalis also shortens the QT interval but produces its characteristic "effects" in leads where R waves predominate. The classical upward concavity of the ST segment is seen in the left chest leads in patients with LVH and in V_1 and V_2 when there is RVH (with predominantly positive deflections in these leads).

Hypocalcemia

The typical ECG pattern of hypocalcemia consists of QT prolongation at the expense of the ST segment.[144] The T wave is usually of normal width but can be narrow-based if there is coexistent (moderate) hyperkalemia (Fig. 12-33B). A very marked injury (with so-called hyperacute ST-T changes) can produce a similar pattern, but in those cases the T wave, though peaked, is not as narrow-based. It has been said that

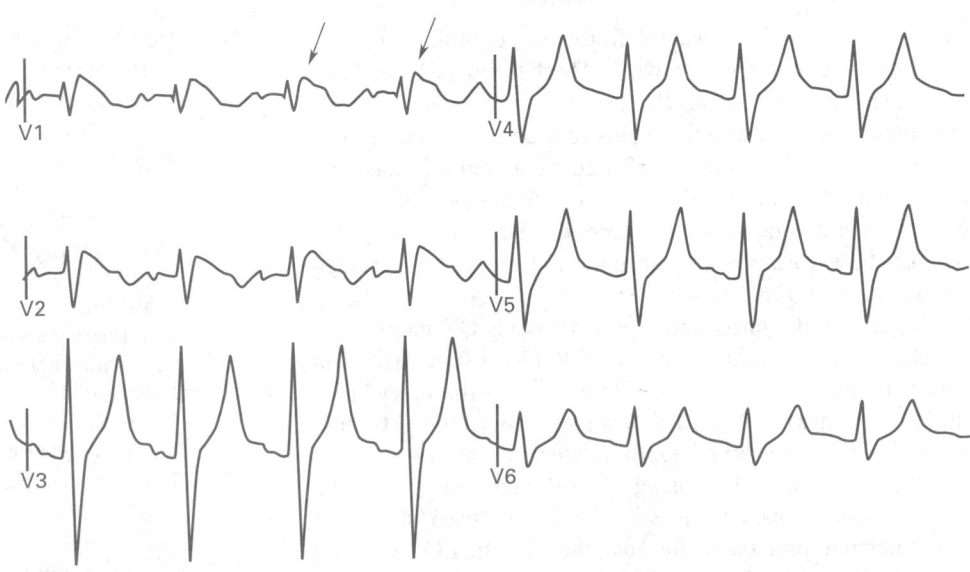

FIGURE 12-34

Advanced hyperkalemia. The wide (0.14 s) QRS complexes are followed by peaked T waves (best seen in lead V_3). The hyperkalemia-induced ST-segment elevation in lead V_1 (*arrows*), known as the "dialyzable current of injury," disappeared after appropriate treatment.

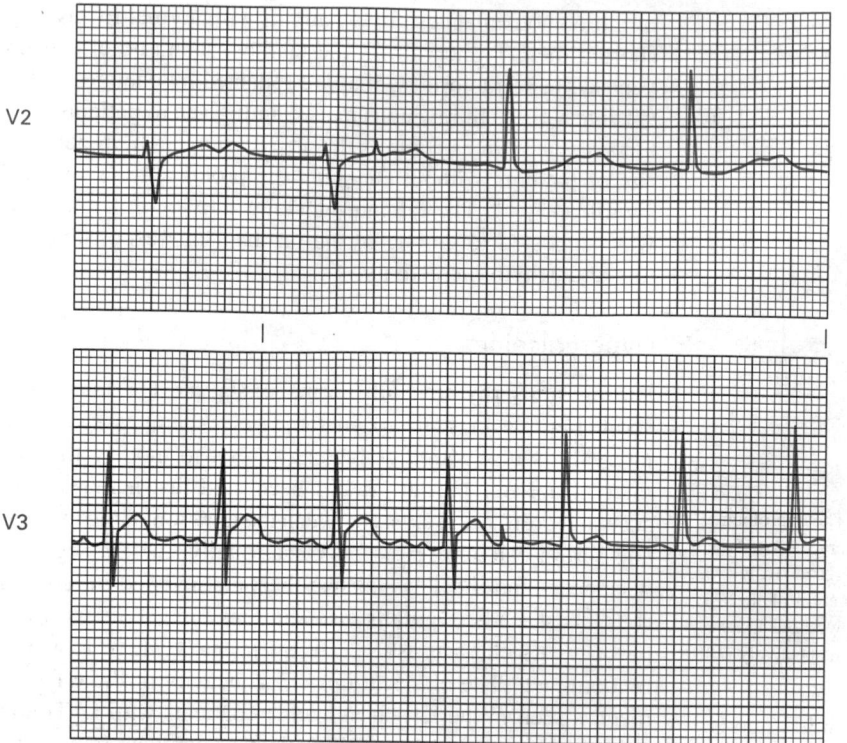

FIGURE 12-35
Electrocardiographic manifestations of hypokalemia (*upper strip*) and of hypercalcemia (*lower strip*).

hypocalcemia per se does produce T-wave inversion. When present, the latter is usually a reflection of coexisting processes such as LVH and incomplete LBBB. An ECG pattern similar to that of hypocalcemia can be produced by some organic abnormalities of the central nervous system and by congenitally prolonged QT intervals (see below).

QT Interval: Normal and Prolonged

The QT interval is measured from the beginning of the q wave to the end of the T wave.[11] The latter may be difficult to define. The point at which the maximal downslope of the T wave crosses the baseline helps to identify the end of this wave.[39] The QT interval is affected by autonomic tone and catecholamines and has day-night difference. It varies with heart rate and gender. Several formulas have been proposed to take these variables into account and provide a corrected measurement (QTc interval).[14]

In general, the unadjusted (noncorrected) QT interval decreases from ±0.42 s at rates of 50/min to 0. ± 0.32 s at 100/min and to ±0.26 s at 150/min.[9,11] On the other hand, during exercise, as the rate becomes faster, the QTc first increases until reaching, approximately, a rate of 120/min and thereafter again decreasing.[149] Although the value of the normal QTc is open to question, it is still used in routine computer interpretations. Because the 12-lead ECG shows a normal degree of QT and QTc dispersion (of repolarization), indexes have been used to quantify the extent of heterogeneity in ventricular repolarization. One is the difference between

the longest and shortest intervals measured in the 12 leads. The second is the relative dispersion of QT or QTc calculated as SD of QT ÷ mean QT × 100.[150]

The QT intervals are shortened with hypercalcemia, pure hyperkalemia, digoxin, and acidosis. Prolongation of the QT interval may be congenital or acquired and is an important marker for malignant ventricular arrhythmias (see Chap. 27). A partial list of conditions causing prolonged QT or Q-U or, in some instances, QU intervals (delayed repolarization) is shown in Table 12-8.[150,151]

Hypothermia

Characteristic ECG changes develop when the body temperature drops to approximately 30° C.[11] The QT interval becomes prolonged. In addition, a deflection, called an *Osborn wave*, appears in a place said to be located between the end of the QRS complex and the beginning of the ST segment (Fig. 12-36).[152,153] This deflection has been attributed to delayed depolarization, to a current of injury, or to "early" repolarization.[153] In leads facing the LV, the deflection is positive and its size is inversely related to body

---

TABLE 12-8

ACQUIRED QT PROLONGATION—USUALLY BRADYCARDIA AND/OR PAUSE-DEPENDENT

1. Electrolyte disturbances
   a. Hypokalemia
   b. Hypocalcemia
   c. Hypomagnesemia
2. Drugs
   a. Class IA antiarrhythmic agents (quinidine, disopyramide, procainamide)
   b. Class III antiarrhythmic agents (amiodarone, sotalol)
   c. Psychotropic drugs
3. Central nervous system diseases
   a. Subarachnoid hemorrhage
   b. Ruptured berry aneurysm
   c. Cryptococcal meningitis
4. Congenital syndromes
5. Electrocardiographic ischemia
6. Arrhythmias
   a. Posttachycardia syndrome
   b. Cardiac arrest of any etiology
   c. Chronic idioventricular rhythms
7. Hypothermia

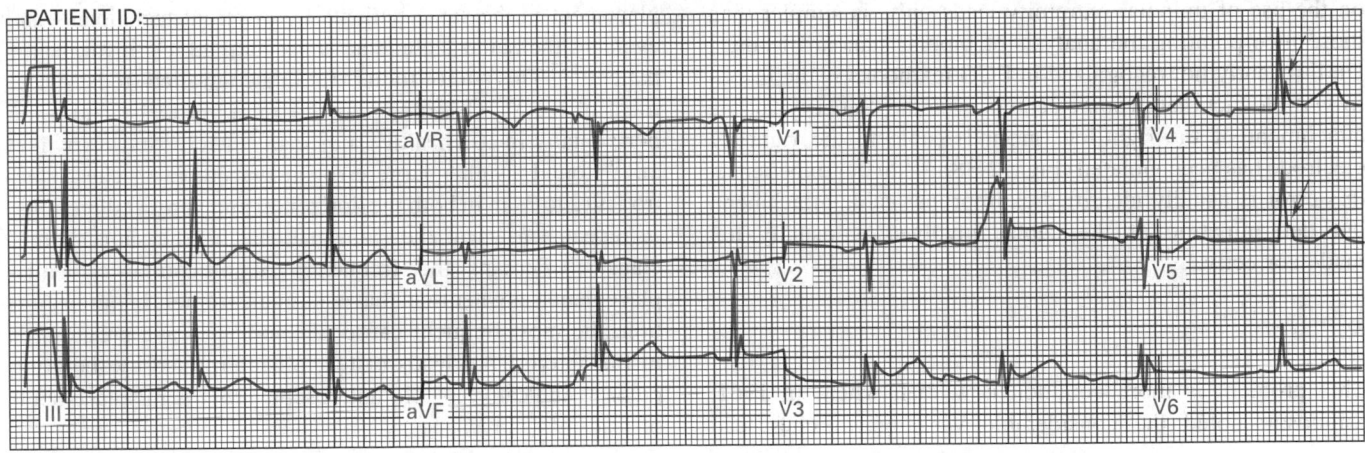

FIGURE 12-36

Electrocardiogram obtained from a patient with hypothermia. The characteristic Osborn wave (*arrows*) is the terminal deflection inscribed between the slender part of the QRS complexes and the beginning of the ST segment. Note that it is not easy to determine where the ST segment starts. In addition, there is marked prolongation of the QT interval.

temperature. The possible role played by the intramyocardial M cells in its genesis has been discussed previously.[41]

ARTIFACTS

During the last few years the number and types of instruments used for noninvasive and invasive (electrical and nonelectrical) study of cardiac functions have multiplied. Naturally, physicians and hospital administrators have concentrated their attention on them. Technicians have been more interested in working in these more lucrative services. Such factors, and others, have downgraded the importance of recording 12-lead ECGs, relegating them to less qualified personnel. Not surprisingly, the quality of technicians and of the ECGs that they record have deteriorated in many centers. Optimal quality can only be achieved if the parties involved understand what is happening. The following are some of the artifacts commonly seen in current routine 12-lead ECGs. They are important since they can confound the interpreter and, worse, the computer program.

Muscle Tremor and Alternating Current Interference

These are the most frequently encountered artifacts because some patients will continue to have disease processes producing tremor and because the amount of electronic equipment causing interference in a hospital environment has increased.

Improper Limb-Lead Positioning

This has become more frequent after relaxation of quality control. It is more frequent in those institutions with inadequate standards for hiring technicians and with poor on-site training. Mixing up the cables from the ECG machine has gone beyond switching the right and left arm cables.[11] Various types of misplacement of only one cable are illustrated in (Fig. 12-37). The method depicted in this illustration, based

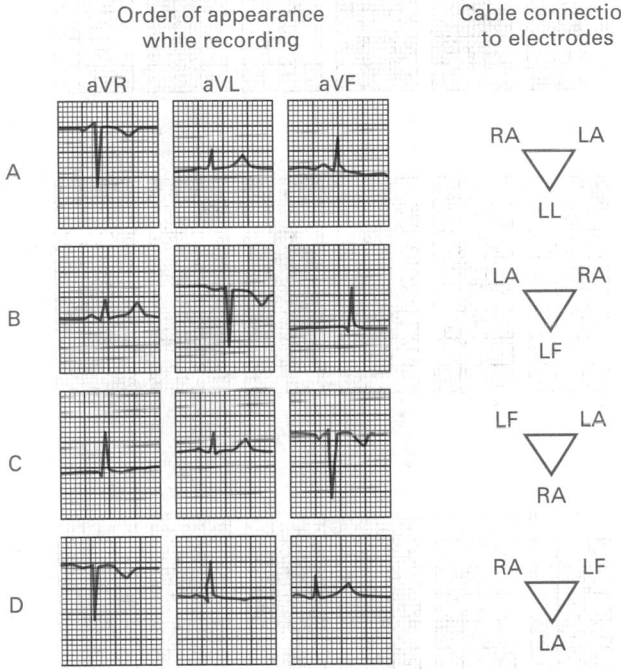

Order of appearance while recording

Cable connection to electrodes

FIGURE 12-37

Indentification of improper connections of a single cable from the ECG machine to the corresponding electrodes placed on the patient's limbs. Note that aV_R, aV_L, and aV_F invariably refer to whatever morphology is recorded when, while the ECG is being obtained, the corresponding knobs are turned in this order (regardless of whether the cables were properly or improperly attached). On the other hand, RA, LA, and LL (or LF) correspond to the normal morphology recorded by the cables so labeled. This method, based solely on the analysis of the unipolar extremity leads, is simpler than the method based on the study of the bipolar standard leads but is useful only when a single cable is misconnected. *A*. Normal. *B*. Since LA appears in aV_R and RA appears in aV_L (with LF being in its normal position), the right and left arm cables must have been switched. *C*. Since LF appears in aV_R and RA appears in aV_F (with LA in its normal position), the right arm and left leg cables must have been switched. *D*. Since LA appears in aV_F and LF appears in aV_L (with RA in its normal position), the left arm and left leg cables must have been switched.

on the use of unipolar extremity leads only, is simpler than those incorporating the analysis of bipolar standard leads.[11] Until recently not recognized in ECG textbooks is the incontrovertible fact that in some centers even the "sanctity" of the attachment of the right-leg (ground) cable to the right-leg electrode has been violated (Fig. 12-38).[154] In our experience, this error is usually identified as improper cable attachment, but determination of the cables involved is usually not made correctly.[154]

Variations in Precordial-Lead Placement

This problem is more common now than when, in 1961, Simonson noted the considerable variation in chest-lead placement in the same patients by different technicians and even by the same technician in several ECGs in the same patient.[155] This author found that in a controlled study, placement of the V_2 electrode varied 10 cm vertically and 8 cm horizontally in 103 healthy subjects.[155] Moreover, Kerwin et al.[156] found a rather large error in placement of chest electrodes (2 to 3 cm in both the horizontal and vertical directions) in repeated trials in the same patients by the same technicians.[156] Perhaps the frequency of precordial-lead misplacement is greater than that of somatic tremor. In our institution, the most frequent cause of "poor" r wave progression in the anteroseptal leads (often, misinterpreted by the computer as indicative of old anteroseptal MI) is misplacements of leads V_2 and V_3.

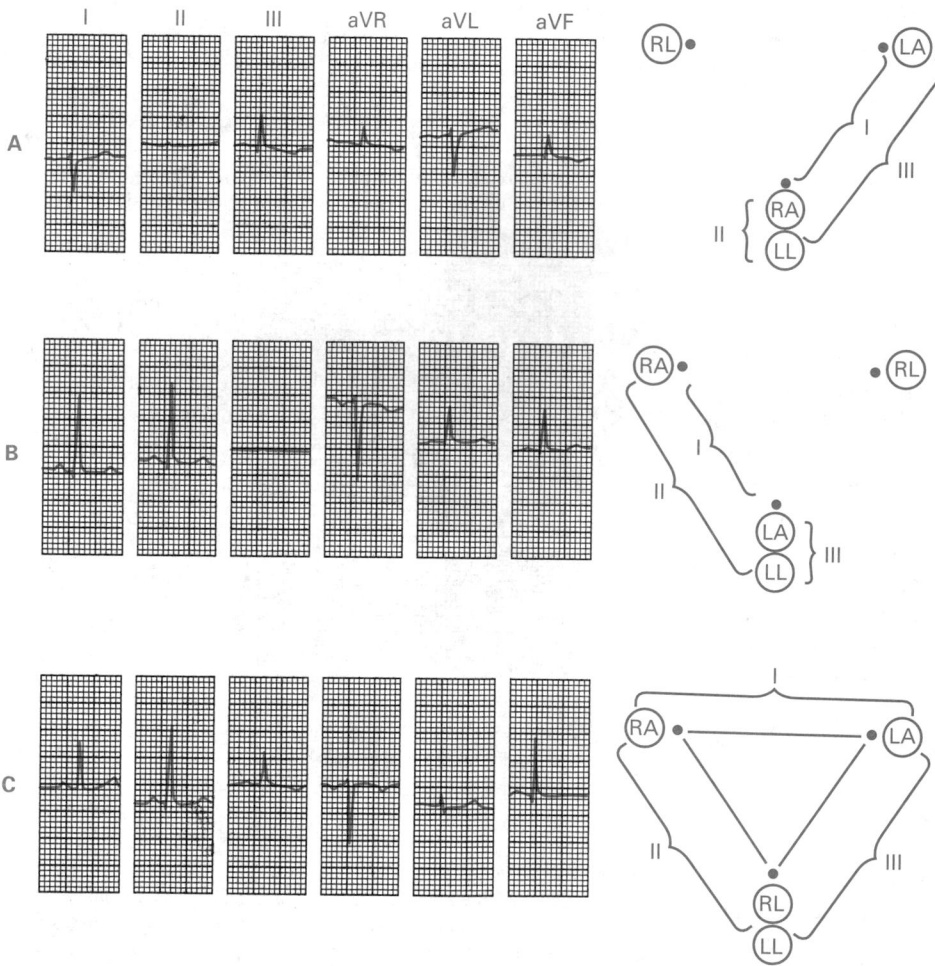

FIGURE 12-38

Identification of improper connections of the right leg (RL) (ground) cable. *C* can be regarded as almost equal to the control tracing, since the RL (ground) and left leg (LL) cables were switched. The corresponding morphologies are not identical to the control morphologies, since a very small difference in potential between both legs does exist. The latter is seen in *A*. Because the RL and RA cables were switched, lead II (RA-LL) records the difference in potential between both legs, which seems to be approximately 0.15 mV. The latter results in an almost straight line interrupted by a small blip. In addition, lead I represents the mirror image of normal lead III and lead III is the normal lead II. In *B*, where the LA and RL cables have been switched, lead III (LA-LL) records almost a straight line. In addition, lead I is the normal lead II and lead II is the normal lead II. [From Castellanos A, Saoudi AN, Schwartz A, et al. Electrocardiographic patterns resulting from improper connection of the right leg (ground) cable. *PACE* 1985; 8:364–368. Reproduced with permission from the publisher and the authors.]

False Variations in Voltage

Garson noticed that in several patients, ECGs taken weeks apart showed markedly different QRS voltages.[157] The latter were sometimes of sufficient magnitude to cause a pseudonormalization of a ventricular hypertrophy pattern. There had been no changes in hemodynamics, but different types of ECGs were used. A study of this problem demonstrated that ECG data had a different voltage depending on whether they were recorded and displayed on an analogue or a digital ECG machine. Thus, if there is a statistically significant difference between ECGs, the serial comparisons must be done with the same machine. Moreover, criteria for voltage are applicable only to the type of instrument with which the data were gathered.

In addition, overshoot, overdamping, and running down of the standardization battery can cause significant changes in QRS voltage and ST segments.

Wandering Baseline

Wandering baseline is usually due to unclean electrodes or electrodal sites.

How Should an ECG Be Performed?

This question is appropriate in view of the many artifacts and technical (machine and human) problems occurring when ECGs are recorded. The Task Force of the American College of Cardiology (ACC)—American Heart Association (AHA) in their *Guidelines for Electrocardiography*[4] have stated that the ECG should be performed and interpreted in accordance with the guidelines for optimal electrocardiography described in the report on the ACC Tenth Bethesda Conference[158]; the guidelines for training described in the ACC Seventeenth Bethesda Conference Report of the ACA[159]; the recommendations for standardization of leads and specifications for instruments in electrocardiography and vectorcardiography of the AHA[160]; and the recommendations for standardization and specifications for automated electrocardiography of the AHA.[161]

COMPUTER APPLICATIONS

It has been almost 40 years since the first attempts were made to apply computer technology to the interpretation of ECGs.[162] During this time, the field has progressed from initial attempts at the recognition of normal tracing to some of today's more sophisticated programs.[1,162–165] In general, computer systems for true analysis of ECGs have, as their main component, a program that usually includes the following four basic functions: (1) the measuring of ECG parameters, which includes an automatic wave front recognition section and a measurement section that extracts the wave fronts, a set of values, and control; (2) the interpretation of previously acquired information, responsible for the final statements generated by the program; (3) the identification of various rhythms, both normal and abnormal; and (4) the comparison with previous ECGs to recognize significant changes. Once a report is generated, a qualified interpreter must correct (if necessary) and edit the computer interpretation. A problem that is not sufficiently emphasized in the literature is the dilemma faced by physicians and hospital administrators who decide to computerize or update their ECG operation. This problem is the decision of selecting among the multiple available programs. Substantial differences exist among available programs in regard to measurement definitions and classification criteria and terminology. As every electrocardiographer knows, there is a lack of standardized, universally agreed upon, diagnostic terms and criteria. This problem, however, is not solely that of computers but is related to all ECG interpretations, whether performed by individuals or machines. It must be remembered that the program used depends on criteria imposed on it by human programmers. Physicians making the selections should be familiar with the diagnostic criteria employed (supplied by the manufacturers) and with the program's practical performance. The latter information can be obtained by communicating directly with other users. Of particular importance is knowledge of the manufacturer's service performance. Finally, the program selected must, at present, be "tuned in" with the operational environment (community hospital or teaching institution, urban center or rural

areas, etc.) in which it must perform. Once a program has been selected and is in use, it requires initial and periodic evaluation. The most practical method consists of accepting as standard constrained human observers, the constrained observers being given a set of measurements or criteria agreed upon before the evaluation. In academic centers, attempts to determine sensitivity and specificities should be made, applying as standards ECG-independent evidence, obtained using *more than one* of the currently available in vivo, noninvasive methods as well as (when possible) postmortem information.

Proper computerization has the following definite advantages: (1) speed in providing reports, with the resulting improved turnaround time; (2) optimal utilization of emergency ECG services; (3) reproducibility of measurements; (4) improvements in quality control; (5) possible decrease in physician's reading time and more consistency in interpretations; (6) enhancement of the capacity to handle large volumes of ECGs; and (7) substantial improvement in record storage and retrieval, with better comparison with previous tracings. Computerized ECG programs must also be evaluated with standard cost-effective methods. That is, the economics involved—initial investment, operational costs, payroll, overhead, and professional fees—must be compared with those of the preexisting system in the same hospital. This is important, since it was estimated that even 10 years ago more than 40 percent of all ECGs recorded in the United States were obtained by some type of automatic system.[162] Presently, this figure is probably reaching 100 percent. Finally, emphasis should be placed on the obvious: All computer ECG interpretations, particularly those of rhythm disturbances, must be checked by a physician qualified to interpret ECGs and who has an in-depth knowledge of the program used. Decisions based on a computerized interpretation may, on occasion, lead to improper patient care. This can also have medicological implications. Of clinical importance was the observation that computer interpretations of ECGs obtained 1 min apart were grossly different in 36 out of 92 (39 percent) of unselected pairs of tracings.[166] The ACC/AHA Task Force on Guidelines for Electrocardiography states, "There is no computer program that can replace the skilled physician."[4] Finally, cardiology fellows in training should preferably interpret ECGs without using a printed computer interpretation rather than having to evaluate the latter.

SPATIAL VECTORCARDIOGRAPHY

Generalities

The following statements, which need reemphasis, should not be considered redundant: (1) Since the ECG deals with electrical forces, it follows that, very strictly speaking, all electrocardiography is necessarily vectorial.[81,167,168] (2) Orthodoxically, a scalar quantity has only magnitude, whereas a vector quantity has magnitude, direction, and sense. In analyzing the vectorcardiogram (VCG), one should consider the activation of each muscle cell as producing an electrical force that can be represented by a vector depicting the spatial orientation and magnitude of this force.[167]

During the spread of the activation process, innumerable electrical forces are generated. These multiple forces vary in magnitude and differ in direction. At any given moment, the resultant of these electrical forces can be represented by a spatial vector possessing magnitude, direction, and sense. This vector is referred to as an *instantaneous vector* and represents the resultant of *all* the forces of the heart acting at that particular moment. Immediately afterward, the wave of accession spreads to different areas of the myocardium, and the new instantaneous vector representing all the forces of the heart now occupies a different spatial position and has a different magnitude. This continues throughout the cardiac cycle, with the succeeding instantaneous vector occupying different spatial positions. If all manifest spatial vectors are diagrammatically represented as having a common point of origin and if the distal points of the vectors are joined, a single spatial loop is formed for ventricular depolarization (QRS), ventricular repolarization (ST-T), and the atrial complex (P). The VCG consists of four different loops. The electrical activity of the atria is recorded as a small loop designated the P loop; the depolarization of the ventricles is recorded as a large loop designated the QRS loop; while the repolarization of the ventricles is recorded as a smaller loop designated the ST-T loop. Finally, at high magnifications, even a small U loop can also be recorded.[169-171]

Space: The Final Frontier

Beyond doubt, the idea of a truly spatial VCG is theoretically attractive. Because the heart is a tridimensional structure (located in space), its electrical activity should be best recorded by a spatial method. Indeed, space, as conceived by physicists through objects and their motion, has three dimensions, and positions are characterized by three numbers. The instant of an event is the fourth number. Four definite numbers correspond to every event; a definite event corresponds to any four numbers. Therefore, the world of events really forms a four-dimensional continuum. Unfortunately, judging by what is being published in the literature, the quest for an optimal method of visualizing the spatial loop has apparently been abandoned. Nevertheless, the spatial VCG is still of importance, especially in children with congenital and acquired heart disease, since in the population the criteria for pressure and volume overloading have proven value.[169] In our opinion, it is also of great value in categorizing the various types of intraventricular conduction defects.[169-171] While this may be attributed to the spatial technique per se, it can also be due to the use of instruments having a higher fidelity than routine ECGs. The VCG has also been found useful in detecting MI and certain types of right ventricular enlargement.[169-171] In practice, it has not been proved that the VCG gives more information than the routine 12-lead ECG, although some

computer programs still use the Frank orthogonal leads X, Y, and Z. These programs thus constitute a 15-lead system. In addition, the time required to obtain a VCG is longer than the time required to record a 12-lead ECG. These are the main reasons for the logarithmic decrease in the use of spatial VCG during recent decades. Other reasons are nonreimbursement and the continuously increasing interest in other noninvasive methods of recording electrical activity (such as signal averaging, body-surface mapping, and heart rate variability) or nonelectrical activity (such as echocardiography or magnetic resonance imaging), which looks at planes from *different* views. To obtain the spatial VCG, electrodes are placed on the body surface so as to record three leads whose planes are at right angles to each other. The true spatial VCG requires three corrected orthogonal leads with the following features[169-172]: (1) Mutual perpendicularity, with each lead being parallel to one of the rectilinear coordinate axes of the human body. Such axes are the horizontal, X (left-to-right and right-to-left) axis; the vertical, Y (inferosuperior or superoinferior) axis; and the sagittal, Z (anteroposterior or posteroanterior) axis. (2) Equal amplitude from the vectorial viewpoint. (3) Retention of the same magnitude and direction for all points where cardiac electromotive forces are generated. For example, even if the leads forming Einthoven's frontal plane were to be spatially correct, Einthoven's theory itself would make any electrodes placed for the purpose of obtaining the horizontal and sagittal planes (such as the tetrahedral system) spatially incorrect. The most widely used, corrected spatial VCG method probably is the one introduced by Frank.[172] Since the spatial loop cannot be analyzed tridimensionally, it is customary to study its planar projections (Fig. 12-39). By proper attachment to the oscilloscope, the X and Y leads are used for the frontal plane, and the X and Z leads for the horizontal plane, and the Z and Y leads for the sagittal plane (of which the right side has been the most popular).

Differences between Electrovectorcardiography and Spatial Vectorcardiography

In comparison with the ECG, the spatial VCG is another method of recording the electrical activity of the heart at the body surface. It is distinctly different from the various vectorial methods of ECG interpretation, such as those of Sodi-Pallares et al.[7] or Grant.[50] In clinical practice and in teaching, both seem to be considered equal, but this is so only for pragmatic and didactic reasons. Although the spatial VCG and the ECG should each be studied as distinct methods, most electrocardiographers either memorize loop patterns or attempt to derive the leads with which they are familiar from the corresponding QRS loops. Thus, bipolar standard and unipolar extremity leads are derived from the frontal plane more or less as when, in clinical ECG, they are derived from electrical axis. To do this in spatial vector loops, the electrical axis is equated with the maximal QRS vector, which extends from the point of origin of the loop to its farthermost point.

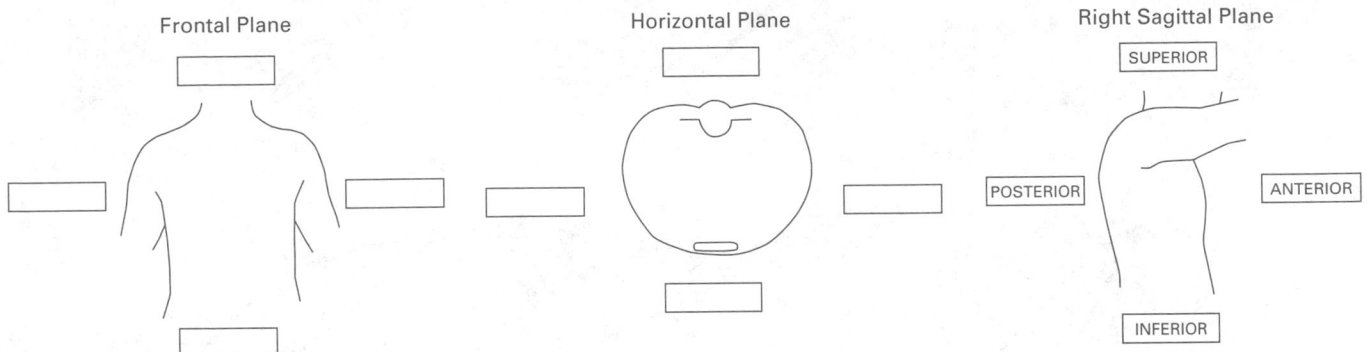

Frontal Plane   Horizontal Plane   Right Sagittal Plane

SUPERIOR

POSTERIOR   ANTERIOR

INFERIOR

FIGURE 12-39

The spatial vectorcardiographic loops cannot be routinely analyzed in space with presently available techniques. Therefore, it is customary to study their projections in three planes seen as depicted in this figure. Note that (1) the frontal plane conforms to Einthoven's view of his equilateral triangle; (2) the horizontal plane is seen in such a way that the anterior surfaces of the heart and sternum are displayed in the inferior portions of the paper (in contrast to other noninvasive, nonelectrical methods); and (3) the sagittal plane is viewed from the right side of the patient. (From Lemberg and Castellanos.[169] Reproduced with permission from the publisher and the authors.)

The unipolar precordial leads are derived from the horizontal plane loops (Fig. 12-40). Leads thus derived are different from the usual ECG leads. It was previously said that the latter recorded electrical forces moving toward or away from them. In the 12-lead ECG (especially when the precordial electrodes are misplaced), however, these forces can move spatially not only in a left-to-right and anteroposterior direction but also in an inferosuperior direction, as in leads V_5 and V_6 of patients with a very superior and leftward deviation of the EA. On the other hand, the theory of spatial vectorcardiography states that the horizontal plane and unipolar leads record only left-to-right and anteroposterior forces. In spatial vectorcardiography, electrical forces oriented superiorly or inferiorly cannot be reflected in the horizontal plane but only in the

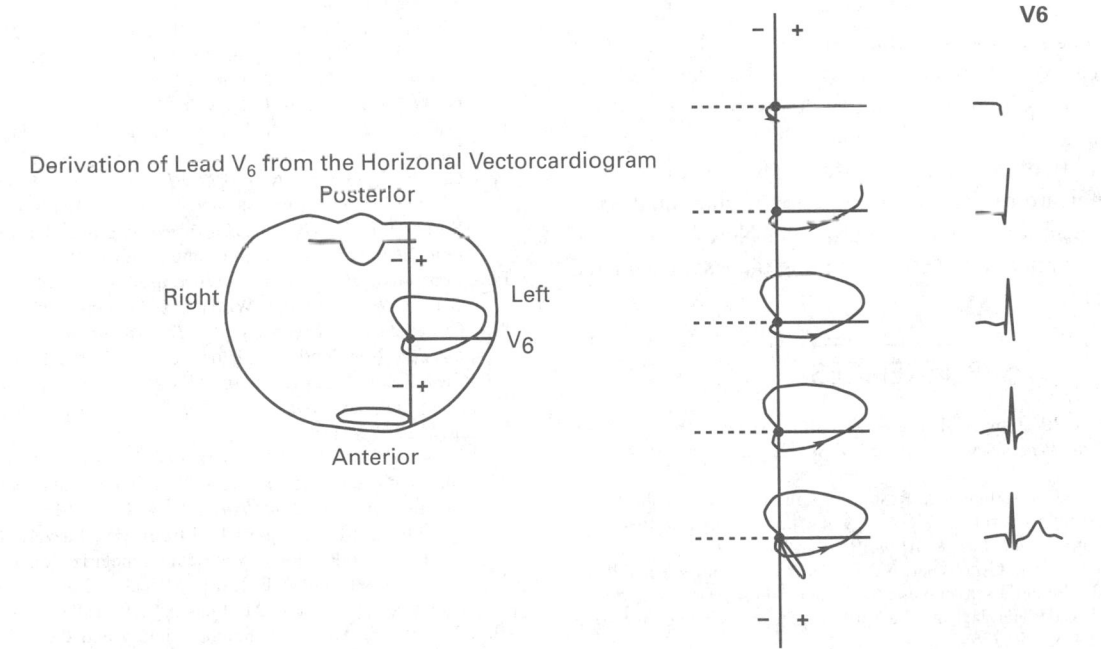

Derivation of Lead V_6 from the Horizontal Vectorcardiogram

Posterior

Right   Left

V_6

Anterior

V_6

FIGURE 12-40

Method used to derive the morphology of a unipolar precordial lead (in this example, lead V_6) from the horizontal plane QRS and ST-T loops. First (*left panel*), a line is drawn from the estimated location of the corresponding electrode to the point of origin of the loops. Thereafter, a perpendicular to this line passing from the point of origin is drawn. This divides the thorax into a negative area (for V_6) that is located beyond the perpendicular line and a positive area that is located between the perpendicular line and the electrode. Thus, in the top right schematic, the small part of the loop located beyond the perpendicular line produces the small q wave in V_6. The other schematics show how progression of depolarization and repolarization produces parts of the QRS loop (and the entire ST-T loop), which are positive in lead V_6. The S wave occurs because the terminal part of the QRS loop is located beyond the perpendicular line. (From Lemberg and Castellanos.[169] Reproduced with permission from the publisher and the authors.)

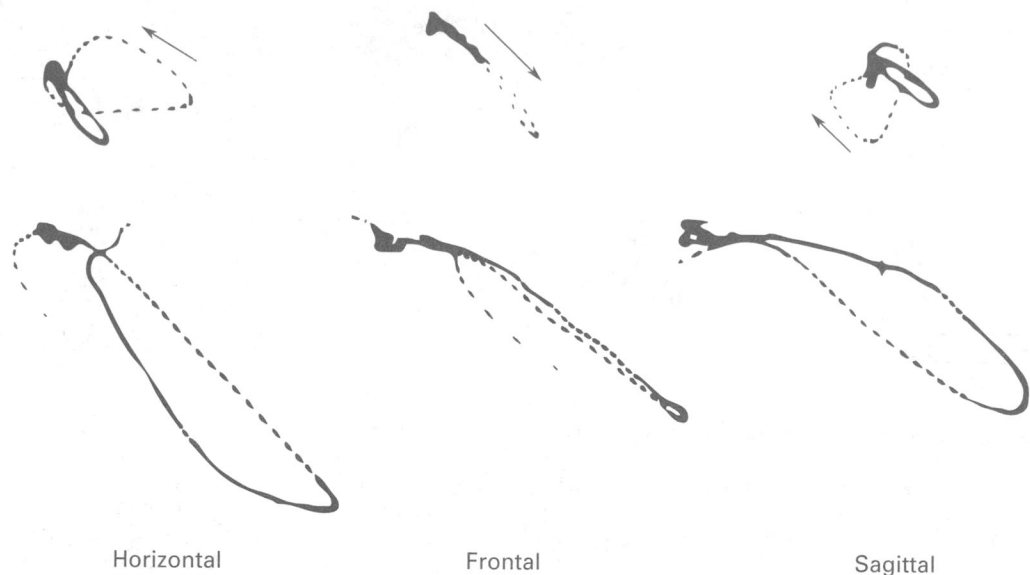

Horizontal   Frontal   Sagittal

FIGURE 12-41

Planar projections of normal spatial VCG obtained with the Frank method. The ST-T loops are enlarged in the bottom view. In the horizontal plane, the QRS loop shows the expected, normal, counterclockwise (CCW) rotation (*arrows*). Although the narrow frontal plane QRS loop has clockwise (CW) rotation, in this plane either CCW, CW, or figure-eight rotations can be normal. In the right sagittal plane, the QRS loop displays its normal (CW) rotation. Enlargement of the ST-T loop clearly shows that its first half is inscribed more slowly. Therefore, the dashes (each representing 0.0025 s, or 25 ms) are closer together. Note that the rotation of the ST-T loop is similar to the rotation of the QRS loop in all planes. (From Lemberg and Castellanos.[169] Reproduced with permission of the publisher and the authors.)

frontal and sagittal planes. Most of the information contained in the sagittal plane is present in the frontal and horizontal planes. In practice, the sagittal plane is useful to act as a "judge" in cases of apparent discrepancy between the other two planes. For example, it serves to determine if a localized delay present in one of the two planes is "real" or is due to perpendicularity of vectors. It also serves for a better evaluation of the upward or downward direction of the initial 0.01- and 0.02-s vectors than the frontal plane. Normal QRS and ST-T loops obtained in the corresponding planes are depicted in Fig. 12-41.

REFERENCES

1. Macfarlane PW, Lawrie TDV, eds. *Comprehensive Electrocardiology: Theory and Practice in Health and Disease.* New York: Pergamon; 1989.
2. Myerburg RJ, Castellanos A. Resolution of nonspecific repolarization patterns from body surface signals: A new horizon of clinical electrocardiography. *J Am Coll Cardiol* 1989; 14:703–704.
3. Einthoven W, Fahr G, de Waart A. Über die Richtung und die manifeste Grosse der Pontetialschwankungen in menschlichen Herzen und über den Einfluss der Herzlage auf die Form des Elecktrokardiograms. *Arch Physiol* 1913; 150:275–315.
4. Task Force Report of the American College of Cardiology and the American Heart Association. ACC/AHA Guidelines for Electrocardiography. *Circulation* 1992; 19:473–481.
5. Castellanos A, Myerburg RJ. Electrocardiography. In: Schlant RC, Alexander RW, Lipton MJ, eds. *Diagnostic Atlas of the Heart.* New York: McGraw-Hill; 1996.
6. Sodi-Pallares D, Calder RM. *New Bases of Electrocardiography.* St. Louis: Mosby; 1956:169, 373.
7. Sodi-Pallares D, Medrano GA, Bisteni A, Ponce de Leon JJ. *Deductive and Polyparametric Electrocardiography.* Mexico: Instituto Nacional Cardiologia Mexico; 1970:36,136.
8. Rosenbaum MB, Elizari MV, Lazzari JO. *The Hemiblocks.* Oldsmar, FL: Tampa Tracings; 1970.
9. Lipman BS, Massie E, Kleiger RE. *Clinical Scalar Electrocardiography,* 6th ed. Chicago: Year Book; 1972:210–215.
10. Schamroth L. *The Electrocardiology of Coronary Artery Disease,* 2d ed. Oxford, England: Blackwell, 1984.
11. Marriott HJL. *Practical Electrocardiography,* 8th ed. Baltimore: Williams & Wilkins; 1988.
12. Cabrera E, Gaxiola A. *Teoria y Practica de la Electrocardiografia,* 2d ed. Mexico: La Prensa Medica Mexicana; 1966.
13. Barker JM. *The Unipolar Electrocardiogram: A Clinical Interpretation.* New York: Appleton-Century-Crofts; 1952.
14. Lepeschkin E. *Modern Electrocardiography:* vol 1. *The P-Q-R-S-T-U Complex.* Baltimore: Williams & Wilkins; 1951.
15. Castellanos A, Myerburg RJ. *The Hemiblocks in Myocardial Infarction.* New York: Appleton-Century-Crofts; 1976.
16. Castellanos A Jr, Lemberg L. *A Programmed Introduction to the Electrical Axis and Action Potential.* Oldsmar, FL: Tampa Tracings; 1974:34,114.
17. Wilson FN, MacLeod AG, Barker PS, Johnston FD. The determination and significance of the areas of the ventricular deflections of the electrocardiogram. *Am Heart J* 1934; 10:46–61.
18. Rosenbaum MB, Blanco HH, Elizari MV, Lazzari JO, Vetulli HM. Electronic modulation of ventricular repolarization and cardiac memory. In: Rosenbaum MB, Elizari MV, eds. *Frontiers of Cardiac Electrophysiology.* Boston: Martinus Nijhoff; 1983:67–99.
19. Bayley RH. An interpretation of injury and the ischemic effects of myocardial infarction in accordance with the laws which determine the flow of electric current in homogenous volume conductors and in accordance with relevant pathologic changes. *Am Heart J* 1942; 24:514–528.
20. Bruyneel KJJ. Use of moving epicardial electrodes in defining ST-segment changes after acute coronary occlusion in the baboon: Relation to primary ventricular fibrillation. *Am Heart J* 1975; 89:731–741.
21. Holland RP, Brooks H. TQ-ST segment mapping: Critical review and analysis of current concepts. *Am J Cardiol* 1977; 40:110–129.
22. Janse MJ. Electrophysiology and electrocardiology of acute myocardial ischemia. *Can J Cardiol* 1986; 2(suppl A):46A–52A.

23. Tzivoni D, Chenzbraun A. The significance of ST abnormalities in myocardial infarction. *Cardiol Clin* 1987; 5:419–426.

24. Mills RM, Young E, Gorlin R, Lesch M. Natural history of S-T segment elevation after acute myocardial infarction. *Am J Cardiol* 1975; 35:609–614.

25. Arvan S, Varat MA. Persistent ST-segment elevation and left ventricular wall abnormalities: A 2-dimensional echocardiographic study. *Am J Cardiol* 1984; 53:1542–1546.

26. Wasserburger RH, Alt WJ. The normal RS-T segment elevation variant. *Am J Cardiol* 1961; 8:184–192.

27. Goldberger AL. ST-segment elevation: Normal variants. Benign (functional ST-segment elevation: "early repolarization variant." In: Goldberger AL, ed. *Myocardial Infarction: ECG Differential Diagnosis.* 3d ed. St Louis: Mosby; 1984:1970–1978.

28. Morace G, Padeletti L, Porciani MC, Fantini F. Effect of isoproterenol on the early repolarization syndrome. *Am Heart J* 1979; 97:343–347.

29. Miyazaki T, Mitamura H, Miyoshi S, Soejima K, Aizawa Y, Ogawa S. Autonomic and antiarrhythmic drug modulation of ST segment elevation in patients with Brugada syndrome. *J Am Coll Cardiol* 1996; 27:1061–1070.

30. Brugada P, Brugada J. Right bundle branch block, persistent ST segment elevation and sudden cardiac death: A distinct clinical and electrocardiographic syndrome. *J Am Coll Cardiol* 1992; 20:1391–1396.

31. Barold SS, Falkoff MD, Ong LS, Heinle RA. Significance of transient electrocardiographic Q waves in coronary artery disease. *Cardiol Clin* 1987; 5:367–380.

32. Timmis GC. Electrocardiographic effects of reperfusion. *Cardiol Clin* 1987; 5:427–446.

33. Braunwald E, Kloner RA. The stunned myocardium: Prolonged post-ischemic ventricular dysfunction. *Circulation* 1982; 66:1146–1149.

34. Bashour TT, Kabbani SS, Brewster HP, Wald SH, Hanna ES, Cheng TO. Transient Q waves and reversible cardiac failure during myocardial ischemia: Electrical and mechanical stunning of the heart. *Am Heart J* 1983; 106:780–783.

35. Rahimtoola SH. A perspective on the three large multicenter randomized clinical trials of coronary bypass surgery for chronic stable angina. *Circulation* 1985; 72(suppl 5):123–135.

36. Braunwald E, Rutherford JD. Reversible ischemic left ventricular dysfunction: Evidence for the "hibernating myocardium." *J Am Coll Cardiol* 1986; 8:1467–1470.

37. Dunn MI, Starr SK. False-positive electrocardiographic findings mimicking myocardial infarction. *Am Coll Cardiol Curr J Rev* 1993; Nov/Dec:74–76.

38. Nelson SD, Kou WH, Annesley T, de Buitleir M, Morady F. Significance of ST segment depression during paroxysmal supraventricular tachycardia. *J Am Coll Cardiol* 1988; 12:383–387.

39. Fisch C. Electrocardiography and vectorcardiography. In: Braunwald E, ed. *Heart Disease*, 4th ed. Philadelphia: Saunders; 1992:116–160.

40. Friedberg CK, Zager A. Nonspecific ST and T-wave changes. *Circulation* 1961; 23:655–661.

41. Antzelevitch C, Sicouri S. Clinical relevance of cardiac arrhythmias generated by afterdepolarizations: Role of M cells in the generation of U waves, triggered activity and torsade de pointes. *J Am Coll Cardiol* 1994; 23:259–277.

42. Spodick DH. Q wave infarction versus ST-T infarction: Nonspecificity of electrocardiographic criteria for differentiating transmural and nontransmural lesion. *Am J Cardiol* 1983; 913–915.

43. Gersh B, Rahimtoola SH. *Acute Myocardial Infarction.* New York: Elsevier; 1991:144.

44. Bayes de Luna A. *Clinical Electrocardiography: A Textbook.* Mt Kisco, NY: Futura; 1993:450–459.

45. Califf RM, Mark DB, Wagner GS. *Acute Coronary Care in the Thrombolytic Era.* Chicago: New York Medical Publishers; 1988.

46. Shah PK, Zahger D, Ganz W. Streptokinase in acute myocardial infarction. In: Francis GS, Alpert JS, eds. *Coronary Care*, 2d ed. Boston: Little Brown; 1995:409–442.

47. Fernandez AR, Sequeira RF, Chakko S, Correa LF, de Marchena E, Chahine RA, et al. ST segment tracking for rapid determination of patency of the infarct-related artery in acute myocardial infarction. *J Am Coll Cardiol* 1995; 26:675–683.

48. Goodman S. Q wave and non–q wave myocardial infarction after thrombolysis (letter). *J Am Coll Cardiol* 1996; 27:1817–1819.

49. The Criteria Committee of the New York Heart Association. *Nomenclature and Criteria for Diagnosis of Diseases of the Heart and Great Vessels,* 8th ed. Boston: Little Brown; 1994:107–109.

50. Grant RP. Spatial vector electrocardiography: A method for calculating the spatial electrical vectors of the heart from conventional leads. *Circulation* 1950; 2:676–695.

51. Grant RP, Estes EH Jr. *Spatial Vector Electrocardiography.* New York: Blakiston; 1951.

52. Kracoff OH, Adelman AG, Marquis JF, Caspi A, Aldridge HE, Schwartz L. Twelve-lead electrocardiogram recording during percutaneous transluminal coronary angioplasty: Analysis of reciprocal changes. *J Electrocardiol* 1990; 23:191–198.

53. Wagner GS. *Marriott's Practical Electrocardiography*, 9th ed. Baltimore: Williams & Wilkins; 1994:141.

54. Braat SH, Brugada P, den Dulk K, van Ommen V, Wellens HJJ. Value of lead V_4R for recognition of the infarct coronary artery in acute inferior myocardial infarction. *Am J Cardiol* 1984; 53:1538–1541.

55. Medrano GA, de Micheli A, Osornio A. Interatrial conduction and STa in experimental atrial damage. *J Electrocardiol* 1987; 20:357–363.

56. Liu CK, Greenspan G, Piccirillo RT. Atrial infarction of the heart. *Circulation* 1961; 23:331–338.

57. Castellanos A, Pino IL, Zaman L, Myerburg RJ. Recent advances in the diagnosis of fascicular blocks. *Cardiol Clin* 1987; 5:469–488.

58. Pruitt RD. Experimental bundle branch block: Fifty years ago. *Circulation* 1967; 36:625–627.

59. Pruitt RD, Watt TB Jr. On block of something less than a bundle branch or of something more. *Circulation* 1971; 43:775–777.

60. Rothberger CJ, Winterberg H. Experimentelle Beitrage zur Kenntnis der Reizleitungstorungen in den Kammern des Saugetierherzens. *Ges Exp Med* 1917; 5:264–284.

61. Watt TB Jr, Pruitt RD. Electrocardiographic findings associated with experimental arborization block in dogs. *Am Heart J* 1965; 69:642–654.

62. Watt TB Jr, Pruitt RD. Left posterior fascicular block in canine and primate hearts: An electrocardiographic study. *Circulation* 1969; 40:677–685.

63. Wilson FN, Johnston FD, Barker PS. Electrocardiograms of an unusual type in right bundle branch block. *Am Heart J* 1934; 9:472–479.

64. Davies MJ. *Pathology of Conducting Tissue of the Heart.* New York: Appleton-Century-Crofts; 1971.

65. Demoulin JC, Kulbertus HE. Histopathological examination of concept of left hemiblock. *Br Heart J* 1972; 34:807–814.

66. Grant RP. Left axis deviation: An electrocardiographic-pathologic correlation study. *Circulation* 1956; 14:233–249.

67. Kulbertus HE. Concept of left hemiblocks revisited: A histopathological and experimental study. *Adv Cardiol* 1975; 14:126–135.

68. Lenegre J. Contribution a l'etude des blocs de branch important notament les contortations electriques et histologiques. *Arch Mal Coeur* 1957; 50(suppl 1):50–63.

69. Massing GK, James TN. Anatomical configuration of the His bundle and bundle branches in the human heart. *Circulation* 1976; 53:609–621.

70. Rosenbaum MB, Elizari MV, Lazzari JO. *Los Hemibloqueos.* Buenos Aires: Ed Paidos, 1968.

71. Tawara S. Variations in the left bundle system. *Circulation* 1970; 41:782.

72. Uhley HM. Some controversy regarding the peripheral distribution of the conduction system. *Am J Cardiol* 1972; 30:919–920.

73. Uhley HN. The quadrifascicular nature of the peripheral conduction system. In: Dreifus LS, Likoff W, eds. *Cardiac Arrhythmias.* New York: Grune & Stratton; 1973:339–348.

74. Rosenbaum MB, Corrado G, Oliveri R, Castellanos A, Elizari MV. Right bundle branch block with left anterior hemiblock surgically induced in tetralogy of Fallot. *Am J Cardiol* 1970; 26:12–19.

75. Dodge HT, Grant RP. Mechanisms of QRS complex prolongation in man: Right ventricular conduction defects. *Am J Med* 1956; 21:534–550.

76. Cohen SI, Lau SH, Stein E, Young MW, Damato AN. Variations of aberrant ventricular conduction in man: Evidence of isolated and combined block within the specialized conduction system. *Circulation* 1968; 38:899–916.

77. Milliken JA. Isolated and complicated left anterior fascicular block: A review of suggested electrocardiographic criteria. *J Electrocardiol* 1983; 16:199–211.

78. Warner RA, Hill NE, Mookerjee S, Smucyan H. Improved electrocardiographic criteria for the diagnosis of left anterior hemiblock. *Am J Cardiol* 1983; 51:723–726.

79. Rosenbaum MB, Elizari MV, Lazzari JO, Nau GJ, Halpern MS, Levi RJ. The differential electrocardiographic manifestations of hemiblocks, bilateral bundle branch blocks and trifascicular blocks. In: Schlant RC, Hurst JW, eds. *Advances in Electrocardiography*. New York: Grune & Stratton; 1972:145–182.

80. Rosenbaum MB, Elizari MV, Lazzari JO, Kretz A, Darvos HO. The clinical causes and mechanisms of intraventricular conduction disturbances. In: Schlant RC, Hurst JW, eds. *Advances in Electrocardiography*. New York: Grune & Stratton; 1972:183–220.

81. Grant RP. Peri-infarction block. *Prog Cardiovasc Dis* 1959; 27:237–247.

82. Oppenheimer BS, Rothschild MA. Electrocardiographic changes associated with myocardial involvement: With special reference to prognosis. *JAMA* 1917; 69:429–431.

83. Castle CH, Keane WM. Electrocardiographic "peri-infarction block": A clinical and pathologic correlation. *Circulation* 1965; 31:403–408.

84. Cotne RA, Parkin TW, Brandenburg RO, Brown AL Jr. Peri-infarction block: Postmyocardial-infarction intraventricular conduction disturbance. *Am Heart J* 1965; 69:150–153.

85. First SR, Bayley RH, Bedford DR. Peri-infarction block. *Circulation* 1950; 2:31–36.

86. Wilson FN, Herrmann GR: Bundle branch block and arborization block. *Arch Intern Med* 1920; 26:153–191.

87. Wilson FN, Hill IGW, Johnston FD. The form of electrocardiogram in experimental myocardial infarction: III. The later effects produced by ligation of the anterior descending branch of the left coronary artery. *Am Heart J* 1935; 10:903–915.

88. Castellanos A Jr. Diagnosis of left anterior hemiblock and left posterior hemiblock in the presence of inferior wall myocardial infarction. *Bull NY Acad Med* 1971; 47:923–930.

89. Jacobson LB, Scheinman M. Catheter-induced intra-Hisian and intrafascicular block during recording of His bundle electrograms: A report of two cases. *Circulation* 1974; 49:579–584.

90. Luck JC, Engel TR. Transient right bundle branch block with "Swan-Ganz" catheterization. *Am Heart J* 1976; 92:263–264.

91. Narula OS. Longitudinal dissociation in the His bundle: Bundle branch block due to asynchronous conduction within the His bundle in man. *Circulation* 1977; 56:996–1006.

92. El-Sherif N, Amat-y-Leon F, Schonfield C, Scherlag BJ, Rosen K, Lazzara R, et al. Normalization of bundle branch block patterns by distal His bundle pacing: Clinical experimental evidence of longitudinal dissociation in the pathologic His bundle. *Circulation* 1978; 57:473–483.

93. Scherlag BJ, El-Sherif N, Hope RR, Lazzara R. The significance of dissociation of conduction in the canine His bundle: Electrophysiological studies in vivo and in vitro. *J Electrocardiol* 1978; 4:343–354.

94. Scherlag BJ, El-Sherif N, Lazzara R. Bundle branch block due to His bundle lesions (abstr). *Am J Cardiol* 1974; 33:169.

95. Nakaya Y, Hiasa Y, Murayama L, Lleda S, Nagao T, Niki T, et al. Prominent anterior QRS forces as a manifestation of left septal fascicular block. *J Electrocardiol* 1978; 11:39–46.

96. Gambetta M, Childers RW. Rate-dependent right precordial Q waves. "Septal focal block." *Am J Cardiol* 1973; 32:196–201.

97. Dhala A, Gonzalez-Zuelgaray J, Deshpande S, Blanck Z, Biehl M, Sra J, et al. Unmasking the trifascicular left intraventricular conduction system by ablation of the right bundle branch. *Am J Cardiol* 1996; 77:706–712.

98. Wilson FN, Herrmann GR. An experimental study of incomplete bundle branch block and of the refractory period of the heart of the dog. In: Johnston FD, Lepeschkin E, eds. *Selected Papers of Dr. Frank N. Wilson*. Ann Arbor, MI: Edwards Brothers; 1954:749–810.

99. Sodi-Pallares D, Bisteni A, Medrano GA. *Electrocardiografia y Vectorcardiografia Deductivas*. Mexico City: La Prensa Medica Mexicana, 1964:419.

100. Barker JM, Valencia F. The precordial electrocardiogram in incomplete right bundle branch block. In: Johnston FD, Lepeschkin E, eds. *Selected Papers of Dr. Frank N. Wilson*. Ann Arbor, MI: Edwards Brothers, 1954:884–914.

101. Grishman A, Scherlis L. *Spatial Vectorcardiography*. Philadelphia: Saunders; 1952:107.

102. Kossman CE, Berger AR, Rader B, Brumlik J, Briller SA, Donnelly JH. Intracardiac and intravascular potentials resulting from electrical activity of the normal human heart. *Circulation* 1950; 2:10–30.

103. Blount SG, Munyan EA Jr, Hoffman MS. Hypertrophy of the right ventricular outflow tract: A concept of the electrocardiographic findings in atrial septal defect. *Am J Med* 1957; 22:784–790.

104. Cabrera E, Gaxiola A. A critical re-evaluation of systolic and diastolic overloading patterns. *Prog Cardiovasc Dis* 1959; 2:219–236.

105. Moore EN, Hoffman BF, Patterson DF, Stuckey JH. Electrocardiographic changes due to delayed activation of the wall of the right ventricle. *Am Heart J* 1964; 68:347–361.

106. Fahr G. Some fundamental principles of electrocardiography. *Arch Intern Med* 1921; 26:126–130.

107. Punja MM, Schneebaum R, Cohen J. Bifascicular block induced by hyperkalemia. *J Electrocardiol* 1973; 6:71–75.

108. Sung RJ, Tamer DM, Agha AS, Castellanos A, Myerburg RJ, Gelband H. Etiology of the electrocardiographic pattern of "incomplete right bundle branch block" in atrial septal defect: An electrophysiologic study. *J Pediatr* 1975; 87:1182–1186.

109. Castellanos A, Ramirez AV, Mayorga-Cortes A, Pefkaros K, Rozanski JJ, Sprung C, et al. Left fascicular blocks during right-heart catheterization using the Swan-Ganz catheter. *Circulation* 1981; 64:1271–1276.

110. Pickoff AS, Wolff GS, Tamer D, Gelband H. Arrhythmias and conduction system disturbances in infants and children—Recent advances and contributions of intracardiac electrophysiology. In: Castellanos A, Brest AN, eds. *Cardiac Arrhythmia—Mechanisms and Management. Cardiovasc Clin* 1980; 11:203–219.

111. Garcia OL, Castellanos A, Sung RJ, Gelband H. Exposure of concealed right bundle branch block in Wolff-Parkinson-White type B by pacing from the vicinity of the A-V node. *Am Heart J* 1978; 96:662–668.

112. Sgarbossa EB. Recent advances in the electrocardiographic diagnosis of myocardiol infarction: Left bundle branch block and pacing. *PACE*. In press.

113. Sodeman WA, Johnston FD, Wilson FN. The Q1 deflection of the electrocardiogram in bundle branch block and axis deviation. *Am Heart J* 1944; 28:271–286.

114. Kindwall KE, Brown JP, Josephson ME. Predictive accuracy of criteria for chronic myocardial infarction in pacing-induced left bundle branch block. *Am J Cardiol* 1986; 57:1255–1260.

115. Wackers FJT. The diagnosis of myocardial infarction in the presence of left bundle branch block. *Cardiol Clin* 1987; 5:393–401.

116. Wolff L, Parkinson J, White PD. Bundle-branch block with short P-R interval in healthy young people prone to paroxysmal tachycardia. *Am Heart J* 1930; 5:685–704.

117. Castillo CA, Castellanos A Jr. His bundle recordings in patients with reciprocating tachycardias and Wolff-Parkinson-White syndrome. *Circulation* 1970; 42:271–285.

118. Rosenbaum FF, Hecht HH, Wilson FN, Johnston FD. The potential variations of the thorax and esophagus in anomalous atrioventricular excitation (Wolff-Parkinson-White syndrome). *Am Heart J* 1945; 29:281–326.

119. Wallace AG, Sealy WC, Gallagher JJ, Kasell J. Ventricular excitation in Wolff-Parkinson-White syndrome. In: Wellens HJJ, Lie KI, Janse MJ, eds. *The Conduction System of the Heart: Structure, Function and Clinical Implications*. Leiden: HE Stenfert Kroese BV; 1976:613–630.

120. Befeler B, Castellanos A, Castillo CA, Agha AS, Vagueiro MC, Myerburg RJ. Arrival of excitation at the right ventricular apical endocardium in Wolff-Parkinson-White syndrome type B. *Circulation* 1973; 48:655–660.

121. Castillo CA, Castellanos A Jr, Befeler B, Myerburg RJ, Agha AS, Vagueiro MC. Arrival of excitation at right ventricular apical endocardium in Wolff-Parkinson-White syndrome type A, with and without right bundle branch block. *Br Heart J* 1973; 35:594–600.

122. Castellanos A, Agha AS, Portillo B, Myerburg RJ. Usefulness of vectorcardiography combined with His bundle recordings and cardiac pacing in evaluation of the pre-excitation (Wolff-Parkinson-White) syndrome. *Am J Cardiol* 1972; 30:623–628.

123. Wellens HJJ: Contribution of cardiac pacing to our understanding of the Wolff-Parkinson-White syndrome. *Br Heart J* 1975; 37:231–241.

124. Gallagher JJ, Sealy WC, Kasell J, Wallace AG. Multiple accessory pathways in patients with the pre-excitation syndrome. *Circulation* 1976; 54:571–591.

125. Milstein S, Sharma AD, Guiraudon GM, Klein GJ. An algorithm for the electrocardiographic localization of accessory pathways in the Wolff-Parkinson-White syndrome. *PACE* 1987; 10:555–563.

126. Gallagher JJ, Smith WM, Kasell JH, Benson DW Jr, Sterba R, Grant AO. Role of Mahaim fibers in cardiac arrhythmias in man. *Circulation* 1971; 64:176–189.

127. Chiang CE, Chen SA, Teo WS, Tsai DS, Wu TJ, Cheng CC, et al. An accurate stepwise electrocardiographic algorithm for localization of accessory pathways in patients with Wolff-Parkinson-White syndrome from a comprehensive analysis of delta waves and r/s ratio during sinus rhythm. *Am J Cardiol* 1995; 76:40–46.

128. Murdock CJ, Leitch JW, Klein GJ, Guiraudon GM, Yec R, Teo WS: Epicardial mapping in patients with "nodoventricular" accessory pathways. *Am J Cardiol* 1991; 68:208–214.

129. Castellanos A Jr, Ortiz JM, Pastis N, Castillo CA. The electrocardiogram in patients with pacemakers. *Prog Cardiovasc Dis* 1970; 13:190–209.

130. Castellanos A Jr, Lemberg L, Salhanick L, Berkovits BV. Pacemaker vectorcardiography. *Am Heart J* 1968; 75:6–18.

131. Munuswamy K, Alpert MA, Martin RH, Whiting RB, Mechlin NJ. Sensitivity and specificity of commonly used electrocardiographic criteria for left atrial enlargement determined by M-mode echocardiography. *Am J Cardiol* 1984; 53:829–832.

132. Josephson ME, ed. *Clinical Cardiac Electrophysiology: Techniques and Interpretations.* 2d ed. Philadelphia: Lea & Febiger; 1993.

133. Surawicz B. Electrocardiographic diagnosis of chamber enlargement. *J Am Coll Cardiol* 1986; 8:711–724.

134. Reichet N, Devereaux RB. Left ventricular hypertrophy: Relationship of anatomic echocardiographic and electrocardiographic findings. *Circulation* 1981; 63:1391–1398.

135. Bommer K, Weinert L, Neumann A, Nief J, Mason DT, De Marias A. Determinations of right atrial and right ventricular size by two-dimensional echocardiography. *Circulation* 1980; 60:91–100.

136. Doxandabaratz J, Fort de Ribot R, Trilla E, Bayes de Luna A, Bosch I, Turull J, et al. Miocardiopatia hipertrofica apical. *Rev Latina Cardiol* 1982; 3:35–41.

137. Romhilt D, Estes E. A point score system for the ECG diagnosis of left ventricular hypertrophy. *Am Heart J* 1968; 75:752–758.

138. Casale PN, Devereaux R, Alonso D, Campo M, Khofiled P. Autopsy validation of improved ECG criteria of left ventricular hypertrophy (abstr.) *J Am Coll Cardiol* 1985; 5:511.

139. Talbot S, Kilpatrick D. Diagnostic criteria for left ventricular hypertrophy. In: McFarlane PW, ed. *Progress in Electrocardiology.* London: Pittman Medical; 1979:534–541.

140. Koito H, Spodick D. Electrocardiographic RV_6/RV_1 voltage ratio for diagnosis of left ventricular hypertrophy. *Am J Cardiol* 1989; 63:352–361.

141. Hernandez Padial L. Usefulness of total 12-lead QRS voltage for determining the presence of left ventricular hypertrophy in systemic hypertension. *Am J Cardiol* 1991; 68:261–262.

142. Kafka H, Burggraf GW, Milliken JA. Electrocardiographic diagnosis of left ventricular hypertrophy in the presence of left bundle branch block: An echocardiographic study. *Am J Cardiol* 1985; 55:103–106.

143. Gertsch M, Theler A, Foglia E. Electrocardiographic detection of left ventricular hypertrophy in the presence of left anterior fascicular block. *Am J Cardiol* 1988; 61:1089–1101.

144. Vander Ark CR, Ballantyne F III, Reynolds EW Jr. Electrolytes and the electrocardiogram. *Cardiovasc Clin* 1973; 5:269–294.

145. Levine HD, Wanzer SH, Merrill JP. Dialyzable currents of injury in potassium intoxication resembling acute myocardial infarction or pericarditis. *Circulation* 1956; 13:29–36.

146. Mosseri M, Porath A, Ovsyshcher I, Stone D. Electrocardiographic manifestations of combined hypercalcemia and hypermagnesemia. *J Electrocardiol* 1990; 23:235–241.

147. Kulick DL, Hong R, Ryzen E, Rude RK, Rubin JN, Elkayam U, et al. Electrophysiologic effects of intravenous magnesium in patients with normal conduction systems and no clinical evidence of significant cardiac disease. *Am Heart J* 1988; 148:367–373.

148. Tzivoni D, Keren A, Cohen AM, Loebel H, Zahavi I, Chenzbraun A, et al. Magnesium therapy for torsades de pointes. *Am J Cardiol* 1984; 53:528–530.

149. Kligfield P, Lax KG, Okin PM. QT_c behavior during treadmill exercise as a function of the underlying QT-heart rate relationship. *J Electrocardiol* 1996; 206–210.

150. Schwartz PJ, Locati EH, Napolitano C, Priori SG. The long QT syndrome. In: Zipes DP, Jalife E, eds. *Cardiac Electrophysiology: From Cell to Bedside,* 2d ed. 1995:788–811.

151. Hashiba K, Moss AJ, Schwartz PJ, eds. QT prolongation and ventricular arrhythmias. *Ann NY Acad Sci* 1992, 644:1–247.

152. Osborn JJ. Experimental hypothermia: Respiratory and blood pH changes in relation to cardiac function. *Am J Physiol* 1953; 175:389–398.

153. Santos EM, Kittle CF. Electrocardiographic changes in the dog during hypothermia. *Am Heart J* 1958; 55:415–420.

154. Castellanos A, Saoudi NC, Schwartz A, Sodi-Pallares D. Electrocardiographic patterns resulting from improper connections of the right leg (ground) cable. *PACE* 1985; 8:364–368.

155. Simonson E. *Differentiation between Normal and Abnormal in Electrocardiography.* St Louis: Mosby; 1961:262.

156. Kerwin AJ, McLean R, Tegelaar H. A method for the accurate placement of chest electrodes in the taking of serial electrocardiographic tracings. *Can Med Assoc J* 1960; 82:258–261.

157. Garson A Jr. Clinically significant differences between the "old" analog and the "new" digital electrocardiograms. *Am Heart J* 1987; 114:194–197.

158. Tenth Bethesda Conference of the American College of Cardiology: Optimal electrocardiography. *Am J Cardiol* 1978; 41:111–191.

159. Seventeenth Bethesda Conference of the American College of Cardiology: Adult cardiology training. *J Am Coll Cardiol* 1986; 7:1192–1218.

160. AHA. Recommendations for standardization of leads and of specifications for instruments in electrocardiography and vectorcardiography: Report of the Committee on Electrocardiography, American Heart Association. *Circulation* 1975; 52:11–31.

161. Bailey JJ, Berson AS, Garson A Jr, Horan LG, Macfarlane PW, Mortara DW, et al. Recommendations for standardization and specifications in automated electrocardiography: Bandwith and digital signal processing. A report for health professionals by an ad hoc writing group of the Committee on Electrocardiography and Cardiac Electrophysiology of the Council on Clinical Cardiology, American Heart Association. *Circulation* 1990; 81:730–739.

162. Taback L, Marden E, Mason HL, Pipberger HV. Digital recording of electrocardiographic data for analysis by a digital computer. *IRE Trans Med Elect* 1959; 6:167–171.

163. Pipberger HV, Cornfeld J. What ECG computer program to choose for clinical application: The need for consumer protection. *Circulation* 1973; 47:918–920.

164. Laks MM, Ginzton L. Computerized electrocardiographic interpretation—A practical adjunct to the electrocardiographer. *Pract Cardiol* 1979; 5:127–144.

165. Proceedings of the Engineering Foundation Conference "Computerized interpretation of the electrocardiogram XII." *J Electrocardiol* 1987; 20(suppl):preface.

166. Spodick DH, Bishop RL. Computer treason: Intraobserver variability of an electrocardiographic computer system. *Am J Cardiol* 1997; 80:102–103.

167. Wilson FN, Johnston FD. The vectorcardiogram. *Am Heart J* 1938; 16:14–28.

168. Mann H. A method of analyzing the electrocardiogram. *Arch Intern Med* 1920; 25:238–294.

169. Lemberg L, Castellanos A Jr. *Vectorcardiography,* 2d ed. New York: Appleton-Century-Crofts; 1975.

170. Massie E, Walsh TJ. *Clinical Vectorcardiography and Electrocardiography.* Chicago: Year Book; 1960.

171. Chou TC, Helm RA, Kaplan S. *Clinical Vectorcardiography,* 2d ed. New York: Grune & Stratton; 1974.

172. Frank E. An accurate, clinically practical system for spatial vectorcardiography. *Circulation* 1956; 13:737–749.

13

THE CHEST ROENTGENOGRAM AND CARDIAC FLUOROSCOPY

James T. T. Chen

On November 8, 1895, Wilhelm Conrad Röntgen discovered x-rays[1] and ushered in the new era of diagnostic roentgenology. With wavelengths only 1/10,000 those of visible light, x-rays can penetrate the human body to produce roentgenograms, thereby revolutionizing the field of medical diagnosis. Chest roentgenography in particular has since become a routine part of medical workup because of the invaluable information it can provide.

Familiarity with the altered anatomy and understanding of the underlying pathophysiology of a diseased heart are the keys to appropriate interpretation of its roentgen manifestations. The conventional four-view cardiac series is tabulated in Table 13 1 and the views are illustrated in Fig. 13-1C, D, E, and F.

The approach to the chest roentgenogram (film, radiograph, or x-ray) should be thorough and objective so that no clue is overlooked and no bias is incorporated in the process of radiographic analysis.[2-5] Rib notching (Fig. 13-1A and B), for example, offers important clues to the diagnosis of coarctation of the aorta.[4,6] To prevent occasional erroneous clinical information from misleading the radiographic interpretation, films should at first be read without any knowledge about the patient. A patient may be referred, for instance, because of "bronchial asthma" refractory to therapy, only to be found later to suffer from cardiac asthma due to critical mitral stenosis. In this case, the classical radiographic manifestations of severe mitral stenosis should help clarify the confusion and prompt the change in patient management.

On other occasions, a secundum atrial septal defect may be misinterpreted as mitral stenosis because of similar physical signs. The split-second sound may be misinterpreted as the opening snap. The diastolic rumble due to increased flow through a normal tricuspid valve may mimic the diastolic murmur of mitral stenosis. The x-ray signs of the two entities, however, are quite different (Figs. 13-2B versus 13-3A).

The final radiologic conclusion, however, should be drawn only after correlating the x-ray findings with clinical information and other laboratory parameters.

ROENTGENOGRAPHIC EXAMINATION FOR ANATOMY

An Overview

The first step is to survey the roentgenogram and look at the entire situation, searching particularly for noncardiac conditions that may reflect heart disease. For instance, a right-sided stomach with an absent image of the inferior vena cava may suggest the possibility of congenital interruption of the inferior vena cava with azygos continuation[7,8] (Fig. 13-4). A narrowed anteroposterior diameter of the thorax may be the cause of an innocent murmur (Fig. 13-5).[9]

Pulmonary Vasculature

The lung may be likened to a mirror that faithfully reflects the underlying pathophysiology of the heart. By careful evaluation of the pulmonary vasculature, one may narrow down the diagnostic possibilities to a manageable level. For example, if uniform dilation of all pulmonary vessels is present, the diagnosis of a left-to-right shunt (Fig. 13-2B) is more likely

TABLE 13-1

CONVENTIONAL FOUR-VIEW CARDIAC SERIES

Posteroanterior (PA) view	With barium
Left lateral (lateral) view	With barium
45° Right anterior oblique (RAO) view	With barium
60° Left anterior oblique (LAO) view	Without barium

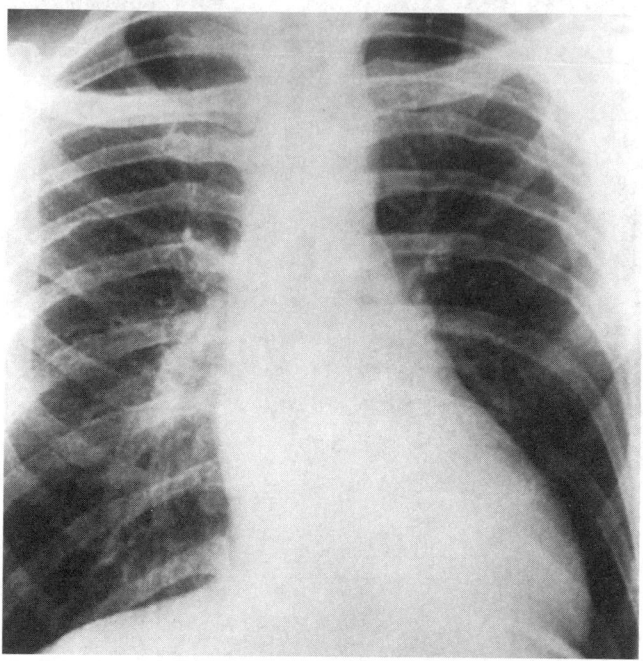

A

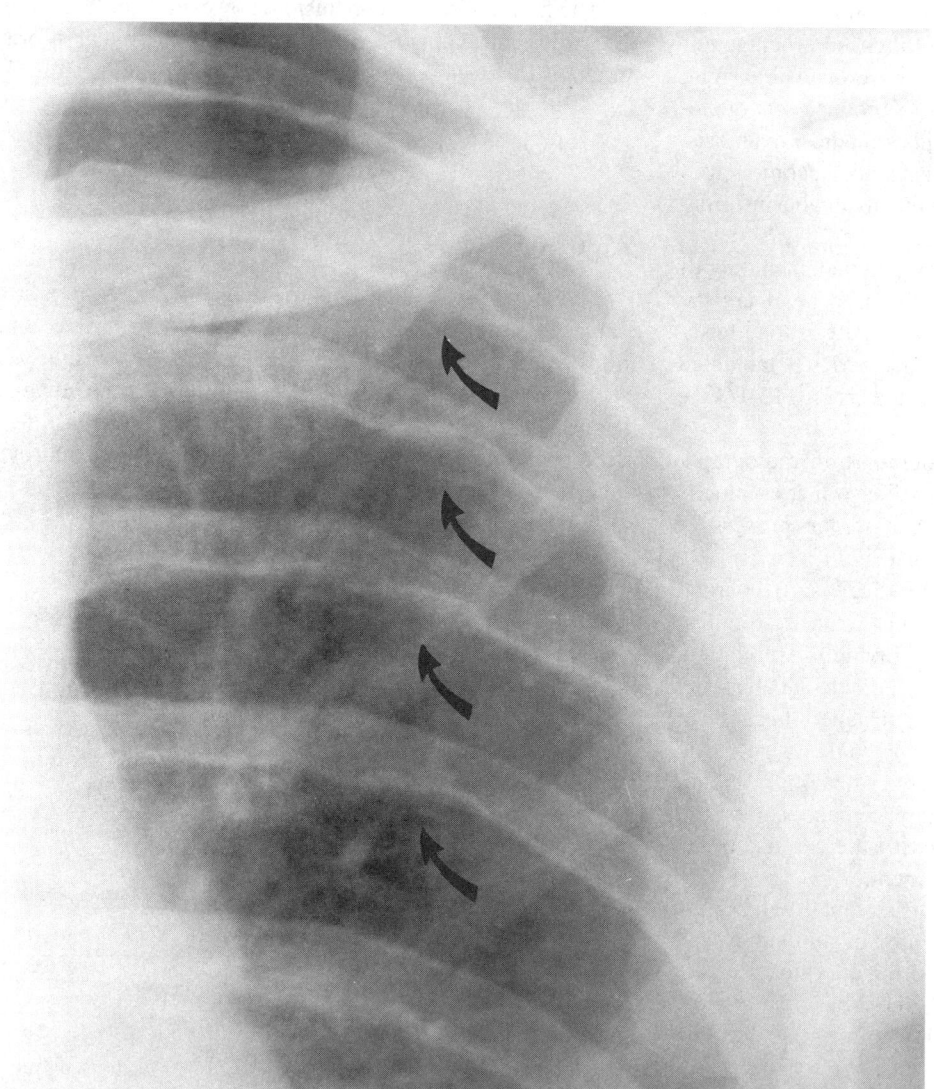

B

FIGURE 13-1

Practical application of four-view cardiac series. *A.* Posteroanterior view in a patient with coarctation of the aorta showing areas of rib notching bilaterally and left ventricular enlargement in the inferior and leftward direction. *B.* Magnified view of the left upper thorax of the same patient showing multiple areas of rib notching (*arrows*). The sclerotic margin of each represents a reparative process by which new bone is laid down in the defect.

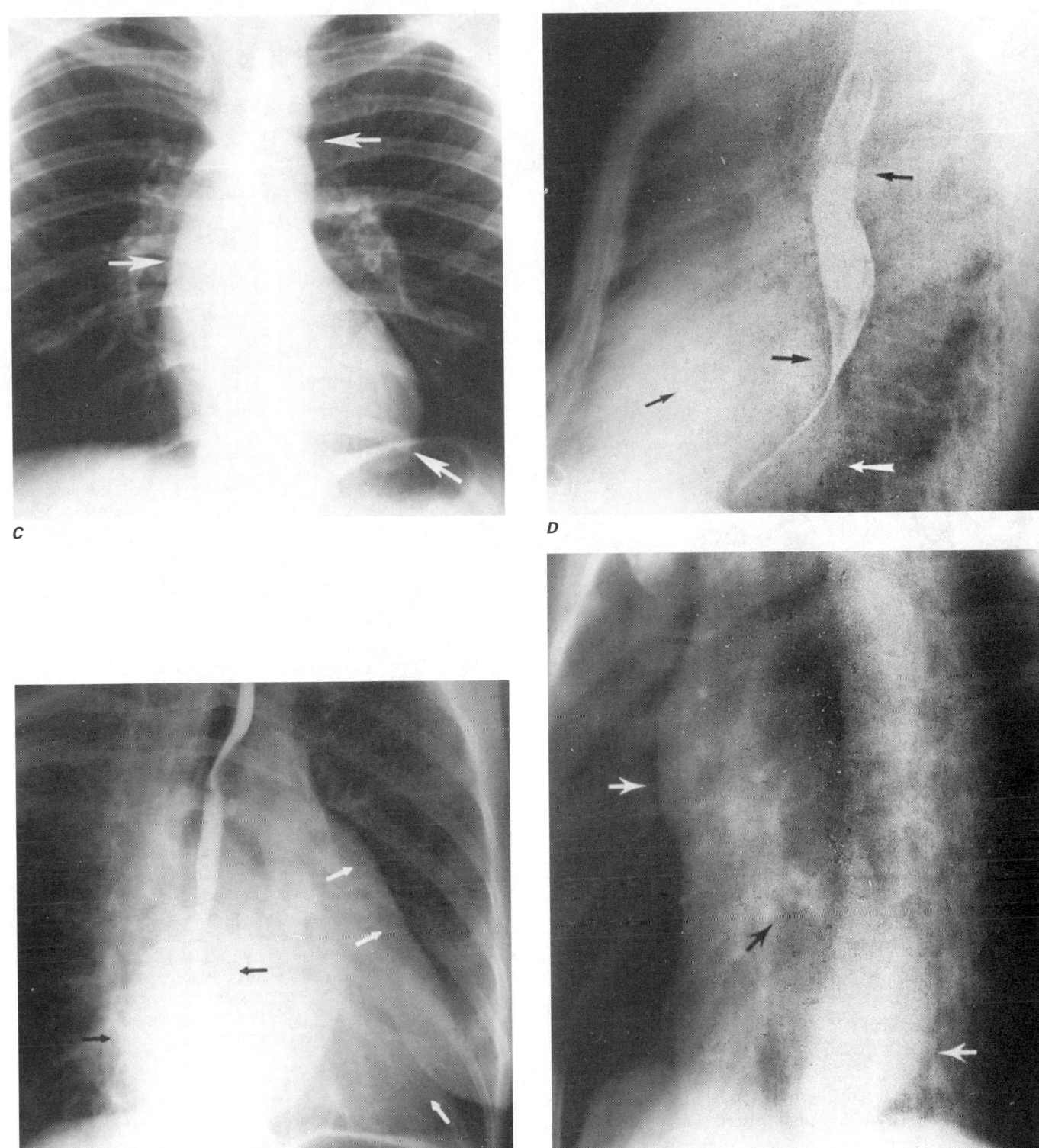

C

D

E

F

FIGURE 13-1 (*Continued*)

C. Posteroanterior view of another patient with aortic coarctation showing "3" sign of the deformed descending aorta and "E" sign on the barium-filled esophagus. The upper arrow (on the patient's left) points to the level of coarctation. The lower arrow (on the patient's left) marks the apex of the enlarged left ventricle. The arrow on the patient's right indicates the dilated ascending aorta. D. Lateral view of a third patient with same disease showing barium-filled esophagus to be pushed forward (*upper arrow*) by the poststenotic dilatation of the descending aorta and pushed backward (*middle arrow*) by the enlarged left atrium. The very large left ventricle (*lower arrow*) simply casts a shadow behind the esophagus without displacing it. The oblique arrow points to the calcified stenotic bicuspid aortic valve. E. Right anterior oblique view of same patient whose posteroanterior view is shown in Fig. 13-7D. Note the huge right atrium casting a triangular density (*lower horizontal arrow*) behind the esophagus without displacing it. The esophagus is deviated posteriorly by the enlarged left atrium (*upper horizontal arrow*). The upper oblique arrows indicate the direction of the enlarging pulmonary trunk and right ventricle. The lower oblique arrow points to the normal left ventricle with the undisturbed left costophrenic sulcus. F. Left anterior oblique view of patient with valvular aortic stenosis. The dilated ascending aorta (*upper white arrow*) is immediately above the flat anterior border of normal right ventricle. The black arrow points to the calcified aortic valve. The lower white arrow marks the enlarged left ventricle.

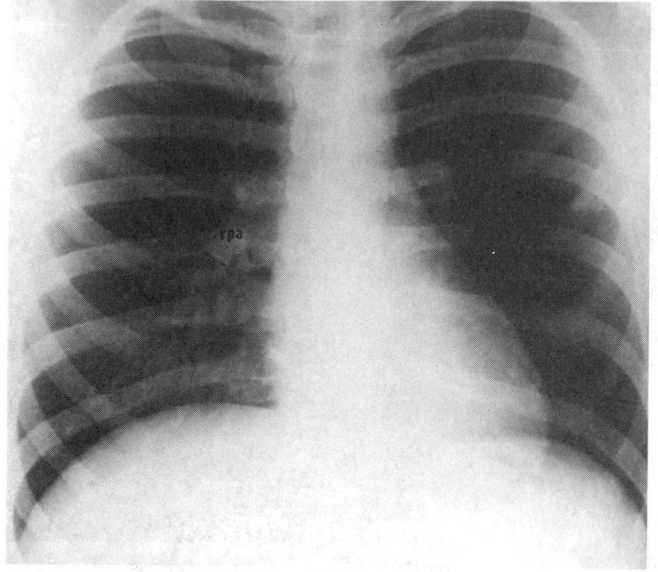

A

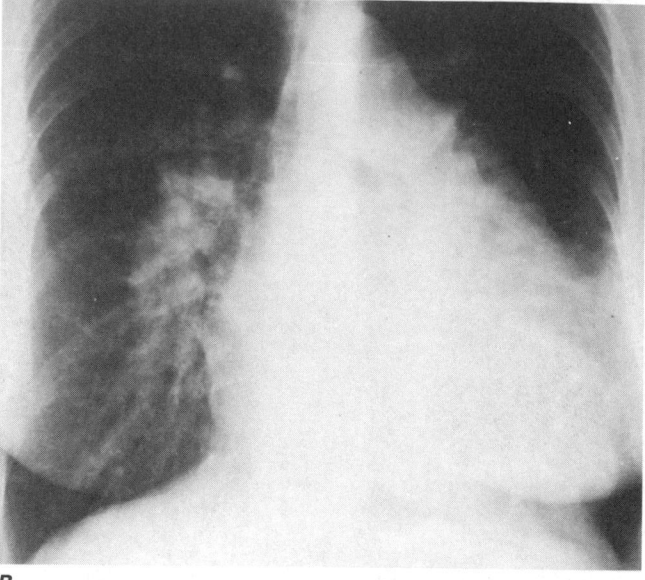

B

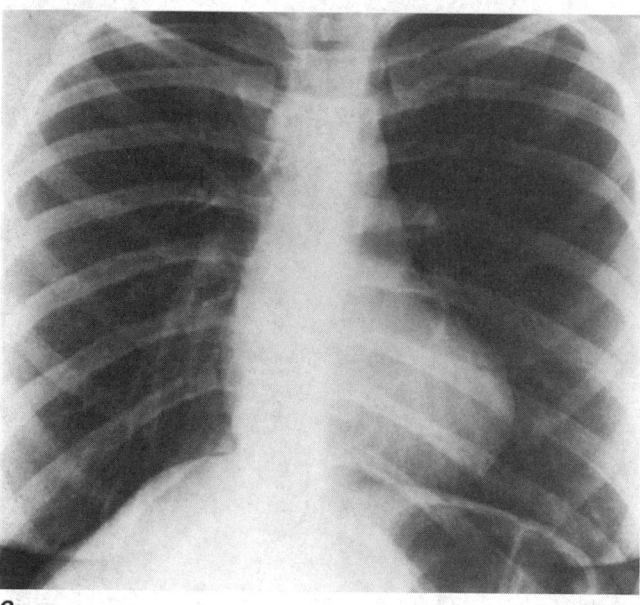

C

FIGURE 13-2

Roentgenographic assessment of the volume of pulmonary blood flow. *A*. Normal: There is caudalization of the pulmonary vascularity due to gravity. The right descending pulmonary artery (rpa) measures 13 mm in diameter in this young man. *B*. Increased: Patient with a secundum atrial septal defect showing uniform increase in pulmonary vascularity bilaterally. The right descending pulmonary artery is markedly enlarged, measuring 27 mm. *C*. Decreased: Patient with tetralogy of Fallot showing a boot-shaped heart and uniform decrease in pulmonary vascularity. The right descending pulmonary artery is markedly decreased, measuring 6 mm.

than a left-sided obstructive lesion. The latter typically shows a cephalic pulmonary blood-flow pattern (Fig. 13-3*A*). More detailed analysis of the pulmonary vascularity will be discussed separately below.

Lung Parenchyma

With right heart failure, the lungs become unusually radiolucent because of decreased pulmonary blood flow (PBF). On the other hand, significant failure on the left side of the heart is characterized by the presence of pulmonary edema and/ or a cephalic blood-flow pattern (Fig. 13-6). Long-standing, severe pulmonary venous hypertension may lead to hemosiderosis and/or ossification of the lung.[10] When right-sided heart failure results from severe left-sided heart failure, the preexisting pulmonary congestion may improve because of the decreased pulmonary blood flow (Fig. 13-6*B*).

Cardiac Size

A significantly enlarged heart is always abnormal; however, mild cardiomegaly may reflect a higher than average cardiac output from a normal heart, as seen in athletes in active training. The cardiothoracic ratio remains the simplest and the most practical yardstick for the assessment of cardiac size.[2] The mean value for adults in upright position in the posteroanterior (PA) view is 44 percent. More accurate roentgen measurements of cardiac size have been well documented[11,12] but are beyond the scope of the present discussion.

The nature of cardiomegaly can usually be determined by the specific roentgen appearance. As a rule, when the PBF pattern remains normal, cardiac lesions with volume overload tend to present a greater degree of cardiomegaly than lesions with pressure overload alone. For example, patients with aortic

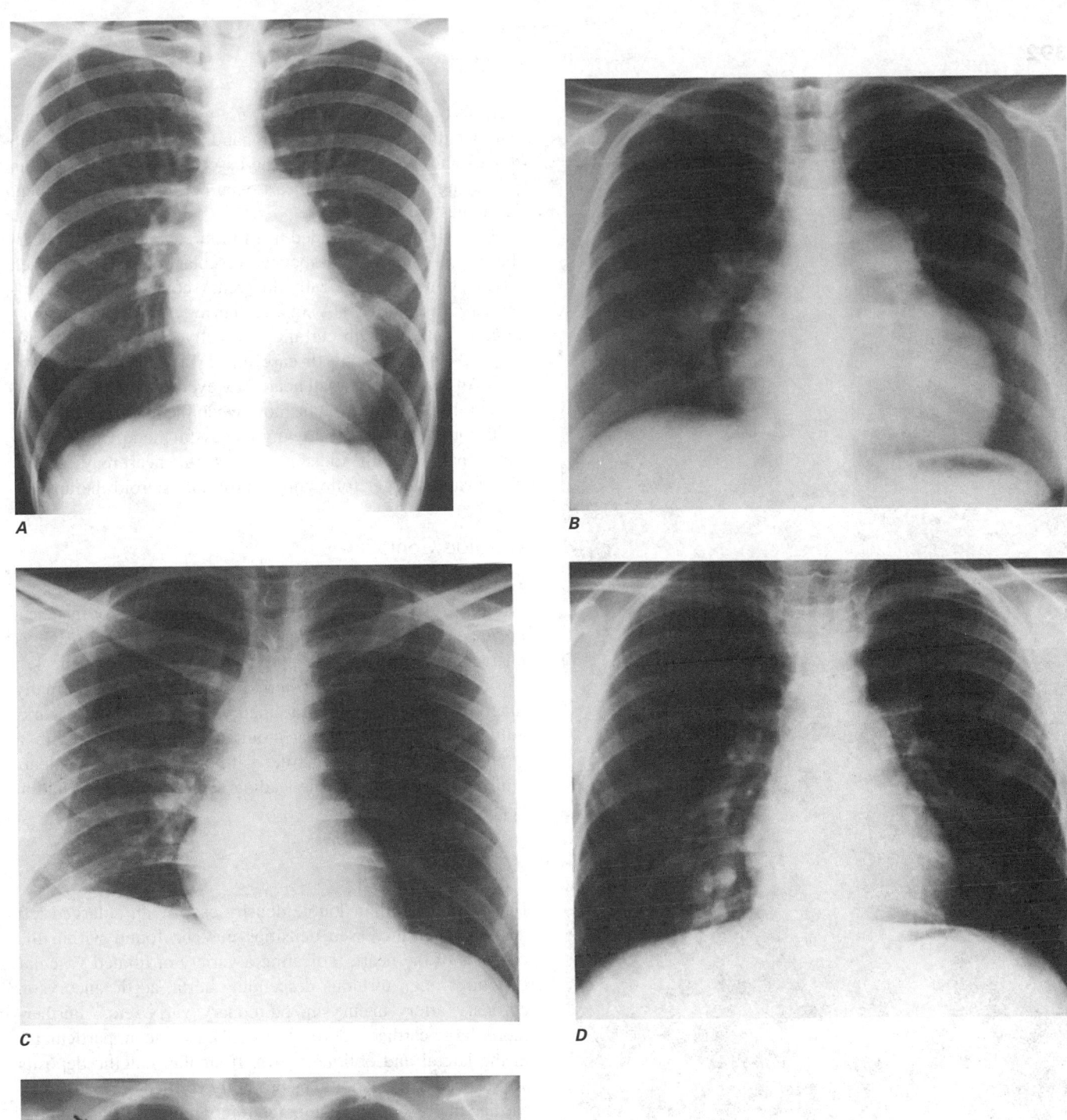

FIGURE 13-3

Abnormal pulmonary blood flow patterns. *A.* Cephalization: Patient with severe mitral stenosis showing dilatation of the upper vessels with constriction of the lower vessels. *B.* Centralization: Patient with primary pulmonary hypertension showing marked dilatation of the pulmonary trunk and the central segments of both pulmonary arteries with pruning of the peripheral branches. *C.* Lateralization: Patient with massive pulmonary embolism obstructing the left main pulmonary artery. Note the uneven distribution of pulmonary blood flow between the two lungs in favor of the right. *D.* Localization: A cyanotic child showing localized vascular changes representing a large pulmonary arteriovenous fistula in the right lower lobe. *E.* Collateralization: A child with pseudotruncus arteriosus with cardiomegaly and a right aortic arch (*small arrow*). Note severe pulmonary oligemia with numerous small tortuous vessels (*large arrow*) in upper medial lung zones, representing bronchial arterial collaterals.

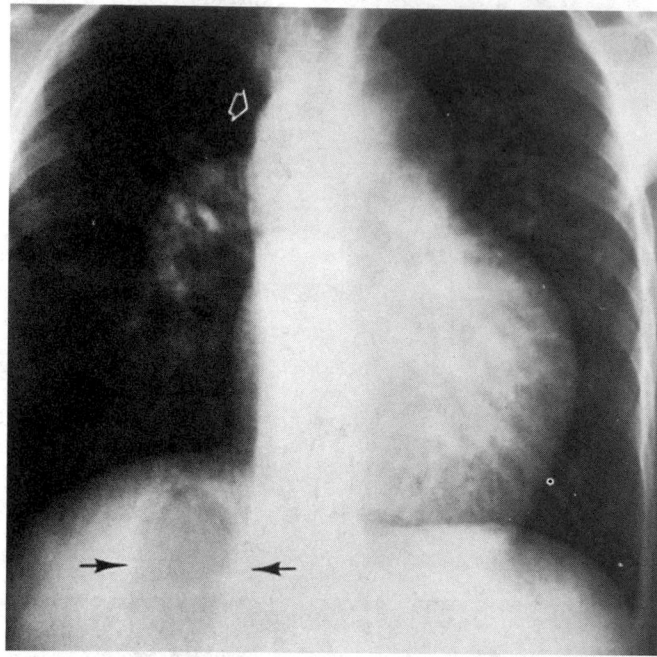

A

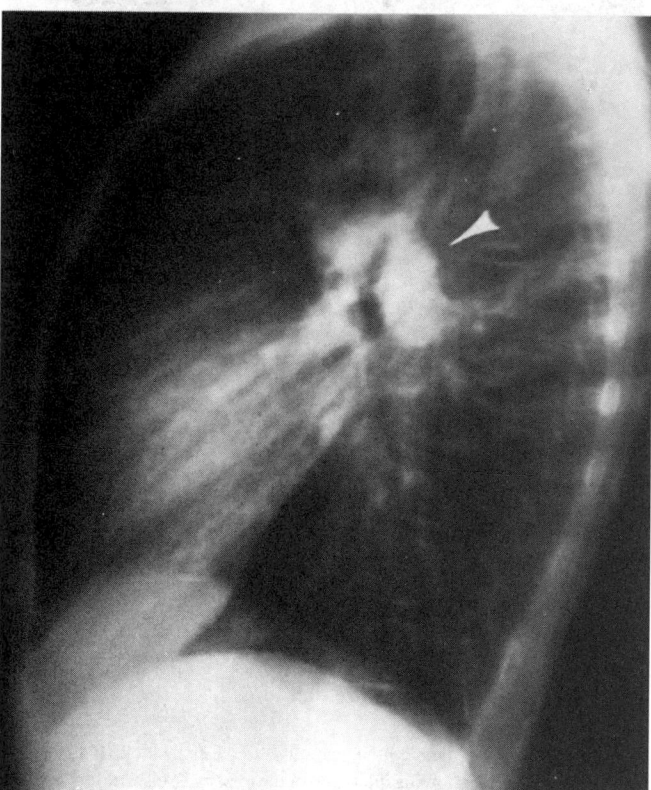

B

FIGURE 13-4

Patient with situs ambiguous, interruption of inferior vena cava, ventricular septal defect, and polysplenia. *A.* Posteroanterior view shows that the aortic arch and the heart are left-sided and the stomach (*lower arrows*) is right-sided. The azygos vein (*upper arrow*) is markedly enlarged. The heart is mildly enlarged and there is moderate increase in pulmonary vascularity. *B.* Lateral view shows an absent image of the inferior vena cava. The azygos arch (*arrow*) is markedly dilated.

stenosis typically show features of left ventricular hypertrophy without dilation. On the other hand, the left ventricle both dilates and hypertrophies in the case of aortic regurgitation, producing a much larger heart even before the development of congestive heart failure.

Both right-and left-sided heart failure can cause gross cardiac enlargement. The associated vascular abnormality in each case is, however, drastically different (see below, under "Pulmonary Vascularity"). A smaller than average heart is encountered in patients with chronic obstructive pulmonary disease (Fig. 13-7A), Addison's disease, anorexia nervosa, and starvation. An abnormally small heart, however, is difficult to define except in a retrospective fashion, when the heart has returned to its normal capacity following successful therapy. For example, in patients with Addison's disease, the heart may become significantly larger following appropriate steroid therapy.

Cardiac Contour

Any significant deviation from the normal cardiovascular contour may serve as a clue to the correct diagnosis. For instance, *coeur en sabot,* or a "boot-shaped heart" (Fig. 13-2C) is characteristic of tetralogy of Fallot. A bulge along the left cardiac border with a retrosternal double density is virtually diagnostic of left ventricular aneurysm (Fig. 13-8). A markedly widened right cardiac contour in association with a straightened left cardiac border is frequently seen in patients with severe mitral stenosis leading to tricuspid regurgitation (Fig. 13-7D).

Abnormal Densities

Besides the familiar double density cast by an enlarged left atrium, other increased densities may be found within the confines of the heart, indicating a variety of dilated vascular structures: e.g., tortuous descending aorta, aortic aneurysm, coronary artery aneurysm, pulmonary varix, etc.[3] Furthermore, large cardiac calcifications are easily seen, particularly in the lateral and oblique views. If smaller calcific deposits are suspected, they should be promptly verified or ruled out by cardiac fluoroscopy or computed tomographic (CT) scanning. Any radiologically detectable calcification in the heart is of clinical importance. The heavier the calcification, the more significant it becomes (Fig. 13-1F). As a rule, the extent of valvular calcification is proportionate to the severity of the valve stenosis regardless of the other roentgen signs of the disease.[2,3,13,14] Calcification of the coronary artery is almost always atherosclerotic in nature. Mönckeberg medial calcification of the coronary system is extremely rare. A fluoroscopically detectable coronary calcification is correlated with major vessel occlusion in 94 percent of patients with chest pain[15]; however, the sensitivity of the test is only 40 percent (see below under "Cardiac Fluoroscopy").

Recently, electron beam CT has proved to be the most sensitive tool for the detection and quantification of coronary

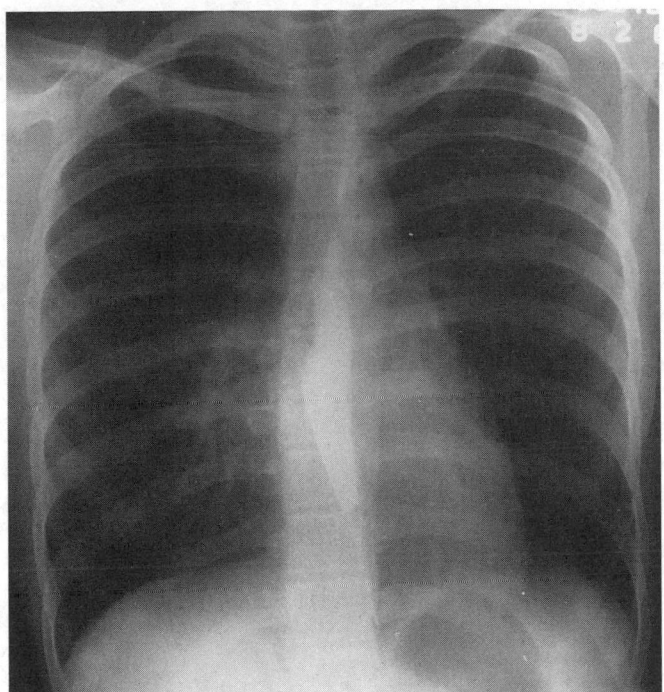

A

FIGURE 13-5

A 16-year-old woman with straight back syndrome. *A*. Posteroanterior radiograph shows normal pulmonary vascularity and normal heart size. Note leftward displacement and rotation of the heart, making its left border unusually prominent. *B*. Lateral view shows that the anteroposterior diameter of the chest is extremely narrow. The heart is squeezed, creating an innocent murmur.

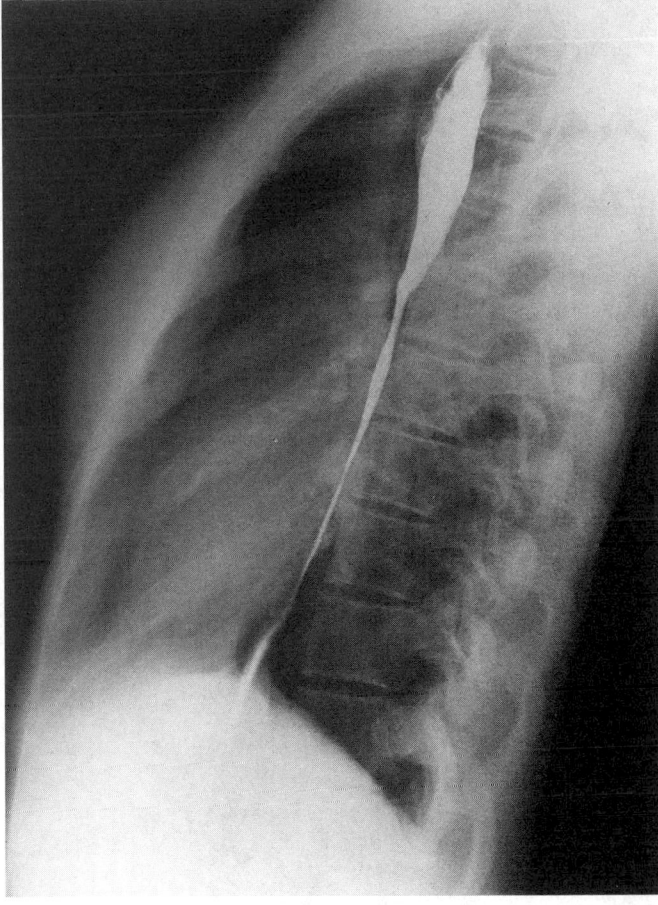

B

calcifications (see Chap. 18). A negative result eliminates the need for further testing in most patients. A positive result, however, does not necessarily denote obstructive coronary artery disease. The sensitivity for detecting significant disease is >95 percent with a specificity of 65 percent. Another advantage of this method is to identify high-risk patients with calcific nonobstructive atherosclerotic lesions. By vigorous therapeutic intervention, one may be able to halt progression or even cause regression of their disease. In fact, the results of such interventions can be correlated with the increase or decrease of coronary calcific plaques[14] (see Chap. 18).

A calcified ascending aortic aneurysm with aortic regurgitation is highly suggestive of syphilitic aortitis (Fig. 13-9).[13]

Abnormal Lucency

The abnormal lucent areas in and about the heart include (1) displaced subepicardial fat stripes caused by effusion or thickening of the pericardium (see Fig. 13-10), (2) pneumopericardium (Fig. 13-11), and (3) pneumomediastinum. Pneumomediastinum is differentiated from pneumopericardium by the fact that the former shows a superior extension of the air strip beyond the confine of the pericardium.

Cardiac Malpositions[7,8]

DEXTROCARDIA WITH SITUS INVERSUS

Recently the term *dextrocardia* has been used to indicate any congenital right-sided heart regardless of the position of abdominal viscera. To specify the kind of dextrocardia under test, one must affix the status of the abdominal viscera. "Dextrocardia with situs inversus" means the mirror image of normal. In this situation, the incidence of congenital heart disease is only 5 percent, which is a ninefold increase over the general population. The combination of dextrocardia, sinusitis, and bronchiectasis is known as *Kartagener's triad*.

DEXTROCARDIA WITH SITUS SOLITUS

This represents an anomaly with normal situs but a right-sided heart. Radiographically, normal situs (situs solitus) is a certainty when both the aortic knob and the gastric air bubble are on the left side. *Situs solitus* also means that both the abdominal viscera and the atria are in the normal position. Under these circumstances, if the ventricles fail to swing from the primitive right-sided position to the normal left-sided position, abnormal relationships between the ventricles and the rest of the cardiovascular structures are bound to develop. This entity was formerly termed *dextroversion*.

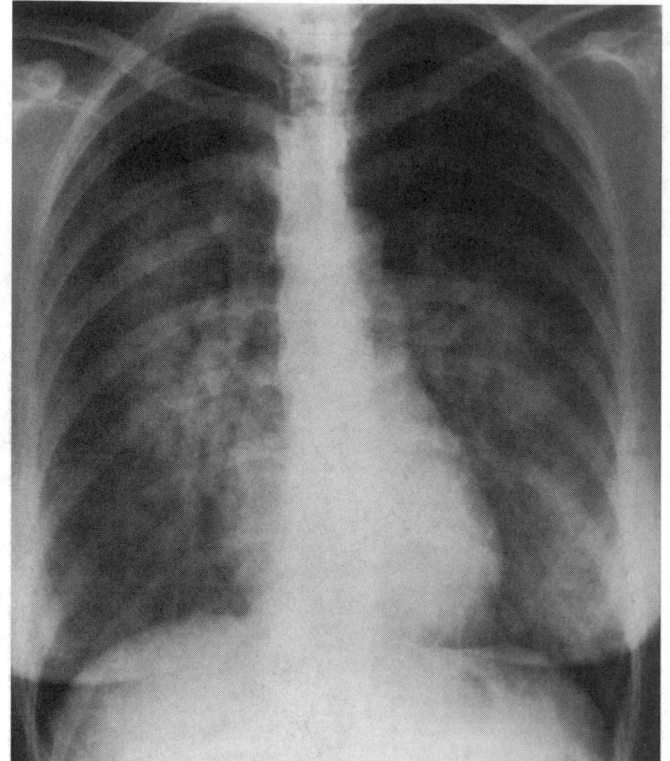

A

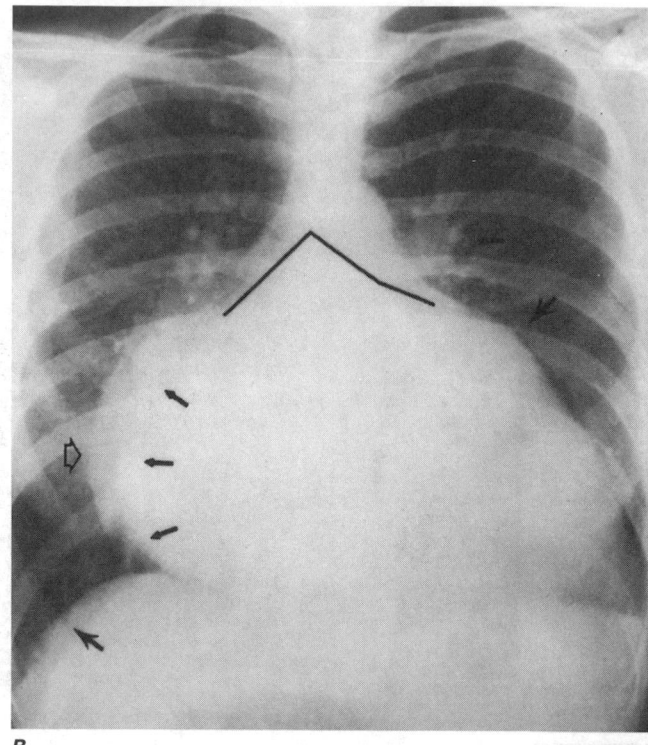

B

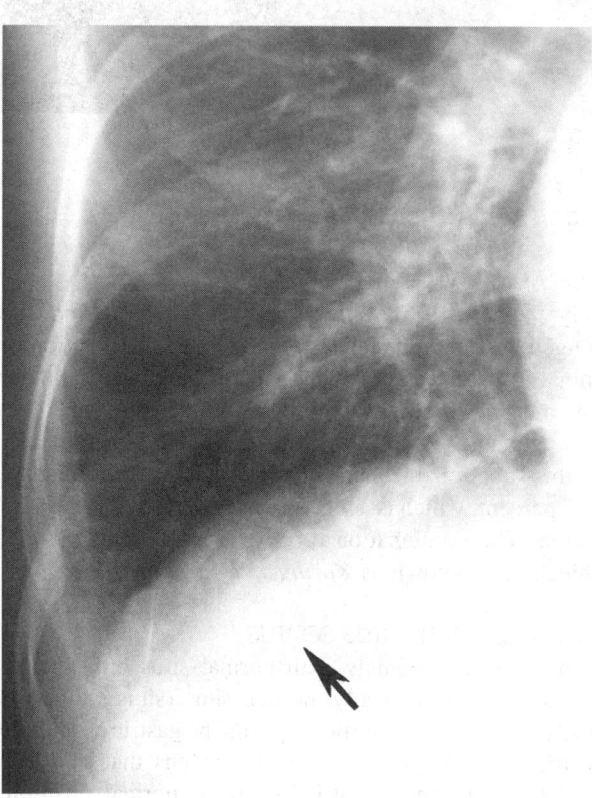

C

FIGURE 13-6

Roentgen appearance of left-sided heart failure. *A.* Acute: Patient with acute mitral regurgitation due to rupture of chordae tendineae, showing "bat wings" appearance of severe alveolar type of pulmonary edema and a normal-sized heart. *B.* Chronic: Patient with severe mitral and tricuspid regurgitation and mild aortic regurgitation. This is a predominantly left-sided failure pattern. Note gross cardiomegaly with striking cephalization and interstitial pulmonary edema. The giant left atrium forms the right cardiac border (*open arrow*), makes its appendage bulge outward on the left side (*upper large arrow*), and splays the mainstem bronchi wide apart (*solid lines*). The huge right atrium forms a double density within the right cardiac border (*three small arrows*). The upper small arrow marks the peribronchial cuffing of edema fluid. The lower large arrow points to multiple Kerley "B" lines. *C.* Magnified view of right costophrenic sulcus showing multiple Kerley "B" lines (*arrow*).

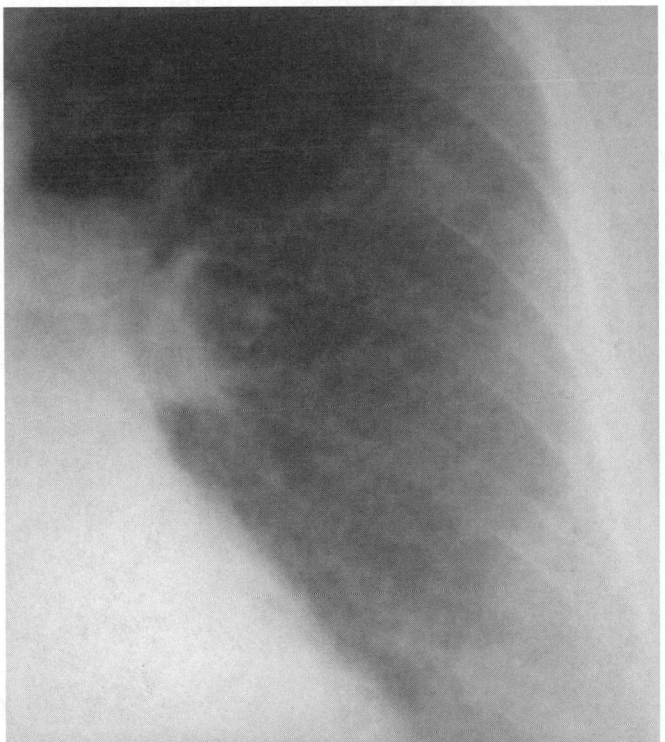

D

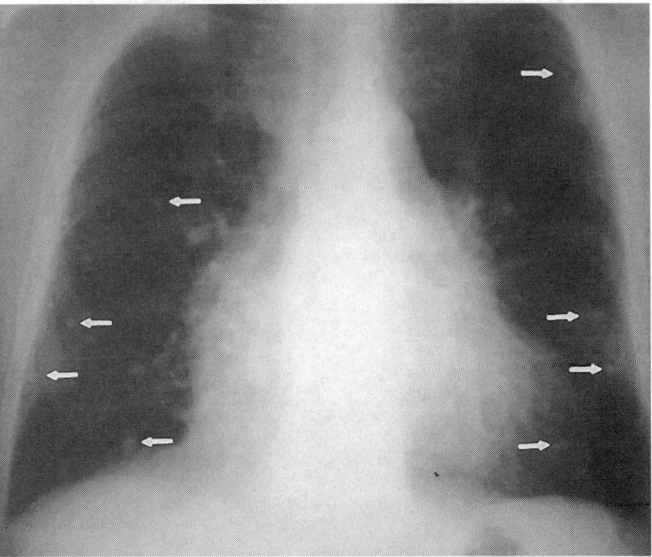

E

FIGURE 13-6 (*Continued*)

D. A 44-year-old woman with severe mitral stenosis. The magnified view of her left middle lung zone shows a diffuse stippling with fine nodules representing hemosiderosis. Hemosiderin-laden macrophages were found in her sputa. *E.* Posteroanterior radiograph of a 63-year-old man with severe mitral stenosis, status post mitral valve replacement, shows multiple scattered bony nodules (*arrows*), 2 to 10 mm in diameter, throughout the lower two-thirds of both lungs, compatible with pulmonary ossification.

In patients with dextroversion, the incidence of congenital heart disease has been estimated at 98 percent. More than 80 percent have congenitally corrected (or L-loop) transposition of great arteries. The next most commonly associated lesions are a combination of ventricular septal defect and pulmonary stenosis, a tetralogy-like pathophysiology (Fig. 13-12). Therefore, from the statistical point of view, it is important to be able to differentiate this entity from dextrocardia with situs inversus, which is associated with a much lower incidence of congenital heart disease (see above and also Chap. 70).

LEVOCARDIA WITH SITUS INVERSUS
This is a mirror image of dextroversion and it is associated with an extremely high incidence (nearly 100 percent) of cyanotic congenital cardiac lesions similar to those seen in dextroversion. This entity was formerly termed *levoversion.*

LEVOCARDIA WITH SITUS SOLITUS
This is entirely normal.

CARDIAC MALPOSITIONS WITH INDETERMINATE SITUS
In this group, the patient's heart may be either left- or right-sided. The situs is ambiguous, with the roentgenogram show-ing aorticogastric bubble discordance. In other words, the aortic knob and the stomach are not on the same side; therefore the situs is unpredictable, though the left atrium tends to be on the side of the aorta. Under these circumstances, interruption of the inferior vena cava with azygos continuation is almost always present (see Fig. 13-4). The next most commonly associated lesions are polysplenia and a left-to-right shunt, most frequently a ventricular septal defect. The only exception to the rule of indeterminate situs is an isolated right-sided aortic arch (see Chaps. 8 and 70).

Other Abnormalities

GREAT VESSELS
The roentgen appearance of the great vessels often provides valuable information for the diagnosis of heart disease.[2,3,16,17] For example, selective dilation of the ascending aorta is the hallmark of valvular aortic stenosis (Fig. 13-13); generalized dilation of the entire thoracic aorta (Fig. 13-14), on the other hand, favors the diagnosis of aortic regurgitation, systemic hypertension, or both, depending on the size of the left ventricle. A larger left ventricle is associated with aortic regurgitation because of volume overload. In atrial septal defect and in mitral stenosis, the pulmonary trunk is quite large and the

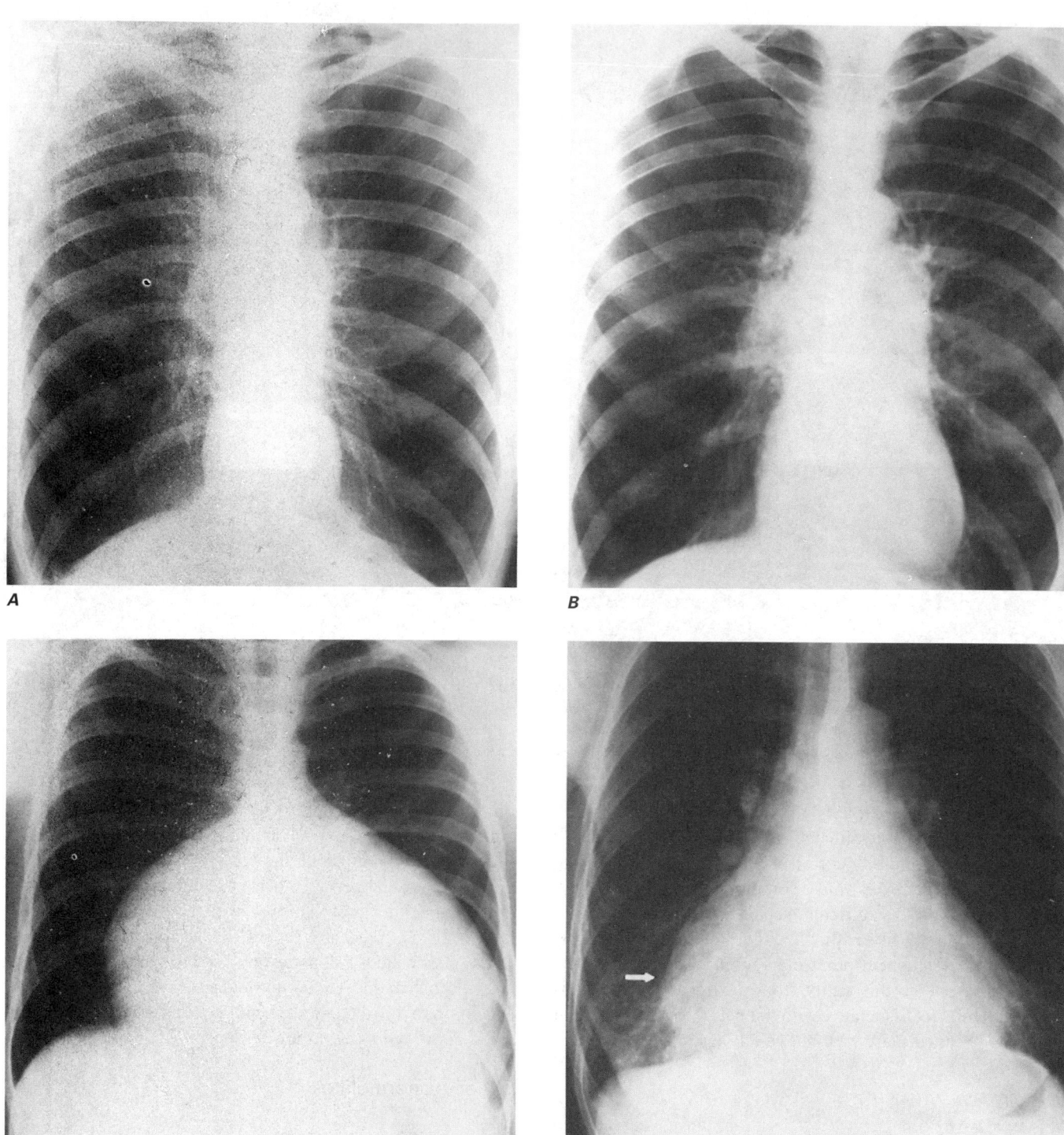

A

B

C

D

FIGURE 13-7

Roentgen appearance of right-sided heart failure. *A.* Patient with severe obstructive emphysema showing overaeration of the lungs, centralized flow pattern, and a small heart size. *B.* Three years later, the patient was in frank right-sided heart failure. Note that the heart got bigger as his emphysema got worse. The centralized flow pattern became more severe. *C.* Patient with Ebstein's anomaly, showing gross cardiomegaly with severe decrease in pulmonary vascularity. The right cardiac border represents the huge right atrium, and the left cardiac border represents the giant right ventricle. *D.* Patient with mitral stenosis showing a giant right atrium (*arrow*) representing severe functional tricuspid regurgitation due to unrelenting left-sided failure. The pulmonary venous congestion had improved following the onset of right-sided heart failure.

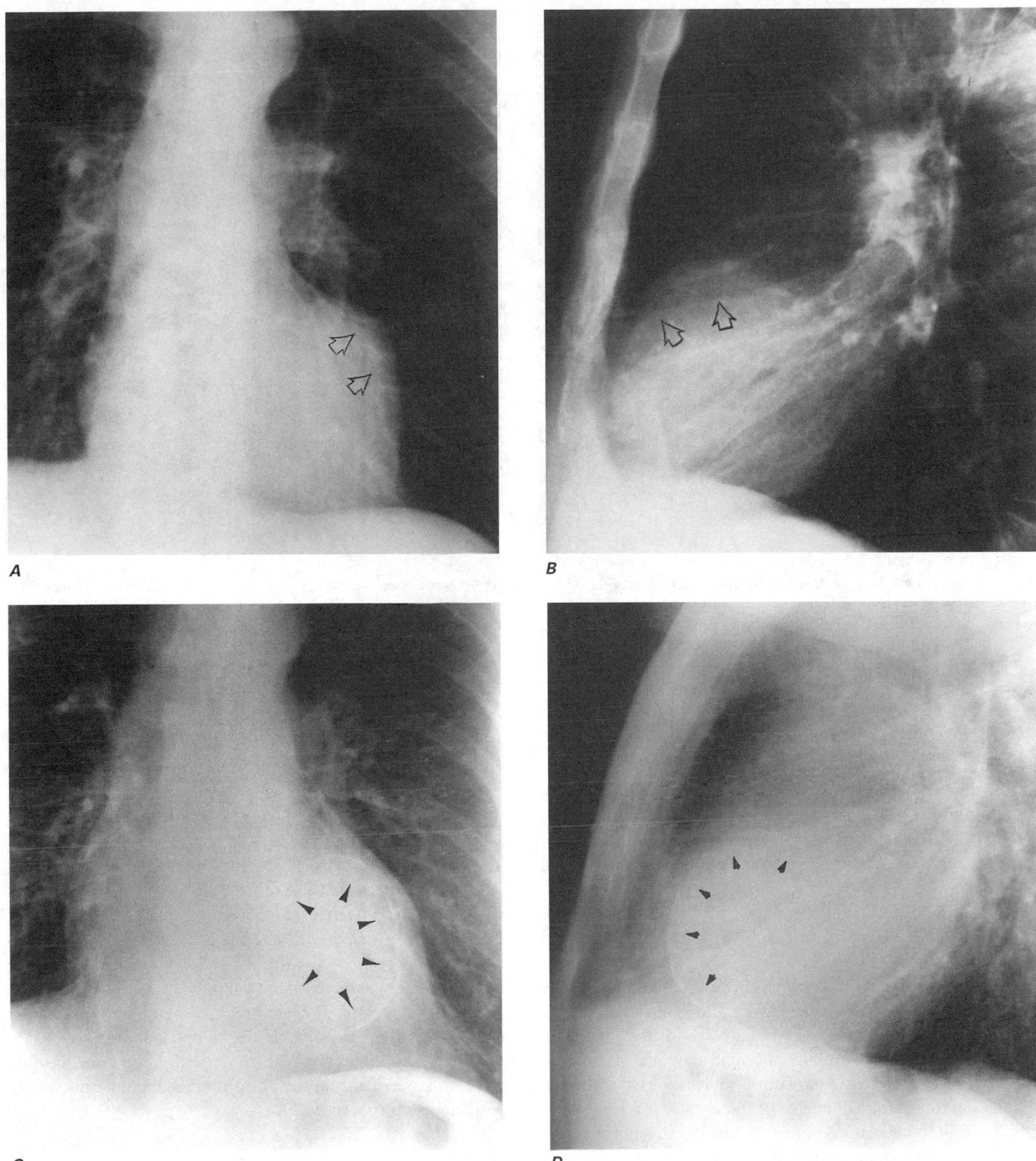

FIGURE 13-8

Left ventricular aneurysms. *A.* Posteroanterior view of patient 1 shows a localized bulge (*arrows*) along the left cardiac border representing a left ventricular aneurysm from the anterolateral wall. *B.* Lateral view shows a double density with sharp borders anteriorly and superiorly (*arrows*). This is the left ventricular aneurysm that casts a shadow on the normal right ventricle. Fluoroscopically, it is easy to confirm its origin and to separate it from the right ventricle by rotating the patient under direct vision. *C.* Posteroanterior view of patient 2, a 69-year-old man, shows total calcification of an anterolateral apical left ventricular aneurysm (*arrows*). *D.* Lateral view shows the same (*arrows*).

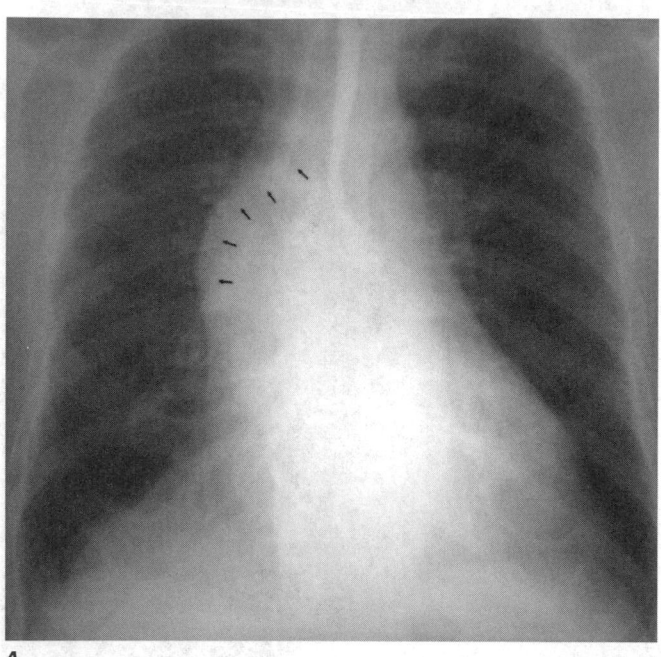

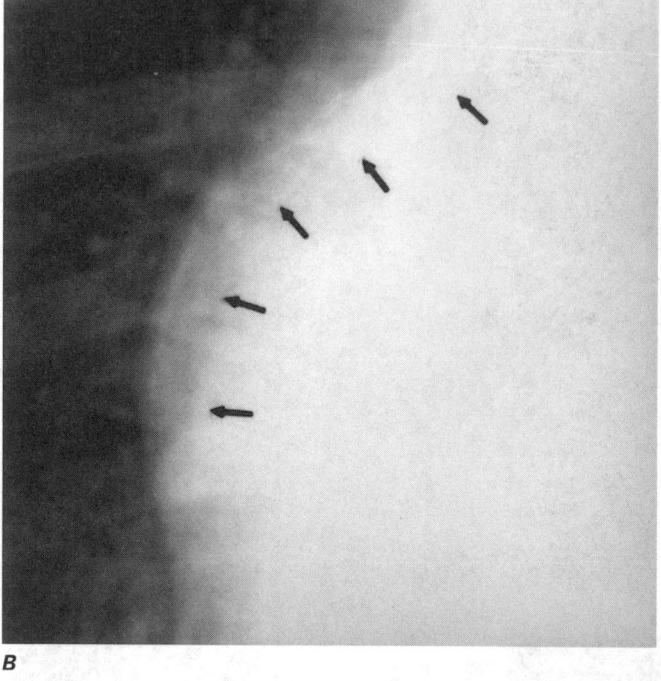

A

B

FIGURE 13-9

A 71-year-old woman had syphilitic aortitis. Her posteroanterior radiograph (*A*) shows a huge, calcified, ascending aortic aneurysm (*arrows*). In addition, the entire aorta and the left ventricle were markedly dilated, compatible with severe aortic regurgitation. (From Chen,[13] with permission.) A magnified view of the ascending aorta (*B*) shows the calcified aneurysm to better advantage.

aortic knob is usually small (see Figs. 13-2*B* and 13-3*A*). This is explained on the basis of a leftward cardiac rotation that occurs when an enlarged right ventricle coexists with a normal-sized left ventricle. When the heart rotates to the left, the aorta folds on itself in the midline and becomes inconspicuous. Meanwhile, the pulmonary trunk is brought laterally and looks larger than it actually is. Aortic aneurysm (Fig. 13-15) and dissection are frequently associated with hypertensive and atherosclerotic disorders.

As already mentioned, prominence of the pulmonary trunk is a reliable secondary sign of right ventricular enlargement (Fig. 13-16; also see Fig. 13-2*B*), with the following exceptions: (1) tetralogy of Fallot with right ventricular hypertrophy but pulmonary trunk hypoplasia, (2) idiopathic dilatation of the pulmonary artery, (3) patent ductus arteriosus with dilated pulmonary trunk but normal right ventricle, and (4) straight back syndrome, pectus excavatum, and scoliosis with narrowed anteroposterior diameter of the chest. Under the latter conditions, the heart is compressed, displaced, and rotated to the left, giving rise to a falsely enlarged pulmonary artery.

In coarctation of the aorta, the engorged aortic knob and the poststenotic dilatation of the descending aorta may cause a "3" sign on the aorta and an "E" sign on the barium-filled esophagus, both depicting the site of coarctation[6] (see Fig. 13-1*C*).

The abnormal size and distribution of both the pulmonary and systemic veins are important clues to the presence of certain conditions, e.g., anomalous pulmonary venous connections and interruption of inferior vena cava with azygos continuation (see Fig. 13-4).

The significance of aortic arch anomalies is discussed under "Statistical Guidance," on page 1316.

MEDIASTINAL STRUCTURES

The mediastinal organs are frequently affected by the cardiovascular structures because of their close spatial interrelationships. An enlarged left atrium not only displaces the esophagus (see Fig. 13-1*C*, *D*, and *E*) and the descending aorta but also elevates and compresses the left stem bronchus. A double aortic arch may compress both the trachea and the esophagus. On the other hand, malignant processes may invade the heart and great vessels, causing cardiac tamponade or the superior vena cava syndrome, for example. Usually, these mediastinal changes are evident on the chest roentgenogram and should be recognized promptly.[16–20]

PLEURA

A right-sided pleural effusion is often present with left heart failure. A bilateral hydrothorax, on the other hand, suggests bilateral heart failure or a noncardiac etiology of the effusion. Congestive heart failure is also known to be associated with a pseudotumor or "vanishing" tumor, representing an interlobar collection of pleural fluid (Fig. 13-17). As congestive heart failure improves, the "tumor" disappears.

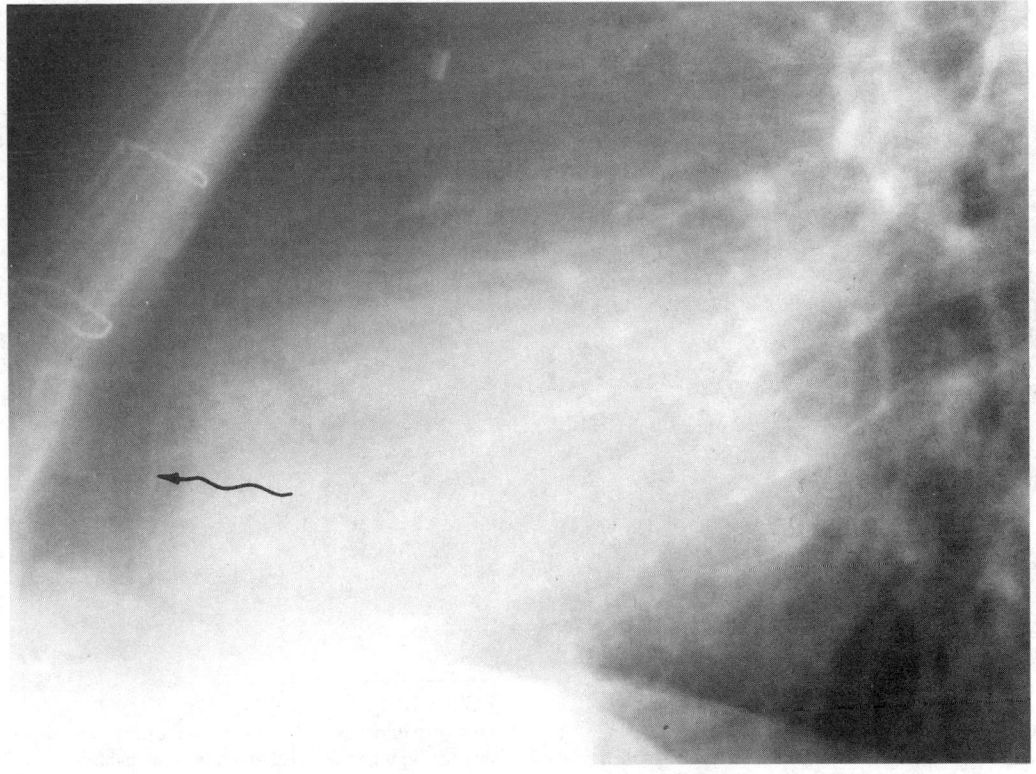

A

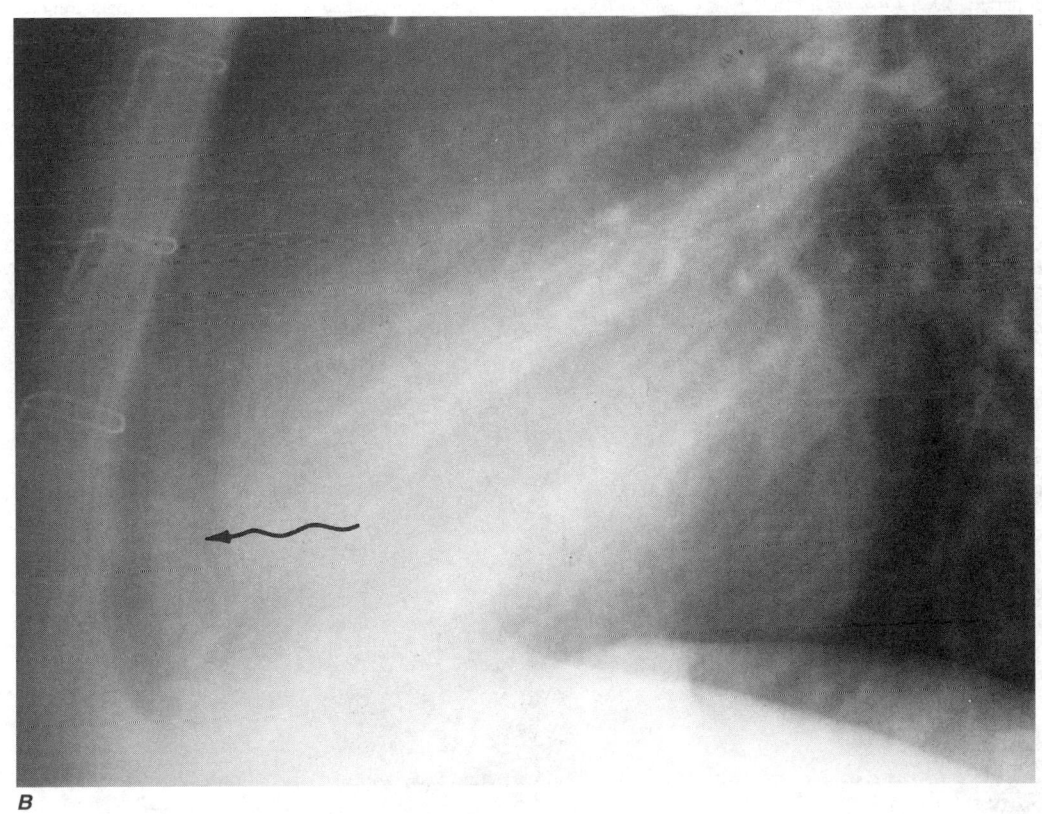

B

FIGURE 13-10

Developing pericardial effusion in 2 weeks. *A.* A magnified view of the retrosternal area showing the hairlike normal pericardium (*arrow*) sandwiched between the subepicardial fat stripe interiorly and the mediastinal fat stripe exteriorly. The maximal width of normal pericardium is 2 mm. *B.* The same patient 2 weeks later, with moderate pericardial effusion. The pericardial cavity now measured >1 cm in width (*arrow*).

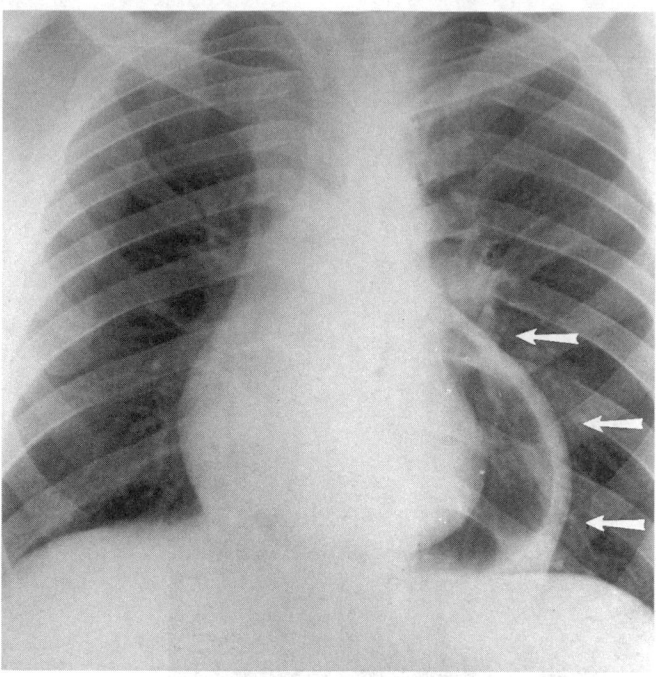

FIGURE 13-11

Traumatic constrictive-effusive pericarditis in a young man. Following emergent pericardiocentesis and injection of air, a radiograph was taken in the supine position. Air is confined to the left side of the pericardium. Note markedly thickened parietal layer (*arrows*).

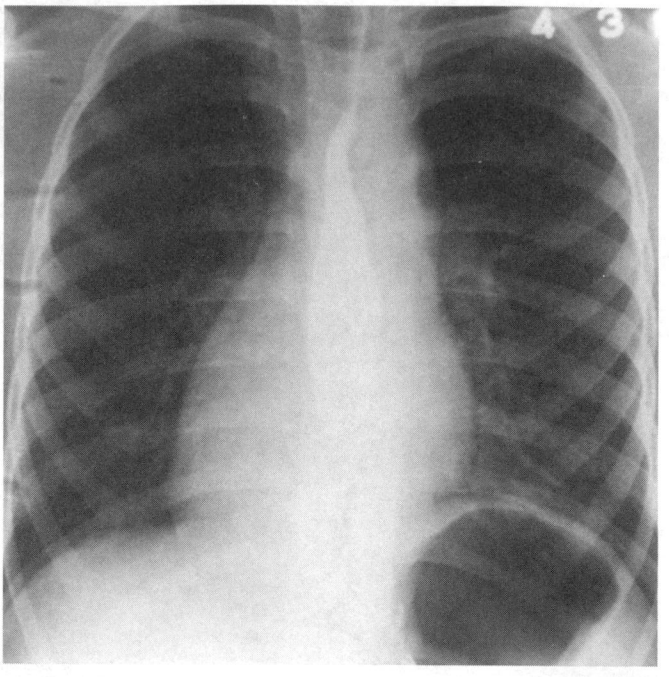

FIGURE 13-12

Posteroanterior view of a patient with dextrocardia and situs solitus. Note that the aortic arch and the stomach air bubble are both on the left (*situs solitus*) and the apex of the ventricles is pointing to the right inferiorly. According to statistics and proved by cardiac catheterization, this patient had the typical combination of congenitally corrected transposition of great arteries, ventricular septal defect, and pulmonary stenosis. He was cyanotic. The pulmonary vascularity appears decreased.

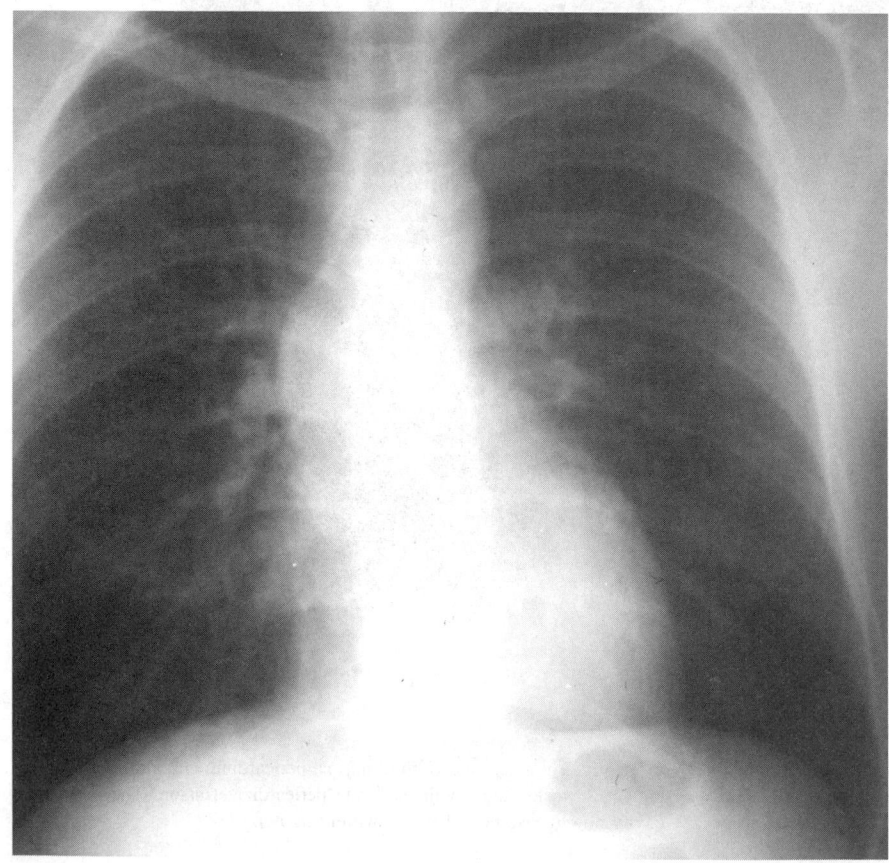

FIGURE 13-13

A 17-year-old man with congenital aortic valve stenosis. Note dilatation of the ascending aorta, increased convexity of the left ventricle, and normal pulmonary vascularity. The systolic aortic pressure gradient was 100 mmHg.

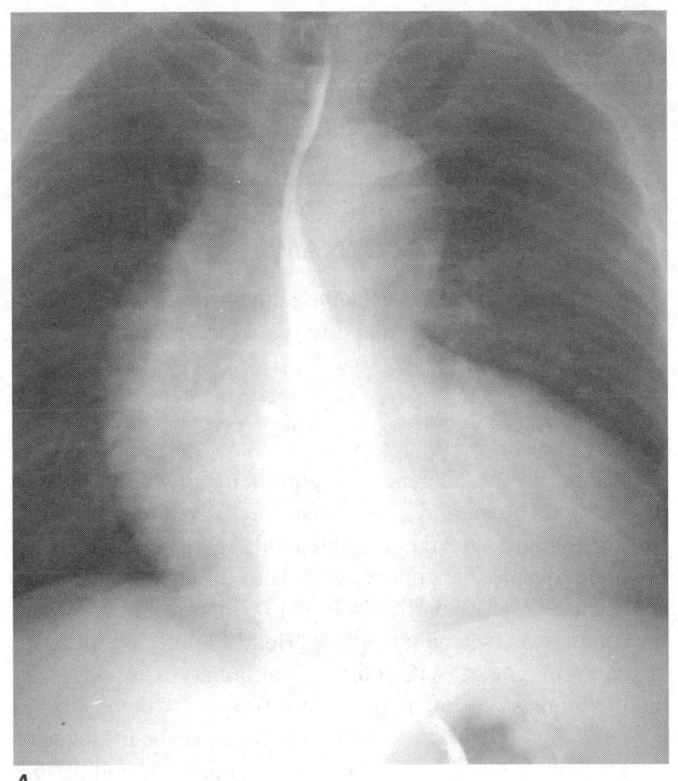

A

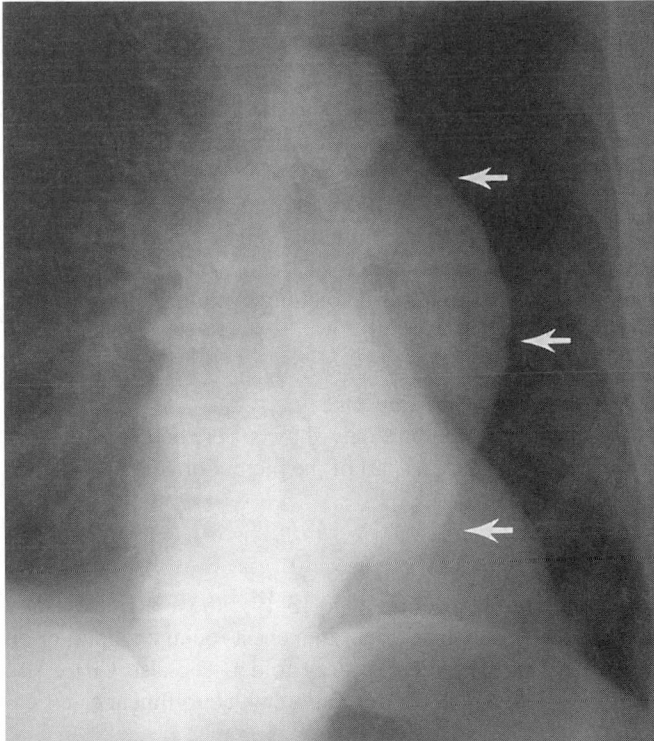

FIGURE 13-15
Posteroanterior view of a 77-year-old man shows a huge descending aortic aneurysm (*arrows*).

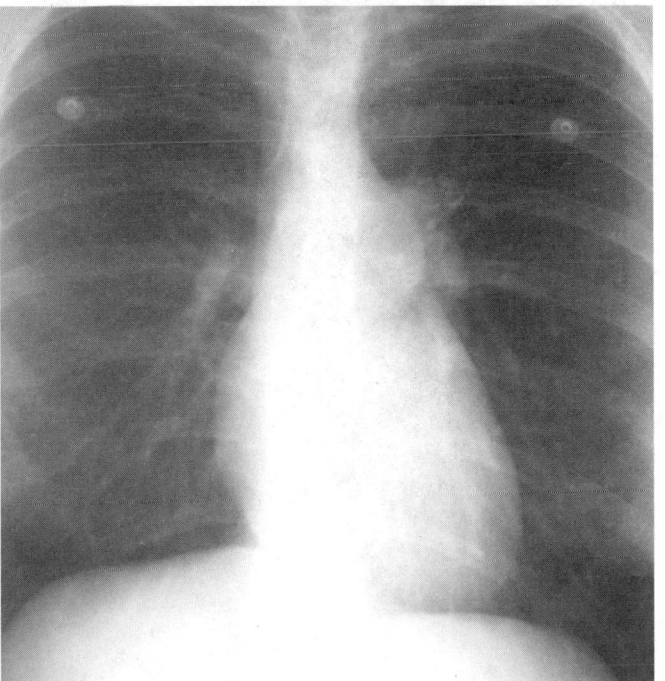

FIGURE 13-14
A 45-year-old man with Marfan's syndrome, severe aortic regurgitation, and proximal aortic dissection into the pericardial cavity. *A*. Posteroanterior view shows a huge left ventricular and aneurysmal dilatation of the ascending aorta. There is no sign of heart failure. *B*. Lateral view shows a small pericardial effusion (*arrow*).

FIGURE 13-16
A 37-year-old woman with congenital valvular pulmonary stenosis. Note enlarged pulmonary trunk and left pulmonary artery versus diminished right pulmonary artery. Also note increased pulmonary blood flow on the left and decreased pulmonary blood flow on the right side.

BONES AND JOINTS

Notching of the ribs has many origins. Basically any of the three major intercostal structures can enlarge, compress, and erode the lower borders of the ribs, producing areas of notching. They are intercostal arteries, veins, and nerves. Co-arctation of the aorta[6] (see Fig. 13-1A) represents the most common cause of rib notching due to dynamic dilation and tortuosity of the arteries. Superior vena cava syndrome may cause a similar phenomenon of venous origin. Neurofibro-matosis can also produce rib notching by numerous intercostal neurofibromas.

SOFT TISSUES OVER THE CHEST

Patients with renal failure may show severe edema in the soft tissues over the chest as part of the picture of general anasarca (Fig. 13-18).

EXTRATHORACIC STRUCTURES

In Holt-Oram syndrome (Fig. 13-19), the upper extremity abnormalities may be evident in a chest roentgenogram or on other films in the patient's x-ray folder (see also Chap. 70). A large arteriovenous malformation with curvilinear calcifica-tions may be seen in the neck, thereby providing a clue as to the etiology of the patient's congestive heart failure. Radiographic evaluation of the patient's abdominal viscera is an integral part of the workup for cardiac malpositions.[7,8]

FLUOROSCOPIC OBSERVATION FOR DYNAMICS

Cardiac fluoroscopy is a valuable adjunct to the chest roent-genogram.[2] Its advantages and limitations are detailed at the end of this chapter.

Comparison

To appreciate the acuteness or chronicity of the disease or its response to therapy, one must carefully compare serial roentgenograms. As demonstrated in Fig. 13-7B, the heart might be considered neither enlarged nor failing if the baseline study made 3 years earlier in Fig. 13-7A were not available for comparison (see below, under "Heart Failure"). Similarly, an enlarging heart with normal pulmonary vascularity is highly suggestive of pericardial effusion. Conversely, a shrinking heart in the presence of normal vascularity is compatible with resolution of a pericardial effusion (Fig. 13-20).

Statistical Guidance

Certain roentgenologic findings are by themselves diagnostic of a disease; other signs are sugges-tive of a diagnosis on the basis of statistics only. Nevertheless, the latter can be quite useful by virtue of their high predictive value of a particular disease or a group of similar diseases. There-fore, one should always keep the statistical information in mind.

In addition to what has been mentioned above, other anatomic settings may also provide useful statistical guidance for making an intelligent radiographic sugges-tion. Different types of aortic arch anomaly are good examples.

The incidence of congenital heart disease in patients with right-sided aortic arch increases 10- to 100-fold, depending on the anatomic details of the anom-aly.[19,20] Of practical importance, there are only two types of right-sided aortic arch. The first has been called the *avian type*, implying a normal status for birds

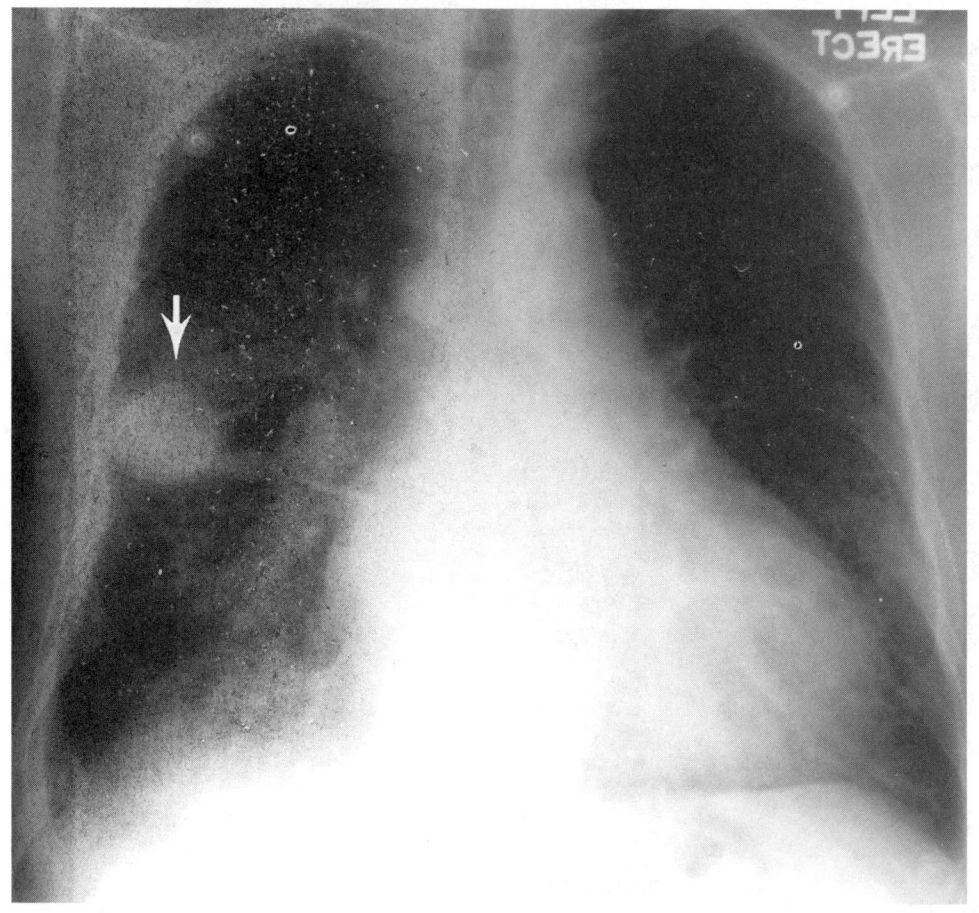

FIGURE 13-17

Patient with congestive heart failure. Note gross cardiomegaly, cephalization, interstitial pulmonary edema, and right-sided pleural effusion. Some of the fluid was loculated in the minor interlobar fissure (*arrow*), which disappeared with improved cardiac function.

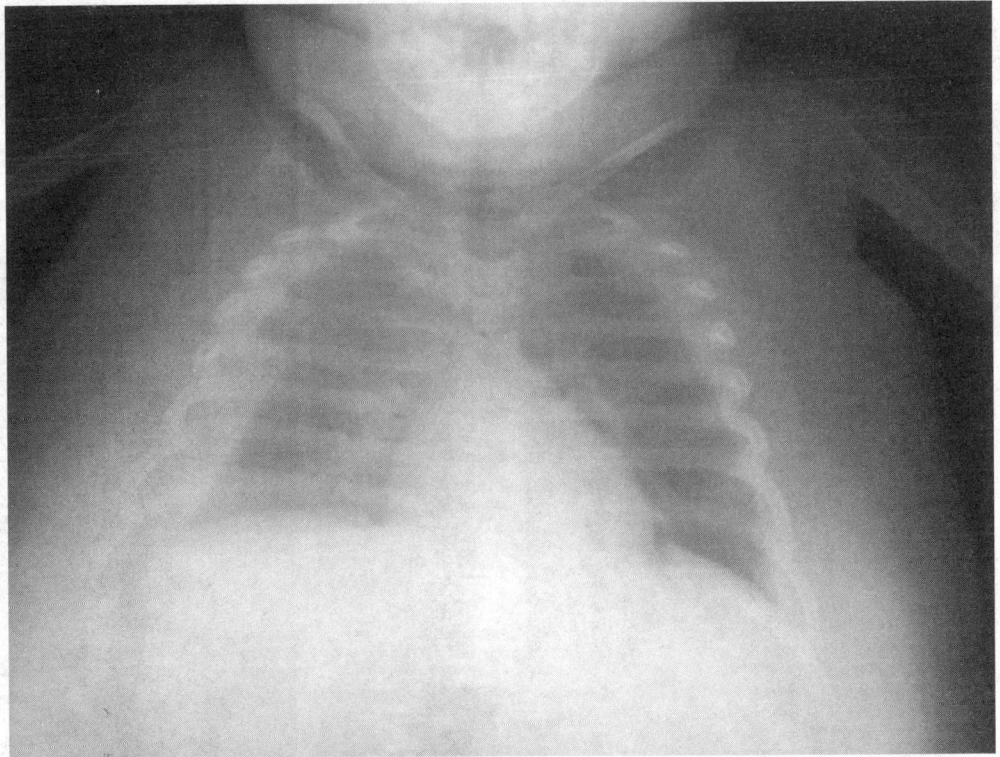

A

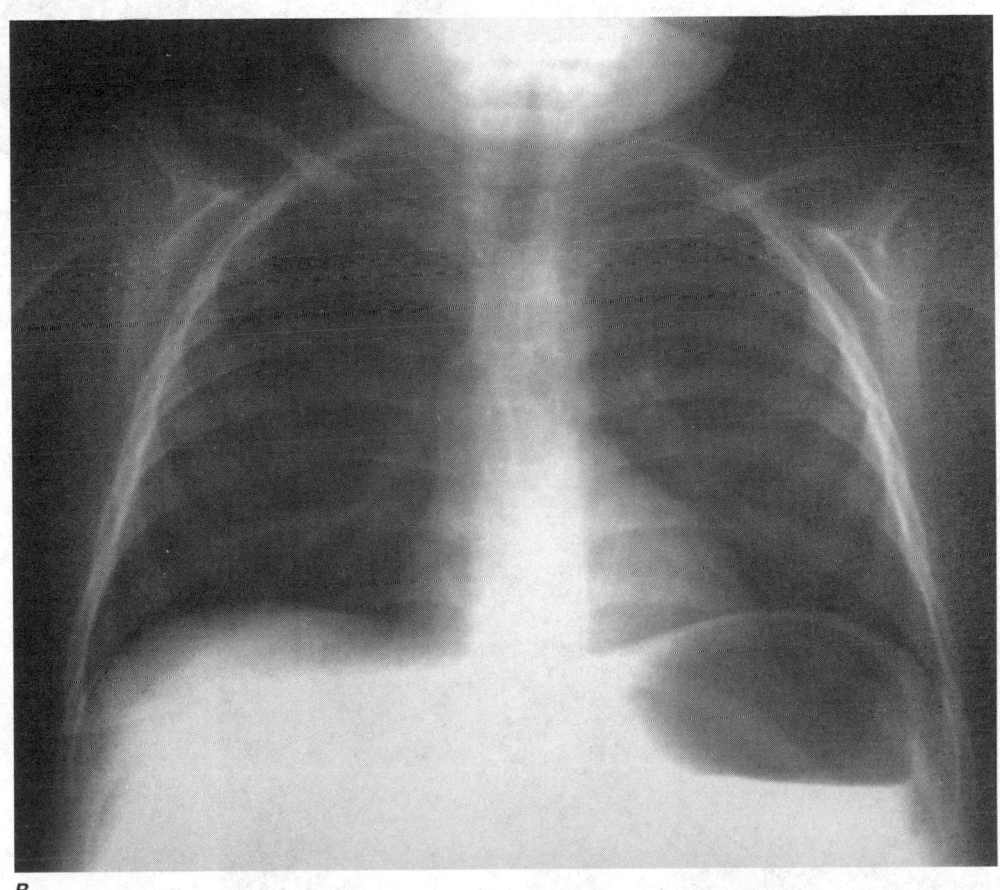

B

FIGURE 13-18

A child suffering from nephrotic syndrome, which was successfully treated. *A*. Posteroanterior view during the worst period of his disease shows general anasarca, pulmonary edema, and pleural effusion. Note considerable soft tissue edema in the chest wall. *B*. With proper treatment, everything returned to normal in 2 weeks.

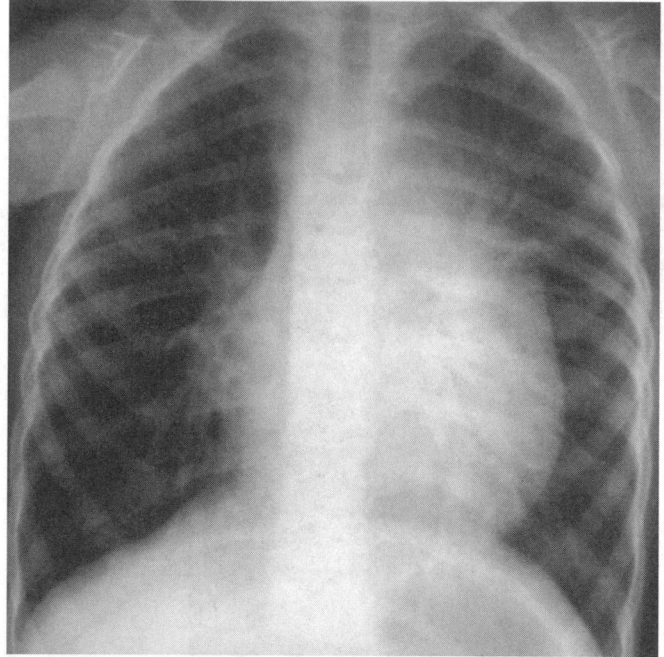

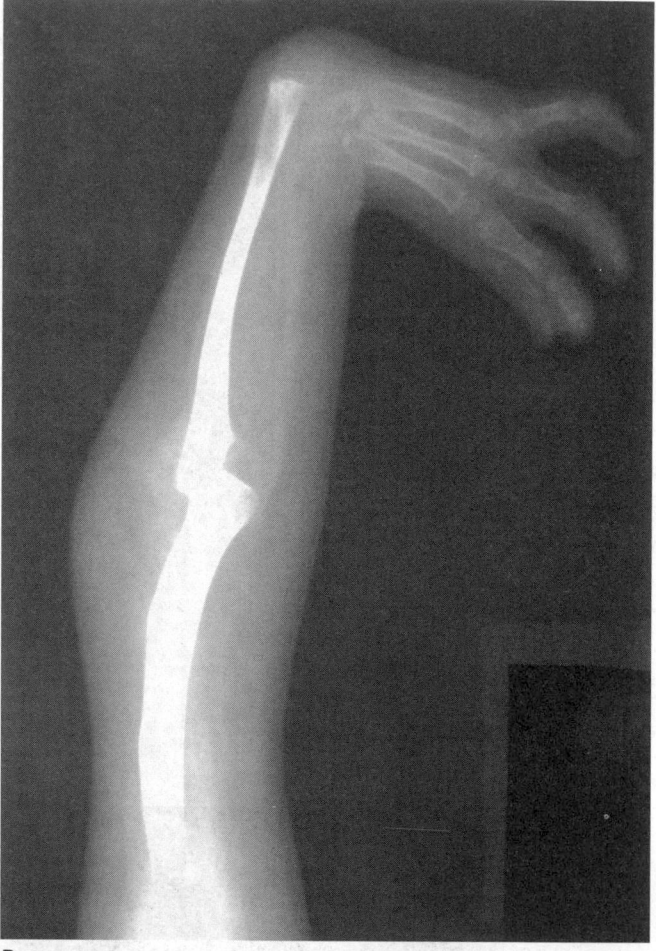

FIGURE 13-19

Patients with Holt-Oram syndrome. *A.* Posteroanterior view of patient 1, a 7-year-old girl, shows a globular cardiac contour with increased pulmonary blood flow. The aortic arch is on the right side. Catheterization diagnosis: 2° atrial septal defect. *B.* Her left arm shows absent radius and thumb with radial clubhand. Her right arm is a mirror image of the left (not shown). *C.* Forearms of patient 2, a 33-year-old woman, with 2° atrial septal defect, show bilateral absence of thumb.

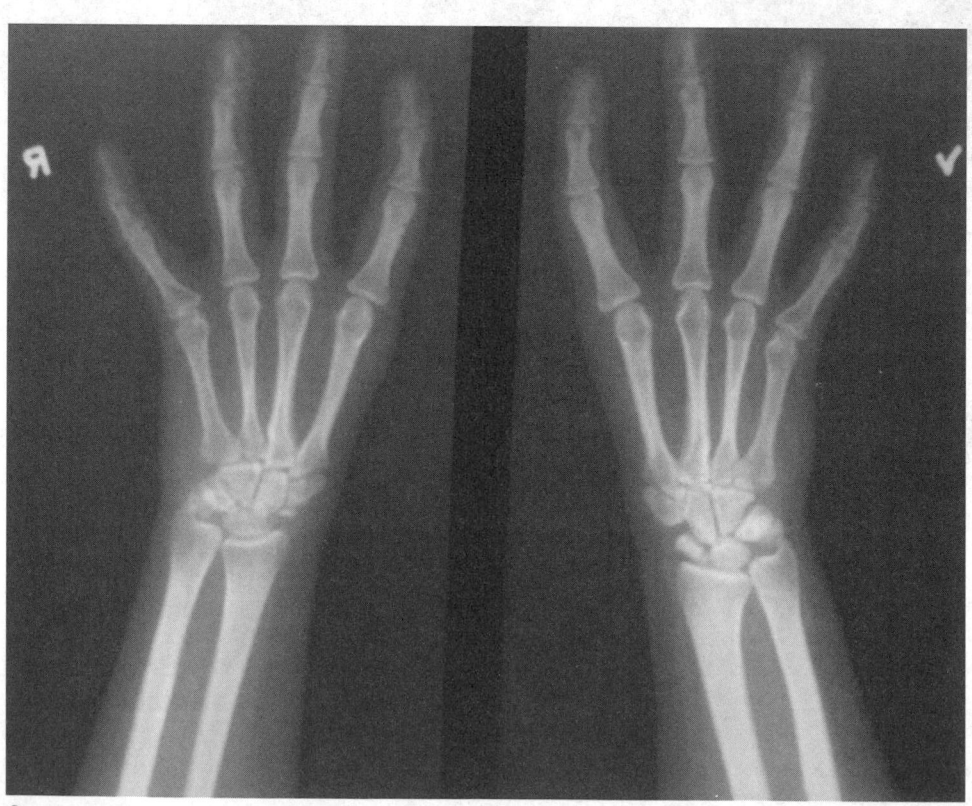

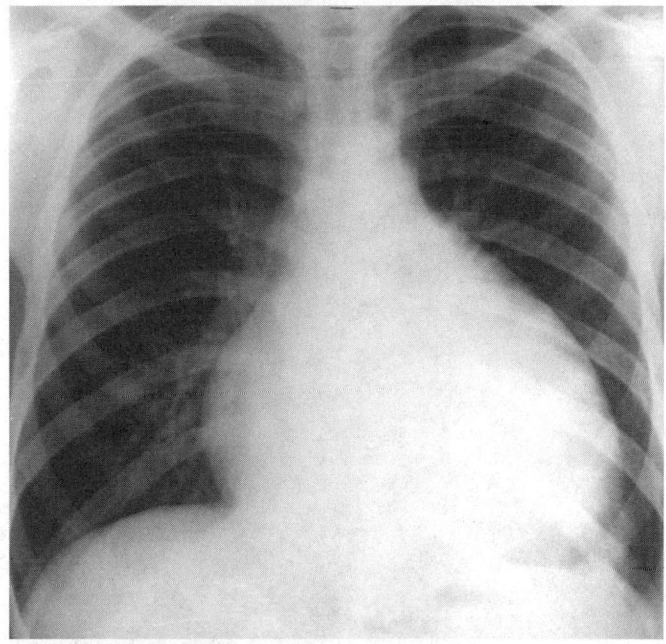

A

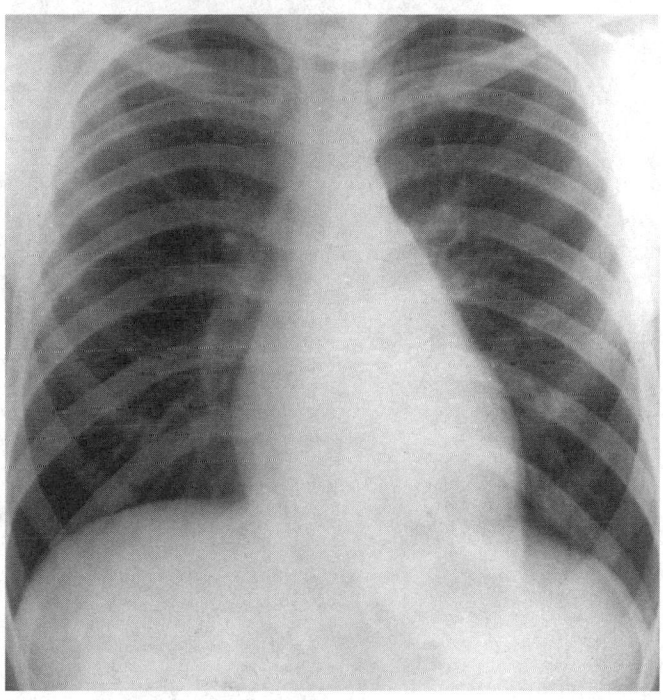

B

FIGURE 13-20

Young man with acute pericarditis with effusion. *A.* Posteroanterior view shows a water bottle–shaped cardiomegaly, clear lungs and normal pulmonary vascularity. *B.* Repeat film taken 5 days later shows excellent response to therapy.

but a detrimental one for humans. The overwhelming majority of patients with this type are born with cyanotic congenital heart disease. The second may be called the *common type* because of its higher incidence in the general population. Most patients with the common type are physiologically normal and have their anomaly incidentally diagnosed on chest radio-

graphs or a barium-meal study. The x-ray findings of the two types are similar in the PA view but are quite different in the lateral view (Fig. 13-21). The incidence and list of congenital heart diseases with each type[18] are shown in Table 13-2. Only 2 percent of patients with the avian type are physiologically normal. Tetralogy of Fallot should be the diagnosis in these patients until proved otherwise.[19,20]

Patients with a double aortic arch, on the other hand, rarely have congenital heart disease, though they tend to be symptomatic in infancy because of a compressing vascular ring.[19]

Clinical Correlation

The next step in the examination is to correlate the roentgenologic findings with the clinical information and other laboratory parameters for the final conclusion. It may become necessary, at this point, to reexamine the radiograph or review the fluoroscopic observation or both. After detailed analysis of some finer points, a wrong impression may be corrected or a correct diagnosis reinforced[2] (Table 13-3).

PULMONARY VASCULARITY

Normal

The normal roentgen appearance of the pulmonary vasculature of an upright human being is typified by a caudal flow pattern because of gravity. The pressure differential between the apex and the base of the lung is approximately 22 mmHg in adults in the upright position.[2,21] Therefore, more flow under higher distending pressure is expected in the lower-lobe vessels than in the upper. Normally one sees very little vascularity above the hilum, whereas more and larger vessels are found below the hilum. Since the pulmonary resistance is normal, all vessels taper gradually in a treelike manner from the hilum toward the periphery of the lung. The right descending pulmonary artery measures 10 to 15 mm in diameter in males and 9 to 14 mm in females (Fig. 13-3).[2,22]

Abnormal

Abnormal pulmonary vascularity can be classified into two categories, either in terms of volume or in terms of distribution[2,10,23] (Table 13-4).

Abnormalities in Volume

In the evaluation of pulmonary vasculature, the caliber of the vessels is more important than the length or the number. As long as the PBF pattern remains normal, with greater amount of flow to the bases than to the apices, the volume of the flow is proportional to the caliber of the pulmonary arteries (see Fig. 13-2). In addition to measuring the right descending pulmonary artery, one may also assess the pulmonary blood volume by comparing the size of the pulmonary artery with

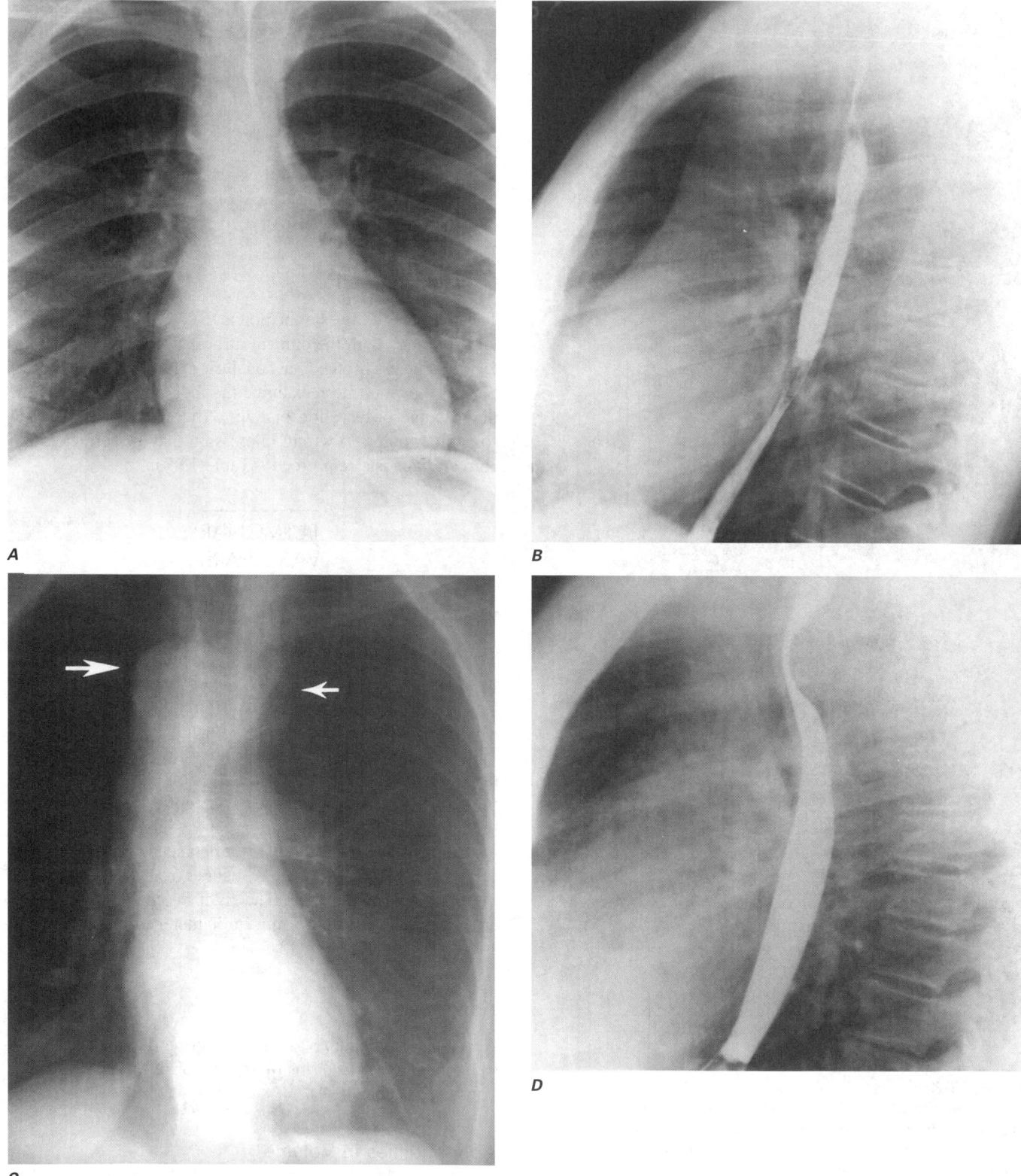

A

B

C

D

FIGURE 13-21

Statistical guidance focusing on the best diagnostic possibilities. *A.* Poster-oanterior view of a patient with tetralogy of Fallot showing a right aortic arch, avian type. Note that the esophagus and trachea are deviated to the left. The cardiovascular structures are otherwise within normal limits. *B.* Lateral view of the same patient showing the aortic arch normally situated, in front of the trachea and esophagus. *C.* Posteroanterior radiograph of a healthy woman shows a right aortic arch (*large arrow*) with a large aortic diverticulum (*small arrow*) that protrudes to the left of the midline. The distal segment of the trachea is deviated to the left side by the right arch. Unlike double aortic arch, the left lateral margin of the trachea is not indented because the diverticulum is posterior and not lateral in position. *D.* Lateral view of similar patient, a healthy man. Note that both the esophagus and the trachea are markedly displaced anteriorly by a huge diverticulum, which invariably gives rise to the aberrant left subclavian artery.

TABLE 13-2

CARDIAC DEFECTS ASSOCIATED WITH EACH TYPE OF RIGHT-SIDED AORTIC ARCH

	Type of Anomaly	
	Avian	Common
Anatomic details	With mirror-image branching; the arch is anterior to the trachea	With aberrant left subclavian artery arising from a large aortic diverticulum that is posterior to the esophagus
Patients with cardiac defects, %	98	12
Type of defects, %		
Tetralogy of Fallot	90	71
Truncus arteriosus	2.5	
Transposition of great arteries	1.5	
Atrial septal defect and/or ventricular septal defect	0.5	21
Coarctation of aorta		7
Others	5.5	1

that of the accompanying bronchus where they are viewed on end. Normally the two structures have approximately equal diameters.[2,24] When the artery/bronchus ratio is greater than unity, increased blood flow is suggested. Conversely, when the ratio is smaller than unity (see Fig. 13-2), decreased flow is likely.

INCREASED PBF

In the case of mild to moderate left-to-right shunts, for example, the vessels dilate in proportion to the increased flow with no significant change in pressure, resistance, or flow pattern. This phenomenon is also called *shunt vascularity* or *equalization*. Equalization of PBF between the upper and lower lung zones is only apparent rather than real, however; the lower lobes still receive a great deal more blood than the upper lobes, although the ratio of PBF between the two zones has changed—e.g., from 5 to 1 to 4 to 1 or 3 to 1. A mild increase in pulmonary vascularity with slight cardiomegaly is commonly found in pregnant women and trained athletes

TABLE 13-3

MAJOR STEPS OF ROENTGENOLOGIC EXAMINATION

Roentgenographic examination for anatomy
  Overview, e.g., rib notching
  Pulmonary vascularity, e.g., shunt vascularity in ASD
  Lung parenchyma, e.g., ossification in critical MS
  Cardiac size, e.g., huge right heart in Ebstein's anomaly
  Cardiac contour, e.g., boot-shaped heart in TOF
  Abnormal densities, e.g., calcification of LV aneurysm
  Abnormal lucency, e.g., conspicuous fat stripes in PE
  Cardiac malpositions, e.g., dextrocardia with SS
  Other abnormalities, e.g., Holt-Oram syndrome
Fluoroscopic observation for dynamics
  Comparison
  Statistical guidance
  Clinical correlation

Abbreviations: ASD = atrial septal defect; MS = mitral stenosis; TOF = tetralogy of Fallot; LV = left ventricle; PE = pericardial effusion; SS = situs solitus.

with increased cardiac output and supernormal performance of the heart (see Chaps. 92 and 95).

DECREASED PBF

Patients with tetralogy of Fallot frequently show decreased pulmonary vascularity with smaller and shorter pulmonary arteries and veins and more radiolucent lungs (see Fig. 13-2*C*). Marked reduction in PBF is also encountered in patients with isolated right-sided heart failure without a right-to-left shunt (Fig. 13-7). This is attributed to the significant decrease in cardiac output from both ventricles.

TABLE 13-4

PULMONARY VASCULARITY

Normal
  Caudal PBF pattern in upright position (PBF controlled by gravity)
  Gradual branching, treelike
  RDPA = 10–15 mm in males
  RDPA = 9–14 mm in females
  A/B ratio = 1
Abnormal
  Volume with normal PBF pattern (distribution)
    Increased, larger vessels, e.g., ASD
    Decreased, smaller vessels, e.g., TOF
  Distribution with abnormal PBF pattern
    Cephalic, e.g., MS
    Centralized, e.g., Eisenmenger syndrome
    Lateralized, e.g., Westermark sign
    Localized, e.g., pulmonary AV fistulas
    Collateralized, e.g., severe TOF
Combined
  Decreased volume and cephalization, e.g., critical MS
  Lateralization and localization, e.g., scimitar syndrome

Abbreviations: RDPA = right descending pulmonary artery; A/B = artery/bronchus; PBF = pulmonary blood flow; ASD = atrial septal defect; TOF = tetralogy of Fallot; AV = arteriovenous; MS = mitral stenosis.

Abnormalities in Distribution

An abnormal distribution of PBF (or an abnormal PBF pattern) always reflects a changed pulmonary vascular resistance, either locally or diffusely.

CEPHALIZATION

In the presence of postcapillary pulmonary hypertension, physiologic disturbances may begin when the total intravascular pressure exceeds the oncotic pressure of the blood. As a result, fluid leaks out of the vessels and collects in the interstitium before pouring into the alveoli.

Pulmonary edema interferes with gas exchange, resulting in a state of hypoxemia. Alveolar hypoxia has a profound influence on the pulmonary vessels to constrict. Since there is greater alveolar hypoxia in the lung bases than in the apices, the basilar vessels constrict significantly, forcing the blood to flow upward. This phenomenon actually represents a reversal of the normal PBF pattern: redistribution or cephalization of the pulmonary vascularity.

Cephalization occurs in any of three conditions: (1) left-sided obstructive lesions, e.g., mitral stenosis (Fig. 13-3A)[22] or aortic stenosis; (2) left ventricular failure, e.g., coronary heart disease or cardiomyopathies; and (3) severe mitral regurgitation even before pump failure of the left ventricle occurs. It should be emphasized that unless there is obvious constriction of the lower-lobe vessels, the diagnosis of cephalization should not be made. Dilation of the upper lobe vessels is of secondary importance and can be found without narrowing of the basilar vessels in a number of entities, most noticeably left-to-right shunts.

CENTRALIZATION

In the presence of precapillary pulmonary hypertension, the pulmonary trunk and central pulmonary arteries dilate, whereas the distal pulmonary arteries constrict in a concentric fashion from the periphery of the lung toward the hilum. This phenomenon is called *centralization of the pulmonary vascularity*. It occurs in patients with primary pulmonary hypertension (Fig. 13-3B), Eisenmenger's syndrome, or severe obstructive emphysema (Fig. 13-7A and B).

LATERALIZATION

Massive unilateral pulmonary embolism may cause a lateralized PBF pattern. Since one major pulmonary artery is obstructed, the blood is forced to flow through the healthy lung only. The paucity of pulmonary vascularity in the diseased lung with the obstructed pulmonary artery is termed the *Westermark sign* (Fig. 13-3). In the case of congenital valvular pulmonary stenosis, a jet effect from the stenotic valve can cause a lateralized PBF pattern in favor of the left side (see Fig. 13-16).

LOCALIZATION

A localized abnormal flow pattern is exemplified by a congenital pulmonary arteriovenous fistula in a cyanotic child (see Fig. 13-3D).

COLLATERALIZATION

Patients with markedly decreased PBF (severe tetralogy of Fallot, for example) tend to show numerous small and tortuous bronchial arterial collaterals in the upper medial lung zones near their origin from the descending aorta. The native pulmonary arteries are extremely small, though smooth and branching gracefully (see Fig. 13-3E).

Combined Abnormalities

In reality, an abnormal pulmonary vascularity is often a mixed type. There is a great variety of possible combinations—e.g., cephalization plus decreased flow in severe mitral stenosis (see Fig. 13-3A) or centralization with increased PBF in Eisenmenger's atrial septal defect (Fig. 13-22).

Summary

Roentgen analysis of the pulmonary vasculature is accomplished in two steps. First, the volume of the pulmonary flow can be estimated by the degree of pulmonary arterial enlargement as long as the flow remains normal. Second, the distribution of the pulmonary flow is assessed by the presence of an abnormal flow pattern. The volume and the distribution of pulmonary blood flow may change singly or in combination depending on the nature and the severity of the underlying heart disease.

HEART FAILURE

In addition to specific chamber enlargement, the pulmonary vasculature uniquely portrays the underlying pathophysiology of heart failure. In the chronic setting, decreased flow with increased pulmonary lucency is the hallmark of right-sided heart failure (see Fig. 13-7); striking cephalization of the pulmonary vasculature is typical for left-sided decompensation (see Figs. 13-3A and 13-6B).

Left-Sided

ACUTE LEFT-SIDED HEART FAILURE

The pulmonary vascular changes associated with acute left ventricular failure are usually not discernible for two reasons: (1) The resultant severe pulmonary edema obscures the pulmonary vasculature and (2) the redistribution of PBF secondary to acute left-sided heart failure is usually relatively mild. The combination of alveolar pulmonary edema and a normal-sized heart is the hallmark of acute left-sided heart failure (see Fig. 13-6A),[10] most commonly seen in acute myocardial infarction. The edema fluid under this circumstance tends to distribute in a butterfly pattern.[25] The reason for this is poorly understood.

CHRONIC LEFT-SIDED HEART FAILURE

Chronic left-sided heart failure is characterized by striking cephalization of the pulmonary vasculature and interstitial pulmonary edema or fibrosis with multiple distinct Kerley

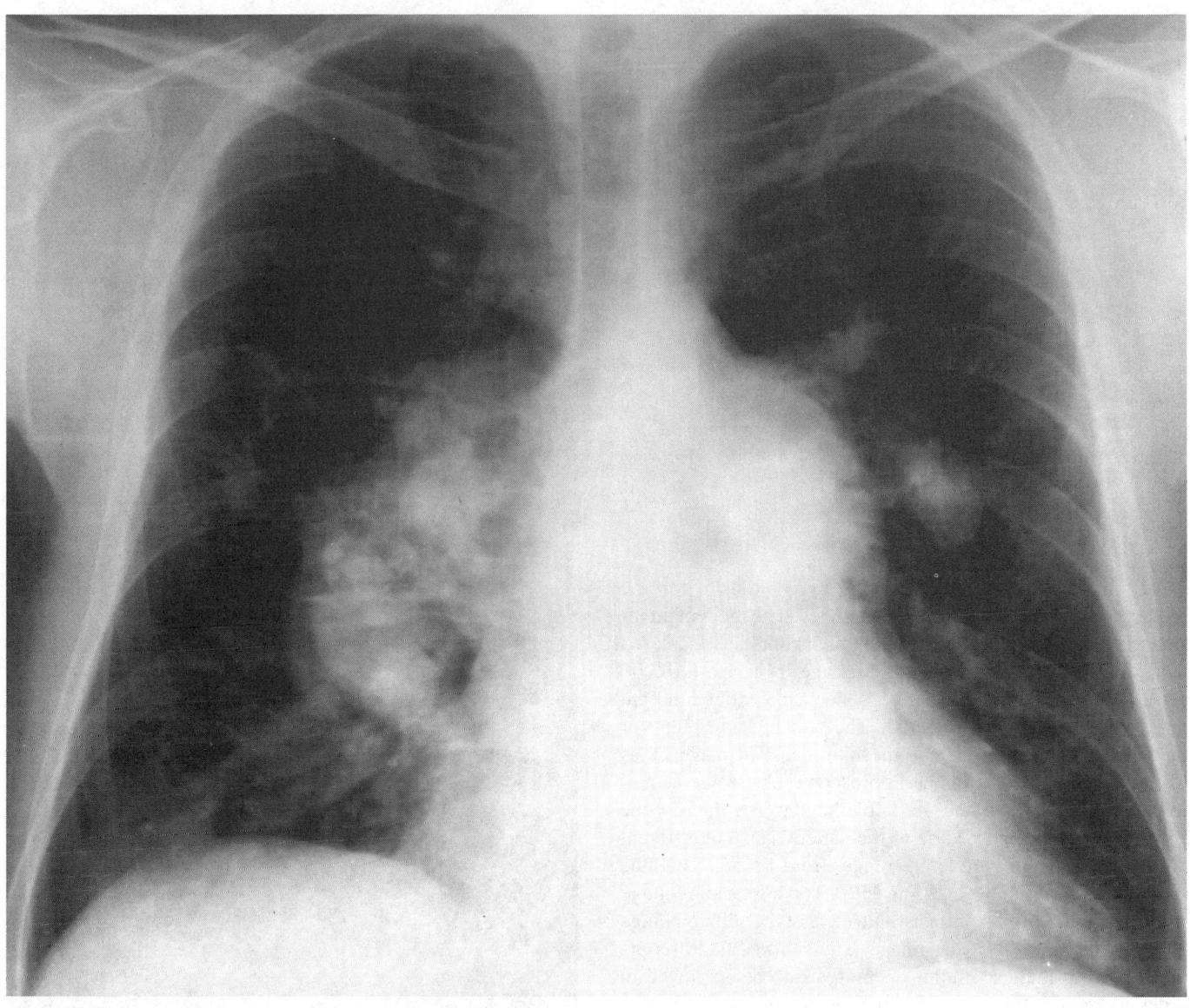

FIGURE 13-22
A 42-year-old man with Eisenmenger's atrial septal defect. Note increased pulmonary blood flow with a centralized pattern.

"B" lines. Pulmonary hemosiderosis, ossification, or both may result from long-standing severe postcapillary pulmonary hypertension (see Figs. 13-6B, C, D, and E).

Right-Sided

ACUTE RIGHT-SIDED HEART FAILURE
Acute right-sided heart failure most commonly results from massive pulmonary embolism. The typical radiographic signs are rapidly developing centralization of the pulmonary vasculature and dilation of the right-sided cardiac chambers and the venae cavae. In addition, the lungs may show localized or lateralized oligemia (see Fig. 13-3C). Eventually, opacities in either or both lungs may develop as a result of pulmonary infarction.

CHRONIC RIGHT-SIDED HEART FAILURE
Chronic right-sided heart failure has a number of causes. The common ones include congenital pulmonary stenosis, Ebstein's anomaly, severe chronic obstructive pulmonary disease, and recurrent pulmonary thromboembolic disease. Diffusely decreased pulmonary vascularity with unusually lucent lungs is seen in patients with right-sided heart failure without pulmonary hypertension (see Fig. 13-7C). Centralized PBF pattern is encountered when the right-sided heart failure is secondary to precapillary pulmonary hypertension (see Fig. 13-7A and B). A cephalized flow pattern with unusually lucent lungs is found in patients with right-sided heart failure (see Fig. 13-7D). The degree of right-sided chamber enlargement is proportional to the severity of tricuspid regurgitation.

Combined

It is generally believed that right-sided heart failure is most often caused by severe left-sided heart failure. This is exemplified by patients with severe mitral stenosis leading to severe tricuspid regurgitation (see Fig. 13-7D). Other examples of bilateral heart failure are cardiac tamponade and constrictive pericarditis, when both sides of the heart are affected (Fig. 13-23).

CARDIAC FLUOROSCOPY

Cardiac radiography deals primarily with anatomic details by filming at short exposure times that stop the motion. Cardiac fluoroscopy, on the other hand, explores the dynamic features of the organ that are discernible only in motion.[26] The two techniques are mutually complementary.

Description[2,17]

A good-quality image intensifier is a prerequisite for the proper performance of cardiac fluoroscopy. The modern intensifier with the use of cesium iodide phosphors has increased the brightness of the fluoroscopic image by at least 10,000 times. Television viewing permits cone vision under dim light with better perception of detail. The attached videotape or videodisk recorder provides a means for instant playback as well as future analysis of the fluoroscopic observation.

The milliamperage and the kilovoltage of the fluoroscope should be adjusted according to the patient's size in different projections. The milliamperage ranges from 1.5 to 3.5 and the kilovoltage varies between 90 and 120. Too high a kilovoltage tends to reduce the contrast, and excessive milliamperage blurs off the margin of the image. The shortest fluoroscopic time and the smallest shutter opening are to be employed in order to reduce the dose of radiation to the minimal. The average examining time for this author is 3 min.

The patient is routinely examined in the erect position with four views. The patient should be asked to stop breathing during the brief moment of fluoroscopy. A barium meal is given only after a thorough search for cardiac calcifications is completed. Occasionally, a recumbent position is used for better visualization of small calcifications as well as for a critical evaluation of cardiac asynergy. The cardiac output increases and the heart rate decreases on assuming recumbency, thereby giving a truer and more representative picture of the left ventricular contractility. In obese patients, the thick layer of soft tissues over the thorax is compressed and pushed aside, thereby improving the fluoroscopic image significantly.

Results

When properly performed, cardiac fluoroscopy is useful in the following areas of investigation: (1) assessment of cardiovascular dynamics; (2) detection of small cardiovascular calcifications; (3) visualization of important anatomic landmarks,

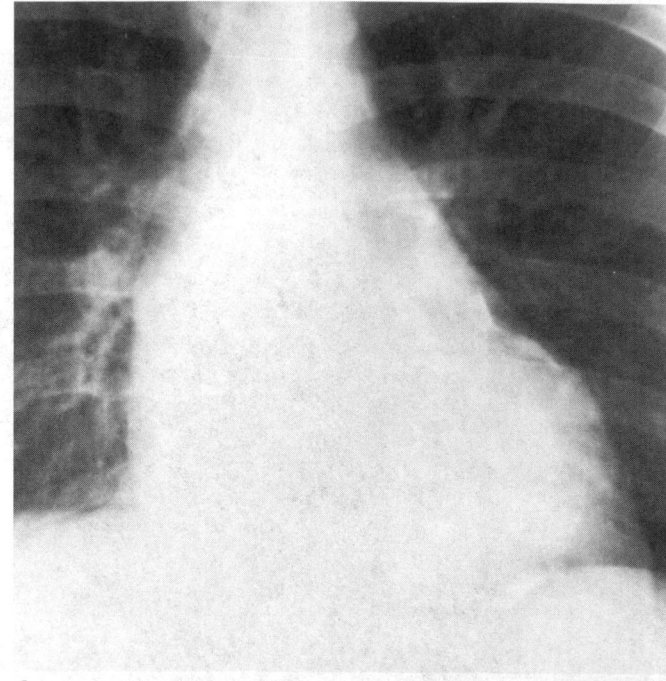

A

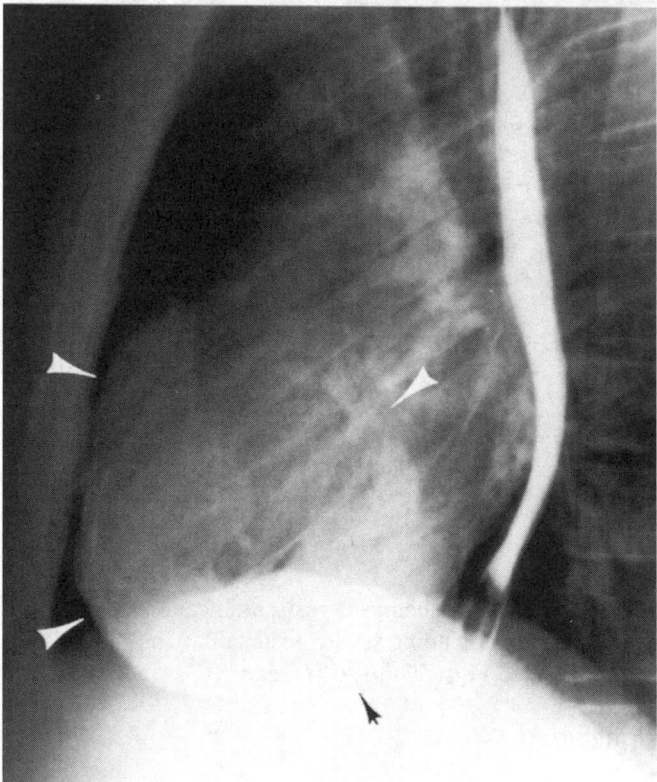

B

FIGURE 13-23

Patient with calcific constrictive pericarditis. Typically there is only mild postcapillary pulmonary hypertension due to left-sided constriction. Severe pulmonary venous congestion is prevented by the concurrent right-sided constriction. *A*. Posteroanterior view shows moderate cardiomegaly and mildly cephalic pulmonary blood flow pattern. *B*. Lateral view shows heavy calcification of the pericardium (*arrows*) and left atrial enlargement deviating the barium-filled esophagus posteriorly.

e.g., subepicardial fat stripes; (4) differentiation of cardiac from noncardiac disease; and (5) evaluation of cardiac valve prostheses, pacemakers, and radiopaque foreign bodies.

Precaution

Although no complication from modern fluoroscopy has been reported, both the patient and the examiner should be protected from excessive radiation. Even with an image intensifier, a routine cardiac fluoroscopy still involves more radiation than does two-view chest roentgenography. Therefore, the fluoroscopist should accomplish the task within the shortest possible period of time. Although all aspects of the heart are briefly surveyed, one should emphasize special areas of interest for each patient as suggested by the baseline radiographs. If coarctation of the aorta is suspected in a patient above 40 years of age, for instance, particular attention should be paid to finding calcium in a stenotic bicuspid aortic valve.

Application

ASSESSMENT OF CARDIOVASCULAR DYNAMICS[2,27–30]
The chest roentgenogram that is taken at random largely records the diastolic image of the heart. Fluoroscopy, on the other hand, provides a continuous vision of the pulsating organ through the entire cardiac cycle. On becoming familiar with the normal cardiovascular movements, the fluoroscopist will find that any deviation from the norm will be obvious.

The telltale x-ray signs of many cardiac lesions manifest themselves only in ventricular systole. Therefore, what may be missed on the film is often readily seen and diagnosed under the fluoroscope. For instance, left ventricular enlargement may be the only radiographic abnormality of severe aortic

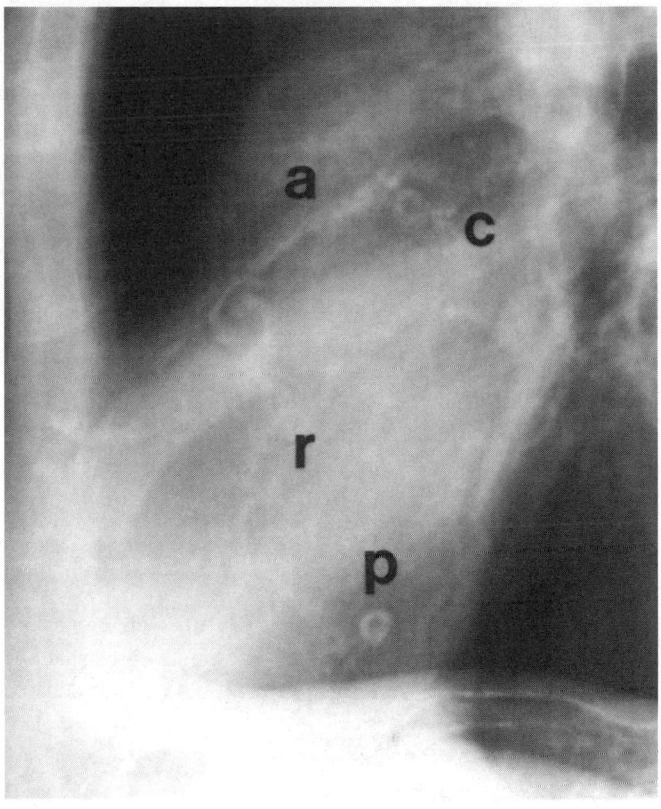

FIGURE 13-25
Lateral view shows heavy railroad track–like calcification of all three major coronary arteries: r = right coronary artery; a = anterior descending; c = circumflex; p = posterior descending. Note the ringlike densities representing vessels viewed on end.

regurgitation in children or young adults. On fluoroscopy, however, the aorta is vigorously expanding in systole and rapidly collapsing in diastole. This dynamic alternation is characteristic of aortic regurgitation (Fig. 13-24). Other examples include mild mitral regurgitation, mitral valve prolapse, left ventricular dyskinesia, and broad-based left ventricular aneurysm.

In valvular pulmonary stenosis, vigorous pulsation of the pulmonary trunk and its left branch is in bold contrast to the diminished pulsation of the right pulmonary artery.[29] Increased pulsation of diffusely enlarged pulmonary arteries is characteristic of left-to-right shunts. When marked discrepancy in size and pulsation is noted between the central and peripheral vessels, Eisenmenger's syndrome should be considered. Exaggerated left atrial expansion in ventricular systole is a reliable sign of mitral regurgitation.[30]

DETECTION OF CARDIOVASCULAR CALCIFICATIONS[3,8]
Heavy calcifications of the heart and vessels are easily detected by chest roentgenography, particularly in the lateral and oblique views (Fig. 13-25). Small calcifications, on the other hand, can be registered only by fluoroscopy by virtue of their rhythmic movements from the pulsating heart. Detection of even tiny coronary artery calcifications is of vital

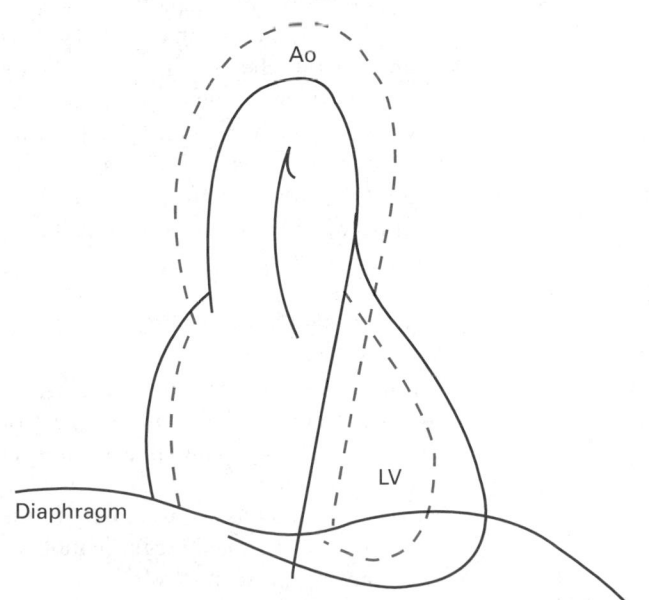

FIGURE 13-24
Schematic representation of dynamic changes of aortic regurgitation. Blue interrupted lines represent images in systole; solid lines, those in diastole.

practical importance. The combination of chest pain and coronary calcification results from major vascular obstruction 94 percent of the time.[15] Since the major coronary arteries are embedded in the subepicardial fat stripes in the grooves between cardiac chambers (Fig. 13-26), such fat stripes can be used effectively to locate the calcified arteries. Under the fluoroscope, the fat stripes present as pulsating radiolucent (bright) lines, in contrast to the accompanying pulsating radiopaque (dark) lines of calcified coronary arteries. If the artery coincides with the fat line within the left atrioventricular groove (aL), it portrays the circumflex coronary artery. The right coronary artery is moving synchronously with the right atrioventricular groove (aR). The anterior descending artery coincides with the anterior interventricular groove (vA), as does the posterior descending artery with the posterior interventricular groove (vP).

The lateral view is the best or the only view for the detection of a calcified right coronary artery. The left anterior oblique view at 20 to 30° is the most suitable for localizing the bifurcation of the left coronary artery. In this view, the left coronary artery is brought into relief between the hilar shadow anteriorly and the spinal column posteriorly. A ringlike density is frequently seen in this view, representing the end-on image of the calcified anterior descending artery. The right anterior oblique angle is used to view a calcified left main coronary artery. If both the anterior descending and the circumflex branches are also calcified, a Y-shaped density may be seen. The calcified cardiac valves, the myocardium, and the pericardium are easily confirmed by fluoroscopy.[2,27]

VISUALIZATION OF SUBEPICARDIAL FAT STRIPES

The subepicardial fat lines are important landmarks in the diagnosis of heart disease. The fat stripe is a cushionlike structure separating the myocardium from the pericardium. Normally it is difficult to see the fat line because of the adjacent similar radiolucency of the air-filled lung. The in-between hairline density of the normal pericardium is delicate and also difficult to see except in the left lateral view (Fig. 13-27A). In the presence of pericardial effusion or thickening, the subepicardial fat line is displaced interiorly and becomes more visible because of the added background of water density (Fig. 13-27B). The subepicardial fat pulsates with the contracting myocardium within the immobile band of pericardial fluid. This is diagnostic of pericardial effusion.[29] In contrast, when pericardial thickening alone is present, the exterior border of the heart pulsates with the fat line. This, in turn, suggests the diagnosis of pericardial constriction.

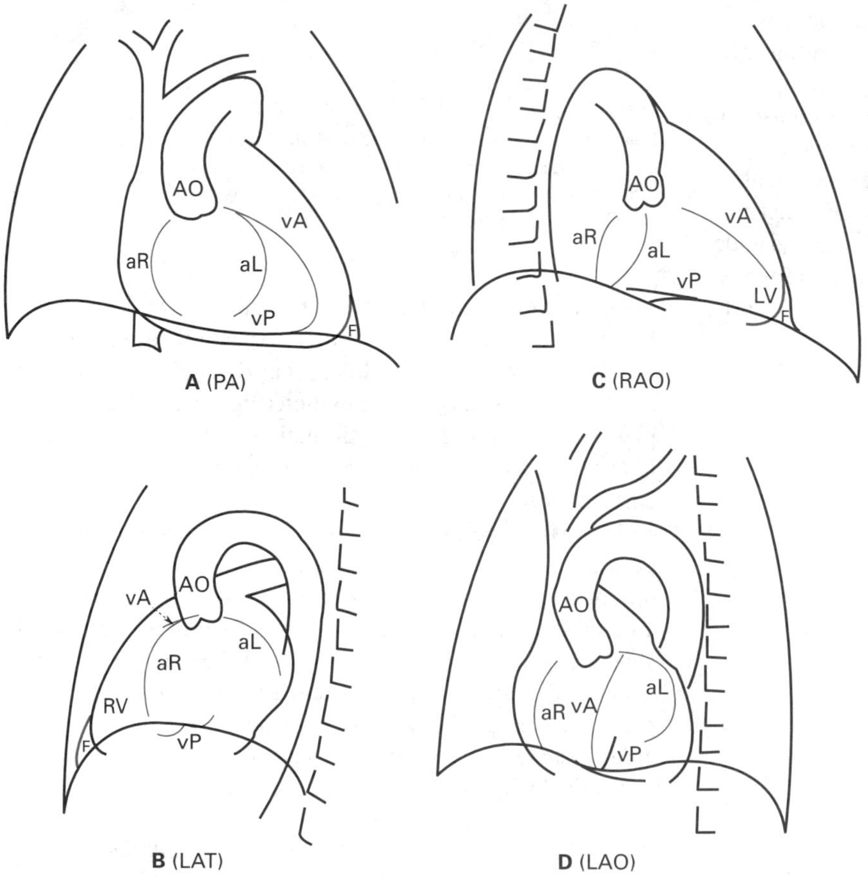

DIFFERENTIATION OF CARDIAC FROM NONCARDIAC DISEASE

When respiration is suspended, any structures that are moving are likely to be cardiovascular in nature. Conversely, noncardiac structures are immobile. This is exemplified by a bullet in the heart versus another in the chest wall. A pulmonary varix or an azygos vein collapses on Valsalva maneuver, with exaggerated pulsation following release of the breath. Enlarged lymph nodes in these areas, on the other hand, will not change with such maneuver.

EVALUATION OF VALVE PROSTHESES AND PACEMAKERS

The normal movements of cardiac valve prostheses are parallel between the two phases of cardiac cycle. If a significant angle of tilt (more than 12°) is formed between the two phases, instability of the valve with associated regurgitation is nearly always present.[2,28,31,32]

The bileaflet St. Jude valve[31] is used in both mitral and aortic positions. The valve is difficult to see radiographically (Fig. 13-28) but is readily detected under

FIGURE 13-26

Schematic representation of the subepicardial fat stripes in relation to major coronary arteries. *A*. Posteroanterior view. *B*. Lateral view. *C*. Right anterior oblique view. *D*. Left anterior oblique view. Abbreviations: aL = left atrioventricular groove (circumflex); aR = right atrioventricular groove (right); vA = anterior interventricular groove (anterior descending); vP = posterior interventricular groove (posterior descending); F = apical fat pad; AO = aorta; LV = left ventricle.

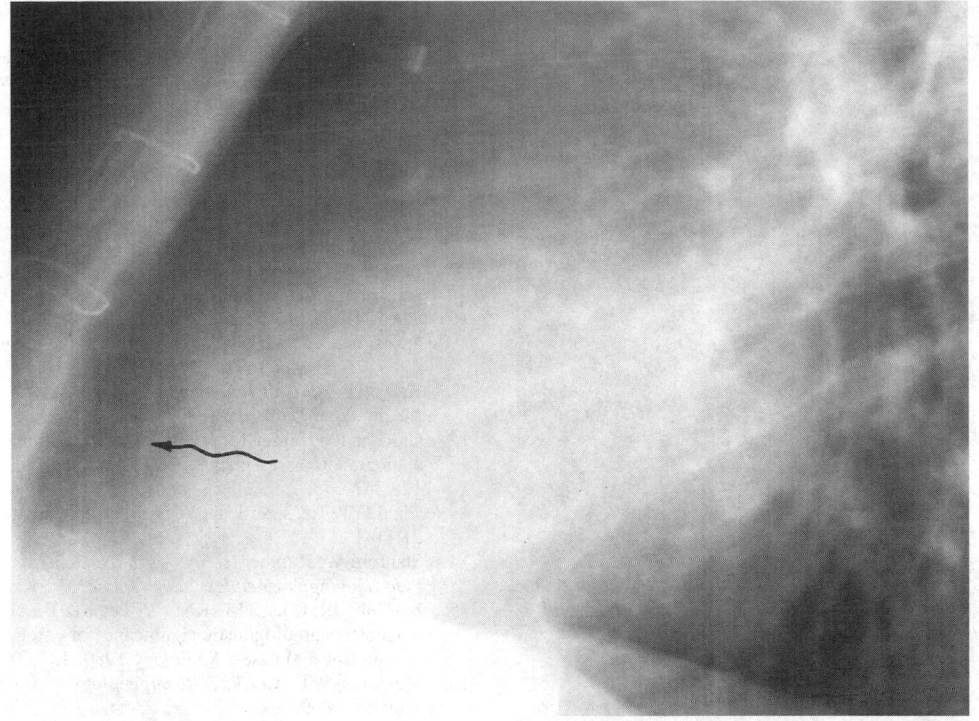

A

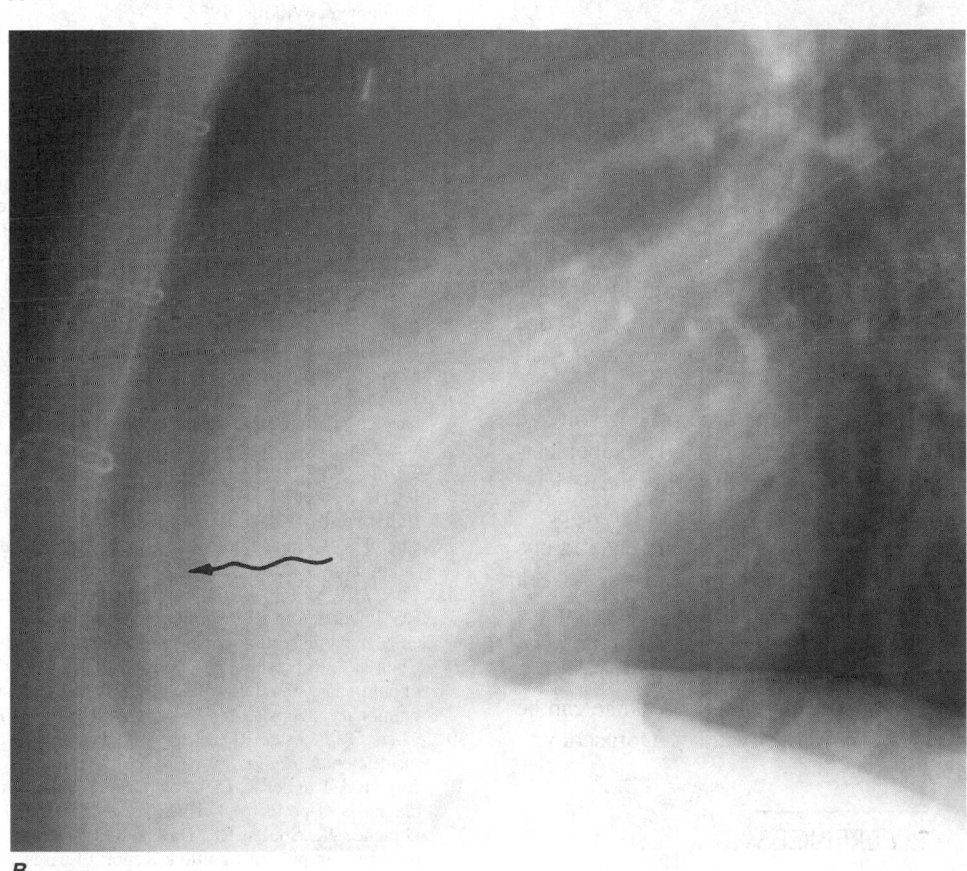

B

FIGURE 13-27

Subepicardial fat stripe in the diagnosis of pericardial effusion. *A*. Lateral view in a patient 3 weeks after coronary bypass procedure showing a normal pericardium as a hairline density (*arrow*) sandwiched between the subepicardial fat stripe interiorly and the mediastinal fat exteriorly. The maximal width of normal pericardium is 2 mm. *B*. Lateral view of same patient, who developed postpericardiotomy syndrome 2 weeks later. Note widening of the pericardium (*arrow*) representing the large pericardial effusion. The fat stripes were now widely separated by the water density and became much more conspicuous.

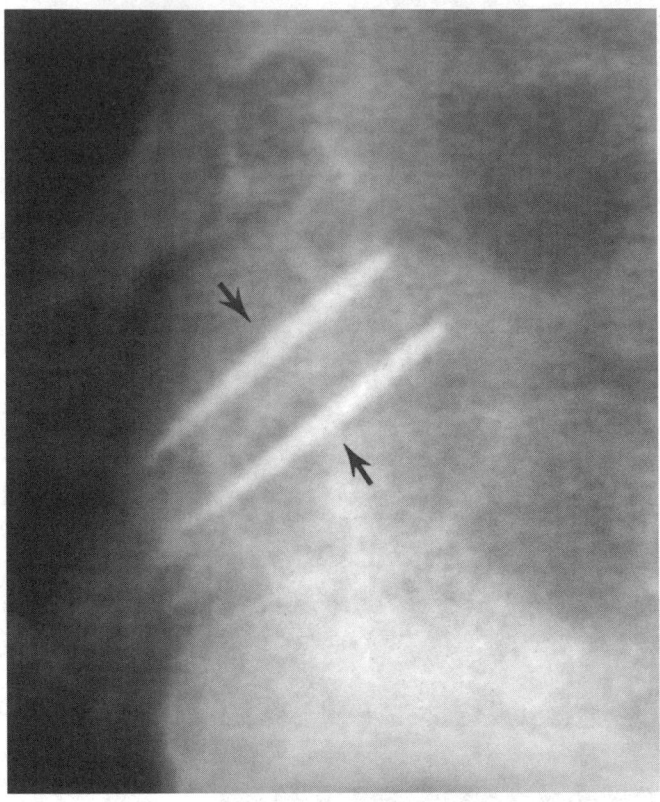

FIGURE 13-28

Patient with congenitally corrected transposition of the great arteries. The left-sided atrioventricular valve was replaced with a St. Jude prosthesis. The valve was caught in the opened position (in diastole), when both leaflets were seen as a pair of parallel lines (*arrows*). The same valve was invisible in the closed position (*not shown*).

the fluoroscope.[1,31] When the leaflets move sluggishly, thrombotic stenosis of the valve should be suspected. Rarely, one leaflet may dislodge and embolize distally, causing acute valvular regurgitation.[33]

The position of the pacemaker can be promptly determined under the fluoroscope and recorded on film.[2,34] The subepicardial fat line overlies the myocardium and underlies the pericardium. If the pacing catheter is found within the fat stripe, it may have passed through the coronary sinus and entered one of the major cardiac veins. If the tip of the catheter is seen outside the fat stripe, however, it may have perforated the myocardium and thus be lying in the pericardium.[2,34] Although the wires and electrodes of a transmediastinal pacemaker may look normal on the films, minor breakage can be appreciated only in ventricular systole by aid of fluoroscopy.[34]

REFERENCES

1. Röentgen WB. *New Forms of Radiation*. Würzburg, Germany: Würzburger Physical Medical Society; December 28, 1895.
2. Chen JTT. *Essentials of Cardiac Roentgenology*. Boston: Little, Brown; 1987.
3. Chen JTT. The plain radiograph in the diagnosis of cardiovascular disease. In: Putnam C, ed. Symposium on cardiopulmonary imaging. *Radiol Clin North Am* 1983; 21:609–621.
4. Juhl JH, Grummy AB. *Essentials of Radiologic Imaging*, 6th ed. Philadelphia: Lippincott; 1993:1065–1138.
5. Meschan I, Formanek A. Roentgenology of the heart inclusive of major vessels. In Meschan I, ed. *Roentgen Signs in Diagnostic Imaging*, 2d ed. Philadelphia: Saunders; 1987:784–925.
6. Figley M. Accessory roentgen signs of coarctation of the aorta. *Radiology* 1954; 62:671–686.
7. Elliott LP, Jue KL, Amplatz K. A roentgen classification of cardiac malpositions. *Invest Radiol* 1966; 1:17–28.
8. Elliott LP, Schiebler GL. *X-ray Diagnosis of Congenital Cardiac Disease*, 2d ed. Springfield, IL: Charles C Thomas; 1979.
9. deLeon AC, Perloff JK, Twigg HL. The straight back syndrome: Clinical and cardiovascular manifestations. *Circulation* 1965; 32:193–203.
10. Chen JTT, Capp MP, Johnsrude IS, Goodrich JK, Lester RG. Roentgen appearance of pulmonary vascularity in the diagnosis of heart disease. *Am J Roentgenol* 1971; 112:559–570.
11. Keats TE. *Atlas of Roentgenographic Measurement*, 6th ed. St Louis, Mosby–Year Book, 1990:393–450.
12. Chickos PM, Figley MM, Fisher L. Correlation between chest film and angiographic assessment of left ventricular size. *J Roentgenol* 1977; 128:367–373.
13. Chen JTT. The significance of cardiac calcifications. *Appl Radiol* 1992; 21:11–19.
14. Stanford W, Rumberger JA. *Ultrafast Computed Tomography in Cardiac Imaging: Principles and Practice*. Mt. Kisco, NY: Futura; 1992.
15. Margolis JR, Chen JTT, Kong Y, Peter RH, Behar VS, Kisslo JA. The diagnostic and prognostic significance of coronary artery calcification: A report of 800 cases. *Radiology* 1980; 137:609–616.
16. Meszaros WT. *Cardiac Roentgenology*. Springfield, IL: Charles C Thomas; 1969.
17. Cooley RN. *Radiology of the Heart and Great Vessels*, 3d ed. Baltimore: Williams & Wilkins; 1978.
18. Swischuck LE. *Plain Film Interpretation in Congenital Heart Disease*, 2d ed. Baltimore: Williams & Wilkins; 1979.
19. Shuford WH, Sybers RG. *The Aortic Arch and Its Malformations*. Springfield, IL: Charles C Thomas; 1974:18.
20. Stewart JR, Kincaid OW, Titus JL. Right aortic arch: Plain film diagnosis and significance. *Am J Roentgenol* 1966; 97:377–389.
21. Fraser RG, Pare JAP, Pare PD, Fraser RS, Genereux GP. Factors influencing pulmonary circulation. In: Fraser RG, Pare JAP, Pare PD, Fraser RS, Genereux GP, eds. *Diagnosis of Diseases of the Chest*, 3d ed. Vol I. Philadelphia: Saunders; 1988:128–129.
22. Chen JTT, Behar VS, Morris JJ, McIntosh HD, Lester RG. Correlation of roentgen findings with hemodynamic data in pure mitral stenosis. *Am J Roentgenol* 1968; 102:280–292.
23. Milne ENC. Some new concepts of pulmonary blood flow and volume. *Radiol Clin North Am* 1978; 16:515–536.
24. Wojtowicz J. Some tomographic criteria for an evaluation of the pulmonary circulation. *Acta Radiol [Diagn] (Stockh)* 1964; 2:215–224.
25. Fleischner FG. The butterfly pattern of acute pulmonary edema. *Am J Cardiol* 1967; 20:39–000.
26. Jeffers K, Rees S, eds. *Clinical Cardiac Radiology*, 2d ed. London: Butterworths; 1980.
27. Chen JTT. Cardiac fluoroscopy. In: Kelley MJ, ed. Symposium on chest radiography for the cardiologist. *Cardiol Clin* 1983; 1:565–573.
28. Chen JTT, McIntosh HD, Capp MP, Morris JJ Jr, Canent RV Jr, Lester RG. Intercalative angiocardiography: A method for recording cardiovascular dynamics on a single film. *Radiology* 1969; 93:499–506.
29. Chen JTT, Robinson AE, Goodrich JK, Lester RG. Uneven distribution of pulmonary blood flow between left and right lungs in isolated valvular pulmonary stenosis. *Am J Roentgenol* 1969; 107:343–350.
30. Chen JTT, Lester RG, Peter RH. Posterior wedging sign of mitral insufficiency. *Radiology* 1974; 113:451–453.
31. Jorgens J, Kundel R, Lieber A. The cinefluorographic approach to the diagnosis of pericardial effusion. *Am J Roentgenol* 1962; 87:911–916.
32. Gimenez JL, Soulen RL, Davila JC. Prosthetic valve detachment: Its roentgenographic recognition: Report of cases. *Am J Roentgenol* 1968; 103:595–600.
33. Kotler MN, Panidis J, Mintz GS, Monaco O, Morris GC, Moschetto A. The role of noninvasive technique in the evaluation of the St. Jude cardiac prosthesis. In: DeBakey ME, ed. *Advances in Cardiac Valves: Clinical Perspectives*. New York: York; 1983:213–226.
34. Sorkin RP, Schuurmann BJ, Simon AB. Radiographic aspects of permanent cardiac pacemakers. *Radiology* 1976; 119:281–286.

14

THE ECHOCARDIOGRAM

Anthony N. DeMaria / Daniel G. Blanchard

The term *echocardiography* refers to the evaluation of cardiac structure and function with images and recordings produced by ultrasound. Although it was not until the early 1970s that echocardiography initially began to diffuse into clinical practice, it has rapidly become a fundamental component of cardiac evaluation. Currently, echocardiography provides essential (and sometimes unexpected) clinical information and has become the second most frequency performed diagnostic procedure after electrocardiography.[1] What began as a one-dimensional method performed from the precordial area to assess cardiac anatomy has evolved into a two-dimensional modality performed from either the thorax or from within the esophagus, capable of also delineating flow and deriving hemodynamic data.[2] Technical developments currently under way promise to extend the capacity of ultrasound to routine three-dimensional visualization[3] as well as to the assessment of myocardial perfusion in conjunction with contrast agents.[4]

Although several attempts to study the heart with ultrasound were carried out earlier, the development of echocardiography is usually credited to Elder and Hertz in 1954.[5] Primitive cross-sectional images of the excised human heart were produced in 1957[6]; however, for nearly two additional decades clinical echocardiography consisted primarily of one-dimensional time-motion (M-mode) recordings as popularized by Feigenbaum.[7] In the mid-1970s, Bom and associates developed a multielement linear array scanner that could produce spatially correct images of the beating heart.[8] Two-dimensional images of superior quality were soon achieved by mechanical sector scanners[9,10] and ultimately by phased-array instruments as developed by Thurston and Von Ramm, which are the present-day standard.[11]

Although efforts to use the Doppler principle to measure flow velocity by ultrasound were begun in the early 1970s by Baker et al.,[12] clinical application of this technique did not blossom until the work of Hatle in the early 1980s.[13,14] Pulsed and continuous-wave Doppler recordings soon were expanded to full two-dimensional color-flow imaging.[15] Most recently, miniaturization of ultrasound transducers has led to their incorporation into gastroscopes and cardiac catheters to achieve transesophageal and intravascular images.[16,17]

PRINCIPLES OF ECHOCARDIOGRAPHY

Physics and Instrumentation

Sound is an energy form that travels through a medium as a series of alternating compressions and rarefactions of the molecules (Fig. 14-1). Sound is typically characterized by its wavelength, which is the distance between any two consecutive phases of the cycle (e.g., peak compression to peak compression), and by its frequency, which is the number of wavelengths per unit time (customarily expressed as cycles per second or Hz). Since the velocity of sound is the product of wavelength and frequency, there is an inverse relationship between these two characteristics; the greater the frequency, the shorter the wavelength. Ultrasound is sonic energy with a frequency above the audible range of the human ear (greater than 20,000 Hz), and is useful for diagnostic imaging, since, like light, it can be directed as a beam that will obey the laws of reflection and refraction.[14–18] Thus, an ultrasound beam will travel in a straight line through a homogeneous medium. If the beam meets an interface of different acoustic impedance, however, part of the energy will be reflected, and the remaining attenuated signal will be transmitted. The reflected energy, or echo, is used to construct an image—in the case of echocardiography, an image of the heart (Fig. 14-2).

The most fundamental component of any echocardiographic instrument is the transducer, which is responsible for both transmitting and receiving the ultrasound signal. The transducer consists of electrodes and a piezoelectric crystal whose ionic structure results in deformation of shape when exposed to an electric current.[18] Thus, piezoelectric crystals are composed of synthetic materials such as barium titanate that, when exposed to electric current from the electrodes, alternately expand and contract to create sound waves. When subjected to the mechanical energy of sound returning from a reflecting surface, the same piezoelectric element changes shape, thereby generating an electrical signal detected by the electrodes (Fig 14-3). In this way, the transducer both produces and receives ultrasonic signals.

As an imaging modality, ultrasound carries with it several unique technical difficulties. Sound energy is poorly transmitted through air and bone, and the ability to record adequate images is dependent upon a thoracic window that gives the

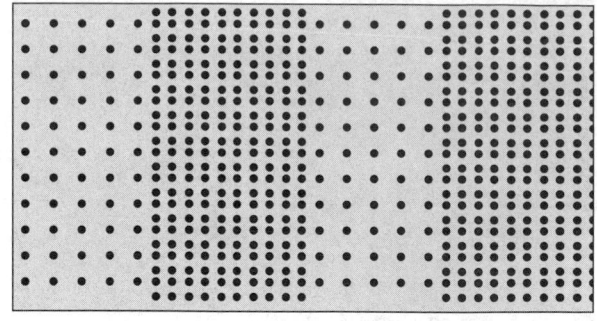

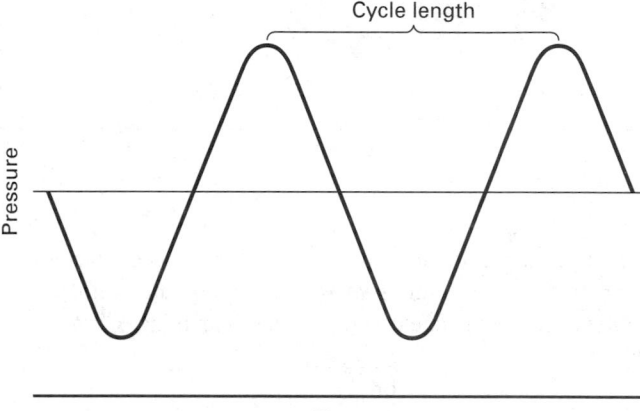

FIGURE 14-1

Sound energy results in alternating compression and rarefaction of particles in a conducting medium. This alternation, which can be plotted against time (or distance), conforms to a sine wave pattern (*bottom panel*). (Modified from Hagan AD, DeMaria AN. *Clinical Applications of Two-Dimensional Echocardiography and Cardiac Doppler.* Boston: Little, Brown; 1989, with permission.)

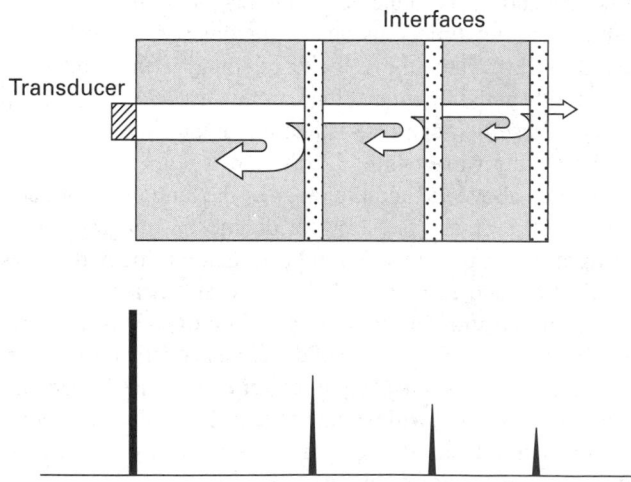

FIGURE 14-2

Upper panel: Attenuation of an ultrasound beam emitted from a transducer. There is reflection and progressive loss of energy at each interface encountered. *Lower panel:* the reflected wavefronts are recorded as signals of varying amplitudes (A-mode) via the piezoelectric crystal. (Upper panel modified from Hagan AD, DeMaria AN. *Clinical Applications of Two-Dimensional Echocardiography and Cardiac Doppler.* Boston: Little, Brown; 1989, with permission).

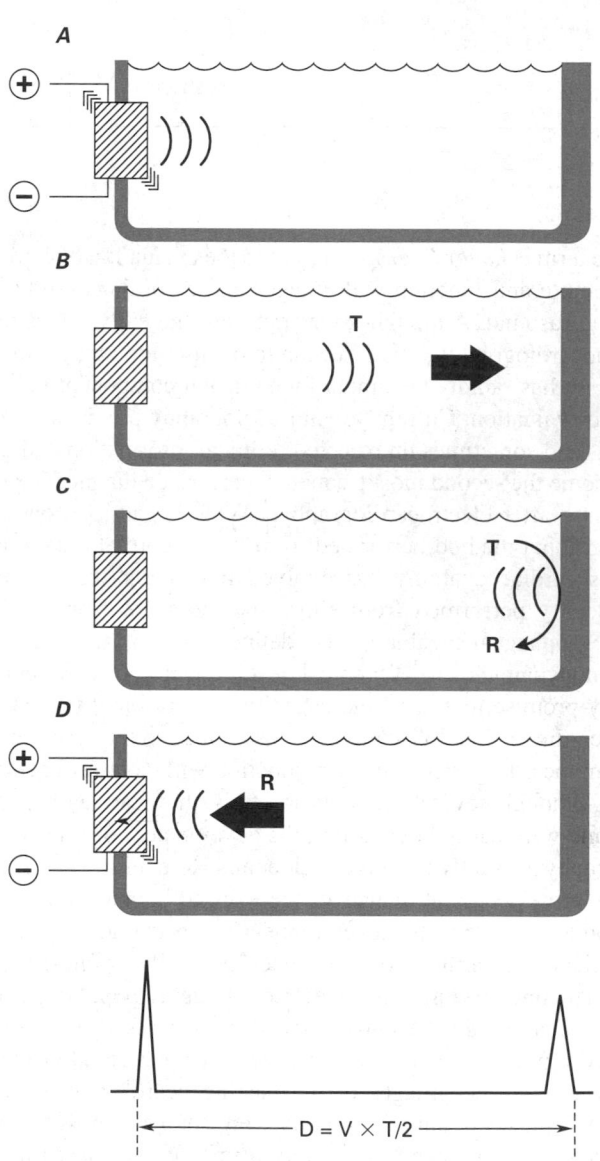

FIGURE 14-3

A through *D:* the basic principle of ultrasonic imaging. The piezoelectric crystal is activated, producing a transmitted pulse (T), which reflects off the interface. The reflected pulse (R) excites the crystal, producing an electric current. As the velocity of the pulse is constant, distance can be calculated based on the transit time. (Because the pulse must travel back and forth from the interface, the time is divided by 2). (Modified from Weyman AE. *Principles and Practice of Echocardiography,* 2d ed. Philadelphia: Lea & Febiger; 1994, with permission.)

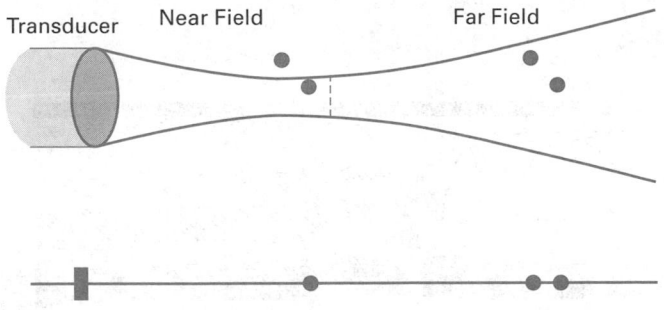

FIGURE 14-4

Upper panel: The transducer emits an ultrasonic beam that has a near field (where the beam is relatively focused) and a far field (where the beam width increases). *Lower panel:* B-mode diagram showing the effect of beam width. In the near field, the beam reflects off only one of two objects in close proximity to each other. In the far field, however, two similarly positioned objects are both within the beam width. Therefore, lateral resolution is compromised and the objects' positions are misrepresented.

interrogating beam adequate access to cardiac structures. The degree to which ultrasonic energy will be reflected when striking an interface of differential impedance is dependent upon how perpendicular the interrogating beam is to the interface. When the ultrasound beam is directed parallel or near parallel to the interface, little or no sound energy will be reflected to the transducer. Therefore, poor signal transmission, a nonorthogonal orientation of the ultrasound beam to the surface, and energy attenuation can result in failure to record signals from cardiac structures—a phenomenon referred to as *echo dropout*.[19] Conversely, some structures may be such strong ultrasonic reflectors—by virtue of being perpendicular to the beam or extremely dense—that sufficient energy returns to the transducer to be reflected and again transmitted into the field. This phenomenon can lead to reverberations, or the reproduction of the echoes of anatomic structures at multiple locations within the image.[20] Finally, since the ultrasound beam diverges with distance from the transducer and always has a finite width, targets lying on the periphery of the beam may be recorded and displayed as if they were located along the central scan line (Fig. 14-4). This problem may be accentuated in the setting of very strong reflectors and result in the formation of *side lobes*.[21] In either case, beam-width problems associated with ultrasound may result in depicting targets in erroneous locations and create problems in interpreting the images.[22]

The construction of a cardiac image from ultrasonic signals is based upon computation of the distance between an anatomic structure and the transducer (Fig. 14-3). Thus, an ultrasound beam is produced by a hand-held transducer positioned on the thorax and directed into the heart. This beam will travel in a straight line until it reaches an interface between structures of different acoustic impedance, such as blood and myocardium. At this point, some ultrasonic energy will be reflected (depending on the density of interface), some will be scattered, and some will continue forward. The amplitude of the propagating signal will be attenuated because of the reduction in energy at the interface (Fig. 14-2). The reflected sound waves return to the transducer and form the basis of the echogram. Electronic circuitry within the echograph measures the time interval required for the transit of the ultrasound beam from the transducer to the interface and back again. Since the velocity of sound in soft tissue is constant (approximately 1540 m/s), the instrument can calculate the total distance traveled to and from the reflecting surface as the product of transit time and velocity of sound. Interface location is derived as one-half of the total transit distance, and a signal is depicted on an oscilloscope or video monitor at that point (Fig. 14-3). The amplitude of ultrasonic energy reflected from each target interface is represented by the brightness of the signal that is displayed.

The one-dimensional ultrasonic B- (or brightness) mode scan line resulting from a single transmitted beam is the cornerstone of echocardiographic imaging. In the most basic form of echocardiography, a single scan line produced by a piezoelectric crystal is passed through the heart (Fig. 14-5). At each structural interface, ultrasonic energy is reflected back and displayed at the appropriate distance as a signal, whose amplitude represents the acoustic impedance or density of the material encountered. These signals are subsequently displayed as dots, whose brightness is proportional to the amplitude of reflected ultrasonic energy. The distance from the transducer of these *B*-mode dots changes as the cardiac structures move during the cardiac cycle. Accordingly, if repetitive B-mode scan lines are produced and swept across the screen

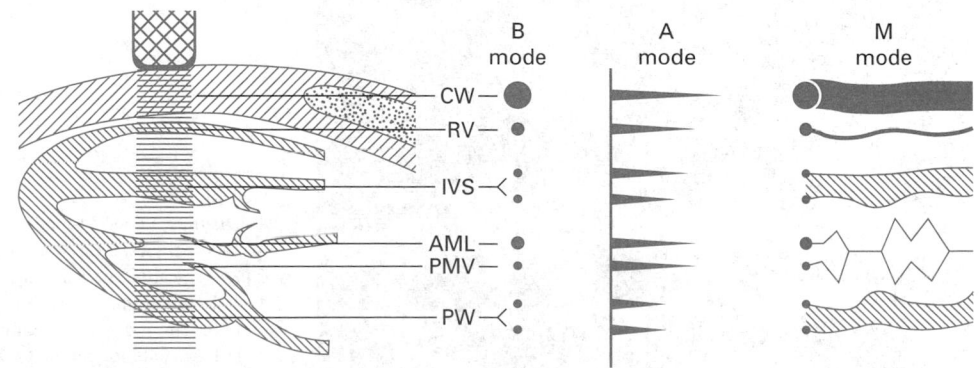

FIGURE 14-5

Formation of A-mode, B-mode, and M-mode echocardiograms. The transducer emits an ultrasound beam, which reflects at each anatomic interface. The reflected wavefronts can be represented as dots (B mode) or spikes (A mode). The dot brightness and spike magnitude vary with the amplitude of the reflected wave. If the B-mode scan is swept from left to right with time, an M-mode image is produced. (Modified from Hagan AD, DeMaria AN. *Clinical Applications of Two-Dimensional Echocardiography and Cardiac Doppler.* Boston: Little, Brown; 1989, with permission.)

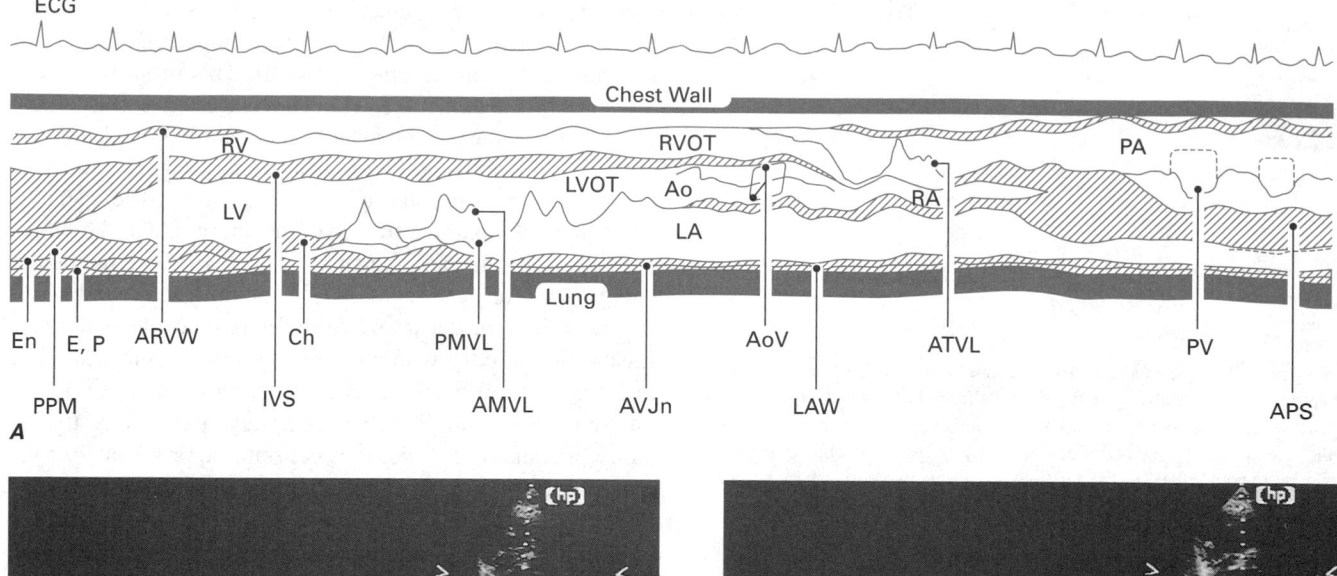

ECG

Chest Wall

RV   RVOT   PA

LV   LVOT   Ao   RA
LA

En   E, P   ARVW   Ch   PMVL   Lung   AoV   ATVL   PV

PPM   IVS   AMVL   AVJn   LAW   APS

A

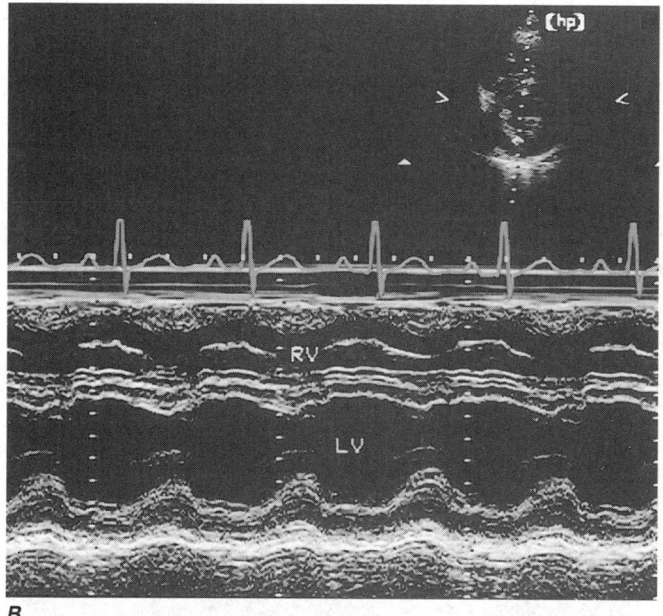

RV

LV

B

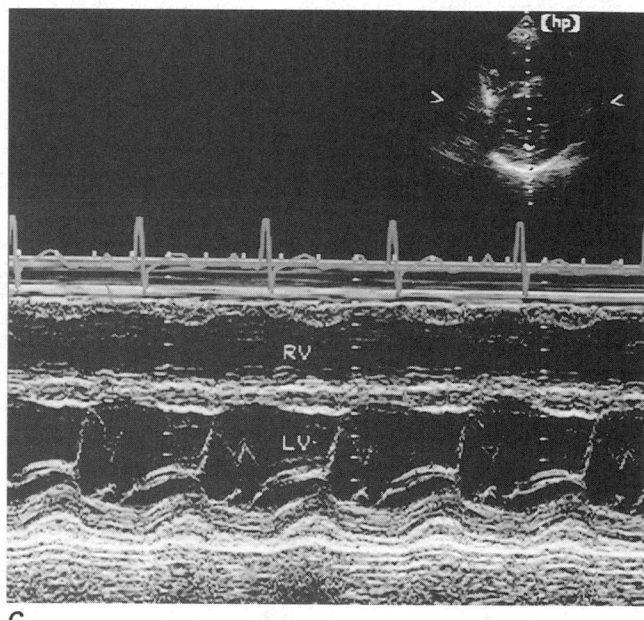

RV

LV

C

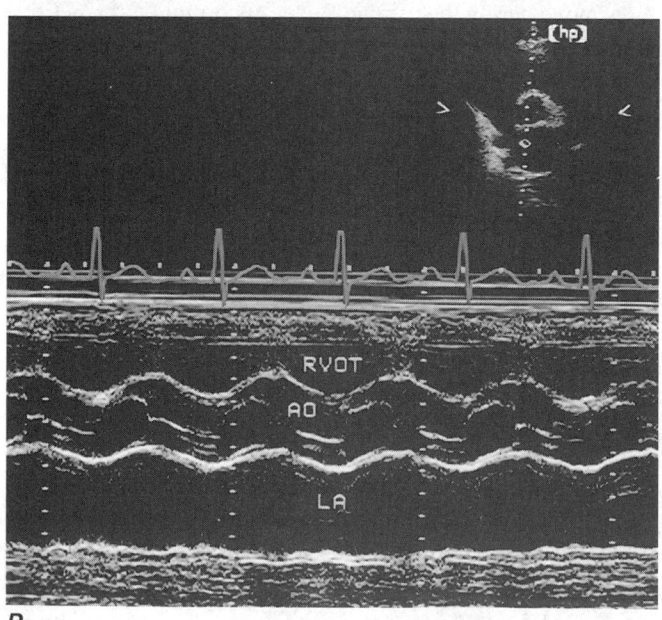

RVOT

AO

LA

D

FIGURE 14-6

A. Diagram of an M-mode sweep from apex to base in a normal heart (parasternal view). En = endocardium; PPM = posterior papillary muscle; E,P = epicardial/pericardial interface; ARVW = anterior right ventricular wall; RV = right ventricle; LV = left ventricle; IVS = interventricular septum; Ch = chordae tendineae; PMVL = posterior mitral valve leaflet; AMVL = anterior mitral valve leaflet; LVOT = left ventricular outflow tract; AV Jn = atrioventricular junction; RVOT = right ventricular outflow tract; Ao = aorta; LA = left atrium; AoV = aortic valve; LAW = left atrial wall; RA = right atrium; ATVL = anterior tricuspid valve leaflet; PA = pulmonary artery; PV = pulmonary valve; APS = atriopulmonic sulcus. (From Felner JM, Schlant RC. *Echocardiography; A Teaching Atlas.* New York: Grune & Stratton; 1976, with permission.) *B–D.* M-mode sweep from apex to base in a normal individual.

over time, the movement of the heart can be obtained as a time-motion (or "M"-mode) recording,[23] providing dynamic rather than merely static cardiac images (Fig. 14-5). In clinical use, the piezoelectric crystal within the transducer is activated by alternating electric current to transient at a rate of approximately 1000 pulses per second. This same crystal also receives the returning echo reflections and actually spends the great majority of the time (>90 percent) in the "receive" rather than "transmit" mode. Because the beam is confined to a single location and transmits ultrasound signals at the pulse rate of the transducer, M-mode echocardiography provides very high temporal resolution. Not surprisingly, M-mode is an excellent modality for timing cardiac events or recording high-velocity motion.

As ultrasound technology advanced and it became possible to determine accurately the spatial orientation of the interrogating beam, multiple B-mode scan lines from different imaging angles were collected and displayed in proper alignment to create a two-dimensional image. As opposed to B- or M-mode recordings, which are unidimensional (on an anterior-posterior axis) two-dimensional echocardiography provides additional information in either superior-inferior or medial-lateral directions. At the current time, M-mode recordings are derived from the two-dimensional images rather than as a stand-alone signal.

Several characteristics of sound energy are of fundamental importance in determining the quality of the images obtained. High-quality images require optimal resolution—that is, the ability to distinguish two individual objects separated in space. Short wavelengths yield excellent resolution in echo imaging, since the shorter the cycle length, the smaller the object that will reflect the signal and be detected by the echo scanner. Since wavelength is inversely related to frequency, transducers that emit a high-frequency signal (3.5 to 7.0 MHZ or greater) yield high-resolution images. High-frequency signals also overcome an important limitation of ultrasonic imaging associated with lateral resolution. Since ultrasonic beams diverge as they propagate away from the transducer, the width of the beam can become sufficiently great to encompass multiple targets and diminish resolution (Fig. 14-4). The degree of beam divergence is less with high-frequency sonic energy than with low-frequency signals. The smaller wavelengths associated with high-frequency signals, however, are subject to greater reflection and scattering (therefore substantially higher attenuation) as the beam propagates through tissue. The re-sultant attenuation is greater than that with low-frequency signals and leads to decreased sensitivity. Therefore, in clinical practice, echocardiographic examinations are performed utilizing the highest-frequency transducer capable of obtaining signals from all potential targets within the ultrasound field.[23]

M-Mode Echocardiography

THE STANDARD M-MODE EXAMINATION

Although largely supplanted by two-dimensional imaging, M-mode echocardiography remains a useful part of a complete ultrasound examination. Figure 14-6A through D shows the typical views obtained when the transducer is placed at the left parasternal area and rocked through the heart from apex to base. Tissue typically reflects ultrasound at its surface (specular reflectors) and from internal inhomogenicity (backscatter), while blood is homogenous and does not produce reflections. Thus, blood is free of ultrasonic signals on the echocardiogram. At the mitral valve level (Fig. 14-6C), the cardiac structure seen closest to the transducer is the right ventricular free wall; it is followed by the right ventricular cavity, the interventricular septum, the mitral valve apparatus, and the left ventricular posterior wall as the beam travels backward. At this level, mitral valve excursion is well seen and is more easily recorded for the longer anterior leaflet. For the anterior leaflet, diastolic mitral opening is bipeaked (M-shaped) with maximal opening during early diastolic filling at the E point, a subsequent reclosure downslope to the F point, and a reopening with atrial contraction at the A point, prior to valve closure at the C point[24] (Fig. 14-7). The posterior leaflet manifests a mirror-image W-shaped pattern. In some

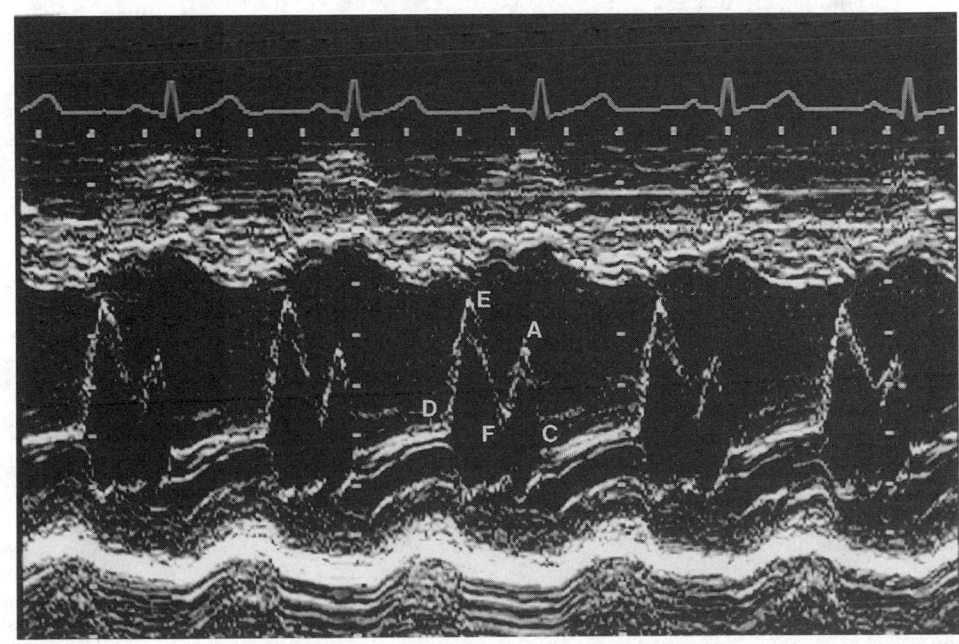

FIGURE 14-7
Standard M-mode image through the left ventricle at the level of the mitral valve. See text for discussion of nomenclature.

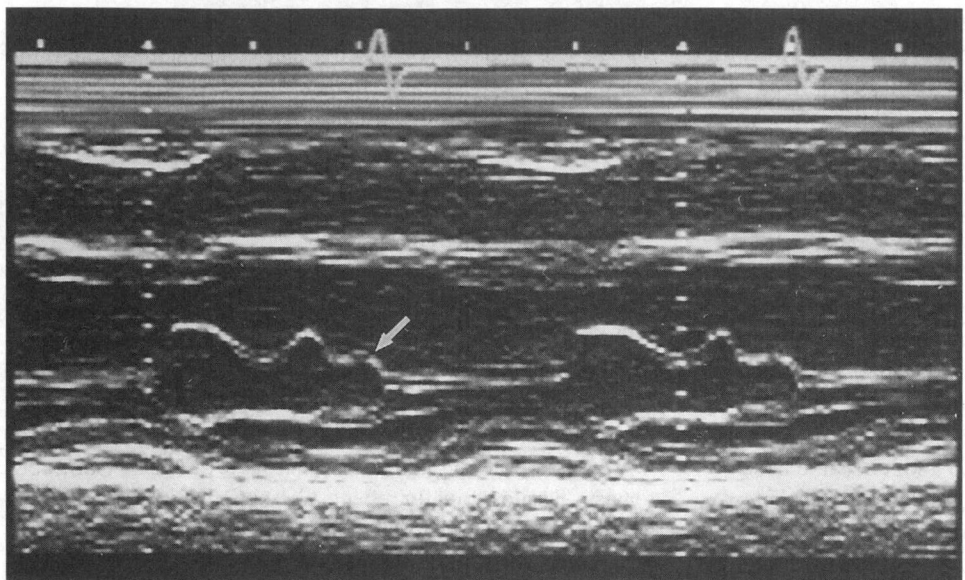

FIGURE 14-8
M-mode image through the mitral valve showing a "B-bump," suggesting high left ventricular diastolic pressure (*arrow*). The E-point septal separation is also increased. (Transducer is in the left parasternal position.)

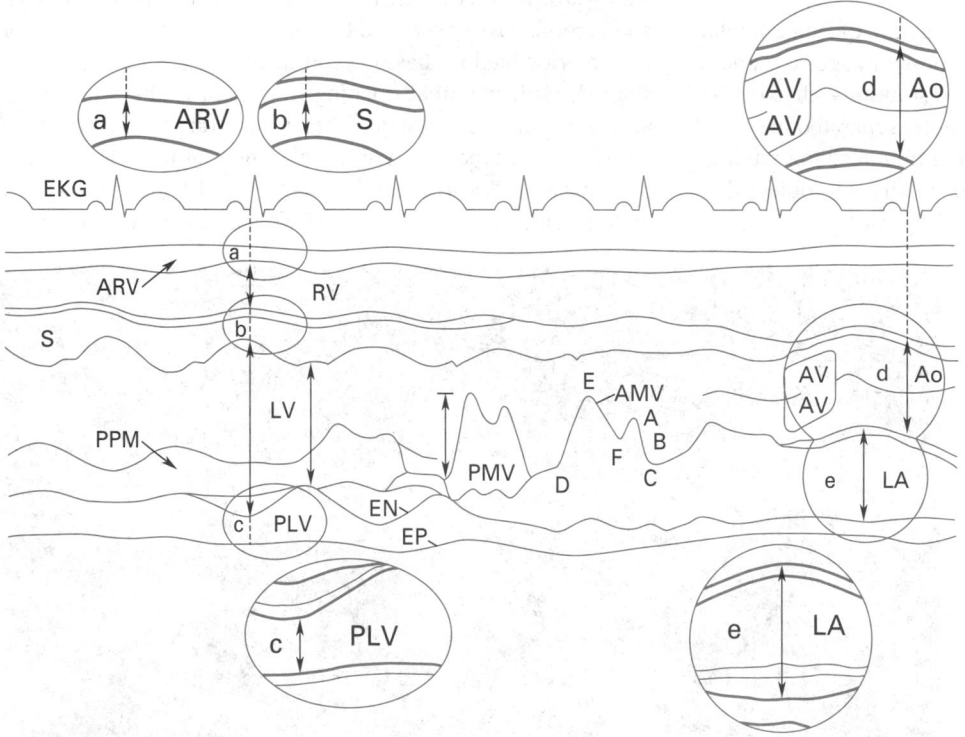

FIGURE 14-9
Recommended criteria for M-mode measurement of cardiac dimensions (see text for details). The figure and the elliptical inserts (a, b, c, d, and e) illustrate the leading edge method. ARV = anterior right ventricular wall; RV = right ventricle; LV = left ventricle; PLV = posterior left ventricular wall; S = septum; PPM = papillary muscle; AMV and PMV = anterior and posterior mitral valve leaflets, EN: endocardium, EP: epicardium; AV = aortic valve; Ao = aorta; LA = left atrium. (Reproduced with permission from Sahn DJ, DeMaria AN, Kisslo J, Weyman AE. Recommendations regarding quantitation in M-mode echocardiography: Results of a survey of echocardiographic measurements. *Circulation* 1978; 58;1072, with permission.)

cases, particularly when left ventricular end-diastolic pressure is elevated, a shoulder (B notch) is present between the A and C points[25] (Fig. 14-8). If the transducer beam is directed inferolaterally from the mitral valve level, the papillary muscles and left ventricular apex will be imaged (Fig. 14-6A). With superior and medial angulation, the left atrium, aortic valve, and aortic root are seen. The tricuspid valve can be imaged by angulating the transducer inferomedially and the pulmonic valve by angulating slightly superiorly and laterally.

ASSESSMENT OF SYSTOLIC FUNCTION BY M-MODE ECHOCARDIOGRAPHY

Measurements of left ventricular (LV) cavity dimension and wall thickness can be readily derived from M-mode recordings (Fig. 14-9) and are usually made according to the recommendations of the American Society of Echocardiography at end diastole (the onset of the QRS complex) and end systole (the point of maximum upward motion of the LV posterior wall endocardium).[26] These measurements should be made from leading edge to leading edge (that is, from the edge of the echo border that is closest to the transducer) to avoid "blooming" artifacts and reverberations; they are accurate if the beam is orthogonal to the long axis of the ventricle. By convention, left atrial dimension is measured at end systole and aortic root diameter is recorded at end diastole at the level of the base of the heart (Fig. 14-9). During systole, opening of the aortic leaflets appears as a parallelogram produced by motion of the right coronary and (usually) the noncoronary aortic valve cusps.[27]

The M-mode LV cavity dimensions can be used to estimate

ventricular volumes and ejection fraction if desired, most simply by merely cubing the value (D^3) but these calculations involve several assumptions regarding geometry that are not uniformly valid.[28,29] In addition, the M-mode dimension may not be representative of the entire ventricle. The fractional shortening

[(end-diastolic dimension − end-systolic dimension)
$\times$ 100% / end-diastolic dimension]

can also be determined.[30] This value is often helpful in assessing systolic function, but it reflects the function of the LV base and can be misleading with asynchronous contraction (for example, left bundle branch block) or segmental dyssynergy.[31] An additional M-mode marker of systolic function is E point–septal separation (EPSS), or the distance between the anterior mitral valve leaflet at its most anterior opening excursion (the E point) and the interventricular septum. A value of 8 mm or greater is abnormal.[32] The normal M-mode measurements are seen in Table 14-1.

Two-Dimensional Echocardiography

A number of technical approaches exist by which multiple individual B-mode scan lines can be rapidly transmitted, received, and displayed in appropriate spatial orientation to construct a two-dimensional image of the heart. The initial approach simply utilized a linear array of 20 piezoelectric crystals placed side by side, each of which transmitted and received signals independently[8] (Fig. 14-10A). The resulting scan lines were displayed simultaneously to yield rectangular images. Unfortunately, transducer size and interaction between the elements resulted in images of unsatisfactory quality.

Current two-dimensional scanners utilize B-mode scan lines that are independently transmitted and received and are directed through a wedge-shaped sector of cardiac anatomy by means of mechanical or electrical beam steering (Fig. 14-10B–D). A variety of motorized devices are available that, by rapidly oscillating or rotating one or more ultrasonic crystals through space, can mechanically direct multiple scan lines through a sector arc of the cardiovascular system.[9,10] The position of the beam in space

is derived by determining the orientation of the piezoelectric crystal. A majority of current two-dimensional scanners utilize a phased-array approach, where multiple ultrasonic crystals are employed in concert to create individual B-mode scan lines.[11] The piezoelectric crystals are activated in a closely coordinated temporal sequence such that the individual wavelets produced by each element merge to form a single beam whose direction is determined by the sequence of crystal firing (Fig. 14-11). Since the direction of the resultant beam is determined by the sequence of activation of the individual elements, the beam can be electrically swept throughout a 90° sector arc. In addition to electronic beam steering, a firing sequence can be employed that results in dynamic focusing of the beam along its length to achieve minimal beam width and increased resolution. Phased-array two-dimensional scanners employ small transducers without moving parts that could require repair. The increased complexity of these scanners, however, makes the systems more costly.

Originally, echocardiographic data were displayed in analog form on a standard oscilloscope, transferred to a video monitor by a television camera, and hard-copied onto videotape or paper. Currently, computerized analog-to-digital scan conversion is standard, so that the polar signals of individ-

TABLE 14-1

NORMAL VALUES

	Mean ± Standard Deviation	Range	Mean ± Standard Deviation	Range
No. of patients	25	—	50	—
Age, years	10 ± 3	4–18	24 ± 6	1.10–2.53
BSA, m²	1.33 ± 0.38	0.72–2.04	1.81 ± .34	1.10–2.53
LVID$_d$, mm,	44 ± 6	32–50	50 ± 3	42–60
LVID$_s$, mm	28 ± 7	32–50	50 ± 3	22–43
FSLV	34 ± 4	25–42	33 ± 3	28–37
IVS thickness, mm	8 ± 2	5–10	9 ± 1	7–12
IVS excursion, mm	7 ± 1	5–9	9 ± 1	7–12
PW$_d$ thickness, mm	7 ± 2	4–9	9 ± 1	7–12
PW$_s$ thickness, mm	12 ± 3	8–17	16 ± 2	13–20
Δ thickening PW	0.70 ± 0.25	0.41–0.95	0.50 ± 0.19	0.32–0.69
PW excursion, mm	9 ± 2	7–14	11 ± 2	9–17
RVD$_d$ supine, mm	—	—	15 ± 6	7–22
RVD$_d$ left lateral, mm	—	—	20 ± 8	10–37
Aorta$_d$ mm	23 ± 4	15–27	28 ± 5	26–36
LAD$_s$ mm	25 ± 5	20–31	27 ± 6	12–35

Key: BSA = Body surface area; LVID$_d$ = left ventricular internal diameter, end diastole; LVID$_s$ = left ventricular internal diameter, end systole; FSLV = fractional shortening of left ventricle; PWV = posterior wall velocity; IVS = interventricular septum; PW = posterior wall; RVD = right ventricular dimension; LAD = left atrial dimension.

Source: Felner JM, Schlant RC. *Echocardiography: A Teaching Atlas.* New York: Grune & Stratton; 1976. Reproduced with permission from the publisher and authors.

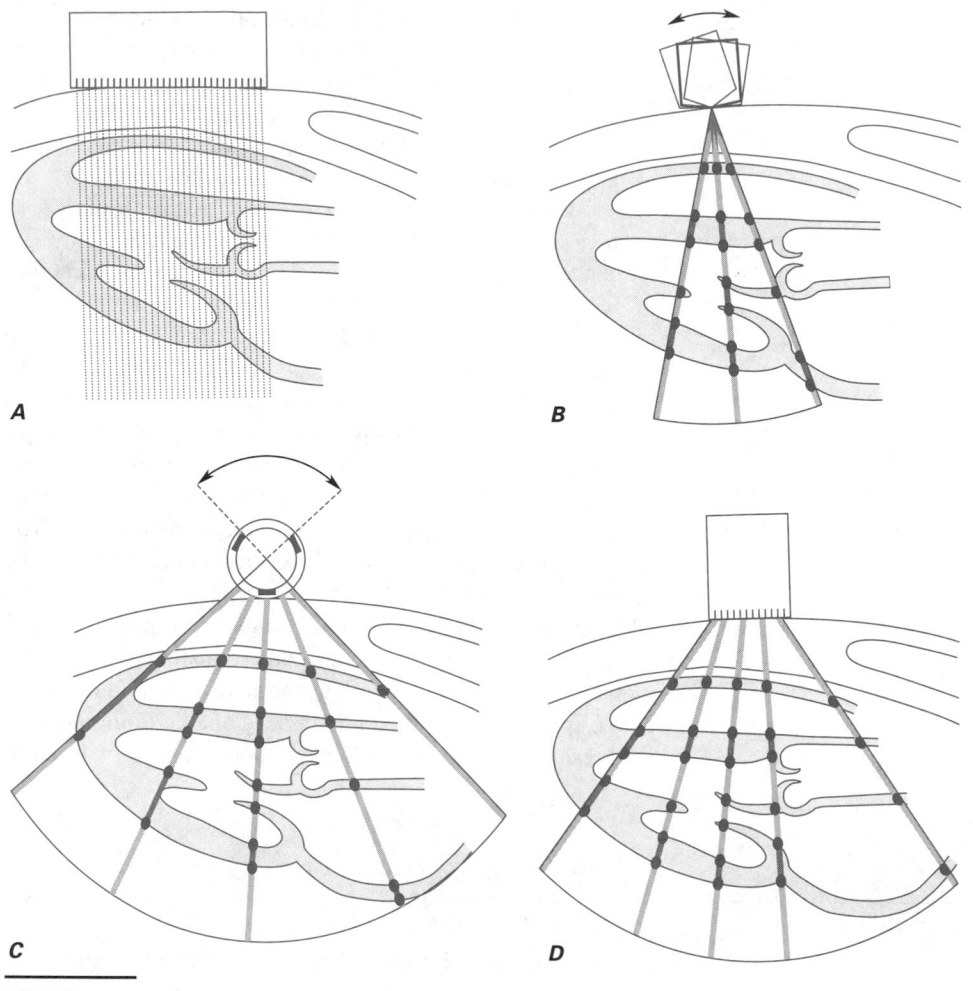

FIGURE 14-10
The four major types of ultrasonic scanners used to acquire 2D echocardiographic images. *A.* Linear array scanner. *B.* Oscillating scanner. *C.* Rotating mechanical scanner. *D.* Phased-array scanner. (From Hagan AD, DeMaria AN. *Clinical Applications of Two-Dimensional Echocardiography and Cardiac Doppler.* Boston: Little, Brown; 1989, with permission.)

THE STANDARD TWO-DIMENSIONAL EXAMINATION

The heart can be imaged through a multitude of planes with two dimensional (2D) echocardiography. To help standardize the 2D examination, the American Society of Echocardiography has recommended that cardiac imaging be performed in three orthogonal planes: long-axis (from aortic root to the apex), short-axis (perpendicular to long axis), and four-chamber (traversing both ventricles and atria through the mitral and tricuspid valves)[34] (Fig. 14-12). It is important to recognize that the long and short axes are those of the heart, not the body. These three planes can be visualized using four basic transducer positions: parasternal, apical, subcostal, and suprasternal[35,36] (Figs. 14-13*A, B,* and *C*). In general, the long-axis plane is best imaged from parasternal, apical, and occasionally the suprasternal positions, while the short-axis plane is best imaged in the parasternal and subcostal positions. The four-chamber views are obtained from the apical and subcostal positions. The American Society of Echocardiography recognizes that these basic positions and planes may be modified somewhat and re-

ual scan lines are converted to a series of numerical gray-level values for individual boxlike picture elements (pixels) aligned along *X-Y* coordinates.[33] The ability of a digital step-gradation technique to reproduce the continuous gradation of analog methods is a function of the density of pixels in the matrix and the shades of gray levels available. No loss of data can be detected in current digitally converted images, and the digital format provides the opportunity for image processing, enhancement, and quantitation. More importantly, storage in digital format can avoid the image degradation inherent in videotape, provide random access and easy comparison of studies, enable rapid image transmission, and prevent deterioration with image copying and prolonged storage. Although available technology is not quite sufficient for fully digital echocardiography, greater standardization with the DICOM format and improved image compression and digital storage modalities will likely enable full digital acquisition and storage of echocardiograms in the near future.

commends that an image obtained within 45° of a basic orthogonal plane be identified with that orthogonal plane. Table 14-2 lists the standard transducer positions and transthoracic echocardiographic views. Anatomic drawings of the various imaging planes are seen in Figs. 14-13 through 14-20.

As opposed to other types of cardiac imaging, such as chest radiography, which are well standardized, the echocardiographic examination is iterative and largely determined by the anatomic characteristics of the patient and manual manipulation of the transducer by the operator. Of paramount importance is the identification of a thoracic site (window) that enables transmission of the ultrasound signal to the heart. In actual practice, the echocardiographic examination is performed with the operator either to the patient's left or right. The patient is in the left lateral decubitus position for the majority of the examination, with the head of the bed elevated 20 to 30°. Alternate positioning may be employed for individual patients and views. Use of a thick foam rubber mattress (made expressly for echocardiography), which has a remov-

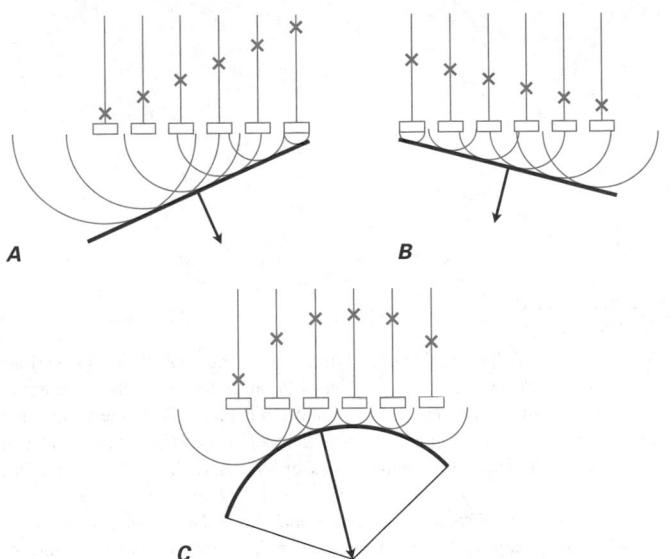

FIGURE 14-11

Electronic "steering" of a phased-array ultrasound beam. *A*. Elements are fired in sequence from left to right, resulting in a beam directed to the left. *B*. Elements are fired in sequence opposite to those in (*A*), producing a beam directed to the right. *C*. Elements are fired from the periphery toward the center, producing a beam that converges on a given focal point. (From Hagan AD, DeMaria AN. *Clinical Applications of Two-Dimensional Echocardiography and Cardiac Doppler.* Boston: Little Brown; 1989, with permission.)

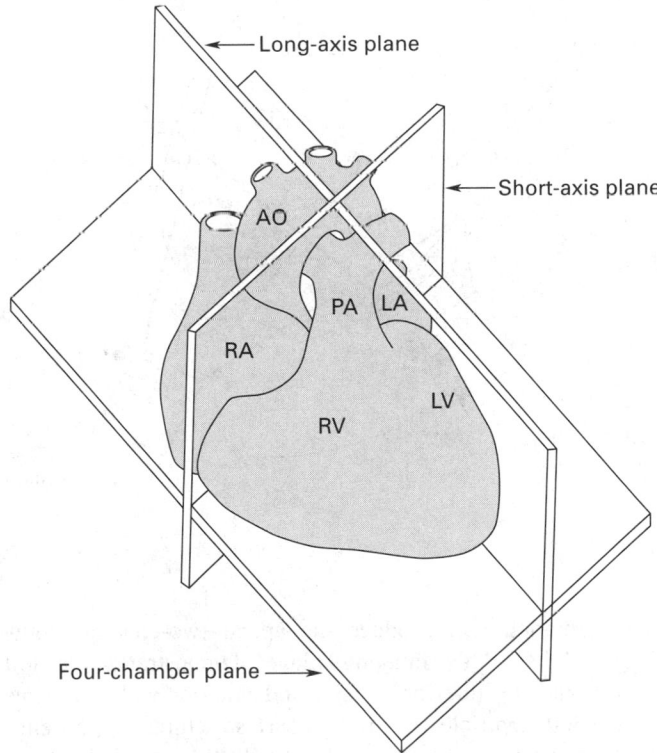

FIGURE 14-12

The three basic tomographic imaging planes used in echocardiography: long-axis, short-axis, and four-chamber. LV = left ventricle; LA = left atrium; RV = right ventricle; RA = right atrium; PA = pulmonary artery; AO = aorta. (From Hagan AD, DeMaria AN. *Clinical Applications of Two-Dimensional Echocardiography and Cardiac Doppler.* Boston: Little, Brown; 1989, with permission.)

TABLE 14-2

STANDARD TWO-DIMENSIONAL ECHOCARDIOGRAPHIC TRANSDUCER POSITIONS

PARASTERNAL POSITION

Long axis
    Left ventricular long axis
    Right ventricular inflow
    Right ventricular outflow
Short axis
    Short axis through the plane of
        The cardiac base
        The mitral valve
        The chordae tendineae
        The papillary muscles
        The apex

APICAL POSITION

Four-chamber plane
Five-chamber plane
    (Four-chamber plane angled superiorly to include the aorta)
Two-chamber plane
Three-chamber plane

SUBCOSTAL POSITION

Four-chamber plane
Short-axis through the plane of
    The mitral valve
    The papillary muscles
    The cardiac base
Posteriorly directed planes through the venae cavae and atria

SUPRASTERNAL POSITION

Long axis (through the ascending and descending aorta)
Short axis

able section under the area of the cardiac apex, may facilitate the examination.

The examination customarily begins with the transducer in the left parasternal position in the long-axis view (Fig. 14-14). This provides excellent images of the left ventricle, aorta, left atrium, and the mitral and aortic valves. By angling the beam slightly rightward and inferiorly (right ventricular inflow view), the right atrium, right ventricle, and tricuspid valve are visualized (Fig. 14-15). If the beam is turned slightly leftward and rotated clockwise from the standard parasternal long-axis view, the right ventricular outflow tract, pulmonic valve, and main pulmonary artery appear (right ventricular outflow view).

A 90° clockwise turn of the transducer produces the parasternal short-axis view. Slight axial angulation of the transducer enables visualization of the left ventricle at various levels of the short axis, including the papillary muscle, mitral leaflets, and aortic valve (Fig. 14-16). With angulation toward the base, the left atrium, right heart structures, main pulmonary artery, and occasionally the left atrial appendage are also recorded.

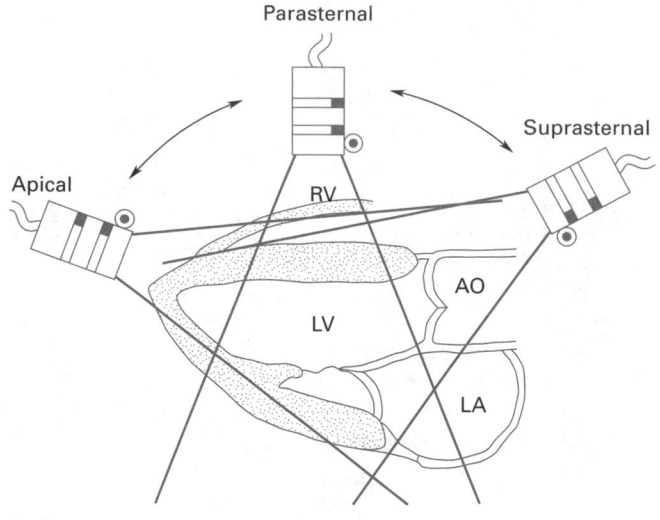

A

FIGURE 14-13

Visualization of the heart's basic tomographic imaging planes by various transducer positions. The long-axis plane (*A*) can be imaged in the parasternal, suprasternal, and apical positions; the short axis plane (*B*) in the parasternal and subcostal positions; and the four-chamber plane (*C*) in the apical and subcostal positions. (From Henry WL, DeMaria AN, Gramiak R, King DL, Kisslo JA, Popp RL, et al. *Report of the American Society of Echocardiography Committee on Nomenclature and Standards in Two-Dimensional Echocardiography.* Reproduced with permission from the American Society of Echocardiography.)

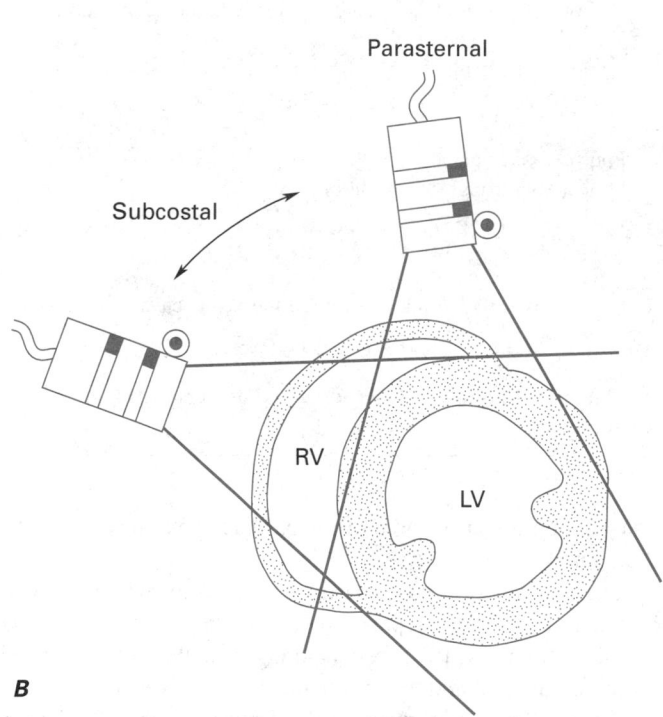

B

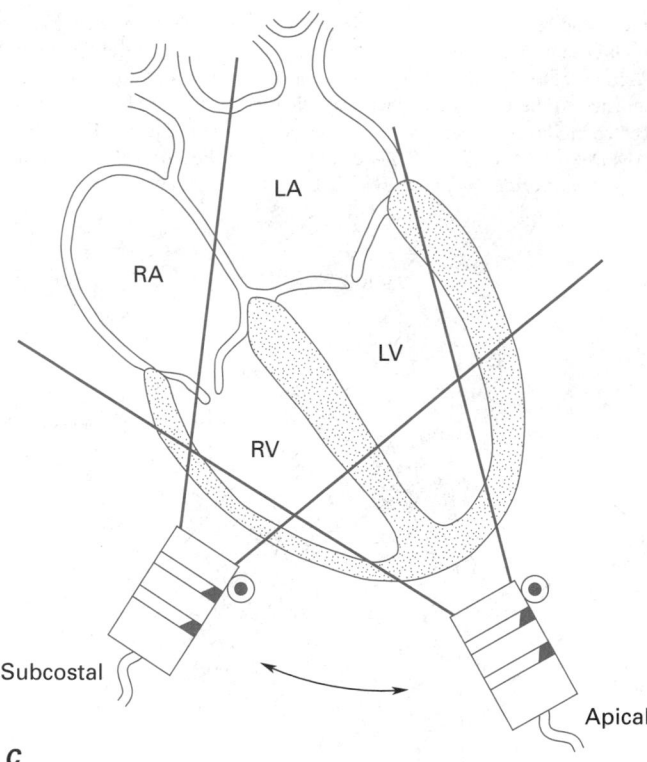

C

The apical views are best acquired with the patient in a steep left lateral decubitus position and the transducer at the point of the apical impulse. The four-chamber view is obtained by turning the transducer so that both ventricles, atrioventricular valves, and atria are visualized (Fig. 14-17). In this view, the septal, apical, and lateral walls of the left ventricle are visualized. Slight superior angulation of the transducer will add the aortic valve and proximal ascending aorta to the echocardiographic image (apical five-chamber view). From the four-chamber view, 90° of counterclockwise trans-

ducer rotation will produce the apical two-chamber view (Fig. 14-18). This imaging plane demonstrates the left atrium and the inferior, apical, and anterior wall segments of the left ventricle (the right heart structures are absent). If the transducer is rotated slightly back toward the four-chamber plane, a three-chamber view similar to the parasternal long-axis view is produced (Fig. 14-18) and provides images of the posterior, apical, and anteroseptal LV wall segments as well as the left atrium, aorta, and mitral and aortic valves.

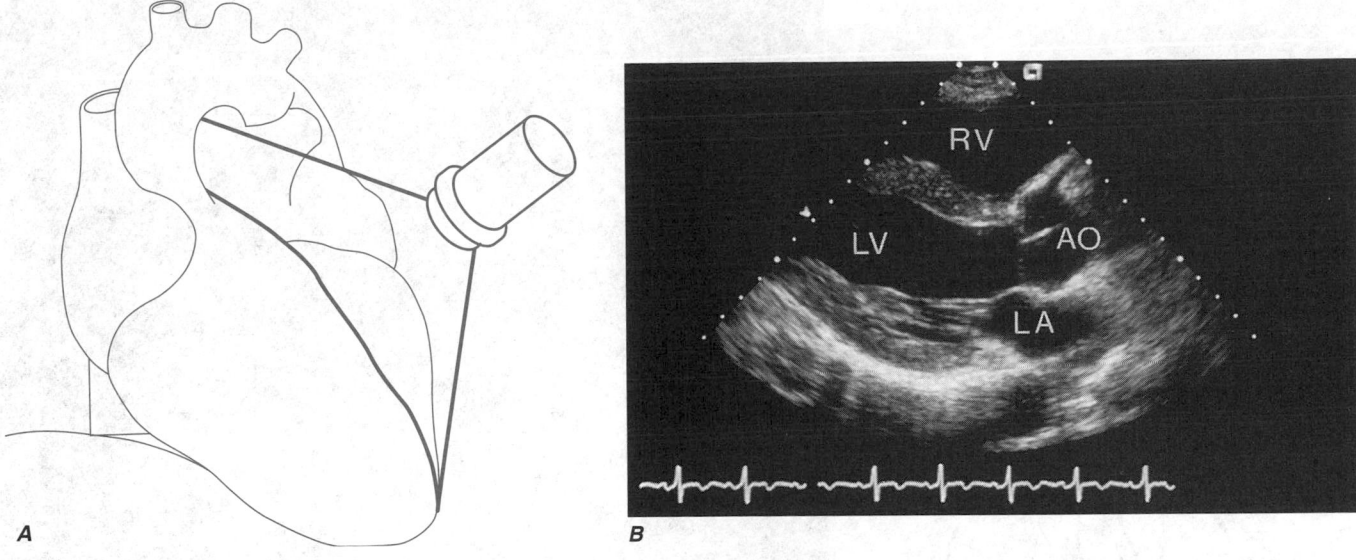

FIGURE 14-14

A. Orientation of the sector beam and transducer position for the parasternal long-axis view of the left ventricle. *B.* Two dimensional image of the heart, parasternal long axis view. LV = left ventricle; LA = left atrium; AO = aorta; RV = right ventricle.

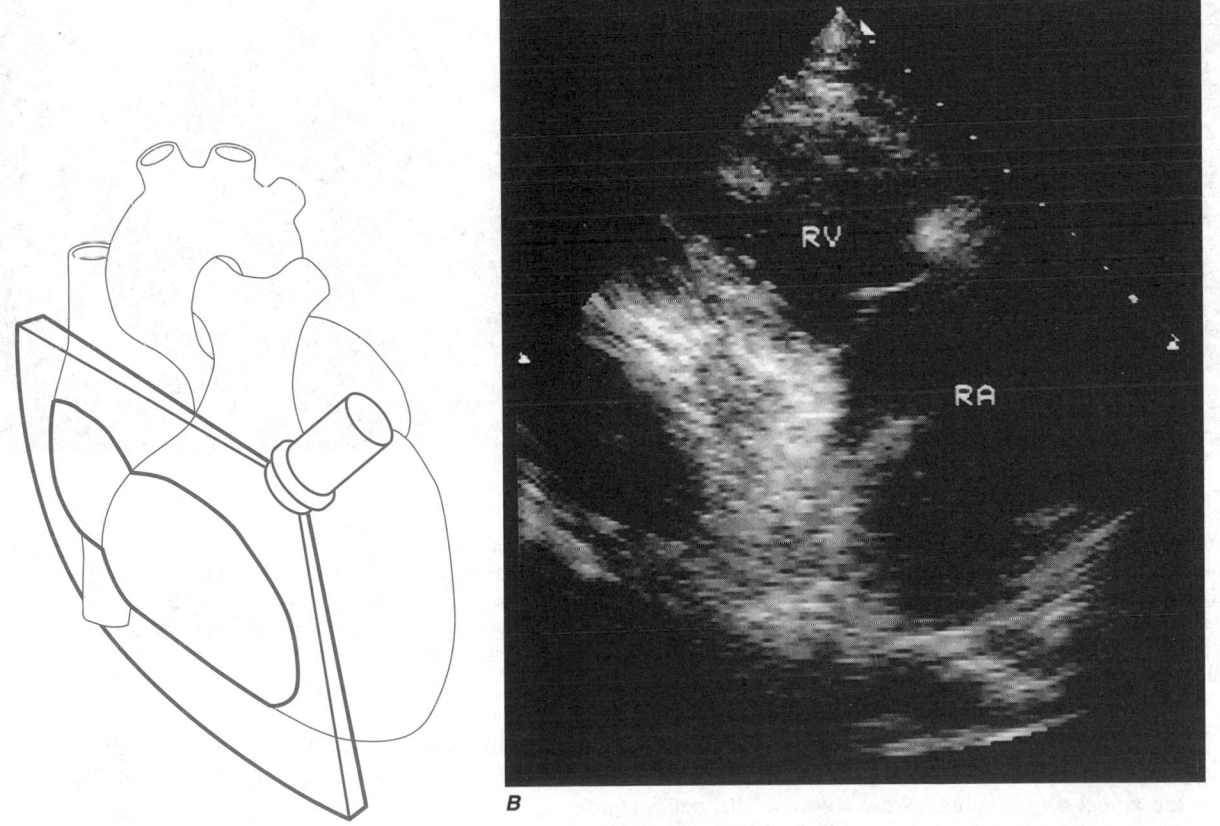

FIGURE 14-15

A. Orientation of the sector beam and transducer position for the parasternal right ventricular inflow plane. (From Hagan AD, DeMaria AN. *Clinical Applications of Two-Dimensional Echocardiography and Cardiac Doppler.* Boston: Little, Brown; 1989, with permission.) *B.* Two-dimensional image of right ventricular inflow plane. RA = right atrium, RV = right ventricle.

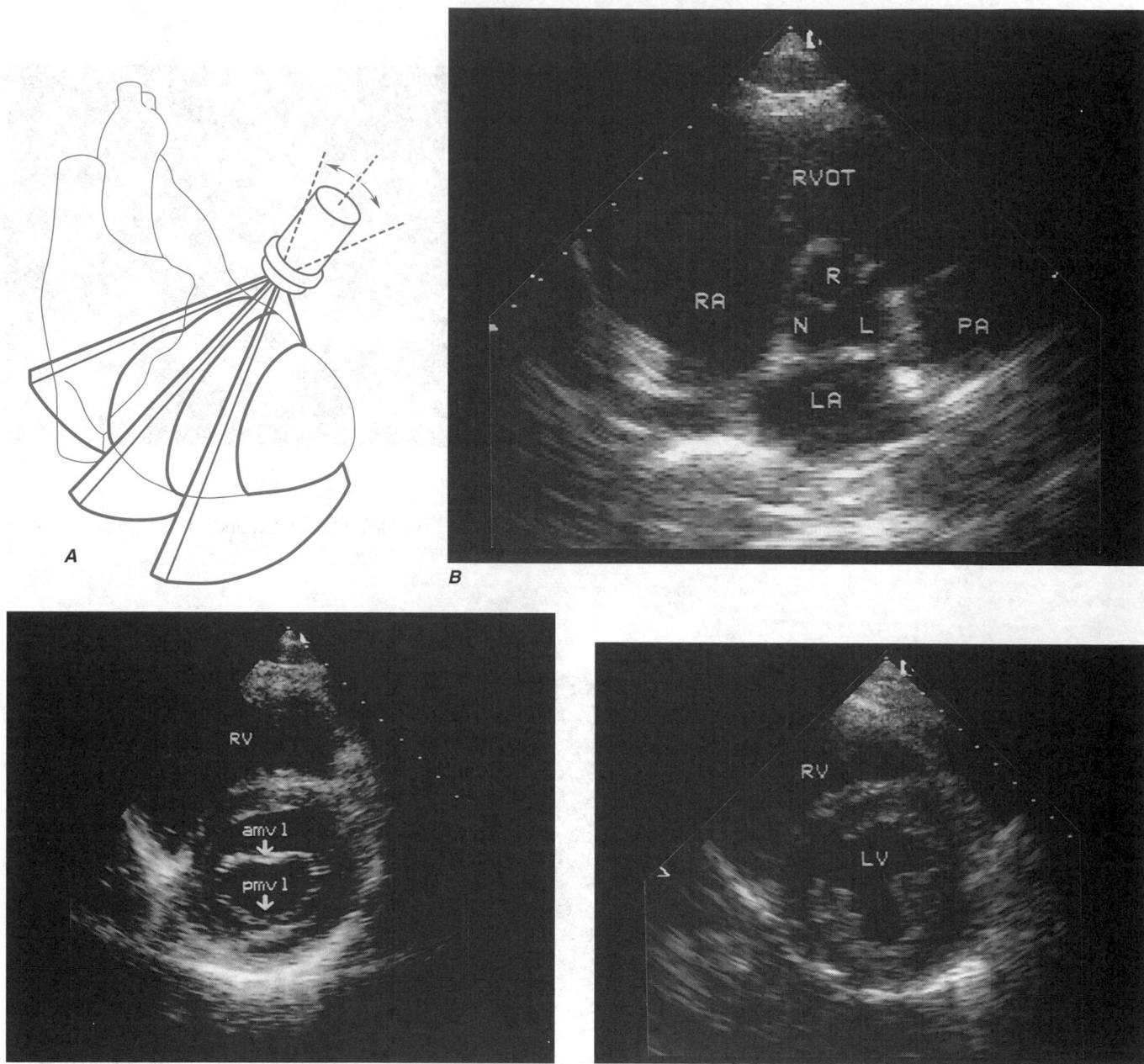

FIGURE 14-16

A. Orientation of various short-axis sector beams through the left ventricle obtained by angling the transducer in the parasternal position. (From Hagan AD, DeMaria AN. *Clinical Applications of Two-Dimensional Echocardiography and Cardiac Doppler.* Boston: Little, Brown; 1989, with permission.) *B.* Short-axis plane through the base of the heart. *C.* At the level of the mitral valve leaflets. *D.* At the papillary muscle level. LV = left ventricle; RV =

right ventricle; LA = left atrium; RA = right atrium; RVOT = right ventricular outflow tract; PA = pulmonary artery; R, L, N = right, left, and noncoronary cusps of the aortic valve. RV = right ventricle; LV = left ventricle; amvl = anterior mitral valve leaflet; pmvl = posterior mitral valve leaflet.

To facilitate subcostal imaging, the patient is moved into a supine position. The subcostal four-chamber view is much like the apical four-chamber view (Fig. 14-19), but because the ultrasound beam is now more perpendicular to the interventricular and interatrial septa, subcostal imaging is often helpful in the examination of these structures. A 90° rotation of the transducer will record a subcostal short-axis view. The

transducer can also be angled to image the right ventricular outflow and pulmonary artery as well as the inferior vena cava (Fig. 14-19).

The long-axis suprasternal imaging plane is shown in Fig. 14-20. In adult echocardiography, the left ventricle is usually not visualized satisfactorily from the suprasternal position, but these imaging planes are well suited for examination

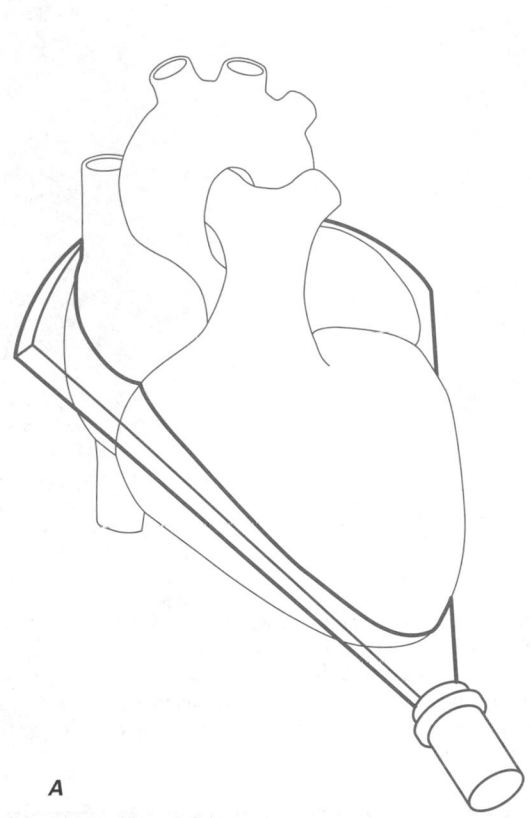

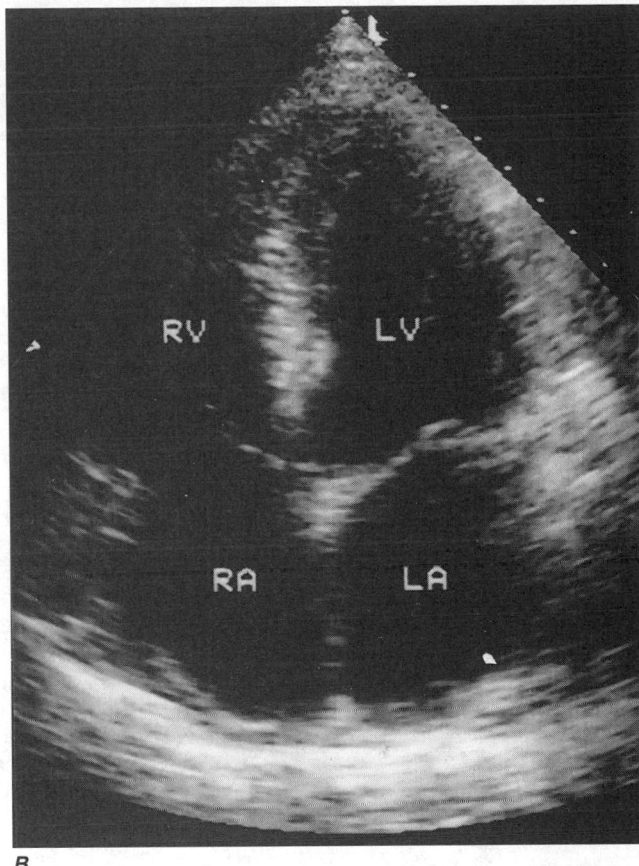

FIGURE 14-17

A. Orientation of the sector beam and transducer position for the apical 4-chamber plane. (From Hagan AD, DeMaria AN. *Clinical Applications of Two-Dimensional Echocardiography and Cardiac Doppler.* Boston: Little, Brown; 1989, with permission.) *B.* Two-dimensional image of the apical four-chamber plane. RA = right atrium; RV = right ventricle; LV = left ventricle; LA = left atrium.

of the thoracic aorta, pulmonary artery, and great vessels. Normal values for 2D echocardiographic measurements are shown in Table 14-3.

ASSESSMENT OF SYSTOLIC FUNCTION BY TWO-DIMENSIONAL ECHOCARDIOGRAPHY

Because 2D echocardiography enables visualization of the entire LV perimeter in multiple planes, it is significantly superior to M-mode approaches for the measurement of cardiac chamber volumes and ejection fraction.[37–40] Numerous algorithms have been applied to calculate LV volumes by echocardiography (Fig. 14-21). Most such algorithms have assumed that the left ventricle conforms to the shape of a prolate ellipsoid and calculated volume by diameter-length or area-length formulas.[38,41] Multiple studies comparing LV volume calculated by area-length methods to those obtained by other techniques have yielded good correlations, with the best results obtained utilizing biplane apical views.[41,42] Other algorithms have assumed an LV cavity configuration that is a combination of geometric shapes, such as a cylinder-cone or a cylinder-hemiellipse.[41,43] Currently, the most commonly used algorithm to calculate LV volumes is based upon the Simpson rule, which derives measurements by dividing the left ventricle by parallel planes into a number of small segments (usually referred to as disks) and the summating the area of the individual disks. This approach has the advantage of making no assumptions about the geometry of the ventricle. A number of modifications of the basic Simpson rule method have been applied to calculate LV volumes. Although all have yielded good results, the optimal correlations have been achieved with a modification that separately quantifies the volume of the apex as an ellipsoid.[40–45]

Regardless of the methodologic approach used, accurate calculations of LV volumes by echocardiography require attention to detail and are critically dependent upon high-quality images to delineate the endocardium and image the entire left ventricular perimeter. As a rule, echocardiographic estimates of LV volumes underestimate those calculated by other techniques and are most accurate in the absence of significant alterations of LV size and contraction. End-systolic measurements are more accurate than those made at end-diastole, probably due to superior endocardial definition. Nevertheless,

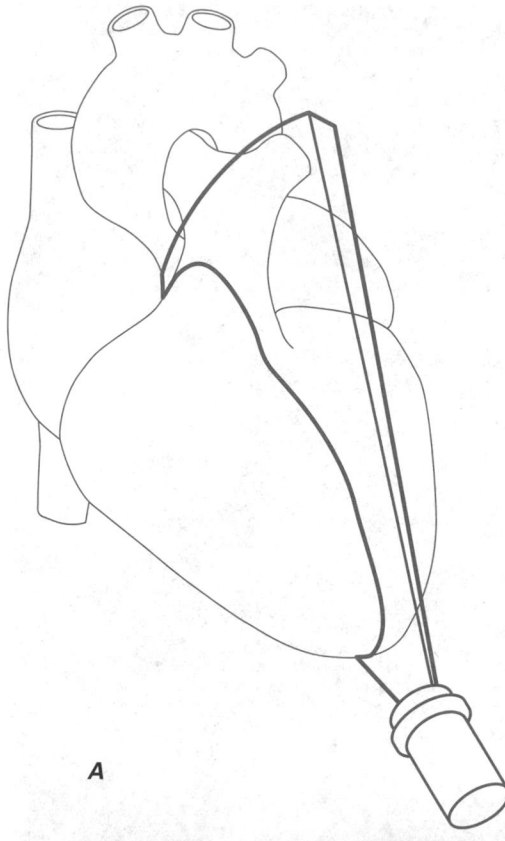

A

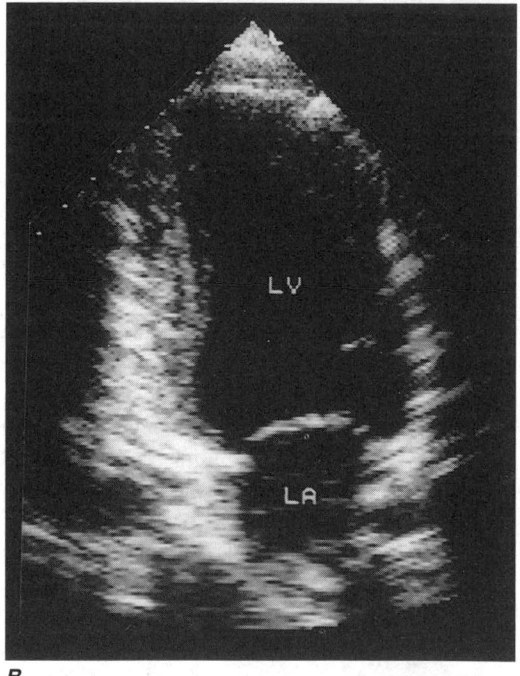

B

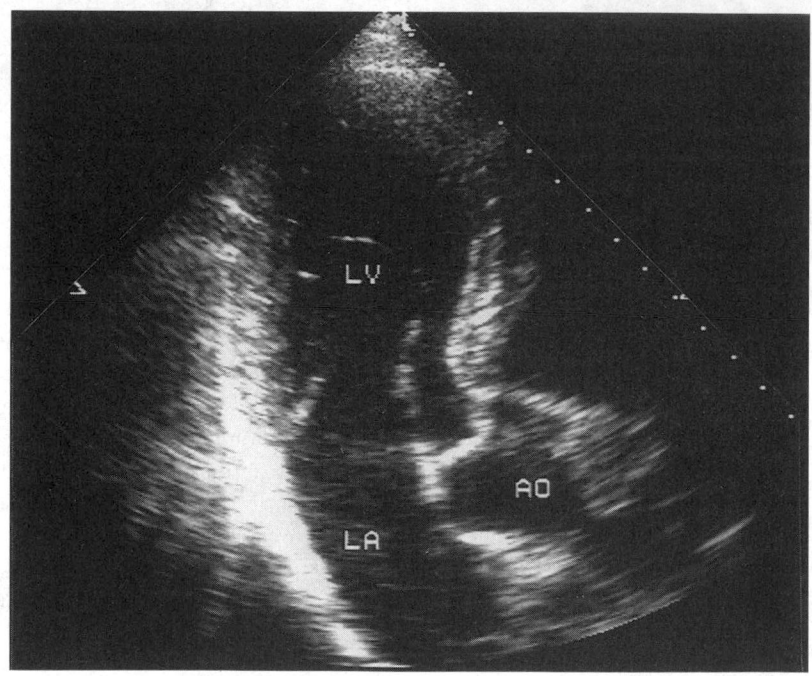

C

FIGURE 14-18

A. Orientation of the sector beam and transducer position for the apical two-chamber plane. (From Hagan AD, DeMaria AN. *Clinical Applications of Two-Dimensional Echocardiography and Cardiac Doppler.* Boston: Little, Brown; 1989, with permission.) *B.* Two-dimensional image of the apical two-chamber plane. LV = left ventricle; LA = left atrium. *C.* Two-dimensional image of the apical three-chamber view. LV = left ventricle; LA = atrium; AO = aorta.

echocardiographic calculations of LV volumes have generally yielded correlation coefficients in excess of 0.75 as compared with radionuclide angiography, cineangiography, and autopsy studies regardless of the algorithm employed.[37–45] Of importance, calculation of LV volumes generally yields values with a standard error of estimate that renders these measurements

suitable for clinical decision making in the care of most patients.

In an attempt to refine and facilitate the derivation of LV volume measurements from echocardiography, a number of technical developments have been evaluated. Images of the power spectrum of the Doppler signal produced by contrac-

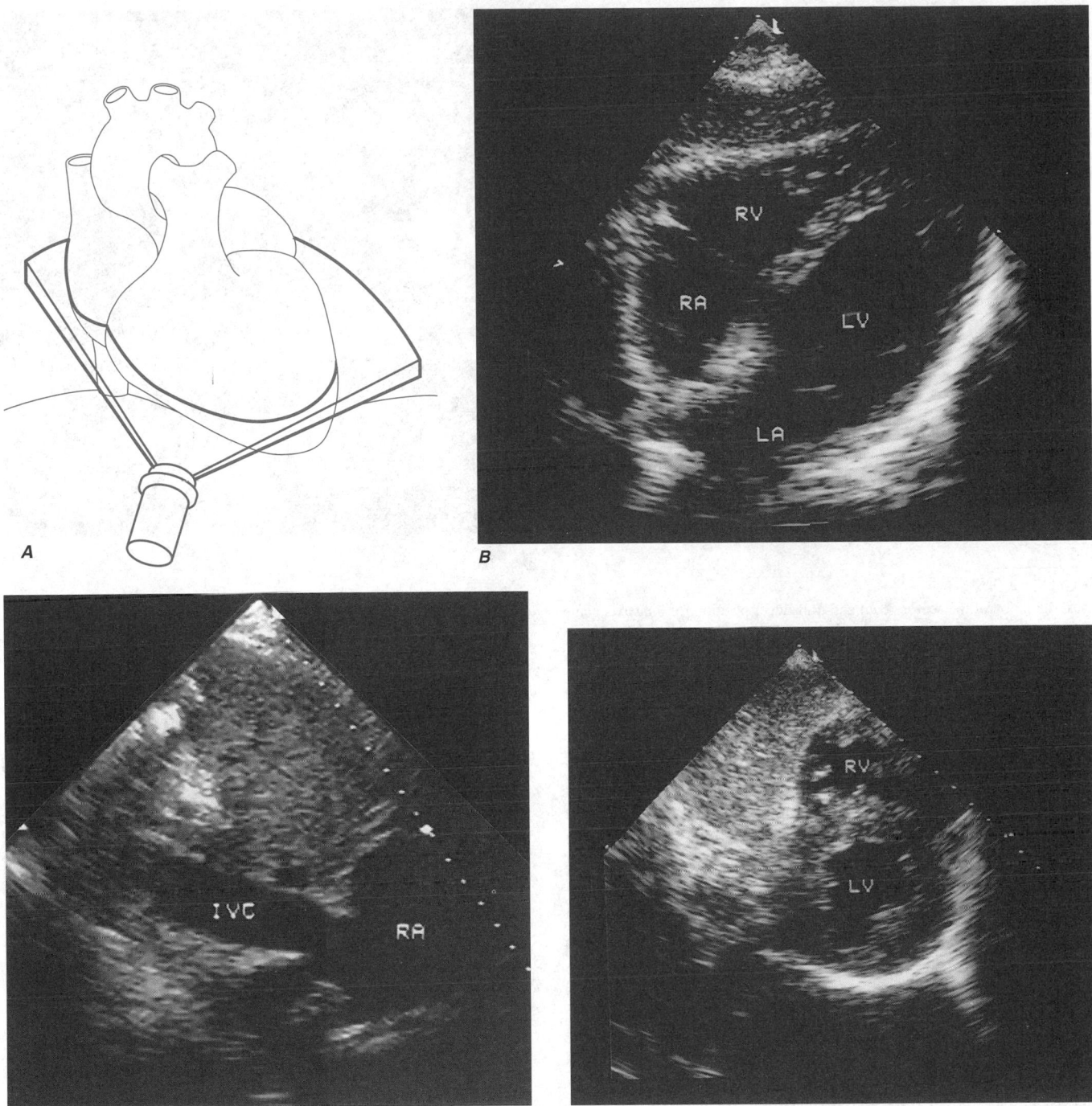

FIGURE 14-19

A. Orientation of the sector beam and transducer position for the subcostal 4-chamber plane. (From Hagen AD, DeMaria AN. *Clinical Applications of Two Dimensional Echocardiography and Cardiac Doppler.* Boston, Little, Brown Publ. Co., 1989, with permission.) *B.* Two-dimensional image of the subcostal four-chamber plane. LV = left ventricle; LA = left atrium; RA = right atrium; RV = right ventricle. *C.* Subcostal 2D image demonstrating the right atrium (RA) and inferior vena cava (IVC). *D.* Two dimensional image of the subcostal short-axis plane. LV = left ventricle; RV = right ventricle.

tion/relaxation have been utilized to visualize the endocardial surface. This technique has been reported to be useful in identifying endocardial signals, particularly in patients with suboptimal tissue images. Colorization of the 2D tissue image ("B-color") has been implemented in some instruments to exploit the ability of the eye to discern more accurately color shades than gray levels, thus enhancing endocardial identification. Little improvement was obtained from this approach, however.[46] A software package that provides instantaneous and automated endocardial border delineation throughout the cardiac cycle has been developed based upon the display of tissue signals as backscatter rather than specular reflection.[47]

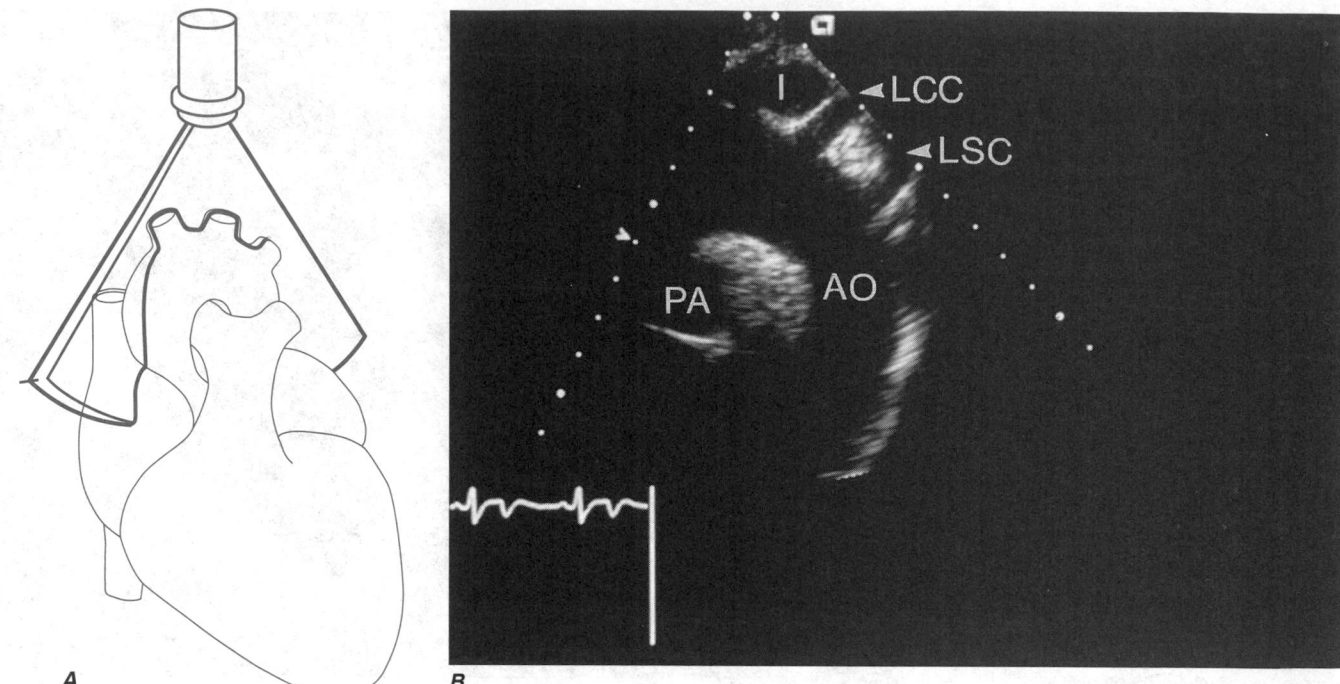

FIGURE 14-20

A. Orientation of the sector beam and transducer position for long axis plane through the aorta from the suprasternal position. *B.* Two-dimensional image of the suprasternal long axis view of the thoracic aorta. AO = aorta; PA = right pulmonary artery; I = innominate artery; LCC = left common carotid artery; LSC = left subclavian artery.

This technique of automated quantitation can yield continuous measurements of LV volume throughout the cardiac cycle and can derive values for ejection fraction, ejection rate, and rate of filling during diastole (Fig. 14-22). This same technology has been utilized to display endocardial excursion throughout systolic contraction or diastolic expansion in a color format superimposed upon the tissue image (Fig. 14-23, Plate 25). This technique has proved to be of value in the recognition of abnormalities of LV contraction and regional disturbances of LV diastolic function.[48,49] Although these technical developments are new, they promise to facilitate the quantitative assessment of LV size and function from routine echocardiograms.

DOPPLER ECHOCARDIOGRAPHY: PRINCIPLES AND APPLICATIONS

The Doppler Principle

Although 2D and M-mode echocardiography provide abundant information about cardiac structure and movement, they supply no direct data concerning blood flow. This is a significant limitation, as the presence and severity of conditions such as valvular regurgitation and intracardiac shunting can be suspected or inferred only indirectly by 2D imaging. Using the principle first delineated by the physicist Johann Christian

Doppler,[50] one can use ultrasound to determine the velocity and direction of blood flow by measuring the change in frequency produced when sound waves are reflected from red blood cells.[51–53] In this way, information regarding the presence, direction, velocity, and turbulence of blood flow can be acquired by cardiac ultrasound.[54]

The Doppler principle states that when a sound (or light) signal strikes a moving object, the frequency of that signal will be altered, and the increase or decrease in frequency will be proportional to the velocity and direction at which the object is moving. This is illustrated in Fig. 14-24. If a stationary transducer at the apex emits a sound wave with a transmitted frequency of *fo* and the wave is reflected by nonmoving RBCs in an isovolumic phase of the cardiac cycle, then the received frequency *fr* will be identical to *fo*. If the signal is reflected by RBCs that are moving toward the transducer, as through the mitral valve in diastole, the returning waves will be compressed so that *fr* will be greater than *fo*. Conversely, if the target red blood cells (RBCs) are moving away from the transducer, as in the outflow tract in systole, the returning sound waves will be elongated and the received frequency will be decreased. Of importance, the magnitude of change in the received frequency is directly related to the velocity at which blood is flowing toward or away from the transducer.[53] If the velocity of sound and the angle θ between the direction of RBC flow and the beam path are known, then the velocity of the RBCs is described by the Doppler equation:

$$v = \frac{fd(c)}{2fo\,(\cos\theta)}$$

FIGURE 14-23
See color Plate 25.

where fd is the frequency shift recorded, fo the transmitted frequency, and c the velocity of sound. Note that the denominator is doubled because the sound wave does not originate with the RBC but must travel back and forth from the transducer. By measuring Doppler shift frequencies, the velocity and direction of blood flow can be calculated, displayed, and recorded.

The angle between the direction of blood flow and the course of the sound beam is a most important factor in Doppler ultrasound Fig. 14-25). Velocity is a vectorial entity, having magnitude and direction, and Doppler will detect only those velocities parallel or near parallel to the interrogating signal. Since the relationship between velocity and the angle is a cosine function and the cosine of angles up to 20° is 0.9, little error is introduced within this range.[53] Because the processor that calculates blood velocity assumes that the angle is 0°, however, considerable errors occur when it is greater than 20°. Moreover, the angle of incidence in 3D space usually cannot be determined with certainty from 2D echocardiographic images. Therefore, in order to obtain accurate velocity determination by Doppler, it is crucial to position and direct the transducer so that the beam is as parallel to flow as possible.

In clinical use, the frequency of transmitted ultrasound is in the range of 2 to 5 MHZ, the velocity of sound in tissue is approximately 1540 m/s, and the Doppler shift frequency is relatively small (approximately 1 to 4 kHz) as compared with the transmitted frequency. As the Doppler shift frequencies are in the audible range, a speaker integrated into the Doppler echocardiography system can present them as an audible signal. Normal signals are tonal or musical. The Doppler

TABLE 14-3

CARDIAC DIMENSIONS BY TWO-DIMENSIONAL ECHOCARDIOGRAPHY

Cardiac Feature	Range	Mean	Index, cm/m²
APICAL FOUR-CHAMBER VIEW			
LV$_d$ major	6.9–10.3 cm	8.6 cm	4.1–5.7
LV$_d$ minor	3.3–6.1 cm	4.7 cm	2.2–3.1
LV$_s$ minor	1.9–3.7 cm	2.8 cm	1.3–2.0
LV$_d$ area	21.2–40.2 cm²	31.2 cm²	
LV$_s$ area	8.0–21.1 cm²	14.2 cm²	
RV major	6.5–9.5 cm	8.0 cm	3.8–5.3
RV minor	2.2–4.4 cm	3.3–3.5 cm	1.0–2.8
RV$_d$ area	12.0–22.2 cm²	18.6–2.1 cm²	
RV$_s$ area	5.4–14.6 cm²	9.9 cm²	
LA major	4.1–6.1 cm	5.1 cm	2.3–3.5
LA minor	2.8–4.3 cm	3.5 cm	1.6–2.4
LA area	10.2–17.8 cm²	14.7 cm²	
RA major (inf-sup)	3.5–5.5 cm	4.3–4.5 cm	2.0–3.1
RA minor	2.5–4.9 cm	3.7 cm	1.7–2.5
RA area	11.3–16.7 cm²	13.8–14 cm²	
APICAL TWO-CHAMBER VIEW			
LV$_d$ major	6.8–9.4 cm	8.0 cm	
LV$_d$ minor	3.8–5.7 cm	4.6 cm	
LV$_d$ area	19.4–48.0 cm²	35.6 cm²	
LV$_s$	8.9–27.0 cm	14.3 cm	
PARASTERNAL LONG-AXIS VIEW			
LV$_d$	3.5–6.0 cm	4.8 cm	2.3–3.1
LV$_s$	2.1–4.0 cm	3.1 cm	1.4–2.1
RV	1.9–3.8 cm	2.8 cm	1.2–2.0
LA (A-P)	2.7–4.5 cm	3.6 cm	1.6–2.4
LA (S-I)	3.1–5.5 cm	4.4 cm	
LA area	9.0–19.3 cm²	13.8 cm²	
Ao	2.2–3.6 cm	2.9 cm	1.4–2.0
PARASTERNAL SHORT-AXIS VIEW			
Ao	2.3–3.7 cm	3.0–2.3 cm	1.6–2.4
RVOT	1.9–2.2 cm	2.7 cm	
RA	1.5–2.5 cm	1.9–2.2 cm	
LA	2.6–4.5 cm	3.6 cm	1.6–2.4
LA area	7.2–13.0 cm²	10.8 cm²	
LV$_d$ (PM level)	3.5–5.8 cm	4.7 cm	2.2–3.1
LV$_s$ (PM level)	2.2–4.0 cm	3.1 cm	1.4–2.2
LV$_d$ area (PM level)	16.0–31.2 cm²	22.2 cm²	
LV$_s$ area (PM level)	5.2–13.4 cm²	8.5 cm²	
LV$_d$ (Ch. level)	3.5–6.2	4.8 cm	2.3–3.2
LV$_s$ (Ch. level)	2.3–4.0 cm	3.2 cm	1.5–2.2
LV$_d$ area (Ch. level)	16.4–32.3 cm²	22.5 cm²	
LV$_s$ area (Ch. level)	6.1–16.8 cm²	10.7 cm²	
SUBCOSTAL VIEW			
IVC diameter		1.8 cm	

Key: LV = left ventricle; LV$_d$ = left ventricle, end diastole; LV$_s$ = left ventricle, end systole; RV = right ventricle; RV$_d$ = right ventricle, end diastole; RV$_s$ = right ventricle, end systole; LA = left atrium; RA = right atrium; Ao = aorta; RVOT = right ventricular outflow tract; PA = pulmonary artery; IVC = inferior vena cava; PM = papillary muscle; Ch = chordal.

Source: The values shown in this table represent a compilation of data from three sources: Schnittinger I, Gordon EP, Fitzgerald PJ, et al. Standardized intracardiac measurements of two-dimensional echocardiography. *J Am Coll Cardiol* 1983; 5:934. Triulzi M, Weyman A. Normal cross-sectional measurements in adults. In: Weyman A, ed. *Echocardiography.*Philadelphia: Lea & Febiger; 1982:497. Hagan AD, DiSessa TG, Bloor CM, et al. *Two-Dimensional Echocardiography: Clinical-Pathological Correlations in adult and Congenital Heart Disease.* Boston: Little, Brown; 1983:553.

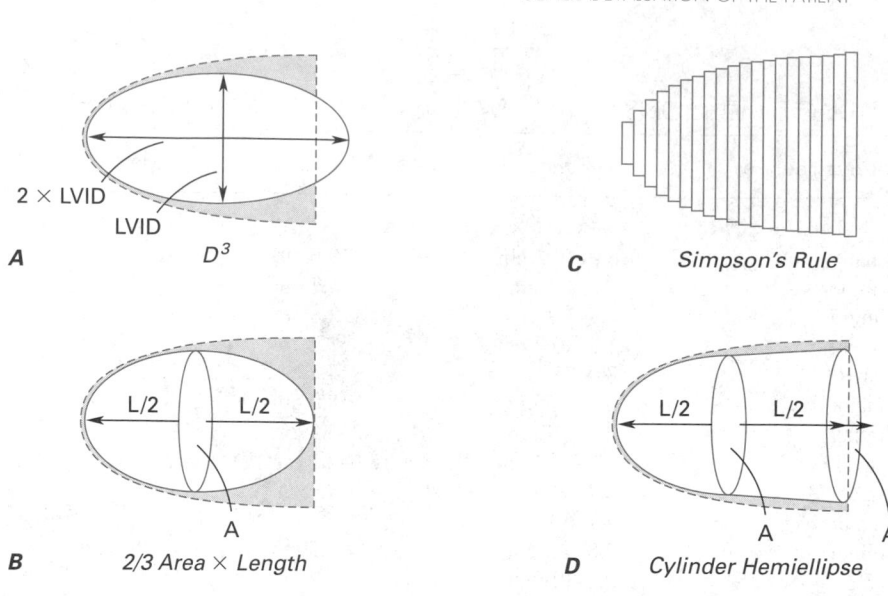

A 2 × LVID LVID D^3

B 2/3 Area × Length

C Simpson's Rule

D Cylinder Hemiellipse

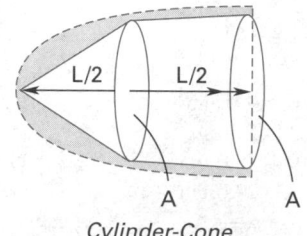

E Cylinder-Cone

FIGURE 14-21

Various models used to estimate left ventricular volume. *A.* "D-cubed." *B.* Two-thirds area × length. *C.* Simpson's rule. *D.* Cylinder-hemiellipse. *E.* Cylinder-cone. A = cross-sectional area; LVID = left ventricular internal dimension (minor axis); L = left ventricular major axis length.

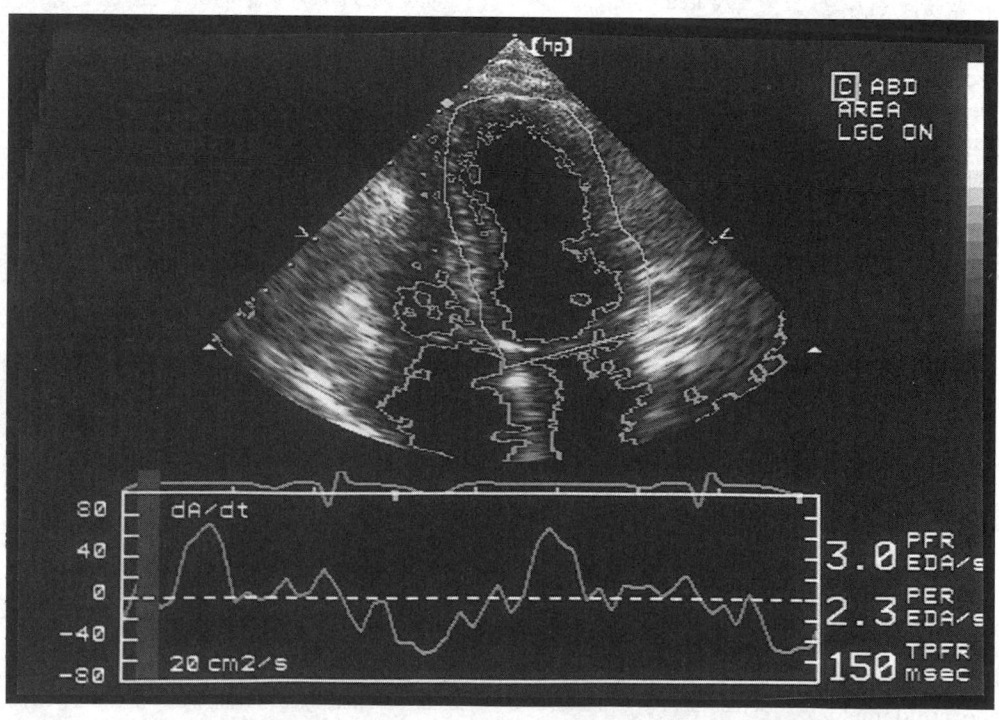

FIGURE 14-22

Example of endocardial border detection and on-line calculation of change in area over time (*dA/dt*).

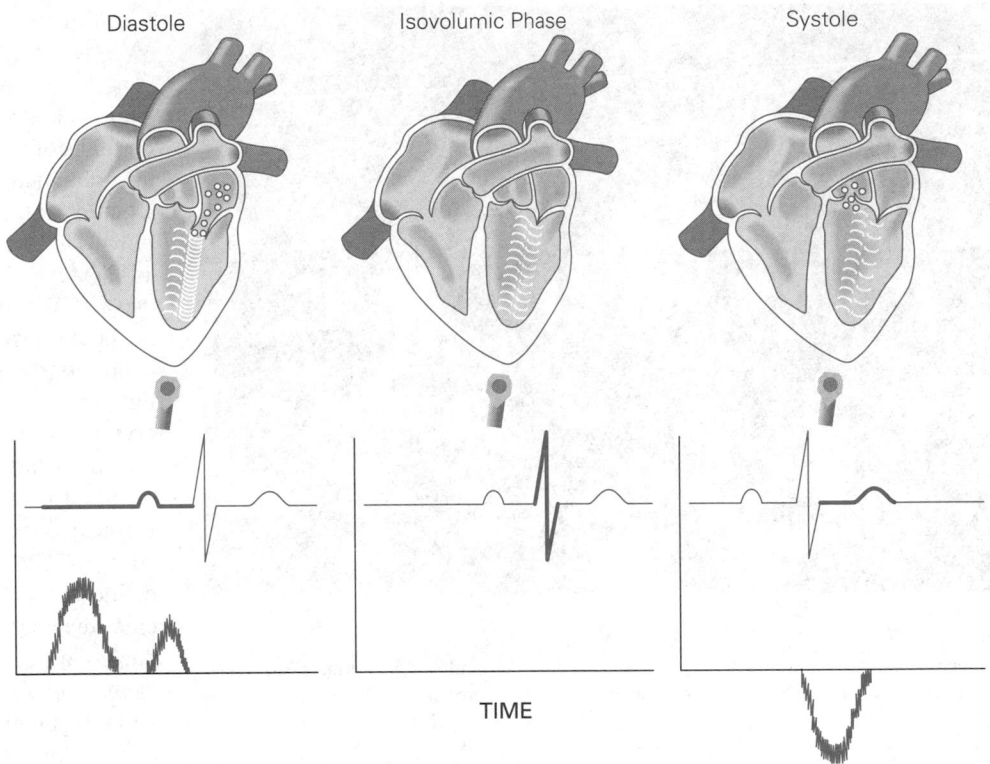

Diastole   Isovolumic Phase   Systole

TIME

FIGURE 14-24

Basic principle of the Doppler shift. During diastole (*left panel*), an ultrasound beam directed toward the junction of the mitral and aortic annuli is reflected by red blood cells moving toward the transducer. The frequency of the received ultrasound is greater than that of the transmitted beam, and the spectral tracing is recorded above the baseline (i.e., flow is toward the transducer). During the isovolumic phase (*middle panel*), both the mitral and aortic valves are closed and little flow occurs within the left ventricle. There-fore, there are no significant changes in the transmitted and received frequencies of the Doppler beam and no spectral tracing is recorded. During systole (*right panel*), the transmitted beam is reflected by red blood cells moving away from the transducer. Therefore, the frequency of the received ultrasound is lower than that of the transmitted beam, and the spectral tracing is recorded below the baseline.

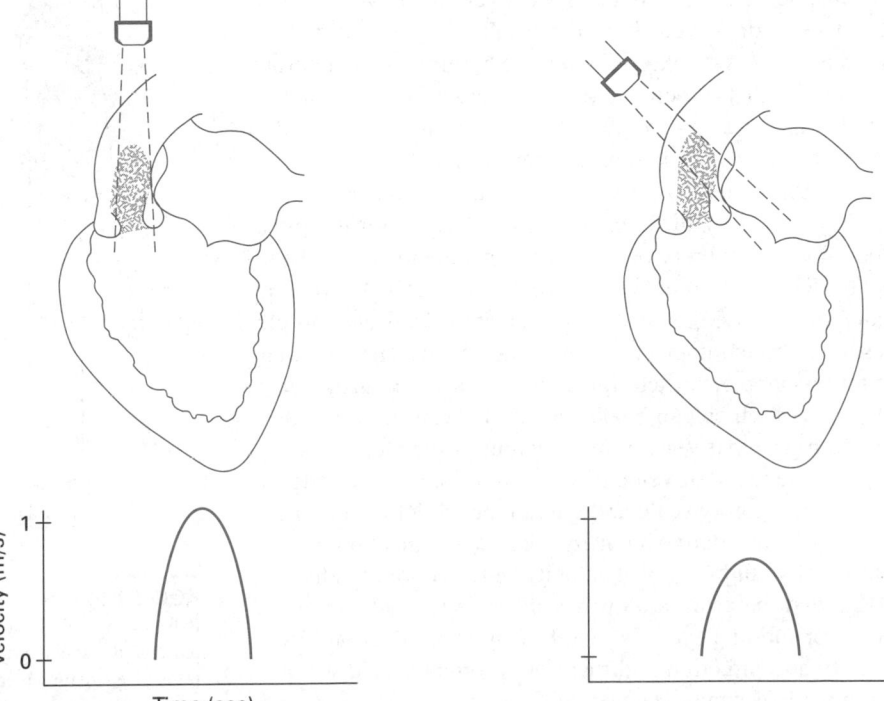

FIGURE 14-25

Effect of the angle of incidence on the velocity recorded with Doppler analysis. The true velocity is underestimated when the ultrasound beam is not parallel to the direction of blood flow. (From Hagan AD, DeMaria AN. *Clinical Applications of Two-Dimensional Echocardiography and Cardiac Doppler.* Boston: Little, Brown; 1989, with permission.)

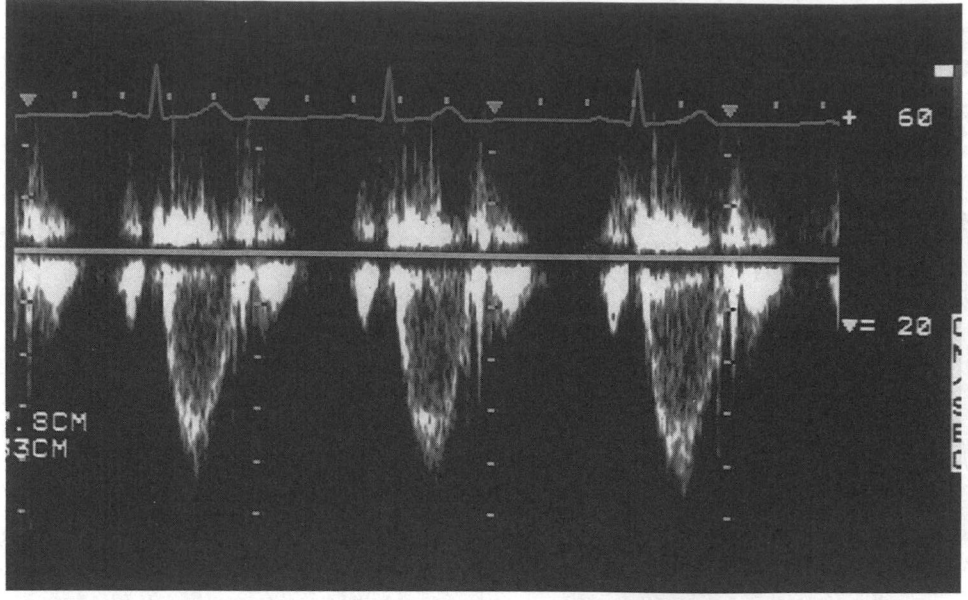

FIGURE 14-26

Doppler spectral envelope of normal blood flow through the right ventricular outflow tract during systole. The transducer is in the parasternal position and the sample volume is placed just proximal to the pulmonic valve.

Continuous and Pulsed-Wave Doppler

Time-velocity spectral recordings of blood flow are generally obtained with two types of Doppler interrogation: *continuous wave* and *pulsed wave* (Fig. 14-27).[54,55] In the continuous-wave (CW) mode, sound waves are both transmitted and received continuously (in clinical practice, this requires two piezoelectric crystals in each transducer, one for transmitting and one for receiving). Because all flow velocities along the beam are recorded, CW Doppler cannot define individual signals at specific distances from the transducer—a problem referred to as *range ambiguity*. Continuous-wave Doppler, however, has no upper limit of velocity that can be accurately recorded. Thus, a CW Doppler beam can accurately measure the direction and velocity of overall flow but cannot discern the precise site of origin of individual components within the signal (Fig. 14-28*B*).

The problem of range ambiguity can be overcome by

shift also can be presented graphically to provide a hard copy printout and enable measurement.

Figure 14-26 shows the typical graphic pulsed Doppler pattern of normal systolic blood flow through the right ventricular outflow tract into the pulmonary artery, with flow velocity on the *y* axis and time on the *x* axis. The location and size of the area from which Doppler recordings are derived is determined by the operator by positioning a sample volume on the echo image. The absence of flow is represented by the zero or no-flow line, termed the *baseline*. By convention, flow toward the transducer is displayed above the baseline and flow away from the transducer is displayed below the baseline. It is important to recognize that velocities above and below baseline represent flow toward or away from the transducer and not forward or backward in the circulation. Because of the effects of viscous friction, the sample volume almost invariably includes RBCs flowing at slightly different velocities. Even normal laminar blood flow in the great vessels varies in velocity across the lumen, as RBCs in the center of the vessel move at higher velocity than those exposed to viscous friction at the wall, and this creates a parabolic rather than a flat flow profile. Therefore, any returning Doppler shifted signal contains a spectrum of velocities, each of which can be displayed by means of fast Fourier transform analysis. The graphic output of the Doppler signal displays the range of velocities within the sample volume site at any time in gray scale and the number of RBCs moving at any velocity as relative intensity. Normal laminar flow is characterized by a uniformity of velocity and direction of individual RBCs, and therefore a narrowly dispersed signal, while disturbed or turbulent low is manifest by marked variability in velocity and direction and therefore a broad signal, which is multitoned, dissonant, and harsh.

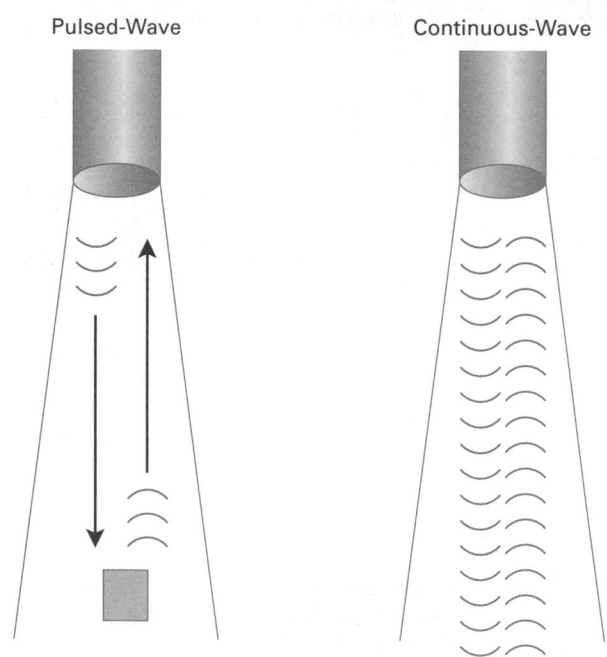

FIGURE 14-27

Pulsed-wave (PW) and continuous-wave (CW) Doppler. With PW, a single pulse of ultrasound energy is emitted and its reflection from a sample volume is received before the following pulse is transmitted. With CW, there is continuous transmission and reception of ultrasound energy.

pulsed-wave Doppler. In this mode, short bursts (rather than a continuous output) of signal are transmitted from the transducer at a given *pulse-repetition frequency* (PRF). The instrument then receives the signal for only a brief period—an interval that corresponds to the time required for sound energy to travel and return from a specific site along the beam path. In practice, the operator selects the location at which flow is to be examined by positioning a sample volume, and the instrument determines the period during which to receive the incoming reflected frequencies. With pulsed-wave Doppler, only a single piezoelectric crystal is needed and flow can be recorded in one small area within the heart or vasculature.[54,55] Unfortunately, pulsed Doppler techniques employ intermittent sampling and are therefore susceptible to a problem of range ambiguity referred to as *aliasing*.[56] By definition, aliasing is the erroneous representation of flow in the direction opposite to that in which it is actually occurring. To correctly record the velocity of blood flow by pulsed Doppler, the pulse repetition frequency (PRF) must be at least double the Doppler shift frequency, a value known as the *Nyquist limit*. If the blood flow examined is of very high velocity or far from the transducer (requiring a long transit time), it may necessitate an unobtainably high PRF. In such cases, aliasing will occur as Doppler signals that depict flow at high velocity in ambiguous or opposite directions compared to actual flow (Fig. 14-28). An intermediate mode between pulsed and CW methods, high-PRF Doppler, is also available.[57,58] This mode enables higher-velocity recordings to be obtained at a compromise of depicting two to four sample sites simultaneously.

Color-Flow Doppler

The major limitation of pulsed and CW Doppler (sometimes referred to as *spectral Doppler*) is that no spatial information regarding the size, shape, and 2D direction of flow is provided.

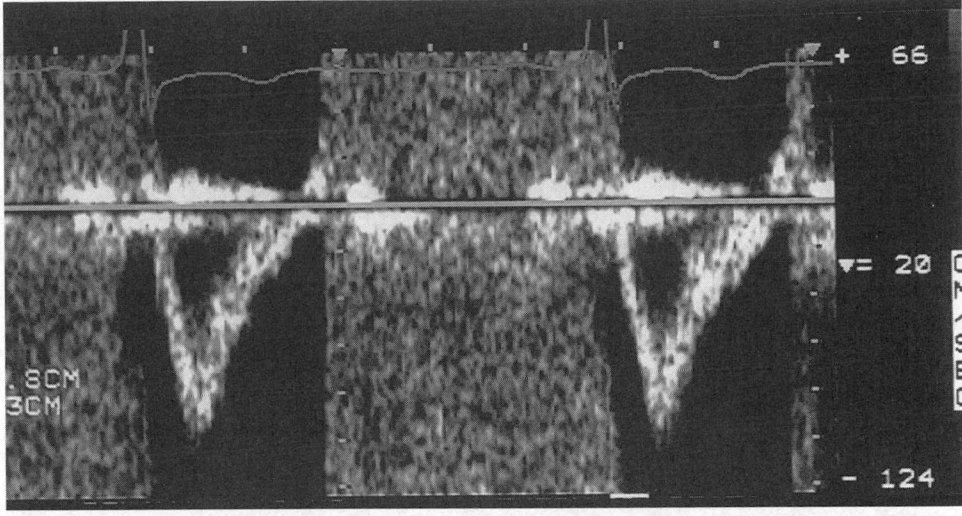

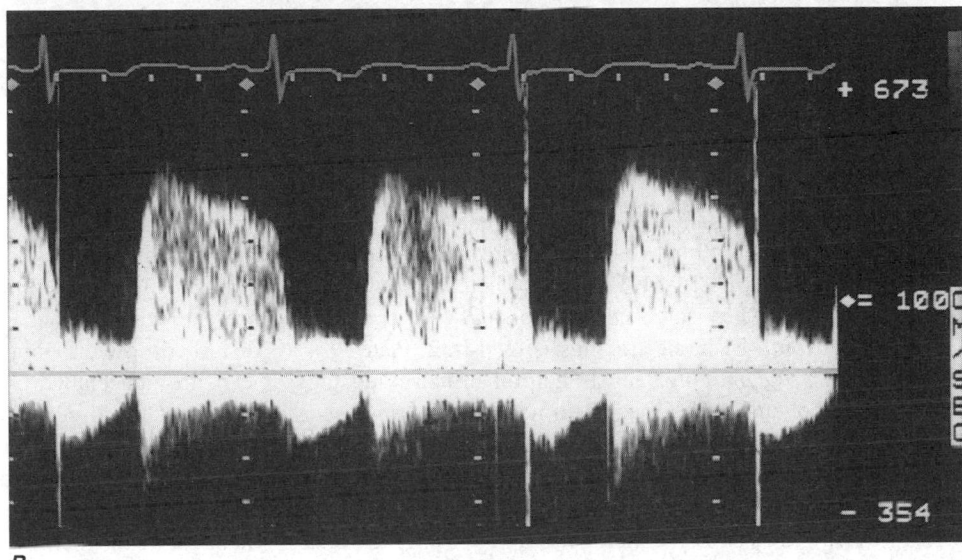

FIGURE 14-28

A. Pulsed-wave Doppler tracing from a patient with aortic regurgitation. The transducer is in the apical position and the sample volume is in the left ventricular outflow tract. A laminar envelope is seen during systole, while aliased flow is present during diastole because of high-velocity flow. *B.* Continuous-wave Doppler tracing through the left ventricular outflow tract (with transducer in the apical position). The maximal velocity of the aortic regurgitation is now measurable, but all other velocities along the Doppler beam are recorded as well.

An extension of pulsed-wave Doppler techniques, *color-flow Doppler* (CFD), provides real-time imaging of blood flow by presenting the velocity and direction of RBC movement as shades of color superimposed upon gray-level 2D tissue structure. Standard pulsed Doppler yields flow signals from a single site along a single scan line. In CFD, rapid pulsed-wave interrogations are performed at multiple sites for multiple scan lines to create a spatially correct and dynamic display of moving blood within the heart and vasculature[59–61] (Fig. 14-29). In light of the quantity of data acquired, Doppler signals are presented as colors assigned to individual sites (Fig. 14-30, Plate 26). Blood flow moving toward the transducer is displayed in red, flow away from the transducer is displayed

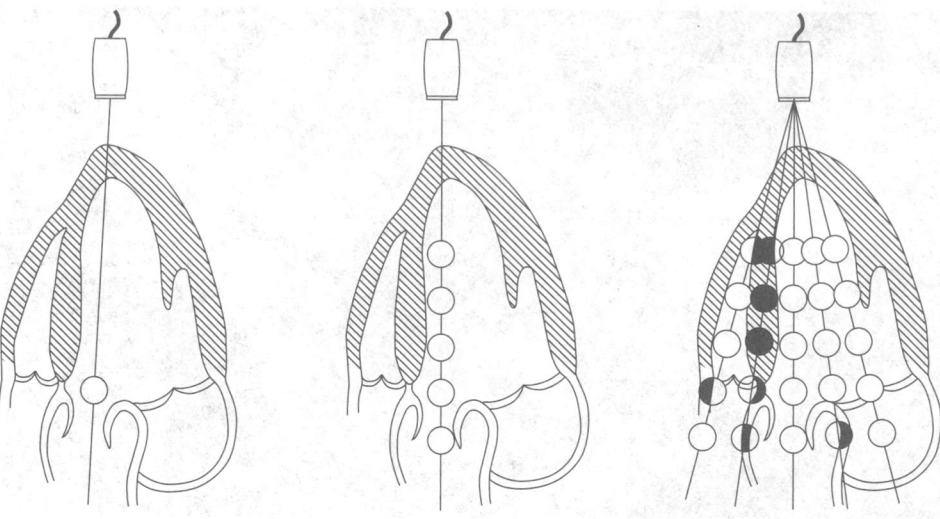

FIGURE 14-29

Simplified mechanism of color-flow Doppler imaging. Single gate (*left*) or multiple-gate pulsed Doppler (*center*) can evaluate flow at points along a single ultrasound beam path. Color-flow imaging (*right*) assesses the velocity and direction of flow for multiple sample volumes along multiple beam paths and assigns a color indicative of velocity and direction at each sample volume site. (From Hagan AD, DeMaria AN. *Clinical Applications of Two-Dimensional Echocardiography and Cardiac Doppler*. Boston: Little, Brown; 1989, with permission.)

in blue, and increasing velocity is depicted in brighter shades of each color. The variance within each signal is calculated as a statistical marker of turbulence and is presented by adding green to the image (Fig. 14-31, Plate 27). Therefore, turbulent flow jets appear as a mosaic mix of colors. CFD also can be superimposed onto M-mode tracings (Fig. 14-32, Plate 28), often termed *M/Q imaging,* and is helpful in clarifying the timing of flow phenomena. Given the time constraints imposed by collecting the large volume of data required by CFD, velocity estimates are performed by autocorrelation techniques that are less accurate than fast Fourier transform analysis.[62] Nevertheless, CFD technology is a major advance that has improved the rapid detection of cardiac pathology, especially valvular regurgitation and intracardiac shunts.

Normal and Abnormal Flow Dynamics

The clinical application of Doppler recordings is based on the fundamental differences between normal and disturbed blood flow. Normal flow is laminar, with all RBCs exhibiting the same velocity and direction of flow. Although some abnormalities involve laminar flow, such as atrial septal defects, most pathologic conditions involve disturbed or turbulent flow and share a common hydrodynamic basis for the resultant flow

dynamics. Specifically, nearly all circulatory disturbances (stenosis, regurgitation, shunt) involve blood flow from a high-pressure chamber to a lower-pressure chamber through a restricted orifice.[53] Aortic valve disease is a perfect example. Aortic stenosis is a forward flow disturbance in which turbulent blood travels from a high-pressure left ventricle to a lower-pressure aorta through a restricted aortic orifice in systole. Aortic regurgitation is a retrograde flow disturbance in which turbulent blood regurgitates from a high-pressure aorta to a lower-pressure left ventricle through a small regurgitant orifice in diastole. In each case, the pressure gradient results in a high velocity jet coursing through a restricted orifice, reaching its maximal velocity at a site just distal to the orifice, designated the *vena contracta,* at which time shear forces produce vortices resulting in flow of varying direction and velocity (Fig. 14-33). In each case, the velocity of the jet is related to the pressure gradient across the orifice. Thus, the hallmark of disturbed flow on Doppler recordings is a very high velocity jet with adjacent vortices of varying direction and velocity of flow. On pulsed Doppler recordings, these hemodynamic abnormalities cause broadening of the spectral signal and aliasing. On CW recordings, high velocity represents the primary abnormality. By color-flow imaging, the disturbance is manifest by the increased variance and higher velocities in the signal. With any of these techniques, of course, inappropriate timing of flow serves to highlight the abnormality (for example, high-velocity left-atrial flow during systole in mitral regurgitation).

FIGURE 14-30
See color Plate 26.

FIGURE 14-31
See color Plate 27.

FIGURE 14-32
See color Plate 28.

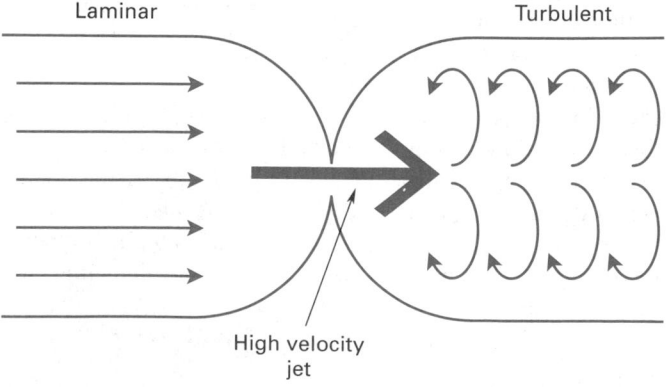

Laminar   Turbulent

High velocity
jet

FIGURE 14-33

Flow characteristics through a stenotic orifice. Proximal to the stenosis, the flow is laminar. Near the point of maximal stenosis, the flow velocity is markedly increased. Turbulent flow is present distal to the stenosis.

The Standard Doppler Examination

A clinical Doppler examination must be performed with full consideration of the three different Doppler modalities available, the types of information each can provide, the multiple sites for flow interrogation, and the spectrum of pathologic lesions that produces flow disturbances. In light of these considerations, it is understandable that the Doppler examination may not be as standardized as the format for 2D cardiac imaging; however, a number of usual practices have emerged. A vast majority of echocardiographic examinations include screening for flow disturbances by CFD. Since Doppler signals are best recorded with the ultrasound beam parallel to flow, screening is typically performed in long-axis or apical views. Any flow disturbances visualized are subsequently examined by CW spectral recordings and, in most laboratories, by pulsed-wave Doppler. Although CW examination is typically reserved for flow disturbances, pulsed-wave Doppler also may be of value in quantifying flow dynamics in the setting of laminar flow. In this regard, pulsed Doppler recordings obtained at the mitral, tricuspid, and aortic valve orifices, pulmonary artery, and pulmonary veins constitute part of a standard echocardiogram in many laboratories (Figs. 14-26 and 14-34 to 14-37).

The normal Doppler examination is characterized by uniformity of flow velocity and the absence of high-velocity turbulent flow. CFD recordings demonstrate laminar flow through the atrioventricular valves in diastole and the semilunar valves in systole. Since the Doppler examination is usually performed with a long-axis or apical transducer orientation, diastolic filling is

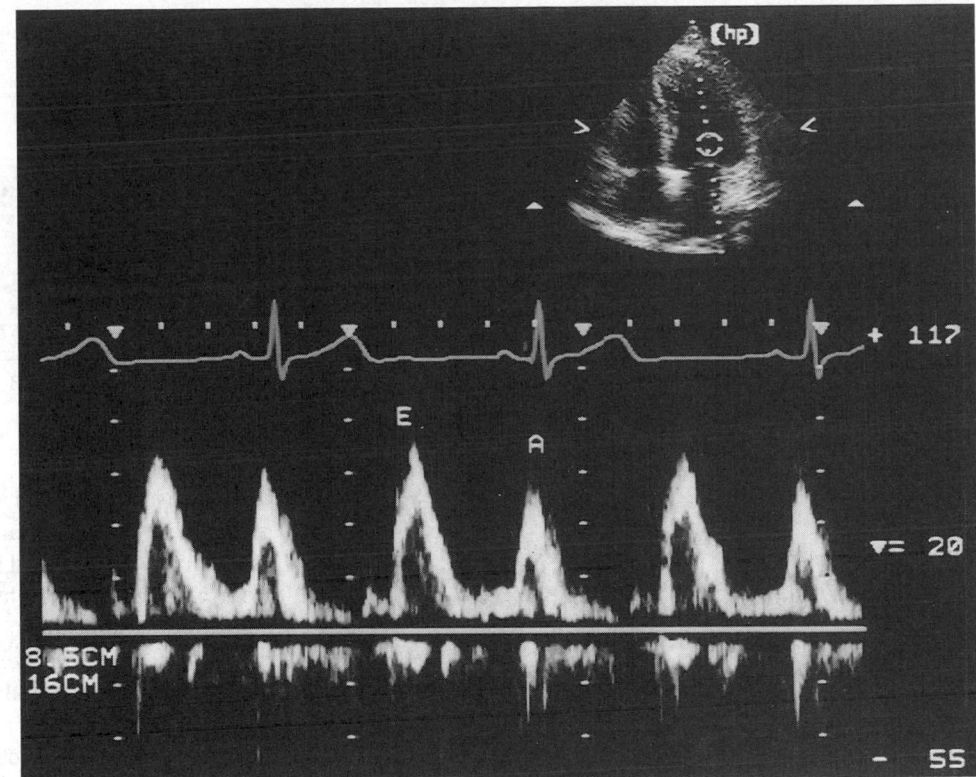

FIGURE 14-34

Normal pulsed-wave Doppler tracing from the left ventricular inflow tract, displaying the early rapid filling (E) and atrial contraction (A) phases of diastolic flow. The transducer is in the apical position and the sample volume is at the mitral leaflet tips.

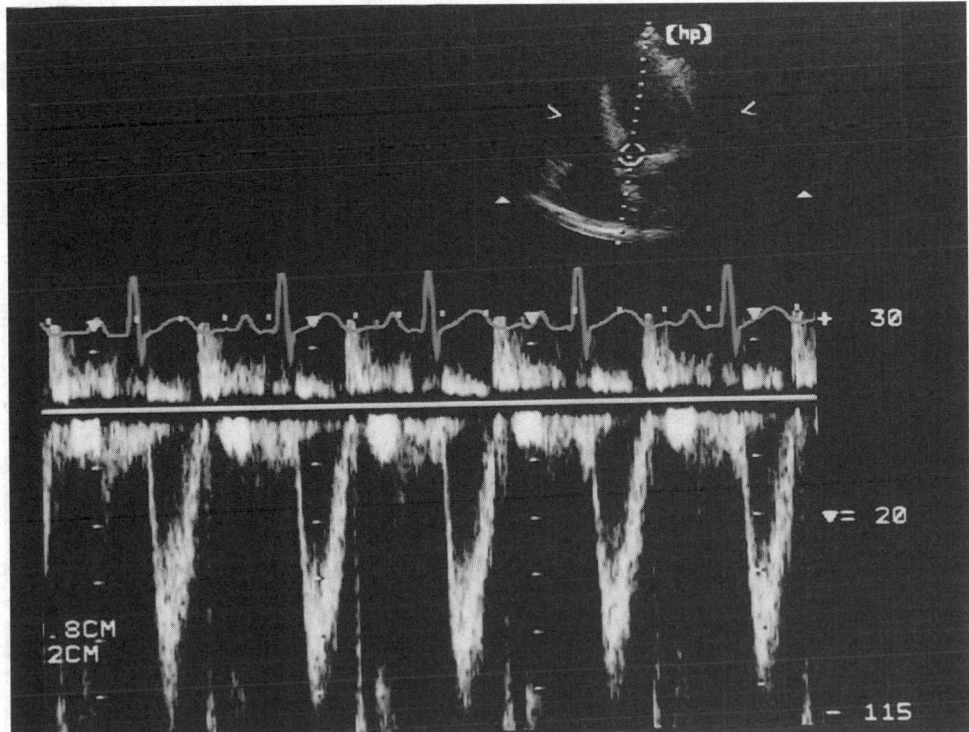

FIGURE 14-35

Normal pulsed-wave Doppler tracing with the sample volume in the left ventricular outflow tract (apical transducer position).

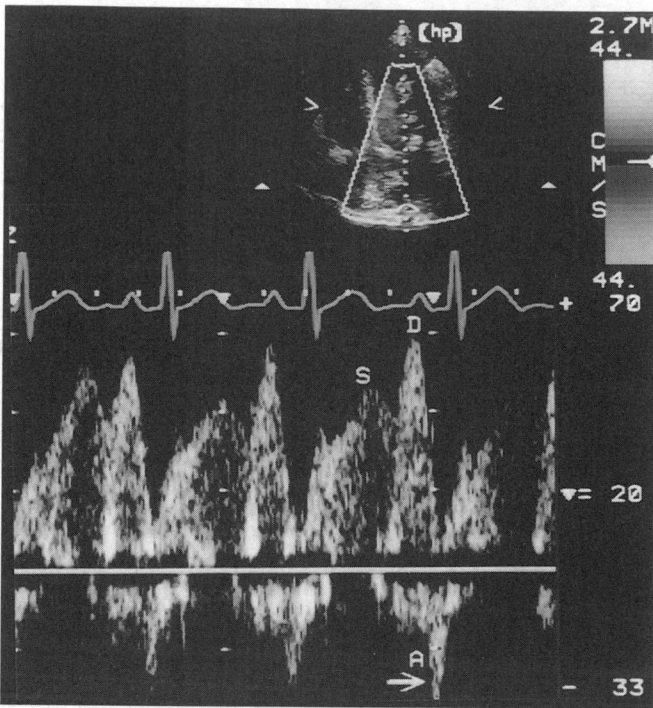

FIGURE 14-36
Pulsed-wave Doppler tracing from the right upper pulmonary vein (recorded from the apical transducer position). Flow toward the heart is biphasic, with peaks in systole (S) and diastole (D). A small amount of reversed flow is seen during atrial contraction (A).

TABLE 14-4

NORMAL INTRACARDIAC DOPPLER VELOCITIES

	Velocity, m/s
Right ventricle	
Tricuspid flow	0.3–0.7
Pulmonary artery	0.6–0.9
Left ventricle	
Mitral flow	0.6–1.3
Aorta	1.0–1.7

Source: Hatle L, Angelsen B. *Doppler Ultrasound in Cardiology,* 2d ed. Philadelphia: Lea & Febiger; 1985.

characteristically encoded in red and ejection in blue (Fig. 14-30, Plate 26). Color aliasing is often observed at the levels of the mitral annulus and LV outflow tract as an abrupt change from bright red to bright blue or vice versa, usually in the center of the flow stream. Pulsed Doppler recordings of transmitral flow velocities are often recorded at the level of both the leaflet tips and annulus. Velocities are higher at the tips, while recordings at the annulus offer the ability to calculate flow through a cross-sectional area that is relatively uniform throughout the cardiac cycle. A sample volume positioned in the right upper pulmonary vein reveals systolic and diastolic emptying flow of nearly equal magnitude followed by a short, low-velocity reversal of flow into the pulmonary veins following atrial contraction (Fig. 14-36). Flow in the LV outflow tract and aortic annulus area is characterized by a progressive increase of velocity peaking in early systole, followed by a more gradual deceleration of flow (Fig. 14-35). Minimal if any flow velocities are detected in the mitral valve orifice and LV outflow tract in systole and diastole, respectively, in normal examinations. Examinations of the tricuspid and pulmonic valves give qualitatively similar results to those of the mitral and aortic valves (Figs. 14-26 and 14-37). Normal values for forward flow velocity are given in Table 14-4. As can be seen, velocity in normal individuals is highest in the aorta and is less than 2 m/s.[63] Other commonly made measurements include the acceleration time (from the beginning of flow to peak velocity of flow in the ascending aorta or pulmonary artery); and the deceleration time, from left ventricular inflow peak

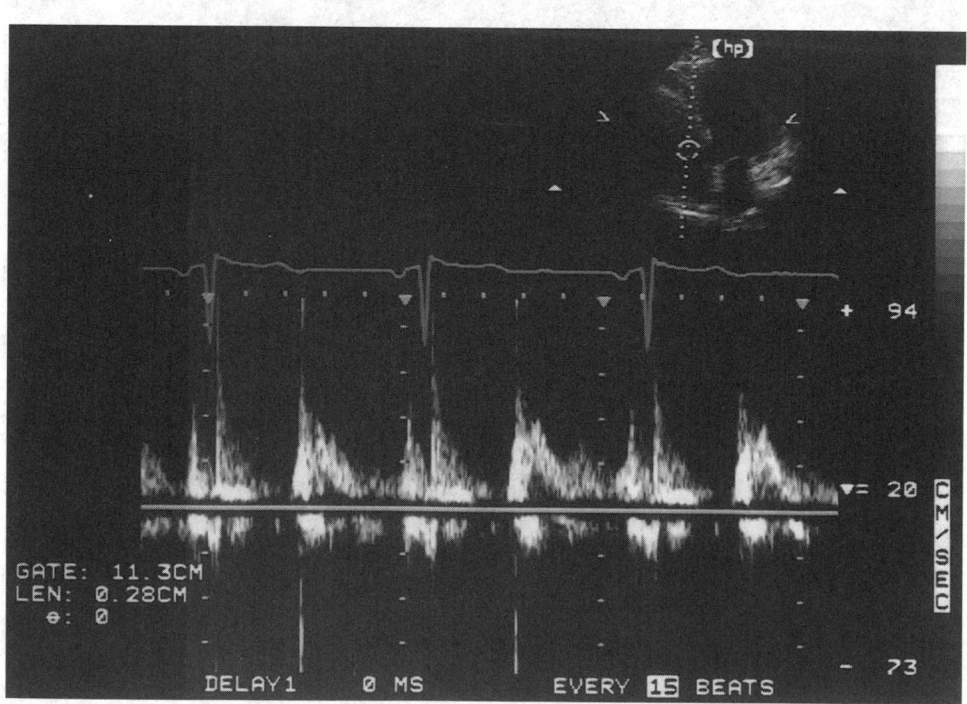

FIGURE 14-37
Pulsed-wave Doppler tracing from the right ventricular inflow tract (apical transducer position).

E-wave velocity extrapolated to baseline zero velocity.

Doppler Assessment of Diastolic Function

In recent years, there has been a great deal of interest in using mitral inflow velocity patterns to evaluate LV diastolic properties.[64–74] Transmitral filling velocities reflect the pressure gradient between the left atrium and left ventricle during diastole[65] (Fig. 14-34). In early diastole, pressure in the left ventricle normally falls below that in the left atrium, producing an increase in velocity due to rapid transmitral inflow (E wave). Flow decelerates as the pressures equilibrate in mid-diastole. In late diastole, left atrial contraction restores a small gradient, causing transmitral flow to accelerate to a second peak (A wave) that is of less magnitude than the E wave. In individuals in whom early LV relaxation is impaired, the transmitral pressure gradient is blunted, resulting in a decrease in both the velocity of early filling and rate of E wave deceleration[66,68,70] (Fig. 14-38). Conversely, in patients with marked increases of left atrial pressure and LV stiffness, early diastolic filling velocities are high, deceleration is rapid, and late filling following atrial contraction is markedly reduced. This is the so-called restrictive pattern of LV filling (Fig. 14-39). Accordingly, an E wave velocity that is substantially less than the A wave velocity and is accompanied by a prolonged deceleration time represents evidence of impaired early diastolic relaxation by Doppler, while an increased E wave velocity and decreased A wave velocity (E/A ratio greater than 2.5 or 3 to 1) accompanied by a diminished deceleration time (less than 100 ms) is indicative of a noncompliant left ventricle with markedly elevated left atrial pressures.[69,70,73] Although a restrictive pattern can be seen with restrictive car-

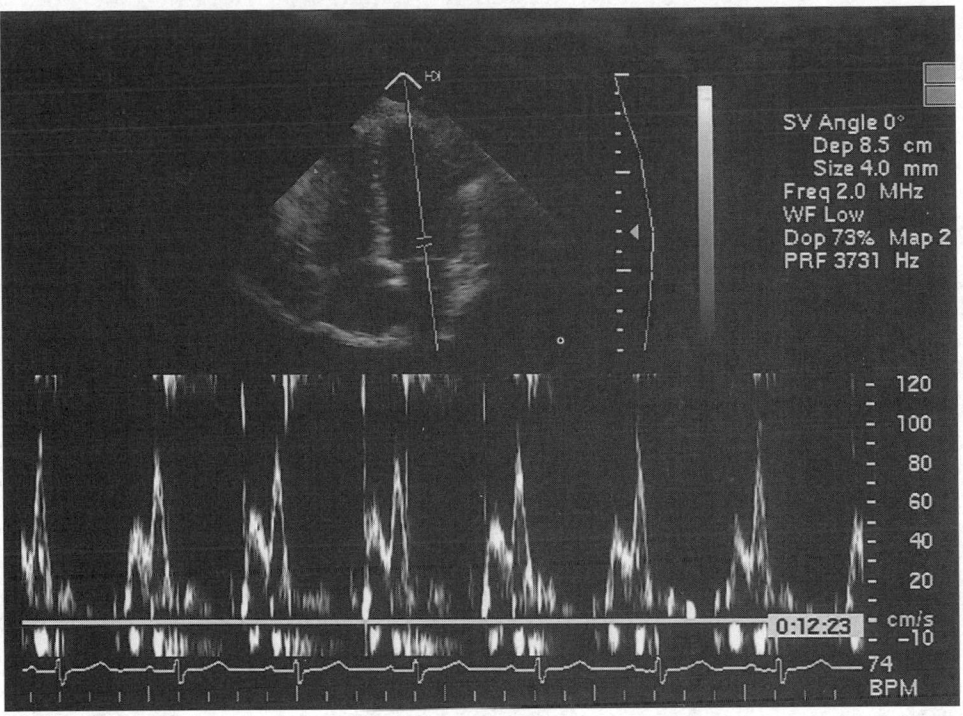

FIGURE 14-38
Pulsed-wave Doppler tracing of diastolic relaxation abnormality (see text for details).

diomyopathy or advanced LV dysfunction of any cause, it also occurs in pericardial disease.[75] Of significance, a restrictive pattern of LV filling has been associated with an increased mortality rate in patients with advanced congestive heart failure,[76] and persistence of this pattern despite

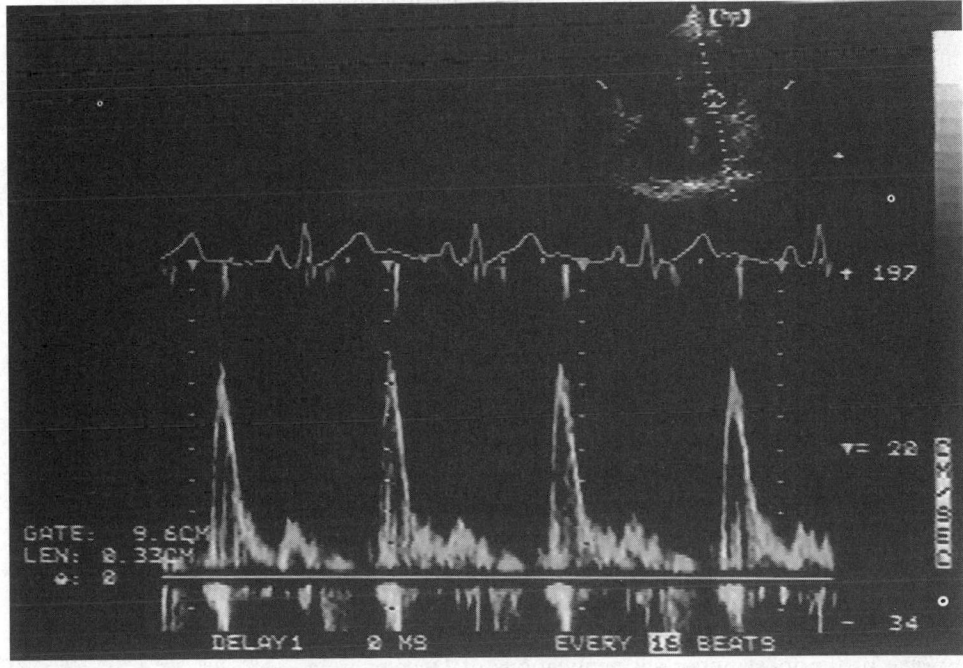

FIGURE 14-39
Pulsed-wave Doppler tracing of diastolic restrictive abnormality (see text for details).

changes in loading condition is an additional poor prognostic sign.[76a]

These abnormal mitral inflow patterns can be clinically useful and, when they are markedly distorted, are generally reliable in identifying and characterizing diastolic dysfunction. A number of variables other than diastolic function, however, are capable of influencing transmitral filling velocities. It has been shown that transmitral Doppler filling dynamics are affected by the age of the patient,[77,78] changes in heart rate,[79,80] respiration,[81] and even the position of the Doppler sample volume within the mitral valve orifice.[82–84] Of greatest significance, transmitral inflow is very sensitive to loading conditions, and reductions in LV preload induced by nitroglycerin and/or lower-body negative pressure can induce a striking decrease in early transmitral filling velocities independent of changes in diastolic properties.[85,86] The influence of LV loading upon transmitral filling is most striking when an increase in left atrial pressure due to cardiac dysfunction restores early diastolic filling velocities and obscures impaired relaxation, thus inducing "pseudonormalization."[68] Therefore, as Doppler transmitral filling dynamics have many limitations in assessing diastolic function, particular filling patterns should not be interpreted as "pathognomonic" findings of diastolic dysfunction but rather as a component of a complete clinical and echocardiographic evaluation.

Recently, attention has focused on velocity recordings from the pulmonary veins as a method to evaluate left atrial pressure and LV diastolic function (Fig. 14-36). An impaired systolic filling wave and increased A-wave flow reversal in the pulmonary veins in the setting of a relatively normal transmitral pattern of diastolic filling may be useful in distinguishing normal from pseudonormal mitral inflow patterns. In addition, an increased amplitude of the pulmonary vein A-wave reversal in comparison with the forward transmitral A-wave velocity, especially in regard to duration, has been found to be of value in estimating LV filling pressures by Doppler.[87,88] These findings, coupled with the value of systolic flow reversal in identifying severe mitral regurgitation, make it likely that recordings from the pulmonary veins will assume an increasingly important role in Doppler examination.

Doppler Assessment of Systolic Function and Cardiac Output

Although measurements of LV volumes and ejection fraction can be obtained by 2D echocardiography, Doppler interrogation provides a unique and complementary noninvasive assessment of systolic function. Thus, LV systolic dysfunction often results in decreased aortic velocity and acceleration time.[89–91] As will be discussed, in the presence of mitral regurgitation (MR) the acceleration of the MR jet can provide information regarding contractile function.[92]

One of the most important applications of Doppler is in the calculation of the stroke volume.[93] The theory involved is relatively simple. The volume of flow through any orifice or tube can be calculated as the product of the cross-sectional

area through which flow occurs and the velocity of that flow (Fig. 14-40). Measures of anatomic cross-sectional area can be derived from echocardiographic images, while velocity can be determined by Doppler. As the annulus of the aortic valve is nearly circular; its cross-sectional area can be estimated from a measurement of diameter, as $\pi(\text{diameter}/2)^2$. The pulsed-wave Doppler envelope also can be recorded at the same level. The *mean* flow velocity through the orifice is calculated by integrating velocity over time (in other words,

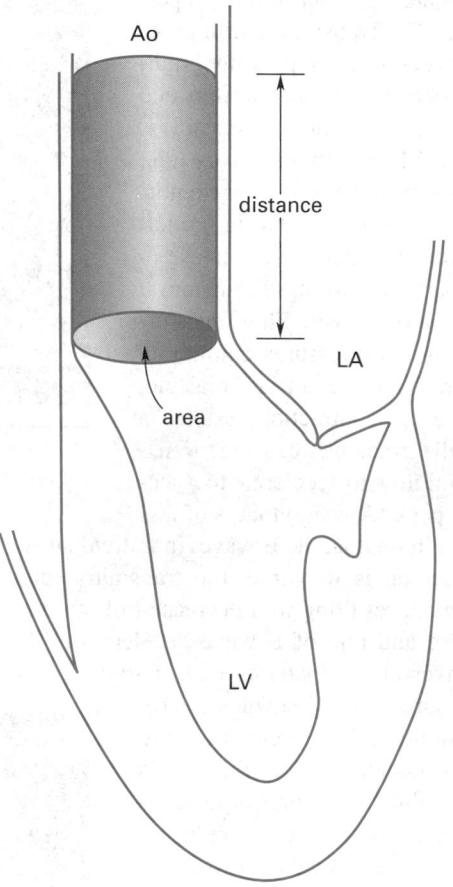

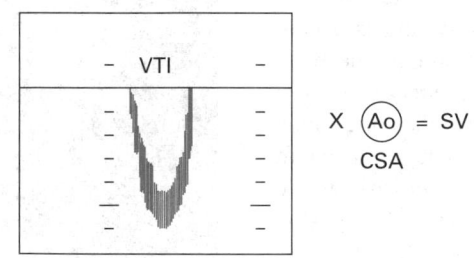

FIGURE 14-40

Calculation of stroke volume. Multiplying the cross-sectional area (CSA) of the blood column in the ascending aorta by the distance the column moves during a single cardiac contraction yields the stroke volume (SV). The velocity-time integral (VTI), expressed in units of length, represents the "stroke distance." (Modified from Pearlman AS. Technique of Doppler and color flow Doppler in the evaluation of cardiac disorders and function. In: Schlant RC, Alexander RW, eds. *The Heart, Arteries, and Veins,* 8th ed. New York: McGraw-Hill; 1994:2229, with permission.)

by measuring the area under the Doppler curve). This velocity-time integral, often called the *stroke distance,* is then multiplied by the cross-sectional area at the level of the Doppler interrogation to obtain the stroke volume.[93–96] The product of the stroke volume and heart rate then yields cardiac output.

Calculation of stroke volume by the Doppler method involves a number of assumptions. The orifice must be circular and constant in size, and the flow velocity must be uniform throughout the cross-sectional area. In addition, the angle between flow and the interrogating beam must be less than 20°. Despite the uncertainty of these assumptions, Doppler-derived measurements of cardiac output and stroke volume have been shown to correspond well with thermodilution, Fick, and the angiographic calculations, though the correlation is not perfect.[93–99]

Theoretically, stroke volume can be calculated at any valve annulus.[96,97,100–102] In clinical practice, however, this is not always possible (for example, it is difficult to obtain an accurate diameter of the pulmonary artery in every patient). Because the measurement of annular radius is squared in the computation of area, it is the most important source of error of Doppler stroke-volume analyses. Stroke-volume analysis through the mitral annulus is cumbersome; it is uncertain whether the mitral annulus is best described as a circle or an ellipse, and the cross-sectional area of the annulus probably changes slightly during diastole. Calculations using the tricuspid annulus are hampered by similar problems. Despite these limitations, measurements of stroke volume through the various cardiac valves are clinically useful and can be used to calculate pulmonary-to-systemic shunt ratios, regurgitant volumes,[103–110] and orifice areas of stenotic valves by the continuity equation[111–115] (see below).

The Bernoulli Equation

One of the most important applications of Doppler echocardiography is the calculation of pressure gradients within the cardiovascular system using a modification of the Bernoulli equation.[116–118] This theorem states that the pressure drop across a discrete stenosis in the heart or vasculature occurs because of energy loss due to three processes: (1) acceleration of blood through the orifice (*convective acceleration*), (2) inertial forces (*flow acceleration*), and (3) resistance to flow at the interfaces between blood and the orifice (*viscous friction*).[119] Therefore, the pressure drop across any orifice can be calculated as the sum of these three variables (Fig. 14-41). In most clinical situations, the contribution of inertial forces and viscous friction are minimal and can be discounted. Since convective acceleration is determined by velocity, the pressure gradient can be calculated from the velocities of blood proximal to and at the level of an orifice as gradient = $4[(\text{orifice velocity})^2 - (\text{proximal velocity})^2]$. If the blood velocity proximal to the stenosis is low (≤ 1.0 m/s), this term can be ignored as well. The resulting modified equation states that the pressure gradient across a discrete orifice

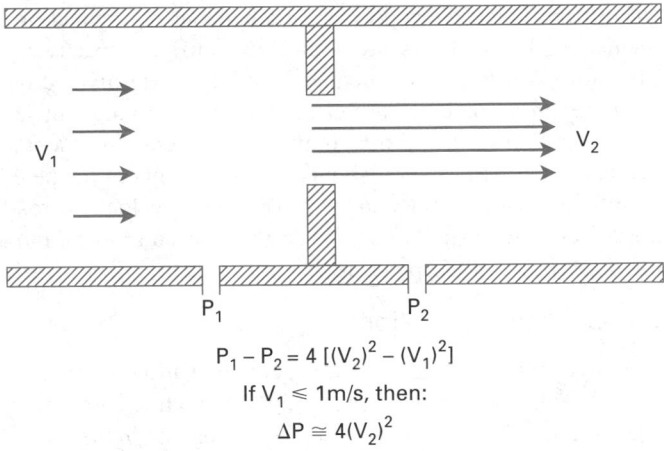

$$P_1 - P_2 = 4[(V_2)^2 - (V_1)^2]$$
If $V_1 \leq 1$ m/s, then:
$$\Delta P \cong 4(V_2)^2$$

FIGURE 14-41

The modified Bernoulli equation. Pressure drop across a small orifice can be estimated as four times the square of the peak velocity (if the proximal velocity is less than 1 m/s). V_1 and P_1 = proximal velocity and pressure; V_2 and P_2 = distal velocity and pressure, respectively. (Modified from Pearlman AS. Technique of Doppler and color flow Doppler in the evaluation of cardiac disorders and function. In: Schlant RC, Alexander RW, eds. *The Heart, Arteries, and Veins,* 8th ed. New York: McGraw-Hill; 1994:2229, with permission.)

is equal to four times the square of the peak velocity (*V*) through the stenosis (PG = $4V^2$).[116–119]

The modified Bernoulli equation can be used to calculate pressure gradients across any flow-limiting orifice and has been validated against invasive measurements.[116–122] The method was originally applied to aortic, mitral, and pulmonic stenosis, but further uses have been identified. If at least trivial valvular regurgitation is present, systolic gradients across the tricuspid and end-diastolic gradients across the pulmonic valve can be calculated.[123,124] If the right ventricular diastolic pressure is known (or estimated as the right atrial or central venous pressure), peak right ventricular and pulmonary artery pressure (assuming pulmonic stenosis is absent) can be computed[125,126]:

$$\text{Peak pulmonary artery pressure} = 4(\text{TR velocity})^2 + \text{RA pressure}$$

End-diastolic pulmonary artery pressure (PAD) also can be calculated:

$$\text{PAD} = 4 \, (\text{end-diastolic pulmonary regurgitation velocity})^2 + \text{RA pressure}$$

In the presence of mitral regurgitation, a variety of calculations can be made. With measurement of peak systolic arterial pressure, systolic left atrial pressure can be estimated[127]:

$$\text{Left atrial systolic pressure} = \text{systolic blood pressure} - 4 \, (\text{MR velocity})^2$$

Further, the acceleration of the MR jet can be used to estimate *dP/dt*.[128] Thus, from the Bernoulli equation, the left atrial-to-left ventricular pressure gradients at regurgitant velocities of 1 and 3 m/s are 4 and 36 mmHg, respectively. Therefore, *dP/dt* can be calculated as: 32 mmHg divided by the time (in seconds) required for the mitral regurgitant jet to accelerate from 1 to 3 m/s. In the case of ventricular septal defects or aortopulmonary shunts, measurements of the peak systolic arterial pressure and the peak Doppler velocity across the defect allows calculation of the right ventricular (or pulmonary arterial) systolic pressure.

The Continuity Equation

Although transvalvular pressure gradients can be calculated from CW Doppler recordings using the modified Bernoulli equation, gradients sometimes can be misleading in the evaluation of valvular stenosis. The transvalvular gradient is determined by both the size of the stenotic orifice and the stroke volume traversing it. Severe aortic stenosis and accompanying LV systolic dysfunction may produce a low transvalvular gradient despite a small valve area, while coexistent aortic regurgitation may result in a large gradient with only mild aortic stenosis. The calculation of orifice area by Doppler echocardiography employs the *continuity equation,* which is derived from the law of the conservation of mass and states that the product of cross-sectional area and velocity is constant in a closed system of flow[129] (Fig 14-42). Thus, in the case of aortic stenosis, the product of the area and velocity of the left LV outflow tract

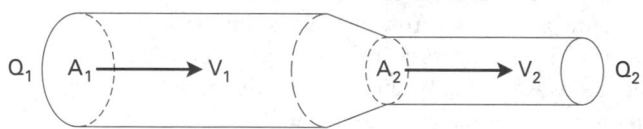

$$(A_1) = \pi r^2 = \pi \left(\frac{D}{2}\right)^2 = 0.785 \, (D^2)$$

$$(A_2)(V_2) = (A_1)(V_1) \text{ or } (A_2) = \frac{(A_1)(V_1)}{(V_2)}$$

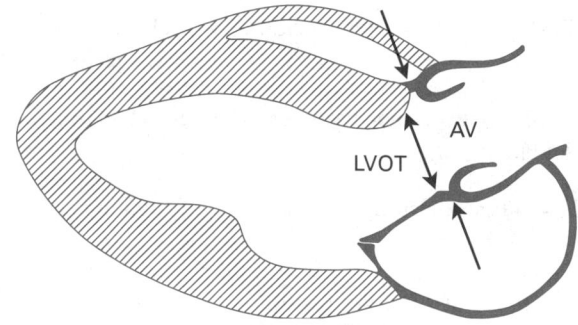

FIGURE 14-42

The continuity equation. In a closed system (*top*) with constant flow, $Q_1 = Q_2$. Therefore, $A_1 \times V_1$ must equal $A_2 \times V_2$. Determination of any three of the variables allows calculation of the fourth. Clinically (*bottom*), the area of the left ventricular outflow tract (LVOT) can be estimated and used to determine aortic valve area. (From Hagan AD, DeMaria AN. *Clinical Applications of Two-Dimensional Echocardiography and Cardiac Doppler.* Boston: Little, Brown; 1989, with permission.)

equals the product of the area and velocity of the aortic valve orifice. Annulus diameter and integrated velocity measurements are derived by the standard volumetric approach, while the velocity across the stenotic orifice is derived by CW Doppler. The equation is then solved for the valve area.[111–116]

The continuity equation is simple and the constituent factors are readily measured, but a number of potential errors can occur. The most common pitfall is an inaccurate estimation of the cross-sectional area proximal to the stenosis. In addition, it is essential that blood velocity proximal to a stenosis be measured outside the area of flow acceleration. Finally, the continuity equation actually solves for the area of the vena contracta, which is usually just distal to the stenotic orifice. Although this area is very similar to the area of the stenotic orifice, occasional discrepancies occur.

Determinants of the Size of Flow Disturbances

Although CFD yields primarily qualitative information, it is unique in its ability to provide measurements of the size of flow disturbances. It seems logical that the size of a turbulent jet should correlate with the volume of blood contained within the flow disturbance. Regardless of the lesion, however, the area of turbulence recorded by CFD has multiple determinants.[130–134] The volume of flow present in the disturbance is, of course, a major factor in its size. The pressure gradient operative in any flow disturbance is also an important determinant of the spatial distribution or "spray area" of turbulence.[134] In addition, studies have demonstrated that the size of a flow disturbance is influenced by the orifice through which flow occurs as well as the size and compliance of the receiving chamber.[130–136] Finally, a number of technical factors can influence jet size as imaged by CFD, including instrument gain, the angle of incidence of the interrogating beam, the frequency and pulse repetition rate of the transducer, and the temporal sampling rate.[137] Therefore, derived from the size of the turbulent jet recorded by color Doppler, are at best semi-quantitative and should not be expected to correlate with the volume of blood contained in the flow disturbance.

TRANSESOPHAGEAL ECHOCARDIOGRAPHY

Transthoracic echocardiography (TTE) usually defines cardiac anatomy and function satisfactorily, often obviating the need for further cardiac imaging. Occasionally, however, TTE does not provide complete or adequately detailed information. This is especially true in the evaluation of posterior cardiac structures (e.g., the left atrium, the left atrial appendage, the interatrial septum, the aorta distal to the root), in the assessment of prosthetic cardiac valves, and in the delineation of cardiac structures less than 3 mm in size (e.g., small vegetations or thrombi). Ultrasonic imaging from the esophagus is uniquely suited to these situations, as the esophagus is adjacent to the left atrium and the thoracic aorta for much of its course[138,139] and affords excellent access of the interrogating beam to these structures.

The earliest transesophageal probes consisted of miniaturized phased-array transducers attached to standard gastroscopes. Over the past decade, a number of technologic advances have occurred in the field of transesophageal echocardiography (TEE), and flexible transesophageal ultrasound probes capable of multiplanar imaging of the heart are now widely available.[140-142] The current generation of probes also provide full pulsed-wave, CW, and CFD capabilities.

Although images can be recorded from a variety of probe positions most authorities recommend three basic positions: (1) posterior to the base of the heart, (2) posterior to the left atrium, and (3) inferior to the heart (transgastric position; Fig. 14-43). Figures 14-44 through 14-47 show TEE images obtained in various planes through the heart. It must be emphasized that, with the transducer in the esophagus, posterior structures appear at the top of the image. With the transducer in the stomach, a short-axis view is standardly obtained, with long-axis and apical views available to a variable degree. Upon withdrawing the transducer to the esophagus, one usually obtains apical-equivalent four-chamber and long-axis views, with multiple intermediate projections. Further withdrawal of the probe to the base yields excellent views of the atria, great vessels and semilunar valves, and pulmonary veins. Of particular value are views that delineate the left atrial appendage, all three leaflets of the aortic valve in short axis, and the transverse and descending aorta.[143]

TEE has become an important imaging modality for the diagnosis and management of infective endocarditis and its complications, including valvular vegetations, chordal rupture, fistulas, perivalvular abscesses, and mycotic aneurysms.[143-148] TEE is more accurate in detecting vegetations and abscesses than TEE[143,149,150] and provides prognostic information as well[150] (Fig. 14-48). In addition, TEE imaging may aid in accurate quantification of valvular disease (particularly mitral regurgitation) if TEE is inconclusive[151] (Fig. 14-49, Plate 29). TEE is especially useful for Doppler interrogation of the pulmonary veins (Fig. 14-50, Plate 30). Flow patterns in these vessels reflect left atrial pressure, and

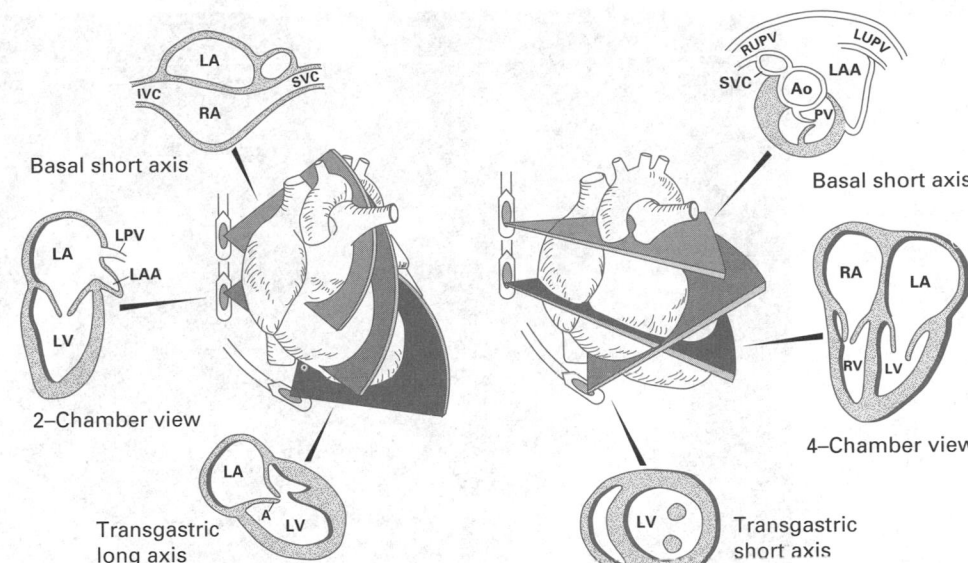

FIGURE 14-43
Standard TEE imaging planes in transverse and longitudinal axes. (From Fisher EA, Stahl JA, Budd JH, Goldman ME. Transesophageal echocardiography: Procedures and clinical applications. *J Am Coll Cardiol* 1991; 18:1333–1348, with permission.)

systolic reversal of pulmonary venous flow has been identified as an accurate marker of mitral regurgitation.[152,153] Although mitral regurgitant color jets are easier to see with TEE than TTE, they are usually larger, and care must be exercised not to overestimate severity of the regurgitation.[154] Multiplane TEE can be used to planimeter the orifice area in aortic stenosis.[155] The technique is also quite helpful in detection of aortic disease, including dissection, aneurysm, congenital malformations, and atherosclerosis.[139,156,157] Because of its portability, accuracy, and short preparation and procedural times, TEE is now recommended as the preferred diagnostic study in many cases of suspected aortic dissection (Fig. 14-51, Plate 31).[139,158]

Thromboemboli may originate from posterior cardiac structures such as the left atrium and appendage, interatrial septum and aorta[159-168]; therefore, TEE has received wide application in the evaluation of possible cardiogenic embolization. Since the most common site of left atrial thrombi is the appendage, the ability of TEE to visualize this structure is of particular value (Fig. 14-52). TEE can also detect spontaneous contrast signals (that appear to represent transient rouleaux formation and predispose to thromboemboli).[169] In addition, TEE has provided unique real-time images of mobile, pedunculated, atherosclerotic "debris" in the thoracic aorta (Fig. 14-53). Although the optimal therapy for this disorder is currently unknown, mobile or protruding aortic atheromas appear to be significant risk factors for embolic events.[167,168,170,171] The optimal role for TEE in the detection of intracardiac sources of emboli is controversial, and clinical trials are

FIGURE 14-49
See color Plate 29.

FIGURE 14-50
See color Plate 30.

FIGURE 14-51
See color Plate 31.

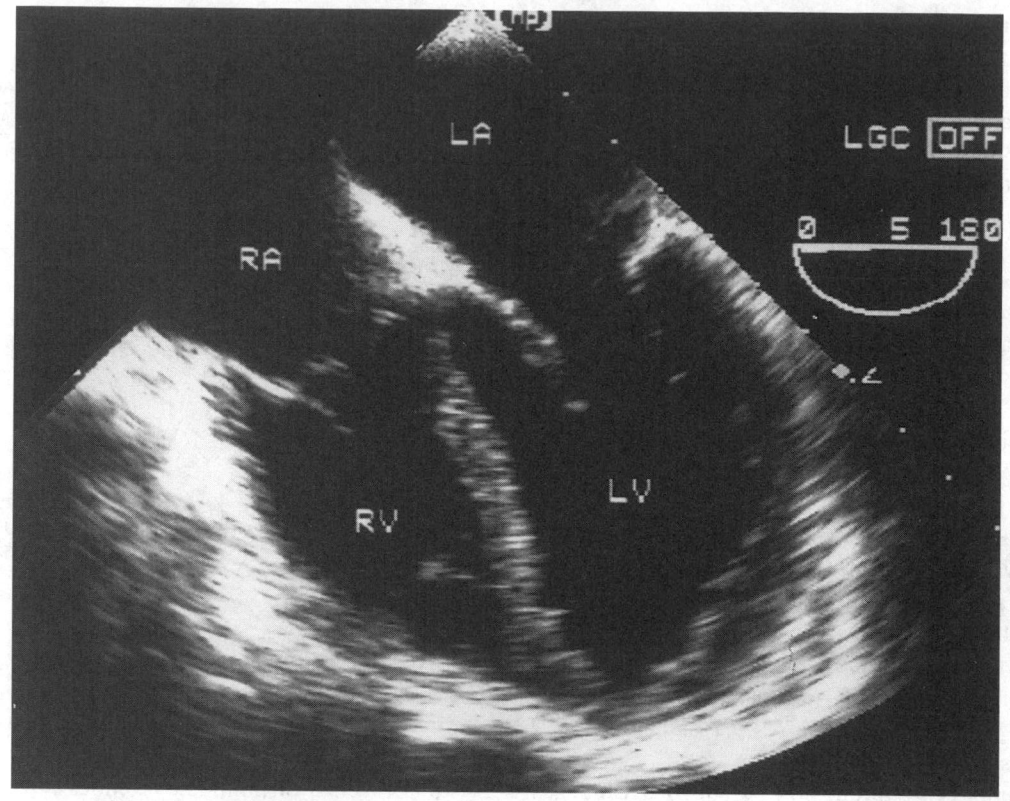

FIGURE 14-44

Transverse four-chamber TEE plane. LA = left atrium; LV = left ventricle; RA = right atrium; RV = right ventricle.

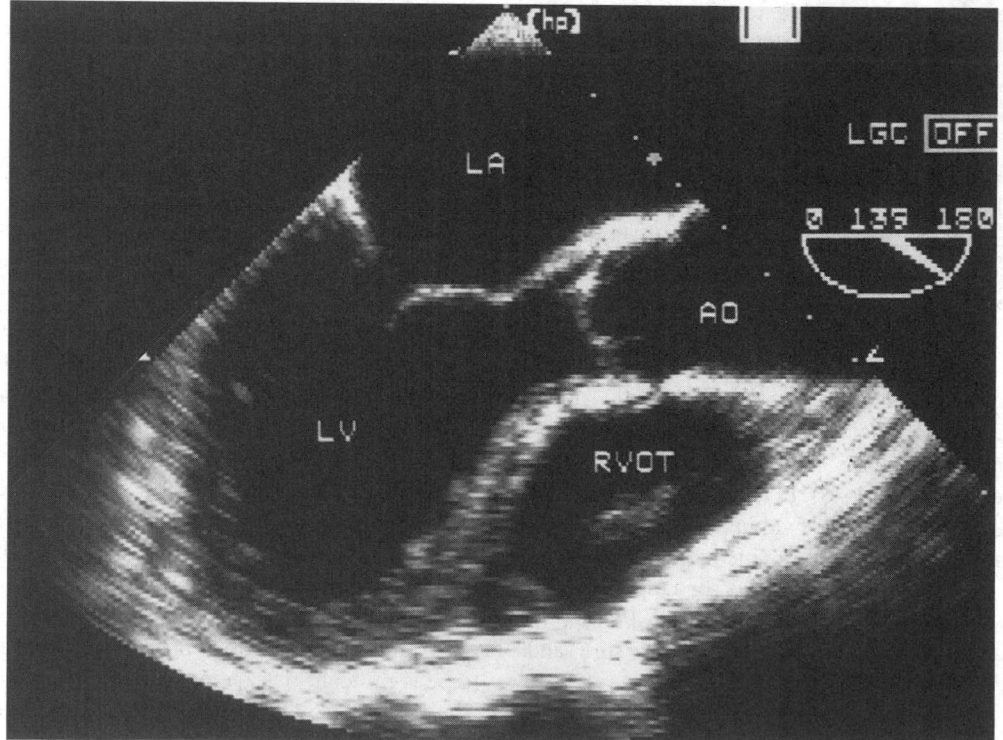

FIGURE 14-45

Modified longitudinal TEE plane (with transducer rotated to approximately 140°), demonstrating a TEE apical "three-chamber" view. AO = ascending aorta; RVOT = right ventricular outflow tract; LA = left atrium; LV = left ventricle.

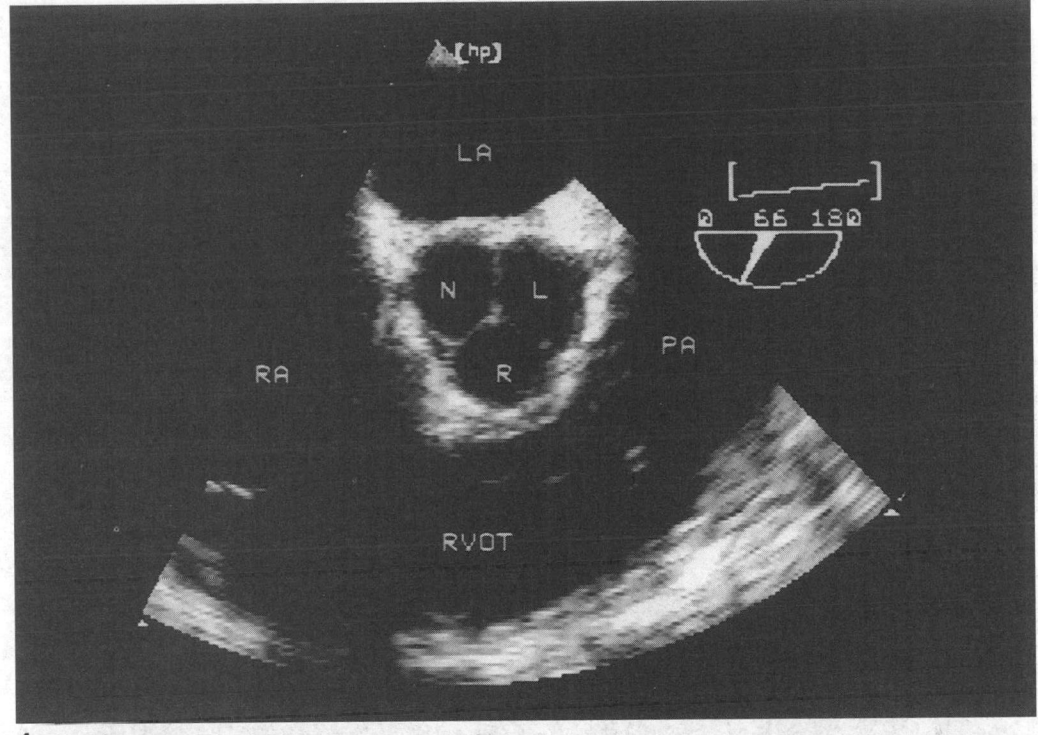

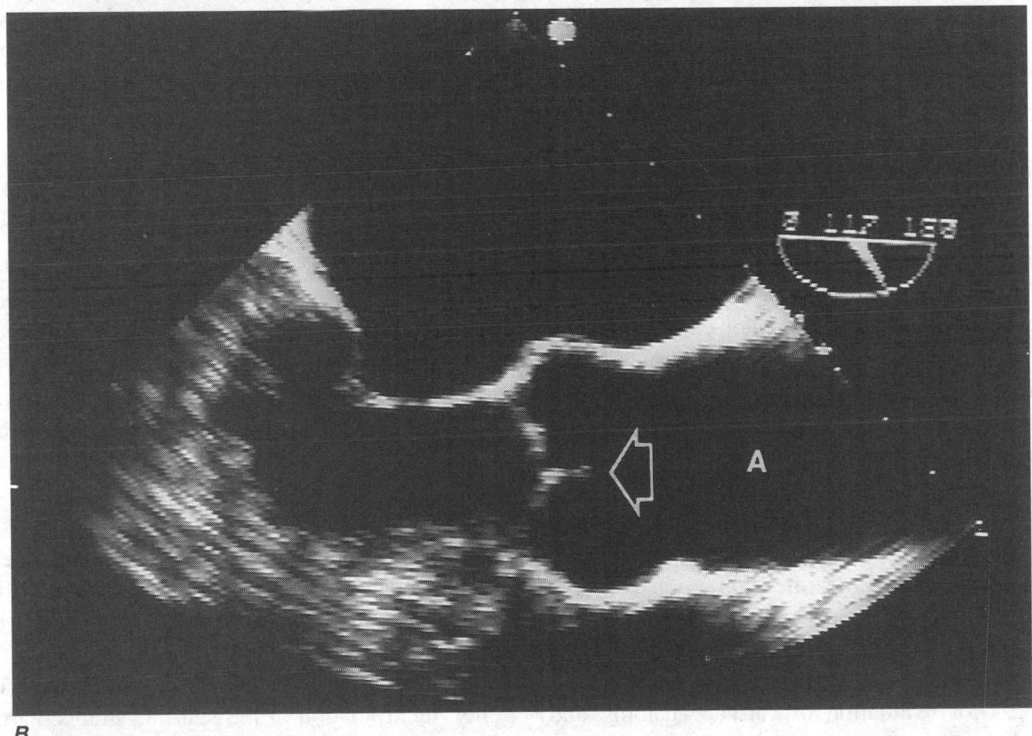

FIGURE 14-46

A. Modified short-axis view through the level of the aortic valve, demonstrating the left (L), right, (R), and noncoronary (N) valvular cusps. LA = left atrium; RA = right atrium; RVOT = right ventricular outflow tract; PA = pulmonary artery. *B*. Magnified longitudinal view of the aortic valve (*arrow*) showing the coaptation of the cusps and the sinuses of Valsalva. A = aorta. (From Blanchard DG, Kimura BJ, Dittrich HC, DeMaria AN. Transesophageal echocardiography of the aorta. *JAMA* 1994; 272:546–551, with permission.)

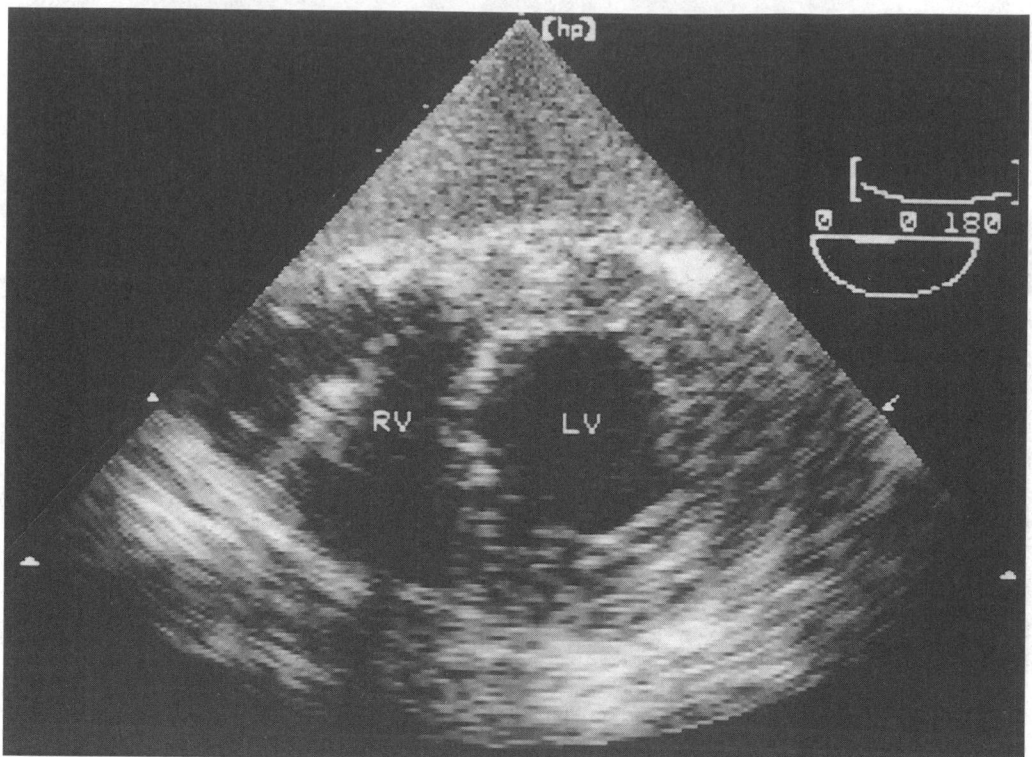

FIGURE 14-47

Short-axis TEE plane through the left ventricle from transgastric position. The inferior wall is closest to the transducer, the anterior wall farthest. The interventricular septum is to the reader's left, the lateral wall to the right. LV = left ventricle; RV = right ventricle.

ongoing to evaluate the effect of treatment after discovery of potential embolic sources.

One of the proven applications of TEE is the evaluation of prosthetic valve dysfunction, particularly mechanical valves in the mitral position.[172–174] Since the materials used in artificial valves are strong reflectors and often cause ultrasonic shadowing, the areas behind prosthetic valves are usually hidden from view when transthoracic imaging is used. Because of its unique window on the heart, TEE is clearly superior to TTE imaging for detection of prosthetic regurgitation, infection, tissue ingrowth, and thrombosis[172,174] (Fig. 14-54).

TEE has also become an important intraoperative tool for the detection of cardiac ischemia, the evaluation of valve function after surgical repair or replacement, and the delineation of congenital heart disease (especially in adults).[175–183] It is not at all uncommon for cardiac surgeons to request intraoperative TEE for evaluation of cardiac anatomy and confirmation of the success of surgical repair before closing the chest. In this regard, TEE has almost completely replaced epicardial echocardiography. When TEE images are inadequate, TEE is helpful in managing critical ill patients[184–187] and also can be used to monitor or guide interventional procedures, such as transseptal catheterization,[185–190] mitral valvuloplasty, pericardiocentesis, and endomyocardial biopsy.[191]

CONTRAST ECHOCARDIOGRAPHY

Opacification of the right heart cavities with dense ultrasonic reflectances during intravenous contrast injection was first applied clinically in 1968.[192] In the ensuing years, it became clear that the origin of the dense intracavitary echoes were microbubbles within the injectate, and that any agitated liquid injected intravenously caused the effect.[193] Since room-air microbubbles with the diameter of pulmonary capillaries persist in blood for less than 1 s before dissolving, agitated agents injected intravenously cannot cross the lungs and enter the left-sided cardiac chambers. Thus, the presence of echocardiographic contrast entering left heart chambers after intravenous injection of an agitated liquid indicates the presence of a right-to-left shunt.[194,195]

Contrast injection can be used to delineate right heart anatomy. Identification of intracardiac shunts, particularly patent foramen ovale in patients with unexplained cerebral ischemia (Fig. 14-55) remains the most frequent indication for contrast echocardiography.[196] Simple agitated normal saline solution remains the most commonly used contrast agent for such studies.

In recent years, many attempts have been made to achieve echocardiographic opacification of the left ventricular cavity and myocardium.[197–200] Initial attempts utilized direct left-

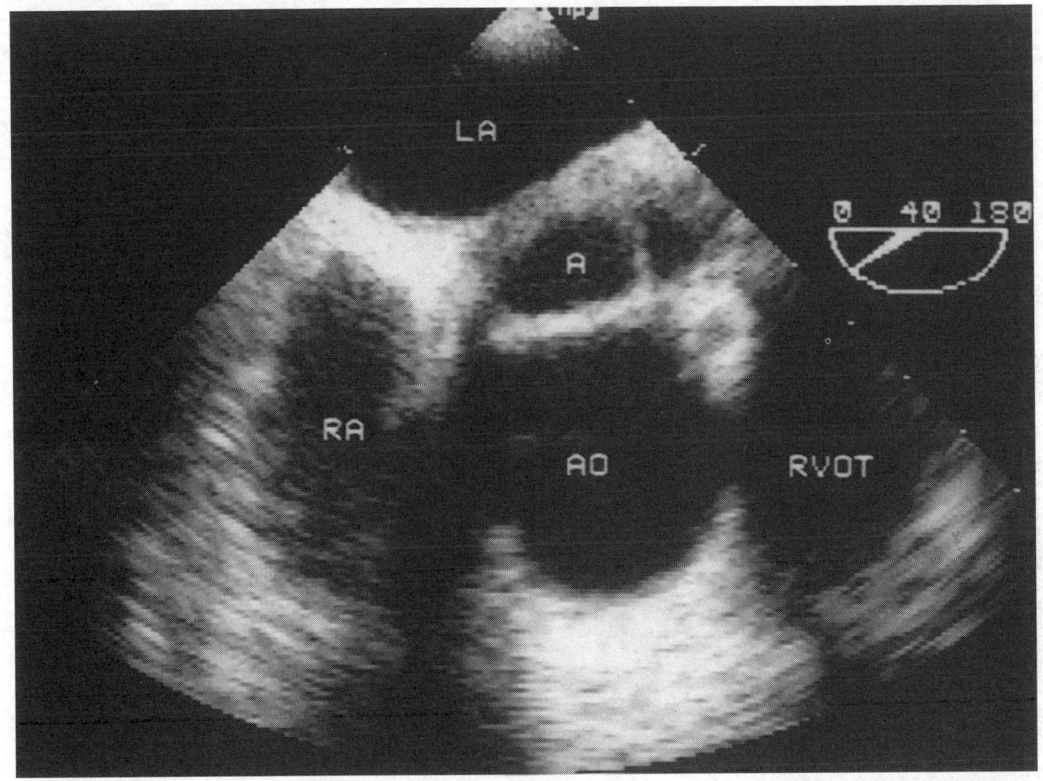

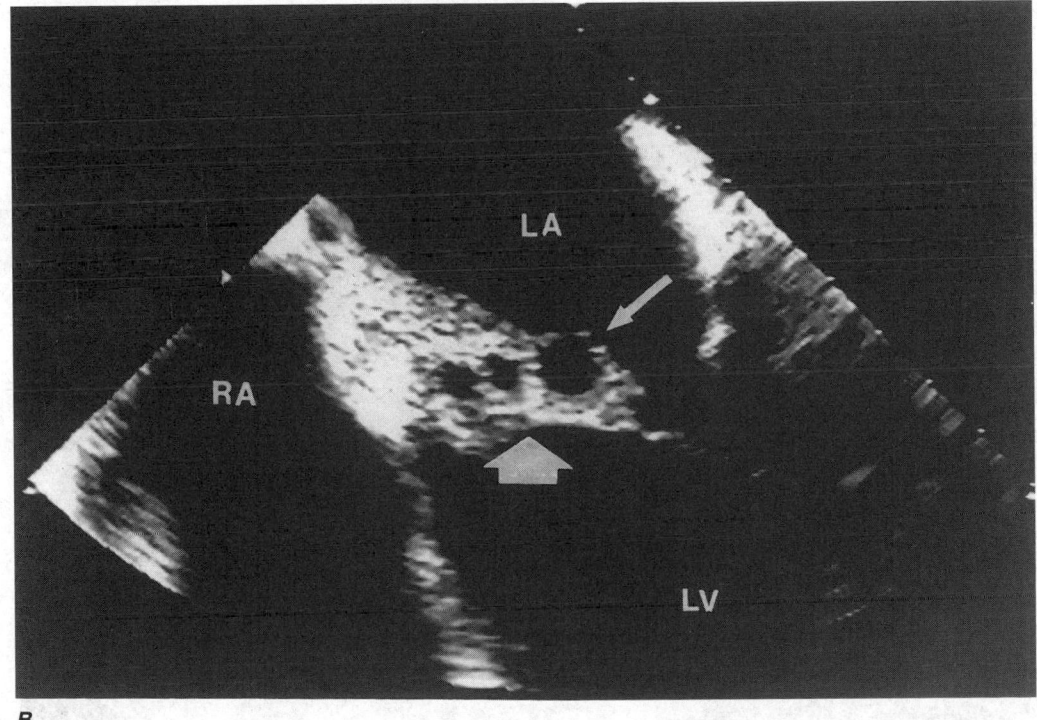

FIGURE 14-48

A. Short-axis plane TEE plane through the cardiac base. A large septated abscess cavity (A) is present between the aortic root (AO) and the left atrium (LA). RA = right atrium; RVOT = right ventricular outflow tract. *B.* Modified transverse four-chamber TEE plane showing a large abscess with several cavitations (*arrows*) involving the anterior mitral valve leaflet and the intervalvular fibrosa. RA = right atrium; LA = left atrium; LV = left ventricle. (From Sobel J, Maisel AS, Tarazi R, Blanchard DG. Gonococcal endocarditis: Assessment by transesophageal echocardiography. *J Am Soc Echocardiogr* 1997; 10:367–370.)

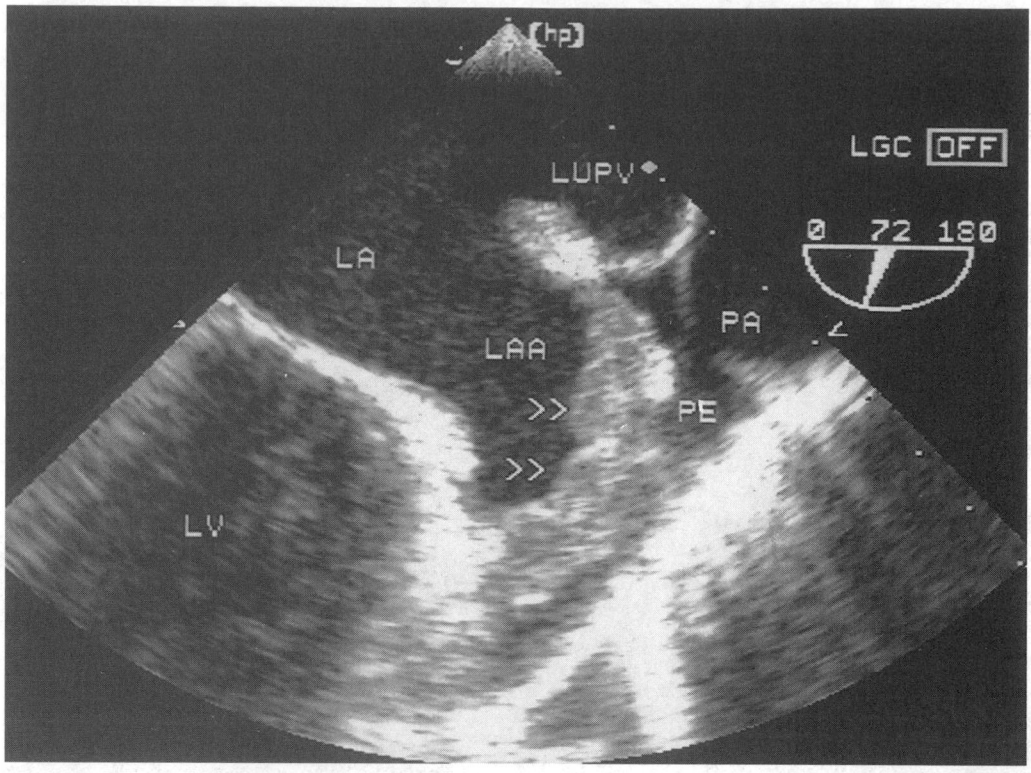

FIGURE 14-52
Transesophageal echocardiography image of a laminar thrombus (*arrows*) within the left atrial appendage (LAA). This thrombus was not visible with transthoracic echocardiography. LA = left atrium; LV = left ventricle; LUPV = left upper pulmonary vein; PA = pulmonary artery; PE = small pericardial effusion.

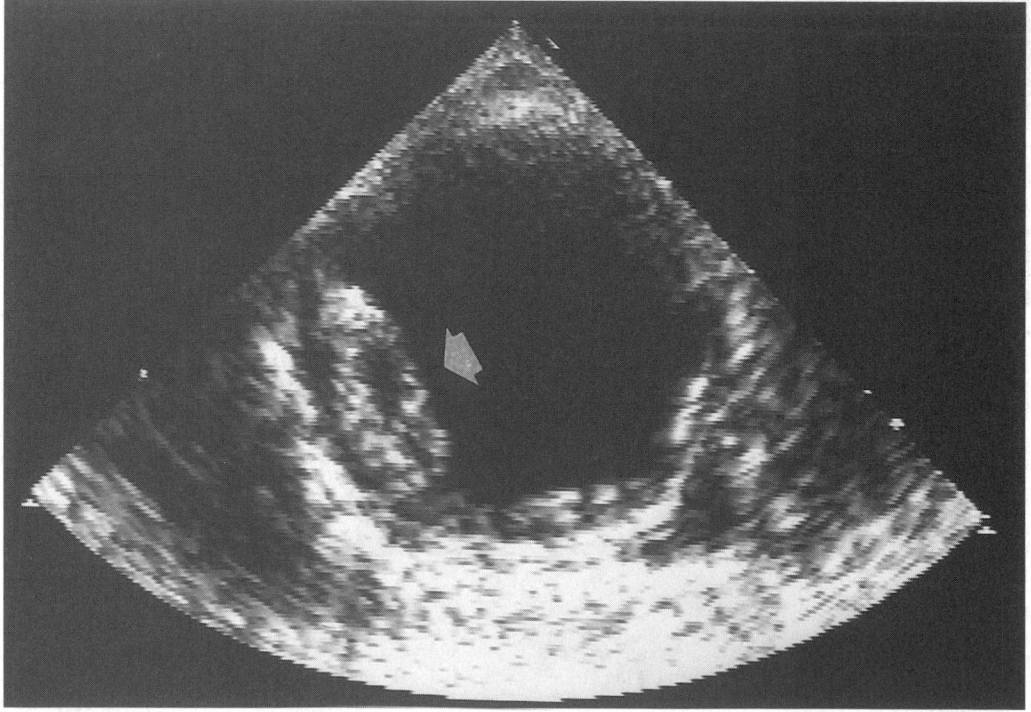

FIGURE 14-53
Transverse TEE image of the descending aorta, demonstrating extensive atherosclerosis and a large atheroma (*arrow*).

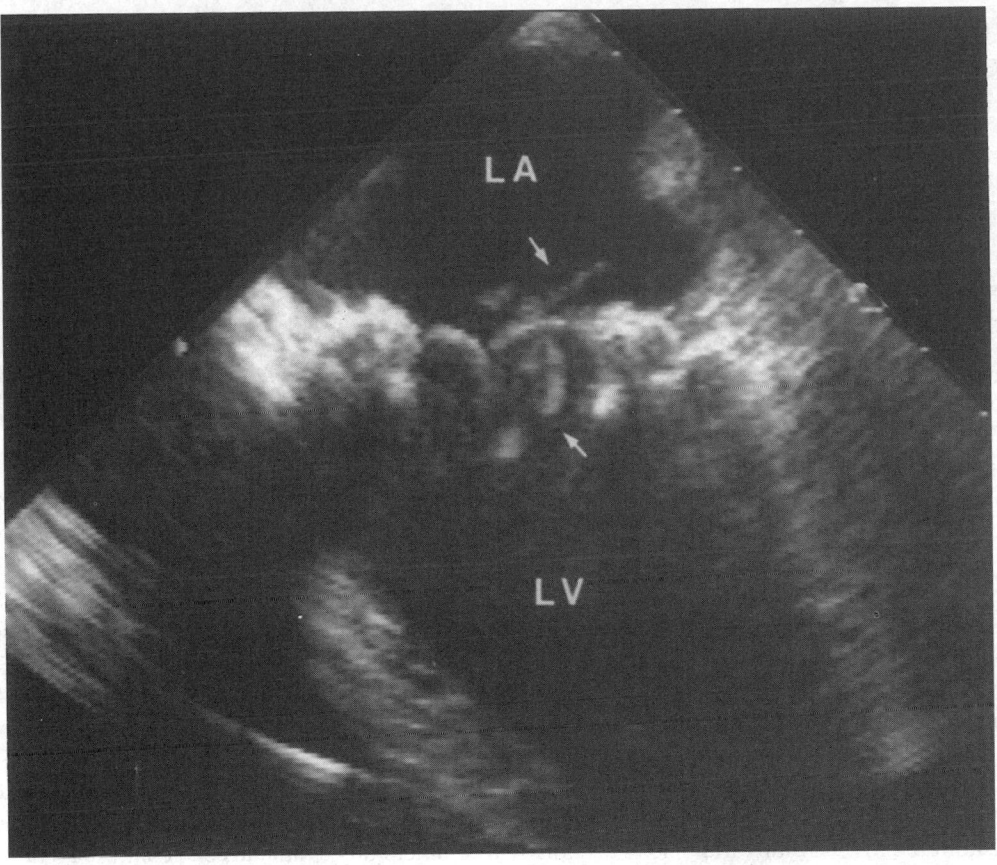

FIGURE 14-54
Transverse four-chamber TEE image of infective vegetations (*arrows*) on a porcine prosthesis in the mitral position. LA = left atrium; LV = left ventricle.

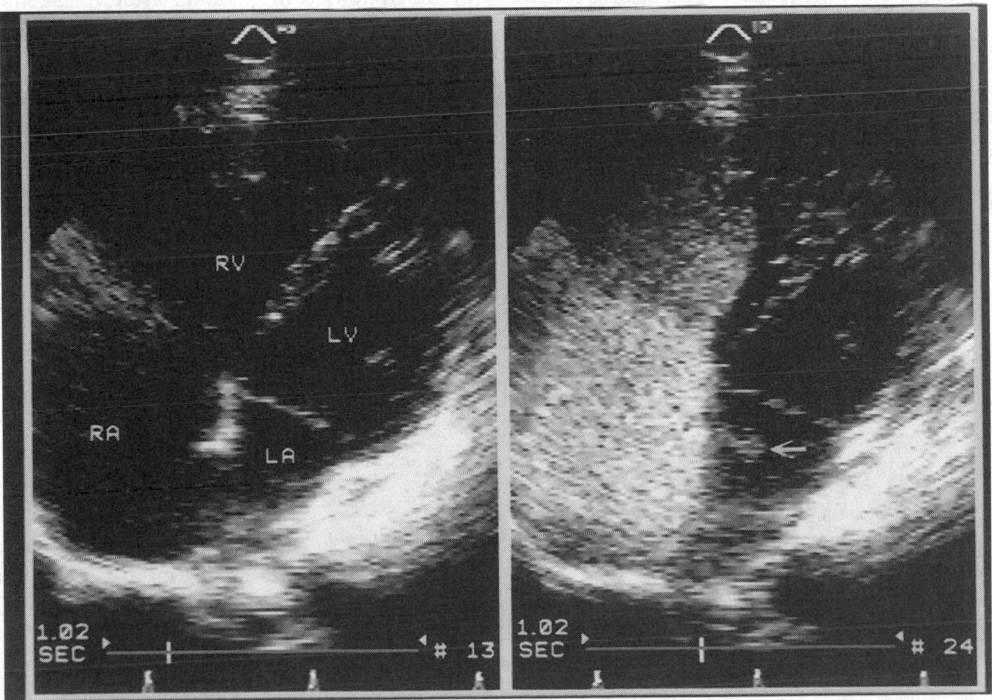

FIGURE 14-55
Contrast microbubble injection demonstrating a shunt (*arrow*) from the right atrium (RA) to left atrium (LA). RV = right ventricle; LV = left ventricle.

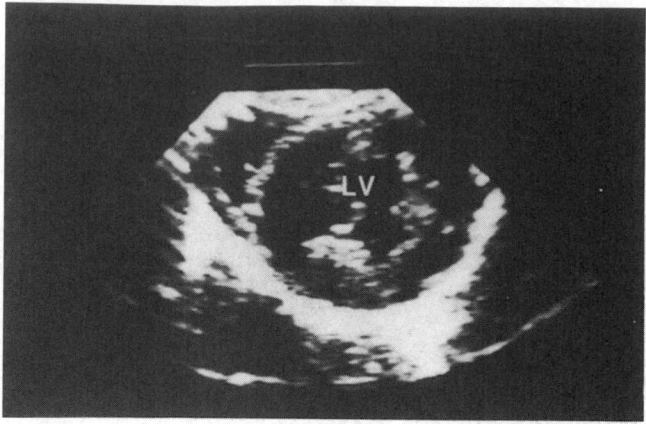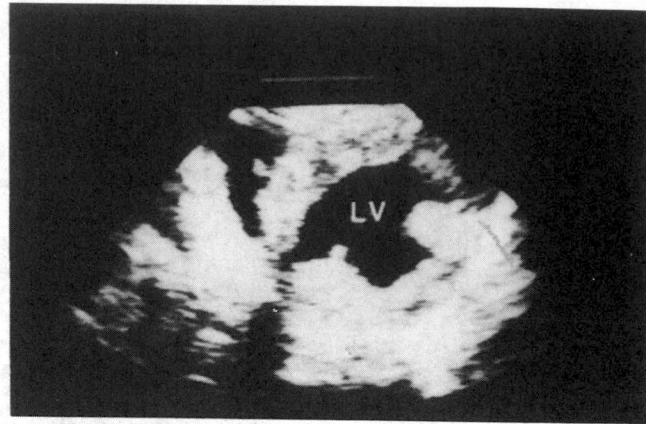

FIGURE 14-56

Short-axis plane through the left ventricle (LV) before (*left*) and after (*right*) injection of microbubbles into the aortic root. The myocardium is densely opacified on the right. (From Hagan AD, DeMaria AN. *Clinical Applications* *of Two-Dimensional Echocardiography and Cardiac Doppler.* Boston: Little, Brown; 1989, with permission.)

sided administration. Injection of agitated saline or other fluids into the left ventricle or aorta causes echocardiographic opacification of those chambers and has been used as an alternative to angiography to evaluate mitral and aortic regurgitation.[194] In addition, injection of sonicated radiographic contrast agents into the aortic root or coronary arteries can produce myocardial opacification[201] (Fig. 14-56). The presence of echocardiographic contrast within the myocardium after such injections reflects the spatial distribution of coronary blood flow[198] and is valuable in identifying coronary collateral blood flow and the absence of reflow following reperfusion therapy of acute myocardial infarction.[202–210] Of significance, the presence of

microcirculatory flow and integrity in these studies was a reliable predictor of viable myocardium.[207–209]

Although direct injection of coronary contrast into the left heart may provide clinically useful information, this technique is limited by its invasive nature. Efforts to produce stabilized solutions of microbubbles that could traverse the pulmonary capillary bed after intravenous injection resulted in the first commercially available echo contrast agent, Albunex.[200] This solution of sonicated human albumin alters the surface tension of room air bubbles, thereby prolonging their persistence prior to dissolving. Injection of Albunex opacifies the left ventricle in the majority of patients after intravenous injection and facilitates identification of the endomyocardial border.[200] This latter capacity has found its greatest application in stress echocardiography, where detection of the endocardium is of fundamental importance in recognizing abnormal contraction produced by ischemia. By intensifying backscatter within the intracardiac cavities, new ultrasonic agents also enhance Doppler imaging.[211] Marginal Doppler spectral tracings in cases of MR, tricuspid regurgitation, and aortic stenosis often improve dramatically after contrast injection, facilitating the quantitation of valvular lesions and pulmonary hypertension.[212,213] Unfortunately, sonicated albumin has not succeeded in opacifying the myocardium after intravenous injection.

The second-generation echocardiographic contrast agents

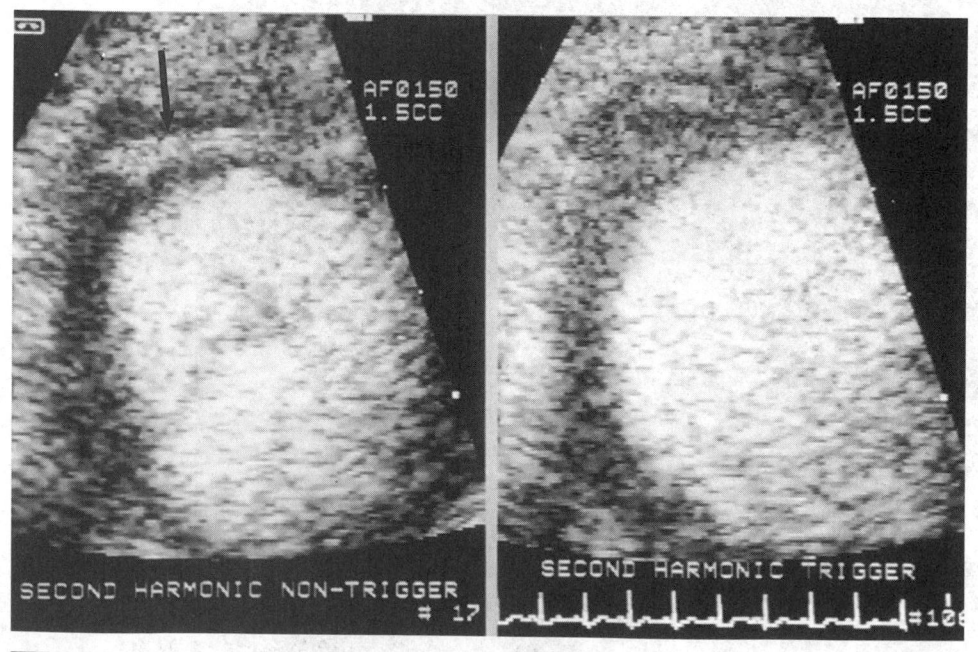

FIGURE 14-57

Transthoracic short-axis views (with second-harmonic imaging) after intravenous injection of a second-generation echocardiography contrast agent. Imaging was continuous on the left and gated ("triggered") on the right. With continuous imaging, an intramyocardial vessel (*arrow*) is visualized.

have been developed to achieve prolonged bubble persistence with the goal of myocardial enhancement by intravenous administration. The persistence time of a bubble prior to dissolving in blood is increased by a greater density of the gas, a reduced capacity to diffuse across the bubble's shell, and a low saturation constant in blood. Therefore, the new agents utilize microbubbles of various perfluorocarbon gases rather than air, as these gases are dense and poorly soluble.[214] Second-generation agents all produce measurable myocardial opacification after intravenous injection, and some actually permit visualization of intramyocardial coronary vessels (Fig. 14-57).[214–217] The ability to delineate regional myocardial perfusion with intravenous echocardiographic contrast agents is a major step forward in noninvasive imaging, and second-generation contrast agents may be routinely used for this purpose in the near future.

In addition to new contrast agents, novel imaging technologies directed to the amplification of contrast signals are also available. For example, second-harmonic imaging enhances the ultrasonic backscatter from contrast microbubbles (which resonate in an ultrasonic field) while decreasing the returning signal from myocardium (which does not resonate)[217–219] (Fig. 14-58). Early after contrast injection, second-harmonic imaging increases the cavity-to-myocardium contrast intensity ratio, improving visualization of the left ventricular cavity. Second-harmonic imaging may also enhance the myocardial contrast phase, which follows LV cavity opacification with second-generation contrast agents.[217–219] As exposure to ultrasound energy can produce microbubble destruction, intermittent rather than continuous ultrasound transmission can also prolong microbubble persistence and amplify contrast signals.[220,221]

DISEASES OF THE AORTIC VALVE AND AORTA

Aortic Stenosis

The aortic valve is best imaged in the parasternal views.[222] The leaflets are thin, linear structures. All three can be visualized in the short-axis view and produce a triangular orifice during systolic opening. The long-axis view exhibits the right and usually the noncoronary leaflets, which normally open to the walls of the aorta. In older adults, acquired aortic stenosis (AS) is manifested by markedly thickened, often calcified, immobile aortic valve leaflets,[223] while doming of the leaflets suggests congenital aortic stenosis and is usually encountered in younger patients (Fig. 14-59).[224] Echocardiography can distinguish valvular from sub- and supravalvular AS, can accurately identify bicuspid valves, and can delineate the presence of LV hypertrophy.[225,226] Subaortic stenosis may be caused by asymmetric septal hypertrophy with systolic anterior mitral motion, a subaortic membrane, or (less commonly) a subaortic tunnel. Bicuspid valves exhibit an oval rather than triangular orifice (Fig. 14-60). Although the severity of stenosis can be assessed semiquantitatively by 2D and M-

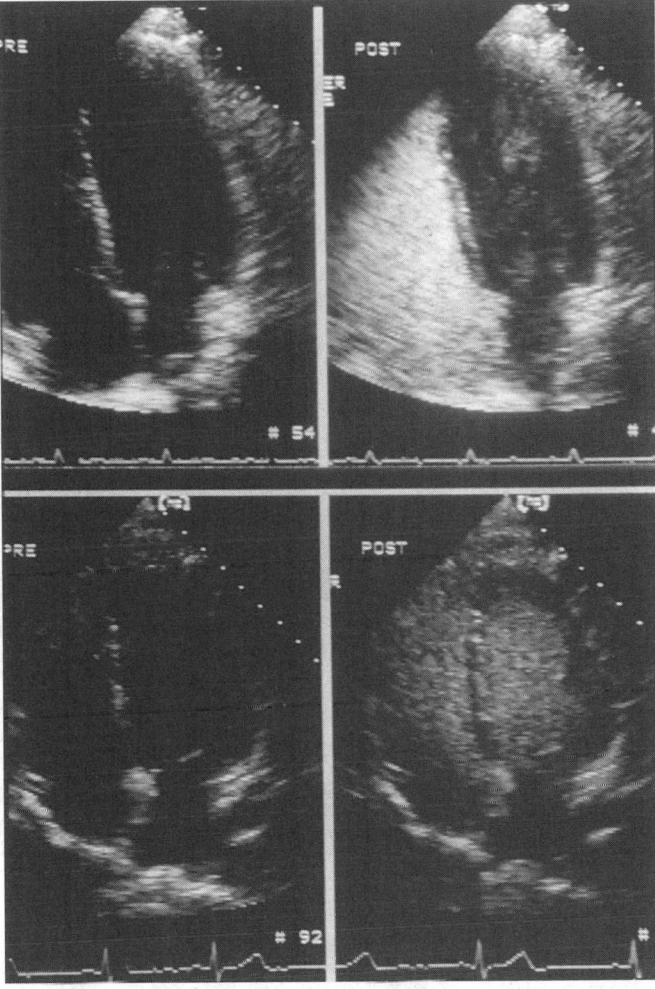

FIGURE 14-58

Utility of second-harmonic imaging. The two upper panels show an apical four-chamber plane before (*left*) and after (*right*) injection of an intravenous echocardiography contrast agent. Opacification of the left ventricle is suboptimal. In the lower panels, a similar injection is recorded with second harmonic imaging. Contrast between the cavity and myocardium is accentuated.

mode images echocardiography, valvular calcification may shadow the leaflets or produce reverberations and obscure their motion.[223] Therefore, attempts to measure valve area by transthoracic planimetry have been unsuccessful, although multiplane TEE has been of greater value[155] (Fig. 14-61). Thus, 2D-echocardiographic imaging accurately detects the presence and etiology of AS but not the severity. Likewise, CFD demonstrates turbulent flow through the aortic valve and may guide continuous wave interrogation but provides little quantitative data.[227] The use of Doppler echocardiography and the modified Bernoulli and continuity equations have now made noninvasive calculation of aortic gradients and valve area routine and have affected utilization of cardiac catheterization in AS patients.[228] (See also Chap. 63).

The cornerstone of the ultrasound evaluation of AS is CW Doppler interrogation through the aortic valve. The calculated gradient using the peak Doppler velocity [$4 \, (\text{AS velocity})^2$]

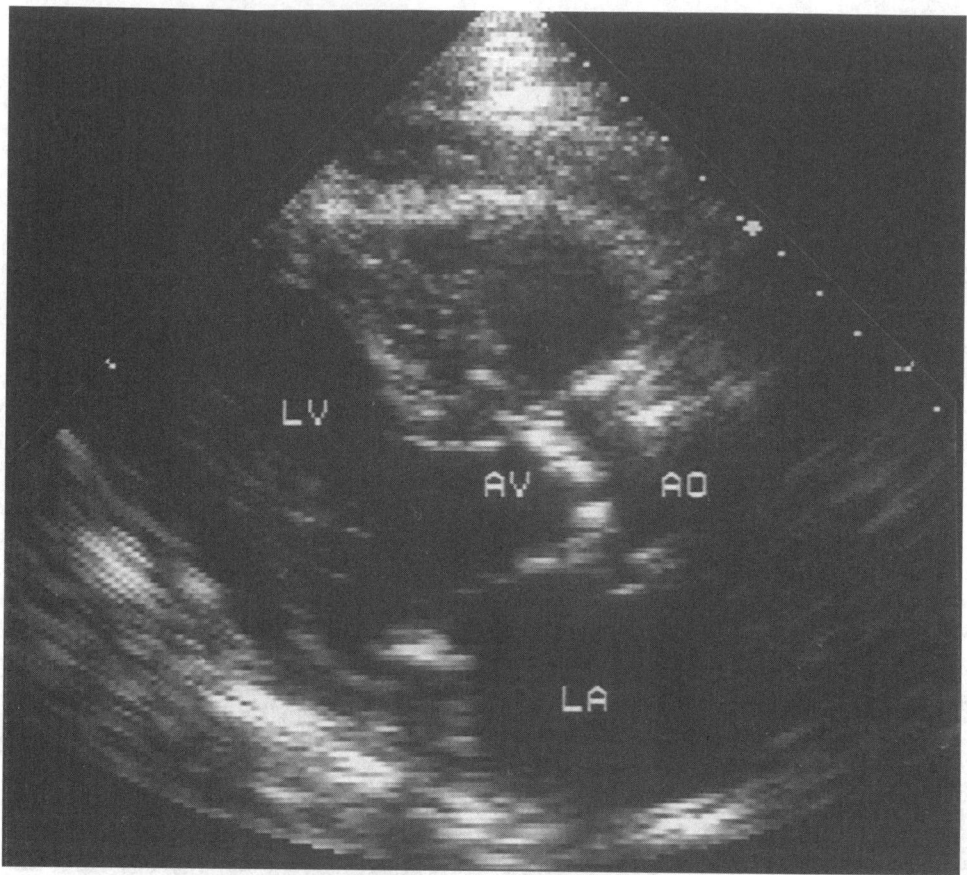

FIGURE 14-59
Parasternal long-axis plane demonstrating a thickened, stenotic aortic valve (AV). AO = aorta; LV = left ventricle; LA = left atrium.

flow velocity in the Bernoulli equation if it is 1.5 m/s or greater. Finally, since some degree of pressure recovery occurs distal to the aortic valve leaflets, it is important to record continuous wave signals as close to these structures as possible.

Values for aortic valve area can be calculated using the continuity equation by measuring the velocity of the jet across the aortic valve with CW Doppler, the velocity in the LV outflow tract just proximal to the valve with pulsed-wave PW Doppler, and by deriving the area of the outflow tract from the diameter of the aortic annulus. Results from the continuity equation have been found to correlate well with the area calculations based on catheterization data and the Gorlin formula.[111–115] As both AS jet velocity and aortic annulus radius are squared in the continuity equation, accurate determination of these parameters is essential for reliable measurements. When atrial fibrillation is present, the peak Doppler velocity still correlates with peak instantaneous gradient through the aortic valve, but calculations of valve area may be problematic, as the outflow tract and peak aortic velocities are not measured simultaneously.

In summary, a comprehensive echocardiographic examination in a patient with AS should establish both the presence and severity of disease. Echocardiographic imaging should identify the structural abnormality involving either the subvalvular, valvular, or supravalvular area; distinguish congenital from acquired etiologies; and evaluate the state of LV hypertrophy and function. CW Doppler recordings should provide accurate measurements of instantaneous and mean transaortic valvular gradients, and the continuity equation should provide reliable estimates of aortic valve area. In cases where the relative roles of orifice stenosis and LV dysfunction are uncertain, TEE imaging or Doppler recordings during inotropic stimulation with dobutamine may be of value.[155,229] Cardiac catheterization is still necessary for the delineation of coronary anatomy.

correlates closely with the peak instantaneous gradient measured at catheterization[117–119] (Fig. 14-62). In interpreting echocardiographic studies, it is important to distinguish between the peak instantaneous pressure gradient, the mean gradient, and the peak-to-peak gradient. The first two physiologic parameters represent simultaneous pressure differences between LV and aorta and can be measured accurately by Doppler echocardiography. The peak-to-peak gradient, commonly used in the catheterization laboratory, compares the highest pressures reached in the LV and aorta (even though not simultaneous) and is uniformly lower than the peak instantaneous gradient recorded by Doppler. Therefore, the maximal Doppler gradient does not correlate with the peak-to-peak catheterization gradient, and comparisons between the two should be avoided.

A number of potential sources of error exist in the estimation of the transvalvular aortic gradient by CW Doppler recordings. It is imperative that Doppler signals from the stenotic jet be obtained with an angle of incidence of less than 20°. Since the direction of the jet rarely can be known with precision from 2D techniques, it is necessary that each examination employ all possible windows and angulations, including apical, parasternal, and suprasternal transducer positions. Also, one must be careful to account for the proximal

Aortic Regurgitation

In contrast to AS, the aortic valve leaflets are often anatomically normal by echocardiography in patients with aortic regurgitation (AR).[230–231] 2D and M-mode echocardiography

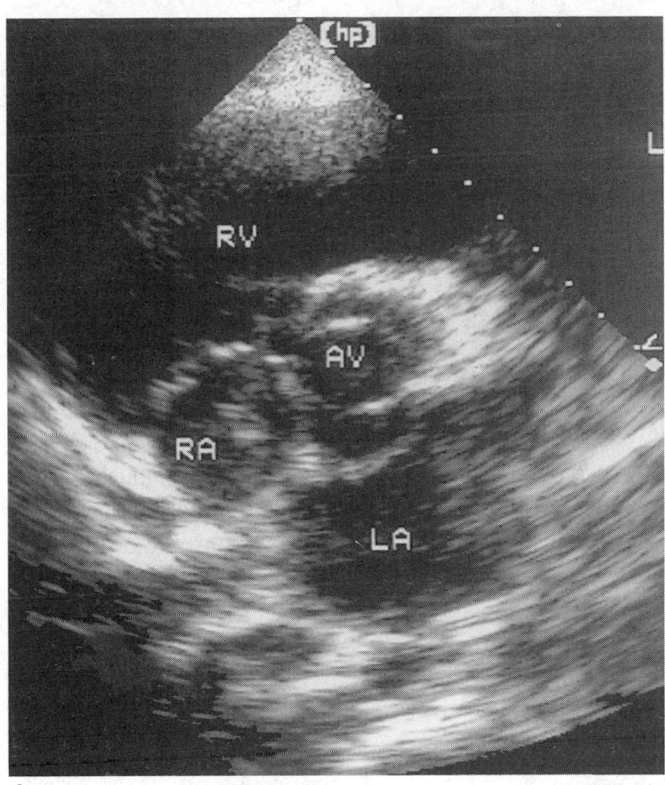

A

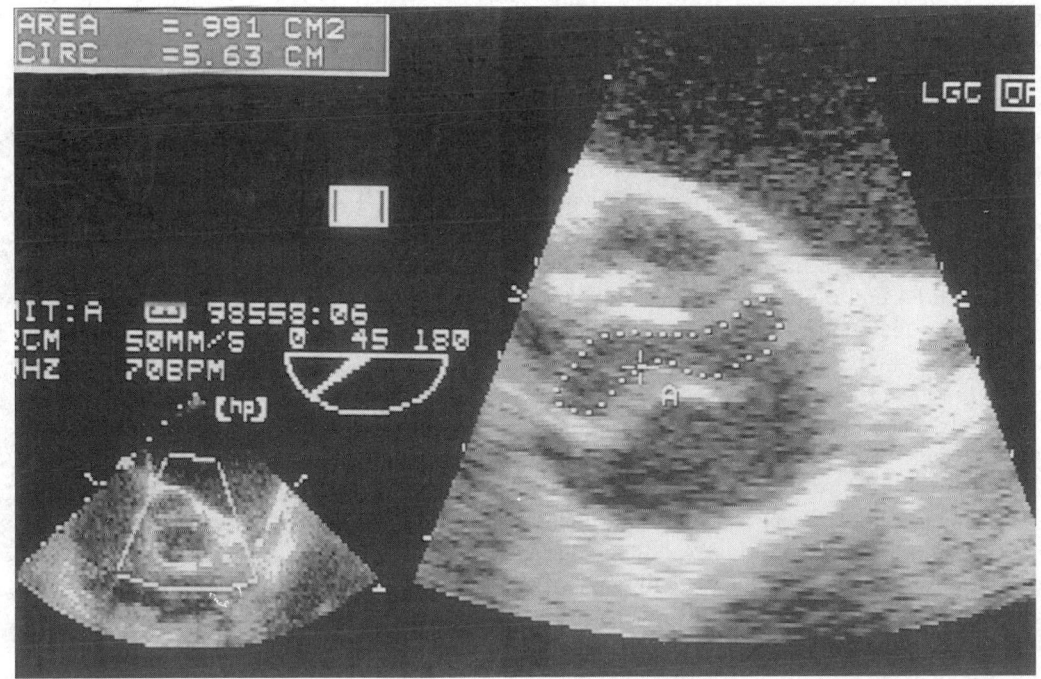

B

FIGURE 14-60

A. Parasternal short-axis image of a bicuspid aortic valve (AV) during systole. RV = right ventricle; RA = right atrium; LA = left atrium. *B*. Transesophageal image of a bicuspid aortic valve (A). LA = left atrium, R = right ventricular outflow tract. (From Blanchard DG, Kimura BJ, Dittrich HC, DeMaria AN. Transesophageal echocardiography of the aorta. *JAMA* 1994; 272:546–551, with permission.)

FIGURE 14-61

Transesophageal image of a stenotic bicuspid aortic valve (A) with superimposed planimetry of the valve area (approximately 1 cm^2).

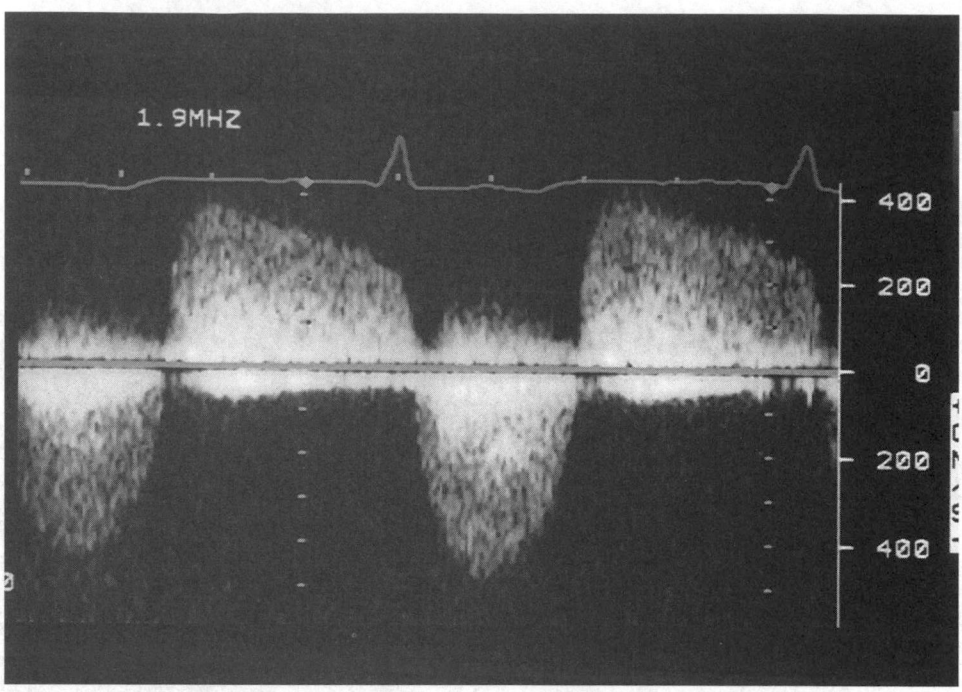

FIGURE 14-62

Continuous-wave Doppler tracing (from the apical transducer position) through the aortic valve in a case of combined aortic stenosis and insufficiency. The peak systolic velocity approaches 5 m/s.

spectral recordings from this jet yield a high-velocity diastolic signal directed toward the apex[237] (Fig. 14-62). Since AR jet velocity accurately reflects the diastolic pressure gradient between aorta and left ventricle, it is maximum at the point of valve closure and decreases throughout diastole.[238] The flow pattern of AR may be readily distinguished from mitral inflow in that it is higher in velocity, begins immediately after aortic valve closure, generally has a much slower deceleration, and does not have an increased velocity following atrial contraction.

Several approaches exist for the quantitation of AR by echocardiography. Conventional echocardiographic imaging can provide evidence of the presence and extent of LV volume overload. More direct evidence of the severity of AR can be derived from the deceleration rate of the jet recorded by CW Doppler (Fig. 14-65).[237–240] In the presence of mild degrees of AR, the transvalvular pressure gradient will be maintained throughout diastole, creating a high-velocity jet with a minimal deceleration rate. Conversely, severe AR reduces aortic pressures and increases LV pressures in diastole, eliminating the pressure

often provide indirect evidence of the presence of AR, including signs of LV volume overload, diastolic fluttering of the anterior mitral valve leaflet, aortic root enlargement, and incomplete coaptation of the aortic valve leaflets.[232,233] The important M-mode finding of premature diastolic closure of the mitral valve prior to the onset of systole due to LV filling by the regurgitant jet signifies acute, severe AR[234] (Fig. 14-63) and the need for surgery.

Perhaps the most important contribution of echocardiographic tissue imaging to the assessment of aortic regurgitation is in identifying the etiology.[235] Thus, thickened leaflets that are restricted in movement are observed in patients with acquired AS, while oval doming of two functional leaflets will be observed in the presence of a bicuspid aortic valve (Fig. 14-60). AR due to infectious endocarditis can be identified by the presence of valvular vegetations, while regurgitation due to diseases of the aorta are manifest by anatomic changes of the vessel. Less common etiologies of AR, such as those associated with subvalvular pathology or ventricular septal defect, may also be recognized by echocardiographic imaging.

Although the findings yielded by echocardiographic imaging are useful, Doppler interrogation is necessary to obtain direct evidence of the presence and severity of AR. Screening with CFD demonstrates turbulent flow in the LV outflow tract during diastole in virtually all views[236] (Fig. 14-64A, B, and C, Plates 32A, B, and C). The jet is typically elliptical and may be located anywhere in the LV outflow tract. CW Doppler

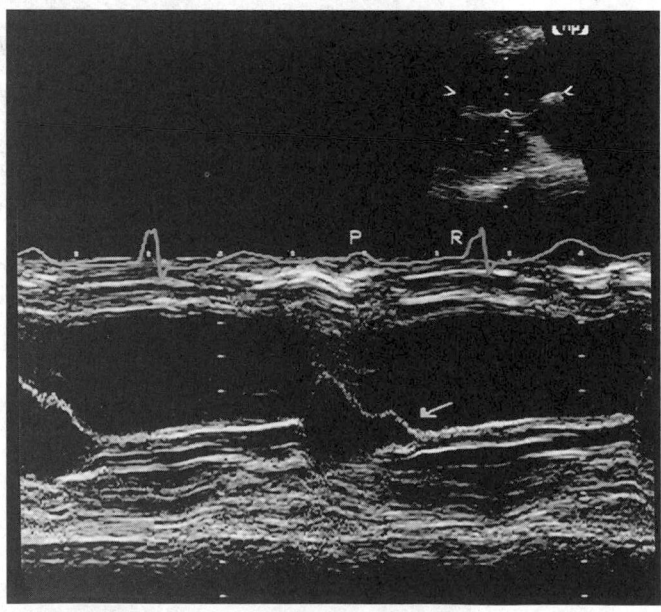

FIGURE 14-63

M-mode tracing (from the parasternal position) in patient with acute severe aortic regurgitation. The mitral valve leaflets close (*arrow*) before ventricular contraction begins. P = p wave, R = QRS complex.

FIGURE 14-64

See color Plate 32.

gradient and creating a rapid jet deceleration to a low velocity (Fig. 14-65). Severe, acute AR can also cause diastolic MR (Fig. 14-64C, Plate 32C). The most common approach to assessing the deceleration rate of the AR jet is by calculating the time required for the velocity to fall to one-half of the maximal pressure equivalent, a technique similar to the pressure half-time measurements performed in the quantitation of mitral stenosis. Previous studies have demonstrated that a pressure half-time of less than 250 ms reliably identifies patients with severe degrees of aortic regurgitation as assessed by invasive methods.[240] Application of the pressure half-time approach to quantifying AR must take into account that, since the deceleration rate is a reflection of pressure gradient, it is determined by both the volume of AR and the com-

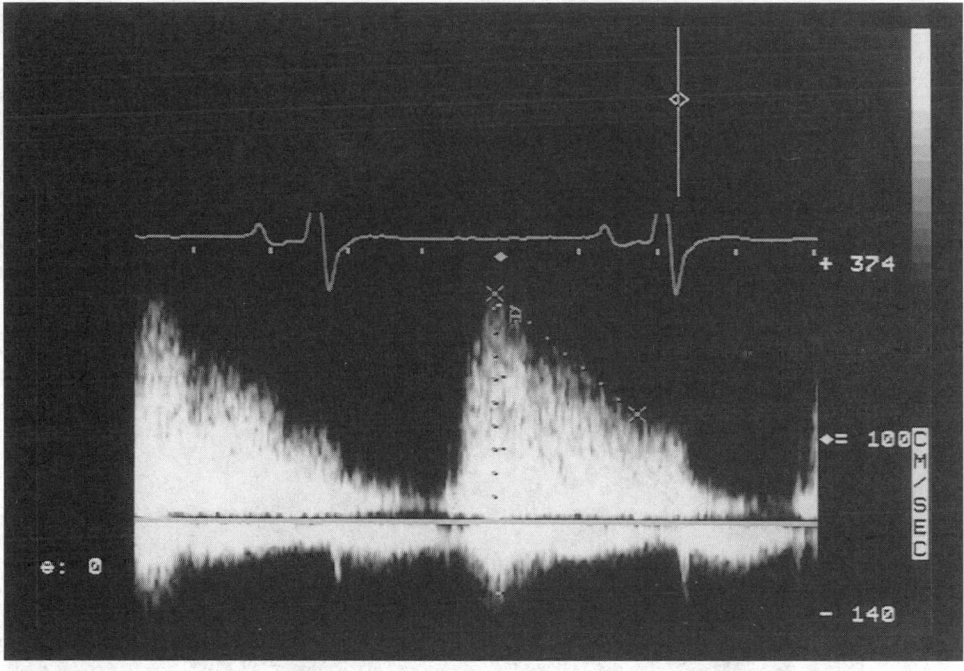

FIGURE 14-65

Continuous-wave Doppler tracing (from the apical transducer position) of severe AR. The pressure half-time of the AR envelope is approximately 200 ms.

pliance of the left ventricle. Accordingly, ventricles that vary greatly in stiffness or distensibility will yield different *AR* deceleration rates for the same regurgitant volume.

The estimate of severity most commonly derived from echocardiography is the size of the AR jet by CFD.[236] Conceptually, jets that are distributed over a small area of the LV outflow tract represent lesser degrees of regurgitation than jets that penetrate widely and to the level of the papillary muscles. Some studies have demonstrated a general correlation between jet length and severity of AR.[241] The optimal results have been obtained when the width of the AR jet just proximal to the valve was expressed as a percentage of the width of the LV outflow tract; a jet occupying 50 percent or more of the outflow tract correlates with severe regurgitation by angiography.[236] Quantitation of AR based upon the size of the flow disturbance is subject to errors induced by the other factors that influence jet area: transvalvular pressure gradient, volume and compliance of the receiving chamber, regurgitant orifice, the Coanda effect (wall effect), and technical factors relating to the operator and instrument settings. In addition, entrainment and displacement of RBCs in the LV outflow tract also influence the size of the regurgitant jet. Finally, convergence of AR with normal transmitral filling may obscure the flow disturbance. Therefore, assessment of the severity of AR by analysis of the size and shape of the flow disturbance is at best semiquantitative.

The AR volume can be estimated by comparing volumetric measurements of LV inflow and LV outflow calculated from annular velocity and cross-sectional area (derived from pulsed Doppler and 2D images respectively).[110] This method is con-

tingent upon the absence of valvular stenosis and of other regurgitant lesions. In the setting of AR, the volume ejected through the aortic annulus represents both systemic flow and regurgitant volume, while the volume coursing through the mitral annulus represents only systemic flow. Thereby, LV outflow will exceed LV inflow by the amount of the regurgitant volume.[110,242–244] This technique can provide useful estimates of regurgitant volume, but with any flow volume calculation by echocardiography, errors in technique and the assumptions involved in volume calculation can result in significant errors. An alternate quantitative approach derives estimates of regurgitant fraction from reverse diastolic flow in the aorta.[245] Assuming a constant cross-sectional aortic area, comparison of integrated flow velocities during forward systolic flow and retrograde diastolic flow should yield an estimate of regurgitant fraction. Although this is somewhat imprecise, the presence of a significant flow reversal in the aorta visualized by color or spectral Doppler is a reliable marker of severe AR (Fig. 14-66).

Determination of the optimal timing of surgical intervention in patients with AR remains a difficult problem in clinical medicine (see also Chap. 63). Several criteria derived from echocardiographic recordings have been proposed to guide this decision.[246–249] Most prominently, an LV end-systolic dimension of 55 mm or greater with a shortening fraction of 25 percent or less have been advocated as sufficient criteria for surgical intervention in the absence of symptoms.[250] Considerable debate continues regarding this issue, however, and no universally accepted echocardiographic criteria exist by which to determine the optimal role for surgical treatment.

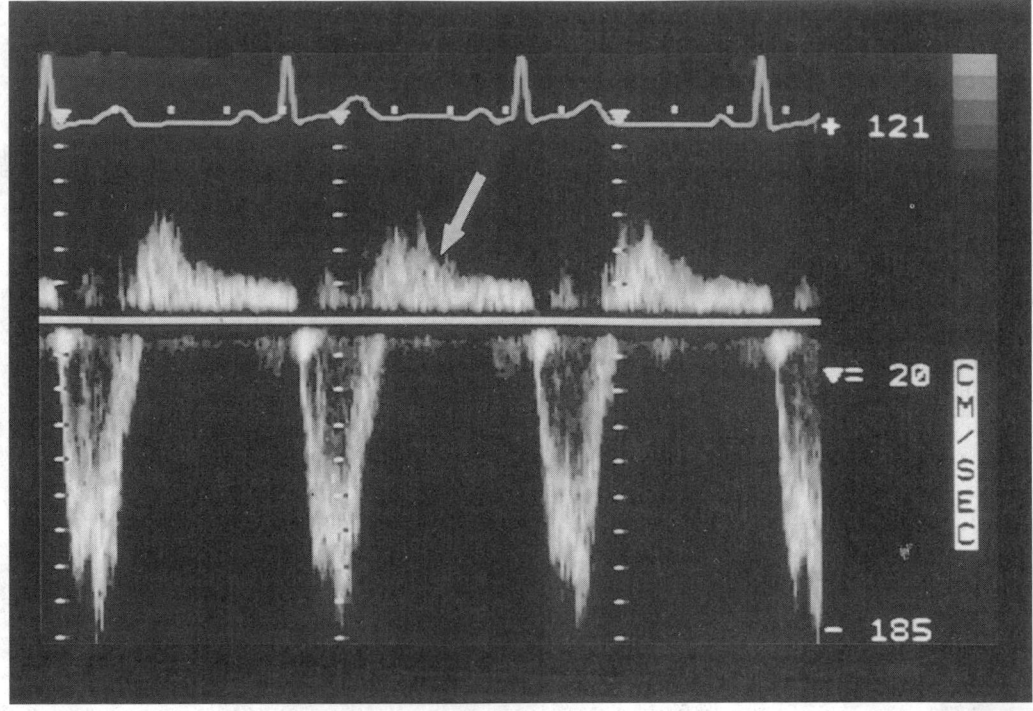

FIGURE 14-66
Pulsed-wave Doppler tracing (from the suprasternal transducer position) in a case of severe aortic regurgitation. The sample volume is in the descending thoracic aorta, and holodiastolic flow reversal (*arrow*) is present.

Diseases of the Aorta

The thoracic aorta is best visualized from the left and right parasternal positions and from the suprasternal notch.[251] The descending aorta may also be imaged from subcostal and modified apical views. Normally, short-axis images of the aortic root yield a circular structure, while long-axis imagines exhibit two parallel linear walls with a maximal diameter of 35 mm.[252] Although 2D imaging is used most commonly, M-mode recordings of the aortic root facilitate precise measurement of its dimensions.

AORTIC DISSECTION

In recent years, 2D echocardiography has dramatically changed the diagnostic approach to aortic dissection. TTE is a convenient screening test (Fig. 14-67) and often enables accurate detection of ascending aortic dissection.[253] The diagnostic findings include a dilated aorta with a mobile intimal flap that presents as a thin, linear signal within the lumen. Transthoracic imaging is unreliable for detection of descending aortic dissection,[254] although it occasionally visualizes the complete length of the thoracic aorta (see also Chap. 98).

Although several noninvasive methods exist to diagnose aortic dissection, TEE has become the procedure of choice in many hospitals because of its accuracy, portability, rapid procedural time, and ability to provide data regarding valvular regurgitation and LV function.[139,158,255–257]

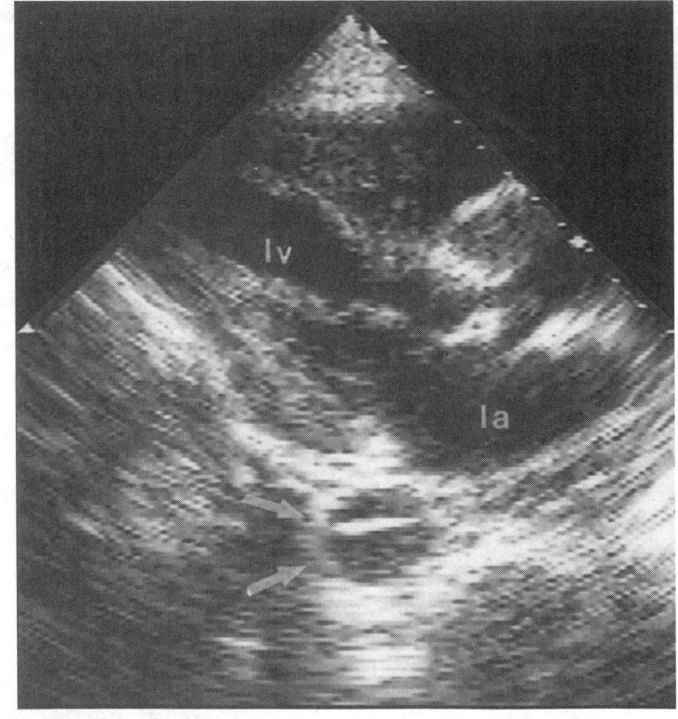

FIGURE 14-67
Transthoracic parasternal long-axis plane demonstrating a dissection of the descending thoracic aorta. The aortic root is dilated, the aortic valve is thickened, and an intimal flap is present in the descending aorta (*arrows*). LV = left ventricle; LA = left atrium.

Except for a short portion of the proximal aortic arch, which is obscured by the bronchus, multiplane TEE provides excellent visualization of the entire thoracic aorta and high accuracy in detecting aortic enlargement, intimal tears, and false lumen thrombus (Fig. 14-68). CFD may reveal communications between true and false channels (Fig. 14-51, Plate 31; Fig. 14-69, Plate 33). TEE also appears useful for the diagnosis of aortic intramural hematoma, an increasingly recognized disorder which has a clinical prognosis similar to that of classic dissection.[258,259]

AORTIC ANEURYSM

Aneurysms of the aorta may be saccular or fusiform and are recognized as localized or circumferential areas of aortic enlargement, often with thin walls. Transthoracic imaging is especially useful in detecting ascending aortic dilatation but can also visualize descending thoracic and abdominal aortic aneurysms.[252,260] Echocardiography has been used extensively to assess aortic pathology in patients with Marfan syndrome.[261] The nature of the lesion is relatively specific in that there is symmetric dilatation of the annulus, sinuses of Valsalva, and aortic root (Fig. 14-70). Aortic leaflet coaptation may be compromised leading to regurgitation. Echocardiography is helpful in determining prognosis and optimal timing of aortic root replacement.[262–264]

Sinus of Valsalva aneurysms are also well visualized by both TTE and TEE.[265,266] These lesions cause asymmetric dilatation of the aortic root and seem to affect the right coronary sinus most frequently. They are prone to rupture, often into the right heart.[267] Doppler echocardiography in such settings demonstrates fluttering of the tricuspid valve, a color jet crossing from the aortic root into the right heart, and occasionally diastolic opening of the pulmonic valve.

Congenital aortic disease, such as supravalvular aortic stenosis (AS), aortic coarctation, patent ductus arteriosus, and truncus arteriosus also can be detected with echocardiography (see Chaps. 70 and 71).[225,268] In these conditions, suprasternal and transesophageal imaging are often helpful. Supravalvular stenosis is recognized as an "hourglass" narrowing just distal to the leaflets, while coarctation presents a more localized, abrupt luminal reduction in the descending aorta. Patent ductus arteriosus and truncus arteriosis are often best identified by virtue of the accompanying flow disturbance on CFD.[269,270]

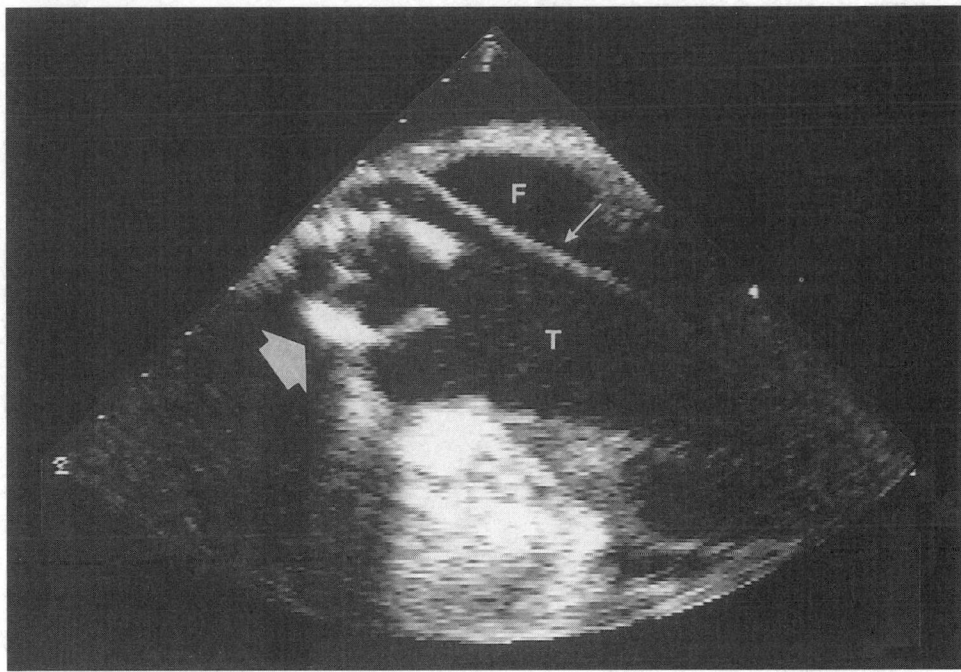

FIGURE 14-68
Longitudinal TEE view of an ascending aortic dissection in a patient with a porcine prosthetic valve in the aortic position (*large arrow*). The false (F) and true (T) lumens are separated by an intimal flap (*small arrow*). (From Blanchard DG, Kimura BJ, Dittrich HC, DeMaria AN. Transesophageal echocardiography of the aorta. *JAMA* 1994; 272:546–551, with permission.)

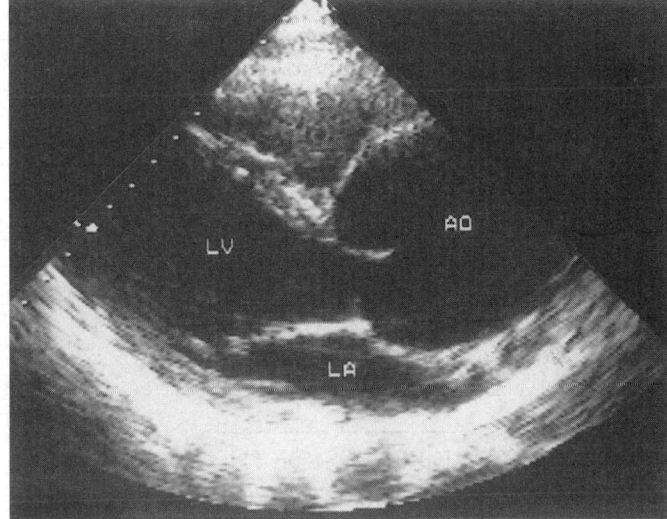

FIGURE 14-70
Parasternal long-axis plane demonstrating severe aortic root (AO) enlargement. LV = left ventricle; LA = left atrium (Courtesy of Kirk L. Peterson, MD.)

FIGURE 14-69
See color Plate 33.

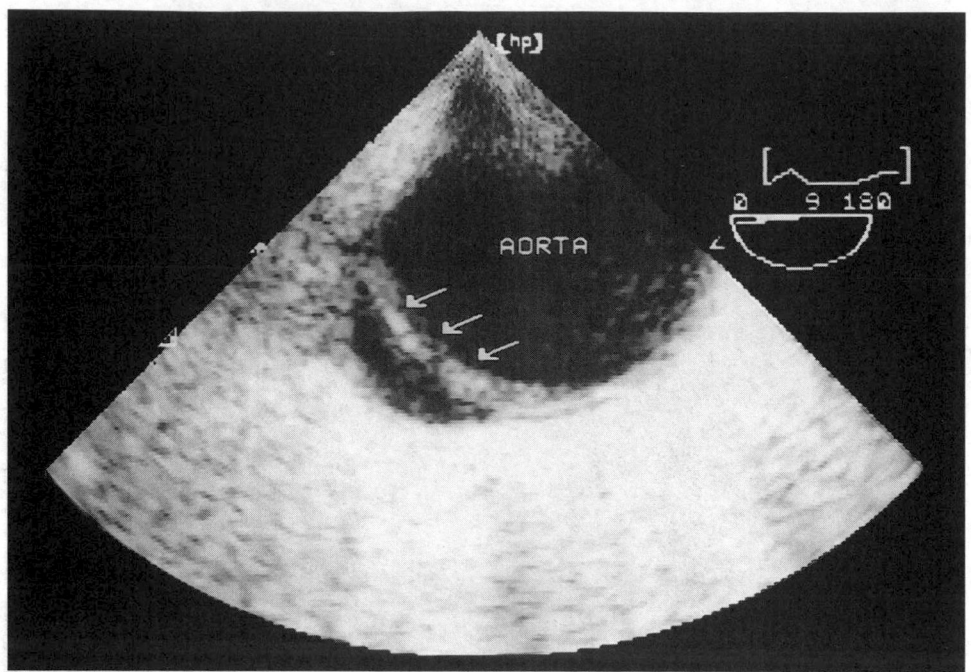

FIGURE 14-72
Transverse TEE image of traumatic aortic disruption and partial transection (*arrows*) involving the distal portion of the aortic arch.

AORTIC ATHEROSCLEROSIS

As mentioned in the section on TEE, recent studies suggest that aortic atherosclerosis is an important cause of stroke and embolic events.[167,168] Mobile and protruding intimal plaques have been detected by TEE (Fig. 14-53) in patients with stroke with a prevalence greater than in controls, a finding not previously appreciated by other imaging techniques.[271] Optimal treatment for extensive aortic atherosclerosis is currently unknown; controlled trials are required. It appears that detection of large aortic arch plaques prior to cardiopulmonary bypass should prompt adjustment of cannula placement to avoid dislodging the aortic debris.[272]

Penetrating aortic ulceration, which affects the descending aorta and mimics the clinical syndrome of acute aortic dissection, may also be diagnosed by TEE (Fig. 14-71, Plate 34).[273] The diagnosis is based upon visualization of a localized defect with protrusion of the ulcer into the vessel wall (in the absence of dissection). This disease entity, which occurs in the setting of atherosclerosis, warrants urgent surgery to avoid aortic rupture. Aortic tears induced by trauma are also accurately detected by TEE[273a,273b] (Fig. 14-72).

DISEASES OF THE MITRAL VALVE

Mitral Stenosis

Detection of mitral stenosis (MS) was one of the earliest clinical applications of echocardiography.[274] In the majority of individuals, the mitral valve leaflets are easily visualized in most views and yield thin linear echoes that exhibit wide bi-peaked excursions as they open in early and late diastole.[24] The characteristic 2D ultrasound findings of MS are seen clearly in nearly all patients with this disorder.[275] The mitral valve leaflets are thickened and often present bright high-intensity reflections indicative of calcification. The process may involve thickening and shortening of the chordal apparatus as well. There are varying degrees of commissural fusion restricting mitral leaflet separation, especially at the distal tips.[276,277] This leads to diastolic "doming" or a right-angle bend of the anterior mitral valve leaflet, as high left atrial pressure creates a bulge in the leaflet's midportion (which is generally more pliable than the distal portion) (Fig. 14-73). The posterior leaflet actually may be pulled anteriorly during diastole because of commissural fusion with the longer anterior leaflet.[278] Mitral doming may also occur in congenital valvular disease, but it is not seen when mitral leaflet opening is reduced due to low-flow states[32] or aortic regurgitant jets. The left atrium is nearly always enlarged with MS.

The effects of stenosis upon mitral valve motion are often best demonstrated by M-mode recordings (Fig. 14-74). Thus, in addition to leaflet thickening and reduced excursion, M-mode tracings also depict a characteristic decrease in the reclosure rate of the anterior mitral leaflet in early diastole (reduced E-F slope) due to a persistent left atrial/left ventricular pressure gradient and a slow rate of LV filling.[276–279] The decrease of the E-F slope has been found to correlate grossly with the severity of mitral stenosis. This finding is not specific for MS, however, and may occur whenever early diastolic filling is reduced.[24,280] Attempts to calculate mitral valve orifice area using the E-F slope have proved unsatisfactory.[281]

The entire perimeter of the mitral valve orifice can be visualized in the 2D parasternal short-axis view, and mitral leaflet excursion normally approaches the endocardial borders of the left ventricle at the mitral tip level. In the setting of mitral stenosis, the thickened leaflets form a fish-mouth orifice, which occupies only a small portion of the cross-sectional area of the left ventricle (see also Chap. 64).[275,282] Measurements of mitral valve area may be obtained by planimetry of the orifice visualized in the parasternal short-axis view and

FIGURE 14-71
See color Plate 34.

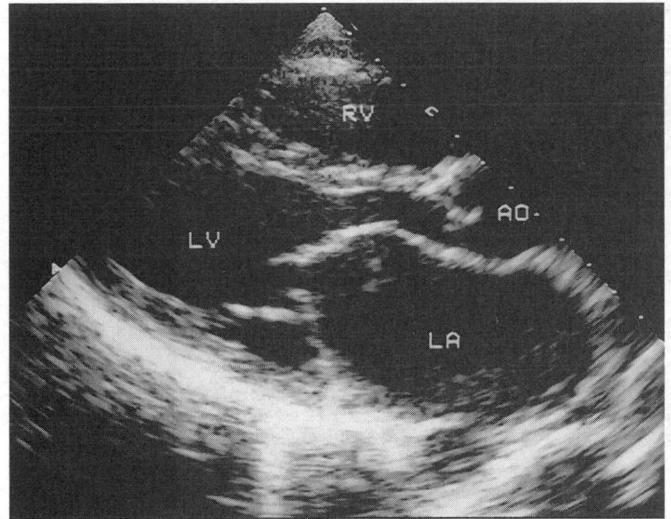

A

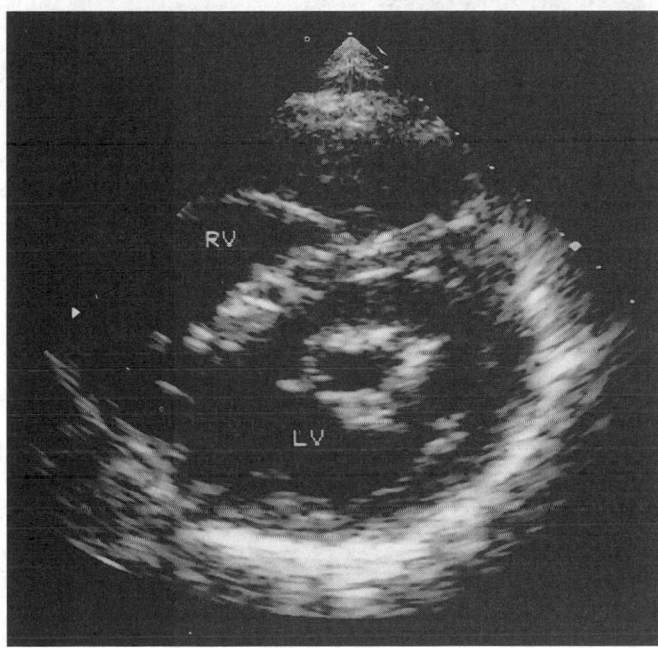

C

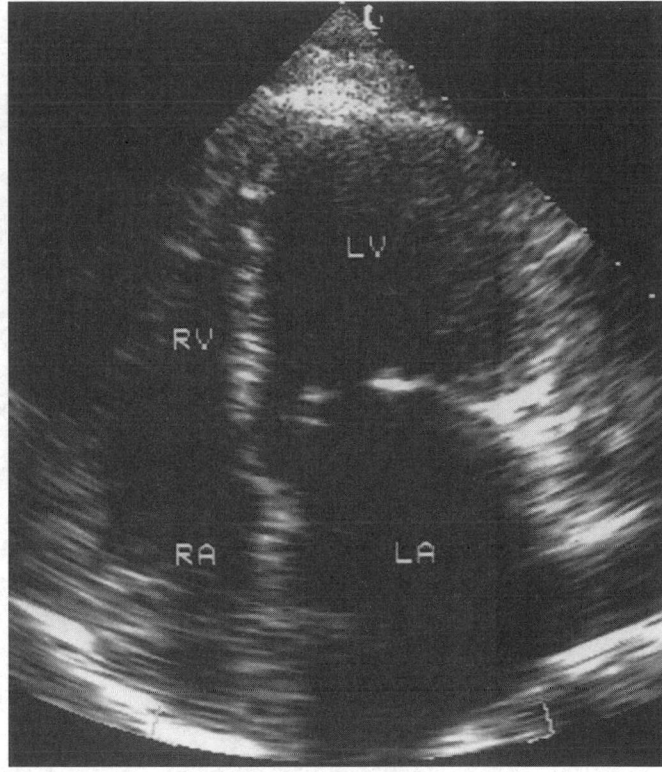

B

FIGURE 14-73

A. Parasternal long-axis view of mitral stenosis. The left atrium (LA) is enlarged, mitral opening is limited, and "doming" of the anterior mitral leaflet is present. LV = left ventricle; RV = right ventricle; AO = aorta. *B.* Apical 4-chamber view in mitral stenosis. The left atrium is markedly dilated. RA = right atrium. *C.* Parasternal short-axis plane in mitral stenosis.

correlate well with those obtained by cardiac catheterization (Fig. 14-73).[282–284] Since the shape of the mitral valve resembles a funnel, it is crucial to identify the smallest cross-sectional area and obtain recordings with orthogonal beam orientation at that point in order to avoid overestimation. Optimal gain settings must be employed to avoid encroachment of tissue signals upon the orifice.[285]

Doppler examination provides additional quantitation of mitral stenosis.[286,287] Interrogation of mitral inflow with either PW or CW modes (depending on velocity and Nyquist limit) reveals elevated diastolic velocities, with a reduction in the rate of deceleration in early diastole yielding a pattern similar to decreased E-F slope seen with M-mode in mitral stenosis (Fig. 14-75). In a fashion similar to that of AS, the maximal gradient across the mitral valve can be calculated from the peak diastolic velocity utilizing the Bernoulli equa-

tion.[286,288] But since the maximal transmitral gradient is very sensitive to changes in heart rate and loading, the mean transmitral gradient obtained as the average of a number of individual gradients derived throughout diastole is customarily utilized to assess the severity of MS.[288] In addition, Doppler technique may provide estimates of mitral valve area by means of the calculation of the pressure half-time.[284,287] The pressure half-time represents the interval required for transmitral velocity to decelerate from its highest point (E) to a velocity that yields one-half of the pressure equivalent (Fig. 14-75). As the severity of mitral stenosis increases, the rate of deceleration decreases, prolonging the pressure half-time. Further, dividing an empiric constant of 220[289] by the pressure half-time yields an estimate of mitral valve area, which correlates with values obtained during cardiac catheterization. Since Doppler estimates of mitral valve area are indirect and involve the use of

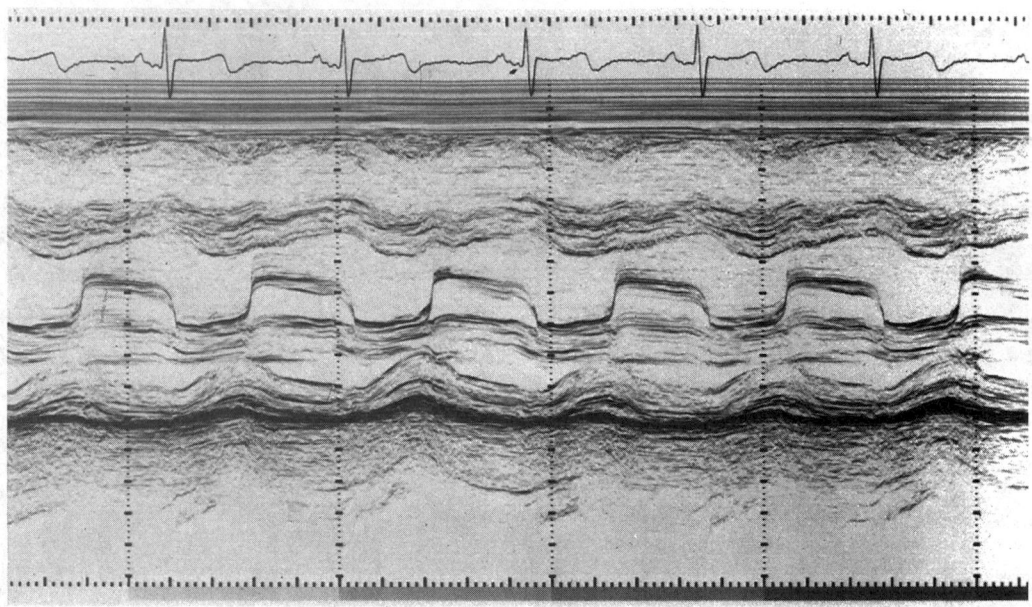

FIGURE 14-74

Parasternal M-mode image through the mitral valve in a patient with mitral stenosis. The normal rapid downslope of the anterior mitral leaflet after early rapid diastolic filling is absent.

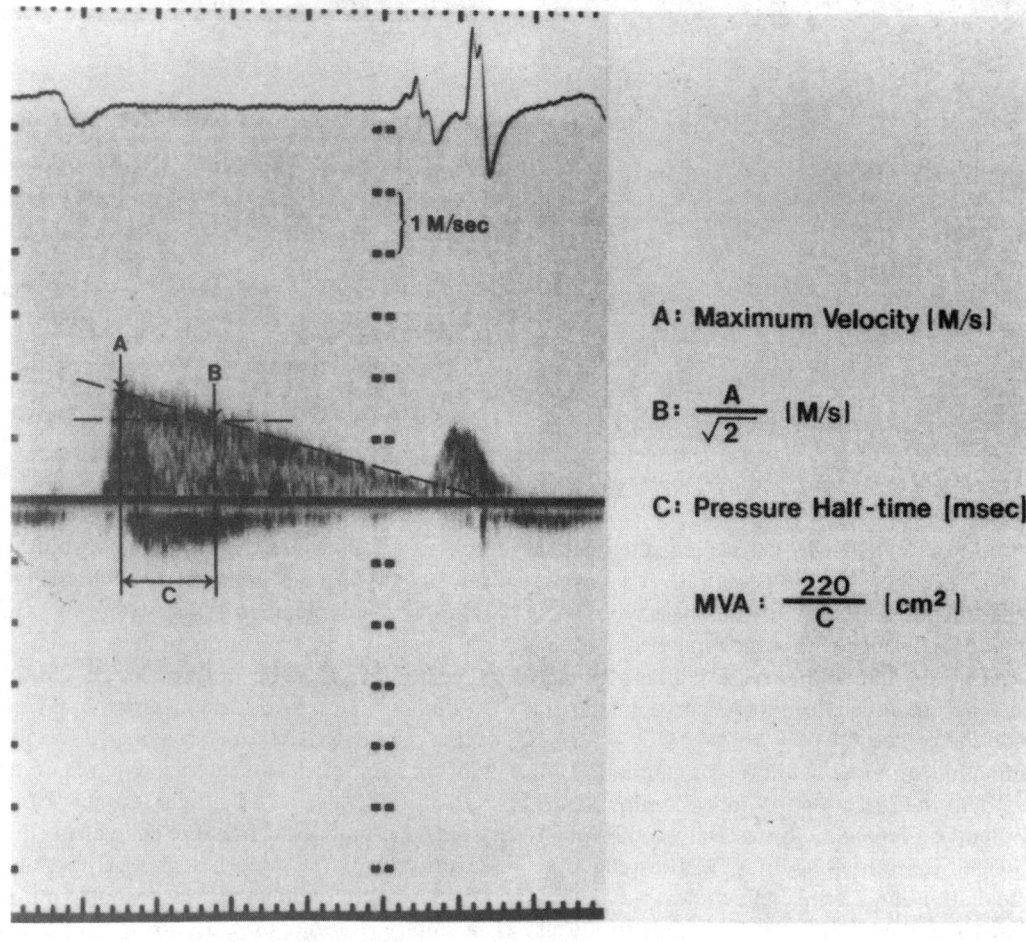

FIGURE 14-75

Pressure half-time method for calculation of mitral valve area (MVA). (From Hagan AD, DeMaria AN. *Clinical Applications of Two-Dimensional Echo-* *cardiography and Cardiac Doppler.* Boston: Little, Brown; 1989, with permission.)

empiric constants, they are considered less accurate than direct measurements of mitral area derived by planimetry of the mitral valve orifice.[290] The pressure half-time method is inaccurate immediately following mitral commissurotomy.[291,292]

Echocardiography can help assess the feasibility and appropriateness of percutaneous catheter balloon mitral valvuloplasty to treat individual patients with MS.[293,294] An echocardiographic scoring system based on evaluation of mitral valvular thickening, calcification, mobility, and subvalvular involvement has been devised. Each variable is assigned a grade of 1 (minimal involvement) to 4 (severe), with a maximal score of 16. Although the prognostic capability of this method is limited, the outcome of balloon valvuloplasty in patients with higher scores, particularly greater than 12, is less satisfactory and involves a higher risk of complications than in patients with lower scores.[293,294] Therefore, echocardiographic analysis is an important part of the decision-making process prior to balloon mitral valvuloplasty. Preprocedural TEE is also often performed to detect left atrial thrombi, which can embolize during transseptal catheterization.[295,296] Following valvuloplasty, echocardiography can identify complications including mitral regurgitation[297] and atrial septal defect.[298]

Mitral Regurgitation

Although echocardiography is extremely accurate in the detection of mitral (and aortic) regurgitation, *quantitation* is more difficult. 2D imaging alone does not provide direct evidence of mitral regurgitation but usually reveals the etiology of the lesion.[299] Thus, 2D echocardiography reveals thickened, restricted leaflets in rheumatic disease, vegetations in infective endocarditis, flail mitral leaflets with torn chordae, and redundant leaflets with abnormal coaptation in mitral valve prolapse.[300] 2D echocardiography can also detect left atrial and LV abnormalities associated with MR, such as myxoma, papillary muscle dysfunction, and dilated cardiomyopathy. In addition, enlargement of these chambers offers indirect evidence of MR severity. In cases of chronic, severe MR, 2D echocardiography can also discern the presence of depressed LV function and decreased ejection fraction (see also Chap. 64).

Doppler echocardiography is the primary method for the detection and evaluation of MR[301–303] and reveals a disturbed flow jet in the left atrium during systole. Spectral Doppler

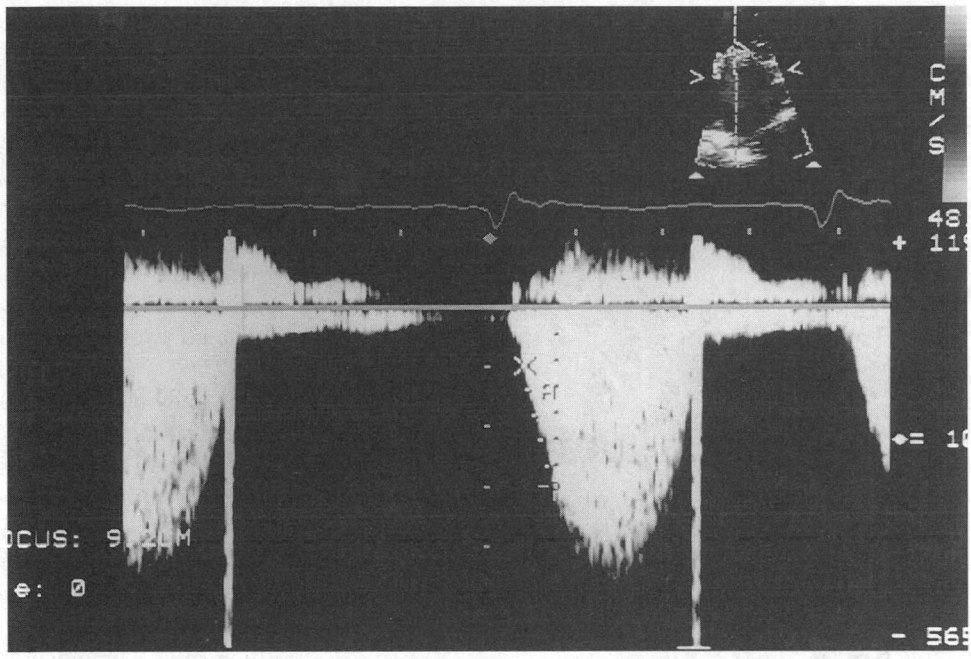

FIGURE 14-76

Continuous-wave tracing of mitral regurgitation with calculation of *dP/dt* (apical transducer position). The time period between velocities of 1 and 3 m/s is 0.07 s; the calculated *dP/dt* is approximately 460 mmHg/s. See text for details.

recordings provide several indexes of severity which are of semiquantitative value. Since the intensity of the Doppler signal is a function of the number of RBCs in the sample volume, the videodensity of the jet correlates in a general way with regurgitant volume.[304] Similarly, an increase in transmitral filling velocities reflects increased forward flow and suggests a large regurgitant volume. Measurements obtainable from the envelope of the CW Doppler recording of the mitral regurgitant jet include a slow rate of acceleration, indicative of a diminished left ventricular *dP/dt*[305] (Fig. 14-76). Early peaking followed by rapid deceleration of the MR jet suggests a large V wave, increased left atrial pressure, and usually acute severe mitral regurgitation.[306]

As in the case of aortic regurgitation, volumetric calculations of LV inflow and outflow by combined pulsed Doppler and 2D-echocardiographic imaging techniques can be used to derive measurements of regurgitant volume.[307,308] In the case of MR, transmitral filling represents both systemic and regurgitant volume, while aortic outflow represents only systemic flow. Therefore, mitral filling should exceed left ventricular ejection, and the difference will be regurgitant volume.

The most commonly applied method for evaluation of MR is assessment of jet size by CFD.[303,309,310] Imaging of the left atrium in systole reveals a turbulent, mosaic jet of varying direction, size, and configuration (Fig. 14-77A and B, Plate 35A and B). Previous studies have demonstrated that a mitral regurgitant jet whose absolute area exceeds 8 cm² [303,310] or

FIGURE 14-77
See color Plate 35.

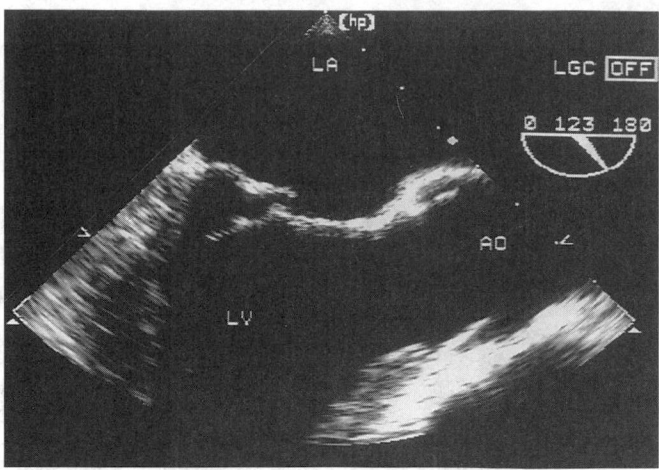

FIGURE 14-78
TEE images from a case of severe mitral regurgitation secondary to a flail posterior mitral valve leaflet. *A.* abnormal coaptation and prolapse of the posterior leaflet is apparent. *B.* See color Plate 36.

fills at least 40 percent of the area of the left atrium[309] is predictive of finding 3+ to 4+ MR by LV angiography. Unfortunately, neither jet size nor angiographic grade correlates closely with measurements of actual regurgitant volume.[310] The lack of correlation between CFD jet area and regurgitant volume is attributable to the additional variables that influence the distribution of the flow disturbance, such

as pressure gradient and the volume and compliance of the left atrium, as well as technical limitations. The Coanda effect is of particular significance in regard to MR, since jets into the left atrium are often eccentric (for example, in cases of mitral valve prolapse and torn chordae tendineae). Due to differential frictional forces and resistance to flow, eccentric MR jets are draw along the walls of the left atrium, resulting in cross-sectional jet areas that are smaller than centrally directed flow disturbances of comparable regurgitant volume (Figs. 14-77 and 14-78). This effect can lead to underestimation of severity of regurgitation.[311,312]

TEE is also useful for assessment of MR, as the close proximity of the probe and its higher-frequency interrogating beam permit imaging of regurgitant jets in greater detail than TTE.[313–315] Eccentric jets and mitral valvular anatomy are well visualized (Fig. 14-78A and Fig. 14-78B, Plate 36), and rightward bulging of the interatrial septum with severe MR is also sometimes apparent. As the regurgitant jets often appear larger with TEE than with TTE, one must avoid overestimation of MR severity.[154] TEE often yields Doppler interrogation of the pulmonary veins that is superior to TTE, and several recent studies have shown that systolic reversal of flow into the pulmonary veins is a reliable sign of severe MR[152] (Fig. 14-79).

Another color Doppler method of flow quantitation involves measurement of the zone of flow convergence proximal to the regurgitant orifice (or the proximal isovelocity surface area, referred to as PISA).[316–319] The mechanism for this

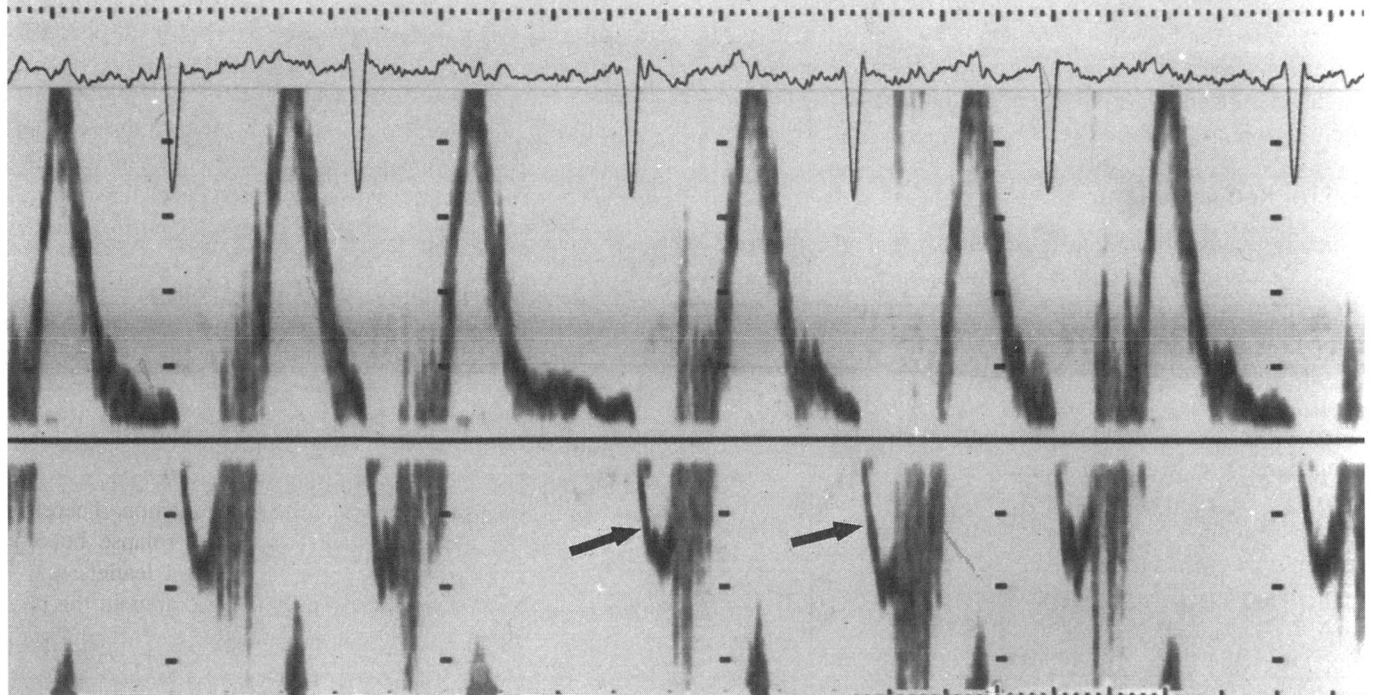

FIGURE 14-79
Pulmonary venous pulsed-wave Doppler in severe mitral regurgitation. Systolic flow reversal (i.e., systolic flow into the pulmonary vein) is present (*arrows*).

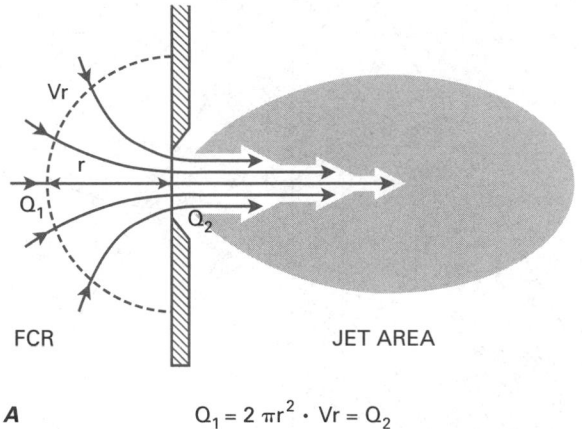

FIGURE 14-80

A. Proximal isovelocity surface area (PISA). See text for details. Q = flow; FCR − flow convergence region; r = radius of isovelocity hemisphere; Vr = velocity of flow at distance r from the orifice. (From Bargiggia GS, Tronconi L, Sahn DJ, et al. A new method for quantitation of mitral regurgitation based on color flow Doppler imaging of flow convergence proximal to regurgitant orifice. *Circulation* 1991; 84:1481–1489, with permission.) B. See color Plate 37.

phenomenon is derived from the hydrodynamic principle that blood flow accelerates before passing through a small orifice under high pressure. If this increase in flow velocity exceeds the Nyquist limit, color aliasing occurs and the velocity aliasing border is equal to the Nyquist limit (Figs. 14-31 and 14-80A; and Fig. 14-80B, Plate 37). If one assumes that the aliasing border conforms to the geometry of a hemisphere around the mitral orifice, then the instantaneous flow rate of blood through the orifice can be calculated as

$$\text{Flow} = 2\,\pi r^2 \cdot V_r$$

where r is the radius of the hemisphere shell (distance from alias border to orifice) and V_r is the velocity of blood at distance r (the Nyquist limit velocity).[316] If the maximal calculated flow rate is divided by the peak regurgitant flow velocity (measured with CW Doppler), the regurgitant orifice area is then obtained.[320] The product of regurgitant orifice area and integrated velocity of the MR jet by CW yields regurgitant volume.

The PISA method avoids the variables associated with jet size and the assumptions and technical limitations of volumetric calculations. Numerous studies have shown a correlation between both flow rate and regurgitant orifice area calculated by PISA and the severity of MR assessed by standard methods.[316,320] In addition, flow convergence calculations have been applied to other valvular lesions, including AR and MS[321,322] (Fig. 14-81, Plate 38), ventricular septal defect,[323] and prosthetic heart valves.[324] The proximal flow convergence

FIGURE 14-81
See color Plate 38.

assumes a hemispheric geometry for the PISA signal and that the plane of the mitral leaflets is flat, two sources of potential error.[325] Despite these limitations, the method holds considerable promise for the clinical evaluation of valvular regurgitation.

Mitral Valve Prolapse

As is true of so many aspects of mitral valve prolapse,[326] the echocardiographic findings in this disorder have been controversial for many years.[327] Recent insights into the anatomy of the mitral annulus and the significance of abnormal leaflet structure have established a central role for echocardiography in the diagnosis and prognosis of mitral valve prolapse.[328] The classic echocardiographic findings in overt mitral valve prolapse syndrome consists of mid- to late-systolic bulging of one or both mitral leaflets across the plane of the mitral valve annulus into the left atrium (Fig. 14-82A to C).[329] The leaflets are often observed to be structurally abnormal, with thickening, elongation, and hooding.[330] Mid- to late-systolic mitral regurgitation is sometimes present, often eccentric, and generally directed away from the prolapsing leaflet.[326] The chordae tendineae may be thickened and elongated, the aortic root may be dilated, and the tricuspid valve leaflets may prolapse as well. LV function is usually normal, although the left atrium and ventricle may be enlarged if mitral regurgitation is significant. The greater temporal resolution of M-mode over 2D echocardiography often yields striking evidence of abrupt midsystolic posterior/superior motion of the mitral valve leaflets in prolapse patients[331] (Fig. 14-82C). Although such M-mode findings, which resemble a question mark on its side, are specific for mitral valve prolapse, patients with classic mitral valve prolapse occasionally may demonstrate diagnostic findings only with 2D imaging.

Although the diagnosis of classic, fully expressed mitral valve prolapse is straightforward by echocardiography, identification of mild prolapse is more difficult, and no absolute diagnostic criteria currently exist.[329] This is largely related to the absence of any gold standard with which to validate findings, including auscultation, angiography, and even pathology.[326] For prolapse to be present, the mitral valve leaflets must cross the plane of the mitral valve annulus after initial systolic coaptation. Recent studies have established that the mitral valve annulus is not flat but rather saddle-shaped.[332] The annulus reaches its nadir in the apical four-chamber view, and even normally coapting mitral valve leaflets may appear to prolapse in this projection. Therefore, current criteria require that mitral valve prolapse be diagnosed only when one or both of the mitral leaflets clearly bulge past the plane of the mitral valve annulus in the parasternal long-axis view.[328] Unfortunately, the degree to which the mitral leaflets must break the plane of the annulus is unclear. The greater the portion of the mitral valve leaflets entering the left atrium, the more likely the existence of signs and symptoms related to this disorder; a peak distance

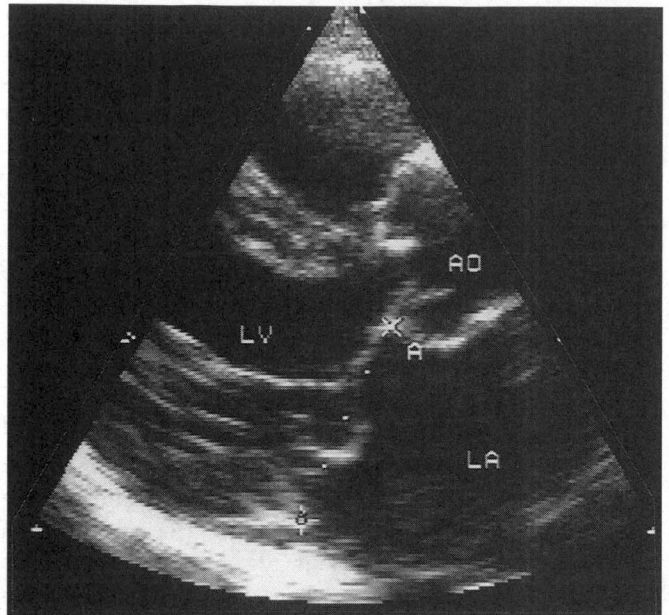

A

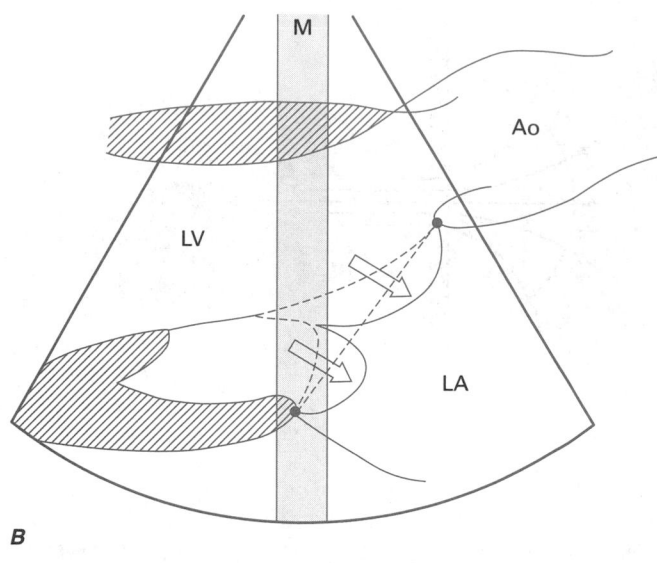

B

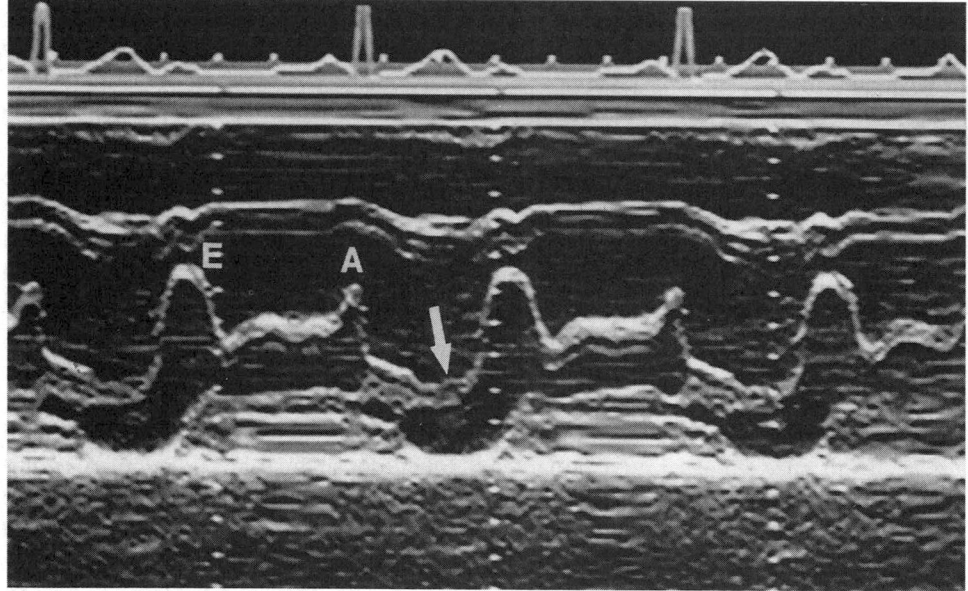

C

FIGURE 14-82

A. Parasternal long-axis plane through the mitral valve in late systole. The plane of the mitral annulus (A) is drawn in a dotted line. The posterior mitral leaflet prolapses past the level of the annulus into the left atrium (LA). AO = aorta; LV = left ventricle. *B*. Diagram of true mitral valve prolapse. The mitral leaflets clearly prolapse (*arrows*) posterior to the plane of the mitral annulus (*straight dotted line*). Ao = aorta; LV = left ventricle; LA = left atrium; M = m-mode imaging beam. (From Devereux RB, Kramer-Fox R, Kligfield P. Mitral valve prolapse: Causes, clinical manifestations, and management. *Ann Intern Med* 1989; 111:305–317, with permission.) *C*. M-mode image through the plane of the mitral valve demonstrating posterior prolapse of the leaflets during systole (*arrow*). E = early diastolic filling; A = atrial component.

behind the annulus of 2 mm almost invariably establishes the presence of prolapse.[329] The diagnosis of mild mitral prolapse may be assisted by examination of the structure of the leaflets and chordae tendineae, since it has been demonstrated that patients with redundant or thickening valve leaflets (greater than 5 mm in midleaflet) are at increased risk of complications, including severe mitral regurgitation and infective endocarditis.[333]

Torn Chordae Tendineae

Rupture of chordae tendineae may occur spontaneously or in conjunction with mitral valve prolapse or endocarditis. This can result in a flail mitral leaflet and severe MR. Although

TTE often detects these lesions, TEE is especially sensitive and accurate and often demonstrates free motion of the leaflet and ruptured chord into the left atrium even when the transthoracic echocardiogram is equivocal (Fig. 14-83A and B).[334] As with mitral valve prolapse, the MR jet in this condition is usually eccentric and directed away from the affected leaflet, often "hugging" the adjacent left atrial wall (Coanda effect). Therefore, the jet's cross-sectional area may be misleadingly small. The findings of mitral valvular anatomy on TEE may also be helpful in predicting the feasibility and success of valve repair surgery.[335]

In the setting of ischemic heart disease, both LV enlargement and papillary muscle dysfunction (from infarction or transient ischemia) may cause MR.[336] Both the MR and the contractile abnormality responsible for it are usually well visualized by 2D echocardiography. In rare cases, papillary muscle rupture (partial or complete) occurs in the postinfarction period.[337] Rapid echocardiographic diagnosis often requires TEE and may be lifesaving in these cases.[334]

Mitral Annular Calcification

The finding of mitral annular calcification is fairly common in adults and occurs more frequently with advancing age. Although ultrasound cannot discern histology, calcification typically appears as thickened extremely high intensity ("bright") signals (Fig. 14-84). The posterior portion of the mitral annulus is affected much more commonly than the anterior segment, and calcification often extends into the posterior mitral leaflet, sometimes restricting its motion.[338–340] The abnormality, best visualized in the parasternal long- and short-axis views, is seen as a bright calcific density at the junction of the posterior mitral leaflet and the annulus. In the short-axis view, the posterior band of calcification often appears crescentic. Rarely, the calcification is extensive enough to cause marked valvular thickening and clinically significant mitral stenosis.[339] Mitral annular calcification also has been implicated as a source of cardiogenic embolization.[341]

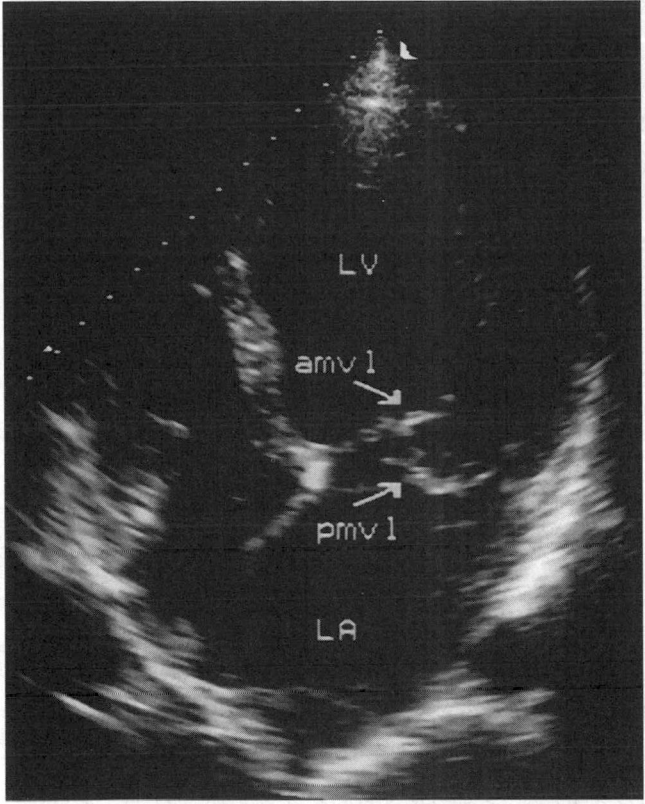

A

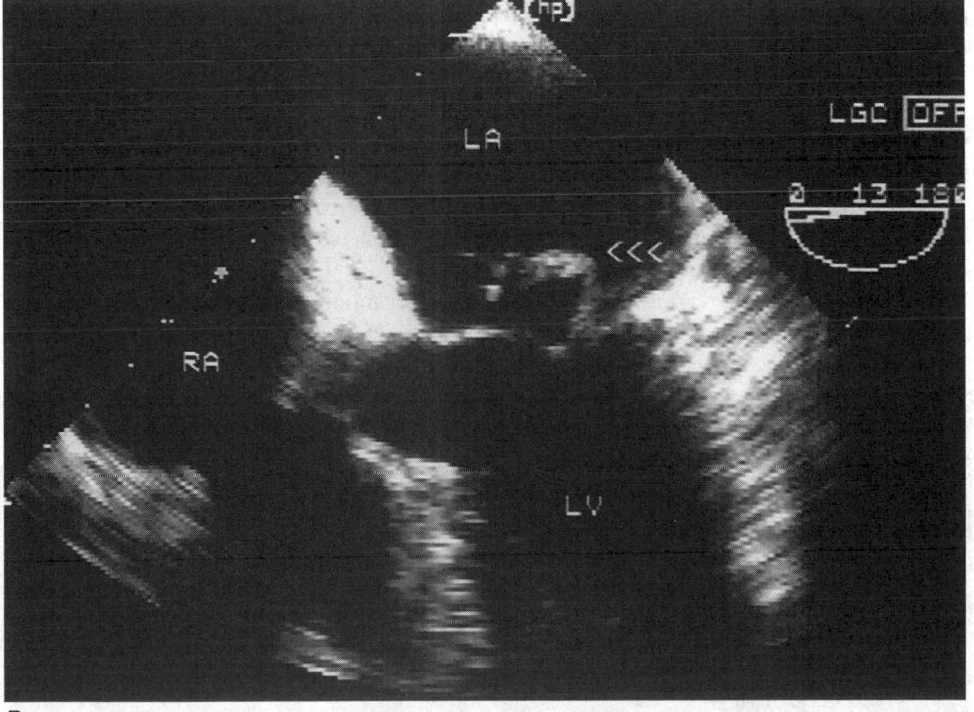

B

FIGURE 14-83

A. Apical four-chamber image of a flail posterior mitral valve leaflet (pmvl). The mitral valve is thickened and myxomatous. amvl = anterior mitral valve leaflet. *B.* Transesophageal echocardiography image (transverse four-chamber plane) of a flail posterior mitral valve leaflet (*arrows*) secondary to ruptured chordae. LA = left atrium; RA = right atrium; LV = left ventricle.

RIGHT-SIDED VALVULAR DISEASE AND PULMONARY HYPERTENSION

Pulmonic Valve

Major structural abnormalities of the pulmonic valve are relatively rare. Pulmonic stenosis (PS) is usually congenital in origin and resembles congenital AS in many respects. The stenotic valve does not open fully and exhibits characteristic thickening and systolic doming on 2D imaging[342] (Fig. 14-85). M-mode recordings of the pulmonic valve often show a large *a* wave, since right ventricular diastolic pressure is often so high and pulmonary artery (PA) pressure so low that the atrial "kick" is sufficient to open the pulmonic valve.[343] Doppler interrogation reveals turbulent flow distal the valve,

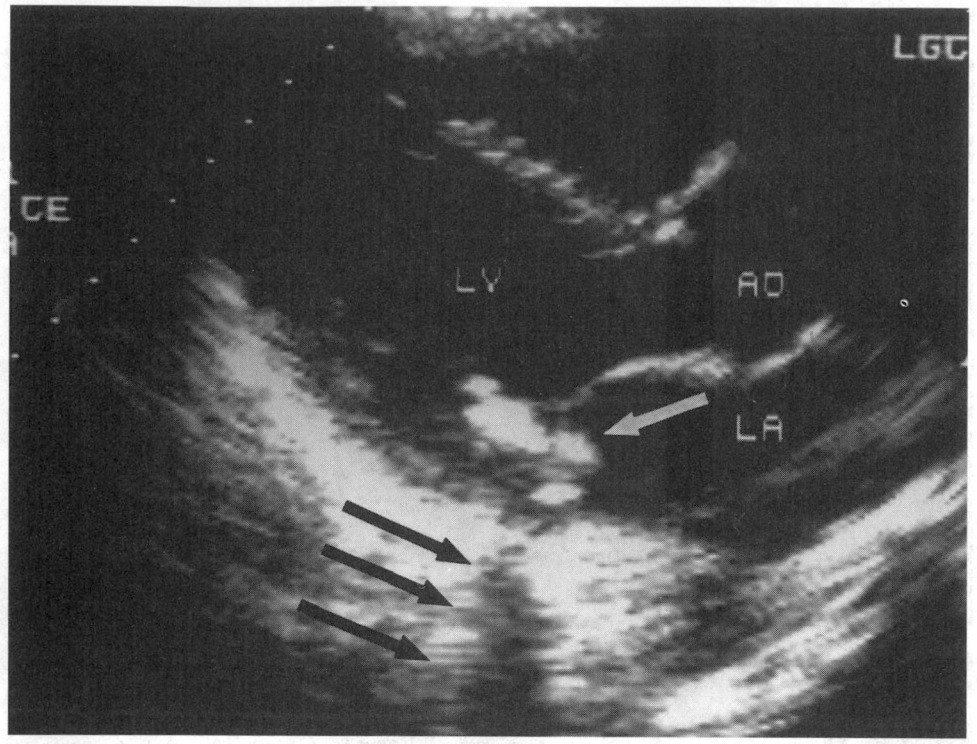

FIGURE 14-84

Parasternal long-axis plane demonstrating mitral annular calcification (*white arrow*) with ultrasonic shadowing posteriorly (*black arrows*). AO = aorta; LV = left ventricle; LA = left atrium. (From Blanchard DG, DeMaria AN. Cardiac and extracardiac masses: Echocardiographic evaluation. In: Skorton DJ, Schelber HR, Wolf GL, Brundage BH, eds. *Marcus' Cardiac Imaging,* 2d ed. Philadelphia: Saunders; 1996:452–480, with permission.)

dynamically significant PR is uncommon; when present, it is usually due to congenital heart disease, valvular tumors, endocarditis, or carcinoid heart disease. The echocardiographic grading of PR is semiquantitative, based on the density of the CW envelope, area of the color Doppler jet, and width of the jet at the valve.[346,347] The PR pressure half-time by CW Doppler may be shorter with more severe PR, but this is not as well investigated as in the case of aortic regurgitation. Measurements derived from the CW Doppler recording also provide estimates of end-diastolic pulmonary artery pressure using the Bernoulli equation as 4 (PR end-diastolic velocity)^2 + central venous pressure (CVP).[348]

Tricuspid Valve

Tricuspid stenosis is usually rheumatic in origin, and coexistent mitral and aortic valvular disease is the rule. Congenital or acquired (nonrheumatic) causes

and CW measurements can be used to calculate gradients and valve areas with the Bernoulli and continuity equations much as in aortic stenosis.[344]

Although severe pulmonic regurgitation (PR) is rare, mild PR is common and appears as a flame shaped flow disturbance in the right ventricular outflow tract (RVOT) in diastole.[345] Many individuals have trivial PR on color Doppler examination; this is a physiologic, normal variant (Fig. 14-86). Hemo-

of tricuspid stenosis are quite uncommon. On rare occasions, tricuspid stenosis may be caused by carcinoid heart disease or by leaflet adhesions to permanent pacemaker leads. Because of the large size of the tricuspid annulus, obstruction by masses, even multiple vegetations, is unlikely to cause stenosis.

Regardless of the etiology, diastolic doming of the valve leaflets suggests stenosis.[349,350] CW Doppler interrogation is also helpful and mimics the findings of MS (high diastolic

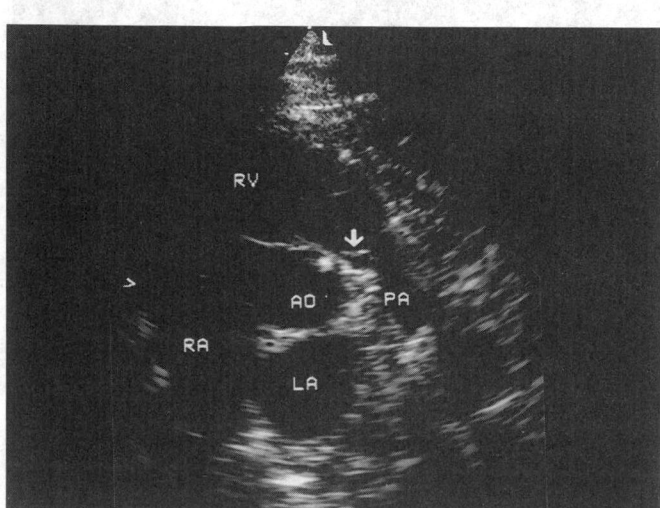

FIGURE 14-85

A. Pulmonic stenosis. The pulmonic valve leaflet is thickened and echoreflective (*arrow*). RA = right atrium; LA = left atrium; AO = aorta; PA = pulmonary artery; RV = right ventricle. *B.* Doppler interrogation reveals increased flow velocity (4 m/s) through the valve orifice.

velocity with prolonged pressure half-time).[349] The pressure half-time equation of mitral valve area calculation cannot be applied directly to the tricuspid valve, and large studies comparing Doppler echocardiography with right heart catheterization in tricuspid stenosis are not available.

Tricuspid regurgitation (TR) is much more common than tricuspid stenosis, and like PR is present to a mild degree in many normal individuals. Hemodynamically significant TR may be caused by endocarditis, rheumatic valvular disease, pulmonary hypertension, congenital heart disease (for example, Ebstein's anomaly), carcinoid heart disease, flail TR leaflet (which can occur as a complication of cardiac trauma or endomyocardial biopsy), and tricuspid valve prolapse. Echo-

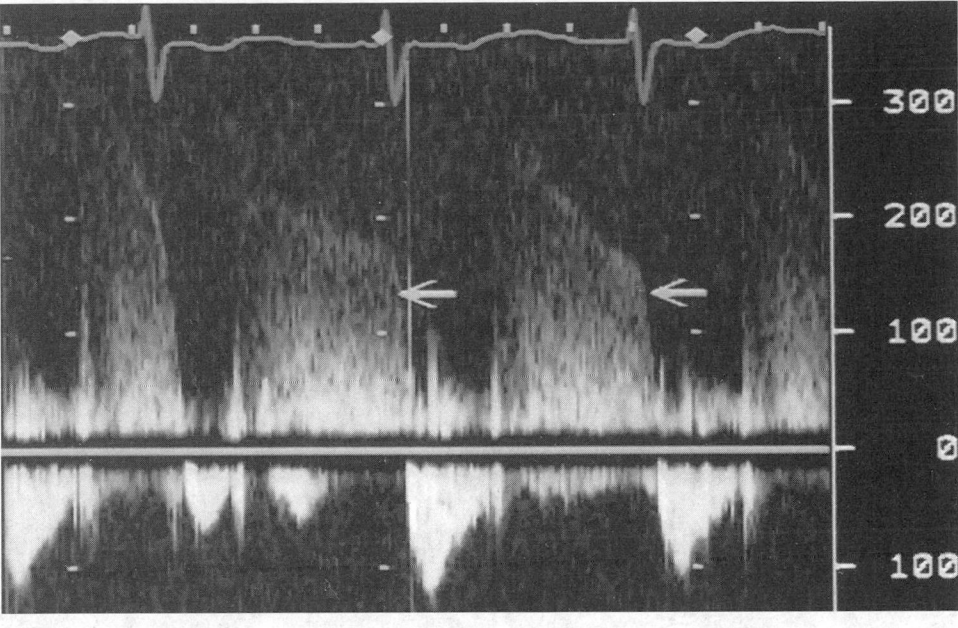

FIGURE 14-86

Continuous-wave Doppler tracing through the right ventricular outflow tract and pulmonary artery (left parasternal transducer position). Mild pulmonic regurgitation is present (*arrows*).

cardiographic findings in patients with TR generally mirror those found in MR.[351] Although 2D imaging can detect abnormalities associated with TR, such as incomplete leaflet coaptation, flail leaflet, and right-sided chamber enlargement, the technique cannot accurately quantify TR grade. Doppler echocardiography, especially color-flow mapping, has become the procedure of choice to detect TR, and has reasonable accuracy for semiquantitation of severity.[352,353] As with MR, severity of TR can be estimated by regurgitant jet area, ratio of jet area to right atrial area, and size of proximal flow convergence zones[354] (Fig. 14-31). Doppler interrogation of the hepatic vein is also useful, as systolic flow reversal within the vein suggests severe TR[355] (Fig. 14-87). Peak right ventricular (and pulmonary artery) pressure can be estimated using measurements of peak TR velocity by CW Doppler (see section on Bernoulli Equation). If necessary, intravenous echocardiographic contrast agents can be injected to accentuate the TR Doppler jet and facilitate more accurate measurements of pulmonary artery pressure.[352–354]

Right Ventricular Function and Pulmonary Hypertension

Right ventricular (RV) enlargement and pulmonary hyperten-

sion can be diagnosed and assessed by echocardiography[355,356] (Fig. 14-88A and B). Because of the asymmetric and crescentic shape of the right ventricle, accurate volume calculations are difficult.[357,358] Nonetheless, 2D imaging provides useful general information regarding RV size and function. In the apical four-chamber view, the RV should appear somewhat smaller than the LV; therefore RV enlargement can be diagnosed qualitatively when the RV cross-sectional area exceeds that of the LV. RV chamber area measurements in the apical four-chamber imaging plane can also be compared to standardized normal values.[359] Although not well

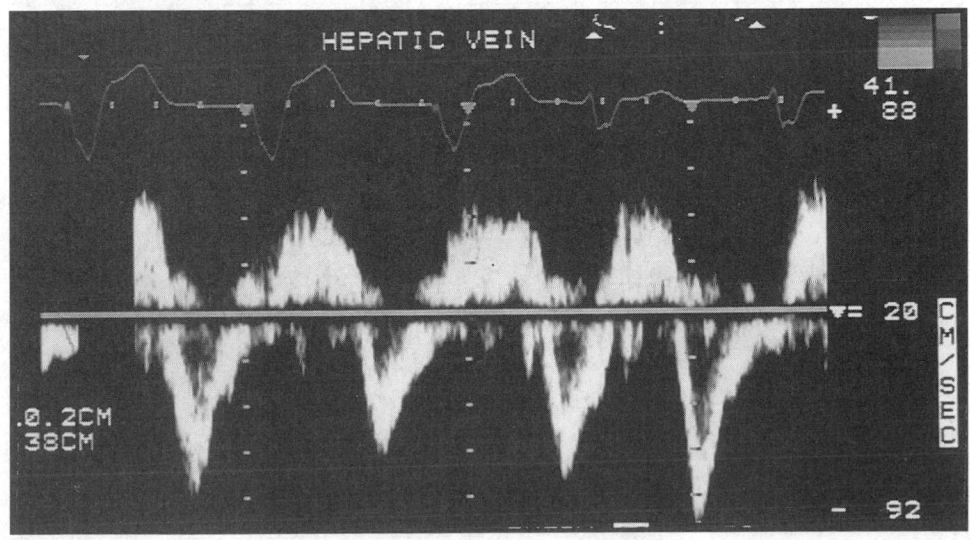

FIGURE 14-87

Pulsed-wave Doppler tracing of the hepatic vein in severe tricuspid regurgitation (TR) subcostal transducer position). Systolic flow reversal into the hepatic vein is present.

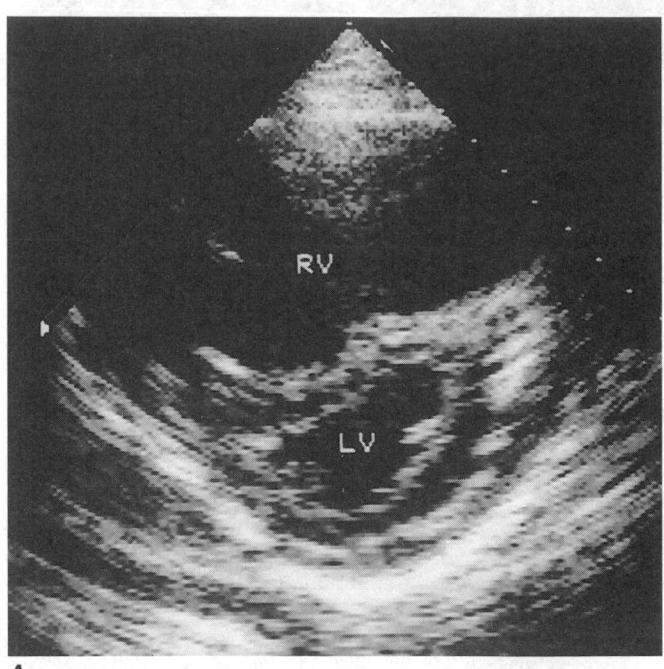

A

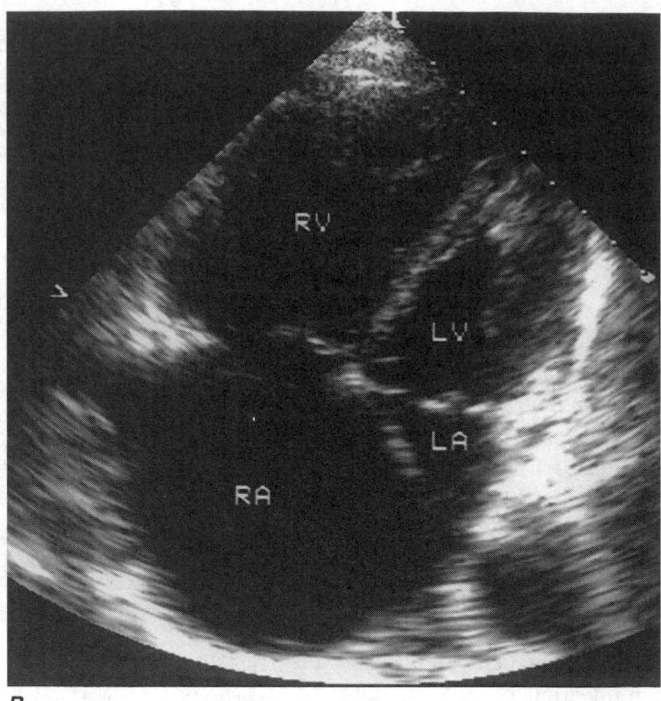

B

FIGURE 14-88

A. Parasternal short-axis view in severe pulmonary hypertension with marked enlargement of the right ventricle (RV). The left ventricle (LV) is small, and the interventricular septum is flattened. *B.* Apical four-chamber view in pulmonary hypertension. The right atrium (RA) and right ventricle (RV) are much larger than the left-sided chambers. LA = left atrium; LV = left ventricle.

standardized, measurements of RV wall thickness can be performed from the parasternal view; a value of 5 mm is generally accepted as the upper limit of normal.[360,361] Systolic motion of the RV free wall and LV lateral wall toward the interventricular septum should be similar and roughly symmetric in normal situations. Asymmetric hypokinesis of the RV free wall indicates RV dysfunction.[362]

RV volume overload can lead to RV hypertrophy, chamber enlargement, and, in advanced stages, depressed RV systolic function. TR can result from or cause RV overload, and the TR Doppler velocity allows estimation of the peak RV systolic pressure. The interventricular septum also becomes abnormal in RV overload and tends to flatten or even bulge toward the LV (Fig. 14-89).[363] The pattern of septal movement can help distinguish between volume and pressure overload: in pure volume overload, the RV diastolic pressure may equal or exceed that of the LV, while the systolic pressure of the LV greatly exceeds that of the RV. Therefore, the interventricular septum flattens during diastole and returns to its normal curvature during systole.[363,364] With RV pressure overload, however, the abnormally high RV pressures persist through the entire cardiac cycle and the interventricular septum remains deformed

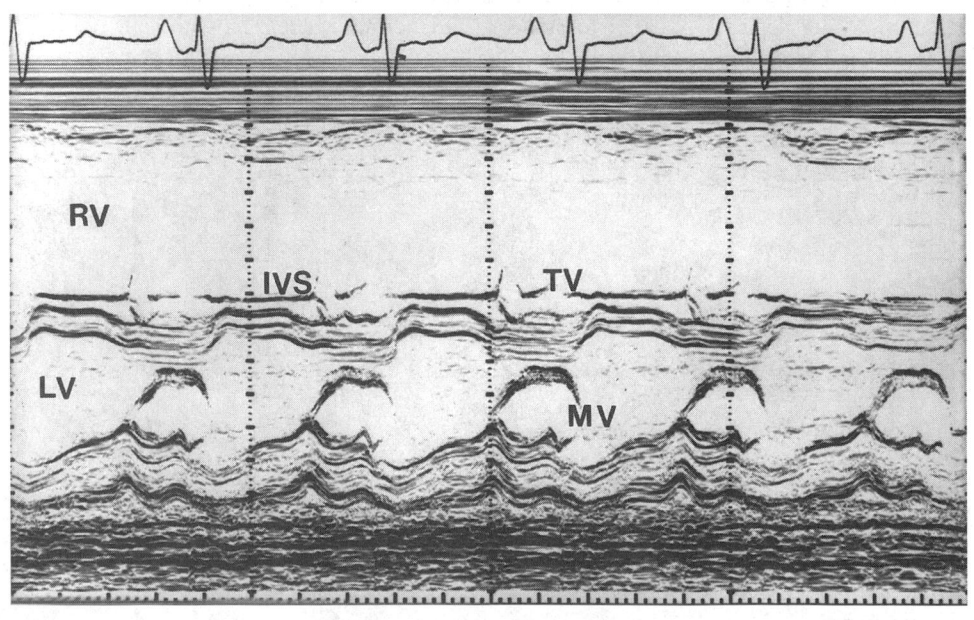

FIGURE 14-89

M-mode in severe pulmonary hypertension. The dimension of the right ventricle (RV) is larger than that of the left ventricle (LV). The interventricular septum (*IVS*) moves paradoxically—i.e., *toward* the mitral valve (MV) during diastole rather than away. TV = tricuspid valve.

during both systole and diastole.[364]

The hallmark of pulmonary hypertension by Doppler echocardiography is a high-velocity TR jet in the absence of pulmonic stenosis. Peak TR jet velocity can be converted to peak systolic PA pressure as $4(\text{TR velocity})^2 + \text{CVP}$.[365] In the setting of severe pulmonary hypertension, the main PA and the inferior vena cava are often dilated. If right atrial pressure is elevated, the inferior vena cava (IVC) does not decrease in diameter with inspiration as normally expected.[366] M-mode examination of the pulmonic valve in pulmonary hypertension may show a characteristic W-shaped motion of the valve leaflet during systole[367–369] (Fig 14-90) and loss of the normal *a* dip caused by partial opening of

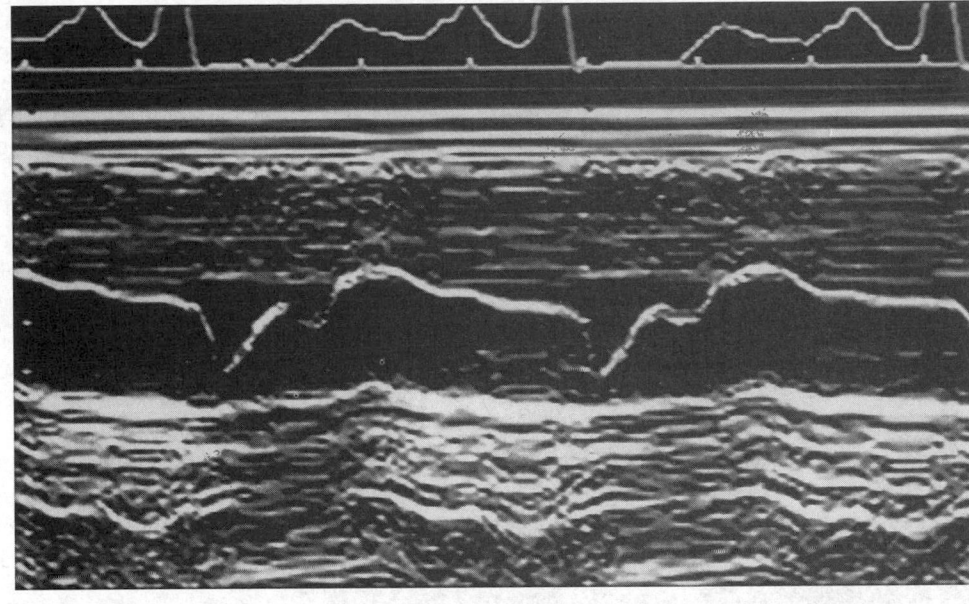

FIGURE 14-90

M-mode image of the pulmonic valve in severe pulmonary hypertension (parasternal transducer position). The a dip is absent, and a characteristic W-shaped motion of the leaflet is present during systole, indicating partial closure of the valve during midsystole followed by reopening prior to diastole.

the valve during atrial contraction. The loss of the a wave is probably due to the large pressure difference between the right ventricle and pulmonary artery during late diastole and the resulting inability of the atrial contraction to partially open the pulmonic valve. The midsystolic closure of the valve and partial reopening in late systole (sometimes called the *flying W*) may be caused by elevated pulmonary vascular resistance and oscillation of a pressure wavefront within the pulmonary artery.[370]

Characteristic pulsed-wave Doppler abnormalities in pulmonary hypertension include a decrease in the velocity-time integral of flow through the pulmonic valve (secondary to depressed RV stroke volume) and a shortening of the acceleration time (measured from beginning of flow through the pulmonic valve to peak velocity). The acceleration time (in milliseconds) can be used to estimate the mean pulmonary artery (PA) pressure[371] as

$$\text{Mean PA pressure} = 80 - \left(\frac{\text{acceleration time}}{2}\right)$$

Pulmonic regurgitation is also common in the setting of pulmonary hypertension and is usually well recorded by pulsed Doppler. As discussed above, the end-diastolic PR velocity can be used to estimate PA end-diastolic pressure by the Bernoulli equation.

PROSTHETIC CARDIAC VALVES

Echocardiography is a critically important tool in the evaluation and serial follow-up of mechanical and bioprosthetic valves.[372] Unfortunately, the increased echo reflectivity of prosthetic valves (especially the mechanical models) causes extensive distal shadowing and reverberations that markedly limit the utility of transthoracic 2D echocardiography (Figs. 14-91 and 14-92). Transthoracic 2D imaging may detect partial ring dehiscence manifest as abnormal "rocking" motion of a prosthetic valve. TTE may also identify reduced movement of the valve disks or leaflets and may occasionally visualize adherent thrombi, tissue ingrowth, and vegetations.[373–375] Leaflet thickening, detachment, and flail motion also may be visualized for bioprosthetic valves.

Doppler interrogation is the cornerstone of the echocardiographic assessment of prosthetic valvular stenosis and regurgitation.[376–379] Color-flow imaging can document the presence, direction, and size of the forward flow stream. Color-flow Doppler can also detect regurgitant flow jets, but like 2D imaging, is limited by acoustic shadowing distal to the prosthesis. Doppler color jets due to prosthetic aortic regurgitation can be readily visualized from the transthoracic apical view, but jets produced by prosthetic mitral and tricuspid regurgitation are often obscured.[380,381] Therefore, although detection of prosthetic regurgitation by transthoracic Doppler is usually feasible, quantitation is often difficult. A small flow signal shortly after valve closure may be observed frequently with prosthetic valves and is likely related to the blood caught behind the occluder as it closes.[382]

Doppler flow velocities and gradients (calculated by the Bernoulli equation) through normal prosthetic valves vary depending upon the type, position, and diameter of the prosthesis.[376–379] The velocities and gradients across prosthetic valves are flow-dependent as well[383] and therefore related to LV function. Given these variables, it is not surprising that a wide range of transvalvular gradients exists for normally functioned prosthetic valves. Nevertheless, "normal" ranges

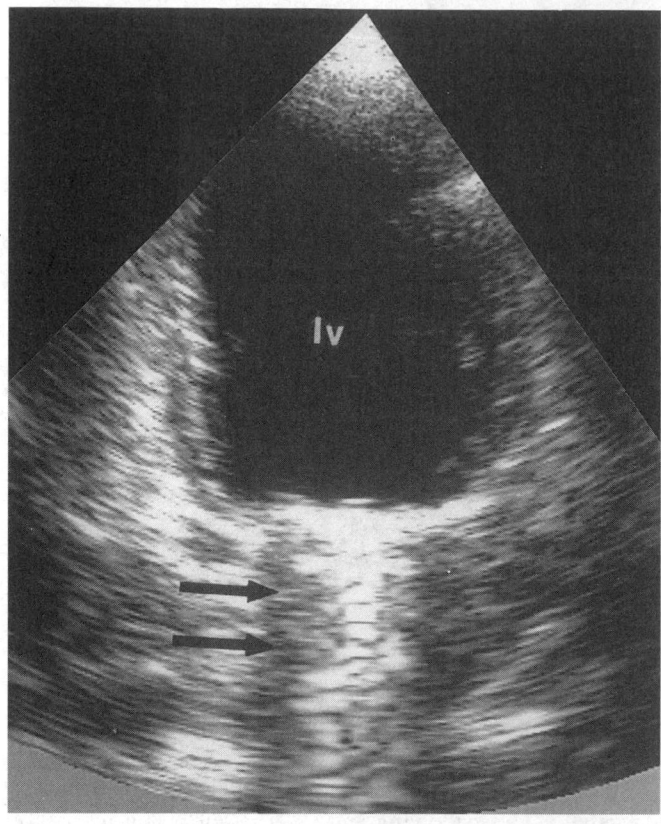

FIGURE 14-91
Apical two-chamber view of a mechanical prosthetic valve (mitral position) during systole. The left atrium is completely obscured by ultrasonic shadowing (*arrows*). LV = left ventricle.

have been reported for various valve types and can be used as a guide to recognize malfunction. Pressure half-time calculation can be performed for prosthetic mitral valves, as in mitral stenosis. High prosthetic valvular gradients due to increased flow volume rather than stenosis can be recognized by high flow velocity across the remaining native valves, a short pressure half-time for mitral prostheses, and a short ejection time for aortic prosthesis. With aortic valve prostheses, peak systolic Doppler velocities may indicate higher systolic pressure gradients than those actually found during cardiac catheterization.[384,385] This problem may be more prevalent with Starr-Edwards (ball-in-cage) and St. Jude (bileaflet tilting disks) valves than with Medtronic-Hall (single tilting disk) and bioprosthetic valves. The inaccuracies with Starr-Edwards and St. Jude valves are probably due to the presence of multiple flow channels (with various orifice areas) and the phenomenon of flow recovery.[385,386] Because of these variabilities, an echocardiographic examination is warranted following prosthetic valve implantation to establish its baseline Doppler characteristics.[387] As opposed to peak gradients, mean transvalvular gradients calculated by Doppler correlate reasonably well with direct catheter measurements.

TEE has dramatically changed the diagnostic approach to prosthetic valve dysfunction.[380,381] Although the technique is useful for the visualization of prosthetic devices implanted

in any valve position, it is especially helpful for mitral prostheses, as it overcomes the problem of left atrial shadowing and reverberation (Fig. 14-93). TEE is extremely accurate in the detection of prosthetic regurgitation and impaired movement of the valve occluder, and it is the diagnostic procedure of choice in most cases of suspected prosthetic valve endocarditis.[388–390] Small thrombi, tissue ingrowth, infected or sterile vegetations, and even sutures in the sewing ring usually can be readily visualized. The enhanced sensitivity of TEE requires operator experience and judgment, as nearly all mechanical prostheses exhibit a normal small amount of regurgitation, which should not be misinterpreted as pathologic.[382] TEE may also visualize thin fibrinous strands sometimes attached to prosthetic valves; these structures appear to be a potential source of cardiogenic embolization.[391,392] The technique is quite accurate in the diagnosis of prosthetic valve thrombosis, a potentially fatal medical emergency, and can assist clinical decision making in this disorder.[393–395]

INFECTIVE ENDOCARDITIS

Infective endocarditis remains an all too common illness, with a significant risk of morbidity and mortality (see also Chap. 82). Traditionally, the diagnosis has been based on either the cumulative results of blood cultures, physical examination, and laboratory findings or on pathologic proof of infected valvular

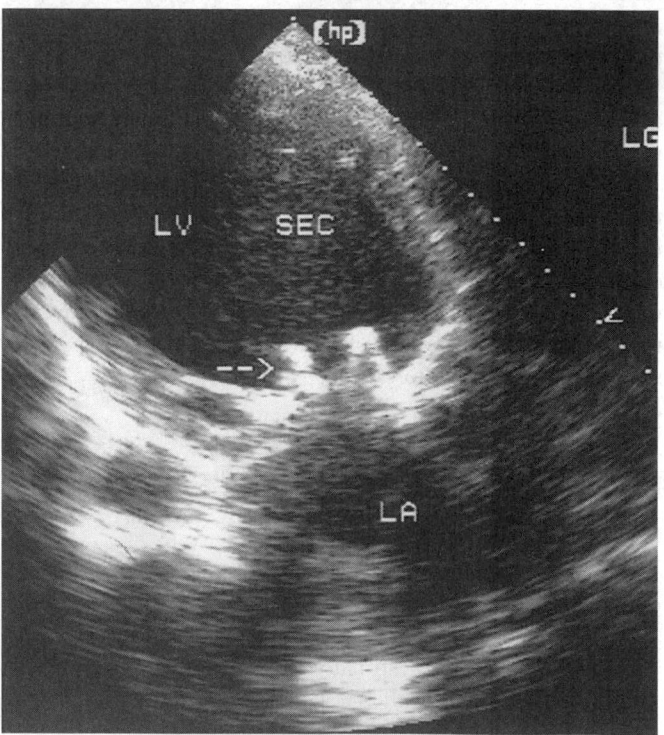

FIGURE 14-92
Apical view of a bioprosthetic valve (*arrow*) in the mitral position (two of the three prosthetic valve struts are apparent). Spontaneous echo contrast (SEC) is also present, secondary to systolic dysfunction and enlargement of the left ventricle (LV); LA = left atrium.

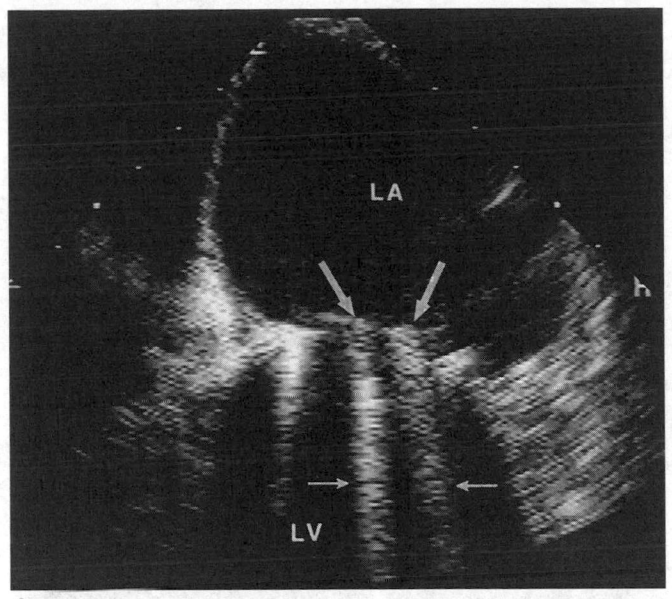

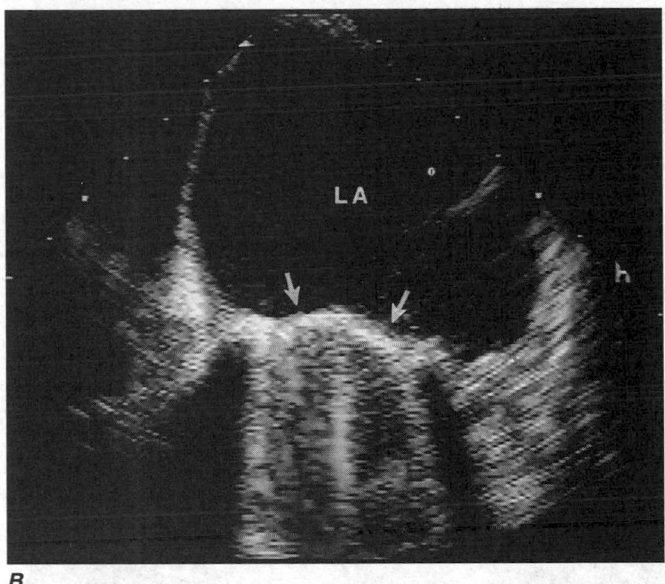

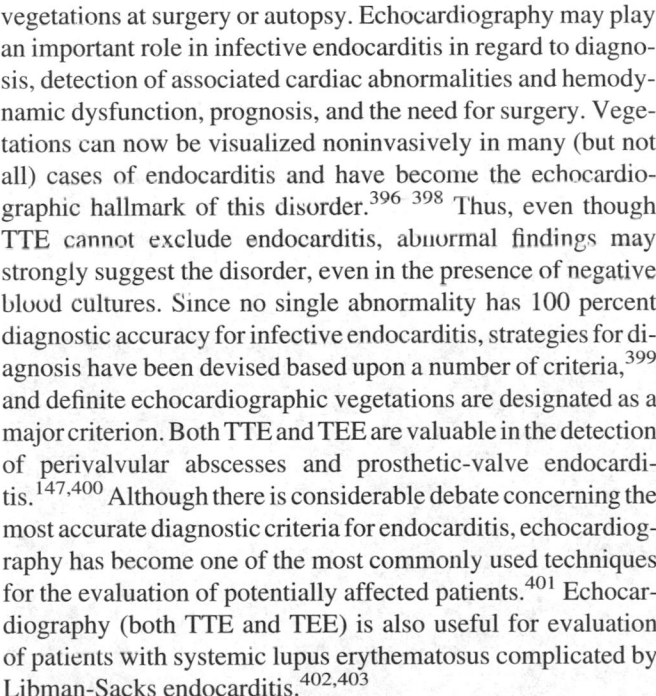

A

B

FIGURE 14-93

TEE images from a patient with a St. Jude prosthetic valve in the mitral position. *A*. Diastolic image. The two struts of the open valve are seen (*large arrows*) as well as their ultrasonic shadows (*small arrows*). LA = left atrium;

LV = left ventricle. *B*. Systolic image. The two prosthetic leaflets are closed (*arrows*) and cast a dense ultrasonic shadow, obscuring the left ventricle.

vegetations at surgery or autopsy. Echocardiography may play an important role in infective endocarditis in regard to diagnosis, detection of associated cardiac abnormalities and hemodynamic dysfunction, prognosis, and the need for surgery. Vegetations can now be visualized noninvasively in many (but not all) cases of endocarditis and have become the echocardiographic hallmark of this disorder.[396-398] Thus, even though TTE cannot exclude endocarditis, abnormal findings may strongly suggest the disorder, even in the presence of negative blood cultures. Since no single abnormality has 100 percent diagnostic accuracy for infective endocarditis, strategies for diagnosis have been devised based upon a number of criteria,[399] and definite echocardiographic vegetations are designated as a major criterion. Both TTE and TEE are valuable in the detection of perivalvular abscesses and prosthetic-valve endocarditis.[147,400] Although there is considerable debate concerning the most accurate diagnostic criteria for endocarditis, echocardiography has become one of the most commonly used techniques for the evaluation of potentially affected patients.[401] Echocardiography (both TTE and TEE) is also useful for evaluation of patients with systemic lupus erythematosus complicated by Libman-Sacks endocarditis.[402,403]

Even though M-mode recordings produced the first echocardiographic description of vegetations,[396] this modality has gradually been largely replaced by 2D imaging. With 2D echocardiography, valvular vegetations typically appear as irregular, usually localized masses of varying echocardiographic density attached to valvular or perivalvular structures (Figs. 14-94 and 14-95) without significantly altering their mobility. The vegetations may be small or quite large and may attach directly to the valve leaflets or the supporting

chordal apparatus.[397,398,404,405] Both small, nonmobile vegetations on a normal valve and large vegetations on a markedly abnormal valve may be difficult or impossible to identify with certainty. Aggressive infections often cause perforation or distortion of the affected leaflet, leading to varying degrees of valvular regurgitation. This is distinctly different from most cases of nonbacterial thrombotic (marantic) endocarditis, where the valvular vegetations are usually nondestructive.[406] In cases of infective endocarditis, the presence of vegetations by TTE increases the risk of heart failure, embolic events, and the ultimate necessity of valve replacement.[407-411] Unfortunately, TTE is not 100 percent sensitive in detecting vegetations, and up to 20 percent of patients with proved native-valve endocarditis may have unremarkable examinations.[412] The sensitivity of TTE in prosthetic valve endocarditis has been found to be even lower (approximately 60 percent) due to technical limitations in imaging.[400]

TEE has proved significantly more sensitive than TTE for detection of infective vegetations and is extremely helpful for the diagnosis of perivalvular abscesses, mycotic diverticula, and prosthetic valve involvement.[147,413] The technique is also useful for assessing valvular regurgitation, fistulas (Fig. 14-96), and other hemodynamic complications of endocarditis.[414] Although a negative TEE examination cannot completely exclude infective endocarditis, it confers a relatively good prognosis in those cases where the diagnosis is eventually confirmed.

The optimal use of TEE in suspected endocarditis remains controversial: some authorities recommend routine TEE in all cases, but many do not.[415] A reasonable approach may be to perform transthoracic echocardiography as the first screening test in patients with suspected endocarditis. If the study

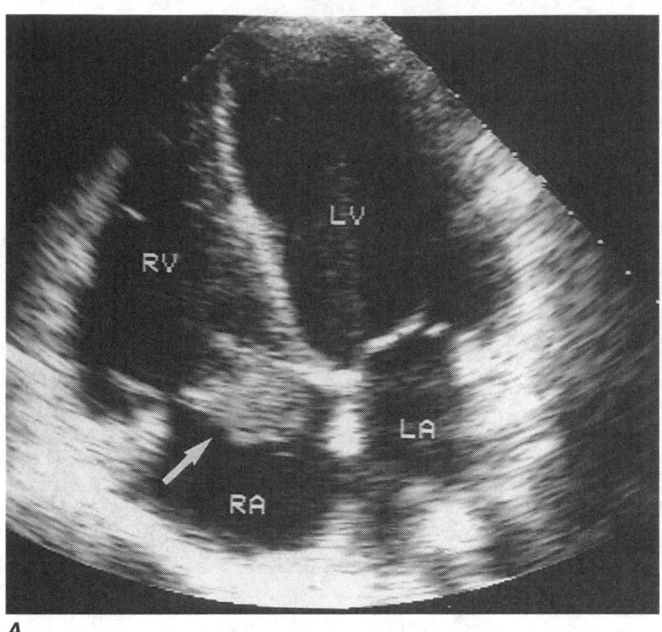

A

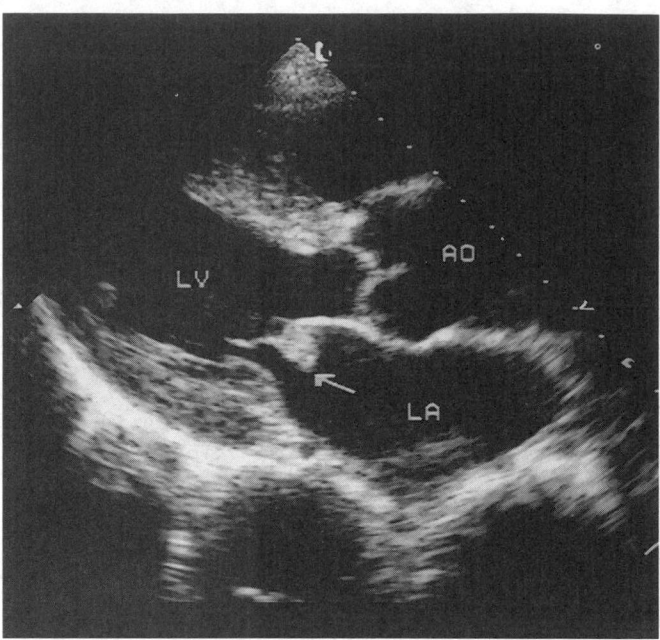

B

FIGURE 14-94

A. Apical four-chamber view demonstrating a large tricuspid valve vegetation (*arrow*) RA = right atrium; LA = left atrium; LV = left ventricle; RV = right ventricle. *B.* Parasternal long axis view demonstrating a vegetation (*arrow*) on the anterior valve leaflet; AO = aorta.

is technically difficult, equivocal, or detects vegetations in patients at high risk for perivalvular complications or hemodynamic compromise, TEE should be performed. If TTE is unremarkable or detects vegetations in patients at low risk for complications, TEE may not be necessary.[149] Exceptions to this last recommendation might include patients with prior antibiotic treatment or those with persistent bacteremia or fever of unknown etiology. In high-risk patients (i.e., with possible prosthetic valve involvement, congenital heart disease, or infection with especially virulent organisms), TEE is recommended even if TTE is normal.[149]

Echocardiographic evaluation of suspected endocarditis is not without pitfalls. It may be quite difficult to detect active vegetations in patients with preexisting valvular abnormalities such as calcification, myxomatous change, rheumatic involvement, and healed vegetations. Despite recent technologic advances, the diagnosis of infective endocarditis remains a clinical one, and over-reliance on echocardiography may cause mistakes. Therefore, echocardiographic results should be integrated with other clinical information to diagnose this disorder accurately.[416]

ISCHEMIC HEART DISEASE

Echocardiography in Coronary Heart Disease

Although originally of greatest value in valvular heart disease and cardiomyopathy, echocardiography has now become one of the most important techniques for the detection and quanti-

tative assessment of myocardial ischemia and infarction. Cardiac ultrasound—because it is rapid, portable, noninvasive, and inexpensive—is especially well suited to the evaluation of ischemic heart disease. Although visualization of coronary artery structure and flow has been achieved by echocardiography,[417–420] the application of this technique in ischemic heart disease continues to revolve primarily about the assessment of LV function.

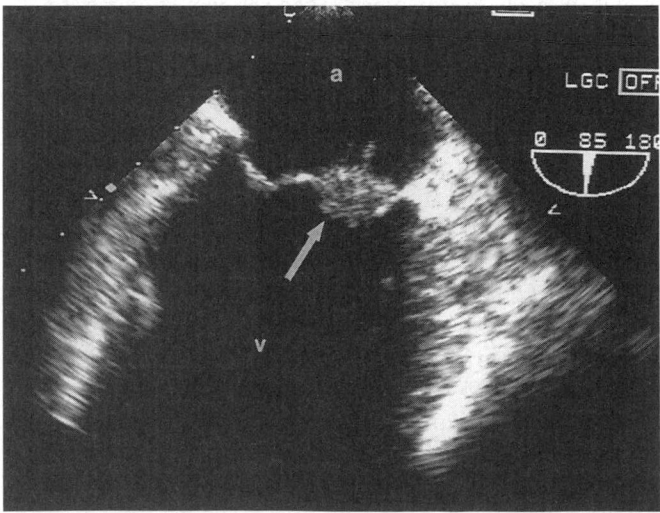

FIGURE 14-95

Longitudinal TEE view of a large mitral valve vegetation (*arrow*). a = left atrium; v = left ventricle. (Courtesy of William D. Keen, Jr., MD.)

Currently, the primary application of echocardiography in patients with coronary heart disease is based upon the detection of the effects of myocardial ischemia and/or infarction upon LV structure and function. Interruption of coronary flow or imposition of an oxygen demand that exceeds oxygen supply quickly leads to impaired systolic thickening and excursion of the affected myocardium. If flow is not restored and transmural infarction occurs, the affected myocardium may become akinetic or dyskinetic and eventually thinned and fibrotic. In addition, myocardial ischemia produces diastolic dysfunction, which may be detected by analysis of transmitral Doppler flow recordings or endocardial expansion profiles. These changes in the structure, contraction, and relaxation of myocardium are often readily detected by echocardiography.

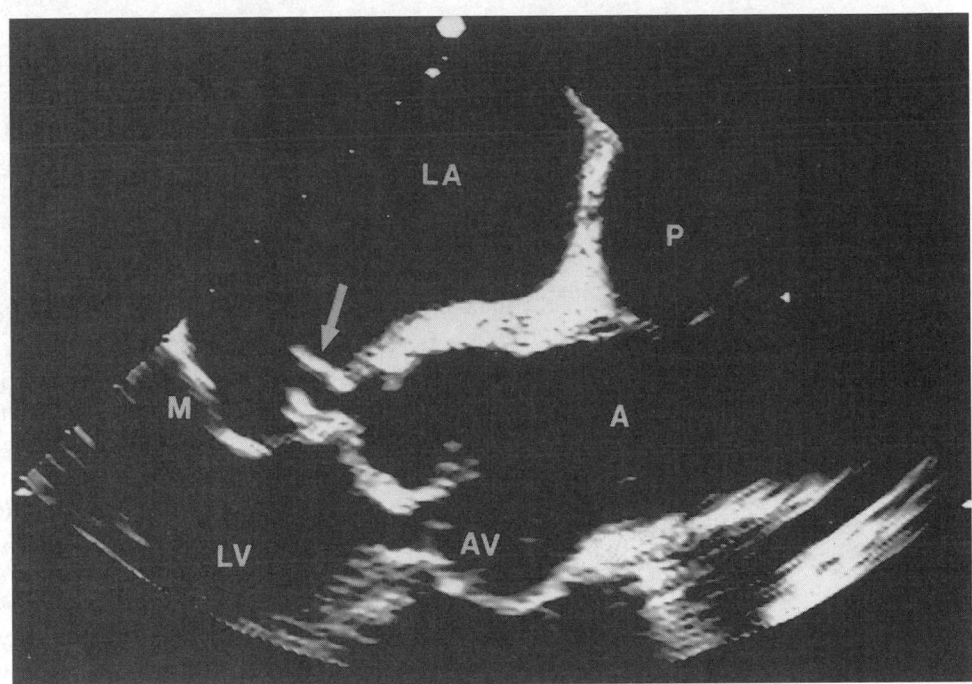

FIGURE 14-96

Longitudinal TEE image demonstrating a fistula between the aorta (A) and left atrium (LA) in a patient with endocarditis. AV = aortic valve; P = pulmonary artery; LV = left ventricle; M = mitral valve. (From Sobel J, Maisel AS, Tarazi R, Blanchard DG. Gonococcal endocarditis: Assessment by transesophageal echocardiography. *J Am Soc Echocardiogr* 1997; 10:367–370.)

The echocardiographic detection of myocardial ischemia was initially described using M-mode echocardiography, and this modality remains useful because of its excellent sensitivity and temporal resolution.[421] 2D imaging, however, has now become the primary technique for the examination of LV size, wall thickness, myocardial thickening, and regional wall motion, since it enables visualization of all LV wall segments. Thereby, in patients with coronary artery disease, standard echocardiographic approaches can be utilized to calculate LV diastolic and systolic volumes as well as ejection fraction.

The echocardiographic manifestations of coronary artery disease, consist of one or more of the following: reduction in systolic thickening, abnormal segmental wall motion during systole or diastole, and alterations in the acoustic properties of the myocardium (usually termed *tissue characterization*).[422] These abnormalities may be expressed as a disturbance in global left ventricular size and function, an increase in LV volume, and a decrease in LV ejection fraction calculated by standard approaches. In addition, using the standard tomographic planes, the left ventricle can be divided into 16 wall segments according to the format recommended by the American Society of Echocardiography (Fig. 14-97).[423] By grading the contraction of each of the 16 segments as hyperkinetic, normal, hypokinetic, akinetic, or dyskinetic (and assigning a numerical value to each grade), a semiquantitative wall motion score can be calculated as the mean numerical value for all segments. Wall motion scores of this kind have been used to assess prognosis in both acute myocardial infarction[424] and chronic coronary artery disease.[425] When LV dysfunction is detected echocardiographically, the specific coronary artery responsible can often be inferred based upon the dyssnergy region(s).[126,427] The echocardiographic findings of akinesis with segmental myocardial thinning can also be used to distinguish coronary artery disease from dilated cardiomyopathy, which typically manifests global hypokinesis and decreased wall thickness. There is overlap in the echocardiographic findings between these two groups, however, as severe ischemic disease may cause global hypokinesis and nonischemic cardiomyopathy may sometimes cause heterogeneous dysfunction.[428]

Myocardial Infarction and Postinfarction Complications

Cardiac ultrasound has achieved an important role in the evaluation of patients with acute myocardial infarction and is frequently used for diagnosis, quantitative functional assessment, risk stratification, and detection of complications[424,429–432] (see also Chap. 47). Echocardiography is especially valuable in *excluding* transmural infarctions, as these are almost always associated with regional akinesis or dyskinesis (Figs. 14-98 to 14-100).[433,434] Non-Q-wave infarctions are more difficult to diagnose with certainty, however, as the echocardiogram may show subtle regional hypokinesis or

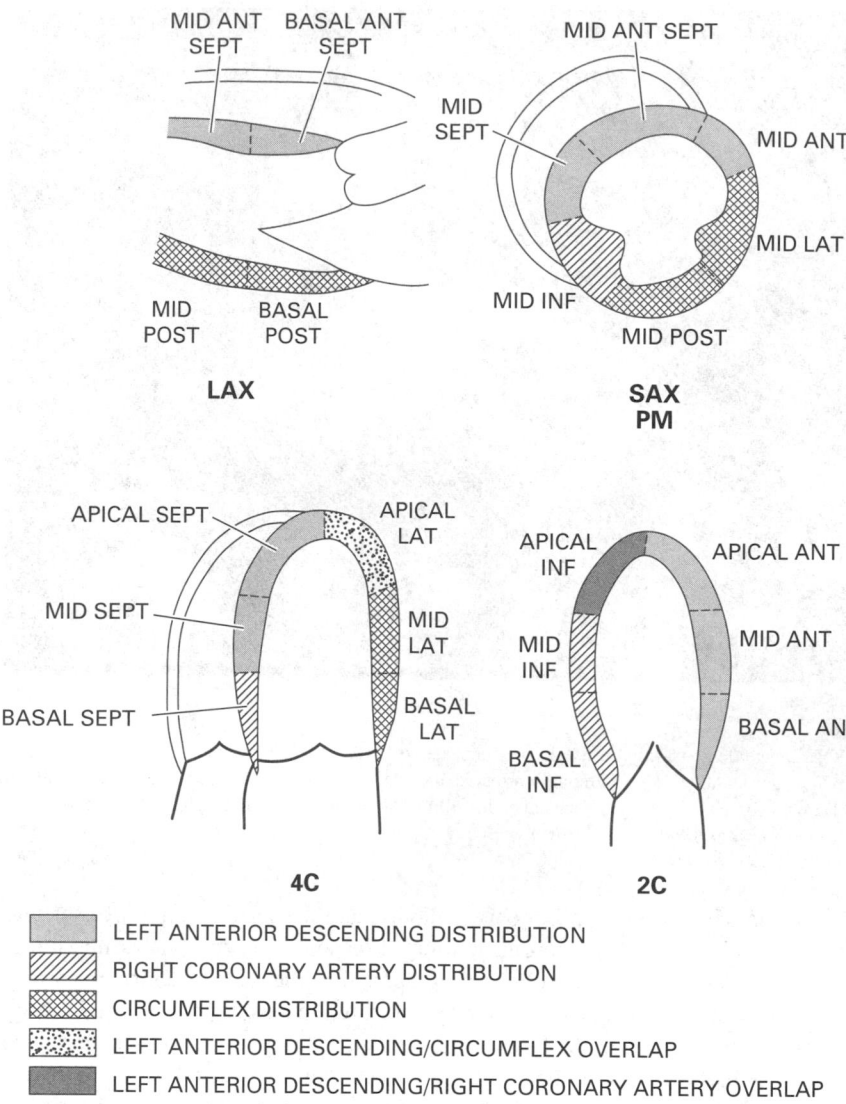

LEFT ANTERIOR DESCENDING DISTRIBUTION

RIGHT CORONARY ARTERY DISTRIBUTION

CIRCUMFLEX DISTRIBUTION

LEFT ANTERIOR DESCENDING/CIRCUMFLEX OVERLAP

LEFT ANTERIOR DESCENDING/RIGHT CORONARY ARTERY OVERLAP

FIGURE 14-97

Sixteen-segment format for identification of left ventricular wall segments. Coronary arterial territories are also included. LAX = parasternal long axis; SAX PM = short axis at papillary muscle level; 4C = apical four-chamber; 2C = apical two-chamber; ANT = anterior; SEPT = septal; POST = posterior; LAT = lateral; INF = inferior. (From Segar D, Brown S, Sawada S, Ryan T, Feigenbaum H. Dobutamine stress echocardiography: Correlation with coronary lesion severity as determined by quantitative angiography. *J Am Coll Cardiol* 1992; 19:1197, with permission.)

even normal wall motion in some cases. Thus, echocardiography has been used to evaluate chest pain in the emergency department and appears to have a reasonable sensitivity and specificity in the diagnosis of myocardial infarction.[433,434] It may also help select patients for thrombolytic therapy.[435] In addition, patients without contractile abnormalities who ultimately exhibit signs of myocardial infarction have a low incidence of complications.[434]

Echocardiography is now the most commonly utilized approach to assess the effects of myocardial infarction upon LV function. Ultrasound imaging studies of LV remodeling have demonstrated that infarct expansion occurs commonly with anterior infarctions, often beginning within the first 10 days, and conveys an adverse prognosis.[436,437] Similarly, calcula-

tion of the wall motion score has identified a cohort of post–myocardial infarction patients at markedly increased risk for in-hospital complications.[434] This prognostic marker appears superior to conventional clinical criteria in predicting events.[434]

Echocardiography is probably of greatest value in the assessment of complications associated with acute myocardial infarction. Most such complications are quickly detected by echocardiography, and the fact that it is portable, rapid, and noninvasive render the technique extremely valuable in these circumstances. As indicated above, severe LV dysfunction resulting in advanced heart failure or shock can be readily identified by echocardiography. In addition, aneurysm formation is usually quite apparent in ultrasonic images.[438] By definition, postinfarction LV aneurysms are recognized as wide-mouthed, thinned-walled myocardial segments that display dyskinetic expansion during systole. Aneurysms are a favored site for development of LV thrombi, which are discussed in detail in the discussion of cardiac masses, below. A less frequent complication is rupture of the LV free wall, which is usually rapidly fatal and therefore rarely imaged by echocardiography.[439] However, the presence of significant pericardial effusion on echocardiography in patients with hemodynamic compromise in the postinfarction period should suggest this condition. If a free wall rupture is sealed off by clot and pericardial inflammation, a pseudoaneurysm is formed[440,441] (Fig. 14-101). This lesion is distinguished from a true aneurysm by its highly localized nature and the presence of a narrow neck connecting it with the ventricle. Pseudoaneurysms frequently have multilayered thrombi within them and exhibit characteristic Doppler flow signals at the junction with the ventricle.[441] Since the risk of rupture is high, accurate diagnosis and prompt surgical repair of pseudoaneurysms is important.

Although postinfarction free wall rupture does not lend itself well to echocardiographic detection, acquired defects of the interventricular septum are more commonly delineated by cardiac ultrasound.[442,443] Acquired ventricular septal defects often consist of a latticework of tissue rather than a discrete orifice, but nevertheless echocardiographic images can depict absence of myocardium and distinct flow jets communicating between the left and right ventricles (Fig. 14-102, Plate 39).[444] These color jets are typically high-velocity and aliased, coursing from the septum into the right ventricle. The echocardiographic location of the defect and jet correlate well with the location by cineangiography, surgery, or autopsy, and an apical location is most amenable to surgical correction.[444]

Mitral regurgitation is a common sequela of acute myocardial infarction; if severe, it may result in profound congestive heart failure and shock. Several mechanisms may be responsible for the occurrence of post-infarction mitral regurgitation including dilation of the LV cavity and mitral annulus, papillary muscle dysfunction, and partial or complete rupture of a papillary muscle (Fig. 14-103).[445–447] Mitral regurgitation from papillary dysfunction may lead to eccentric color jets within the left atrium. In general, the recognition and quantitation of mitral regurgitation occurring in the postin-

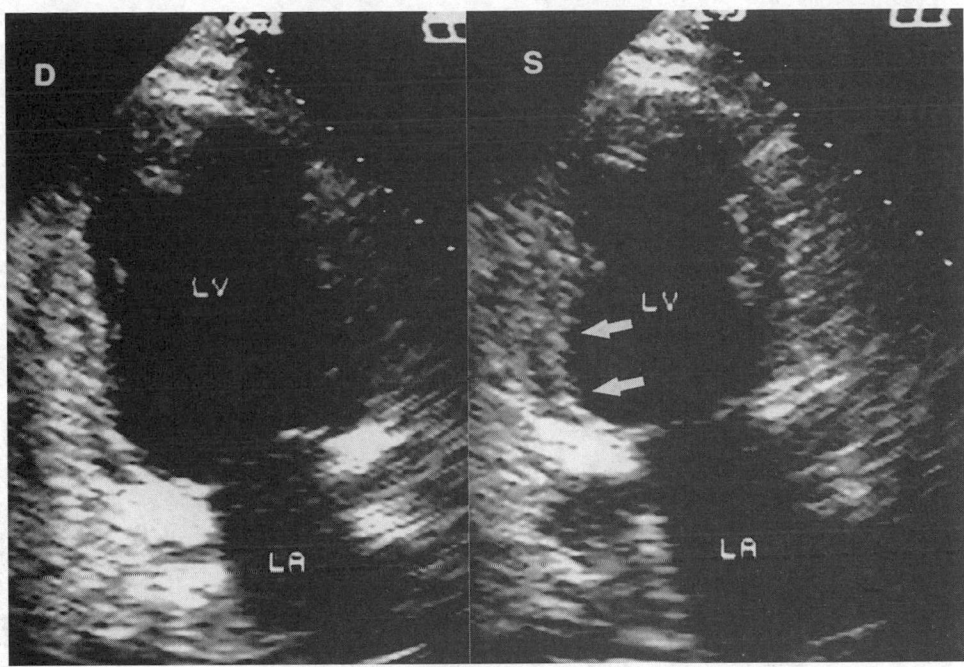

FIGURE 14-98

Diastolic (*left*) and systolic (*right*) images (apical two-chamber plane) from a patient with an inferior wall myocardial infarction. The inferobasal segment is dyskinetic (*arrows*). LV = left ventricle; LA = left atrium.

farction period is no different from that of any other type of MR. Acute ischemic MR, however may cause a smaller flow disturbance by color Doppler than comparable grades of chronic MR, particularly with transthoracic imaging. Therefore, TEE may play an important role in the identification and quantitative assessment of this complication, as well as in ensuring adequate operative repair.[447]

In the setting of inferior wall infarction due to occlusion of the proximal right coronary artery, right ventricular myocardial infarction may occur. The most specific echocardiographic sign of right ventricular infarction is a regional wall motion abnormality, which is usually best visualized in the right ventricular free wall (Fig. 14-104).[448] Right ventricular infarction is typically accompanied by right ventricular enlargement and tricuspid regurgitation; associated inferior or posterior left ventricular wall motion abnormalities are virtually always present.

Pericarditis is a common complication of acute myocardial infarction, typically occurring during the acute phase of the illness and much less often in the late phases as part of Dressler syndrome. Postinfarction pericarditis, however, is not typically associated with marked echocardiographic abnormalities. If a pericardial effusion is present at all, the amount of fluid is usually quite small. Therefore, the absence of pericardial fluid on echocardiogram cannot rule out pericarditis, and the presence of a large effusion with tamponade should raise the suspicion of a left ventricular free wall rupture.

TEE has recently assumed a central role in the evaluation of patients with significant hemodynamic abnormalities in the postinfarction period. When TTE is technically suboptimal, transesophageal images can rapidly identify LV dyssynergy,

valvular dysfunction, and other abnormalities associated with infarction. TEE may enable direct visualization of acquired ventricular septal defects when the lesion is not obvious or seen only as a disturbed flow stream in the right ventricle with transthoracic imaging. Perhaps of greatest significance,

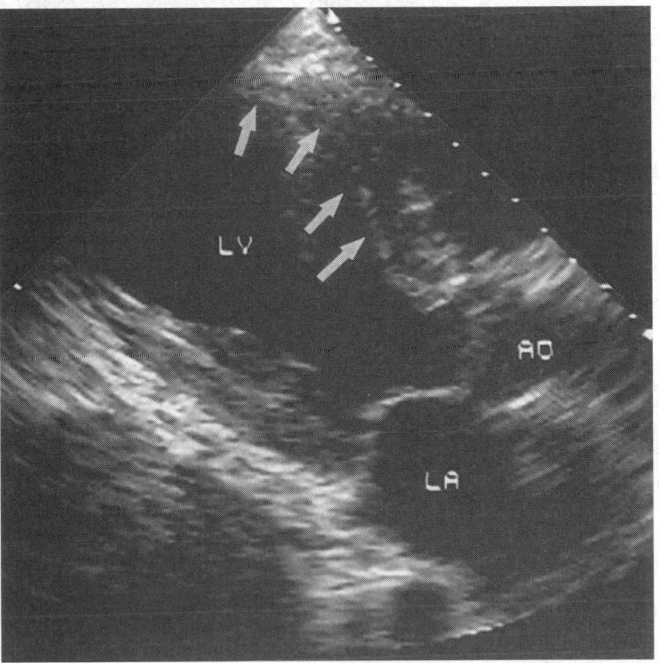

FIGURE 14-99

Parasternal long-axis view of a large anteroseptal myocardial infarction, with thinning and dyskinesis of the anteroseptal wall (*arrows*). LV = left ventricle; LA = left atrium; AO = aorta.

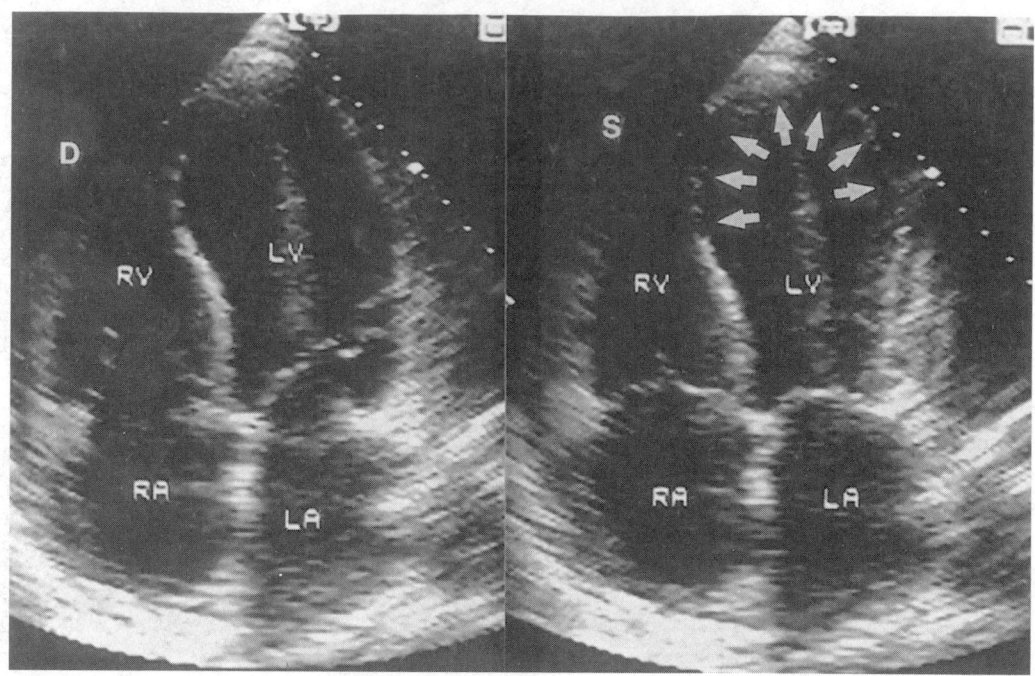

FIGURE 14-100
Apical four-chamber images of a large apical infarction. Diastole (D) is displayed on the left, systole (S) on the right. During systole, the base of the ventricle contracts, but the apex is dyskinetic (*arrows*).

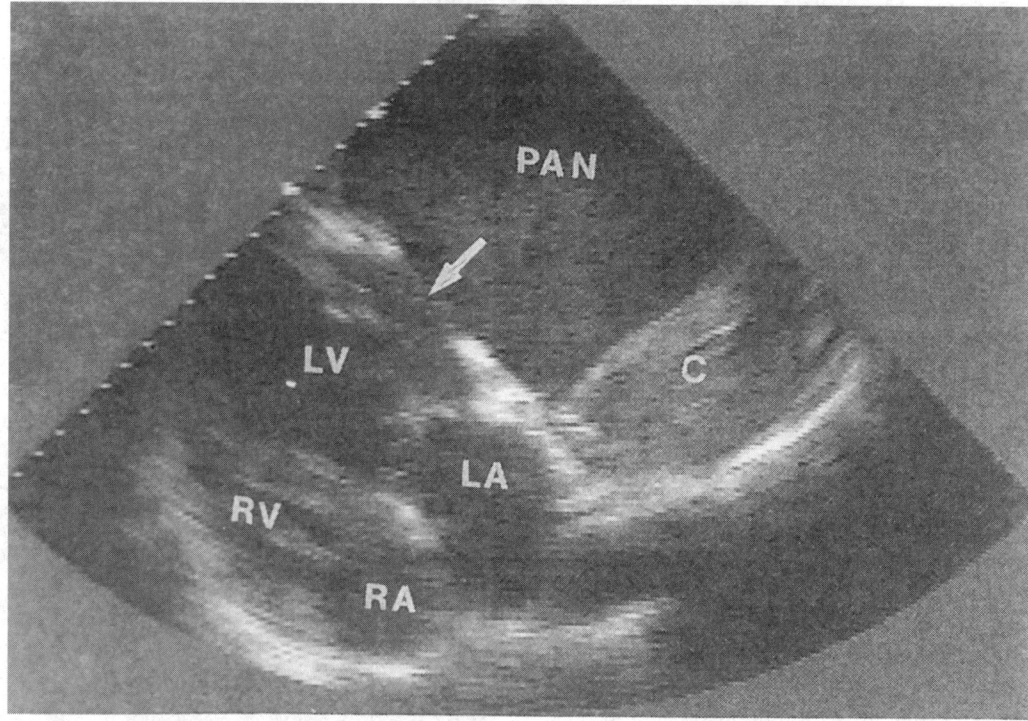

FIGURE 14-101
Modified apical four-chamber view of a large pseudoaneurysm (PAN) communicating with the left ventricle (LV). The rupture site is apparent (*arrow*); clot (C) is present within the aneurysm. (From Yucel G, Steinberg E, O'Reilly M, Kronzon I. Giant left ventricular pseudoaneurysm. *Circulation* 1996; 94:848, with permission.)

FIGURE 14-102
See color Plate 39.

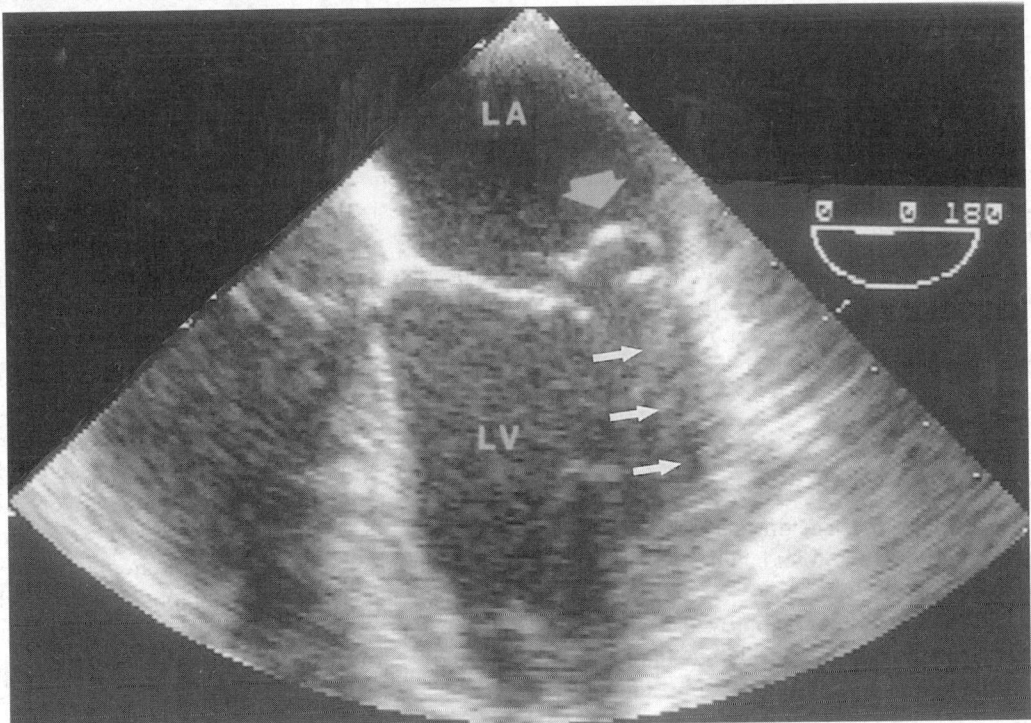

FIGURE 14-103
Transverse four-chamber TEE image of a posterolateral infarction causing posterior papillary muscle ischemia and partial rupture. The posterior mitral leaflet (*large arrow*) is poorly supported (but not actually flail) and prolapses into the left atrium (LA). The basal lateral wall segment (*small arrows*) of the left ventricle (LV) is dyskinetic.

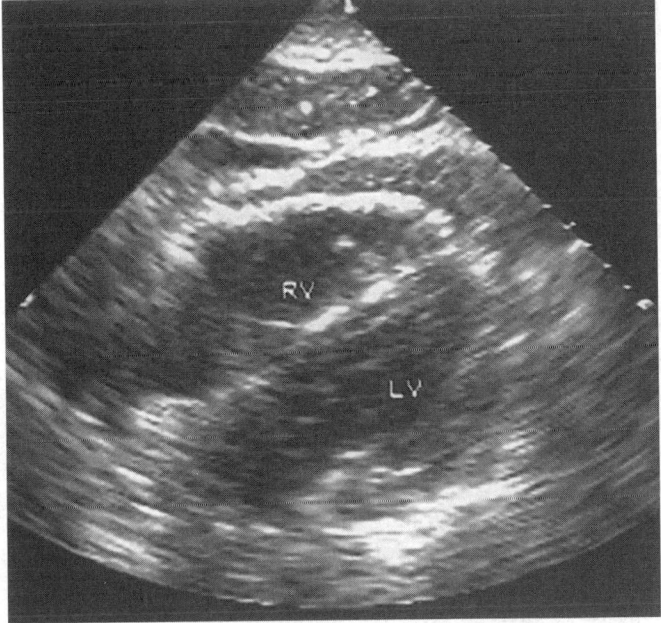

A

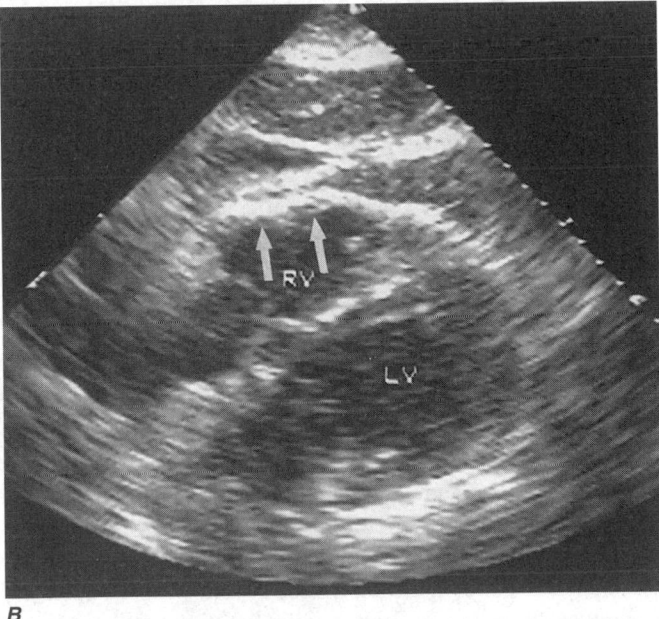

B

FIGURE 14-104
Diastolic (*A*) and systolic (*B*) subcostal four-chamber images of right ventricular (RV) myocardial infarction. The RV free wall is dyskinetic (*arrows*) during systole (*B*).

TEE can provide definitive identification of a ruptured papillary muscle and a quantitative assessment of postinfarction mitral regurgitation.

Echocardiography has been used to evaluate the extent of reperfusion after thrombolytic or interventional therapy for acute myocardial infarction. Several reports have demonstrated that LV systolic function assessed by 2D imaging improved within 24 h to 10 days of successful thrombolysis.[449,450] More recently, contrast echocardiograms obtained by direct intracoronary injection have shown that reperfusion of the infarct-related epicardial coronary artery by angiography is not necessarily accompanied by evidence of normal flow in the downstream microcirculation. In addition, this "no-reflow" phenomenon on echocardiography heralds a poor prognosis, including failure of improvement of LV performance as well as increased late complications.[208–210]

Stress Echocardiography

Recently, the combination of stress testing and echocardiography (stress echocardiography) has found an important role in the diagnosis of coronary artery disease.[451–453] (See also Chap. 45.) The utility of this technique improved dramatically when technologic advances permitted side-by-side viewing of rest and stress images together in a cine-loop format.[454] The application of stress echocardiography is based upon the concept that a stress-induced imbalance in the myocardial supply/demand ratio will produce regional ischemia and resultant abnormalities of regional contraction, which can be readily identified by echocardiography (Fig. 14-105). The location of wall motion abnormalities may be used to predict the stenosed coronary vessel(s), while the ratio of dyssynergic to normal myocardium can provide a quantitative assessment of LV ischemia.[426,427] Although the digital techniques currently employed limit the number of views available and restrict the examination to eight frames during systole, this process does not seem to impair the ability to identify contractile dysfunction.[455,456]

The types of stress employed fall into two basic groups, exercise and pharmacologic.[426,427] Other forms, such as mental stress and atrial pacing, are not widely used. Exercise testing can be performed either on a treadmill or a stationary bicycle (either upright or supine).[457] Treadmill testing involves a familiar activity, uses equipment that is widely available, and achieves a greater oxygen consumption than bicycle ergometry. Echo imaging usually can be accomplished only before and after treadmill exercise, however, whereas bicycle exertion facilitates the acquisition of images during the exercise protocol. Thus far, treadmill has been the preferred exercise modality. Of importance, all postexertional images should be obtained within a 2-min window following exercise to avoid recording normal contractile function after recovery from ischemia.

Pharmacologic stress has the advantages of reducing the motion artifact of exercise, enabling continuous imaging throughout the protocol, and assessing myocardial viability.[458–469] Pharmacologic stress echocardiography can employ vasodilator agents such as dipyridamole or adenosine, which induce a heterogeneity of myocardial perfusion in ischemic heart disease, or inotropic agents such as dobutamine and arbutamine, which increase myocardial oxygen demand and directly produce ischemia.[458–469] As with exercise stress, diagnostic criteria include induction of regional wall motion abnormalities and LV dilatation. It is important to recognize that the normal response to exercise is hyperkinesis, and wall motion abnormalities may take the form of a lesser degree of hyperkinesis of a given segment in comparison with the rest of the LV myocardium. Dobutamine stress echocardiography appears to be of particular value in for detecting myocardial viability.[455–463,466–469]

The safety and accuracy of stress echocardiography for the diagnosis of myocardial ischemia has been examined in a number of studies.[453,469–472] Both exercise and pharmacologic stress carry an extremely low risk of arrhythmia or infarction, although dobutamine can result in hypotension or systolic anterior motion of the mitral valve (SAM) with resultant LV outflow obstruction.[453,473,474] In general, stress echocardiography and nuclear scintigraphy yield similar results, although stress echocardiography may be slightly less sensitive and slightly more specific than scintigraphy.[455,464,475] In a study performed in an institution with high volumes and expertise in both ultrasound and radionuclide stress imaging, the two techniques were found to be comparable in their accuracy of detecting coronary artery disease.[455]

The most common clinical application of stress echocardiography is in the diagnosis of coronary artery disease (CAD), and it appears especially useful in cases where exercise electrocardiography (ECG) may be inaccurate or falsely positive (e.g., abnormal baseline ECG, LV hypertrophy, or chronic digitalis administration).[453,472,476,477] In this regard, stress echocardiography appears especially useful for detection of ischemia in women,[478,478a] in whom stress ECG yields a high incidence of false-positive results. Stress echocardiography also adds independent prognostic information to exercise ECG, even in multivessel CAD.[479] Dobutamine echocardiography may aid in the detection of ischemia in patients with cardiac transplantation and allograft vasculopathy (chronic rejection).[480] In patients with known CAD, exercise echocardiography may facilitate localization and quantitation of ischemia, guide revascularization procedures, and assess the functional severity of coronary artery stenoses.[481] Stress echocardiography can also demonstrate resolution of regional ischemia after successful coronary artery bypass surgery or angioplasty.[482–485]

Stress echocardiography can play an important role in determining the prognosis of patients with CAD.[486–494] Both exercise and pharmacologic stress echocardiography appear superior to exercise ECG for identification of patients at high risk of recurrent ischemic events after myocardial infarction.[486–491] In addition, dobutamine stress echocardiography is useful in predicting perioperative ischemic complications in patients undergoing noncardiac surgery and appears to have a very strong negative predictive value.[492–494]

In patients with chronic coronary heart disease, dobutamine

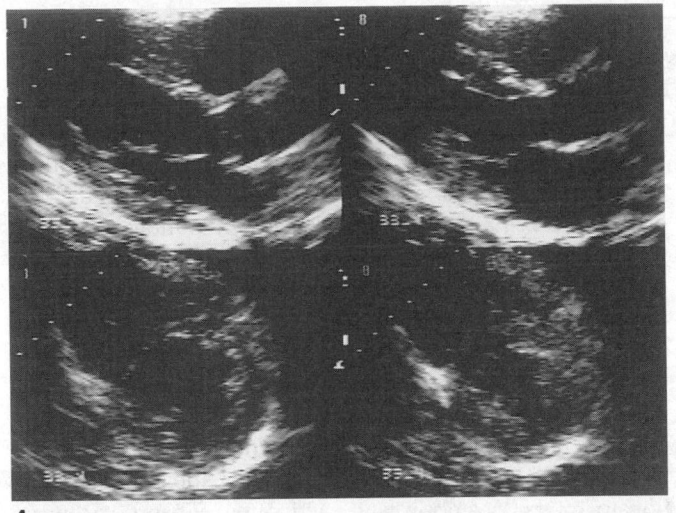

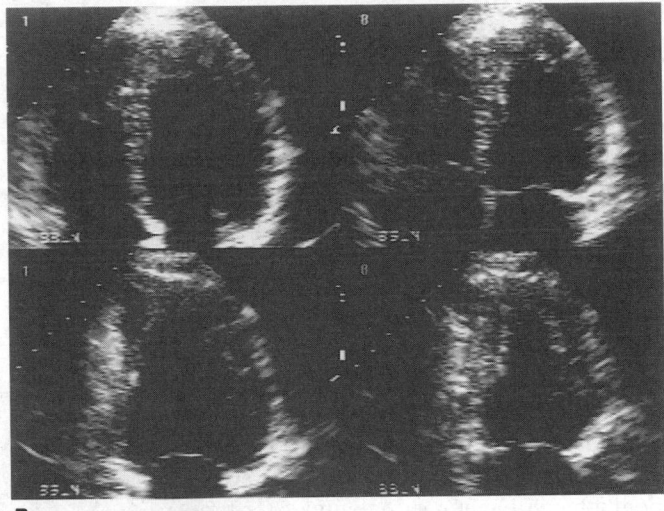

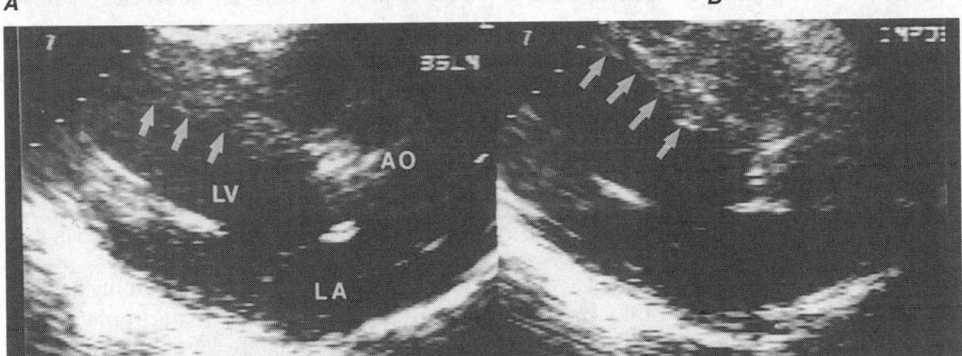

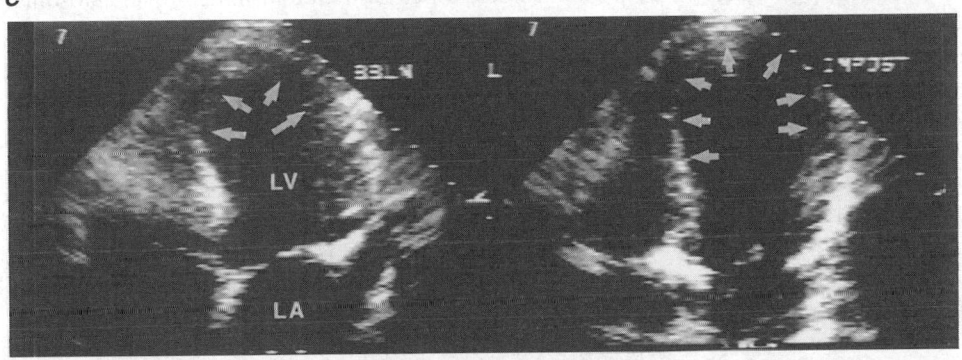

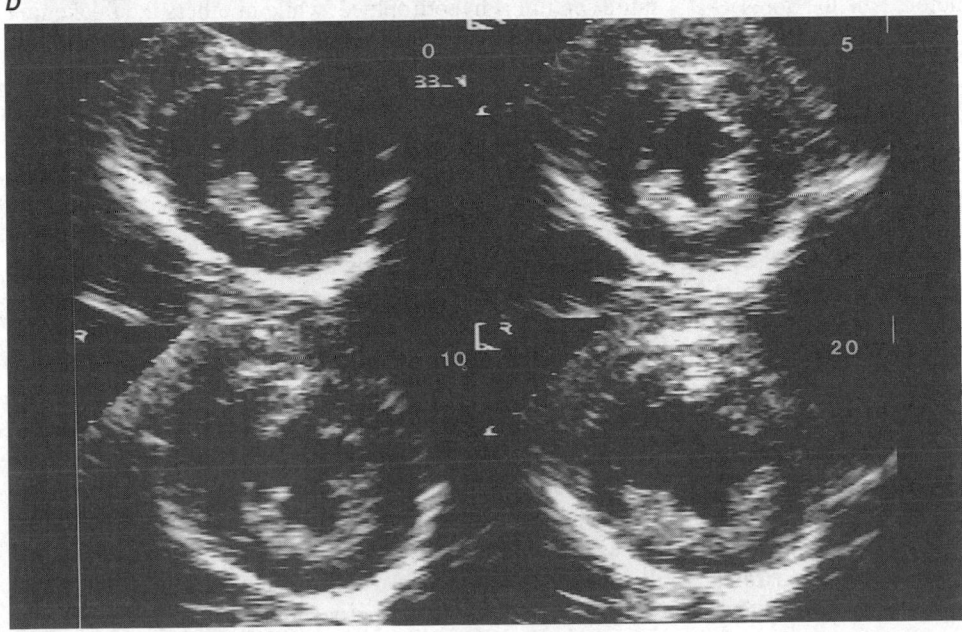

FIGURE 14-105

A. Digitized parasternal views during diastole (*left*) and systole (*right*) from a normal individual. *Upper panels:* long-axis plane; *lower panels:* short-axis plane. *B.* Digitized apical views during diastole (*left*) and systole (*right*) from a normal individual. *Upper panels:* four-chamber plane; *lower panels:* two-chamber plane. *C.* Digitized parasternal long-axis views at peak systole before (*left*) and immediately after exercise (*right*). The anteroseptal wall moves normally at rest (*arrows*) but becomes dyskinetic with exercise. LV = left ventricle; LA = left atrium; AO = aorta. *D.* Digitized apical 4-chamber views at peak systole before (*left*) and immediately after exercise (*right*). The apical septal, apical, and apical lateral walls become dyskinetic with exercise, suggesting inducible ischemia in the left anterior descending artery territory. LA = left atrium; LV = left ventricle. *E.* Digitized parasternal short axis views (all recorded at peak systole) during dobutamine echocardiography in a patient with 3-vessel coronary artery disease. At baseline (*upper left panel*), the left ventricular systolic function is normal. With low-dose dobutamine (5 μg/kg/min, *upper right panel*), function improves. With 10 μg/kg/min, however (*lower left panel*), function is similar to that at baseline. At 20 μg/kg/min (*lower right panel*), systolic function deteriorates and the left ventricle dilates. This response suggests global ischemia induced by dobutamine infusion.

stress echocardiography can identify hypokinetic yet viable myocardium and predicts improvement in function after successful revascularization.[457–463,467–470] Functional improvement in a hypokinetic segment with low-dose dobutamine infusion which then progresses to hypokinesis or akinesis with higher dobutamine dose (the so-called biphasic response) correlates well with the presence of ischemic yet viable ("hibernating") myocardium. Studies have suggested that dobutamine stress echocardiography compares well with positron emission tomography and thallium single-photon emission computed tomography (SPECT) imaging in this regard.[466–468,495–501] It is likely that this application of echocardiography will continue to evolve over time, particularly for pharmacologic stress testing.

There is evidence that exercise echocardiography can provide useful information regarding the hemodynamic status and functional severity of valvular heart disease.[502–505] Specifically, stress echocardiography has been used to assess the degree of obstruction in patients with mitral stenosis[503] and to quantitate the severity of aortic stenosis in patients with advanced LV dysfunction.[505] These data may help guide the timing of surgical valve repair or replacement.

As is true of all diagnostic modalities, stress echocardiography has certain limitations. High-quality ultrasound images may be difficult to acquire in some patients, a situation which may be exacerbated by exertion and the time constraints inherent to exercise stress testing. In addition, considerable expertise is required to interpret stress echocardiographic images accurately, and this learning curve precludes the use of stress echocardiography by all but experienced echocardiographers. Nevertheless, stress echocardiography has many advantages over alternate diagnostic approaches such as radionuclide scintigraphy and coronary angiography, including its noninvasive and relatively inexpensive nature, rapid acquisition and interpretation times, and freedom from ionizing radiation. Therefore, it is anticipated that the use of stress echocardiography will continue to increase in the foreseeable future.

THE CARDIOMYOPATHIES

The evaluation of cardiomyopathy is complicated by the fact that few specific diagnostic criteria exist, and identification is often a process of exclusion. Further, many potential etiologies may be responsible for the myopathic process, and it may be possible to identify a specific etiology in only the minority of patients. accordingly, a diagnostic strategy has evolved that initially seeks to place patients into one of three pathophysiologic categories: dilated, hypertrophic, or restrictive; then, the specific etiologies recognized as producing the individual pathophysiologic state are pursued.[506] Thus, dilated cardiomyopathies are associated with myocyte loss and necrosis, a marked increase in LV volume, thinning of the myocardium, and profound systolic dysfunction.[507] Hypertrophic cardiomyopathy (HCM) is recognized by increased myocardial thickness, particularly involving the interventricular septum,

with preserved systolic function.[508] Restrictive cardiomyopathies may be due to infiltration of the myocardium by abnormal substances or fibrotic tissue; these cause symmetric degrees of wall thickening with modest or no diminution of systolic function and little change in cavity size.[509] Echocardiography customarily serves as the cornerstone of such evaluations and provides data on cavity size, wall thickness, and systolic function. Thus, on echocardiogram, patients with dilated cardiomyopathy exhibit a marked increase in left LV and volume, little change in wall thickness, and severe contractile dysfunction.[507] Patients with HCM exhibit a dramatic increase in LV wall thickness, with the septum characteristically disproportionate to the posterior wall, and often subaortic stenosis induced by systolic anterior motion of the anterior mitral valve leaflet. Patients with restrictive cardiomyopathy are identified by a symmetric increase in wall thickness accompanied by modest changes in contractile function and LV cavity size.[509]

Hypertrophic Cardiomyopathy

HCM is a primary abnormality of the myocardium that exhibits myocyte disarray and unprovoked hypertrophy, often affecting the septum disproportionately[508] (see also Chap. 74). The disorder, which is often transmitted in an autosomal dominant pattern, has been linked to a number of abnormalities in genes that code for myocardial proteins.[510,511] A number of classic echocardiographic findings occur in HCM (Fig. 14-106). The fundamental abnormality on echocardiogram in HCM is LV hypertrophy, which is often severe. Although the hypertrophy may be confined to the septum, it may be concentric or involve any other portion of the left ventricle.[512] The customary classic finding is asymmetric septal hypertrophy (ASH), defined as a disproportionate thickness of the interventricular septum compared to the posterobasal wall with a ratio of greater than 1.3 to 1.[513,514] In some cases the entire septum is hypertrophied, while in others the thickening may be localized to the proximal, mid-, or distal (apical) septum.[515] Asymmetric hypertrophy of the proximal interventricular septum may lead to dynamic LV outflow tract obstruction—hypertrophic obstructive cardiomyopathy (HOCM) or idiopathic hypertrophic subaortic stenosis (IHSS). Although ASH is almost always present cases of dynamic LV outflow tract obstruction, it is not a specific marker for HCM and may occur in some patients with right ventricular hypertrophy, inferior myocardial infarction, and a minority with hypertensive LV hypertrophy.[516] In general, the more extensive the hypertrophic process, the more severe the symptoms. Extent of hypertrophy, however, does not appear to correlate well with risk of sudden death, as patients with minimal hypertrophy may still be at significant risk.[517]

The second characteristic finding of HCM is systolic anterior motion of the mitral valve, or SAM, which usually involves the anterior mitral valve leaflet. Posterior-leaflet SAM also has been reported in HCM, as have a variety of mitral valve deformities.[518,519] Encroachment of the pathologically thickened septum upon the LV outflow tract creates a pressure drop by a Venturi effect, which draws the mitral leaflets toward the septum, creating dynamic (subaortic) LV outflow obstruction (Fig. 14-106). Recent work has also demonstrated the important effects of papillary muscle position and chordal tension on systolic mitral morphology and SAM.[520] Because of distorted mitral coaptation during systole, SAM generally causes mitral regurgitation of variable severity. The severity and duration of SAM directly influence the degree of both outflow tract obstruction and mitral regurgitation.[521] Like asymmetric septal hypertrophy, SAM (especially systolic motion of the chordae) is not pathognomonic for HCM, having been reported in other conditions such as hypovolemia, anemia, and states where LV outflow tract narrowing and hyperdynamic contraction are present.[522,523]

The third manifestation of classic HCM is midsystolic closure of the aortic valve.[524] This finding is best seen on M-mode recordings, occurs only in the presence of outflow tract obstruction, and is probably a manifestation of the sudden pressure drop during mid- and late systole caused by SAM. As with ASH and SAM, midsystolic aortic closure is not specific for HCM and can occur in MR, aortic root dilatation, ventricular septal defect, and discrete subaortic stenosis.[525,526] When HCM is present, however, midsystolic aortic valve closure suggests significant outflow tract obstruction.

The fourth important abnormality of HCM is observed on Doppler examination of the LV outflow tract (LVOT). Normally, Doppler interrogation of this area produces a spectral tracing that peaks early in systole and has a maximum velocity of less than 1.7 m/s. In many patients, HCM creates

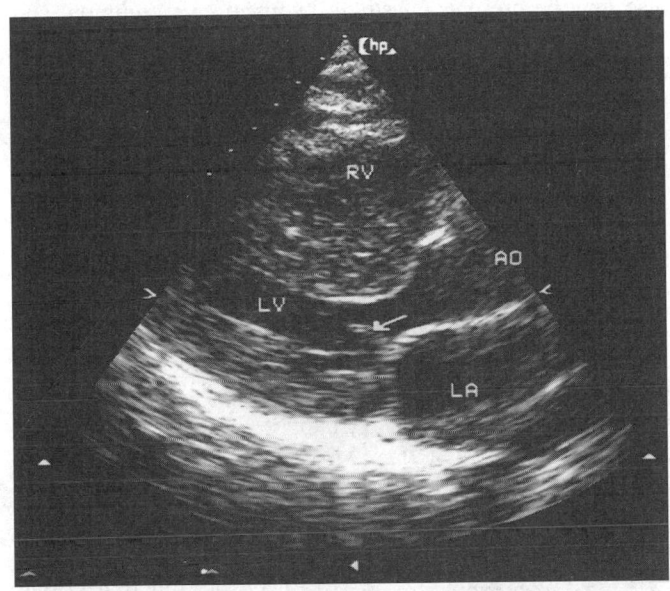

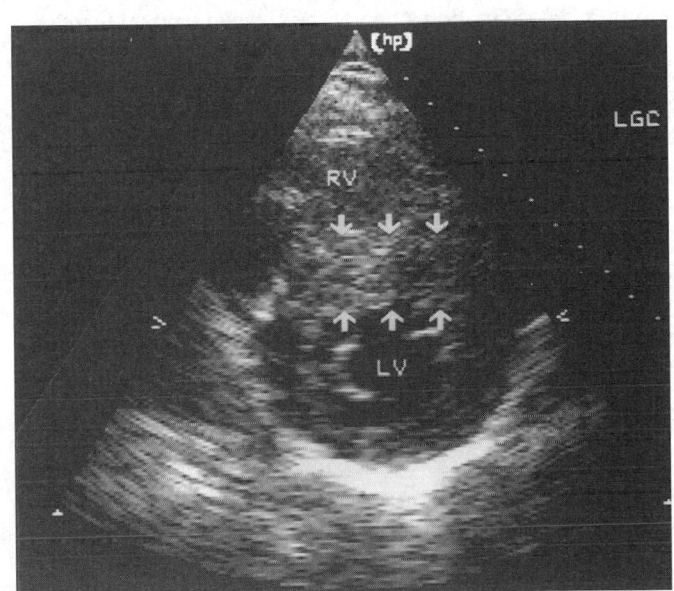

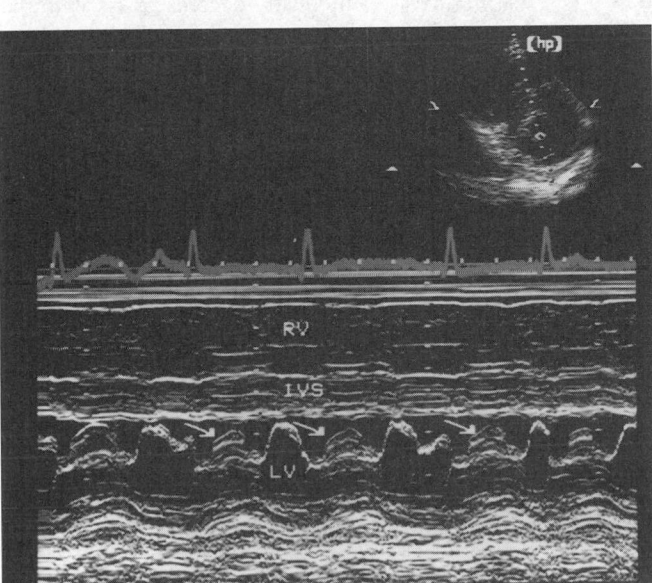

FIGURE 14-106

A. Parasternal long-axis view (during systole) of hypertrophic cardiomyopathy (HCM). Asymmetric septal hypertrophy is present, as is systolic anterior motion of the anterior mitral valve leaflet (*arrow*). LV = left ventricle; LA = left atrium; RV = right ventricle; AO = aorta. *B.* Parasternal short-axis view of HCM. Asymmetric septal hypertrophy is present (*arrows*). RV = right ventricle; LV = left ventricle. *C.* Parasternal M-mode image from a patient with HCM, demonstrating systolic anterior motion of the anterior mitral valve leaflet (*arrows*). RV = right ventricle; IVS = interventricular septum; LV = left ventricle.

a high-pressure gradient coincident with SAM, which is detected by Doppler as a high-velocity systolic jet in the LVOT. As opposed to valvular aortic stenosis, however, the maximal velocity in obstructive HCM peaks late in systole, creating a characteristic "saber-tooth" pattern (Fig. 14-107).[527–530] Although the subaortic gradient can be estimated using the modified Bernoulli equation,[529,530] the assumptions used in this equation may not apply to HCM, as intraventricular gradient calculations can be spuriously high because of the phenomenon of pressure recovery.[531] Similar Doppler patterns also may be seen occasionally within the LV in patients with HCM if systolic obliteration of the hypertrophied left ventricle causes localized areas of high flow velocity in the more distal portions of the ventricular cavity.[527]

Diastolic dysfunction has been long recognized in HCM. Doppler interrogation of LV inflow often reveals a relaxation abnormality, with a reduced early diastolic (E) velocity, a prolonged deceleration slope of the E wave, and an increased velocity of the atrial systolic (A) component.[532,533] Color Doppler imaging can be used to demonstrate intraventricular flow characteristics.[534]

Dilated Cardiomyopathy

In cases of dilated cardiomyopathy (DCM), the heart is typically greatly enlarged and systolic function is markedly depressed (see also Chap. 73).[535] Four-chamber dilatation is a common but not uniform finding, as some patients may have relatively preserved RV size (this may confer an improved prognosis).[536] Marked LV enlargement and generalized dysfunction can also be caused by severe ischemic heart disease, chronic alcohol abuse, various infectious myocarditides, anthracyclines and other cardiotoxic agents, nutritional deficiencies, and hereditary myopathies.[537,538] Severe ischemic disease is often segmental and has been reported to spare the posterior wall frequently,[539] while the LV dysfunction of DCM is usually global. The typical constellation of echocardiographic findings in DCM include an increased LV end-diastolic diameter and volume with decreased fractional shortening, thinning of the LV walls (Fig. 14-108), increased E point–septal separation, left atrial enlargement, and limited mitral and aortic valve opening (due to low stroke volume).[535,540] Intracardiac thrombi are frequently observed and are most often found in the LV apex.[540] M-mode imaging of the mitral leaflets may demonstrate a "B bump," or notch just before systolic valve closure, indicating elevated LV diastolic pressure (Fig. 14-8). The cardiac valves are usually normal, but mitral annular dilatation and secondary MR are common.

Doppler echocardiography often reveals an abnormally low-velocity time integral in the LV outflow or inflow tracts.[541] Diastolic MR due to elevated LV diastolic pressure also may be present. Diastolic dysfunction is common, and pulsed-wave Doppler interrogation of mitral inflow may show an abnormal relaxation, restrictive, or pseudonormal pattern depending on LV diastolic pressures and loading conditions.[541] A restrictive pattern of mitral inflow Doppler confers a poor prognosis in patients with DCM.[542,543]

Restrictive Cardiomyopathy

Restrictive cardiomyopathy may be idiopathic or secondary to infiltrative diseases such as amyloidosis, hemochromatosis, hypereosinophilic syndrome and Löffler endocarditis, sarcoidosis, radiation toxicity, glycogen storage diseases, and Gaucher disease[544] (see also Chap. 75). Typical 2D echocardiographic features of these diseases include (1) a diffuse increase of ventricular thickness in the absence of marked ventricular chamber dilation and (2) marked biatrial enlargement,[509,545–549] (Fig. 14-109). Systolic function is often modestly decreased. As with the other cardiomyopathies, these echocardiographic findings are nonspecific. Doppler examination may show a mitral inflow relaxation abnormality early in the course of restrictive cardiomyopathy, but restrictive pattern (E much greater than A, with shortened E deceleration time) is a more classic finding, which often evolves with time and indicates both a high left atrial pressure and poor prognosis.[550]

Amyloidosis is generally the most commonly encountered restrictive cardiac disease. In addition to biventricular hypertrophy, amyloidosis is also associated

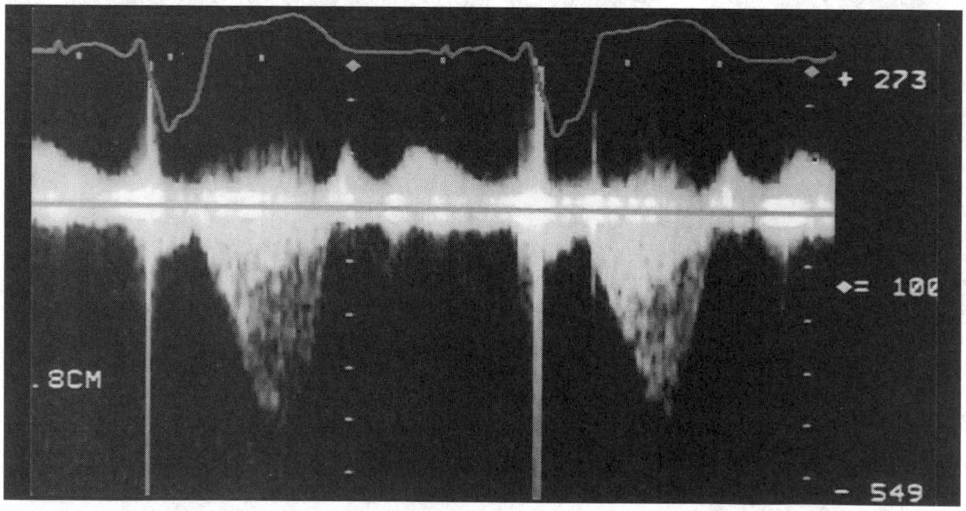

FIGURE 14-107

Continuous-wave Doppler tracing through the left ventricular outflow tract (from the apical transducer position) in hypertrophic obstructive cardiomyopathy (HOCM). In comparison to valvular aortic stenosis, the rise in velocity is delayed (reflecting dynamic rather than fixed outflow obstruction).

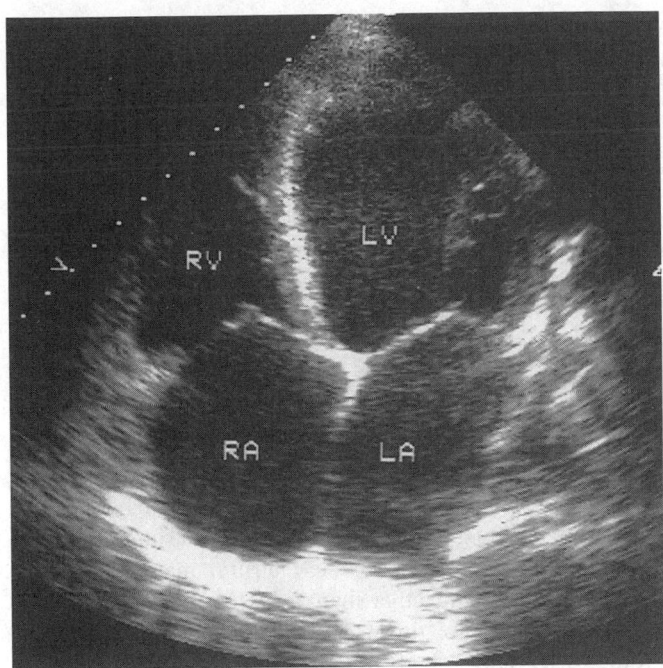

FIGURE 14-108

Apical four-chamber image of dilated cardiomyopathy. There is four-chamber enlargement as well as left ventricular (LV) spontaneous echo contrast. RV = right ventricle; RA = right atrium; LA = left atrium.

with diffuse thickening of the interatrial septum and cardiac valves.[549] In advanced disease, depressed systolic function is also common. An abnormal "speckled" pattern or "ground-glass" appearance of the myocardium has been described on 2D echocardiography, but this sign is absent in many cases and therefore has minimal clinical usefulness.[547,549] The finding of a restrictive mitral inflow pattern (and an abnormally high diastolic component of pulmonary vein inflow) on Doppler echocardiography has been identified as a marker of advanced disease and poor prognosis.[551,552] In addition to increased myocardial thickness, endocardial thickening and fibrosis and restricted atrioventricular leaflet motion are common features of Löffler endocarditis and endomyocardial fibroelastosis.[548] Intraventricular thrombi are also common in these processes.[553]

CONGENITAL HEART DISEASE

Echocardiographic Identification of Congenital Cardiac Anomalies

2D and Doppler echocardiography has had a major impact on the diagnosis and management of patients with congenital heart disease (see also Chaps. 70 and 71). From isolated congenital lesions to complex, extensive cardiac malformations, echocardiographic imaging (often with intravenous con-

trast injection) is usually sufficient to delineate cardiac anatomy. Transesophageal imaging is an important adjunctive technique as well[554]; in many cases, a thorough echocardiographic evaluation may obviate the need for cardiac catheterization and angiography.[555–557]

The ultrasound diagnosis of a simple intracardiac shunt is usually straightforward, but the task of defining complex congenital cardiac abnormalities can be daunting. In these cases, it is useful to remember a few basic anatomic rules. The venae cavae and pulmonary veins generally empty into the morphologic right atrium and left atrium, respectively. The atrioventricular valves uniformly follow their ventricles through embryologic development: a tricuspid valve accompanies the morphologic right ventricle and a mitral valve accompanies the left. Similarly, the semilunar valves follow the great vessels. The aorta and pulmonary artery can be distinguished, regardless of their position, by the bifurcation of the pulmonary artery.

Several features aid identification of the morphologic right and left ventricles. The right ventricle has a tricuspid atrioventricular valve; in comparison with the mitral annulus, the tricuspid annulus is positioned slightly closer to the cardiac apex.[558] The right ventricle also has a moderator band, coarser trabeculations than those in the left ventricle, and an infundib-

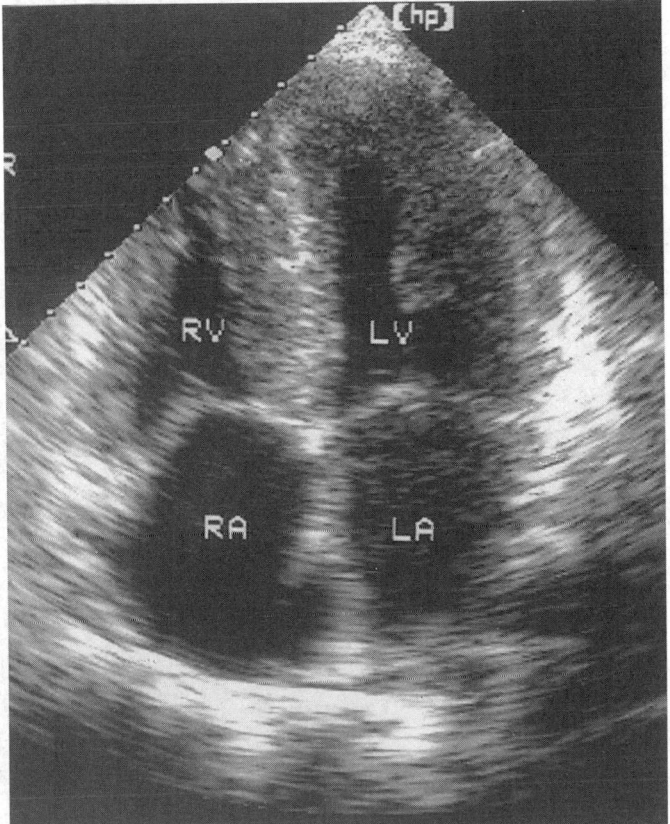

FIGURE 14-109

Apical four-chamber image of cardiac amyloid. RV = right ventricle; RA = right atrium; LA = left atrium; LV = left ventricle.

ulum that separates the inlet area from the right ventricular outflow tract.

Cardiovascular Shunts

ATRIAL SEPTAL DEFECT

Most secundum and primum primum atrial septal defects (ASD) are easily visualized by echocardiography, although sinus venous defects are often difficult to detect without transesophageal imaging.[559,560] Apical echocardiographic views often show artifactual "dropout" in the region of the fossa ovalis, since the interatrial septum is thin in this area and runs parallel to the ultrasound beam. Therefore, the subcostal view provides the optimal imaging plane to detect lesions of the atrial septum.[561] Ostium secundum defects are the most common form of ASD, and 2D imaging shows a localized absence of septal tissue in the midportion of the interatrial septum (Fig. 14-110A, Plate 40). Lack of any interatrial septal tissue between the defect and the base of the interventricular septum characterizes an ostium primum defect (Figure 14-110B). Although ostium secundum defects are usually isolated, ostium primum (or partial atrioventricular canal) defects are often accompanied by other lesions, such as cleft anterior mitral valve leaflet, MR, and atrioventricular canal ventricular septal defect.[562] Sinus venosus defects are strongly associated with partial anomalous pulmonary venous return (for example, drainage of the right upper pulmonary vein into the right atrium or superior vena cava) (Fig. 14-111). Rarely, the atrial septum may be completely absent (Fig. 14-112). With all but small atrial septal defects, the right atrium is enlarged and RV volume overload is present, with a dilated RV and paradoxical septal motion.[563]

Intravenous contrast injection generally demonstrates shunting across the ASD, frequently with bidirectional flow.[564] Therefore, "negative jets" of unopacified flow from the left atrium into the contrast-filled right atrium may alternate with the appearance of contrast bubbles flowing through the defect into the left atrium. When an ASD is present, contrast should appear quickly (within three to five heartbeats) in the left atrium after entering the right atrium. Delayed appearance of contrast in the left atrium may indicate an intrapulmonary shunt rather than an ASD.

Color Doppler imaging is also useful for detecting flow through ASDs (Fig. 14-110A, Plate 40), although the pressure drop between atria often does not produce turbulence. Inflow from the inferior vena cava and right-sided pulmonary veins

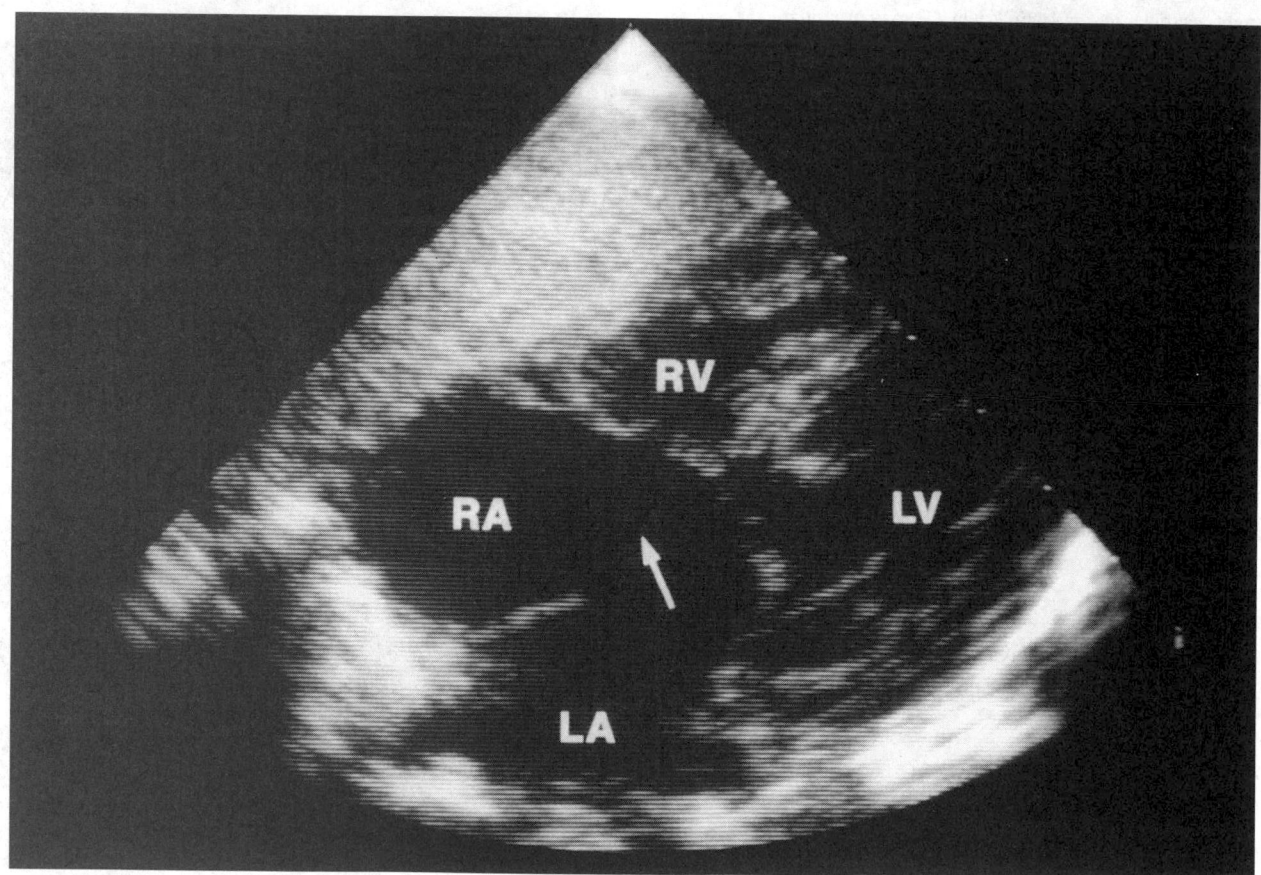

FIGURE 14-110

A. See color Plate 40. B. Subcostal 4-chamber view of a large ostium primum atrial septal defect (*arrow*). RA = right atrium; LA = left atrium; LV = left ventricle; RV = right ventricle. (Reproduced with permission of Joseph A. Kisslo, MD.)

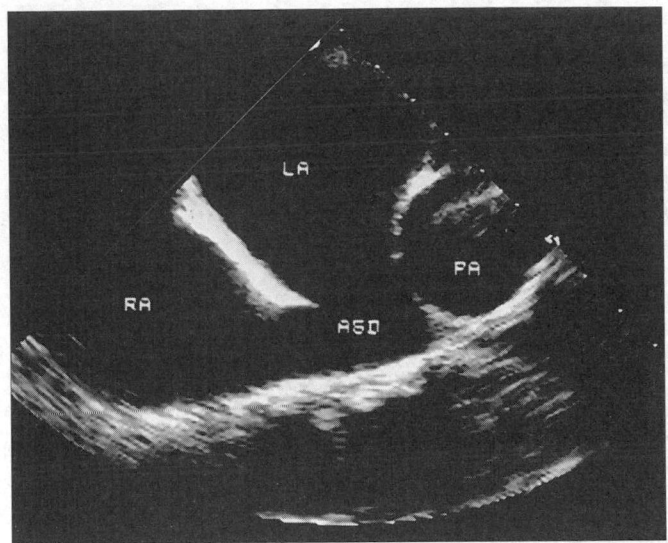

FIGURE 14-111

Transesophageal image of a sinus venosus atrial septal defect (ASD) (longitudinal plane). The defect is present in the superior portion of the interatrial septum. RA = right atrium; LA = left atrium; ASD = atrial septal defect; PA = pulmonary artery.

may be prominent in normals and can be misinterpreted as a shunt.[565,566] Pulsed-wave Doppler recordings usually reveal continuous flow, which peaks in late systole. Pulmonary-to-systemic flow ratios can be estimated in ASD (and ventricular septal defects) by comparing volumetric flow measurements through the LV and right ventricular out-flow tracts. Such calculations are only moderately accurate in adults.[567,568]

VENTRICULAR SEPTAL DEFECT

Ventricular septal defects (VSDs) may be classified as perimembranous, inlet, outlet, or trabecular. Echocardiography is quite useful for the detection and classification of VSDs.[569–571] The defect itself is sometimes visible with 2D imaging alone (Fig. 14-113A), but smaller VSDs are easily missed. Complete absence of the interventricular septum (single ventricle) is quite rare (Fig. 14-113B). Pulsed- or continuous-wave Doppler interrogation often reveals discrete areas of high-velocity flow across the interventricular septum. Measurement of the peak CW velocity through the shunt allows calculation of the interventricular pressure gradient (via the modified Bernoulli equation); subtraction of this gradient from the systolic blood pressure (in the absence of aortic valve disease) approximates the RV systolic pressure.

Overall, color-flow imaging is the most useful Doppler technique for the diagnosis of VSDs.[571] Typically, a high-velocity systolic color jet is seen traversing the interventricular septum, although the velocity is lower with large defects and in the presence of pulmonary hypertension (Fig. 14-114, Plate 41). The appearance of the color jet in the standard imaging planes can be used to determine the type of VSD. Intravenous contrast injection may reveal a negative contrast jet in the right ventricle, and contrast may cross the defect and partially opacify the left ventricle. In the absence of MR, contrast will not enter the left atrium, distinguishing an isolated VSD from

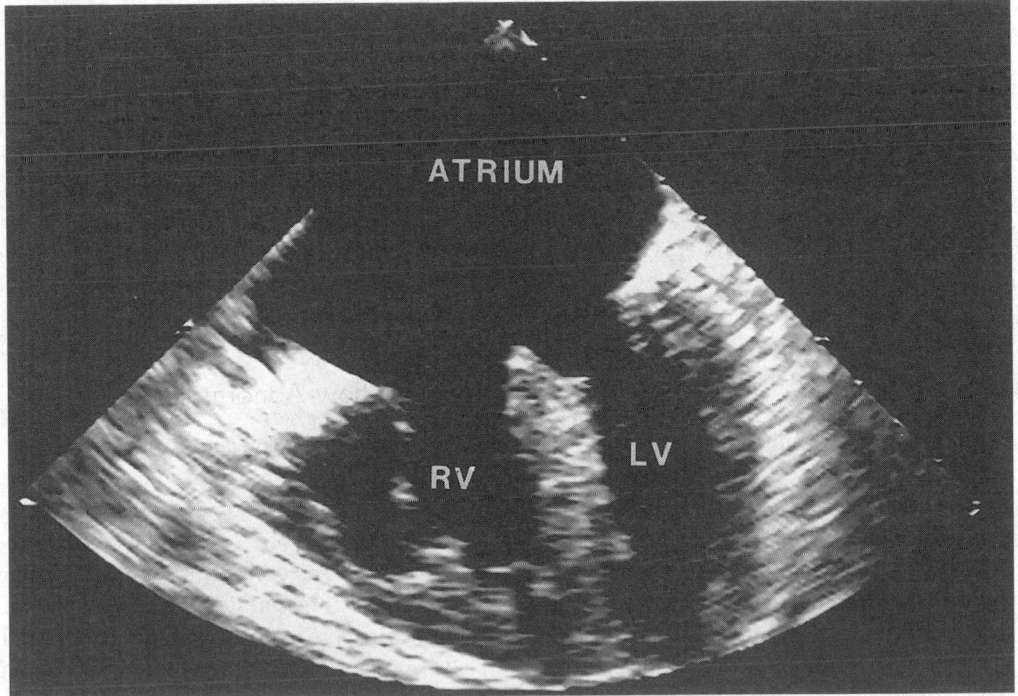

FIGURE 14-112

Transverse transesophageal image of single atrium. RV = right ventricle; LV = left ventricle. (From Blanchard DG, Scott ED. Single atrium. *Circulation* 1997; 95:273, with permission.)

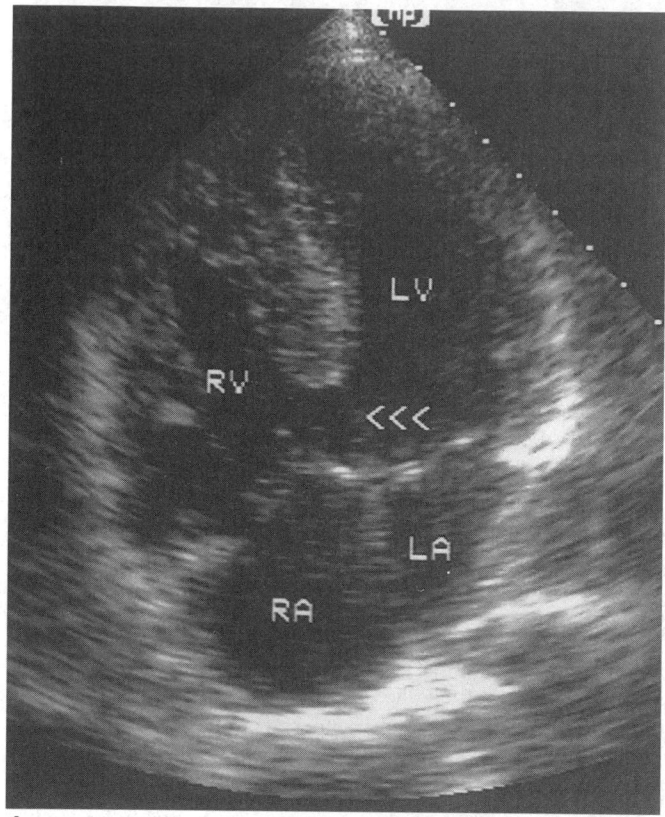

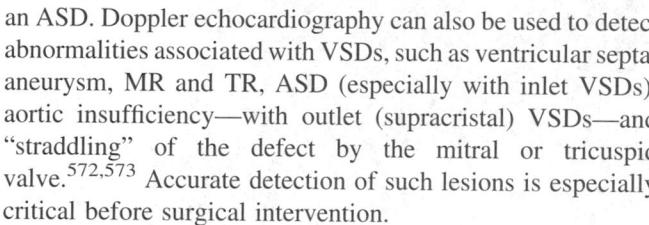

A

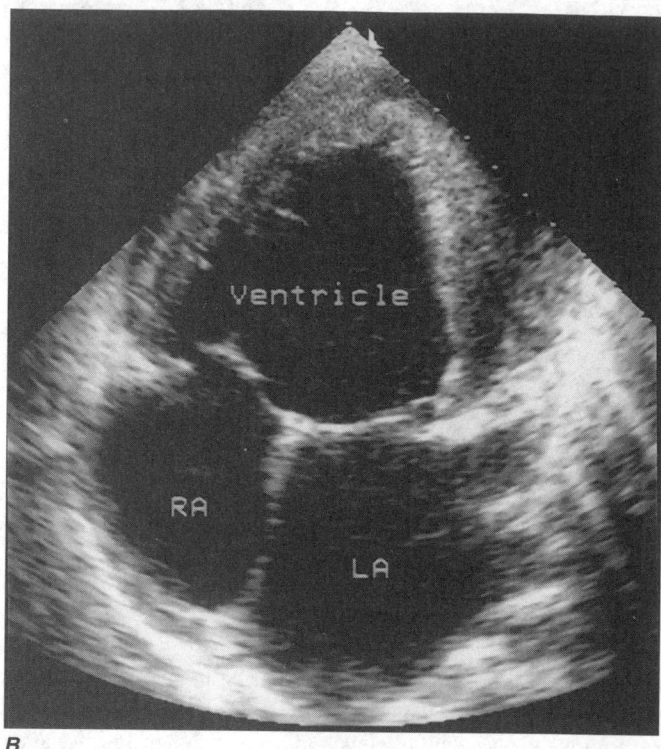

B

FIGURE 14-113

A. Apical four-chamber image of an inlet ventricular septal defect (VSD). The defect (*arrows*) is situated more inferiorly than the typical position of a perimembranous VSD. RV = right ventricle; RA = right atrium; LA = left atrium; LV = left ventricle. *B.* Apical image of single ventricle. RA = right atrium; LA = left atrium.

an ASD. Doppler echocardiography can also be used to detect abnormalities associated with VSDs, such as ventricular septal aneurysm, MR and TR, ASD (especially with inlet VSDs), aortic insufficiency—with outlet (supracristal) VSDs—and "straddling" of the defect by the mitral or tricuspid valve.[572,573] Accurate detection of such lesions is especially critical before surgical intervention.

PATENT DUCTUS ARTERIOSUS

The ductus arteriosus originates just to the left of the PA bifurcation and inserts into the aorta slightly distal to and opposite from the ostium of the left subclavian artery. Given this posterior location, it is difficult to image a patent ductus arteriosus (PDA) itself with 2D TTE alone, and TEE is usually superior for direct visualization of the lesion[574] (Fig. 14-115*A* and *B*, Plates 42*A* and *B*). In most cases, 2D imaging of the communication is not essential, as color-flow Doppler reliably detects high-velocity diastolic flow within the PA in nearly all non-Eisenmenger patients.[575–577] The flow jet characteristically enters the distal left region of the main PA

and streams anterior along the medial wall of the vessel (Fig. 14-115*B*, Plate 42*B*). With large shunts, volume overload and subsequent dilation of the left ventricle occurs. Aortopulmonary window is a much rarer shunt involving the great vessels which presents as a communication anteriorly between the ascending aorta and proximal PA.[578,579] It is embryologically distinct from a PDA and more closely related to a truncus arteriosus defect.

Venous Inflow Abnormalities

Anomalous pulmonary venous return (APVR) may be partial or total. Partial APVR is present in 80 percent of sinus venosus ASD cases and is a feature of the Scimitar syndrome.[580,581] The usual finding on TTE is RV volume overload. TEE is quite useful in detecting these abnormal venous connections. In total APVR, the pulmonary veins may empty directly into the right atrium or into a common posterior chamber or vein. This structure and its connection with the right atrium may be visualized echocardiographically, along with the obligatory

FIGURE 14-114
See color Plate 41.

FIGURE 14-115
See color Plate 42.

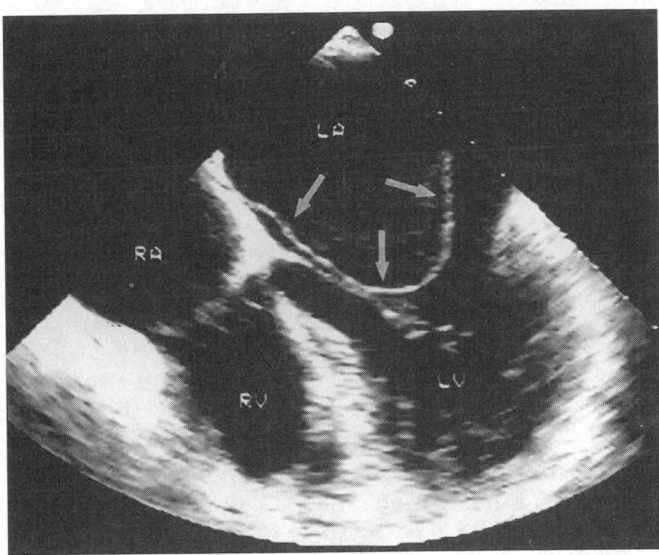

FIGURE 14-116

Transverse transesophageal image of cor triatriatum. A membrane (*arrows*) is present in the left atrium. RV = right ventricle; RA = right atrium; LA = left atrium; LV = left ventricle. (From Blanchard DG, DeMaria AN. Cardiac and extracardiac masses: Echocardiographic evaluation. In: Skorton DJ, Schelbert HR, Wolf GL, Brundage BH, eds. *Marcus' Cardiac Imaging,* 2d ed. Philadelphia: Saunders; 1996:452–480, with permission.)

ASD.[582–585] In some cases, the collecting chamber posterior to the left atrium may mimic the appearance of *cor triatriatum,* an entity characterized by a membrane in the posterior left atrium which may obstruct pulmonary venous inflow, causing symptoms similar to those of mitral stenosis[586] (Fig. 14-116).

Persistent left superior vena cava occurs in 0.5 percent of the normal population.[587,588] In most cases, the anomalous vein empties into the coronary sinus, which then drains into the right atrium (Fig. 14-117). Unless the coronary sinus is unroofed and drains into the left atrium, no shunting occurs. The typical echocardiographic finding is a large coronary sinus, which is especially well seen on transesophageal or parasternal transthoracic views. The diagnosis may be confirmed by intravenous contrast injection from the left arm, as this will opacify the coronary sinus shortly before filling the right atrium.[587,588]

Conotruncal and Aortic Abnormalities

Tetralogy of Fallot is one of the more common conotruncal abnormalities, and affected individuals may sometimes survive to adulthood without surgical intervention. The classic echocardiographic features include a large perimembranous VSD, an anteriorly displaced aorta which overrides the VSD, RV enlargement and dysfunction, and pulmonic stenosis (either infundibular, valvular, or suprevalvular) (Fig. 14-118).[589,590] The VSD and aorta are well visualized in the parasternal long-axis view, while the RV outflow tract and proximal PA are best seen in the parasternal short-axis view at the base of the heart. Doppler interrogation can provide

evaluation of the severity of pulmonic stenosis, both before and after surgery. Echocardiography may aid detection of infants with tetralogy who will require early surgical intervention as well as patients who are at high risk for sudden death after surgical repair.[591,592]

Although *double-outlet right ventricle* (DORV) shares several clinical characteristics with tetralogy of Fallot (VSD and

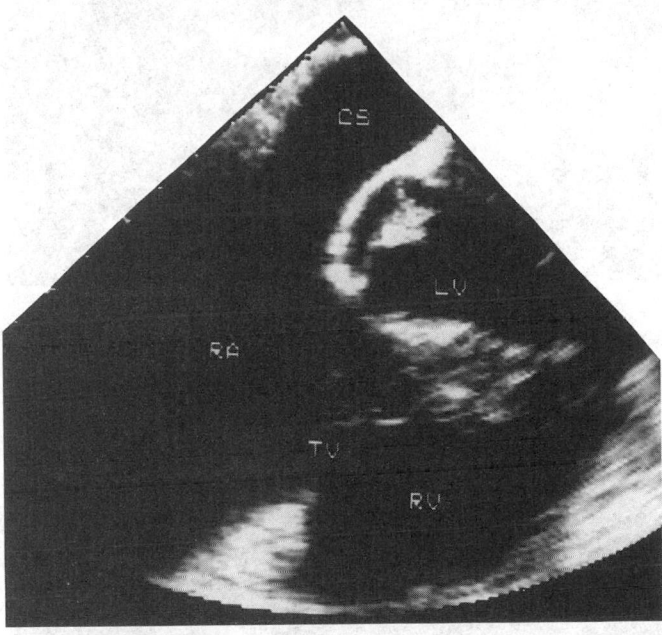

A

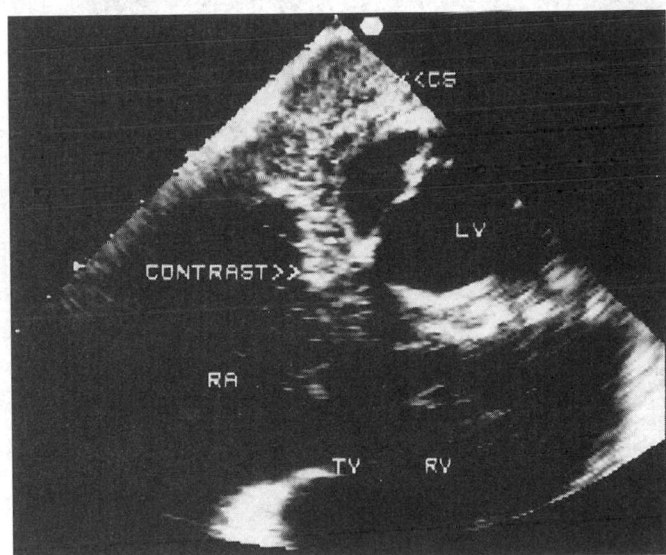

B

FIGURE 14-117

A. Transesophageal image (transverse plane) fro a patient with persistent left superior vena cava. The coronary sinus (CS) is dilated. *B.* After injection of agitated saline into the left antecubital vein, contrast is seen entering the right atrium (RA) via the CS. TV = tricuspid valve; RV = right ventricle; LV = left ventricle. (From Blanchard DG, DeMaria AN. Cardiac and extracardiac masses: Echocardiographic evaluation. In: Skorton DJ, Schelbert HR, Wolf GL, Brundage BH, eds. *Marcus' Cardiac Imaging,* 2d ed. Philadelphia: Saunders; 1996:452–480, with permission.)

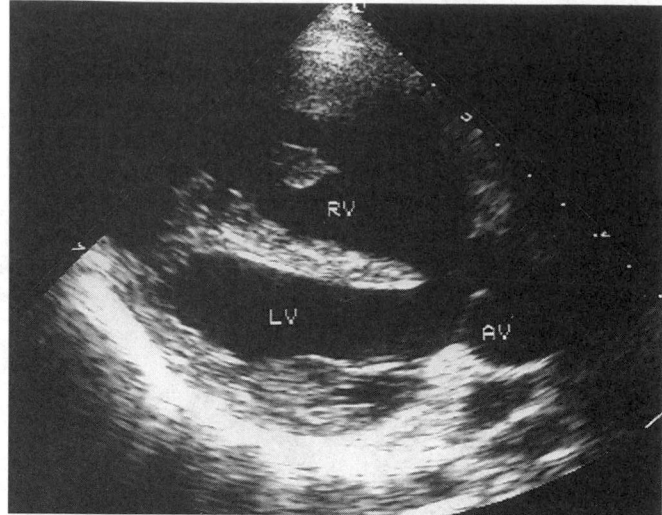

A

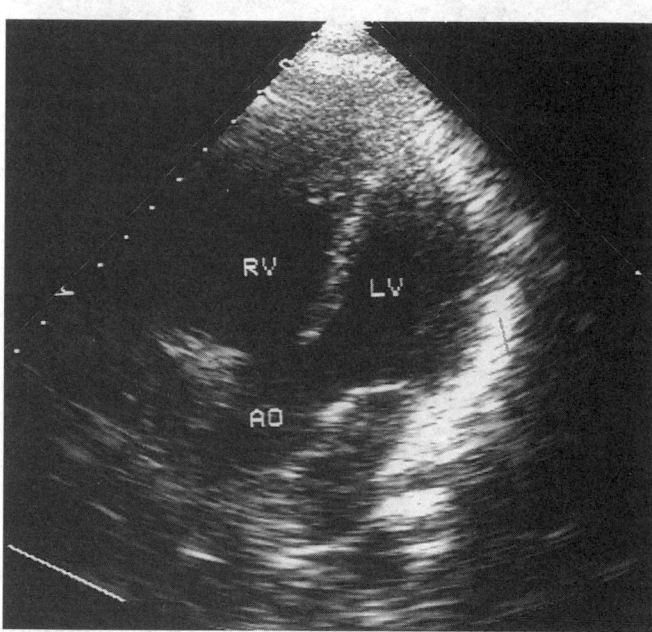

B

FIGURE 14-118

Parasternal long-axis (*A*) and apical four-chamber (*B*) images of tetralogy of Fallot. The right ventricle (RV) is enlarged, and a large VSD is present. The aorta (AO) overrides the interventricular septum. LV = left ventricle. (Courtesy of Reinaldo W. Beyer, MD.)

anterior aortic displacement are invariably present, and pulmonic valvular stenosis and ASD are common in both), it is morphologically distinct (Fig. 14-119). Normal continuity of the posterior aortic wall with the anterior mitral valve leaflet (always present in tetralogy of Fallot) is absent in DORV, and an interposed mass of fibrous tissue between the left atrium and the nearest great vessel is seen on 2D imaging.[593,594] In addition, the great vessels may be transposed in DORV, resulting in a characteristic side-by-side appearance of the aorta and PA on parasternal short-axis images.[595]

Echocardiography has become a valuable tool for detec-

tion, management, and postoperative follow-up of patients with *transposition of the great arteries*. Attention to the anatomic rules mentioned earlier is essential for accurate diagnosis of both D (classic) and L ("congenitally corrected") transposition. In D-transposition, the aorta arises from the RV, the PA arises from the LV, and one or more obligatory shunts are present. With L-transposition, the morphologic right and left ventricles are switched, and associated anomalies such as VSD and pulmonic stenosis are common. In both types of transposition, the normal echocardiographic orientation of the great vessels on parasternal short-axis images (a sausage-shaped RVOT and PA draped over a circular aorta) is no longer present, and the two great vessels are typically side by side and parallel (Fig. 14-120).[596,597] In general, the aorta is anterior and to the right of the PA in D-transposition and anterior and to the left in L-transposition. Both TTE and TEE are an important part of continuing care after surgical repair or palliation of transposition; they can detect valvular insufficiency, outflow tract narrowing, and stenosis of the atrial baffle systems used to palliate D-transposition surgically.[598–600]

Truncus arteriosus is a rare anomaly characterized by a large VSD, a single semilunar valve, and a single great vessel that divides into the ascending aorta and PA.[601,602] Ultrasound imaging can determine the anatomy of the great vessels and assist in defining the various subsets of truncus arteriosus.

Coarctation of the aorta is associated with a bicuspid aortic valve and is best visualized from the suprasternal position. 2D imaging may identify the site of coarctation, but the natural mild curving of the descending aorta can occasionally lead to a false-positive diagnosis. Clear visualization of narrowing in the proximal descending aorta with poststenotic dilatation,

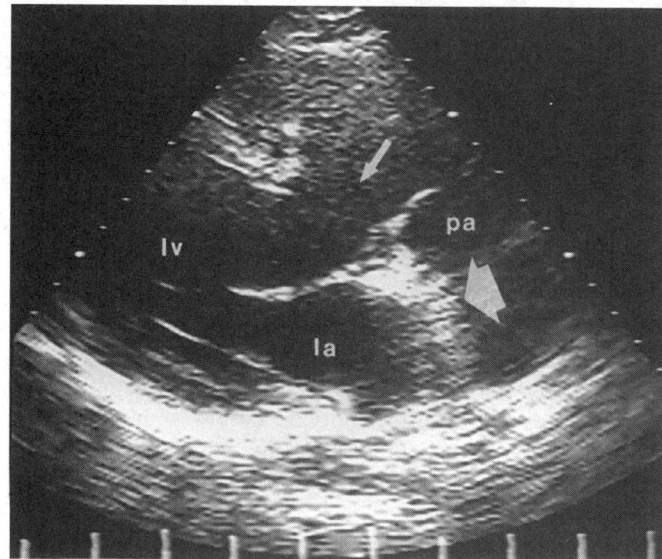

FIGURE 14-119

Parasternal long-axis image of double-outlet right ventricle. A large VSD is present (*small arrow*) and the normal continuity between the posterior aortic wall and the anterior mitral leaflet is absent. Fibrous tissue is seen (*large arrow*) between the left atrium (LA) and the nearest great vessel (in this case, the pulmonary artery (PA). LV = left ventricle.

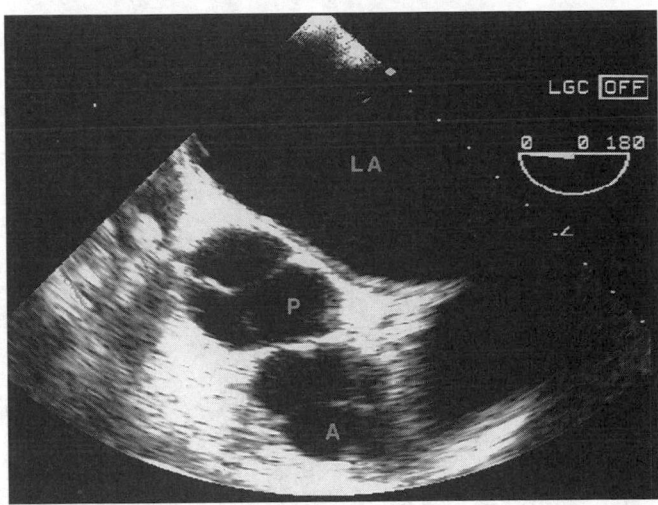

FIGURE 14-120

Transverse transesophageal image through the semilunar valves in L-transposition. The aortic valve (A) is anterior and to the left of the pulmonic valve (P). LA = left atrium.

however, is pathognomonic of coarctation.[603,604] Doppler interrogation from the suprasternal notch demonstrates increased systolic velocity in the descending aorta and may also reveal a persistent flow gradient throughout diastole in cases of severe coarctation (Fig. 14-121).[605] Color imaging often displays flow acceleration and aliasing proximal to the site of coarctation. The maximum velocity through the coarctation can be used to estimate the pressure gradient, and this measurement can be particularly valuable for the detection of restenosis after surgical repair or percutaneous balloon aortic dilation.[606,607]

Supravalvular aortic stenosis, either isolated or associated with Williams syndrome, is generally imaged best from the suprasternal and superior parasternal positions. Echocardiography reveals either an hourglass-shaped stenosis of the aorta above the sinuses of Valsalva, diffuse hypoplasia of the ascending aorta, or a focal fibrous ridge at the sinotubular junction.[608] Doppler imaging can help estimate the gradient across the stenosis, and marked aliasing of color-flow imaging in the ascending aorta should raise suspicion of the diagnosis. Thickening of the aortic valve leaflets and stenoses of the coronary ostia are important associated findings that may be detectable by echocardiography.

Ventricular Outflow Tract and Semilunar Valve Abnormalities

RIGHT VENTRICLE

Infundibular stenosis is rare outside the setting of tetralogy of Fallot and is much less common than valvular pulmonic stenosis. On 2D imaging, muscular hypertrophy is often visualized proximal to the pulmonary artery, while Doppler interrogation reveals increased flow velocities through the infundibulum.[609] *Pulmonic valve stenosis* is reasonably common and may be either isolated or associated with other congenital lesions (such as VSD, transposition, and tetralogy of Fallot). Typical echocardiographic features include thickening of the leaflets, restricted leaflet motion, systolic doming of the valve, and elevated systolic flow velocity on Doppler[610] (Fig. 14-85). As with other stenotic lesions, the gradient can be estimated using the modified Bernoulli equation. The pulmonic valve is best visualized in the parasternal short-axis view through the base (or a modified parasternal view of the RVOT). In children, the subcostal position frequently provides excellent visualization of the RVOT and pulmonic valve. When TTE is suboptimal, TEE can provide detailed images of the pulmonic valve. In pulmonic stenosis, the valve leaflets

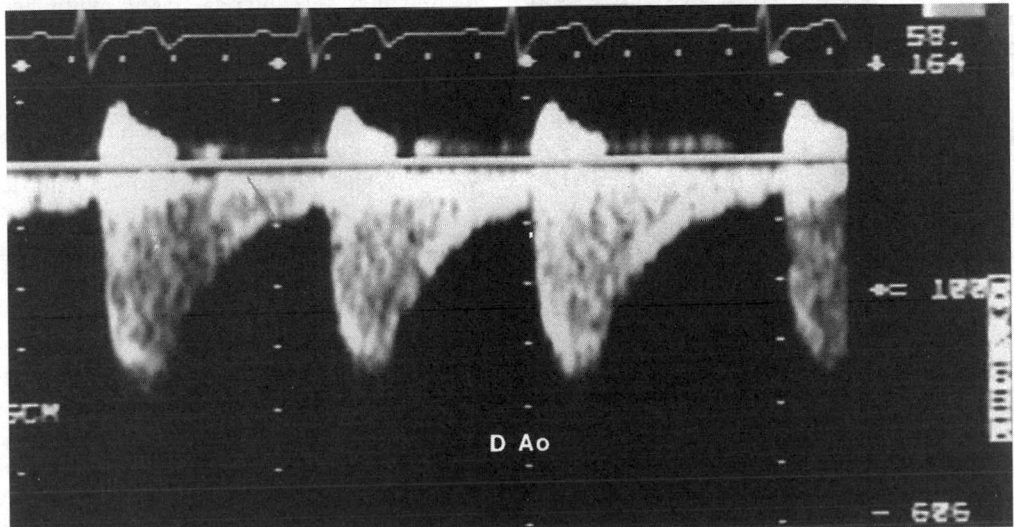

FIGURE 14-121

Continuous-wave Doppler tracing of the descending aorta (from the suprasternal position) in aortic coarctation. Peak systolic velocity is approximately 3.6 m/s, and there is persistent flow during diastole, suggesting severe coarctation. D Ao = descending aorta.

may calcify over time, and poststenotic dilatation of the pulmonary artery is often present.

LEFT VENTRICLE

Subvalvular obstruction may be dynamic or fixed. *Hypertrophic cardiomyopathy,* which may present at any age, is discussed earlier in this chapter. *Discrete subaortic stenosis* may be caused by a thin membrane in the LV outflow tract, a fibromuscular ridge, or diffuse muscular narrowing of the outflow tract (Figs. 14-122A and 14-122B, Plate 43).[611] 2D echocardiographic imaging can distinguish these various forms of discrete subvalvular stenosis, and Doppler analysis permits estimation of the systolic gradient.[612] Color-flow imaging demonstrates increased turbulence in the LVOT as well as aortic valvular regurgitation in about 50 percent of cases. Apical views are sometimes more useful for detecting thin subaortic membranes, as these structures are parallel to the ultrasound beam on parasternal images (Fig. 14-122). Subaortic fibromuscular ridges are sometimes associated with anomalous mitral valve chordae connecting the papillary muscles or the anterior mitral valve leaflet to the septum.[613,614] M-mode imaging may reveal midsystolic partial closure of the aortic valve, differentiating subvalvular from valvular AS.

Bicuspid aortic valve is the most common congenital cardiac lesion in adults and is present in 1 to 2 percent of all individuals (men are affected more often than women).[615,616]

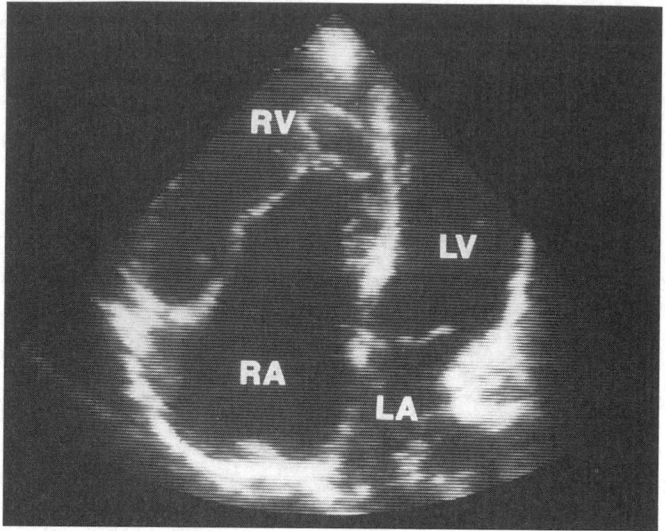

FIGURE 14-123
Apical four-chamber image of Ebstein's anomaly. The right heart is enlarged, and the insertion of the septal leaflet of the tricuspid valve is displaced apically. The anterior tricuspid leaflet (to the patient's right) is abnormally elongated. RV = right ventricle; RA = right atrium; LA = left atrium; LV = left ventricle. (Reproduced with permission of Joseph A. Kisslo, MD.)

Initially, eccentric diastolic coaptation of the aortic cusps was reported on M-mode in patients with bicuspid valves. However, M-mode findings are less accurate than 2D imaging, and the parasternal short-axis view is generally best for defining the fish-mouthed systolic aortic valvular anatomy (Figs. 14-60 and 14-61). Bicuspid valves are sometimes easy to detect in diastole as well, but raphes and remnants of commissures may obscure the diagnosis and mimic a trileaflet valve. In general, asymmetry of the aortic leaflets suggests congenital deformation. In equivocal cases, multiplane TEE is usually diagnostic (Fig. 14-61).

Ventricular Inflow Tract Abnormalities

Ebstein's anomaly is a congenital deformity of the tricuspid valve in which the leaflets are displaced into the right ventricle. Associated findings include TR, right atrial enlargement, and ASD.[617,618] 2D imaging typically shows abnormal apical displacement of the septal leaflet insertion, with variable deformity of the leaflet (Fig. 14-123). The anterior leaflet originates from the tricuspid annulus but is elongated and often tethered to the RV free wall by abnormal chordal attachments. The tricuspid deformity and regurgitation are best visualized in the apical four-chamber view, although the subcostal and modified parasternal views also may be helpful.

Atrioventricular valvular atresia is usually accompanied by hypoplasia of the corresponding ventricle. Echocardiographic images of tricuspid atresia characteristically show a small, nonfunctional right ventricle, an interatrial communication of variable size, and a normally developed left ventricle.

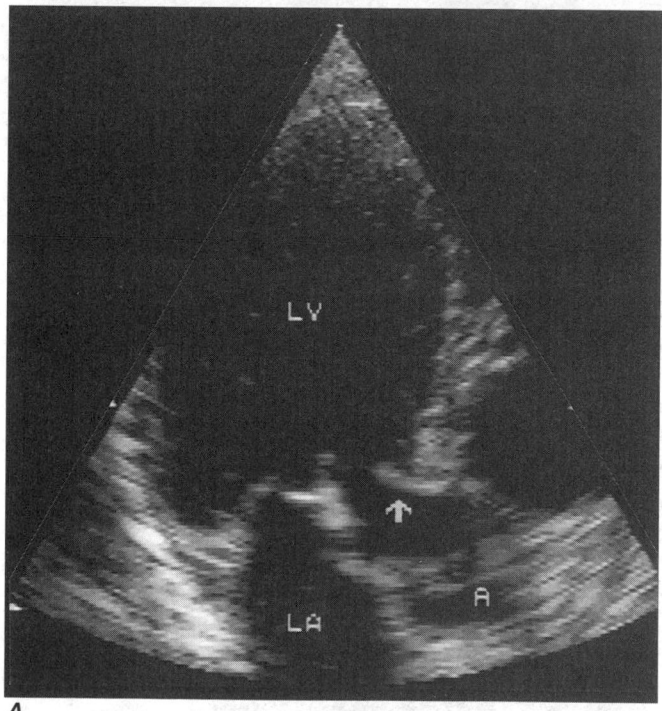

A

FIGURE 14-122
Apical three-chamber view of discrete subaortic stenosis. *A.* Fibromuscular ridge (*arrow*) is present in the left ventricular outflow tract. LV = left ventricle; LA = left atrium; A = aortic root. *B.* See color Plate 43.

Associated lesions include VSD, transposition, and RV outflow obstruction. Echocardiography is an important tool in the management of patients with tricuspid atresia after palliation with the Fontan procedure. Mitral atresia is associated with a hypoplastic left ventricle. Additional rare congenital mitral anomalies imaged by echocardiography include parachute mitral valve and congenital mitral stenosis.

Fetal Echocardiography

The average risk for significant heart disease in the fetus is approximately 0.4 to 0.8 percent. Fetal echocardiography has evolved over the past 14 years into a sophisticated method for intrauterine detection of cardiac abnormalities[619] (Fig. 14-124). The technique has been advocated for the preterm diagnosis of congenital heart disease, especially in higher-risk cases [for example, maternal congenital heart disease or diabetes mellitus, maternal teratogen exposure or toxoplasmosis, other intrauterine infections, rubella, cytomegalovirus, and herpes virus (TORCH) infection, and familial syndromes that may affect the heart].[620] Fetal echocardiography has successfully identified a variety of congenital lesions including atrial and ventricular septal defect, pulmonic stenosis, transposition, tetralogy of Fallot, hypoplasic left heart, Ebstein's anomaly, and tricuspid atresia.[621] Prenatal detection of these lesions may improve prognosis and guide therapy. Although some have recommended routine limited fetal echocardiography during the second or third trimester,[620] recent reports have suggested a low yield and limited diagnostic accuracy.[622–624] Like many imaging techniques, fetal echocardiography is evolving, and further study is required to define its optimal clinical use.

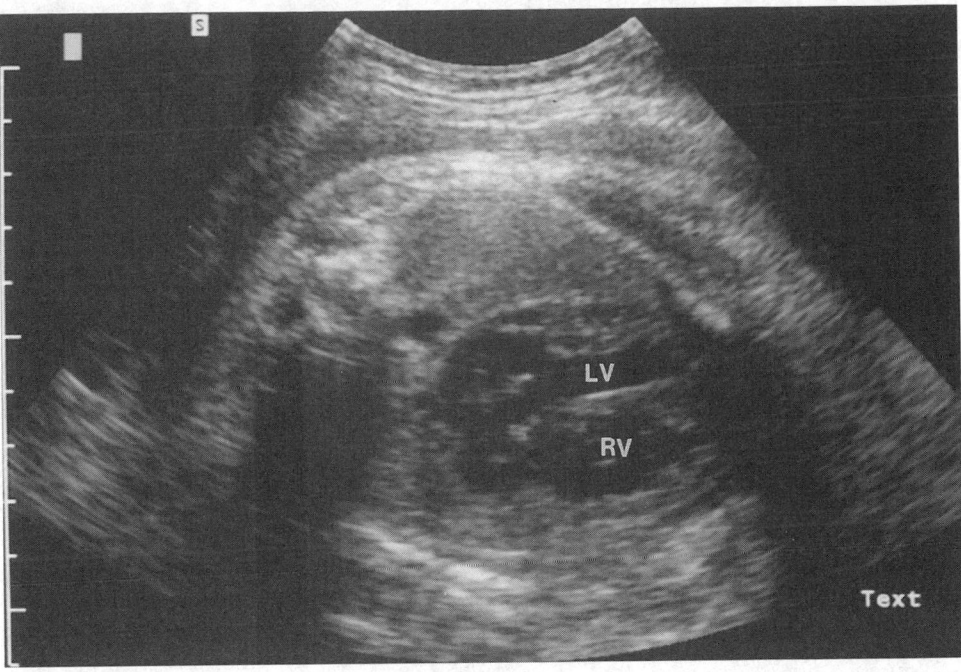

FIGURE 14-124
Fetal echocardiogram (four-chamber view). LV = left ventricle; RV = right ventricle.

CARDIAC MASSES, THROMBI, AND TUMORS

Normal Variants and Masses of Uncertain Significance

When an abnormally localized accumulation of dense reflectances appears on the echocardiogram, it is said to represent a mass. Echocardiographic masses may be caused by technical artifacts or anomalous structures, but they are of greatest significance in representing true lesions of the heart such as tumors, thrombi, and vegetations. Echocardiography is the procedure of choice for the detection and evaluation of cardiac mass lesions; often, it is the only modality capable of delineating small lesions such as papillary fibroelastomas.[625] Accordingly, echocardiographic examinations are commonly performed to search for embolic sources, particularly in patients with cerebral ischemic events.

A number of technical artifacts are capable of appearing as masses on echocardiogram. For example, side lobe signals, reverberations, and noise artifact may lead to accumulations of ultrasonic reflectance within the cavities or adjacent to the myocardium of the heart.[20,21] Such structures usually lack distinct borders, do not move appropriately through the cardiac cycle, lack identifiable attachments to endocardial surfaces, and cannot be visualized in all views and at all depth settings. In seeking a way to distinguish artifacts from LV thrombi (a common clinical dilemma) the absence of wall motion abnormalities is of particular value.[626]

A number of benign normal variant findings can be observed during echocardiographic examination and must be distinguished from pathologic lesions. Thus, many adults manifest persistence of the eustachian valve (Fig. 14-125), a thin ridge of tissue at the junction of the inferior vena cava and right atrium.[627,628] The eustachian valve appears as a long, linear, freely mobile structure in the right atrium at the mouth of the inferior vena cava and is nearly always benign (although infective involvement has been reported).[629,630] An additional embryonic remnant that may be seen in the posterior right atrium is the Chiari network, which typically appears as a weblike mobile structure.[631,632] In some individuals, RV

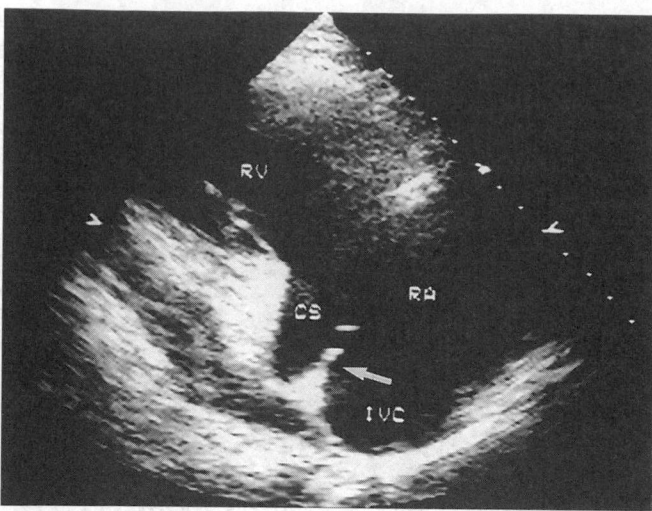

FIGURE 14-125

Right ventricular inflow view showing a prominent eustachian valve (*arrow*) at the junction of the inferior vena cava (IVC) and the right atrium (RA). RV = right ventricle; CS = coronary sinus. (From Blanchard DG, DeMaria AN. Cardiac and extracardiac masses: Echocardiographic evaluation. In: Skorton DJ, Schelbert HR, Wolf GL, Brundage BH, eds. *Marcus' Cardiac Imaging,* 2d ed. Philadelphia; Saunders; 1996:452–480, with permission.)

hypertrophy may produce significant enlargement of the RV moderator band coursing along the interventricular septum to the apex of the RV.[633] Similarly, false chordae tendineae ("heartstrings") can occasionally be visualized as linear structures spanning the LV cavity attached to endomyocardium at both ends (Fig. 14-126).[634,635] Neither of the foregoing lesions has been conclusively associated with morbidity or mortality. On occasion, LV hypertrophy or hypertrophied papillary muscles may simulate cardiac mass lesions.[633] Although

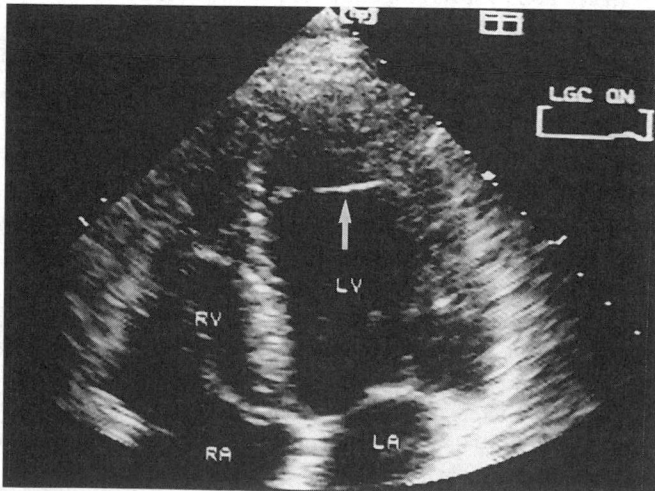

FIGURE 14-126

Apical four-chamber view demonstrating a false chord (*arrow*) within the left ventricle (LV). LA = left atrium; RA = right atrium; RV = right ventricle. (From Blanchard DG, DeMaria AN. Cardiac and extracardiac masses: Echocardiographic evaluation. In; Skorton DJ, Schelbert HR, Wolf GL, Brundage BH, eds. *Marcus' Cardiac Imaging,* 2d ed. Philadelphia: Saunders; 1996:452–480, with permission.)

TEE provides enhanced sensitivity and resolution in the delineation of cardiac mass lesions, this technique may be associated with variants and artifacts of its own.[636,637]

A variety of foreign bodies and iatrogenically induced anatomic alterations may be visualized on echocardiogram and must be distinguished from pathologic lesions. Intracardiac catheters, pacemaker leads (Fig. 14-127), prosthetic valves or patches, and atrial suture lines after cardiac transplantation can be visualized during echocardiographic examination.[638,639] These structures are usually easily recognized due to the highly reflective properties of the foreign material, which result in bright echoes, reverberations, and shadowing behind the structures. In this regard, endomyocardial biotomes and pericardiocentesis catheters can be readily visualized by cardiac ultrasound, and echocardiography can be employed to guide procedures utilizing these instruments in lieu of fluoroscopy.[640,641] Last, a variety of manufactured objects that have penetrated the heart have been described on echocardiography, including bullets, pellets, and nails.[642]

Several morphologic changes involving the interatrial septum are often considered under the classification of cardiac mass lesions of uncertain significance. Aneurysms of the interatrial septum have been reported in about 1 percent of the population and are recognized on echocardiogram as a protrusion of the interatrial septum of at least 1.5 cm from its longitudinal plane dividing the left and right atrium

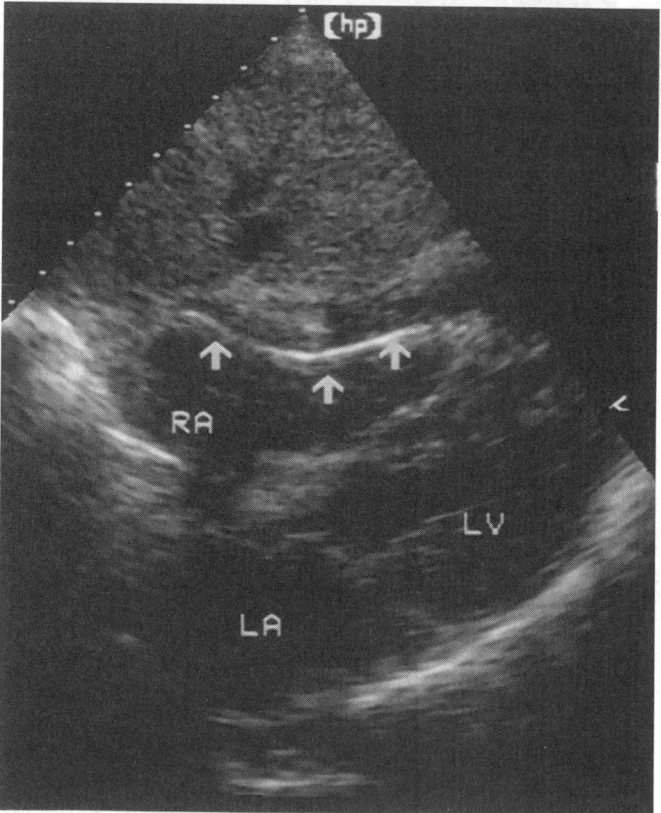

FIGURE 14-127

Subcostal four-chamber image demonstrating a pacemaker wire (*arrows*) in the right heart. RA = right atrium; LA = left atrium; LV = left ventricle.

(Fig. 14-128).[643,644] Although usually benign, interatrial septal aneurysms are often associated with a patent foramen ovale and have been implicated as a source of cardiogenic emboli.[645] Interatrial septal aneurysms may be detected by TTE, but they are more readily imaged by the transesophageal approach.[644] Lipomatous hypertrophy of the interatrial septum, or accumulation of adipose tissue within this structure, is not an uncommon findings in elderly individuals. Lipomatous hypertrophy appears as a highly reflective thickening of the interatrial septum that typically spares the foramen ovale, thereby creating a characteristic dumbbell echocardiographic appearance.[646,647] No significant consequences or sequelae have been attributed to lipomatous infiltration of the interatrial septum.

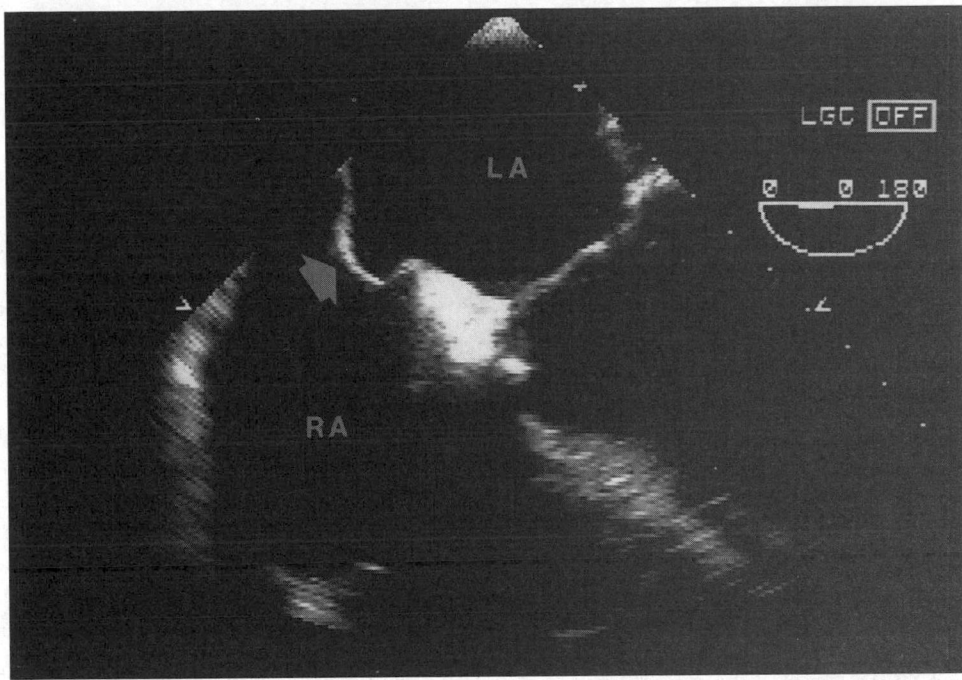

FIGURE 14-128

Transverse transesophageal image of an interatrial septal aneurysm (*arrow*). RA = right atrium; LA = left atrium. (From Blanchard DG, DeMaria AN. Cardiac and extracardiac masses: Echocardiographic evaluation. In: Skorton DJ, Schelbert HR, Wolf GL, Brundage BH, eds. *Marcus' Cardiac Imaging,* 2d ed. Philadelphia: Saunders; 1996:452–480, with permission.)

Intracardiac Thrombi

Intracardiac thrombi occur commonly in a variety of cardiovascular disorders, may be visualized in any chamber of the heart, and frequently result in embolic events.[648] The major factors that predispose to the formation of intracardiac thrombi include localized stasis of flow, low cardiac output, and cardiac injury. In addition, migration of venous thrombi may also result in intracardiac clots.[649,650] The appearance of intracardiac thrombi may vary considerably, and although they are typically attached to the endocardium, unrestricted and freely mobile thrombi occasionally may be encountered (particularly in the setting of valvular stenosis which prevents exit of the thrombus from the heart).[651] Thrombi typically have identifiable borders and may be layered and homogeneous or heterogeneous, with areas of central liquefaction (Figs. 14-129 and 14-130).[651,652]

RIGHT HEART

Thrombi within the right heart chambers may form locally or migrate from the venous circulation; they are found most commonly in the right atrium.[653] As opposed to the laminar, relatively immobile nature of right atrial thrombi that form in situ, venous thromboemboli trapped in the right atrium tend to be serpentine and mobile.[649] The potential for pulmonary embolism is high.[654] Thrombi also can be seen within the main pulmonary arteries, although they are less well visualized by TTE than TEE.[655] RV thrombi are rare but may occur with RV infarction and endomyocardial fibrosis.[656,657] Their appearance is similar to that of LV thrombi.

LEFT ATRIUM

Left atrial thrombi occur in the setting of low cardiac output, mitral valvular disease (particularly mitral stenosis), atrial fibrillation, and left atrial enlargement. Both TTE and TEE can detect thrombi within the main cavity of the left atrium (Fig. 14-131), but TEE is clearly superior for visualizing

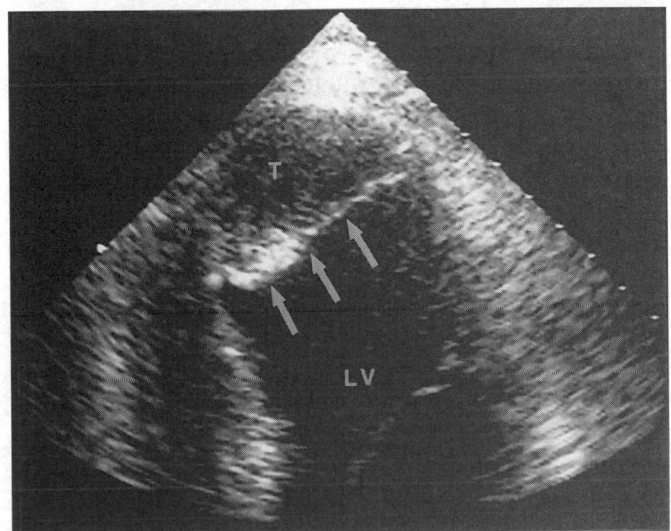

FIGURE 14-129

Magnified apical view of a large thrombus (T) in the apex of the left ventricle (LV). Although the thrombus is fairly homogeneous, its border is more echodense (*arrows*).

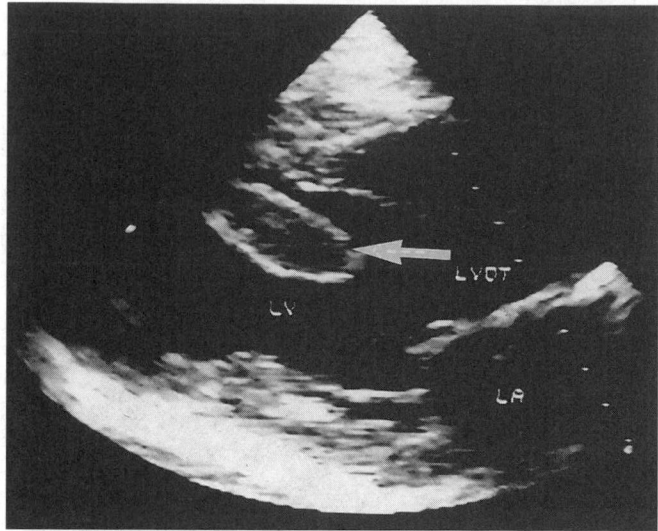

FIGURE 14-130

Parasternal long-axis view of a large mobile thrombus (*arrow*) attached to the anteroseptal segment of the left ventricle (LV). LVOT = left ventricular outflow tract; LA = left atrium. (From Blanchard DG, DeMaria AN: Cardiac and extracardiac masses: Echocardiographic evaluation. In: Skorton DJ, Schelbert HR, Wolf GL, Brundage BH, eds. *Marcus' Cardiac Imaging,* 2d ed. Philadelphia: Saunders; 1996:452–480, with permission.)

thrombi within the left atrial appendage.[658–660] Since approximately 50 percent of left atrial thrombi are limited to the appendage, TEE is the diagnostic procedure of choice to detect this lesion.[652,661] Left atrial thrombi appear as discrete masses, either fixed or mobile, and are usually of homogeneous echo density[659] (Fig. 14-52). On TEE, normal pectinate muscular ridges in the appendage must be distinguished from small thrombi. In addition, the left atrial appendage may occasionally be multilobed. Although this anatomic variant may be a risk factor for appendage thrombi, the atrial tissue separating the lobes should not be mistaken for clot.[662]

Left atrial thrombi are often accompanied by spontaneous echo contrast (or "smoke") within the left atrium. This finding, probably produced by transient aggregation of erythrocytes and plasma proteins,[663] indicates stagnant blood flow and can occur in any cardiac chamber or the aorta. Left atrial spontaneous echo contrast, like left atrial thrombus, has been associated with embolic events[664,665] and may be a marker of regional prothrombotic activity.[666] On 2D imaging, the contrast signals are in constant motion and can be missed if gain settings are inappropriately low.

LEFT VENTRICLE

Most LV thrombi occur in settings of abnormal systolic contraction (dilated cardiomyopathy, acute myocardial infarction, and chronic LV ventricular aneurysm).[667–669] LV Thrombi have been reported in up to one-half of patients with large myocardial infarctions and occur more frequently in anterior infarctions (up to 30 to 40 percent of such patients).[668] Most thrombi are located in the apex[626] and thus are best visualized in the apical views (Fig. 14-129). Although echocardiography

is the procedure of choice for detecting LV thrombi,[669] the technique's true sensitivity and specificity remains uncertain, since most patients included in validating studies had LV aneurysms and the echocardiographic criteria applied were subjective.[668–670]

LV thrombi may be laminar an fixed or protruding and mobile, and they may have a heterogeneous echo density (Figs. 14-129 and 14-130). Studies suggest that "immature" thrombi are often filamentous, with irregular borders, while older thrombi tend to be echodense and fixed.[626,648,671] The echocardiographic characteristics of thrombi may influence the risk of cardiogenic embolization, as irregularly shaped, mobile, and protruding thrombi are more likely to embolize than laminar, immobile clots.[648] True LV thrombi have a density distinct from the underlying myocardium, appear in multiple imaging planes, and move concordantly with the underlying myocardium.[669] Suspected masses in areas of normally functioning myocardium are rarely thrombi.

Cardiac Tumors

Although diagnosed infrequently, cardiac tumors often are included in the differential diagnosis of cardiac problems because of their protean clinical manifestations. Cardiac tumors may be intracavitary or intramural, and the location

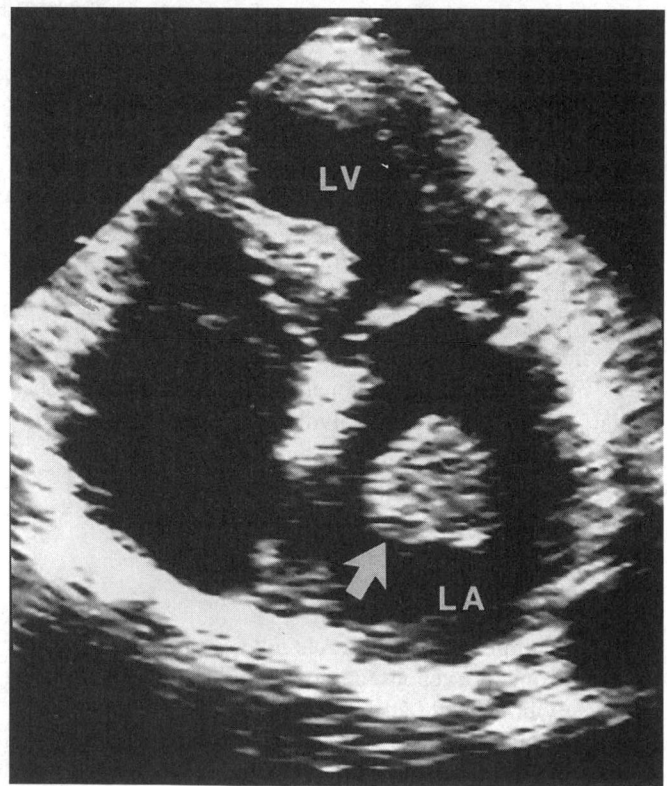

FIGURE 14-131

Apical four-chamber image of a large mobile "ball" thrombus (*arrow*) in the left atrium (LA). LV = left ventricle. (From Blanchard DG, DeMaria AN. Cardiac and extracardiac masses: Echocardiographic evaluation. In: Skorton DJ, Schelbert HR, Wolf GL, Brundage BH, eds. *Marcus' Cardiac Imaging,* 2d ed. Philadelphia: Saunders; 1996:452–480, with permission.)

determines their echocardiographic appearance. Intracavitary tumors appear as sessile or mobile echo densities attached to the mural endocardium while intramural tumors appear as localized thickening of the LV wall.[672] The pericardium also may be involved with cardiac tumors, with or without the presence of concomitant effusion.

MYXOMAS

Myxomas are the most common primary cardiac tumors, accounting for about 25 percent of all such lesions.[673–675] Myxomas can occur in any cardiac chamber, but 75 percent are found in the left atrium.[675] On 2D imaging, myxomas usually appear as gelatinous, speckled, sometimes globular masses with frondlike projections (Figs. 14-132 and 14-133). Tissue heterogeneity is common, but calcification is rare.[673] Although they may be sessile, myxomas are usually attached to the endocardial surface by a pedicle. Typically, they are attached to the interatrial septum, but they can originate from the posterior or anterior atrial wall, the appendage, or even the cardiac valves.[676,677] Large tumors are almost always mobile to some degree, and a sizable left atrial mass that appears fixed in position is therefore less likely to be a myxoma. Large left atrial myxomas may move back and forth into the mitral valve annulus during the cardiac cycle, entering the orifice in diastole and the left atrium in systole. Accordingly, Doppler interrogation may demonstrate either obstruction of flow, valvular regurgitation, or both.[678,679] Most myxomas are visible on TTE, but TEE is superior for the delineation of tumor attachments and detection of small myxomas.[680] Since approximately 5 percent of myxomas are biatrial, careful evaluation of the right atrium is mandatory.[675]

ADDITIONAL PRIMARY TUMORS

Benign

Rhabdomyomas are rare cardiac tumors associated with tuberous sclerosis.[681,682] There is a strong tendency for multiple tumors to occur within an affected heart (90 percent of cases).[681,683] Fibromas are found most often in children and affect the left ventricle most frequently. The tumor may grow within the myocardium rather than expanding into a cardiac chamber.[684,685] Papillary fibroelastomas are usually quite small in size (less than 1 cm in diameter) and often grow on cardiac valves or chordae. These rare tumors typically have multiple small fronds that tend to embolize.[625,686,687] Echocardiographic differentiation from vegetations can be difficult.

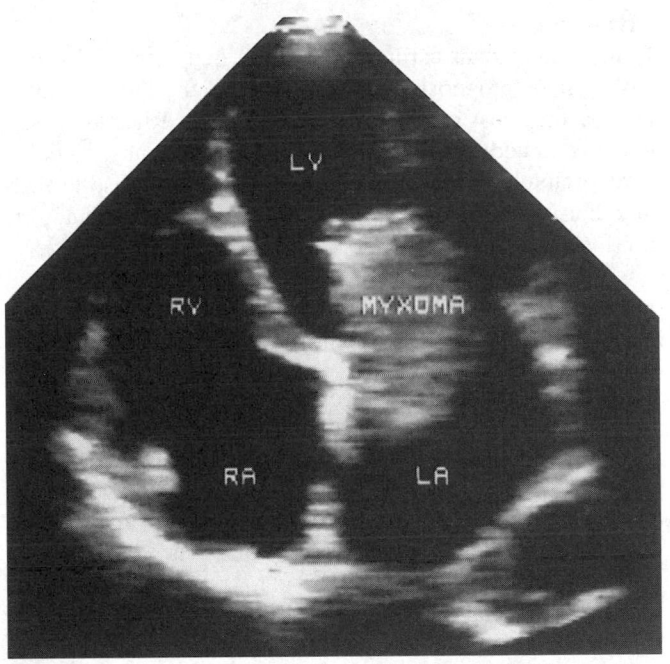

FIGURE 14-132
Apical four-chamber image of a left atrial myxoma which is attached to the interatrial septum and prolapses through the mitral valve. LA = left atrium; RA = right atrium; RV = right ventricle; LV = left ventricle. (From Blanchard DG, DeMaria AN. Cardiac and extracardiac masses: Echocardiographic evaluation. In: Skorton DJ, Schelbert HR, Wolf GL, Brundage BH, eds. *Marcus' Cardiac Imaging,* 2d ed. Philadelphia: Saunders, 1996:452–480, with permission.)

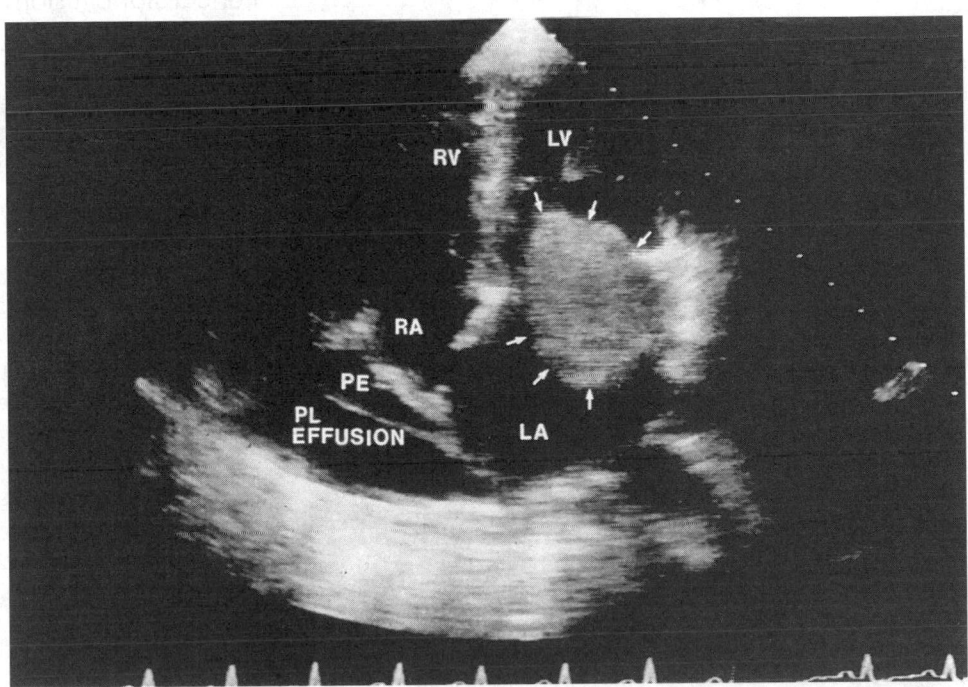

FIGURE 14-133
Apical four-chamber image of a large left atrial myxoma (*arrows*) which is attached to the lateral wall of the atrium. LA = left atrium; RA = right atrium; RV = right ventricle; LV = left ventricle; PE = pericardial effusion; PL = pleural.

Malignant

Primary malignant cardiac tumors are quite rare and confer a very poor prognosis. Angiosarcoma is the most common and occurs most often in the right atrium. Rhabdomyosarcoma is an additional primary cardiac malignancy.[688] Echocardiography can be useful in monitoring response to therapy, but its diagnostic utility is limited, as most findings are nonspecific.

Metastatic and Secondary Tumors of the Heart and Pericardium

Metastatic tumors to the pericardium and heart occur 20 to 40 times more often than primary cardiac tumors (Fig. 14-134).[689] Tumors that commonly involve the heart and pericardium include breast and lung carcinoma, melanoma, and lymphoma. Involvement may be secondary to hematogenous, lymphatic, or contiguous spread. Tumors such as hepatoma and renal carcinoma can also extend to the heart via the venae cavae.[690] In these cases, tumor is often visible in the inferior vena cava and right atrium. Metastatic disease affects the pericardium more frequently than the heart itself, and pericardial effusion is the most common echocardiographic manifestation in patients with cardiac metastases.[689,691,692] Intracavitary and pericardial masses are easily visualized with 2D imaging, although intramural tumors are sometimes difficult to image. Echocardiographic findings are nonspecific, and metastatic tumors may be mistaken for primary cardiac neoplasms, vegetations, thrombi, or even prominent muscular trabeculations.

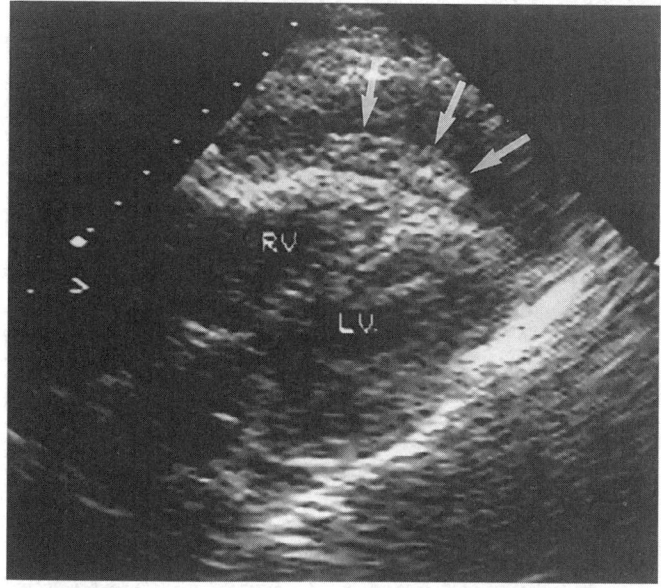

FIGURE 14-134
Modified subcostal image showing a metastatic tumor on the epicardium (*arrows*) and a malignant pericardial effusion. RV = right ventricle; LV = left ventricle. (From Blanchard DG, DeMaria AN. Cardiac and extracardiac masses: Echocardiographic evaluation. In: Skorton DJ, Schelbert HR, Wolf GL, Brundage BH, eds. *Marcus Cardiac Imaging*, 2d ed. Philadelphia: Saunders; 1996:452–480, with permission.)

Additional Cardiac Masses

The heart is rarely involved in echinococcal disease (<2 percent of cases), but intracardiac or intrapericardial rupture of a cyst can lead to anaphylaxis and cardiac tamponade, respectively.[693] Echocardiographic detection of a multiseptated cyst in the left ventricle or interventricular septum suggests cardiac echinococcal disease.[694]

Simple pericardial cysts usually occur in the right costophrenic angle (posterior to the right atrium) and have a benign prognosis. The structures are nonseptated and fluid-filled; they do not compress the cardiac chambers.[695]

PERICARDIAL DISEASE

In normal subjects, the pericardium is difficult to visualize since the pericardial cavity is only a potential space and visceral and parietal pericardial layers appear as a single echo.[696] In the setting of pericardial effusion, the fluid appears as a sonolucent area (or clear space) separating epicardium from pericardium.[697] Pericarditis may be unaccompanied by pericardial effusion and in such cases may be undetectable by echocardiography.[698] In addition, thickening and/or calcification of the pericardium may be detectable by echocardiography in patients with constrictive pericarditis, cardiac ultrasound is limited in this capability.[699,700] Therefore, the evaluation of constrictive pericarditis by echocardiography primarily involves Doppler flow recordings.[701]

Pericardial Effusion

Echocardiography is the diagnostic procedure of choice for detection of pericardial fluid[696,697] (Fig. 14-135), and early M-mode studies demonstrated that volumes as small as 20 to 30 mL could be detected reliably.[702] As both myocardium and pericardium are echo-reflective and pericardial fluid is not, a sonolucent area between the epicardium and pericardium is diagnostic of a pericardial effusion. Although epicardial-pericardial separation may be seen during systole in normal cases, separation throughout the cardiac cycle is abnormal.[702] Descending aorta, coronary sinus, pleural effusion, pericardial cyst, and left ventricular pseudoaneurysm occasionally may be mistaken for pericardial effusion.[703]

Echocardiography can be used to identify pericardial loculations, fibrous strands, and pericardial tumors as well as to assess the size of effusions[692,696,697,699,700] (Fig. 14-136). Pericardial effusions may be concentric or loculated (the latter type is especially common with postoperative, infective, and malignant effusions). As pericardial tissue reflects upon itself behind the left atrium between the pulmonary veins (the oblique sinus), fluid is rarely seen in this area. Small, nonloculated effusions may move depending on patient position and thus are often drawn posteriorly and inferiorly by gravity during routine imaging. A rim of pericardial fluid surrounding the heart is evidence of a moderate or large effusion, and the heart can sometimes be seen "swinging" back and forth within

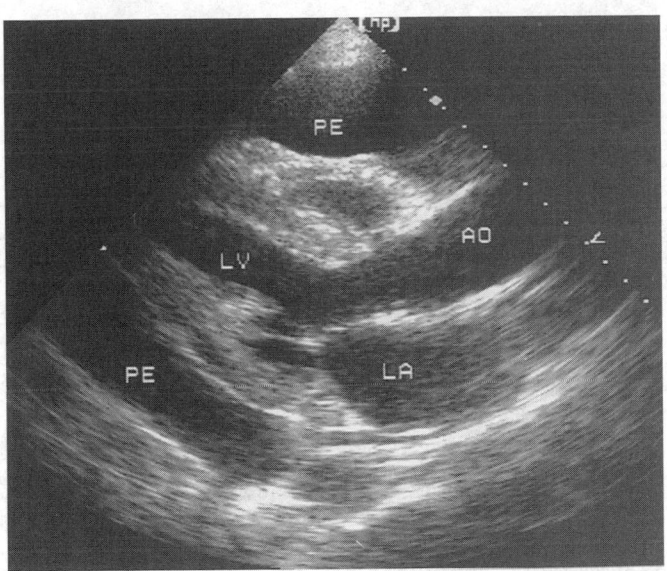

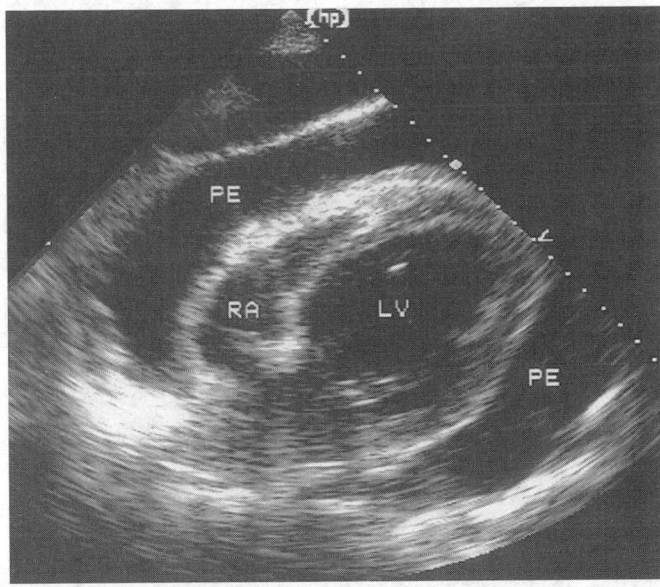

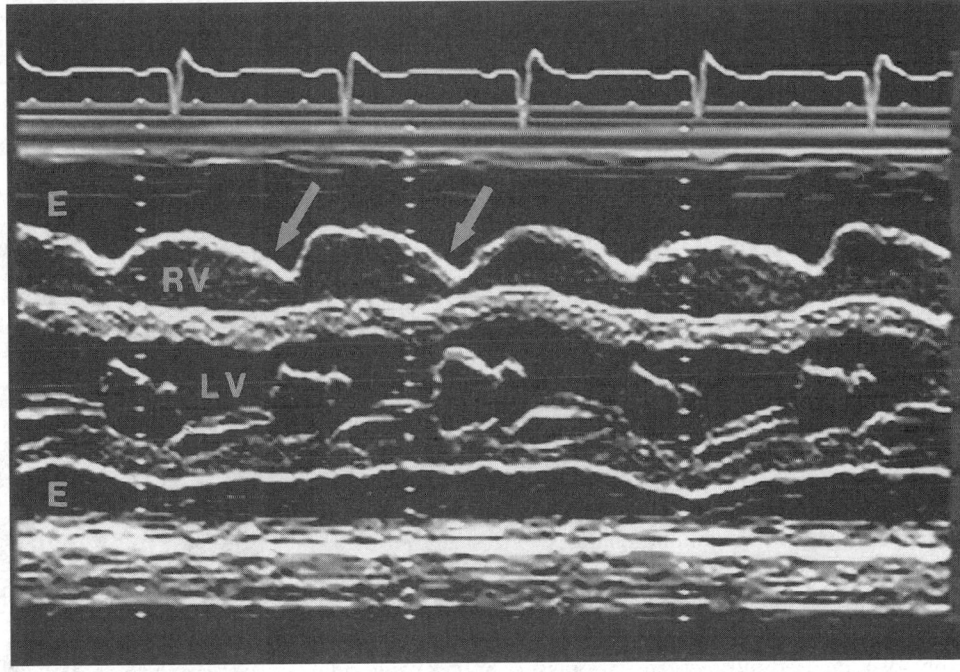

FIGURE 14-135

A. Moderate pericardial effusion (PE) on parasternal long-axis imaging. AO = aorta; LV – left ventricle; LA = left atrium. *B.* Right ventricular compression in cardiac tamponade (subcostal plane). RA = right atrium; LV = left ventricle; PE = pericardial effusion. *C.* M-mode image of cardiac tamponade and right ventricular diastolic collapse. The right ventricular (RV) free wall (*arrows*) moves posteriorly toward the interventricular septum during diastole. E = effusion; LV = left ventricle.

the pericardial space, creating the mechanism of electrical alternans.[704] In general, small effusions are seen posteriorly rather than anteriorly on supine imaging.[696] Moderate-sized (100 to 500 mL) nonloculated effusions are present both anterior and posterior to the heart.[696] Large nonloculated effusions (>500 mL) are circumferential and frequently allow free motion of the heart within the fluid-filled space.[696,697]

Distinguishing between pericardial and pleural effusions is occasionally difficult with echocardiography.[705] If these conditions coexist, the pericardium usually can be identified as a linear density separating fluid in the two spaces. The parasternal long-axis view is often helpful in differentiating the disorders. The descending aorta is a mediastinal structure;

therefore pericardial effusions will often separate the heart and descending aorta, while pleural effusions are seen inferior and posterior to the aorta[705] (Fig. 14-137). In cases of large pleural effusions, atelectatic lung tissue also may be present (Fig. 14-137). Subcostal views are often valuable and may yield the only satisfactory transthoracic images in postoperative or posttraumatic cases. The inferior vena cava also can be imaged in this view; if the vessel does not display inspiratory collapse greater than 50 percent of its maximum diameter, elevated right atrial pressure is present.[366]

On parasternal images, a echolucent space is sometimes visualized anterior to the RV.[706] Although this finding may represent pericardial fluid, it usually is caused by epicardial

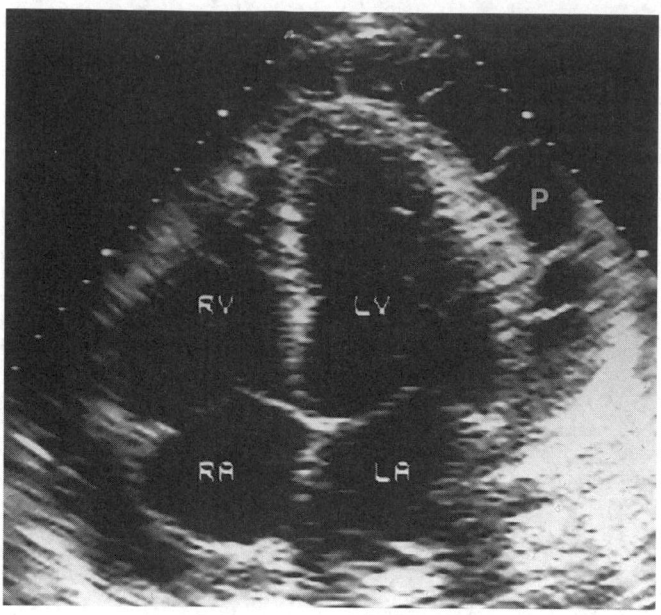

FIGURE 14-136

Apical four-chamber image in a case of malignant pericardial effusion (P). Numerous fibrinous strands are seen within the effusion. LA = left atrium; RA = right atrium; RV = right ventricle; LV = left ventricle. (From Blanchard DG, DeMaria AN. Cardiac and extracardiac masses: Echocardiographic evaluation. In: Skorton DJ, Schelbert HR, Wolf GL, Brundage BH, eds. *Marcus' Cardiac Imaging,* 2d ed. Philadelphia: Saunders, 1996:452–480, with permission.)

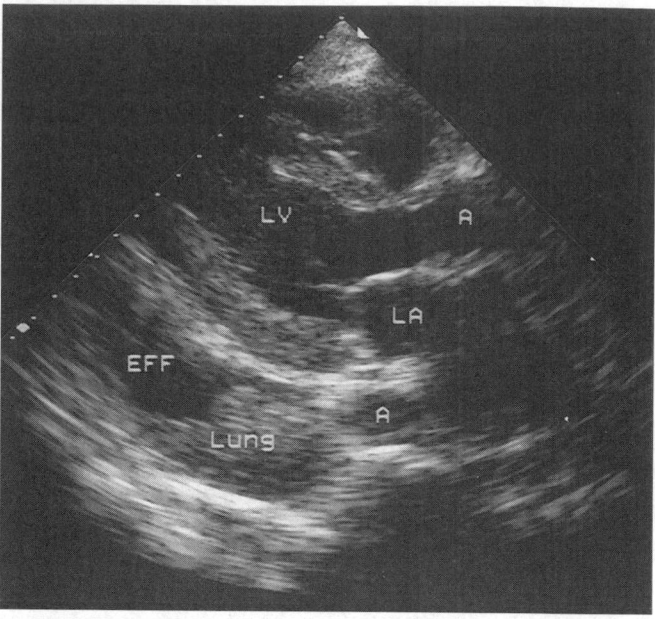

FIGURE 14-137

Parasternal long-axis view in a patient with a pleural effusion (EFF) posterior to the heart. Atelectatic lung tissue is present within the effusion. LA = left atrium; LV = left ventricle; A = aorta.

fat (without effusion) and has no pathologic significance. Therefore, the diagnosis of pericardial effusion based solely on the presence of this anterior clear space should be avoided.

Cardiac Tamponade

As the pericardium is a relatively noncompliant membrane that adapts slowly to volume changes, pericardial effusions (especially those that accumulate rapidly) may limit cardiac filling and cause cardiac tamponade. Echocardiography can help diagnose this condition by detecting (1) morphologic signs of increased intrapericardial pressure and (2) abnormal intracardiac flow patterns caused by tamponade and enhanced ventricular interdependence.[707,708]

As diastolic pressures are slightly lower in the right heart than the left, the right atrium and ventricle are usually the first chambers to exhibit evidence of increased intrapericardial pressure. High intrapericardial pressure can cause compression or collapse of right heart chambers.[707,709,710] Invagination of the right atrial wall during atrial systole is a sensitive (but not specific) sign of tamponade (Fig. 14-138).[709] Diastolic collapse or "buckling" of the RV free wall is a more specific sign of tamponade, and can be visualized both on 2D and M-mode imaging[707,710] (Fig. 14-135*B* and *C*). In cases of localized tamponade or severe RV hypertrophy, left atrial or ventricular diastolic collapse may be the first sign of tamponade.[711,712]

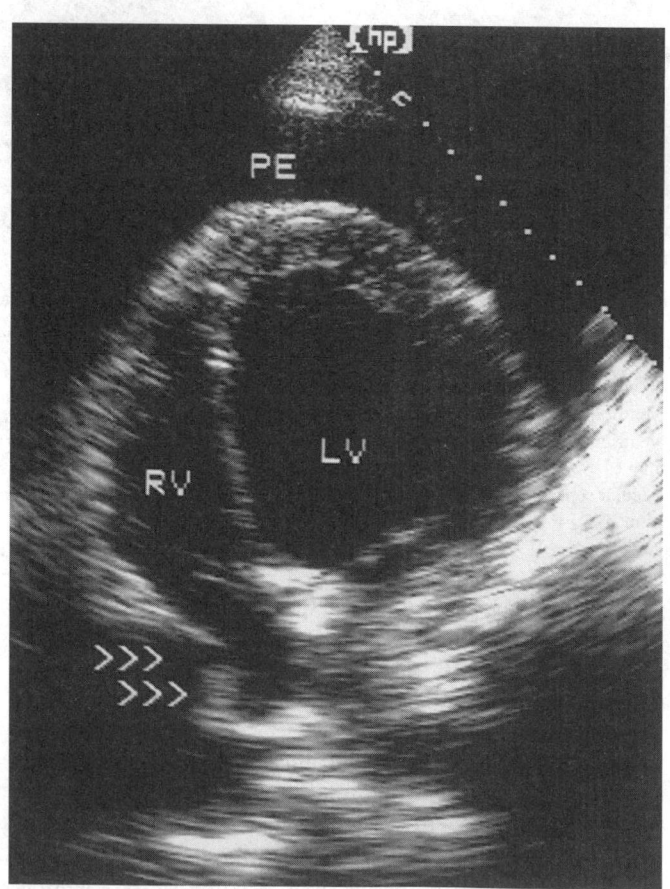

FIGURE 14-138

Right atrial collapse (*arrows*) in cardiac tamponade. PE = pericardial effusion; LV = left ventricle; RV = right ventricle.

Doppler echocardiographic recordings in patients with tamponade have demonstrated an enhancement or exaggeration of the normal respiratory variation in ventricular inflow and outflow.[708,713] Thus, transmitral and LVOT velocities decrease significantly with inspiration, probably because of enhanced ventricular interdependence and a marked decrease in the transmitral diastolic gradient during inspiration (Fig. 14-139). The latter is caused both by high intrapericardial pressure as well as leftward motion of the interventricular septum from increased RV filling.[708] Although cardiac tamponade remains a clinical diagnosis, echocardiography has significantly improved the detection of hemodynamic effects from pericardial fluid, especially in early and equivocal cases. Studies have also indicated that when echocardiography is used to direct pericardiocentesis to the site of greatest fluid accumulation, the risks associated with blind pericardial puncture are decreased.[714]

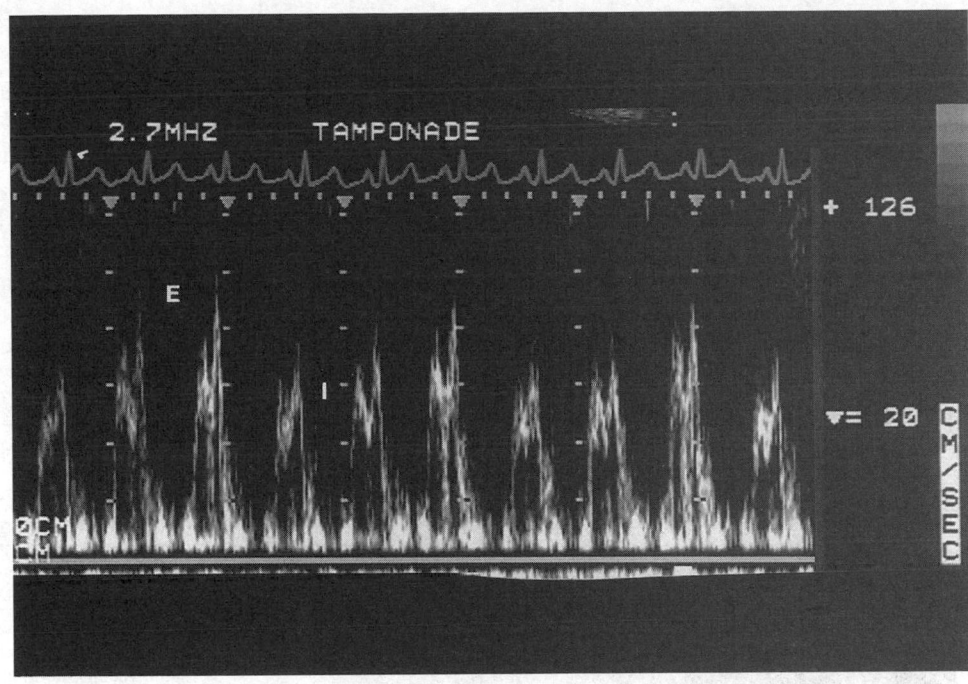

FIGURE 14-139

Pulsed-wave Doppler tracing of left ventricular inflow in cardiac tamponade (apical transducer position). There is abnormal respiratory variation in the peak E wave velocity (which varies from 60 to 80 cm/s). E = expiration; I = inspiration.

Constrictive Pericarditis

The diagnosis of constrictive pericarditis is sometimes difficult to establish, even by cardiac catheterization. 2D and M-mode echocardiography may provide evidence of thickened pericardial tissue by demonstrating increased reflectivity and multiple parallel moving echoes in the area of the pericardium.[699,700] The criteria for pericardial thickening on echocardiogram are imperfect, however, as the normal pericardium is an echodense, highly reflective structure with a gain-dependent signal.[715] Paradoxical septal motion may be seen on M-mode with constriction, as can an abnormal inspiratory interventricular septal "bounce"[716] and limited diastolic motion of the posterior LV wall.[717] A dilated inferior vena cava that does not collapse on deep inspiration is indicative of high right atrial pressure and may be observed on 2D imaging in constrictive pericarditis.[716]

The utility of Doppler recordings in evaluating constrictive pericarditis has been shown in several recent studies.[550,701,718–723] As with cardiac tamponade, pericardial constriction produces exaggerated respiratory variation in the isovolumic relaxation time and in flow velocities within right and left ventricles, pulmonary veins, and hepatic vein.[701,718,722] A respiratory variation of >20 percent in peak mitral E velocity favors the diagnosis of constriction over restrictive cardiomyopathy, while little respiratory variation and a shortened E deceleration time favor restrictive physiology.[701] Doppler echocardiographic criteria for constriction have been validated prospectively and may help predict clinical response to pericardiectomy.[721] Unfortunately, exaggerated respiratory flow variation is not specific for pericardial constriction and also can be seen in chronic obstructive pulmonary disease and asthma.[724] In these cases, Doppler examination of superior vena cava flow is useful: patients with asthma will have increased flow toward the heart during inspiration, while limited forward flow will be seen in constriction (the echocardiographic equivalent of Kussmaul's sign).[724] Recently, respiratory variation in the peak velocity and duration of continuous-wave Doppler TR spectral envelopes has been shown to reflect accurately the enhanced ventricular interaction seen in constrictive pericarditis.[725]

IMAGING OF THE CORONARY ARTERIES

The ability to visualize the proximal segments of the left and right coronary arteries was initially demonstrated by Weyman et al.[417] Subsequent studies established the ability of color and spectral Doppler examination to image and record the velocity of flow from transthoracic and transesophageal approaches, particularly with regard to the left anterior descending coronary artery.[418–420] However, visualization of the coronary arteries by echocardiography has not achieved a significant role in clinical practice because the resolution of the technique is at the limit of vessel size and the vessels are circuitous and move vigorously, often coursing in and out of

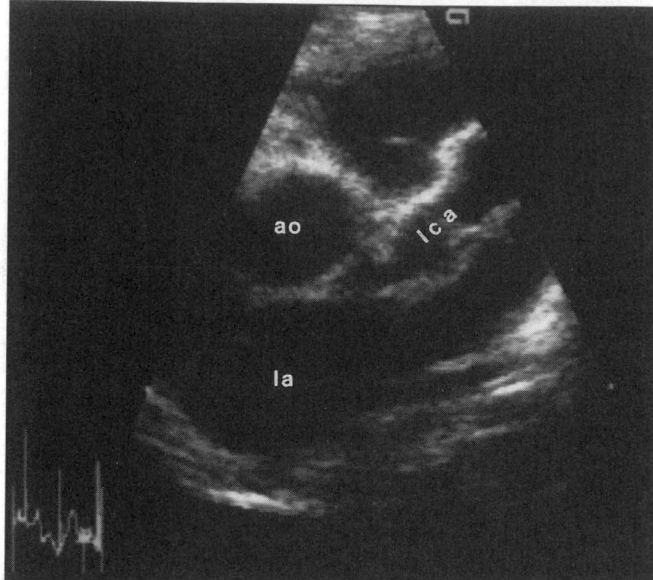

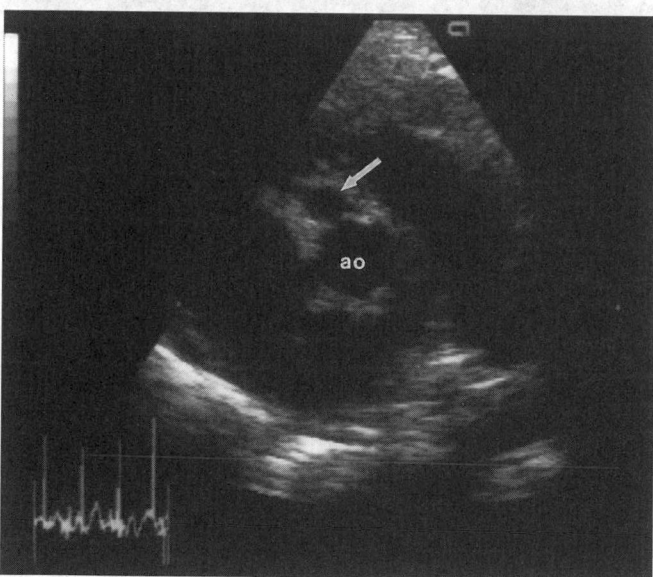

FIGURE 14-140

Parasternal short-axis images of coronary artery aneurysms associated with Kawasaki's disease. In *A*, the proximal left coronary artery (LCA) is diffusely dilated and aneurysmal. A proximal right coronary artery aneurysm (*arrow*) is shown in *B*. AO = aorta, LA = left atrium. (Courtesy of Victor Lucas, MD and Paul Grossfeld, MD.)

the beam path. Despite these limitations, transthoracic imaging has proven useful for the diagnosis and follow-up of patients with Kawasaki disease and coronary involvement[726-728] (Fig. 14-140) and may also help distinguish normal from atherosclerotic coronary arteries.[729]

The coronary arteries are routinely imaged with TEE, which can detect proximal stenoses, atherosclerosis, and con-

genital abnormalities of the coronaries more accurately than surface imaging.[730-732] Doppler TEE analysis also has been used to determine coronary low reserve.[733,734]

Visualization of mid- and distal coronary arteries is problematic with both TTE and TEE. Recent advances in technology and contrast agents, however, may significantly improve capabilities in this area. Figure 14-141 (Plate 44) shows color flow within a septal coronary artery. This image was produced by an instrument utilizing a carrier frequency range of 5 to 7 MHz, rather than the more commonly used range of 2.5 to 3.5 MHz. This area of echocardiography is expanding rapidly and clinical applications will grow in the future.[735,736]

FIGURE 14-141
See color Plate 44.

REFERENCES

1. Krumholz HM, Douglas PS, Goldman L, Waksmonski C. Clinical utility of transthoracic two-dimensional and Doppler echocardiography. *J Am Coll Cardiol* 1994; 24:125–231.
2. Daniel WG, Mügge A. Transesophageal echocardiography. *N Engl J Med* 1995; 332:1268–1279.
3. Handschumacher MD, Lethor JP, Siu SC, Mele D, Rivera JM, Picard MH, et al. A new integrated system for three-dimensional echocardiographic reconstruction: Development and validation for ventricular volume with application in human subjects. *J Am Coll Cardiol* 1993; 21:743–753.
4. Rovai D, DeMaria AN, L'Abbate A. Myocardial contrast echo effect: The dilemma of coronary blood flow and volume. *J Am Coll Cardiol* 1995; 26:12–17.
5. Elder I, Hertz CH. The use of ultrasonic reflectoscope for the continuous recording of movement of heart walls. *Kungl Fysiorgr Sallski Fund Forhandl* 1954; 24:40–45.
6. Wild JJ, Crawford HD, Reid JM. Visualization of the excised human heart by means of reflected ultrasound or echocardiography. *Am Heart J* 1958; 54:903–906.
7. Feigenbaum H, Zaky A. Use of diagnostic ultrasound in clinical cardiology. *J Indiana State Med Assoc* 1966; 49:140–152.
8. Bom N, Lancee CT Jr, Van Zwieten G, Kloster FE, Roelandt J, et al. Multiscan echocardiography: I. Technical description. *Circulation* 1973; 48;1066–1073.
9. Griffith JM, Henry WL. A sector scanner for real time two-dimensional echocardiography. *Circulation* 1974; 49:1147–1152.
10. Eggelton RC, Johnston KW. Real time mechanical scanning system compared with array techniques. *IEEE Proc Sonics Ultrasounds* 1974; Cat. No. 74-CH0896-1:16.
11. VonRamm OT, Thurstone FL. Cardiac imaging using a phased array ultrasound system. I: System design. *Circulation* 1976; 53:258–262.
12. Baker DW. Pulsed ultrasonic Doppler blood-flow sensing. *IEEE Trans Sonics Ultrasonics* 1970; SU-17(3).
13. Hatle L, Angelsen B, Tromsdal A. Noninvasive assessment of atrioventricular pressure half-time by Doppler ultrasound. *Circulation* 1979; 60:1096–1104.
14. Hatle L, Angelsen BA, Tromsdal A. Noninvasive assessment of aortic stenosis by Doppler ultrasound. *Br Heart J* 1980; 3:284–292.
15. Omoto R. *Color Atlas of Real-Time Two-Dimensional Doppler Echocardiography,* 2d ed. Tokyo: Sindan-to-Chiryo; 1987.
16. Hanrath P, Kremer P, Langenstein BA, Matsumoto M, Bleifield W. Transoesophageale Eckokardiographie: Ein neues Verfahren zur dynamischen Ventrikelfunktionsanalyse. *Dtsch Med Wochenschr* 1981; 106:523–525.
17. Seward JB, Khanderia BK, Oh JK, Hughes RW, Edwards WD, Nichols BA, et al. Transesophageal echocardiography: Technique, anatomic correlations, implementation and clinical applications. *Mayo Clin Proc* 1988; 63:649–680.
18. Wells, PNT. *Ultrasonics in Clinical Diagnosis,* 2d ed. New York: Churchill Livingstone; 1977.
19. Kremkau FW, Taylor KJW. Artifacts in ultrasound imaging. *J Ultrasound Med* 1986; 15:227–237.
20. Yeh E. Reverberations in echocardiograms. *J Clin Ultrasound* 1977; 5:84–86.

21. Weyman AE. Physical principles of ultrasound. In: Weyman AE, ed. *Principles and Practice of Echocardiography,* 2d ed. Philadelphia: Lea & Febiger; 1994:3–28.

22. Mann DL, Gillam LD, Weyman AE. Cross-sectional echocardiographic assessment of regional left ventricular performance and myocardial perfusion. *Prog Cardiovac Dis* 1986; 29:1–52.

23. Rose JL, Goldberg BB. *Basic Physics in Diagnostic Ultrasound.* New York: Wiley; 1979.

24. DeMaria AN, Miller RR, Amsterdam EA, Markson W, Mason DT. Mitral valve early diastolic closing velocity in the echocardiogram: Relation to sequential diastolic flow and ventricular compliance. *Am J Cardiol* 1976; 37:693–700.

25. Konecke L, Feigenbaum H, Chang S. Abnormal mitral valve motion in patients with elevated left ventricular end diastolic pressure. *Circulation* 1973; 47:989–996.

26. Sahn DJ, DeMaria A, Kisslo J, Weyman AE. Recommendations regarding quantitation in M-mode echocardiography: Results of a survey of echocardiographic measurements. *Circulation* 1978; 58:1072–1083.

27. Nanda NC, Gramiak R, Manning EB. Echocardiographic recognition of the congenital bicuspid aortic valve. *Circulation* 1974; 49:870–875.

28. Rasmussen S, Corya BC, Phillips JF, Black MJ. Unreliability of M-mode left ventricular dimensions for calculating stroke volume and cardiac output in patients without heart disease. *Chest* 1982; 81:614–619.

29. Teichholz LE, Kreulen T, Herman MV, Gorlin R. Problems in echocardiographic volume determinations: Echocardiographic-angiographic correlations in the presence or absence of synergy. *Am J Cardiol* 1976; 37:7–11.

30. McDonald IG, Feigenbaum H, Chang S. Analysis of left ventricular wall motion by reflected ultrasound: Application to assessment of myocardial function. *Circulation* 1972; 46:14–25.

31. Feigenbaum H: Echocardiographic examination of the left ventricle. *Circulation* 1975; 51:1–7.

32. Massie BM, Schiller NB, Ratshin RA, Parmley WW. Mitral-septal separation: New echocardiographic index of left ventricular function. *Am J Cardiol* 1977; 39:1008–1016.

33. Ophir J, Maklad NF. Digital scan converters in diagnostic ultrasound imaging. *Proc IEEE* 1979; 67.

34. Henry WL, DeMaria A, Gramiak R, King DL, Kisslo JA, Popp RL, et al. Report of the American Society of Echocardiography: Nomenclature and standards in two-dimensional echocardiography. *Circulation* 1980; 62:212–217.

35. Feigenbaum H. The echocardiographic examination. In: Feigengaum H. *Echocardiography,* 5th ed. Philadelphia: Lea & Febiger; 1994:68–133.

36. Weyman AE. *Principles and Practice of Echocardiography,* 2d ed. Philadelphia: Lea & Febiger; 1994.

37. Teichholtz LE, Kreulen T, Herman MV, Gorlin R. Problems in echocardiographic volume determinations: Echocardiographic-angiographic correlations in the presence or absence of asynergy. *Am J Cardiol* 1976; 37:7–11.

38. Wyatt HL, Heng MK, Meerbaum S, Gueret P, Hestenes J, Dula E, et al. Cross-sectional echocardiography: II. Analysis of mathematic models for quantifying volume of formalin fixed left ventricle. *Circulation* 1980; 61:1119–1125.

39. Wyatt HL, Meerbaum S, Heng MK, Gueret P, Corday E. Cross-sectional echocardiography: III. Analysis of mathematic models for quantifying volume of symmetric and asymmetric left ventricles. *Am Heart J* 1980; 100:821–828.

40. Schiller NB, Acquatella H, Ports TA, Drew D, Goerke J, Ringertz H, et al. Left ventricular volume from paired biplane two-dimensional echocardiography. *Circulation* 1979; 60:547–555.

41. Folland ED, Parisi AF, Moynihan PF, Jones DR, Feldman CL, Tow DE. Assessment of left ventricular ejection fraction and volumes by real-time, two-dimensional echocardiography and radionuclide techniques. *Circulation* 1979; 60:760–766.

42. Stamm RB, Carabello BA, Mayers DL, Martin RP. Two-dimensional echocardiographic measurement of left ventricular ejection fraction: Prospective analysis of what constitutes an adequate determination. *Am Heart J* 1982; 104:136–144.

43. Gueret P, Corday E. Etude quantitative de la fonction ventriculaire gauche par l'echocardiographie bidimensionnelle. *Arch Mal Coeur* 1981; 74:329–336.

44. Starling MR, Crawford MH, Sorensen SG, Levi B, Richards KI, O'Rourke RA. Comparative accuracy of apical biplane cross-sectional echocardiography and gated equilibrium radionuclide angiography for estimating left ventricular size and performance. *Circulation* 1981; 63:1075–1084.

45. Erbel R, Schweizer P, Lambertz H, Henn G, Meyer J, Krebs W, et al. Echoventriculography—A simultaneous analysis of two-dimensional echocardiography and cineventriculography. *Circulation* 1983; 67;205–215.

46. Huang ZH, Long WY, Xie G-Y, Kwan OL, DeMaria AN. Comparison of gray-scale and B-color ultrasound images in evaluating left ventricular systolic function in coronary artery disease. *Am Heart J* 1992; 123:395.

47. Perez JE, Waggoner AD, Barzilai B, Melton HE, Miller JG, Sobel BE. On-line assessment of ventricular function by automatic boundary detection and ultrasonic backscatter imaging. *J Am Coll Cardiol* 1992; 19:313.

48. Lang RM, Vignon P, Weinert L, Bednarz J, Korcarc C, Sandelsky J, et al. Echocardiographic quantification of regional left ventricular wall motion with color kinesis. *Circulation* 1996; 93:1877–1885.

49. Duong AM, Blanchard DG, Cotter B, Wheeler K, Donaghey L, Kwan OL, et al. Endomyocardial movement in patients with disturbed diastolic filling dynamics: assessment by acoustic quantitation color kinesis (abstr). *J Am Soc Echocardiogr* 1996; 9:365.

50. Doppler JC. Ueber das farbige Licht der Dopplesterne und einiger anderer Gestirne des Himmels. *Abhandlungen der Konigl, Bohmischen Gesellschaft der Wissenschaften,* 5th ser. 1842; 2:465.

51. Franklin DL, Schlegal W, Rushmer RF. Blood flow measured by Doppler frequency shift of backscattered ultrasound. *Science* 1961; 134:564.

52. Baker DW. Pulsed ultrasonic Doppler flow sensing. *IEEE Trans Sonics Ultrasonics* 1970; 17:170.

53. Hatle L, Angelsen B. *Doppler Ultrasound in Cardiology: Physical Principles and Clinical Applications,* 2d ed. Philadelphia: Lea & Febiger; 1984.

54. Baker DW, Rubenstein SA, Lorch GS. Pulsed Doppler echocardiography: Principles and applications. *Am J Med* 1977; 63:69–80.

55. Burns PM. The physical principles of Doppler and spectral analysis. *J Clin Ultrasound* 1987; 15:567–590.

56. Bom K, deBoo J, Rijsterborgh H. On the aliasing problem in pulsed Doppler cardiac studies. *J Clin Ultrasound* 1984; 12:559–567.

57. Steward WJ, Galvin KA, Gillam LD, Guyer DE, Weyman AE. Comparison of high pulse repetition frequency and continuous wave Doppler echocardiography in the assessment of high flow velocity in patients with valvular stenosis and regurgitation. *J Am Coll Cardiol* 1985; 6:565–571.

58. Otto CM, Pearlman AS. Measurement of high flow velocities using pulsed Doppler echocardiography. *Echocardiography* 1985; 2:141–152.

59. Omoto R. *Color Atlas of Real-Time Two-Dimensional Doppler Echocardiography,* 2d ed. Tokyo, Shindan-to-Chiryo, 1987.

60. Bommer W, Miller L. Real time two-dimensional color flow Doppler-enhanced imaging in the diagnosis of cardiovascular disease. (abstract) *Am J Cardiol* 1982; 49:944.

61. Stevenson JG. Appearance and recognition of basic concepts in color flow imaging. *Echocardiography* 1989; 6:451.

62. Omoto R, Kasai C. Physics and instrumentation of Doppler color flow mapping. *Echocardiography* 1987; 4:467.

63. Feigenbaum H. Appendix: Echocardiographic measurements and normal values. In: Feigenbaum H, ed. *Echocardiography,* 5th ed. Philadelphia, Lea & Febiger, 1994:658–683.

64. Rakowski H, Appleton C, Chan K-L, Dumesnil JG, Honos G, Jue J, et al. Canadian consensus recommendations for the measurement and reporting of diastolic dysfunction by echocardiography. *J Am Soc Echocardiogr* 1996; 9:736–760.

65. Nishimura RA, Housmans PR, Hatle LK, Tajik AJ. Assessment of diastolic function of the heart: Background and current applications of Doppler echocardiography: Part I. Physiologic and pathophysiologic features. *Mayo Clin Proc* 1989; 64:71–81.

66. Nishimura RA, Hatle LK, Abel MD, Tajik AJ. Assessment of diastolic function of the heart: Background and current applications of Doppler echocardiography: Part II. Clinical studies. *Mayo Clin Proc* 1989; 4:181–204.

67. Stoddard MF, Pearson AC, Kern MJ, Ratcliff J, Mrosek DG, Labovitz AJ. Left ventricular diastolic function: Comparison of pulsed Doppler echocardiographic and hemodynamic indexes in subjects with and without coronary artery disease. *J Am Coll Cardiol* 1989; 13:327–336.

68. Klein AL, Hatle L, Burstow DJ, Seward JB, Kyle RA, Bailey KR. Doppler characterization of left ventricular diastolic function in cardiac amyloidosis. *J Am Coll Cardiol* 1989; 13:1017–1026.

69. Cohen GI, Pietrolungo JF, Thomas JD, Klein AL. A practical guide to assessment of ventricular diastolic function using Doppler echocardiography. *J Am Coll Cardiol* 1996; 27;1753–1760.

70. Thomas JD, Weyman AE. Echocardiographic Doppler evaluation of left ventricular diastolic function: Physics and physiology. *Circulation* 1991; 84:977–990.

71. Chen C, Rodriguez L, Levine RA, Weyman AE, Thomas JD. Noninvasive measurement of the time constant of left ventricular relaxation using the continuous-wave Doppler velocity of mitral regurgitation. *Circulation* 1992; 86:272–278.

72. Nishimura RA, Schwartz RS, Tajik AJ, Holmes DR Jr. Noninvasive measurement of rate of left ventricular relaxation by Doppler echocardiography: validation with simultaneous cardiac catheterization. *Circulation* 1993; 88:146–55.

73. Pai RG, Suzuki M, Heywood JT, Ferry DR, Shah PM. Mitral A velocity wave transit time to the outflow tract as a measure of left ventricular diastolic stiffness: Hemodynamic correlations in patients with coronary artery disease. *Circulation* 1994; 84:553–7.

74. Yamamoto K, Masuyama T, Doi Y, et al. Noninvasive assessment of left ventricular relaxation using continuous-wave Doppler aortic regurgitant velocity curve: Its comparative value to the mitral regurgitation method. *Circulation* 1995; 91:192–200.

75. Appleton CP, Hatle LK, Popp RL. Cardiac tamponade and pericardial effusion: Respiratory variation in transvalvular flow velocities studied by Doppler echocardiography. *J Am Coll Cardiol* 1988; 11:1020–1030.

76. Xie G-Y, Berk MR, Smith MD, Gurley JC, DeMaria AN. Prognostic value of Doppler transmitral flow patterns in patients with congestive heart disease. *J Am Coll Cardiol* 1994; 24:132–139.

76a. Pozzoli M, Traversi E, Cioffi G, Stenner R, Sanarico M, Tavazzi L. Loading manipulations improve the prognostic value of Doppler evaluation of mitral flow in patients with chronic heart failure. *Circulation* 1997; 95:1222–1230.

77. Miyatake K, O'Kamoto M, Knoshita N, Owa M, Nakasone I, Sakakibara H. Augmentation of atrial contribution to left ventricular inflow with aging as assessed by intracardiac Doppler flowmetry. *Am J Cardiol* 1984; 53:586–589.

78. Bryg RJ, Williams GA, Labovitz AJ. Effect of aging on left ventricular diastolic filling in normal subjects. *Am J Cardiol* 1987; 59:971–974.

79. Harrison M, Clifton G, Pennell A, DeMaria A. Effect of heart rate on left ventricular diastolic transmitral flow velocity patterns assessed by Doppler echocardiography in normal subjects. *Am J Cardiol* 1991; 67:622–627.

80. Appleton C, Carucci M, Henry C, Olajos M. Influence of incremental changes in heart rate on mitral flow velocity: assessment of lightly sedated, conscious dogs. *J Am Coll Cardiol* 1991; 17:227–236.

81. Dabestani A, Takenaka K, Allen B, Gardin JM, Fischer J, Russell D, et al. Effects of spontaneous respiration on left ventricular filling assessed by pulsed Doppler echocardiography. *Am J Cardiol* 1988; 61:1356–1358.

82. Drinkovic N, Smith MD, Wisenbaugh T, Friedman B, Kwan OL, DeMaria AN. Influence of sampling site upon the ratio of atrial to early diastolic transmitral flow velocities by Doppler (abstr). *J Am Coll Cardiol* 1987; 9:16A.

83. Pearson AC, et al. Effect of sample volume location on pulsed Doppler-echocardiographic evaluation of left ventricular filling. *Am J Cardiac Imaging* 1988; 24:40.

84. Dittrich HC, Blanchard DG, Wheeler K, McCann HA, Donaghey L. Influence of Doppler sample location on the assessment of changes in mitral inflow velocity profiles. *J Am Soc Echocardiogr* 1990; 3:303–309.

85. Choong CY, Abascal VM, Thomas JD, Guerrero JL, McGlow S, Weyman AE. Combined influence of ventricular loading and relaxation on the transmitral flow velocity profile in dogs measured by Doppler echocardiography. *Circulation* 1988; 78:672–683.

86. Berk MR, Xie G, Kwan OL, Knapp C, Evans J, Kotchen T, et al. Reduction of left ventricular preload by lower body negative pressure alters Doppler transmitral filling patterns. *J Am Coll Cardiol* 1990; 16:1387–1392.

87. Appleton CP, Galloway JM, Gonzalez MS, Gabella M, Basnight MA. Estimation of left ventricular filling pressures using two dimensional and Doppler echocardiography in adult patients with cardiac disease: Additional value of analyzing left atrial size, left atrial ejection fraction and the difference in duration of pulmonary venous and mitral flow velocity at atrial contraction. *J Am Coll Cardiol* 1993; 22:1972–1982.

88. Rossvoll O, Hatle LK. Pulmonary venous flow velocities recorded by transthoracic Doppler ultrasound: Relation to left ventricular diastolic pressures. *J Am Coll Cardiol* 1993; 21:1687–1696.

89. Gardin JM. Doppler measurements of aortic blood flow velocity and acceleration: Load-independent indexes of left ventricular performance? *Am J Cardiol* 1989; 64:935–936.

90. Harrison MR, Smith ND, Nissen SE, Grayburn PA, DeMaria AN. Use of exercise Doppler echocardiography to evaluate cardiac drugs: Effects of propranolol and verapamil on aortic blood flow velocity and acceleration. *J Am Coll Cardiol* 1988; 11:1002–1009.

91. Gardin JM, Tobis J, Henry WL. Evaluation of dilated cardiomyopathy by pulsed Doppler echocardiography. *Am Heart J* 1983; 106:1057–1065.

92. Chen C, Rodriguez L, Guerrero JL, Marshall S, Levine RA, Weyman AE, et al. Noninvasive estimation of the instantaneous first derivative of left ventricular pressure using continuous-wave Doppler echocardiography. *Circulation* 1991; 83:2101–2110.

93. William GA, Labovitz AJ. Doppler estimation of cardiac output: Principles and pitfalls. *Echocardiography* 1987; 4:355–374.

94. Huntsman LL, Stewart DK, Barnes SR, Franklin SB, Colocousis JS, Hessel EA. Noninvasive Doppler determination of cardiac output in man—Clinical validation. *Circulation* 1983; 67:593–602.

95. Ihlen H, Amlie JP, Dale J, Forgang K, Nitter-Hauge S, Otterstad JA. Determination of cardiac output by Doppler echocardiography. *Br Heart J* 1984; 51:54–60.

96. Sahn DJ. Determination of cardiac output by echocardiographic Doppler methods: Relative accuracy of various sites for measurement. *J Am Coll Cardiol* 1985; 6:663–664.

97. Lewis JF, Kuo KC, Nelson JG, Limacher MC, Quinones MS. Pulsed Doppler echocardiographic determination of stroke volume and cardiac output: Clinical validation of two new methods using the apical window. *Circulation* 1984; 70:425–431.

98. Huntsman LL, Stewart DK, Barnes SR, Franklin SB, Colocousis JS, Hessel EA. Noninvasive Doppler determination of cardiac output in man—Clinical validation. *Circulation* 1983; 67:593–602.

99. Looyenga DS, Liebson PR, Bone RC, Balk RA, Messer JV. Determination of cardiac output in critically ill patients by dual beam Doppler echocardiography. *J Am Coll Cardiol* 1989; 13:340–347.

100. Meijboom EJ, Horowitz S, Valdes-Cruz LM, Sahn DJ, Larson DF, Lima CO. A Doppler echocardiographic method for calculating volume flow across the tricuspid valve: Correlative laboratory and clinical studies. *Circulation* 1985; 71:551–556.

101. Zhand Y, Nitter-Hauge N, Ihlen H, Myhre E. Doppler echocardiographic measurement of cardiac output using the mitral orifice method. *Br Heart J* 1985; 53:130–136.

102. Valdes-Cruz LM, Horowitz S, Goldberg SJ, Allen HD. The mitral valve orifice method for noninvasive two-dimensional echo Doppler determinations of cardiac output. *Circulation* 1983; 67:872–877.

103. Kitabatake A, Inoue M, Asao M, Ito H, Mauyami T, Tanouchi J, et al. Noninvasive evaluation of the ratio of pulmonic to systemic flow in atrial septal defect by duplex Doppler echocardiography. *Circulation* 1984; 69:73–79.

104. Kurokawa S, Takahashi M, Katoh Y, Muramitsu J, Kikawada R, et al. Noninvasive evaluation of the ratio of pulmonary to systemic flow in ventricular septal defect by means of Doppler two-dimensional echocardiography. *Am Heart J* 1988; 116:1033–1044.

105. Barron JV, Sahn DJ, Valdes-Cruz LM, Lima CO, Goldberg SJ, Grenadier E, Allen HD. Clinical utility of two-dimensional Doppler echocardiographic techniques for estimating pulmonary to systemic flow ratios in children with left to right shunting, atrial septal defect, ventricular septal defect and patent ductus arteriosus. *J Am Coll Cardiol* 1984; 3:169–178.

106. Cloez JL, Schmidt KG, Birk E, Silverman NH. Determination of pulmonary to systemic blood flow ratio in children by a simplified Doppler echocardiographic method. *J Am Coll Cardiol* 1988; 11:825–830.

107. Nichol PM, Boughner DR, Persaud J. Noninvasive assessment of mitral insufficiency by Doppler ultrasound. *Circulation* 1976; 54:656–661.

108. Zhang Y, et al. Quantification of mitral regurgitation by Doppler echocardiography. *Eur Heart J* 1987; 8:59–62.

109. Blumlein S, Bouchard A, Schiller NB, Dae M, Byrd BF, Posts T, Botvinick EH, et al. Quantitation of mitral regurgitation by Doppler echocardiography. *Circulation* 1986; 74:306–314.

110. Xie G-Y, Berk MR, Smith ND, DeMaria AN. A simplified method for determining regurgitant fraction by Doppler echocardiography in patients with aortic regurgitation. *J Am Coll Cardiol* 1994; 24:1041–1045.

111. Skjaerpe T, Hegrenaes L, Hatle L. Noninvasive estimation of valve area in patients with aortic stenosis by Doppler ultrasound and two-dimensional echocardiography. *Circulation* 1985; 72:810–818.

112. Warth DC, Stewart WJ, Block PC, Weyman AE. A new method to calculate aortic valve area without left heart catheterization. *Circulation* 1984; 70:978–983.

113. Oh JK, Taliercio CP, Holmes DR, Reeder GS, Bailey KR, Seward JB. Prediction of the severity of aortic stenosis by Doppler aortic valve area determination: Prospective Doppler-catheterization correlation in 100 patients. *J Am Coll Cardiol* 1988; 11:1227–1234.

114. Richards KL, Cannon SR, Miller JF, Crawford MH. Calculation of aortic valve area by Doppler echocardiography: A direct application of the continuity equation. *Circulation* 1986; 73:964–969.

115. Zoghbi WA, Farmer KL, Soto JG, Nelson JG, Quinones MA. Accurate noninvasive quantitation of stenotic aortic valve area by Doppler echocardiography. *Circulation* 1986; 73:452–459.

116. Hegrenaes L, Hatle L. Aortic stenosis in adults: Non-invasive estimation of pressure differences by continuous wave Doppler echocardiography. *Br Heart J* 1985; 54:396–404.

117. Currie PJ, Seward JB, Reeder GS, Vlictstra RE, Bresnahan DR, Bresnahan JF, et al. Continuous wave Doppler echocardiographic assessment of severity of calcific aortic stenosis: A simultaneous Doppler-catheter correlative study in 100 adult patients. *Circulation* 1985; 71:1162–1169.

118. Smith MD, Dawson PL, Elion JL, Booth DC, Handshoe R, Kwan OL, et al. Correlation of continuous wave Doppler velocities with cardiac catheterization gradients: An experimental model of aortic stenosis. *J Am Coll Cardiol* 1985; 6:1306–1314.

119. Holen J, Waag RC, Gramiak R, Violante MR, Roes A. Doppler ultrasound in orifice flow: In vitro studies of the relationship between pressure difference and fluid velocity. *Ultrasound Med Biol* 1985; 11:261–266.

120. Currie PJ, Hagler DJ, Seward JB, Reeder GS, Fyfe DA, Bove AA, et al. Instantaneous pressure gradient: A simultaneous Doppler and dual catheter correlative study. *J Am Coll Cardiol* 1986; 7:800–806.

121. Hatle L, Brubakk A, Tromsdal A, Angelsen B. Noninvasive assessment of pressure drop in mitral stenosis by Doppler ultrasound. *Br Heart J* 1978; 40:131–140.

122. Stamm RB, Martin RP. Quantification of pressure gradients across stenotic valves by Doppler ultrasound. *J Am Coll Cardiol* 1983; 2:707–718.

123. Perez JE, Ludbrook PA, Ahumada GG. Usefulness of Doppler echocardiography in detecting tricuspid valve stenosis. *Am J Cardiol* 1985; 55:601–602.

124. Lee RT, Lord CP, Plappert T, Sutton MS. Prospective Doppler echocardiographic evaluation of pulmonary artery diastolic pressure in the medical intensive care unit. *Am J Cardiol* 1989; 64:1366–1370.

125. Berger M, Haimowitz A, van Tosh A, Berdoff RL, Goldberg E. Quantitative assessment of pulmonary hypertension in patients with tricuspid regurgitation using continuous wave Doppler ultrasound. *J Am Coll Cardiol* 1985; 6:359–365.

126. Yock PG, Popp RL. Noninvasive estimation of right ventricular systolic pressure by Doppler ultrasound in patients with tricuspid regurgitation. *Circulation* 1984; 70:657–662.

127. Nishimura RA, Tajik AJ. Determination of left-sided pressure gradients by utilizing Doppler aortic and mitral regurgitant signals. Validation by simultaneous dual catheter and Doppler studies. *J Am Coll Cardiol* 1988; 11:317–321.

128. Pai RG, Bansal RC, Shah PM. Doppler-derived rate of left ventricular pressure rise: Its correlation with the postoperative left ventricular function in mitral regurgitation. *Circulation* 1990; 84:514–520.

129. Requarth JA, Goldberg SJ, Vasko SD, Allen HD, et al. In vitro verification of Doppler prediction of transvalve pressure gradient and orifice area in stenosis. *Am J Cardiol* 1984; 53:1369–1373.

130. Krabill KA, Tamura T, Phil C, Sahn DJ, Chung KJ, Yoganathan AP, et al. The shape of regurgitant jets: In vitro flow visualization and color flow Doppler studies (abstr). *J Am Coll Cardiol* 1987; 9:110A.

131. Thomas JD, Davidoff R, Wilkins GT, Choong CX, Svizzero T, Weyman AE. The volume of a color flow jet varies directly with flow rate and inversely with orifice size: A hydrodynamic in vitro assessment (abstr). *J Am Coll Cardiol* 1988; 11:19A.

132. Thomas JD, O'Shea JP, Rodriguez L. The impact of orifice geometry on the shape of jets: An in vitro color Doppler flow study. *J Am Coll Cardiol* 1991; 17:901–908.

133. Wong M, Matsumura M, Suzuki K, Omoto R. Technical and biologic sources of variability in the mapping of aortic, mitral and tricuspid color flow jets. *Am J Cardiol* 1987; 60:847–851.

134. Simpson IA, Valdes-Cruz LM, Sahn DJ, Murillo A, Tamura T, Chung KJ. Color Doppler flow mapping of simulated in vitro regurgitant jets: Evaluation of the effects of orifice size and hemodynamic variables. *J Am Coll Cardiol* 1989; 13:1195.

135. Chao K, Moises VA, Shandas R, Elkadi T, Sahn DJ, Weintraub R. Influence of the Coanda effect on color Doppler jet area and color encoding; In vitro studies using color Doppler flow mapping. *Circulation* 1992; 85:333–341.

136. Chen C, Thomas JD, Anconina J, Harrigan P, Mueller L, Picard MH. Impact of impinging wall jet on color Doppler quantification on mitral regurgitation. *Circulation* 1991; 84:712–720.

137. Matsumura M, Wong M, Omoto R. Assessment of Doppler color flow mapping in quantification of aortic regurgitation—Correlations and influencing factors. *Jpn Circ J* 1989; 53:735–746.

138. Dittrich HC, ed. *Clinical Transesophageal Echocardiography.* St. Louis: Mosby Year Book; 1992.

139. Blanchard DG, Kimura BJ, Dittrich HC, DeMaria AN. Transesophageal echocardiography of the aorta. *JAMA* 1994; 272:546–551.

140. Freeman WK, Seward JB, Khanderia BK, Tajik AJ, eds. *Transesophageal Echocardiography.* Boston: Little, Brown; 1994.

141. Seward JB, Khanderia BK, Edwards WD, Oh JK, Freeman WK, et al. Biplanar transesophageal echocardiography: Anatomic correlations, image orientation, and clinical applications. *Mayo Clin Proc* 1990; 65:1193–1213.

142. Roelandt JRTC, Thomsom IR, Vletter WB, Brommersma P, Bom N, Linker DT. Multiplane transesophageal echocardiography: Latest evolution in an imaging revolution. *J Am Soc Echocardiogr* 1992; 5:361–367.

143. Daniel WG, Mügge A. Transesophageal echocardiography. *N Engl J Med* 1995; 332:1268–1279.

144. Taams MS, Gussenhoven EJ, Bos E, De Jaegere P, Roelandt J, Sutherland G, et al. Enhanced morphological diagnosis in infective endocarditis by transesophageal echocardiography. *Br Heart J* 1990; 63:109–113.

145. Shively BK, Gurule FT, Roldan CA, Leggett JH, Schiller NB. Diagnostic value of transesophageal compared with transthoracic echocardiography in infective endocarditis. *J Am Coll Cardiol* 1991; 18:391–397.

146. Bansal RC, Graham BM, Jutzy KR, Shakudo M, Shah PM. Left ventricular outflow tract to left atrial communication secondary to rupture of mitral-aortic intervalvular fibrosa in infective endocarditis: Diagnosis by transesophageal echocardiography and color flow imaging. *J Am Coll Cardiol* 1990; 15:499–504.

147. Daniel WG, Mügge A, Martin RP, Lindert O, Hausmann D, Nonnast-Daniel B, et al. Improvement in the diagnosis of abscesses associated with endocarditis by transesophageal echocardiography. *N Engl J Med* 1991; 324:795–800.

148. Erbel R, Rohmann S, Drexler M, Mohr-Kahaly S, Gerharz CD, Iversen S, et al. Improved diagnostic value of echocardiography in patients with infective endocarditis by transesophageal approach: A prospective study. *Eur Heart J* 1988; 9:43–53.

149. Yvorchuk KJ, Chan K-L. Application of transthoracic and transesophageal echocardiography in the diagnosis and management of infective endocarditis. *J Am Soc Echocardiogr* 1994; 14:294–308.

150. Mügge A, Daniel WG, Frank G, Lichtlen PR. Echocardiography in infective endocarditis: Reassessment of prognostic implications of vegetation size determined by the transthoracic and the transesophageal approach. *J Am Coll Cardiol* 1989; 14:631–638.

151. Yoshida K, Yoshikawa J, Yamaura Y, Hozumi T, Akasaka T, Fukaya T. Assessment of mitral regurgitation by biplane transesophageal color Doppler flow mapping. *Circulation* 1990; 82:1121–1126.

152. Klein AL, Obarski TP, Stewart WJ, Casale PN, Pearce GL, Husbands K, et al. Transesophageal Doppler echocardiography of pulmonary venous flow: A new marker of mitral regurgitation severity. *J Am Coll Cardiol* 1991; 18:518–526.

153. Castello R, Pearson AC, Lenzen P, Labovitz AJ. Effect of mitral regurgitation on pulmonary venous velocities derived from transesophageal echocardiography and color-guided pulsed Doppler imaging. *J Am Coll Cardiol* 1991; 17:1499–1605.

154. Smith MD, Harrison MR, Pinton R, Kandil H, Kwan OL, DeMaria AN. Regurgitant jet size by transesophageal compared with transthoracic Doppler color flow imaging. *Circulation* 1991; 83:79–86.

155. Hoffmann R, Flachskampf FA, Hanrath P. Planimetry of orifice area in aortic stenosis using multiplane transesophageal echocardiography. *J Am Coll Cardiol* 1993; 22:529–534.

156. Freeman WK. Diseases of the thoracic aorta: utility of transesophageal echocardiography. In: Freeman WK, Seward JB, Khanderia BK, Tajik AJ, eds. Transesophageal Echocardiography. Boston: Little, Brown; 1994:425–467.

157. Keren A, Kim CB, Hu BS, Eyngoria I, Billingham ME, Mitchell RA et al. Accuracy of biplane and multiplane transesophageal echocardiography in diagnosis of typical acute aortic dissection and intramural hematoma. *J Am Coll Cardiol* 1996; 28:627–636.

158. Cigarroa JE, Isselbacher EM, DeSanctis RW, Eagle KA. Diagnostic imaging in the evaluation of suspected aortic dissection. *N Engl J Med* 1993; 328:35–43.

159. Pearson AC. Transthoracic echocardiography vs. transesophageal echocardiography in detecting cardiac source of embolism. *Echocardiography* 1993; 10:397–403.

160. Hoffman T, Kasper W, Meinertz T, Geibel A, Just H. Echocardiographic evaluation of patients with clinically suspected arterial emboli. *Lancet* 1990; 336:1421–1424.

161. DeRook FA, Comess KA, Albers GW, Popp RL. Transesophageal echocardiography in the evaluation of stroke. *Ann Intern Med* 1992; 117:922–932.

162. Manning WJ, Weintraub RM, Waksmonski CA, Haering JM, Rooney PS, Maslow AD, et al. Accuracy of transesophageal echocardiography for identifying left atrial thrombi: A prospective, intraoperative study. *Ann Intern Med* 1995; 123:817–822.

163. Kronzon I, Tunick PA. Transesophageal echocardiography as a tool in the evaluation of patients with embolic disorders. *Prog Cardiovasc Dis* 1993; 36:39–60.

164. Daniel WG, Kronzon I, Mügge A, eds. *Cardiogenic Embolism.* Baltimore: Williams & Wilkins; 1996.

165. Click RL, Espinosa RE, Khanderia BK. Source of embolism: Utility of transesophageal echocardiography. In: Freeman WK, Seward JB, Khanderia BK, Tajik AJ, eds. *Transesophageal Echocardiography.* Boston: Little, Brown; 1994:469–499.

166. Zenker G, Erbel R, Krämer G, Mohr-Kahaly S, Drexler M, Harnoncourt K. Transesophageal two-dimensional echocardiography in young patients with cerebral ischemic events. *Stroke* 1988; 19:345–348.

167. Amarenco P, Cohen A, Tzourio C, Bertrand B, Hommel M, Besson G. Atherosclerotic disease of the aortic arch and the risk of ischemic stroke. *N Engl J Med* 1994; 331:1474–1479.

168. Amarenco P, Duyckaerts C, Tzourio C, Henin D, Bousser M-G, Hauw J-J. The prevalence of ulcerated plaques in the aortic arch in patients with stroke. *N Engl J Med* 1992; 326:221–5.

169. Merino A, Haupman P, Badimon L, Badimon JJ, Cohen M, Fuster V, et al. Echocardiographic "smoke" is produced by an interaction of erythrocytes and plasma proteins modulated by shear forces. *J Am Coll Cardiol* 1992; 20:1661–1668.

170. The French Study of Aortic Plaques in Stroke Group. Atherosclerotic disease of the aortic arch as a risk factor for recurrent ischemic stroke. *N Engl J Med* 1996; 334:1216–1221.

171. Khatibzadeh M, Mitusch R, Stierle U, Gromoll B, Sheikhzadeh A. Aortic atherosclerotic plaques as a source of systemic embolism. *J Am Coll Cardiol* 1996; 27:664–669.

172. Dittrich HC, McCann HA, Walsh TP, Blanchard DG, Oppenheim GE, Waack TC, et al. Transesophageal echocardiography in the evaluation of prosthetic and native aortic valves. *Am J Cardiol* 1990; 66:758–760.

173. Van den Brink RBA, Visser CA, Basart DCG, Duren DR, De Jong AP, Dunning AJ. Comparison of transthoracic and transesophageal color Doppler flow imaging in patients with mechanical prostheses in the mitral valve position. *Am J Cardiol* 1989; 63:1471–1474.

174. Nellessen U, Schnittger I, Appleton CP, Masuyama T, Bolger A, Fishell TA, et al. Transesophageal two-dimensional echocardiography and color Doppler flow velocity mapping in the evaluation of cardiac valve prostheses. *Circulation* 1988; 78:848–855.

175. Kronzon I, Tunick PA, Freedberg RS, Trehan N, Rosenzweig BP, Schwinger ME. Transesophageal echocardiography is superior to transthoracic echocardiography in the diagnosis of sinus venous atrial septal defect. *J Am Coll Cardiol* 1991; 17:537–542.

176. Fyfe DA. Transesophageal echocardiography for congenital heart disease. *J Invasive Cardiol* 1992; 4;459–67.

177. Joffe II, Jacobs LE, Lampert C, Owen AA, Loli AW, Kotler MN. Role of echocardiography in perioperative management of patients undergoing open heart surgery. *Am Heart J* 1996; 131:162–176.

178. Dan M, Bonato R, Mazzucco A, Bortolotti U, Faggian G, Giron G, et al. Value of transesophageal echocardiography during repair of congenital heart defects. *Ann Thorac Surg* 1990; 50:637–643.

179. Fyfe DA, Kline CH. Transesophageal echocardiography for congenital heart disease. *Echocardiography* 1991; 8:573–586.

180. Mehta RH, Helmcke F, Nanda NC, Hsiung M, Pacifo AD, Hsu TL. Transesophageal Doppler color flow mapping assessment of atrial septal defect. *J Am Coll Cardiol* 1990; 16:1010–1016.

181. Kremer P, Calahan M, Beaupre P, Schroeder E, Hanrath P, Keinrich H, et al. Intraoperative monitoring by two-dimensional echocardiography. *Anesthetist* 1985; 34:111–117.

182. Smith JS, Cahalan MK, Benefiel DJ, Byrd BF, Lurz FW, Shapiro WA, et al. Intraoperative detection of myocardial ischemia in high risk patients: Electrocardiography versus two-dimensional transesophageal echocardiography. *Circulation* 1985; 72:1015–1021.

183. Dahm M, Iverson S, Schmidt FS, Drexler M, Erbel R, Oelert H. Intraoperative evaluation of reconstruction of the atrioventricular valves by transesophageal echocardiography. *Thorac Cardiovasc Surg* 1987; 35(special issue 2):140–142.

184. Chan KL, Seward JB, Khandheria BK, Gersh BJ, McGregor CGA, et al. Transesophageal echocardiography in critically ill patients. *Am J Cardiol* 1990; 61:1492–1495.

185. Alam M. Transesophageal echocardiography in critical care units: Henry Ford hospital experience and review of the literature. *Prog Cardiovasc Dis* 1996; 38:315–328.

186. Foster E, Schiller NB. The role of transesophageal echocardiography in critical care: The UCSF experience. *J Am Soc Echocardiogr* 1992; 5:368–374.

187. Oh JK, Seward JB, Khanderia BK, Gersh BJ, McGregor CGA, Freeman WK, et al. Transesophageal echocardiography in critically ill patients. *Am J Cardiol* 1990; 66;1492–1495.

188. Hellenbrand WE, Fahey JT, McGowan FX, Weltin GG, Kleinman CS. Transesophageal echocardiographic guidance of transcatheter closure of atrial septal defect. *Am J Cardiol* 1990; 66:207–213.

189. Tong AD, Rothman A, Shiota T, Rice M, Blanchard DG, Hellenbrand W, et al. Interventional cardiac catheterization under transesophageal echocardiographic guidance. *Am Heart J* 1995; 129:827–831.

190. Ballal RS, Mahan EF III, Nancy NC, Dean LS. Utility of transesophageal echocardiography in interatrial septal puncture during percutaneous mitral balloon commissurotomy. *Am J Cardiol* 1990; 66:230–232.

191. Jaarsma W, Visser CA, Suttorp MJ, Haagen FDH, Ernest S. Transesophageal echocardiography during percutaneous balloon mitral valvuloplasty. *J Am Soc Echocardiogr* 1990; 3:384–391.

192. Gramiak R, Shah PM: Echocardiography of the aortic root. *Invest Radiol* 1968; 3:356–366.

193. Meltzer RS, Tichner EG, Shaines TP, Popp RL. The source of ultrasonic contrast effect. *J Clin Ultrasound* 1980; 8:121–127.

194. Kerber RE, Kioschos JM, Lauer RM: Use of an ultrasonic contrast method in the diagnosis of valvular regurgitation and intracardiac shunts. *Am J Cardiol* 1974; 34:722–727.

195. Valdes-Cruz LM, Sahn DJ: Seminar on contrast two-dimensional echocardiography: applications and new developments: Part II. *J Am Coll Cardiol* 1984; 3:978–985.

196. Lechat P, Mas JL, Lascault G, Loron PH, Thread M, Klimczac M. Prevalence of patent foramen ovale in patients with stroke. *N Engl J Med* 1988; 318:1148–1152.

197. DeMaria AN. Echocardiographic visualization of myocardial perfusion by left heart and intracoronary injection of echo contrast agents (abstr). *Circulation* 1980; 60(suppl 3):II-143.

198. Armstrong WF, Mueller TM, Kinney EL, Tickner EG, Dillon JC, Feigenbaum H. Assessment of myocardial perfusion abnormalities with contrast enhanced two-dimensional echocardiography. *Circulation* 1982; 66:166–173.

199. Kaul S, Jayaween AR, Glasheen WP, Villanueva FS, Gutgesell HP, Spotnitz WD. Myocardial contrast echocardiography and the transmural distribution of flow: A critical appraisal during myocardial ischemia not associated with infarction. *J Am Coll Cardiol* 1992; 20:1005–1016.

200. Crouse LJ, Cheirif J, Hanly DE, Kisslo JA, Labovitz AJ, Raichlen JJ. Opacification and border delineation improvement in patients with suboptimal endocardial border definition in routine echocardiography: Results of the phase III Albunex multicenter trial. *J Am Coll Cardiol* 1993; 22:1494–1500.

201. Moore CA, Smucker ML, Kaul S. Myocardial contrast echocardiography in humans: I. Safety—a comparison with routine coronary arteriography. *J Am Coll Cardiol* 1986; 8:1066–1072.

202. Sabia PJ, Powers ER, Jayaweera AR, Ragosta M, Kaul S. Functional significance of collateral blood flow in patients with recent acute myocardial infarction. *Circulation* 1992; 85:2080–2089.

203. Lim Y-J, Nanto S, Masuyama T, Kodama K, Ikedu T, Kitabatake A. Visualization of subendocardial myocardial ischemia with myocardial contrast echocardiography in humans. *Circulation* 1989; 79:233–244.

204. Agati L, Voci P, Bilotta F, Luongo R, Autone C, Penco M, et al. Influence of residual perfusion within the infarct zone on the natural history of left ventricular dysfunction after acute myocardial infarction: A myocardial contrast echocardiographic study. *J Am Coll Cardiol* 1994; 24:336–342.

205. Perchet H, Dupouy P, Duval-Moulin A-M, Hittinger LUC, Pelle G, Brun P, Castaigne H, et al. Improvement of subendocardial myocardial perfusion after percutaneous transluminal coronary angioplasty: A myocardial contrast echocardiography study with correlation between myocardial contrast reserve and Doppler coronary reserve. *Circulation* 1995; 91:1419–1426.

206. Ismail S, Jayaweera AR, Goodman NC, Camarano GP, Skyba DM, Kaul S. Detection of coronary stenoses and quantification of the degree and spatial extent of blood flow mismatch during coronary hyperemia with myocardial contrast echocardiography. *Circulation* 1995; 91:821–830.

207. Sabia PJ, Powers ER, Ragosta M, Sarembock IJ, Burwell LR, Kaul S. An association between collateral blood flow and myocardial viability in patients with recent myocardial infarction. *N Engl J Med* 1992; 327:1825–1831.

208. Ito H, Tomooka T, Sakai N, Yu H, Higashino Y, Fuji K, et al. Lack of myocardial perfusion immediately after successful thrombolysis: A predictor of poor recovery of left ventricular function in anterior myocardial infarction. *Circulation* 1992; 85:1699–1705.

209. Ito H, Maruyama A, Iwakura K, Takiuchi J, Masuyama T, Hori M, et al. Clinical implications of "no reflow" phenomenon: A predictor of complications and left ventricular remodeling in reperfused anterior wall myocardial infarction. *Circulation* 1996; 93:223–228.

210. Villanueva FS, Camarano G, Ismail S, Goodman NC, Sklenar J, Kaul S. Coronary reserve abnormalities in the infarcted myocardium: Assessment of myocardial viability immediately versus late after reflow by contrast echocardiography. *Circulation* 1996; 94:748–754.

211. vonBibra H, Becher H, Firschke C, Schlief R, Emslander HP, Schomig A. Enhancement of mitral regurgitation and normal left atrial color Doppler flow signals with peripheral venous injections of a saccharide-based contrast agent. *J Am Coll Cardiol* 1993; 22:521–528.

212. Himelman RB, Stulbarg MS, Lee E, Kuecherer HF, Schiller NB. Noninvasive evaluation of pulmonary artery systolic pressure during dynamic exercise by saline-enhanced Doppler echocardiography. *Am Heart J* 1990; 119:685–688.

213. Nakatani S, Imanishi T, Terasawa A, Beppu S, Nagata S, Miyatake K. Clinical application of transpulmonary contrast enhanced Doppler technique in the assessment of severity of aortic stenosis. *J Am Coll Cardiol* 1992; 20:973–975.

214. Cotter B, Kwan OL, Cha YM, Dittrich H, Bhargava V, DeMaria AN. Dose-response characteristics, time-course, and hemodynamic responses to QW3600, an ultrasonic contrast agent capable of myocardial opacification by intravenous injection (abstr). *J Am Coll Cardiol* 1994; 23:393A.

215. Dittrich HC, Bales GL, McFerran BA, Kuvelas MT, Hunt RM. Reproducibility of myocardial opacification using FS069, a new intravenously administered ultrasound contrast agent (abstr). *J Am Coll Cardiol* 1995; 25:204A.

216. Porter TR, Xie F, Kresfeld A, Kilzer K. Noninvasive identification of acute myocardial ischemia and reperfusion with contrast ultrasound using intravenous perfluoropropane-exposed sonicated dextrose albumin. *J Am Coll Cardiol* 1995; 26:33–40.

217. Mulvagh SL, Foley DA, Aeschbacher BC, Klarich KK, Seward JB. Second harmonic imaging of an intravenously administered echocardiographic contrast agent: Visualization of coronary arteries and measurement of coronary blood flow. *J Am Coll Cardiol* 1996; 27;1519–1525.

218. Cotter B, Kwan OL, Cha YM, Mahmud E, Kimura B, Calisi C, et al. augmentation of contrast enhancement by second harmonic imaging: Experimental studies with new agents (abstr). *J Am Soc Echocardiogr* 1995; 8:345.

219. Porter TR, Xie F, Kricsfeld D, Armbruster RW. Improved myocardial contrast with second harmonic transient ultrasound response imaging in humans using intravenous perfluorocarbon-exposed sonicated dextrose albumin. *J Am Coll Cardiol* 1996; 27:1497–1501.

220. Ohmori K, Cotter B, Kwan OL, DeMaria AN. Relation of flow velocity and signal intensity to the amplification of contrast opacification produced by intermittent ultrasound emission (abstr). *J Am Soc Echocardiogr* 1996; 9:384.

221. Mottley JG, Giakoumopoulos M, Porter T, Xie F, Meltzer R. Acoustic bubble destruction is a possible mechanism for transient response imaging (abstr). *J Am Soc Echocardiogr* 1996; 9:385.

222. Tajik AJ, Seward JB, Hagler DJ, Mair DD, He JJ. Two-dimensional real-time ultrasonic imaging of the heart and great vessels. Technique, image orientation, structures, identification, and validation. *Mayo Clin Proc* 1978; 53:271–303.

223. DeMaria AN, Bommer W, Joye JA, Lee G, Bouteller J, Mason DT. Value and limitations of cross-sectional echocardiography of the aortic valve in the diagnosis and quantification of valvular aortic stenosis. *Circulation* 1980; 62:304–312.

224. Nanda NC, Gramiak R. Evaluation of bi-cuspid valves by two-dimensional echocardiography. *Am J Cardiol* 1978; 41:372 (abstract).

225. Weyman AE, Feigenbaum H, Hurwitz RA. Localization of left ventricular outflow obstruction by cross-sectional echocardiography. *Am J Med* 1976; 60:33–38.

226. Williams DE, Sahn DJ, Friedman WF. Cross-sectional echocardiographic localization of sites of left ventricular outflow obstruction. *Am J Cardiol* 1976; 37:250–255.

227. Fan PH, Kapur KK, Nanda NC. Color-guided Doppler echocardiographic assessment of aortic valve stenosis. *J Am Coll Cardiol* 1988; 12:441–449.

228. Roger VL, Tajik AJ, Reeder GS, Hayes SN, Mullany CJ, Bailey KR, et al. Effect of Doppler echocardiography on utilization of hemodynamic cardiac catheterization in the preoperative evaluation of aortic stenosis. *Mayo Clin Proc* 1996; 71:141–149.

229. DeFilippi CR, Willett DL, Brickner ME, Appleton CP, Yancy CW, Eichhorn CJ, et al. Usefulness of dobutamine echocardiography in distinguishing severe from nonsevere valvular aortic stenosis in patients with depressed left ventricular function and low transvalvular gradients. *Am J Cardiol* 1995; 75:191–194.

230. Ciobanu M, Abbasi AS, Allen M, Hermer A, Spellberg R. Pulsed Doppler echocardiography in the diagnosis and estimation of severity of aortic insufficiency. *Am J Cardiol* 1982; 49:339–343.

231. Klein AL, Davison MB, Vonk G, Tajik AJ. Doppler echocardiographic assessment of aortic regurgitation: Uses and limitations. *Cleve Clin J Med* 1992; 59:359–368.

232. Robertson WS, Stewart J, Armstrong WF, Dillon JC, Feigenbaum H. Reverse doming of the anterior mitral leaflet with severe aortic regurgitation. *J Am Coll Cardiol* 1984; 3:431–436.

233. Grayburn PA, Smith MD, Handshoe R, Friedman BJ, DeMaria AN. Detection of aortic insufficiency by standard echocardiography, pulsed Doppler echocardiography and auscultation. *Ann Intern Med* 1986; 104:599–605.

234. Pridie RB, Beham R, Oakley CM. Echocardiography of the mitral valve in aortic valve disease. *Br Heart J* 1971; 33:296–304.

235. Guiney TE, Davies MJ, Parker DJ, Leech GJ, Leathan A. The etiology and course of isolated severe aortic regurgitation; a clinical, pathological and echocardiographic study. *Br Heart J* 197; 53:358–368.

236. Perry GJ, Nelmcke F, Nanda NC, Byard C, Soto B. Evaluation of aortic insufficiency by Doppler color flow mapping. *J Am Coll Cardiol* 1987; 9:952–959.

237. Masuyama T, Kodama K, Kitabatake A, Nanto S, Sato H, Uematsu M, et al. Noninvasive evaluation of aortic regurgitation by continuous-wave Doppler echocardiography. *Circulation* 1986; 73:460–466.

238. Grayburn PA, Handshoe R, Smith MD, Harrison MR, DeMaria AN. Quantitative assessment of the hemodynamic consequences of aortic regurgitation. *J Am Coll Cardiol* 1987; 10:135–141.

239. Beyer RW, Ramirez M, Josephson MA, Shah PM. Correlation of continuous wave Doppler assessment of chronic aortic regurgitation with hemodynamics and angiography. *Am J Cardiol* 1987; 60:852–856.

240. Samstad SO, Hegrenaes L, Skjaerpe T, Hatle L. Half time of the diastolic aortoventricular pressure difference by continuous wave Doppler ultrasound: A measure of the severity of aortic regurgitation? *Br Heart J* 1989; 61:336–343.

241. Omoto R, Yokote Y, Takamoto S, Kyo S, Ueka K, Asano H, et al. The development of real-time two-dimensional Doppler echocardiography and its clinical significance in acquired valvular disease. *Jpn Heart J* 1984; 25:325–340.

242. Quinones MA, Young JB, Waggoner AD, Ostojic MC, Ribeiro LG, Miller RR: Assessment of pulsed Doppler echocardiography in detection and quantification of aortic and mitral regurgitation. *Br Heart J* 1980; 44:612–620.

243. Touch T, Prasquier R, Nitenberg A, Zuttere DD, Gourgon R. Assessment and follow-up of patients with aortic regurgitation by an updated Doppler echocardiographic measurement of the regurgitant fraction in the aortic arch. *Circulation* 1985; 72:819–824.

244. Takenaka K, Dabelstani A, Gardin JM, Russell D, Clark S, Allfie A, et al. A simple Doppler echocardiographic method for estimating severity of aortic regurgitation. *Am J Cardiol* 1986; 57:1340–1343.

245. Perlman AS, Otto CM. Quantification of valvular regurgitation. *Echocardiography* 1987; 4:271–287.

246. Fioretti P, Roelandt J, Sclavo M, Domeniccucci S, Haalebos M, Bos E, Hugenholtz PG. Postoperative regression of left ventricular dimensions in aortic insufficiency: A long-term echocardiographic study. *J Am Coll Cardiol* 1985; 5:856–861.

247. Siemienzuk D, Greenberg B, Morris C, Massie B, Wilson RA, Topic N, et al. Chronic aortic insufficiency: Factors associated with progression to aortic valve replacement. *Ann Intern Med* 1989; 110:587–592.

248. Bonow RO, Dodd JT, Maron BJO, Gara PT, White GG, McIntosh CC, et al. Long-term serial change in left ventricular function and reversal of ventricular dilatation after valve replacement for chronic aortic regurgitation. *Circulation* 1988; 78:1108–1120.

249. Kodas E, Enriquez-Sarano M, Tajik AJ, Mullany CJ, Bailey KR, Seward JB. Surgery for aortic regurgitation in women: Contrasting indications and outcomes compared with men. *Circulation* 1996; 94:2472–2478.

250. Henry WL, Bonow RO, Borer JS, Ware JH, Kent KM, Redwood DR, et al. Observations on the optimum time for operative intervention for aortic regurgitation: I. Evaluation of the results of aortic valve replacement in symptomatic patients. *Circulation* 1980; 61:471–483.

251. Seward JB, Tajik AJ. Non-invasive visualization of the entire thoracic aorta: A new application of wide-angle two dimensional sector echocardiographic technique. *Am J Cardiol* 1979; 43:387. (abstract)

252. DeMaria AN, Bommer W, Newmann A, Weinert L, Bogren H, Mason DT. Identification and localization of aneurysms of the ascending aorta by cross-sectional echocardiography. *Circulation* 1979; 59:755–761.

253. Granato JE, Dee P, Gibson RS. Utility of two-dimensional echocardiography in suspected aortic dissection. *Am J Cardiol* 1985; 56:123–129.

254. Eagle KA, DeSanctis RW. Aortic dissection. *Curr Prob Cardiol* 1989; 14:231–278.

255. Ballal RS, Nanda NC, Gatewood R, D'Arcy B, Samdarshi TE, Holman WL, et al. Usefulness of transesophageal echocardiography in assessment of aortic dissection. *Circulation* 1991; 84:1903–1914.

256. Nienaber CA, Spielman RP, von Kodolitsch Y, Siglow V, Piepho A, Jaup T, et al. Diagnosis of thoracic aortic dissection: Magnetic resonance imaging versus transesophageal echocardiography. *Circulation* 1992; 85:434–447.

257. Nienaber CA, von Kodlitsch Y, Nicolas V, Siglow V, Piepho A, Brochoff C, et al. The diagnosis of thoracic aortic dissection by noninvasive imaging procedures. *N Engl J Med* 1993; 328:1–9.

258. Robbins RC, McManus RP, Mitchell RS, Latter DR, Moon MR, Olinger GN, et al. Management of patients with intramural hematoma of the thoracic aorta. *Circulation* 1993; 88(part 2):1–10.

259. Nienaber CA, von Kodolitsch Y, Petersen B, Loose R, Helmchen U, Haverich A, et al. Intramural hemorrhage of the thoracic aorta: Diagnostic and therapeutic implications. *Circulation* 1995; 92:1465–1472.

260. Eisenberg MJ, Geraci SJ, Schiller NB. Screening for abdominal aortic aneurysms during transthoracic echocardiography. *Am Heart J* 1995; 130:109–115.

261. Come PC, Fortuin NJ, White RI Jr McKusick VA. Echocardiographic assessment of cardiovascular abnormalities in the Marfan syndrome. *Am J Med* 1983; 74:465–474.

262. Roman MJ, Rosen SE, Kramer-Fox R, Devereux RB. Prognostic significance of the pattern of aortic root dilation in the Marfan syndrome. *J Am Coll Cardiol* 1993; 22:1470–1476.

263. Shores J, Berger KR, Murphy EA, Pyeritz RE. Progression of aortic dilatation and the benefit of long-term beta-adrenergic blockade in Marfan's syndrome. *N Engl J Med* 1994; 30:1335–1341.

264. Recchia D, Sharkey AM, Bosner MS, Kouchoukos NT, Wickline SA. Sensitive detection of abnormal aortic architecture in Marfan syndrome with high-frequency ultrasonic tissue characterization. *Circulation* 1994; 91:1036–1043.

265. Kiefaber RW, Tabakin BS, Coffin LH, Gibson TC. Unruptured sinus of Valsalva aneurysm with right ventricular outflow obstruction diagnosed by two-dimensional and Doppler echocardiography. *J Am Coll Cardiol* 1986; 7:438–442.

266. Lewis RS, Agathangelou NE. Echocardiographic diagnosis of unruptured sinus of Valsalva aneurysm. *Am Heart J* 1984 107:1025–1027.

267. Chia BL, Ee BK, Choo MH, Yan PC. Ruptured aneurysm of sinus of Valsalva: Recognition by Doppler color flow mapping. *Am Heart J* 1988; 115:686–688.

268. Alboliras E, Seward J, Hagler D, Danielson GK, Puga FJ, Tajik AJ. Impact of two-dimensional and Doppler echocardiography on care of children aged two years and younger. *Am J Cardiol* 1988; 61:166–169.

269. Rice MJ, Seward JB, Hagler DJ, Mair DD, Tajik AJ. Definitive diagnosis of truncus arteriosus by two-dimensional echocardiography. *Mayo Clin Proc* 1982; 57:476–481.

270. Swensson RE, Valdes-Cruz LM, Sahn DJ, Sherman FS, Chung KJ, Scagnelli S, et al. Real-time Doppler color flow mapping for detection of patient ductus arteriosus. *J Am Coll Cardiol* 1986; 8:1105–1112.

271. Tunick PA, Perez JL, Kronzon I. Protruding atheromas in the thoracic aortic and systemic embolization. *Ann Intern Med* 1991; 115:423–427.

272. Katz ES, Tunick PA, Rusinek H, Ribakove G, Spencer RC, Kronzon I. Protruding atheromas predict stroke in elderly patients undergoing cardiopulmonary bypass: Experience with intraoperative transesophageal echocardiography. *J Am Coll Cardiol* 1992; 20:70–77.

273. Cooke JP, Kazmeier FJ, Orszulak TA. The penetrating aortic ulcer: Pathologic manifestations, diagnosis, and management. *Mayo Clin Proc* 1988; 63:718–725.

273a. Smith MD, Cassidy M, Souther S, Morris EJ, Sapin PM, Johnson SB, et al. Transesophageal echocardiography in the diagnosis of traumatic rupture of the aorta. *N Engl J Med* 1995; 332:356–362.

273b. Vignon P, Gueret P, Vedrinne J-M, Lagrange P, Cornu E, Abrieu O, et al. Role of transesophageal echocardiography in the diagnosis and management of traumatic aortic disruption. *Circulation* 1995; 92:2959–2968.

274. Edler I. The diagnostic use of ultrasound in heart disease. *Acta Med Scand* 1955; 308:32.

275. Nichol PM, Gilbert BW, Kisslo JA. Two-dimensional echocardiographic assessment of mitral stenosis. *Circulation* 1977; 55:120–128.

276. Zaky A, Nasser WK, Feigenbaum H. Study of mitral valve action recorded by reflected ultrasound and its application in the diagnosis of mitral stenosis. *Circulation* 1988; 37:789–799.

277. Glover MU, Warren SE, Vieweg WVR, Ceretto WJ, Samtoy LM, Hagan AD. M-mode and two-dimensional echocardiographic correlation with findings at catheterization and surgery in patients with mitral stenosis. *Am Heart J* 1983; 105:98–102.

278. Duchak JM Jr, Chang S, Feigenbaum H. The posterior mitral valve echo and the echocardiographic diagnosis of mitral stenosis. *Am J Cardiol* 1972; 29:628–632.

279. Segal BL, Likoff W, Kingsley B. Echocardiography: Clinical application in combined mitral stenosis and mitral regurgitation. *Am J Cardiol* 1967; 19:42–49.

280. Quinones MA, Gaasch WH, Waisser E, Alexander J. Reduction in the rate of diastolic descent of the mitral valve echogram in patients with altered left ventricular diastolic pressure-volume relations. *Circulation* 1974; 49:246–254.

281. Gustafson A: The correlation between ultrasound cardiology, hemodynamics, and surgical findings in mitral stenosis. *Am J Cardiol* 1967; 19:32–41.

282. Henry WL, Griffith JM, Michaelis LL, McIntosh CL. Measurement of mitral orifice area in patients with mitral valve disease by real-time two-dimensional echocardiography. *Circulation* 1975; 51:827–831.

283. Wann LS, Weyman AE, Feigenbaum H, Dillon JC, Johnson KW. Determination of mitral valve area by cross-sectional echocardiography. *Ann Intern Med* 1978; 88:337–341.

284. Smith MD, Handshoe R, Handshoe S, Kwan OL, DeMaria AN. Comparative accuracy of two-dimensional echocardiography and Doppler pressure half-time methods in assessing severity of mitral stenosis in patients with and without prior commissurotomy. *Circulation* 1986; 73:100–107.

285. Martin RP, Rakowski H, Kleinman JH, Beaver W, London E, Popp RL. Reliability and reproducibility of two-dimensional echocardiography measurement of the stenotic mitral valve orifice area. *Am J Cardiol* 1979; 43:560–568.

286. Holen J, Simonsen S: Determination of pressure gradient in mitral stenosis with Doppler echocardiography. *Br Heart J* 1979; 41:529–535.

287. Hatle L, Angelsen B, Tromsdal A. Noninvasive assessment of atrioventricular pressure half-time by Doppler ultrasound. *Circulation* 1979; 60:1096–1104.

288. Hatle A, Brubakk A, Tromsdal A, Angelsen B. Noninvasive assessment of pressure drop in mitral stenosis by Doppler ultrasound. *Br Heart J* 1978; 40:131–140.

289. Libanoff AJ, Rodbard S. Atrioventricular pressure half-time: measure of mitral valve area. *Circulation* 1968; 38:144.

290. Loyd D, Ask P, Wranne B. Pressure half-time does not always predict mitral valve area correctly. *J Am Soc Echocardiogr* 1988; 1:313–321.

291. Thomas JD, Wilkins GT, Choong CYP, Abascal VM, Pakacios IF, Block PC, et al. Inaccuracy of mitral pressure half-time immediately after percutaneous mitral valvulotomy. *Circulation* 1988; 78:980–993.

292. Chen C, Wang Y, Guo B, Lin Y. Reliability of the Doppler pressure half-time method for assessing effects of percutaneous mitral balloon valvuloplasty. *J Am Coll Cardiol* 1989; 13:1309–1313.

293. Wilkins GT, Weyman AE, Abascal VM, Block PC, Palacios IF. Percutaneous balloon dilatation of the mitral valve: An analysis of echocardiographic variables related to outcome and the mechanism of dilatation. *Br Heart J* 1988; 60:299–308.

294. Palacios IF, Block PC, Wildins GT, Weyman AE. Follow-up of patients undergoing percutaneous mitral balloon valvotomy. *Circulation* 1989; 79:573–579.

295. Manning WJ, Reis GJ, Douglas PS. Use of transesophageal echocardiography to detect left atrial thrombi before percutaneous balloon dilatation of the mitral valve: A prospective study. *Br Heart J* 1992; 67:170–173.

296. Chen W-J, Chen MF, Liau C-S, Wu C-C, Lee Y-T. Safety of percutaneous transvenous balloon mitral commissurotomy in patients with mitral stenosis and thrombus in the left appendage. *Am J Cardiol* 1992; 70:117–119.

297. Abascal VM, Wilkins GT, Choong CY, Block PC, Palacios IF, Weyman AE. Mitral regurgitation after percutaneous balloon valvuloplasty in adults: Evaluation by pulsed Doppler echocardiography. *J Am Coll Cardiol* 1988; 11:257–263.

298. Yoshida K, Yoshikawa J, Akasaka T, Yamaura Y, Shadudo M, Nozumi T, et al. Assessment of left-to-right atrial shunting after percutaneous mitral valvuloplasty by transesophageal color Doppler flow-mapping. *Circulation* 1989; 80:1521–1526.

299. Roberts WC, Perloff JK. Mitral valvular disease: A clinicopathologic survey of the conditions causing the mitral valve to function abnormally. *Ann Intern Med* 1972; 77:939–975.

300. Mintz GS, Kotler MN, Segal BL, Parry WR Two-dimensional echocardiographic evaluation of patients with mitral insufficiency. *Am J Cardiol* 1979; 44:670–678.

301. Abbasi AS, Allen MW, DeCristofara D, Ungar T. Detection and estimation of the degree of mitral regurgitation by range-gated pulsed Doppler echocardiography. *Circulation* 1980; 61:143–147.

302. Matsuo H, Morita H, Senda S, Kitabatake A, Asao M, Tanouchi J, et al. Detection and visualization of regurgitant flow in valvular diseases by pulsed Doppler technique. *Jpn Circ J* 1982; 46:377–388.

303. Miyatake K, Izumi S, Okamoto M, Kinoshita N, Asnuma H, Nakagawa H. Semiquantitative grading of severity of mitral regurgitation by real-time two-dimensional Doppler flow imaging. *J Am Coll Cardiol* 1986; 7:82–88.

304. Utsunomiya T, Patel D, Doshi R, Quan M, Gardin JM. Can signal intensity of the continuous wave Doppler regurgitant jet estimate severity of mitral regurgitation? *Am Heart J* 1992; 123:166–171.

305. Pai RG, Bansal RC, Shah PM: Doppler-derived rate of left ventricular pressure rise: Its correlation with the postoperative left ventricular function in mitral regurgitation. *Circulation* 1990; 84:514.

306. Kisanuki A, Tei C, Minagoe S, Natsugoe K, et al. Continuous wave Doppler echocardiographic evaluations of the severity of mitral regurgitation. *J Cardiol* 1989; 19:831.

307. Rokey R, Sterling LL, Zoghbi WA, Sorton MP, Limacher MC, Kuo LC et al. Determination of regurgitant fraction in isolated mitral or aortic regurgitation by pulsed Doppler two-dimensional echocardiography. *J Am Coll Cardiol* 1986; 7:1273.

308. Enriques-Sarano M, Bailey KR, Seward JB, Tajik AJ, Krohn MJ, May MJ. Quantitative Doppler assessment of valvular regurgitation. *Circulation* 1993; 87:841–848.

309. Helmeke R, Nanda N, Hsiung MC, Soto B, Adey CK, Goyal RC et al. Color Doppler assessment of mitral regurgitation with orthogonal planes. *Circulation* 1987; 75:175.

310. Spain MG, Smith MD, Grayburn PA, Horlamert EA, DeMaria AN, O'Brien M et al. Quantitative assessment of mitral regurgitation by Doppler color flow imaging: Angiographic and hemodynamic correlations. *J Am Coll Cardiol* 1989; 13:585.

311. Chao K, Moises VA, Shandas R, Elkadi T, Sahn DJ, Weintraub R. Influence of the Coanda effect on color Doppler jet area and color encoding: In vitro studies using color Doppler flow mapping. *Circulation* 1992; 85:333–341.

312. Chen C, Thomas JD, Anconina J, Harrison P, Mueller L, Picard MH, et al. Impact of impinging wall jet on color Doppler quantification on mitral regurgitation. *Circulation* 1991; 84:712–720.

313. Klein AL, Stewart WJ, Bartlett J, Cohen GI, Kahan F, Pearce G, et al. Effects of mitral regurgitation on pulmonary venous flow and left atrial pressure: An intraoperative transesophageal echocardiographic study. *J Am Coll Cardiol* 1992; 20:1345–1352.

314. Castello R, Lenzen P, Aguirre F, Labovitz AJ. Quantitation of mitral regurgitation by transesophageal echocardiography with color flow mapping: Correlation with cardiac catheterization. *J Am Coll Cardiol* 1992; 19;1516–1521.

315. Pieper EPG, Hamer HPM, Sluijs RAP, Ravelli ACJ, Tijssen JGP, Crijns H, et al. Usefulness of multiplane transesophageal echocardiography to improve the assessment of severity of mitral regurgitation. *Am J Cardiol* 1996; 78:1132–1139.

316. Bargiggia GS, Tronconi L, Sahn DJ, Recusani F, Raisaro A, DeServis, et al. A new method for quantitation of mitral regurgitation based on color flow Doppler imaging of flow convergence proximal to regurgitant orifice. *Circulation* 1991; 84:1481–1489.

317. Xie G-Y, Berk MB, Hixson CS, Smith AC, DeMaria AN, Smith MD. Quantification of mitral regurgitation volume by the color Doppler proximal isovelocity surface area method: A clinical study. *J Am Soc EchocarDiogr* 1995; 8:48–54.

318. Enriquez-Sarano M, Miller FA, Hayes SN, Bailey KR, Tajik AJ, Seward JB. Effective mitral regurgitant orifice area: clinical use and pitfalls of the proximal isovelocity surface area method. *J Am Coll Cardiol* 1995; 25:703–709.

319. Utsunomiya T, Doshi R, Patel D, Nguyen D, Mehta K, Gardin JM. Regurgitant volume estimation in patients with mitral regurgitation: Initial studies using the color Doppler "proximal isovelocity surface area" method. *Echocardiography* 1992; 9:63–70.

320. Vandervoort PM, Rivera JM, Mele D, Palacios IF, Dinsmore RE, Weyman AE, et al. Application of color Doppler flow mapping to calculate effective regurgitant orifice area: An in vitro study and initial clinical observations. *Circulation* 1993; 88:1150–1156.

321. Rodriguez L, Thomas JD, Monterroso V, Weyman AE, Harrison P, Mueller LN, Levine RA. Validation of the proximal flow convergence method: Calculation of orifice area in patients with mitral stenosis. *Circulation* 1993; 88:1157–1165.

322. Rivera JM, et al. Quantification of tricuspid regurgitation using proximal flow convergence methods: Clinical validation (abstr). *J Am Soc Echocardiogr* 1992; 5:318.

323. Moises VA, Maciel BC, Hornberger LK, Murillo-Olivas A, Valdez-Cruz LM, Sahn DJ, et al. A new method for noninvasive estimation of ventricular septal defect shunt flow by Doppler color flow mapping: Imaging of the laminar convergence region on the left septal surface. *J Am Coll Cardiol* 1991; 18:824–832.

324. Yoshida K, Yoshikawa J, Akasaka T, Nishigami K, Minagoe S. Value of acceleration flow signals proximal to the leaking orifice in assessing the severity of prosthetic mitral valve regurgitation. *J Am Coll Cardiol* 1992; 19:333–338.

325. Simpson IA, Shiota T, Gharib M, Sahn DJ. Current status of flow convergence for clinical applications: Is it a leaning tower of "PISA"? *J Am Coll Cardiol* 1996; 27;504–509.

326. Devereux RB, Kramer-Fox R, Kligfield P. Mitral valve prolapse: Causes, clinical manifestations, and management. *Ann Intern Med* 1989; 111:305–317.

327. DeMaria AN, King JF, Bogren HG, Lies JE, Mason DT. The variable spectrum of echocardiographic manifestations of the mitral valve prolapse syndrome. *Circulation* 1974; 50:33–41.

328. Levine RA, Triulzi MO, Harrigan P, Weyman AE. The relationship of mitral annular shape to the diagnosis of mitral valve prolapse. *Circulation* 1987; 75:756–767.

329. Levine RA, Stathogiannis E, Newell JB, Harrigan P, Weyman AE. Reconsideration of echocardiographic standards for mitral valve prolapse: Lack of association between leaflet displacement isolated to the apical four-chamber view and independent echocardiographic evidence of abnormality. *J Am Coll Cardiol* 1988; 11:1013–1019.

330. Chun PKC, Sheehan MW. Myxomatous degeneration of mitral valve M-mode and two-dimensional echocardiographic findings. *Br Heart J* 1982; 47:404–408.

331. Dillon JC, Haine CL, Chang S, Feigenbaum H. Use of echocardiography in patients with prolapsed mitral valve. *Circulation* 1971; 43:503–507.

332. Levine RA, Handschumacher MD, Sanfilippo AJ, Hagege AA, Harrigan P, Marshall JE, et al. Three-dimensional echocardiographic reconstruction of the mitral valve with implications for the diagnosis of mitral valve prolapse. *Circulation* 1989; 80:589–598.

333. Nishimura RA, McGowon MD, Shub C, Miller FA, Ilstru DM, Tajik AJ. Echocardiographically documented mitral valve prolapse: Long term follow-up of 232 patients. *N Engl J Med* 1985; 313:1305–1309.

334. Himelman RB, Kusumoto R, Oken K, Lee E, Cahalan MK, Shah PM, et al. The flail mitral valve: Echocardiographic findings by precordial and transesophageal imaging and Doppler color flow imaging. *J Am Coll Cardiol* 1991; 17:272–279.

335. Marwick TH, Stewart WJ, Currie PJ Cosgrove DM. Mechanisms of failure of mitral valve repair: An echocardiographic study. *Am Heart J* 1991; 122:149–156.

336. Boltwood CM, Tei C, Wong M, Shah PM. Quantitative echocardiography of the mitral complex in dilated cardiomyopathy: The mechanism of functional mitral regurgitation. *Circulation* 1983; 68:498–508.

337. Nishimura RA, Shub C, Tajik AJ. Two dimensional echocardiographic diagnosis of partial papillary muscle rupture. *Br Heart J* 1982; 48:598–600.

338. D'Cruz I, Panetta F, Cohen H, Glock G. Submitral calcification or sclerosis in elderly patients: M-mode and two-dimensional echocardiography in "mitral annulus calcification." *Am J Cardiol* 1979; 44:31–38.

339. Nair CK, Aronow WS, Sketch MH, Mohiuddin SM, Ragano T, Esterbrookes DJ, et al. Clinical and echocardiographic characteristics of patients with mitral annular calcification. *Am J Cardiol* 1983; 51:992–995.

340. Nair CK, Thompson W, Ryschon K, Cook C, Hee TT, Sketch MH. Long-term follow-up of patients with echocardiographically detected mitral annular calcium and comparison with age- and sex-matched control subjects. *Am J Cardiol* 1989; 63:465–470.

341. Benjamin EJ, Plehn JF, D'Agostino RB, Belanger AJ, Comai K, Fuller DL, et al. Mitral annular calcification and the risk of stroke in an elderly cohort. *N Engl J Med* 1992; 327:374–379.

342. Weyman AE, Hurwitz RA, Gilrod DA, et al. Cross-sectional echocardiographic visualization of the stenotic pulmonary valve. *Circulation* 1977; 56:769–774.

343. Weyman AE, Dillon JC, Feigenbaum H, Chang S. Echocardiographic patterns of pulmonic valve motion in pulmonic stenosis. *Am J Cardiol* 1974; 34:644–651.

344. Johnson GL, Kwan OL, Handshoe S, Noonan JA, DeMaria AN. Accuracy of combined two-dimensional echocardiography and continuous wave Doppler recordings in the estimation of pressure gradient in right ventricular outlet obstruction. *J Am Coll Cardiol* 1984; 3:1013–1018.

345. Chandraratna PA, Wilson D, Imaizumi T, Ritter WS, Arnow WS. Invasive and noninvasive assessment of pulmonic regurgitation: Clinical, angiographic, phonocardiographic, echocardiographic, and Doppler ultrasound correlations. *Clin Cardiol* 1982; 5:360–365.

346. Waggoner AD, Quinones MA, Young JB, Brandon TA, Shah AB, Verani MS, et al. Pulsed Doppler echocardiographic detection of right-side valve regurgitation. *Am J Cardiol* 1981; 47:279–286.

347. Miyatake K, Okamoto M, Kinoshita N, Matsuhi SM, Nagata S, Beppu S, et al. Pulmonary regurgitation studied with the ultrasonic pulsed Doppler technique. *Circulation* 1982; 65:969–976.

348. Lee RT, Lord CP, Plappert T, Sutton MS. Prospective Doppler echocardiographic evaluation of pulmonary artery diastolic pressure in the medical intensive care unit. *Am J Cardiol* 1989; 64:1366–1370.

349. Parris TM, Panidis IP, Ross J, Mintz GS. Doppler echocardiographic findings in rheumatic tricuspid stenosis. *Am J Cardiol* 1987; 60:1414–1416.

350. Guyer DE, Gillam LD, Foale RA Clark MC, Dinsmore R, Palacios I, et al. Comparison of the echocardiographic and hemodynamic diagnosis of rheumatic tricuspid stenosis. *J Am Coll Cardiol* 1984; 3:1135–1144.

351. Miyatake K, Okamoto M, Kinoshita N, Ohta M, Kozuka T, Sakakibara H, et al. Evaluation of tricuspid regurgitation by pulsed Doppler and two-dimensional echocardiography. *Circulation* 1982; 66:777–784.

352. Curtius MM, Thyssen M, Breuer HWM, Loogen F. Doppler versus contrast echocardiography for diagnosis of tricuspid regurgitation. *Am J Cardiol* 1985; 56:333–336.

353. Suzuki Y, Kambara H, Kadota K, Tamaki S, Yamazato A, Nohara R. Detection and evaluation of tricuspid regurgitation using a real-time, two-dimensional, color-coded, Doppler flow imaging system: Comparison with contrast two-dimensional echocardiography and right ventriculography. *Am J Cardiol* 1986; 57:811–815.

354. Skjaerpe T, Hatle L. Diagnosis of tricuspid regurgitation. Sensitivity of Doppler ultrasound compared with contrast echocardiography. *Eur Heart J* 1985; 6:429–436.

355. Pennestri F, Loperfido F, Salvatori MP, Mongiardo R, Ferrazza A, Guccione P, et al. Assessment of tricuspid regurgitation by pulsed Doppler ultrasonography of the hepatic veins. *Am J Cardiol* 1984; 54:363–368.

356. Dittrich HC, McCann HA, Blanchard DG. Cardiac structure and function in chronic thromboembolic pulmonary hypertension. *Am J Cardiac Imaging* 1994; 8:18–27.

357. Levine R, Gibson T, Aretz T, Gillam LD, Guyer DE, King ME, et al. Echocardiographic measurement of right ventricular volume. *Circulation* 1984; 69:497–505.

358. Gibson TC, Miller SW, Aretz T, Hardin NJ, Weyman AE. Method for estimating right ventricular volume by planes applicable to cross-sectional echocardiography: Correlation with angiographic formulas. *Am J Cardiol* 1985; 15:1584–1588.

359. Weyman AE. Appendix A: Normal cross-sectional echocardiographic measurements. In: Weyman AE, ed. *Principles and Practice of Echocardiography,* 2d ed. Philadelphia: Lea & Febiger; 1994:1289–1298.

360. Cacho A, Prakash R, Sarma R, Kaushik VS. Usefulness of two-dimensional echocardiography in diagnosing right ventricular hypertrophy. *Chest* 1983; 84:154–157.

361. Baker BJ, Scovil JA, Kane JJ, Murphy MG. Echocardiographic detection of right ventricular hypertrophy. *Am Heart J* 1983; 105:611–614.

362. D'Arcy B, Nanda NC. Two-dimensional echocardiographic features of right ventricular infarction. *Circulation* 1982; 65:167–173.

363. Weyman AE, Wann LS, Feigenbaum H, Dillon JC. Mechanism of abnormal septal motion in patients with right ventricular volume overload. *Circulation* 1976; 54:179.

364. Ryan T, Petrovic O, Dillon J, Feigenbaum H, Conley M, Armstrong W. An echocardiographic index for separation of right ventricular volume and pressure overload. *J Am Coll Cardiol* 1985; 5:918–924.

365. Yock PG, Popp RL. Noninvasive estimation of right ventricular systolic pressure by Doppler ultrasound in patients with tricuspid regurgitation. *Circulation* 1984; 70:657–662.

366. Himelman RB, Kircher B, Rockey DC, Schiller NB. Inferior vena cava plethora with blunted respiratory response: A sensitive echocardiographic sign of cardiac tamponade. *J Am Coll Cardiol* 1988; 12:470–477.

367. Weyman AE, Dillon JC, Feigenbaum H, Chang S. Echocardiographic patterns of pulmonary valve motion with pulmonary hypertension. *Circulation* 1974; 50:905–910.

368. Tukelvich D, Groves BM, Micco A, Trapp JA, Reeves JT. Early partial systolic closure of the pulmonic valve relates to severity of pulmonary hypertension. *Am Heart J* 1988; 115:409–418.

369. Hirshfeld S, Meyer R, Schwartz DC, Kofhagen J, Kaplan S. The echocardiographic assessment of pulmonary artery pressure and pulmonary vascular resistance. *Circulation* 1975; 52:642–650.

370. Tahara M, Tanaka H, Nakao S, Yoshimura H, Sakurai S, Tei C, et al. Hemodynamic determinants of pulmonary valve motion during systole in experimental pulmonary hypertension. *Circulation* 1981; 64:1249–1256.

371. Beard JT, Newman JH, Loyd JE, Byrd BF III. Doppler estimation of changes in pulmonary artery pressure during hypoxic breathing. *J Am Soc Echocardiogr* 1991; 4:121–130.

372. Zabalgoitia M. Echocardiographic assessment of prosthetic heart valves. *Curr Prob Cardiol* 1992; 17:271–325.

373. Mehta A, Kessler KM, Tamer D, Pefkaros K, Kessler R, Myerburg RJ. Two-dimensional echocardiographic observations in major detachment of a prosthetic aortic valve. *Am Heart J* 1981; 101:231–233.

374. Ledain LD, Onayon JP, Colle JP, Lorient-Roudaut FM, Roudaut RP, Beese PM. Acute thrombotic obstruction with disc valve prostheses: Diagnostic considerations and fibrinolytic treatment. *J Am Coll Cardiol* 1986; 7:743–751.

375. Come PC, Riley MF. Echocardiographic recognition of perivalvular infection complicating aortic bacterial endocarditis. *Am Heart J* 1984; 108:166–168.

376. Williams GA, Labovitz AJ. Doppler hemodynamic evaluation of prosthetic (Starr-Edwards and Bjork-Shiley) and bioprosthetic (Hancock and Carpentier-Edwards) cardiac valves. *Am J Cardiol* 1985; 56:325–332.

377. Cooper DM, Stewart WJ, Schiavone WA, Lombardo HP, Lytle BW, Loop FD, et al. Evaluation of normal prosthetic valve function by Doppler echocardiography. *Am Heart J* 1987; 114:576–582.

378. Reisner SA, Meltzer RS: Normal values of prosthetic valve Doppler echocardiographic parameters: A review. *J Am Soc Echocardiogr* 198; 1:201–210.

379. Panadis IP, Ross J, Mintz GS. Normal and abnormal prosthetic valve function as assessed by Doppler echocardiography. *J Am Coll Cardiol* 1986; 8:317–326.

380. Nellessen U, Schnittger I, Appleton CP, Masuyama T, Bolder A, Fischell TA, et al. Transesophageal two-dimensional echocardiography and color Doppler flow velocity mapping in the evaluation of cardiac valve prostheses. *Circulation* 1988; 78:848–855.

381. Khandheria BK, Seward JB, Oh JK, Freeman WK, Nichols BA, Sinak LJ, et al. Value and limitations of transesophageal echocardiography in assessment of mitral valve prostheses. *Circulation* 1991; 83:1956–1968.

382. Flachskampf FA, O'Shea JP, Griffin BP, Vuerrero L, Weyman AE, Thomas JD. Patterns of normal transvalvular regurgitation in mechanical valve prostheses. *J Am Coll Cardiol* 1991; 18:1493–1498.

383. Baumgartner H, Khan S, DeRobertis M, Czer L, Maurer G. Effect of prosthetic aortic valve design on the Doppler-catheter gradient correlation: An in vitro study of normal St. Jude, Medtronic-Hall, Starr-Edwards and Hancock valves. *J Am Coll Cardiol* 1992; 19:324–332.

384. Burstow DJ, Nishimura RA, Bailey KR, Reeder GS, Holmes DR, Seward JB, et al. Continuous wave Doppler echocardiographic measurement of prosthetic valve gradients: A simultaneous Doppler-catheter correlative study. *Circulation* 1980; 8:504–514.

385. Vandervoort PM, Greenberg NL, Pu M, Powell KA, Cosgrove DM, Thomas JD. Pressure recovery in bileaflet heart valve prostheses: Localized high velocities and gradients in central and side orifices with implications for Doppler-catheter gradient relation in aortic and mitral position. *Circulation* 1995; 92:3464–3472.

386. Voelker W, Reul J, Stelzer T, Schmidt A, Karsch KR. Pressure recovery in aortic stenosis: An in vitro study in a pulsatile flow model. *J Am Coll Cardiol* 1992; 20:1585–1593.

387. Wiseth R, Hegrenaes L, Rossvoll O, Skjaerpe T, Hatle L. Validity of an early postoperative baseline Doppler recording after aortic valve replacement. *Am J Cardiol* 1991; 7:869–872.

388. Dittrich HC, McCann HA, Walsh T, Blanchard DG, Oppenheim G, Waack TC, et al. Transesophageal echocardiography in the evaluation of prosthetic and native aortic valves. *Am J Cardiol* 1990; 66:758–761.

389. Alam M, Serwin JB, Rosman HS, Polanco GA, Sun I, Silverman NA. Transesophageal echocardiographic features of normal and dysfunctioning bioprosthetic valves. *Am Heart J* 1991; 121:1149–1155.

390. Alam M, Serwin JB, Rosman HS, Shethm, Sun I, Silverman NA, et al. Transesophageal color flow Doppler and echocardiographic features of normal and regurgitant St. Jude medical prostheses in the mitral valve position. *Am J Cardiol* 1990; 66:871–873.

391. Orsinelli DA, Pearson AG. Detection of prosthetic valve strands by transesophageal echocardiography: Clinical significance in patients with suspected cardiac source of embolism. *J Am Coll Cardiol* 1995; 26:1713–1718.

392. Freedberg RS, Goodkin GM, Perez JL, Tunick PA, Kronzon I. Valve strands are strongly associated with systemic embolization: A transesophageal echocardiographic study. *J Am Coll Cardiol* 1995; 26:1709–1712.

393. Dzavik V, Cohen G, Chan KL. Role of transesophageal echocardiography in the diagnosis and management of prosthetic valve thrombosis. *J Am Coll Cardiol* 1991; 18:1829–1833.

394. Currie P, Sutherland GR, Starkey IR. Thrombolysis as an emergency treatment for a thrombosed prosthetic mitral valve diagnosed by transesophageal echocardiography. *Br Heart J* 1993; 70:198–200.

395. Hurrell DG, Schaff HV, Tajik AJ. Thrombolytic therapy for obstruction of mechanical prosthetic valves. *Mayo Clin Proc* 1996; 71:605–613.

396. Dillon LC, Feigenbaum H, Konecke LL, Davis RF, Chang S. Echocardiographic manifestations of valvular vegetations. *Am Heart J* 1973; 86:698–704.

397. Wann LS, Dillon JC, Weyman AE, Feigenbaum H. Echocardiography in bacterial endocarditis. *N Engl J Med* 1976; 295:135–139.

398. Gilbert BW, Haney RS, Crawford F, McClellan J, Gallis HA, Johnson ML, et al. Two-dimensional echocardiographic assessment of vegetative endocarditis. *Circulation* 1977; 55:346–353.

399. Durack DT, Lukes AS, Bright DK. New criteria for diagnosis of infective endocarditis: Utilization of specific echocardiographic findings. *Am J Med* 1994; 96:200–209.

400. Pedersen WR, Walker M, Olson JD, Gobel F, Lange HW, Daniel JA, et al. Value of transesophageal echocardiography as an adjunct to transthoracic echocardiography in evaluation of native and prosthetic valve endocarditis. *Chest* 1991; 100:351–356.

401. von Reyn CF, Arbeit RD. Case definitions for infective endocarditis. *Am J Med* 1994; 96:220–222.

402. Galve E, Candell-Riera J, Pigrau C, Permanyer-Miralda G, Garcia-Del-Castillo H, Soler-Soler J. Prevalence, morphologic types, and evolution of cardiac valvular disease in systemic lupus erythematosus. *N Engl J Med* 1988; 319:817–823.

403. Roldan CA, Shively BK, Crawford MH. An echocardiographic study of valvular heart disease associated with systemic lupus erythematosus. *N Engl J Med* 1996; 335:1424–1430.

404. Martin RP, Meltzer RS, Chia BL, Stinson EB, Rakowski H, Popp RL. Clinical utility of two-dimensional echocardiography in infective endocarditis. *Am J Cardiol* 1980; 46:379–385.

405. Stewart JS, Silimpert D, Harris P, Wise NK, Fraker TD, Kisslo J. Echocardiographic documentation of vegetative lesions in infective endocarditis: Clinical implications. *Circulation* 1980; 61:374–380.

406. Blanchard DG, Ross RS, Dittrich HC. Nonbacterial thrombotic endocarditis: Assessment by transesophageal echocardiography. *Chest* 1992; 102:954–956.

407. Mügge A, Daniel WG. Echocardiographic assessment of vegetations in patients with infective endocarditis: Prognostic implications. *Echocardiography* 1995; 12:651–661.

408. Buda AJ, Zotz RJ, LeMire MS, Bach DS. Prognostic significance of vegetations detected by two-dimensional echocardiography in infective endocarditis. *Am Heart J* 1986; 112:1291–1296.

409. Sanfillipo AJ, Picard MH, Newell JB, Rosas E, Davidoff R, Thomas J, et al. Echocardiographic assessment of patients with infectious endocarditis: Prediction of risk for complications. *J Am Coll Cardiol* 1991; 18:1191–1199.

410. Jaffe WM, Morgan DE, Perlman AS, Otto CM. Infective endocarditis, 1983–1988: Echocardiographic findings and factors influencing morbidity and mortality. *J Am Coll Cardiol* 1990; 15:1127–1233.

411. Steckelberg JM, Murphy JG, Ballard D, Bailey K, Tajik AJ, Taliercio CP, et al. Emboli in infective endocarditis: The prognostic value of echocardiography. *Ann Intern Med* 1991; 114:635–640.

412. Klodas E, Edwards WD, Khanderia BK. Use of transesophageal echocardiography for improving detection of valvular vegetations in subacute bacterial endocarditis. *J Am Soc Echocardiogr* 1989; 2:386–289.

413. Birmingham GD, Rahko PS, Ballantyne F. Improved detection of infective endocarditis with transesophageal echocardiography. *Am Heart J* 1992; 123:774–781.

414. Karalis DG, Bansal RC, Hauck AJ, Ross JJ, Applegate PM, Jutzy KR. Transesophageal echocardiographic recognition of subaortic complications in aortic valve endocarditis: Clinical and surgical implications. *Circulation* 1992; 86:353–362.

415. Khanderia BK. Suspected bacterial endocarditis: To TEE or not to TEE. *J Am Coll Cardiol* 1993; 21:222–224.

416. Lindner JR, Case RA, Dent JM, Abbott RD, Scheld WM, Kaul S. Diagnostic value of echocardiography in suspected endocarditis: An evaluation based on pretest probability of disease. *Circulation* 1996; 93:730–736.

417. Weyman AE, Feigenbaum H, Dillon JL, Johnston KW, Eggleton RC. Noninvasive visualization of the left main coronary artery by cross-sectional echocardiography. *Circulation* 1976; 54:169.

418. Raisinghani A, Ohmori K, Cotter B, Mahmud E, Calisi C, Kwan OL, et al. Does flow reversal within intramyocardial coronary vessels occur

systole? Detection of biphasic flow in intramyocardial vessels by transthoracic echo (abstr). *J Am Coll Cardiol* 1997; 29;365A.

419. Ryan T, Armstrong WF, Feigenbaum H. Prospective evaluation of the left main coronary artery using digital two-dimensional echocardiography. *J Am Coll Cardiol* 1986; 7:807–812.

420. Yamagishi M, Miyatake K, Beppu S, Kumon K, Suzuki S, Tanaka N, et al. Assessment of coronary blood flow by transesophageal two-dimensional pulsed Doppler echocardiography. *Am J Cardiol* 1988; 62: 641–644.

421. Kerber R, Abboud F. Echocardiographic detection of regional myocardial infarction. *Circulation* 1973; 47:997.

422. Franklin TD Jr, Cuddeback JK, Sanghn NT, Weyman AE, Avery KS, Fry FJ. Differentiation of A-mode ultrasound signals from normal and ischemic myocardium by multivariate discriminant analysis of waveform parameters. *Am J Cardiol* 1980; 45:403. (abstract)

423. Bourdillon PDV, Broderick TM, Sawada SG, Armstrong WF, Ryan T, Dillon JC, et al. Regional wall motion index for infarct and noninfarct regions after reperfusion in acute myocardial infarction: Comparison with global wall motion index. *J Am Soc Echocardiogr* 1989; 2:398–407.

424. Nishimura RA, Tajik AJ, Shub C, Miller FA, Ilstrup DM, Harrison CE. Role of two-dimensional echocardiography in the prediction of in-hospital complications after acute myocardial infarction. *J Am Coll Cardiol* 1984; 4:1080–1087.

425. Feigenbaum H. Coronary artery disease. In: *Echocardiography,* 5th ed. Philadelphia: Lea & Febiger; 1994:452.

426. Crouse LJ, Harbrecht JJ, Vacek JL, Rosamond TL, Kramer PH. Exercise echocardiography as a screening test for coronary artery disease and correlation with coronary arteriography. *Am J Cardiol* 1991; 67;1213–1218.

427. Segar DS, Brown SC, Sawada SG, Ryan T, Feigenbaum H. Dobutamine stress echocardiography: Correlation with coronary lesions severity as determined by quantitative angiography. *J Am Coll Cardiol* 1992; 19:1197–1202.

428. Corya BC, Feigenbaum H, Rasmussen S, Black MJ. Echocardiographic features of congestive cardiomyopathy compared with normal subjects and patients with coronary artery disease. *Circulation* 1974; 49:1153–1159.

429. Heger J, Weyman AE, Wann S, Rogers EW, Dillon JC, Feigenbaum H. Cross-sectional echocardiographic analysis of the extent of left ventricular asynergy in acute myocardial infarction. *Circulation* 1980; 61:1113–1118.

430. Weiss JL, Buckley BH, Hutchins GM, Mason SJ. Two-dimensional echocardiographic recognition of myocardial injury in man: Comparison with postmortem studies. *Circulation* 1981; 63:401–408.

431. Horowitz RS, Morganroth J, Parrotto C, Chen CC, Soffer J, Pauletto FJ. Immediate diagnosis of acute myocardial infarction by two-dimensional echocardiography. *Circulation* 1982; 65:323–329.

432. Gibson RS, Bishop HL, Stamm RB, Crampton RS, Beller GA, Martin RP. Value of early two-dimensional echocardiography in patients with acute myocardial infarction. *Am J Cardiol* 1982; 49:1110–1119.

433. Peels CH, Visser CA, Kupper AJF, Visser FC, Ross J. Usefulness of two-dimensional echocardiography for immediate detection of myocardial ischemia in the emergency room. *Am J Cardiol* 1990; 65:687–691.

434. Sabia P, Abbott RD, Afrookteh A, Keller MW, Touchstone DA, Kaul S. Importance of two-dimensional echocardiographic assessment of left ventricular systolic function in patients presenting to the emergency room with cardiac-related symptoms. *Circulation* 1991; 84:1615–1624.

435. Oh JK, Miller FA, Shub C, Reeder GS, Tajik AJ. Evaluation of acute chest pain syndromes by two-dimensional echocardiography: Its potential application in the selection of patients for acute reperfusion therapy. *Mayo Clin Proc* 1987; 62:59–66.

436. Eaton L, Weiss JL, Bulkley BH, Garrison JB, Weisfeldt ML. Regional cardiac dilatation after acute myocardial infarction. *N Engl J Med* 1979; 300:57–62.

437. Picard MH, Wilkins GT, Ray PA, Weyman AT. Progressive changes in ventricular structure and function during the year after acute myocardial infarction. *Am Heart J* 1992; 124:24–31.

438. Matsumoto M, Watanabe F, Gotto A, Hamano Y, Yasui K, Minamino T, et al. Left ventricular aneurysm and the prediction of left ventricular enlargement studied by two-dimensional echocardiography: Quantitative assessment of aneurysm size in relation to clinical course. *Circulation* 1985; 72:280–286.

439. VanTassel RA, Edwards JE. Rupture of the heart complicating myocardial infarction: analysis of 40 cases including nine examples of left ventricular false aneurysms. *Chest* 1972; 61:104–116.

440. Catherwood E, Mintz GS, Kotler MN, Parry WR, Segal BL. Two-dimensional echocardiographic recognition of left ventricular pseudoaneurysm. *Circulation* 1980; 62:294–303.

441. Roelandt J, Sutherland GR, Yoshida K, Yoshikawa J. Improved diagnosis and characterization of left ventricular pseudoaneurysm by Doppler color imaging. *J Am Coll Cardiol* 1988; 12:807–411.

442. Miyatake K, Okamoto M, Kinoshita N, Park Y-D, Nagata S, Izumi S, et al. Doppler echocardiographic features of ventricular septal rupture in myocardial infarction. *J Am Coll Cardiol* 1985; 5:182–187.

443. Helmcke F, Mahan EF, Nanda NC, Jain SP, Soto B, Kirklin JK, et al. Two-dimensional echocardiography and Doppler color flow mapping in the diagnosis and prognosis of ventricular septal rupture. *Circulation* 1990; 81:1775–1783.

444. Harrison MR, MacPhail B, Gurley JC, Harlamert EA, Steinmertz JE, Smith MD, et al. Usefulness of color Doppler flow imaging to distinguish ventricular septal defect from acute mitral regurgitation complicating acute myocardial infarction. *Am J Cardiol* 1989; 64:697–701.

445. Kono T, Sabbah HN, Rosman H, Slam H, Jafri S, Stein PD, et al. Mechanism of functional mitral regurgitation during acute myocardial infarction. *J Am Coll Cardiol* 1992; 9:1101–1105.

446. Nishimura RA, Schaff HV, Shub C, Gersh BJ, Edwards WD, Tajik AJ. Papillary muscle rupture complicating acute myocardial infarction. Analysis of 17 patients. *Am J Cardiol* 1983; 51:373–377.

447. Stoddard MF, Keedy DL, Kupersmith J. Transesophageal echocardiographic diagnosis of papillary muscle rupture complicating acute myocardial infarction. *Am Heart J* 1990; 120:690–692.

448. D'Arcy B, Nanda NC: Two-dimensional echocardiographic features of right ventricular infarction. *Circulation* 1982; 65:167–173.

449. Otto CM, Stratton JR, Maynard C, Althouse R, Johannessen KA, Kennedy W. Echocardiographic evaluation of segmental wall motion early and late after thrombolytic therapy in acute myocardial infarction: The Western Washington issue plasminogen activator emergency room trial. *Am J Cardiol* 1990; 65:132–138.

450. Bourdillon PDV, Broderick TM, Williams ES, Dillon JC, Armstrong WF. Early recovery of regional left ventricular function after reperfusion in acute myocardial infarction assessed by serial two-dimensional echocardiography. *Am J Cardiol* 63:641–642.

451. Wann LS, Faris JV, Childress RH, Dillon JC, Weyman AE, Feigenbaum H. Exercise cross-sectional echocardiography in ischemic heart disease. *Circulation* 1979; 60:1300–1308.

452. Armstrong WF, O'Donnell J, Ryan T, Feigenbaum H. Effect of prior myocardial infarction and extent and location of coronary disease on accuracy of exercise echocardiography. *J Am Coll Cardiol* 1987; 10:531–538.

453. Marwick T, Nemec J, Pashkow F, Stewart WJ, Salcedo E. Accuracy and limitations of exercise echocardiography in a routine clinical setting. *J Am Coll Cardiol* 1992; 19:74–81.

454. Feigenbaum H. Exercise echocardiography. *J Am Soc Echocardiogr* 1988; 1:161–166.

455. Quinones MA, Verani MS, Haichin RM, Mamarian JJ, Suarez J, Zoghbi WA. Exercise echocardiography versus T1-201 single photon emission computerized tomography in evaluation of coronary artery disease: Analysis of 292 patients. *Circulation* 1992; 85:1026–1031.

456. Roger VL, Pellikka PA, Oh JK, Bailey KR, Tajik AJ. Identification of multivessel coronary artery disease by exercise echocardiography. *J Am Coll Cardiol* 1994; 24:109–114.

457. Ryan T, Segar DS, Sawada SG, Berkowitz KE, Whang D, Dohan AM, et al. Detection of coronary artery disease with upright bicycle exercise echocardiography. *J Am Soc Echocardiogr* 1993; 6:186–197.

458. Cigarroa CG, deFilippi CR, Brickner ME, Alvarez LG, Wait MA, Grayburn PA. Dobutamine stress echocardiography identifies hibernating myocardium and predicts recovery of left ventricular function after coronary revascularization. *Circulation* 1993; 88:430–436.

459. Marcowitz P, Armstrong WF. Accuracy of dobutamine stress echocardiography in detecting coronary artery disease. *Am J Cardiol* 1992; 69:1269–1273.

460. Sawada SG, Segar DS, Ryan T, Brown SE, Dohan AM, Williams R, et al. Echocardiographic detection of coronary artery disease during dobutamine infusion. *Circulation* 1991; 83:1605–1614.

461. Picano E. Stress echocardiography: From pathophysiologic toy to diagnostic tool. *Circulation* 1992; 85:1604–1612.

462. Sun KT, Czernin J, Krivokapich J, Lau Y-K, Böttcher M, Maurer G, et al. Effects of dobutamine stimulation on myocardial blood flow, glucose metabolism, and wall motion in normal and dysfunctional myocardium. *Circulation* 1996; 94:3146–3154.

463. Pierard LA, De Landsheere CM, Berthe C, Rigo P, Kulbertus HE. Identification of viable myocardium by echocardiography during dobutamine infusion in patients with myocardial infarction after thrombolytic therapy: Comparison with positron emission tomography. *J Am Coll Cardiol* 1990; 15:1021–1031.

464. Smart SC, Sawada S, Ryan T, Segar D, Atherton L, Berkowitz K, et al. Low-dose dobutamine echocardiography detects reversible dysfunction after thrombolytic therapy of acute myocardial infarction. *Circulation* 1993; 88:405–415.

465. Forster T, McNeill AJ, Salustri A, Reijs AE, El-Said ES, Roelandt JR. Simultaneous dobutamine stress echocardiography and echocardiography and technetium-99m isonitrile single-photon emission computed tomography in patients with suspected coronary artery disease. *J Am Coll Cardiol* 1993; 21:1591–1596.

466. Attenhoffer CH, Pellikka PA, Oh JK, Roger VL, Sohn DW, Seward JB. Comparison of ischemic response during exercise and dobutamine echocardiography in patients with left main coronary artery disease. *J Am Coll Cardiol* 1996; 27:1171–1177.

467. Bax JJ, Cornel JH, Visser FC, Fioretti PM, van Lingen A, Reijs AE, et al. Prediction of recovery of myocardial dysfunction after revascularization: Comparison of fluorine-18 fluorodeoxyglucose/thallium-201 SPECT, thallium-201 stress-reinjection SPECT and dobutamine echocardiography. *J Am Coll Cardiol* 1996; 28:558–564.

468. Afridi I, Main ML, Grayburn PA. Accuracy of dobutamine echocardiography for detection of myocardial viability in patients with occluded left anterior descending coronary artery. *J Am Coll Cardiol* 1996; 28:455–459.

469. Vanoverschelde J-LJ, D'Hount A-M, Marwick T, Gerber BL, DeKock M, Dion R, et al. Head-to-head comparison of exercise-redistribution-reinjection thallium single-photon emission computed tomography and low dose dobutamine echocardiography for prediction of reversibility of chronic left ventricular ischemic dysfunction. *J Am Coll Cardiol* 1996; 28:432–442.

470. Baer FM, Voth E, Deutsch HJ, Schneider CA, Schicha H, Sechtem U. Assessment of viable myocardium by dobutamine transesophageal echocardiography and comparison with fluorine-18 fluorodeoxyglucose positron emission tomography. *J Am Coll Cardiol* 1994; 24:343–353.

471. Mertes H, Sawada SG, Ryan T, Segar DS, Kovacs R, Foltz J, et al. Symptoms, adverse effects, and complications associated with dobutamine stress echocardiography: Experience in 1118 patients. *Circulation* 1993; 88;15–19.

472. Bach DS, Muller D, Gros BJ, Armstrong WF. False positive dobutamine stress echocardiograms: Characterization of clinical, echocardiographic, and angiographic findings. *J Am Coll Cardiol* 1994; 24:928–933.

473. Anthopoulos LP, Bonou MS, Kardaras FG, Sioras EP, Kardara DN, Sideris AM, et al. Stress echocardiography in elderly patients with coronary artery disease. *J Am Coll Cardiol* 1996; 28:52–59.

474. Pellikka PA, Oh JK, Bailey KR, Nichols BA, Monahan KH, Tajik AJ. Dynamic intraventricular obstruction during dobutamine stress echocardiography: A new observation. *Circulation* 1992; 86:1429–1432.

475. Tanimoto M, Pai RG, Jintapakorn W, Shah PM. Mechanisms of hypotension during dobutamine stress echocardiography in patients with coronary artery disease. *Am J Cardiol* 1995; 76:26–30.

476. Marwick T, Wilemart B, D'Hondt AM, Baudhuin T, Wijins W, Detry JM, et al. Selection of the optimal non-exercise stress for the evaluation of ischemic regional myocardial dysfunction and malperfusion: Comparison of dobutamine and adenosine using echocardiography and Tc-99m MIBI single photon emission computerized tomography. *Circulation* 1993; 87:345–354.

477. Mairesse GH, Marwick TH, Arnese M, Vanoverschelde J-LJ, Cornel JH, Detry J-MR, et al. Improved identification of coronary artery disease in patients with left bundle branch block by use of dobutamine stress echocardiography and comparison with myocardial perfusion tomography. *Am J Cardiol* 1995; 76:321–325.

478. Sawada SG, Ryan T, Feinberg NS, Armstrong WF, Judson WE, McHenry PL, et al. Exercise echocardiographic identification of coronary artery disease in women. *J Am Coll Cardiol* 1989; 14:1440–1447.

478a. Marwick TH, Anderson T, Williams J, Haluska B, Melin JA, Pashkow F, et al. Exercise echocardiography is an accurate and cost-effective technique for detection of coronary artery disease in women. *J Am Coll Cardiol* 1995; 26:335–341.

479. Roger VL, Pellikka PA, Oh JK, Bailey K,. Tajik AJ. Identification of multivessel coronary artery disease by exercise echocardiography. *J Am Coll Cardiol* 1994; 24:109–114.

480. Spes CH, Mudra H, Schnaak SD, Klauss V, Reichle FM, Uberfuhr P, et al. Dobutamine stress echocardiography for noninvasive diagnosis of cardiac allograft vasculopathy: A comparison with angiography and intravascular ultrasound. *Am J Cardiol* 1996; 78:168–174.

481. Davila-Roman VG, Wong AK, Li D, Shelton ME, Lasala JM, Hopkins WE, et al. Usefulness of dobutamine stress echocardiography for the prospective identification of the physiological significance of coronary narrowings of moderate severity in patients undergoing evaluation for percutaneous transluminal coronary angioplasty. *Am J Cardiol* 1995; 76:245–249.

482. Kafka H, Leach AJ, Fitzgibbon GM. Exercise echocardiography after coronary artery bypass surgery: Correlation with coronary angiography. *J Am Coll Cardiol* 1995; 25:1019–1023.

483. Elhendy A, Geleijnse ML, Roelandt J, Cornel JH, van Domburg RT, El-Refare M, et al. Assessment of patients after coronary artery bypass grafting by dobutamine stress echocardiography. *Am J Cardiol* 1996; 77:1234–1237.

484. Labovitz AJ, Lewen M, Kern WJ, Vandormael M, Mrosek DG, Byers SL, et al. The effects of successful PTCA on left ventricular function: Assessment by exercise echocardiography. *Am Heart J* 1989; 117:1003–1008.

485. Crouse LJ, Vacek JL, Beauchamp GD, Porter CB, Rosamond TL, Kramer PH. Exercise echocardiography after coronary artery bypass grafting. *Am J Cardiol* 1992; 70:572–576.

486. Ryan T, Armstrong WF, O'Donnell JA, Feigenbaum H. Risk stratification after acute myocardial infarction by means of exercise two-dimensional echocardiography. *Am Heart J* 1987; 114:1305–1316.

487. Picano E, Pingitore A, Sicari R, Minardi G, Gandolfo N, Seveso G, et al. Stress echocardiographic results predict risk of reinfarction early after uncomplicated acute myocardial infarction: large-scale multicenter study. *J Am Coll Cardiol* 1995; 26:908–913.

488. Quintana M, Lindvall K, Ryden L, Brolund F. Prognostic value of predischarge exercise stress echocardiography after acute myocardial infarction. *Am J Cardiol* 1995; 76:1115–1121.

489. Williams MJ, Odabashian J, Lauer MS, Thomas JD, Marwick TH. Prognostic value of dobutamine echocardiography in patient with left ventricular dysfunction. *J Am Coll Cardiol* 1996; 27:132–139.

490. Smart SC, Sawada S, Ryan T, Segar D, Atherton L, Berkovitz K, et al. Low-dose dobutamine echocardiography detects reversible dysfunction after thrombolytic therapy of acute myocardial infarction. *Circulation* 1993; 88:405–415.

491. Kamaran M, Teague SM, Finkelhor RS, Dawson N, Bahler RC. Prognostic value of dobutamine stress echocardiography in patients referred because of suspected coronary artery disease. *Am J Cardiol* 1995; 76:887–891.

492. Davila-Roman VG, Waggoner AD, Sicard GA, Geltman EM, Schechtman KB, Perez JE. Dobutamine stress echocardiography predicts surgical outcome in patients with an aortic aneurysm and peripheral vascular disease. *J Am Coll Cardiol* 1993; 21:957–963.

493. Poldermans D, Fioretti PM, Forster T, Thomson IR, Boersma E, El-Said EM, et al. Dobutamine stress echocardiography for assessment of perioperative cardiac risk in patients undergoing major vascular surgery. *Circulation* 1993; 87:1506–1512.

494. Lane RT, Sawada DS, Segar DS, Ryan T, Lalka SG, Williams R, et al. Dobutamine stress echocardiography for assessment of cardiac risk before noncardiac surgery. *Am J Cardiol* 1991; 68:976–977.

495. Chen C, Li L, Chen LL, Prada JV, Chen MH, Fallon JT, et al. Incremental doses of dobutamine induce a biphasic response in dysfunctional left ventricular regions subtending coronary stenoses. *Circulation* 1995; 92:756–766.

496. Afridi I, Kleiman NS, Raizner AE, Zoghbi WA. Dobutamine echocardiography in myocardial hibernation: Optimal dose and accuracy in predicting recovery of ventricular function after coronary angioplasty. *Circulation* 1995; 91:663–670.

497. Perrone-Filardi P, Pace L, Prastaro M, Piscione F, Betocchi S, Squane F, et al. Dobutamine echocardiography predicts improvement of hypoperfused dysfunctional myocardium after revascularization in patients with coronary artery disease. *Circulation* 1995; 91:2556–2565.

498. Arnese M, Cornel JH, Salustri A, Maat A, Elhendy A, Reijs AE, et al. Prediction of improvement of regional left ventricular function after surgical revascularization: A comparison of low-dose dobutamine echocardiography with thallium-201 single-photon emission computed tomography. *Circulation* 1995; 91:2748–2752.

499. Watada H, Ito H, Oh H, Masuyama T, Aburaya M, Hori M, et al. Dobutamine stress echocardiography predicts reversible dysfunction and quantitates the extent of irreversibly damaged myocardium after reperfusion of anterior myocardial infarction. *J Am Coll Cardiol* 1994; 24:624–630.

500. La Canna G, Alfieri O, Giubbini R, Gargano M, Ferrari R, Visioli O. Echocardiography during infusion of dobutamine for identification of reversible dysfunction in patients with chronic coronary artery disease. *J Am Coll Cardiol* 1994; 23:617–626.

501. Baer FM, Voth E, Deutsch HJ, Schneider CA, Horst M DeVivieer, et al. Predictive value of low dose dobutamine transesophageal echocardiography and fluorine-18 fluorodeoxyglucose positron emission tomography for recovery of regional left ventricular function after successful revascularization. *J Am Coll Cardiol* 1996; 28:60–69.

502. Tischler MD, Plehn JF. Applications of stress echocardiography: Beyond coronary artery disease. *J Am Soc Echocardiogr* 1995; 8:185–197.

503. Leavitt JI, Coats MH, Falk RH. Effects of exercise on transmitral gradient and pulmonary artery pressure in patients with mitral stenosis or a prosthetic mitral valve: A Doppler echocardiographic study. *J Am Coll Cardiol* 1991; 17:1520–1526.

504. Tunick PA, Freedberg RS, Gargiulo A, Kronzon I. Exercise Doppler echocardiography as an aid to clinical decision making in mitral valve disease *.J Am Soc Echocardiogr* 1992; 5:225–230.

505. deFilippi CR, Willett DL, Brickner ME, Appleton CP, Yancy CW, Eichhorn CJ, et al. Usefulness of dobutamine echocardiography in distinguishing severe from nonsevere valvular aortic stenosis in patients with depressed left ventricular function and low transvalvular gradients. *Am J Cardiol* 1995; 75:191–194.

506. Abelmann WH. Classification and natural history of primary myocardial disease. *Prog Cardiovasc Dis* 1984; 27:73–94.

507. Rihal CS, Nishimura RA, Hatle LK, Bailey KR, Tajik AJ. Systolic and diastolic dysfunction in patients with clinical diagnosis of dilated cardiomyopathy: Relation to symptoms and prognosis. *Circulation* 1994; 90:2772–2779.

508. Wigle ED, Rakowski H, Kimball BP, Williams WG. Hypertrophic cardiomyopathy: Clinical spectrum and treatment. *Circulation* 1995; 92:1680–1692.

509. Siegel RJ, Shah PK, Fishbein MC. Idiopathic restrictive cardiomyopathy. *Circulation* 1984; 70:165–169.

510. Watkins H, McKenna WJ, Thierfelder L, Suk HJ, Anan R, O'Donoghue A, et al. Mutations in the genes for cardiac troponin T and a-tropomyosin in hypertrophic cardiomyopathy. *N Engl J Med* 1995; 332:1058–1064.

511. Solomon S, Wolff S, Watkins H, Ridker PM, Come P, McKenna WJ, et al. Left ventricular hypertrophy and morphology in familial hypertrophic cardiomyopathy associated with mutations of the beta-myosin heavy chain gene. *J Am Coll Cardiol* 1993; 22:498–505.

512. Louie EK, Maron BJ. Apical hypertrophic cardiomyopathy: Clinical and two-dimensional echocardiographic assessment. *Ann Intern Med* 1987; 106:663–670.

513. Maron BJ. Asymmetry in hypertrophic cardiomyopathy: The septal to free wall ratio revisited. *Am J Cardiol* 1985; 55:835–838.

514. Henry WL, Clark CE, Epstein SE. Asymmetric septal hypertrophy (ASH): Echocardiographic identification of the pathonomonic anatomic abnormality of IHSS. *Circulation* 1973; 47:225–233.

515. Maron BJ, Gottdiener JS, Epstein SE. Patterns and significance of distribution of left ventricular hypertrophy in hypertrophic cardiomyopathy: A wide angle, two dimensional echocardiographic study of 125 patients. *Am J Cardiol* 1981, 48:418–428.

516. Maron BJ, Epstein SE. Hypertrophic cardiomyopathy: Recent observations regarding the specificity of three hallmarks of the disease: Asymmetric septal hypertrophy, septal disorganization and systolic anterior motion of the anterior mitral leaflet. *Am J Cardiol* 1980; 45:141.

517. Blanchard DG, Ross J Jr. Hypertrophic cardiomyopathy: Prognosis with medical or surgical therapy. *Clin Cardiol* 1991; 14:11–19.

518. Maron BJ, Harding AM, Spirito P, Roberts WC, Waller BF. Systolic anterior motion of the posterior mitral leaflet: A previously unrecognized cause of dynamic subaortic obstruction in patients with hypertrophic cardiomyopathy. *Circulation* 1983; 68:282–293.

519. Klues HG, Roberts WC, Maron BJ. Morphologic determinants of echocardiographic patterns of mitral valve systolic anterior motion in obstructive hypertrophic cardiomyopathy. *Circulation* 1993; 87:1570–1579.

520. Jiang L, Levine RA, King ME, Weyman AE. An integrated mechanism for systolic anterior motion of the mitral valve in hypertrophic cardiomyopathy based on echocardiographic observations. *Am Heart J* 1987; 113:633–644.

521. Henry WL, Clark CE, Griffith JM, Epstein SE. Mechanism of left ventricular outflow obstruction in patients with obstructive asymmetric septal hypertrophy (idiopathic hypertrophic subaortic stenosis). *Am J Cardiol* 1975; 35:337–345.

522. Gardin JM, Talano JV, Stephanides L, Fizzano J, Lesch M. Systolic anterior motion in the absence of asymmetric septal hypertrophy: A buckling phenomenon of the chordae tendineae. *Circulation* 1981; 63:181–188.

523. Maron BJ, Gottdiener JS, Perry LW. Specificity of systolic anterior motion of anterior mitral leaflet for hypertrophic cardiomyopathy. *Br Heart J* 1981 45:206–212.

524. Gilbert BW, Pollick C, Adelman AG, Wigle ED. Hypertrophic cardiomyopathy: Subclassification by M mode echocardiography. *Am J Cardiol* 1980; 45:861–872.

525. Gardin J, Tommaso CL, Talano JV. Echocardiographic early systolic partial closure (notching) of the aortic valve in congestive cardiomyopathy. *Am Heart J* 1984; 107:135–142.

526. Eldar M, Motro M, Rath S, Schy N, Neufeld HN. Systolic closure of aortic valve in patients with prosthetic mitral valves. *Br Heart J* 1982; 48:48–53.

527. Zoghbi WA, Haichin RN, Quinones MA. Mid-cavity obstruction in apical hypertrophy: Doppler evidence of diastolic intraventricular gradient with higher apical pressure. *Am Heart J* 1988; 116:1469–1474.

528. Maron BJ, Gottdiener JS, Arce J, Rosing DR, Wesley YE, Epstein SE. Dynamic subaortic obstruction in hypertrophic cardiomyopathy: Pulsed Doppler echocardiography. *J Am Coll Cardiol* 1985; 6:1–15.

529. Sasson Z, Yock PG, Hatle LK, Alderman EL, Popp R. Doppler echocardiographic determination of the pressure gradient in hypertrophic cardiomyopathy. *J Am Coll Cardiol* 1988; 11:752–756.

530. Panza JA, Petrone RK, Fananapazir L, Maron BJ. Utility of continuous wave Doppler echocardiography in the noninvasive assessment of left ventricular outflow tract pressure gradient in patients with hypertrophic cardiomyopathy. *J Am Coll Cardiol* 1992; 19:91–99.

531. Baumgartner H, Schima H, Tulzer G, Kühn P. Effect of stenosis geometry on the Doppler-catheter gradient relation in vitro: A manifestation of pressure recovery. *J Am Coll Cardiol* 1993; 21:1018–1025.

532. Spirito P, Maron BJ. Relation between extent of left ventricular hypertrophy and diastolic filling abnormalities in hypertrophic cardiomyopathy. *J Am Coll Cardiol* 1990; 15:808–813.

533. Keren A, Popp RL. Assignment of patients into the classification of cardiomyopathies. *Circulation* 1992; 86:1622–1633.

534. Hoit BD, Penonen E, Dalton N, Sahn DJ. Doppler color flow mapping studies of jet formation and spatial orientation in obstructive hypertrophic cardiomyopathy. *Am Heart J* 1989; 117:1119.

535. Douglas PS, Morrow R, Ioli A, Reichek N. Left ventricular shape afterload in survival in idiopathic dilated cardiomyopathy. *J Am Coll Cardiol* 1989; 13:311–315.

536. Lewis JF, Webber JD, Sutton LL, Chesoni S, Curry CL. Discordance in degree of right and left ventricular dilation in patients with dilated cardiomyopathy: Recognition and clinical implications. *J Am Coll Cardiol* 1993; 21:640–654.

537. Blanchard DG, Hagenhoff C, Chow LC, McCann HA, Dittrich HC. Reversibility of cardiac abnormalities in human immunodeficiency virus (HIV) infected individuals: A serial echocardiographic study. *J Am Coll Cardiol* 1991; 17:1270–1276.

538. Frishman WH, Sung HM, Yee HCM, Liu LL, Einzig AL, Dutcher J, et al. Cardiovascular toxicity with cancer chemotherapy. *Curr Prob Cardiol* 1996; 21:225–288.

539. Corya BC, Feigenbaum H, Rasmussen S, Black MJ. Echocardiographic features of congestive cardiomyopathy compared with normal subjects and patients with coronary artery disease. *Circulation* 1974; 49:1153–1159.

540. Shah PM. Echocardiography in congestive or dilated cardiomyopathy. *J Am Soc Echocardiogr* 1988; 1:20–27.

541. Rihal CS, Nishimura RA, Hatle LK, Bailey KR, Tajik AJ. Systolic and diastolic dysfunction in patients with clinical diagnosis of dilated

cardiomyopathy: Relation to symptoms and prognosis. *Circulation* 1994; 90:2772–2779.

542. Pinamonti B, Di Lenarda A, Sinagra G, Camerini F. Restrictive left ventricular filling pattern in dilated cardiomyopathy assessed by Doppler echocardiography: Clinical, echocardiographic, and hemodynamic correlations and prognostic implications. *J Am Coll Cardiol* 1993; 22:808–815.

543. Nishimura RA, Tajik AJ. Quantitative hemodynamics by Doppler echocardiography: A noninvasive alternative to cardiac catheterization. *Prog Cardiovasc Dis* 1994; 36:309–342.

544. Shabetai R. The role of the pericardium in the pathophysiology of heart failure. In: Hosenpud JD, Greenberg BH, eds. *Congestive Heart Failure: Pathophysiology, Diagnosis, and Comprehensive Approach to Management.* New York: Springer-Verlag; 1994:95–125.

545. Borer JS, Henry WL, Epstein SE. Echocardiographic observations in patients with systemic infiltrative disease involving the heart. *Am J Cardiol* 1977; 39:184–188.

546. Gross DM, Williams JC, Caprioli CC, Dominguez B, Howell RR. Echocardiographic abnormalities in the mucopolysaccharide storage diseases. *Am J Cardiol* 1988; 61:170–176.

547. Picano E, Pinamonti B, Ferdeghini EM, Ferdeghini EM, Landini L, Slavich G. Two-dimensional echocardiography in myocardial amyloidosis. *Echocardiography* 1991; 8:253–262.

548. Acquatella H, Schiller NB, Puigbo JJ, Gomez-Mancebo JR, Suarez C, Acquatella G. Value of two dimensional echocardiography in endomyocardial disease with and without eosinophilia. *Circulation* 1983; 67:1219–1226.

549. Siqueira-Filho AG, Cunha CLP, Tajik AJ, Seward JB, Schattenberg TT, Giuliani ER. M-mode and two-dimensional echocardiographic features in cardiac amyloidosis. *Circulation* 1981; 63:188–196.

550. Klein AL, Cohen GI. Doppler echocardiographic assessment of constrictive pericarditis, cardiac amyloidosis, and cardiac tamponade. *Cleve Clin J Med* 1992; 59:278–290.

551. Klein AL, Hatle LK, Taliercio CP, Taylor CL, Kyle RA, Bailey KR, et al. Serial Doppler echocardiographic follow-up of left ventricular diastolic function in cardiac amyloidosis. *J Am Coll Cardiol* 1990; 16:1135–1141.

552. Klein AL, Hatle LK, Taliercio CP, Oh JK, Kyle RA, Gertz MA, et al. Prognostic significance of Doppler measures of diastolic function in cardiac amyloidosis. *Circulation* 1991; 83:808–816.

553. Acquatella H, Schiller NB. Echocardiographic recognition of Chagas' disease and endomyocardial fibrosis. *J Am Soc Echocardiogr* 1988; 1:60–68.

554. Fyfe DA, Kline CH. Transesophageal echocardiography for congenital heart disease. *Echocardiography* 1991; 8:573–586.

555. Huhta JC, Glasow P, Murphy DJ, Gutgesell HP, Otto A, McNamara DG, et al. Surgery without catheterization for congenital heart defects: Management of 100 patients. *J Am Coll Cardiol* 1987; 9:823–829.

556. Lipschulz SE, Sanders SP, Mayer JE, Colan SD, Lock JE. Are routine preoperative cardiac catheterization and angiography necessary before repair of ostium primum atrial septal defect? *J Am Coll Cardiol* 1988; 11:373–378.

557. Shub C, Tajik J, Seward JB, Hagler DJ, Danielson GK. Surgical repair of uncomplicated atrial septal defect without "routine" operative cardiac catheterization. *J Am Coll Cardiol* 1985; 6:49–54.

558. Hagler DJ, Tajik AJ, Seward JB, Edwards WD, Mair DD, Ritter DG. Aterioventricular and ventriculoarterial discordance (corrected transposition of the great arteries): Wide-angle two-dimensional echocardiographic assessment of ventricular morphology. *Mayo Clin Proc* 1981; 56:591–600.

559. Nasser FN, Tajik AJ, Stewart JB, Hagler DJ. Diagnosis of sinus venous atrial septal defect by two-dimensional echocardiography. *Mayo Clin Proc* 1981; 6:568–572.

560. Mehta RH, Helmcke F, Nanda NC, Hsiung M, Pacifico AD, Hsu TL. Transesophageal Doppler color flow mapping assessment of atrial septal defect. *J Am Coll Cardiol* 1990; 16:1010–1016.

561. Shub C, Dimopoulos IN, Seward JB, Cullahan JA, Tancredi RG, Schattenberg TT, et al. Sensitivity of two-dimensional echocardiography in the direct visualization of atrial septal defect utilizing the subcostal approach: Experience with 154 patients. *J Am Coll Cardiol* 1983; 2:127–135.

562. Hagler DJ, Tajik AJ, Seward JB, Mair D, Riter DG. Real-time wide-angle sector echocardiography: Atrioventricular canal defects. *Circulation* 1979; 59:140–150.

563. Mehta RH, Helmcke F, Nanda NC, Pinheiro L, Samdarshi TE, Shah VK. Uses and limitations of transthoracic echocardiography in the assessment of atrial septal defect in the adult. *Am J Cardiol* 1991; 67:288–294.

564. Franker TD, Harris PJ, Behar VS, Kisslo JA. Detection and exclusion of interatrial shunts by two-dimensional echocardiography and peripheral venous injections. *Circulation* 1979; 59:379–384.

565. Pollick C, Sullivan H, Cujec B, Wilansky S. Doppler color-flow imaging assessment of shunt size in atrial septal defect. *Circulation* 1988; 78:522–528.

566. Minagoe S, Tei C, Kisanuki A, Arikawa K, Nakazono Y, Yoshimura H, et al. Noninvasive pulsed Doppler echocardiographic detection of the direction of shunt flow in patients with atrial septal defect. *Circulation* 1985; 71:745–753.

567. Dittman H, Jacksch R, Voelker W, Karsch KR, Seipel L. Accuracy of Doppler echocardiography in quantification of left to right shunts in adult patients with atrial septal defect. *J Am Coll Cardiol* 1988; 11:338–342.

568. Jenni R, Ritter M, Vieli A, Hirzel HO, Schmidt ER, Grimm JG, et al. Determination of the ratio of pulmonary blood flow to systemic blood flow by deviation of amplitude weighed mean velocity from continuous wave Doppler spectra. *Br Heart J* 1989; 61:167–171.

569. Sutherland GR, Godman MJ, Smallhort JF, Guiterras P, Anderson RH, Hunter S. Ventricular septal defects: Two-dimensional echocardiographic and morphological correlations. *Br Heart J* 1982; 47:316–328.

570. Capelli H, Andrade JL, Somerville J. Classification of the site of ventricular septal defect by two-dimensional echocardiography. *Am J Cardiol* 1983; 51:1474–1488.

571. Linker DT, Rossvoll O, Chapman JV, Angelsen B. Sensitivity and speed of color Doppler flow mapping compared with continuous wave Doppler for the detection of ventricular septal defects. *Br Heart J* 1991; 65:201–203.

572. Baron JV, Sahn DJ, Valdes-Cruz LM, Grenadier E, Allen HD, Goldberg SJ. Two-dimensional echocardiographic features of ventricular septal aneurysm paradoxically bulging into the left ventricular outflow tract. *Am Heart J* 1982; 104:156–158.

573. Schmidt KG, Cassidy SC, Silverman NH, Stanger P. Doubly committed subarterial ventricular septal defects: Echocardiographic features and surgical implications. *J Am Coll Cardiol* 1988; 12:1538–1546.

574. Takenaka K, Sakmoto T, Shiota T, Amano W, Igarshi T, Sugimoto T. Diagnosis of patent ductus arteriosus in adults by biplane transesophageal color Doppler flow mapping. *Am J Cardiol* 1991; 68:691–693.

575. Snider AR, Silverman NH. Suprasternal notch echocardiography: a two-dimensional technique for evaluating congenital heart disease. *Circulation* 1982; 63:165–173.

576. Liao P-K, Su W-J, Hung J-S. Doppler echocardiographic flow characteristics of isolated patent ductus arteriosus: Better delineation by Doppler color flow mapping. *J Am Coll Cardiol* 1988; 12:1285–1291.

577. Swensson RE, Valdes-Cruz LM, Sahn DJ, Sherman FS, Chung KJ, Scagnelli S, et al. Real-time Doppler color flow mapping for detection of patient ductus arteriosus. *J Am Coll Cardiol* 1896; 8:1105–1112.

578. Alboliras ET, Chin AJ, Barbar G, Helton JG, Piggot J. Detection of aortopulmonary window by pulsed and color Doppler echocardiography. *Am Heart J* 1988; 115:900–902.

579. Balaji S, Burch M, Sullivan ED. Accuracy of cross-sectional echocardiography in diagnosis of aortopulmonary window. *Am J Cardiol* 1991; 67:650–653.

580. Gao Y-A, Burrows PE, Benson LN, Rabinovitch M, Freedom RM. Scimitar syndrome in infancy. *J Am Coll Cardiol* 1993; 22:873–882.

581. Oakley D, Naik D, Verel D, Rajan S. Scimitar vein syndrome: Report of nine new cases. *Am Heart J* 1984; 107:596–598.

582. Huhtas JC, Gutgesell HP, Nihill MR. Cross-sectional echocardiographic diagnosis of total anomalous pulmonary venous connection. *Br Heart J* 1985 53:525–534.

583. Sahn DJ, Allen HD, Lange LW, Goldberg SJ. Cross-sectional echocardiographic diagnosis of the sites of total anomalous pulmonary venous drainage. *Circulation* 1979; 60:1317–1325.

584. Smallhorn JF, Burrows P, Wilson G, Cols J, Gilday DL, Fredom RM. Two-dimensional and pulsed Doppler echocardiography in the postoperative evaluation of total anomalous pulmonary venous connection. *Circulation* 1987; 76:289–305.

585. Sreeram N, Walsh K: Diagnosis of total anomalous pulmonary venous drainage by Doppler color flow imaging. *J Am Coll Cardiol* 1992; 19:1577–1582.

586. Lengyel M, Arvay A, Biro V. Two-dimensional echocardiographic diagnosis of cor triatriatum. *Am J Cardiol* 1987; 59:484–485.

587. Snider AR, Port TA, Silverman NH. Venous anomalies of the coronary sinus: detection by M-mode, two-dimensional, and contrast echocardiography. *Circulation* 1979; 60:721–727.

588. Chaudhry F, Zabalgoitia M: Persistent left superior vena cava diagnosed by contrast transesophageal echocardiography. *Am Heart J* 1991; 122:1175–1177.

589. Flanagan MF, Foran RB, VanPraagh R, Jonas R, Sanders SP. Tetralogy of Fallot with obstruction of the ventricular septal defect: Spectrum of echocardiographic findings. *J Am Coll Cardiol* 1988; 11:386–395.

590. Musewe NN, Smallhorn JF, Moes CAF, Freedom RM, Trusler GA. Echocardiographic evaluation of obstructive mechanism of tetralogy of Fallot with restrictive ventricular septal defect. *Am J Cardiol* 1988; 61:664–668.

591. Geva T, Ayres NA, Pac FA, Pignatelli R. Quantitative morphometric analysis of progressive infundibular obstruction in tetralogy of Fallot: A prospective longitudinal echocardiographic study. *Circulation* 1995; 9:886–892.

592. Bricker JT. Sudden death and tetralogy of Fallot: Risks, markers, and causes. *Circulation* 1995; 92:158–159.

593. Macartney FJ, Rigby ML, Anderson RH, Stark J, Silverman NH. Double outlet right ventricle: Cross-sectional echocardiographic findings their anatomical explanation and surgical relevance. *Br Heart J* 1984; 52:164–177.

594. DiSessa TG, Hagman AD, Pope C, Samtoy L, Friedman WF. Two-dimensional echocardiographic characteristics of double outlet right ventricle. *Am J Cardiol* 1979; 44:1146–1154.

595. Roberson DA, Silverman NH. Malaligned outlet septum with subpulmonary ventricular septal defect and abnormal ventriculoarterial connection: A morphologic spectrum defined echocardiographically. *J Am Coll Cardiol* 1990; 16:459–468.

596. Chin AJ, Yeager SB, Sanders SP, Williams RG, Bierman FZ, Burger BM, et al. Accuracy of prospective two-dimensional echocardiographic evaluation of left ventricular outflow tract in complete transposition of the great arteries. *Am J Cardiol* 1985; 55:759–764.

597. Daskalopoulos DA, Edwards WD, Driscoll DJ, Seward JB, Tajik AJ, Hagler DJ. Correlation of two-dimensional echocardiographic and autopsy findings in complete transposition of the great arteries. *J Am Coll Cardiol* 1983; 3:1151–1157.

598. Smallhorn J, Grow R, Freedom R, Trusler G, Olley P, Pacquet M, et al. Pulsed Doppler echocardiographic assessment of the pulmonary venous pathway after the Mustard or Senning procedure for transposition of the great arteries. *Circulation* 1986; 73:765–774.

599. Kaulitz R, Stümper OFW, Geuskens R, Sreeram N, Elzenga NJ, Chan CK, et al. Comparative values of the precordial and transesophageal approaches in the echocardiographic evaluation of atrial baffle function after an atrial correction procedure. *J Am Coll Cardiol* 1990; 16:686–694.

600. Mahoney LT, Knoedel Dl, Skorton DJ. Echocardiographic postoperative assessment of patients with transposition of the great arteries. *Echocardiography* 1995; 12:545–557.

601. Rice MJ, Seward JB, Hagler DJ, Mair DD, Tajik AJ. Definitive diagnosis of truncus arteriosus by two-dimensional echocardiography. *Mayo Clin Proc* 1982; 57:476–481.

602. Marin-Garcia J, Tonkin ILD. Two-dimensional echocardiographic evaluation of persistent truncus arteriosus. *Am J Cardiol* 1982; 50:1376–1379.

603. Simpson IA, Sahn DJ, Valdes-Cruz LM, Chung KJ, Sherman FS, Swenson RE. Color Doppler flow mapping in patients with coarctation of the aorta: New observations and improved evaluation with color flow diameter and proximal acceleration as predictors of severity. *Circulation* 1988; 77:736–744.

604. Rao PS, Carey P. Doppler ultrasound in the prediction of pressure gradients across aortic coarctation. *Am Heart J* 1989; 118:299–307.

605. Shaddy RE, Snider AR, Silverman NH, Lutin W. Pulsed Doppler findings in patients with coarctation of the aorta. *Circulation* 1986; 73:82–88.

606. Nihoyannopoulos P, Karas S, Sapsford RN, Hallidie-Smith K, Foale R. Accuracy of two-dimensional echocardiography in the diagnosis of aortic arch obstruction. *J Am Coll Cardiol* 1987; 10:1072–1077.

607. Marx GR, Allen HD. Accuracy and pitfalls of Doppler evaluation of the pressure gradient in aortic coarctation. *J Am Coll Cardiol* 1986; 7:1379–1385.

608. Vogt J, Rupprath G, Grimm T, Beuren AJ. Qualitative and quantitative evaluation of supravalvular aortic stenosis by cross-sectional echocardiography: A report of 80 patients. *Pediatr Cardiol* 1982; 3:13–17.

609. Johnson GL, Kwan OL, Handshoe S, Noonan JA, DeMaria AN. Accuracy of combined two-dimensional echocardiography and continuous wave Doppler recordings in the estimation of pressure gradient in right ventricular outlet obstruction. *J Am Coll Cardiol* 1984; 3:1013–1018.

610. Weyman AE, Hurwitz RA, Girod DA, Dillon JC, Feigenbaum H, Green D. Cross-sectional echocardiographic visualization of the stenotic pulmonary valve. *Circulation* 1977; 56:769–774.

611. Choi JY, Sullivan ID. Fixed subaortic stenosis: Anatomical spectrum and nature of progression. *Br Heart J* 1991; 65:280–286.

612. Valdes-Cruz LM, Jones M, Scagnelli S, Sahn DJ, Tomizuka FM, Pierce JE. Prediction of gradients in fibrous subaortic stenosis by continuous wave two-dimensional Doppler echocardiography: Animal studies. *J Am Coll Cardiol* 1985; 5:1363–1367.

613. Wu JR, Huang TY, Chen YF, Lin YT, Roan HR. Aortico-left ventricular tunnel: Two-dimensional echocardiographic and angiocardiographic features. *Am Heart J* 1989; 117:697–699.

614. Zielinsky P, Rossi M, Haertel JC, Vitola D, Luchese FA, Rodrigues R. Subaortic fibrous ridge and ventricular septal defect: Role of septal malalignment. *Circulation* 1987; 75:1124–1129.

615. Zema JJ, Caccavano M. Two-dimensional echocardiograpic assessment of aortic morphology: Feasibility of bicuspid valve detection. *Br Heart J* 1982; 48:428–433.

616. Brandenberg J, Tajik AJ, Edwards WD, Reeder GS, Shub C, Seward JB. Accuracy of two-dimensional echocardiographic diagnosis of congenitally bicuspid aortic valve: Echocardiographic-anatomic correlation in 115 patients. *Am J Cardiol* 1983; 51:1469–1473.

617. Shiina A, Seward JB, Edwards WD, Hagler DJ, Tajik AJ. Two-dimensional echocardiographic spectrum of Ebstein's anomaly: Detailed anatomic assessment. *J Am Coll Cardiol* 1984; 3:356–370.

618. Quaegebeur JM, Sreeram N, Fraser AG, Bogers A, Stumper OFW, Hess J, et al. Surgery for Ebstein's anomaly: The clinical and echocardiographic evaluation of a new technique. *J Am Coll Cardiol* 1991; 17:722–728.

619. Copel JA, Pilu G, Green J, Hobbins JC, Kleinman CS. Fetal echocardiographic screening for congenital heart disease: The importance of the four-chamber view. *Am J Obstet Gynecol* 1987; 157:648–655.

620. Tan A, Kleinman C, Copel J. Does prenatal diagnosis of congenital heart disease make a difference? *Ultrasound Obstet Gynecol* 1995; 6:76S.

621. Sharland GK, Chita SK, Allan LD. The use of color Doppler in fetal echocardiography. *Int J Cardiol* 1990; 28:229–236.

622. Ewingman BG, Crane JP, Frigoletto F, Lefevre ML, Bair RP, McNellis D. Effect of prenatal ultrasound screening on perinatal outcome. *N Engl J Med* 1993; 329:821–827.

623. Buskens E, Grobbee DE, Frohn-Mulder IME, Stewart PA, Juttmann RE, Wladimiroff JW, et al. Efficacy of routine fetal ultrasound screening for congenital heart disease in normal pregnancy. *Circulation* 1996; 94:67–72.

624. Chang AC, Huhta JC, Yoon GY, Wood DC, Tulzer G, Cohen A. Diagnosis, transport, and outcome in fetuses with left ventricular outflow tract obstruction. *J Thorac Cardiovasc Surg* 1991; 102:841–848.

625. Hicks KA, Kovack JA, Frishberg DP, Wiley TM, Gurczak PB, Vernalis MN. Echocardiographic evaluation of papillary fibroelastoma: A case report and review of the literature. *J Am Soc Echocardiogr* 1996; 9:353–360.

626. DeMaria AN, Bommer W, Neumann A, Weinert L, Grehl T, Amsterdam EA, et al. Left ventricular thrombi identified by cross-sectional echocardiography. *Ann Intern Med* 1979; 90:14–18.

627. Limacher M, Gutgesell HP, Vick GW, Cohen MH, Huhta JA. Echocardiographic anatomy of the eustachian valve. *Am J Cardiol* 1986; 57:363–365.

628. Orita Y, Meno H, Kanarck M, Koiwayg Y, Tajimit T, Tongka J, et al. Echocardiographic features of persistent right sinus venosus valve in adults. *J Clin Ultrasound* 1982; 10:461.

629. Georgeson R, Liu M, Bansal RC. Transesophageal echocardiographic diagnosis of eustachian valve endocarditis. *J Am Soc Echocardiogr* 1996; 9:206–208.

630. Palakodeti V, Keen WD, Rickman L, Blanchard DG. Eustachian valve endocarditis: Detection by transesophageal echocardiography. *Clin Cardiol* 1997; 20:579–580.

631. Panidis IP, Kotler MN, Mintz GS, Ross J. Clinical and echocardiographic features of right atrial masses. *Am Heart J* 1984 107:745–758.

632. Werner JA, Cheitlin MD, Gross BW, Speck JM, Iwey TD. Echocardiographic appearance of the Chiari network: Differentiation from right-heart pathology. *Circulation* 1981; 63:1104–1109.

633. Keren A, Billingham ME, Popp RL. Echocardiographic recognition and implications of ventricular hypertrophic trabeculations and aberrant bands. *Ciculation* 1984; 70:836–842.

634. Perry LW, Ruckman RN, Shapiro SR, Kuehl KS, Galioto FM, Scott LP. Left ventricular false tendons in children: Prevalence as detected by two dimensional echocardiography and clinical significance. *Am J Cardiol* 1983; 52:1264–1266.

635. Vered Z, Melzer RS, Benjamin P, Motro M, Neufeld HN. Prevalence and significance of false tendons in the left ventricle as determined by echocardiography. *Am J Cardiol* 1984; 53:330–332.

636. Seward JB, Khanderia BK, Oh JK, Freeman WK, Tajik AJ. Critical appraisal of transesophageal echocardiography: Limitations, pitfalls, and complications. *J Am Soc Echocardiogr* 1992; 5:288–305.

637. Blanchard DG, Dittrich HC, Mitchell M, McCann HA. Diagnostic pitfalls in transesophageal echocardiography. *J Am Soc Echocardiogr* 1992; 5:525–540.

638. Starling RC, Baker PB, Hirsch SC, Myerowitz PD, Galbraith TA, Binkley PF. An echocardiographic and anatomic description of the donor-recipient atrial anastomosis after orthotopic cardiac transplantation. *Am J Cardiol* 1989; 64:109–111.

639. Drinkovic N. Subcostal echocardiography to determine right ventricular pacing catheter position and control advancement of electrode catheters in intracardiac electrophysiologic studies: M-mode and two-dimensional studies. *Am J Cardiol* 1981; 47:1260–1265.

640. Bierard L, Allaf DE, D'Orio V, Demoulin J-C, Carlier J. Two-dimensional echocardiographic guiding of endomyocardial biopsy. *Chest* 1984; 85:759–762.

641. French JW, Popp RL, Pitlick PT. Cardiac localization of transvascular biotome using two-dimensional echocardiography. *Am J Cardiol* 1983; 51:219–223.

642. Reeves WC, Movahed A, Chitwood R, Williams M, Jolly SR, Jordan JC, et al. Utility of precordial, epicardial and transesophageal two-dimensional echocardiography in the detection of intracardiac foreign bodies. *Am J Cardiol* 1989; 64:406–409.

643. Hanley PC, Tajik AJ, Hynes JK, Edwards WD, Reeder GS, Hagler DT, et al. Diagnosis and classification of atrial septal aneurysm by two-dimensional echocardiography: Report of 80 consecutive cases. *J Am Coll Cardiol* 1985; 6:1370–1382.

644. Pearson AC, Nagelhout D, Castello R, Gomez CR, Labovitz AJ. Atrial septal aneurysm and stroke: A transesophageal echocardiographic study. *J Am Coll Curdiol* 1991; 18:1223–1229.

645. Zabalgoitia-Reyes M, Herrera C, Gandhi DK, Mehlman DJ, McPherson DD, Talano JV. A possible mechanism for neurologic ischemic events in patients with atrial septal aneurysm. *Am J Cardiol* 1990; 66:761–764.

646. Fyke III FE, Tajik AJ, Edwards WD, Seward JB. Diagnosis of lipomatous hypertrophy of the interatrial septum by two-dimensional echocardiography. *J Am Coll Cardiol* 1983; 1:1352–1357.

647. Pochis WT, Saeian K, Sager KB. Usefulness of transesophageal echocardiography in diagnosing lipomatous hypertrophy of the atrial septum with comparison to transthoracic echocardiography. *Am J Cardiol* 1992; 70:396–398.

648. Haugland JM, Asinger RW, Mikell FL, Elsperger J, Hodges M. Embolic potential of left ventricular thrombi detection by two-dimensional echocardiography. *Circulation* 1984; 70:588–598.

649. Hunter JJ, Johnson KR, Karagianes TG, Dittrich HC. Detection of massive pulmonary embolus-in-transit by transesophageal echocardiography. *Chest* 1991; 100:1210–1214.

650. Pasierski TJ, Alton ME, Van Fossen DB, Pearson AC. Right atrial mobile thrombus: Improved visualization by transesophageal echocardiography. *Am Heart J* 1991; 123:802–803.

651. Armbruster RW, Labovitz AJ. Mitral stenosis. In: Daniel WG, Kronzon I, Mügge A, eds. *Cardiogenic Embolism*. Baltimore: Williams & Wilkins; 1996:81–92.

652. Aschenberg W, Schluter M, Kremer P, Schroder E, Siglow V, Bleifeld W. Transesophageal two-dimensional echocardiography for the detection of left atrial appendage thrombus. *J Am Coll Cardiol* 1986; 7:163–166.

653. Torbicki A, Pasierski T, Uchman B, Miskiewicz A. Right atrial mobile thrombi: Two-dimensional echocardiographic diagnosis and clinical outcome. *Cor Vasa* 1987; 29:293–303.

654. Goldberg SM, Pizzarello RA, Goldman MA, Padmanabhan VT. Echocardiographic diagnosis of right atrial thromboembolism resulting in massive pulmonary embolization. *Am Heart J* 1984; 108:1371–1372.

655. Klein AL, Stewart WC, Cosgrove DM III, Mick MJ, Salcedo E. Visualization of acute pulmonary emboli by transesophageal echocardiography. *J Am Soc Echocardiogr* 1990; 3:412–415.

656. Wiseman MN, Giles MS, Camm AJ. Unusual echocardiographic appearance of intracardiac thrombi in a patient with endomyocardial fibrosis. *Br Heart J* 1986; 56:179–181.

657. Stowers SA, Leiboff RH, Wasserman AG, Katz RJ, Bren GB, Hsu I. Right ventricular thrombus formation in association with acute myocardial infarction: Diagnosis by 2-dimensional echocardiography. *Am J Cardiol* 1983; 52:912–913.

658. Herzog CA, Bass L, Kane M, Asinger R. Two-dimensional echocardiographic imaging of left atrial appendage thrombi. *J Am Coll Cardiol* 1984; 3:1340–1344.

659. Manning WJ, Reis GJ, Douglas PS. Use of transesophageal echocardiography to detect left atrial thrombi before percutaneous balloon dilatation of the mitral valve: A prospective study. *Br Heart J* 1992; 67:170–173.

660. Olson JD, Goldenberg IF, Pedersen W, Brandt D, Kane M, Daniel JA, et al. Exclusion of atrial thrombus by transesophageal echocardiography. *J Am Soc Echocardiogr* 1992; 5:52–56.

661. Feltes TF, Friedman RA. Transesophageal echocardiographic detection of atrial thrombi in patients with nonfibrillation atrial tachyarrhythmias and congenital heart disease. *J Am Coll Cardiol* 1994; 24:1365–1370.

662. Galzerano D, Tucillo B, Lama D, Mirra G, Giasi M, Varricchio M, et al. Does multilobularity of left atrial appendage represent an additional risk for thrombus formation in atrial fibrillation? (abstr). *J Am Coll Cardiol* 1997; 29:212A.

663. Merino A, Hauptman P, Badimon L, Badimon JJ, Cohen M, Fuster V, et al. Echocardiographic "smoke" is produced by an interaction of erythrocytes and plasma proteins modulated by shear forces. *J Am Coll Cardiol* 1992; 20:1661–1668.

664. Castello R, Pearson AC, Labovitz AJ. Prevalence and clinical implications of atrial spontaneous contrast in patients undergoing transesophageal echocardiography. *Am J Cardiol* 1990; 65:1149–1153.

665. Daniel WG, Nellessen U, Schroder E, Nonnast-Daniel B, Bednarski P, Nikutta P. Left atrial spontaneous echo contrast in mitral valve disease: An indicator for an increased thromboembolic risk. *J Am Coll Cardiol* 1988; 11:1204–1211.

666. Peverill RE, Harper RW, Gelman J, Gan TE, Harris G, Smolich JJ. Determinants of increased regional left atrial coagulation activity in patients with mitral stenosis. *Circulation* 1996; 94:331–339.

667. Keating EC, Gross SA, Schalmatitz RA, Glassman J, Mazur JH, Pitt WA, et al. Mural thrombi in myocardial infarctions: Prospective evaluations by two-dimensional echocardiography. *Am J Med* 1983; 74:989–995.

668. Asinger RW, Mikell FL, Elsperger J, Hodges M. Incidence of left ventricular thrombosis after acute transmural myocardial infarction: Serial evaluation by two-dimensional echocardiography. *N Engl J Med* 1981; 305:297–302.

669. Visser CA, Kan G, David G, Ve KI, Durrer D. Two-dimensional echocardiography in the diagnosis of left ventricular thrombus: A prospective study of 67 patients with anatomic validation. *Chest* 1983; 83:228–232.

670. Takamoto T, Kim D, Murie P, Gurthaner DF, Gordon HJ, Keren A. Comparative recognition of left ventricular thrombi by echocardiography and cineangiography. *Br Heart J* 1985; 53:36–42.

671. Meltzer RS, Visser CA, Kan G, Roelandt J. Two-dimensional echocardiographic appearance of left ventricular thombi with systemic emboli after myocardial infarction. *Am J Cardiol* 1984; 53:1511–1513.

672. Edwards LC III, Louie EK. Transthoracic and transesophageal echocardiography for the evaluation of cardiac tumors, thrombi, and valvular vegetations. *Am J Cardiac Imaging* 1994; 8:45–58.

673. Meller J, Teichholz LE, Pichard AD, Matta R, Litwak R, Heiman MV. Left ventricular myxoma: Echocardiographic diagnosis and review of the literature. *Am J Med* 1977; 63:816.

674. Peters MN, Hall RJ, Cooley DA, et al. The clinical syndrome of atrial myxomas. *JAMA* 1974; 230:695.

675. Reynen K. Cardiac myxomas. *N Engl J Med* 1995; 1610–1617.

676. Gosse P, Herpin D, Roudault R, Malergue M-C, Lorgn M, Baudet E, et al. Myxoma of the mitral valve diagnosed by echocardiography. *Am Heart J* 1986; 111:803–805.

677. Suri RK, Pattnkar VL, Singh H, Aikat BK, Gunral JS. Myxoma of the tricuspid valve. *Aust NZ J Surg* 1978; 48:429–432.

678. Goli VD, Thadani U, Thomas SR, Voyles WF, Teague SM. Doppler echocardiographic profiles in obstructive right and left atrial myxomas. *J Am Coll Cardiol* 1987; 9:701–703.

679. Gorcsan J III, Blanc MS, Reedy PS, Marrone GC. Hemodynamic diagnosis of mitral valve obstruction by left atrial myxoma with transesophageal continuous wave Doppler. *Am Heart J* 1992; 124:1109–1112.

680. Obeid AI, Marvasti M, Parker F, Rosenberg J. Comparison of transthoracic and transesophageal echocardiography in diagnosis of left atrial myxoma. *Am J Cardiol* 1989; 63:1006–1008.

681. Nir A, Tajik AJ, Freeman WK, Seward JB, Offord KP, Edwards WD. Tuberous sclerosis and cardiac rhabdomyoma. *Am J Cardiol* 1995; 76:419–421.

682. Fenoglio JJ, McAllister HA, Fernas VJ. Cardiac rhabdomyoma: A clinicopathologic and electron microscopic study. *Am J Cardiol* 1976; 38:241–251.

683. Smythe JF, Dick JD, Smallhorn JF, Freedon RM. Natural history of cardiac rhabdomyoma in infancy and childhood. *Am J Cardiol* 1990; 66:1247–1249.

684. deRuiz M, Potter JL, Stavinoha J. Real-time ultrasound diagnosis of cardiac fibroma in a neonate. *J Ultrasound Med* 1985; 4:367–369.

685. Parmley LF, Salley RK, William JP, Head GB. The clinical spectrum of cardiac fibroma with diagnostic and surgical considerations: Noninvasive imaging enhances management. *Ann Thorac Surg* 1988; 45:455–465.

686. Topol EJ, Biern RO, Reitz BA. Cardiac papillary fibroelastoma and stroke. *Am J Med* 1986; 80:129–132.

687. Brown RD, Khanderia BK, Edwards WD. Cardiac papillary fibroelastoma: A treatable cause of transient ischemic attack and ischemic stroke detected by transesophageal echocardiography. *Mayo Clin Proc* 1995; 70:863–868.

688. Hui KS, Green LK, Schmidt WA. Primary cardiac rhabdomyosarcoma: Definition of a rare entity. *Am J Cardiovasc Pathol* 1988; 2:19–29.

689. Hanfling SM. Metastatic cancer to the heart. *Circulation* 1960; 22:474.

690. Riggs T, Paul MH, DeLeon S, Ilbawi M. Two-dimensional echocardiography in evaluation of right atrial masses: Five cases in pediatric patients. *Am J Cardiol* 1981; 48:961–966.

691. Roberts WC, Glancy DL, DeVita VT. Heart in malignant lymphoma (Hodgkins' disease, lymphosarcoma, reticulum cell sarcoma and mycosis fungoides): A study of 196 autopsy cases. *Am J Cardiol* 1968; 22:85–107.

692. Chandraratna PAN, Arnow WS. Detection of pericardial metastases by cross-sectional echocardiography. *Circulation* 1981; 63:197–199.

693. Limacher MC, McEntee CW, Attart M, Nelson JG, DeBakey ME, Quinones MA. Cardiac echinococcal cyst: Diagnosis by two dimensional echocardiography. *J Am Coll Cardiol* 1983; 2:574–577.

694. Rey M, Alfonso F, Torricella EG. Diagnostic valve of two-dimensional echocardiography in cardiac hydatid disease. *Eur Heart J* 1991; 12:1300.

695. McAllister HA Jr. Primary tumors and cysts of the heart and pericardium. *Curr Probl Cardiol* 1979; 4:1–51.

696. Martin RP, Rakowski H, French J, Popp RL. Localization of pericardial effusion with wide angle phased-array echocardiography. *Am J Cardiol* 1978; 42:904–912.

697. Martin RP, Bowden R, Filly K. Intrapericardial abnormalities in patients with pericardial effusion: Findings by two-dimensional echocardiography. *Circulation* 1980; 61:568–572.

698. Luft FC, Gilman JK, Weyman AE. Pericarditis in the patient with uremia: Clinical and echocardiographic evaluation. *Nephron* 1980; 25:160–166.

699. Schnittger I, Bowden RE, Abrams J, Popp RL. Echocardiography: Pericardial thickening and constrictive pericarditis. *Am J Cardiol* 1978; 42:388–395.

700. Lewis BS. Real time two dimensional echocardiography in constrictive pericarditis. *Am J Cardiol* 1982; 49:1789–1793.

701. Hatle LK, Appleton CP, Popp RL. Differentiation of constrictive pericarditis and restrictive cardiomyopathy by Doppler echocardiography. *Circulation* 1989; 79:357–370.

702. Horowitz MS, Schultz CS, Stinson EB. Sensitivity and specificity of echocardiographic diagnosis of pericardial effusion. *Circulation* 1974; 50:239–247.

703. Come PC, Riley MF, Fortuin NJ. Echocardiographic mimicry of pericardial effusion. *Am J Cardiol* 1981; 47:365–370.

704. Gabor GE, Winsberg F, Bloom HS. Electrical and mechanical alternation in pericardial effusion. *Chest* 1971; 59:341–344.

705. Haaz WS, Mintz GS, Kotler MN, Parry W, Segal BL. Two dimensional echocardiographic recognition of the descending thoracic aorta: Value in differentiating pericardial from pleural effusion. *Am J Cardiol* 1980; 46:739–743.

706. Isner JM, Carter BL, Roberts WC, Bankoff MS. Subepicardial adipose tissue producing echocardiographic appearance of pericardial effusion. *Am J Cardiol* 1983; 51:565–569.

707. Schiller NB, Botvinick EH. Right ventricular compression as a sign of cardiac tamponade: An analysis of echocardiographic ventricular dimensions and their clinical implications. *Circulation* 1977; 56:774–779.

708. Appleton CP, Hatle LK, Popp RL. Cardiac tamponade and pericardial effusion: Respiratory variation in transvalvular flow velocities studied by Doppler echocardiography. *J Am Coll Cardiol* 1988; 11:1020–1030.

709. Gillam LD, Guyer DE, Gibson TC, King ME, Marshall JE, Weyman AE. Hydrodynamic compression of the right atrium: A new echocardiographic sign of cardiac tamponade. *Circulation* 1983; 68:294–301.

710. Armstrong WF, Schilt BF, Helper DJ, Dillon JC, Feigenbaum H. Diastolic collapse of the right ventricle with cardiac tamponade: An echocardiographic study. *Circulation* 1982; 65:1491–1503.

711. Conrad SA, Byrnes TJ. Diastolic collapse of the left and right ventricles in cardiac tamponade. *Am Heart J* 1988; 115:475–478.

712. Brodyn NE, Rose MR, Prior FP, Haft JI. Left atrial diastolic compression in a patient with a large pericardial effusion and pulmonary hypertension. *Am J Med* 1990; 88:1–8.

713. Leeman DE, Levine MJ, Come PC. Doppler echocardiography in cardiac tamponade: Exaggerated respiratory variation in transvalvular blood flow velocity integrals. *J Am Coll Cardiol* 1988; 11:572–578.

714. Callahan JA, Seward JB, Tajik AJ. Cardiac tamponade: Pericardiocentesis directed by two-dimensional echocardiography. *Mayo Clin Proc* 1985; 60:344–347.

715. Pandian NG, Skorton DJ, Kieso RA, Kerber RE. Diagnosis of constrictive pericarditis by two-dimensional echocardiography: Studies in a new experimental model and in patients. *J Am Coll Cardiol* 1984; 4:1164–1173.

716. Himelman RB, Lee S, Schiller NB. Septal bounce, vena cava plethora, and pericardial adhesion: Informative two-dimensional echocardiographic signs in the diagnosis of pericardial constriction. *J Am Soc Echocardiogr* 1988; 1:333–340.

717. Morgan JM, Raposo L, Clague JC, Chow WH, Oldershaw PJ. Restrictive cardiomyopathy and constrictive pericarditis: Non-invasive distinction by digitized M mode echocardiography. *Br Heart J* 1988; 59:629. (abstract)

718. Schiavone WA, Calafiore PA, Currie PJ, Lytle BW. Doppler echocardiographic demonstration of pulmonary venous flow velocity in three patients with constrictive pericarditis before and after pericardioectomy. *Am J Cardiol* 1989; 63:145–147.

719. vonBibra H, Schober K, Jenni R, Busch R, Sebening H, Blomer H. Diagnosis of constrictive pericarditis by pulsed Doppler echocardiography of the hepatic vein. *Am J Cardiol* 1989; 63:483–488.

720. Schiavone WA, Calafiore PA, Salcedo EE. Transesophageal Doppler echocardiographic demonstration of pulmonary venous flow velocity in restrictive cardiomyopathy and constrictive pericarditis. *Am J Cardiol* 1989; 63:1286–1288.

721. Oh JK, Hatle LK, Seward JB, Danielson GK, Schaff HV, Reeder GS, Tajik AJ. Diagnostic role of Doppler echocardiography in constrictive pericarditis. *J Am Coll Cardiol* 1994; 23:154–162.

722. Klein AL, Cohen GI, Pietrolungo JF, White RD, Bailey A, Pearce GL, et al. Differentiation of constrictive pericarditis from restrictive cardiomyopathy by Doppler transesophageal echocardiographic measurements of respiratory variations in pulmonary vein flow. *J Am Coll Cardiol* 1993; 22:1935–1943.

723. Garcia MJ Rodriquez L, Ares M, Griffin BP, Thomas JD, Klein AL. Differentiation of constrictive pericarditis from restrictive cardiomyopathy: Assessment of left ventricular diastolic velocities in longitudinal axis by Doppler tissue imaging. *J Am Coll Cardiol* 1996; 27:108–114.

724. Izumi S, Mariyama K, Kobayashi S, Toda H, Ohta T, Matsuno V, et al. Phasic venous return abnormality in chronic pulmonary diseases: Pulsed Doppler echocardiographic study. *Intern Med* 1994; 33:326–333.

725. Kodas E, Nishimura RA, Appleton CP, Redfield MM, Oh JK. Doppler evaluation of patients with constrictive pericarditis: Use of tricuspid

regurgitation velocity curves to determine enhanced ventricular interaction. *J Am Coll Cardiol* 1996; 28;652–657.

726. Capannari TE, Daniels SR, Meyer RA, Schwartz DC, Kaplan S. Sensitivity, specificity, and predictive value of two-dimensional echocardiography in detecting coronary artery aneurysms in patients with Kawasaki disease. *J Am Coll Cardiol* 1986; 7:355–360.

727. Noto N, Ayusawa M, Karasawa K, Yamaguchi H, Sumitomo N, Okada T, et al. Dobutamine stress echocardiography for detection of coronary artery stenosis in children with Kawasaki disease. *J Am Coll Cardiol* 1996; 27:1251–1256.

728. Burns JC, Shike H, Gordon JB, Malhotra A, Schoenwetter M, Kawasaki T. Sequelae of Kawasaki disease in adolescents and young adults. *J Am Coll Cardiol* 1996; 28:253–257.

729. Petrovic O, Elsner GB, Wilensky RL, Swanson ST, Feigenbaum H. Transthoracic echocardiographic detection of coronary atherosclerosis. *Am J Cardiol* 1996; 77:569–574.

730. Fernandes F, Alam M, Smith S, Khaja F. The role of transesophageal echocardiography in identifying anomalous coronary arteries. *Circulation* 1993; 88:2532–2540.

731. Samdarshi TE, Nanda NC, Gatewood RP Jr, Ballal RS, Chang LK, Singh HP, et al. Usefulness and limitations of transesophageal echocardiography in the assessment of proximal coronary artery stenosis. *J Am Coll Cardiol* 1992; 19:572–580.

732. Yamagishi M, Yasu T, Ohara K, Kuro M, Miyatake K. Detection of coronary blood flow associated with left main coronary artery stenosis by transesophageal Doppler color flow echocardiography. *J Am Coll Cardiol* 1991; 17:87–93.

733. Redberg RF, Sobol Y, Chou TM, Malloy M, Kumar S, Botvinick E, et al. Adenosine-induced coronary vasodilatation during transesophageal Doppler echocardiography: Rapid and safe measurement of coronary flow reserve ratio can predict significant left anterior descending coronary stenosis. *Circulation* 1995; 92:190–196.

734. Zehetgruber M, Mundigler F, Christ G, Mortl D, Probst P, Baumgartner H, et al. Estimation of coronary flow reserve by transesophageal coronary sinus Doppler measurements in patients with syndrome X and patients with significant left coronary artery disease. *J Am Coll Cardiol* 1995; 25:1039–1045.

735. Raisinghani A, Ohmori K, Blanchard D, Cotter B, Kwan OL, Calisi C, et al. Non-invasive visualization and measurement of coronary blood flow by transthoracic Doppler echocardiography: Initial results. *Circulation* 1996; 94(I):I-561. (abstract)

736. Raisinghani A, Cotter B, Ohmori K, Kwan OL, Calisi C, DeMaria AN. Assessment of the effects of sublingual NTG upon intramyocardial blood flow velocity in normals by transthoracic echocardiography. *Circulation* 1996; 94(I):I-503. (abstract)

15

THE EXERCISE TEST

Gerald F. Fletcher / Robert C. Schlant

Exercise testing defines the body's reaction to measured increases in acute exercise. The changes in heart rate, blood pressure, respiration, and perceived level of exertion provide data for quantitative estimation of cardiovascular conditioning and function. These data also correlate with more general aspects of conditioning, such as flexibility and musculoskeletal strength. In addition to "numerical" data, exercise tests provide an opportunity to observe a person during exercise. By monitoring heart rate and blood pressure and continually observing the electrocardiogram (ECG), one can detect alterations in the hemodynamic response and ECG ST-segment changes and identify disturbances in cardiac rate, rhythm, and conduction associated with exercise.

THE CARDIOVASCULAR RESPONSE TO EXERCISE

Exercise, a common physiologic stress, elicits cardiovascular abnormalities not present at rest and can be used to assess function of the cardiovascular system. Exercise is only one of the many stresses to which humans are exposed; therefore, it is frequently more appropriate to refer to an "exercise" test and not a "stress" test. Several types of muscular contraction (activity) can be used as an exercise test of the cardiovascular system: isometric (static), isotonic (dynamic), or resistance.[1] *Isometric (static) exercise*, defined as a constant muscular contraction without movement (e.g., handgrip), provokes more pressure load than volume load on the left ventricle in relation to the body's ability to supply oxygen. The cardiovascular response to isometric exercise, however, is difficult to grade since the response to activation of a small muscle group is similar to the response of a large muscle group. In addition, cardiac output is not increased as much as is resistance. *Isotonic (dynamic) exercise*, defined as muscular contraction of larger muscle groups resulting in movement, primarily provides a volume load to the left ventricle, and the cardiovascular response is proportional to the degree of the exercise. *Resistance exercises* are combinations of both isometric and iso-

tonic; for example, lifting a free weight, as in doing an "arm curl."

Maximum Oxygen Uptake

When dynamic exercise begins, oxygen uptake by the lungs increases. After several minutes, oxygen uptake usually remains relatively stable (steady state) at each intensity of exercise. During the steady state, heart rate (HR), cardiac output, blood pressure, and pulmonary ventilation are maintained at reasonably constant levels.[1]

Maximal oxygen consumption ($\dot{V}_{O_2max}$) is the greatest amount of oxygen a person can utilize while performing dynamic exercise involving large components of total muscle mass[2] and represents the amount of oxygen transported and used in cellular metabolism. It is appropriate to express oxygen uptake in multiples of sitting/resting requirements. The metabolic equivalent (MET) is a unit of sitting/resting oxygen uptake [3.5 mL O_2 per kilogram of body weight per minute (mL kg^{-1} min^{-1})]. Rather than determining each person's true resting oxygen uptake, one MET is designated as this average. $\dot{V}_{O_2max}$ is significantly related to age, gender, exercise habits, heredity, and clinical cardiovascular status.

Maximum values of $\dot{V}_{O_2max}$ occur between the ages of 15 and 30 years and decrease progressively with age. At age 60, mean $\dot{V}_{O_2max}$ in men is approximately three-fourths that at age 20. Individuals with a sedentary lifestyle have a 9 percent decrease per decade versus less than 5 percent per decade in those with an active lifestyle. Up to age 12 to 16, there is no significant difference in $\dot{V}_{O_2max}$ among children. At ages 12 to 14, however, a decrease is observed in girls. The reduced $\dot{V}_{O_2max}$ in women is related to less muscle mass, lower hemoglobin and blood volume, and smaller stroke volume than men.

Physical activity level has an important influence on $\dot{V}_{O_2max}$. After 3 weeks of bed rest, there is a 25 percent decrease in $\dot{V}_{O_2max}$ in healthy men. In moderately active young men, $\dot{V}_{O_2max}$ is about 12 METs, whereas individuals performing aerobic training such as distance running can have a $\dot{V}_{O_2max}$ as high as 18 to 24 METs (60 to 85 mL kg^{-1} min^{-1}). There appears to be a natural variation in $\dot{V}_{O_2max}$ related to genetic factors; in addition, $\dot{V}_{O_2max}$ is affected by the degree of impairment from cardiovascular disease.

It is difficult to predict $\dot{V}_{O_2max}$ accurately based on exercise habits and age. Table 15-1 lists average levels of METs for various activities and the prognostic value of different levels of METs.[3]

Maximum $\dot{V}_{O_2}$ is equal to maximum cardiac output times maximum arteriovenous (AV) oxygen (AV_{O_2}) difference. Since cardiac output is equal to the product of stroke volume and HR, $\dot{V}_{O_2}$ is directly related to HR. The maximum AV_{O_2} difference during exercise has a physiologic limit of 15 to 17 mL/dL; therefore, if maximum effort is achieved, $\dot{V}_{O_2max}$ can be used to estimate maximum cardiac output.

Myocardial Oxygen Uptake

Myocardial oxygen uptake (M_{O_2}) is determined by intramyocardial wall tension [left ventricular (LV) systolic pressure times end-diastolic volume, divided by LV wall thickness], contractility, and HR. Other less important factors include the external work performed by the heart, energy necessary for activation, and the basal metabolism of the myocardium (see also Chap. 3).

The accurate measurement of M_{O_2} requires cardiac catheterization; however, M_{O_2} can be estimated during exercise testing by the product of HR and systolic blood pressure, called the *rate-pressure product*. In general, there is a linear relation between M_{O_2} and coronary blood flow. During exercise, coronary blood flow increases as much as fivefold above the resting value. A patient with obstructive coronary disease, however, may not have adequate coronary blood flow to supply the metabolic demands of the myocardium during vigorous

exercise; as a consequence, myocardial ischemia occurs (see also Chap. 43).

RESPONSE TO DYNAMIC EXERCISE

The response to dynamic exercise consists of a complex series of cardiovascular adjustments to provide active muscles with blood appropriate for metabolic needs, dissipate heat generated by muscles, and maintain blood supply to essential organs such as the brain and heart. As cardiac output increases with dynamic exercise, vascular resistance decreases in active muscles but increases in tissues that are not functional during exercise.[4]

Heart Rate Response

An increase in HR due to a decrease in vagal outflow is an immediate response of the cardiovascular system to exercise. This is rapidly followed by an increase in sympathetic outflow to the heart and systemic blood vessels, which also contributes to the increase in HR. During dynamic exercise, HR increases linearly with workload and $\dot{V}_{O_2}$. During low levels of exercise and at a constant work rate, HR will reach a steady state within several minutes; however, as workload increases, the time to stabilize progressively lengthens.

Heart rate response is influenced by several factors including age, sex, subject motivation, body habitus, and type of exercise. There is a decline in mean maximum HR with age,[5] which seems related to intrinsic cardiac changes rather than neural influences (see Chap. 96). Dynamic exercise increases HR more than isometric exercise, and an accentuated HR response is observed after extended bed rest. Other factors that influence HR include body position, general state of health, blood volume, and environment.

Arterial Blood Pressure Response

Systolic blood pressure increases with dynamic work as a result of increasing cardiac output, while diastolic pressure usually remains about the same or decreases slightly. An inadequate rise in systolic blood pressure (20 to 30 mmHg or less) can result from aortic valve or outflow obstruction, left ventricular dysfunction, or myocardial ischemia. Patients who develop hypotension during exercise frequently have severe heart disease. Changes of blood pressure are strongly influenced by changes in peripheral resistance.

After maximum exercise, there is normally a decrease in systolic blood pressure, usually reaching resting levels in 6 min and then often remaining lower than preexercise levels for several hours. In some patients with coronary artery disease (CAD), higher levels of systolic blood pressure, at times even exceeding peak exercise values, may develop in the recovery phase. When exercise is terminated abruptly, some healthy persons have precipitous drops in systolic blood pressure due to venous pooling. Figure 15-1 shows the physiologic response to submaximum and maximum treadmill exercise

TABLE 15-1

CLINICALLY SIGNIFICANT METABOLIC EQUIVALENTS FOR MAXIMUM EXERCISE

1 MET[a]	Resting
2 METs	Level walking at 2 mph
4 METs	Level walking at 4 mph
<5 METs	Poor prognosis; usual limit immediately after myocardial infarction; peak cost of basic activities of daily living
10 METs	Prognosis with medical therapy as good as coronary artery bypass surgery
13 METs	Excellent prognosis regardless of other exercise responses
18 METs	Elite endurance athletes
20 METs	World-class athletes

[a] MET = metabolic equivalent, or a unit of sitting resting oxygen uptake. 1 MET = 3.5 mL kg^{-1} min^{-1} oxygen uptake.

Source: From Fletcher GF, Balady G, Froelicher VF, Hartley LH, Haskell WL, Pollock ML. Exercise standards: A statement for health professionals from the American Heart Association Writing Group. *Circulation* 1995; 91:580–615. Reproduced with permission from the publisher and the authors.

based on tests of more than 700 apparently healthy men aged 25 to 54. Maximum rate-pressure product ranges from a 10th percentile value of 25,000 to a 90th percentile value of 40,000.

The arterial blood supply to the myocardium and other muscles and organs is usually adequate for maximal perfusion. If obstructive coronary artery disease is present, only minimal reduction in maximal blood flow will take place until the degree of arterial obstruction becomes quite advanced[6] (see Chap. 3). If the subject engages only in sedentary behavior, it is possible for an advanced degree of coronary arterial obstruction to develop without clinically significant underperfusion of the myocardium. The predictive importance of exertional myocardial ischemia is related to the intensity of cardiac activity at which the ischemia becomes apparent.[7] For example, if there is no evidence of ischemia at 75 percent of maximum exercise but there is such evidence at 90 to 100 percent of maximal exercise, it would likely be associated with a less severe degree of coronary obstruction than if the ischemia had been detectable at only 25 to 50 percent of maximal exercise.

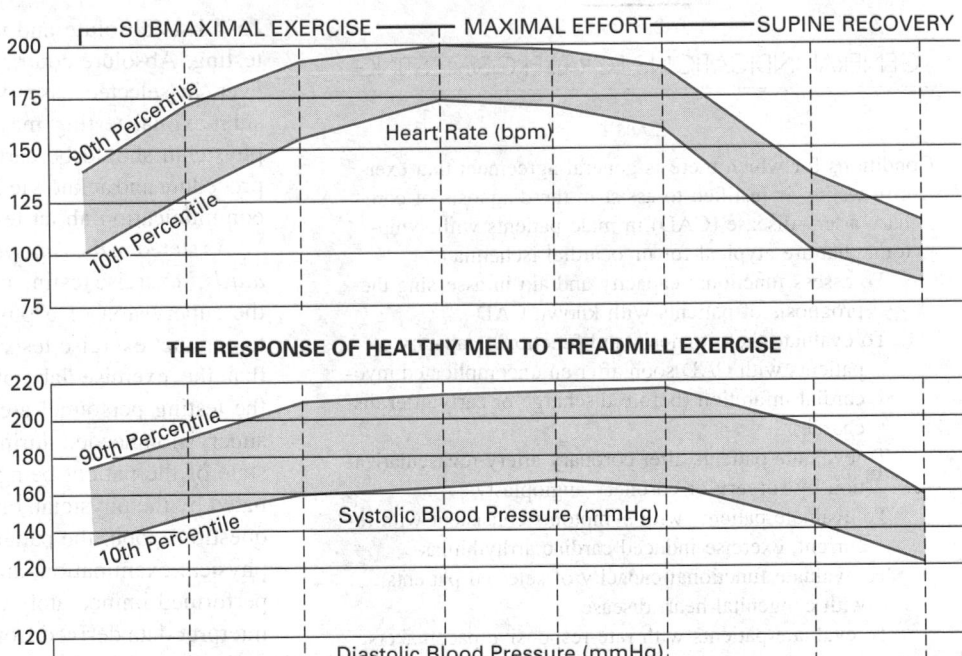

FIGURE 15-1

Normal response to progressive treadmill protocol in healthy subjects. (From Froelicher VF. *Exercise and the Heart: Clinical Concepts.* Chicago: Year Book; 1987. Reproduced with permission from the publisher and the author.)

TESTING PROCEDURES

Exercise testing of patients should be conducted only by well-trained personnel with a basic knowledge of exercise physiology and electrocardiography. In general, only physicians and other health professionals (especially nurses) familiar with normal and abnormal responses during exercise and qualified in Advanced Cardiac Life Support have the skills needed to perform exercise tests.[8] Equipment, medications, and personnel trained to provide cardiopulmonary resuscitation (CPR) must be readily available. Although exercise testing of patients is considered safe, there are reports of acute myocardial infarction and death related to the procedure. Several surveys confirm that up to 10 myocardial infarctions, deaths, or both can be expected per 10,000 tests. The risk is greater in post-myocardial infarction patients and in those being evaluated for malignant ventricular arrhythmias. Table 15-2 lists three classes of complications secondary to exercise tests.

Good clinical judgment is imperative in determining indications for and contraindications to exercise testing.[9] Table 15-3 lists the general indications for exercise testing and Table

TABLE 15-2

COMPLICATIONS SECONDARY TO EXERCISE TESTS

CARDIAC COMPLICATIONS

Bradyarrhythmias
  Sinus
  Atrioventricular junctional
  Ventricular
  Atrioventricular block
  Asystole
Sudden death (ventricular tachycardia/fibrillation)
Myocardial infarction
Congestive heart failure
Hypotension and shock

NONCARDIAC COMPLICATIONS

Musculoskeletal trauma

ILL-DEFINED AND MISCELLANEOUS COMPLICATIONS

Severe fatigue, dizziness, fainting, general malaise, body aches, delayed ill feelings, and fatigue sometimes persisting for days

Source: From Fletcher GF, Balady G, Froelicher VF, Hartley LH, Haskell WL, Pollock ML. Exercise standards: A statement for health professionals from the American Heart Association Writing Group. *Circulation* 1995; 91:580–615. Reproduced with permission from the publisher and the authors.

TABLE 15-3
GENERAL INDICATIONS FOR EXERCISE TESTING

CLASS I

Conditions for which there is general agreement that exercise testing is justified to assist in the diagnosis of coronary artery disease (CAD) in male patients with symptoms that are atypical for myocardial ischemia

To assess functional capacity and aid in assessing the prognosis of patients with known CAD

To evaluate the prognosis and functional capacity of patients with CAD soon after an uncomplicated myocardial infarction (before discharge or early after discharge)

To evaluate patients after coronary artery revascularization by surgery or coronary angioplasty

To evaluate patients with symptoms consistent with recurrent, exercise-induced cardiac arrhythmias

To evaluate functional capacity of selected patients with congenital heart disease

To evaluate patients with rate-responsive pacemakers

CLASS II

Conditions for which exercise testing is frequently performed but in which there is a divergence of opinion with respect to its value and appropriateness

To evaluate asymptomatic male patients over the age of 40 with special occupations (pilots, air traffic controllers, firefighters, police officers, critical process operators, bus or truck drivers, and railroad engineers)

To evaluate asymptomatic males over the age of 40 with two or more risk factors for CAD

To evaluate sedentary male patients >40 years who plan to enter a vigorous exercise program

To assist in the diagnosis of CAD in women with a history of typical or atypical angina pectoris

To assist in the diagnosis of CAD in patients who are taking digitalis or who have complete right bundle branch block

To evaluate the functional capacity and response to therapy with cardiovascular drugs in patients with CAD or heart failure

To evaluate patients with variant angina

To follow up serially (at 1-year intervals or longer) patients with known CAD

To evaluate patients with a class I indication who have baseline ECG changes or coexisting medical problems that limit the value of the test (In some of these patients, exercise testing may still yield clinically useful information, such as duration of exercise, blood pressure response, and production of chest discomfort.)

To evaluate patients who have sustained a complicated myocardial infarction but who have subsequently "stabilized" (before discharge or early after discharge)

Source: From Schlant RC, Blomqvist CG, Brandenburg RO, DeBusk R, Ellestad MH, Fletcher GF, et al. Special report. In: Guidelines for exercise testing. A report of the Joint American College of Cardiology/American Heart Association Task Force on Assessment of Cardiovascular Procedures (Subcommittee on Exercise Testing). *Circulation* 1986; 74:653A–667A. Reproduced with permission from the publisher and the authors.

15-4 lists absolute and relative contraindications to exercise testing. Absolute contraindications are quite definitive; however, in selected cases with relative contraindications, even submaximal testing may provide valuable information. The physician should be certain that the subject understands the procedure and acknowledges the risks. Good physician-patient communication about testing and its risks is essential.

As stated in the *American Heart Association Exercise Standards*,[3] exercise testing of patients should be performed under the supervision of a physician who is appropriately trained to conduct exercise tests and who is responsible for ensuring that the exercise laboratory is properly equipped and that the testing personnel are appropriately trained. The level of supervision needed during a test is determined by the clinical state of the patient being tested. Supervision must be designated by the physician or physician's staff, who ask pertinent questions about the patient's medical history, perform a brief physical examination, and review the standard 12-lead ECG performed immediately before testing. The physician should interpret data derived from testing, suggest further evaluation or therapy, and aid in providing effective and timely advanced CPR when necessary. A defibrillator and appropriate medications should be immediately available. Table 15-5 details safety measures for exercise testing.

TABLE 15-4
ABSOLUTE AND RELATIVE CONTRAINDICATIONS TO EXERCISE TESTING

Absolute	Relative[a]
Acute myocardial infarction or recent change on resting ECG	Less serious noncardiac disorder
Active unstable angina	Significant arterial or pulmonary hypertension
Serious cardiac arrhythmias	Tachyarrhythmias or bradyarrhythmias
Acute pericarditis	Moderate valvular or myocardial heart disease
Endocarditis	Drug effect or electrolyte abnormalities
Severe aortic stenosis	Left main coronary obstruction or its equivalent
Severe left ventricular dysfunction	Hypertrophic cardiomyopathy
Acute pulmonary embolus or pulmonary infarction	Psychiatric disease
Acute or serious noncardiac disorder	Severe physical handicap or disability

[a] Under certain circumstances and with appropriate precautions, relative contraindications can be superseded.

Source: From Schlant RC, Blomqvist CG, Brandenburg RO, DeBusk R, Ellestad MH, Fletcher GF, et al. Special report. In: Guidelines for exercise testing. A report of the Joint American College of Cardiology/American Heart Association Task Force on Assessment of Cardiovascular Procedures (Subcommittee on Exercise Testing). *Circulation* 1986; 74:653A–667A. Reproduced with permission from the publisher and the authors.

TABLE 15-5

SAFETY MEASURES FOR EXERCISE TESTING

1. Definite plan of emergency action, including the duties of each member of the team. In addition to direct patient care, the plan should include notification of appropriate individuals and provision of other necessities for patient transfer.
2. Prompt admission to a coronary care unit.
3. All members of team trained in cardiopulmonary resuscitation.
4. Defibrillator within cable reach of treadmill, turned on and charged (200 J) during test. Full tube of electrode paste on top of unit.
5. Emergency drug kit.
6. Intravenous solutions, administration sets, needles, and syringes.
7. Oropharyngeal airways, laryngoscope, endotracheal tubes, ventilation bag, and suction machine.
8. Equipment for the administration of oxygen.

Source: From Fletcher GF, ed. *Exercise in the Practice of Medicine*, 2d ed. Mt. Kisco, NY: Futura, 1988. Reproduced with permission from the publisher and the author.

The degree of supervision of an exercise test can range from assigning monitoring of the test to a properly trained nonphysician (i.e., nurse or exercise specialist) for testing apparently healthy younger persons (less than 40 years old) or assigning patients with stable chest discomfort syndromes to the physician who directly monitors the patient's status throughout exercise and recovery. The latter is the ideal for testing patients for diagnostic or prognostic purposes and is a requirement for testing all patients at increased risk for an exercise-induced complication. A physician should be immediately available during all exercise tests on patients.

Patient Preparation

Preparations for exercise testing include the following:

- The patient should be instructed not to eat or smoke for 2 to 3 h before the test and to dress appropriately for exercise. No strenuous physical efforts should be made for at least 12 h before testing.
- Cessation of medications may sometimes be considered, since some drugs interfere with exercise responses, complicating the interpretation of exercise testing. Most patients, however, are tested on their medications. Specific questioning is important to determine which drugs have been taken so that the physician can be aware of possible electrolyte abnormalities and other effects.
- A brief history should be taken and physical examination done to rule out contraindications to testing or detect important clinical signs such as murmurs, gallop sounds, pulmonary bronchospasm, or rales. Patients with a history of increasing or unstable angina or uncontrolled heart failure should not undergo exercise testing until their condition stabilizes. A cardiac physical examination should indicate which patients have valvular or congenital heart disease, particularly adult patients with severe aortic stenosis, who generally should not undergo exercise testing.

- A detailed explanation of the testing procedure should be given, outlining risks and possible complications. The patient should be told how to perform the exercise test, and the testing procedure should be demonstrated.
- A standard resting 12-lead ECG should be obtained, since it may differ from the resting preexercise ECG. This is essential, particularly in patients with known heart disease, since an abnormality or change may contraindicate testing. Recording the ECG before starting the exercise test and after hyperventilation at another time may be helpful in detecting false-positive (indeterminate) ECG changes, particularly in women.
- Standing ECG and blood pressure should be recorded to determine vasoregulatory abnormalities, particularly ST-segment depression.

Electrocardiographic Recording

The most important aspect of the electrode-amplifier-recording system is the interface between the electrodes and the skin. Removing the superficial layer of skin significantly lowers resistance, decreasing the signal-to-noise ratio. The areas for electrode application are first shaved (if necessary) and then rubbed with an alcohol-saturated gauze. After the skin dries, it is marked with a felt-tipped pen and rubbed with a fine sandpaper or other rough material to reduce skin resistance.

Many electrode systems are available for performing exercise testing; silver plate or silver chloride crystal pellets are preferred, since they have the lowest offset voltage. The electrodes should have a metal interface that is sunken, creating a column to be filled with either an electrolyte solution or a saturated sponge. Connecting cables between the electrodes and recorder should be light, flexible, and properly shielded. Cables generally have a life span of a year or so, depending on use. Cables can eventually become a source of both noise and electrical discontinuity, so that replacement is required.

Bipolar lead systems are advantageous in recording ECG changes during exercise. The relatively short placement time, freedom from motion artifacts, and ease with which noise problems can be located are all factors favoring their use. The usual positive reference is one electrode placed in the same position as the positive reference for V_5 (the fifth intercostal space at the midclavicular line) and the negative reference at Wilson's central terminal. Figure 15-2 illustrates negative electrode placement for most bipolar lead systems. CM_5 is the most sensitive for ST-segment changes. CC_5 excludes the vertical component included in CM_5 and decreases influence of atrial repolarization (Ta), reducing false-positive responses.[10]

Since a standard 12-lead ECG with electrodes placed on the limbs cannot be effectively obtained during exercise, other electrode placements have been used. Differences can be minimized by placing arm electrodes close to the shoulders and leg electrodes below the umbilicus. Any modification of lead placement should be recorded on the tracing.

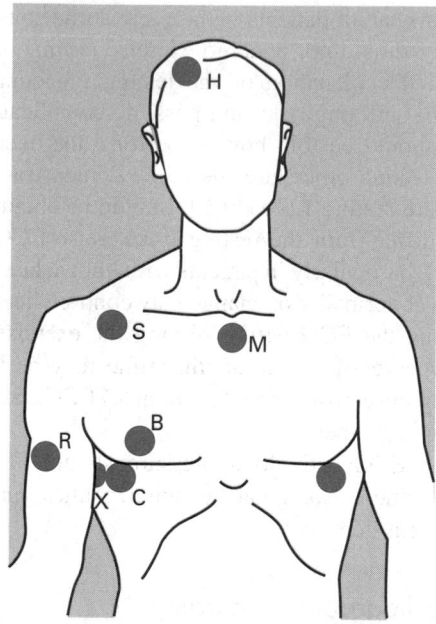

FIGURE 15-2

Negative electrode placement for most bipolar lead systems. B, on back, subscapular; M, top of manubrium; X, midaxillary line, fifth intercostal level; C, anterior axillary line, fifth intercostal level; H, above shoulders (neck or above); S, right clavicular edge; R, right arm; +, positive electrode placement for C_5 bipolar electrodes. (From Froelicher VF. *Exercise and the Heart: Clinical Concepts.* Chicago: Year Book; 1987. Reproduced with permission from the publisher and the author.)

The lateral precordial leads (V_4 through V_6) are capable of detecting 90 percent of all ECG ST depression observed in multiple lead systems. A more extensive lead system, however, is preferred in certain patients with a high prevalence of previous myocardial infarction or symptoms suggesting coronary artery spasm. ST depression in five leads or more usually predicts multivessel disease. A three-lead system (V_2, II, and V_5) is usually adequate for localizing ischemia related to spasm and is also helpful for characterization of arrhythmias.

There are various recorders designed to provide high-quality ECG data during exercise. Many use microprocessors to generate average waveforms and make ECG measurements; however, computer processing is not completely reliable because of software limitations in handling noise and inadequacy of the available algorithms. The physician must, therefore, compare the raw analog data with computer-generated output to validate its accuracy.

EQUIPMENT AND PROTOCOLS

Figure 15-3 illustrates the relation of METs to stages in the commonly used testing protocols. Numerous devices have been used to provide dynamic exercise for testing; however, the treadmill and the cycle ergometer remain the most commonly used dynamic exercise testing devices.

The treadmill should have front and side rails for patients to steady themselves; however, they should not grasp the front or side rails tightly, as this decreases $\dot{V}_{O_2}$ and work while increasing exercise time and muscle artifact. Most patients can walk without aid of the hand rails; however, older and poorly coordinated subjects may need such support. It is helpful if patients take their hands off the rails and place one or two fingers on the rails to maintain balance after they have become accustomed to walking on the treadmill. The treadmill should have both variable speed and grade capability and must be accurately calibrated.

Mechanical or electrically braked cycles are calibrated in kiloponds (kpm) or watts and are capable of varying the force to the pedaling speed (rate-independent ergometers). This permits more precise control of power output, since it is common for uncooperative or fatigued patients to decrease their pedaling speed. The highest values of $\dot{V}_{O_2}$ and HR are obtained with pedaling speeds of 60 to 80 rpm. One watt is equivalent to approximately 6 kpm, and since exercise on a cycle ergometer is non-weight-bearing, kiloponds or watts can be converted to oxygen uptake in milliliters per minute. METs are obtained by dividing $\dot{V}_{O_2}$ in milliliters per minute by the product of body weight in kilograms multiplied by 3. The cycle ergometer is usually less expensive and occupies less space than a treadmill. Upper-body motion is usually reduced, making it easier to obtain blood pressure measurements and to record the ECG; however, care must be taken to prevent isometric or resistive exercise of the arms.

There is a considerable difference between the body's response to acute exercise in the supine and erect positions. In healthy persons during supine cycle exercise, stroke volume and end-diastolic volume change relatively little, perhaps 10 to 20 percent, from volumes at rest; whereas during cycle exercise in the erect position, stroke volume increases (and may double during severe exercise) and then plateaus during mild work. In patients with intrinsic cardiac abnormalities, left ventricular filling pressure is more likely to increase during exercise in the supine than in the erect position. When patients with angina pectoris perform identical submaximal cycle work in the supine and erect positions, HR is higher in the supine position. Maximum work performed, however, is lower in the supine position, and angina develops at a lower rate-pressure product. ST changes are more frequently detected during exercise in the upright position; however, ST-segment changes are usually greater in magnitude during exercise in the supine position because of the greater LV volume.

Protocols for clinical exercise testing should include an initial low load (warmup), progressive uninterrupted exercise with an adequate duration in each level, and a recovery period. For cycle ergometry, the initial power output is usually 10 or 25 W (150 kpm/min), usually followed by increases of 25 W every 2 or 3 min until symptomatic or objective end points are reached. If arm ergometry is substituted for cycle leg ergometry, a similar protocol may be used except that initial power output and incremental increases are lower. Two-minute stages are most popular with arm ergometry.[11,12]

Several different treadmill protocols are in use, the most popular of which is the Bruce. The advantages of the Bruce

Functional class	Clinical status	O₂ cost mL/kg/min	METS	Bicycle ergometer	Treadmill protocols — Bruce 3-min stages		Balke-Ware %GR at 3.3 mph 1-min stages	Ellestad 3/2/3 min stages		McHenry		Naughton 2-min stages 3.0 mph %GR	METS
					mph	%GR		mph	%GR	mph	%GR		
				1 watt = 6 kpds	5.5	2.0							
Normal and I	Healthy, dependent on age, activity	56.0	16	For 70 kg body weight, kpds	5.0	18		6	15			32.5	16
		52.5	15									30.0	15
		49.0	14	1500			26 25 24	5	15	mph %GR		27.5	14
		45.5	13		4.2	16	23 22			3.3	21	25.0	13
		42.0	12	1350			21 20			3.3	18	22.5	12
		38.5	11	1200			19 18 17	5	10	3.3	15	20.0	11
	Sedentary healthy	35.0	10	1050	3.4	14	16 15 14					17.5	10
		31.5	9	900			13 12					15.0	9
		28.0	8				11 10	4	10	3.3	12	12.5	8
		24.5	7	750	2.5	12	9 8	3	10	3.3	9	10.0	7
II	Limited	21.0	6	600			7 6					7.5	6
		17.5	5	450	1.7	10	5 4	1.7	10	3.3	6	5.0	5
III	Symptomatic	14.0	4	300	1.7	5	3					2.5	4
		10.5	3	150			2			2.0	3	0.0	3
		7.0	2		1.7	0	1						2
IV		3.5	1										1

FIGURE 15-3

Treadmill protocols with approximate oxygen uptakes. mph = miles per hour; %GR = percent grade; kpds = kiloponds. (Modified from Froelicher VF. *Exercise and the Heart: Clinical Concepts.* Chicago: Year Book; 1987. Reproduced with permission from the publisher and the author.)

protocol include a seventh or final stage (which cannot be completed by most individuals) and its use in many published studies, thus providing extensive data for comparison. Its disadvantages include large increments in workload that make estimation of $\dot{V}_{O_2max}$ less accurate. In addition, the fourth stage can be either run or walked, probably resulting in different oxygen costs. Some subjects are forced to stop prematurely because of musculoskeletal difficulties or inability to tolerate the high workload increments. Initial stages of zero and one-half (1.7 mph at 0 percent, then 5 percent grade) may be used for some patients. Regardless of technique used, *the optimum exercise testing protocol should last 6 to 12 min and should be adjusted to the type of patient being tested.* Performance can be estimated with the oxygen cost of maximum workload or power output achieved rather than by total treadmill time if hand rails are not used for support. This allows comparison of performance in different protocols.

Since there is strong evidence that the level of exercise required to produce ischemia is the most important part of the exercise test result, there is concern as to how the exercise test workload is selected. There is overwhelming agreement on use of a progressively increasing exercise protocol beginning with a stage low enough to be tolerated by the "weakest"

candidate for testing and ending with a stage sufficiently difficult to challenge the "strongest" candidate. Each stage should be long enough in duration for the subject to reach or closely approach steady state, and the work increments from one stage to the next should be small enough to permit the desired degree of precision in estimating work capacity.[13,14] The Bruce treadmill protocol is widely used (Table 15-6). Typical work output requirements for each stage in terms of oxygen consumption have been determined, and the range of stages is adequate both for sedentary individuals and athletes.[15] To increase applicability, two easier stages may be added below stage 1 in order to accommodate virtually all ambulatory individuals.[15] In order for measurement of treadmill performance, exercise time, or rate-pressure response to be directly related to the actual cardiac work involved, the subject must have reached or closely approached a "steady state." This implies that if the subject continued to exercise at this same intensity, cardiac output, HR, and other indices would remain essentially the same until the point of fatigue. Steady-state attainment requires at least 3 min, and perhaps longer on the treadmill, and exercise times shorter than this will not yield a reliable reflection of cardiovascular capacity.

TABLE 15-6

SCHEDULE OF TREADMILL EXERCISE FOR THE GRADED EXERCISE TEST

Stage Number	Time per Stage, min	Elapsed Time at End of Stage	Speed km/h	Speed mph	Treadmill Slope Grade, %	Treadmill Slope Elevation, degrees
Zero[a]	3	3[b]	2.7	1.7	0 (level)	0 (level)
One-half[a]	3	3[b]	2.7	1.7	5	2.8
First	3	3	2.7	1.7	10	5.7
Second	3	6	4.0	2.5	12	6.8
Third	3	9	5.5	3.4	14	8.0
Fourth	3	12	6.8	4.2	16	9.0
Fifth	3	16	8.0	5.0	18	10.0
Sixth	3	18	8.9	5.5	20	11.0
Seventh	3	21	9.6	6.0	22	12.4

[a] Begin with stage zero or stage one-half if appearance and demeanor of subject suggest that walking capacity is severely limited.

[b] Exercise time in these preliminary stages is not counted when tabulating functional capacity.

Source: From Fletcher GF, ed. *Exercise in the Practice of Medicine*, 2d ed. Mt. Kisco, NY: Futura; 1988. Reproduced with permission from the publisher and the author.

Rather than assign a certain stage of exercise protocol as a goal for an individual (whether based on age, history of exercise participation, or level of conditioning), it is preferable to require the subject to exercise progressively through the protocol until it becomes excessively uncomfortable or impossible to continue—that is, to an end point of exhaustion unless other terminating end points occur. As discussed below, there are several means of determining whether or not the subject makes a good effort so that the exercise time is a true representation of physical capacity. The most obvious criterion is HR, which can be predicted with about 90 percent accuracy.[16–18] Failure to attain an exercise tachycardia reasonably close to a predicted maximum may not, however, provide an adequate indication of the degree of effort (Table 15-7).

SUBMAXIMAL VERSUS MAXIMAL EXERCISE TESTING

In some cases, testing is terminated when the patient reaches 90 percent of predicted maximal HR for age and level of

training. The designated target HR, however, may be maximal for some subjects, beyond the limit of others, or submaximal for others. A test is considered maximal when the patient appears to give a true maximal effort (point of overall bodily exhaustion) or when other clinical end points are reached.

Perceived Exertion

The subjective rating of exertion is a good indicator of relative fatigue and is used to quantify effort. Rather than using HR alone to clinically determine intensity of exercise, the 6- to 20-point Borg scale of perceived exertion[19] is useful in some patients (Table 15-8). Although there is some variation among patients in their actual rating of fatigue, individual patients rate consistently from test to test. Thus, the Borg scale can assist the clinician in judging the degree of fatigue with testing and in correlating the level of fatigue during testing with that experienced during daily activities.

Indications for Terminating Exercise Testing

Indications for discontinuing an exercise test include absolute and relative indications (Table 15-9).

Postexercise Period

Some abnormal responses occur only in recovery after exercise. For maximum sensitivity, patients should be supine in the postexercise period; however, the seated position may be utilized effectively. Monitoring of blood pressure and ECG should continue for at least 6 to 8 min after exercise. An abnormal ECG response occurring only in the recovery period is not unusual, as mechanical dysfunction and electrophysiologic abnormalities in the ischemic ventricle after exercise can persist for minutes to hours.

INTERPRETATION

Clinical Responses

Classical anginal chest discomfort induced by the exercise test is strongly predictive of CAD and is even more predictive in the presence of ST depression. The patient's general appearance is also helpful. A decrease in skin temperature, cool perspiration, and peripheral cyanosis during

TABLE 15-7

PREDICTED EXERCISE HEART RATE: MEN/WOMEN

Age	30	35	40	45	50	55	60	65
Maximal predicted heart rate								
(M)	193	191	189	187	184	182	180	178
(W)	190	185	181	177	172	168	163	159
80% of maximal predicted heart rate (HRi = 0.80)								
(M)	154	153	151	150	147	146	144	142
(W)	152	148	145	142	138	134	130	127

Source: From Fletcher GF, ed. *Exercise in the Practice of Medicine*, 2d ed. Mt. Kisco, NY: Futura; 1988. Reproduced with permission from the publisher and the author.

TABLE 15-8
BORG SCALE FOR RATING PERCEIVED EXERTION

15-Grade Scale		10-Grade Scale	
6		0	Nothing
7	Very, very light	0.5	Very, very weak (just noticeable)
8		1	Very weak
9	Very light	2	Weak (light)
10		3	Moderate
11	Fairly light	4	Somewhat strong
12		5	Strong (heavy)
13	Somewhat hard	6	
14		7	Very strong
15	Hard	8	
16		9	
17	Very hard	10	Very, very strong (almost maximum)
18			
19	Very, very hard	°	Maximum
20			

Source: From Pollock ML, Wilmore JH. *Exercise in Health and Disease: Evaluation and Prescription for Prevention and Rehabilitation*, 2d ed. Philadelphia: Saunders; 1990:290. Reproduced with permission from the publisher and the authors.

exercise may indicate poor tissue perfusion due to inadequate cardiac output with secondary vasoconstriction. In such instances, higher workloads are not encouraged. Neurologic manifestations such as light-headedness or vertigo can also indicate inadequate cardiac output.

Physical Examination

Cardiac examination immediately after exercise can provide information about ventricular function. A precordial bulge or gallop rhythm can result from LV dysfunction. A mitral regurgitant murmur suggests papillary muscle dysfunction related to transient ischemia.

Exercise or Functional Capacity

The maximal oxygen consumption ($\dot{V}_{O_2max}$) is the best index of maximal exercise capacity. A decrease in maximum cardiac output (which correlates with $\dot{V}_{O_2max}$) may be a consequence of CAD, and exercise may be limited by either anginal pain or an acute reduction in LV output. An increase in LV diastolic filling pressure and increasing pulmonary artery pressure will also limit exercise. A mean exercise capacity of 10 METs has been observed in nonathletic, middle-aged, healthy men. If patients with CAD reach 13 METs, their prognosis is good, regardless of other exercise test responses. As expected, patients with an exercise capacity of less than 5 METs have a higher mortality during follow-up than patients with higher capacities.

A normal exercise capacity does not exclude severe cardiac impairment. Mechanisms proposed to explain a normal exer-

cise performance in such patients include increased peripheral oxygen extraction, preservation of chronotropic reserve, ability to tolerate elevated pulmonary wedge pressures without dyspnea, and increased levels of plasma norepinephrine at rest and during exercise.[3]

HEMODYNAMIC RESPONSES

Blood pressure is a function of cardiac output and peripheral resistance. Although some normal subjects have a transient drop in systolic blood pressure at maximal exercise, this finding is frequently associated with severe CAD and ischemic dysfunction of the myocardium. Exercise-induced hypotension also identifies patients at increased risk for ventricular fibrillation in the exercise laboratory. Figure 15-4 illustrates normal and abnormal systolic blood pressure responses to exercise tests.

A relatively rapid HR during submaximal exercise or recovery could be due to decreased vascular volume or peripheral resistance, prolonged bed rest, anemia, or metabolic disorders; therefore, it may not reflect intrinsic cardiac disease. This finding is also relatively frequent in patients soon after myocardial infarction or coronary artery surgery. A relatively low HR at any point during submaximal exercise may be due to lack of training or drugs such as beta blockers. Conditions that affect the sinus node can also attenuate the normal

TABLE 15-9
INDICATIONS FOR TERMINATING EXERCISE TESTING

ABSOLUTE INDICATIONS

Drop in systolic blood pressure (persistently below baseline) despite an increase in workload
Onset of new or increasing anginal chest discomfort
Central nervous system symptoms (ataxia, dizziness, or near syncope)
Evidence of poor peripheral perfusion (cyanosis or pallor)
Serious arrhythmias (i.e., high-grade ventricular, such as multiform complexes, triplets, and runs)
Technical difficulties in monitoring the ECG or systolic blood pressure
Patient's request to stop

RELATIVE INDICATIONS

ST or QRS changes such as excessive (≥ 3–4 mm) ST displacement, junctional depression, or marked QRS axis shift
Increasing chest discomfort
Fatigue, shortness of breath, wheezing, leg cramps, or intermittent claudication
General appearance (see discussion)
Less serious arrhythmias, including supraventricular tachycardias
Development of bundle branch block that cannot be distinguished from ventricular tachycardia

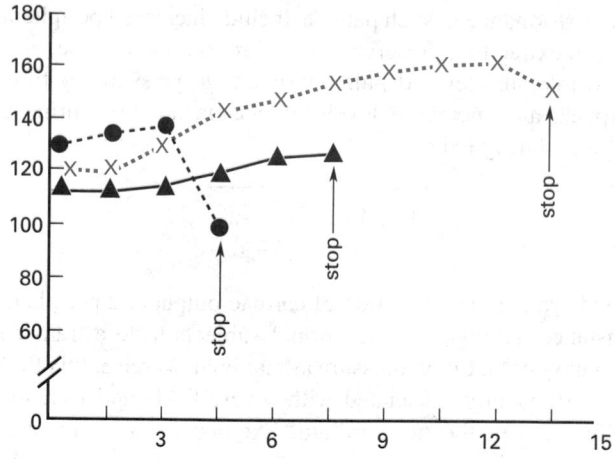

FIGURE 15-4

Normal and abnormal systolic blood pressure responses to exercise tests. X = Normal response. Subject able to exercise 13 1/2 min, drops blood pressure at peak of normal exercise capacity. ● = abnormal. Subject increases systolic pressure initially, but pressure drops early in exercise before normal exercise capacity is reached. ▲ = abnormal. Subject fails to raise systolic pressure to 130 mmHg or higher, even though exercise duration may be nearly normal. (From Fletcher GF, ed. *Exercise in the Practice of Medicine*, 2d ed. Mt. Kisco, NY: Futura; 1988. Reproduced with permission from the publisher and the author.)

response of HR during exercise testing. Table 15-7 shows predicted exercise HR in normals.

Electrocardiographic Responses in Subjects with Normal Resting Electrocardiograms

During exercise, the P-wave vector tends to become more vertical and the P-wave magnitude increases in the inferior leads. The PR segment (interval) shortens and slopes downward in the inferior leads. The change, which has been attributed to atrial repolarization (Ta wave), may cause false-positive or indeterminate ST depression in the inferior leads. Changes in R-wave amplitude are noted near maximal effort with a decrease in the R wave in the lateral leads (V_5) at maximal exercise and 1 min into recovery. In the lateral and vertical leads (V_5 and aVF), the S wave becomes greater in depth, showing a greater deflection at maximal exercise, and then gradually returning to resting values in recovery.

The J junction is depressed in the lateral leads at maximum exercise and then gradually returns to preexercise values in recovery. A dramatic increase in J-junctional depression may be observed in all leads and may be greatest at 1 min into recovery. Subjects with resting J-junction elevation may develop an isoelectric J junction with exercise as a normal finding. These changes revert in recovery. The normal ST segment vector response to both tachycardia and exercise is a shift rightward and upward in the frontal plane; however, there appears to be considerable biological variation in the degree of this shift. A gradual decrease in T-wave amplitude is observed in all leads during early exercise. At maximum exercise the T wave begins to increase, and at 1-min recovery the amplitude is equivalent to resting values in the lateral leads.[3]

Abnormal Responses

The ST-segment level is measured relative to the PR segment, for with the increased HR during exercise, the U-P segment is usually unclear. ST elevation is measured as the deviation from the baseline ST level. If the baseline ST segment is depressed, the deviation from that level to the level during exercise or recovery is measured. The point for measuring the ST level is the J junction; points 60 or 80 ms beyond this are usually used when the ST-segment slope is horizontal or downsloping. Considering a rapidly upsloping ST depression to be abnormal increases test sensitivity but decreases specificity. Various ST scores have been recommended, but none have been validated as superior to standard "visual" measurements. Exercise-induced myocardial ischemia can result in one of three ST-segment changes on the surface ECG: depression, elevation, and normalization.

ST-segment depression is the most common manifestation of exercise-induced myocardial ischemia. It usually reflects diffuse subendocardial ischemia, with vector direction determined largely by the area of ischemia and the position of the heart in the thoracic cavity. The standard criterion for this abnormal response is horizontal or downsloping ST-segment depression of 0.10 mV (1.0 mm) or more for 80 ms in at least three consecutive "isoelectric" or level complexes. As shown in Fig. 15-5, however, other criteria have been considered. Downsloping (divergent) ST-segment depression usually reflects more ischemia than horizontal depression. In the presence of baseline abnormalities (especially in patients on digitalis), exercise-induced ST-segment depression is less specific for ischemia. Factors related to the probability and severity of CAD include the degree, time of appearance, duration, persistence in recovery, and number of leads with ST-segment depression. The lower the workload and the double product at which the ST change occurs, the worse the prognosis and the more likely the presence of multivessel CAD. ST elevation must be judged by whether or not it occurs in the presence of Q waves from a previous myocardial infarction. ST-segment elevation is more frequently observed in anterior leads (V_1 and V_2) with Q waves.[20]

Previous myocardial infarction is the most frequent cause of ST-segment elevation during exercise and seems to be related to dyskinetic areas or ventricular aneurysms. Approximately 50 percent of patients with recent anterior and 15 percent with inferior myocardial infarction exhibit this finding during exercise.[20] Patients with elevation usually have a lower left ventricular ejection fraction (LVEF) than those without such ST-segment elevation in leads with abnormal Q waves from prior myocardial infarction. These changes may result in reciprocal ST depression simulating ischemia in other leads. The development of both ST-segment elevation and depression during the same test may indicate multivessel CAD.

In patients without previous myocardial infarction (absence of Q waves on the resting ECG), ST-segment elevation during exercise frequently reflects severe transient ischemia resulting from significant proximal CAD or spasm.

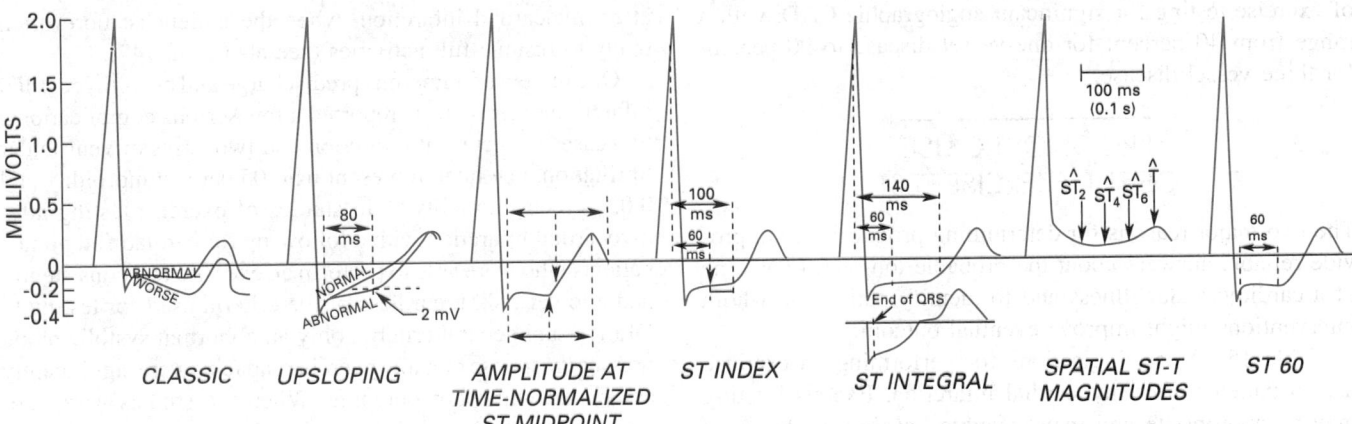

FIGURE 15-5

Types of abnormal ST responses. (From Froelicher VF. *Exercise and the Heart: Clinical Concepts*. Chicago: Year Book; 1987. Reproduced with permission from the publisher and the author.)

In patients with variant angina (often indicating coronary spasm), ST-segment elevation usually occurs during spontaneous anginal episodes, frequently at rest. During exercise, ST-segment elevation has been reported in about 30 percent of these patients and a reversible thallium-201 perfusion defect usually corresponds to the site of ST elevation. Another manifestation of ischemia may be the normalization of an ST-segment. ECG abnormalities at rest, including T-wave inversion and ST-segment depression, may return to normal during attacks of angina and during exercise in some patients with myocardial ischemia. This can also be observed in subjects with a "persistent juvenile pattern" on the resting ECG.[3]

The R-wave amplitude may increase during exercise in certain subjects with cardiac disease; however, exercise-induced changes in R-wave amplitude have not improved diagnostic accuracy despite use of several lead systems, clinical subsets of patients, and different criteria for an abnormal response.

In normals, a gradual decrease in T-wave amplitude is observed in all leads during early exercise, although the T wave begins to increase with maximum exercise. At 1-min recovery, T-wave amplitude usually returns to resting values. U-wave inversion may be associated with LV hypertrophy, CAD, or aortic and mitral regurgitation. Exercise-induced U-wave inversion in patients with a normal resting ECG appears to be a marker of myocardial ischemia and suggests left anterior descending CAD. U-wave changes may, however, be difficult to assess during exercise, which increases HR and the proximity of the T and P waves.

Plasma potassium increases with maximal exercise testing and, in subjects on atenolol and propranolol therapy, increases more after training.[21] In addition (in sedentary individuals), both plasma potassium and magnesium increase significantly with maximal exercise, and these increases are unaffected by atenolol and propranolol blockade. To the contrary, propranolol, but not atenolol and placebo, prolongs the time of return to baseline of potassium (compared with magnesium) after the acute exercise.[22] Such changes must be considered with

exercise testing because of electrolyte effects on ST-T, and U waves.

Exercise tests can be performed with radionuclide imaging to further evaluate myocardial perfusion (see Chap. 17). Echocardiographic images and Doppler flow measurements (Chap. 14) can also be made during and after exercise, and LVEF, wall motion, and valvular function can be assessed with these techniques.

DIAGNOSTIC VALUE OF THE EXERCISE TEST

Sensitivity and Specificity

Sensitivity and specificity define how effectively a test detects disease. *Sensitivity* is the percentage of those with a disease who will have an abnormal test. *Specificity* is the percentage of those without the disease who will have a normal test. This may be affected by drugs, baseline ECG patterns, and whether a test is submaximal or maximal. Sensitivity and specificity are inversely related; when sensitivity is the highest, specificity is lowest, and vice versa.

If the population studied has a greater prevalence of disease, the test will have a higher sensitivity. For instance, the exercise test has a higher sensitivity in individuals with triple-vessel CAD than in those with single-vessel disease. A test can also have a lower specificity if it is used in individuals who are more likely to give false-positive (indeterminate) results, such as some women or individuals with mitral valve prolapse.

Sensitivity and specificity of exercise-induced ST-segment depression can be demonstrated by comparing the results of exercise testing and coronary angiography.[23] In these studies, the exercise test with 0.1-mV horizontal or downsloping ST-segment depression has approximately 84 percent specificity for angiographically significant CAD; that is, 84 percent of those without significant angiographic disease had a normal exercise test. These studies had a mean 66 percent sensitivity of exercise testing for significant angiographic CAD, with a range from 40 percent for one-vessel disease to 90 percent for three-vessel disease.

PROGNOSTIC USE OF THE EXERCISE TEST

The two major reasons for determining prognosis are to provide reliable answers about the probable long-term outcome of a cardiovascular illness and to identify patients in whom interventions might improve eventual outcome.

Table 15-10 lists indications for performing an exercise test in patients after myocardial infarction. Exercise testing may be appropriate and may expedite hospital discharge of patients recovering from a myocardial infarction. Ventricular arrhythmias not present at rest may be provoked during exercise, and the patient's reaction to exercise at the time of discharge from the hospital can be assessed. An exercise test before discharge is important to provide guidelines for activity at home, reassurance of physical status, determination of risk of complications, and a basis for advising the patient to resume or increase activity level and return to work. Because of the shortened hospital stay for many patients, however, there is often not time to include such testing.

Some investigators perform exercise tests using symptom- or sign-limited end points 2 or 3 weeks after myocardial infarction. A HR limit of 130 to 140 beats per minute and a MET level of 5 to 7 can be arbitrarily used, or a Borg perceived exertion level in the range of 13 to 15 can be used as a test end point, particularly for patients receiving beta blockers. A maximum test is probably more appropriate 3 weeks or more after myocardial infarction, when the patient is more often ready to resume full activities (see also Chap. 47).

One review of numerous predischarge and post–myocardial infarction exercise tests reported a few serious complications: two cases of recurrent infarction and two cases of ventricular fibrillation, one fatal, representing 0.05 percent morbidity and 0.02 percent mortality.[24] In studies of exercise testing after myocardial infarction with a follow-up for cardiac end points, patients who were able to perform an exercise test consistently had a lower risk, regardless of the criteria used for testing.[24] Of the usual general criteria, only an abnormal systolic blood pressure response or a low exercise capacity were significantly associated with poor outcome. When the studies were subgrouped by whether testing was done before or after discharge from the hospital, a significant proportion of predischarge test results indicated poor outcome. Submaximal testing resulted in the highest proportion of positive associations and the highest risk ratios, and abnormal responses at higher workloads were not as predictive as those at lower workloads.[24]

Studies using exercise testing of patients with stable CAD have provided data to predict angiographic findings, cardiac events in those with silent ischemia, or improved survival with coronary artery bypass surgery (CABG). Exercise testing has also been used to predict left main or triple-vessel coronary artery disease or both, with varying results.[25]

Exertional Hypotension

In most studies, exercise-induced hypotension indicates a poor prognosis and has a predictive value of 50 percent for left main/triple-vessel disease.[26] Exercise-induced hypotension can occur in patients with CAD, valvular heart disease, or cardiomyopathy. Occasionally, however, subjects without clinically significant heart disease will exhibit exercise-induced hypotension during or at maximal exercise related to antihypertensive therapy or prolonged strenuous exercise.

Cardiac Events in Patients with Silent Ischemia

The prognostic implication of asymptomatic ("silent") ischemia detected during exercise testing is controversial. It has been suggested that those with silent ischemia are at greater risk for cardiac death; however, in three large studies of patients with a high prevalence of CAD who underwent exercise testing, those with ST-segment depression, with or without angina during testing, had similar prognoses.[27] Ischemia is asymptomatic in approximately 60 percent of patients with CAD and ischemic ST-segment depression, and silent ischemia occurring with testing does not appear to confer an increased risk for death relative to patients experiencing angina with signs of ischemia. Table 15-11 itemizes exercise test findings associated with a poor prognosis in patients with CAD, and Table 15-12 shows data from eight studies in the prediction of cardiac events.[28-35] (see Chap. 45).

In patients with CAD, exercise-induced ventricular arrhythmias are not an independent risk factor for subsequent

TABLE 15-10
PURPOSES OF EXERCISE TESTING IN PATIENTS AFTER MYOCARDIAL INFARCTION

PREDISCHARGE SUBMAXIMUM TEST

Setting safe exercise levels (exercise prescription)
Optimizing discharge
Altering medical therapy
Triaging for intensity of follow-up
Assuring, encouraging patient (first step in rehabilitation)
Reassuring spouse
Recognizing exercise-induced ischemia and arrhythmias

MAXIMUM TEST FOR RETURN TO NORMAL ACTIVITIES

Determining limitations (including exercise prescription)
Prognostication
Reassuring employers
Determining levels of disability
Triaging for invasive studies
Selecting medications

Source: From Fletcher GF, Balady G, Froelicher VF, Hartley LH, Haskell WL, Pollock ML. Exercise standards: A statement for health professionals from the American Heart Association Writing Group. *Circulation* 1995; 91:580–615. Reproduced with permission from the publisher and the authors.

TABLE 15-11

EXERCISE TEST PARAMETERS ASSOCIATED WITH POOR
PROGNOSIS AND/OR INCREASED SEVERITY
OF CORONARY ARTERY DISEASE

Duration of symptom-limiting exercise
  Failure to complete stage II of Bruce protocol or equivalent workload (≤6.5 METs)[a] with other protocols
Exercise heart rate (HR) at onset of limiting symptoms
  Failure to attain HR ≥120/min (off beta blockers)
Time of onset, magnitude, morphology, and postexercise duration of abnormal horizontal or downsloping ST-segment depression
  Onset at HR <120/min or ≤6.5 METs
  Magnitude ≥2.0 mm
  Postexercise duration ≥6 min
  Presence in multiple leads
Systolic BP response during or following progressive exercise
  Sustained decrease of >10 mmHg or flat BP response (≤130 mmHg) during progressive exercise
Other potentially important determinants
  Exercise-induced ST-segment elevation in leads other than aVR
  Angina pectoris during exercise
  Exercise-induced U-wave inversion
  Exercise-induced ventricular tachycardia

[a] Energy expenditure at rest, equivalent to an oxygen uptake of approximately 3.5 mL O_2/kg body weight per minute.

Source: From Schlant RC, Blomqvist CG, Brandenburg RO, DeBusk R, Ellestad MH, Fletcher GF, et al. Special report. In: Guidelines for exercise testing. A report of the Joint American College of Cardiology/American Heart Association Task Force on Assessment of Cardiovascular Procedures (Subcommittee on Exercise Testing). *Circulation* 1986; 74:653A–667A. Reproduced with permission from the publisher and the authors.

mortality or coronary events. Some studies, however, suggest that these arrhythmias may add independent prognostic information to thallium-201 ST-segment changes[36,37] and that they are associated with severe CAD and wall motion abnormalities. In selected subjects with CAD, exercise testing may be of considerable value in the evaluation of drug therapy of ventricular arrhythmias.

One study suggests that patients with multivessel CAD, cardiomegaly, exercise capacity of less than 5 METs, or a maximum systolic blood pressure of less than 130 mmHg have a more favorable outcome if treated with surgery.[38] In another trial, patients who had an exercise test response of 1.5 mm of ST-segment depression showed enhanced survival with surgery, which also improved survival in patients with baseline ST-segment depression or claudication.[39] In another study,[40] the benefit of surgery was greatest in patients with 1 mm ST-segment depression at less than 5 METs.

In several studies evaluating coronary bypass graft occlusion and recurrence of symptoms, exercise-induced ST depression did not predict prognosis after CABG. *An exercise capacity of 9 METs or more, however, indicates a good prognosis, regardless of other responses.*[41]

Exercise testing may be of value in the routine (6- to 12-month) follow-up of patients who have undergone percutaneous transluminal coronary angioplasty (PTCA), especially in the evaluation of chest discomfort and the detection of restenosis. Testing is of particular benefit in patients in cardiac rehabilitation programs (Chap. 55). It may be especially helpful in the patient with symptoms suggestive of ischemia or the patient whose progress in rehabilitation is limited.

There is substantial support for the use of exercise testing as the first noninvasive procedure after the history, physical examination, and resting ECG in the prognostic evaluation of patients with CAD (Chap. 45). Exercise testing accomplishes both purposes of prognostic testing by providing information about the patient's clinical status and in helping provide recommendations for proper management. Exercise testing also helps select patients who should undergo further evaluation, as by radionuclear or echocardiographic studies and coronary angiography. Since the exercise test can be performed as an outpatient procedure and provides valuable information about activity levels, response to therapy, and disability, it is a reasonable first choice for prognostic assessment. Because of its widespread availability, the exercise test can have a substantial impact on cost-effective delivery of cardiovascular care. The exercise test is not usually recommended for screening apparently healthy persons without risk factors since it has a high rate of false-positive results.[42,43]

OTHER USES OF THE EXERCISE TEST

Exercise testing has been used in patients with valvular heart disease to evaluate exercise-induced symptoms, quantify disability, and evaluate the response to medical and surgical therapy.[44] It has also been used to identify concurrent CAD in such patients; however, there is a high prevalence of false-positive responses because of frequently seen baseline ECG abnormalities and LV hypertrophy.

In selected patients with valvular heart disease, exercise testing may be useful to determine when surgery is indicated (see Chaps. 63 and 64). Effort syncope in patients with *aortic stenosis*[45,46] is an important symptom. Most guidelines for exercise testing list moderate to severe aortic stenosis as a contraindication for testing because of concerns about syncope and cardiac arrest. Therefore, exercise testing of patients with aortic stenosis should be restricted to those with mild to moderate gradients. Four proposed mechanisms for exercise-induced syncope in patients with aortic stenosis include carotid hyperactivity, LV failure, arrhythmias, and LV baroreceptor stimulation. Exercise testing, however, is relatively safe in both the pediatric and adult patient with mild to moderate aortic stenosis when performed very carefully and with experienced supervision. Attention should focus on the patient's symptoms, minute-by-minute response of blood pressure, slowing HR, and both ventricular and atrial arrhythmias. In the presence of an abnormal blood pressure response, the patient with aortic stenosis should take at least a 2-min cool-

TABLE 15-12

POPULATION DESCRIPTORS INCLUDING CLINICAL VARIABLES, EXERCISE TESTING, AND CORONARY ANGIOGRAPHY FROM STUDIES OF MULTIVARIATE PREDICTION OF CARDIAC EVENTS

	LBVAMC	VACABS	CASS	Duke	Italian	German	Seattle	Buenos Aires
Years entered	1984–1990	1970–1974	1974–1979	1969–1981	1976–1979	1975–1978	1971–1974	1972–1982
Population size	592	245	4,083	2,842	1,083	1,034	733	180
Exercise test % with 1 mm ST Depression	58	72	44	35	—	—	—	65
Cardiac cath Findings 3V left Main disease (%)	21	68	23	27	20	45	12	44
Follow-up Years	5	7	5	5	5.5	5	3.5	6
Annual CV Mortality (%)	2.7	NA	1.0	—	1.54	—	—	4.6
Independent predictors of mortality	CHF Q waves <5 METs	E-I PVCs Max HR >140 bpm >2 mm ST depression	CHF Treadmill stage ST depression	ST depression Angina index Treadmill time	Q wave Prior MI Effort ischemia Poor Ex capacity	Ex capacity Angina MHR	CHF Maximal DP Maximal SBP Angina frequency Resting ST depression	Max SBP 130 ST Elevation <4 METs

Abbreviations: LBVAMC = Long Beach Veterans Administration Medical Center; VACABS = Veterans Administration Coronary Artery Bypass Study; CASS = Coronary Artery Surgical Study; V = vessel; CV = cardiovascular; CHF = congestive heart failure; METs = metabolic equivalents; E-I = exercise induced; PVC = premature ventricular contractions; MI = myocardial infarction; Ex = exercise; MHR = maximal heart rate; DP = diastolic pressure; SBP = systolic blood pressure.

Source: Reproduced with permission from Refs. 28 through 35.

down walk at a lower stage of exertion to avoid acute LV volume overload, which may occur when the patient assumes the supine position (see Chap. 63).

Patients with *aortic regurgitation*[47] usually maintain a normal exercise capacity for a longer time than those with aortic stenosis, as volume workload of the myocardium requires less oxygen than pressure work. During exercise, there is a decrease in the duration of diastole and regurgitant volume and a decrease in peripheral vascular resistance, favoring forward output. As the left ventricle fails, both LVEF and stroke volume decrease, with an increase in both end-diastolic and end-systolic ventricular diameter. Exercise testing is useful for monitoring selected patients with aortic regurgitation, using onset of ST-segment depression, a reduction of HR response to each workload, and decrease in $\dot{V}_{O_2max}$ as markers for decreasing LV function (see Chap. 63).

Patients with *mitral stenosis*[48] may have either a normal or excessive increase in HR during exercise. As stroke volume cannot be increased, the usual increase in cardiac output is less and may fall during exercise, frequently accompanied by

exercise-induced hypotension. The increase in HR and right ventricular pressure results in an increase in right ventricular myocardial oxygen demand. In patients with mitral stenosis, chest discomfort and ST-segment depression during exercise may occur either due to CAD or secondary to pulmonary hypertension. ST depression during exercise is attributed both to a decrease in coronary perfusion secondary to tachycardia and a fall in cardiac output and to an increase in myocardial oxygen demand secondary to right ventricular overload. The shortening of diastole associated with tachycardia and the increase in pulmonary blood flow associated with exercise act to increase left atrial pressure and may cause pulmonary congestion (see Chap. 64).

Patients with mild to moderate *mitral regurgitation*[49] maintain normal cardiac output during exercise. Blood pressure, HR, and ECG responses are usually also normal. When transient mitral regurgitation occurs suddenly during exercise as a result of ischemic papillary muscle dysfunction, however, a flat response in systolic blood pressure can occur. Patients with severe mitral regurgitation usually have decreased cardiac output and limited exercise capacity. ST-segment depression during exercise is infrequent in these patients; however, a hypotensive response can develop, and arrhythmias are frequent (see Chap. 64).

Several mechanisms have been suggested to explain the ST depression noted in some patients with *mitral valve prolapse,*[50] including regional ischemia of the papillary muscle, CAD, compression of the anterior descending artery, coronary spasm, and primary cardiomyopathy, ECG ST changes can be normalized by propranolol or other nonselective beta blockers, improving the specificity of the exercise test (see Chap. 65).

An exercise test is often used to evaluate the safety of an exercise training program and to formulate an exercise prescription. In general, an exercise test is often advised for a sedentary individual who at or about the age of 40 decides to enter an exercise program of a higher intensity than walking at 50 to 60 percent of maximal HR reserve. Testing should also be done in younger individuals with coronary risk factors or a strong family history of CAD. It is preferable to determine an individual's maximal HR rather than to give a predicted value for maximal HR to be attained during training because of the wide scatter of maximal HR when plotted against age. An exercise test can be used in adult exercise or cardiac rehabilitation programs to safely advance an individual to a higher intensity. An improvement in exercise capacity on an exercise test can also be an effective incentive to continue the program and to encourage risk-factor modification.

Exercise testing is used to determine the degree of impairment and disability of patients with various forms of cardiovascular disease. Patients who "exaggerate" their symptoms or who have a psychological impairment can often be identified. $\dot{V}_{O_{2max}}$ is the best noninvasive measurement of the exercise capacity of the cardiovascular system. Inability to reach 5 METs (below 18 mL kg^{-1} min^{-1}) without signs or symptoms is a criterion of disability used by the Social Security Administration. The determination of a patient's exercise capacity affords an objective measurement of the degree of cardiac impairment[51] (see also Chap. 104).

The results of exercise testing do not add significantly to the risk stratification provided by the resting ECG in patients without known CAD who are candidates for major elective noncardiac surgery.[52] Therefore, exercise testing is not routinely recommended before major elective noncardiac surgery under general anesthesia (see also Chap. 83). The efficacy of angioplasty or surgery for peripheral vascular disease can, however, be assessed effectively by exercise testing.[53]

DRUGS AND EXERCISE TESTING

Beta Blockers

Maximum HR and systolic blood pressure product during exercise may be reduced by beta blockers. Patients with angina who receive beta blockers may have a greater exercise capacity with less ST-segment depression and less angina if the drugs prevent their reaching the ischemic rate-pressure product. In some individuals, however, angina disappears, but ST depression occurs if the ischemic product can still be reached (see also Chap. 54).

Vasodilators

Vasodilators can increase exercise capacity in patients with angina, heart failure, or both.[54] To date, however, there are no good data that long-acting nitrates increase exercise capacity in patients with angina when they are tested after chronic administration.

Angiotensin-Converting Enzyme Inhibitors

Angiotensin-converting enzyme inhibitors decrease blood pressure both at rest and during exercise and can increase exercise capacity in patients with chronic heart failure.

Calcium Antagonists

Calcium antagonists have multiple hemodynamic effects. They can delay time to ischemia, improve exercise capacity, and delay ST-segment depression until workloads are higher. Heart rate and systolic blood pressure are decreased for a given level of exercise (see also Chap. 54).

Digitalis

ST-segment depression can be induced or accentuated during exercise in individuals who are taking digitalis, including both normal subjects and patients with CAD.[55] Profound ST-segment depression (>2 mm more) compared to baseline usually indicates ischemia, even in patients who are taking digitalis. Exercise-induced ST-segment depression related to digitalis has been said to persist for 2 weeks or more after the drug is discontinued.

Other Drugs

Quinidine can cause prolongation of phase 2 of the ventricular action potential, decreasing the repolarization gradient during the ST segment and thus decreasing the magnitude of ST depression. A decrease of 20 beats per minute in maximum exercise HR has been reported in patients taking amiodarone, which also increases duration of the QRS complex during exercise. Diuretics can cause hypokalemia, producing muscle fatigue, ventricular ectopy, and (rarely) ST-segment depression with exercise.

SPECIAL CASES OF EXERCISE TESTING INTERPRETATION

The difference in the predictive accuracy of exercise testing between men and women can be explained in part by the difference in the prevalence of CAD[56]; however, the specificity of exercise testing is also lower in women. Several mechanisms have been suggested to explain the high false-positive (indeterminate) rate of ST depression in women, including estrogens and resting ST-T abnormalities. Since estrogens have a similar chemical structure to digitalis, it has been suggested that they may be partially responsible for the high prevalence of false-positive exercise test results in women.

Although exercise testing may detect labile hypertensives or individuals who will eventually become hypertensive, there is little objective support for this hypothesis.[57,58] Hypertensive patients frequently have ECG abnormalities (LV hypertrophy) and myocardial hypertrophy, both of which may result in false-positive ST responses.

Exercise testing has been used in patients with idiopathic dilated cardiomyopathy to determine exercise capacity, pulmonary response to LV dysfunction, grade of ventricular ectopy, and effectiveness of treatment.[59] Patients with LV dysfunction usually have reduced exercise capacity due to an inadequate increase in cardiac output during exercise, which limits $\dot{V}_{O_2max}$ and exercise tolerance. Initially, stroke volume may increase normally during upright exercise despite a decrease in LVEF; however, if there is limited chronotropic reserve with increasing exercise, the stroke volume and cardiac output cannot continue to meet the increased demands. A few patients may have normal exercise tolerance despite severe LV dysfunction. Several peripheral compensatory mechanisms have been proposed to explain the poor correlation between LV function and exercise capacity (see also Chap. 73).

Exercise may result in sudden death due to arrhythmias in hypertrophic cardiomyopathy.[60,61] Chest discomfort, an abnormal resting ECG, and exercise-induced ST-segment depression are frequent. In this condition, exercise testing under very careful supervision may be helpful to demonstrate the level at which significant events occur, such as the presence or severity of arrhythmias, myocardial ischemia, murmurs indicating obstruction in LV outflow, and presyncopal manifestations (see Chap. 74).

Intracardiac conduction blocks can either develop or resolve during exercise. Rate-dependent intraventricular blocks that occur during exercise often precede the appearance of chronic blocks present at rest.[62-64] The diagnosis of ischemia from the exercise ECG is not usually reliable when there is left bundle branch block, which can be associated with a marked degree of ST-segment depression with exercise in addition to that found at rest. Left bundle branch block occurring with HR below 125 beats per minute in patients with typical angina is frequently associated with CAD. The presence of intraventricular blocks and their disappearance during exercise are rare. Rarely, patients with left bundle branch block develop a normal QRS pattern during exercise. Preexisting right bundle branch block[65-69] does not influence interpretation of the exercise test except in the anterior (V_{1-2}) precordial leads; however, the sensitivity of exercise testing in these patients is uncertain.

In addition to left or right bundle branch block, left anterior or posterior hemiblock and bifascicular block (a combination of right bundle branch block and either left anterior or posterior hemiblock) may be induced by exercise. The presence of such blocks is primarily a rate-related phenomenon occur-

ring as the sinus rate increases beyond a critical point. Intraventricular block during exercise may be difficult to distinguish from ventricular tachycardia.

First-degree AV block occasionally occurs at the end of exercise or during the recovery phase. Medications or conditions that may produce prolonged AV conduction time (e.g., digitalis, propranolol, myocarditis) may predispose the individual to lengthening of the PR interval.

Second-degree AV block—Wenckebach (Mobitz type I) AV block—during exercise is rare. The clinical significance of exercise-induced Mobitz II AV block is not known, but it may also be a rate-related phenomenon, appearing as the sinus rate is accelerated beyond a critical level. It has been seen in patients with CAD.

Complete AV block at rest is a relative contraindication to exercise testing, but with very careful supervision, exercise testing may be performed in selected patients. Exercise testing can also be performed in patients with congenital complete AV block provided that there are no coexisting significant congenital anomalies.

Rarely, patients develop long periods of sinus arrest and sinoventricular conduction immediately after exercise. This usually occurs in patients with severe myocardial ischemia. Exercise may provoke, abolish, or not affect anomalous AV conduction in individuals with known preexcitation such as Wolff-Parkinson-White syndrome (WPW).[70] Exercise usually does not abolish anomalous AV conduction; when it does occur, these individuals are thought to be in less danger of exercise-induced ventricular tachycardia. With anomalous AV conduction (as with WPW), significant ST depression can be observed during exercise testing; this may not be due to ischemia but rather represent a false-positive (indeterminate) change. In general, there is a low prevalence of tachyarrhythmias during or after exercise in WPW patients (see also Chap. 27).

Exercise may induce cardiac arrhythmias under several conditions, especially with diuretic and digitalis therapy.[71-73] The recent ingestion of alcohol or caffeine may also exacerbate exercise-induced arrhythmias. Since exercise increases myocardial oxygen demand, the presence of CAD can predispose some patients to arrhythmias during exercise. It appears that subendocardial ischemia (ST depression) is not as arrhythmogenic as transmural ischemia (ST elevation). Exercise-induced arrhythmias are generated by enhanced sympathetic tone and catecholamines, increased myocardial oxygen demand, or both. The immediate postexercise period is of particular concern because of high catecholamine levels in combination with generalized vasodilation. The combination of peripheral arteriolar dilation induced by exercise and reduced cardiac output from diminished venous return secondary to the sudden termination of muscular activity may lead to a reduction in coronary perfusion while HR is elevated. The associated increased sympathetic tone may stimulate ectopic Purkinje pacemaker activity in the myocardium by accelerating phase 4 of the action potential, provoking spontaneous discharge and leading to increased automaticity.

Exercise can suppress cardiac arrhythmias present in patients at rest. This phenomenon has been attributed to the overdrive suppression of the ectopic impulse formation by sinus tachycardia induced by exercise-vagal withdrawal and increased sympathetic stimulation (see also Chap. 26).

Ventricular ectopy is the most frequent typed cardiac arrhythmia that develops during exercise, followed by supraventricular arrhythmias. Their prevalence is directly related to age and the presence of cardiac abnormalities. In general, ventricular arrhythmias are of concern in patients with a family history of cardiomyopathy, valvular heart disease, or known severe ischemia.

Sinus arrhythmias with periods of sinus bradycardia and wandering atrial pacemaker are relatively common during exercise and the immediate recovery phase. Atrial ectopy can occur in either normal or diseased hearts. Exercise-induced transient atrial fibrillation and flutter occur in less than 1 percent of individuals who undergo exercise testing.[74] These arrhythmias may be induced by exercise in both healthy individuals and patients with rheumatic heart disease, hyperthyroidism, WPW syndrome, or cardiomyopathy. Paroxysmal AV junctional tachycardia is rarely observed during exercise. Exercise-induced supraventricular arrhythmias alone are usually not related to CAD but are more often related to pulmonary disease, recent alcohol ingestion, or excessive caffeine.[75]

COST CONSIDERATIONS IN EXERCISE TESTING

Many "adjunct" investigations are widely utilized with basic exercise testing. These include echocardiography (Chap. 14), gated-blood-pool imaging, myocardial perfusion imaging (Chap. 17), and various types of pharmacologic exercise studies. The basic ECG monitored exercise test with recording of blood pressure is the least expensive of all exercise tests. If one assumes basic unit of one (X), the relative costs of several types of exercise tests can be approximated as follows:

Testing with ECG monitoring	X
Pharmacologic exercise studies	1.7 X
Exercise echocardiography	2.2 X
Gated-blood-pool exercise imaging	2.2 X
Exercise myocardial perfusion imaging	5.2 X

As is noted, there is a considerable increase in cost—as much as fivefold—when more than basic exercise testing with hemodynamic recording and ECG monitoring is utilized. Although more sophisticated studies such as nuclear and echocardiographic assessment with exercise may yield improved sensitivity and specificity, the value of this (versus the cost increase) must be considered with reference to the population being tested.

REFERENCES

1. Rowell LB. *Human Circulation: Regulation During Physical Stress.* New York: Oxford University Press; 1986.

2. Cohn JN, ed. Quantitative exercise testing for the cardiac patient: The value of monitoring gas exchange: Introduction. *Circulation* 1987; 76 (suppl VI):VI-1–VI-2.

3. Fletcher GF, Balady G, Froelicher VF, Hartley LH, Haskell WL, Pollock ML. Exercise standards: A statement for healthcare professionals from the American Heart Association Writing Group. *Circulation* 1995; 91:580–615.

4. Higginbotham MB. Cardiac performance during submaximal and maximal exercise in healthy persons. *Heart Failure* 1988; 4:68–76.

5. Londeree BR, Moeschberger ML. Influence of age and other factors on maximal heart rate. *J Cardiac Rehabil* 1984; 4:44–49.

6. Gould KL, Lipscomb K. Effects of coronary stenoses on coronary flow reserve and resistance. *Am J Cardiol* 1974; 34:48–55.

7. Froelicher VF Jr. The detection of asymptomatic coronary artery disease. *Annu Rev Med* 1977; 28:1–12.

8. ACP/ACC/AHA Task Force on Exercise Testing. *J Am Coll Cardiol* 1990; 16:1061–1065.

9. Schlant RC, Blomqvist CG, Brandenburg RO, DeBusk R, Ellestad MH, Fletcher GF, et al. Special report. In: Guidelines for exercise testing: A report of the Joint American College of Cardiology/American Heart Association Task Force on Assessment of Cardiovascular Procedures (Subcommittee on Exercise Testing). *Circulation* 1986; 74:653A–667A.

10. Becker RC, Alpert JS. Electrocardiographic ST segment depression in coronary heart disease. *Am Heart J* 1988; 115:862–868.

11. Balady GJ, Weiner DA, McCabe CH, Ryan TJ. Value of arm exercise testing in detecting coronary artery disease. *Am J Cardiol* 1985; 55:37–39.

12. Franklin BA. Exercise testing, training and arm ergometry. *Sports Med* 1985; 2:100–119.

13. Dalke B, Ware RW. An experimental study of "physical fitness" of Air Force personnel. *U.S. Armed Forces Med J* 1959; 10:675–688.

14. Fletcher GF, ed. *Exercise in the Practice of Medicine.* 2d ed. Mt. Kisco, NY: Futura, 1988.

15. Bruce RA, Blackmon JR, Jones JW, Strait G. Exercise testing in adult normal subjects and cardiac patients. *Pediatrics* 1963; 32:742–756.

16. Sheffield LT, Roitman D. Stress testing methodology. *Prog Cardiovasc Dis* 1976; 19:33–49.

17. Lester FM, Sheffield LT, Reeves TJ. Electrocardiographic changes in clinically normal older men following near maximal and maximal exercise. *Circulation* 1967; 36:5–14.

18. Sheffield LT, Maloof JA, Sawyer JA, Roitman D. Maximal heart rate and treadmill performance of healthy women in relation to age. *Circulation* 1978; 57:79–84.

19. Borg GA. Psychophysical bases of perceived exertion. *Med Sci Sports Exerc* 1982; 14:377–381.

20. Bruce RA, Fisher LD, Pettinger M, Weiner DA, Chaitman BR. ST segment elevation with exercise: A marker for poor ventricular function and poor prognosis: Coronary Artery Surgery Study (CASS) confirmation of Seattle Heart Watch results. *Circulation* 1988; 77:897–905.

21. Fletcher GF, Fletcher BJ, Sweeney ME. Effects of exercise testing, training and beta blockade on serum potassium in normal subjects. *Am J Cardiol* 1990; 65:1242–1245.

22. Fletcher GF, Sweeney ME, Fletcher BJ. Blood magnesium and potassium alterations with maximal treadmill exercise testing: Effects of beta-adrenergic blockade. *Am Heart J* 1991; 121:105–110.

23. Gianrossi R, Detrano R, Mulvihill D, Lehmann K, Dubach P, Colombo A, et al. Exercise-induced ST depression in the diagnosis of coronary artery disease: A meta-analysis. *Circulation* 1989; 80:87–98.

24. Froelicher VF, Perdue S, Pewen W, Risch M. Application of meta-analysis using an electronic spread sheet to exercise testing in patients after myocardial infarction. *Am J Med* 1987; 83:1045–1054.

25. Lee TH, Cook EF, Goldman L. Prospective evaluation of a clinical and exercise-test model for the prediction of left main coronary artery disease. *Med Decision Making* 1986; 6:136–144.

26. Dubach P, Froelicher VF, Klein J, Oakes D, Grover-McKay M, Friis R. Exercise-induced hypotension in a male population: Criteria, causes, and prognosis. *Circulation* 1988; 78:1380–1387.

27. Dagenais GR, Rouleau JR, Hochart P, Magrina J, Cantin B, Dumesnil JG. Survival with painless strongly positive exercise electrocardiogram. *Am J Cardiol* 1988; 62:892–895.

28. Klein J, Froelicher VF, Detrano R, Dubach P, Yen R. Does the rest electrocardiogram after myocardial infarction determine the predictive value of exercise-induced ST depression? A 2 year follow-up study in a veteran population. *J Am Coll Cardiol* 1989; 14:305–311.

29. Krone RJ, Dwyer EM Jr, Greenberg H, Miller JP, Gillespie JA. Risk stratification in patients with first non-Q wave infarction: Limited value of the early low level exercise test after uncomplicated infarcts. The Multicenter Post-Infarction Research Group. *J Am Coll Cardiol* 1989; 14:31–37; discussion 38–39.

30. Hammermeister KE, DeRouen TA, Dodge HT. Variables predictive of survival in patients with coronary disease: Selected by univariate and multivariate analyses from the clinical, electrocardiographic, exercise, arteriographic, and quantitative angiographic evaluations. *Circulation* 1979; 59:421–430.

31. Mark DB, Hlatky MA, Harrell FE Jr, Lee KL, Califf RM, Pryor DB. Exercise treadmill score for predicting prognosis in coronary artery disease. *Ann Intern Med* 1987; 106:793–800.

32. Brunelli C, Cristofani R, L'Abbate A. Long-term survival in medically treated patients with ischaemic heart disease and prognostic importance of clinical and electrocardiographic data (the Italian CNR Multicentre Prospective Study ODI). *Eur Heart J* 1989; 10:292–303.

33. Weiner DA, Ryan TJ, McCabe CH, Chaitman BR, Sheffield LT, Ferguson JC, et al. Prognostic importance of a clinical profile and exercise test in medically treated patients with coronary artery disease. *J Am Coll Cardiol* 1984; 3:772–779.

34. Gohlke H, Samek L, Betz P, Roskamm H. Exercise testing provides additional prognostic information in angiographically defined subgroups of patients with coronary artery disease. *Circulation* 1983; 68:979–985.

35. Peduzzi P, Hultgren H, Thomsen J, Angell W. Veterans Administration Cooperative Study of medical versus surgical treatment for stable angina—Progress report. Section 8. Prognostic value of baseline exercise tests. *Prog Cardiovasc Dis* 1986; 28:285–292.

36. Kaul S, Lilly DR, Gascho JA, Watson DD, Gibson RS, Oliner CA, et al. Prognostic utility of the exercise thallium-201 test in ambulatory patients with chest pain: Comparison with cardiac catheterization. *Circulation* 1988; 77:745–758.

37. Marieb MA, Beller GA, Gibson RS, Lerman BB, Kaul S. Clinical relevance of exercise-induced ventricular arrhythmias in suspected coronary artery disease. *Am J Cardiol* 1990; 66:172–178.

38. Bruce RA, Fisher LD, Hossack KF. Validation of exercise-enhanced risk assessment of coronary heart disease events: Longitudinal changes in incidence in Seattle community practice. *J Am Coll Cardiol* 1985; 5:875–881.

39. Anonymous. Long-term results of prospective randomised study of coronary artery bypass surgery in stable angina pectoris. European Coronary Surgery Study Group. *Lancet* 1982; 2:1173–1180.

40. Weiner DA, Ryan TJ, McCabe CH, Chaitman BR, Sheffield LT, Fisher LD, et al. The role of exercise testing in identifying patients with improved survival after coronary artery bypass surgery. *J Am Coll Cardiol* 1986; 8:741–748.

41. Dubach P, Froelicher V, Klein J, Detrano R. Use of the exercise test to predict prognosis after coronary artery bypass grafting. *Am J Cardiol* 1989; 63:530–533.

42. McHenry PL, O'Donnell J, Morris SN, Jordan JJ. The abnormal exercise electrocardiogram in apparently healthy men: A predictor of angina pectoris as an initial coronary event during long-term follow-up. *Circulation* 1984; 70:547–551.

43. Sox HC Jr, Littenberg B, Garber AM. The role of exercise testing in screening for coronary artery disease. *Ann Intern Med* 1989; 110:456–469.

44. Hochreiter C, Borer JS. Exercise testing in patients with aortic and mitral valve disease: Current applications. *Cardiovasc Clin* 1983; 13:291–300.

45. Areskog NH. Exercise testing in the evaluation of patients with valvular aortic stenosis. *Clin Physiol* 1984; 4:201–208.

46. Atwood JE, Kawanishi S, Myers J, Froelicher VF. Exercise testing in patients with aortic stenosis. *Chest* 1988; 93:1083–1087.

47. Misra M, Thakur K, Bhandari K, Puri VK. Value of the treadmill exercise test in asymptomatic and minimally symptomatic patients with chronic severe aortic regurgitation. *Int J Cardiol* 1987; 15:309–316.

48. Vacek JL, Valentin-Stone P, Wolfe M, Davis WR. The value of standardized exercise testing in the noninvasive evaluation of mitral stenosis. *Am J Med Sci* 1986; 292:335–343.

49. Weber KT, Janicki JS, McElroy PA. Cardio-pulmonary exercise testing in the evaluation of mitral and aortic valve incompetence. *Herz* 1986; 11:88–96.

50. Broustet JP, Douard H, Mora B. Exercise testing in arrhythmias of idiopathic mitral valve prolapse. *Eur Heart J* 1987; 8:37–42.

51. Lee TH, Shammash JB, Ribeiro JP, Hartley LH, Sherwood J, Goldman L. Estimation of maximum oxygen uptake from clinical data: Performance of the Specific Activity Scale. *Am Heart J* 1988; 115:203–204.

52. Carliner NH, Fisher ML, Plotnick GD, Garbart H, Rapoport A, Kelemen MH, et al. Routine preoperative exercise testing in patients undergoing major noncardiac surgery. *Am J Cardiol* 1985; 56:51–58.

53. McPhail N, Calvin JE, Shariatmadar A, Barber GG, Scobie TK. The use of preoperative exercise testing to predict cardiac complications after arterial reconstruction. *J Vasc Surg* 1988; 7:60–68.

54. Sullivan M, Savvides M, Abouantoun S, Madsen EB, Froelicher V. Failure of transdermal nitroglycerin to improve exercise capacity in patients with angina pectoris. *J Am Coll Cardiol* 1985; 5:1220–1223.

55. Sullivan M, Atwood JE, Myers J, Feuer J, Hall P, Kellerman B, et al. Increased exercise capacity after digoxin administration in patients with heart failure. *J Am Coll Cardiol* 1989; 13:1138–1143.

56. Guiteras P, Chaitman BR, Waters DD, Bourassa MG, Scholl JM, Ferguson RJ, et al. Diagnostic accuracy of exercise ECG lead systems in clinical subsets of women. *Circulation* 1982; 65:1465–1474.

57. Exercise hypertension: A symposium issue. *Herz* 1987; 12:76–149.

58. Liao Y, Emidy LA, Gosch FC, Stamler R, Stamler J. Cardiovascular responses to exercise of participants in a trial on the primary prevention of hypertension. *J Hypertens* 1987; 5:317–321.

59. Wilson JR, Fink LI, Ferraro N, Dunkman WB, Jones RA. Use of maximal bicycle exercise testing with respiratory gas analysis to assess exercise performance in patients with congestive heart failure secondary to coronary artery disease or idiopathic dilated cardiomyopathy. *Am J Cardiol* 1986; 58:601–606.

60. Losse B, Kuhn H, Loogen F, Schulte HD. Exercise performance in hypertrophic cardiomyopathies. *Eur Heart J* 1983; 4:197–208.

61. Savage DD, Seides SF, Maron BJ, Myers DJ, Epstein SE. Prevalence of arrhythmias during 24-hour electrocardiographic monitoring and exercise testing in patients with obstructive and nonobstructive hypertrophic cardiomyopathy. *Circulation* 1979; 59:866–875.

62. Heinsimer JA, Irwin JM, Basnight LL. Influence of underlying coronary artery disease on the natural history and prognosis of exercise-induced left bundle branch block. *Am J Cardiol* 1987; 60:1065–1067.

63. Vasey C, O'Donnell J, Morris S, McHenry P. Exercise-induced left bundle branch block and its relation to coronary artery disease. *Am J Cardiol* 1985; 56:892–895.

64. Whinnery JE, Froelicher VF Jr, Stewart AJ, Longo MR Jr, Triebwasser JH, Lancaster MC. The electrocardiographic response to maximal treadmill exercise of asymptomatic men with left bundle branch block. *Am Heart J* 1977; 94:316–324.

65. Williams MA, Esterbrooks DJ, Nair CK, Sailors MM, Sketch MH. Clinical significance of exercise-induced bundle branch block. *Am J Cardiol* 1988; 61:346–348.

66. Wayne VS, Bishop RL, Cook L, Spodick D. Exercise-induced bundle branch block. *Am J Cardiol* 1983; 52:283–286.

67. Whinnery JE, Froelicher VF. Exercise testing in right bundle-branch block (letter). *Chest* 1977; 72:684–685.

68. Whinnery JE, Froelicher VF Jr, Longo MR Jr, Triebwasser JH. The electrocardiographic response to maximal treadmill exercise of asymptomatic men with right bundle branch block. *Chest* 1977; 71:335–340.

69. Whinnery JE, Froelicher VF. Acquired bundle branch block and its response to exercise testing in asymptomatic air crewmen: A review with case reports. *Aviat Space Environ Med* 1976; 46:69–78.

70. Sharma AD, Yee R, Guiraudon G, Klein GJ. Sensitivity and specificity of invasive and noninvasive testing for risk of sudden death in Wolff-Parkinson-White syndrome. *J Am Coll Cardiol* 1987; 10:373–381.

71. Allen BJ, Casey TP, Brodsky MA, Luckett CR, Henry WL. Exercise testing in patients with life-threatening ventricular tachyarrhythmias: Results and correlation with clinical and arrhythmia factors. *Am Heart J* 1988; 116:997–1002.

72. Ryan M, Lown B, Horn H. Comparison of ventricular ectopic activity during 24-hour monitoring and exercise testing in patients with coronary heart disease. *N Engl J Med* 1975; 292:224–229.

73. Sami M, Chaitman B, Fisher L, Holmes D, Fray D, Alderman E. Significance of exercise-induced ventricular arrhythmia in stable coronary artery disease: A coronary artery surgery study project. *Am J Cardiol* 1984; 54:1182–1188.

74. Atwood JE, Myers J, Sullivan M, Forbes S, Friis R, Pewen W, et al. Maximal exercise testing and gas exchange in patients with chronic atrial fibrillation. *J Am Coll Cardiol* 1988; 11:508–513.

75. Froelicher VF. *Exercise and the Heart: Clinical Concepts*. Chicago: Year Book; 1987.

16

CARDIAC CATHETERIZATION AND CORONARY ARTERIOGRAPHY

Robert H. Franch / John S. Douglas, Jr. / Spencer B. King III

In 1929, Werner Forssman, a resident surgeon at Eberswalde, catheterized his right atrium from a left antecubital vein cutdown, utilizing self-fluoroscopy with a mirror. The position of the catheter tip was verified by a roentgenogram.[1] The extensive use of the right heart catheter by Cournand in the early 1940s in the study of human cardiovascular physiology led his group and others to explore the use of this technique for the study of heart disease.[2] In 1945, Brannon, Weens, and Warren described the hemodynamics of atrial septal defect in four patients.[3] From these beginnings steady advances in methods occurred.[4,5] Catheterization then spread from the laboratory to the bedside, to yield physiologic data and to guide treatment. Now, palliative or even corrective interventions involving valves, arteries, veins, and septal defects may accompany the catheterization study.[4–6]

PREPARATIONS FOR CARDIAC CATHETERIZATION

A relaxed meeting with the patient and the patient's family serves to lessen apprehension, correct any misunderstanding, and establish rapport. Since catheterization is frequently the first major step on the road to cardiac surgery, a tolerable experience fosters an optimistic attitude in the patient and family toward future events. The patient should be examined, and the history, a current chest x-ray, an electrocardiogram, and past catheterizations reviewed along with surgical records and angiocardiograms. The site of optimal vascular access is chosen while reviewing past documentation of a failed site. Nearly all balloon catheters and many gloves contain latex, and it should be added to the list of allergens sought in the history.[7] Old operative notes are noted especially for complex palliation or repair. A clinical diagnosis is made, and a catheterization protocol is designed to answer pertinent specific questions. The catheterization protocol may also be modified as data become available during the procedure.

The patient's education booklet about the procedure is usually read by the patient and the family prior to securing informed consent. Absolute contraindications include the refusal of a competent adult or the absence of a qualified operator and/or a suitable facility[8] (Table 16-1). Anticoagulants are stopped, and the prothrombin time is brought to less than 18 s (INR < 2) before a percutaneous arterial catheterization. Dimethyl biguanide, an oral hypoglycemic drug, is not given for 1 to 2 days prior to angiography. Serum levels of creatinine, urea nitrogen, and potassium are noted. A patient with chronic renal disease is hydrated; prophylaxis for past allergy to contrast media is given.[9] Breakfast is withheld for a morning procedure; for an afternoon procedure, coffee or juice is permitted and lunch is withheld. In the authors' experience, prophylactic antibiotics are not necessary. Conscious sedation for diagnostic catheterization involves the incremental use of intravenous drugs that are titrated to each patient's response. Pulse oximeter monitors require accuracy to within 3 percent in the 70 to 100 percent saturation range. Diazepam (Valium) or midazolam (Versed) is given intravenously; intravenous fentanyl may be added for more sedation. Intravenous hydromorphone (Dilaudid) is used if analgesia is required. Subcutaneous 1% lidocaine (Xylocaine) is used locally. If there is a history of allergy, intradermal or subcutaneous testing is done with serial dilutions of a preservative-free, local anaesthetic agent.[10] Occasionally, particularly in adults, vagal slowing of the pulse, nausea, and perspiration are noted, for which intravenous atropine is the antidote. Systemic anticoagulation is achieved via a bolus of heparin at the start of a diagnostic study that uses the brachial artery, but not routinely if the femoral artery is used.

It is desirable that the laboratory be fully involved daily in diagnostic work. General efficiency is increased, costly equipment and space are utilized, and, most important, all

TABLE 16-1

CONTRAINDICATIONS TO CARDIAC CATHETERIZATION

THE ONLY ABSOLUTE CONTRAINDICATIONS

1. Refusal of a mentally competent adult (>16 years of age) patient, or of the parent(s) (guardians) of children, infants, or neonates to consent to the procedure
2. Absence of an experienced cardiac angiography and/or suitable laboratory facilities

RELATIVE CONTRAINDICATIONS TO BE CAUTIOUSLY APPLIED TO INDIVIDUAL PATIENT

1. Significant electrolyte abnormalities or digitalis toxicity
2. Uncontrolled hypertension
3. Febrile illness (not related to endocarditis)
4. Decompensated congestive heart failure
5. Bleeding diathesis: includes patients receiving anticoagulation therapy whose prothrombin time is >18 s (INR > 2)
6. Presence of a noncardiac disease that precludes long-term survival
7. Refusal to undergo surgical or interventional curvative or palliative procedures regardless of the outcome of the catheterization (angiogram)
8. Previous history of severe contrast reaction
9. Active gastrointestinal bleeding
10. Pregnancy, especially during first trimester

Source: From Ruiz et al.,[8] with permission from the authors and publisher.

personnel become confident and knowledgeable with experience. Certainly the most important ingredient in the laboratory is the thoroughly experienced technical-professional team. The procedure must move briskly. The primary objective is to make an accurate diagnosis at one sitting, with the least possible risk and discomfort to the patient. After the procedure, a preliminary, labeled single-page diagram in the patient's chart can accurately present the essence of the catheterization findings.

Outpatient left-sided heart and coronary artery studies require careful selection of patients and an experienced support team.[11,12] The clinical profiles of patients who are not suitable candidates for outpatient catheterization have been published.[13] Others have stated that if a patient is stable enough to be at home before cardiac catheterization, an outpatient catheterization can be considered and a decision following the procedure can be made based on the patient's tolerance of the procedure and the catheterization findings. This approach is most relevant when a catheterization laboratory is in or adjacent to a hospital. The cost savings per case with outpatient procedures remain significant. Although some physicians have performed cardiac catheterization of stable, low-risk patients in freestanding facilities, the lack of support in this environment is a potential liability and is not recommended.

TECHNIQUES

Catheterization of the Right Side of the Heart: Percutaneous Venous

Percutaneous femoral or median cubital vein catheterization usually permits reuse of the vein. The femoral vein is entered medial to the common femoral artery pulse. Puncture may be facilitated by a Valsalva maneuver to increase femoral vein size. To extend the range of the percutaneous technique, a thin tubular sheath is advanced over a short introducer catheter into the lumen of the vein. This temporary conduit may then be used to introduce a variety of catheters. Two catheters can be inserted through a single femoral vein puncture site by initially placing two guidewires through the femoral vein sheath; the maneuver is repeated to insert an additional catheter.[14] If the hepatic portion of the inferior vena cava (IVC) is absent, the azygos vein channels the catheter tip into the right superior vena cava (SVC) and thence into the right atrium (Fig. 16-1), or the azygos vein may enter a persistent left SVC and thence through the coronary sinus to the right atrium (Fig. 16-2). In order to cross the tricuspid valve from the IVC, bending the catheter tip against the right atrial wall may be required. If atrial ectopy occurs, the catheter tip can be looped in a hepatic vein and then advanced into the right atrium. The tip is then rotated from the lateral right atrial wall clockwise across the anterior atrial wall and through the tricuspid valve, followed by a slight counterclockwise turn

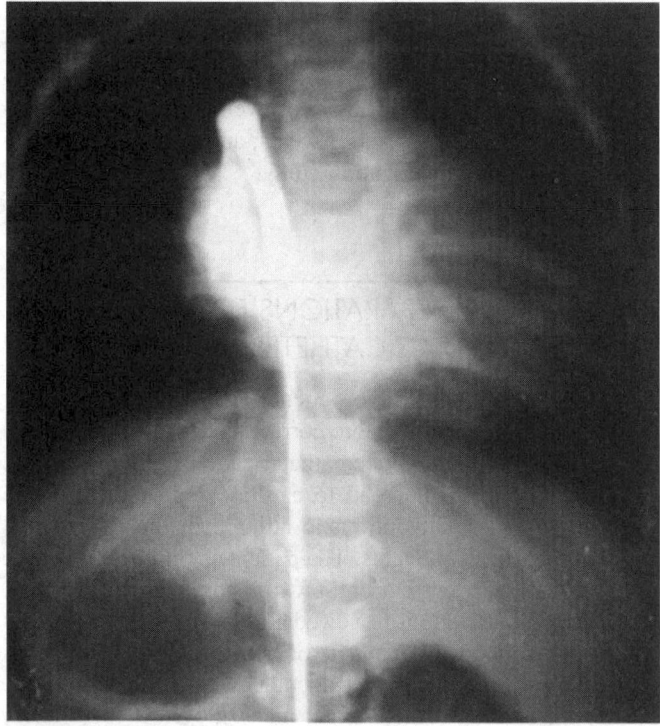

FIGURE 16-1

Selective injection of a right azygos vein. The hepatic portion of the inferior vena cava is absent. The catheter tip enters the right atrium superiorly through the right superior vena cava via the azygos vein.

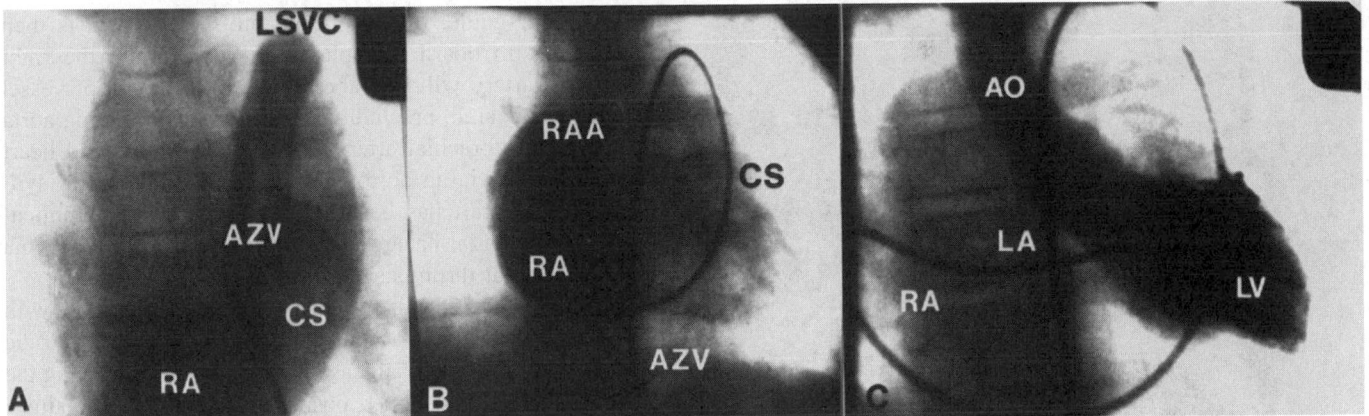

FIGURE 16-2

A–C. Progression of a catheter from the femoral vein. The hepatic portion of the inferior vena cava is absent. The systemic venous return is via a left azygos vein (AZV) to the left superior vena cava (LSVC), thence via the coronary sinus (CS) to the right atrium (RA). The catheter tip passes from the RA to the left atrium (LA) via an atrial septal defect, thence across the mitral valve into the left atrium (LV). RAA, right atrial appendage.

to the anterolateral position in the right ventricle and then clockwise to place the tip via the outflow tract into the main pulmonary artery and then into the left pulmonary artery, its direct continuation. The foramen ovale is entered with the tip pointed leftward and 45° posteriorly. The SVC lies posteriorly and is entered by making a 60° counterclockwise turn from the lateral right atrial border with a straight catheter tip. The foramen ovale is probe patent in approximately 20 to 35 percent of adults.

The internal jugular vein or the subclavian vein may also be used to insert a balloon catheter percutaneously. The latter catheter produces little ectopy since the advancing force is distributed over the surface of the balloon. The tricuspid valve is easily crossed from this approach. If a right-to-left shunt is present, the balloon should be filled with CO_2, and the side arm of the sheath flushed regularly. In children who lack conventional venous access, transhepatic venous catheterization via a right mid-axillary approach is safe and effective.[15]

Rarely if a venous cutdown is necessary, the right basilic or right median cubital (but not the cephalic) vein is preferred. Care should be taken not to mistake the superficial radial, ulnar, or accessory brachial arteries for veins. From the left arm, the catheter tip may enter a persistent left SVC, exiting via the coronary sinus into the right atrium in an awkward position for entering the right ventricle. A deep inspiration often enables the catheter tip to pass the subclavian vein–brachiocephalic vein junction. The seating of a conventional catheter tip in the pulmonary artery wedge position may be difficult if severe pulmonary artery hypertension or extreme enlargement of the right side of the heart is present. A flow-directed balloon catheter may then be used. Clues to inadvertent coronary sinus catheterizations are (1) the acute angle that the catheter shaft makes as it enters the coronary sinus, especially in the right anterior oblique position; (2) the marked desaturation of coronary sinus blood; and (3) the posterior position of the catheter in the lateral view.

In order to enter the pulmonary artery in patients with transposition of the great arteries and an intact ventricular septum, a balloon catheter is passed across the inevitably present interarterial communication to the left atrium and then superiorly looped in the left ventricular (LV) outflow tract, from which it enters the PA readily. In postsurgical patients with pulmonary valve atresia, the PA may also be entered via a subclavian (Blalock) or aorticopulmonary (Waterston or Potts) shunt.

Catheterization of the Left Side of the Heart

PERCUTANEOUS TECHNIQUE

In 1953, Seldinger described the use of a flexible metal leader to introduce a polyethylene tube into the artery. The Seldinger technique is used in the common femoral and less often in the axillary or brachial arteries in carrying out catheterization of the left side of the heart. The common femoral artery, 4 cm in length, begins at the inguinal ligament and ends at its bifurcation into the deep and superficial femoral arteries at the inferior cortical margin of the head of the femur. The inguinal crease, especially in an obese patient, tends to be inferior to the ligament. In this case, a puncture at or below the crease may involve the superficial femoral artery, and lack of posterior bony support results in poor compression with the chance of bleeding and pseudoaneurysm formation[16,17] (Fig. 16-3). A skin puncture site chosen 3 cm below the inguinal ligament (not the crease) allows the common femoral artery to be entered at a point where it is compressible against the head of the femur. External rotation of the leg and slight adduction help fixate the artery. The artery is punctured with a nonstylet needle at a 45° angle, transfixing the anterior wall. The guidewire is inserted only when the needle spurt is maximal. Resistance to insertion usually indicates an intramural or extravascular position of the needle or entry into a side

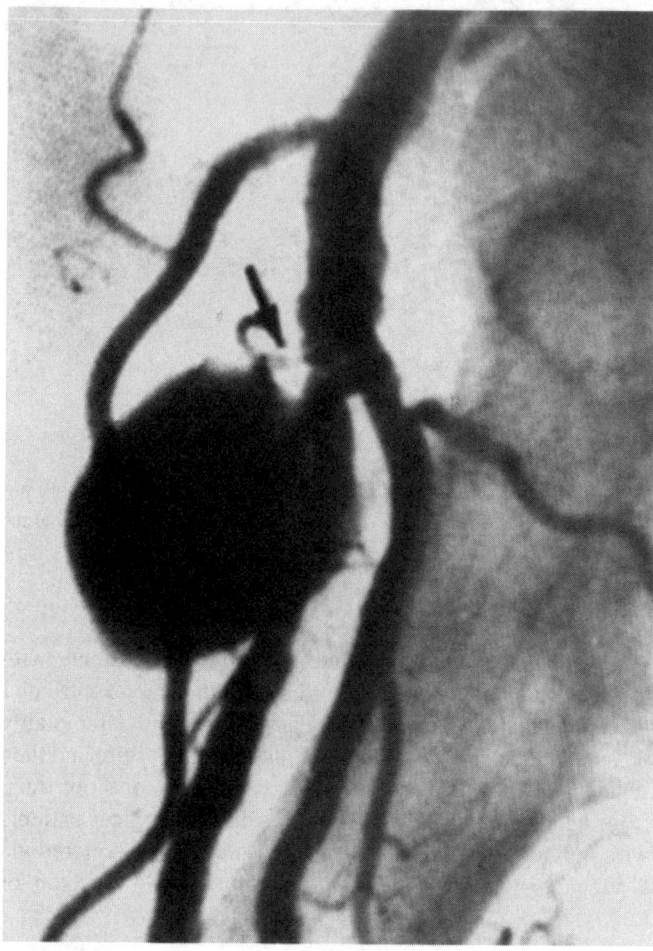

FIGURE 16-3

The femoral arteriogram shows the neck (*arrow*) of an oval pseudoaneurysm (pulsating hematoma) arising from the right superficial femoral artery (*arrow*) at the site of the previous catheter entry. (Reproduced with permission from Rapoport et al.[16] and the Radiological Society of North America, Inc., Supervisory Publisher.)

branch artery by the guide. The catheter is inserted into the artery over the guidewire, or a sheath assembly may be used, facilitating catheter introduction in a very obese patient or if scar tissue is superficial to the artery. The catheter sheath reduces bleeding during manipulation and reduces discomfort during catheter changes. Arterial pressure may be monitored through a side port in the sheath. Guidewires with torsional control of a flexible distal tip aid passage through a tortuous iliac artery, as does a right Judkins catheter, alone or with a guide. The guide tip is kept at the level of the diaphragm, and the catheter is advanced to this level. The catheter is aspirated and then flushed with heparinized saline solution. To avoid added manipulation of the catheter tip in the transverse arch, the guidewire is placed in the aortic root.[18] The femoral and foot pulses are palpated prior to withdrawal. The artery is compressed for 10 to 15 min, maintaining normal ankle pulses. The brachial artery is punctured with an 18-gauge needle, a sheath is inserted and a no. 6 French 80-cm multipurpose catheter is advanced to the ascending aorta over

a 0.032-in. J-guide. Five thousand units of heparin is then given. An arm board is applied for 6 h. Rarely, the right subclavian artery will rise aberrantly as the last root vessel of a left aortic arch, precluding access to the ascending aorta from the right brachial artery. Percutaneous left-sided heart catheterization via an aortofemoral or axillary-femoral synthetic bypass graft has been surprisingly free of complications.[19] A potential hazard is disruption of the pseudointima with subsequent thrombosis.

The normal aortic valve is easily crossed retrogradely with the catheter tip. Even in aortic valve stenosis, the left ventricle can be entered in nearly all cases. By slowly withdrawing the catheter tip from its looped position in the left aortic sinus, one may perform wall-to-wall exploration of the severely stenotic valve. A straight-tip guidewire may enhance this maneuver. Left and right Judkins, left Amplatz, and pigtail catheters have all been used to center the guidewire in the aortic root to achieve more effective probing of the stenotic orifice.[20,21]

In selected patients who have aortic and mitral valve disk or ball-valve prosthesis, a brief direct percutaneous puncture through the palpable apex of the left ventricle is surprisingly free of complications. LV angiography can be performed through the cannula. Retrograde catheterization of the left ventricle via a prosthetic aortic disk valve is not difficult but should be avoided if possible. Valvular incompetence is induced, and the catheter may become entrapped in the disk valve mechanism. In contrast, tissue valves can be crossed without significant hazard.

In cases with both femoral and axillary artery disease, selective coronary arteriography can be performed via a translumbar aortic approach, utilizing a sheath,[22] or via a transseptal approach.[23]

ARTERIAL CUTDOWN

The cutdown technique for left-sided heart study usually utilizes the brachial artery. After the administration of 100 units/kg of heparin intravenously, the anterior wall of the exposed artery is punctured with the tip of an 18-gauge needle. The opening is enlarged slightly with a small forceps, permitting insertion of the tapered catheter. The arteriotomy is closed either by a previously placed, very small purse string loop or by one or two interrupted sutures. If brisk bleeding does not occur from both proximal and distal artery segments, thrombectomy is performed with a balloon catheter.

Transseptal Approach

Transseptal catheterization may be used to enter the left atrium.[24,25] From the right femoral vein percutaneously, a 71-cm-long needle is advanced inside a dilator catheter-sheath system to a position beneath the ledge of the limbus fossae ovalis in the right atrium. The needle is then bared to puncture the atrial septum.[26–28] Entry into the left atrium is confirmed by a clear continuous pressure tracing. The dilator is then pushed across the septum. The needle tip is pulled back into the dilator, and when both are well in the left atrium (Fig. 16-4),[25] the sheath is slid over them to also enter the left

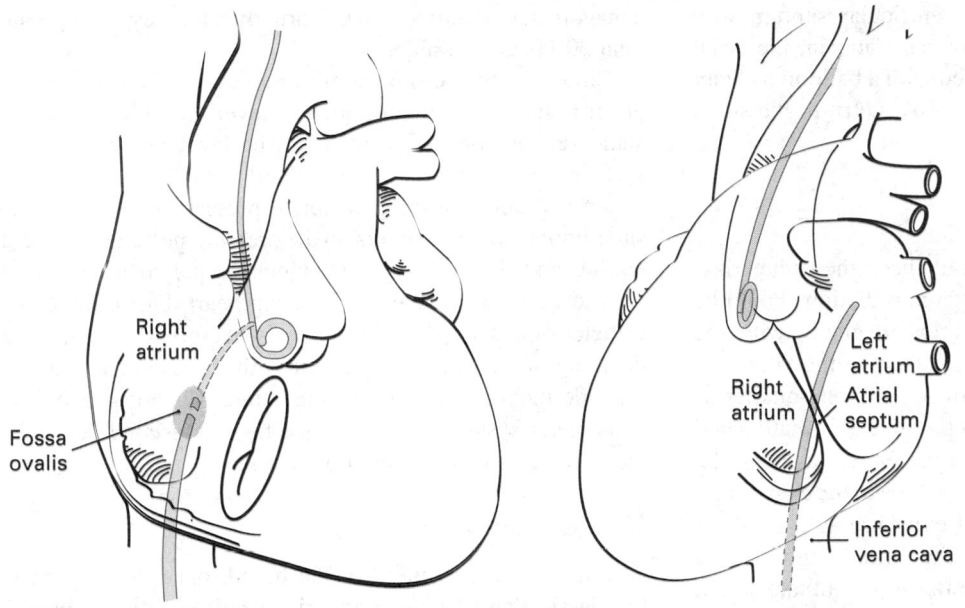

FIGURE 16-4

Anteroposterior (*left*) and lateral (*right*) views of a sheath and dilator positioned in the left atrium following needle puncture of the interatrial septum. The aortic root is defined by a pigtail catheter. Note that the septum is safely crossed posterior and inferior to the aortic valve. (Reproduced with permission from the publisher and authors: Roelke M, Conrad, Smith AJ, Palacios IF. The technique and safety of transseptal left heart catheterization. *Cathet Cardiovasc Diagn* 1994; 32:332–339.)

atrium; needle and dilator are then withdrawn. The sheath permits various preformed open- or closed-tip catheters or large guidewires to be passed into the left atrium and left ventricle. A CO_2-filled balloon catheter may be passed from the left atrium to the left ventricle to the ascending aorta. Biplane fluoroscopy, continuous pressure recording, a catheter in the aortic root, and knowledge of the size and position of the left atrium following pulmonary artery angiography are helpful in positioning the transseptal needle. The left atrium is difficult to enter if there is deformity of the thoracic or lumbar spine or if there is a very large right atrium. Other relative contraindications to transseptal catheterization include marked dilatation of the aortic root and other anatomic distortions of the inferior cava or atria. The procedure is not done if there is intraatrial thrombus or tumor.

Retrograde catheterization of the left atrium from the left ventricle in the right anterior obligue (RAO) projection utilizes a tapered flexible catheter that forms a clockwise loop in the left ventricle as it passes to the left atrium. A pigtail catheter has been similarly used.[29]

EQUIPMENT

Catheters

Disposable single-use catheters in a wide range of sizes, shapes, and lengths with end and/or side holes are available for diagnostic use. The ideal nonpreformed catheter is soft enough to permit bending as required, has memory to hold its shape, and has enough strength or body to permit the curve

of the tip to be advanced intact. Torque control is improved by incorporating a thin wire braid in the walls. Transmission of torque to the catheter tip in the ascending aorta is damped by a tortuous iliac artery. The torque is received instead by the proximal part of the catheter, resulting in coiling or potential knotting in the iliac artery. Preformed catheters are made to serve a specific function with a minimum of manipulation. Catheters should have smooth, regular surfaces to reduce thrombogenicity. Atrial septostomy with a fluid-filled balloon catheter or with a controlled folding surgical blade at the catheter tip improves shunting and increases systemic arterial saturation in patients with transposition of the great arteries.[30] A precompressed ivalon plug or thrombogenic coils inserted by catheter have been used to close the patent ductus arteriosus. Loop-snare or jawed biopsy catheters are used for nonthoracotomy retrieval of intraluminal cardiovascular foreign bodies. A small Doppler crystal mounted on a thin guidewire serves as an intraluminal probe to measure coronary artery blood flow velocity.[31] A catheter-tip electromagnetic probe can be used to measure aortic blood flow velocity. A Doppler pulmonary artery catheter can provide continuous instantaneous stroke output values,[32] assuming a flat velocity profile.

An intracoronary artery ultrasound imaging catheter system can provide a cross-sectional, two-dimensional image of good anatomic detail (see Chap. 49). The coronary artery lumen may also be visualized by fiberoptic angioscopic catheters.[33] Inhaled hydrogen gas is detected within 4 s of inhalation with extreme sensitivity by a pacing catheter electrode positioned at the site of a left-to-right shunt or downstream from it.

Used in treating valvular pulmonic stenosis and coarctation of the aorta,[34] pulmonary valvuloplasty and aortic angioplasty balloons up to 4 cm long with an inflation diameter up to 20 mm are made of high-tensile-strength polyethylene. Inflation to 3 to 4 atm with a 20-mL plastic syringe is usual. The lumen between the no. 8 or 9 French catheter and the balloon is large, permitting deflation in less than 7 s, decreasing the occlusion time. A short bilobed balloon catheter (two layers with a polyester micromesh between) permits stable positioning across the stenotic valve, stepwise dilation, and a short deflation time.[35] A balloon catheter is used to size a secundum atrial septal defect, especially if umbrella closure is to be done.[36] Test balloon occlusion of aortopulmonary collaterals mimics the effects of planned surgical closure. In patients with pulmonary atresia and intact ventricular septum who have had surgical relief of the pulmonary atresia, the atrial septal defect can be temporarily closed with a balloon catheter in order to direct all the systemic venous return to the small right ventricle, testing its response.

Radiation Exposure

A qualified radiologic physicist should check the catheterization facilities, and secondary or scattered radiation should be minimized.[37] Radiation intensity varies inversely with the square of the distance; i.e., if the distance to the source is doubled, the amount of radiation will be only one-quarter as much. One should select the smallest possible collimation and keep the image intensifier as close to the patient as possible. The U-arm position that places the x-ray tube to the examiner's side of the table causes the greatest exposure as a result of scattered radiation from the patient. Two film badges should be worn, one at the belt beneath the 0.5-mm equivalent lead apron and the other at the collar level outside the apron. The eyes, gonads, and red bone marrow have a whole-body limit of 5 rem (roentgen equivalent man) per year; any specific organ, such as the thyroid or skin, has a yearly limit of 15 rem. Lead glass spectacles and a thyroid collar reduce radiation to the eye and to the thyroid. Both a floating and a table-to-floor screen are needed for added shielding. The maximal permissible dose, or "safe" exposure, for catheterization laboratory personnel is 100 mrem/week monitored by an unshielded left collar badge. If possible, women of childbearing age should have studies done within 10 days after the onset of menstruation.

Pressure-Recording System

If the heart rate is 60 to 120 beats per minute, the fundamental frequency of the basic wave is 1 to 2 per s. The tenth harmonic or sine wave component of the pressure wave then occurs at a frequency of 10 to 20 Hz; it is important to detect these components without phase lag or amplitude distortion since their sum represents the rising and falling contours of the native pressure curve. A properly responding pressure-recording system should have a high natural frequency and optimal damping. A high natural frequency is obtained by using a bubble-free, saline solution–filled system of minimum length whose catheter and connector tubings have stiff walls and wide bores. Many catheter-tubing transducer systems are underdamped. To achieve optimal damping, a damping needle or tube is placed between the catheter and the transducer. This extends the output-input ratio of the pressure wave in a nearly uniform manner (unity + 5 percent) to as close as possible to the natural frequency of the system. The values for both frequency response and damping coefficient are obtained by introducing a square-wave pressure input to the catheter system and by measuring the amplitude ratio of any two successive peak pressure amplitudes and the time interval between peaks (Fig. 16-5). For clinical cardiac catheterization,

a manometer system with a uniform dynamic response greater than 20 Hz is desirable.

Clinically, the zero position for an external pressure transducer is set at the lateral midchest level. Specifically, hydrostatic zero is considered to be at the level of most anterior surfaces of the left ventricular blood pool.[38]

An additional limiting factor in pressure recording is the superimposition of artifacts on the pressure pulse by the accelerating and decelerating movements imparted to the fluid-filled cardiac catheter by the beating heart. Distortion of the catheter-obtained phasic pressure waveform by motion or damping artifact can be avoided with the use of a catheter-tip, side-mounted, ultraminiature semiconductor gauge. This manometer system is required for first- or second-derivative measurements of the pressure curve.

Oxygen Analysis

The total oxygen content of the blood, once determined by the classic Van Slyke manometric technique, is now obtained by gas chromatography or mass spectrometry. The percent oxyhemoglobin saturation is measured from a small sample of whole blood in a disposable plastic curvette by direct photooximetry or, after hemolysis, by a precision spectrophotometer.[39] A fiberoptic reflection oximeter catheter permits intracardiac oxygen saturation measurements without withdrawal of blood.[40]

Analysis of expired air, from collecting bag or breath by breath, for oxygen and carbon dioxide may be made by gas analyzers or infrared or mass spectroscopy.[41] Oxygen consumption can also be measured throughout the procedure using a flow-through hood technique.[42] Oxygen consumption

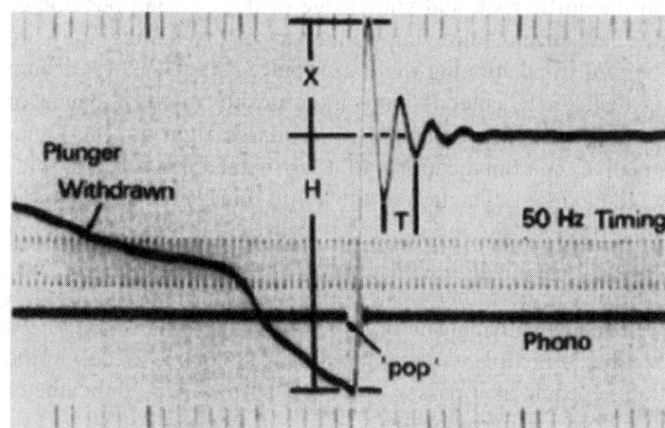

FIGURE 16-5

In order to measure the dynamic frequency response of a catheter transducer system, an abrupt transient input dynamic pressure is applied to the catheter tip (a plunger is pulled free of an air-filled syringe); the pressure oscillations are recorded at a fast paper speed and measured. X, height of the initial overshoot; H, end height of the recorded deflection; T, period of a free oscillation, 0.08 s. The natural frequency is 13 Hz; the useful range is 4 Hz. The amplitude ratio of two successive peak amplitudes is 0.59, and the damping coefficient is 0.17. This underdamped system is optimally damped to a coefficient around 0.64 by the addition of a narrow-bore tube between catheter and transducer. (Reproduced with permission of Irex Corporation.)

can also be estimated with a 10 to 25 percent variation from measured values.[43]

DATA OBTAINED AT CATHETERIZATION

Pressure Measurements

High-fidelity phasic pressure curves are not obtained from the ventricles or great arteries by fluid-filled catheter recording systems. The underdamped curve gives falsely high systolic and falsely low diastolic readings, and the overdamped curve has a smooth shape with disappearance of the incisura. The shape of the ventricular or great-artery pressure trace is occasionally of diagnostic aid. An abrupt fall in pressure in early diastole (early diastolic dip) followed by a sudden rise to a high end-diastolic pressure plateau occurs in both ventricles in abnormal compliance states such as constrictive pericarditis and restrictive cardiomyopathy. In patients with constriction, the LV and right ventricular (RV) pressures have a respiratory reciprocal (discordant) relationship, whereas with heart failure, the relationship is concordant.[44] In isolated pulmonary stenosis, the configuration of the RV pressure curve is frequently peaked or triangular.

In valvular pulmonary stenosis, the pulse pressure is frequently greater in the left PA than in the right PA, because flow is preferentially directed into the left PA and kinetic energy is translated into lateral pressure. A systolic dip is noted in the main PA due to pressure loss from the Bernoulli effect (Fig. 16-6). In bilateral branch pulmonary artery stenosis, the proximal main PA shows a wide pulse pressure with a low dicrotic notch. In supravalvular aortic stenosis, the coanda effect makes the right brachial and right carotid artery peak pressures greater than those on the left. A large A wave in the right atrium is characteristic of valvular pulmonary stenosis but not of tetralogy of Fallot. A large V wave on the pulmonary artery wedge ("pulmonary capillary") pressure tracing may or may not mean that severe mitral regurgitation is present.[45]

Left ventricular end-diastolic pressure (LVEDP) is recorded on a high-sensitivity scale and is measured where the downslope of the A wave in the left ventricle coincides with the initial upstroke of the left ventricular pressure. The LVEDP may also be measured at the peak of the R wave of the electrocardiogram. An elevated LVEDP reflects an alteration in the ventricular pressure-volume relation or a decrease in diastolic compliance of the ventricle. An increased LVEDP occurs commonly with a dilated failing left ventricle but may also be noted in a small ventricular cavity with thick walls or in a normal-size LV cavity during an acute ischemic attack.

In order to measure the maximal rate of rise of LV pressure, or peak dP/dt, a high-fidelity pressure record is needed, obtained ideally via a catheter-tip transducer. This value is influenced by preload and afterload in addition to the contractile state. The preejection phase index, $(dP/dt)/P$, where P is the

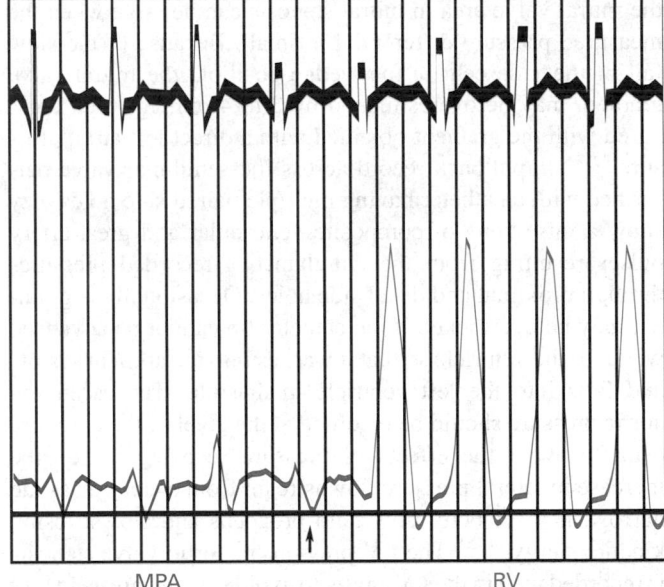

FIGURE 16-6

Pullback continuous pressure tracing from the main pulmonary artery (MPA) to the right ventricle (RV) recorded in a 27-year-old male with moderate valvular pulmonic stenosis. RV systolic pressure is 84 mmHg. MPA pressure is 16/7 mmHg. Note the systolic dip (*arrow*) in the MPA pressure tracing, due to the pressure loss from the Bernoulli effect. (From Franch RH. Recognition and management of valvular pulmonic stenosis. *Heart Dis Stroke* 1994; 3:365–370. Reproduced with permission from the author and publisher.)

LV pressure during isovolumic systole, reflects the velocity of shortening of contractile elements but also responds to changes in preload. In daily practice, ejection phase indexes derived from the conventional LV angiogram are used to assess LV function.[46] The ejection fraction is commonly employed as an index of ventricular contractility but is sensitive to changes in preload and afterload as well (see Chap. 22).

A satisfactory pulmonary artery wedge mean pressure provides a good estimate of left atrial mean pressure. Some damping in waveform and phase shift (0.06-s time delay) occurs in the transmitted wedge pressure when compared with the direct left atrial pressure record. During diastole, pulmonary artery wedge diastolic mean pressure tends to be higher than the left atrial diastolic mean pressure, especially in the presence of a prosthetic or abnormal mitral valve. End-expiratory pulmonary artery diastolic pressure agrees within 2 to 4 mmHg with mean pulmonary artery wedge pressure in the absence of increased pulmonary arteriolar resistance. In contrast, pulmonary vein wedge pressure does not give an accurate estimate of the pulmonary artery pressure in the presence of pulmonary artery hypertension.

Pressure recording permits measurement of either the peak or the mean pressure differential across a stenotic semilunar or atrioventricular (AV) valve or a segmentally narrowed blood vessel. If possible, simultaneous pressure recordings across a valve should be obtained, especially if there is atrial fibrillation. If the pulmonary artery wedge is used as an estimate of left atrial mean pressure, the waveform and amplitude should be confirmed at a second site. The error in assessing the mitral valve area in mitral stenosis can be large when the measured pressure differential is small. Because of the slow fall of the *y* descent in the wedge position, the mitral valve gradient may be overestimated by 3 to 4 mmHg when compared with the gradient obtained with a direct left atrial pressure.[47,48] A pullback record across the semilunar valve performed with a catheter having multiple paired side holes may show a false zone of composite ventricular and great-artery pulses resulting from the simultaneous recorded pressures through proximal and distal side holes. Occasionally, a gradient may be overlooked if the catheter tip cannot be advanced well into the ventricle so that it washes into the aorta in systole and falls into the left ventricle in diastole. The ascending aortic pressure should be recorded at the level of the coronary ostia to avoid the effects of pressure recovery[49]; i.e., the increase in lateral pressure downstream from a stenosis as the narrow, high-velocity flow field broadens and slows, losing kinetic energy.[50,51] The LV pressure in aortic valve stenosis is recorded well in the LV cavity to avoid systolic pressure loss due to tapering high-velocity flow in the subaortic area.[49,52] In a case of proximal infundibular pulmonary stenosis, if the pullback is at the cranial aspect of the tricuspid valve, the catheter may fall back into the right atrium from the RV outflow tract very quickly, missing the gradient.

Left ventricular cavity obliteration with catheter entrapment may result in spurious pressure gradient. To detect an intraventricular gradient, the LV pressure should be checked in the inflow and outflow, i.e., submitral and subaortic, positions simultaneously and in the apical versus the inflow or outflow positions simultaneously. These recordings enable one to detect any delay in the fall of LV systolic pressure that may occur when the catheter is entrapped.

Interventions during Catheterization

A bicycle ergometer used by the authors provides loads of 0 to 450 watts (W) in steps of 5 W; the level of effort remains constant by maintaining a monitor pointer at a neutral position. The regression equation for oxygen consumption in milliliters per minute for a given load in watts on this ergometer is $V_{O_2} = 13.16\,W + 254$ mL. An increase in cardiac output of 0.6 L/min or greater for each 100 mL of oxygen consumed presumes a normal response. If the oxygen consumption is increased 200 to 250 mL/min by supine use of a bicycle ergometer, an increase in arteriovenous oxygen content difference greater than 30 mL/L is considered abnormal. When the pulmonary artery oxygen saturation falls to substantially less than 30 percent during exercise, the upper limit of circulatory stress is being approached. Normally, during moderate exercise, LVEDP actually falls and stroke work increases; if LV performance is only moderately impaired, LVEDP rises and stroke work rises; but in severe dysfunction, stroke work fails to increase despite an increase in LVEDP. Isometric hand-grip exercise increases heart rate, systemic mean pressure, and cardiac output. A fall in LV stroke work and a sharp rise

in LVEDP during the grip test is evidence of poor LV reserve (see also Chap. 22).

All patients with mitral stenosis who have normal or mildly increased pulmonary artery and wedge pressures at rest should have the mitral gradient and cardiac output rechecked during exercise. In normal patients during exercise, pulmonary artery pressure rises minimally, usually no higher than 25 mmHg mean. In a patient with a repaired ventricular septal defect and residual pulmonary vascular disease, the pulmonary artery pressure may be at the upper limits of normal or slightly increased at rest but may double with low-level exercise.

Rapid atrial pacing may also be used as a stress intervention. In normal individuals, LVEDP falls as the heart rate is increased. If a paced patient with coronary artery disease is unable to meet the increased myocardial oxygen demand, the LVEDP rises in the early postpacing period and excess lactate is noted in coronary sinus blood. In patients with tetralogy of Fallot, spontaneous or drug-induced increases in heart rate or atrial pacing produce a drop in arterial oxygen saturation and an increase in right-to-left shunting by increasing dynamic right ventricular outflow tract obstruction.

In hypertrophic obstructive cardiomyopathy, isoproterenol, amyl nitrite, exercise, tilting, and the Valsalva maneuver, which tends to decrease diastolic ventricular volume, can intensify or provoke a systolic outflow tract pressure gradient, whereas a purely vasopressor amine, phenylephrine, which enlarges ventricular volume, tends to decrease the outflow tract pressure gradient[53] (see Chap. 74).

The response of cardiac output to vasodilator drugs in a patient with heart failure can be assessed. In patients with primary pulmonary artery hypertension (Chsp. 59), a 30 percent decrease in pulmonary vascular resistance and a 10 percent decrease in mean pulmonary artery pressure are the usual criteria for a positive response to pulmonary vasodilator drugs.[54]

Blood Oxygen Measurements

An increase in the oxygen content of blood from the chambers of the right side of the heart in excess of the normal variation in oxygen content on serial sampling is used as evidence of a left-to-right shunt.[55,56] Thus an oxygen step-up from the SVC to the right atrium (RA) >1.9 volume percent indicates shunting into the RA; a step-up from the RA to the right ventricle (RV) ≥0.9 volume percent and a step-up from the RV to the PA ≥0.5 volume percent indicates a left-to-right shunt at the right ventricular and PA levels, respectively. By these criteria, false-positive results are rare, but false-negative results can occur in patients with small shunts. In an anemic or polycythemic patient, the detection of shunting is best reflected by the step-up in percentage oxygen saturation rather than the step-up in volume percent, since the latter is dependent on the hemoglobin concentration.[57,58]

Studies show that sensitivity in detecting left-to-right shunts is improved if numerous serial blood samples are withdrawn in rapid succession for oximetry. If two sets of interrupted samples are taken from the SVC, RA, RV, and PA, a 9 percent saturation increase between the SVC and the RA indicates a large atrial shunt; a 5 percent saturation increase between the RA and the RV a ventricular shunt; and a 3 percent saturation increase between the RV and the PA a pulmonary artery shunt. Sensitivity can be improved if blood samples are obtained in multiple pairs in a rapid serial sweep without flushing with saline solution between samples. The rise in oxygen saturation step-up for a given left-to-right shunt is related to the saturation of mixed venous blood (MVB). For example, if the MVB is 85 percent, a 5 percent step-up represents a 2:1 shunt; if MVB is 75 percent, a 10 percent step-up is needed; if the MVB is 65 percent, a 15 percent step-up indicates a 2:1 shunt. The results of the blood oxygen analysis should be reviewed before the catheterization is completed. Left-to-right shunts less than 20 percent of pulmonary flow are not detectable by oximetry. Since no oximetric criteria exist for exclusion of a shunt, selective angiography and/ or the use of a hydrogen (platinum) electrode provide maximal sensitivity and reliability in excluding small shunts.[59] The presence of an increased oxygen step-up in the right side of the heart should be closely correlated with angiographic findings.

Catheter Position

The catheter position may be useful in identifying the anatomic location of an intracardiac defect or an anomalous vein (Fig. 16-7). In crossing a membranous ventricular septal defect in the anteroposterior view, the catheter inserted from the arm passes into the ascending aorta from the RV in a hairpin loop and enters the PA from the RV in a wider U loop. A patent ductus arteriosus is entered by pointing the tip of the catheter toward the "roof" of the junction of the main and left PAs. Failing direct catheter passage, a flexible-spring guidewire, introduced while the venous catheter tip rests in the main PA, readily passes through the ductus into the descending aorta; in aorticopulmonary septal defect, the tip passes directly up the ascending aorta from the main PA. When the catheter tip enters a pulmonary vein within the heart shadow, angiography is necessary to ascertain whether the pulmonary vein drains into the left or the right atrium. A secundum atrial septal defect is more easily crossed from the leg approach, a sinus venosus defect from an arm approach, and an ostium primum defect from either approach. If the tricuspid valve is congenitally displaced into the RV, the pressure transition from the RV to the RA may occur while the catheter tip is far to the left of the spine. Simultaneous intracardiac electrocardiography is confirmatory (see also Chap. 70).

Flow and Shunt Calculations

FICK METHOD; CARDIAC OUTPUT

In 1870, Adolph Fick expounded a theory for the measurement of blood flow that he never used in the laboratory: "The total uptake or release of a substance by an organ is the product of the blood flow to the organ and of the arteriovenous concen-

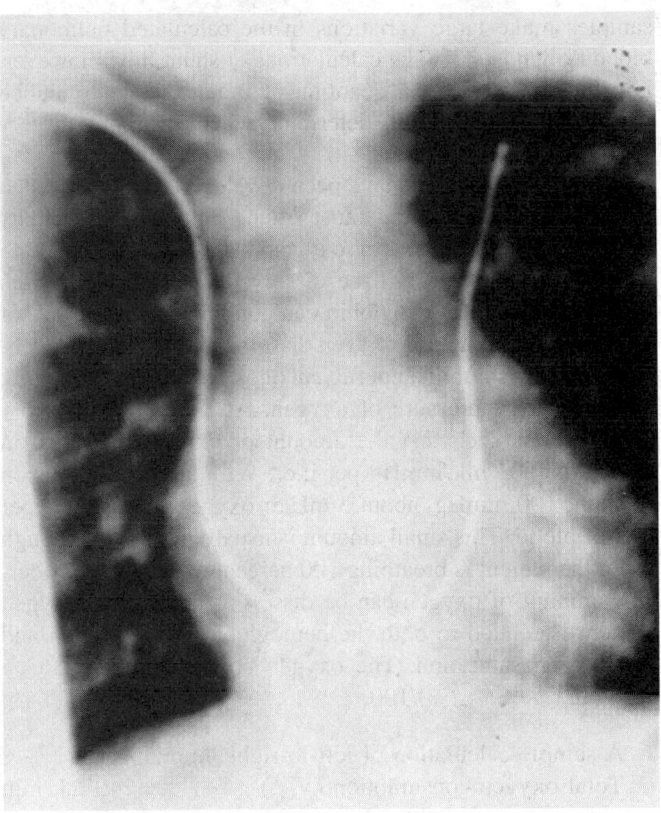

FIGURE 16-7
The catheter tip passes from the right superior vena cava to the right atrium, thence to the coronary sinus, thence to the left superior vena cava, and thence to an anomalous left upper lobe pulmonary vein.

tration of the substance." In the following example the cardiac output may be calculated given the following three values: total oxygen consumption of 300 mL/min, arterial blood oxygen content of 19 mL per 100 mL of blood, and mixed venous blood oxygen content of 14 mL per 100 mL of blood. The cardiac output, in liters per minute, is equal to the oxygen consumption divided by the arteriovenous oxygen difference multiplied by 10 (to convert the latter to liters). In this case the cardiac output equals 6.0 L/min. Cardiac output may be related to the body surface area (BSA) as the *cardiac index*. If one assumes a BSA of 2.0 m^2, the cardiac index would be 3 L/min per square meter. Because of laminar flow from the coronary sinus and the cavae and in the RA, MVB is best obtained from the PA. Under conditions of exercise, a minimum of 3 min is usually required to obtain a steady-state preliminary to expired air and blood collection. In a given person, repeated measurements of the cardiac output at rest by the Fick technique may vary to a maximum of ±17 percent, presuming a continued steady state.

SHUNT CALCULATIONS

Shunt calculations utilizing the Fick principle tend to be approximations since complete mixing of venous and shunted blood may not occur. Also, as the arteriovenous oxygen narrows, small errors in the analysis or in the collection of blood samples make large variations in the calculated pulmonary blood flow possible. The calculations of shunt flow, however, is useful; it provides a quantitative index that is combined with clinical findings to determine whether or not surgery is advisable.

Numerous formulas have been developed, but those listed below are the ones used most often. The *oxygen capacity* is the maximal amount of oxygen that will combine with hemoglobin and that will be dissolved in plasma at a high P_{O_2}. One gram of hemoglobin can combine with 1.36 mL of oxygen. The amount of oxygen dissolved in plasma is dependent upon the solubility coefficient of oxygen, the temperature, and the partial pressure of oxygen. At 37°C, the solubility coefficient is such that the amount of oxygen dissolved in plasma is 0.03 mL/mmHg per liter. With an oxygen tension of about 100 mmHg, about 3 mL of oxygen is dissolved per liter of blood. This small amount is usually ignored, although when the patient is breathing 100 percent oxygen, a considerable amount of oxygen can be dissolved in plasma. Oxygen content is related to both the hemoglobin concentration and the oxygen saturation. The oxygen content equals $1.36 \times$ Hb(g/dL) $\times$ $Sa_{O_2}(\%)/100$.

1. A sample calculation of left-to-right shunt:

Total oxygen consumption (V_{O_2})	240 mL/min
Pulmonary artery blood oxygen content ($P_{A_{O_2}}$)	17 mL/100 mL
Mixed venous blood oxygen content (MV_{O_2})	15 mL/100 mL
Arterial blood oxygen content (Sa_{O_2}) (assumed to equal pulmonary venous oxygen content)	19 mL/100 mL

$$\text{Pulmonary flow } (Q_p) = \frac{V_{O_2}}{Sa_{O_2} - P_{A_{O_2}}}$$
$$= \frac{240}{19 - 17(10)}$$
$$= 12 \text{ L/min}$$

$$\text{Systemic flow } (Q_s) = \frac{V_{O_2}}{Sa_{O_2} - MV_{O_2}}$$
$$= \frac{240}{19 - 15(10)}$$
$$= 6 \text{ L/min}$$

a. Pulmonary flow/systemic flow ratio = Q_p/Q_s = $\frac{12}{6} = 2$.

b. If one substitutes for Q_s and Q_p in the above formula and reduces to a common denominator, the *pulmonary flow–systemic flow ratio* is obtained from a formula requiring only the oxygen saturation. Assuming an oxygen capacity of 20 volumes percent, the following blood oxygen saturations for the above

samples are Sa = 95 percent, P_A = 85 percent, and MV = 75 percent.

$$\frac{Q_p}{Q_s} = \frac{Sa_{O_2}\% - MV_{O_2}\%}{Sa_{O_2}\% - Pa_{O_2}\%} = \frac{95 - 75}{95 - 85} = 2$$

c. Left-to-right shunt may also be expressed as the percentage of total pulmonary flow that is shunted blood. The 2:1 Q_p/Q_s ratio above then represents a 50 percent left-to-right shunt.

2. Calculation of right-to-left shunt:

$$V_{O_2} = 240 \text{ mL/min}$$
$$MV_{O_2} = 13 \text{ mL/100 mL blood}$$
$$Sa_{O_2} = 17 \text{ mL/100 mL blood}$$

Pulmonary vein blood oxygen content is as follows:

$$PV_{O_2} = 19 \text{ mL/100 mL blood}$$

(assumed to be 98 percent of oxygen capacity + 0.3 mL of dissolved oxygen)

$$Q_p = \frac{V_{O_2}}{PV_{O_2} - MV_{O_2}} = \frac{240}{19 - 13(10)}$$
$$= 4 \text{ L/min}$$

$$Q_s = \frac{V_{O_2}}{Sa_{O_2} - MV_{O_2}} = \frac{240}{17 - 13(10)}$$
$$= 6 \text{ L/min}$$

Pulmonary/systemic flow ratio = Q_p/Q_s = 0.7. Right-to-left shunt may also be expressed as the percentage of total systemic flow that is shunted blood. The 0.66 Q_p/Q_s ratio above represents a 33 percent right-to-left shunt.

3. Calculation of bidirectional shunt*

$$V_{O_2} = 240 \text{ mL/min}$$
$$P_{A_{O_2}} = 15 \text{ mL/100 mL blood}$$
$$MV_{O_2} = 13 \text{ mL/100 mL blood}$$
$$Sa_{O_2} = 18 \text{ mL/100 mL blood}$$
$$PV_{O_2} = 19 \text{ mL/100 mL blood}$$

$$Q_p = \frac{V_{O_2}}{PV_{O_2}} - \frac{240}{19 - 15(10)}$$

$$Q_s = \frac{V_{O_2}}{Sa_{O_2} - MV_{O_2}} = \frac{240}{18 - 13(10)}$$
$$= 4.8 \text{ L/min}$$

$$Q_{ep} = \frac{V_{O_2}}{PV_{O_2} - MV_{O_2}} = \frac{240}{19 - 13(10)}$$
$$= 4.0 \text{ L/min}$$

---

* Effective pulmonary flow Q_{ep} is that volume of systemic venous blood that, after returning to the right atrium, actually reaches the pulmonary capillaries. It is equal to effective systemic blood flow Q_{es}.

$$\text{Left-to-right shunt} = Q_p - Q_{ep} = 6 - 4$$

$$= 2 \text{ L/min}$$

$$\text{Right-to-left shunt} = Q_s - Q_{es} = 4.8 - 4.0$$

$$= 0.8 \text{ L/min}$$

INDICATOR-DILUTION TECHNIQUE

Cardiac Output: Dye Method

The cardiac output, or the mean volume rate of flow, may be determined by using a modification of the standard concentration equation used for the determination of a static fluid volume such as the blood volume:

$$V = \frac{I}{C}$$

where V = fluid volume, mL
I = indicator added to fluid, mg
C = concentration of indicator in each milliliter of fluid, mg/mL

For determination of a moving fluid volume,

$$\text{Cardiac output} = \frac{I}{Ct}$$

where t = time required for all indicator-fluid mixture to pass sampling site once

If the indicator particles are injected into the circulation as a bolus and measured in the initial passage at a downstream site, they distribute themselves in a time-concentration plot of grossly predictable form called an *indicator-dilution curve* (Fig. 16-8). The descending limb of the indicator-dilution curve is distorted by indicator-blood mixture that has begun a second circulation. To exclude recirculating indicator, the concentration is plotted logarithmically against time. The early portion of the disappearance slope is extrapolated linearly on semilogarithmic paper to obtain a primary curve, on the premise that if indicator-blood mixing is complete, the washout of indicator is an exponential function of time. A cuvette densitometer is used to obtain a continuous arterial time-concentration curve. Thus

$$\text{Cardiac output (in L/min)} = \frac{I \times 60 \text{ s}}{Ct}$$

where

C = mean concentration of indicator in one circulator passage, mg/L
t = time, s

The cardiac output is falsely high if an indicator is lost. If an indicator is counted twice, i.e., if undetected recirculation

occurs, the cardiac output is falsely low. An analogue computer provides rapid calculation of cardiac output from dye-dilution curves and detects whether or not logarithmic decay of indicator concentration has occurred. The Stewart-Hamilton formula assumes constant heart rate and stroke volume and a linear runoff in the pulmonary artery. Values for cardiac output obtained with the indicator-dilution technique compare closely with those obtained by the Fick method.[60]

In the absence of shunt, the indicator-dilution curve shows an uninterrupted buildup slope, a sharp concentration peak, a steep disappearance slope, and a prominent recirculation peak. Two major types of distortion are produced by central shunting. In a left-to-right shunt, there is decreased peak concentration of dye, a gentle disappearance slope (prolonged disappearance time), and absence of the recirculation peak. These alterations are produced by the recirculation of indicator particles through the lungs, resulting in a slow release of indicator to the peripheral circulation. The typical curve produced by a venoarterial, or right-to-left, shunt shows deformity of the buildup slope by an abnormal or early-appearing hump, or reflection, representing indicator that has been shunted from right to left. The distortion in contour of the indicator-dilution curve in valvular regurgitation is similar to that occurring with left-to-right shunts. Efforts have been made to predict all or part of the curve from certain other curve components. The cardiac output obtained by the forward-triangle method compares favorably with the classic Hamilton method. In this technique, the initial portion of the indicator-dilution curve is considered to be a triangle. The area of this triangle multiplied by a constant gives the area of the primary dilution curve. Intracardiac shunts can be detected and quantified by indicator dilution curves.[61]

Cardiac Output: Thermodilution Technique

The thermodilution technique was introduced by Fegler in 1953 to measure volume flow rate.[62] A multiple-lumen, balloon-tipped flow-directed thermistor catheter is placed in the pulmonary artery. Ten milliliters of room temperature (22°C) 5% dextrose or normal saline solution is injected rapidly (<4 s) through a second lumen into the RA. As the injectate blood mixture initially passes from the RV, the pulmonary artery blood temperature drops maximally and then progressively rises in a beat-to-beat disappearance slope as the residual injectate-blood mixture is washed out of the RV. The recirculation phase is negligible. Recording the curve allows assessment of the technical adequacy of the study. The area under the time-temperature curve is electronically integrated, and the cardiac output is computed by the Stewart-Hamilton formula. The difference between successive determinations should be less than 10 percent. Since there is no "gold standard" for cardiac output, the results have been compared with the dye dilution and Fick techniques and have been noted to correlate well,[63] except in low cardiac output states where the Fick method is preferable. If severe tricuspid or pulmonary regurgitation or significant left-to-right shunting is present, the peak is attenuated and the downslope of the curve is prolonged, so the thermal dilution cardiac output will likely be unreliable.[4,64] In general, when one uses thermal dilution, a true directional change in cardiac output is reflected by an observed change of ±10 percent.

Ventricular Volume Measurements

Left ventricular volume is estimated by selective injection of contrast medium into the left ventricle or left atrium. The image of the opacified LV cavity is obtained by cineventriculography. Biplane view image pairs used include frontal and lateral, right and left anterior oblique, or half-axial left anterior oblique and conventional right anterior oblique (RAO).[65–67] A single-plane mode using the frontal or the RAO projection is often adequate.[68,69] In the classic biplane technique, each shadow of the LV cavity is treated as an ellipse. The long axis of the ventricle (L_m) and the two mutually perpendicular short axes at its midpoint (D_a and D_l) are measured, and the volume (V) is calculated from the formula for volume of an ellipsoid:

$$V = \frac{4}{3}\pi \times \frac{D_a}{2} \times \frac{D_l}{2} \times \frac{L_m}{2}$$

or

$$V = \frac{\pi}{6} \times D_a \times D_l \times L_m$$

In the single-lane method, the long axis and one short axis are measured; the second nonvisible short axis is assumed to equal the first; thus

$$V = \frac{\pi}{6} \times L_m \times D_l^2$$

More often, in either the biplane or single-plane method, the short-axis dimension is derived from the measured long axis and the area (A) of the LV shadow, treated as an ellipse (area-length method of Dodge) (Fig. 16-9):

$$A = \pi L_m \frac{D}{4}$$

Corrections are made for magnification due to the divergence of the x-ray beam.[70] A calibrated grid or circular reference marker is filmed at the estimated level of the left ventricle. The true grid size equals the size measured on the projected film times a correction factor. More magnification may occur in the periphery than in the center of the field (pincushion effect) due to spherical aberration in the lens system. Digital ventriculography provides rapid computer-derived ventricular volumes. Geometric and nongeometric count-based radionuclide techniques for calculation of ventricular volumes are well validated.

By the use of magnetic resonance imaging (MRI) in each case, LV volume obtained by the biplane long-axis method and LV volume obtained from multiple short-axis plane images (using Simpson's rule) agree closely.[71] If the left ventricle of a postmortem heart specimen is filled with contrast material and filmed, the calculated estimate of the volume of the left ventricle is higher than the known volume of the left ventricle. An appropriate regression equation for both single-plane[68,69] and biplane[65,67] techniques has been derived to adjust for this initial overestimate. The

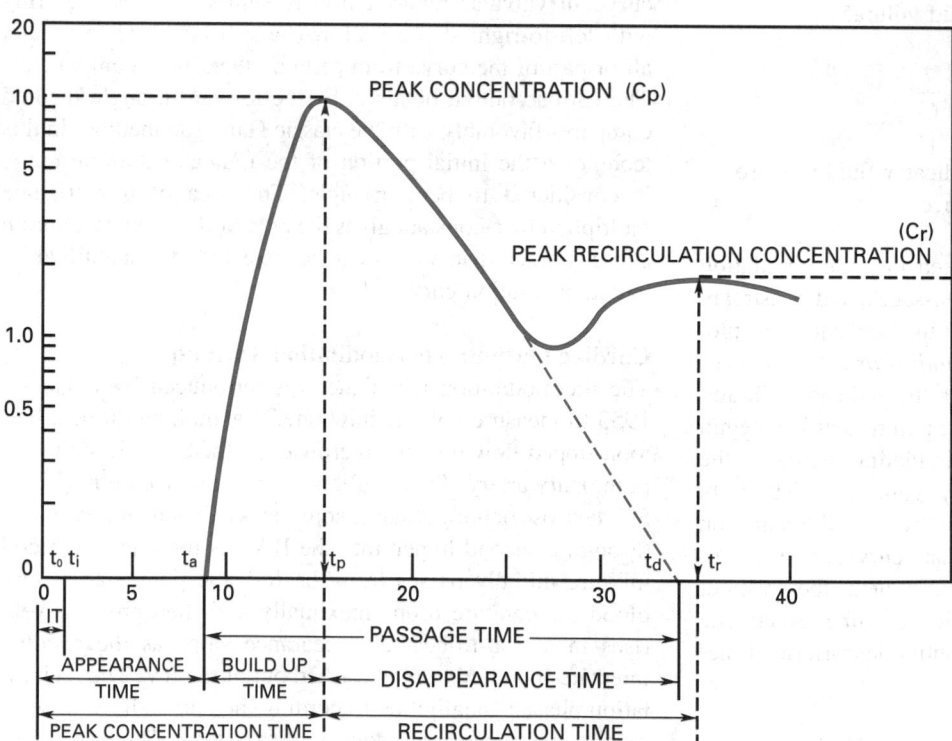

FIGURE 16-8

Time and concentration components of a normal indicator-dilution curve that has been replotted semilogarithmically, with the extrapolation of the declining slope of concentration to eliminate the effect of recirculated indicator. The logarithm of the concentration on the ordinate is plotted against time on the abscissa. t_o, time of onset of injection of the indicator slug; t_i, time from t_o to the end of the injection; t_a, time from t_o to the first detectable appearance of indicator at the sampling site; t_p, time from t_o to the peak (maximal) concentration of the indicator; t_d, time when the declining concentration of indicator reaches a minimally detectable value; t_r, time from t_o to the time of the secondary concentration peak due to systemic recirculation of indicator; IT, the injection time. (From Wood EH, Swan HJC. Definition of terms and symbols for description of circulatory dilution curves. *J Appl Physiol* 1954; 6:797. Modified and reproduced with permission from the publisher and authors.)

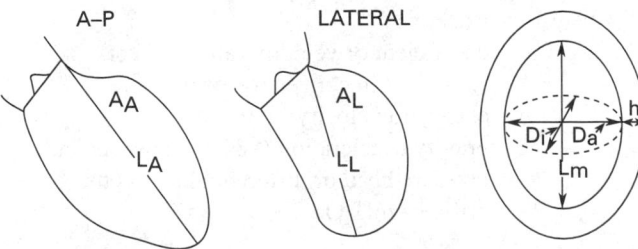

FIGURE 16-9

Dimensions of the left ventricular (LV) cavity in end diastole used for the calculation of the ventricular volume by the area-length method, biplane technique. A-P, anteroposterior plane; A_a, A_l, area, A-P and area lateral plane (planimetry); L_a, L_l, length or long axis of the left ventricle (measured); D_a, D_l, diameter of short axis, A-P lateral plane (derived; L_m, maximum length or long axis whether from the lateral A-P or lateral plane; h, wall thickness, LV. See text for formulas. (Left and middle portion of figures from Sandler and Dodge.[68] Right portion of figure from Dodge HT. Hemodynamic aspects of cardiac failure. *Hosp Pract* January 1971, p. 91. Illustration by Tagawa B, Miller A. Reproduced with permission from the publishers and authors.)

left ventricular end-diastolic volume is normally 70 ± 20 mL/m², and the end-systolic volume is 24 ± 10 mL/m². The forward stroke volume obtained by left ventriculography agrees well with indicator dilution and Fick determinations. The ejection fraction of the left ventricle is 0.67 ± 0.08; values below 0.55 are usually considered abnormal. Diastolic LV wall thickness measured by angiography is 9 mm for women and 12 mm for men, and LV wall mass is 76 g/m² for women and 99 g/m² for men.[72]

The total stroke volume obtained by left ventriculography is used to assess the severity of mitral and aortic valve regurgitation. Total stroke volume minus forward stroke volume equals regurgitant stroke volume. The regurgitant fraction equals regurgitant stroke volume divided by total stroke volume. Severe valvular regurgitation has a regurgitant fraction of 0.50 or greater. Direct measurement of aortic regurgitation in milliliters per stroke in a pulsatile circulation model agrees closely with MRI-derived phase velocity encoding data in the model. The technique is clinically applicable (Fig. 16-10).

Right ventricular volume is estimated by applying Simpson's rule or the area-length method to the cavity silhouettes after biplane angiography.[73] The end-diastolic volume of the right ventri-

cle in normal persons is 81 ± 12 mL/m².[74] The opacified left atrial shadow is represented as an ellipsoid so that left atrial volume can also be calculated in the biplane mode; the normal left atrial maximal volume is 63 ± 16 mL with a mean volume of $35 + 8.7$ mL.[75]

Resistance

By Poiseuille's law, the flow varies directly with the fourth power of the radius of a tube; resistance varies inversely with the fourth power of the radius. Vascular resistance to blood flow in systemic, pulmonary, or regional vascular beds is estimated by analogy to Ohm's law:

$$\text{Resistance} = \frac{\text{Pressure (or volts)}}{\text{Mean blood flow (or amperes)}}$$

or resistance = mean pressure differential across the vascular bed divided by the blood flow (see also Chap. 3).

To obtain the pressure difference across the pulmonary bed, subtract the pulmonary artery wedge (or left atrial) pressure from the pulmonary artery mean pressure; for the systemic pressure difference, subtract the mean central venous or right atrial pressure from the mean aortic pressure. Conversion into centimeter-gram-second (cgs) units (dyn•s/cm⁵) is usual, but it does not add to the intrinsic significance of the measurements. Resistance can also be expressed simply as R in units

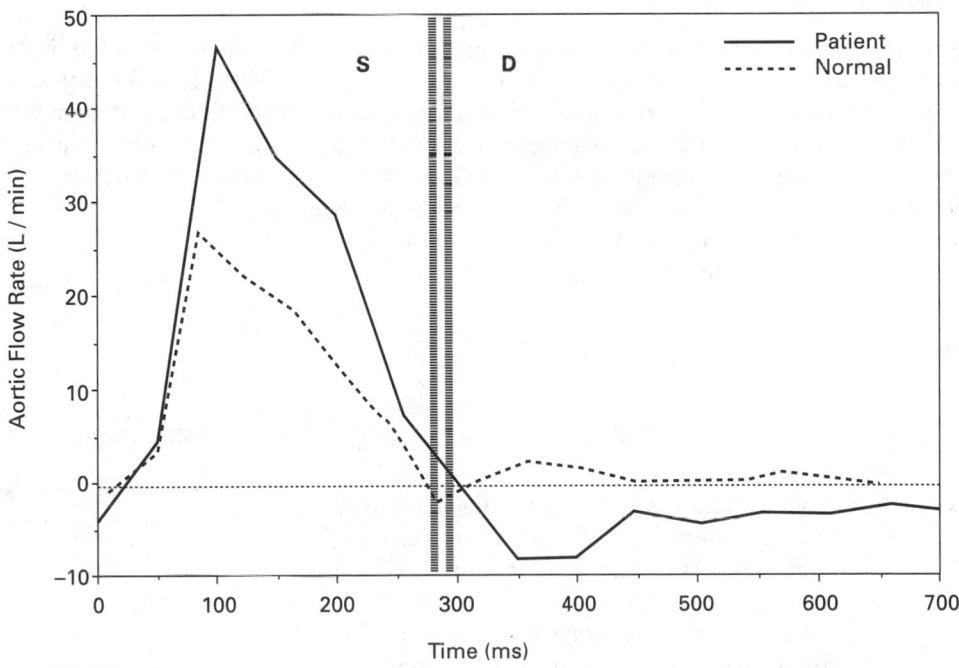

FIGURE 16-10

Using magnetic resonance phase-velocity mapping, aortic flow waveforms are obtained from an imaging slice placed in the aortic root. In a patient with moderate aortic valve regurgitation, increased forward flow occurred in systole and significant negative (regurgitant) flow rate occurred in diastole. The regurgitant volume was 32 mL per beat. No significant reverse flow is seen in the normal subject. (With permission of Chatzimavroudis GP, Walker PG, Oshinski JN, Franch RH, Pettigrew RI, and Yoganathan AP. Institute for Bioengineering and Biosciences, Georgia Institute of Technology, and F. Phillips Magnetic Resonance Research Center, Emory University Hospital, Atlanta, GA.)

= mean pressure difference (mean flow in millimeters of mercury) divided by the cardiac output (in liters per minute). In infants and children, the pressure drop is related to the flow index; thus, R in units $\times$ m^2 = pressure difference divided by cardiac index. Pulmonary resistance calculations in adults are usually not indexed, although there is an increasing tendency to do so. The normal pulmonary vascular resistance index is 1 to 2 units. Generally, 1 resistance unit is approximately equal to 80 dyn·s/c^5. In a physiologic sense, the term *resistance* avoids specific definition. A change in resistance usually implies a change in a cross-sectional area of the vascular bed but does not indicate the mechanism behind the change. Passive widening of the vessels by increases in intravascular flow as well as the opening of previously closed channels may produce changes in resistance similar to those of active vasomotion. Subnormal calculated pulmonary vascular resistance is found in the patient who has a large atrial septal defect with normal pulmonary artery pressure. Clinically, the resistance figure is useful in quantitating the extent of pulmonary vascular disease; thus a patient with a pulmonary vascular resistance of 10 units/m^2 probably would not benefit from closure of a septal defect (see Chap. 70). The total resistance to blood flow in a pulsatile system is defined as *impedance*. Its clinical use is limited, however, since the accurate calculation of impedance requires high-fidelity pressure and velocity or flow recordings.

Calculation of Valve Areas

The equation for calculation of valve area (Torricelli's orifice equation) uses a standard hydrokinetic formula for a rounded-edge orifice or a short tube. When flow occurs across a narrow orifice, the pressure differential is related to the conversion of pressure energy into kinetic energy. The Gorlin formula for calculation of valve area is derived by combining two standard orifice formulas, one describing the volume rate of flow and the second, the velocity of flow.[76]

FORMULA I

$$F = AVC_c$$

where F = volume rate of flow during the time the valvular orifice is open, mL/s of diastole or systole
A = area of fixed orifice, cm^2
V = velocity flow, cm/s
C_c = coefficient of orifice contraction compensating for the physical phenomenon of reduction of the orifice stream to an area less than the area of the actual orifice.

FORMULA II

$$V^2 = C_v{}^2\,2\,gh \quad \text{or} \quad V = C_v\sqrt{2gh}$$

where V = as above
C_v = coefficient of velocity (allowing for some loss in conversion of pressure energy to velocity)
g = gravity acceleration (980 cm/s per second)
h = pressure head or differential across the orifice, cmH$_2$O

COMBINING I AND II

$$A = \frac{F}{C_c \times C_v\sqrt{2gh}} \qquad A = \frac{F}{C \times 44.3\sqrt{P_1 - P_2}}$$

where C = discharge coefficient (an orifice constant obtained by comparing calculated with measured valve areas at postmortem, which combines C_c, C_v, conversion factor, mmHg to cmH$_2$O, other unknown factors)

$$44.3 = \sqrt{2g} = \sqrt{1960}$$
$$h = P_1 - P_2$$
= pressure differential across the orifice, mmHg

The duration of ventricular filling or emptying is calculated in seconds per minute from pullback or simultaneous pressure records obtained immediately upstream and downstream from the valve. The systolic or diastolic time per beat multiplied by the heart rate gives the number of seconds in each minute during which either filling or emptying occurs across the atrioventricular or semilunar valve, respectively. Thus, the volume rate of flow in milliliters per second of systole or diastole is the mean volume rate of flow (cardiac output in milliliters per minute) divided by the filling or emptying time in seconds per minute. A sample calculation of mitral valve area is as follows:

Cardiac output (CO) = 5000 mL/min

Diastolic filling period (DFP) beat = 0.38 s/beat

Pulse rate = 90 beats/min

DFP/min = 34 s/min

Left atrial mean diastolic pressure (LAP) = 30 mmHg

Left ventricular mean diastolic pressure (LVDP)
= 5 mmHg

C = 0.85 (orifice constant for the mitral valve)[77]

$$\text{Mitral valve flow (MVF)} = \frac{CO}{DFP/\min}$$

$$= \frac{5000 \text{ mL/min}}{34 \text{ s/min}}$$

$$= 147 \text{ mL/s of diastole}$$

Mitral valve orifice area (MAV)

$$= \frac{MVF}{0.85 \times 44.5\sqrt{LAP - LVDP}}$$

$$= \frac{147}{38\sqrt{25}} = 0.8 \text{ cm}^2$$

The calculation for the aortic valve area is as follows:

$$AVA \text{ (in cm}^2) = \frac{F}{C \times 44.5\sqrt{P_1 - P_2}}$$

$$= \frac{\text{aortic valve flow (mL/s of systole)}}{1 \times 44.5\sqrt{LVS - ASP}}$$

where LVS = left ventricular systolic mean
pressure, mmHg
ASP = aortic systolic mean pressure, mmHg
C = orifice constant coefficient (value of
1 for the aortic valve)

If the femoral artery is used, the aortic gradient from the simultaneous left ventricular–femoral artery pressure tracing should be averaged with the gradient obtained from the tracing that is realigned to correct for the central to peripheral time lag of the femoral pulse.[78] Other modifications have also been proposed.[79,80]

Similarly, orifice areas may be calculated for the tricuspid and pulmonary valves, using an orifice constant of 1.0. In a pulsatile flow model, the Gorlin valve area predicted the severity of aortic stenosis better than valvular resistance or stroke-work loss measurements.[81] The approximations and systemic errors in the formula do not detract from its usefulness in providing objectivity in the classification of patients with valvular disease.[82] The valve orifice, and thus the calculated valve area, may not be fixed and may be flow- and pressure-dependent. The orifice constant, too, may vary with the square root of the mean pressure gradient. Modifications of the widely used Gorlin formula have been made. To estimate aortic valve area, the Bache formula uses either the peak-to-peak or the maximum systolic gradient, thus avoiding planimetry.[83] Hakki omits the ejection or filling period and the empiric constant. He uses the square root of either the mitral mean, aortic mean, or aortic peak pressure gradients divided into the cardiac output. The Hakki mitral or aortic valve area generally agrees with the Gorlin areas[84]; a correction factor for heart rate has been proposed.[85] If flow is normal, reducing a valve orifice diameter to less than half or the cross-sectional area to one-fourth is generally required to offer significant obstruction. A significantly reduced mitral valve area is 1 cm^2; aortic valve area is 0.7 cm^2 (see Chap. 64). The transmitral pressure gradient is somewhat overestimated if the pulmonary artery wedge pressure is used rather than the left atrial pressure.[86] Calculation of the orifice area of a stenotic valve in the presence of associated valvular regurgitation must take into consideration the added regurgitant flow or the severity of the stenosis will be overestimated. To obtain an estimate of mitral or aortic regurgitant volume, the forward stroke volume should be subtracted from total angiographic LV stroke volume.

SELECTIVE ANGIOGRAPHY

Since 1947, when contrast medium was first injected through a rubber catheter placed in the right ventricle,[87] the technique of selective angiography has been continually refined. In the patient with valvular or congenital heart disease, the diagnosis is often made initially by noninvasive imaging. Catheterization and angiography are then performed as directed studies in order to provide physiologic data and additional anatomic detail. A catheter with a large lumen facilitates rapid low-pressure delivery of a single bolus of the contrast agent. A catheter with a coiled open tip and multiple laterally directed openings reduces recoil. A balloon-tipped angiographic catheter with proximal side holes is easy to manipulate and induces less ectopy than do conventional catheters. A power injector delivers the desired volume of contrast medium at a preselected maximal flow rate. In adults with complex cyanotic congenital heart disease, a large closed-end catheter with multiple side holes inserted via the femoral vein can deliver 70 mL of contrast medium in 2 s without recoil. Positioning the catheter in the apex of the right ventricle is done by using a guidewire or a tip deflector wire when a large-diameter catheter is used.

Contrast Media

In 1923, Osborn noted that the urinary bladder of luetic patients treated with oral and intravenous sodium iodide became opaque to x-rays because of the absorption of photons by iodine. All contrast media contain three iodine molecules attached to a fully substituted benzene ring. The fourth position in the standard ionic agent is taken up by sodium or methylglucamine as cation; the remaining two positions of the benzene ring have side chains of diatrizoate or metatrizoate or iothalamate. All media are excreted predominantly by glomerular filtration. The normal half-time of excretion is 20 min; biliary excretion is 1 percent. A dose of 0.5 to 1.0 mL/kg of medium may be scaled up or down in relation to total body weight, size of the heart chambers, systemic blood flow, degree of left-to-right shunting, severity of pulmonary vascular disease, and clinical status of the patient. If significant hemodynamic changes rapidly follow the administration of contrast medium, subsequent large-volume injections ideally should be spaced in time as the clinical status of the patient dictates. Marked systemic vasodilatation occurs within 30 s, accompanied by a transient decrease in arterial pressure that returns to control or slightly higher levels within 1 or 2 min.[88] The vasodilator effect and the transient decrease in systemic vascular resistance are directly related to the degree of osmolality of the contrast medium used. Transient hypervolemia and depressed contractility are in part responsible for the elevation of left atrial and LV end-diastolic pressure.

To reduce the osmotic effects of contrast medium, the number of dissolved particles must be decreased or the molal concentration of iodine per particle must be increased (Fig. 16-11). New-generation, nonionic, monomer, and ionic dimer contrast agents have approximately the same viscosity and iodine concentration but have only one-half or less the osmolality of the ionic agents, e.g., iopamidol and ioxaglic acid (ioxaglate), 796 and 560 mosmol/kg H_2O, respectively, versus 1689 mosmol/kg H_2O for diatriozate sodium.[89] The advantages of the new agents include less hemodynamic loading,[90,91] patient discomfort, binding of ionic calcium,[92] depression of myocardial function and blood pressure,[93] and possibly less anaphylactoid reaction. A disadvantage is the high cost that leads to a policy of selected use.[94,95] Also, while standard contrast media have a moderate anticoagulant effect, nonionic media have only a slight anticoagulant effect, and the catheter and syringe containing them should thus be kept free of blood.[95,96] The principal use of the new agents may be in very ill patients, especially in adults with extremely poor LV function; in patients with renal disease, especially those with diabetes; and in patients with a history of serious reaction to contrast media or with multiple allergies. If standard high-osmolality agents are used, those that are non–

CONTRAST MEDIA

Structure	Standard Agents	New Generation Agents	
	High Osmolality	Low Osmolality	
	Ionic Monoacid Monomer	Non-Ionic Monomer	Ionic Monoacid Dimer
Benzene Rings	One	One	Two
Cation	One	None	One
Moles of Iodine	Three	Three	Six
Particles in Solution	Two	One	Two
Molal Concentration Of Iodine Per Particle	1.5	3.0	3.0
Side Chains	Ditrizoate[1] Metrizoate[2] Iothalamate[3]	Metrizamide[4] Iopamidol[5] Iohexol[6]	Ioxaglate[7]
Proprietary Names	[1]Renografin 76 Angiovist Hypaque [2]Isopaque [3]Conray	[4]Amipaque [5]Isovue [6]Omnipaque	[7]Hexabrix

FIGURE 16-11

Comparison of structure, iodine per particle, and side chain between standard and new contrast media. The number next to the proprietary name identifies the side chain it contains.

calcium binding may produce less negative inotropic effect and less ventricular fibrillation.[97]

Filming Methods

Cineangiography uses intensification and amplification fluoroscopy and filming by a 35-mm movie camera as well as television monitoring and disk recording.[98] Perfection in image quality is achieved when each point in the object is recorded as a point on the film. In practice, this reproduction is hindered by the diffusion of light by intensifying screens interfering with sharpness and resolving power. Though the detail of the individual cine frame lacks the spatial resolution of the cut-film screen angiogram, the motion itself increases visual perception by noise averaging and use of the integrating (5 frames per second) or persistence ability of the eye (0.2 s). The circular image of the phosphor is usually overframed on relatively slow 35-mm film with an 18×24 mm useful film area. Meticulous attention to film processing and the film type is essential to obtain the desired contrast and image detail. Radiographic contrast or the difference in density or grayness between areas depends in part on the proper x-ray photon penetration of the subject, film contrast, and scatter radiation. The latter is minimized by a collimation of the x-ray beam. For coronary angiography, short-scale, high-contrast, sharp, white images on a dark gray background are desired; in the congenital heart patient, a long scale of shades of gray helps to define the entire cardiac anatomy. Biplane cineangiography is highly desirable in the study of complex congenital heart defects, especially in infancy. The total amount of contrast medium is significantly reduced, and chamber and great-vessel relations are better defined.

To perform computer-enhanced digital angiography, the catheterization laboratory image intensifier and video camera are linked to an analogue-to-digital converter, computer system, and digital storage device. The analogue video signal is digitized into a series of discrete numerical values that represent continuous voltage fluctuation and can be stored on disks. The images are acquired in the standard cineradiographic mode and simultaneously are stored on film via the cine camera and digitized from the video image. The digital information is enhanced for display by a real-time image processor and is stored on a digital disk for further processing. In single-lane acquisition, exposure rates of 15, 30, and 60 frames per second in a 512×512 or 1024×1024 matrix are available. In simultaneous biplane acquisition, 7.5, 15, and 30 frames per second are possible. Enhanced images can be recalled and reviewed to allow selection of a freeze frame. The selected image can be stored and displayed on a separate monitor. A real-time image processor enhances and smooths the fluoroscopic image. For difficult projections, pulsed fluoroscopy is available on demand at approximately half the cine dose level, the last 5 s of which can be stored on digital disk for instant review. Varying degrees of enhancement, frame rates, and exposure times can be selected from a preprogrammed push-button module. Analytical programs include subtraction capabilities, ventricular ejection fraction, edge enhancement, and regional and global wall motion. An image mask is made electronically by reversing the polarity of the background image of bone and tissue. The mask is then superimposed on the angiographic image. The positive and negative images of the competing tissue background cancel, leaving the digital subtraction angiogram. Arterial stenosis quantification and $2\times$ zoom magnification can be performed in postprocessing. A hand-held infrared control device permits image review and freeze-frame storage during the study. It can be placed in a sterile bag and operated by the cardiologist at tableside. Postcase review and additional image processing are accomplished via the view panel. Hard-copy images of selected frames, which are particularly useful for interventional procedures, can be recorded via video paper, x-ray film, or laser copier. In practice, the resolution of the digital arteriogram from the hard disk approaches that of cine film. Unacceptable image degradation occurs when the digital angiogram is transferred to videocassette tape. Thus, once a practical way of permanent digital image archiving is established and if a standard compatible system for exporting image data is developed, digital angiography is likely to replace film in the catheterization laboratory.[99] The compact disc–recordable (CD-R) format and a universal interchange standard set by users and makers, i.e., Digital Imaging and Communications in Medicine (DICOM), appears promising.

Positioning

Universal positioning capability of the x-ray and intensifier tubes by using stands of L-, U-, or C-arm configuration permits angled views of a supine patient. Two profile views of the curved ventricular septum are needed. They are made in degrees of axial obliquity and cranial angulation as follows: (1) The 40° left anterior oblique (LAO) and 30° cranial position (four-chamber view) outlines the posterior third of the ventricular septum, the valve plane in AV canal defects, and the four heart chambers without superimposition. (2) The 60° LAO and 30° cranial position (long-axial view) outlines the anterior two-thirds of the ventricular septum, the membranous ventricular septal defect, and the LV outflow tract (Fig. 16-12*A,B*). An elongated RAO view, which is useful for seeing the right ventricular infundibulum and supracristal ventricular septal defect, is obtained by 30° axial RAO and 40° cranial angulation. The main PA and its bifurcation

are seen in the frontal position with 30° of cranial angulation; a steep LAO position with marked cranial angulation is also used.[100]

A successful procedure results when a rapid injection of the proper volume of contrast medium is made through an adequate-sized catheter, properly positioned, with detailed attention to radiologic technique and to the position of the x-ray tube or tubes. Complete opacification of the LV cavity without inducing ventricular ectopy defines a satisfactory LV angiogram.[101]

Uses of Angiography

Right atrial angiography is useful in defining the following: (1) the tricuspid valve in Ebstein's anomaly and tricuspid atresia or stenosis, (2) myxoma or thrombus, (3) juxtaposition of right atrial appendage in cyanotic congenital heart disease, (4) the right atrial border in pericardial effusion or tumor, and (5) atrial septal defect with right-to-left shunting or occasionally the site entrance of an anomalous pulmonary vein by reflux. In the lateral position, a right ventricular injection is used in order to study the caliber and the level of obstruction to right ventricular outflow and the relation of the great vessels to the right ventricle (Fig. 16-13). A pulmonary artery injection may be used to fill the left side of the heart in order to detect a left-to-right shunt and to detect the site of partial (Fig. 16-14) or total anomalous venous drainage of the pulmonary veins and to visualize the PA and its branches (Fig. 16-15). An atrial septal defect is best defined by selectively injecting the right upper-lobe pulmonary vein rather than the left atrium itself. In patients with an endocardial cushion defect and an ostium primum atrial defect, selective LV angiography shows relative elongation (Swan's neck) of the LV outflow tract and shortening of the LV inflow tract due to

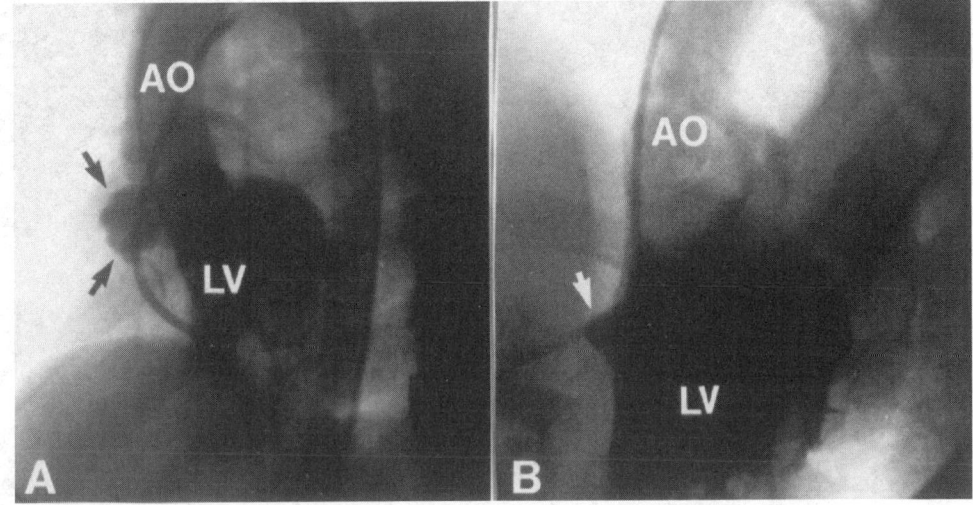

FIGURE 16-12
Selective left ventricular angiography. *A.* 60° left anterior oblique (LAO) and 30° cranial position demonstrates closed membranous ventricular septal defect (VSD) at the site of a large septal aneurysm (*arrows*). *B.* 40° LAO and 30° cranial position outlines a closing muscular VSD. A jet of contrast media exits the funnel-shaped defect (*arrow*).

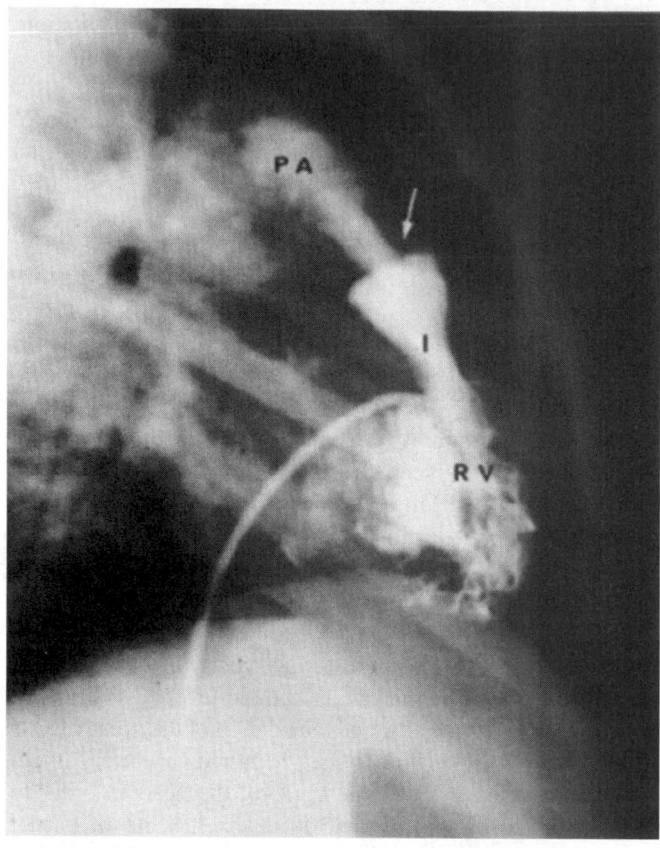

FIGURE 16-13
Valvular pulmonary stenosis (lateral view). Right ventricular injection of opaque medium. Contrast material exits through central orifice of pulmonary valve in form of a jet (*arrow*). RV, right ventricle; I, infundibulum of right ventricle; PA, pulmonary artery.

deficiency of the upper part of the inlet ventricular septum (Fig. 16-16). To identify the PAs in cases of pulmonary atresia with ventricular septal defect or to identify one PA in cases where a shunt procedure has inadvertently produced discontinuity between right and left branches, a hand injection of contrast medium into an end-hole balloon catheter occluding a pulmonary vein or into a conventional catheter in the pulmonary vein wedge position will frequently opacify the ipsilateral PA retrogradely back to its main confluence.[102,103] The size and origin of systemic artery-to-pulmonary artery collaterals arising from the descending aorta, the patent ductus, and the subclavian arteries should be defined in the patient with pulmonary atresia (Fig. 16-17).

Valve Regurgitation

Injections made above the aortic valve serve to detect and qualitatively assess aortic regurgitation. In milder degrees of aortic regurgitation, a fine regurgitant jet or puff is noted; opacification is limited to the LV outflow tract, clearing with each systole (grade 1), or faint, persistent, incomplete opacification of the LV cavity (grade 2) occurs. In grades 3 and 4, no distinct jet is seen, and dense complete opacification of the left ventricle occurs either progressively or in one or two diastolic cycles, and LV density exceeds aortic density in the severe case. After an aortic injection, the size and mobility of a stenotic aortic valve may be visualized by negative-contrast washout of the opacified aorta with nonopaque ventricular blood. In the LAO view, the mouthlike opening of a bicuspid aortic valve is seen when fusion of the commissure between the right and the left aortic sinus leaflets occurs. An

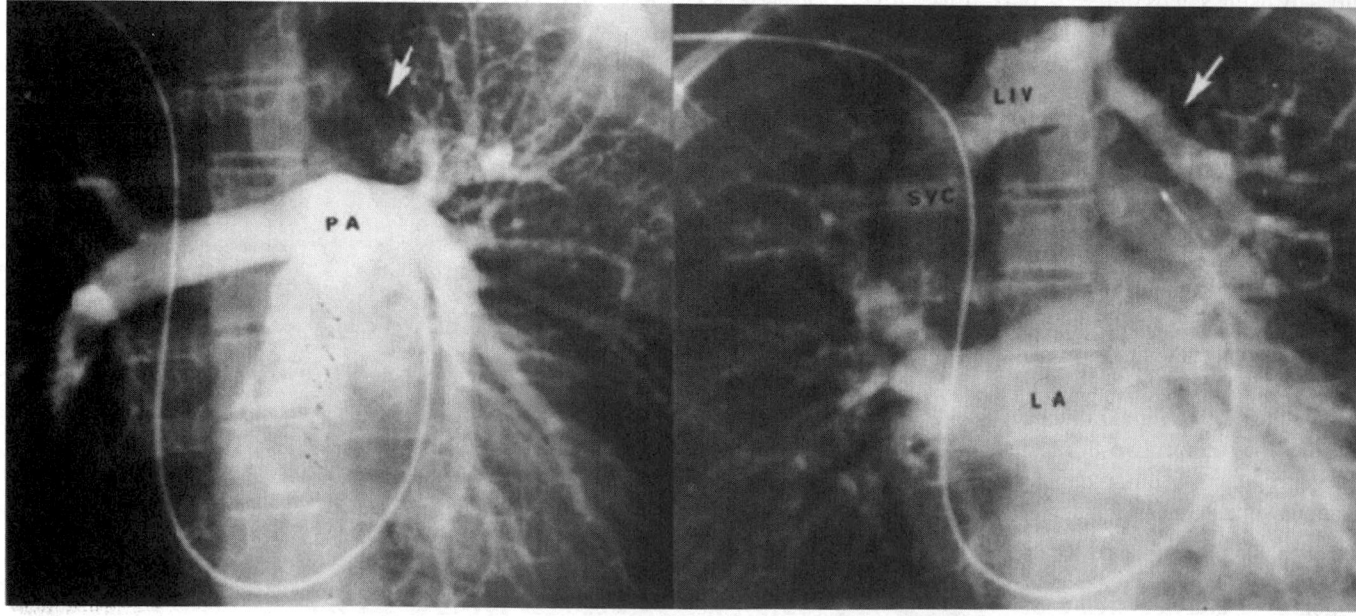

A   *B*

FIGURE 16-14
Partial anomalous drainage of pulmonary veins (*frontal view*). *A*. The catheter has been introduced into the right atrium and ventricle and positioned in the main pulmonary artery (PA) where selective injection is performed.

B. Pulmonary venous phase. A large pulmonary vein (*arrow*) drains the upper lobe of the left lung, with anomalous venous return to the left innominate vein (LIV). SVC, superior vena cava; LA, left atrium.

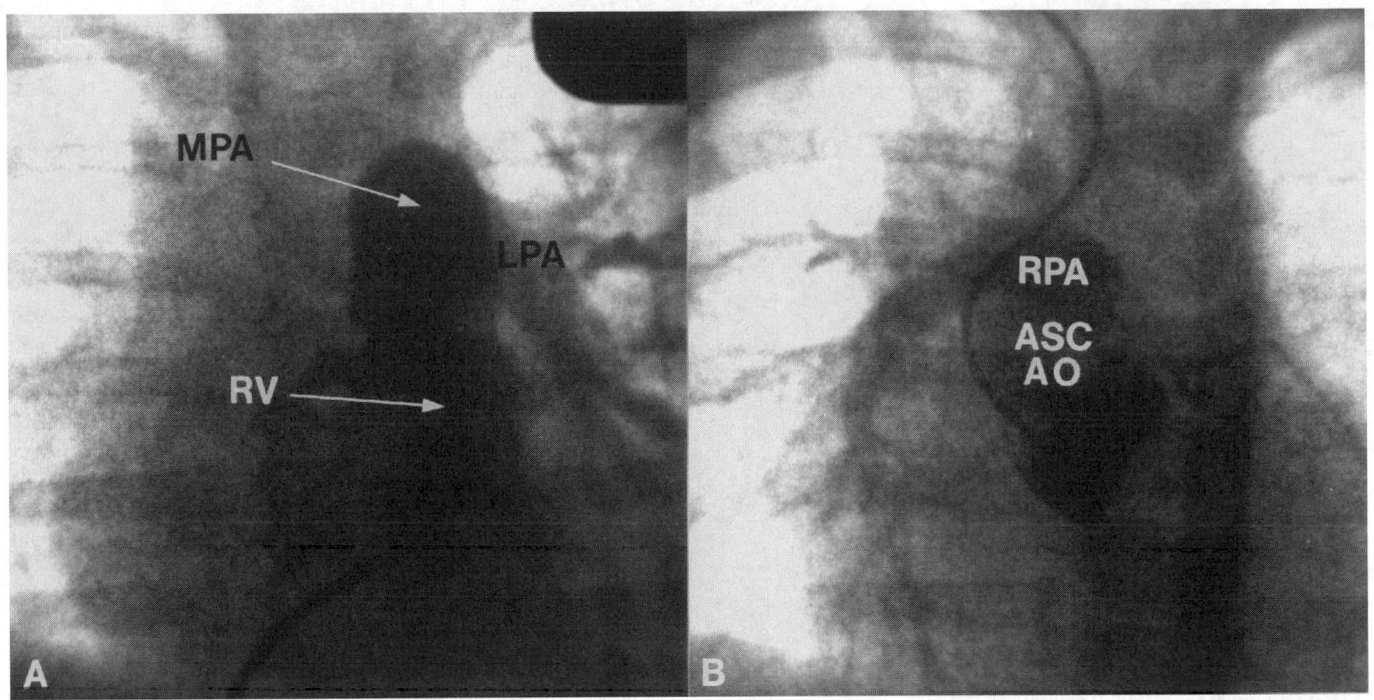

FIGURE 16-15

A. Selective right ventricular (RV) injection, frontal view opacifying the main pulmonary artery (MPA) and the left PA (LPA). The right PA does not opacify. *B.* Selective injection of the aortic root in the frontal view opacifies the aberrant right PA (RPA) originating from the medial side of the ascending aorta (ASC AO).

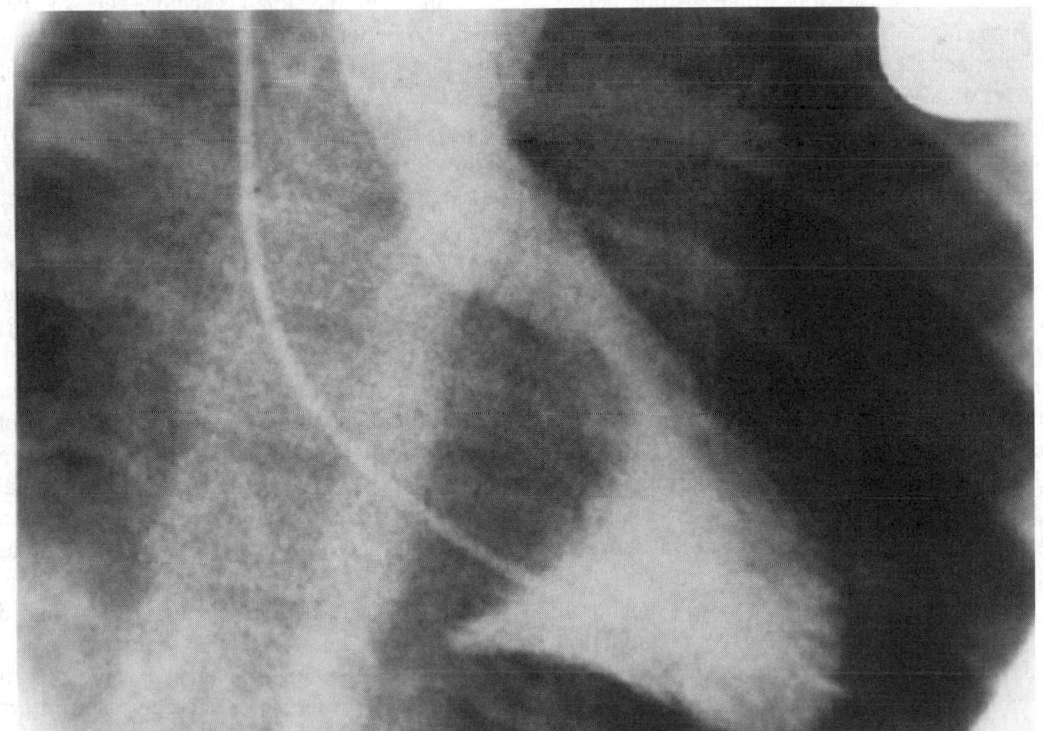

FIGURE 16-16

The frontal view of the left ventricular (LV) cineangiogram of a young girl with partial atrioventricular canal shows the typical swan's neck contour of the LV outflow tract. Note the shorter than normal mitral valve annulus to LV apex distance (the LV inflow tract) in comparison to the LV apex to aortic valve distance (LV outflow tract).

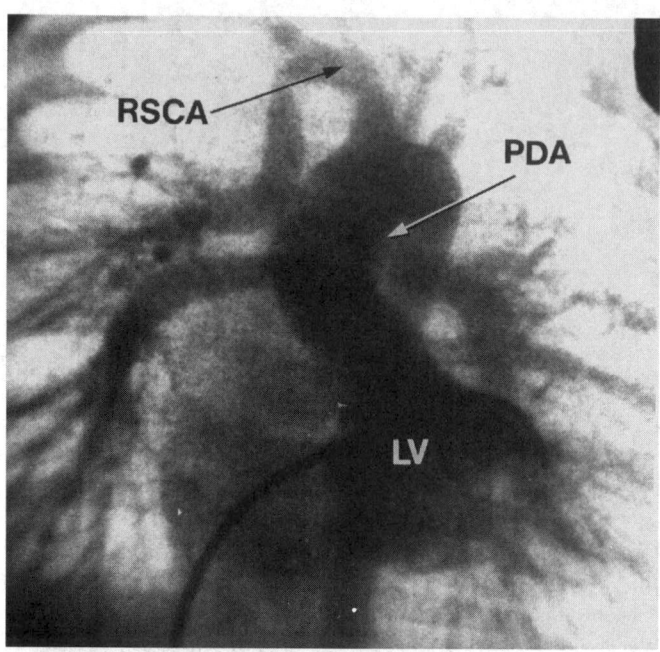

FIGURE 16-17

Selective left ventricular angiogram in a patient with ventricular septal defect and pulmonary atresia, frontal view. The right and left pulmonary arteries are supplied by a patent ductus arteriosus (PDA). A branch from the right subclavian artery (RSCA) fills a separate right pulmonary artery supplying the right middle and upper lobe.

LV injection may display the level of subaortic obstruction to LV outflow. In patients with endocardial cushion defect, the frontal view may show a radiolucent notch in the anterior mitral valve leaflet or between the superior and inferior bridging leaflets of the AV valve.

Left ventricular injection in the RAO view is used to detect and grossly quantitate mitral regurgitation. Forty five milliliters of contrast media is delivered at 15 ml/s via a pigtail catheter positioned to avoid ventricular ectopy. The angiographic criteria for grading mitral regurgitation are somewhat subjective, and so disagreement may arise between observers in assessing the degree of reflux. In grades 1 and 2 mitral regurgitation, a narrow- to moderate-width regurgitant jet of slight to moderate density is noted; minimum to moderate opacification of the left atrium clears quickly. In grades 3 and 4, a well-defined jet is absent and left atrial opacification is intense, immediate, and lingering; thus the left atrium appears denser than the left ventricle or aorta in grade 4 mitral regurgitation. In mitral valve prolapse, which is shown best in a lateral projection with slight cranial angulation, all or a portion of one or both leaflets balloon above the mitral annulus in systole, with or without associated mitral valve regurgitation. A normal mitral valve may leak if ectopic beating occurs. Unlike disk or ball valves, prosthetic tissue valves can be crossed with the catheter tip without interfering with valve function. Selective right ventricular angiography in the RAO or lateral position via a pigtail catheter lying in the apex of the RV gives adequate evaluation of tricuspid regurgitation.[104] Reflux into the superior vena cava and inferior vena cava

is associated with severe tricuspid regurgitation. A properly placed main pulmonary artery catheter will detect significant pulmonary regurgitation.

COMPLICATIONS OF CARDIAC CATHETERIZATION AND ANGIOGRAPHY

An experienced operator can carry out catheterization of the right side of the heart without difficulty in practically all cases. Complications may include knotting of the catheter; breakage of the guidewire; perforation of the atrium, ventricle, or coronary vein; and pulmonary infarction or pulmonary artery rupture associated with balloon catheter inflation.[105] Complete heart block may be induced if left bundle branch block is already present or if prolonged catheter manipulation is required in a cyanotic patient. Prolonged ventricular or atrial arrhythmia may occur.

In the catheterization of the left side of the heart, thrombosis or hematoma may occur at the percutaneous arterial puncture site and blood may migrate into fascial and retroperitoneal planes.[106] Perforation may occur at a tortuous subclavian or pelvic arterial site. The commonest vascular complication is femoral arterial pseudoaneurysm or pulsating hematoma, in part due to the increased use of heparin postcatheterization (see Fig. 16-3). Pseudoaneurysm following catheterization may be detected by color Doppler flow imaging. In systole, a high-velocity flow signal moves into the sac of the pseudoaneurysm from the small puncture site in the superficial or common femoral artery; in diastole, there is a low-flow velocity from the sac into the femoral artery retrogradely. In the presence of the femoral artery to femoral vein fistula, there is a constant-flow signal from the artery to the vein.[107–109] Ultrasound-guided compression obliteration of these communications has been helpful. Among approximately 23,000 patients (72 percent males) at Emory University Hospital who have had coronary artery angiography via the percutaneous femoral approach using a no. 8 French multipurpose catheter, 14 patients (12 females and 2 males) required femoral artery thrombectomy. The smaller femoral artery of the female is more prone to thrombotic occlusion than is that of the male. Cerebral embolism results primarily from plaque material dislodgment in the ascending aorta and less often from a fibrin clot on catheters.[110] Isolated persistent diplopia or hemianopia may occur. In 30,000 coronary artery and LV catheterizations, 35 patients had central nervous system complications (carotid distribution in 15, vertebrobasilar in 20, and diffuse encephalopathy in 2). The deficit resolved in one-half of all cases and persisted in one-half. There were two deaths. Cholesterol crystal embolization shower syndrome may follow catheter manipulation in the aorta and can result in progressive renal failure. Transseptal puncture may result in inadvertent perforation of the aorta or the free wall of the atrium, with resultant cardiac tamponade.

Nausea with or without vomiting may develop immediately after the initial injection of contrast media, probably related to direct stimulation of serotonin receptors in the brain. Adverse reactions also include sneezing, chills, low-grade fever, hives, itching, angioedema, bronchospasm, and shock. Since no anticontrast media immunoglobulin E (IgE) is found, these reactions are anaphylactoid rather than being true anaphylaxis. The mechanism may be related to activation of the kallikrein, classic or alternate complement, or intrinsic coagulation systems or to direct hyperosmolar or chemical cytoxocity.[111] Rare reactions include parotitis (iodide mumps), glossitis, and pancreatic edema. A two-dose oral glucocorticoid regimen (methylprednisolone, 32 mg) given 12 and 2 h before standard contrast medium injection significantly reduces acute allergic reactions. Diphenhydramine hydrochloride, cimetidine hydrochloride, epinephrine, or hydrocortisone, singly or combined, have been added to a treatment protocol outlined in Table 16-2. Patients at high risk for contrast media nephropathy usually have preexisting renal insufficiency and diabetes. An increase in serum creatinine levels of 0.5 to 1.0 mg/dL or a

TABLE 16-2

GUIDELINES FOR MANAGEMENT OF ANAPHYLACTOID REACTIONS IN THE CARDIAC CATHETERIZATION LABORATORY

Condition	Therapy
Urticaria and skin itching	1. No treatment 2. Diphenhydramine, 25–50 mg, PO or IV 3. Unresponsive to therapy: Epinephrine, 0.3 mL of 1:1000 solution, SQ q 15 min up to 1 mL Cimetidine, 300 mg, or ranitidine, 50 mg in 20 mL normal saline, IV over 15 min
Bronchospasm	1. O_2 by mask Oximetry 2. *Mild*: albuterol inhaler—2 puffs *Moderate*: epinephrine, 0.3 mL of 1:1000 solution sq, q 15 min up to 1 mL *Severe*: epinephrine IV as bolus(es)[a] of 10 μg/min, then infusion[b] of 1 to 4 μg/min; observe for desired effect with blood pressure and ECG monitoring 3. Diphenhydramine, 50 mg IV 4. Hydrocortisone, 200–400 mg IV 5. Optional: H_2 blocker as outlined
Facial and laryngeal edema	1. Call anesthesia 2. Assess airway O_2 Intubation Tracheostomy tray 3. *Mild*: epinephrine SQ as outlined *Moderate/severe*: epinephrine IV as outlined above 4. Diphenhydramine, 50 mg IV 5. Oximetry/arterial blood gases 6. H_2 blocker as outlined
Hypotension/shock	1. Simultaneous administration: a. Epinephrine IV as bolus(es) of 10 μg/min until desired blood pressure response obtained, then infusion of 1–4 μg/min to maintain desired blood pressure b. Large volumes of 0.9% normal saline IV (1–3 L in the first hour) 2. O_2 by mask Intubation 3. Diphenhydramine, 50–100 mg IV 4. Hydrocortisone, 400 mg IV 5. Central venous pressure/Swan-Ganz 6. Oximetry/arterial blood gases 7. Unresponsive to therapy: H_2 blocker as outlined Dopamine, 2–15 μg/kg per min IV Advanced cardiac life support

[a] Bolus dose: 0.1 mL of 1:1000 solution or 1 mL of 1:10,000, diluted to 10 mL (10 μg/mL).

[b] Infusion dose: 1 mL of 1:1000 or 10 mL in 250 mL normal saline (4 μg/mL).

Note: ECG, electrocardiographic; IV, intravenous; PO, by mouth; SQ, subcutaneous.

Source: From Goss JE, Chambers CE, Heupler FA, members of the Laboratory Performance Standards Committee of the Society for Cardiac Angiography and Interventions. *Cathet Cardiovasc Diagn* 1995; 34: 99–104. With permission of the authors and publisher.

rise of 25 to 50 percent over baseline at 24 to 48 h postangiography is noted in 2 to 7 percent of an unselected population and is considered to reflect contrast media–induced renal injury. Good hydration is essential in preventing or diminishing renal injury: 0.45% normal saline at a rate of 1 mL/kg per hour is begun 12 h before and is continued for 12 h after the procedure.[113] The mechanism of contrast nephrotoxicity is related in part to renal cortical vasoconstriction and to tubular cell toxicity[114–117] (Fig. 16-18). Renal insult in a high-risk group subset in a randomized trial was diminished with the use of low-osmolality media. There is little difference in the rate in serum creatinine levels postangiography in low-risk groups whether ionic or nonionic contrast media are used.[116,118,119] Pulmonary edema following angiography may be caused by volume overload and a negative inotropic effect.

In desperately ill patients and in those with marked ventricular dysfunction or severe valvular obstruction, the desire for films that display the cardiac anatomy spectacularly should be tempered by the potential consequences of large doses of contrast medium in this setting.

CORONARY ARTERIOGRAPHY AND LEFT VENTRICULOGRAPHY

Coronary arteriography remains the standard by which all methods of diagnosing coronary artery disease are measured. It is the primary method of defining coronary anatomy in living patients. To accomplish this in a safe, reliable, and reproducible manner, adherence to certain principles of performance and interpretation is required.[120–122]

Coronary arteriography provides not only an anatomic map of the coronary arteries, including the site, severity, and shape of stenotic lesions, but also the characteristics of distal vessels in terms of size, presence of atherosclerotic disease, mass of myocardium served, a rough index of differential coronary

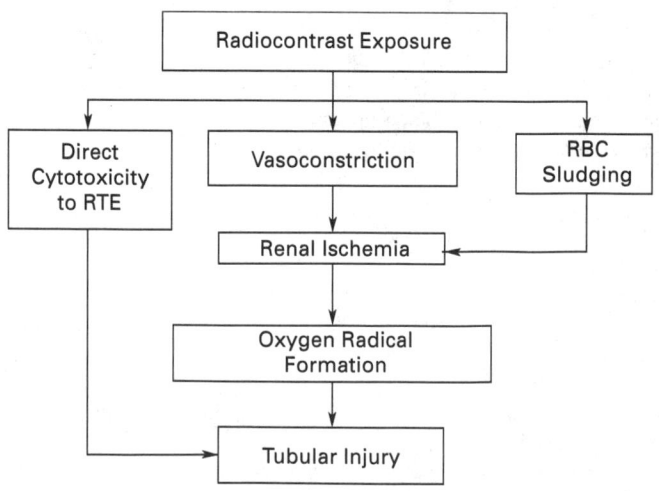

FIGURE 16-18
Proposed mechanisms of contrast media–induced acute renal injury. RBC, red blood cells; RTE, renal tubular epithelial cells. (From Rocher.[116] Reproduced with permission of the author and publisher.)

flow, identification of collateral vessels, and an estimate of their functional importance.[123–126] Intracoronary thrombi can be recognized, although it is clear from angioscopic studies that coronary arteriography is relatively insensitive in the detection of thrombi. In addition, the presence of coronary spasm can be ascertained by using provocative maneuvers.[127–129] The functional significance of a coronary stenosis can be assessed by measuring coronary flow directly, both at rest and during an intense coronary dilator stimulus. The difference between resting and maximal coronary flow is the coronary flow reserve capacity of the coronary bed. Coronary flow reserve can be measured in the coronary arteriography laboratory by using digital subtraction or intracoronary Doppler techniques.[130]

Left ventricular catheterization makes possible measurements of LV pressure at rest, with exercise, or after pharmacologic agents. Left ventriculography enables one to make a visual analysis of wall motion. Ventricular systolic and diastolic volume and ejection fraction can be calculated. Careful correlation of the coronary arteriogram and left ventriculogram permits identification of stenotic and potentially bypassable arteries serving viable myocardium. LV wall motion can be further evaluated by the addition of stress such as atrial pacing, pharmacologic agents, or exercise.

Augmenting LV contraction by the use of nitrates, catecholamines, or postextrasystolic beats may permit the identification of LV wall segments that have a potential for improved function after revascularization surgery.[131–133] The presence of associated valvular heart disease may be determined. In patients who have previously undergone surgery, patency of grafts and status of the native coronary arteries can be ascertained. In certain children with congenital heart disease, the location of the coronary arteries can be determined as an aid to planning surgical correction.[134]

Techniques of Coronary Arteriography

Sones ushered in the modern era of coronary arteriography in 1958 when he developed a safe and reliable method of selective coronary arteriography.[123] The Sones technique utilizes an antecubital incision over the brachial artery. The artery is exposed, and a woven Dacron catheter (Sones USCI) is passed into the brachial artery and maneuvered through the axillary and subclavian arteries into the ascending aorta. Manipulation techniques depend on deflecting the soft, tapered catheter tip off the aortic valve cusps up to the coronary orifices. The Sones technique has stood the test of time. The advantages are that it requires only one catheter, aortoiliac disease is avoided, and the operator is close to the aortic root and therefore has a good feel of the catheter tip. The disadvantages of antecubital dissection, arteriotomy, and arterial closure have been nearly entirely overcome by percutaneous entry of the brachial artery. Manipulation skills and precise knowledge of the aortic root anatomy are required. A detailed description of the Sones technique has been published.[135]

Percutaneous arterial catheterization, described in 1953 by Seldinger,[136] was first used to study the coronary arteries, as reported by Ricketts and Abrams in 1962.[137] Modification of catheters was made by Amplatz et al.[138] and by Judkins[139] in 1967. The Judkins technique requires three preformed catheters: one for each coronary artery and a pigtail catheter for the left ventricular injection. The Judkins technique is much easier to learn; paradoxically, this may be its major drawback. The femoral artery is punctured below the inguinal ligament, and a left coronary artery catheter is passed over the guidewire into the aorta. After the catheter is flushed and good pressure tracings are obtained from the tip, the catheter is advanced until it engages the left coronary orifice. The preformed shape of the catheter holds it against the inside of the aortic curve, enabling the tip to spring into the left coronary orifice. The tip is made in four lengths for use with different-sized aortic roots. After the left catheter is removed, the appropriate-sized right coronary catheter is inserted over a guidewire and positioned above the right coronary orifice, where it is rotated clockwise. The tip will descend and will be held against the outside curve of the aorta, causing it to spring into the right coronary orifice. LV studies are performed by replacing the coronary catheters with the pigtail catheter. A detailed description of the Judkins technique has also been published.[140]

This technique has the advantages of a percutaneous approach; the disadvantages are the requirement for multiple catheter exchanges and a potential increased risk of emboli to the coronary or cerebral circulation. Complications may arise from the ease of entry of the catheter tip into the coronary arteries. Some poorly trained angiographers have applied this technique without proper appreciation of the devastating consequences of catheter obstruction of the left main coronary artery. Methods of avoiding serious complications of catheter emboli, including systemic heparinization and catheter-debriding techniques, have reduced complications in active centers.

In an attempt to combine the advantages of the Sones and Judkins techniques, the single-catheter percutaneous femoral approach was first applied by Schoonmaker in 1968, and the use of this technique was reported by Schoonmaker and King.[141] This technique has been employed at Emory University Hospital in over 80,000 studies since 1972.

Performance of Coronary Arteriography

The description of the authors' technique of coronary arteriography is brief; a more detailed description has been published.[142] It is the authors' belief that one cannot become expert in performing coronary arteriography by reading. Only through training in an active laboratory and performing hundreds of coronary arteriograms under close supervision can the physician gain a proper appreciation of the potential hazards of coronary arteriography so that they can be avoided.[143] A close physician-patient relationship is essential to reduce fear of the examination. The patient is seen before the procedure, and a thorough history, physical examination, and description

of the procedure are completed. Patients with mild or stable symptoms may undergo coronary arteriography as outpatients, unless noninvasive studies indicate the likely presence of severe anatomic problems such as left main coronary artery stenosis. In most laboratories, outpatient catheterization studies are performed with smaller diameter catheters of a no. 5 or no. 6 French size. Propranolol and nitrates are usually continued up to and through the procedure. An intravenous line is routinely started for administration of midazolam for conscious sedation. The intravenous line is also essential as a port for the administration of additional drugs during the procedure, as needed, if pain or hypotension occurs or if congestive failure is aggravated. Electrocardiographic and pulse oximetry monitoring are performed throughout the procedure. Atropine, lidocaine, propranolol, furosemide, glucocorticoids, and antihistamine, nitroglycerin, epinephrine and other vasopressors, and narcotics should be readily available for intravenous administration. Heparin and antibiotics are not routinely administered in the authors' laboratory. Patients with a history of anaphylactoid reactions to contrast media are pretreated with antihistamines and glucocorticoids.

A three-way stopcock manifold is connected to lines for pressure monitoring, contrast medium, and heparinized saline solution. A clear catheter is maintained by intermittent flushing with saline solution and contrast medium. The femoral artery is catheterized by the Seldinger technique, and a multipurpose polyurethane catheter is inserted into the descending aorta, where it is flushed before being advanced around the aortic arch without a guidewire. The catheter is advanced to the left ventricle, where, following pressure measurements and test injections to exclude catheter-tip entrapment, 32 to 40 mL of contrast medium is injected over 4 s. This slow injection allows adequate visualization without recoil of the end-hole and side-hole catheter. Filming is routinely done in the RAO view or in a biplane mode using RAO and LAO views.

Essential to any coronary arteriographic technique is a thorough knowledge of aortic root anatomy (Fig. 16-19). Usu-

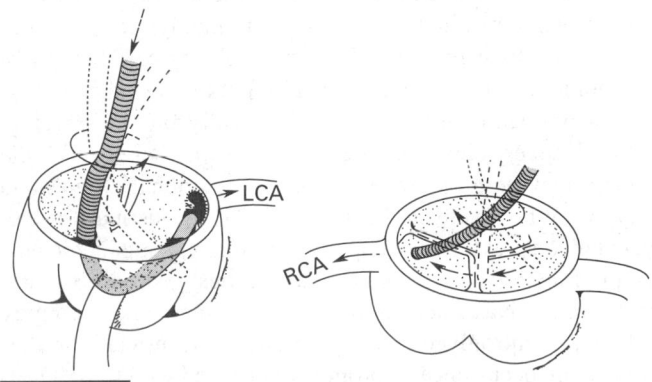

FIGURE 16-19

Left. A 30° right anterior oblique view of the aortic root demonstrating the left coronary orifice. *Right.* A 60° left anterior oblique view of the aortic root demonstrating location of the right coronary orifice. (From Schoonmaker and King.[141] Reproduced with permission from the American Heart Association, Inc., and the authors.)

ally the left coronary orifice arises from the left sinus of Valsalva, which is posterior and to the left. The right coronary artery usually arises from the right sinus of Valsalva, which is anterior. Because of extensive variation in the position, size, and number of orifices, considerable experience is required to avoid failure to identify and study one of the arteries. Left coronary cannulation is performed in the following manner: The tip of the catheter is placed in the noncoronary cusp, which lies posterior and to the left (toward the spine in the RAO view). As the catheter is advanced with a slight clockwise rotation, the tip flips up into the left coronary ostium or into the left cusp. From the left coronary cusp, the catheter tip can be rotated posteriorly and advanced superiorly into the left coronary ostium (see Fig. 16-19). Right coronary artery catheterization is done by positioning the tip of the catheter above the left coronary cusp and rotating clockwise so that the tip sweeps along the anterior aortic root until it reaches the right coronary ostium (see Fig. 16-19). An alternative method is to advance the catheter tip in the right cusp; it curves into the right orifice. When the operator is unsuccessful in reaching one or the other coronary orifices, the catheter is removed and replaced by an appropriate Judkins or other preformed catheter.

All injections into the coronary arteries are preceded by aspiration of a small amount of contrast medium into the hand-held syringe (to exclude the possibility of air embolism) and are monitored visually until the contrast medium clears. Pressure monitoring is done after these injections. Hypotension following coronary injection usually clears spontaneously or with coughing, which transiently increases aortic pressure and enhances clearing of contrast medium. If hypotension lasting more than a few seconds occurs, especially in a patient with severe proximal coronary artery disease, a pressor agent in an adequate dose to obtain a quick response is started promptly. Adequate coronary perfusion pressure is essential. If congestive heart failure is aggravated by the effect of contrast medium, the first drug used is sublingual nitroglycerin; furosemide may be needed, however. When chest pain occurs, nitrates are given sublingually or intravenously and the catheter is repositioned in the left ventricle to monitor left ventricular end-diastolic pressure. If pain continues or ST-segment elevation occurs, coronary injection may reveal coronary spasm. Intracoronary nitroglycerin usually provides prompt relief. If severe elevation of end-diastolic pressure occurs, the patient may be propped up and given additional nitrates and oxygen. When tachycardia accompanied by adequate or elevated blood pressure develops during angina, 1-mg increments of propranolol may be given intravenously, producing dramatic relief. Narcotics are used for pain that is not promptly relieved by nitroglycerin and propranolol. Ventricular fibrillation, a rare occurrence, is promptly corrected with the defibrillator. All laboratory personnel must be thoroughly trained in cardiopulmonary resuscitation, as unstable patients may develop life-threatening arrhythmias before, during, and after angiography.[143] Minor anaphylactoid reactions are treated with antihistamines; more serious reactions are treated with

the addition of epinephrine and glucocorticoids.[144] Maximal safety is obtained when an expert angiographer performs a brief but complete study, obtaining all clinically pertinent information with a minimal number of injections. Because of the osmotic diuresis induced by the contrast media, intravenous and oral fluid supplements are required after catheterization, and postural hypotension must be checked for when the patient is allowed up.

Interpretation of the Coronary Arteriogram

Once of interest to angiographers and surgeons only, the viewing and interpretation of coronary arteriograms should now be of vital interest to cardiologists if they are to make informed decisions about their patients. The coronary arteriogram should be viewed in a systematic fashion. Because coronary anatomy can be quite variable, one needs to view the films with an eye toward making sure the entire LV epicardial surface and septum are adequately supplied and that no gaps exist. If significant gaps are found, an occluded or anomalous artery is likely. The coronary arteries should be viewed one at a time, and some division of arterial segments such as the one suggested by the American Heart Association[145] should be made (Fig. 16-20). Areas of foreshortening and overlap should be examined in other views to convince the observer that there is not a hidden lesion. It is helpful for several observers to study the arteriogram. As each segment is viewed, a systematic scoring and recording system is mandatory if consistency is to be maintained and no segments are to be overlooked.

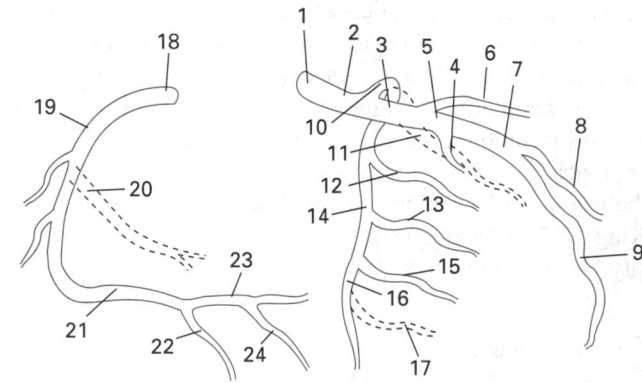

FIGURE 16-20

Diagram of the coronary circulation. Each arterial segment is evaluated carefully in all views and the degree of stenosis is determined. Left main coronary artery 1, 2; left anterior descending coronary artery 3, 5, 7, 9; diagonal branches 6, 8; major septal perforating branch 4; circumflex coronary artery in the atrioventricular groove 10, 14, 16; ramus intermedius 11; obtuse marginal branches 12, 13, 15; posterior descending branch of the circumflex coronary artery, if present 17; right coronary artery in the atrioventricular groove 18, 19, 21, 23; large right ventricular branch of the right coronary artery 20; posterior descending branch of the right coronary artery 22; left ventricular branch of the right coronary artery 24. (From King SB III, Douglas JS Jr. *Coronary Arteriography and Angioplasty.* New York: McGraw-Hill; 1985, p 363. Reproduced with permission from the publisher and authors.)

Angiographic Views

Filming is done in a number of projections so that all coronary arteries can be visualized throughout their lengths and significant disease can be detected and quantified. Multiple views in the transverse plane (Figs. 16-21 to 16-23) were utilized until 1973, when Bunnell reported the advantages of obtaining views incorporating sagittal angulation of the x-ray beam along the long axis of the body (Fig. 16-24). The use of these views (Figs. 16-25 and 16-26) greatly enhances the ability to visualize the proximal left coronary artery, unmasking lesions that would otherwise be missed in up to 20 percent of patients and significantly improving diagnosis in an additional 30 to 40 percent.[146–148] The evolution of a new generation of x-ray equipment to obtain these views has revolutionized coronary arteriography. In most laboratories, standard views of the left coronary artery are the frontal view, 30° RAO, 45° LAO, 45° LAO with 30° cranial angulation, 30° RAO with 30° cranial angulation, and 30° RAO with 15° caudal angulation. Other

views may be needed to separate overlapping vessels or to focus on a particular problem area. The right coronary artery is usually visualized in the right and left oblique projections, and sagittally angulated views are frequently helpful in evaluating the proximal posterior descending artery (Figs. 16-27 and 16-28). The use of sagittally angulated views also provides for improved visualization of LV wall motion and mitral valve motion and for evaluation of the LV outflow tract.[149]

THE LEFT CORONARY ARTERY

The ostium of the left coronary artery originates from the left sinus of Valsalva near the sinotubular ridge. The main left coronary usually courses to the left and slightly anterior. After a quite variable length, it gives rise at near right angles to the circumflex artery and continues in a straight line as the anterior descending artery (Figs. 16-29 and 16-30). The left orifice and the left main coronary artery are best seen in a direct frontal view or in a shallow LAO or RAO projection or a shallow LAO with 30° cranial angulation. The diagonal artery

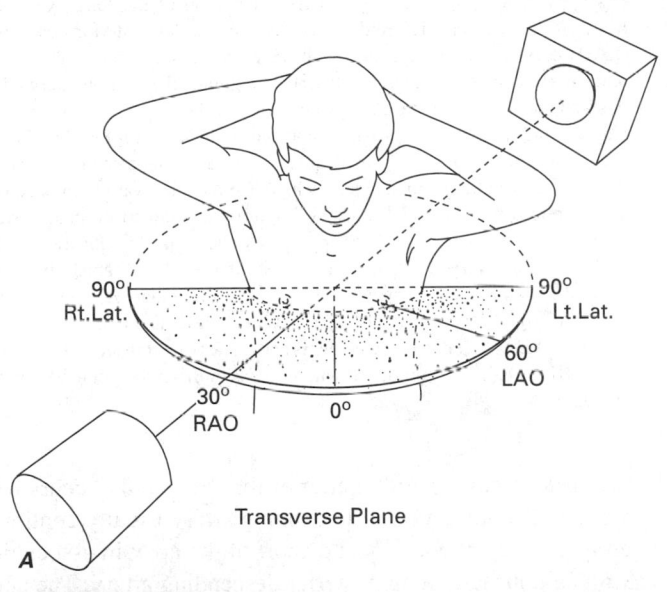

A

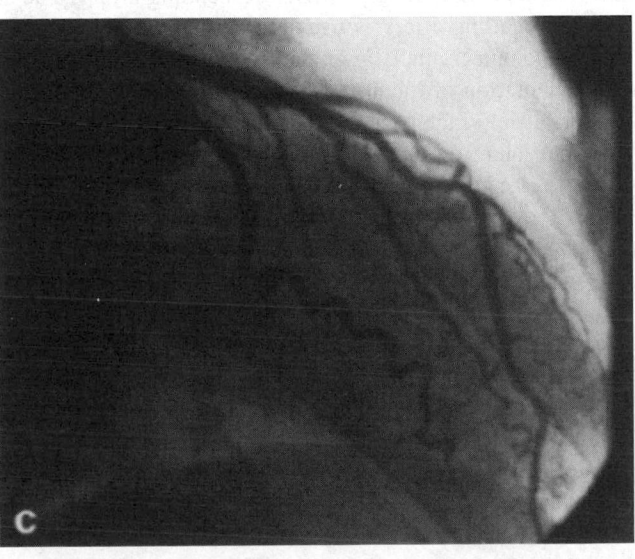

C

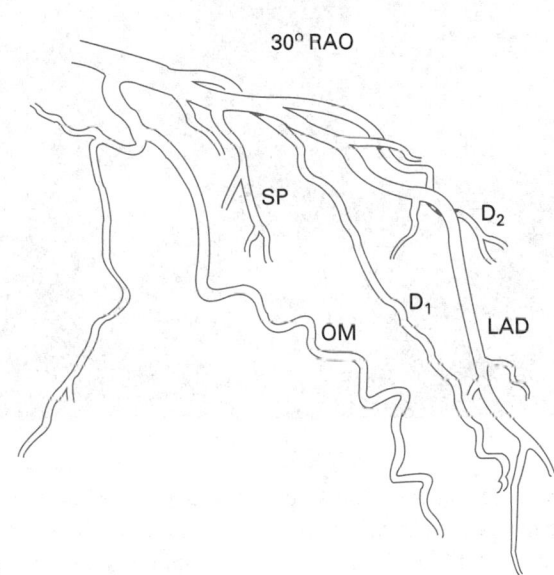

B

FIGURE 16-21

Diagrammatic representation of the standard right anterior oblique (RAO) view of the left coronary angiogram, the direction of the x-ray beam, and the position of the overhead image intensifier. Most of the left coronary artery is well visualized in this projection, although there is considerable overlap of the mid-left anterior descending artery and the diagonal branches. When the left main, circumflex, and diagonal branches have a leftward initial course, the long axis of these arterial segments is projected away from the image intensifier, preventing optimal visualization from the RAO view. The image intensifier is placed anteriorly in an RAO position relative to the patient. (From King et al.[149] Reproduced with permission from the publisher, editor, and authors.)

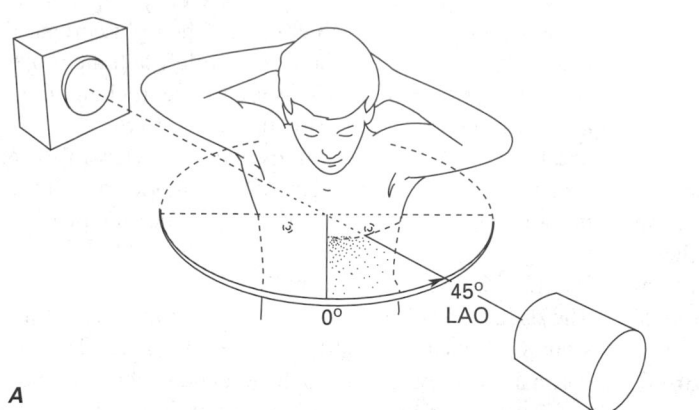

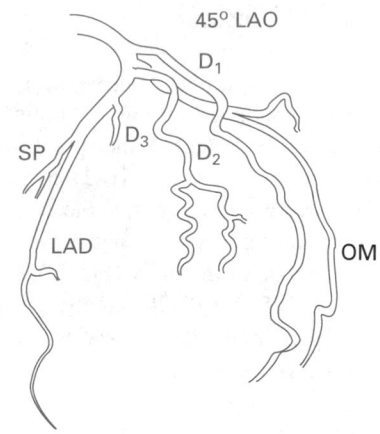

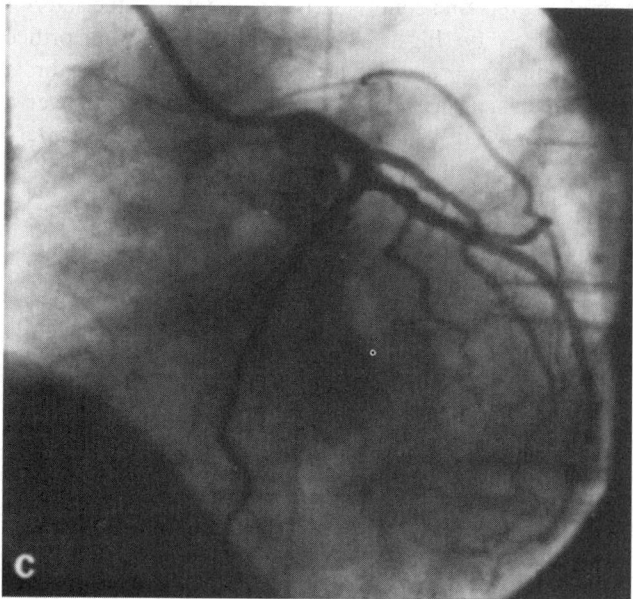

FIGURE 16-22

Diagrammatic representation of the left anterior oblique (LAO) left coronary angiogram and the direction of the x-ray beam in this view. The value of this view depends in large part on the orientation of the long axis of the heart. When the heart is relatively horizontal, the left anterior descending (LAD) coronary artery and diagonal branches are seen end-on throughout much of the course. In this illustration, the longitudinal axis is an intermediate position and there is moderate foreshortening of the anterior descending and diagonal branches in their proximal portions (compare with Fig. 16-25). The LAO projection is frequently inadequate to visualize the proximal LAD and its branches; the left main segment, which is directed toward the image tube and therefore foreshortened; and the proximal circumflex coronary artery, which may be obscured by overlapping vessels, as in this illustration. The LAO projection is frequently used to visualize the distal LAD and its branches, the mid-circumflex coronary artery in the atrioventricular (AV) groove, and the distal right coronary artery that is filling via collaterals from the left coronary artery. The image intensifier is above the patient in an LAO position. (From King et al.[149] Reproduced with permission from the publisher, editor, and authors.)

may arise between the circumflex and anterior descending arteries as a trifurcation of the left main coronary artery, or the diagonal branch may originate from the anterior descending artery and course over the anterolateral free wall of the left ventricle. The diagonal branches are seen on the side in the RAO view; however, the origin is obscured by overlap with the anterior descending artery (see Figs. 16-29 and 16-30). The LAO view separates the anterior descending artery and diagonals somewhat; however, because of the frequent horizontal orientation of these arteries, there may be considerable foreshortening. Cranial angulation of the overhead intensifier with shallow LAO or RAO rotation is most helpful in separating the proximal anterior descending artery and its diagonal branches (see Figs. 16-25 and 16-26). The anterior descending artery continues in the interventricular groove toward the apex, giving rise at nearly right angles to the septal perforating arteries that go deep into the muscular septum. The first septal perforator may arise before or after the first diagonal and is usually the largest septal artery. The septal vessels differ from the epicardial arteries in that they are straighter and move little with cardiac action, in contrast to

the buckling of epicardial arteries that frequently occurs with systole. The left anterior descending artery usually continues around the apex but may end short of the apex in association with an unusually long posterior descending artery. The anterior descending artery is usually best visualized in the RAO view and in a cranially angulated shallow oblique view unless the orientation of the anterior descending artery is unusually superior, in which case a caudally angulated LAO view or a straight lateral view may be helpful.

The circumflex coronary artery, after its right-angle origin from the left anterior descending artery, travels in the AV groove. Its course is quite variable. The artery may terminate in one or more large, obtuse marginal branches that course over the lateral to posterolateral LV free wall, or it may continue as a large artery in the interventricular groove and, in 10 to 15 percent of cases, give rise to a posterior descending artery, which more often arises from the right coronary artery (Fig. 16-31). When the circumflex artery supplies the major posterior descending artery, it is commonly referred to as a *dominant circumflex artery*. The circumflex artery in the AV groove is best seen in the LAO view, but surgically more

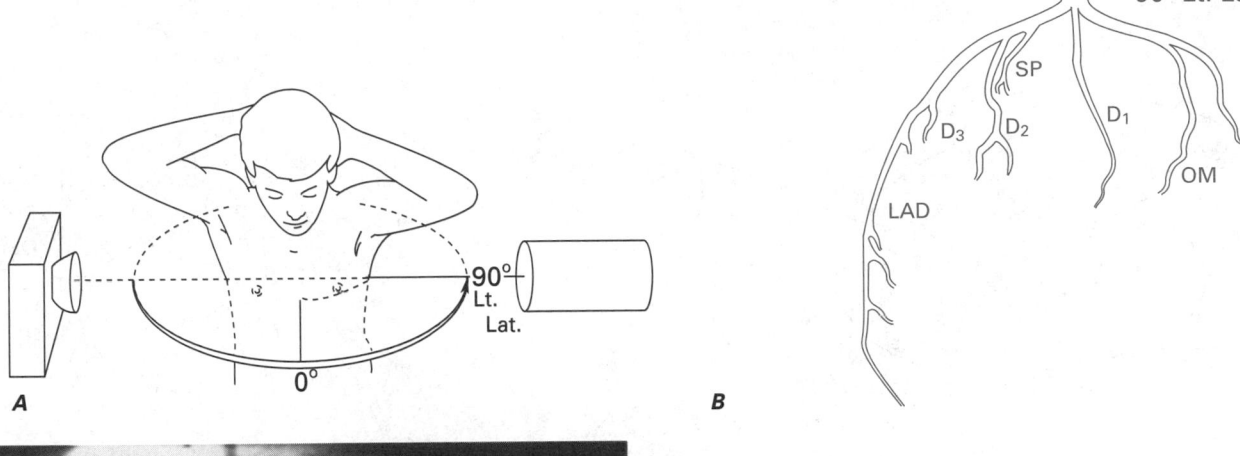

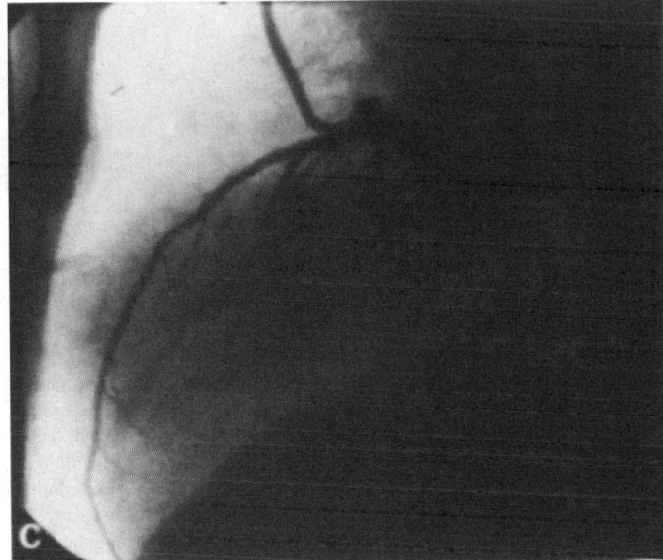

FIGURE 16-23
Diagrammatic illustrations of the left lateral or 90° LAO view of the left coronary arteriogram and direction of the x-ray beam. The left lateral view of the left coronary artery is most useful for analyzing the proximal and mid-LAD by avoiding overlap with the diagonal branches, which commonly take an inferior course from the LAD in this projection. The most proximal portion of the diagonal branches may not be well visualized since the long axis of these segments may be in the direction of the x-ray beam. The leftward-directed left main segment is foreshortened in this view (compare with Fig. 16-22). In this view, the image intensifier is placed on the patient's left, and the x-ray beam has a right-to-left direction in the horizontal plane. (From King et al.[149] Reproduced with permission from the publisher, editor, and authors.)

important marginal branches are visualized best in the RAO view. Occasionally, proximal stenoses in the circumflex artery are best viewed in an RAO view with 15° caudal angulation, which produces a view as though looking from the superior aspect of the liver toward the left shoulder.

THE RIGHT CORONARY ARTERY

The right coronary artery orifice is normally located in the right sinus of Valsalva. It may be high near the sinotubular ridge or above it, in the midsinus, or occasionally low near the aortic valve. The artery commonly courses upward from the plane of the aortic valve and then travels in the right AV groove as a conduit to reach the posterior LV wall (Figs. 16-32 and 16-33). Along the way, several vessels arise. The conus branch and sinus node branches arise first, followed by small right ventricular branches. At the acute margin of the heart, there is usually a large branch that courses over the right ventricle. In some cases this may supply the apical portion of the interventricular septum and therefore be of greater importance. The posterior descending artery usually arises before the right coronary artery reaches the crux of the heart

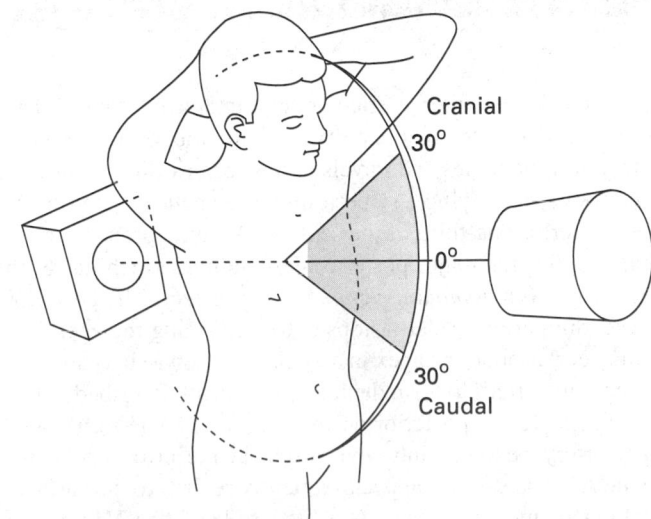

FIGURE 16-24
Illustration of sagittal angulation of x-ray beam in coronary arteriography. (From King et al.[149] Reproduced with permission from the publisher, editor, and authors.)

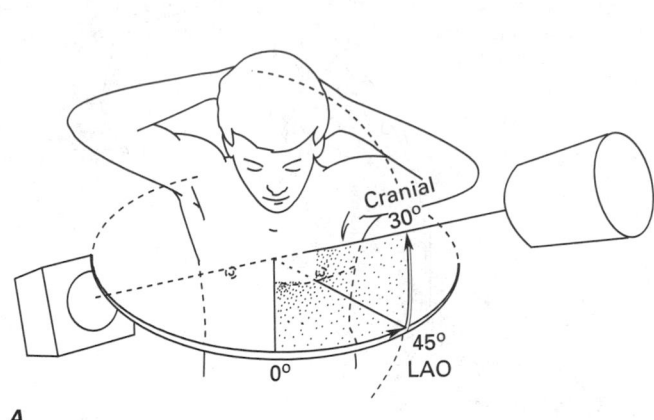

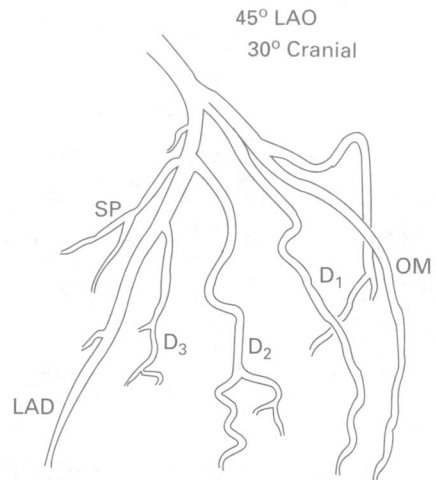

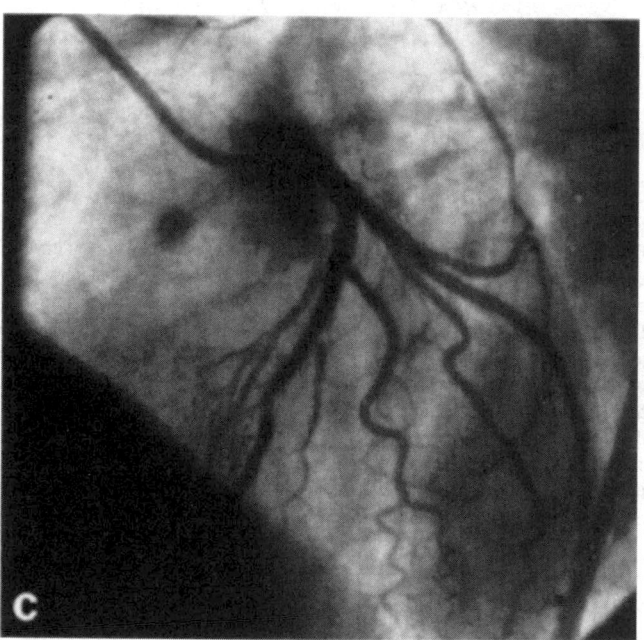

FIGURE 16-25

Diagrammatic illustration of the left coronary angiogram in the 45° left anterior oblique (LAO) with 30° cranial angulation and the direction of the x-ray beam used to produce this view. This is the most valuable view of the left coronary artery in most patients. Foreshortening of the left main and proximal left anterior descending and diagonal branches present in the LAO view is usually overcome by cranial angulation of the image intensifier. The proximal left coronary arterial segments are frequently visualized at an angle almost perpendicular from their long axis. The ostium of the left main coronary artery, the most proximal portion of the LAD, and the origin of the diagonal branches are usually well visualized without overlap (compare with Fig. 16-22). Some overlap may occur with branches of the proximal circumflex coronary artery, and this is frequently overcome by using a 60° LAO with 30° cranial angulation. The value of the LAO with cranial angulation is considerably less when the proximal left coronary artery is superiorly directed, in which case caudal angulation of the image intensifier is frequently helpful. The direction of the x-ray beam in the 45° LAO with 30° angulation is demonstrated. (From King et al.[149] Reproduced with permission from the publisher, editor, and authors.)

(junction of the interventricular and interatrial septa). The posterior descending artery arises from the right coronary artery at right angles and travels in the posterior interventricular groove, supplying the perforating branches to the basal and posterior one-third of the septum. A right coronary artery that supplies the major posterior descending branch has been referred to as a *dominant right coronary artery*. The posterior descending artery usually stops before reaching the apex, but it may curl around the apex in association with a short anterior descending artery to form the loop previously described. After giving rise to the posterior descending artery, the right coronary artery becomes intramyocardial at the crux, gives rise to the AV node artery, and subsequently returns to the surface, making an inverted U curve (see Fig. 16-33). The LV branches of the right coronary artery are variable and cover the same area as the posterolateral branches of a large circumflex system. The proximal conduit portion of the right coronary artery is well seen in standard RAO and LAO views. Because of its horizontal orientation, however, the origin of the posterior descending artery is well seen in the RAO view but foreshortened in the LAO view; to overcome this, cranial angulation of the intensifier is necessary. Pathologic studies indicate that lesions at the takeoff of the posterior descending artery are frequently overlooked if standard oblique views in the transverse plane are used.

Grading Stenoses

Visual inspection of the coronary arteriogram has traditionally been used to assess the severity of coronary artery stenosis. In the authors' laboratory, a system of analyzing each arterial segment has been used, and the degree of stenosis is recorded as a reduction in lumen diameter expressed as a percentage, with total occlusion being 100 percent. Measurement of cineangiograms has been done with a programmable digital caliper system. In each available projection, the frame show-

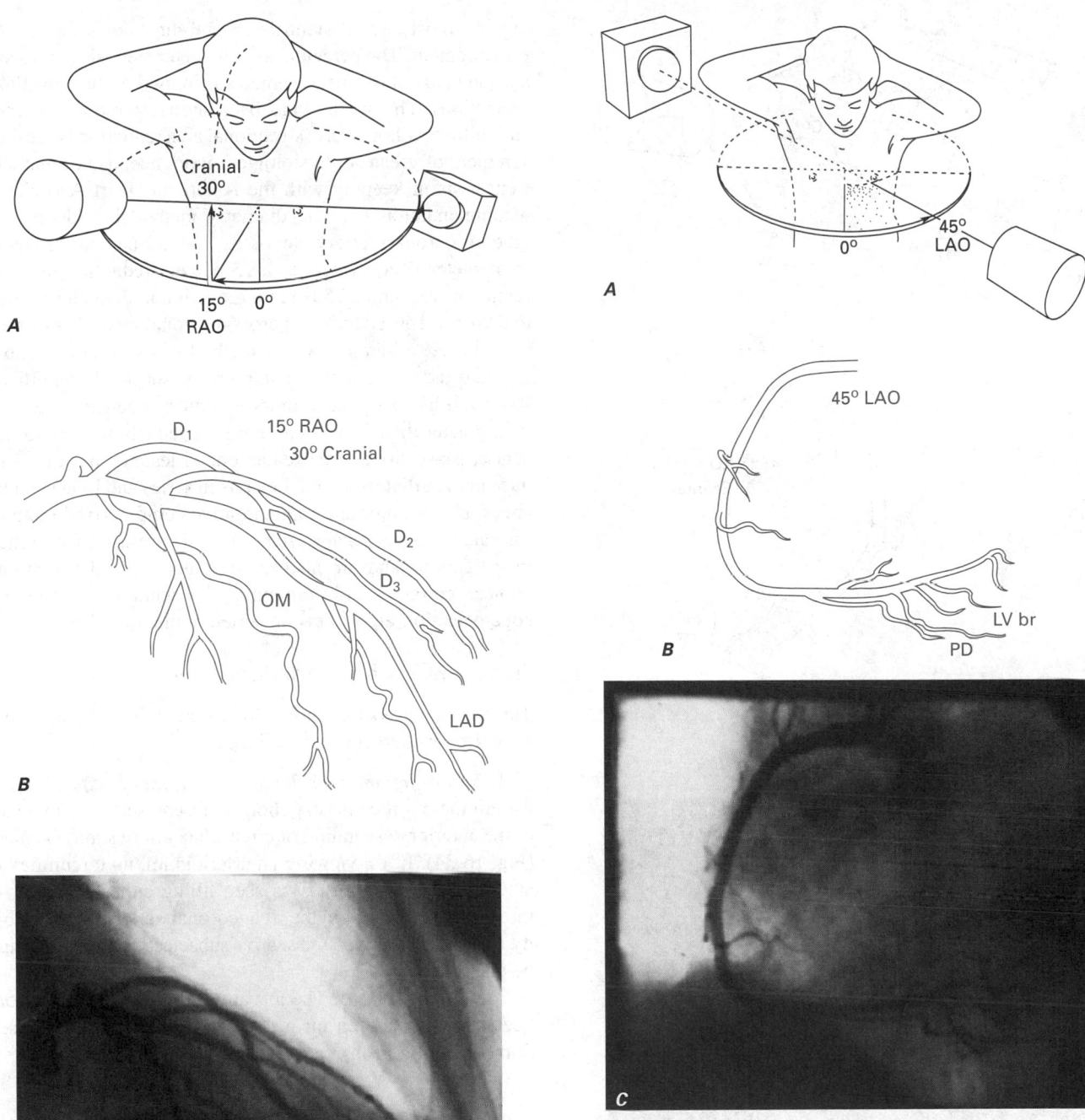

FIGURE 16-26
Diagrammatic illustration of the direction of the x-ray beam and the left coronary angiogram in the 15° RAO with 30° cranial angulation. This view is particularly helpful in analyzing the mid-left anterior descending artery and the diagonal branch points. Overlap with diagonal branches is usually avoided. The origin of the circumflex artery may be well seen, as in this illustration. (From King et al.[149] Reproduced with permission from the publisher, editor, and authors.)

FIGURE 16-27
Diagrammatic illustration of the direction of the x-ray beam and the right coronary artery in the 45° LAO projection. This view is excellent for visualizing the proximal mid and distal right coronary artery in the AV groove since the direction of the x-ray beam is perpendicular to these arterial segments. Ostial lesions of the right coronary artery are now well visualized if the proximal right coronary artery takes an anterior direction from the aorta and therefore originates in a direction parallel to the x-ray beam. This can usually be overcome by turning to a more severe left oblique projection. The posterior descending and left ventricular branches of the right coronary artery, which pass down the posterior aspect of the heart toward the apex, are severely foreshortened since the long axis of these vessels is in the same direction as the x-ray beam. The proximal posterior descending branches can be visualized by cranial angulation of the overhead intensifier (see Fig. 16-28) or from a right oblique view. The image intensifier is in the standard LAO position. (From King et al.[149] Reproduced with permission from the publisher, editor, and authors.)

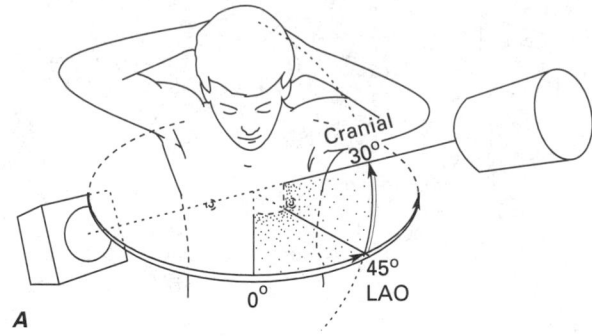

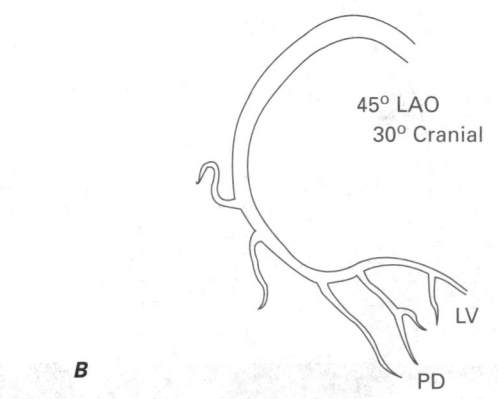

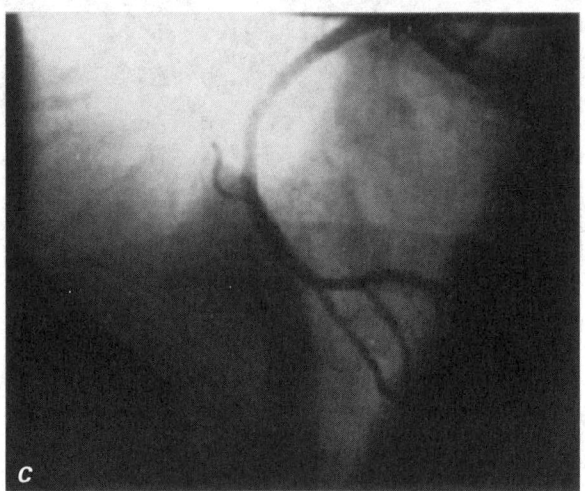

ing the most severe stenosis in end-diastole is chosen for measurement. The percentage of diameter stenosis recorded is a mean value of the measurements from two or three available projections. This method has been shown to reduce observer variability. Although cross-sectional area reduction is the measurement of greatest physiologic importance, use of diameter stenosis is in keeping with the American Heart Association recommendation that the diameter method be adopted for grading coronary artery stenoses.[145] A 50 percent reduction in diameter is equivalent to a 75 percent reduction in cross-sectional area, and a 75 percent reduction in diameter is equal to a 90 percent reduction in cross-sectional area. It is of great importance to identify which method of expressing stenosis is being used. From the standpoint of surgically significant lesions, it has been the authors' practice to consider stenoses with greater than 50 percent diameter reduction, or >75 percent cross-sectional area reduction, as lesions that may produce myocardial ischemia. Lesions in series and long stenoses are of added importance. Quantitative computerized methods for calculating coronary artery stenosis are used for clinical investigations and are also increasingly utilized for routine clinical coronary arteriography.[150] Techniques employing edge-detection algorithms are often applied clinically.

Pitfalls in Coronary Arteriography

There are a number of pitfalls in coronary arteriography that should be looked for and avoided.

1. *Short left main or double left coronary orifices.* When the left main orifice is very short or absent, selective injection of the anterior descending or circumflex arteries may be made (Fig. 16-34). If, on viewing an arteriogram, no circumflex or anterior descending artery is seen filling either primarily or through collaterals from the right coronary artery, the possibility that the artery was missed by subselective injection must be entertained.

2. *Orifice lesions.* The left and right coronary artery orifices need to be seen on a tangent with the aortic sinuses. Some backflow from the orifices is needed if the catheter is

FIGURE 16-28
Diagrammatic illustration of the direction of the x-ray beam and the right coronary artery in 30° LAO with 30° cranial angulation. Cranial angulation of the image intensifier overcomes the problem of foreshortening of the posterior descending and left ventricular branches observed in Fig. 16-27. Lesions in the posterior descending or left ventricular branches can be well visualized. When the right coronary artery originates anteriorly from the aorta, the proximal portion of the vessel is frequently well seen in this projection. With anomalous origin of the left anterior descending artery from the right coronary artery, this view is helpful since the standard LAO view produces considerable foreshortening of the anomalous artery. The direction of the x-ray beam is the same as in Fig. 16-25. (From King et al.[149] Reproduced with permission from the publisher, editor, and authors.)

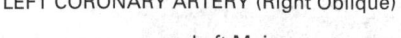

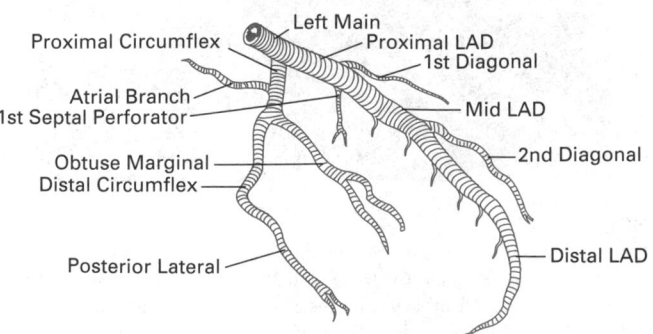

FIGURE 16-29
Anatomy of the left coronary tree in the right oblique view.

lying within the left main or proximal right coronary artery to avoid missing an orifice lesion.

3. *Myocardial bridges.* The anterior descending, diagonal, and marginal branches not uncommonly dip intramyocardially, and the overlying myocardium may act to compress the artery during systole (Fig. 16-35). If the coronary artery is not viewed carefully in diastole, this bridging may give the appearance of an area of stenosis.[151]

4. *Foreshortening.* When possible, avoid reading lesions in segments that are seen only coming toward or away from the image intensifier. Dense opacification of segments seen end-on may produce the appearance of a lesion in an intervening segment.

5. *Coronary spasm.* Catheter-induced spasm may give the appearance of a lesion (Fig. 16-36). When spasm is suspected (usually at the catheter tip in the right coronary artery), nitrates should be given and the injection should be repeated in 5 to 10 min. Spontaneous coronary artery spasm is a separate problem, and when this is suspected, nitrates and atropine are avoided since the atropine may play a role in blocking coronary artery spasm. Provocation with ergot derivatives will identify most patients with spontaneous coronary artery spasm.[127-129]

6. *Anomalous coronary arteries.* Coronary arteries may arise from ectopic locations, or a single coronary artery may be present.[152] Only by ensuring that the entire epicardial surface has an adequate arterial supply can one be confident that all branches have been visualized.

7. *Totally occluded arteries or vein grafts.* Absence of vascularity in a portion of the heart may indicate total occlusion of its arterial supply. Usually, however, collateral channels permit visualization of the distal occluded artery unless it is an acute occlusion. Vessels filled solely by collaterals have very little pressure supporting their walls and may appear smaller than their actual lumen size, giving a false sense of pessimism about the possibilities for surgical anastomosis.

Limitations of Coronary Arteriography

In spite of significant improvements in the quality of coronary arteriographic studies as a result of improved x-ray imaging systems, there remain a number of limitations of the method. Film interpretation is subjective. Different angiographers may interpret the same film differently, and the same angiographer may render a different interpretation at a time remote from

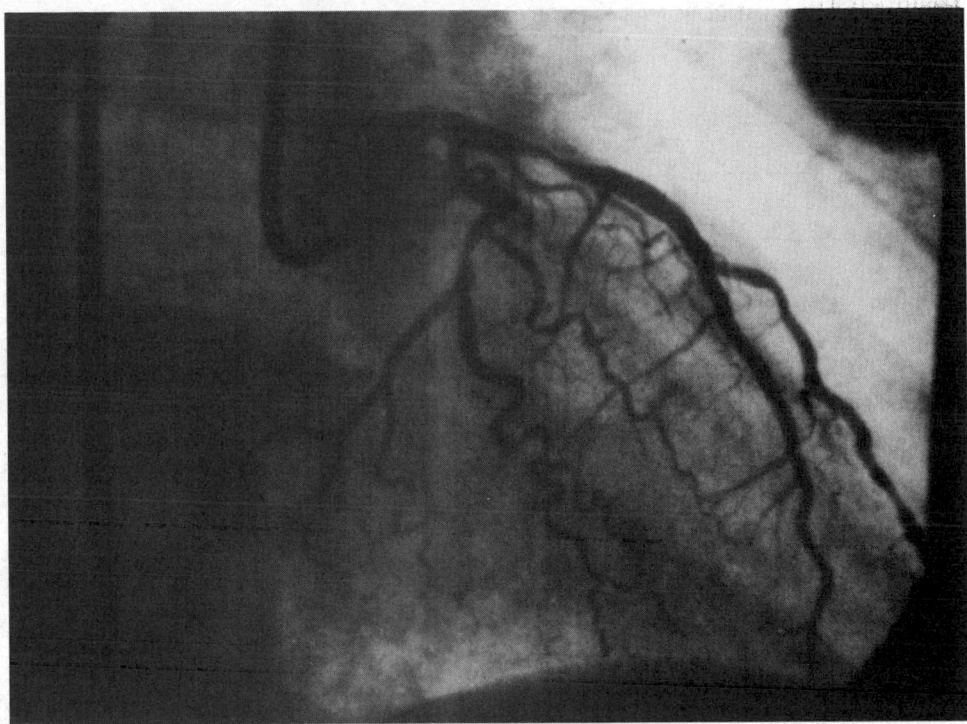

FIGURE 16-30
Right anterior oblique view of the left coronary artery showing high-grade stenosis of the left anterior descending proximal to the first septal perforating branch.

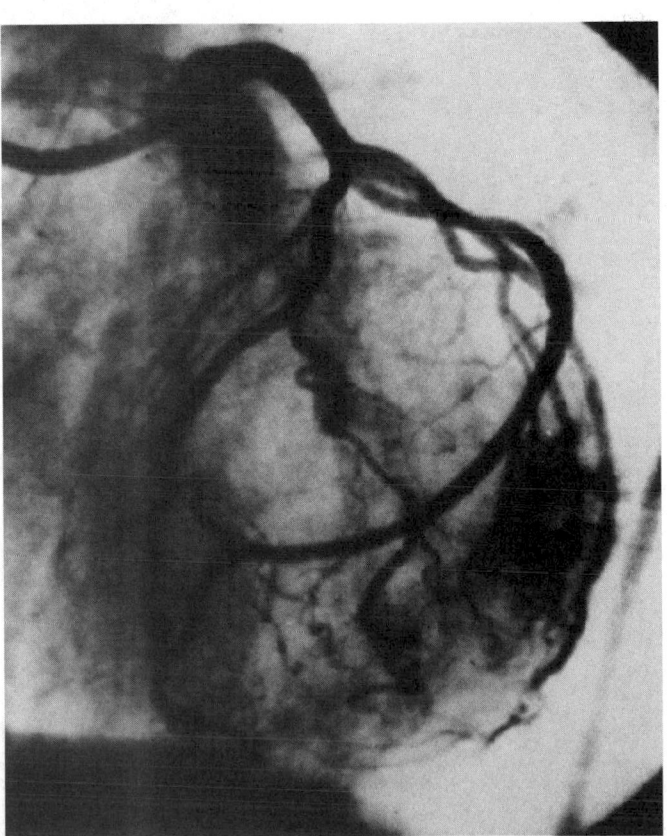

FIGURE 16-31
LAO view of the left coronary artery demonstrating dominant circumflex coronary artery giving rise to the posterior descending artery.

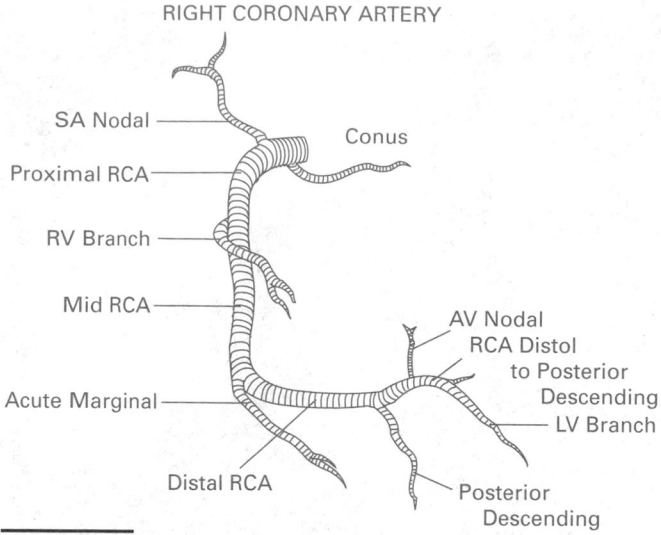

RIGHT CORONARY ARTERY

FIGURE 16-32
Anatomy of the right coronary tree.

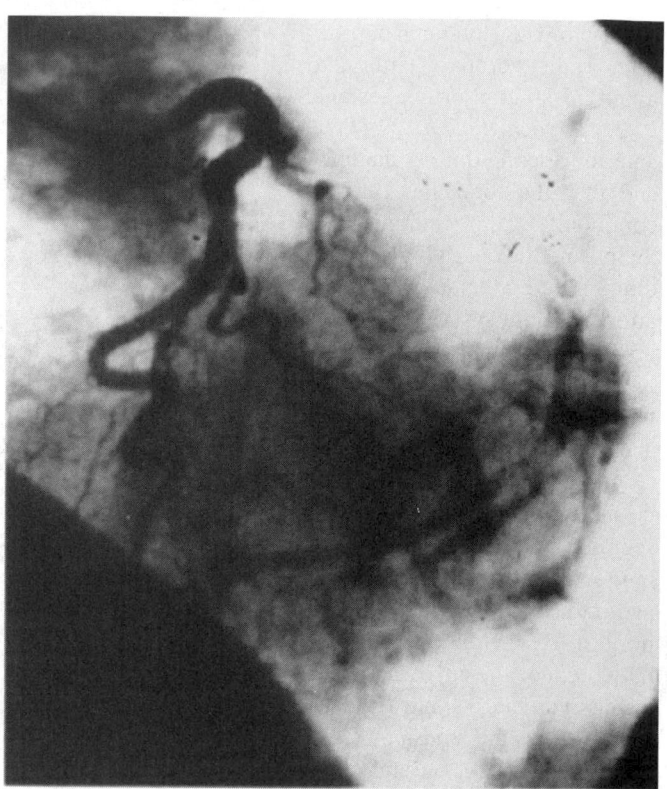

the first reading.[153,154] It has been reported that the average standard deviation of estimation of any segmental stenosis by experienced angiographers may be as high as 20 percent and that disagreement about the number of major vessels with 70 percent stenosis may occur 30 percent of the time.[155] These reported studies, however, utilized only views in the transverse

A

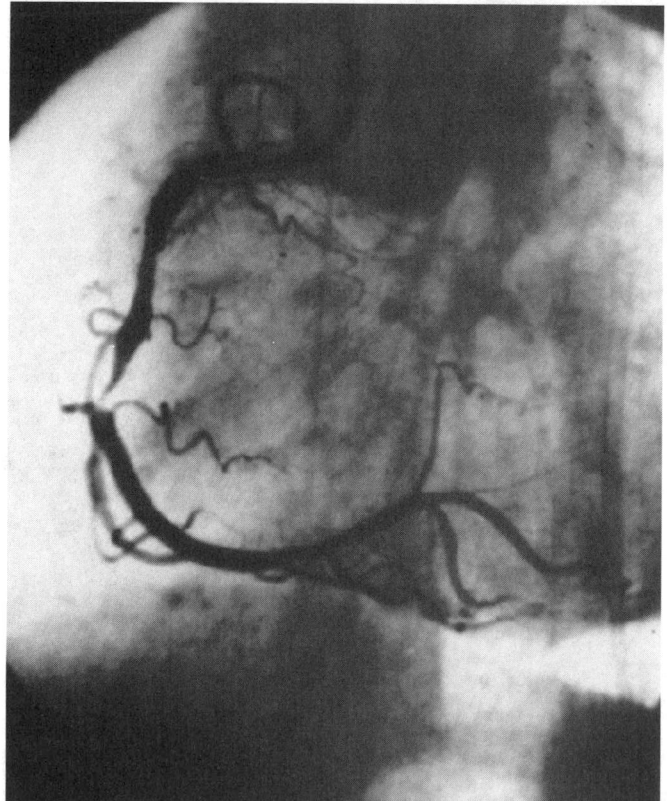

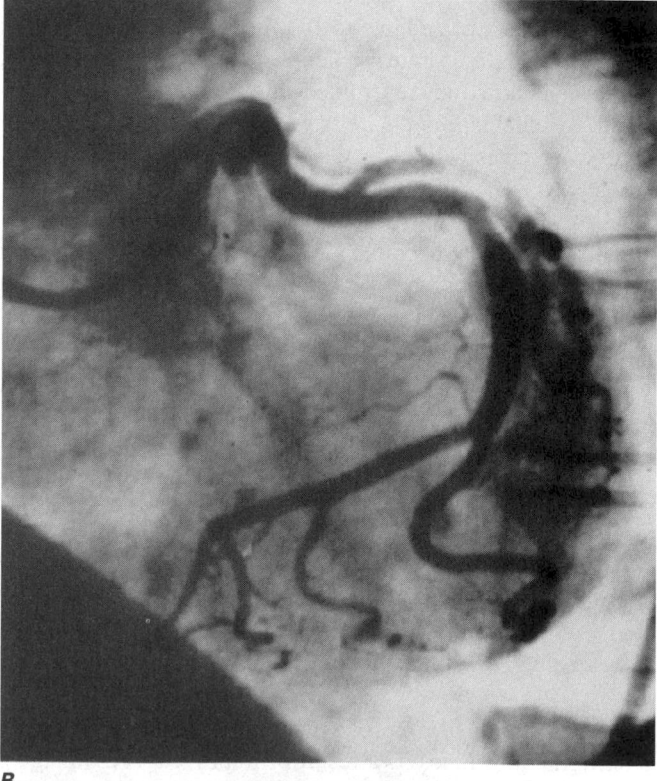

B

FIGURE 16-33
LAO view of the right coronary artery (RCA) with high-grade lesion in its midportion.

FIGURE 16-34
A. LAO view of selective injection into left anterior descending (LAD) artery.
B. LAO view of selective injection into circumflex artery.

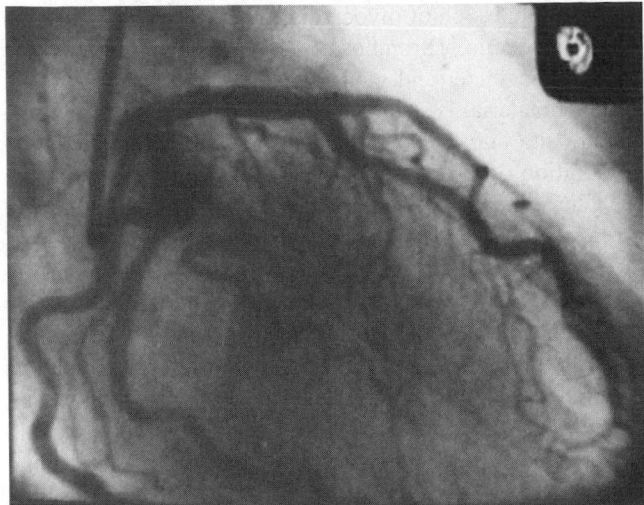

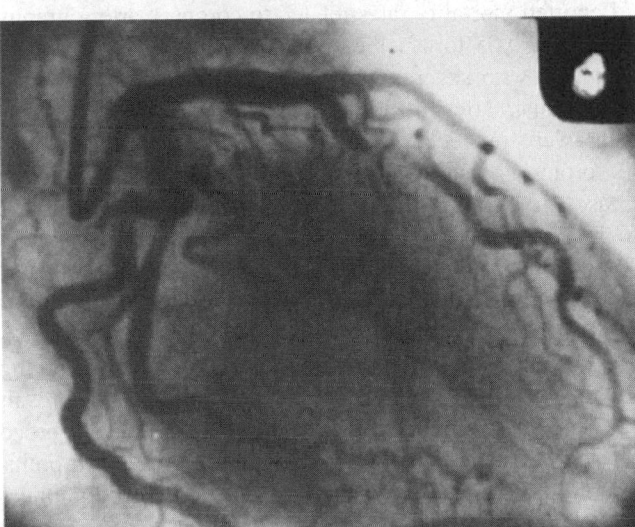

FIGURE 16-35
RAO view of left coronary artery system. *A.* Diastolic appearance of anterior descending artery showing smooth lumen. *B.* Systolic appearance showing obliteration of the lumen by an overriding muscular bridge.

segment for comparison or may choose for comparison an apparently normal segment that in fact has diffuse tubular narrowing.[158–160] This leads to underestimation of the degree of stenosis present. Pathologic studies currently available probably overestimate the frequency of this problem since the pathologic material available for study represents the severest end of the spectrum of the disease. Eccentric atherosclerotic plaques also may be underestimated unless the minor axis of the stenotic lumen is visualized. Sagittally angulated views are particularly valuable in this regard. Very discrete membrane-like lesions, which fortunately are rare, may be missed unless they are visualized directly in the plane of

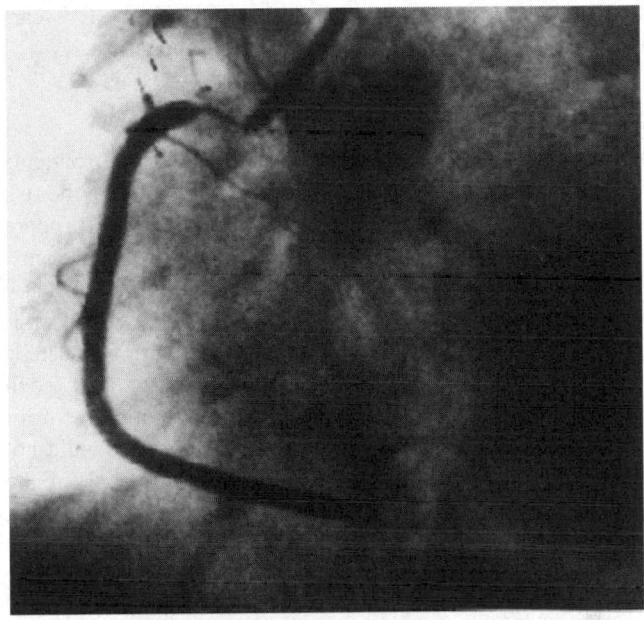

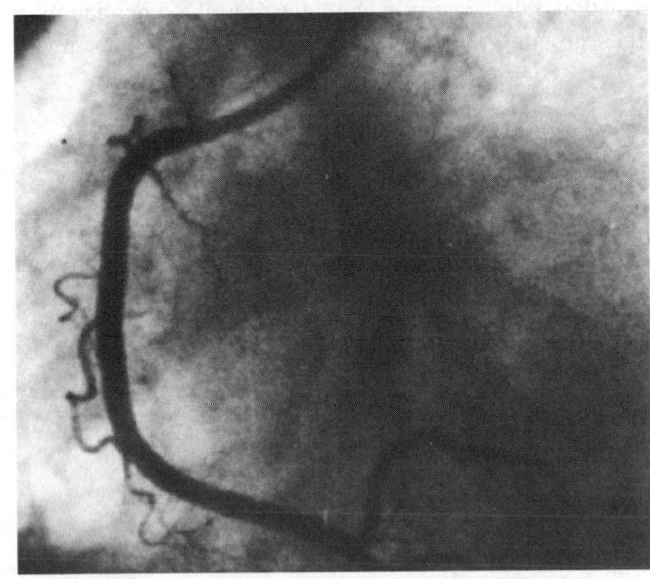

FIGURE 16-36
A. LAO view of right coronary injection showing pericatheter spasm.
B. Same view following nitroglycerin, showing relief of spasm.

plane, imposing greater interpretive burdens than are encountered when sagittally angulated views are obtained. Further studies using sagittally angulated views would be expected to show less variability in interpreting coronary arteriograms. Inter- and intraobserver variability in interpreting coronary arteriograms is not unlike interpretive differences in chest x-rays or other diagnostic studies involving human error and judgment. Routine use of several readers has been shown to reduce interpretive error.[154] Although correlation of angiography with postmortem findings has been acceptable in most studies,[155–161] certain coronary pathologic-anatomic factors may favor angiographic underestimation of the degree of stenosis present in any arterial segment. In large part, this is due to the tendency for diffuse atheromatous narrowing of the coronary arteries to occur. In attempting to grade stenosis of an obviously narrow segment, one may not have a normal

the lesion. Pathologic studies have shown poor correlation between left main coronary stenosis at autopsy and that at angiography, especially in the presence of a short left main coronary artery, and point out the importance of sufficient angiographic views and excellent interpretive skills in evaluating this critical portion of the coronary circulation.[161] Quantitative computer techniques have shown excellent correlation between the cross-sectional luminal area of stenotic lesions at arteriography and direct planimetered measurements of distended postmortem specimens.[162] Dynamic phenomena that are not active at the time of the study may be important. "Hit and run" events such as coronary embolization or thrombosis with subsequent resolution, coronary artery spasm, and even primary coronary artery dissection may leave LV scars but not result in coronary angiographic findings.

Risk of Coronary Arteriography

As with any invasive procedure, there is a finite risk to patients undergoing coronary arteriography. The magnitude of the risk is influenced by certain factors definable prior to the procedure (skill of the angiographer and instability of clinical symptoms) but primarily by the extent of the disease found at coronary arteriography and left ventriculography.[124,141,163–169] Physicians referring patients for coronary arteriograms must be aware of the complication rate in a given laboratory and, when practical, should achieve stability of clinical symptoms prior to study. That is not to say that unstable patients should not be studied, but the physician must balance the risk of the procedure and potential benefit against the risk of not doing the procedure. The frequency of major complications has decreased in active centers (Table 16-3).

Major complications are of two types: Local arterial complications consist of arterial occlusion or stenosis, hematoma formation, false aneurysm, and infection; the other and more lethal group of complications relates to thromboembolic events or depression of myocardial function due to infarction or acute ischemia. Thromboemboli are more commonly due to multiple catheter and guidewire exchanges, during which thrombus material is stripped from the catheter surface at the puncture site only to be deposited on a subsequent catheter. The addition of systemic heparinization was felt to have reduced thromboembolic complications in some laboratories. The early CASS report[164] and that by Abrams and Adams,[163] however, found that the use of heparin did not influence complication rates. Of equal or greater importance may be the routine use of catheter debriding techniques, with vigorous aspiration and flushing of the catheter in the abdominal aorta to dislodge any retained thrombus material. Minor allergic reactions to contrast media in the form of urticaria occur commonly, but anaphylactic and pyrogenic reactions are exceedingly rare. Radiation exposure to the patient, estimated as 20 to 45 rem, has little risk unless multiple restudies are needed.

Reported mortality rates related to coronary arteriography range from 0.05 to 4 percent, and virtually all deaths occur in patients with severe, multivessel coronary disease or left main coronary artery stenosis.[139,163–166] Of 30 patients whose deaths were related to diagnostic cardiac catheterization at the Toronto hospital, 18 (60 percent) had left main coronary disease. In 89 percent (16/18) of left main disease deaths and in 50 percent (4/8) of coronary disease patients without apparent left main disease, death was related to catheter-induced left main trauma. A widely quoted acceptable mortality rate for coronary arteriography is 0.1 percent. Case selection, however, may play an important role in determining mortality. Studies in predominantly stable patients will result in a very low mortality rate. On the other hand, if a broad spectrum of patients is studied—including those with preinfarction angina; acute myocardial infarction; and complications of myocardial infarction such as heart failure, cardiogenic shock, ruptured interventricular septum, and ruptured papillary muscle—complication rates will be higher, depending on the frequency with which sicker patients are studied. The overall mortality rate in the CASS and Society for Cardiac Angiography and Interventions reports was 0.07 to 0.1 percent. It was 0.05 percent for single-vessel disease, 0.07 percent for double-vessel disease, 0.012 percent for triple-vessel disease, and 0.8 percent in patients with left main coronary artery stenosis.[164,167] The point to be made is that laboratory and surgical teams must be prepared to act in the best interest of severely ill patients and not be overly concerned with an arbitrary mortality figure.

Left Ventriculography

Left ventriculography is the standard method for evaluating LV performance in the coronary angiography laboratory. The normal pattern of LV contraction is a uniform and almost concentric inward movement of all points along the endocardial surface during systole. Harrison introduced the term *asynergy*, which has been used to indicate a disturbance of the normal contraction pattern. The Ad Hoc Committee for Grad-

TABLE 16-3
COMPLICATIONS OF CORONARY ARTERIOGRAPHY

	CASS[a]		SCAI,[b] 1990–
	1979[164]	1983[167]	1995[168]
Death	0.0020	0.0007	0.001 each year
Myocardial infarction	0.0025	0.0027	<0.001 each year
Cerebral emboli	0.0003	0.0007	<0.001 each year
Arterial complications	0.0080	0.0082	—
Ventricular fibrillation	0.0063	0.0038	0.003 (0.002 in 1995)

[a] Coronary Artery Surgery Study.
[b] Society for Coronary Angiography and Interventions.

LEFT VENTRICULOGRAM — WALL SEGMENTS

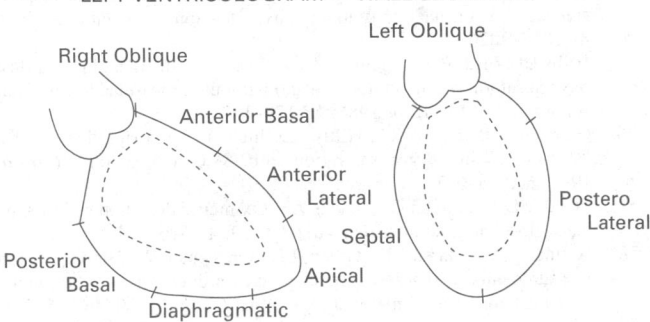

FIGURE 16-37
Left ventricular wall silhouette in RAO and LAO views.

ing of Coronary Artery Disease of the American Heart Association[145] has recommended that five RAO segments and two LAO left ventricular segments be defined and characterized as to wall motion (Fig. 16-37). Herman and coworkers classified LV asynergy according to the severity of the contractile abnormality, and a similar classification of LV wall motion was recommended by the Ad Hoc Committee:

Normal: normal wall motion of the indicated ventricular segment
Reduced: reduced velocity and/or amplitude of indicated wall segment
None: absence of appropriate wall motion of indicated ventricular segment
Dyskinetic: paradoxical wall motion of the indicated segment
Aneurysmal: bulging during systole and diastole with sharply defined margins of indicated ventricular segment
Undefined

Many angiographers use the term *akinesis* when no wall motion is present and the term *hypokinesis* when wall motion is reduced.

The ability of the left ventricle to function as a pump is best analyzed by LV volume determinations. Single-plane and biplane volume determinations may differ significantly in patients with coronary artery disease and nonhomogeneous contraction patterns. In particular, the single-plane RAO or lateral left ventriculogram frequently underestimates overall LV contraction because it selectively visualizes the anterior and inferior free walls of the left ventricle, which are most commonly involved in myocardial infarction. Vogel and associates[170] found that the single-plane RAO left ventriculogram underestimated ejection fraction in 70 percent of patients with coronary artery disease. For this reason, biplane left ventriculography is frequently desirable in evaluating patients with coronary artery disease.

REFERENCES

1. Forssman W. Die Sondierung des rechten Herzens. *Berl Klin Wochenschr* 1929; 8:2085–2087.
2. Cournand A. Cardiac catheterization: Development of the technique, its contribution to experimental medicine and its initial application to man. *Acta Med Scand* 1975; 579(suppl):7–32.
3. Brannon ES, Weens HS, Warren JV. Atrial septal defect: Study of hemodynamics by the technique of right heart catheterization. *Am J Med Sci* 1945; 214:248–251.
4. Grossman W, Baim DS, eds. *Cardiac Catheterization, Angiography and Intervention*, 5th ed. Baltimore: Williams & Wilkins; 1996.
5. Pepine CJ, Hill JA, Lambert CR. *Diagnostic and Therapeutic Cardiac Catheterization*, 2d ed. Baltimore: Williams & Wilkins; 1994.
6. Allen HD (chairman). AHA guidelines for pediatric therapeutic cardiac catheterization. *Circulation* 1991; 84:2248–2258.
7. Myers GE, Crick WF, King WS, Mumma M, Friedberg HD, Jamieson DM, et al. Latex versus iodinated contrast media anaphylaxis in the cardiac cath lab. *Cathet Cardiovasc Diagn* 1995; 35:228–231.
8. Ruiz CE, Mullins CE, Rochini AP, Radtke WAK, Hijazi ZM, O'Laughlin MP, et al. Core curriculum for the training of pediatric invasive interventional cardiologists. *Cathet Cardiovasc Diagn* 1996; 37:409.
9. Lasser EC, Berry CC, Talner LB, Santini LC, Lang EK, Gerber FH, et al. Pretreatment with corticosteroids to alleviate reactions to intravenous contrast material. *N Engl J Med* 1987; 317:845–849.
10. Feldman T, Moss J, Teplinsky K, Carroll JD. Cardiac catheterization in the patient with a history of allergy to local anesthesia. *Cathet Cardiovasc Diagn* 1990; 20:165–167.
11. Clements SD, Gatlin S. Outpatient cardiac catheterization: A report of 3000 cases. *Clin Cardiol* 1991; 14:477–480.
12. Block PC, Ockene I, Goldberg RJ, Butterly J, Block EH, Degon C, et al. A prospective randomized trial of outpatient versus inpatient cardiac catheterization. *N Engl J Med* 1988; 319:1251–1256.
13. Ad Hoc Task Force, Pepine CJ (chairman). ACC/AHA guidelines for cardiac catheterization and cardiac catheterization laboratories. *J Am Coll Cardiol* 1991; 18:1149–1182.
14. Cooper MW. A simple method for insertion of multiple catheters through a single venipuncture site. *Cathet Cardiovasc Diagn* 1982; 8:305–310.
15. Shim D, Lloyd TR, Cho KJ, Moorehead CD, Beekman III RH. Transhepatic cardiac catheterization in children. *Circulation* 1995; 92:1526–1530.
16. Rapoport S, Sniderman KW, Morse SS, Proto MH, Ross GR. Pseudoaneurysm: A complication of faulty technique in femoral artery puncture. *Radiology* 1985; 154:529–530.
17. Kim D, Oaron DE, Skillman JJ, Kent C, Porter DH, Schlam BW, et al. Role of superficial femoral artery puncture in the development of pseudoaneurysm and arteriovenous fistula complicating percutaneous transferred cardiac catheterization. *Cathet Cardiovasc Diagn* 1992; 25:91–97.
18. Montgomery DH, Veveris JJ, McGorisk G, Frohwein S, Martin RP, Taylor WR. Natural history of severe atheromatous disease of the thoracic aorta: A transesophageal echocardiographic study. *J Am Coll Cardiol* 1996; 27:95–101.
19. Lesnefsky EJ, Carrea FP, Groves BM. Safety of cardiac catheterization via peripheral vascular grafts. *Cathet Cardiovasc Diagn* 1993; 29:113–116.
20. Laskey WK. Percutaneous retrograde left ventricular catheterization in aortic valve stenosis. *Cathet Cardiovasc Diagn* 1986; 12:75–79.
21. MacDonald RG, Feldman RL, Pepine CJ. A modified catheter system for retrograde left ventricular catheterization in aortic valve stenoses. *Cathet Cardiovasc Diagn* 1985; 11:433–439.
22. Nath PH, Soto B, Holt JH, Satler LF. Selective coronary angiography by translumbar aortic puncture. *Am J Cardiol* 1983; 52:425–426.
23. Pearce AC, Schwengal RH, Simione LM, Patrick CJ, Santiago C, Ziskind AA. Antegrade selective coronary angiography via the transseptal approach in a patient with severe vascular disease. *Cathet Cardiovasc Diagn* 1992; 26:300–303.
24. O'Keefe JH, Vlietstra RE, Hanley PC, Seward JB. Revival of the transseptal approach for catheterization of the left atrium and ventricle. *Mayo Clin Proc* 1985; 60:790–795.
25. Chen CR, Cheng TO, Huang T, Zhou YL, Chen JY, Huang YG, et al. Percutaneous balloon valvuloplasty for pulmonic stenosis in adolescents and adults. *N Engl J Med* 1996; 335:21–25.
26. Mullins CE. Transseptal left heart catheterization: Experience with a new technique in 520 pediatric and adult patients. *Pediatr Cardiol* 1983; 4:239–246.
27. Laskey WK, Kusiak V, Untereker WJ, Hirshfeld JW. Transseptal left heart catheterization: Utility of a sheath technique. *Cathet Cardiovasc Diagn* 1982; 8:535–542.
28. Croft CH, Lipscomb K. Modified technique of transseptal left heart catheterization. *J Am Coll Cardiol* 1985; 5:904–910.

29. Iskandrian AS, Bemis CE, Kimbiris D, Owens J. Retrograde catheterization of left atrium. *Br Heart J* 1979; 42:715–718.

30. Ali Kahn MA, Bucher JT, Mullins CE, Yousef AL, Nihill MR, Varga TA, et al. Blade atrial septostomy: Experience with the first 50 procedures. *Cathet Cardiovasc Diagn* 1991; 23:257–262.

31. Doucette JW, Corl PD, Payne HM. Validation of a Doppler guidewire for intravascular measurement of coronary artery. *Circulation* 1992; 85:1899–1911.

32. Segal J, Nasse M, Ford AJ Jr, Schuenemeyer TD. Instantaneous and continuous cardiac output in humans obtained with a Doppler pulmonary artery catheter. *J Am Coll Cardiol* 1990; 16:1398–1407.

33. Mizuno K, Satomura K, Miyamoto A. Angioscopic evaluation of coronary artery thrombi in acute coronary artery syndromes. *N Engl J Med* 1992; 326:287–291.

34. Rocchini AP, Kveselis DA, Crowley D, Dick M, Rosenthal A. Percutaneous balloon valvuloplasty for treatment of congenital pulmonary valvular stenosis in children. *J Am Coll Cardiol* 1984; 3:1005–1012.

35. Mitchell SE, White RI Jr, Kan J, Tolkoff J. Improved balloon catheters for large vessel and valvular angioplasty. *Am J Roentgenol* 1984; 142:571–572.

36. Sievert H, Babic UU, Ensslen R, Scherer D, Spies H, Wiederspahn T, et al. Transcatheter closure of large atrial septal defects with the Babic system. *Cathet Cardiovasc Diagn* 1995; 36:232–240.

37. Johnson LW, Moore RJ, Balter S. Review of radiation safety in the cardiac catheterization laboratory. *Cathet Cardiovasc Diagn* 1992; 25:186–194.

38. Courtois M, Faltal PG, Kovacs SJ, Tiefenbrunn AJ, Ludbrook PA. Anatomically and physiologically based reference levels for measurement of intracardiac pressures. *Circulation* 1995; 92:1994–2000.

39. Shepherd AP, McMahan CA. Role of oximeter error in the diagnosis of shunts. *Cathet Cardiovasc Diagn* 1996; 37:435–446.

40. Krovetz LJ, Brenner JI, Polanyi M. Application of an improved intracardiac fiberoptic system. *Br Heart J* 1978; 40:1010–1013.

41. Dehmer GJ, Firth BG, Hillis LD. Oxygen consumption in adult patients during cardiac catheterization. *Clin Cardiol* 1982; 5:436–540.

42. Lange RA, Dehmer GJ, Wells PJ. Limitations of the metabolic rate meter for measuring oxygen consumption and cardiac output. *Am J Cardiol* 1989; 64:783–786.

43. Crocker RH, Ockene IS, Alpert JS, Pape LA, Dalen JE. Determinants of total body oxygen consumption in adults undergoing cardiac catheterization. *Cathet Cardiovasc Diagn* 1982; 8:363–372.

44. Hurrell DG, Nishamura RA, Higano ST, Appleton CP, Danielson GK, Holmes Jr, et al. Value of dynamic respiratory changes in left and right ventricular pressures for the diagnosis of constrictive pericarditis. *Circulation* 1996; 93:2007–2013.

45. Snyder RW II, Glamann DB, Lange RA, Willard JE, Laundau C, Negus BH, et al. Predictive value of prominent pulmonary arterial wedge V waves on assessing the presence and severity of mitral regurgitation. *Am J Cardiol* 1994; 73:568–570.

46. Dodge HT, Sheehan FH. Quantitative contrast angiography for assessment of ventricular performance in heart disease. *J Am Coll Cardiol* 1983; 1:73–81.

47. Lange RA, Moore DM Jr, Cigarroa RG, Hillis LD. Use of pulmonary capillary pressure to assess severity of mitral stenosis. Is true left atrial pressure needed in this condition. *J Am Coll Cardiol* 1989; 13:825–829.

48. Nishimura R, Rihal CS, Tajik AJ, Holmes DR. Accurate measurement of the transmitral gradient in patients with mitral stenosis: A simultaneous catheterization and Doppler echocardiographic study. *J Am Coll Cardiol* 1994; 24:152–158.

49. Assey ME, Zile MR, Usher BW, Karavan MP, Carabello BA. Effect of catheter positioning on the variability of measured gradient in aortic stenosis. *Cathet Cardiovasc Diagn* 1993; 30:287–292.

50. Laskey WK, Kussmoul WG. Pressure recovery in aortic stenosis. *Circulation* 1984; 89:116–121.

51. Vandervoort DM, Greenberg NL, Pu M, Powell KA, Cosgrove DM, Thomas JD. Pressure recovery in bileaflet heart valve prosthesis. *Circulation* 1995; 92:3464–3472.

52. Baumgartner H, Schima H, Tulzer G, Kuhn P. Effect of stenosis geometry on the Doppler-catheter gradient relation in vitro: A manifestation of pressure recovery. *J Am Coll Cardiol* 1993; 21:1018–1025.

53. Fananapazir L, Epstein ND, Curiel RV, Panza JA, Tripodi D, McAreavey D. Long-term results of dual chamber (DDD) pacing in the obstructive cardiomyopathy. *Circulation* 1994; 90:2731–2742.

54. Palevsky HI, Long W, Crow J, Fishman AP. Prostacyclin and acetyl-choline as screening agents for acute pulmonary vasodilator responsiveness in primary pulmonary hypertension. *Circulation* 1990; 82:2018–2026.

55. Hillis DL, Firth BG, Winniford MD. Variability of right-sided cardiac oxygen saturations in adults with and without intracardiac left-to-right shunting. *Am J Cardiol* 1986; 58:129–132.

56. Glamann DB, Lange RA, Hillis LD. Incidence and significance of a "step-down" in oxygen saturation from SVC to PA. *Am J Cardiol* 1991; 68:695–697.

57. Freed MD, Miettinen OS, Nadas AS. Oximetric detection of intracardiac left-to-right shunts. *Br Heart J* 1979; 42:690–694.

58. Autman EM, Marsh JD, Green LH, Grossman W. Blood oxygen measurements in the assessment of intracardiac left-to-right shunts: A critical appraisal of methodology. *Am J Cardiol* 1980; 46:265–271.

59. Glamman DB, Lange RA, Willard JE, Landau C, Hillis LD. Hydrogen inhalation for detecting intracardiac left-to-right shunting in adults. *Am J Cardiol* 1993; 72:711–714.

60. Bloomfield DA. *Dye Curves: The Theory and Practice of Indicator Dilution.* Baltimore: University Park Press; 1974.

61. Hillis DL, Winniford MD, Jackson JA, Firth BG. Measurement of left-to-right intracardiac shunting in adults: Oximetric versus indicator dilution techniques. *Cathet Cardiovasc Diagn* 1985; 11:467–472.

62. Levett JM, Replogle RL. Thermodilution cardiac output: A critical analysis and review of the literature. *J Surg Res* 1979; 27:392–404.

63. Fischer AP, Benis AM, Jurado RA, Seely E, Teirstein P, Litwak RS. Analysis of errors in measurement of cardiac output by simultaneous dye and thermal dilution in cardiothoracic surgical patients. *Cardiovasc Res* 1978; 12:190–199.

64. Hamilton MA, Stevenson LW, Woo RN, Child JS, Tillisch JH. Effect of tricuspid regurgitation on the reliability of the thermodilution cardiac output technique in congestive heart failure. *Am J Cardiol* 1989; 64:945–948.

65. Dodge HT, Sandler H, Ballew DW, Lord JD Jr. The use of biplane angiocardiography for the measurement of left ventricular volume in man. *Am Heart J* 1960; 60:762–776.

66. Als AV, Paulin S, Aroesty JM. Biplane angiographic volumetry using the right anterior oblique and half-axial left anterior oblique technique. *Radiology* 1978; 126:511–514.

67. Wynne J, Green LH, Mann T, Levin D, Grossman W. Estimation of left ventricular volumes in man from biplane cineangiograms filmed in oblique projections. *Am J Cardiol* 1978; 41:726–732.

68. Sandler H, Dodge HT. The use of single plane angiocardiograms for the calculation of left ventricular volume in man. *Am Heart J* 1968; 75:325–334.

69. Kennedy JW, Trenholme SE, Kasser IS. Left ventricular volume and mass from single plane cineangiocardiograms. *Am Heart J* 1970; 80:343–352.

70. Sheehan FH, Mitten-Lewis S. Factors influencing accuracy in left ventricular volume determination. *Am J Cardiol* 1989; 64:661–664.

71. Lawson MA, Blackwell GG, Doves ND, Roney M, Dell'Italia LJ, Pohost GM. Accuracy of biplane long-axis left ventricular volume determined by cine magnetic resonance imaging in patients with regional and global dysfunction. *Am J Cardiol* 1996; 77:1098–1104.

72. Kennedy JW, Baxley WA, Figley MM, Dodge HT, Blackmon JR. Quantitative angiocardiography. I. The normal left ventricle in man. *Circulation* 1966; 34:272–278.

73. Shimazaki Y, Kawashima Y, Mori T, Beppu S, Yokota K. Angiographic volume estimation of right ventricle. *Chest* 1980; 77:390–395.

74. Gentzler RO II, Briselli MF, Gault JH. Angiographic estimation of right ventricular volume in man. *Circulation* 1974; 50:324–330.

75. Murray JA, Kennedy JW, Figley MM. Quantitative angiocardiography. II. The normal left atrial volume in man. *Circulation* 1968; 37:800–804.

76. Gorlin R, Gorlin G. Hydraulic formula for calculation of area of stenotic mitral valve, other cardiac valves and central circulatory shunts. *Am Heart J* 1951; 41:1–29.

77. Cohen MV, Gorlin R. Modified orifice equation for the calculation of mitral valve area. *Am Heart J* 1972; 84:839–840.

78. Folland ED, Parisi AF, Carbone C. Is peripheral arterial pressure a satisfactory substitute for ascending aortic pressure when measuring aortic valve gradients? *J Am Coll Cardiol* 1984; 4:1207–1212.

79. Vaitkus PT, Higgins C, Watkins MW, Brown KA, Battle RW. Accuracy of quantitation of aortic stenosis using femoral artery recording corrected for both temporal delay and systolic amplification. *Am J Cardiol* 1995; 76:725–728.

80. Krueger SK, Orme EC, King CS, Barry WH. Accurate determination of the transaortic valve gradient using simultaneous left ventricular and femoral artery pressure. *Cathet Cardiovasc Diagn* 1989; 16:202–206.

81. Voelker W, Reul H, Niehaus G, Stelzer T, Schmitz B, Steegers A, et al. Comparison of valvular resistance, stroke work loss and Gorlin valve area for quantification of aortic stenosis. *Circulation* 1995; 91:1196–1204.

82. Roger VL, Tajik AJ, Reeder GS, Hayes SN, Mullany CJ, Bailey KR, et al. Effect of Doppler echocardiography on utilization of hemodynamic cardiac catheterization in the preoperative evaluation of aortic stenosis. *Mayo Clin Proc* 1996; 71:141–149.

83. Bache RJ, Jorgensen CR, Wany Y. Simplified estimation of aortic valve area. *Br Heart J* 1972; 34:408–411.

84. Hakki AH. A simplified valve formula for the calculation of stenotic cardiac valve areas. *Circulation* 1981; 63:1050–1055.

85. Angel J, Soler-Soler J, Anivarro I, Domingo E. I. Hemodynamic evaluation of stenotic cardiac valves. II. Modification of the simplified formula for mitral and aortic valve area calculation. *Cathet Cardiovasc Diagn* 1985; 11:127–138.

86. Hosenpud JD, McAnulty JH, Morton MJ. Overestimation of mitral valve gradients obtained by phasic pulmonary artery wedge pressure. *Cathet Cardiovasc Diagn* 1983; 9:283–290.

87. Chavez I, Dorbecker N, Celis A. Direct intracardiac angiocardiography: Its diagnostic value. *Am Heart J* 1947; 33:560–593.

88. Brown R, Rahimtoola SH, Davis GD, Swan HJC. The effects of angiocardiographic contrast medium on circulatory dynamics in man: Cardiac output during angiocardiography. *Circulation* 1965; 31:234–290.

89. Bettmann MA. Angiographic contrast agents: Conventional and new media compared. *Am J Roentgenol* 1982; 139:787–794.

90. Kern MJ. Selection of radiocontrast media in cardiac catheterization. Comparative physiology and clinical effects of nonionic and ionic dimeric formulations. *Am Heart J* 1991; 122:195–201.

91. Gertz EW, Wisneski JA, Chiu D, Akin JR, Hu C. Clinical superiority of a new nonionic contrast agent (iopamidol) for cardiac angiography. *J Am Coll Cardiol* 1985; 5:250–258.

92. Morris TW, Sahler LG, Violante M, Fischer HW. Reduction of calcium activity by radiopaque contrast media. *Radiology* 1983; 148:55–59.

93. Werner GS, Schmidt T, Scholz KH, Figulla HR, Kreuzer H. Comparison of hemodynamic and Doppler echocardiographic effects of new low osmolar non-ionic and a standard ionic contrast agent after left ventriculography. *Cathet Cardiovasc Diagn* 1994; 33:11–19.

94. McClennan BL. Ionic and nonionic iodinated contrast media: Evolution and strategies for use. *Am J Roentgenol* 1990; 155:225–233.

95. Ritchie JL, Nissen SE, Douglas JS, Dreifus LS, Gibbons RJ, Higgins CB, et al. Use of non-ionic or low osmolar contrast agents in cardiovascular procedures. *J Am Coll Cardiol* 1989; 21:269–273.

96. Brogan WC III, Hillis LD, Lange RA. Contrast agents for cardiac catheterization: Conceptions and misconceptions. *Am Heart J* 1991; 122:1129–1135.

97. Hirshfield JW Jr. Cardiovascular effects of contrast agents. *Am J Cardiol* 1990; 66(suppl):9F–17P.

98. Curry III TS, Dowdey JE, Murray RC Jr, (eds). *Christensen's Physics of Diagnostic Radiology*, 4th ed. Philadelphia: Lea & Febiger; 1990:77.

99. Nissen SE, Pepine CJ, Bashore TM, Block PC, Boncheck LI, Brinker JA, et al. Cardiac angiography without cine film: Erecting a "Tower of Babel" in the cardiac catheterization laboratory. *J Am Coll Cardiol* 1994; 24:834–837.

100. Soto B, Pacifico AD. *Angiocardiography in Congenital Heart Malformations*. Mount Kisco, NY: Future; 1990.

101. Delegonul U, Jones S, Shurmur S, Oskarsson H. Contrast cine left ventriculography. *Cathet Cardiovasc Diagn* 1996; 37:428–433.

102. Nihill MR, Mullins CE, McNamara DG. Visualization of the pulmonary arteries in pseudotruncus by pulmonary vein wedge angiography. *Circulation* 1978; 58:140–147.

103. Keane JF, McFaul R, Fellows K, Lock J. Balloon occlusion angiography in infancy: Methods, uses and limitations. *Am J Cardiol* 1985; 56:495–497.

104. McGrath LB, Chen C, Bailey BN, Cha SD, Fernandez J, Lamb GW, et al. Determination of the need for tricuspid valve replacement value of pre-operative right ventricular angiography. *J Invas Cardiol* 1991; 3:35–40.

105. Fraser RS. Catheter-induced pulmonary artery perforation: Pathologic and pathogenic features. *Hum Pathol* 1987; 18:1246–1251.

106. Trerotola SO, Kuhlman JE, Fishman EK. Bleeding complications of femoral catheterization: CT evaluation. *Radiology* 1990; 174:37–40.

107. Cohen GI, Chan KL. Physical examination and echo Doppler study in the assessment of femoral artery complications following cardiac catheterization. *Cathet Cardiovasc Diagn* 1990; 21:137–143.

108. Schaub F, Theiss W, Heinz M, Zagel M, Shomig A. New aspects of ultrasound-guided compression repair of postcatheterization femoral artery injuries. *Circulation* 1994; 90:1861–1865.

109. Chatterjee T, Do D, Kaufmann U, Mahler F, Meier B. Ultrasound-guided repair for treatment of femoral artery pseudoaneurysm. *Cathet Cardiovasc Diagn* 1996; 38:335–340.

110. Lazar JM, Uretsky BF, Denys BG, Reddy PS, Counihan PJ, Ragosta M. Predisposing risk factors and natural history of acute neurologic complications of left-sided cardiac catheterization. *Am J Cardiol* 1995; 75:1056–1060.

111. Cohan RH, Dunnick NR. Intravascular contrast media: Adverse reactions. *Am J Roentgenol* 1987; 149:665–670.

112. Greenberger PA, Patterson R, Tapio CM. Prophylaxis against repeated radiocontrast media reactions in 857 cases. *Arch Intern Med* 1985; 145:2197–2200.

113. Solomon R, Wenner C, Mann D, D'Elia J, Silva P. Effects of saline, mannitol, and furosemide on acute decreases in renal function induced by radiocontrast agents. *N Engl J Med* 1994; 331:1416–1420.

114. Dawson P. Contrast agent nephrotoxicity: An appraisal. *Br J Radiol* 1985; 58:121–124.

115. Dawson P. Chemotoxicity of contrast media and clinical adverse effects: A review. *Invest Radiol* 1985; 20(suppl):84–91.

116. Rocher L. Radiocontrast-induced acute renal failure. *Am Coll Cardiol Curr J Rev* 1996; 5:75–78.

117. Barrett BJ. Contrast nephrotoxicity. *J Am Soc Nephrol* 1994; 125–137.

118. Parfrey PS, Griffiths SM, Barrett MB, Paul MD, Genge M, Withers J, et al. Contrast material–induced renal failure in patients with diabetes mellitus, renal insufficiency or both. *N Engl J Med* 1989; 320:143–149.

119. Schwab SJ, Hlatky MA, Pieper KS. Contrast nephrotoxicity: A randomized controlled trial of a nonionic and an ionic contrast agent. *N Engl J Med* 1989; 320:149–153.

120. Ross J Jr (chairman). Guidelines for coronary angiography: A report of the American College of Cardiology/American Heart Association Task Force on assessment of diagnostic and therapeutic cardiovascular procedures (Subcommittee on Coronary Arteriography). *Circulation* 1987; 76(4):963A–977A.

121. Pepine CJ, Allen HD, Bashore TM, Brinker JA, Cohn LH, Dillon JC, et al. ACC/AHA Guidelines for Cardiac Catheterization Laboratories. *Circulation* 1991; 84:2213–2247.

122. Bashore TM. State of the art of coronary angiography. *J Invas Cardiol* 1991; 3(suppl B):47B–59B.

123. Sones FM Jr, Shirey EK. Cine coronary arteriography. *Mod Concepts Cardiovasc Dis* 1962; 31:735–738.

124. Conti ER. Coronary arteriography. *Circulation* 1977; 55:227–237.

125. Nohara R, Kambara H, Murakami T, Kadota K, Tamaki S, Kawai C. Collateral function in early acute myocardial infarction. *Am J Cardiol* 1983; 52:955–959.

126. Helfant RH, Vokonas PS, Gorlin R. Functional importance of the human coronary collateral circulation. *N Engl J Med* 1971; 284:1277–1281.

127. Heupler FA Jr. Syndrome of symptomatic coronary arterial spasm with nearly normal coronary arteriograms. *Am J Cardiol* 1980; 45:873–881.

128. Conti CR, Curry RC, Christie LG, Pepine CJ. Clinical use of provocative pharmacoangiography in patients with chest pain. *Adv Cardiol* 1979; 26:44–54.

129. Waters DD, Szlachcic J, Bonan R. Comparative sensitivity of exercise, coldpressor and ergonovine testing in provoking attacks of variant angina in patients with active disease. *Circulation* 1983; 67:310–315.

130. Donohue TJ, Kern MJ, Aguirre FV, Bach RG, Wolford T, Bell CA, et al. Assessing the hemodynamic significance of coronary artery stenoses: Analysis of translesional pressure-flow velocity relations in patients. *J Am Coll Cardiol* 1993; 22:449–458.

131. Helfant RH, Pine R, Meister SG, Feldman MS, Trout RG, Banka VS. Nitroglycerin to unmask reversible asynergy: Correlation with post coronary bypass ventriculography. *Circulation* 1974; 50:108–113.

132. Horn HR, Teichholz LE, Cohn PF, Herman MV, Gorlin R. Augmentation of left ventricular contraction pattern in coronary artery disease by inotropic catecholamine: The epinephrine ventriculogram. *Circulation* 1974; 49:1063–1071.

133. Dyke SH, Cohn PF, Gorlin R, Sonnenblick EH. Detection of residual myocardial function in coronary artery disease using post extrasystolic potentiation. *Circulation* 1974; 50:694–699.

134. Formanek A, Nath PH, Zollikofer C, Moller JH. Selective coronary arteriography in children. *Circulation* 1980; 61:84–95.

135. Heupler FA Jr. Coronary arteriography and left ventriculography: Sones technique. In: King SB III, Douglas JS Jr, eds. *Coronary Arteriography*. New York: McGraw-Hill; 1984:137–181.

136. Seldinger SI. Catheter replacement of the needle in percutaneous arteriography: A new technique. *Acta Radiol* 1953; 39:368–376.

137. Ricketts HJ, Abrams HL. Percutaneous selective coronary cine arteriography. *JAMA* 1962; 181:620–626.

138. Amplatz K, Formanek G, Stranger P, Wilson W. Mechanics of selective coronary artery catheterization via femoral approach. *Radiology* 1967; 89:1040–1047.

139. Judkins MP. Selective coronary arteriography. I. A percutaneous transfemoral technique. *Radiology* 1967; 89:815–824.

140. Judkins MP, Judkins EJ. The Judkins technique. In: King SB III, Douglas JS Jr, eds. *Coronary Arteriography*. New York: McGraw-Hill; 1984:182–217.

141. Schoonmaker FW, King SB III. Coronary arteriography by the single catheter percutaneous femoral techniques: Experience with 6,800 cases. *Circulation* 1974; 50:735–740.

142. King SB III, Douglas JS Jr. Catheterization techniques in coronary arteriography and left ventriculography: Multipurpose techniques: In: King SB III, Douglas JS Jr, eds. *Coronary Arteriography*. New York: McGraw-Hill; 1984:239–274.

143. Heupler FA, Chambers CE, Dear WE, Angello DA, Heisler M. Guidelines for internal peer review in the cardiac catheterization laboratory. *Cathet Cardiovasc Diagn* 1997; 40:21–32.

144. Douglas JS Jr, King SB III. Complications of coronary arteriography: Management during and following the procedure. In: King SB III, Douglas JS Jr, eds. *Coronary Arteriography*. New York: McGraw-Hill; 1984:302–313.

145. Austin WG, Edwards JE, Frye RL, Gensini GC, Gott VL, Griffith LSC, et al. A reporting system on patients evaluated for coronary artery disease: Report of the ad hoc committee for grading coronary artery disease, Council on Cardiovascular Surgery, American Heart Association. *Circulation* 1975; 51(suppl 4):5–40.

146. Bunnell IL, Greene DG, Tandom RN, Arani DT. The half-axial projection: A new look at the proximal left coronary artery. *Circulation* 1973; 48:1151–1156.

147. Aldridge HE, McLoughlin MJ, Taylor KW. Improved diagnosis in coronary cine arteriography with routine use of oblique views and cranial and caudal angulations. *Am J Cardiol* 1975; 36:468–473.

148. Frederick PR, Fry WH, Russell JG, Marshall HW. Longitudinal angulation in coronary arteriography: Apparatus and evaluation. *Cathet Cardiovasc Diagn* 1977; 3:305–311.

149. King SB III, Douglas JS Jr, Morris DC. New angiographic views for coronary arteriography. In: Hurst JW, ed. *The Heart, Update IV*. New York: McGraw-Hill; 1980:275–287.

150. Hermiller JB, Cusma JT, Spero LA, Fortin DF, Harding MB, Bashore TM. Quantitative and qualitative coronary angiographic analysis. Review of methods, utility and limitations. *Cathet Cardiovasc Diagn* 1992; 25:110–131.

151. Kramer JR, Kitazume H, Proudfitt WL, Sones FM Jr. Clinical significance of isolated coronary bridges: Benign and frequent condition involving the left anterior descending artery. *Am Heart J* 1982; 103:283–288.

152. Douglas JS Jr, Franch RH, King SB III. Coronary artery anomalies. In: King SB III, Douglas JS Jr, eds. *Coronary Arteriography and Angioplasty*. New York: McGraw-Hill; 1985:33–85.

153. Zir LM, Miller SW, Dinsmore RE, Gilbert JP, Harthorne JW. Interobserver variability in coronary arteriography. *Circulation* 1976; 53:627–630.

154. DeRouen TA, Murray JA, Owen W. Variability in the analysis of coronary arteriograms. *Circulation* 1977; 55:324–328.

155. Schwartz JN, King Y, Hackel DB, Bartel AG. Comparison of angiographic and postmortem findings in patients with coronary artery disease. *Am J Cardiol* 1975; 36:174–178.

156. Kemp HG, Evans H, Elliott WC, Gorlin R. Diagnostic accuracy of selective coronary cinearteriography. *Circulation* 1967; 36:526–533.

157. Grandin CM, Dyrda I, Pastemac A, Campeau L, Bourassa MG, Lesperance J. Discrepancies between cineangiographic and postmortem findings in patients with coronary artery disease and recent myocardial revascularization. *Circulation* 1974; 49:703–708.

158. Roberts WC. The coronary arteries and left ventricle in clinically isolated angina pectoris: A necropsy analysis. *Circulation* 1976; 54:388–390.

159. Arnett EN, Isner JM, Redwood DR, Kent KM, Baker WP, Ackerstein H, et al. Coronary artery narrowing in coronary heart disease: Comparison of cine angiographic and necropsy findings. *Ann Intern Med* 1979; 91:350–356.

160. Roberts CS, Roberts WC. Cross-sectional area of the proximal portions of the three major epicardial coronary arteries in 98 patients with different coronary events: Relationship to heart, weight, age, and sex. *Circulation* 1980; 62:953–959.

161. Isner JM, Kishel J, Kent KM, Ronan JA Jr, Ross AM, Roberts WC. Inaccuracy of angiographic determination of left main coronary arterial narrowing: Angiographic-histologic correlative analysis of 29 patients. *Circulation* 1979; 59,60(suppl 2):II–161.

162. Brown BG, Bolson E, Frimer M, Dodge HT. Quantitative coronary arteriography: Estimation of dimensions, hemodynamic resistance, and atheroma mass of coronary artery lesions using the arteriogram and digital computation. *Circulation* 1977; 55:329–337.

163. Abrams HL, Adams DF. The complications of coronary arteriography (abstr). *Circulation* 1975; 52(suppl 2):27.

164. Davis K, Kennedy JW, Kemp HG, Judkins MP, Gosselin AJ, Killip T. Complications of coronary arteriography from the Collaborative Study of Coronary Artery Surgery (CASS). *Circulation* 1979; 59:1105–1112.

165. Johnson LW, Lozner EC, Johnson S, Krone R, Pichard AD, Vetrovec GW, et al. Coronary arteriography 1984–1987: A report of the Registry of the Society for Cardiac Angiography and Interventions. 1. Results and complications. *Cathet Cardiovasc Diagn* 1989; 17:5–10.

166. Devlin G, Lazzam LM, Schwartz L. Current mortality rate of diagnostic cardiac catheterization: The importance of left main coronary artery disease and catheter-induced trauma (abstr). *Circulation* 1995; 92(suppl I):I–602.

167. Gersh BJ, Kronmal RA, Frye RL, Schaff HV, Ryan TJ, Gosselin AJ, et al. Coronary arteriography and coronary bypass surgery: Morbidity and mortality in patients ages 65 years or older: A report from the coronary artery surgery study. *Circulation* 1983; 67:483–491.

168. Krone RJ, Johnson L, Noto T. Five year trends in cardiac catheterization: A report from the Registry of the Society for Cardiac Angiography and Interventions. *Cathet Cardiovasc Diagn* 1996; 39:31–35.

169. Takaro T, Hultgren HN, Littmann D, Wright EC. An analysis of deaths occurring in association with coronary arteriography. *Am Heart J* 1973; 86:587–597.

170. Vogel JHK, Cornish D, McFadden RB. Underestimations of ejection fraction with single plane angiography in coronary artery disease: Role of biplane angiography. *Chest* 1973; 64:217–221.

C H A P T E R

17

NUCLEAR CARDIOLOGY

Randolph E. Patterson / Robert L. Eisner / Byron R. Williams, Jr.

The past quarter century has witnessed the transformation of radioactive tracers in cardiovascular disease from being tools for research to being tools that help guide clinical decisions.[1-5] This chapter reviews the uses of radiopharmaceutical imaging to indicate its advantages and limitations in order to help guide management decisions in cardiac patients. The chapter is organized around three main areas related to imaging of conventional gamma-emitting radionuclides: (1) myocardial perfusion imaging (MPI); (2) cardiac blood pool imaging (BPI) for ventricular function by gated equilibrium and first-pass methods; and (3) other radionuclide cardiovascular imaging procedures, which include acute myocardial infarct (MI) "hot spot" imaging, imaging of cardiac neural function, imaging of cardiovascular thrombus, imaging of radionuclide-labeled components of atherosclerotic plaque, and ventilation-perfusion lung imaging. Positron emission tomography is covered in Chap. 20.

Each section of the chapter will discuss the relevant aspects of instrumentation (camera systems and computers), radiopharmaceuticals, clinical procedures, image processing and analysis, clinical validation and applications of the methods, and future developments that are likely to influence clinical utility of the procedure. There is no long continuous section on instrumentation, radiopharmaceuticals, or image processing and analysis; instead, this information is placed within the sections on clinical applications, where it might be easier to understand how the methodology influences the clinical value of the procedure.

The focus of nuclear cardiology has changed and matured over the past several years. No longer is the major objective just to identify the presence or absence of cardiac disease, e.g., by showing agreement with cardiac catheterization findings. Rather, nuclear cardiology is proving its usefulness in guiding the management of patients because it provides independent and incremental value to the other clinical information and diagnostic tests.

MYOCARDIAL PERFUSION IMAGING

Imaging Instrumentation and Physics

This section is provided as a brief introduction to how nuclear camera/computer systems make images of the heart. The information here is the basis for the clinical use of nuclear methods, and it will be helpful to the physician who is involved in quality assurance so that the images will provide accurate clinical information. This information should also help the physician who is involved in planning acquisition of new equipment for a hospital or office.

All of the clinically useful radioisotopes (e.g., ^{201}Tl, ^{99m}Tc) injected into the body emit gamma rays. The nuclear detector system, called a *gamma camera* or *Anger camera,* furnishes a two-dimensional "picture" of the three-dimensional distribution of the radioisotope by imaging those gamma rays that emerge from the heart and pass through lung, ribs, and other tissues to reach the camera. The gamma camera consists of a lead collimator, a thallium-activated sodium-iodide [NaI(Tl)] crystal, a light pipe, and a set of photomultiplier tubes (Fig. 17-1). The collimator consists of a honeycomb of hollow openings in the lead to "focus" the gamma rays. For cardiac imaging, the holes are usually aligned parallel to each other (i.e., parallel-hole collimator). In this configuration, gamma rays that are emitted in a direction that is not perpendicular to the camera surface are stopped by the lead in the collimator. The location of the gamma ray interaction in the NaI crystal corresponds to the site of origin of the gamma ray in the body. Most of the gamma rays that pass through the holes of the collimator are stopped in the NaI crystal. When stopped, the energy of each gamma ray is converted into quanta of light. The higher the energy of the gamma ray, the greater the number of light quanta that are created (to produce images with better spatial and energy resolution). The light quanta

Top view

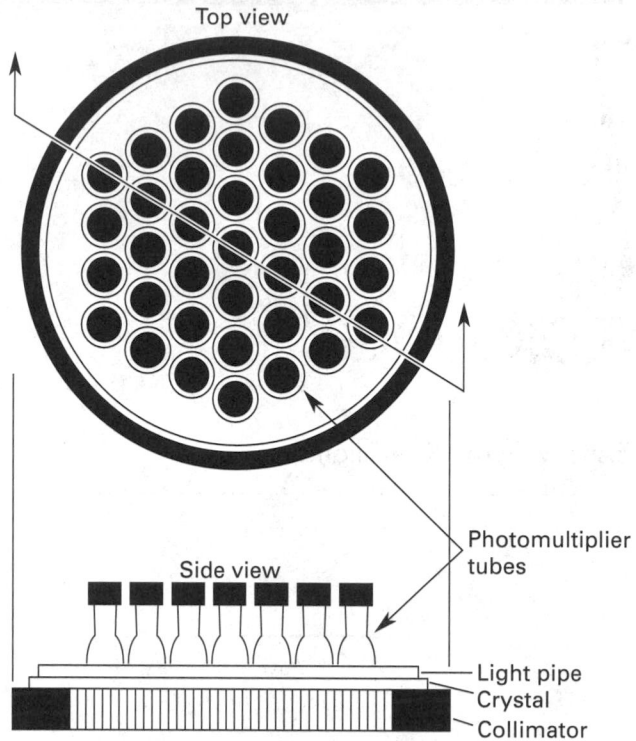

Side view

Photomultiplier
tubes

Light pipe
Crystal
Collimator

FIGURE 17-1

Schematic diagram of a gamma camera showing the arrangement of the 37 photomultiplier tubes, light pipe, NaI crystal, and lead collimator. (From Rollo.[10] Reproduced with permission of the publisher and author.)

pass through the light pipe and impinge on the front (photocathode) of the photomultiplier tubes.[6]

Each photomultiplier tube converts the light energy into an electrical current. Older cameras took the analogue signals from the photomultiplier tubes and used Anger-camera logic to calculate the (x, y) position of the gamma ray interaction in the NaI crystal and the energy of the incident gamma ray. Present-day digital cameras convert the signals to a digital representation and use digital logic to evaluate the location and energy of the incident gamma ray. The imaging parameters (resolution, uniformity, energy resolution, etc.) of the newer gamma cameras are superior to the older cameras, and the newer cameras are also able to acquire data accurately at much higher count rates. In the authors' experience, however, the older analogue cameras are still able to provide high quality planar and tomographic cardiac scans if preventive maintenance, quality control, and service procedures are performed carefully.

The design of a gamma camera is partly art and partly science. The choice of which trade-offs should be made depends on how the camera will be used. Newer gamma cameras are approaching the "theoretical" limit for performance capabilities. Unfortunately, the lead collimator degrades the spatial resolution of the image significantly. The collimator cannot be removed from the imaging system since that would produce chaotic images by exposing the NaI crystal to gamma rays from all sources and angles (rather than from perpendicular

paths as dictated by the collimator holes), and camera images would provide no usable information.

There are trade-offs between the maximum number of counts obtained per unit time (*sensitivity*) and the image resolution. High-resolution collimators provide better spatial resolution but fewer counting statistics than general purpose or high-sensitivity collimators. While there is no general rule, some literature[7] and the authors' experience suggest that the collimators with better resolution represent the appropriate trade-off compared to collimators that provide more count statistics.

There are two basic acquisition techniques, planar imaging and single photon emission computed tomography (SPECT), used in nuclear cardiology.[8,9] In planar imaging, the gamma camera is placed over the heart in several positions (views).[10] Depending on the clinical application, images are acquired for a preset time or for total counts or number of heart beats. Much like data acquisition in x-ray computed tomography (CT), SPECT data are acquired from multiple views or projections about the body. In order to produce a CT-like image of the heart, the SPECT reconstruction program requires that the gamma camera collect data from at least a 180° arc about the patient.

Radiopharmaceuticals for MPI (See Table 17-1)

Radioactive tracers are distributed throughout the body in proportion to blood flow. Thallium (^{201}Tl) replaced potassium as the preferred agent because of its availability, physical half-life, photon energy level, and its extraction from blood to myocardial tissue.[11,12] The underlying physiologic processes involved in the transport of radiolabeled agents from blood to cells have been studied with great interest.[11–17] *For MPI, the ideal radiotracer would be extracted from blood to tissue with identical efficiency at any value of blood flow velocity. In fact, the fraction of most tracers that is extracted from blood to tissues varies dramatically at different levels of blood flow.*[17] The extraction of ^{201}Tl from blood to myocardium is high (85 percent) during the first pass at rest but increases somewhat at slower flow rates, related to a longer residence time for ^{201}Tl to cross from blood in capillaries to the tissues. The more significant clinical problem is that the fraction of ^{201}Tl in the blood that is extracted to tissues decreases at high flow rates, related to a shorter residence time available for ^{201}Tl to cross from blood to tissues.[17]

The mechanisms of ^{201}Tl transport into cells are not clearly defined.[12,14–17] There have been conflicting results concerning whether ^{201}Tl uptake requires ATP[14,15] or whether it is inhibited by digitalis glycosides.[14] It does seem clear that necrotic cardiac cells do not take up ^{201}Tl in vitro.[15–17] Radioactive decay of ^{201}Tl yields photons with energies between 68 and 80 keV (>90 percent of photon emissions) and at 167 keV (<10 percent of the emitted photons). The physical half-life ($t_{1/2}$) of ^{201}Tl is 73 h, and it is eliminated from the body primarily by the kidney with a biologic $t_{1/2}$ in the heart of 3 to 4 h in normal individuals after exercise. When injected

TABLE 17-1

RADIOPHARMACEUTICALS FOR SINGLE PHOTON EMISSION COMPUTED TOMOGRAPHIC MYOCARDIAL
PERFUSION IMAGING (SPECT MPI)

Radiopharmaceutical	Physical $t_{1/2}$, h	Energy Peak, keV	Ex.F. on First Transit	Change in Ex.F. as Flow Increases	Dose (Rest and Stress), mCi	Primary Route of Excretion	Biologic $t_{1/2}$, h
Thallium 201 chloride	73	68–80, 167	0.85	Small	3.5	Renal	3
Technectium 99m sestamibi	6	140	0.60	Large	20–30	Liver, bile	6
Technetium 99m teboroxine	6	140	0.95	Negligible	20–30	Liver	Biphasic 30 s, h

Note: Ex.F., extraction fraction.

into a peripheral vein, ^{201}Tl clears from the blood to tissue with a $t_{1/2}$ of 40 to 50 s, and 90 to 95 percent of the injected dose clears from the blood to tissue in 2 min. With higher levels of exercise and a higher cardiac output, the clearance rate is faster.[13,17,18] In order to establish a perfusion defect during stress, the critical variable is the duration of time that coronary blood flow (CBF) remains increased after injection of [201]Tl.[19,20] If the duration of the stress-induced increase in CBF after ^{201}Tl injection is too brief, then not enough ^{201}Tl is deposited in myocardium to form a "footprint" of the relative distribution of CBF during stress.[20] Continued deposition of a large amount of ^{201}Tl into the heart after CBF returns to normal will diminish the difference between ^{201}Tl concentrations in myocardium supplied by patent versus stenotic arteries.[20] *This issue is crucial for the clinician, because the physician supervising the stress test needs to encourage the patient to provide at least a 1-min warning so that ^{201}Tl can be injected to circulate during at least 1 min of exercise to maintain the relative flow differences—if it seems safe for the patient.*[19]

As soon as any ^{201}Tl is deposited in the heart, the CBF begins "washing out" [201]Tl into venous blood in a bidirectional exchange, i.e., wash-in versus wash-out.[13,18,19] The net effect of ^{201}Tl delivery and wash-out is its biologic $t_{1/2}$ in the heart of 3 to 4 h, but wash-out is faster from myocardium receiving elevated or normal CBF than from myocardium receiving lower CBF.[1,18] Thus the footprint of the MPI defect will disappear over time as more ^{201}Tl washes out by the normal blood flow rates through patent arteries compared to less ^{201}Tl wash-out by slower flow rates through a stenotic artery. Long delays between ^{201}Tl injection and image acquisition could obscure defects due to the wash-in versus wash-out effect.[1,2,19,20] This limitation requires rapid transfer of the patient from the stress test to the camera for image acquisition—once it is clear that the patient is medically stable.[1,19,20]

Wash-out analysis over 2 to 6 h has been used to assess myocardial viability, as will be described later.[12] Wash-out may also be analyzed to determine whether a patient might

have balanced reductions in CBF to different regions of the left ventricle due to left main coronary stenosis or similar severity of stenoses in all three coronary arteries, i.e., "balanced ischemia."[13]

TECHNETIUM 99m SESTAMIBI FOR MPI (See Table 17-1)

For many years there has been an interest in developing a radiopharmaceutical for MPI that could be labeled with [99m]Tc. The advantages of ^{99m}Tc are the low cost of its production by the molybdenum generator and the fact that the generator can be "milked" at any time for a clinical dose.[1,2] [99m]Tc is used for most nuclear medicine studies, so the generators are widely available in the radiopharmacies of hospitals or commercial suppliers. Most sites now prefer receiving "unit doses" from commercial suppliers to reduce radiation exposure to staff and to guarantee quality control. [99m]Tc has a shorter physical $t_{1/2}$ than [201]Tl (6 versus 73 h), so that one can employ much (tenfold) higher doses of ^{99m}Tc with similar radiation exposure to the patient and acquire many more counts than with ^{201}Tl in the same imaging time.[12,21] In general, myocardial images can be limited by the total number of counts acquired.[6] Radioisotopic decay follows a Poisson distribution. Based on the Poisson nature of the decay, the standard deviation (SD) can be estimated as the square root of the number of acquired counts, and the coefficient of variation, or "noise," is estimated as SD/(total counts acquired), which is equal to (total counts acquired)$^{-1/2}$.[6] Accordingly, images with fewer counts appear to be noisier (i.e., have a larger coefficient of variation) than images with better counting statistics. The counting statistics of ^{201}Tl are adequate for good quality clinical planar or SPECT imaging, but ^{99m}Tc-based radiopharmaceutical images are less noisy and visually more pleasing because counts are greater (e.g., by sixfold for ^{99m}Tc sestamibi) for the same acquisition time.[21,22]

Another advantage of a ^{99m}Tc-based radiopharmaceutical is its higher energy peak (140 keV) compared to [201]Tl (68 to 80 keV). The higher energy photon emissions by ^{99m}Tc are clearly an advantage over ^{201}Tl, but it would be an oversimplification to attribute all differences between radiopharmaceuticals to differences in energy peaks. The following comments show how the differences in energies interact with other factors to produce differences in the clinical uses between ^{99m}Tc and ^{201}Tl. This higher gamma ray energy allows for the following:

1. There is a small decrease in the attenuation coefficient in tissues to provide somewhat less attenuation-related image degradation (artifact) in SPECT imaging[23] (Fig. 17-2), but, as discussed in detail below, attenuation remains a major issue for SPECT ^{99m}Tc MPI.[8]

2. ^{99m}Tc shows better intrinsic camera resolution but little difference in the system resolution with the same collimator, so that the image resolution is only changed slightly.[23–25]

3. ^{99m}Tc shows less scatter to produce better defect contrast between normal and abnormal regions of uptake.[23,24]

4. With some ^{99m}Tc agents, however, there may be decreased defect contrast in the inferior wall of the heart due to scatter from prominent visceral uptake (e.g., liver and gall bladder uptake with ^{99m}Tc sestamibi). These effects of visceral ^{99m}Tc-tracer uptake are more prominent using pharmacologic stress and vary among different patients.

5. The advantages in image quality and defect contrast using ^{99m}Tc agents are offset considerably by limitations associated with greater decrease in extraction fraction at high flow.[26–29]

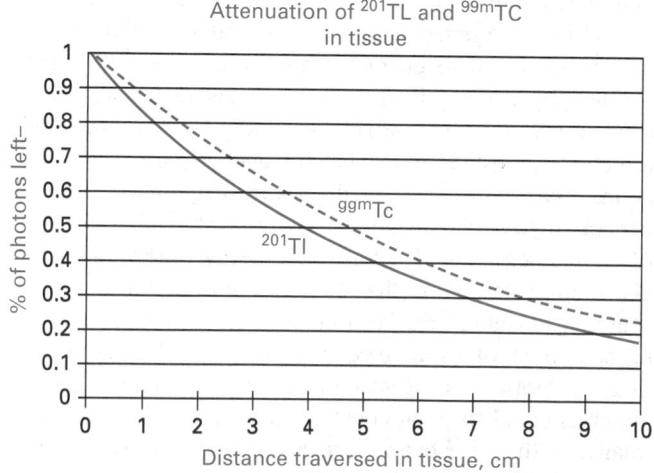

FIGURE 17-2

The effect of attenuation on photons as they traverse tissue is depicted. The percentage of photons remaining (vertical axis) is plotted against the distance traversed in tissue (horizontal axis). The dashed curve is for ^{99m}Tc, and the solid curve is for ^{201}Tl. The curves were generated using the exponential decay law: (percent of photons left) = (number at $x = 0$) $\exp(-\mu x)$, where x is the distance in tissue and μ is the attenuation coefficient with a unit of cm^{-1}; $\mu(^{201}$Tl$) = 0.18$ cm^{-1}; and $\mu(^{99m}$Tc$) = 0.15$ cm^{-1}. At each depth, there are relatively more ^{99m}Tc photons remaining since the 140 keV photons from the ^{99m}Tc decay suffer less attenuation; however, the differences are small (5 to 15 percent for tissue depths of 2 to 6 cm).

The first ^{99m}Tc-based radiopharmaceutical was ^{99m}Tc sestamibi, which has the advantage of a much longer residence time in the heart after intravenous injection,[30] i.e., a "stay-put" indicator. ^{99m}Tc sestamibi is trapped in cytoplasm of cells by the negative charge generated by the mitochondrial ion gradient,[31] so that it washes out very slowly from the heart (10 to 15 percent over 2 h).[30,32] This stay-put behavior of ^{99m}Tc sestamibi is one of its greatest assets, particularly for the logistics of performing the stress test.[30,32] It allows the patient to have a stress test with a variable delay in the time between ^{99m}Tc sestamibi injection and image acquisition from 20 to 240 min, but optimally, 45 to 60 min.[33] *This flexibility in time between the stress test and the actual acquisition of stress images means that one physician can perform stress tests for several patients without having to wait for the imaging system to become free after completing scans for previous patients, as with ^{201}Tl.*

There are, however, certain disadvantages of ^{99m}Tc sestamibi relative to ^{201}Tl. First, it is excreted primarily via the gall bladder and liver so that these organs show intense activity immediately after injection, and this activity declines gradually and variably over hours.[21–23] This visceral activity contributes scattered photons to the nearby regions of the heart—particularly the inferior wall of the left ventricle. A longer wait between ^{99m}Tc sestamibi injection and image acquisition may be required for the visceral activity to clear sufficiently to produce adequate quality images. Ingesting some fat, such as milk, can also stimulate gall bladder emptying to clear the ^{99m}Tc sestamibi more quickly.[33] The major disadvantage of ^{99m}Tc sestamibi is its limited extraction from blood to tissues at high CBF.[26–29] The extraction fraction at rest is lower (60 percent) than for ^{201}Tl (85 percent), and it decreases more dramatically than ^{201}Tl when CBF is increased during stress.[26–29,34] In one animal study, it was found that ^{99m}Tc sestamibi concentration in the heart increased to its maximum after only a twofold increase in CBF and showed no further increase even when CBF increased from two to four times the resting value.[28] Two clinical studies of patients having exercise tests to the same levels of heart rate and blood pressure with ^{201}Tl and ^{99m}Tc sestamibi showed more severe defects on images with the former than the latter. The authors' group, working with dogs, found large differences in defect area and contrast: *^{99m}Tc sestamibi defect area = 47 percent of ^{201}Tl defect area, and ^{99m}Tc sestamibi contrast = 116 percent of ^{201}Tl contrast* (i.e., less severe), even though the measured (twofold) increase in CBF by adenosine was the same for ^{201}Tl and ^{99m}Tc sestamibi.[29] Using dobutamine to elicit regional differences in blood flow in dogs with coronary stenoses, another group found little correlation between flow (measured by radioactive microspheres) and ^{99m}Tc sestamibi uptake in normal and moderately underperfused myocardium.[37] These differences are most likely due to the marked decrease in extraction fraction at high CBF, which decreases ^{99m}Tc sestamibi concentration in the normal zone.[26,27,38] Decreased ^{99m}Tc sestamibi in the normal zone decreases the contrast between normal and defect zones.[26–29] In fact, total myocardial counts after stress ^{99m}Tc sestamibi usually increase fivefold, even though the radioactivity doses increase tenfold. Clinical studies often show similar sensitivities for ^{99m}Tc sestamibi and ^{201}Tl in detecting coronary artery disease (CAD),[39–43] due in part to the large number of patients (over 50 percent) in the studies who had prior MI.[39–43] Patients with prior MI have severe defects on stress and rest ^{99m}Tc sestamibi imaging that make it easy to detect CAD. In fact, the severe defects on resting ^{99m}Tc sestamibi after MI make it harder to detect myocardial viability,[44] which encouraged the development of a protocol for MPI using ^{201}Tl at rest and ^{99m}Tc sestamibi during a subsequent stress test.[45]

Another limitation of ^{99m}Tc sestamibi is that relative heart-to-lung uptake does not reflect stress-induced pulmonary edema in the way that ^{201}Tl does. The fivefold higher count rate on ^{99m}Tc sestamibi studies, however, allows better electrocardiogram (ECG)-gated acquisitions than ^{201}Tl to analyze cardiac contraction and myocardial wall thickening.[46,47] Also, the higher count rate with ^{99m}Tc sestamibi allows performance of first-pass radionuclide cardiac BPI to quantitate left ventricular (LV) and/or right ventricular ejection fractions during stress and rest.[48] Thus, there are methodologic advantages and disadvantages for ^{201}Tl versus ^{99m}Tc sestamibi; the latter, however, is more expensive than ^{201}Tl.

OTHER RADIOPHARMACEUTICALS FOR MPI
(See Table 17-1)
There are other ^{99m}Tc-labeled agents similar to sestamibi, such as tetrofosmin, some of which have been approved for clinical use.[49] One ^{99m}Tc-labeled radiopharmaceutical, teboroxime, differs considerably from ^{99m}Tc sestamibi.[38,50–52] Teboroxime is cleared very rapidly from the blood.[52] Its extraction fraction changes very little at different levels of CBF, so that it has almost ideal characteristics as a blood flow tracer, nearly equal to radioactive plastic microspheres.[38,50–52] The disadvantage of teboroxime, however, is its very rapid decrease in activity, which requires early and very fast (complete acquisition in less than 2 min following injection) imaging at a time when it still shows considerable visceral activity and some blood pool.[50] *Most laboratories have found it to be too difficult to use teboroxime for clinical studies.*

Procedures and Protocols for MPI

The main emphasis of this section will be to explain procedures for stress/rest ^{201}Tl SPECT MPI and to explain briefly how these procedures are modified for planar imaging, rest ^{201}Tl MPI, and protocols using other radiopharmaceuticals. The protocol favored by most and used in the authors' laboratory utilizes exercise with either delay rest-redistribution or rest-reinjection ^{201}Tl SPECT MPI.[53] The nuclear technologists or nurses first review the patient's orders for the test, the patient's ability to exercise, and any recent change in the patient's symptoms. It is imperative to ask women of appropriate age about the possibility of pregnancy.

The dose of ^{201}Tl is drawn into a shielded syringe and placed near the treadmill for exercise, 3.0 to 3.5 mCi, or more if the patient is very large. The patient is then interviewed and examined by a physician or a physician-extender to assess appropriateness of exercise and radioactive material exposure (Table 17-2). *Particular attention is directed to the symptoms of chest discomfort, blood pressure, and findings suggestive of LV outflow obstruction and to the standard resting 12-lead ECG.* It is essential to have at least two people with the patient during exercise: a technologist (or nurse or technician) to operate the treadmill, check the intravenous catheter operation, and inject ^{201}Tl; and a physician (or physician-extender) to monitor the patient's overall condition, symptoms, blood pressure, and ECG rhythm and ST segments (see Chap. 15). It is very important that the patient should indicate when he or she thinks it is possible to exercise for only one more minute so that ^{201}Tl can be injected and allowed to distribute for 1 min during conditions of stress. The physician should stay close enough to the patient to prevent injury in case of a fall on the treadmill. As soon as the patient stops exercise, he or she should be assisted to a chair or stretcher for 2 to 3 min before going to the imaging room. If the patient has chest discomfort or severe dyspnea, then the physician may want to give nitroglycerin.

The patient should be positioned comfortably under the camera on a padded table no later than 10 to 15 min after stopping exercise. For single-headed SPECT camera systems, the camera head is positioned in the 45° right anterior oblique (RAO) position to rotate 180° anteriorly to the left posterior oblique (LPO) position. For dual-headed systems, the second head begins its 90° rotation in the left anterior oblique (LAO) position 90° to the left of the first camera head. Planar ^{201}Tl imaging is clearly inferior to SPECT.[54] It is performed in three views: anterior, LAO, and left lateral, usually performed in that sequence for 5 to 10 min per image.

PHARMACOLOGIC STRESS AGENTS FOR MPI
(See Table 17-2)
If the patient cannot exercise or fails to achieve 85 percent of age-predicted maximum heart rate, then he or she should receive a pharmacologic stress agent. If the patient does not achieve an adequate level of cardiac stress, then CBF (and ^{201}Tl delivery) through patent arteries will not achieve maximal levels for that patient. This submaximal CBF stimulus decreases sensitivity of MPI because the contrast or difference in CBF (and ^{201}Tl delivery) between myocardium supplied by patent versus stenotic coronary arteries may not be large enough to be detected. If the difference in ^{201}Tl concentrations in normal versus underperfused myocardium is too small, the contrast on MPI will be too small to be detected as a defect.[55] *If there is no evidence of a reversible defect on MPI but the exercise level did not produce 85 percent of age-predicted maximum heart rate, the images should be interpreted as nondiagnostic—not as normal.* If the patient fails to achieve 85 percent of age-predicted maximum heart rate but develops symptoms or ECG ST abnormalities to suggest ischemia, then

TABLE 17-2

MODES OF STRESS FOR MYOCARDIAL PERFUSION IMAGING (MPI)

Stress Mode	Mechanism	Dose	Major Risk	Reversal Agents	Advantages
Exercise	Increases myocardial oxygen demand (MVO_2) and coronary blood flow (CBF)	Bruce treadmill protocol increases in stages of 3 (from 4 to 23) metabolic equivalents of exercise (METS)	Ischemia/MI Physical injury Arrhythmia Hypertension	Rest, NTG Response suppressed by some drugs	Only way to get meaningful correlation between symptoms and MPI
Dipyridamole	Primary coronary vasodilation (by preventing degradation of adenosine)[57,58]	0.142 μg/kg per min for 5 min, or 0.56–0.84 mg[59]	Asthma Ischemia/MI	Aminophylline 125 mg, IV, over 1–2 min Caffeine blocks	For people who cannot exercise
Adenosine	Primary vasodilation Binds adenosine (A_2) receptor	0.142 μg/kg per min for 6 min	Asthma Ischemia (brief)	Same, but rarely needed due to $t_{1/2}$	Shorter $t_{1/2}$ than dipyridamole for safety
Dobutamine	Increases MVO_2 and CBF	Increases in steps of 2.5–5, to maximum of 40 μg/kg per min (2–3 min per stage)	Ischemia/MI Arrhythmia Hypotension Hypertension	Metoprolol 2.5 mg IV and may repeat Response suppressed by some drugs	For people who cannot exercise and have asthma

Note: MI, myocardial infarction; NTG, nitroglycerin.

it is quite reasonable to inject ^{201}Tl at that time to correlate the MPI with other findings. SPECT ^{201}Tl images will show very reproducible defects on separate stress tests if the patient achieves similar peak heart rates and blood pressures.[56]

The first pharmacologic stress agent to be used widely was dipyridamole.[57] The mechanism of action of dipyridamole is blockade of the facilitated transport of adenosine from extracellular fluid (where it causes vasodilatation) to intracellular fluid (where it is phosphorylated by 5′-nucleotidase to adenosine-5′-monophosphate, which cannot leave the cell).[57,58] Thus, dipyridamole results in increased adenosine concentration near the coronary arterioles where it binds to the adenosine-2 (A_2) receptor to produce vasodilatation. Intravenous administration of dipyridamole appears to result in a relatively selective dilation of coronary arteries more than other arteries. The drug usually decreases systolic and/or diastolic blood pressure by at least 10 mmHg and/or causes a reflex increase in heart rate of at least 10 beats per minute.[58,59] Gould and others have shown that CBF measured by an electromagnetic flow probe in dogs decreased after the arterial lumen area measured directly was narrowed by 75 percent or more (corresponding to a 50 percent reduction in lumen diameter)[59] (Fig. 17-3). Thus, dipyridamole produces the MPI defect due to differential dilation of normal versus stenotic arteries, but the drug does not usually produce myocardial ischemia (as reflected in the absence of coronary venous lac-

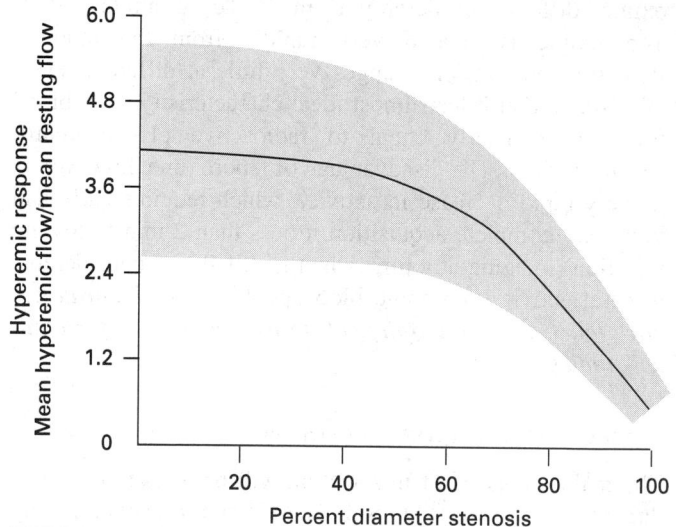

FIGURE 17-3

Relation of percent diameter narrowing of a single stenosis of the circumflex artery to hyperemic responses after intracoronary injection of contrast medium in 10 consecutive dogs. Hyperemic responses are expressed as the ratio of hyperemic mean flow after injection of contrast medium to resting basal mean flow before each injection. The solid line is the best fit curve, and the shaded area indicates the limits of the relations plotted for individual dogs. Resting flow would be equivalent to 1.0 on the vertical axis, with a decrease to zero after stenosis reaches 85 percent. (From Gould and Lipscomb.[59] Reproduced with permission of the publisher and authors.)

tate production), even in patients with reversible defects.[60] The hemodynamic effects of dipyridamole include arterial vasodilatation, decreased systemic vascular resistance, increased cardiac output, and, often, a small increase in LV dimensions and filling pressures.[61]

Dipyridamole has a duration of action of 20 to 30 min so that vasodilatation is sustained for sufficient time for radionuclide deposition.[57,62,63] The side effects of dipyridamole include chest discomfort (usually not due to myocardial ischemia), dyspnea, headache, abdominal discomfort, flushing, fatigue, and heaviness in the legs.[57] One of the most serious side effects of dipyridamole is the exacerbation of asthma, which may be due to a direct effect of dipyridamole or to discontinuation of theophylline therapy.[62] *Any patient presenting for dipyridamole testing should be excluded if there is a history of severe bronchospastic lung disease or if wheezes are heard on examination, because deaths have been reported in such patients.*[62,63] Caffeinated beverages can block the vasodilation from dipyridamole,[64] and aminophylline, 125 mg intravenously over 3 to 5 min, will reverse side effects within 2 to 4 min by blocking the A_2 receptor. Unless the patient seems unstable, one should allow about 2 min after ^{201}Tl injection before giving the aminophylline, in order to allow ^{201}Tl deposition during maximal vasodilation (see Table 17-2).

Dipyridamole can produce myocardial ischemia, but only in the presence of very severe coronary stenoses that make the underperfused myocardium dependent on collateral coronary arteries[62,63] (by creating "coronary steal"[64–66]). Coronary steal is explained most clearly in terms of the perfusion pressure in the coronary arteries at the origin of the collateral vessels.[66] Arteriolar vasodilation increases the velocity of CBF in the normal artery. This increase in flow velocity (or kinetic energy) leads to a decrease in perfusion pressure (or potential energy), according to physical laws of conservation of energy.[66] Clinically, arteriolar vasodilators would be much more likely to produce myocardial ischemia if the patient has multivessel CAD and a large decrease in diastolic blood pressure.[66]

Adenosine has been used clinically in recent years to dilate the coronary arteries for MPI[67] (see Table 17-2). The main advantage of adenosine over dipyridamole is its brief duration of action (<2 min), which reduces the duration of side effects. There has been more limited clinical experience with the use of adenosine, and its brief duration of action makes it difficult to measure blood pressure effects of the drug. Atrioventricular conduction block is particularly common with adenosine, but its duration is so brief that it is rarely necessary to give aminophylline.[67] As with dipyridamole, adenosine is contraindicated in patients with asthma, and it should not be used in patients as a substitute for exercise.

For patients with asthma who cannot exercise, dobutamine (Table 17-2) has been used as a stress agent for MPI.[68] The mechanism of action of dobutamine is stimulation of beta-adrenergic receptors.[69] At low to intermediate doses of dobutamine, there is some increase in heart rate, an increase in

cardiac contractile performance, a decrease in diastolic blood pressure, and, usually, an increase in systolic blood pressure. At higher doses, blood pressure increases moderately and heart rate increases, but the heart rate often does not increase to 85 percent of the age-predicted maximum, the target stress level to increase CBF sufficiently for diagnostic purposes. The supplemental use of atropine has been advocated to increase heart rate.[70] Measured CBF in animals increases with dobutamine but not to maximal levels.[70]

Dobutamine can cause ventricular and supraventricular tachycardias.[70] The drug predictably causes myocardial ischemia, which is essential for detecting regional wall motion abnormalities and, thus, diagnosing CAD by stress echocardiography[69] (see Chap. 14). Patients who experience symptoms of myocardial ischemia cannot willfully regulate the intensity of the stressful stimulus with dobutamine as they can with exercise, so the *physician must be hypervigilant to detect the earliest evidence of ischemia in any patient receiving this powerful inotropic agent.*

Other side effects of dobutamine include palpitations, sweating, nausea, chest discomfort, dyspnea, dysphoria, and arterial hypotension.[68,70] These side effects are reversible with beta-adrenergic blocking drugs.[70] One potential advantage of using dobutamine, in contrast to dypyridamole or adenosine,[70] for MPI is that the resulting wall motion abnormality may accentuate the severity of the defect contrast on MPI to enhance detection of CAD.[71]

For stress testing, exercise is strongly preferred because it is the form of stress that occurs naturally and allows the best correlation between symptoms and objective evidence of myocardial ischemia. Exercise testing also saves the cost and side effects of the pharmacologic agents used for stress. For patients who cannot achieve 85 percent of maximum heart rate or evidence of ischemia during exercise, the authors prefer dipyridamole to adenosine because of the extensive experience with the agent and its somewhat milder (although more prolonged) side effects. Since most patients with reactive airway disease show an early increase in heart rate during exercise, dobutamine is only occasionally necessary as a stress agent.

PROTOCOLS TO ASSESS MYOCARDIAL VIABILITY BY MPI
(See Table 17-3)

Initially, stress/rest ^{201}Tl MPI was performed with separate injections of ^{201}Tl several days apart to avoid contamination of the stress and/or rest MPI. [201]Tl imaging became much more efficient after the demonstration that rest MPI could be provided by "redistribution" images obtained 3 to 6 h after injection of ^{201}Tl at stress.[11] In recent years, studies have shown that 3- to 6-h redistribution MPI failed to detect reversibility of stress defects in patients who did have viable myocardium, indicated by improved regional function after revascularization.[72–74] Next, studies found improved ability to detect viable myocardium if redistribution MPI were acquired after allowing a longer (16 to 48 h) delay for redistribution of

TABLE 17-3

COMPARISON OF SOME SPECT MPI PROTOCOLS

Protocol	Radiopharmaceutical	Images to Acquire	Time Needed, h	Advantages	Disadvantages	Costs
^{201}Tl stress/ redistribution	1. ^{201}Tl 3.5 mCi at stress	1. Stress 2. Rest-redistribution	4.5	1. Simplest 2. Lowest cost 3. Best for left main CAD (wash-out delay)	1. Time 2. Low counts	+
^{201}Tl stress/ reinjection at rest	1. ^{201}Tl 3.5 mCi at stress + 2. 1.5 mCi at rest	1. Stress 2. Rest reinjection	4.5	1. Best for viability	1. Time and cost of reinjection	+ +
^{99m}Tc sestamibi rest/stress	1. ^{99m}Tc sestamibi 9 mCi at rest 2. 22 mCi at stress	1. Rest 2. Stress	3	1. More counts for image quality 2. More counts for gated studies 3. Can do all stress tests with no waiting for image acquisition, and acquire images later	1. Extraction fraction of sestamibi decreases as flow increases 2. Poor for viability 3. Cannot interpret lung uptake	+ + +
Dual isotope	1. ^{201}Tl 3.0 mCi at rest 2. ^{99m}Tc sestamibi 20–30 mCi at stress	1. Rest (^{201}Tl) 2. Stress (^{99m}Tc)	1.5	1. Fastest 2. ^{201}Tl rest for viability 3. More counts on stress	1. Cost 2. Extraction fraction of sestamibi 3. Lung uptake 4. Compare rest/stress—potential technical problems	+ + + +

Note: CAD, coronary artery disease.

^{201}Tl to occur, i.e., wash-out of ^{201}Tl from the body to the bloodstream and subsequent deposition of ^{201}Tl under resting conditions. Later, other investigators found improved detection of *viable myocardium* by observing amelioration of the severity of ^{201}Tl-imaged defects between stress images and 4-h redistribution images, and between images acquired 10 min after *reinjection* of ^{201}Tl and the redistribution images.[72–74] One group has indicated that a small (5 to 8 percent) group of patients show more improvement between MPI acquired 10 min after reinjection of ^{201}Tl at rest and "late redistribution" MPI acquired 12- to 24 h after reinjection at rest, to allow more time for delivery of ^{201}Tl to viable myocardium.[75] Other evidence from studies of ^{201}Tl kinetics[11,17,19,20] suggests that the 12- to 24-h delay images may be less necessary if rest reinjection images are acquired 20 to 30 min (instead of 10 min) after rest-reinjection of ^{201}Tl. *In the authors' protocol, the ^{201}Tl stress images are processed and reinjection at rest is performed 2.5 to 3.0 h later only if the stress defect involves 10 percent or more of the left ventricle; otherwise, 3-h redistribution images are acquired. When a significant stress defect is present (>10 percent of the left ventricle), rest reinjection images are acquired 20 to 30 min following reinjection of ^{201}Tl without acquiring redistribution images.*

PROCEDURAL MODIFICATIONS FOR OTHER RADIOPHARMACEUTICALS (See Table 17-3)

^{99m}Tc Sestamibi Rest/Stress

Because ^{99m}Tc sestamibi shows little redistribution after injection,[30,32] it allows more flexibility in designing protocols than does ^{201}Tl.[33] ^{99m}Tc sestamibi has been used in a 2-day protocol where the stress study is done 1 day, and if there is a heterogeneous uptake of the tracer to suggest a defect on stress images, then the patient is brought back on another day for a second injection of ^{99m}Tc sestamibi at rest. Each image set is acquired 30 to 60 min after injecting 20 to 30 mCi ^{99m}Tc sestamibi. This protocol allows stress and rest images to be performed with essentially no background activity from a prior injection, and the order of stress/rest can be reversed. It frequently is inconvenient, however, for the patient to come to the department on two separate days. For a same-day protocol, a rest/stress sequence has advantages.[33] After an initial small (8 to 10 mCi) dose for the rest study, one injects a large (25 to 30 mCi) dose for the stress study with only modest background contamination from the initial injection after 2 to 6 h.[39]

A third protocol has increased in popularity in recent years.

This dual-isotope study uses an initial ^{201}Tl injection at rest and a subsequent ^{99m}Tc sestamibi injection during stress.[76] The advantage of this protocol is that it requires less total time because the stress study can begin immediately after the rest ^{201}Tl MPI study. Also, the differences in energy level between isotopes means that ^{99m}Tc sestamibi can be imaged with only negligible contamination from the downscattered ^{201}Tl high-energy (167 keV) emissions. The disadvantages of this clinical protocol are associated with the differences in imaging and physiologic properties of the two radiopharmaceuticals, which make it somewhat more difficult to compare severity of defects on rest and stress to distinguish ischemia from MI.

Thus, for using ^{99m}Tc sestamibi, the protocols differ from those for ^{201}Tl in several ways. Patients should be fasting for several hours before ^{201}Tl to minimize visceral activity but might even ingest some fatty food (e.g., whole milk) to stimulate gall bladder function to clear sestamibi from its main site of excretion, the gall bladder.[39] The other major difference between the radiopharmaceuticals is the time between injection and image acquisition. ^{201}Tl image acquisition should begin at least 20 to 30 minutes *after a rest injection* to minimize activities in the cardiac blood pool and viscera and to allow time for delivery of ^{201}Tl to regions with low CBF. ^{201}Tl image acquisition should begin no more than 15 min after a *stress injection* to minimize redistribution of ^{201}Tl from other tissues to the myocardial regions dependent on stenotic coronary arteries to decrease contrast between normal and ischemic regions. It appears, however, that SPECT ^{201}Tl MPI should not begin before about 10 min after exercise in order for the heart to stabilize its position in the body, i.e., avoiding "upward creep"[77] of the heart. SPECT acquisition during upward creep of the heart following a stress test, independent of body motion, can produce imaging artifacts because the tomographic reconstruction algorithms assume that the heart remains in the same position for the entire SPECT scan.[77,78]

^{99m}Tc sestamibi image acquisition should begin at least 1 h after injection at rest in order to minimize visceral activity. After exercise, which decreases visceral activity, it is possible to begin acquisition somewhat earlier (30 min).[33] Dipyridamole and adenosine stress images are better if there is an interval of at least 1 h. It is certainly possible to wait longer (3 to 4 h) if this is needed to meet the schedules of the physician and others in the laboratory. There is a decrease in count rate due to the physical $t_{1/2}$ of ^{99m}Tc (6 h) and the cumulative effect of the slow redistribution over a prolonged period,[30,32] which will decrease image quality and contrast after several hours.

^{99m}Tc Teboroxime

^{99m}Tc teboroxime is an excellent indicator of CBF due to its high extraction fraction, which changes little over a wide range of flow rates.[38,50–52,79] Despite this major advantage, however, there are serious disadvantages due to the rapid wash-out from the heart (6 to 11 min biologic $t_{1/2}$).[38,50–52,79]

An interaction with red blood cells decreases the apparent extraction of ^{99m}Tc teboroxime.[80] Many laboratories using ^{99m}Tc teboroxime MPI position the patient on the imaging bed, perform pharmacologic stress using dypridamole or adenosine,[81] and immediately image the patient using a multidetector imaging system. A multicenter trial, however, reported good results using treadmill exercise and single-headed detector systems.[82] In this study, stress ^{99m}Tc teboroxime imaging (10 to 30 mCi) was begun 1.5 to 2 min following injection. Average imaging time was 6 min. Images at rest were acquired 1 to 2 h later. The logistical problems with ^{99m}Tc teboroxime have caused most clinical laboratories to avoid its use for MPI.

SPECT FOR MPI

SPECT images provide a three-dimensional picture of the radioactivity in the myocardium and afford excellent localization of perfusion defects and substantially better contrast than planar images. Similar to planar imaging, there are many factors that degrade SPECT MPI image quality to decrease sensitivity and specificity.[1–4,8,9,83] The increased image contrast on SPECT versus planar images allows better visualization of artifactual defects on SPECT images due to the attenuation of the photons emitted from the radioisotope in the myocardium.[2–9] *These attenuation artifacts are the major cause of decreased specificity in SPECT MPI.*[2–9,83] Artifacts arise because the conventional SPECT reconstruction program, called *filtered backprojection,* assumes that the same number of counts should be present in each projection or view of the SPECT acquisition.[6–9] In fact, for SPECT MPI, each view sees a variable number of cardiac counts because of variable attenuation through the thorax.[6–9] For example, fewer counts are acquired in LPO views than in the LAO views because of the relatively longer pathlength and resulting greater attenuation from the heart to the gamma camera in these views. Accordingly, variation in the view-to-view counts acquired from the heart means that images reconstructed with the SPECT program will not reflect the true distribution of radioactivity in the myocardium.[6–9] To a lesser degree, the degrading effects due to changes in resolution at different depths, in association with the view-to-view variation in resolution, cause image distortion to decrease specificity.[6–9] Inclusion of scattered photons in the image serves to decrease SPECT tomographic image contrast, which decreases sensitivity.[23–25]

Most of the technical limitations of SPECT result in artifactual decreases in myocardial counts, which may mimic actual perfusion defects. Observers tend to compensate for this problem by ignoring mild and/or small defects—in effect, setting more stringent threshold criteria (requiring larger and/or more severe defects) for defining a defect as abnormal. This change in threshold criteria helps reduce the rate of false-positive results (improved specificity). Understanding this approach to diagnosis is important in all areas of medicine, i.e., history, physical examinations, or interpreting any type of images. The danger of this shift to more stringent threshold criteria for defining abnormal is that it will cause the observer to miss more true-positive defects that are actually due to underperfusion (worsen sensitivity). This trade-off between the true- versus false-positive rates of a diagnostic test based on the threshold criteria for defining abnormal has been referred to as a *receiver-operator characteristic* (ROC) curve.[84,85] The false-positive rates with different criteria are usually plotted along the horizontal axis, with the corresponding true-positive rates resulting from the change in criteria plotted going up the vertical axis.[84,85] These ROC curves describe a very fundamental approach to any diagnostic maneuver in medicine—*if one tries to identify all abnormalities (true-positive), one will identify too many false-positive results.*

Acquisition Issues for SPECT MPI

The 180° anterior arc acquisition is better than the 360° acquisition because data from the highly attenuated posterior views actually degrade the SPECT image.[8,9] Images acquired from circular orbits differ from those from elliptical orbits because the distance between the camera and heart varies more in elliptical orbits.[8,9,86] Acquisition with the patient lying prone rather than supine on the imaging table appears to decrease patient motion and inferior attenuation,[87] but many obese patients do not tolerate the position, and the images of normal patients are not completely homogeneous. Accordingly, the authors have not imaged patients in the prone position for clinical purposes.

Processing Issues for SPECT MPI

SPECT Reconstruction Filter As in x-ray CT, the SPECT reconstruction algorithm uses a mathematical "filter" to create two-dimensional transaxial slices from the acquired (projection or view) data. The type of filter selected in the reconstruction program affects SPECT image quality significantly. The problem is that the physician must choose from a large number of possibilities, and a trade-off has to be made between filters that produce substantial smoothing of images to decrease noise at the expense of resolution versus "sharp" filters that produce more noise but preserve resolution. Phantom studies that evaluated the effect of different filters on defect contrast (i.e., signal/background ratio) have always favored high-resolution filters.[9] It is the authors' experience, however, that physicians like to read smoother, less noisy images. In order to balance the noise and resolution content for clinical interpretation of MPI, the authors and others have selected "intermediate" filters that produce moderate smoothing between the two extremes.

^{99m}Tc versus ^{201}Tl Because of its higher energy (140 keV versus 68 to 80 keV), ^{99m}Tc has better imaging properties than ^{201}Tl.[21–26] As mentioned above, without compensation for the attenuation of photons by the body, MPI is severely distorted,[6–9,24,25,83] and MPI in women differs from that in men.[88] Although there is less attenuation with ^{99m}Tc, the differences compared with ^{201}Tl are quite small (see Fig. 17-2). It is crucial to understand that both isotopes are affected by attenuation. As such, ^{201}Tl and ^{99m}Tc images reconstructed with conventional methodologies are distorted similarly. In fact, analysis of stress ^{99m}Tc and rest ^{201}Tl bull's-eye normal files show no significant differences (Fig. 17-4). If all other things are the same (ignoring the differences in extraction fraction), defect contrast should be better with ^{99m}Tc because it has better scatter properties and slightly better resolution than ^{201}Tl.[24,25]

Attenuation Correction The implementation of methods to

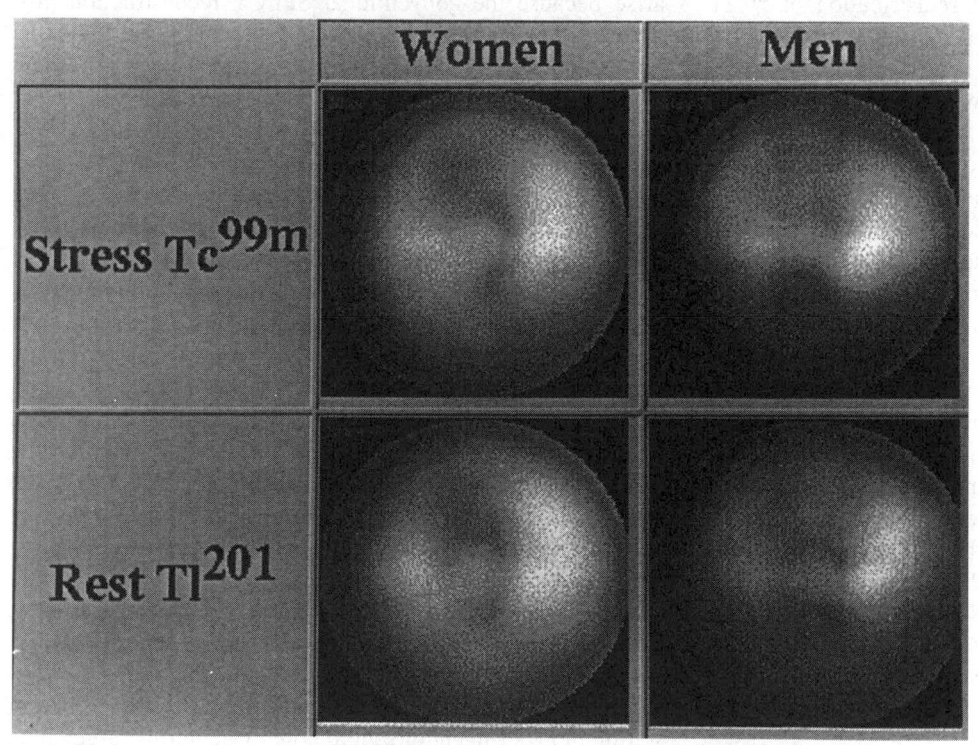

FIGURE 17-4

The bull's-eye display synthesizes the count data from the reconstructed SPECT short-axis slices. Information about the count distribution at the apex appears at the center of the bull's-eye, and information about the counts at the base are shown at the peripheral edge. The lateral wall is on the right, the septal wall on the left, the anterior wall on top, and the inferior wall on the bottom of the display. The figure shows dual-isotope normal file bull's-eye displays from 25 men and 29 women with low probability of coronary artery disease. For each gender, the rest SPECT ^{201}Tl and stress SPECT ^{99m}Tc sestamibi normal files are virtually identical. (R. L. Eisner, personal communication.)

compensate for the degrading effects of photon attenuation inside the body (i.e., attenuation correction) should improve SPECT MPI, as shown by the fact that attenuation-corrected positron emission tomography (PET) MPI has much higher sensitivity and specificity than SPECT MPI, according to the literature[89,90] and the authors' own experience.[91–93] Attenuation correction has been studied for many years,[24,25,94–96] and several manufacturers have now introduced attenuation correction software. The attenuation correction process requires two sets of data to be acquired: (1) the conventional MPI dataset (called the *emission dataset*), and (2) a dataset (called the *transmission dataset*) acquired using a radioactive source whose photon emissions pass through the patient and into the gamma camera. The SPECT MPI emission data (i.e., conventional MPI scan) are acquired either simultaneously or close in time to the transmission data. The transmission data from each slice are reconstructed to produce an image, or map, of the attenuation coefficients for that slice.[94,95] This image resembles an x-ray CT image. Reconstruction of attenuation-compensated images uses the attenuation map to correct the emission image for the degrading effects of attenuation. The reconstruction program for attenuation correction is much more complicated than the conventional reconstruction (filtered backprojection) program.[94,95] Basically, the program "guesses" initially at the radioactivity distribution in the myocardium, simulates the SPECT imaging process, and projects this distribution through the attenuating medium (as determined by the reconstruction of the transmission data) to produce a first guess about the count distribution in each view of the SPECT study. Then, the differences between the actual data and simulated projected data are backprojected through the attenuating medium to produce a better guess for the radioactivity distribution in the myocardium. This process of projection and backprojection is repeated over and over (iteratively) until the actual data agree with the projected data.[95] Initial results with attenuation compensation are quite encouraging[94,95] (see "Future Developments," below).

Processing/Quantitative Analysis for MPI

The revolution in computer technology has been a great boon to handling radionuclide myocardial images. Processing of 32 to 64 planar views acquired at known angles to reconstruct a tomographic (SPECT) three-dimensional image of the heart is now accomplished quickly (seconds). Continued improvements are reducing the subjectivity of operator interaction, e.g., automatic slice selection for SPECT reconstruction of the left ventricle and automatic oblique angle reconstruction to produce short-axis and vertical and horizontal long-axis slices. Counts per picture element (pixel) in the left ventricle on rest and stress can be normalized systematically to show the same brightness for the pixel with the most counts. Normalization of images allows the use of human skills and experience for synthesizing large amounts of visual information to compare two images.[97]

The major benefit of computers for SPECT MPI is the ability to quantitate counts in different regions of the heart.[98,99] This quantitation allows one to define precisely the range of normal[88] and the criteria for distinguishing normal from abnormal.[85,88,98,99] As discussed previously, without appropriate compensation, SPECT images of the heart are degraded due to the effects of attenuation, resolution, and scatter.[6–9] Thus, independent of variations in cardiac physiologic (e.g., blood flow) or anatomic (e.g., myocardial wall thickness) parameters in patients, differences in SPECT MPI are expected because differences in body habitus create differences in attenuation. In lieu of correcting the data for the degrading effects, it has proven quite valuable to compare the patient images to a normal database of individuals without heart disease.[88,98,99] *The authors found that the normal reference databases for SPECT ^{201}Tl imaging had to be gender-specific (i.e., one normal database for women and another for men) due to gender differences in images of normal persons.*[88,98] Such normal databases must be derived from individuals who can be classified as free of heart disease, based on criteria that are completely independent of the myocardial images per se.[85,88] It is customary to use the history, physical examination, resting ECG, and, preferably, also exercise ECG data, which can be compared to previous large-scale experiences such as the Framingham Heart Study to define a probability of CAD (Fig. 17-5).[85,88,100,101] These criteria can define individuals as "normal" (<5 percent or 10 percent probability

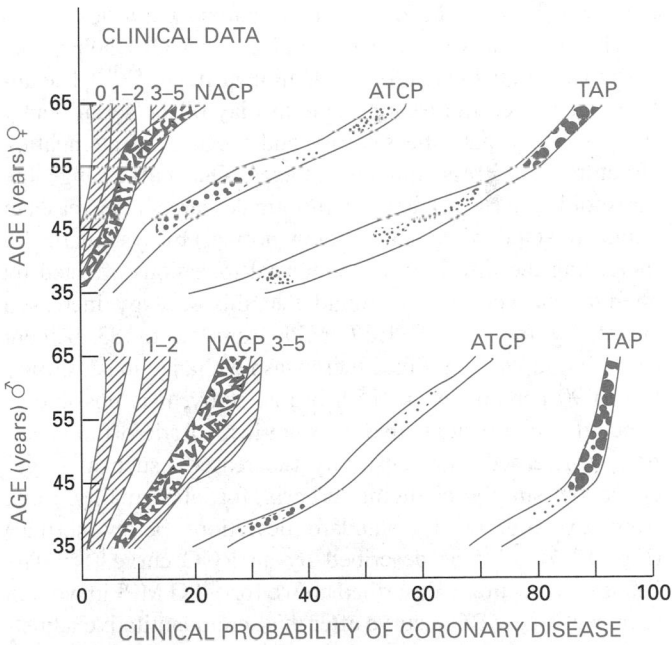

FIGURE 17-5

Use of clinical data to estimate the probability of coronary artery disease (CAD). Women are shown in the upper panel, men are shown in the lower panel with age (increasing up the vertical axis). Number of risk factors for asymptomatic people (0 to 5 of the following: diabetes mellitus, hyperlipidemia, hypertension, smoking, and resting ECG ST-T abnormality). Symptoms are chest pain that is nonanginal (NACP), atypical (ATCP), or typical angina pectoris (TAP). The probability of CAD increases from left to right, and 95 percent confidence intervals are shown as the widths of the bar based on data from the Framingham study. (From Patterson and Horowitz.[85] Reproduced with permission of the publisher and authors.)

of CAD) to define the expected range of distributions of myocardial counts (usually expressed as the mean ± standard deviations).

Each individual new patient's MPI, then, can be compared pixel by pixel with the gender-specific normal file, and defects defined as those regions that fall a predetermined number of standard deviations (e.g., 2 to 4) below the mean value in the normal file.[98,99] The advantage of using standard deviations rather than percent decrease in counts compared to the normal region in that patient is that the standard deviation accounts for expected decreases in counts in regions usually influenced by attenuation in persons of the same gender.[98,99] For example, for men and women it has been shown that SPECT MPI (both ^{201}Tl and ^{99m}Tc) normal files show a relative decrease of counts in the septum compared to the lateral wall (i.e., "hot" lateral wall),[88] consistent with predictions based on the physics of SPECT imaging.[7,8] Men show a decrease of counts in the inferior wall, usually due to the diaphragm, which is not seen in normal women, due to offsetting anterior attenuation by breast tissue.[88] Expressing reversibility in terms of the percent change in counts, or the change in standard deviations away from normal, between stress and rest can assist in assessing myocardial viability.[88,102,103] Quantitative algorithms can also help identify regions with different defect severity and/or different degrees of reversibility to help distinguish whether one defect might contain myocardium dependent on one, two, or more different stenotic coronary arteries.

The quantitative grading of defects can also help make systematic adjustments for attenuation artifacts.[93,104] The authors have used the rotating cine display of the serial planar images to estimate the severity and location of attenuating structures on stress and rest images. One can change the threshold criteria for abnormal/normal (percent decrease in counts or standard deviation below normal) by systematically increasing the threshold for abnormal in regions affected by attenuation. The authors found that this strategy increased specificity of ^{201}Tl SPECT MPI from 58 to 83 percent ($p < .05$) in women. Since there was no change in sensitivity (95 to 90 percent, p = N.S.) in this study, it is possible to conclude that this maneuver was not just a trade-off of specificity (increased) for sensitivity (decreased), such as might occur by simply changing criteria for abnormality (e.g., from 2.0, 3.0, or 4.0 standard deviations below normal) (Fig. 17-6),[93,104] as described by an ROC curve.[84,85] The changes in accuracy described above for ^{201}Tl MPI in women represent a new ROC curve after this semiquantitative adjustment for attenuation—not just moving from one point to another along the same ROC curve.[84,85,93,104]

The display of this quantitative information about myocardial perfusion requires simplification, rather than showing the overwhelming number of oblique angle–reconstructed tomographic slices or table after table of numbers. One of the most useful displays is a bull's-eye display (Fig. 17-4), which represents the count distribution of the serial short-axis slices with the apex at the center to the base at the peripheral edge in a polar map representation.[53,98] Figures

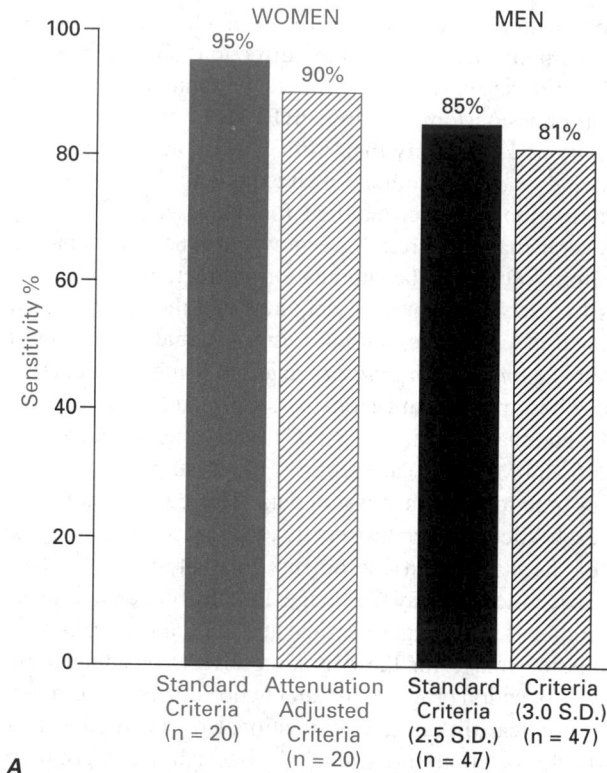

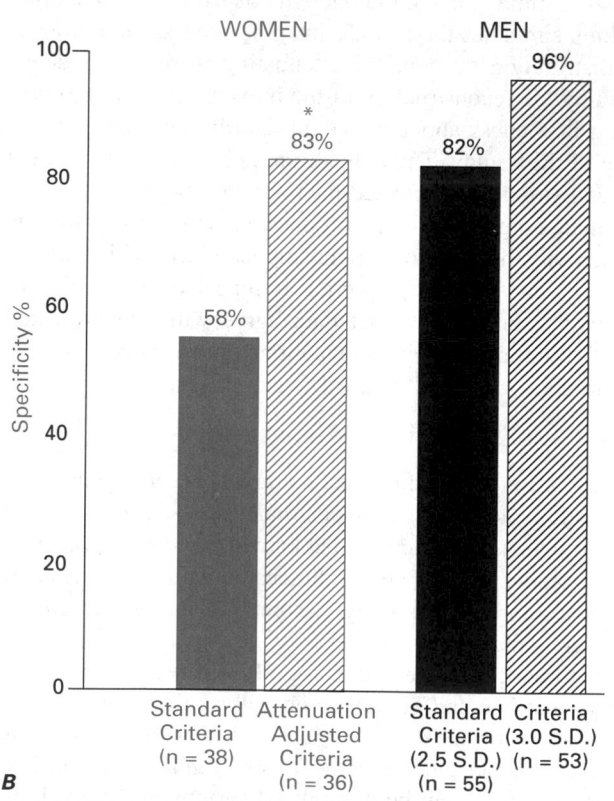

FIGURE 17-6

Effect of semiquantitative correction for attenuation on sensitivity (*A*) and specificity (*B*) of exercise SPECT ^{201}Tl, based on adjusting criteria for defining an abnormality based on estimated severity (0 to 4+) and location of attenuation artifacts. Note the large increase in specificity (*B*) in women without changing sensitivity (*A*). (From Patterson et al.[104] Reproduced with permission of the publisher and authors.)

17-7; 17-8, colorPlate 45; 17-9, color Plate 46; and 17-10, color Plate 47 explain the quantitative bull's-eye displays and show results from representative patient studies using a modern quantitative processing and display program that uses the bull's-eye display format.

^{201}Tl MPI also provides useful information about cardiac size and function. Analysis of ^{201}Tl uptake by lung relative to heart on stress versus rest can identify exercise-induced LV dysfunction and a poor prognosis.[105] If LV diastolic pressure rises during exercise, it will transmit backward to the left atrium, pulmonary veins, and pulmonary capillaries. At a certain level of pulmonary capillary pressure, fluid and ^{201}Tl will leak from the vascular to the extracellular fluid space, where it is recorded as an increase in ^{201}Tl activity in lung relative to the heart.[105] Increased lung ^{201}Tl uptake is often associated with enlargement of the LV cavity on immediate postexercise images, in comparison to the resting images—another sign of LV dysfunction and a poor prognosis.[106,107]

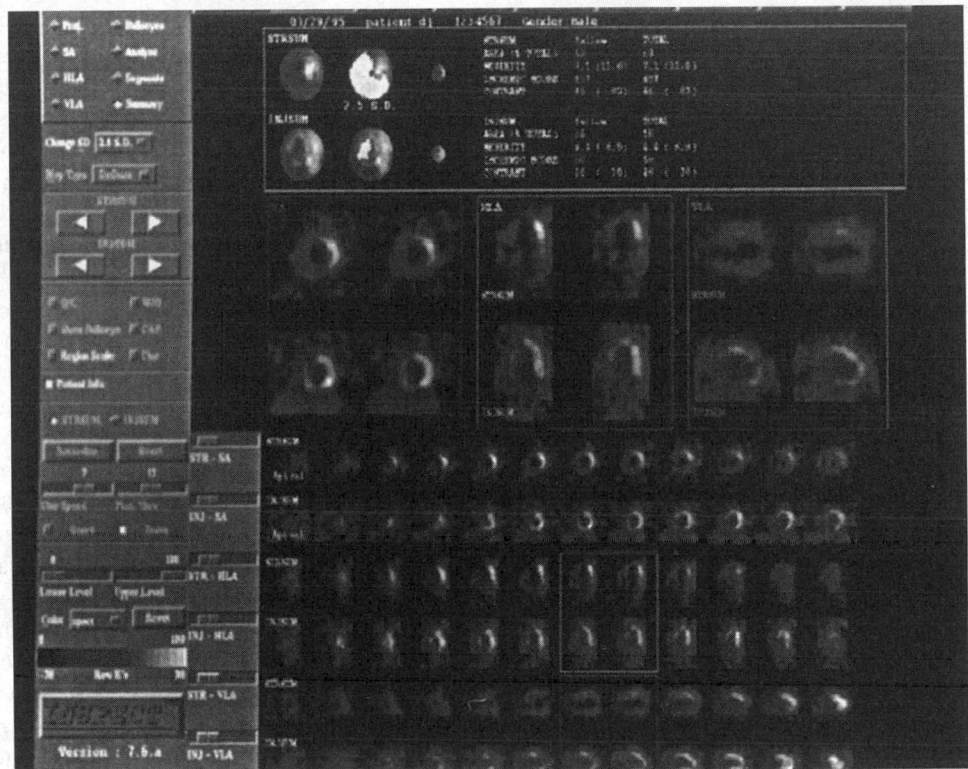

FIGURE 17-7
Summary review screen from INSPECT program for quantitative analysis and display of SPECT Tl^{201} myocardial perfusion images (MPI). Bull's-eye displays are shown (*top left*) along with quantitative information on extent and severity of defects (*top right*). Short-axis, vertical long-axis, and horizontal long-axis slices are displayed in subsequent rows, with stress images on top and reinjection images on the bottom. These images show a large, severe anterior-septal and inferior defect on stress, involving 65 percent of the left ventricle, that improves dramatically at rest.

ECG-Gated Acquisition of SPECT MPI

Gated MPI to create 8 to 16 sequential images over each cardiac cycle can create a display to analyze global and regional contraction and myocardial wall thickening of the left and right ventricles.[46,47,108] These images resemble echocardiographic or magnetic resonance images of the ventricular wall, and they can be viewed qualitatively or quantitatively to measure regional wall motion and wall thickening (change in counts between the end-diastolic and the end-systolic frames).[46,47,108] Global left ventricular ejection fraction (LVEF) can also be quantitated by measurements of cavity size in three-dimensional SPECT, and these measurements

FIGURE 17-8
See color Plate 45.

FIGURE 17-9
See color Plate 46.

FIGURE 17-10
See color Plate 47.

correlate with other methods.[109] The gated MPI are often superior to echocardiographic images, gated blood pool images (GBPI), or contrast x-ray ventriculography for measurement of right ventricular function.

Gated SPECT myocardial images are better with ^{99m}Tc sestamibi than with ^{201}Tl due to the higher count rate and statistical reliability. Gated SPECT or gated planar myocardial images, however, can be acquired and analyzed with SPECT ^{201}Tl. Addition of the data at each time in the cardiac cycle for each planar view of the tomographic acquisition provides images as if they had been acquired in the conventional ungated mode. Thus, the conventional SPECT acquisition is not compromised when gated SPECT data are acquired, and no additional acquisition time is needed.

Gated SPECT images can be reconstructed using conventional software to produce transaxial, short-axis, and vertical and horizontal long-axis slices. The software must have the option that all reconstruction and reorientation parameters (e.g., angles, slice limits), defined by the operator, for a set of images from one phase of the cardiac cycle can be transposed automatically by the software to the other phases of the cardiac cycle in order to avoid having to process each of the 8 to 16 sets of images separately. Even though the spatial resolution of nuclear SPECT imaging is poor (on the order of 16 mm),

SPECT-gated studies provide data about wall thickening. Actually, the gated studies provide information about count changes over the cardiac cycle, which is related to wall thickening over the cardiac cycle.[46,47,86]

Analysis of regional LV wall thickening provides a potential way to assess viability within a defect on MPI.[47] The problem for myocardial perfusion tracers is the very low count rate in the defect due to the low flow rates, which makes it difficult to acquire adequate images of the wall. Indeed, one preliminary study has shown that measurement of regional wall thickening within fixed defects was absent in about half the gated SPECT ^{99m}Tc sestamibi images that actually showed the presence of wall thickening on gated magnetic resonance imaging.[110] The analysis of SPECT MPI during each phase of the cardiac cycle may also improve the accuracy of SPECT by eliminating artifacts due to motion of the heart. Also, fixed defects on stress and rest imaging, which show count changes (wall thickening) over the cardiac cycle, are most likely artifacts caused by attenuation.

It is important to remember that, even though the radiopharmaceutical is injected under conditions of stress, the "stress"-gated SPECT images are actually acquired under resting conditions, several minutes to a few hours after stress. Thus, wall motion abnormalities elicited by stress may recover by the time the gated SPECT images are obtained.[71]

Clinical Applications of MPI

MPI DURING STRESS AND REST (See Table 17-4)

In patients with known or suspected CAD, stress/rest MPI has been found to be a remarkably powerful tool to answer the following clinical questions.[85] (1) Does the patient have myocardial ischemia or infarction? To explain symptoms? Or silent? (2) Is the anatomic coronary artery stenosis (seen angiographically) physiologically significant? (3) Is there sufficient viable myocardium to justify invasive revascularization of the myocardium? (4) Does the patient have a good or poor prognosis? (5) Has a therapeutic measure improved MPI?

Question 1 Does the patient have myocardial ischemia or infarction (Table 17-5)? SPECT MPI with stress and rest has shown a good sensitivity and specificity to answer this question in women and men (Figs. 17-6, 17-11, 17-12).[1-5,43,93,123-127] A wide range of values of sensitivity and specificity are likely to have been reported for any test. It is essential to analyze critically several aspects of the design of any study performed to determine accuracy of the test.[85] The impact of the most important aspects of study design are shown in Table 17-5.

The physician must know the test result, the sensitivity and specificity of the test in that institution, and the patient's clinical history. Figure 17-12 shows sensitivity and specificity values for SPECT ^{201}Tl from the literature, and Fig. 17-6 shows values obtained in the authors' laboratory. It is helpful to estimate quantitatively the patient's pretest probability of disease, based on the individual patient's risk factors and clinical history (Fig. 17-5).[85,100,105] Then, the physician can estimate the predictive value of a positive or negative result of the test in the individual patient[85] (Fig. 17-13) using Bayes' theorem, assuming that sensitivity and specificity are not influenced by prevalence of disease.[85,100,128-131] Alternatively, one can use a nomogram based on multivariate analysis of a large data base, but this approach assumes that the individual patient resembles the population in the data base used to develop the nomogram.[101] One can even use these methods (Bayes' theorem or tables reflecting multivariate analysis) to combine the results of the exercise ECG and exercise SPECT to predict the final probability of CAD in the individual patient[85,100,132,133] (see Fig. 17-13). *Before ordering the test, the physician should consider what step might be recommended if the patient has a particular result, e.g., whether to refer the patient for coronary angiography if the final probability of CAD is over 10, 20, 40, or 80 percent.* For example, the 55-year-old man with typical angina pectoris (pretest likelihood of CAD of 90 percent) should proceed directly to coronary angiography. On the other hand, the 45-year-old man with no symptoms or risk factors should have no tests for CAD. *Stress/rest MPI is obviously most useful for patients with intermediate likelihoods of CAD.* The physician would, appropriately, be more likely to recommend coronary angiography if the defect size is large (over 15 percent of the left ventricle), if symptoms require hospital admission, if functional aerobic capacity is low, and if the patient's occupation could place other people at risk (bus driver) and if the patient is relatively healthy otherwise.

Question 2 Is an anatomic stenosis physiologically significant? This question has obvious clinical importance because it helps to determine whether to recommend revascularization.[85,134] It is particularly useful to correlate symptoms and functional aerobic capacity for exercise with the objective results of SPECT MPI. Especially in this situation, it is very useful for the physician to interpret the SPECT MPI without knowing the clinical, angiographic, or exercise test data, i.e., the physician is "blinded."[85,97] Some studies show greater benefit of revascularization in patients with objective evidence of ischemia, and, indeed, *demonstrating objective evidence of ischemia has been recommended as a prerequisite to percutaneous transluminal coronary angioplasty (PTCA).*[135] SPECT MPI is more accurate in identifying ischemia than is exercise ECG.[54] Several studies show that patients with MPI evidence of ischemia show greater benefit of revascularization than do patients without MPI evidence of ischemia[135]—partly because those patients with no ischemia on MPI have a better prognosis without revascularization than do patients with ischemia on MPI.[136-139] Other approaches to assessing the functional significance of anatomic lesions have been tried, but they also have drawbacks. Invasive measurement of coronary pressure[140] and blood flow velocity reserve[141] are elegant physiologically, but the catheter across the lesion may obstruct flow, and the measurements need correlation with symptoms and outcomes. Third-party payers have shown interest in the

TABLE 17-4

CLINICAL QUESTIONS IN CORONARY ARTERY DISEASE (CAD) TO BE ANSWERED BY STRESS/REST SPECT MPI

Question	Specific Needs	Comparison with Other Modalities	Clinical Value
Diagnosis of presence of coronary atherosclerotic heart disease (myocardial ischemia)	Need adequate stress	1. Exercise ECG is much less accurate 2. Stress echo is less sensitive 3. Angiogram is more accurate (more risk)	1. Best (after PET MPI) for patients with CAD $p = .1-.7$ 2. Attenuation problems in women and large people
Physiologic significance of anatomic CAD	Exercise is best to correlate symptoms	1. Exercise ECG is less accurate 2. Stress echo is difficult during exercise	1. Best to decide on PTCA or CABG 2. Correlate symptoms
Viability of myocardium	1. ^{201}Tl rest is best (except PET ^{18}FDG) 2. Gated for regional LV contraction	1. Stress echo requires capturing regional LV contraction increase at low level stress and decrease at higher level stress 2. Less accurate	1. Best to decide on PTCA or CABG 2. Correlate LV function on gated MPI
Prognosis of CAD	1. Best with exercise 2. Gated for global LV function	1. Exercise ECG is more variable 2. Stress echo has limited validation 3. Angiogram shows similar prediction of prognosis	1. Excellent 2. Correlate with exercise capacity and LV function
Response to therapy	1. Best with exercise (compare hemodynamic responses) 2. Best if compared with similar, prior study	1. Exercise ECG can be helpful 2. Stress echo has limited validation	1. Correlate with symptoms, exercise capacity, LV function, and hemodynamics

Note: ECG, electrocardiogram; echo, echocardiography; PET, positron emission tomography; PTCA, percutaneous transluminal coronary angiography; CABG, coronary artery bypass graft.

indications for revascularization, and some seek documentation of ischemia as an indication for elective revascularization.

Question 3 *Does the patient have sufficient viable myocardium to justify revascularization?* In patients with prior MI and/or congestive heart failure (CHF) and CAD, this question is pivotal to deciding whether or not to recommend revascularization.[72–75,103] Viable myocardium is the surviving tissue in the subepicardium overlying the infarcted (nonviable) tissue in the subendocardium[103,117,142,143] (Fig. 17-14). Only viable myocardium can improve its function after blood flow is restored. Even a "transmural" MI rarely extends its "wavefront" through the full thickness of the wall of the left ventricle, and the key question is how much myocardium remains viable.[103,117,142,143] The viable myocardium may consist of one or a mixture of three categories: (1) acutely ischemic (which over time will evolve and change to a different category), (2) "stunned" (the prolonged abnormality of regional contraction that follows reperfusion after a brief period of ischemia[144] or (3) "hibernating" (the chronic impairment of cardiac contraction that reduces myocardial metabolic demands to a level that matches the reduced myocardial oxygen supply to prevent ischemia)[145] (see Chap. 43).

All three of these categories of viable myocardium show reduced contractile performance, reduced utilization of free fatty acids for aerobic metabolism, and increased utilization of glucose for anaerobic metabolism.[103,104–146] The abnormalities of ischemic myocardium return toward normal gradually after blood flow is restored, and the myocardium has been termed *stunned* during this recovery phase by Braunwald and Kloner.[144] These abnormalities are easily demonstrated in animal models. Hibernating myocardium, on the other hand, is corrected almost immediately after restoration of blood flow, e.g., during coronary artery bypass graft (CABG) surgery.[145] Hibernating myocardium, however, is a concept used to explain clinical events but has remained difficult to demonstrate experimentally.[103,145]

These categories and concepts about myocardial viability help explain why some—but not all—patients with CAD and CHF show improved LV function after successful PTCA or

TABLE 17-5

FACTORS INFLUENCING REPORTED ACCURACY OF DIAGNOSTIC TEST (DxT)

Patient selection	
Referral bias	If patients are selected because they had the DxT plus a reference or "gold standard" test (GST), e.g., SPECT plus coronary angiogram, then
	Patients with negative (−) results of DxT will rarely be referred for GST, thus
	Reported sensitivity (SENS) will increase (small effect), and
	Reported specificity (SPCF) will decrease (large effect), and
	Rate of equivocal or nondiagnostic (Ndx) results of DxT will increase
Prevalence of disease in population tested	Changes in prevalence have no effect on SENS and SPCF of the DxT, unless:
	DxT is interpreted by observers who are not blinded;
	Criteria of normal vs. abnormal results were developed in a population that is very different from the patient
	Prevalence has a major impact on (+) or (−) predictive value (PV):
	Increasing prevalence:
	Increases (+) PV
	Decreases (−) PV
Blinded observers	If observers who interpret DxT or GST are not blinded, then the results may be influenced unintentionally, i.e., unblinded observers would be more likely to interpret a test as (+) in a patient with a higher pretest likelihood of disease
Criteria for normal vs. abnormal, equivocal or nondiagnostic (Ndx) results	Need to be defined explicitly, e.g., qualitative, quantitative
	Need to know if SENS and SPCF are calculated after excluding Ndx results
	Need to know frequency of Ndx results
	If Ndx results are excluded before calculating SENS and SPCF, and Ndx rate increases, then calculated SENS and SPCF will both increase
Number (n) of patients tested	Too small a number (n) of patients can render calculations meaningless
	Calculate confidence intervals (CI) to show the range of values to be expected
Multicenter trial	Readers often believe that a study involving more than one center will have more explicit criteria and built-in "watchdogs" to assure validity
Population selection	Excluding women, large people, and older people may help apparent test accuracy
	Including prior myocardial infarction helps apparent test SENS
Sponsorship and the appearance of bias	If results show merit for a product that sponsors the trial, then authors need extra precautions to avoid even the appearance of bias

CABG.[72–75,103,145,146] The "gold standard" method for clinical definition of myocardial viability is to observe improved regional LV contraction after revascularization.[72–75,103,146] The goal is to assess myocardial viability to help decide which patient with CAD and CHF is likely to benefit from revascularization. In patients with only a small amount of viable myocardium, LV function will derive little or no benefit despite restoring blood flow (Fig. 17-14B). CABG, especially, poses such a stress that patients with little viable myocardium will derive little benefit and are likely to suffer the highest rate of perioperative complications and death.[150,209] Conversely, patients with a large amount of viable myocardium (Fig. 17-14A) will derive a large benefit from PTCA or CABG[110–113,147–151] (see Chap. 20). These patients are likely to suffer lower rates of complications and death because their LV function will improve. Even those patients with CHF after MI who have classic angina pectoris may need viability assessment because the angina may be arising from a small

amount of viable myocardium, e.g., <10 percent of the left ventricle that is dependent on one small but stenotic arterial branch, while the CHF results from a prior large MI with little viable myocardium. In such cases, one might revascularize the small branch by PTCA to alleviate angina, but one would not recommend CABG designed to revascularize the infarct-related arteries in addition to the small branch.

As discussed above, ^{201}Tl MPI after stress with 3- to 6-h delay rest (redistribution) images may detect fewer than one-half of the LV segments that will actually show improved contraction after successful revascularization.[72–75,103] If ^{201}Tl is reinjected at rest after 2 to 3 h this "booster dose" delivers more ^{201}Tl to the viable myocardium overlying the MI defect and decreases the contrast on MPI between the defect and the normal zone, compared to stress or 3- to 6-h delay rest (redistribution) images.[110–113] This method appears to detect improvement between stress and rest in half or more of the LV segments that showed no improvement between stress

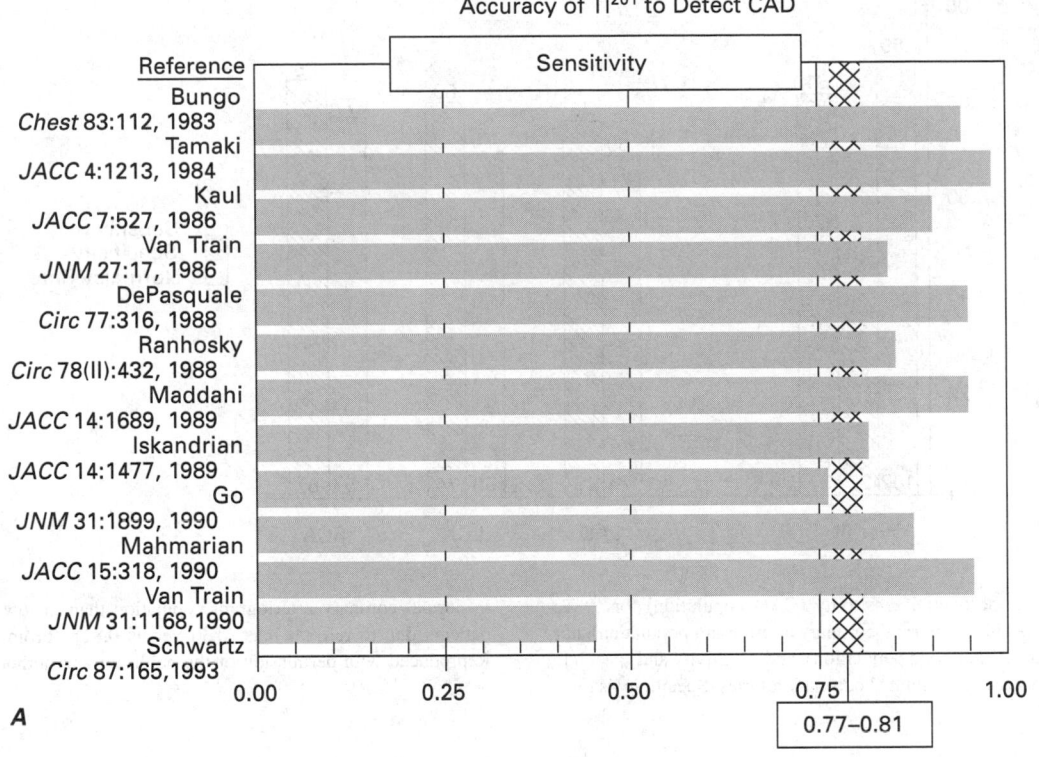

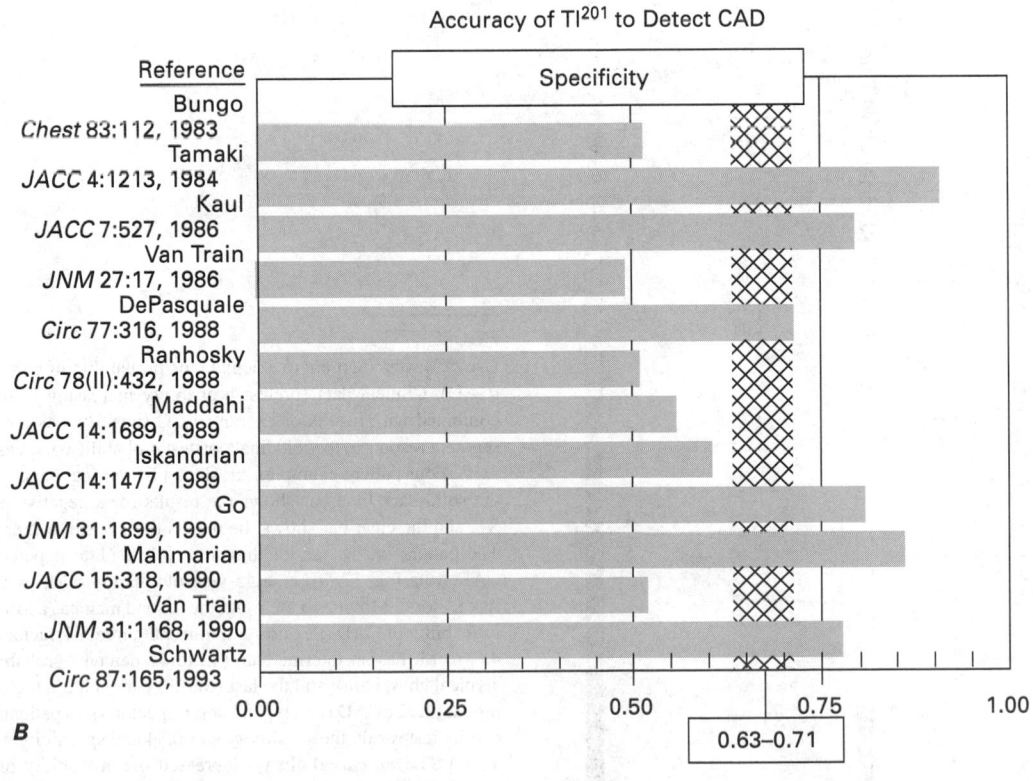

FIGURE 17-11

Comparison of the sensitivity (*A*) and specificity (*B*) of SPECT ^{201}Tl to detect coronary artery disease. The first author and reference are shown on the left, and the horizontal bar graph shows the percent value. The 95 percent confidence interval is shown by the width of the vertical line. (From Patterson et al.[104] Reproduced with permission of the publisher and author.)

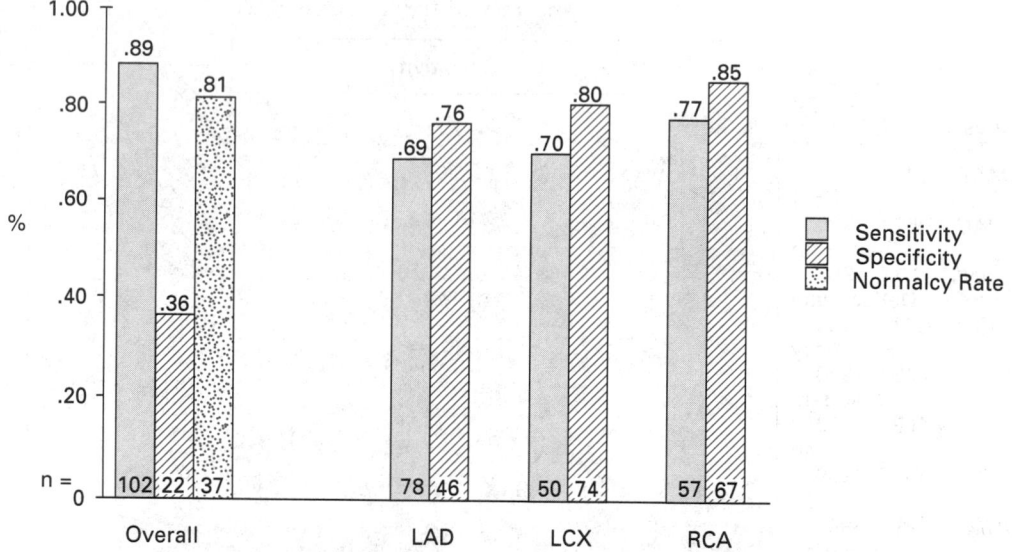

FIGURE 17-12

Combined results for the overall sensitivity (CAD population) for ⁹⁹ᵐTc-sestamibi SPECT, specificity (normal coronary arteriogram population), normalcy rate (low clinical likelihood population), and sensitivity and specificity for localization of disease in individual coronary arteries. Specificity is lower in normal coronary arteriogram population than in low clinical likelihood patients due to referral bias (0.36 versus 0.81). (From Van Train et al.[43] Reproduced with permission of the publisher and authors.)

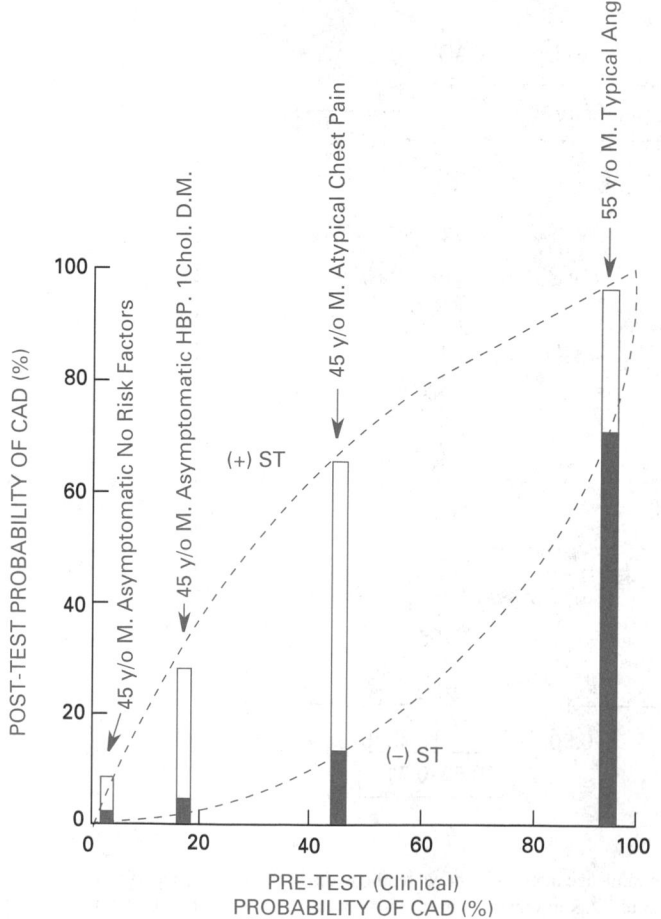

FIGURE 17-13

Use of Bayes' theorem to calculate the probability of coronary artery disease (CAD). Clinical data (pretest probability increasing from left to right) are combined with results of exercise ECG [positive (+) or negative (−) ST-segment response] to yield final posttest probability (increasing up the vertical axis). Four patient examples are shown by vertical bars, where the height of the solid dark blue bar shows the results for a negative exercise ECG (−) ST, and the clear bar shows the results for a positive exercise ECG (+) ST. The patient on the far left has a very low (1 to 4 percent) probability of CAD from Fig. 17-5 [i.e., a 45-year-old man (y/o M.) with no symptoms or risk factors]. Moving to the right, the second man has a low (15 to 18 percent) probability of CAD (i.e., no symptoms but three risk factors). The next (third) 45 y/o M. has an intermediate (42 to 47 percent) probability of CAD (i.e., atypical chest pain); and the last (fourth) patient has a high (89 to 92 percent) probability of CAD (i.e., typical angina pectoris). In patients with a diagnostic quality test result, the sensitivity was 0.84 and specificity was 0.62. Although a (+) ST (*top curve*) always increased the probability of CAD above that found with a (−) ST (*lower curve*), the posttest or final probability of CAD was much higher when the clinical data suggested a higher pretest probability of disease. (From Patterson et al.[85] Reproduced with permission of the publisher and authors.)

and 3- to 6-h redistribution images. An alternative approach has been to acquire late-delay (late-redistribution) images 16 to 24 h after a single injection during stress. This approach requires prolonged acquisition times in order to get reasonable counting statistics, and it requires another trip to the department on a different day. Neither is popular with patients. Most importantly, this method appears to detect improvement in the MPI defect less often than does reinjection at rest.[72–75,103] Improvement in the ^{201}Tl MPI defect on late delay (late redistribution) at 16 to 24 h can occur after the reinjection dose at 3 to 4 h after the stress injection.[72,73] It is possible that the improvement between the initial and late reinjection images was due to image acquisition beginning too early, i.e., 10 min after reinjection. Image acquisition beginning 30 min after ^{201}Tl reinjection at rest would be expected to show more improvement than the 10-min image and reduce the need for the 16- to 24-h delay (redistribution) image.[103]

Reinjection protocols[72–75] present a challenge to devise the most efficient strategy.[103] Is it necessary to acquire delay-redistribution images on everyone after stress ^{201}Tl, first, and then decide whether reinjection is needed? This strategy will minimize the number of reinjection procedures but will require delays for the patient, physician, and staff so as to acquire, process, and interpret stress and redistribution images promptly in order to perform reinjection procedures in a timely fashion. Even so, delays are unavoidable, and availability of ^{201}Tl reinjection doses is problematic. Keeping doses always available will lead to wasting unused doses, and getting doses only when needed will lead to more delays and probably missing some reinjection procedures that would have been helpful. On the other hand, if all patients are reinjected without first checking the redistribution image, there will be many unnecessary rein-

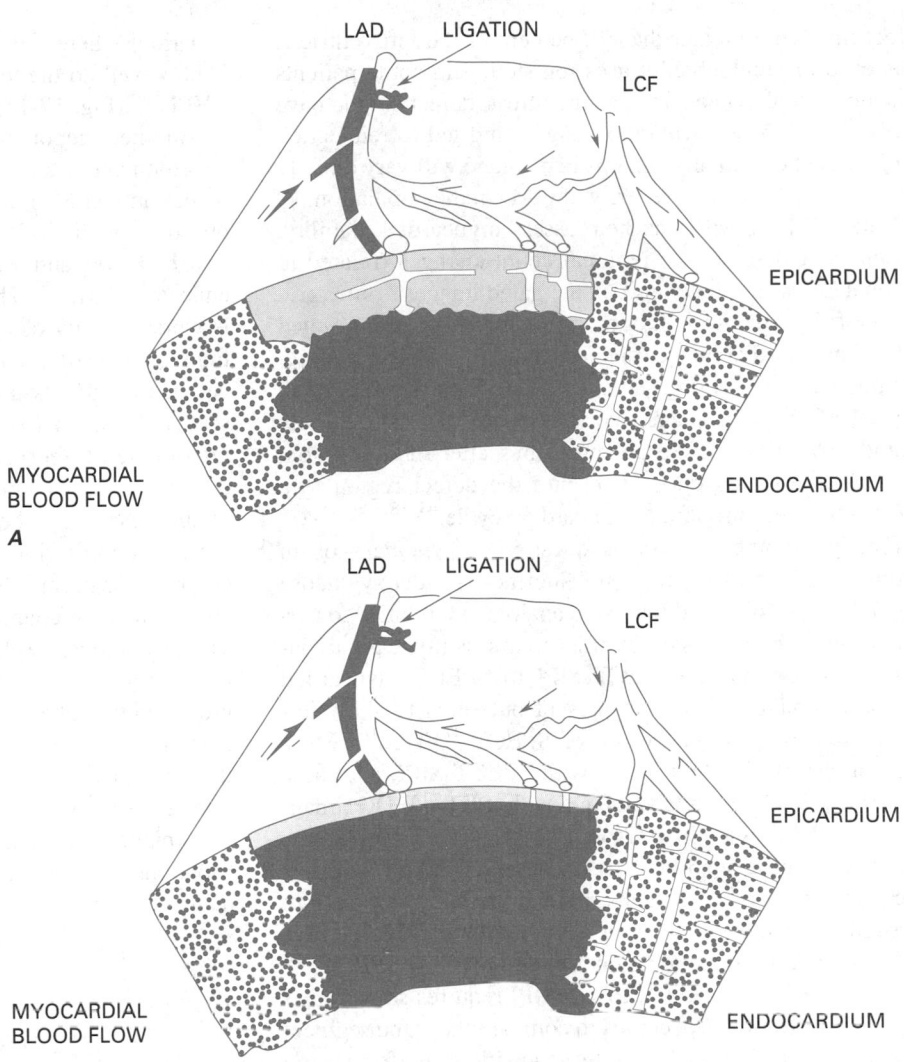

FIGURE 17-14

These diagrams of the left ventricular wall show the three-dimensional geometry of myocardial infarction (MI) that is the basis for understanding myocardial viability. The left anterior descending (LAD) coronary artery on the epicardial surface has been occluded to create MI. The MI is shown as the solid blue area, beginning at the endocardial surface and progressing over 50 percent of the wall thickness toward the epicardium in *A* and about 90 percent of the wall thickness toward the epicardial surface in *B*. Viable myocardium is the tissue shown between the darkly shaded MI and the epicardial surface. The dots shown in the tissue on either side of the MI represent microspheres used to measure blood flow, and their density is proportional to blood flow. Density is lower (to indicate reduced flow) in the viable myocardium in the epicardial distribution of the occluded LAD artery compared to the surrounding normal tissue. The presence of a larger region receiving perfusion in the epicardial viable tissue overlying the MI in *A* would produce a milder defect on resting myocardial perfusion images and much more flourine-18-deoxyglucose uptake as measured by PET, indicating viable myocardium (see Chap. 20). The diagram shows much more viable myocardium in the epicardium overlying the MI in *A* than in *B*, so that successful revascularization should cause much more recovery of contraction of the wall in *A* than in *B*. LCF, left circumflex. (Modified from Kirk and Jennings.[142] Reproduced with permission of the publisher and authors.)

jection procedures. We assessed the 3-h redistribution images in 300 consecutive patients in our laboratory and found that reinjection images were needed in 19 to 26 percent, depending on criteria for the size of the fixed defect on the redistribution images and the presence and severity of attenuation artifacts.[103] Criteria could be developed from the stress images to predict which patients might need reinjection, e.g., a stress defect involving greater than 10 percent of the left ventricle. This criterion undoubtedly uses reinjection in some patients who don't really need it, i.e., the stress defect might have resolved on 3-h redistribution images, and led to reinjection in 35 percent of patients, but this percentage will vary directly with the prevalence and severity of CAD in the population.[103]

Gated SPECT MPI can help assess myocardial viability, especially if one can see regional count changes (related to regional LV wall thickening) on the gated images.[47] Interpretation of regional wall motion and thickening using gated SPECT myocardial images depends not only on local contraction but also on counting statistics, the motion of the heart in and out of the slice plane, the rotation of the left ventricle around its long axis, and problems from scatter and resolution, which blur normal zone counts into the defect region to a different degree throughout the cardiac cycle.[47,48,109]

Finally, another important question is whether—or in whom—imaging metabolism [of fluorine-18 2-deoxyglucose (^{18}FDG) or radiolabeled fatty acid analogues], relative to perfusion, might be necessary in order to assess myocardial viability. Comparisons of SPECT MPI to SPECT myocardial metabolic images are few at present but seem to show improved sensitivity with the use of SPECT ^{18}FDG.[147] More data compare PET ^{18}FDG MPI with SPECT MPI, and these data show a clear-cut advantage with PET ^{18}FDG imaging[72–75,148–151] (see Chap. 20).

Some of these viability studies deserve careful analysis. One good study of 14 patients divided the left ventricle into 27 segments, and the relative distribution of ^{18}FDG PET was compared to the relative distribution of ^{201}Tl SPECT.[150] Comparing PET ^{18}FDG to SPECT MPI requires some rather difficult registration procedures to compare the same segment of the left ventricle on separate acquisitions performed on the different imaging modalities used for SPECT, PET, and contraction measurements. The study measured perfusion by oxygen-15-water PET studies that provide an excellent flow tracer to measure absolute CHF per gram of myocardium.[150] The oxygen-15-water PET myocardial images, however, are of low quality, partly due to the need to subtract activity from the cardiac chambers, and these studies are difficult to compare with studies using PET ^{18}FDG. Substantial agreement was found between relative distributions of ^{201}Tl and ^{18}FDG.[150] It appeared that only 22 percent of segments with fixed defects on ^{201}Tl showed much ^{18}FDG activity to suggest viability. Very few patients (3 to 5 percent) showed severely decreased ^{18}FDG activity in regions with substantial ^{201}Tl activity.[150] Other studies[146,151] define viability on PET as a mismatch between perfusion and metabolism—rather than comparing relative counts in different regions for ^{18}FDG versus ^{201}Tl[150]—which does not utilize the main benefit of metabolic imaging.[146,151] In reviewing studies that compare different modalities to assess myocardial viability, it is important to recall the clinical relevance of the study. If a patient has a small defect and/or normal or only mild impairment of LV function, then viability is not the important question. It appears that most modalities perform best to assess viability in those

situations where it is least necessary. The real question, then, is how well do the tests perform in patients with the poorest LVEF[139] (Fig. 17-15)? The answer is not yet clearly known.

Another phenomenon that has been discussed is the initial development of a new defect or the worsening of an existing defect on rest MPI compared to no defect or a milder defect on stress MPI. This phenomenon has been called *reverse redistribution,* and it has been suggested as representing subendocardial MI.[152] This phenomenon of a defect on MPI that is worse or only observed at rest usually has other explanations: (1) oversubtraction of background activity[153]; (2) attenuation that affects a region more at rest than at stress; (3) scattered counts from "hot" bowel on stress (to mask an inferior wall defect) and from farther away at rest (to unmask the defect); or (4) when using quantitative programs, a region of the heart may show a decrease in counts that falls just outside the criterion for normal at rest but just within the criterion for normal on stress, even though the actual difference in relative counts between stress and rest is very small. The physiologic explanation proposed[153] to explain reverse redistribution is that the relative increment in blood flow is greater in the subepicardial myocardium overlying the infarct than in the subepicardium in the normal region. Although this explanation is directionally correct, the magnitude of difference in subepicardial blood flow to the normal versus abnormal regions is much too small to produce reverse redistribution, as shown by a large body of experimental data.[103,117,154]

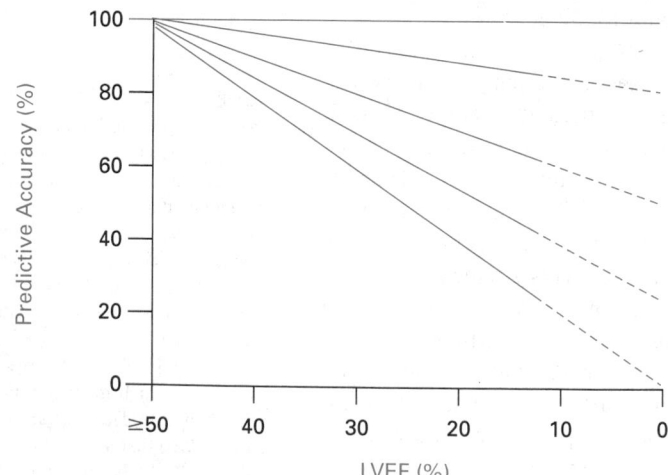

FIGURE 17-15

Assessment of myocardial viability depends on the degree of left ventricular (LV) dysfunction. Schematic presentation of predictive accuracy of various methods to assess myocardial viability. In patients with normal LV ejection fraction, all methods should theoretically be 100 percent accurate. In patients with mild LV dysfunction, the accuracy is similar for all methods. It appears that the accuracy of various methods differs in patients with more severe LV dysfunction. There are not yet sufficient data to draw firm conclusions as to which line represents which test modality. 2-DE, two-dimensional echocardiography. (From Iskandrian.[139] Reproduced with permission from the publisher and author.)

SPECT ^{201}Tl assessment of myocardial viability has been compared to SPECT ^{99m}Tc sestamibi and shows that the latter underestimates viability relative to ^{201}Tl with reinjection.[44]

In summary, myocardial viability is a crucial clinical issue, but it is difficult to assess. The best method is PET ^{18}FDG (see Chap. 20) compared to MPI for mismatch between defects (perfusion defect on MPI that shows uptake of ^{18}FDG indicating viability).[103,146,150,151] If PET and ^{18}FDG are not available, then SPECT ^{201}Tl stress with reinjection at rest appears to be the best validated method; however, SPECT ^{18}FDG compared to SPECT MPI is a promising approach that deserves intensive study.

Question 4 ***Does the patient have a good or poor prognosis?*** Assessment of patient prognosis is unquestionably the most important information available from any test, and stress/rest ^{201}Tl MPI has an outstanding track record for predicting prognosis in patients with known or suspected CAD (Figs. 17-16 and 17-17).[105,112–114,127,136–139,155–159] Several facts have been established: Normal MPI with adequate exercise stress yields a cardiac event rate in patients of 0.4 to 1.0 percent per year, with an especially low event rate for the first 2 years after the scan[105,112–114,127,136–139,155–159] (Figs. 17-16 to 17-18). The presence of MPI defects predicts a higher cardiac event rate, and the event rate is related to the size and the reversibility of the defect.[136,156,159] A high-risk MPI scan vis-à-vis a low-risk scan provides greater discrimination for predicting event-free survival than either exercise ECG or coronary angiography (Fig. 17-19). Defect size on MPI is closely related to the relative

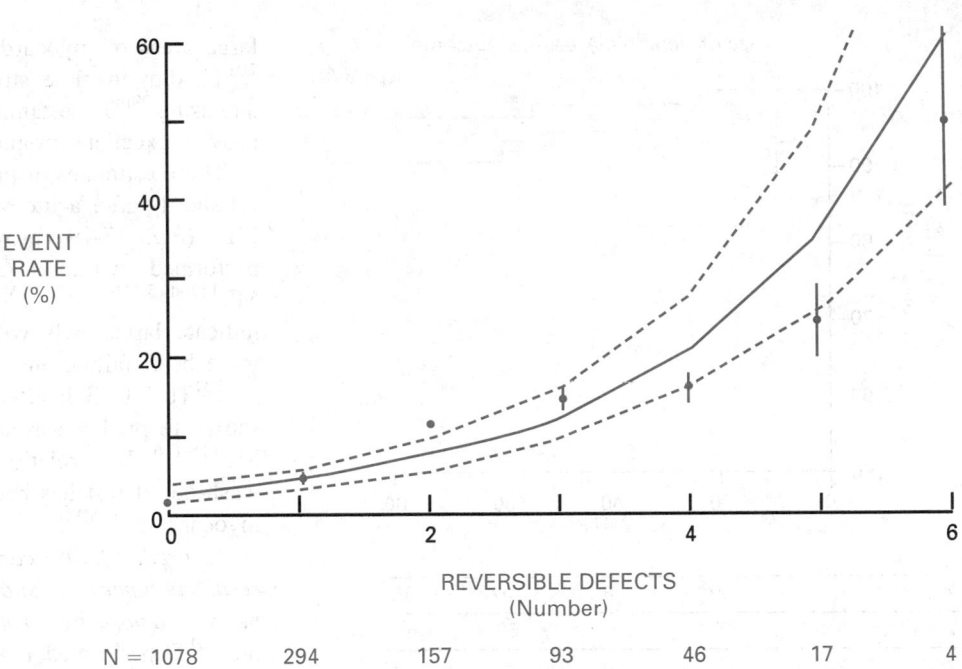

FIGURE 17-16

Thallium 201 results predict patient prognosis, as shown by the strong correlation between the development of coronary events in the future and extent of hypoperfusion on stress planar ^{201}Tl (estimated as the number of hypoperfused regions that reverse by a score of at least 1). The extent of reversible ^{201}Tl defects (extent) is exponentially related to event rate ($r = 0.97, p < .001$). (From Ladenheim et al.[136] Reproduced with permission from the publisher and authors.)

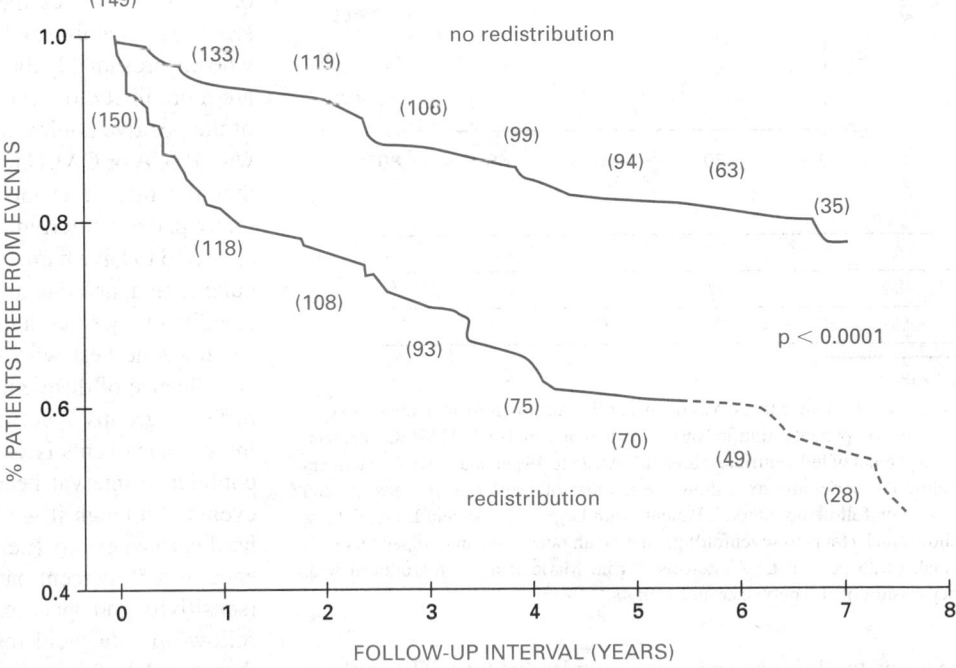

FIGURE 17-17

The survival of patients with redistribution of defects on stress/delayed rest planar ^{201}Tl images is lower than in patients without redistribution. The numbers in parentheses indicate the number of patients still at risk at that time during the follow-up. The mean (± 1 SEM) 5-year event-free survival is 82 ± 3 percent for patients with no redistribution versus 60 ± 4 percent for those with redistribution ($p < .0001$). (From Kaul et al.[156] Reproduced with permission of the publisher and authors.)

Size of Ischemic Area and Outcome

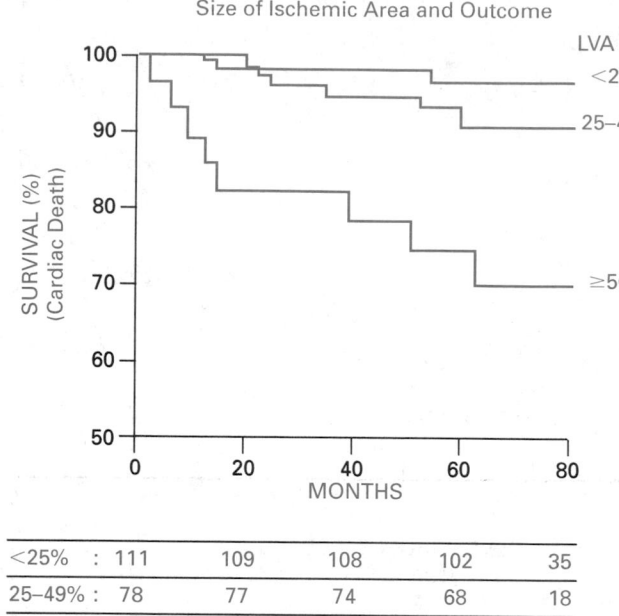

<25% :	111	109	108	102	35
25-49% :	78	77	74	68	18
≥50% :	28	23	21	20	12

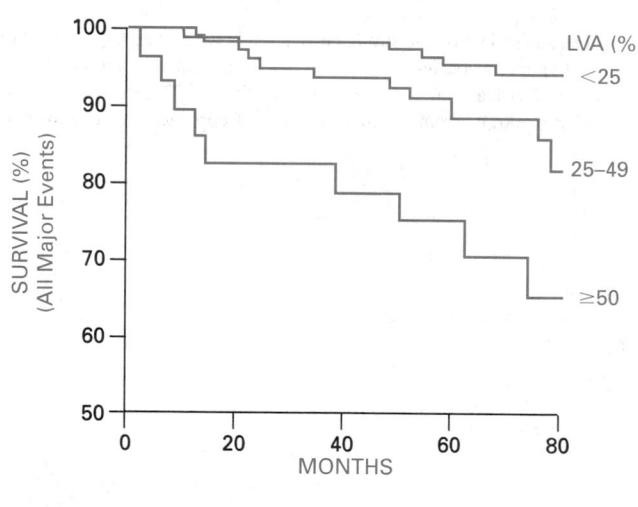

<25% :	111	109	108	102	34
25-49% :	78	76	73	67	15
≥50% :	28	23	21	20	11

FIGURE 17-18

Actuarial survival curves based on cardiac death (*top*) and major events (*bottom*) for patients stratified by total extent of exercise ^{201}Tl SPECT defects: <25 percent of left ventricular area (LVA), 25 to 49 percent of LVA. Numbers below the horizontal axis show the number of event-free patients at each 20-month follow-up interval. Patients with large (≥50 percent LVA) defects show much (four- to sevenfold) greater death rates compared to patients with small (≤25 percent LVA) defects. (From Marie et al.[159] reproduced with permission of the publisher and authors.)

mass of the left ventricle that is underperfused. The outlook is also much worse for patients with exercise-induced LV dysfunction indicated by increased lung ^{201}Tl uptake and/or LV cavity dilation on exercise versus rest[105,106,112–114,127,136–139,155–159] (Figs. 17-20 and 17-21). These changes, which reflect ischemia-induced LV dysfunction, correlate with

large areas of myocardium at risk. In addition to exercise ^{201}Tl, dipyridamole stress/rest acquired with dipyridamole and using ^{99m}Tc sestamibi or rest ^{201}Tl/stress ^{99m}Tc sestamibi provide excellent prognostic evaluation.

These estimates of prognosis by ^{201}Tl are also quite useful shortly after acute MI. Even resting and low-level stress MPI (Fig. 17-19) provide indicators of prognosis when performed within a few days of the onset of the MI.[111–115,119,121,127,138,155] The larger, more severe defects indicate larger MIs with poorer LV function and predict more heart failure and sudden cardiac death. The wash-out of [201]Tl 2 to 3 h after resting MPI defect has also been shown to predict cardiac events in the first few days after MI.[115,116] This relationship between prognosis and ^{201}Tl wash-out at rest has been attributed to viable and ischemic myocardium.[115,116]

To predict future cardiac events, knowing the ^{201}Tl MPI results is superior to knowing the number of vessels with >50 percent stenosis by coronary angiography,[116] and dipyridamole ^{201}Tl performed 1 week after MI predicted events quite well.[155] As indicated above, studies of large numbers of patients show that "hard" end-points (death or acute MI) or "soft" end-points (referral for PTCA or CABG) are more likely to occur when the following results are seen on MPI: size and/or reversibility of MPI defects are greater, there is evidence of LV dysfunction, or reversible defects occur at low levels of exercise. One must analyze critically several key aspects of the study of how well any diagnostic test can predict prognosis. Inclusion of soft events such as PTCA or CABG increases the number of patients with events for statistical reliability and helps account for outcomes in patients who are presumably the sickest. The problem is that physicians are more likely to refer patients for PTCA or CABG because of the positive noninvasive test. If the study excludes patients with PTCA or CABG to calculate only hard events, it is likely that the rate of events will be very low for two reasons: many patients referred for PTCA or CABG would have been expected to have hard events if they had not undergone revascularization, and the number of cardiac events is (fortunately) usually a very small number. Comparisons of patient prognosis are done best with statistical procedures to compute the significance of differences in the frequency of events among different groups over time.[138] The proportion of patients having cardiac events is virtually always associated with a wide confidence interval because of the small number of cardiac events. Although it is always preferable for a test to predict hard cardiac events (i.e., prognosis) rather than just the presence of a 50 percent narrowing of coronary arterial diameter (sensitivity and specificity), the uncertainties associated with follow-up data yield results that are inherently less reliable than are data for sensitivity and specificity. Thus prognosis studies must inevitably sacrifice some statistical reliability of the data for their gain in clinical relevance.

Numerous studies have shown the remarkable ability of stress ^{201}Tl or ^{99m}Tc sestamibi with exercise or dipyridamole (Fig. 17-22) to predict prognosis.[104,112,113,127,136–139,155–160]

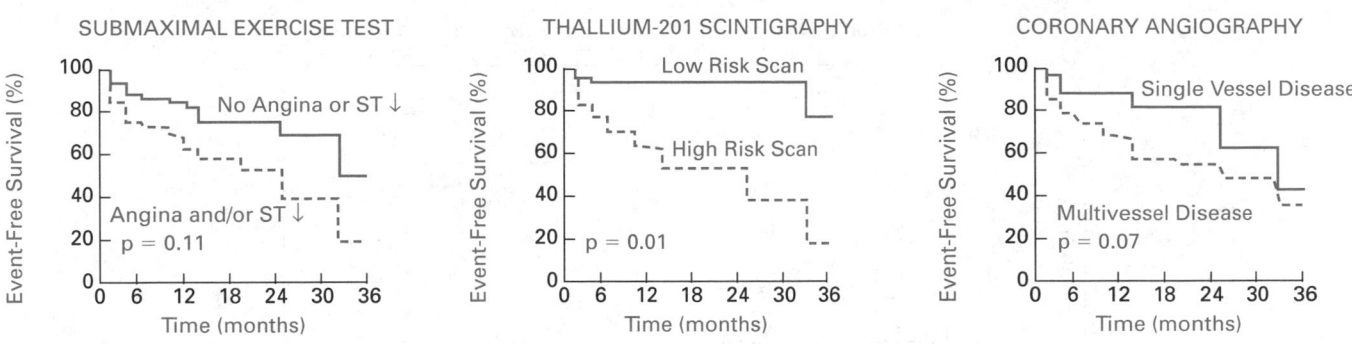

FIGURE 17-19

Event-free survival after myocardial infarction is predicted by the results of tests performed before hospital discharge. The best separation between high- and low-risk patients is provided by low-level exercise planar ^{201}Tl scintigra- phy, compared to exercise ECG or the number of stenotic arteries on coronary arteriography. (From *Circulation* 1991; 84(suppl 1):148. Reprinted with per- mission from the American Heart Association.)

More importantly, it has also been shown that stress MPI provides *incremental* information that is truly independent of other data to predict prognosis, i.e., MPI adds signifi- cantly to the information already available from the history, rest and exercise ECG, and even cardiac catheteriza- tion[127,138,139,156,160–164] (Figs. 17-23 to 17-27). The most demanding criterion by which to judge any one test is whether it can add significantly to all other clinical and test data. Studies of prognosis are valuable because the ability to predict patient outcome is justifiably becoming the most important issue for everyone who evaluates the quality and cost of health

care.[165] Stress MPI also provides an excellent way to assess preoperatively the risk of noncardiac surgery, providing incre- mental information to the clinical risk profile[164] (Fig. 17-27) (see Chap. 83). Over the years, the selection of patients for surgery and the perioperative care have improved to reduce the rates of morbidity and mortality with most surgical proce- dures. Applying any test to a population at relatively lower risk makes it appear less effective than in high-risk popula- tions.[85,93,165] This phenomenon probably explains some re-

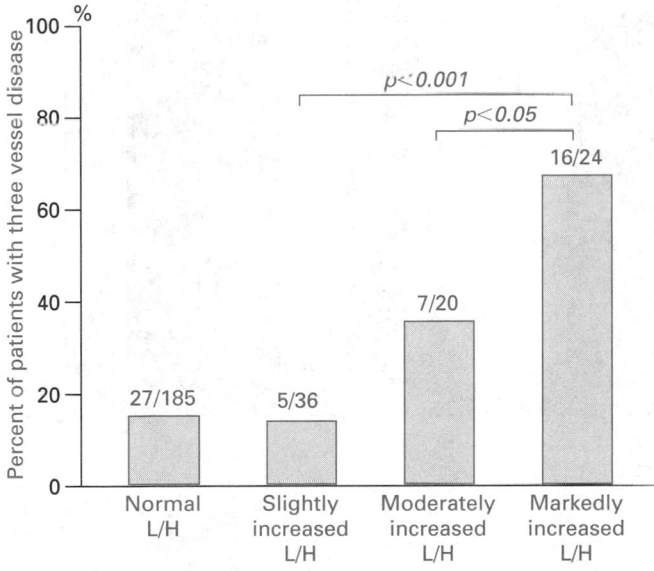

FIGURE 17-20

In addition to ^{201}Tl defect area, severity, and redistribution, ^{201}Tl images provided indirect assessment of LV dysfunction on exercise (lung ^{201}Tl uptake). Comparison of the number of patients with three-vessel disease among those with normal, slightly increased, moderately increased, and mark- edly increased lung/heart (L/H) ^{201}Tl ratios in group 3 subjects. The fraction shown above each column represents the total number of subjects in each subgroup (denominator) and the number of those with three-vessel disease in the subgroup (numerator), e.g., 16 of 24 subjects with a markedly increased L/H ratio have three-vessel disease—far right column. (From Kurata et al.[105] Reproduced with permission of the publisher and authors.)

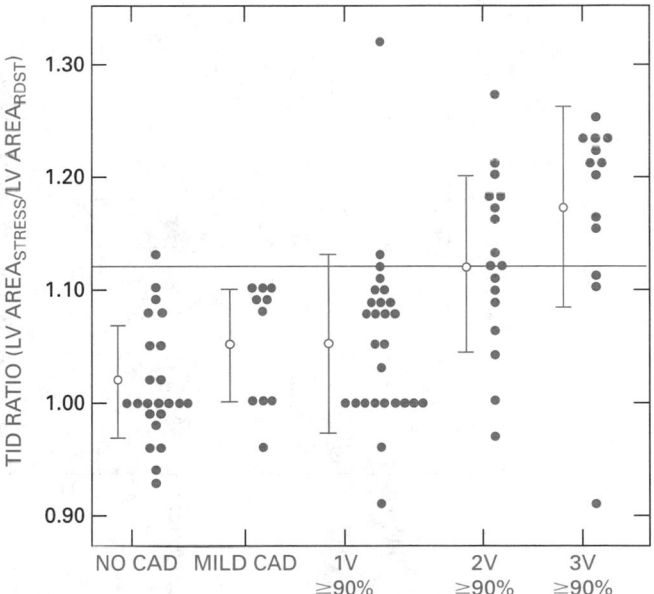

FIGURE 17-21

[201]Tl can also estimate change in average LV cavity size on ungated images at stress and rest. The average LV cavity size is strongly influenced by LV end-systolic volume, so that an increase in cavity size correlates with de- creased ejection fraction on stress. Relation is depicted between the increase in LV cavity size on stress versus rest, i.e., the transient ischemic dilation ratio (TID) and the presence and extent/severity of coronary artery disease (CAD). Mean ± 1 SD values are shown to the left of the individual values in the group. Horizontal line: Upper normal for TID ratio. LV, left ventricular; RDST, redistribution; 1V, 2V, 3V, one-, two-, and three-vessel disease; ≥90 percent, ≥90 percent coronary artery stenosis. (From Weiss et al.[106] Reproduced with permission from the publisher and authors.)

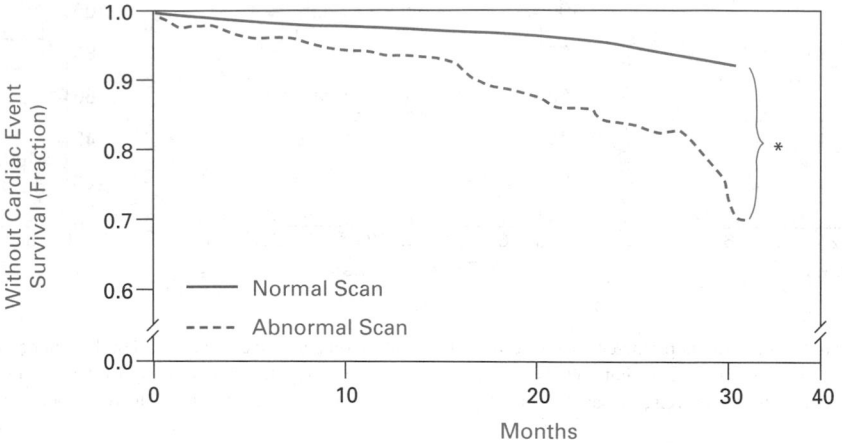

Life Table Analysis of I.V. Dipyridamole Thallium-201 Imaging

N = 506
*p < 0.005
Hendel R. et al. *JACC* 1990:15,109

FIGURE 17-22

[201]Tl can predict prognosis even in patients who cannot exercise, as shown by these results with dipyridamole. Cardiac death or myocardial infarction occurred more frequently in patients with abnormal dipyridamole-thallium scintigrams (dashed line, *n* = 332) than in those with normal scans (solid line, *n* = 172) (*p* < .005). (From Hendel R et al. *J Am Coll Cardiol* 1990; 15:109. Reprinted with permission from the American College of Cardiology.)

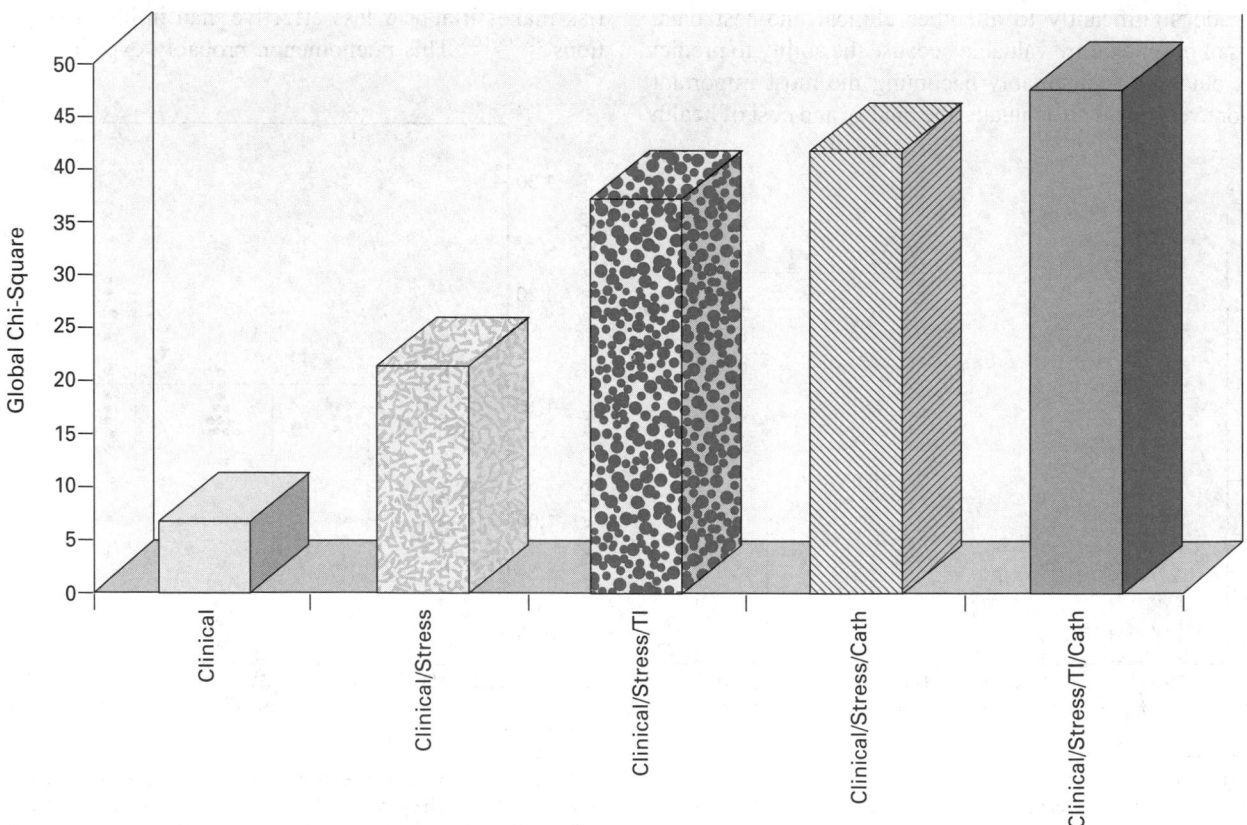

FIGURE 17-23

The most demanding statistical test of the ability of a test to predict prognosis is to determine whether the test can add significantly (incrementally) to all the other information available. Incremental prognostic value of tests performed in a hierarchical order is assessed by the global chi-square. There is incremental value when exercise ECG test variables (stress) are added to clinical information (clinical). There is a further increase in prognostic information when the number of defects on planar ^{201}Tl interpreted qualita- tively is added to clinical and ECG stress test information. Prognostic informa- tion provided by adding cardiac catheterization (Cath.) to clinical and stress variables is only slightly greater than the prognostic information provided by adding ^{201}Tl to clinical and stress variables in this study. Chi-square for each column is *p* < .01 compared to chi-square of adjacent column. (From Pollock et al.[138] Reproduced with permission of the publisher and authors.)

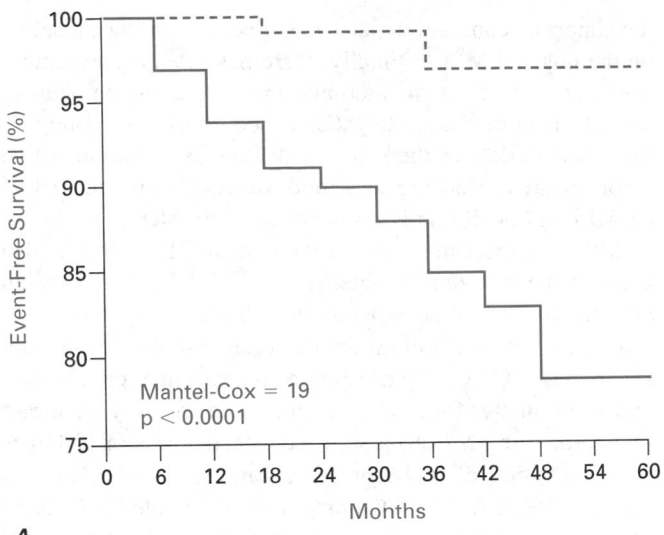

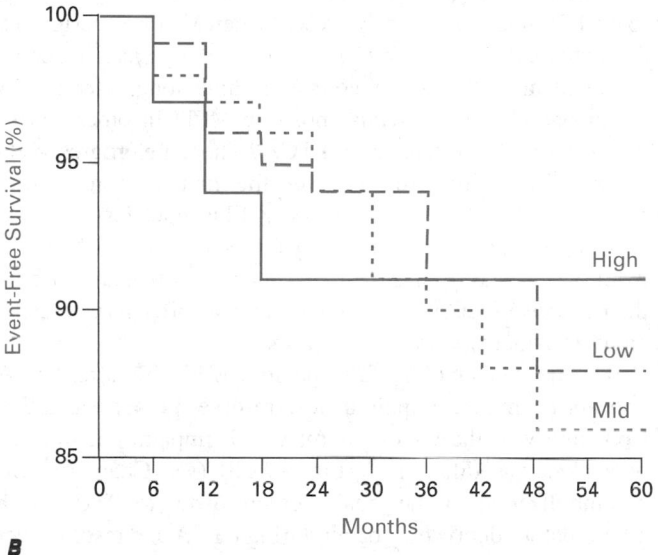

B

FIGURE 17-24

A. Event-free survival in patients with a large perfusion abnormality (solid line ≥ 15 percent of left ventricle) was much poorer than for patients with small or no perfusion abnormality (broken line < 15 percent of left ventricle) on myocardial perfusion imaging. *B.* In the same patients, the exercise ECG failed to distinguish high-risk versus low-risk patients, using the treadmill exercise score. (From Iskandrian et al.[160] Reproduced with permission of the publisher and authors.)

cent reports to indicate less benefit from MPI before major surgery, but for patients who are at risk, MPI is clearly an effective tool to assess risk and guide management.[1,2,5,164] *The authors currently suggest the use of MPI before major noncardiac surgery (such as vascular surgery on the aorta or lower extremities and some other major procedures such as thoracotomy and major intraabdominal procedures) for patients with multiple risk factors (especially diabetes), restricted physical activity (to avoid symptoms), and prior diagnosis of CAD.*

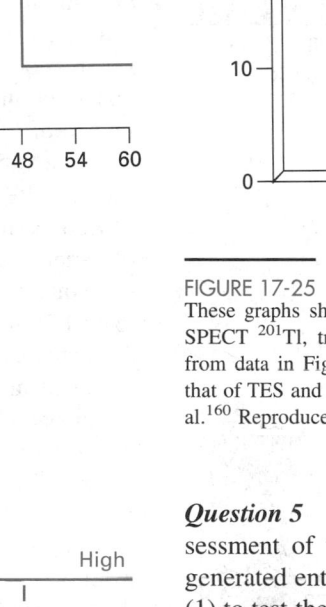

FIGURE 17-25

These graphs show the independent and incremental prognostic power of SPECT ^{201}Tl, treadmill exercise score (TES), and coronary angiography from data in Fig. 17-24. SPECT provided independent information above that of TES and equal to that of coronary angiography. (From Iskandrian et al.[160] Reproduced with permission of the publisher and authors.)

Question 5 *Has a therapeutic measure improved MPI?* Assessment of the response to therapy demonstrated by MPI generated enthusiasm a number of years ago for two reasons: (1) to test the robustness of the methodology, since MPI was expected to improve after patent CABG[160–162]; and (2) to evaluate the adequacy of revascularization after intervention. Since PTCA, particularly, seemed to need documentation of improved perfusion, MPI played an important role in detecting restenosis in patients with atypical symptoms.[166–168] MPI was a major tool used to compare benefits of CABG versus PTCA in a large trial at Emory (EAST).[169] MPI offered advantages for such a trial by objective documentation of whether a borderline anatomic lesion was physiologically significant by quantitating the size of perfusion defects (superior to angiographic techniques), documenting the role of collateral coronary arteries in total perfusion, and distinguishing infarcted versus ischemic myocardium.[166–169] Thus, MPI could serve as a common end point for any type of therapy.

Some special problems are encountered in the use of MPI to assess the effects of CABG. First, the region of myocardium dependent on a graft to a small branch artery, e.g., obtuse marginal branch of the circumflex, may be so small that it is difficult to detect graft occlusion by SPECT MPI.[170] Second, MPI reflects only total perfusion and does not distinguish among the following sources of blood flow: antegrade through a partially occluded native coronary artery, antegrade through a CABG, retrograde through collateral arteries, or a combination of the three.[171] Third, the variable distributions of coronary arteries can make it difficult or impossible to assign a particular defect on MPI to the vascular distribution of a single coronary artery branch or CABG. Elegant methods, however,

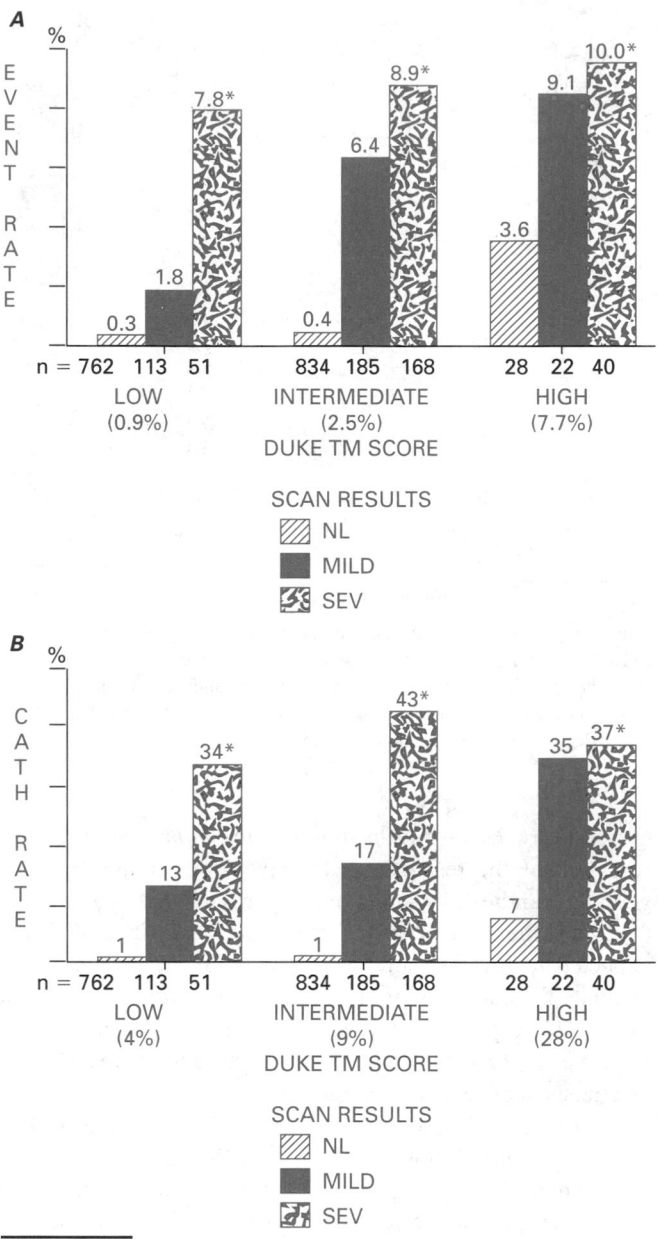

FIGURE 17-26

A. Duke treadmill (TM) score category (low, intermediate, and high risk) and myocardial perfusion scan results are shown versus hard events in patients in low, intermediate, and high Duke TM score categories with scans that were either normal (NL), mildly abnormal (MILD), or severely abnormal (SEV). Parentheses under Duke treadmill subgroups show hard event rates in these groups. *p* < .05 across all scan results. *B.* Duke TM score category and scan result are plotted versus the rate of referral to catheterization within 60 days after the scan. These results show that myocardial perfusion scans provide dramatic differentiation of the level of risk, in each exercise ECG (TM) categories. The scan result profoundly influences the management decisions, e.g., which patients are referred to cardiac catheterization. (From Hachamovitch et al.[163] Reproduced with permission of the publisher and authors.)

have been developed to superimpose the coronary angiogram on the three-dimensional MPI to solve this problem for a patient where both studies are available.[172] Fourth, if the patient has had open-heart surgery, there is usually an abnormal contraction pattern of the interventricular septum, and

the abnormal contraction pattern, per se, can produce a defect on the ungated MPI.[71] Finally, there has often been speculation that even a patent internal mammary artery implant to the left anterior descending (LAD) coronary artery may be too small to deliver the same peak flow as a normal native coronary artery, leading to a mild, reversible anterior defect on MPI, although this is not a common problem.[173]

MPI is important in the evaluation of PTCA but is also associated with some problems.[167–169,174] First, it is often difficult to determine whether a SPECT MPI defect was caused by a stenosis in an arterial branch that is technically suitable for PTCA or by a lesion in an adjacent arterial branch that is not suitable for PTCA. A unique and critically important feature of using MPI to assess the effectiveness of PTCA is the observation of transient defects in the distribution of a successful PTCA.[167,168] Cloninger et al.[167] noted defects on SPECT performed 1 to 2 days after PTCA in about one-third of patients where the PTCA was proven to be successful by subsequent angiography. The MPI defects in the region distal to the PTCA site were rarely present when MPI was performed 6 months later.[167] The key question for the physician seeing a patient after PTCA, of course, is how long after PTCA might one observe this false-positive MPI? In other words, when can MPI be trusted after PTCA? There are progressively fewer false-positive results over the first 6 months after PTCA.[167,168,174,175] False-positive MPI is much less common at 4 to 6 weeks versus 1 to 7 days after PTCA.[167,168,174,175] SPECT ^{201}Tl has been shown to be more sensitive and specific than exercise ECG in detecting restenosis after PTCA, especially in patients without symptoms.[174]

The mechanism of the false-positive MPI early after PTCA appears to involve impaired flow reserve, perhaps resulting from injury to the endothelium, which impairs endothelial-dependent vasodilation[175] (Fig. 17-28) (see Chap. 4). Microembolization of the small vessels distal to PTCA with atheromatous debris may occur during PTCA and resolve over time. Whether follow-up SPECT MPI is needed after PTCA depends on the patient's symptoms. *If patients have a return of the same symptoms typical of angina that were present before PTCA, then coronary angiography is preferable.*[165,168] *If patients develop symptoms not typical of either angina pectoris or of their own symptoms before PTCA, then exercise SPECT MPI would be most useful.*[165,168] On the other hand, for patients with no symptoms after PTCA, MPI may be useful under selected circumstances: (1) the patient who is diabetic or had no symptoms or very atypical symptoms before PTCA or CABG; (2) the patient who wants to return to or begin high-level stress activities for recreational reasons (e.g., mountain-climbing or competitive sports) or for occupational reasons (e.g., pilot or bus driver); (3) the patient who had a difficult PTCA of a very proximal lesion in a large coronary artery, even if the patient is asymptomatic; or (4) the patient who travels or lives at a considerable distance from health care facilities that offer PTCA or CABG who needs extraordinarily careful follow-up. On the other hand, the patient who had definite symptoms before PTCA but becomes asymptomatic, even during exercise, after PTCA of a medium- or small-sized artery does not necessarily need "routine" follow-up MPI. Multivessel PTCA creates a higher risk situation because the probability of restenosis of at least one PTCA site is high, and these patients have greater need for objective assessment after multiple PTCA procedures.[168]

Perhaps the most exciting new role for MPI in assessing the response to therapy is to monitor selected patients on medical therapy. MPI can document improvement in patients on nitrates[176] or calcium channel blockers.[177] The most intriguing results, however, have been the improvement in evidence of ischemia over several months in patients on cholesterol-lowering therapy.[178,179] *Improvements in defects documented by MPI have greatly exceeded the improvement in relative or absolute diameter of the lesions documented by quantitative coronary angiography, in part because of the exponential relationship between diameter and flow[179] but also, perhaps more importantly, because of the healing of the vasodilator function of the endothelium[178]* (see Chaps. 4 and 44).

In view of the proven clinical benefits of cholesterol-lowering drugs[178,179] and the need to reduce medical costs,[175] aggressive medical therapy has become the standard of care for most patients with CAD, and the relative values of drug therapy and interventional procedures are being reassessed. Stress/rest MPI will help define those patients in whom medical therapy—including aggressive lipid lowering—is ameliorating or eliminating myocardial ischemia.

MPI IN DISEASES THAT DO NOT AFFECT LARGE CORONARY ARTERIES (See Tables 17-6 and 17-7)

MPI defects have been reported in several conditions that do not affect primarily large, epicardial coronary arteries, e.g., hypertrophic cardiomyopathy (HCM); end-stage renal disease with hypertensive cardiomyopathy; left bundle branch block

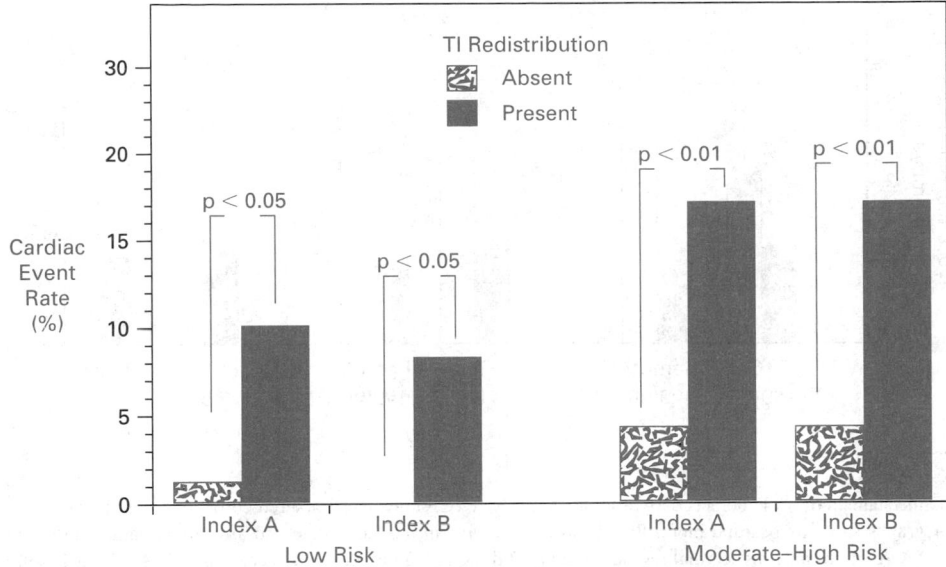

A

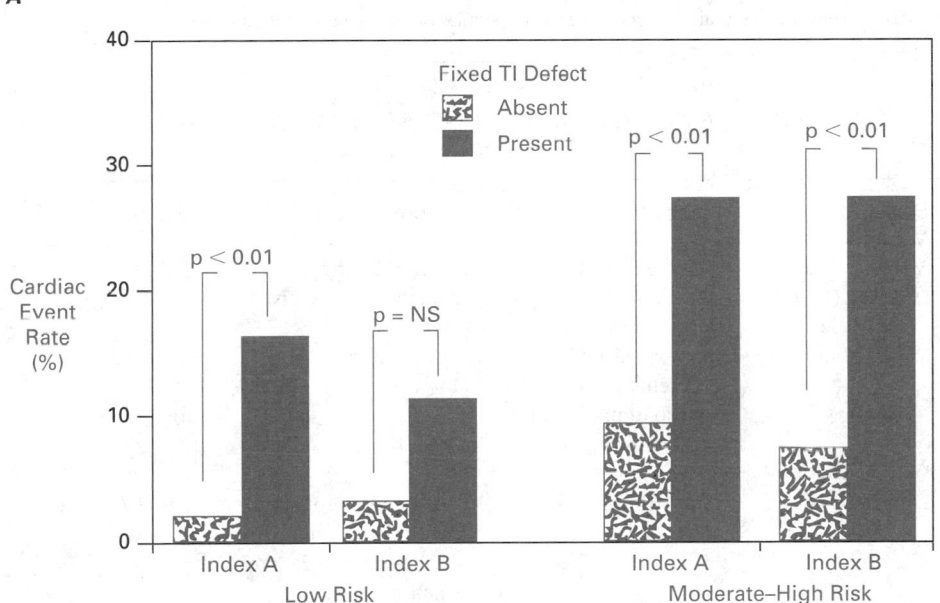

B

FIGURE 17-27

^{201}Tl predicts perioperative risk for noncardiac surgery and adds significantly to the other data (clinical indexes). Incidence of perioperative cardiac events is shown by the height of the bars, based on clinical risk indexes (low versus moderate to high) and presence or absence of ^{201}Tl defects, whether they show redistribution (*A*) or remain fixed (*B*). Marked increase in cardiac event rates is noted for each index and within each risk group when thallium redistribution was noted (*A*). Perioperative risk also increased, even when the ^{201}Tl defects were fixed (*B*). (From Hendel and Leppo.[164] Reproduced with permission of the publisher and authors.)

(LBBB); and a variety of cardiomyopathies related to sarcoidosis, Duchenne's type muscular dystrophy, scleroderma, myocarditis, and, probably, essential arterial hypertension and diabetes mellitus. In general, any cardiomyopathy that causes regional wall motion abnormalities can cause defects on the ungated MPI,[71] although the defects in nonischemic cardiomyopathies are generally smaller than those in ischemic cardiomyopathies.[180] In fact, if clinical MPI results show defects, it can be very helpful to comment that the defects are too

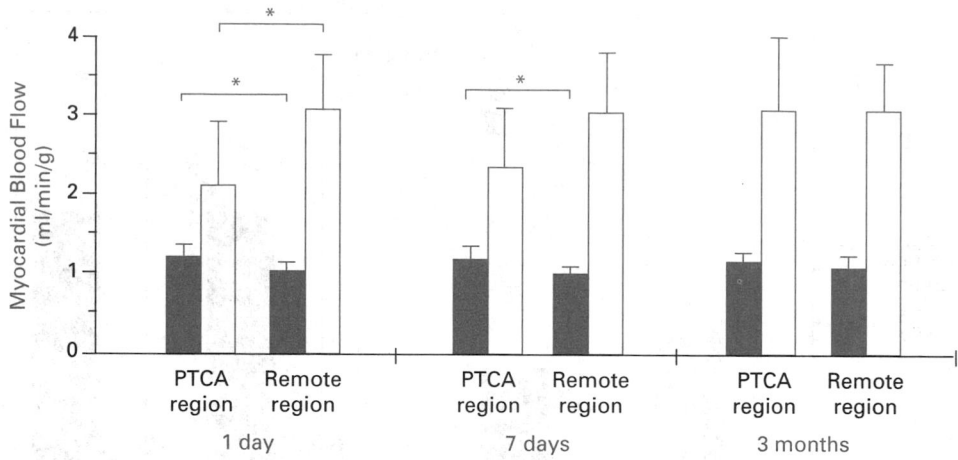

FIGURE 17-28

The mechanism of ^{201}Tl defects early after angioplasty (PTCA) involves impaired coronary blood flow reserve. Bar graphs show myocardial blood flow measured by PET in the basal state and after dipyridamole effect in the PTCA and remote myocardial regions at 1 day, 7 days, and 3 months after successful PTCA. $p < .01$; solid bars, basal state; open bars, peak dipyridamole effect. Coronary flow reserve improves over the first 3 months after PTCA. (From Uren et al.[175] Reproduced with permission of the publisher and authors.)

TABLE 17-6

CLINICAL VALUE OF SPECT MPI IN DISEASES THAT DO NOT INVOLVE LARGE CORONARY ARTERIES

Disease	Special Needs	Purpose	Value (?/ + + +)
Valvular heart disease (mitral and aortic regurgitation)	1. [201]Tl for lung uptake 2. Exercise 3. Careful with aortic stenosis (AS) (contraindicated if significant AS at rest)	To provide objective evidence of exercise-induced LV dysfunction	+/+ + +
Dilated cardiomyopathy	1. [201]Tl for viability 2. Gated helps	To rule out coronary artery disease as etiology if defects are small or absent	+ + +/+ + +
		To look for viable myocardium as treatable	+ + +/+ + +
Hypertrophic cardiomyopathy	1. Careful if LV outflow obstruction	To look for ischemia	+/+ + +

that maximum CBF per gram of myocardium (CBF/g) is reduced in hypertrophy,[181] MPI detects only *regional* differences in CBF/g. *The disease process, therefore, would need to have asymmetric effects in different large myocardial segments, if it is to explain MPI defects.* The observation of microscopic abnormalities distributed uniformly throughout the heart[182,183] would not be expected to cause MPI defects.

Several studies have reported MPI defects in *HCM*.[184,185] Reversible MPI defects were found in 74 percent of one group of 50 patients and showed excellent sensitivity (87 percent) but poor specificity (47 percent) in predicting myocardial ischemia (excess coronary venous lactate production during rapid atrial pacing).[185] Verapamil[186] and surgical myotomy/myomectomy[187] improved reversible MPI defects in many HCM patients.

End-stage renal disease is sometimes associated with lateral wall defects,[188] and *LBBB* is sometimes (10 to 35 percent) associated with septal defects.[189] The LBBB defect in some patients may be related to abnormally delayed contraction of the septum,[71] which may be accentuated during exercise because the septum remains thin while the other LV walls show increased thickening during systole. Dipyridamole stress may reduce the likelihood of a defect on MPI because it would not accentuate the differences in systolic thickening between septum and other walls,[190] but the clinician does not gain information about exercise-induced symptoms and functional aerobic capacity from dipyridamole. The MPI defect due to LBBB is usually located in the septum per se, where MPI defects due to CAD would require an unusual distribution of lesions, specifically isolated to the septal perforating arteries. CAD rarely involves only these branches unless there has been revascularization of the LAD coronary artery. CABG can restore flow to the mid-LAD artery but allow progression of disease to occlude the LAD artery proximal to the insertion of the graft and

small to explain the evidence of cardiac dysfunction, i.e., even if the patient has some CAD, it is not likely to explain the cardiac dysfunction (cavity dilation, lung ^{201}Tl uptake on stress, or impaired global contraction on gated MPI). Such patients may have some CAD, but, more importantly, their major problem appears to be a generalized cardiomyopathy that would not benefit from revascularization.

One must be very cautious before concluding that perfusion is impaired in all conditions in which MPI defects have been reported, e.g., some early studies used planar ^{201}Tl with subjective, unblinded interpretations. Although it has been proven

proximal to the origin of septal perforators. In contrast, LAD coronary artery stenosis proximal to the first septal perforator has been shown to cause defects in the septum plus the anterior wall.[191] PTCA of the proximal LAD artery can sacrifice septal perforators, although this complication is less common than it was several years ago. One experimental study reported reduced blood flow to the septum relative to the other walls during pacing-induced LBBB.[192]

Sarcoidosis was reported to produce MPI defects in the base of the interventricular septum by planar ^{201}Tl, interpreted qualitatively, in the site found in other studies to have the most histologic involvement at autopsy[193] (see Chap. 76). Exercise ^{201}Tl MPI performed significantly better than exercise ECG to predict prognosis after acute MI (Fig. 17-19). MPI defects have been reported in *hypertension*,[188,194] but the authors' study of patients with low probability of CAD ($n = 24$) found only a minimal (5 percent) decrease in ^{201}Tl counts in the lateral wall of the left ventricle compared to normal men ($n = 50$).[195] None of the 24 patients with hypertension had MPI defects, although their LV wall thickness was 14 ± 3 mm.[195] From a clinical perspective, hypertension per se should not be used to explain MPI defects.[5]

The presence of *marked left ventricular hypertrophy* (LVH) in hypertension, end-stage renal disease, HCM, or valvular heart disease creates the potential for lateral wall MPI defects due to an interesting mechanism.[196] Usually the left lung wraps around the lateral wall, but not the septal wall, of the left ventricle, and the lung tissue has a lower attenuation coefficient than muscle. Thus, normally lateral wall counts suffer less attenuation than do septal wall counts.[196] The simulation study by DiBella et al. used PET transmission and emission images to demonstrate that the relative difference between lateral and septal wall attenuation can explain the relative increase ("hot spot") in counts in the lateral wall versus the septum found in SPECT studies of normal subjects without evidence of CAD. If LVH is severe, the left ventricle can rotate to fill the space between chest wall and heart, leading to more lateral wall attenuation and a relative decrease in counts due to the lack of lung wrapping around the lateral wall of the left ventricle compared to normal findings.[196]

Valvular heart disease can be associated with LVH and, perhaps, inadequate maximum CBF/g, but regional MPI defects would not be expected in the absence of CAD. Mitral valve prolapse (MVP) has been reported to produce occasional positive planar ^{201}Tl MPI interpreted qualitatively.[197] In the authors' experience, SPECT MPI defects occurred in only 5 of 70 male patients with MVP, and 2 of these 5 patients had prior endocarditis requiring mitral valve replacements. A 7 percent positive rate on SPECT ^{201}Tl in MVP certainly does not exceed the expected rate of false-positive results for SPECT in men. Thus, it would be inaccurate to attribute SPECT MPI defects to MVP.

Another possible use of MPI in valvular heart disease might be evaluation of ^{201}Tl lung uptake and LV dilation immediately after exercise to detect exercise-induced LV dysfunction[107] in mitral or aortic valve regurgitation. Demonstration of lung uptake, LV dilation, and impaired functional aerobic capacity for exercise limited by dyspnea would indicate impaired LV functional reserve capacity. In these valvular regurgitant lesions, the changes indicated above might be more convincing than changes in LVEF, because LVEF is profoundly influenced by changes in regurgitant fraction associated with changes in blood pressure, heart rate, and cardiac volumes.[198,199]

CLINICAL APPLICATIONS OF MPI AT REST

Most MPI is performed during both stress and rest, but there are some applications for resting MPI as an indicator of MI and to estimate its size and severity. In one study, the sensitivity of resting planar ^{201}Tl MPI to detect acute MI was excellent during the first 6 h after the onset of chest pain.[111] Sensitivity decreased during the period 6 to 24 h after onset, with a further decrease when imaging was performed more than 24 h later.[111] Thus, for patients who have been in the hospital 2 or more days with equivocal studies for acute MI, a resting ^{201}Tl MPI is not a very sensitive test, and a negative result cannot rule out MI with these late images.[111] On the other hand, if a defect is present on resting MPI, it is not possible to determine the age of the defect, i.e., whether the MI occurred within minutes or years earlier. MPI can estimate MI size, which helps predict prognosis.

A potentially more important clinical use of MPI is to assess patients with chest pain in emergency departments.[112–114] [201]Tl, or more frequently ^{99m}Tc sestamibi, is

TABLE 17-7
EFFECTS OF VARIOUS (NONCORONARY) CONDITIONS ON SPECT MPI

Condition	Change in MPI	Magnitude of Problem	Solution
LBBB	Defect isolated to septum (fixed or reversible)	10–30% of patients	Perhaps using dipyridamole or gating
End-stage renal disease	Defect in lateral wall (fixed or reversible)	15–40% of patients	?
Left mastectomy	Inferior defect	All women	Change criterion for abnormality in inferior wall i.e., 3.5 vs 2.5 SD, or compare to male file
Asymmetric septal hypertrophy	Lateral wall defect (fixed)	Most	

injected to determine whether the chest pain is due to myocardial ischemia or MI. Patients who were carefully preselected based on clinical criteria and who also have a negative MPI at rest during pain have an excellent short-term prognosis, while patients with positive MPI during pain have a high likelihood of acute MI and other cardiac events.[112–115]

Another use of resting MPI is to distinguish whether there is sufficient viable myocardium overlying a region of MI to justify revascularization. The wash-out after ^{201}Tl injection at rest is a predictor of prognosis and response to revascularization, apparently because it indicates viable, potentially ischemic myocardium.[116] Studies in experimental MI[117] support the logic that the severity of the resting defect would be closely related to the transmural extent of MI, from endocardium to epicardium. In fact, this result has been found both in animal studies[118] and in patients with MI.[119,120] The area of the defect has been studied more extensively, and the mass of MI relative to the mass of the left ventricle correlates closely with the defect size relative to the LV size on the resting MPI.[118–120]

Prognosis in unstable angina is worse if there is a resting perfusion defect,[121] and MPI during chest pain has also been used to detect evidence of coronary artery spasm.[122] In summary, resting MPI is mainly useful to identify acute MI early and to detect viable myocardium. *Resting MPI is less helpful in determining whether a patient with equivocal history, ECG, and cardiac enzymes actually has had a recent MI.*

Coronary Spasm/Syndrome X

Myocardial ischemia and angina can result from *spasm* of a large epicardial coronary artery.[122] There had been debate concerning whether ischemia could result from dynamic constriction of small-resistance arteries because of compensatory vasodilator mechanisms, but experimental[200] and clinical[201] studies have now demonstrated myocardial ischemia due to constriction of these resistance arteries. The clinical syndrome associated with ischemia and angina in the absence of critical fixed lesions or spasm in large, epicardial coronary arteries has been called *syndrome X* (see Chap. 45), while spasm of epicardial coronary arteries, which usually reflects underlying atherosclerosis that may or may not be apparent angiographically, can be associated with a spectrum of clinical manifestations that range from contributing to subendocardial ischemia by partial occlusion to total occlusion, transmural ischemia, and even sudden death (Prinzmetal's variant angina) (see Chaps. 44 to 46). [201]Tl MPI has been used to document defects during spontaneous episodes of coronary artery spasm,[122] but, from a clinical perspective, it would not be practical to have ^{201}Tl ready to inject and to acquire images during episodes of suspected spasm. Since ^{99m}Tc sestamibi will stay put longer after injection,[30,32] it permits image acquisition within 2 to 4 h rather than within 15 to 30 min as for [201]Tl.[11,20] It should be noted that ^{99m}Tc sestamibi is an excellent flow tracer over the range of flows expected in coronary spasm (normal to severely reduced).[17,21,22,29]

Syndrome X, on the other hand, poses a different prob-lem.[201] If there is diffuse constriction of numerous small coronary arteries throughout the heart,[182,183,201] then one would expect uniform reduction in CBF/g in all parts of the heart. Such an abnormality would not be expected to produce the regional differences in flow that would be required to create MPI defects. Most reports of positive MPI in patients with chest pain and normal coronary arteriograms represent false-positive results.[3,5,126,127] Consistent with this interpretation, one study that reported MPI defects in syndrome X found no relationship among the defect size and other evidence of ischemia.[202] Methods such as PET [13]NH$_3$ or [82]Rb, that can measure absolute CBF/g, or measures of global LV function[200,201] may be the best way to diagnose these diffusely distributed abnormalities of small coronary arteries.

Future Developments in MPI

By far the most important and exciting new development in SPECT myocardial radionuclide imaging is *attenuation correction.*[94–96] Hardware and software have been developed, and clinical trials are underway. This technology holds great promise for reducing artifactual defects due to attenuation of SPECT images, leading to a decrease in frequency of false-positive results. If true, then there might also be a secondary benefit, i.e., a decrease in false-negative SPECT MPI because one could apply stricter criteria for abnormal versus normal results, shifting the ROC curve.[84] If these developments can be validated in clinical trials, then attenuation-corrected SPECT could provide much more accurate testing for CAD with only a small increase in costs. Attenuation-compensated SPECT images, however, will show a lower quality than PET images because of inherent differences in spatial resolution, scatter correction, and counting statistics and the fact that the attenuation compensation methodology is far more compli-cated in SPECT compared to PET imaging[89,90,95] (see Chap. 20).

Other exciting developments provide reasonable SPECT images of positron-emitting radiopharmaceuticals that have previously required true PET cameras, e.g., [18]FDG.[203–205] The most straightforward method is with a 511-keV collimator attached to a traditional SPECT imaging system with a thick NaI crystal. Compared to [18]FDG images with a dedicated PET camera system (i.e., detection of the two 511-keV photons simultaneously with a ring detector system with bismuth ger-manate crystals), 511-keV-collimated SPECT images have much lower resolution (18 mm versus 5 mm) and much more noise due to the poor stopping power of the NaI crystal and the use of the collimator. The most elegant method for SPECT imaging of positron-emitting radionuclides employs a two-headed SPECT detector system, without collimators, and, as with "true" PET, the two 511-keV photons from the [18]FDG decay are detected simultaneously. Spatial resolution of the system (order of 5 mm) is excellent, and early results with this method are promising. A crucial limitation of SPECT [18]FDG images is that they are not corrected for photon attenua-tion. These "poor-man's PET imaging devices," however, produce reasonable [18]FDG images.[203–205] Some groups have used the 511-keV SPECT imaging systems for simultaneous assessment of myocardial viability (with [18]FDG) and perfusion (with ^{99m}Tc sestamibi),[204] but downscatter of the 511-keV photons into the ^{99m}Tc sestamibi energy window can distort the SPECT sestamibi MPI.

CARDIAC BLOOD POOL IMAGING FOR VENTRICULAR FUNCTION

Instrumentation

Left and right ventricular global function can be assessed by the change in volume of the chamber during the cardiac cycle.[206,207] The basic principle is that when the radioactive tracer is mixed in the blood, the counts arising from the chamber are proportional to the volume of blood in the chamber at that point in time (assuming no effects of attenuation, resolution, or scatter). Thus, it is necessary for the tracer to be mixed adequately and for the camera to be able to count accurately during a brief period of time (1/16 to 1/64 fraction of the cardiac cycle). The first method used for this cardiac BPI was the *first pass,* where the camera recorded counts during the first pass of the tracer through the heart after injection into a large vein.[207] This method produces very high levels of radioactivity in the heart for a brief period of time, so that it requires a camera to perform at very high count rates. Conventional, single-crystal nuclear medicine analogue cameras are too "slow" and cannot record the high count rates required to perform high-quality first-pass studies. A camera with multiple individual NaI crystals to detect the high count rates from the first-pass studies can detect the highest count rates, although newer, single-crystal digital cameras that digitize information from each photomultiplier tube can record high count rates and are "faster" than the older analogue cameras.

One can also assess ventricular function by *ECG-GBPI.*[208] In this method, the blood pool is labeled by a tracer, and the camera/computer system acquires events with their location indicated by their (*x, y*) coordinates on the computer digital matrix or picture element (pixel), along with the timing signal recorded by the ECG.[205] The computer system acquires the data in either list mode or frame mode. In *list mode acquisition,* each (*x, y*) event along with an R-wave marker and interspersed time markers (usually at 1-ms time intervals) are stored on the hard disk of the computer system. Following image acquisition, the average R-R wave time interval is divided into 16, 32, or 64 segments to determine the time window for each frame in the gated study. Next, each event is placed into one of the 16 to 64 image frames depending on the time at which that event occurred after the R wave for that beat. Beats with an R-R interval that is either too short or too long are not included in the reformatted frame data.[206] Most laboratories do not use list mode acquisition because: (1) the hard disk must have a large amount of free space (for most systems it has to be contiguous disk space) to hold the

large number of acquired events, and (2) several minutes (longer, on the older computers) are required to reformat the list mode data into frame data. In *frame mode acquisition,* the events are placed into one of the 16 to 64 frames as they are acquired. Based upon the average heart rate, the time interval for each frame is determined as the duration of the average cardiac cycle divided by a number between 16 and 64. The larger the number of frames, from 16 to 64, the better the temporal resolution; however, each of the frames will have proportionally fewer counts. As events are recorded, they are stored in the frame corresponding to the appropriate time from the start of the R wave so that several hundred cardiac cycles can be used to construct the average cardiac cycle. It is important for the patient to have a regular—not necessarily sinus—rhythm in order for the gating mechanism to work well. The computer system interfaced to the camera/ECG must discard data from a cardiac cycle if the interval between R waves varies by more than a preset percentage of the total interval between beats—usually 10 to 20 percent. Optimal computer systems have a buffer that holds data from one beat of the cardiac cycle and only adds data from this beat to the average dataset if the beat length is within the preset interval.

The "nuclear stethoscope," or probe, is a small NaI gamma ray detector that does not use a collimator and does not create images, but it can detect extremely high count rates even at equilibrium when the probe is pointed at the cardiac chamber of interest. A small probe can be worn in a vest to record LVEF continuously during a person's normal daily activities.[209]

Radiopharmaceuticals for Cardiac BPI

[99m]Tc is the only radionuclide used for practical purposes, and it can be linked to almost any carrier compound for the first-pass BPI method,[210] including ^{99m}Tc sestamibi. For the GBPI method, ^{99m}Tc is linked to a compound that will stay in the vascular space for as long as possible in order to permit GBPI for multiple studies over 4 to 6 h. Over the years, compounds have been developed to link ^{99m}Tc to red blood cells, which remain stable in the vascular space for many hours. Only a few other radiopharmaceuticals have been used for first pass; such as gold derived from an iridium generator, which has such a short physical half-life that it allows multiple first-pass studies.[210]

Procedures for Cardiac BPI

First-pass BPI at rest requires insertion of a large (18 or 19 gauge) plastic catheter in a vein in order to deliver a bolus of radioactivity rapidly.[207,210] The goal is to inject so rapidly into such a large vein that the bolus will travel, intact, sequentially to the right and left ventricles. The patient is positioned so that the camera acquires images in an anterior view. The acquisition is started as the bolus is injected, usually 10 mCi intravenously. If a second view is needed, then the patient is positioned for an LAO or left lateral view. This study takes very little time, and one can choose whether to process images of the left and/or right ventricles in one or more views. In fact, first-pass BPI is superior to other radionuclide methods or echocardiography for evaluation of RV function. Images are usually acquired to allow ECG gating to add three to eight cardiac cycles into one summed, representative cycle.

PROCEDURE FOR ECG-GBPI AT REST

GBPI is obtained after an ECG rhythm strip shows a regular rhythm for purposes of gating. Then the intravenous catheter is inserted to inject 20 to 35 mCi of ^{99m}Tc-labeled red blood cells. Images are acquired after equilibrium has been obtained to yield equal concentrations of radioactivity throughout the blood volume.[206,208] Reliability of GBPI depends on positioning of the camera over the patient in order to isolate the left or right ventricle and minimize overlap from other cardiac chambers. During first pass, either ventricle can be isolated using images acquired during the time when the bolus arrives in the particular chamber of interest. It is difficult to isolate the right ventricle in GBPI for quantitative analysis, primarily due to overlap of the right atrium. These procedures at rest can be repeated during stress.

PROCEDURES FOR CARDIAC BPI DURING EXERCISE

The GBPI can be acquired during 30 to 240 s (usually 1 to 2 min) at each level of stress after a single injection of ^{99m}Tc-labeled red blood cells.[211] First pass is acquired during two to eight cardiac cycles with up to two to four acquisitions, and each first-pass acquisition requires a separate injection of ^{99m}Tc. *A major advantage of first pass and GBPI for stress imaging of ventricular function is that it is much easier to acquire images during exercise than it is with echocardiography.*[210] A bicycle can be used in the supine, semisupine, or upright position.[212] For first pass, a treadmill can be used that requires a special program to correct for patient motion during the study.[48,210] Isometric handgrip, the cold pressor test, and the stress of mental arithmetic[213] have also been used. Pharmacologic stress is not usually necessary for GBPI or first pass, but several drugs have been used, such as isoproterenol and dobutamine.[210]

Processing/Quantitative Analysis of Cardiac BPI

The first task in analysis of the first-pass BPI is to select the portion of the curve describing measured radioactivity counts (vertical axis) versus time (horizontal axis), the time-activity curve, which represents the time when radioactivity is located in the chamber of interest.[206,210] Then the operator selects the region of interest for the left and/or right ventricle and background. Next, the computer calculates the change in counts over time in the region of interest. The ejection fraction is calculated from the individual curves derived from the regions of interest:

$$EF = \frac{(EDC - EDB) - (ESC - ESB)}{(EDC - EDB)}$$

where EF = ejection fraction; EDC = end-diastolic counts in the region of interest for the left ventricle; EDB = end-

diastolic background counts; ESC = end-systolic counts in the region of interest for the left ventricle; and ESB = end-systolic background counts. Regional ventricular function is assessed by inspection of the cine display of serial images over time and by a variety of quantitative images: (1) ventricular cavity edges displayed at different points in time over the cardiac cycle, (2) edge images related to regional stroke volume or ejection fraction displayed at different points in time over the cardiac cycle, (3) images where gray scale or color of each pixel is related to the ejection fraction or stroke volume, (4) images of the amplitude of the first harmonic (similar to stroke-volume maps) from sinusoidal fits to the time-activity curve for each pixel, and (5) gray-scale or color-phase images related to the temporal location of the maximum count in each pixel.[206–208,210,214,215]

First pass is unique in its ability to measure intracardiac shunts, based on the transit time of the bolus of radioactivity.[216] In an experienced laboratory, this method can equal the accuracy of cardiac catheterization. This feature and the optimal assessment of RV function make first pass uniquely valuable to the practice of pediatric cardiology or follow-up of congenital heart disease in adults.

For GBPI, computer programs that detect the LV edges and background regions on each frame automatically or semi-automatically have made the method more objective and reproducible. It is critical that the physician interpreting the test review appropriate images and information (e.g., diastolic and systolic images with boundaries and background regions) to confirm that the edges and background regions were chosen correctly. The physician is responsible for confirming that LV edges do not overlap with the right ventricle or left atrium and that the background region was not placed on inappropriate hot areas (e.g, descending aorta). Errors in edge positions or background placement can lead to incorrect values of ejection fraction and regional parameters. The regional function analysis is similar to that of first pass.[210,214,215] Lung counts can be measured as an index of pulmonary blood volume,[217,218] and diastolic function can be analyzed by the peak rate of diastolic filling of the chamber (best when compared to peak systolic emptying rate) and the relative contribution of the atrial contraction to ventricular filling (amplitude of the *a* wave—late diastolic filling—relative to total end-diastolic counts).[218–220] Valvular regurgitation (aortic or mitral) has been measured by the ratios of stroke counts (LV/RV) and found to correlate with regurgitant fraction measured in the cardiac catheterization laboratory.[199,220,221] The critical issue here is that the region of interest for each chamber (left and right ventricles) must include all of the counts from that chamber and essentially no counts from other regions, such as the atria. Sometimes the optimal position requires caudal tilt of the camera in the LAO view in order to isolate the left ventricle from the left atrium by imaging perpendicular to the plane of the mitral valve. The right ventricle is even more difficult to isolate and is the major reason why the ratio of LV/RV stroke counts always exceeds 1.00 by more than the 5 to 10 percent of stroke counts that go to coronary blood flow, i.e., means of 1.15 to 1.35 with ranges of 1.00 to 1.75. This method also assumes no significant tricuspid valve regurgitation, which would increase RV stroke volume.[199,220,221]

Clinical Application of Cardiac BPI in Coronary Artery Disease

Global LV function measured as LVEF has been shown to be the major determinant of prognosis in the case of either CAD or valvular heart disease.[210,222–225] Although the Coronary Artery Surgery Study (CASS) used a highly selected population, it emphasized the good prognosis of stable patients with CAD and good LVEF during either medical or surgical therapies, and thus reliable estimation of LVEF is critical to clinical decision-making.[223] Part of the interest in stress echocardiography for detecting and assessing CAD has been its estimate of global LV function.[226–228] First pass and GBPI provide more consistently reliable estimates of LVEF than does echocardiography because they are less dependent on chest wall anatomy and skill of the operator in acquiring an adequate image of the entire left and right ventricles.[228,229] Interpretation of global LV function is less objective by echocardiography than by first pass or GBPI, particularly because of difficulty in identifying the critical endocardial edges. In fact, first pass FP or GBPI are often regarded as the reference methods for assessment of LVEF when new modalities are evaluated.[1,2]

GBPI provides very well validated assessment of LV diastolic function which is frequently abnormal in CAD[218,219] related primarily to regional LV dysfunction and which worsens with age, even in the absence of manifest CAD[219,230] (Fig. 17-29). Regional LV contraction is often abnormal in CAD, usually due to prior MI, but perhaps also due to ischemic,[230] stunned,[144] or hibernating[145] myocardium in the distribution of a diseased coronary artery. In fact, if a patient with an apparent dilated cardiomyopathy is found to have a regional wall motion abnormality, then CAD is the most likely etiology.[180]

The first pass and GBPI are also quite useful in detecting complications of acute MI. First, if a patient with suspected acute MI had completely normal global and regional LV function by first pass or GBPI within the first several hours, then one should reconsider the diagnosis of acute MI. Normal global and regional LV function acutely could not abso-

lutely rule out an acute MI. If present, however, any acute MI must be confined to the subendocardial layers of a small area of the left ventricle.[231] As with echocardiography, it is crucial that all walls of the left ventricle be seen in order to exclude a regional wall motion abnormality. Certainly, the prognosis of a patient after acute MI is strongly correlated with global LVEF. The relationship is nonlinear; e.g., if LVEF is under 0.20 at 1 month, a 50 percent death rate is predicted, while an LVEF over 0.50 predicts a death rate of less than 5 percent.[232] As expected, the LVEF at rest predicts complications such as death and disability—reflecting established damage[210,222,223,232]—better than it predicts subsequent acute MI, which would require initially viable myocardium and an artery diseased with unstable atherosclerotic plaque.[233,234]

If a patient with acute MI has heart failure but a normal or near-normal LVEF, then one should search for other diagnoses or complications, most of which should have manifestations on physical examination: mitral valve regurgitation,[199,220] ventricular septal defect,[235] or problems not specifically due to the acute MI, e.g., arteriovenous (AV) fistula (especially in trauma patients or patients with recent cardiac catheterization). First pass or GBPI, under these circumstances, should show an LVEF better than expected, based on the evidence of heart failure, and some enlargement of the left ventricle and left atrium. LV stroke volume should exceed RV stroke volume in proportion to the severity of mitral regurgitation.[199,220]

First pass and GBPI are the best widely available tests for RV involvement by acute MI.[236] During the first 1 to

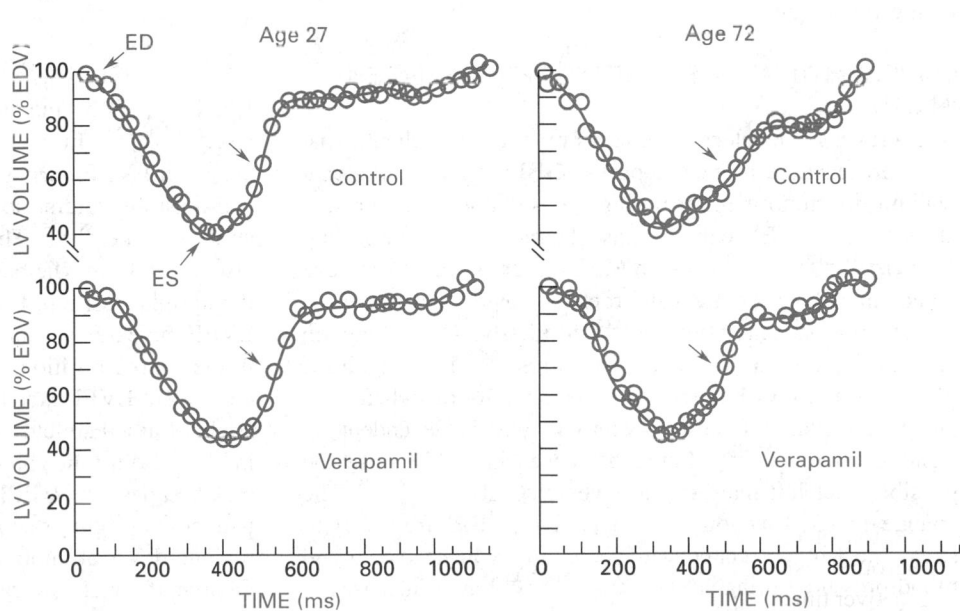

FIGURE 17-29

Gated blood pool scans can guide in diagnosis and management of diastolic left ventricular (LV) dysfunction. LV time-activity curves in a younger (*left panel*) and an older (*right panel*) normal subject. In the younger subject, LV diastolic filling rate at baseline is faster (*top left*) and is unaffected by verapamil (*bottom left*). In the older subject, LV diastolic filling rate is slower at baseline (*top right*) and improves with verapamil (*bottom right*). ED, end-diastole; ES, end-systole; % EDV, percentage of end-diastolic volume; *arrows* indicate rapid diastolic filling portion of curve. (From Arrighi et al.[219] Reproduced with permission of the publisher and authors.)

2 days after RV MI, the right ventricle appears dilated, with a global and regional wall motion abnormality. After a few days, the right ventricle usually decreases in size and contracts better. The prognosis may be poor if RV cavity size and contraction remain markedly abnormal. Thus, for a patient with a low output state after acute MI, the first pass or GBPI can be most helpful. A dilated, hypokinetic right ventricle points toward RV MI,[236] while a poor LVEF and large regional LV wall motion abnormality with relatively normal right ventricle would indicate a large LV MI as the etiology of the low cardiac output.[234] The presence of a surprisingly good LVEF raises the possibility of acute mitral regurgitation, ventricular septal defect, or AV fistula in addition to the possibility of major RV involvement.[234] If the post-MI patient is too ill and unstable to move, echocardiography is frequently useful in this setting (see Chaps. 14 and 47). Another complication of MI, LV aneurysm, is typically recognized after the acute phase. The first pass or GBPI will show regional akinesis or dyskinesis in systole and an abnormal shape of the left ventricle in diastole.[234,237]

The resting first pass or GBPI can also help predict the outcome of surgery for CAD. The prognosis for surviving CABG is strongly correlated with resting LVEF.[210,222,238] If the RV function is poor after RV MI, then surgery is likely to be complicated by severe RV dysfunction.[236] If some contraction is preserved in an abnormal region, then contraction in that region and LVEF are likely to improve after CABG. The absence of contraction in a region, however, does not mean that revascularization cannot improve its regional function[145,146,238] (see previous discussion on stunned and hibernating myocardium).

CLINICAL APPLICATIONS OF STRESS/REST CARDIAC BPI IN CAD

Stress testing can detect evidence of myocardial ischemia that is not present at rest. The first pass or GBPI can detect regional wall motion abnormalities during stress that were not present at rest, and LVEF can decrease from rest to stress (Fig. 17-30).[210–212,239–243] As with MPI, it is important to achieve an adequate level of stress in order to provoke consequences of ischemia that can be detected.[244] Similarly, RV dysfunction can develop due to ischemia during stress.[245] The magnitude of decrease in LVEF is related to the severity of ischemia[200] and to the mass of the left ventricle that is dependent on stenotic arteries.[246,247] Large decreases in LVEF raise the possibility of left main or three-vessel CAD.[210,246–249] The change in LV function on first pass or GBPI from rest to stress must be correlated with the changes in heart rate and blood pressure during stress.[210,212,214,244] Large increases in blood pressure, particularly diastolic, during stress raise afterload and decrease LVEF.[212,244,250] Small increases in heart rate or systolic blood pressure may not increase myocardial oxygen demand enough to exceed its supply and, thus, provoke no evidence of ischemia during stress.[210,212,244,248,249]

It is important to understand the normal changes in LV function during exercise. For men who are not trained athletes,

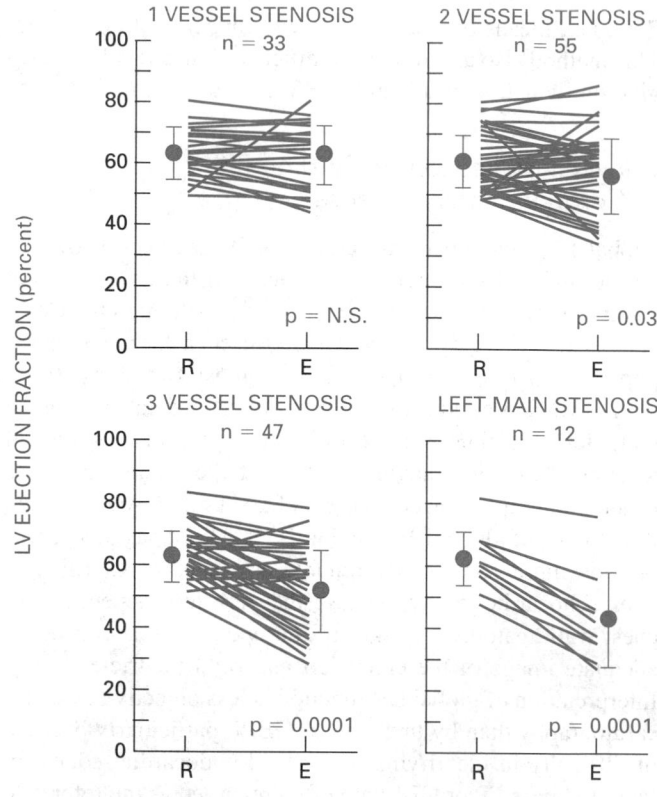

FIGURE 17-30

Radionuclide angiography shows more severe abnormalities in left ventricular ejection fraction (LVEF) during exercise in patients with more extensive coronary artery disease ($n = 147$). LVEF decreases more from rest (R) to exercise (E) and to lower values in patients with more coronary arteries obstructed. (From Jones et al.[243] Reproduced with permission of the publisher and authors.)

LVEF typically increased by at least 0.05 during exercise.[211,239–243] In contrast, women may show less or no increase in LVEF during exercise but show an increase in LV end-diastolic volume so that they achieve the same increase in stroke volume.[251,252] The response of LVEF to bicycle exercise also depends on whether the person is upright or supine.[212] In the upright position, LV end-diastolic volume decreases and LVEF increases substantially during exercise.[212] In contrast, in the supine position, LV end-diastolic volume tends to increase and LVEF increases less or not at all during exercise. Highly trained athletes, on the other hand, can show increases in LV end-diastolic volume even in the upright position. In general, first pass and GBPI are useful to assess CAD whether the patient is upright or supine.[253] Thus the LVEF increases and regional LV wall motion remains symmetric during exercise. Of note, if LVEF is very high at rest in normal subjects, it may show no change or even a small decrease, but to normal values, i.e., over 0.55, during exercise. For most people, however, a decrease in LVEF to a value below 0.55 would be an abnormal response. *One can be most confident in diagnosing myocardial ischemia if global and regional LV function improve during low to moderate levels of stress, deteriorate at the highest level achieved, and improve during recovery.*[210,211,235–243]

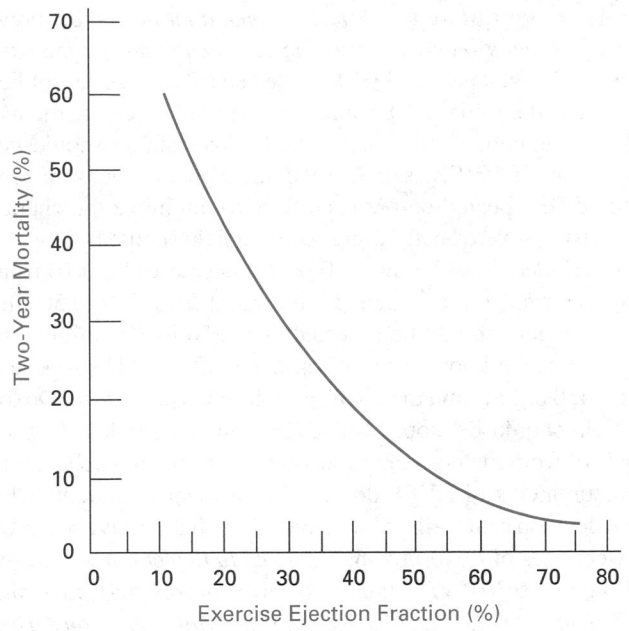

FIGURE 17-31

Two-year mortality rates after acute myocardial infarction are much lower in patients with higher left ventricular ejection fraction during exercise. (From Morris et al.[234] Reproduced with permission of the publisher and authors.)

Using first pass or GBPI, the change in LVEF from rest to exercise shows a sensitivity of 0.80 to 0.90 and a specificity of 0.75 to 0.85 for patients referred to coronary angiography and a "normalcy rate" of 0.90 to 0.95 ("specificity" in people with low clinical probability of CAD and normal blood pressures who were not referred to coronary angiography).[210,211,235–243] Using the criterion that ischemia can be diagnosed by either a failure to increase LVEF by 0.05 or the development of a new regional wall motion abnormality, sensitivity increases but specificity decreases. If one requires both a failure to increase LVEF and a new regional wall motion abnormality to diagnose myocardial ischemia, then sensitivity decreases and specificity increases, as expected for an ROC curve with stricter criteria for abnormality.[84] Exercise LVEF and the change in LVEF from rest to exercise provide outstanding predictions of prognosis in patients with CAD[210,234,249,253–258] (Figs. 17-31 and 17-32). The response of LVEF and regional wall motion to exercise also predicts which patients will respond most favorably to CABG.[259,260] The LVEF during exercise and often at rest increases after CABG.[222,259,260] The LVEF during exercise has also been shown to increase in patients with CAD after success-

ful PTCA[261] and after a program to change lifestyle by diet, relaxation techniques, and moderate exercise.[262] The authors and others have found higher exercise LVEF several months after acute anterior MI if the infarct-related artery was opened early.[231]

Clinical Application of Cardiac BPI in Noncoronary Heart Disease

In *valvular heart disease,* resting LVEF can be decreased due to decrease in preload as in mitral stenosis or because of increased afterload in aortic stenosis.[198] When resting LVEF begins to decrease basally or especially in response to exercise in mitral or aortic valve regurgitation, the patient needs to be considered for surgery (Fig. 17-33).[224,225,263] RV ejection fraction may also decrease from rest to exercise in patients with mitral regurgitation who could benefit from surgery.[264] In aortic regurgitation, the response to exercise is more predictable than it is in mitral regurgitation. As heart rate increases, the degree of aortic regurgitation decreases, and if aortic diastolic blood pressure increases, the degree of aortic regurgitation increases.[198,264] In most patients with significant aortic regurgitation, LVEF decreases from rest to exercise (Fig. 17-33), but this finding, per se, does not mean that the time has come for the patient to have aortic valve surgery.[199,225,264,265] Surgery for mitral regurgitation, however, actually produces a decrease in LVEF because the left ventricle can no longer empty into the low-pressure left atrium.[198,224] Resting and exercise LVEF usually increase after surgery for aortic regurgitation[222,225,263] (Fig. 17-33). Clinically, first pass and GBPI are most useful in following the asymptomatic patient with mitral or aortic regurgitation. Exercise first pass or GBPI is most useful in the patient with aortic regurgitation because an increase in LVEF from rest to exercise essentially excludes severe aortic regurgitation. A decrease in LVEF from rest to exercise, however, does not

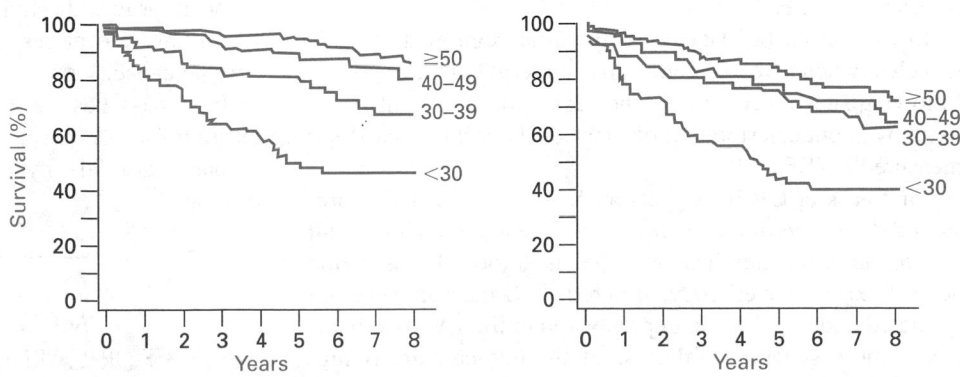

FIGURE 17-32

Radionuclide angiographic left ventricular ejection fraction (LVEF) during exercise predicted prognosis in patients with coronary artery disease. Kaplan-Meier curves for cardiovascular (CV) survival (*left*) and infarction-free (MI) survival (*right*) for groups of patients stratified by exercise LVEF. (From Lee et al.[257] Reproduced with permission of the publisher and authors.)

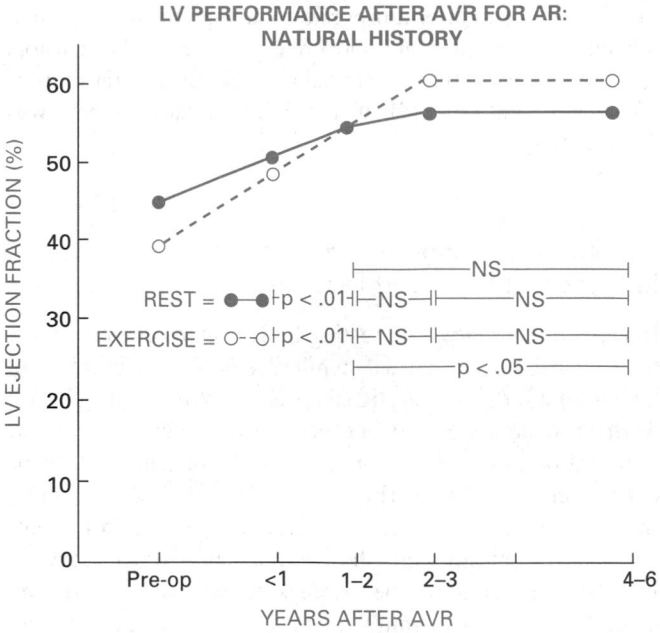

FIGURE 17-33

Left ventricular ejection fraction at rest and during exercise before (Pre-op) and during 5 years (average) after aortic valve replacement (AVR) for aortic regurgitation (AR). NS, not significant. (From Borer et al.[264] Reproduced with permission of the publisher and authors.)

indicate that surgery is needed. The most frequent use of first pass or GBPI in valvular heart disease is to make sequential measurements of LVEF over time to detect early deterioration of LV function. Since the physician may recommend valve surgery—with its 5 percent risk—for an asymptomatic person with severe aortic regurgitation, it seems best to document functional aerobic capacity by treadmill testing and to measure LVEF by first pass or GBPI regularly. Because of the magnitude of the clinical decision, one may want to supplement these LVEF data with measurements of LV dimensions by echocardiography, but first pass or GBPI provides the most accurate measuring tool to detect an early, small decline in LVEF, especially when LV volumes may increase without a decline in LVEF.

In asymptomatic patients with mitral regurgitation, it is less clear when to recommend valve surgery, but the physician following such a patient over the years would certainly want to know about deterioration of functional aerobic capacity or measured LVEF.

First pass or GBPI can be very helpful in evaluating presumed *dilated cardiomyopathy*. The presence of regional wall motion abnormalities increases the likelihood that ischemic heart disease is the etiology, as noted.[180] If the right ventricle is dilated and hypokinetic in proportion to the LV abnormalities, a more generalized disease of the myocardium is suggested. In a person with recent onset of clinical evidence of severe CHF and cardiomegaly, but relatively normal or increased LVEF, one must consider other problems, such as hyperthyroidism, AV fistulas, and severe diastolic LV dysfunction (see Chap. 23).

Assessing resting LVEF has become a mainstay for monitoring patients receiving doxorubicin chemotherapy for cancer.[266,267] First pass and GBPI have been used in serial studies to define the initial LVEF and suggest guidelines for the use of doxorubicin.[267] If LVEF < 0.30, doxorubicin should not be given. If LVEF is 0.30 to 0.50, then the measurement should be repeated before each dose to minimize the chance of causing severe heart failure. Doxorubicin should be stopped if LVEF decreases below 0.30 or if it decreases by 0.10 from the abnormal initial value. If the initial LVEF > 0.50, the measurement should be repeated after 250 to 300 mg/m². In the absence of known heart disease, LVEF should be repeated after 450 mg/m² and then before each subsequent dose. Doxorubicin should be stopped if LVEF decreases below 0.50 or by 0.10 from the normal initial value.[267] Unfortunately, serial measurements of LVEF do not always identify patients who will develop heart failure later, even though they have received lower doses of doxorubicin. *The need to detect a quantitative change of 0.10 LVEF units, however, makes first pass and GBPI more valuable than echocardiography in monitoring chemotherapy.*[228,229]

Exercise LVEF has been tested as a possible predictor of CHF due to doxorubicin.[266] It is often difficult to measure exercise LVEF accurately in patients who need chemotherapy for cancer because of their general debilitation. It is also not clear that exercise LVEF improves prediction of doxorubicin-induced cardiomyopathy.[266]

The LVEF in HCM is usually elevated at rest, and the diastolic filling rate is markedly impaired, particularly when normalized to systolic ejection rate or the heart rate and LVEF[268] (see Chap. 74). The hypertrophied septum and/or other walls of the left ventricle can be identified on LAO GBPI as a larger-than-usual area where muscle attenuated the counts from the LV and RV cavities. The abnormal shape of the left ventricle at end systole with midcavity obliteration is characteristic of HCM with LV outflow obstruction. The most consistent finding with HCM, however, is abnormal diastolic LV function (decreased peak LV diastolic filling rate and increased contribution of the atrium to the LV filling). Verapamil improves diastolic LV filling rate, and the change in LV filling rate at rest correlates with improved functional aerobic capacity on a treadmill test.[269]

First pass has been used to show improvement in RV ejection fraction during oxygen therapy in patients with pulmonary arterial hypertension and chronic pulmonary disease.[270]

OTHER RADIONUCLIDE IMAGING PROCEDURES FOR CARDIOVASCULAR DISEASE

Acute Myocardial Infarction "Hot Spot" Imaging

Instrumentation initially involved planar imaging, but later studies have shown that SPECT improves on planar images of acute MI with infarct-avid imaging agents. The first radio-pharmaceutical used for infarct-avid imaging was ^{99m}Tc-pyro-phosphate (PYP), which binds to calcium released from necro-tic cells in acute MI.[271] PYP binds even more avidly to bone in ribs, vertebrae, and sternum. SPECT improves on planar images for diagnosis of acute MI because it permits a clearer image of the heart, unobstructed by ribs and sternum.[271]

The clinical role of PYP imaging for acute MI is limited.[272] Clinically, ^{99m}Tc-PYP has shown good sensitivity and speci-ficity to detect acute Q-wave MI if the patient has two ^{99m}Tc-PYP SPECT studies 2 to 5 days apart.[271] The patients in whom the clinical diagnosis of acute MI by symptoms, ECG, and enzymes is most confusing, however, are the same patients for whom the diagnosis of acute MI by ^{99m}Tc-PYP is also most difficult. Patients with non-Q-wave acute MI often show moderate PYP uptake in the LV region where MI is suspected, and patients with unstable angina but no ECG or serum en-zyme evidence of acute MI sometimes show mild PYP uptake in the left ventricle.[272] Many patients with heart failure also have mild, diffuse PYP uptake, which may be related to residual cardiac blood pool activity in patients with slow circulation times. Thus, in the patients for whom the clinical story, ECG, and serum enzymes are inconclusive, the results of PYP myocardial imaging appear to be less helpful for clinical diagnosis[272] than in the populations of patients in whom PYP was initially validated (patients with classic find-ings for acute Q-wave MI versus patients with extremely low clinical probability of acute MI).

Recent developments of other infarct-avid imaging agents has resulted in other approaches. Monoclonal antibodies tar-geted to myosin have been labeled with indium 111 and, more recently, ^{99m}Tc.[273] These antibodies bind selectively to myosin chains that are exposed when cardiac cell membranes break down. The antibodies appear to provide more accurate diagnosis of acute MI than does PYP.[273–275] Monoclonal antibodies, however, are also taken up by the liver, which can complicate detection of hot spots in the heart,[274,275] and their cost is much greater than that of PYP. Antimyosin-antibody myocardial imaging has been reported in different groups of patients to be more sensitive for acute Q-wave MI, and for non-Q-wave MI, compared to PYP.[273–275] Patients with unstable angina also frequently have more positive im-ages recorded with antimyosin antibodies compared with PYP. Specificity of antimyosin imaging has been reported to be excellent in patients with very low clinical probability of acute MI.[273–275] Despite some improvement in accuracy, the clini-cal role for antimyosin imaging seems limited. If the clinical history, ECG, and serum enzymes show inconclusive evidence for acute MI, then the antimyosin study is likely to yield indeterminate or equivocal results.

Patients most likely to benefit from infarct-avid myocar-dial imaging to diagnose acute MI would include those with the following conditions: diabetes mellitus (chest discomfort history less reliable), LBBB (ECG less useful), missing or lost blood samples for serum enzymes at the critical times,

and, perhaps, known prior MI with abnormal rest ECG and wall motion.

One novel approach to imaging acute MI or ischemia has been the development of agents that bind selectively to hyp-oxic tissue. Developed originally to identify and kill tumors nitroimidazole derivatives labelled with iodine 123 or ^{99m}Tc are taken up by hypoxic myocardium after experimental coro-nary ligation.[276] Their clinical role remains uncertain but should be clarified by clinical trials.

One area in which infarct-avid imaging agents may prove useful is in predicting prognosis after acute MI. In an effort to predict patient outcomes, ^{201}Tl (first) has been combined with ^{99m}Tc-PYP or antimyosin antibody (second). This dual-isotope approach allows estimation of the size of the acute MI (hot spot image) as a percentage of the left ventricle (from ^{201}Tl MPI).[274] The larger the hot spot, the worse the prognosis for heart failure or death in the next several months, and LVEF is reduced in rough proportion to the size of the hot spot.[274,275] Comparison of evidence of underperfusion (^{201}Tl defects at rest) and acute necrosis (^{99m}Tc-PYP or ^{111}In-anti-myosin hot spot) on myocardial images has been described as showing one of three results: "matching" defects (to indicate necrosis), "mismatch" (^{201}Tl defect is larger than the hot spot in one region or involves an additional coronary arterial distribution), and "overlapping" (a mild-to-moderate ^{201}Tl defect in a region with mild-to-moderate increase in antimyo-sin uptake).[274] Patients with matching defects appear to have completed infarcts since they have fewer ischemic events in the subsequent few weeks compared to patients with mis-matched or overlapping abnormalities. Patients with old plus acute MI may have mismatched abnormalities but little in-crease in risk of new ischemic events.[274–276] This approach remains investigational.

Perhaps the major strength of nuclear cardiology has been its solid foundation in the anatomy, physiology, and biochem-istry of cardiovascular disease and the physics of imaging. Sometimes, however, the imaging of acute MI has produced interpretations that require careful analysis of their basic sci-ence background. Myocardial images have shown a central hot spot from an infarct-avid imaging agent, surrounded by a larger area of a cold spot on an MPI agent.[274] This appear-ance is explainable by the physical limitations of resolution inherent in nuclear imaging.[6–9,87] More importantly, the bio-logic evidence refutes the possibility that the three-dimen-sional geometry of the MI could create a true "lateral border zone" of ischemia (cold spot on MPI) surrounding the central area of necrosis (hot spot on infarct-avid agent).[103,277] The lateral border between infarcted and normal tissue is deter-mined by the vascular distributions of the occluded and patent coronary arterial branches as shown by Kirk, Factor, and their group[117,278–281] and by others.[103,277,282–284] A narrow (3 to 5 mm) region of overlap exists between the distributions of the occluded and patent arteries, but each cell depends on only one artery,[279,280,282] and the severity of ischemia or infarction is uniform from one lateral border to the other.[278,279,281–284] The true border zone, including a gradient of severity of ischemia injury, is transmural, i.e., endocardial (severe) to epicardial (mild) (Fig. 17-14).[103,117,154,200,277–284] Thus, nuclear imaging can show greater severity of a perfusion defect when the abnormality extends farther from the endocardium towards the epicardium, but there is no biologic basis for its showing a lateral border zone of intermediate level of severity of ischemic injury.

In summary, infarct-avid myocardial imaging agents play only a minor role in clinical cardiology because they cannot assess the relative extents of established myocardial necrosis versus ongoing ischemia in viable myocardium—*within the time frame (minutes) required to decide on thrombolytic therapy, direct PTCA, CABG, or conservative therapy for acute MI. Chiefly for this reason, current infarct-avid myocardial imaging agents offer only limited clinical usefulness.*

Evaluation of Cardiac Neural Function by Radionuclide Imaging

Several radiopharmaceuticals have been used to develop noninvasive images of the integrity of the sympathetic nervous system. Most of these agents have required production in a cyclotron using the positron-emitting radionuclide carbon 11 (^{11}C) incorporated into analogues of norepinephrine.[285] The chemical specificity of binding sites for norepinephrine has led to a preference for using radioligands that are chemically the same as the native neurotransmitters or their metabolites, because radioligands that include ^{99m}Tc, ^{123}I, ^{111}In, or ^{18}F cause a major chemical change in the ligand, affecting its binding specificity. The radiopharmaceutical that has been used most widely for planar and SPECT imaging of cardiac neural function is ^{123}I-methyliodobenzyl guanidine (MIBG).[286] Developed initially to identify pheochromocytoma, MIBG has shown regional defects that match perfusion defects due to transmural MI, consistent with the idea that MIBG uptake is related to the integrity of cardiac nerves.[286] The MIBG defect usually exceeds the size of the resting perfusion defect in acute MI.[286] Subendocardial MI creates smaller sized MIBG defects than does transmural MI, consistent with there being less damage to the nerves that are located in the epicardium when the ischemic injury is located in the subendocardium.[287] The risk of cardiac arrhythmias appears to be increased when the areas of MIBG defect are larger, especially if the same region has relatively normal perfusion.[288] Thus, MIBG defects have been reported in the abnormal cardiac regions in patients with arrhythmogenic RV dysplasia, the long QT interval syndromes, and other causes of ventricular tachycardia without CAD, for example, valvular aortic stenosis and HCM.[288,289]

The most straightforward studies are those that show essentially no MIBG activity immediately after cardiac transplant, which denervates the heart, with gradual increase in MIBG activity near the base of the heart by 2 years after the transplant to indicate reinnervation.[287] Others have found rapid wash-out and/or decreased uptake of MIBG in doxorubicin-induced cardiomyopathy.[290] The MIBG abnormalities appear to occur earlier than the decrease in LVEF, which suggests a possible approach to early detection of the abnormality before doxorubicin causes frank CHF.[288,290]

In CHF, chronically high-level adrenergic stimulation leads to decreased concentrations of norepinephrine in myocardium[291] and increased concentrations in blood.[292] In fact, any condition that leads to greater sympathetic stimulation of the heart would be expected to increase wash-out of MIBG from the heart.[293] It may be too simplistic to equate MIBG uptake by the heart with myocardial norepinephrine stores, because the two do not change in parallel during reinnervation of the heart after severing cardiac nerves in the dog.[293] Studies with MIBG in animals and in patients with CHF have shown abnormalities in MIBG wash-out and/or uptake.[293–296] One particularly important study in this area studied patients with CHF due to CAD (*n* = 24) or to unknown causes (*n* = 66).[297] MIBG uptake 4 h after injection (thus allowing time for wash-out) was a more powerful independent predictor of patient survival than was radionuclide LVEF or echocardiographic end-diastolic dimensions.[297]

In summary, nuclear medicine research efforts need to focus more attention on the unique strengths of radionuclide imaging, such as labeling a variety of chemical compounds to assess different aspects of cardiac innervation.[298] Studies are needed using pharmacologic probes to stimulate reflex-mediated release of norepinephrine (e.g., vasodilators), or to inhibit cardiac stimulation by adrenergic nerve activity (e.g., ganglionic blocker), or to block neuronal uptake of norepinephrine (e.g., desipramine) to reveal how much cardiac uptake is due to nonneuronal, (e.g., nonspecific) norepinephrine uptake.[299] Further progress in SPECT imaging of cardiac sympathetic neural innervation will require better radiopharmaceuticals. This is a most important area for cardiology, however, because other methodologies provide little or no information about cardiac innervation. An elegant series of studies used serial RV myocardial biopsies to show decreased beta-adrenergic receptor activity, measured in vitro, and impaired responses to catecholamines, in vivo, in patients with CHF, presumably due to compensatory sympathetic stimulation and downregulation of beta-receptor activity.[300] Beta-adrenergic blocking drugs can reverse this process and upregulate beta-adrenergic receptor activity.[300] If the beta-receptor activity and norepinephrine concentration in the heart could be defined noninvasively for each individual patient with CHF, then this might allow better prediction of the risk of sudden cardiac death[297] and the risks and benefits of such diametrically opposed treatments as beta-adrenergic blocking drugs or beta stimulants, such as dobutamine. *The clinical usefulness of currently available radionuclide images to assess the autonomic nervous system is very limited.* The magnitude of the clinical and economic problems posed by CHF, the preliminary physiologic information, and the need for more answers suggest that cardiac neural imaging deserves further intensive research efforts.

Imaging Cardiac Inflammation

Early radiopharmaceuticals designed to image cardiac inflammation included gallium 67 (^{67}Ga) imaging.[301] Active myocarditis and sarcoidosis have been associated with positive cardiac gallium scans,[301] but the method has not proven to be a useful clinical diagnostic procedure for these conditions. More recently, ^{111}In-antimyosin-antibody images have been found to be positive quite frequently during active myocarditis[302] and transplant rejection.[303,304] These cardiac images appear to be quite sensitive but only moderately specific when compared to myocardial biopsy evidence of cardiac inflammation.[302,303] Some studies, however, indicate that the positive antimyosin cardiac images may actually be correct—true positive rather than false positive—in identifying inflammation in some patients with negative myocardial biopsies.[304] Presumably, the biopsy needle samples may have missed regions of the heart with active inflammation that could be detected on cardiac ^{111}In-antimyosin images. The evidence that the positive antimyosin images were true and the negative myocardial biopsies were false in identifying inflammation came from using a different reference method to define myocardial inflammation, i.e., clinical follow-up rather than histology. Thus, follow-up studies of patients with newly diagnosed dilated cardiomyopathy have identified myocarditis, based on subsequent spontaneous recovery. Also, studies of cardiac transplant patients have identified some who progressed rapidly to clear-cut episodes of acute rejection to indicate rejection/inflammation despite the negative myocardial biopsy.[303,304] In either case, the scan may be more useful if it can predict the patient's clinical outcome accurately. This area is still under development. Current development of antibodies directed to granulocytes, adhesion molecules, and other markers of acute inflammation seem likely to produce better radiopharmaceuticals for identification and quantitation of inflammatory activity, e.g., in infective endocarditis.[305] Such a test would also be most welcome for transplant patients who undergo multiple and frequent myocardial biopsy procedures during their first year after cardiac transplantion.

Imaging Platelets and Thrombus in the Heart and Blood Vessels

Imaging cardiac thrombus can be performed with the following radiopharmaceuticals: labeled platelets,[306] clotting factors,[307] and recombinant tissue plasminogen activator.[308] ^{111}In-labeling procedures are difficult for platelets, but these studies have shown intriguing clinical results.[309] Identification of LV thrombus can be accomplished by ^{111}In-labeled platelets with images acquired 48 to 72 h after injection.[309,310] A positive ^{111}In-labeled platelet cardiac image has been reported to be a more powerful predictor of subsequent embolic events than is the echocardiogram. The result seems explainable by comparing the abilities of anatomic (echocardiographic) versus physiologic (^{111}In-labeled platelet) images to predict the subsequent physiologic event of thromboembolism. Given the importance of cardiac thrombus in producing cerebral vascular events, such studies deserve greater emphasis and wider availability and study. Labeling problems appear to explain the limited use of these studies at present.[310] Recent development of labeled antibodies and other agents directed toward receptors that are exposed only when the platelets are activated to create aggregates[310] may yield even more selective and readily produced radiopharmaceuticals. Labeling thrombus in blood vessels can be performed with radiopharmaceuticals used for imaging cardiac thrombus. Most of these studies imaged thrombus in veins and, less often, in arteries.[310,311] Imaging thrombus in lower extremity veins and pulmonary arteries has been combined with ventilation-perfusion ($\dot{V}/\dot{Q}$) imaging of the lung. The main contribution of venous radionuclide imaging may be in the identification of pelvic vein thrombosis and differentiating old (low risk for emboli) versus new (high risk for emboli) thrombus in patients with chronic venous disease.[310] Some studies have demonstrated pulmonary arterial thrombus which enhances the accuracy of $\dot{V}/\dot{Q}$ imaging to detect patients at increased risk of pulmonary emboli[310,311] (see Chap. 60).

Imaging Atherosclerotic Plaque in Arteries

Labeling atherosclerotic plaque in arteries by radionuclide imaging must be considered experimental at this time, but it could potentially provide a major breakthrough for guiding treatment of atherosclerosis and prevention of complications of CAD.[312] The most widely used radiopharmaceuticals to date have been ^{123}I- or ^{99m}Tc-labeled low-density lipoprotein cholesterol,[313–315] some of its synthetic analogues,[316,317] and antibodies to other plaque components.[318] These agents have demonstrated atherosclerotic plaque in carotid arteries.[313] The accuracy of a radionuclide imaging procedure in detecting atherosclerosis requires an understanding of the goal of the imaging study and the appropriate "gold standard," or reference method. If the goal is to detect early evidence of atherosclerosis[312,316] in order to help motivate the patient to change lifestyle and to help the physician decide whether to recommend lipid-altering drugs,[319] then the imaging method to be developed needs to be referenced against the observation of lumen irregularities on a contrast angiogram or, better, plaque seen on intravascular ultrasound or angioscopic images.[320] If the goal is to detect unstable atherosclerotic plaque that could cause unstable angina or acute MI,[233] then one might use clinical events such as acute MI or unstable angina as the reference method with which to compare radionuclide imaging agents. Radiopharmaceuticals are currently in their infancy for the purpose of identifying atherosclerotic lesions, but the rapid progress in vascular biology[321] should lead to selective markers for different components of atherosclerotic plaque: platelets, clotting factors, oxidized low-density lipoprotein, or markers of active inflammatory processes in the arterial wall. A major rationale for developing these radiopharmaceuticals is to prevent clinical manifestations of CAD by targeting the most aggressive interventions against the early stages of the atherosclerotic process per se.[322]

Ventilation-Perfusion (V/Q̇) Lung Imaging for Pulmonary Embolism

Acute pulmonary embolism is a common problem that is serious but frequently difficult to diagnose.[323,324] The symptoms, physical signs, and laboratory studies are usually inconclusive, although in recent years, it has been shown that patients with negative plasma D-dimer levels are unlikely to have acute pulmonary embolism (<10 percent of false-negative results in patients suspected of pulmonary embolism)[325] (see Chaps. 52 and 60). The problem with this test is its very high rate of (false) positive results in patients with recent surgery, acute MI, or other illnesses.[323,324] Arterial P_{O_2} values appear to be virtually useless, and the chest x-ray is helpful mainly when used to clarify nuclear imaging.[326,327] The ECG can be helpful but is not definitive[328]; ultrasound[329] and nuclear[309] and contrast radiographic techniques can demonstrate evidence of peripheral venous thrombosis, but this diagnosis does not prove pulmonary embolism. Echocardiographic or nuclear BPI and right heart catheterization can show abnormal RV function due to massive pulmonary embolism but can be normal with smaller pulmonary emboli.[330] Newer, noninvasive three-dimensional imaging techniques such as spiral volumetric CT,[331] magnetic resonance imaging and angiography (see Chap. 19),[332] and ultrafast electron beam CT (see Chap. 18)[333] are all quite promising but need wider validation and availability to make a major clinical impact. Contrast pulmonary angiography is justifiably considered the gold standard reference method to diagnose acute pulmonary embolism,[323,324] but it can be misinterpreted and/or dangerous.[334] Newer invasive approaches include imaging pulmonary arterial thrombus with ultrasonic[335] or angioscopic[336] instruments mounted in catheters.

The above discussion indicates the continuing need for a widely available noninvasive test for acute pulmonary embolism, especially since the condition is quite common.[323,324] Pulmonary perfusion scans are acquired after injecting ^{99m}Tc-macroaggregated albumin, but perfusion is reduced in regions with many types of lung pathology.[337] Images of the regional distribution of ventilation can detect many of the local areas of lung pathology where decreased perfusion might be expected. Ventilation is generally normal in a region with acute embolic occlusion of its blood supply. Thus imaging a region of segment size or greater with decreased perfusion but normal ventilation indicates a high probability of acute pulmonary embolism.[337,338]

Radiopharmaceuticals are usually ^{99m}Tc-macroaggregated albumin microspheres, 10 to 60 μm in diameter, and xenon 133 (^{133}Xe) for ventilation.[337] ^{99m}Tc-DTPA aerosolized particles have also been used for ventilation. Planar images are acquired for ^{99m}Tc radiopharmaceuticals in six projections. For ^{133}Xe, one can image wash-out related to ventilation, usually in the posterior oblique projections.[337,338]

The diagnostic accuracy of V/Q̇ lung imaging is limited and has led to reporting the results as normal or nearly normal, or as one of three probabilities of abnormality: low, intermediate, or high probability, based on the appearance of the lung images and the chest x-ray (see Table 17-8).[323,324,337–339] A truly normal V/Q̇ image excludes the diagnosis of pulmonary embolism with considerable (96 percent) confidence,[339] but few patients (14.5 percent) suspected of acute pulmonary embolism have these truly normal results because they have atelectasis, heart failure, pneumonia, or other processes. A high probability V/Q̇ lung image allows a very confident diagnosis of the presence of pulmonary embolism (87 percent), but few patients (13 percent) have this result. The more common results are low (33 percent) and intermediate (39 percent) probability V/Q̇ images—to indicate likelihoods of pulmonary embolism of 14 percent and 30 percent, respectively.[339] These results can be improved by using revised criteria for classifying V/Q̇ scans as intermediate instead of low probability.[340] This revised classification scheme may help solve the problem for patients with (erroneously) "low" probability V/Q̇ scan results but with considerable likelihood

TABLE 17-8

PROBABILITY OF PULMONARY EMBOLISM (PE) ON PULMONARY ANGIOGRAPHY (ANGIO) RELATED TO V/Q̇ SCAN AND CLINICAL PROBABILITY IN PIOPED STUDY (n = 887 PATIENTS WITH ANGIO)[339]

V/Q̇ Lung Scan Result	Clinical Probability of Pulmonary Embolism							
	Low (<20%)		Intermediate (20–79%)		High (>79%)		All Patients	
	%Popul.	%PE	%Popul.	%PE	%Popul.	%PE	%Popul.	%PE
Normal (or nearly)	6.9	2	7.0	6	0.6	0	14.5	4
Low probability	10.1	4	21.5	16	1.7	40	33.3	14
Intermediate probability	7.7	16	26.6	28	4.6	66	38.9	30
High probability	1.0	56	9.0	88	3.3	96	13.3	87
All patients	25.7	9	64.1	30	10.2	68	100.0	28

Note: %Popul., percent of population that has the particular clinical or V/Q̇ probabilities indicated.

of acute pulmonary embolism[341,342] (4 to 40 percent, depending on the clinical setting in one large multicenter study).[339] Some interesting studies suggest that an even better way to increase the accuracy of diagnosis of acute pulmonary embolism may be the use of labeled agents to identify thrombus in the pulmonary arteries.[310,311]

REFERENCES

1. Pohost GM, O'Rourke RA, ed. *Principles and Practice of Cardiovascular Imaging.* Boston: Little-Brown; 1991.
2. Zaret BL, Wackers FJ. *Nuclear cardiology. N Engl J Med* 1993; 329:775–783, 855–863.
3. Skorton DJ, Schelbert HR, Wolf GL, Brundage BH, ed. *Marcus' Cardiac Imaging: A Companion to Braunwald's "Heart Disease."* Philadelphia: Saunders; 1996.
4. De Puey EE, Berman DS, Garcia EV. *Cardiac SPECT Imaging.* Philadelphia: Lippincott-Raven; 1996.
5. Beller GA. *Clinical Nuclear Cardiology.* Philadelphia: Saunders; 1996.
6. Sorensen JA, Phelps ME. *Physics in Nuclear Medicine.* Philadelphia: Saunders; 1987.
7. Garcia EV, Van Train K, Maddahi J, Prigent F, Friedman J, Areeda J, et al. Quantification of rotational thallium-201 myocardial tomography. *J Nucl Med* 1985; 26:17–26.
8. Eisner RL. Principles of Instrumentation in SPECT. *J Nucl Med Tech* 1985; 13:23–31.
9. Eisner RL, Nowak DJ, Pettigrew RI, Fajman WA. Fundamentals of 180 acquisition and reconstruction in SPECT imaging. *J Nucl Med* 1986; 27:1717–1728.
10. FD Rollo (ed). *Nuclear Medicine: Physics, Instrumentation and Agents.* St. Louis: Mosby; 1977:234.
11. Pohost GM, Zir LM, Moore RH, McKusick KA, Guiney TE, Beller GA. Differentiation of transiently ischemic from infarcted myocardium by serial imaging after a single dose of thallium-201. *Circulation* 1977; 55:294–302.
12. Gerry JL Jr, Becker LC, Flaherty JT, Weisfeldt ML. Evidence for a flow-independent contribution to the phenomenon of thallium redistribution. *Am J Cardiol* 1980; 45:58–61.
13. Nielsen AP, Morris KG, Murdock R, Bruno FP, Cobb FR. Linear relationship between the distribution of thallium-201 and blood flow in ischemic and nonischemic myocardium during exercise. *Circulation* 1980; 61:797–801.
14. Krivokapich J, Shine KI. Effects of hyperkalemia and glycoside on thallium exchange in rabbit ventricle. *Am J Physiol* 1981; 240:H612–619.
15. Goldhaber SZ, Newell JB, Alpert NM, Andrews E, Pohost GM, Ingwall JS. Effects of ischemic-like insult on myocardial thallium-201 accumulation. *Circulation* 1983; 67:778–786.
16. McCall D, Zimmer LJ, Katz AM. Kinetics of thallium exchange in cultured rat myocardial cells. *Circ Res* 1985; 56:370–376.
17. Dahlberg ST, Leppo JA. Myocardial kinetics of radiolabelled perfusion agents: Basis for perfusion imaging. *J Nucl Cardiol* 1994; 1:189–197.
18. Kaul S, Chesler DA, Pohost GM, Strauss HW, Okada RD, Boucher CA. Influence of peak exercise heart rate on normal thallium-201 myocardial clearance. *J Nucl Med* 1986; 27:26–30.
19. Wharton TP Jr, Neill WA, Oxendine JM, Painter LN. Effect of duration of regional myocardial ischemia and degree of reactive hyperemia on the magnitude of the initial thallium-201 defect. *Circulation* 1980; 62:516–521.
20. Patterson RE, Halgash DA, Horowitz SF, Miceli K, Eng C, Goldsmith SJ. Physiological influences on perfusion imaging in transient myocardial ischemia: Importance of early distribution of thallium-201. *Cardiovasc Res* 1982; 16:47–54.
21. Berman DS, Kiat H, Van Train K, Garcia E, Friedman J, Maddahi J. Technetium-99m sestamibi in the assessment of chronic coronary artery disease. *Semin Nucl Med* 1991; 21:190–212.
22. Leppo JA, DePuey KG, Johnson LL. A review of cardiac imaging with sestamibi and teboroxime. *Nucl Med* 1991; 32:2012–2022.
23. Garcia EV, Cooke CD, Van Train KF, Folks R, Peifer J, DePuey EG, et al. Technical aspects of myocardial SPECT imaging with technetium-99m sestamibi. *Am J Cardiol* 1990; 66:23E–31E.

24. Galt JR, Cullom SJ, Garcia EV. SPECT quantification: A simplified method of attenuation and scatter correction for cardiac imaging. *J Nucl Med* 1992; 33:2232–2237.
25. Tsui BMW, Hu HB, Gilland DR, Gullberg GT. Implementation of simultaneous attenuation and detector response correction in SPECT. *IEEE Trans Nucl Sci* 1988; 35:778–783.
26. Marshall RC, Leidholdt EM Jr, Zhang DY, Barnett CA. Technetium-99m hexakis 2-methoxy-2-isobutyl isonitrile and thallium-201 extraction, washout, and retention at varying coronary flow rates in rabbit heart. *Circulation* 1990; 82:998–1007.
27. Leppo JA, Meerdink DJ. Comparison of the myocardial uptake of a technetium-labeled isonitrile analogue and thallium. *Circ Res* 1989; 65:632–639.
28. Glover DK, Okada RD. Myocardial kinetics of Tc-MIBI in canine myocardium after dipyridamole. *Circulation* 1990; 81:628–637.
29. Leon AR, Eisner RL, Martin SE, Schmarkey LS, Aaron AM, Boyers AS, et al. Comparison of single photon emission computed tomographic (SPECT) myocardial perfusion imaging with thallium-201 and technetium-99m sestamibi in dogs. *J Am Coll Cardiol* 1992; 20:1612–1625.
30. Li QS, Solol G, Frank TL, Wagner HN Jr, Becker LC. Myocardial redistribution of technetium-99m methoxyisobutyl isonitrile (sestamibi). *J Nucl Med* 1990; 31:1069–1076.
31. Piwnica-Worms D, Kronauge JF, Chiu ML. Uptake and retention of hexakis (2-methoxyisobutyl isonitrile) technetium in cultured chick myocardial cells. Mitochondrial and plasma membrane potential dependence. *Circulation* 1990; 82:1826–1838.
32. Sinusas A, Bergin JD, Edwards N, Watson DD, Ruiz M, Makuch RW, et al. Redistribution of ^{99m}Tc-sestamibi and ^{201}Tl in the presence of a severe coronary stenosis. *Circulation* 1994; 89:2332–2341.
33. Berman DS, Kiat HS, Van Train KF, Germano G, Maddahi J, Friedman JD. Myocardial perfusion imaging with technetium-99m sestamibi: Comparative analysis of available imaging protocols. *J Nucl Med* 1994; 35:681–688.
34. Canby RC, Silber S, Pohost GM. Relations of the myocardial imaging agents ^{99m}Tc-MIBI and ^{201}Tl to myocardial blood flow in a canine model of myocardial ischemic insult. *Circulation* 1990; 81:289–296.
35. Narahara KA, Villanueva-Meyer J, Thompson CJ, Brizendine M, Mena I. Comparison of thallium-201 and technetium-99m hexakis 2-methoxyisobutyl isonitrile single-photon emission computed tomography for estimating the extent of myocardial ischemia and infarction in coronary artery disease. *Am J Cardiol* 1990; 66:1438–1444.
36. Maublant JC, Marcaggi X, Lusson JR, Boire JY, Cauvin JC, Jacob P, et al. Comparison between thallium-201 and technetium-99m methoxyisobutyl isonitrile defect size in single-photon emission computed tomography at rest: Exercise and redistribution in coronary artery disease. *Am J Cardiol* 1992; 69:183–187.
37. Glover DK, Ruiz M, Cunningham M, Edwards NC, Simanis JP, Smith W, et al. Comparison between thallium-201 and Tc-99m sestamibi uptake during adenosine-induced vasodilation as a function of coronary stenosis severity. *Circulation* 1995; 91:813–820.
38. Di Rocco RJ, Rumsey WL, Kuczynski BL, Linder KE, Pirro JP, Narra RK, et al. Measurement of myocardial blood flow using a co-injection technique for technetium-99m-teboroxime, technetium-99m-sestamibi and thallium-201. *J Nucl Med* 1992; 33:1152–1159.
39. Taillefer R, Lambert R, Dupras G, Gregoire J, Leveille J, Essiambre R, et al. Clinical comparison between thallium-201 and Tc99m-methoxy isobutyl isonitrile (hexamibi) myocardial perfusion imaging for detection of coronary artery disease. *Eur J Nucl Med* 1989; 15:280–286.
40. Kahn JK, McGhie I, Akers MS, Sills MN, Faber TL, Kulkarni PV, et al. Quantitative rotational tomography with ^{201}Tl and ^{99m}Tc 2-methoxy-isobutyl-isonitrile: A direct comparison in normal individuals and patients with coronary artery disease. *Circulation* 1989; 79:1282–1293.
41. Iskandrian AS, Heo J, Kong B, Lyons E, Marsch S. Use of technetium-99m isonitrile (RP-30A) in assessing left ventricular perfusion and function at rest and during exercise in coronary artery disease, and comparison with coronary arteriography and exercise thallium-201 SPECT imaging. *Am J Cardiol* 1989; 64:270–275.
42. Maisey MN, Lowry A, Bischof-Delaloye A, Fridrich R, Inglese E, Khalil MN, et al. European multi-centre comparison of thallium-201 and technetium-99m methoxyisobutyl isonitrile in ischaemic heart disease. *Eur J Nucl Med* 1990; 16:869–872.
43. Van Train KF, Maddahi J, Areeda J, Cooke CD, Kiat H, Silagan G, et al. Multicenter trial validation for quantitative analysis of same-

day rest-stress technetium-99m-sestamibi myocardial tomograms. *J Nucl Med* 1994; 35:609–618.

44. Cuocolo A, Pace L, Ricciardelli B, Chiariello M, Trimarco B, Salvatore M. Identification of viable myocardium in patients with chronic coronary artery disease: Comparison of thallium-201 scintigraphy with reinjection and technetium-99m-methoxyisobutyl isonitrile. *J Nucl Med* 1992; 33:505–511.

45. Berman DS, Kiat H, Friedman JD, Wang FP, Van Train K, Matzer L, et al. Separate acquisition rest thallium-201/technetium-99m sestamibi dual-isotope myocardial perfusion single photon emission computed tomography. A clinical validation study. *J Am Coll Cardiol* 1993; 22:1455–1464.

46. Cooke CD, Garcia EV, Cullom J, Faber TL, Pettigrew RI. Determining the accuracy of calculating systolic wall thickening using a fast Fourier transform approximation: A stimulation study based on canine and patient data. *J Nucl Med* 1994; 35:1185–1192.

47. Chua T, Kiat H, Palmas W, Maurer G, Rubin P, Friedman J, et al. Can assessment of stress/perfusion/rest function by single injection gated SPECT Tc-99m sestamibi substitute for separate injection stress/rest perfusion studies? *Circulation* 1992; 86:I-507.

48. Borges-Neto S, Coleman RE, Potts JM, Jones RH. Combined exercise radionuclide angiocardiography and single photon emission computed tomography perfusion studies for assessment of coronary artery disease. *Semin Nucl Med* 1991; 21:223–229.

49. Sinusas AJ, Shi QX, Saltzberg MT, Vitals P, Jain D, Wackers FJ, et al. Technetium-99m-tetrofosmin to assess myocardial blood flow: Experimental validation in an intact canine model of ischemia. *J Nucl Med* 1994; 35:664–671.

50. Stewart RE, Heyl B, O'Rourke RA, Blumbardt R, Miller DD. Demonstration of differential post-stenotic myocardial technetium-99m teboroxime clearance kinetics after experimental ischemia and hyperemic stress. *J Nucl Med* 1991; 32:2000–2008.

51. Smith AM, Gullberg GT, Christian PK, Datz FL. Kinetic modeling of teboroxime using dynamic SPECT imaging in a canine model. *J Nucl Med* 1994; 35:484–495.

52. Chiao P-C, Ficaro EP, Dayanikili F, Rogers WL, Schwaiger M. Compartmental analysis of technetium-99m-teboroxime kinetics employing fast dynamic SPECT at rest and stress. *J Nucl Med* 1994; 35:1265–1273.

53. Eisner RL, Churchwell A, Noever T, Nowalk DJ, Cloninger KG, Dunn DW, et al. Quantitative analysis of the tomographic thallium-201 myocardial bullseye display: Critical role of correcting for patient motion. *J Nucl Med* 29:91–97, 1988.

54. Fintel DJ, Links JM, Brinker IA, Frank TL, Parker M, Becker LC. Improved diagnostic performance of exercise thallium-201 single photon emission computed tomography over planar imaging in the diagnosis of coronary artery disease: A receiver operating characteristic analysis. *J Am Coll Cardiol* 1989; 13:600–612.

55. Iskandrian AS, Heo I, Kong B, Lyons E. Effect of exercise level on the ability of thallium-201 tomographic imaging in detecting coronary artery disease: Analysis of 461 patients. *J Am Coll Cardiol* 1989; 14:1477–1486.

56. Alazraki NP, Krawczyaska KG, DePuey KG, Ziffer JA, Vansant JP, Pettigrew RI, et al. Reproducibility of thallium-201 exercise SPECT studies. *J Nucl Med* 1994; 35:1237–1244.

57. Gould KL, Goldstein RA, Mullani NA, Kirkoeide RL, Wong WH, Tewson TJ, et al. Noninvasive assessment of coronary stenoses by myocardial perfusion imaging during pharmacologic coronary vasodilation. Clinical feasibility of positron cardiac imaging without a cyclotron using generator-produced rubidium-82. *J Am Coll Cardiol* 1986; 7:775–789.

58. Feldman RL, Nichols WW, Pepine CJ, Conti CR. Acute effect of intravenous dipyridamole on regional coronary hemodynamics and metabolism. *Circulation* 1981; 64:333–344.

59. Gould KL, Lipscomb K. Effects of coronary stenoses on coronary flow reserve and resistance. *Am J Cardiol* 1974; 34:48–55.

60. McLaughlin DP, Beller GA, Linden J, Ayers CR, Ripley ML, Taylor H, et al. Hemodynamic and metabolic correlates of dipyridamole-induced myocardial thallium-201 perfusion abnormalities in multivessel coronary artery disease. *Am J Cardiol* 1994; 74:1159–1164.

61. Klein HO, Ninio R, Eliyahu S, Bakst A, Levi A, Dean H, et al. Effects of the dipyridamole test on left ventricular function in coronary artery disease. *Am J Cardiol* 1992; 69:482–488.

62. Homma S, Gilliland Y, Guincy TE, Slrauss HW, Boucher CA. Safety of intravenous dipyridamole for stress testing with thallium imaging. *Am J Cardiol* 1987; 59:152–154.

63. Ranhosky A, Kempthome-Rawson J. The safety of intravenous dipyridamole thallium myocardial perfusion imaging. Intravenous dipyridamole thallium imaging study group. *Circulation* 1990; 81:1205–1209.

64. Bottcher M, Czermin J, Sun KT, Phelps ME, Schelbert HR. Effect of caffeine on myocardial blood flow at rest and during pharmacological vasodilation. *J Nucl Med* 1995; 36:2016–2021.

65. Fam WM, McGregor M. Effect of nitroglycerin and dipyridamole on regional coronary resistance. *Circ Res* 1968; 22:640–657.

66. Patterson RE, Kirk ES. Coronary steal mechanisms in dogs with single vessel occlusion and other arteries normal. *Circulation* 1983; 67:1009–1015.

67. Cerqueira MD, Verani M, Schwaiger M, Heo I, Iskandrian A. Safety profile of adenosine stress perfusion imaging: Results from the adenoscan multicenter trial registry. *J Am Coll Cardiol* 1994; 23:384–389.

68. Elliott BM, Robison JG, Zeilner JL, Hendrix GH. Dobutamine ^{201}Tl imaging. Assessing cardiac risks associated with vascular surgery. *Circulation* 1991; 84:III54–III60.

69. Fung AY, Gallagher KP, Buda AJ. The physiologic basis of dobutamine as compared with dipyridamole stress interventions in the assessment of critical coronary stenosis. *Circulation* 1987; 76:943–951.

70. Martin TW, Seaworth JF, Johns JP, Pupa LE, Condos WR. Comparison of adenosine, dipyridamole, and dobutamine in stress echocardiography. *Ann Intern Med* 1992; 116:190–196.

71. Eisner RL, Schmarkey LS, Martin SE, Carey D, Worthy MA, Chu TH, et al. Defects on SPECT "perfusion" images can occur due to abnormal segmental contraction. *J Nucl Med* 1994; 35:638–643.

72. Rocco TP, Dilsizian V, McKusick KA, Fischman AJ, Boucher CA, Strauss HW. Comparison of thallium redistribution with rest "reinjection" imaging for the detection of viable myocardium. *Am J Cardiol* 1990; 66:158–163.

73. Dilsizian V, Rocco TP, Freedman NM, Leon MB, Bonow RO. Enhanced detection of ischemic but viable myocardium by the reinjection of thallium after stress-redistribution imaging. *N Engl J Med* 1990; 323:141–146.

74. Dilsizian V, Perrone-Filardi P, Arrighi JA, Bacharach SL, Quyyumi AA, Freedman NMT, et al. Concordance and discordance between stress-redistribution-reinjection and rest-redistribution thallium imaging for assessing viable myocardium. *Circulation* 1993; 88:941–952.

75. Dilsizian V, Freedman NM, Bacharach SL, Perrone-Filardi P, Bonow RO. Regional thallium uptake in irreversible defects. Magnitude of change in thallium activity after reinjection distinguishes viable from nonviable myocardium. *Circulation* 1992; 85:627–634.

76. Berman DS, Kiat H, Friedman JD, Wang FP, Van Train K, Matzer L, et al. Separate acquisition rest thallium-201/technetium-99m sestamibi dual-isotope myocardial perfusion single photo emission computed tomography. A clinical validation study. *J Am Coll Cardiol* 1993; 22:1455–1464.

77. Friedman J, Van Train K, Maddahi J, Rozanski A, Prigent F, Bietendorf J, et al. Upward creep of the heart: A frequent source of false-positive reversible defects during thallium-201 stress-redistribution SPECT. *J Nucl Med* 1989; 30:1718–1722.

78. Eisner RL, Aaron AM, Worthy MR, Boyers AS, Leon AR, Fajman WA, et al. Apparent change in cardiac geometry during single-photon emission tomography thallium-201 acquisition: A complex phenomenon. *Eur J Nucl Med* 1993; 20:324–329.

79. Leppo JA, DePuey G, Johnson LL. A review of cardiac imaging with sestamibi and teboroxime. *J Nucl Med* 1991; 32:2012–2022.

80. Dahlberg ST, Gilmore MP, Leppo JA. Interaction of technetium-99m-labeled teboxime with red blood cells reduces the compound's extraction and increases apparent cardiac washout. *J Nucl Cardiol* 1994; 1:270–279.

81. Iskandrian AD, Heo J, Nyuyen T, Mercuro J. Myocardial imaging with teboroxime: Technique and initial results. *Am Heart J* 1991; 121:889–894.

82. Burns RJ, Illes S, Fung AY, Wright LM, Daigneault L. The Canadian exercise technetium-99m-labeled teboroxime single-photon emission computed tomographic study. *J Nucl Cardiol* 1995; 2:117–125.

83. DePuey KG. How to detect and avoid myocardial perfusion SPECT artifacts. *J Nucl Med* 1994; 35:699–702.

84. Metz CE. Basic principles of ROC analysis. *Semin Nucl Med* 1978; 8:283–298.

85. Patterson RE, Horowitz SF. Importance of epidemiology and biostatistics in deciding clinical strategies for using diagnostic tests: A simplified approach using examples from coronary artery disease. *J Am Coll Cardiol* 1989; 13:1653–1665.

86. Hoffman EJ, Huang SC, Phelps ME. Quantitation in positron emission computed tomography: 1. Effect of object size. *J Comput Assist Tomogr* 1979; 3:299–308.

87. Kiat H, Van Train K, Friedman, Germano G, Silagan G, Wang FP, et al. Quantitative stress-redistribution thallium-201 SPECT using prone imaging: Methodologic development and validation. *J Nucl Med* 1992; 33:1509–1515.

88. Eisner RL, Tamas MJ, Cloninger K, Shonkoff D, Oates JA, Gober AM, et al. The normal SPECT thallium-201 bullseye display: Gender differences. *J Nucl Med* 1989; 29:1901–1909.

89. Schelbert HR. Current status and prospects of new radionuclides and radiopharmaceuticals for cardiovascular nuclear medicine. *Semin Nucl Med* 1987; 17:145–181.

90. Gould KL. Clinical cardiac positron emission tomography: State of the art. *Circulation* 1991; 84:122–136.

91. Williams BR, Mullani NA, Jansen DE, Anderson BA. A retrospective study of the diagnostic accuracy of the first community hospital based positron emission tomography center for the detection of coronary artery disease using rubidium-82. *J Nucl Med* 1994; 35:1586–1593.

92. Churchwell KB, Pilcher WC, Eisner RL, Barclay AB, Patterson RE. Quantitative analysis of PET: The women's test for coronary artery disease. *J Nucl Med* 1995; 36:79P.

93. Patterson RE, Horowitz SF, Eisner RL. Comparison of modalities to diagnose coronary artery disease. *Semin Nucl Med* 1994; 24:286–310.

94. King MA, Tsui BMW, Pan TS, Glock SJ, Soares EJ. Attenuation compensation for cardiac single-photon emission computed tomographic imaging: Part 2: Attenuation compensation algorithms. *J Nucl Cardiol* 1996; 3:55–63.

95. Bacharach SL, Buvat I. Attenuation correction in cardiac positron emission tomography and single-photon emission computed tomography. *J Nucl Cardiol* 1995; 2:246–255.

96. Ficaro EA, Fessler JA, Shreve PD, Kritzman JN, Rose PA, Corbett JA. Simultaneous transmission/emission myocardial perfusion tomography: Diagnostic accuracy of attenuation corrected Tc-99m sestamibi single-photon emission computed tomography. *Circulation* 1996; 93:463–473.

97. Kundel HL, Hendee WR. The perception of radiologic image information. *Invest Radiol* 1985; 20:874–881.

98. Caldwell JH, Williams DL, Harp GL, Stratton JR, Ritchie JL. Quantitation of size of relative myocardial perfusion defect by single photon emission computed tomography. *Circulation* 1984; 70:1048–1056.

99. Garcia EV, Van Train K, Maddahi J, Prigent F, Friedman J, Areeda J, et al. Quantification of rotational thallium-201 myocardial tomography. *J Nucl Med* 1985; 26:17–26.

100. Diamond GA, Forrester JS. Analysis of probability as an aid in the clinical diagnosis of coronary artery disease. *N Engl J Med* 1979; 300:1350–1358.

101. Pryor DB, Harrell FE, Lee KL Califf RM, Rosati RA. Estimating the likelihood of significant coronary artery disease. *Am J Med* 1983; 75:771–780.

102. Garcia EV, DePuey KG, Sonnemaker RE, Neely HR, DePasquale EE, Robbins WL, et al. Quantification of the reversibility of stress-induced thallium-201 myocardial perfusion defects: A multicenter trial using bull's-eye polar maps and standard normal limits. *J Nucl Med* 1990; 31:1761–1765.

103. Patterson RE, Pilcher WC. Assessing myocardial viability to help select patients for revascularization to improve left ventricular dysfunction due to coronary artery disease. *Semin Thorac Cardiovasc Surg* 1995; 7:214–226.

104. Patterson RE, Cloninger K, Churchwell KJ, Shonkoff D, Sullivan KS, Williams BR, et al. Special problems with cardiovascular imaging to assess coronary artery disease in women. In Julian J, Wenger NK, eds. *Women and Heart Disease.* London: Martin Dunitz, 1997:91–115.

105. Kurata C, Tawarahara K, Taguchi T, Sakata K, Yamazaki N, Narith Y. Lung thallium-20 uptake during exercise emission computed tomography. *J Nucl Med* 1991; 32:417–423.

106. Weiss AT, Berman DS, Lew AS, Nielsen I, Potkin B, Swan HJ, et al. Transient ischemic dilation of the left ventricle on stress thallium-201 scintigraphy: A marker of severe and extensive coronary artery disease. *J Am Coll Cardiol* 1987; 9:752–729.

107. Mannting F. Pulmonary thallium uptake: Correlation with systolic and diastolic left ventricular function at rest and during exercise. *Am Heart J* 1990; 119:1137–1146.

108. Marcassa C, Marzullo P, Pandi O, Sambuceti G, L'Abbate A. A new method for noninvasive quantitation of segmental myocardial thickening using 99mTc-sestamibi: Results in normal subjects. *J Nucl Med* 1990; 31:173–177.

109. Germano G, Kiat H, Kavanagh P, Moriel M, Mazzanti M, Su HT, et al. Automatic quantification of left ventricular ejection fraction from gated myocardial perfusion SPECT. *J Nucl Med* 1995; 36:2138–2147.

110. Leyendecker J, Vansant J, Pettigrew RI. Cine MRI for myocardial scar and viability in the non acute setting: Correlation with SPECT-sestamibi. Book of abstracts. Soc Mag Res Med 1992; 2502.

111. Wackers FJ, Sokole EB, Samson G, Schoot JB, Lie KI, Liem KL, et al. Value and limitations of thallium-201 scintigraphy in the acute phase of myocardial infarction. *N Engl J Med* 1976; 295:1–5.

112. Varetto T, Cantalupi D, Altieri A, Orlandi C. Emergency room technetium-99m sestamibi imaging to rule out acute myocardial ischemic events in patients with nondiagnostic electrocardiogram. *J Am Coll Cardiol* 1993; 22:1804–1808.

113. Hilton TC, Thompson RC, Williams HJ, Saylors R, Fulmer H, Stowers SA. Technetium-99m sestamibi myocardial perfusion imaging in the emergency room for evaluation of chest pain. *J Am Coll Cardiol* 1994; 23:1016–1022.

114. Weissman IA, Dickinson CZ, Sworkin HJ, O'Neill WW, Juni JE. Cost-effectiveness of myocardial perfusion imaging with SPECT in the emergency department evaluation of patients with unexplained chest pain. *Radiology* 1996; 199:353–357.

115. Gewirtz H, Beller GA, Strauss HW, Dinsmore RE, Zir LM, McKusick KA, et al. Transient defects of resting thallium scans in patients with coronary artery disease. *Circulation* 1979; 59:707–713.

116. Berger BC, Watson DD, Burwell LR, Crosby IK, Wellons HA, Teates CD, et al. Redistribution of thallium at rest in patients with stable and unstable angina and the effect of coronary artery bypass surgery. *Circulation* 1979; 60:1114–1125.

117. Hirzel HO, Nelson GR, Sonnenblock EH, Kirk ES. Redistribution of collateral blood flow from necrotic to surviving myocardium following coronary occlusion in the dog. *Circ Res* 1976; 39:214–221.

118. Okada RD, Lim YL, Chesler DA, Kaul S, Pohost GM. Quantitation of myocardial infarct size from thallium-201 images: Validation of a new approach in an experimental model. *J Am Coll Cardiol* 1984; 3:948–955.

119. Perez-Gonzalez J, Botvinick E, Dunn R, Rahimtoola S, Ports T, Chatterjee K, et al. The late prognostic value of acute scintigraphic measurement of myocardial infarct size. *Circulation* 1982; 66:960–971.

120. Mahmarian JJ, Pratt CM, Borges-Neto S, Cashion WR, Roberts R, Verani MS. Quantification of infarct size by ^{201}Tl single-photon emission computed tomography during acute myocardial infarction in humans. Comparison with enzymatic estimates. *Circulation* 1988; 78:831–839.

121. Wackers FJ, Lie KI, Liem KL, Sokole EB, Samson G, van der Schoot IB, et al. Thallium-201 scintigraphy in unstable angina pectoris. *Circulation* 1978; 57:738–742.

122. Maseri A, Parodi O, Sevcri S, Pesola A. Transient transmural reduction of myocardial blood flow demonstrated by thallium-201 scintigraphy, as a cause of variant angina. *Circulation* 1976; 54:280–288.

123. Tamaki N, Yonekura Y, Mukai T, Kodama S, Kadota K, Kambara H, et al. Stress thallium-201 transaxial emission computed tomography: Quantitative versus qualitative analysis for evaluation of coronary artery disease. *J Am Coll Cardiol* 1984; 4:1213–1221.

124. DePasquale EE, Nody AC, DePuey KG, Garcia EV, Pilche G, Bredlau C, et al. Quantitative rotational thallium-201 tomography for identifying and localizing coronary artery disease. *Circulation* 1988; 77:316–327.

125. Van Train KF, Maddahi J, Berman DS, Kiat H, Areeda I, Prigent F, et al. Quantitative analysis of tomographic stress thallium-201 myocardial scintigrams: A multicenter trial. *J Nucl Med* 1990; 31:1168–1179.

126. Kotler TS, Diamond GA. Exercise thallium-201 scintigraphy in the diagnosis and prognosis of coronary artery disease. *Ann Intern Med* 1990; 13:684–702.

127. Beller GA. Myocardial perfusion imaging with thallium-201. *J Nucl Med* 1994; 35:674–680.

128. Patterson RE, Horowitz SF, Eng C, et al. Can exercise electrocardiography and thallium-201 myocardial imaging exclude the diagnosis of

coronary artery disease? Bayesian analysis of the clinical limits of exclusion and indications for coronary angiography. *Am J Cardiol* 1982; 49:1127–1135.

129. Rozanski A, Diamond G, Forrester JS, Morris D, Swan HJC. Declining specificity of exercise radionuclide ventriculography. *N Engl J Med* 1983; 309:518–522.

130. Diamond GA. Reverend Bayes' silent majority: An alternative factor affecting sensitivity and specificity of exercise electrocardiography, (editorial). *Am J Cardiol* 1986; 57:1175–1180.

131. Patterson RE. Value of objective assessment of new radiopharmaceuticals. *J Nucl Med* 1995; 36:1086–1087.

132. Weintraub WS, Madeira SW Jr, Bodenheimer MM, Seelaus PA, Katz RI, Feldman MS, et al. Critical analysis of the application of Bayes' theorem to sequential testing in the noninvasive diagnosis of coronary artery disease. *Am J Cardiol* 1984; 54:43–49.

133. Patterson RE, Eng C, Horowitz SF. Practical diagnosis of coronary artery disease: A Bayes' theorem nomogram to correlate clinical data with noninvasive exercise test. *Am J Cardiol* 1984; 53:252–256.

134. Gould KL. Identifying and measuring severity of coronary artery stenosis quantitative coronary arteriography and positron emission tomography. *Circulation* 1988; 78:237–245.

135. Ryan TJ, Reeves TJ, Faxon DP. ACC/AHA task force on the assessment of diagnostic and therapeutic cardiovascular procedures: Guidelines for percutaneous transluminal coronary angioplasty. *J Am Coll Cardiol* 1988; 12:529–545.

136. Ladenheim ML, Pollock BH, Rozanski A, Berman DS, Staniloff HM, Forrester JS, et al. Extent and severity of myocardial hypoperfusion as predictors of prognosis in patients with suspected coronary artery disease. *J Am Coll Cardiol* 1986; 7:464–471.

137. Brown KA. Prognostic value of thallium-201 myocardial perfusion imaging. A diagnostic tool comes of age. *Circulation* 1991; 83:363–381.

138. Pollock SG, Abbott RD, Boucher CA, Beller CA, Kaul S. Independent and incremental prognostic value of tests performed in hierarchical order to evaluate patients with suspected coronary artery disease. Validation of models based on these tests. *Circulation* 1992; 85:237–248.

139. Iskandrian AS. Myocardial viability. Unresolved issues. *J Nucl Med* 1996; 37:794–797.

140. De Bruyne B, Bartunek J, Pijls NHJ. Coronary pressure measurements in evaluation of coronary stenoses. In: Marwick TH, ed. *Cardiac Stress Testing and Imaging: A Clinician's Guide*. New York: Churchill Livingstone, 1996:281–298.

141. Tuzcu EM, DeFranco AC, Brener SJ, Nissen SE. Intravascular ultrasound and coronary Doppler flow measurements. In: Marwick TH, *Cardiac Stress Testing and Imaging: A Clinician's Guide*. New York; Churchill Livingstone, 1996:299–322.

142. Kirk ES, Jennings RB. Pathophysiology of myocardial ischemia. In: Hurst JW, Logue RB, Rackley CE, et al., eds. *The Heart, Arteries, and Veins*. New York: McGraw-Hill; 1992:976–1008.

143. Reimer KA, Jennings RB. The "wave-front phenomenon" of myocardial ischemic cell death. II. Transmural progression of necrosis within the framework of ischemic bed size (myocardium at risk) and collateral flow. *Lab Invest* 1979; 40:633–643.

144. Braunwald E, Kloner RA. The "stunned myocardium." Prolonged postischemic ventricular dysfunction. *Circulation* 1982; 66:1146–1149.

145. Rahimtoola SH. The hibernating myocardium. *Am Heart J* 1989; 117:211–221.

146. Schelbert HR. Metabolic imaging to assess myocardial viability. *J Nucl Med* 1994; 35(suppl):85–145.

147. Delbeke D, Videlefsky S, Patton J, Campbell NG, Martin WH, Ohana I, et al. Rest myocardial perfusion/metabolism imaging using simultaneous dual isotope acquisition SPECT with technetium-99m MIBI/flourine-18-FDG. *J Nucl Med* 1995; 36:2110–2119.

148. Kayden DS, Sigal S, Soufer R, Mattera J, Zaret BL, Wackers FJ. Thallium-201 for assessment of myocardial viability: Quantitaive comparison of 24-hour redistribution imaging with imaging after reinjection at rest [published erratum appears in *J Am Coll Cardiol* 1991 Apr, 19(5):1121]. *J Am Coll Cardiol* 1991; 18:1480–1486.

149. Ragosta M, Beller G, Watson D, Kaul S, Gimple L. Quantitative planar rest-redistribution Tl-201 imaging in detection of myocardial viability and prediction of improvement in left ventricular function after coronary bypass surgery in patients with severely depressed left ventricular function. *Circulation* 1993; 87:1630–1641.

150. Bonow RO, Dilsizian V, Cuacolo A, Bacharach SL. Identification of viable myocardium in patients with chronic coronary artery disease and left ventricular dysfunction. Comparison of thallium scintigraphy with reinjection and PET imaging with 18F-fluorodeoxyglucose. *Circulation* 1991; 83:26–37.

151. Maddahi J, Schelbert H, Brunken R, Di Carli M. Role of thallium-201 and PET imaging in evaluation of myocardial viability and management of patients with coronary artery disease and left ventricular dysfunction. *J Nucl Med* 1994; 35:707–715.

152. Hecht HS, Hopkins JM, Rose JG, Blumfield DE, Wong M. Reverse redistribution: Worsening of ^{201}Tl myocardial images from exercise to redistribution. *Radiology* 1981; 140:177–181.

153. Lear JL, Rarf U, Jain R. Reverse and pseudo-redistribution of thallium-201 in healed myocardial infarction and normal and negative thallium-201 washout in ischemia due to background oversubtraction. *Am J Cardiol* 1988; 62:543–550.

154. Patterson RE, Jones-Collins BA, Aamodt R. Impaired collateral blood flow reserve early after nontransmural myocardial infarction in dogs. *Am J Cardiol* 1982; 50:1133–1140.

155. Leppo JA, O'Brien J, Rothendler JA, Getchell JD, Lee VW. Dipyridamole-thallium-201 scintigraphy in the prediction of future cardiac events after acute myocardial infarction. *N Engl J Med* 1984; 310:1014–1018.

156. Kaul S, Lilly DR, Gascho JA, Watson DD, Gibson RS, Olivier CA, et al. Prognostic utility of the exercise thallium-201 test in ambulatory patients with chest pain: Comparison with cardiac catheterization. *Circulation* 1988; 77:745–758.

157. Wilson WW, Gibson RN, Nygaard TW, Cradduck GB, Watson DD, Crampton RS, et al. Acute myocardial infarction associated with single vessel coronary artery disease: An analysis of clinical outcome and the prognosotic importance of vessel patency and residual myocardial ischemia. *J Am Coll Cardiol* 1988; 11:223–234.

158. Machecourt J, Longere P, Fagret D, Vanzetlo G, Wolf JE, Polidori C, et al. Prognostic value of thallium-201 single-photon emission computed tomographic myocardial perfusion imaging according to extent of myocardial defect. Study in 1,926 patients with a follow-up at 33 months. *J Am Coll Cardiol* 1994; 23:1030–1106.

159. Marie YP, Danchin N, Durand JF, Feldmann L, Grentzinger A, Olivier P, et al. Long term prediction of major ischemic events by exercise thallium-201 single photon emission computed tomography. *J Am Coll Cardiol* 1995; 26:879–886.

160. Iskandrian AS, Johnson J, Tung TL, Wasserleben RN, Cave V, Heo J, et al. Comparison of the treadmill exercise score and single-photon emission computed tomographic thallium imaging in risk assessment. *J Nucl Cardiol* 1994; 2:144–149.

161. Stratmann HG, Williams GA, Wittry MD, Chaitman BR, Miller DD. Exercise technetium-99m sestamibi tomography for cardiac risk stratification of patients with stable chest pain. *Circulation* 1994; 89:615–622.

162. Raikes K, Sinusas AJ, Wackers FJTh, Zaret BL. One-year prognosis of patients with normal planar or single-photon emission computed tomographic technetium-99m labeled sestamibi exercise imaging. *J Nucl Cardiol* 1994; 1:449–456.

163. Hachamovitch R, Berman DS, Kiat H, Cohen I, Cabico JA, Friedman J, et al. Exercise myocardial perfusion SPECT in patients without known coronary artery disease. Incremental prognostic value and use in risk stratification. *Circulation* 1996; 93:905–914.

164. Hendel RC, Leppo JA. The value of perioperative clinical indexes and dipyridamole thallium scintigraphy for the prediction of myocardial infarction and cardiac death in patients undergoing vascular surgery. *J Nucl Cardiol* 1995; 2:18–25.

165. Patterson RE, Eng C, Horowitz SF, Gorlin R, Goldstein SR. Bayesian comparison of cost-effectiveness of different clinical approaches to diagnose coronary artery disease. *J Am Coll Cardiol* 1984; 4:276–289.

166. Greenberg BH, Han R, Bolvinick EH, Wemer JA, Brundage BH, Shames DM, et al. Thallium-201 myocardial perfusion scintigraphy to evaluate patients after coronary bypass surgery. *Am J Cardiol* 1978; 42:167–176.

167. Cloninger KG, DePuey KG, Garcia EV, Roubin GS, Robbins WL, Nody A, et al. Incomplete redistribution in delayed thallium-201 single photon emission computed tomographic (SPECT) images: An overestimation of myocardial scarring. *J Am Coll Cardiol* 1988; 12:955–963.

168. Miller DD, Verani MS. Current status of myocardial perfusion imaging after percutaneous transluminal coronary angioplasty. *J Am Coll Cardiol* 1994; 24:260–266.

169. King SB III, Lembo NJ, Weintraub WS, Kosinski AS, Barnhart HX, Kutner MH, et al., for the Emory Angioplasty versus Surgery Trial (EAST). A randomized trial comparing coronary angioplasty with coronary bypass surgery. *N Engl J Med* 1994; 331:1044–1051.

170. Mueller TM, Marcus ML, Ehrhardt JC, Chaudhuri T, Abboud FM. Limitations of thallium-201 myocardial perfusion scintigrams. *Circulation* 1976; 54:640–646.

171. Gregg DE, Patterson RE. Functional importance of the coronary collateral circulation. *N Engl J Med* 1980; 303:1404–1406.

172. Klein JL, Peifer JW, Garcia EV. Three dimensional coronary angiography. *Am J Card Imaging* 1993; 7:187–194.

173. Johnson AM, Kron IL, Watson DD, Gibson RS, Nolan SP. Evaluation of postoperative flow reserve in internal mammary artery bypass grafts. *J Thorac Cardiovasc Surg* 1986; 92:822–826.

174. Stuckey TD, Burwell LR, Nygaard TW, Gibson RS, Watson DD, Beller GA. Quantitative exercise thallium-201 scintigraphy for predicting angina recurrence after percutaneous transluminal coronary angioplasty. *Am J Cardiol* 1989; 63:517–571.

175. Uren NG, Crake T, Lefroy DC, de Silva R, Davies GJ, Maseri A. Delayed recovery of coronary resistive vessel function after coronary angioplasty. *J Am Coll Cardiol* 1993; 21:612–621.

176. Mahmarian JJ, Fenimorl NL, Marks GF, Francis MJ, Morales-Ballejo H, Merani MS, et al. Transdermal nitroglycerin patch therapy reduces the extent of exercise-induced myocardial ischemia: Results of a double-blind, placebo-controlled trial using quantitative thallium-201 tomography. *J Am Coll Cardiol* 1994; 24:25–32.

177. Zacca NM, Verani MS, Chahine RA, Miller RR. Effect of nifedipine on exercise-induced left ventricular dysfunction and myocardial hypoperfusion in stable angina. *Am J Cardiol* 1982; 50:689–695.

178. Harrison DG, Armstrong ML, Frieman PC, Heistad DD. Restoration of endothelium-dependent relaxation by dietary treatment of atherosclerosis. *J Clin Invest* 1987; 80:1801–1811.

179. Gould KL, Martucci JP, Goldberg DI, Hess MJ, Edens RP, Latifi R, et al. Short-term cholesterol lowering decreases size and severity of perfusion abnormalities by positron emission tomography after dipyridamole in patients with coronary artery disease. *Circulation* 1994; 89:1530–1538.

180. Greenberg JM, Murphy JH, Okada RD, Pohost GM, Strauss WH, Boucher CA. Value and limitations of radionuclide angiography in determining the cause of reduced left ventricular ejection fraction: Comparison of idiopathic dilated cardiomyopathy and coronary artery disease. *Am J Cardiol* 1985; 55:541–544.

181. Bache RJ, Vrobel TR, Arentzen CE, Ring WS. Effect of maximal coronary vasodilation on transmural perfusion during tachycardia in dogs with left ventricular hypertrophy. *Circ Res* 1981; 48:76–85.

182. Maron BJ, Wolfson JK, Epstein SE, Roberts WC. Intramural ("small vessel") coronary artery disease in hypertrophic cardiomyopathy. *J Am Coll Cardiol* 1986; 8:545–557.

183. Factor SM, Sonnenblick EH. Pathogenesis of clinical and experimental congestive cardiomyopathies: Recent concepts. *Prog Cardiovasc Dis* 1985; 27:395–420.

184. Bulkley BH, Huiehins GM, Gailey I, Strauss HW, Pitt B. Thallium-201 imaging and gated cardiac blood pool scans in patients with ischemic and idiopathic congestive cardiomyopathy. A clinical and pathologic study. *Circulation* 1977; 55:753–760.

185. Cannon RO, Dilsizian V, O'Gara PT, Udelson JE, Schenke WH, Quyyumi A, et al. Myocardial metabolic, hemodynamic, and electrocardiographic significance of reversible thallium-201 abnormalities in hypertrophic cardiomyopathy. *Circulation* 1991; 83:1660–1667.

186. Udelson JE, Bonow RO, O'Gara PT, Maron BJ, van Lingen A, Bacharach SE, et al. Verapamil prevents silent myocardial perfusion abnormalities during exercise in patients with hypertrophic cardiomyopathy. *Circulation* 1989; 79:1052–1060.

187. Cannon RO, Dilsizian V, O'Gara PT, Udelson JE, Tucker E, Panza JA, et al. Impact of surgical relief of outflow obstruction on thallium perfusion abnormalities in hypertrophic cardiomyopathy. *Circulation* 1992; 85:1039–1045.

188. DePuey EG, Guertler-Krawczynska E, Perkins JV. Alterations in myocardial thallium-201 distribution in patients with chronic systemic hypertension undergoing single photon emission computed tomography. *Am J Cardiol* 198; 62:234–238.

189. DePuey KG, Guenler-Krawczyuska E, Robbins WL. Thallium-201 SPECT in coronary artery disease patients with left bundle branch block. *J Nucl Med* 1988; 29:1479–1485.

190. Burns RJ, Galligan, Wright LM, Lawand S, Burke RJ, Gladstone PJ. Improved specificity of myocardial thallium-201 single-photon emission computed tomography in patients with left bundle branch block by dipyridamole. *Am J Cardiol* 1991; 68:504–508.

191. Pichard AD, Maritinez E, Wiener I, Patterson RE, Goldsmith SJ, Horowitz SF, et al. Regional myocardial perfusion imaging with thallium-201 in the diagnosis of left anterior descending coronary artery disease. *Am Heart J* 1981; 102:30–36.

192. Hirzel HO, Senn M, Nuesch K, Buettner C, Pfeiffer A, Hess OM, et al. Thallium-201 scintigraphy in patients in complete left bundle branch block. *Am J Cardiol* 1984; 53:764–769.

193. Makler PT, Lavine SI, Denenberg BS, Bove AA, Idell S. Redistribution on the thallium scan in myocardial sarcoidosis: Concise communication. *J Nucl Med* 1981; 22:428–432.

194. Tubau JF, Szalchcic J, Hollenbeg M, Massie BM. Usefulness of thallium-201 scintigraphy in predicting the development of angina pectoris in hypertensive patients with left ventricular hypertrophy. *Am J Cardiol* 1989; 66:45–49.

195. Cecil MP, Pilcher WC, Eisner RL, Chu TH, Merlino JD, Patterson RE. Absence of defects in SPECT thallium-201 myocardial images in patients with systemic hypertensiona and left ventricular hypertrophy. *Am J Cardiol* 1994; 74:43–46.

196. DiBella EVR, Eisner RL, Barclay AB, Patterson RE, Nowalk DJ. Attenuation artifacts in SPECT: Effect of wrap-around lung in 180-degree cardiac studies. *J Nucl Med* 1996; 37:1891–1896.

197. Gaffney FA, Wohl AJ, Blomqvist CG, Parkey RW, Willerson JT. Thallium-201 myocardial perfusion studies in patients with the mitral valve prolapse syndrome. *Am J Med* 1978; 64:21–26.

198. Schlant RC, Nutter DO. Heart failure in valvular heart disease. *Medicine* 1971; 50:421–451.

199. Urquhart J, Patterson RE, Horowitz SF, Packer M, Litwak R, Gorlin R. Quantification of valvular regurgitation before and after surgery by radionuclide angiocardiography. *Am J Cardiol* 1981; 47:287–291.

200. Maturi MF, Greene R, Speir E, Burrus C, Dorsey LMA, Markle DR, et al. Neuropeptide-Y. A peptide recently found in human coronary arteries causes coronary vasoconstriction severe enough to produce myocardial ischemia in dogs. *J Clin Invest* 1989; 83:1217–1224.

201. Cannon RO. Chest pain with normal coronary angiograms. In: Fuster V, Ross R, Topol FJ, eds. *Atherosclerosis and Coronary Artery Disease.* Philadelphia: Lippincott-Raven; 1996:1577–1590.

202. Tweddel AC, Martin W, Hutton I. Thallium scans in syndrome X. *Br Heart J* 1992; 68:48–50.

203. Bax JJ, Visser FC, van Lingen A, Groeneveld AB, Huitnk JM, Teule GJ, et al. Relation between myocardial uptake of thallium-201 and fluorine-18-fluorodeoxyglucose imaged with single photon emission computed tomography in normal individuals. *Eur J Nucl Med* 1995; 22:56–63.

204. Burt RW, Perkins OW, Oppenheim BE, Schauwecker DS, Stein L, Wellman HN. Direct comparison of fluorine-18-FDG SPECT, FDG PET and rest thallium-201 SPECT for detection of myocardial viability. *J Nucl Med* 1995; 36:176–179.

205. Martin WH, Delbelke D, Patton JA, Sandler MP. FDG-SPECT: Correlation with FDG-PET. *J Nucl Med* 1995; 36:988–995.

206. Bacharach SL, Green MV, Borer JS, Douglas MA, Ostrow HG, Johnston GS. A real-time system for multi-image gated cardiac studies. *J Nucl Med* 1977; 18:79–84.

207. Marshall RC, Berger HJ, Costin JC Freedman GS, Wolberg J, Cohen LS, et al. Assessment of cardiac performance with quantitative radionuclide angiography: Sequential left ventricular ejection fraction, normalized left ventricular ejection rate and regional wall motion. *Circulation* 1977; 56:820–829.

208. Burow RD, Strauss HW, Singleton R, Pond M, Rehn T, Bailey IK, et al. Analysis of left ventricular function from multiple gated acquisition cardiac blood pool imaging. Comparison to contrast angiography. *Circulation* 1977; 56:1024–1028.

209. Zaret BL, Jain D. Continuous monitoring of left ventricular function with miniaturized nonimaging detectors. In: Zaret BL, Beller GA, eds. *Nuclear Cardiology: State of the Art and Future Directions.* St. Louis: CV Mosby; 1993:111–145.

210. Port S. First-pass radionuclide angiography. In: Skorton DJ, Schelbert HR, Wolf GL, Brundage BH, eds. *Marcus' Cardiac Imaging: A Companion to Braunwald's Heart Disease,* 2d ed. Philadelphia: Saunders; 1996:923–941.

211. Borer J, Kant K, Bacharach S, Green M, Rosing D, Sedes S, et al. Sensitivity, specificity and predictive accuracy of radionuclide cineangiography during exercise in patients with coronary artery disease.

Comparison with exercise electrocardiography. *Circulation* 1979; 60:572–580.

212. Steingart R, Wexler J, Slagle S, Scheuer J. Radionuclide ventriculographic responses to graded supine and upright exercise: Critical role of the Frank-Starling mechanism at submaximal exercise. *Am J Cardiol* 1984; 53:1671–1678.

213. Rozanski A, Bairey CN, Krantz DS, Friedman J, Resser KJ, Morell M, et al. Mental stress and the induction of silent myocardial ischemia in patients with coronary artery disease. *N Engl J Med* 1988; 818:1005–1012.

214. Maddox DE, Wynne J, Uren R, Parke JA, Idoine J, Siegel LC, et al. Regional ejection fraction: A quantitative radionuclide index of regional left ventricular performance. *Circulation* 1979; 59:1001–1009.

215. Botvinick EH, Frais MA, Shosa DW, O'Conneil JW, Pacheco-Alvarez IA, Scheinman M, et al. An accurate means of detection, and characterizing abnormal patterns of ventricular activation by phase image analysis. *Am J Cardiol* 1982; 50:289–298.

216. Maltz DL, Treves S. Quantitative radionuclide angiocardiography: Determination of $Q_p:Q_s$ in children. *Circulation* 1973; 47:1049–1056.

217. Okada RD, Osbakken MD, Boucher CA, Strauss HW, Block PC, Pohost GM. Pulmonary blood volume ratio response to exercise: A noninvasive determination of exercise-induced changes in pulmonary capillary wedge pressure. *Circulation* 1982; 65:126–133.

218. Bonow RO, Bacharach SL, Green MV, Kent KM, Rosing DR, Lipson LC, et al. Impaired left ventricular diastolic filling in patients with coronary artery disease: Assessment with radionuclide angiography. *Circulation* 1981; 65:315–323.

219. Arrighi JA, Soufer R. Left ventricular diastolic function: Physiology, methods of assessment and clinical significance. *J Nucl Cardiol* 1995; 6:525–543.

220. Gerson MD, ed. *Cardiac Nuclear Medicine.* New York: McGraw-Hill; 1991:191–218.

221. Rigo P, Alderson PO, Robertson RM, Becker LC, Wagner HN Jr. Measurement of aortic and mitral regurgitation by gated cardiac blood pool scans. *Circulation* 1979; 60:306–312.

222. Cohn PF, Gorlin R, Cohn LH, Collins JJ Jr. Left ventricular ejection fraction as a prognostic guide in surgical treatment of coronary and valvular heart disease. *Am J Cardiol* 1974; 34:136–141.

223. Mock MB, Ringqvist L, Fisher LD, Davis KB, Chaitman BR, Kouchoukos NT, et al. Survival of medically treated patients in the coronary artery surgery study (CASS) registry. *Circulation* 1982; 66:562–568.

224. Phillips HR, Levine FH, Carter JE, Boucher CA, Osbakken MD, Okada RD, et al. Mitral valve replacement for isolated mitral regurgitation: Analysis of clinical course and late postoperative left ventricular ejection fraction. *Am J Cardiol* 1981; 48:647–654.

225. Bonow RO. Radionuclide angiography in the management of asymptomatic aortic regurgitation. *Circulation* 1991; 84:1296–1302.

226. Sawada SG, Ryan T, Conley MI, Corya BC, Feigenbaum H, Armstrong WF. Prognostic value of a normal exercise echocardiogram. *Am Heart J* 1990; 120:49–55.

227. Hecht HS, DeBord L, Shaw R, Dunlap R, Ryan C, Stertzer SH, et al. Digital supine bicycle stress echocardiography: A new technique for evaluating coronary artery disease. *J Am Coll Cardiol* 1993; 21:950–956.

228. Verani MS. Myocardial perfusion imaging versus two-dimensional echocardiography: Comparative value in the diagnosis of coronary artery disease. *J Nucl Cardiol* 1994; 1:299–314.

229. Schelbert HR. Integrated clinical approach to diagnosis using imaging methods: Coronary artery disease. In: Skorton DJ, Schelbert HR, Wolf GL, Brundage BH, eds. *Marcus' Cardiac Imaging: A Comparison to Braunwald's "Heart Disease".* Philadelphia: Saunders; 1996:81–84.

230. Green MV, Jones-Collins BA, Bacharach SL, Findley SL, Patterson RE, Larson SM. Prolongation of regional time to left ventricular end-systole during acute myocardial ischemia: A scintigraphic study in the dog. *J Am Coll Cardiol* 1984; 4:72–79.

231. Little T, Crenshaw MH, Liberman HA, Battey LL, Warner R, Churchwell AL, et al. Effects of time required for reperfusion (thrombolysis or angioplasty, or both) and location of acute myocardial infarction on left ventricular functional reserve capacity several months later. *Am J Cardiol* 1991; 67:797–805.

232. Multicenter Postinfarction Research Group. Risk stratification and survival after myocardial infarction. *N Engl J Med* 1983; 303:331–336.

233. Falk E, Shah PK, Furster V. Coronary plaque disruption. *Circulation* 1995; 92:657–671.

234. Morris KG, Palmeri ST, Califf RM, McKinnis RA, Higginbotham MB, Coleman RE, et al. Value of radionuclide angiography for predicting specific cardiac events after acute myocardial infarction. *Am J Cardiol* 1985; 55:318–324.

235. Alazaraki NP, Ashburn WL, Hagan A, Friedman WF. Detection of left to right cardiac shunts with the scintillation camera pulmonary dilution curve. *J Nucl Med* 1972; 13:142–149.

236. Berger PB, Ruocco NA Jr, Ryan TJ, Jacobs AK, Zaret BL, Wackers FJ, et al. Frequency and significance of right ventricular dysfunction during inferior wall left ventricular myocardial infarction treated with thrombolytic therapy (results from the thrombolysis in myocardial infarction [TIMI] II trial). The TIMI Research Group. *Am J Cardiol* 1993; 71:1148–1152.

237. Sorensen SG, Crawford MH, Richards KL, Chaudhuri TK, O'Rourke RA Noninvasive detection of ventricular aneurysm by combined two-dimensional echocardiography and equilibrium radionuclide angiography. *Am Heart J* 1982; 104:145–152.

238. Rahimtoola S. Clinical overview of management of chronic ischemic heart disease. *Circulation* 1991; 84(suppl I):I81–I84.

239. Berger HJ, Reduto LA, Johnstone DE, Borkowski H, Sands JM, Cohen LS, et al. Global and regional left ventricular response to bicycle exercise in coronary artery disease. Assessment by quantitative radionuclide angiocardiography. *Am J Med* 1979; 66:13–21.

240. Jengo JA, Oren V, Conant R, Brizendine M, Nelson T, Uszler IM, et al. Effects of maximal exercise stress on left ventricular function in patients with coronary artery disease using first pass radionuclide angiocardiography: A rapid, noninvasive technique for determining ejection fraction and segmental wall motion. *Circulation* 1979; 59:60–65.

241. Bodenheimer MM, Banka VS, Fooshee CM, Helfant RH. Comparative sensitivity of the exercise electrocardiogram, thallium imaging and stress radionuclide angiography to detect the presence and severity of coronary heart disease. *Circulation* 1979; 60:1270–1278.

242. Caldwell JH, Hamilton GW, Sorenson SG, Ritchie JL, Williams DL, Kennedy JW. The detection of coronary artery disease with radionuclide techniques: A comparison of rest-exercise thallium imaging and ejection fraction response. *Circulation* 1980; 61:610–619.

243. Jones RH, McEwan P, Newman GE, Pon S, Rerych SK, Scholz PM, et al. Accuracy of diagnosis of coronary artery disease by radionuclide management of left ventricular function during rest and exercise. *Circulation* 1981; 64:586–601.

244. Brady TJ, Thrall JH, Lo K, Pitt B. The importance of adequate exercise in the detection of coronary heart disease by radionuclide ventriculography. *J Nucl Med* 1980; 21:1125–1130.

245. Johnson LL, McCarthy DM, Sciacca RR, Cannon PI. Right ventricular ejection fraction during exercise in patients with coronary artery disease. *Circulation* 1979; 60:1284–1291.

246. DePaee NL, Iskandrian AS, Hakki AH, Kane SA, Segal BL. Value of left ventricular ejection fraction during exercise in predicting the extent of coronary artery disease. *J Am Coll Cardiol* 1983; 1:1002–1010.

247. Weintraub WS, Schneider Rm, Seelaus PA, Wiener DH, Agarwal JB, Helfant RH. Prospective evaluation of the severity of coronary artery disease with exercise radionuclide angiography and electrocardiography. *Am Heart J* 1986; 111:537–542.

248. Gibbons RJ, Zinsmeister AR, Miller TD, Clements IP. Supine exercise electrocardiography compared with exercise radionuclide angiography in noninvasive identification of severe coronary artery disease. *Ann Intern Med* 1990; 112:743–749.

249. Bonow RO. Prognostic assessment in coronary artery disease: Role of radionuclide angiography. *J Nucl Cardiol* 1994; 1:280–291.

250. Wasserman AG, Katz RJ, Varghese PJ, Leiboff RH, Bren GG, Schieselman S, et al. Exercise radionuclide ventriculographic responses in hypertensive patients with chest pain. *N Engl J Med* 1984; 311:1276–1280.

251. Higginbotham MB, Morris KG, Coleman RE, Cobbs FR. Sex-related differences in the normal cardiac response to upright exercise. *Circulation* 1984; 70:357–366.

252. Hanley PC, Zinsmeister AR, Clements IP, Bove AA, Brown ML, Gibbons RJ. Gender-related differences in cardiac response to supine exercise assessed by radionuclide angiography. *J Am Coll Cardiol* 1989; 13:624–629.

253. Gibbons RJ. Rest and exercise radionuclide angiography for diagnosis in chronic ischemic heart disease. *Circulation* 1991; 84:193–199.

254. Pryor DB, Harrell FE, Lee KL, Rosati RA, Coleman RE, Cobb FR, et al. Prognostic indicators from radionuclide angiography in medically treated patients with coronary artery disease. *Am J Cardiol* 1984; 53:18–22.

255. Iskandrian AS, Hakki AH, Schwartz JS, Kay H, Mattleman S, Kane S. Prognostic implications of rest and exercise radionuclide ventriculography in patients with suspected or proven coronary heart disease. *Int J Cardiol* 1984; 6:707–718.

256. Mazzotta J, Bonow RO, Pace L, Brittain E, Epstein SE. Relation between exertional ischemia and prognosis in mildly symptomatic patients with single or double vessel coronary artery disease and left ventricular dysfunction at rest. *J Am Coll Cardiol* 1989; 13:567–573.

257. Lee KL, Pryor DB, Pieper KS, Harrell FE Jr, Califf RM, Mark DB, et al. Prognostic value of radionuclide angiography in medically treated patients with coronary artery disease. A comparison with clinical and catheterization variables. *Circulation* 1990; 82:1705–1717.

258. Iqbal A, Gibbons RJ, Zinsmeister AR, Mock MB, Ballard DJ. Prognostic value of exercise radionuclide angiography in a population based cohort of patients with known or suspected coronary artery disease. *Am J Cardiol* 1994; 74:119–124.

259. Kronenberg MW, Pederson RW, Harston WE, Born ML, Bender HW Jr, Friesinger GC. Left ventricular performance after coronary artery bypass surgery. Prediction of functional benefit. *Ann Intern Med* 1983; 99:305–313.

260. Jones RH, Floyd RD, Austin EH, Sabirson DC. The role of radionuclide angiocardiography in the preoperative prediction of pain relief and prolonged survival following coronary artery bypass grafting. *Ann Surg* 1983; 197:743–754.

261. DePuey KG, Leathemian LL, Leachman RD, Dear WE, Massin EK, Mathur VS, et al. Restenosis after transluminal coronary angioplasty detected with exercise-gated radionuclide ventriculography. *J Am Coll Cardiol* 1984; 4:1103–1113.

262. Schuler G, Schlierf G, Wirth A, Mautner HP, Scheurlen H, Thumm M, et al. Low-fat diet and regular, supervised physical exercise in patients with symptomatic coronary artery disease: Reduction of stress-induced myocardial ischemia. *Circulation* 1988; 77:172–181.

263. Greves J, Rahimtoola SH, McAnulty JH, DeMots H, Clark W, Greenberg B, et al. Preoperative criteria predictive of late survival following valve replacement for severe aortic regurgitation. *Am Heart J* 1981; 101:300–308.

264. Borer JS, Wencker D, Hochreiter C. Management decisions in valvular heart disease. The role of radionuclide-based assessment of ventricular function and perfusion. *J Nucl Cardiol* 1996; 3:72–79.

265. Borer JS, Rosing DR, Kent KM, Bacharach SL, Green MV, Macintosh CJ, et al. Left ventricular function at rest and during exercise after aortic valve replacement in patients with aortic regurgitation. *Am J Cardiol* 1979; 44:1297–1305.

266. Palmeri S, Bonow R, Myers C, Seipp C, Jenkins J, Green M, et al. Prospective evaluation of doxorubicin cardiotoxicity by rest and exercise radionuclide angiography. *Am J Cardiol* 1985; 58:607–613.

267. Schwartz RG, McKenzie WB, Alexander J, Sager P, D Souza A, Manatunga A, et al. Congestive heart failure and left ventricular dysfunction complicating doxorubicin therapy. Seven-year experience using serial radionuclide angiocardiography. *Am J Med* 1987; 82:1109–1118.

268. Bonow RO, Rosing DR, Bacharach SL, Green MV, Kent KM, Lipson LC, et al. Effects of verapamil on left ventricular systolic function and diastolic filling in patients with hypertrophic cardiomyopathy. *Circulation* 1981; 64:787–796.

269. Bonow RO, Dilsizian V, Rosing DR, Maron BJ, Bacharach SL, Green MV. Verapamil-induced improvement in left ventricular diastolic filling and increased exercise tolerance in patients with hypertrophic cardiomyopathy: Short- and long-term effects. *Circulation* 1985; 72:853–864.

270. Matthay RA, Berger HJ, Davies RA, Loke J, Mahler DA, Gottschalk A, et al. Right and left ventricular exercise performance in chronic obstructive pulmonary disease: Radionuclide assessment. *Ann Intern Med* 1980; 93:234–239.

271. Corbett JR, Lewis M, Willerson JT, Nicod PH, Huxley RL, Simon T, et al. 99m-Tc-pyrophosphate imaging in patients with acute myocardial infarction: Comparison of planar imaging with single-photon tomography with and without blood pool overlay. *Circulation* 1984; 69:1120–1128.

272. Massie BM, Botvinick EH, Werner JA, Chatterjee K, Parmley WW. Myocardial scintigraphy with technetium-99m stannous pyrophosphate: An insensitive test for nontransmural myocardial infarction. *Am J Cardiol* 1979; 43:186–192.

273. Johnson LL, Seldin DW, Becker LC, LaFrance N, Liberman HA, James C, et al. Antimyosin imaging in acute transmural myocardial infarctions: Results of a multicenter clinical trial. *J Am Coll Cardiol* 1979; 43:186–192.

274. Khaw B-A, Narula I. Antibody imaging in the evaluation of cardiovascular diseases. *J Nucl Cardiol* 1994; 1:457–476.

275. Maddahi I. Clinical applications of antimyosin monoclonal antibody imaging. *Am J Card Imaging* 1994; 8:249–260.

276. Martin GV, Caldwell JH, Graham MM, Grierson JR, Kroll K, Cowan MJ, et al. Noninvasive detection of hypoxic myocardium using fluorine-18-fluoroisonidazole and positron emission tomography. *J Nucl Med* 1992; 33:2202–2207.

277. Marcus ML, Harrison DG. Physiologic basis for myocardial perfusion imaging. In: Marcus ML, Schelbert HR, Skorton DJ, Wolf GL, eds. *Cardiac Imaging.* Philadelphia: Saunders; 1992:8–23.

278. Factor SM, Okun E, Kirk ES. The histologic lateral border zone of canine myocardial infarction: A function of microcirculation. *Circ Res* 1981; 48:640–649.

279. Okun E, Factor SM, Kirk ES. End-capillary loops in the heart: An explanation for discrete myocardial infarctions without border zones. *Science* 1979; 206:565–567.

280. Patterson RE, Kirk ES. Analysis of coronary collateral structure, function, and ischemic border zone in pigs. *Am J Physiol Heart Circ Physiol* 1983; 13:H23–H31.

281. Factor SM, Okun E, Minase T, Kirk ES. The microcirculation of the human heart: End-capillary loops with discrete perfusion fields. *Circulation* 1982; 66:1241–1249.

282. Patterson RE, Weintraub WS, Halgash DA, Miao J, Rogers JR, Kupersmith J. Spatial distribution of 14-C-lidocaine and blood flow in transmural and lateral border zones of ischemic canine myocardium. *Am J Cardiol* 1982; 50:63–73.

283. Conolly C, Apstein CS. Effects of reperfusion at different times on extent and location of myocardial infarction in the rabbit. *Am J Physiol Heart Circ Physiol* 1983; 12:H200–H206.

284. Minardo ID, Tuli MM, Mock BH, Weiner RE, Pride HP, Wellman HN, et al. Scintigraphic and electrophysiological evidence of canine myocardial sympathetic denervation and reinnervation produced by myocardial infarction or phenol application. *Circulation* 1988; 78:1008–1019.

285. Schwaiger M, Kalff V, Rosenspire K, Haka MS, Molina E, Hutchin GD, et al. Noninvasive evaluation of sympathetic nervous system in human heart by positron emission tomography. *Circulation* 1990; 82:457–464.

286. Stanton MS, Tuli MM, Radtke NL, Heger JJ, Miles WM, Mock BH, et al. Regional sympathetic denervation after myocardial infarction in humans detected noninvasively using I-123-metaiodobenzylguanidine. *J Am Coll Cardiol* 1989; 14:1519–1526.

287. Dai MW, Herre IM, O'Connell IW, Botvinick EH, Newman D, Munoz L. Scintigraphic assessment of sympathetic innervation after transmural versus nontransmural myocardial infarction. *J Am Coll Cardiol* 1991; 17:1416–1423.

288. Hutchins GD, Zipes DP. Imaging the cardiac autonomic nervous system. In: Skorton DJ, Schelbert HR, Wolf GL, Brundage BR, eds. *Marcus' Cardiac Imaging: A Companion to Braunwald's Heart Disease,* 2nd ed. Philadelphia: Saunders; 1996:1052–1061.

289. Nakajima K, Bunko H, Taki J, Shimizu M, Muramori A, Hisada K. Quantitative analysis of I-123-MIBI uptake in hypertrophic cardiomyopathy. *Am Heart J* 1990; 119:1329–1337.

290. Carrio I, Estorch M, Bern L, Lopez-Pousa J, Tabernero J, Torres G. Indium-111-antimyosin and iodine-123-MIBG studies in early assessment of doxorubicin cardiotoxicity. *J Nucl Med* 1995; 36:2044–2049.

291. Chidsey CA, Braunwald E, Morrow AG. Catecholamine excretion and cardiac stores of norepinephrine in congestive heart failure. *Am J Med* 1965; 39:442–451.

292. Cohn JN, Levine TB, Olivari MT, Garberg V, Lura D, Francis GS, et al. Plasma norepinephrine as a guide to prognosis in patients with chronic congestive heart failure. *N Engl J Med* 1984; 311:819–823.

293. Glowniak JV. Cardiac studies with metaiodobenzylguanidine: A critique of methods and interpretation of results. Critical review. *J Nucl Med* 1995; 36:2133–2137.

294. Henderson EB, Kahn JK, Corbett JR, Jansen DE, Pippin JJ, Kulkarni P, et al. Abnormal ^{123}I metaiodobenzylguanidine myocardial washout and distribution may reflect myocardial adrenergic derangement in patients with congestive cardiomyopathy. *Circulation* 1988; 78:1192–1199.

295. Schofer J, Spielmann R, Schuchert A, Weber K, Schluter M. Iodine-123 metaiodobenzylguanidine scintigraphy: A noninvasive method to demonstrate myocardial adrenergic nervous system disintegrity in patients with idiopathic dilated cardiomyopathy. *J Am Coll Cardiol* 1988; 12:1252–1258.

296. Yamakado K, Takeda K, Kitano T, Nakagawa T, Futagami T, Konishi T, et al. Serial change of iodine-123 metaiodobenzylguanidine myocardial concentration in patients with dilated cardiomyopathy. *Eur J Nucl Med* 1992; 19:265–270.

297. Merlet P, Valette H, Dubois-Rande IL, Moyse D, Duboc D, Dove P, et al. Prognostic value of cardiac metaiodobenzylguanidine imaging in patients with heart failure. *J Nucl Med* 1992; 33:471–477.

298. Mhnch G, Ziegler S, Nguyen N, Hartman F, Watzlowik P, Schawaiger M. Scintigraphic evaluation of cardiac innervation. *J Nucl Cardiol* 1996; 3:265–277.

299. Goldstein DS, Chang PC, Eisenhofer G, Miletich R, Finn R, Bacher I, et al. Positron emission tomographic imaging of cardiac sympathetic innervation and function. *Circulation* 1990; 81:1606–1621.

300. Heilbrunn SM, Shah P, Bristow MR, Valantine HA, Ginsburg R, Fowler MB. Increased beta-receptor density and improved hemodynamic response to catecholamine stimulation during long-term metoprolol therapy in heart failure from dilated cardiomyopathy. *Circulation* 1989; 79:483–490.

301. O'Connell JB, Robinson JA, Subramanian R, Scanlon PJ. Gallium-67 imaging in patients with dilated cardiomyopathy and biopsy proven myocarditis. *Circulation* 1984; 70:58–62.

302. Dec GW, Palacios I, Yasuda T, Fallon JT, Khaw BA, Strauss HW, et al. Antimyosin antibody cardiac imaging: Its role in the diagnosis of myocarditis. *J Am Coll Cardiol* 1990; 16:97–104.

303. Johnson LL, Cannon PI. Antimyosin imaging in cardiac transplant rejection. *Circulation* 1991; 84:1273–1279.

304. Chow LH, Radio SJ, Sears TD, McManus BM. Insensitivity of right ventricular endomyocardial biopsy in the diagnosis of myocarditis. *J Am Coll Cardiol* 1989; 14:915–920.

305. Morguet AJ, Munz DL, Ivancevic V, Wemer GS, Sandrock D, Biokemeier M, et al. Immunoscintigraphy using technetium-99m-labeled anti-NCA-95 antigranulocyte antibodies as an adjunct to echocardiography in subacute infective endocarditis. *J Am Coll Cardiol* 1994; 23:1171–1178.

306. Lister-James J, Knight LC, Maurer AH, Bush LR, Moyer BR, Dean RT. Thrombus imaging with a technetium-99m-labelled, activated platelet receptor-binding peptide. *J Nucl Med* 1996; 37:775–780.

307. Knight LC. Scintigraphic methods for detecting vascular thrombus. *J Nucl Med* 1993; 34:554–561.

308. Butler SP, Boyd SJ, Parkes SL, Quinn RJ. Technetium-99m-modified recombinant tissue plasminogen activator to detect deep venous thrombosis. *J Nucl Med* 1996; 37:744–747.

309. Ezekowitz MD, Wilson DA, Smith EO, Burow RD, Harrison LH, Parker DE, et al. Comparison of indium-111 platelet scintigraphy and two-dimensional echocardiography in the diagnosis of left ventricular thrombi. *N Engl J Med* 1982; 306:1509–1513.

310. Stratton JR. Thrombosis imaging with indium-111-labeled platelets. In: Skorton DJ, Schelbert HR, Wolf GL, Brundage BR, eds. *Marcus' Cardiac Imaging: A Companion to Braunwald's Heart Disease,* 2d ed. Philadelphia: Saunders; 1996:1034–1051.

311. Kanke M, Matsueda GR, Strauss HW, Yasuda T, Liau CS, Khaw BA. Localization and visualization of pulmonary emboli with radiolabelled fibrin specific monoclonal antibody. *J Nucl Med* 1991; 32:1254–1260.

312. Strauss HW. Imaging of atherosclerosis: A worthy challenge (editorial). *J Nucl Cardiol* 1996; 3:278–280.

313. Lees AM, Lees RS, Strauss HW, Gallon JT, Taveras J, Kopiwoda S. Selective accumulation flow density lipoproteins in damaged arterial wall. *J Lipid Res* 1983; 24:1160–1167.

314. Lees RS, Lees AM, Strauss HW. External imaging of human atherosclerosis. *J Nucl Med* 1983; 24:154–156.

315. Ginsberg HN, Goldsmith SJ, Vallabhajosula S. Noninvasive imaging of 99m-techntium-labeled low density lipoprotein uptake by tendon xanthomas in hypercholesterolemic patients. *Arteriosclerosis* 1990; 10:256–262.

316. Borer JS. Atherosclerosis imaging: Pathophysiological assessment for a new era. *J Nucl Med* 1993; 34:1321–1325.

317. Hardoff R, Zanzonico P, Braegelmann F, Herrold EM, Lees RS, Lees AM, et al. Localization of 99m-Tc-labeled ApoB synthetic peptide in arterial lesions of an experimental model of spontaneous atherosclerosis. *Am J Therapeutics* 1995; 2:88–89.

318. Narula J, Petrov A, O'Donnel SM, Ditlow C, Pieslak I, Dilley J, et al. Gamma imaging of atherosclerotic lesions: The role of antibody affinity in vivo target localization. *J Nucl Cardiol* 1996; 3:231–241.

319. Carleton RA, Bazzare T, Drake J, Dunn A, Fisher EB Jr, Grundy SM, et al. American Heart Association Special Report. Report of the expert panel on awareness and behavior change to the board of directors, American Heart Association. *Circulation* 1996; 93:1768–1772.

320. Alfonso F, Goicolea J, Hernandez R. Findings of coronary angioscopy in angiographically normal coronary segments of patients with CAD. *Am Heart J* 1995; 130:987–993.

321. Bender JR. To harness the revolution in molecular biology. *J Nucl Cardiol* 1994; 1:307–308.

322. The Expert Panel II. Summary of the second report of the National Cholesterol Education Program (NCEP) Expert Panel on detection, evaluation and treatment of high blood cholesterol in adults. *JAMA* 1993; 269:3015–3023.

323. Goldhaber SZ, Morpurgo M, for the WHO/ISFC Task Force on Pulmonary Embolism: Diagnosis, treatment and prevention of pulmonary embolism: Report of the WHO/International Society and Federation of Cardiology Task Force. *JAMA* 1992; 268:1727–1733.

324. Stein PD, Hull RD, Saltzman HA, Pineo G. Strategy for diagnosis of patients with suspected acute pulmonary embolism. *Chest* 1993; 103:1553–1559.

325. Bounameaux H, de Moerloose P, Perrier A, Reber G. Plasma measurement of D-dimer as diagnostic aid in suspected venous thromboembolism: An overview. *Thromb Haemost* 1994; 71:1–6.

326. Stein PD, Athanasoulis C, Greenspan PH, Henry JW. Relation of plain chest radiographic findings to pulmonary arterial pressure and arterial blood oxygen levels in patients with acute pulmonary embolism. *Am J Cardiol* 1992; 69:394–396.

327. Stein PD, Goldhar SZ, Henry JW. Alveolar-arterial oxygen gradient in the assessment of acute pulmonary embolism. *Chest* 1995; 17:139–143.

328. Sreeram N, Cheriex EC, Smeets JL, Gorgels AP. Value of the 12-lead electrocardiogram at hospital admission in the diagnosis of pulmonary embolism. *Am J Cardiol* 1994; 73:298–303.

329. Lensing AWA, Prandoni P, Brandjes D, Huisman PM, Vigo M, Tomasella G, et al. Detection of deep vein thrombosis by real time B-mode ultrasonography. *N Engl J Med* 1989; 320:342–345.

330. Lualdi JC, Goldhaber SZ. Right ventricular dysfunction after acute pulmonary embolism: Pathophysiologic factors, detection and therapeutic implications. *Am Heart J* 1995; 130:1276–1282.

331. Remy-Jardin M, Remy J, Wattinne L, Giread F. Central pulmonary thromboembolism: Diagnosis with spiral volumetric CT with the single-breath-hold technique—comparison with pulmonary angiography. *Radiology* 1992; 185:381–387.

332. Wielopolski PA. Pulmonary arteriography. *MRI Clin North Am* 1993; 1:295–313.

333. Geraghty JJ, Stanford W, Landas SK, Galvin JR. Ultrafast computed tomography in experimental pulmonary embolism. *Invest Radiol* 1992; 27:60–63.

334. Tapson VF, Davidson CJ, Kisslo KB, Stack RS. Rapid visualization of massive pulmonary emboli utilizing intravascular ultrasound. *Chest* 1994; 105:888–890.

335. Uchida Y, Oshima T, Hirose T, Sasaki T, Morizuki S, Morita T. Angioscopic detection of residual pulmonary thrombin in the differential diagnosis of pulmonary embolism. *Am Heart J* 1995; 130:854–859.

336. Stein PD, Athanasoulis C, Alavi A, Greenspan RH, Hales CA, Saltzman HA, et al. Complications and validity of pulmonary angiography in acute pulmonary embolism. *Circulation* 1992; 85:462–468.

337. Wellman HN. Pulmonary thromboembolism: Current status report of the role of nuclear medicine. *Semin Nucl Med* 1986; 16:236–274.

338. Biello DR. Radiological (scintigraphic) evaluation of patients with suspected pulmonary thromboembolism. *JAMA* 1987; 257:3257–3259.

339. The Pioped Investigators. Value of the ventilation/perfusion scan in acute pulmonary embolism—results of the prospective investigation of pulmonary embolism diagnosis. *JAMA* 1990; 263:2753–2759.

340. Gottschalk A, Sostman HD, Coleman RD, Juni JE, Thrall J, McKusick KA, et al. Ventilation-perfusion scintigraphy in the PIOPED study. Part II. Evaluation of the scintigraphic criteria and interpretations. *J Nucl Med* 1993; 34:1119–1126.

341. Hull RD, Raskob GE, Pineo GF, Brant RF. The low-probability lung scan: A need for change in nomenclature. *Ann Intern Med* 1995; 155:1845–1851.

342. Bone RC. The low-probabability lung scan. A potentially lethal reading. *Arch Intern Med* 1993; 153:2621–2622.

18

COMPUTED TOMOGRAPHY OF THE HEART

Bruce H. Brundage

In 1983, the introduction for clinical use of electron beam computed tomography (EBCT), previously known as ultrafast computed tomography (CT), opened a new area of cardiac imaging. Previous attempts to use conventional x-ray transmission CT to evaluate the heart had been severely limited because of motion artifact created by cardiac contraction and relaxation. Some modicum of success was achieved with conventional CT in the evaluation of aortic disease.[1] The relative lack of aortic motion permitted reasonable imaging of aortic dissection and aortic aneurysms.[2] There was also some success in the evaluation of patency of coronary artery bypass grafts using this technique.[3] The advent of EBCT, however, has relegated conventional CT to a relatively secondary role in many aspects of the diagnosis of cardiovascular disease.

TECHNOLOGY

EBCT is a unique technology that utilizes a powerful electron beam and has a scanner with no moving parts. Conventional CT is limited in its evaluation of the heart because an x-ray tube is mechanically rotated around the thorax, which requires 1 to 2 s. The newer spiral CT scanner is capable of subsecond scan speeds, but it still requires rotation of the x-ray tube and is not fast enough for adequate cardiac imaging. The EBCT scanner projects an electron beam that passes through a magnetic coil; this coil focuses and bends the electron beam to strike a series of fixed tungsten targets that encircle the thorax (Fig. 18-1). The beam is swept magnetically along the tungsten targets in an arc of 210°. The x-radiation generated from the tungsten target passes through the thorax and is attenuated by the intervening structures before striking the twin fixed-detector array opposite the targets. The electron beam can be swept along the tungsten target in 50 ms, and after an 8-ms interscan delay, the procedure can be repeated. This sequence translates into a scanning frequency of 17 scans per second. The x-ray generated by each tungsten target is collimated to strike the twin adjacent detector arrays. Thus, for each beam sweep, two adjacent 8-mm sections of anatomy are imaged. Since there are four tungsten targets, the electron beam can be cascaded across each target in sequence so that in a period of seven heart beats, eight adjacent slices are obtained. There is a 4-mm gap between targets such that eight adjacent scan levels represent 8 cm of anatomy. Each 50-ms scan gives a skin entry x-ray dose of approximately 0.5 Gy.

IMAGING PROTOCOLS

Three imaging protocols are employed for cardiac imaging with EBCT. One commonly employed protocol, known as the *cine mode* because the images obtained can be displayed on a television screen in a movie format, creates real-time, cross-sectional views of the beating heart. This imaging mode is particularly useful for assessing ventricular function as well as valve motion (Fig. 18-2).

The *flow mode* imaging protocol is used to evaluate blood flow. In this mode each scan is gated to the electrocardiogram, assuring that sequential images are obtained at the same point in the cardiac cycle. This assures that there will be excellent anatomic registration of the images when a scan series is obtained following the intravenous injection of an iodine contrast medium. The entrance, progressive enhancement, and egress of the iodine through the various cardiac chambers or within the myocardium itself can then be analyzed by time-density curves (Fig. 18-3). Each image is usually acquired in 50 ms, and up to 20 images can be obtained at each anatomic level during one imaging sequence. Interscan interval is a function of heart rate.

The *volume imaging* protocol is very similar to traditional imaging protocols employed with conventional CT scanners. Single images, usually gated to the electrocardiogram, are acquired, and the patient couch is then moved 1.5, 3, or 8

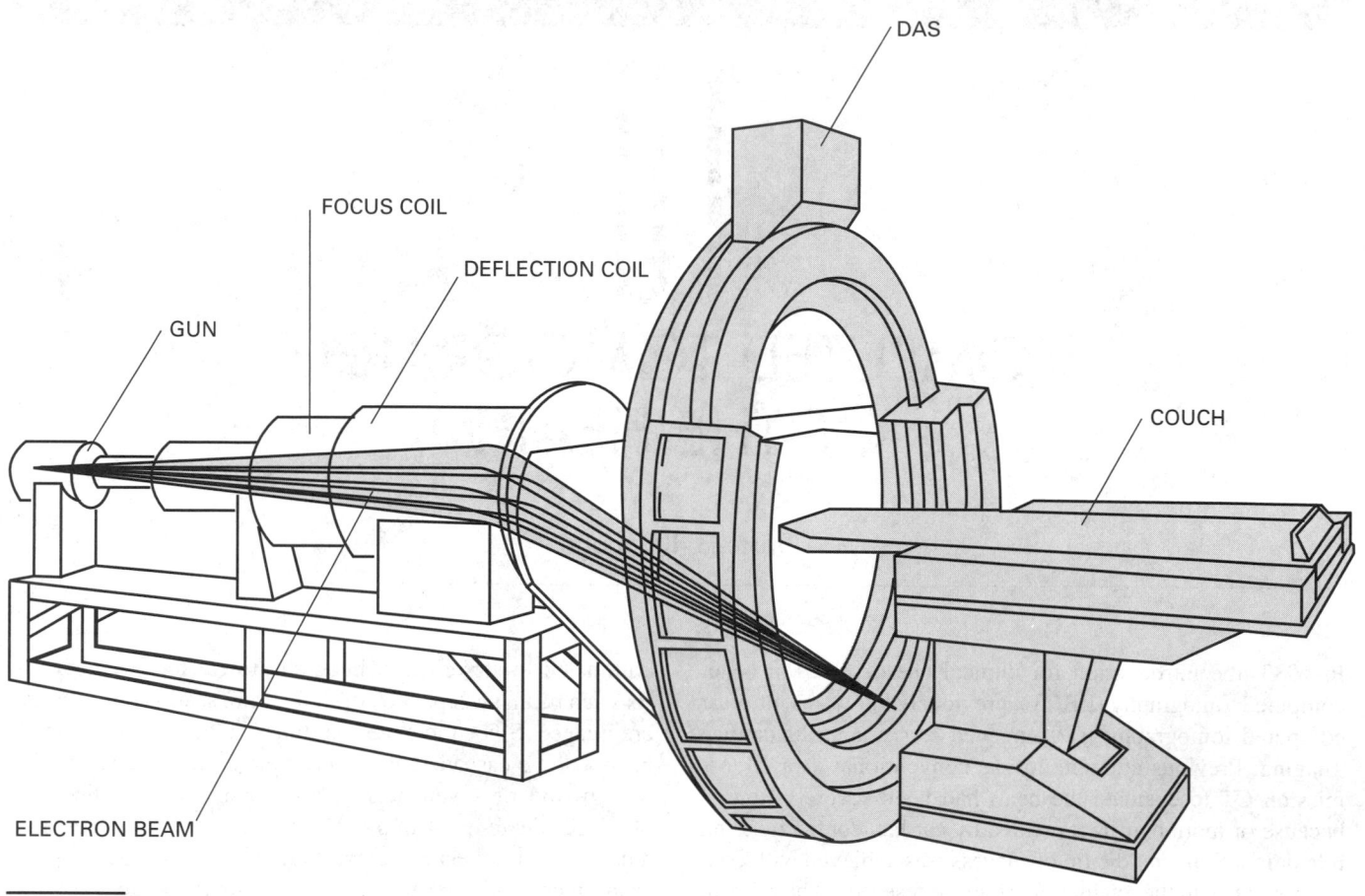

FIGURE 18-1
Cutaway diagram of the ultrafast CT scanner depicts the electron beam emitting from the electron gun and
being focused on the tungsten target by the magnetic deflection coil. DAS = immediate memory.

mm (usually depending on slice thickness desired) and another single gated scan is obtained. This sequence can be repeated for up to 40 contiguous scans, axially encompassing 12 to 32 cm of anatomy (see Fig. 18-8 as example). The acquisition time for each scan is 50 ms or multiples of that interval if high image resolution is desired. Commonly, 100-ms scanning times are used to provide high-resolution cardiac images. In this case the skin entry x-ray dose is approximately 1 Gy. The spatial resolution is 1.6 mm^2 in the 50-ms mode and 0.8 mm^2 in the 100-ms mode.

The cine mode imaging protocol is used to provide precise assessment of right and left ventricular global and regional systolic and diastolic function (Fig. 18-4A).[4-6] Multiple images of the entire right and left ventricle are obtained during intravenous contrast enhancement of the cavities throughout one cardiac cycle. Measurements of ejection fraction and cardiac volumes are obtained by computing end-systolic and end-diastolic volumes from the summation of the individual volumes of each slice[5,7] (Fig. 18-2). Usually eight slices (averaging 1 cm in thickness) will encompass the left and right ventricles. When cardiac enlargement is present, however, 12 slices may be required. This is accomplished by summating images from two and occasionally three scanning periods. As long as the heart rate is the same during each imaging sequence, accurate cardiac volumes and ejection fractions are obtainable.

A radial area technique has been developed for determining regional left ventricular function.[8] Each slice of the left ventricle is divided into 12 equal regions, and the wall motion is displayed graphically or numerically (Fig. 18-4B). With the same analysis program it is also possible to quantify regional systolic wall thickening. Border definition of the endocardium and epicardium for this program can be determined visually by the operator or with a computer-assisted edge-detection method. Assessment of global and regional ventricular function can be obtained at rest and during bicycle exercise.[8] The configuration of the scanner couch and gantry facilitates assessment of cardiac function during bicycle exercise (Fig. 18-5). Function can also be assessed by EBCT during various pharmacologic stresses, including intravenous inotropic drugs and dipyridamole.[9,10] Frame-by-frame analysis of cardiac volumes during diastole provides an accurate depiction of the ventricular volume curve. Maximum peak filling rate, time to maximum peak filling rate, and dv/dt can be computed.[6] The results are comparable to those obtained by radioisotope techniques. The cine mode imaging protocol can also be used to measure myocardial, i.e., muscle, volume accurately.[11] Assuming a uniform specific gravity for myocardium of 1.005, myocardial mass can be computed from myocardial volume. Several investigators have demonstrated remarkable precision for the measurement of both right and left ventricular mass with excellent intraobserver, interobserver, and interstudy reproducibility.[12,13] EBCT may well be a new standard for the measurement of myocardial mass.

The flow mode imaging protocol is employed to measure cardiac output and myocardial blood flow. Following the intravenous injection of a known amount of iodinated contrast material, analysis of the time-density curves in the pulmonary artery, left ventricle, or aorta will provide an accurate estimate of cardiac output, provided the dead space between the injection site and the central circulation is known. Several investigators have verified accurate measurement of cardiac output using EBCT.[14,15] The most important use of flow mode imaging protocol, however, is the assessment of tissue perfusion, in particular, myocardial blood flow. Myocardial blood flow is quantified by analysis of the myocardial time-density curves. Wolfkiel et al.[16] demonstrated that intravenous injections of small amounts of contrast medium (0.35 mL/kg) could be employed to measure regional myocardial blood flow accurately in resting or basal states and during temporary regional ischemia (Fig. 18-6). During high blood flow states such as produced with pharmacologic vasodilation, however, EBCT measurements of blood flow were inappropriately low when compared with radioactive microsphere flow measurement. This underestimation at high flows appears to be due to the washout of the iodinated indicator from the myocardium before all indicator has reached it. Several methods have been proposed for analyzing the myocardial time-density curves. The simplest measures the change in myocardial density and relates that to the blood pool time-density curves:

$$\frac{F}{V} = \frac{C_m}{\int_0^\infty C_i(t)\, dt}$$

where F = flow; V = volume of myocardium; C_m = contrast density in myocardium; C_i = contrast density in aorta or left ventricle; and t = time. Several corrections or modifications have been suggested to overcome underestimation at high

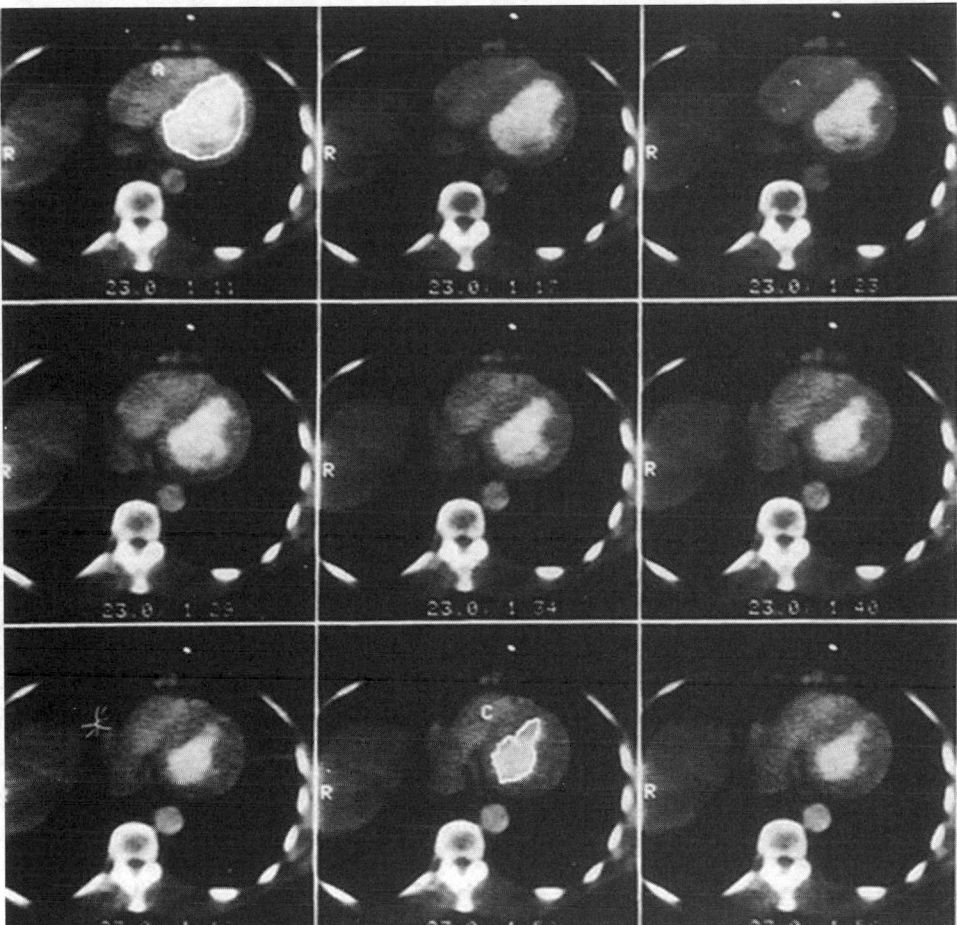

FIGURE 18-2
An 8-mm CT slice of the mid-left ventricle imaged for one complete cardiac cycle at 58-ms intervals. A = end diastole; C = end systole.

flows, but at present this problem remains unsolved.[17,18] In an attempt to circumvent the problems of early washout and beam hardening, several investigators have employed direct intraaortic injection of the contrast medium and have demonstrated excellent correlation between EBCT and radioactive microsphere flow measurement over a wide range of flows including those following pharmacologic vasodilation.[18,19] Obviously, the requirement of intraaortic injection of contrast medium seriously limits the clinical usefulness of this technique for measuring myocardial blood flow at the present time. Research in progress, however, suggests that myocardial blood flow may be measurable over a wide range of flows using intravenous contrast injections.[20] Similar flow measurement techniques have been tested for the evaluation of pulmonary lung perfusion as well.[21] Much more work needs to be done in this area before the clinical value of EBCT for assessing pulmonary tissue perfusion is known.

The volume imaging protocol is employed primarily when detailed evaluation of cardiovascular anatomy is required. High-resolution scanning (0.8 mm² spatial resolution) with thin, 3-mm slices is usually employed with this imaging protocol; however, 1.5-mm slice capability is also available.

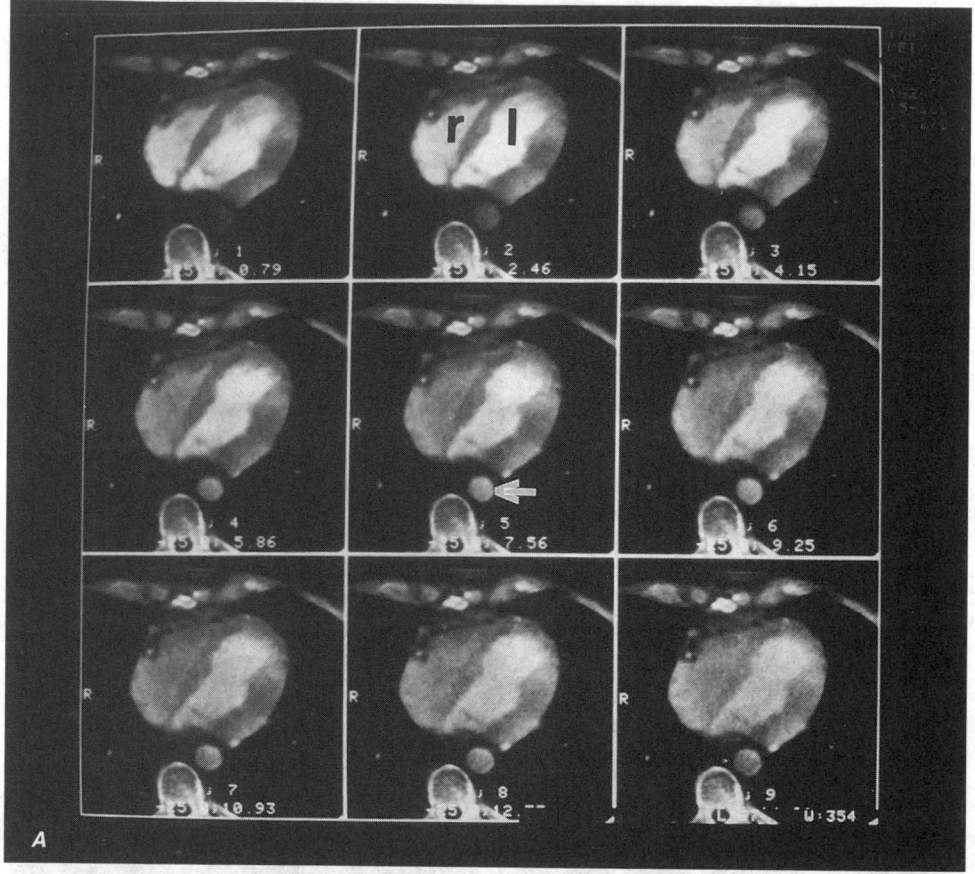

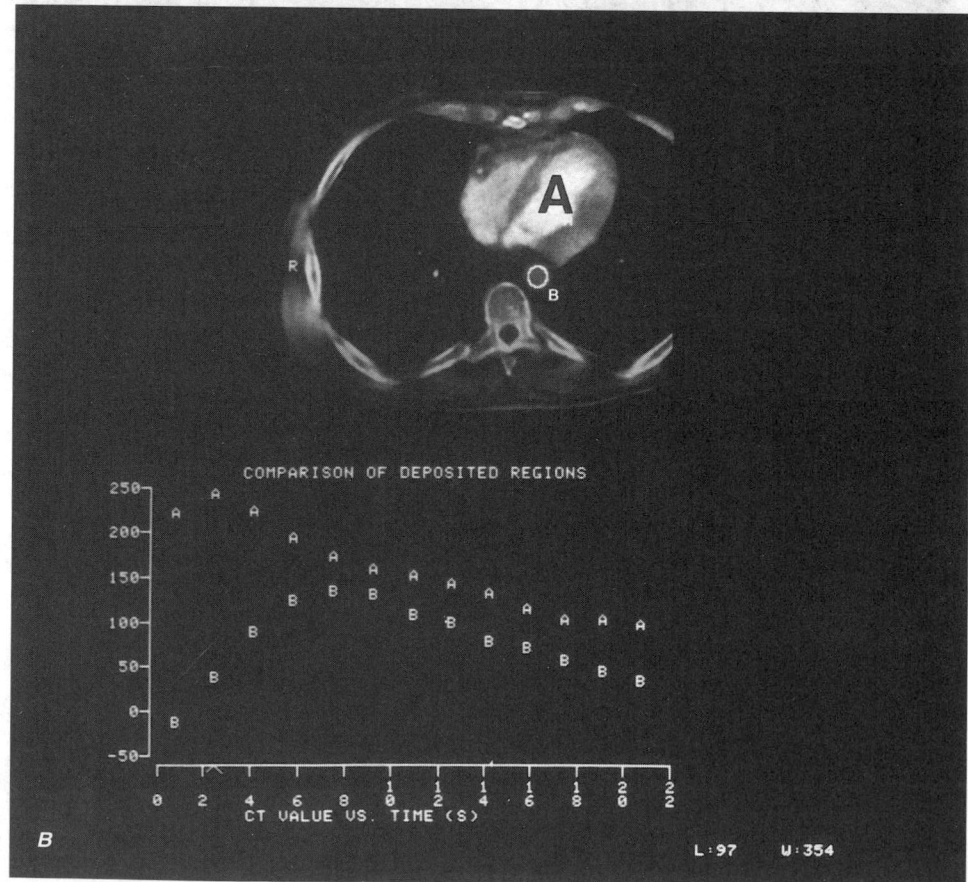

FIGURE 18-3

A. A flow mode study of right (r) and left (l) ventricle demonstrates sequential contrast enhancement of each chamber followed by enhancement of the descending aorta (*white arrow*). *B.* The density (CT number in Hounsfield units) of the ventricle (A) and the descending aorta (B) is plotted over time quantifying the changes visualized in *A*.

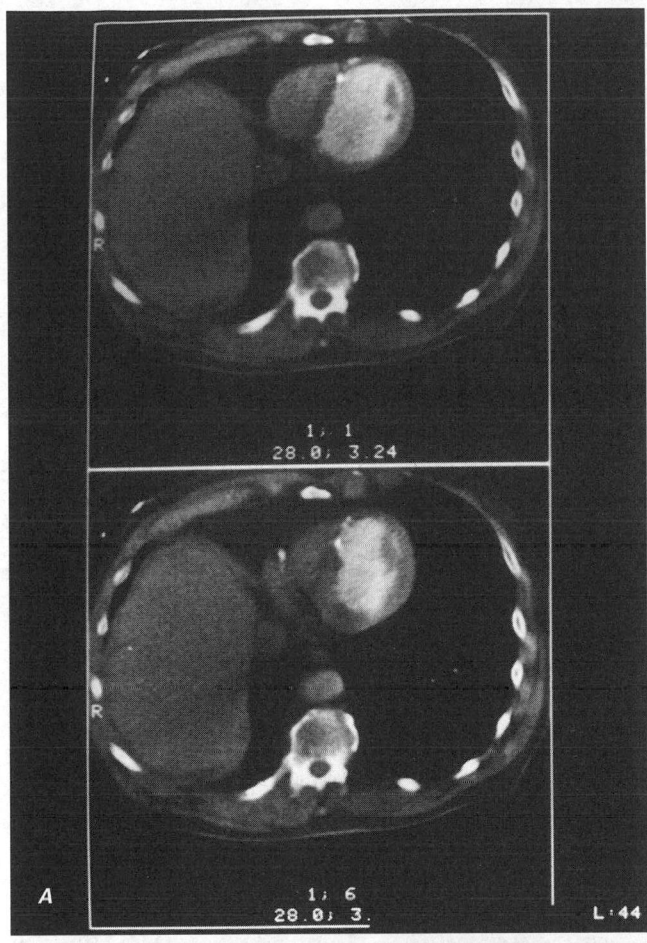

Coronary artery calcification, aortic intimal dissection, and pulmonary artery embolization (see below) are examples of conditions for which this protocol can be used.

CORONARY ARTERY DISEASE

The greatest clinical experience with the use of EBCT has been in the evaluation and study of patients with coronary artery disease (CAD). Based on successes with conventional CT to assess coronary artery bypass graft patency, EBCT was evaluated for this use soon after its clinical availability (Fig. 18-7A). A multicenter prospective study evaluated the accuracy of EBCT compared with graft angiography and demonstrated a sensitivity of 89 percent, a specificity of 96 percent, and a predictive accuracy exceeding 92 percent.[22] The technique appears to work equally well for saphenous vein grafts and internal mammary artery grafts. A major drawback of EBCT in evaluating bypass grafts has been the difficulty in differentiating fully patent grafts from those that are partially obstructed. Several approaches to this problem have been suggested, including measurement of graft flow velocity and comparison of graft time-density curves to aortic curves before and after pharmacologic vasodilation,[23,24] but none has proven to be clinically useful. Recently, the development of software capable of three-dimensional reconstruction of the EBCT slices may enhance the clinical utility of this application. Combining the high-resolution volume imaging mode with the three-dimensional reconstruction technique, excellent

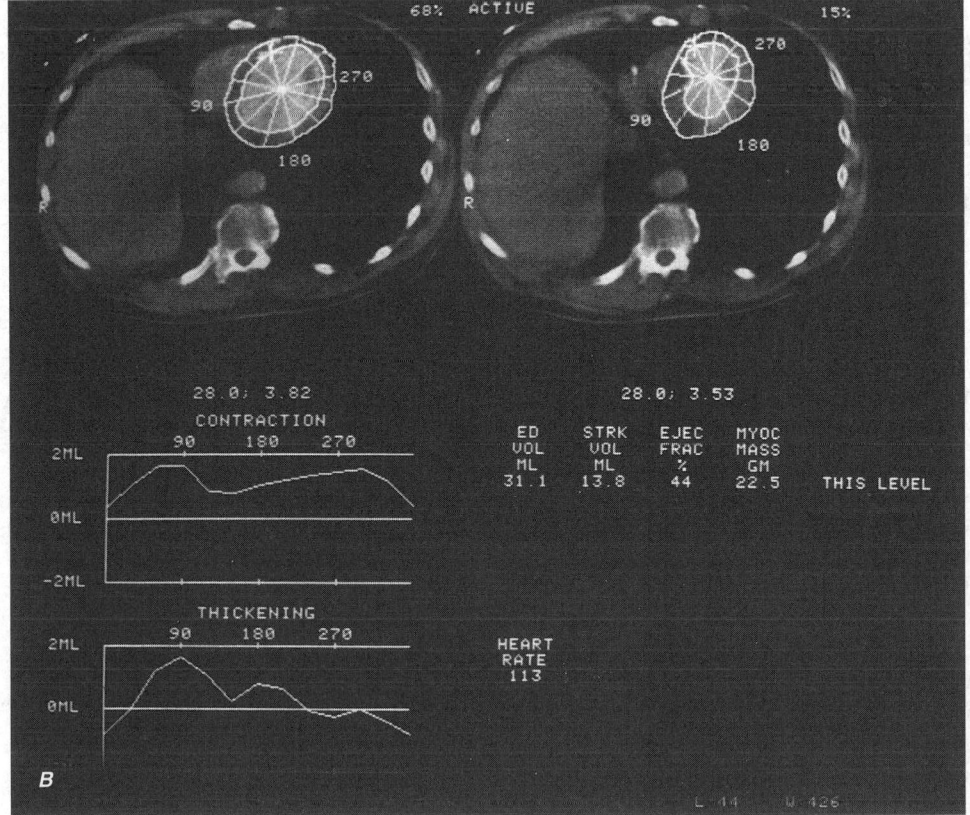

FIGURE 18-4

A. Comparison of an end-diastolic frame of the mid-left ventricle from a cine mode study with an end-systolic frame defines an anteroseptal wall motion abnormality. Also note the absence of systolic wall thickening in the same region. *B.* Quantitative wall motion and wall thickening analysis of the images shown in *A.*

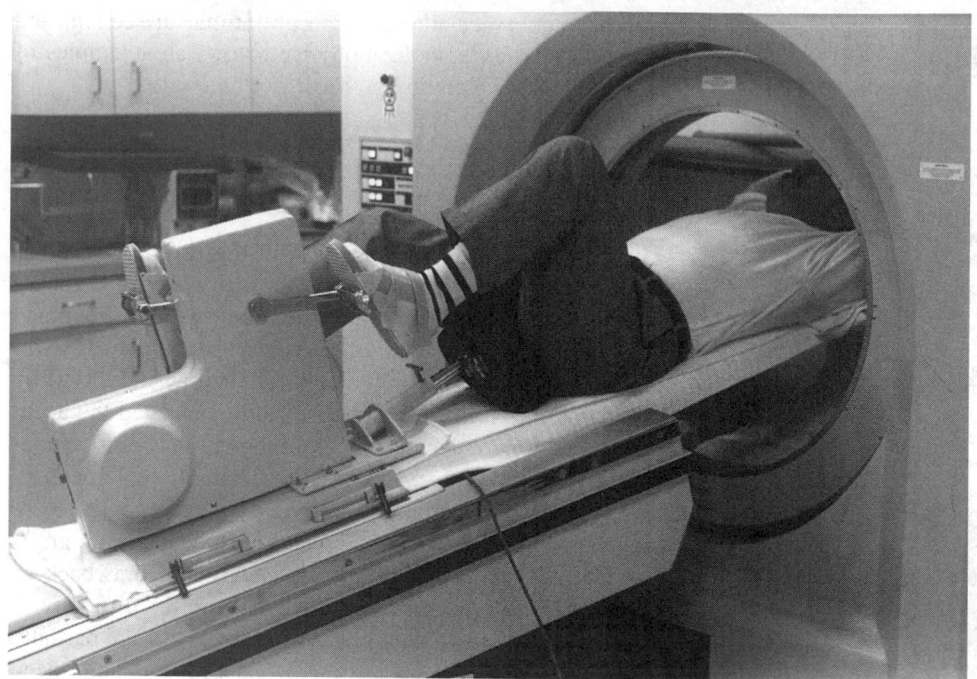

FIGURE 18-5

A patient performs bicycle exercise while cine CT images are obtained of the right and left ventricle.

representations of bypass grafts are possible (Fig. 18-7B). Image resolution appears sufficient to identify areas of graft stenosis and to assess the multiple distal anastomoses of sequential grafts. Clinical studies are required, however, to confirm this potentially new application.

EBCT can identify acute myocardial infarction as a region of absent or markedly reduced resting myocardial blood flow (Fig. 18-8). Imaging the left ventricle using the flow mode protocol is the best technique for this purpose. Relatively few data are available regarding the accuracy of this technique, but in one small study of 20 patients, comparison of EBCT, thallium perfusion scintigraphy, and technetium pyrophosphate scanning demonstrated EBCT to be the most sensitive and specific of the three modalities.[25] Several investigators have reported the value of EBCT for the evaluation of ventricular remodeling following acute myocardial infarction.[26,27] The combination of regional wall motion analysis using the cine mode protocol and assessment of myocardial blood flow by the flow mode protocol may prove useful in determining residual risk area after acute infarction. Equivalent areas of hypokinesis/akinesis and resting hypoperfusion indicate completed infarction. Conversely, a large area of hypokinesis with only a small central area of hypoperfusion suggests substantial myocardium is at risk. EBCT is a relatively untapped imaging resource for the assessment of acute myocardial infarction and holds significant promise in this regard. The excellent spatial and temporal resolution of EBCT make it an ideal method for evaluating left ventricular aneurysm and associated thrombus.[28,29] Regional wall motion abnormalities characteristic of ventricular aneurysms are easily detected, as is the intracavitary filling defect of the often-associated throm-

bus (Fig. 18-9). One study suggests that EBCT may be superior to transthoracic echocardiography in the detection of left ventricular thrombus.[28]

EBCT is useful in the evaluation of patients with chest pain and suspected CAD. In one study of patients presenting with chest pain and undergoing coronary arteriography, the ejection fraction response to exercise (Fig. 18-10) and the presence or absence of exercise-induced wall motion abnormalities were used successfully for differentiating patients with chest pain and CAD from those with chest pain and no CAD.[8] The positive predictive accuracy was 92 percent for ultrafast CT, compared to 63 percent for stress electrocardiography and 70 percent for thallium-201 myocardial scintigraphy.

One of the more promising applications of ultrafast CT is the detection of coronary calcium as a surrogate for the presence and amount of coronary atherosclerosis (Fig. 18-11). Several groups have demonstrated that the presence of coronary calcium detected by ultrafast CT is predictive of obstructive coronary artery disease.[31–33] A recently reported large multicenter study comparing the detection and qualification of coronary calcium by EBCT with coronary angiography demonstrated that the presence of coronary calcium was 95 percent sensitive for predicting the presence of obstructive coronary artery disease.[33] The few

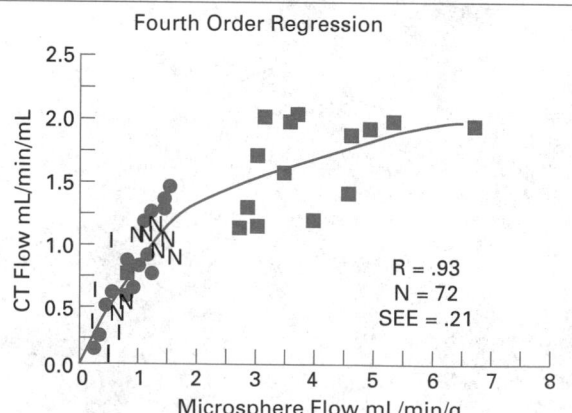

ALL FLOW ANALYSIS

Fourth Order Regression

R = .93
N = 72
SEE = .21

FIGURE 18-6

Ultrafast CT measurement of myocardial flows in dogs are correlated with radioisotope microsphere measurements. (●) Baseline state; (■) pharmacologic vasodilation. I = ischemic myocardium; N = nonischemic myocardium. (From Wolfkiel et al.[16] Reproduced with permission from the publisher and the author.)

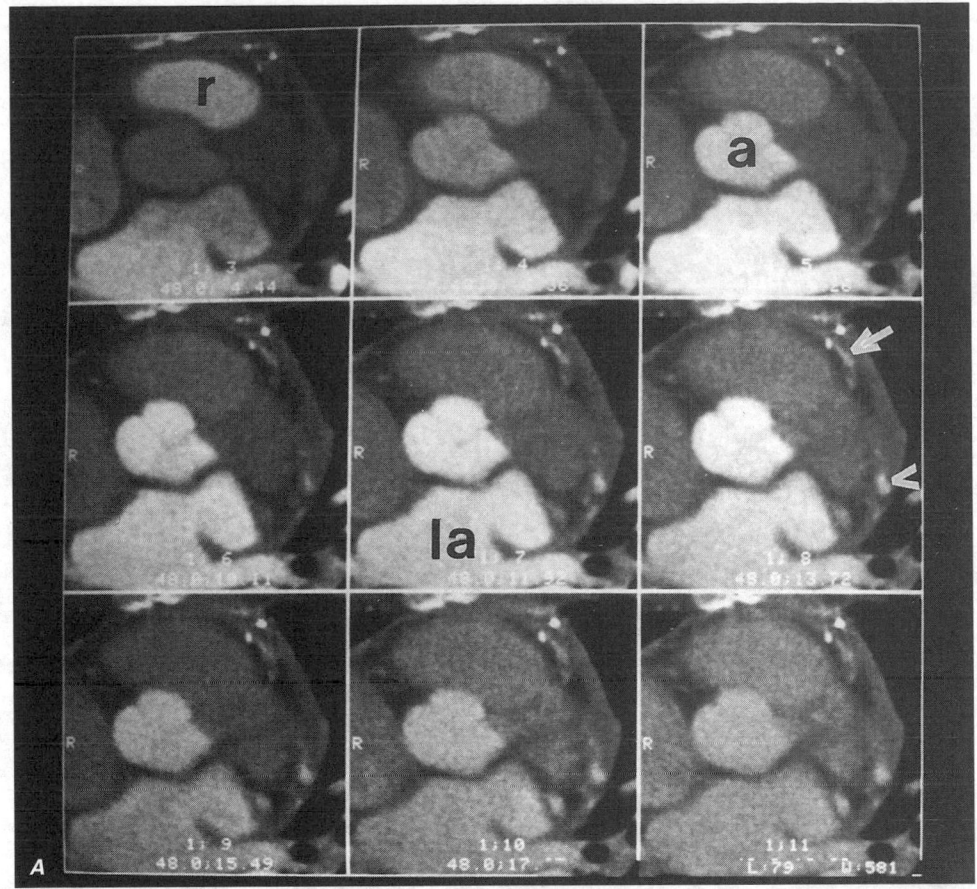

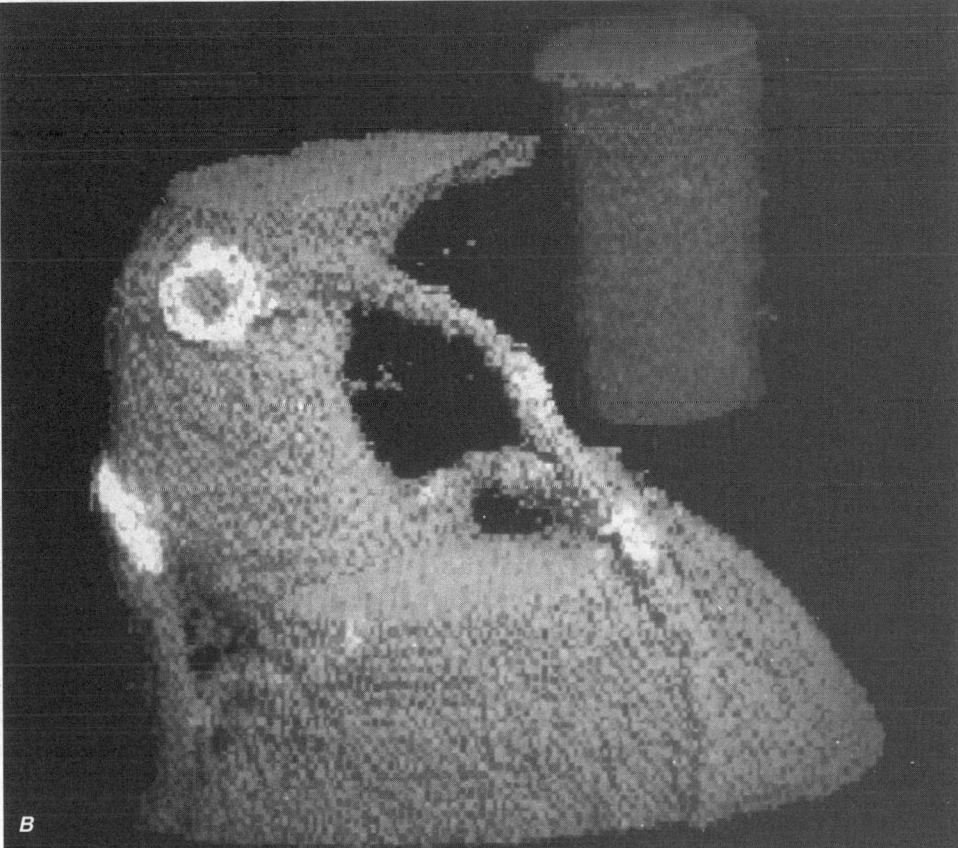

FIGURE 18-7

A. A flow mode study at the level of the aortic valve (a) demonstrates progressive contrast enhancement of a left internal mammary artery graft to the left anterior descending coronary artery (*white arrow*) and a saphenous vein graft to the circumflex (*white arrowhead*). R = right ventricle, la = left atrium. *B.* A single view of a three-dimensional reconstruction of contrast-enhanced EBCT scans demonstrates the courses of patent saphenous vein grafts to the left anterior descending and right coronary arteries. The aortic anastomosis of each graft is identified by a radiopaque "doughnut."

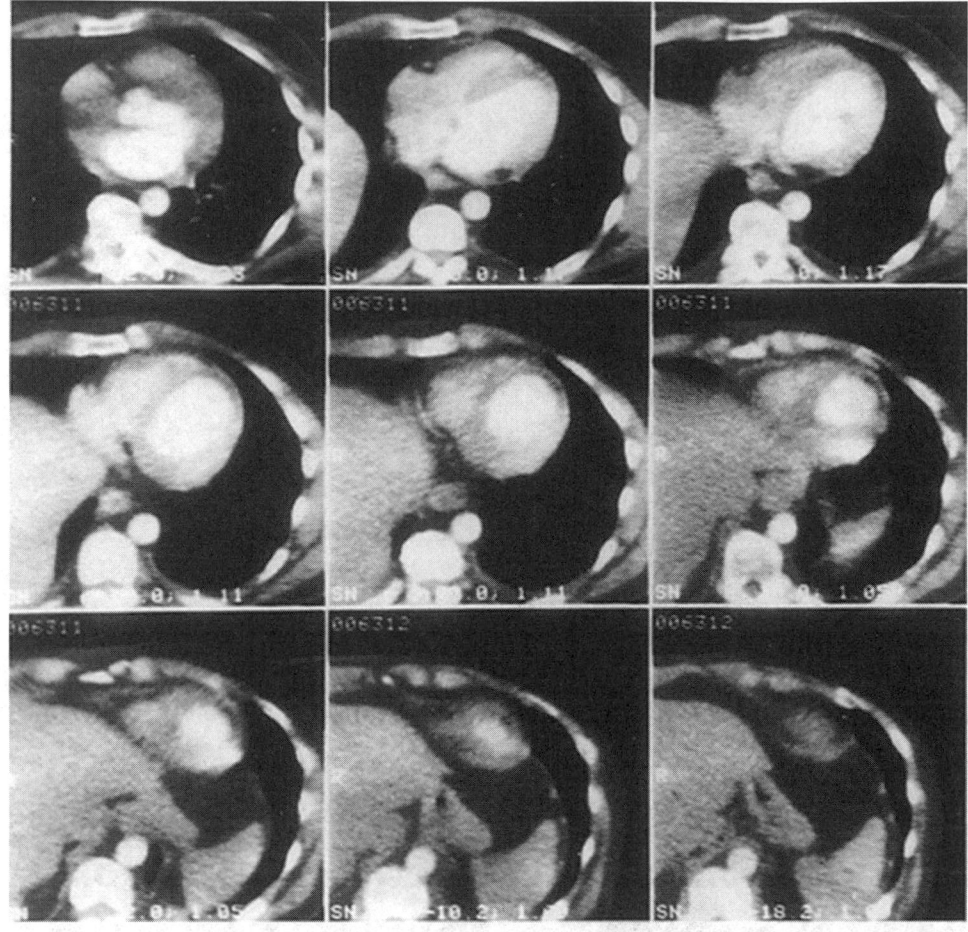

FIGURE 18-8

Fifty-millisecond contrast-enhanced EBCT scans gated to end-diastole include the left ventricle from base (*top left*) to apex (*bottom right*). An acute myocardial infarction identified by the absence of myocardial enhancement is seen in panel 6 but is also apparent in several adjacent scans. (From Brundage BH, Chomka E. Evaluation of acute myocardial infarction by computed tomography. In: Brundage BH, ed. *Comparative Cardiac Imaging.* Rockville, MD, Aspen, 1990:223–229. Reproduced with permission from the publisher and the authors.)

is the presence of coronary calcium the most effective predictor of future coronary events, even in a predominantly symptomatic group of patients,[39,40] but that it is a better predictor of future coronary events than all other coronary risk factors combined.[41,42] The progression of coronary artery calcification has been shown to be more rapid in patients with symptomatic CAD than in those with coronary artery calcium but no symptoms.[43] Another, more recent follow-up of asymptomatic subjects also indicates that those individuals demonstrating the greatest rate of calcium increase are at greatest risk for having a coronary event.[44] Studies in progress are evaluating the value of serial quantification of coronary artery calcium to track the progression of CAD and to determine if risk factor–prevention strategies are effective in slowing or reversing the progression of the disease, as marked by the calcium content. The potential clinical value of EBCT detection of coronary calcium has been recently summarized by an American Heart Association Medical/Scientific statement.[45] Understandably, this organiza-

false-negative results were associated with single-vessel disease in young individuals, usually under the age of 45 years. While the specificity of any detected coronary calcium was relatively low (44 percent) for obstructive disease, the quantity of calcium and the number of calcified vessels greatly enhanced the specificity (Fig. 18-12). Autopsy studies have also confirmed the good correlation between the amount of coronary calcium and the amount and severity of coronary atherosclerosis.[34,35] In asymptomatic populations, EBCT may be useful for identifying patients at risk for future coronary events, so that clinicians can focus their risk factor–reduction strategies on the most appropriate patients. Two studies have demonstrated that the presence and amount of coronary calcium detected by EBCT is predictive of future coronary events, including nonfatal myocardial infarction, need for coronary revascularization, and development of stable and unstable angina.[36,37] The report by Detrano et al. also suggests that coronary death will likely be predicted when their more than 1400 asymptomatic subjects have been followed long enough.[38] Other studies have provided evidence that not only

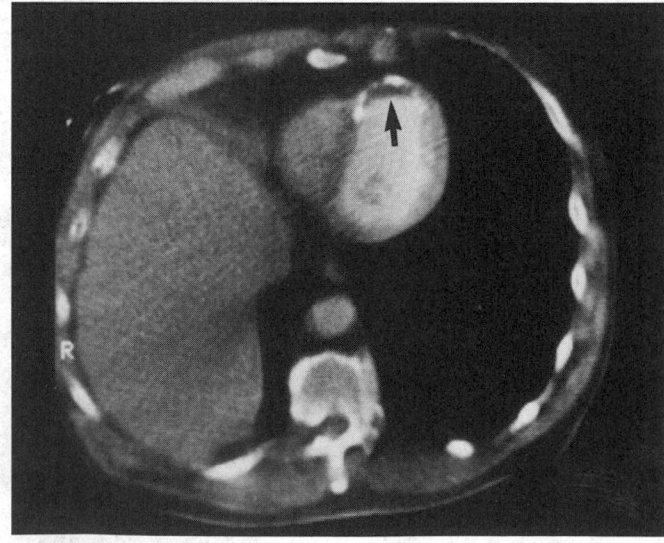

FIGURE 18-9

A single frame from a contrast-enhanced cine CT demonstrates thrombus in a left ventricular aneurysm. Also note that the wall of the aneurysm is calcified.

tion was conservative in making recommendations about the clinical use of EBCT detection of coronary calcium. The recommendations from that report (outlined in Tables 18-1 and 18-2), however, contain clinically useful applications. Clearly high- and low-risk individuals for developing coronary events can be differentiated. This information should be helpful in planning therapeutic approaches to risk factor modification, particularly in the use of expensive cholesterol-lowering drugs.

Recently, Moshage et al. have reported experience with the use of EBCT to perform intravenous coronary angiography.[46] While this application is still in development, the images currently being obtained are quite promising (Fig. 18-13). The diagnosis of Kawasaki's disease or anomalous origin of the coronary artery is also possible with current EBCT technology[47] (Fig. 18-14). Future improvements in spatial resolution and slice thickness may soon make it feasible to perform diagnostic coronary angiography with EBCT and intravenous contrast administration.

VALVULAR HEART DISEASE

Echocardiography remains the standard for the evaluation of valvular heart disease; however, EBCT offers several possible advantages in selected patients. Precise and accurate measurement of cardiac volumes has been demonstrated by several investigators. Reiter and coworkers[5] demonstrated in animals that ultrafast CT measurements of aortic regurgitant volume correlate well with measurements made by electromagnetic flow probes. In patients with isolated aortic or mitral regurgitation, determination of right ventricular and left ventricular volumes provides an

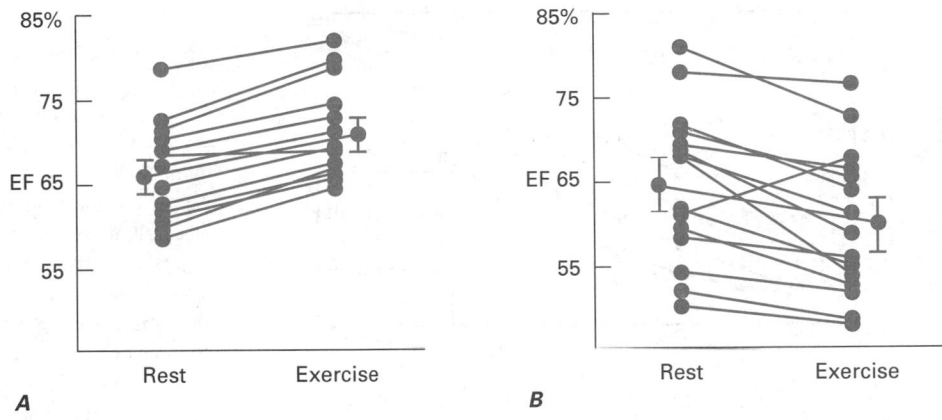

FIGURE 18-10

Ejection fraction (EF) response to bicycle exercise determined by ultrafast CT scanning is contrasted between chest pain patients with normal coronary arteries (*A*) and those with coronary artery disease (*B*) as defined by coronary arteriography. (From Roig et al.[8] Reproduced with permission from the publisher and the author.)

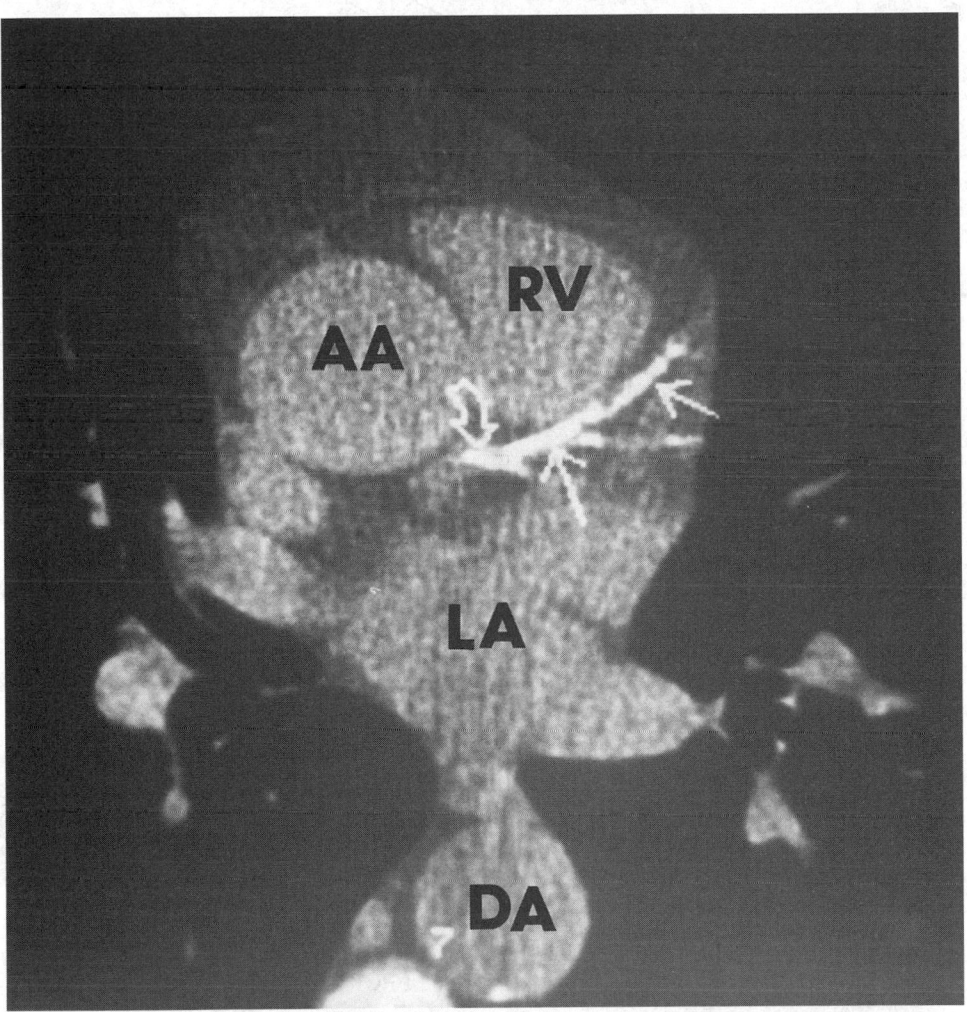

FIGURE 18-11

The entire proximal left coronary artery is calcified. The left main (*open arrow*) and left anterior descending coronary arteries (*stick arrows*) are well seen in this scan; also, the proximal circumflex and diagonal vessels are easily identified. AA = ascending aorta; DA = descending aorta; LA = left atrium; RV = right ventricular outflow tract. (From Brundage BH, Mao SS. In: Schlant RC et al., eds. *Diagnostic Atlas of the Heart*. New York: McGraw-Hill, 1996:236. Reproduced with permission from the publisher and authors.)

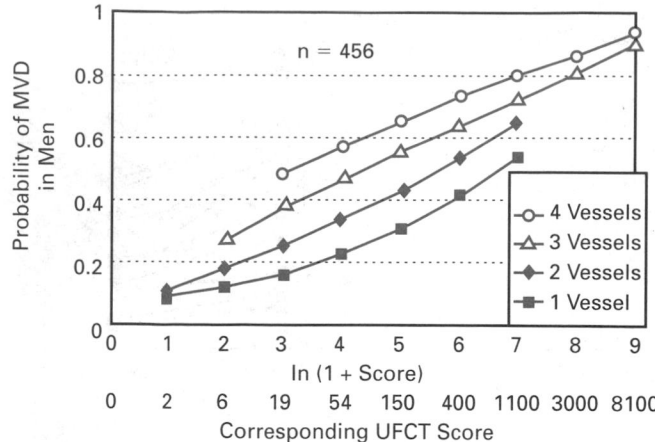

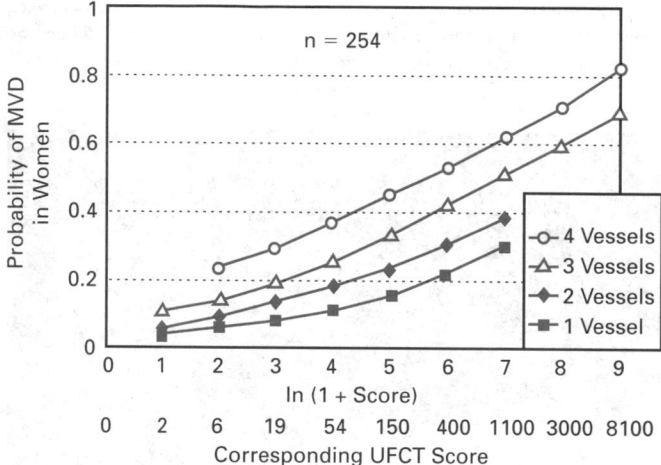

FIGURE 18-12

Increasing amounts of coronary calcium (*score*) correlate with increasing probability of multivessel angiographic obstruction in men and women. Increasing number of vessels calcified further increases the probability of multivessel obstruction. (From Budoff et al.[33] Reproduced with permission from the publisher and the authors.)

TABLE 18-1

ABSENCE OF DETECTABLE CORONARY ARTERY CALCIFICATION USING ELECTRON BEAM COMPUTED TOMOGRAPHY (NEGATIVE TEST)

Does not absolutely rule out the presence of atherosclerotic plaque, including unstable plaque.

Highly unlikely in the presence of significant luminal obstructive disease.

Observation made in the majority of patients who have had both angiographically normal coronary arteries and EBCT scanning.

Testing is gender independent.

May be consistent with a low risk of a cardiovascular event in the next 2–5 years.

Source: From Wexler et al.,[45] reproduced with permission by the American Heart Association.

TABLE 18-2

PRESENCE OF DETECTABLE CORONARY ARTERY CALCIFICATION USING ELECTRON BEAM COMPUTED TOMOGRAPHY (POSITIVE TEST)

Confirms the presence of coronary atherosclerotic plaque.

The greater the amount of calcification (i.e., calcium area or calcium score), the greater the likelihood of obstructive disease, but there is no one-to-one relation, and findings may not be site specific.

Total amount of calcification correlates best with total amount of atherosclerotic plaque, although the true "plaque burden" is underestimated.

A high calcium score may be consistent with moderate to high risk of a cardiovascular event within the next 2–5 years.

Source: From Wexler et al.,[45] reproduced with permission by the American Heart Association.

accurate measurement of regurgitant volume. The degree of accuracy achieved has not been possible with other imaging techniques, including biplane ventriculography. Several studies have demonstrated that CT can identify left atrial thrombus successfully[28,48] (Fig. 18-15). One study comparing EBCT with echocardiography suggests that EBCT may be more

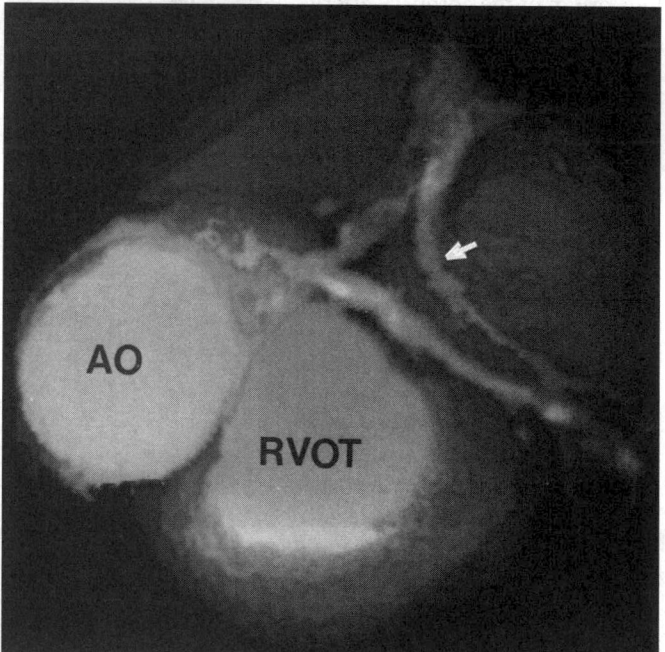

FIGURE 18-13

A top-down view of a three-dimensional reconstruction of contrast-enhanced EBCT scans shows the origin of the left main coronary artery from the aorta (AO). The left anterior interventricular vein (*white arrow*) parallels the left anterior descending coronary artery and then passes over the circumflex coronary artery to join the coronary sinus. Note the calcium in the left anterior descending and circumflex coronary arteries. RVOT = right ventricular outflow tract. (From Brundage BH. What is the current role of ultrafast CT in coronary imaging? In Reiber JHC, Van der Wall EE, eds. *Cardiovascular Imaging*. Boston: Kluwer, 1996: 540. Reproduced with permission from the publisher and the author.)

sensitive than transthoracic echocardiography.[28] to date, there have been no comparisons of transesophageal echocardiography and EBCT, but EBCT is less invasive than transesophageal echocardiography. Valve function and anatomy can be imaged by EBCT, but echocardiography remains the procedure of choice if an adequate acoustic window is available. In those patients in whom body habitus, obesity, or hyperinflation of the lungs prevents adequate images by echocardiography, EBCT is a reasonable alternative (Fig. 18-16). Prosthetic valve function can be assessed by EBCT because the streak artifacts created by motion are minimized. Detection of valve ring abscess has also been reported.[49,50]

DISEASES OF THE GREAT VESSELS

Conventional CT has been widely employed for the assessment of aortic dissection (see also Chap. 98). Movement due to aortic pulsation and patient respiration, however, sometimes creates a motion artifact that may conceal torn intima. EBCT with its rapid image acquisition overcomes this drawback (Fig. 18-17). To date there are no comparisons of EBCT with conventional CT, nuclear magnetic resonance imaging, or echocardiography. Stanford[51] demonstrated excellent results when comparing EBCT images with findings at surgery or autopsy. EBCT has advantages of speed, minimal invasiveness, and tomographic format over conventional angiography. Comparative studies with transesophageal echocardiography and nuclear magnetic resonance imaging are needed, but the speed with which EBCT can be performed may well make it the procedure of choice for diagnosing aortic dissection. EBCT is also useful in assessing thoracic and abdominal atherosclerotic aortic aneurysms.[51] Excellent definition of the extent of the aneurysm and the amount of intraaneurysmal thrombus has been demonstrated

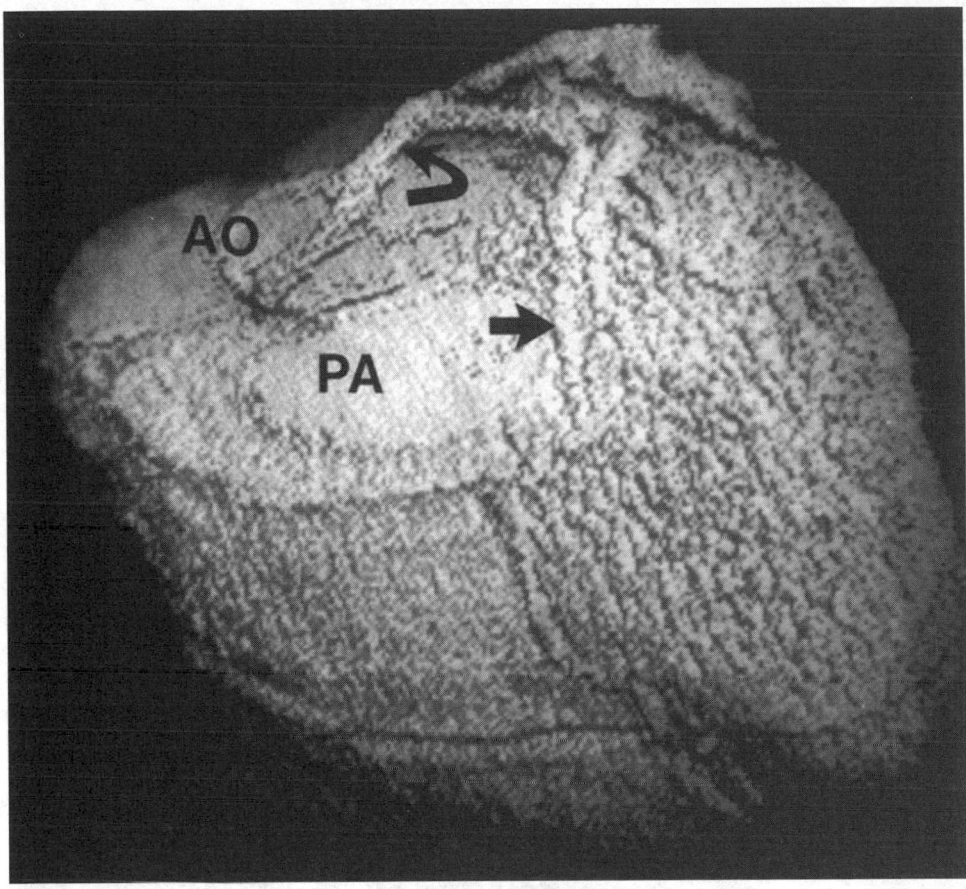

FIGURE 18-14

A selected view of a three-dimensional reconstruction of coronary arteries demonstrates the abnormal origin of the right coronary artery (*curved arrow*) from the left anterior descending coronary artery (*straight arrow*) and its course between the pulmonary artery (PA) and the aorta (AO). (From Brundage BH. What is the current role of ultrafast CT in coronary imaging? In Reiber JHC, Van der Wall EE, eds. *Cardiovascular Imaging.* Boston: Kluwer, 1996:541. Reproduced with permission from the publisher and the authors.)

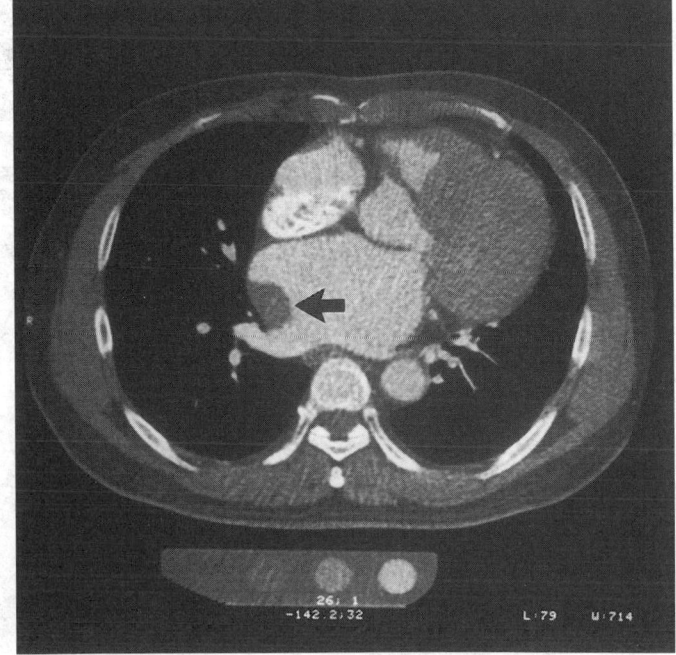

FIGURE 18-15

A left atrial thrombus (*arrow*) anterior to the right superior pulmonary vein is well described in this contrast enhanced EBCT scan. The transthoracic echocardiogram did not detect any left atrial thrombus.

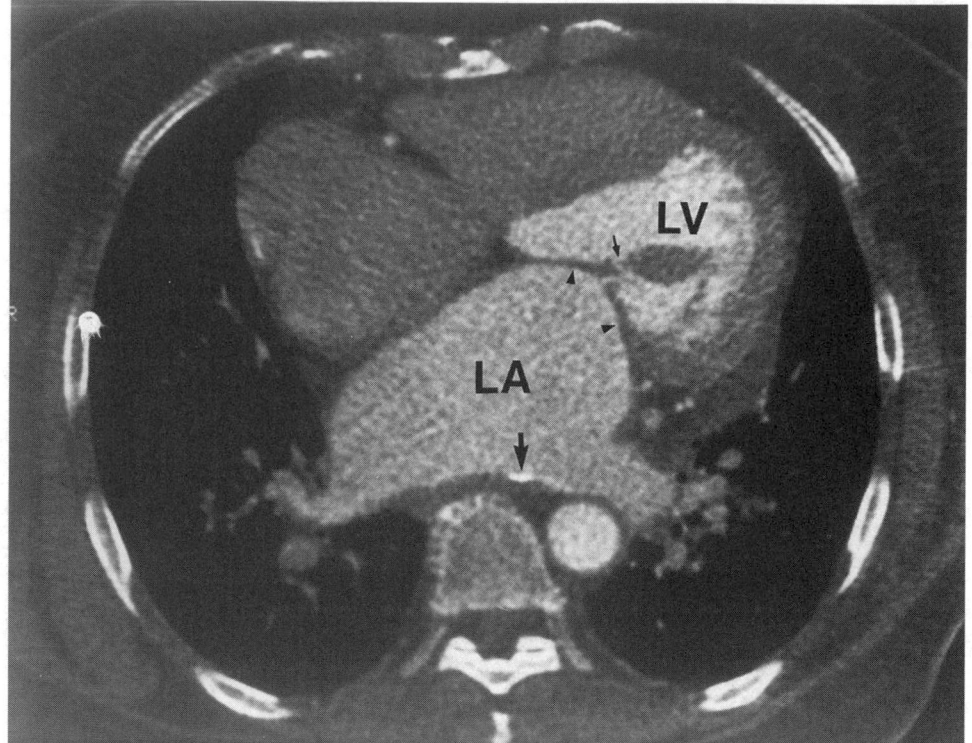

FIGURE 18-16
A contrast-enhanced scan at the level of the mitral valve depicts anterior and posterior valve thickening (*arrowheads*), chordal shortening (*small arrow*), and left atrial (LA) and pulmonary vein enlargement. Also note the calcification of the posterior left atrial wall (*large arrow*). LV = left ventricle. (From Brundage BH, Mao SS. In: Schlant RC et al., eds. *Diagnostic Atlas of the Heart*. New York: McGraw-Hill, 1996:238. Reproduced with permission from the publisher and authors.)

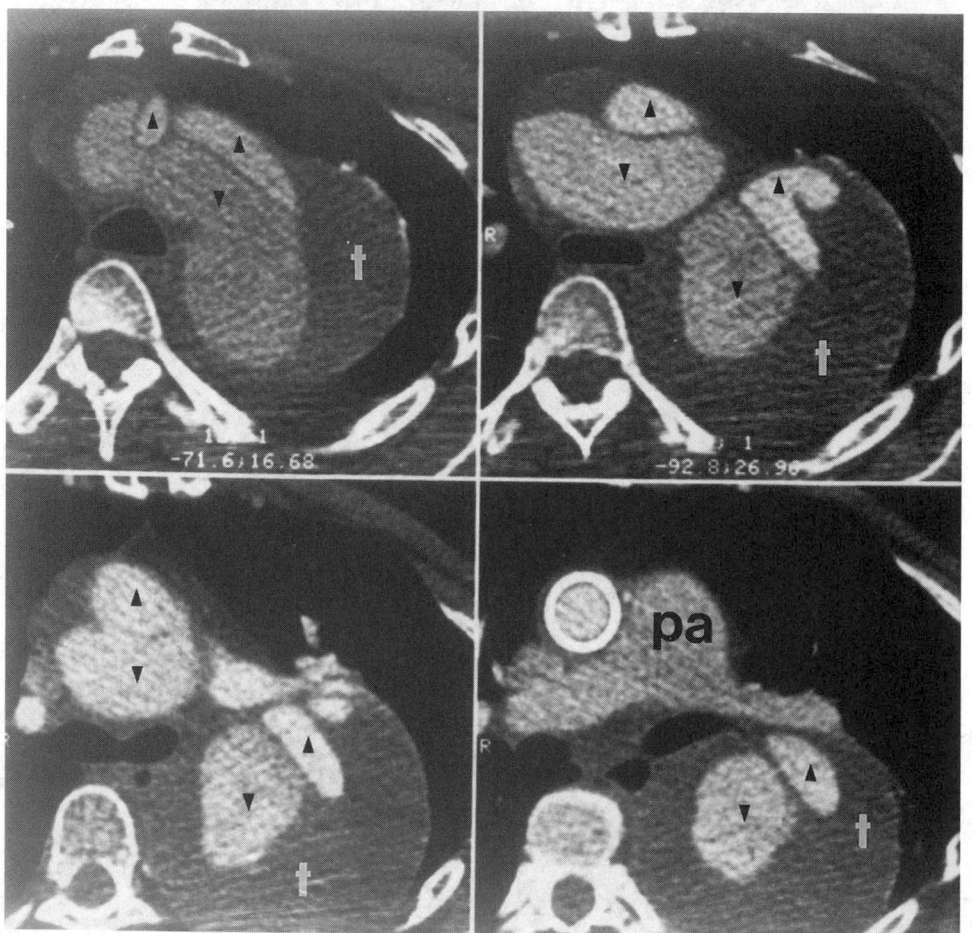

FIGURE 18-17
Postoperative evaluation of a patient with Marfan's syndrome by EBCT delineates the status of a type I dissection. Four selected contrast-enhanced scans of the ascending and descending aorta detail the anatomy of the true lumen (▲), false lumen (▼), and associated thrombus (t). The dense ring in the fourth panel is a graft conduit used to repair the ascending aorta. pa = pulmonary artery. (From Brundage BH, Mao SS. In: Schlant RC et al, eds. *Diagnostic Atlas of the Heart*. New York: McGraw-Hill, 1996:247. Reproduced with permission from the publisher and authors.)

(Fig. 18-18). Other abnormalities of the aorta, such as sinus of Valsalva aneurysm, supervalvular aortic stenosis, and coarctation, have been well demonstrated by this technique.[52,53] Abnormalities of the pulmonary artery are also well visualized by EBCT. Chronic pulmonary artery thromboembolism can be diagnosed, and the determination of the proximal extent of the thrombus, which is critical in planning surgical therapy, is well delineated (Fig. 18-19). Recent reports suggest that EBCT may also be a useful tool in the detection of acute pulmonary thromboembolism and that relatively small emboli are detectable.[54,55] Furthermore, tissue perfusion imaging techniques provide a type of "lung scan" that is a useful adjunct to the anatomic information provided.[21]

PERICARDIAL DISEASE

EBCT is well suited to the assessment of pericardial disease because of its tomographic representation of cardiac anatomy, high spatial resolution, and excellent density resolution.[56] Calcific constrictive pericarditis is easily diagnosed by ultrafast CT, and the distribution of the calcification, its thickness, and its extension into the visceral pericardium and myocardium are well defined (Fig. 18-20). Such geographic demonstration is helpful in planning the surgical treatment. The surgeon can focus on those areas of pericardium where the removal of the calcified pericardium is feasible. As with two-dimensional echocardiography and radionuclide angiography, diastolic properties of the left ventricle can be evaluated using the cine mode.[6,57] Alterations in early and late diastolic filling are easily detected. Superior and inferior vena cava cross-sectional

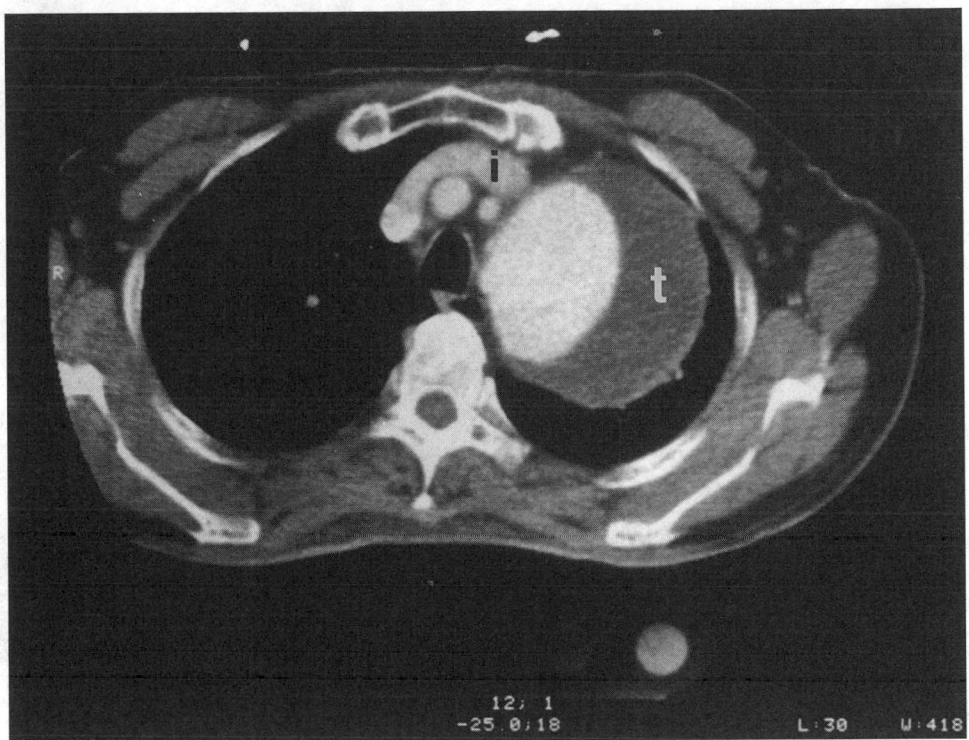

FIGURE 18-18
A large thrombus (t)-filled aneurysm of the aortic arch occupies most of the upper left thoracic cavity. The innominate vein (i) courses anterior to the innominate and left common carotid artery.

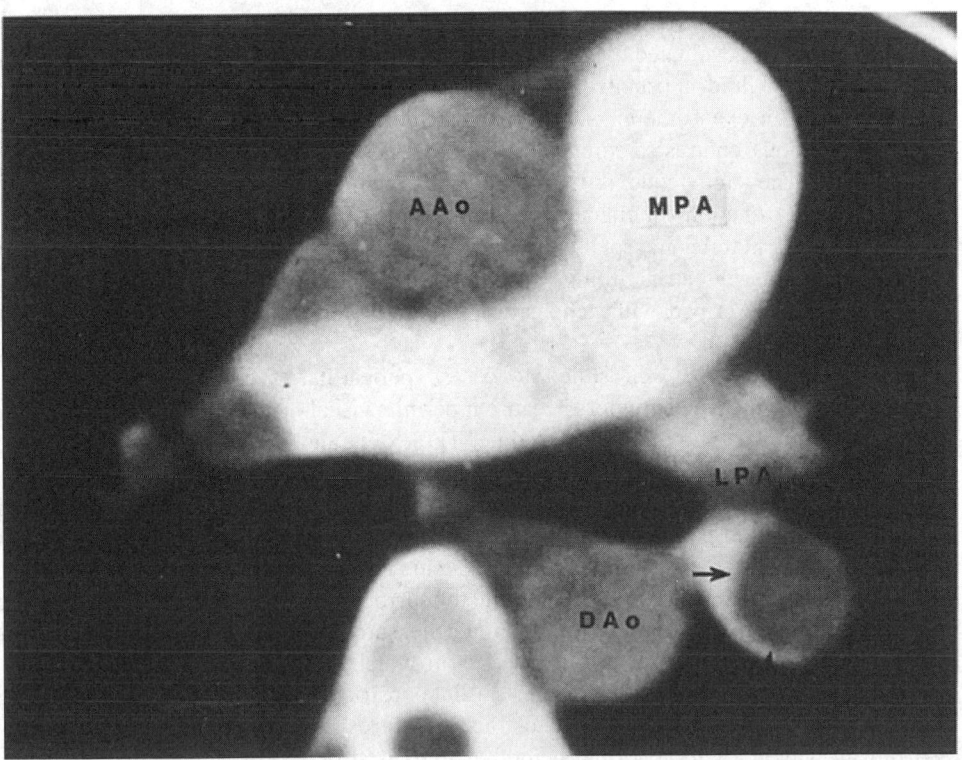

FIGURE 18-19
Large left pulmonary artery (LPA) chronic thrombus (*arrows*) is outlined by contrast medium on this high-resolution ultrafast CT scan. AAo = ascending aorta; DAo = descending aorta; MPA = main pulmonary artery.

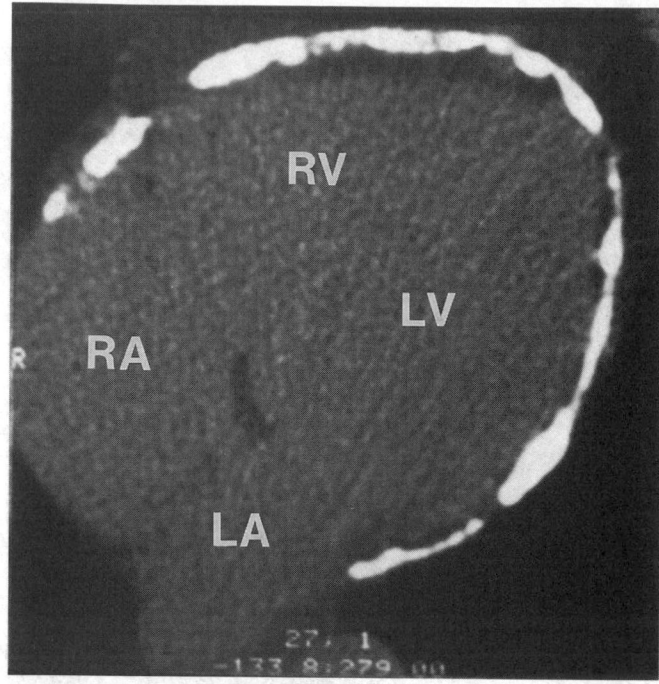

FIGURE 18-20
Densely calcified pericardium is easily identified in this scan of the mid-heart. LA = left atrium; LV = left ventricle; RA = right atrium; RV = right ventricle. (From Brundage BH, Mao SS. In: Schlant RC et al, eds. *Diagnostic Atlas of the Heart.* New York: McGraw-Hill, 1996:243. Reproduced with permission from the publisher and authors.)

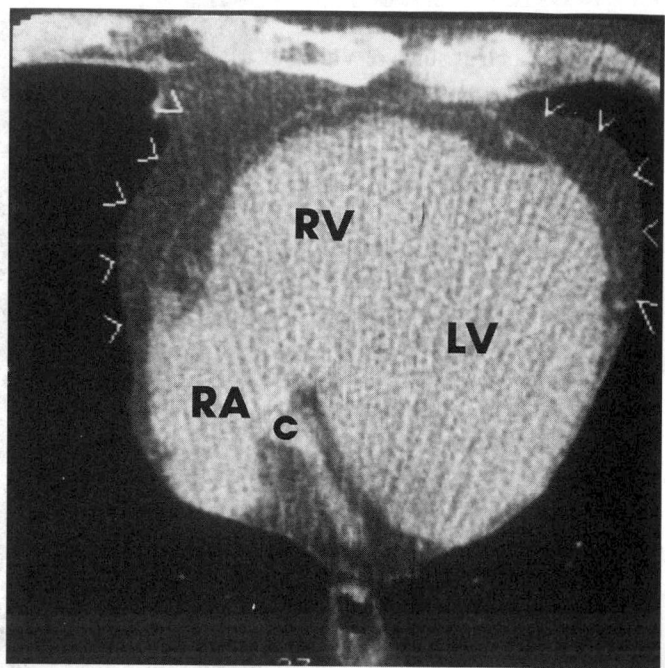

FIGURE 18-21
The fat that resides both inside and outside (*arrowheads*) the pericardium provides sufficient contrast to outline the normal pericardium, which is only 1 to 2 mm thick. Contrast enhancement with iodine agents is unnecessary. c = coronary sinus; LV = left ventricle; RA = right atrium; RV = right ventricle. (From Brundage BH, Mao SS. In: Schlant RC et al, eds. *Diagnostic Atlas of the Heart.* New York: McGraw-Hill, 1996:243. Reproduced with permission from the publisher and authors.)

areas are good indicators of the degree of elevation of right ventricular diastolic and atrial filling pressures. Pericardial effusion can also be evaluated by EBCT, although the density of the pericardial fluid is usually very similar to that of the myocardium so the exact amount of fluid cannot be determined unless intravenous contrast medium is used to enhance the myocardium. The cine mode is used to evaluate left and right ventricular function simultaneously. Tamponade can be detected by abnormalities in septal and right ventricular free-wall motion and right atrial filling characteristics that are similar to those described with echocardiography (see also Chaps. 14 and 81).

EBCT is particularly well suited to assess pericardial involvement with metastatic tumors because it permits visualization of the mediastinum at the same time. The extent and location of pericardial involvement are therefore easily determined. The high spatial resolution of ultrafast CT makes it possible to determine pericardial thickness, particularly over the anterior wall of the right ventricle (Fig. 18-21). The pericardium is silhouetted by the epicardial fat and the surrounding lung tissue. This approach allows an accurate measurement of pericardial thickness and is useful in cases in which it is difficult to determine whether there is pericardial constriction or myocardial restriction. A pericardial thickness in excess of 4 mm in patients with abnormal hemodynamics is strong evidence for pericardial constriction. Pericardial cysts and lipomas are also easily identified by EBCT.

MYOCARDIAL DISEASE

The myocardium of both the right and left ventricle can be visualized in its entirety with EBCT. Therefore, both precise measurement of myocardial mass and evaluation of right and left ventricular function are possible, and evaluation of diseases of the myocardium is optimized.[4,5,11–13] Ventricular hypertrophy of any cause can be quantified and serially evaluated, as in the case of regression of left ventricular hypertrophy following the treatment of hypertensive heart disease or correction of aortic valve stenosis. Since both ventricular volumes and wall thickness can be determined accurately, when coupled with pressure analysis, global and regional wall stresses can be measured. In patients with hypertrophic cardiomyopathy, the distribution and severity of the hypertrophic process can be quantified.[58] Also, systolic and diastolic ventricular function can be measured. Furthermore, assessment of mitral valve motion is also possible.

In idiopathic dilated cardiomyopathy, quantitation of systolic and diastolic ventricular function and measurement of chamber volumes and wall stress before and after vasodilator treatment may be useful (see also Chaps. 23 and 73). Clues to the etiology of the dilated cardiomyopathy may also be acquired. Arrhythmogenic right ventricular dysplasia may be identified by careful analysis of right ventricular endocardial anatomy.[59] Magnetic resonance imaging is probably the superior modality for diagnosing this entity (see Chap. 19). Furthermore, phase analysis of the left ventricular and right ventricular activation-contraction sequence can be used to identify the focus of ventricular tachycardia.[60] EBCT has also been used to identify previously undetected cardiac abnormalities in patients with lone atrial fibrillation.[61]

CONGENITAL HEART DISEASE

The use of EBCT to diagnose congenital heart disease is well described.[62,63] In addition to the obvious advantages of cross-sectional high-resolution imaging for defining cardiac structural abnormalities, EBCT can also be used to quantify intracardiac shunts,[64,65] assess right and left ventricular function,[4,5] measure myocardial mass,[11–13] and evaluate valvular function (Fig. 18-22). With the indicator-dilution technique, quantification of cardiac shunts by EBCT has an accuracy equivalent to that of radioisotope methods.[64]

EBCT has been used to diagnose atrial septal defect,[65] supravalvular aortic stenosis,[53] Ebstein's anomaly,[66] congenital arteriovenous fistulae,[52] cor triatriatum,[67] and other complex congenital anomalies.[63] The experience with EBCT in diagnosing congenital heart disease is limited, but its ability to acquire images rapidly; its high spatial resolution; and its capacity to evaluate function, flow, and anatomy during a single diagnostic test offer great promise. The ability to acquire very thin 1.5-mm slices should further enhance its utility.

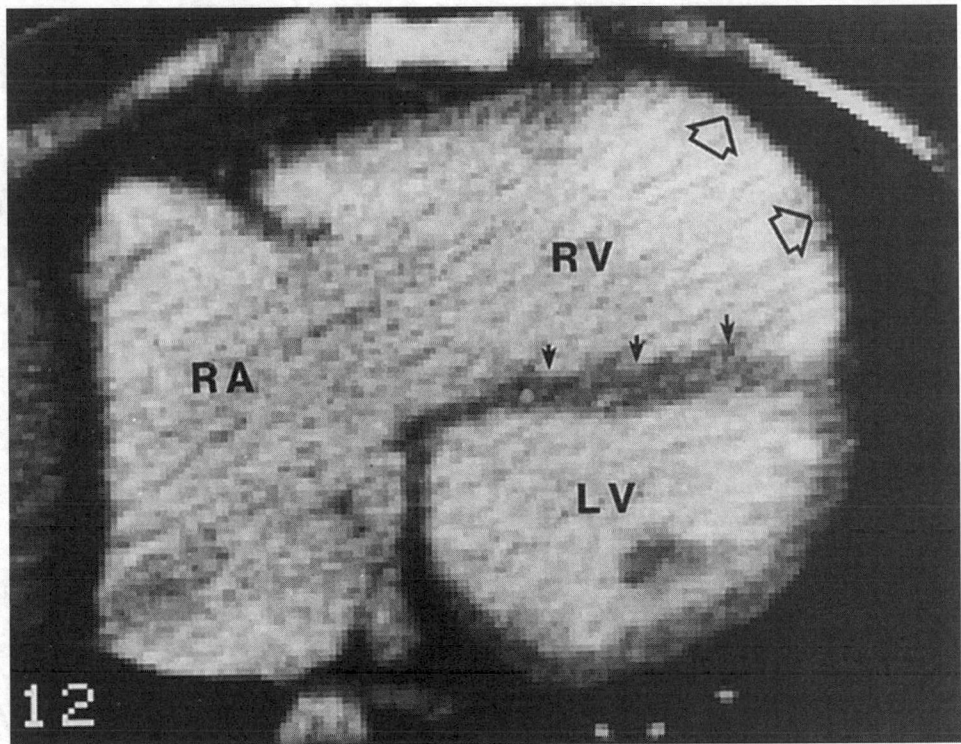

A

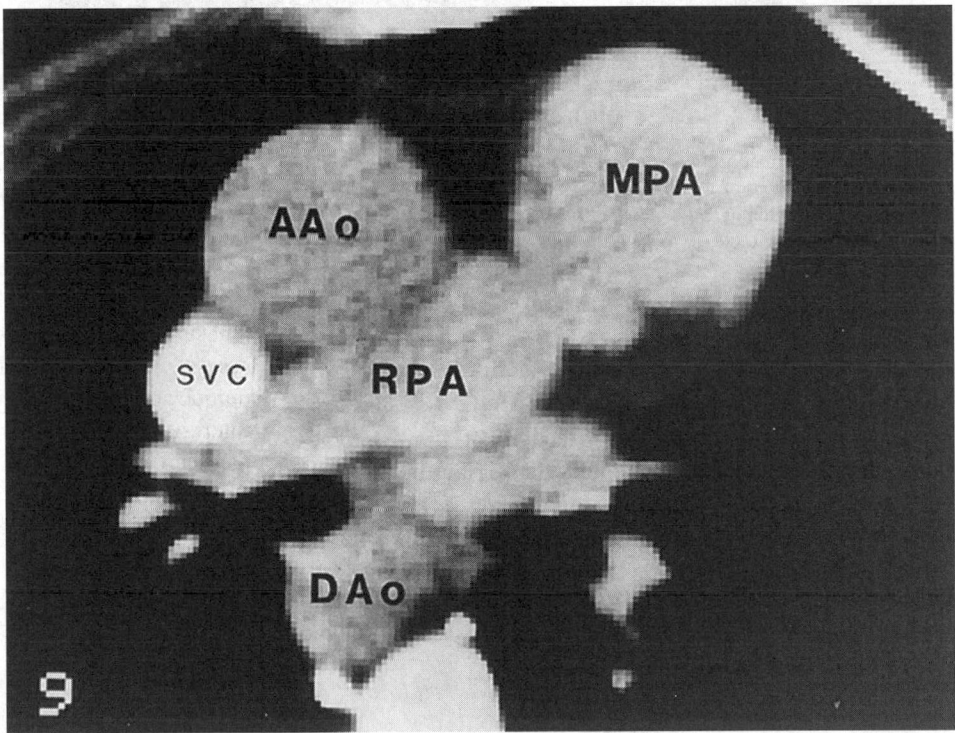

B

FIGURE 18-22

Postoperative ultrafast CT study of a patient operated for tetralogy of Fallot demonstrates (*A*) right ventricular dilation and aneurysm (*open arrows*) with paradoxical diastolic flattening of the interventricular septum due to severe tricuspid regurgitation. The same study (*B*) revealed residual stenosis of the right pulmonary artery (RPA). AAo = ascending aorta; DAo = descending aorta; LV = left ventricle; MPA = main pulmonary artery; RA = right atrium; SVC = superior vena cava.

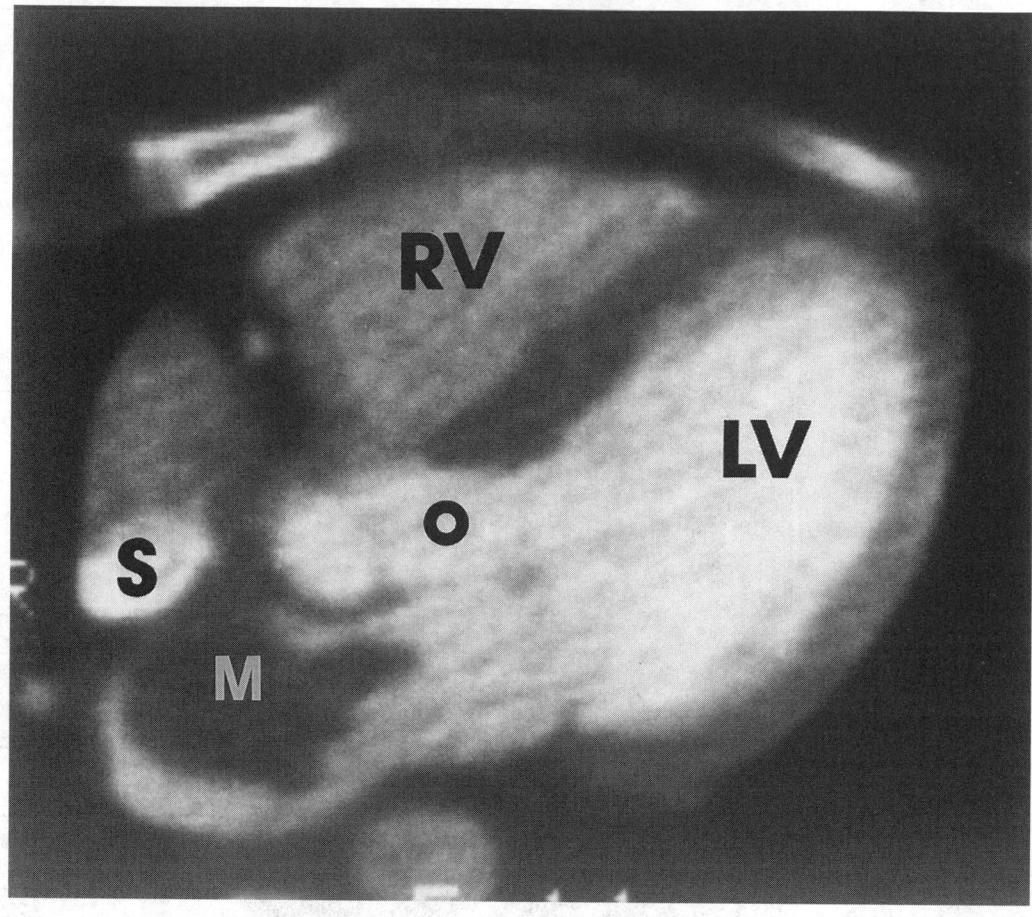

FIGURE 18-23

A single diastolic frame from a contrast-enhanced cine CT defines the left atrial septal attachment of a myxoma (M). The frondlike excrescences are characteristic of this tumor. LV = left ventricle; O = left ventricular outflow tract; RV = right ventricle; S = superior vena cava. (From Brundage BH, Mao SS. In: Schlant RC et al, eds. *Diagnostic Atlas of the Heart*. New York: McGraw-Hill, 1996:244. Reproduced with permission from the publisher and authors.)

CARDIAC TUMORS

Intracardiac tumors are well visualized by EBCT with intravenous contrast enhancement. Reports diagnosing both right[68] (Fig. 18-23) and left[69] atrial myxomas have been published. EBCT can also be useful for the evaluation of cardiac metastatic tumor. The excellent visualization of adjacent mediastinal, pulmonary, and chest wall structures makes it useful in staging the tumor as well as suggesting its primary source (see also Chap. 86).

SUMMARY

EBCT is a new technology that has been clinically available only for a relatively short time. In this interval it has been demonstrated to be useful in evaluating most forms of cardiac disease. In addition to providing excellent definition of normal and pathologic anatomy, its ability to evaluate both right and left ventricular global and regional function, provide precise

measurements of cardiac volumes and myocardial mass, and assess myocardial tissue perfusion makes it a particularly unique and potentially powerful diagnostic tool. There is great interest in defining its role in detecting the presence of coronary artery disease, particularly in asymptomatic, high-risk patients, through the ability to image coronary artery calcium. In the coming years, EBCT can be expected to receive much wider utilization.

REFERENCES

1. Gonda RL, Gutierrez OH, Azodo MVU. Mycotic aneurysms of the aorta: Radiologic features. *Radiology* 1988; 168:343–346.
2. Godwin JD, Herfkens RJ, Skioldebrand CG, Federle MP, Lipton MJ. Evolution of dissections and aneurysms of the thoracic aorta by conventional and dynamic CT scanning. *Radiology* 1980; 136:125–136.
3. Brundage BH, Lipton MJ, Herfkens RJ, Berninger WH, Redington RW, Chatterjee K, et al. Detection of patent coronary bypass grafts by computed tomography: A preliminary report. *Circulation* 1980; 61:826–831.
4. Feiring AJ, Rumberger JA, Reiter SJ, Collins SM, Skorton DJ, Rees M, et al. Sectional and segmental variability of left ventricular function: Experimental and clinical studies using ultrafast computed tomography. *J Am Coll Cardiol* 1988; 12:415–425.

5. Reiter SJ, Rumberger JA, Feiring AJ, Stanford W, Marcus ML. Precision of measurements of right and left ventricular volume by cine computed tomography. *Circulation* 1986; 74:890–900.

6. Rumberger JA, Weiss RM, Feiring AJ, Stanford W, Hajduczok ZD, Rezai K, et al. Patterns of regional diastolic function in the normal human left ventricle: An ultrafast computed tomographic study. *J Am Coll Cardiol* 1989; 14:119–126.

7. Rich S, Chomka EV, Stagl R, Shanes JG, Kondos GT, Brundage BH. Determination of left ventricular ejection fraction using ultrafast computed tomography. *Am Heart J* 1986; 112:392–396.

8. Roig E, Chomka EV, Castaner A, Campo A, Heras M, Rich S, et al. Exercise ultrafast computed tomography for the detection of coronary artery disease. *J Am Coll Cardiol* 1989; 13:1073–1081.

9. Lanzer P, Garrett J, Sievers R, O'Connell WO, Botvinick E, Higgens CB. Quantitation of regional myocardial function by cine computed tomography: Pharmacologic changes in wall thickness. *J Am Coll Cardiol* 1986; 8:682–692.

10. Rumberger JA, Bell MR. Measurement of myocardial perfusion and cardiac output using intravenous injection methods by ultrafast (cine) computed tomography. *Invest Radiol* 1992; 27:S40–S46.

11. Feiring AJ, Rumberger JA, Reiter SJ, Skorton DJ, Collins SM, Lipton MJ, et al. Determination of left ventricular mass in dogs in rapid acquisition cardiac computed tomography. *Circulation* 1985; 72:1355–1364.

12. Roig E, Georgiou D, Chomka EV, Wolfkiel C, Logalbo-Zak C, Rich S, et al. Reproducibility of left ventricular myocardial volume and mass measurements by ultrafast computed tomography. *J Am Coll Cardiol* 1991; 18:990–996.

13. Hajduczok ZD, Weiss RM, Stanford W, Marcus ML. Determination of right ventricular mass in humans and dogs with ultrafast computed tomography. *Circulation* 1990; 82:202–212.

14. Wolfkiel CJ, Ferguson JL, Chomka EV, Law WR, Brundage BH. Determination of cardiac output by ultrafast computed tomography. *Am J Physiol Imaging* 1986; 1:117–123.

15. Garrett J, Lanzer P, Jaschke W, Botvinick E, Sievers R, Higgens CB, et al. Measurement of cardiac output by cine computed tomography. *Am J Cardiol* 1985; 56:657–661.

16. Wolfkiel CJ, Ferguson JL, Chomka EV, Law WR, Labin IN, Tenzer ML, et al. Measurement of myocardial blood flow by ultrafast computed tomography. *Circulation* 1987; 76:1262–1273.

17. Rumberger JA, Feiring AJ, Lipton MJ, Higgins CB, Ell SR, Marcus ML. Use of ultrafast computed tomography to quantitate regional myocardial perfusion: A preliminary report. *J Am Coll Cardiol* 1987; 9:59–69.

18. Wang T, Wu X, Cheng N, Ritman EL. Myocardial blood flow estimated by synchronous, multislice, high-speed computed tomography. *IEEE Med Imaging* 1989; 8:70–77.

19. Weiss RM, Otoadese EA, Noel MP, DeJong SC, Heery SD. Quantitation of absolute regional myocardial perfusion using cine computed tomography. *J Am Coll Cardiol* 1994; 23:1186–1193.

20. Wolfkiel CJ, Brundage BH. Transfer function analysis of UFCT myocardial time-density curves by time varying recursive least squares analysis. *IEEE Trans Biomed Eng* 41:1, 69–76, 1994.

21. Hoffman EA, Tajik JK, Kugelmass SD. Matching pulmonary structure and perfusion via combined dynamic multislice CT and thin-slice high-resolution CT. *Comput Med Imag Graph* 1995; 19:101–112.

22. Stanford W, Brundage BH, MacMillan R, Bateman TM, Chomka EV, Lipton MJ, et al. Sensitivity and specificity of assessing coronary bypass graft patency with ultrafast computed tomography: Results of a multicenter study. *J Am Coll Cardiol* 1988; 12:1–7.

23. Bateman TM, Whiting JS, Forrester JS. Determination of coronary bypass graft patency with ultrafast CT. *New Concepts Cardiac Imag* 1988; 4:217–230.

24. Rumberger JA, Feiring AJ, Hiratzka LE, Reiter SJ, Stark CA, Stanford W, et al. Quantitation of coronary artery bypass flow reserve in dogs using cine computed tomography. *Circ Res* 1987; 61:5-II, 117–123.

25. Brundage BH, Hart K, Chomka E, Kieras K, Pietras RJ, Pavel D. Detection, location and sizing of acute myocardial infarction by fast, computed tomography. (Abstract) *Clin Res* 1985; 33:172A.

26. Rumberger JA, Behrenbeck T, Breen JR, Reed JE, Gersh BJ. Nonparallel changes in global left ventricular chamber volume and muscle mass during the first year after transmural myocardial infarction in humans. *J Am Coll Cardiol* 1993; 21:673–682.

27. Chareonthaitawee P, Christian TF, Hirose K, Gibbons RJ, Rumberger JA. Relation of initial infarct size to extent of left ventricular remodeling in the year after acute myocardial infarction. *J Am Coll Cardiol* 1995; 25:567–573.

28. Helgason CM, Chomka E, Louie E, Rich S, Zajoc E, Roig E, et al. The potential role for ultrafast cardiac computed tomography in patients with stroke. *Stroke* 1989; 20:465–472.

29. Lessick J, Sideman S, Azhari H, Marcus M, Orenadir E, Beyer R. Regional three-dimensional geometric ventricle with fibrous aneurysms: A cine computed tomography study. *Circulation* 1991; 84:1172–1186.

30. Tannenbaum SR, Kondos GT, Veselick KE, Pendergast MR, Brundage BH, Chomka EV. Detection of calcific deposits in coronary arteries by ultrafast computed tomography and correlation with angiography. *Am J Cardiol* 1989; 63:870–871.

31. Agatston AS, Janowitz WR, Hildner FJ, Zusmer AR, Viamonte M, Detrano R. Quantification of coronary artery calcium using ultrafast computed tomography. *J Am Coll Cardiol* 1990; 15:827–832.

32. Breen JF, Sheedy PF, Schwartz RS, Stanson AW, Kaufmann RB, Moll PP, et al. Coronary artery calcification detected with ultrafast CT as an indication of coronary artery disease. *Radiology* 1992; 185:435–439.

33. Budoff MJ, Georgiou D, Brody A, Agatston AS, Kennedy J, Wolfkiel C, et al. Ultrafast computed tomography as a diagnostic modality in the detection of coronary artery disease. A multicenter study. *Circulation* 1996; 93:898–904.

34. Rumberger JA, Schwartz RS, Simons DB, Sheedy PF, Edwards WD, Fitzpatrick LA. Relation of coronary calcium determined by electron beam tomography and lumen narrowing determined by autopsy. *Am J Cardiol* 1994; 73:1169–1173.

35. Mautner GC, Mautner SL, Froehlich J, Feuerstein IM, Proschan MA, Roberts WC, et al. Coronary artery calcification: Assessment with electron beam CT and histomorphometric correlation. *Radiology* 1995; 192:619–623.

36. Detrano RC, Wong ND, Tang W, French WJ, Georgiou D, Young E, et al. Prognostic significance of cardiac cinefluoroscopy for calcific deposits in asymptomatic high risk subjects. *J Am Coll Cardiol* 1994; 24:354–358.

37. Arad Y, Spadero LA, Goodman K, Lledo-Perez A, Sherman S, Lerner G, et al. Predictive value of electron beam computed tomography of the coronary arteries—19 month follow-up of 1173 asymptomatic subjects. *Circulation* 1996; 93.1951–1953.

38. Detrano R, Tang W, Wong N, Puentes G, French W, Narahara K, et al. Coronary calcium predicts myocardial infarction in asymptomatic subjects after two years of follow-up. (Abstract) *J Am Coll Cardiol* 1995; 25:(suppl):901A.

39. Margolis JR, Chen JT, Kong Y, Peter RH, Behar VS, Kisslo JA. The diagnostic and prognostic significance of coronary artery calcification. A report of 800 cases. *Radiology* 1980; 137:609–616.

40. Detrano R, Hsiai T, Wang S, Puentes G, Fallavollita J, Shields P, et al. Prognostic value of coronary calcification and angiographic stenoses in patients undergoing coronary angiography. *J Am Coll Cardiol* 1996; 27:285–290.

41. Spadero LA, Lledo A, Roth M, Lerner G, Guerci AD. Comparison of electron beam tomography and conventional risk factors in the prediction of coronary artery disease. (Abstract) *J Am Coll Cardiol* 1996; 27(suppl):758A.

42. Kennedy JM, Budoff MJ, Georgiou D, Agatston AS, Romano MA, Detrano RC, et al. Coronary calcification by ultrafast computed tomography is an independent predictor of obstructive coronary artery disease: A multivariate risk factor analysis. (Abstract) *J Am Coll Cardiol* 1995; 25(suppl):387A.

43. Janowitz WR, Agatston AS, Viamonte M. Comparison of serial quantitative evaluation of calcific coronary artery plaque by ultrafast computed tomography in persons with and without obstructive coronary artery disease. *Am J Cardiol* 1991; 68:1–6.

44. Eusebio J, Chomka EV, Daniels T, Rick S, Brundage BH, Wolfkiel CJ. Five-year changes in coronary calcification by ultrafast computed tomography. (Abstract) *J Am Coll Cardiol* 1995; 25(suppl):386A.

45. Wexler L, Brundage B, Crouse J, Detrano R, Fuster V, Maddahi J, et al. Coronary artery calcification pathophysiology, epidemiology, imaging methods, and clinical implications. *Circulation* 1996; 94:1175–1192.

46. Moshage WE, Achenback S, Seese B, Bachmann K, Kirchgeorg M. Coronary artery stenoses: Three-dimensional imaging with electrocardiographically triggered, contrast agent–enhanced, electron-beam CT. *Radiology* 1995; 196:707–714.

47. Frey EE, Matherne GP, Mahoney LT, Soto Y, Stanford W, Smith WL. Coronary artery aneurysms due to Kawasaki disease: Diagnosis with ultrafast CT. *Radiology* 1988; 167:725–726.

48. Tomada H, Hoshiai M, Tagawa R, Koide S, Kawada S, Shotsu A, et al. Evolution of left atrial thrombus with computed tomography. *Am Heart J* 1980; 100:306–310.

49. Paramesworam R, Roman C, Eldredge WJ, Maranhao V. Detection of valve ring abscess by ultrafast computed tomography. *Am J Card Imaging* 1988; 2:229–231.

50. Bleiweis MS, Milliken JC, Baumgartner FJ, Georgiou D, Brundage BH. Application of the ultrafast CT for diagnosis of perivalvular abscesses: Surgical implications. *Chest* 1994; 106:629–632.

51. Stanford W. Ultrafast computed tomography in the diagnosis of aortic aneurysms and dissections. *J Thorac Imaging* 1990; 5:32–39.

52. Scagliotti D, Fisher EA, Deal BJ, Gordon D, Chomka EV, Brundage BH. Congenital aneurysm of the left sinus of Valsalva and aortopulmonary tunnel. *J Am Coll Cardiol* 1986; 7:443–445.

53. Bertch MJ, Chomka EV, Brundage BH. Ultrafast CT in the diagnosis and evaluation of supravalvular aortic stenosis. *Am J Card Imaging* 1988; 1:47–54.

54. Geraghty JJ, Stanford W, Landas SK, Galvin JR. Ultrafast computed tomography in experimental pulmonary embolisms. *Invest Radiol* 1992; 27(1):60–63.

55. Teigen CL, Maus TP, Sheedy PF, Stanson AW, Johnson CM, Breen JF, et al. Pulmonary embolism diagnosis with contrast-enhanced electron-beam CT and comparison with pulmonary angiography. *Radiology* 1995; 194:313–319.

56. Rees M, MacMillan R, Flicker S, Fender B, Clark D. Rapid-acquisition computed tomography demonstration of chronic calcified pericardial constriction. *J Comput Tomogr* 1986; 10:183–186.

57. Oren RM, Grover-McKay M, Stanford W, Weiss RM. Accurate preoperative diagnosis of pericardial constriction using cine computed tomography. *J Am Coll Cardiol* 1993; 22:832–838.

58. Chomka EV, Wolfkiel CJ, Rich S, Shanes JG, Tamboli H, Brundage BH. Ultrafast computed tomography: A new method for the evaluation of hypertrophic cardiomyopathy. *Am J Noninvas Cardiol* 1987; 1:140–151.

59. Dery R, Lysbon MJ, Garrett JS, Abbott J, Higgins CB, Sheinman MM. Cine-computed tomography of arrhythmogenic right ventricular dysplasia. *J Comput Assist Tomogr* 1986; 10:120–123.

60. Martins JB, Fisher DJ, Collins SM, Stanford W. Phase analysis of cine computed tomography identifies sites of origin of ventricular tachycardia in patients. (Abstract) *J Am Coll Cardiol* 1991; 17:284A.

61. Hopson JR, Weiss RM, Stanford W, Kringle G. Cine computed tomographic abnormalities in "lone" atrial fibrillation. (Abstract) *Circulation* 1990; 82(suppl III):III-58.

62. Eldredge WJ, Flicker S. Evaluation of congenital heart disease using cine-CT. *Am J Cardiac Imaging* 1987; 1:38–50.

63. Husayni TS. Ultrafast computed tomography evaluation of congenital cardiovascular disease in children and adults. In: Skorton DJ, Schelbert HR, Wolf GL, Brundage BH, eds. *Marcus Cardiac Imaging: A Companion to Braunwalds Heart Disease*, 2d ed. Philadelphia: Saunders; 1996; pp 871–886.

64. MacMillan RM, Rees MR, Eldredge WJ, Maranhao V, Clark D. Quantitation of shunting at the atrial level using rapid acquisition computed tomography with comparison to cardiac catheterization. *J Am Coll Cardiol* 1986; 7:946–948.

65. Skotvicki R, Maranhao V, Clark D, Flicker S, Eldredge J. Detection of atrial septal defect by cine CT scanning. *Cathet Cardiovasc Diagn* 1986; 12:103–106.

66. Garrett JS, Schiller NB, Botvinick EH, Higgins CB, Lipton MJ. Cine-computed tomography of Ebstein's anomaly. *J Comput Assist Tomogr* 1986; 10:664–666.

67. MacMillan RM, Rees MR, Maranhao V, Clark DL. Cine-computed tomography of cor triatriatum. *J Comput Assist Tomogr* 1986; 10:124–125.

68. Seifert P, Chomka EV, Stagl R, Swarner D, Brundage BH, Levitsky S. Application of the cine computed tomographic scan for precise localization of the origin of an atrial myxoma: Surgical implications. *Ann Thorac Surg* 1986; 42:467–470.

69. Bateman TM, Sethna DH, Whiting JS, Chaux A, Berman DS, Forrester JS. Comprehensive non-invasive evaluation of left atrial myxoma using cardiac cine-computed tomography. *J Am Coll Cardiol* 1987; 9:1180–1183.

19

MAGNETIC RESONANCE IMAGING OF THE HEART AND GREAT VESSELS

Robert E. Foster / Gerald M. Pohost

Nuclear magnetic resonance (NMR) was discovered more than 50 years ago and initially applied by chemists to define chemical structure and composition by spectroscopic methods.[1,2] Although NMR spectroscopy has been invaluable in providing metabolic information in a variety of different states, it is currently used as a research tool. The concept of using NMR to obtain images was introduced by Lauterbur[3] in the early 1970s, when he discovered that an inhomogeneous magnetic field could localize nuclei in space and produce an image. Now with advances in computer technology and superconducting magnets, the concepts are applied to humans to obtain images with exquisite morphologic detail, in any tomographic plane, in a nondestructive, noninvasive manner.

As NMR entered mainstream clinical practice, the public concerns regarding a "nuclear" technology were suppressed by using the term *magnetic resonance imaging* (MRI). Now patient and physician acceptance as well as the immense versatility of MRI have allowed this imaging technique to become the "gold standard" of noninvasive imaging in many diagnostic and management areas of cardiac and other diseases. MRI has the potential to become an invaluable tool for the cardiologist to evaluate cardiovascular morphology, function, perfusion, and viability.

This chapter focuses on the basic principles and practices of applying MRI to the evaluation of normal cardiovascular structures and for the diagnosis of diseases that affect cardiac and related vascular systems.

PRINCIPLES OF NMR

Magnetism and Vectors

To fully understand NMR, one must have extensive knowledge of quantum and nuclear physics; however, the basic theory of NMR is easily comprehended. Certain atoms possess a unique property whereby the nucleus spins and the spinning motion produces angular momentum. Since the nucleus is a charged particle, the spinning is equivalent to an electric current traveling through a small loop of wire, which produces a small magnetic field resembling a tiny bar magnet (Fig. 19-1). The strength of the magnetic field is expressed in terms of a magnetic moment.

Within the body, naturally occurring nuclei orient themselves randomly in space and thus have no net magnetization; however, positioning the body within a strong magnetic field creates a net magnetic moment. Intuitively, one might expect all of the nuclei to align parallel to the magnetic field (B_0); however, two energy states are created: parallel and antiparallel to B_0. Since the parallel alignment is at a lower energy level, slightly more nuclei are aligned parallel, causing the body to become weakly magnetized and generating a weak magnetization vector (Fig. 19-2). The strength of the vector is proportional to the strength of B_0, energy difference between spin states, and temperature. The fractional excess in the lower energy state is extremely small [i.e., about 3 in 1 million for hydrogen nuclei at room temperature at a 1.0-tesla (T) system at body temperature].

The magnetic moment itself is too small to measure, so a perturbation is created such that the spins deviate from alignment, and thus a torque is created on the magnetic moment. The result is similar to a gyroscope tilted out of alignment with the earth's gravitational field, which when perturbed will wobble or precess. Similarly, the magnetic vector precesses about B_0 at a frequency (ω_0) proportional to B_0, related by a constant (γ) called the *gyromagnetic ratio*, unique for each nuclear species. This precession rate is defined by the Larmor equation: $\omega_0 = \gamma B_0$ (Fig. 19-3).

The Resonance Phenomenon

To displace the spins from alignment with B_0, a secondary magnetic field (B_1) is applied that rotates in a plane perpendic-

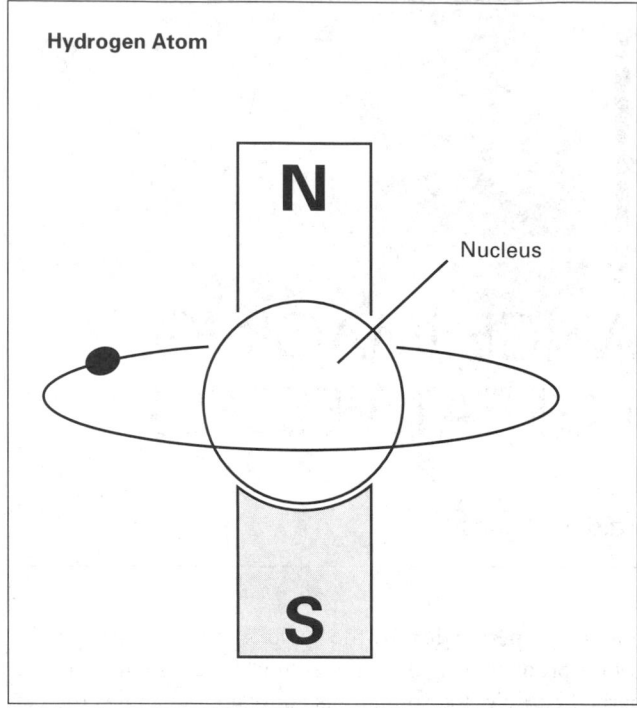

Hydrogen Atom

N

Nucleus

S

FIGURE 19-1
The positively charged nucleus of the hydrogen atom spins and creates a magnetic field.

ular to B_0. The B_1 field rotates around B_0 at the Larmor frequency, maximally affecting the spin magnetization of the net magnetic moment of the nuclei by the resonance phenomenon. The rotational frequency of the B_1 field is in the radiofrequency (RF) range. Thus, applying RF pulses at the Larmor

Magnetization Vector

S N   N S   S N   S N
S N   S N   N S   S N

B_0 ⟶

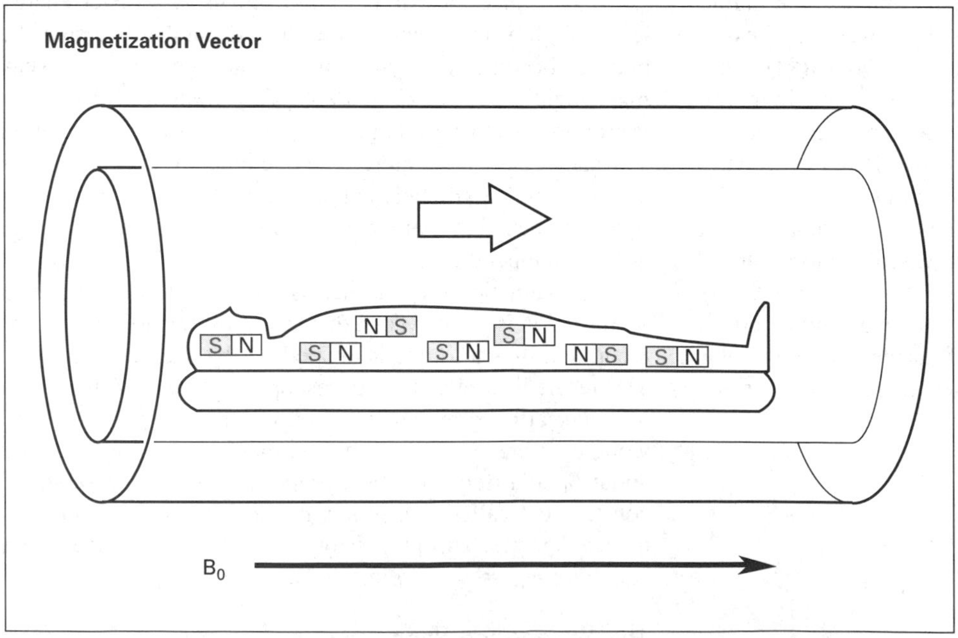

FIGURE 19-2
The nuclei of the hydrogen atoms within the body align parallel and antiparallel to the magnetic field (B_0) created by a superconducting magnet. Slightly more nuclei align parallel (represented by the bar magnets labeled N-S or S-N) to the B_0, creating a net magnetization vector (*open arrow*).

frequency to perturb the spin contributes the term *resonance* to MRI. The degree, or angle (θ), of displacement from the B_0 direction is proportional to the time (t) of the application of the rotating field: $\theta = \gamma\beta_1 \cdot t$. When B_1 is turned off, the spins are free to precess under the influence of the static magnetic field. This magnetic environment is not perfectly homogeneous, and thus the spins gradually dephase, causing a detrimental loss of signal known as the *free induction decay* (Fig. 19-4). In addition to magnetic field imperfection, the macromolecular environment also influences the rate of signal decay.

Relaxation

The free induction decay signal gradually decays due to the "relaxation" phenomenon. The gradual return of nuclei to their equilibrium position following perturbation by an RF pulse involves the release of energy into the surroundings; it is affected by interaction of adjacent nuclei, local chemical and electrical environments, and the strength of the external magnetic field. There are two distinct relaxation parameters frequently used: T1 and T2.

T1 RELAXATION

Nuclei in the body are surrounded by a network of other structures collectively known as the *lattice*. The lattice absorbs energy, and thus the nuclei lose the energy initially released from the RF pulse, resulting in the decay of signal as the magnetic moment realigns with B_0 in an exponential manner. The T1 parameter relates to the time constant for this exponential decay of the spins as energy is absorbed by the lattice. T1 is frequently referred to as the *spin-lattice relaxation time*.

The time constant, T1, for a particular sample is the time needed for 63 percent of the nuclei to return to the equilibrium value.

T2 RELAXATION

Aside from the lattice, neighboring spins also result in relaxation and progressive loss of signal from the transverse plane (*xy*). These interactions are referred to as *spin-spin relaxation* or *T2 relaxation*. This occurs since the precession frequency is not uniform for each spin, and the spins gradually lose phase coherence. In this context, unlike T1, T2 is a loss of phase coherency rather than a transfer of energy. The T2 for a sample is the time interval for the transverse magnetization process to decay to 37 percent of its original value. In clinical practice, B_0 fields are not homogeneous. Thus, nuclei

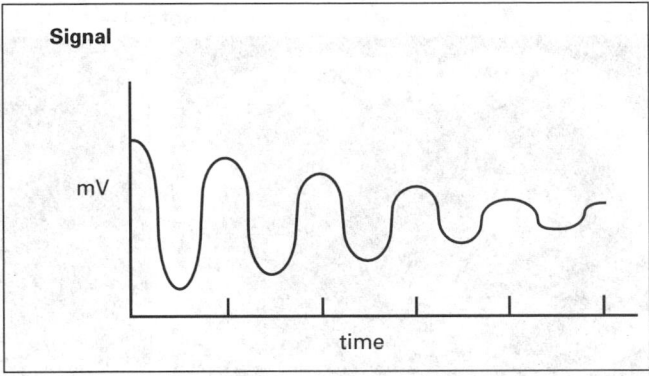

FIGURE 19-4
Oscillating signal with free induction decay.

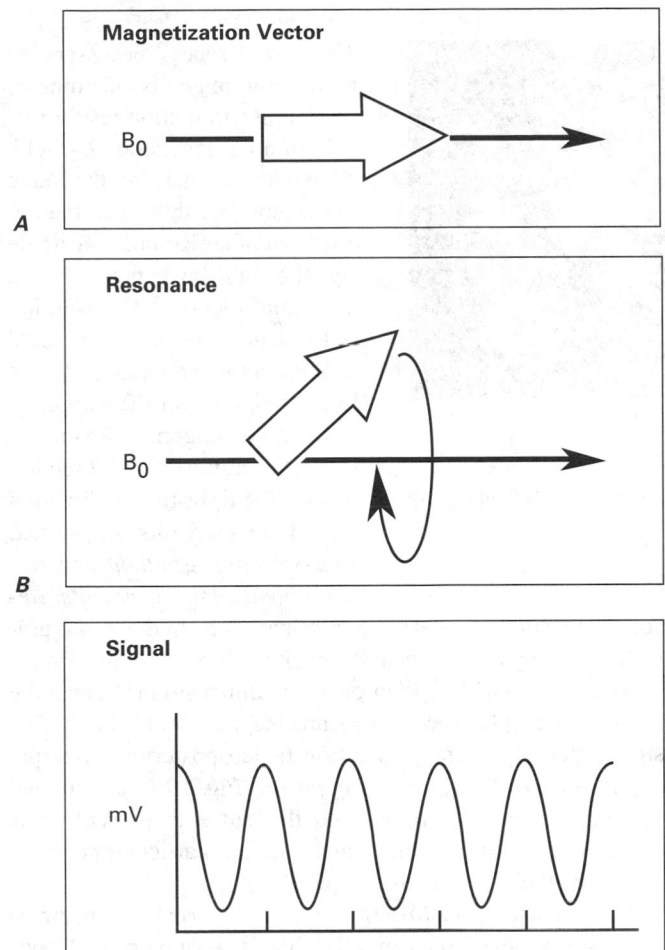

FIGURE 19-3
The net magnetization vector aligns with B_0 (*A*). A radiofrequency (RF) pulse causes the vector to precess out of B_0 alignment (*B*). The RF pulse is then discontinued and the vector resonates, producing a signal (*C*) with a characteristic frequency dependent on the field strength (B_0) and the atomic species producing the signal (usually hydrogen).

within a sample are exposed to slightly different magnetic fields and, as a result, will precess at slightly different frequencies. The free induction decay signal obtained in such a field will decay faster than what would be expected. This more rapid rate of decay is termed *T2** ("T2 star").

Tissues of various types have different T1 and T2 relaxation times due to a variety of conditions: fluid or solid state, the effects of molecules in the surrounding environment, hydrogen concentration of the tissue, and exposure to different magnetic fields, termed *field gradient*. In addition, MRI utilizes various RF pulse sequences to enhance a particular relaxation time, and the images produced are thus termed *T1-* or *T2-weighted images*. Furthermore, saturating imaging fields with rapid pulse sequences will enhance the contrast between static tissue in an imaging slice and unsaturated blood moving into the imaging plane. These are a few of the techniques used clinically to image cardiovascular structures without the need for administration of intravenous contrast agents.

MAGNETIC RESONANCE IMAGE FORMATION

Technical Considerations

HARDWARE AND SOFTWARE
A general misconception exists that clinical magnetic resonance (MR) systems, commonly used for brain and musculoskeletal imaging, cannot perform cardiovascular imaging, and thus a separate cardiovascular-dedicated system is needed. In fact, most clinical systems have cardiovascular software such that cardiovascular MRI can be performed. Typically, the only additional hardware requirements are cardiac and respiratory gating devices, which are available for most systems. Clinical MR systems use superconducting magnets with field strengths ranging from 0.5 to 1.5 T. The tesla is the equivalent of 10,000 gauss (G). To put this into perspective, the earth's magnetic field is between 0.3 and 0.7 G, and a refrigerator magnet has about 100 G ($= 0.01$ T). Higher field strength magnets result in increased signal-to-noise ratio and, as a consequence, clearer images; however, these higher field strength magnets often exaggerate artifacts due to cardiac, respiratory, and blood flow motion. Most clinical systems operate at 1.5 T, but magnets with field strengths of 5 T are being used in areas of research.

Pulse Sequences

As mentioned previously, if a single RF pulse is applied to a sample and then discontinued, simple T1 and T2 relaxation rates can be determined; however, the maximal amount of signal occurs immediately after the RF pulse is terminated. Application of a second pulse of 180° causes the spins to reverse direction and realign, emitting a signal remote from the RF pulse and correcting for effects of field inhomogeneity that caused the spins to relax at different frequencies. This refocusing phenomenon is termed the *echo*, and the time for the maximal signal to occur is called the *echo time* (TE). The sequence can be repeated, and the time between successive applications of excitation RF pulses is termed the *repetition*

Normal

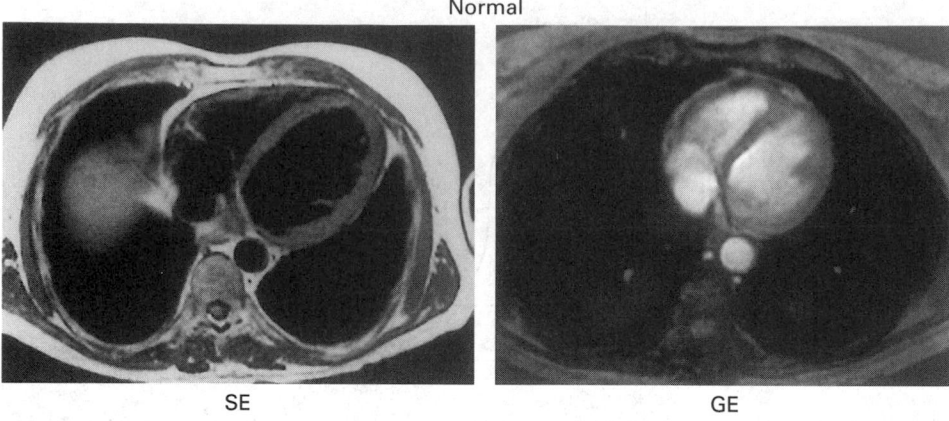

SE   GE

FIGURE 19-5

A transverse image of the thorax using spin-echo (SE) and gradient-echo (GE) techniques. Note the sharp contours between the blood and the cardiac structures in the spin-echo images.

time (TR). The operator can vary these two parameters, resulting in images that are T1 weighted (short TE and TR) or T2 weighted (long TE and TR). Much of the contrast, however, on spin-echo images occurs as a result of rapidly flowing blood. Since most flowing blood has moved out of the imaging plane between applications of RF pulses, the region of blood flow returns little, if any, signal. Thus, within vascular lumens and cardiac chambers, signal void is present in spin-echo images (also termed *dark blood* images). This sequence highlights cardiovascular wall morphology (Fig. 19-5).

Another widely used method to generate clinical images involves applying a magnetic gradient across the sample then reversing the polarity of the gradient, which refocuses the spins into an echo, rather than applying a 180° pulse (as in spin-echo). This method typically uses rapidly repeated RF pulses and causes partial saturation of spins. Thus, decreased signal from the static tissues results from the rapid sampling rates. Blood flowing into the imaging plane has not been exposed to the train of RF pulses, thus not experiencing signal saturation and resulting in a more intense blood signal relative to the static tissue signal (Fig. 19-5). Consequently, flowing blood appears bright. Thus, gradient-echo sequences are also termed *bright blood* sequences. This type of imaging is extremely useful to the cardiologist since these images may be placed in a cine/movie mode to view cardiac and blood dynamics. One might now appreciate that turbulent flow causes dephasing of spins, due to chaotic motion, and thus signal loss. As a result, this technique is used to evaluate regurgitant, stenotic, or shunt lesions within the cardiovascular system.

Many creative pulse sequences to highlight morphology, function, or blood flow are based on variants of gradient-echo or combinations of spin-echo and gradient-echo pulse sequences. These include techniques used for MR angiography, blood flow velocity measurements, and tagging myocardial structures. Clinical application of these will be discussed in detail below.

Gradients

The next process necessary to produce an image is encoding of spatial discrimination resolution. Within a homogeneous B_0 field, all nuclei resonate at the same frequency, and thus after the application of an RF pulse, a single signal would be generated with no spatial identity. The solution is to change the magnetic field slightly below and above B_0 in a linear fashion over the sample in different orthogonal directions; i.e., in the cranio-caudal direction (z) and the right-to-left direction (x). These gradients are termed *slice-selection gradient* and *frequency-encoding gradients*, respectively (Fig. 19-6). Using information from these two gradients, a single slice can be excited; however, the image obtained for that slice is in only one dimension (x) since the nuclei in the y plane are to the same magnetic field. To resolve signal spatially in the y direction (anteroposterior), multiple applications of *phase-encoding pulses* (Fig. 19-6) are applied by varying the length of time the pulse is present, thus changing the phase of the signal within a particular segment or line of the image map (K space).

In conclusion, an MR image can be formed with three-dimensional capabilities, highlighting tissue or blood and identifying turbulent flow and flow velocity, in a noninvasive, nonradioactive manner and without the need for a contrast agent.

PATIENT CONSIDERATIONS

Patient Comfort

Most patients tolerate the procedure without the need for sedation. Claustrophobia limits scan completion in approximately 5 percent of patients. Although rarely necessary, gentle sedation may be required so the patient may relax and then remain motionless during scan acquisition. Methods more commonly used to decrease anxiety include removing the patient from the magnet bore between scans and allowing a friend or family member to be positioned at the head of the bore and talk to the patient during scanning. Earphones are also placed on the patient to minimize the noise, allowing many patients to sleep during the scan.

Scan preparation and imaging time vary, depending on the complexity of the clinical situation. For example, if only ventricular function is required, the scan can be performed in approximately 30 min; on the other hand, complex congenital cases may require more than 1 h of total patient time to complete the imaging. As magnet and software technologies improve, the imaging times will be reduced.

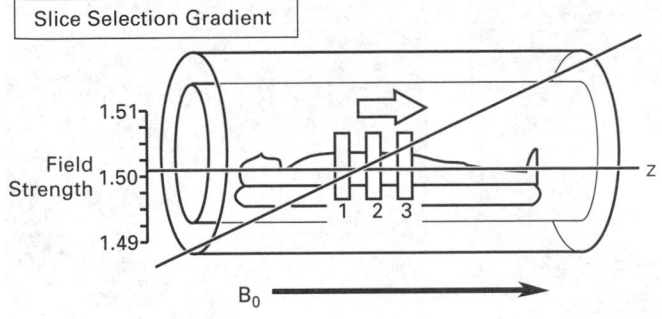

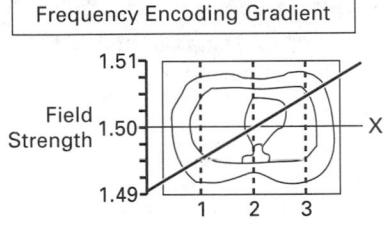

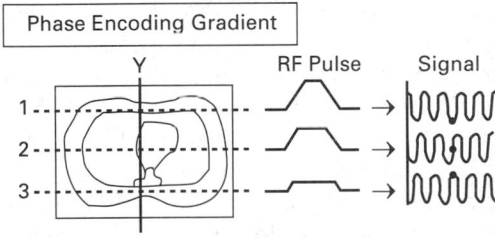

FIGURE 19-6

Gradients used for spatial information. To image a specific slice, a linear field gradient is applied in the *z* direction so that the atoms in each slice are exposed to a slightly different magnetic field strength than atoms in an adjacent slice and thus have a slightly different resonance frequency (*top*). Similarly, a gradient is applied across the patient to encode frequency information from columns of atoms along the *x* axis (*center*). Linear changes in the amplitude of the radiofrequency (RF) pulse in the *y* direction alter the resonance phase, which is then used for spatial resolution in this direction (*bottom*).

Patient Safety

Safety, as for all techniques, is a critical issue, and safety procedures and rules should be familiar to the physician ordering the scan and the technician performing the scan. In particular, two main areas of safety must be addressed *prior* to the patient entering the magnetic field: implanted or external patient devices and surrounding metal objects. For cardiology patients, the most common implanted devices that exclude the patient from having an MRI scan are a pacemaker (permanent or temporary), automated implantable cardiovascular defibrillator, or an internal hemodynamic monitoring catheter. Prosthetic heart valves and annular rings are MR-safe with the exception of the pre-600 series Starr-Edwards valve, a caged-ball device used clinically several decades ago. The presence of sternal wires and bypass graft clips are not hazardous to the patient but result in MR signal artifact. Within several weeks of implantation, intravascular coils, stents, and filters are unlikely to dislodge but result in MR signal loss in the region of the metallic device. Other major internal structures that are MR-unsafe include aneurysm clips and certain metallic ocular, cochlear, and penile prostheses.

External devices that may cause harm to the patient by causing skin burns include pulse oximetry and electrocardiogram cables. MR-safe cables are available and must be used in the MR facility. In addition, all metal cables and detection devices must be removed from the patient prior to the scan. Technicians must also be aware of the metallic devices that may accompany the patient such as IV poles, oxygen tanks, and iron shot–filled hemostatic "sandbags." These may become dangerous projectiles when near a superconducting magnet.

CLINICAL APPLICATION

The heart is a complex geometric structure; in the normal or diseased state, it can have a variety of geometric, positional, or functional changes. Since MRI can image in any tomographic plane, MRI becomes a unique tool for adequate and complete imaging of this organ with excellent spatial and temporal resolution. In addition, two- and three-dimensional temporally resolved functional imaging allows MRI to replace invasive and nuclear techniques under certain conditions. The following is an overview of the current clinical application of MRI as it applies to the cardiovascular system.

Image Acquisition

SLICE ORIENTATION

Cardiac MRI studies begin with standard spin-echo images in the axial planes of the body: transverse, coronal, and sagittal. To evaluate cardiac function, image planes are oriented to the intrinsic axes of the heart. Accordingly, cine cardiac MR images are obtained in the two-chamber (right anterior oblique), four-chamber, and short-axis views (Fig. 19-7). Consequently, the resultant image orientation is familiar and comparable with other imaging techniques. Both static spin-echo and dynamic cine MR images allow comprehensive measurements of a wide variety of cardiac dimensions and volumes.

MEASUREMENTS

Computer calipers are a standard feature of clinical MR systems and allow point-to-point linear measurements similar to those used on echocardiographic equipment. Since spin-echo images highlight morphologic detail, these images are used to evaluate the size of vascular structures and cardiac chambers,[4–6] ventricular wall thickness,[7] left ventricular (LV) mass, pericardial thickness, cardiac and paracardiac masses, and congenital anomalies.

MRI generally provides precise definition of endocardial contours, allowing ready measurement of end-diastolic and end-systolic size within each myocardial slice. By using area-length calculations or summating serial short-axis slices of the ventricle (Simpson's rule), end-systolic, end-diastolic, and stroke volumes can be determined. From these measurements, one can easily calculate cardiac output and ejection fraction.

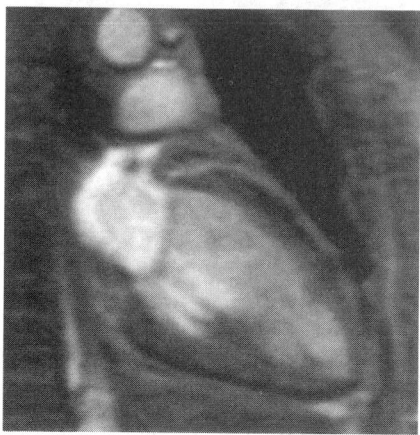

2 Chamber

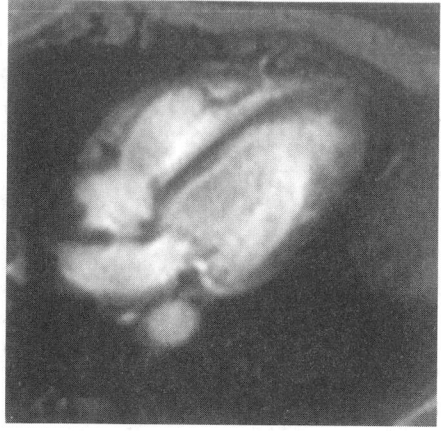

4 Chamber

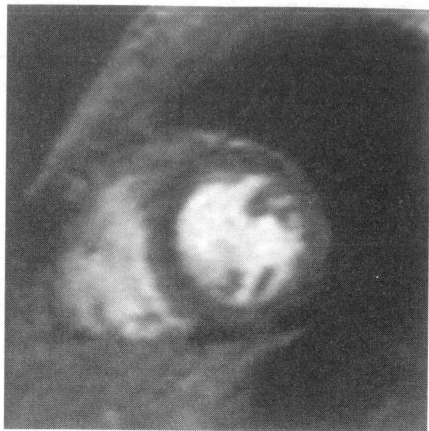

Short Axis

FIGURE 19-7
Gradient-echo images acquired in the two-chamber, four-chamber, and midventricular short-axis tomographic planes.

These volume and functional measurements correlate well with those of other imaging techniques.[8–16] MRI allows routine quantitative assessment of regional LV function with complete visualization of all myocardial segments. In a similar fashion, the epicardial contour also may be outlined, and thus the volume of myocardium between the epi- and endocardial surface calculated. By multiplying the volume of the myocardium by the value for the density of myocardial tissue, determination of myocardial mass is determined without geometric assumptions.[17–21]

Using a technique called *phase-contrast MRI* (phase velocity mapping, velocity flow mapping, or velocity-encoded cine MR), blood flow velocity can be determined (Fig. 19-8). With this technique, a phase-encoding gradient is placed in the direction of flowing blood to produce a controlled dependence of phase shift on velocity. Resultant information can be visualized using a phase-sensitive image reconstruction technique to calculate the velocity of blood flow directly. Validation of this method has been confirmed by its performance in a variety of in vivo models.[22–26] Using this technique, blood flow in both the ascending aorta and pulmonary artery can be determined simultaneously, allowing calculation of the pulmonary to systemic flow ratio (Q_p/Q_s) for assessment of shunt size.[27]

Ischemic Heart Disease

MYOCARDIAL ISCHEMIA
There are several approaches for using MR to detect myocardial ischemia or ischemic damage. These include myocardial tissue characterization, stress-induced segmental dysfunction, MR perfusion imaging, and ischemia-induced changes in high-energy phosphate metabolism using MR spectroscopic methods.

Myocardial Tissue Characterization
Changes in the biophysical properties of ischemic myocardium during an ischemic insult can be

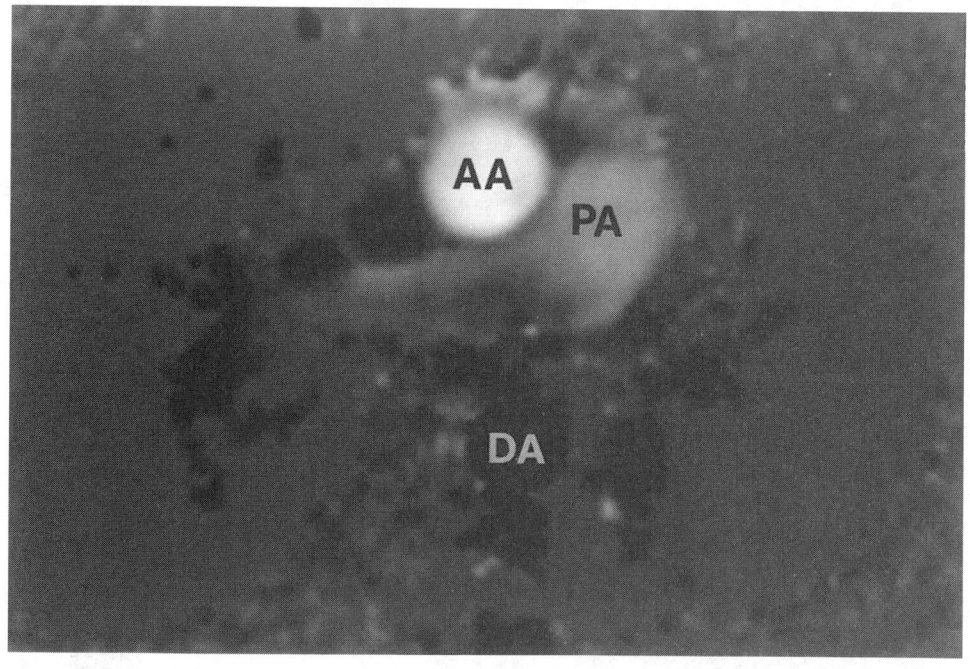

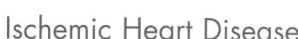

FIGURE 19-8
Phase-encoded image in the transverse plane at the level of the right pulmonary artery. Note the bright signal of blood flowing in the cranial direction in the ascending aorta (AA) and pulmonary artery (PA) compared to dark signal from blood flowing in the caudal direction in the descending aorta (DA).

readily detected using MR imaging. The relaxation times, T1 and T2, increase with several ischemic insults and are largely related to an increase in water content.[28–31] In animal models, the largest increase in relaxation times occurs in the ischemic zones with moderate to severely reduced blood flow; whereas in the zones in which the ischemia is total, there is little, if any, increase in myocardial T1 and T2.[28] Other factors, of less importance than edema, that contribute to such changes in relaxation times include the presence of free radicals, the change in magnetic susceptibility related to the paramagnetic effects of deoxyhemoglobin as a result of hemorrhage, and, finally, lipid accumulation.[32,33] Spin-echo images with long echo times will emphasize T1 increases, depicting them as zones of increased intensity.

Stress-Induced Segmental Dysfunction

It has been well established that stress-induced impairment of regional LV function is an early and reliable sign of significant coronary artery stenosis, generally preceding the development of ST-segment depression and angina pectoris.[34,35] Dobutamine provides a pharmacologic means to stress the myocardium which has been useful in detecting coronary artery disease using electrocardiographic,[36] radionuclide ventriculography,[37] echocardiography,[38–41] and thallium perfusion imaging.[42,43] MRI offers noninvasive imaging with high spatial resolution, leading to accurate assessment of regional LV dysfunction.[44] Van Rugge and colleagues[45] performed dobutamine stress MRI on 45 patients with chest pain, 37 of whom had angiographically significant coronary artery disease. During peak dobutamine infusion, segmental dysfunction occurred in 30 patients, yielding an overall sensitivity for detection of coronary artery disease of 81 percent and a specificity of 100 percent. Furthermore, the sensitivity of detecting single-, double-, and triple-vessel disease was 75 percent, 80 percent, and 100 percent, respectively. The total duration of the examination was approximately 1 h.

Myocardial Perfusion Imaging Using MR Contrast Agents

Paramagnetic compounds cause a decrease of both the T1 and T2 relaxation times. The magnitude of the change in relaxation time is influenced by both the magnetic field strength and the concentration of the paramagnetic agent.[46] Such agents injected intravenously as a bolus provide a means to assess myocardial perfusion using MR imaging. Currently there are three classes of paramagnetic agents: extracellular, blood pool, and intracellular agents. The most commonly used is the extracellular agent gadolinium diethylenetriamine pentacetic acid (Gd DTPA), which actually distributes in the blood pool and the extracellular space. The imaging technique records the first pass of the paramagnetic agent and uses the pulse sequence, which optimally reduces the signal intensity of the myocardium. Thus, the myocardium with the highest content of contrast agent (normally perfused) appears bright while the myocardium with reduced content of contrast agent (underperfused or ischemic myocardium) appears dark (Fig.

19-9). Manning et al.[47] used Gd DTPA to assess myocardial perfusion at rest in patients with severe coronary artery disease. As anticipated, the time to peak signal intensity was delayed, and peak signal intensity decreased in regions of the myocardium perfused by a severely stenosed coronary artery.

Using dipyridamole infusion, Matheijssen et al. compared perfusion MRI to sestamibi single photon emission computed tomography (SPECT).[48] Agreement in localization of the stenosed artery was 80 percent between angiography and SPECT, 70 percent between angiography and MRI, and 90 percent between SPECT and MRI. MR perfusion studies have been limited by the need to use first-pass acquisition, resulting in the depiction of only one[47] or two[48] slices at the level of the mid-left ventricle. Walsh et al. have developed a method to acquire up to four tomographic slices through the ventricle on a conventional MR scanner, allowing a more extensive evaluation of perfusion within the short duration of the first pass of the paramagnetic bolus.[49,50] Contrast agents are under development that include blood pool agents and intracellular agents. The kinetics of paramagnetic contrast agents that remain within the blood pool are less complex to analyze since they involve only one compartment. Iron particles have been under investigation, since they remain within the blood pool. Finally, Simor et al. have described an agent that appears to enter and remain within the intracellular space, like thallium or sestamibi.[51] Such agents, when clinically available, would allow acquisitions over numerous cardiac cycles rather than only one, as in the first-pass approach. This would take full advantage of the high resolution available using MRI.

MR Spectroscopy

Cardiac metabolism and energy reserve can be assessed using spectroscopic methods to identify changes in the high-energy phosphates within the myocardium. Studies in isolated and surgically exposed animals demonstrate a decrease in phosphocreatine (PCr) soon after coronary occlusion. The PCr to adenosinetriphosphate (ATP) ratio is frequently used to express changes in these bioenergetic markers with ischemic insult.[52–54] In addition, spectroscopic methods have been applied to human hearts noninvasively to measure phosphorus metabolites in localized areas of the myocardium.[55,56] Using isometric hand-grip stress, Weiss et al.[57] and Yabe et al.[58] reported significant decreases in PCr/ATP ratios with myocardial ischemia in patients with known coronary artery disease. MR spectroscopic methods are currently a research tool but may soon be a clinically useful modality.

MYOCARDIAL INFARCTION

Many facets of MR imaging can be useful in evaluating patients with recent or remote myocardial infarction. MR methods can be used to assess infarct size, regional and global function, and viability and to evaluate the sequelae of myocardial infarction.

Infarct Size

Studies show that within an hour of a myocardial infarction, the T1 and T2 relaxation times are generally increased within

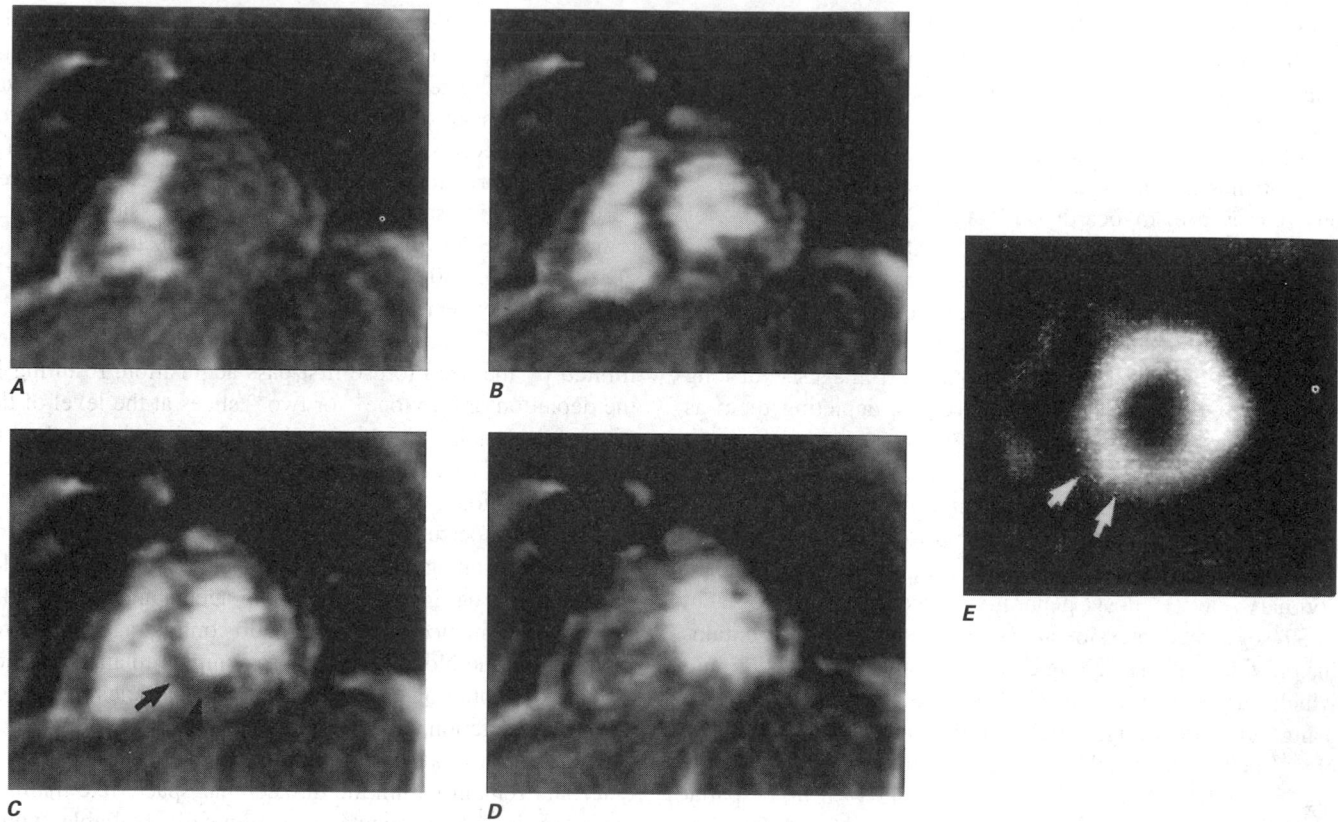

FIGURE 19-9

First-pass magnetic resonance perfusion study images are shown (*A–D*) compared to the midventricular short-axis thallium image of the same patient (*E*). The images *A–D* are temporally related. In the initial image (*A*), the contrast agent has entered the right ventricular chamber and results in a high signal intensity within that region. In *B*, the contrast agent enters the left ventricle, resulting in high signal intensity from both the right and left ventricular chambers. The contrast agent then enters the myocardium and the region of lower signal intensity (*arrow*) defines a region of compromised blood flow. For comparison, note the decrease in signal intensity in the same region on the thallium image (*E*).

infarcted myocardium, and that these prolonged relaxation times allow imaging for determination of the location and the extent of the infarction.[59,60] Although some investigators claim that localization using T1- or T2-emphasized imaging is nonspecific for infarcted tissue,[61] studies by Krauss et al. showed good correlation between the extent of increased signal intensity and infarct size and location when compared to defects demonstrated by resting thallium 201 scintigraphy.[62,63] Using spin-echo imaging sequences, increased signal intensity has been noted in regions of infarcted tissue, and this technique may be used to size the infarct.[64,65] Furthermore, wall thinning may also be of some value in assessing the extent of myocardial tissue damage.[66]

Contrast agents have been reported to be of some additional value in differentiating between infarcted and noninfarcted myocardium. Delayed imaging after contrast administration can further enhance the signal intensity of the infarcted tissue and improve the image quality and ability to size the infarct.[67–69] The enhancement of signal with contrast agents is most pronounced if administered within the first 2 weeks after the acute event.[70] Such enhancement is most likely related to the ability of the paramagnetic contrast agent to enter the infarcted cellular debris and the low blood flow of the territory.

Global and Regional Function

Wall thickening, as quantified by MR imaging using a cine technique, distinguishes patients with global and regional ventricular contractile abnormalities from normal individuals[71–73] (Fig. 19-10). Regionally impaired wall thickening after myocardial infarction can be readily demonstrated by MR imaging and correlates well with sites of dysfunction shown by x-ray ventriculography.[74] End-diastolic wall thickness and the degree of systolic wall thickening demonstrated by MRI may be used as markers for predicting myocardial viability. Using technetium 99m sestamibi SPECT imaging, Sechtem et al. showed that an end-diastolic wall thickness of greater than 6 mm or systolic wall thickening greater than 1 mm represented viable myocardium.[75] This is further supported by correlating positron emission tomography imaging with ^{18}F-fluorodeoxyglucose (Chap. 20) and cine MR imaging of wall thickness and wall thickening to define viability.[76,77]

Complications of Myocardial Infarction

MR imaging provides exquisite morphologic and functional detail of cardiovascular structures. Accordingly, it can be used to detect short- and long-term sequelae of myocardial injury. The most commonly occurring MR-detectable complications include ventricular aneurysms, mitral valve dysfunction due to papillary muscle necrosis, ventricular septal perforation, LV thrombus, and pericardial effusion. In addition to regional wall thinning of infarcted segment, compensatory regional wall thickening and hypertrophy as well as LV chamber enlargement (remodeling) may also be evaluated. Furthermore, pleural and pericardial effusions suggestive of cardiac decompensation are readily detected, and this information may assist in the proper management of these patients.

MR Imaging of the Coronary Arteries

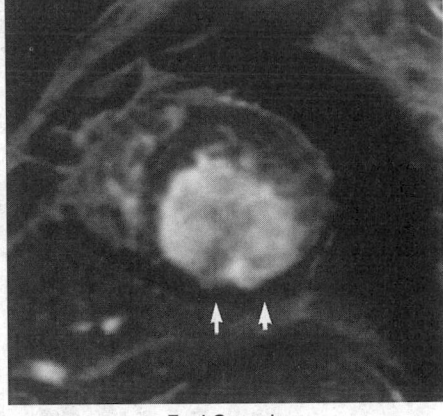

End Diastole   End Systole

FIGURE 19-10

Regional left ventricular dysfunction. Midventricular short-axis end-diastolic and end-systolic gradient-echo images are shown. Note the normal thickening of the anteroseptal anterior and anterolateral walls, with akinesis and thinning of the inferior and inferoseptal regions (*arrows*).

ANOMALOUS CORONARY ARTERIES

Although major anomalies of the coronary arteries are found in fewer than 1 percent of the population,[78–81] proximal coronary artery segments coursing between the aorta and pulmonary artery may affect myocardial perfusion, with life-threatening consequences.[82–85] Delineating the proximal course of the coronary arteries by conventional coronary angiography may be difficult because of the inability to visualize surrounding structures, and thus there may be uncertainty as to the complex three-dimensional pathway of the coronary artery. Inability to visualize aberrant coronary arteries has been reported to occur in as many as 16 to 50 percent of the cases using coronary angiography.[86,87] Because of the virtually unlimited number of tomographic planes and rapid gradient-echo imaging, the proximal portions of the coronary arteries can be visualized noninvasively by MR. Recently, two independent investigators compared MRI with conventional coronary angiography to discern the origin and proximal course of anomalous coronary arteries.[87,88] Remarkably, in one study, the sensitivity and specificity of MRI in detecting the proximal coronary artery path was 100 percent with an intraobserver agreement of 100 percent, whereas in 3 of the 36 patients studied by x-ray coronary angiography, inaccurate interpretation of the coronary position resulted.[88] Other authors have also reported imaging of coronary artery aneurysms[89] and fistulas[90,91] by MR techniques.

CORONARY ARTERY DISEASE

If MR could image the native coronary arteries and detect stenotic lesions accurately, it would provide a noninvasive, less expensive alternative to coronary angiography. Accordingly, MR could be an ideal approach in a managed-care environment. The physiologic and anatomic characteristics of the coronary arteries present a number of technical challenges that must be overcome before MR coronary angiography be-

comes a realistic clinical tool.[92,93] Aside from the problems presented by respiratory and cardiac motion, the coronary arteries are anatomically small and tortuous.[94] Many of these problems have been overcome by using a variety of innovative techniques to produce a three-dimensional angiogram. In addition, the fat that surrounds the coronary arteries can interfere with MRI. Pulse sequences for fat suppression have been developed to reduce the fat signal effectively. Breathholding[95,96] and innovative gating methods can reduce blurring caused by respiratory motion.[97–99] In addition, cardiac gating is required until images can be acquired with a single heart cycle. Thus, high-quality images of the proximal coronary arteries are now possible. Using fat-suppression, breathholding, and cardiac gating methods, Manning et al. were able to image the first 10 cm of each coronary artery, with vessel dimension correlating well with contrast angiography[100]; however, the left circumflex artery could be identified in only 76 percent of the subjects. In another study, these investigators studied 39 patients with coronary artery disease and were able to identify individual vessels with >50 percent angiographic stenosis, with positive and negative predictive values of 85 and 95 percent, respectively.[101] Undoubtedly, these techniques will continue to improve and ultimately will provide means to evaluate the coronary arteries noninvasively. Localization of the proximal portions of the native coronary arteries is performed and coronary artery bypass graft patency routinely examined in centers with advanced cardiac MR capability (Fig. 19-11).

Valvular Heart Disease

The ideal imaging techniques for evaluating patients with valvular heart disease must include accurate assessment of the valvular morphology and valve function and the means to assess cardiovascular structure and function. The structural

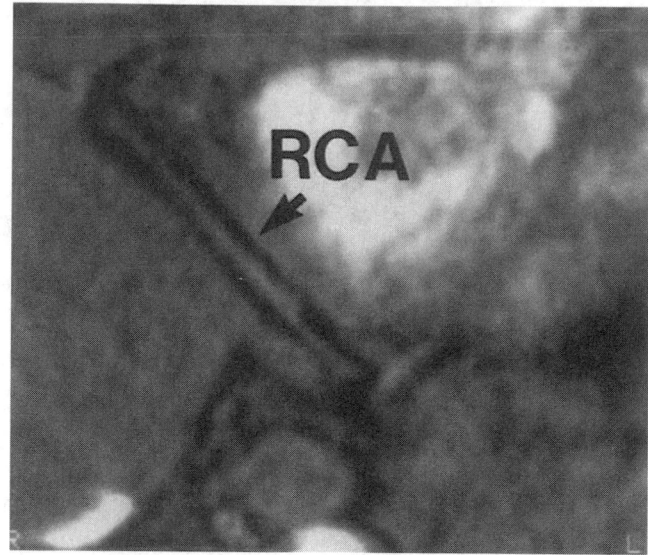 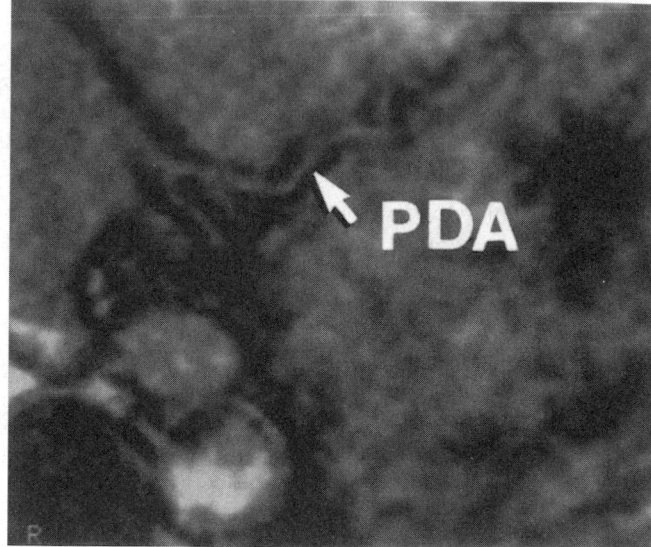

FIGURE 19-11

An image of the distal right coronary artery (RCA) (*left panel*) and its continuation into the posterior descending artery (PDA) shown (*right panel*).

and functional changes as a result of valve dysfunction include atrial or ventricular chamber enlargement, ventricular wall thickening, poststenotic dilatation of the aorta and pulmonary artery, and atrial and/or ventricular thrombus.

ANATOMY

The thickness of normal valve leaflets is 1 to 2 mm, and they are highly mobile throughout the cardiac cycle. Echocardiography images the valve leaflets with high spatial and temporal resolution (Chap. 14). Since the slice thickness of MR images ranges from 5 to 10 mm, spatial resolution is not adequate to assess the valve leaflets accurately and reproducibly. Spin-echo and gradient-echo images allow a crude assessment of the number of leaflets, degree of excursion, and leaflet thickness.

Unlike valve anatomy, the ventricular and atrial morphology and function can be accurately assessed without geometric assumptions. In this manner, MR imaging can assist the clinician to determine the appropriate timing for replacement of an abnormal valve by defining chamber size, volumes, and function. It is well established that preoperative LV size and performance are excellent predictors of LV function after valve replacement for aortic and mitral regurgitation.

VALVE FUNCTION

The severity of valvular dysfunction can be assessed by two MR methods: cine gradient-echo imaging and velocity-encoded imaging. In the former, the chaotic motion of turbulent flow results in dephasing and consequently in MR signal loss. Thus, a signal void is present within a normally signal-intense blood pool. The area of the MR signal void correlates with the area of color Doppler signal by echocardiography[102–105] (Fig. 19-12). The signal void, however, may be altered by changing acquisition parameters such as TE, TR, sampling size of imaged volume element (voxel), and orienta-

tion to flow.[106,107] Thus, consistency of these parameters must be maintained to assure accuracy of interpretation. Similar to echocardiography, proximal flow convergence, identified as a small wedge-shaped MR signal void on the opposite side of the valve to the direction of regurgitation, predicts the severity of regurgitation.[108,109] Investigators have used MR to measure regurgitant volumes and regurgitant fraction directly by measuring right ventricular (RV) and LV stroke volumes and thus determining the severity of regurgitation.[110–112]

Gradient-echo imaging may be used to approximate the degree of aortic stenosis by observing the extent of turbulent flow in the ascending aorta.[113] On the other hand, it is possible to use a method termed *phase-velocity imaging* to assess flow velocities to 5 m/s.[114] In this way the severity of the aortic stenosis is better assessed.

In summary, MRI represents a noninvasive method for assessing valvular and ventricular function to assist in determining the appropriate timing for valve replacement. Phase-velocity mapping may be useful for quantification of valve dysfunction.

Pericardial Disease

The pericardium stabilizes the heart by extending from the great arteries to a tendinous attachment on the diaphragm. In addition, there are pericardial ligamentous attachments anteriorly to the sternum and posteriorly to the spine. Between the visceral and parietal pericardium, a potential space exists containing 15 to 50 mL of proteinaceous fluid.[115,116] On multislice spin-echo MR images, the pericardium appears as a thin, low-intensity signal (<3 mm) between the high-intensity signal of mediastinal and epicardial fat and the medium-intensity signal of myocardial tissue.[117,118] The low signal intensity of the pericardium is a result of the amount of fibrous tissue

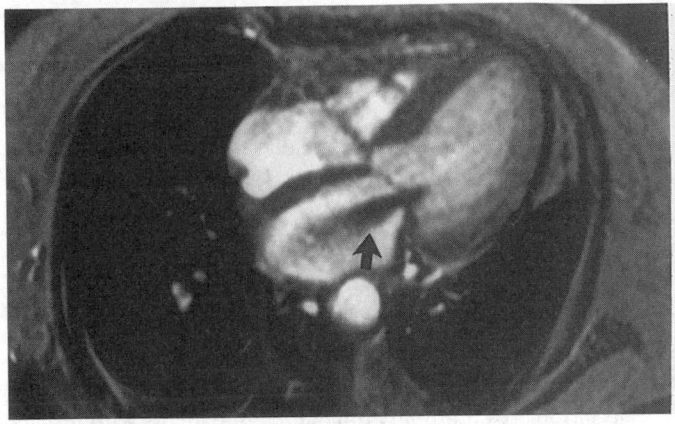 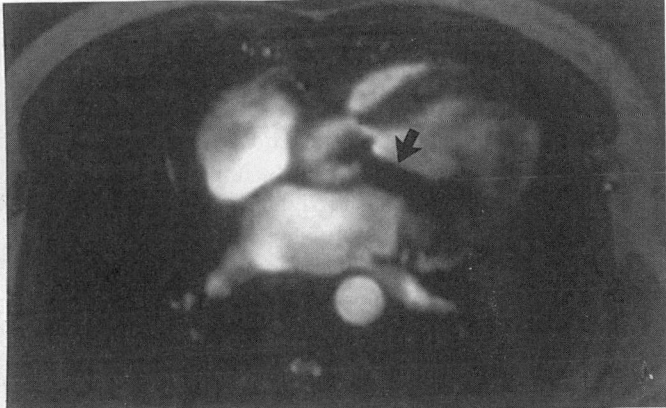

FIGURE 19-12

Transverse gradient-echo images are shown depicting mitral regurgitation (*left*) and aortic insufficiency (*right*). In each case, turbulent flow caused by the regurgitant lesion results in loss of MR signal (*arrow*). Also in each case, note the proximal flow convergence on the ventricular side of the mitral valve in the patient with mitral regurgitation and the aortic side of the aortic valve in the patient with aortic insufficiency.

(with long T1 and short T2 relaxation times) (Fig. 19-13). Sechtem et al. reported that the pericardium adjacent to the right ventricle could be visualized by MR in 100 percent of subjects studied, whereas the pericardium along the lateral wall of the left ventricle could be visualized in only 61 percent of subjects.[119]

PERICARDIAL EFFUSION

Normally, pericardial fluid has a low signal intensity on spin-echo images. Such fluid leads to a zone of reduced signal intensity separating the pericardium from the myocardium and from the epicardial fat. It is postulated that the appearance is dark because of the nonlaminar flow of fluid within the pericardial sac as a consequence of cardiac motion. Such nonlaminar flow changes the spin phase and causes MR signal loss.[120] In gradient-echo images, the pericardial fluid appears bright due to this flow clearly separating the parietal pericardium from the myocardium (Fig. 19-13).

The capability of MR to detect moderate or large pericardial effusions is comparable to that of echocardiography. However, MR is able to detect small fluid collections better than echocardiography, especially in areas at the medial border of the right atrium or posterior to the LV apex.[121]

Thus, because of its lower cost and portability, echocardiography should be used first to assess patients for pericardial effusion; however, MR imaging should be performed when a clinically suspected pericardial effusion is not detected on echocardiography. MR is also useful for localizing loculated or smaller pericardial effusions.

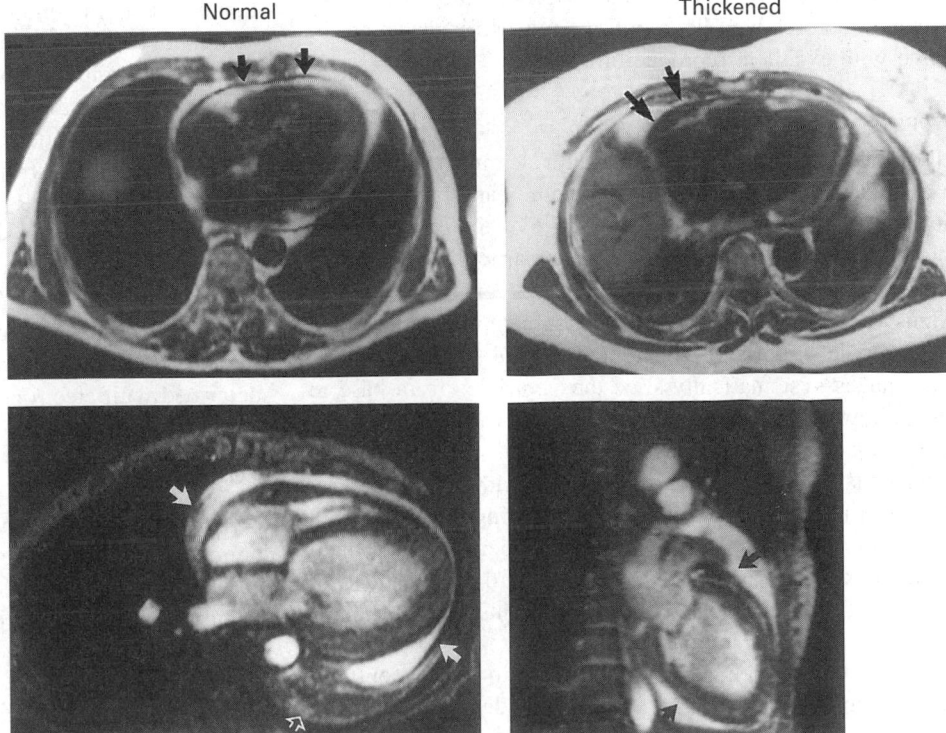

Pericardial Effusion

FIGURE 19-13

The upper panels are transverse spin-echo images depicting the normal pericardium (*left*) and a patient with a thickened pericardium (*right*). In the lower two panels are four-chamber (*left*) and two-chamber (*right*) images of a patient with a large pericardial effusion. Due to the motion of the pericardial fluid, the effusion appears bright (➡); a left pleural effusion is also noted in this patient (⇨).

PERICARDIAL THICKENING

In both MR and computed x-ray tomography, a pericardial thickness of more than 4 mm is considered abnormal.[122] The pericardium as imaged by MRI varies in thickness in different regions of the heart, and thus a standard imaging plane must be established. For this reason, transverse images at the anatomic levels of the right atrium and right and left ventricles are recommended. The thickness of the pericardial line in *any* section greater than 7 mm is abnormal by computed x-ray tomography[123] and probably by MRI.

MRI can help distinguish between constructive pericarditis and restrictive cardiomyopathy by revealing the presence or absence of a thickened pericardium. Patients examined by MRI who had proven constructive pericarditis had associated pericardial thickening of greater than 5 mm.[124] In addition, calcification of the pericardium, which has reduced signal intensity, also aids in the diagnosis of a probable pericardial rather than a myopathic disorder.

Cardiomyopathy

Evaluation of global and regional wall thickness, ventricular function, and chamber size is crucial for the diagnosis and prognosis of cardiomyopathy. For example, a dilated cardiomyopathic ventricle with substantial regional wall motion abnormalities suggests an "ischemic" process. Further, valve dysfunction, ventricular outflow tract obstruction, and caval dilatation are also readily detectable signs of cardiomyopathy. As stated before, MRI is an optimal means for detecting the above with excellent reproducibility.

HYPERTROPHIC CARDIOMYOPATHY

All of the myocardium of the left ventricle must be visualized to exclude the diagnosis of hypertrophic cardiomyopathy in view of its wide phenotypic variability (Chap. 74). The most common patterns are asymmetric and particularly heterogeneous. Most patterns of wall thickening can be seen, from extensive and diffuse to limited and segmental, with no single morphologic expression considered typical.[125] Serial short-axis images systematically slice the ventricles from base to apex, allowing complete measurements of wall thickness and thickening during the cardiac cycle (Fig. 19-14). This method is particularly useful and correlates well with echocardiography and x-ray ventriculography in delineating the precise site and extent of the hypertrophy.[126–128] Hypertrophy confined to the apex is a variant of hypertrophic cardiomyopathy that may be difficult to visualize by conventional echocardiography but is readily distinguished by MRI.[129–131] By defining the extent of turbulent flow (signal loss) in the LV outflow tract, a semiquantitative assessment of the degree of dynamic LV outflow tract obstruction can be made with gradient-echo MRI.

DILATED CARDIOMYOPATHY

The typical appearance of a dilated cardiomyopathy is that of biventricular enlargement with depressed systolic function

(Fig. 19-15). MRI provides a noninvasive method for accurately determining RV and/or LV end-systolic and end-diastolic volumes, stroke volume, ejection fraction, thrombus, and/or valve dysfunction. Segmental wall thinning and dysfunction may suggest an ischemic etiology, although the apex is frequently akinetic in idiopathic dilated cardiomyopathy.

RESTRICTIVE CARDIOMYOPATHY

The classic appearance of restrictive cardiomyopathy is that of a thickened myocardium with reduced chamber volumes and normal or depressed LV systolic function. In addition, due to restricted diastolic ventricular filling, the atria and venae cavae are commonly dilated.[132] In patients with restrictive/constrictive hemodynamics, MRI can frequently distinguish between a restrictive cardiomyopathy, which is managed medically, and constrictive pericarditis, which is managed surgically,[132] by the presence or absence of a thickened pericardium.

ARRHYTHMOGENIC RIGHT VENTRICULAR DYSPLASIA

Because of the geometric shape of the right ventricle, segmental analysis is exceedingly difficult using current imaging technologies. Segmental morphology and function of the right ventricle can be extensively evaluated using serial contiguous slices of the heart by spin-echo and gradient-echo imaging. The hallmark of arrhythmogenic RV dysplasia is fatty infiltration with extreme thinning of the RV free wall. Fat is readily identified on T1-weighted MR images. The RV free wall, however, is normally 3 mm in thickness, and spatial resolution limits visualizing the free wall. In addition, the right ventricle is normally surrounded by epicardial fat, which makes distinguishing epicardial from intramyocardial lipid more difficult.[133] Analysis of RV function using gradient-echo MRI provides a means of observing focal RV free wall aneurysms and segmental dyskinesis[134] (Fig. 19-16). The morphologic detail afforded by MRI allows other characteristics of arrhythmogenic RV dysplasia such as conspicuous trabeculations and scalloping of the RV free wall to be visualized, as has been described with electron-beam computed tomography.[135]

Vascular Imaging

MRI has emerged as an important means for evaluating acquired and congenital vascular pathology because of the inherent sensitivity of MR to flow. Pulse sequences can be designed to either enhance or suppress the blood flow signal intensity. Enhancement is achieved by suppressing stationary tissue signal with rapid pulse sequences (bright blood angiography). Suppression uses long echo times to shorten the T2 (dark blood angiography). Recall that dark blood techniques are best for evaluating morphologic detail. Thus vascular wall anatomy, identifying anomalous vascular connections and their relation to other vital thoracic structures, is optimally visualized. More typically, bright blood techniques are used clinically to form MR angiograms. Generally, MR angiograms

End Diastole   End Systole

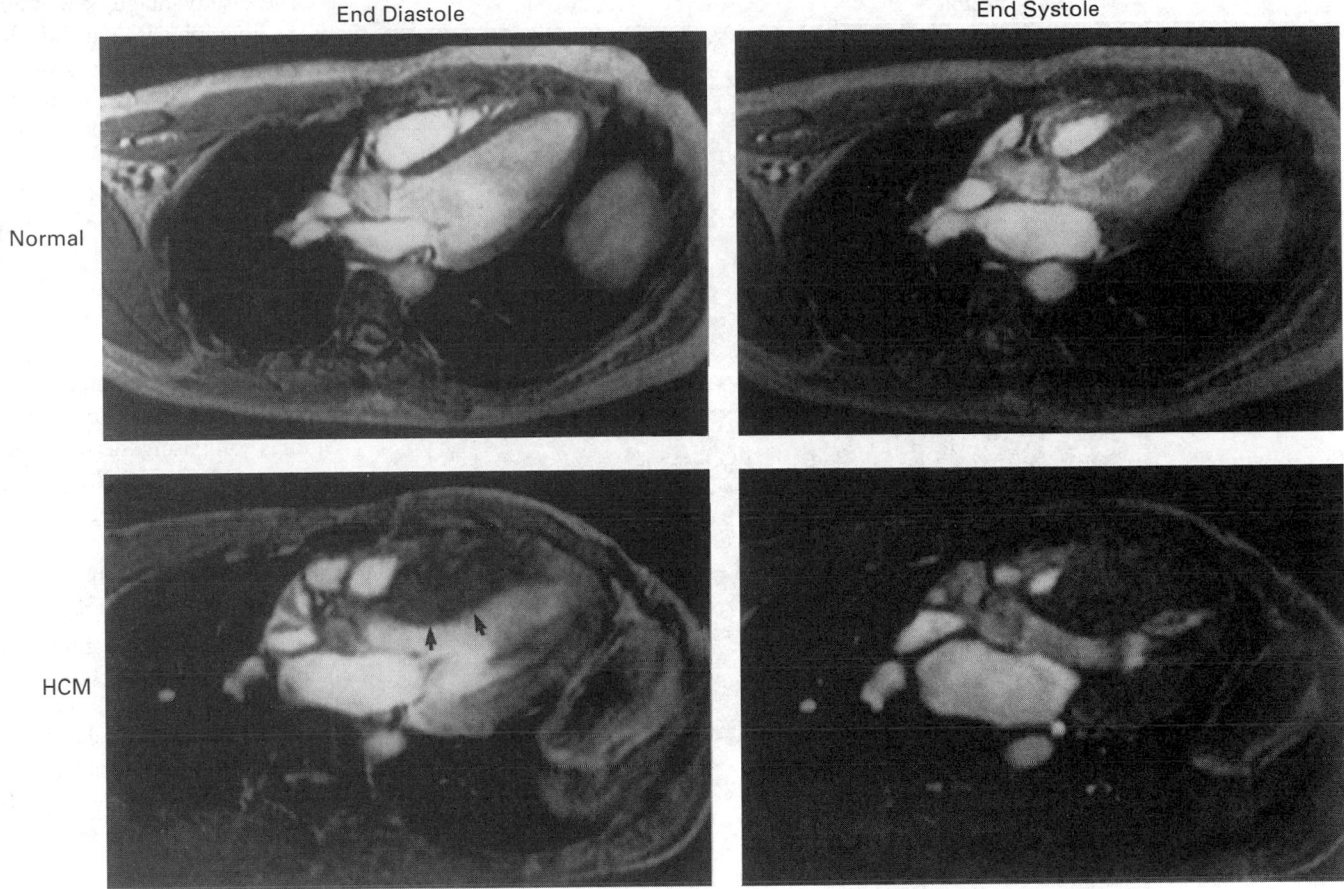

Normal

HCM

FIGURE 19-14

End-diastolic and end-systolic gradient-echo images are shown of a normal patient (*top*) and a patient with hypertrophic cardiomyopathy (HCM) (*bottom*). Note the marked thickening of the interventricular septum in the patient with HCM (*arrows*). With systole, there is near obliteration of the left ventricular cavity.

are acquired in two-dimensional, overlapping axial slices that are then stacked and projected onto the screen. The resultant image is called a *maximal intensity projection*, since the computer forms the image only from pixels with the highest signal, i.e., the vessels. These projections produce an angiogram that can be rotated, giving a three-dimensional perspective for improved interpretation. The vessels seen in these two-dimensional time-of-flight images may also be outlined manually to form a three-dimensional surface image, allowing color coding for further delineation of structures such as the false lumen of an aortic dissection. Tortuous vessels are best imaged using a three-dimensional technique obtained by imaging a thick "slab" of tissue. To enhance visualization of either venous or arterial structures, a saturation pulse is applied either above or below the imaging field, thus selectively eliminating either the arterial or the venous blood signal to produce a separate arteriogram or venogram without contamination from the other vascular system. MR angiography may be used to image virtually any moderate to large vessel. In current clinical practice, it is most often used to evaluate the aorta; however, carotid, renal, and iliofemoral arterial MR images can be obtained, and they replace those obtained by conven-

tional diagnostic angiography. The following discussion will concentrate on aortic imaging.

AORTIC MR ANGIOGRAPHY

MRI has been shown to be useful in both acquired and congenital abnormalities of the aorta. The noninvasive and high-resolution nature of MR makes it an ideal tool for imaging the deep structures of the thorax.

Aortic Dissection

MR angiography allows rapid detection of the presence of acute thoracic aortic dissection in stable patients. Such imaging is quite useful to the surgeon for planning the repair (Chap. 98). Usually, involvement of the coronary ostia, extent of the dissection, entry and exit sites, aortic valve function, and presence of flow in the false channel can be assessed[136-138] (Fig. 19-17). Although a type A dissection will require immediate surgical attention, MRI may assist in deciding whether an acute type B dissection should be treated medically or would have better long-term results with a surgical approach. For example, Kato et al.[139] reported improved outcome if patients were treated surgically for type B dissection when

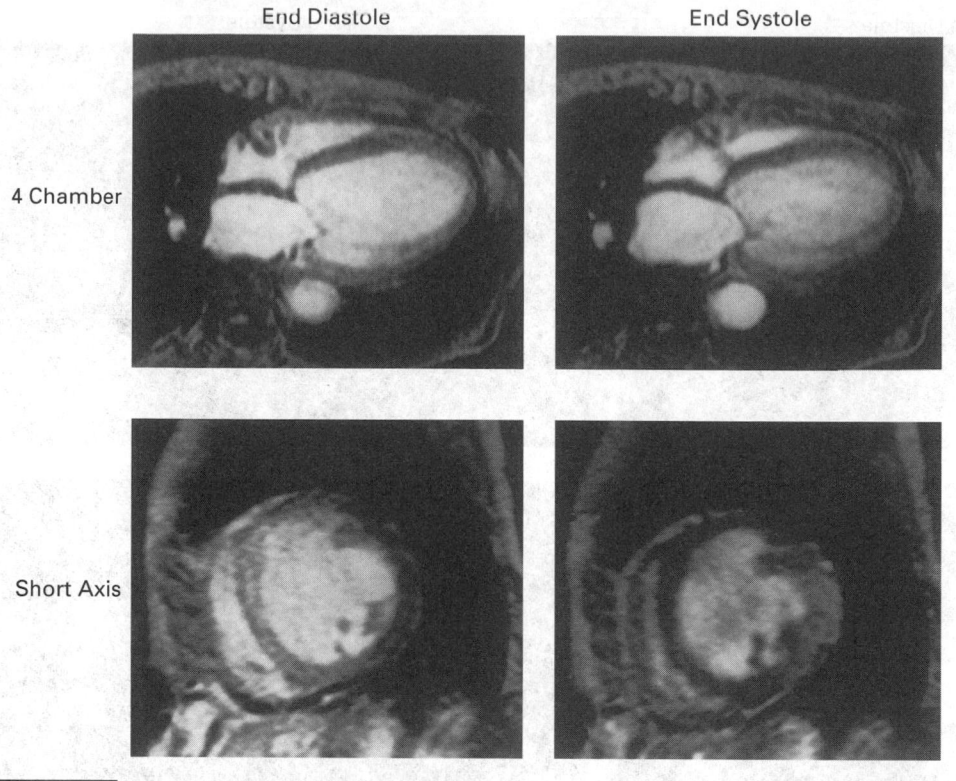

End Diastole   End Systole

4 Chamber

Short Axis

FIGURE 19-15
End-diastolic and end-systolic four-chamber and midventricular short-axis images are shown of a patient with dilated cardiomyopathy.

The disadvantage of MR aortic angiography is that only hemodynamically stable patients may be imaged safely. Although pulse oximetry, blood pressure, respiratory, and heart rate monitoring are routinely performed throughout the scan procedure, rapid access to the patient can be delayed by one or more minutes. In the stable patient, MR angiography is the most accurate noninvasive method for detecting the presence of aortic dissection. Studies comparing the sensitivity and specificity of MR angiography, transesophageal echocardiography (TEE), transthoracic echocardiography (TTE), and computed tomography revealed that MR angiography is superior for detecting aortic dissection. Furthermore, involvement of branch vessels, whose presence may elude other techniques, is also provided by MR angiography.[140,141]

the aortic dimension was large (≥40 mm) and a primary entry site was present in the thorax. In addition, MR angiography is particularly useful in patients with previously repaired aortic disease, who often have a poor transthoracic echocardiographic window.

Aortic Aneurysms

The applications applied to the detection of aortic dissection are readily applicable to aortic aneurysms.[142–144] Luminal dimensions, the extent of the aneurysm, and the branch vessels involved can help pinpoint the timing for surgical repair

ARVD

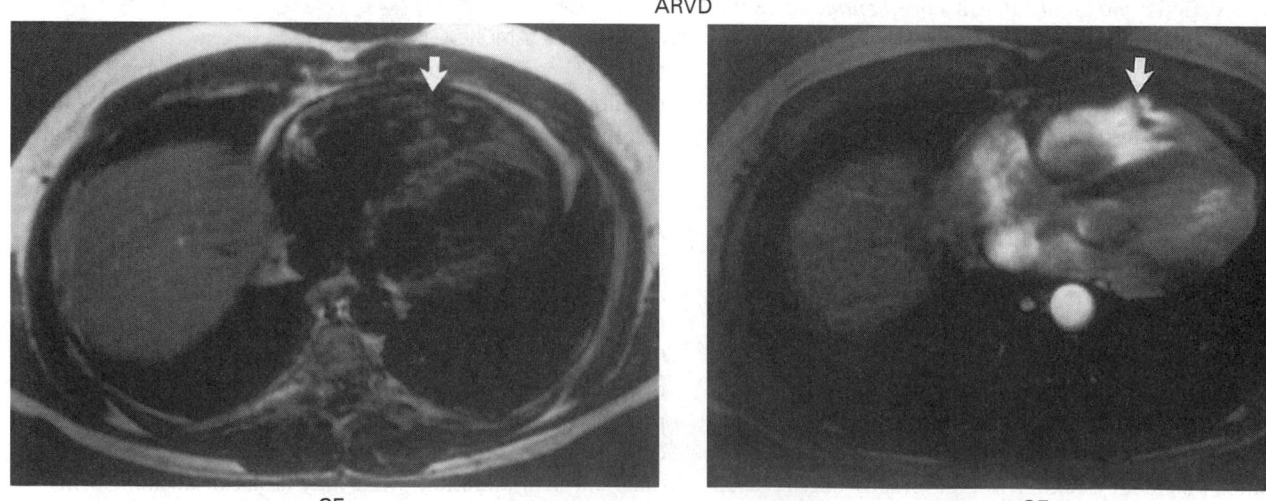

SE   GE

FIGURE 19-16
Spin-echo (SE) and gradient-echo (GE) images are shown of a patient with arryhythmogenic RV dysplasia (ARVD). Note the focal region of thinning of the right ventricular free wall (*arrows*).

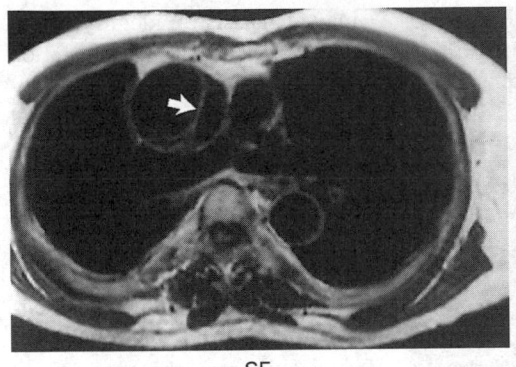
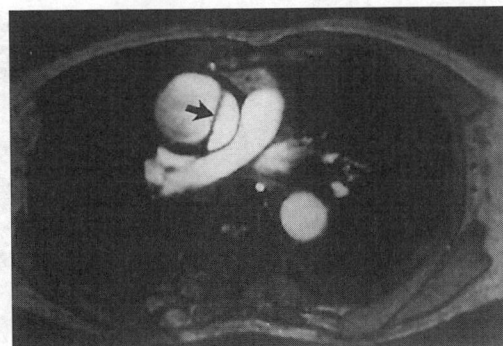
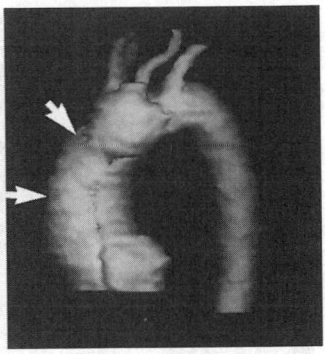

SE   GE   3D

FIGURE 19-17

Spin-echo (SE), gradient-echo (GE), and three-dimensional (3D) reconstruction of the thoracic aorta of a patient with a type II aortic dissection. Note in the transverse SE and GE images, the dissection flap (*arrows*) is easily identified with a larger false lumen and smaller, compressed true lumen. In the 3D image, the large, laterally located false lumen extends to the aortic arch vessels (*arrows*).

(Fig. 19-18). Ultrasound remains an excellent screening tool for abdominal aortic aneurysms; however, it may be less reliable in determining the relationship between complex aneurysm and aortic branch vessel involvement.[145]

Congenital Aortic Anomalies

Echocardiographic assessment of the vascular structures is excellent in infants and children, but in adults with congenital vascular anomalies, MR is the imaging technique of choice because of its large field of view and lack of need for administration of contrast medium. MR angiography is useful for assessing the presence and severity of aortic coarctation. It is also useful for evaluation of potential postoperative complications, i.e., aneurysms or dissections.[146,147] The luminal dimensions of the aorta can be serially reproduced to assess risk for aortic aneurysm ruptures, such as in patients with Marfan's syndrome.[148,149] Occasional concurrent problems such as pectus excavatum and scoliosis limit echo windows; even so, several studies have concluded that MR angiography provides more complete anatomic detail than echocardiography and can be utilized to assess and follow virtually all those with Marfan's syndrome. Lastly, anomalous aortic configurations such as vascular rings, right-sided aortas, and anomalous origins of branch vessels may be delineated by MR, not only to generate morphologic information but also to determine blood flow.

Congenital Heart Disease

Transthoracic echocardiography is an excellent clinical tool in infants and young children for noninvasive evaluation of congenital cardiovascular anomalies since this technique often requires no sedation, and the ultrasound is not obstructed by bone and has a nearer target than in older children, adolescents, and adults. As a child approaches adolescence or has a surgical repair, the echo assessment may become more difficult and sometimes incomplete. More often, invasive techniques must be performed to assess cardiac, vascular, conduit, or baffle structures adequately. Because of the morphologic detail afforded by MRI methods, almost every common congenital anomaly has been reported in the MRI literature.[150–153]

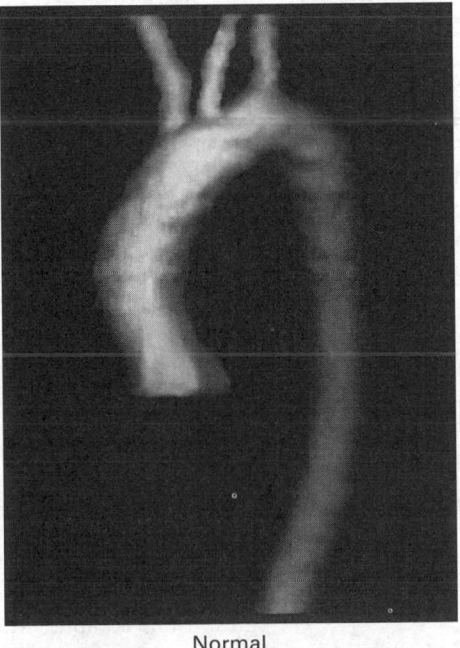
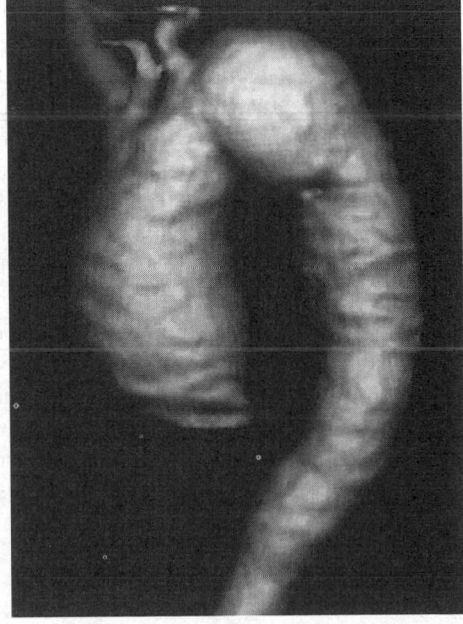

Normal   Aneurysmal

FIGURE 19-18

Three-dimensional MR images of a normal (*left*) and aneurysmally dilated (*right*) thoracic aorta.

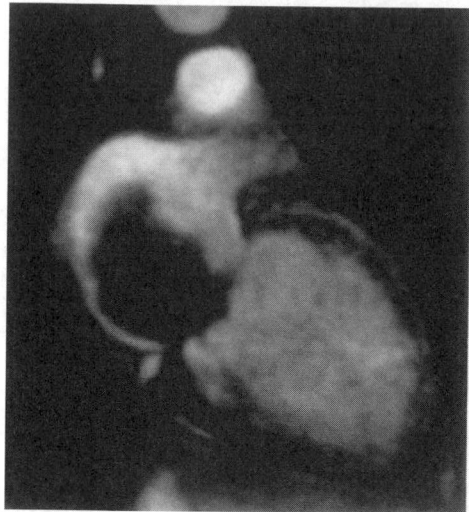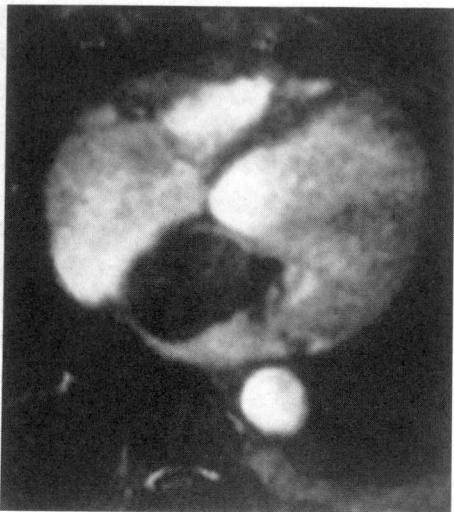

FIGURE 19-19

Two-chamber and four-chamber gradient-echo images are shown of a patient with a large left atrial mass. Note the mass has a similar signal intensity as the myocardium and fills the majority of the left atrial cavity. This mass is a left atrial myxoma and is attached to the interatrial septum.

Hence, many patients do not require invasive procedures to identify complex anatomy accurately.

MRI can obtain the five necessary anatomic parameters for the initial evaluation of a patient with complex congenital heart disease: situs, ventricular loop, atrioventricular connection, location of the apex, and the ventriculoarterial connections. Because MRI is not influenced by body habitus and scar tissue, deep vascular structures such as the central pulmonary arteries and ductus arteriosus are imaged well, even in the postoperative patient. Baffles and conduit size and function can be completely assessed by MR, provided no metallic (conductor or ferromagnetic) materials were used at the sites, which would interfere with image integrity due to substantial signal loss. As stated earlier, RV size and function are determined more accurately by MRI, which is most relevant in the management of patients with disorders such as transposition of the great arteries or interventricular and interatrial shunts or after repair of tetralogy of Fallot. In patients with coarctation of the aorta, with or without aortic hypoplasia, the need for angiography is no longer required unless knowledge of coronary anatomy is also desired.[154–157] Measurements of flow and velocity across shunts and within baffles and conduits have also been performed using phase-velocity mapping. From these measurements, one can determine the severity of the shunt (Q_p/Q_s) or the stenosis noninvasively.[158,159] In addition, using phase-contrast cine MR, the size of an atrial septal defect can be defined accurately, thus assisting in planning optimal operative intervention.[160]

Intracardiac Masses/Thrombi

A mass within a chamber of the heart is identified with either spin-echo (dark blood) or gradient-echo (bright blood) imaging. The signal intensity of the mass in the spin-echo image

may also assist in identifying the pathology based on T1 relaxation time; for example, cysts and lipomas will have very high signal intensity, whereas the signal intensity for lymphoma and myxoma will be less intense[161–165] (Fig. 19-19). Thrombus is more difficult to identify since it is usually present in an area of segmental wall dysfunction in the ventricule or the atrial appendages.[166] Within a cardiac chamber, slow-moving blood within the area of the akinetic or dyskinetic region will possess signal and appear as a mass; thus, gradient-echo and/or phase-velocity images must be obtained to aid in the distinction. The atrial appendages, especially in patients with atrial fibrillation, may also resemble thrombus since the blood movement is typically sluggish. Currently, definitive assessment of atrial thrombi is provided by another imaging modality such as TEE.

SUMMARY

Cardiovascular MR methods have now emerged beyond the status of a research tool to become a diagnostic method of choice in many circumstances related to the care of the patient with a cardiovascular disease or anomaly. Its major strengths are that it is noninvasive, that unlimited tomographic planes can be acquired, that operator interaction is not necessary, and that there is no imaging radiation exposure. Weaknesses include the lack of portability and the maintenance expense of the instrument. Nevertheless, reimbursement for cardiac MRI is not substantially higher than that for a two-dimensional echo/Doppler study. Currently, the utilization of MR imaging and angiography is most cost-effective when they either replace an invasive procedure (e.g., aortography, TEE) or are performed when multiple diagnostic techniques would otherwise be required (e.g., TTE and angiography, TTE and computed tomography, TTE and radionuclide perfusion imaging). For complex congenital heart disease in the adult, aortic pathology, and cardiac/paracardiac masses, MRI is the imaging modality of choice. As MRI becomes more widely used in clinical practice and research, the physician will discover a most amazing diagnostic technology capable of answering questions that were heretofore unanswerable and of providing improvement in the information provided by other technologies. If one compiles ventricular and valve function, myocardial perfusion, viability, and coronary anatomy imaging into a single package, there will be no better way to evaluate a patient with suspected cardiovascular pathology.

REFERENCES

1. Bloch R, Hensen WW, Packard ME. Nuclear induction. *Phys Rev* 1946; 69:127.

2. Purcell EM, Torrey HC, Pound RV. Resonance absorption by nuclear magnetic moments in a solid. *Phys Rev* 1946; 69:37–38.

3. Lauterbur PC. Image formation by induced local interactions: Examples employing nuclear magnetic resonance. *Nature* 1973; 242:190–191.

4. Friedman BJ, Waters J, Kwan OL, Demaria AN. Comparison of magnetic resonance imaging and echocardiography in determination of cardiac dimensions in normal subjects. *J Am Coll Cardiol* 1985; 5:1369–1376.

5. Byrd BF III, Schiller NB, Botvinick EH, Higgins CB. Normal cardiac dimensions by magnetic resonance imaging. *Am J Cardiol* 1985; 55:1440–1442.

6. Kaul S, Wismer G, Brady TJ, Johnston DL, Weyman AE, Okadad RD, et al. Measurements of normal left heart dimensions using optimally oriented MR images. *AJR* 1986; 146:75–79.

7. Fisher MR, vonSchulthess GK, Higgins CB. Multi-phase cardiac magnetic resonance imaging: Normal regional left ventricular wall thickening. *AJR* 1985; 145:27–30.

8. Van Rossum AC, Visser FC, Sprenger M, van Eenige MJ, Valk J, Ross JP, et al. Evaluation of magnetic resonance imaging for determinations of left ventricular ejection fraction and comparison with angiography. *Am J Cardiol* 1988; 62:628–633.

9. Buser PT, Auffermann W, Holt WW, Wagner S, Kircher B, Wolfe C, et al. Noninvasive evaluation of global left ventricular function with use of cine nuclear magnetic resonance. *J Am Coll Cardiol* 1989; 13:1294–1300.

10. Dilworth LR, Aisen AM, Mancini J, Lande Y, Buda AJ. Determination of left ventricular volumes and ejection fraction by nuclear magnetic resonance imaging. *Am Heart J* 1987; 113:24–32.

11. Cranney GB, Lotan CS, Dean L, Baxley W, Bouchard A, Pohost GM. Left ventricular volume measurement using cardiac axis nuclear magnetic resonance imaging. Validation by calibrated ventricular angiography. *Circulation* 1990; 82:154–163.

12. Matsouka H, Hamada M, Honda T, Kobayashi T, Suzuki M, Ohtani T, et al. Measurement of cardiac chamber volumes by cine magnetic resonance imaging. *Angiology* 1993; 44(4):321–327.

13. Buser PT, Auffermann W, Holt WW, Wagner S, Kircher B, Wolfe C, et al. Noninvasive evaluation of left global left ventricular function with use of cine nuclear magnetic resonance. *J Am Coll Cardiol* 1989; 13:1294–1300.

14. Rehr RB, Malloy CR, Filichuck NG, Peshock RM. Left ventricular volumes measured by MR imaging. *Radiology* 1985; 156:717–719.

15. Semeika RC, Tomei E, Wagner S, Mayo J, Caputo GR, O'Sullivan M, et al. Normal left ventricular dimensions and functions: Interstudy reproducibility of measurements of cine MR imaging. *Radiology* 1990; 174:763–768.

16. Van Rossum AC, Visser FC, Sprenger M, Van Eenige MJ, Valk J, Ross JP, et al. Evaluation of magnetic resonance imaging for determinations of left ventricular ejection fraction and comparison with angiography. *Am J Cardiol* 1988; 62:628–633.

17. Ostrzega E, Maddahi J, Honma H, Crues JV III, Resser JK, Charuzi Y, et al. Quantification of left ventricular myocardial mass in humans by nuclear magnetic resonance imaging. *Am Heart J* 1989; 117:444–452.

18. Yamaoka O, Yabe T, Okada M, Endoh S, Nakamura Y, Mitsunami K, et al. Evaluation of left ventricular mass: Comparison of ultrafast computed tomography, magnetic resonance imaging, and contrast left ventriculography. *Am Heart J* 1993; 126:1372–1379.

19. Aurigemma G, Davidoff A, Silver K, Boehmer J. Left ventricular mass quantitation using single-phase cardiac magnetic resonance imaging. *Am J Cardiol* 1992; 70:259–262.

20. Keller A, Peshock R, Mally C, Buja LM, Nunnally R, Parkey R, et al. In vivo measurements of myocardial mass using MR imaging. *J Am Coll Cardiol* 1986; 8:113–117.

21. Allison JD, Flickinger FW, Wright JC, Falls DG, Prisant LM, VonDohlen, et al. Measurement of left ventricular mass in hypertrophic cardiomyopathy using MRI: Comparison with echocardiography. *Magn Reson Imaging* 1993; 11(3):329–334.

22. Bryant DJ, Payne JA, Firmin DN, Longmore DB. Measurement of flow with NMR imaging using gradient pulses and phase difference technique. *J Comput Assist Tomogr* 1984; 8:588–593.

23. Firmin DN, Nayler GL, Klipstein RH, Underwood SR, Rees RSO, Longmore DB. In vivo validation of MR velocity imaging. *J Comput Assist Tomogr* 1987; 11:751–756.

24. Van Rossum A, Sprenger KH, Peels FC. In vivo validation of quantitative flow imaging in arteries and veins using magnetic resonance phase-shift techniques. Proceedings of the Society of Magnetic Resonance in Medicine, Amsterdam, 1989; 205.

25. Kondo C, Caputo GR, Semelka R, Shimakawa M, Higgins CB. Right and left ventricular slope volume measurements with velocity encoded cine and MR imaging: In vitro and in vivo evaluation. *AJR* 1991; 157:9–16.

26. Hundley WG, Li HF, Hillis LD, Meshack BM, Lange RA, Willard JE, et al. Quantitation of cardiac output with velocity-encoded, phase-difference magnetic resonance imaging. *Am J Cardiol* 1995; 75(17):1250–1255.

27. Brenner LD, Caputo GR, Mostbeck G, Steiman D, Delce M, Cheitlin MD, et al. Quantification of left to right atrial shunts with velocity-encoded cine nuclear magnetic resonance imaging. *J Am Coll Cardiol* 1992; 20:1246–1250.

28. Canby RC, Reeves RC, Evanochko WT, Elgavish GA, Pohost GM. Proton nuclear magnetic resonance relaxation times in severe myocardial ischemia. *J Am Coll Cardiol* 1987; 10:412–420.

29. Scholz TD, Martins JB, Skortin DJ. NMR relaxation times and acute myocardial ischemia: Relative influence of tissue water and fat content. *Magn Reson Med* 1992; 23:89–95.

30. Higgins CB, Herfkins R, Lipton MJ, Sievers R, Sheldon P, Kaufman L, et al. Nuclear magnetic resonance imaging of acute myocardial infarction in dogs: Alterations in magnetic relaxation times. *Am J Cardiol* 1983; 52:184–188.

31. Williams ES, Kaplan JI, Thatcher F, Zimmerman G, Knobel SB. Prolongation of proton spin lattice times in regionally ischemic tissue from dog hearts. *J Nucl Med* 1980; 21:449–453.

32. Pflugfelder PW, Wisenberg G, Prato FS, Carrol SE. Serial imaging of canine myocardial infarction by in vivo nuclear magnetic resonance. *J Am Coll Cardiol* 1986; 7:843–849.

33. Lotan CS, Miller SK, Bouchard A, Cranney GB, Reeves RC, Bishop SB, et al. Detection of intramyocardial hemorrhage using high-field proton nuclear magnetic resonance imaging. *Cathet Cardiovasc Diagn* 1990; 20:205–211.

34. Sugishita J, Koscki S, Matsido M, Tamura T, Yamaguchi I, Ito I. Dissociation between regional myocardial dysfunction and EKG changes during myocardial ischemia induced by exercise in patients with angina pectoris. *Am Heart J* 1993; 106:1–8.

35. Upton MT, Rerych SK, Newman GE, Port S, Cobb FR, Jones RH. Detecting abnormalities in left ventricular function during exercise before angina, and ST segment depression. *Circulation* 1980; 62:341–349.

36. Coma-Canella I. Sensitivity and specificity of dobutamine-electrocardiography test to detect multivessel disease after acute myocardial infarction. *Eur Heart J* 1990; 11:249–257.

37. Freeman ML, Palac RT, Mason J, Barnes WE, Eastman G, Virupannavar S, et al. A comparison of dobutamine infusion and supine bicycle exercise for radionuclide cardiac stress testing. *Clin Nucl Med* 1984; 9:251–255.

38. Cohen JL, Green TO, Ottenweller J, Binenbaum SZ, Wilchfort SD, Kim CS. Dobutamine digital echocardiography for detecting coronary artery disease. *Am J Cardiol* 1991; 67:1311–1318.

39. Marcovitz PA, Armstrong WF. Accuracy of dobutamine stress echocardiography in detecting coronary artery disease. *Am J Cardiol* 1992; 69:1269–1273.

40. Sawada SG, Segar DS, Ryan T, Brown SE, Dohan AM, Williams R, et al. Echocardiography detection of coronary disease during dobutamine infusion. *Circulation* 1991; 83:1605–1614.

41. Mazeika PK, Nadazdin A, Oakley CM. Dobutamine stress echocardiography for detection and assessment of coronary disease. *J Am Coll Cardiol* 1992; 19:1203–1211.

42. Pennell DJ, Underwood SR, Swanton H, Walker M, Lell PJ. Dobutamine thallium myocardial perfusion tomography. *J Am Coll Cardiol* 1990; 18:1471–1479.

43. Mason JR, Palac RT, Freeman ML, Virupannavar S, Loeb HS, Kaplan E, et al. Thallium scintigraphy during dobutamine infusion: Nonexercise-dependent screening test for coronary disease. *Am Heart J* 1984; 107:481–485.

44. Lotan CS, Cranney CB, Bouchard A, Bittner V, Pohost GM. The value

of cine magnetic resonance imaging for assessing regional ventricular function. *J Am Coll Cardiol* 1989; 14:1721–1729.

45. van Rugge FP, van der Wall EE, de Roos A, Bruschke AVG. Dobutamine stress magnetic resonance imaging for detection of coronary artery disease. *J Am Coll Cardiol* 1993; 22:431–439.

46. Brown JJ, Higgins CB. Myocardial paramagnetic contrast agents for MR imaging. *AJR* 1988; 151:865–872.

47. Manning WJ, Atkinson DJ, Grossman W, Paulin S, Edelman RR. First-pass nuclear magnetic resonance imaging studies using gadolinium-DTPA in patients with coronary artery disease. *J Am Coll Cardiol* 1991; 18:59–65.

48. Matheijssen NA, Louwerenburg HW, van Rugge FP, Arens R, Kauer B, De Roos A, et al. Comparison of ultrafast dipyridamole magnetic resonance imaging with dipyridamole sestamibi SPECT for detection of profusion abnormalities in patients with one-vessel coronary artery disease: Assessment by quantitative model fitting. *Magn Reson Med* 1996; 35:221–228.

49. Walsh EG, Doyle M, Lawson MA, Blackwell GG, Pohost GM. Multislice first-pass myocardial perfusion imaging on a conventional clinical scanner. *Magn Reson Med* 1995; 34:39–47.

50. Walsh EG, Doyle M, Lawson MA, Pohost GM. Multislice myocardial perfusion imaging using BRISK (abstr). Proceedings of the Society of Magnetic Resonance, Fourth Scientific Meeting, Vancouver, 1996.

51. Simor T, Chu W-J, Johnson L, Safranko A, Doyle M, Pohost G, et al. In vivo MRI visualization of acute myocardial ischemia and reperfusion in ferrets by the persistent action of contrast agent Gd (BME-DTTA). *Circulation* 1995; 92:3549–3559.

52. Flaherty JT, Weisfeldt ML, Bulkley BH, Gardner TJ, Gott VL, Jacobus WE. Mechanisms of ischemic myocardial damage assessed by phosphorous-31 nuclear magnetic resonance. *Circulation* 1982; 65:561–570.

53. Nunnally RL, Bottomley PA. Assessment of pharmacological treatment of myocardial infarction by phosphorous-31 NMR with surface coils. *Science* 1981; 211:177–180.

54. Jacobus WE, Taylor GJ, Hollis DP, Nunnally RL. Phosphorous nuclear magnetic resonance of perfused working rat hearts. *Nature* 1977; 265:756–758.

55. Bottomley PA, Herfkins RJ, Smith LS, Brazcamano S, Blinder R, Hedlund LW, et al. Noninvasive detection of monitoring of regional myocardial ischemia in situ using depth-resolved ^{31}P NMR spectroscopy. *Proc Natl Acad Sci USA* 1985; 82:8747–8751.

56. Bottomley PA. Noninvasive study of high-energy phosphate metabolism in human heart by depth-resolved ^{31}P NMR spectroscopy. *Science* 1985; 229:769–772.

57. Weiss RG, Bottomley PA, Hardy CJ, Gerstenblith G. Regional metabolism of high-energy phosphates during isometric exercise in patients with coronary artery disease. *N Engl J Med* 1990; 323:1593–1600.

58. Yabe T, Mitsunami K, Okada M, Morikawa S, Inubushi T, Kinoshita M. A detection of myocardial ischemia by ^{31}P magnetic resonance spectroscopy during handgrip exercise. *Circulation* 1994; 89:1709–1716.

59. Fisher MR, McNamara MT, Higgins CB. Acute myocardial infarction: MR evaluation in 29 patients. *AJR* 1987; 148:247–251.

60. Johnston DL, Thompson RC, Liu P, Dinsmore RE, Wismer GL, Saini S, et al. Magnetic resonance imaging during acute myocardial infarction. *Am J Cardiol* 1986; 57:1059–1065.

61. Ahmad M, Johnson RF, Fawcett HD, Schreiber MH. Magnetic resonance imaging in patients with unstable angina: Comparison with acute myocardial infarction and normals. *Magn Reson Imaging* 1988; 6:527–534.

62. Krauss XH, van der Wall EE, Doornbos J, Blokland JAK, Postema S, De Roos A, et al. The value of nuclear magnetic resonance imaging in patients with a recent myocardial infarction: Comparison with planar thallium-201 scintigraphy. *Cardiovasc Intervent Radiol* 1989; 12:119–124.

63. Krauss XH, van der Wall EE, van der Laarse A, Doornbos J, Matheijssen NAA, De Roos A, et al. Magnetic resonance imaging of myocardial infarction: Correlation with enzymatic angiographic and radionuclide findings. *Am Heart J* 1991; 122:1274–1283.

64. Johns JA, Leavitt MB, Newell JB, Yasuda T, Leinbach RC, Gold HK, et al. Quantitation of acute myocardial infarction size by nuclear magnetic resonance imaging. *J Am Coll Cardiol* 1990; 15:143–149.

65. Turnbull LW, Ridgeway JP, Nicoll JJ, Bell D, Best JJK. Estimating the size of myocardial infarction by magnetic resonance imaging. *Br Heart J* 1991; 66:359–363.

66. White RD, Holt WW, Cheitlin MD, Cassidy MM, Ports TA, Lim AD, et al. Estimation of the functional and anatomic extent of myocardial infarction using magnetic resonance imaging. *Am Heart J* 1988; 115:740–748.

67. Matheijssen NAA, de Roos A, van der Wall EE, Doornbos J, van Dijkman PRM, Bruschke AVG, et al. Acute myocardial infarction: Comparison of T2-weighted and T1-weighted gadolinium-DTPA enhanced MR imaging. *Magn Reson Med* 1991; 17:460–469.

68. Eichstaedt HW, Felix R, Dougherty FC, Langer M, Rutsch W, Schmutzler H. Magnetic resonance imaging (MRI) in different stages of myocardial infarction using contrast agent gadolinium-DTPA. *Clin Cardiol* 1986; 9:527–535.

69. van Dijkman PRM, Doornbos J, De Roos A, van der Laarse A, Postema S, Matheijssen NAA, et al. Improved detection of acute myocardial infarction by magnetic resonance imaging using gadolinium-DTPA. *Int J Cardiac Imaging* 1989; 5:1–8.

70. Nishimura T, Kobayashi H, Ohra Y, Yamada N, Haze K, Takamiya M, et al. Serial assessment of myocardial infarction using gated MR imaging and Gd-DTPA. *AJR* 1989; 153:715–720.

71. Higgins CB, Sakuma H. Heart disease: Functional evaluation with MR imaging. *Radiology* 1996; 199:307–315.

72. Sechtem U, Sommerhoff BA, Markiewicz W, White RD, Cheitlin MD, Higgins CB. Regional left ventricular wall thickening by magnetic resonance imaging: Evaluation in normal persons and persons with global and regional dysfunction. *Am J Cardiol* 1987; 59:145–151.

73. Pflugfelder PW, Sechtem UP, White RD, Higgins CB. Quantification of regional myocardial function by rapid cine MR imaging. *AJR* 1988; 150:523–529.

74. Underwood SR, Rees RSO, Savage PE, Klipstein RH, Firmin DN, Fox KN, et al. Assessment of regional left ventricular function by magnetic resonance. *Br Heart J* 1986; 56:334–340.

75. Sechtem U, Baer F, Voth E, Schneider C, Theissen P, Schicha H. Assessment of residual viability in patients with myocardial infarction using magnetic resonance imaging. *Int J Cardiac Imaging* 1993; 9:931–940.

76. Baer FM, Smolarz K, Jungehulsing M, Buckwilm J, Theissen P, Sechtem U, et al. Chronic myocardial infarction: Assessment of morphology, function and perfusion by gradient echo magnetic resonance imaging and ^{99}m Tc-methoxyisobutyl-isonitrile SPECT. *Am Heart J* 1992; 123:636–645.

77. Baer FM, Voth E, Schneider CA, Theissen P, Schicha H, Sechtem U. Comparison of low-dose dobutamine-gradient-echo magnetic resonance imaging and positron emission tomography with [^{18}F] fluorodeoxyglucose in patients with chronic coronary artery disease. *Circulation* 1995; 91:1006–1015.

78. Kimbiris D, Iskandrian AS, Segal BL, Bemis CE. Anomalous aortic origin of coronary arteries. *Circulation* 1978; 58:606–615.

79. Click RL, Holmes DR, Vlietstra RE, Kosinski AS, Kronmal RA, CASS Participants. Anomalous coronary arteries: Location, degree of atherosclerosis and effect on survival: A report from the Coronary Artery Surgery Study. *J Am Coll Cardiol* 1989; 13:531–537.

80. Yamanaka O, Hobbs RE. Coronary artery anomalies in 126,595 patients undergoing coronary arteriography. *Cathet Cardiovasc Diagn* 1990; 21:28–40.

81. Chaitman BR, Lesperance J, Saltiel J, Bourassa MG. Clinical, angiographic, and hemodynamic findings in patients with anomalous origin of the coronary arteries. *Circulation* 1976; 53:122–131.

82. Isner JM, Shen EM, Martin ET, Fortin RV. Sudden unexpected death as a result of anomalous origin of the coronary artery from the left sinus of Valsalva. *Am J Med* 1984; 76:155–158.

83. Liberthson RR, Dinsmore RE, Fallon JT. Aberrant coronary artery origin from the aorta: Report of 18 patients, review of the literature and delineation of natural history of management. *Circulation* 1978; 58:748–754.

84. Cheitlin MD, DeCastro CM, McAllister HA. Sudden death as a complication of anomalous left coronary origin from anterior sinus of Valsalva: A not-so-minor congenital anomaly. *Circulation* 1974; 58:780–787.

85. Kragel AH, Roberts WC. Anomalous origin of either the right or left main coronary artery from the aorta with subsequent coursing between the aorta and pulmonary trunk: Analysis of 32 necropsy cases. *Am J Cardiol* 1988; 62:771–777.

86. Ischikawa T, Brandt PWT. Anomalous origin of the left coronary artery from the right anterior aortic sinus: Angiographic definition of anomalous course. *Am J Cardiol* 1985; 55:770–776.

87. Post JC, van Rossum AC, Bronzwar JGF, de Cock CC, Hofman MBM, Valk J, et al. Magnetic resonance angiography of anomalous coronary arteries. *Circulation* 1995; 92:3163–3171.

88. McConnell MV, Ganz P, Selwyn AP, Li W, Edelman R, Manning WJ. Identification of anomalous coronary arteries and their anatomic course by magnetic resonance coronary angiography. *Circulation* 1995; 92:3158–3162.

89. Bisset GS III, Strife JL, McCloskey J. MR imaging of coronary artery aneurysms in a child with Kawasaki's disease. *AJR* 1989; 152:805–807.

90. Kubota S, Suzuki T, Murata K. Cine magnetic resonance imaging for diagnosis of right coronary arterial-ventricular fistula. *Chest* 1991; 100:735–737.

91. Pucillo AL, Schechter AG, Moggio RA, Kay RH, Baum SJ, Herman MV. MR imaging in the definition of coronary artery anomalies. *J Comput Assist Tomogr* 1990; 14:171–174.

92. Paschal CB, Haacke EM, Adler LP, Fineli DA. Coronary artery imaging. *Cardiovasc Intervent Radiol* 1992; 15:23–31.

93. Paschal CB, Haacke EM, Adler LP. Three-dimensional MR imaging of the coronary arteries: Preliminary clinical experience. *J Magn Reson Imaging* 1993; 3:491–500.

94. Spiller P, Schmiel FK, Politz B, Block M, Fermor U, Hackbarth W, et al. Measurement of systolic and diastolic flow rates in the coronary artery system by x-ray densitometry. *Circulation* 1983; 68:337–347.

95. Edelman RR, Manning WJ, Burstein D, Paulin S. Coronary arteries: Breath-hold MR angiography. *Radiology* 1991; 181:641–643.

96. Wang Y, Grimm RC, Rossman PJ, Debbins JP, Riederer SJ, Ehman RL. 3D coronary MR angiography and multiple breath-holds using a respiratory feedback monitor. *Magn Reson Med* 1995; 34:11–16.

97. Hofman MBM, Paschal CB, Li D, Haacke EM, van Rossum AC, Sprenger M. MRI of coronary arteries, 2D breath-hold versus 3D respiratory gating acquisition. *J Comput Assist Tomogr* 1995; 19:56–62.

98. Korin HW, Ehman RL, Riederer SJ, Felmlee JP, Grimm RC. Respiratory kinematics of the upper abdominal organs: A quantitative study. *Magn Reson Med* 1992; 23:172–178.

99. Wang Y, Christy PS, Korosec FR, Alley MT, Grist TM, Polzin JA, et al. Coronary MRI with respiratory feedback monitor: The 2D imaging case. *Magn Reson Med* 1995; 33:116–121.

100. Manning WJ, Li W, Boyle NG, Edelman R. Fat-suppressed breath-hold magnetic resonance coronary angiography. *Circulation* 1993; 87:94–104.

101. Manning WJ, Li W, Edelman RR. A preliminary report comparing magnetic resonance coronary angiography with conventional angiography. *N Engl J Med* 1993; 328:828–832.

102. Schiebler N, Axel L, Reichek N, Aurigemma G, Yeager B, Douglas P, et al. Correlation of cine MR imaging with two-dimensional pulse Doppler echocardiography in valvular insufficiency. *J Comput Assist Tomogr* 1987; 11:627–632.

103. Utz JA, Herfkens RJ, Heinsimer JA, Shimakawa A, Glover G, Pelc N. Valvular regurgitation: Dynamic MR imaging. *Radiology* 1988; 168:91–94.

104. Pflugfelder PW, Landzberg JS, Cassidy MN, Cheitlin MD, Schiller NB, Auffermann W, et al. Comparison of cine MR imaging with Doppler echocardiography for the evaluation of aortic regurgitation. *Am J Roentgenol* 1989; 152:729–735.

105. Underwood SR, Klepstein RH, Firmin DN, Fox KM, Poole-Wilson PA, Rees RSO, et al. Magnetic resonance assessment of aortic and mitral regurgitation. *Br Heart J* 1986; 56:455–462.

106. Bryant DJ, Payne JA, Firman DN, Longmore DB. Measurement of flow with NMR imaging using a gradient pulse and phase difference technique. *J Comput Assist Tomogr* 1984; 8:588.

107. Podolak MJ, Hedlund LW, Evans AJ, Herfkens RJ. Evaluation of flow through simulated vascular stenosis with gradient echo magnetic resonance imaging. *Invest Radiol* 1989; 24:184.

108. Recusani F, Bargiggia G, Yaganathan AP, Valdez-Cruz L, Raisaro A, Simpson IA, et al. Color flow quantitation of regurgitant flow using flow convergence proximal to the orifice of the regurgitant jet. *Circulation* 1991; 83:594–604.

109. Shandas R, Golebiovski P, Elkadi T, Mrosko B, Moises V, Valdez-Cruiz L, et al. Influence of complex "valve" surface geometry on flow convergence methods for calculating flow rate by color Doppler (abstr). *Circulation* 1990; 82(suppl III):III-63.

110. Hundley WG, Li HF, Willard JE, Landau C, Lang RA, Meshack BM, et al. Magnetic resonance imaging assessment of the severity of mitral regurgitation: Comparison with invasive techniques. *Circulation* 1995; 92:1151–1158.

111. Fugita N, Chazauilleres AF, Hartiala JJ, O'Sullivan M, Heidenrich P, Kapla JD, et al. Quantification of mitral regurgitation by phase-encoded cine nuclear magnetic resonance imaging. *J Am Coll Cardiol* 1994; 23:951–958.

112. Sechtem U, Pflugfelder PW, Cassidy MM, White RD, Cheitlin MD, Schiller MB, et al. Mitral and aortic regurgitation: Quantification of regurgitant volumes with cine MR imaging. *Radiology* 1988; 167:425–430.

113. de Roos A, Reichek N, Axel L, Kressel HY. Cine MR imaging in aortic stenosis. *J Comput Assist Tomogr* 1989; 13:421–425.

114. Kilner JP, Manzara KG, Mohaiddin RH, Pennell DJ, St John Sutton MG, Firmin DN, et al. Magnetic resonance jet velocity mapping in mitral and aortic stenosis. *Circulation* 1993; 87:1279–1298.

115. Roberts WC, Spray TL. Pericardial disease: A study of its causes, consequences and morphologic features. In: Spodlick D, ed. *Pericardial Disease.* Philadelphia: Davis; 1976:17.

116. Bluemic DA, Lund JT, Lipton MJ. *Nuclear Magnetic Resonance Assessment of Pericardial Disease.* In Marcus ML, Schelbert HR, Skorton DJ, Wolf GL, eds. *Cardiac Imaging.* Philadelphia: Saunders; 1991:938.

117. Stark DD, Higgins CB, Lanzer P, Lipton MJ, Schiller N, Crooks LE, et al. Magnetic resonance imaging of the pericardium: Normal and pathologic findings. *Radiology* 1984; 151:469–474.

118. White CS. MR evaluation of the pericardium. *Top Magn Reson Imaging* 1995; 7(4):258–266.

119. Sechtem U, Tscholakoff D, Higgins CB. MRI of the normal pericardium. *AJR* 1986; 147:239.

120. vonSchulthess GK, Higgins CB. Blood flow imaging with MR: Spin phase phenomena. *Radiology* 1985; 157:687.

121. Mulvagh SL, Rokey R, Vick GW, Johnston DL. Usefulness of nuclear magnetic resonance imaging for evaluation of pericardial effusions, in comparison with two-dimensional echocardiography. *J Am Coll Cardiol* 1989; 64:1002–1009.

122. Sechtem U, Tscholakoff D, Higgins CB. MRI of the abnormal pericardium. *AJR* 1986; 147:245.

123. Moncada R, Baker M, Salinas M, Demos TC, Churchill R, Love L, et al. Diagnostic role of computed tomography and pericardial heart disease. Congenital defects, thickening, neoplasms, and effusions. *Am Heart J* 1982; 103:263–282.

124. Soulen RL, Stark DD, Higgins CB. Magnetic resonance imaging of constrictive pericardial disease. *Am J Cardiol* 1995; 55:480–484.

125. Klues HG, Schiffers A, Maron BJ. Phenotypic spectrum and patterns of left ventricular hypertrophy and hypertrophic cardiomyopathy: Morphologic observations and significance as assessed by 2-dimensional echocardiography in 600 patients. *J Am Coll Cardiol* 1995; 26:1699–1708.

126. Thompson RC, Lavine RA, Mille S, Dinsmore RE. Magnetic resonance imaging along the left ventricular axis in hypertrophic heart disease: Accurate characterization of cardiac hypertrophy. *Circulation* 1985; 72(suppl III):122.

127. Higgins CB, Byrd BF III, Stark D, McNamara M, Lanzer P, Lipton MJ, et al. Magnetic resonance imaging in hypertrophic cardiomyopathy. *Am J Cardiol* 1985; 55:1121–1126.

128. Higgins CB, Byrd BF III, Stark D, McNamara M, Lanzer P, Lipton MJ, et al. Magnetic resonance imaging in hypertrophic cardiomyopathy. *Am J Cardiol* 1985; 55:1121–1126.

129. Webb JG, Sasson Z, Rakowski H, Liu P, Wigle ED. Apical hypertrophic cardiomyopathy: Clinical follow-up and diagnostic correlates. *J Am Coll Cardiol* 1990; 15:83–90.

130. Suzuki J, Watanabe F, Takenaka K, Amano K, Amano W, Igarashi T, et al. New subtype of apical hypertrophic cardiomyopathy identified with nuclear magnetic resonance imaging as an underlying cause of markedly inverted T waves. *J Am Coll Cardiol* 1993; 22:1175–1181.

131. Guado C, Pelliccia FTA, Nzilli G, Mazzarotto P, Cianfrocca C, Marino B. Magnetic resonance imaging for assessment of apical hypertrophy in hypertrophic cardiomyopathy. *Clin Cardiol* 1992; 15:164–168.

132. Sechtem U, Higgins CB, Summerhoff BA, Lipton MJ, Huycke EC. Magnetic resonance imaging of restrictive cardiomyopathy. *Am J Cardiol* 1987; 59:480–482.

133. Blake LM, Scheinman MM, Higgins CB. MR features of arrhythmogenic right ventricular dysplasia. *AJR* 1994; 162:809–812.

134. Ricci C, Longo R, Pagnan L, Dalla Palma L, Pinamonti B, Camerini F, et al. Magnetic resonance imaging in right ventricular dysplasia. *Am J Cardiol* 1992; 70:1589–1595.

135. Hamada S, Takamiya M, Ohe T, Ueda H. Arrhythmogenic right ventricular dysplasia: Evaluation with electron-beam CT. *Radiology* 1993; 187:723–727.

136. Amparo EG, Higgins CB, Hricak H. Aortic dissection: Magnetic resonance imaging. *Radiology* 1985; 155:399.

137. Gensinger MA, Risuis B, O'Donnell JA, Zelch MG, Moodie DS, Graor RA, et al. Thoracic aortic dissections: Magnetic resonance imaging. *Radiology* 1985; 155:407–412.

138. Kersting-Sommerhoff BA, Higgins CB, White RD, Sommerhof CP, Lipton MI. Aortic dissection: Sensitivity and specificity of MR imaging. *Radiology* 1988; 166:651–655.

139. Kato M, Bai H, Sato K, Kawamoto S, Kaneko M, Ueda T, et al. Determining surgical indications for acute type B dissection based on enlargement of the aortic diameter during the chronic phase. *Circulation* 1995; 92(suppl II):II107–II112.

140. Nienaber CA, VonKodolitsch Y, Nicholas V. The diagnosis of thoracic aortic dissection by non-invasive imaging procedures. *N Engl J Med* 1993; 328:1–9.

141. Nienaber CA, von Kodolitsch Y, Brockhoff CJ. Comparison of conventional and transesophageal echocardiography with magnetic resonance imaging for anatomical mapping of thoracic aortic dissection. A visual non-invasive imaging study with anatomical and/or angiographic validation. *Int J Cardiol Imaging* 1994; 10:1–14.

142. Dinsmore RE, Liberthson RR, Wismer GL, Miller SW, Liu P, Thompson R, et al. Magnetic resonance imaging of thoracic aortic aneurysms: Comparison with other imaging methods. *Am J Roentgenol* 1986; 146:309–314.

143. Valk PE, Hale JD, Kaufman L, Crooks LE, Higgins CB. MR imaging of the aorta with 3-dimensional vessel reconstruction: Validation by angiography. *Radiology* 1985; 157:721–725.

144. Webb WR, Sostman HD. MR imaging of thoracic disease: Clinical uses. *Radiology* 1992; 182:621–630.

145. Lee JKT, Ling D, Heiken JP, Glazer HS, Sicard GA, Totty WG, et al. Magnetic resonance imaging of abdominal aortic aneurysms. *AJR* 1984; 143:1197.

146. VonSchulthess G, Higashino SM, Higgins SS, Didier D, Fisher MR, Higgins CB. Coarctation of the aorta: MR imaging. *Radiology* 1986; 158:469–474.

147. Simpson IA, Chung KJ, Glass RF. Cine magnetic resonance imaging for evaluation of anatomy and flow relations in infants and children with coarctation of the aorta. *Circulation* 1988; 78:142.

148. Boxer RA, LaCorte MA, Singh S, Davis J, Goldman M, Stein HL. Evaluation of the aorta in the Marfan's syndrome by magnetic resonance imaging. *Am Heart J* 1986; 111:1001–1002.

149. Schaefer S, Peshock RM, Malloy CR, Katz J, Parkey RW, Willersom JT. Nuclear magnetic resonance imaging in Marfan's syndrome. *J Am Coll Cardiol* 1987; 9:70–74.

150. Higgins CB, Byrd BF, Farmer D, Silverman N, Kheitlin M. Magnetic resonance imaging in patients with congenital heart disease. *Circulation* 1984; 70(5):851–860.

151. Didier D, Higgins CB, Fisher MR, Osaki L, Silverman NH, Cheitlin MD. Congenital heart disease: Gated MR imaging in 72 patients. *Radiology* 1986; 158:227.

152. Kersting-Summerhoff BA, Sechtem UP, Fisher MR, Higgins CB. MR of congenital anomalies of the aortic arch. *AJR* 1987; 149:9.

153. Fletcher BD, Jacobstein MD, Nelson AD, Riemenschneider TA, Alfidi RJ. Gated magnetic resonance imaging of congenital cardiac malformations. *Radiology* 1984; 150:137–140.

154. vonSchulthess G, Higashino SM, Higgins SS, Dier D, Fisher MR, Higgins CB. Coarctation of the aorta: MR imaging. *Radiology* 1986; 158:469–474.

155. Amparo EG, Higgins CB, Shafton EP. Demonstration of coarctation of the aorta by magnetic resonance imaging. *AJR* 1984; 143:1192–1194.

156. Gomes AS, Lois JF, George B, Alpan G, Williams RG. Congenital abnormalities of the aortic arch: MR imaging. *Radiology* 1987; 165:691–695.

157. Nyman R, Hallberg M, Sunnegardh J, Thuren J, Henze A. Magnetic resonance imaging and angiography in the assessment of coarctation of the aorta. *Acta Radiol* 1989; 30:481–485.

158. Rees S, Firmin D, Mohiaddin R, Underwood R, Longmore D. Application of flow measurements and magnetic resonance velocity mapping to congenital heart disease. *Am J Cardiol* 1989; 64:953–956.

159. Brenner LD, Caputo GR, Mostbeck G, Steiman D, Dulce M, Cheitlin MD, et al. Quantitation of left to right atrial shunts with velocity-encoded cine nuclear magnetic imaging. *J Am Coll Cardiol* 1992; 20:1246–1250.

160. Holmvang G, Palacios I, Vlahakes G, Dinsmore R, Miller S, Liberthson RR, et al. Imaging and sizing of atrial septal defects by magnetic resonance. *Circulation* 1995; 92:3473–3480.

161. Go R, O'Donnell JK, Underwood DA, Feiglin DH, Salcedo EE, Pantoja M, et al. Comparison of gated cardiac MRI and 2D echocardiography of intracardiac neoplasm. *AJR* 1985; 145:21–25.

162. Freedberg RS, Krozon I, Runnancik WN, Liebeskind D. The contribution of magnetic resonance imaging to the evaluation of intracardiac tumors, diagnosed by echocardiography. *Circulation* 1988; 77:96–103.

163. Lund JT, Ehman RL, Julsrud PR, Sinak LJ, Tajik AJ. Cardiac masses: Assessment by MR imaging. *AJR* 1989; 152:469–473.

164. Casolo F, Biasi S, Balzarii L, Borroni M, Ceglia E, Petrillo R, et al. MRI as an adjunct to echocardiography for the diagnostic imaging of cardiac masses. *Eur J Radiol* 1988; 88:226–230.

165. Winkler M, Higgins CB. Suspected intracardiac masses: Evaluation with MR imaging. *Radiology* 1987; 165:117–122.

166. Dooms GC, Higgins CB. MR imaging of cardiac thrombi. *J Comput Assist Tomogr* 1986; 10:415–420.

20

POSITRON EMISSION TOMOGRAPHY

Heinrich R. Schelbert

Positron emission tomography (PET) exceeds the capability of conventional single photon emission computed tomography (SPECT). It offers the opportunity to probe and to define in absolute units regional functional processes in the human heart, including blood flow to biochemical reaction rates, substrate fluxes, and neuronal activity. The many positron-emitting, biologically active tracers, the truly quantitative imaging capability, and the in vivo application of tracer kinetic principles are unique to PET. They permit a comprehensive characterization of the physiology and pathophysiology of the human heart that might offer novel insights into its function and that can aid in the diagnosis and management of patients with cardiovascular disease.

This chapter describes how PET can be applied to the diagnosis and characterization of coronary artery disease (CAD) and to the evaluation of the effect of CAD on regional myocardial tissue function and how PET can decisively affect patient management.

DIAGNOSIS AND CHARACTERIZATION OF CORONARY ARTERY DISEASE

General Considerations

Unlike more conventional radionuclide approaches, PET relies almost exclusively on pharmacologic stress for the detection of CAD, the determination of its extent, and the assessment of the functional significance of coronary stenoses. This requirement exists because the transmission images, essential for correction of photon attenuation, must be acquired with the patient in exactly the same position as during the emission images.

The most frequently used pharmacologic stress agents are dipyridamole and adenosine. Both agents afford the determination of the myocardial flow reserve as the ratio of hyperemic to resting blood flows. The now classic study by Gould and coworkers[1] demonstrated a curvilinear, inverse correlation between severity of stenosis and hyperemic blood flows or

flow reserve. Thus, the magnitude of an attenuated response of blood flow during dipyridamole-induced hyperemia depends on the hemodynamic severity of the stenosis. As demonstrated by quantitative flow measurements with either ^{15}O-water or ^{13}N-ammonia, both dipyridamole and adenosine, which are direct vascular smooth muscle dilators, evoke variable hyperemic responses among different patients, although on average they increase blood flow four- to fivefold.[2-5] This increase in flow with stimulation has been termed *flow reserve*. Both vasodilator agents evoke comparable hyperemic flow responses.[5] Higher doses of dipyridamole, for example, at rates of 0.84 mg per kilogram of body weight (as compared to the standard dose of 0.56 mg/kg), do not augment hyperemic blood flows further, nor do they reduce the variability of the flow responses between individuals.[6]

There is increasing evidence that the myocardial flow reserve declines progressively with age (Fig. 20-1).[7-9] While a decline in vasodilator capacity appears to be one contributing factor, the major determinant is an age-dependent rise in baseline blood flow in response to a progressive increase in the rate-pressure product, which is a major determinant of blood flow at rest.[7] A progressive decline in vascular compliance with age possibly accounts for the increase in the rate-pressure product.

Increases in the mean arterial blood pressure and, thus, the coronary driving pressure, due to either isometric handgrip exercise or supine bicycle exercise during pharmacologically induced hyperemia, had been predicted to augment the hyperemic response. Both interventions attenuate the maximum flow response, however, presumably as a consequence of increased extravascular resistive forces.[6,10] These factors may also contribute to the less than maximal increases in flow during physical exercise where flow increases in proportion to oxygen demand. These observations suggest further that pharmacologically induced hyperemia might not necessarily prove to be more accurate than exercise in identifying functionally significant coronary stenoses. Even though flows in remote myocardium may rise less with exercise, depending

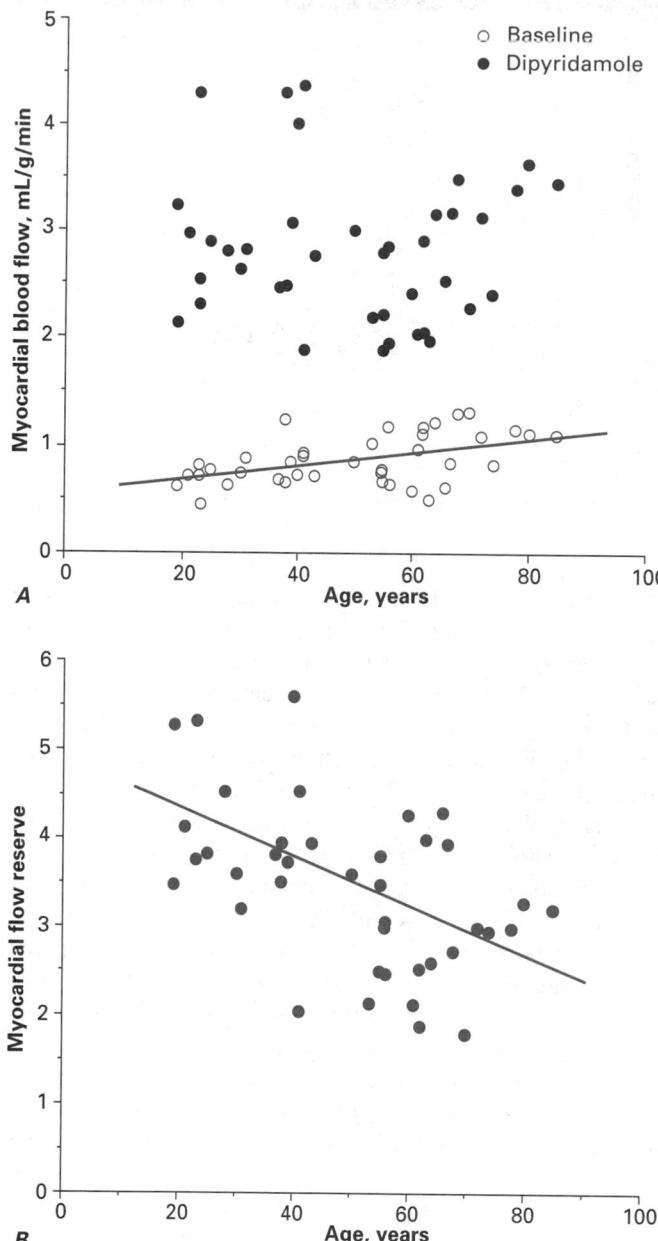

FIGURE 20-1

A. Resting (baseline) and hyperemic (dipyridamole) myocardial blood flows as a function of age determined in 40 normal volunteers. Note the progressive increase in resting blood flow with increasing age, while no statistically significant correlation was noted between hyperemic blood flows and age. *B.* Myocardial flow reserve as the ratio of blood flows determined during hyperemia and at rest as a function of age. (Reproduced with permission of the American Heart Association from Czernin et al.[29])

on the level of cardiac work achieved, both higher intracavitary left ventricular pressures and higher regional wall stress in ischemic or dysfunctional myocardium enhance the extravascular resistive forces so that flow responses in stenosis-dependent myocardium may be even more attenuated or suppressed. Finally, given these differences between ischemia induced pharmacologically or by physical stress, the vasodilator reserve as determined pharmacologically may not neces-

sarily reflect the myocardium's true ability to increase flow during physical exercise.

Detection of Coronary Artery Disease

For the detection of CAD, the relative distribution of myocardial blood flow is examined with the flow tracers ^{82}Rb or ^{13}N-ammonia, initially at rest and then again during pharmacologic vasodilation. Both flow tracers are retained in myocardium in proportion to blood flow. The resulting images depict the distribution of myocardial blood flow at rest and during hyperemia (Fig. 20-2).

Several investigations have confirmed the high diagnostic performance of PET for the detection of CAD.[11–17] Sensitivities range from 87 to 97 percent, and specificities from 78 to 100 percent. Most studies have employed visual analysis of stress and rest images and compared the image findings to the presence or absence of narrowing in lumen diameter of at least 50 to 70 percent found with coronary angiography. One study graded coronary flow reserve by quantitative coronary arteriography.[13] On a scale of 1 to 4, coronary stenoses were classified as moderate to severe if the angiographically predicted coronary flow reserve was less than 3, as intermediate if the coronary flow reserve ranged from 3 to 4, and as minimal for coronary flow reserves of greater than 4. According to this classification, 94 percent of vessels with moderate to severe, 49 percent of vessels with intermediate, and 5 percent of vessels with minimal stenoses were accurately identified with PET and pharmacologic vasodilator stress.

Comparison of PET and SPECT

An early study that used supine bicycle stress and ^{13}N-ammonia in 48 patients with CAD failed to demonstrate significant differences in the diagnostic performance between PET and SPECT.[12] A subsequent report explored the accuracy of PET and SPECT in 202 patients during the same pharmacologic stress.[14] Myocardial blood flow was evaluated with ^{82}Rb at baseline and again 4 min after dipyridamole infusion. About 8 to 9 min later, i.e., 12 to 13 min after the end of the dipyridamole infusion, ^{201}Tl was injected and SPECT imaging performed within 10 min. Both imaging approaches exhibited comparable specificities, whereas PET demonstrated a higher sensitivity than SPECT. When only the 132 patients without prior cardiac events such as angioplasty or bypass grafting were analyzed, the results remained similar. Another study[15] reported somewhat different findings in 81 patients. Again, all patients underwent rest and dipyridamole stress imaging with ^{82}Rb and PET; for the ^{201}Tl SPECT study, 38 (or 47 percent) of the patients underwent treadmill stress testing and the remaining 43 (or 53 percent) received pharmacologic stress with dipyridamole. That study demonstrated comparable sensitivities for PET and SPECT but a higher specificity for PET. The findings were similar for patients submitted to treadmill stress testing and for patients with pharmacologically induced hyperemia.

Both of these studies indicate PET's higher diagnostic accuracy yet differ in terms of higher sensitivities or specificities. In the one study that employed only one hyperemic stress for the administration of both ^{82}Rb and ^{201}Tl,[14] the lower sensitivity for SPECT has been ascribed to a possible dissipation of the hyperemic response from the time of the ^{82}Rb injection to the time of the ^{201}Tl administration, which occurred about 8 to 9 min later. As the hyperemic response to dipyridamole decays with an average half-time of 33 min,[18] hyperemic flows at the time of the ^{201}Tl injection would have been about 17 percent lower than at the time of the ^{82}Rb administration. This modest decline might not explain fully the lower sensitivity of the SPECT approach. While the reason for the higher sensitivity of ^{82}Rb PET therefore remains uncertain, image analysis at different points of the receiver operating curve might provide one explanation. The higher specificity of PET in the second study[15]

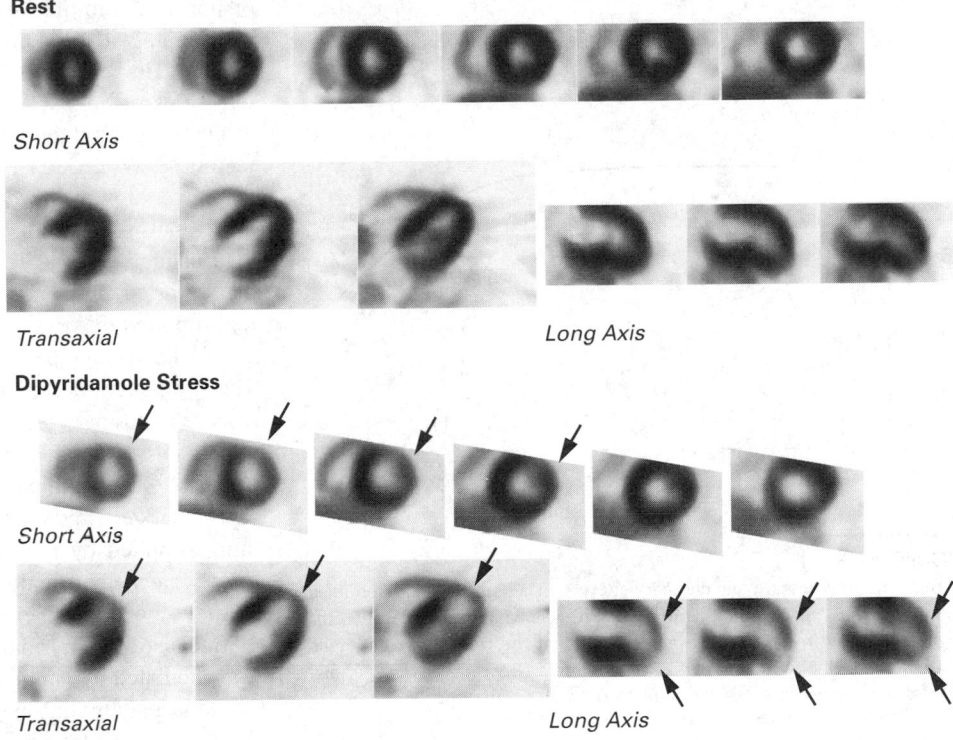

FIGURE 20-2

Rest and dipyridamole stress myocardial perfusion images obtained with ^{13}N-ammonia and PET in a patient with coronary artery disease. In the upper panel, homogeneous tracer uptake at rest is seen on the short axis (*upper row*) and in the transaxial and vertical long axis cuts in the second row. In contrast, the dipyridamole stress images in the lower panels depict a reduction in tracer uptake in the anterior wall consistent with disease of the left anterior descending coronary artery.

most likely resulted from the correction of the images for photon attenuation. The latter can frequently account for false-positive flow defects on ^{201}Tl SPECT images and thus for their lower specificity. Lastly, the absence of a significant difference in diagnostic accuracy in the first of the three comparative studies[12] might be attributed to the use of a first-generation, less advanced PET system and the use of supine bicycle exercise rather than pharmacologic vasodilation.

Taken together, the reported studies demonstrate a statistically significant gain in diagnostic accuracy for the detection of CAD by PET. Although larger clinical trials, especially in previously undiagnosed patients with normal blood flow and normal wall motion at baseline, will be needed for defining the diagnostic gain more clearly, the improved diagnostic accuracy as reported by PET might eliminate additional diagnostic procedures such as coronary arteriography and thus may prove to be cost effective.

Myocardial Blood Flow and Stenosis Severity

Most intriguing for the characterization of human CAD has been the capability of PET to measure regional myocardial blood flow in absolute units. The attainment of accurate and reproducible measurements of regional myocardial blood flow with dynamic PET imaging and flow tracers like ^{15}O-water

and ^{13}N-ammonia has been well established and validated in experimental animals and in humans.[2,3,19–24] This capability allows exploration and definition of the relationships among the angiographic stenosis severity, hyperemic flow responses, and vasodilator capacity.[25–27] Statistically significant correlations were observed between the severity of anatomic stenosis and attenuation of hyperemic response to pharmacologic vasodilation. An inverse, though nonlinear, correlation has been noted between the reduction in cross-sectional area of the stenosis and the myocardial flow reserve in the dependent myocardium (Fig. 20-3),[26] which resembles that observed in animals by Gould and coworkers.[1] To explore the existence of a similar correlation in human CAD, confounding factors such as coronary stenoses in series or stenosis-dependent myocardium also supplied by collateral vessels were excluded from the analysis.[26] Several factors may contribute to the scatter in such data, including possible inaccuracies in regional flow measurements, the variability of the hyperemic response to pharmacologic vasodilation, age-dependent differences in the hyperemic flow response, or differences in the hemodynamic state at baseline. The scatter of the data may also point to a disparity between the anatomic and the functional assessment of the hemodynamic consequences of human coronary artery stenoses. Unlike the controlled and idealized coronary stenosis in the experimental setting,[1] human coronary

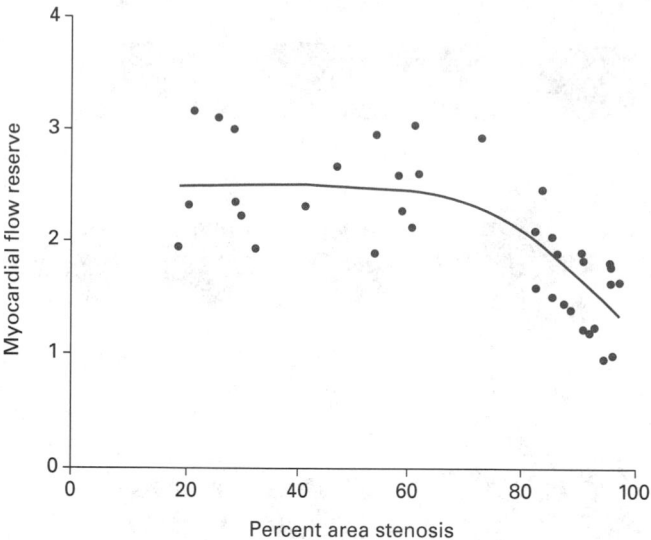

FIGURE 20-3

Myocardial flow reserve and coronary artery stenosis severity as determined by quantitative angiography. Note the curvilinear relationship between the myocardial flow reserve as determined quantitatively from hyperemic and rest blood flow measurements with ^{13}N-ammonia. (Reproduced with permission of the American Heart Association from Di Carli et al.[26])

stenoses reveal remarkably greater morphologic complexities such as eccentricity, differences in inflow and outflow angles of the stenosis, variable lengths, and irregular surfaces. These features may not be fully appreciated by angiographic criteria alone or may not be adequately accounted for by assumptions underlying model-based estimates of stenosis severity. It seems probable that the evaluation of blood flow, either semi-quantitatively or quantitatively, provides accurate information on the functional severity of coronary stenoses and, more broadly, on CAD. Moreover, estimates of an attenuated flow reserve obtained from static images of the relative distribution of myocardial blood flow during hyperemic stress clearly offer invaluable information on the functional significance of a coronary stenosis. In view of the nonlinear increase in the myocardial net uptake of flow tracers in response to increasing myocardial blood flow, however, "semiquantitative" estimates tend to be less accurate than those available from quantitative measurements of blood flow.

Abnormal Coronary Vasomotion and Preclinical Disease

The ability to measure regional myocardial blood flow offers the intriguing possibility of uncovering vasomotor abnormalities that might exist in the early stages of CAD, which would allow the detection of disease during its preclinical stage. Such measurements further offer the prospect of monitoring progression of disease as well as the responses to interventions aimed at regression of disease or slowing or halting its progression. Several lines of evidence support such a possibility.

Flow reserves in myocardial territories subtended by coronary arteries with minimal disease (irregular luminal surfaces) or non-flow-limiting lesions have been found to be reduced in patients with CAD. For example, one study in 12 patients with single-vessel disease reported a flow reserve in such territories of only 2.9 ± 0.9 as compared to 4.1 ± 1.0 in a group of normal healthy volunteers without coronary risk factors.[28] While consistent with a vasomotor abnormality, the lower flow reserve in these patients relative to normal individuals may also be attributable to the normal, age-dependent change.[29] This limitation also applies to another study that reported an average flow reserve of about 2.5 for territories supplied by vessels with less than 50 percent area stenosis.[26] The average patient age in this study was 66 ± 8 years. The previously described correlation between age and flow reserve in normal volunteers[29] predicts a flow reserve of 2.82, which is comparable with the above value noted in these patients. Other studies in patients with single-vessel disease report markedly reduced hyperemic flow responses in myocardium supplied by normal coronary arteries when compared to age-matched normal volunteers.[30] Thus, studies with dipyridamole-induced hyperemia have remained inconclusive.

Because the dipyridamole test primarily explores vasodilation mediated by smooth muscle, interventions designed to examine endothelial-mediated flow increases may be more suitable for the detection of preclinical or minimal CAD. For example, cold pressor testing has been shown to uncover abnormalities in endothelial function.[31] Further, in minimally diseased coronary arteries, this intervention caused constriction or no changes in the diameter of epicardial vessels as compared to a consistently observed dilation of normal vessels.[32] Used in conjunction with flow measurements and PET, cold pressor testing produced regional flow reductions in clinically diseased coronary territories and blunted flow responses in mildly diseased coronary territories in patients with CAD.[33] These intriguing observations are based on only a small patient sample, however, and await further confirmation.

In patients with hypercholesterolemia, hyperemic flows induced by dipyridamole averaged 2.6 ± 4 mL/min per gram as compared to 4.3 ± 0.5 mL/min per gram for normal age-matched controls (Fig. 20-4).[34] This diminished response resulted in significantly lower flow reserves in the hypercholesterolemia patients than in normal individuals (2.9 ± 0.9 vs. 4.3 ± 0.5; $p < .001$). Also, a significant inverse correlation occurs between the flow reserve and the ratio of total cholesterol to high-density lipoprotein cholesterol (Fig. 20-5). Although other factors such as differences in blood viscosity might have contributed to the observed differences, the high plasma cholesterol levels may have caused endothelial dysfunction with impaired nitric oxide formation, which, in turn, would account for a lack of flow-mediated, endothelial-dependent augmentation of hyperemic blood flows (see also Chaps. 4 and 44).

Measurements of myocardial blood flow can reveal the effects of cardiovascular conditioning on the coronary microcirculation. In one study, cardiovascular conditioning included regular exercise, lipid-lowering diet, weight loss, and lifestyle changes.[35] As depicted in Fig. 20-6, myocardial flow reserve improved (even over a 6-week period) by 20 percent from 2.8 ± 1.1 to 3.4 ± 0.9. The improvement resulted from both a decline in resting blood flow and an increase in hyperemic blood flow. Lower rate-pressure products after cardiovascular conditioning accounted for the decreased blood flows at rest. The reasons for the increased vasodilator capacity are less certain. They might include less extravascular resistive forces, changes in blood viscosity, increases in capillary densities, or an improved endothelial function as a consequence of lower cholesterol levels.

Similar mechanisms, together with direct effects on the coronary stenoses and their structural elements and configuration, may have accounted for the changes in the extent and severity of flow defects on perfusion imaging with PET reported in patients with CAD who had undergone a 5-year program of rigorous risk-factor modification.[36] In this randomized control trial, patients changed to a very low fat vegetarian diet, underwent daily mild to moderate exercise and stress management, and received group support. As depicted in Fig. 20-7, the extent and severity of flow defects in the control group increased during the 5-year period, while the study group revealed mild though statistically significant reductions in the severity and the extent of stress-induced flow defects.

ASSESSMENT
OF MYOCARDIAL VIABILITY

Chronic Coronary Artery Disease and Ischemic Cardiomyopathy

GENERAL CONSIDERATIONS
Distinguishing viable myocardium from nonviable myocardium or scar tissue in areas of impaired contractile function is a problem of considerable clinical importance, but it remains diagnostically challenging. Since both types of functionally compromised myocardium share several common features, including similar degrees of abnormal systolic wall motion, reduced regional blood flow, and electrocardiographic changes, their differentiation can be difficult.[37] What may distinguish a potentially reversible from an irreversible impairment of regional contractile function is the preserved cellular homeostasis, including transmembranous gradients in ion concentrations. Viability requires energy and thus hinges upon the continued production of high-energy phosphates that can be sustained only in the presence of residual blood flow for the continued delivery of substrates and, importantly, re-

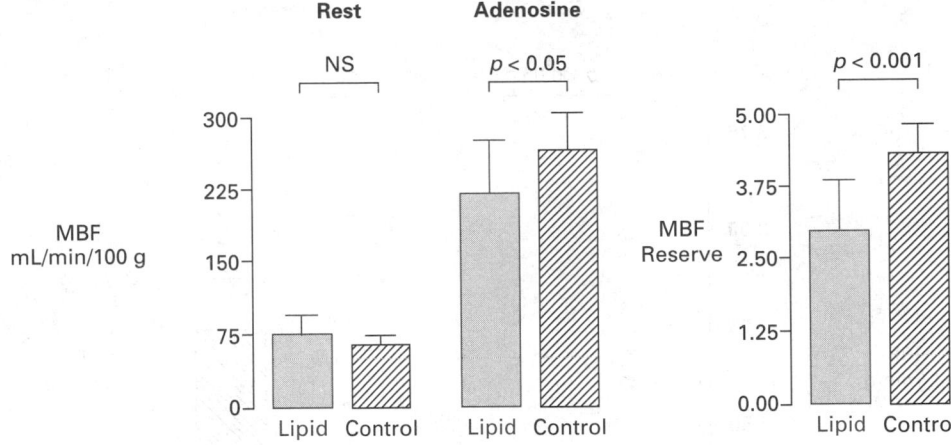

FIGURE 20-4
Myocardial blood flow at rest and during adenosine-induced hyperemia as well as myocardial blood flow (MBF) reserve in patients with hypercholesterolemia (lipid) as compared to normal (control) volunteers. Note the significantly lower hyperemic flows in the hypercholesteremia patients, which result in a markedly attenuated myocardial flow reserve. (Reproduced with permission of the American Heart Association from Dayanikli et al.[34])

moval of inhibitory metabolites such as lactate and hydrogen ions. PET affords the assessment of each of these three aspects of tissue function critical for survival or viability. Cellular homeostasis and ion concentration gradients can be explored with radioactive positron emitting cations,[38,39] such as $^{82}Rb^+$ or $^{38}K^+$, or with the *water perfusable tissue index* as a measure of the fractional tissue volume that is still capable of rapidly exchanging water. The perfusable tissue index can be assessed with ^{15}O-water and ^{15}O-labeled carbon monoxide and red blood cell labeling. The index assumes that only viable myocardium retains the ability to exchange water rapidly. Its potential utility for identifying myocardial viability has been demonstrated in patients early after myocardial infarction and in patients with chronic CAD.[40,41]

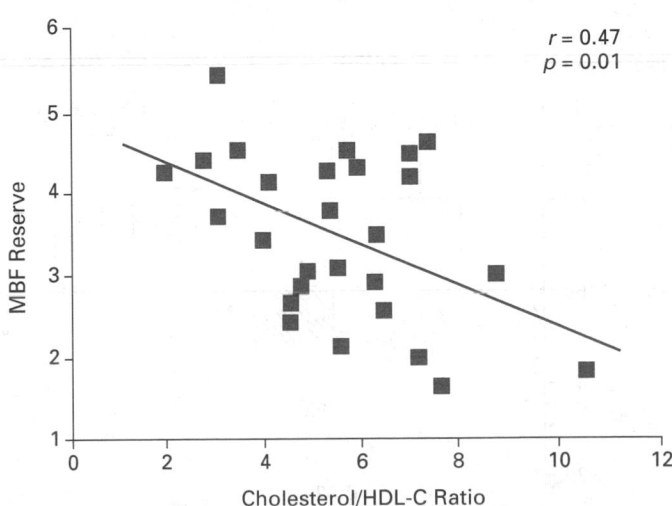

FIGURE 20-5
Correlation between the myocardial blood flow (MBF) reserve and the ratio of total cholesterol to HDL-cholesterol. Note the statistically significant inverse correlation. (Reproduced with permission of the American Heart Association from Dayanikli et al.[34])

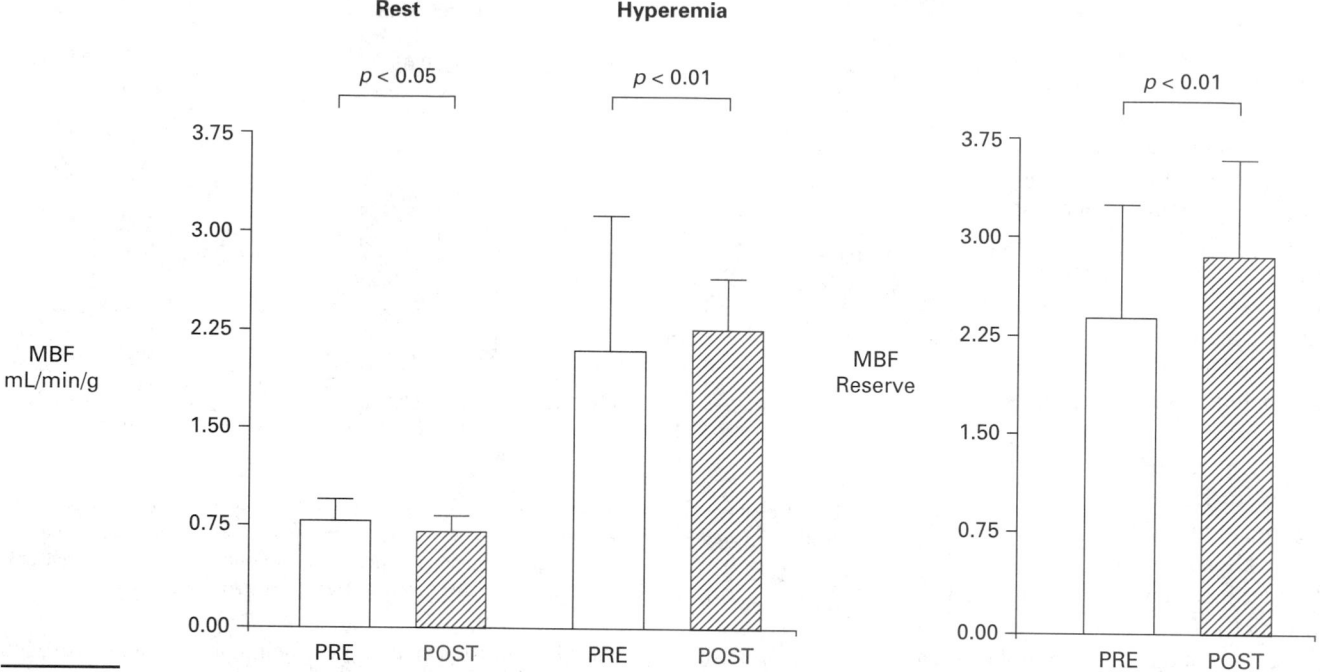

FIGURE 20-6

Effects of 6 weeks of cardiovascular conditioning on myocardial blood flow (MBF) and myocardial flow reserve. The measurements prior to entering the cardiovascular conditioning (pre) are compared to those after 6 weeks (post).

After conditioning, note the significantly lower myocardial blood flows at rest and higher blood flows during hyperemia, resulting in a significant increase in the myocardial flow reserve. (Data plotted from Czernin et al.[7])

The presence of residual blood flow can be determined and its magnitude be quantitated with flow tracers like ^{15}O-water, ^{82}Rb, or ^{13}N-ammonia. As mentioned above and discussed in detail below, however, flow reductions per se discriminate unreliably between viable and nonviable myocardium. Therefore, most PET approaches for identifying viable myocardium rely on probing regional myocardial metabolic activity.

Before discussing metabolic approaches to the assessment of myocardial viability, a short description of the human myocardium's substrate metabolism and the assessment of its various facets with PET radiotracers follows.

MYOCARDIAL SUBSTRATE METABOLISM

Figure 20-8 depicts the major aspects of myocardial substrate metabolism. According to this highly simplified presentation, the myocardium can choose among various substrates, foremost of which are free fatty acids, glucose, lactate, and ketone bodies. Selection of a given fuel substrate depends largely on its concentration in plasma and the overall hormonal milieu.[42,43] These factors in turn are governed by the dietary state, the level of physical activity, and the plasma concentrations of catecholamines and insulin. For example, circulating free fatty acid levels are high and insulin levels are low in the fasting state, and as much as 70 to 80 percent of the myocardium's oxygen consumption can be accounted for by oxidation of free fatty acids.[44] Conversely, oral glucose intake elevates the plasma glucose level

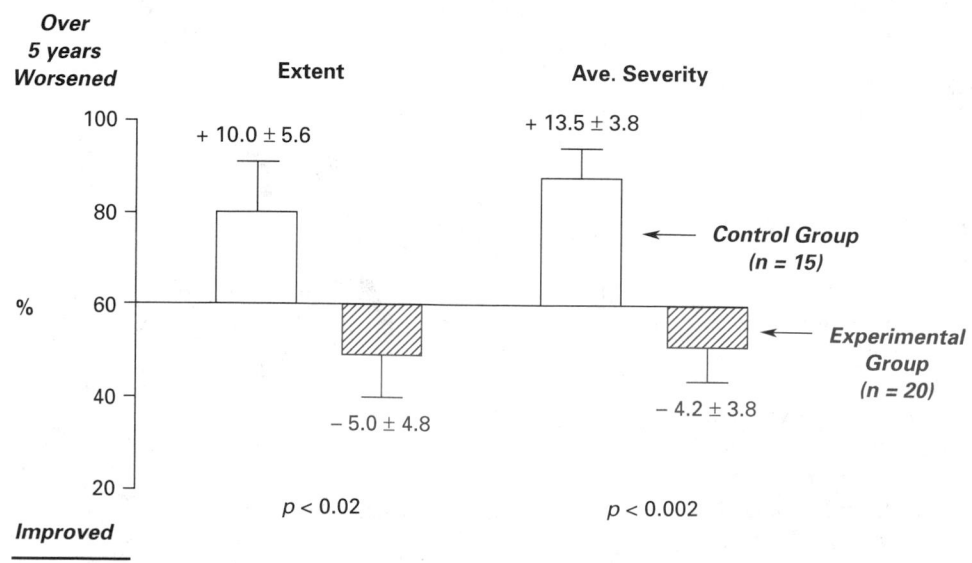

FIGURE 20-7

Changes in the extent and the average severity of flow defects during hyperemia as determined by PET in a control group and a study group submitted to a 5-year coronary risk modification program (see text). (Data taken from Gould et al.[36])

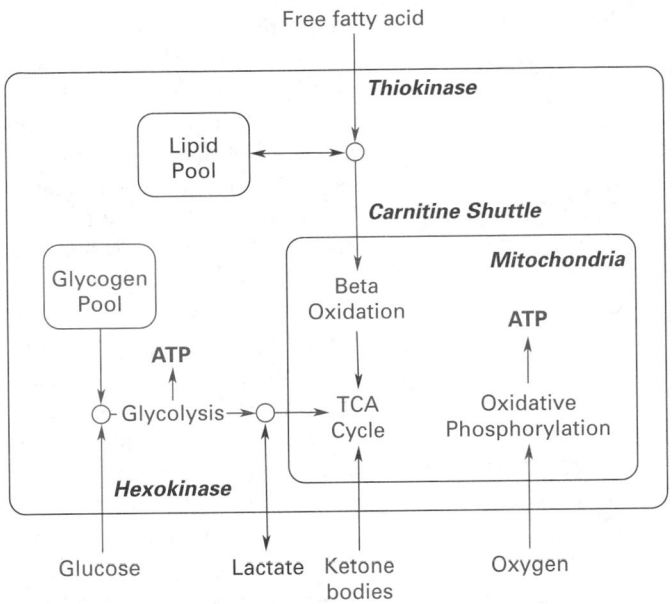

FIGURE 20-8
Highly simplified depiction of the myocardium's substrate metabolism.
(TCA = tricarboxylic acid; ATP = adenosine triphosphate.)

and, in response, the insulin level while it lowers free fatty acid levels; as a result, the myocardium shifts its fuel selection to glucose.[42,45,46] Strenuous physical exercise is associated with increased release of lactate from skeletal muscle. Plasma lactate levels therefore rise, and lactate can become the major fuel substrate.[47] In fact, as much as 60 percent of the oxygen consumption can be accounted for by oxidation of lactate.[47] On the other hand, catecholamines accelerate lipolysis, increasing the concentration of circulating free fatty acids and shifting the heart's substrate selection to free fatty acids.

The hexokinase reaction phosphorylates glucose to glucose-6-phosphate, which may then be used in the synthesis of glycogen, or it may enter glycolysis with pyruvate as its end product. Converted to lactate, it may then leave the myocardium or, if activated to acyl-CoA, it enters the tricarboxylic acid (TCA) cycle as the final oxidative pathway common to most fuel substrates. Exogenous lactate can be converted to pyruvate, which, after esterification to acyl-CoA, enters the TCA cycle.

Free fatty acids, like glucose, enter two different metabolic pathways. Upon entering the cells, they are esterified by the thiokinase reaction to acyl-CoA and then either enter an endogenous lipid pool, consisting mostly of glycerides and phospholipids, or proceed via the carnitine shuttle to the inner mitochondrial membrane, where two-carbon fragments are cleaved from the long chain acyl-CoA units by β-oxidation and engage in the TCA cycle. The TCA cycle metabolizes the 2-carbon acyl-CoA units into CO_2 and H_2O. The rate of flux through the TCA cycle is coupled closely to oxidative phosphorylation, where the energy resulting from the processing of oxygen and hydrogen ions is stored in the high-energy phosphate bonds of adenosine triphosphate (ATP). The latter is shuttled into the cytosol with transfer of energy

to the high-energy phosphate bond of creatine phosphate as a readily available source of energy. Other sites of high-energy production include glycolysis. The energy yields in terms of ATP relative to oxygen differ between the various substrates. For example, for 1 mol of oxygen, glucose yields 6.3 mol ATP, lactate yields 6 mol ATP, and free fatty acids yield 5.7 mol ATP.[48]

Assessment of Glucose Utilization

The initial metabolic step of exogenous glucose metabolism can be evaluated and quantified with [18]F 2-fluoro-2-deoxyglucose. This radiolabeled glucose analogue exchanges across the capillary and sarcolemmal membranes in proportion to glucose, with which it then competes for hexokinase for phosphorylation to ^{18}F-deoxyglucose-6-phosphate.[49–52] Unlike its natural counterpart, the phosphorylated glucose analogue is a poor substrate for glycogen formation, glycolysis, and the fructose-pentose shunt; its rate of dephosphorylation is low in the myocardium. Also, it is relatively impermeable to the cell membrane. Thus, the phosphorylated tracer becomes virtually trapped in the cell, allowing images of the myocardial ^{18}F activity concentrations acquired about 40 to 60 min after tracer injection to reflect the relative distributions of exogenous glucose utilization rates. Because the compound traces only the initial steps of glucose utilization (up to the branch point between glycogen synthesis and glycolysis; Fig. 20-8), it offers no direct information on glycolytic rates, glucose oxidation, or glycogen synthesis. In states of glycogen depletion, for example, during ischemia, exogenous glucose serves as the major source of glycolytic flux, and ^{18}F-deoxyglucose appears to offer an estimate of the rate of glycolysis.

The tissue kinetics of ^{18}F-deoxyglucose have been described by a unidirectional transport model,[49–52] which affords the quantification of regional rates of myocardial glucose utilization through relatively simple, rapid, and computationally efficient analyses.[53,54] With this tracer approach, rates of exogenous glucose utilization of 0.64 ± 0.18 μmol/min per gram have been reported for the post-glucose absorption state and of 0.24 ± 0.18 μmol/min per gram for the fasted state.[55]

Myocardial Fatty Acid Metabolism

This aspect of the heart's metabolism can be evaluated qualitatively with ^{11}C-labeled palmitate.[56–60] The labeled long-chain fatty acid participates fully in the metabolic rate of its natural counterpart (Fig. 20-8). Once esterified to acyl-CoA, a fraction of tracer label proceeds via the carnitine shuttle into mitochondria for β-oxidation and oxidation via the TCA cycle. The radiolabel is released from the myocardium in the form of [11]CO_2.[61,62] The remaining fraction of the initially extracted and activated tracer enters the intracellular lipid pool mainly in the form of di- and triglycerides and phospholipids. The biexponential morphology of the recorded tissue-time activity curve reflects the metabolic fate of the tracer (Fig. 20-9). The slow turnover rate of the intracellular lipid pool accounts for the slow-clearance phase, while the rapid-clearance curve

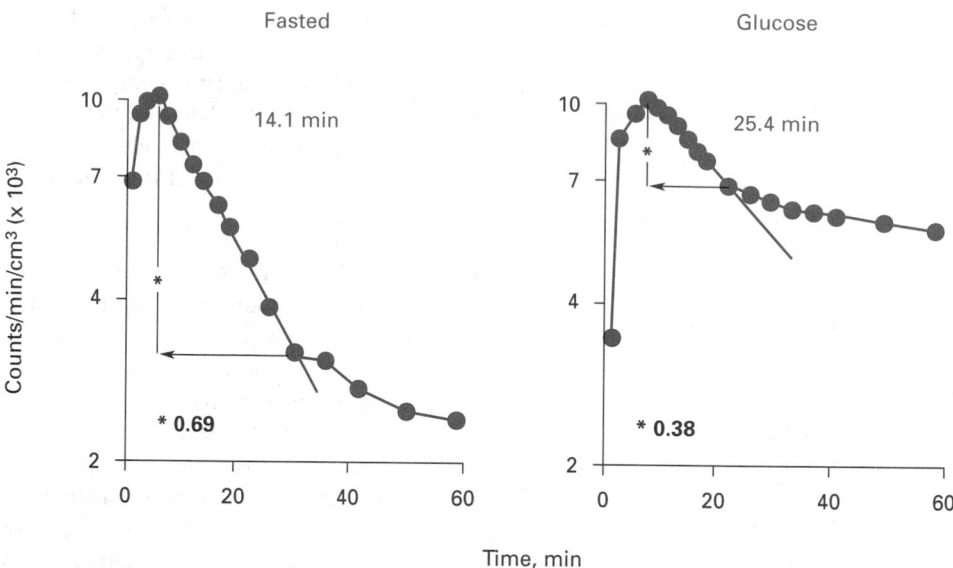

FIGURE 20-9

Myocardial time-activity curves derived from serially acquired images following the intravenous administration of ^{11}C-palmitate. Both time-activity curves were obtained in a normal volunteer. The curve shown on the left was recorded with the volunteer in the fasting state, the one on the right after oral administration of 100 g glucose. Note the biexponential clearance curve morphology for both time-activity curves. In the fasting state, however, the clearance half-time is markedly shorter than after glucose loading, while the relative size of the rapid clearance curve component declines from the fasting to the glucose-loaded state. The change in the clearance curve morphology is consistent with a change in the myocardium's substrate utilization from primarily free fatty acid to glucose when, during the same amount of cardiac work, disproportionately less glucose is oxidized after glucose loading.

component corresponds to the fraction of tracer that has entered oxidative pathways directly and to its rate of oxidation.

A change in the myocardium's preferential substrate utilization as a result of changing plasma substrate concentrations can be demonstrated with either ^{11}C-palmitate, ^{18}F-deoxyglucose, or both.[45,50,54] In the presence of high free fatty acid and low glucose and insulin levels in plasma, the preferential metabolism of free fatty acid is reflected in the ^{11}C-palmitate myocardial tissue curve by the relatively large size of the rapid-clearance phase and its steep slope (both corresponding to increased fatty acid oxidation) and by the low or even undetectable ^{18}F-deoxyglucose uptake in the myocardium. Ingestion of carbohydrates raises plasma glucose levels, stimulates insulin secretion, and depresses fatty acid plasma levels. In response, the myocardium shifts to glucose as its preferred substrate. This shift is reflected on the tissue clearance curve by a decline in the size and slope of the rapid-clearance phase of ^{11}C-palmitate and by an increase in myocardial ^{18}F-deoxyglucose uptake.

Myocardial Oxygen Consumption

Preliminary studies have demonstrated the possibility of measuring myocardial oxygen consumption directly using molecular ^{15}O-oxygen administered by inhalation. PET measures the extraction of labeled oxygen; if multiplied by myocardial blood flow,[63,64] the mass of oxygen consumed per minute per gram of myocardium can be obtained. More widely applied is ^{11}C-labeled acetate as a tool for probing myocardial oxidative

metabolism and, thus, oxygen consumption. The radiotracer rapidly clears from blood into the myocardium and produces high signal-to-background images.[65-71] The rate of clearance of ^{11}C activity from the myocardium, as derived from serially acquired images, corresponds to the TCA cycle activity. Since the latter is closely coupled to oxidative phosphorylation, ^{11}C-acetate clearance rates reflect rates of oxidative metabolism and myocardial oxygen consumption. It should be emphasized that the tracer does not yield mass fluxes but only rate constants. These, however, can be converted into units of O_2 per minute per gram of myocardium. Unlike ^{11}C-palmitate or ^{18}F-deoxyglucose, the clearance rate of ^{11}C-acetate from the myocardium is relatively insensitive to changes in myocardial preferential utilization of substrate. A tracer compartment model, based on biochemical assays of the tracer tissue kinetics in isolated rat hearts,[72] has been tested in vivo in animal experiments and promises to yield estimates of myocardial oxygen consumption in absolute units in the human heart.[73]

METABOLIC ALTERATIONS IN MYOCARDIAL ISCHEMIA AND VIABILITY

Observations in experimental animals provide the foundation for the detection of myocardial viability. These early studies indicate that alterations in substrate metabolism in response to acute myocardial ischemia could be demonstrated noninvasively with positron emitting tracers of myocardial substrate metabolism. Consistent with the known impairment in fatty acid oxidation,[74,75] the initial uptake of ^{11}C-palmitate and its subsequent rate of clearance from the myocardium were markedly diminished in acutely ischemic myocardium.[60,76] Additionally, the known increase in glucose extraction and glucose utilization[42,74] was reflected by a regional increase in ^{18}F-deoxyglucose uptake.[77] Initial studies in patients with clinical evidence of acute myocardial ischemia revealed findings that were virtually identical to those in animals, e.g., enhanced ^{18}F-deoxyglucose uptake in hypoperfused dysfunctional myocardial regions. The observation of a similar pattern in patients with chronic CAD who did not have clinical signs of acute ischemia was unexpected (Fig. 20-10). This finding has raised the question as to whether or not the blood flow–metabolism pattern is unique to acute ischemia or whether it represents a more general metabolic pattern in chronically dysfunctional and hypoperfused myocardium. Observations in other patients with CAD were no less intriguing as they had a segmentally reduced ^{18}F-deoxyglucose uptake that paralleled the reduction in regional myocardial blood flow (Fig. 20-11).[78] A more systematic exploration of these findings in patients slated for surgical coronary artery bypass grafting confirmed the hypothesis that the regionally enhanced ^{18}F-deoxyglucose uptake, in contrast to a reduction, reflected sustained glucose utilization and, thus, metabolic activity that was evidence of viability in myocardium despite complete or partial loss of contractile function.[79] These studies demonstrated that the *restoration of tissue perfusion resulted in an improvement or even normalization of contractile function in myocardium with persistent glucose metabolic activity but not in myocardium without such activity* (Fig. 20-12).

MECHANISMS OF THE BLOOD FLOW–METABOLISM PATTERN

The observations described above support the clinical relevance of these PET findings, although their mechanisms remain uncertain. Patients with CAD undergoing supine bicycle stress who had stress-induced flow defects have demonstrated an augmented ^{18}F-deoxyglucose uptake when the radiotracer was administered 20 to 30 min after exercise and after the stress-induced flow defect had resolved.[80] This implies that such enhanced tracer uptake represents "stunned myocardium," as supported by earlier animal experimental observations.[81] These latter studies demonstrated the evolution of a blood flow–metabolism pattern in chronically reperfused myocardium: an immediate postreperfusion decrease in glucose uptake that was followed by an increase

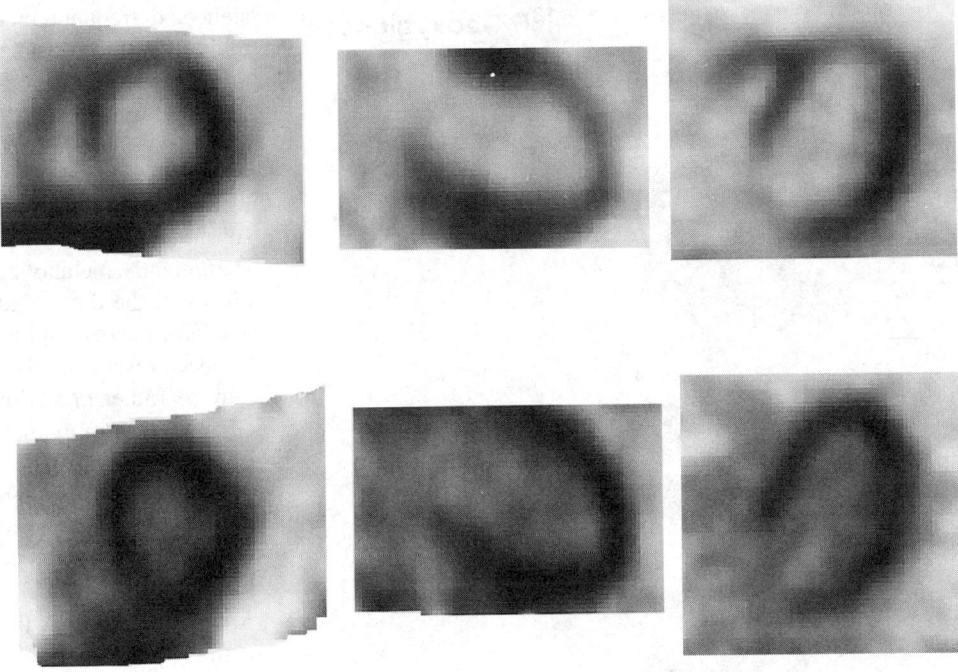

FIGURE 20-10

Myocardial blood flow imaging in a patient with depressed left ventricular function and advanced coronary artery disease. The upper panel depicts myocardial blood flow at rest (resting perfusion), and the lower panel depicts the myocardial uptake of ^{18}F-deoxyglucose (metabolism). Short-axis images are shown on the left, vertical long-axis images in the center, and horizontal long-axis images on the right. Note the reduced flow in the anterior wall and the intraventricular septum, while glucose uptake is normally preserved.

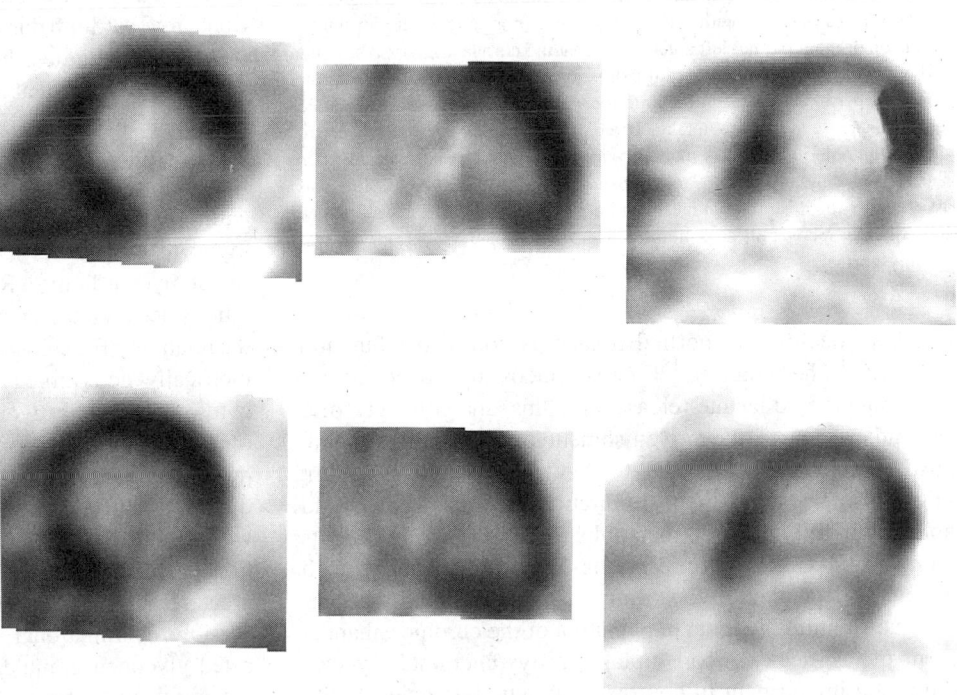

FIGURE 20-11

Blood flow and ^{18}F-deoxyglucose imaging in a patient with ischemic cardiomyopathy. Again, short- and long-axis images are shown as in Fig. 20-10. Note the extensive perfusion defect in the inferolateral and posterolateral wall, which is associated on the ^{18}F-deoxyglucose study with a concordant reduction in glucose utilization.

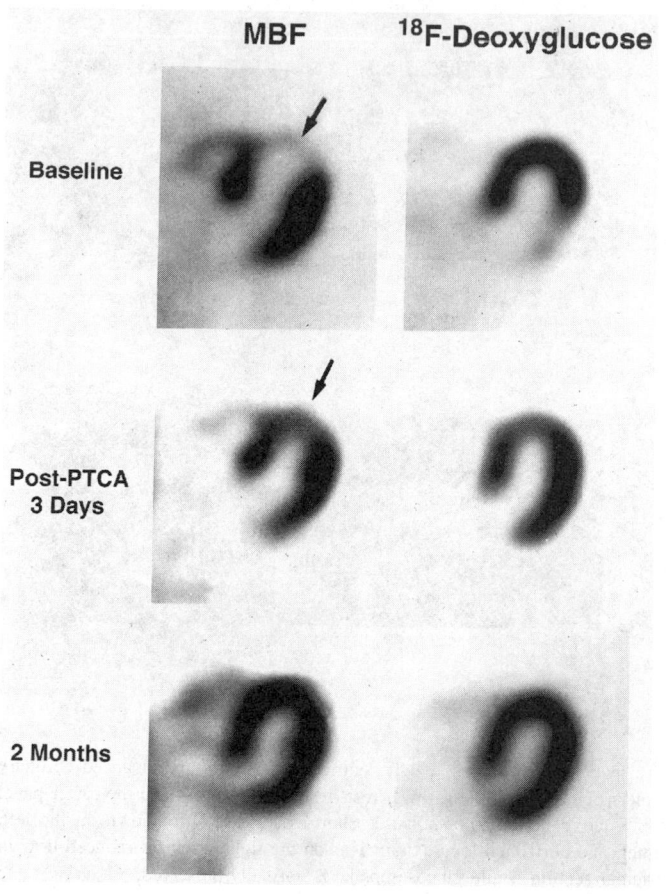

MBF ^{18}F-Deoxyglucose

Baseline

Post-PTCA
3 Days

2 Months

FIGURE 20-12

Serial blood flow images obtained with ^{13}N ammonia (MBF) and glucose uptake images obtained with ^{18}F-deoxyglucose in a patient with a subtotal occlusion of the proximal left anterior descending coronary artery at baseline and 3 days and 2 months following coronary angioplasty (PTCA). Note the extensive perfusion defect in the anterior wall at baseline associated with a marked increase in glucose uptake. Three days following angioplasty, perfusion to the anterior wall has markedly improved and has normalized when reexamined 2 months later. The extensive perfusion defect at baseline was associated with severe hypokinesis and akinesis of the anterior wall, which subsequently recovered; at 2 months, wall motion of the anterior wall was entirely normal.

that later declined to normal uptake as contractile function returned.[81] The enhanced ^{18}F-deoxyglucose uptake was attributed to increased lactate release and, thus, anaerobic glycolysis, rather than to the replenishment of glycogen stores in postischemic myocardium.[82,83] Such a metabolic pattern might also be found in postinfarction patients[84] but would not explain fully the flow-metabolism observations in patients with chronic CAD. More recent observations in patients with collateral-dependent myocardium raise the possibility of "repetitive stunning"[85] as an explanation of the chronic enhancement of ^{18}F-deoxyglucose uptake in dysfunctional myocardium. An impairment in contractile function associated with enhanced glucose utilization has been noted in collateral-dependent myocardium only if its flow reserve were markedly restricted.[86] Such a loss of flow reserve would limit the ability of the coronary circulation to respond appropriately to tran-

sient and frequent increases in oxygen demand, producing multiple transient ischemic episodes, each followed by stunning and further hindering the recovery of contractile function.

In addition to repetitive stunning, "myocardial hibernation" is also possible.[87,88] This postulated downregulation of contractile function in response to diminished resting blood flow would then be associated with a change in the myocardium's substrate metabolism with a dominant role for glucose, which is efficiently metabolized. *Hibernation* in its truest sense implies that the downregulated energy requirements match the available energy supply. Thus, a new supply-demand balance has been reset at a lower level. Such a new balance, however, may be rather precarious as modest increases in demand or decreases in supply may unsettle this steady state and produce ischemia. It is possible and likely that in many patients both hibernation and stunning coexist to varying extents. Recent observations in experimental animals suggest that reductions in both blood flow and contractile function can be maintained for as long as 1 week without significant necrosis but with structural alterations that resemble those observed in patients with chronic CAD.[89–91] The sustained reduction in flow was found to be associated with an initial, transient increase in lactate release but a persistent increase in glucose utilization. Thus, these studies might provide an underpinning for the concept of hibernation (see also Chap. 43).

ULTRASTRUCTURAL AND HISTOCHEMICAL OBSERVATIONS

Other attempts to gain mechanistic insights into the enhanced ^{18}F-deoxyglucose uptake include morphometric and histochemical analyses of biopsy specimens obtained from dysfunctional myocardium during surgical revascularization. Based on prior autopsy studies, there exists a general correlation between the degree of regional myocardial fibrosis and the severity of the impairment of regional contractile function, although there are exceptions.[92] In some instances dyskinetic myocardium is free of fibrosis or, conversely, some normally contracting myocardium contains as much as 40 percent fibrosis.[93] "Abnormal" myocytes (Fig. 20-13) also are present in chronically dysfunctional myocardium.[94] Recent investigations have noted correlations between the externally determined relative blood flow, the relative ^{18}F-deoxyglucose concentrations, and the morphometrically determined fractions of fibrosis, abnormal myocytes, and normal myocardium.[86,95,96] Various studies agree on a general correlation between relative blood flow and the percentage of tissue fibrosis (Fig. 20-14) but differ in regard to the fraction of abnormal myocytes. In one study, this fraction was virtually the same in reversibly and irreversibly dysfunctional myocardium,[95] while another study noted a significantly greater fraction of abnormal myocytes in reversibly than in irreversibly dysfunctional myocardium.[96] Because centrally located glycogen granules are one of the key features of such abnormal myocytes and because of a statistically significant correlation between the fraction of such abnormal myocytes and the relative ^{18}F-deoxyglucose uptake, those abnormal myocytes have been thought of as the ultrastructural correlate of the enhanced ^{18}F-deoxyglucose uptake.

Other observations, however, argue against such an explanation. Electron microscopy and histochemistry of biopsy samples retrieved from the center of the dysfunctional myocardial wall during surgical bypass grafting have demonstrated a more heterogeneous pattern of morphologic alterations in myocardium with blood flow–metabolism mismatches.[97] Despite identical flow-metabolism findings, nearly half of the 24 patients in this study exhibited minimal, if any, significant morphologic changes, while others demonstrated abnormalities consistent with those described earlier. Such heterogeneity in morphologic alterations argue against the structurally abnormal myocyte and, especially, the glycogen granules as an explanation of the enhanced ^{18}F-deoxyglucose uptake.

ABNORMAL MYOCYTES IN CHRONICALLY DYSFUNCTIONAL MYOCARDIUM

At present, it remains uncertain whether abnormal myocytes are unique to a particular pathophysiologic mechanism underlying the chronic, though potentially reversible, impairment of contractile function. Some investigators postulate that they can result from the following: (1) contractile unloading, (2) increased wall stress (stretch), or (3) a metabolic substrate switch to preferential glucose utilization.[98] The expression and distribution patterns of other cellular constituents, such as of α-smooth muscle actin, cardiotin, and titin, as well as an increased expression of glucose transporter I (GLUT I) mRNA,[99] features that resemble those in embryonic and/or neonatal myocytes, led to the notion that such abnormal myocytes might represent "dedifferentiation."[98] Histochemical analysis revealed alterations in the extracellular matrix, with increased amounts of collagen and fibronectin surrounding the abnormal myocytes. The absence of true degenerative changes has lent further claim to support the possibility of myocyte differentiation. Other evidence, on the other hand, suggests a progressive deterioration of the morphology and metabolism of the cell, initially with few if any structural changes but with a switch in substrate selection to glucose, either because of its greater oxygen efficiency or because of loss of enzymes essential for fatty acid oxidation; this is followed by loss of sarcomeres and sarcoplasmatic

reticulum, accumulation of glycogen, and mitochondrial and nuclear alterations, ultimately leading to cell death and scar tissue formation.[97] Several investigations point to the high prevalence of blood flow—metabolism mismatch patterns in patients with prior myocardial infarctions.[78,100] The decline in the incidence of these mismatches as a function of time after an acute myocardial infarction[101] seems to support such progression and raises the question whether or not a new supply-demand balance reset at a lower level can be sustained permanently. If not, then the blood flow–metabolism mismatch represents a transient rather than permanent state of reversibly dysfunctional myocardium. Consequently, prompt restoration of adequate tissue perfusion via interventional revascularization would be essential clinically, regardless of whether the abnormal myocytes represent dedifferentiation or degeneration. As it remains uncertain at what stage the structural alterations become irreversible, it would seem that the return of contractile function may ultimately depend upon the amount of connective tissue. As another clinical implication, the presence of structural changes in viable myocardium as demonstrated with blood flow–metabolism imaging implies

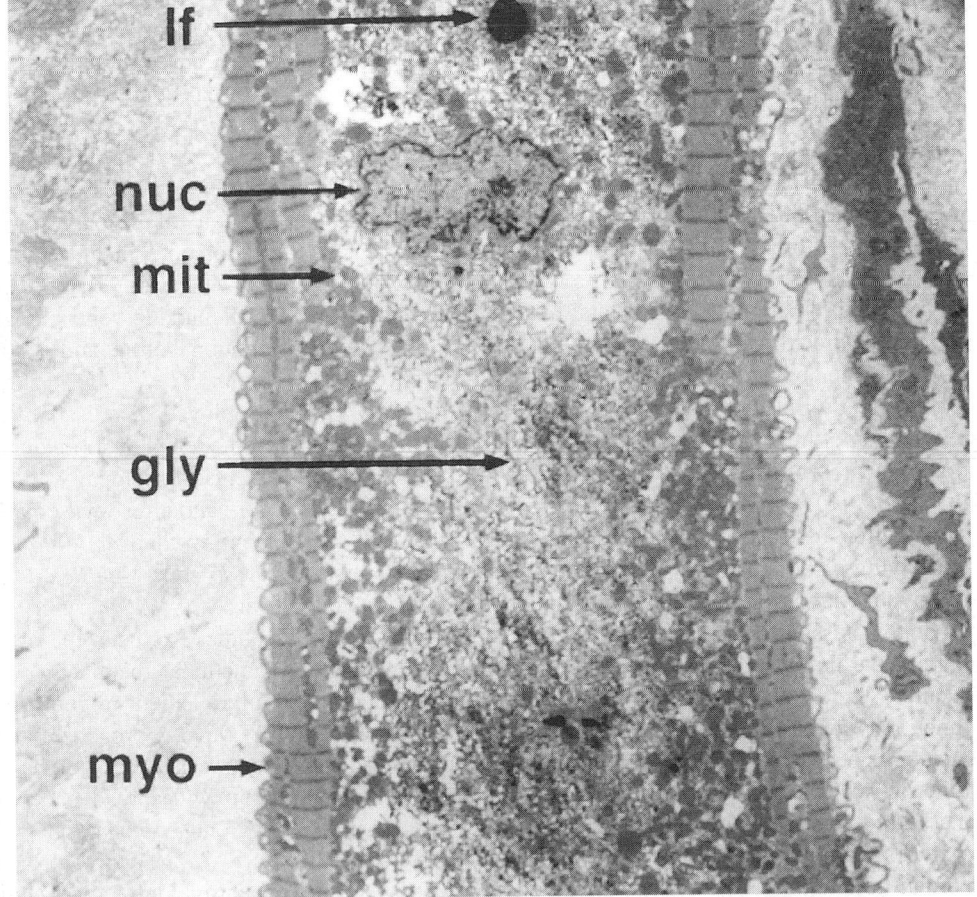

FIGURE 20-13

Abnormal myocyte as found in a biopsy sample from a patient with chronic dysfunction of the anterior wall. Note the irregularly shaped nucleus (nuc), the central loss of myofibrils (myo), and the extensive deposition of glycogen (gly). In addition, lipofuscin (lf) droplets and the numerous small mitochondria (mit) are noted. (Courtesy of M. Borgers, Maastricht, The Netherlands.)

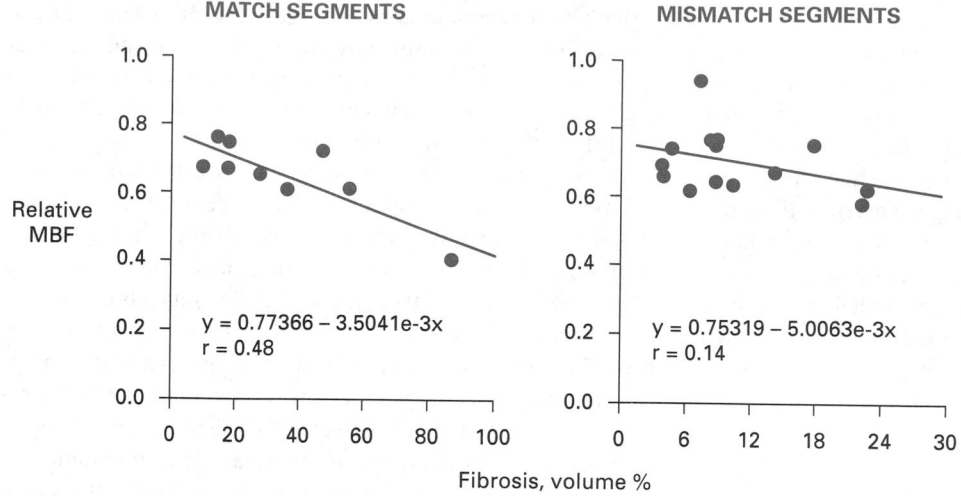

MATCH SEGMENTS

MISMATCH SEGMENTS

$y = 0.77366 - 3.5041\text{e-}3x$
$r = 0.48$

$y = 0.75319 - 5.0063\text{e-}3x$
$r = 0.14$

Fibrosis, volume %

FIGURE 20-14

Correlation between the relative myocardial blood flow (MBF) and the fraction of tissue fibrosis as determined from transmural biopsy samples obtained during bypass grafting. (Data plotted from Maes et al.[95])

that if the contractile machinery in abnormal or dedifferentiated myocytes can be reconstructed, the recovery of contractile function will not be immediate but rather will occur slowly, as clinical investigations have demonstrated.[102,103]

Viability Assessment in the Clinical Setting

Imaging of blood flow and metabolism with PET offers several approaches to the assessment of myocardial viability. The most widely applied approach entails evaluation of the relative distribution of blood flow and of the utilization of exogenous glucose with ^{18}F-deoxyglucose. The initial studies exploring this concept in patients with regional myocardial dysfunction have uncovered the following three distinct patterns: (1) blood flow and metabolism are normal, (2) blood flow is reduced but glucose utilization is enhanced or at least markedly exceeds flow ("mismatch"), and (3) blood flow and glucose uptake are both decreased concordantly ("match").[79] While the terms *match* and *mismatch* are purely operational, they might infer, at least to some extent, some insights into the underlying pathophysiology. Normal flow and/or metabolism in a hypocontractile area might represent stunned myocardium while the classic mismatch might be consistent with hibernating myocardium. Both patterns predict with a 74 to 92 percent accuracy a postrevascularization improvement in contractile function, whereas the concordant reduction in blood flow and metabolism predicts with a 74 to 88 percent accuracy that function will not improve.[79,104,105] It should be emphasized that the reduction in regional flow for both matches and mismatches may vary considerably between patients. Modest concordant reductions in both blood flow and ^{18}F-deoxyglucose uptake would indicate a prior nontransmural infarction as compared to the more severe reduction of both following transmural infarction. Also, flow reductions in mismatches may vary considerably as a reflection of varying degrees of transmural involvement.

Another conceptually identical approach evaluates regional myocardial blood flow with ^{99m}Tc-sestamibi and SPECT and evaluates glucose metabolism with ^{18}F-deoxyglucose and PET. The predictive accuracy of this hybrid approach matches that of the pure PET approach. More recent developments indicate that both blood flow (with either ^{99m}Tc-sestamibi or ^{201}Tl) and metabolism with ^{18}F-deoxyglucose can be evaluated with SPECT, using either high-energy photon collimation[106–108] or coincidence detection SPECT systems.[109,110]

Lastly, another approach entails the assessment of glucose utilization only. This approach derives from comparative studies with gated magnetic resonance imaging and PET and assumes that regional reductions in ^{18}F-deoxyglucose greater than 50 percent relative to remote myocardium represent irreversible contractile dysfunction, whereas mildly reduced or normal uptake indicates the presence of reversible dysfunction.[111,112] While this has been used for some time as a benchmark for defining the accuracy of ^{201}Tl-based techniques for assessing myocardial viability,[111] recent studies have tested the validity of this particular approach against the postrevascularization outcome in regional contractile function.[113]

Most studies have employed either echocardiography or radionuclide ventriculography for evaluating segmental wall motion before and 1 to 3 months following revascularization.[79,104,105,112–117] A majority of these investigations have employed visual analysis of regional wall motion, whereas some relied on more quantitative approaches such as measurements of regional wall motion from cineventriculograms before and after revascularization.[97,118,119] These studies again confirm that *blood flow–metabolism mismatches are associated with a significant postrevascularization improvement in regional wall motion.* One particular aspect of these latter studies has been the observation that the most severely dysfunctional mismatches demonstrated the greatest benefit or improvement in contractile function.

Other approaches for the assessment of myocardial viability are available or have been proposed but have failed to gain widespread acceptance. One such approach evaluates regional myocardial oxidative metabolism with ^{11}C-acetate.[120] The approach has been reported to predict an improvement in contractile function with an 85 percent accuracy and to predict irreversibility of contractile function in severely dysfunctional segments following revascularization in patients with chronic CAD with an 87 percent accuracy.[120] It was found to be similarly accurate in early postinfarction patients.[121]

In synthesizing the currently available information, it appears that ultimately the total fraction of scar tissue in a given myocardial segment largely determines whether or not contractile function will improve. Because of the linear correlation between scar tissue and relative blood flow,[86,95,96] evaluation or even quantitation of regional blood flow offers information on potential reversibility. On the other hand, if blood flow is also reduced in viable though functionally compromised myocardium, the augmented glucose utilization as evidenced by the enhanced ^{18}F-deoxyglucose uptake offers additional and critical information. This observation has prompted some investigators to predict the ultimate functional outcome from a combined assessment of blood flow and ^{18}F-deoxyglucose uptake (Fig. 20-15).[122,123] Further, the temporal recovery of contractile function after revascularization appears to depend on the degree of ultrastructural changes of myocytes as well as the fractional distribution between myocytes with only mild and those with severe ultrastructural changes.[122] If, as postulated, only mild structural changes are associated with a full functional recovery within 3 months, more severe structural changes may require substantially longer time periods and, further, may account for the persistence of increased ^{18}F-deoxyglucose uptake for many months following revascularization.[124]

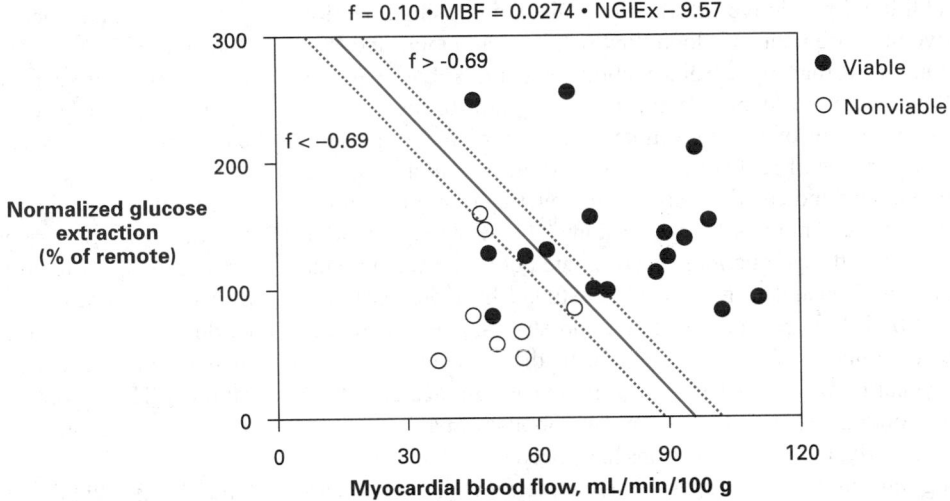

$$f = 0.10 \cdot MBF = 0.0274 \cdot NGIEx - 9.57$$

FIGURE 20-15

Relation between the normalized glucose extraction (NG1Ex) and myocardial blood flow (MBF) and superimposition of the discriminate function and its 95 percent confluence limits. (Reproduced with permission of the Journal of Nuclear Medicine from Grandin et al.[123])

Alternative Approaches to the Identification of Myocardial Viability

A series of studies has reported a high accuracy of ^{18}F-deoxyglucose PET imaging in predicting the postrevascularization outcome in regional left ventricular wall motion.[79,104,105,112–117] Even though some investigations employed permutations of the initially described blood flow–metabolism approach or relied only on the evaluation of regional ^{18}F-deoxyglucose uptake in dysfunctional myocardium,[112,113] the predictive accuracy, both positive and negative, continued to be high. Of note, comparably high predictive accuracies have been reported for the more conventional ^{201}Tl stress-redistribution and/or reinjection or the rest-redistribution approaches.[125] A comparison of both approaches in the same patients consistently demonstrated a higher predictive accuracy for the metabolic approach.[107,126] Other studies with ^{201}Tl rest-redistribution imaging revealed a relatively low predictive accuracy for segmental wall motion changes in patients with severely depressed left ventricular function.[127] This low accuracy appears consistent with observations made in comparison studies

that indicated that the conventional ^{201}Tl approach may falsely identify as many as 50 percent of segments as either viable or nonviable.[100] Additionally, among 29 of 46 patients with an average left ventricular ejection fraction of only 23 ± 6 percent with a fixed or equivocal ^{201}Tl defect, blood flow–metabolism imaging with ^{15}O-water and ^{18}F-deoxyglucose uncovered substantial amounts of viable myocardium in 18 patients.[128] The mean ejection fraction in this group of patients with viability either by ^{201}Tl or ^{18}F-deoxyglucose improved to 39 ± 13 percent at 4 to 6 months following revascularization. The latter comparison study again points to a considerable limitation of the conventional and widely employed ^{201}Tl approach in its ability to distinguish reliably between reversibly and irreversibly compromised myocardium in patients with severely depressed left ventricular function. In 62 percent of 29 patients with equivocal evidence of viability on ^{201}Tl SPECT imaging, blood flow–metabolism imaging with PET uncovered substantial amounts of viable myocardium that resulted in a significant postrevascularization improvement in global left ventricular function. These together with other findings demonstrate a clearly superior diagnostic accuracy of PET blood flow–metabolism imaging relative to the more conventional SPECT approaches in patients with severely compromised left ventricular function who, if substantial amounts of viable myocardium are present, are likely to benefit most from interventional revascularization.

As another approach to determining myocardial viability, the extent to which the severity of regional flow reductions can discriminate between viable and nonviable myocardium has been explored. Because the amount of connective tissue formation in a given myocardial region has been reported to be a major determinant of whether or not contractile function can recover and because the fraction of scar tissue appears to correlate inversely with regional blood flow,[95,96] the severity of regional flow reductions would be expected to yield additional predictive information. One study using quantitative measurements of blood flow with ^{13}N-ammonia and PET concluded that myocardial viability was unlikely if regional flows were less than 0.25 mL/min per gram (or less than 30 to 35 percent of that in remote myocardium).[129] In general, comparisons of relative regional flows to the amount of scar tissue have indicated a considerable overlap of regional flows in viable and nonviable myocardium.[95–97] As a result, mild to moderate flow reductions discriminate poorly between viable myocardium and scar tissue. Other studies have demonstrated that both flow reductions at rest and stress-induced flow defects contain information relative to the presence of viable myocardium, but that this information is less accurate than that obtainable with blood flow–metabolism imaging.[126]

Clearly, these investigations have been important in exploring various approaches to the assessment of viable myocardium. They have pointed out limitations of the more conventional ^{201}Tl for assessing flow reductions alone and, at the same time, have firmly established the value of metabolic imaging for predicting postrevascularization changes in segmental myocardial wall motion. As yet, these investigations have not established the importance of viability assessment in the clinical setting.

Clinical Role of PET Viability Assessment

Among the various PET approaches, the blood flow–glucose metabolism approach has gained the greatest clinical acceptance. Thus, most of the information related to the clinical assessment of myocardial viability using PET is based on this approach. There are two conditions where PET viability assessments can decisively affect the therapeutic strategies in patients with CAD. One is in patients with chronic CAD and ischemic cardiomyopathy (Chap. 45), while the second is in patients early after an acute myocardial infarction (Chap. 47).

CHRONIC CORONARY ARTERY DISEASE

Patients who are likely to benefit most from the assessment of myocardial viability are those with ischemic cardiomyopathy. The therapeutic options in these patients range from aggressive medical management to surgical revascularization and cardiac transplantation. While conservative pharmacologic approaches to the management of such patients have markedly improved over the past decade, the long-term survival of medically treated patients remains relatively poor.[130] Cardiac transplantation offers better long-term survival and an improvement in the quality of life; yet the supply of suitable donor hearts has not kept pace with the increasing demand so that this therapeutic option remains limited. The annual number of cardiac transplantations has remained fairly constant at 2300 over the past several years, while the incidence of cardiomyopathy appears to be on the rise (see also Chap. 73). At present, the prevalence of ischemic cardiomyopathy in the United States alone amounts to about 2.5 million cases, thus affecting roughly 1 percent of the U.S. population (*Heart Facts,* American Heart Association). The same statistics indicate an annual incidence of ischemic cardiomyopathy of about 400,000, with 200,000 deaths resulting from ischemic cardiomyopathy each year (see also Chap. 38).

Interventional revascularization through either surgical bypass grafting or transcutaneous coronary angioplasty often remains the third choice. The approach, however, is associated with a relatively high perioperative mortality, while the potential benefits often remain difficult to predict presurgically. The decision to revascularize is therefore predicated on the answers to the following questions: (1) Is there enough myocardium so that revascularization will result in an improvement in left ventricular performance? (2) Will congestive heart failure (CHF) symptoms improve? (3) Will revascularization avert future catastrophic cardiac events and prolong survival?

GLOBAL LEFT VENTRICULAR FUNCTION

Several studies have demonstrated an inverse correlation between the extent of myocardial flow defects and the left ventricular ejection fraction.[131,132] Therefore, if it were possible to identify myocardium as opposed to scar tissue and the extent to which revascularization would restore its blood flow, it should become possible to predict, at least to some extent, the magnitude of an improvement in global left ventricular ejection fraction. In a highly selected group of patients with chronic CAD, percutaneous coronary angioplasty promptly restored flow to hypoperfused but metabolically mismatched regions.[103] The extent of the prerevascularization mismatch correlated linearly with the postrevascularization improvement in regional myocardial wall motion.

Other studies, though only semiquantitative ones, have similarly demonstrated some correlation between the extent of the blood flow–metabolism mismatch and the postrevascularization gain in left ventricular ejection fraction.[79] Patients with blood flow–metabolism mismatches that occupied at least two or more of a total of seven myocardial segments had a statistically significant increase in the left ventricular ejection fraction following coronary bypass grafting.[79] No such improvement was observed in patients with only one mismatch segment or with only matches. Subsequent studies have confirmed these initial observations or have reported a significant improvement in the response of the postrevascularization left ventricular ejection fraction to physical exercise or in the exercise capacity.[96,97,105,116,117] Improvements in global left ventricular function, as reported in these studies, ranged from 8 to 18 percent ejection fraction units in patients with large mismatches as compared to no significant change in patients without mismatches. Therefore, the extent of blood flow–metabolism mismatches or of viable myocardium contains predictive information on the postrevascularization gain in global left ventricular function.

It is important to emphasize that an improvement in regional and especially global left ventricular function may not occur immediately but, rather, may occur slowly and progressively following revascularization. Again, in one highly selected patient group, blood flow was shown to recover promptly following revascularization by angioplasty, whereas contractile function initially remained unchanged.[103] On reexamination 67 ± 19 days later, no further improvements in regional blood flow were observed although there was a significant increase in systolic wall motion. The disparity between the recovery of blood flow and of contractile function might be attributed to stunning, yet it also may be related to a progressive rebuilding of the contractile machinery in abnormal myocytes. In one group of 15 patients, the left ventricular ejection fraction recovered slowly over a period of 6 months, paralleled by a progressive decline in the end-diastolic volume.[102] Consistent with such rebuilding of the contractile machinery are other preliminary observations that indicate that contractile function appears to recover or improve more promptly in myocardial regions without marked ultrastructural abnormalities or with a lesser fraction of abnormal myocytes.[122]

CHF-RELATED SYMPTOMS

Several retrospective studies indicate that such symptomatic improvement is possible. For example, two groups of investigators concluded that patients with blood flow–metabolism mismatches undergoing surgical revascularization demonstrated a significantly higher incidence of improvement in functional class (New York Heart Association Congestive Heart Failure class) than either patients without mismatches or patients with matches but not submitted to surgical revascularization.[133,134] Among the 52 patients with mismatches and CHF in class III or IV, 81 percent of the 26 patients undergoing revascularization revealed a significant improvement in CHF class (by at least one class) as compared to an improvement in only 23 percent of the 26 patients treated conservatively.[134]

The amount of viable myocardium as determined by blood flow–[18]F-deoxyglucose imaging apparently contains information on the magnitude of the postrevascularization improvement in CHF symptoms.[135] The level of physical activity performed by patients prior to and 24 ± 14 months following coronary artery bypass grafting was graded on a specific activity scale and expressed in metabolic equivalents.[136] Among the 36 patients in this study with an average left ventricular ejection fraction of only 28 ± 6 percent, the extent of the blood flow–metabolism mismatch ranged from 0 to 74 percent (mean 23 ± 22 percent) on polar map analysis. When the patients were grouped according

to the extent of the mismatch, 11 patients with a mismatch occupying less than 5 percent of the left ventricular myocardium had a statistically significant (though only mild) improvement in functional status (34 percent increase in metabolic equivalents). Intermediate-sized mismatches (5 to 17 percent) in eight patients were associated with a 42 percent increase in metabolic equivalents, whereas large mismatches, i.e., greater than 18 percent, in 17 patients were followed after revascularization by an average increase of 107 percent in metabolic equivalents. Furthermore, as seen in Fig. 20-16, there was a statistically significant correlation between the improvement in functional status and the anatomic extent of the blood flow–metabolism mismatch. Finally, blood flow–metabolism mismatches equal to or greater than 18 percent were 70 percent sensitive and 78 percent specific in predicting an improvement in physical activity or functional status following successful surgical revascularization.

IMPROVEMENT IN LONG-TERM SURVIVAL

Several studies have examined the long-term fate of patients after being evaluated for myocardial blood flow and metabolism by PET.[126,133,134,137] These studies have presented compelling evidence for the notion of an increased incidence of cardiac events in patients with blood flow–metabolism mismatches who were not submitted to interventional revascularization. They also implied that revascularization of patients with blood flow–metabolism mismatches might avert future nonfatal and fatal cardiac events.

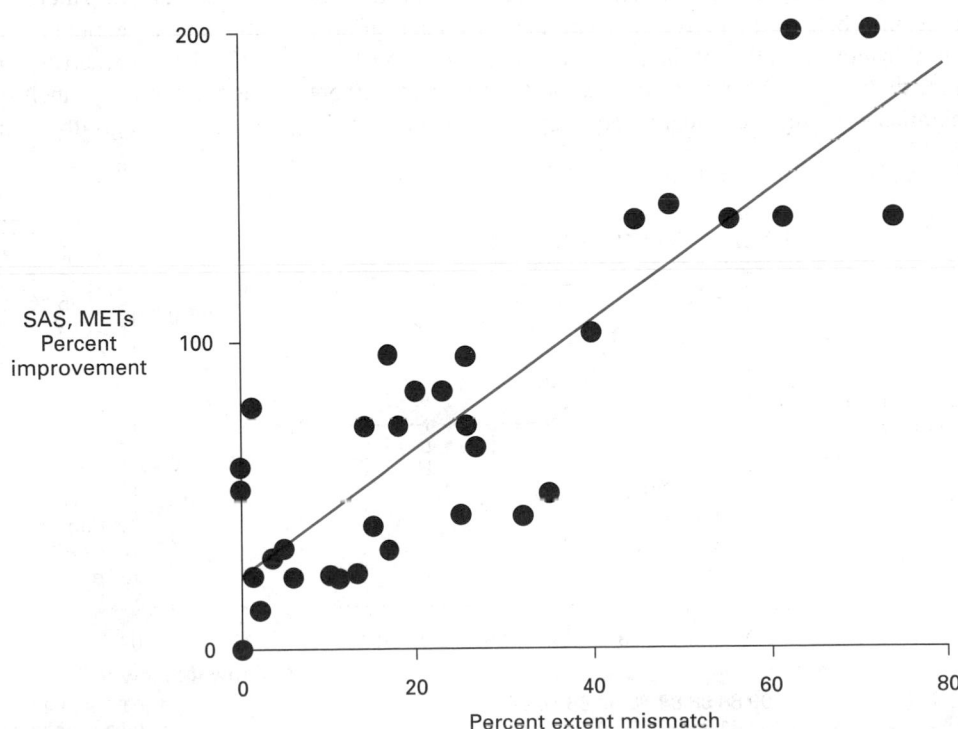

FIGURE 20-16

Correlation between the postrevascularization improvement in daily physical activities and the preoperative extent of a blood flow–metabolism mismatch. The physical activity was determined by a specific activity scale and expressed in metabolic equivalents (METs). (Reproduced with permission of the American Heart Association from Di Carli et al.[135])

Despite this general agreement, important differences emerge from these studies. One study of 129 chronic CAD patients followed clinically for an average time period of 17 ± 19 months found the presence of mismatches in the absence of revascularization to be an independent predictor of the 17 nonfatal ischemic events.[137] On the other hand, the left ventricular ejection fraction and the patient's age contained the highest predictive values for the 13 cardiac deaths in this patient group. The left ventricular ejection fraction in this patient group, however, averaged 38 ± 16 percent; the large standard deviation implies considerable interpatient differences in left ventricular ejection fractions. In view of the well-established relationship between long-term survival and left ventricular ejection fraction, the high prognostic value of this parameter for future cardiac mortality in this more heterogeneous patient group is of great interest. On the other hand, as was true for the two other investigations, when left ventricular ejection fractions were more homogeneously depressed in all patients, the predictive value of a low ejection fraction applied equally to all groups. This affords an analysis of other factors as prognosticators of cardiac mortality. As shown in Fig. 20-17, the cumulative long-term survival was lowest in the patient subgroup with blood flow–metabolism mismatches who were on medical treatment. Of note, all four subgroups were similar in terms of age and clinical and hemodynamic characteristics. There were no significant intergroup differences in the left ventricular ejection fraction, which for the whole patient group averaged 25 ± 7 percent. Patients with mismatches who underwent revascularization had a significantly better cumulative survival that no longer differed significantly from that of the patients without mismatches. In this study, the left ventricular ejection fraction was without significant predictive value, whereas by Cox model analysis,

the extent of a mismatch had a significant negative effect on survival ($p < .02$) and revascularization of mismatch patients positively affected survival ($p < .04$).[134] Although submitted to a less rigorous statistical analysis, a second study in patients with a similar uniform depression of the left ventricular ejection fractions reached similar conclusions.[133] Among the patient groups with and without mismatches, the subgroup of patients with mismatches had a 33 percent incidence of cardiac death during the 12-month follow-up period as compared to only a 4 percent mortality in patients with mismatches who underwent revascularization.

In summary, these observations imply that the presence of blood flow–metabolism mismatches identifies patients who are at high risk for a nonfatal cardiac event and, in instances of severely depressed left ventricular function, for sudden cardiac death. The observations further suggest that revascularization may significantly lower these risks and markedly improve long-term survival. If large enough, a mismatch may also contain predictive information on the improvement in CHF-related symptoms after revascularization and, further, on the improvement in global left ventricular function. The ability of blood flow–metabolism imaging with PET to provide clinically predictive information on the long-term outcome of patients with ischemic cardiomyopathy, therefore, can decisively impact the risk-benefit ratio of surgical revascularization and thus more generally affect therapeutic strategies. The absence of viability can affirm the decision to proceed with medical management or cardiac transplantation. Conversely, in patients with large amounts of viable myocardium, interventional revascularization represents a true and effective alternative. Indeed, in the setting of ischemic cardiomyopathy, inclusion of PET as a key feature in the diagnostic algorithm can be cost effective and, at the same

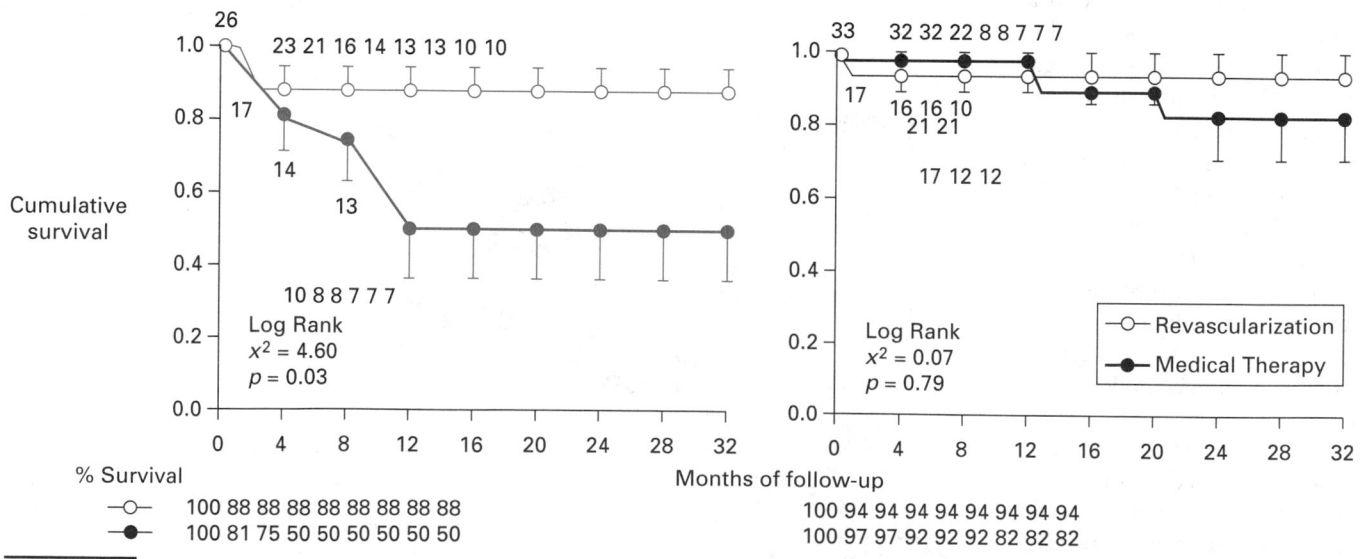

FIGURE 20-17

Cumulative survival of cardiomyopathy patients submitted to blood flow–metabolism imaging with PET. Patients are grouped according to the presence (panel A) or absence (panel B) of blood flow–metabolism mismatches. Note the significantly better cumulative survival in patients with mismatches who underwent revascularization. (Reproduced with permission from the American Journal of Cardiology from Di Carli et al.[134])

time, cost saving.[138,139] Clinical criteria for deciding on coronary artery bypass grafting in patients with ischemic cardiomyopathy have already been developed.[140] In addition to the left ventricular diastolic dimension, the left ventricular ejection fraction, and the presence of suitable target vessels, the criteria include the presence of viable myocardium affecting at least 15 to 20 percent of the left ventricular myocardium (see also Chap. 45).

ACUTE MYOCARDIAL INFARCTION

Early investigations in the prethrombolytic era explored the consequences of an acute myocardial infarction on regional myocardial blood flow and glucose metabolism. In 13 patients examined 54 ± 12 h after the onset of acute symptoms, PET consistently revealed flow reductions in the myocardium subtended by the infarct vessel.[84] Half of the hypoperfused segments exhibited concordant reductions in ^{18}F-deoxyglucose uptake, whereas mismatches were noted in the remaining eight segments. The severity of both flow reductions and wall motion abnormalities were similar for match and mismatch regions. The assessment of blood flow or of wall motion alone, therefore, would not have discriminated between truly infarcted and still viable myocardium. Reexamination of regional wall motion 6.0 ± 4.6 weeks later demonstrated a persistent impairment in all eight segments with early postinfarction matches and in four of the eight segments with mismatches. Repeat imaging of blood flow and metabolism in some patients suggested that the mismatch present initially had, on follow-up, reverted to a match, suggesting that ischemia had progressed to necrosis and scar tissue formation (Fig. 20-18). The persistent impairment in wall motion in all match segments implied that an irreversible injury had already occurred early after the myocardial infarction. Importantly, however, four of the eight segments with early postinfarction mismatches demonstrated a significant improvement in systolic wall motion.

These findings suggest that myocardium may survive the initial ischemic event and may be salvageable by restoration of blood flow. On the other hand, if blood flow remains severely compromised, it may be inadequate to sustain cell viability, and the cells may progress to necrosis. Thus, there may be a period of time for rescuing myocardium

at risk, the concept underlying the treatment of acute myocardial infarction with thrombolytics and acute angioplasty (Chap. 47). PET may have a role in determining whether tissue perfusion has been adequately restored and whether there is residual compromised myocardium that may be salvageable through additional interventional revascularization.

Measurements of blood flow, exogenous glucose utilization, and oxidative metabolism with PET in 22 early postinfarction patients pointed to several compensatory mechanisms that might explain the survival of myocytes in the presence of reduced blood flow.[141] In these patients, regional rates of oxidative metabolism and, thus, of oxygen consumption correlated with regional blood flow in a linear, though piecewise, fashion. In regions with blood flows in excess of 0.56 mL/min per gram, oxidative metabolism declined disproportionately less than flow. As depicted in Fig. 20-19, once blood flows declined below 0.56 mL/min per gram, oxidative metabolism declined precipitously. Consistent with observations in experimental animals,[142] such piecewise correlation implicates a progressive rise in the extraction of oxygen in response to declining blood flows as one compensatory mechanism available to the myocardium. A second mechanism is an increased reliance on glucose as a more oxygen-efficient substrate; that is, for the same amount of oxygen, more ATP can be generated by metabolizing glucose rather than free fatty acid. This hypothesis is supported by the presence of blood flow–metabolism mismatches, that is, a relative increase in glucose extraction, as observed in these patients in 93 percent of the segments with less than 25 percent reduction in oxidative metabolism.

Stunning serves as another possible explanation for the regionally enhanced glucose utilization.[143] It is consistent

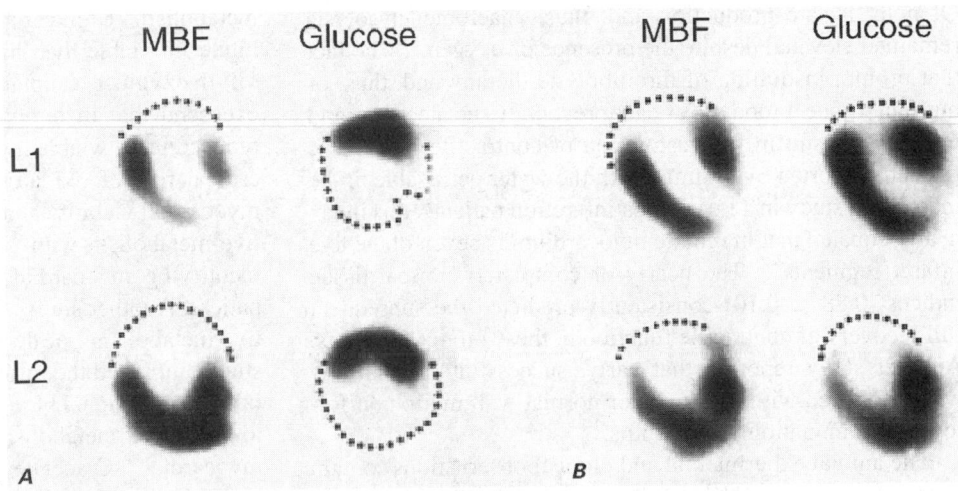

FIGURE 20-18

Blood flow (MBF) and glucose metabolism imaging in a patient following an acute myocardial infarction. The initial study (*A*) was performed during the early postinfarction period, the follow-up study (*B*) 6 weeks later. L1 and L2 indicate two selected transaxial cuts of the left ventricle. Note the profound perfusion defect in the anterior wall, which shows markedly enhanced glucose utilization om the ^{18}F-deoxyglucose images. On follow-up, the flow defect persists, associated with a concordant reduction in glucose utilization. Thus, an initial blood flow–metabolism mismatch reverted to a blood flow–metabolism match. (Reproduced with permission of the Journal of the American College of Cardiology from Schwaiger et al.[84])

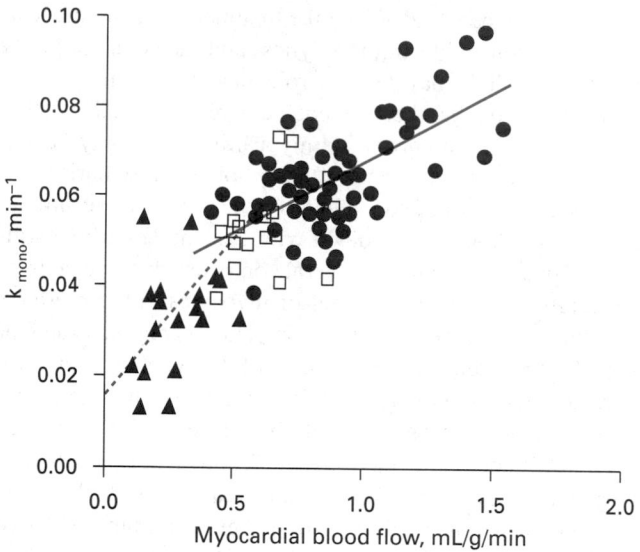

FIGURE 20-19

Correlation between myocardial blood flow and oxidative metabolism as determined from the clearance rate of ^{11}C-acetate from the myocardium (k_{mono}). Note the piecewise correlation. The solid circles indicate normal myocardium; the open rectangles, myocardium with mismatches; and the solid triangles, myocardium with matches. (Reproduced with permission from the American Heart Association from Czernin et al.[141])

with observations in experimental animals[81]; upon reperfusion following a 3-h coronary occlusion, ^{18}F-deoxyglucose uptake was found to be initially depressed but to be markedly increased above that in remote myocardium when reexamined after 24 h of reperfusion. Evaluation of glucose metabolism in reperfused myocardium with ^{14}C-labeled glucose and ^{13}C-labeled lactate demonstrated that glucose oxidation in reperfused myocardium equaled that in remote myocardium. Of note, lactate production and, thus, anaerobic glycolysis remained elevated despite the presence of oxygen.[83] The fact that prompt institution of thrombolytic therapy and, thus, of nutrient tissue blood flow can prevent tissue necrosis and ultimately result in full restoration of contractile function is further supported by findings with the water perfusable tissue index. In a study in 11 early postinfarction patients, this index nearly equaled that in remote myocardium in seven of the five infarct segments.[40] The nearly or completely normal tissue indices (0.88 ± 0.10) consistently predicted the subsequent full recovery of contractile function in these infarct segments. Another study reported that early, successful thrombolysis was associated with improved or normal wall motion on follow-up examination at 3 months.[144]

The animal experimental and clinical observations contain several implications. Normal blood flow and/or a normal water perfusable tissue index identify so-called infarcted myocardium as stunned. Even though wall motion remains initially impaired, it is likely to recover spontaneously. Conversely, reductions in blood flow associated with severe decreases in oxidative metabolism and/or glucose utilization identify myocardium as truly infarcted or irreversibly injured. The

severity of the reductions in flow and metabolism may vary between patients yet depends on whether the infarct is transmural or nontransmural. Finally, the presence of oxidative metabolism and/or glucose utilization implies the existence of myocardium that has survived the ischemic event, is viable, and thus potentially salvageable.

It remains uncertain, however, as to how long such initially viable myocardium can survive. For example, one study in 15 patients noted mismatches in 11 regions in 10 patients studied within 3 months after an acute myocardial infarction.[78] There were also 14 match regions in these 11 patients. Another study in 65 patients with prior Q-wave myocardial infarctions implied that the presence of blood flow–metabolism mismatches and, thus, of salvageable myocardium declines with time.[101] The infarct region revealed match defects in 26 and mismatch defects in 39 patients. The incidence of mismatches declined as a function of time after the acute event. For example, none of the infarctions that had occurred more than 500 days prior to the metabolic study exhibited viable myocardium, whereas virtually all patients examined within 90 days after the acute event demonstrated mismatches.

Several studies have explored the predictive value of blood flow, oxidative metabolism, and glucose utilization rates for salvaging ischemically injured myocardium or for predicting the long-term outcome in contractile function. One study in 11 patients defined *viable* and *truly infarcted* myocardial regions according to the postrevascularization outcome in contractile function following angioplasty or coronary artery bypass grafting.[121] Blood flow, oxidative metabolism, and glucose utilization were determined at an average of 6 days after the myocardial infarction but prior to revascularization. Compared to remote myocardium, viable and nonviable myocardial regions revealed both reduced blood flow and oxidative metabolism. Unlike blood flow, oxidative metabolism was higher in viable than in nonviable myocardial regions. Last, ^{18}F-deoxyglucose uptake in viable myocardium equaled or exceeded that in remote myocardium but was significantly reduced in nonviable myocardium. The study emphasized the critical role of oxidative metabolism for the persistence of myocardial viability and implies that the assessment of oxidative metabolism with ^{11}C-acetate is an important means for identifying myocardial viability in the early postinfarction patient. Another study[145] confirmed the importance of oxidative metabolism but derived more complex conclusions. The study employed the initial uptake of ^{11}C-acetate as a measure of relative regional blood flow[146] and compared relative flows to oxidative metabolism, as determined from the regional myocardial ^{11}C-acetate clearance. Proportional reductions in both flow and oxidative metabolism reflected nonviable myocardium and a lack of long-term improvement in contractile function. Such concordance might imply the coexistence of irreversibly injured myocardium with normal myocardium. Importantly, however, disparities between flow and metabolism, which were mostly due to a disproportionately greater suppression of oxidative metabolism than blood flow, appeared predictive of long-term improvement in contractile function.

Finally, persistent glucose metabolism is also important. Uptake of ^{18}F-deoxyglucose in viable myocardium equaled or even exceeded that in remote myocardium but was reduced in nonviable myocardium.[121] Although the ratio of ^{18}F-deoxyglucose uptake to blood flow did not differ between viable and nonviable myocardial regions, the magnitude of tracer uptake alone may have correctly identified viable myocardium, as proposed for chronic CAD.[147] One preliminary report noted the presence of 11 blood flow–metabolism mismatch regions in 10 patients examined at 3.4 days after the acute event.[148] Matches were observed in 10 segments. The finding of a blood flow–metabolism mismatch in the infarct territory led to interventional revascularization in some patients, with an improvement in wall motion on follow-up. Reexamination of regional wall motion in seven patients by echocardiography failed to demonstrate a significant improvement in contractile function in match regions, whereas wall motion had significantly improved in all mismatch regions. These observations are consistent with recent findings[144] that interventional revascularization of infarct territories resulted in a long term improvement in contractile function only if blood flow–metabolism mismatches were present during the early postinfarction period. This study in 30 acute infarct patients further demonstrated a failure of wall motion to improve on late follow-up if regional blood flow was severely reduced early after the acute infarct, despite successful thrombolysis. In contrast, the finding of normal regional blood flow was associated with improved wall motion at 3 months.

Several conclusions can be drawn from these findings. *First, prompt restoration of blood flow to the infarct region predicts a long-term improvement in contractile function. Second, persistent flow reductions associated with either enhanced glucose utilization or suppressed though persistent oxidative metabolism contain considerable predictive information for the long-term improvement in regional systolic wall motion if blood flow can be restored successfully. Third, myocardium may survive the initial ischemic attack and remain viable for some time. Since such ischemically compromised, though potentially viable, myocardium may slowly progress to necrosis, myocardial blood flow should be restored as soon as possible.*

DIAGNOSTIC STRATEGIES FOR DEMONSTRATING MYOCARDIAL VIABILITY

The clinical information available for blood flow and metabolism imaging with PET permits the formulation of diagnostic strategies for the assessment of myocardial viability. Clearly, observations with such tracers of fatty acid of oxidative metabolism as, for example, ^{11}C palmitate or ^{11}C acetate have provided important insights into the pathophysiology of viable myocardium and have been found useful for the assessment of myocardial viability. The use of these tracers, however,

has remained limited in the clinical settings, as is true for the water perfusable tissue index. Therefore, the proposed diagnostic strategies include only the assessment of regional myocardial blood flow and exogenous glucose utilization with ^{18}F-deoxyglucose.

The first step in this diagnostic approach entails the assessment of regional myocardial blood flow, which can be accomplished with either ^{82}Rb or ^{13}N-ammonia and PET. If neither tracer is available (as is true for the PET satellite concept with only ^{18}F-deoxyglucose available from a regional distribution center), myocardial blood flow can also be evaluated with ^{201}Tl or ^{99m}Tc-sestamibi. Blood flow images alone may, in some patients, be sufficient to separate reversibly from irreversibly injured myocardium. For example, normal or near-normal blood flow in a dysfunctional myocardial region implies the presence of stunned myocardium and, thus, of myocardial viability. It indicates successful restoration of coronary blood flow in postinfarction patients. Therapeutic approaches would then depend on the status of the corresponding coronary vessel. As examples, a persistent coronary stenosis in early postinfarction patients or the presence of significant coronary stenosis in patients with chronic CAD could then be identified either by coronary angiography or, noninvasively, with stress myocardial blood flow imaging. Conversely, severely reduced blood flows in dysfunctional myocardial regions would almost entirely exclude the presence of viable myocardium, at least in amounts that would be of any consequence in regard to a potential improvement in regional contractile function. Flows in such nonrecovering myocardium will typically be less than 25 percent of that in normally contracting, remote myocardium. Intermediate flow reductions, however, distinguish only poorly between viable and nonviable myocardium and require further exploration with tracers of myocardial metabolism.

The second step in the diagnostic approach then entails the assessment of exogenous glucose utilization in dysfunctional myocardial regions with intermediate flow reductions. Glucose metabolic imaging is performed best after an oral glucose load or during the euglycemic, hyperinsulinemic clamp. Glucose loading and/or insulin administration will typically result in images of markedly better diagnostic quality than those obtained in the fasting state. Reductions in regional ^{18}F-deoxyglucose uptake that are proportional to flow reductions signify the absence of viability; conversely, ^{18}F-deoxyglucose uptake that is increased either relative to that in remote myocardium or to myocardial blood flow indicates the presence of viable myocardium.

Quantitative image analysis techniques, including polar map displays, have become available and offer estimates of the extent and severity of flow defects as well as of blood flow–metabolism matches and mismatches. Estimates of the latter are of particular importance in the prediction of potential benefits of surgical revascularization. Quantitative image analysis approaches are also frequently useful for a more objective, less operator-dependent assessment of regional blood flow metabolism patterns.

SUMMARY AND CONCLUSIONS

PET offers the opportunity for probing and quantifying a wide range of functional processes in the human heart. While of considerable interest in the research environment, the utility and potential value of these probes in the diagnosis and characterization of human cardiovascular disease remains largely unexplored. Clinical investigations, however, have demonstrated the impressive accuracy with which PET detects CAD, provides estimates of its severity, offers a means to uncover preclinical CAD, and permits characterization of its metabolic and functional consequences. It is in these areas where this new technology begins to play an increasingly important role in patient management. At the same time, PET offers numerous possibilities to explore other cardiac disorders, to contribute to a better understanding of their underlying pathophysiology, to improve their characterization in the clinical environment, and to monitor responses to therapy.

ACKNOWLEDGMENTS

The author wishes to acknowledge Eileen Rosenfeld's skillful secretarial assistance in preparing this manuscript and Diane Martin for preparing the illustrations.

REFERENCES

1. Gould KL, Lipscomb K, Hamilton GW. Physiologic basis for assessing critical coronary stenosis. Instantaneous flow response and regional distribution during coronary hyperemia as measures of coronary flow reserve. *Am J Cardiol* 1974; 33:87–94.
2. Bergmann SR, Herrero P, Markham J, Weinheimer CJ, Walsh MN. Noninvasive quantitation of myocardial blood flow in human subjects with oxygen-15-labeled water and positron emission tomography. *J Am Coll Cardiol* 1989; 14:639–652.
3. Araujo L, Lammertsma A, Rhodes C, McFalls E, Iida H, Rechavia E, et al. Noninvasive quantification of regional myocardial blood flow in coronary artery disease with oxygen-15-labeled carbon dioxide inhalation and positron emission tomography. *Circulation* 1991; 83:875–885.
4. Hutchins G, Schwaiger M, Rosenspire K, Krivokapich J, Schelbert H, Kuhl D. Noninvasive quantification of regional blood flow in the human heart using N-13 ammonia and dynamic positron emission tomographic imaging. *J Am Coll Cardiol* 1990; 15:1032–1042.
5. Chan S, Brunken R, Czernin J, Porenta G, Kuhle W, Krivokapich J, et al. Comparison of maximal myocardial blood flow during adenosine infusion with that of intravenous dipyridamole in normal men. *J Am Coll Cardiol* 1992; 20:979–985.
6. Czernin J, Auerbach M, Sun K, Phelps M, Schelbert H. Effects of modified pharmacologic stress approaches on hyperemic myocardial blood flow. *J Nucl Med* 1995; 36:575–580.
7. Czernin J, Barnard J, Sun K, Krivokapich J, Nitzsche E, Dorsey D, et al. Effect of short term cardiovascular conditioning and low fat diet on myocardial blood flow and flow reserve. *Circulation* 1995; 92:197–204.
8. Senneff M, Geltman E, Bergmann S, Hartman J. Noninvasive delineation of the effects of moderate aging on myocardial perfusion. *J Nucl Med* 1991; 32:2037–2042.
9. Uren N, Camici P, Melin J, Bol A, de Bruyne B, Radvan J, et al. Effect of aging on myocardial perfusion reserve. *J Nucl Med* 1995; 36:2032–2036.
10. Müller P, Czernin J, Choi Y, Aguilar F, Nitzsche E, Buxton D, et al. Effect of exercise supplementation during adenosine infusion on hyperemic blood flow and flow reserve. *Am Heart J* 1994; 128:52–60.
11. Schelbert HR, Wisenberg G, Phelps ME, Gould KL, Henze E, Hoffman EJ, et al. Noninvasive assessment of coronary stenoses by myocardial imaging during pharmacologic coronary vasodilation. VI. Detection of coronary artery disease in man with intravenous N-13 ammonia and positron computed tomography. *Am J Cardiol* 1982; 49:1197–1207.
12. Tamaki N, Yonekura Y, Senda M, Yamashita K, Koide H, Saji H, et al. Value and limitation of stress thallium-201 single photon emission computed tomography: Comparison with nitrogen-13 ammonia positron tomography. *J Nucl Med* 1988; 29:1181–1188.
13. Demer LL, Gould KL, Goldstein RA, Kirkeeide RL, Mullani NA, Smalling RW, et al. Assessment of coronary artery disease severity by positron emission tomography. Comparison with quantitative arteriography in 193 patients. *Circulation* 1989; 79:825–835.
14. Go R, Marwick T, MacIntyre W, Saha G, Neumann D, Underwood D, et al. A prospective comparison of rubidium-82 PET and thallium-201 SPECT myocardial perfusion imaging utilizing a single dipyridamole stress in the diagnosis of coronary artery disease. *J Nucl Med* 1990; 31:1899–1905.
15. Stewart R, Schwaiger M, Molina E, Popma J, Gacioch G, Kalus M, et al. Comparison of rubidium-82 positron emission tomography and thallium-201 SPECT imaging for detection of coronary artery disease. *Am J Cardiol* 1991; 67:1303–1310.
16. Williams B, Millani N, Jansen D, Anderson B. A retrospective study of the diagnostic accuracy of a community hospital–based PET center for the detection of coronary artery disease using rubidium-82. *J Nucl Med* 1994; 35:1586–1592.
17. Simone G, Mullani N, Page D, Anderson B Sr. Utilization statistics and diagnostic accuracy of a nonhospital-based positron emission tomography center for the detection of coronary artery disease using rubidium-82. *Am J Physiol Imaging* 1992; 7:203–209.
18. Brown BG, Josephson MA, Peterson RB, Pierce CD, Wong M, Hecht HS, et al. Intravenous dipyridamole combined with isometric handgrip for near maximal acute increase in coronary flow in patients with coronary artery disease. *Am J Cardiol* 1981; 48:1077–1085.
19. Krivokapich J, Smith GT, Huang SC, Hoffman EJ, Ratib O, Phelps ME, et al. N-13 ammonia myocardial imaging at rest and with exercise in normal volunteers: Quantification of absolute myocardial perfusion with dynamic positron emission tomography. *Circulation* 1989; 80:1328–1337.
20. Kuhle W, Porenta G, Huang S-C, Buxton D, Gambhir S, Hansen H, et al. Quantification of regional myocardial blood flow using ^{13}N-ammonia and reoriented dynamic positron emission tomographic imaging. *Circulation* 1992; 86:1004–1017.
21. Bellina C, Parodi O, Camici P, Salvadori P, Taddei L, Fusani L, et al. Simultaneous in vitro and in vivo validation of a nitrogen-13-ammonia for the assessment of regional myocardial blood flow. *J Nucl Med* 1990; 31:1335–1343.
22. Muzik O, Beanlands RSB, Hutchins GD, Mangner TJ, Nguyen N, Schwaiger M. Validation of nitrogen-13-ammonia tracer kinetic model for quantification of myocardial blood flow using PET. *J Nucl Med* 1993; 34:83–91.
23. Nagamachi S, Czernin J, Kim A, Sun K, Phelps M, Schelbert H. Reproducibility of measurements of regional resting and hyperemic myocardial blood flow assessed with positron emission tomography. *J Nucl Med* 1996; 37:1626–1631.
24. Nitzsche E, Choi Y, Czernin J, Hoh C, Huang S-C, Schelbert H. Noninvasive quantification of myocardial blood flow in humans. A direct comparison of the $[^{13}N]$ ammonia and the $[^{15}O]$ water techniques. *Circulation* 1996; 93:2000–2006.
25. Uren N, Melin J, De Bruyne B, Wijns W, Baudhuin T, Camici P. Relation between myocardial blood flow and the severity of coronary-artery stenosis. *N Engl J Med* 1994; 330:1782–1788.
26. Di Carli M, Czernin J, Hoh C, Gerbaudo V, Brunken R, Huang S, et al. Relation among stenosis severity, myocardial blood flow, and flow reserve in patients with coronary artery disease. *Circulation* 1995; 91:1944–1951.
27. Beanlands R, Schwaiger M. Changes in myocardial oxygen consumption and efficiency with heart failure therapy measured by ^{11}C acetate PET. *Can J Cardiol* 1995; 11:293–300.
28. Uren N, Marraccini P, Gistri R, de Silva R, Camici P. Altered coronary vasodilator reserve and metabolism in myocardium subtended by normal arteries in patients with coronary artery disease. *J Am Coll Cardiol* 1993; 22:650–658.

29. Czernin J, Müller P, Chan S, Brunken R, Porenta G, Krivokapich J, et al. Influence of age and hemodynamics on myocardial blood flow and flow reserve. *Circulation* 1993; 88:67–69.

30. Sambuceti G, Parodi O, Marcassa C, Neglia D, Salvadori P, Giorgetti A, et al. Alteration in regulation of myocardial blood flow in one-vessel coronary artery disease determined by positron emission tomography. *Am J Cardiol* 1993; 72:538–543.

31. Zeiher A, Drexler H, Wollschläger H, Just H. Endothelial dysfunction of the coronary microvasculature is associated with impaired coronary blood flow regulation in patients with early atherosclerosis. *Circulation* 1991; 84:1984–1992.

32. Nabel E, Ganz P, Gordon J, Alexander R, Selwyn A. Dilation of normal and constriction of atherosclerotic coronary arteries caused by the cold pressor test. *Circulation* 1988; 77:43–52.

33. Drzezga A, Blasini R, Ziegler S, Picker W, Neumann F, Schömig A, et al. Quantitative flow measurement using N-13 ammonia positron emission tomography during rest and stress by cold pressor test in normal subjects and patients with dilated cardiomyopathy. *J Nucl Med* 1995; 36:3P. Abstract.

34. Dayanikli F, Grambow D, Muzik O, Mosca L, Rubenfire M, Schwaiger M. Early detection of abnormal coronary flow reserve in asymptomatic men at high risk for coronary artery disease using positron emission tomography. *Circulation* 1994; 90:808–817.

35. Czernin J, Barnard J, Sun K, Krivokapich J, Brunken R, Porenta G, et al. Beneficial effect of cardiovascular conditioning on myocardial blood flow and coronary vasodilator capacity. *Circulation* 1993; 88:I-51. Abstract.

36. Gould K, Ornish D, Scherwitz L, Brown S, Edens R, Hess M, et al. Changes in myocardial perfusion abnormalities by positron emission tomography after long-term, intense risk factor modification. *JAMA* 1995; 274:894–901.

37. Brunken R, Tillisch J, Schwaiger M, Child JS, Marshall R, Mandelkern M, et al. Regional perfusion, glucose metabolism and wall motion in chronic electrocardiographic Q-wave infarctions. Evidence for persistence of viable tissue in some infarct regions by positron emission tomography. *Circulation* 1986; 73:951–963.

38. Gould L, Yoshida K, Hess M, Haynie M, Mullani N, Smalling R. Myocardial metabolism of fluorodeoxyglucose compared to cell membrane integrity for the potassium analogue rubidium-82 for assessing infarct size in many by PET. *J Nucl Med* 1991; 32:1–9.

39. Pierard L, De Landsheere C, Berthe C, Rigo P, Kulbertus H. Identification of viable myocardium by echocardiography during dobutamine infusion in patients with myocardial infarction after thrombolytic therapy: Comparison with positron emission tomography. *J Am Coll Cardiol* 1990; 15:1021–1031.

40. Yamamoto Y, De Silva R, Rhodes C, Araujo L, Iida H, Rechavia E, et al. A new strategy for the assessment of viable myocardium and regional myocardial blood flow using ^{15}O-water and dynamic positron emission tomography. *Circulation* 1992; 86:167–178.

41. De Silva R, Yamamoto Y, Rhodes CG, Iida H, Nihoyannopoulos P, Davies GJ, et al. Preoperative prediction of the outcome of coronary revascularization using positron emission tomography. *Circulation* 1992; 86:1738–1742.

42. Liedtke AJ. Alterations of carbohydrate and lipid metabolism in the acutely ischemic heart. *Prog Cardiovasc Dis* 1981; 23:321–336.

43. Opie LH. Metabolism of the heart in health and disease. *Am Heart J* 1968; 76:685–698.

44. Bing RJ. The metabolism of the heart. Harvey Lectures. Series L. New York: Academic Press; 1954–1955:27–70.

45. Schelbert HR, Henze E, Schön HR, Keen R, Hansen HW, Selin C, et al. C-11 palmitate for the noninvasive evaluation of regional myocardial fatty acid metabolism with positron computed tomography. III. In vivo demonstration of the effects of substrate availability on myocardial metabolism. *Am Heart J* 1983; 105:492–504.

46. Nuutila P, Koivisto V, Knuuti J, Ruotsalainen U, Teras M, Haaparanta M, et al. Glucose-free fatty acid cycle operates in human heart and skeletal muscle in vivo. *J Clin Invest* 1992; 89:1767–1774.

47. Keul J, Doll E, Steim H, Homburger H, Kern H, Reindell H. Uber den Stoffwechsel des menschlichen Herzens. I. Substratversorgung des gesunden Herzens in Ruhe, während und nach körperlicher Arbeit. *Pflugers Arch* 1965; 282:1–27.

48. Taegtmeyer H. Myocardial metabolism. In: Phelps M, Mazziotta J, Schelbert H eds. *Positron Emission Tomography and Autoradiography*. New York: Raven; 1986:149–195.

49. Sokoloff L, Reivich M, Kennedy C, Des Rosiers MH, Patlak CS, Pettigrew KD, et al. The [^{14}C]-deoxyglucose method for the measurement of local cerebral glucose utilization: Theory, procedure and normal values in the conscious and anesthetized albino rat. *J Neurochem* 1977; 28:897–916.

50. Phelps ME, Hoffman EJ, Selin CE, Huang SC, Robinson G, MacDonald N, et al. Investigation of [18F] 2-fluoro-2-deoxyglucose for the measure of myocardial glucose metabolism. *J Nucl Med* 1978; 19:1311–1319.

51. Ratib O, Phelps ME, Huang SC, Henze E, Selin CE, Schelbert HR. Positron tomography with deoxyglucose for estimating local myocardial glucose metabolism. *J Nucl Med* 1982; 23:577–586.

52. Gambhir SS, Schwaiger M, Huang SC, Krivokapich J, Schelbert HR, Nienaber CA, et al. Simple noninvasive quantification method for measuring myocardial glucose utilization in humans employing positron emission tomography and fluorine-18 deoxyglucose. *J Nucl Med* 1989; 30:359–366.

53. Choi Y, Hawkins R, Huang S, Gambhir S, Brunken R, Phelps M, et al. Parametric images of myocardial metabolic rate of glucose generated from dynamic cardiac PET and 2-[18F]fluoro-2-deoxy-D-glucose studies. *J Nucl Med* 1991; 32:733–738.

54. Choi Y, Hawkins R, Brunken R, Huang S, Kuhle W, Chen K, et al. Evaluation of regional heterogeneity of myocardial glucose metabolism in normal humans using dynamic FDG-PET. *J Nucl Med* 1991; 32:938. Abstract.

55. Choi Y, Brunken R, Hawkins R, Huang S-C, Buxton D, Hoh C, et al. Factors affecting myocardial 2-[F-18]fluoro-2-deoxy-D-glucose uptake in positron emission tomography studies of normal humans. *Eur J Nucl Med* 1993; 20:308–318.

56. Hoffman EJ, Phelps ME, Weiss ES, Welch MJ, Coleman RE, Sobel BE, et al. Transaxial tomographic imaging of canine myocardium with ^{11}C-palmitic acid. *J Nucl Med* 1977; 18:57–61.

57. Klein MS, Goldstein RA, Welch MJ, Sobel BE. External assessment of myocardial metabolism with ^{11}C-palmitate in rabbit hearts. *Am J Physiol* 1979; 237:H51–H58.

58. Weiss ES, Hoffman EJ, Phelps ME, Welch MJ, Henry PD, Ter-Pogossian MM, et al. External detection and visualization of myocardial ischemia with ^{11}C-substrates in vitro and in vivo. *Circ Res* 1976; 39:24–32.

59. Schön HR, Schelbert HR, Najafi A, Robinson G, Huang SC, Barrio J, et al. C-11 labeled palmitic acid for the noninvasive evaluation of regional myocardial fatty acid metabolism with positron computed tomography. I. Kinetics of C-11 palmitic acid in normal myocardium. *Am Heart J* 1982; 103:532–547.

60. Schelbert HR, Henze E, Schön HR, Najafi A, Hansen H, Huang SC, et al. C-11 palmitic acid for the noninvasive evaluation of regional myocardial fatty acid metabolism with positron computed tomography. IV. In vivo demonstration of impaired fatty acid oxidation in acute myocardial ischemia. *Am Heart J* 1983; 106:736–750.

61. Wyns W, Schwaiger M, Huang SC, Buxton DB, Hansen H, Selin C, et al. Effects of inhibition of fatty acid oxidation on myocardial kinetics of C-11 labeled palmitate. *Circ Res* 1989; 65:1787–1797.

62. Rosamond TL, Abendschein DR, Sobel BE, Bergmann SR, Fox KAA. Metabolic fate of radiolabeled palmitate in ischemic canine myocardium: Implications for positron emission tomography. *J Nucl Med* 1987; 28:1322–1329.

63. Merlet P, Mazoyer B, Dubois-Rande J, Raynaud L, Valette H, Crouzel C, et al. Assessment of coronary reserve in man using intravenous bolus ^{15}O-water and positron emission tomography (PET): A comparison with intracoronary doppler study. *J Nucl Med* 1991; 32:998. Abstract.

64. Bol A, Iida H, Essamri B, Vanbutsele R, Labar D, Grandin C, et al. Assessment of myocardial oxidative reserve with PET: Comparison of C-11 acetate kinetics with quantitation of metabolic rate of oxygen (MV$_{O_2}$) using O-15 O$_2$. *J Nucl Med* 1991; 32:988–989.

65. Brown M, Marshall DR, Burton BS, Sobel BE, Bergmann SR. Delineation of myocardial oxygen utilization with carbon-11-labeled acetate. *Circulation* 1987; 76:687–696.

66. Brown MA, Myears DW, Bergmann SR. Noninvasive assessment of canine myocardial oxidative metabolism with ^{11}C-acetate and positron emission tomography. *J Am Coll Cardiol* 1988; 12:1054–1063.

67. Buxton DB, Schwaiger M, Nguyen A, Phelps ME, Schelbert HR. Radiolabeled acetate as a tracer of myocardial tricarboxylic acid cycle flux. *Circ Res* 1988; 63:628–634.

68. Buxton DB, Nienaber CA, Luxen A, Ratib O, Hansen H, Phelps ME, et al. Noninvasive quantitation of regional myocardial oxygen consumption in vivo with [1-^{11}C] acetate and dynamic positron emission tomography. *Circulation* 1989; 79:134–142.

69. Armbrecht JJ, Buxton DB, Schelbert HR. Validation of [1-^{11}C] acetate as a tracer for noninvasive assessment of oxidative metabolism with positron emission tomography in normal, ischemic, post-ischemic and hyperemic canine myocardium. *Circulation* 1991; 81:1594–1605.

70. Armbrecht JJ, Buxton DB, Brunken RC, Phelps ME, Schelbert HR. Regional myocardial oxygen consumption determined noninvasively in humans with [1-^{11}C] acetate and dynamic positron tomography. *Circulation* 1989; 80:863–872.

71. Henes CG, Bergmann SR, Walsh MN, Sobel BE, Geltman EM. Assessment of myocardial oxidative metabolic reserve with positron emission tomography and carbon-11 acetate. *J Nucl Med* 1989; 30:1489–1499.

72. Ng C, Huang S-C, Schelbert H, Buxton D. Validation of a model for [1-11C] acetate as a tracer of cardiac oxidative metabolism. *Am J Physiol* 1994; 266:H1304–H1315.

73. Sun KT, Chen K, Huang SC, Buxton DB, Hansen HW, Kim AS, et al. Compartment model for measuring myocardial oxygen consumption using[1-11]acetate. *J Nuc Med* 1997; 38:459–466.

74. Opie LH, Owen P, Riemersma RA. Relative rates of oxidation of glucose and free fatty acids by ischemic and non-ischemic myocardium after coronary artery ligation in the dog. *Eur J Clin Invest* 1973; 3:419–435.

75. Opie LH. Myocardial ischemia—metabolic pathways and implications of increased glycolysis. *Cardiovasc Drugs Ther* 1990; 4:777–790.

76. Schön HR, Schelbert HR, Najafi A, Hansen H, Robinson GR, Huang SC, et al. C-11 labeled palmitic acid for the noninvasive evaluation of regional myocardial fatty acid metabolism with positron computed tomography. II. Kinetics of C-11 palmitic acid in acutely ischemic myocardium. *Am Heart J* 1982; 103:548–561.

77. Schelbert HR, Phelps ME, Selin C, Marshall RC, Hoffman EJ, Kuhl DE. Regional myocardial ischemia assessed by ^{18}fluoro-2-deoxyglucose and positron emission computed tomography. In: Heiss HW, ed. Quantification of Myocardial Ischemia; Kreuzer H, Parmley WW, Rentrop P, Heiss HW: *Advances in Clinical Cardiology*. New York: G Witzstrock, 1980, 437–447.

78. Marshall RC, Tillisch JH, Phelps ME, Huang SC, Carson RC, Henze E, et al. Identification and differentiation of resting myocardial ischemia and infarction in man with positron computed tomography 18F-labeled fluorodeoxyglucose and N-13 ammonia. *Circulation* 1983; 67:766–778.

79. Tillisch J, Brunken R, Marshall R, Schwaiger M, Mandelkern M, Phelps M, et al. Reversibility of cardiac wall motion abnormalities predicted by positron tomography. *N Engl J Med* 1986; 314:884–888.

80. Camici P, Araujo LI, Spinks T, Lammertsma AA, Kaski JC, Shea MJ, et al. Increased uptake of ^{18}F-fluorodeoxyglucose in postischemic myocardium of patients with exercise-induced angina. *Circulation* 1986; 74:81–88.

81. Schwaiger M, Schelbert HR, Ellison D, Hansen H, Yeatman L, Vinten-Johansen J, et al. Sustained regional abnormalities in cardiac metabolism after transient ischemia in the chronic dog model. *J Am Coll Cardiol* 1985; 6:336–347.

82. Camici P, Bailey IA. Time course of myocardial glycogen repletion following acute transient ischemia. *Circulation* 1984; 70:II-85.

83. Schwaiger M, Neese RA, Araujo L, Wyns W, Wisneski JA, Sochor H, et al. Sustained nonoxidative glucose utilization and depletion of glycogen in reperfused canine myocardium. *J Am Coll Cardiol* 1989; 13:745–754.

84. Schwaiger M, Brunken R, Grover-McKay M, Krivokapich J, Child J, Tillisch JH, et al. Regional myocardial metabolism in patients with acute myocardial infarction assessed by positron emission tomography. *J Am Coll Cardiol* 1986; 8:800–808.

85. Bolli R, Triana F, Jeroudi MO. Postischemic mechanical and vascular dysfunction (myocardial "stunning" and microvascular "stunning") and the effects of calcium-channel blockers on ischemia/reperfusion injury. *Clin Cardiol* 1989; 12:III-16–III-25.

86. Vanoverschelde J-L, Wijns W, Depré C, Essamri B, Heyndrickx GR, Borgers M, et al. Mechanisms of chronic regional postischemic dysfunction in humans: New insights from the study of noninfarcted collateral-dependent myocardium. *Circulation* 1993; 87:1513–1523.

87. Rahimtoola SH. A perspective on the three large multicenter random-ized clinical trials of coronary bypass surgery for chronic stable angina. *Circulation* 1987; 72:V-123–V-135.

88. Rahimtoola SH. The hibernating myocardium. *Am Heart J* 1989; 117:211–221.

89. Schulz R, Rose J, Martin C, Brodde O-E, Heusch G. Development of short-term myocardial hibernation—its limitation by the severity of ischemia and inotropic stimulation. *Circulation* 1993; 88:684–695.

90. Chen C, Gillam L, Chen L, Knibb D, Knight D, Waters D. Temporal hierarchy in functional and ultrastructural recoveries between short-term and chronic hibernating myocardium after reperfusion. *Circulation* 1995; 92:I-552.

91. Chen C, Chen L, Fallon J, May L, Bow L, Knibbs D, et al. Functional and structural alterations with 24-hour myocardial hibernation and recovery after reperfusion. *Circulation* 1996; 94:507–516.

92. Stinson E, Billingham M. Correlative study of regional left ventricular histology and contractile function. *Am J Cardiol* 1977; 39:378–383.

93. Cabin HS, Soni Clubbs K, Vita N, Zaret BL. Regional dysfunction by equilibrium radionuclide angiography: A clinicopathologic study evaluating the relation of degree of dysfunction to the presence and extent of myocardial infarction. *J Am Coll Cardiol* 1987; 10:743–747.

94. Flameng W, Suy R, Schwarz F, Borgers M, Piessens J, Thone F, et al. Ultrastructural correlates of left ventricular contraction abnormalities in patients with chronic ischemic heart disease: Determinants of reversible segmental asynergy post-revascularization surgery. *Am Heart J* 1981; 102:846–857.

95. Maes A, Flameng W, Nuyts J, Borgers M, Shivalkar B, Ausma J, et al. Histological alterations in chronically hypoperfused myocardium: Correlation with PET findings. *Circulation* 1994; 90:735–745.

96. Depré C, Vanoverschelde J-LJ, Melin J, Borgers M, Bol A, Ausma J, et al. Structural and metabolic correlates of the reversibility of chronic left ventricular ischemic dysfunction in humans. *Am J Physiol* 1995; 268:H1265–H1275.

97. Schwarz E, Schaper J, vom Dahl J, Altehoefer C, Grohmann B, Schoendube F, et al. Myocyte degeneration and cell death in hibernating human myocardium. *J Am Coll Cardiol* 1996; 27:1577–1585.

98. Borgers M, Ausma J. Structural aspects of the chronic hibernating myocardium in man. *Basic Res Cardiol* 1995; 90:44–46.

99. Schwaiger M, Sun D, Deeb G, Nguyen N, Haas F, Sebening F, et al. Expression of myocardial glucose transporter (GLUT) mRNAs in patients with advanced coronary artery disease (CAD). *Circulation* 1994; 90:I-113.

100. Brunken R, Mody F, Hawkins R, Nienaber C, Phelps M, Schelbert H. Metabolic imaging with positron emission tomography detects viable tissue in myocardial segments with persistent defects on twenty-four hour tomographic thallium-201 scintigraphy. *Circulation* 1992; 86:1357–1369.

101. Fragasso G, Chierchia S, Lucignani G, Landoni C, Conversano A, Gilardi M, et al. Time dependence of residual tissue viability after myocardial infarction assessed by [18F] fluorodeoxyglucose and positron emission tomography. *Am J Cardiol* 1993; 72:131G–139G.

102. Vanoverschelde J, Melin J, Depré C, Borgers M, Dion R, Wijns W. Time-course of functional recovery of hibernating myocardium after coronary revascularization. *Circulation* 1994; 90:I-378. Abstract.

103. Nienaber C, Brunken R, Sherman C, Yeatman L, Gambhir S, Krivokapich J, et al. Metabolic and functional recovery of ischemic human myocardium after coronary angioplasty. *J Am Coll Cardiol* 1991; 18:966–978.

104. Tamaki N, Yonekura Y, Yamashita K, Saji H, Magata Y, Senda M, et al. Positron emission tomography using fluorine-18 deoxyglucose in evaluation of coronary artery bypass grafting. *Am J Cardiol* 1989; 64:860–865.

105. Carrel T, Jenni R, Haubold-Reuter S, Von Schulthess G, Pasic M, Turina M. Improvement of severely reduced left ventricular function after surgical revascularization in patients with preoperative myocardial infarction. *Eur J Cardiothorac Surg* 1992; 6:479–484.

106. Burt R, Perkins O, Oppenheim B, Schauwecker D, Stein L, Wellman H, et al. Direct comparison of fluorine-18-FDG SPECT, fluorine-18-FDG PET and rest thallium-201 SPECT for detection of myocardial viability. *J Nucl Med* 1995; 36:176–179.

107. Bax J, Cornel J, Visser F, Fioretti P, van Lingen A, Kamp O, et al. Quantitative analysis of FDG and Tl-201 SPECT for the prediction of functional outcome after revascularization. *J Nucl Med* 1995; 36:36P. Abstract.

108. Bax J, Visser F, Blanksma P, Veening M, Tan E, Willemsen A, et al. Comparison of myocardial uptake of fluorine-18-fluorodeoxyglucose imaged with PET and SPECT in dyssynergic myocardium. *J Nucl Med* 1996; 37:1631–1636.

109. Miyaoka R, Costa W, Lewellen T, Kaplan M, Kohlmyer S, Jansen F. Coincidence mode imaging using a standard dual-headed gamma camera. *J Nucl Med* 1996; 37:223P. Abstract.

110. Glass E, Nelleman P, Hines H, Mandelkern M, Blahd W. Initial coincidence imaging experience with a SPECT/PET dual head camera. *J Nucl Med* 1996; 37:53P. Abstract.

111. Bonow R, Dilsizian V, Cuocolo A, Bacharach S. Identification of viable myocardium in patients with chronic coronary artery disease and left ventricular dysfunction: Comparison of thallium scintigraphy with reinjection and PET imaging with F-18-fluorodeoxyglucose. *Circulation* 1991; 83:26–37.

112. Knuuti M, Saraste M, Nuutila P, Harkonen R, Wegelius U, Happanen A, et al. Myocardial viability: Fluorine-18-deoxyglucose positron emission tomography in prediction of wall motion recovery after revascularization. *Circulation* 1994; 90:2356–2366.

113. Baer F, Voth E, Deutsch H, Schneider C, Horst M, de Vivie E, et al. Predictive value of low dose dobutamine transesophageal echocardiography and fluorine-18 fluorodeoxyglucose positron emission tomography for recovery of regional left ventricular function after successful revascularization. *J Am Coll Cardiol* 1996; 28:60–69.

114. Tamaki N, Ohtani H, Yamashita K, Magata Y, Yonekura Y, Nohara R, et al. Metabolic activity in the areas of new fill-in after thallium-201 reinjection: Comparison with positron emission tomography using fluorine-18-deoxyglucose. *J Nucl Med* 1991; 32:673–678.

115. Gropler RJ, Geltman EM, Sampathkumaran K, Perez JE, Schechtman KB, Conversano A, et al. Comparison of carbon-11-acetate with fluorine-18-fluorodeoxyglucose for delineating viable myocardium by positron emission tomography. *J Am Coll Cardiol* 1993; 22:1587–1597.

116. Lucignani G, Paolini G, Landoni C, Zuccari M, Paganelli G, Galli L, et al. Presurgical identification of hibernating myocardium by combined use of technetium-99m hexakis 2-methoxyisobutylisonitrile single photon emission tomography and fluorine-18 fluoro-2-deoxy-D-glucose positron emission tomography in patients with coronary artery disease. *Eur J Nucl Med* 1992; 19:874–881.

117. Marwick T, Nemec J, Lafont A, Salcedo E, MacIntyre W. Prediction by postexercise fluoro-18 deoxyglucose positron emission tomography of improvement in exercise capacity after revascularization. *Am J Cardiol* 1992; 69:854–859.

118. vom Dahl J, Altehoefer C, Sheehan F, Buechin P, Uebis R, Messmer B, et al. Recovery of regional left ventricular dysfunction after coronary revascularization: Impact of myocardial viability assessed by nuclear imaging and vessel patency at follow-up angiography. *J Am Coll Cardiol* 1996; 28:948–958.

119. vom Dahl J, Eitzman D, Al-Aouar A, Kanter H, Hicks R, Deeb G, et al. Relation of regional function, perfusion, and metabolism in patients with advanced coronary artery disease undergoing surgical revascularization. *Circulation* 1994; 90:2356–2366.

120. Gropler R, Geltman E, Sampathkumaran K, Perez J, Moerlein S, Sobel B, et al. Functional recovery after coronary revascularization for chronic coronary artery disease is dependent on maintenance of oxidative metabolism. *J Am Coll Cardiol* 1992; 20:569–577.

121. Gropler R, Siegel B, Sampathkumaran K, Perez J, Sobel B, Bergmann S, et al. Dependence of recovery of contractile function on maintenance of oxidative metabolism after myocardial infarction. *J Am Coll Cardiol* 1992; 19:989–997.

122. Shivalkar B, Maes A, Borgers M, Ausma J, Scheys I, Nuyts J, et al. Only hibernating myocardium invariably shows early recovery after coronary revascularization. *Circulation* 1996; 94:308–315.

123. Grandin C, Wijns W, Melin J, Bol A, Robert A, Heyndrickx G, et al. Delineation of myocardial viability with PET. *J Nucl Med* 1995; 36:1543–1552.

124. Marwick T, MacIntyre W, Lafont A, Nemec J, Salcedo E. Metabolic responses of hibernating and infarcted myocardium to revascularization: A follow-up study of regional perfusion, function, and metabolism. *Circulation* 1992; 85:1347–1353.

125. Dilsizian V, Rocco T, Freedman N, Leon M, Bonow R. Enhanced detection of ischemic but viable myocardium by the reinjection of thallium after stress-redistribution imaging. *N Engl J Med* 1990; 323:141–146.

126. Tamaki N, Kawamoto M, Takahashi N, Yonekura Y, Magata Y, Nohara R, et al. Prognostic value of an increase in fluorine-18 deoxyglucose uptake in patients with myocardial infarction: Comparison with stress thallium imaging. *J Am Coll Cardiol* 1993; 22:1621–1627.

127. Ragosta M, Beller GA, Watson DD, Kaul S, and Gimple LW. Quantitative planar rest-redistribution ^{201}Tl imaging in detection of myocardial viability and prediction of improvement in left ventricular function after coronary bypass surgery in patients with severely depressed left ventricular function. *Circulation* 1993; 87:1630–1641.

128. Dreyfus G, Duboc D, Blasco A, Vigoni F, Dubois C, Brodaty D, et al. Myocardial viability assessment in ischemic cardiomyopathy: Benefits of coronary revascularization. *Ann Thorac Surg* 1994; 57:1402–1408.

129. Gewirtz H, Fischman A, Abraham S, Gilson M, Strauss H, Alpert N. Positron emission tomographic measurements of absolute regional myocardial blood flow permits identification of nonviable myocardium in patients with chronic myocardial infarction. *J Am Coll Cardiol* 1994; 23:851–859.

130. Stevenson W, Stevenson L, Middlekauff H, Fonarow G, Hamilton M, Woo M, et al. Improving survival for patients with advanced heart failure: A study of 737 consecutive patients. *J Am Coll Cardiol* 1995; 26:1417–1423.

131. Czernin J, Porenta G, Müller P, Vaghaiwalla Mody F, Brunken R, Tillisch J, et al. Perfusion defect extent determines LV function in patients with PET ischemia. *Circulation* 1991; 84:II-474. Abstract.

132. Yoshida K, Gould K. Quantitative relation of myocardial infarct size and myocardial viability by positron emission tomography to left ventricular ejection fraction and 3-year mortality with and without revascularization. *J Am Coll Cardiol* 1993; 22:984–997.

133. Eitzman D, Al-Aouar Z, vom Dahl J, Kirsh M, Schwaiger M. Clinical outcome of patients with advanced coronary artery disease after viability studies with positron emission tomography. *J Am Coll Cardiol* 1992; 20:559–565.

134. Di Carli M, Davidson M, Little R, Khanna S, Mody F, Brunken R, et al. Value of metabolic imaging with positron emission tomography for evaluating prognosis in patients with coronary artery disease and left ventricular dysfunction. *Am J Cardiol* 1994; 73:527–533.

135. Di Carli M, Farbod A, Schelbert H, Brunken R, Laks H, Phelps M, et al. Quantitative relation between myocardial viability and improvement in heart failure symptoms after revascularization in patients with ischemic cardiomyopathy. *Circulation* 1995; 92:3436–3444.

136. Goldman L, Hashimoto B, Cook E, Loscalzo A. Comparative reproducibility and validity of systems for assessing cardiovascular functional class: Advantages of a new specific activity scale. *Circulation* 1981; 64:1227–1234.

137. Lee K, Marwick T, Cook S, Go R, Fix J, James K, et al. Prognosis of patients with left ventricular dysfunction, with and without viable myocardium after myocardial infarction. *Circulation* 1994; 90:2687–2694.

138. Duong T, Hendi P, Fonarow G, Asgarzadie F, Stevenson L, Di Carli M, et al. Role of positron emission tomographic assessment of myocardial viability in the management of patients who are referred for cardiac transplantation. *Circulation* 1995; 92:I-123. Abstract.

139. Duong T, Fonarow G, Laks H, Hendi P, Czernin J, Phelps M, et al. Cost effectiveness of positron emission tomography (PET) in the management of ischemic cardiomyopathy patients who are referred for cardiac transplantation. *J Am Coll Cardiol* 1996; 27:144A. Abstract.

140. Louie H, Laks H, Milgalter E, Drinkwater D, Hamilton M, Brunken R, et al. Ischemic cardiomyopathy: Criteria for coronary revascularization and cardiac transplantation. *Circulation* 1991; 84:III-290–III-295.

141. Czernin J, Porenta G, Brunken R, Krivokapich J, Chen K, Bennett R, et al. Regional blood flow, oxidative metabolism, and glucose utilization in patients with recent myocardial infarction. *Circulation* 1993; 88:884–895.

142. Feigl E, Neat G, Huang A. Interrelations between coronary artery pressure, myocardial metabolism and coronary blood flow. *J Mol Cell Cardiol* 1990; 22:375–390.

143. Braunwald E, Kloner RA. The stunned myocardium: Prolonged, postischemic ventricular dysfunction. *Circulation* 1982; 66:1146–1149.

144. Maes A, Van de Werf F, Nuyts J, Bormans G, Desmet W, Mortelmans L. Impaired myocardial tissue perfusion early after successful thrombolysis: Impact on myocardial flow, metabolism, and function at late follow-up. *Circulation* 1995; 92:2072–2078.

145. Hicks R, Melon P, Kalff V, Wolfe E, Dick R, Popma J, et al. Metabolic imaging by positron emission tomography early after myocardial infarction as a predictor of recovery of myocardial function after reperfusion. *J Nucl Cardiol* 1994; 1:124–137.

146. Chan S, Brunken R, Phelps M, Schelbert H. Use of the metabolic tracer C-11 acetate for evaluation of regional myocardial perfusion. *J Nucl Med* 1991; 32:665–672.

147. Knuuti M, Nuutila P, Ruotsalainen U, Teräs M, Saraste M, Härkönen R, et al. The value of quantitative analysis of glucose utilization in detection of myocardial viability by PET. *J Nucl Med* 1993; 34:2068–2075.

148. Czernin J, Porenta G, Brunken R, Bennet R, Tillisch J, Phelps M, et al. Metabolic and functional fate of viable myocardium by PET early after acute infarction. *J Am Coll Cardiol* 1991; 17:120A. Abstract.

THREE

HEART FAILURE

21
PATHOPHYSIOLOGY OF HEART FAILURE

Robert C. Schlant / Edmund H. Sonnenblick / Arnold M. Katz

DEFINITIONS

The subject of heart failure requires a number of definitions to denote pathology, hemodynamic alterations, and clinical symptoms. The following definitions and classification (Table 21-1) are presented, although more precise analysis and classification of heart failure in the future might be based on differences in pathology and biochemistry.[1–10]

Circulatory Failure

Circulatory failure is a general term that refers to an inadequacy of the cardiovascular system in performing its basic functions of providing nutrition to and removing metabolic products from the cells of the body. It may be caused primarily by either cardiac or noncardiac (peripheral) conditions. Noncardiac conditions that can cause circulatory failure include inadequate blood volume, decreased venous return, increased capacity of the vascular system, peripheral vascular abnormalities or disease, and inadequate oxyhemoglobin.

Circulatory overload or *congestion* is a general term referring to excess blood volume from either cardiac or noncardiac causes.[1] *Noncardiac circulatory overload* may be divided into two categories: (1) conditions where the primary defect appears to be an increase in blood volume, as may occur with the accumulation of excess salt and water due to salt-retaining steroids, excess blood or fluid administration, acute glomerulonephritis, oliguria, or anuria; and (2) conditions where the primary defect appears to be an increased venous return and/or decreased peripheral resistance, as may occur with arteriovenous fistulas, beriberi, cirrhosis, or severe anemia, in which the increase in blood volume is secondary. Many patients with noncardiac circulatory overload eventually develop secondary "high-output" heart failure.

Heart Failure

Heart failure is a clinical syndrome that arises when the heart is unable to pump sufficient blood to meet the metabolic needs of the body at normal filling pressures, provided the venous return to the heart is normal. It is often preceded by ventricular dysfunction, which is characterized by loss of overload of the myocardium accompanied by the compensations of ventricular hypertrophy and/or dilatation. This syndrome, however, involves more than a circulatory disorder caused by impaired pump function, and heart failure is generally associated with a very poor prognosis, even when symptoms are mild.[11,12]

Systolic left ventricular dysfunction or *failure* reflects a decrease in normal emptying capacity [usually with an ejection fraction (EF) of ≤45 percent] that is usually associated with a compensatory increase in diastolic volume, whether or not symptoms or limitation of function are present. *Isolated diastolic ventricular dysfunction* or *failure* is present when the filling of one or both ventricles is impaired while the emptying capacity is normal. It may be due to a thickened (hypertrophied) ventricular wall, infiltrative cardiomyopathies, and/or tachycardia, which limits the time for diastolic filling, resulting in increased ventricular filling pressures and eventually pulmonary edema.

Congestive heart failure (CHF) denotes a syndrome with complex and variable symptoms and signs, including dyspnea and increased fatigability, tachypnea, tachycardia, pulmonary rales, cardiomegaly, ventricular gallop sounds, and peripheral edema. In most patients, CHF and abnormal circulatory congestion occur as a result of both heart failure and subsequent changes in the peripheral circulation, accompanied by activation of the sympathetic nervous system and the renin-angiotensin system. In most patients with clinical CHF due to mechanical or myocardial abnormalities, the heart (pump) failure is

TABLE 21-1

CLASSIFICATION OF CIRCULATORY FAILURE AND CIRCULATORY OVERLOAD

Circulatory failure
  Heart (cardiac) failure
  Noncardiac (peripheral) circulatory failure
    Decreased return of blood to heart, inadequate blood volume
    Increased capacity of vascular bed
    Peripheral vascular abnormalities or disease
    Inadequate oxyhemoglobin
Circulatory congestion
  Cardiac circulatory overload
    Heart (cardiac) failure
  Noncardiac circulatory overload
    Increase in blood volume
    Increase in venous return and/or decrease in peripheral vascular resistance

preceded by a substantial period of *myocardial* dysfunction during which cardiac *pump* function and cardiac output (at least while at rest) may be maintained by compensatory mechanisms that include myocardial hypertrophy and ventricular dilatation. For this reason, in the early stages the patient may have little or no limitation or symptoms. Initially, the cardiac output may be within the range of normal at rest but fails to increase or may even decline during exercise or stress. Ultimately, the cardiac output is decreased even at rest. Associated changes include an increase in peripheral vascular resistance (PVR) at rest and a failure of the PVR to decrease with increased metabolic needs.

When intravascular circulatory congestion is present for any length of time with elevation of left ventricular diastolic and pulmonary venous pressures, fluid transudation from the capillaries into the interstitial spaces increases. In the pulmonary circulation, pulmonary edema develops if the rate of transudation exceeds the rate of lymphatic drainage. Pulmonary edema is often detected initially by x-ray examination, and only later are audible rales detected on physical examination. In the systemic venous system, elevated jugular venous pressure is often visible and may be accompanied by dependent peripheral edema and hepatomegaly. In the majority of patients, CHF develops chronically and is associated with the retention of sodium and water by the kidneys (see Chap. 94).

Acute heart failure can develop during acute ischemia of the ventricle, following a myocardial infarction, tachycardia, or the rupture of a cardiac valve or structure. An acute shift of blood from the systemic to the pulmonary circulation can occur before the retention of significant sodium or water. The term *congestive heart failure* should not be used unless there is congestion of cardiac origin. When the cause of the pulmonary or peripheral congestion is not clear, however, it is usually preferable to describe the symptoms or signs, which are nonspecific, and to avoid improperly diagnosing heart failure.

Forward and Backward Failure

Classically, the hemodynamic consequences of heart failure are conceptually simple because, like any pump, the heart has only two ways to fail: inadequate emptying of the venous reservoirs (backward failure), and reduced ejection of blood under pressure into the aorta and pulmonary artery (forward failure). Backward failure of the left heart can be caused by mitral stenosis, where narrowing of the mitral valve orifice reduces blood flow into a normal left ventricle, or a hypertrophic cardiomyopathy, where reduced left ventricular cavity volume impairs diastolic filling. Forward failure of the left heart can occur when aortic stenosis mechanically obstructs ejection or when myocarditis or a large myocardial infarction reduces ejection.

The usefulness of the concepts of forward and backward failure is limited because a heart that empties poorly retains an excessive end-systolic volume that reduces filling during the subsequent diastole, and a heart that does not fill adequately cannot eject a normal stroke volume. For these reasons, backward and forward failure invariably coexist. The hemodynamic patterns of backward and forward failure are also modified by circulatory adjustments such as salt and water retention and vasoconstriction, which influence the extent to which impaired left ventricular ejection (forward failure) leads to a fall in blood pressure or a fall in cardiac output. In most patients with heart failure, reflex vasoconstriction maintains blood pressure at the expense of reduced ejection; as a result, cardiac output is reduced in most patients with heart failure, whereas arterial pressure generally remains at or near normal levels.

Forward failure is commonly equated with depressed ventricular contractility whether due to loss of myocardium or to reduced myocardial function secondary to sustained overloading, and backward failure with impaired relaxation (decreased lusitropy) (Table 21-2). These properties of the

TABLE 21-2

CLASSIFICATION OF IMPAIRED VENTRICULAR FUNCTION

Forward and Backward Failure
  Forward failure: (depressed inotropy, impaired ejection)
  Backward failure: (depressed lusitropy, impaired filling)
Systolic and diastolic dysfunction
  Systolic dysfunctions (eccentric hypertrophy)
  Diastolic dysfunctions (concentric hypertrophy)

Forward and backward failure are related conceptually to systolic and diastolic dysfunction, respectively. These relationships are often obscured, however, because neurohumoral responses and therapy commonly obscure any relationship between systolic dysfunction, depressed inotropy, and impaired ejection (forward failure), and between diastolic dysfunction, depressed lusitropy, and impaired filling (backward failure). Systolic dysfunction refers to a pathophysiologic abnormality in which heart failure is associated with a dilated, often eccentrically hypertrophied ventricle, while diastolic dysfunction is seen most commonly in patients with a thick-walled, concentrically hypertrophied ventricle.

myofibrils, however, are not closely linked to altered hemodynamics; instead, reflex changes in the peripheral circulation and alterations in the architecture of the failing ventricle, rather than depressed contractility and relaxation, are often the major determinants of the extent of forward and backward failure.

Therapy also determines the extent of forward and backward failure. Vasodilator therapy, by reducing the afterload of a failing left ventricle, alleviates the symptoms of forward failure without directly affecting either inotropy or lusitropy, while diuresis, by depleting vascular volume, improves backward failure by lowering venous pressure but at the same time may worsen forward failure by decreasing cardiac output. For these reasons, the severity of either forward or backward failure, as evaluated in terms of reduced cardiac output and increased venous pressure, generally provides little information as to whether the primary hemodynamic abnormality is impaired relaxation or depressed contractility.

Systolic and Diastolic Dysfunction

A more useful distinction in ventricular failure is that between systolic and diastolic dysfunction (Table 21-2). These terms, however, are most appropriately defined in terms of altered ventricular architecture, rather than systemic hemodynamics. *Systolic dysfunction* describes a ventricle whose output is limited by impaired ejection (forward failure), whereas *diastolic dysfunction* refers to a ventricle in which filling is limited (backward failure). Because the manifestations of forward and backward failure are influenced by circulatory dynamics (see above), it is appropriate to reserve the term *systolic dysfunction* for a dilated, often eccentrically hypertrophied ventricle, and *diastolic dysfunction* for the thick-walled, concentrically hypertrophied ventricle with a normal or small cavity.

Generally, systolic ventricular dysfunction is characterized by an increase in end-diastolic volume (EDV) and a normal or somewhat reduced stroke volume (SV), resulting in a decrease in ejection fraction (EF). This relationship of SV to EDV is normally described by the Frank-Starling relationship (Fig. 3-14). The increase in EDV is associated with an increase in ventricular end-diastolic pressure (EDP) in consonance with the resting pressure-volume curve. As will be discussed, the filling pressures may be further elevated for a given EDV by concentric hypertrophy or a fibrotic wall or be actually decreased by chronic overdistension (eccentric hypertrophy).

In patients with mild heart failure, the ventricular EDP and the cardiac output may be normal at rest, but the former may become elevated to abnormal levels during stress such as exercise or an increase in afterload. The increase in cardiac output relative to the increase in oxygen consumption is also decreased (see below and Chap. 22). In patients with more severe systolic dysfunction, both the early- and the end-diastolic pressures may be elevated even at rest. The elevated left ventricular diastolic pressure increases pulmonary venous and capillary pressures and contributes to increased dyspnea,

as a result of changes in pulmonary compliance due to pulmonary congestion and edema. It is also apparent that before one reaches this stage of clinical heart failure, the body has utilized many compensatory mechanisms after the onset of the initial abnormality or stress and that these compensatory mechanisms eventually have failed to maintain the needs for cardiac output (see below).

Since the fundamental clinical manifestations of heart failure reflect inability of the heart as a pump to supply the demands of the body at normal filling pressures adequately, it is apparent that this term could be applicable in a very general sense whenever the demands for increased cardiac output are not met as a result of cardiac disease. This implies that any heart would eventually "fail" if the demands were increased sufficiently. In fact, this might rarely occur in persons with apparently normal hearts during extreme exertion. In most individuals, however, exertion is stopped prior to heart failure by fatigue or breathlessness, although these symptoms might be related to a limitation of cardiac output.

The causes of overall heart pump failure may be classified in three main categories: (1) failure primarily related to work overloads or mechanical abnormalities, (2) failure primarily related to primary myocardial abnormalities, and (3) failure related to abnormal cardiac rhythm or conduction disturbances (Table 21-3). Myocardial infarction resulting in a quantitative loss of myocardium creates a special type of work overload. During the acute infarction, the EF falls as the EDV is increased to sustain a reduced SV, and the fall in EF is approximately proportional to the amount of myocardium lost. With time, the EF tends to remain at this reduced level. With healing of the infarction, the akinetic infarcted region becomes a scar that not only cannot contribute to ventricular emptying but may even contribute to the load. Thus, the entire load falls on the remaining nonischemic myocardium. This load is further increased by the increased diastolic volume, which causes wall tension to be increased for any given pressure even though the nonischemic myocardium hypertrophies in proportion to the amount of myocardium that is lost. Heart failure may ensue months or years later as a so-called ischemic cardiomyopathy that results from progressive ventricular dilatation and reactive hypertrophy, termed *ventricular remodeling*, in the remaining nonischemic myocardium (see Chap. 73). Although heart failure is usually considered to be due to ventricular failure, atrial failure (see below) can contribute significantly.

There are several causes of both "primary" and "secondary" myocardial failure (Table 21-3). Myocardial failure is said to be *primary* when it is caused by any of the following: (1) idiopathic cardiomyopathy (dilated, hypertrophic, or restrictive; Chaps. 73 to 75); (2) cardiomyopathy associated with a primary neuromuscular disease, such as Friedreich's ataxia, myotonic dystrophy, or Duchenne's muscular dystrophy (Chap. 69); (3) myocarditis (Chap. 76); (4) metabolic deficiencies that may affect the myocardium, such as diabetes mellitus, beriberi, and possibly hyper- or hypothyroidism (Chap. 78); (5) toxic effects of radiation, electricity, or chemi-

TABLE 21-3

GENERAL CAUSES OF OVERALL HEART PUMP FAILURE

Mechanical abnormalities
  Increased pressure load
    Central (aortic stenosis, etc.)
    Peripheral (systemic arterial hypertension, etc.)
  Increased volume load (valvular regurgitation, shunts,
    increased venous return, etc.)
  Obstruction to ventricular filling (mitral or tricuspid
    stenosis)
  Pericardial constriction, tamponade
  Endocardial or myocardial restriction
  Ventricular aneurysm
  Ventricular dyssynergy
Myocardial (muscular) abnormalities or loss of myocytes
  Primary abnormalities or loss of myocytes
    Cardiomyopathy
    Neuromuscular disorders
    Myocarditis
    Metabolic (diabetes mellitus, etc.)
    Toxic (alcohol, cobalt, etc.)
    Presbycardia
  Secondary myocardial abnormalities or loss of myocytes
    Dysdynamic (secondary to mechanical abnormalities)
    Ischemia (coronary heart disease)
    Metabolic
    Inflammation
    Infiltrative diseases
    Systemic diseases
    Chronic obstructive lung disease
    Myocardial depression due to drugs
Altered cardiac rhythm or conduction disturbances
  Standstill
  Fibrillation
  Extreme tachycardia or bradycardia
  Chronic tachycardia
  Electrical asynchrony, conduction disturbances

cals, such as alcohol or cobalt (Chaps. 77 and 80); or (6) the process of aging, where myocytes are lost diffusely and progressively with reactive hypertrophy and focal fibrosis (Chap. 96).

Myocardial failure is said to be *secondary* when it is produced by any of the following: (1) "dysdynamic" myocardial failure (see below); (2) myocardial ischemia, which may produce either an acute, dysdynamic myocardial failure or chronic, static failure due to a specific heart muscle disease with loss of myocytes and myocardial fibrosis, as noted above (Chaps. 38 and 43), (3) metabolic disorders, such as acromegaly, hypoparathyroidism, pheochromocytoma, and occasionally thyroid disease or toxins (Chap. 78); (4) myocardial inflammation (Chap. 76); (5) myocardial infiltrative disorders and restrictive cardiomyopathies (Chap. 75); (6) systemic diseases (Chaps. 76, 78, 79, 85, 93, 94); (7) acute or chronic lung disease (Chaps. 59 to 61); or (8) depression due to drugs, such as adriamycin (Chap. 80). The distinction between primary and secondary myocardial failure is frequently diffi-

cult and occasionally arbitrary. For example, in diabetes mellitus, heart muscle disease or cardiomyopathy may develop, most commonly associated with hypertension and diffuse myocyte loss (Chap. 78). This loss may be due to microvascular spasm and focal ischemia.

The cause of left ventricular systolic dysfunction in patients with chronic obstructive lung disease in unknown, although the combination of hypoxia and hypercapnia may be important. Left ventricular diastolic dysfunction in such patients is, in part, secondary to the pronounced right ventricular hypertrophy and dilatation with secondary elevation of left ventricular diastolic pressure due to ventricular interdependence. The latter phenomenon is also important in the pathophysiology of acute pulmonary edema occasionally encountered in patients with acute pulmonary embolus.

Dysdynamic myocardial failure is a general term used to refer to secondary myocardial failure that commonly develops after a period of increased ventricular preload or afterload. In response to an increased load, myocytes hypertrophy in accord with the Laplace relationship, as discussed below. When this adaptation is inadequate, ventricular dilatation ensues. These changes, together with any myocyte loss and resultant fibrosis, are termed *ventricular remodeling*; myocardial failure is a late stage in the process. Dysdynamic failure is frequently associated with hypokinesis, akinesis, and dyskinesis, denoting focal wall abnormalities or loss of contraction. Dysdynamic (i.e., with impaired force or power) myocardial failure implies that the *systolic* mechanical performance, or myocardial contractility per unit mass, is significantly decreased; initially, however, the overall cardiac (pump) function may be maintained by the compensatory mechanisms noted above, and the cardiac output at rest may not be abnormally decreased.

Dysdynamic heart failure can be viewed as a load-induced cardiomyopathy, or a "cardiomyopathy of overload."[13] The mechanism by which chronic overload leads to the progressive deterioration of the myocardium remains unclear but may involve cell death due to energy starvation, apoptosis, and/or a maladaptive growth response[14] (Fig. 21-1).

In general, it is important to note that patients' symptoms are related to CHF, whereas patient survival is related to progressive deterioration of the failing myocardium.

Myocardial or Ventricular Failure

Ventricular (myocardial) dysfunction is a term used to denote performance that is reduced, while *ventricular (myocardial) failure* refers to a more markedly decreased performance of the myocardium. When used in reference to myocardium, *function* has usually referred to systolic or shortening function, although there may also be diastolic abnormalities in the presence of minimal or no significant systolic abnormalities. In many patients with moderate or more marked myocardial dysfunction or myocardial failure, the decreased myocardial function can be detected by studies of overall cardiac pump function, whereas milder dysfunction in other patients may

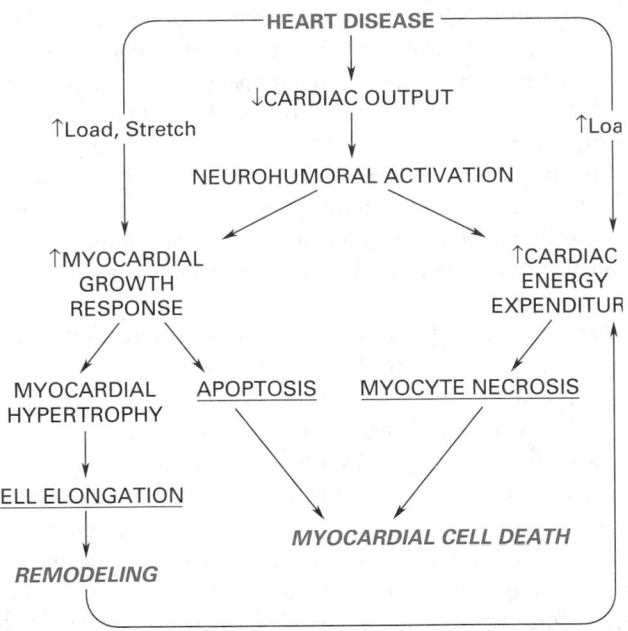

HEART DISEASE

↓CARDIAC OUTPUT

↑Load, Stretch   ↑Loa

NEUROHUMORAL ACTIVATION

↑MYOCARDIAL GROWTH RESPONSE   ↑CARDIAC ENERGY EXPENDITUR

MYOCARDIAL HYPERTROPHY   APOPTOSIS   MYOCYTE NECROSIS

ELL ELONGATION

MYOCARDIAL CELL DEATH

REMODELING

FIGURE 21-1

Possible mechanisms by which overloading can cause progressive deterioration of the heart ("cardiomyopathy of overload"). Several mechanisms, including myocyte stretch, activate a growth response that initiates myocardial hypertrophy in the overloaded heart (*left*). The same growth response may also activate signal transduction systems that cause programmed cell death (apoptosis). The hypertrophic response to overload, by causing sarcomeres to be added in series, can also lead to cell elongation and so accelerate remodeling; the resulting increase in wall tension, along with the overload itself (*right*), increases cardiac energy expenditure that, in the overloaded heart, can accelerate myocyte necrosis. Reduced cardiac output activates neurohumoral responses (*center*), which, by increasing afterload and β-adrenergic stimulation of the heart, also increase cardiac energy expenditure. Because many mediators of the neurohumoral response to a fall in cardiac output promote myocardial cell growth, neurohumoral activation can also accelerate both apoptosis and remodeling.

be detected only by more specific and sensitive indices of myocardial contractility (see Chap. 22). In many patients with myocardial dysfunction failure, the overall cardiac pump function (and cardiac output at rest) may be maintained reasonably well by compensatory mechanisms such as increased ventricular filling (preload) with dilatation and/or cardiac hypertrophy.

Myocardial failure may develop from many causes (Table 21-3). It may evolve from pressure overloads in which myocytes hypertrophy to meet the load. Hypertrophied cells contract and relax more slowly[15] and may be subject to metabolic limitations. In addition, hypertrophied myocardial cells appear to have a shortened life span.[13,14] This is of considerable prognostic importance because cardiac myocytes appear to have little or no capacity to proliferate. When age-related myocyte loss is added, particularly in association with a late decrease in myocyte contractile activity, failure may ensue with ventricular dilatation. Loss of myocytes—whether segmental, as in acute myocardial infarction, or diffuse, as in myocarditis—sets up a vicious cycle that leads to reactive hypertrophy in remaining myocytes. As compensatory hyper-

trophy becomes more marked in some disease states, the unit contractility of the myocardium often declines because of molecular changes in the heart's contractile proteins and activation system. This is especially likely to occur in response to pressure overload, as in systemic arterial hypertension or aortic stenosis, but also ensues when myocytes are lost.

Ultimately, the myocardial failure (plus mechanical abnormalities that may be present) often leads to a decrease in systolic pump function that is sufficient to produce overall pump or heart failure. In most patients, significant dysfunction and failure of the myocardium occurs before heart (pump) dysfunction or failure and the clinical syndrome of CHF become apparent (see Chap. 22).

Although both systolic and diastolic dysfunction or failure are present in the majority of patients with heart failure, and contraction and relaxation of the ventricle are coupled in patients with and without heart failure,[16] it is useful to consider the systolic and the diastolic properties of the myocardium and of the ventricle separately.[17] Thus, some patients may have marked *systolic ventricular dysfunction or failure* at a time when they do not have significant, if any, elevation of ventricular diastolic pressures. On the other hand, some patients have marked elevation of left ventricular diastolic pressure and pulmonary congestion (*diastolic dysfunction of the ventricle*) at a time when the systolic or pumping function of the ventricle, as characterized by a normal (≥50 percent) EF, is well maintained. The latter situation is especially likely to occur in some patients with hypertrophic cardiomyopathy, systemic hypertension, or aortic stenosis. In these patients the elevated ventricular diastolic pressure may be present due to a combination of the effects of concentric ventricular hypertrophy and myocardial diastolic dysfunction at a time when the EF is normal or slightly elevated, and systolic function or cardiac may be nearly normal. In patients with severe pressure overload hypertrophy, the duration of contraction is prolonged and relaxation is delayed.[15] As a result, systole occupies a greater proportion of time. This effect is amplified by tachycardia, which may produce a high filling pressure for any given diastolic volume (i.e., diastolic dysfunction) despite well-maintained contractile force and EF. Acute, transient diastolic dysfunction may also occur in patients with coronary artery disease, with or without angina pectoris.[18–25] In general, most, but not all, patients with acute diastolic failure of the myocardium also have some systolic abnormalities of contraction, and a ventricle that fills poorly will have a reduced SV.

High-Output Failure

Some patients with high-output states or primary noncardiac circulatory overload may develop pulmonary congestion and edema secondary to an abnormal elevation of ventricular diastolic pressure at a time when the total cardiac output (systolic, or pump, function) and EF of the left ventricle are normal or even increased. The latter syndrome can also occur in conditions associated with an increase in blood volume from the accumulation of excess salt and water due to salt-retaining steroids, excess blood or fluid administration, acute glomerulonephritis, oliguria, or anuria. In other patients, it may occur with an abnormally increased venous return and/or decreased peripheral resistance, as might occur in patients with arteriovenous fistulas, beriberi, hyperthyroidism, cirrhosis, severe anemia, and large vascular tumors. Under such conditions, the chronic volume and/or pressure load on the ventricle may eventually produce myocardial and ventricular systolic (pump) dysfunction or failure. Ultimately, this can both increase diastolic pressures and reduce cardiac output to abnormally low levels. When symptoms of pulmonary congestion or pulmonary edema secondary to elevated diastolic pressure occur while the cardiac output is still normal or elevated, the syndrome is sometimes referred to as *high-output failure*.

"Left-" and "Right-Heart" Failure

"Left-heart" (left-sided) failure and *"right-heart" (right-sided) failure* are clinical terms for conditions in which the primary impairment is of the left side of the heart or of the right side of the heart, respectively. Since both sides of the heart are in a circuit, it is apparent that one side cannot pump significantly more blood than the other side for any length of time in the absence of abnormal shunts, communications, or regurgitation. Furthermore, experimentally produced failure of one ventricle may produce significant hemodynamic and biochemical abnormalities of the other ventricle, even without the usual hemodynamic manifestations of ventricular failure. Abnormal function of the left ventricle not only overloads the right ventricle from augmented pulmonary pressures but may also affect the right ventricle via the shared septum and the phenomenon of ventricular interdependence, or interaction (see below). Altered elastic recoil of the left ventricle in diastole may also affect the right ventricle. Accordingly, when the pumping ability of one ventricle is primarily impaired, the output of the contralateral ventricle can be secondarily decreased; the biochemistry and hemodynamics of the contralateral ventricle can also be abnormal even in "pure" one-sided failure.

Right-sided heart failure commonly follows left-sided heart failure. In most situations, the expression *left-sided heart failure* is clinically used in reference to symptoms and signs of elevated pressure and congestion in the pulmonary veins and capillaries, whereas *right-sided heart failure* is used in reference to symptoms and signs of elevated pressures and congestion in the systemic veins and capillaries. Actually, significant amounts of sodium and water retention, with subsequent peripheral edema formation, may occur with pure left-sided heart failure without hemodynamic evidence of right-sided heart failure. As noted previously, an increase in the diastolic pressure in either ventricle can increase the diastolic pressure or decrease the distensibility of the contralateral ventricle, especially if the pericardium is intact.

Compensated Heart Failure

Compensated heart failure is that condition in which the symptoms of heart failure are relieved by neurohumoral responses or therapy, although the EDV and EDP often remain elevated and the EF remains reduced. As noted below and in Table 21-4, the usual "compensatory" mechanisms include increased sympathetic adrenergic stimulation of the heart, activation of the renal renin-angiotensin system, increased vasoconstriction, fluid retention by the kidney with increased venous return and increased ventricular preload, and cardiac dilatation and hypertrophy. Clinically, myocardial compensation and a decrease in congestion may be produced by improved ventricular performance, and a decrease in congestion may be produced by digitalis glycosides, diuretics, or vasodilator drugs. The term *compensated heart failure* is frequently used in reference to patients with CHF whose symptoms and signs of pulmonary or peripheral congestion have been

TABLE 21-4

COMPENSATORY MECHANISMS INITIATED BY LOW CARDIAC OUTPUT[a]

Mechanism	Short-Term Adaptive Response	Long-Term Maladaptive Response
Salt and water retention	⇑ Preload ⇑ Cardiac output[b]	Edema, anasarca, pulmonary congestion
Vasoconstriction	⇑ Afterload Maintained blood pressure	⇓ Cardiac output, ⇑ cardiac energy expenditure Cell death[b]
⇑ Cardiac, adrenergic drive	⇑ Contractility, ⇑ relaxation, ⇑ heart rate ⇑ Cardiac output[b]	Arrhythmias, ⇑ cardiac energy expenditure Cell death[b]
Transcription factor activation, cell growth	Adaptive hypertrophy ⇑ Sarcomere number ⇑ Cardiac output[b]	Maladaptive hypertrophy Apoptosis, mitochondrial DNA abnormalities Cell death[b]

[a] The compensatory mechanisms initiated by a short-term fall in cardiac output, as occurs following hemorrhage, generate an adaptive response. However, when sustained, as in the chronically overloaded heart, these same mechanisms cause maladaptive responses that further reduce cardiac output, exacerbate symptoms, and appear to accelerate cell death.
[b] Secondary responses.
Source: Adapted with permission from Katz AM.[14]

relieved by therapy. In many such patients, reduced myocardial function and cardiac output persist, although symptoms are relieved by an improvement in peripheral circulation and the reduction in edema and congestion.

Atrial Failure

Although isolated atrial failure rarely, if ever, produces failure of the normal heart, the development of atrial fibrillation or flutter can precipitate clinical heart failure in patients with compensated cardiac function, especially when marked ventricular hypertrophy or diastolic dysfunction is present and when an "atrial kick" is important in maintaining cardiac output (see below). In the presence of severe hypertrophy of the left ventricle, the left atrium may play an important role in augmenting late diastolic filling and thus reducing mean filling pressures. Further, rapid ventricular response in the presence of atrial flutter or fibrillation may limit the time for ventricular filling and lead to elevated diastolic pressures with eventual pulmonary edema.

Stages of Heart Failure

Heart failure is a progressive disease, both in terms or cardiac function and the development of CHF. Later, the peripheral circulatory changes may become the dominant factor in the development of CHF and the evolution of symptoms (see below).

BASIC MECHANISMS OF MYOCARDIAL FAILURE

The basic mechanisms of myocardial failure remain a very active area of investigation. No single mechanism is present in all cases but, rather, mechanisms (Table 21-5) may contribute to myocardial failure under various circumstances and at different points in time. Moreover, many adaptive processes have been identified within the process of heart failure. It is not clear which of these processes are central and primarily responsible for the progression of the disease and which are secondary. The fall in cardiac output in patients with heart failure evokes powerful neurohumoral responses, such as α-adrenergic stimulation that causes vasoconstriction, several mechanisms that increase circulating blood volume by retaining salt and water, and β-adrenergic stimulation that increases both heart rate and stroke volume.[26,27] Increased sympathetic tone and decreased parasympathetic tone occurring early in the process tend to produce sinus tachycardia. Whereas all provide valuable short-term compensation for a transient decrease in cardiac output, they are generally harmful when sustained in the patient with heart failure (Table 21-4). Adverse effects occur when vasoconstriction (increased overload) exacerbates the low-output state in patients with heart failure, when salt and water retention increase filling pressure (preload) and thereby worsen the manifestations of backward failure (see below), and when β-adrenergic stimulation, along with the increased afterload and ventricular dilatation, increases the energy demands of the failing heart. Growing evidence that many of the chemical transmitters that mediate these responses (notably α- and β-adrenergic agonists and angiotensin II) also stimulate maladaptive hypertrophy and even further diffuse myocyte loss suggests that these responses also contribute to the poor prognosis in these patients, and thus may provide an important therapeutic opportunity.

The major primary causes of heart failure have already been noted (Table 21-3). In general, the initiating cause is either related to loss of myocardium, as occurs following an acute myocardial infarction coronary artery disease, or to an excessive overload, i.e., hypertension or valve disease, or both. These primary problems result in compensatory adaptations including hypertrophy and dilatation (ventricular remodeling) and activation of neurohumoral systems (sympathetic and renin-angiotensin). As noted below, continuation of the primary events combined with the progressive alterations of the compensatory adaptions in time result in progressive ventricular failure. As discussed in Chap. 78, diabetes mellitus adds to these problems through development of small-vessel disease, accelerated atherosclerosis, and, in some patients, cardiomyopathy.

TABLE 21-5

POSSIBLE MECHANISMS OF MYOCARDIAL FAILURE

Loss of myocytes
Hypertrophy of remaining myocytes
Energy production and utilization
    Oxygen and energy supply
    Substrate utilization and energy storage
    Inadequate mitochondria mass and function
Ventricular remodeling
Contractile proteins
    Abnormal myofibrillar or myosin ATPase
    Abnormal myocardial proteins
    Defective protein synthesis
    Nonuniformity of contraction and function
Activation of contractile elements
    Membrane Na^+, K^+-ATPase defects
    Abnormal sarcoplasmic reticulum function
        Abnormal Ca^{2+} release
        Abnormal Ca^{2+} uptake
Abnormal myocardial receptor function
    Downregulation of beta adrenoreceptors
    Decreased β_1 receptors
    Decreased G_s protein
    Increased G_1 protein
Autonomic nervous system
    Abnormal myocardial norepinephrine function or kinetics
    Abnormal baroreceptor function
Increased myocardial fibroblast growth and collagen
  synthesis
Aging changes, presbycardia
Sustained tachycardia
Miscellaneous

Energy Production and Utilization

OXYGEN AND ENERGY SUPPLY

Oxygen deprivation, which is most often due to coronary artery disease, results in impaired relaxation and weakened contraction, as may be seen in angina pectoris. When transient, these are readily reversible. With prolonged ischemia, decreased contraction (dyskinesis) may persist for hours beyond return of blood flow and is termed *stunning*. If coronary blood flow is chronically reduced, myocardium may fail to contact ("hibernation") even if necrosis does not ensue. With more serious loss of flow, infarction can occur. All of these states may produce substantial dyskinesia for which the remaining myocardium must sustain the load. The result is hypertrophy of the nonischemic portion of the ventricle; if this is inadequate, an increase in ventricular volume occurs using the Frank-Starling mechanism to sustain stroke volume.

In patients with heart failure, the total amount of oxygen consumed by the heart may be significantly increased because of the increased total mass, the increase in myocardial systolic wall tension due to the Laplace relationship, and perhaps some wasted contractile energy. This increase may result in the extraction of a greater amount of oxygen from each unit or coronary blood flow and a widening of the coronary arteriovenous oxygen difference. Many patients with heart failure are able to increase coronary blood flow during exercise; however, some patients with a dilated ventricle that increases in diameter during exercise may have a further widening of the coronary arteriovenous oxygen difference during exercise and a decrease in coronary blood flow reserve (Chaps. 3 and 22). In the presence of severe left ventricular hypertrophy, coronary blood flow per unit mass of myocardium is usually normal. On the other hand, the capacity of the coronary vascular bed to dilate during reactive hyperemia, which is normally four- to fivefold, is reduced. While reduced perfusion is probably common in end-stage heart failure, a deficit in coronary blood flow or oxygen delivery has not been clearly demonstrated to be a primary cause of heart failure associated with hypertrophy, except in the presence of obstructive coronary disease (see below).

SUBSTRATE UTILIZATION AND ENERGY STORAGE

Although the myocardial uptake of fatty acids and glucose per 100 g of myocardium is normal in heart failure,[28] there is conflicting evidence on whether or not there is a primary decrease in energy liberation by mitochondrial oxidative phosphorylation.[13,14,28–32] The reductions in stores of myocardial high-energy phosphate, creatine phosphate, and/or adenosine triphosphate (ATP) generally found in heart failure are usually thought to be secondary and to be the consequence of the failure rather than the primary cause of the failure.[4,5,13,14,28–34] There also may be reduced levels of creatine kinase and changes in the isoenzymes of creatine kinase in heart failure.[35–37]

The major consequences of the state of energy starvation that is probably seen in many, if not most, failing hearts are due to attenuation of important allosteric (regulatory) effects of ATP, rather than reduction in the supply of substrate for the many energy-consuming reactions involved in contraction, relaxation, and excitation-contraction coupling. Because the normal cytosolic ATP concentration is around 5 to 10 mM, whereas the substrate-binding sites of most ATP-hydrolizing systems are saturated at ATP concentrations less than $1\mu M$, it is unlikely that ATP concentrations fall to levels below those needed to saturate known energy-consuming reactions except in the dying heart. These allosteric effects of high ATP concentrations, which do not require that the nucleotide be hydrolyzed, resemble those of a "lubricant" in that ATP accelerates ion pumps, ion exchangers, and passive ion fluxes through membrane channels. By facilitating the many calcium fluxes involved in excitation-contraction coupling and relaxation, these allosteric effects of ATP exert both inotropic and lusitropic effects.[31]

MITOCHONDRIA MASS AND FUNCTION

There are conflicting data on whether or not there is a significant decrease in the mass of mitochondria relative to the mass of myofibrils that occurs in experimental cardiac hypertrophy.[38–44] It is possible that this is one of the limitations of severe hypertrophy. Defects in mitochondrial oxidative phosphorylation and in mitochondrial calcium metabolism may also be associated with myocardial failure.[13,28–31,45–47] Except in circumstances where coronary flow is limited, such as with large vessel obstructive disease (Chap. 43) or purported microvascular obstructive or vasospastic disease, a primary role of energy limitation in the evolution of heart failure has yet to be demonstrated.[48] It is possible that it may play a role during periods of higher metabolic demand, such as tachycardia.[49]

Ventricular Remodeling (Hypertrophy and Dilatation)

When one portion of the ventricle is disabled, an *increase in intraventricular volume* occurs, presumably in response to a sustained venous return. This involves increased myocyte length, with the limit being the sarcomere at 2.2 μm. With time, compensatory hypertrophy occurs with myocytes becoming longer as well as thicker.

Acute dilatation is limited by the sarcomere, which at 2.2 μm attains maximum force. Beyond this point, stiffness of the sarcomere and the myocardium becomes very large and resting tension rises to high levels. When distending forces become chronic, addition of new sarcomeres in series and dilatation of the ventricle add the load of the Laplace relation, whereby tension in the wall rises with increased volume at the same pressure. In addition, functional mitral regurgitation may occur from excessive ventricular volume.

When increased systolic tension occurs, myocyte *hypertrophy* occurs with the laying down of sarcomeres in parallel. This is accomplished by biochemical alterations in both the contractile proteins and activating membrane systems (see Chap. 6).

In addition to the synthesis of sarcomeres in series with preexisting sarcomeres, "slippage" of myofibrils and myocardial fibers and rearrangement of myocardial fibers along cleavage planes of the left ventricle occur.[2,50–56] Thus, although overstretch of sarcomeres may rarely be present very transiently, it does not appear to be an important primary mechanism of chronic heart failure. There is evidence, however, that excessive stretch of myocytes can lead to myocyte death, apparently by the process of *apoptosis* (programmed cell death), which may lead to further heart failure. The effects of the law of Laplace with ventricular dilatation have been noted above. Nonuniformity of myocardial contraction and functional mitral regurgitation also contribute to pump (heart) failure.[15,57]

Structural and Bichemical Alterations Occurring With Adaptive Hypertrophy and Evolving Failure

CONTRACTILE PROTEINS
Myofibrillar and myosin adenosine triphosphatase (ATPase) are decreased as hypertrophy occurs, both in experimental animals and the atria of patients with heart failure.[29,58–67] A smaller, but probably significant, fall in ventricular myosin ATPase is also seen in clinical heart failure. This correlates with a reduction in the velocity of shortening of the myocardium, and hence a decrease in myocardial contractility, associated with hypertrophy. At the same time, duration of contraction is prolonged and relaxation slowed, although the force of contraction is largely maintained. Thus, these changes may be viewed as an adaptation to load and not a cause of systolic failure. Slowed relaxation, however, can contribute to diastolic dysfunction.

In small animals, the decrease in myosin ATPase is associated with increased synthesis of the slower β (fetal) component of myosin heavy chain isoform and a decrease in the faster α (adult) component. In the human ventricle, the β isoform predominates,[68] so that the decreased myofibrillar ATPase activity may result from other alterations, perhaps in the troponin-tropomyosin system..

ACTIVATION OF CONTRACTILE ELEMENTS

Sarcolemma ATPase and Activating Ca^{2+}
Heart failure may also be associated with defects in the activity of the membrane transport enzyme Na^+, K^+-ATPase or the sarcolemmal transport of Ca^{2+},[2,69–71] although the role of these changes in the pathogenesis of myocardial failure is less definite.[29] In the human ventricle, whose V_3 isoenzyme system predominates, changes in the enzyme systems of the sarcolemma and sarcoplasmic reticulum (SR)[72–74] may be central to the slowing of contraction and relaxation seen in hypertrophy and heart failure.(Table 21-5).

Sarcoplasmic Reticulum Function
There is substantial evidence of defects in both Ca^{2+} release and Ca^{2+} uptake by SR, which is accomplished by a Ca^{2+}, Mg^{2+}-dependent ATPase under the influence of phospholamban or by mitochondria in many types of clinical or experimental hypertrophy and heart failure.[4,7,29,45,75–96] Several studies have shown that this is at least partially due to quantitative alterations of gene expression of SR Ca^{2+}-transport proteins, and particularly the sarco(endo)plasmic reticulum Ca^{2+}-ATPase (SERCA). These abnormalities of calcium metabolism appear to be of primary importance in some types of failure, whereas they may be secondary in other types. Intracellular acidosis decreases the affinity of the troponin complex for Ca^{2+} and may contribute to some forms of heart failure, especially those associated with ischemia.[97] Patients with coronary artery disease may also have transient episodes of abnormal diastolic relaxation of the myocardium with acute changes in diastolic compliance that can produce an acute "stiff heart syndrome" and pulmonary edema.[15,25] These episodes, which may occur with or without angina pectoris, are thought to be caused by abnormalities of the intracellular uptake of Ca^{2+} by SR.[19–25] The amount of activator Ca^{2+} available for contraction can also be reduced by alterations in either intracellular Na^+ or K^+.[2,79,80,92,98]

The significance of abnormalities in the release of Ca^{2+} from SR in chronic myocardial failure is uncertain. As noted in Chap. 3, calcium release from SR is triggered by the increase of Ca^{2+} that crosses the plasma membrane via L-type calcium channels. Most abnormalities of myocardial activation have been demonstrated only in the very late stages of the heart failure process. Thus, alterations in these systems may be the result of maladaptive hypertrophy rather than primary cause of heart failure.

Myocardial Receptor Function
Myocardial β-adrenergic receptor density is downregulated and the production of "second-messenger" cAMP is decreased in heart failure.[99–113] These may be the result of increased circulating catecholamines that are not buffered (i.e., removed from receptor sites) by dysfunctional sympathetic nerve terminals. Indeed, in severe heart failure, norepinephrine (NE) stores in sympathetic nerve endings are depleted, and these nerves neither synthesize, store, nor normally release catecholamines. Thus, the failing myocardium becomes functionally denervated, leaving exposed β_1-receptors. In the nonfailing human ventricular myocardium, the total β-receptor density is approximately 90 fmol/mg, with the β_1 and β_2 proportions being 80 and 20 percent, respectively. In failing myocardium most of the decrease in total β-receptor density results from a selective decrease in β_1-receptors.[99,103,114–119] As a consequence, β_2-receptors constitute about 40 percent of the total β-receptors in the failing human myocardium. The decrease in β_1-receptor density and β-adrenoreceptor downregulation probably account for much of the decrease in inotropic potential under the influence of β-adrenergic receptors.

Although β_2-receptor density is relatively well preserved, the maximal adenylate cyclase response is decreased about 30 to 35 percent.[104] The H_2 histamine, the A_1 adenosine, and the α-receptor pathways appear to be relatively normal in heart failure.[120–122] There is evidence that the vasoactive intestinal peptide receptors are decreased in heart failure but have increased receptor affinity, with a supersensitive dose-responsive curve.

Heart failure is associated with altered levels of G proteins (guanine nucleotide–binding regulatory proteins), which couple a variety of receptors to effector enzymes and either stimulate or inhibit adenylate cyclase.[117,123–133] Thus, there is evidence of a decrease in stimulatory guanyl nucleotide–binding protein (G_s)[117,124,134] and of an increase in inhibitory guanyl nucleotide–binding protein (G_i).[132,133,135–137] In terms of the changes in G_s and G_i, there are potentially important differences between patients with heart failure due to coronary artery disease and patients with failure due to idiopathic dilated cardiomyopathy.[133] Adenylate cyclase activity may also be decreased in heart failure.[110,138] G_h, which transfers the signal from the α_1-adrenergic receptor to the 69-kDa phospholipase C, is also downregulated in heart failure.[139]

Autonomic Nervous System

In CHF, there are defects both in cardiac sympathetic neurotransmitters and in the cardiac parasympathetic control system.[5,99,140–162] At relatively early stages in the evolution of CHR, augmentation of generalized sympathetic nervous system activity is observed with a concomitant decrease in parasympathetic tone. This results in increased circulating levels of NE. At the same time, there is increased activity of the sympathetic nerves to the heart with augmented NE release. Ultimately, this results in marked decrements in myocardial NE stores. As discussed below, these changes may contribute importantly to progression of the disease.

Heart failure is associated with significant impairment of baroreceptor reflexes that control both sympathetic and parasympathetic nervous system activity to the systemic arteries and veins and to the heart.[144,148,150–166]

STRUCTURE

Connective Tissue

Collagen and other connective tissues increase during the process of hypertrophy and also following the loss of myocytes.[167–177] These changes in the cardiac skeleton, which have been termed *interstitial heart disease*,[173] can contribute to the impairment of both diastolic and systolic function in the failing myocardium.[13,176] It may be significant that connective tissue hypertrophy regresses more slowly than myocyte hypertrophy in experimental studies of hypertrophy due to pressure loading. In addition, the collagen of the hypertrophied, pressure-overloaded myocardium apparently differs from that of normal myocardium. It is difficult, however, to separate alterations of loading due to increased fibrous tissue from changes reflecting myocyte loss. The increase in collagen not only increases myocardial stiffness but may also predispose to reentrant arrhythmia caused by abnormal electrical dispersion.[172] Quantitative and qualitative changes in the connective tissue framework of the heart probably play a significant role

in the ventricular remodeling process associated with various types of congestive heart failure.

Senile Cardiomyopathy, Presbycardia, or Senile Heart Disease

With aging, many organs have diminished function, and the heart is no exception. In some elderly individuals, involutional changes of the myocardium may be associated with decreased elasticity of the skeleton of the heart and with mild fibrotic changes of the valves. In rats, myocytes appear to be lost as a process of aging, and the same process occurs in humans.[178] Thus, reactive hypertrophy may occur in the aged from the loss of cells and also as a consequence of the systolic hypertension resulting from decreased compliance of both the aging heart and aorta (see Chap. 96). The chemical basis of these aging changes and of the associated brown pigmentation of the heart is not known. This condition, known as *presbycardia*, *senile heart disease*, or *senile cardiomyopathy*, probably only rarely produces heart failure by itself; however, it probably plays an important role in causing heart failure in the elderly by decreasing contractility, the rate of relaxation, and the adaptive reserve capacity of the heart.[179–184] Myocyte hypertrophy secondary to myocyte loss or systolic hypertension may result in delayed relaxation of the ventricle, which, in the presence of either a tachycardia and/or loss of the atrial "kick" in atrial fibrillation, can result in acute pulmonary edema in the elderly (acute diastolic dysfunction), even when systolic function is still preserved. Accordingly, patients with this condition more readily develop heart failure in the presence of other forms of heart disease or occasionally even from the increased demands of fever, moderate anemia, excess tachycardia, mild hyperthyroidism, excess fluid administration, myocardial ischemia, or a relatively small myocardial infarction. Aged myocardium has also been shown to have a diminished inotropic response to catecholamines[185,186](see Chap. 96).

Sustained Tachycardia

Experimentally, right ventricular pacing of dogs and pigs, usually at rates of about 240 to 260 beats per minute, produces a syndrome of heart failure after a few weeks that is similar to heart failure from idiopathic dilated cardiomyopathy in human beings and that may be reversible.[187–209] Clinically, sustained tachycardia can produce heart failure, especially in older patients or patients with coronary artery disease or marked ventricular hypertrophy. Such tachycardia can also produce substantial subendocardial ischemia and myocyte necrosis and may explain the deterioration of fibrillating atria.

Miscellaneous Mechanisms

Several other factors occur in heart failure that may contribute secondarily to myocardial heart failure. These factors include an increase in free radical production,[210] myocardial interstital edema,[211] and direct toxic effects on myocardial cells from NE[212] and angiotensin II.[213]

COMPENSATORY MECHANISMS IN HEART FAILURE

Many of the adjustments and adaptations to heart failure are similar to the homeostatic mechanisms utilized by the body in response to circulatory failure from any cause, such as acute blood loss and acute myocardial infarction. Many of these neurohumoral compensatory mechanisms (Table 21-6) are also utilized by normal individuals during exercise or during periods of increased stress (see Chap. 3). In human beings with heart failure, it is often impossible to separate the many complex mechanisms of adjustment, many of which affect and modify one another. It is important to stress that the alterations in heart failure usually occur over a relatively long period of time. Following initial damage, e.g., after acute myocardial infarction, pump function may be markedly reduced while the patient remains asymptomatic. Indeed, in many patients, heart failure tends to become manifest only with evidence of activation of the neurohumoral "compensatory" adaptations. In patients with mild heart failure, these compensatory mechanisms are often able to restore to normal or near normal the arterial blood pressure, the organ perfusion, and the cardiac output at rest and at times during moderate exercise. When the failure is mild, no symptoms or clinically apparent organ dysfunction may result from these "compensa-

tory" mechanisms. Eventually, however, many of the symptoms, signs, and organ dysfunction (and even death) that occur in patients with heart failure result from some of these same adaptive mechanisms (Fig. 21-2; see also Chaps. 10 and 22).

Autonomic Nervous System

One of the more important acute adjustments to heart failure is a reflex increase in autonomic sympathetic excitation of the heart and most arteries and veins.[2,139,140,214–219] Generalized arterial vasoconstriction and an increase in venous tone are produced by the increased sympathetic activity, in combination with increased plasma concentrations of NE,[26,214,220] angiotensin II,[6] vasopressin,[149,221,222] endothelin-1,[223–230] neuropeptide Y,[231–234] cytokines such as tumor necrosis factor,[235–238] and with reduced endothelial-dependent vasodilatation.[239–242] These last two changes commonly herald the end stage in the progression of heart failure with a state of malnutrition, muscle loss, and a marked decrease in exercise capacity, i.e., progression to class III and IV heart failure. Calcitonin gene–related peptide[243] and plasma aldosterone levels are frequently elevated.[244,245] Table 21-7 summarizes the neurohumoral changes that may occur in heart failure. The increased platelet activity reported in patients with heart failure[246,247] may result from these changes.

The increased sympathetic adrenergic stimulation of the heart is associated with an inhibition of cardiac parasympathetic activity.[140] An acute increase in sympathetic impulses to the heart normally stimulates the local release of NE and thereby produces β-adrenergic stimulation with an increase in heart rate and in myocardial contractility. NE also increases the rate of ventricular relaxation, which further contributes to increased ventricular filling. In addition, the generalized increased sympathetic activity and the release of NE from the adrenal medulla and the peripheral blood vessels contribute to increasing myocardial contractility.

Patients with chronic CHF have a significant decrease in the myocardial concentration of NE.[2,145,248,249] The cause of this decrease is controversial. Studies in humans have shown increased NE "spillover" from rapid turnover and release of NE. Other studies suggest that these overstimulated nerves cease to function adequately, mimicking cardiac denervation. This is associated with decreased activity of myocardial tyrosine hydroxylase, which is the rate-limiting enzyme in the synthesis of NE.[146] When right ventricular hypertrophy and failure are produced experimentally, the myocardial NE concentration is decreased in both the right and the left ventricle.[147] In experimental chronic heart failure, there are a decrease in the amount of mycardial NE released per nerve impulse and defects in the synthesis, uptake, and binding of NE.[145] On the other hand, net myocardial NE release may be markedly increased in patients with early heart failure,[250,251] perhaps related to a defective reuptake mechanism at the nerve endings for locally released NE.[252,253]

In general, the arterial concentrations of NE and dopamine in patients with moderate to severe CHF are elevated at rest

---

TABLE 21-6
COMPENSATORY MECHANISMS IN HEART FAILURE

Autonomic nervous system
  Heart
    Increased heart rate
    Increased myocardial contractile stimulation
    Increased rate of relaxation
  Peripheral circulation
    Arterial vasoconstriction (increased afterload)
    Venous vasoconstriction (increased preload)
Kidney (renin-angiotensin-aldosterone)
  Arterial vasoconstriction (increased afterload)
  Venous vasoconstriction (increased preload)
  Sodium and water retention (increased preload and afterload)
  Increased myocardial contractile stimulation
Endothelin-1 (increased preload and afterload)
Arginine vasopressin (increased preload and afterload)
Atrial and brain natriuretic peptides (decreased afterload)
Prostaglandins
Peptides
Frank-Starling law of the heart
  Increased end-diastolic fiber length, volume, and pressure (increased preload)
Hypertrophy
Peripheral oxygen delivery
  Redistribution of cardiac output
  Altered oxygen-hemoglobin dissociation
  Increased oxygen extraction by tissues
Anaerobic metabolism

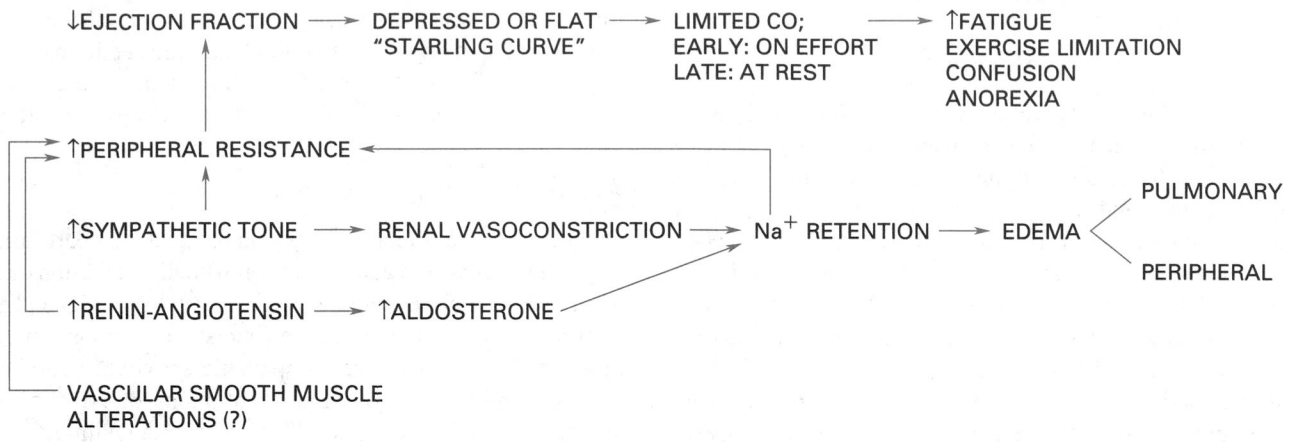

FIGURE 21-2

Schema of events in congestive heart failure leading to symptoms. Note that fatigue and other symptoms of limited cardiac output are primarily related to decreased ejection, whereas peripheral and pulmonary edema are related to Na$^+$ and water retention from increased sympathetic tone and increased renin-angiotensin-aldosterone. See text for details.

and increase more than normally during mild or moderate exercise.[254–257] This elevation of NE appears to be due predominantly to an increased synthesis in the peripheral vasculature and the adrenal medulla.[220] There is, however, a blunted response of plasma NE release during a 60 percent upright tilt.[258] The high plasma levels of NE and angiotensin II may potentiate the hypertrophic response of the remaining myocytes. Plasma epinephrine concentrations are only inconsistently increased in patients with heart failure.[256] Importantly, increased serum NE levels may also produce myocellular damage per se and further the progression of heart failure.[212]

TABLE 21-7

NEUROHUMORAL CHANGES IN HEART FAILURE

Changes that increase vascular systemic resistance
  Increased sympathetic nervous system activity (increased
    norepinephrine, epinephrine)
  Increased endothelin
  Increased arginine vasopressin
  Increased renin and angiotensin II
  Increased aldosterone
  Increased neuropeptide Y
  Increased tumor necrosis factor
  Reduced endothelial-dependent vasodilatation
  Reduced parasympathetic nervous system activity
  Impaired baroreceptor activity
  Increased vasoconstrictor prostaglandins, kinines
Changes that decrease systemic vascular resistance
  Increased atrial and brain natriuretic peptides
  Increased dopamine
  Increased vasodilator prostaglandins (PGI$_2$, PGE$_2$)
  Increased vasodilator peptides, (e.g., bradykinin,
    kalliden)

Note: Changes in individual patients vary significantly and changes may not always be present.

Although the myocardial synthesis of NE is impaired in CHF, the myocardium can still respond to exogenous NE.[147] As noted above, there is a decreased catecholamine sensitivity and β-adrenergic receptor density (downregulation) in failing human hearts.[99,249,259] In general, however, the failing heart is responsive and in severe failure pump function may even be dependent upon extracardiac circulating NE. As a result, CHF is sometimes made somewhat worse by the acute administration of drugs such as beta blockers, guanethidine, or reserpine, all of which may interfere with the myocardial sympathetic adrenergic system. In many patients, especially when failure is mild, this effect is modest, transient, and does not prevent their use (e.g., following acute myocardial infarction). In addition, there is growing evidence that the cautious use of beta blockers may improve ventricular performance in selected patients with heart failure.[260–280] Some studies have found no benefit,[281–284] whereas others found a clinical benefit and reduced mortality in patients with dilated cardiomyopathy but a limited benefit in heart failure due to coronary artery disease[266] (see Chap. 23).

In general, however, the defective synthesis and the depletion of myocardial NE do not appear to be major, primary causes of myocardial failure, although they may be important contributing mechanisms. Patients with chronic CHF may also have a significant depression of the normal parasympathetic nervous control of the heart.[141]

In patients with heart failure, the complex reflex actions of the autonomic nervous system and the local autoregulatory mechanisms tend to preserve circulation to the brain and heart while decreasing blood flow to the skin, skeletal muscles, splanchnic organs, and kidneys.[285–287] The increased adrenergic stimulation of the peripheral arteries and the increased concentrations of circulating NE, angiotensin II, endothelin-1, and vasopressin contribute to arteriolar vasoconstriction, the maintenance of arterial pressure, and an increase in venous tone, which together help to maintain venous return and ventricular filling and to support cardiac performance by Starling's law of the heart.[216] The arterial and arteriolar resistance of patients with CHF may also be increased by an increased sodium and water content of the vessel walls, which increases their "stiffness."[288] The generalized increase in sympathetic nervous system activity also appears to play a facilitative role in sodium and water retention in heart failure.[286]

The increased systemic arteriolar vasoconstriction associated with heart failure is an example of a compensatory mechanism that probably evolved in response to an inadequate cardiac output from other causes, such as traumatic hemorrhage or an inadequate blood volume. In such an acute situation, the reflex maintains arterial pressure and perfusion of the brain and heart. On the other hand, in the patient with chronic heart failure, the chronic compensatory increase in arteriolar resistance may actually make it more difficult for the failing heart to eject blood. One of the major cornerstones of the therapy of heart failure is the reduction of peripheral vascular resistance by converting enzyme inhibitors and other vasodilator drugs (see below and Chap. 23).

The Kidney

The compensatory, homeostatic adjustments that occur when the heart fails tend to maintain cardiac output, although often at the price of increased diastolic pressures in the involved ventricle and the venous system filling the involved ventricle. A major compensatory mechanism is the increase in ventricular filling volume and pressures produced by an increase in plasma volume as the result of salt and water retention by the kidneys.[214,215,289] Ultimately, the mechanisms leading to an increase in plasma volume and capillary pressure may contribute to the formation of interstitial edema and may also contribute to increased peripheral resistance (Fig. 21-3).[290] The mechanisms or stimuli for the initial changes in the kidneys that produce salt and water retention in heart failure are still not clear.[286,289,291–294] Possible mechanisms include a decrease in the "effective" arterial blood volume sensed by arterial volume receptors; by decreased distending pressure in the carotid sinus and other cardiothoracic mechanoreceptors in the great arteries and veins; or by sensors in the thorax, kidneys, atria, and possibly the ventricles, liver, and central nervous system.[163,286,295,296] Increased renal venous pressure or decreased arterial perfusion pressure may also contribute to sodium retention by the kidneys (see also Chap. 94).

During the phase of edema formation, patients with heart failure have a significantly delayed ability to excrete a load of either sodium chloride or water. In patients with very mild heart failure, if normal renal perfusion is restored by the expansion of blood volume, the handling of additional small amounts of sodium may return toward normal; however, patients with severe failure remain unable to excrete solute and water normally despite a marked expansion of blood volume and interstitial fluid volume.

Renal vasoconstriction in CHF is thought to result primarily from increased activity of both the sympathetic nervous

system and the renin-angiotensin system.[216,289,293,294,297] Local redistribution of renal blood flow is also important. Prostaglandins (PG) and vasoactive peptides, especially neuropeptides and other endothelial products, may also be involved. In addition to a reduction in total renal blood flow, there is a redistribution of flow that produces a greater reduction of flow in the outer renal cortex with a relative maintenance of perfusion in the juxtamedullary areas.[286,289,294,298]

Patients with mild heart failure may have a normal glomerular filtration rate despite a reduced renal blood flow. This results from an increased filtration fraction due to marked vasoconstriction of efferent renal arterioles and decreased hydrostatic pressure in the peritubular capillaries.[299,300] In patients with more severe heart failure, total renal blood flow is further decreased, along with the glomerular filtration rate, even though the filtration fraction may increase further. In this situation, "prerenal azotemia" is often present with an increase in the blood urea concentration.

The sympathetic nervous system, which can be activated by lowering of the arterial blood pressure or by direct stimulation of the renal nerves, plays a facilitative role in the renal retention of sodium and water. The increased tubular reabsorption of sodium and water is aided by the marked redistribution of renal blood flow described above.[286,291,298] In addition, the uptake of fluid from the interstitium into the peritubular capillaries is enhanced by the efferent renal arteriolar vasoconstriction, which increases colloid osmotic pressure in the peritubular capillaries. These hemodynamic mechanisms work synergistically to increase sodium and water reabsorption in failure.

Patients with heart failure have significantly decreased excretion rates of sodium chloride due to increased tubular reabsorption, even when the glomerular filtration rate is normal. About 60 to 70 percent of the glomerular filtrate is normally reabsorbed in the proximal convoluted tubules. Sodium appears to diffuse into proximal tubular cells, from which it is pumped into the lateral and basal intercellular spaces, with chloride and water following passively.[286,291,301] At present, it is uncertain whether or not proximal tubular reabsorption of sodium is increased in heart failure[291] (see Chaps. 24 and 94).

About 25 percent of sodium reabsorption normally occurs in the ascending limb in the loop of Henle. In the thick ascending limb, the absorption of chloride is active with sodium following passively.[286] It is probable that there is increased reabsorption of sodium and water in the thick ascending limb in heart failure.[298,302]

Most of the remaining 10 percent of filtered sodium is normally reabsorbed in the distal convoluted tubules and collecting ducts by active sodium transport.[298,303] This is linked to the action of *aldosterone*, which also enhances the excretion of potassium and hydrogen ions. In experimental heart failure, the reabsorption of sodium in the collecting ducts is increased significantly.[291,298,301] The sensitivity of the cells of the distal tubules and collecting ducts to aldosterone may also be increased by an unidentified factor.[286]

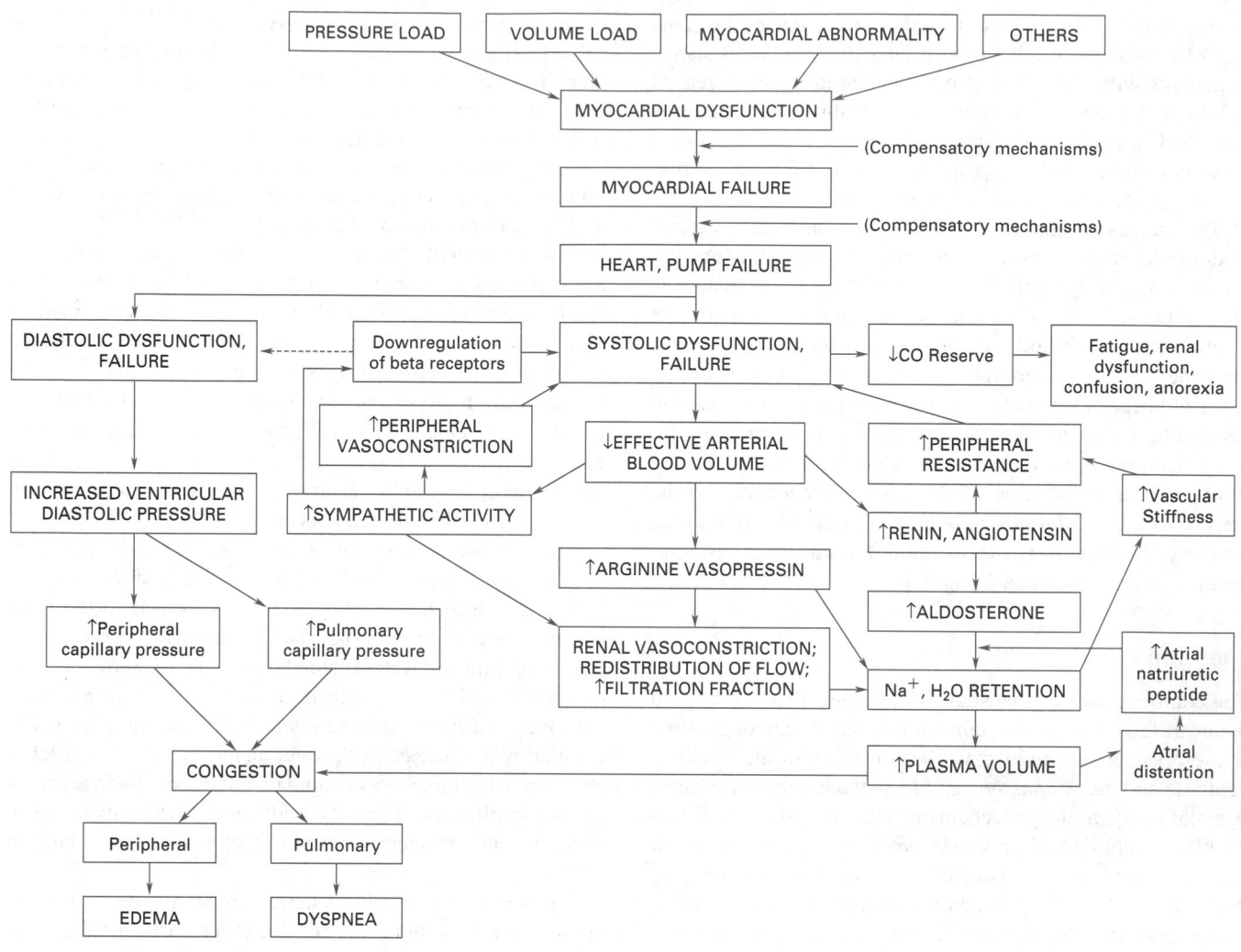

FIGURE 21-3

Schema of the sequence of events in heart failure. An increased load or myocardial abnormality leads to myocardial failure and eventually to heart failure. This results in increased sympathetic activity, increased levels of renin-angiotensin-aldosterone, pulmonary and peripheral congestion and edema, and decreased cardiac output reserve. Endothelial dysfunction also occurs, with decreased endothelial-dependent vasodilatation and with increased plasma levels of endothelin-1, a very strong vasoconstrictor. See text for details.

Renin, Angiotensin, and Aldosterone

Renin is released by the kidneys whenever diuretics are given, even in a normal individual. Within hours after the production of acute heart failure, the kidneys secrete increased amounts of renin.[216,292,304,305] The secretion of renin is controlled by at least four mechanisms: (1) changes in wall tensions in renal afferent arterioles, (2) a macula densa receptor that detects changes in the rate at which sodium and/or chloride reaches the distal tubule, (3) a negative feedback effect from the elevated plasma levels of angiotensin II, and (4) the central nervous system, which influences renin secretion by the renal nerves, adrenal medulla, and the posterior pituitary gland.[306] Carotid sinus or atrial distension may also influence renin secretion.[291,292,296,306,307] In general, decreased renal perfusion pressure, decreased renal blood flow, and decreased sodium load at the distal tubule result in the release of renin.

It is uncertain whether or not the increased levels of arginine vasopressin (AVP), often present in heart failure, influence renin release.[307]

The enzyme *renin* acts upon angiotensinogen, which is produced mainly in the liver, to produce pharmacologically inactive angiotensin I, which is then converted to *angiotensin II*.[304,305] Angiotensin II produces potent arterial vasoconstriction and contributes to the increase in peripheral vascular resistance and the maintenance of blood pressure in heart failure when "effective" filling of the arterial circulation decreases.[286,308] Angiotensin II further constricts renal efferent arterioles; in the brain, it stimulates thirst; while in the adrenal gland, it stimulates secretion of aldosterone, which promotes the reabsorption of sodium and the excretion of potassium in the distal tubules and collecting ducts of the kidney. Plasma concentrations of both angiotensin II and aldosterone are usually elevated in patients with symptomatic CHF. Angiotensin

II also has some direct, albeit minor, inotropic properties and may also augment the release of NE from nerve endings. Glomerular mesangial cells have angiotensin II receptors, which may influence mesangial cell contraction and thereby the glomerular surface area available for filtration.[309] In mild experimental heart failure, the secretion of renin and the elevated plasma concentrations of angiotensin II and aldosterone may return to or toward normal after the retention of sodium and water has produced expansion of the blood volume and interstitial fluid volume.[244,245,286,304]

Angiotensin II is not only a vasoconstrictor but also a growth factor, so that activation of angiotensin II receptors in the myocardium contributes to myocyte hypertrophy[310] as well as fibroblast growth. Angiotensin II, like NE, can also lead to myocyte death, which can add importantly to disease progression.

There is good evidence of a renin-angiotensin system in the myocardium itself, although its full significance is not yet fully established.[311,312] Other evidence supports the existence of renin-angiotensin systems in many other tissues, some of which may also play a role in heart failure.[313-315]

Endothelial Dysfunction

The normal and abnormal functions of the endothelium are discussed in detail in Chaps. 4 and 44. Heart failure, like other conditions such as hyperlipidemia, atherosclerosis, and systemic arterial hypertension, is associated with significant endothelial dysfunction.[239-242] Thus, symptomatic heart failure is associated with diminished endothelial-dependent vasodilatation resulting in decreased exercise capacity.[239] Normally, endothelium-derived relaxing factor, which is now thought to be nitric oxide, is a local (paracrine) hormone that is released from endothelial cells, from which it diffuses to underlying smooth muscle cells and produces dilatation by binding to the heme moiety of soluble guanylate cyclase, thereby increasing guanosine-5-monophosphate (cGMP) production.[316,317]

One of the more important physiologic stimulants of endothelium-derived relaxing factor release is the longitudinal shear force on endothelial cells produced by changes in flow rate. The endothelium also releases endothelin-1, which is one of the most potent vasoconstrictor substances known. Patients with heart failure have increased circulating levels of endothelin-1.[223-230] It has also been suggested that the endocardial endothelium is capable of influencing the duration of cardiac contraction.[318-320] The importance of the latter phenomenon in human heart failure is unknown (see also Chaps. 4 and 44).

Arginine Vasopressin

In severe heart failure, secretion of pituitary antidiuretic hormone, or AVP, is increased, particularly in patients with hyponatremia.[149,222,321-325] Although AVP may contribute to the decreased ability of some patients to secrete a water load, it does not appear to play a major primary role in edema formation.[286,326] AVP is also a strong vasoconstrictor and contributes to the increase in systemic vascular resistance in heart failure.

Atrial and Ventricular Natriuretic Peptides (Factors)

Atrial natriuretic peptides (ANPs) are made and stored in specialized atrial cells, from which they are released by the stimulus of atrial distension.[327-330] Brain natriuretic peptides (BNPs) are released largely by ventricular myocytes.[331,332] Both families of vasoactive peptides have both a natriuretic and a diuretic effect, and some relax vascular smooth muscle and/or intestinal smooth muscle.[333-340]

The plasma concentrations of ANP and BNP are increased in heart failure.[327-338] Their role in heart failure, if any, is unclear.[339-342] They produce a natriuresis by a direct renal action, and ANP also decreases the production of aldosterone, renin, and AVP.[339,342-344] In heart failure, however, it appears that the homeostatic control of circulatory blood volume by this mechanism is inadequate to overcome the stronger forces tending to retain sodium and water.

The importance of ANPs and BNPs in the pathogenesis of the syndrome of congestive heart failure is unclear.[340-343] Patients with severe heart failure may have downregulation of the ANP receptor coupled to guanylate cyclase in their pulmonary vasculature.[345]

Prostaglandins

The kidneys synthesize prostaglandins PGE_2 and $PGF_{2\alpha}$ in the interstitium and collecting duct cells of the medulla. These substances are released into the renal interstitial fluid and renal venous blood and are metabolized in both the renal cortex and the lungs. Prostacyclin (PGI_2) and PGE_2 can be synthesized by renal vascular and smooth muscle cells.[346] Their role in the maintenance of normal sodium balance or in heart failure is still unclear.[286,347] They may help maintain glomerular filtration in the presence of marked efferent arteriolar vasoconstriction.[348] PGI_2 and PGE_2 may stimulate the release of renin.[347,348]

Some patients with heart failure have increased levels of the metabolites of vasodilator prostaglandins, which may oppose the vasoconstriction produced by the renin-angiotensin-aldosterone system.[347,348] Those patients with heart failure in whom the vasodilating effects of prostaglandins are important in opposing the many vasoconstricting influences are susceptible to a worsening of their clinical condition when they are given agents that inhibit prostaglandin synthesis, such as indomethacin.[347,348] The negative inotropic effects of furosemide noted experimentally appear to be prostaglandin-mediated.[349]

Peptides

The vasodilator peptides bradykinin and kalliden, which are formed by the kallidrein-kinin system, may be involved in the intrarenal distribution of blood flow and the excretion of sodium,[350,351] but their importance in heart failure is unclear. It should be noted that the angiotensin-converting enzyme inhibitors not only inhibit the formation of the vasoconstrictor angiotensin II but also the breakdown of bradykinin. The neuropeptide tyrosin (NPY), a 36-amino acid peptide, may be important in the control of myocardial contractility and the regulation of myocardial perfusion.[352] Increased plasma levels of neuropeptide Y217-220 and substance P219 have been found in some patients with heart failure.

Frank-Starling Law of the Heart

When the ventricle fails acutely, the Frank-Starling law of the heart is immediately brought into play. When the normally filled ventricle fails to eject a normal quantity of blood during one beat, its end-systolic volume increases. Consequently, this increased volume remains and is added to the blood entering the ventricle during the next diastole. The net result is an increased EDV for the next beat. This increased "preload" produces an increased SV during the next contraction in accordance with the Frank-Starling law of the heart. This increase in contractile force is related to sarcomere lengthening, which is mediated by increasing the Ca^{2+} sensitivity of the myofilament and thus enhancing cross-bridge formation for a given amount of Ca^{2+} released into the myocyte.[353–361] (see Chap. 3).

Over a period of time, the ventricle may be able to maintain normal or nearly normal stroke volume and work at an increased end-diastolic fiber length and EDV (Fig. 21-4). In many patients with a chronic increase in preload, as may be produced by aortic or mitral regurgitation, the ventricle dilates markedly and, by a process called "remodeling," increases its EDV strikingly without an increase in diastolic pressure. This reflects a shift in the passive pressure-volume curve to the right as the wall of the ventricle dilates. As ventricular failure progresses, the increase in SV that is associated with an increase in EDV or EDP is reduced. A relatively sustained SV, with an increased EDV, results in a reduced ratio of SV/EDV, the ejection fraction. Due to the increased stiffness of the ventricle as volume is increased, increases in EDP may produce very little further increase in diastolic volume, and thus the SV-EDP curve becomes flattened. With further increases in EDP, effective SV may decline, due not to a descending limb of the myocardial force curve but to increased functional mitral regurgitation and/or increased afterload via the Laplace relationship. Thus, the function curve of the intact heart does not have a true "descending limb."[362,363] In general, because of the flattened Starling curve, the chronically dilated left ventricle subjected to additional volume load is unable to utilize the Frank-Starling mechanism to a significant degree[50,56] and the stroke volume is relatively fixed (Fig. 21-4).

In patients with CHF, the retention of salt and water by the kidneys increases effective blood volume, which tends to increase ventricular filling volume. This mechanism may return stroke output to normal or near normal but at the expense of both increased wall tension, which is energetically wasteful, and increased venous pressure in the pulmonary or the sys-

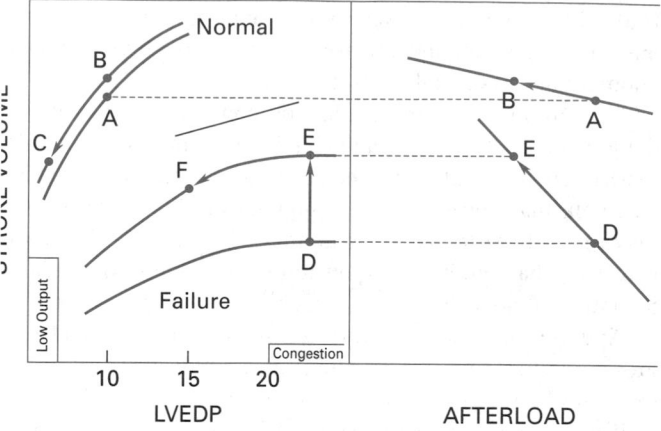

FIGURE 21-4

Relationship between stroke volume and left ventricular end-diastolic pressure (LVEDP) (*left*) and afterload (*right*). Normally, the ventricle operates on a sharply rising Frank-Starling curve with an LVEDP less than 12 mmHg (point A), where small changes in filling pressure yield large changes in stroke volume. Further, stroke volume is largely independent of the afterload. When failure occurs, ventricular function is characterized by a shift of the curve relating stroke volume to LVEDP to the right and downward. Low output may ensue if the curve is sufficiently depressed, while pulmonary congestion occurs as the LVEDP is increased. At the same time, this failing ventricle is now highly afterload-dependent, in that small changes in afterload produce large changes in stroke volume. When afterload is reduced in the normal heart (point A to point B, *right*), stroke volume rises very slightly. If, at the same time, venodilation reduces filling pressure, stroke volume falls to point C (*left*). The net result is a decrease in cardiac output. On the contrary, when afterload is reduced in the presence of severe ventricular failure, stroke volume is increased (point D to point E, *right*). Since the Frank-Starling curve is relatively flattened, a simultaneous decrease in filling pressure leads to a decrease in LVEDP with only a small decrease in stroke volume (point E to point F, *left*). The net reult of these opposing consequences can increase stroke volume. These results are observed clinically when a vasodilator is administered along with a diuretic in treating the failing ventricle.

temic veins. In some patients in whom increased filling pressure is necessary for a reasonable cardiac output, symptoms of systemic hypotension and decreased cardiac output may appear if the ventricular filling pressure is excessively decreased by diuretics or arterial vasodilators. This "preload dependence" is particularly likely to occur in patients with pericardial constriction, aortic stenosis, restrictive cardiomyopathy, or hypertrophic cardiomopathy (see Chaps. 63, 74, 75, and 81).

Another characteristic of the dilated, failing heart is that it becomes less influenced by preload and more afterload-dependent (Figs. 21-4 and 21-5). The normal heart can sustain large changes in systolic loading or afterload with relatively little change in cardiac output and with only minor changes in diastolic volume. When myocardial failure is present and the diastolic volume is increased and the heart is dilated, however, any further increase in afterload may lead to a substantial decrease in SV. Conversely, a decrease in afterload may substantially increase the cardiac output (Fig. 21-4). Ventricular dilatation, although a compensation that helps to sustain SV, has other adverse effects on ventricular function. With dilatation, functional mitral regurgitation can occur and

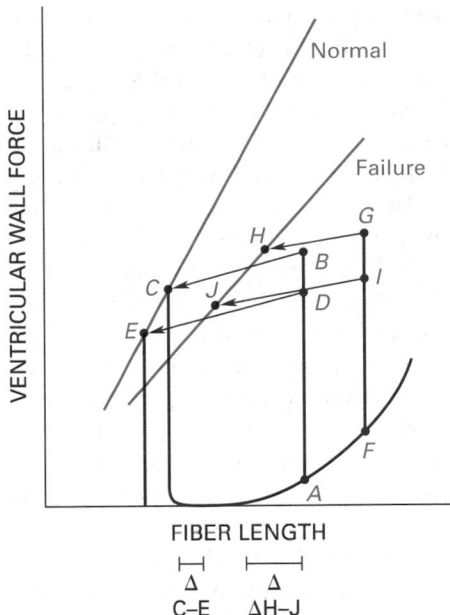

FIGURE 21-5

Relationship between LV wall force and fiber length. Hypothetical contractile cycles have been portrayed for the normal and failing ventricle. In the normal heart, contraction starts at point *A*, LV pressure rises until the aortic valve is opened (point *B*), the ventricle empties (point *B* to *C*), and relaxation ensues. When arterial pressure (afterload) is reduced (e.g., to point *D*), ejection starts at point *D* and proceeds to point *E*, which increases stroke volume. When the ventricle fails, the fiber length in diastole is increased, and ventricular contraction starts at point *F*. With systolic contraction, ventricular pressure rises to point *G*, and with ventricular emptying, fiber length decreases to point *H*. With a similar decrease in the afterload, wall force only needs to reach point *I* when ventricular emptying occurs to point *J*. As a result, for the same relative change in afterload, the increase in shortening is greater in the failing ventricle (Δ*H–J*) than in the normal heart (Δ*C–E*).

become very severe. Overstretch of the myocardium can also lead to diffuse death of myocytes, which could add to disease progression.[364]

Hypertrophy of the Heart

Hypertrophy is one of the major adaptations of the heart to chronically increased systolic stress, but it may itself contribute to the progression of heart failure. Experimentally, metabolic evidence of hypertrophy appears within a few hours after an increase in cardiac work.[7,168,169,365] Hyperplasia, or an actual increase in the total number of myocardial cells, has generally been thought to occur in human beings only if the increased stress occurs within the first few months of life. Some evidence, however, suggests that hyperplasia can also occur later in life under conditions of excessive loading or myocyte loss[366,367]; however, any capacity for cell division is limited and new cells may not function normally. Cardiac Hypertrophy is associated with a significant increase in the number of sarcomeres within each myocardial cell. In general, chronic pressure loads tend to result in thicker myocardial cells with replication of sarcomeres in parallel, whereas chronic

volume loads result in longer and somewhat thicker individual myocardial cells with replication of sarcomeres both in series and in parallel.[366,368–373] In addition, significant hyperplasia can occur in myocardial interstitial cells, which outnumber myocytes three to one in the normal adult myocardium (see below).[170–177]

Two classic types of left ventricular hypertrophy are recognized: concentric and eccentric. In pure *concentric hypertrophy* of the left ventricle, there is an increase in the thickness of the ventricular wall, but the ventricular chamber does not increase in diameter. In some instances, the ventricular chamber may actually decrease in size. In concentric hypertrophy that results from increased systolic loading, myocytes increase in diameter rather than in length. This is classically present with isolated valvular aortic stenosis or arterial hypertension. In experimental models of pressure overload hypertrophy, capillary growth is less than the increase in muscle mass.[374–378]

In pure *eccentric hypertrophy*, the thickness of the left ventricular wall and the internal diameter of the ventricle increase proportionately. This may be seen in normal growth, in endurance athletes, or in patients with volume overload of the left ventricle, as in isolated mitral regurgitation.[368–370,379] In these circumstances, myocytes elongate as well as thicken. As noted previously, *reactive hypertrophy* of remaining myocytes can occur in response to loss of myocytes after myocardial infarction.[373,380]

Although the stimuli and signal transduction pathways involved in myocardial hypertrophy are not completely known,[5,168,169,355,381–383] it has been suggested that an increase in systolic wall tension of the ventricle in conditions associated with increased afterload stimulates the synthesis of sarcomeres in parallel to existing sarcomeres and thereby produces concentric hypertrophy[368–370] (see also Chap. 6). Conversely, it has been suggested that an increase in diastolic wall tension under conditions of increased preload primarily stimulates the synthesis of sarcomeres in series with preexisting sarcomeres and produces eccentric hypertrophy. In so-called compensated hypertrophy, the increase in wall thickness is such that the tension in the wall is maintained in a normal range. It should be emphasized that hypertrophy of the remaining myocytes is very common in heart failure, and that the increased stress on the remaining myocytes may result in their early loss and initiate a vicious cycle with even greater stress upon the surviving myocytes.[178,372,373,383,384] Local activation of the autocrine/paracrine renin-angiotensin system related to myocyte load may participate in the hypertrophic process[310] and may also contribute to continued myocyte loss.

As noted above, there is evidence that in some species there may be differences in the myosin present at various ages and synthesized in response to a stimulus to hypertrophy; these differences are more marked in atrial myosin.[68,380,385–387] In the rat and the rabbit, the myosin synthesized in response to pressure loading may have more of the slow β myosin heavy chain than does myosin synthesized in response to volume loading.[388]

It is significant that the increase in individual myocardial cell length produced by the increase in the number of sarcomeres in patients with chronically dilated hearts is not adequate to explain the increase in heart size frequently encountered. In such patients, there is also myocardial "slippage" or rearrangement at the level of myofibrils, myocardial fibers, and muscle bundles. There may also be a significant increase in the amount of interstitial tissue.[171-177,368,389]

In general, the compensatory hypertrophy in patients with chronic pressure or volume overload can initially return the calculated systolic wall tension to normal, although diastolic wall stress may remain abnormal in patients with volume overload (see Chap. 22).[4,56,368-370,390-394] In contrast, uncompensated failure is commonly characterized by an increase in systolic wall tension despite the compensatory hypertrophy. Many factors, including growth hormone, thyroid hormone, cortisol, angiotensin, and increased sympathetic stimulation of the heart, contribute to the development of cardiac hypertrophy in response to stress[394] (see Chap. 6).

Hypertrophy is a natural adaptation to a systolic overload of the ventricle. Reactive hypertrophy occurs when myocardium is lost following a myocardial infarction or with a cardiomyopathy. Moreover, the hypertrophic response to overload returns the tension per cell in the wall toward normal. As myocardial hypertrophy occurs, physiologic and biochemical alterations also ensue. The rate of contraction of the myocardium decreases, the time to attain peak tension is delayed, and relaxation is slowed. Nevertheless, if enough time is available for contraction, peak force and shortening are maintained. As noted above, in some species, these physiologic alterations have a correlate in biochemical changes wherein, with hypertrophy, a slower myosin heavy chain, the fetal β isoform, is synthesized instead of the faster adult α isoform.[380,381,385,386,388] A similar reversion to the fetal isoform of myosin tends to occur as a function of aging itself. With aging, however, myocytes are also lost, so that the effects of aging and hypertrophy are additive. In addition, other enzyme systems that are associated with the control of activating Ca^{2+} for the heart are also slowed. In human beings, the latter changes appear to be major biochemical alterations in heart failure (see above).

EFFECT OF CARDIAC HYPERTROPHY ON DIASTOLIC COMPLIANCE

The diastolic compliance, or distensibility, of ventricles of patients with concentric hypertrophy due to pressure overload is typically much less than that of patients with eccentric hypertrophy due to volume overload in the absence of severe myocardial failure. Elastic recoil and the rate of relaxation may also be impaired. Thus, the extremely thick, hypertrophied ventricle of a patient with concentric hypertrophy from aortic stenosis, systemic arterial hypertension, or hypertrophic cardiomyopathy may require a high left ventricular EDP for normal filling due to the hypertrophy itself.[395-399] In such preload-dependent hearts, an elevation of ventricular diastolic pressure is not necessarily evidence for systolic myocardial failure (Fig. 21-6).

These alterations form the substrate for "diastolic ventricular dysfunction," which is characterized by an elevated ventricular filling pressure with a normal SV and EDV and thus a normal (50 to 75 percent) EF. Hypertrophy and delayed left ventricular relaxation may limit the time for diastolic filling and elevate filling pressure, producing pulmonary congestion, pulmonary edema, and the clinical picture of diastolic heart failure. This is amplified by tachycardia and salt and water retention.[73,395-406] Figure 21-7 illustrates the major parameters of diastolic dysfunction evaluated by noninvasive studies. Early left ventricular filling has multiple determinants in addition to muscle relaxation, such as elastic recoil forces, viscoelastic effects, left ventricular filling pressure, left atrial pressure, left ventricular stiffness, ventricular interaction (interdependence), and pericardial constraint.[407,408] Obesity can be associated with impaired diastolic function even in normotensive subjects.[409] (see Chap. 93).

In contrast, many patients with eccentric hypertrophy from mitral or aortic regurgitation may have markedly increased EDV, with relatively normal diastolic pressures, often in the presence of significant myocardial and ventricular systolic dysfunction. These findings limit the value of ventricular EDP as an index of left ventricular performance, especially if the diastolic pressure is not correlated with other data (see Chap. 22).[410-418] Nevertheless, an elevated EDP is one of the hallmarks of left ventricular dysfunction.[73,399,401-406,419-421]

Left ventricular diastolic pressure-volume relationships may be significantly influenced by the phenomenon of ventricular interaction (interdependence) and by elevated right ventricular pressure and volume, particularly if the pericardium is intact.[407,422-430]

The acute decrease in left ventricular distensibility produced by ischemia or hypoxia is greater in ventricles with chronic pressure overload hypertrophy than in normal ventricles.[431] The effects of myocardial ischemia upon ventricular systolic and diastolic function are discussed in more detail in Chap. 45. Reduced left ventricular distensibility is frequently a contributing factor to left ventricular diastolic dysfunction. Factors influencing ventricular distensibility include alterations in the composition and geometry of the left ventricle, pericardial constraint, and coronary turgor from blood in the coronary circulation.[170,171,432-434] The possible mechanisms of impaired relaxation in ventricular hypertrophy include increased wall thickness, increased wall stress (afterload mismatch), fibrosis, and impaired myocardial relaxation caused by subendocardial ischemia or diastolic calcium overload intrinsic to hypertrophy.[395,397,399] Normally, in early diastole, the pressure in the left ventricle rapidly falls below the pressure in the left atrium and accelerates the flow of blood into the left ventricle.[433,435] "Ventricular suction," which results from the active elastic recoil of the myocardium in early relaxation, normally contributes to rapid ventricular filling and is frequently markedly impaired in patients with left ventricular failure. With ventricular dilatation, this elastic recoil is decreased and early filling is reduced. As a result, late filling is increased along with increased filling pressures. The

SYSTOLIC FAILURE

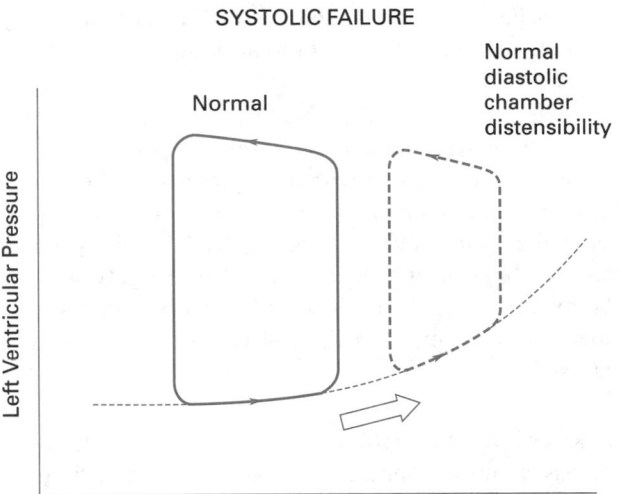

DIASTOLIC FAILURE

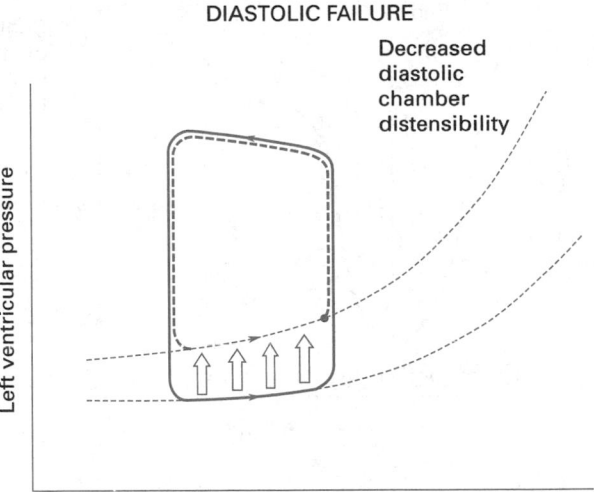

FIGURE 21-6

The left panel shows a schematized left ventricular pressure-volume loop from a patient with primary systolic failure. A normal left ventricular pressure-volume loop (*solid loop*) is shown on the left portion of the curve, and the transition to inotropic failure (*dashed loop*) is shown on the right. Systolic failure is manifested as an increase in LV end-systolic volume and as a reduction in the extent of shortening (stroke volume). LVEDP is increased because left ventricular volume is increased. As indicated by the arrow, the diastolic portion of the pressure-volume loop has simply shifted to the right along the same diastolic pressure-volume relationship, thus no change in the distensibility of the left ventricle has occurred. The right panel shows a left ventricular pressure-volume loop from a patient with primary diastolic failure

(*dashed loop*). Note that the LVEDP is the same as that in the patient with primary inotropic failure, as denoted by the heavy dot on both pressure-volume loops. In the right panel, however, this is caused by an upward shift of the left ventricular diastolic pressure-volume relationship (*arrows*), which indicates a decrease in left ventricular diastolic distensibility such that a higher diastolic pressure is required to achieve the same diastolic volume. In this patient, no change in end-diastolic volume or systolic shortening has occurred. (From BH Lorell: Left ventricular diastolic pressure-volume relations: Understanding and managing congestive heart failure. *Heart Failure* 1988; 4:206–223. Reproduced with permission from the publisher and author.)

term *lusitrophy* is used to refer to the diastolic relaxation and compliance properties of the ventricles.[87]

EFFECTS OF EXPERIMENTAL CARDIAC HYPERTROPHY ON INDICES OF MYOCARDIAL CONTRACTILITY

The evaluation of contractility may depend on the particular index used and the setting in which it is employed.[436] When the heart is experimentally caused to become hypertrophied by increasing ventricular preload (volume overload), the myocardial contractility per unit mass is usually not decreased initially but is decreased later with severe pump failure.[2,56,437] In contrast, with the development of hypertrophy that is experimentally produced by increased ventricular afterload (pressure overload), namely, the experimental hypertrophy of aortic or pulmonic stenosis, contractile behavior is altered but cannot be said to be depressed. Thus, the speed of contraction is slowed and the duration of contraction is prolonged in association with slowed relaxation. Force development and shortening capacity, however, remain normal. Only in late failure does contractile force decline.[2,147,438,439] This altered contractility may be reversible if the experimental hypertrophy is reversed by unbanding before the onset of failure.[440] Some studies of pressure-induced hypertrophy have found that myocardial contractility per unit mass may also return to normal if the elevated pressure load is maintained for 24 weeks,[441] whereas other investigators have found normal ventricular

function at rest in animals with stable hypertrophy from either volume or pressure overload.[422]

Overall, it appears that alterations in myocardial contractility with associated experimental cardiac hypertrophy are extremely variable and depend on the inciting stimulus, the experimental design and species studied, the particular index of contractility utilized, and the duration of the disease process that initiated the hypertrophic response.[15,438–442] For example, left ventricular hypertrophy induced by high-altitude hypoxia is not associated with a decrease in the indexes of contractility, whereas there is a decrease in the indexes in experimental chronic coarctation of the aorta.[443] Some of these discrepancies among experimental studies may also depend on the acuteness and severity of the overload or preload, the extent of resultant hypertrophy, the extent of myocyte loss and whether or not it is progressive, and the age of the individual when it occurs (see Chap. 22).

Heart Rate

The normal heart responds to an increase in heart rate by a positive inotropic effect, which is known as *frequency treppe* or the *Bowditch effect*.[444] In the failing heart, however, an increase in heart rate may produce a reduction in or even a reversal of the normally positive force frequently effect (*reversed* or *negative treppe*).[445–447] This phenomenon is

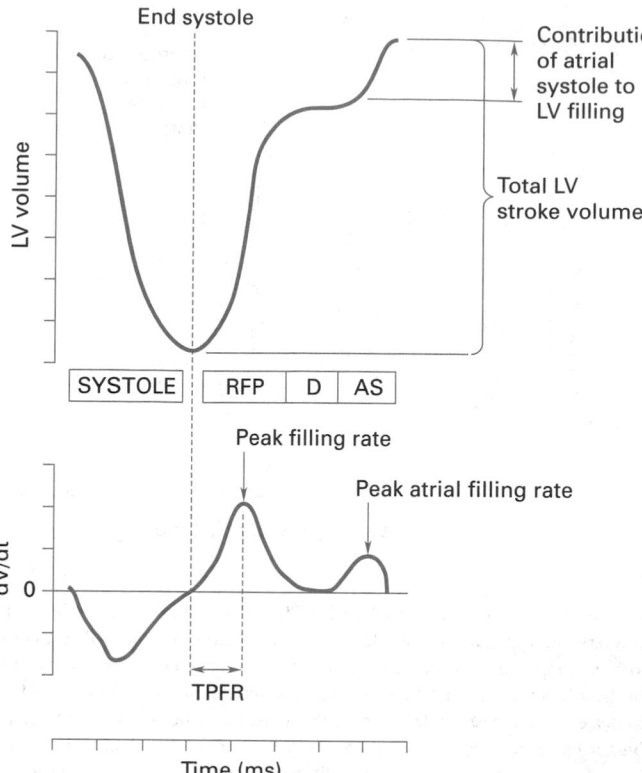

FIGURE 21-7

Idealized plot of left ventricular volume versus time (*top*) and the rate of change of volume (*dV/dt*) versus time (*bottom*), such as might be obtained from contrast or radionuclide ventriculographic studies. The representative cardiac cycle begins at end diastole. Subsequent events as depicted by the bars in the center of the figure are (1) systole, during which left ventricular volume decreases to a minimum and −*dV/dt* reaches its maximum; and (2) diastole, the beginning of which is signaled by the opening of the mitral valve and the onset of left ventricular filling. Diastole has three distinct phases in normal individuals: (1) the rapid filling phase (RFP), during which the left ventricle fills rapidly but passively and the peak filling rate occurs; (2) diastasis (D), during which relatively little left ventricular volume change occurs; and (3) atrial systole (AS), in which active atrial contraction fills the left ventricle to its end-diastolic volume. The diastolic parameters that have been derived from such analysis are the peak filling rate, the time to peak filling rate (TPFR), the percent contribution of atrial systole, and the first third filling fraction. (From AJ Labovitz, AC Pearson. Evaluation of left ventricular diastolic function: Clinical relevance and recent Doppler echocardiographic insights. *Am Heart J* 1987; 114:836–849. Reproduced with permission from the publisher and authors.)

likely responsible for some of the deterioration of ventricular performance associated with tachycardia.

Peripheral Oxygen Delivery

REDISTRIBUTION OF BLOOD FLOW

Patients with heart failure redistribute their diminished cardiac output. In general, perfusion of the brain and heart is maintained at the expense of circulation to the kidney, splanchnic area, and skin. The peripheral tissues in heart failure extract more oxygen per unit of blood flow, and this produces an increase in the arteriovenous oxygen difference of the whole body. This "venous oxygen reserve" is potentially less useful to the myocardium,

which even normally extracts about 65 to 75 percent of the oxygen coming to it (see Chap. 3), or to the brain.

OXYGEN-HEMOGLOBIN DISSOCIATION

The usual decrease in blood flow to the peripheral tissues in heart failure is associated with a progressive decline in the affinity of hemoglobin for oxygen, which is caused by an increase in 2,3-diphosphoglycerate (DPG).[448] This change in affinity for oxygen, which is reflected in a rightward shift in the oxygen-hemoglobin dissociation curve, facilitates the release of oxygen in the peripheral capillaries of underperfused tissues.

ANAEROBIC METABOLISM

Some tissues utilize anaerobic metabolism during transient periods of increased stress, such as exercise. Unfortunately, this reserve mechanism is of limited value to myocardium or the brain.

Peripheral Vascular Resistance

Patients with heart failure have an increase in peripheral vascular resistance due to multiple mechanisms, including increased sympathetic adrenergic vasoconstrictor activity and increased plasma concentrations of NE, angiotensin II, endothelin-1, and AVP. In addition, the sodium and water retention in heart failure tends to make the arterioles "stiff" from an increased content of sodium and water. An increase in tissue turgor can compress blood vessels and contribute to the increased peripheral vascular resistance at rest as well as to the important failure of the peripheral vascular resistance to decrease normally during exertion. In the later stages of heart failure, hypertrophy of arteriolar smooth muscle may also contribute to the limitation of normal metabolically mediated vasodilatation.

In the early stages of heart failure, cardiac output and arterial vascular resistance are generally normal, despite marked reductions in EF. When symptoms develop, cardiac output may be somewhat reduced at rest, while peripheral vascular resistance is elevated; nevertheless, with reactive hyperemia and during exercise, cardiac output may increase three- to fourfold with concomitant falls in vascular resistance. In patients with late, highly symptomatic heart failure, a further important abnormality develops in the peripheral arterial circulation. At this stage, cardiac output is reduced at rest with an increased peripheral vascular resistance. During exercise, nitric oxide–mediated arterial vascular dilatation is impaired and blood flow to the exercising organ does not increase normally. There is little increase in cardiac output, and exercise performance becomes limited, in part due to lack of skeletal muscle blood flow. This is accompanied by decreased muscle mass as well. Skeletal muscle metabolism may also be altered.[449–453] This abnormality of dilatation may result from a reduction of the release by the vascular endothelium of endothelium-derived relaxing factor (nitric oxide), which normally mediates dilatation. This abnormality is partially reversible with increased exercise training[453–456] or with long-term drug therapy for heart failure.[457]

THE LAW OF LAPLACE

The law of Laplace and the effects of ventricular dilatation on the mechanics and energetics of myocardial contraction are important factors in heart failure. On first thought, it might seem that ventricular dilatation is advantageous. With an increased ventricular EDV and sarcomere length, each sarcomere would have to shorten less to eject a given volume of blood, and each myocardial fiber would be able to perform more work by virtue of greater preload (the Frank-Starling law of the heart). These seeming advantages, however, are negated by other consequences of dilatation. The more important of these is the need for the myocardial fibers in the wall of a dilated ventricle to develop greater tension in order to produce a given pressure within the ventricle. Because wall tension is a major determinant of the internal work of the heart, which is degraded to heat during diastole, dilatation decreases cardiac efficiency. These energetic consequences of the law of Laplace probably play an important role in the progressive deterioration of energy-starved myocytes in the failing heart.

Ventricular myocardial wall tension is calculated by employing the law of Laplace, which actually applies to a distensible membrane with a spherical or cylindrical shape, and by assuming that the ventricle has a spherical cavity. In general, calculations of myocardial tension can be expressed in terms of tension (T) per unit of cross-sectional area; for a thick-walled cylinder, $T = P \cdot r/2h$, where P is transmural pressure, r is average radius, and h is wall thickness.[390] It is apparent that, as the radius increases acutely, more tension must be developed by each fiber to produce or maintain a given intraventricular pressure, while increased thickness of the ventricular wall tends to decrease the required systolic tension per cross-sectional area.

The law of Laplace expresses an additional disadvantage of the dilated ventricle. In a normal ventricle, the decrease in average radius of the ventricle during ejection is relatively large; consequently, the effect of this decrease in diameter on instantaneous wall tension is normally greater than the opposite effect of the increasing pressure in the ventricle. As a result, the myocardial fiber tension, or force, may actually *decrease* soon after the beginning of ejection from a normal-sized ventricle, and the wall tension is usually less at the moment of peak systolic pressure in the ventricle than at the beginning of ejection. On the other hand, if the ventricle is markedly dilated and the contractility and the shortening capacity of the myocardial fibers are reduced, both the relative and the absolute decrease in average radius are much less during the ejection of an equal volume. In a markedly dilated ventricle, therefore, the average tension in the myocardial fibers may continue to increase from the beginning of ejection up to the peak systolic pressure.[390,458–460] In a sense, this is an additional type of "afterload" encountered during ejection

by ventricles that are significantly dilated. A further disadvantage of dilatation is that the increased force, or tension, in the myocardial fibers required to develop a given pressure inside a dilated ventricle results in a decrease in the *rate* of myocardial fiber shortening (see Chap. 3), further limiting the ability of the ventricle to eject blood.[2,49,390,461,462] In mitral regurgitation, the early reduction in afterload (impedance) produced by the relatively rapid early emptying of the left ventricle into the low-pressure left atrium helps to maintain left ventricular function for many years.[463] When the ventricle dilates and left atrial pressure is high, the unloading effect of rapid emptying may be lost, thus adding to decompensation.

HEART FAILURE DUE TO PRESSURE OVERLOAD OR VOLUME OVERLOAD

Most types of congenital and acquired heart disease result in mechanical stress on the heart and myocardium. The two most common general types of mechanical cardiac stress are that resulting from an increased resistance to ventricular emptying of increased afterload (e.g., aortic stenosis, systemic hypertension) and that resulting from an increased preload or increased ventricular filling (e.g., aortic or mitral regurgitation, ventricular septal defect). The hemodynamics of several other specific types of mechanical abnormalities are described in more detail elsewhere: mitral stenosis (Chap. 64), pericardial tamponade or constriction (Chap. 81), endocardial restriction (Chap. 75), and the several varieties of ventricular dysynergy and aneurysm (Chap. 47). Figure 21-8 diagrams the progression from myocardial damage to left ventricular dysfunction to congestive heart failure.

In some patients with severe acute mechanical abnormalities, such as the acute rupture of a mitral chordae tendineae or an aortic valve leaflet, the overall capacity of the heart as a pump may be unable to meet the massive overload, although contractility of the myocardium may initially be normal. Similarly, some chronic mechanical abnormalities can prevent the heart from pumping an adequate amount of blood even without the development of myocardial failure. In most patients with a chronic pressure or volume load on the left ventricle, however, the development of either clinical CHF or pump failure is associated with the development of myocardial systolic dysfunction and eventually myocardial failure. This may be referred to as "dysdynamic" systolic dysfunction or failure. As noted previously, some patients with marked hypertrophy from hypertrophic cardiomyopathy, systemic hypertension, or aortic stenosis may develop diastolic dysfunction or failure with pulmonary congestion before the development of systolic failure of the ventricle.

Myocardial Compensatory Mechanisms in Heart Failure Due to Increased Afterload (Pressure Overload)

The basic reaction of isolated myocardium to an increased afterload is to contract more forcefully but more slowly. In

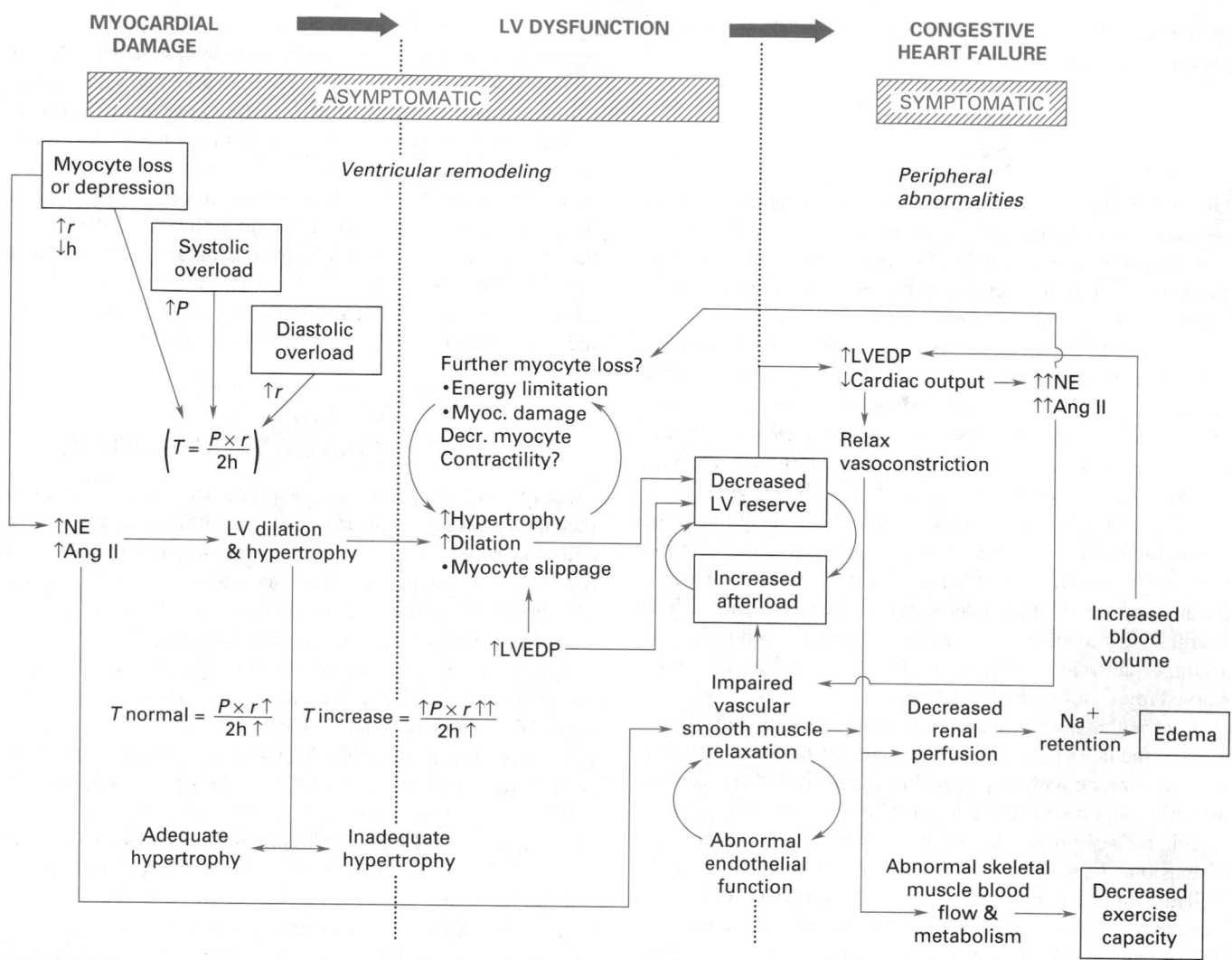

FIGURE 21-8

Evolution of myocardial damage to left ventricular function and ultimate congestive heart failure. The syndrome of congestive heart failure is the end result of processes that evolve in response to initial myocardial damage and/or cardiac overloads. The initiating event may be myocyte loss, either segmental, as with acute myocardial infarction, or diffuse, as with idiopathic cardiomyopathies and myocarditis; systolic overload, such as hypertension or aortic stenosis; or diastolic overload, such as mitral regurgitation or aortic regurgitation. Major loss of myocytes may also stimulate the renin-angiotensin and adrenergic systems, which may contribute to ventricular and vascular remodeling. All of these overloads create an increased workload for the heart, as characterized by Laplace relationship, where tension (T) is equal to the product of pressure (P) and ventricular radius (r) divided by twice the wall of thickness (h). The initial adaptations to these overloads, termed *ventricular remodeling*, are an increase in both myocyte length and diameter as well as an increase in ventricular volume to maintain adequate stroke volume and hence cardiac output. If hypertrophy is adequate to normalize the tension load, a relatively steady state may be maintained. Myocytes continue to be lost as a function of aging per se, however, and this tends to lead to further myocyte hypertrophy and cardiac dilatation. Moreover, the aging process may be amplified by hypertrophy. Should there be a sudden increase in end-diastolic pressure within the ventricle, an added factor of relative myocyte slippage within the wall tends to occur, which may lead to a further decrease in myocytes across the ventricular wall, further increasing ventricular wall tension. This may create a downward spiral in which progressive cell loss leads to further ventricular remodeling and continued ventricular dilation. As noted above, the entire process of ventricular remodeling may occur asymp-

tomatically, and myocardial damage progresses to left ventricular dysfunction, which is characterized by an increasing diastolic volume and thus a reduced ventricular ejection fraction. Symptoms associated with congestive heart failure occur when decreased left ventricular reserve limits cardiac output response to exercise. As the process of heart failure evolves, abnormalities of endothelial function in the peripheral arterioles lead to reduced ability of the peripheral vasculature to dilate in response to metabolic need. As these abnormalities occur, abnormal skeletal muscle blood flow occurs in response to exercise and decreased exercise tolerance. In addition decreased renal perfusion leads to further activation of the renin-angiotensin-aldosterone system (RAAS), with increased aldosterone secretion and sodium retention. The combination of these two events leads to decreased exercise capacity and peripheral edema, important components of the symptom complex of congestive heart failure. Decreased cardiac performance promotes neurohumoral responses characterized by activation of the sympathetic nervous system and the renin-angiotensin-aldosterone system, leading to peripheral vasoconstriction and sodium accumulation. These factors feed back to increase the ventricular remodeling process and to amplify cardiac damage. Thus, initial myocardial damage progresses to ventricular dysfunction and ultimately to congestive heart failure. It is important to note that the myocardial damage and left ventricular dysfunction are often asymptomatic, and by the time symptomatic heart failure ensues, the disease process is far advanced. (Revised from LeJemtel TH, Sonnenblick EH. Heart failure and maladaptive processes: Introduction. *Circulation* 1993; 87(suppl VII):VII1–VII4. Reproduced with permission from the American Heart Association and the authors.)

addition, when the heart of an experimental animal is acutely subjected to increased afterload, there is metabolic evidence of hypertrophy within a few hours.[168,169,352–356] The biochemical signal is unknown but may be related to a chronic increase in systolic wall tension (see Chaps. 3 and 6).[169,354,368,369] As noted previously, the classic type of cardiac hypertrophy associated with aortic stenosis is concentric hypertrophy, in which there is marked thickening of the left ventricular wall (including the ventricular septum) but no increase in the size of the left ventricular cavity, which may even get smaller. Increased afterload effects myocardial thickening by replication of sarcomeres in parallel.[365] Although the contractility of the myocardium subjected to pressure overload may be decreased per unit mass later in the process (see above), overall ventricular compensation may be maintained by the increase in myocardial mass. Systolic wall tension is generally returned to normal by the concentric hypertrophy and the spherical shape, although diastolic wall stress remains elevated.[2,5,30,354,365,368,388–392] During this phase of adaptive hyperfunction, function of the left ventricle is compensated, although the reserve may be reduced. Eventually, however, systolic, in addition to diastolic, myocardial dysfunction occurs and myocardial failure develops. Left ventricular diastolic volume increases in association with cardiac pump dysfunction and failure, or "hyperadaptation" of Meerson.[353–356,443] Some of the possible structural and biochemical mechanisms responsible for myocardial failure are discussed above. Programmed cell death (apoptosis) has recently been suggested as playing an important role in the progressive deterioration of the failing heart.[464,465] Apoptosis generally occurs without scarring, however, whereas fibrosis is a prominent feature in end-state heart failure. For this reason, other causes of cell death such as free radical damage and energy starvation are also likely to play a major role in heart failure.

In aortic stenosis, there may be special difficulties with the delivery of adequate amounts of oxygen to the myocardial cells, particularly in the endocardium. Some of the factors responsible for inadequate oxygen delivery in aortic stenosis (and other conditions associated with marked concentric hypertrophy, such as hypertrophic cardiomyopathy and systemic hypertension) include the elevated myocardial oxygen requirements and the very high intramyocardial pressure, which throttles systolic coronary blood flow even more than usual, especially with tachycardia.[466–469] An elevated ventricular diastolic pressure, which may be necessary to fill the hypertrophied ventricle, can further impede diastolic coronary blood flow to the endocardium (see Chap. 3).[470] In addition, the growth of capillaries may be relatively less than the growth of myocytes, and the diffusion distance from myocardial capillaries to the center of the hypertrophied myocardial cells may be significantly increased.[471] Thus, there is a reduction in the relative increase in coronary blood flow during reactive hyperemia (decreased coronary reserve), which can be limiting during periods of stress. Patients with marked concentric hypertrophy from aortic stenosis or other causes frequently have an elevation of left ventricular diastolic filling pressure

(and a decreased rate of left ventricular relaxation and decreased left ventricular compliance or distensibility) due to the hypertrophy itself rather than to cardiac failure (see "Hemodynamic Characteristics of Heart Failure" below).[391,392,394–418,472]

Myocardial Compensatory Mechanisms in Patients with Increased Left Ventricular Preload (Volume Overload)

With increased left ventricular preload (volume overload), eccentric hypertrophy develops, and the ventricular chamber and the left ventricular wall increase in size proportionately.[168,169,352–357,368–370] It has been suggested that this type of hypertrophy is produced by a chronic increase in diastolic wall stress and is associated with the synthesis of additional sarcomeres, predominantly in series.[370] Since increased preload also increases systolic wall stress and afterload by the law of Laplace, some replication of sarcomeres in parallel also occurs and helps to normalize systolic stress.

When the ventricle is subjected acutely to an increased preload, the ventricle dilates and functions on a higher portion of the "ascending limb" of its length-tension function curve, with the sarcomere length ultimately increasing to about 2.2 μm in the midwall of the left ventricle. This length approximates L_{max}, the sarcomere length at which the maximal performance is achieved on the sarcomere length-tension function curve.[51–54] In experimental animals subjected to chronic left ventricular volume loading, the left ventricle continues to work on the ascending limb of a function curve. When the ventricle is subjected to increased preload, however, there does not appear to be any additional increase in sarcomere length in the midwall of the left ventricle beyond about 2.2 μm, although there is some additional recruitment in sarcomere length up to about 2.2 μm in the left ventricular endocardial and epicardial area.[50–56] At this point, sarcomeres are very stiff, and any further increase in diastolic volume produces a very large increase in diastolic pressure. Normally, the functioning sarcomere lengths are somewhat less in the endocardium and the epicardium than in the midwall of the left ventricle.[50] The marked ventricular dilatation of chronic volume loading is produced by several mechanisms, including an increase in individual sarcomere length, the synthesis of new sarcomeres in series and parallel with previous sarcomeres so that the myocytes are longer, "slippage" between and within myofibrils and fibers, and the rearrangement of myocardial fibers along the normal cleavage planes of the ventricle.[2,50–55,365,443] Taken together, these changes have been terms *ventricular remodeling*.

The performance of the ventricle with mitral regurgitation is aided by the fact that during systole the left ventricle empties relatively rapidly by regurgitation into the low-pressure left atrium as well as by aortic ejection. This rapid decrease in the mean left ventricular diameter has the effect of rapidly decreasing the systolic wall tension and afterload (impedance) and thus increasing the velocity of contraction.[56,436,472] The diastolic capacity of the ventricle with chronically increased volume loads is much increased to accommodate a large volume without excess elevation of diastolic pressure,[56,353] although any additional volume loading may produce a precipitous elevation of diastolic pressure, indicative of reduced compliance.[473] When the myocardial contractility eventually becomes markedly decreased in patients with chronic volume overload, the many compensatory mechanisms, including ventricular dilatation and hypertrophy, are no longer able to maintain normal compensation. Mitral regurgitation commonly occurs or worsens at this point, and overall heart pump function fails.

ATRIAL FAILURE AND HEART FAILURE[474,475]

The atria normally function as pumps and reservoirs.[474,475] In addition, the atria are the source of ANPs.[328,329,338,342] Normally, the atria contribute approximately 15 to 20 percent of Ventricular filling but the relative contribution increases markedly with tachycardia. In normal individuals or patients with mild heart disease, loss of the atrial pumping function may result in no change in cardiac output at rest, although the response to exercise may be diminished. On the other hand, in patients with heart disease and limited cardiac reserve, atrial fibrillation or atrial flutter can product *atrial failure* with severe detrimental effects on ventricular filling and on the total pump function of the heart. This is particularly likely in patients with moderate or marked concentric cardiac hypertrophy from aortic stenosis, hypertrophic cardiomyopathy, or system arterial hypertension, where the stiffness of the ventricle is already increased.

The more common forms of atrial failure are due to arrhythmia (e.g., atrial fibrillation), mechanical abnormalities (e.g., mitral or tricuspid stenosis), or "dysdynamic" failure of the atrial myocardium. In some patients with compensated heart disease, CHF may be precipitated by the onset of atrial fibrillation, at times even when the ventricular rate is controlled by digitalis. In these patients, the restoration of normal sinus rhythm may result in a marked improvement in their hemodynamics, presumably by restoration of the normal "primer-pump" function of the atria. In some patients following cardioversion and the restoration of normal sinus rhythm, effective atrial contraction may not return for several days.[476] Very rarely, atrial fibrillation has been reported to produce heart failure in patients with otherwise apparently normal hearts.[477]

Left Atrial Compliance and Heart Failure

The compliance of the left atrium is of great importance in determining the level of left atrial pressure produced by disease of the left side of the heart and especially by mitral regurgitation. Thus, a given volume of mitral regurgitation in a patient with a lax, capacious left atrium, as is common in severe mitral regurgitation of long duration, may produce only slight elevation of left atrial pressure, whereas the same

volume regurgitated into a smaller left atrium with less distensibility, as occurs with acute mitral regurgitation due to chordae tendineae rupture, produces marked elevation of left atrial pressure and severe pulmonary congestion (see Chaps. 47 and 64).[56,478]

HEMODYNAMIC CHARACTERISTICS OF HEART FAILURE

The major hemodynamic alterations and several of the major compensatory mechanisms produced by myocardial and subsequent pump failure are diagrammatically shown in Fig. 21-9. Also indicated are the sites of action of major therapeutic interventions.

As described in Chaps. 3 and 22 the systolic performance of the intact heart should generally be assessed at two levels. The first type of analysis is an evaluation of the overall *cardiac pump function* as indicated by the relationship between stroke work (or cardiac output) and ventricular EDV (or EDP). Ideally, these or other systolic indexes of pump performance are measured at rest and again during exercise or after induced changes in preload or afterload in order to construct a "function curve," although such measurements are seldom obtained clinically. The second type of assessment is of systolic *myocardial function* (*myocardial contractility* or *inotropic state*). Although decreases in myocardial contractility can sometimes be inferred from studies of overall cardiac function (i.e., when the cardiac output and SV are significantly decreased despite a markedly increased ventricular EDV greater than 110 mL/m^2 and the presence of normal afterload and heart rate), more specific and more sensitive quantitative evidence of changes in myocardial contractility in patients is obtained from other special types of analyses. These include the following: (1) *isovolumic phase indexes* utilizing the rate of rise of ventricular pressure (dP/dt) or a derivative, (2) *ejection phase indexes* of contractility utilizing circumferential fiber shortening rate (V_{cf}), and (3) *end-systolic indexes*, including analysis of ventricular end-systolic pressure or wall stress–volume relationships.[479] The techniques used clinically for evaluation of cardiac function and myocardial contractility are reviewed in Chap. 22.

Changes in the Contralateral Ventricle

The diastolic filling pressures of one ventricle affect the other across the common ventricular septum. Thus, elevated right ventricular filling pressure may produce an increase in left ventricular filling pressure (i.e., "reversed" Bernheim effect).[426,480–483] These effects are much more apparent with an intact pericardium, which can substantially affect the left ventricular diastolic pressure-volume relationships.[483] In general, whenever there is moderate or marked ventricular hypertrophy of one ventricle, the diastolic pressure-volume relationships of the opposite ventricle may be altered.[407,422–428,484] This ventricular interdependence, or interaction, may occur chronically or acutely, as in patients with acute pulmonary embolus. In addition, in experimental heart failure models, the contralateral left ventricle may have decreased NE concentration,[147,485] decreased myofibrillar ATPase activity,[59] and increased amounts of collagen.[167]

Secondary (Functional) Mitral or Tricuspid Regurgitation

"Functional" mitral valve regurgitation may develop secondary to left ventricular dilatation, and a similar form of tricuspid regurgitation occurs secondary to right ventricular dilatation. This may be a very major hemodynamic deficit in heart failure. In both instances the regurgitation is principally the result of failure of the papillary muscles and chordae tendineae of the dilated ventricle to anchor or constrain the atrioventricular valve leaflets. A secondary mechanism, which is present in chronic lesions, is dilatation of the valve annulus and its failure to constrict properly during systole. If the regurgitation is moderate or severe, the atrial pressure tracings may have a large regurgitant R wave ("giant V wave"). Heart failure is frequently associated with changes in left ventricular shape manifested by increased sphericity.[486–489] Functional mitral regurgitation may be more likely with a spherical left ventricle.[488,489]

Pulsus Alternans

Pulsus alternans may occur in patients with very severe heart failure, particularly from aortic stenosis. It may be associated with an alteration of EDV or fiber length, with or without an alteration of either EDV or EDP.[490–492] The latter cases appear to be associated with an isolated alteration of myocardial contractility. Pulsus alternans is probably related to a defect in the Ca^{2+} transport systems involved in excitation-contraction coupling. It may occur briefly in some apparently normal hearts during or following marked tachycardia.

The Pulmonary Circulation

In moderate or severe left ventricular failure, elevated left ventricular diastolic pressure increases left atrial, pulmonary capillary, and pulmonary artery diastolic pressures. Initially, the pulmonary artery pressure and right ventricular systolic

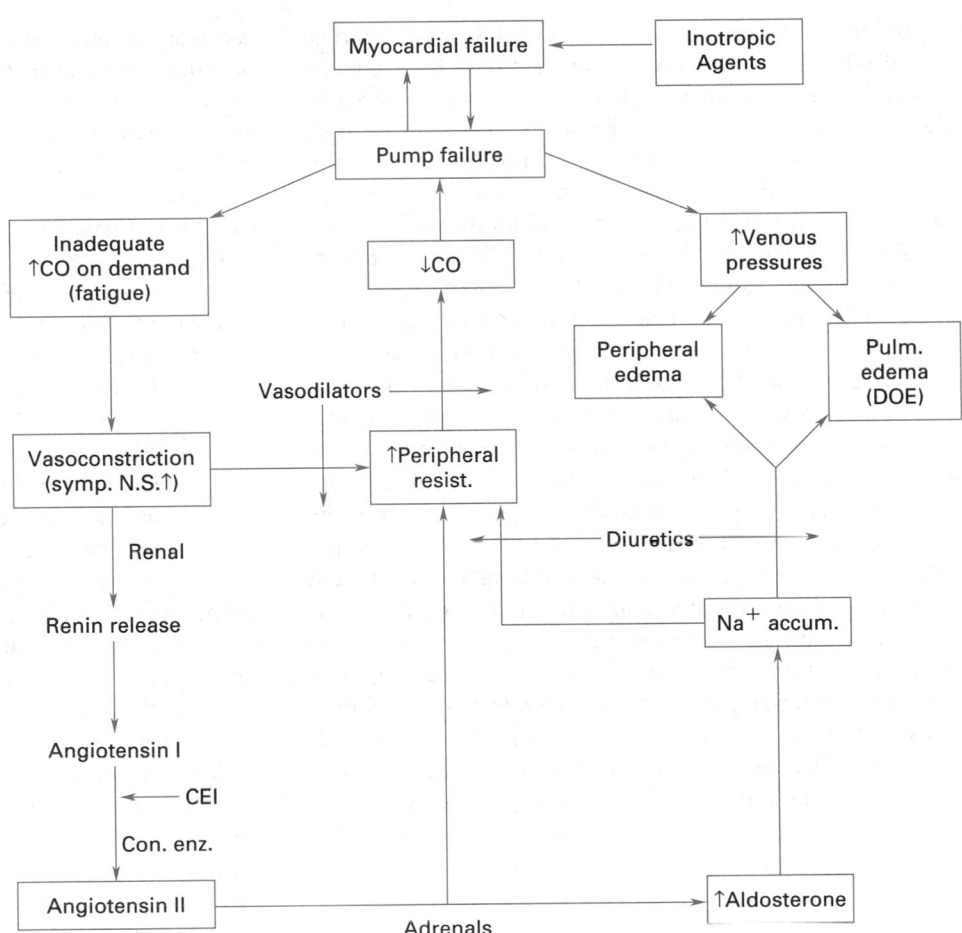

FIGURE 21-9

Schematic diagram of the major hemodynamic alterations and several of the major compensatory mechanisms that result from the development of myocardial failure and pump (heart) failure. Also shown are the sites of action of major therapeutic interventions: administration of inotropic agents, diuretics, converting enzyme inhibitors (CEI), and vasodilators.

pressure are abnormally elevated only during exercise, although later they may be chronically elevated to systemic levels at rest, particularly in patients with mitral disease (see Chap. 64). In the absence of significant pulmonary vascular disease or tachycardia, the pulmonary artery diastolic pressure can be used as a reasonably good reflection of mean left atrial pressure.

The Right Ventricle

Right ventricular dilatation and failure, with a decreased EF and rate of ejection, most often occur secondary to left ventricular failure, perhaps as a result of the pressure load created by elevated pulmonary pressures but also from interactions across the ventricular septum that vitiate diastolic elastic recoil and may also slow emptying. There may also be secondary biochemical changes in the right ventricular myocardium.[2,59,147,167,485] Right ventricular failure may be reflected in a decreased right ventricular SV and EF, despite an abnormal elevation of the right ventricular EDV and EDP, the mean right atrial pressure, and the mean systemic venous pressure. If the failure is mild, these abnormalities may be absent at rest but apparent during exercise. Failure of the right ventricle may also be associated with development of right ventricular pulsus alternans, auscultatory alternans, and a right ventricular diastolic gallop (S_3) sound. The sequence of severe right ventricular failure secondary to left ventricular failure is frequently associated with the development of tricuspid regurgitation, especially in patients with atrial fibrillation, or occasionally with the development of functional pulmonary regurgitation due to dilatation of the pulmonary valve ring. Severe pulmonary regurgitation can produce an equalization of the pulmonary artery and right ventricular pressures during mid- or late diastole, although this rarely occurs with functional pulmonary regurgitation. Secondary, or so-called functional, tricuspid regurgitation is caused by the inability of the papillary muscles and chordae tendineae of the dilated right ventricle to anchor and to maintain adequate closure of the tricuspid valve. Dilatation, or overstretch, of the tricuspid valve ring also contributes to the regurgitation when right ventricular dilatation is severe and chronic. Tricuspid regurgitation may produce large regurgitant R (or V waves during systole in the right atrium and systemic veins (see Chap. 10). Clinically, the development of marked right ventricular failure in association with tricuspid regurgitation in a patient with severe left-sided heart failure may, very rarely, be associated with a significant decrease in the clinical symptoms of pulmonary congestion. More often, however, it is associated with a worsening of the pulmonary congestion.

Effects of Exercise

During exercise in the supine position, the normal ventricle increases its cardiac output predominantly by an increase in rate, although SV may increase 10 to 20 percent.[493] The increased SV occurs from an unchanged or slightly smaller EDV and a decreased end-systolic volume[494,495]; consequently, the EF and SV may increase. The ventricular EDP normally stays the same or slightly decreases, whereas the systolic ejection period shortens and the mean systolic ejection rate and the rate of relaxation increase.[493–506] In contrast, during exercise in the upright position, SV may double,[507,508] and during maximal exercise the EDV may increase.[2] The calculated efficiency (ratio of external work to oxygen consumed by the heart) increases during exercise in normal individuals, perhaps in part as the result of the decreased average ventricular radius throughout systole.

Conversely, in patients with heart failure due to dysdynamic myocardial failure, exercise may result in the following changes: an elevation of the EDP above 12 mmHg, only a slight increase or an actual decrease in SV despite an increased EDV, a decreased EF,[509] an increased end-systolic volume, and a prolonged preejection phase.[2,496,509] The calculated ventricular efficiency decreases as the result of no increase (or an actual decrease) in SV despite an increased ventricular EDV. The latter increases the mean radius of the ventricle and, by the Laplace relationship, increases the sarcomere tension

necessary to produce a given intraventricular pressure. Not only does the increased tension required by the dilated ventricle increase the myocardial oxygen consumption ($M\dot{V}_{O_2}$), it also decreases the velocity of shortening, further limiting the performance of the ventricle.[2,365,390,391, 458–461,510] Exercise may also increase functional atrioventricular valvular regurgitation (see Chap. 22).

In patients with heart failure during dynamic exercise, the cardiac output either does not increase or does not increase adequately relative to the increased oxygen requirements of the body. One of the mechanisms for this is a failure of the peripheral vascular resistance to decrease normally during exertion.[511] Usually, the increase in blood flow to exercising limbs is less than normal in clinical heart failure, while there are marked decreases in the already diminished flow to skin, kidneys, and splanchnic organs. Coronary flow usually increases, whereas cerebral flow remains unchanged.[287] The excessive increase in venous tone and central venous pressure during exercise in heart failure may be in part related to a reflex with the afferent limb in the exercising muscle and the efferent limb in the sympathetic nervous system.[503] In addition, the plasma concentration of NE, which is often increased in moderate or severe CHF, is further increased. High plasma concentrations of angiotensin II, endothelin-1, and AVP may also contribute to the increase in arterial and venous tone. In general, exercise capacity in heart failure appears to be more closely related to the diastolic filling pattern of the left ventricle than to indices of left ventricular systolic function.[512]

The fact that the peripheral blood vessels of patients with heart failure have increased sodium and water content and are relatively stiff and relatively unresponsive to local metabolic vasodilator influences during exercise may have a protective influence in some patients with severe mitral stenosis. For example, if cardiac output did not increase or even decreased during extensive exercise, vasodilatation of large skeletal muscle groups could produce an excess fall in the mean arterial pressure. On the other hand, the increased stiffness tends to maintain arteriolar resistance and systemic blood pressure, although at the expense of increased total impedance to left ventricular emptying.

The Peripheral Circulation

Increased muscle fatigue in patients with heart failure is related not only to decreased blood flow during exertion but also to intrinsic changes in the skeletal muscles, including fiber atrophy and significant ultrastructure abnormalities that reflect a depressed oxidative capacity.[513–519] Altered skeletal muscle metabolism has been demonstrated by magnetic resonance spectroscopy.[515,516,520] Many patients appear to have a favorable training response.[521–525]

In heart failure associated with a diminished cardiac output, there is a significant redistribution of blood flow that in part resembles the normal redistribution occurring during exercise

(Chap. 3).[287] Thus, in heart failure, the renal and skin blood flows are disproportionately reduced early, whereas the decreases in blood flow to the cerebral, splanchnic, and skeletal muscle areas are approximately proportional to the decrease in total cardiac output until the failure is severe. Coronary blood flow per 100 g of tissue tends to remain normal or nearly normal in most patients in heart failure. The decreased skin circulation contributes to the heat intolerance and even mild temperature elevations in heart failure, while the decreased flow to the brain and kidneys contributes significantly to the deranged functions of these organs.

As noted above, the increased sympathetic impulses to the kidney and the high blood levels of NE and angiotensin II produce a redistribution of intrarenal blood flow and lead to further retention of sodium and water.

In addition to a redistribution of blood flow in heart failure, the tissues extract more oxygen per unit of blood flow and utilize anaerobic metabolism to a greater extent than normal, particularly during acute exertion. The increased oxygen extraction results in a widening of the arteriovenous oxygen differences for most organs and for the body as a whole. The pulmonary arteriovenous oxygen difference, which indicates the average of the whole body, is one of the better parameters for judging the adequacy of the heart as a pump to provide oxygen to the tissues.

PHYSIOLOGIC BASIS OF THERAPY FOR HEART FAILURE

As discussed in Chap. 23, appropriate therapy and anticipated benefits depend on the phase of the disease. Early, a specific diagnosis is sought in order to treat the primary damaging factor or factors, whether it is systolic overload, volume abnormalities, or ischemic myocardium. The primary goals of therapy should be twofold. Traditionally, emphasis has been on relief of symptoms, using such approaches as diuresis, vasodilatation, and inotropic stimulation of the failing heart. While all are appropriate, it must be kept in mind that each can have detrimental effects. Excess diuresis can reduce preload to levels that cannot sustain a reasonable cardiac output, vasodilators can lower blood pressure to dangerous levels, and overly vigorous inotropic stimulation can lead to arrhythmias and myocardial cell death. Even when used judiciously, each can be harmful. Prolonged diuresis can lead to electrolyte abnormalities and worsening renal and hepatic function, afterload reduction that lowers blood pressure rapidly can evoke harmful neurohumoral responses, while inotropic therapy can accelerate the deterioration of the failing heart. The need to tailor therapy to the manifestations of this syndrome that appear in individual patients has become more apparent as our understanding of the pathophysiology of heart failure has increased. The important differences between short- and long-term effects of the neurohumoral responses to impaired cardiac performance (see above) require that therapeutic strategies balance both the immediate and chronic needs of the individual patient. For example, when using vasodilators or inotropic agents to alleviate symptoms, the ability of both classes of drugs to worsen long-term prognosis must be kept in mind. Once ventricular dysfunction is present, one seeks to limit the adaptive mechanisms that may become damaging, such as progressive ventricular dilatation (remodeling), while controlling salt and water accumulation. To prevent progression, it is important to prevent both further myocyte loss and continued dilatation. Late in the course of failure, while one still seeks these effects, major symptomatic improvement is gained by increasing peripheral organ perfusion and improving skeletal muscle performance.

It is useful in selecting the therapy for a patient with heart failure to consider each determinant of myocardial performance separately. In general, an excessive increase in preload is treated with either diuretics or venous vasodilators. The relative increase in afterload associated with heart failure is treated with arterial vasodilators that inhibit the conversion of angiotensin I to angiotensin II or compounds that block angiotensin II receptors (Chap. 23), while the excess sodium retention with peripheral or pulmonary edema or circulatory congestion is treated with diuretics (see Chap. 24). Some of the benefits of therapy with angiotensin-converting enzyme (ACE) inhibitors in patients with mild to moderate heart failure or with left ventricular dysfunction without overt heart failure may be due to the effects of (ACE) inhibitors in slowing progression of cardiac deterioration, possibly mediated by inhibition of myocardial or tissue renin-angiotensin system activity (see also Chap. 23).

Myocardial systolic failure is present in most patients with systolic pump (heart) failure, either as a primary or as a secondary event. Direct therapy for a decrease in myocardial contractility includes the administration of digitalis (see Fig. 21-9) and other inotropic agents (Chap. 23) in addition to therapy to decrease afterload.[526,527] Theoretically, inotropic agents used to treat mild myocardial failure might hasten the progression of the disease.[528] Improvement in central pump function permits progressive rehabilitation of the patient, which over several weeks is associated with a return toward normal of endothelial-dependent vascular vasodilatation and improved peripheral muscle blood flow during exercise. This permits increased exercise performance and, in terms of the inhibition of the renin-angiotensin system, improved quality of life. Digitalis may also have significant sympathoinhibitory actions in patients with heart failure.[529] (See Chap. 23 for further details of the treatment of heart failure.) Beta-blocking agents may play a role in preventing progression by reducing myocyte loss, controlling heart rate, increasing diastolic filling time, and perhaps reducing arrhythmias (see Chaps. 23 and 54).

Diastolic dysfunction is treated acutely by the restoration, if necessary, of atrial contraction, the cautious use of diuretics to decrease pulmonary congestion, and the avoidance of myocardial ischemia and tachycardia. Chronically, the aim of therapy is to induce regression of the left ventricular hypertrophy.

PULMONARY FUNCTION AND PULMONARY EDEMA

Pulmonary Function

The ventilatory functions of the lungs are frequently impaired due to pulmonary congestion from left ventricular failure or mechanical obstruction at the mitral valve.[530–532] The amount of intrathoracic space available for ventilation may be decreased by fluid in the interstitial, perivascular, and alveolar spaces; by hydrothorax; or, in some patients, by an increase in pulmonary blood volume.[533] The increased amount of fluid and congestion in the lungs decreases the compliance (increases the stiffness) of the lungs and increases the work and oxygen cost of breathing. Alveolar fluid decreases pulmonary compliance by altering the normal surface tension characteristics, while pericapillary thickening and interstitial edema interfere with alveolar-capillary diffusion of oxygen. The respiratory muscles, which have an increased workload because of the decreased pulmonary compliance, may suffer from relative ischemia and, rarely, may produce pain difficult to distinguish from pain of myocardial origin. As heart failure becomes severe, the oxygen consumption of the work of breathing becomes an increasing part of overall oxygen consumption and may ultimately become an overwhelming burden.[534]

Many patients with moderate pulmonary congestion have compensatory hyperventilation with respiratory alkalosis, although some patients with severe pulmonary edema can have metabolic and respiratory acidosis.[535] Pulmonary congestion alters many pulmonary function tests, and it is often difficult to distinguish by such tests between dyspnea due to cardiac causes and dyspnea due to pulmonary causes. In clear-cut instances, however, such a separation is often possible (see Chap. 22).[531,532]

Pulmonary Edema[536–540]

GENERAL

The hydrostatic pressure in the pulmonary capillaries is normally 7 to 12 mmHg at rest in the supine position. When this pressure exceeds plasma oncotic pressure, which is normally 25 to 30 mmHg, net transudation of fluid from the pulmonary capillaries occurs. Pulmonary edema occurs when this rate of transudation exceeds the rate of lymphatic drainage from the tissues. If the plasma oncotic pressure is low due to a decreased serum protein concentration, transudation of fluid across the pulmonary capillaries occurs at even lower pressure.[541] There is little evidence that altered capillary permeability due to central nervous system influences or hypoxia is ordinarily an important factor in the production of pulmonary edema in most patients, although changes in capillary permeability can be important in some specialized forms of pulmonary edema due to the "capillary leak syndrome"[542] or in some patients with virus infections of the respiratory tract. The major factor

in cardiac pulmonary edema is the pulmonary capillary pressure.[532] The pulmonary capillaries have a significant "reserve" compared to systemic capillaries, since the pulmonary capillary pressure can ordinarily increase by 10 to 20 mmHg before significant transudation occurs.

An important consideration in the pulmonary circulation is the normal increase in hydrostatic pressure in both the arteries and veins in the dependent areas of the lungs. This increased pressure accounts, in part, for the initial appearance of pulmonary edema in the lower lobes in many patients with congestive failure. In normal persons in the upright position, relatively little pulmonary blood flow goes to the upper areas of the lungs. In patients with severe mitral stenosis or in severe left ventricular failure, however, the relative blood flow to the upper lobes may be equal or even exceed that to the lower lobes. It is uncertain whether this change in distribution of pulmonary blood flow is caused by local vasoconstriction produced by alveolar hypoxia, by a reactive hypertrophy and increased vascular tone of small arteries in the lower lobes secondary to the elevation of pulmonary arterial pressure, or by reflexes from the left atrium or pulmonary veins. Patients with marked elevation of left atrial pressure for long periods of time may often withstand elevations of pulmonary capillary pressure reasonably well, whereas the same level of pulmonary capillary pressure can produce severe, fulminating pulmonary edema in 5 to 10 min in a patient whose pulmonary circulation is not accustomed to these high pressure levels. The explanation for this difference may be that patients with chronic transudation of fluid from pulmonary capillaries often develop capacious lymphatic channels capable of removing large quantities of fluid from the pulmonary interstitial spaces.[543] In addition, the pericapillary thickening and the perivascular edema associated with chronic pulmonary capillary hypertension tend to decrease the rate of fluid transudation.[544] Since pulmonary lymphatic drainage empties into systemic veins, an elevation of central systemic venous pressure tends to decrease pulmonary lymphatic drainage and to worsen pulmonary edema.

It is probable that the occurrence of localized pulmonary edema in areas of acute infection or of previous infection is partially related to permanent alterations in local lymphatic drainage. The relative rarity of pulmonary rales in infants with left ventricular failure may be, in part, related to the presence of a pulmonary lymphatic system unscarred by respiratory tract infection. Patients with severe, chronic pulmonary disease may have such marked destruction of their pulmonary lymphatic vessels that they develop interstitial pulmonary edema much more readily than do normal individuals.

MORPHINE IN PULMONARY EDEMA

The beneficial effects of morphine in acute pulmonary edema are in part produced by decreased arterial resistance and pressure secondary to a reduction of centrally mediated sympathetic neural tone, which decreases ventricular afterload; by a decrease in venous return, perhaps aided by depression of the respiratory pump; and by "pharmacologic phlebotomy" resulting from an increase in the capacity of the peripheral vascular beds with perfusion of unperfused areas and venous pooling.[545,546]

Noncardiac Pulmonary Edema

HIGH-ALTITUDE PULMONARY EDEM

High-altitude pulmonary edema (HAPE) is apparently associated with marked pulmonary artery hypertension and pulmonary arteriolar vasoconstriction but with normal pulmonary artery wedge ("pulmonary capillary") pressure.[547–553] The mechanism of pulmonary edema in this rare syndrome is uncertain, although it is possible that the development of HAPE is related to an unusually marked, nonuniform vasoconstriction of the terminal pulmonary arterioles in response to decreased partial pressure of oxygen in the alveoli. As a consequence, there is excessive blood flow in the other areas of the lung, and the capillary bed may be relatively "unprotected" from the high pulmonary arterial pressure. An additional factor that may be important is the presence of preterminal arterioles, which are short, nonmuscular vessels that arise at right angles from small and medium-sized pulmonary arteries, bypass the pulmonary arterioles, and empty directly into the venous side of the pulmonary capillary bed.[554] These arterioles may be important in transmitting the strikingly elevated pulmonary artery pressure directly to the capillary bed in subjects with HAPE. Acute pulmonary hypertension may also damage the arterial walls and lead to direct transarterial leakage of plasma or even blood and allow the formation of microthrombi that may shower the distal capillary bed.[547] Postmortem studies have also suggested that pulmonary vascular obstruction by thrombi may occur in some cases.

MISCELLANEOUS FORMS OF PULMONARY EDEMA

The occasional occurrence of pulmonary edema secondary to pulmonary emboli may be related to "overperfusion edema" similar to that described for HAPE,[555] acute left ventricular failure, or an acute "reversed" Bernheim effect. The mechanism of pulmonary edema in patients with opiate-induced pulmonary edema or heroin intoxication is uncertain, although it may be due to acute apnea with hypoxic pulmonary edema from high-pressure damage to the pulmonary vascular endothelium.[547,556] Acute depression of ventricular function may also occur.[557] Changes in pulmonary capillary permeability appear to occur in some forms of pulmonary edema associated with infection, inhalation of toxic gases, or chemicals, such as ethchlorvynol or ingested paraquat.[547] Vasoconstriction of the pulmonary veins may be an important factor in the pulmonary edema produced by certain endotoxins.[558] Multiple small pulmonary venous thrombi may also produce acute pulmonary edema. Neurogenic pulmonary edema appears to be associated with intensive elevations in systemic arterial and venous pressures and pulmonary arterial, capillary, and

venous pressures. The abrupt elevation of pulmonary vascular pressure and volume may damage the vascular endothelium, altering reactivity and permeability and allowing pulmonary edema to develop.[547,559]

MORTALITY IN HEART FAILURE

The prognosis of patients with heart failure is generally poor; in several series, 50 percent of the patients with severe symptoms died within 12 months. In less severe heart failure, mortality approaches 50 percent in 3 to 4 years.[11,560–563] The primary factor that predicts prognosis is left ventricular function, as reflected in the EF. Other factors that have been shown to have prognostic value include functional classification; electrolyte abnormalities such as hyponatremia; elevated levels of plasma catecholamines, angiotensin II, aldosterone, and atrial natriuretic factor; poor exercise tolerance; presence of atrial fibrillation; and coronary artery disease as the etiology of the heart failure.[564,565] Many patients with heart failure, perhaps 30 to 40 percent, die suddenly, presumably from ventricular arrhythmias. Moreover, increasing heart failure is associated with an increased incidence of ventricular arrhythmias, which may be decreased by aggressive, successful therapy for heart failure or by the prevention of hypokalemia or hypomagnesemia. In patients surviving myocardial infarction, the prognosis is strongly related to the left ventricular EF, in addition to the amount of myocardium that becomes ischemic during stress and the amount of ventricular ectopy (see Chaps. 23 and 47).

REFERENCES

1. Eichna LW. Circulatory congestion and heart failure. *Circulation* 1960; 68:864–882.
2. Braunwald E, Ross J Jr, Sonnenblick EH. *Mechanisms of Contraction of the Normal and Failing Heart*, 2d ed. Boston: Little, Brown; 1976:1–417.
3. Weber KT, Janicki JS. The heart as a muscle-pump system and the concept of heart failure. *Am Heart J* 1979; 98:371–384.
4. Braunwald E, Mock MB, Watson J, eds. *Congestive Heart Failure: Current Research and Clinical Applications*. New York: Grune & Stratton; 1982:1–384.
5. Alpert NR, ed. *Myocardial Hypertrophy and Failure: Perspectives in Cardiovascular Research*, vol. 7. New York: Raven; 1983:1–682.
6. Levine HJ, Gaasch WH. *The Ventricle: Basic and Clinical Aspects*. Boston: Martinus Nijhoff; 1985:1–345.
7. Rupp H, ed. *Regulation of Heart Function: Basic Concepts and Clinical Applications*. Stuttgart: Thieme; 1986:1–446.
8. Fozzard HA, Haber E, Jennings RB, Katz AM, Morgan HE, eds. *The Heart and Cardiovascular System: Scientific Foundations*, 2d ed. New York: Raven; 1991.
9. Hosenpud JD, Greenberg BH, eds. *Congestive Heart Failure*. New York: Springer; 1994:1–769.
10. McCall D, Rahimtoola SH, eds. *Heart Failure*. New York: Chapman & Hall; 1995:1–436.
11. Cowie MR, Mosterd A, Wood DA, Deckers JW, Poole-Wilson PA, Sutton GC, et al. The epidemiology of heart failure. *Eur Heart J* 1997; 18:208–225.
12. Ho KKL, Anderson KM, Kannel WB, Grossman W, Levy D. Survival

after the onset of congestive heart failure in Framingham heart study objects. *Circulation* 1993; 88:107–115.

13. Katz AM. Cardiomyopathy of overload. A major determinant of prognosis in congestive heart failure. *N Engl J Med* 1990; 322:100–110.

14. Katz AM. Cardiomyopathy of overload. An unnatural growth response in the hypertrophied heart. *Ann Intern Med* 1994; 121:363–371.

15. Skelton CL, Sonnenblick EH. Heterogeneity of contractile function in cardiac hypertrophy. *Circ Res* 1974; 35(suppl 2):83–96.

16. Eichhorn EJ, Willard JE, Alvarez L, Kim AS, Glamann DB, Risser RC, et al. Are contraction and relaxation coupled in patients with and without congestive heart failure? *Circulation* 1992; 85:2132–2139.

17. Mirsky I, Pfeffer JM, Pfeffer MA. Mechanical properties of normal and hypertrophied myocardium: Is there a relationship between diastolic and systolic function. In: Alpert NR, ed. *Perspectives in Cardiovascular Research*, vol 7. New York: Raven; 1983:39–52.

18. Dodek A, Kassenbaum DG, Bristow JD. Pulmonary edema in coronary-artery disease without cardiomegaly. *N Engl J Med* 1972; 286:1347–1350.

19. McLaurin LP, Rolett EL, Grossman W. Impaired left ventricular relaxation during pacing-induced ischemia. *Am J Cardiol* 1973; 32:751–757.

20. Barry WH, Brooker JZ, Alderman EL, Harrison DC. Changes in diastolic stiffness and tone of the left ventricular during angina pectoris. *Circulation* 1974; 49:255–263.

21. Mann T, Brodie BR, Grossman W, McLaurin LP. Effect of angina on the left ventricular diastolic pressure-volume relationship. *Circulation* 1977; 55:761–766.

22. Bourdillon PD, Lorell BH, Mirsky I, Paulus WJ, Wynne J, Grossman W. Increased regional myocardial stiffness of the left ventricle during pacing-induced angina in man. *Circulation* 1983; 67:316–323.

23. Carroll JD, Hess OM, Hirzel HO, Krayenbuehl HP. Exercise-induced ischemia: The influence of altered relaxation on early diastolic pressures. *Circulation* 1983; 67:521–528.

24. Sasayama S, Nonoogi H, Miyazaki S, Sakurai T, Kawai C, Eihos S, et al. Changes in diastolic properties of the regional myocardium during pacing-induced ischemia in human subjects. *J Am Coll Cardiol* 1985; 5:599–606.

25. Pantley GA, Bristow JD. Ischemic cardiomyopathy. *Prog Cardiovasc Dis* 1984; 27:95–114.

26. Francis GS, Goldsmith SR, Levine TB, Olivari MT, Cohn JN. The neurohumoral axis in congestive heart failure. *Ann Intern Med* 1984; 101:370–377.

27. Parker M. The neurohumoral hypotheses: A theory to explain the mechanism of disease progression in heart failure. *J Am Coll Cardiol* 1992; 20:248–254.

28. Scheuer J. Metabolism of the heart in heart failure. *Prog Cardiovasc Dis* 1970; 13:24–54.

29. Schwartz A, Sordahl LA, Entman ML, Allen JC, Reddy YS, Goldstein MA, et al. Abnormal biochemistry in myocardial failure. In: Mason DT, ed. *Congestive Heart Failure: Mechanisms, Evaluation and Treatment.* New York: Yorke Medical; 1976:25–44.

30. Badeer HS. *Cardiovascular Physiology.* Basel: Karger; 1984:1–276.

31. Katz AM. *Physiology of the Heart*, 2d ed. New York: Raven; 1992:1–687.

32. Katz AM. Is the failing heart an energy-starved organ? (editorial). *J Card Failure* 1996; 2:267–272.

33. Alpert NR, Hamrell BB. Cardiac hypertrophy: A compensatory and anticompensatory response to stress. In: Vassalle M, ed. *Cardiac Physiology for the Clinician.* New York: Academic; 1976: 174–201.

34. Feldman MD, Copelas L, Gwathmey JK, Phillips P, Warren SE, Schoen FJ, et al. Deficient production of cyclic AMP: Pharmacologic evidence of an important case of contractile dysfunction in patients with end-stage heart failure. *Circulation* 1987; 75:331–339.

35. Meerson FZ, Javich MP. Isozyme pattern and activity of myocardial creatine phosphokinase under heart adaptation to prolonged overload. *Basic Res Cardiol* 1982; 77:349–358.

36. Sievers R, Parmley WW, James T, Wikman-Coffelt J. Energy levels at systole and diastole in normal hamster hearts vs. myopathic hamster hearts. *Circ Res 1983;* 53:759–766.

37. Ingwall JS, Kramer MF, Fifer MA, Lovell BH, Shemin R, Grossman W, et al. The creatine kinase system in normal and diseased human myocardium. *N Engl J Med* 1985; 313:1050–1054.

38. Rabinowitz M, Zak R. Mitochondria and cardiac hypertrophy. *Circ Res* 1975; 36:367–376.

39. Anversa P, Ricci R, Olivetti G. Quantitative structural analysis of the myocardium during physiologic growth and induced cardiac hypertrophy: A review. *J Am Coll Cardiol* 1986; 7:1140–1149.

40. Hyatt PY. Morphological approach to the mechanism of heart failure. *Cardiology* 1988; 75(suppl 1):3–7.

41. Sabbah HN, Sharov V, Riddle JM, Kono T, Lesch M, Goidstein S. Mitochondrial abnormalities in myocardium of dogs with chronic heart failure. *J Mol Cell Cardiol* 1992; 24:1333–1347.

42. Kunkel B, Schneider M. Myocardial structure and left ventricular function in hypertrophic and dilative cardiomyopathy and aortic valve disease. In: Kaltenbach M, Hopf R, Kunkel B, eds. *New Aspects of Hypertrophic Cardiomyopathy.* Damstadt: Steinkopff; 1987.

43. Schaper J, Froede R, Hein S, Buck A, Friedl A, Hashizume H, et al. Impairment of myocardial ultrastructure and changes of the cytoskeleton in dilated cardiomyopathy. *Circulation* 1991; 83:504–514.

44. Scholz J, Hein S, Scholz D, Mollnau H. Multifaceted morphological alterations are present in the failing human heart. *J Mol Cell Cardiol* 1995; 27:857–861.

45. Lentz RW, Harrison CE Jr, Dewey JD, Barnhorst DA, Danielson GK, Pluth JR. Functional evaluation of cardiac sarcoplasmic reticulum and mitochondria in human pathologic states. *J Mol Cell Cardiol* 1978; 10:3–30.

46. Unverfeth DV, Lee SW, Wallick ET. Human myocardial adenosine triphosphatase activities in health and heart failure. *Am Heart J* 1988; 115:139–146.

47. Schulze K, Becker BF, Schultheiss HP. Antibodies to the ADP/ATP carrier, an autoantigen in myocarditis and dilated cardiomyopathy, penetrate into myocardial cells and disturb energy metabolism in vivo. *Circ Res* 1989; 64:179–192.

48. Scheuer J. Metabolic factors in myocardial failure. *Circulation* 1993; 87(suppl VII):VII54–VII57.

49. Markiewicz W, Wu S, Sievers R, Parmley WW, Higgins CB, James TL, et al. Influence of heart rate on metabolic and hemodynamic parameters in the Syrian hamster cardiomyopathy. *Am Heart J* 1987; 114:362–368.

50. Ross J Jr, Sonnenblick EH, Taylor RR, Spotnitz HM, Covell J. Diastolic geometry and sarcomere lengths in the chronically dilated left ventricle. *Circ Res* 1971; 28:49–61.

51. Charney RH, Takahashi S, Zhao M, Sonnenblick EH, Eng C. Collagen loss in the stunned myocardium. *Circulation* 1992; 85:1483–1490.

52. Spotnitz HM, Sonnenblick EH. Structural conditions in the hypertrophied and failing heart. *Am J Cardiol* 1973; 32:398–406.

53. Yoran C, Covell JW, Ross J Jr. Structural basis for the ascending limb of left ventricular function. *Circ Res* 1973; 32:297–303.

54. Sonnenblick EH, Skelton CL. Reconsideration of the ultrastructural basis of cardiac length-tension relations. *Circ Res* 1974; 35:517–526.

55. Spotnitz HM, Sonnenblick EH. Structural conditions in the hypertrophied and failing heart. In: Mason DT, ed. *Congestive Heart Failure: Mechanisms, Evaluation and Treatment.* New York: Yorke Medical; 1976:13–24.

56. Ross J Jr. Adaptations of the left ventricle to chronic volume overload. *Circ Res* 1974; 35(suppl 2):64–70.

57. Brutsaert DL. Nonuniformity: A physiologic modulator of contraction and relaxation of the normal heart. *J Am Coll Cardiol* 1987; 9:341–348.

58. Alpert NR, Gordon MS. Myofibrillar adenosine triphosphate activity in congestive heart failure. *Am J Physiol* 1962; 202:940–946.

59. Chandler BM, Sonnenblick EH, Spann JF Jr, Pool PE. Association of depressed myofibrillar adenosine triphosphatase and reduced contractility in experimental heart failure. *Circ Res* 1967; 21:717–725.

60. Luchi RJ, Kritcher EM, Thyrum PT. Reduced cardiac myosin adenosine-triphosphatase activity in dogs with spontaneously occurring heart failure. *Circ Res* 1969; 24:513–519.

61. Conway G, Heazlitt RA, Montag J, Mattingly SF. The ATPase activity of cardiac myosin from failing and hypertrophied hearts. *J Mol Cell Cardiol* 1975; 7:817–826.

62. Wikman-Coffelt J, McPherson J, Salel AF, Kamiyama T, Mason DT. Mechanism of impaired contractile protein function in aortic stenosis: Alterations in myosin ATPase activity in the chronically pressure overload canine left ventricle (abstr). *Am J Cardiol* 1975; 35:177.

63. Wikman-Coffelt J, Walsh R, Fenner C, Kamiyama T, Salel A, Mason DT. Effects of severe hemodynamic pressure overload on the properties of canine left ventricular myosin: Mechanisms by which myosin ATPase activity is lowered during chronic increased hemodynamic stress. *J Moll Cell Cardiol* 1976; 8:263–270.

64. Wikman-Coffelt J, Mason DT. Mechanism of decreased contractility in chronic hemodynamic overload. In: Mason DT, ed. *Advances in Heart Diseases*, vol. 1. New York: Grune & Stratton; 1977:491–504.

65. Leclercq JF, Swynghedauw B. Myofibrillar ATPase, DNA, and hydroxyproline content of human hypertrophied heart. *Eur J Clin Invest* 1976; 6:27–33.

66. Cummins P. Contractile proteins in muscle disease. *J Muscle Res Cell Motil* 1983; 4:5–24.

67. Pagani ED, Alonsi AA, Grant AM, Older TM, Dziuban SW, Allen PD. Changes in myofibrillar content and Mg-ATPase activity in ventricular tissues from patients with heart failure caused by coronary artery disease, cardiomyopathy, or mitral valve insufficiency. *Circ Res* 1988; 63:380–385.

68. Gorza L, Mercadier JJ, Schwartz K, Thronell LE, Sartore S, Schiaffino S. Myosin types in the human heart: An immunofluorescence study of normal and hypertrophied atrial and ventricular myocardium. *Circ Res* 1984; 54:694–702.

69. Mead RJ, Peterson MB, Welty JD. Sarcolemmal and sarcoplasmic reticular ATPase activities in the failing canine heart. *Circ Res* 1971; 29:14–20.

70. Dubois-Randé JL, Comoy E, Merlet P, Benvenuti C, Carville C, Hittinger L, et al. Relationship among neuropeptide Y, catecholamines and haemodynamics in congestive heart failure. *Eur Heart J* 1992; 13:1233–1238.

71. Beller GA, Conroy J, Smith TW. Ischemia-induced alterations in myocardial (Na$^+$ and K$^+$) ATPase and cardiac glycoside binding. *J Clin Invest* 1976; 57:341–350.

72. Mercadier JJ, Lompre A-M, Duc P, Boheler KR, Fraysse J-B, Wisnewsky C, et al. Altered sarcoplasmic reticulum Ca^{++}-ATPase gene expression in the human left ventricle during endstage heart failure. *J Clin Invest* 1990; 85:305–309.

73. Grossman W. Diastolic dysfunction in congestive heart failure. *N Engl J Med* 1991; 325:1557–1564.

74. Arai M, Alpert NR, MacLennan DH, Barton P, Periasamy M. Alterations in sarcoplasmic reticulum gene expression in human heart failure: A possible mechanism for alterations in systolic and diastolic properties of the failing myocardium. *Circ Res* 1993; 72:463–469.

75. Sordahl LA, McCollum WB, Wood WG, Schwartz A. Mitrochondria and sarcoplasmic reticulum function in cardiac hypertrophy and failure. *Am J Physiol* 1973; 224:497–502.

76. Ito Y, Suko J, Chidsey CA. Intracellular calcium and myocardial contractility: V. Calcium uptake of sarcoplasmic reticulum fraction in hypertrophied and failing rabbit hearts. *J Moll Cell Cardiol* 1974; 6:237–247.

77. Reuter H. Exchange of calcium ions in the mammalian myocardium: Mechanisms and physiological significance. *Circ Res* 1974; 34:599–605.

78. Katz AM. Congestive heart failure: Role of altered myocardial cellular control. *N Engl J Med* 1975; 293:1184–1191.

79. Dhalla NS, Das PK, Sharma GP. Subcellular basis on cardiac contractile failure. *J Mol Cell Cardiol* 1978; 10:363–385.

80. Factor SM, Sonnenblick EH. Pathogenesis of clinical and experimental congestive cardiomyopathies: Recent concepts. *Prog Cardiovasc Dis* 1985; 27:395–420.

81. Staley NA, Noren GR, Einzig S. Early alterations in the function of sarcoplasmic reticulum in a naturally occurring model of congestive cardiomyopathy. *Cardiovasc Res* 1981; 15:276–281.

82. Dhalla NS, Alto LE, Heyliger CE, Pierce GN, Panagia V, Singal PK. Sarcoplasmic reticular Ca^{2+}-pump adaptation in cardiac hypertrophy due to pressure overload in pigs. *Eur Heart J* 1984; 5(suppl F):323–328.

83. Felin FS, Sonnenblick EH. Diabetic cardiomyopathy. *Prog Cardiovasc Dis* 1985; 4:255–270.

84. Fizel A, Turcani M, Fizelova A, Maasovad D, Simko F. Calcium transport by intracellular membrane structures in the myocardium of hypertrophied and failing hearts. *Cor Vasa* 1986; 28:373–383.

85. Smith VE, Katz AM. Inotropic and lusitropic abnormalities in the genesis of heart failure. *Eur Heart J* 1983; 4(suppl A):7–17.

86. Limas CJ, Olivari M, Goldenberg IF, Levine TB, Benditt DG, Simon A. Calcium uptake by cardiac sarcoplasmic reticulum in human dilated cardiomyopathy. *Cardiovasc Res* 1987; 21:601–605.

87. Gwathmey JK, Copelas L, MacKinnon R, Schoen FJ, Feldman MD, Grossman W, et al. Abnormal intracellular calcium handling in myocardium from patients with end-stage heart failure. *Circ Res* 1987; 61:70–76.

88. Movsesian MA, Bristow MR, Krall J. Ca^{2+} uptake by cardiac sarcoplasmic reticulum from patients with idiopathic dilated cardiomyopathy. *Circ Res* 1989; 65:1141–1144.

89. Morgan JP, Erny RE, Allen PD, Grossman W, Gwathmey JK. Abnormal intracellular calcium handling: A major cause of systolic and diastolic dysfunction in ventricular myocardium from patients with heart failure. *Circulation* 1990; 81:III21–III32.

90. Langer GA, ed. *Calcium and the Heart*. New York: Raven; 1990; 1–387.

91. Morgan JP. Abnormal intracellular modulation of calcium as a major cause of cardiac contractile dysfunction. *N Engl J Med* 1991; 325:625–632.

92. Siri FM, Krueger J, Nordin C, Ming Z, Aronson R. Depressed intracellular calcium transients and contraction in myocytes from hypertrophied and failing guinea pig hearts. *Am J Physiol* 1991; 261(*Heart Circ Physiol* 30):H514–H530.

93. Beuckelmann DJ, Näbauer M, Erdmann E. Intracellular calcium handling in isolated ventricular myocytes from patients with terminal heart failure. *Circulation* 1992; 85:1046–1055.

94. Hasenfuss G, Mulieri LA, Leavitt BJ, Allen PD, Haeberle JR, Alpert NR. Alteration of contractile function and excitation-contraction coupling in dilated cardiomyopathy. *Circ Res* 1992; 70:1225–1232.

95. Wankerl M, Schwartz K. Calcium transport proteins in the nonfailing and failing heart: Gene expression and function. *J Mol Med* 1995; 73:487–496.

96. Schwartz K, Mercadier JJ. Molecular and cellular biology of heart failure. *Curr Opin Cardiol* 1996; 11:227–236.

97. Katz AM, Hecht HH. The early pump failure of the ischemic heart. *Am J Med* 1969; 47:497–502.

98. Van Winkle WB, Schwartz A. Ions and ionotropy. *Annu Rev Physiol* 1976; 38:247–272.

99. Bristow MR, Ginsburg R, Minobe W, Cubicciotti RS, Sageman WS, Lurie K, et al. Decreased catecholamine sensitivity and β-adrenergic-receptor density in failing human hearts. *N Engl J Med* 1982; 307:205–211.

100. Bristow MR, Kantrowitz NE, Ginsburg R, Fowler MB. β-adrenergic function in heart muscle disease and heart failure. *J Mol Cell Cardiol* 1985; 17(suppl 2):41–52.

101. Vatner DE, Vatner SF, Fuzii AM, Homcy CJ. Loss of high affinity cardiac beta-adrenergic receptors in dogs with heart failure. *J Clin Invest* 1985; 76:2259–2264.

102. Fowler MB, Laser JA, Hopkins GL, Minobe W, Bristow MR. Assessment of the beta-adrenergic receptor pathway in the intact failing human heart: Progressive β-receptor down-regulation and specific pharmacologic subsensitivity to agonist response. *Circulation* 1986; 74:1290–1302.

103. Bristow MR, Ginsburg R, Umans V, Fowler M, Minobe W, Rasmussen R, et al. β$_1$ and β$_2$-adrenergic receptor subpopulations in normal and failing human ventricular myocardium: Coupling of both receptor subtypes to muscle contraction and selective β$_1$ receptor down-regulation in heart failure. *Circ Res* 1986; 59:297–309.

104. Bristow MR, Ginsburg R, Gilbert EM, Herschberger RE. Heterogeneous regulatory changes in cell surface membrane receptors coupled to a positive inotropic response in the failing human heart. *Basic Res Cardiol* 1987; 82(suppl 2):369–376.

105. Colucci WS, Leatherman GF, Ludmer PL, Gauthier DF. Beta-adrenergic inotropic responsiveness of patients with heart failure: Studies with intracoronary dobutamine infusion. *Circ Res* 1987; 61(suppl I):I82–I86.

106. Bohm M, Beukelmann D, Brown L, Feiler G, Lorenz B, Nabaver M, et al. Reduction of beta-adrenoreceptor density and evaluation of positive inotropic responses in isolated, diseased human myocardium. *Eur Heart J* 1988; 9:844–852.

107. Feldman MD, Copelas L, Gwathmey JK, Phillips P, Warren SE, Schoen FJ, et al. Deficient production of cyclic AMP: Pharmacologic evidence of an important cause of contractile dysfunction in patients with end-stage heart failure. *Circulation* 1987; 75:331–339.

108. Bristow MR, Port JD, Herschberger RE, Gilbert EM, Feldman AM. The β-adrenergic receptor–adenylate cyclase complex as a target for therapeutic intervention in heart failure. *Eur Heart J* 1989; 10(suppl B):45–54.

109. Denniss AR, Marsh J, Quigg RJ, Gordon JB, Colucci WS. Beta-adrenergic receptor number and adenylate cyclase function in denervated transplanted and cardiomyopathic human hearts. *Circulation* 1989; 79:1028–1034.

110. Feldman AM: The receptor-G protein-adenylate cyclase complex in heart failure. In: Rapaport E, ed. *Cardiology Update: Reviews for Physicians.* New York: Elsevier; 1990; 213–233.

111. Stiles GL. Adrenergic receptor responsiveness and congestive heart failure. *Am J Cardiol* 1991; 67:13C–17C.

112. Bogaert MG, Fraeyman N. Receptor function in heart failure. *Am J Med* 1991; 90(suppl 5B):S10–S13.

113. Bristow MR, Minobe W, Rasmussen R, Larrabee P, Skerl L, Klein JW, et al. β-adrenergic neuroeffector abnormalities in the failing human heart are produced by local rather than systemic mechanisms. *J Clin Invest* 1992; 89:803–815.

114. Brodde OS, Schüler S, Kretsch R, Brinkmann M, Borst HG, Hetzer R, et al. Regional distribution of β-adrenoceptors in the human heart: Coexistence of functional β1- and β2-adrenoceptors in both atria and ventricles in severe congestive cardiomyopathy. *J Cardiovasc Pharmacol* 1986; 8:1235–1242.

115. Boehm M, Benchelmann D, Brown L, Feiler G, Lorenz B, Näbauer M, et al. Reduction of beta-adrenoceptor density and evaluation of positive inotropic responses in isolated diseased human myocardium. *Eur Heart J* 1988; 9:844–852.

116. Brodde OE, Zerkowski HR, Borst HG, Maier W, Michel MC. Drug- and disease-induced changes of human cardiac β1- and β2-adrenoceptors. *Eur Heart J* 1989; 10(suppl B):38–44.

117. Gopalakrishnan M, Triggle DJ. The regulation of receptors, ion channels, and G proteins in congestive heart failure. *Cardiovasc Drug Rev* 1990; 8:255–302.

118. Steinfath M, Lavicky J, Schmitz W, Scholz H, Döring V, Kalmár P: Regional distribution of β1- and β2-adrenoceptors in the failing and nonfailing human heart. *Eur J Clin Pharmacol* 1992; 42:607–612.

119. Homcy CJ, Vatner SF, Vatner DE. β-Adrenergic receptor regulation in the heart in pathophysiologic states: Abnormal adrenergic responsiveness in cardiac disease. *Annu Rev Physiol* 1991; 53:137–139.

120. Bristow MR, Ginsburg R, Harrison DC. Histamine and the human heart: The other receptor system. *Am J Cardiol* 1982; 49:249–251.

121. Baumann G, Mercader D, Busch U, Felix SB, Loher J, Ludwig L, et al. Effects of the H2-receptor agonist impromidine in human myocardium from patients with heart failure due to mitral and aortic valve disease. *J Cardiovasc Pharmacol* 1983; 5:618–625.

122. Hershberger RE, Bristow MR. The A1 adenosine receptor pathway in failing and nonfailing human heart. *Circulation* 1987; 76(suppl 4):443.

123. Fedida D, Braun AP, Giles WR. α1-Adrenoceptors in myocardium: Functional aspects and transmembrane signaling mechanisms. *Physiol Rev* 1993; 73:469–487.

124. Horn EM, Corwin ST, Steinberg SF, Chow YK, Neuberg GW, Cannon PJ, et al. Reduced lymphocyte stimulatory guanine nucleotide regulatory protein and β-adrenergic receptors in congestive heart failure and reversal with angiotensin converting enzyme inhibitor therapy. *Circulation* 1988; 78:1373–1379.

125. Bilezikian JP, Steinberg SF, Horn EM, Robinson RB, Rosen MR. G protein-adrenergic interactions in the heart. *Mol Cell Biochem* 1988; 82:5–11.

126. Majerus PW, Connolly TM, Deckmyn H, Ross TS, Bross TE, Ishii H, et al. The metabolism of phosphoinositide-derived messenger molecules. *Science* 1986; 234:1519–1526.

127. Kikkawa U, Nishizuka Y. The role of protein kinase C in transmembrane signaling. *Annu Rev Cell Biol* 1986; 2:149–178.

128. Hunter T. A thousand and one protein kinases. *Cell* 1987; 50:823–829.

129. Feldman AM, Cates AE, Baumgartner W, Baughman KL, Van Dop C. Alterations of the M$_r$ 40,000 pertussin toxin substrate (AG1) in human heart failure. *Circulation* 1987; 76(suppl 4):IV432.

130. Feldman AM, Cates AE, Veazey WB, Hershberger RE, Bristow MR, Baughman KL. Increase of the 40,000-mol wt pertussis toxin substrate (G protein) in the failing human heart. *J Clin Invest* 1988; 82:189–197.

131. Feldman AM. Modulation of adrenergic receptors and G-transduction proteins in failing human ventricular myocardium. *Circulation* 1993; 83(suppl IV):IV27–IV34.

132. Feldman AM. Experimental issues in assessment of G protein function in cardiac disease. *Circulation* 1991; 84:1852–1861.

133. Feldman AM. Alterations of the β-adrenergic signaling pathway in cardiac failure and its role in pathophysiology and treatment. *Curr Opin Cardiol* 1992; 7:367–373.

134. Longabaugh J, Vatner D, Vatner S, Homey C. Decreased stimulatory guanosine triphosphate binding protein in dogs with pressure-overload left ventricular failure. *J Clin Invest* 1988; 81:420–424.

135. Neumann J, Scholz H. Döring V, Schmitz W, Meyerinck L, Kalmar P. Increase in myocardial G1-proteins in heart failure. *Lancet* 1988; 2:936–937.

136. Boehm M, Gierschik P, Jacobs KH, Pieske B, Schnabel P, Ungerer M, et al. Increase of G1 in human hearts with dilated but not ischemic cardiomyopathy. *Circulation* 1990; 82:1249–1265.

137. Bristow MR, Hershberger RE, Port JD, Sandoval A, Rasmussen R, Cates AE, et al. β-Adrenergic pathways in nonfailing and failing human ventricular myocardium. *Circulation* 1990; 82(suppl I):I12–I25.

138. Bristow M, Ginsburg R, Strosberg A, Montgomery W, Minobe W. Pharmacology and inotropic potential of forskolin in the human heart. *J Clin Invest* 1984; 74:212–223.

139. Hwang KC, Gray CD, Sweet WE, Moravec CS, Im M-J. α1-Adrenergic receptor coupling with G$_h$ in the failing human heart. *Circulation* 1996; 94:718–726.

140. Higgins CB, Vatner SF, Braunwald E. Parasympathetic control of the heart. *Pharmacol Rev* 1973; 25:119–155.

141. Eckberg DL, Drabinsky M, Braunwald E. Defective cardiac parasympathic control in patients with heart disease. *N Engl J Med* 1971; 285:877–883.

142. Rutenberg HL, Spann JF Jr. Alterations of cardiac sympathetic neurotransmitter activity in congestive heart failure. *Am J Cardiol* 1973; 32:472–480.

143. Braunwald E. Regulation of the circulation. *N Engl J Med* 1974; 290:1420–1425.

144. Goldstein RE, Beiser GD, Stampfer M, Epstein SE. Impairment of autonomically mediated heart rate control in patients with cardiac dysfunction. *Circ Res* 1975; 36:571–578.

145. Rutenberg HL, Spann JF Jr. Alterations of cardiac sympathetic neurotransmitter activity in congestive heart failure. In: Mason DT, ed. *Congestive Heart Failure: Mechanisms, Evaluation and Treatment.* New York: Yorke Medical; 1976:85–95.

146. Pool PE, Covell JW, Levitt M, Gibb J, Braunwald E. Reduction of cardiac tyrosine hydroxylase activity in experimental congestive heart failure: Its role in the depletion of cardiac norepinephrine stores. *Circ Res* 1967; 20:349–353.

147. Spann JF Jr, Buccino RA, Sonnenblick EH, Braunwald E. Contractile state of cardiac muscle obtained from cats with experimentally produced ventricular hypertrophy and heart failure. *Circ Res* 1967; 21:341–354.

148. White CW: Abnormalities in baroreflex control of heart rate in canine failure. *Am J Physiol* 1981; 240:H793–H799.

149. Goldsmith SR, Francis GS, Cowley AW Jr, Levine TB, Cohn JN. Increased plasma arginine vasopressin levels in patients with congestive heart failure. *J Am Coll Cardiol* 1983; I:1385–1390.

150. Kubo SH, Cody RJ. Circulatory autoregulation in chronic congestive heart failure: Responses to head-up tilt in 41 patients. *Am J Cardiol* 1983; 52:512–518.

151. Levine TB, Francis GS, Goldsmith SR, Cohn JN. The neurohumoral and hemodynamic responses to orthostatic tilt in patients with congestive heart failure. *Circulation* 1983; 67:1070–1075.

152. Ferguson DW, Abboud FM, Mark AL. Selective impairment of baroreflex-mediated vasoconstrictor responses in patients with ventricular dysfunction. *Circulation* 1984; 69:451–460.

153. Hirsh AT, Dzau J, Creager MA. Baroreceptor function in congestive heart failure: Effect of neurohormonal activity and regional vascular resistance. *Circulation* 1987; 75(suppl IV):36–48.

154. Vatner DE, Lee DL, Schwarz K, Longabaugh JP, Fuji AM, Vatner SF, et al. Impaired cardiac muscarinic receptor function in dogs with heart failure. *J Clin Invest* 1988; 81:1836–1842.

155. Ellenbogen KA, Mohanty PK, Szentpetery S, Thames MD. Arterial baroreflex abnormalities in heart failure. *Circulation* 1989; 79:51–58.

156. Mohanty PK, Arrowood JA, Ellenbogen KA, Thames MD. Neurohumoral and hemodynamic effects of lower body negative pressure in patients with congestive heart failure. *Am Heart J* 1989; 118:78–85.

157. Sopher SM, Smith ML, Eckberg DL, Fritsch JM, Dibner-Dunlap ME. Autonomic pathophysiology in heart failure: Carotid baroreceptor-cardiac reflexes. *Am J Physiol* 1990; 259(*Heart Circ Physiol* 28):H689–H696.

158. Ferguson DW, Berg WJ, Roach PJ, Oren RM, Mark AL, Kempf JS. Effects of heart failure on baroreflex control of sympathetic neural activity. *Am J Cardiol* 1992; 69:523–531.

159. Dibner-Dunlap ME, Thames MD. Control of sympathetic nerve activity by vagal mechanoreflexes is blunted in heart failure.*Circulation* 1992; 86:1929–1934.

160. Goldsmith SR, Hasking GJ. Dissociation of sympathetic responses to baroreceptor loading and unloading in compensated congestive heart failure secondary to ischemic or nonischemic dilated cardiomyopathy. *Am J Cardiol* 1992; 69:646–649.

161. Creager MA. Baroreceptor reflex function in congestive heart failure. *Am J Cardiol* 1992; 69:10G–16G.

162. Mancia G, Seravalle G, Giannattasio C, Bossi M, Preti L, Cattaneo BM, et al. Reflex cardiovascular control in congestive heart failure. *Am J Cardiol* 1992; 69:17G–23G.

163. Bishop VS, Malliani A, Thoren P. Cardiac mechanoreceptors. In: Shepherd JT, Abboud FA, eds. *Handbook of Physiology.* Bethesda, MD: American Physiological Society; 1983:497–556.

164. Goldsmith SR, Francis GS, Levine TB, Cohn JN. Regional blood flow responses to orthostasis in patients with congestive heart failure. *J Am Coll Cardiol* 1983; 1:1391–1395.

165. Zucker IH, Gilmore JP, eds. *Reflex Control of the Circulation.* Boca Raton, FL: CRC Press; 1991:1–1053.

166. Nolan J, Flapan AD, Capewell S, MacDonald TM, Neilson JMM, Ewing DJ. Decreased cardiac parasympathetic activity in chronic heart failure and its relation to left ventricular function. *Br Heart J* 1992; 67:482–485.

167. Buccino RA, Harris E, Spann JF Jr, Sonnenblick EH. Response of myocardial connective tissue to development of experimental hypertrophy. *Am J Physiol* 1969; 216:425–428.

168. Alpert NR, ed. *Cardiac Hypertrophy.* New York: Academic; 1971:1–223.

169. Zak R, ed. *Growth of the Heart in Health and Disease.* New York: Raven; 1984:1–463.

170. Weber KT, Clark WA, Janicki JS, Shroff SG. Physiologic versus pathologic hypertrophy and the pressure-overloaded myocardium. *J Cardiovasc Pharmacol* 1987; 10(suppl 6):537–550.

171. Weber KT, Janicki JS, Shroff SG, Pick R, Abrahams C, Chen RM, et al. Collagen compartment remodeling in the pressure overloaded left ventricle. *J Appl Cardiol* 1988; 3:37–46.

172. Weber KT, Janicki JS, Shroff SG, Pick R, Chen RM, Bashey RI. Collagen remodeling of the pressure-overloaded hypertrophied nonhuman primate myocardium. *Circ Res* 1988; 62:757–765.

173. Weber KT. Cardiac interstitium in health and disease: The fibrillar collagen network. *J Am Coll Cardiol* 1989; 13:1637–1652.

174. Zhao M, Zhang H, Robinson TF, Factor SM, Sonnenblick EH, Eng C. Profound structural alterations of the extracellular collagen matrix in post-ischemic dysfunctional but viable myocardium. *J Am Coll Cardiol* 1987; 10:1322–1334.

175. Weber KT, Pick R, Silver MA, Moe GW, Janicki JS, Zucker IH, et al. Fibrillar collagen and remodeling of dilated canine left ventricle. *Circulation* 1990; 82:1387–1401.

176. Weber KT, Brilla CG. Pathological hypertrophy and cardiac interstitium: Fibrosis and renin-angiotensin-aldosterone system. *Circulation* 1991; 83:1849–1865.

177. Weber KT, Brilla CG, Janicki JS. Myocardial fibrosis: Functional significance and regulatory factors. *Cardiovasc Res* 1993; 27:341–348.

178. Olivetti G, Melissari M, Capasso JM, Anversa P. Cardiomyopathy of the aging human heart: Myocyte loss and reactive cellular hypertrophy. *Circ Res* 1991; 68:1560–1568.

179. Dock W. How some hearts age. *JAMA* 1966; 195:442–444.

180. Burch G, Giles T. Senile cardiomyopathy. *J Chronic Dis* 1971; 24:1–3.

181. Dock W. Cardiomyopathies of the senescent and senile. In: Burch GE, ed. *Cardiomyopathy.* Philadelphia: FA Davis; 1972:361–373.

182. Miller TR, Grossman SJ, Schectman KB, Biello DR, Ludbrook PA, Ehsani AA. Left ventricular diastolic filling and its association with age. *Am J Cardiol* 1986; 58:531–535.

183. Bryg RJ, Williams GA, Labovitz AJ. Effect of aging on left ventricular diastolic filling in normal subjects. *Am J Cardiol* 1987; 59:971–974.

184. Lie JT, Hammond PI. Pathology of the senescent heart: Anatomic observations on 237 autopsy studies of patients 90 to 105 years old. *Mayo Clin Proc* 1988; 63:552–564.

185. Lakatta EG, Gerstenblith G, Angell CS, Shock NW, Weisfeldt ML. Diminished inotropic response of aged myocardium to catecholamines. *Circ Res* 1975; 36:262–269.

186. Lakatta EG. Cardiovascular regulatory mechanisms in advanced age. *Physiol Rev* 1933; 73:413–467.

187. Whipple GH, Sheffield LT, Woodman EG, Theophilis C, Friedman S. Reversible congestive heart failure due to chronic rapid stimulation of the normal heart. *Proc N Engl Cardiovasc Soc* 1962; 20:39–40.

188. Coleman HN III, Taylor RR, Pool PE, Whipple GH, Covell JW, Ross J Jr, et al. Congestive heart failure following chronic tachycardia. *Am Heart J* 1971; 81:790–798.

189. Riegger AJG, Liebau G. The renin-angiotensin-aldosterone system: Antidiuretic hormone and sympathetic nerve activity in an experimental model of congestive heart failure in the dog. *Clin Sci* 1982; 62:465–469.

190. Armstrong PW, Stopps TP, Ford SE, DeBold AJ. Rapid ventricular pacing in the dog: Pathophysiologic studies of heart failure. *Circulation* 1986; 74:1075–1084.

191. Packer DL, Bardy GH, Worley SJ, Smith MS, Cobb FR, Coleman RE, et al. Tachycardia-induced cardiomyopathy: A reversible form of left ventricular dysfunction. *Am J Cardiol* 1986; 57:563–570.

192. Wilson JR, Douglas P, Hickey WF, Lanoce V, Ferraro N, Muhammad A, et al. Experimental congestive heart failure produced by rapid ventricular pacing in the dog: Cardiac effects. *Circulation* 1987; 75:857–867.

193. Damiano RJ, Tripp HF, Asano T, Small KW, Jones RH, Lowe JE. Left ventricular dysfunction and dilatation resulting from chronic supraventricular tachycardia. *J Thorac Cardiovasc Surg* 1987; 94:135–143.

194. Riegger GA, Elsner D, Kromer EP, Daffner C. Atrial natriuretic peptide in congestive heart failure in the dog: Plasma levels, cyclic guanosine monophosphate, ultrastructure of atrial myoendocrine cells, and hemodynamic, hormonal, and renal effects. *Circulation* 1988; 77:398–406.

195. Moe GW, Stopps TP, Howard RJ, Armstrong PW. Early recovery from heart failure: Insights into the pathogenesis of experimental chronic pacing-induced heart failure. *J Lab Clin Med* 1988; 112:426–432.

196. Moe GW, Stopps TP, Angus C, Forster C, De Bold AJ, Armstrong PW. Alterations in serum sodium in relation to atrial natriuretic factor and other neuroendocrine variables in experimental pacing-induced heart failure. *J Am Coll Cardiol* 1989; 13:173–179.

197. Morgan DE, Tomlinson CW, Qayumi AK, Toleikis PM, McConville B, Jamieson WRE. Evaluation of ventricular contractility indexes in the dog with left ventricular dysfunction induced by rapid atrial pacing. *J Am Coll Cardiol* 1989; 14:489–495.

198. Vaitkus PT, Curtis M, Marchlinski FE, Mancini DM. Incessant atrial tachycardia and heart failure. *Heart Failure* 1990; 6:183–188.

199. Spinale FG, Hendrick DA, Crawford FA, Smith AC, Hamada Y, Carabello BA. Chronic supraventricular tachycardia causes ventricular dysfunction and subendocardial injury in swine. *Am J Physiol* 1990; 259:H218–H229.

200. Calderone A, Bouvier M, Li K, Juneau C, de Champlain J, Rouleau JL. Dysfunction of the β- and α-adrenergic systems in a model of congestive heart failure: The pacing-overdrive dog. *Circ Res* 1991; 69:332–342.

201. Tomita M, Spinale FG, Crawford FA, Zile MR. Changes in left ventricular volume, mass and function during development and regression of supraventricular tachycardia-induced cardiomyopathy; Disparity between recovery of systolic versus diastolic function. *Circulation* 1991; 83:635–644.

202. Shannon RP, Komamura K, Stambler BS, Bigaud M, Manders WT, Vatner SF. Alterations in myocardial contractility in conscious dogs with dilated cardiomyopathy. *Am J Physiol* 1991; 260:H1903–H1911.

203. Spinale FG, Pearce AP, Crawford FA, Schulte BA. Ventricular function and NA$^+$,K$^+$-ATPase activity and distribution with chronic supraventricular tachycardia. *Cardiovasc Res* 1991; 25:138–144.

204. Spinale FG, Tomita M, Zellner JL, Cook JC, Crawford FA, Zile MR. Collagen remodeling and changes in LV function during development and recovery from supraventricular tachycardia. *Am J Physiol* 1991; 261:H308–H318.

205. Spinale FG, Zellner JL, Tomita M, Tempel GE, Crawford FA, Zile MR. Reduced myocardial blood flow and altered capillary structure occur with chronic supraventricular tachycardia-induced cardiomyopathy. *Am J Physiol* 1991; 261:H140–H148.

206. Zellner JL, Spinale FG, Eble DK, Hewett KW, Crawford FA Jr. Alterations in myocyte shape and basement membrane attachment with tachycardia-induced heart failure. *Circ Res* 1991; 69:590–600.

207. Moe GW, Angus C, Howard RJ, Parker TG, Armstrong PW. Evaluation of indices of left ventricular contractility and relaxation in evolving canine experimental heart failure. *Cardiovasc Res* 1992; 26:362–366.

208. Spinale FG, Fulbright M, Mukherjee R, Tanaka R, Hu J, Crawford FA, et al. Relation between ventricular and myocyte function with tachycardia-induced cardiomyopathy. *Circ Res* 1992; 71:174–187.

209. Juneau C, Calderone A, Rouleau J-L. Myocardial β-adrenergic and mechanical properties in pacing-induced heart failure in dogs. *Am J Physiol* 1992; 262 (*Heart Circ Physiol* 31):H1458–H1467.

210. Belch JJF, Budges AB, Scott N, Chopra M. Oxygen free radicals and congestive heart failure. *Br Heart J* 1991; 65:245–248.

211. Laine GA, Allen SJ. Left ventricular myocardial edema: Lymph flow, interstitial fibrosis, and cardiac function. *Circ Res* 1991; 68:1713–1721.

212. Mann DL, Kent RL, Parsons B, Cooper G. Adrenergic effects on the biology of the adult mammalian cardiocyte. *Circulation* 1992; 85:790–804.

213. Tan LB, Jalil JE, Pick R, Janicki JS, Weber KT. Cardiac myocyte necrosis induced by angiotensin II. *Circ Res* 1991; 69:1185–1195.

214. Francis GS. Neurohumoral mechanisms involved in congestive heart failure. *Am J Cardiol* 1985; 55(suppl A):A15–A21.

215. Cody RJ. Neurohormonal influences in the pathogenesis of congestive heart failure. In: Weber K, ed. *Heart Failure Cardiology Clinics.* Philadelphia: Saunders; 1989; 7:73–86.

216. Forfar JC. Neuroendocrine activation in congestive heart failure. *Am J Cardiol* 1991; 67(suppl C):3C–15C.

217. Zucker IH. Baro and cardiac reflex abnormalities in chronic heart failure. In: Zucker IH, Gilmore JP, eds. *Reflex Control of the Circulation.* Boca Raton, FL: CRC Press; 1991:849–873.

218. Katz AM. Heart failure. In: Fozzard HA, Haber E, Jennings RB, Katz AM, Morgan HE, eds. *The Heart and Cardiovascular System. Scientific Foundations,* 2d ed. New York: Raven; 1991:333–353.

219. Alton M, Cody RJ. Neurohormonal mechanisms in congestive heart failure. *Curr Opin Cardiol* 1992; 7:374–380.

220. Ferrari R, Anand IS, Ceconi C, De Giuli F, Poole-Wilson PA, Harris P. Neuroendocrine response to standing and mild exercise in patients with untreated severe congestive heart failure and chronic constrictive pericarditis. *Heart* 1996; 76:50–55.

221. Creager MA, Faxon DP, Cutler SS, Kohlman O, Ryan TJ, Gavras H. Contribution of vasopressin to vasoconstriction in patients with congestive heart failure: Comparison with the renin-angiotensin system and the sympathetic nervous system. *J Am Coll Cardiol* 1986; 7:758–765.

222. Manthey J, Kietz R, Opherk D, Osterziel KJ, Leinberger H, Kübler W. Baroreceptor-mediated release of vasopressin in patients with chronic congestive heart failure and defective sympathetic responsiveness. *Am J Cardiol* 1992; 70:224–228.

223. Margulies KB, Hildebrand FL, Lerman A, Perrella MP, Burnett JC Jr. Increased endothelin in experimental heart failure. *Circulation* 1990; 82:2226–2230.

224. Cavero PG, Miller WL, Heublein DM, Margulies KB, Burnett JC Jr. Endothelin in experimental congestive heart failure in the anesthetized dog. *Am J Physiol* 1990; 259:F312–F317.

225. Cody RJ, Haas GJ, Binkley PF, Caper Q, Kelley R. Plasma endothelin correlates with the extent of pulmonary hypertension in patients with chronic congestive heart failure. *Circulation* 1992; 58:504–509.

226. Rodeheffer RJ, Lerman A, Heublein DM, Burnett JC Jr. Increased plasma concentrations of endothelin in congestive heart failure in humans. *Mayo Clin Proc* 1992; 67:719–724.

227. Lerman A, Kubo SH, Tschumperlin LK, Burnett JC Jr. Plasma endothelin concentrations in humans with end-stage heart failure and after heart transplantation. *J Am Coll Cardiol* 1992; 20:849–853.

228. Cody RJ. The potential role of endothelin as a vasoconstrictor substance in congestive heart failure. *Eur Heart J* 1992; 13:1573–1578.

229. Stewart DJ, Cernacek P, Costello KB, Rouleau JL. Elevated endothelin-1 in heart failure and loss of normal response to postural change. *Circulation* 1992; 85:510–517.

230. McMurray JJ, Ray SG, Abdullah I, Dargie HJ, Morton JJ. Plasma endothelin in chronic heart failure. *Circulation* 1992; 85:1374–1379.

231. Maisel AS, Scott NA, Motulsky HJ, Michel MC, Boublik JH, Rivier JE, et al. Elevation of plasma neuropeptide Y levels in congestive heart failure. *Am J Med* 1989; 86:43–48.

232. Hulting J, Sollevia A, Ullman B, Franco-Cereceda A, Lundberg JM. Plasma neuropeptide Y on admission to a coronary care unit: Raised levels in patients with left heart failure. *Cardiovasc Res* 1990; 24:102–108.

233. Edvinsson L, Ekman R, Hedner P, Valdemarsson S. Congestive heart failure: Involvement of perivascular peptides reflecting activity in sympathetic, parasympathetic and afferent fibres. *Eur J Clin Invest* 1990; 20:85–90.

234. Valdemarsson S, Edvinsson L, Edman R, Hedner P, Sjöholm A. Increased plasma level of substance P in patients with severe congestive heart failure treated with ACE inhibitors. *J Intern Med* 1991; 230:325–331.

235. Levine B, Kalman J, Mayer L, Fillit HM, Packer M. Elevated circulating levels of tumor necrosis factor in severe chronic heart failure. *N Engl J Med* 1990; 323:236–241.

236. Torre-Amione G, Kapadia S, Benedict C, Oral H, Young JB, Mann DL. Proinflammatory cytokine levels in patients with depressed left ventricular ejection fraction: A report from the Studies of Left Ventricular Dysfunction (SOLVD). *J Am Coll Cardiol* 1996; 27:1201–1206.

237. Kelly RA, Smith TW. Cytokines and cardiac contractile function (editorial). *Circulation* 1997; 95:778–781.

238. Shah K, Kurrelmeyer K, Seta Y, Wang F, Zibbs Z, Deswal A, et al. The role of cytokines in disease progression in heart failure. *Curr Opin Cardiol* 1997; 12:218–223.

239. Drexler H, Lu W. Endothelial dysfunction of hindquarter resistance vessels in experimental heart failure. *Am J Physiol* 1992; 262 (*Heart Circ Physiol* 31):H1640–H1645.

240. Drexler H, Hayoz D, Münzel T, Hornig B, Just H, Brunner HR, et al. Endothelial function in chronic congestive heart failure. *Am J Cardiol* 1992; 69:1596–1601.

241. Katz SD, Biasucci L, Sabba C, Strom JA, Jondeau G, Galvao M, et al. Impaired endothelium-mediated vasodilatation in the peripheral vasculature of patients with congestive heart failure. *J Am Coll Cardiol* 1992; 19:918–925.

242. Taquet H, Komajda M, Grenier O, Belas F, Landault C, Carayon A, et al. Plasma calcitonin gene–related peptide decreases in chronic congestive heart failure. *Eur Heart J* 1992; 13:1473–1476.

243. Katz S. Mechanisms and implications of endothelial dysfunction in congestive heart failure. *Curr Opin Cardiol* 1997; 12:259–264.

244. Anand IS, Ferrari R, Kalra GS, Wahi PL, Poole-Wilson PA, Harris PC. Edema of cardiac origin: Studies of body water and sodium, renal function, hemodynamic indexes and plasma hormones in untreated congestive cardiac failure. *Circulation* 1989; 80:299–305.

245. Weber KT, Villarreal D. Aldosterone and antialdosterone therapy in congestive heart failure. *Am J Cardiol* 1993; 71(suppl A):3A–11A.

246. Mehta J, Mehta P. Platelet function studies in heart disease: Enhanced platelet aggregate formation in congestive heart failure. *Circulation* 1979; 60:497–503.

247. Jafri SM, Ozawa T, Mammen E, Levine TB, Johnson C, Goldstein S. Platelet function, thrombin and fibrinolytic activity in patients with heart failure. *Eur Heart J* 1993; 14:205–212.

248. Chidsey CA, Braunwald E, Morrow AG, Mason DT. Myocardial norepinephrine concentration in man. *N Engl J Med* 1963; 269:653–658.

249. Bristow MR. The adrenergic nervous system in heart failure. *N Engl J Med* 1984; 311:850–851.

250. Swedberg K, Viquerat C, Rouleau J-L. Comparison of myocardial catecholamine balance in chronic congestive heart failure and in angina pectoris without failure. *Am J Cardiol* 1984; 54:783–786.

251. Hasking GJ, Esler MD, Jennings GL, Barton D, Johns JA, Korner PI. Norepinephrine spillover to plasma in patients with congestive heart failure: Evidence of increased overall and cardiorenal sympathetic nervous activity. *Circulation* 1986; 73:615–621.

252. Lund DD, Schmid PG, Johansen J, Roskoski R Jr. Biochemical indices of cholinergic and adrenergic automatic innervation in dog heart: Disparate alterations in chronic right heart failure. *J Mol Cell Cardiol* 1982; 14:419–425.

253. Rose CP, Burgess JH, Cousineau D. Tracer norepinephrine kinetics in coronary circulation of patients with heart failure secondary to chronic pressure and volume overload. *J Clin Invest* 1985; 76:1740–1747.

254. Chidsey CA, Harrison C, Braunwald E. Augmentation of the plasma norepinephrine response to exercise in patients with congestive heart failure. *N Engl J Med* 1962; 267:650–654.

255. Minami M, Yasuda H, Yamazaki N, Kojima S, Nishijima H, Matsumura N, et al. Plasma norepinephrine concentration and plasma dopamine-beta-hydroxylase activity in patients with congestive heart failure. *Circulation* 1964; 67:1324–1329.

256. Francis GS, Goldsmith SR, Ziesche S, Cohn JN. Response of plasma

norepinephrine and epinephrine to dynamic exercise in patients with congestive heart failure. *Am J Cardiol* 1982; 49:1152–1156.

257. Hasking GJ, Esler MD, Jennings GL, Dewar E, Lambert G. Norepinephrine spillover to plasma during steady-state supine bicycle exercise: Comparison of patients with congestive heart failure and normal subjects. *Circulation* 1988; 78:516–521.

258. Levine TB, Francis GS, Goldsmith SR, Cohn JN. The neurohumoral and hemodynamic response to orthostatic tilt in patients with congestive heart failure. *Circulation* 1983; 67:1070–1075.

259. Bristow MR. Myocardial beta-adrenergic receptor down regulation in heart failure. *Int J Cardiol* 1984; 5:648–652.

260. Waagstein F, Hjalmarson A, Varnaysclas E, Wallentin I. Effect of chronic β-adrenergic receptor blockade in congestive cardiomyopathy. *Br Heart J* 1975; 37:1022–1036.

261. Swedberg K, Waagstein F, Hjalmarson A, Wallentin I. Prolongation of survival in congestive cardiomyopathy in β-receptor blockade. *Lancet* 1979; 1:1374–1376.

262. Heidenreich PA, Lee TT, Massie BM. Effect of beta-blockade on mortality in patients with heart failure: A meta-analysis of randomized clinical trials. *J Am Coll Cardiol* 1997; 30:27–34.

263. Engelmeier RS, O'Connell JB, Walsh R, Rad N, Scanlon PJ, Funnar R. Improvement in symptoms and exercise tolerance by metoprolol in patients with dilated cardiomyopathy: A double-blind, randomized, placebo-controlled trial. *Circulation* 1985; 72:536–546.

264. Heilbrunn SM, Shah P, Bristow MR, Valantine HA, Ginsburg R, Fowler MB. Increased beta-receptor density and improved hemodynamic response to catecholamine stimulation during long-term metoprolol therapy in heart failure from dilated cardiomyopathy. *Circulation* 1989; 79:483–490.

265. Eichhorn EJ, Bedotto JB, Malloy CR, Hatfield BA, Deitchman D, Brown M, et al. Effect of β-adrenergic blockade on myocardial function and energetics in congestive heart failure: Improvements in hemodynamic, contractile, and diastolic performance with bucindolol. *Circulation* 1990; 82:473–483.

266. Anderson JL, Gilbert EM, O'Connell JB, Renlund D, Yanowitz F, Murray M, et al. Long-term (2 year) beneficial effects of beta-adrenergic blockade with bucindolol in patients with idiopathic dilated cardiomyopathy. *J Am Coll Cardiol* 1991; 17:1373–1381.

267. Andersson B, Blomström-Lundqvist C, Hedner T, Waagstein F. Exercise hemodynamics and myocardial metabolism during long-term beta-adrenergic blockade in severe heart failure. *J Am Coll Cardiol* 1991; 18:1059–1066.

268. Eichhorn EJ. The paradox of β-adrenergic blockade for the management of congestive heart failure. *Am J Med* 1992; 92:527–538.

269. Bristow MR. Pathophysiologic and pharmacologic rationales for clinical management of chronic heart failure with beta-blocking agents. *Am J Cardiol* 1993; 71(suppl C):12C–22C.

270. Swedberg K. Initial experience with beta blockers in dilated cardiomyopathy. *Am J Cardiol* 1993; 71(suppl C):30C–38C.

271. Fowler MB. Controlled trials with beta blockers in heart failure: Metoprolol as the prototype. *Am J Cardiol* 1993; 71(suppl C):45C–53C.

272. Ikram H, Fitzpatrick D, Crozier IG. Therapeutic controversies with use of beta-adrenoceptor blockade in heart failure. *Am J Cardiol* 1993; 71(suppl C):54C–60C.

273. CIBIS Investigators and Committees: A randomized study of beta-blockade in heart failure: The Cardiac Insufficiency Bisoprolol Study (CIBIS). *Circulation* 1994; 90:1765–1773.

274. Eichhorn E, Heesch C, Barnett J, Alvarez LG, Fass SM, Grayburn PA, et al. Effects of metoprolol on myocardial infarction and energetics in patients with non-ischemic dilated cardiomyopathy: A randomized, double-blind, placebo-controlled study. *J Am Coll Cardiol* 1994; 24:1310–1320.

275. Packer M, Bristow MR, Cohn JN, Colucci WS, Fowler MB, Gilbert EM, et al, for the US Carvedilol Heart Failure Study Group. The effect of carvedilol on morbidity and mortality in patients with chronic heart failure. *N Engl J Med* 1996; 334:1349–1355.

276. Packer M, Bristow MR, Cohn JN, Colucci WS, Fowler MB, Gilbert EM, et al, for the US Carvedilol Heart Failure Study Group. Carvedilol inhibits clinical progression in patients with mild symptoms of heart failure. *Circulation* 1996; 94:2800–2806.

277. Parker M, Colucci WS, Sackner-Bernstein JD, Liang C-S, Goldscher DA, Freeman I, et al. Double-blind, placebo-controlled study of the effects of carvedilol in patients with moderate to severe heart failure. The PRECISE Trial. *Circulation* 1996; 94:2793–2799.

278. Bristow MR, Gilbert EM, Abraham WT, Adams KF, Fowler MB, Hershberger RE, et al, for the MOCHA Investigators. Carvedilol produces dose-related improvements in left ventricular function and survival in subjects with chronic heart failure. *Circulation* 1996; 94:2807–2816.

279. Gilbert EM, Abraham WT, Olsen S, Hattler B, White M, Bristow MR, et al. Comparative hemodynamic, left ventricular functional, and antiadrenergic effects of chronic treatment with metoprolol versus carvedilol in the failing heart. *Circulation* 1996; 94:2817–2825.

280. Demopoulos L, Yeh M, Gentilucci M, Testa M, Bijou R, Katz SD, et al. Nonselective β-adrenergic blockade with carvedilol does not hinder the benefits of exercise training in patients with congestive heart failure. *Circulation* 1997; 95:1764–1767.

281. Ikram H, Fitzpatrick D. Double-blind trial of chronic oral beta-blockade in congestive cardiomyopathy. *Lancet* 1981; 2:490–493.

282. Ikram H, Fitzpatrick MA. Beta-blockade for dilated cardiomyopathy: The evidence against therapeutic benefit. *Eur Heart J* 1983; 4(suppl A):179–180.

283. Currie PJ, Kelly MJ, McKenzie A, Harper RW, Lim YL, Federman J, et al. Oral beta-adrenergic blockade with metoprolol in chronic severe dilated cardiomyopathy. *J Am Coll Cardiol* 1984; 3:203–209.

284. Brinkley PF, Lewe RF, Lima JJ, Al-Awwa A, Unverferth DV, Leier CV. Hemodynamic-inotropic response to beta-blockers with intrinsic sympathomimetic activity in patients with congestive cardiomyopathy. *Circulation* 1986; 74:1390–1398.

285. Vanhoutte PM. Adjustments in the peripheral circulation in chronic heart failure. *Eur Heart J* 1983; 4(suppl A):67–83.

286. Cannon P, Martinez-Maldonado M. The pathogenesis of cardiac edema. *Semin Nephrol* 1983; 3:211–224.

287. Leier CV. Regional blood flow in human congestive heart failure. *Am Heart J* 1992; 124:726–738.

288. Zelis R, Delea CS, Coleman HN, Mason DT. Arterial sodium content in experimental congestive heart failure. *Circulation* 1970; 41:213–216.

289. Raine AEG. Renal abnormalities in congestive heart failure. In: Fozzard HA, Haber E, Jennings RB, Katz AM, Morgan HE, eds. *The Heart and Cardiovascular System. Scientific Foundations*, 2d ed. New York: Raven; 1991:1379–1391.

290. Casley-Smith JR. Mechanisms in the formation of lymph. In: Guyton AC, Halls JE, eds. *Cardiovascular Physiology IV, International Review of Physiology*, vol 26. Baltimore: University Park Press; 1982: 147–187.

291. deWardener H. The control of sodium excretion. In: Orloff J, Berliner RW, eds. *Handbook of Physiology*, sec 8, *Renal Physiology*. Bethesda, MD: American Physiological Society; 1973:677–720.

292. Laragh JH, Scaley JE. The renin-angiotensin-aldosterone hormonal system and regulation of sodium, potassium, and blood pressure homeostasis. In: Orloff J, Berliner RW, eds. *Handbook of Physiology*, sec 8, *Renal Physiology*. Bethesda, MD: American Physiological Society; 1973: 831.

293. Hall JE. Regulation of renal hemodynamics. In: Guyton AC, Halls JE, eds. *Cardiovascular Physiology IV, International Review of Physiology*, vol 26. Baltimore: University Park Press; 1982:243–321.

294. Schrier RW. Pathogenesis of sodium and water retention in high-output and low-output cardiac failure, nephrotic syndrome, cirrhosis, and pregnancy. *N Engl J Med* 1988; 319:1127–1134.

295. Peterson TV. Cardiac reflexes and control of renal function in primates. In: Zucker IH, Gilmore JP, eds. *Reflex Control of the Circulation*. Boca Raton FL: CRC Press; 1991:313–358.

296. Shepherd JT. Cardiac mechanoreceptors. In: Fozzard HA, Haber E, Jennings RB, Katz AM, Morgan HE, eds. *The Heart and Cardiovascular System. Scientific Foundations*, 2d ed. New York: Raven; 199:1481–1504.

297. Hasking GJ, Esler MD, Jennings GL, Burton D, Korner PI. Norepinephrine spillover to plasma in patients with congestive heart failure: Evidence of increased overall and cardiorenal sympathetic nervous activity. *Circulation* 1986; 73:615–621.

298. Stein JH, Boinjarern S, Wilson CB, Ferris TF. Alterations in intrarenal blood flow distribution. *Circ Res* 1973; 32(suppl):61–72.

299. Warren JV, Stead EA Jr. Fluid dynamics in chronic congestive heart failure. *Arch Intern Med* 1944; 73:138–147.

300. Merrill AJ. Edema and decreased renal blood flow in patients with chronic congestive heart failure: Evidence of forward failure as the primary cause of edema. *J Clin Invest* 1946; 25:389–400.

301. deWardener HE. Mechanisms influencing urinary sodium excretion. In: Dickinson CJ, Marks J, eds. *Developments in Cardiovascular Medicine*. Baltimore: University Park Press; 1978:179–190.

302. Mandin H. Cardiac edema in dogs: I. Proximal tubular and renal function (abstr). *Kidney Int* 1976; 10:591.

303. Skorecki KL, Brenner BM. Body fluid homeostasis in man. *Am J Med* 1981; 70:77–88.

304. Dzau VJ, Collucci WS, Hollenberg NK, Williams GH. Relation of the renin-angiotensin-aldosterone system to clinical state in congestive heart failure. *Circulation* 1981; 63:645–651.

305. Dzau VJ, Pratt RE. Renin-angiotensin system. In: Fozzard HA, Haber E, Jennings JB, Katz AM, Morgan HE, eds. *The Heart and Cardiovascular System*, 2d ed. New York: Raven; 1991:1817–1849.

306. Linden RJ. Neurocirculatory control of sodium and water excretion. In: Dickinson CJ, Marks J, eds. *Developments in Cardiovascular Medicine*. Baltimore: University Park Press; 1978:191–203.

307. Kiowski W, Julius S. Renin response in stimulation of cardio-pulmonary mechanoreceptors in man. *J Clin Invest* 1978; 62:656–663.

308. Curtiss C, Cohn JN, Vrobel T, Franciosa JA. Role of the renin-angiotensin system in the systemic vasoconstriction of chronic congestive heart failure. *Circulation* 1978; 58:763–770.

309. Ausiello DA, Kreisberg JI, Roy C, Karnovsky MJ. Contraction of cultured rat glomerular cells of apparent mesangial origin after stimulation with angiotensin II and arginine vasopressin. *J Clin Invest* 1980; 65:754–760.

310. Sadoshima J, Malhotra R, Izumo S. The role of the cardiac renin-angiotensin system in load-induced cardiac hypertrophy. *J Cardiac Failure* 1996; 2(suppl 4):S1–S6.

311. Dzau VJ. Cardiac renin-angiotensin system: Molecular and functional aspects. *Am J Med* 1988; 84(suppl 3A):22–27.

312. Lindpainter K, Ganten D. The cardiac renin-angiotensin system: An appraisal of present experimental and clinical evidence. *Circ Res* 1991; 68:905–921.

313. Dzau VJ, Hirsch AT. Emerging role of the tissue renin-angiotensin systems in congestive heart failure. *Eur Heart J* 1990; 11(suppl B):65–71.

314. Dzau VJ. Tissue renin-angiotensin system in myocardial hypertrophy and failure. *Arch Intern Med* 1993; 153:937–942.

315. Lee MA, Böhm M, Paul M, Ganten D. Tissue renin-angiotensin systems. Their role in cardiovascular disease. *Circulation* 1993; 87(suppl 5):IV7–IV13.

316. Ignarro LJ. Biological actions and properties of endothelium-derived nitric oxide formed and released from artery and vein. *Circ Res* 1989; 65:1–21.

317. Moncada S, Palmer RMJ, Higgs EA. Nitric oxide: Physiology, pathophysiology and pharmacology. *Pharmacol Rev* 1991; 43:109–142.

318. Brutsaert DL, De Keulenaer GW, Fransen P, Mohan P, Kaluza GL, Andries LJ, et al. The cardiac endothelium: Functional morphology, development, and physiology. *Prog Cardiovasc Dis* 1996; 39:239–262.

319. Brutsaert DL. Role of endocardium in cardiac overloading and failure. *Eur Heart J* 1991; 11(suppl G):8–16.

320. Shah AM, Grocott-Mason RM, Pepper CB, Mebazza A, Henderson AH, Lewis MJ, et al. The cardiac endothelium: Cardioactive mediators. *Prog Cardiovasc Dis* 1996; 39:263–284.

321. Cohn JN, Levine TB, Francis GS, Goldsmith S. Neurohumoral control mechanisms in congestive heart failure. *Am Heart J* 1981; 102:509–514.

322. Riegger GAJ, Liebau G, Kochsie K. Antidiuretic hormone in congestive heart failure. *Am J Med* 1982; 72:49–52.

323. Preibisz JJ, Sealey JE, Laragh JH. Plasma and platelet vasopressin in essential hypertension and congestive heart failure. *Hypertension* 1983; 5(suppl 1):1-129–1-138.

324. Pruszczynski W, Vahanian A, Ardaillou R, Acar J. Role of antidiuretic hormone in impaired water excretion of patients with congestive heart failure. *J Clin Endocrinol Metab* 1984; 58:599–605.

325. Share L. Role of vasopressin in cardiovascular regulation. *Physiol Rev* 1988; 68:1248–1284.

326. Cowley AW Jr. Vasopressin and cardiovascular regulation. In: Guyton AC, Halls JE, eds. *Cardiovascular Physiology IV, International Review of Physiology*, vol 26. Baltimore: University Park Press; 1982:189–248.

327. Nakaoka H, Imataka K, Amano M, Fujii J, Ishibashi M, Yamaji T. Plasma levels of atrial natriuretic factor in patients with congestive heart failure. *N Engl J Med* 1985; 313:892–893.

328. Cody RJ, Atlas SA, Laragh JH, Kubo SH, Covitt AB, Ryman KS. Atrial natriuretic factor in normal subjects and heart failure patients: Plasma levels and renal, hormonal, and hemodynamic responses to peptide infusion. *J Clin Invest* 1986; 78:1362–1374.

329. Raine AEG, Erne P, Burgisser E, Muller FB, Bolli P, Burkart F. Atrial natriuretic peptide and atrial pressure in patients with congestive heart failure. *N Engl J Med* 1986; 315:553–557.

330. Ogawa K, Ito T, Hashimoto H, Ito Y, Ohno O, Tsuboi H, et al. Plasma atrial natriuretic factor in congestive heart failure. *Lancet* 1986; 1:106.

331. Yamamoto K, Burnett M, Jouqasaki M, Nishimura RA, Bailey KR, Saito Y, et al. Superiority of brain natriuretic peptide as a hormonal marker of ventricular systolic and diastolic function and ventricular hypertrophy. *Hypertension* 1996; 28:988–994.

332. Tsutamoto T, Wada A, Maeda K, Hisanago T, Maeda Y, Fukai D, et al. Attenuation of endogenous cardiac natriuretic peptide system in chronic heart failure. Prognostic role of plasma brain natriuretic peptide concentration in patients with chronic symptomatic left ventricular dysfunction. *Circulation* 1997; 96:509–516.

333. Bates ER, Shenker Y, Grekin RJ. The relationship between plasma levels of immunoreactive atrial natriuretic hormone and hemodynamic function in man. *Circulation* 1986; 73:1155–1161.

334. Pettersson A, Hedner J, Hedner T, Held P, Swedberg K, Towle AC. Increased plasma levels of atrial natriuretic peptide in patients with congestive heart failure. *Eur Heart J* 1986; 7:693–696.

335. Tsutamoto T, Bito K, Kinoshita M. Plasma atrial natriuretic polypeptide as an index of left ventricular end-diastolic pressure in patients with chronic left-sided heart failure. *Am Heart J* 1989; 117:599–606.

336. Donckier JE, De Coster PM, Vanoverschelde J-L, Brichant C, Cauwe F, Installe E, et al. Atrial natriuretic factor, cardiac volumes and filling pressures during exercise in congestive heart failure. *Eur Heart J* 1991; 12:322–327.

337. Nicholls DP, Riley M, Elborn JS, Stanford CF, Shaw C, McKillop JM, et al. Regulatory peptides in the plasma of patients with chronic cardiac failure at rest and during exercise. *Eur Heart J* 1992; 13:1399–1404.

338. Abraham WT, Hensen J, Kim JK, Dürr J, Lesnefsky EJ, Groves BM, et al. Atrial natriuretic peptide and urinary cyclic guanosine monophosphate in patients with chronic heart failure. *J Am Soc Nephrol* 1992; 2:1697–1703.

339. Atarashi K, Mulrow PJ, Franco-Saenz R, Mulrow PJ, Snajclar RM, Rapp JP. Inhibition of aldosterone production by an atrial extract. *Science* 1984; 224:992–994.

340. de Bold AJ, Borenstein HB, Veress AT, Sonnenberg H. A rapid and potent natriuretic response to intravenous injection of atrial myocardial extract in rats. *Life Sci* 1981; 28:89–94.

341. Ballerman BJ, Brenner BM. Role of atrial peptides in body fluid homeostasis. *Circ Res* 1986; 58:619–623.

342. Maack T, Marion DN, Camargo MJF, Kleinert HO, Laragh JH, Jaughan EO Jr. Effects of auriculin (atrial natriuretic factor) on blood pressure, renal function, and the renin-aldosterone system in dogs. *Am J Med* 1984; 77:1069–1071.

343. Wildey GM, Misono KS, Graham RM. Atrial natriuretic factor: Biosynthesis and mechanisms of action. In: Fozzard HA, Haber E, Jennings RB, Katz AM, Morgan HE, eds. *The Heart and Cardiovascular System. Scientific Foundations*, 2d ed. New York: Raven; 1991; 1777–1796.

344. Samson WK. Atrial natriuretic factor inhibits dehydration and hemorrhage-induced vasopressin release. *Neuroendocrinology* 1985; 40:277–279.

345. Tsutamoto T, Kanamori T, Wada A, Kinoshita M. Uncoupling of atrial natriuretic peptide extraction and cyclic guanosine monophosphate production in the pulmonary circulation in patients with severe heart failure. *J Am Coll Cardiol* 1992; 20:541–546.

346. Levenson DJ, Simmons CE Jr, Brenner BM. Arachidonic acid metabolism, prostaglandins and the kidney. *Am J Med* 1982; 72:354–374.

347. Zusman RM. Eicosanoids: Prostaglandins, thromboxane and prostacyclin. In: Fozzard HA, Haber E, Jennings JB, Katz AM, Morgan HE, eds. *The Heart and Cardiovascular System*, 2d ed. New York: Raven; 1991; 1797–1815.

348. Dzau VJ, Packer M, Lilly LS, Swartz SL, Hollenberg NK, Williams GH. Prostaglandins in severe congestive heart failure: Relation to activation of the renin-angiotensin system and hyponatremia. *N Engl J Med* 1984; 310:347–352.

349. Feldman AM, levine MA, Gerstenblith G, Kaufman KO, Baughman KL. Negative inotropic effects of furosemide in the isolated rabbit

heart: A prostaglandin-mediated event. *J Cardiovasc Pharmacol* 1987; 9:493–499.

350. Margolius HS, Horwitz D, Pisano JJ, Keiser HR. Relationships among urinary kallikrein, mineralocorticoids and human hypertensive disease. *Fed Proc* 1976; 35:203–206.

351. Carretero OA, Scicli AG. The kallikrein-kinin system. In: Fozzard HA, Haber E, Jennings RB, Katz AM, Morgan HE, eds. *The Heart and Cardiovascular System. Scientific Foundations*, 2d ed. New York: Raven; 1991; 1851–1874.

352. Gu J, Adrian TE, Tatemoto K, Bloom SR. Neuropeptide tyrosine (NPY): A major cardiac neuropeptide. *Lancet* 1983; 1008–1010.

353. Meerson FZ, Javitz MP, Breger AM, Lerman MI. The mechanism of the heart's adaptation to prolonged load and dynamics of RNA synthesis in the myocardium. *Basic Res Cardiol* 1974; 484–499.

354. Allen DG, Kentish JG. The cellular basis of the length-tension relation in cardiac muscle. *J Mol Cell Cardiol* 1985; 17:821–840.

355. Meerson FZ. Development of modern components of the mechanism of cardiac hypertrophy. *Circ Res* 1974; 35(suppl 2)11:58–63.

356. Meerson FZ, Katz AM, ed. *The Failing Heart: Adaptation and Deadaptation.* New York: Raven; 1983:1–323.

357. LaKatta EG. Length modulation of muscle performance: Frank-Starling Law of the Heart. In: Fozzard HA, Haber E, Jennings RB, Katz AM, Morgan HE, eds. *The Heart and Cardiovascular System: Scientific Foundations*, 2d ed. New York: Raven Press; 1991:1325–1351.

358. LaKatta EG. Starling's law of the heart is explained by an intimate interaction of muscle length and myofilament calcium activation. *J Am Coll Cardiol* 1987; 10:1157–1164.

359. Babu A, Sonnenblick E, Gulati J. Molecular basis for the influence of muscle length on myocardial performance. *Science* 1988; 240:74–76.

360. Hofmann PA, Fuchs F. Bound calcium and force development in skinned cardiac muscle bundles: Effect of sarcomere length. *J Mol Cell Cardiol* 1988; 20:667–677.

361. Hoh JF, Rossmanith GH, Kwan LJ, Hamilton AM. Adrenaline increases the rate of cycling of crossbridges in rat cardiac muscle as measured by pseudo-random binary noise–modulated perturbation analysis. *Circ Res* 1988; 62:452–461.

362. Katz AM. The descending limb of the Starling curve and the failing heart. *Circulation* 1965; 32:871–875.

363. MacGregor DC, Covell JW, Mahler F, Dilley RJ, Ross J. Relations between afterload, stroke volume, and the descending limb of Starling's curves. *Am J Physiol* 1974; 227:884–890.

364. Cheng W, Li B, Kajstura J, Li P, Wolin MS, Sonnenblick EH, et al. Stretch-induced programmed myocyte cell death. *J Clin Invest* 1995; 96:2247–2259.

365. Grossman W, Carabello BA, Gunther S, Fifer MA. Ventricular wall stress and the development of cardiac hypertrophy and failure. In: Alpert NR, ed. *Perspectives in Cardiovascular Research*, vol 7. New York: Raven; 1983: 1–18.

366. Anversa P, Ricci R, Olivetti G. Quantitative structural analysis of the myocardium during physiological growth induced cardiac hypertrophy: A review. *J Am Coll Cardiol* 1986; 7:1140–1149.

367. Anversa P, Capasso JM, Olivetti G, Sonnenblick EH. Cellular basis of ventricular remodeling in hypertensive cardiomyopathy. *Am J Hypertens* 1992; 5:758–770.

368. Linzbach AJ. Heart failure from the point of view of quantitative anatomy. *Am J Cardiol* 1960; 5:370–382.

369. Badeer HS. Biological significance of cardiac hypertrophy. *Am J Cardiol* 1964; 14:133–138.

370. Grossman W, Jones D, McLaurin LP. Wall stress and patterns of hypertrophy in the human left ventricle. *J Clin Invest* 1975; 56:56–64.

371. Marino TA, Kent RL, Uboh CI, Fernandez E, Thompson EW, Cooper G. Structural analysis of pressure versus volume overload hypertrophy of cat right ventricle. *Am J Physiol* 1985; 18:H371–H379.

372. Olivetti G, Ricci R, Lagrasta C, Maniga E, Sonnenblick EH, Anversa P. Cellular basis of wall remodeling in long-term pressure overload-induced right ventricular hypertrophy in rats. *Circ Res* 1988; 63:648–657.

373. Olivetti G, Capasso JM, Meggs LG, Sonnenblick EH, Anversa P. Cellular basis of ventricular remodelling after myocardial infarction in rats. *Circ Res* 1991; 68:856–869.

374. Breisch EA, Houser SR, Carey RA, Spann JF, Bove AA. Myocardial blood flow and capillary density in chronic pressure overload of the feline left ventricle. *Cardiovasc Res* 1980; 14:469–475.

375. Anversa P, Ricci R, Olivetti G. Quantitative structural analysis of the myocardium during physiologic growth and induced cardiac hypertrophy: A review. *J Am Coll Cardiol* 1986; 7:1140–1149.

376. Tomanek RJ, Palmer PJ, Peiffer GL, Schreiber KL, Eastham CL, Marcus ML. Morphometry of canine coronary arteries, arterioles, and capillaries during hypertension and left ventricular hypertrophy. *Circ Res* 1986; 58:38–46.

377. Anversa P, Beghi C, Kikkawa Y, Olivetti G. Myocardial infarction in rats: Infarct size, myocyte hypertrophy, and capillary growth. *Circ Res* 1986; 58:26–37.

378. Bache RJ. Effects of hypertrophy on the coronary circulation. *Prog Cardiovasc Dis* 1988; 31:403–440.

379. Schaper J. Hypertrophy in the human heart: Evaluation by qualitative and quantitative light and electron microscopy. In: Alpert NR, ed. *Perspectives in Cardiovascular Research*, vol 7. New York: Raven; 1983:177–196.

380. Anversa P, Sonnenblick EH. Ischemic cardiomyopathy: Pathophysiologic mechanisms. *Prog Cardiovasc Dis* 1990; 33:49–70.

381. Jacob R, Kissling G, Rupp H, Vogt M. Functional significance of contractile proteins in cardiac hypertrophy and failure. *J Cardiovasc Pharmacol* 1987; 10(suppl 6):S2–S12.

382. Swynghedauw B, Schwartz K, Lecarpentier Y, Clapier-Ventura R, Perennec J, Waldenstron A, et al. Species-specificity of the isomyosin shift in cardiac overload. *J Appl Cardiol* 1988; 3:133–143.

383. Kitsis RN, Scheuer J. Correlations and dissociations between myosin isoenzymes and cardiac function. *J Appl Cardiol* 1988; 327–335.

384. Anversa P, Palackal T, Sonnenblick EH, Olivetti G, Meggs LG, Capasso J. Myocyte cell loss and myocyte cellular hyperplasia in the hypertrophied aging rat heart. *Circ Res* 1990; 67:871–885.

385. Jacob R, Ebrecht G, Kissling G, Rupp H, Takeda N. Functional consequences of cardiac myosin isoenzyme redistribution. In: Rupp H, ed. *Regulation of Heart Function: Basic Concepts and Clinical Applications.* Stuttgart: Thieme; 1986:305–326.

386. Mercadier J-J, Lompre A-M, Wisnewsky C, Samuel JL, Bereovici J, Swynghedauw B, et al. Myosin isoenzymatic changes in several models of rat cardiac hypertrophy. *Circ Res* 1981; 49:525–532.

387. Horowits R, Winegrad S. cAMP regulation of myosin ATPase activity in the maturing rat heart. *Circ Res* 1987; 61:914–924.

388. Cummins P, Lambert SJ. Myosin transitions in the bovine and human heart: A developmental and anatomical study of heavy and light chain subunits in the atrium and ventricle. *Circ Res* 1986; 58:846–858.

389. Olivetti G, Capasso JM, Sonnenblick EH, Anversa P. Side-to-side slippage of myocytes participates in ventricular wall remodeling acutely after myocardial infarction in rats. *Circ Res* 1990; 67:23–24.

390. Badeer HS. Contractile tension in the myocardium. *Am Heart J* 1963; 66:432–434.

391. Hood WP Jr, Rackley CE, Rolett EL. Wall stress in the normal and hypertrophied human left ventricle. *Am J Cardiol* 1968; 22:550–558.

392. Grossman W, McLaurin LP, Moos SP, Stefadouros M, Young DT. Wall thickness and diastolic properties of the left ventricle. *Circulation* 1974; 49:129–135.

393. Sasayama S, Ross J Jr, Franklin D, Bloor CM, Bishop S, Dilley RB. Adaptations of the left ventricle to chronic pressure overload. *Circ Res* 1976; 38:172–178.

394. Cohen J. Role of endocrine factors in the pathogenesis of cardiac hypertrophy. *Circ Res* 1974; 35(suppl II):II49–II57.

395. Lorell BH, Grossman, W. Cardiac hypertrophy: The consequences for diastole. *J Am Coll Cardiol* 1987; 9:1189–1193.

396. Harizi RC, Bianco JA, Alpert JS. Diastolic function of the heart in clinical cardiology. *Arch Intern Med* 1988; 148:99–109.

397. Grossman W, Lorell BH, eds. *Diastolic Relaxation of the Heart: Basic Research and Applications for Clinical Cardiology.* Boston: Martinus Nijhoff; 1988:1–310.

398. Gaasch WH, LeWinter MM, eds. *Left Ventricular Diastolic Dysfunction and Heart Failure.* Philadelphia: Lea & Febiger; 1993.

399. Perreault CL, Williams CP, Morgan JP. Cytoplasmic calcium modulation and systolic versus diastolic dysfunction in myocardial hypertrophy and failure. *Circulation* 1993; 87(suppl VII):VII31–VII37.

400. Dougherty AH, Naccarelli GV, Gray EL, Hicks CH, Goldstein RA. Congestive heart failure with normal systolic function. *Am J Cardiol* 1984; 54:778–782.

401. Soufer R, Wohlgelernter D, Vita NA, Amuchestegui M, Sostman HD, Berger HL, et al. Intact systolic left ventricular function in clinical congestive heart failure. *Am J Cardiol* 1985; 55:1032–1036.

402. Kessler KM. Heart failure with normal systolic function: Update of prevalence, differential diagnosis, prognosis, and therapy. *Ann Intern Med* 1988; 148:2109–2111.

403. Grossman W. Diastolic dysfunction and congestive heart failure. *Circulation* 1990; 81(suppl III):III1–III7.

404. Yellin EL, Nikolic S, Frater RWM. Left ventricular filling dynamics and diastolic function. *Prog Cadiovasc Dis* 1990; 32:247–271.

405. Stauffer J-C, Gaasch WH. Recognition and treatment of left ventricular diastolic dysfunction. *Prog Cardiovasc* 1990; 32:319–332.

406. Gaasch WH. Congestive heart failure in patients with normal left ventricular systolic function: A manifestation of diastolic dysfunction. *Herz* 1991; 16:22–32.

407. Glantz SA, Misbach GA, Moores WY, Mathey DG, LeKven J, Stowe DF. The pericardium substantially affects the left ventricular diastolic pressure-volume relationship in the dog. *Circ Res* 1978; 42:433–441.

408. Gilbert JC, Glantz SA. Determinants of left ventricular filling and of the diastolic pressure-volume relation. *Circ Res* 1989; 64:827–852.

409. Scaglione R, Dichiara MA, Indovina A, Lipari R, Ganguzza A, Parrinello G, et al. Left ventricular diastolic and systolic function in normotensive obese subjects: Influence of degree and duration of obesity. *Eur Heart J* 1992; 13:738–742.

410. Braunwald E, Ross J Jr. The ventricular end-diastolic pressure: Appraisal of its value in the recognition of ventricular failure in man. *Am J Med* 1963; 34:147–150.

411. Rackley CE, Hood WP Jr, Rolett EL, Young DT. Left ventricular end-diastolic pressure in chronic heart disease. *Am J Med* 1970; 48:310–319.

412. Levine HJ. Compliance of the left ventricle. *Circulation* 1972; 46:423–426.

413. Covell JW, Ross J Jr. Nature and significance of alterations in myocardial compliance. *Am J Cardiol* 1973; 32:449–455.

414. Grossman W, McLaurin LP. Diastolic properties of the left ventricle. *Ann Intern Med* 1976; 84:316–326.

415. Gaasch WH, Levine HJ, Quinones MA, Alexander JK. Left ventricular compliance: Mechanisms and clinical implications. *Am J Cardiol* 1976; 38:645–653.

416. Wisneski JA, Bristow JD. Left ventricular stiffness. *Annu Rev Med* 1978; 29:475–483.

417. Grossman W, Barry WH. Diastolic pressure-volume relations in diseased heart. *Fed Proc* 1980; 39:148–155.

418. Lewis BS, Gotsman MS. Current concepts of ventricular relaxation and compliance. *Am Heart J* 1980; 99:101–112.

419. Gaasch WH, Levine HJ, Quinones MA, Alexander JK. Left ventricular compliance: Mechanisms and clinical implications. *Am J Cardiol* 1976; 38:645–653.

420. Gaasch WH, Zile MR. Evaluation of myocardial function in cardiomyopathic states. *Prog Cardiovasc Dis* 1984; 27:115–132.

421. Bonow RO, Udelson JE. Left ventricular diastolic dysfunction as a cause of congestive heart failure. *Ann Intern Med* 1992; 117:502–510.

422. Hefner LL, Coghlan CH, Jones WB. Distensibility of the dog left ventricle. *Am J Physiol* 1961; 201:97–101.

423. Janicki JS, Weber KT. The pericardium and ventricular interaction, distensibility, and function. *Am J Physiol* 1980; 238:H494–H503.

424. Bove A, Santamore W. Ventricular interdependence. *Prog Cardiovasc Dis* 1981; 23:365–388.

425. Maruyama Y, Ashikawa K, Isoyama S, Kanatsuka H, Ino-Oka E, Takishima T. Mechanical interactions between four heart chambers with and without the pericardium in canine hearts. *Circ Res* 1982; 50:86–100.

426. Little WC, Badke FR, O'Rourke RA. Effect of right ventricular pressure on the end-diastolic left ventricular pressure-volume relationship before and after chronic right ventricular pressure overload in dogs without pericardia. *Circ Res* 1984; 54:719–730.

427. Santamore WP, Constantinescu M, Vinten-Johansen J, Johnston WE, Little WC. Alterations in left ventricular compliance due to changes in right ventricular volume, pressure and compliance. *Cardiovasc Res* 1988; 22:768–776.

428. Santamore WP, Shaffer T, Hughes D. A theoretical and experimental model of ventricular interdependence. *Basic Res Cardiol* 1986; 81:529–538.

429. Janicki JS. Influence of the pericardium and ventricular interdependence on left ventricular diastolic and systolic function in patients with heart failure. *Circulation* 1990; 82(2 suppl):III15–III20.

430. Hoit BD, Dalton N, Bhargava V, Shabetai R. Pericardial influences on right and left ventricular filling dynamics. *Circ Res* 1991; 68:197–208.

431. Lorell BH, Wexler LF, Momomura S, Weinberg E, Apstein CS. The influence of pressure overload left ventricular hypertrophy on diastolic properties during hypoxia in isovolumically contracting rat hearts. *Circ Res* 1986; 58:653–663.

432. Grossman W, McLaurin LP, Moos SP, Stefadouras MA, Young DT. Wall thickness and diastolic properties of the left ventricle. *Circulation* 1974; 49:129–135.

433. Thiedemann KU, Holubarsch CH, Medugorac I, Jacob R. Connective tissue content and myocardial stiffness in pressure overload hypertrophy: A combined study of morphologic, morphometric, biochemical and mechanical parameters. *Basic Res Cardiol* 1983; 78:140–155.

434. Lorell BH. Significance of diastolic dysfunction of the heart. *Annu Rev Med* 1991; 42:411–436.

435. Cheng CP, Freeman GL, Santamore WP, Constantinescu MS, Little WC. Effect of loading conditions, contractile state, and heart rate on early diastolic left ventricular filling in conscious dogs. *Circ Res* 1990; 66:814–823.

436. Brutsaert DL, Sonnenblick EH. Cardiac muscle mechanics in the evaluation of myocardial contractility and pump function: Problems, concepts and directions. *Prog Cardiovasc Dis* 1973; 16:337–361.

437. Taylor RR, Hopkins BE. Left ventricular response to experimentally induced chronic aortic regurgitation. *Cardiovasc Res* 1972; 6:404–414.

438. Spann JF Jr, Covell JW, Eckberg DL, Sonnenblick EH, Ross J Jr, Braunwald E. Contractile performance of the hypertrophied and chronically failing cat venticle. *Am J Physiol* 1972; 223:1150–1157.

439. Spann JF. Contractile and pump function of the pressure-overloaded heart. In: Alpert NR, ed. *Perspectives in Cardiovascular Research*, vol 7. New York: Raven; 1983:19–38.

440. Cooper G IV, Satava RM, Harrison CE, Coleman HN 3d. Normal myocardial function and energetics after reversing pressure-overload hypertrophy. *Am J Physiol* 1974; 226:1158–1165.

441. Williams JF Jr, Potter RD. Normal contractile state of hypertrophied myocardium following pulmonary artery constriction in the cat. *J Clin Invest* 1974; 54:1266–1272.

442. Malik AB, Abe T, O'Kane HO, Geha AS. Cardiac performance in ventricular hypertrophy induced by pressure and volume overloading. *J Appl Physiol* 1974; 37:867–874.

443. Meerson FZ, Kapelko VI. The contractile function of the myocardium in two types of cardiac adaptation to a chronic load. *Cardiology* 1972; 57:183–199.

444. Noble MIM, Seed WA, eds. *The Interval-Force Relationship of the Heart: Bowditch Revisited.* Cambridge: Cambridge University Press; 1992:1–368.

445. Hasenfuss G, Holubarsch C, Hermann H-P, Astheimer K, Pieske B, Just H. Influence of the force-frequency relationship in haemodynamics and left ventricular function in patients with non-failing hearts and in patients with dilated cardiomyopathy. *Eur Heart J* 1944; 15:164–170.

446. Schmidt U, Schwinger RHG, Böhm M, Erdmann E. Alterations of the force-frequency relation depending on stages of heart failure in humans. *Am J Cardiol* 1994; 74:1066–1068.

447. Ross J Jr, Miura T, Kamboyashi M, Eising GP, Ryu K-H. Adrenergic control of the force-frequency relation. *Circulation* 1995; 92:2327–2332.

448. Valeri CR, Fortier NL. Red-cell 2,3-diphosphoglycerate and creatine levels in patients with red-cell mass deficiency or with cardiopulmonary insufficiency. *N Engl J Med* 1969; 281:1452–1455.

449. Massie BM, Conway M, Rajagopalan B, Yonge R, Frostick S, Ledingham J, et at. Skeletal muscle metabolism during exercise under ischemic conditions in congestive heart failure. Evidence for abnormalities unrelated to blood flow. *Circulation* 1988; 78:320–326.

450. Drexler H, Riede U, Münzel T, König H, Funke E, Just H. Alterations of skeletal muscle in chronic heart failure. *Circulation* 1992; 85:1751–1759.

451. Supinski G, Di Marco A, Dibner-Dunlap M. Alterations in diaphragm strength and fatiguability in congestive heart failure. *J Appl Physiol* 1994; 76:2707–2713.

452. Walsh JJ, Andrews R, Johnson P, Phillips L, Cowley AJ, Kinnear WJM. Inspiratory muscle endurance in patients with chronic heart failure. *Heart* 1996; 76:332–336.

453. Tikunov B, Levine S, Mancini D. Chronic congestive heart failure elicits adaptations of endurance exercise in diaphragmatic muscle. *Circulation* 1997; 95:910–916.

454. Hornig B, Maier V, Drexler H. Physical training improves endothelial function in patients with chronic heart failure. *Circulation* 1996; 93:210–214.

455. Kiilavuori K, Sovijärvi A, Näveri H, Ikonen T, Leinonen H. Effect of physical training on exercise capacity and gas exchange in patients with chronic heart failure. *Chest* 1996; 985–991.

456. Gordon A, Tyni-Lenné R, Jansson E, Kaijser L, Theodorsson-Norheim E, Sylvén C. Improved ventilation and decreased sympathetic stress in chronic heart failure patients following local endurance training with leg muscles. *J Cardiac Failure* 1997; 3:3–12.

457. Drexler H, Kurz S, Jeserich M, Münzel T, Hornig B. Effect of chronic angiotensin-converting enzyme inhibition on endothelial function in patients with chronic heart failure. *Am J Cardiol* 1995; 76:13E–18E.

458. Mancini DM, LeJemtel TH, Factor S, Sonnenblick EH. Central and peripheral components of cardiac failure. *Am J Med* 1986; 80(suppl 2B):2–13.

459. Burch GE, Ray CT, Cronvich JA. Certain mechanical peculiarities of the human cardiac pump in normal and diseased states. *Circulation* 1952; 5:504–513.

460. Burch GE. Theoretic considerations of the time course of pressure developed and volume ejected by the normal and dilated left ventricle during systole. *Am Heart J* 1955; 50:352–355.

461. Burch GE, DePasquale NP, Cronvich JA. Influence of ventricular size on the relationship between contractile and manifest tension. *Am Heart J* 1965; 69:624–628.

462. Mason DT, Spann JF Jr, Zelis R, Amsterdam EA. Alterations of hemodynamics and myocardial mechanics in patients with congestive heart failure: Pathophysiologic mechanisms and assessment of cardiac function and ventricular contractility. *Prog Cardiovasc Dis* 1970; 12:507–557.

463. Winegrad S. Mechanism of contraction in cardiac muscle. In: Guyton AC, Halls JE, eds. *Cardiovascular Physiology IV, International Review of Physiology*, vol 26. Baltimore: University Park Press; 1982:87–117.

464. Sharov VG, Sabbah HN, Shimogama H, Goussev AV, Lesch M, Goldstein S. Evidence of cardiocyte apoptosis in myocardium of dogs with chronic heart failure. *Am J Pathol* 1996; 148:141–149.

465. Narula J, Haider N, Virmani R, DiSalvo TG, Kolodgie FD, Hajjar RJ, et al. Apoptosis in myocytes in end-stage heart failure. *N Engl J Med* 1996; 335:1182–1189.

466. Olivetti G, Abbi R, Quaini F, Kajstura J, Cheng W, Nitahara JA, et al. Apoptosis in the failing heart. *N Engl J Med* 1997; 336:1131–1141.

467. Vincent WR, Buckberg GD, Hoffman JIE. Left ventricular subendocardial ischemia in severe valvular and supravalvular aortic stenosis: A common mechanism. *Circulation* 1974; 49:326–333.

468. Brazier JR, Buckberg GD. Effects of tachycardia on the adequacy of subendocardial oxygen delivery in experimental aortic stenosis. *Am Heart J* 1975; 90:222–230.

469. Downey JM, Kirk ES. Inhibition of coronary blood flow by a vascular waterfall mechanism. *Circ Res* 1975; 36:753–760.

470. Brazier J, Cooper N, Buckberg G. The adequacy of subendocardial oxygen delivery: The interaction of determinants of flow, arterial oxygen content, and myocardial oxygen need. *Circulation* 1974; 49:968–977.

471. Honig CR, Bourdeau-Martini J. Extravascular component of oxygen transport in normal and hypertrophied hearts with special reference to oxygen therapy. *Circ Res* 1974; 35(suppl II):II97–II103.

472. Shapiro LM, Gibson DG. Patterns of diastolic dysfunction in left ventricular hypertrophy. *Br Heart J* 1988; 59:438–451.

473. McCullagh WH, Covell JW, Ross J Jr. Left ventricular dilatation and diastolic compliance changes during chronic volume overload. *Circulation* 1972; 45:943–951.

474. Michell JH, Gilmore JP, Sarnoff SJ. The transport function of the atrium: Factors influencing the relation between mean left atrial pressure and left ventricular end diastolic pressure. *Am J Cardiol* 1962; 9:237–247.

475. Braunwald E. Hemodynamic significance of atrial systole. *Am J Med* 1964; 37:665–669.

476. Ikram H, Nixon PGF, Arcan T. Left atrial function after electrical conversion to sinus rhythm. *Br Heart J* 1968; 30:80–83.

477. Brill IC, Rosenbaum EE, Flanery JR. Congestive failure due to auricular fibrillation in an otherwise normal heart. *JAMA* 1960; 173:784–785.

478. Suga H. Importance of atrial compliance in cardiac performance. *Circ Res* 1974; 35:39–43.

479. Borow KM, Green LH, Grossman W, Braunwald E. Left ventricular end-systolic stress-shortening and stress-length relations in humans: Normal values and sensitivity to inotropic state. *Am J Cardiol* 1982; 50:1301–1308.

480. Taylor RR, Covell JW, Sonnenblick EH, Ross J Jr. Dependence of ventricular distensibility on filling of the opposite ventricle. *Am J Physiol* 1967; 213:711–718.

481. Kelly DT, Spotnitz HM, Beiser GD, Pierce JE, Epstein SE. Effects of chronic right ventricular volume and pressure loading on left ventricular performance. *Circulation* 1971; 44:403–412.

482. Bemis CE, Serur JR, Borkenhagen D, Sonnenblick EH. Influence of right ventricular filling pressure on left ventricular pressure and dimension. *Circ Res* 1974; 34:498–504.

483. Glantz SA, Misbach GA, Moores WY, Mathey DG, Lekuen J, Stowe DF. The pericardium substantially affects the left ventricular diastolic pressure-volume relationship in the dog. *Circ Res* 1978; 42:433–441.

484. Little WC, Badke FR, O'Rourke RA. Effect of right ventricular pressure on the end-diastolic left ventricular pressure-volume relationship before and after chronic right ventricular pressure overload in dogs without pericardia. *Circ Res* 1984; 54:719–730.

485. Chidsey CA, Kaiser GA, Sonnenblick EH, Spann JF, Braunwald E. Cardiac norepinephrine stores in experimental heart failure in the dog. *J Clin Invest* 1964; 43:2386–2393.

486. Burton AC. The importance of the shape and size of the heart. *Am Heart J* 1957; 54:801–809.

487. Kono T, Sabbah HN, Stein PD, Brymer JF, Khaja F. Left ventricular shape as a determinant of functional mitral regurgitation in patients with severe heart failure secondary to either coronary artery disease or idiopathic dilated cardiomyopathy. *Am J Cardiol* 1991; 68:355–359.

488. Sabbah HN, Knon T, Stein PD, Mancini GBJ, Goldstein S. Left ventricular shape changes during the course of evolving heart failure. *Am J Physiol* 1992; 263(*Heart Circ Physiol* 32):H266–H270.

489. Sabbah HN, Knon T, Rosman H, Jafri S, Stein PD, Goldstein S. Left ventricular shape: A factor in the etiology of functional mitral regurgitation in heart failure. *Am heart J* 1992; 123:961–966.

490. Mitchell JH, Sarnoff SJ, Sonnenblick EH. The dynamics of pulsus alternans: Alternating end-diastolic fiber length as a causative factor. *J Clin Invest* 1963; 42:55–63.

491. Hada Y, Wolfe C, Craige E. Pulus alternans determined by biventricular simultaneous systolic time intervals. *Circulation* 1982; 65:617–626.

492. Hess OM, Surber EP, Ritter M, Krayenbuehl HP. Pulsus altenans: Its influence on systolic and diastolic function in aortic valve disease. *J Am Coll Cardiol* 1984; 4:1–7.

493. Braunwald E, Goldblatt A, Harrison DC, Glick EP, Mason DT. Studies on cardiac dimensions in intact, unanesthetized man: III. Effects of muscular exercise. *Circ Res* 1963; 13:460–467.

494. Gorlin R, Cohen LS, Elliott WC, Klein MD, Lane FJ. Effect of supine exercise on left ventricular volume and oxygen consumption in man. *Circulation* 1965; 32:361–371.

495. Braunwald E. The control of ventricular function in man. *Br Heart J* 1965; 27:1–16.

496. Chapman CB, ed. Physiology of muscular exercise. *Circ Res* 1967; 20(suppl I):I1–I226.

497. Bevegard BS, Shepherd JT. Regulation of the circulation during exercise in man. *Physiol Rev* 1967; 47:178–213.

498. Horwitz LD, Atkins JM, Leshin SJ. Role of the Frank-Starling mechanism in exercise. *Cir Res* 1972; 31:868–875.

499. Vatner SF, Pagani M. Cardiovascular adjustments to exercise: Hemodynamics and mechanisms. *Prog Cardiovasc Dis* 1976; 19:91–108.

500. Bertrand ME, Carre AG, Ginestet AP, Lefebvre JM, Desplanaque LA, Lekieffre JP. Maximal exercise in normal subjects. *Eur J Cardiol* 1977; 516:481–491.

501. Astrand P-O, Rodahl K. *Textbook of Work Physiology: Physiological Basis of Exercise*, 3d ed. New York: McGraw-Hill; 1986.

502. Christensen NJ, Galbo H. Sympathetic nervous activity during exercise. *Annu Rev Physiol* 1983; 45:139–153.

503. Ludbrook J. Reflex control of blood pressure during exercise. *Annu Rev Physiol* 1983; 45:155–168.

504. Brengelmann GL. Circulatory adjustments to exercise and heat stress. *Annu Rev Physiol* 1983; 45:191–212.

505. Mitchell JH, Kaufman MP, Iwamoto GA. The exercise pressor reflex: Its cardiovascular effects, afferent mechanisms, and central pathways. *Annu Rev Physiol* 1983; 45:229–242.

506. Schlant RC. Physiology of exercise. In: Fletcher GF, ed. *Exercise in the Practice of Medicine*, 2d ed. Mount Kisco, NY: Futura; 1988; 1–47.

507. Epstein SE, Robinson BF, Kahler RL, Braunwald E. Effects of beta-adrenergic blockade on the cardiac response to maximal and submaximal exercise in man. *J Clin Invest* 1965; 44:1745–1753.

508. Robinson BF, Epstein SE, Kahler RL, Braunwald E. Circulatory effects of acute expansion of blood volume: Studies during maximal exercise and at rest. *Circ Res* 1966; 19:26–32.

509. Bristow JD, Kloster FE, Farrehi C, Brodeur MT, Lewis RP, Griswold HE. The effects of supine exercise on left ventricular volume in heart disease. *Am Heart J* 1966; 71:319–329.

510. Skelton CL, Sonnenblick EH. Physiology of cardiac muscle. In: Levine HJ, ed. *Clinical Cardiovascular Physiology*. New York: Grune & Stratton; 1976:57–120.

511. Zelis R, Nellis SH, Longhurst J, Lee G, Mason DT. Abnormalities in the regional circulations accompanying congestive heart failure. *Prog Cardiovasc Dis* 1975; 18:181–199.

512. Davies SW, Fussell AL, Jordan SL, Poole-Wilson PA, Lipkin DP. Abnormal diastolic filling patterns in chronic heart failure—relationships to exercise capacity. *Eur Heart J* 1992; 13:749–757.

513. Wiener DH, Fink LI, Maris J, Jones RA, Chance B, Wilson JR. Abnormal skeletal muscle bioenergetics during exercise in patients with heart failure: Role of reduced muscle blood flow. *Circulation* 1986; 73:1127–1136.

514. Massie BM, Conway M, Yonge R, Frostick S, Ledingham J, Sleight P, et al. Skeletal muscle metabolism in patients with congestive heart failure: Relation to clinical severity and blood flow. *Circulation* 1987; 76:1009–1019.

515. Massie BM, Conway M, Yonge R, Frostick S, Sleight P, Ledingham J, et al. ³¹P nuclear magnetic resonance evidence of abnormal skeletal muscle metabolism in patients with congestive heart failure. *Am J Cardiol* 1987; 60:309–315.

516. Masie BM, Conway M, Rajagopalan B, Yonge R, Frostick S, Ledingham J, et al. Skeletal muscle metabolism during exercise under ischemic conditions in congestive heart failure: Evidence for abnormalities unrelated to blood flow. *Circulation* 1988; 78:320–326.

517. Sullivan MJ, Green HJ, Cobb FR. Altered skeletal muscle metabolic response to exercise in chronic heart failure: Relation to skeletal muscle aerobic enzyme activity. *Circulation* 1991; 84:1597–1607.

518. Minotti JR, Christoph I, Oka R, Weiner MW, Wells L, Massie BM. Impaired skeletal muscle function in patients with congestive heart failure: Relationship to systemic exercise performance. *J Clin Invest* 1991; 88:2077–2082.

519. Minotti JR, Pillay P, Chang L, Wells L, Massie BM. Neurophysiological assessment of skeletal muscle fatigue in patients with congestive heart failure. *Circulation* 1992; 86:903–908.

520. Wilson JR, Fink L, Maris J, Ferraro N, Power-Vanwart J, Eleff S, et al. Evaluation of energy metabolism in skeletal muscle of patients with heart failure with gated phosphorus-31 nuclear magnetic resonance. *Circulation* 1985; 71:57–62.

521. Clausen JP. Circulatory adjustments to dynamic exercise and effect of physical training in normal subjects and in patients with coronary artery disease. *Prog Cardiovasc Dis* 1976; 18:459–495.

522. Sullivan MJ, Higginbotham MB, Cobb FR. Exercise training in patients with severe left ventricular dysfunction: Hemodynamic and metabolic effects. *Circulation* 1988; 78:506–515.

523. Sullivan MJ, Higginbotham MB, Cobb FR. Exercise training in patients with chronic heart failure delays ventilatory anaerobic threshold and improves submaximal exercise performance. *Circulation* 1989; 79:324–329.

524. Dubach P, Froelicher VF. Cardiac rehabilitation for heart failure patients. *Cardiology* 1989; 76:368–373.

525. Drexler H, Riede U, Münzel T, König H, Funke E, Just H. Alterations of skeletal muscle in chronic heart failure. *Circulation* 1992; 85:1751–1759.

526. Colucci WS, Wright RF, Braunwald E. New positive inotropic agents in the treatment of congestive heart failure: Mechanisms of action and recent clinical developments. *N Engl J Med* 1986; 314:349–358.

527. Weber KT, Gill SK, Janicki JS, Maskin CS, Jain MC. Newer positive inotropic agents in the treatment of chronic cardiac failure: Current status and future directions. *Drugs* 1987; 33:503–519.

528. LeJemtel TH, Sonnenblick EH. Should the failing heart be stimulated? *N Engl J Med* 1984; 310:1384–1385.

529. Ferguson DW, Berg WJ, Sanders JS, Roach PJ, Kempf JS, Kienzle MG. Sympathoinhibitory responses to digitalis glycosides in heart failure patients: Direct evidence from sympathetic neural recordings. *Circulation* 1989; 80:65–77.

530. Fishman AP, Renkin EM, eds. *Pulmonary Edema.* Bethesda, MD: American Physiology Society; 1979:1–261.

531. Murray JF, Nadel JA, eds. *Textbook of Respiratory Medicine.* Philadelphia: Saunders; 1988.

532. Rapaport E. Dyspnea: Pathophysiology and differential diagnosis. *Prog Cardiovasc Dis* 1971; 13:532.

533. Luepker R, Liander B, Korsgren M, Varnauskas E. Pulmonary intravascular and extravascular fluid volumes in exercising cardiac patients. *Circulation* 1971; 44:626–637.

534. Myers J, Salleh A, Buchanan N, Smith D, Neutel J, Bowes E, et al. Ventilatory mechanisms of exercise intolerance in chronic heart failure. *Am Heart J* 1992; 124:710–718.

535. Aberman A, Fulop M. The metabolic and respiratory acidosis of acute pulmonary edema. *Ann Intern Med* 1972; 76:173–184.

536. Lee G de J. Pulmonary oedema. In: Yu PN, Goodwin JF, eds. *Progress in Cardiology,* vol 1. Philadelphia: Lea & Febiger; 1972:261.

537. Fishman AP. Pulmonary edema: The water-exchanging function of the lung. *Circulation* 1972; 46:390–408.

538. Robin ED, Cross CE, Zelis R. Pulmonary edema. *N Engl J Med* 1973; 288:292–304.

539. Staub NC. Pulmonary edema. *Physiol Rev* 1974; 54:678–811.

540. Schreiner BF, Yu PN. Pulmonary circulation and edema: Anatomic and physiologic considerations. In: Levine HJ, ed. *Clinical Cardiovascular Physiology.* New York: Grune & Stratton; 1976:635–706.

541. Gaar KA Jr, Taylor AE, Owens LJ, Guyton AC. Development of pulmonary edema. *Am J Physiol* 1967; 213:79–82.

542. Robin ED, Carey LC, Grenvik A, Glauser F, Gaudio R. Capillary leak syndrome with pulmonary edema. *Arch Intern Med* 1972; 130:66–71.

543. Uhley HN, Leeds SE, Sampson JJ, Friedman M. Right duct lymph flow in experimental heart failure following acute elevation of left atrial pressure. *Circ Res* 1967; 20:306–310.

544. Davies SW, Bailey J, Keegan J, Balcon R, Rudd RM, Lipkin DP. Reduced pulmonary microvascular permeability in severe chronic left heart failure. *Am Heart J* 1992; 124:137–142.

545. Zelis R, Mansour EJ, Capone RJ, Mason DT. The cardiovascular effects of morphine: The peripheral capacitance and resistance vessels in human subjects. *J Clin Invest* 1974; 54:1247–1258.

546. Vismara LA, Learman DM, Zelis R. Effects of morphine on venous tone in patients with acute pulmonary edema. *Circulation* 1976; 54:335–337.

547. Overland ES, Severinghaus JW. Noncardiac pulmonary edema. *Annu Rev Med* 1978; 23:307–326.

548. Hultgren HN, Grover RF. Circulation adaptation to high altitude. *Annu Rev Med* 1968; 19:119–152.

549. Jerome EH, Severinghaus JW. High-altitude pulmonary edema. *N Engl J Med* 1996; 334:662–663.

550. Viswanathan R, Jain SK, Subramanian S. Pulmonary edema of high altitude: III. Pathogenesis. *Am Rev Respir Dis* 1969; 100:324–349.

551. Vogel JHK, ed. *Hypoxia, High Altitude and the Heart. Advances in Cardiology,* vol 5. Basel: Karger: 1970.

552. Severinghaus JW. Transarterial leakage: A possible mechanism of high altitude pulmonary edema. In: Porter R, Knight J, eds. *High Altitude Physiology: Cardiac and Pulmonary Aspects.* London: Churchill Livingstone; 1971:61–77.

553. Kleiner JP, Nelson WP. High altitude pulmonary edema: A rare disease? *JAMA* 1975; 234:491–495.

554. Recavarren S. The preterminal arterioles in the pulmonary circulation of high altitude natives. *Circulation* 1966; 33:177–180.

555. Hultgren HN, Robinson MC, Wuerflein RD. Over-perfusion pulmonary edema. *Circulation* 1966; 34(suppl 3):132–138.

556. Duberstein JL, Kaufman DM. A clinical study of an epidemic of heroin intoxication and heroin-induced pulmonary edema. *Am J Med* 1971; 51:704–714.

557. Paranthaman SK, Khan F. Acute cardiomyopathy with recurrent pulmonary edema and hypotension following heroin overdosage. *Chest* 1976; 69:117–119.

558. Kuida H, Hinshaw LB, Bilbert RP, Gilbert RP, Visscher MB. Effect of gram-negative endotoxin on pulmonary circulation. *Am J Physiol* 1958; 192:335–344.

559. Theodore J, Robin ED. Pathogenesis of neurogenic pulmonary edema. *Lancet* 1975; 2:749–751.

560. Packer M, ed. Physiologic determinants of survival in congestive heart failure. *Circulation* 1987; 75(suppl IV):IV1–IV3.

561. McKee PA, Castelli WP, McNamara PM, Kannel WB. The natural history of congestive heart failure: The Framingham Study. *N Engl J Med* 1971; 285:1441–1446.

562. Kannel WB, Savage D, Castelli WP. Cardiac failure in the Framingham Study: Twenty-year follow-up. In: Braunwald E, Mock MB, Watson JT, eds. *Congestive Heart Failure: Current Research and Clinical Applications.* New York: Grune & Stratton; 1982;15–30.

563. Rector TS, Cohn JN. Chronic heart failure: Incidence, prognosis, and the effects of medical interventions. In: Kapoor AS, Singh BN, eds. *Prognosis and Risk Assessment in Cardiovascular Disease.* New York: Churchill Livingstone; 1993:283–289.

564. Cohn JN, Levine TB, Olivari MT, Garberg V, Lura D, Francis GS, et al. Plasma norepinephrine as a guide to prognosis in patients with chronic congestive heart failure. *N Engl J Med* 1984; 311:819–823.

565. Swedberg K, Eneroth P, Kjekshus J, Wilhelmsen L. Hormones regulating cardiovascular function in patients with severe congestive heart failure and their relations to mortality. *Circulation* 1990; 82:1730–1736.

22

ASSESSMENT OF CARDIAC FUNCTION AND MYOCARDIAL CONTRACTILITY

John Ross, Jr.

In evaluating the patient with cardiac dysfunction, a high index of suspicion about the underlying pathophysiologic process (after careful clinical examination and routine tests) will aid greatly in the selection of any additional procedures that may be needed to establish a diagnosis or to direct therapy. Before discussing the use of special tests and their application to selected clinical problems, we shall consider first some general concepts about overall failure of the heart, myocardial failure, and the effects of altered loading conditions on cardiac function.

IS HEART FAILURE PRESENT OR NOT?

Failure of the heart as a pump (*overall heart failure*) is not synonymous with *myocardial failure*.

Overall Heart Failure (Failure of the Pump)

Ideally, at least two measures are desirable to determine the effects of heart failure on the tissues of the body: (1) the amount of blood pumped per minute relative to body surface area (the cardiac index) and (2) the pressures behind the pumping chambers (ventricular "filling pressures," reflected either by the mean atrial or the ventricular end-diastolic pressures) both at rest and during stress.

In clinical terms, failure of the right side of the heart at rest is evidenced by the presence of an elevated right-sided filling pressure (mean venous pressure 8 cmH_2O or greater) in the resting state, which may be associated with signs of congestion (peripheral edema, hepatomegaly, ascites). Left-sided heart failure at rest is evidenced by the presence of an abnormally elevated filling pressure on the left side of the heart, sufficient to cause pulmonary venous congestion on the chest roentgenogram; this may be associated with pulmonary rales or pleural effusion. A low cardiac index (2.4 L/min per square meter or less) would provide supportive evidence of overall heart failure at rest.

Further identification of overall heart failure is provided by inability of the heart to produce a normal increase in cardiac output during exercise with a reduction of maximum oxygen uptake ($\dot{V}_{O_2max}$).[1] Such impaired responses to exercise are often associated with an abnormal increase in the right- or left-sided filling pressures or both during exercise. The finding of impaired functional capacity, reflected by a reduced maximal oxygen consumption determined noninvasively during exercise, also signifies overall heart failure, since this measure correlates with the cardiac output and indicates that *cardiac reserve* is impaired.[2] However, it has been shown that some patients with poor left ventricular function at rest (ejection fraction below 30 percent) can exhibit good exercise capacity and oxygen uptake during a graded treadmill exercise test, whereas others with normal resting ventricular function can have impaired exercise performance.[2] Therefore, the presence of *abnormal ventricular function* at rest does not necessarily indicate that overall heart failure is present, nor does the absence of overall cardiac failure necessarily mean that ventricular function is normal.

The above descriptions of overall, or circulatory, heart failure say nothing about the *cause* of the failure; with such a broad description, heart failure may be due to such diverse etiologies as generalized myocardial disease, mitral stenosis, chronic pulmonary disease, or constrictive pericarditis. Nevertheless, such descriptions provide a starting point for the identification of right- and left-sided heart failure or both, from which one may proceed to determine whether or not signs of overall heart failure are due to myocardial disease, mechanical factors, or both. Regardless of cause, the manifestations of heart failure may be aggravated by other conditions such as fever, anemia, dysrhythmia, fluid overload, or metabolic disorders (see also Chap. 23).

Myocardial Failure

Depression of myocardial function (reduced myocardial contractility or inotropic state) constitutes *one cause* of overall heart failure. Myocardial failure has been described using various frameworks.[3] It can be defined as the inability of each unit of muscle in the ventricle to shorten a normal distance at a normal velocity against a normal level of systolic load (afterload); it can also be described as the inability of the left ventricle to develop pressure or tension to a normal level and at a normal rate during isovolumetric contraction. The direct causes of most forms of myocardial failure remain unknown, but a few can be identified, such as acute depression of contractility produced by myocarditis, certain drugs, acidosis, or ischemia; chronic depression of contractility can be caused by scarring or patchy myofibrillar loss or damage to muscle cells caused by inflammation and other processes. Myocardial failure ensues from sustained overloads on the myocardium due to either loss of myocardium (e.g., myocardial infarction) or abnormal pressure or volume overload on the ventricles.

Most commonly, the clinical problem is to determine whether or not *basal myocardial contractility is depressed* in hearts of greatly differing sizes or in the same heart at different points in time under different loading conditions (for example, in serial studies after cardiac valve replacement).[4] To compare one heart with another, it is necessary to "normalize," or to correct for a given initial heart size. Therefore, when used to detect depressed contractility, systolic function is usually expressed as percentage change of the diastolic volume produced by systole (the ejection fraction), as discussed subsequently.

Ideally, systolic loading on the ventricles (afterload) should also be known and expressed in normalized terms, since the afterload affects wall shortening. Systolic pressure in the aorta or the left ventricle is often used to provide an index of afterload, but a variation of the Laplace equation should be applied, if possible, to define force per unit of cross-sectional area of the ventricular wall (wall stress). Thus, it is generally recognized that a large, thin-walled ventricle maintaining a normal systolic pressure in the resting state is carrying a higher than normal systolic wall stress, whereas a ventricle that is concentrically hypertrophied may be creating a very high systolic pressure but carrying a normal level of systolic wall stress. Under some circumstances, excessive cardiac loading conditions alone can produce failure of the heart as a pump, as in aortic stenosis, even though myocardial contractility may not be depressed.[4] Under other circumstances, favorable loading conditions and/or compensatory events may *mask* the presence of depressed myocardial contractility, as in mitral regurgitation.[4] In addition, impaired cardiac filling due to a variety of causes (e.g., diastolic dysfunction) can produce changes in overall cardiac performance without impaired myocardial systolic function. Finally, severe segmental contraction disorders can coexist with areas of supranormal regional contraction to yield normal overall cardiac function.

These general categories of *dissociation* between cardiac pump function and myocardial contractility are summarized in Table 22-1.

Heart Failure without Myocardial Failure

MECHANICAL OVERLOAD AND AFTERLOAD MISMATCH

The level of contractility or inotropic state of the myocardium significantly affects the behavior of the heart. It is useful to distinguish *cardiac performance* from *myocardial contractility* per se, since performance is also importantly influenced by the interplay between preload and afterload. In making this distinction, however, it is important to recognize that changes in resting fiber length can directly affect contractility—so-called length-dependent activation.[5] Examples of how cardiac performance can be greatly impaired by mechanical overload are severe acute hypertension or sudden aortic regurgitation, which can quickly lead to left ventricular pump failure without myocardial depression (Table 22-1); this situation can be described within a framework termed *afterload mismatch with limited preload reserve*.[6] Afterload mismatch can be simply defined as inability of the ventricle operating at any stable level of inotropic state to maintain a normal forward stroke volume against the prevailing systolic load.

Afterload mismatch tends to occur when preload reserve is unavailable and the ventricle is therefore unable to compensate for altered afterload (Table 22-2). Thus, when the normal

---

TABLE 22-1

DISSOCIATIONS BETWEEN PUMP FUNCTION AND MYOCARDIAL FUNCTION

OVERALL HEART FAILURE WITHOUT MYOCARDIAL FAILURE

Acute mechanical overload
    Acute cor pulmonale
    Malignant hypertension
    Acute volume overload (valvular regurgitation)
Chronic severe overload
    High cardiac output states (Paget's disease, beriberi)
    Valvular and congenital heart disease
Impaired cardiac filling
    Pericardial restriction
    Restrictive myocardial disease
    Mechanical obstruction (mitral and tricuspid stenosis, tumor)
    Tachycardias
Low cardiac output due to heart block or bradycardia

MYOCARDIAL FAILURE WITHOUT OVERALL HEART FAILURE

Systolic unloading of the ventricle
    Mitral regurgitation
    Vasodilator drugs
Compensated myocardial failure
Segmental contraction disorders
    Transient myocardial ischemia
    Myocardial infarction

TABLE 22-2

FACTORS CAUSING LIMITED PRELOAD RESERVE THAT PREDISPOSE TO AFTERLOAD MISMATCH

Peripheral	Cardiac
Venous return held constant experimentally	Acute volume loading to limit of ventricular filling
Venous return limited by peripheral factors	Chronic cardiac dilation
	Increased impedance to cardiac filling

heart is pushed to the limit of its preload reserve, a further increase in afterload (as by acute hypertension, which leads to augmentation of systolic wall stress) can produce a reduction in wall shortening and in the forward stroke volume of the left ventricle (Fig. 22-1). This situation resembles that in the normal heart under experimental circumstances, where the preload is controlled and held constant and only the afterload is varied; there is an *inverse* relation between the systolic pressure and the stroke volume.[7] Similarly, if aortic pressure is increased in the failing heart when preload reserve is fully utilized, the ventricle cannot compensate and stroke volume falls,[8] yielding an apparent descending limb of function due to afterload mismatch (Fig. 22-1). That is, the failing ventricle behaves *as if its preload were fixed,* and any increase in systolic pressure induces afterload mismatch. Afterload mismatch can also occur in the normal heart when a vasopressor drug is administered and the venous return is inadequate to allow the ventricle to maintain stroke volume.[9] Reflex venodilation or other peripheral regulatory factors may be responsible for such responses, which in the normal or failing heart can lead to displacement of the function curve relating stroke volume to end-diastolic volume upward or downward by decreases or increases in afterload, respectively, rather than by changes in myocardial contractility.[9] Finally, afterload mismatch can occur even without intervention when the failing ventricle is unable to deliver a normal stroke volume at the prevailing level of normal aortic pressure.[4,6] Thus, under conditions in which the reserve provided by increasing preload is limited or unavailable, the *stroke volume becomes inversely related to the afterload.* An apparent "descending limb" of ventricular function under these conditions is undoubtedly due primarily to excess afterload (afterload mismatch) rather than to sarcomere overstretch.[4–6] These principles are illustrated in Fig. 22-1, using two different schemes for describing cardiac function (ventricular function curves and pressure-volume loops with end-systolic pressure-volume relations). Of course, all of these responses, which reflect alterations in ventricular performance due to induced changes in loading, can be altered by inducing changes in the inotropic state. In *acute* overall heart failure due to *afterload mismatch* (apparent descending limb, point *D,* Fig. 22-1), reduction of the overload by vasodilator therapy or by replacement of a defective valve with a prosthesis should promptly reverse the pump failure,

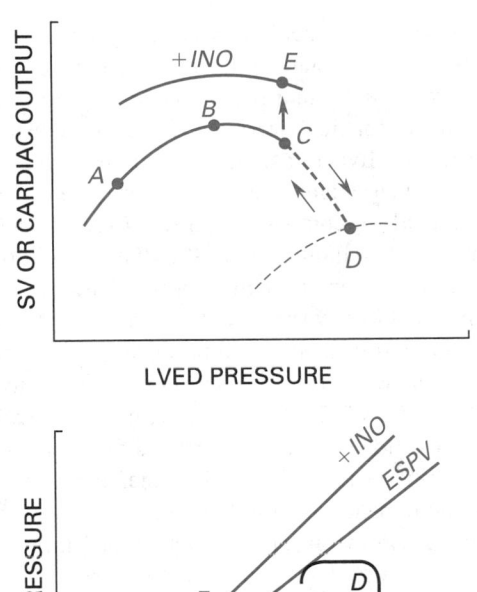

FIGURE 22-1

Two different frameworks for describing ventricular function and the effects of afterload mismatch and alterations in contractility. *Upper panel:* Relation between left ventricular (LV) end-diastolic (LVED) pressure and stroke volume (SV) or cardiac output in the presence of mild depression of ventricular function but with considerable preload reserve. Points *A* to *B* show the effects of a volume load: the stroke volume and cardiac output increase. Points *B* to *C* show the response to a small dose of a vasopressor, such as angiotensin II or phenylephrine, and points *C* to *D* show the effect of a high dose of vasopressor: a marked increase in LV systolic pressure and an apparent descending limb of cardiac function [increased LVED pressure with decreased stroke volume, as the LV reaches the limit of preload reserve (heavy dashed line to point *D*)]. Reduction of the aortic pressure (correction of afterload mismatch) would move the ventricle back to point *C.* Point *D* may also be seen as operation of the ventricle on a downwardly displaced "cardiac output curve," the curve being displaced by the effects of increased resistance to ventricular ejection. Also seen are the effects of a positive inotropic drug (+INO), administered at point *C,* which shifts the function curve upward, allowing the delivery of a larger stroke volume or cardiac output from the same LVED pressure (point *E*). *Lower panel:* Diagram of the same responses in another framework: LV pressure-volume loops and the linear end-systolic pressure-volume relation (ESPVR).[7] The curved lower line represents the diastolic pressure-volume relation. Beat *A* is a control contraction (corresponding to point *A* in upper diagram), showing the counterclockwise loop during LV isovolumetric contraction, ejection, and isovolumetric relaxation; the stroke volume (SV) is indicated. With volume loading, there is a mild pressure increase as the ventricle moves to beat *B.* With infusion of a vasopressor in low dose, the ventricle moves to point *C* and continues to reach the linear ESPV relation at end ejection; the stroke volume drops slightly (point *C*). With a marked pressor stress (beat *D*), the ventricle reaches the limit of its preload reserve; it cannot compensate for the increased systolic pressure and the stroke volume drops markedly (beat *D,* corresponding to point *D* in the upper panel). This response is due to afterload mismatch and not to change in myocardial contractility. The effect of a positive inotropic agent (+INO) to shift the linear ESPVR upward and to the left is shown, and the stroke volume increases (beat *E* compared to beat *C*); notice that the slope of the ESPVR (E_{max}) is increased by augmentation of contractility.

since myocardial contractility is basically intact.[6] Augmentation of the inotropic state with a positive inotropic drug will further improve ventricular performance (Fig. 22-1, point *E*).

In *chronic* mechanical overload, such as that due to valvular heart disease or hypertension, adaptations occur primarily through the development of concentric or eccentric hypertrophy, which tends to compensate for the overload and to prevent overall cardiac failure. In most of these conditions, heart failure does not occur until myocardial damage supervenes due to long-standing overload and hypertrophy. As discussed subsequently, aortic stenosis can produce afterload mismatch and heart failure *without* irreversible depression of myocardial contractility (Fig. 22-2). Less is known about heart failure due to the overload of high-output states, such as Paget's disease or beriberi, although it is likely that in these conditions, altered sodium balance with fluid retention can lead to a congested state in the absence of myocardial failure.

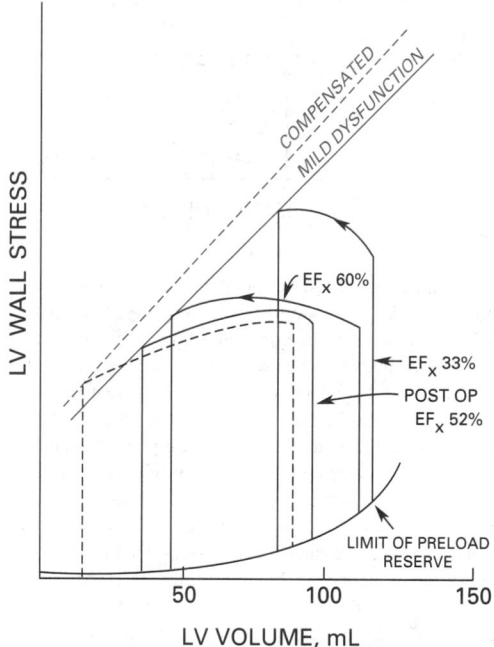

FIGURE 22-2

Diagrammatic examples of left ventricular (LV) function in valvular aortic stenosis. Loops of LV volume versus wall stress are shown during single contractions. The curved relation between diastolic LV volume and wall stress is also shown, along with the linear end-systolic wall stress–volume relation. In compensated aortic stenosis (*dashed lines*), the LV volume and the LV wall stress–volume loop are normal, with a fall of wall stress during ejection and a normal level of systolic wall stress despite elevated systolic pressure, due to concentric LV hypertrophy (see text). With development of mild depression of myocardial contractility, the linear end-systolic relation is shifted somewhat to the right, the left ventricle enlarges to encroach on its preload reserve, and the wall stress rises somewhat during ejection, although the ejection fraction (EF_x) is well maintained at 60 percent. With further progression of critical stenosis, the ventricle reaches the limit of its preload reserve, the wall stress rises markedly during ejection as the ventricle is unable to unload itself, and the stroke volume drops sharply ($EF_x = 33$ percent). This response is due to afterload mismatch, not to further depression of myocardial contractility. Following aortic valve replacement, there is persistence of mild depression of myocardial contractility, but the afterload mismatch is corrected and the ejection fraction returns to near normal postoperatively ($EF_x = 52$ percent).

IMPAIRED CARDIAC FILLING

There is ample evidence that impaired cardiac filling of various types can lead to heart failure (Table 22-1).

Pericardial Restraint

It has been well documented that decreased forward cardiac output and elevation of cardiac filling pressures are often associated with normal systolic function in chronic constrictive pericarditis and in acute cardiac tamponade.[10] There is also experimental evidence that acute volume overload, as by overtransfusion, can cause elevated cardiac filling pressures and impaired filling of the left side of the heart due to limitation of pericardial expansion as the right side of the heart overfills.[10] This response is associated with elevation of the *intrapericardial pressures,* with *apparent* depression of the ventricular function curve. It also leads to a shift upward of the entire diastolic pressure-volume relation of the left and right ventricles, due to changes of intrapericardial pressure, and the shift can be corrected by the use of a vasodilator such as nitroprusside.[10] Such responses may explain acute shifts downward of the left ventricular diastolic pressure-volume relation observed clinically with vasodilators,[11] and elevated intrapericardial pressures could play a role in producing the high filling pressures in severe acute heart failure (see Chap. 21).

Diastolic Myocardial Dysfunction

Ventricular relaxation reflects an active process of Ca^{2+} reuptake that is also influenced by loading conditions and nonuniformity.[12] When abnormally slow, it affects primarily early ventricular filling, reflected on the Doppler tracing by reduction of peak early mitral inflow velocity, often with a compensatory increase in the late velocity during atrial contraction (i.e., a decrease in the E to A ratio) (see Chap. 14).[13] Increased ventricular chamber stiffness (reduced compliance) also diminishes peak early inflow velocity, but it also reduces peak late velocity during atrial contraction due to the increased impedance to atrial emptying.[13] Impaired relaxation shifts the early portion of the ventricular diastolic pressure-volume curve upward, in association with a decreased maximum rate of left ventricular pressure fall during isovolumetric relaxation, as occurs in acute regional ischemia of the left ventricle induced by exercise.[14] On the other hand, increased chamber stiffness typically steepens and displaces the entire ventricular diastolic pressure-volume curve upward, as in severe left ventricular hypertrophy or chronic coronary heart disease.[13] Noninvasive techniques may allow differentiation between myocardial restrictive and pericardial constrictive disease, but sometimes cardiac catheterization is required[15] (see also Chap. 21). Restrictive disease of the ventricular chambers, such as in amyloidosis, can lead to elevated diastolic ventricular and atrial pressures, often with normal systolic contractile function of the myocardium[15] (Chap. 75).

Mechanical Obstruction to Ventricular Filling

Mitral and tricuspid valve stenosis, cor triatriatum, fibrosing mediastinitis, and intraatrial clots or tumors can cause impaired ventricular filling and lead to pulmonary or systemic venous hypertension.

Arrhythmias

Very rapid ventricular and atrial tachyarrhythmias, including atrial fibrillation, can cause marked reduction of the time per minute for diastolic ventricular filling along with inappropriate timing or loss of atrial systole, which can lead to elevated cardiac filling pressures and a fall in cardiac output. Also, marked bradyarrhythmias can impair the cardiac output. All of these conditions, which impair or limit cardiac filling in diastole (Table 22-1), can produce signs of overall heart failure despite relatively normal systolic function of the ventricular myocardium—that is, a dissociation between cardiac pump function and myocardial contractility—a condition termed *diastolic dysfunction* or *diastolic heart failure*.

Myocardial Failure without Heart Failure

As might be anticipated, the converse of afterload mismatch can occur when the preload is adequate but the afterload or wall stress on the myocardial fibers is abnormally low. This may occur in mitral regurgitation, in which the low-impedance leak into the left atrium early in systole may result in maintenance of a normal ejection fraction until late in the clinical course, when depression of myocardial contractility has already occurred.[16] As the ventricle ejects blood into the atrium, volume decreases, which reduces load and speeds contraction further. Thus, favorable loading conditions can mask depressed contractility, which, under normal loading conditions, would produce a low ejection fraction (Fig. 22-3).

Favorable loading conditions can be produced by treatment of the failing heart with a vasodilator drug that lowers the afterload during ejection[17] (Table 22-1). Experimental studies indicate that in acute heart failure, favorable effects of a vasodilator such as nitroprusside on the cardiac output result from both decreased afterload and peripheral circulatory effects. In this setting, left ventricular unloading by nitroprusside produces a large shift of blood volume from the distended central circulation to the peripheral bed, which is sufficient to counterbalance the peripheral pooling of blood due to the drug's dilating action on the veins. This shift of blood volume allows the venous return to increase and, when coupled with reduced resistance to ventricular ejection and afterload, which shift the ventricular function curve upward, leads to an increase in the output of the failing heart by the vasodilator.[18] Overall heart failure may thereby be relieved, despite severe persistent depression of myocardial contractility.

WHICH SPECIAL PROCEDURE SHOULD BE SELECTED?

Special diagnostic procedures to identify and quantify cardiac dysfunction or myocardial failure must be selected with careful regard to the question being asked as well as the overall safety, usefulness, and cost of each procedure (Table 22-3). For example, if the question can be answered by an extremely safe, noninvasive procedure such as echocardiography or treadmill exercise testing, there is little reason to use a more expensive procedure that requires intravenous injection of a radioisotope. If the problem is to evaluate symptoms and the degree of functional impairment in a patient with heart disease of known etiology, then an exercise test for functional capacity or for ischemic changes on the electrocardiogram (ECG) may be all that is needed to guide therapy. If the problem is to confirm a suspected diagnosis of depressed left ventricular function due to primary myocardial disease, an echocardiogram may provide an adequate answer as well as information about whether valvular heart disease, hypertrophic cardiomyopathy, pericardial disease, or restrictive myocardial disease can be implicated. Doppler studies with color mapping can

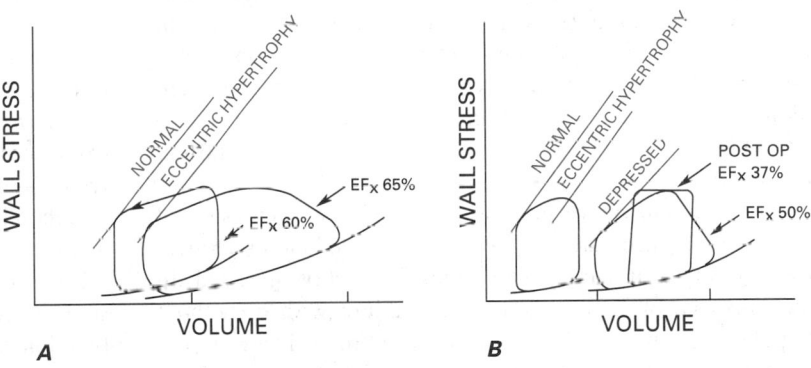

FIGURE 22-3

Diagrammatic examples of left ventricular (LV) function in mitral regurgitation. *A.* Volume overload hypertrophy (eccentric hypertrophy) causes displacement to the right of the curved diastolic pressure–volume relation and the linear end-systolic volume–wall stress relation, and the loop of a single LV contraction (volume versus wall stress) shows delivery of a very large total stroke volume. Because of the low-impedance leak into the left atrium, the ejection fraction is maintained at high-normal level (EF_x = 65 percent). *B.* The development of markedly and irreversibly depressed myocardial contractility shifts the linear end-systolic volume–wall stress relation downward and to the right. In this setting, prior to mitral valve replacement, the ventricle can still maintain a relatively low mean systolic wall stress, wall stress being reduced in particular early and late during ejection because of the regurgitant leak; therefore the total stroke volume remains high and ejection fraction is only mildly reduced (EF_x = 50 percent). Following mitral valve replacement, despite some reduction in end-diastolic volume in this example, the LV must now eject entirely into the aorta with its high impedance of the aorta, the wall stress early and late during ejection rises, and the ejection fraction falls (postoperative EF_x = 37 percent). This postoperative response, the opposite of that in the patient with aortic stenosis (Fig. 22-2), may be due to altered systolic loading conditions rather than a change in myocardial contractility produced by the operation. However, recent studies in patients generally having less severe LV myocardial dysfunction indicate that mitral valve replacement with chordal preservation, as well as primary mitral valve repair, may preserve LV function postoperatively without a significant fall in the LV ejection fraction. (From Ross J Jr. Left ventricular function and the timing of surgical treatment of valvular heart disease. *Ann Intern Med* 1981; 94:498. Modified and reproduced with permission from the publisher and author.)

TABLE 22-3

POTENTIAL STEPS IN ASSESSING VENTRICULAR DYSFUNCTION

Exercise capacity
Echocardiography
   Two-dimensional, M mode for ventricular size; ejection phase indexes; Doppler studies
Radionuclide angiography for ejection fraction
Balloon catheterization of right side of the heart
   Cardiac output, filling pressures, systemic vascular resistance
Formal cardiac catheterization
   Hemodynamic variables; quantitative ventriculography; ejection fraction (isovolumic phase indexes); coronary arteriography

also provide quantitative information about the location and severity of valve lesions. If, for technical reasons, the echocardiogram is not conclusive for evaluating the degree of left ventricular dysfunction, a radionuclide angiographic determination of the ejection fraction provides an appropriate next step. If assessment of the level of global left ventricular dysfunction in coronary artery disease is necessary when regional wall motion abnormalities are present or suspected, the nongeometric technique of radionuclide ventriculography is a more reliable first step. The noninvasive tomographic technique of magnetic resonance imaging of the ventricle is used in some centers for assessing global and regional ventricular function.[19]

If such noninvasive tests do not provide a diagnosis that is sufficiently accurate to allow effective medical or surgical therapy, then cardiac catheterization is usually indicated. In the presence of acute, severe heart failure with or without hypotension and sometimes in severe chronic heart failure, right-sided heart catheterization with measurement of pulmonary artery wedge pressure in the intensive care setting may be highly useful, both in the diagnosis of causative factors and in guiding the responses to acute therapy. A common problem in this regard is to decide how much overall ventricular dysfunction is due to primary myocardial failure and how much is due to an excessive load that might be relieved by surgical intervention.

Assessment of Overall Heart Failure

In evaluating symptoms of severe dyspnea, orthopnea, or edema, special procedures are usually not required for identifying the presence of right- or left-sided heart failure at rest. Knowledge of the cardiac output is generally not required, and filling pressures can be estimated from the venous pressure and chest radiograph.

EXERCISE CAPACITY

By the use of a treadmill or bicycle ergometer, exercise capacity can be determined from the maximum workload that the patient is able to achieve. The $\dot{V}_{O_2}$ when the patient performs a truly maximum effort is the best indicator of overall cardiac function, since it equals the product of the maximum cardiac output and the maximum arteriovenous O_2 difference. Noninvasive measurement of respiratory gas exchange during exercise has provided a useful approach for characterizing cardiac functional class based on the $\dot{V}_{O_2\text{max}}$; class A (normal) exceeds 20 mL/min per kilogram; class B is 16 to 20 mL/min per kilogram; class C is 10 to 15 mL/min per kilogram; and class D is below 10 mL/min per kilogram.[20] In class D patients, for example, there is an inability to increase the stroke volume during exercise, although the resting cardiac output is reduced to the same degree as in class C patients.[20] $\dot{V}_{O_2\text{max}}$ in METS (multiple of resting $\dot{V}_{O_2}$) can also be estimated from the workload performed, and this can provide a useful clinical estimate of functional capacity. Determination of the exercise capacity can be highly useful for objectively evaluating the significance of symptoms in patients with chronic cardiomyopathy or chronic valvular heart disease, even though it is not possible in the latter instance to determine the relative contributions of myocardial dysfunction, hemodynamic abnormalities due to the valve disease, or inadequate peripheral vasodilatation, as occurs in late failure. (In severe aortic stenosis exercise testing is usually avoided.) Exercise testing can also be valuable for following responses to various forms of treatment, such as vasodilator therapy in chronic heart failure, or for reaching decisions concerning cardiac transplantation.[20]

The response to exercise is determined primarily by the exercise-induced increase in cardiac output, but many other factors—including adaptations in the skeletal muscles and the peripheral vascular bed, cardiovascular reflexes, motivation, and drug therapy—also are operative. It is therefore not surprising that good functional capacity has been reported in some individuals who have markedly impaired left ventricular function at rest and vice versa.[2,21] For example, Franciosa et al.[21] reported some patients with ejection fractions of only 25 percent who were able to exercise for 17 min and others with normal ejection fractions who had exercise times of less than 5 min (see also Chap. 15).

RIGHT-SIDED HEART CATHETERIZATION

Catheterization of the pulmonary artery by the Swan-Ganz technique may be useful for evaluation and management of severe overall heart failure in certain clinical settings. This approach is frequently employed for evaluating severe heart failure and guiding therapy in acute myocardial infarction,[22] particularly when it is complicated by hypotension. For example, exclusion of relative hypovolemia as a cause of hypotension and low cardiac output together with a test of left ventricular function can be performed by using a small volume load (a 200- to 300-mL dextrose infusion) and measuring the response of the cardiac output, stroke volume, or stroke work index relative to the accompanying rise in pulmonary artery wedge pressure. A flat or descending relation indicates that left ventricular function is severely depressed with maximum use of the preload reserve. Catheterization of the right side of the heart in the intensive care unit is also sometimes indicated to quantitate chronic refractory heart failure; it may be invaluable for selecting an appropriate vasodilator or other agent and monitoring its initial hemodynamic effects.[22]

ASSESSMENT OF MYOCARDIAL FAILURE

The most common type of ventricular dysfunction is depressed systolic contraction due to reduced shortening of myocardial fibers. The first step is the *detection* of such an abnormality; then further steps may be needed to define its cause (e.g., overload due to valvular disease or primary myocardial failure). In chronic disease, such an abnormality is almost always accompanied by diastolic enlargement of the ventricle. Less commonly, systolic function is preserved and diastolic dysfunction (increased myocardial stiffness, pericardial disease) is responsible for high filling pressures. Often, the basic problem is to distinguish reduced ventricular performance due to mechanical abnormalities from that due to myocardial failure. Several measures of ventricular function, obtained by a variety of methods, can be used for this purpose.

CONTRACTILITY INDICES

For evaluating *basal contractility* in many types of heart disease, it is *not* necessary to rely on hemodynamic indices of contractility that are independent of preload and afterload. In effect, when preload reserve has been fully utilized, depressed myocardial contractility will result in an "afterload mismatch" in the resting state, which will be expressed by inability of the ventricle to maintain normal performance *per unit* of its circumference or volume. In this setting, the afterload (wall stress) may be somewhat increased (and may contribute further to impaired performance), but this increase occurs *because* depressed myocardial function has produced chamber enlargement. Therefore, measurement of normalized ejecting performance will effectively detect depressed myocardial contractility.

In the resting state, the so-called indices of the ejection phase based on measurements of the left ventricular chamber size are perhaps the *most useful and practical* means of detecting depressed myocardial function. Such indices include the percentage of the end-diastolic volume that is ejected (the *ejection fraction,* for which 55 percent is the lower limit of normal), the percentage shortening of the ventricular end-diastolic diameter (the *fractional shortening,* for which the lower limit of normal is 28 percent), and the mean velocity of internal diameter or circumferential fiber (CF) shortening, the *mean* V_{CF} (lower limit of normal is 1.2 circumferences per second). The ejection fraction is most commonly employed, and a reduced value measured in the resting state can usually detect depressed basal ventricular contractility. Like all of the "ejection phase" measures, it is particularly sensitive to *changes in afterload* and under some conditions may not reflect depressed basal myocardial contractility when the level of afterload is *low* or *high.* In the absence of excessive loading, the ejection phase indices effectively separate normal patients

from patients with clear-cut left ventricular myocardial disease.[23] The ejection phase measures have the advantage that they can be determined noninvasively by echocardiography or radionuclide angiography, and good agreement with measurements made from angiograms has been found.

Analyses of right ventricular function have been limited, primarily because of the complex shape of this chamber and the difficulty of computing right ventricular volumes angiographically. However, function can be estimated by echocardiography, and radionuclide techniques (nongeometric) have permitted assessment of the left and right ventricular ejection fractions at rest and during stress. At rest, the lower limit of normal of the right ventricular ejection fraction is approximately 40 to 43 percent.[24]

In chronic, compensated valvular heart disease or chronic hypertension, the left ventricular wall undergoes hypertrophy of the volume or pressure overload type, so that the mean systolic wall stress is often maintained at relatively normal or only mildly elevated levels.[25] In sudden aortic or mitral regurgitation, in acute hypertension, or with long-standing severe hypertension, the ejection phase measures may become unreliable for evaluating myocardial contractility, since a reduced ejection fraction can be due to afterload mismatch (Table 22-1). Alternatively, the systolic unloading of the left ventricle in chronic mitral regurgitation may yield a normal or near normal ejection fraction even when myocardial contractility is depressed (Fig. 22-3).[16] Under such circumstances, *limitations* of the ejection phase measures for identifying impaired myocardial contractility *must be recognized.* If measurement of the degree of depression of myocardial contractility or lack thereof is desired, normalized ventricular performance can be examined at the operating level of systolic *wall stress* and compared with the performance of the normal ventricle at a comparable level of wall stress.

Calculation of wall stress remains largely a research technique,[25,26] although it can be done in simple terms noninvasively using echocardiography.[27] On the other hand, it is rarely necessary to determine wall stress for effective clinical management if one keeps in mind the above caveats about loading conditions. Several techniques have been described for assessing myocardial contractility under abnormal loading conditions using analysis of wall stress. Some involve determining the inverse relation between afterload and a normalized measure of systolic function (such as velocity or stroke volume) over a range of loading conditions in the normal heart and then comparing the function of the heart in question with the normal relationship.[6] One such approach used clinically compares a given value of end-systolic wall stress and fractional shortening to a plot of the normal inverse relationship measured in a large group of normal subjects (Fig. 22-4).[28] Also, the slope of the linear relationship between left ventricular end-systolic volume and end-systolic pressure (E_{max}) or wall stress determined by acutely changing loading conditions with nitroprusside, phenylephrine, or angiotensin has been used to define normal and depressed basal contractility (see Fig. 22-2).[26,29-31]

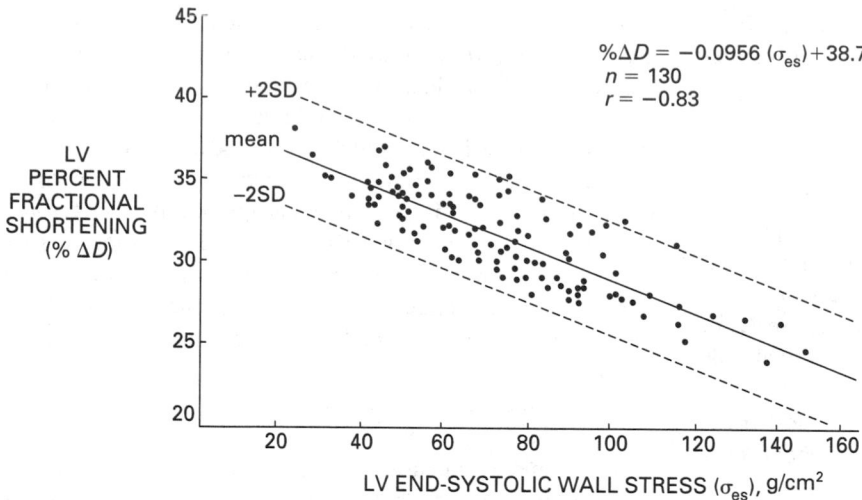

FIGURE 22-4

Example of one approach, employed by Borow et al.,[28] for defining basal myocardial contractility when systolic loading conditions are abnormal. Shown are the relations between left ventricular (LV) fractional shortening (percentage change of LV internal diameter, *D*, determined by echocardiography) over a range of LV end-systolic wall stress values. The LV systolic pressure and wall stress were varied in these normal patients by graded infusions of phenylephrine to produce the linear regression shown (standard deviations indicated). Using such a plot, a patient with normal end-systolic wall stress (70 g/cm², for example) in the resting state could be characterized as having myocardial failure if the fractional shortening were below approximately 30 percent. Alternatively, in a patient with aortic stenosis in whom the end-systolic wall stress is elevated (120 g/cm²), fractional shortening might be below 25 percent, but this reduction is due to afterload mismatch rather than to depressed myocardial contractility (see also Fig. 22-1). (From Borow RM, Greene LH, Grossman W, Braunwald E. Left ventricular end-systolic stress-shortening and stress-length relations in humans. *Am J Cardiol* 1982; 50:1301. Reproduced with permission from the publisher and author.)

NONINVASIVE METHODS

Echocardiography (two-dimensional and M-mode) is the most common method employed for assessing global and regional myocardial function; it also allows identification of mechanical cardiac disorders and provides clues to impaired filling. Diastolic dysfunction is signaled by abnormal Doppler indexes, as described earlier; reduced E-F slope of the mitral valve on echo; and by left atrial enlargement. Chamber enlargement can be confirmed (left ventricular end-diastolic size is increased if the dimension is over 5.6 cm or 3.2 cm/m² body surface area). All of the above-mentioned ejection phase indexes of contractility can be calculated, including fractional shortening and ejection fraction, together with chamber wall thickness, left ventricular end-diastolic volume, and myocardial mass (Chap. 14). Radionuclide angiography (Chap. 17) is particularly suitable for determining the ejection fraction of the ventricles,[32] and it correlates well with angiography. Measurements of absolute ventricular volumes and diastolic filling rates have also been reported.[33] Radionuclide ventriculography is a reliable approach for obtaining serial ejection fraction values when needed [as in following a patient under treatment with doxorubicin (Adriamycin)]. This approach is valuable when technically adequate echo studies cannot be obtained, as, for example, in chronic obstructive pulmonary disease or when assessment of global function independent of ventricular geometry and regional wall motion is needed

in the presence of coronary heart disease, as in the predischarge assessment of a patient following acute myocardial infarction. An abnormal response (less than 5 percent increase) in the left or right ventricular ejection fraction during exercise occurs during regional myocardial ischemia in patients with coronary heart disease, but it may not be specific for ischemia.[32]

CARDIAC CATHETERIZATION AND ANGIOGRAPHY

In the evaluation of cardiac and myocardial dysfunction, because of expense and some risk to the patient (Chap. 16), formal cardiac catheterization and coronary arteriography are undertaken only when a precise diagnosis is critical to the selection of appropriate medical or surgical therapy and when that diagnosis cannot be achieved by noninvasive techniques. Selective ventriculography using single or biplane left ventriculographic studies to calculate the ejection fraction or other ejection phase measures (Chap. 16) has long provided the standard for accurately quantifying the basal level of left ventricular size and function.[34] The normal ejection fraction is 0.55 or greater, and chamber enlargement can be identified, the upper limit of normal of left ventricular end-diastolic volume being 110 mL/m² body surface area (2 SD).[35]

High-fidelity pressure measurements together with volume and wall thickness calculations have also been used, largely as research tools, to study systolic wall stress,[36] diastolic filling rates,[37] diastolic stress-strain abnormalities,[38] and "isovolumic-phase indexes" of contractility.[39] Calculation of E_{max} as a load-independent measure of contractility (the slope of the relation between end-systolic pressure and end-systolic volume determined at several points by changing loading conditions) also remains largely a research tool, particularly for assessing chronic changes in myocardial contractility.[29–31] The simplest isovolumic index of myocardial contractility is the maximum rate of rise of left ventricular pressure (dP/dt_{max}), which should be determined with a catheter-tip micromanometer; when it is reduced below about 1400 mmHg/s, myocardial contractility is usually depressed. This measure is affected by other factors, particularly the preload. In the author's view, various other contractile indexes derived from isovolumic systole are generally less reliable than ejection phase indexes such as the ejection fraction in the individual patient. High-fidelity pressure tracings also allow the detection of impaired isovolumic left ventricular relaxation using the maximum rate of pressure fall ($-dP/dt_{min}$), or calculating the time constant of relaxation (tau).

MYOCARDIAL BIOPSY

When cardiac catheterization studies fail to reveal a specific cause for unexplained severe cardiac failure, myocardial biopsy (Chap. 25) can sometimes reveal evidence of an unsuspected infiltrative cardiomyopathy, microvascular disease, or evidence of inflammation. In the past the diagnostic yield of such myocardial biopsies has been relatively low, but more recently, with the use of electron microscopy and special staining techniques, a considerable number of patients with unexplained congestive heart failure have shown evidence of inflammation.[40]

HOW SHOULD SPECIAL PROCEDURES BE USED TO SOLVE SPECIFIC CLINICAL PROBLEMS?

Recognition of Mechanical Factors Sufficient to Cause Heart Failure

In assessing the patient who has clinical signs of acute or chronic overall heart failure, it is important to consider the possibility that *mechanical factors* rather than myocardial depression are primarily responsible (Table 22-1). Impaired cardiac filling due to pericardial disease, myocardial disease, or other cause should be carefully excluded, as discussed subsequently under "Recognition and Evaluation of Primary Myocardial Disease," below. In some patients, a mechanical cause for secondary heart failure may be relatively obvious, as in severe systemic hypertension, coarctation of the aorta, arteriovenous fistula due to trauma or other cause, or other high-output states such as hyperthyroidism (see Table 22-1). In those settings, extensive evaluation of the associated cardiac dysfunction may not be necessary, since treatment of the primary disorder will correct the cardiac problem. In other patients, a congenital defect or acquired valvular lesion capable of producing an excessive flow or pressure load on one or both ventricles may be suspected. If mechanical overload is present, it is then necessary to establish whether or not there is a *sufficiently severe* mechanical overload to cause secondary myocardial dysfunction.

Once the presence of a significant mechanical problem is established, it is usually possible to exclude or detect the presence of associated depressed myocardial contractility by noninvasive methods. The most useful screening approach is echocardiography, in which direct measurements of the left-sided chamber dimensions, and sometimes right ventricular size, are made. The left or right ventricular ejection fraction can also be determined by radionuclide angiography. In the presence of chronic volume overload, the finding of normal systolic contractile function by echocardiography or a normal radionuclide ejection fraction, despite the presence of a moderately increased ventricular end-diastolic dimension, usually indicates the absence of significant depression of myocardial contractility. An important exception occurs in chronic mitral regurgitation, as discussed in the next section, "Recognition of Myocardial Failure in Chronic Valvular Heart Disease," below. If

coronary artery disease and regional wall motion abnormalities coexist with valvular heart disease, the M-mode echocardiogram can be unreliable and calculation of left ventricular volumes by echocardiography may be feasible, or the ejection fraction may be determined by the radionuclide technique.

In heart failure due to sudden, severe volume overload that may occur consequent to infective endocarditis of the aortic or mitral valves, ruptured chordae tendineae, infarction of a papillary muscle, or ruptured interventricular septum, noninvasive studies should be performed and may provide clues to the mechanical cause of the heart failure as well as to the presence of severe ventricular dysfunction. Echocardiographic (by transthoracic or transesophageal techniques) studies may allow the identification of a flail mitral valve leaflet, ventricular septal defect, or vegetations on the aortic, mitral, or tricuspid valves (Chap. 14); when these investigations are coupled with pulsed color Doppler studies, the location of regurgitant leaks or ventricular septal rupture can be identified (Chap. 14). Diastolic fluttering of the anterior mitral valve leaflet may be noted in aortic valve regurgitation; with acute severe aortic regurgitation, preclosure of the mitral valve in middiastole may be identified (Chap. 14).

The echocardiogram or radionuclide ventriculogram will also allow identification of the reduction in fractional shortening and ejection fraction of the left ventricle that usually accompanies severe acute overload. This is often due primarily to full utilization of the preload reserve with acute afterload mismatch rather than to significant depression of myocardial contractility[6] and can occur with acute pressure overload (e.g., uncontrolled hypertension) as well as sudden volume overload (e.g., sudden aortic regurgitation). In the further diagnosis and treatment of heart failure due to sudden cardiac overload in the intensive care setting, the insertion of a balloon (Swan-Ganz) catheter is usually advisable to measure the wedge pressure, cardiac output, and vascular resistance; to search for a left-to-right shunt; and to guide vasodilator and other therapy.

Before one considers surgical treatment, full cardiac catheterization should usually be performed to ascertain the severity of the mechanical lesion and the state of the left ventricle as well as to examine the coronary arteries.[41]

Recognition of Myocardial Failure in Chronic Valvular Heart Disease

Valvular lesions that overload the left ventricle, such as aortic stenosis, aortic regurgitation, and mitral regurgitation, can, over time, produce severe left ventricular hypertrophy. Eventually, this is associated with myocardial fibrosis or other subcellular changes and left ventricular dysfunction.[42] Such dysfunction may persist even after surgical correction of the valve defect; patients with chronic valvular heart disease must therefore be carefully managed to avoid irreversible left ventricular dysfunction.[43] The types of special studies on the left ventricle and the frequency with which they should be performed vary somewhat among the three valvular lesions.

VALVULAR AORTIC STENOSIS

The adult with clinical features of significant aortic stenosis who develops symptoms of left ventricular dysfunction, syncope, or angina pectoris and in whom echocardiographic studies, including Doppler assessment of the aortic flow velocity (Chap. 14), suggest significant stenosis should have cardiac catheterization performed promptly (Chap. 63). Cardiac catheterization should document whether or not the aortic valve narrowing is significant (valve orifice area less than 0.75 cm^2 or 0.6 cm/m^2 body surface area are approximate guidelines)[43] and whether or not there is depressed left ventricular function. In male patients over 35 years of age and females over age 40, coronary angiography is usually indicated to search for significant coronary atherosclerosis.[41] Generally, if the stenosis is severe and symptoms are present, operation is undertaken, since the outlook with medical therapy is poor.[44] The adult patient who, following initial evaluation including echocardiography with Doppler study, does not have significant symptoms can be followed by clinical examination and watched closely for onset of symptoms, with the proviso that in some very active individuals with severe stenosis but few or no symptoms, operation may be warranted (see also Chap. 63).

If left ventricular function is found to be moderately depressed preoperatively, early studies found that ventricular function tends to return toward normal during the first 6 months postoperatively. In recent studies of patients with severe aortic stenosis and a left ventricular (LV) ejection fraction preoperatively below 50 percent (average, 38 percent), which included patients with coronary artery disease, the average LV ejection fraction did not improve at 1 week despite a fall in the average peak systolic wall stress, but the ejection fraction was normal at 6 months.[45] In a larger series with similarly low LV ejection fractions, 75 percent of patients showed improvement in the LV ejection fraction postoperatively, but the improvement was inversely related to the extent of coronary artery disease.[46] Late normalization of LV diastolic dysfunction, i.e., after 2 years and up to 7 years, has been shown to occur after correction of aortic stenosis and to correlate both with regression of hypertrophy and with the degree of interstitial fibrosis assessed by myocardial biopsy.[47]

Even in patients with severely depressed ventricular function preoperatively, the average ejection fraction can return to near normal or normal, although in some patients it remains depressed.[46] These findings suggest that effects due to mechanical overload per se (*afterload mismatch*), rather than irreversibly depressed myocardial contractility, are often primarily responsible for the reduced left ventricular function preoperatively.[43] The development of some dilation of the left ventricular chamber at end-diastole, with relative thinning of the ventricular wall and reduced fractional shortening, may be due to increasing severity of critical aortic stenosis as well as to early left ventricular decompensation with full utilization of the preload reserve. Further progression of the critical aortic stenosis will then result in afterload mismatch with a fall in the ejection fraction (Fig. 22-2).[43] In some patients, marked hypertrophy may result in impaired ventricular filling because of reduced ventricular compliance, so that the preload reserve is not fully utilized.[6] Aortic valve replacement allows the ventricle to eject more normally, with marked improvement of the ejection fraction in many instances (correction of afterload mismatch) (Fig. 22-2).

The current criteria for surgical treatment, based on the development of significant symptoms rather than the development of left ventricular dysfunction, remain appropriate. Thus, clinical results showing marked improvement of functional status at about 3 years after operation tend to be independent of the pre- and postoperative ejection fractions in patients with aortic stenosis, although most late deaths do tend to occur in patients with low pressure gradients.[48] Therefore, operation for aortic stenosis need not be considered *solely* to protect the left ventricle from irreversible myocardial damage. In addition, the data suggest that even in the patient with severe left ventricular dysfunction and an ejection fraction as low as 12 to 15 percent, operation should *not be denied,* since ventricular function will frequently improve postoperatively.[43] Nevertheless, operation should be carried out before patients develop severe ventricular dysfunction with cardiac enlargement and class III or IV symptoms, since even though symptoms improve, operative mortality is somewhat higher and 10-year survival is markedly reduced[48] (see also Chap. 63).

AORTIC REGURGITATION

In the adult patient with clinically severe aortic regurgitation (Chap. 63) and symptoms of LV dysfunction or angina pectoris, it is generally advisable to proceed directly with cardiac catheterization, including coronary angiography when indicated, and consideration of surgical treatment. Such studies will characterize the severity of the regurgitation, the status of LV function, and the presence or absence of associated coronary artery disease. Initial echocardiographic or radionuclide studies in such individuals may help to confirm the need for catheterization studies (see below).

In the patient without symptoms who has severe aortic regurgitation (regurgitant fraction over 40 percent or angiographic grade III or IV) and whose heart size is increased on the chest roentgenogram and by physical examination, a baseline echocardiogram should be obtained for measurement of the LV dimensions. If moderate enlargement of the left ventricle (end-diastolic dimension less than 70 mm) with normal fractional shortening and calculated ejection fraction is found and the patient remains asymptomatic, serial echocardiographic studies about every 1 to 1.5 years can be recommended. In patients without symptoms with LV enlargement more marked and systolic function near the lower limit of normal (ejection fraction 45 to 50 percent), echocardiographic follow-up every 6 months to 1 year should be advised, since recent studies suggest that the proper timing of surgery can be identified. Bonow et al.[49] have shown in late follow-up studies from 3 to 7 years, in patients who have undergone aortic valve replacement for aortic regurgitation, that many patients who show improvement in LV function early postoperatively show continued improvement at late study. If both

LV function and exercise capacity were impaired preoperatively, however, or LV dysfunction (ejection fraction below 45 percent) had persisted preoperatively for more than 1 or 2 years, little postoperative improvement occurred.[49] Most of the few patients with a preoperative ejection fraction below 30 percent failed to show improvement in LV function postoperatively.[49] That patients with severe aortic regurgitation who are asymptomatic and have normal LV function can safely be followed has been confirmed in a series of 101 patients followed for 10 years. No deaths occurred and surgery was required in only 24 percent of patients by the end of the 10-year follow-up either because of the onset of symptoms or the occurrence of LV dysfunction; postoperatively, LV function normalized in all patients.[50] The vasodilator nifedipine can delay the onset of LV dysfunction and postpone surgery in patients with severe aortic regurgitation without risk of postoperative LV dysfunction,[51] but the onset of symptoms should lead to prompt surgical treatment.

When there is normal or only moderate depression of LV function, the heart size diminishes, hypertrophy regresses, and LV function returns toward normal by 6 months to 1 year after aortic valve replacement.[52] This sequence most likely reflects, at least in part, correction of afterload mismatch by the operation,[43] since the high systolic aortic pressure and volume overload preoperatively in aortic regurgitation make the systolic wall stress elevated (and higher than in mitral regurgitation).[53] In support of this view, other studies showing that early improvement in the ejection fraction at 2 years after valve replacement for aortic regurgitation can be explained entirely by lowered end-systolic wall stress postoperatively[54] (correction of afterload mismatch),[4] with some patients exhibiting persistent depression of contractility[54]; nevertheless, all patients exhibited improved functional class.[55] Extreme LV dilation with an echocardiographic end-diastolic dimension ≥ 80 mm was found not to be a contraindication to operation, but among this population the degree of depression of LV function preoperatively predicted the postoperative LV ejection fraction and late mortality.[56] It would clearly be desirable to avoid persistent left ventricular dysfunction and potentially increased late mortality, and there is a growing tendency to consider earlier operation, particularly if there is evidence of progressive LV dysfunction,[43,49] as discussed above (see also Chap. 63).

MITRAL REGURGITATION

In the patient with moderate chronic mitral regurgitation (Chap. 64) who has limiting symptoms of LV failure that are refractory to medical treatment and in whom echocardiographic studies support the presence of severe regurgitation, cardiac catheterization may be performed to confirm the severity of the regurgitation, assess its etiology, evaluate the degree of LV dysfunction, and determine whether or not associated disease of other valves or the coronary arteries[41] is contributory. In such patients, surgical repair or replacement of the mitral valve is usually undertaken.

In the relatively asymptomatic patient with severe mitral regurgitation, the possibility of developing "silent" irreversible myocardial dysfunction poses an important problem.[43] As discussed earlier, mitral regurgitation places relatively favorable systolic loading conditions on the left ventricle, and eccentric hypertrophy coupled with the low-impedance leak early and late in systole yields a high normal ejection fraction when contractility is not reduced (Fig. 22-3A). Even when myocardial contractility becomes severely depressed, a relatively normal ejection fraction can be maintained (Fig. 22-3B). Thus, if significant cardiomegaly is seen on the chest roentgenogram or found on physical examination in such patients, a baseline echocardiographic study should be obtained to assess LV performance.

Despite the limitations of the LV ejection fraction as a measure of myocardial contractility in chronic mitral regurgitation, in an early study it was found that 5-year survival after surgery was 89 percent if the preoperative LV ejection fraction was greater than 50 percent but only 38 percent if it was below 40 percent.[57] In a more recent study using echocardiography, the best preoperative predictors of postoperative LV dysfunction after mitral valve repair or replacement were LV end-systolic diameter greater than 45 mm and an LV ejection fraction below 60 percent.[58]

When there is a marked increase in LV end-diastolic and particularly end-systolic dimensions preoperatively, with the fractional shortening and ejection fraction at low-normal or depressed levels, ventricular function may deteriorate further at 6 months to 1 year following mitral valve replacement. The fall in the ejection fraction following mitral valve replacement in these patients suggests that the ejection fraction was maintained at an artificially high value preoperatively, masking depression of myocardial function (Fig. 22-3B).[43] Following correction of the low-impedance leak, some of which occurs at low wall stress *early* in systole even though peak and mean wall stress values may be elevated,[36] the depression of ventricular function becomes manifest. This occurs since with relief of the regurgitant leak, all of ventricular ejection is now into the aorta, with its high impedance, and the ejection fraction falls, reflecting afterload mismatch and revealing irreversibly depressed myocardial contractility (Fig. 23-3B).

In contrast to aortic valve disease, since further deterioration of ventricular function may occur postoperatively in patients with significantly depressed LV function, operation should be undertaken with caution if the ejection fraction is reduced below 40 percent. Nevertheless, if such patients survive operation, it appears that they often show improved functional status for many years despite ejection fraction values postoperatively of 30 to 40 percent.[57]

Recent studies indicate a changing pattern of mitral valve pathology from rheumatic to degenerative and suggest that up to 70 percent of adult patients are now candidates for mitral valve repair.[59] In contrast to earlier studies with mitral valve replacement, following mitral valve repair, the LV ejection fraction appears to be preserved.[60] Some of this difference may reflect recent improvements in myocardial preservation during surgery. Also, chordal preservation in patients with mitral regurgitation undergoing mitral valve replacement appears to prevent the fall in the LV ejection fraction postoperatively that often occurs with standard replacement methods.[61] Thus, operation in patients with severe chronic mitral regurgitation and few or no symptoms may be recommended to prevent postoperative LV dysfunction when the LV end-systolic dimension reaches 45 to 50 mm and the LV ejection fraction falls below 55 to 60 percent (see also Chap. 64).

RECOGNITION OF MYOCARDIAL FAILURE AFTER HEART SURGERY

Signs of left or right ventricular failure in the early or late postoperative period after aortic or mitral valve replacement can be due to irreversible myocardial disease existing preoperatively. Occasionally, the failure is due to intraoperative myocardial infarction or damage due to inadequate myocardial preservation of the hypertrophied heart, although the advent of hypothermic cardioplegia has made these complications less common. Heart failure in this setting can also be due to a paravalvular leak causing severe regurgitation or to prosthetic valve dysfunction due to clotting or fibrosis producing obstruction or regurgitation. It is very important to identify a mechanical cause of the heart failure so that reoperation can be considered. In the postoperative setting, however, physical findings are often not definitive; for example, a severe paravalvular leak around a prosthetic mitral valve can occur with little or no systolic murmur. Echocardiography or radionuclide ventriculography are useful for detecting severe LV dysfunction or cardiac compression, and pulsed and color Doppler studies may point to a prosthetic valve abnormality (Chap. 14). To definitively establish the cause of postoperative heart failure, it is often advisable to proceed with diagnostic cardiac catheterization and ventriculography together with coronary arteriography.

Recognition and Evaluation of Primary Myocardial Disease

In suspected myocardial disease, the initial goal should be to establish by the simplest possible methods whether or not myocardial dysfunction is present. The physiologic pattern of the disease and its cause should then be sought, although information obtained by invasive studies may *not* be necessary to decide on appropriate treatment.

IS MYOCARDIAL DISEASE PRESENT?

The most useful initial screening test is echocardiography. If such studies are technically unsatisfactory or inconclusive, a radionuclide angiogram can be performed to detect a depressed ejection fraction of either the left or right ventricle.

If the diameter of the LV end-diastolic chamber is increased on the echocardiogram without a significant increase in wall thickness and the fractional shortening or calculated ejection fraction is reduced, it is likely that a cardiomyopathy (or myocarditis) of the dilated type is present (Chap. 73); the right ventricular internal diameter may also be increased in

this condition. This diagnosis is particularly likely in the absence of a heart murmur, hypertension, prior myocardial infarction, or other cause for secondary ventricular enlargement and dysfunction.

In some endurance-trained athletes, the internal chamber diameter of the right or left ventricle or both may be abnormally large and associated with ECG evidence of ventricular hypertrophy. On the other hand, measures of systolic contractile function by echocardiography (fractional shortening, calculated ejection fraction, and V_{CF}) are normal in such individuals[62] (see Chap. 95). If the echocardiogram shows an abnormally thickened LV wall but the diameter of the chamber at end-diastole and systolic function is normal, hypertrophic cardiomyopathy is likely, provided that hypertension and aortic stenosis are absent (Chap. 74). The echocardiogram will usually allow further differentiation into the symmetric or asymmetric type of hypertrophy; if systolic anterior motion of the mitral valve is associated with a heart murmur, hypertrophic obstruction to LV outflow should be considered (see Chap. 74).

If there is a significantly reduced ejection fraction slope of an otherwise normal mitral valve and decreased initial filling velocity on Doppler studies, together with significant left atrial enlargement, a restrictive pathophysiology is suggested. Such patients may have normal end-diastolic ventricular dimensions, with normal or depressed ventricular function.[15] A granular sparkling appearance to the myocardium with other features may suggest amyloidosis.[63] The diagnostic value of this finding has subsequently been found to be less than previously thought (see Chap. 75). Echocardiography may detect a thickened pericardium or pericardial effusion, valvular abnormalities, or unexpected wall motion disorders. The use of x-ray computed tomography[64] (Chap. 18) or magnetic resonance imaging[65] (Chap. 19) has been useful in excluding or confirming the presence of a thickened pericardium.[19] In some patients with cardiomyopathy, radionuclide angiography (Chap. 17) during exercise can demonstrate an abnormal decrease of ejection fraction or a failure to increase it, even when coronary heart disease is absent. Thus, for simply establishing the presence or absence of significant myocardial disease, cardiac catheterization is rarely necessary.

WHEN SHOULD CARDIAC CATHETERIZATION BE DONE?

Whenever the patient with myocardial disease is refractory to therapy or there is a deteriorating clinical course, as complete a pathophysiologic diagnosis as possible should be reached by cardiac catheterization. When diagnostic cardiac catheterization is undertaken, right- and left-sided heart catheterization, left ventriculography, and coronary arteriography[41] should generally be done, since even if a specific etiology is not identified, such studies often assist in management. In some patients, endomyocardial biopsy of either the right or the left ventricle may be performed to search for a tissue diagnosis (see Chap. 16).

One major goal of the cardiac catheterization study is to exclude the presence of surgically treatable disease, such as unsuspected congenital heart disease with a left-to-right shunt (atrial septal defect and anomalous venous connection are often missed clinically), unexpectedly severe valvular aortic stenosis or mitral regurgitation, a severe obstructive component of hypertrophic cardiomyopathy, constrictive pericarditis, or a significant contribution from unsuspected coronary atherosclerosis (see below).

Another major goal is to establish the pathophysiologic pattern of the myocardial disease in order to allow more rational selection of therapy. Basically, there are three patterns to myocardial disease: dilated, hypertrophic, and restrictive (or several of these patterns may coexist) (Chaps. 73 through 75). The dilated type is most common, and the pure restrictive type is quite rare. A restrictive pattern can be mimicked by constrictive pericarditis, and that condition should be carefully excluded (Chaps. 75 and 81). Selective ventriculography and analysis of pressure tracings from the right and left ventricles and atria will generally establish whether the disorder is primarily due to dilated cardiomyopathy with dilation of the chambers, wall thinning, and reduced systolic function or to restrictive disease. In restrictive disease, the chamber size and systolic function may be normal, although this is not always the case.[15] There may be a thickened left ventricular wall, and there is evidence of reduced ventricular diastolic compliance with impaired filling of the left ventricle.[37] Characteristically, there is an early diastolic dip followed by a rapid rise and then a plateau of pressure during diastasis, a prominent *a* wave with an elevated end-diastolic pressure, and a delayed *y* descent on the pulmonary artery wedge pressure or left atrial tracing, indicating impaired atrial emptying into the diseased ventricle.[15,37] The right ventricle may also exhibit these phenomena. These features resemble constrictive pericarditis (Chap. 81), although typically in restrictive disease, the right- and left-sided diastolic pressures do not equilibrate as they do in the former case. In dilated cardiomyopathy, the above features are generally absent, although the ventricular end-diastolic pressure is usually elevated and the early-diastolic pressure is also high. Thus, the dominant physiologic pattern, dilated or restrictive, can usually be identified. Which pattern is present carries important implications for therapy, since vigorous use of diuretics and positive inotropic stimuli are appropriate for the dilated pattern, whereas such therapy in the patient with restrictive pathophysiology can lead to decreased ventricular filling pressures and volumes, with further impairment of the filling of the stiffened ventricle and a reduction of cardiac output. Likewise, afterload reduction therapy by vasodilators is more appropriate in the congestive setting, since, in restrictive cardiomyopathy, ventricular systolic emptying may already be near maximum, and dilating properties of these agents on the veins may also lead to reduced diastolic filling (see Chap. 75).

The restrictive type of pathophysiology may blend with that due to outflow tract obstruction in hypertrophic cardiomyopathy, and surgical relief by myomectomy of a severe resting outflow gradient identified at cardiac catheterization may become necessary in occasional patients who are refractory to

medical therapy[66] (see Chap. 74). Coronary arteriography should accompany diagnostic studies to exclude the possibility of silent ischemia in the patient with cardiomyopathy.[41] Ischemic heart muscle disease ("cardiomyopathy") sometimes cannot be distinguished from other types of cardiomyopathy without such studies.

There are some settings in which limited cardiac catheterization should be considered. In the patient with established myocardial disease associated with severe heart failure refractory to treatment, it may be advisable to undertake balloon catheterization of the right side of the heart in order to characterize the hemodynamic setting if vasodilator therapy is being considered.[22] Moreover, serial measurements following single oral doses of the proposed therapeutic regimen can allow selection of the most appropriate drugs.[17] Alternatively, the finding of an unexpectedly low cardiac filling pressure with a normal cardiac output together with lack of response to a therapeutic test of vasodilators may contraindicate the use of chronic vasodilator therapy.

Recognition and Evaluation of Ischemic Myocardial Dysfunction

The LV ejection fraction determined noninvasively by radionuclide ventriculography, echocardiography, or intravenous digital or direct cine left ventriculography is highly useful in detecting global depression of cardiac function due to myocardial ischemia or infarction in patients with coronary artery disease. Since ischemic heart disease typically produces abnormalities of regional contraction,[67] a normal LV ejection fraction or a normal fractional shortening by echocardiography does not imply the absence of myocardial dysfunction. Thus, regional hypokinesia or even dyskinesia in one region can lead to compensatory hyperfunction in a normal region, with maintenance of a normal global ejection fraction.[67] Quantitative cine left ventriculography during cardiac catheterization is frequently used to measure regional wall motion precisely, as, for example, when studying the reversibility of ischemic dysfunction after therapeutic interventions such as thrombolysis in acute myocardial infarction.[68] Noninvasive approaches are also available for assessing regional wall motion abnormalities, including two-dimensional echocardiography for endocardial motion or regional systolic wall thickening (Chap. 14), assessing regional ejection fraction by radionuclide ventriculography (Chap. 17), or intravenous digital contrast angiography.[69]

LEFT VENTRICULAR FUNCTION IN CHRONIC CORONARY HEART DISEASE

In patients with chronic coronary heart disease, the level of *global* LV function has been found to be more important than the number of diseased coronary arteries in assessing mortality trends.[70] Thus, a depressed ejection fraction significantly reduces life expectancy regardless of the number of coronary vessels involved by significant stenoses, and it predicts a reduction in life expectancy even when one or two coronary arteries are diseased—a setting that has only a minor effect on annual mortality rate in the absence of depressed left ventricular function.[70] In some studies, coronary bypass surgery has been found to improve life expectancy compared to medical treatment only in patients with left main disease or those with three-vessel disease who have a depressed ejection fraction.[71–73] There is other evidence, however, that in patients with significant symptoms, coronary bypass surgery may improve survival in those with three-vessel disease even when left ventricular function is normal[74] (see also Chaps. 45 through 47 and 50).

VENTRICULAR FUNCTION AFTER MYOCARDIAL INFARCTION

The ejection fraction has found increasing application in risk stratification of patients following acute myocardial infarction, along with a number of variables including age, prior history of myocardial infarction, persistent ischemic pain, congestive heart failure in the hospital, and exercise-induced ischemia or limited exercise capacity near the time of hospital discharge. The presence of such prognostic indicators often leads to coronary angiography to determine whether or not myocardial revascularization by surgery or coronary angioplasty should be performed in an effort to reduce the increased risk.[41]

The LV ejection fraction, often determined by radionuclide angiography, is an independent determinant of mortality during the first 1 or 2 years following acute myocardial infarction,[75,76] and it has been used alone or in combination with several other variables for risk stratification. An ejection fraction below 45 percent at the time of hospital discharge provides both optimum sensitivity and specificity for identifying patients at increased risk[76] but does not have high predictive accuracy in identifying patients who will die, since a relatively large number of patients with a low ejection fraction will survive 1 year.[76] Nevertheless, the *sensitivity* of a reduced ejection fraction (<45 percent) for predicting 1-year mortality is relatively good (approximately 60 to 65 percent); the sensitivity for sudden death is somewhat higher (over 70 percent).[76]

The usefulness of the ejection fraction in prognosis after myocardial infarction can be considerably enhanced if clinical variables indicative of heart failure in the hospital are also considered.[75,76] For example, in our data base, when two out of three variables (pulmonary congestion on x-ray examination, pulmonary rales, and S_3 gallop) were present during hospitalization or if the roentgenogram alone was positive, there was a three- to fourfold enhancement of the usefulness of a depressed ejection fraction for predicting 1-year mortality compared to use of the ejection fraction alone; in the absence of these variables, the ejection fraction lost a considerable degree of its predictive ability for 1-year mortality.[77] Among the many variables predicting outcome after acute myocardial infarction, heart failure and the predischarge ejection fraction continue to predict mortality after thrombolytic treatment.[78]

ISCHEMIC HEART MUSCLE DISEASE (CARDIOMYOPATHY)

In the patient with a clinical diagnosis of cardiomyopathy, the clinical symptoms and the ECG may not suggest prior myocardial infarction or recurrent ischemia, yet coronary heart disease may be the underlying process.[79–81] In some patients, attacks of dyspnea without pain or with atypical pain may reflect recurrent myocardial ischemia or subendocardial infarction, and "silent" or painless myocardial ischemia is being recognized with increasing frequency.[82] The finding of coronary artery calcification on image intensification fluoroscopy may be very helpful in suggesting the diagnosis; among a group of younger patients with heart muscle disease, an ischemic cardiomyopathy as shown by coronary arteriography was associated with calcification of either two or three coronary arteries.[79] Perfusion imaging during and after exercise may also indicate the presence of myocardial scar at rest or show transient exercise-induced perfusion defects, and a fall in the radionuclide ejection fraction with exercise has been reported to be more indicative of ischemic heart muscle disease than of idiopathic dilated cardiomyopathy. Generally, if this diagnosis is suspected, cardiac catheterization with coronary arteriography will be required to fully characterize the degree of coronary atherosclerosis. In the more typical patient with ischemic heart muscle disease or "ischemic cardiomyopathy," a clear history of previous myocardial infarction and angina pectoris is obtained. Such patients should usually undergo cardiac catheterization as well, even if heart failure without angina pectoris is the presenting picture, since myocardial revascularization can result in improvement of dyspnea and heart failure or transient attacks of myocardial ischemia in some patients with ischemic heart muscle disease. Also, patients with coronary heart disease and an ejection fraction below 25 percent who usually have ischemic symptoms appear to show improved life expectancy following coronary artery bypass surgery[83] (see also Chaps. 38, 45 through 47, and 50).

REVERSIBILITY OF MYOCARDIAL DYSFUNCTION

Periods of partial ischemia lasting several hours, although followed by *myocardial stunning,* can be completely reversible with reperfusion.[84,85] During such conditions of low coronary flow, contraction is reduced in proportion to the reduction of regional myocardial blood flow, a condition that has been termed *perfusion-contraction matching.*[86] Such reversibility of contractile dysfunction (either complete or partial) has been demonstrated after coronary bypass surgery or balloon angioplasty in patients with unstable angina pectoris.[87]

Following thrombolysis for acute myocardial infarction, improved LV function has been well documented.[88–90] The degree of recovery of ventricular function depends on many factors, including variables affecting infarct size—including the risk area, the duration of coronary occlusion, and the level of residual coronary blood flow via collaterals or a partially patent vessel—late or unsuccessful reperfusion, inadequate reflow, residual coronary stenosis, and coronary reocclusion.[91]

Reversibility of contractile dysfunction has also been demonstrated to occur in some patients with chronic, stable coronary heart disease (without acute ischemia) after balloon angioplasty[92] or coronary bypass surgery.[93] This type of chronic dysfunction may represent either stunning consequent to repeated episodes of ischemia or the occurrence of very prolonged low-flow perfusion-contraction matching or both[85]; the latter has been termed *myocardial hibernation*.[84,94] In a recent study, surgical biopsy tissue was taken from patients with symptomatic coronary heart disease at the time of coronary artery bypass surgery from regions with chronic regional dysfunction that showed mismatch at rest between perfusion and metabolic imaging.[95] Among the findings were varying degrees of myocardial fibrosis and alterations in contractile material, with ultrastructural changes in nuclei, mitochondria and t tubules considered to represent changes associated with hibernation; 6 months after myocardial revascularization, the left ventricular ejection fraction and regional function had improved, but the improvement was not correlated with the degree of histologic changes.[95] The detection of such poorly contracting but viable regions is important in patients having coronary artery disease and LV dysfunction in whom revascularization might be beneficial, and it has been accomplished with combined perfusion imaging with metabolic imaging (^{18}F deoxyglucose) using positron emission tomography (Chap. 20)[96] or rest perfusion imaging techniques alone[97,98] (see also Chaps. 17 and 45).

VENTRICULAR ANEURYSM

Sometimes heart failure or low cardiac output due to a left ventricular aneurysm is suggested by the ECG or the chest roentgenogram, and echocardiography has proved reliable in detecting the presence of an aneurysm (Chap. 14). If a ventricular aneurysm is seriously suspected in a patient who has significant symptoms due to heart failure, cardiac catheterization should be carried out to define the extent of the aneurysm and to assess the degree of coronary artery disease prior to considering corrective operation (Chap. 50).

REFERENCES

1. Weber KT, Janicki JS, McElroy PA. Determination of aerobic capacity and the severity of chronic cardiac and circulatory failure. *Circulation* 1987; 76(suppl VI):VI40–VI45.
2. Benge W, Litchfield RL, Marcus ML. Exercise capacity in patients with severe left ventricular dysfunction. *Circulation* 1980; 61:955–959.
3. Ross J Jr, Covell JW. Frameworks for analysis of ventricular and circulatory function. Integrated responses. In: West JB, ed. *Best and Taylor's Physiological Basis of Medical Practice,* 12th ed. Baltimore: Williams & Wilkins; 1991:291–306.
4. Ross J. Cardiac function and myocardial contractility: A perspective. *J Am Coll Cardiol* 1983; 1:52–62.
5. LaKatta EG. Starling's law of the heart is explained by an intimate interaction of muscle length and myofilament calcium activation. *J Am Coll Cardiol* 1987; 10:1157–1164.
6. Ross J Jr. Afterload mismatch and preload reserve: A conceptual framework for the analysis of ventricular function. *Prog Cardiovasc Dis* 1976; 18:255–264.
7. MacGregor DC, Covell JW, Mahler F, Dilley RB, Ross R Jr. Relations between afterload, stroke volume, and descending limb of Starling's curve. *Am J Physiol* 1974; 227:884–890.
8. Ross J Jr, Braunwald E. The study of left ventricular function in man by increasing resistance to ventricular ejection with angiotensin. *Circulation* 1964; 29:739–749.
9. Lee JD, Tajimi T, Patritti J, Ross J Jr. Preload reserve and mechanisms of afterload mismatch in the normal conscious dog. *Am J Physiol* 1986; 19:H464–H473.
10. Shabetai R. Disease of the pericardium. In: Bennett JC, Plum F, eds. *Cecil Textbook of Medicine,* 20th ed. Philadelphia: Saunders; 1996:336–342.
11. Alderman EL, Glantz SA. Acute hemodynamic interventions shift the diastolic pressure-volume curve in man. *Circulation* 1976; 54:662–671.
12. Brutsaert DL, Rademakers FE, Sys SU. Triple control of relaxation: Implications in cardiac disease. *Circulation* 1984; 69:190–196.
13. Stoddard MF, Pearson AC, Kern MJ, Ratcliff J, Mrosek DG, Labovitz AJ. Left ventricular diastolic function: Comparison of pulsed Doppler echocardiographic and hemodynamic indices in subjects with and without coronary heart disease. *J Am Coll Cardiol* 1989; 13:327–336.
14. Miyazaki S, Guth BD, Miura T, Indolfi C, Schulz R, Ross J Jr. Changes of left ventricular diastolic function in exercising dogs without and with ischemia. *Circulation* 1990; 81:1058–1070.
15. Vaitkus PT, Kussmaul WG. Constrictive pericarditis versus restrictive cardiomyopathy: A reappraisal and update of diagnostic criteria. *Am Heart J* 1991; 122:1431–1441.
16. Schuler G, Peterson K, Johnson A, Francis G, Dennish G, Utley J, et al. Temporal response of left ventricular performance to mitral valve surgery. *Circulation* 1979; 59:1218–1231.
17. Chatterjee K, Parmley WW. Vasodilator therapy for acute myocardial infarction and chronic congestive heart failure. *J Am Coll Cardiol* 1983; 1:133–153.
18. Pouleur H, Covell JW, Ross J Jr. Effects of nitroprusside on venous return and central blood volume in the absence and presence of acute heart failure. *Circulation* 1980; 61:328–337.
19. Higgins CB, Lanzer P, Stark D, Botvinick E, Schiller NB, Lipton MJ, et al. Assessment of cardiac anatomy using nuclear magnetic resonance imaging. *J Am Coll Cardiol* 1985; 5:775–815.
20. Weber KT, Kinasewitz GT, Janicki JS, Fishman AP. Oxygen utilization and ventilation during exercise in patients with chronic cardiac failure. *Circulation* 1982; 65:1213–1223.
21. Franciosa JA, Park M, Levine TB. Lack of correlation between exercise capacity and indexes of resting left ventricular performance in heart failure. *Am J Cardiol* 1981; 47:33–39.
22. Swan HJC, Ganz W: Hemodynamic measurements in clinical practice: A decade in review. *J Am Coll Cardiol* 1983; 1:103–113.
23. Peterson KL, Sklovan D, Ludbrook P, Uther JB, Ross J Jr. Comparison of isovolumetric and ejection phase indices of myocardial performance in man. *Circulation* 1974; 49:1088–1101.
24. Berger HJ, Johnstone DE, Sands JM, Gottschalk A, Zaret BL. Response of right ventricular ejection fraction to upright bicycle exercise in coronary artery disease. *Circulation* 1979; 60:1292–1299.
25. Grossman W, Jones D, McLaurin LP. Wall stress and patterns of hypertrophy in the human left ventricle. *J Clin Invest* 1975; 56:56–64.
26. Lee J, Tajimi T, Widman TF, Ross J Jr. Application of end-systolic pressure-volume and pressure-wall thickness relations in conscious dogs. *J Am Coll Cardiol* 1987; 9:136–146.
27. Takahashi M, Sasayama S, Kawai C, Kotoure H. Contractile performance of the hypertrophied ventricle in patients with systemic hypertension. *Circulation* 1980; 62:116–126.
28. Borow KM, Green LH, Grossman W, Braunwald E. Left ventricular end-systolic stress-shortening and stress-length relations in humans. *Am J Cardiol* 1982; 50:1301–1308.
29. Mehmel HC, Stockins B, Ruffmann K, von Olshausen K, Schuler G, Kubler W. The linearity of the end-systolic pressure-volume relationship in man and its sensitivity for assessment of left ventricular function. *Circulation* 1981; 63:1216–1222.
30. McKay RG, Aroesty JM, Heller GV, Royal HD, Warren SE, Grossman W. Assessment of the end-systolic pressure-volume relationship in human beings with the use of a time-varying elastance model. *Circulation* 1986; 74:97–104.
31. Kass DA, Maughan WC. From "E_{max}" to pressure-volume relations: A broader view. *Circulation* 1988; 77:1203–1211.
32. Pitt B, Kalff V, Rabinovitch MA, Buda AJ, Colfen HT, Vogel RA. Impact of radionuclide techniques on evaluation of patients with ischemic heart disease. *J Am Coll Cardiol* 1983; 1:63–72.

33. Starling MR, Dell'Italia LJ, Walsh RA, Little WC, Benedetto AR, Nusynowitz ML. Accurate estimates of absolute left ventricular volumes from equilibrium radionuclide angiographic count data using a simple geometric attenuation correction. *J Am Coll Cardiol* 1984; 3:789–798.

34. Dodge HT, Sheehan FH. A quantitative contrast angiography for assessment of ventricular performance in heart disease. *J Am Coll Cardiol* 1983; 1:73–81.

35. Kennedy JW, Baxley WA, Figley MM, Dodge HT, Blackman JR. Quantitative angiocardiography: I. The normal left ventricle in man. *Circulation* 1966; 34:272–278.

36. Corin WJ, Monrad ES, Murakami T, Nonogi-Ho, Hess OM, Krayenbuehl HP. The relationship of afterload to ejection performance in chronic mitral regurgitation. *Circulation* 1987; 76:59–67.

37. Tyberg TL, Goodyer AVN, Hurst VW III, Alexander J, Langou RA. Left ventricular filling in differentiating restrictive amyloid cardiomyopathy and constrictive pericarditis. *Am J Cardiol* 1981; 47:791–796.

38. Peterson KL, Tsuji J, Johnson A, DiDonna J, LeWinter M. Diastolic left ventricular pressure-volume and stress-strain relations in patients with valvular aortic stenosis and left ventricular hypertrophy. *Circulation* 1978; 58:77–89.

39. Mahler F, Ross JP Jr, O'Rourke RA, Cavell JW. Effects of changes in preload, afterload and inotropic state on ejection and isovolumic phase measures of contractility in the conscious dog. *Am J Cardiol* 1975; 35:626–634.

40. Mason JW, O'Connell JB. Clinical merit of endomyocardial biopsy. *Circulation* 1989; 79:971–979.

41. Ross J Jr, Brandenburg R, Dinsmore R, Friesinger GC II, Holtgren HH, and the Subcommittee on Coronary Angiography. Guidelines for coronary angiography: A report of the American College of Cardiology/American Heart Association Task Force on Assessment of diagnostic and therapeutic cardiovascular procedures (Subcommittee on Coronary Angiography). *J Am Coll Cardiol* 1987; 10:935–950. Also *Circulation* 1987; 76:963A–977A.

42. Schwarz F, Schaper J, Kittstein D, Flameng W, Walter P, Schaper W. Reduced volume fraction of myofibrils in myocardium of patients with decompensated pressure overload. *Circulation* 1981; 63:1299–1303.

43. Ross J Jr. Afterload mismatch in aortic and mitral valve disease: Implications for surgical therapy. *J Am Coll Cardiol* 1985; 5:811–826.

44. Carabello BA. Indications for valve surgery in symptomatic patients with aortic and mitral stenosis. *Chest* 1995; 108:1678–1682.

45. Robiolio PA, Rigolin VH, Hearne SE, Baker WA, Kisslo KB, Pierce CH, et al. Left ventricular performance improves late after aortic valve replacement in patients with aortic stenosis and reduced ejection fraction. *Am J Cardiol* 1995; 76:612–615.

46. Roger VL. Left ventricular function in aortic stenosis: A clinical review. *J Heart Valve Dis* 1995; 4(suppl II):S230–S235.

47. Villari B, Vassalli G, Monrad ES, Chiariello M, Turina M, Hess OM. Normalization of diastolic dysfunction in aortic stenosis late after valve replacement. *Circulation* 1995; 91:2353–2358.

48. Lund O, Jensen FT. Functional status and left ventricular performance late after valve replacement for aortic stenosis: Relation to preoperative data. *Eur Heart J* 1988; 9:1234–1243.

49. Bonow RO, Dodd JT, Maron BJ, O'Gara PT, White GG, McIntosh CL, et al. Long-term serial changes in left ventricular function and reversal of ventricular dilatation after valve replacement for chronic aortic regurgitation. *Circulation* 1988; 78:1108–1120.

50. Tornos MP, Olona M, Permanyer-Miralda G, Herrejon P, Camprecios M, Evangelista A, et al. Clinical outcome of severe symptomatic chronic aortic regurgitation: A long-term prospective follow-up study. *Am Heart J* 1995; 130:333–339.

51. Scognamiglio R, Rahimtoola SH, Pasoli G, Nisirt S, Volta SD. Nifedipine in asymptomatic patients with severe aortic regurgitation and normal left ventricular function. *N Engl J Med* 1994; 331:689–694.

52. Schuler G, Peterson KL, Johnson AD, Francis G, Ashburn W, Dennish G, et al. Serial non-invasive assessment of left ventricular hypertrophy and function after surgical correction of aortic regurgitation. *Am J Cardiol* 1979; 44:585–594.

53. Wisenbaugh T, Spann JF, Carabello BA. Differences in myocardial performance and load between patients with similar amounts of chronic aortic versus chronic mitral regurgitation. *J Am Coll Cardiol* 1984; 3:916–923.

54. Taniguchi K, Nakano S, Kawashima Y, Sakai K, Kawamoto T, Sakaki S, et al. Left ventricular ejection performance, wall stress, and contractile state in aortic regurgitation before and after aortic valve replacement. *Circulation* 1990; 82:798–807.

55. Taniguchi K, Nakano S, Matsuda H, Shimazaki Y, Sakai K, Kawemoto T, et al. Timing of operation for aortic regurgitation: Relation to postoperative contractile state. *Ann Thorac Surg* 1990; 50:779–785.

56. Klodas E, Enriquez-Sarano M, Tajik AJ, Mullany CJ, Bailey KR, Seward JB. Aortic regurgitation complicated by extreme left ventricular dilation: Long-term outcome after surgical correction. *J Am Coll Cardiol* 1996; 27:670–677.

57. Phillips HR, Levine RH, Carter JE, Boucher CA, Osbakken MD, Okada RD, et al. Mitral valve replacement for isolated mitral regurgitation: Analysis of clinical course and late postoperative left ventricular function. *Am J Cardiol* 1981; 48:647–654.

58. Enriquez-Sarano M, Tajik AJ, Hertzell V, et al. Echocardiographic prediction of left ventricular function after correction of mitral regurgitation: Results and clinical implications. *Am J Cardiol* 1994; 24:1536–1543.

59. Rozich JD, Carabello BA, Usher BW, et al. Mitral valve replacement with and without chordal preservation in patients with chronic mitral regurgitation. *Circulation* 1992; 86:1718–1726.

60. Cosgrove DJ, Stewart WJ. Mitral valvuloplasty. *Curr Probl Cardiol* 1989; 14:353–416.

61. Krishman P, Schaff HV, Orszulak TA, Odell JA, Enriquez-Sarano M. Surgical management of asymptomatic patients with severe mitral valve regurgitation: Rationale and early outcome (abstr) *Circulation* 1995; 92:I-515.

62. Gilbert CA, Nutter DO, Felner JM, Perkins JV, Heymsfield SB, Schlant RC. Echocardiographic study of cardiac dimensions and function in the endurance-trained athlete. *Am J Cardiol* 1977; 40:528–533.

63. Siquera-Filho AG, Cunha CLP, Tajik AJ, Seward JB, Schattenberg TT, Giuliani ER. M-mode and two-dimensional echocardiographic features in cardiac amyloidosis. *Circulation* 1980; 63:188–196.

64. Isner JM, Carter BL, Bankoff MS, Pastore JO, Ramaswasny K, McAdam KP, et al. Differentiation of constrictive pericarditis from restrictive cardiomyopathy by computed tomographic imaging. *Am Heart J* 1983; 105:1019–1025.

65. Soulen RL, Stark DD, Higgins CB. Magnetic resonance imaging of constrictive pericardial disease. *Am J Cardiol* 1985; 55:480–484.

66. Maron BJ, Bonow RO, Cannon RO III, Leon BG, Epstein SE. Hypertrophic cardiomyopathy: Interrelations of clinical manifestations, pathophysiology, and therapy. *N Engl J Med* 1987; 316:844–852.

67. Ross J Jr. Perspective: Assessment of ischemic regional myocardial dysfunction and its reversibility. *Circulation* 1986; 74:1186–1190.

68. Dodge HT, Sheehan FH, Mathey DG, Brown BG, Kennedy JW. Usefulness of coronary artery bypass graft surgery or percutaneous transluminal angioplasty after thrombolytic therapy. *Circulation* 1985; 72:V-39–V-45.

69. Chappuis FP, Widmann TF, Nicod P, Peterson KL. Densitometric regional ejection fraction: A new three-dimensional index of regional left ventricular function. Comparison with geometric methods. *J Am Coll Cardiol* 1988; 11:72–82.

70. Mock MB, Ringqvist I, Fisher LD, Davis KB, Chaitman BR, Kouchoukos NT, et al. Survival of medically treated patients in the coronary artery surgery study (CASS) registry. *Circulation* 1982; 66:562–568.

71. Takaro T, Hultgren H, Lipton M, Thomsen J, Takaro T. VA cooperative randomized study for coronary arterial occlusive disease: II. Left main disease. *Circulation* 1976; 54(suppl III):III107–III117.

72. Murphy M, Hultgren H, Detre K, et al. Treatment of chronic stable angina: A preliminary report of survival data of the randomized Veterans Administration cooperative study. *N Engl J Med* 1977; 297:621–628.

73. CASS principal investigations and their associates. Coronary artery surgery study (CASS): A randomized trial of coronary artery bypass surgery. *Circulation* 1983; 68:939–950.

74. European Coronary Surgery Study Group. Long-term results of prospective randomized study of coronary artery bypass surgery in stable angina pectoris. *Lancet* 1982; 2:1173–1180.

75. Moss AJ, Bigger TJ, Case RB, Gillespie JA, Goldstein RE, Greenberg HM, et al. The multicenter postinfarction research group: Risk stratification and survival after myocardial infarction. *N Engl J Med* 1983; 309:331–336.

76. Ahnve S, Gilpin E, Henning H, Curtis G, Collins D, Ross R Jr. Limitations and advantages of the ejection fraction for defining high risk after acute myocardial infarction. *Am J Cardiol* 1986; 58:872–878.

77. Nicod P, Gilpin E, Dittrich H, Chappuis F, Ahnve S, Engler R, et al. Influence on prognosis and morbidity of left ventricular ejection fraction with and without signs of left ventricular failure after acute myocardial infarction. *J Am Coll Cardiol* 1988; 61:1165–1171.

78. Volpe A, De Vita C, Franzosi MG, Maggioni AP, Mauri F, Negri E, et al. Determinants of 6-month mortality in survivors of myocardial infarction after thrombosis. *Circulation* 1993; 88:416–429.

79. Johnson AD, Laiken SL, Shabetai R. Noninvasive diagnosis of ischemic cardiomyopathy by fluoroscopic detection of coronary artery calcification. *Am Heart J* 1978; 96:521–524.

80. Burch GE, Giles TD, Colclough HL. Ischemic cardiomyopathy. *Am Heart J* 1970; 79:291–292.

81. Dash H, Johnson RA, Dinsmore RE, Francis CK, Harthorne JW. Cardiomyopathic syndrome due to coronary artery disease: I. Relation to angiographic extent of coronary disease and to remote myocardial infarction. *Br Heart J* 1977; 39:733–739.

82. Chierchia S, Lazzari M, Freedman B, Brunelli C, Maseri A. Impairment of myocardial perfusion and function during painless myocardial ischemia. *J Am Coll Cardiol* 1983; 1:924–930.

83. Alderman EL, Fisher LD, Litwin P, Kaiser GC, Myers WO, Maynard C, et al. Results of coronary artery surgery in patients with poor left ventricular function (CASS). *Circulation* 1983; 68:785–795.

84. Heusch G, Schulz R, eds. *New Paradigms of Coronary Artery Disease: Hibernation, Stunning, Ischemic Preconditioning.* New York: Darmstadt; Germany: Steinkopff; 1996.

85. Matsuzaki M, Gallagher KP, Kemper WS, White F, Ross J Jr. Sustained regional dysfunction produced by prolonged coronary stenosis: Gradual recovery after reperfusion. *Circulation* 1983; 68:170–182.

86. Ross J Jr. Myocardial perfusion contraction matching circulation: Implications for coronary heart disease and hibernation. *Circulation* 1990; 83:1076–1083.

87. Renkin J, Wijns W, Ladha Z, Col J. Reversal of segmental hypokinesis by coronary angioplasty in patients with unstable angina, persistent T wave inversion and left anterior descending stenosis. *Circulation* 1990; 82:913–921.

88. White HD, Norris RM, Brown MA, Takayama M, Maslowski A, Bass NM, et al. Effect of intravenous streptokinase on left ventricular function and early survival after acute myocardial infarction. *N Engl J Med* 1987; 317:850–855.

89. Martin GV, Sheehan FH, Stadius M, Maynard C, Davis KB, Ritchie JL, et al. Intravenous streptokinase for acute myocardial infarction: Effects on global and regional systolic function. *Circulation* 1988; 78:258–275.

90. Schröder R, Neuhaus K-L, Leizorovicz A, Linderer T, Tebbe U for the ISAM Study Group. A prospective trial of intravenous streptokinase in acute myocardial infarction (ISAM): Mortality, morbidity, and infarct size at 21 days. *N Engl J Med* 1986; 314:1465–1471.

91. Ross J Jr. Left ventricular function after coronary artery reperfusion. *Am J Cardiol* 1993; 72:91G–97G.

92. van den Berg EK Jr, Popma JJ, Dehmer GJ, Snow FR, Lewis SA, Vetrovec GW, et al. Reversible segmental left ventricular dysfunction after coronary angioplasty. *Circulation* 1990; 81:1210–1216.

93. Dilsizian V, Bonow RO, Cannon RO III, Tracy CM, Vitale AF, McIntosh CL, et al. The effect of coronary artery bypass grafting on left ventricular systolic function at rest: Evidence for preoperative subclinical myocardial ischemia. *Am J Cardiol* 1988; 61:1248–1254.

94. Rahimtoola SH. A perspective on the three large multicenter randomized clinical trials of coronary bypass surgery for chronic stable angina. *Circulation* 1985; 72(suppl V):V123–V135.

95. Schwarz ER, Schaper J, vom Dahl J, Altehoefer C, Grohmann B, Schoendube F, et al. Myocyte degeneration and cell death in hibernating human myocardium. *J Am Coll Cardiol* 1996; 27:1577–1585.

96. Altehoefer C, Kaiser HJ, Doerr R, et al. Fluorine-18 deoxyglucose PET for assessment of viable myocardium in perfusion defects in 99^mTc-MIBI SPECT: A comparative study in patients with coronary artery disease. *Eur J Nucl Med* 1992; 19:334–342.

97. Bonow RO, Dilsizian V, Cuocolo A, Bacharach SL. Identification of viable myocardium in patients with chronic coronary artery disease and left ventricular dysfunction: Comparison of thallium scintigraphy with reinjection and PET imaging with ^{18}F-fluorodeoxyglucose. *Circulation* 1991; 83:26–37.

98. Kauffman GJ, Boyne TS, Watson DD, Smith WH, Beller GA. Comparison of rest thallium-201 imaging and rest technetium-99m sestamibi imaging for assessment of myocardial viability in patients with coronary artery disease and severe left ventricular dysfunction. *J Am Coll Cardiol* 1996; 27:1592–1597.

23

DIAGNOSIS AND MANAGEMENT
OF HEART FAILURE

Thierry H. LeJemtel / Edmund H. Sonnenblick / William H. Frishman

The diagnosis and treatment of patients with chronic heart failure is a difficult undertaking, as congestive heart failure (CHF) is not one specific disease requiring specific therapy but a syndrome representing the end result of many cardiovascular, pulmonary, or systemic diseases.[1] Moreover, ventricular dysfunction generally precedes clinical symptoms by months or years[2] (see Chap. 21). Nevertheless, despite the multiplicity of etiologies, clinical presentations, and variable rates of progression that characterize this syndrome, a general approach can be employed to diagnose and treat these patients. This general approach to management rests on an in-depth knowledge of the pathophysiology of the syndrome of CHF and of the common problems encountered during initiation and maintenance of therapy; this can be summarized in relation to three guiding principles requiring constant consideration.

The first guiding principle in CHF management is the concomitant, continuous, and aggressive pursuit and treatment of the underlying disease(s) that led to the development of CHF. For example, when CHF is due to obstruction of the coronary arteries, demonstration of reversible myocardial ischemia, even in the absence of angina, could lead to a coronary revascularization procedure that in turn could lead to an improvement in myocardial function. Similarly, slowing the progression of coronary artery disease, by the use of both antithrombotic and lipid-lowering therapies along with cessation of cigarette smoking, is as important as the treatment of the clinical symptoms of ischemic CHF.

The second guiding principle in managing patients with CHF is to define precisely the stage of the disease when therapy begins. The syndrome of CHF is a dynamic process, and the therapeutic goals and endpoints vary with the stage of the process. In that respect, management of patients with CHF should resemble that of patients having malignancy, where the evaluation of the extent and stage of the disease process dictates therapy. Further, the extent of ventricular

dysfunction, as measured by the ejection fraction (EF) (see Chap. 22), and clinical symptoms, as judged by exercise performance,[3] are poorly correlated. Thus, symptoms and their relief may not foretell survival. While the prevention of sudden death is an important therapeutic outcome in patients with asymptomatic or mildly asymptomatic left ventricular (LV) systolic dysfunction, it may be a limited therapeutic goal in extremely symptomatic patients who are not candidates for cardiac transplantation or LV assist devices.

The third guiding principle in managing patients with severe CHF is the recognition that a key determinant of successful therapy is the quality of care; this requires frequent visits, in-home monitoring, and meticulous attention given to management details such as diet, daily activity level, and the dosages of medications being used, with an appreciation for their adverse effects.[4,5] The importance of this third guiding principle is illustrated by the careful approach that is required to both successfully initiate and increase the dosage of β-adrenergic blockade therapy in patients with symptomatic LV systolic dysfunction.

In order to plan an appropriate therapy, an accurate clinical diagnosis is necessary, with an understanding of the pathophysiology involved. Details of diagnostic approaches are presented elsewhere (see Chap. 21).

PATHOPHYSIOLOGY AND DIAGNOSIS OF CONGESTIVE HEART FAILURE

The dynamic process by which ventricular dysfunction evolves into CHF can be conveniently described in three phases[6] (Fig. 23-1). The clinical characteristics of each phase and its duration depend heavily on the specific primary etiology involved. Myocardial damage with massive myocyte loss and fibrotic repair may be rapid, as occurs with an acute transmural myocardial infarction or a viral myocarditis, or

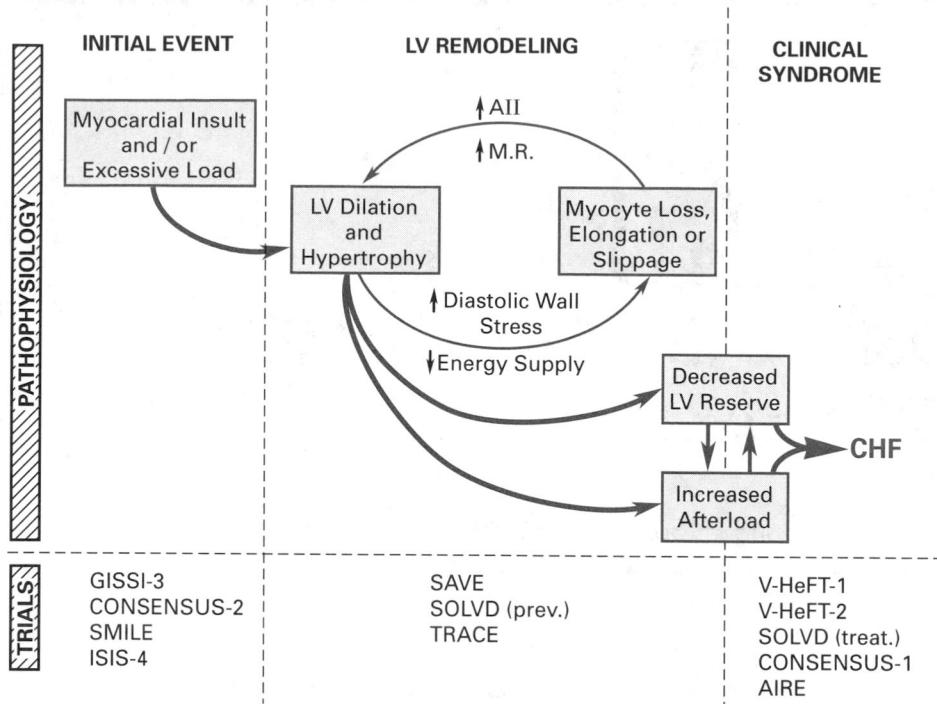

FIGURE 23-1

The pathophysiology of heart failure progressing with time from the initial event, related to a loss of myocardium and/or a persistent overload, to the adaptive responses, including myocardial hypertrophy, and ultimately ventricular dilatation. Left ventricular (LV) dilatation augments diastolic wall stress that produces deformations of the ventricular wall and functional mitral regurgitation (MR), as well as further myocyte loss (apoptosis). Neurohumoral responses become activated with increased sympathetic tone, reduced parasympathetic tone, and activation of the renin-angiotensin system. These structural alterations comprise what is termed *ventricular remodeling*. With progression of these latter processes, and with decreased ventricular capacity to augment cardiac output as required along with renal retention of sodium, central and peripheral edema ensue, with limitation of exercise performance. Thus, the syndrome of congestive heart failure (CHF) finally becomes manifest. Shown at the bottom of the figure are various studies addressing these phases of heart failure in terms of morbidity and mortality. GISSI, Gruppo Italiano per lo Studio dell a Sopravivenza nell'Infarto Miocardio; CONSENSUS, Cooperative North Scandinavian Enalapril Study; SMILE, Survival of Myocardial Infarction; ISIS, International Study of Infarct Survival; SAVE, Survival and Ventricular Enlargement Trial; SOLVD, Studies of Left Ventricular Dysfunction; TRACE, Trandolapril Cardiac Evaluation: V-HeFT, Veterans Administration Cooperative Vasodilator Heart Failure Trial; AIRE, Acute Infarction Ramipril Efficacy Study.

may evolve over years, as occurs with overloads resulting from systemic hypertension or valvular disease.[7] In the absence of overt clinical symptoms, such as chest pain with a myocardial infarction or sudden (flash) pulmonary edema, the initial damage may go on undiagnosed. In this situation, a two-dimensional echocardiogram can be helpful in documenting the presence and extent of LV dysfunction (see Chap. 14). Ventricular dilatation may argue for a more chronic underlying disease process in largely asymptomatic patients.

The second stage in the evolution of heart failure involves an adaptation to the initial myocardial damage, termed *ventricular remodeling*. This involves myocardial hypertrophy in response to myocardium that is lost or overloaded and ventricular dilatation, which helps to sustain cardiac output (Fig. 23-2). At the same time, neurohumoral activation occurs.[8] Activation of the sympathetic nervous system with parasympathetic withdrawal leads to tachycardia and peripheral vasoconstriction. Activation of the renin-angiotensin systems

causes further vasoconstriction and salt accumulation via stimulated aldosterone secretion. Both these latter factors, along with excessive stretch of the myocardium, can lead to further myocyte loss while ventricular dilatation may induce functional mitral and/or tricuspid insufficiency and an additional hemodynamic load (Fig. 23-2).[9]

The third phase in the evolution of heart failure evolves from these adaptive changes, with development of the symptoms of CHF: decreased exercise tolerance, pulmonary and systemic congestion, and central and peripheral edema.

The interval between initiation of ventricular dysfunction and the onset of symptoms, during which ventricular remodeling occurs, may extend over a long time period, but should the damage be related to an acute myocardial infarction, this period can be very short. With more chronic processes, such as those that occur with hypertension or idiopathic cardiomyopathies, this period may extend over months or years. Indeed, when patients were first identified with asymptomatic LV dysfunction in the Studies of Left Ventricular Dysfunction (SOLVD) trial (discussed below), their average EF was already reduced to 28 percent, indicating that extensive ventricular damage had already occurred (Fig. 23-3). At this point, exercise performance, as represented by peak oxygen consumption, was moderately reduced but not to such an extent as to limit exercise performance or produce symptoms. Circulating norepinephrine was increased slightly, while plasma renin levels (slashed lines) were not, except when diuretics had been administered (open bars). Once symptoms occurred, there was a progressive increase in circulating norepinephrine and plasma renin. A progressive decline in exercise capacity was documented as patients progressed from New York Heart Association (NYHA) class I to class IV. The reduction in exercise performance was relatively greater than the decrease in the EF. This relates to the finding that with inactivity, the capacity for peripheral vasodilatation is reduced, which limits skeletal muscle performance.

Abnormalities of ventricular function may involve the left or right ventricles, or both. In addition, such abnormalities may be amplified by overloads created by valvular insufficiency (e.g., mitral or tricuspid) or systolic overloads (e.g., aortic stenosis, arterial or pulmonary hypertension). Separating the effects of myocardial dysfunction from such imposed overloads is difficult (see Chap. 22). Moreover, functional mitral and/or tricuspid insufficiency resulting from ventricular dilatation imposes a further volume load on an already damaged myocardium.

Abnormalities of ventricular function can be usefully divided into problems of ventricular filling (diastole) and ventricular emptying (systole). Diastolic filling of the left ventricle, in turn, can be analyzed in terms of three phases: (1) rapid ventricular filling following ventricular relaxation, which involves substantial diastolic recoil in the normal heart; (2) passive filling during the middle of diastole; and (3) late diastolic filling augmented by atrial contraction. In general, diastolic filling can be evaluated from noninvasive Doppler measurements of early (E wave) versus later (A wave) filling or from invasive measurements of ventricular filling pressures just prior to ventricular contraction (see Chap. 14).

Even in the presence of normal systolic ventricular performance, abnormalities of ventricular filling, termed *diastolic dysfunction*, may

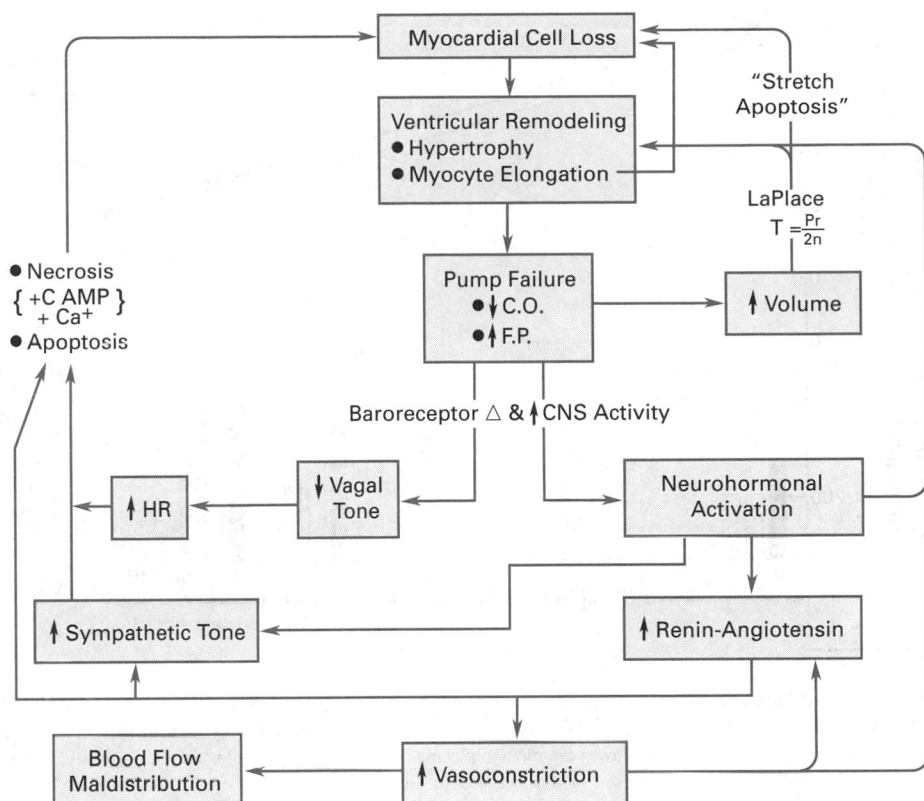

FIGURE 23-2

Ventricular remodeling and progression of ventricular dysfunction. Myocardial cell loss leads to ventricular remodeling, characterized by myocyte hypertrophy and elongation. An increase in ventricular volume (the Starling effect) helps to maintain cardiac output (CO) but at the cost of increasing ventricular filling pressures. The increase in diastolic stretch and pressure produces further damage, including stretch-induced myocyte death (apoptosis), which amplifies the process of remodeling. With inadequate pump function, neurohumoral activation occurs with decreased vagal tone and enhanced sympathetic tone. With activation of the renin-angiotensin system and increased sympathetic tone, arterial vasoconstriction occurs with resultant maldistribution of blood flow. Decreased vagal and increased sympathetic stimulation induce tachycardia, and the latter system along with the activated renin-angiotensin system via angiotensin II can produce further myocyte death. In this manner, the process is self-perpetuating, in that ventricular damage leads to remodeling, which, in turn, leads to further damage. These interrelated cycles thus provide therapeutic opportunities.

be observed, which require specific therapeutic consideration (Fig. 23-4). These are characterized by an increased ventricular filling pressure for any end-diastolic volume (EDV) due to reduced compliance of the ventricle. Thus, with normal EDV and stroke volume (SV), filling pressures may be markedly increased, leading to signs of pulmonary congestion despite a normal EF. Such a situation may occur with LV hypertrophy, especially when associated with a rapid heart rate, which further limits the time for ventricular filling. It can also occur with the aging heart where diffuse myocyte loss can occur with replacement fibrosis and reactive myocyte hypertrophy.[10]

Systolic function is characterized by the ability to generate pressure isovolumically, as measured by high-fidelity recording of LV pressure rise, dP/dt, which is followed by the ejection of blood into the aorta. As is known from classic physiology, the SV depends on the diastolic volume as well as the afterload, which is directly related to the arterial pressure. If the afterload is reasonably normal, there is a linear relation between SV and EDV, and the resultant slope (SV/EDV) is termed the *ejection fraction*. Should the slope of the relation linking end-systolic pressure and LV volume be reduced, as occurs when the ventricle is depressed, the SV at any EDV is reduced, resulting in a decreased EF. If the afterload is approximately normal, this reduced EF can serve as a measure of reduced ventricular performance. Since the extent of shortening of myocardium is reduced as afterload is increased, an increased systolic ventricular pressure can by itself reduce SV and hence tend to decrease EF, as can occur in severe aortic stenosis. Similarly with severe mitral insufficiency, which decreases afterload via a low impedance pathway into the left atrium, an increased SV tends to occur, yielding an artificially increased EF. Thus, with these considerations in mind, the EF can provide a useful indicator of systolic ventricular performance (see Chap. 22).

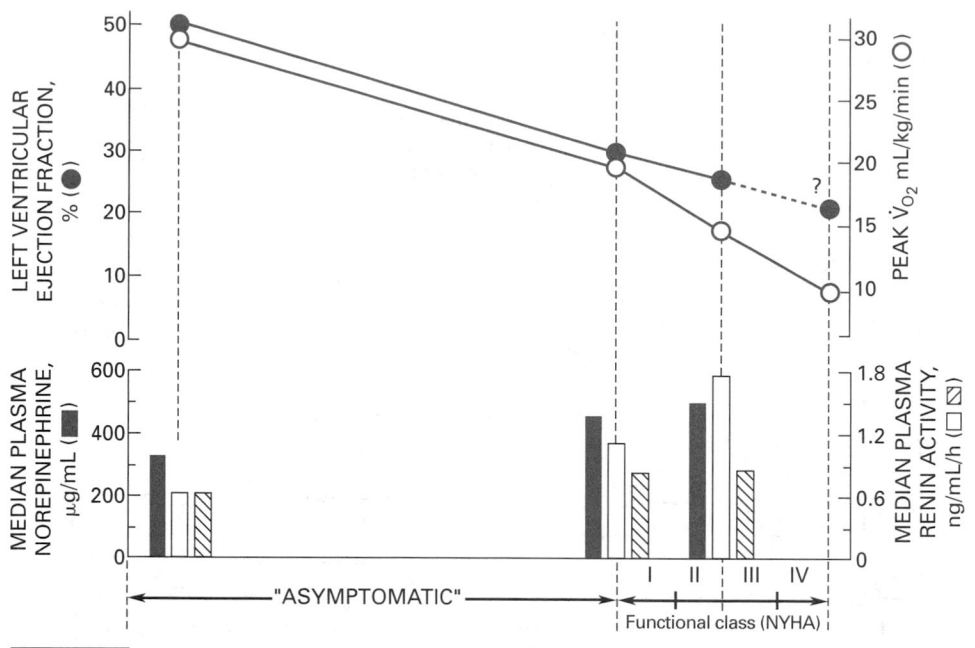

FIGURE 23-3

Progression of initial ventricular damage to sympathetic congestive heart failure. Data from the SOLVD trial of enalapril therapy; plotted in terms of LV ejection fraction and exercise capacity measured in terms of peak oxygen consumption ($\dot{V}_{O_2}$). Also shown are median plasma norepinephrine and plasma renin activity. The latter is shown in terms of patients who did or did not receive diuretics.

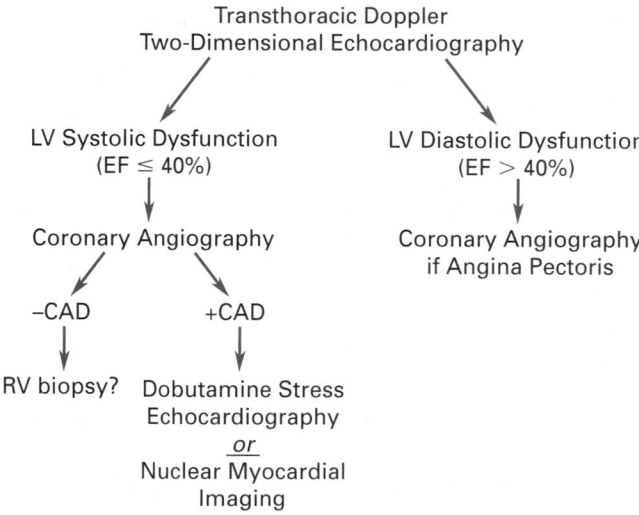

FIGURE 23-4

Evaluation of patients with congestive heart failure. Transthoracic Doppler and two-dimensional echocardiography provide a central modality to evaluate ventricular function and valvular abnormalities. Ventricular wall thickness and both end-diastolic and end-systolic volumes can be determined. With an ejection fraction (EF) more than 40 percent, coronary angiography is indicated in the presence of angina pectoris or evidence of significant ischemia. With an EF less than 40 percent, coronary arteriography is indicated since the underlying ischemic depression may be amenable to reperfusion by either angioplasty or coronary bypass surgery. Nuclear imaging techniques are used to define viable ischemic myocardium, while stimulation of such myocardium with dobutamine or extrasystolic potentiation may indicate recoverable hibernating myocardium. Right ventricular biopsy may be indicated in the absence of coronary artery disease to rule out processes such as amyloid or sarcoid.

Although complex indices of systolic ventricular function have been described on the basis of myocardial muscle function,[11] the measurement of EF has served as the clinical standard, whether determined noninvasively by echocardiography (see Chap. 14) and nuclear imaging techniques (see Chap. 17) or invasively with angiography (see Chap. 16). In addition to an overall depression of myocardial function, focal abnormalities of ventricular wall motion, described in terms of hypokinesis and akinesis, may produce major alterations in overall LV function, as seen in coronary artery disease (see Chaps. 44 and 45). While a segment of the LV wall may be replaced by fibrotic scar, focal abnormalities of contraction may occur in viable myocardium when coronary perfusion is transiently reduced, leading to prolonged decrease in contraction; this is termed *stunning*. Alternatively, with a sustained reduction in coronary blood flow that is still adequate to sustain viability, contraction can be persistently reduced or absent; this is termed *hibernation*.[12,13] These important alterations can occur simultaneously in a given patient and are hard to separate.[13] Defining these abnormalities in coronary heart disease with heart failure is extremely important, since reversal of transient or persistent ischemia with vascular reperfusion may be vital for restoring segmental contraction and improving overall ventricular function.[12,14] Various techniques have been employed to identify such tissue, including echocardiographic studies using a catecholamine stress[15–18] and angiographic studies using nitroglycerin[19] or extrasystolic potentiation following a premature ventricular contraction.[12,20,21]

Once ventricular dysfunction is manifest, abnormalities of reflex control of the circulation ensue. As CHF progresses, decreased baroreceptor sensitivity occur with augmented sympathetic tone and reduced parasympathetic tone (Fig. 23-2).[8] This results in an increase in heart rate along with reduced beat-to-beat heart rate variability (see Chap. 27) and loss of the Valsalva overshoot. These changes also help to establish the diagnosis of heart failure.

With reduced ventricular function, exercise performance tends to be reduced as measured by a reduced maximum O_2 uptake on a treadmill ($\dot{V}_{O_2}$). However, this reduction in exercise performance does not always correlate with a reduced EF,[3] since it also reflects the *training* state of the peripheral circulation.

Clinical Assessment

Clinically, the diagnosis of heart failure is made by the patient's history, by physical findings on clinical examination, and by data obtained from routine chest x-rays and electrocardiogram. The history obtained from patients tends to reflect either pulmonary or systemic congestion, or both, with complaints of shortness of breath, initially with effort and on lying down, generally associated with easy fatiguability and, commonly, peripheral edema. Common factors in the history will often include diabetes mellitus, coronary events, and hypertension. On physical examination, peripheral vasoconstriction and tachycardia are common, along with the presence of pulmonary rales and physical signs of pleural effusion. Cardiac findings may include a fourth heart sound (S_4), reflecting a stiffened or hypertrophied ventricle, and a third heart sound reflecting more profound LV failure. A pulsus paradoxus may be present. Murmurs can be auscultated that may relate to valvular organic abnormalities, although functional mitral and tricuspid insufficiency can occur as a function of LV and/or right ventricular (RV) dilatation per se. Peripheral venous engorgement and an enlarged liver, along with peripheral edema, will be detected as RV failure ensues. If RV failure is severe, clinical symptoms associated with LV failure, such as severe shortness of breath, may actually be lessened.

Precipitant factors for developing CHF should be looked for, such as anemia, infection, dietary indiscretion, acute arrhythmias (especially atrial fibrillation), poor treatment compliance, pulmonary embolism, and occult myocardial infarction.

Nuclear imaging techniques (see Chap. 17), computed tomography (see Chap. 18), and magnetic resonance imaging (see Chap. 19) have been useful in assessing ventricular volume, shapes, and motion and have provided an excellent assessment of ventricular function. However, two-dimensional echocardiography will provide much of the necessary information in a practical and cost-effective manner and remains the clinical standard. Its accuracy and usefulness depend on the care expended in performing the procedure and the professional oversite that is utilized in both detecting and interpreting the findings that are obtained. Echo-Doppler examination not only provides information about systolic and diastolic volumes, and thus EF, but also allows for the evaluation of valve structure and function, including regurgitation and stenosis (see Chap. 14). Reasonably accurate measurements of gradients, and thus valvular orifices, can be made, which can help direct therapy.

In defining the etiology of heart failure, segmental wall motion abnormalities with hypokinetic and contralateral hyperkinetic segments suggest an ischemic etiology. Indeed, following an acute myocardial infarction, a two-dimensional echocardiogram obtained within a few days is essential. The finding of ventricular dilatation within a few days of an acute anterior wall infarction tends to predict progressive LV dilatation with a falling EF. In patients sustaining an anterior wall infarction without initial ventricular dilatation, approximately one-third will show ventricular dilatation at 3 months. In contrast, ventricular dilatation rarely occurs following inferior wall infarctions, except when the region involved is large, extending from the base of the heart to the apex. After an acute myocardial infarction,[22] LV enlargement, as measured by two-dimensional echocardiography, is associated with an increased incidence of adverse cardiovascular events. When LV diastolic volumes of patients with infarction are divided into quartiles, patients in the fourth quartile have a mortality rate of 45.5 percent, while patients in the third quartile have a mortality rate of 21.1 percent and patients in the first and second quartiles have the same mortality rate of 16.7 percent.[23] If LV dilatation occurs much later, however, two-dimensional echocardiography will not differentiate between the cause of heart failure, i.e., coronary artery disease or other etiologies. Moreover, patients with a primary cardiomyopathy may also exhibit segmental wall motion abnormalities. As noted above, stimuli that elicit latent contraction, such as low-dose dobutamine, stress, or premature ventricular contractions, may help identify patients with dilated left ventricles and severe coronary artery disease who also have *hibernating* or *stunned* myocardium.[13,24,25]

THE TREATMENT OF CONGESTIVE HEART FAILURE

As noted initially, the treatment of heart failure requires close attention to both the primary etiology and the relief of symptoms, while attempting to reduce the risk of death from the process. This includes control of hypertension, if present, and an evaluation for treatment of myocardial ischemia. As noted above and discussed further relative to surgical approaches to heart failure (see below), noncontractile but viable myocardium, whether due to stunning or hibernation, requires definition with consideration of coronary reperfusion.[13] Valvular disease that imposes an excessive volume or pressure overload must be considered relative to the need for surgical correction (see Chaps. 63, 64, and 65). For example, critical aortic stenosis with heart failure is a very urgent indication for valve replacement when possible, not medical therapy. To those ends, there is a multifactorial approach to therapy[13] depending on the etiology and stage of the heart failure process (Fig. 23-5).

Nonpharmacologic Aspects of Treatment

Nonpharmacologic factors contribute to the overall efficacy of care. Weight reduction by dieting is generally advisable when obesity is present. Often, however, nutritional status is compromised and cachexia is present.[26] Limitation of salt intake is important and may delay the time when diuretics may be necessary as well as reduce the amount required. In advanced heart failure, strict salt limitation is essential, although it is difficult to maintain. A diet containing less than 20 g/d of salt is desirable. Intake of fluids should be reduced

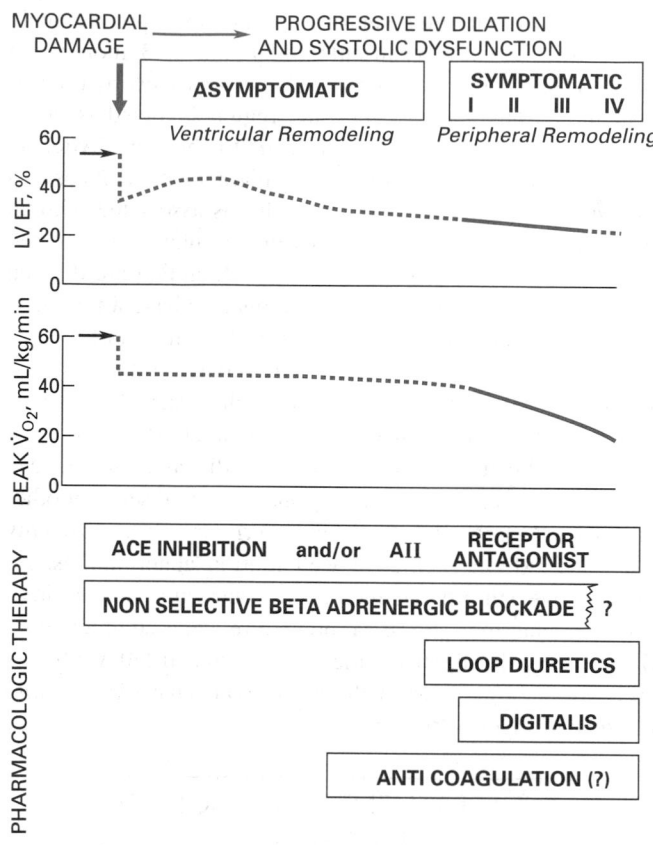

MYOCARDIAL DAMAGE → PROGRESSIVE LV DILATION AND SYSTOLIC DYSFUNCTION

ASYMPTOMATIC

Ventricular Remodeling

SYMPTOMATIC
I   II   III   IV

Peripheral Remodeling

ACE INHIBITION   and/or   AII   RECEPTOR ANTAGONIST

NON SELECTIVE BETA ADRENERGIC BLOCKADE   ?

LOOP DIURETICS

DIGITALIS

ANTI COAGULATION (?)

FIGURE 23-5

Staged use of therapeutic agents in heart failure. Initial approaches include control of factors that may cause progression of heart failure and/or augment its manifestations. Hypertension requires control. Unanticipated tachycardia may augment oxygen needs while reducing the time in diastole for coronary flow to take place. The reduction in the diastolic time can lead to marked elevations of left ventricular (LV) diastolic pressure as well as increased ischemia. Moreover, atrial fibrillation will deprive ventricular filling of the "atrial kick" and lead to further elimination of diastolic pressures. These considerations are of special importance with ventricular hypertrophy and resultant diastolic dysfunction. During the "remodeling" phase of ventricular failure, the patient may be asymptomatic. Nevertheless, inhibition of the renin-angiotensin system is indicated to reduce the rate of ventricular remodeling and slow ventricular dilation. β-Adrenergic blockade shows increasing promise in reducing progression and perhaps mortality in heart failure, especially in nonischemic dilated cardiomyopathies. Once symptoms ensue, loop diuretics are generally needed for fluid control. Digitalis glycosides are also indicated for neurohumoral benefits in reducing sympathetic tone and enhancing parasympathetic tone while providing modest inotropic support. These actions appear to improve morbidity, without necessarily altering mortality.

to 1 to 1.5 L every 24 h in patients with advanced heart failure, with or without hyponatremia, except in warm climates. As will be stressed in relation to the use of diuretics, a readable weight scale is essential, and daily weights are of great value in judging therapy.

Smoking should be strongly discouraged in all patients, especially in the presence of obstructive vascular disease. Alcohol is a cardiac depressant in general and should be forbidden if an alcoholic cardiomyopathy is suspected. In all other cases, daily intake of alcohol probably should not exceed 40 g day in men and 30 g day in women, although there are,

as yet, insufficient data on the effects of alcohol in patients with mild heart failure to support these recommendations.[27]

Patients should routinely receive vaccinations against influenza and pneumococcal pneumonia.

Deconditioning related to muscular inactivity in association with muscular atrophy and decreased metabolic vascular dilatation is a major factor in reducing exercise performance as heart failure progresses.[28] The 6-min walk test is a semiquantitative assessment tool for assessing functional capacity before and after treatment.[29] Low-level exercise, such as walking, should be encouraged, whereas strenuous isometric activities should be discouraged. Specific exercise training needs to be tailored to the appropriate level of the patient's disease and always performed under medical guidance. Isometric exercise should be avoided. In patients with stable heart failure, there is evidence that appropriate physical exercise and exercise training can lead to improvements in both exercise capacity and the quality of life of the patient, although the effect of this intervention on prognosis is unknown.[30–32] Specific recommendations include dynamic aerobic exercise (walking) three to five times a week for 20 to 30 min, or cycling for 20 min at 70 to 80 percent of peak heart rate five times a week.[30,31]

In patients with acute heart failure or in those with exacerbations of chronic heart failure, rest is advisable. Prolonged rest, however, should not be encouraged in patients with stable chronic heart failure.

Pharmacologic Treatment

In general, pharmacologic treatment is directed to three demonstrable hemodynamic endpoints: (1) to reduce volume overloads and maintain a stable volume state, (2) to reduce preload and afterload to enhance ventricular performance, and (3) to improve ventricular contractility when necessary. An additional pharmacologic aim is to reduce heightened neurohumoral activity, which is seen in patients with heart failure, with the hope of limiting abnormal loading created by these systems and preventing the progression of the heart failure process. The ultimate aim is to reduce morbidity and perhaps extend life.

DIURETICS

Sodium accumulation tends to occur in the early stages of CHF, with peripheral edema accompanied by weight gain. Diuretics, along with salt restriction, remain the best therapeutic tool for treating the edematous state in heart failure. Despite the advent of new agents for treating symptomatic CHF, diuretics continue to be among the most commonly prescribed drugs in the world.

The mechanism for edema is generally multifactorial and includes renal vasoconstriction, increased aldosterone, and/or increased venous pressures (see Chap. 21). Increased sympathetic nervous system activity (tone) tends to occur early in the course of heart failure. Activation of the renin-angiotensin axis tends to occur somewhat later in time, commonly when diuretics are begun.[33] This leads to increased aldosterone, leading to sodium accumulation and potassium loss. Even with asymptomatic LV dysfunction, avidity of the kidneys for sodium and water is greatly enhanced, and peripheral edema comprises an early physical sign that brings the problem of CHF to the physician's attention. Salt and water retention lead to an expanded intravascular volume, with an increase in LV filling pressures in order to maintain cardiac output.[34] With continued worsening of LV function, progressive volume expansion continues and LV end-diastolic pressure rises along with venous hydrostatic pressure in both the systemic and pulmonary beds. This alteration in Starling forces favors transudation of intravascular fluid into the interstitial compartment, culminating in edema formation.[35] Eventually a point is reached at which additional increases in LV filling pressure fail to augment cardiac output, and with progressive increases in peripheral arterial vasoconstriction, renal perfusion is reduced. By this time, overt heart failure is established, and the kidney's ability to excrete a salt load severely impaired.[34] Important mediators in this process are: (1) activation of the renin-angiotensin-aldosterone axis; (2) stimulation of the sympathetic nervous system; (3) increased levels of antidiuretic hormone leading to water retention and hyponatremia; and (4) resistance to atrial natriuretic peptide (ANP), which is an endogenous hormonal vasodilator and diuretic.

Loop Diuretics

The most potent diuretics are those whose action is in the medullary thick ascending limb of Henle, because of the percentage of filtrate reabsorption that occurs at this segment of the nephron. In the euvolemic state, about 20 percent of filtered sodium load is reabsorbed in the thick ascending limb, compared with only 7 percent in the distal tubule and 5 percent in the collecting duct.[36] Drugs in this diuretic class include furosemide, bumetanide, torsemide, and ethacrynic acid. The loop diuretics are more than 98 percent protein-bound and therefore not freely filtered by the glomerulus. Rather, they access the tubular lumen, where they act by secretion via an organic anion transporter.[37] This secretion of loop diuretic may be impaired and their action limited by the presence of elevated levels of endogenous organic acids, such as occurs in renal failure, and by probenecid, salicylates, and nonsteroidal anti-inflammatory agents (NSAIDs). Once in the lumen of the tubule, the loop diuretics compete with chloride for binding to the $Na^+/K^+/2Cl$ cotransporter situated on the apical membrane of cells of the medullary thick ascending limb, thereby inhibiting the reabsorption of both sodium and chloride.[38] The urinary diuretic concentration best represents the fraction of drug delivered to the thick ascending limb and significantly correlates with the natriuretic response following diuretic administration.[39]

Furosemide is the most widely used loop diuretic. In normal patients, the oral bioavailability of furosemide is 50 percent. Following an oral dose, the onset of action occurs within 30 to 60 min, peaks at 1 to 2 h, and has a duration of action of 6 h, with a half-life of 50 min.[37,40] Furosemide may be given

intravenously over 1 to 2 min; following intravenous administration, diuresis begins within 15 min and peaks at 30 to 60 min. The duration of action is up to 2 h when given intravenously. Sixty percent of furosemide is excreted unchanged in the urine; the rest is conjugated with glucuronic acid in the kidney.[37,40] In renal insufficiency [glomerular filtration rate (GFR) <30 mL/min], the elimination half-life is prolonged, although the diuretic response is impaired, largely owing to reduced drug delivery to its site of action within the tubule.[41]

In CHF, the pharmacokinetics of oral furosemide are also altered; furosemide absorption is delayed, which leads to a delay in the time at which peak concentration occurs.[39] Altered furosemide pharmacodynamic properties occur independent of the route of administration, due to adaptations within the glomerular microcirculation and renal tubule that are present during chronic diuretic administration.[39]

Bumetanide is 40 times more potent than furosemide and is available in both oral and intravenous formulations. In normal patients, the bioavailability is 80 percent following an oral dose, and the onset of diuretic effects occurs within 30 min and peaks within 1 h. The duration of action of oral bumetanide is between 3 and 6 h, with a half-life between 1 and 3.5 h.[40,42] Similar to furosemide, the delayed absorption of oral bumetanide in heart failure results in lower peak concentrations as well as in a delayed time to peak concentration.

Torsemide is a new loop diuretic that differs from others in its class in that 80 percent of a dose undergoes hepatic metabolism. Because only 20 percent of the drug is excreted unchanged in the urine, its half-life is minimally altered in renal failure.[43] Torsemide is rapidly absorbed and is 80 to 90 percent bioavailable. In patients with chronic renal insufficiency or with cirrhosis, the natriuretic response following torsemide is unaffected by route of administration.[44] Maximal sodium excretion occurs within the first 2 h after either routine. In healthy individuals, the half-life of torsemide is 3.3 h but is prolonged to 8 h in cirrhosis.[43,45] When selecting an oral agent in patients with heart failure, the physician may find oral torsemide to be advantageous since its absorption is unimpaired and is less variable than that with oral furosemide.[46] In fact, the pharmacokinetics of torsemide in CHF are comparable to those in normal persons. As is the case with all loop diuretics, however, dose-response curves for torsemide in patients with CHF are shifted downward and to the right, suggesting altered drug pharmacodynamics and a diminished diuretic response.

The efficacy of loop diuretics is often significantly reduced in decompensated heart failure. Impaired drug absorption has been implicated as one cause of variable efficacy. Reduced gastric and intestinal motility, edematous bowel wall, and decreased splanchnic blood flow may delay absorption. The total amount of furosemide absorbed over 24 h, however, is similar to that found in normal individuals.[47–49]

In patients with stable, compensated heart failure given oral furosemide, the time to peak urinary excretion is prolonged to about 190 min (normal, 90 min) and peak urinary excretion rate is reduced by 50 percent.[39] Furosemide and bumetanide, when given in doses of equivalent potency, induce a similar natriuretic response in patients with heart failure.[39] The pharmacokinetic properties of intravenous furosemide are unaltered in heart failure patients compared with normal individuals.[50]

The effectiveness of loop diuretics is limited by two phenomena in patients with chronic heart failure and normal renal function. The *rebound phenomenon* consists of a decrease in sodium excretion below baseline after the effect of the loop diuretic has worn off. The *braking phenomenon* refers to an increase in tubular sodium reabsorption by the distal tubule, which occurs during long-term administration of loop diuretics.

In decompensated heart failure, the intravenous route of administration is preferable when possible, since the onset of diuresis is shorter and more predictable (Fig. 23-6). In patients with CHF refractory to standard doses of intravenous furosemide, higher doses may be efficacious. In 20 patients with severe CHF previously resistant to lower intravenous doses of furosemide,[51] intravenous furosemide was administered at doses of 500 to 2000 mg daily for a mean of 10 days, with increased diuresis, weight reduction, and symptomatic improvement. Other investigators observed a similar clinical improvement, as assessed by NYHA classification criteria, in 17 of 21 patients using high-dose oral furosemide (>500 mg daily) for 1 month.[52]

Continuous intravenous rather than intermittent administration of loop diuretics is an effective method of overcoming diuretic resistance in heart failure. In a randomized crossover study comparing continuous versus bolus bumetanide in patients with chronic renal failure (mean GFR, 17 mL/min), a greater net sodium excretion was observed during continuous infusion despite comparable drug excretion.[53] In CHF, continuous infusion of furosemide produces a similar natriuresis at serum concentrations 20 times lower than after a comparable effective bolus dose.[54] Only one prospective, randomized crossover study is available that compares the continuous infusion of furosemide (loading dose 30 to 40 mg followed by infusion at a rate of 2.5 to 3.3 mg/h for 48 h) with intermittent intravenous bolus administration (30 to 40 mg every 8 h for 48 h) in NYHA class III and IV heart failure.[55] When infused continuously, furosemide's pattern of delivery produced more effective drug utilization, that is, sodium excretion relative to total furosemide excretion, whereas with intermittent bolus furosemide, wide fluctuations in urine output and sodium excretion were observed. Theoretically, an infusion of furosemide at a constant rate may be safer than using intermittent intravenous dosing, although a larger study is needed to confirm this.[56]

In summary, loop diuretics with salt restriction monitored by weight measurement by scale remains the basis for treatment of edema. As CHF progresses, increasing oral doses of loop diuretics tend to be needed. In severe CHF with hospitalization, intravenous loop diuretics, commonly at higher doses, become essential. As will be discussed below, other agents, such as metolazone, may be required as well to increase and sustain sodium loss. Limitations to diuretic use remain hyponatremia and a progressive increase in serum creatinine, which may require careful dose reductions (Table 23-1).

Thiazides

The thiazide diuretics may be reasonable first-line natriuretic agents in early LV dysfunction when renal perfusion is not yet significantly compromised. In overt ventricular failure, however, thiazides are usually ineffective or inadequate. Thiazides are 50 percent protein-bound, and more than 95 percent

---

TABLE 23-1

STEPWISE APPROACH TO LOOP DIURETIC RESISTANCE

1. Enforce strict low-sodium diet.
2. Use effective doses of loop diuretic.
3. Combination administration of long-acting thiazide with loop diuretic to offset the antinatriuretic rebound effect observed after administration of short-acting loop diuretic.
4. Constant intravenous infusion of loop diuretic.

STEPWISE APPROACH TO THERAPY OF DECOMPENSATED CONGESTIVE HEART FAILURE

Fluid Retention	Low Flow State
IV Boluses of Loop Diuretics	Dobutamine (No β block.)
Continuous IV Infusion of Loop Diuretics	Milrinone (On β block.)
Metolazone and/or Spironolactone	Dobutamine and Milrinone
Extracorporeal Ultrafiltration	LVAD

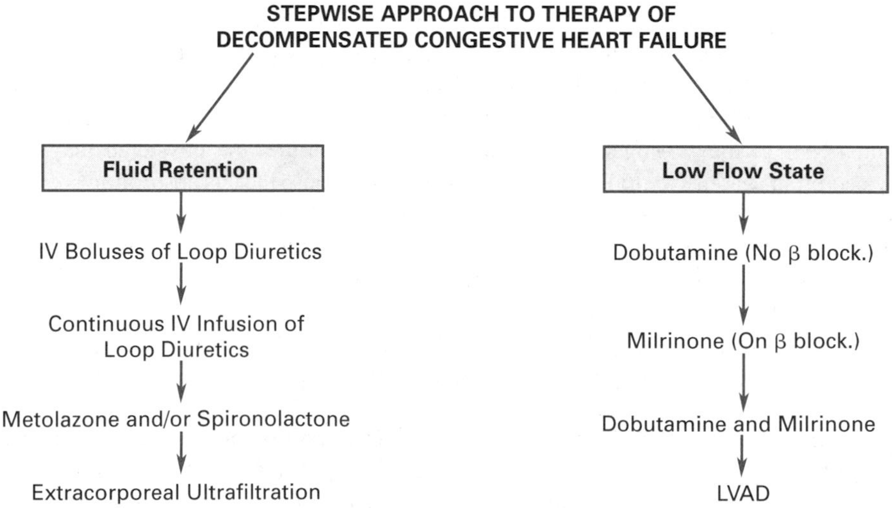

FIGURE 23-6

Treatment of congestive heart failure is directed toward controlling salt and water retention (central or peripheral edema) and/or relieving a low-flow state by increasing cardiac output while reducing very increased filling pressures. Dobutamine is useful to augment cardiac output except when β-adrenergic blockade is present. Milrinone, which stimulates the adenyl cyclase system beyond the beta receptor, acts well in this circumstance to augment the effects of dobutamine while serving as an arterial and venous dilator. When inadequate cardiac output can no longer be maintained, surgical implantation of a left ventricular assist device (LVAD) may be used to pump blood from the left ventricle to the aorta as a temporary support or bridge to transplantation.

of the dose is excreted unchanged in the urine.[40] They gain access into the tubular lumen by both glomerular filtration and tubular secretion. In the kidney, they inhibit sodium chloride reabsorption in the early distal tubule where they compete for the chloride site on the apically located Na^+/Cl cotransporter.[57,58]

Hydrochlorothiazide is the most widely prescribed drug in this class of diuretics. Seventy-one percent of an oral dose is absorbed. The onset of diuresis is within 2 h, peaks between 3 and 6 h, and continues for up to 12 h.[40] Hydrochlorothiazide's pharmacokinetics follow a two-compartment model of elimination (α phase, 5 h; β phase, 6 to 15 h), and the half-life is prolonged in patients with decompensated heart failure and in those with renal insufficiency.

Metolazone is a quinazoline diuretic and is similar to the thiazides in structure and mechanism of action.[40,59] Although its major effect is in the cortical diluting segment, metolazone has a minor inhibitory effect on proximal tubular sodium reabsorption. Metolazone is lipid-soluble and easily accesses the tubular lumen during states of renal insufficiency, unlike the thiazides.[60] Another advantage of metolazone is its longer duration of action (12 to 24 h).[40,59]

Potassium-Sparing Diuretics

Aldosterone, an endogenous adrenal hormone, normally increases Na^+ reabsorption with the simultaneous excretion of K^+, which may induce hypokalemia. Spironolactone, a lipid-soluble potassium-sparing diuretic, competes with aldosterone for binding to its receptor in the principal cell of the collecting duct and thus leads to diuresis.[40] Spironolactone is particularly advantageous during states of reduced renal perfusion because the drug's delivery to its site of action is not dependent on GFR. Moreover, aldosterone levels are increased in heart failure, to some degree due to its augmented secretion induced by angiotensin II.

The dose of spironolactone is 25 mg twice daily. Since the exchange of Na^+ for K^+ is reduced, K^+ loss is reduced and hypokalemia may be corrected. Indeed, K^+ supplements given for hypokalemia should generally be stopped in order to avoid hyperkalemia.

Amiloride and triamterene are similar to spironolactone in that they are potassium-sparing and act on the principal cell; however, they must be delivered intralumenally to be effective. More specifically, they reduce Na^+ flux into principal cells by blocking the apically located sodium channel.[40] When used alone, the potassium-sparing diuretics are relatively weak. In heart failure, they are useful when used in combination with a loop diuretic to overcome diuretic resistance and to reduce potassium wasting.[61]

Combined Use of Diuretics

Numerous reports have demonstrated a rapid, profound diuresis (1 to 2 L daily within 24 to 48 h), accompanied by clinical improvement, following the addition of metolazone to furosemide in patients with CHF (Fig. 23-6) who were previously resistant to furosemide alone.[62-69] Metolazone, a thiazide-like

diuretic, is particularly advantageous since it has a prolonged duration of action, is lipophilic, and remains effective in states of renal impairment. In a study comparing metolazone with a thiazide, however, when either was used in combination with a loop diuretic, no significant difference in sodium excretion or urine output was observed between the two drugs.[69] Spironolactone, when used in combination with a loop diuretic (Fig. 23-6), has also been associated with an improvement in diuretic response in patients with CHF previously resistant to loop diuretics.[61]

In summary, thiazides, potassium-sparing diuretics, aldosterone inhibitors (e.g., spironolactone), along with loop diuretics, provide potent tools to reduce salt accumulation in CHF. Early in CHF, their use is mainly to reduce or eliminate peripheral edema and help relieve pulmonary congestion. Once dry weight is approximated, intermittent and reduced diuretic use is advisable to avoid electrolyte problems. Daily weights are the best guide to adequacy of this therapy. Early in CHF, thiazides and potassium-sparing diuretics may be all that are necessary, although loop diuretics provide increased diuresis. Indeed, loop diuretics can be used intermittently on top of thiazides, when needed.

It is possible that the early use of diuretics can hasten the evolution of CHF by increasing reflex neurohumoral responses that may have adverse consequences, such as activation of the renin-angiotensin system.[33] As CHF progresses, the loop diuretics in increasing amounts are generally required. Here again, a scale for weight provides guidance for dose. With excessive diuresis in very severe CHF, increasing renal insufficiency may be induced by hypovolemia, and this, in itself, may increase loop diuretic dose, its use intravenously, and the need for concomitant use of thiazides (metalazone) or spironolactone.

INOTROPIC AGENTS

The use of inotropic agents in the treatment of CHF is predicated on the finding that a major contributing factor in reducing ventricular performance results from depression of myocardial contractility and that this can be reversed, or at least improved, by inotropic drugs. That there is reduced myocardial contractility in failing heart muscle, whether from a sustained work overload of pressure or in response to losing myocardium, has been well demonstrated and appears to be largely due to inadequate Ca^{2+} availability for activation (see Chap. 22). All inotropic agents currently available act to increase Ca^{2+} for activation in both normal and failing myocardium. This is the case whether the mechanism of action is via the cyclic AMP system excitation (e.g., catecholamines) or by sarcolemmal Na^+-K^+-ATPase inhibition (e.g., digitalis glycosides). The problem remains whether this increase in intracellular Ca^{2+} will benefit pump function while doing no harm, such as enhancing the propensity for arrhythmia or theoretically producing further myocyte loss. Moreover, agents that reduce afterload may enhance ventricular emptying without these potential hazards. In end-stage, severely decompensated CHF, inotropic agents (e.g., dobutamine) may be temporarily lifesaving (Fig. 23-6), and at somewhat earlier stages, they may reduce morbidity (e.g., digitalis glycosides). In earlier stages of CHF, benefits of inotropic agents may not outweigh risk, and their use is relegated to later stages in the disease process (Figs. 23-5 and 23-6).

Digitalis Glycosides

Digitalis glycosides have had a long and venerable history in the treatment of CHF and are the only oral inotropic agents available currently for this purpose (Fig. 23-7). In 1785, William Withering[70] reported on his use of the digitalis leaf as a purported diuretic agent to treat anasarca, presumably due to CHF. Indeed, the major effects of digitalis were initially thought to be on the kidneys, although important effects on heart rate were noted. Only during the latter part of the nineteenth century did it become apparent that there was a direct action of digitalis glycosides to increase cardiac contractility,[71] while in the earlier part of the twentieth century the effects of digitalis on the peripheral circulation and the autonomic nervous system were noted.[72] Despite this long history, the risks and benefits of digitalis administration on patients with sinus rhythm have remained controversial. The controversy has been partially addressed in a large randomized, placebo-controlled clinical trial of digoxin use in CHF.[73] Overall, digoxin was shown to be safe with a significant reduction in morbidity, expressed in terms of less need for hospitalization, but not in mortality. The benefit on hospitalization for heart failure appears greatest in those with lower EFs. As discussed later, with serum digoxin levels below 1 μg/mL, the neurohumoral and autocrine effects of digoxin predominate over the inotropic effects.

Digitalis glycosides have important effects on multiple systems in addition to augmenting the contractility of the myocardium.[74,75] Electrophysiologically, digitalis glycosides speed conduction in the atrium while inhibiting conduction at the atrioventricular node. This has made them useful in rate control in atrial fibrillation (see Chap. 30). In the normal circulation, digitalis glycosides also produce generalized arteriolar vasoconstriction, while affecting the central nervous system to enhance parasympathetic tone and reduce sympathetic nervous system activation. Digitalis glycosides sensitize baroreflexes to decrease efferent sympathetic activity, which acts to reduce sinus node activity and thus reduce heart rate. The precise mechanism for these effects is still unclear. The increase in baroreflex sensitization also increases parasympathetic tone, even in mild heart failure, while central vagal nuclei are also stimulated. The broad enhancement of parasympathetic activity with digitalis glycosides helps to explain the sinus heart rate slowing observed with digitalis glycosides even with sinus rhythm, as well as their therapeutic efficacy in control of supraventricular arrhythmias. As discussed below, in the failing state, the effects of sympathetic withdrawal may be dominant so as to reduce arterial vascular resistance, while in the normal circulation, arterial vasoconstriction may be dominant. Integration of these various actions adds to the inotropic activity and therapeutic usefulness of digitalis glycosides.

The positive inotropic action of digitalis glycosides to increase contractility and alter electrophysiology of heart muscle occurs through binding to and inhibition of the enzyme Na^+, K^+-ATPase on the surface membrane of myocardial cells, which results in an increase in the cytocyclic Ca^{2+} concentration.[76,77] The Na^+, K^+-ATPase is an energy-requiring "sodium pump" that extrudes three Na^+ ions, which enter the cell during depolarization in exchange for two K^+ ions, thus creating an electrical current and a negative resting potential.[78] Contraction is initiated with an action potential that depolarizes the surface membrane of the cell. This is created by a rapid inward current of Na^+ into the cell that opens sarcolemmal Ca^{2+} channels, permitting Ca^{2+} to enter the cell. This Ca^{2+} releases substantially more Ca^{2+} from stores in the sarcoplasmic reticulum within the cell, which in turn activates the contractile mechanism by binding to a component of the troponin-tropomyosin system that had been maintaining the resting state. With Ca^{2+} bound to troponin, actin and myosin can interact to produce force and shortening. The greater the amount of activating Ca^{2+}, the greater the force and shortening.[77,78] When Ca^{2+} is released from troponin and taken up by the sarcoplasmic reticulum, relaxation occurs.[77] The relatively small amount of Ca^{2+} that enters the cell with activation is ultimately removed by an electrogenic Na^+/Ca^{2+} exchange, which extrudes one Ca^{2+} for three Na^+ ions. When intracellular Na^+ is increased, less exchange occurs and the net amount of intracellular Ca^{2+} is increased. Thus, by inhibiting the Na^+, K^+-ATPase, digitalis glycosides produce a decrease in intracellular K^+ and an increase in intracellular Na^+ that increases intracellular Ca^{2+} (Fig. 23-8).[77,78] In general, the main way in which all inotropic agents, including digitalis glycosides, increase contractility is by increasing the amount of Ca^{2+} available for activation.[79] This is the case in both normal and failing myocardium. In the failing heart, there is also a decrease in the Ca^{2+} released into the cytosol with activation.[80,81] Digitalis glycosides increase this intracellular Ca^{2+} that augments Ca^{2+} stores in the sarcoplasmic

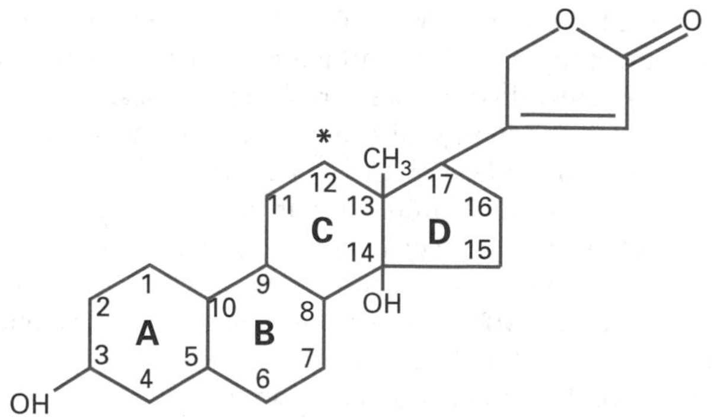

FIGURE 23-7
Structure of digitalis molecule. *Digitoxin becomes digoxin with OH placement at C_{12}. (From Sonnenblick EH, LeJemtel TH, Frishman WH. Digitalis preparations and other inotropic agents. In: Frishman WH, Sonnenblick EH, eds. *Cardiovascular Pharmacotherapeutics*. New York: McGraw-Hill; 1997:241. Reproduced with permission from the publisher and authors.)

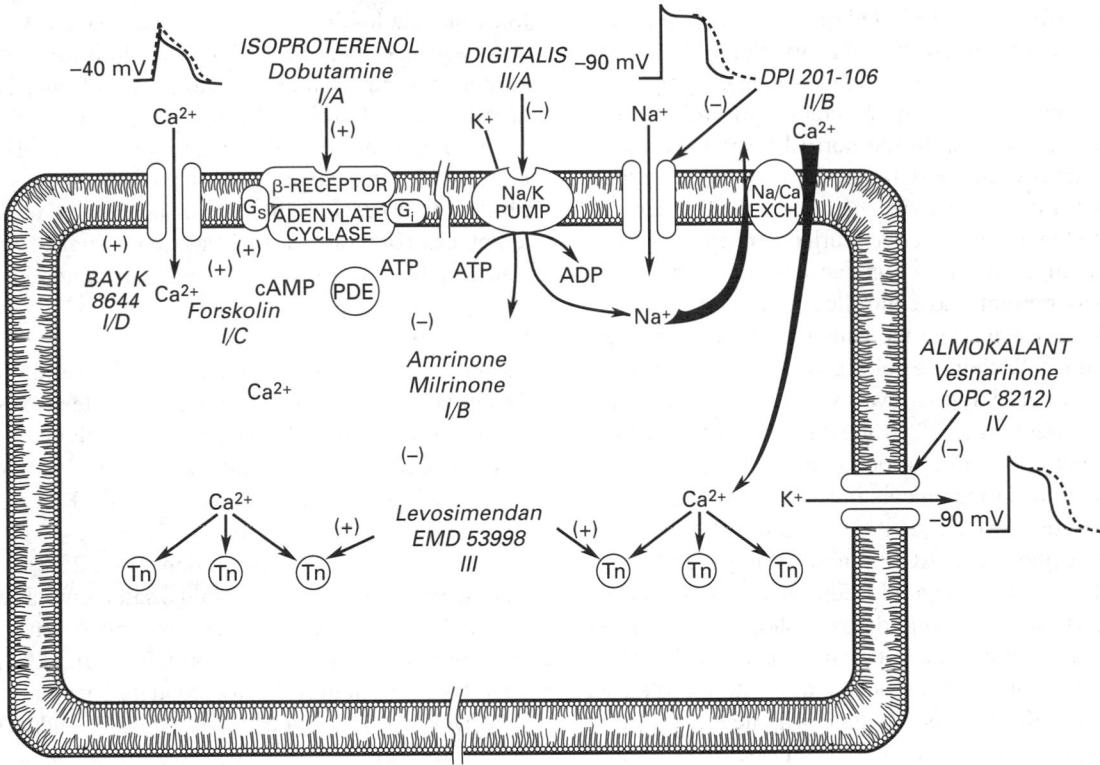

FIGURE 23-8

Diagram of various inotropic sites of action on and within the cardiac cell. While catecholamines act at cell surface receptors, agents such as amrinone and milrinone (PDE III inhibitors) act within the cell to augment adenylate cyclase. Calcium sensitizers increase Ca^{2+} sensitivity of troponin (Tn) in reticulum, resulting in a subsequent increase in previously reduced myocyte contraction. the contractile system itself. (From Varro A, Papp JG: Classification of positive inotropic actions based on electrophysiologic characteristics: Where should calcium sensitizers be placed? *J Cardiovasc Pharmacol* 1995; 26(suppl 1):S32. Reproduced with permission from the publisher and authors.)

Digoxin

Although there are numerous digitalis glycosides with varying duration of action and metabolic fate, digoxin has relatively rapid onset and intermediate duration of action. Digoxin has its most beneficial hemodynamic actions when substantial ventricular depression is evident along with CHF. In this circumstance, it augments myocardial performance while reflexly reducing peripheral resistance.[82] Acutely, digoxin also reduces cardiac norepinephrine spillover and reduces efferent sympathetic nerve activity in skeletal muscles in the patient with CHF.[82] Slowing of the heart rate, whether via enhanced parasympathetic tone and reduced sympathetic activity to reduce sinus rate or via control of heart rate in atrial fibrillation (as discussed below), will greatly benefit ventricular filling and reduce pulmonary congestion.[83] In the treatment of CHF, digoxin is generally employed along with diuretics and vasodilator agents. Thus, by reducing peripheral resistance, digoxin and peripheral vasodilators act in a complementary manner.

In acute heart failure, either due to massive sudden loss of myocardium, as may occur with a myocardial infarction, or with increasing decompensation in severe chronic CHF, characterized by acute pulmonary edema, severe limitations of cardiac output, and perhaps hypotension, more rapidly acting inotropic agents such as intravenous dobutamine or milrinone (discussed below) may be required (Fig. 23-6) together with loop diuretics and vasodilators. This situation may occur in the setting of rapid deterioration of the patient with more chronic heart failure or following a large myocardial infarction.[84] In this circumstance, the main aim is to increase cardiac output and reduce filling pressures as a setting for longer term stabilization. While rapidly acting inotropic agents are being used, digitalization may be begun cautiously for its longer term effects. In the setting of myocardial infarction, the situation is more complex. Due to a fear that arrhythmias may be induced or oxygen consumption increased, which might be detrimental, digoxin is generally avoided in the first few days following infarction,[84] although in a longer term treatment of CHF, digitalization, especially if dosing is carefully controlled, may be of value along with other agents, especially angiotensin-converting enzyme (ACE) inhibitors (see below).

For chronic CHF, digoxin is of use over the long term when administered in association with loop diuretics and ACE inhibitors. Benefits are most evident in patients with NYHA class III or IV CHF. In this circumstance, the response of the circulation is characterized by a decrease in venous pressures and ventricular filling pressures and an increase in cardiac output. Heart rate is slowed and EF tends to rise, while peripheral resistance falls with little or no change in arterial pressure.

These salutary effects are attributed to a combination of augmented myocardial contractility and restoration of baroreceptor sensitivity, which results in enhanced parasympathetic and decreased sympathetic tone. Whereas myocardial oxygen consumption may increase in the normal heart from the increased contractility, in heart failure it tends to be reduced due to a decrease in heart size, and thus ventricular wall tension, and a slowing of heart rate. Earlier concepts supported the view that digoxin was of greatest benefit when atrial fibrillation was present and controlled. It is now clear that efficacy is also present when the patient with heart failure is in sinus rhythm.[85] Withdrawal of digoxin from such patients has led to rapid deterioration, even when both diuretics and ACE inhibitors were used.[86,87] While digoxin has been associated with an increase in EF, vasodilators have been shown to cause more significant increments in exercise performance.[88] These considerations would justify the combined use of these agents. Whereas the use of ACE inhibitors may well be indicated when the ejection fraction is reduced and symptoms are limited (class I, II), however, digoxin should probably be reserved for use with more overt symptoms (class III, IV).

While digoxin can be given once a day without tolerance or tachyphylaxis, the dose is a matter of issue.[89] In general, a serum level of 0.5 to 1.5 mg/L is felt to be therapeutic.[90] This level may vary from patient to patient, and a clear dose-response relation has not been established. Indeed, some of the greatest benefits may be gained from lower doses (e.g., 0.125 mg/d), which may induce the neurohumoral benefits of lower sympathetic and higher parasympathetic tone while reducing the incidence of possible toxic side effects,[89] as discussed below. There appear to be no adverse effects from digoxin usage in terms of mortality in patients with CHF,[73] and substantially increased morbidity noted when the drug is withdrawn[86,91,92] suggests such a result. Effects on mortality with digoxin are complicated by the fact that the nature and progression of the underlying process, which led to failure in the first place, may well be the ultimate determinant of mortality. If morbidity is reduced substantially with digoxin, as demonstrated,[73] a neutral effect on ultimate mortality would be acceptable. This was recently demonstrated in the Digitalis Investigation Group (DIG) Study (sponsored by the National Institutes of Health), a controlled trial in patients with CHF, which showed no effect on survival compared to placebo, a reduction in hospitalizations, and a low incidence of digoxin toxicity.[73]

Digoxin has been shown to be of limited value in treatment of right-sided heart failure, which can occur in cor pulmonale or with left-to-right shunts. Digoxin also has limited value in acute LV failure due to acute myocardial infarction, although it is useful in the subsequent treatment of ischemic-related CHF. Nevertheless, since mortality may be increased after infarction by digoxin, especially when clear evidence of heart failure is absent, its use is best reserved for patients with overt CHF.

Toxicities from digitalis glycosides can be numerous and are somewhat dependent on serum level. Central nervous symptoms include loss of appetite and nausea and visual changes may be seen. Cardiac limitations include atrioventricular block, premature ventricular extra systoles, and ultimately ventricular tachycardia and fibrillation. Monitoring serum levels may be useful in the patient with sinus rhythm, while the ventricular rate provides an adequate guide to dose in the presence of atrial fibrillation. Except in dire circumstances, such as a suicide attempt, cessation of therapy is adequate. In the former circumstance, antibodies to digoxin may be indicated.

Catecholamines

As noted above, positive inotropism is based on enhancing the delivery of Ca^{2+} to the contractile system so as to increase force and shortening. Increasing Ca^{2+} in the serum will effect this transiently, while digitalis glycosides increase Ca^{2+} for activation by inhibiting sarcolemmal Na^+-K^+-ATPase. Catecholamines increase activating Ca^{2+} via β-adrenergic receptors and the adenyl cyclase system (Fig. 23-8).

Beta receptors are located in the sarcolemma and comprise a complex structure that spans the membrane.[93] The beta receptor is connected with G proteins (Fig. 23-8) that either activate (G_s) or inhibit (G_i) a secondary enzyme system, adenylate cyclase, which, when activated by G_s, induces the formation of $3'$-$5'$ cyclic adenosine-monophosphate (cyclic AMP). Cyclic AMP in turn activates certain protein kinases, which lead to intracellular phosphorylation of proteins that both enhance the entry and removal of intracellular Ca^{2+}.[94] By providing more Ca^{2+} to the troponin-tropomyosin system, a greater interaction between actin and myosin occurs, increasing force and shortening. Increasing the rate of Ca^{2+} removal from the cytoplasm speeds the rate of relaxation.

In the normal heart, norepinephrine is synthesized and stored in the sympathetic nerve endings that invest the entire heart, including atria, conduction system, and ventricle.[95] When these nerve endings are depolarized, norepinephrine is released from granules in nerve endings into myocardial clefts containing β-adrenergic receptors, which, when activated, turn on the sequence of events noted above. Not only does this enhance Ca^{2+} entry into the myocyte to augment contraction, but it also phosphorylates phospholambam, which enhances relaxation.[94] Subsequently, most of the released norepinephrine is taken back up and re-stored in the sympathetic nerve endings. Released norepinephrine is also inactivated by two enzymes, catechol O-methyltransferase (COMT) and monoamine oxidase (MAO), and the products are excreted largely by the kidneys.[94]

In very severe heart failure, stores of norepinephrine in the ventricle are largely depleted and the sympathetic nerve endings fail to take up norepinephrine normally.[96] Rapid turnover of whatever norepinephrine stores remain is suggested by increased cardiac norepinephrine spillover in CHF. At the same time, circulating norepinephrine released from peripheral sympathetic nerve endings may be increased, especially in severe failure.[97] In less severe heart failure, the serum norepinephrine levels tend to be normal despite increased sympathetic nerve activity.[98]

In both the normal and failing myocardium, activation of the adenyl cyclase system can augment contractility. Agents that do this may be divided into two categories. The first comprises the catecholamines (e.g., norepinephrine, epinephrine) and their synthetic derivatives (e.g., dobutamine, isoproterenol), which act via cell-surface adrenergic receptors (Fig. 23-8).[94] The second includes agents that inhibit the breakdown of cyclic AMP by inhibition of phosphodiesterase type III (e.g., amrinone, milrinone, and pimobendan), resulting in an increase in cyclic AMP.[98] Some of these agents, such as pimobendan, may also increase myofibril sensitivity to calcium and then further augment contraction.[99]

Catecholamines constitute an endogenous hormonal system exerting reflex control of the heart and circulation. Their effects depend on localized, controlled neural release and receptor specificity in terms of action. Dopamine is the naturally occurring precursor of both norepinephrine and epinephrine (Fig. 23-9).[100] While epinephrine is released from the adrenal medulla, norepinephrine is the primary mediator in the heart and peripheral circulation.[94]

The actions of both endogenous and exogenous catecholamines depend on their activation of specific α- and β-adrenergic receptors (Tables 23-2 and 23-3).[94] Alpha receptors include alpha$_1$ receptors, which are postsynaptic and are located in vascular smooth muscle and in the myocardium (see Chap. 54). In smooth muscle, they mediate vasoconstriction; in the heart, weak positive inotropic and negative chronotropic effects. Alpha$_2$ receptors are presynaptic and, when stimulated, decrease norepinephrine release from peripheral nerve endings as well as sympathetic outflow from the central nervous system. Alpha$_2$ receptors may also mediate vasoconstriction in specific peripheral vascular beds.

β-Adrenergic receptors can be divided into β_1 and β_2 subtypes (see Chap. 54). Beta$_1$ receptors are located in the myocardium where they mediate positive inotropic, chrono-

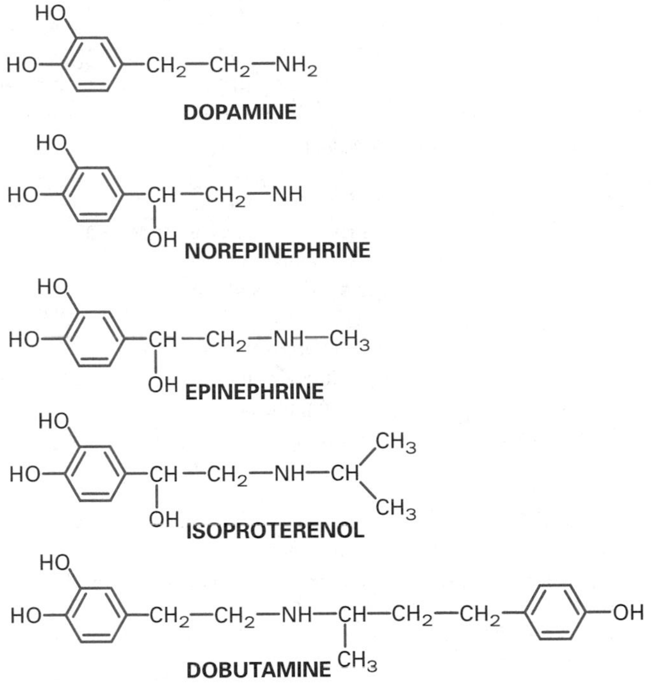

FIGURE 23-9

Structure of catecholamines.

tropic, and dromotropic effects.[98] Their activation occurs primarily by norepinephrine released from neurons in the heart. Beta$_2$ receptors are located in vascular smooth muscle, where they mediate vasodilatation, and in the sinoatrial node, where they are chronotropic. In general, beta$_2$ receptors are activated by circulating catecholamines released from peripheral sites such as the adrenal medulla.

Another type of receptor, which has been termed the *dopaminergic receptor*, is localized to the mesenteric and renal

TABLE 23-2

ADRENERGIC RECEPTOR ACTIVITY OF SYMPATHOMIMETIC AMINES

	α_1	β_1	β_2	Dopaminergic	Dose
Dopamine	+ + +	+ +	+	+ + + +	<2 (μg/kg)/min: vasodilation effects on peripheral dopaminergic receptors 2–10 (μg/kg)/min: inotropic effects, β_1 receptor activation; 5–20 (μg/kg)/min: peripheral vasoconstriction, α effects
Norepinephrine	+ + + +	+ + + +	0	0	Initiate with 8–12 μg/min; maintain 2–4 μg/min
Epinephrine	+ + +	+ + + +	+ +	0	
Isoproterenol	0	+ + + +	+ + + +	0	0.5–5 μg/min
Dobutamine	+ + +	+ + + +	+ +	0	Start at 2–3 (μg/kg)/min and titrate upward

Source: From Sonnenblick EH, LeJemtel TH, Frishman WH. Digitalis preparations and other inotropic agents. In: Frishman WH, Sonnenblick EH, eds. *Cardiovascular Pharmacotherapeutics*. New York: McGraw-Hill; 1997:246. Reproduced with permission from the publisher and authors.

TABLE 23-3

PHYSIOLOGIC AND PHARMACOLOGIC ACTIONS
OF CATECHOLAMINE RECEPTORS

Receptor	Receptor Activity	Primary Location
β_1	Positive inotropic and chronotropic action; increased AV conduction	Heart (atria, ventricle, AV node)
β_2	Peripheral vasodilation	Arterioles, arteries, veins, bronchioles
α_1	Arteriolar vasoconstriction	Arterioles
α_2	Presynaptic inhibition of norepinephrine release	Sympathetic nerve endings, CNS
Dopaminergic-1	Renal and mesenteric vasodilation, natriuresis, diuresis	Kidneys

Note: AV, atrioventricular; CNS, central nervous system.
Source: From Sonnenblick EH, LeJemtel TH, Frishman WH. Digitalis preparations and other inotropic agents. In: Frishman WH, Sonnenblick EH, eds. *Cardiovascular Pharmacotherapeutics*. New York: McGraw-Hill; 1997:246. Reproduced with permission from the publisher and authors.

circulation and mediates arterial vasodilatation. The physiologic and pharmacologic action of various catecholamines depend on which receptor they activate, both in the heart and in the periphery (Tables 23-2 and 23-3).

Norepinephrine has potent alpha$_1$ and beta$_1$ activity. When norepinephrine is released from cardiac nerve endings, as occurs in normal exercise, myocardial contractility and heart rate are augmented. When norepinephrine is administered exogenously, its major action is to stimulate alpha$_1$ receptors, leading to marked peripheral arterial vasoconstriction. Thus, norepinephrine has been used to increase arterial blood pressure in the presence of severe hypotension so as to maintain blood flow to vital organs. Long-term renal vasoconstriction from continued norepinephrine administration may produce ischemic renal damage, including acute tubular necrosis, so that prolonged use, i.e., more than 24 to 48 h, is usually untenable. For the failing heart, this peripheral vasoconstriction also provides an undesirable added pressure load (afterload), which tends to vitiate the potential benefits of beta$_1$ stimulation.

Dopamine[100] has both alpha$_1$ and beta$_1$ activity but also stimulates dopaminergic receptors in the renal vasculature to produce arterial dilation and increased renal blood flow. Its beta$_1$ effects in the heart occur largely through the release of endogenous norepinephrine, which may be largely depleted in the failing heart. As doses of dopamine are increased, conversion to norepinephrine also occurs, which tends to produce relatively more pressor effects than myocardial inotropic stimulation (Table 23-2). As such, the benefits of dopamine administration, if any, are at low doses (e.g., 0.02 mg/kg per minute) where it may induce renal arterial vasodilatation. In general, it is employed in association with more potent inotropic agents (e.g., dobutamine).

Dobutamine[101,102] is a synthetic variant of the catecholamines whose structure has been altered to optimize hemody-

namic response in the dog, characterized by an increase in cardiac output and a decrease in ventricular filling pressure with little change in heart rate. Since arterial pressure also rises modestly, peripheral vascular resistance must of necessity fall. The positive inotropic activity of dobutamine is mediated by direct stimulation of beta$_1$-adrenergic receptors in the myocardium (Table 23-2). It is unclear why a concomitant increase in heart rate does not always occur. One possibility is that an increase in cardiac output that increases arterial pressure serves to buffer any heart rate increase reflexly. Given its capacity to increase cardiac output and reduce filling pressures without substantial heart rate change, dobutamine has been widely used to treat severe acute LV failure in the absence of profound hypotension, which is poorly responsive to diuretics and vasodilators (Fig. 23-6). This may be seen following a very large myocardial infarction or in acute decompensation in the course of chronic CHF. In the presence of severe hypotension, the beta$_2$ stimulation of dobutamine may be harmful, and administration of an alpha$_1$-stimulating vasoconstrictor, such as norepinephrine or higher dose dopamine, may also be necessary in order to increase arterial peripheral resistance.

Dobutamine infusion is generally begun at 2 μg/kg per minute and titrated to optimize cardiac output while reducing LV filling pressure. Tachycardia is carefully avoided so as not to increase myocardial oxygen demands and induce ischemia. The effects on myocardial oxygen consumption ($M\dot{V}_{O_2}$) are complex.[102] While the increase in contractility will increase $M\dot{V}_{O_2}$, a decrease in heart size will tend to reduce it. The end result is generally a modest increase in $M\dot{V}_{O_2}$ induced by dobutamine. With a better maintained arterial pressure and reduced LV diastolic pressure in the absence of tachycardia, coronary perfusion pressure may also be increased. The major side effects of dobutamine are an excessive increase in heart rate with high doses and ventricular arrhythmias, both of which may mandate dose reduction and even drug discontinuation. Tachyphylaxis may also occur to a variable degree. In general, once hemodynamic benefits are attained, dobutamine is slowly withdrawn. In some cases, this has not been possible and sustained administration becomes necessary, which may require portable pumps for administration at home. The outcome in this circumstance is generally dire.

In chronic CHF, the patient is commonly maintained on vasodilators such as ACE inhibitors, loop diuretics, and digoxin. Nevertheless, episodes of acute decompensation may intervene, characterized by increased pulmonary congestion and edema and reduced renal function with increasing fluid accumulation (Fig. 23-6). In-hospital addition of dobutamine, with or without milrinone (see below), using a Swan-Ganz catheter to monitor hemodynamics, provides for an increase in cardiac output with a decrease in filling pressures, which, with added diuretics, may help to restore a steady state for a variable period of time. Dopamine, at a low dose, is commonly used concomitantly to augment renal blood. this generally requires a short hospitalization and temporary hemodynamic monitoring. In CHF, norepinephrine would only be used for a limited time to treat severe hypotension and shock unresponsive to dopamine and dobutamine, and then the outcome is generally very poor.

Phosphodiesterase Inhibitors and Other Agents

The adenyl cyclase–cyclic AMP system can also be activated beyond the beta receptor. Hormones such as glucagon activate the system and can increase myocardial contractility acutely despite beta$_1$ blockade.[103] While intravenous glucagon administration is useful in overcoming β-adrenergic blockade when necessary, glucagon may induce gastric atony and nausea, and this has limited its more generalized use.

Amrinone and milrinone are prototypes of cardiotonic agents that activate the adenyl cyclase system through inhibition of the enzyme that breaks down cyclic AMP, phosphodiesterase (PDE) III.[104,105] Type III PDE inhibitors decrease the breakdown of cyclic AMP in the myocardium and increase cyclic guanidine monophosphate (cyclic GMP) in vascular smooth muscle, resulting in an increase in myocardial contractility as well as arterial and venous vasodilatation. Other members of this class of drugs include enoximone and pimobendan, although only intravenous amrinone and milrinone have been approved by the U.S. Food and Drug Administration (FDA) for treatment of acute heart failure. The mechanisms by which vasodilatation occurs are not completely understood. Increased cyclic GMP induces phosphorylation of myosin light-chain kinase, which decreases sensitivity to calcium and calmodulin. In the heart, inotropism may relate not only to increased cyclic AMP–mediated calcium availability for contraction and increased rates of its removal for relaxation but also to increased sensitivity of the contractile system for calcium.[106] Both amrinone and milrinone,[105] which are available as intravenous agents, have substantial ability to augment cardiac output while reducing both RV and LV filling pressures. The lowering of filling pressures is greater than that seen with dobutamine. Dilatation of the pulmonary arterial vasculature is also a very useful therapeutic effect. Arterial pressure tends to be reduced, while an increase in heart rate may occur. Since dobutamine increases cyclic AMP and milrinone reduces its breakdown, the combination of these agents is substantially more potent than either agent alone.[105] When either dobutamine or milrinone are utilized, ectopic activity may be increased, which requires careful supervision in their use.

PDE III inhibitors are also orally active and produce the same hemodynamic improvement as seen with intravenous use. In longer-term oral use, however, increased mortality was seen with the use of milrinone, especially in the presence of class IV heart failure.[107] This increased mortality may have been due to the relatively short action of this agent (90-min half-life), which leads to large peaks and valleys in dosing and concomitant arrhythmias. For the time being, this has vitiated clinical study of these agents in oral formulations, but more stringent control of the use of this class of agents as adjuncts to other agents may ultimately increase their value, especially in improving quality of life in the terminal and short-term outcome of very severe CHF.

NEWER INOTROPIC AGENTS

Agents under investigation include the inodilatory benzimidazoline PDE inhibitors, such as levosimendan, which acutely increase cardiac output and reduce filling pressure while improving exercise tolerance in patients with CHF.[108] Levosimendan, and other drugs in this class (MCI-154, EMD 53998, EMD 57033), may have additional effects to enhance calcium binding to troponin-C, a calcium-sensitizing action (Fig. 23-8).[108–110] Theoretically, this could enhance contractile response for a given amount of cytolytic Ca^{2+}, which could lead to less arrhythmogenicity. This may be an important consideration since the activation of the cyclic AMP system may be detrimental in inducing tachycardia and arrhythmias. Clinical trials of efficacy and safety of levosimendan are currently in progress. The critical issues to be addressed, now that acute efficacy is apparent, are whether these agents will improve symptoms, i.e., reduce morbidity, and/or will they improve mortality.

VASODILATION: INHIBITION OF THE RENIN-ANGIOTENSIN SYSTEM

As described earlier, with the evolution of progressive heart failure accompanied by ventricular remodeling, neurohumoral activation occurs. Following initial increases in sympathetic tone and decreases in parasympathetic tone, the renin-angiotensin system is activated.[33] This generally occurs when diuretics are initiated or, in their absence, with the onset of clinical symptoms of CHF. With release of renin from the kidneys, angiotensinogen, which is circulating in the blood, is converted to inactive angiotensin I, which in turn is converted to the highly active angiotensin II by a converting enzyme that is ubiquitously located along vascular walls. Angiotensin II in turn stimulates aldosterone secretion by the adrenals, which results in sodium accumulation and also produces marked arteriolar constriction, which augments peripheral vascular resistance. Both phenomena, which increase ventricular preload (filling pressure) and afterload (systolic pressure), contribute to the clinical picture of CHF. In addition to these actions, angiotensin II serves as a growth factor, adding to myocardial hypertrophy and apparently fostering fibrosis. It may also contribute to subtle myocyte loss through enhancing apoptosis.[111]

Angiotensin-Converting Enzyme Inhibitors

In the late 1970s, manipulation of cardiac preload and afterload with combined administration of nitroglycerin, as a venodilator, and hydralazine, as a pure arteriolar dilator, received increasing attention for the treatment of patients with CHF by producing reduction in ventricular filling pressures with an increased cardiac output.[112] In the context of these effects, the development of captopril, an orally active ACE inhibitor that exerted both arteriolar and venous vasodilatation, appeared extremely promising. Initial hemodynamic studies demonstrated substantial lowering of ventricular filling pressures, a modest increase in cardiac output, and a reduction in arterial pressure without a reactive tachycardia.[113] In a landmark trial in heart failure, oral administration of captopril over a 3-month period produced sustained improvement in LV systolic performance, improved functional class, and increased maximal exercise duration.[114] In the first few weeks of the study, exercise performance improved in placebo patients as well, probably due to recovered conditioning. Beyond that time, patients on captopril were substantially better relative to the placebo group. Of note, 12 of 42 patients randomized to placebo died during the 3-month study, while only 2 of 49 patients randomized to captopril died, suggesting, but not proving, an effect on mortality as well.[115] Although the acute hemodynamic effects of captopril were similar to those noted with combined nitrate/hydralazine, the clinical benefits, in terms of symptomatic improvement and long-term outcome, appeared superior with captopril. This dissociation between acute hemodynamic effects and long-term clinical benefit pointed out mechanisms underlying the benefits of ACE inhibition that could be related to multiple factors, including reconditioning of the peripheral vasculature.[116]

Several aspects of long-term therapy with ACE inhibitors in patients with CHF are worthy of mention.

1. The magnitude of the initial hemodynamic change does not predict the long-term clinical response. Some of the beneficial effects to lower filling pressures and perhaps improve peripheral circulation may relate to increased levels of kinins.[117] This is due to their decreased enzymatic destruction when ACE, which normally breaks down kinins, is inhibited.

2. The impact of long-term ACE inhibition on LV systolic function appears to be modest, in that the absolute percent increase in LV EF has ranged from 1 to 3 percent.[118] Although long-term use of enalapril in the SOLVD trial was shown to reduce LV end-diastolic and -systolic volumes, most LV volumes increased substantially as early as 2 weeks after discontinuation of therapy.[119] Thus, the enalapril-induced reduction in LV volume appears more related to changes in loading conditions, i.e., reduction in cardiac preload and afterload, than to persistent reversal of the functional and structural abnormalities that are responsible for LV dilatation. While long-term ACE inhibition may reverse existing LV dysfunction only modestly, it appears to delay the progression of LV dysfunction significantly.[120]

3. Long-term use of ACE inhibitors has significant natriuretic effects. From a hormonal point of view, a decrease in angiotensin II leads to less aldosterone secretion, with resultant lessening of sodium accumulation and reduced potassium loss. Increased diuresis with the consequent need to reduce doses of loop diuretics have been reported during long-term therapy with captopril.[121] This natriuretic effect of captopril is also related to the increase in renal blood flow demonstrated after administration of captopril despite reduction in mean systemic arterial pressure.[122] The natriuretic effect of ACE inhibition was subsequently demonstrated in patients with dilated cardiomyopathy and mild heart failure during volume loading with a saline solution, where ACE inhibition produced a threefold higher urinary sodium excretion.[123]

4. The long-term benefits of ACE inhibition to increase peak exercise duration and oxygen consumption ($\dot{V}_{O_2}$, ml/kg per minute) are directly related to the enhanced vasodilatory response to exercise of the skeletal muscle beds.[28] Such enhancement of the vasodilatory response of the skeletal muscle beds to exercise takes weeks to occur and thereby explains the delayed response to ACE inhibition in terms of functional class and exercise capacity.[124] While ACE inhibition has been shown to improve LV performance at rest and at peak exercise immediately, the improvement in functional capacity and exercise duration takes weeks to months to reach a peak.[125] The importance of the changes in the periphery and particularly the peripheral circulation in mediating the effects of ACE inhibition on functional capacity may explain the unimpressive early results of ACE inhibition in patients who develop CHF acutely as a result of a myocardial infarction.[126] Due to the abrupt decrease in ventricular function in these patients, substantial peripheral abnormalities have not had time to evolve, and thus their exercise capacity is limited by central components, i.e., LV systolic performance itself, which consistently increases during long-term ACE inhibition. The time differential between the acute hemodynamic and delayed functional benefits also points out that cellular effects of ACE inhibition rather than just afterload reduction appear to mediate the clinical effects.

The mechanism by which peripheral vasodilatation and enhanced peripheral blood flow occur is complex and poorly understood. ACE inhibitors not only reduce angiotensin II vasoconstriction acutely but, over a longer period, tend to normalize peripheral vascular structure,[127] improve endothelial dysfunction, and reduce levels of circulating endothelin, another vasoconstrictor substance.[128–130] Angiotensin II is also a smooth muscle growth factor, and its reduction may also reduce smooth muscle mass, which produces enhanced vascular tone.[131]

The effects of an ACE inhibitor on mortality in patients with CHF was first demonstrated with enalapril. The results of the Cooperative North Scandinavian Enalapril Study (CONSENSUS) involving 253 patients with symptoms compatible with NYHA functional class IV showed that after an average follow-up of 188 days, 68 of the 126 patients randomized to placebo died, while only 50 of 127 patients randomized to enalapril died, a reduction in mortality of 27 percent ($p = .003$).[132] The entire reduction in total mortality was found to be among patients with progressive heart failure, whereas no difference was observed in the incidence of sudden death. After the initial dose of enalapril was reduced from 10 mg to 2.5 mg, only 3.2 percent of the patients could not tolerate enalapril because of symptomatic hypotension.

The second Veterans Administration Cooperative Vasodilator Heart Failure Trial (V-HeFT II) randomized 804 men with peak aerobic capacity <25 ml/kg per minute to enalapril or to hydralazine plus isosorbide dinitrate. At 2 years, the mortality was lower in the enalapril group than in the hydralazine plus isosorbide dinitrate group (18 versus 25 percent, $p = .016$; reduction in mortality, 28 percent).[133] The reduction in mortality, particularly in patients with less severe symptoms (NYHA classes I and II), was attributable to a reduction in sudden death. V-HeFT II also confirmed previous findings that treatment with long-term ACE inhibitor was associated with a minimal absolute increase in the LV EF, i.e., 2 percent.

The SOLVD trial assessed the effect of ACE inhibition with enalapril in patients with symptomatic and asymptomatic LV systolic dysfunction as evidenced by an EF <35 percent.[134,135] 2569 patients who had CHF as defined by the need for therapy and mean EF of 24.8 percent were enrolled in the *treatment arm* of SOLVD and randomized to placebo or enalapril. Over a period of 48 months, 510 of the 1284 patients randomized to placebo died, while only 452 of the 1285 patients randomized to enalapril died [risk reduction, 10 percent; 95 percent confidence interval (CI), 5 to 26 percent; $p = .0036$]. The chief difference in mortality was mostly due to progressive heart failure, as the number of deaths classified as arrhythmogenic without worsening CHF was similar in the placebo and enalapril arms. 4228 patients, who were not treated for CHF and thus considered asymptomatic, had a mean EF of 28 percent and were enrolled in the *prevention arm* of SOLVD. Over a period of 37.4 months, 334 of the 2117 patients randomized to placebo and 313 of the 2111 patients randomized to enalapril died (risk reduction, 8 percent; 95 percent CI, 8 to 21 percent; $p = .030$). In the placebo group, 818 patients developed heart failure or died as compared to only 630 patients in the enalapril group, i.e., 38.1 versus 29.8 percent (risk reduction, 29 percent; 95 percent CI, 21 to 30 percent; $p < .001$). Of great note, a common effect of enalapril in both the treatment and prevention arms of the SOLVD trials was to reduce the incidence of recurrent myocardial infarction, i.e., 288 in the enalapril group versus 362 in the placebo group (risk reduction, 23 percent; 95 percent CI, 11 to 34 percent; $p < .001$).[136] Similarly, 499 in the enalapril group and 595 in the placebo group developed unstable angina (risk reduction, 20 percent; 95 percent CI, 9 to 29 percent; $p < .001$). Whether this reduction in the incidence of acute coronary events in patients with coronary artery disease is associated with long-term ACE inhibition with enalapril or related to the improvement in endothelium vasomotor dysfunction, which was subsequently demonstrated with quinapril, another ACE inhibitor, is not known.[137] It is also

possible that ACE inhibition plays a role in stabilizing atherosclerotic plaques, perhaps by reducing smooth muscle growth. Importantly, as noted below, the same considerations have been raised by the Survival and Ventricular Enlargement (SAVE) trial of ACE inhibition in the depressed heart following myocardial infarction.

As previously stated, the initial impetus toward the use of orally active converting enzyme inhibitors for the treatment of CHF was to improve LV systolic performance by reducing cardiac loading. The work of Pfeffer and Braunwald[138] provided the second impetus for the use of ACE inhibitors in patients with LV systolic dysfunction and heart failure. Using the LV changes that follow ligation of left anterior descending coronary artery in rats as a paradigm for LV deterioration, long-term therapy with captopril reduced ventricular dilatation and shifted the pressure volume to the left after acute myocardial infarction. The process of LV enlargement is largely dependent on the size and location of the myocardial infarct as well as the patency of the infarct-related coronary artery. It was theorized that by lowering LV diastolic wall stress, long-term therapy with an ACE inhibitor could favorably alter the loading conditions of a left ventricle and reduce LV enlargement, thereby enhancing survival of patients after a myocardial infarction. In an initial randomized study of 59 patients with their first anterior wall myocardial infarction and a reduced LV EF, administration of captopril or placebo for 12 months produced significant reductions in ventricular filling pressures and appeared to attenuate ventricular dilatation, especially when the initial infarction was associated with a large akinetic area.[139] Subsequently, the ACE inhibitor–induced reduction in LV enlargement was found to be associated with a reduced morbidity and mortality in patients in the SAVE trial.[140] 2231 patients with an EF of 40 percent or less were randomized to captopril or placebo within 3 to 16 days after an acute myocardial infarction. Mortality from all causes was found to be significantly reduced by captopril (20 versus 25 percent; risk reduction, 19 percent; 95 percent CI, 3 to 32 percent; $p = .019$). It is also important to note that, in general, the major reduction in mortality after infarction, which amounts to 25 to 30 percent, is obtained during the first year with use of beta-blocking agents, especially in the presence of a very reduced EF. The benefits of ACE inhibition are largely apparent in the second year and beyond.

As documented in the SOLVD trials, the incidence of nonfatal cardiovascular events and development of heart failure were significantly reduced by captopril in the SAVE trial when compared to placebo. The benefits of ACE inhibition after acute myocardial infarction were also demonstrated in patients who had received thrombolytic therapy, aspirin, and beta-blocking agents during the acute event. Of added importance, the reinfarction rate was also reduced 25 percent, which itself may have reduced mortality. This remarkable finding is in parallel to that observed in the SOLVD trial noted above. The mechanism for this important finding is currently being explored and may involve effects to stabilize atherosclerotic plaques in obstructed coronaries.

In another study of ACE inhibition following acute myocardial infarction, enalapril failed to improve survival at 6 months, when compared to placebo, in the 6090 patients enrolled in the CONSENSUS II trial when the drug was started within 24 h of the event.[141] It is probable that this was due to the very short period of study, since the major benefits of SAVE occurred beyond 6 months. Since the negative results of CONSENSUS II, several large randomized studies of ACE inhibition after acute myocardial infarction have confirmed the findings of the SAVE trial. In the AIRE Trial (Acute Infarction Ramipril Efficacy Study), with an average follow-up of 15 months, mortality from all causes was significantly lower for those patients with myocardial infarction and clinical evidence of failure randomized to ramipril than for those randomized to placebo (risk reduction, 27 percent; 95 percent CI, 11 to 40 percent; $p = .002$).[142] In the Gruppo Italiano per lo Studio della Sopravivenza nell' Infarto Miocardio III trial (GISSI-3), lisinopril started within 24 h of an acute myocardial infarction reduced overall mortality significantly when compared to placebo (odds ratio, 0.88; 95 percent CI, 0.79 to 0.99; $p = .03$).[143] When administered within 24 h of an acute myocardial infarction, the ACE inhibitor zofenopril reduced the incidence of death or severe CHF.[144] At 6 weeks, zofenopril reduced the cumulative risk of death or severe CHF by 34 percent (95 percent CI, 8 to 54 percent; $p = .018$); after 1 year, the cumulative risk was reduced by 29 percent (95 percent CI, 6 to 51 percent; $p = .011$).

Lastly, the benefits of ACE inhibition on all-cause mortality, sudden death, and the development of severe CHF were confirmed with trandolapril in patients with LV dysfunction after a myocardial infarction.[145] Trandolapril was administered 3 to 7 days after the myocardial infarction. The relative risk of death in the trandolapril group, as compared with the placebo group, was 0.78 (95 percent CI, 0.67 to 0.91; $p = .001$). Progression to severe heart failure was also less frequent in the trandolapril group (relative risk, 0.71; 95 percent CI, 0.56 to 0.89; $p = .003$). In contrast to the findings of the SAVE trial, however, the risk of recurrent myocardial infarction was not significantly reduced (risk reduction, 0.86; 95 percent CI, 0.66 to 1.13; $p = .29$).

From the above-mentioned studies conducted in patients with acute myocardial infarction with and without LV dysfunction, and in patients with CHF and without symptoms, it is clear that ACE inhibition is indicated in all patients with LV systolic dysfunction, whether or not symptoms are present. ACE inhibition is currently the cornerstone in the treatment of LV dysfunction, with or without clinical CHF. The lack of effect of enalapril on mortality in the prevention arm of the SOLVD trials does mean that ACE inhibition does not prolong survival in this patient population. The failure to reach statistical significance appears related to the relatively short duration of the study, since mortality develops over many years in an asymptomatic patient population. Moreover, delaying the development of symptoms for 1 to 2 years in this patient population may be clinically more meaningful than prolonging life by a few months in patients with class IV symptoms.

At this juncture, six ACE inhibitors are approved for the treatment of patients with CHF (Table 23-4). There is as yet no study to show an advantage of one of these drugs over another.

Although the efficacy of ACE inhibitors has been established beyond doubt in the treatment of CHF, many patients with CHF do not benefit from this therapy for three major reasons. First, the fall in systemic arterial pressure below 90 mmHg leads physicians to discontinue administration of ACE inhibitor. In the absence of symptoms, a fall in systemic arterial pressure is not an indication to discontinue therapy. In most patients, the fall in systemic arterial pressure is extremely well tolerated and even desirable. When associated with symptoms, the fall in systemic arterial pressure should first lead to reducing or temporarily discontinuing diuretic therapy.[146] In patients not treated with diuretics, the dose of ACE inhibitor may be reduced, with a long-acting agent administered at

---

TABLE 23-4

FDA APPROVED INDICATIONS FOR ACE INHIBITORS

ACE Inhibitor	Proprietary Name	Hypertension	CHF	Post MI-CHF	Diabetic Nephropathy	Asymptomatic LV Dysfunction
Benazepril	Lotensin	+				
Captopril	Capoten	+	+	+	+	
Enalapril	Vasotec	+	+			+
Fosinopril	Monopril	+	+			
Lisinopril	Prinivil, Zestril	+	+			
Moexipril	Univasc	+				
Quinipril	Accupril	+	+			
Ramipril	Altace	+	+			
Trandolapril	Mavik	+				

Note: ACE, angiotensin-converting enzyme; CHF, congestive heart failure; LV, left ventricular; MI, myocardial infarction.
Source: From Ruddy MC, Kostis JB, Frishman WH. Drugs that affect the renin-angiotensin system. In: Frishman WH, Sonnenblick EH, eds. *Cardiovascular Pharmacotherapeutics*. New York: McGraw-Hill; 1997; 161.

bedtime being the drug of choice. In view of the well-documented benefits of ACE inhibitors, other vasodilators, such as hydralazine, nitrates, and α-adrenergic blockers, if taken, should be discontinued.

The second limit in ACE inhibitor benefit is worsening of renal function. Several risk factors for ACE inhibition–induced worsening of renal function have been identified, which include hyponatremia, hypotension, intravascular depletion, diabetes, the use of NSAIDS, and baseline renal insufficiency. Close monitoring of renal function during initiation and uptitration of ACE inhibition in patients with risk factors for renal insufficiency is essential. Overall, increases in creatinine level of 0.5 to 1.0 mg/dL reflect dilation of the glomerular efferent arteries and not renal damage. When the rise in creatinine levels stabilizes, ACE inhibitor therapy need not be altered. In fact, the resultant lower intraglomerular pressure may help to explain the benefits of ACE inhibition on the natural course of diabetic nephropathy.[147]

The third limit to the benefit of ACE inhibition is the development of a drug-related persistent cough resulting from elevated bradykinin levels. ACE inhibition–induced cough may occur in up to 20 percent of patients, but it is severe enough to require discontinuation of therapy in fewer than 5 percent of patients. Cough may occur or be more severe during respiratory infections, during which the drug may be withdrawn and reinstituted later. Changing ACE inhibitor does not prevent this generic problem.

Several issues concerning the use of ACE inhibition in patients with chronic heart failure have not yet been thoroughly determined. They include what degree, if any, of renal insufficiency contraindicates ACE inhibition therapy; the clinical relevance of the ACE inhibitor escape phenomenon in patients with CHF; and the importance of inhibiting tissue versus systemic ACE inhibition. With regard to the degree of renal insufficiency, definitive data are not available, as most ACE inhibitor trials have excluded patients with creatinine levels >2.5 mg/dL. Nevertheless, providing there is extremely close monitoring of renal function and potassium levels, renal insufficiency, per se, cannot be considered a contraindication to ACE inhibition therapy. While renal function is more likely to deteriorate and hyperkalemia is most likely to occur in patients with baseline renal insufficiency, these patients deserve a trial of ACE inhibitor at low dose. In view of its hepatic elimination, fosinopril may be the preferred agent in this clinical situation, while the dosage of other ACE inhibitors has to be adjusted to creatinine clearance.

The phenomenon of ACE inhibitor escape has been reported in hypertensive patients during long-term ACE inhibition.[148] After several weeks of therapy, plasma angiotensin II levels returned to baseline values. Whether such a phenomenon occurs and is clinically relevant in patients with CHF is currently unknown. Preliminary experience, however, points to the safety and benefits of combined ACE inhibition and angiotensin II type I receptor blockade in patients with severe CHF.[149]

Lastly, the vast majority, i.e., 90 percent, of ACE is tissue-bound. Whether the clinical effects of ACE inhibition relate to the individual drug's ability to interfere with tissue ACE levels has not been thoroughly investigated. The relative potency of individual ACE inhibition to inhibit tissue-converting enzyme varies. This issue may be most relevant when ACE inhibitors are administered at less than the recommended doses because of symptomatic hypotension or worsening renal function.

Angiotensin II Receptor Antagonists

Angiotensin II receptor antagonists, a new class of pharmacologic blockers of the renin-angiotensin system, have recently been shown to be safe and effective antihypertensive agents in human studies.[150–171] Given the fact that they inhibit the angiotensin receptor and not the converting enzyme, they do not increase bradykinin levels and do not produce cough. Losartan and valsartan are angiotensin II receptor blockers currently being marketed for hypertension, and these drugs and others in this class are under investigation for the treatment of patients with CHF.

Angiotensin receptors may be differentiated into two distinct subtypes by radioligand receptor–binding studies using the specific, nonpeptide antagonists, losartan (DuP753) and PD 123177,[172–174] as well as by their sensitivity to reducing agents. The type 1 angiotensin receptor (AT_1) is inactivated by pretreatment with the reducing agent dithiothreitol (DTT), and it has a high affinity for losartan but a low affinity for PD 123177 (Fig. 23-10). AT_1 mediates its physiologic functions by coupling to a transmembrane G protein[169,175–177] and can be inhibited by guanine nucleotides.[169,177] The type 2 angiotensin receptor (AT_2) is resistant to DTT inactivation and is PD 123177 sensitive. Both receptor subtypes appear to be found in different tissues in varying proportions.[174,178,179] The AT_1 receptor predominates in virtually all vascular tissue and is the only type present in the liver and in rat spleen and largely in the heart.[180,181] A number of new oral nonpeptide angiotensin II receptor antagonists, similar to losartan and valsartan, are currently being tested, including irbesartan, eprosartan, candesartan, tasosartan, telmisartan, forasartan, and ripisartin.[182–191]

While ACE inhibitors have been proven safe and effective in the treatment of hypertension and CHF, the ability of an AT_1 receptor blocker to inhibit the receptor directly provides the opportunity for more complete inhibition of the effects of angiotensin II without the added effects of increased bradykinin, whether it is beneficial or not. Directly blocking the effect of angiotensin II with losartan has shown similar hemodynamic response to those of ACE inhibitors, although the effects on lower filling pressures appear somewhat less, probably due to lack of increased bradykinin. Experimental hemodynamic studies in ischemic heart failure have shown that losartan and captopril cause similar acute hemodynamic, hormonal, and renal effects without changing the LV weight/body weight ratio, mean aortic pressures, or heart rates when compared with placebo.[192–195] In CHF, favorable hemody-

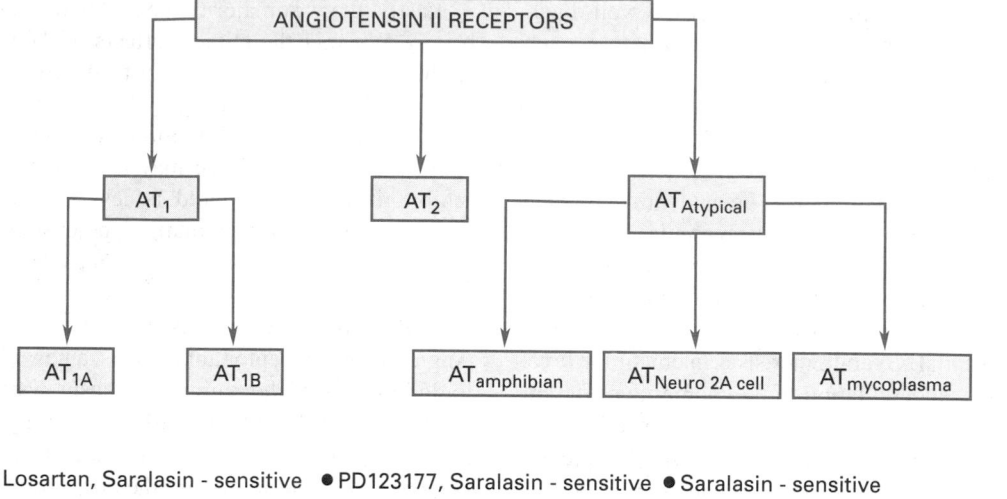

FIGURE 23-10

The classification and characteristics of angiotensin II receptors. DTT, dithiothreitol. (From Kang et al.[170] Reproduced with permission from the publisher and authors.)

namic effects from direct angiotensin II receptor blockade and reductions in LV volume, LV mass, and collagen content have been demonstrated.[196]

Relative to the treatment of patients with CHF, Gottlieb et al.[197] demonstrated reductions in systemic vascular resistance and mean arterial pressure in 66 patients with NYHA class II to III CHF and mean EF <40 percent, but they were not able to demonstrate more than a trend in the reduction in pulmonary capillary wedge pressure (PCWP) or increases in cardiac index. Crozier et al.[198] in 134 patients with NYHA class II to III CHF and a mean EF ≤ 24 percent demonstrated significant improvement in hemodynamics associated with angiotensin receptor antagonism, characterized by reductions in PCWP, heart rate, systemic vascular resistance, and norepinephrine levels and an increase in cardiac index. Patients who received either of the direct renin antagonists, remikiren[199] or enkiren,[200] alone experienced increased cardiac index, reduced LV filling pressures, and reduced systemic vascular resistance. Remikiren and enalaprilat, when given individually, result in nearly identical hemodynamic changes. The addition of enalapril to remikiren did not result in additional hemodynamic changes.[199] Thus, selective inhibition of the effects of angiotensin II can result in favorable hemodynamic changes in heart failure that largely parallel those seen with ACE inhibition. Elevated levels of bradykinin may or may not produce clinically significant hemodynamic changes. Whether angiotensin blockade will produce the same reduction in filling pressures as ACE inhibitors has yet to be widely demonstrated.

In a rat model of heart failure induced by myocardial infarction, captopril and losartan produce comparable effects on LV volume, LV end-diastolic pressure, and venous compliance.[201] When given for 2 weeks in the period following ligation of the left anterior descending coronary artery, both captopril and losartan reduced LV volume, LV end-diastolic pressure, and central venous pressure, although no significant differences in infarct size and LV mass were noted. With ligation of the left anterior descending coronary artery in rats,[202] treatment with losartan led to a decrease in collagen content of the noninfarcted myocardium, although only blood pressure was significantly changed. Taken together, limited data support the beneficial effects of angiotensin II receptor antagonism in the treatment of severe heart failure following myocardial infarction.[203–205] Comparisons of angiotensin II receptor blockade to ACE inhibitors are, as yet, limited.[206]

Lastly, the autocrine-paracrine renin-angiotensin system has been defined at the myocyte level, and a non-ACE tissue, chymase, which can generate angiotensin II, has been localized within the myocardium.[207,208] Although the importance of tissue ACE is controversial, this chymase may be responsible for 80 percent of the angiotensin II produced in the human heart.[209] Thus, this tissue-based renin-angiotensin system might be a further specific target for therapy in contrast to ACE inhibition, angiotensin II receptor blockade should be effective regardless of the pathway through which the angiotensin II is generated. Angiotensin II receptor blockade combined with ACE inhibition might produce more complete angiotensin II blockade, while maintaining the favorable effects of ACE on bradykinin and prostaglandin. Indeed, preliminary studies do suggest an additive beneficial hemodynamic action when ACE inhibitors are combined with angiotensin II receptor blockers in heart failure.[149,210] The long-term clinical implications of this combined treatment approach need to be defined.

The extent to which bradykinin and prostaglandin mediate some of the beneficial effects of ACE inhibition in heart failure is uncertain. Sources of ambiguity arise from species-specific effects of ACE inhibitors on the endothelium or vascular reactivity of laboratory animals[211–215] and the small number of studies in humans. Evidence supports an important role for postglandins and bradykinin and an intact and normal endothelial function in patients with LV dysfunction and ischemic heart disease. The role of angiotensin in the pathogenesis of LV remodeling, however, should not be diminished. The available evidence demonstrates hemodynamic and potential effects of angiotensin inhibition on myocardial growth and LV dilatation after myocardial infarction in the absence of changes in bradykinin metabolism. A large-scale trial comparing traditional ACE inhibition with angiotensin receptor inhibition appears warranted and safe. An initial study evaluating mortality in elderly patients receiving the angiotensin II receptor blocker losartan compared to the ACE inhibitor captopril in patients with CHF demonstrated greater efficacy with losartan.[216] Other studies relative to this important questions are in progress. These findings, to date, demonstrate that inhibition of the renin-angiotensin system creates favorable hemodynamic changes in heart failure and suggests that losartan should be as effective in the treatment of heart failure as ACE inhibitors.

Other Vasodilators

Vasodilator agents may be used as adjunctive therapy in the management of heart failure. The combination of hydralazine and isosorbide dinitrate is an alternative therapy when ACE inhibitors are contraindicated or cannot be tolerated. Daily doses of hydralazine, up to 300 mg, in combination with isosorbide dinitrate, 160 mg, in the presence of cardiac glycosides and diuretics probably have some effect in reducing mortality of patients with chronic heart failure but not in reducing hospitalization for heart failure.[217] At these doses, the combination increased exercise performance more than with enalapril.[133] The effects of hydralazine and nitrates, alone or in combination, when added to ACE inhibitors are unknown. There is no evidence of proven benefit when either nitrates or hydralazine are used alone, but nitrates are often prescribed without hydralazine. Nitrates also may be used effectively for the treatment of concomitant angina. Early development of hemodynamic tolerance (tachyphylaxis) to nitrates may occur with frequent dosing (every 4 to 6 h) but is less with intervals of 8 to 12 h[218] or in conjunction with ACE inhibition. Also, hemodynamic tolerance may be less during coadministration with hydralazine.[219]

VASODILATION: CALCIUM ANTAGONISTS

Calcium antagonists are not recommended for the treatment of CHF due to their negative inotropic effects. However, second-generation dihydropyridine-type calcium antagonists such as amlodipine and felodipine may be considered for the treatment of concomitant arterial hypertension or angina (see Chap. 54). Some second-generation calcium antagonists are still under investigation with respect to their long-term effect on mortality in chronic heart failure, in addition to baseline therapy including ACE inhibition. Preliminary data indicate either no effect[220] or a positive outcome in restricted patient populations, i.e., in patients with idiopathic dilated cardiomyopathy.[221] Although in these studies the second-generation dihydropyridine agents evaluated appeared to be safe and not to increase mortality, there are as yet no reasons to recommend these agents for the treatment of heart failure due to systolic dysfunction, but rather they can be recommended as adjunctive medication for ischemia. Due to the potential benefits of beta blockers, noted below, however, these agents should be preferable to the calcium blockers for patients with CHF and ischemia.

Studies are in progress evaluating the dihydropyridine agent amlodipine in patients with congestive cardiomyopathy and the selective T-channel calcium antagonist mibefradil, a drug having no apparent effect on myocardial function.[222]

The use of calcium blockers in patients with diastolic dysfunction (e.g., verapamil) has been reported, but there are no long-term outcome studies with this form of treatment. The use of calcium channel blockers in the treatment of patients with hypertrophic cardiomyopathy has been well defined.[222]

BETA-ADRENERGIC BLOCKADE

The potential clinical benefits of using β-adrenergic blockade for the treatment of chronic heart failure were first reported on in 1975 by Waagstein et al. in seven patients with dilated cardiomyopathy.[223] While being treated with alprenolol or practolol for an average of 5.4 months, the functional capacity of the patients increased and heart size decreased. Subsequently, in a large group of patients with nonischemic dilated cardiomyopathies, significant improvement in EF was observed from an average of 33 to 42 percent; functional status was also improved significantly. With continuous use of β-adrenergic blockade, however, benefits were both variable and unpredictable.[224] Further, the initial enthusiasm for the use of β-adrenergic blockade for the treatment of congestive cardiomyopathy was tempered by the apparently negative results of two placebo-controlled, double-blind trials.[225,226] In retrospect, it is now recognized that these studies were too short in duration, i.e., 1 month, for patients with CHF to derive benefits of β-adrenergic blockade. At present, multiple studies[227–239] lend strong support to the view that careful initiation and long-term administration of β-adrenergic blocking agents to patients with a dilated cardiomyopathy already receiving conventional therapy offer substantial benefits in improving ventricular function, relieving symptoms, and perhaps prolonging life. The latter issue awaits further study. Moreover, as will be discussed further, improvement in ventricular function generally precedes symptomatic benefit, and these effects are unpredictable in any given patient. Further, nonischemic myopathies benefit to a greater extent than ischemic myopathies,[237] and beta blockers with additional vasodilatory action may demonstrate an even greater efficacy.[240–243]

Subsequent to these initial confusing results noted above, the benefits of metoprolol were clearly demonstrated by Engelmeier et al. in a double-blind randomized, placebo-controlled trial.[227] These investigators emphasized that in CHF, β-adrenergic blockers should be introduced in progressively, increasing doses over a 6 to 8 weeks period. With such progressive increase of the dose of metoprolol, only 1 of their 21 patients was unable to tolerate beta blockade, despite markedly depressed ventricular function at baseline. These promising results have also been affirmed by Anderson et al.[228]

During the first weeks of therapy, the signs and symptoms of CHF may worsen, particularly in very symptomatic patients. Initiation of β-adrenergic blockade tends to reduce depressed LV systolic function further, which in patients with very limited LV reserve may precipitate or exacerbate symptoms. Deterioration of LV function at initiation of β-adrenergic blockade can most often be prevented by initial administration of very small doses of beta-blocking agents (e.g., metoprolol 5 mg twice daily) and increasing the dose gradually over several weeks to achieve full β-adrenergic blockade. If symptomatic deterioration of CHF occurs, it is most often transient and can be controlled by increased use of loop diuretics. Once the dose of beta blocker has been titrated (e.g., metoprolol 50 to 100 mg twice daily), it should be maintained continuously. The need for continuous therapy in order to maintain the beneficial effects of β-adrenergic blockade was first documented by Waagstein et al.[223] Two-thirds of their patients who experienced symptomatic improvement on metoprolol deteriorated when the drug was withdrawn, as evidenced by a return of symptoms and a fall in LV EF. The deterioration during withdrawal of metoprolol, which argues in favor of a cause-effect relationship between clinical improvement and metoprolol therapy, supports the view that long-term β-adrenergic blockade is, at best, palliative and does not cure primary disease.

An indirect proof of the efficacy of long-term β-adrenergic blockade in patients with LV systolic dysfunction has also come from the Multicenter Diltiazem Post Infarction Study.[244] In the placebo group, the likelihood of developing CHF requiring treatment was significantly lower in patients receiving β-adrenergic blocking agents than in those patients who were not, i.e., 46 versus 61 percent (relative risk, 0.75; 95% CI, 0.48 to 1.19).

The effects of long-term adrenergic blockade on LV systolic and diastolic performance have been extensively investigated by Eichhorn et al.[231] After 3 months of therapy with bucindolol, a nonselective β-adrenergic blocking agent with vasodilatory properties, myocardial contractility and diastolic relaxation were enhanced, while myocardial chamber stiffness was unchanged. The improvement in contractile function was not associated with an increase in myocardial oxygen extraction and consumption, although increased carbohydrate utilization was noted. Similar results were reported with metoprolol, a selective beta$_1$-blocking agent.[232] The time course of the improvement in LV function, mass, and geometry was also studied in patients with CHF treated with metoprolol.[233] After a brief decline in EF, which is observed during the first 24 h of therapy, LV EF was increased at 3 months, while LV mass was reduced and LV shape became less spherical after 18 months of therapy.

The benefits of bucindolol on LV systolic function were subsequently confirmed by Gilbert et al. in a double-blind, randomized trial involving 24 patients with idiopathic dilated cardiomyopathy.[236] The response to long-term β-adrenergic blockade also appears to be, in part, determined by the etiology of the cardiomyopathy responsible for the syndrome of CHF.[237] During long-term therapy with bucindolol, patients with idiopathic dilated cardiomyopathy experienced a much greater improvement in LV performance and functional class than patients with ischemic cardiomyopathy, despite a similar degree of β-adrenergic blockade.[237] Subsequently, different degrees of β-adrenergic receptor downregulation and uncoupling of beta receptors from mechanical response have been documented by Bristow et al. in patients with idiopathic dilated and ischemic cardiomyopathy.[245] Whether such differences contribute to variable clinical responses to β-adrenergic blockade of patients with ischemia and idiopathic-dilated cardiomyopathy is uncertain. Indeed, in contrast to their previous findings, Bristow et al. reported that the clinical effect of long-term therapy with bucindolol did not differ in patients with idiopathic dilated and ischemic cardiomyopathy.[238] Similarly, it has been shown that patients with dilated cardiomyopathy due to coronary artery disease benefit from long-term β-adrenergic blockade with metoprolol.[239]

The magnitude of improvement in LV systolic function induced by long-term β-adrenergic blockade varies from patient to patient. Among all the hemodynamic indices at baseline, only peak systolic LV pressure is an independent predictor of the magnitude of improvement. Patients with the highest peak systolic LV pressure are likely to benefit the most from long-term β-adrenergic blockade. In contrast to earlier findings, an initial tachycardia has not predicted a beneficial response to β-adrenergic blockade.[234]

The mechanism by which β-adrenergic blockade can improve ventricular function and ameliorate CHF in dilated cardiomyopathies remains controversial and obscure (see Chap. 54). This also reflects the fact that the initial cause of a dilated cardiomyopathy is unknown, although the compensatory responses of the process, including ventricular remodeling (dilation and hypertrophy) and neurohumoral activation, have been well described. These latter processes are also accompanied by further myocyte loss and fibrosis, which, together with the compensatory changes, may lead to disease progression. Waagstein has entertained the concept that beta blockers may improve energy balance that may be limited in the failing myocardium.[223] Bristow et al. have suggested that multiple mechanisms may mediate the clinical benefits derived from long-term β-adrenergic blockade.[245] Bucindolol-induced improvements in LV EF appear to be dose-related, while prevention of LV deterioration is not. Thus, beta blockade–related improvement in ventricular function may be mediated by different mechanisms than those responsible for prevention of deterioration. Alternatively, the sensitivities for these effects are different. The clinical benefits of long-term β-adrenergic blockade in patients with dilated cardiomyopathy associated with coronary artery disease have been demonstrated with metoprolol by Fisher et al. in a double-blind, randomized trial.[239] When compared to patients receiving placebo, patients receiving metoprolol experienced a significant reduction in hospital admission and an increase in functional class, EF, and exercise duration. In this situation, limitation of ischemia, per se, may have had a beneficial effect.

Clinical experience with long-term β-adrenergic blockade in heart failure has recently focused on carvedilol, a nonselective β-adrenergic blockade with mild vasodilatory action due to α-adrenergic blockade, which has additional antioxidant properties.[246] The drug recently received FDA approval for reducing the progression of heart failure in class II and III CHF patients. In an early experience, patients with severe CHF due to idiopathic and ischemic dilated cardiomyopathy, who were treated with digitalis, loop diuretics, and ACE inhibitors, demonstrated substantial improvement with 6 months' administration of carvedilol.[240] LV EF was increased from an average of 17 to 27 percent, while functional capacity was improved, as evidenced by a reduction in one functional class of the NYHA from 2.8 to 1.9. Improvement occurred in patients with ischemic and idiopathic cardiomyopathies, although the improvement was significantly less in the ischemic group. These results in a mixed patient population of ischemic and nonischemic dilated cardiomyopathy have confirmed the earlier experience of Metra et al. with long-term administration of carvedilol in patients with idiopathic dilated cardiomyopathy.[242] The Australian-New Zealand Heart Failure Research Collaboration Group[243] showed that after 6 months of therapy with carvedilol, LV EF was significantly improved by an absolute value of 5.2 percent in patients with ischemic cardiomyopathy, while symptoms were not significantly altered. Moreover, only 27 of the 442 patients failed to tolerate carvedilol.

The benefits of carvedilol on mortality and hospitalization for cardiovascular causes have been demonstrated in 1094 patients with CHF who were entered in four double-blind, placebo-controlled protocols.[240] The overall 6-month mortality was 7.8 percent for the placebo group and 3.2 percent for the carvedilol group, a reduction of 65 percent (95 percent CI, 39 to 80 percent; $p < .001$). The risk of hospitalization was reduced by 27 percent by carvedilol, i.e., from 19.6 to 14.1 percent; $p = .036$. The progression of heart failure, as defined by death or hospitalization due to heart failure, or the need for a sustained increase in heart failure medication was also significantly reduced by carvedilol in patients with mild symptoms of heart failure.[247] Clinical progression of heart failure occurred in 21 percent of patients receiving placebo and in only 11 percent of patients

receiving carvedilol, a reduction of 48 percent (relative risk, 0.52; CI, 0.32 to 0.85). Similar clinical benefits of carvedilol have also been observed in patients with mild to moderate stable chronic heart failure.[248] In addition, the carvedilol-induced reductions in mortality and hospitalization rate, as well as improvement in LV function, were related to dose. In patients with moderate to severe heart failure, carvedilol, when compared to placebo, increased the frequency of symptomatic improvement and lowered the risk of clinical deterioration. As evaluated by physicians, 53 percent of patients receiving placebo and 81 percent of patients receiving carvedilol showed symptomatic improvement, whereas 12 percent of the placebo group and 2 percent of the carvedilol group evidenced deterioration.[249]

In summary, the clinical benefits derived from carvedilol appear to differ in magnitude and/or nature from those reported with first-generation β-adrenergic blocking agents, which are nonselective, and second-generation beta blockers such as metoprolol and bisoprolol, which are beta$_1$-selective. Based on the available clinical data, carvedilol has been approved by the FDA for preventing further disease progression in patients with class I and III heart failure. The drug is not approved for class IV heart failure, although it is currently being evaluated in clinical trials.

In contrast to the studies with carvedilol, bisoprolol did not reduce mortality in patients with ischemic cardiomyopathy and did not reduce the incidence of sudden death in the Cardiac Insufficiency Bisoprolol Study (CIBIS).[250] The benefits of carvedilol on 6-month mortality have far exceeded those noted with metoprolol and have led to a 35 percent reduction in the combined morbidity/mortality endpoints.[249]

The exact mechanisms responsible for the apparent superiority of carvedilol over metoprolol are not fully understood. From a pharmacologic standpoint, carvedilol differs from metoprolol (Table 23-5). While carvedilol is relatively nonselective for blockade of beta$_1$ and beta$_2$ receptors, it is an alpha$_1$ blocker, which results in arterial vasodilatation. Moreover, it has antioxidant properties that may play a role in improving myocyte viability.[251]

The hemodynamic and antiadrenergic effects of long-term treatment with metoprolol and carvedilol have been compared by Gilbert et al.[251] Hemodynamically, carvedilol tends to

TABLE 23-5

PHARMACOLOGIC CHARACTERISTICS OF SOME BETA BLOCKERS USED IN CONGESTIVE HEART FAILURE

	β$_1$	β$_2$	α	Direct VSMC Relaxant	Antioxidant
Metoprolol	+	−	−	−	−
Bisoprolol	+	−	−	−	−
Bucindolol	+	+	±	+	−
Carvedilol	+	+	+	−	+

Note: VSMC, vascular skeletal muscle cells.

produce greater improvements in LV EF, SV, and stroke work than metoprolol.[251] In regard to antiadrenergic activity, carvedilol lowers coronary sinus norepinephrine levels, an index of cardiac adrenergic activity, whereas metoprolol does not. Conversely, carvedilol does not change cardiac beta-receptor expression while metoprolol leads to an increase in cardiac beta-receptor density. Neither carvedilol nor metoprolol alter systemic norepinephrine levels, although in another study,[252] sympathetic nerve activity was reduced substantially after several months of metoprolol therapy. However, as pointed out by Gilbert et al.[251] current comparison between metoprolol and carvedilol is weakened by several issues: (1) the study design was not a three-way comparison of metoprolol, carvedilol, and placebo but a comparison of two concurrently performed placebo-controlled trials; (2) the limited and variable duration of follow-up, which was 6 months for metoprolol and 4 months for carvedilol; and (3) lack of coronary sinus blood flow measurements, which could have influenced coronary sinus norepinephrine levels.

Thus, while the impressive results of the carvedilol trials and intrinsic pharmacologic and functional properties of carvedilol suggest important differences between carvedilol and other beta-blocking agents, the question whether long-term therapy with carvedilol leads to greater clinical benefits than long-term therapy with other beta-blocking agents will only be answered by comparative large randomized trials, which are currently ongoing. While the evidence from previous beta-blocking agent trials in heart failure point to a class effect of β-adrenergic blockade by agents in the progression of heart failure, their individual therapeutic efficacy appears to vary to a much greater extent than does the therapeutic efficacy of ACE inhibitors.

As with other β-adrenergic blockers, the mechanism by which carvedilol beneficially affects the failing heart is controversial. Energy needs are reduced through a decreased heart rate from beta$_1$-receptor blockade and reduced peripheral resistance, and blood pressure through alpha$_1$-receptor blockade. One suspects that myocyte loss is also reduced, which may help prevent further deterioration. The antioxidant action of the agent may be useful in this regard. Integration of these effects may prevent remodeling from progressing and even permit some regression, resulting in improved ventricular performance and reduced mortality.

The benefits of long-term β-adrenergic blockade in patients with chronic heart failure are summarized in Table 23-6. It is also important to remember that beta blockers reduce mortality very substantially in patients following an acute myocardial infarction, in the presence of very reduced EFs.[253]

At present, carvedilol is the only β-adrenergic blocker approved by the FDA for the treatment of patients with CHF who have symptoms compatible with functional class II to III of the NYHA. Whether stable patients with symptoms compatible with functional class IV can also benefit from nonselective β-adrenergic blockade is currently unclear. This issue is being addressed by the Beta-Blocker Evaluation Survival Trial (BEST), which has randomized patients with CHF

TABLE 23-6

POSSIBLE MECHANISMS BY WHICH β-ADRENERGIC BLOCKERS IMPROVE VENTRICULAR FUNCTION IN CHRONIC CONGESTIVE HEART FAILURE

1. Upregulation of β receptors
2. Direct myocardial protective action against catecholamine toxicity
3. Improved ability of noradrenergic sympathetic nerves to synthesize norepinephrine
4. Decreased release of norepinephrine from sympathetic nerve endings
5. Decreased stimulation of other vasoconstrictive systems including renin-angiotensin-aldosterone, vasopressin, and endothelin
6. Potentiation of kalikrein-kinin system and natural vasodilatation (increase in bradykinin)
7. Antiarrhythmic effects raising ventricular fibrillation threshold
8. Protection against catecholamine-induced hypokalemia
9. Increase in coronary blood flow by reducing heart rate and improving diastolic perfusion time; possible coronary dilation with vasodilator–β blocker
10. Restoration of abnormal baroreflex function
11. Prevention of ventricular muscle hypertrophy and vascular remodeling
12. Antioxidant effects (carvedilol?)
13. Shift from free fatty acid to carbohydrate metabolism (improved metabolic efficiency)
14. Vasodilation (e.g., bucindolol, carvedilol)
15. Antiapoptosis effect
16. Improved left atrial contribution to left ventricular filling

in functional classes III and IV to bucindolol, a third-generation beta-blocking agent, or placebo. In any event, while compensated patients in functional class IV may benefit from administration of carvedilol, this should be administered with great care. In decompensated class IV patients, carvedilol may be poorly tolerated, and for the present is best avoided. If contemplated in stable patients with compensated functional class IV CHF, carvedilol therapy is best initiated by clinicians who have experience with carvedilol, and with close monitoring. During the first weeks of carvedilol therapy, symptomatic deterioration is expected. This requires increasing the dose of loop diuretics and occasionally the initiation of temporary inotropic support with a type III-specific PDE inhibitor such as milrinone. The management of patients in functional class IV who continue to decompensate without a clear precipitating factor while being treated with conventional therapy along with carvedilol remains a challenge. One approach is to initiate inotropic support with milrinone while continuing therapy with carvedilol, and to discontinue carvedilol only in patients who can be weaned from milrinone therapy but remain decompensated. In order to use dobutamine in decompensated patients treated with carvedilol, this beta blocker, as with others, must be reduced or withdrawn.

In summary, nonselective β-adrenergic blockade has finally gained wide acceptance for the treatment of patients with CHF.[254] In view of the substantive benefits of carvedilol therapy on LV dimension and function, this agent appears the most effective. It should be started early in the syndrome of symptomatic CHF, when ventricular remodeling with dilatation is the least and extensive ventricular fibrosis has yet to occur.

ADJUNCTIVE THERAPIES

As mentioned earlier, patients with heart failure require treatment of underlying disease processes that may be aggravating the myopathic process. Systemic hypertension should be treated vigorously. In diabetes, hyperglycemia should be controlled. Aspirin prophylaxis and cholesterol-lowering drugs should be used in patients with coronary artery disease. It is not known if estrogen replacement therapy in postmenopausal women can modify the course of heart failure.[255]

Beta blockers should be considered in all patients who survive a myocardial infarction, with or without ventricular dysfunction. As described earlier, carvedilol should probably be the beta blocker of choice in patients with symptomatic mild to moderate CHF of ischemic and nonischemic origin. Propranolol, metoprolol, atenolol, or timolol should be used in myocardial infarction survivors who are asymptomatic, with and without LV dysfunction.

Patients with CHF are liable to develop venoembolic disease and systemic emboli from intracardiac mural thrombi. These embolic events are major causes of morbidity and mortality in CHF. In patients with atrial fibrillation and CHF, with and without mitral stenosis, anticoagulation is indicated. In patients with normal sinus rhythm and cardiomyopathy, the role of prophylactic anticoagulation with warfarin is not defined. It is more difficult to anticoagulate patients with CHF because of drug-drug interactions, malabsorption of medications, varying perfusion of the liver, and malnutrition. Patients with CHF who have developed a phlebothrombotic process or who have definite evidence of ventricular mural thrombi and systemic embolism should receive warfarin despite the potential problems with regulation of anticoagulation in these patients.

Patients with heart failure have a markedly increased prevalence of ventricular ectopy and incidence of sudden death. Patients should be assessed for hypokalemia, hypomagnesemia, hypoxia, infection, and the use of antidepressant drugs. Many antiarrhythmic drug regimens have negative inotropic actions and may aggravate the heart failure process. Amiodarone and beta blockers have been used in patients with LV dysfunction with less risk involved and are probably the drugs of choice when treatment of ventricular ectopy is considered.[256,257] There is little evidence to show that antiarrhythmic drug therapy changes the natural history of advanced CHF.[257] Amiodarone can also be used to treat atrial arrhythmias, with and without digoxin and calcium channel blockers.

DIASTOLIC DYSFUNCTION

Diastolic dysfunction of the left and right ventricles will often lead to all the signs and symptoms of systolic dysfunction,

but the therapeutic approach varies for these two conditions. Often, there is significant LV hypertrophy present, and aggressive management of systemic hypertension is required.[256,258] These patients will develop significant congestion, so that diuretics are often necessary. With hypovolemia from other diseases, however, patients are prone to develop hypotension. The effects of diuretics in these patients should be carefully monitored. Digoxin is probably of no use unless the patient is in atrial fibrillation, and vasodilating drugs with peripheral venodilator actions may cause hypotension. The role of ACE inhibitors, angiotensin II receptor blockers, and other vasodilator drugs are not well defined in this condition, and they may cause hypotension. Tachycardia needs to be avoided, and the rate-lowering calcium blockers (verapamil, diltiazem) are probably the drugs of choice for reducing elevated blood pressure, keeping the heart rate under control, and improving ventricular compliance.[259] β-Adrenergic blockers may also be of help, but their effects on ventricular compliance are not as well defined. Both verapamil and beta blocker can be used with caution in patients with heart failure due to hypertrophic cardiomyopathy.

DRUG THERAPIES UNDER INVESTIGATION

Natriuretic Peptides

Conventional diuretics are associated with undesirable stimulation of the renin-angiotensin axis, sympathetic nervous system, and vasopressin. ANP and brain natriuretic peptide (BNP), on the other hand, induce a diuresis and natriuresis while concomitantly suppressing the renin-angiotensin axis with dilating of peripheral vascular beds.[260–264] In heart failure, despite high endogenous ANP and BNP levels, a state of intense sodium avidity prevails.[260,261,264,265] Attempts at restoring the efficacy of ANP in heart failure include infusing ANP intravenously and administering a neutral endopeptidase inhibitor. Prolonged infusion of ANP in patients with moderate CHF (NYHA class II to III) has been associated with doubling of the urine flow rate and a three- to fourfold increase in sodium excretion.[266] When ANP is infused in patients with moderate to severe CHF (NYHA class II to IV), however, the natriuretic and diuretic response is attenuated.[261,262]

Favorable hemodynamic responses have been observed after ANP infusion, including a fall in PCWP, plasma renin activity, and systemic vascular resistance and an increase in cardiac output.[261,262,267] When ANP and furosemide are administered concomitantly, urine volume and sodium excretion are not augmented, although in this setting ANP does maintain its inhibitory effect on the renin-angiotensin axis and on sympathetic discharge.[268]

Neutral endopeptidase inhibitor administration is associated with a rise in endogenous ANP levels due to the inhibition of ANP metabolism.[264,269–273] In a canine model of CHF, Cavero et al. reported that, at similar ANP levels, neutral endopeptidase inhibitor treatment was associated with a better diuretic and natriuretic effect than with an ANP infusion.[269] In human studies, however, the two modalities appear to have similar natriuretic and diuretic effects. In 1989, Northridge and colleagues were the first to report a diuresis following neutral endopeptidase inhibitor infusion in six patients with mild CHF (mean EF 37 percent).[272] A 60 percent increase in the 4-h urine sodium excretion was observed, associated with a three- to fivefold rise in ANP levels.[272] The same investigators compared the renal and hemodynamic effects of neutral endopeptidase inhibitor administration to low-dose furosemide in mild CHF.[274] Eighteen patients were randomized to receive either a neutral endopeptidase inhibitor, candoxatrilat 200 mg twice daily, candoxatrilat 400 mg twice daily, or furosemide 20 mg twice daily. The administration of a neutral endopeptidase inhibitor was associated with a diuresis; however, the change in urine flow rate and sodium excretion from baseline was greater in the low-dose furosemide group. Although its diuretic effect was modest, the neutral endopeptidase inhibitor was associated with desirable hemodynamic effects, including marked preload reduction (PCWP decreased by 40 percent), and with no stimulation of plasma renin activity. In comparison, the group given furosemide experienced only a 15 percent reduction in PCWP and a threefold rise in plasma renin activity.

The natriuretic properties of neutral endopeptidase inhibitors are mediated by inhibition of sodium reabsorption within the renal tubule, since they do not significantly alter renal hemodynamics (GFR or renal plasma flow). This is supported by their association with an increased fractional excretion of lithium, a marker of proximal tubular reabsorption.[269,271] In addition to inhibiting ANP degradation, the neutral endopeptidase inhibitors inhibit the breakdown of bradykinin and BNP. They have also been shown to enhance prostacyclin synthesis, another mechanism by which they may exert a natriuretic effect.[275,276] In the most severe stages of CHF (NYHA class III to IV; EF, 22 percent), an impaired renal response to neutral endopeptidase inhibitor treatment can be expected. Munzel and colleagues[263] reported an unpredictable natriuretic response to candoxatrilat in nine patients with severe CHF. Three patients had no diuresis, five had a minimal response, and one (cardiac index > 2.5 L/min) had a good diuresis. The natriuretic response correlated closely with the cardiac output, which, theoretically, was most likely related to renal perfusion status.

In contrast to ANP, the natriuretic effect of BNP infusion is surprisingly and significantly more pronounced in patients with CHF than in normal patients, even when similar BNP levels are infused.[264] Yoshimura et al. infused BNP in normal patients and in those with NYHA class II to IV CHF and observed a fivefold rise in urine flow rate and a tenfold increase in sodium excretion in the CHF group.[264] In normal patients, diuresis and natriuresis were only three- to fourfold that of baseline, respectively. BNP infusion was also associated with a reduction in PCWP, systemic vascular resistance, and aldosterone levels as well as with a rise in ANP levels.

It is unclear why high-dose BNP infusion is not associated with an attenuated natriuretic response in CHF, as is seen with ANP infusion. Like the process in ANP, inhibition of neutral endopeptidase 24.11 with candoxatril prevents the metabolism of BNP, increasing BNP levels by about 50 percent.[276] Because of its enhanced natriuretic effect at high infusion rates and its prolonged duration of action compared with ANP, BNP appears to be the most promising natriuretic peptide candidate for future investigation and potential clinical therapeutic use.

Endothelin Inhibitors

Endothelin-1 exhibits potent inotropic activity in isolated hearts, cardiac muscle strips, isolated cells, and in instrumented intact animals.[277] High-affinity receptors for endothelin have been demonstrated in both the atria and ventricles.[278–280] Intravenous endothelin-1 produces a delayed prolonged augmentation of LV performance in addition to its biphasic vasoactive effects of a transient vasodilation followed by a sustained vasoconstriction.[277]

Endothelin is also a potent secretagogue of atrial natriuretic factor, which is a naturally occurring antagonist of endothelin that acts by inhibiting its release.[281] The endothelin-A receptor appears to mediate endothelin's actions of vasoconstriction and the stimulation of the ANP secretion, and the endothelin-B receptor mediates endothelin-induced vasodilatation and activation of the renin-angiotensin-aldosterone system. Urinary water excretion is mediated through both receptors, but sodium excretion is mediated through the endothelin-A receptor.

Increased endothelin levels have been described in patients with CHF[282–287] that are predictive of increased mortality risk.[283] It has also been suggested that increased endothelin levels may be playing an important role in the increased systemic vascular resistance observed in CHF.[282,288,289] Endothelin-1 levels decrease with therapy and have been found to correlate significantly with symptomatic improvement. It therefore appears that endothelin-1 is an independent, noninvasive predictor of functional and hemodynamic response to therapy in patients with CHF.[290]

Increased endothelin levels have also been observed in the plasma and hearts of cardiomyopathic Syrian hamsters[291] and in the cells of endothelial cells infected with *Trypanosoma cruzi* in experimental Chagas' cardiomyopathy.[292]

There is early clinical evidence that treatment with endothelin-A receptor antagonists and endothelin-converting enzyme inhibitors can influence the course of human heart failure favorably.[293] Some of these agents are being investigated in clinical heart failure trials.[294,295] ACE inhibitors may also be benefiting patients with heart failure because of their antiendothelin actions.[128,296]

Vasopressin Antagonists

The first peptide vasopressin antagonists (V2 receptor specific) were developed in the early 1980s.[297] Although initially found to induce a water diuresis in rats and dogs, this did not occur in humans owing to a component of V2 receptor agonist effect.[298] Recently, a nonpeptide V2 receptor antagonist, OPC 31260 (Otsuka Pharmaceutical Co., Japan), has been shown to promote a diuresis in humans. In normal subjects under water-restricted conditions, where antidiuretic hormone concentrations were elevated and the urine was maximally concentrated, stimulating the state of CHF,[299] intravenous administration of OPC 31260 produced an eightfold increase in urine volume within 1 h, which returned to baseline within 4 h. Urine volume was decreased, while urine osmolality declined from 918 + 60 to 99 + 2 mOsm/kg. These findings suggest potential therapeutic utility of aquaretic agents in edematous states such as CHF.[300]

Adenosine Receptor Antagonism

Blockade of adenosine (A1) receptors in animals can induce a brisk natriuresis without a kaliuretic effect,[301] an observation that has been confirmed in humans in short-term studies using FK 4531, a selective A1 receptor antagonist.[302–304] The mechanism for this lack of kaliuretic action has not been elucidated, neither has the safety and efficacy of this drug class in long-term clinical trials.

Oral Dopamine Receptor Agonists

The unique, selective vasodilatory and inotropic actions of intravenous dopamine are limited by the lack of oral formulation. This has led investigators to develop newer dopamine agonists that are orally effective. Unlike L-dopa, which has been used in heart failure, these new drugs do not cross the blood-brain barrier but maintain most of the pharmacologic activity of dopamine.[305]

Ibopamine, which is an orally active derivative of dopamine, has dopaminergic D_1 and D_2 activity with α- and β-adrenergic actions. In therapeutic doses, it is a peripheral vasodilator and appears to have favorable cardiovascular and renovascular actions in patients with heart failure. The results of the recent Prospective Randomized Study of Ibopamine on Mortality and Efficacy in Heart Failure (PRIM-2), however, raised serious questions about the safety of ibopamine and agents of this class[306] in patients with heart failure. Fenoldopam is a selective D_1 agonist that has been used to treat patients with CHF and hypertension. Because of bioavailability problems with the oral formulation, only the intravenous form is used in patients with severe hypertension. Dopexamine is an intravenous D_1 and beta$_2$-receptor agonist that is being studied in patients with CHF and low cardiac output states.

Inhibition of Immune Activation

Cytokines are a group of small pleiotropic endogenous peptides produced by a variety of cell types in response to a variety of different stimuli. Tumor necrosis factor alpha (TNFα), interleukin 1α and 1β, and interleukin 6 are classified as "proinflammatory" cytokines. These substances are responsible for initiating the primary host response to bacterial infections as well as initiating the repair of injured tissues.[307]

Cytokines are involved in augmenting the expression of adhesion molecules and for enhanced cell-to-cell interactions involved in inflammation. In addition, the proinflammatory cytokines are able to affect cardiovascular functioning by promoting LV remodeling, causing ventricular dysfunction,

and uncoupling myocardial beta receptors.[307] They are elevated in the serum in various cardiovascular disorders and are often a marker of the severity of disease.[308]

TNFα was originally discovered in 1975 as a protein with necrotizing effects in certain transplantable mouse tumors.[309] More recently, this cytokine has been shown to exert a spectrum of pleiotropic effects in many different cell types.[310] The major biologic role of TNFα is thought to be a host response to systemic infections, most notably gram-negative sepsis.[311] In fact, TNFα levels are considerably elevated in patients with septic shock, and TNFα has been implicated as an important mediator in the lethal effect of endotoxin, possibly causing the symptoms characteristic of the "shock state."

Many experimental and clinical studies have shown there is an association between depressed myocardial function and elevated levels of TNFα.[312] The basis of this association is not yet clear; however, there are studies suggesting that elevated levels of TNFα play a major role in causing myocardial depression, whereas other studies conclude that TNFα is likely to play a part in the alleviation of this condition.[313] A third school of thought suggests that the elevated levels of TNFα are merely a marker that may indicate the stage of progression of the disease. Thus, although it is clear there are elevated levels of TNFα in various cardiac diseases, the reasons for these increased levels and the mechanisms of their effects are not agreed on. Since there is a strong association and possibly a causative relationship exists between TNFα and CHF, various drug trials are looking at TNFα and its possible metabolic pathways as a therapeutic target in the treatment of heart disease.[314]

Nitric Oxide

Preliminary work is now being done investigating inhaled nitric oxide, a vasodilator substance produced by the endothelium, as a possible treatment for CHF.[315–318] Arginine, a nitric oxide precursor, and agents that potentiate nitric oxide synthesis are potential new directions for new heart failure therapies. Nitric oxide donor substances are also being evaluated.[318]

Surgical Treatment

IMPLANTABLE CARDIOVERTER DEFIBRILLATORS

In patients with documented sustained ventricular tachycardia or ventricular fibrillation, the implantable cardioverter defibrillator is highly effective in treating recurrences of these arrhythmias by antitachycardia pacing or cardioversion-defibrillation, thereby reducing morbidity and the need for rehospitalization. There is some evidence that the efficacy of this device in terminating ventricular tachycardia or ventricular fibrillation may translate into improved survival,[319] but in the absence of randomized trials, no definite proof exists. The benefit of implantable cardioverter defibrillation therapy may decrease with increasing degrees of heart failure.[320] Preliminary data suggest improved survival compared to conventional antiarrhythmic therapy, including amiodarone, in patients with asymptomatic LV dysfunction or mild to moderate heart failure.[321] For patients with severe heart failure and documented sustained ventricular tachyarrhythmias, implantable cardioverter defibrillators at present should be considered as a bridge to transplantation, but their effectiveness in this setting has not been proven either.

HEART TRANSPLANTATION

Heart transplantation is now an accepted mode of treatment for endstage CHF (see Chap. 25). Transplantation significantly increases survival, exercise capacity, return to work, and quality of life compared to conventional treatment, provided proper selection criteria are applied. Recent results in patients on triple immunosuppressive therapy have shown a 5-year survival of approximately 70 to 80 percent[322] and return to full- or part-time work or seeking employment after 1 year in about two-thirds of the patients in the best series.[323]

Patients who should be considered for transplantation are those with severe CHF with no alternative form of treatment. Predictors of poor survival are taken into account. The patient must be willing and capable to undergo intensive medical treatment and be emotionally stable so as to withstand the many uncertainties likely to occur both before and after transplantation.

Besides shortage of donor hearts, the main problem of heart transplantation is rejection of the allograft, which is responsible for a considerable percentage of deaths in the first postoperative year. The long-term outcome is limited predominantly by the consequences of immunosuppression (infection, hypertension, renal failure, malignancy, accelerated progression of atherosclerotic vascular disease) and by transplant coronary artery disease.

In the patient who cannot be sustained with medical therapy and for whom ultimate cardiac transplantation is anticipated, a left ventricular mechanical support device (LVAD) has been successful, serving to maintain ventricular function as a bridge to transplantation (see Chap. 25).

CORONARY REVASCULARIZATION SURGERY

A major and important surgical approach to ischemic cardiomyopathies is reperfusion of ischemic tissue by coronary bypass surgery.[324] This is based on the concept that transiently ischemic myocardium (stunning) and myocardium with reduced flow (hibernating) have reduced contractility, which may return to normal with restoration of an adequate coronary blood flow. Moreover, revascularization of ischemic regions of the ventricle may prevent recurrent infarction in this area, and so help prevent further deterioration of ventricular function. In such patients, it is necessary to establish that significant amounts of viable tissue remain in an akinetic or hypokinetic zone; this can be accomplished with nuclear techniques such as a 24-h thallium perfusion study or positron emission tomographic scanning[325] (see Chap. 20). If contractile activity can also be elicited, as shown in echo studies with low-dose dobutamine stimulation[13] or postextrasystolic potentiation, coronary bypass surgery provides a good chance to stabilize or

improve ventricular function[324] and enhance survival.[326] In this era, every patient with an ischemic cardiomyopathy should be evaluated for possible revascularization and assumed to be a candidate until proven otherwise.

OTHER PROCEDURES

Other surgical approaches to the dilated heart have included the recent concept of removing a segment of the left ventricular wall, the "Baptista operation," so as to reduce LV volume and thus wall stress. The surgical risk is immense, and specific benefits have yet to be established.

Immunoabsorption procedures have been directed against β_1-adrenergic receptor antibodies with clinical improvement found in patients with heart failure.[327]

The General Approach to Therapy in Congestive Heart Failure

Appropriate therapy in CHF depends on the stage of the disease process (Table 23-7, Figs. 23-11 and 23-12). While one seeks to define and treat the factors that initiated the process, one also attempts to reduce symptoms and prolong life. Thus, with initial damage, e.g., following a large myocardial infarction, ACE inhibition or angiotensin II receptor blockade is indicated. β-Adrenergic receptor blockers are also indicated at this stage because of mortality reduction. As failure progresses to more symptomatic phases, beta blockers also appear indicated, along with ACE inhibition. Once symptoms increase and edema and central congestion occur, loop diuretics become useful to maintain dry weight. In order to prevent further ischemic tissue loss, other measures, such as cessation of smoking and appropriate lipid control, are essential. Digitalis glycosides, especially in modest doses, are indicated when class II to III symptoms occur.

In acute decompensation, such as may occur following a massive myocardial infarction or intermittently in class III to IV chronic heart failure, more aggressive therapy may be required, along with hospitalization for Swan-Ganz catheter monitoring. In this circumstance, short-term stimulation of the myocardium with dobutamine and/or milrinone, along with increasing amounts of intravenous diuretics, may be required for short periods of time to regain a stable state. At present there are no oral agents of this nature available to extend this care to the out-patient, and if dobutamine cannot be withdrawn, occasional administration by an external pump is required. Such therapy presents a short outcome of days or months.

In summary, the therapy of heart failure seeks the reversal or attenuation of the processes that initiated the syndrome while treating the patient to relieve symptoms and prolong life. The latter end is best achieved early in the disease process through prevention of further loss of myocardium (e.g., reperfusion) or reduction of loading (e.g., appropriate valve surgery or treatment of hypertension). In very late stages of the disease, relief of symptoms can now be accomplished with modest gains in life expectancy.

TABLE 23-7

CHRONIC HEART FAILURE—CHOICE OF PHARMACOLOGICAL THERAPY

	ACE Inhibitor	Diuretic	Potassium-Sparing Diuretic	Cardiac-glycosides	Vasodilator (Hydralazine/ISDN)	Beta Blocker
Systolic dysfunction						
Asymptomatic LV dysfunction	Indicated in some	Not indicated (unless ↑ BP)	Not indicated	Only with atrial fibrillation	Not indicated	Post MI
Symptomatic HF (NYIIA II)	Indicated			(a) When atrial fibrillation is present, or (b) when improved from more severe HF in sinus rhythm[a]	If ACE inhibitors are not tolerated	Indicated (under specialist care)
− fluid retention		Indicated in some	Not indicated			
+ fluid retention		Indicated	Persisting hypokalaemia			
Worsening/severe HF (NYHA III–IV)	Indicated	Indicated, combinations of diuretics	Persisting hypokalaemia; spironolactone for efficacy	Indicated	If ACE inhibitors are not tolerated or insufficient	Indicated (under specialist care)
Endstage HF (persisting NHYA IV)	Indicated	Indicated, combinations of diuretics	Persisting hypokalaemia; spironolactone for efficacy	Indicated	If ACE inhibitors are not tolerated or insufficient	Indicated (under specialist care)

[a] Preliminary data from the DIG (Digitalis Investigation Group) trial suggest that digoxin may also be indicated in NYHA II heart failure and sinus rhythm.
Note: ACE, angiotensin-converting enzyme; BP, blood pressure; HF, heart failure; ISDN, isosorbide dinitrate; LV, left ventricular; MI, myocardial infarction; NYHA, New York Heart Association.
Source: From Task Force of the Working Group on Heart Failure of the European Society of Cardiology. The treatment of heart failure. *Eur Heart J* 1997; 18.748. Reproduced with permission from the publisher and authors.

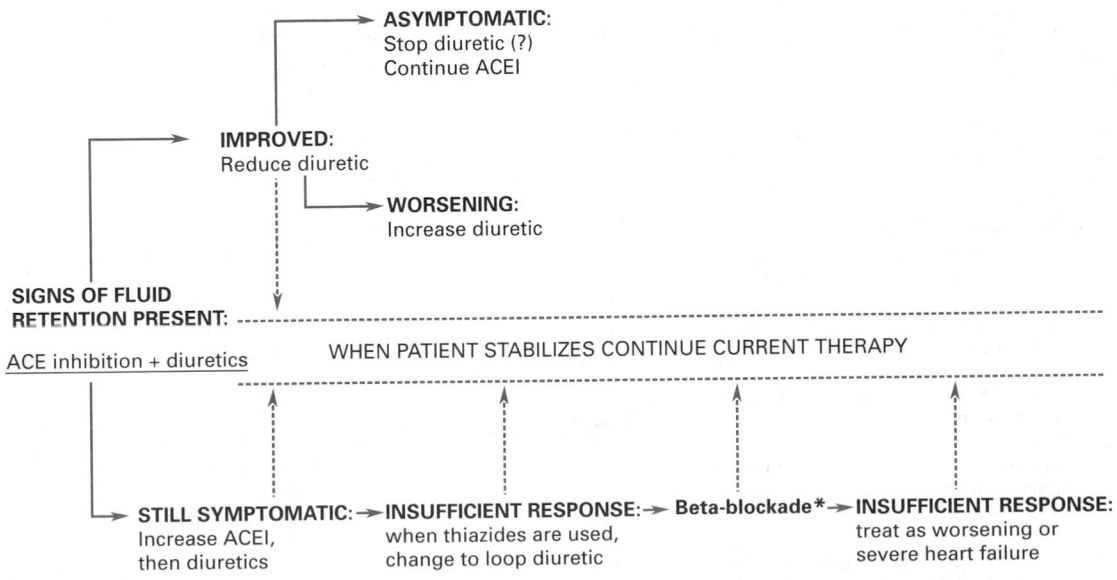

FIGURE 23-11
Flowchart of pharmacologic treatment of mild symptomatic systolic left ventricular (LV) dysfunction, NYHA II, and signs of fluid retention. *Data available only for carvedilol. (From Task Force of the Working Group on Heart Failure of the European Society of Cardiology. The treatment of heart failure. *Eur Heart J* 1997; 18:746. Reproduced with permission from the publisher and authors.)

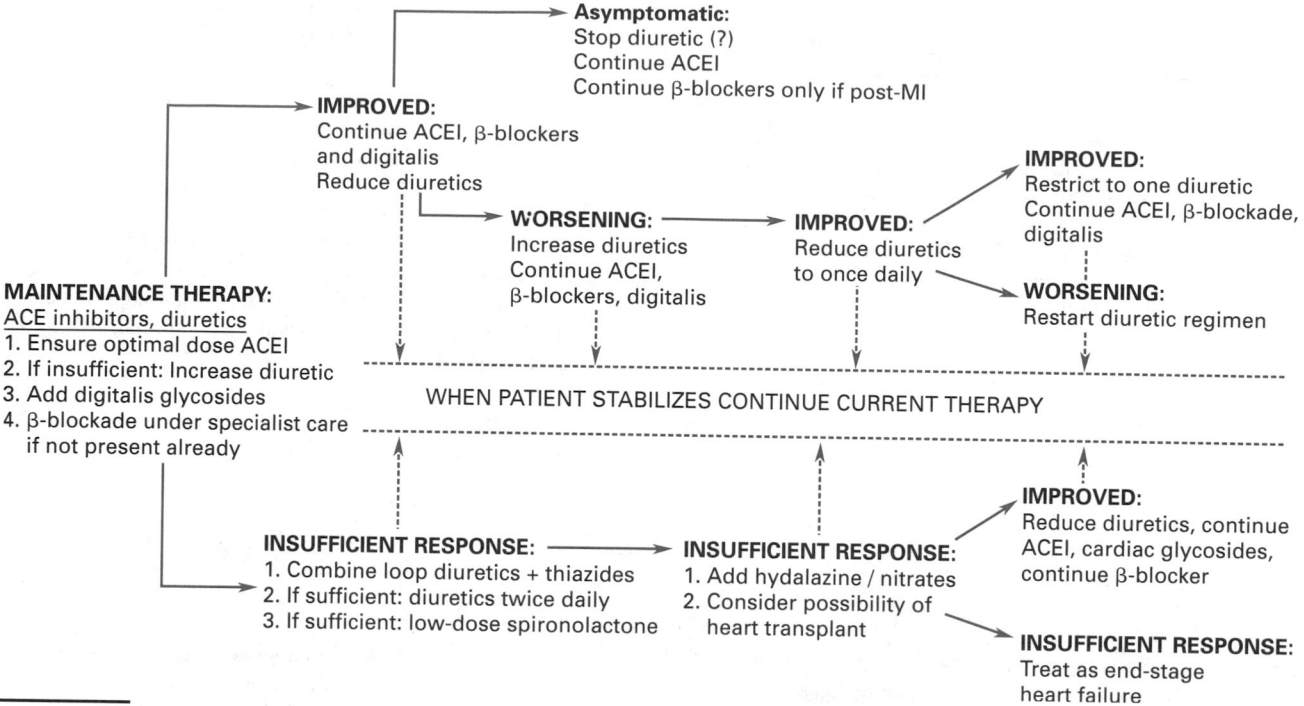

FIGURE 23-12

Flowchart of pharmacologic treatment of symptomatic left ventricular dysfunction and worsening heart failure (NYHA III to IV). (From Task Force of the Working Group on Heart Failure of the European Society of Cardiology.

The Treatment of heart failure. *Eur Heart J* 1997; 18:747. Reproduced with permission from the publisher and authors.)

REFERENCES

1. Guidelines for Evaluation and Management of Heart Failure. *Circulation* 1995; 92:2764–2784.
2. Sonnenblick EH, LeJemtel TH. Heart failure: Its progression and its therapy. *Hosp Pract* 1993; 28:121–130.
3. Benge W, Litchfield RL, Marcus ML. Exercise capacity in patients with severe left ventricular dysfunction. *Circulation* 1980; 61:955–959.
4. Rickenbacher PR, Trindade PT, Haywood GA, Vagelos RH, Schroeder JS, Willson K, et al. Transplant candidates with severe left ventricular dysfunction managed with medical treatment: Characteristics and survival. *J Am Coll Cardiol* 1996; 27:1192–1197.
5. Rich MW, Beckham V, Wittenberg C, Leven CL, Freedand KE, Carney RM. A multidisciplinary intervention to prevent the readmission of elderly patients with congestive heart failure. *N Engl J Med* 1995; 333:1190–1195.
6. LeJemtel TH, Sonnenblick EH. Heart failure: Adaptive and maladaptive processes. *Circulation* 1993; 87(suppl VII):1–4.
7. Carabello BA, Crawford FA. Valvular heart disease. *N Engl J Med* 1997; 337:32–41.
8. Floras JS. Clinical aspects of sympathetic activation and parasympathetic withdrawal in heart failure. *J Am Coll Cardiol* 1993; 22(suppl A):72A–84A.
9. Olivetti G, Abbi R, Quaini F, Kajstura J, Cheng W, Nitahara JA, et al. Apoptosis in the failing human heart. *N Engl J Med* 1997; 336:1131–1141.
10. LeJemtel TH, Sonnenblick EH. Heart failure in elderly patients. In, Aronow W, Tresch DD, eds. *Cardiovascular Disease in the Elderly Patient.* New York: Marcel Dekker; 1993:473–484.
11. Brutsaert DL, Sonnenblick EH. Cardiac muscle mechanics in the evaluation of myocardial contractility and pump function. Problems, concepts and directions. *Prog Cardiovasc Dis* 1973; 16:337–361.
12. Hendel RC, Chandhry FA, Bonow RO. Myocardial viability. *Curr Probl Cardiol* 1996; 21:145–224.
13. Bonow RO. Identification of viable myocardium. *Circulation* 1996; 94:2674–2680.
14. Vanoverschelde J-LJ, Wijns W, Borgers M, Heyndrickx G, Depre C, Flameng W, et al. Chronic myocardial hibernation in humans. *Circulation* 1996; 95:1961–1971.
15. Perrone-Filardi P, Pace L, Prastaro M, Piscione F, Betocchi S, Squame F, et al. Dobutamine echocardiography predicts improvement in hypoperfused dysfunctional myocardium after revascularization in patients with coronary artery disease. *Circulation* 1995; 91:2556–2565.
16. La Canna G, Alfiero O, Giubbini R, Gargano M, Ferrari R, Visioli O. Echocardiography during infusion of dobutamine for identification of reversible dysfunction in patients with chronic coronary artery disease. *J Am Coll Cardiol* 1994; 23:617–626.
17. Cigarroa CG, deFilippi CR, Bricker E, Alvarez LG, Wait MA, Grayburn PA. Dobutamine stress echocardiography identifies hibernating myocardium and predicts recovery of left ventricular function after coronary revascularization. *Circulation* 1993; 88:430–436.
18. Nesto RW, Cohn LH, Colins JJ Jr, Wynne J, Holman L, Cohn PF. Inotropic contractile reserve: A useful predictor of increased 5 year survival and improved postoperative left ventricular function in patients with coronary artery disease and reduced ejection fraction. *Am J Cardiol* 1982; 50:39–44.
19. Helfant RH, Pine R, Meister SG, Fieldman MS, Trout RG, Banks VS. Nitroglycerin to unmask reversible asynergy. Correlation with post coronary bypass ventriculography. *Circulation* 1974; 50:108–113.
20. Rahimtoola SH. Hibernating myocardium has reduced blood flow at rest that increases with low-dose dobutamine. *Circulation* 1996; 94:3055–3061.
21. Popio KA, Gorlin R, Bechtel D, Levine JA. Postextrasystolic potentiation as a predictor of potential myocardial viability: Preoperative analyses compared with studies after coronary bypass surgery. *Am J Cardiol* 1977; 39:944–953.
22. Picard MH, Wilkins GT, Ray PA, Weyman AE. Natural history of left ventricular size and function after acute myocardial infarction. Assessment and prediction by echocardiographic endocardial surface mapping. *Circulation* 1990; 82:484–494.
23. St. John Sutton M, Pfeffer MA, Plappert T, Rouleau J-L, Moyé LA, Dagenais GR, et al. for the SAVE Investigators. Quantitative two-dimensional echocardiographic measurements are major predictors of

adverse cardiovascular events after acute myocardial infarction. The protective effects of captopril. *Circulation* 1994; 89:68–75.

24. Marmor A, Raphael T, Marmor M, Blondheim D. Evaluation of contractile reserve by dobutamine echocardiography: Noninvasive estimation of the severity of heart failure. *Am Heart J* 1996; 132:1195–1201.

25. Horn HR, Teichholz LE, Cohn PF, Herman MV, Gorlin R. Augmentation of left ventricular contraction pattern in coronary artery disease by an inotropic catecholamine. The epinephrine ventriculogram. *Circulation* 1974; 49:1063–1071.

26. Ankers S, Ponikowski P, Varney S, Chua YP, Clark AL, Webb-Peploe KM, et al. Wasting as an independent risk factor for mortality in chronic heart failure. *Lancet* 1997; 349:1050–1053.

27. DelVecchio A, Frishman WH, Fadel A, Ismail A. Cardiovascular manifestations of substance abuse. In: Frishman WH, Sonnenblick EH, eds. *Cardiovascular Pharmacotherapeutics*. New York: McGraw-Hill; 1997:1115–1149.

28. Mancini DM, Davis L, Wexler JP, Chadwick B, LeJemtel TH. Dependence of enhanced maximal exercise performance on increased peak skeletal muscle perfusion during long-term captopril therapy in heart failure. *J Am Coll Cardiol* 1987; 10:845–850.

29. Guyatt GH, Sullivan MJ, Thompson PJ, Fallen EL, Pugsley SO, Taylor DW, et al. The six-minute walk: A new measure of exercise capacity in patients with chronic heart failure. *Can Med Assoc J* 1985; 132:919–923.

30. Coats AJS, Adamopoulos S, Meyer TE, Conway J, Sleight P. Effects of physical training in chronic heart failure. *Lancet* 1990; 335:63–66.

31. Coats AJS, Adamopoulos S, Radeaelli A, McCance A, Meyer TE, Bernardi L. Controlled trial of physical training in chronic heart failure. Exercise performance, hemodynamics, ventilation and autonomic function. *Circulation* 1992; 85:2119–2131.

32. Hambrecht R, Niebauer J, Fiehn E, Kalberer B, Offner B, Hauer K, et al. Physical training in patients with stable chronic heart failure: Effects on cardiorespiratory fitness and ultra-structural abnormalities of leg muscles. *J Am Coll Cardiol* 1995; 25:1239–1249.

33. Francis GS, Benedict C, Johnstone DE, Kirlin PC, Nicklas J, Liang C-S, et al. Comparison of neuroendocrine activation in patients with left ventricular dysfunction with and without congestive heart failure. A Substudy of the Studies of Left Ventricular Dysfunction (SOLVD). *Circulation* 1990; 82:1724–1729.

34. Schlant RC, Sonnenblick EH. Pathophysiology of heart failure. In: Hurst JW, Schlant RC, Rackly CE, eds. *The Heart*, 7th ed. New York: McGraw Hill; 1990:387–397.

35. Bichet DG, Schrier RW. Cardiac failure, liver disease and nephrotic syndrome. In: Schrier RW, Gottschalk CW, eds. *Diseases of the Kidney*, 5th ed. Boston: Little, Brown; 1993:2453–2465.

36. Koeppen B, Stanton B. Regulation of extracellular fluid volume. In: Koeppen BM, Stanton BA, eds. *Renal Physiology*. St. Louis: Mosby Year Book; 1992:91–109.

37. Boles Ponto LL, Schoenwald RD. Furosemide: A pharmacokinetic/pharmacodynamic review. *Clin Pharmacokinet* 1990; 18:381–408.

38. O'Grady SM, Palfrey HC, Field M. Characteristics and function of Na-K-2Cl cotransport in epithelial tissues. *Am J Physiol* 1987; 253 (2 pt 1):C177–192.

39. Brater DC, Day B, Burdette A, Anderson S. Bumetidine and furosemide in heart failure. *Kidney Int* 1984; 26:183.

40. Knoben JE, Anderson PO, eds. Diuretics. In: *Clinical Drug Data*, 6th ed. Illinois: Drug Intelligence Publications; 1988.

41. Voelker JR, Brown-Cartwright D, Anderson S, Leinfelder J, Sica DA, Kokko JP, et al. Comparison of loop diuretics in patients with chronic renal insufficiency: Mechanism of difference in response. *Kidney Int* 1987; 32:572–578.

42. Ward A, Heel RC. Bumetadine: A review of its pharmacokinetic and pharmacodynamic properties and therapeutic use. *Drugs* 1984; 28:426–464.

43. Brater DC. Clinical pharmacology of loop diuretics in health and disease. *Eur Heart J* 1992; 13(suppl G):10–14.

44. Rudy DW, Gehr TWB, Matzke GR, Kramer WG, Sica DA, Brater DC. The pharmacodynamics of IV and oral torsemide in patients with chronic renal insufficiency. *Clin Pharmacol Ther* 1994; 56:39–47.

45. Schwartz S, Brater C, Pound D, Green PK, Kramer WG, Rudy D. Bioavailability, pharmacokinetics, and pharmacodynamics of torsemide in patients with cirrhosis. *Clin Pharmacol Ther* 1993; 54:90–97.

46. Vargo DL, Kramer WG, Black PK, Smith WB, Serpas T, Brater DC. Bioavailability, pharmacokinetics, and pharmacodynamics of torse-mide and furosemide in patients with congestive heart failure. *Clin Pharmacol Ther* 1995; 57:601–609.

47. Benet LZ, Greither A, Meister W. Gastrointestinal absorption of drugs in patients with cardiac failure. In: Benet LZ, ed. *The Effect of Disease States on Drug Pharmacokinetics*. Washington, DC: American Pharmaceutical Association Academy of Pharmaceutical Sciences; 1976:33–50.

48. Vasko MR, Brown-Cartwright D, Knochel JP, Nixon JV, Brater DC. Furosemide absorption altered in decompensated congestive heart failure. *Ann Intern Med* 1985; 102:314–318.

49. Van Meyel JJM, Gerlag PGG, Smits P, Russel FGM, Tan Y, Van Ginneken CAM, et al. Absorption of high dose furosemide in congestive heart failure. *Clin Pharmacokinet* 1992; 22:308–318.

50. Brater DC. Resistance to loop diuretics: Why it happens and what to do about it. *Drugs* 1985; 30:427–443.

51. Marangoni E, Oddone A, Surian M, Panciroli C, Galloni G, Masa A, et al. Effect of high-dose furosemide in refractory congestive heart failure. *Angiology* 1990; 41:862–868.

52. Kuchar DL, O'Rourke MF. High dose furosemide in refractory cardiac failure. *Eur Heart J* 1985; 6:954–958.

53. Rudy DW, Voelker JR, Greene PK, Esparzo FA, Brater DC. Loop diuretics for chronic renal insufficiency: A continuous infusion is more efficacious than bolus therapy. *Ann Intern Med* 1991; 115:360–366.

54. Lawson DH, Gray J, Henry DA, Tilstone WJ. Continuous infusion of frusemide in refractory oedema. *Br Med J* 1978; 2:476.

55. Lahav M, Regev A, Ra'Anani P, Theodor E. Intermittent administration of furosemide vs continuous infusion preceded by a loading dose for congestive heart failure. *Chest* 1992; 102:725–731.

56. Rybak LP. Pathophysiology of furosemide ototoxicity. *J Otolaryngol* 1982; 11:127–133.

57. Tran JM, Farrell MA, Fanestil DD. Effect of ions on binding of the thiazide-type diuretic metolazone to kidney membrane. *Am J Physiol* 1990; 258:F908–915.

58. Ellison DH, Morrisey J, Desir GV. Solubilization and partial purification of the thiazide diuretic receptor from rabbit renal cortex. *Biochem Biophys Acta* 1991; 1069:241.

59. Stern A. Metolazone, a diuretic agent. *Am Heart J* 1976; 91:262–263.

60. Craswell PW, Ezzat E, Kopstein J, Varghese Z, Moorhead JF. Use of metolazone, a new diuretic, in patients with renal disease. *Nephron* 1973; 12:63–73.

61. Van Vliet AA, Donker AJM, Nauta JJP, Verheught FWA. Spironolactone in congestive heart failure refractory to high-dose loop diuretic and low-dose angiotensin converting enzyme inhibitor. *Am J Cardiol* 1993; 71:21A–28A.

62. Epstein M, Lepp BA, Hoffman DS, Levinson R. Potentiation of furosemide by metolazone in refractory edema. *Curr Ther Res* 1977; 21:656–667.

63. Olesen KH, Sigurd B. The supra-additive natriuretic effect addition of quinethazone or bendroflumethiazide during long-term treatment with furosemide and spironolactone. *Acta Med Scand* 1971; 190:233–240.

64. Asscher AW. Treatment of frusemide resistant oedema with metolazone. *Clin Trials* 1974; 11:134–137.

65. Ram CVS, Reichgott MJ. Treatment of loop diuretic resistant edema by the addition of metolazone. *Curr Ther Res* 1977; 22:686–691.

66. Furrer J, Hess OM, Kuhlmann U, Satz N, Siegenthaler W. Furosemid und Metolazon: Eine hochwirksame Diuretikakombination. *Schweiz Med Wschr* 1980; 110:1825–1829.

67. Channer KS, Richardson M, Crook R, Jones JV. Thiazides with loop diuretics for severe congestive heart failure. *Lancet* 1990; 335:922–923.

68. Kiyingi A, Field MJ, Pawsey CC, Yiannikis J, Lawrence JR, Arter WJ. Metolazone in treatment of severe refractory congestive cardiac failure. *Lancet* 1990; 335:29–31.

69. Channer KS, McLean KA, Lawson-Matthew P, Richardson M. Combination diuretic treatment in severe heart failure: Randomized controlled trial. *Br Heart J* 1994; 71:146–150.

70. Withering W. *An Account of the Foxglove, and Some of Its Medical Uses: With Practical Remarks on Dropsy and Other Diseases*. London: G.G.J. and J. Robinson; 1785.

71. Fothergill JM, *Digitalis: Its Mode of Action*. London, 1871.

72. Dock W, Tainter ML. The circulatory changes after full therapeutic doses of digitalis, with critical discussion of views on cardiac output. *J Clin Invest* 1929; 8:467–484.

73. The Digitalis Investigation Group. The effect of digoxin on mortality and morbidity in patients with heart failure. *N Engl J Med* 1997; 336:525–533.

74. Fisch C, Withering W: An account of the foxglove and some of its medical uses, 1785–1985. *J Am Coll Cardiol* 1985; 5:1A–2A.

75. Gillis RA, Quest JA. The role of the nervous system in the cardiovascular effects of digitalis. *Pharmacol Rev* 1980; 31:19–97.

76. Skou JC. Enzymatic basis for active transport of Na$^+$ and K$^+$ across cell membrane. *Physiol Rev* 1965; 45:596–617.

77. Fozzard HA, Sheets MF. Cellular mechanism of action of cardiac glycosides. *J Am Coll Cardiol* 1985; 5:10A–15A.

78. Charlemagne D. Molecular and cellular level of action of digitalis. *Herz* 1993; 18:79.

79. Scholz H. Inotropic drugs and their mechanisms of action. *J Am Coll Cardiol* 1984; 4:389–397.

80. Siri FM, Krueger JW, Nordin C, Ming Z, Aronson RS. Depressed intracellular calcium transients and contraction in myocytes from hypertrophied and failing guinea pig hearts. *Am J Physiol* 1991; 261:H514–530.

81. Li P, Park C, Micheletti R, Li B, Cheng W, Sonnenblick EH, et al. Myocyte performance during evolution of myocardial infarction in rats: Effects of propionyl-L-carnitine. *Am J Physiol* 1995; 268:H1702–1713.

82. Mason DT, Braunwald E, Karsh RB, Bullock FA. Studies on digitalis. X: Effects on ouabain on forearm vascular resistance and venous tone in normal subjects and in patients with heart failure. *J Clin Invest* 1964; 43:532–543.

83. Van Veldhuisen DJ, de Graeff PA, Remme WJ, Lie KI. Value of digoxin in heart failure and sinus rhythm: New features of an old drug? *J Am Coll Cardiol* 1996; 28:813–819.

84. Muller JE, Turi ZG, Stone PH, et al. for the MILIS Group. Digoxin therapy and mortality following confirmed or suspected myocardial infarction: Experience in the MILIS Study. In: Erdmann E, Greeff JC, Skou JC, eds. *Update in Cardiac Glycosides 1785–1985.* New York: Springer-Verlag; 1986:493–508.

85. Kraus F, Rudolph C, Rudolph W. Efficacy of digitalis in patients with chronic congestive heart failure and sinus rhythm: An overview of randomized, double-blind, placebo-controlled studies. *Herz* 1993; 18:95.

86. Packer M, Gheorghiade M, Young JB, Costantini PJ, Adams KF, Cody RJ, et al. Withdrawal of digoxin from patients with chronic heart failure treated with angiotensin-converting-enzyme inhibitors. RADIANCE Study. *N Engl J Med* 1993; 329:1–7.

87. Adams KF Jr, Gheorghiade M, Uretsky BF, Young JB, Ahmed S, Tomasko L, et al. Patients with mild heart failure worsen during withdrawal from digoxin therapy. *J Am Coll Cardiol* 1997; 30:42–48.

88. Captopril-Digoxin Multicenter Research Group. Comparative effects of therapy with captopril and digoxin in patients with mild to moderate heart failure. *JAMA* 1988; 259:539–544.

89. Slatton ML, Irani WN, Hall SA, Marcoux LG, Page RL, Grayburn PA, et al. Does digoxin provide additional hemodynamic and autonomic benefit at higher doses in patients with mild to moderate heart failure and normal sinus rhythm? *J Am Coll Cardiol* 1997; 29:1206–1213.

90. Wirth KE. Relevant metabolism of cardiac glycosides. In: Erdmann E, Greeff K, Skou JC, eds. *Update in Cardiac Glycosides, 1785–1985.* New York: Springer-Verlag; 1986:257–262.

91. Uretsky BF, Young JB, Shahidi FE, Yellin LG, Harrison MC, Jolly MK. Randomized study assessing the effect of digoxin withdrawal in patients with mild to moderate chronic congestive heart failure: Results of the PROVED Trial. *J Am Coll Cardiol* 1993; 22:955–962.

92. Tauke J, Goldstein S, Gheorghiade M. Digoxin for chronic heart failure: A review of the randomized controlled trials with special attention to the PROVED and RADIANCE Trials. *Prog Cardiovasc Dis* 1994; 37:49–58.

93. Benovic JL, Bouvier M, Caron MG, Lefkowitz RJ. Regulation of adenylyl cyclase–coupled β-adrenergic receptors. *Am Rev Cell Biol* 1988; 4:405–428.

94. Lefkowitz RJ, Hoffman BB, Taylor P. Neurotransmission. In: *Goodman & Gilman's The Pharmacological Basis of Therapeutics,* 9th ed. New York: McGraw-Hill; 1996:105–139.

95. Kelley RB. Storage and release of neurotransmitters. *Cell/Neuron* 1993; 72/10(suppl):43–53.

96. Spann JF, Sonnenblick EH, Cooper T, Chidsey CA, William VL,

Braunwald E. Cardiac norepinephrine stores and the contractile state of the heart. *Circ Res* 1966; 19:317–325.

97. Francis GS, Goldsmith SR, Levine TB, Olivari MT, Cohn JN. The neurohumoral axis in congestive heart failure. *Ann Intern Med* 1984; 101:370–377.

98. Insel PA. Adrenergic receptors—evolving concepts and clinical implications. *N Engl J Med* 1996; 334:580–585.

99. Haikala H, Linden I. Mechanisms of action of calcium-sensitizing drugs. *J Cardiovasc Pharm* 1995; 26(suppl 1):S10–S19.

100. Goldberg LI, Raifer SI. Dopamine receptors: Applications in clinical cardiology. *Circulation* 1985; 72:245–248.

101. Ruffolo RR Jr. Review: The pharmacology of dobutamine. *Am J Med Sci* 1987; 294:244–248.

102. Sonnenblick EH, Frishman WH, LeJemtel TH. Dobutamine: A new synthetic cardioactive sympathetic amine. *N Engl J Med* 1979; 300:17–22.

103. Parmley WW, Sonnenblick EH. A role for glucagon in cardiac therapy (editorial). *Am J Med Sci* 1969; 258:224–229.

104. Braunwald E, Sonnenblick EH, Chakrin LW, Schwarz RP Jr, eds. *Milrinone Investigation: A New Inotropic Therapy for Congestive Heart Failure.* New York: Raven; 1984.

105. Grose R, Strain J, Greenberg M, LeJemtel TH. Systemic and coronary effects of intravenous milrinone and dobutamine in congestive heart failure. *J Am Coll Cardiol* 1986; 7:1107–1113.

106. Nielsen-Kudsk JE, Aldershville J. Will calcium sensitizers play a role in the treatment of heart failure? *J Cardiovasc Pharmacol* 1995; 26(suppl 1):S77–S84.

107. Packer M, Carver JR, Rodeheffer RJ, Ivanhoe RJ, DiBianco R, Zeldis SM, et al. for the PROMISE Study Research Group. Effect of oral milrinone on mortality in severe chronic heart failure. *N Engl J Med* 1991; 325:1468–1475.

108. Rector TW, Cohn JN with the Pimobendan Multicenter Research Group. Assessment of patient outcome with the Minnesota Living with Heart Failure questionnaire: Reliability and validity during a randomized, double-blind, placebo-controlled trial of pimobendan. *Am Heart J* 1992; 124:1017–1025.

109. Lilleberg J, Sundberg S, Nieminen MS. Dose-range study of a new calcium sensitizer, levosimendan, in patients with left ventricular dysfunction. *J Cardiovasc Pharmacol* 1995; 26(suppl 1):S63–S69.

110. Pagel PS, Haikala H, Pentikainen PJ, Toivonen M-L, Nieminen MS, Lehtonen L, et al. Pharmacology of levosimendan: A new myofilament calcium sensitizer. *Cardiovasc Drug Rev* 1996; 14:286–316.

111. Kajstura J, Cigola E, Malhotra A, Li P, Cheng W, Meggs LG, et al. Angiotensin II induces apoptosis of adult ventricular myocytes in vitro. *J Mol Cell Cardiol* 1997; 29:859–870.

112. Remme WJ. Vasodilator therapy without converting-enzyme inhibition in congestive heart failure—usefulness and limitations. *Cardiovasc Drugs Ther* 1989; 3:375–396.

113. Davis R, Ribner HS, Keung E, Sonnenblick EH, LeJemtel TH. Treatment of chronic congestive heart failure with captopril, an oral inhibitor of angiotensin-converting enzyme. *N Engl J Med* 1979; 301:117–121.

114. Captopril Multicenter Research Group. A placebo-controlled trial of captopril in refractory chronic congestive heart failure. *J Am Coll Cardiol* 1983; 2:755–763.

115. Newman TJ, Maskin CS, Dennick LG, Meyer JH, Hallows BG, Cooper WH. Effects of captopril on survival in patients with heart failure. *Am J Med* 1988; 84(suppl 3A):140–144.

116. Massie BM, Kramer BL, Topic N. Lack of relationship between the short-term hemodynamic effects of captopril and subsequent clinical responses. *Circulation* 1984; 69:1135–1141.

117. Vanhoutte PM, Auch-Schwelk A, Biondi ML, Lorenz RR, Schini VB, Vidal MJ. Why are converting enzyme inhibitors vasodilators? *Br J Clin Pharmacol* 1989; 28:95A–104S.

118. Giles TD, Katz R, Sullivan JM, Wolfson P, Haugland M, Kirlin P, et al. Short- and long-acting angiotensin converting enzyme inhibitors: A randomized trial of lisinopril versus captopril in the treatment of congestive heart failure. *J Am Coll Cardiol* 1989; 13:1240–1247.

119. Konstam MA, Rousseau MF, Kronenberg MW, Udelson JE, Melin J, Stewart D, et al. Effects of the angiotensin converting enzyme inhibitor enalapril on the long-term progression of left ventricular dysfunction in patients with heart failure. *Circulation* 1992; 86:431–438.

120. Cohn JN. The prevention of heart failure—a new agenda (editorial). *N Engl J Med* 1992; 327:725–727.

121. Good JM, Brady AJB, Noormohamed FH, Oakley CM, Cleland JGF. Effect of intense angiotensin II suppression on the diuretic response

to furosemide during chronic ACE inhibition. *Circulation* 1994; 90:220–224.

122. LeJemtel TH, Maskin CS, Chadwick B. Effects of acute angiotensin converting enzyme inhibition on renal blood flow in patients with stable congestive heart failure. *Am J Med Sci* 1986; 292(3):123–127.

123. Volpe M, Tritto C, DeLuca N, Rubattu S, Mele AF, Lembo G, et al. Angiotensin converting enzyme inhibition restores cardiac and hormonal responses to volume overload in patients with dilated cardiomyopathy and mild heart failure. *Circulation* 1992; 86:1800–1809.

124. Drexler H, Banhardt U, Meinertz T, Wollschläger H, Lehmann M, Just H. Contrasting peripheral short-term and long-term effects of converting enzyme inhibition in patients with congestive heart failure. A double-blind, placebo-controlled trial. *Circulation* 1989; 79:491–502.

125. Kramer BL, Massie BM, Topic N. Controlled trial of captopril in chronic heart failure: Rest and exercise hemodynamic study. *Circulation* 1983; 67:807–816.

126. Dickstein K, Barvik S, Aarsland T. Effects of long-term enalapril therapy on cardiopulmonary exercise performance after myocardial infarction. *Circulation* 1991; 83:1895–1904.

127. Lonn EM, Yusuf S, Jha P, Montague TJ, Teo KK, Benedict CR, et al. Emerging role of angiotensin-converting enzyme inhibitors in cardiac and vascular protection. *Circulation* 1994; 90:2056–2069.

128. Galatius-Jensen S, Wroblewski H, Emmeluth C, Bie P, Haunsø S, Kastrup J. Plasma endothelin in congestive heart failure: Effect of the ACE inhibitor, fosinopril. *Cardiovasc Res* 1996; 32:1148–1154.

129. Mancini GBJ, Henry GC, Macaya C, O'Neill BJ, Pucillo AL, Carere RG, et al. Angiotensin-converting enzyme inhibition with quinapril improves endothelial vasomotor dysfunction in patients with coronary artery disease. The TREND (Trial on Reversing Endothelial Dysfunction) Study. *Circulation* 1996; 94:258–265.

130. Desideri G, Ferri C, Bellini C, DeMattia G, Santucci A. Effects of ACE inhibition on spontaneous and insulin-stimulated endothelin-1 secretion. *Diabetes* 1997; 46:81–86.

131. Editorial. Angiotensin II: Hemodynamic regulator or growth factor? *J Mol Cell Cardiol* 1990; 22:739–747.

132. The CONSENSUS Trial Study Group. Effect of enalapril on mortality in severe congestive heart failure: Results of the Cooperative North Scandinavian Enalapril Survival Study (CONSENSUS). *N Engl J Med* 1987; 316:1429–1435.

133. Cohn JN, Johnson G, Ziesche S, Cobb F, Francis G, Tristani F, et al. A comparison of enalapril with hydralazine-isosorbide dinitrate in the treatment of chronic congestive heart failure. *N Engl J Med* 1991; 325:303–310.

134. The SOLVD Investigators. Effect of enalapril on survival in patients with reduced left ventricular ejection fraction and congestive heart failure. *N Engl J Med* 1991; 325:293–302.

135. The SOLVD Investigators. Effect of enalapril on mortality and the development of heart failure in asymptomatic patients with reduced left ventricular ejection fractions. *N Engl J Med* 1992; 327:685–691.

136. Yusuf S, Pepine CJ, Garces C, Pouleur H, Salem D, Kostis J, et al. Effect of enalapril on myocardial infarction and unstable angina in patients with low ejection fractions. *Lancet* 1992; 340:1173–1178.

137. Rajagopalan S, Harrison DG. Reversing endothelial dysfunction with ACE inhibitors. A new TREND? *Circulation* 1996; 94:240–243.

138. Pfeffer MA, Braunwald E. Ventricular remodeling after myocardial infarction. Experimental observations and clinical implications. *Circulation* 1990; 81:1161–1172.

139. Pfeffer MA, Lamas GA, Vaughan DE, Parisi AF, Braunwald E. Effect of captopril on progressive ventricular dilatation after anterior myocardial infarction. *N Engl J Med* 1988; 319:80–86.

140. Pfeffer MA, Braunwald E, Moyé LA, Basta L, Brown EJ Jr, Cuddy TE, et al. on behalf of the SAVE Investigators. Effect of captopril on mortality and morbidity in patients with left ventricular dysfunction after myocardial infarction. *N Engl J Med* 1992; 327:669–677.

141. Swedberg K, Held P, Kjekshus J, Rasmussen K, Rydén L, Wedel H on behalf of the CONSENSUS II Study Group. Effects of the early administration of enalapril on mortality in patients with acute myocardial infarction. Results of the Cooperative North Scandinavian Enalapril Survival Study II (CONSENSUS II). *N Engl J Med* 1992; 327:678–684.

142. The Acute Infarction Ramipril Efficacy (AIRE) Study Investigators. Effect of ramipril on mortality and morbidity of survivors of acute myocardial infarction with clinical evidence of heart failure. *Lancet* 1993; 342:821–828.

143. Gruppo Italiano per lo Studio della Sopravvivenza nell-Infarto Miocardico: GISSI-3. Effects of lisinopril and transdermal glyceryl trinitrate singly and together on 6 week mortality and ventricular function after acute myocardial infarction. *Lancet* 1994; 343:1115–1122.

144. Ambrosioni E, Borghi C, Magnani B for the Survival of Myocardial Infarction Long-Term Evaluation (SMILE) Study Investigators. The effect of the angiotensin converting enzyme inhibitor zofenopril on mortality and morbidity after anterior myocardial infarction. *N Engl J Med* 1995; 332:80–85.

145. Køber L, Torp-Pedersen C, Carlsen JE, Bagger H, Eliasen P, Lyngborg K, et al. for the Trandolapril Cardiac Evaluation (TRACE) Study Group. A clinical trial of the angiotensin converting enzyme inhibitor trandolapril in patients with left ventricular dysfunction after myocardial infarction. *N Engl J Med* 1995; 333:1670–1676.

146. Hood WB Jr, Youngblood M, Ghali JK, Reid M, Rogers WJ, Howe D, et al. Initial blood pressure response to enalapril in hospitalized patients (Studies of Left Ventricular Dysfunction [SOLVD]). *Am J Cardiol* 1991; 68:1465–1468.

147. Lewis EJ, Hunsiker LG, Bain RP, Rohde RD. The effect of angiotensin converting enzyme inhibition on diabetic nephropathy. *N Engl J Med* 1993; 329:1456–1462.

148. Sassano P, Chatellier G, Billaud E, Alhenc-Gelas F, Corvol P, Menard J. Treatment of mild to moderate hypertension with or without the converting enzyme inhibitor enalapril. Results of a six month double-blind trial. *Am J Med* 1987; 83:227–235.

149. Hamroff G, Blaufarb I, Mancini D, Katz S, Bijou R, Jondeau G, et al. Angiotensin II receptor blockade further reduces afterload safely in patients maximally treated with angiotensin converting enzyme inhibitors in heart failure. *J Cardiovasc Pharmacol* 1997 in press.

150. Timmermans PB, Wong PC, Chiu AT, Herblin WF. Non-peptide angiotensin II receptor antagonists. *Trends Pharmacol Sci* 1991; 12:55–62.

151. Timmermans PB, Carini DJ, Chiu AT, Duncia DV, Price WA Jr, Wells GJ, et al. Angiotensin II receptor antagonists: From discovery to antihypertensive drugs. *Hypertension* 1991; 18(suppl):III136–142.

152. Wong PC, Price WA Jr, Chiu AT, Duncia DV, Carini DJ, Wexler RR, et al. Nonpeptide angiotensin II receptor antagonists: VIII. Characterization of functional antagonism displayed by DuP 753, an orally active antihypertensive agent. *J Pharmacol Exp Ther* 1990; 252:719–725.

153. Wong PC, Price WA Jr, Chiu AT, Duncia VA, Carini DJ, Wexler RR, et al. In vivo pharmacology of DuP 753. *Am J Hypertens* 1991; 4.288s–302s.

154. Wong PC, Price WA Jr, Chiu AT, Duncia DV, Carini DJ, Wexler RR, et al. Nonpeptide angiotensin II receptor antagonists. IX. Antihypertensive activity in rats of DuP 753, an orally active antihypertensive agent. *J Pharmacol Exp Ther* 1990; 252:726–732.

155. Tofovic SP, Pong AS, Jackson EK. Effects of angiotensin subtype 1 and subtype 2 receptor antagonists in normotensive versus hypertensive rats. *Hypertension* 1991; 18:774–782.

156. Abdelrahman A, Pang CC. Competitive antagonism of pressor responses of angiotensin II and angiotensin III by the angiotensin II-1 receptor ligand losartan. *Can J Physiol Pharmacol* 1992; 70:716–719.

157. Mizuno K, Nimura S, Tani M, Haga H, Gomibuchi T, Sanada H, et al. Antihypertensive and hormonal activity of MK 954 in spontaneously hypertensive rats. *Eur J Pharmacol* 1992; 215:305–308.

158. Morton JJ, Beattie ED, MacPherson F. Angiotensin II receptor antagonist losartan has pesistent effects on blood pressure in the young spontaneously hypertensive rat: Lack of relation to vascular structure. *J Vasc Res* 1992; 29:264–269.

159. Christen Y, Waeber B, Nussberger J, Lee RJ, Timmermans PBMWM, Brunner HR. Dose-response relationship following oral administration of DuP 753 to normal humans. *Am J Hypertens* 1991; 4:350s–353s.

160. Christen Y, Waeber B, Nussberger J, Porchet M, Borland RM, Lee RJ, et al. Oral administration of DuP753, a specific angiotensin II receptor antagonist, to normal volunteers: Inhibition of pressor response to exogenous angiotensin I and II. *Circulation* 1991; 83:1333–1342.

161. Brunner HR, Christen Y, Munafo A, Lee RJ, Waeber B, Nussberger J. Clinical experience with angiotensin II receptor antagonists. *Am J Hypertens* 1992; 5:243s–246s.

162. Munafo A, Christen Y, Nussberger J, Shum LY, Borland RM, Lee RJ, et al. Drug concentration response relationships in normal volunteers after oral administration of losartan, an angiotensin II receptor antagonist. *Clin Pharmacol Ther* 1992; 51:513–521.

163. Hagino T, Abe K, Tsunoda K, Yoshinaga K. Antihypertensive effect on a non-peptide angiotensin II receptor antagonist, MK 954, in patients with essential hypertension. *Nippon Jinzo Gakkai Shi* 1992; 34:133–140.

164. Tsunoda K, Abe K, Hagino T, Omata K, Misawa S, Imai Y, et al. Hypotensive effect of losartan, a nonpeptide angiotensin II receptor antagonist, in essential hypertension. *Am J Hypertens* 1993; 6:28–32.

165. Nelson E, Arcuri K, Ikeda L, Snavely D, Sweet C. Efficacy and safety of losartan in patients with essential hypertension (abstr). *Am J Hypertens* 1992; 5:19A.

166. Weber MA. Clinical experience with the angiotensin II receptor antagonist losartan: A preliminary report. *Am J Hypertens* 1992; 5:247S–251S.

167. Carr AA, Prisant LM. Losartan: First of a new class of angiotensin antagonists for the management of hypertension. *J Clin Pharmacol* 1996; 36:3–12.

168. Goa KL, Wagstaff AJ. Losartan potassium: A review of its pharmacology, clinical efficacy and tolerability in the management of hypertension. *Drugs* 1996; 51:820–845.

169. Goodfriend TL, Elliott ME, Catt KJ. Angiotensin receptors and their antagonists. *N Engl J Med* 1996; 334:1649–1654.

170. Kang PM, Landau AJ, Eberhardt RT, Frishman WH. Angiotensin II receptor antagonists: A new approach to blockade of the renin-angiotensin system. *Am Heart J* 1994; 127:1388–1401.

171. Bauer JH, Reams GP. The angiotensin II type 1 receptor antagonists: A new class of antihypertensive drugs. *Arch Intern Med* 1995; 155:1361–1368.

172. Chiu AT, Herblin WF, McCall DE, Ardecky RJ, Carini DJ, Duncia JV, et al. Identification of angiotensin II receptor subtypes. *Biochem Biophys Res Commun* 1989; 165:196–203.

173. Herblin WF, Chiu AT, McCall DE, Ardecky RJ, Carini DJ, Duncia JV, et al. Angiotensin II receptor heterogeneity. *Am J Hypertens* 1991; 4:299s–302s.

174. Timmermans PB, Chiu AT, Herblin DM, Wong PC, Smith RD. Angiotensin II receptor subtypes. *Am J Hypertens* 1992; 5:406–410.

175. Bergsma DJ, Ellis C, Kumar C, Nuthulaganti P, Kersten H, Elshourbagy N, et al. Cloning and characterization of a human angiotensin II type 1 receptor. *Biochem Biophy Res Commun* 1992; 183:989–995.

176. Sasamura H, Hein L, Krieger JE, Pratt RE, Kobika BK, Dzau VJ. Cloning, characterization and expression of two angiotensin receptor (AT-1) isoforms from the mouse genome. *Biochem Biophys Res Commun* 1992; 185:253–259.

177. Ernsberger P, Zhou J, Damon TH, Douglas JG. Angiotensin II receptor subtypes in cultured rat renal mesangial cells. *Am J Physiol* 1992; 263:F411–F416.

178. Peach MJ, Dostal DE. The angiotensin II receptor and the actions of angiotensin II. *J Cardiovasc Pharm* 1990; 16(suppl 4):S25–S30.

179. Timmermans PB, Benfield P, Chiu AT, Herblin WF, Wong PC, Smith RD. Angiotensin II receptors and functional correlates. *Am J Hypertens* 1992; 5:221s–235s.

180. Smith RD, Chiu AT, Wong PC, Herblin WF, Timmermans PBMWM. Pharmacology of nonpeptide angiotensin II receptor antagonists. *Annu Rev Pharmacol Toxicol* 1992; 32:135–165.

181. Tsutsumi K, Stromberg C, Saavedra JM. Characterization of angiotensin II receptor subtypes in the rat spleen. *Peptides* 1992; 13:291–296.

182. Brooks DP, Fredrickson TA, Weinstock J, Ruffolo RR Jr, Edwards RM, Gellai M. Antihypertensive activity of the non-peptide angiotensin II receptor antagonist SK&F 108566, in rats and dogs. *Naunyn Schmiedeberg Arch Pharmacol* 1992; 345:673–678.

183. Edwards RM, Aiyar N, Ohlstein EH, Weidley EF, Griffin E, Ezekiel M, et al. Pharmacological characterization of the nonpeptide angiotensin II receptor antagonist, SK&F 108566. *J Pharmacol Exp Ther* 1992; 260:175–181.

184. Zhang J, Entzeroth M, Wienen W, Van Meel JC. Characterization of BIBS39 and BIBS222: Two new nonpeptide angiotensin II receptor antagonists. *Eur J Pharmacol* 1992; 218:35–41.

185. Robertson MJ, Barnes JC, Drew GM, Clark KL, Marshall FH, Michel A, et al. Pharmacological profile of GR117289 in vitro: A novel, potent and specific non-peptide angiotensin AT1 receptor antagonist. *Br J Pharmacol* 1992; 107:1173–1180.

186. Chang RS, Siegl PK, Clineschmidt BV, Mantlo NB, Chakravarty PK, Greenlee WJ, et al. In vitro pharmacology of L-158,809, a new highly potent and selective angiotensin II receptor antagonist. *J Pharmacol Exp Ther* 1992; 262:133–138.

187. Siegl PK, Chang RS, Mantlo NB, Chakravarty PK, Ondeyka DL, Greenlee WJ, et al. In vivo pharmacology of L-158,809 a new highly potent and selective non-peptide angiotensin II receptor antagonist. *J Pharmacol Exp Ther* 1992; 262:139–144.

188. Chen TB, Lotti VJ, Chang RS. Characterization of the binding of [3H]L-158,809, a new potent and selective nonpeptide angiotensin II receptor (AT1) antagonist radioligand. *Mol Pharmacol* 1992; 42:1077–1082.

189. Olins GM, Corpus VM, McMahon EG, Palomo MA, Schuh JR, Blehm DJ, et al. In vitro pharmacology of a nonpeptide angiotensin II receptor antagonist, SC 51316. *J Pharmacol Exp Ther* 1992; 261:1037–1043.

190. Mizuno K, Niimura S, Tani M, Saito I, Sanada H, Takahashi M, et al. Hypotensive activity of TCV-116, a newly developed angiotensin II receptor antagonist in spontaneously hypertensive rats. *Life Sci* 1992; 51:PL183–187.

191. De B, Winn M, Zydowsky TM, Kerkman DJ, DeBernardis JF, Buckner JLS, et al. Discovery of a novel class of orally active, non-peptide angiotensin II antagonists. *J Med Chem* 1992; 35:3714–3717.

192. Raya TE, Fonkin SJ, Lee RW, Daughtery S, Goldman S, Wong PC, et al. Hemodynamic effects of direct angiotensin II blockade compared to converting enzyme inhibition in rat model of heart failure. *Am J Hypertens* 1991; 4:334s–340s.

193. Fitzpatrick MA, Rademaker MT, Charles CJ, Yandle TG, Espiner EA, Ikram H. Angiotensin II receptor antagonism in bovine heart failure: Acute hemodynamic, hormonal and renal effects. *Am J Physiol* 1992; 263:H250–256.

194. Werrman JG, Cohen SM. Use of losartan to examine the role of the cardiac renin-angiotensin system in myocardial dysfunction during ischemia and reperfusion. *J Cardiovasc Pharmacol* 1996; 27:177–182.

195. Milavetz A, Raya TE, Johnson CS, Morkin E, Goldman S. Survival after myocardial infarction in rats: Captopril versus losartan. *J Am Coll Cardiol* 1996; 27:714–719.

196. Blaufarb IS, Sonnenblick EH. The renin-angiotensin system in left ventricular remodeling. *Am J Cardiol* 1996; 77:8C–16C.

197. Gottlieb SS, Dickstein K, Fleck E, Kostis J, Levine TB, LeJemtel T, et al. Hemodynamic and neurohormonal effects of the angiotensin II antagonist losartan in patients with congestive heart failure. *Circulation* 1993; 88:1602–1609.

198. Crozier I, Ikram H, Awan N, Cleland J, Stephen N, Dickstein K, et al. Losartan in heart failure: Hemodynamic effects and tolerability. Losartan Hemodynamic Study Group. *Circulation* 1995; 91:691–697.

199. Kiowski W, Beermann J, Rickenbacher P, Haemmerli R, Thomas M, Burkart F, et al. Angiotensinergic versus nonangiotensinergic hemodynamic effects of converting enzyme inhibition in patients with chronic heart failure: Assessment by acute renin and converting enzyme inhibition. *Circulation* 1994; 90:2748–2756.

200. Neuberg GW, Kukin ML, Penn J, Medina N, Yushak M, Packer M. Hemodynamic effects of renin inhibition by enalkiren in chronic congestive heart failure. *Am J Cardiol* 1991; 67:63–66.

201. Raya TE, Fonkin SJ, Lee RW, Daughtery S, Goldman S, Wong PC, et al. Hemodynamic effects of direct angiotensin II blockade compared to converting enzyme inhibition in rat model of heart failure. *Am J Hypertens* 1991; 4:334s–340s.

202. Smits JFM, Van Krimpen C, Schoemaker RG, Cleutjens JPM, Daemen MJA. Angiotensin II receptor blockade after myocardial infarction in rats: Effects on hemodynamics, myocardial DNA synthesis, and interstitial collagen content. *J Cardiovasc Pharmacol* 1992; 20:772–778.

203. Awan NA, Mason DT. Direct selective blockade of the vascular angiotensin II receptors in therapy for hypertension and severe congestive heart failure. *Am Heart J* 1996; 131:177–185.

204. Rush JE, Rajfer SI. Theoretical basis for the use of angiotensin II antagonists in the treatment of heart failure. *J Hypertens* 1993; 3(suppl 11):S69–S71.

205. Bonarjee VV, Dickstein K. Novel drugs and current therapeutic approaches in the treatment of heart failure. *Drugs* 1996; 51:347–358.

206. Dickstein K, Chang P, Willenheimer R, Haunso S, Remes J, Hall C, et al. Comparison of the effects of losartan and enalapril on clinical status and exercise performance in patients with moderate or severe chronic heart failure. *J Am Coll Cardiol* 1995; 26:438–445.

207. Sadoshima J, Xu Y, Slayter HS, Izumo S. Autocrine release of angiotensin II mediates stretch-induced hypertrophy of cardiac myocytes in vitro. *Cell* 1993; 75:977–984.

208. Urata H, Boehm KD, Philip A, Kinoshita A, Gabrovsek J, Bumpus FM,

et al. Cellular localization and regional distribution of an angiotensin II-forming chymase in the heart. *J Clin Invest* 1993; 91:1269–1281.

209. Urata H, Hoffmann S, Ganten D. Tissue angiotensin II system in the human heart. *Eur Heart J* 1994; 15(suppl D):68–78.

210. Spinale FG, DeGasparo M, Whitebread S, Hebbar L, Clair MJ, Melton M, et al. Chronic combined angiotensin converting enzyme inhibition and angiotensin type 1 receptor blockade: Unique effects in congestive heart failure (abstr). *Circulation* 1996; 94(suppl V):I-429.

211. Mombouli JV, Illiano S, Nagao T, Scott-Burden T, Vanhoutte PM. The potentiation of endothelium-dependent relaxation to bradykinin by angiotensin I converting enzyme in canine coronary artery involves both endothelium-derived relaxing and hyperpolarizing factor. *Circ Res* 1992; 71:137–144.

212. Mombouli JV, Vanhoutte PM. Heterogeneity of endothelium-dependent vasodilator effects of angiotensin converting enzyme inhibitors: Role of bradykinin generation during ACE inhibition. *J Cardiovasc Pharmacol* 1992; 20(suppl 9):S74–S82.

213. Feletou M, Teisseire B. Converting enzyme inhibition in isolated porcine resistance arteries potentiates bradykinin relaxation. *Eur J Pharmacol* 1990; 190:159–166.

214. Okamura T, Okunishi H, Ayajiki K, Toda N. Conversion of angiotensin I to angiotensin II in dog isolated renal artery: Role of two different angiotensin II-generating enzymes. *J Cardiovasc Pharmacol* 1990; 15:353–359.

215. Nagao T, Vanhoutte PM. Hyperpolarization as a mechanism for endothelium-dependent relaxations in the porcine coronary artery. *J Physiol (London)* 1992; 445:355–367.

216. Pitt B, Segal R, Martinez FA, Meurers G, Cowley AJ, Thomas I, et al. Randomised trial of losartan versus captopril in patients over 65 with heart failure. Evaluation of Losartan in the Elderly Study (ELITE). *Lancet* 1997; 349:747–752.

217. Cohn JN, Archibald DG, Ziesche S, Franciosa JA, Harston WE, Tristani FE, et al. Effect of vasodilator therapy on mortality in chronic congestive heart failure. Results of a Veterans Administration Cooperation study. *N Engl J Med* 1986; 314:1547–1552.

218. Packer M, Lee WH, Kessler PD, Gottlieb SS, Medina N, Yushak M. Prevention and reversal of nitrate tolerance in patients with congestive heart failure. *N Engl J Med* 1987; 317:799–804.

219. Gogia H, Mehra A, Parikh S, Raman M, Ajit-Uppal J, Johnson JV, et al. Prevention of tolerance to hemodynamic effects of nitrates with concomitant use of hydralazine in patients with chronic heart failure. *J Am Coll Cardiol* 1995; 26:1575–1580.

220. Cohn JN, Ziesche SM, Loss LE, Anderson GT. Effects of felodipine on short-term exercise and neurohormones and long-term mortality in heart failure. Results of V-HeFT III (abstr). *Circulation* 1995; 92(suppl I):I-143.

221. O'Connor CM, Belkin RN, Carson PE, Cropp AB, Frid DJ, Miller AB, et al. for PRAISE Investigators. Effect of amlodipine on mode of death in severe chronic heart failure: The PRAISE trial (abstr). *Circulation* 1995; 92(suppl I):I-143.

222. Frishman W. Calcium channel blockers. In: Frishman WH, Sonnenblick EH, eds. *Cardiovascular Pharmacotherapeutics*. New York: McGraw-Hill; 1997:101–130.

223. Waagstein F, Hjalmarson A, Varnauskas E, Wallentin I. Effect of chronic beta-adrenergic receptor blockade in congestive cardiomyopathy. *Br Heart J* 1975; 37:1022–1036.

224. Swedberg K, Hjalmarson A, Waagstein F, Wallentin I. Beneficial effects of long-term beta blockade in congestive cardiomyopathy. *Br Heart J* 1980; 44:117–133.

225. Ikram H, Fitzpatrick D. Double-blind trial of chronic oral beta blockade in congestive cardiomyopathy. *Lancet* 1981; 2:490–493.

226. Currie PJ, Kelly MJ, McKenzie A, Harper RW, Lim YL, Federman J, et al. Oral beta-adrenergic blockade with metoprolol in chronic severe dilated cardiomyopathy. *J Am Coll Cardiol* 1984; 3:203–209.

227. Engelmeier RS, O'Connell JB, Walsh R, Rad N, Scanlon PJ, Gunnar RM. Improvements in symptoms and exercise tolerance by metoprolol in patients with dilated cardiomyopathy: A double-blind, randomized, placebo-controlled trial. *Circulation* 1985; 72:536–546.

228. Anderson JL, Lutz JR, Gilbert EM, Sorensen SG, Yanowitz FG, Menlove RL, et al. A randomized trial of low-dose beta blockade therapy for idiopathic dilated cardiomyopathy. *Am J Cardiol* 1985; 55:471–475.

229. Waagstein F, Caidahl K, Wallentein I, Bergh C-H, Hjalmarson Å. Long-term β blockade in dilated cardiomyopathy. Effects of short- and long-term metoprolol treatment followed by withdrawal and re-administration of metoprolol. *Circulation* 1989; 80:551–563.

230. Lichstein E, Hager WD, Gregory JJ, Fleiss JL, Rolnitzky LM, Bigger JT Jr, for the Multicenter Diltiazem Post-Infarction Research Group. Relation between beta-adrenergic blocker use, various correlates of left ventricular function and the chance of developing congestive heart failure. *J Am Coll Cardiol* 1990; 16:1327–1332.

231. Eichhorn EJ, Bedotto JB, Malloy CR, Hatfield BA, Deitchman D, Brown M, et al. Effect of β-adrenergic blockade on myocardial function and energetics in congestive heart failure. Improvements in hemodynamic, contractile, and diastolic performance with bucindolol. *Circulation* 1990; 82:473–483.

232. Eichhorn EJ, Heesch CM, Barnett JH, Alvarez LG, Fass SM, Grayburn PA, et al. Effect of metoprolol on myocardial function and energetics in patients with nonischemic dilated cardiomyopathy: A randomized, double-blind, placebo-controlled study. *J Am Coll Cardiol* 1994; 24:1310–1320.

233. Hall SA, Cigarroa CG, Marcoux L, Risser RC, Grayburn PA, Eichhorn EJ. Time course of improvement in left ventricular function, mass and geometry in patients with congestive heart failure treated with beta-adrenergic blockade. *J Am Coll Cardiol* 1995; 25:1154–1161.

234. Eichhorn EJ, Heesch CM, Risser RC, Marcoux L, Hatfield B. Predictors of systolic and diastolic improvement in patients with dilated cardiomyopathy treated with metoprolol. *J Am Coll Cardiol* 1995; 25:154–162.

235. Wisenbaugh T, Katz I, Davis J, Essop R, Skoularigis J, Middlemost S, et al. Long-term (3 month) effects of a new beta blocker (nebivolol) on cardiac performance in dilated cardiomyopathy. *J Am Coll Cardiol* 1993; 21:1094–1100.

236. Gilbert EM, Anderson JL, Deitchman D, Yanowitz FG, O'Connell JB, Renlund DG. Long-term β blocker vasodilator therapy improves cardiac function in idiopathic dilated cardiomyopathy: A double-blind, randomized study of bucindolol versus placebo. *Am J Med* 1990; 88:223–229.

237. Woodley SL, Gilbert EM, Anderson JL, O'Connell JB, Deitchman D, Yanowitz FG, et al. β Blockade with bucindolol in heart failure caused by ischemic versus idiopathic dilated cardiomyopathy. *Circulation* 1991; 84:2426–2441.

238. Bristow MR, O'Connell JB, Gilbert EM, French WJ, Leatherman G, Kantrowitz NE, et al. Dose-response of chronic β blocker treatment in heart failure from either idiopathic dilated or ischemic cardiomyopathy. *Circulation* 1994; 89:1632–1642.

239. Fisher ML, Gottlieb SS, Plotnick GD, Greenberg NL, Patten RD, Bennett SK, et al. Beneficial effects of metoprolol in heart failure associated with coronary artery disease: A randomized trial. *J Am Coll Cardiol* 1994; 23:943–950.

240. Packer M, Bristow MR, Cohn JN, Colucci WS, Fowler MB, Gilbert EM, et al. The effect of carvedilol on morbidity and mortality in patients with chronic heart failure. *N Engl J Med* 1996; 334:1349–1355.

241. Krum H, Sackner-Bernstein JD, Goldsmith RL, Kukin ML, Schwartz B, Penn J, et al. Double-blind, placebo-controlled study of the long-term efficacy of carvedilol in patients with severe chronic heart failure. *Circulation* 1995; 92:1499–1506.

242. Metra M, Nardi M, Giubbini R, Dei Cas L. Effects of short- and long-term carvedilol administration on rest and exercise hemodynamic variables, exercise capacity and clinical conditions in patients with idiopathic dilated cardiomyopathy. *J Am Coll Cardiol* 1994; 24:1678–1687.

243. Australia–New Zealand Heart Failure Research Collaborative Group. Effects of carvedilol, a vasodilator-β-blocker, in patients with congestive heart failure due to ischemic heart disease. *Circulation* 1995; 92:212–218.

244. The Multicenter Diltiazem Post Infarction Trial Research Group. The effect of diltiazem on mortality and reinfarction after myocardial infarction. *N Engl J Med* 1988; 319:385–392.

245. Bristow MR, Anderson FL, Port JD, Skerl L, Hershberger RE, Larrabee P, et al. Differences in β-adrenergic neuroeffector mechanisms in ischemic versus idiopathic dilated cardiomyopathy. *Circulation* 1991; 84:1024–1039.

246. Dunn CJ, Lea AP, Wagstaff AJ. Carvedilol: A review of its pharmacological properties and therapeutic potential in congestive heart failure. *Drugs* 1997; 54:161–185.

247. Colucci WS, Packer M, Bristow MR, Gilbert EM, Cohn JN, Fowler MB, et al. for the US Carvedilol Heart Failure Study Group. Carvedilol inhibits clinical progression in patients with mild symptoms of heart failure. *Circulation* 1996; 94:2800–2806.

248. Bristow MR, Gilbert EM, Abraham WT, Adams KF, Fowler MB, Hershberger RE, et al. for the MOCHA Investigators. Carvedilol produces dose-related improvements in left ventricular function and survival in subjects with chronic heart failure. *Circulation* 1996; 94:2807–2816.

249. Packer M, Colucci WS, Sackner-Bernstein JD, Liang C-S, Goldscher DA, Freeman I, et al. for the PRECISE Study Group. Double-blind, placebo-controlled study of the effects of carvedilol in patients with moderate to severe heart failure. The PRECISE trial. *Circulation* 1996; 94:2793–2799.

250. CIBIS Investigators and Committees. A randomized trial of β blockade in heart failure. The Cardiac Insufficiency Bisoprolol Study (CIBIS). *Circulation* 1994; 90:1765–1773.

251. Gilbert EM, Abraham WT, Olsen S, Hattler B, White M, Mealy P, et al. Comparative hemodynamic, left ventricular functional, and antiadrenergic effects of chronic treatment with metoprolol versus carvedilol in the failing heart. *Circulation* 1996; 94:2817–2825.

252. Rahman MA, Hara K, Daly PA, Wygle ED, Floras JS. Reductions in muscle sympathetic nerve activity after long-term metoprool for dilated cardiomyopathy: Preliminary observations. *Br Heart J* 1995; 74:431–436.

253. Yusuf S, Sleight P, Held P, McMahon S. Routine medical management of acute myocardial infarction. Lessons from overviews of recent randomized controlled trials. *Circulation* 1990; 82(suppl II):II117–II134.

254. Heidenreich PA, Lee TT, Massie BM. Effect of beta blockade on mortality in patients with heart failure: A meta-analysis of randomized clinical trials. *J Am Coll Cardiol* 1997; 30:27–34.

255. Gomberg-Maitland M, Frishman WH, Karch S, Schwartz J, Freeman R, Shapiro J. Hormones as cardiovascular drugs: Estrogens, progestins, thyroxine, growth hormone, corticosteroids, and testosterone. In: Frishman WH, Sonnenblick EH, eds. *Cardiovascular Pharmacotherapeutics.* New York: McGraw-Hill; 1997:787–835.

256. McAlister FA, Teo KT. The management of congestive heart failure. *Postgrad Med J* 1997; 73:194–200.

257. Singh SN, Fletcher RD, Fisher SG, Singh BN, Lewis HD, Deedwania PC, et al. Amiodarone in patients with congestive heart failure and asymptomatic ventricular arrhythmia. *N Engl J Med* 1995; 333:77–82.

258. Gottdiener JS, Reda DJ, Massie BM, Materson BJ, Williams DW, Anderson RJ, for the VA Cooperative Study Group of Antihypertensive Agents. Effect of single-drug therapy on reduction of left ventricular mass in mild to moderate hypertension. comparison of six antihypertensive agents. The Department of Veterans Affairs Cooperative Study Group on Antihypertensive Agents. *Circulation* 1997; 95:2007–2014.

259. Nul DR, Doval HC, Grancelli HO, Varini SD, Soifer S, Perrone SV, et al. Heart rate is a marker of amiodarone mortality reduction in severe heart failure. *J Am Coll Cardiol* 1997; 29:1199–1205.

260. Cogan MG. Atrial natriuretic peptide. *Kidney Int* 1990; 37:1148–1160.

261. Cody RJ, Atlas SA, Laragh JH, Kubo SH, Covit AB, Ryman KS, et al. Atrial natriuretic factor in normal subjects and heart failure patients. Plasma levels and renal, hormonal, and hemodynamic responses to peptide infusion. *J Clin Invest* 1986; 78:1362–1374.

262. Molina CR, Fowler MB, McCrory S, Peterson C, Myers BD, Schroeder JS, et al. Hemodynamic, renal and endocrine effects of atrial natriuretic peptide infusion in severe heart failure. *J Am Coll Cardiol* 1988; 12:175–186.

263. Munzel T, Kurz S, Holtz J, Busse R, Steinhauer H, Just H, et al. Neurohumoral inhibition and hemodynamic unloading during prolonged inhibition of ANP degradation in patients with severe chronic heart failure. *Circulation* 1992; 86:1089–1098.

264. Yoshimura M, Yasue H, Morita E, Sakaino N, Jougasaki M, Kurose M, et al. Hemodynamic, renal and hormonal responses to brain natriuretic peptide infusion in patients with congestive heart failure. *Circulation* 1991; 84:1581–1588.

265. Brandt RR, Wright RS, Redfield MM, Burnett JC. Atrial natriuretic peptide in heart failure (abstr). *J Am Coll Cardiol* 1993; 22(suppl A):86A.

266. Elsner D, Muders F, Muntze A, Kromer EP, Forssmann WG, Riegger GA. Efficacy of prolonged infusion of urodilatin [ANP (95-126)] in patients with congestive heart failure. *Am Heart J* 1995; 129:766–773.

267. Giles TD, Quiroz AC, Roffidal LE, Marder H, Sander GE. Prolonged hemodynamic benefits from a high-dose bolus injection of human atrial natriuretic factor in congestive heart failure. *Clin Pharmacol Ther* 1991; 50:557–563.

268. Connelly TP, Francis GS, Williams RN, Beltran AM, Cohn JN. Interac-tion of intravenous atrial natriuretic factor with furosemide in patients with heart failure. *Am Heart J* 1994; 127:392–399.

269. Cavero PG, Margulies KB, Winaver J, Seymour AA, Delaney NG, Burnett JC Jr. Cardiorenal actions of neutral endopeptidase inhibition in experimental congestive heart failure. *Circulation* 1990; 82:196–201.

270. Northridge DB, Jardine AG, Findlay IN, Archibald M, Dilly SG, Dargie HJ. Inhibition of the metabolism of atrial natriuretic factor causes diuresis and natriuresis in chronic heart failure. *Am J Hypertens* 1990; 3:682–687.

271. Good JM, Peters M, Wilkins M, Jackson N, Oakley CM, Cleland JG. Renal response to candoxatrilat in patients with heart failure. *J Am Coll Cardiol* 1995; 25:1273–1281.

272. Northridge DB, Jardine AG, Alabaster CT, Barclay PL, Connell JMC, Dargie HJ, et al. Effects of UK 69 578: A novel atriopeptidase inhibitor. *Lancet* 1989; 2:591–593.

273. Frishman WH, Goldman A. Inhibitors of neutral endopeptidase. In: Frishman WH, Sonnenblick EH, eds. *Cardiovascular Pharmacotherapeutics.* New York: McGraw-Hill; 1997:611–617.

274. Northridge DB, Jackson NC, Metcalfe MJ, MacFarlane N, Dargie HJ. Effects of candoxatril, a novel endopeptidase inhibitor, compared with frusemide in mild chronic heart failure. Proceedings of the British Pharmacological Society, University of Glasgow, July 10–12, 1991. *Br J Clin Pharmacol* 1991; 32:645.

275. Ura N, Carretero OA, Erdos EG. Role of renal endopeptidase 24.11 in kinin metabolism in vitro and in vivo. *Kidney Int* 1987; 32:507–513.

276. Lang CC, Motwani J, Coutie W, Struthers AD. Influence of candoxatril on plasma brain natriuretic peptide in heart failure. *Lancet* 1991; 338:255.

277. Ohno M, Li W, Cheng C-P. Effects of endothelin-1 on left ventricular performance in conscious dogs: Assessment by pressure-volume analysis (abstr). *Circulation* 1994; 90(4, pt 2):I-16.

278. Gu X-H, Casley D, Nayler W. Specific high affinity binding sites for 125I-labelled porcine endothelin in rat cardiac membranes. *Eur J Pharmacol* 1989; 167:281–290.

279. Galron R, Kloog Y, Bdolah A, Sokolovsky M. Functional endothelin/sarafotoxin receptors in rat heart myocytes: Structure activity relationships and receptor subtypes. *Biochem Biophys Res Commun* 1989; 163:936–943.

280. Hirata Y. Endothelin-1 receptors in cultured vascular smooth muscle cells and cardiocytes of rats. *J Cardiovasc Pharmacol* 1989; 13:s157–s158.

281. Moe GW, Ferrazzi S, Naik G, Howard RJ. Endothelin in heart failure: Temporal evolution, source of production and interaction with atrial natriuretic peptide (abstr). *Circulation* 1994; 90(4, pt 2):I-592.

282. Teerlink JR, Hess P, Clozel M, Clozel J-P, Hoffman F. Role of endothelin in conscious rats with chronic heart failure (abstr). *Circulation* 1994; 90(4, pt 2):I-261.

283. Galatius-Jensen S, Wroblewski H, Emmeluth C, Bie P, Haunso S, Kastrup J. Plasma endothelin-1 in chronic heart failure-a predictor of cardiac death? *Circulation* 1994; 90(4, pt 2):I-379.

284. Pacher R, Stanek B, Hulsmann M, Koller-Strametz J, Berger R, Schuller M, et al. Prognostic impact of big endothelin-1 plasma concentrations comapred with invasive hemodynamic evaluation in severe heart failure. *J Am Coll Cardiol* 1996; 27:633–641.

285. Colucci WS. Myocardial endothelin. Does it play a role in myocardial failure? (editorial). *Circulation* 1996; 93:1069–1072.

286. Sakai S, Miyauchi T, Sakurai T, Kasuya Y, Ihara M, Yamaguchi I, et al. Endogenous endothelin-1 participates in the maintenance of cardiac function in rats with congestive heart failure. Marked increase in endothelin-1 production in the failing heart. *Circulation* 1996; 93:1214–1222.

287. Nootens M, Kaufman E, Rector T, Toher C, Judd D, Francis GS, et al. Neurohormonal activation in patients with right ventricular failure from pulmonary hypertension: Relation to hemodynamic variables and endothelin levels. *J Am Coll Cardiol* 1995; 26:1581–1585.

288. Webb DJ. Evidence for endothelin-1-mediated vasoconstriction in severe chronic heart failure. Endothelin antagonism in heart failure. *Circulation* 1995; 92:3372.

289. Cannan CR, Burnett JC Jr, Lerman A. Enhanced coronary vasoconstriction to endothelin-B-receptor activation in experimental congestive heart failure. *Circulation* 1996; 93:646–651.

290. Krum H, Gu A, Wilshire Clement M, et al. Changes in plasma endothelin-1 levels reflect clinical response to beta blockade in chronic heart failure. *Am Heart J* 1996; 131:337–341.

291. Inada T, Tanaka M, Hasegawa K, Ohtani S, Doyama K, Fujiwara T. Increased levels of endothelin-1 in plasma and heart tissue of cardiomyopathic Syrian hamsters (abstr). *Circulation* 1994; 90(4, pt 2):I-260.

292. Wittner M, Morris SA, Christ GJ, Hatcher VB, Zeballos GA, Bilezikian JP, et al. Infection of cultured human endothelial cells increases endothelin levels (abstr). *Circulation* 1994; 90(4, pt 2):I-293.

293. Love MP, Haynes WG, Webb DJ, McMurray JJV. Anti-endothelin therapy is of potential benefit in heart failure (abstr). *Circulation* 1994; 90(4, pt 2):I-547.

294. Teerlink JR, Loffler BM, Hess P, Maire J-P, Clozel M, Clozel J-P: Role of endothelin in the management of blood pressure in conscious rats with chronic heart failure: Acute effects of the endothelin receptor antagonist RO 47-0203 (bosentan). *Circulation* 1994; 90:2510–2518.

295. Frishman WH, Tamirisa P, Kumar A. Endothelin and endothelin antagonism. In: Frishman WH, Sonnenblick EH, eds. *Cardiovascular Pharmacotherapeutics*. New York: McGraw-Hill; 1997:689–701.

296. Clavell AL, Mattingly MM, Nir A, Aarhus LL, Heublein DM, Burnett JC Jr. Angiotensin converting enzyme inhibition modulates circulating and tissue endothelin activity in experimental heart failure (abstr). *Circulation* 1994; 90(4, pt 2):I-452.

297. Manning M, Sawyer WH. Discovery, development and some uses of vasopressin and oxytocin antagonists. *J Lab Clin Med* 1989; 114:617–632.

298. Kinter LB, Caltabiano S, Huffman F. Anomalous antidiuretic activity of antidiuretic hormone antagonists. *Biochem Pharmacol* 1993; 45:1731–1737.

299. Shimizu K. Aquaretic effects of the nonpeptide V2 antagonist OPC-31260 in hydropenic humans. *Kidney Int* 1995; 48:220–226.

300. Frishman WH, Mayerson AB. Vasopressin and vasopressin receptor antagonists in cardiovascular disease. In: Frishman WH, Sonnenblick EH, eds. *Cardiovascular Pharmacotherapeutics*. New York: McGraw-Hill; 1997:769–785.

301. Kuan CJ, Herzer WA, Jackson EK. Cardiovascular and renal effects of blocking A1 adenosine receptors. *J Cardiovasc Pharmacol* 1993; 21:822–828.

302. Balakrishnan VS, Coles GA, Williams JD. A potential role for endogenous adenosine in control of human glomerular and tubular function. *Am J Physiol* 1993; 265:F504–510.

303. VanBuren M, Bijlsma JA, Boer P, van Rijn HJ, Koomans HA. Natriuretic and hypotensive effect of adenosine-1 blockade in essential hypertension. *Hypertension* 1993; 22:728–734.

304. Somer DG, Frishman WH. Adenosine and its pharmacologic manipulation in cardiovascular disease. In: Frishman WH, Sonnenblick EH, eds. *Cardiovascular Pharmacotherapeutics*. New York: McGraw-Hill; 1997; 703–726.

305. Frishman WH, Hotchkiss H. Selective and non-selective dopamine receptor agonists: An innovative approach to cardiovascular disease treatment. *Am Heart J* 1996; 132:861–870.

306. Frishman WH, Hotchkiss H. Selective and nonselective dopamine receptor agonists. In: Frishman WH, Sonnenblick EH, eds. *Cardiovascular Pharmacotherapeutics*. New York: McGraw-Hill; 1997; 727–737.

307. Mann DL, Young JB. Basic mechanisms in congestive heart failure: Recognizing the role of proinflammatory cytokines. *Chest* 1994; 105:897–904.

308. Biasucci LM, Vitelli A, Liuzzo G, Altamura S, Caligiuri G, Monaco C, et al. Elevated levels of interleukin-6 in unstable angina. *Circulation* 1996; 94:874–877.

309. Carswell EA, Old LJ, Kassel RL, Green S, Fiore N, Williamson B. An endotoxin-induced serum factor that causes necrosis of tumors. *Proc Natl Acad Sci* 1975; 72:3666–3670.

310. Yokoyama T, Vaca L, Rossen RD, Durante W, Hazarika P, Mann DL. Cellular basis for the negative inotropic effects of tumor necrosis factor-alpha in the adult mammalian heart. *J Clin Invest* 1993; 92:2303–2312.

311. Bazzoni F, Beutler B. The tumor necrosis factor ligand and receptor families. *N Engl J Med* 1996; 334:1717–1725.

312. Frishman WH, Weisen S, Lerro KA, Retter A, Fadel A, Hussain J, et al. Innovative drug targets for treating cardiovascular disease: Adhesion molecules, cytokines, neuropeptide Y and bradykinin. In: Frishman WH, Sonnenblick EH, eds. *Cardiovascular Pharmacotherapeutics*. New York: McGraw-Hill; 1997; 881–905.

313. Katz SD, Rao R, Berman JW, Schwarz M, LeJemtel TH. Pathophysiological correlates of increased serum tumor necrosis factor in patients with congestive heart failure: Relation to nitric oxide dependant vasodilation in the forearm circulation. *Circulation* 1994; 90:12–16.

314. Mohler ER III, Sorensen LC, Ghali JK, Schocken DD, Willis PW, Bowers JA, et al. Role of cytokines in the mechanism of action of amlodipine: The PRAISE Heart Failure Trial. *J Am Coll Cardiol* 1997; 30:35–41.

315. Hayward CS, Kalnins WV, Rogers P, Feneley MP, Macdonald PS, Kelly RP. Effect of inhaled nitric oxide on normal human left ventricular function. *J Am Coll Cardiol* 1997; 30:49–56.

316. Hare JM, Sherman SK, Body SC, Graydon E, Collucci WS, Cooper G. Influence of inhaled nitric oxide on systemic flow and ventricular filling pressure in patients receiving mechanical circulatory assistance. *Circulation* 1997; 95:2250–2253.

317. Matsumoto A, Momomura S, Hirata Y, Aoyagi T, Sugiura S, Omata M. Inhaled nitric oxide and exercise capacity in congestive heart failure. *Lancet* 1997; 349:999–1000.

318. Helisch A, Frishman WH, Hays RM, Loskove JA. Nitric oxide donors in the treatment of cardiovascular disease. In: Frishman WH, Sonnenblick EH, eds. *Cardiovascular Pharmacotherapeutics*. New York: McGraw-Hill; 1997; 739–756.

319. Bocker D, Block M, Isbruch F, Wietholt D, Hammel D, Borggrefe M, et al. Do patients with an implantable defibrillator live longer? *J Am Coll Cardiol* 1993; 21:1638–1644.

320. Breithardt G, Camm AJ, Campbell RWF. Guidelines for the use of implantable cardioverter defibrillators. *Eur Heart J* 1992; 13:1304–1310.

321. Moss AJ, Hall WJ, Cannom DS, Daubert JP, Higgins SL, Klein H, et al. on behalf of the MADIT Investigators. Multicenter Automatic Defibrillator Implantation Trial (abstr). *Circulation* 1996; 94:I-567.

322. The Registry of the International Society of Heart and Lung Transplantation. Ninth Official Report 1992. *J Heart Lung Transplant* 1992; 11:599–606.

323. Paris W, Woodbury A, Thompson S, Levick M, Nothegger S, Arbuckle P, et al. Returning to work after heart transplantation. *J Heart Lung Transplant* 1993; 12:46–54.

324. Milano CA, White WD, Smith LR, Jones RH, Lowe JE, Smith PK, et al. Coronary artery bypass in patients with severely depressed ventricular function. *Ann Thorac Surg* 1993; 56:487–493.

325. Maddahi J, Schelbert H, Brunken R, DiCarli M. Role of thallium-201 and PET imaging in evaluation of myocardial viability and management of patients with coronary artery disease and left ventricular dysfunction. *J Nucl Med* 1994; 35:707–715.

326. Elefteriades JA, Tolis G Jr, Levi E, Mills LK, Zaret BL. Coronary artery bypass grafting in severe left ventricular dysfunction: Excellent survival with improved ejection fraction and functional state. *J Am Coll Cardiol* 1993; 22:1411–1417.

327. Dörffel WV, Felix SB, Wallukat G, Brehme, Bestvater K, Hofmann T, et al. Short-term hemodynamic effects of immunoabsorption in dilated cardiomyopathy. *Circulation* 1997; 95:1994–1997.

24

DIURETICS

Juha P. Kokko

Diuretics increase excretion of salt and water. While the primary clinical indication for their use is to decrease extracellular fluid volume, they have other uses not strictly related to their diuretic properties. This chapter deals initially with a description of the nephrologic sites affected and the molecular mechanism(s) of action of the various diuretics. The second part discusses the use and complications of the five major diuretic families. Finally, the clinical circumstances of special interest to the cardiologist are emphasized. These include use in congestive heart failure and as prophylaxis to prevent nephrotoxicity during radiocontrast infusions.

SEGMENTAL NEPHRON TRANSPORT OF SALT AND WATER AND THE SITE OF DIURETIC ACTION

Figure 24-1 shows schematically the various segments of the mammalian nephron and summarizes the principal transport mechanisms across these sites. The figure also contains an inset listing the various families of diuretics, with associated numbers indicating those nephron segments where they exert their major effect.

Proximal Convoluted Tubule

The proximal convoluted tubule reabsorbs some two-thirds of the glomerular filtrate.[1] Since this tubule is highly permeable to water,[2–7] the net fluid reabsorption across it occurs isoosmotically.[8–13] This reabsorption is complicated and occurs by both active and passive mechanisms. The proximal convoluted tubule reabsorbs most of the filtered glucose,[14–18] amino acids,[19–24] and other organic constituents as well as most of the bicarbonate.[14,25–31] With the reabsorption of the organic solutes and sodium bicarbonate early in the tubule, the remaining constituents are changed so that passive transport processes then contribute in a major way to net fluid reabsorption.[32]

One of the primary active transport processes contributing to net fluid reabsorption across the proximal convoluted tubule is that of reabsorption of sodium bicarbonate by carbonic anhydrase–dependent mechanisms.[33–37] This explains the fact that net reabsorption of salt and fluid in the proximal convoluted tubule can be inhibited to a major extent by carbonic anhydrase inhibitors, such as acetazolamide (Diamox).[34,36] Similarly, since this segment is highly permeable to water and not permeable to solutes such as mannitol, it is also the primary site of action where tubular fluid reabsorption is inhibited by osmotic diuretics such as mannitol. It should be appreciated, however, that inhibition of proximal tubule fluid reabsorption has relatively a small effect on net fluid homeostasis, since nephron segments distal to the proximal tubule have tremendous unused capacity to reabsorb more salt and water if increased amounts are delivered to them. As a result, *diuretics that have their major effect across the proximal tubule are weak diuretics.*

Pars Recta

The pars recta is the straight component of the proximal tubule and is also highly permeable to water.[38,39] Thus, net fluid reabsorption across this segment, as is the case with the proximal convoluted segment, occurs isoosmotically. Since its capacity to reabsorb salt and water is roughly one-third that of the proximal convoluted tubule,[40,41] inhibition of net salt and fluid reabsorption across the pars recta is clinically insignificant.

The pars recta is functionally important for the organic anion transport mechanism, since it secretes many organic anions and cations, including diuretics.[42–44] These secretory processes are important, since all diuretics except spironolactone have their major effect from the urinary side of the tubule. It should be noted that diuretics are not filtered to a significant degree, since they are carried in plasma by various nonfilterable proteins, and that these secretory processes are critically

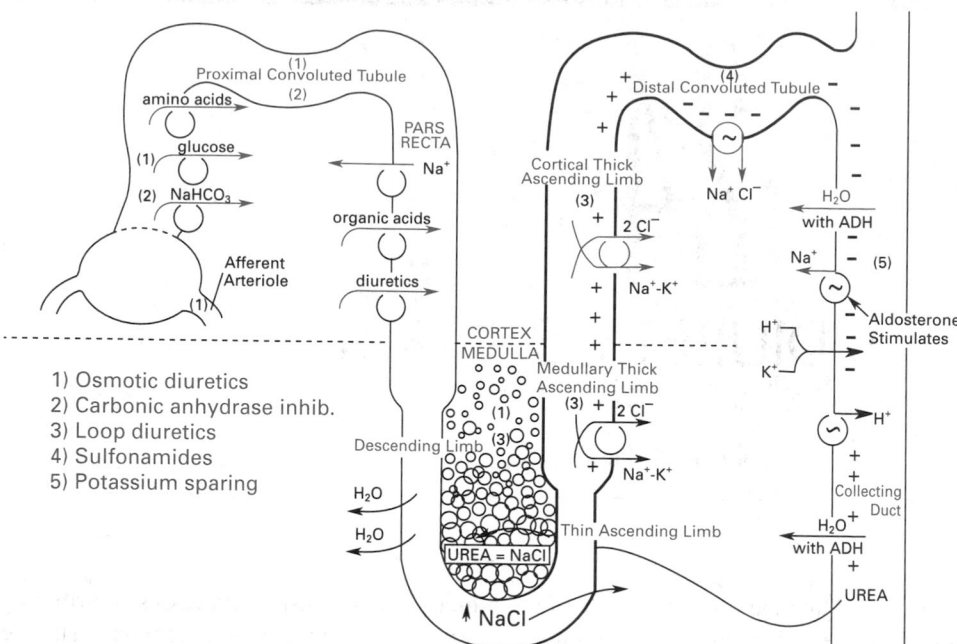

FIGURE 24-1

Major transport processes along the various segments of the mammalian nephron. The numbers refer to the respective sites of action of the various diuretics. Blue lines represent active transport processes.

important in obtaining clinically significant urinary concentrations of diuretics. The exact molecular mechanism of diuretic secretion has not been established, but membrane interactive processes on luminal as well as basolateral membranes play a role. Since organic anions and cations compete, respectively, with diuretics that are organic acids (thiazides, loop diuretics, acetazolamide) or organic bases (amiloride and triamterene) for secretory sites, it is not surprising that in clinical circumstances such as uremia and organic acidosis there is a lower concentration of organic acid diuretic in the urine for any given concentration of diuretic in the blood.[45–47] The urinary concentration of diuretics (determined by the pars recta) correlates more closely with the degree of induced natriuresis than do their blood concentrations.[48]

Descending Limb of Henle

Various lengths of descending limbs of Henle (DLH) descend toward the papillary tip into a normally progressively hypertonic environment (Fig. 24-1). Since all lengths of DLH are highly water-permeable,[49–51] a significant amount of the fluid delivered to them from the proximal tubule is reabsorbed as a consequence of osmotic equilibration.[49] This segment does not possess any active transport processes to be inhibited by diuretics.[49] If loop diuretics obliterate the papillary hypertonicity by inhibiting active transport in segments generating this hypertonicity, net water reabsorption will decrease significantly across the DLH. Indeed, *a significant component of the increased water diuresis caused*

by diuretics is the result of decreased water reabsorption across the thin DLH.

Thin Ascending Limb of Henle

While the thin ascending limb of Henle is important for the countercurrent multiplication system, it does not have a major role in diuretic action, since it is water-impermeable and does not actively transport solutes transepithelially.[52–55]

Thick Ascending Limb of Henle

Both the cortical and the medullary thick ascending limb of Henle have important roles in diuretic function. The cortical thick ascending limb forms dilute urine, while the function of the medullary thick ascending limb is to generate surroundings allowing formation of concentrated urine. Salt transport mechanisms are similar in both segments and are affected similarly by loop diuretics. Figure 24-2 summarizes schematically a secondary active chloride transport mechanism in these segments. Chloride is transported across epithelium against an electrochemical gradient,[56,57] but transport is dependent on the energy generated by the sodium potassium adenosinetriphosphatase (ATPase) on the blood side. Thus, active chloride transport is considered secondary.[58] In this model, the lumen positive potential difference (largely created by back diffusion of potassium into the lumen)[59] creates an electrochemical driving force for passive reabsorption of sodium through paracellular routes.[56,57] Thus, sodium is reabsorbed transcellularly and paracellularly, while all chloride transport appears to be transcellular.[60] The loop diuretics act luminally to inhibit the Na-K-2Cl cotransporter, thus decreasing the lumen positive potential difference toward zero.[61–67] The mechanism is competitive inhibition of the chloride binding sites as a pseudosubstrate,[68,69] thus preventing the translocation of the electrolytes from the urinary side into the cell.

The thick ascending limb of Henle transports not only sodium and chloride by the cotransporter but also divalent cations due to diffusion down the electrochemical gradient. While active calcium and magnesium transport mechanisms may exist in these segments, significant amounts of the cations are reabsorbed due to lumen positive potential differences.[70] Thus, loop diuretics that inhibit the lumen positive potential difference cause increased urinary loss of magnesium[71] as well as calcium.[72]

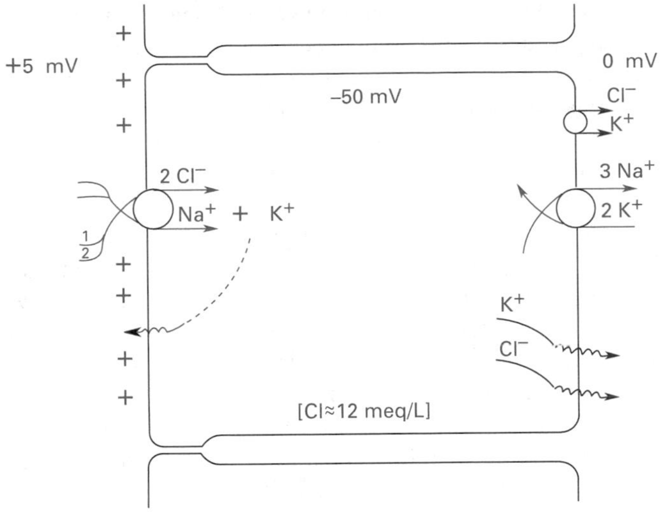

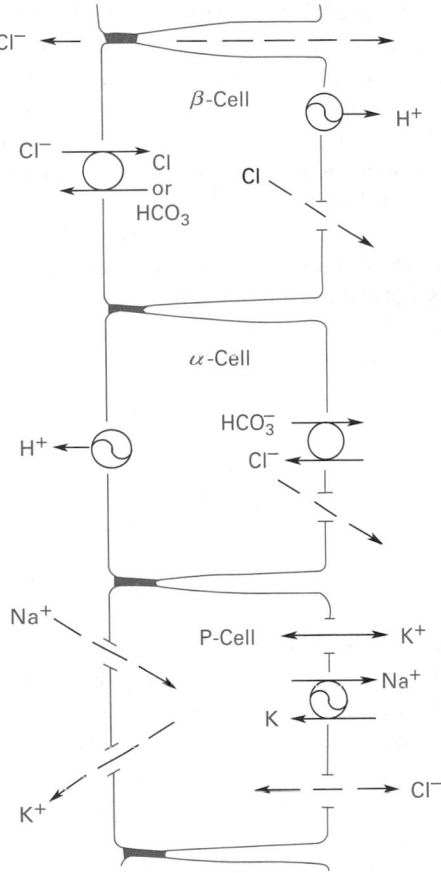

FIGURE 24-2

Cellular model of secondary active chloride transport across the thick ascending limb of Henle. The left side of the figure represents the luminal side with lumen-positive +5 mV potential; the middle section is intracellular cytoplasm with −50 mV potential; the right side of the figure is the blood side at 0 mV potential. In this model, there are four ionic binding sites on the cotransport protein existing on the luminal surface. These binding sites must be occupied by sodium, potassium, and two chloride ions before translocation of these ions can take place from the luminal side into the intracellular space. The lumen-positive potential occurs in large part by potassium diffusing back into the lumen; it is this lumen-positive potential difference that is responsible for a significant amount of passive sodium transport by paracellular routes. The loop diuretics compete for occupancy and act as a pseudosubstrate for one of the chloride transport sites, thus preventing the normal transport of chloride across this segment. Blue lines indicate membrane interactive transport processes.

FIGURE 24-3

Schematics of the three cell types existing in the mammalian cortical collecting tubules. In each case the lumen is on the left side of the figure, while the right side represents the blood side. The top two cells represent the two types of intercalated cells responsible for bicarbonate secretion (*beta cell*) and that are involved with acid secretion (*alpha cell*). The bottom cell illustrates the primary transport processes of the *principal cell*, which is responsible for salt transport and is the target organ for aldosterone. It is this cell that is primarily affected by the potassium-sparing diuretics. Blue lines indicate membrane interactive transport processes. (From Schuster V, Stokes J. *Am J Physiol* 1987; 22:F203–F212. Reproduced with permission from the publisher and the author.)

Distal Convoluted Tubule

The primary importance of the distal convoluted tubule in diuretic action is the presence of a luminal surface-neutral sodium chloride transport mechanism[73,74] that is inhibited by thiazides.[73–77] The process by which salt transport occurs out of the distal convoluted tubule is depicted in Fig. 24-1. Since this segment is impermeable to water with or without antidiuretic hormone,[78] it follows that it is also a diluting segment. Thus, thiazide diuretics inhibit the formation of dilute urine, which is the basis of thiazide-induced hyponatremia.[79] While some hydrogen and potassium secretion occurs, the capacity for transport of these ions is lower than that in the collecting duct.[80]

The Collecting Duct

The collecting duct traverses the cortex, outer medulla, and papilla, while expressing functional differences in each area. The cortical collecting duct, however, is the most important of these segments, physiologically and pharmacologically, in the final urinary excretion of salt and acid base in that it can be modified by the potassium-sparing diuretics. The cortical collecting tubule is composed of three primarily different types of cells depicted in Fig. 24-3.[81] The *principal* cell is involved with salt transport, while the *alpha* and *beta* intercalated cells are involved with acid-base transport.

Aldosterone is the main determinant of the net transport of sodium across the principal cell.[78] In this cell sodium gains access from lumen to intracellular space by traversing through sodium channels down electrochemical gradients.[82–87] The primary movement of sodium from lumen to cell creates a luminal electronegativity. Once the sodium is in the cell, it is pumped out by the peritubular sodium potassium ATPase, the activity of which is modulated by aldosterone levels.[88–95] Thus, increasing the sodium potassium ATPase activity by aldosterone increases net transport of sodium across this cell and creates a more lumen-negative potential difference that favors passive secretion of hydrogen and potassium.

The primary effects of those diuretics affecting the collecting duct are upon the principal cell. Three different types of diuretics affect this segment. Amiloride and triamterene decrease the conductance of sodium channels and inhibit sodium reabsorption by that mechanism.[87,96] Spirolactones inhibit sodium reabsorption by competitive inhibition of the mineralocorticoid action.[97] Each of these compounds not only inhibits sodium reabsorption but also, secondarily, decreases the generation of lumen negative potential difference and therefore is potassium-sparing. These diuretics do not have clinically significant effects on salt and acid-base homeostasis across the more distal outer medullary or papillary collecting duct segments.

DIURETIC CLASSES

Benzothiazides

MECHANISM OF ACTION

While the thiazide diuretics were initially developed as inhibitors of carbonic anhydrase, studies in animals and humans led to the conclusion that their primary effect is to inhibit the function of the cortical diluting segment,[98–101] with no effect on sodium chloride transport in the medullary thick ascending limb of Henle.

The cortical diluting segment, however, includes epithelia of the cortical thick ascending limb of Henle, distal convoluted tubule, connecting tubule, and early segments of the cortical collecting duct. While there may be some species differences with respect to the exact site of action, thiazides appear to inhibit the electroneutral sodium-dependent chloride transport mechanism on the luminal side. The exact molecular mechanism of this inhibition is unknown.

The thiazide diuretics can be given orally and intravenously. Their oral effectiveness is one of their principal advantages. The choice of thiazides is based primarily on the cost and desired duration of effect. The various thiazide diuretics seem to be quite similar in their effect at their respective equivalent dose levels (see Table 24-1). The effects of these diuretics are relatively slow in onset (around 30 min), but their duration of action is quite long (up to 24 h).

COMPLICATIONS

The complications of the benzothiazides can be classified as those that are idiosyncratic and those that derive from their metabolic consequences. The reported hypersensitivity reactions include purpura, urticaria, rash, photosensitivity, and pancreatitis. Except for photosensitivity, these other reactions are rare. The metabolic complications include effects on potassium, calcium, glucose, and lipid abnormalities.

Hypokalemia

The kaliuresis induced by thiazides results from increased delivery of sodium chloride to the potassium secretory seg-

ments of the nephron distal to the connecting segments. The resultant kaliuresis is highly dependent on the patient's aldosterone level. The higher the aldosterone level, the greater the potassium secretion.[102,103] While kaliuresis is an accepted consequence of thiazide therapy and reductions in serum potassium of 0.4 to 0.8 meq/L are not uncommon, significant total-body potassium deficiency (greater than 10 percent) is less common.[104–109] Approximately 20 to 30 percent of patients receiving normal doses of thiazides become hypokalemic to levels below 3.5 meq/L and total-potassium deficient to amounts greater than 10 percent of total-body potassium stores. It is interesting that the incidence of hypokalemia appears to be greater with thiazides than with loop diuretics, even though loop diuretics cause a higher fractional excretion of potassium.[108] This differential effect occurs because thiazides have a more prolonged effect than do the loop diuretics. The shorter-acting loop diuretics will have a longer nondiuretic compensatory period when the kidney can readjust to potassium deficits by increasing potassium reabsorption. It appears that those patients at highest risk for developing potassium deficiency are those with the highest aldosterone levels, especially if coupled with a decreased potassium intake.

Thiazide-induced hypokalemia is causally associated with a number of untoward clinically significant side effects, including decreased insulin release (abnormal carbohydrate tolerance),[110–112] increased incidence of arrhythmias both with and without digitalis,[113–120] decreased blood pressure with increased incidence of postural hypotension,[121–125] and potentiation of rhabdomyolysis.[126–130] Thus, *potassium repletion should be considered in patients receiving thiazides, but by no means should this be a routine practice.*[109,131] There are significant differences of opinion as to when to treat asymptomatic hypokalemia; however, it seems prudent that patients who are diabetic, have congestive heart failure, or are receiving digitalis should not be allowed to become total-body potassium-deficient and that their serum potassium should be kept at levels above 3.5 meq/L. Furthermore, patients who are at risk for developing arrhythmias, whether they are on digitalis or not, should also receive therapy to prevent their potassium levels from falling below 3.5 meq/L.[109,131] It has also been suggested that patients who are hospitalized with acute myocardial infarction have an increased mortality if their serum potassium levels fall below 3.5 meq/L.

Patients who are symptomatic from a decreased potassium concentration should be supplemented with potassium chloride.[109,131] There are numerous potassium supplements that are preferable to potassium-sparing diuretics, since renal potassium regulatory processes are left unaltered with such supplementation.[132] In patients who refuse to take potassium supplements, it may be necessary to utilize a combination of potassium-sparing diuretics with thiazides.

Hyperglycemia

Glucose intolerance may be associated with thiazides. Both in vitro and in vivo studies now suggest that the major reason

TABLE 24-1

ORAL DIURETIC AGENTS

Generic Name	Trade Name	Usual Daily Dosage, mg	Onset of Action, h	Peak Effect, h	Duration of Action, h
THIAZIDE AND RELATED DIURETICS					
Bendroflumethiazide	Naturetin	2.5–15	2	4	6–12
Benzthiazide	Aquatag, Exna, Marazide	50–200	2	4–6	6–12
Chlorothiazide	Diuril, Diachlor, Diurigen	500–2000	1–2	4	6–12
Chlorthalidone	Hygroton, Hylidone	25–100	2	2–6	24–72
Cyclothiazide	Anhydron	2	Within 6	7–12	18–24
Hydrochlorothiazide	Esidrix, HydroDIURIL	25–100	2	4–6	6–12
Hydroflumethiazide	Diucardin, Saluron	50–200	2	4	6–12
Indapamide	Lozol	2.5–5	1–2	Within 2	Up to 36
Methylclothiazide	Enduron, Ethon	2.5–5	2	4–6	24
Metolazone	Diulo, Zaroxolyn	2.5–5	1	2	12–24
Polythiazide	Renese	2–4	2	6	24–48
Quinethazone	Hydromox	50–100	2	6	18–24
Trichlormethiazide	Metahydrin, Naqua	2–4	2	6	24
LOOP DIURETICS					
Bumetanide	Bumex	0.5–2	0.5–1	1–2	4–6
Ethacrynic acid	Edecrin	50–100	Within 0.5	2	6–8
Furosemide	Lasix	20–80	Within 1	1–2	6–8
Torsemide	Demadex	5–20	Within 1	1–2	6–8
POTASSIUM-SPARING DIURETICS					
Amiloride	Midamor	5–20	2	6–10	24
Spironolactone	Aldactone	25–200	24–48	48–72	48–72
Triamterene	Dyrenium	200–300	2–4	6–8	12–16
COMBINATION DIURETICS					
Amiloride and hydrochlorothiazide	Moduretic	5–10(A) 50–100(H)	See individual agents above	See individual agents above	See individual agents above
Spironolactone and hydrochlorothiazide	Aldactazide, Alazide	25–200(S) 25–200(H)	See individual agents above	See individual agents above	See individual agents above
Triamterene and hydrochlorothiazide	Maxide, Dyazide	37.5–100(T) 25–50(H)	See individual agents above	See individual agents above	See individual agents above

Source: Compiled by Clyde Buchanan from *Facts and Comparisons Drug Information*, 1992.

is decreased beta-cell sensitivity to glucose during thiazide-induced hypokalemia with a fall of plasma potassium concentrations of greater than approximately 1.0 meq/L.[110–112] If potassium deficiency is prevented, glucose intolerance is not noted.[112]

Hyperuricemia

Hyperuricemia is common in thiazide-treated patients, primarily due to circulatory volume contraction.[133,134] Volume contraction can cause proximal tubule reabsorption of all solutes, including uric acid. The hyperuricemia with thiazides is usually mild (increases of 1 to 2 mg/dL) and of no clinical

significance except in those patients with gout.[132] In nongouty patients, the diuretic-induced hyperuricemia requires no therapy if uric acid levels are below 15 mg/dL.[135] The hyperuricemia usually responds rapidly to expansion of the effective arterial blood volume and discontinuation of thiazide diuretics. Probenecid can be given to lower uric acid if thiazides are needed in gouty patients.

Hypercalcemia

Thiazides cause a 40 to 50 percent reduction in urinary excretion of calcium.[136–138] The hypocalciuria is due to a direct effect of thiazides to increase calcium reabsorption by the early portion of the distal tubule.[73] The reciprocal result of hypocalciuria, however, is a mild degree of hypercalcemia. Acutely, the rise may be 0.5 to 1.5 mg/dL; but with chronic use, the expected rise in total serum calcium is often less than 0.2 mg/dL.[139,140] Clearly these changes are of no clinical significance unless they are superimposed on underlying hypercalcemia.

Hyperlipidemia

Thiazide diuretics can increase total serum cholesterol by up to 10 percent.[141–147] Thiazides increase serum triglycerides, very low density lipoprotein (VLDL), and low-density lipoprotein (LDL) cholesterol concentrations by unknown mechanisms. Any changes in high-density lipoprotein (HDL) cholesterol are quite small or nonexistent.[148,149] Although this issue is controversial, some feel that even modest increases in cholesterol concentration can increase the rate of progression of atherosclerosis. In patients with hyperlipidemia or established atherosclerotic vascular disease, it is prudent to choose diuretics that do not induce hyperlipidemia.

ADVANTAGES

Thiazides have the advantages of being relatively inexpensive, orally active, and effective over an extended period.

DISADVANTAGES

The primary disadvantages of thiazides are their relatively frequent metabolic side effects and their lower potency than loop diuretics in inducing salt and water excretion.

USE

Thiazides are indicated in those clinical states in which mild diuresis is desired if no contraindications exist.[150] Low doses of thiazides are especially useful as antihypertensives. The antihypertensive effects can be obtained at such low doses that the expected adverse biochemical effects can be minimized.[151] *Thiazide diuretics are not effective and are often contraindicated in chronic renal failure.*

Loop Diuretics

The loop diuretics act by inhibiting transport of salt in the thick ascending limb of Henle. The four major diuretics in this group are furosemide, ethacrynic acid, bumetanide, and torsemide. A number of newer loop diuretics are currently being developed but appear to have effects similar to those of currently available agents in clinically equivalent doses.

MECHANISM OF ACTION

As noted, the loop diuretics compete with chloride for occupancy of the luminal Na-K-2Cl cotransporter in the thick ascending limb of Henle (Fig. 24-2) and thus inhibit the translocation of sodium chloride from the luminal side to intracellular space.[152] In in vitro studies, the inhibition of salt transport across this segment occurs almost instantaneously, and once the diuretic is removed from the luminal fluid, the reabsorptive rate of chloride rapidly returns toward normal.[62,64,66,68] Since

TABLE 24-2

TITRATION TO DEFINE A SINGLE EFFECTIVE DOSE OF LOOP DIURETIC IN PATIENTS WITH CHRONIC RENAL INSUFFICIENCY

Creatinine clearance, mL/min	20–50	< 20
Starting dose		
Furosemide	40 mg IV	80 mg IV
Furosemide	80 mg PO	160 mg PO
Bumetanide	1 mg IV or PO	4 mg IV or PO
Ceiling dose		
Furosemide	120–160 mg IV	160–200 mg IV
Furosemide	240–320 mg PO	320–400 mg PO
Bumetanide	4–6 mg IV or PO	8–10 mg IV or PO

Source: From Brater.[48]

both the cortical and medullary thick ascending limbs of Henle are affected, it follows that both the diluting and concentrating capacities of the kidney are decreased. In vivo, these diuretics generally have a very rapid onset of action within minutes when given intravenously and within 30 min when given orally. They have a short duration of action, with most of the diuresis occurring within 4 h. As noted, the loop diuretics are secreted into the urine by the pars recta by mechanisms that compete with endogenous organic acids.[45–47] Thus, under circumstances of organic acidosis, especially in the setting of chronic uremia, these diuretics have to be administered at higher than normal levels to achieve the same desired urinary concentration (see Table 24-2). Intravenous furosemide also produces venous vasodilatation, which may be beneficial in acute heart failure.

COMPLICATIONS OF LOOP DIURETIC THERAPY

Loop diuretics as a group are quite well tolerated. Complications or adverse reactions generally can be classified into those due to hypersensitivity reactions to the drugs and those due to inhibition of the Na-K-2Cl cotransport mechanism. Hypersensitivity reactions are unpredictable and primarily dermatologic, with rare episodes of necrotizing angiitis, photosensitivity, exfoliative dermatitis, and pruritus. Rarely, hematologic reactions have been reported, with thrombocytopenia and generalized suppression of the bone marrow. The predictable complications of loop diuretics are due to inhibition of the Na-K-2Cl cotransport mechanism. With this inhibition, there is an increased delivery of sodium and fluid to the cortical collecting tubule, resulting in increased kaliuresis. Usually, the decline in serum potassium concentration with loop diuretics is modest—0.3 to 0.4 meq/L.[104,105,107,108,153] Only approximately 10 percent of patients who receive once-a-day doses of loop diuretics develop hypokalemia of less than 3.5 meq/L.[154,155] This degree of hypokalemia is less than that seen with thiazides—20 to 30 percent. The lower incidence of hypokalemia with the loop diuretics is due to their short duration of action, as noted. If the loop diuretics are combined with a chlorthalidone or other diuretic with a longer duration of action, the incidence of hypokalemia is increased significantly.[156,157]

Hypomagnesemia occurs with the loop diuretics, since they inhibit magnesium reabsorption across the thick ascending limb of Henle and increase urinary magnesium excretion[158-161]; however, symptomatic hypomagnesemia is relatively rare except in the setting of chronic alcoholism or after prolonged use of the diuretics. Ventricular ectopy may occur as a consequence of decreased serum magnesium concentration, and magnesium deficiency should be corrected in patients with ventricular ectopy.[162,163] In some patients it is difficult to correct potassium deficiency until magnesium deficiency has been corrected.

Metabolic alkalosis may occur with loop diuretics but is usually mild and of no clinical significance.[132] Hyperuricemia and hypoglycemia have also been reported with loop diuretics, but less commonly than with the longer-acting thiazide diuretics, where the degree of hypokalemia may be greater. The mechanisms of these metabolic abnormalities are similar to those induced by the thiazide diuretics discussed above.

One of the unique complications of loop diuretics has been ototoxicity. Ototoxicity has been reported with all the loop diuretics but was much more common in the past, when very high doses were utilized.[164-168] Indeed, cochlear function has been checked by audiometry before and after normal doses of loop diuretics and no adverse effects were noted in a small study.[169] If the loop diuretics are given at high concentrations or if they are given with aminoglycosides or other ototoxic drugs, it is prudent to decrease or discontinue them if patients complain of buzzing in their ears or decreased hearing activity. In most circumstances, ototoxicity is reversible, but irreversible ototoxicity has been reported.

ADVANTAGES
The advantages of the loop diuretics are their potency and rapid onset of action. They also exert their effect in most clinical states with metabolic abnormalities; however, increased doses must be given during organic acidosis.

DISADVANTAGES
The two primary disadvantages of loop diuretics are cost and short duration of action. They should be discontinued if idiosyncratic reactions occur and should be discontinued or their dose reduced if major metabolic consequences occur.

USE
The loop diuretics can be used alone in essentially all instances where diuresis is indicated. Because of their bioavailability, in most circumstances there is no difference if doses are given orally or intravenously. They also are indicated in the first-line defense against hypercalcemia, since these diuretics induce rapid calciuria.[158,159,170,171] This effect is due to inhibition of calcium reabsorption by the thick ascending limb of Henle, as noted.[172]

Potassium-Sparing Diuretics

As noted previously, spironolactone, amiloride, and triamterene cause natriuresis and antikaliuresis through effects across the cortical collecting tubule. As a group, these drugs induce a relatively mild natriuresis, and often the primary indication for their use is to produce potassium retention. The principal but not sole reason for the antikaliuresis is inhibition of the normally negative transepithelial potential difference across the cortical collecting tubule, which is the primary driving force for potassium secretion.[82-87] These diuretics have a relatively slow onset of action, especially the aldosterone receptor inhibitors. Transepithelial effects are not expressed until 3 or 4 h after administration in experimental studies, and it is usual for the maximal clinical effects of spirolactones to be seen only after several days. The effects of amiloride and triamterene are seen somewhat earlier, and their duration of action is in the intermediate range of 8 to 16 h.

COMPLICATIONS
A potential complication of the potassium-sparing diuretics is life-threatening hyperkalemia. In one study,[173] hyperkalemia occurred in 8.6 percent of hospitalized patients receiving spironolactone. Life-threatening hyperkalemia has been reported in patients who have received these diuretics in a setting of renal insufficiency and diabetes, especially with the coadministration of potassium supplements.[174-178] Physicians should carefully follow the serum potassium concentration, especially in the initial phases of potassium-sparing diuretic use, and should avoid the concurrent administration of potassium supplements and angiotensin converting enzyme (ACE) inhibitors. In addition, concurrent use of beta blockers and noninflammatory agents with potassium-sparing diuretics should be approached with some caution.[179]

Since the potassium-sparing diuretics also inhibit hydrogen ion secretion, one might expect that metabolic acidosis would be a common complication of their use. Clinical experience, however, has shown that metabolic acidosis is a relatively rare complication.[132]

A unique complication of spironolactone is gynecomastia.[180,181] The mechanism is not clear. This side effect has not been reported with sodium channel blockers. Various hypersensitivity reactions have been seen with the sodium channel blockers, and nonspecific gastrointestinal symptoms such as nausea and anorexia occur in some patients.

ADVANTAGES
The primary advantage of this group of diuretics is to conserve potassium in patients with an intolerance to potassium supplementation or in whom potassium supplementation is not practical. Spironolactone may have other beneficial effects in the treatment of congestive heart failure, including decreased urinary magnesium excretion; reduced ventricular arrhythmias; and increased cardiac norepinephrine uptake.[182,183] Spironolactone is especially useful in those clinical states such as cirrhosis that are characterized by high concentrations of circulating aldosterone.

DISADVANTAGES
The principal disadvantage of this group of diuretics is their lack of diuretic potency.

USE

The primary use of potassium-sparing diuretics is in the setting where potassium retention is desired. They may also be used as adjunctive agents to potentiate other diuretics. Recent studies have also suggested that the addition of spironolactone to ACE inhibitors may improve mortality rates in congestive heart failure.[182] Spironolactone is often indicated in patients with secondary aldosteronism, as in cirrhosis and ascites.

Carbonic Anhydrase Inhibitors

MECHANISM OF ACTION

The principal diuretic effect of carbonic anhydrase inhibitors results from inhibition of carbonic anhydrase–mediated fluid reabsorption across the proximal convoluted tubule.[31–36] They also affect carbonic anhydrase–mediated processes in the distal tubule, but their primary diuretic effect (in contrast to their effect on hydrogen secretion) is through their action on the proximal tubule. As a consequence, there is increased bicarbonate excretion and free-water formation. Because of a decrease in hydrogen ion excretion and an increase in delivery of bicarbonate to the collecting tubule, there is increased loss of potassium across the cortical collecting tubule. The onset of effect of carbonic anhydrase inhibitors occurs within minutes if they are given intravenously or within 30 min if given orally. The maximum effect occurs in several hours; the duration of action is 8 to 12 h.

COMPLICATIONS

Carbonic anhydrase inhibitors are remarkably nontoxic in both animals and humans. If acetazolamide is given at doses greater than 1 g/day, patients may complain of drowsiness and occasional numbness and tingling of the fingers. At more clinically appropriate doses, however, this group of diuretics is well tolerated.

Carbonic anhydrase inhibitors have predictable metabolic complications. Metabolic acidosis is a necessary side effect, since their primary effect is to increase excretion of bicarbonate; however, bicarbonate concentrations generally do not fall below 18 to 20 meq/L.[184,185] If more severe acidosis is demonstrated, other causes besides carbonic anhydrase inhibitors should be sought.[186,187] Since these diuretics increase distal delivery of nonreabsorbable bicarbonate, it is not surprising that kaliuresis is a common phenomenon and frank hypokalemia may occur, especially in the setting of increased aldosterone levels. Patients who are on maintenance levels of high doses of carbonic anhydrase inhibitors should have their serum potassium monitored regularly.

ADVANTAGES

Carbonic anhydrase inhibitors are generally not used for their diuretic effects. In metabolic alkalosis, they may have the advantage of promoting increased excretion of bicarbonate.

DISADVANTAGES

Carbonic anhydrase inhibitors as a group are relatively ineffective diuretics.

USE

A primary use of carbonic anhydrase inhibitors is to alkalinize the urine. This is especially useful when it is desirable to increase the excretion of those drugs or toxins that are more soluble in alkaline urine when they have been taken in excess (overdose). Carbonic anhydrase inhibitors may also increase excretion of endogenous compounds such as uric acid. Some physicians use carbonic anhydrase inhibitors and volume expansion in the treatment of hematopoietic disorders in which high uric acid excretion rates are anticipated. They may also be useful in decreasing metabolic alkalosis—for example, in patients being weaned from a respirator.

Osmotic Diuretics

MECHANISM OF ACTION

Mannitol is the prototype osmotic diuretic. Under normal physiologic conditions, mannitol has beneficial effects on both renal plasma flow and on the tubules, causing decreased absorption of filtrate. The increase in renal plasma flow occurs as a consequence of at least three factors: increased plasma volume, increased release of atrial natriuretic peptide, and decreased resistance to renal plasma flow.[188–193] With increased renal plasma flow and a decrease in the glomerular oncotic pressure caused by mannitol, there is a resultant increase in glomerular filtration rate.[192] Once this glomerular filtrate reaches the proximal tubule, there is a nonspecific inhibition of the proximal tubule reabsorption due to the osmotic effects of mannitol.[188] The onset of action of mannitol is immediate and its duration of action is only as long as the mannitol remains in the circulation.

COMPLICATIONS

No specific complications are associated with osmotic diuretics with the exception of increased blood volume.

ADVANTAGES

Mannitol is the most effective diuretic in restoring glomerular filtration rate during transient hypotension.[193,194]

DISADVANTAGES

Mannitol must be given intravenously. Another disadvantage is that if it does not increase glomerular filtration rate, there is a danger of overexpansion of the blood volume with hyponatremia. Pulmonary edema can be produced or worsened.

USE

Osmotic diuretics are useful in many clinical settings with transiently decreased renal plasma flow. A decrease in renal plasma flow may occur during the induction phases of anesthesia or during the use of radiocontrast materials.[193] The dose of mannitol is 25 to 50 g as a single intravenous bolus in a 20% solution. If the urine flow does not increase within 10 min, further doses of mannitol are contraindicated. In those patients who respond favorably, a continuous infusion of a

10 to 15% solution may be started and continued as long as deemed necessary.

USE OF DIURETICS IN SPECIFIC CIRCUMSTANCES

Congestive Heart Failure

GENERAL ISSUES

The primary reason for salt and water retention in acute congestive heart failure is the activation of the renin-angiotensin-aldosterone axis in a setting of low cardiac output with decreased blood flow to the kidney (Fig. 24-4).[195] The decrease in effective arterial blood volume increases proximal tubule reabsorption of salt and water and sodium reabsorption is further increased by aldosterone-dependent mechanisms across the cortical collecting tubule.[88–95] Thus the therapeutic approaches to increasing natriuresis are fourfold: use of diuretics to increase salt excretion, use of ACE inhibitors to reduce afterload and increase renal blood flow, reduction of salt and water intake, and increase of cardiac output by the use of inotropic agents (see Chaps. 21 and 23).

Generally speaking, the loop diuretics are the most effective of the various diuretics in moderate or severe congestive heart failure. They have the advantage of being potent natriuretic agents and of being effective in patients with a wide variety of electrolyte abnormalities. Satisfactory diuresis can

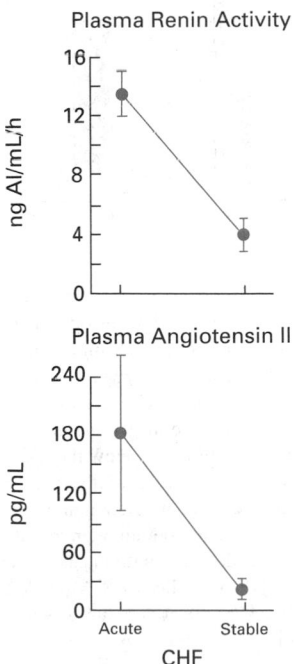

FIGURE 24-4

This figure demonstrates that in acute congestive heart failure, the renin-angiotensin system is activated (*left*) and that values return to normal once stabilization of congestive heart failure occurs (*right*). (From Dzau VJ, Colucci WS, Hollenberg NK, et al. *Circulation* 1981; 63:645–651. Reproduced with permission from the publisher and the author.)

usually be obtained in patients with normal renal function with furosemide, 40 mg intravenously twice a day; ethacrynic acid, 50 mg intravenously twice a day; bumetanide, 1 mg twice a day intravenously; or torsemide, 20 mg intravenously twice a day. It should be noted, however, that oral and intravenous routes are essentially equally efficacious because of the effective gastrointestinal absorption and high bioavailability of loop diuretics. If renal disease is present, the maximum necessary intravenous doses should be increased, as summarized in Table 24-1.[48] If adequate diuresis is not achieved by the loop diuretics, a more proximally acting diuretic, such as metalazone, or a more distally acting diuretic, such as a potassium-sparing diuretic, can be added. Since the combination of metalazone and loop diuretics can lead to life-threatening hypokalemia, it is important to monitor the serum potassium concentrations carefully.[156,157]

One of the recent advances in the treatment of congestive heart failure is the appreciation of the importance of inhibiting the renin-angiotensin system.[196–199] Cardiologists are very aware that further forced decreases in effective arterial blood volume by diuretics in the setting of prerenal azotemia can worsen the degree of azotemia.[196] This adverse outcome can often be prevented with the simultaneous use of ACE inhibitors.[196] While the initial studies were conducted with captopril, similar beneficial effects on renal function in congestive heart failure have been seen with other ACE inhibitors.[200] In contrast to some speculation, there is no compelling evidence that ACE inhibitors adversely affect natriuresis induced by loop diuretics. Indeed, a recent study has demonstrated that ACE inhibitors did not significantly alter either urinary excretion of furosemide or its natriuretic effects.[201]

In summary, improved cardiac and renal function have been shown with the use of the combination of ACE inhibitors and diuretics both acutely (Fig. 24-5)[196] and chronically.[198,200,202] When ACE inhibitors are used in congestive heart failure and in the setting of presumed high angiotensin levels, it is prudent to use a low dose initially to be certain that an untoward hypotensive episode will not occur.[203] The potential for an inappropriate large decrease in blood pressure is more likely in patients who acutely or subacutely have elevated angiotensin II levels than in patients who are in a steady state with elevated angiotensin II levels—for example, those patients with high renin hypertension.

As noted in Chap. 23, salt restriction is a key component of treatment of congestive heart failure even with the use of diuretics and ACE inhibitors. Indeed, well-controlled studies have demonstrated that *with a high sodium intake, loop diuretics given once a day fail to achieve a negative sodium balance.*[204,205] The reason is that even though there is an impressive natriuresis for 3 h after the furosemide administration, there is a compensatory increase in sodium reabsorption in the remaining 24-h period that exactly matches the earlier losses (Fig. 24-6).[204] Thus, *it is essential to limit the sodium intake to ensure negative sodium balances. Balance studies on normal humans have demonstrated that significant negative sodium balance can be predictably obtained with loop diuret-*

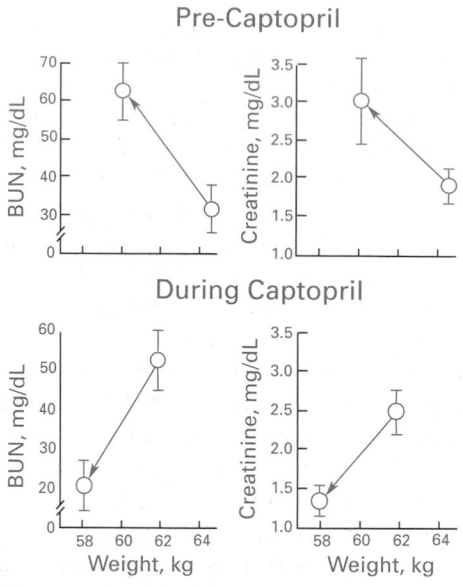

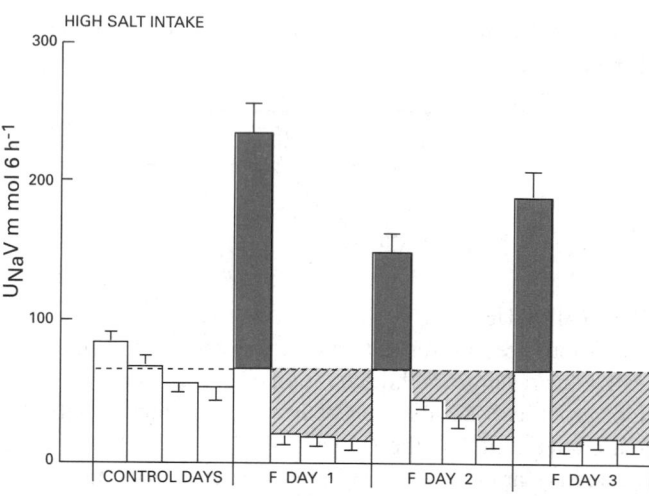

FIGURE 24-5

Studies in congestive heart failure patients demonstrating the frequent finding whereby blood urea nitrogen (BUN) and creatinine increase with diuretics without the use of captopril, whereas with the additional use of captopril, the BUN and creatinine can decrease with diuretics together with a reduction of edema and reduction of circulatory volume. (From Dzau VJ, Colucci WS, Williams GH, et al. *N Engl J Med* 1980; 302:1373–1379. Reproduced with permission from the publisher and the author.)

ics if sodium intake is limited to 20 meq/day (equivalent to 460 mg sodium or 1.2 g sodium chloride per day).

DEVELOPING ISSUES

Combination Diuretics

There are two reasons to consider the use of more than one family of diuretics: (1) to improve the degree of natriuresis and (2) to improve the patient's metabolic status.

Generally, one cannot expect to increase the degree of natriuresis if another diuretic is added to the regimen from the same family of diuretics. Judicious use of diuretics that act on different nephron segments, however, can induce increased natriuresis provided that the cardiovascular system is presenting the kidney with sufficient substrate (salt and water). It is better practice to add another family of diuretics than to increase the dose of a given diuretic above its ceiling level. Diuretic "resistance" in the presence of normal kidneys is not a consequence of unfavorable pharmacokinetics[206] but generally a manifestation of poor cardiac output with resultant poor renal perfusion.

The most common metabolic complication of diuretics is hypokalemia, which can be ameliorated by use of potassium-sparing diuretics. The conventional wisdom, however, supports the use of potassium supplements rather than potassium-sparing diuretics because the collecting duct has an enormous capacity to secrete extra potassium if faced with hyperkalemia. This capacity is lost if it is blocked by the use of potassium-sparing diuretics. There are patients, however, in whom this

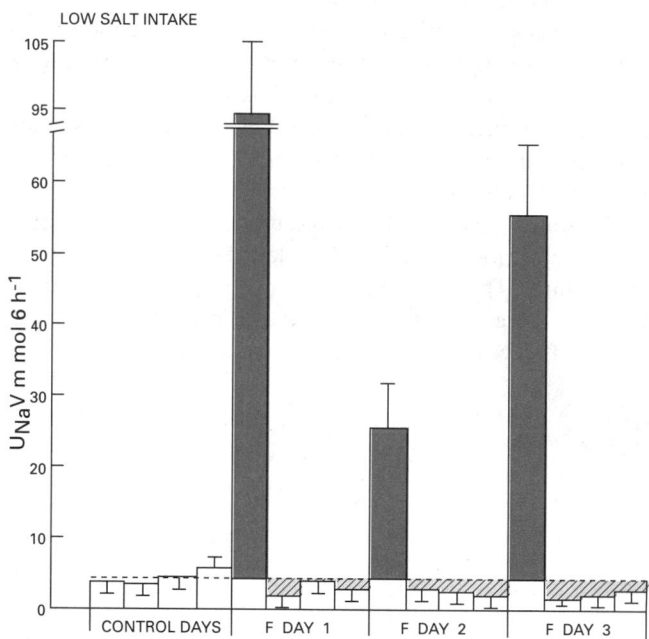

FIGURE 24-6

Mean 6-h balance studies of six normal subjects given 40 mg of furosemide (f) on sodium intakes of 20 mmol (460 mg) per day, equivalent to 1.2 g NaCl per day (*low salt, lower panel*) and 270 mmol (6.2 g) per day, equivalent to 15.8 g NaCl per day (*high salt, upper panel*). The horizontal line in both panels represents balance of intake and excretion of sodium for that time period. Bars above the line show the magnitude of negative sodium balance for that 6 h, while the distance of a bar below the horizontal line represents positive retention of sodium. The area of the dark blue bars above the horizontal line represents the amount of sodium excretion, while the light blue area below the line represents sodium retention. It should be noted that only during low salt intake do these individuals achieve negative sodium balance for a 24-h period. (From Wilcox CS, Mitch WE, Kelly RA, et al. *J Lab Clin Med* 1983; 102:450–458. Reproduced with permission from the publisher and the author.)

approach must be taken, since they may be intolerant of oral potassium preparations or otherwise noncompliant with potassium supplements. The recent recognition that the increased aldosterone levels present in congestive heart failure can have untoward effects (in addition to increasing sodium reabsorption) has provided a further rationale for the use of diuretic combinations that include an aldosterone antagonist, since aldosterone may increase loss of magnesium, may increase cardiac sympathetic activity, and may increase the incidence of ventricular arrhythmias. Thus, it is interesting to note that combined use of spironolactone with an ACE inhibitor has both short- and long-term benefits.[182,183]

Continuous versus Intermittent Bolus Administration

Recently, there has been increased interest in giving continuous infusions of diuretics because of the ease of administering the drug in this manner in the setting of an intensive care unit and because of the theoretical argument that it provides a consistent urine flow and thus a more gentle shift in body fluids.[207,212] The degree of natriuresis induced by continuous diuretic infusion, however, is not significantly greater than that caused by equivalent doses given by bolus.[212] Furthermore, if potassium reabsorption is blocked continuously, it theoretically should lead to increased potassium deficiency. Indeed, at least two studies have demonstrated this to be the case.[208,209] Thus, while the continuous infusion of diuretics may be a viable option, I personally prefer bolus doses, since the expected metabolic complications will be diminished.

Dopamine Agonist

While dopamine is not a diuretic per se, it has been shown to increase renal blood flow and glomerular filtration rate in animals in some circumstances. It is therefore logical that when an oral dopaminergic agonist, ibopamine, was developed, trials would be undertaken to see if it would increase natriuresis in patients with congestive heart failure. Recent studies, however, showed only minimal effects on renal blood flow and natriuresis even though cardiac output was increased.[213–215]

Diuretics during Radiocontrast Infusion

Radiocontrast-induced renal failure is rare in individuals with normal renal function. Acute renal failure following coronary angiography may occur, however,[193,216–224] because of direct tubular toxicity from radiocontrast materials,[225] intrarenal tubular obstruction,[226] and decreased renal blood flow.[193,227–233] These factors are clinically important in the pathogenesis of acute renal failure in individuals who have underlying renal disease and in those who have effective arterial blood volume contraction, as in congestive heart failure.[223,230,234]

The most important risk factor for radiocontrast-induced renal failure is diabetic nephropathy. Patients with multiple myeloma are also at increased risk. Clearly, prophylactic measures to prevent renal failure are indicated. The easiest preventive step is to keep the patient in a somewhat volume-expanded state with a saline infusion. Volume expansion will clearly decrease the induction of renal vasoconstriction by contrast agents. Whether saline is better alone or in combination with mannitol is still an open question. In one study of the issues 20 consecutive patients with renal failure who received a

mannitol infusion before and during catheterization, no decrease in renal blood flow was seen,[193] while in a more recent, well-conducted, randomized trial on 78 patients, infusion of 0.45% saline alone was associated with a lower incidence of renal failure than if mannitol or furosemide were infused with the saline.[234] It is not clear why mannitol did not add further protection from renal failure.

The conclusion from all of these studies is that prevention of volume contraction is perhaps the most important factor in the prevention of nephrotoxicity. Except for mannitol, other diuretics do not seem to be of benefit and may in fact be harmful when used during infusion of radiocontrast materials.[234–236]

REFERENCES

1. Maddox DA, Gennari JF. The early proximal tubule: A high-capacity delivery-responsive reabsorptive site. *Am J Physiol* 1987; 252: F573–F584.
2. Ullrich KJ, Rumrich G, Fuchs G. Wasserpermeabilitat und transtubularer Wasserfluss corticaler Nephronabschnitte bei verschiedenen Diuresezustanden. *Pflugers Arch* 1964; 280:99–119.
3. Stolte H, Brecht JP, Wiederholt M, Hierholzer K. Einfluss von Adrenalektomie und Glucocorticoiden auf die Wasser-permeabilitat Cortikaler Nephronabschnitte der Rattenniere. *Pflugers Arch* 1968; 299:99–127.
4. Kokko JP, Burg MB, Orloff J. Characterization of NaCl and water transport in the renal proximal tubule. *J Clin Invest* 1971; 50:69–76.
5. Preisig PA, Berry CA. Evidence for transcellular osmotic water flow in rat proximal tubules. *Am J Physiol* 1985; 249:F124–F131.
6. DiBona GF. Effect of magnesium on water permeability of the rat nephron. *Am J Physiol* 1972; 223:1324–1326.
7. Green R, Giebisch G. Reflection coefficients and water permeability in rat proximal tubule. *Am J Physiol* 1989; 257:F658 F668.
8. Fromter EE, Rumrich G, Ullrich KJ. Phenomenological description of Na, Cl, and HCO_3 absorption from proximal tubules in the rat kidney. *Pflugers Arch* 1973; 343:189–220.
9. Green R, Giebisch G. Luminal hypotonicity: A driving force for fluid absorption from the proximal tubule. *Am J Physiol* 1984; 246: F167–F174.
10. Hierholzer K, Kawamura S, Seldin DW, Kokko JP, Jacobson HR. Reflection coefficients of various substrates across superficial and juxtamedullary proximal convoluted segments of rabbit nephrons. *Miner Electrolyte Metab* 1980; 3:172–180.
11. Jacobson HR, Kokko JP. Intrinsic differences in various segments of the proximal convoluted tubule. *J Clin Invest* 1976; 57:818–825.
12. Whittembury G, Oken DE, Windhager EE, Solomon AK. Single proximal tubules of Necturus kidney: IV. Dependence of H_2O movement on osmotic gradients. *Am J Physiol* 1959; 197:1121–1127.
13. Whittembury G, Paz-Aliaga A, Broudi A, Carpi-Medina P, Gonzales E, Linares H. Pathways for volume flow and volume regulation in leaky epithelia. *Pflugers Arch* 1985; 405:S17–S22.
14. Walker AM, Bott PA, Oliver J, MacDowell MC. The collection and analysis of fluid from single nephrons of the mammalian kidney. *Am J Physiol* 1941; 134:580–595.
15. Frohnert PP, Hohmann B, Zweibel R, Baumann K. Free flow micropuncture studies of glucose transport in the rat nephron. *Pflugers Arch* 1970; 315:66–85.
16. Barfuss DA, Schafer JA. Differences in active and passive glucose transport along the proximal tubule. *Am J Physiol* 1981; 240: F322–F332.
17. McKeown JW, Brazy PC, Dennis VW. Intrarenal heterogeneity for fluid, phosphate, and glucose absorption in the rabbit. *Am J Physiol* 1979; 237:F312–F318.
18. Tune BM, Burg MB. Glucose transport by proximal renal tubules. *Am J Physiol* 1971; 221:580–585.
19. Lingard J, Rumrich G, Young JA. Reabsorption of L-glutamine and L-histidine from various regions of the rat proximal convolution studied by stationary microperfusion: Evidence that the proximal convolution is not homogeneous. *Pflugers Arch* 1973; 342:1–12.

20. Bergeron M, Morel F. Amino acid transport in rat renal tubules. *Am J Physiol* 1969; 216:1139–1149.

21. Wright LA, Nicholson TF. The proximal tubular handling of amino acids and other ninhydrin-positive substances. *Can J Physiol Pharmacol* 1966; 44:183–193.

22. Eisenbach GM, Weise M, Stolte H. Amino acid reabsorption in the rat nephron. *Pflugers Arch* 1975; 357:63–76.

23. Silbernagl S. Tubular reabsorption of L-glutamine studied by free-flow micropuncture and microperfusion of rat kidney. *Int J Biochem* 1980; 12:9–16.

24. Lingard J, Rumrich G, Young JA. Kinetics of l-histidine transport in the proximal convolution of the rat nephron studied using the stationary microperfusion technique. *Pflugers Arch* 1973; 342:13–28.

25. Liu F-Y, Cogan MG. Axial heterogeneity in the rat proximal convoluted tubule: I. Bicarbonate, chloride, and water transport. *Am J Physiol* 1984; 247:F816–F821.

26. Liu F-Y, Cogan MG. Axial heterogeneity of bicarbonate, chloride and water transport in the rat proximal convoluted tubule. *J Clin Invest* 1986; 78:1547–1557.

27. Maddox DA, Atherton LJ, Deen WM, Gennari FJ. Proximal HCO$_3^-$ reabsorption and the determinants of tubular and capillary P$_{CO_2}$ in the rat. *Am J Physiol* 1984; 247:F73–F81.

28. Maddox DA, Gennari FJ. Load dependence of HCO$_3$ and H$_2$O reabsorption in the early proximal tubule of the Munich-Wistar rat. *Am J Physiol* 1985; 248:F113–F121.

29. Maddox DA, Gennari FJ. Load dependence of proximal tubular bicarbonate reabsorption in chronic metabolic alkalosis in the rat. *J Clin Invest* 1986; 77:709–716.

30. Maddox DA, Horn JF, Famiano FC, Gennari FJ. Load dependence of proximal tubular fluid and bicarbonate reabsorption in the remnant kidney of the Munich-Wistar rat. *J Clin Invest* 1986; 77:1639–1649.

31. Jacobson HR. Effects of CO$_2$ and acetazolamide on bicarbonate and fluid reabsorption in rabbit proximal tubules. *Am J Physiol* 1981; 240:F54–F62.

32. Neumann KH, Rector FC. Mechanism of NaCl and water reabsorption in the proximal convoluted tubule of the rat kidney. *J Clin Invest* 1976; 58:1110–1118.

33. Rector FC, Carter NW, Seldin DW. The mechanism of bicarbonate reabsorption in the proximal and distal tubules of the kidney. *J Clin Invest* 1965; 44:278–290.

34. Lucci MS, Tinker JP, Weiner IM, DuBose TD. Function of proximal tubule carbonic anhydrase defined by selective inhibition. *Am J Physiol* 1983; 245:F443–F449.

35. Rector FC. Sodium bicarbonate, and chloride absorption by the proximal tubule. *Am J Physiol* 1983; 244:F461–F471.

36. Cogan MG, Maddox DA, Warnock DG, Lin ET, Rector FC. Effect of acetazolamide on bicarbonate reabsorption in the proximal tubule of the rat. *Am J Physiol* 1979; 237:F447–F454.

37. Aronson PS. Mechanisms of active H$^+$ secretion in the proximal tubule. *Am J Physiol* 1983; 245:F647–F659.

38. Schafer JA, Patlak CS, Troutman SL, Andreoli TE. Volume absorption in the pars recta: II. Hydraulic conductivity coefficient. *Am J Physiol* 1978; 234:F340–F348.

39. Schafer JA. Mechanisms coupling the absorption of solute and water in the proximal nephron. *Kidney Int* 1984; 25:708–716.

40. Kawamura S, Imai M, Seldin DW, Kokko JP. Characteristics of salt and water transport in superficial and juxtamedullary straight segments of proximal tubules. *J Clin Invest* 1975; 55:1269–1277.

41. Schafer JA, Troutman SL, Andreoli TE. Volume reabsorption, trans-epithelial potential differences and ionic permeability properties in mammalian superficial proximal straight tubules. *J Gen Physiol* 1974; 64:582–607.

42. Weiner IM. Organic acids and bases and uric acid. In: Seldin DW, Giebisch G, eds. *The Kidney: Physiology and Pathophysiology*. New York: Raven Press; 1985: 1703–1724.

43. Wright SH, Wunz TM. Amiloride transport in rabbit renal brush-border membrane vesicles. *Am J Physiol* 1989; 256:F462–F468.

44. Dantzler WH, Wright SH, Chatsudthipong V, Brokl OH. Basolateral tetraethylammonium transport in intact tubules: Specificity and trans-stimulation. *Am J Physiol* 1991; 261:F386–F392.

45. Rose HJ, O'Malley K, Pruitt AW. Depression of renal clearance of furosemide in man by azotemia. *Clin Pharmacol Ther* 1976; 21:141–146.

46. Rose HJ, Pruitt AW, Dayton PG, McNay JL. Relationship of urinary furosemide excretion rate to natriuretic effect in experimental azotemia. *J Pharmacol Exp Ther* 1976; 199:490–497.

47. Rose HJ, Pruitt AW, McNay JL. Effect of experimental azotemia on renal clearance of furosemide in the dog. *J Pharmacol Exp Ther* 1976; 196:238–248.

48. Brater DC. Use of diuretics in chronic renal insufficiency and nephrotic syndrome. *Semin Nephrol* 1988; 8:333–341.

49. Kokko JP. Sodium chloride and water transport in the descending limb of Henle. *J Clin Invest* 1970; 49:1838–1846.

50. Imai M, Hayashi M, Araki M. Functional heterogeneity of the descending limbs of Henle's loop. I. Internephron heterogeneity in the hamster kidney. *Pflugers Arch* 1984; 402:385–392.

51. Imai M, Taniguchi J, Yoshitomi K. Transition of permeability properties along the descending limb of long-loop nephron. *Am J Physiol* 1988; 254:F323–F328.

52. Imai M, Kokko JP. Sodium, chloride, urea, and water transport in the thin ascending limb of Henle. *J Clin Invest* 1974; 53:393–402.

53. Morgan T, Berliner RW. Permeability of the loop of Henle, vasa recta, and collecting duct to water, urea, and sodium. *Am J Physiol* 1968; 215:108–115.

54. Imai M. Function of the thin ascending limbs of Henle of rats and hamsters perfused in vitro. *Am J Physiol* 1977; 232:F201–F209.

55. Kondo Y, Imai M. Effect of glutaraldehyde on renal tubular function: II. Selective inhibition of Cl$^-$ transport in the hamster thin ascending limb of Henle's loop. *Pflugers Arch* 1987; 408:484–490.

56. Burg M, Green N. Function of the thick ascending limb of Henle's loop. *Am J Physiol* 1973; 224:659–668.

57. Rocha AS, Kokko JP. Sodium chloride and water transport in the medullary thick ascending limb of Henle. Evidence for active chloride transport. *J Clin Invest* 1973; 52:612–623.

58. Kedem O. Criteria of active transport. In: Kleinzeller A, Kityk A, eds. *Membrane Transport and Metabolism*. Prague: Czechoslovak Academy of Sciences; 1961:87–93.

59. Greger R, Schlatter E. Properties of the lumen membrane of the cortical thick ascending limb of Henle's loop of rabbit kidney. *Pflugers Arch* 1983; 396:315–324.

60. Hebert SC, Andreoli TE. Control of NaCl transport in the thick ascending limb. *Am J Physiol* 1984; 246:F745–F756.

61. Burg M, Green N. Effect of ethacrynic acid on the thick ascending limb of Henle's loop. *Kidney Int* 1973; 4:301–308.

62. Burg M, Stoner L, Cardinal J, Green N. Furosemide effect on isolated perfused tubules. *Am J Physiol* 1973; 225:119–224.

63. Greger R. Coupled transport of Na$^+$ and Cl$^-$ in the thick ascending limb of Henle's loop of rabbit nephron. *Scand J Audiol* 1981; 14:1–15.

64. Greger R, Schlatter E. Cellular mechanism of the action of loop diuretics on the thick ascending limb of Henle's loop. *Klin Wochenschr* 1983; 61:1019–1027.

65. Kokko JP. Membrane characteristics governing salt and water transport in the loop of Henle. *Fed Proc* 1974; 33:25–30.

66. Imai M. Effect of bumetanide and furosemide on the thick ascending limb of Henle's loop of rabbits and rats perfused in vitro. *Eur J Pharmacol* 1977; 41:409–416.

67. Wangemann P, Wittner M, DiStefano A, Englert HC, Lang HJ, Schlatter E, et al. Cl$^-$ channel blockers in the thick ascending limb of the loop of Henle. *Pflugers Arch* 1986;407:S128–S141.

68. Greven J. Studies on the renal receptors of loop diuretics. *Clin Exp Hypertens Theory Pract* 1983; A5:193–208.

69. Greven J. The pharmacological basis of the action of loop diuretics. In: Puschett JB, Greenberg A, eds. *Diuretics II*. New York: Elsevier Science; 1986:173–181.

70. Quamme GA. Control of magnesium transport in the thick ascending limb. *Am J Physiol* 1989; 256:F197–F210.

71. Quamme GA. Effect of furosemide on calcium and magnesium transport in the rat nephron. *Am J Physiol* 1981; 241:F340–F347.

72. Suki WN, Rouse D, Ng RCK, Kokko JP. Calcium transport in the thick ascending limb of Henle: Heterogeneity of function in the medullary and cortical segments. *J Clin Invest* 1980; 66:1004–1009.

73. Costanzo LS, Windhager EE. Calcium and sodium transport by the distal convoluted tubule of the rat. *Am J Physiol* 1978; 235:F493–F506.

74. Shimizu T, Yoshitomi K, Nakamura M, Imai M. Site and mechanism of action of trichlormethiazide in rabbit distal nephron segments perfused in vitro. *J Clin Invest* 1988; 82:721–730.

75. Stokes J, Lee I, D'Amico M. Sodium chloride absorption by the urinary bladder of the winter flounder: A thiazide-sensitive, electrically neutral transport system. *J Clin Invest* 1984; 74:7–16.

76. Ellison DH, Velazquez H, Wright FS. Thiazide-sensitive sodium chloride cotransport in early distal tubule. *Am J Physiol* 1987; 253:F546–F554.

77. Kunau RT, Weller DR, Webb HL. Clarification of the site of action of chlorothiazide in the rat nephron. *J Clin Invest* 1975; 56:401–407.

78. Gross JB, Imai M, Kokko JP. A functional comparison of the cortical collecting tubule and the distal convoluted tubule. *J Clin Invest* 1975; 55:1284–1294.

79. Ashraf N, Locksley R, Arieff A. Thiazide-induced hyponatremia associated with death or neurologic damage in outpatients. *Am J Med* 1981; 70:1163–1168.

80. Lucci MS, Pucacco LR, Carter NW, DuBose TD. Evaluation of bicarbonate transport in rat distal tubule: Effects of acid-base status. *Am J Physiol* 1982; 243:F335–F341.

81. Schuster VL, Stokes JB. Chloride transport by the cortical and outer medullary collecting duct. *Am J Physiol* 1987; 253:F203–F212.

82. Koeppen BM, Biagi BA, Giebisch G. Intracellular microelectrode characterization of the rabbit cortical collecting duct. *Am J Physiol* 1983; 244:F35–F47.

83. O'Neil RG, Helman SI. Transport characteristics of renal collecting tubules: Influences of DOCA and diet. *Am J Physiol* 1977; 233:F544–F558.

84. O'Neil RG, Sansom SC. Characterization of apical cell membrane Na$^+$ and K$^+$ conductances of cortical collecting duct using microelectrode techniques. *Am J Physiol* 1984; 247:F14–F24.

85. O'Neil RG, Sansom SC. Electrophysiological properties of cellular and paracellular conductive pathways of the rabbit cortical collecting duct. *J Membr Biol* 1984; 82:281–295.

86. Palmer LG, Frindt G. Amiloride-sensitive Na channels from the apical membrane of the rat cortical collecting tubule. *Proc Natl Acad Sci USA* 1986; 83:2767–2770.

87. Ling BN, Hinton CF, Eaton DC. Amiloride-sensitive sodium channels in rabbit cortical collecting tubule primary cultures. *Am J Physiol* 1991; 261:F933–F944.

88. Doucet A, Morel F, Katz AI. Microdetermination of Na-K-ATPase in single tubules: Its application for the localization of physiologic processes in the nephron. *Int J Biochem* 1980; 12:47–52.

89. El Mernissi G, Chabardes D, Doucet A, Hus-Citharel A, Imbert-Teboul M, Le Bouffiant F, et al. Changes in tubular basolateral membrane markers after chronic DOCA treatment. *Am J Physiol* 1983; 245:F100–F109.

90. Garg LC, Knepper MA, Burg MB. Mineralocorticoid effects on Na-K-ATPase in individual nephron segments. *Am J Physiol* 1981; 240:F536–F544.

91. Horster M, Schmid H, Schimidt V. Aldosterone in vitro restores nephron Na-K-ATPase of distal segments from adrenalectomized rabbits. *Pflugers Arch* 1980; 384:203–206.

92. LeHir M, Kaissling B, Dubach UC. Distal tubular segments of the rabbit kidney after adaptation to altered NA- and K-intake: II. Changes in Na-K-ATPase activity. *Cell Tissue Res* 1982; 224:493–504.

93. Mujais SK, Chekal MA, Jones WJ, Hayslett JP, Katz AI. Regulation of renal Na-K-ATPase in the rat. *J Clin Invest* 1984; 73:13–19.

94. O'Neil RG, Hayhurst RA. Sodium-dependent modulation of the renal Na-K-ATPase: Influence of mineralocorticoids on the cortical collecting duct. *J Membr Biol* 1985; 85:169–179.

95. Petty KJ, Kokko JP, Marver D. Secondary effect of aldosterone on Na-K-ATPase activity in the rabbit cortical collecting tubule. *J Clin Invest* 1981; 68:1514–1521.

96. Helman SI, Kizer NL. Apical sodium ion channels of tight epithelia as viewed from the perspective of noise analysis. *Cur Top Membr Transp* 1990; 37:117–155.

97. Fanestil DD. Mechanism of action of aldosterone blockers. *Semin Nephrol* 1988; 8:240–263.

98. Early LE, Kahn M, Orloff J. The effects of infusions of chlorothiazide on urinary dilution and concentration in the dog. *J Clin Invest* 1961; 40:857–866.

99. Suki W, Rector FC, Seldin DW. The site of action of furosemide and other sulfonamide diuretics in the dog. *J Clin Invest* 1965; 44:1458–1469.

100. Seldin DW, Eknoyan G, Suki WN, Rector FC. Localization of diuretic action from the pattern of water and electrolyte excretion. *Ann NY Acad Sci* 1966; 139:328–343.

101. Velazquez H, Wright FS. Effect of diuretic drugs on Na, Cl, and K transport by rat renal distal tubule. *Am J Physiol* 1986; 250:F1013–F1023.

102. Schwartz GJ, Burg MB. Mineralocorticoid effects on cation transport by cortical collecting tubules in vitro. *Am J Physiol* 1978; 235:576–585.

103. Field MJ, Stanton BA, Giebisch G. Differential acute effects of aldosterone, dexamethasone, and hyperkalemia on distal tubule potassium secretion in the rat kidney. *J Clin Invest* 1984; 74:1792–1802.

104. Finnerty FA, Maxwell MH, Kuhn J, Moser M. Long-term effects of furosemide and hydrochlorothiazide in patients with essential hypertension. *Angiology* 1977; 28:125–133.

105. Morgan DB, Davidson C. Hypokalemia and diuretics: An analysis of publications. *Br Med J* 1980; 280:905–908.

106. Multicenter Cooperative Study Group. Multiclinic comparison of amiloride, hydrochlorothiazide, and hydrochlorothiazide plus amiloride in essential hypertension. *Arch Intern Med* 1981; 141:482–486.

107. Araoye MA, Chang MY, Khatri IM, Freise D. Furosemide compared with hydrochlorothiazide. *JAMA* 1978; 240:1863–1866.

108. Anderson J, Godfrey BE, Hill DM, Munro-Faure AD, Sheldon J. A comparison of the effects of hydrochlorothiazide and furosemide in the treatment of hypertensive patients. *Q J Med* 1971; 15:541–560.

109. Schnaper HW, Freis ED, Friedman RG, Garland WT, Hall WD, Hollifield J, et al. Potassium restoration in hypertensive patients made hypokalemic by hydrochlorothiazide. *Arch Intern Med* 1989; 149:2677–2681.

110. Gorden P. Glucose intolerance with hypokalemia. *Diabetes* 1973; 22:544–551.

111. Sagild U, Andersen V, Andreasen PB. Glucose tolerance and insulin responsiveness in experimental potassium depletion. *Acta Med Scand* 1961; 169:243–251.

112. Helderman JH, Elahi D, Andersen DK, Raizes GS, Tobin JD, Schocken D, et al. Prevention of the glucose intolerance of thiazide diuretics by maintenance of body potassium. *Diabetes* 1983; 32:106–111.

113. Dyckner T, Helmers C, Lundman T, Wester PO. Initial serum potassium level in relation to early complications and prognosis in patients with acute myocardial infarction. *Acta Med Scand* 1975; 197:207–210.

114. Dyckner T, Helmers C, Wester PO. Cardiac dysrhythmias in patients with acute myocardial infarction: Relation to serum potassium level and prior diuretic therapy. *Acta Med Scand* 1984; 216:127–132.

115. Solomon RJ, Cole AG. Importance of potassium in patients with acute myocardial infarction. *Acta Med Scand* 1981; 647(suppl):87–93.

116. Nordrehaug JR, von der Lippe G. Hypokalemia and ventricular fibrillation in acute myocardial infarction. *Br Heart J* 1983; 50:525–529.

117. Johansson BW, Dziamski R. Malignant arrhythmias in acute myocardial infarction: Relationship to serum potassium and effect of selective and nonselective beta-blockade. *Drugs* 1984; 28(suppl 1):77–85.

118. Steiness E, Olesen KH. Cardiac arrhythmias induced by hypokalemia and potassium loss during maintenance digoxin therapy. *Br Heart J* 1976; 38:167–172.

119. Jelliffe RW. Effect of serum potassium level upon risk of digitalis toxicity. *Ann Intern Med* 1973; 78:821.

120. Seller RH. The role of magnesium in digitalis toxicity. *Am Heart J* 1971; 82:551–556.

121. Tannen RL. Potassium and blood pressure control. *Ann Intern Med* 1983; 98:773–780.

122. Paller MS, Linas SL. Hemodynamic effects of alterations in potassium. *Hypertension* 1982; 4:III20–III26.

123. Paller MS, Douglas JG, Linas SL. Mechanism of decreased vascular reactivity to angiotensin II in conscious, potassium-deficient rats. *J Clin Invest* 1984; 73:74–79.

124. Linas SL, Dickmann D. Mechanism of the decreased renal blood flow in the potassium-depleted conscious rat. *Kidney Int* 1982; 21:757–764.

125. Abbrecht PH. Cardiovascular effects of chronic potassium deficiency in the dog. *Am J Physiol* 1972; 223:555–560.

126. Knochel JP, Schlein EM. On the mechanism of rhabdomyolysis in potassium depletion. *J Clin Invest* 1972; 51:1750–1758.

127. Dominic JA, Koch M, Guthrie CP, Gallas JH. Primary aldosteronism presenting as myoglobinuric acute renal failure. *Arch Intern Med* 1978; 138:1433–1434.

128. Nadel SM, Jackson JW, Ploth DW. Hypokalemic rhabdomyolysis and acute renal failure: Occurrence following total parenteral nutrition. *JAMA* 1979; 241:2294–2296.

129. Bierbach H, Bohl J, Goldner HJ, Majdandzic J. Hypokalemic rhabdomyolysis associated with Barter's syndrome. *Klin Wochenschr* 1983; 61:183–186.

130. Patterson RE, Haut MJ, Montgomery CA, Lowensohn HS, McQuilken CT, Djuh YY, et al. Natural history of potassium-deficiency myopathy in the dog: Role of adrenocorticosteroid in rhabdomyolysis. *J Lab Clin Med* 1983; 102:565–576.

131. Kaplan NM, Carnegie A, Raskin P, Heller JA, Simmons M. Potassium supplementation in hypertensive patients with diuretic-induced hypokalemia. *N Engl J Med* 1985; 12:746–749.

132. Nader PC, Thompson JR, Alpern RJ. Complications of diuretic use. *Semin Nephrol* 1988; 8:365–387.

133. Suki WN, Hull AR, Rector FC. Mechanism of the effect of thiazide diuretics on calcium and uric acid. *J Clin Invest* 1967; 46:1121.

134. Manuel MA, Steele TH. Changes in renal urate handling after prolonged thiazide treatment. *Am J Med* 1974; 57:741–746.

135. Langford HG, Blaufox MD, Borhani NO, Curb JD, Molteni A, Schneider KA, et al. Is thiazide-produced uric acid elevation harmful? *Arch Intern Med* 1987; 147:645–649.

136. Brickman AS, Massry SG, Coburn JW. Changes in serum and urinary calcium during treatment with hydrochlorothiazide: Studies on mechanisms. *J Clin Invest* 1972; 51:945–954.

137. Seitz H, Jaworski ZF. Effect of hydrochlorothiazide on serum and urinary calcium and urinary citrate. *Can Med Assoc J* 1964; 90:414–420.

138. Duarte CG, Winnacker JL, Becker KL, Pace A. Thiazide-induced hypercalcemia. *N Engl J Med* 1971; 284:828–830.

139. Yendt ER, Guay GF, Garcia DA. The use of thiazides in the prevention of renal calculi. *Can Med Assoc J* 1970; 102:614–620.

140. Ljunghall S, Backman U, Danielson BG, Fellstrom B, Johansson G, Wikstrom B. Calcium and magnesium metabolism during long-term treatment with thiazides. *Scand J Urol Nephrol* 1981; 15:257–262.

141. Ames RP, Hill P. Antihypertensive therapy and the risk of coronary heart disease. *J Cardiol Pharm* 1982; 4:206–212.

142. Boehringer K, Weidmann P, Mordasini R, Schiffl H, Bachmann C, Riesen W. Menopause-dependent plasma lipoprotein alterations in diuretic-treated women. *Ann Intern Med* 1982; 97:206–209.

143. Gluck Z, Weidmann P, Mordasini R, Bachmann C, Riesen W, Peheim E, et al. Increased serum low-density lipoprotein cholesterol in men treated short term with the diuretic chlorthalidone. *Metabolism* 1980; 29:240–245.

144. Grimm RH, Leon AS, Hunninghake DB, Lenz K, Hannan P, Blackburn H. Effects of thiazide diuretics on plasma lipids and lipoproteins in mildly hypertensive patients. *Ann Intern Med* 1981; 94:7–11.

145. Ames RP, Hill P. Elevation or serum lipid levels during diuretic therapy of hypertension. *Am J Med* 1976; 61:748–757.

146. Chrysant SG, Neller GK, Dillard B, Frohlich ED. Effects of diuretics on lipid metabolism in patients with essential hypertension. *Angiology* 1976; 27:707–711.

147. Goldman AI, Steele BW, Schnaper HW, Fitz AE, Frohlich ED, Perry HM Jr. Serum lipoprotein levels during chlorthalidone therapy. A Veterans Administration–National Heart, Lung, and Blood Institute Cooperative Study on Antihypertensive Therapy: Mild Hypertension. *JAMA* 1980; 244:1691–1695.

148. Lasser NL, Grandits G, Caggiula AW, Cutler JA, Grimm RH Jr, Kuller LH, et al. Effects of antihypertensive therapy on plasma lipids and lipoproteins in the multiple risk factor intervention trial. *Am J Med* 1984; 76:52–66.

149. Middeke M, Weisweiler P, Schwandt P, Holzgreve H. Serum lipoproteins during antihypertensive therapy with beta blockers and diuretics: A controlled long-term comparative trial. *Clin Cardiol* 1987; 10:94–98.

150. Black HR. Metabolic considerations in the choice of therapy for the patient with hypertension. *Am Heart J* 1991; 121:707–715.

151. Carlsen JE, Kober L, Torp-Pedersen C, Johansen P. Relation between dose of bendrofluazide, antihypertensive effect, and adverse biochemical effects. *Br Med J* 1990; 300:975–978.

152. Kinne R. Molecular properties of the sodium-potassium-chloride cotransport system in the kidney. In: Puschett JB, Greenberg A, eds. *Diuretics II: Chemistry, Pharmacology, and Clinical Applications.* New York: Elsevier; 1987:138–144.

153. Dargie HJ, Boddy K, Kennedy AC, King PC, Read PR, Ward DM. Total body potassium and long term furosemide therapy: Is potassium supplementation necessary? *Br Med J* 1974; 4:316–319.

154. Manner RJ, Brechbill DO, Dewitt K. Prevalence of hypokalemia in diuretic therapy. *Clin Med* 1972; 79:15–18.

155. Licht JH, Haley RJ, Pugh B, Lewis SB. Diuretic regimens in essential hypertension: A comparison of hypokalemia effects, BP control, and cost. *Arch Intern Med* 1983; 143:1694–1699.

156. Black WD, Shiner PT, Roman J. Severe electrolyte disturbances associated with metolazone and furosemide. *South Med J* 1978; 71:380–385.

157. Epstein M, Lepp BA, Hoffman DS, Levinson R. Potentiation of furosemide by metolazone in refractory edema. *Curr Ther Res* 1977; 21:656–667.

158. Eknoyan G, Suki WN, Martinez-Maldonado M. Effect of diuretics on urinary excretion of phosphate, calcium, and magnesium in thyroparathyroidectomized dogs. *J Lab Clin Med* 1970; 76:257–266.

159. Davies DL, Lant AF, Millard NR, Smith AJ, Ward JW. Renal action, therapeutic use, and pharmacokinetics of the diuretic bumetanide. *Clin Pharm Ther* 1974; 15:141–155.

160. Shareghi GR, Agus ZS. Magnesium transport in the cortical thick ascending limb of Henle's loop of the rabbit. *J Clin Invest* 1982; 69:759–769.

161. Quamme GA. Effect of furosemide on calcium and magnesium transport in the rat nephron. *Am J Physiol* 1981; 241:340–347.

162. Hollifield JW. Potassium and magnesium abnormalities: Diuretics and arrhythmias in hypertension. *Am J Med* 1984; 77:28–32.

163. Dyckner T, Wester PO. Ventricular extrasystoles and intracellular electrolytes before and after potassium and magnesium infusions in patients on diuretic treatment. *Am Heart J* 1979; 97:12–18.

164. Rybak LP. Pathophysiology of furosemide ototoxicity. *J Otolaryngol* 1982; 11:127–133.

165. Meriwether WD, Mangi RJ, Serpick AA. Deafness following standard intravenous dose of ethacrynic acid. *JAMA* 1971; 216:795–798.

166. David DS, Hitzig P. Diuretics and ototoxicity. *N Engl J Med* 1971; 284:1328–1329.

167. Schwartz GH, David DS, Riggio RR, Stenzel KH, Rubin AL. Ototoxicity induced by furosemide. *N Engl J Med* 1970; 282:1413–1414.

168. Lloyd-Mostyn RH, Lord IJ. Ototoxicity of intravenous furosemide. *Lancet* 1971; 2:1156–1157.

169. Clasen W, Kindler J, Khartabil T, Imm S, Frisch J, Sieberth HG. Torasemide versus furosemide in patients with advanced chronic renal failure—Effect on saliuresis, renin-aldosterone-system and cochlear function. In: Puschett JB, Greenberg A, eds. *Diuretics II: Chemistry, Pharmacology, and Clinical Applications.* New York: Elsevier; 1987:53–57.

170. Suki WN, Yium JJ, Von Minden M, Saller-Hebert C, Eknoyan G, Martinez-Maldonado M. Acute treatment of hypercalcemia with furosemide. *N Engl J Med* 1970; 283:836–840.

171. Gadbow PA, Hanson TJ, Popovtzer MM, Schrier RW. Furosemide-induced reduction in ionized calcium in hypoparathyroid patients. *Ann Intern Med* 1977; 85:579–581.

172. Bourdeau JE, Buss SL, Vurek GG. Inhibition of calcium absorption in the cortical thick ascending limb of Henle's loop by furosemide. *J Pharm Exp Ther* 1982; 221:815–819.

173. Greenblatt DJ, Koch-Wester J. Adverse reactions to spironolactone. A report from the Boston collaborative drug surveillance program. *JAMA* 1973; 225:40–43.

174. McNay JL, Oran E. Possible predisposition of diabetic patients to hyperkalemia following administration of potassium-retaining diuretic, amiloride (MK 870). *Metabolism* 1970; 19:58–70.

175. Crosley AP, Ronquillo LM, Strickland WH, et al. Triamterene, a new natriuretic agent. *Ann Intern Med* 1962; 56:241–251.

176. Whiting GFM, McLaran CJ, Bochner F. Severe hyperkalemia with Moduretic. *Med J Aust* 1979; 1:409.

177. Cohen AB. Hyperkalemic effects of triamterene. *Ann Intern Med* 1966; 65:521–527.

178. Walker BR, Capuzzi DM, Alexander F, Familiar RG, Hoppe RC. Hyperkalemia after triamterene in diabetic patients. *Clin Pharm Ther* 1972; 13:643–651.

179. Ponce SP, Jennings AE, Madias NE, Harrington JT. Drug-induced hyperkalemia. *Medicine* 1985; 64:357–370.

180. Rose LI, Underwood RH, Newmark SR, Kisch ES, Williams GH. Pathophysiology of spironolactone-induced gynecomastia. *Ann Intern Med* 1977; 87:398–403.

181. Huffman DH, Kampmann JP, Hignite CE, Azarnoff DL. Gynecomastia induced in normal males by spironolactone. *Clin Pharmacol Ther* 1978; 24:465–473.

182. Dahlstrom U, Karlsson E. Captopril and spironolactone therapy for refractory congestive heart failure. *Am J Cardiol* 1993; 71:29A–33A.

183. Barr CS, Lang CC, Hanson J, Arnott M, Kennedy N, Struthers AD. Effects of adding spironolactone to an angiotensin-converting enzyme inhibitor in chronic congestive heart failure secondary to coronary artery disease. *Am J Cardiol* 1995; 76:1259–1265.

184. Counihan TB, Evans BM, Milne MD. Observations on the pharmacology of the carbonic anhydrase inhibitor "Diamox." *Clin Sci* 1954; 13:583–598.

185. Epstein DL. Carbonic anhydrase inhibitor side effects. Serum chemical analysis. *Arch Ophthalmol* 1977; 95:1378–1382.

186. Siklos P, Henderson RG. Severe acidosis from acetazolamide in a diabetic patient. *Curr Med Res Opin* 1979; 6:284–286.

187. O'Sullivan PJ, Crowley JG, Muldowney FP. A case of acetazolamide induced (Diamox) acidotic coma in polycystic renal disease. *J Irish Med Assoc* 1967; 60:382–384.

188. Seely JF, Dirks JH. Micropuncture study of hypertonic mannitol diuresis in the proximal and distal tubule of the dog kidney. *J Clin Invest* 1969; 48:2330–2340.

189. Blantz RC, Israelit AH, Rector FC, Seldin DW. Relation of distal tubular NaCl delivery and glomerular hydrostatic pressure. *Kidney Int* 1972; 2:22–32.

190. Goldberg AH, Lilienfield LS. Effects of hypertonic mannitol on renal vascular resistance. *Proc Soc Exp Biol Med* 1965; 119:635–642.

191. Flores J, DiBona DR, Beck CH, Leaf A. The role of cell swelling in ischemic renal damage and the protective effect of hypertonic solute. *J Clin Invest* 1972; 51:118–226.

192. Blantz RC. Effect of mannitol on glomerular ultrafiltration in the hydropenic rat. *J Clin Invest* 1974; 54:1135–1143.

193. Kurnik BRC, Weisberg LS, Cuttler IM, Kurnik PB. Effects of atrial natriuretic peptide versus mannitol on renal blood flow during radiocontrast infusion in chronic renal failure. *J Lab Clin Med* 1990; 116:27–35.

194. Morris CR, Alexander EA, Bruns FJ, Levinsky MG. Restoration and maintenance of glomerular filtration by mannitol during hypoperfusion of the kidney. *J Clin Invest* 1972; 51:1555–1564.

195. Dzau VJ, Colucci WS, Hollenberg NK, Williams GH. Relation of the renin-angiotensin-aldosterone system to clinical state in congestive heart failure. *Circulation* 1981; 63:645–651.

196. Dzau VJ, Colucci WS, Williams GH, Curfman G, Meggs L, Hollenberg NK. Sustained effectiveness of converting-enzyme inhibition in patients with severe congestive heart failure. *N Engl J Med* 1980; 302:1373–1379.

197. Ader R, Chatterjee K, Ports T, Brundage B, Hiramatsu B, Parmley W. Immediate and sustained hemodynamic and clinical improvement in chronic heart failure by an oral angiotensin-converting enzyme inhibitor. *Circulation* 1980; 61:931–937.

198. Captopril Multicenter Research Group. A placebo-controlled trial of captopril in refractory congestive heart failure. *J Am Coll Cardiol* 1983; 2:755–763.

199. Odemuyiwa O, Gilmartin J, Kenny D, Hall RJC. Captopril and the diuretic requirements in moderate and severe chronic heart failure. *Eur Heart J* 1989; 10:586–590.

200. SOLVD Investigators. Effect of enalapril on survival in patients with reduced left ventricular ejection fractions and congestive heart failure. *N Engl J Med* 1991; 325:293–302.

201. Reed S, Greene P, Ryan T, Cerimele B, Schwertschlag U, Weinberger M, et al. The renin angiotensin aldosterone system and furosemide response in congestive heart failure. *Br J Clin Pharmacol* 1995; 39:51–57.

202. Davis R, Ribner HS, Keung B, Sonnenblick EH, LeJemtel TH. Treatment of chronic congestive heart failure with captopril, an oral inhibitor of angiotensin-converting enzyme. *N Engl J Med* 1979; 102:117–121.

203. Kokko JP. The role of the kidney in acute congestive heart failure: Treatment. *Cardiovasc Rev Rep* 1987; 8:60–63.

204. Wilcox CS, Mitch WE, Kelly RA, Skorecki K, Meyer TW, Friedman PA, et al. Response of the kidney to furosemide: I. Effects of salt intake and renal compensation. *J Lab Clin Med* 1983; 102:450–458.

205. Kelly RA, Wilcox CS, Mitch WE, Meyer TW, Souney PF, Rayment CM, et al. Response of the kidney to furosemide: II. Effect of captopril on sodium balance. *Kidney Int* 1983; 24:233–239.

206. Cook JA, Smith DE, Cornish LA, Tankanow RM, Nicklas JM, Hyneck ML. Kinetics, dynamics, and bioavailability of bumetanide in healthy subjects and patients with congestive heart failure. *Clin Pharmacol Ther* 1988; 44:487–500.

207. Martin S, Danziger LH. Continuous infusion of loop diuretics: pharmacodynamic concepts and clinical applications. *Clin Trends Pharm Pract* 1994; 8:10–13.

208. Singh NC, Kissoon N, Al Mofada S, Bennett M, Bohn DJ. Comparison of continuous versus intermittent furosemide administration in postoperative pediatric cardiac patients. *Crit Care Med* 1992; 20:17–21.

209. Copeland JG, Campbell DW, Plachetka JR, Salomon NW, Larson DF. Diuresis with continuous infusion of furosemide after cardiac surgery. *Am J Surg* 1983; 146:796–799.

210. Alvan G, Holleday J, Lindholm A, Sanz E, Villen T. Diuretic effect and diuretic efficiency after intravenous dosage of furosemide. *Br J Clin Pharmacol* 1990; 29:215–219.

211. Yelton SL, Gaylor MA, Murray KM. The role of continuous infusion loop diuretics. *Ann Pharmacother* 1995; 29:1010–1014.

212. Kramer WG, Smith WB, Ferduson J, Serpas T, Grant AG, Black PK, et al. Pharmacodynamics of torsemide administered as an intravenous injection and as a continuous infusion to patients with congestive heart failure. *J Clin Pharmacol* 1996; 36:265–270.

213. Dei Cas L, Metra M, Visioli O. Effects of acute and chronic ibopamine administration on resting and exercise hemodynamics, plasma catecholamines and functional capacity of patients with chronic congestive heart failure. *Am J Cardiol* 1992; 70:629–634.

214. Lieverse AG, van Veldhuisen DJ, Smit AJ, Zijlstra JG, Meijer S, Reitsma WD, et al. Renal and systemic hemodynamic effects of ibopamine in patients with mild to moderate congestive heart failure. *J Cardiovasc Pharmacol* 1995; 25:361–367.

215. Lieverse AG, Girbest ARJ, van Veldhuisen DJ, Smit AJ, Zulstra JG, Meuer S, et al. The effects of ibopamine on glomerular filtration rate and plasma norepinephrine remain preserved during prolonged treatment in patients with congestive heart failure. *Eur Heart J* 1995; 16:937–942.

216. D'Elia JA, Gleason RE, Alday M, Malarick C, Godley K, Warram J, et al. Nephrotoxicity from angiographic contrast material. *Am J Med* 1982; 72:719–725.

217. Eisenberg RL, Bank WO, Hedgcock MW. Renal failure after major angiography. *Am J Med* 1980; 68:43–46.

218. Hou SH, Bushinsky DA, Wish JB, Cohen JJ, Harrington JT. Hospital acquired renal insufficiency: A prospective study. *Am J Med* 1983; 74:243–247.

219. Weinrauch LA, Healy RW, Leland OS, Goldstein HH, Kassissieh SD, Libertino JA, et al. Coronary angiography and acute renal failure in diabetic azotemic nephropathy. *Ann Intern Med* 1977; 86:56–59.

220. Martin-Paredero V, Dixon SM, Baker JD, Takiff H, Gomes AS, Busutil RW, et al. Risk of renal failure after major angiography. *Arch Surg* 1983; 118:1417–1420.

221. Kumar S, Hull J, Lathi S, Cohen AJ, Pletka PG. Low incidence of renal failure after angiography. *Arch Intern Med* 1981; 141:1268–1270.

222. Gomes AS, Baker JD, Martin-Paredero V, Dixon SM, Takiff H, Machleder HI, et al. Acute renal dysfunction after major arteriography. *Am J Radiol* 1985; 145:1249–1253.

223. Taliercio CP, Vlietstra RE, Fisher LD, Burnett JC. Risks for renal dysfunction with cardiac angiography. *Ann Intern Med* 1986; 104:501–504.

224. Schwab SJ, Hlatky MA, Pieper KS, Davidson CJ, Morris KG, Skelton TN, et al. Contrast nephrotoxicity: A randomized controlled trial of a nonionic and an ionic radiographic contrast agent. *N Engl J Med* 1989; 320:149–153.

225. Humes HD, Hunt DA, White MD. Direct toxic effect of the radiocontrast agent diatrizoate on renal proximal tubule cells. *Am J Physiol* 1987; 252:F246–F255.

226. Zager RA, Timmerman TP, Merola AJ. Effects of immediate blood flow enhancement on the post ischemic kidney: Functional, morphologic and biochemical assessments. *J Lab Clin Med* 1985; 106:360–368.

227. Aperia A, Broberger O, Ekengren K. Renal hemodynamics during selective renal angiography. *Invest Radiol* 1968; 3:389–396.

228. Talner LB, Davidson AJ. Effect of contrast media on renal extraction of PAH. *Invest Radiol* 1968; 3:301–309.

229. Norby LH, DiBona GF. The renal vascular effects of meglumine diatrizoate. *J Pharm Exp Ther* 1975; 193:932–940.

230. Margulies KB, Hildebrand FL, Lerman A, Perella MA, Burnett JC.

Increased endothelin in experimental heart failure. *Circulation* 1990; 82:2226–2230.

231. Margulies KB, McKinley LJ, Cavero PG, Burnett JC. Induction and prevention of radiocontrast-induced nephropathy in dogs with heart failure. *Kidney Int* 1990; 38:1101–1108.

232. Talner LB, Davidson AJ. Renal hemodynamic effects of contrast media. *Invest Radiol* 1968; 3:310–317.

233. Margulies KB, Hildebrand FL, Heublein DM, Burnett JC. Radiocontrast increases plasma and urinary endothelin. *J Am Soc Nephrol* 1991; 2:1041–1045.

234. Solomon R, Werner C, Mann D, D'Elia J, Silva P. Effects of saline, mannitol, and furosemide on acute decreases in renal function induced by radiocontrast agents. *N Engl J Med* 1994; 331:1416–1420.

235. Rudnick MR, Goldfarb S, Murphy MJ. Mannitol and other prophylactic regimens in contrast media-induced acute renal failure. *Coron Artery Dis* 1991; 2:1047–1052.

236. Weinstein JM, Heyman S, Brezis M. Potential deleterious effect of furosemide in radiocontrast nephropathy. *Nephron* 1992; 62:413–415.

25

CARDIAC TRANSPLANTATION, MECHANICAL VENTRICULAR SUPPORT, AND ENDOMYOCARDIAL BIOPSY

Sharon A. Hunt / John S. Schroeder / Gerald J. Berry / Margaret E. Billingham

HISTORY/OVERVIEW

Although a number of advances in therapy for failing myocardium have saved or at least prolonged the lives of many patients with previously terminal myocardial dysfunction, there remains a sizable number of young patients who are fated to die or be severely disabled because of irreversible myocardial disease. In patients with such end-stage disease, biologic replacement of the heart has come to be a standard therapy and is currently widely accepted as a modality for prolonging life and improving its quality in carefully selected patients. As technological and engineering advances occur, mechanical replacement of the heart and xenotransplantation (transplantation of animal organs) may well become very competitive or complementary modalities for treatment of such patients, but biologic replacement with human donor hearts is the current standard of therapy.

Interest in developing the surgical techniques to interpose a functioning heart into a recipient's circulation dates back at least to the early part of the twentieth century. In 1905, Alexis Carrel[1] first described heterotopic transplantation of a functioning donor heart into the neck of a dog. The heart in this model functioned in sequence with the recipient's heart in the circulation and was not actually capable of supporting the circulation. Although the exact anatomic connections were not described in detail, this apparently nonworking model of heterotopic transplantation beat regularly for approximately 2 h before the blood clotted in all chambers. Carrel's initial interest was in the concept of performing vascular anastomoses, an interest reportedly stimulated by his distress at the inability of the best French surgeons of the time to avert the death by exsanguination from a severed portal vein of the president of the French republic.[2] Carrel and his colleague Guthrie developed innovative surgical techniques for vascular anastomoses at the University of Chicago, and these set the stages for the anastomoses leading to organ transplantation. This work was a major part of the body of work for which Dr. Carrel was awarded the Nobel Prize for Medicine and Physiology in 1912.

Work in the field lay dormant until Dr. Frank Mann and coworkers from the Mayo Clinic published their seminal report in 1933 of a technique for heterotopic heart transplantation with circulatory loading of the right ventricle.[3] Presumably because this was a working model, the chambers did not clot immediately, and the hearts in his dogs beat for a mean of 4 days. Mann perceived several important surgical points, including the importance of avoiding ventricular distension and air embolism and the prevention of thrombosis by heparin, but his most incisive and critical observation was that failure of the transplanted heart was, in fact, not always due to faulty surgical technique "but to some biologic factor which is probably identical to that which prevents survival of other homotransplanted tissues and organs." In what was undoubtedly the first description of acute allograft rejection, Mann recounts: "When the heart was removed just before it became quiescent . . . the surface of the heart was covered with mottled areas of ecchymoses . . . histologically the heart was completely infiltrated by large mononuclears and polymorphonuclears." Although various other animal models for surgical techniques for heterotopic heart transplantation were described in subsequent years,[4–7] it took another 30 years to better understand and manipulate the "biologic factor" which Mann described as limiting the survival of allografted organs. In 1960, Norman Shumway and Richard Lower performed orthotopic heart transplants in dogs using cardiopulmonary bypass and topical hypothermia for donor heart preservation.[8] The dogs survived

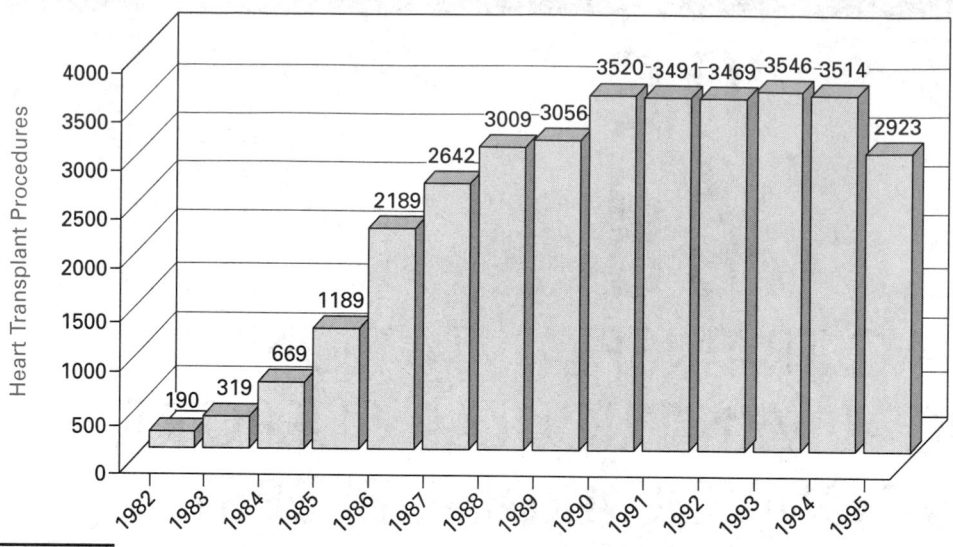

FIGURE 25-1

Data from International Society for Heart and Lung Transplantation: numbers of heart transplant procedures per calendar year. (From Hosenpud et al.,[13] with permission.)

between 6 and 21 days and died of rejection. Shumway and Lower also recognized the limiting "biologic factor" and stated that "if the immunologic mechanisms of the host were prevented from destroying the graft, in all likelihood it would continue to function adequately for the normal lifespan of the animal." Their technique, involving anastomoses at the mid-atrial level and the supravalvular level in the great vessels, remains the basis of cardiac transplant technique in the 1990s.

In the early 1960s, the concept of pharmacologic immuno-suppression was introduced; it ushered in the marriage of surgical and medical technology that is today known as the field of organ transplantation. Immunosuppression was, of course, seen as a means to mitigate the "biologic factor" that otherwise limited organ graft survival. The first clinical transplants were of the kidney, a logical choice since hemodi-alysis was then available as a backup system should the graft fail, and the field has flourished since the early 1960s.[9]

The first human heart allograft procedure was performed in South Africa in 1967,[10] followed shortly by the first U.S. transplant by Shumway at Stanford in 1968 and then by a flurry of transplant activity in many centers. This initial enthusiasm subsided as it became evident that postoperative survival was limited by a variety of complex medical problems, including opportunistic infections and graft rejection. Most major centers discontinued performing heart transplantation in the early 1970s, and it was not until the introduction of cyclosporine-based immunosuppression at Stanford in 1980 and the demon-stration of the attendant improvement in survival rates[11] that the procedure reemerged as widely accepted therapy for end-stage heart disease. In the 1990s many tertiary care centers provide programs for heart transplantation, and most medical care payers in the United States, including the federal govern-ment, provide coverage for such care.

Cardiopulmonary transplantation was introduced at Stan-ford in 1981,[12] and subsequent experience with heart/lung and with both single- and double-lung transplantation in many cen-ters has proven these procedures to be valid therapy for a wide variety of primary lung diseases and end-stage cardiopulmonary disorders.[13]

Current Status

The most accurate data on vol-ume and outcomes of thoracic or-gan transplantation is provided by the Registry of the Interna-tional Society for Heart and Lung Transplantation, which is up-dated yearly and published in the journal of that society. Since 1994, the Registry has been ad-ministered by the United States' donor allocation organization, the United Network for Organ Sharing (UNOS), but it includes data on the vast majority of non-U.S. programs as well as all U.S. programs. As of the most recent Registry report,[13] there has been a plateau of heart transplant operations at approxi-mately 3500 procedures worldwide on an annual basis since the late 1980s, a level generally accepted to be due to limita-tions of donor availability (Fig. 25-1). This most recent report includes data on 34,326 transplant procedures reported since the Registry's inception in 1982 and documents overall patient survival rates of 79, 71, and 63 percent, at 1, 3, and 5 years respectively (Fig. 25-2). After the first year, there is a linear attrition to a survival of about 40 percent at 10 years.

According to this Registry, there are currently 271 pro-grams in clinical heart transplantation, of which 165 are in the United States. According to data published in 1994, a large number of these U.S. programs have very low volume, and low volume is associated with inferior survival rates.[14,15] Thus, survival rates to be expected at major, high-volume programs should be somewhat in excess of the overall re-ported rates.

RECIPIENT SELECTION AND MANAGEMENT

As is the case with any surgical procedure, careful selection of patients for heart transplantation results in optimum postop-erative survival rates. In contrast, however, to the quality-of-life or prolongation-of-life issues involved in decisions regarding more conventional heart surgery, decisions regard-ing candidacy for heart transplantation must take into consid-eration a limited donor supply and the necessity of following a highly complex medical regimen for the rest of the patient's posttransplant life. These considerations can make selecting recipients most difficult. Major guidelines for recipient selec-tion have been developed and are intended to provide the maximum benefit from the limited resource of donor organs.[16] Selection criteria are in a state of change worldwide, and criteria for acceptance at one center may not match exactly those at another center. The criteria generally reflect our experiences with the selection of patients who are most likely to survive and benefit, with a return to a normal life post transplant. Nevertheless, some basic or general criteria can be described that are universally accepted; these are summarized in Table 25-1. They include the most basic criterion: the existence of end-stage cardiac disease irremediable by other more conventional forms of medical or surgical therapy. The term *end stage* is, of course, difficult to define exactly, but in general it refers to cardiac disease associated with New York Heart Association (NYHA) Functional Class IV symptomatic status despite optimum medical management. In the past, one criterion was an estimated life expectancy of 6 months or less; however, the increasingly long waiting times for a suitable donor because of increased patient numbers on the transplant waiting list now require the much more difficult task of estimating 1- to 2-year mortality in potential candidates. *With the recent major advances in heart failure therapy has come the realization that many transplant operations in patients referred for transplant can be avoided by utilizing aggressive medical therapies.* Many transplant centers have found that as many as 30 to 50 percent of patients referred for heart transplant can be stabilized or even have their heart failure

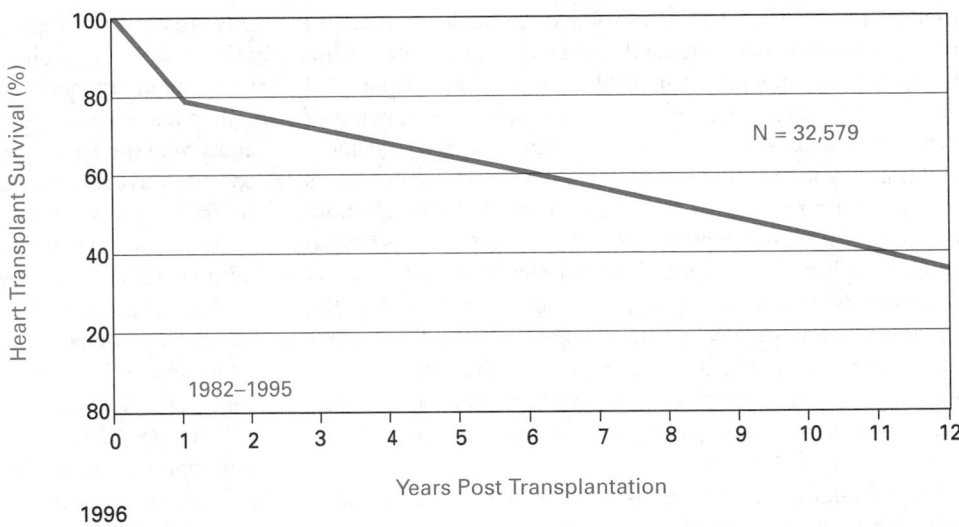

FIGURE 25-2
Data from International Society for Heart and Lung Transplantation: overall cardiac transplant recipient postoperative survival rates. (From Hosenpud et al.,[13] with permission.)

reversed by aggressive, well-organized medical approach using angiotensin-converting enzyme (ACE) inhibitors or angiotensin II receptor blockade, combination diuretics, beta blockers, and meticulous monitoring of the patient's weight, general status, electrolytes, and renal function.[17,18] Thus, most heart transplant centers have evolved into centers for heart failure management as well as transplantation. Table 25-2 lists a typical drug regimen for a patient with advanced heart failure waiting for a donor. The frequency of clinic visits for monitoring ranges from every 1 to 4 weeks, depending on the status of the patient. Furthermore, the introduction of transvenously placed antitachycardia/defibrillation devices and the increasing use of new beta blockers have all contributed to this ability to stabilize patients in order to avoid or delay heart transplantation. We have also realized that a small percentage of patients may have their left ventricular dysfunction reversed by high-risk percutaneous interventional procedures or coronary bypass surgery in order to restore blood flow to areas of "hibernating myocardium." Positron emission tomography (Chap. 20) or 24-h thallium scanning (Chap. 17) is utilized

TABLE 25-1

CRITERIA FOR ACCEPTANCE OF CARDIAC TRANSPLANT RECIPIENT

- Unacceptable heart failure that has not responded to an aggressive medical or surgical regimen
- Unacceptable prognosis for survival of 1–2 years
- Biologic age less than 55–60 years
- Absence of irreversible pulmonary hypertension
- Absence of other systemic diseases that would limit long-term survival
- Medically compliant, with the ability to follow a complex medical regimen
- Adequate psychosocial support to assure compliance with medical directions and office visits
- Absence of self-abusive behavior that would interfere with the postoperative course

TABLE 25-2

TYPICAL PHARMACOLOGIC REGIMEN FOR THE ADVANCED HEART FAILURE PATIENT

ACE inhibitor/angiotensin II blocker
Loop diuretic
Triamterene/hydrochlorothiazide
Digoxin (low dose)
Coumadin
Enteric-coated aspirin if CAD
HMG-CoA reductase inhibitor if CAD
Beta-blocker trial

Note: ACE = angiotensin-converting enzyme; CAD = coronary artery disease.

to identify potential candidates for such procedures. It is also important to identify potentially reversible causes of cardiomyopathy as summarized in Table 25-3 (see also Chaps. 73 and 76). Cessation of excessive alcohol intake or slowing of ventricular rate with drugs or atrioventricular (AV) nodal ablation in patients with rapid heart rates occasionally results in a dramatic reversal of the heart failure.[19] Although more controversial, some centers continue to treat biopsy-proven acute lymphocytic myocarditis with high-dose steroids. This approach is also used for sarcoid cardiomyopathy. Finally, the introduction of newer beta blockers with alpha-receptor blocking effects has resulted in dramatic improvement in preliminary survival statistics. Their use is associated with improved left ventricular ejection fraction over time as well[20,21] (see also Chap. 23).

Age limits for cardiac transplant recipients are a second criterion for acceptance, and these limits have been expanded considerably in both directions over the past several years. In the early years of experience with cardiac transplantation, older patients experienced very inferior survival rates and the upper limit of eligibility was set at age 50. Since the advent of cyclosporine-based immunosuppression in 1980, it has become apparent that survival rates are no longer inferior in older age groups.[22] In the most recent year in which such data were analyzed in the Registry of the International Society for Heart Transplantation, the 30-day mortality rates according to age were identical (at 10 percent) for all ages between 10 and 69.[23] Reports from several centers have also attested to the excellence of both early and late postoperative survival rates in older patients.[24–27] Based on such data, most centers have now advanced the official age of acceptability to 55 and may accept patients up to age 60 as well as highly selected patients over age 60. The lower age limits for transplantation eligibility have also been expanded recently, with a number of major centers embarking on programs involving neonates and young children.

Potential cardiac transplant recipients are also screened for the existence of any other systemic disease that independently is likely to limit their survival. The coexistence of an active malignancy and the potentially increased tendency for its advancement in the presence of immunosuppression is one obvious problem, and such patients are routinely excluded. How to deal with a patient with end-stage heart disease and a remote history of malignancy is a more difficult problem.

TABLE 25-3

IDENTIFICATION OF POTENTIALLY REVERSIBLE CAUSES
OF CONGESTIVE HEART FAILURE

Ischemic left ventricular dysfunction reversible with interventional or surgical reperfusion
Cardiomyopathy secondary to
    Lymphocytic myocarditis
    Sarcoidosis
    Tachycardia
    Ethanol

Edwards et al.[28] reported a small group of patients with a prior history of malignancy who were considered to have been cured of their malignant disease and were otherwise candidates for cardiac transplantation. Seven such patients underwent transplantation; six had a remote history of lymphoproliferative disease and one had had adenocarcinoma of the colon. Only the patient with colon cancer has had recurrence of malignancy during follow-up averaging over 2 years. Thus, cautious acceptance of such patients may be justified.

The coexistence of one other major systemic disease, insulin-requiring diabetes, has been considered to be a contraindication to cardiac transplantation in otherwise acceptable patients. The rationale for this has been the well-known increase in incidence of early peripheral and cerebrovascular disease and nephropathy in these patients as well as their generally poor ability for wound healing and the difficulty of diabetic control during the period of constantly varying steroid doses in the early postoperative period. As steroid requirements have become lower, there has been discussion about relaxing this requirement to allow inclusion of stable (as opposed to "brittle") insulin-requiring diabetic patients, and in recent years, several reports have attested to the safety and efficacy of heart transplantation in very carefully selected diabetic patients.[29–31] Human immunodeficiency virus (HIV) positivity is generally considered an absolute contraindication to heart transplantation.

Other comorbid conditions must be considered on an individual basis, but irreversible organ dysfunction such as emphysema, severe peripheral vascular disease, and hepatic or renal dysfunction out of proportion to that predictable as a consequence of severe congestive heart failure are strong relative contraindications. The presence of an active infection is an (often temporary) absolute contraindication to transplantation because of the mandatory posttransplant institution of immunosuppression. Early in the years of clinical experience with heart transplantation, it was found that a normal donor right ventricle is unable to increase its external work load acutely to overcome an elevated pulmonary vascular resistance (PVR). Because of this, patients who have end-stage heart disease with an elevated PVR often experience acute right-sided heart failure and cardiogenic shock after the transplantation of a normal heart with a right ventricle not conditioned to pump against high resistance. This problem was a major cause of intraoperative deaths in the early years of transplantation and led to the setting of an upper limit of 4 Wood units of PVR (approximately 320 dynes·s/cm⁵) as the cutoff point or fourth criterion for suitability for cardiac transplantation. In recent years, the concept of reactivity of the pulmonary vasculature and potential reversibility of elevated PVR has gained acceptance. Because of this, potential candidates with PVR greater than 4 Wood units (320 dynes·s/cm⁵) at baseline are usually subjected to pharmacologic maneuvers during hemodynamic monitoring, using nitroprusside and/or prostaglandin E₁ to determine whether or not the elevated PVR is reversible; such patients are accepted as candidates for transplantation if the PVR can be reduced to acceptable levels while systemic arterial pressure remains adequate.

The last criterion that is accepted by most centers is the absence of unresolved pulmonary infarction. In spite of systemic anticoagulation, pulmonary infarcts due to emboli from the dilated right ventricle or leg or pelvic veins are common complications in patients with biventricular congestive heart failure awaiting transplantation. *Experience has shown that pulmonary infarcts have a high probability of becoming pulmonary abscesses after institution of immunosuppression.* For this reason, waiting recipients who sustain pulmonary infarction usually are removed temporarily from the waiting list until the infarct resolves radiographically. Unfortunately, such resolution can be quite slow in this severely ill group of patients, and many never survive to return to the waiting list.

Based on these criteria, a group of patients is selected who are believed to have the best chance of benefiting from the operation and the attendant substantial commitment of medical resources. The type of underlying heart disease in the adult population selected for the procedure is nearly evenly split between idiopathic cardiomyopathy and ischemic disease, and in the pediatric population, predictably, there is a higher percentage with congenital heart disease.

DONOR SELECTION AND MANAGEMENT

Acceptance of the concept of brain death, both legally and medically, has been central to the emergence of organ transplantation (and particularly transplantation of unpaired organs such as the heart) in the modern era. The mandatory warm ischemic time involved if cardiopulmonary death were the only accepted criterion of death would make heart transplantation impossible. Acceptance of the concept of irreversible brain death has been a perhaps surprisingly recent phenomenon. In 1970, Kansas became the first state in the United States to pass legislation recognizing the legal concept of brain death. Several states followed suit, and the medical and legal criteria for brain death have been refined over the years. The most recent and widely accepted set of guidelines was set out in the President's Commission Report in 1980.[32] It has been estimated that only 15 to 20 percent of persons who qualify as brain dead and have usable or transplantable organs become organ donors in the United States.[33] The reasons for this are complex and include public unawareness of the potential to donate organs as well as reticence among medical staff to make the request for donation. Efforts are being made in many areas to improve the percentage of organs recovered for transplantation from potential donors, but even with much higher recovery rates, heart transplantation will likely be a donor-limited field for the foreseeable future.

To be considered suitable donors for cardiac transplantation, brain-dead individuals must meet certain minimum criteria. Age criteria vary in different programs, but most cardiac donors have been under age 40. The donor should obviously not have had any significant cardiac disease, malignant disease, or acute or chronic infection. Risk factors for cardiovascular disease such as diabetes or severe hypertension or hypercholesterolemia are relative exclusion factors. Donors are routinely screened serologically for HIV and for hepatitis B and C. Baseline serology for a number of other infectious diseases such as cytomegalovirus (CMV) is obtained in many programs but is usually not used prospectively in donor-recipient matching. If there is any suspicion of cardiac disease in the donor, appropriate diagnostic studies (including echocardiography, cardiac catheterization, and coronary angiography) to assure the normalcy of the potential cardiac graft are pursued.

Once a potential donor is identified, the procurement process is initiated by contacting and referring to the local organ procurement organization (OPO), which maintains a registry of waiting recipients and coordinates equitable distribution of donor organs within a geographic area. Donor-recipient matching is fairly straightforward and requires ABO blood group compatibility as well as overall body size comparability, with ±20 percent body weight considered to be an acceptable discrepancy. Human leukocyte antigen (HLA) matching is not attempted prospectively because of the difficulty in obtaining HLA typing promptly as well as the relatively small numbers of donors and recipients, which severely limits choices

Most donor hearts currently are "harvested," or removed, from the donor by a transplant donor team from a transplant center and transported back to the center for implantation. A cold ischemic time of 4 h in adults is generally considered safe; this requirement limits the distance from which hearts can be transported and leads to the rationale for geographic subdivision into OPOs.

SURGICAL TECHNIQUE

As noted above, the surgical technique used in most centers today differs little from that described by Lower and Shumway in 1960.[8] With this procedure, both the donor and recipient hearts are removed by transecting the atria at the mid-atrial level, leaving the multiple pulmonary venous connections to the left atrium intact in the posterior wall of the left atrium, and then transecting the aorta and pulmonary artery just above their respective semilunar valves (Fig. 25-3).

As noted above, the donor heart is usually explanted, or harvested, by a surgical team at a hospital remote from the transplant center, and this surgery most often needs to be coordinated with the requirements of other surgical teams procuring nonthoracic organs for transplantation at other centers. The donor heart is arrested with cold crystalloid or blood cardioplegic solution, and the explanted heart is then cooled topically by being placed in an iced preservation solution; it is then placed in a secure container and transported expeditiously to the transplant center. Ischemic times average 3 to 4 h. Implantation of the heart in the orthotopic position begins with reanastomosis at the mid-atrial level beginning with the atrial septum (Fig. 25-4). Efforts are made to include a generous cuff of donor right atrium so that the sinoatrial node will be included. The great vessels are reanastomosed just above the semilunar valves.

In recent years, there has been a move to alter the surgical

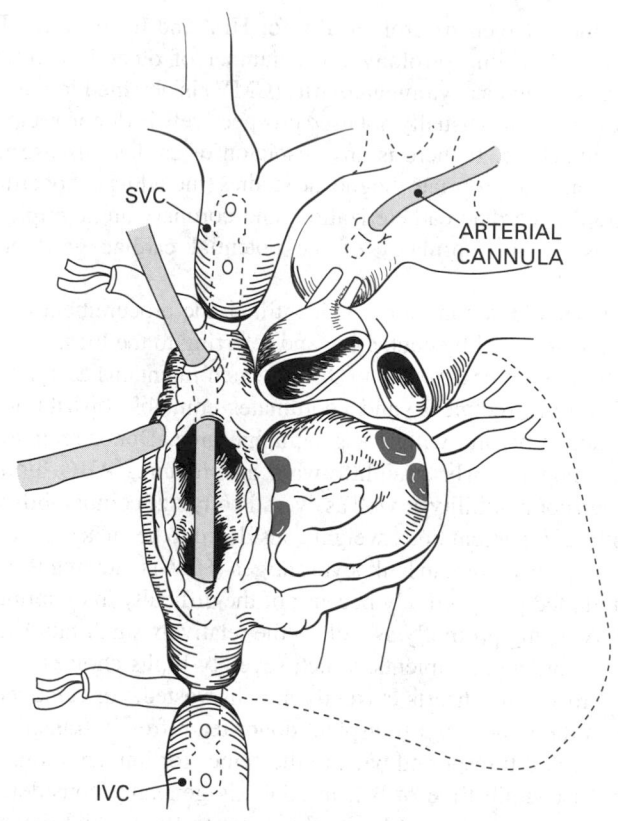

FIGURE 25-3
Diagram of recipient mediastinum, with heart resected and arterial and venous cannulae in place.

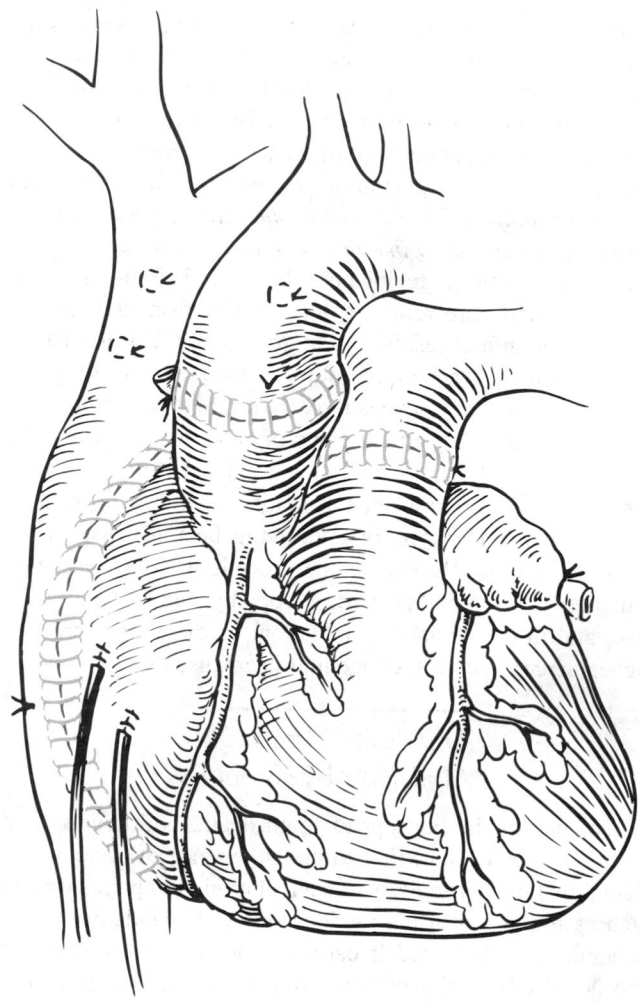

FIGURE 25-4
Diagram of donor heart anastomosed in the orthotopic position. Suture lines at mid-atrial level and aorta and pulmonary artery above semilunar valves.

technique by leaving the donor atria intact and making anastomoses at the level of the superior and inferior venae cavae and pulmonary veins[34]—the *technique of bicaval anastomosis*.[35,36] There is evidence that this modified technique is associated with a decreased requirement for pacemaker placement for donor sinus node malfunction as well as with less AV valve regurgitation,[37,38] most likely as a result of preservation of the geometric configuration and anatomic size of the atria and the preserved integrity of the sinoatrial node.

Immediate postoperative care differs little from that after more routine heart surgery, except for the institution of immunosuppression (described below) and the need for chronotropic support of the donor sinoatrial node for the first 2 to 3 postoperative days, usually with temporary pacemaker support but occasionally with infusion of isoproterenol. Uncomplicated patients may be discharged from the hospital 7 to 10 days postoperatively.

POSTOPERATIVE MANAGEMENT

Immunosuppression

GENERAL

The need to suppress the normal immune response to the presence of a solid organ allograft begins immediately at the time of surgery and continues for the life of the graft, which is generally concurrent with the life of the patient in the field of cardiac transplantation. Historically, most clinically used immunosuppressive regimens have consisted of a combination of several agents used concurrently and sequentially. This multiple-drug approach continues to be considered the state of the art: the number of drugs and timing of their administration varies from institution to institution, but several general principles are commonly adhered to.

The first general principle is that immune reactivity and the tendency to graft rejection are highest early after graft implantation and decrease with time, although they likely never disappear entirely. Thus, most regimens employ the highest levels of immunosuppression immediately after surgery and decrease later, eventually settling on the lowest maintenance levels of suppression compatible with preventing recurrent graft rejection. The second general principle is reminiscent of that originated in oncology chemotherapy regimens, using low doses of several drugs without overlapping toxicities in preference to higher (and more toxic) doses of fewer drugs whenever feasible. The third general principle is that too much or too intense immunosuppression is undesirable because it leads to myriad undesirable effects such as susceptibility to infection and malignancy, but too little is equally undesirable because it permits graft rejection. Finding the right balance between over- and underimmunosuppression in an individual patient is truly an art that utilizes science. As newer immunosuppressive agents and modalities are developed, the possible array of drug regimens can be expected to multiply accordingly, but these principles will likely remain, and the process of tailoring an individual patient's immunosuppressive regimen will likely continue to be an art as well as a science.

There is currently a relatively limited repertoire of approved agents for immunosuppression after organ transplantation, but their numbers can be expected to increase. Most programs employ a long-term two- or three-drug regimen and roughly half additionally use a brief early postoperative course of "induction" cytolytic therapy. Most programs employ glucocorticoids as one of the agents, usually in relatively high doses early postoperatively and then tapering to low doses or discontinuing the drug during the first postoperative year. The commonly used drugs and their toxicities are outlined in Table 25-4.

In managing patients on these drugs, it is most important to be aware of the potential for drug interactions when other agents are added to or deleted from the patient's regimen. A list of the most common and clinically important drug interactions is shown in Table 25-5. It is also important to keep in mind the potential for changing drug concentrations in the face of intercurrent hepatic or renal dysfunction.

SURVEILLANCE AND THERAPY FOR REJECTION

There are rarely any striking physical signs or symptoms of rejection until it is far advanced. Cardiac allograft rejection is diagnosed almost exclusively by examining histologic findings in surveillance right ventricular endomyocardial biopsies. The technique used and pathologic criteria for diagnosis are described below. A wide variety of noninvasive methods to diagnose rejection have been investigated, but none has yet been determined to have sufficient sensitivity and specificity to replace the biopsy. Protocols for timing of surveillance endomyocardial biopsies are generally chosen to match the observed frequency of rejection episodes, which is clearly highest in the early postoperative period. Most programs perform surveillance biopsies on a weekly basis for the first 4 to 6 postoperative weeks, then with diminishing frequency in the stable patient but, at a minimum, every 3 months for the first postoperative year. The need for continued surveillance biopsies after the first year in clinically stable patients has been questioned,[39,40] but most centers do continue them every 4 to 6 months.

Rejection episodes are treated with augmented immunosuppression, the intensity of which is matched to the histologic, or occasionally clinical, severity of the episode. Early or first rejection episodes are usually treated with methylprednisolone, given intravenously in a dose of 1 g daily for 3 days followed by a repeat biopsy in 7 to 10 days. Episodes after 3 months that are not clinically severe can be treated safely with an increase in the oral steroid dose.[41] More severe rejection is treated with glucocorticoids and the addition of cytolytic therapy, with either polyclonal antithymocyte globulin (commonly of rabbit or equine origin) or the murine monoclonal anti-CD3 preparation OKT3. Such treatment is highly effective,[42] but sensitization can limit its use.[43]

Several strategies are currently employed as adjunctive therapy for repetitive or recalcitrant rejection episodes. They include the use of two modalities with proven efficacy in the therapy of autoimmune disease, namely, total lymphoid irradiation[44] and low-dose methotrexate.[45] Both have been shown to be of benefit in patients with frequent or difficult-to-treat cardiac allograft rejection.[46–49] A recent analysis suggests that the two modalities are both reasonably effective in this setting.[50] Tacrolimus (FK506), when substituted for cyclosporine, has been reported to benefit several heart transplant recipients with resistant rejection[51] as well as to be safe and effective as a primary agent in a cohort of patients[52]; there is a larger body of experience with its use in resistant renal graft rejection.[53] Studies are currently under way to evaluate several other drugs, modalities, and immunologic manipulations in the setting of resistant graft rejection.

If all such strategies fail and severe graft dysfunction super-

TABLE 25-4

CURRENTLY AVAILABLE IMMUNOSUPPRESSIVE AGENTS

Agent	Toxicities	Avoid Toxicity
Cyclosporine	Renal dysfunction	Follow blood levels
	Hypertension	Antihypertensive medication
	Neurotoxicity	?
Tacrolimus (FK506)	Renal dysfunction	Follow blood levels
	Neurotoxicity	?
Mycophenolate mofetil	Gastrointestinal disturbances	Reduce dose
	Marrow toxicity (mild)	Follow CBC
Azathioprine	Marrow toxicity	Follow CBC
	Hepatotoxicity	Discontinue drug
Glucocorticoids	Cushingoid habitus	Minimize dose
	Glucose intolerance	
	Osteoporosis	
Methotrexate	Marrow toxicity	Follow CBC

Note: CBC = complete blood count.

TABLE 25-5

DRUG INTERACTIONS WITH AZATHIOPRINE AND/OR CYCLOSPORINE

Medication	Effects	Mechanism	Management	Onset	Severity
Allopurinol	Neutropenia 2° bone marrow suppression	Competitive inhibition of azathioprine metabolism	1. *Don't use* allopurinol unless absolutely necessary 2. If used, monitor WBC count and adjust azathioprine dose accordingly	Delayed 2–3 weeks	Major
Amphotericin	Increased nephrotoxicity	Possible synergism with cyclosporine	Follow renal function; titrate dose accordingly	Delayed 1–2 weeks	Moderate
Barbiturates	Decreased cyclo levels	Increased hepatic metabolism	Follow cyclo levels carefully; increase cyclo doses PRN	Delayed 1 week	Moderate
Diltiazem (?? other Ca²⁺ antagonists)	Increased cyclo levels	Unknown	Follow cyclo levels carefully; decrease cyclo doses PRN	Delayed 1–2 weeks	Moderate
Erythromycin	Increased cyclo levels	Decreased hepatic metabolism	Decrease cyclo dose by approximately *half*; follow levels carefully during and after therapy	Rapid	Major
Hydantoins	Decreased cyclo levels	Increased hepatic metabolism	Increase cyclo dose by 25%; follow levels carefully	Rapid	Major
Imipenem	Increased CNS effects	Unknown	Avoid the antibiotic	Rapid	Moderate
Ketoconazole or itraconazole	Increased cyclo levels	Unknown	Follow levels carefully; decrease cyclo doses PRN	Delayed 1–2 weeks	Moderate
Metoclopramide	Increased cyclo levels	Increased cyclo bioavailability	Follow cyclo levels carefully; decrease cyclo doses PRN	Delayed 1–2 weeks	Moderate
Rifampin	Decreased cyclo levels	Increased hepatic metabolism	Increase cyclo dose by 100%; follow levels carefully	Delayed 1 week	Major
Sulfamethoxazole/ trimethoprim	Increased nephrotoxicity Increased marrow suppression Neutropenia	Unknown	Follow WBC count and renal function; adjust cyclo and azathioprine doses PRN	Delayed 2–3 weeks	Moderate

Note: WBC = white blood cell; cyclo = cyclosporine; 2° = secondary.

venes, retransplantation is the only remaining option and is offered in many centers. The results of retransplantation in this setting are, however, disappointing, with only 33 percent 1-year survival in one registry.[54]

Infectious Complications

Although their incidence has decreased in the cyclosporine "era," infections, often with unusual and opportunistic organisms, are the major cause of death during the first postoperative year and remain a threat throughout the life of the chronically immunosuppressed patient. Effective therapy demands an extremely aggressive approach to obtaining a specific diagnosis and a background of experience in recognizing the commoner clinical presentations of CMV, *Aspergillus*, and other opportunistic infectious agents. Transplant cardiologists generally have expertise in infectious disease management but usually require the availability of both infectious disease consultation for the more unusual problems and a high-quality infectious disease laboratory. Several well-proven regimens for infection prophylaxis are commonly used and are outlined in Table 25-6. Infection surveillance is mainly clinical, but the routine chest radiograph will often detect infections, especially fungal and mycobacterial ones, at an early and asymptomatic stage.

Posttransplant Malignancy

Any program of chronic immunosuppression is associated with a subsequent increased risk of lymphoproliferative malignancy, the earliest cases being noted after a period of immunosuppressive therapy for chronic hepatitis.[55] Organ transplantation has proven to be no exception, and the incidence of posttransplant lymphoproliferative disease (PTLD) has been documented in a registry based at the University of Cincinnati. The incidence of PTLD in heart transplant recipients is somewhat higher than in kidney transplant recipients but is not as high as in liver recipients (Table 25-7), which is probably

TABLE 25-6
INFECTION PROPHYLAXIS REGIMENS

Pathogen/Disease	Strategy
Aspergillus	? Air filtration
	? Prophylactic antifungals
Bacterial endocarditis	Standard subacute bacterial endocarditis prophylaxis
Cytomegalovirus	Blood product selection
	Prophylactic ganciclovir
	Prophylactic immunoglobulin
Influenza	None recommended
Pneumococcus	Preoperative vaccine
Pneumocystis	Sulfamethoxazole/trimethoprim
	Inhaled pentaminide
Toxoplasma	Pyrimethamine if donor seropositive

related to the intensity of immunosuppression required after the various allograft procedures.[56] According to the most recent registry report, malignancy accounts for 11.8 percent of deaths after heart transplantation.[13]

There is convincing evidence that most PTLDs are related to infection (either primary or reactivation) with the Epstein-Barr virus (EBV).[57–59] They frequently occur in unusual, extranodal locations and may respond to reduction in immunosuppression,[60] although such reduction is clearly a "double-edged sword" with a cardiac allograft for which there is no alternative system, such as dialysis in renal transplantation, if the graft is rejected. PTLDs are usually quite radiosensitive, and both radiotherapy and surgical resection can play a major role in therapy when there is a single lesion.

There is anecdotal evidence that use of the antiviral agent acyclovir may be useful in therapy of PTLD,[61] and most centers employ it as adjunctive therapy. In recent years, there has been interest in the use of interferon for these malignancies,[62] and a multicenter oncology group protocol is currently underway to evaluate its efficacy. Recently, there has been interest in the use of infusions of donor leukocytes[63] and donor-derived EBV-specific cytotoxic lymphocytes for this

TABLE 25-7
POSTTRANSPLANT LYMPHOPROLIFERATIVE DISORDER INCIDENCE IN ORGAN TRANSPLANTATION

Organ	Incidence, %
Kidney	1.0
Heart	1.8
Liver	3.0
Heart/lung	4.6

Source: Reproduced from Penn I. Roundtable report: Immunosuppression and lymphoproliferative disorders, 1992. (With permission of the author and Pro/Com International, Parsippany, NJ.)

disease in bone marrow transplant recipients.[64] The technology may well be transferred to organ transplant recipients but would require maintenance of donor tissue lines prospectively.

Allograft Vasculopathy

INCIDENCE

When clinical heart transplantation was introduced, the complications discussed above were all anticipated problems, given the nonspecific nature of available immunosuppression, but the frequent development of diffuse and often rapidly progressive obliterative coronary artery disease in young donor hearts was not expected. It occurs angiographically in approximately 10 percent of cardiac transplant recipients by the first postoperative year and in 50 percent by 5 years postoperatively,[65,66] and its incidence did not decrease after the introduction of cyclosporine-based immunosuppression in the early 1980s.[67] *The ischemic sequellae of this vasculopathy account for the vast majority of late posttransplant deaths, and it is currently the main factor limiting truly long-term survival.*[13]

MORPHOLOGY

The angiographic morphology of cardiac allograft vasculopathy has been well described,[68,69] and its main features are summarized in Table 25-8. The very diffuseness of the disease makes it easy to underestimate angiographically, even when, as is usually recommended, similar angiographic views from serial angiograms are reviewed simultaneously with side-by-side projectors.

In recent years, the use of intravascular ultrasound has gained acceptance as a sensitive and early detector of the intimal thickening that characterizes graft vasculopathy.[70–72] Intravascular ultrasound measurements of the extent of coronary intimal thickening currently serve as surrogate end points for prevention of vasculopathy in several trials of new immunosuppressive agents that have shown promise of lessening the incidence of vasculopathy in animal models.

PATHOLOGY

The morphologic features of accelerated transplant vasculopathy and the principal differences from conventional atherosclerosis have been described previously.[73–75] In transplant arteriopathy, the major epicardial vessels, their branches, and often the intramyocardial divisions display uniform, diffuse involvement extending along their entire length. The arteries are cordlike in texture, and cross sections show uniform, concentric luminal narrowing (Fig. 25-5). The asymmetric

TABLE 25-8
ANGIOGRAPHIC FEATURES OF CARDIAC ALLOGRAFT CORONARY ARTERY DISEASE

Distribution: diffuse, distal, concentric, longitudinal obliterative lesions
May coexist with focal proximal lesions
Collateral vessel formation uncommon

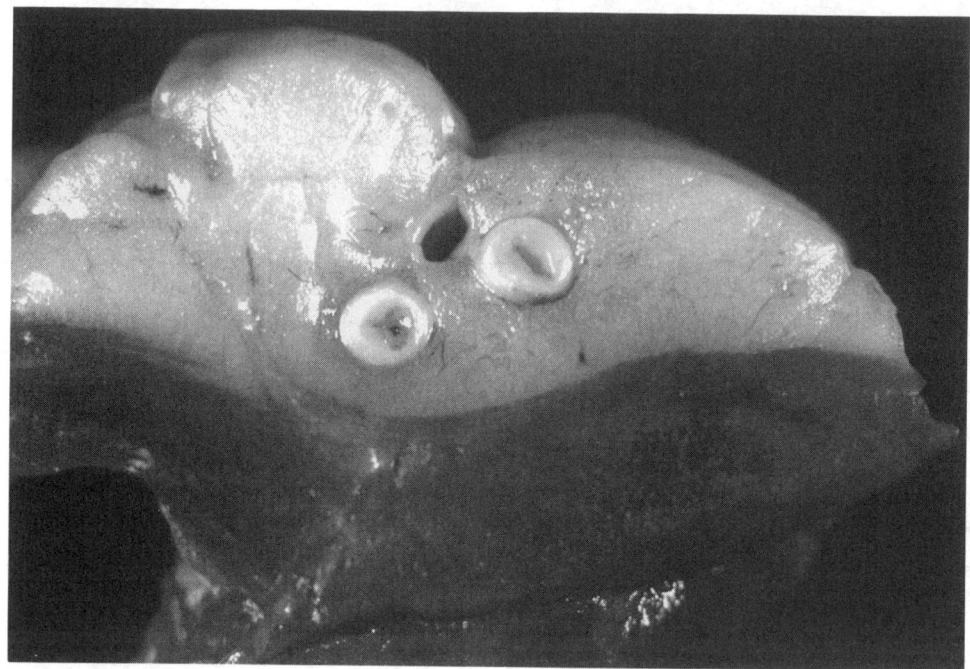

FIGURE 25-5

The mid-left anterior descending artery at autopsy in a 63-year-old man with advanced graft coronary disease.

cytes within a connective tissue matrix that ranges from loose, edematous, and myxoid in early lesions to densely hyalinized and fibrotic in older lesions (Fig. 25-6). The internal elastic membrane is usually preserved, with only focal interruptions and reduplications. The medial layer is generally intact but may show atrophy in advanced lesions. Intraluminal thrombosis is uncommon. While these changes are rarely seen on endomyocardial biopsy samples, signs of ischemia or infarction seen in the endomyocardial biopsy should alert the pathologist and the clinician to the possibility of the insidious presence of graft coronary disease.[76]

CLINICAL PRESENTATION, SCREENING, AND PROGNOSIS

and calcified plaques or lesions composed of cholesterol characteristic of conventional atherosclerosis are not found in uncomplicated lesions of vessels affected by transplant vasculopathy. Histopathologic sections show a thickened intimal layer composed of modified smooth muscle cells, foamy macrophages, and variable numbers of histiocytes and lympho-

Because most cardiac transplant recipients have a persistent state of both afferent and efferent cardiac denervation, most are incapable of experiencing the subjective sensation of angina pectoris. Clinical presentations of ischemia in this patient population are usually related to sequellae of the ischemia, such as arrhythmias or left ventricular dysfunction. In recent years, it has been convincingly shown that some cardiac transplant recipients do have physiologic evidence of reinnervation[77,78] and may experience angina pectoris.[79]

The usual lack of angina and the diffuseness of the disease have made the standard clinical and noninvasive screening for native coronary artery disease fairly insensitive in detecting this form of coronary vasculopathy.[80] Most such technology is designed to detect uneven myocardial perfusion due to focal lesions and is less good at detecting the global ischemia of diffuse obliterative disease. Several recent reports have suggested that dobutamine stress echocardiography may, in fact, be the one noninvasive technique to offer reasonable sensitivity and specificity in screening for this disease,[81,82] and it offers an attractive alternative to the usual annual coronary angiography performed in these patients.

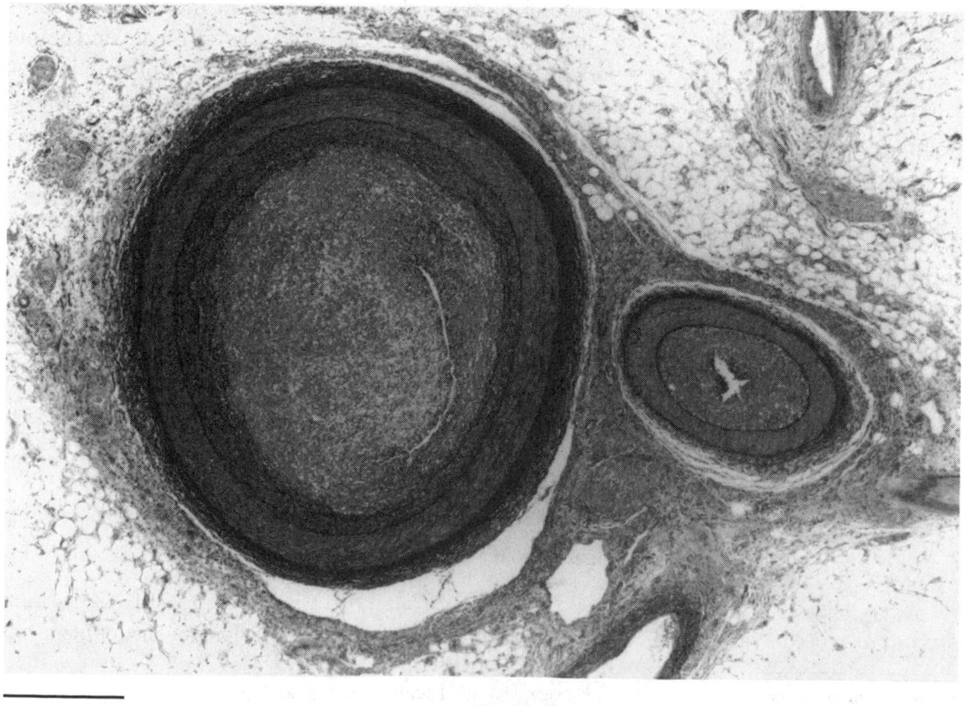

FIGURE 25-6

A main epicardial artery and division vessel showing occlusive graft coronary disease. Note the concentric intimal proliferation with a slitlike lumen. The internal elastica of both vessels is intact. (EUG × 10)

The prognosis for survival once significant graft vasculopathy is detected angiographically is generally poor. In one study, the 1- and 2-year survival rates after detection of any 40 percent coronary artery stenosis were 67 and 44 percent, respectively.[83] After an ischemic event such as congestive heart failure or myocardial infarction, 1-year survival was only 18 to 20 percent in this study.

APPROACHES TO PREVENTION

A number of approaches to prevention of allograft vasculopathy have been proposed, and several show some promise. As noted above, a decreased incidence of vasculopathy is one of the desired endpoints in all preclinical and clinical trials of new immunosuppressive agents, and several such trials are in progress. In addition, two studies have shown some decrease in the incidence and sequellae of vasculopathy with the use of other agents—one with a calcium channel blocker added to the patient regimen early after surgery and another with the lipid-lowering agent pravastatin added. In the former, diltiazem was used in a randomized study involving a total of 106 patients, and those taking diltiazem had little change in overall coronary diameter on quantitative angiography over a 3-year follow-up period and displayed a trend toward a decreased incidence of angiographic coronary stenosis and clinical events due to ischemia.[84] In the other study,[85] also randomized and involving a total of 97 patients, the use of the pravastatin (regardless of lipid levels) was associated with a markedly decreased incidence of allograft vasculopathy seen both at angiography and at autopsy.

The mechanism of action for either of these agents remains speculative. It is to be hoped that since, as described below, the etiology of allograft vasculopathy is most likely immunologic, improved methods of inducing specific graft tolerance in the future may lead to disappearance of this disease and permit truly long-term survival rates after heart and other organ transplantation.

APPROACHES TO THERAPY

The choice of treatment of established cardiac allograft vasculopathy is often difficult and controversial. No agent or modality has as yet been shown to reverse the process. Its very diffuseness makes the disease only infrequently amenable to otherwise standard revascularization procedures such as angioplasty or surgical bypass grafting. A recent registry of revascularization procedures performed on heart transplant recipients in 13 large transplant centers in the United States documented 97 balloon angioplasty procedures in 66 patients prior to November, 1991.[86] There was an angiographic 94 percent success rate and an acceptable complication rate. There was, however, a 55 percent restenosis rate at a mean of 8 months postangioplasty, and 19 patients underwent 31 repeat angioplasty procedures for 24 restenoses and 30 new lesions. Only 61 percent of the patients were alive without retransplantation at a mean of 19 months after coronary angioplasty. In the same registry, 12 surgical coronary bypass procedures were reported; four of these died in hospital, a fifth died suddenly 2 months postoperatively, and a sixth has required

further palliative angioplasty. Revascularization is clearly, at best, short-term palliation for this highly lethal disease.

The most definitive form of therapy for graft failure due to severe vasculopathy is obviously retransplantation, and this procedure has been offered in many centers to highly selected patients with advanced allograft vasculopathy. Survival rates after retransplantation, however, are clearly inferior to those after primary transplants, averaging only 52 percent at 1 year in the most recent Registry data.[13] In data analyzed from a group of the highest volume U.S. centers, even the most ideal retransplant candidates had only a 68 percent 1-year postoperative survival.[54] While this clearly represents an improvement in the individual patient's prognosis, these lower survival rates plus the increased costs involved[87] have led some to question the ethics of performing retransplantation.[88] Nevertheless, most large programs do continue to offer the option to highly selected patients.

ALTERNATIVES TO TRANSPLANTATION

Mechanical Support

TEMPORARY: PERCUTANEOUS INTRAAORTIC BALLOON PUMP

When aggressive medical therapy for severe heart failure no longer provides adequate organ perfusion in either the acute or the chronic setting, several mechanical devices are available to support the failing circulation on a temporary basis until either myocardial recovery ensues or an appropriate cardiac donor for transplantation is procured. The intraaortic balloon pump (IABP), first described by Mouloupoulos in 1962,[89] is the most widely used device for such mechanical circulatory assistance. The device consists of a nonocclusive balloon catheter positioned in the descending aorta, with the balloon cyclically inflated during diastole (to provide diastolic pressure augmentation and increase coronary blood flow) and deflated during systole (to provide reduced arterial impedance or afterload reduction during ejection), a rhythmic sequence termed *counterpulsation*. These devices are widely used for circulatory support in acute situations, such as cardiogenic shock or refractory ischemia after myocardial infarction or cardiac surgery, as well as to support patients awaiting cardiac transplantation who become refractory to pharmacologic therapy.

Technique

A number of IABP systems are commercially available for either surgical or percutaneous insertion. Most have a second lumen that permits balloon insertion over a guidewire and later provides monitoring of central aortic pressure. Percutaneous insertion systems generally require 9F femoral introducer sheaths. Retrograde insertion of the IABP system through a sheath in the femoral artery is the most commonly used method of insertion and can be accomplished under local anesthesia in the intensive care unit setting. When femoral pulses are absent or when percutaneous femoral cannulation is felt to be hazardous, surgical exposure of the common femoral artery enables the operator to cannulate the artery under direct vision. The existence of severe aortoiliac occlusive disease occasionally mandates insertion of the IABP from the upper extremities or from a graft attached to the ascending aorta.

Timing

Proper timing of inflation and deflation is necessary for IABP counterpulsation to provide effective ventricular assistance. Ideally, the balloon should inflate immediately after aortic valve closure and deflate at the onset of the subsequent systole. When initiating support, it is often helpful to begin with the balloon augmenting every other beat (the 2:1 mode) to be able to compare an unaugmented beat with an augmented beat as one adjusts the timing of the balloon, the aim being to maximize the height of the augmented diastolic peak and minimize the height of the systolic peak following the augmented diastole.

Weaning

The balloon is generally used for augmentation of all beats (1:1 mode) until the patient's ventricular function improves and allows stepwise reduction of the assist mode to the 2:1 and later 3:1 mode over a period of 6 to 12 h.[90] When hemodynamic independence from the IABP is established, the balloon may be removed.

Complications

Complications have been reported to occur in 5 to 35 percent of IABP insertions.[91,92] Ischemia of the extremity distal to the femoral insertion site is the most common complication and may be more common when the percutaneous technique is used.[93] Severe ischemia requiring amputation of the toes, foot, or lower leg has been reported in 1 to 2 percent of cases.[90–92] Wound infection at the groin insertion site is the second most common complication, occurring in 3 to 4 percent of patients and usually presenting several days after catheter removal. Most resolve with topical care and systemic antibiotics. Other reported complications of IABP use include dissection or perforation of the distal aorta or its branches and peripheral or visceral embolization due to thrombus formation. The incidence of the latter is decreased by the routine use of therapeutic doses of heparin.

TEMPORARY: VENTRICULAR ASSIST DEVICES

Mechanical support for the failing heart that becomes refractory even to IABP support is available in the form of ventricular assist devices (VADs) or replacement artificial ventricles. Since the first report of successful use of a VAD in 1965,[94] the technology has progressed a great deal. Most such assist devices function by diverting blood out of the left ventricle through a large inflow conduit inserted into the left ventricular apex, into a pump-drive system, and back through a large outflow conduit into the ascending aorta. Figure 25-7 is an example of a typical VAD system in situ.

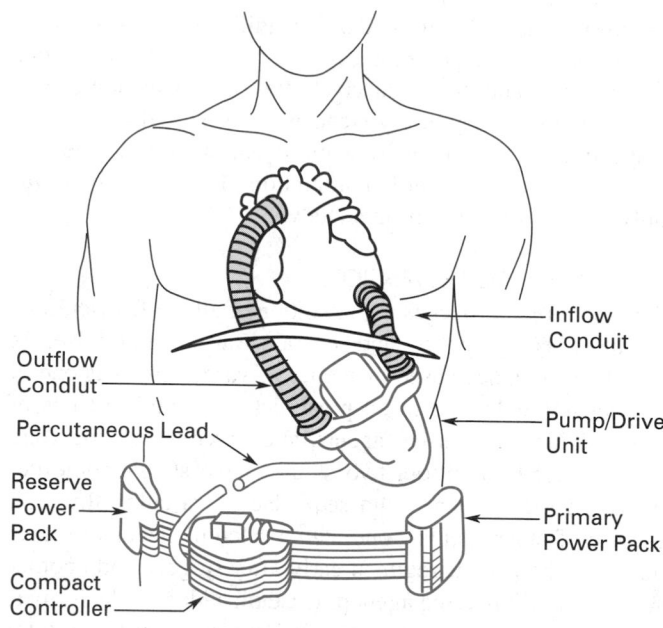

Outflow Conduit
Percutaneous Lead
Reserve Power Pack
Compact Controller
Inflow Conduit
Pump/Drive Unit
Primary Power Pack

FIGURE 25-7

Diagram of wearable Novacor left ventricular assist device in situ, showing inflow conduit inserted in apex of left ventricle leading to body of electrically driven pump, with outflow conduit returning blood to the ascending aorta. (Courtesy of Novacor Division, Baxter Healthcare Corporation, Oakland, CA.)

In the United States, VADs are currently approved for two indications. The first is that of temporary support of potentially reversible cardiac dysfunction, and substantial myocardial salvage has been achieved in postcardiotomy[95,96] and, less frequently, in postinfarction[97] cardiogenic shock. The second approved indication for VAD support is as a "bridge" to transplantation in waiting transplant recipients (who, by definition, have irreversible myocardial dysfunction) who deteriorate severely before a donor becomes available. Successful bridging with a VAD was first reported in 1984 using the Novacor implantable electrical VAD (Novacor Division, Baxter Healthcare Corporation, Oakland, CA) in a patient with end-stage ischemic heart disease.[98] Success with replacement artificial ventricles (an orthotopic artificial heart) was reported a year later in a patient with cardiomyopathy.[99] The artificial heart technology, however, was fraught with high complication rates and has not been used for a number of years. There has been some resurgence of interest in the use of total artificial hearts as bridges to transplantation recently,[100] and their future remains to be seen.

Because of the progressive "mismatch" between the increasing demand for donor hearts and the stable donor supply rate, increasing numbers of patients on transplant waiting lists are deteriorating and requiring the use of such bridge devices to survive until a donor becomes available. The use of mechanical technology in this situation is associated with excellent posttransplant survival rates for supported patients,[101,102] but it does add a substantial level of pretransplant expense and, of course, does not increase the overall size of the donor pool.

The Future: Permanent Ventricular Assist Devices

With the growing shortage of donor organs, there is an increasing need for a mechanical device as an alternative to biologic transplantation of the failing heart. The ultimate goal of the evolving technology first used for temporary ventricular assistance has been to develop a completely implantable electrical system with rechargeable batteries (allowing the patient freedom from tethering to a power supply) to serve as a permanent assist to left ventricular function. The first clinical trials of such devices are about to commence and will involve patients with end-stage heart disease who, for reasons of age or other comorbid conditions, are not considered to be transplant candidates. If their safety and efficacy is established in this patient population, then clinical trials comparing VAD support directly with transplantation can proceed and address many endpoints, such as quality of life, in addition to survival.

The Future: Xenotransplantation

Work on development of a mechanical alternative to biologic cardiac transplantation has proceeded simultaneously with immunologic research aimed at making it possible to use animal organs in humans—a field known as *xenotransplantation*. There are formidable anatomic, physiologic, and immunologic barriers to be overcome before xenotransplantation can become a solution to the shortage of donor organs.[103] Anatomically, transplanted organs must be of appropriate size and structure to replace the native organ. Physiologically, the transplanted organ must perform a complex set of tasks, to accomplish which it must receive and often send appropriate hormonal and metabolic signals. Such needs require reasonable homology of both the involved hormones and cell surface receptors between the human and donor species. Technically and biologically, primates would be the obvious choice for a donor species. However, the supply of primates is much too small to fill the potential demand; ethical considerations also remain a drawback to the use of primates as organ donors. The pig has emerged as the most likely species to provide the appropriate size, anatomic structure, and available numbers for human organ transplantation. Unfortunately, swine are quite phylogenetically distant from humans, and this distance is associated with a formidable immunologic barrier. Humans universally possess so-called natural antibodies directed against swine antigens, primarily against carbohydrate moieties that are present on endothelial and other cells. These antibodies lead to hyperacute rejection of a swine organ, through activation of the complement system initiated by the antibodies binding to donor endothelial cells, a process which occurs within an hour after implantation and leads to rapid destruction of the graft.[104,105]

Several means have been investigated to prevent hyperacute rejection. Depletion of xenogeneic natural antibodies against the donor organ as a way of modifying the host's humoral immunity is one approach.[106,107] Transient inhibition of complement activity with cobra venom factor or soluble complement receptor delays hyperacute rejection and attests to the central role of the complement system in this process.[108] The activation and activity of complement are ordinarily regulated and limited by several endothelial cell–associated proteins. These proteins may function less effectively against heterologous than against native complement, making xenografts potentially more susceptible to complement-mediated injury. The production of transgenic swine bred to express human complement regulatory proteins in order to decrease the xenograft's susceptibility to complement-mediated injury has been an area of active research.[109,110] Such genetic alterations of the donor species hold some promise, at least for overcoming this first immunologic barrier to xenotransplantation. The later occurrences of acute and chronic rejection, however, are problems that remain to be solved. With current technology, the prevention of acute rejection of xenografts would require unacceptably intense regimens of immunosuppression, and prevention of chronic rejection, as noted earlier, is inadequate with current technology, even in allograft.

The prospect of using animal tissues in transplantation has raised concern about the potential for transmission of zoonotic pathogens from animal to human.[111] Since the likelihood of an organism causing disease in humans may be independent of its disease-causing potential in the donor species, the issue becomes a major one for the individual recipient and is potentially an issue with wide public health implications. When clinical trials begin, it will be extremely important to monitor recipients of xenogeneic tissue for the occurrence of unexplained illness; it has been suggested that creation of a national or international registry of exposure to xenogeneic tissue would facilitate identification of clusters of events or illness.[111]

ENDOMYOCARDIAL BIOPSY

The Instrument

A percutaneous transvascular approach to biopsy of the beating heart was first described by Drs. Sakakibara and Konno in Japan in 1962,[112] and modifications of their instrument are still widely used. They are generally introduced from a femoral or brachial vein. This technology to permit nonsurgical biopsy of the myocardium was further developed in response to the need to obtain tissue from the transplanted heart in order to assess the presence and severity of graft rejection and monitor response to antirejection therapy. Cardiac allograft rejection had initially been recognized by means of clinical observation of phenomena such as emergence of heart failure, a gallop rhythm, or declining electrocardiogram voltage. Such phenomena often did not occur, however, until rejection was quite severe, and biopsy offered a means of early and objective assessment of rejection. In 1973, Caves et al. at Stanford introduced a new, shorter (and therefore, more controllable) bioptome, which was introduced from the jugular rather than the femoral vein and allowed easy and repeated serial biopsy procedures under fluoroscopic guidance.[113] The Caves-

Schultz-Scholten instrument was improved by Mason[114] and for years was the most commonly used bioptome in the United States. This bioptome is reusable, but its cleaning procedure is costly and labor-intensive, and several disposable instruments have been developed and have gained widespread use in recent years. An example of one of the most widely used is shown in Fig. 25-8 with the standard percutaneous approach from the right internal jugular vein. Longer bioptomes are also available for use from the femoral approach (usually through a long guiding sheath) in patients without internal jugular access.

The Technique

The right ventricle is usually the ventricle of choice for obtaining biopsy material because of the relative convenience and safety of approach to the right, as opposed to the left, ventricle as well as the usually homogeneous distribution of myocardial inflammatory and rejection processes. The procedure is performed with the patient supine, usually in the cardiac catheterization laboratory or in a procedure room or in the operating room if facilities are available. For the internal jugular approach, positioning with the feet elevated increases central venous pressure and facilitates cannulation of the vein. After introduction of an intravascular sheath with standard percutaneous technique, the bioptome can be advanced through it down to the right atrium, across the tricuspid valve, and into the right ventricle pointed toward the septal wall. The stimulation of some premature ventricular contractions by the instrument serves as confirmation of its presence in the ventricular chambers. Once it is safely within the ventricle and directed toward the septum, the jaws of the bioptome are opened, the instrument is advanced gently against the wall, and the jaws are closed, "biting off" a piece of septal myocardium 1 to 3 mm in diameter. The bioptome is then withdrawn, and the specimen is retrieved and placed in appropriate me-

dium for pathologic examination. The process is repeated until three to five adequate specimens are obtained.

Endomyocardial biopsy procedures are generally performed on an outpatient basis without any requirement for sedation or for concomitant measurement of right heart pressures, unless these are clinically indicated. The procedure is usually done under fluoroscopic guidance,[115] but many centers perform them safely[116] and potentially with less cost[117] under echocardiographic guidance.

Complications

Large series have documented the low morbidity and mortality of endomyocardial biopsy, with major complications such as cardiac perforation and tamponade occurring in <0.5 percent of procedures.[118,119] More minor, and generally transient, complications include bundle branch block and arrhythmias. Fistulae between the coronary artery and right ventricle have been described in a number of transplant patients who have had multiple biopsy procedures, but these generally seem to have no hemodynamic consequence.[120,121] With increasing lengths of survival of cardiac transplant recipients and the continued use of surveillance myocardial biopsies, complications related to the sheer numbers of biopsies performed are becoming more apparent. Chief among these is damage to the tricuspid valve and its subvalvular structures. This complication was first reported in 1990,[122] when a series of five patients with tricuspid valve chordal rupture as a complication of endomyocardial biopsy was reported. None of these had hemodynamically significant tricuspid regurgitation. Subsequently, there have been reports suggesting that signs of right heart failure eventually appear in some patients, and several patients are known to have required tricuspid valve replacement because of intractable right heart failure. The incidence of tricuspid valve injury may be decreased with the use of a sheath across the valve during biopsy.[123]

Role in the Evaluation and Diagnosis of Cardiac Disease

TISSUE HANDLING AND PROCESSING

Correct handling of retrieved biopsy specimens is essential for obtaining high quality pathology results and interpretability. To limit crush distortion of the tissue, the biopsy specimen should be gently teased from the bioptome with a needle and immediately placed in an appropriate fixative. Neutral buffered 10% formalin is the standard fixative for light microscopy, and gluteraldehyde-based solutions are used for transmission electron microscopy (TEM). The specific clinical circumstances will usually determine how

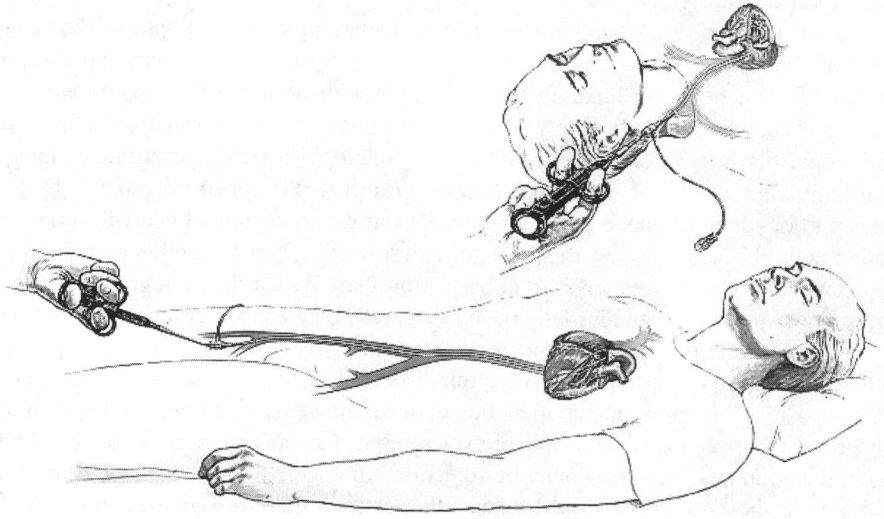

FIGURE 25-8
Diagrams of bioptomes inserted from right internal jugular or femoral approach. (Courtesy of Cordis Corporation, Miami, FL.)

the specimen is to be fixed and processed and which histochemical stains are to be selected. For the evaluation of myocarditis, cardiomyopathy, and specific heart muscle diseases, at least four biopsy pieces are recommended for light microscopy; one piece may be retained for TEM, and an unfixed piece may be frozen for immunofluorescence or immunohistochemical studies (optional). At least four pieces are required for light microscopy for adequate sampling in the grading of acute rejection; one piece may be frozen for immunofluorescence studies if acute vascular rejection is suspected. All the tissue samples (four to five pieces) should be placed in gluteraldehyde when grading of anthracycline cardiotoxicity is the clinical issue.

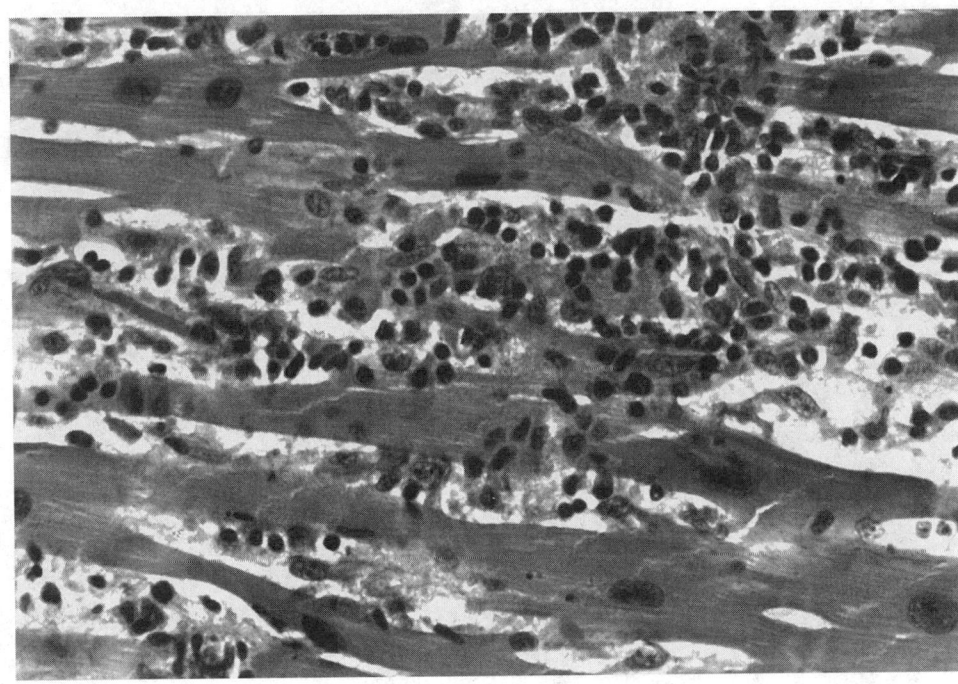

FIGURE 25-9
Lymphocytic myocarditis in a young man presenting with sudden-onset congestive heart failure. Dense interstitial infiltrates of lymphocytes are seen in association with myocyte damage. (H&E × 400)

INDICATIONS FOR ENDOMYOCARDIAL BIOPSY

since the successful application of the endomyocardial biopsy for the diagnosis and monitoring of acute rejection in the early 1970s, the indications for the procedure have expanded. The right ventricle is usually selected for technical reasons, including safety, although left ventricular biopsy is occasionally performed for the diagnosis of endomyocardial fibrosis, infantile fibroelastosis, left-sided irradiation effects, and cardiac involvement by scleroderma. The current indications for endomyocardial biopsy are listed in Table 25-9.

Myocarditis

As an inflammatory or immunologic process, myocarditis is defined by the presence of an inflammatory infiltrate in association with nonischemic damage or necrosis of the adjacent myocytes,[124] features termed *the Dallas criteria* (see Chap.

TABLE 25-9

POSSIBLE INDICATIONS
FOR ENDOMYOCARDIAL BIOPSY

Diagnosis and grading of acute rejection
Diagnosis of myocarditis
Evaluation of idiopathic cardiomyopathy
Diagnosis of specific heart muscle diseases
Distinguish restrictive versus constrictive heart disease
Evaluation and grading of anthracycline cardiotoxicity
Diagnosis of primary and secondary cardiac neoplasms
Evaluation of idiopathic arrhythmias
Evaluation of atypical chest pain

---

76). The different types of inflammatory cells help define possible etiologies in myocarditis. Predominantly lymphocytes are seen in idiopathic (postviral) myocarditis (Fig. 25-9), sarcoidosis, Lyme disease, Kawasaki disease, polymyositis, and AIDS-myocarditis (see Chap. 79). Eosinophils are commonly found in drug hypersensitivity but may also indicate parasitic infection or a hypereosinophilic syndrome. Myocyte necrosis associated with multinucleated giant cells is characteristic of giant cell myocarditis (Fig. 25-10). Epithelioid histiocytes forming granulomas are seen in cardiac sarcoidosis.

Idiopathic Cardiomyopathy

The morphologic diagnosis of idiopathic dilated cardiomyopathy including familial and postpartum types is primarily one of exclusion, as a variety of storage and infiltrative heart muscle diseases and myocarditis may mimic dilated cardiomyopathy (see Chaps. 69, 73–76, 92). Hypertensive, ischemic, and valvular heart disease must also be excluded. The endomyocardial biopsy is used routinely in some institutions in evaluating dilated cardiomyopathy of unknown causes. The morphologic features of idiopathic cardiomyopathy are nonspecific and include myocyte hypertrophy and interstitial fibrosis (Fig. 25-11). Hypertrophic cardiomyopathy is the second most common type of cardiomyopathy. It cannot be reliably diagnosed by endomyocardial biopsy since the characteristic histologic features are mainly found in the midportion of the ventricular septum.[125] Mimics of hypertrophic cardiomyopathy such as amyloidosis can be delineated by biopsy.

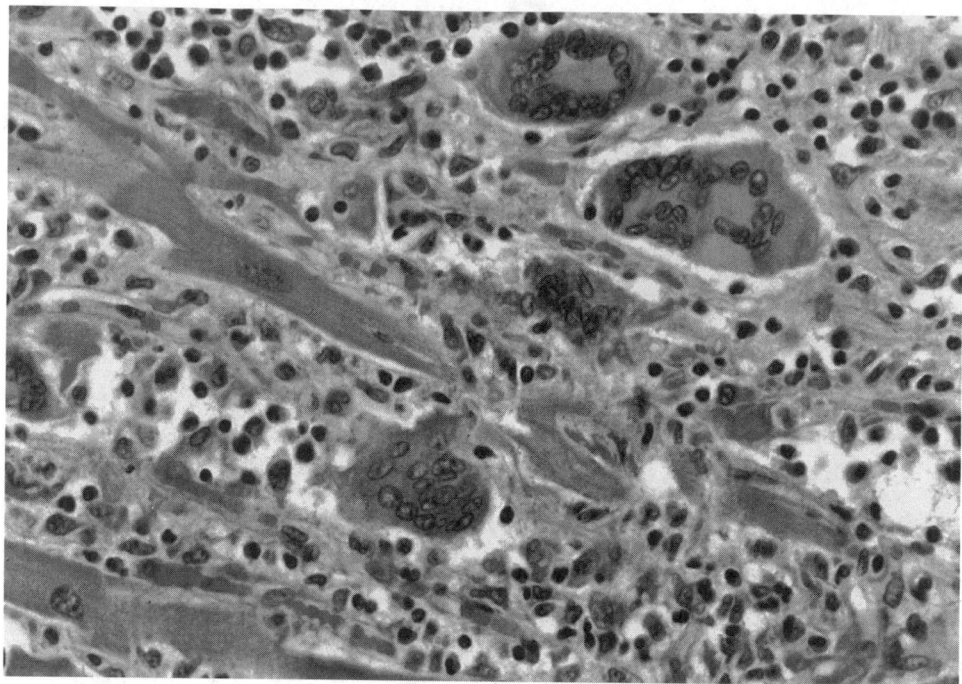

FIGURE 25-10

Giant cell myocarditis showing an inflammatory infiltrate composed of lymphocytes, histiocytes, and eosinophils admixed with multinucleated giant cells. Myocyte damage is conspicuous in this case. (H&E × 400)

Specific Heart Muscle Diseases

A variety of infiltrative diseases and storage disorders of the myocardium can be readily diagnosed by endomyocardial biopsy (see Chap. 75). Cardiac amyloidosis may be seen with primary amyloidosis, plasma cell dyscrasias, and chronic inflammatory conditions and in elderly patients (senile amyloid).

The histologic appearance includes interstitial, subendocardial, or vascular deposits of finely fibrillar, eosinophilic material (Fig. 25-12). Senile amyloid is often characterized by nodular deposits of transthyretin. Histochemical stains such as Congo red or trichrome are useful to distinguish amyloid from collagen.

Disorders of iron metabolism (hemochromatosis) and iron overload states (hemosiderosis) result in perinuclear accumulations of iron pigment within the myocytes. Special stains such as the Prussian blue stain highlight the pigment (Fig. 25-13). In advanced disease, marked myocyte hypertrophy and interstitial fibrosis are found. The diagnosis of metabolic enzyme deficiencies, including glycogen storage diseases, Gaucher's disease, and Fabry's disease (see Chap. 69), may also be established by endomyocardial biopsy.

Restrictive versus Constrictive Heart Disease

The clinical distinction of restrictive heart disease from constrictive pericardial disease can be difficult, and the therapeutic implications are significant. In some cases, imaging and hemodynamic studies may not provide a definitive diagnosis. Specific heart muscle diseases resulting in restrictive physiologic profiles, including amyloidosis, carcinoid heart disease, endocardial fibrosis, and radiation-induced interstitial fibrosis, can be diagnosed by biopsy[126] (see Chaps. 75 and 81).

Anthracycline Cardiotoxicity

Anthracyclines such as doxorubicin are commonly used in the treatment of solid tumor and hematologic malignancies. Cardiac toxicity in the form of congestive heart failure is the most significant side effect of these agents and may develop months to years after completion of therapy. The condition is dose-related and generally occurs after a cumulative dose of 550 mg/m^2. Individual patient variation and factors

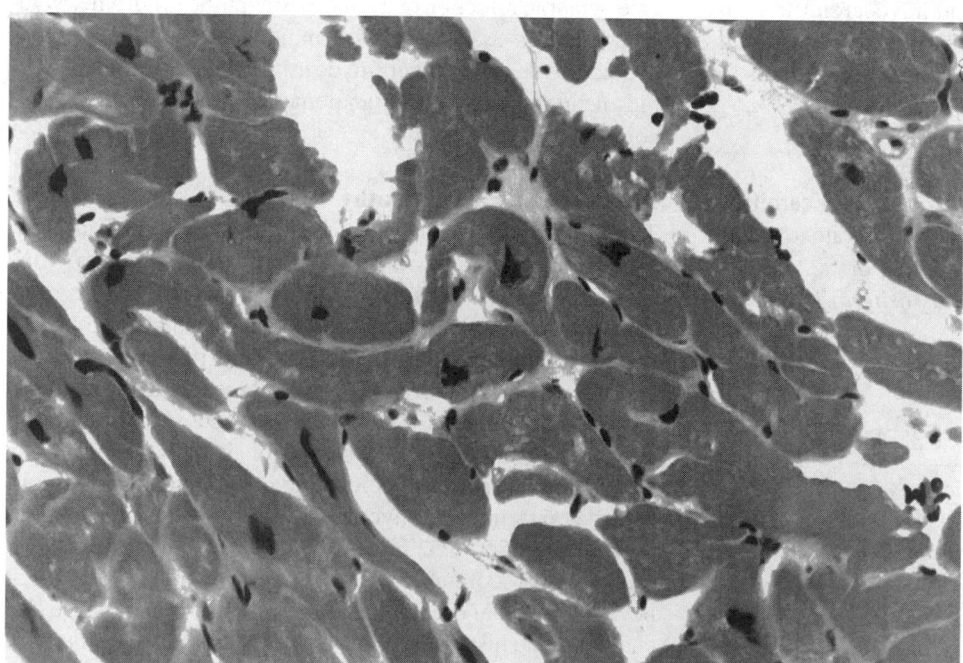

FIGURE 25-11

A young woman presenting with congestive heart failure. Myocyte hypertrophy characterized by large, irregular nuclei are seen. The findings are compatible with dilated cardiomyopathy. (H&E × 400)

such as prior mediastinal irradiation, hypertension, and increased age may potentiate cardiotoxicity at lower cumulative doses.[127] TEM of heart biopsies remains the "gold standard" for the diagnosis and grading of doxorubicin toxicity.[128]

The Billingham grading scheme for doxorubicin toxicity is based on the percentage of myocytes demonstrating doxorubicin effect. Grades 0 through 3 are used, and these are associated with specific therapeutic recommendations.[129] The characteristic changes include myofibrillar loss with Z band remnants and sarcotubular dilatation within the myocytes (Fig. 25-14). This approach to drug toxicity has provided a valuable method of monitoring patients and preventing irreversible cardiac failure.

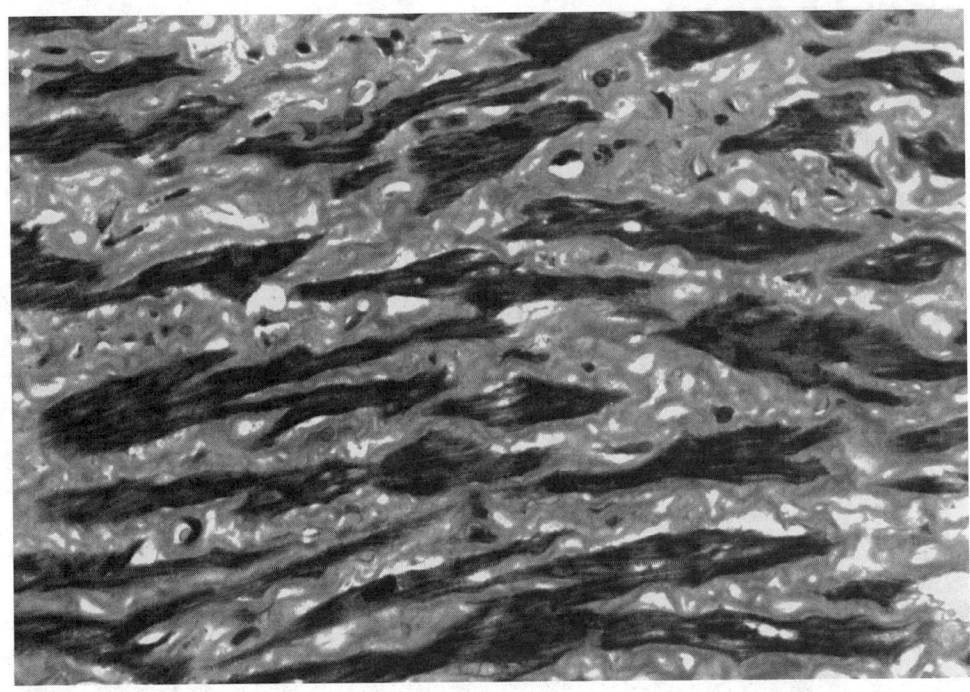

FIGURE 25-12
Severe interstitial amyloidosis showing the fibrillar deposits along the sarcolemma with constriction of the myocytes. (H&E × 400)

Primary and Metastatic Neoplasms

The endomyocardial biopsy has been used to provide morphologic confirmation and classification of benign and malignant primary cardiac tumors and to document the presence of metastatic malignancies[130] (see Chap. 86). Cardiac myxomas, fibromas, and rhabdomyomas as well as sarcoma, lymphoma, leukemia, and malignant mesothelioma have been diagnosed. Secondary neoplasms such as metastatic carcinoma and melanoma may also be found in right ventricular specimens (Fig. 25-15).

Idiopathic Arrhythmias

In the absence of a documented anatomic abnormality such as ischemic heart disease, cardiomyopathy, or mitral valve prolapse as an explanation for ventricular or supraventricular rhythm disturbances, the endomyocardial biopsy may be helpful. Lesions of the conduction system can result in nonspecific myocyte hypertrophy and interstitial fibrosis. Lymphocytic myocarditis, sarcoidosis, and giant cell myocarditis all may present with arrhythmias. In a study of 27 patients with unexplained ar-

rhythmias from the Mayo Clinic, a third of the biopsies showed features of cardiomyopathy, 15 percent had clinically unsuspected myocarditis, and 55 percent had essentially normal biopsies.[131] An uncommon cause of arrhythmia is arrhythmogenic right ventricular dysplasia (see Chap. 36). It should be suspected in biopsy specimens showing hypertrophy

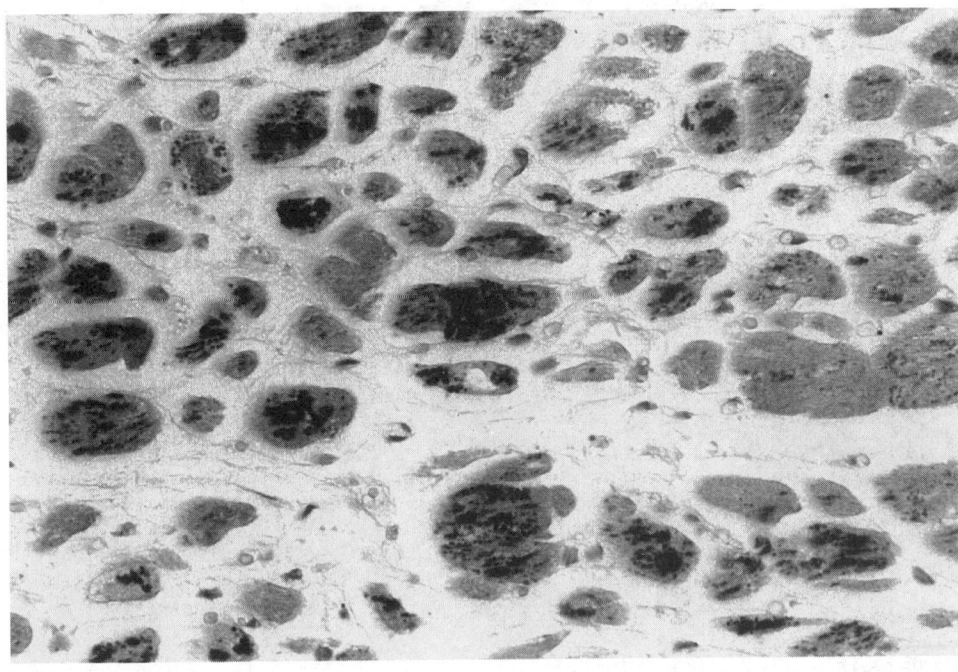

FIGURE 25-13
Cardiac hemochromatosis in a young man. Dense accumulations of iron pigment are seen in a perinuclear location. (Prussian blue × 400)

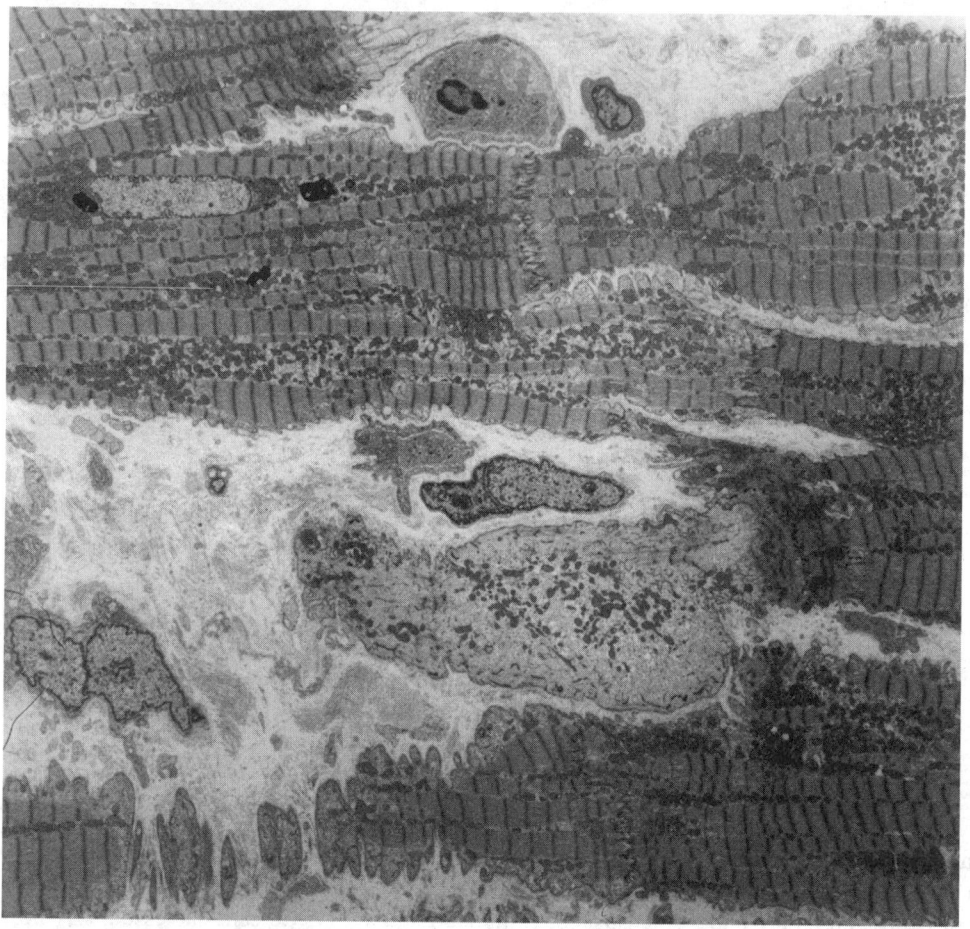

FIGURE 25-14
Transmission electron micrograph of adriamycin cardiotoxicity. Note the atrophic myocyte with myofibrillar loss surrounded by normal myocytes. (TEM × 3200)

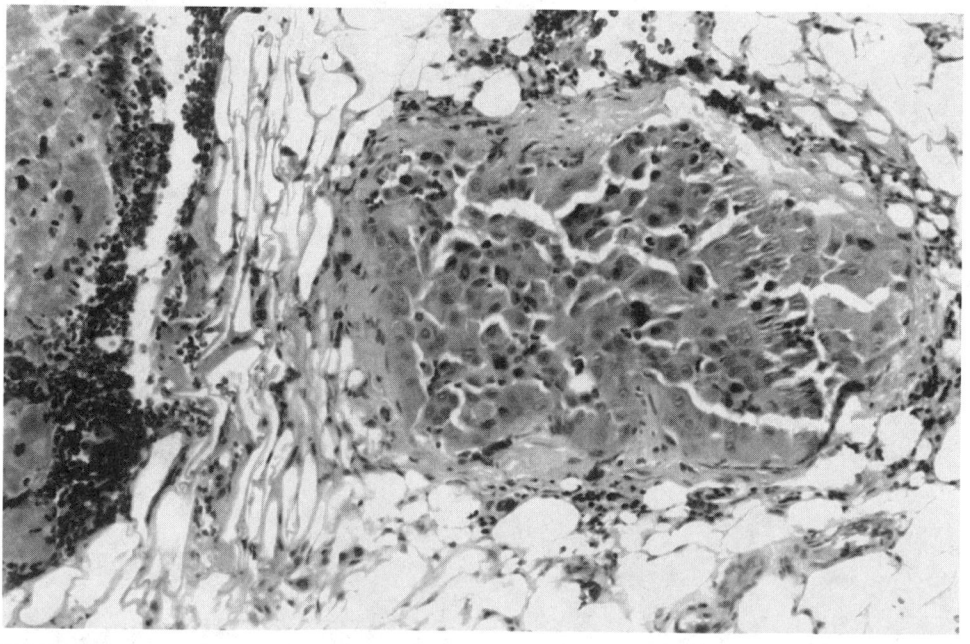

FIGURE 25-15
Metastatic adenocarcinoma in a 51-year-old woman with sudden-onset congestive heart failure and tamponade. (H&E × 400)

and fibrosis in association with abundant myocardial deposits of adipose tissue. Clinicopathologic correlation is required for the diagnosis, as myocardial accumulations of fat are normally found in the right ventricle.

Pathology of Acute Rejection

MACROSCOPIC PATHOLOGY

In advanced cardiac rejection, the heart is larger than normal, stiff, and noncompliant. In the early posttransplant period, a fibrinous pericarditis may be seen. The heart appears edematous and hemorrhagic with a dark plum color. Along the atrial sutures a sharp tinctorial delineation between the hemorrhagic myocardium of the donor heart and the pale tan myocardium of the recipient heart is a characteristic of severe rejection. Less commonly, the valves may be swollen and turgid. The trabecular muscles are prominent and often demonstrate subendocardial hemorrhages.

MICROSCOPIC PATHOLOGY

Hyperacute Rejection

This rare pattern of allograft rejection occurs in the setting of preformed circulating antibodies such as ABO blood group incompatibility or, rarely, antibodies against specific endothelial antigens or HLA.[132] The myocardium is globally edematous and hemorrhagic as a result of diffuse interstitial hemorrhages. Neutrophils and fibrin thrombi may be seen within the microvasculature (Fig. 25-16). Hyperacute rejection manifests as severe graft failure immediately or within the first few hours following transplantation. Without mechanical cardiopulmonary support, plasmapheresis, and emergent retransplantation, the recipient does not usually survive.

Acute Cellular Rejection

The principal histopathologic features of acute cellular rejection are the distribution and extent of inflammation and the presence or absence of myocyte damage. The severity of the rejection process reflects these features along a morphologic continuum. In 1973, the Stanford grading scheme of mild-moderate-severe rejection was introduced,[133] and modifications were developed by other programs.[134–136] As a result, comparison of results between institutions and in multicenter clinical trials were not feasible. In 1990, a consensus was reached establishing a uniform and standardized grading system.[137] Currently a numerical and descriptive grade is assigned to each biopsy sample. This scheme requires at least four pieces of myocardium using a standard bioptome, 50 percent of which must be evaluable myocardium, i.e., not a biopsy site or scar. If a smaller bioptome (7F or smaller) is used, at least six pieces of myocardium are required.

Six patterns of acute rejection have been described (Table 25-10). Mild acute rejection is divided into two patterns on the basis of the cytoarchitectural features. Focal mild rejection (grade IA) represents a circumscribed, usually perivascular arrangement of lymphocytes in one or more sites that is not associated with myocyte damage. In diffuse mild rejection

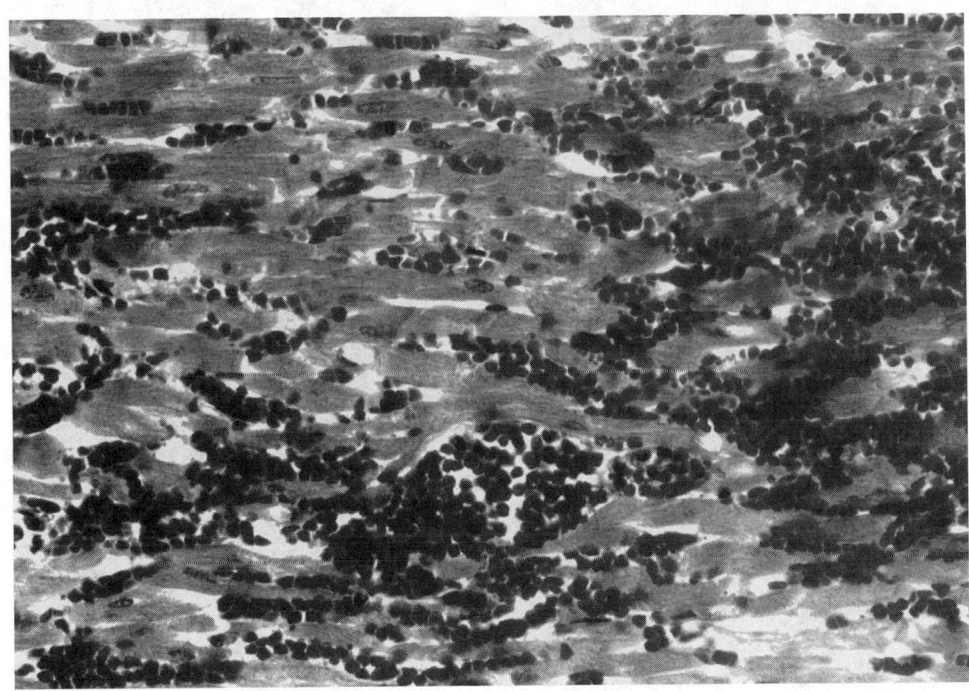

FIGURE 25-16
Hyperacute rejection is characterized by diffuse interstitial hemorrhage. (H&E × 400)

(grade IB), the infiltrates are arranged in a more diffusely interstitial architectural pattern; myocyte damage is not found. Focal moderate rejection (grade II) is characterized by a solitary, sharply circumscribed inflammatory focus that is associated with myocyte damage. The other biopsy pieces may be free of rejection or have a lesser grade. In multifocal moderate rejection (grade IIIA), at least two foci of inflammatory infiltrate display myocyte damage. These foci are often in different pieces of myocardium. Diffuse moderate rejection (grade IIIB) is represented by diffuse interstitial infiltrates in most or all

TABLE 25-10

STANDARDIZED CARDIAC BIOPSY GRADING (MODIFIED)

"Old" Nomenclature	Grade	"New" Nomenclature
No rejection	0	No rejection
Mild rejection	I	A = Focal (perivascular or focal interstitial infiltrate without myocyte damage)
		B = Sparse focal interstitial infiltrate without myocyte damage
"Focal" moderate rejection	II	One focus only with activated lymphocytes and myocyte damage
"Low" moderate rejection	III	A = Multifocal lymphocytic infiltrates with myocyte damage
"Borderline/severe" rejection		B = Diffuse (sometimes polymorphous) inflammatory process
"Severe/acute" rejection	IV	Diffuse, polymorphous infiltrate with myocyte necrosis ± edema ± hemorrhage ± vasculitis
"Resolving" rejection	Denoted by a lesser grade	Healing tissue with fibroblasts and pigmented macrophages
"Resolved" rejection	0	Mature scar tissue

Source: From Billingham et al.,[137] with permission.

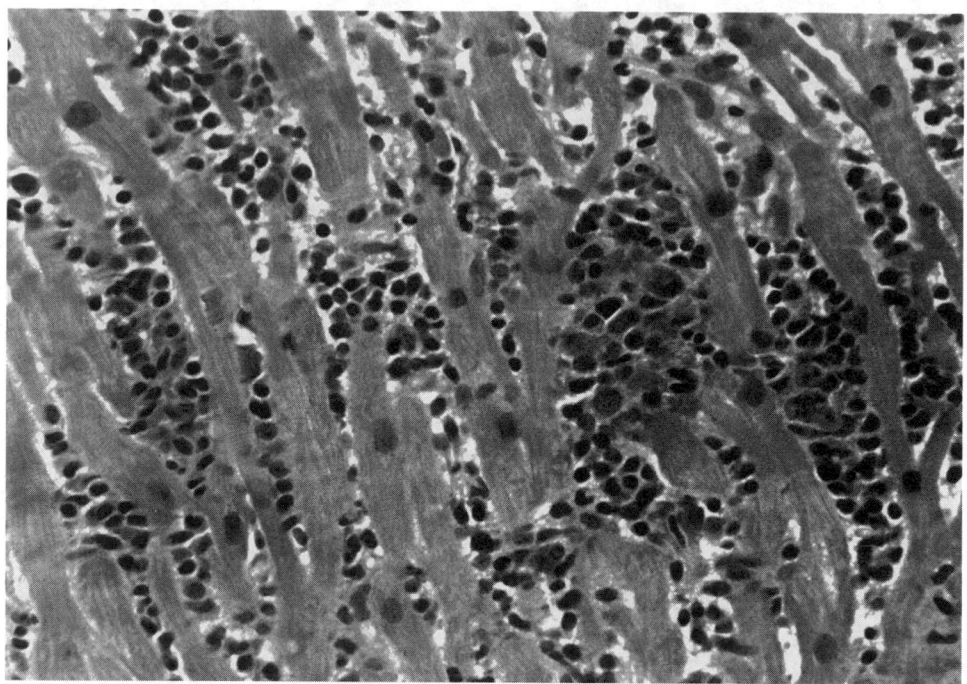

FIGURE 25-17
Diffuse moderate acute rejection (grade IIIB) showing activated lymphocytes within the interstitium and myocyte damage. (H&E × 400)

of the biopsy pieces. Myocyte damage is significant, and the findings may be classified as borderline severe rejection (Fig. 25-17). In severe rejection (grade IV), a dense polymorphous infiltrate that includes lymphocytes, neutrophils, and eosinophils is present diffusely in the interstitium. Myocyte damage, edema, and hemorrhage are conspicuous as a result of injury of the microvasculature. Resolving or resolved acute rejection is denoted by a lesser grade on the biopsy than was denoted on the previous biopsy.

Morphologic Mimics of Acute Rejection

Inflammatory infiltrates and myocyte damage of the allograft may be found in conditions other than cardiac rejection. The diagnosis of acute rejection should be made after the careful exclusion of these histologic mimics (Table 25-11). Within the first 3 weeks after transplantation, biopsies often show evidence of ischemia or preservation injury. Reperfusion of the allograft contributes to myocyte damage. Likewise, the use of pressor agents for hemodynamic support either prior to or following transplantation may result in small circumscribed

TABLE 25-11

HISTOPATHOLOGIC MIMICS OF ACUTE REJECTION

Reperfusion/ischemic injury
Quilty effect
Infectious myocarditis (cytomegalovirus/toxoplasmic)
Previous biopsy site
Posttransplant lymphoproliferative disorder

foci of myocyte damage. The infiltrates are composed of neutrophils in the initial stages and are replaced by granulation tissue. Sharply delineated endocardial infiltrates composed of lymphocytes and a delicate vascular stroma have been designated as the "*Quilty effect*" and may be confused with rejection when the infiltrate extends into the subadjacent myocardium. Infectious myocarditis, particularly toxoplasmic and CMV myocarditis, can resemble acute rejection. The infiltrates are usually polymorphous (lymphocytes, neutrophils, and eosinophils), and the organisms themselves may be found. Immunohistochemical or molecular techniques are useful in difficult cases.[138] The granulation tissue and inflammation associated with previous biopsy sites may be confused with acute rejection. PTLDs uncommonly involve the cardiac allograft. Both polyclonal and monoclonal lesions have been reported, and histopathologic analysis and clonality studies are essential for classification and prognosis. The presence of atypical lymphocytes, plasmacytoid or immunoblastic cell infiltrates, abundant tissue necrosis, and frequent mitotic figures should suggest the possibility of PTLD.[139]

Acute Vascular (Humoral) Rejection

Most episodes of rejection in the posttransplant period are mediated by lymphocytes and histiocytes and are examples of "cellular" rejection. Hammond and her colleagues have found cases of allograft dysfunction occurring in the first 6 weeks after transplantation in which the classic features of cellular rejection are absent.[140] Immunofluorescence studies on fresh-frozen myocardial samples demonstrate the presence of immunoglobulin, complement, and fibrinogen, suggesting a humoral immune response mediated by endothelial and B cells. The myocardium displays large prominent endothelial cells in venules and capillaries, perivascular inflammation, and interstitial edema. Currently, the diagnosis requires both the histologic and immunofluorescence findings. Infection and ischemic changes must also be excluded. A number of studies have suggested that these patients are at higher risk for developing accelerated graft coronary disease.[141] The etiology, incidence, optimum treatment strategies, and natural history of this form of rejection warrant further clinical studies.

REFERENCES

1. Carrel A, Guthrie CC. The transplantation of veins and organs. *Am J Med* 1905; 10:1101.

2. Edwards WS, Edwards PD. *Alexis Carrel: Visionary Surgeon*. Springfield, IL: Charles C Thomas; 1974.

3. Mann FC, Priestly JT, Markowitz J, Yater WM. Transplantation of the intact mammalian heart. *Arch Surg* 1933; 26:219–224.

4. Marcus E, Wong SNT, Luisida AA. Homologous heart grafts: Transplantation of the heart in dogs. *Surg Forum* 1951; 2:212–214.

5. Neptune WB, Cookson BA, Bailey CP. Complete homologous heart transplantation. *Arch Surg* 1953; 66:174–177.

6. Downie HG. Homotransplantation of the dog heart. *Arch Surg* 1953; 66:624–626.

7. Demikhov VP. *Experimental Transplantation of Vital Organs*, Haigh B (trans). New York: Consultants Bureau; 1962.

8. Lower RR, Shumway NE. Studies of orthotopic homotransplantation of the canine heart. *Surg Forum* 1960; 11:18–19.

9. Starzl TE, Marchioro RI, Waddell WR. The reversal of rejection in human renal homografts with subsequent development of homograft tolerance. *Surg Gynecol Obstet* 1963; 117:385–395.

10. Barnard CN. The operation. *S Afr Med J* 1967; 41:1271–1274.

11. Oyer PE, Stinson EB, Jamieson SW, Hunt SA, Billingham ME, Scott W, et al. Cyclosporine A in cardiac allografting: A preliminary experience. *Transplant Proc* 1983; 15:1247–1252.

12. Reitz BA, Wallwork JL, Hunt SA, Pennock JL, Billingham ME, Oyer PE, et al. Heart-lung transplantation: Successful therapy for patients with pulmonary vascular disease. *N Engl J Med* 1982; 306:557–564.

13. Hosenpud JD, Novick RJ, Bennett LE, Keck BM, Fiod B, Daily OP. The Registry of the International Society for Heart and Lung Transplantation: Thirteenth official report—1996. *J Heart Lung Transplant* 1996; 15:655–674.

14. Laffel GL, Barrett AI, Finkelstein S, Kaye ML. The relation between experience and outcome in heart transplantation. *N Engl J Med* 1992; 327:1220–1225.

15. Hosenpud JD, Breen TJ, Edwards EB, Daily OP, Hunsicker LG. The effect of transplant center volume on cardiac transplant outcome. A report of the United Network for Organ Sharing Scientific Registry. *JAMA* 1994; 271:1844–1849.

16. Costanzo MR, Augustine S, Bourge R, Bristow M, O'Connell JB, Driscoll D, et al. Selection and treatment of candidates for heart transplantation: A statement for health professionals from the Committee on Heart Failure and Cardiac Transplantation of the Council on Clinical Cardiology, American Heart Association. *Circulation* 1995; 92:3593–3612.

17. Stevenson WG, Stevenson LW, Middlekauff HR, Fonarow GC, Hamilton MA, Woo MA, et al. Improving survival for patients with advanced heart failure: A study of 737 consecutive patients. *J Am Coll Cardiol* 1995; 26:1417–1423.

18. Stevenson LW. Heart transplant centers: No longer the end of the road for heart failure. *J Am Coll Cardiol* 1996; 27:1198–2000.

19. Packer DL, Bardy GH, Worley SJ, Smith MS, Cobb FR, Coleman RE, et al. Tachycardia-induced cardiomyopathy: A reversible form of left ventricular dysfunction. *Am J Cardiol* 1986; 57:563–570.

20. Olsen SL, Gilbert EM, Renlund DG, Taylor DO, Yanowitz FD, Bristow MR. Carvedilol improves left ventricular function and symptoms in chronic heart failure: A double-blind randomized study. *J Am Coll Cardiol* 1995; 25:1225–1231.

21. Australia–New Zealand Heart Failure Research Collaborative Group. Effects of carvedilol, a vasodilator-β-blocker, in patients with congestive heart failure due to ischemic heart disease. *Circulation* 1995; 92:212–218.

22. Bull DA, Karwande SV, Hawkins JA, Neumayer LA, Taylor DO, Jones KW, et al. Older transplant recipients still do less well. *J Thorac Cardiovasc Surg* 1996; 111:423–428.

23. Heck CF, Shumway SJ, Kaye MP. The Registry of the International Society for Heart Transplantation: Sixth official report, 1989. *J Heart Transplant* 1989; 8:271–276.

24. Aravot DJ, Banner NR, Khanghani A, Fitzgerald M, Radley-Smith R, Mitchell AG, et al. Cardiac transplantation in the seventh decade of life. *Am J Cardiol* 1989; 63:90–93.

25. Olivari MT, Antolick A, Kaye MP, Jamieson SW, Ring WS. Heart transplantation in elderly patients. *J Heart Transplant* 1988; 7:258–264.

26. Miller LW, Vitale-Naedel N, Pennington G, McBride L, Kanter KR. Heart transplantation in patients over age fifty-five years. *J Heart Transplant* 1988; 7:254–257.

27. Carrier M, Emery RW, Riley JE, Levinson MM, Copeland JG. Cardiac transplantation in patients over 50 years of age. *J Am Coll Cardiol* 1986; 8:285–288.

28. Edwards BS, Hunt SA, Fowler MB, Valantine HA, Stinson EB, Schroeder JS. Cardiac transplantation in patients with preexisting malignant disease. *Am J Cardiol* 1990; 65:501–504.

29. Rhenman MJ, Rhenman B, Icenogle T, Christensen R, Copeland J. Diabetes and heart transplantation. *J Heart Transplant* 1988; 7:356–358.

30. Badellino MM, Cavarocchi B, Narins M, Jessup M, Alpern JB, McClurken JB, et al. Cardiac transplantation in diabetic patients. *Transplant Proc* 1990; 22:2384–2388.

31. Ladowski JS, Kormos RL, Uretsky BP, Griffith BP, Armitage JM, Hardesty RL. Heart transplantation in diabetic patients. *Transplantation* 1990; 49:303–305.

32. Report of the medical consultants on the diagnosis of death to the President's Commission for the Study of Ethical Problems in Medicine and Biomedical and Behavioral Research: Guidelines for the determination of death. *JAMA* 1981; 246:2184–2186.

33. Evans RW, Manninen DL, Garrison LP, Maier MA. Donor availability as the primary determinant of the future of heart transplantation. *JAMA* 1986; 255:1892–1898.

34. Dreyfus G, Jebara V, Mihaileanu MD, Carpentier A. Total orthotopic heart transplantation: An alternative to the standard technique. *Ann Thorac Surg* 1991; 52:1181–1184.

35. Yacoub M, Mankad P, Ledingham S. Donor procurement and surgical techniques for cardiac transplantation. *Semin Thorac Cardiovasc Surg* 1990; 2:153–161.

36. El Gamel A, Yonan NA, Grant S, Deiraniya AK, Rahman AN, Sarsam MAI, et al. Orthotopic cardiac transplantation: A comparison of standard and bicaval Wythenshawe techniques. *J Thorac Cardiovasc Surg* 1995; 109:721–730.

37. Deleuze PH, Benvenuti C, Mazzucotelli MD, Perdrix C, Le Besnerais P, Mourtada A, et al. Orthotopic cardiac transplantation with direct caval anastomosis: Is it the optimal procedure? *J Thorac Cardiovasc Surg* 1995; 109:731–737.

38. Trento A, Czer LSC, Blanche C. Surgical techniques for cardiac transplantation. *Semin Thorac Cardiovasc Surg* 1996; 8:126–132.

39. Sethi GK, Kosaraju S, Arabia FA, Rosado LJ, McCarthy MS, Copeland JG. Is it necessary to perform surveillance endomyocardial biopsies in heart transplant recipients? *J Heart Lung Transplant* 1995; 14:1047–1051.

40. White JA, Guiraudon C, Pflugfelder PW, Kostuk WJ. Routine surveillance myocardial biopsies are unnecessary beyond one year after heart transplantation. *J Heart Lung Transplant* 1995; 14:1052–1056.

41. Michler RE, Smith CR, Drusin RE. Reversal of cardiac transplant rejection without massive immunosuppression. *Circulation* 1986; 74(suppl III):III68–III74.

42. Costanzo-Nordin MR, Silver MA, O'Connell JB. Successful reversal of cardiac allograft rejection with OKT3 monoclonal antibody. *Circulation* 1987; 76(suppl V):V71–V79.

43. Macris MP, Frazier OH, Lammermeier D, Radovancevic B, Duncan MJ. Clinical experience with Muromonab-CD3 monoclonal antibody (OKT3) in heart transplantation. *J Heart Transplant* 1989; 8:281–287.

44. Strober S. Total lymphoid irradiation in alloimmunity and autoimmunity. *J Pediatr* 1987; 111(6, part 2):1051–1055.

45. Weinblatt ME. Methotrexate for chronic diseases in adults. *N Engl J Med* 1995; 332:330–331.

46. Hunt SA, Strober S, Hoppe RT, Stinson EB. Total lymphoid irradiation for treatment of intractable cardiac allograft rejection. *J Heart Lung Transplant* 1991; 10:211–216.

47. Levin B, Bohannon L, Warvariv V, Bry W, Collins G. Total lymphoid irradiation (TLI) in the cyclosporine era—use of TLI in resistant cardiac allograft rejection. *Transplant Proc* 1989; 21:1793–1795.

48. Costanzo-Nordin MR, Grusk BB, Silver MA. Reversal of recalcitrant cardiac allograft rejection with methotrexate. *Circulation* 1988; 78(suppl III):III47–III57.

49. Bouchart F, Gundry SR, Van Schaack-Gonzales J, Razzouk AJ, Marsa RJ, Kawauchi M, et al. Methotrexate as rescue/adjunctive immunotherapy in infant and adult heart transplantation. *J Heart Lung Transplant* 1993; 12:427–433.

50. Ross HJ, Gullestad L, Pak J, Slauson S, Valantine HA, Hunt SA. Methotrexate or total lymphoid irradiation for treatment of persistent or recurrent allograft cellular rejection: A comparative study. *J Heart Lung Transplant* 1997; 16:179–189.

51. Armitage JM, Kormos RL, Griffith BL, Hardesty RL, Fricker FJ, Stuart RS, et al. A clinical trial of FK506 as primary and rescue

immunosuppression in cardiac transplantation. *Transplant Proc* 1991; 23:1149–1152.

52. Pham SM, Kormos RL, Hattler BG, Kawai A, Tsamandas AC, Demetris AJ, et al. A prospective trial of tacrolimus (FK506) in clinical heart transplantation: Intermediate term results. *J Thorac Cardiovasc Surg* 1996; 111:1–9.

53. Jordan ML, Shapiro R, Vivas CA, Scantlebury VP, Rhandhawa P, Carrieri G, et al. FK506 "rescue" for resistant rejection of renal allografts under primary cyclosporine immunosuppression. *Transplantation* 1994; 57:860–865.

54. Ensley RD, Hunt S, Taylor DO, Renlund DG, Menlove RL, Karwande SV, et al. Predictors of survival after repeat heart transplantation. *J Heart Lung Transplant* 1992; 11:S142–S158.

55. Silvergleid AJ, Schrier S. Acute myelogenous leukemia in two patients treated with azathioprine for non-malignant diseases. *Am J Med* 1974; 57:885–888.

56. Penn I. Cancers after cyclosporine therapy. *Transplant Proc* 1988; 20(suppl I):276–279.

57. Young L, Alfieri C, Hennessy K, Evans H, O'Hara C, Anderson KC, et al. Expression of Epstein-Barr virus transformation-associated genes in tissues of patients with EBV lymphoproliferative diseases. *N Engl J Med* 1989; 321:1080–1085.

58. Hanto DW, Frizzera G, Gail-Peczalska KJ, Purtillo DT, Klein G, Simmons RL, et al. The Epstein-Barr virus (EBV) in the pathogenesis of post transplant lymphoma. *Transplant Proc* 1981; 13:756–760.

59. Hanto DW. Classification of Epstein-Barr virus-associated post transplant lymphoproliferative diseases: Implications for understanding their pathogenesis and developing rational treatment strategies. *Annu Rev Med* 1995; 46:381–394.

60. Starzl TE, Porter FA, Iwatsuki S, Rosenthal JT, Shaw BW, Atchison RW, et al. Reversibility of lymphoma and lymphoproliferative lesions developing under cyclosporine-steroid therapy. *Lancet* 1984; 1:583–587.

61. Hanto DW, Frizzera G, Gail-Peczalska KJ, Sakamoto J, Purtillo DT, Balfour HH, et al. Epstein-Barr virus induced B-cell lymphoma after renal transplantation. *N Engl J Med* 1982; 306:913–918.

62. Shapiro RS, Chauvenet A, McGuire W, Pearson A, Craft AW, McGlave P, et al. Treatment of B-cell lymphoproliferative disorders with interferon alpha and intravenous gamma globulin. *N Engl J Med* 1988; 318:1334.

63. Papdopoulos EB, Ladanyi M, Emanuel D, Mackinnon S, Bonlad F, Carbasi MH, et al. Infusions of donor leukocytes to treat Epstein-Barr virus-associated lymphoproliferative disorders after allogeneic bone marrow transplantation. *N Engl J Med* 1994; 330:1185–1191.

64. Rooney CM, Smith CA, Ng CYC, Lofitin S, Li C, Krance RA, et al. Use of gene-modified virus-specific T lymphocytes to control Epstein-Barr-virus related lymphoproliferation. *Lancet* 1995; 345:9–13.

65. Gao SZ, Schroeder JS, Alderman EL, Hunt SA, Silverman JF, Wiederhold V, et al. Clinical and laboratory correlates of accelerated coronary artery disease in the cardiac transplant patient. *Circulation* 1987; 76(suppl V):56–61.

66. Uretsky BF, Murali S, Reddy PS, Rabin B, Lee A, Griffith BP, et al. Development of coronary artery disease in cardiac transplant patients receiving immunosuppressive therapy with cyclosporine and prednisone. *Circulation* 1987; 76:827–834.

67. Gao SZ, Schroeder JS, Alderman EL, Hunt SA, Valantine HA, Wiederhold V, et al. Prevalence of accelerated coronary artery disease in heart transplant survivors: Comparison of cyclosporine and azathioprine regimens. *Circulation* 1989; 80(suppl III):III100–III105.

68. Gao SZ, Alderman EL, Schroeder JS, Silverman JF, Hunt SA. Accelerated coronary vascular disease in the heart transplant patient: Coronary arteriographic findings. *J Am Coll Cardiol* 1988; 12:334–340.

69. Newton M, Vetrovec G, Hastillo A. Coronary angiographic characteristics of chronic cardiac transplant rejection, abstract. *Circulation* 1984; 70(suppl II):174.

70. St. Goar FG, Pinto FJ, Alderman EL. Intracoronary ultrasound in cardiac transplant recipients: In vivo evidence of "angiographically silent" intimal thickening. *Circulation* 1992; 85:979–987.

71. Heroux AL, Silvermann P, Costanzo MR, O'Sullivan J, Johnson MR, Lino Y, et al. Intracoronary ultrasound assessment of morphological and functional abnormalities associated with cardiac allograft vasculopathy. *Circulation* 1994; 89:272–277.

72. Rickenbacher PR, Pinto FJ, Lewis NP, Hunt SA, Alderman EL, Schroeder JS, et al. Prognostic importance of intimal thickness as measured by intracoronary ultrasound after cardiac transplantation. *Circulation* 1995; 92:3445–3452.

73. Billingham ME. Cardiac transplant atherosclerosis. *Transplant Proc* 1987; (suppl 5):19–25.

74. Pucci AM, Forbes RDC, Billingham ME. Pathologic features in long-term cardiac allografts. *J Heart Lung Transplant* 1990; 9:385–388.

75. Berry GJ, Rizeq MN, Weiss LM, Billingham ME. Graft coronary disease in pediatric heart and combined heart-lung transplant recipients: A study of 15 cases. *J Heart Lung Transplant* 1993; 12:S309–S319.

76. Palmer DC, Tsai CC, Roodman ST, Codd JE, Miller LW, Sarafian JE, et al. Heart graft atherosclerosis: An ominous finding on endomyocardial biopsy. *Transplantation* 1985; 39:385–388.

77. Kaye DM, Esler M, Kingwell B, McPherson G, Esmore D, Jennings G. Functional and neurochemical evidence for partial cardiac sympathetic reinnervation after cardiac transplantation in humans. *Circulation* 1993; 88:1110–1118.

78. Bernardi L, Bianchini B, Spadacini G, Leuzzi S, Valle F, Marchasi E, et al. Demonstrable cardiac reinnervation after human heart transplantation by carotid baroreflex modulation of RR interval. *Circulation* 1995; 92:2895–2903.

79. Stark RP, McGinn AL, Wilson RF. Chest pain in cardiac transplant recipients: Evidence of sensory reinnervation after cardiac transplantation. *N Engl J Med* 1991; 324:1791–1794.

80. Smart FW, Ballantyne CM, Cocanougher B, Farmer JA, Sekela ME, Noon GP, et al. Insensitivity of noninvasive tests to detect coronary artery vasculopathy after heart transplant. *Am J Cardiol* 1991; 67:243–247.

81. Akosah KO, Mohanty PK, Funai JT. Noninvasive detection of transplant coronary artery disease by dobutamine stress echocardiography. *J Heart Lung Transplant* 1994; 13:1024–1038.

82. Derumeaux G, Redonnet M, Mouton-Schliefer D. Dobutamine stress echocardiography in orthotopic heart transplant recipients. *J Am Coll Cardiol* 1995; 25:1665–1672.

83. Keogh AM, Valantine HA, Hunt SA, Schroeder JS, McIntosh N, Oyer PE, et al. Impact of proximal or midvessel discrete coronary artery stenosis on survival after heart transplant. *J Heart Lung Transplant* 1992; 11:892–901.

84. Schroeder JS, Gao SZ, Alderman EL, Hunt SA, Johnstone I, Boothroyd DB, et al. A preliminary study of diltiazem in the prevention of coronary artery disease in heart transplant recipients. *N Engl J Med* 1993; 328:164–170.

85. Kobashigawa JA, Katznelson S, Laks H, Johnson JA, Yeatman L, Wang XM, et al. Effect of pravastatin on outcomes after cardiac transplantation. *N Engl J Med* 1995; 333:621–627.

86. Halle AA, DiSciascio G, Massin EK, Wilson RF, Johnson MR, Sullivan HJ, et al. Coronary angioplasty, atherectomy and bypass surgery in cardiac transplant recipients. *J Am Coll Cardiol* 1995; 26:120–128.

87. Smith JA, Ribakove GH, Hunt SA, Miller J, Stinson EB, Oyer PE, et al. Heart retransplantation: The 25 year experience at a single institution. *J Heart Lung Transplant* 1995; 14:832–839.

88. Ubel PA, Arnold RM, Caplan AL. Rationing failure: The ethical issues of the retransplantation of scarce vital organs. *JAMA* 1993; 270:2469–2474.

89. Mouloupoulos SD, Topaz S, Kolff WJ. Diastolic balloon pumping (with carbon dioxide) in the aorta: Mechanical assistance to the failing circulation. *Am Heart J* 1962; 63:669–675.

90. Kaplan JA, Grover JM. Assisted circulation. In: Kaplan JA, ed. *Cardiac Anesthesia*. New York: Grune & Stratton; 1979:441–469.

91. Creswell L, Rosenbloom M, Cox JL, Fergusson TB, Kouchoukas NT, Spray TL. Intraaortic balloon counterpulsation: Patterns of usage and outcome in cardiac surgery patients. *Ann Thorac Surg* 1992; 54:11–20.

92. Miller JF, Dodson TF, Salan AA, Smith RB. Vascular complications following intraaortic balloon pump insertion. *Am Surg* 1992; 58:232–238.

93. McEnany MT, Kay HR, Buckley MJ, Daggett WM, Endman AJ, Mundth ED. Clinical experience with intra-aortic balloon pump support in 728 patients. *Circulation* 1978; 58(suppl I):124–132.

94. Spencer FC, Eiseman UG, Trinkle JK. Assisted circulation for cardiac failure following intracardiac surgery with cardiopulmonary bypass. *J Thorac Cardiovasc Surg* 1965; 45:56–59.

95. Pierce WS, Parr GVS, Myers JL, Pae WE, Bull AP, Waldenhausen JA. Ventricular assist pumping in patients with cardiogenic shock after cardiac operations. *N Engl J Med* 1981; 305:1606–1610.

96. Pennington DG, Samuels LD, Williams G, Palmer D, Swartz MT, Codd JE, et al. Experience with the Pierce-Donachy ventricular assist device in postcardiotomy patients with cardiogenic shock. *World J Surg* 1985; 9:37–46.

97. Pae WE, Pierce WS. Temporary left ventricular assistance in acute myocardial infarction and cardiogenic shock: Rationale and criteria for utilization. *Chest* 1981; 79:692–695.

98. Portner PM, Oyer PE, McGregor CGA. First human use of an electrically powered implantable ventricular assist system. *Artif Organs* 1985; 9(A):36–38.

99. Copeland JD, Levinson MM, Smith R, Icenogle TB, Vaughn C, Cheng K, et al. The total artificial heart as a bridge to transplantation: A report of two cases. *JAMA* 1986; 256:2991–2995.

100. Copeland JG, Pavie A, Duveau D, Keon WJ, Masters R, Pifarre R, et al. Bridge to transplantation with the CardioWest total artificial heart: The international experience 1993 to 1995. *J Heart Lung Transplant* 1996; 15:94–99.

101. Kormos RL, Borovetz HS, Armitage JM, Hardesty RL, Marrone GC, Griffith BP. Evolving experience with mechanical circulatory support. *Ann Surg* 1991; 214:471–475.

102. Pifarre R, Sullivan H, Montoya A, Bahkos M, Grieco J, Foy BK, et al. Comparison of results after heart transplantation: Mechanically supported versus nonsupported patients. *J Heart Lung Transplant* 1992; 11:235–239.

103. Hammer CR. Nature's obstacles to xenotransplantation. *Transplant Rev* 1994; 8:174–184.

104. Dalmasso AP, Vercellotti GM, Fischel RJ, Bach FH, Platt JL. Mechanism of complement activation in the hyperacute rejection of porcine organs transplanted into primate recipients. *Am J Pathol* 1992; 140:1157–1166.

105. Platt JL, Fischel RJ, Matas AJ, Reif SA, Bolman RM, Bach FH. Immunopathology of hyperacute xenograft rejection in a swine-to-primate model. *Transplantation* 1990; 52:214–220.

106. Cooper DKC. Depletion of natural antibodies in non human primates—a step toward successful discordant xenografting in humans. *Clin Transplant* 1992; 6:178–184.

107. Henry ML, Han MK, Davies EA, Sedmak DD, Ferguson RM. Antibody depletion prolongs xenograft survival. *Surgery* 1994; 115:355–361.

108. Leventhal JR, Delmasso AP, Cromwell JW, Platt JL, Mantivel CJ, Bolman RM, et al. Prolongation of cardiac xenograft survival by depletion of complement. *Transplantation* 1993; 55:857–866.

109. Cary N, Moody J, Yannoutsos N, Wallwork J, White D. Tissue expression of human decay accelerating factor, a regulator of complement activation expressed in mice: A potential approach to inhibition of hyperacute xenograft rejection. *Transplant Proc* 1993; 25:400–401.

110. McCurry KR, Kooyman DL, Alvarado CG, Cotterell AH, Martin MJ, Logan JS, et al. Human complement regulatory proteins protect swine-to-primate cardiac xenografts from humoral injury. *Nature Med* 1995; 1:423–427.

111. Chapman LE, Folks TM, Salomon DR, Patterson AP, Eggerman TE, Noguchi PD. Xenotransplantation and xenogeneic infections. *N Engl J Med* 1995; 333:1498–1501.

112. Sakakibara S, Konno S. Endomyocardial biopsy. *Japan Heart J* 1962; 3:537–543.

113. Caves PK, Stinson EB, Billingham ME, Shumway NE. Percutaneous transvenous endomyocardial biopsy in human heart recipients (experience with a new technique). *Ann Thorac Surg* 1973; 16:325–336.

114. Mason JW. Techniques for right and left ventricular endomyocardial biopsy. *Am J Cardiol* 1978; 41:887–892.

115. Fowles RE, Anderson JS. Instruments and techniques for cardiac biopsy. In: Fowles RE, ed. *Cardiac Biopsy.* New York: Futura Publishing; 1992:71–77.

116. Miller LW, Labovitz AJ, McBride LA, Pennington DG, Kanter K. Echocardiography-guided endomyocardial biopsy: A 5-year experience. *Circulation* 1988; 78(suppl III):III99–III102.

117. Weston MW. Comparison of costs and charges for fluoroscopic- and echocardiographic-guided endomyocardial biopsy. *Am J Cardiol* 1994; 74:839–840.

118. Fowles RE, Mason JW. Endomyocardial biopsy. *Ann Intern Med* 1982; 97:885–894.

119. Deckers JW, Hare JM, Baughman KL. Complications of transvenous right ventricular endomyocardial biopsy in patients with cardiomyopathy: A seven-year survey of 546 consecutive diagnostic procedures in a tertiary referral center. *J Am Coll Cardiol* 1992; 19:43–47.

120. Henslova MJ, Nath H, Bucy RB, Bourge RC, Kirklin JK, Rogers WJ. Coronary artery to right ventricle fistula in heart transplant recipients: A complication of endomyocardial biopsy. *J Am Coll Cardiol* 1989; 14:258–261.

121. Sandhu JS, Uretsky BF, Zerbe TR, Goldsmith AS, Reddy PS, Kormos RL, et al. Coronary artery fistula in the heart transplant patient: A potential complication of endomyocardial biopsy. *Circulation* 1989; 79:350–356.

122. Braverman AC, Coplen SE, Mudge GH, Lee RT. Ruptured chordae tendinae of the tricuspid valve as a complication of endomyocardial biopsy in heart transplant patients. *Am J Cardiol* 1990; 66:111–113.

123. Williams MJA, Lee MY, DiSalvo TG, Dec W, Picard MH, Palacios IF, et al. Biopsy-induced flail tricuspid leaflet and tricuspid regurgitation following orthotopic cardiac transplantation. *Am J Cardiol* 1996; 77:1339–1344.

124. Aretz HT, Billingham ME, Edwards WD, Factor SM, Fallon JF, Fenoglio JJ, et al. Myocarditis: A histopathologic definition and classification. *Am J Cardiovasc Pathol* 1986; 1:3–14.

125. Tazelaar HD, Billingham ME. The surgical pathology of hypertrophic cardiomyopathy. *Arch Pathol Lab Med* 1987; 111:257–260.

126. Schoenfeld MH, Supple EW, Dec GW, Fallon JF, Palacios IF. Restrictive cardiomyopathy versus constrictive pericarditis: Role of endomyocardial biopsy in avoiding unnecessary thoracotomy. *Circulation* 1987; 75:1012–1016.

127. Billingham ME, Bristow MR, Glatstein E, Mason JW, Masek MA, Daniels JR. Adriamycin cardiotoxicity: Endomyocardial biopsy evidence of enhancement by irradiation. *Am J Surg Pathol* 1977; 1:17–23.

128. Mason JW, Bristow MR, Billingham ME, Daniels JR. Invasive and noninvasive methods of assessing adriamycin cardiotoxic effects in man: Superiority of histopathologic assessment using endomyocardial biopsy. *Cancer Treat Rep* 1978; 2:857–864.

129. Billingham ME, Bristow MR. Evaluation of anthracycline cardiotoxicity: Predictive ability and functional correlation of endomyocardial biopsy. *Cancer Treat Symp* 1984; 3:71–75.

130. Tazelaar HD, Locke TJ, McGregor CG. Pathology of surgically excised primary cardiac tumor. *Mayo Clin Proc* 1992; 67:957–965.

131. Sugrue DD, Holmes DR, Gersh BJ, Edwards WD, McLaren CJ, Wood DL, et al. Cardiac histologic findings in patients with life-threatening ventricular arrhythmias of unknown origin. *J Am Coll Cardiol* 1984; 4:952–957.

132. Trento A, Hardesty T, Griffith BP, Zerpe T, Kormos RL, Bahnson HT. Role of the antibody to vascular endothelial cells in hyperacute rejection in patients undergoing cardiac transplantation. *J Thorac Cardiovasc Surg* 1988; 95:37–41.

133. Caves PK, Stinson EB, Billingham ME, Shumway NE. Percutaneous transvenous endomyocardial biopsy in human heart recipients (experience with a new technique). *Ann Thorac Surg* 1973; 16:325–336.

134. Kemnitz J, Cohnert T, Schafer H, Helmke M, Wahlers T, Hermann G, et al. A classification of acute allograft rejection. *Am J Surg Pathol* 1987; 7:503–515.

135. McAllister HA. Histologic grading of cardiac allograft rejection: A quantitative approach. *J Heart Transplant* 1990; 9:277–282.

136. Zerbe TR, Arena V. Diagnostic reliability of endomyocardial biopsy for assessment of cardiac allograft rejection. *Hum Pathol* 1988; 19:1307–1314.

137. Billingham ME, Carey NRB, Hammond EH, Kemnitz J, Marboe C, McAllister HA, et al. A working formulation for the standardization of nomenclature in the diagnosis of heart and lung rejection: Heart rejection study group. *J Heart Transplant* 1990; 9:587–592.

138. Weiss LM, Movahed LA, Berry GJ, Billingham ME. In situ hybridization studies for CMV viral nucleic acids in heart and lung allograft biopsies. *Am J Clin Pathol* 1990; 93:675–679.

139. Randhawa PS, Yousem SA, Paradis IL, Dauber JA, Griffith BP, Locker J. The clinical spectrum, pathology and clonal analysis of Epstein-Barr virus-associated lymphoproliferative disorders in heart-lung transplant recipients. *Am J Clin Pathol* 1989; 92:177–185.

140. Hammond EH, Hansen JK, Spenser LS, Ensley RD. Vascular rejection in cardiac transplantation: Histologic, immunopathologic and ultrastructural features. *Cardiovasc Pathol* 1993; 2:21–34.

141. Hammond EH, Yowell RI, Price GD, Merilove MR, Olsen SL, O'Connell JB, et al. Vascular rejection of human cardiac allografts and the role of humoral immunity in chronic allograft rejection. *Transplant Proc* 1991; 23(suppl 2):26–30.

FOUR

RHYTHM AND CONDUCTION DISORDERS

26

MECHANISMS OF CARDIAC ARRHYTHMIAS AND CONDUCTION DISTURBANCES

Albert L. Waldo / Andrew L. Wit

OVERVIEW OF MECHANISMS OF CARDIAC ARRHYTHMIAS AND CONDUCTION DISTURBANCES

Introduction

Because of the increasing availability of sophisticated electro-physiologic techniques for the study of cardiac tissues, both in vivo and in vitro, and the ability to study arrhythmias and conduction disturbances in both experimental models and in patients, our knowledge of the mechanisms of arrhythmias and conduction disturbances has increased greatly in recent times. While much is now known, much still remains to be understood. Arrhythmias are due to normal or abnormal impulse generation, abnormal impulse conduction, or a combination of simultaneous abnormalities of impulse generation and conduction.[1] In this chapter, we first provide an overview of these mechanisms and identify the clinical arrhythmias with which they are thought to be associated. Then we provide a much more detailed discussion of these mechanisms as they are currently understood. The detailed discussion requires that the reader have a rudimentary knowledge of basic cellular electrophysiology of the heart, including the ionic channels and membrane currents causing the resting potential and the cardiac action potential, as well as the mechanisms for automaticity and conduction. However, much of this material is also included in our detailed discussion on the mechanisms of arrhythmias, since we consider how alterations in normal electrophysiology lead to abnormal cardiac rhythms.

Causes of Arrhythmias

NORMAL OR ABNORMAL IMPULSE INITIATION

Automatic Rhythms

Normal Mechanism Cardiac cells normally capable of developing spontaneous diastolic (phase 4) depolarization are called *pacemaker cells*. When pacemaker cells manifest spontaneous diastolic depolarization (Fig. 26-1) and thereby are responsible for generating the cardiac rhythm, the rhythm is classified as an *automatic rhythm*. Normally, the dominant pacemaker of the heart is in the sinus node, which, in adults, fires at a rate of 60 to 100 beats per minute. Cells capable of developing spontaneous diastolic depolarization (i.e., of manifesting automaticity) also are normally found in the specialized fibers in the atria, in the atrioventricular (AV) junc-

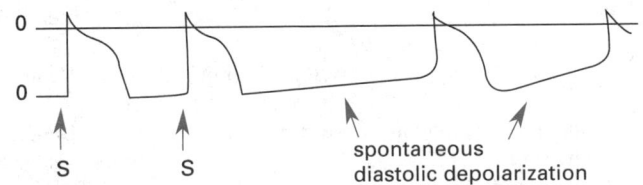

FIGURE 26-1

Arrhythmias may be caused by normal automaticity. Transmembrane potential recorded from a Purkinje fiber stimulated at a regular rate is shown. When the stimulus is turned off, spontaneous diastolic depolarization develops to cause automatic firing.

tion, and in the His-Purkinje system. The normal rate of impulse formation in adults by these ectopic pacemakers is 40 to 60 beats per minute in the AV junction (the AV node and His bundle). Normal rates of more distally located ectopic pacemakers are uncertain but are probably 20 to 40 beats per minute in the bundle branches. These ectopic (i.e., nonsinus) pacemakers are also called *latent* or *escape* pacemakers for two related reasons: (1) the normal intrinsic rate of these pacemakers is less than that of the dominant pacemaker, the sinus node, and (2) spontaneous diastolic depolarization of these latent or escape pacemakers is normally suppressed by the more rapid rate of the sinus node pacemaker by the active process of overdrive suppression. It is only when the sinus rate slows below the intrinsic rate of these ectopic pacemakers

that "the next one in line" warms up and fires (see also "Automaticity," below).

Arrhythmias of the Sinus Node

An arrhythmia occurs when the sinus node pacemaker fires at a rate greater than 100 beats per minute (sinus tachycardia) (Table 26-1) or at a rate less than 60 beats per minute (sinus bradycardia) and is still the dominant pacemaker of the heart. We call these *arrhythmias resulting from normal automaticity*, since the ionic mechanism causing the pacemaker depolarization is unchanged from normal sinus rhythm. A sinus tachycardia is usually an appropriate response to a precipitating factor (e.g., exercise, fever, hypotension, etc.), although, on occa-

TABLE 26-1

TYPES OF TACHYCARDIAS AND THEIR SELECTED CHARACTERISTICS AND DOCUMENTED OR PRESUMED MECHANISM

Tachycardia	Mechanism	Origin	Rate Range, bpm	AV or VA Conduction
Sinus tachycardia	Automatic (normal)	Sinus node	≥100	1:1
Sinus node reentry	Reentry	Sinus node and right atrium	?110–180	1:1 or variable
Atrial fibrillation	Reentry	Atria	260–450, usually >300	Variable
Atrial flutter	Reentry	Right atrium, left atrium (rare)	240–350, usually 300 ± 20	2:1 or variable
Atrial tachycardia	Reentry	Atria	150–240	1:1, 2:1, or variable
	Automatic (normal or abnormal)	Atria	?	?
	Triggered (DADs) 2° to digitalis toxicity	Atria	150–240	1:1, 2:1, or variable
AV nodal reentry tachycardia	Reentry	AV node (? atrial component)	120–250, usually 150–220	1:1
AV reentry (WPW or concealed accessory AV connection)	Reentry	Circuit includes accessory AV connection, atria, AV node, His, Purkinje system, ventricles	140–250, usually 150–220	1:1
Accelerated AV junctional tachycardia	Automatic or ? triggered (? digitalis toxicity)	AV junction (AV node and His bundle)	61–200, usually 80–130	1:1 or variable
Accelerated idioventricular rhythm	Abnormal automaticity	Purkinje fibers	>60–?	Variable, 1:1, or AV dissociation
Ventricular tachycardia	Reentry	Ventricles	120–300, usually 140–240	AV dissociation, variable, or dissociation
	Automatic (rare) (normal or abnormal)	Ventricles	?	Variable, 1:1, or AV dissociation
Bundle ranch reentrant tachycardia	Reentry	Bundle branches and ventricular septum	160–250, usually 195–240	AV dissociation, variable, or 1:1
Right ventricular outflow tract	? Triggered (DADs)	Right ventricular outflow tract	120–220	AV dissociation, variable, or 1:1
Torsades de pointes tachycardia	? Triggered (EADs) (with reentry)	Ventricles	>200	AV dissociation

Key: DAD = delayed afterdepolarization; WPW = Wolff-Parkinson-White syndrome; EAD = early afterdepolarization; bpm = beats per minute.

sion, it may be inappropriate, as in the presence of a sympathetic dysautonomia (inappropriate sinus tachycardia). On the other hand, sinus bradycardia often reflects an abnormality not only of the sinus node pacemakers (they are too slow) but also of the latent or escape pacemakers (when the sinus rate slows abnormally, they do not escape). Sinus bradycardia may be due to an intrinsic abnormality of pacemaker cells, a parasympathetic dysautonomia (inappropriate sinus bradycardia), or an extrinsic factor such as suppression of automaticity by drug therapy (e.g., a beta blocker, a Ca^{2+} channel blocker, or an antiarrhythmic agent). For some patients, sinus bradycardia, particularly when present only at rest, may simply reflect a normal response to increased vagal tone, as in the well-trained athlete. Marked beat-to-beat variations in cycle length of the sinus rhythm, due virtually always to the influence of vagal tone on the pacemaker cells of the sinus node, is also considered an arrhythmia (sinus arrhythmia), even if the overall sinus rate is normal.

Ectopic Automatic Rhythms The arrhythmias occur when the site of the dominant pacemaker shifts to a site other than the sinus node (Table 26-1). The site of impulse initiation may shift from the sinus node to an ectopic (latent or escape) pacemaker if (1) the intrinsic rate of the sinus node decreases—e.g., when pacemaker dysfunction is limited to the sinus node; (2) the intrinsic rate of the ectopic (latent or escape) pacemaker increases—e.g., due to enhanced automaticity of latent pacemakers (during such rhythms, the sinus node is normally automatic, but overdrive suppression of the sinus node pacemaker usually occurs because the ectopic pacemaker fires at a more rapid rate. Alternatively, if the rate of the ectopic pacemaker is very fast, there may be entrance block into the sinus node, in which case exit block of the sinus impulses rather than overdrive suppression occurs); or (3) the normal sinus impulse is prevented from being the dominant pacemaker of the heart, either because of sinus node exit block or sinoatrial block (i.e., the impulse cannot exit from the sinus node to excite the atria and subsequently the ventricles) or AV block (i.e, the impulse cannot excite the ventricles because of conduction block in the specialized AV conduction system, i.e., the AV node, His bundle, or both bundle branches) (see also Chaps. 12 and 27).

Abnormal Mechanism Typically, normal working atrial and ventricular myocardial cells do not develop automaticity. Thus, when they manifest normal transmembrane potentials, no evidence of spontaneous diastolic (phase 4) depolarization is present. Under certain conditions, however, these cardiac muscle fibers, as well as specialized atrial and ventricular fibers, can develop an abnormal type of automatic firing. This occurs when the cell is relatively depolarized, such that maximum diastolic potential is reduced to levels much lower than normal, usually by intrinsic cardiac disease. When this occurs, spontaneous diastolic (phase 4) depolarization may occur (Fig. 26-2). Such abnormal automaticity is caused by a pacemaker current that is different from the pacemaker

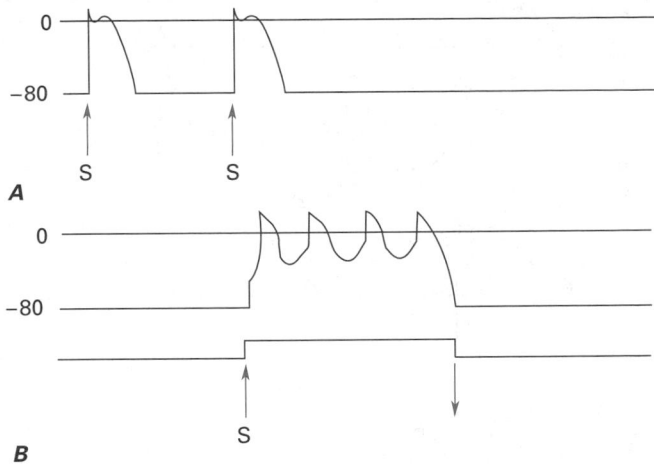

FIGURE 26-2

Arrhythmias may be caused by abnormal automaticity. The figure shows how abnormal automaticity may develop in a ventricular muscle fiber. *A.* Transmembrane potentials recorded from a muscle fiber with a normal resting potential are shown. When the fiber is not stimulated, phase 4 depolarization and automatic firing do not occur (compare with Fig. 26-1). *B.* At arrow, the membrane potential is reduced to −50 mV by a current pulse passed through a microelectrode. Automatic firing occurs at this low level of membrane potential. In the heart, certain abnormal states may cause similar decrease in membrane potential.

current of normally automatic cells. The transmembrane action potentials associated with abnormal automaticity may be of the slow response type; i.e., the transmembrane action potential upstroke may depend on the slow inward (L-type) Ca^{2+} current because of inactivation of Na^+ channels at the reduced level of membrane potential. Arrhythmias caused by abnormal automaticity will not be evident unless the rate of the abnormal focus is greater than that of the dominant automatic pacemaker (usually the sinus node) of the heart. Accelerated idioventricular rhythms after myocardial infarction may sometimes be caused by abnormal automaticity in Purkinje cells in the ischemic region (Table 26-1) (see also Chap. 47).

Triggered Rhythms

These arrhythmias are caused by afterdepolarizations (Table 26-1).

Early afterdepolarizations (*EADs*) are associated with a prolongation of the duration of the action potential and occur during repolarization of a transmembrane action potential that has been initiated from a normal level of membrane potential. They appear as a shift in membrane potential in a positive direction relative to the membrane potential expected during normal repolarization (Fig. 26-3*A* and *B*). Repetitive depolarizations may originate from the low level of membrane potential that occurs during the afterdepolarization (Fig. 26-3*B*). A clinical example of a triggered rhythm thought to be initiated by EADs is *torsades de pointes* associated with a toxic response to class IA or III antiarrhythmic agents or any other agents that prolong the duration of the action potential. Torsades de pointes is associated with other syndromes character-

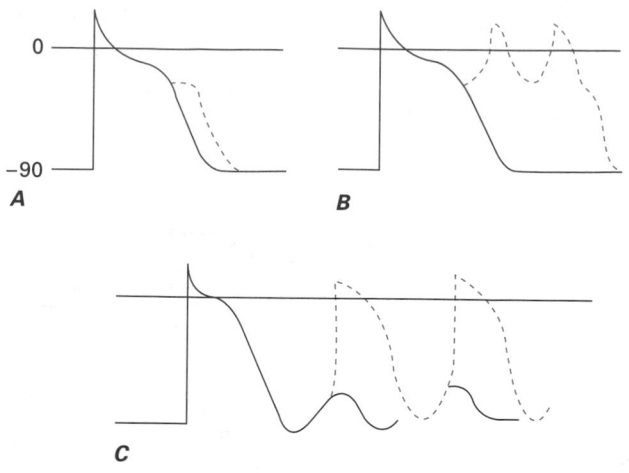

FIGURE 26-3

Triggered activity is caused by afterdepolarizations. *A.* A solid trace shows the normal transmembrane potential from a Purkinje fiber. The dashed trace shows an EAD that is subthreshold. *B.* Early afterdepolarization reached the threshold for the slow inward current, causing repetitive firing during the plateau of the Purkinje fiber action potential. *C.* Solid trace shows a transmembrane action potential followed by a subthreshold DAD. The dashed trace shows the triggered action potentials that occur when the afterdepolarization reaches threshold potential.

ized by a prolonged QT interval and are also thought to be initiated by EADs (Table 26-1).

Delayed afterdepolarizations (DADs) are transient depolarizations that occur after repolarization of the transmembrane action potential (Fig. 26-3*C*). Triggered impulses occur when the DADs reach threshold potential for activation of the inward current responsible for the upstroke of the transmembrane action potential. Delayed afterdepolarizations have been recorded from atrial and ventricular cells exposed to catecholamines, digitalis, or abnormally high levels of Ca^{2+} and are caused by abnormally high intracellular Ca^{2+}. The ionic mechanism causing DADs is the transient inward current, a current caused by oscillatory changes in intracellular Ca^{2+} concentrations. Some digitalis toxic rhythms are thought to be due to delayed afterdepolarizations as well as some idiopathic ventricular tachycardias originating in the right ventricular outflow tract (Table 26-1).

ABNORMAL IMPULSE CONDUCTION

Prolongation of Conduction Time

Prolongation of conduction time of the cardiac impulse may occur anywhere in the heart. It may result from slow conduction and be generalized, as in response to a class IC antiarrhythmic agent, or the slow conduction may be localized to a portion of the heart, e.g., a portion of the specialized AV conduction system or in ventricular myocardium injured by a myocardial infarction or by other kinds of cardiac disease. Prolongation of conduction time resulting from slow conduction may also occur as a normal response of cardiac tissue, as in prolongation of AV nodal conduction time associated with a propagated premature beat. In addition to slow conduc-

tion, prolongation of conduction time may also occur when the cardiac impulse takes longer than normal to get from one place to another, even though conduction velocity of the impulse along the route is normal. An example of the latter is found in patients with an endocardial cushion defect in which the sinus impulse takes an abnormally long time to reach the AV node. This occurs because the location of the ostium primum defect forces the activation wavefront generated by the sinus impulse to take a longer route to reach the AV node.[2] As shown below, however, perhaps the most important role of prolongation of conduction time is in the genesis and maintenance of most tachycardias due to circus movement or reentrant excitation.

Block of Conduction

Block of the propagating impulse may occur for any number of reasons. It may block because the impulse arrives at tissue that is inexcitable, either because the tissue is still in its effective refractory period after a recent depolarization or because it has an abnormally low resting potential caused by disease. Block may also occur because the strength of the propagating wavefront is insufficient to excite the tissue ahead of it despite the fact that that tissue is fully excitable (decremental conduction and block). Block may also occur because the propagating impulse encounters tissue intrinsically unable to conduct the cardiac impulse, e.g., scar tissue associated with a prior myocardial infarction or surgical incision. If there is conduction block of the cardiac impulse, disturbances of cardiac rhythm may occur in several different ways. If the sinus impulse fails to propagate to the right atrium (sinus node exit block or sinoatrial block), normally an ectopic (latent or escape) pacemaker will emerge and assume the role of cardiac pacemaker. If propagation of the cardiac impulse is impaired in the specialized AV conduction system, so that the ventricles are not activated at a sufficiently rapid rate, an ectopic pacemaker (latent or escape) distal to the site of block will often emerge and assume the role of cardiac pacemaker. When either sinoatrial or AV block occurs, however, an ectopic pacemaker may not emerge quickly enough and/or at a clinically adequate rate under some circumstances. Thus, either a period of asystole, marked bradycardia, or both may occur. If either or both happen, the clinical problem may be quite serious and even life-threatening. Block may also occur in one of the bundle branches, causing either left or right bundle branch block. Bundle branch block per se is rarely a clinical problem of any consequence except when the block occurs simultaneously in both bundle branches.

Unidirectional Block and Reentry

During normal sinus rhythm, the conducted impulse from the sinus node pacemaker dies out after orderly and sequential activation of the atria, the specialized AV conduction system, and the ventricles because the impulse is prevented from reactivating the myocardium by the refractoriness of the tissue that has just been activated. The heart must then wait for a new impulse from the sinus node pacemaker for each subsequent activation. The phenomenon of reentry occurs when the propagating impulse does not die out but rather continues to propagate and reactivate the heart, because the activation wavefront continuously encounters excitable cardiac tissue. Almost all clinically important tachyarrhythmias are due to reentry (Table 26-1). For reentry to occur, several conditions must be met. First, there must exist a substrate in the cardiac tissue capable of supporting reentry, i.e., a region in the heart with the appropriate electrical properties in which reentry can occur. Second, the excitation wavefront must encounter unidirectional block. Third, the activation wavefront must be able to circulate around a central area of block.

Figure 26-4*A, B,* and *C* illustrates a simple model of reentry in a loop of excitable tissue, as actually first demonstrated by Mayer in 1906 in the excitable ring of a jellyfish[3] and later by Mines in rings of cardiac tissue cut from the tortoise heart.[4] The center of the loop is a hole, and this serves as a central area of block around which the reentrant wavefront can circulate. If the loop of excitable tissue is stimulated at a single point, two wavefronts of excitation circulate in the ring in opposite directions from this point (Fig. 26-4*A*). Since the wavefronts collide, they die out. If block of one of the circulating wavefronts occurs (e.g., in the shaded area), however, an excitation wavefront can circulate in only one direction around the loop—i.e., unidirectional block of the stimulated wavefront has occurred (Fig. 26-4*B*). If either conduction of the nonblocked impulse around the loop is slow enough (e.g., because of a region or regions of slow conduction) or, in the presence of normal conduction, the loop is long enough so that by the time the circulating wavefront has returned to its site of origin, this latter region has recovered excitability, the wavefront can then reexcite (i.e., reenter) tissue it has previously excited and continue to circulate (Fig. 26-4*C*). In order for this to occur, however, the region of block must manifest unidirectional block, i.e., block in the right-to-left direction but conduction in the left-to-right direction (Fig. 26-4*C*). If the region of previous block remains unexcitable, then bidirectional block at this site has prevented reentry. Since the block is unidirectional, reentry occurs. In the presence of myocardium manifesting unidirectional block and a central inexcitable area around which an excitation wavefront can circulate, as long as the wavelength (the product of the conduction velocity of the circulating wavefront and the effective refractory period of the tissue of the reentrant circuit) of the circulating wavefront is shorter than the length of the pathway in which it is traveling, the wavefront will continue to circulate. In other words, as long as myocardium in the reentrant circuit ahead of the propagating reentrant excitation wave has sufficient time to recover excitability after its prior excitation, reentry can continue. The result is classical circus movement or reentrant excitation. Thus, an area of slow conduction is not an absolute requisite for reentrant excitation to occur.

Reentry can occur at normal conduction velocities if the path length is sufficiently long. Most reentrant circuits, however, require the presence of an area of slow conduction. This is because in most circumstances, despite the presence of unidirectional block, the length of the potential reentrant circuit is too short, so that without the presence of an area or areas of slow conduction, the nonblocked wavefront would otherwise travel around the circuit so quickly that it would arrive at the point of origin of the wavefront (the stimulus site in Fig. 26-4) before this site had recovered sufficiently to become excitable again. In fact, presumably for this very reason, an area (or areas) of slow conduction is part of the reentrant circuit for virtually all clinical reentrant rhythms. Reentrant circuits may be located almost anywhere in the heart, and they can assume many sizes and shapes.

Reentry in which the circulating wavefront continuously reenters over the same stable pathway to generate the reentrant rhythm is called *ordered reentry*.[1] The circuit may comprise a well-defined anatomic pathway, an anatomic circuit. One such example is the reentrant circuit in AV reentrant tachycardia (atrium, AV node, His-Purkinje system, ventricle, accessory AV connection). Functional circuits, which depend on cellular electrophysiologic properties rather than anatomy, can also be associated with ordered reentry if the electrophysiologic properties crucial for reentry are confined to a specific location, and reentry occurs only in that location. Ordered reentry can also involve a combination of anatomic and functional pathways. Examples of ordered reentry include atrial flutter, most monomorphic ventricular tachycardias, AV nodal reentrant tachycardia, AV reentrant tachycardia involving an accessory AV connection, and sinus node reentrant tachycardia (Table 26-1) (see also Chap. 27). During random reentry,[1] propagation occurs in reentrant pathways that continuously change their size and location with time. For this to occur, circuits must, at least to a significant degree, be functional. Random reentry need not depend on any special electrophysiologic abnormality in the heart, although electrophysiologic abnormalities may also lead to random reentry. Examples of random reentry are atrial and ventricular fibrillation (Table 26-1).

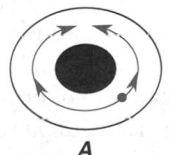 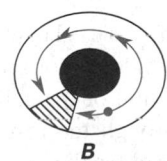 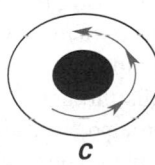

| A | B | C |

FIGURE 26-4

Schematic representation of reentry in a ring of excitable tissue. *A.* Ring was stimulated in the area indicated by the black dot. Impulses propagated away from the point of stimulation in both directions and collided; no reentry occurred. *B.* Cross-hatched area was compressed while the ring was stimulated, again at the black dot. The impulse propagated around the ring in only one direction, having been blocked in the other direction by an area of compression. Then, immediately after stimulation, the compression was relieved. *C.* Circulating impulse is shown returning to its point of origin and then continuing around the ring. Identical reentry would occur if the crosshatched area were a region of unidirectional conduction block with block in the right-to-left direction.

Reflection

The term *reflection* has been used to describe a form of reentry in a linear bundle in which two excitable regions are separated by an area of depressed conduction.[5] During reflection, excitation occurs slowly in one direction along the bundle and is followed by continued propagation and excitation occurring in the opposite direction. One form of reflection may, in fact, be microreentry based on functional longitudinal dissociation within the depressed segment.[6–8] How this might occur is diagrammed in Fig. 26-5. The diagram at the top of the figure depicts two adjacent fibers in a bundle. The entire shaded area is depressed (reduced membrane potential and slow action potential upstrokes), the darker area in the upper fiber indicating more severe depression than the lighter area in the lower fiber. Unidirectional conduction block occurs in the more severely depressed region. Arrows labeled I show the impulse entering the two fibers from the left end. Conduction of the impulse (I) blocks in the fiber at the top, in the severely depressed region, but continues in the fiber at the bottom, which is not as depressed. The impulse conducts transversely from the bottom fiber to the top fiber once past the region of severe depression. It then conducts retrogradely through this severely depressed region in the top bundle. Arrows labeled II show the reflected impulse returning to reexcite the left end of the bundle. Action potentials that were recorded from sites a, b, and c in the bottom fiber are shown below: action potentials labeled I were recorded as the impulse conducted from left to right; action potentials labeled II were recorded as the impulse conducted from right to left, returning to its origin. It is thought that such reentry may occur in the His bundle, one of the bundle branches or peripheral branches of Purkinje fiber bundles.

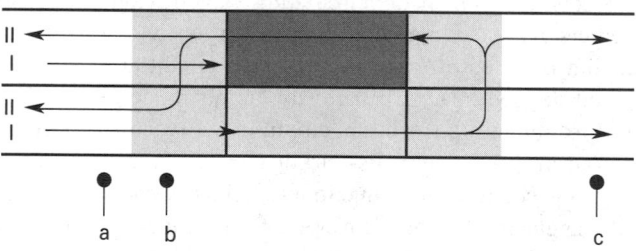

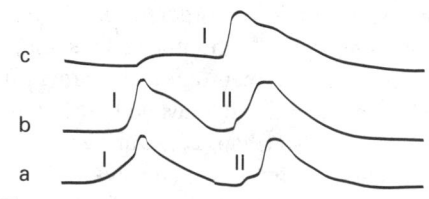

FIGURE 26-5

Diagram of reflection based on microentry. *Top:* Schematic representation of two adjacent myocardial fibers. The shaded region indicates an area of depressed conduction. Arrows show the pattern of activation: Arrow I is a wavefront conducting in an antegrade direction, and arrow II is a reflected wavefront conducting in a retrograde direction. Action potentials shown below were recorded at sites a, b, and c on the diagram. (Modified from Wit AL, Bigger JT Jr. Possible electrophysiological mechanisms for lethal arrhythmias accompanying myocardial ischemia and infarction. *Circulation* 1975; 52(Suppl):III96–III115. Reproduced with permission from the publisher and authors.)

SIMULTANEOUS ABNORMALITIES OF IMPULSE GENERATION AND CONDUCTION PARASYSTOLE

Parasystole

At times, an ectopic pacemaker may be connected to the remainder of the heart through tissue(s) in which there is unidirectional block. The unidirectional block prevents the dominant rhythm, usually a sinus rhythm, from entering the region where the ectopic pacemaker is located. As a result, the ectopic pacemaker is not suppressed by the dominant rhythm of the heart. At the same time, because the block is unidirectional, impulses generated by the ectopic pacemaker can be conducted out to other regions of the heart provided that they are not refractory, causing premature beats or even a tachycardia. This kind of rhythm is called *parasystole*. Thus, parasystole is a rhythm due to impulse generation (presumed to be due to an ectopic pacemaker, but it could be due to any mechanism) in a protected focus. The focus is protected because there is entrance block into the focus (due to unidirectional block). An impulse may exit the focus and excite the heart if the impulse generated by the parasystolic focus finds tissue that is excitable, i.e., not in the effective refractory period.

Phase 4 Block

Block of an impulse may occur if the impulse arrives at a site—e.g., in the His bundle or one of the bundle branches—that is partially depolarized during spontaneous phase 4 depolarization but has not yet reached threshold. This spontaneous diastolic depolarization can sufficiently depolarize the tissue so that the fast Na^+ channels are inactivated enough to cause failure of propagation.[9]

DETAILED DISCUSSION OF MECHANISMS OF ARRHYTHMIAS AND CONDUCTION DISTURBANCES

Arrhythmias Caused by Impulse Initiation

INTRODUCTION

The term *impulse initiation* is used to indicate that an electrical impulse can arise in a single cell or group of closely coupled cells through depolarization of the cell membrane and, once initiated, can spread through the rest of the heart. Impulse initiation occurs because of localized changes in ionic currents that flow across the membranes of single cells. There are two major causes for the impulse initiation that may result in arrhythmias: automaticity and triggered activity. Each has its own unique cellular mechanism resulting in membrane depolarization.

AUTOMATICITY

It is convenient to subdivide automaticity into two kinds: normal and abnormal. Normal automaticity is found in the primary pacemaker of the heart, the sinus node, as well as in certain subsidiary or latent pacemakers that can become the pacemaker under conditions described later. Impulse initiation is a normal property of these latent pacemakers. On the other hand, abnormal automaticity, whether the result of experimental interventions or disease, occurs in cardiac cells only when there are major abnormal changes in their transmembrane potentials, in particular in steady-state depolarization of the membrane potential. This property of abnormal automaticity is not confined to any specific latent pacemaker cell type but may occur almost anywhere in the heart.

Normal Automaticity: Pacemaker Mechanisms

The normal site of impulse initiation is the sinus node. The cause of normal automaticity in the sinus node is a spontaneous decline in the transmembrane potential during diastole, referred to as the *pacemaker potential, phase 4,* or *diastolic depolarization* (the terms are interchangeable). Diastolic depolarization is that part of the sinus node membrane potential labeled dd in the top panel (*A*) of Fig. 26-6. When the depolarization reaches threshold potential (dashed line labeled TP), the upstroke of the spontaneous action potential is initiated. In the case of the sinus node, this upstroke is caused mainly by an inward-directed calcium current through L-type calcium channels. This fall in membrane potential during phase 4 reflects a gradual shift in the balance between inward and outward membrane currents in the direction of net inward (depolarizing) current.

Studies have been done to elucidate and characterize the membrane currents that cause diastolic (phase 4) depolarization in the sinus node using voltage clamp techniques in small tissue preparations and in single dissociated sinus node cells. The cause of the pacemaker potential is still controversial. There is some evidence that diastolic depolarization results from the turning on of an inward current, called i_f, which is activated after repolarization of the sinus node action potential. The net inward i_f current is carried largely by Na^+.[10] From the voltage clamp studies, it is known that the i_f channels are inactivated at positive membrane potentials, begin to activate after hyperpolarization to around -40 mV, and are fully activated after hyperpolarization to around -100 mV.[11–13] Since the maximum diastolic potential of the sinus node pacemaker cells is between -60 and -70 mV, the i_f current is turned on during repolarization to this level, although it is not fully activated at the maximum diastolic potential. Activation of the i_f conductance also has a time dependency; therefore, the inward current continues to increase after complete repolarization, causing the progressive fall in the membrane potential during phase 4. Important roles for other membrane currents, including the potassium current i_K and the T and L Ca^{2+} currents causing spontaneous diastolic depolarization, have also been proposed.[14–22] Therefore, there may be no single pacemaker current in the sinus node but rather a number of currents may contribute to the occurrence of automaticity.[18]

The intrinsic rate at which sinus node pacemaker cells initiate impulses is determined by the interplay of three factors[23]: (1) the maximum diastolic potential; (2) the threshold

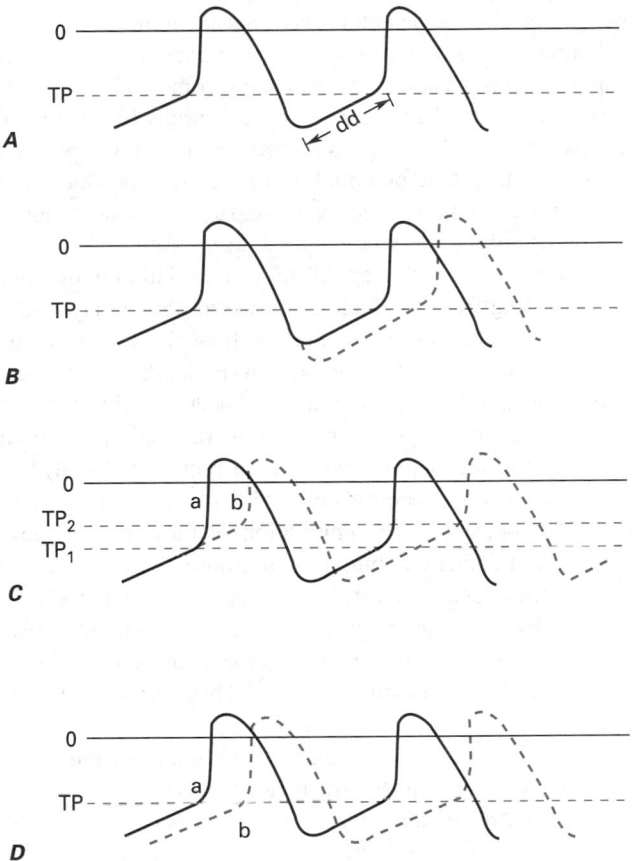

FIGURE 26-6

Diagrams of sinus node action potentials illustrating normal automaticity caused by spontaneous diastolic depolarization and the factors that change the rate of impulse initiation. *A.* Typial sinus node action potential with spontaneous diastolic depolarization (dd). *B.* Change in the rate when the maximum diastolic potential is shifted to a more negative level (from a to b). *C.* Change in rate caused by change in threshold potential to a less negative level (from TP1 to TP2). *D.* Change in rate that occurs when the slope of phase 4 depolarization is decreased (from a to b). (Modified after Wit AL, Janes MJ. *The Ventricular Arrhythmias of Ischemia and Infarction: The Electrophysiological Mechanisms.* Mt Kisco, NY: Futura; 1992. Reproduced with permission from the publisher and authors.)

potential; and (3) the rate or slope of phase 4 depolarization. The third factor is related to the properties of the pacemaker current(s). A change in any one of these factors will alter the time required for phase 4 depolarization to carry the membrane potential from its maximum diastolic level to threshold and thereby alter the rate of impulse initiation. For example, if the maximum diastolic potential increases (becomes more negative) going from solid trace a to dashed trace b in Fig. 26-6*B*, spontaneous depolarization to threshold potential will take longer and the rate of impulse initiation will fall. Conversely, a decrease in the maximum diastolic potential will tend to increase the rate of impulse initiation (going from trace b to trace a). Similarly, changes in threshold potential or changes in the slope of phase 4 depolarization will alter the rate of impulse initiation. In Fig. 26-6*C*, a change in threshold potential from TP1 to the less negative TP2 causes spontaneous diastolic depolarization to proceed for a longer time (dashed action potential trace) before an impulse is initiated, slowing the rate. In Fig. 26-6*D*, a decrease in the slope of spontaneous diastolic depolarization from a to b also results in a longer interval between action potentials (dashed trace) because of the longer time required for membrane potential to reach the threshold potential. In Fig. 26-6*C* and *D*, changes of threshold potential or slope of diastolic depolarization in the opposite direction would speed up the rate.

The alterations in the rate of impulse initiation in the sinus node resulting from the factors discussed above may lead to arrhythmias. They are often the result of the actions of the autonomic nervous system on the sinus node. Parasympathetic stimulation and the resultant release of acetylcholine hyperpolarize the membrane potential through stimulation of muscarinic receptors and activation of a K current (Fig. 26-6*B*).[24,25] Acetylcholine also decreases inward Ca^{2+} current and the i_f pacemaker current.[26] A combination of these effects slows the rate. Sympathetic stimulation and norepinephrine release increase the slope of diastolic depolarization and therefore sinus rate by increasing L-type Ca^{2+} current[27] and by increasing activation of the inward i_f current at the completion of action potential repolarization.[12,13,28] These effects are mediated through β_1-receptor stimulation.

In addition to the sinus node, cells with pacemaking capability in the normal heart are located in some parts of the atria and ventricles, although they are not pacemakers while the sinus node is functioning normally. These are latent or subsidiary pacemakers. Since spontaneous diastolic depolarization is a normal property, the automaticity generated by these cells is classified as normal. In the atria, cells with well-polarized membrane potentials (resting potentials of around -80 mV) and action potentials characterized by fast upstrokes, a plateau phase of repolarization, and spontaneous diastolic depolarization are located along the crista terminalis (Fig. 26-7*A*).[29] Subsidiary atrial pacemakers with somewhat lower maximum diastolic potentials (-75 to -70 mV) and prominent phase 4 depolarization are located at the junction of the inferior right atrium and inferior vena cava, near or on the Eustachian ridge (a remnant of the Eustachian valve of the inferior vena cava) (Fig. 26-7*B*.)[30–32] Other potential atrial pacemakers are at the orifice of the coronary sinus (Fig. 26-7*C*)[33] and in the atrial muscle that extends into the tricuspid and mitral valves (Fig. 26-7*D*).[34–36] Action potentials of cells in the valves have slow upstrokes that are probably caused to a significant extent by L-type Ca^{2+} current. In the AV junction, AV nodal cells possess the intrinsic property of automaticity (Fig. 26-7*E*),[37] although there is still some uncertainty as to the exact location of these pacemakers in the node.[38] The intrinsic rate of the atrial pacemakers is greater than that of AV junctional pacemakers.[39] Both atrial and AV junctional subsidiary pacemakers are under autonomic control, with the sympathetics enhancing pacemaker activity through β_1-adrenergic stimulation and the parasympathetics inhibiting pacemaker activity through muscarinic receptor stimulation.[40–43] In the ventricles, latent or subsidiary pacemakers are found in the His-Purkinje system, where Purkinje fibers have the property of spontaneous diastolic depolariza-

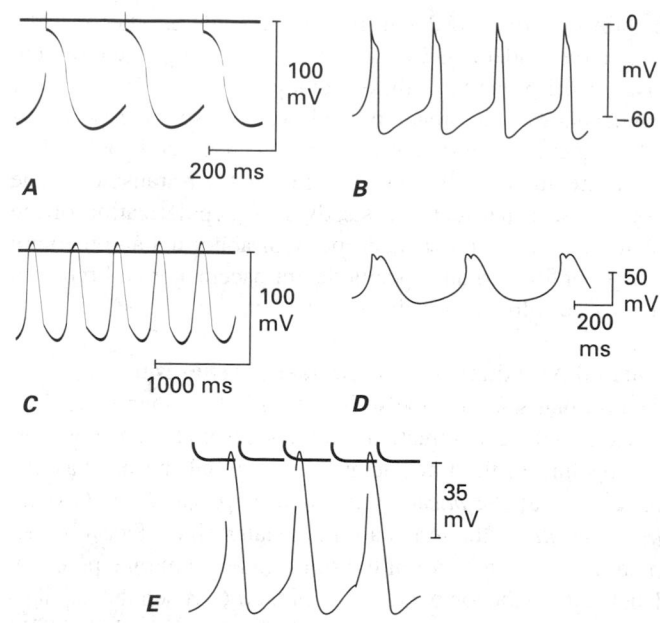

FIGURE 26-7

Transmembrane potentials recorded in isolated superfused preparations from some subsidiary pacemaker cells with the property of normal automaticity. Spontaneous diastolic depolarization that developed in the absence of overdrive suppression is shown in each panel. *A.* Atrial fiber in crista terminalis in the presence of isoproterenol. *B.* Atrial fiber in the inferior right atrium. *C.* Atrial fiber in ostium of coronary sinus in the presence of norepinephrine. *D.* Atrial fiber in stretched mitral valve leaflet. *E.* Atrioventricular nodal fiber of the rabbit heart after the AV node was separated from the atrium. (From Wit AL, Janse MJ. *The Ventricular Arrhythmias of Ischemia and Infarction: The Electrophysiological Mechanisms.* Mt Kisco, NY: Futura; 1992. Reproduced with permission from the publisher and authors.)

tion (Fig. 26-8).[23,44] The intrinsic Purkinje fiber pacemaker rate in general is less than the rate of atrial and AV junctional pacemakers and decreases from the His bundle to the distal Purkinje branches.[45] The spontaneous diastolic depolarization in this region is also under similar autonomic control. As in the atria, sympathetic activation enhances automaticity,[46] while parasympathetic activation can reduce it, mostly through inhibition of sympathetic influences.[47,48]

The membrane currents causing the normal spontaneous diastolic depolarization at ectopic sites have also been studied. The most thorough analyses have been done on the pacemaker current in Purkinje cells using voltage clamp techniques. These studies have shown the presence of an i_f pacemaker current, as in the sinus node.[28,49,50] The i_f channels are deactivated during the action potential upstroke and initial plateau phase of repolarization but begin to activate as repolarization brings the membrane potential to levels more negative than about -60 mV. Since the activation kinetics are slow, the channels continue to activate throughout diastole, leading to an increasing net inward current carried mostly by Na^+ and diastolic depolarization.[49,50] Other currents are also likely to contribute to the pacemaker potential in Purkinje cells.[28,51–53] It is likely that the net increase in inward current during diastole causing spontaneous diastolic depolarization in Purkinje fibers is a result of an increase in an inward current i_f and a decrease in outward current (i_{K_1} and i_K). In the coming years, the relative contributions of each of these currents are sure to be elucidated.

Abnormal Automaticity: Pacemaker Mechanisms

Working atrial and ventricular myocardial cells do not normally have spontaneous diastolic depolarization and do not initiate spontaneous impulses even when they are not excited for long periods of time by propagating impulses. When the resting potentials of working atrial or ventricular myocardial cells are reduced sufficiently, however, spontaneous diastolic depolarization may occur and cause repetitive impulse initiation, a phenomenon called *depolarization-induced automaticity* or *abnormal automaticity*. The level of membrane potential at which abnormal automaticity occurs is often in a range between −70 and −30 mV (see Fig. 26-2).[54] Likewise, cells in the Purkinje system, which are normally automatic at high levels of membrane potential, also show abnormal automaticity when the membrane potential is reduced.[55] As discussed before, the i_f channels that participate in normal pacemaker activity in Purkinje fibers have a gating mechanism controlling channel opening and closing that is dependent on the transmembrane voltage. At membrane potentials positive to about −60 mV, as after the upstroke and during the early phases of repolarization, the channels are closed. In response to the negative potentials occurring after complete repolarization, the channels reopen, generating the inward pacemaker current.[49,50] For this reason, when the steady-state membrane potential of Purkinje fibers is reduced to around −60 mV or less, as may sometimes occur in ischemic regions of the heart, these normal pacemaker channels are not functional, and automaticity is not caused by the normal pacemaker mechanism. It can, however, be caused by an "abnormal" mechanism (described below).

In Fig. 26-9, the transmembrane potential recorded from a spontaneously firing Purkinje fiber with normal automaticity is shown in panel *A*, and abnormal

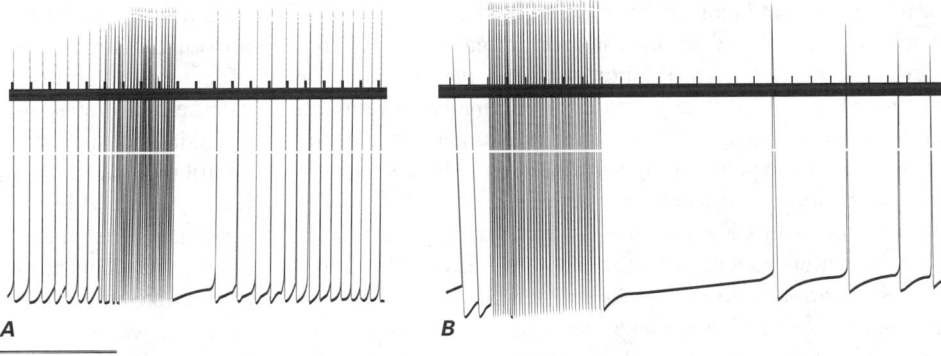

FIGURE 26-8

Overdrive suppression of normal automaticity in a canine Purkinje fiber. The action potentials are displayed at a slow oscilloscopic sweep speed so the time course of repolarization cannot be seen. Note the warmup of the spontaneous pacemaker following termination of pacing. (From Cranefield PF. *The Conduction of the Cardiac Impulse: The Slow Response and Cardiac Arrhythmia.* Mt Kisco, NY: Futura; 1975. Reproduced with permisson from the publisher and author.)

automatic activity occurring while the membrane potential is depolarized to progressively lower membrane potentials is shown in panel *B:* 1, 2, and 3. The abnormal automatic rate increased as membrane potential became more positive. This is a general characteristic of abnormal automaticity in atrial and ventricular cells as well. A low level of membrane potential is not the only criterion for defining abnormal automaticity. If this were so, the automaticity of the sinus node would have to be considered abnormal. Therefore, an important distinction between abnormal and normal automaticity is that

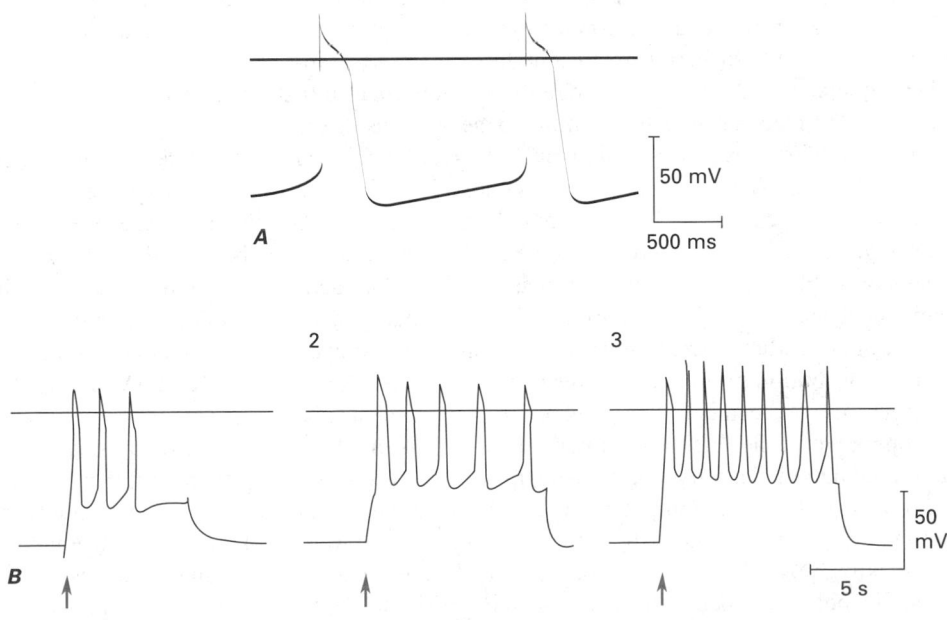

FIGURE 26-9

Normal and abnormal automaticity in a canine Purkinje fiber. *A.* Transmembrane potential recording from a Purkinje fiber with a normal maximum diastolic potential −85 mV and spontaneous diastolic depolarization. *B.* Abnormal automaticity that occurred when membrane potential was decreased: (1) fiber was depolarized (*at arrow*) to a membrane potential of −45 mV by injecting a long-lasting current pulse through a microelectrode; (2) membrane potential was reduced to −40 mV (*at arrow*); (3) membrane potential was reduced to −30 mV (*at arrow*). (Reproduced from Wit AL, Friedman PF. Basis for ventricular arrhythmias accompanying myocardial infarction: alterations in electrical activity of ventricular muscle and Purkinje fibers after coronary artery occlusion. *Arch Intern Med* 1975; 135:459. Reproduced with permission from the publisher and author.)

the membrane potentials of fibers showing the abnormal type of activity are reduced from their own normal level. For this reason, we do not classify automaticity in the AV node or valves, where membrane potential is normally low, to be abnormal automaticity. A likely cause of automaticity at depolarized membrane potentials in ventricular muscle is activation and deactivation of the delayed rectifier K current.[56,57] The conductance of this K channel is activated during the normal action potential plateau, and the outward current that flows through it normally contributes to repolarization. The channel then deactivates during diastole. No significant outward current flows through this channel at normal diastolic potentials, since the resting potential lies near the reversal potential and the driving force is negligible.[57] When the membrane potential is depolarized, however, an outward current flows through this channel, which is activated at the depolarized membrane potentials. This current hyperpolarizes the membrane potential. As the channel then deactivates at the hyperpolarized potentials, spontaneous diastolic depolarization occurs. If either Na or Ca channels have been reactivated since the preceding action potential, the spontaneous depolarization caused by K-channel deactivation may lead to an upstroke caused by current flowing through one of these channels (depending on the level of the membrane potential).[57] A similar mechanism might cause abnormal automaticity in partially depolarized Purkinje fibers.

Experiments on depolarized human atrial myocardium from dilated atria indicate that Ca^{2+}-dependent processes may also contribute to abnormal pacemaker activity at low membrane potentials.[58,59] It was proposed that intracellular Ca^{2+} released from the sarcoplasmic reticulum controls membrane permeability to an inward current during diastole, leading to spontaneous diastolic depolarization and abnormal automaticity. The mechanism may be similar to the one causing the transient inward current responsible for DADs (see "Triggered Rhythms," above). An increase in intracellular Ca^{2+} is also expected to cause an inward Na^+ current through Na^+–Ca^{2+} exchange. In summary, therefore, several different mechanisms probably cause abnormal automaticity, including activation and deactivation of K^+ currents, Ca^{2+}-dependent activation of an inward current, inward Ca^{2+} currents, and even some contribution by the pacemaker current i_f.

It has not yet been determined which of these mechanisms are operative in the different pathologic conditions in which abnormal automaticity may occur. The upstrokes of the spontaneously occurring action potentials generated by abnormal automaticity may be caused by either Na^+ or Ca^{2+} inward currents or, possibly, a mixture of the two. In the range of diastolic potentials between approximately -70 and -50 mV, repetitive activity is dependent on extracellular Na^+ concentration and can be decreased or abolished by the Na^+ channel blockers lidocaine and tetrodotoxin, indicating that the Na^+ inward current is involved. In a diastolic potential range of approximately -50 to -30 mV, repetitive activity depends on extracellular Ca^{2+} concentration and is reduced by the Ca^{2+} channel blockers, Mn^{2+}, and verapamil, indicating a role for the L-type Ca^{2+} inward current.[5,60] The

decrease in membrane potential of cardiac cells required for abnormal automaticity to occur may be induced by a variety of factors related to cardiac disease. Although an increase in extracellular potassium concentration can reduce membrane potential, normal or abnormal automaticity in working atrial, ventricular, and Purkinje fibers usually does not occur when $[K]_o$ is elevated because of the increase in K^+ conductance (and, hence, net outward current) that results from an increase in $[K]_o$.[61,62] This argues against abnormal automaticity being responsible for arrhythmias arising in acutely ischemic myocardium, where cells are partially depolarized by increased extracellular K^+.[63–65] A decrease in $[K]_i$, which also causes a decreased membrane potential, has been shown to occur in the Purkinje fibers that survive on the endocardial surface of infarcts, and this decrease persists for at least 24 h after the coronary occlusion.[66] The reduction in $[K]_i$ contributes to the low membrane potential[67] and the accompanying abnormal automaticity.[68,69] Isolated preparations of diseased atrial and ventricular myocardium from human hearts superfused with Tyrode's solution show phase 4 depolarization and abnormal automaticity at membrane potentials in the range of -50 to -60 mV.[70–72] It has been proposed that a decrease in membrane potassium conductance is an important cause of the low membrane potentials in the atrial fibers.[71]

Suppression of Normal and Abnormal Automatic Subsidiary Pacemakers

During sinus rhythm in the normal heart, the intrinsic rate of impulse initiation due to automaticity of cells in the sinus node is higher than that of the other potentially automatic cells, and the latent pacemakers are excited by propagated impulses from the sinus node before they can depolarize spontaneously to threshold potential. Not only are latent pacemakers prevented from initiating an impulse because they are depolarized before they have a chance to fire, but also the diastolic (phase 4) depolarization of the latent pacemaker cells with the property of normal automaticity is actually inhibited because they are repeatedly depolarized by the impulses from the sinus node.[73,74] This inhibition can be demonstrated by suddenly stopping the sinus node, e.g., by vagal stimulation (vagal stimulation also inhibits subsidiary pacemakers in the atria and AV junction) or in the tissue bath following termination of overdrive pacing (Fig. 26-8). Impulses then usually arise from a subsidiary pacemaker in the ventricular Purkinje system, but that impulse initiation is generally preceded by a long period of quiescence.[75,76] Impulse initiation by the Purkinje fiber pacemaker then begins at a low rate and only gradually speeds up to a final steady rate that is, however, still slower than the original sinus rhythm. The quiescent period following abolition of the sinus rhythm reflects the inhibitory influence exerted on the subsidiary pacemaker by the dominant sinus node pacemaker. This inhibition is called *overdrive suppression*. Similarly, the sinus node also overdrive-suppresses subsidiary atrial pacemakers.[77]

The mechanism of overdrive suppression has been characterized in microelectrode studies on isolated Purkinje fiber bundles exhibiting pacemaker activity.[73] It is mostly mediated by enhanced activity of the Na^+–K^+ exchange pump that results from driving a pacemaker cell faster than its intrinsic spontaneous rate. During normal cardiac rhythm, the sinus node drives the latent pacemakers at a faster rate than their normal (intrinsic) automatic rate. As a result, the intracellular Na^+ of the latent pacemakers is increased to a higher level than would be the case were the pacemakers firing at their own intrinsic rate. This is the result of Na^+ entering the cells during each action potential upstroke. The rate of activity of the Na^+ pump is largely determined by the level of intracellular Na^+ concentration,[78] so that pump activity is enhanced during high rates of stimulation.[73] The increased pump activity prevents intracellular Na^+ from rising to very high levels, although there is some increase in the steady-state Na^+ concentration at high rates of firing. Since the Na^+ pump moves more Na^+ outward than K^+ inward, it generates a net outward (hyperpolarizing) current across the cell membrane.[79] When subsidiary pacemaker cells are driven faster than their intrinsic rate by the sinus node, the enhanced outward pump current hyperpolarizes the membrane potential and suppresses spontaneous impulse initiation in these cells, which, as described before, is dependent on the net inward current. When the dominant (overdrive) pacemaker is stopped, this suppression continues because the Na^+ pump continues to generate the outward current as it reduces the intracellular Na^+ levels toward normal. The continued Na^+ pump-generated outward current is responsible for the period of quiescence, which lasts until the intracellular Na^+ concentration, and hence the pump current, becomes small enough to allow subsidiary pacemaker cells to depolarize spontaneously to threshold. Intracellular Na^+ concentration decreases during the quiescent period because Na^+ is constantly being pumped out of the cell and little is entering.[60] Intracellular Na^+ and pump current continue to decline even after spontaneous firing begins because of the slow rate, causing a gradual increase in the discharge rate of the subsidiary pacemaker.

The higher the overdrive rate, or the longer the duration of overdrive, the greater the enhancement of pump activity, so that the period of quiescence following the cessation of overdrive is directly related to the rate and duration of overdrive.[73] The sinus node itself can also be overdrive-suppressed if it is driven at a rate more rapid than its intrinsic rate. Thus, there may be a quiescent period after termination of either overdrive pacing or a rapid ectopic arrhythmia before the sinus rhythm resumes.[80-83] When overdrive suppression of the normal sinus node occurs, however, it is of lesser magnitude than that of subsidiary pacemakers overdriven at comparable rates.[30,80] The sinus node action potential upstroke is largely dependent on slow inward current carried by Ca^{2+} through the L-type Ca^{2+} channels, and far less Na^+ enters the fiber during the upstroke than in latent pacemaker cells such as Purkinje fibers. As a result, the activity of the Na^+ pump is probably not increased to the same extent in sinus node cells after a period of overdrive; therefore, there is less overdrive suppression caused by enhanced Na^+ pump current. The relative resistance of the normal sinus node to overdrive suppression may be important in enabling it to remain as

the dominant pacemaker even when its rhythm is transiently perturbed by external influences (such as transient shifts of the pacemaker to an ectopic site). The diseased sinus node, however, may be much more easily overdrive-suppressed.[84]

There is an important distinction between the effects of the dominant sinus pacemaker on the two kinds of automaticity, as abnormal automaticity at reduced levels of membrane potential is not overdrive-suppressed to the same extent as the normal automaticity that occurs at high levels of membrane potential.[85-87] The amount of suppression of spontaneous diastolic depolarization causing abnormal automaticity by overdrive is directly related to the level of membrane potential at which the automatic rhythm occurs.[86,87] For example, Purkinje fibers showing automaticity at moderately depolarized membrane potentials of -60 to -70 mV still manifest some overdrive suppression, although less than those fibers with automaticity at -90 mV. Automaticity in Purkinje fibers with membrane potentials less than -60 mV is only slightly suppressed by overdrive if at all. These differences in the effects of overdrive may be related to the reduction in the amount of Na^+ entering the cell as membrane potential decreases, as we described for overdrive of the sinus node. At low levels of membrane potential, Na^+ channels are inactivated, decreasing the fast inward Na^+ current; therefore, there is a reduction in the amount of Na^+ entering the cells during overdrive and the degree of stimulation of the sodium-potassium pump.[88]

In addition to overdrive suppression being of paramount importance for maintenance of normal rhythm, the characteristic response of automatic pacemakers to overdrive, as discussed in the previous paragraphs, is often useful for identifying mechanisms of arrhythmias in the in situ heart, where arrhythmia mechanisms cannot be identified by recording transmembrane potentials because of the technical difficulties. Not all mechanisms of arrhythmogenesis respond in the same way to overdrive as automatic pacemakers, and the differences in response can sometimes be used to distinguish among mechanisms. These differences are described in detail later in this chapter. In addition to overdrive suppression, another mechanism that may suppress subsidiary pacemakers is the electrotonic interaction between the pacemaker cells and nonpacemaker cells in the surrounding myocardium.[89] This mechanism may be particularly important in preventing AV nodal automaticity[90,91] or automaticity in the distal Purkinje system, where the pacemaking Purkinje fibers are in contact with nonpacemaking working ventricular muscle.[89,92,93]

Arrhythmias Caused by Automaticity

Arrhythmias caused by either normal or abnormal automaticity of cardiac fibers may occur for several different reasons. Such arrhythmias might result simply from an alteration in the rate of impulse initiation by the normal sinus node pacemaker without a shift of impulse origin to a subsidiary pacemaker at an ectopic site. Sinus bradycardia and tachycardia are such arrhythmias. The cellular mechanisms that can change the rate of impulse initiation in the sinus node are described in Fig. 26-6. During alterations in sinus rate, there may be shifts of the pacemaker site within the sinus node.[23,94] A shift in the site of impulse initiation to one of the regions where either normal or abnormal subsidiary pacemakers are located also results in arrhythmias. This would be expected to happen when any of the following occurs: (1) the rate at which the sinus node activates subsidiary pacemaker falls considerably below the intrinsic rate of the subsidiary pacemakers; (2) inhibitory electrotonic influences between nonpacemaker and pacemaker cells are interrupted; or (3) impulse initiation in subsidiary pacemakers is enhanced.

The rate at which the sinus node activates subsidiary pacemakers may be decreased in a number of situations. Impulse initiation by the sinus node may be slowed or inhibited altogether by heightened activity in the parasympathetic nervous system[95] or as a result of sinus node disease.[96] Alternatively, there may be block of impulse conduction from the sinus node to the atria or block of conduction from the atria to the ventricles. A latent pacemaker might also be protected from being overdriven by the sinus node if it is surrounded by a region in which impulses of sinus origin block (entrance block) prior to reaching the pacemaker cells. Such block, however, must be unidirectional, so that activity from the pacemaker can propagate into surrounding myocardium whenever the surrounding regions are excitable. Some possible mechanisms for unidirectional block are discussed later in this chapter.

The protected pacemaker is said to be a *parasystolic focus*.[97] In general, under these conditions, such a protected focus of automaticity can fire at its own intrinsic frequency. Electronic current flow from surrounding regions may also influence the cycle length of a protected focus, either prolonging or abbreviating it, depending on whether the surrounding activity occurs during the early or late stage of diastolic depolarization.[98–100] Under any of the above conditions (sinus slowing, sinoatrial or AV block, parasystolic focus), there may be "escape" of a subsidiary pacemaker. There is a natural hierarchy of intrinsic rates of subsidiary pacemakers having normal automaticity, with atrial pacemakers having faster intrinsic rates than AV junctional pacemakers, and AV junctional pacemakers having faster rates than ventricular pacemakers.[45,74] Once overdrive suppression is removed by sinus node inhibition, the pacemaker with the fastest rate becomes the site of impulse origin.[74] Sometimes mechanisms responsible for the suppression of impulse initiation in the sinus node also suppress pacemaker activity in the atria. Following experimental studies in which the sinus node is damaged or removed, the most prevalent atrial pacemaker site is at the junction of the inferior vena cava and posterior wall of the right atrium.[30,101–103] These atrial pacemakers may cause atrial arrhythmias if the sinus node or its arterial supply is damaged.[104]

Ectopic impulse initiation may occur in the AV junction. In fact, an AV junctional pacemaker may become the dominant rhythm in the absence of normal sinus node function. Atrioventricular junctional pacemakers may be located either in the AV node or His bundle. These different sites have somewhat different properties, including their intrinsic rate (faster in the node than in the His bundle) and response to autonomic nerve activity (parasympathetic activity suppresses AV nodal pacemakers to a greater extent than His bundle pacemakers). Atrioventricular junctional rhythms may occur during AV block, since the site of block is often proximal to the AV junctional pacemaker location.[38] If AV junctional pacemakers are also suppressed or if the site of disease causing AV block is in the His bundle or bundle branches, subsidiary pacemaker location is in the His-Purkinje system. The His bundle at the proximal end of the specialized AV conduction system has a faster intrinsic rate than the more distally located Purkinje fibers.[45] The electrocardiogram (ECG) during idioventricular rhythm in patients with complete heart block is often characterized by a wide, aberrant QRS complex, suggesting impulse initiation in the distal Purkinje system.[105]

In acute myocardial ischemia, particularly when it occurs in the inferior wall, parasympathetic activity may be enhanced, depressing sinus rate, AV conduction, or both.[106] Ectopic impulse initiation then may arise in the ventricular specialized conduction system.[107] Any event that decreases intercellular coupling between latent subsidiary pacemaker cells and surrounding nonpacemaker cells may remove the inhibitory influence of electrotonic current flow of the latent pacemakers and allow them to fire at their intrinsic rate.[89] Coupling might be reduced by fibrosis, which can separate myocardial fibers. For example, fibrosis in the atrial aspect of the AV junctional region that results in heart block might release nodal pacemakers from electrotonic suppression by surrounding atrial cells and permit them to become the dominant pacemakers driving the ventricles. Uncoupling might also be caused by factors that increase the intracellular Ca^{2+},[108] since elevated intracellular Ca^{2+} levels decrease coupling between myocardial cells by decreasing the conductance of gap junction channels (*connexons*). This might result, for example, from treatment with digitalis,[109] which inhibits Na^+ extrusion and thus increases Ca^{2+} levels in the cell.[110] In myocardial infarction, Purkinje fiber pacemakers may be uncoupled from damaged ventricular muscle cells, allowing the Purkinje fibers to fire at their intrinsic rates.

Some inhibition of the sinus node is still necessary for the site of impulse initiation to shift to an ectopic site that is no longer inhibited because of uncoupling from surrounding cells, since, as explained above, the intrinsic firing rate of subsidiary pacemakers is still slower than that of the sinus node. Subsidiary pacemaker activity also may be enhanced, causing impulse initiation to shift to ectopic sites even when sinus node function is normal. One cause may be enhanced sympathetic nerve activity. Norepinephrine released locally from sympathetic nerves steepens the slope of diastolic depolarization of latent pacemaker cells[23,33,34,111,112] and diminishes the inhibitory effects of overdrive.[113] The increase in slope of spontaneous diastolic depolarization may result from effects of norepinephrine on the i_f current, as described before, as well as from an increase in inward Ca^{2+} current in those cells in which this current participates in pacemaker activity.

Localized effects on subsidiary pacemakers may occur in the absence of sinus node stimulation.[114] Therefore, sympathetic stimulation may enable membrane potential of ectopic pacemakers to reach threshold before they are activated by an impulse from the sinus node, resulting in ectopic premature impulses or automatic rhythms. There is evidence that in the subacute phase of myocardial ischemia, increased activity of the sympathetic nervous system may enhance automaticity of Purkinje fibers, enabling them to escape from sinus node domination. Enhanced subsidiary pacemaker activity also may not require sympathetic stimulation. The flow of current between partially depolarized myocardium and normally polarized latent pacemaker cells might enhance automaticity.[115] This mechanism has been proposed to be a cause of some of the ectopic beats that arise at the borders of ischemic areas in the ventricle.[93]

Inhibition of the electrogenic sodium-potassium pump results in a net increase in inward current during diastole because of the decrease in outward current normally generated by the pump and, therefore, may increase automaticity in subsidiary pacemakers sufficiently to cause arrhythmias. This might occur after adenosine triphosphate (ATP) is depleted during prolonged hypoxia or ischemia or in the presence of toxic amounts of digitalis.[116,117] A decease in the extracellular potassium level also enhances normal automaticity,[75] as does acute stretch.[118] Stretch can induce rapid automatic rates in Purkinje fibers with normal maximum diastolic potentials.[119,120] Stretch of the ventricles can also induce arrhythmias in the intact heart,[121] although the site of origin of the ectopic impulses has not yet been localized. Stretch of the Purkinje system might occur in akinetic areas after acute ischemia or in ventricular aneurysms in hearts with healed infarcts. At normal sinus rates, there may be little overdrive suppression of pacemakers with abnormal automaticity. As a result of the lack of overdrive suppression, even transient sinus pauses or occasional long sinus cycle lengths may permit an ectopic focus with a slower rate than the sinus node to capture the heart for one or more beats. On the other hand, ectopic pacemakers with normal automaticity would probably be quiescent during relatively short, transient sinus pauses because they are overdrive-suppressed.

It is also possible that the depolarized level of membrane potential at which abnormal automaticity occurs might cause entrance block into the focus and prevent it from being overdriven by the sinus node, even when impulses initiated in the focus could leave it (unidirectional block).[122] This would lead to parasystole, an example of an arrhythmia caused by a combination of an abnormality of impulse conduction and initiation. All these features of abnormal automaticity are evident in the Purkinje fibers that survive in regions of transmural myocardial infarction and cause ventricular arrhythmias during the subacute phase.[68] The firing rate of an abnormally automatic focus might also be enhanced above that of the sinus node, leading to arrhythmias in the absence of sinus node suppression or conduction block between the focus and surrounding myocardium. The automatic rate is a direct function of the level of membrane potential—the greater the depolarization, the faster the rate.[5,55,57,123,124] Experimental studies have shown firing rates in muscle and Purkinje fibers of 150 to 200/min at membrane potentials less than -50 mV, and these rates should be sufficiently rapid to enable these pacemakers sometimes to control the rhythm of the heart. Catecholamines also increase the rate of firing caused by abnormal automaticity[125] and, therefore, may contribute to a shift in the pacemaker site from the sinus node to a region with abnormal automaticity. Among these clinical arrhythmias that are likely to be caused by abnormal automaticity is accelerated idioventricular rhythm after myocardial infarction (see also Chap. 47).

TRIGGERED ACTIVITY

Triggered activity is a term used to describe impulse initiation in cardiac fibers that is dependent on afterdepolarizations.[126–128] Afterdepolarizations are oscillations in membrane potential that follow the upstroke of an action potential. There are two kinds of afterdepolarizations that may cause triggered activity. One occurs early, i.e., during repolarization of the action potential (EADs), and the other is delayed until repolarization is complete or nearly complete (DADs). When either kind of afterdepolarization is large enough to reach the threshold potential for activation of a regenerative inward current, action potentials result that are referred to as "triggered." Therefore, a key characteristic of triggered activity, discriminating it from automaticity, is that for triggered activity to occur, at least one action potential must precede it (the trigger). Automatic rhythms can arise de novo in the absence of any prior electrical activity, such as following long periods of quiescence, whereas triggered activity cannot.[5,128] Triggered activity will cause arrhythmias when the site of impulse initiation shifts from the sinus node to the triggered focus. In order for this to occur, the rate of triggered impulses should be faster than the sinus rate, either transiently or persistently. This might result when firing of the sinus node is slowed or inhibited, when there is block of sinus impulses, or when the rate of triggered activity is faster than normal sinus node impulse initiation. The factors causing the shift in the site of impulse initiation should be very similar to those we described in our discussion of automaticity.

Delayed Afterdepolarizations and Triggered Activity

Figure 26-10 shows an example of a DAD recorded with a microelectrode in a superfused preparation of atrial muscle exposed to catecholamines. The DAD is an oscillation in membrane potential that occurs after repolarization of the action potential (indicated in the figure by the unfilled arrow). The DAD is caused by events occurring during the action potential that will be described later. Figure 26-10A also shows that a DAD may be preceded by an afterhyperpolarization (black arrow), in which case the membrane potential transiently becomes more negative after the action potential than it was just before it. Afterhyperpolarizations, however, do not always precede DADs. The transient nature of the DAD

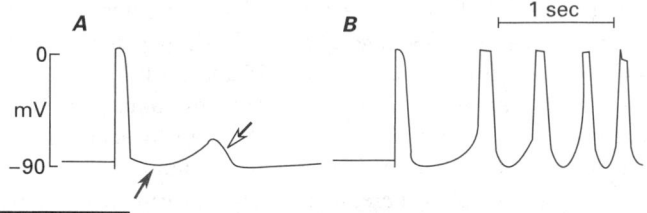

FIGURE 26-10

An example of a DAD (*white arrow*) recorded with a microelectrode from an atrial fiber in the canine coronary sinus. The black arrow indicates an afterhyperpolarization. *B.* The onset of triggered activity is shown. [From Wit AL, Rosen MR. After depolarizations and triggered activity: distinction from automaticity as an arrhythmogenic mechanism. In: Fozzard HA, Haber E, Jennings RB, Katz AM, Morgan HE (eds). *The Heart and Cardiovascular System.* Scientific Foundations. 2nd ed. New York, Raven Press, 1991:2113–2163. Reproduced with permission from the publisher and author.]

clearly distinguishes it from normal spontaneous diastolic (pacemaker) depolarization, during which the membrane potential declines almost monotonically until the next action potential occurs (compare Fig. 26-10*A* with Fig. 26-6). In addition to microelectrode recordings such as the one shown in Fig. 26-10*A,* DADs can also be identified using techniques for recording extracellular potentials.[129,130] A major problem that exists when this technique is used in situ to locate DADs in the heart, however, is discriminating the extracellular voltage deflections caused by afterdepolarizations from deflections that are a result of the motion of the heart, since movement alone can mimic DADs in extracellular recordings.[131] A second important problem is a possible difficulty in locating focal sites at which afterdepolarizations and triggered activity may be originating. Nevertheless, extracellular electrodes have been used to demonstrate what appear to be DADs occurring in the in situ heart.[132,133]

A triggered impulse is initiated when a DAD depolarizes the membrane potential to the threshold potential for activation of the inward current responsible for the upstroke of the action potential. Triggered impulses are shown in Fig. 26-10*B.* Afterdepolarizations do not always reach threshold, so that triggerable fibers may sometimes be stimulated at a regular rate without becoming rhythmically active, e.g., the stimulated action potential in Fig. 26-10*A.* Probably the most important influence that causes subthreshold DADs to reach threshold is a decrease in the cycle length (an increase in the rate) at which action potentials occur. Therefore, arrhythmias triggered by DADs can be expected to be initiated by either a spontaneous or a pacing-induced increase in the heart rate. A triggered action potential is also followed by an afterdepolarization that may or may not reach threshold. When it does not reach threshold, only one triggered action impulse occurs. Quite often, the first triggered action potential is followed by a short or long "train" of additional triggered action potentials, each arising from the afterdepolarization caused by the previous action potential (Fig. 26-10*B*). The merging of the rising phase of the afterdepolarization with the upstroke of the action potential during triggered activity may be smooth, and, as a result, the fiber may show phase 4 depolarization that is indistinguishable from the phase 4 depolarization seen during automatic activity.

Causes of Delayed Afterdepolarizations and Triggered Activity

Delayed afterdepolarizations usually occur under a variety of conditions in which there is an increase in Ca^{2+} in the myoplasm and the sarcoplasmic reticulum above normal levels (sometimes referred to as *Ca overload*). Abnormalities in the sequestration and release of Ca^{2+} by the sarcoplasmic reticulum may also contribute to their occurrence. On depolarization of the membrane during an action potential, the intracellular free Ca^{2+} normally increases, primarily by Ca^{2+} influx through the L-type Ca^{2+} channels. Initially, this rapid rate of change of intracellular Ca^{2+} triggers Ca^{2+} release from the sarcoplasmic reticulum, which causes a further rise in intracellular free Ca^{2+} and contraction[134] (see also Chap. 3). Repolarization then induces synchronous Ca^{2+} uptake by the sarcoplasmic reticulum in the cell and relaxation. If intracellular Ca^{2+} is very high or if catecholamines or cyclic adenosine monophosphate (AMP) is present, both of which enhance Ca^{2+} uptake by the sarcoplasmic reticulum, the Ca^{2+} in the sarcoplasmic reticulum may rise during repolarization to a critical level, at which a secondary spontaneous release of Ca^{2+} from the sarcoplasmic reticulum occurs after the action potential and relaxation of contraction.[134] This secondary release of Ca^{2+} generates an aftercontraction as well as the transient inward (TI) current and the afterdepolarization. The TI current is an oscillatory membrane current that is distinct from the pacemaker currents.[135–142] After one or several afterdepolarizations, myoplasmic Ca^{2+} may decrease because Na^+–Ca^{2+} exchange extrudes Ca^{2+} from the cell, and membrane potential stops oscillating.

The exact mechanism by which the secondary rise in myoplasmic Ca^{2+} after repolarization causes the TI current is unclear. Two possibilities have been considered. The first is that the Ca^{2+} released from the sarcoplasmic reticulum after repolarization acts on the sarcolemma to increase its conductance to ions (mainly Na^+) that flow into the cell down a concentration gradient through membrane channels. The second mechanism proposed for the origin of the TI current is that the rise in Ca^{2+} causes the TI current through an electrogenic (rheogenic) exchange of Ca^{2+} for Na^+. According to this hypothesis, the transient rise in myoplasmic Ca^{2+} released from the sarcoplasmic reticulum after the action potential is expected to result in "transport" of Ca^{2+} out of the cell across the sarcolemma by the Na^+–Ca^{2+} exchanger. Such an efflux is coupled to a Na^+ influx. If more than two Na^+ ions are exchanged for each Ca^{2+} ion, a net inward current occurs.[143–145]

The most widely recognized cause of DAD-dependent triggered activity is digitalis toxicity.[116,117,145–151] Afterdepolarizations caused by digitalis may sometimes reach threshold to cause triggered action potentials, particularly if the rate of stimulation is sufficiently rapid. Ventricular arrhythmias (repetitive responses) caused by digitalis in the heart in situ can also be initiated by pacing at rapid rates.[152] As toxicity progresses, the duration of the trains of repetitive responses induced by pacing increases.[153–155] We assume that these arrhythmias are caused by DADs. In addition, spontaneously occurring accelerated ventricular rhythms and ventricular tachycardia that occur during digitalis toxicity are likely to be caused by DADs.

Cardiac glycosides cause DADs by inhibiting the Na^+–K^+ pump. In toxic amounts, this effect results in a measurable increase in intracellular Na^+.[156,157] An increase in intracellular Na^+, in turn, causes an increase in intracellular Ca^{2+}.[158] When intracellular Na^+ is increased, the concentration-dependent driving force for Na^+ across the sarcolemma is decreased, which, in turn, diminishes Ca^{2+} extrusion from the cell by Na^+–Ca^{2+} exchange. Hence, there is a net inward Ca^{2+} movement.[44,159,160]

Catecholamines are probably the next most widely recognized cause of DADs. Delayed afterdepolarizations and triggered activity caused by catecholamines have been recorded with microelectrodes in atrial fibers of the mitral valve,[161] atrial fibers lining the coronary sinus,[33] atrial fibers in the inferior right atrium,[31] and atrial fibers from hearts with cardiomyopathy.[162] The DADs in Fig. 26-10 were caused by catecholamines in atrial fibers of the canine coronary sinus. Infusion of catecholamines through a catheter into the coronary sinus in the dog causes atrial tachycardia that has all the characteristics of triggered activity[163]; therefore, some naturally occurring atrial tachycardias caused by triggered activity are probably induced by the sympathetic nervous system. Ventricular muscle and Purkinje fibers can also develop DADs in the presence of catecholamines.[164,165] Sympathetic stimulation may therefore also cause triggered ventricular arrhythmias, possibly some of the ventricular arrhythmias that accompany exercise[166] and some ventricular arrhythmias during ischemia and infarction.[167,168]

Catecholamines may cause DADs by increasing the slow inward L-type Ca^{2+} current through stimulation of beta-adrenergic receptors.[169,170] The net effect is an increase in transsarcolemmal Ca^{2+} entry into cardiac cells. In addition to increasing the inward Ca^{2+} current, catecholamines enhance uptake of Ca^{2+} by the sarcoplasmic reticulum leading to increased Ca^{2+} stored in the sarcoplasmic reticulum and the subsequent release of an increased amount of Ca^{2+} from the sarcoplasmic reticulum during contraction.[134,171,172] The increased Ca^{2+} in the sarcoplasmic reticulum induced by catecholamines may also lead to the occurrence of DADs. Delayed afterdepolarizations and triggered activity may also occur in the absence of pharmacologic agents, catecholamines, or an increase in extracellular Ca^{2+}. Triggerable fibers have been found in the upper pectinate muscles bordering the crista terminalis in the rabbit heart, in branches of the sinoatrial ring bundle or in transitional fibers between the ring bundle and ordinary pectinate muscle,[173] in apparently normal fibers in human atrial myocardium,[174] in human atrial fibers with very low membrane potentials (below −60 mV) and slow response action potentials,[70,71,174] in rat ventricular muscle that is hypertrophic secondary to renovascular hypertension

(7.2 to 12.0 mM),[175] and in ventricular myocardium from diabetic rats.[176]

Properties of Delayed Afterdepolarizations The TI current that causes DADs is maximal at around −60 mV and diminishes at more positive and more negative membrane potentials.[138,140,177] As a result of the dependence of the TI current on the level of membrane potential, the amplitude of DADs and, therefore, the possibility of triggered activity are influenced by the level of membrane potential at which the action potentials occur. In the digitalis-toxic Purkinje system, there is a "window" of membrane voltage for maximum diastolic potential, which is approximately between −75 and −80 mV, at which the amplitude of DADs tend to be greatest.[178,179] When DADs occur at the membrane potentials that favor a maximum amplitude, any intervention that hyperpolarizes or depolarizes the membrane tends to reduce their magnitude and to suppress any rhythms the afterdepolarizations might induce. Similarly, when there are no DADs in the presence of digitalis and the membrane potential is at a voltage less than or greater than the window, interventions that bring membrane potential into this voltage range often induce DADs. A similar dependence on membrane potential has been shown for DADs in atrial fibers of the coronary sinus[180] and in Purkinje fibers from infarcts.[181,182]

Delayed afterdepolarizations are influenced by the action potential duration, with longer action potential durations favoring the occurrence of DADs.[180] When action potential duration is longer, more Ca^{2+} is able to enter the cell. Drugs like quinidine, which prolong action potential duration, may increase DAD amplitude,[183] while drugs like lidocaine, which shorten action potential duration, may decrease DAD amplitude.[184] The amplitude of DADs is dependent on the number of action potentials that precede them; i.e., after a period of quiescence, the initiation of a single action potential may be followed by either no afterdepolarization or only a small one. With continued stimulation, the afterdepolarizations increase in amplitude, and triggered activity may eventually occur.[33,117,147,161,185] The amplitude of DADs and their coupling interval to the previous action potentials are also dependent upon the cycle length at which action potentials are occurring, and triggered activity can be induced by a critical decrease in the drive cycle length.[117,147,161,168,173,175,176] This is illustrated by the effects of the stimulus cycle length on the amplitude of DADs recorded from an atrial fiber in the canine coronary sinus, shown in Fig. 26-11. The transmembrane potentials at the left were recorded when the stimulus cycle length was 2000 ms; the afterdepolarization amplitude following the last stimulated impulse is 5 mV. In the center, the stimulus cycle length was 1500 ms, and afterdepolarization amplitude after the last stimulated impulse is 15 mV. At the right, at a stimulus cycle length of 1200 ms, afterdepolarization amplitude reached 20 mV after the third stimulated action potential before triggered activity was initiated. Digitalis-induced DADs occur either singly or as two or more "damped" oscillations following the action potential.[117,147] When two

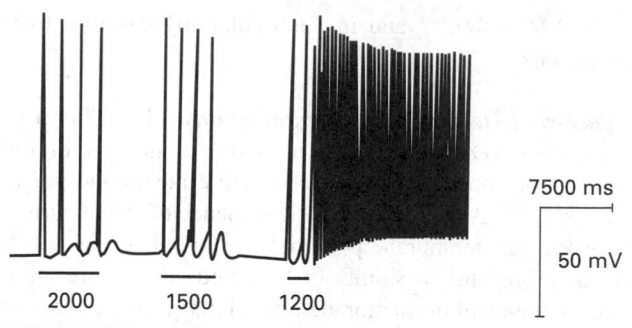

FIGURE 26-11

Effects of stimulation rate on DADs and triggered activity. Transmembrane action potentials were recorded from an atrial fiber in the canine coronary sinus superfused with Tyrode's solution containing norepinephrine. The stimulus cycle lengths and the periods of stimulation are indicated by the black bars. Sustained triggered activity occurred following stimulation at a cycle length of 1200 ms. The rate of triggered activity is so rapid that the individual action potentials cannot be seen at the slow oscilloscopic sweep speed. (From Wit AL, Cranefield PF. Triggered and automatic activity in the canine coronary sinus. *Circ Res* 1977; 41:435. Reproduced with permission from the publisher and author.)

or more afterdepolarizations are present, their relationship to the drive cycle length is complex. As drive cycle length decreases, the amplitude of the first afterdepolarization increases, reaching a peak at a cycle length of about 500 ms, and triggered activity may occur. If it does not, at shorter drive cycle lengths the magnitude of this first afterdepolarization decreases. The second DAD, however, continues to increase in magnitude as drive cycle length shortens further and may eventually reach threshold and induce triggered activity. A decrease in the length of even a single drive cycle (i.e., a premature impulse) also results in an increase in the amplitude of the DAD that follows the premature cycle.

The premature coupling interval at which triggered activity occurs is also dependent on the basic drive cycle length. As the basic drive cycle length decreases, the premature coupling interval needed to induce triggered activity increases.[186] Decreasing the drive cycle length, in addition to increasing amplitude, also tends to decrease the coupling interval of DADs to the action potential upstroke or terminal phase of repolarization by increasing the rate of depolarization of the afterdepolarization.[33,117,147,173] As a result, there is a direct relationship between the drive cycle length at which triggered impulses are initiated and the coupling interval between the first triggered impulse and the last stimulated impulse that induced them; i.e., as the drive cycle length is reduced, the first triggered impulse occurs earlier with respect to the last driven action potential. This characteristic property forms the basis for one of the indirect ways that triggered activity induced by a decrease in the drive cycle length in the whole heart is sometimes distinguishable from reentrant activity induced by a decrease in the drive cycle length, since the relationship for reentrant impulses initiated by rapid stimulation is often the opposite; i.e., as drive cycle length is reduced, the first reentrant impulse occurs later with respect to the last driven action potential because of rate dependent conduction slowing in the reentrant

pathway (described in more detail later in the chapter). The increased time during which the membrane is in the depolarized state at shorter stimulation cycle lengths or after premature impulses increases Ca^{2+} in the myoplasm and the sarcoplasmic reticulum, thereby increasing the TI current responsible for the increased afterdepolarization amplitude and causing the current to reach its maximum amplitude more rapidly, decreasing the coupling interval of triggered impulses. The repetitive depolarizations can increase intracellular Ca^{2+} because of repeated activation of the inward Ca^{2+} current that flows through L-type Ca^{2+} channels.

We have discussed how triggered activity caused by DADs is initiated by stimulation. These characteristics may be of use in identifying triggered activity in the in situ heart (described later). Also of importance in identifying triggered arrhythmias in situ are the effects of electrical stimulation on established triggered activity. In general, triggered activity is markedly influenced by overdrive pacing (i.e., pacing at a rate faster than the rate of the triggered rhythm). The effects of overdrive pacing on triggered activity have been studied only in several experimental situations: in atrial fibers in which triggered activity is caused by catecholamines and in Purkinje fibers in which triggered activity is caused by digitalis or myocardial infarction. These effects are dependent both on the rate and duration of overdrive pacing.[187,188] When overdrive pacing is done for a critical duration of time and at a critical rate during a catecholamine-dependent triggered rhythm, the maximum diastolic potential following the overdrive pacing increases to levels more negative than before; during the increase in membrane potential, the rate of triggered activity slows until the triggered rhythm stops. When triggered activity stops after a period of overdrive pacing at a moderate rate, some 10 to 50 impulses may occur after termination of the overdrive pacing before termination of the triggered activity occurs. The increase in maximum diastolic potential and the slowing and termination of triggered activity following a period of overdrive pacing are caused by an enhanced activity of the electrogenic Na^+ pump.[187] During a period of overdrive pacing, there is a transient increase in intracellular Na^+ because the increased number of action potentials stimulates the pump to generate increased outward current.[73,189]

In digitalis-toxic Purkinje fibers, overdrive pacing can also terminate triggered activity, and this effect is dependent on the overdrive pacing cycle length but not on the overdrive pacing duration.[186,190] Termination occurs more frequently at more rapid overdrive pacing rates and may not be immediate; i.e., several triggered impulses may continue to occur after stimulation is stopped before triggered activity stops.[186] When overdrive pacing is not rapid enough to terminate the triggered rhythm, it can cause overdrive acceleration. Termination by overdrive pacing is not accompanied by hyperpolarization of the maximum diastolic potential and is probably not caused by increased Na^+–K^+ pump activity, since the pump is partially inhibited by digitalis. The exact mechanism for termination has not been elucidated. Premature stimuli may also terminate triggered rhythms, as shown in digitalis-toxic Purkinje fibers,[186] Purkinje fibers in myocardial infarcts,[191] or atrial fibers exposed to catecholamines,[161,188] although termination is much less frequent than by overdrive pacing.[190] It has not been demonstrated that the premature impulse must occur at a critical point in the cycle length of triggered activity.

Early Afterdepolarizations and Triggered Activity

Early afterdepolarizations are manifest as a sudden change in the time course of repolarization of an action potential such that membrane potential does not follow the trajectory characteristic of normal repolarization but suddenly shifts in a depolarizing direction. This is illustrated in the example of an EAD recorded with an intracellular microelectrode in a superfused Purkinje fiber shown in Fig. 26-12. The normal time course of repolarization of the action potential is shown in panel *A*. The arrow in panel *B* shows the deviation in membrane potential that constitutes the EAD. Early afterdepolarizations may appear at the plateau level of membrane potential, which is usually more positive than −60 mV, as in Fig. 26-12*B*, or they may appear later, during phase 3 of repolarization. In Fig. 26-13*B*, trace 1 shows the normal time course of repolarization of a Purkinje fiber action potential, while trace 2 shows a deviation from this normal time course late during phase 3, which is the EAD. Early afterdepolarizations occurring late in repolarization occur at membrane potentials more negative than −60 mV in atrial, ventricular, or Purkinje cells that have normal resting potentials. Normally, a net outward membrane current shifts membrane potential progressively in a negative direction during repolarization of the action potential. An EAD occurs when, for some reason, the current-voltage relationship is altered to cause outward current during repolarization to approach or attain 0, at least transiently. Such a shift can be caused by any factors that either decrease outward current, mostly carried by K^+, or increase inward current, carried by Na^+ or Ca^{2+}. If the change in the current-voltage relationship results in a region of net inward current during the plateau range of membrane potentials,[192] it could lead to a secondary depolarization (a triggered action potential) during the plateau or phase 3 by activating a regenerative inward current.

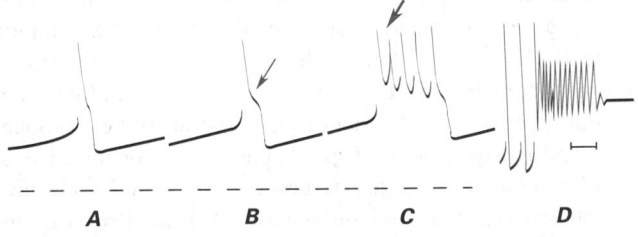

FIGURE 26-12

Early afterdepolarizations and triggered activity during repolarization in a Purkinje fiber. *A.* Transmembrane potential with normal repolarization of a spontaneously active Purkinje fiber. *B.* Early afterdepolarization (*arrow*) occurring during the plateau phase of the action potential. *C.* Triggered action potentials (*arrow*) during the plateau. *D.* Arrest of repolarization at a low level of membrane potential after a period of triggered activity. (From Cranefield PF. Action potentials, afterpotentials and arrhythmias. *Circ Res* 1977; 41:415–425. Reproduced with permission from the publisher and author.)

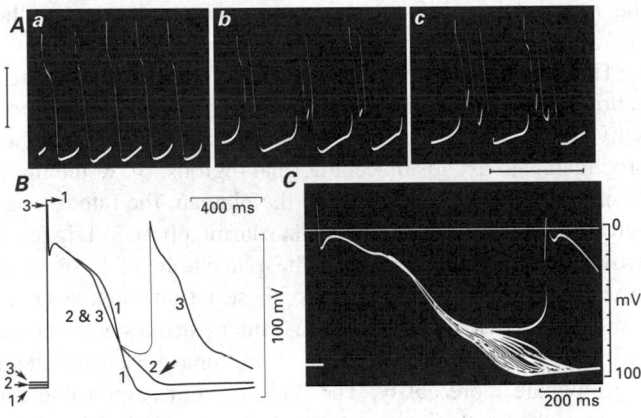

FIGURE 26-13

Early afterdepolarizations and triggered activity during late repolarization in a Purkinje fiber. *A.* Three panels are shown: (*a*) a spontaneously firing Purkinje fiber with prominent phase 4 depolarization; (*b*) occurrence of a single triggered action potential caused by an EAD, occurring during repolarization of each spontaneous action potential; (*c*) two triggered action potentials caused by an EAD occurring during repolarization of each spontaneous action potential. *B.* Development of an EAD and a triggered action potential in three superimposed traces: (1) normal Purkinje fiber action potential; (2) alteration in the time course of late repolarization leading to the occurrence of an EAD (*arrow*); (3) further alteration in alte repolarization, leading to a triggered action potential. *C.* Superimposed traces recorded from a Purkinje fiber in the course of developing EADs and a triggered action potential. [From Coulombe A et al. Role of the "Na window" current and other ionic currents in triggering early after-depolarizations and re-excitation in Purkinje fibers. In: Zipes DP, Jalife J (eds). *Cardiac Electrophysiology and Arrhythmias.* New York: Grune & Stratton; 1985:43–49. Reproduced with permission from the publisher and author.]

Under certain conditions, EADs can lead to "second upstrokes"[5,127] or action potentials; when an EAD is large enough, the decrease in membrane potential leads to an increase in net inward (depolarizing) current, and a second action potential occurs prior to complete repolarization of the first, as shown in panel *C* (arrow) of Fig. 26-12 and by trace 3 in panel *B* of Fig. 26-13. The second action potential occurring during repolarization is triggered in the sense that it is evoked by an EAD, which, in turn, is induced by the preceding action potential. The second action potential may also be followed by other action potentials, all occurring at the low level of membrane potential characteristic of the plateau (Fig. 26-12*C*) or at the higher level of membrane potential of later phase 3 (Fig. 26-13, panels *Ab, Ac,* and *B*). Without the initiating action potential, there could be no triggered action potentials. The sustained rhythmic activity may continue for a variable number of impulses and terminates when repolarization of the initiating action potential returns membrane potential to a high level (Fig. 26-12*C*). As repolarization occurs, the rate of the triggered rhythm slows because the rate is dependent on the level of membrane potential in the same way as is abnormal automaticity. Sometimes repolarization to the high level of membrane potential may not occur, and membrane potential may remain at the plateau level or at a level intermediate between the plateau level and the resting potential[62] (Fig. 26-12*D*). The sustained rhythmic activity may then continue at the reduced level of membrane potential and assumes the characteristics of abnormal automaticity.[127]

The level of membrane potential at which the triggered action potentials occur determines both the rate of triggered activity and whether or not the triggered action potentials can propagate and excite adjacent normal regions.[193] At the more positive membrane potentials of the plateau, the rate of triggered activity is more rapid than late during phase 3. Triggered action potentials occurring at the plateau level have slow upstrokes; therefore, conduction of these action potentials may sometimes block,[194,195] while the faster upstrokes of triggered action potentials occurring later during phase 3 enable them to propagate more easily. The ionic current responsible for the upstrokes of the action potentials during triggered activity caused by EADs is determined by the level of membrane potential at which the action potentials occur. Triggered action potentials occurring during the plateau phase and early during phase 3, at a time when most fast Na^+ channels are still inactivated, most likely have upstrokes caused by the inward L-type Ca^{2+} current.[5,196] At higher membrane potentials during late phase 3 of repolarization, where there is partial reactivation of the first 3 channels, the upstrokes are caused by the fast inward Na^+ current. Current flowing through both L-type Ca^{2+} channels and partially reactivated fast Na^+ channels may be involved over intermediate ranges of membrane potential.

Causes of Early Afterdepolarizations and Triggered Activity

Early afterdepolarizations and triggered activity have been produced in experimental studies under a variety of conditions, some of which would never be expected to be associated with naturally occurring arrhythmias in the in situ heart. Most of these conditions somehow delay repolarization of the action potential by increasing inward current or by decreasing outward current during the plateau and repolarization phases. Most often, EADs occur more readily in Purkinje fibers than in ventricular or atrial muscle although EADs can readily occur in the so-called M cells, which are ventricular muscle cells with a prominent plateau phase.[197] Early afterdepolarizations may occur when the rate of stimulation is markedly slowed, reducing the outward current generated by the Na^+-K^+ pump, especially when K^+ in the extracellular environment is lower than normal, also reducing outward current.[128]

At a "physiologic range" of cycle lengths (a range that encompasses the normal sinus rhythm of the adult human heart, 1000 to 700 ms), EADs have rarely occurred in the studies on isolated preparations of cardiac fibers. As cycle length is increased and repolarization prolongs, EADs and triggered activity are more likely to occur.[198] The result is a bradycardia-induced tachycardia during which there may be very slow conduction. Another important characteristic is that the longer the basic drive cycle length, the greater the number of impulses that are triggered by EADs.[198] Once EADs have achieved a steady-state magnitude at a constant drive cycle length, any event which shortens drive cycle length tends to reduce their amplitude.[198] Hence, initiation of a single

premature depolarization, which is associated with an acceleration of repolarization, will reduce the magnitude of the EADs that accompany the premature action potential; as a result, triggered activity is not expected to follow premature stimulation. Polymorphic ventricular tachycardias that sometimes resemble torsades de pointes have been induced in dogs by infusion cesium, which blocks i_{K_i} to cause EADs.[199] Occurrence of tachycardia is preceded by Q-T interval prolongation, a consequence of delayed repolarization, as is characteristically seen in patients with torsades de pointes.[200] The initial beat of the tachycardia caused by cesium often occurs during repolarization, i.e., during the T wave.

Early depolarizations and triggered activity have been seen in monophasic action potentials recorded from the ventricles in dogs with cesium-induced ventricular tachycardia.[201,202] Because the experimental arrhythmias caused by agents such as cesium, which are known to induce EADs, do resemble torsades de pointes, it has been proposed that clinically occurring torsades de pointes may sometimes be caused by EADs. Other agents which can cause EADs and triggered activity are used therapeutically, and, therefore, arrhythmias associated with their use may result from triggered activity. Antiarrhythmic drugs that prolong the duration of the action potential of Purkinje fibers or ventricular muscle (e.g., sotalol,[203,204] N-acetylprocainamide,[205] and quinidine[206,207]) can cause EADs and triggered activity when administered to isolated preparations, particularly when the rate of stimulation is low and the extracellular K^+ concentration is less than normal, e.g., <4 mM/L.

The mechanisms by which these effects are exerted have been studied in detail for only some of these drugs. Both the d (no beta receptor blockade) and the 1 (beta blocking) forms of sotalol prolong the action potential duration by inhibiting the repolarizing K current, i_{K_i}.[204] Similarly, the prolongation of the action potential by quinidine, which may lead to EADs, is related to quinidine's blocking effect on the outward membrane repolarizing K^+ current and not to quinidine's well-known blocking effect on the Na^+ channel.[208] It is known that quinidine may cause ventricular tachyarrhythmias in patients undergoing antiarrhythmic therapy with the drug. Interestingly, the arrhythmias may occur at low plasma quinidine concentrations that do not cause widening of the QRS complex in the ECG,[209] consistent with observations in superfused Purkinje fibers that afterdepolarizations due to quinidine occur without depression of the action potential upstroke. Hypokalemia and bradycardia both predispose to the occurrence of quinidine-induced torsades de pointes,[200,210] and both have been shown to potentiate induction of EADs in vitro by quinidine.[206,207] Torsades de pointes has also been associated with the administration to patients of N-acetylprocainamide[209] and sotalol.[212] Magnesium has been shown to abolish EAD-dependent triggered activity in experimental studies.[207,213] Magnesium also has been shown to provide effective therapy when used to treat some clinical cases of drug-induced torsades de pointes,[214,215] further evidence that this clinical arrhythmia may be a manifestation of triggered activity (see also Chap. 27).

Arrhythmias Caused by Reentry

INTRODUCTION

As discussed previously, the excitation wavefront originating in the sinus node normally activates the cardiac tissues in an orderly sequence and then dies out. Thus, during normal sinus rhythm, each heartbeat is generated by a new pacemaker impulse in the sinus node. There are, however, arrhythmias in which, in the presence of a requisite set of circumstances, an excitation wavefront does not die out but rather can propagate continuously and thereby continue to excite the heart because it always encounters excitable tissue. Such an arrhythmia is called reentrant.

REQUISITES FOR REENTRANT EXCITATION

Perhaps the easiest way to illustrate this is to discuss again, but in more detail, the earliest description of reentrant excitation by Mayer[3] in 1906 in the excitable subumbrella ring of tissue of the scyphomedusae (jellyfish), as in Fig. 26-4. This example well illustrates the requisites for reentrant excitation. First, a substrate must be present that would support reentrant excitation, in this case the subumbrella ring of excitable tissue of the jellyfish. Second, the excitation wavefront propagating in this substrate must encounter unidirectional block (Fig. 26-4B). Unidirectional block must be present, or else the excitation wavefronts traveling around the ring will collide and extinguish each other (Fig. 26-4A). If the site of unidirectional block instead manifests bidirectional block, reentrant excitation also will not occur because the circulating excitation wavefront will be unable to propagate through the area of block to reexcite the tissue initially excited. Third, there must be a central area of block around which the reentrant excitation wavefront can circulate. In this example, it is the hole in the center of the ring that clearly is inexcitable. Without a central area of block, the excitation wavefront will not necessarily be conducted around the ring of excitable tissue. Rather it could take a shortcut, permitting the circulating excitation wavefront to arrive quite early at the site where it originated. If it arrives sufficiently early, the latter tissue will still be refractory, and reentrant excitation would not be possible. But even with the presence of a central area of block and without the presence of a shortcut, the circulating wavefront will manifest reentrant excitation only if the tissue it initially activated has had sufficient time to recover its excitability by the time the reentrant wavefront returns. Thus, conduction of the circulating excitation wavefront in the rest of the circuit must take long enough for this to happen, and there must always be a gap of excitable tissue (either fully or partially excitable) ahead of the circulating wavefront (the so-called excitable gap). In the case of the experiment by Mayer on the subumbrella ring of excitable tissue of the jellyfish, conduction velocity was constant and the length of the ring long enough so that conduction time around the ring was longer than the effective refractory period of the excitable tissue comprising the ring, permitting reentry. Had the length of the ring been critically shorter or had conduction velocity been critically

faster, the circulating excitation wavefront would have arrived at the site of initial excitation before sufficient recovery of excitability had occurred, preventing reexcitation.

From these sorts of observations grew the concept of the wavelength of the circulating impulse.[4,216,217] The wavelength is the product of the conduction velocity of the circulating excitation wavefront and the effective refractory period of the tissue in which the excitation wavefront is propagating. It quantifies how far the impulse travels relative to the duration of the refractory period. Thus, the wavelength of the reentrant excitation wavefront must be shorter than the length of the pathway of the potential reentrant circuit for reentrant excitation to occur, i.e., the impulse must travel a distance during the refractory period that is less than the complete reentrant path length in order to allow myocardium ahead of it sufficient time to recover excitability.

For virtually all clinically important reentrant arrhythmias due to ordered reentry, however, in the presence of uniform, normal conduction velocity along the reentrant pathway, the wavelength would be too long to permit reentrant excitation. Thus, virtually all these arrhythmias must have and, in fact, do have one or more areas of slow conduction as a part of the reentrant circuit. The associated changes in conduction velocity (as well as associated changes in refractory periods) actually cause the wavelength to change in different parts of the circuit. However, the presence of one or more areas of slow conduction permits the average wavelength of reentrant activation to be shorter than the path length.

The fact that the reentrant circuit of virtually all clinically important reentrant arrhythmias has one or more areas of slow conduction serves to emphasize that the electrophysiologic properties of the cardiac tissue making up the reentrant circuit are not uniform. In fact, there may be, and usually are, variations of conduction velocity and refractoriness along the course of the reentrant circuit. An additional requisite for random reentry is the necessity of a critical mass of tissue in order to sustain the one or usually more simultaneously circulating reentrant excitation wavefronts.[218] Thus, it is essentially not possible to achieve sustained fibrillation of ventricles of very small normal mammalian hearts and equally difficult to achieve sustained fibrillation of the normal atria of humans or smaller mammals.

Finally, another requisite for reentrant excitation to occur is often (but not always) the presence of an initiating trigger. The trigger, usually the occurrence of one or more premature beats, frequently is required because it elicits or brings to a critical state one or more of the conditions necessary to achieve reentrant excitation. Thus, a premature impulse initiating reentry may arrive at one site in the potential reentrant circuit sufficiently early that it encounters unidirectional block because that tissue has had insufficient time to recover excitability following excitation by the prior beat (Fig. 26-4). Furthermore, in the other limb of the potential reentrant circuit, the premature arrival of the excitation wavefront either causes slow conduction or results in further slowing of conduction of the excitation wavefront through an area of already slow conduction. The resulting increase in conduction time around this limb of the potential reentrant circuit serves to allow the region of unidirectional block in the tissue in the other limb activated initially by the premature beat to recover excitability. Thus, when the circulating excitation wavefront of the premature beat arrives at these tissue sites, the excitation wavefront can reexcite the tissue, thereby manifesting reentrant excitation (Fig. 26-4).

It should be noted that the mechanism causing the premature beat may be different than the reentrant mechanism causing the tachycardia. Thus, the premature beat may be caused by automaticity or triggered activity. An example of the latter may be torsade de pointes, in which the initiating beat or beats is the result of triggered activity due to early afterdepolarization, but the remainder of the beats in this rhythm (it is frequently nonsustained) are now thought to be due to reentry.[219] Another example may occur during cardiac catheterization, where the premature beat may be due to the catheter forcefully hitting the heart wall, i.e., a mechanical cause. However, the trigger to initiate reentrant excitation need not be a premature beat. The trigger to initiate reentrant excitation may be the normal sinus beat. One example is the rhythm known as permanent nonparoxysmal AV junctional reentrant tachycardia.[220,221] In this example, the potential reentrant circuit contains an area of permanent unidirectional block in an antegrade direction. Moreover, the potential reentrant circuit also has a relatively stable area of very slow conduction, causing the wavelength of the propagating excitation wavefront to be shorter than the length of the potential reentrant circuit. In this circumstance, the normal sinus beat propagates around the reentrant circuit with sufficient delay that when it arrives in a retrograde direction at the area of permanent antegrade unidirectional block, the tissue at that site has recovered excitability. Furthermore, the conduction time around the reentrant circuit is such that the excitation wavefront continually encounters excitable tissue in the direction in which it is propagating, resulting in continuous reentrant excitation and an incessant tachycardia. Another example where a premature beat is not necessary is reentrant premature ventricular beats as in ventricular bigeminy (see also Chap. 27).

COMPONENTS OF THE REENTRANT CIRCUIT

The Substrate

The cardiac tissue that constitutes the substrate for reentrant excitation can be located almost anywhere in the heart. Furthermore, the reentrant circuit may be a variety of sizes and shapes and may comprise a number of different kinds of myocardial cells, e.g., atrial, ventricular, nodal, Purkinje. The reentrant circuit may be an anatomic structure, such as a loop of fiber bundles in the Purkinje system.[222] The reentrant circuit may be a functionally rather than an anatomically defined pathway, with its existence, size, and shape determined by the electrophysiologic properties of cardiac tissues in which the reentrant wavefront circulates, such as has been shown in some models of atrial flutter.[223,224] Or it may be an anatomic-

functional combination, as has been suggested for some intra-atrial reentrant rhythms such as atrial flutter or ventricular tachycardia.

The Area(s) of Slow Conduction

As we have discussed, a condition necessary for reentry is that the impulse be delayed sufficiently in the alternate pathway(s) to allow elements proximal to the site of unidirectional block to recover excitability. If reentry is to succeed, the impulse traveling around the reentrant circuit in one direction due to the unidirectional block must not return to this site of block before it and regions around it recover excitability. In the presence of normal conduction, sufficient time to allow recovery of excitability might occur if the alternate pathway is sufficiently long. Reentry is facilitated when conduction in all or a part of the alternate pathway is slow, since long pathways that are often not present in the heart are then not necessary. The area(s) of slow conduction may be an anatomic structure normally expected to manifest slow conduction, such as the AV node. Thus, the AV node is the area of slow conduction in AV reentrant tachycardia (a reentrant tachycardia in which the circuit involves the atria, the AV node, the His-Purkinje system, the ventricles, and an accessory AV connection). The area of slow conduction may be in cardiac tissue that normally does not manifest slow conduction. Such an area is not present during sinus rhythm (in contrast to the AV node) but is functionally present during the tachycardia. These areas may develop as a result of premature excitation or may evolve during a rapid transitional rhythm as during atrial flutter.[224,225] An example of a functionally determined area of slow conduction is found in an isthmus in the posterior-inferior right atrium during atrial flutter in patients[226] or in the free wall of the right atrium of the canine sterile pericarditis mode of atrial flutter.[224] Yet another example may be found in tissue that has been damaged, as following a myocardial infarct. Such tissue normally would not manifest slow conduction, but, following the injury, may become an area of slow conduction even during sinus rhythm.[227] Slow conduction can be a consequence of active membrane properties determining the characteristics of inward currents depolarizing the membrane during the action potential, or it can be a consequence of passive properties governing the flow of current between cardiac cells.

Depression of Resting Membrane Potential An important feature of the transmembrane action potential of atrial, ventricular, and Purkinje fibers that governs the speed of propagation is the magnitude of the inward Na^+ current flowing through the fast Na^+ channels in the sarcolemma during the upstroke. The magnitude of this current flow is reflected in the rate at which the cell depolarizes (V_{max} of phase 0)[228] and the overshoot of the upstroke (the positive level of depolarization). The depolarization phase or upstroke of the action potential results from the opening of specific membrane channels (fast Na^+ channels) through which Na^+ ions rapidly pass from the extracellular fluid into the cell.

During conduction of the impulse, the inward transmembrane Na^+ current flowing during the depolarization phase (phase 0) of the action potential results in the flow of axial current along the cardiac fiber through the cytoplasm and the gap junctions of the intercalated disks connecting the cardiac cells. The current flows out of the cells through the membrane ahead as resistive and capacitive current. The conduction velocity depends both on how much capacitive current flows out of the cell at unexcited sites ahead of the propagating wavefront and the distance at which the capacitive current can bring membrane potential to threshold. One important factor that influences the amount of current flowing through the sarcoplasm of a muscle fiber (axial current), and therefore capacitive current, is the amount of fast inward current causing the propagating action potential. A reduction in this inward current, leading to a reduction in the rate or amplitude of depolarization during phase 0, may decrease axial current flow, slow conduction, and lead to conduction block. Such a reduction may result from inactivation of Na^+ channels. The intensity of the inward Na^+ current depends on the fraction of Na^+ channels that open when the cell is excited and the size of the Na^+ electrochemical potential gradient (relative concentration of Na^+ in the extracellular space compared to Na^+ concentration inside the cell[229]). The fraction of Na^+ channels available for opening is determined largely by the level of membrane potential at which an action potential is initiated.[229] The Na^+ channels are inactivated either after the upstroke of an action potential or if the steady-state resting membrane potential is reduced. Immediately after the upstroke, cardiac fibers are inexcitable because of Na^+ channel inactivation at the positive level of membrane potential.

During repolarization, progressive removal of inactivation allows increasingly large Na^+ currents to flow through the still partially inactivated Na^+ channels when the cells are excited. The inward Na^+ current, amplitude, and rate of rise of premature action potentials initiated during this relative refractory period is reduced because the Na^+ channels are only partly reactivated.[229] In Fig. 26-14B, premature action potentials *a, b,* and *c* have low amplitudes and slow rates of depolarization because they were initiated prior to full repolarization of the action potential. Hence, the conduction velocity of these premature action potentials is low. Premature activation of the heart may, therefore, induce reentry because premature impulses conduct slowly in regions of the heart where the cardiac fibers are not completely repolarized (where Na^+ channels are to some extent still inactivated).

Conduction slow enough to facilitate reentry might also occur in cardiac cells with persistently low levels of resting potential (which may be between -60 and -70 mV) caused by disease. At these resting potentials, a significant percentage of the Na^+ channels are inactivated[229]; therefore, they are unavailable for activation by a depolarizing stimulus. Also, at these resting membrane potentials, recovery from inactivation is markedly prolonged and extends beyond complete repolarization.[230] The magnitude of the inward current during phase 0 of the action potential is reduced; consequently, both

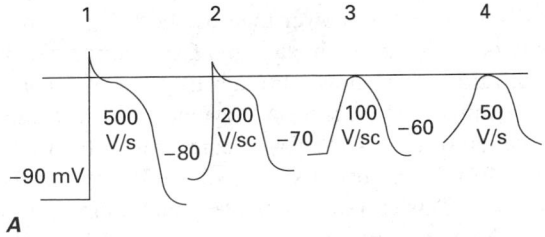

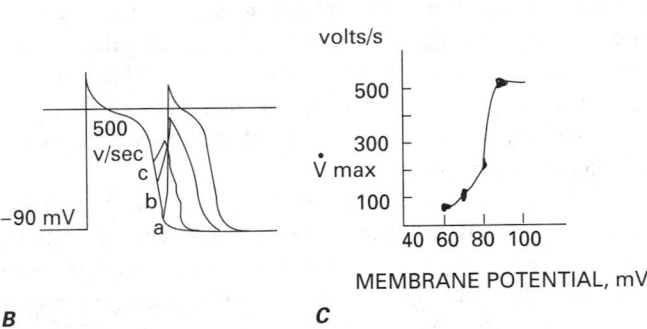

FIGURE 26-14

Diagrammatic representation of the relationship between the level of membrane potential at the onset of phase 0 and the maximum rate of depolarization during phase 0 (dv/dt_{max} or $\dot{V}_{max}$). *A.* Fiber has been depolarized by progressively increasing the extracellular potassium concentration. As resting membrane potential decreases, the rate of depolarization of the action potential upstroke decreases. *B.* Fiber is activated by premature stimuli that occur at different times during phase 3 (*a, b,* and *c*). The premature action potentials have reduced rates of depolarization because they arise at reduced membrane potentials. *C.* For both types of experiments, the general relationship between $\dot{V}_{max}$ and membrane potential is shown.

the speed and amplitude of the upstroke is diminished (Fig. 26-14A, action potentials 2, 3, and 4), decreasing axial current flow and slowing conduction significantly. Such action potentials with upstrokes dependent on inward current flowing via partially inactivated Na^+ channels are sometimes referred to as *depressed fast responses.* Further depolarization of the resting membrane potential and further inactivation of the Na^+ channel may decrease the excitability of cardiac fibers to such an extent that they may become a site of unidirectional conduction block.[231] Thus, in a diseased region with partially depolarized fibers, there may be some areas of slow conduction and some areas of conduction block, depending on the level of resting potential and the amount of Na^+ channels that are inactivated. This combination may cause reentry. The chance for reentry in such fibers is even greater during premature activation or during rhythms at a rapid rate because slow conduction or the possibility of block is increased even further, owing to the prolonged time for the Na^+ channels to recover from inactivation when the resting potential is partially depolarized.

After the upstroke of the normal action potential of atrial, ventricular, or Purkinje cells, membrane potential begins to return to the resting level because the Na^+ channels are inactivated and the fast (depolarizing) Na^+ current ceases to flow. This return, however, is slowed by a second inward current that is smaller and slower than the fast Na^+ current and probably is carried by both Na^+ and Ca^{2+} ions.[232] This secondary inward current flows through L-type Ca^{2+} channels that are distinct from the fast Na^+ channels.[20] The threshold for activation of the L-type Ca^{2+} current is in the range of -30 to -40 mV compared with about -70 mV for the fast Na^+ current. This current inactivates much more slowly than the fast Na^+ current and gradually diminishes as the cell repolarizes. It causes much of the plateau phase of the action potential. Under special conditions, this Ca^{2+} current may also underlie the occurrence of the slow conduction that causes reentrant arrhythmias.[5] Although the fast Na^+ channel may be largely inactivated at membrane potentials near -50 mV, the L-type Ca^{2+} channel is not inactivated and is still available for activation.[5,232]

Under certain conditions, when the resting potential is reduced to levels less than -60 mV (as when membrane conductance is very low or when catecholamines are present), this normally weak inward Ca^{2+} current may give rise to regenerative action potentials that propagate very slowly and are prone to block. The propagated action potential, dependent on inward Ca^{2+} current, is referred to as the *slow response*.[5] Slow-response action potentials can occur in diseased cardiac fibers with low resting potentials, but they also occur in some normal tissue of the heart, such as cells of the sinus and AV nodes, where the maximum diastolic potential is normally about -60 mV or less.[5,233] In fact, slow conduction is a normal property of both the sinus and AV nodes. Thus, it should be of no surprise that either of these nodes may be a critical area of slow conduction in some reentrant circuits, e.g., the AV node in AV reentrant tachycardia involving an accessory AV connection.

Anisotropy   The slow conduction that facilitates the occurrence of reentry can also be caused by factors other than a decrease in inward current during the upstroke of the transmembrane action potential. An increased resistance to axial current flow, which can be expressed as *effective axial resistance* (defined as resistance to current flow in the direction of propagation[234,235]) decreases the magnitude and spread of axial current of the propagating impulse among the myocardial fiber and may decrease conduction velocity. During conduction of the impulse, axial current flows from one myocardial cell to the adjacent cell through the gap junctions of the intercalated disks, which form a major source of intercellular resistance to current flow between fiber bundles.[228] Therefore, the structure of the myocardium that governs the extent and distribution of these gap junctions has a profound influence on axial resistance and conduction. This influence can be seen in normal atrial or ventricular myocardium, although the structure is different in different regions.

The atria (crista terminalis) and certain regions of the ventricles (except for the subepicardial muscle) are composed of bundles of myocardial cells that have been called *unit bundles* by Sommer and Dolber.[236] Such bundles are made up of 2 to 30 cells surrounded by a connective tissue sheath. Within a unit bundle, cells are tightly connected or coupled to each other through intercalated disks that contain the gap junctions. All the cells of a unit bundle are connected to each other within the space of 30 to 50 μm down the length of a strand.[236] An individual cardiac myocyte may be connected to as many as nine other myocytes through one or more intercalated disks.[237] These connections are mainly at the ends of the myocytes rather than along their sides, but the overlapping nature of the junctions effectively connects myocytes within a bundle in the transverse as well as the longitudinal direction. Therefore, as a consequence of the many intercellular connections, the myocytes in a unit bundle are activated uniformly and synchronously as an impulse propagates along the bundle. The unit bundles are also connected to each other. Unit bundles lying parallel to each other in normal atrial and ventricular muscle are connected in a lateral (transverse) direction at intervals in the range of 100 to 150 μm.[236] As a consequence of this structure, the myocardium in regions in which unit bundles occur is better coupled in the direction of the long axis of its cells and bundles (because of the high frequency of the gap junctions within a unit bundle) than the direction transverse to the long axis (because of the low frequency of interconnections between the unit bundles). This is reflected in a lower axial resistivity in the longitudinal direction than in the transverse direction in cardiac tissues that are composed of many unit bundles.[238,239]

The structure of the interconnections between muscle fibers is somewhat different in the subepicardial regions of the ventricles (and possibly other regions as well) but is still a cause of lower longitudinal axial resistance than transverse axial resistance. The subepicardial region is not made up of unit bundles.[240] Each ventricular muscle cell is connected to approximately 11 to 12 other muscle cells in three dimensions. The junctions that connect the cells occur at both the ends and sides of cells in roughly equivalent numbers; approximately half of all connections are side-to-side and half are end-to-end. Therefore, activation wavefronts can conduct equally well between individual cells in both the longitudinal and transverse directions because there are equal numbers of gap junctions. In the transverse direction, however, a wavefront encounters more gap junctions than over an equivalent distance in the longitudinal direction because cell diameter is much less than cell length; therefore, the wavefront must traverse more cells transversely. Thus, there is a greater resistance transversely than longitudinally because of the increased number of gap junctions per unit distance traveled.[238]

As stated above, the effective axial resistivity is an important determinant of the conduction velocity; therefore, conduction through atrial and ventricular myocardium is much more rapid in the longitudinal direction, owing to the lower resistivity, than in the transverse direction. Thus, cardiac muscle is anisotropic; its conduction properties vary depending on the direction in which they are measured.

Spach et al.[234,235,241,242] have classified anisotropy into two major subdivisions: uniform and nonuniform. Uniform anisotropy is characterized by an advancing wavefront that is smooth in all directions (longitudinal and transverse to fiber orientation), indicating relatively tight coupling between groups of fibers in all directions. Uniform anisotropy is exemplified by the conduction properties of normal septal ventricular muscle, as shown in Fig. 26-15A. The muscle in the diagram was stimulated in the center (pulse symbol), and activation spread away from this site in all directions. In the direction of the longitudinal axis of the fibers (from top to bottom) the activation isochrones are widely spaced, indicating rapid conduction—in this case, 0.51 m/s. There is a relatively broad area of fast conduction with an elliptic shape of the isochrones that is characteristic of uniform anisotropy.[241] In the direction transverse to the long axis (to the right and to the left), the isochrones are spaced close together, indicating slower conduction, 0.17 m/s in this example. As the direction of propagation changes between these two axes, the apparent conduction velocity changes monotonically from fast to slow, another characteristic of uniform anisotropy.[234]

The slow conduction in the direction transverse to the longitudinal fiber axis occurs despite action potentials with normal resting potentials and upstroke velocities and is caused by the higher transverse axial resistance. Associated with the differences in conduction velocity based on direction of propagation, however, are unexpected changes in the action potentials. Thus, when going from fast longitudinal conduction to slow transverse conduction, the rate of depolarization during the upstroke of the action potential (V_{max}) increases and the time constant of the foot of the upstroke decreases without any change in the resting potential, as shown in Fig. 26-15C; the upstroke that is dashed was recorded from a cell during longitudinal propagation, while the upstroke indicated by the solid line was recorded from the same cell during transverse propagation.[234] These characteristics are opposite to the changes in the action potentials associated with slowing of conduction when the membrane currents are altered (as by membrane depolarization).[243,244] Despite the increase in V_{max}, when conduction is slowed in the transverse direction, the slowing of conduction is associated with a decrease in the amplitude of the extracellular electrogram, showing that there is a decrease in the extracellular current flow as a result of the increased axial resistivity.

In uniformly anisotropic tissue, the extracellular unipolar waveform has a large-amplitude, smooth biphasic, positive-negative morphology during propagation in the fast longitudi-

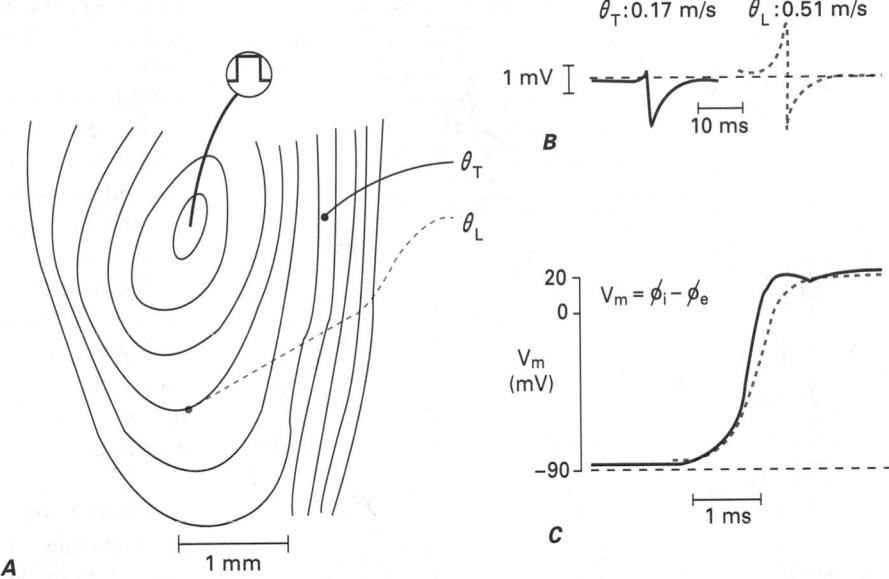

FIGURE 26-15

Relationship between the spread of excitation in uniform anisotropic ventricular muscle (A) and extracellular (B) and transmembrane potential waveforms (C). The excitation sequence in A was constructed from the extracellular waveforms measured at 100 positions on the endocardial surface of the right ventricular septum. The extracellular waveforms in B were measured at the sites indicated by the solid dots superimposed on the isochrones of A. The direction of propagation at the single transmembrane recording site was altered by initiating propagation at different locations, one to produce propagation along the longitudinal axis of the impaled fiber and the other to produce propagation along the transverse axis. Panel C shows the effects of the different directions of propagation on the upstroke of the action potential. [From Spach MS, Dolber PC. The relation between discontinuous propagation in anisotropic cardiac muscle and the "vulnerable period" of reentry. In: Zipes DP, Jalife J (eds). *Cardiac Electrophysiology and Arrhythmias*. New York: Grune & Stratton, 1985:241–252. Reproduced with permission from the publisher and author.]

nal direction (Fig. 26-15B, dashed line) and a low-amplitude, smooth triphasic (negative-positive-negative) morphology in the transverse direction (Fig. 26-15B, solid line). The initial negativity of the electrogram in the transverse direction is a reflection of distant activity rapidly propagating along the longitudinal axis.[245]

Nonuniform anisotropy has been defined[235] as tight electrical coupling between cells in the longitudinal direction but recurrent areas in the transverse direction in which side-to-side electrical coupling of adjacent groups of parallel fibers is absent. Therefore, propagation of normal action potentials transverse to the long axis is interrupted such that adjacent bundles are excited in a markedly irregular sequence, or *zigzag conduction*.[235,241] In nonuniformly anisotropic muscle, there may also be abrupt transition in conduction velocity from the fast longitudinal direction to the slow transverse direction, unlike the case with uniform anisotropic muscle, in which intermediate velocities occur between the two directions. This pattern of excitation in nonuniform anisotropic atrial pectinate bundles from older patients is diagrammed in Fig. 26-16A. The white arrow on the outline of the preparation indicates the narrow region of fast conduction down the long axis of the fibers when the bundle was excited at the asterisk. The zigzag arrow indicates the irregular course of excitation across

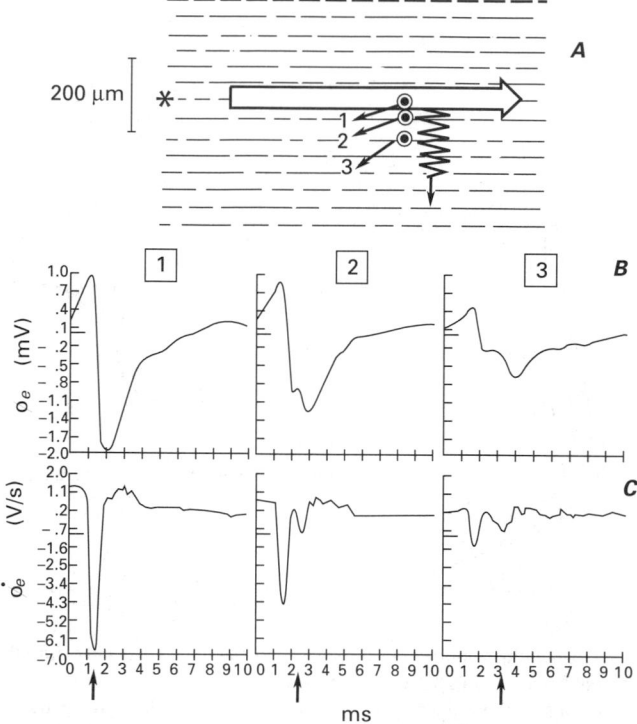

FIGURE 26-16

A. Diagram of a nonuniform anisotropic atrial muscle bundle with the long axis of the myocardial fibers indicated by the dashed lines. The bundle was stimulated at the asterisk. Propagation of the longitudinal wavefront is shown by the large white arrow. Transverse propagation occurred as diagrammed by the zigzag arrow. *B.* Electrograms recorded from sites 1, 2, and 3 on the diagram. *C.* The first derivative of these electrograms is shown. (From Spach MS, Dolber PC. Relating extracellular potentials and their derivatives to anisotropic propagation at a microscopic level in human cardiac muscle: Evidence for uncoupling of side-to-side fiber connections with increasing age. *Circ Res* 1986; 58:356. Reproduced with permission from the publisher and author.)

the fibers, which occurred all along the length of the zone of fast conduction. Conduction in the transverse direction in these nonuniformly anisotropic bundles was nearly as slow at the slowest conduction associated with membrane depolarization and slow-response action potentials.[5] In pectinate muscles from older patients, mean fast velocity was 0.69 m/s and slow velocity was 0.07 m/s, a ratio of almost 10,[241] despite the normal resting potential and the fast action potential upstroke of the atrial cells. As in uniform anisotropy, the upstroke velocity of the action potential is more rapid in the slow direction transverse to the long axis of the fibers than in the fast direction parallel to the long axis.

The morphologic basis for the nonuniform anisotropic properties in human atrial muscle is that the fascicles of muscle bundles are separated in the transverse direction by fibrous tissue that proliferates with aging to form longitudinally oriented insulting boundaries. Intercellular connections cannot occur where the cardiac fibers are separated by connective tissue septa and there is uncoupling between parallel-oriented groups of fibers.[235,241] Part of the reduction of the conduction velocity in this transverse direction may be a result of the

tortuous path length necessary for the wavefront to propagate transversely from one bundle to another because of these septa, accounting for the zigzag activation pattern. Similar connective tissue septa cause nonuniform anisotropy in other normal cardiac tissues, such as the crista terminalis and the interatrial band in adult atria or ventricular papillary muscle, as well as pathologic situations such as chronic ischemia or a healing myocardial infarction, in which fibrosis in the myocardium occurs.

The irregular activation transversely is evident in the extracellular electrogram, which is characterized by a sequence of multiple deflections, each representing activation of a separate bundle of fibers, with the largest, most rapid intrinsic deflection produced by local excitation and less rapid and lower amplitude deflections produced by excitation of adjacent fascicles.[235] In Fig. 26-16*B,* the multiple deflections can be seen in electrograms recorded from sites 2 and 3 in the atrial pectinate muscle and are even more prominent in the derivatives of these electrograms (Fig. 26-16*C*). Similarly fractionated electrogram can also be recorded from diseased regions of the ventricles. During longitudinal propagation, large biphasic electrograms are still evident (electrogram at site 1).

Anisotropy on a macroscopic scale can also influence conduction at sites where a bundle of cardiac fibers branches or where separate bundles coalesce. Marked slowing can occur when there is a sudden change in the fiber direction, causing an abrupt increase in the effective axial resistivity.[235] Figure 26-17 illustrates this point. The drawings show a small branch of an atrial pectinate muscle from the crista terminalis. The general direction of the fiber orientation is indicated by the thin broken lines, and the pattern of propagation is illustrated by the thick solid lines with arrows. In *A* (1) at the left, wavefronts initiated by stimulation at the top propagate throughout the crista and its branch along the longitudinal axis of the fibers throughout, so that there is no conduction delay entering the branch. At the right in *A* (2), wavefronts initiated by stimulation at the bottom propagate up the crista and into the branch, but they encounter a marked change in direction of the fibers from longitudinal to transverse while entering the branch, resulting in a slowing of conduction because of the sudden increase in axial resistance. Conduction block, which sometimes may be unidirectional, may occur at such junction sites, particularly when the inward current is decreased, as we describe later.

In addition to the structural features of the cellular interconnections influencing axial current flow and conduction as expressed in the anisotropic properties of cardiac muscle, the intercellular resistance may also increase because of an increase in gap junctional resistance that results from a decrease in the conductance of the junctions—i.e., a decrease of the ease with which the ions that carry axial current move through the junctions. In a computer model, conduction velocity could be reduced by a factor of 20 by increasing disk resistance, and decremental conduction and block result.[246,247]

Perhaps the most important influence on gap junctional resistance in pathologic situations is the level of intracellular

Ca^{2+}. A significant rise increases resistance to current flow through the junctions and eventually leads to physiologic uncoupling of the cells.[248,249] Intracellular Ca^{2+} increases during ischemia and may be a factor causing slow conduction and reentry. Thus, there are several causes for slow conduction that may lead to reentry: (1) slow responses that are a normal property of some regions of the heart, such as the sinus and AV node; (2) depressed fast responses or slow responses caused by pathology-induced partial depolarization of the membrane potential; (3) anisotropy; and (4) changes in gap junctional resistance.

Unidirectional Block

Unidirectional block occurs when an impulse cannot conduct in one direction along a bundle of cardiac fibers but can conduct in the opposite direction. This condition is necessary for the occurrence of classical reentrant rhythms. Thus, unidirectional block in part of the circuit leaves a return pathway through which

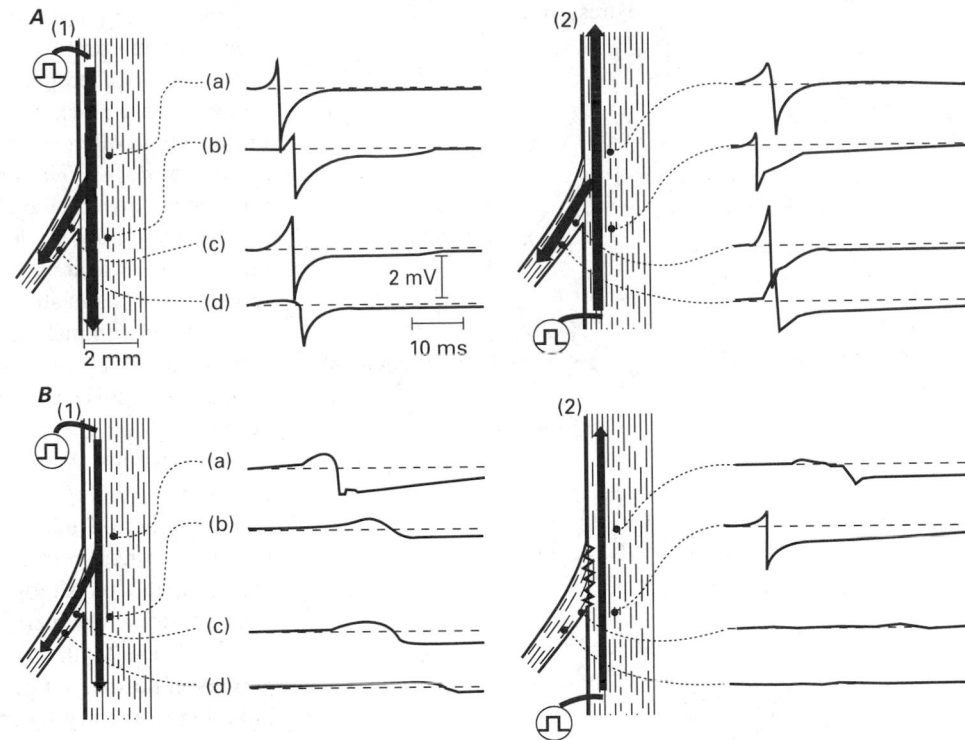

FIGURE 26-17

Conduction characteristics and unidirectional block at branch sites. The drawings represent a small branch formed by the origin of a pectinate muscle from the larger crista terminalis. The general direction of the fiber orientation is indicated by the broken lines. The patterns of propagation are shown by the solid arrows. Extracellular waveforms recorded at sites indicated by the dashed lines are also shown. (From Spach MS et al. The functional role of structural complexities in the propagation of depolarization in the atrium of the dog: Cardiac conduction disturbances due to discontinuities of effective axial resistivity. *Circ Res* 1982; 50:175. Reproduced with permission from the publisher and authors.)

the impulse conducts to reenter previously excited areas. There are a number of mechanisms, involving both active and passive electrical properties of cardiac cells that might cause unidirectional block.

Regional Differences in Recovery of Excitability   One cause of unidirectional block that enables the initiation of reentry is regional differences in recovery of excitability. When differences in the duration of the effective refractory period occur in adjacent areas, conduction of an appropriately timed premature impulse may be blocked in the region with the longest refractory period, which then becomes a site of unidirectional block, while conduction continues through regions with a shorter refractory period. Figure 26-18 is a schematic representation of the initiation and continuation of circus movement in an anatomically defined circuit, with differences in effective refractory period duration resulting from differences in the time course of action potential repolarization being the cause for unidirectional block in one of the pathways. The action potentials in various parts of the circuit are shown. In the upper panel (*A*), conduction of a premature impulse (extrasystole), which can either be induced by electrical stimulation or may occur "spontaneously," is blocked in the pathway with the long action potential duration and, therefore, long effective

refractory period (to the left), referred to as the *blocked pathway*. The premature impulse, however, conducts in the other pathway with shorter action potential durations and refractory periods (to the right). This pattern of activation is indicated by the arrows. In order for block to occur, the premature impulse must also arise in a region with a short effective refractory period so that it occurs before repolarization of the action potentials in the left pathway occurs. In the lower panel (*B*), which shows the continuation of these events, the blocked pathway is retrogradely invaded by the impulse conducting from the right, thereby causing the second action potential (arrow at the left). The proximal region where the premature impulse originated is then reexcited (reentry), as the impulse once again enters the right pathway and continues around the reentrant circuit, causing another action potential in the right pathway (large arrow). For successful reexcitation to occur in the region where the premature impulse was initiated, elements in the circuit at the region of block and proximal to it (toward the site of origin) must have regained their excitability by the time the cardiac impulse arrives there. Continuation of reentry induced by a premature impulse is also facilitated because the duration of the effective refractory period associated with conductance of the premature impulse is shortened. Therefore, on the next excursion of the reentrant impulse

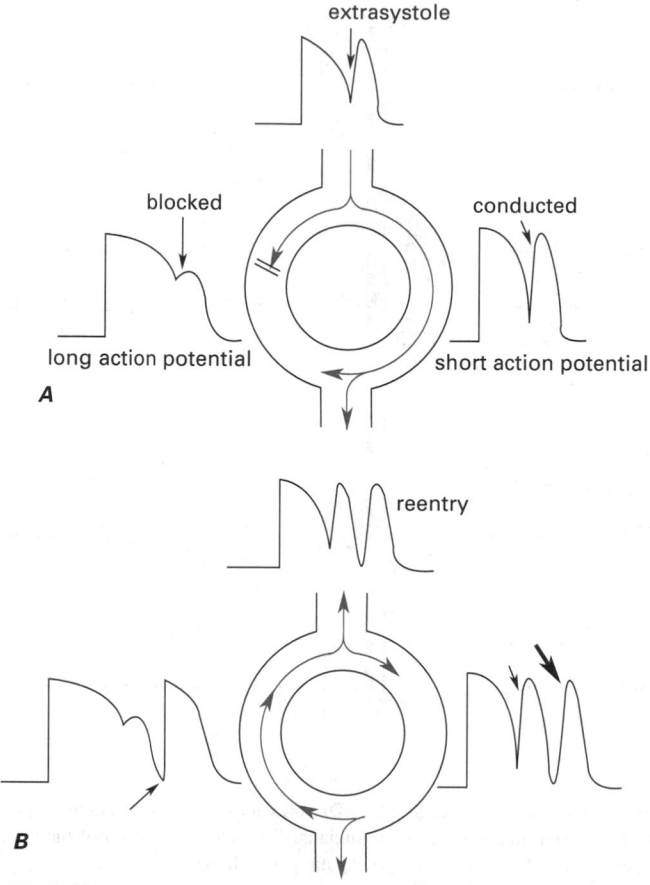

FIGURE 26-18
Diagram of reentry caused by dispersion in refractory periods. A ring of cardiac tissue is shown and the pattern of conduction is indicated by the arrows. Action potentials with different durations located in different regions of the ring are diagrammed. (From Wit AL, Janse MJ. *The Ventricular Arrhythmia of Ischemia and Infarction: The Electrophysiological Mechanisms.* Mt. Kisco, NY: Futura; 1992. Reproduced with permission from the publisher and authors.)

around the circuit, conduction occurs in a circuit with a shorter effective refractory period. Finally, conduction velocity of premature impulses may be decreased, shortening the wavelength[250,251] and facilitating successful excitation of the region proximal to the unidirectional block.

Therefore, unidirectional block caused by regional differences in excitability is actually a result of transient block. Block occurs in the antegrade direction in the left pathway while conduction is successful in the retrograde direction. This kind of unidirectional block can cause initiation of reentry not only in anatomic circuits, as shown in Fig. 26-18, but also in functional circuits. For reentrant arrhythmias to arise because of regional differences in effective refractory periods, a premature impulse that initiates reentry is as necessary a requirement as the conditions allowing perpetuation of reentrant activation. Thus, both a "trigger" (the premature impulse) and a "substrate" (the reentrant circuit) are needed. The mechanism causing the premature impulse may be quite different from the arrhythmia it initiates. It might arise spontaneously by automaticity or it might be a result of triggered activity. The premature impulse might also be induced by an electrical

stimulus during a programmed stimulation protocol. The degree of nonuniformity in effective refractory period duration necessary for a properly timed premature stimulus to cause unidirectional block may be quite small. This degree of non-uniformity is often referred to as the *dispersion in refractory periods* or *dispersion in recovery of excitability,* meaning the difference between the shortest and longest refractor period.

When stimuli were delivered in the region with the shortest refractor period at the border of two areas with different refractor periods in atrial tissue in the experiments of Allessie et al.,[252] the minimal difference in effective refractory period needed to cause block of an appropriately timed stimulated premature impulse was between 11 and 16 ms, well within the normal physiological range of variation of effective refractory period durations. A properly timed single premature stimulus can initiate reentry in the atria because the differences in refractory period may cause unidirectional block.[252] In the ventricles, where refractory periods are much longer than in the atria, the physiologic differences between longest and shortest refractory period duration is on the order of 40 ms.[253,254] Unlike the case in the atria, dispersion of refractor periods in normal ventricles is not sufficiently large to allow initiation of reentry by premature impulses.

In experiments in which dispersion of refractory periods was increased by local cooling of the ventricles and a critical difference between shortest and longest effective refractory period ranging from 95 to 145 ms was reached, premature stimuli delivered at the site with the shortest effective refractory period induced repetitive activity in the canine left ventricle, presumably because block of the premature impulses in the regions with a long effective refractory period created unidirectional block and permitted reentry.[255,256] Similarly, critical increases in the dispersion of refractory periods that are caused by acute or prolonged ischemia result in reentrant arrhythmias. The difference between the longest and shortest refractory period is not the only factor determining whether premature stimuli will induce reentry.[252] If the regions of long and short refractory periods are separated by a large distance, an early premature impulse arising in a region of short refractoriness may not be able to arrive in the region of long refractoriness sufficiently early to cause block because conduction between the regions may be slow. Regions of long refractory periods must, therefore, be relatively close to a region of shorter refractory periods where the premature impulse arises for block to occur. In addition, if block does occur, the size of the area of unidirectional block is of crucial importance, particularly in a functionally determined reentrant circuit. Even in the presence of large differences in effective refractory period duration, reentry may not occur when the area with long effective refractory periods resulting in unidirectional block is small, because the impulse can travel around the area of unidirectional block along an alternate pathway or pathways and will not be delayed sufficiently to allow reexcitation of the point of origin at the end of the latter's effective refractory period. This cannot occur in an anatomic circuit such as the one shown in Fig. 26-18. Thus, *dispersion in recovery of excitability* is, by itself, not sufficient for describing the propensity for induction of reentrant arrhythmias. The regional differences in recovery of excitability that lead to unidirectinal conduction block might also occur in the absence of regional differences in action potential duration. Computer models have shown that the activation sequence of a propagating impulse can lead to asynchronous repolarization and refractoriness even when membrane properties are homogeneous.[89,247] A stimulated premature impulse can block in a region that has been depolarized most recently by a prior wave of excitation and is therefore still refractory, but it may conduct into another region that was excited much earlier by the prior wave of excitation if it has had time to recover excitability. The conducting premature excitation wave then can later return to excite the area of block after it recovers, resulting in reentry.

Asymmetric Depression of Excitability Unidirectional conduction block in a reentrant circuit can also be persistent and independent of premature activation. Persistent unidirectional block is often associated with depression of the transmembrane potentials and excitability of cardiac fibers.[257] There are several possible mechanisms for the persistent unidirectional block in a region where action potentials are depressed. One mechanism is asymmetrical depression of excitability. Such asymmetric depression might occur because of asymmetric distribution of a pathologic event. As a simple example, the action potential upstrokes in a bundle of fibers may be diminished as a result of a reduction of perfusion after coronary occlusion, but the depression of the upstroke may be more severe toward one end of the bundle than the other. This situation is diagrammed in Fig. 26-19. A propagating impulse consisting of an action potential with a normal upstroke velocity (site 1) enters the poorly perfused region (stippled in the diagram) and propagates through this region with decrement (from left to right or from site 1 to 4), i.e., as it conducts from the less depressed end (1) to the more severely depressed end (4), the action potential upstroke velocity and amplitude progressively decrease, as does the axial current flowing to-

ward cells to be excited by the upstroke (as indicated by the decreasing size of the striped arrows). When the impulse arrives at the opposite end of the depressed segment of the bundle where there is suddenly a normally perfused bundle with normal action potentials (between action potential 4 and 5), the action potential amplitude is markedly reduced and the weak axial current from site 4 is not sufficient to depolarize the normal membrane to threshold at site 5. Conduction, therefore, blocks in the left-to-right direction even though the normally perfused region is excitable. Conduction in the opposite direction (from right to left), however, might still succeed. The large axial current generated by the normal action potential at site 5 can flow for a considerable distance through the depressed region and may depolarize to threshold fibers at some distance from the most severely depressed region (perhaps as far as site 3). These cells, in turn, may be able to excite adjacent fibers in the direction of propagation (from right to left), and as a result, the impulse successfully propagates from site 3 to site 1, as indicated by the black arrows.

Geometric Factors Causing Unidirectional Block Geometric factors related to tissue architecture may also influence impulse conduction and under certain conditions lead to unidirectional block. An impulse can conduct rapidly in either direction along the length of a bundle of atrial, ventricular, or Purkinje fibers with normal electrophysiologic properties. There is usually some asymmetry in the conduction velocity, however, meaning that conduction in one direction may take slightly longer than in the other direction.[5,228,231] This is usually of no physiologic significance. The asymmetry of conduction can be the result of several factors. Bundles of cardiac muscle are composed of interconnecting myocardial fibers with different diameters packed in a connective tissue matrix. These bundles branch frequently (although the individual myocardial fibers do not branch). An impulse conducting in one direction encounters a different sequence of changes in fiber diameter, branching, and frequency and distribution of gap junctions than it does when traveling in the opposite direction. The configuration of pathways in each direction is not the same.[231] These structural features influence conduction by affecting the axial currents that flow ahead of the propagating wavefront.

Results of theoretical analyses indicate that the conduction velocity of an impulse passing abruptly from a fiber of small diameter to one of large diameter transiently slows at the junction because the larger cable results in a larger sink for the longitudinal axial current (there is more membrane for this current to depolarize to threshold if conduction of the impulse is to continue).[228,231,247,258,259] A similar slowing occurs when an impulse conducts into a region where there is an abrupt increase in branching of the myocardial syncytium; conduction transiently slows because of the larger current sink provided by the increased membrane area that must be depolarized.

In the opposite direction, it can be predicted that conduction will speed transiently as the impulse moves from a larger to a smaller cable because the small sink for axial current results

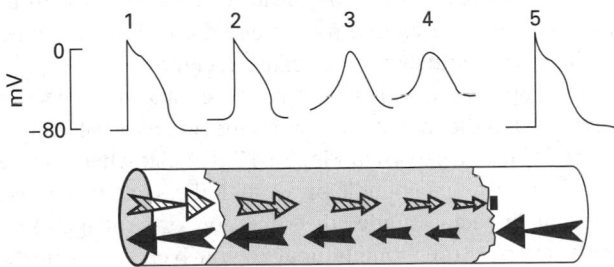

FIGURE 26-19

Asymmetric depression of excitability as a mechanism for unidirectional conduction block in a bundle of cardiac muscle fibers. Action potentials shown above were recorded from sites on the fiber bundle. The stippled part of the bundle is depressed. Conduction from left to right along the bundle is indicated by the striped arrows, conduction from right to left by the black arrows. (Modified from Wit AL, Rosen MR. Cellular electrophysiological mechanisms of cardiac arrhythmias. In: MacFarlane PW, Veitch Lawrie TD (eds). *Comprehensive Electrocardiology: Theory and Practice in Health and Disease*, vol. 2. New York: Pergamon Press; 1989:801–841. Reproduced with permission from the publisher and authors.)

in more rapid depolarization of the membrane to threshold.[228,258,259] Theoretically, if there is a large enough difference in the diameter of the two cables, an impulse conducting from the small cable to the large cable should block at the junction, while conduction in the opposite direction (from large cable to small cable) is maintained.

A probable example of unidirectional block based on this geometric factor in the normal heart is at the junctions between Purkinje and muscle cells. At certain sites, propagation from muscle to Purkinje fibers is possible, while propagation from Purkinje fibers to muscle is not.[260] This asymmetry of conduction results from the difference in mass of the Purkinje and muscle layers. The smaller mass Purkinje fiber bundle is the small-diameter cable while the larger mass muscle is the larger diameter cable. It is unlikely that in normal circumstances these localized sites of unidirectional block predispose to reentry since the myocardium is quickly excited via the many other Purkinje-to-muscle junctions where the geometric differences are not sufficient to cause block. It is possible, however, when conduction in ischemic myocardium is slow and coupling resistance at the junctional increases, that such sites of unidirectional block may become important in initiating reentry.[261–263]

It is doubtful that abrupt changes in geometric properties such as fiber diameter of the magnitude required to cause block of the *normal* action potential often exist (except at some Purkinje fiber–muscle junctions as described above) because the safety factor for conduction is large, i.e., there is a large excess of activating current over the amount required for propagation.[228] Dodge and Cranefield[231] have pointed out that "only if an action potential is a relatively weak stimulus and the unexcited area is not easily excited will plausible changes in membrane resistance, cell diameter, or intercellular coupling procedure block." There is a necessity for interaction of abnormal action potentials and decreased excitability with the preexisting anatomic impediments, such as will occur in acute ischemia. When the resting potential of fibers in a muscle or Purkinje bundle is decreased, the reduced action potential upstroke results in a decreased axial current, and therefore, the action potential is a weak stimulus. The normal directional differences in conduction are then exaggerated.

At a critical degree of depression of the action potential upstroke, conduction may fail in one direction while being maintained in the other (although it may be markedly slowed). At this critical degree of depression, the reduced axial current might not be sufficient to depolarize the membrane to threshold where the current sink is increased because of the structural changes described above (increased fiber diameter), but the axial current is still more than adequate during conduction in the opposite direction.

The anisotropic properties of cardiac muscle also represent a geometric factor that may sometimes contribute to the occurrence of unidirectional block. Spach et al.[234] have indicated that in anisotropic muscle, the safety factor for conduction is lower in the longitudinal direction of rapid conduction than in the transverse direction of slow conduction (opposite to that predicted on the basis of continuous cable theory). The

low safety factor longitudinally is a result of a large current load on the membrane associated with the low axial resistivity and large membrane capacitance in the longitudinal direction. This low safety factor may result in preferential conduction block of premature impulses in the longitudinal direction relative to the transverse direction under certain conditions. In uniformly anisotropic muscle, a decrease in inward current during the depolarization phase of an action potential, as might result from premature activation, results in slowing of conduction in the longitudinal direction more than in the transverse direction, but propagation still continues as a spatially smooth process. Conduction block of early premature impulses occurs in both longitudinal and transverse directions nearly simultaneously in uniformly anisotropic muscle.[242]

In nonuniformly anisotropic muscle, however, premature activation can result in conduction block in the longitudinal direction even when the impulse is conducting from a region with a long refractory period into a region of shorter refractory period, while conduction in the transverse direction continues.[242] The site of block in the longitudinal direction can become a site of unidirectional block that leads to reentry, much like the block of premature impulses caused by a sudden increase in action potential duration and effective refractory period. It can be excited by an impulse propagating in the opposite direction, i.e., by the wavefront initially launched successfully in the transverse direction and that later propagates to the distal side of the region of the block. In contrast to the propensity of premature impulses to block in the longitudinal direction in nonuniformly anisotropic myocardium because of the decreased depolarizing current and low safety factor, when coupling resistance between cells is increased, conduction of all impulses will block first in the transverse direction. Preferential block in this direction occurs because an increase in coupling resistance will reduce the safety factor for longitudinal conduction below the critical level needed to maintain transverse conduction before the safety factor for longitudinal conduction is reduced to this critical level.[265,265] Unlike longitudinal block of a premature impulse, which is transient block and which may lead to reentry, block in the transverse direction caused by increased coupling resistance is bidirectional and should not cause reentry.

Anisotropy can also result in unidirectional block at sites of muscle bundle branching or at the junction of muscle bundles.[235] It was shown in Fig. 26-17A(2) that when a wavefront propagating in a bundle of parallel fibers enters a branch formed at an acute angle, the direction of propagation is quickly altered from longitudinal to transverse, causing an abrupt increase in the effective axial resistance in the direction of propagation and a slowing of conduction velocity. If the inward current is also reduced by partial depolarization such as after premature stimulation or elevation of extracellular K^+, conduction block may occur.[235] This is shown in Fig. 26-17B(2), where extracellular K^+ concentration was increased from 4.6 to 9.0 meq/L. Failure of the stimulated impulse to enter the branch is shown by the absence of electrical activity at sites c and d. On the other hand, as shown in Fig. 26-17B(1), propagation from the other direction into the branch does not involve a change in the direction of the wavefront relative to the fiber orientation since it continues in a parallel direction; therefore, there is no block in this direction.[235] These sites can become areas of unidirectional block that are instrumental in the occurrence of reentry.

Alterations in Refractory Period

Alterations of the effective refractory period may contribute to the occurrence of reentry. A decrease in the effective refractory period decreases the wavelength of the reentrant impulse and, therefore, the necessary size of the reentrant circuit. If the refractory period is decreased, the degree of slow conduction needed for successful reentry is diminished. The effective refractory period of cardiac fibers in a reentrant circuit may be decreased during rapid tachycardias because of rate-dependent shortening of the action potential duration.[247,266] The computer model of Quan and Rudy[247] predicts that in circuits with a small or no excitable gap, electrotonic interaction between the head and the tail of the reentrant wavefront can also shorten action potential duration and the refractory period. If the effective refractory period is decreased sufficiently, more than one reentrant circuit can exist at a time in some regions.[267,268] The effective refractory period of atrial muscle, for example, is decreased by the acetylcholine released during vagal stimulation. As a result, reentry in atrial muscle causing atrial fibrillation is more easily induced during vagal stimulation.[269] Several reentrant circuits exist simultaneously during this arrhythmia.[268,270] Action potential duration and effective refractory period are decreased in the ventricle during reperfusion after brief periods of ischemia or in some of the ventricular muscle cells in chronically ischemic areas, probably contributing to the occurrence of reentry.

The Central Area of Block

The central area of block around which the reentrant wavefront circulates may be anatomic, functional, or a combination of the two. Anatomic block is the result of a nonconductive medium in the center of the circuit. An example of an anatomically determined central area of block is in the tricuspid ring reentrant circuit found in a canine model of atrial flutter[266] and perhaps present in a clinical counterpart, atrial flutter found commonly in patients who have previously had a Mustard procedure to repair transposition of the great vessels.[271] The animal model depends critically on large incisions made in the right atrial free wall, which, in fact, are similar to those made by the surgeon during the Mustard procedure. Functional block at the center of a circuit occurs when there is block of impulses in otherwise excitable cardiac muscle. An example of a functional center of block was first described by Allessie[272] in a model of reentrant excitation in the rabbit left atrium called the leading circle mechanism of reentry. Functional block has subsequently been described in several other models of atrial flutter.[223,224,273,274] The central area of functional block develops during the initiation of the reentrant circuit by the formation of a line of block most likely due to refractoriness. When the reentrant circuit forms, the line of block is then sustained by centripetal activation from the circu-

lating reentrant wavefront which, by repeatedly bombarding the central area of block, maintains the state of refractoriness of this region. A combination of an anatomic and functional central area of block in the reentrant circuit has been described in some models of atrial flutter (e.g., the orifice of one or both of the cavae and an area of functional block continuous with or adjacent to either or both of the caval orifices).[275]

The Excitable Gap

The excitable gap in a reentrant circuit is the region of excitable myocardium that immediately precedes the head of the reentrant wavefront and moves around the circuit in advance of the reentrant wavefront. The occurrence of a gap is dependent on the recovery of excitability of the myocardium from its previous excitation by the reentrant wavefront. There are two different measurements of the excitable gap. One is the spatial gap, which is the distance in the circuit ahead of the wavefront that is excitable. The spatial gap may be comprised of only partially excitable and fully excitable myocardium depending on the time interval between successive excitations of the circuit. The size of the spatial gap changes in different parts of the circuit as the wavelength of the reentrant impulse changes because of changes in conduction velocity, refractory periods, or both as previously described.

The second measurement of the excitable gap is the temporal excitable gap. This is the time period during the cardiac cycle that a stimulus can excite the region ahead of the reentrant wavefront. As for the spatial gap, the temporal gap in different parts of the reentrant circuit also can have both partially excitable and fully excitable components and varies in different parts of the circuit because of the changes in the wavelength. The characteristics of the excitable gap may be quite different in reentrant circuits caused by different mechanisms. For example, some anatomically determined circuits have been shown to have large excitable gaps with a fully excitable component, although even in anatomically determined circuits, the gap may only be partially excitable.[276] By comparison, functional reentrant circuits caused by the leading circle mechanism have very small gaps that are only partially excitable,[273] although parts of some functionally determined reentrant circuits may have a small fully excitable gap during part of the reentrant cycle. The latter may occur because of differences in conduction velocity in different portions of the reentrant circuit.

TYPES OF REENTRY

We have previously indicated that there are two types of reentry: ordered and random.[1] The reentrant circuits can be anatomically determined, functionally determined, or both anatomically and functionally determined. In anatomically determined circuits, the pathway is fixed and the characteristics of the reentrant circuit are determined by the characteristics of the anatomic components of the circuit. Anatomic circuits are, therefore, associated with ordered reentry. Perhaps the best example is that of AV reentrant tachycardia in which the reentrant circuit is composed of atrium, the AV node, the His-Purkinje system, ventricle, and an accessory AV connection.

In functionally determined circuits, the pathway is formed because of the electrophysiological properties of the cardiac cells and not by a predetermined anatomic pathway. Functional circuits can be associated with ordered or random reentry. Mechanisms for functionally determined reentrant circuits include the leading cycle type of reentry,[272] anisotropic reentry, and spiral wave reentry.[277] Allessie and coworkers[252,272,278] were able to induce stable reentrant tachycardia in small pieces of isolated rabbit left atrium by precisely timed premature impulses in regions that were activated normally at regular rates of stimulation. Initiation of reentry was made possible by the different refractory periods of atrial fibers in close proximity to one another. The premature impulse that initiated reentry blocked in fibers with long refractory periods and conducted in fibers with shorter refractory periods, eventually returning to the initial region of block after excitability recovered there. The impulse then continued to circulate around a central area that was kept refractory because it was constantly bombarded by impulses propagating toward it from all sides of the circuit. This central area provides a functional obstacle that prevents excitation from propagating across the fulcrum of the circuit. No anatomic obstacles or anatomically defined conducting pathways are present in the leading circle, and the reentrant circuit is completely defined by the electrophysiological properties of the tissue involved. The circumference of the leading circle around a functional obstacle may be as little as 6 to 8 mm and represents a pathway in which the efficacy of stimulation of the circulating wavefront is just sufficient to excite the tissue ahead, which is still in its relative refractory phase. Conduction through the functional reentrant circuit is slowed, therefore, because impulses are propagating in partially refractory tissue (a partially excitable gap). Reentrant excitation that has been mapped in the atria of canine models of atrial flutter may be caused by the leading circle mechanism.[223,273] The reentrant circuit remains in the same place during the flutter and is therefore ordered reentry. Functional reentrant circuits of the leading circle type may also change their size and location and, if they do, would fall under the general category of random reentry. This may occur when leading circle reentry causes fibrillation.

Anisotropy can cause conduction slow enough to result in reentry in small anatomic circuits. Reentrant circuits caused by anisotropy can also occur without well-defined anatomic pathways and might be classified as functional. Unlike the functional characteristic that leads to the leading circle type of reentry (local differences in membrane properties causing a difference in effective refractory periods in adjacent areas), in functional reentry caused by anisotropy, the functional characteristic that is important is the difference in effective axial resistance to impulse propagation dependent on fiber direction. This mechanism has been classified as *anisotropic reentry*.[277] In its pure form, both the unidirectional conduction block and slow conduction in the reentrant circuit are a result of anisotropic, discontinuous propagation, and there is no need for variations in membrane properties such as regional differences in effective refractory periods or depression of the resting and action potential.[242]

On the basis of the longitudinal and transverse conduction velocities of premature impulses in nonuniform anisotropic muscle and of measurements of refractory periods in these experiments, Spach et al.[242] calculated that circuits in nonuniform anisotropic bundles can be as small as 2 to 4 mm^2 (transverse velocity of 0.5 m/s, dissociated longitudinal velocity of 0.2 m/s) in the absence of nonuniformities in repolarization. Furthermore, anisotropic circuits are elliptical or rectangular because of the directional differences in conduction velocities with the long axis of the ellipse in the fast, longitudinal direction. Circuits with this shape can have a smaller dimension than circular circuits such as the leading circle.[242] Anisotropic reentrant circuits usually remain in a fixed position to cause ordered reentry.[279] The degree of anisotropy (ratio of longitudinal to transverse conduction velocity) varies in different regions of the heart, and the circuit can only reside in a region where the conduction transverse to the longitudinal axis is sufficiently slow to allow reentry. Stability of anisotropic reentrant circuits is also assisted by the presence of an excitable gap that does not occur in the leading circle functional circuit. The excitable gap is caused by the sudden slowing of conduction velocity and decrease in the wavelength of excitation as the reentrant impulse turns the corner from the fast longitudinal direction to the slow transverse direction and from the slow transverse direction to the fast longitudinal direction.[280,281]

Another type of functional reentrant excitation, called spiral waves, does not require any inhomogeneities of refractory periods like in leading circle reentry, inhomogeneities in conduction properties like in aniostropic reentry, nor a central obstacle, be it functional or anatomic. Spiral waves were originally initiated in computer models of homogeneous elements or in various kinds of homogeneous excitable media (properties do not vary throughout the media), an example of which is molecular diffusion in a chemical system. Under appropriate circumstances, a pulse in two-dimensional, homogeneous, excitable media can be made to circulate as a rotor with a wavelength that is proportional to the square root of the diffusion coefficient of the media.[282–284]

Preexisting functional heterogeneities in conduction (or diffusion) properties or refractoriness (time course of recovery of excitability) are not prerequisites for the initiation of spiral wave in excitable media. The heterogeneity that allows initiation can be the result of a previous excitation wave and the pattern of recovery from that wave. When heterogeneities in recovery exist, the application of a second stimulus over a large geometric area to initiate a second excitation wave only excites a region where there has been sufficient time for recovery from the previous excitation and not regions that are not yet recovered. An excitation wave is elicited at the excitable site which is in the form of a rotor because the wave cannot move in the direction of the wake of the previous wave but only in the opposite direction, moving into adjacent regions as they, in turn, recover. The inner tip of the wavefront circulates around a disk of quiescent medium instead of a region of conduction block. The size of this disk expands as the medium is made less excitable.[282–284] The rotor, by definition, has a marked curvature, and this curvature slows down its propagation. A similar pattern of excitation can be induced in cardiac muscle.[285,286]

In the case of a curved depolarization wavefront (rotor) in excitable tissue such as cardiac muscle, slow conduction is the result of an increased electrical load, e.g., a curved wavefront must depolarize not only cells in front of it in the direction of propagation but current also flows to cells on its sides. The slow activation by a rotor is not dependent on conduction in relatively refractory myocardium; therefore, there is an excitable gap despite the functional nature of reentry.[282] The location of the rotor can occur any where the second stimulated excitation encounters the wake of the first excitation with the appropriate characteristics.[287] Reentrant excitation that occurs during the initiation of ventricular fibrillation by strong electrical shocks[288,289] has characteristics consistent with spiral waves or rotors. These small circulating rotors are not stable and meet the criteria of random reentry. Spiral waves might also cause other kinds of arrhythmias. Even though nonuniform dispersions of refractoriness or anisotropy are not necessary for the initiation of reentrant excitation caused by rotors in excitable media, the myocardium, even when normal, is never homogeneous and the heterogeneities may modify the characteristics of the spiral waves.

Methods to Identify Mechanisms of Arrhythmias

INTRODUCTION

Since the early and classic experiments of Mayer[3,290] on reentry in the Medusa ring and later studies by Mines[4,291] on reentry in ring preparations cut from dogfish auricles or from canine right ventricles, it has been thought that mapping of the sequence of activation of the heart during a tachycardia should provide the best evidence for the presence of a reentrant circuit. Even so, the admonition of Mines[291] that "the chief error to be guarded against is that of mistaking a series of automatic beats originating in one point of a ring [substitute apparent reentrant circuit] and traveling around it in one direction only owing to a complete block close to the point of origin of the rhythm on one side of this point" for reentrant beats must be kept in mind. The point, of course, is that even sequence of activation mapping may not provide definitive proof of the presence of reentry even though it provides evidence consistent with reentry. Mines suggested that severing the ring (again, substitute the critical portion of the apparent reentrant circuit) and then demonstrating that no further reentrant excitation could occur was required for proof that reentrant excitation had been present. This, of course, has been accomplished in the example of AV reentrant tachycardia, with cure of the arrhythmia following catheter or surgical ablation of the accessory AV connection. Nevertheless, while "severing the ring" is both diagnostic and therapeutic when it can be accomplished to treat a tachyarrhythmia, it is virtually always clinically impractical as a diagnostic tool. Furthermore, until recently, precise sequence of activation cardiac mapping to identify reentry has been quite difficult to perform, particularly in patients.

Although it is now possible to obtain remarkably precise maps of the sequence of cardiac activation in vivo using simultaneous multisite mapping techniques, it is only possible with use of sophisticated recording techniques that require the chest to be open and the heart exposed. In fact, for the study of arrhythmias in the in situ heart, it is not routinely possible to obtain the direct electrical recordings (microelectrode studies, simultaneous multisite mapping, etc.) from the arrhythmogenic source that enable one to determine the electrophysiologic mechanism causing the arrhythmias. Therefore, indirect approaches have evolved that can provide information that suggests the mechanism of an arrhythmia. These approaches include (1) characterizating the arrhythmia from the ECG; (2) analyzing the response of the arrhythmia to selected forms of cardiac pacing; and (3) analyzing the effects of selected pharmacologic agents on the arrhythmia. Since cardiac pacing has long been an important tool in the study of mechanisms of both clinical and experimental arrhythmias and since it is also usually rather easy to apply, we present here a discussion of the use of this technique to identify the mechanism of an arrhythmia.

CARDIAC PACING TO DETERMINE ARRHYTHMOGENIC MECHANISMS

The mechanism of an arrhythmia in the in situ heart can sometimes be deduced from the response of the arrhythmia to cardiac pacing. Our knowledge of the response of the different arrhythmogenic mechanisms to pacing is based largely on studies in which the effects of electrical stimulation were determined on transmembrane action potentials recorded with microelectrodes in isolated and superfused cardiac tissues. Critical to the ability to use the response to electrical stimulation to determine arrhythmia mechanisms is that the stimulated impulse(s) must reach the site of origin of the arrhythmia. There are many reasons why this might not happen. The stimulated impulse(s) might not reach the site at which the arrhythmia arises because of the electrophysiologic properties of the intervening tissue between the stimulus site and the site of arrhythmia origin. An intervening region of prolonged refractoriness or depressed conduction might cause stimulated impulses to block before they reach the site of origin. If conduction time from the stimulation site to the site of arrhythmia origin is prolonged for any reason, impulses generated in the arrhythmogenic focus also may be able to leave that focus and depolarize large regions of myocardium around it, preventing the stimulated impulse from reaching the site of arrhythmia origin. Even when the stimulation site is close to the site of arrhythmia origin, areas of depressed conduction may prevent the stimulated impulses from reaching the arrhythmogenic cells.

Two basic patterns of stimulation are generally used to study the mechanisms of arrhythmias: (1) overdrive pacing (pacing at a rate or rates faster than the spontaneous rate of the arrhythmia) and (2) introduction of a premature beat or beats using programmed stimulation. With either technique, the effects of the stimulated impulses on the spontaneous rhythm are observed. Overdrive pacing is generally used during the arrhythmia to determine if the overdrive can terminate it or, if it does not, to determine the effect of the overdrive on characteristics of the arrhythmia. Overdrive pacing is sometimes used during sinus rhythm to determine whether or not the period of stimulation can induce an arrhythmia that has previously occurred spontaneously.

Introduction of a premature beat or beats at selected intervals during electrical diastole by programmed stimulation of the heart can be performed either during the spontaneous arrhythmia to test the effects of the premature beats or during sinus rhythm or fixed rate pacing to see if the arrhythmia can be induced.

EFFECTS OF ELECTRICAL STIMULATION ON ARRHYTHMIAS CAUSED BY AUTOMATICITY

The prior discussion of automaticity as an arrhythmogenic mechanism included a consideration of how the sinus node pacemaker and electrical stimulation (pacing) influence subsidiary pacemakers with different automatic mechanisms. Overdrive either by the sinus node or by electrical stimuli exerts an inhibitory effect on the normal automatic mechanism of subsidiary or latent pacemakers (overdrive suppression) that is primarily the result of enhanced Na^+–K^+ pump activity but has less inhibitory effects on the abnormal automatic mechanism of subsidiary pacemakers. These known effects of overdrive on pacemaker mechanisms are sometimes useful in distinguishing automatic arrhythmias from arrhythmias caused by reentry or triggered activity in the in situ heart. The effects of overdrive pacing can also be of use in distinguishing arrhythmias caused by normal automaticity from those caused by abnormal automaticity.[86] Based on the results of experimental studies, it can be assumed that arrhythmias caused by normal automaticity in the in situ heart cannot be initiated by overdrive pacing. Arrhythmias caused by normal automaticity can be suppressed transiently, but cannot be terminated by overdrive pacing. Based on microelectrode studies on isolated superfused pacemaker tissues, when overdrive pacing is applied during an ongoing arrhythmia caused by normal automaticity, the arrhythmia is expected to be transiently suppressed immediately after the overdrive pacing is stopped. This is manifest by a transient pause after overdrive and should be followed by a gradual speeding up of the rhythm (so-called warmup) until the original rate of the automatic rhythm is resumed. The duration of the transient pause and the time required for resumption of the original rate is expected to be directly related to the rate and duration of the overdrive. This behavior is mainly the result of the increased activity of the Na^+–K^+ pump, which is dependent both on the rate and duration of stimulation. This characteristic behavior of normally automatic pacemakers has been demonstrated in some clinical and experimental electrophysiological studies of both atrial and ventricular tachycardias.[181,292,293]

Like normal automaticity, arrhythmias caused by abnormal automaticity can neither be initiated nor terminated by overdrive pacing. On the other hand, arrhythmias caused by abnormal automaticity should not be suppressed by overdrive pacing unless the overdrive period is long and the rate of overdrive

is fast.[86] The difficulty in suppressing such arrhythmias stems from the lesser amount of Na^+ entering the cells during the upstroke of the action potential and, therefore, less intense Na^+ pump stimulation by overdrive. Short periods of overdrive can even result in a transient speeding of the rate of impulse generation (overdrive acceleration).[86] Accelerated idioventricular tachycardia in myocardial infarction is not easily overdrive-suppressed and, therefore, may be caused by abnormal automaticity.

The response of automatic arrhythmias to premature stimulation is also sometimes useful in distinguishing automaticity from other arrhythmogenic mechanisms. Of major importance, automatic rhythms caused by either normal or abnormal automaticity can neither be initiated nor terminated by premature stimuli, in contrast to reentry and triggered activity (discussed later). Other than that, premature impulses induced at different times during diastole may transiently perturb an automatic rhythm for a few cycles. The characteristics of the perturbation may sometimes distinguish automaticity from other arrhythmogenic mechanisms. The response of normal and abnormal automaticity to premature stimulation may be somewhat similar. The characteristic response of an automatic pacemaker to premature stimulation is best exemplified by the response of the sinus node to atrial premature stimulation.[294] In Fig. 26-20 is plotted the normalized return cycle

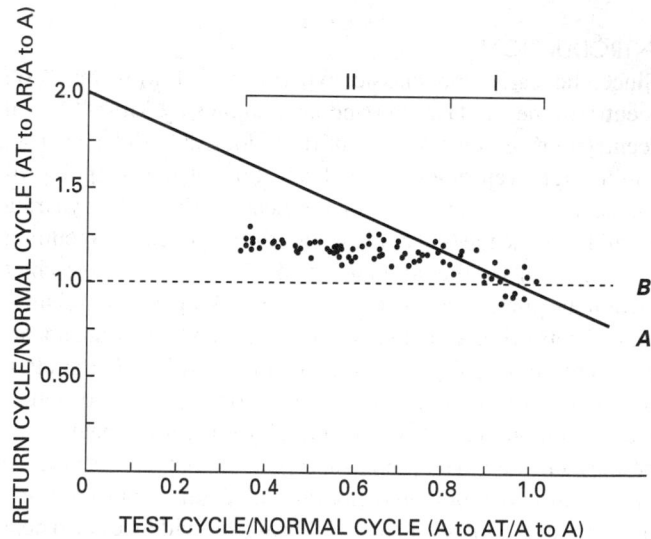

FIGURE 26-20
Return cycles as a function of premature stimulated cycles during premature atrial stimulation in a patient in sinus rhythm. The graph depicts the relationship of the normalized return cycle to the degree of prematurity of the test cycle, which is also normalized. Points falling on line A represent nonreset of the sinus pacemaker (fully compensatory pause) and are in zone I. Premature stimulated atrial beats introduced earlier in atrial diastole fall in zone II. Line B, projected from the y axis, is a reference line indicating the spontaneous sinus cycle length. The distance the zone II points (reset points) are above line B is interpreted to indicate conduction time into and out of the sinus node, assuming the sinus node pacemaker cycle length immediately following the stimulated premature atrial beat is identical to the preceding sinus node pacemaker cycle length. (From Strauss HC, et al. Premature atrial stimulation as a key to the understanding of sinoatrial conduction in man. A presentation of data and critical review of the literature. *Circulation* 1973; 47:86. Reproduced with permission from the publisher and author.)

(cycle following the premature impulse) on the y axis versus the normalized premature cycle (test cycle) on the x axis for a study in which premature stimuli were applied to the atria of the human heart during sinus rhythm. The solid line (A) represents the line of identity; points falling on this line are compensatory (the sum of the premature cycle and the return cycle is equal to the sum of two spontaneous cycles). Premature impulses delivered late in the cycle length are followed by a compensatory pause and fall on this line (as the test cycle shortens, the return cycle lengthens in a reciprocal manner) because the premature impulses collide with the impulse emanating from the sinus node pacemaker without reaching and resetting the pacemaker. Therefore, the pacemaker discharge following the premature impulse occurs exactly on time. As the premature coupling interval is decreased, a point is reached in the basic cycle where the premature impulse reaches the pacemaker before it has spontaneously depolarized to threshold and depolarizes it early. The pacemaker is reset. When this occurs, the postextrasystolic cycle (which is a result of the stimulated or reset pacemaker cells spontaneously depolarizing to threshold) is less than compensatory and the points fall below the line of identity. For the most part, the postextrasystolic cycle length is expected to be equal to the unperturbed spontaneous cycle length. The dashed line (B) on the graph in Fig. 26-20 indicates the cycle length of the basic rhythm, so that the return cycle length relative to the basic cycle length can be seen to be somewhat longer in this study. The prolonged return cycle has been proposed to result from slowed conduction of both the premature impulse into the pacemaker site and the pacemaker impulse out of this site.[294] It might also result, at least partly, from depression of the rate of spontaneous diastolic depolarization. Further shortening of the premature coupling interval to midcycle results in points parallel to the dashed line and possibly slightly above it, which indicates no change in the postextrasystolic cycle length over a wide range of coupling intervals. Finally, conduction of very early premature impulses might block prior to reaching the pacemaker, and the next pacemaker discharge would again occur on time and be compensatory. Of course, this relationship might be upset by changes in conduction of impulses into and out of the pacemaker site. This same relationship between premature and return cycle length found in studies on sinus rhythm has also been shown in studies on some ectopic tachycardias and, when found, indicates that the tachycardias are likely to be caused by automaticity.[292,293,295]

Ectopic pacemakers might also exist in an extensive region of slow conduction, much as the pacemaker in the sinus node, and conduction delays into and out of the pacemaker site may influence to some extent the relationship between return cycle and premature cycle. Conduction delays might cause some prolongation of the return cycle. When the above relationship is seen, however, it is probably indicative of automaticity (either normal or abnormal), since triggered activity and reentry are expected to show a different behavior. In addition to the atrial arrhythmias discussed, some ventricular arrhythmias are likely to be caused by automaticity. Idioventricular rhythms in patients with complete heart block respond in the manner shown

in microelectrode studies on slowly beating Purkinje fibers; the postextrasystolic cycle following late premature impulses is longer than the cycle length of the basic rhythm but less than compensatory, while it is shorter than the basic cycle length following early premature impulses (and obviously less than compensatory).[296] Some exercise-provoked ventricular tachycardia might also be caused by normal automaticity.[297,298] On the other hand, there is some evidence that accelerated idioventricular rhythms in the clinical setting of myocardial infarction might be caused by abnormal automaticity.

EFFECTS OF ELECTRICAL STIMULATION OF REENTRANT EXCITATION

A hallmark feature of a reentrant rhythm is that it usually can be induced and terminated by electrical stimuli (either overdrive pacing, introduction of premature stimuli or both), unlike automaticity. Initially it was thought sufficient to show that an arrhythmia could be initiated or terminated by overdrive pacing or programmed stimulation to demonstrate a reentrant mechanism.[299] That is because until the 1970s, the only other mechanism that was widely considered a cause of arrhythmias was automaticity, and automatic rhythms can neither be initiated nor terminated by pacing. After the 1970s, when the concept of afterdepolarization-induced arrhythmias was revived and expanded, these criteria alone were no longer sufficient, because triggered activity caused by DADs can also be initiated and terminated by pacing.

The induction of arrhythmias by overdrive pacing or introduction of a premature beat or beats can be used as an indicator of a reentrant mechanism if other characteristics are also present that eliminate the probability of triggered activity dependent on DADs. The ability to demonstrate directly that induction of an arrhythmia is related to a critical amount of slow conduction in the region where the arrhythmia originates adds credence to the interpretation that the arrhythmia is caused by reentry. The sudden large increase in the A–H interval associated with pacing induction of AV nodal reentrant tachycardia is one such example. The induction of triggered activity caused by DADs is not dependent on slowed conduction and should not show this relationship. Also, when a tachycardia is initiated by introduction of a premature beat over a wide range of coupling intervals, there may be an inverse relationship between the coupling interval of the premature impulse and the interval from the premature impulse to the first impulse of tachycardia.[300–302] As the premature impulse occurs earlier in the cycle, its conduction through the reentrant pathway is slower, causing the return cycle to prolong. This, too, is not found with the induction of triggered activity due to DADs. Failure to initiate an arrhythmia by stimulated impulses does not, per se, eliminate reentry as a mechanism for the arrhythmia.

Another feature of reentrant arrhythmias is that they can be terminated by overdrive pacing or premature stimulation. This is not specific for reentry, since triggered activity caused by DADs can also be terminated. As with initiation, termination by overdrive pacing requires a critical rate and duration of the stimulation train, while termination with stimulated premature impulses requires a critical coupling interval between the premature impulse and the previous impulse of the tachyarrhythmia. Failure to terminate an arrhythmia by stimulated impulses does not, per se, eliminate reentry as a mechanism for the arrhythmia. Termination of reentry requires that the stimulated impulse enter the reentrant circuit to cause the block of the reentrant wavefront, and this usually requires that the circuit have a fairly large excitable gap. Some reentrant circuits, particularly if caused by the leading circle mechanism of reentry, may not have a gap of excitability large enough to allow a premature impulse to penetrate readily into the circuits. If a tachycardia is very rapid, the excitable gap also may be very small, again preventing ready entry into the circuit by stimulated impulses.

Entrainment

In this context, the demonstration of transient entrainment of a tachycardia with or without its subsequent interruption is a relatively easy and reliable way to identify reentry as the mechanism of a tachyarrhythmia. Transient entrainment of a tachycardia was first described in 1977 during rapid pacing to interrupt type I atrial flutter.[303] At that time, although transient entrainment was not well understood, it was recognized as representing an increase in the rate of the tachycardia to the faster pacing rate, with resumption of the intrinsic rate of the tachycardia upon either abrupt cessation of pacing or slowing of the pacing rate below the intrinsic rate of the tachycardia.[303] On the basis of a series of clinical studies during rapid pacing of atrial flutter,[303–306] ventricular tachycardia,[307–309] AV reentrant tachycardia involving an accessory AV connection,[310,311] AV nodal reentrant tachycardia,[299] and intraatrial reentrant tachycardia,[313] it was proposed that transient entrainment represents capture of a reentrant circuit by wavefronts generated by the pacing impulse without

causing interruption of the tachycardia. This was confirmed during studies of transient entrainment in animal models of ventricular tachycardia[314–316] and atrial flutter[317,318] that utilized multiplexing techniques to record simultaneously from large numbers of electrodes in direct contact with cardiac tissue. During transient entrainment of a reentrant tachycardia, the wavefront from each pacing impulse enters into the excitable gap of the reentrant circuit. Once there, it travels in two directions: (1) antidromically, i.e., in the opposite direction of the circulating reentrant wavefront of the spontaneous tachycardia, where it collides with the orthodromic wavefront of the preceding beat, and (2) orthodromically, i.e., in the same direction as the circulating reentrant wavefront of the spontaneous tachycardia, thereby both continuing the tachycardia and resetting it to the pacing rate. This explanation is universal for transient entrainment of any tachycardia due to reentry with an excitable gap and is diagrammatically illustrated in Fig. 26-21.

The left panel is a diagrammatic representation of the reentrant circuit during a ventricular tachycardia (VT) at an assumed rate of 145 beats per minute. The Xs represent the orthodromic wavefronts of the reentrant rhythm. The arrows indicate the direction of spread of the impulse, the box represents an area of slow conduction in the reentrant circuit, the serpentine line indicates slow conduction of the impulse in this latter area, and the dots represent recording sites along the course of the double arc of reentry from which ventricular electrograms (VEGs) are recorded.

The middle panel is a diagrammatic representation of the introduction of the first pacing impulse $(X + 1)$ during ventricular pacing at a rate of 150 beats per minute during the ventricular tachycardia. The antidromic (anti) wavefronts $(X + 1)$ collide with the orthodromic wavefronts from the previous reentrant beat (X), resulting in fusion of ventricular activation. The orthodromic wavefront (ortho) from the pacing impulse $(X + 1)$ continues the ventricular tachycardia, resetting it to the pacing rate.

The right panel shows a diagrammatic representation of the introduction of the second pacing impulse $(X + 2)$ during ventricular pacing at a rate of 150 beats per minute during the ventricular tachycardia. The antidromic wavefronts $(X + 2)$ collide with the orthodromic wavefronts from the previous paced beat $(X + 1)$, again resulting in ventricular fusion. Once again, the orthodromic wavefront $(X + 2)$ from the pacing impulse continues the ventricular tachycardia, resetting it to the pacing rate.

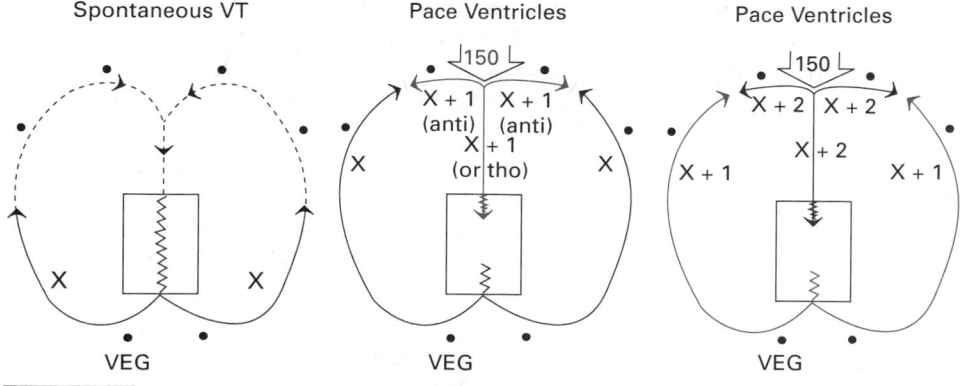

FIGURE 26-21

Diagrammatic representation of the reentrant circuit during spontaneous ventricular tachycardia (VT) and the first two beats of entrainment of the ventricular tachycardia at a rate of 150 beats per minute (*middle and right panels, respectively*). Each X represents the orthodromic wavefronts of the reentrant rhythm. In this and subsequent diagrams, the arrows indicate the direction of spread of the impulse, the box represents an area of slow conduction, the serpentine line indicates slow conduction of the impulse in the area of slow conduction, the dots represent recording sites along the course of the double arc of reentry from which ventricular electrograms (VEGs) are recorded, and the large arrow indicates the wavefront from the pacing impulse entering into the ventricular tachycardia reentry circuit, where it is conducted orthodromically (ortho) and antidromically (anti). (From Waldo AL, Henthorn RW. Use of transient entrainment during ventricular tachycardia to localize a critical area in the reentry circuit for ablation. *PACE* 1981; 12:231. Reproduced with permission from the publisher and authors.)

Criteria to Establish Transient Entrainment Four criteria are

TABLE 26-2

CRITERIA TO ESTABLISH THE PRESENCE OF TRANSIENT ENTRAINMENT

1. The demonstration of constant fusion beats in the ECG during the period of rapid pacing at a constant rate except for the last captured beat, which is entrained but not fused (i.e., the last entrained beat demonstrates the ECG morphology of the spontaneous tachycardia)
2. The demonstration of constant fusion beats in the ECG during rapid pacing at any constant rate but different degrees of constant fusion at different rapid rates, i.e., progressive fusion
3. Interruption of the tachycardia associated with localized conduction block to a site(s) for one beat, followed by subsequent activation of that site(s) from a different direction, manifest by a change in morphology of the electrogram at the blocked site(s) and with a shorter conduction time
4. A change in conduction time to and electrogram morphology at one recording site when pacing from another site at two different constant pacing rates, each of which is faster than the spontaneous rate of the tachycardia but fails to interrupt it

established (Table 26-2), any one of which, if demonstrated, establishes the presence of transient entrainment and thereby the presence of a reentrant rhythm with an excitable gap. Figures 26-22 to 26-24 demonstrate the four criteria in diagrammatic fashion for the same ventricular tachycardia illustrated in Fig. 26-21. In Fig. 26-22, which illustrates the first criterion (Table 26-2), the left panel is a diagrammatic representation of the termination of ventricular pacing illustrated in Fig. 26-21. In the left panel, the large arrow indicates the wavefront from the last pacing impulse delivered at a rate of 150 beats per minute entering into the reentrant circuit of the ventricular tachycardia, where it is conducted orthodromically

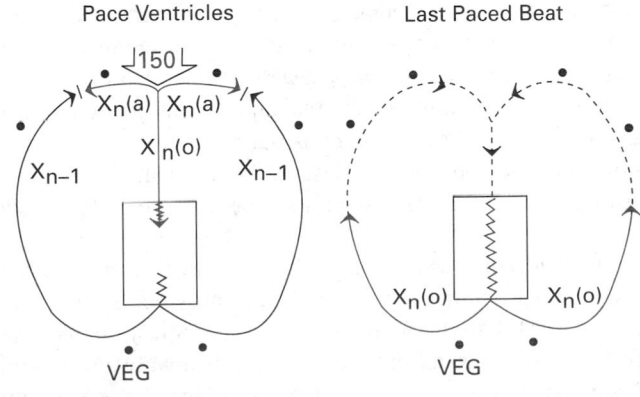

FIGURE 26-22
Diagrammatic representation of the first entrainment criterion during termination of ventricular pacing illustrated in Fig. 26-21. (From Waldo AL, Henthorn RW. Use of transient entrainment during ventricular tachycardia to localize a critical area in the reentry circuit for ablation. *PACE* 1989; 12:231. Reproduced with permission from the publisher and authors.)

and antidromically. The antidromic wavefronts ($X_n[a]$) collide with the orthodromic wavefronts ($X_n[o]$) of the previous beat (X_{n-1}), resulting in the fusion of ventricular activation, but the orthodromic wavefront from the last pacing impulse continues and resets the tachycardia. The right panel shows that the orthodromic wavefronts from the last pacing impulse are now unopposed by any antidromic wavefronts because there is no subsequent pacing impulse. Thus, no fusion of ventricular activation occurs despite the presence of transient entrainment. This last entrained beat travels around the reentrant circuit, continuing the tachycardia.

Figure 26-23 is a diagrammatic representation of entrainment in the same ventricular tachycardia during pacing from the same site proximal to the area of slow conduction of the reentrant circuit at a rate of 150 (left panel), 155 (middle panel), and 160 beats per minute (right panel), demonstrating both the second and fourth entrainment criteria. When pacing at a rate of 155 beats per minute, the pacing cycle length is shorter than at 150 beats per minute, so that the antidromic wavefront from each pacing impulse will penetrate the excitable gap of the reentrant circuit to a further degree in an antidromic direction compared to 150 beats per minute, resulting in a different degree of fusion of the QRS complex in the ECG than at a rate of 150 beats per minute. As a result, the QRS complex morphology in the ECG during pacing at 155 beats per minute will be different than at 150 beats per minute. This, then, is the demonstration of progressive fusion (Table 26-2). When pacing at 160 beats per minute, once again the antidromic wavefront from each pacing impulse will collide with the orthodromic wavefront, but at yet a different site. This occurs because the pacing cycle length is shorter than pacing at the previous rates, permitting greater penetration of the excitable gap by the antidromic wavefront of the pacing impulse, illustrating yet more progressive fusion.

These diagrams also illustrate the fourth criterion (Table 26-2): a site or sites activated by the orthodromic wavefront of each pacing impulse during entrainment at one pacing rate will be activated by the antidromic wavefront of each pacing impulse during entrainment at a faster pacing rate. This will be manifest both by a change in the morphology of the electrogram recorded at the site in question (it will have the same morphology during the tachycardia as during pacing at the rate that results in activation of the site by the orthodromic wavefront but a different morphology when activated by the antidromic wavefront of the pacing impulse at a faster pacing rate) and a change in conduction time to the recording site from the pacing site (the stimulus-to-recording site interval will be longer when activated by the orthodromic wavefront of each pacing impulse than when activated by the antidromic wavefront of each pacing impulse). Thus, note that the two middle recording sites denoted by black dots on each side of the reentrant circuit become activated in turn from a different direction and with a shorter conduction time when the pacing rate is increased from 150 to 155 beats per minute and then to 160 beats per minute.

Figure 26-24 is a diagrammatic representation of the third criterion and shows the events during interruption of the ven-

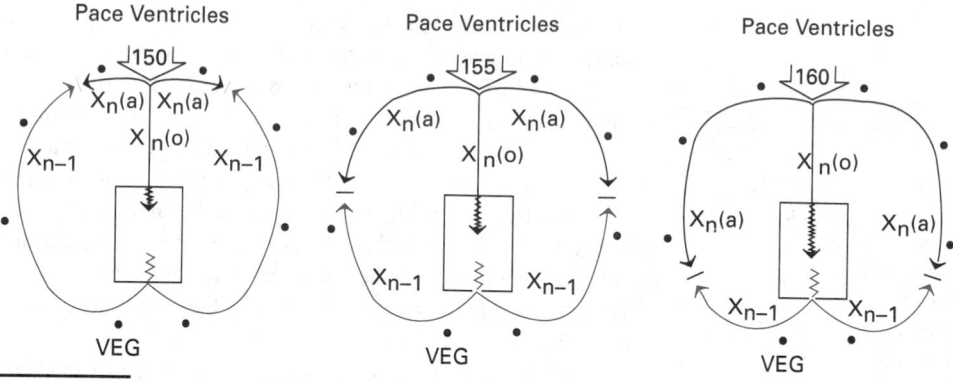

FIGURE 26-23

Diagrammatic representation of the second and fourth entrainment criteria during entrainment of the same spontaneous ventricular tachycardia shown in Fig. 26-21 by ventricular pacing at a rate of 150 (*left panel*), 155 (*middle panel*), and 160 (*right panel*) beats per minute. (From Waldo AL, Henthorn RW. Use of transient entrainment during ventricular tachycardia to localize a critical area in the reentry circuit for ablation. *PACE* 1989; 12:231. Reproduced with permission from the publisher and authors.)

tricular tachycardia by ventricular pacing at a rate of 165 beats per minute. In the left panel, the large arrow indicates the wavefront from the pacing impulse delivered at a rate of 165 beats per minute entering into the reentrant circuit of the ventricular tachycardia, where it is conducted orthodromically ($X + 1[o]$) and antidromically ($X + 1[a]$). The antidromic wavefronts collide with the orthodromic wavefronts from the previous beats (X_n), resulting in fusion of ventricular activation. Note that this fusion of ventricular activation is at still a different site than during pacing at the previous pacing rates (Fig. 26-23). Thus, initially there is still more progressive fusion of the QRS complex morphology in the ECG. This time, however, the orthodromic wavefront does not reset the tachycardia to the pacing rate. Rather, it too is blocked, presumably in the area of slow conduction, during the same beat. Note that each recording site on each of the two arcs of reentry immediately distal to the area of slow conduction is activated by the orthodromic wave front of the previous beat (X) but is not activated by $X + 1$ because the orthodromic wavefront

$(X + 1[o])$ never reaches either site (there is localized conduction block for one beat). In the right panel, the large arrows indicate the next pacing impulse ($X + 2$) delivered at the same pacing rate (165 beats per minute) from the same pacing site as in the left diagram. The dashed lines indicate the reentrant circuit present during the previous periods of ventricular tachycardia and transient entrainment of the ventricular tachycardia. Because the ventricular tachycardia has been interrupted by the previous pacing impulse ($X + 1$), the sequence of ventricular activation of the next pacing impulse ($X + 2$) is as one would expect during overdrive pacing of sinus rhythm from that same ventricular pacing site. Therefore, the two electrogram recording sites immediately distal to the previous (but no longer present) area of slow conduction are now activated from a different direction than during transient entrainment. In addition, because the presumed area of slow conduction is no longer functionally present, the stimulus-to-right-ventricular conduction time is shorter. Thus, the requirements for the third criterion of entrainment are fulfilled (Table 26-2).

Although these illustrative diagrams show the example of transient entrainment and interruption of ventricular tachycardia, the principles are the same for all the putative reentrant rhythms. For AV nodal reentrant tachycardia, however, only the third criterion has been demonstrated,[312] presumably because there is no electrocardiographic manifestation of AV nodal activation, and recording directly from the AV node using surface electrograms has not been reliably demonstrated. Although the phenomena associated with transient entrainment of a tachycardia with or without its subsequent interruption are best explained by reentry, it still must be asked whether or not any or all of the criteria for the demonstration of transient entrainment can be explained by another mechanism. Present understanding of the response of automatic and triggered rhythms to rapid pacing is not consistent with the phenomena observed during transient entrainment (Table 26-2). Automatic rhythms also should not be interrupted by pacing.

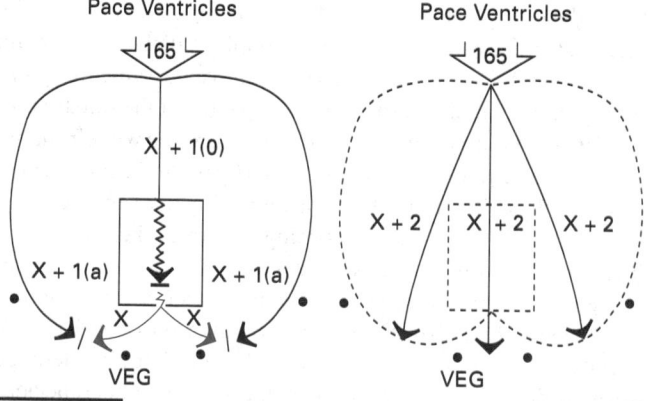

FIGURE 26-24

Diagrammatic representation of the third entrainment criterion durng interruption of the ventricular tachycardia by ventricular pacing at a rate of 165 beats per minute. (From Waldo AL, Henthorn RW. Use of transient entrainment during ventricular tachycardia to localize a critical area in the reentry circuit for ablation. *PACE* 1989; 12:231. Reproduced with permission from the publisher and authors.)

Concealed Entrainment While the ability to demonstrate transient entrainment of a tachycardia provides an important and powerful tool for identification and study of reentrant tachyarrhythmias, a limitation is that it is not always possible to demonstrate any of the transient entrainment criteria despite the fact that rapid pacing may indeed have entrained and even interrupted the tachycardia. This phenomenon, called *concealed entrainment*,[309,311] can result when pacing is performed from a site that is orthodromically distal to the area of slow conduction in the reentry circuit, when pacing from a site that is rather distant from the reentrant circuit, or when pacing from an area of slow conduction in the reentrant circuit.[309,311,319–321]

In order to label a response of a tachycardia to rapid pacing as concealed entrainment, except in the example of pacing from an area of slow conduction in the reentry circuit, one must also show that transient entrainment can be demonstrated when pacing from another site. Thus, it is clear that unless one is able to pace from an appropriate site, a reentrant circuit with an excitable gap may be present, but entrainment, though present, will not be demonstrable.

Resetting

The response of an arrhythmia to a prematurely stimulated impulse that does not terminate the arrhythmia may still provide information useful for determining the mechanism of the arrhythmia. Information on the effects of stimulated premature impulses on reentry comes from studies on experimental preparations of isolated tissues or hearts in which reentrant excitation has been mapped. Other predictions concerning the effects of premature impulses on reentry are based mainly on theoretical considerations using a model of a reentrant circuit with a fixed pathway in which the circuit cannot change its dimensions and in which there is an excitable gap. Such circuits may have a single entrance and exit pathway leading into and out of the circuit, as illustrated in Fig. 26-25, or the entrance and exit pathways may be separate. These characteristics will influence the characteristics of the resetting response as seen on the ECG.

The theoretically possible responses of a tachycardia caused by reentrant excitation to premature stimulation are explained in the diagram in Fig. 26-25. An anatomic circuit with fixed dimensions and a single entrance pathway is diagrammed. In this diagram, the entrance pathway also serves as an exit pathway for the reentrant wavefront to enter surrounding myocardium, but other models may have separate entrance and exit pathways. The black arrow in the reentrant circuit represents the reentrant impulse, with the arrow point being the crest of the depolarizing wave and the end of the arrow being the tail. The length of the arrow is the absolutely refractory part of the circuit, the dotted area that trails it is the relatively refractory part, and the clear region is the fully excitable gap (in some instances there may be no fully excitable gap in the reentrant circuit). The transit time of the reentrant impulse around the circuit determines one cycle length of the tachycardia (the R_1–R_1 interval).

In panel $A(1)$ a stimulated premature impulse (R_2) (black arrow from above) is shown to reach the circuit and enter it in the region of the fully excitable gap. The stimulated premature wavefront may then propagate both in the orthodromic (to the right) and antidromic (to the left) direction in the reentrant pathway. In the antidromic direction, it collides with the oncoming reentrant wavefront, extinguishing both stimulated and reentrant impulses at the point of collision. In the orthodromic direction, the stimulated impulse becomes the reentrant impulse and propagates through the circuit in completely excitable tissue of the gap (which also moves around the circuit), shown in panel $A(2)$. This stimulated reentrant wave-

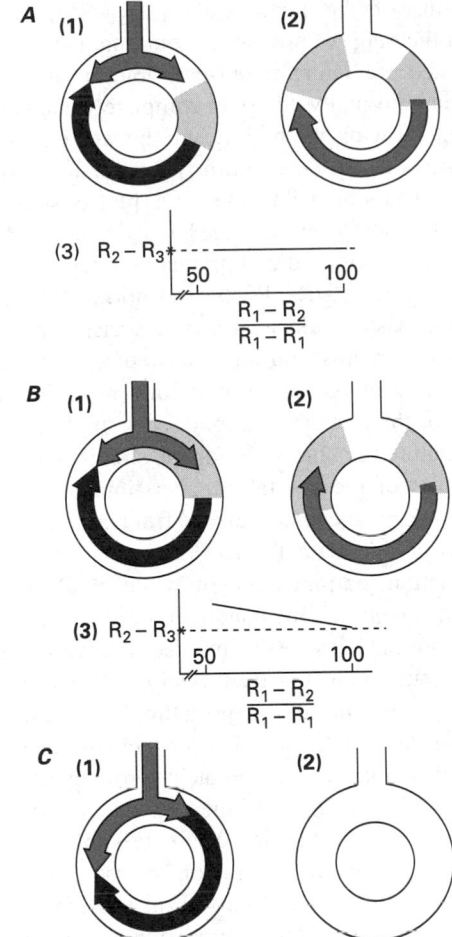

FIGURE 26-25

Effects of premature impulses on reentrant circuit with an excitable gap. In each panel, diagrams are shown of an anatomic circuit with a single entrance route from above. In $A(1)$, $B(1)$, and $C(1)$ black arrows in the circuit represent the reentrant impulse causing tachycardia. The length of the arrow is the wavelength of the impulse and shows the part of the circuit that is completely refractory. The part of the circuit that is stippled is relatively refractory and the part of the circuit that is clear is completely excitable (the fully excitable gap). Black arrows entering the circuit from above represent a prematurely stimulated impulse initiated outside the circuit. $A(2)$ and $B(2)$ show conduction of the premature impulse in the circuit. Graphs show the expected relationship between the return (premature impulse) cycle length (R_2–R_3) and premature coupling interval (R_1–R_2/R_1–R_1) for premature impulses conducting in the fully excitable gap $A(3)$ and in the relatively refractory tissue of a partially excitable gap $B(3)$. (Modified after Wit AL, Janse MJ. *The Ventricular Arrhythmias of Ischemia and Infarction: The Electrophysiological Mechanisms*. Mt. Kisco, NY: Futura; 1992. Reproduced with permission from the publisher and authors.)

front would leave the circuit through the normal exit route and become the next tachycardia impulse.

Since the stimulated impulse traveled through the circuit in completely excitable tissue at normal conduction velocity, the interval between the stimulated impulse (R_2) and the next impulse of tachycardia (R_3) is equal to the normal transit time around the circuit or the normal tachycardia cycle length (R_1–R_1). The rhythm, however, is reset, i.e., the sum of the curtailed (premature) cycle length and the return cycle length (R_1–R_2 + R_2–R_3) (first poststimulus cycle) is less than two cycle lengths of the tachycardia $[2(R_1-R_1)]$. This holds throughout the range of premature coupling intervals at which the stimulated premature impulse is able to conduct around the circuit at a normal velocity in completely excitable tissue. Thus, a plot showing the relationship between the premature coupling intervals and the return (poststimulus) cycles over this range appears as a flat line. This plot is shown in Fig. 26-25A(3). The poststimulus cycle length is the R_2–R_3 interval on the y axis. The normalized premature coupling interval is represented by R_1–R_2/R_1–R_1 on the horizontal axis where R_1–R_1 is the basic cycle length of the tachycardia. In this graph, R_2–R_3 remains constant (and equal to R_1–R_1) over the entire range of premature coupling intervals, indicating conduction of the premature impulse in completely excitable tissue. Premature impulses entering the circuit in the relatively refractory part of the excitable gap (stippled region in the circuit) shown by the black arrow from above in Fig. 26-25B(1) also collide with the reentrant impulse in the antidromic direction, extinguishing it while conducting in the orthodromic direction. But conduction around the circuit is slower than normal because the impulse is activating relatively refractory tissue, indicated by the stippled area in Fig. 26-25B(2). Therefore, the return (poststimulus) cycle, which is dependent on the conduction time of the stimulated impulse in the circuit, is longer than the tachycardia cycle.

As the coupling interval of the stimulated premature impulse is decreased and this impulse enters the circuit earlier and earlier in the relatively refractory period of the excitable gap, conduction time around the circuit and the return cycle progressively increase. Thus, a plot showing the relationship between the premature coupling interval and the return cycle length appears as shown in Fig. 26-25B(3). The line representing the R_2–R_3 interval increases as the normalized premature coupling interval (R_1–R_2/R_1–R_1) decreases. It is also apparent on the graph that conduction time of the premature impulse around the circuit as measured by the R_2–R_3 interval is greater than conduction time of the normal tachycardia impulse around the circuit, which is indicated by the dashed line. The sum of the premature and return cycle may either be less than compensatory or greater than compensatory depending on how slow conduction of the premature impulse is around the circuit. More often, despite slowing of conduction of the premature impulse in the circuit, the prolonged return cycle does not compensate for the shortened premature cycle.[322–325]

Panel C shows what happens when an earlier premature impulse, indicated by the black arrow from above, reaches the circuit when it is even less excitable. It conducts antidromically into the circuit and collides with the wavefront of the reentrant impulse but cannot excite the orthodromic path because it blocks in refractor tissue (black tail of the reentrant impulse). Thus, reentry is terminated, C(2). The range of coupling intervals over which there is evidence that the premature impulse entered the reentrant circuit to reset the tachycardia prior to termination of reentry is a rough measurement of the duration of the excitable gap at the entrance route into the circuit if the premature stimuli are applied close to the circuit.[325] Therefore, fixed reentrant circuits with excitable

gaps have patterns of responses to premature stimulation that are characteristic for this mechanism.

In sum, the stable tachycardia cycle length (R_1–R_1) is determined by the time it takes the reentrant wavefront to travel one complete revolution around the circuit and reach an exit pathway to the ventricles. When such a circuit is the cause of a tachycardia, premature depolarizations delivered late in the cycle length are often followed by a postextrasystolic pause that is compensatory for the same reason as described for automatic tachycardias, i.e., the stimulated impulse may not be able to reach the reentrant circuit, possibly due to collision between the stimulated impulse and the impulse coming from the circuit. The next tachycardia impulse then comes precisely on time. In this case, the tachycardia is not reset since the sum of the premature cycle length and the return cycle length is equal to two successive premature cycle lengths. Over the range of premature coupling intervals that do not reset the tachycardia, the relationship between the premature coupling interval and the following (return) cycle falls along the line of identity (see Fig. 26-20).

Premature impulses delivered earlier in the tachycardia cycle might have several different effects that are dependent on some of the characteristics of the reentrant circuit. If there is virtually no excitable gap, as might be expected of some functional circuits, no resetting of the tachycardia will occur, since the stimulated impulse cannot enter the circuit and the return cycle will remain compensatory. If the excitable gap is partially excitable, e.g., composed of relatively refractory tissue, premature impulses that succeed in entering the circuit and traveling around it will do so at reduced conduction velocities, as diagrammed in Fig. 26-25B.[326] When they emerge from the circuit, they cause the first postextrasystolic (tachycardia) impulse. As a result of the slowing of conduction of the premature impulse around the circuit, the postextrasystolic cycle is longer than the basic cycle [represented by the dashed line in Fig. 26-25B(3)].

Conduction time of the premature impulse around the circuit should continue to increase as the premature impulse is delivered earlier and earlier in the cycle, since the premature impulse conducts in more refractory tissue, causing an inverse relationship between the premature coupling interval and the postextrasystolic cycle [Fig. 26-25B(3)]. In the study of Bigger and Goldreyer[301] on AV nodal reentrant tachycardia, the prolongation of the postextrasystolic cycle over the entire range of premature coupling intervals was sufficient to result in a greater than compensatory pause following the premature impulse. On the other hand, the postextrasystolic cycle length can be less than compensatory. An inverse relationship between the premature interval and the return cycle interval caused by slowing of conduction of the premature impulse in the reentrant circuit, as shown in Fig. 26-25B(3), is indicative of reentry since this type of response does not occur with automaticity or triggered activity. Recall that for automatic impulse initiation, the return cycle length is fairly constant over a wide range of premature coupling intervals. If there is a large fully excitable gap, premature impulses reaching the circuit are expected to conduct around the circuit with the same velocity as the reentrant wavefront that is causing the tachycardia, and the postextrasystolic cycle would be equal to the tachycardia cycle and less than compensatory [Fig. 26-25A(1) and A(2)]. This could occur over a relatively wide range of coupling intervals, resulting in a relationship similar to that expected from a pacemaker over the intermediate range of coupling intervals; the line describing the relationship of the return cycle to the premature cycle would be flat [Fig. 26-25A(3)]. Eventually, it is expected that stimulated extrasystoles that are sufficiently premature would invade the circuit when it is relatively refractory, resulting in prolonged return cycles, inversely related to the premature coupling intervals.

The prolongation of the postextrasystolic cycle after early premature impulses is opposite to that which occurs during automaticity. Thus a curve might be plotted that consists of a segment that is compensatory at long premature coupling intervals (because the stimulated impulse does not reach the circuit), a segment that is less than compensatory and flat at intermediate premature coupling intervals (when the stimulated impulse is conducting in completely excitable tissue in the circuit), and a segment that is ascending at short premature coupling intervals (when the stimulated impulse is conducting in relatively refractory tissue in the circuit). Still earlier premature impulses might block prior to reaching a circuit, resulting in interpolation, as described for an automatic focus. A sufficiently early premature impulse could also terminate the tachycardia by blocking in the circuit and causing block of the reentrant wavefront. This is not expected of automatic impulse initiation.

As mentioned above, the entrance route that a stimulated impulse takes into a reentrant circuit and the exit route from the circuit may be separate. When this occurs, the return cycle following a premature impulse may be less than the tachycardia cycle because the premature impulse, after entering the circuit, need not conduct around the entire circuit before exiting. The return cycle may still show any of the relationships to the premature cycle that is described in Fig. 26-25; i.e., it may be flat or show an inverse relationship to the premature coupling interval depending on whether it is conducting in partially or fully excitable tissue. This expected effect of premature impulses on the cycle length of reentry might also be altered in a functional circuit if the premature impulse can somehow cause a change in the size or shape of the circuit. It is not possible to predict easily what the effects would be.

In summary, the relationship between the postextrasystolic cycle and the curtailed cycle when premature impulses are introduced during a tachycardia caused by reentry may be different than during automaticity. Therefore, premature stimulation during the study of a tachycardia may provide useful information that helps to determine whether or not reentry is the mechanism. There are, however, a number of confounding influences that, if present, can upset the theoretically predicted relationships. They include the absence of a fully excitable gap and properties of intervening tissue between the stimulus site and the site of the circuit that can slow or block conduction of premature impulses into and out of the circuit. Therefore, failure to find the relationships expected for a reentrant mechanism does not necessarily mean that the arrhythmia is caused by a mechanism other than reentry.

EFFECTS OF ELECTRICAL STIMULATION ON ARRHYTHMIAS CAUSED BY TRIGGERED ACTIVITY

Arrhythmias Caused by Delayed Afterdepolarizations

The amplitude of DADs increases with a decrease in the cycle length at which the action potentials occur until the afterdepolarizations reach threshold to cause triggered activity. Therefore, triggered arrhythmias caused by DADs in the in situ heart should be initiated by either overdrive pacing or programmed premature stimulation. Since automatic arrhythmias are not initiated by pacing, they should be readily distinguished from triggered arrhythmias caused by DADs. Reentrant arrhythmias can also be induced by the same stimulation protocols, however, so whether or not there are any other characteristics during arrhythmia induction by pacing that might distinguish between triggered activity and reentry is important. An attempt to distinguish between the two mechanisms is further complicated by the fact that triggered activity caused by DADs may be due to different causes, e.g., digitalis and catecholamines, each with somewhat different characteristics.

The following guidelines have been proposed to assist in distinguishing DAD-induced triggered activity from other causes of arrhythmias.[327,328] The guidelines are based on the characteristics of triggered activity determined from in vitro studies with microelectrodes. Triggered activity caused by DADs has been more easily induced by rapid pacing or by several successive premature stimuli than by a single premature stimulus in studies on isolated tissue preparations. This characteristic, which should be expected to occur in the in situ human heart, is probably explained by the fact that rapid pacing or introduction of a number of premature stimuli are more effective than a single premature stimulus in increasing intracellular Ca^+ levels. The Ca^+ levels control the afterdepolarization amplitude. Also, arrhythmias caused by triggered activity should be more easily induced by premature stimuli superimposed on a rapid drive rate than on a slow one because during rapid pacing, the afterdepolarization amplitude is larger and membrane potential at the peak of the afterpolarization is closer to threshold. In contrast, ordered reentrant rhythms in humans (with the exception of atrial flutter) seem more easily and reproducibly induced by premature impulses than by rapid pacing, although several premature impulses in succession are sometimes necessary. One reason may be that premature impulses block more effectively in areas with long refractory periods than do impulses during rapid pacing because rapid pacing can shorten refractory period duration. This, of course, is important because block is a prerequisite for initiation of reentry.

Both extrasystoles and the first beat of a tachycardia, when caused by DAD-dependent triggered activity initiated by pacing, are predicted to occur late in the cardiac cycle.[327] This proposal is based on experimental data from studies on isolated tissue that show that DADs rarely reach their peak amplitude at less than 50 percent of the cardiac cycle when the drive cycle length is shorter than 1000 ms. In contrast, reentrant beats often occur early in the cycle. One would expect a direct relationship between the pacing cycle length that induces triggered activity due to DADs and the coupling interval from the last stimulated impulse to the first beat of the induced tachycardia. As the pacing cycle length decreases, the coupling interval from the last stimulated impulse to the first impulse of tachycardia should decrease because at short cycle lengths, the coupling interval of the afterdepolarizations to the proceeding action potential decreases.

A direct relationship between pacing cycle length and coupling interval of the first impulse of the tachycardia has been shown to occur in arrhythmias caused by digitalis toxicity.[329] This relationship might sometimes be complicated by the presence of two afterdepolarizations and the possibility of a triggered impulse arising from either one.[330] No comparable data are available from pacing studies on digitalis-toxic human hearts. The direct relationship has also been shown in some cases of idiopathic ventricular tachycardia believed to be caused by triggered activity.[166] Such a direct relationship is not expected during initiation of reentrant arrhythmias. Failure to show the direct relationship, however, cannot be taken as proof that the arrhythmia is not caused by triggered activity, since slow conduction into or out of the triggerable focus can distort it. In microelectrode studies, during initiation of triggered activity with premature stimuli, no significant effects of the premature stimulus coupling interval were observed on the relationship (coupling interval) of the first triggered impulse to the premature stimulus.[188] On the basis of these data, it is expected that during initiation of arrhythmias caused by triggered activity in situ with programmed premature stimulation, the coupling interval of the first beat of tachycardia should remain relatively constant over a range of coupling intervals of introduced premature impulses. The response to premature stimulation is also contrary to that expected during initiation of reentrant arrhythmias, where an inverse relationship is expected between the premature stimulus coupling interval and the coupling interval between the premature impulse and the first impulse of tachycardia.

Triggered arrhythmias, unlike automatic arrhythmias but like reentrant arrhythmias, are predicted to be terminated by cardiac pacing. Single premature impulses may terminate triggered arrhythmias, but based on the results of microelectrode studies, termination should be infrequent and not usually reproducible at the same critical premature cycle length. In contrast, single premature impulses often terminate reentrant arrhythmias in a reproducible manner and over a consistent range of premature cycle length in any one individual as long as the reentrant circuit has an excitable gap.[331,332] Therefore, an arrhythmia that is readily terminated by a single prematurely stimulated impulse is more likely to be caused by reentry than by triggered activity.

The effects of premature impulses that do not terminate sustained triggered activity have also been determined.[191] The response is almost identical to that of automaticity. The return cycle length remains fairly constant over a wide range of premature coupling intervals and nearly the same as the cycle length of the basic triggered rhythm (less than compensatory). On the other hand, overdrive pacing should terminate triggered arrhythmias due to afterdepolarizations. Such termination requires a critical rate and duration of overdrive,[186–188] just as it does with reentry.[302,303,307] Overdrive stimulation may cause acceleration of triggered arrhythmias followed by gradual slowing and termination or rapid overdrive may cause abrupt termination. Although reentrant rhythms might be accelerated by overdrive pacing, a gradual slowing of the rate prior to termination is not expected. Overdrive pacing that does not terminate triggered activity, such as when the cycle length of the overdrive is too long or when the trains of stimuli are too short, does not entrain the arrhythmia either.[333] In fact, none of the characteristics of entrainment are expected during overdrive pacing of triggered activity caused by DADs.

It is therefore apparent that although the response of triggered arrhythmias caused by DADs to stimulation can be predicted from the experimental studies, there is no single feature that would positively enable a triggered rhythm to be distinguished from reentry except entrainment. Since the characteristics of initiation and termination of triggered rhythms by stimulation are very different from the characteristics of automatic rhythms, it should be easier to distinguish between these mechanisms by pacing techniques. This differentiation may be made more difficult when an arrhythmia is persistent and the initiation cannot be studied. Also, entrance block of stimulated impulses into arrhythmogenic foci, whether automatic, triggered, or reentrant, may negate the use of pacing techniques to distinguish between these mechanisms.

The characteristics of some clinical arrhythmias occasionally conform to those expected of DAD-dependent triggered activity.[128,334] In addition to digitalis toxicity, an example is some cases of exercise-induced ventricular tachycardia in patients with no structural heart disease.[166,298] This tachycardia, which occurs spontaneously during exertion, can sometimes be initiated by overdrive pacing or programmed premature stimulation. An isoproterenol infusion during stimulation may be required for successful initiation. Lerman et al.[160] have proposed that the tachycardias are caused by a catecholamine-induced increase in cyclic AMP, which is known to cause DADs. Evidence supporting this hypothesis is the termination of tachycardias by intravenous injection of adenosine, which antagonizes the electrophysiological effects of catecholamines mediated through the adenylate cyclase-cyclic AMP system. Jackman et al.[335] have proposed that some forms of ventricular tachycardia associated with the congenital long QT syndrome and dependent on adrenergic stimulation are a result of triggered activity caused by DADs. Cranefield and Aronson[128] have provided a detailed review of the clinical arrhythmias that may be caused by triggered activity (see also Chap. 27).

Arrhythmias Caused by Early Afterdepolarizations

Arrhythmias caused by EADs should not be inducible by overdrive pacing, similar to automatic arrhythmias and unlike arrhythmias caused by DADs or reentry. Likewise, triggered activity dependent on EADs is not expected immediately to follow the short cycle length of one or several prematurely stimulated impulses. As shown in the experimental studies, the appearance of EAD-induced triggered activity is facilitated by long cycle lengths. Therefore, this kind of triggered activity should be initiated by slowing the basic heart rate. Of course, if an increase in heart rate caused by pacing resulted in entrance block into a focus where EADs occur, the block could cause a prolongation of the cycle length in that focus that might result in triggered activity.[128] Prematurely stimulated impulses might also initiate triggered activity if there is a long compensatory pause following the stimulated impulse. The long cycle might trigger an arrhythmia that would follow it.[128] In the absence of such entrance block, bursts of tachycardia caused by EADs should occur more frequently when the heart rate is slowed, and pacing the heart at rates faster than the basic underlying rhythm is predicted to cause disappearance of the period of tachycardia. Increasing the basic heart rate shortens action potential duration and thereby suppresses EADs. When the pacing is stopped, arrhythmias should reappear, as the action potential returns to its original duration. The reappearance of the arrhythmias may not be immediate, however, since it requires some time for the action potential duration to lengthen owing to the enhanced pump current that follows a period of rapid stimulation.

Many of these characteristics have been shown to apply to the experimental triggered arrhythmias caused by cesium in the in situ canine heart[199] and have been demonstrated in some cases of torsades de pointes in patients. Acquired forms of the syndrome (e.g., prolonged QT and torsades de pointes by quinidine) exhibit all the features expected of triggered activity caused by EADs, whereas other forms (e.g., congenital) may not be due to this mechanism.[336] Torsades de pointes invariably occurs after a preceding long R-R interval,[200] is unlikely to be initiated by programmed stimulation,[337] and can be prevented from occurring by pacing the heart at a rapid rate.[200,337] Parenthetically, it has recently been suggested that such rhythms are initiated by EADs but maintained by reentrant excitation.[219] In contrast, triggered arrhythmias caused by DADs may become more frequent at heart rate increases,[327] and the effect of increasing the heart rate on extrasystoles caused by reentry is variable; i.e., reentry might be exacerbated or it might stop.[222]

There may be some difficulty in distinguishing EAD-dependent triggered arrhythmias from automatic arrhythmias only on the basis of their response to electrical stimulation, however, since the occurrence of automatic arrhythmias is facilitated by slow heart rates and increasing the basic heart rate by overdrive pacing may cause disappearance of automatic arrhythmias during the periods of pacing. The electrocardiographic characteristics of arrhythmias caused by triggered activity due to EADs and by automaticity might be of additional help. The triggered rhythms are more likely to occur in bursts or salvos of different lengths with the first few cycle lengths of a burst decreasing progressively and the last few cycle lengths increasing progressively.

Triggered arrhythmias caused by EADs might not only occur in bursts but might also be sustained. When sustained, their response to single premature stimuli or overdrive pacing can be predicted on the basis of the results of in vitro studies. Some arrhythmias might be terminated by premature stimuli, but this should be a relatively rare occurrence. The effects of premature stimulated impulses that do not terminate the arrhythmia are expected to be the same as their effects on automatic impulse initiation. Some arrhythmias also might be terminated by overdrive pacing, but termination should not be the usual effect. When termination occurs, it is expected to follow the overdrive immediately, whereas termination of triggered activity caused by DADs may sometimes be preceded by up to 10 triggered "afterbeats."[186,187] When termination does not occur, overdrive is not expected to cause any significant effect on the rhythm; the response should be more like that of an arrhythmia caused by abnormal automaticity[191] than normal automaticity, which is readily overdrive-suppressed.[73] Because of this variability of response, stimulation during a sustained tachycardia caused by EADs is not much help in determining the mechanism.

Therefore, like the triggered arrhythmias caused by DADs, there is no single feature in the response to cardiac pacing that would positively enable EAD-induced triggered rhythms to be distinguished from other arrhythmogenic mechanisms. Early afterdepolarization-induced nonsustained arrhythmias can usually be differentiated from rhythms induced by DADs or automaticity at high membrane potentials and sometimes from reentry by pacing, but the response of sustained triggered activity to pacing is often indistinguishable from abnormal automaticity at low membrane potentials.

SUMMARY OF EFFECTS OF ELECTRICAL STIMULATION

Despite the fact that there are exceptions and inconsistencies to virtually all the rules that can be proposed to distinguish among the different arrhythmogenic mechanisms using pacing techniques, determining the effects of electrical stimulation is really quite useful. The following is a summary of the most important points: (1) Initiation of a tachycardia by stimulation indicates that the arrhythmia is caused either by reentry or delayed afterdepolarization-induced triggered activity. Other characteristics of initiation are then useful in distinguishing between the two. Other mechanisms of arrhythmias—such as automaticity and triggered activity caused by early afterdepolarizations—are eliminated when a tachycardia is induced by cardiac pacing. (2) Termination of a tachycardia by overdrive pacing or premature stimulation is expected of reentry or triggered activity caused by delayed afterdepolarizations but not of automaticity and early afterdepolarization-dependent triggered activity. Overdrive suppression is expected of arrhythmias caused by normal automaticity, and overdrive acceleration may occur with arrhythmias caused by abnormal automaticity. (3) Demonstration of entrainment of a tachycardia during overdrive pacing is indicative of a reentrant mechanism and is not expected of other mechanisms. (4) The response to premature stimulation is different during arrhythmias caused by automaticity and those caused by reentry. During automatic arrhythmias, the return cycle length should not increase as the premature coupling interval decreases. The return cycle should be less than compensatory. During reentrant arrhythmias, the return cycle length should increase as the premature impulse occurs earlier in the dominant cycle. The increase may sometimes begin to occur with late coupled premature impulses or it may not occur until premature impulses are early coupled. The return cycle length is often less than compensatory.

REFERENCES

1. Hoffman BF, Rosen MR. Cellular mechanisms for cardiac arrhythmias. *Circ Res* 1981; 49;1–15.
2. Waldo AL, Kaiser GA, Bowman OF Jr, Malm JR. Etiology of prolongation of the P-R interval in patients with an endocardial cushion defect: Further observations on internodal conduction and the polarity of the retrograde P wave. *Circulation* 1973; 48:19–27.
3. Mayer AG. Rhythmical pulsation in Scyphomedusae. Publication no. 47. Washington, DC: Carnegie Institution of Washington; 1906:1–62.
4. Mines GR. On dynamic equilibrium in the heart. *J Physiol* (Lond) 1913; 46:349–383.
5. Cranefield PF. *The Conduction of the Cardiac Impulse: The Slow Response and Cardiac Arrhythmia.* Mount Kisco, NY: Futura Publishing; 1975.
6. Schmitt OF, Erlanger J. Directional differences in the conduction of the impulse through the heart muscle and their possible relation to extrasystolic and fibrillary contractions. *Am J Physiol* 1928–1929; 87:326–347.
7. Wit AL, Hoffman BF, Cranefield PF. Slow conduction and reentry in the ventricular conduction system: I. Return extrasystole in canine Purkinje fibers. *Circ Res* 1972; 30:1–10.
8. Cranefield PF, Wit AL, Hoffman BF. Genesis of cardiac arrhythmias. *Circulation* 1973; 47;190–204.
9. Singer DH, Lazzara R, Hoffman BF. Interrelationships between automaticity and conduction in Purkinje fibers. *Circ Res* 1967; 21:537–558.
10. Di Francesco D. The hyperpolarization-activated current, i_f, and cardiac pacemaking. In: Rosen MR, Janse MJ, Wit AL (eds). *Cardiac Electrophysiology: A Textbook.* Mount Kisco, NY: Futura; 1990:117–132.
11. Yanagihara K, Irisawa H. Potassium current during the pacemaker depolarization in rabbit sinoatrial node cell. *Pflugers Arch* 1980; 388:255–260.
12. Di Francesco D. Characterization of single pacemaker channels in cardiac sinoatrial node cells. *Nature* 1986; 324:470–473.
13. Di Francesco D, Ferroni A, Massanti M, Tromba C. Properties of the hyperpolarizing-activated current i_f in cells isolated from the rabbit sino-atrial node. *J Physiol* 1986; 37:61–88.
14. Brown HF. Electrophysiology of the sinoatrial node. *Physiol Rev* 1982; 52:505–530.
15. Brown HF, Kimura K, Noble SJ. The relative contributions of various time-dependent membrane currents to pacemaker activity in the sino atrial node. In: Bouman LN, Jongsma HJ (eds). *Cardiac Rate and Rhythm: Physiological, Morphological and Developmental Aspects.* Boston: Martinus-Nijhoff; 1982:53–68.
16. Nakayama T, Kurachi Y, Noma A. Action potential and membrane currents of single pacemaker cells of the rabbit heart. *Pflugers Arch* 1984; 402:248–257.
17. Shibasaki T. Conductance and kinetics of delayed rectifier potassium channels in nodal cells of the rabbit heart. *J Physiol* 1987; 387:227–250.
18. Irisawa H, Giles WR. Sinus and atrioventricular node cells: Cellular electrophysiology. In: Zipes DP, Jalife J (eds). *Cardiac Electrophysiology: From Cell to Bedside.* Philadelphia: Saunders; 1990:95–102.
19. Reuter H. Ion channels in cardiac cell membranes. *Annu Rev Physiol* 1984; 46:473–484.
20. Bean BP. Two kinds of calcium channels in canine atrial cells. *J Gen Physiol* 1985; 85:1–30.
21. Hagiwara N, Irisawa H, Kameyama M. Contribution of two types of calcium currents to the pacemaker potentials of rabbit sino-atrial node cells. *J Physiol* 1988; 409:121–141.
22. Doerr T, Denger R, Trautwein W. Calcium currents in single SA nodal

cells of the rabbit heart studied with action potential clamp. *Pflugers Arch* 1989; 413:599–603.
23. Hoffman BF, Cranefield PF. *Electrophysiology of the Heart.* New York: McGraw-Hill, 1960.
24. Trautwein W. Effects of acetylcholine on the SA node of the heart. In: Carpenter O (ed). *Cellular Pacemakers: Mechanisms of Pacemaker Generation.* New York: Wiley; 1981:127–160.
25. Soejma M, Noma A. Mode of regulation of the ACh-sensitive K channel by the muscarinic receptor in rabbit atrial cells. *Pflugers Arch* 1984; 400:424–431.
26. Di Francesco D, Tromba C. Inhibition of the hyperpolarizing-activated current, i_f, induced by acetylcholine in rabbit sino-atrial node myocytes. *J Physiol* 1988; 405:477–491.
27. Noma A, Kotake H, Irisawa H. Slow inward current and its role mediating the chronotropic effect of epinephrine in the rabbit sinoatrial node. *Plfugers Arch* 1980; 388:1–9.
28. Di Francesco D. The cardiac-hyperpolarizing activated current, i_f. Origins and developments. *Prog Biophys Mol Biol* 1985; 46:163–183.
29. Hogan PM, David LD. Evidence for specialized fibers in the canine atrium. *Circ Res* 1968; 23:387–396.
30. Jones SB, Euler DE, Hardie E, Randall WC, Brynjolfsson G. Comparison of SA nodal and subsidiary pacemaker function and location in the dog. *Am J Physiol* 1978; 234:H471–H476.
31. Rozanski GJ, Lipsius SL. Electrophysiology of functional subsidiary pacemakers in canine right atrium. *Am J Physiol* 1985; 249:H594–H603.
32. Rozanski GJ, Lipsius SL, Randall WD. Functional characteristics of sinoatrial and subsidiary pacemaker activity in the canine right atrium. *Circulation* 1983; 67:1378–1387.
33. Wit AL, Cranefield PF. Triggered and automatic activity in the canine coronary sinus. *Circ Res* 1977; 41:435–445.
34. Wit AL, Fenoglio JJ Jr, Wagner BM, Bassett AL. Electrophysiological properties of cardiac muscle in the anterior mitral valve leaflet and the adjacent atrium in the dog: Possible implications for the genesis of atrial dysrhythmias. *Circ Res* 1973; 32:731–745.
35. Bassett AL, Fenoglio JJ, Wit AL, Myerburg RJ, Gelband H. Electrophysiologic and ultrastructural characteristics of the canine tricuspid valve. *Am J Physiol* 1976; 230:1366–1377.
36. Rozanski GJ. Electrophysiological properties of automatic fibers in rabbit atrioventricular valves. *Am J Physiol Heart Circ Physiol* 1987; 22:H720–H727.
37. Kokobun S, Nishimura M, Noma A, Irisawa H. The spontaneous action potential of rabbit atrioventricular node cells. *Jpn J Physiol* 1980; 30:529–540.
38. James TN, Isobe JH, Urthaler JH. Correlative electrophysiological and anatomical studies concerning the site of origin of escape rhythm during complete atrioventricular block in the dog. *Circ Res* 1979; 45:108–119.
39. Jones SB, Euler DE, Randall WC, Brynjolfsson G, Hardie EL. Atrial ectopic foci in the canine heart: Hierarchy of pacemaker automaticity. *Am J Physiol Heart Circ Physiol* 1980; 238:H788–H793.
40. Randall WC, Talano J, Kaye MP, Euler DE, Jones SB, Brynjolfson G. Cardiac pacemakers in the absence of the SA node: Responses to exercise and autonomic blockade. *Am J Physiol* 1978; 234:H465–H470.
41. Wallick DW, Levy MN, Felder DS, Zieske H. Effects of repetitive bursts of vagal activity on atrioventricular junctional rate in dogs. *Am J Physiol* 1979; 237:H275–H281.
42. Spear JF, Moore EN. Influence of brief vagal and stellate nerve stimulation on pacemaker activity and conduction within the atrioventricular conduction system of the dog. *Circ Res* 1973; 32:27–40.
43. Rozanski GJ, Jalife J. Automaticity in atrioventricular valve leaflets of rabbit heart. *Am J Physiol Heart Circ Physiol* 1986; 19:H397–H406.
44. Weidmann S. *Elektrophysiologie Der Herzmuskelfaser.* Bern und Stuttgart: Medizinischer Verlag Hans Huber; 1956.
45. Hope RR, Scherlag BJ, El-Sherif N, Lazzara R. Hierarchy of ventricular pacemakers. *Circ Res* 1976; 39:883–888.
46. Vassalle M, Levine MJ, Stuckey JH. On the sympathetic control of ventricular automaticity. The effects of stellate ganglia stimulation. *Circ Res* 1968; 23:249–258.
47. Levy MN. Sympathetic-parasympathetic interactions in the heart. *Circ Res* 1971; 29:437–445.
48. Levy MN, Blattberg B. Effect of vagal stimulation on the overflow of norepinephrine into the coronary sinus during cardiac sympathetic nerve stimulation in the dog. *Circ Res* 1976; 38:81–85.

49. Di Francesco D. A new interpretation of the pacemaker current in calf Purkinje fibers. *J Physiol* 1981; 314:359–376.

50. Di Francesco D. A study of the ionic nature of the pacemaker current in calf Purkinje fibers. *J Physiol* 1981; 314:377–393.

51. Noble D. The surprising heart: A review of recent progress in cardiac electrophysiology. *J Physiol* 1984; 353:1–50.

52. Di Francesco D, Noble D. A model of cardiac electrical activity incorporating ionic pumps and concentration changes. *Phil Trans R Soc Lond B* 1985; 307:353–398.

53. Gintant GA, Coehn IS. Advances in cardiac cellular electrophysiology: Implications for automaticity and therapeutics. *Annu Rev Pharmacol Toxicol* 1988; 28:61–81.

54. Hauswirth O, Noble D, Tsien RW. The mechanism of oscillatory activity at low membrane potentials in cardiac Purkinje fibers. *J Physiol* 1969; 200:255–265.

55. Imanishi S. Calcium-sensitive discharge in canine Purkinje fibers. *Jpn J Physiol* 1971; 21:443–463.

56. Noble D, Tsien RW. The kinetics and rectifier properties of the slow potassium current in cardiac Purkinje fibers. *J Physiol* 1968; 195:185–214.

57. Katzung BG, Morgenstern JA. Effects of extracellular potassium on ventricular automaticity and evidence for a pacemaker current in mammalian ventricular myocardium. *Circ Res* 1977; 40:105–111.

58. Escande D, Coraboeuf E, Planche C. Abnormal pacemaking is modulated by sarcoplasmic reticulum in partially depolarized myocardium from dilated right atria in humans. *J Mol Cell Cardiol* 1987; 19:231–241.

59. Kimura T, Imanishi S, Atria M, Hadama T, Shirabe J. Two differential mechanisms of automaticity in diseased human atrial fibers. *Jpn J Physiol* 1988; 38:851–867.

60. January CT, Fozzard HA. The effects of membrane potential, extracellular potassium and tetrodotoxin on the intracellular sodium ion activity in sheep cardiac muscle. *Circ Res* 1984; 54:652–665.

61. Carmeliet EE. Chloride and Potassium in Cardiac Purkinje Fibers. Thesis, Editions ARSCI, S.A. Brussels: Presses Academiques Europeennes; 1961.

62. Gadsby DC, Cranefield PF. Two levels of resting potential in cardiac Purkinje fibers. *J Gen Physiol* 1977; 70:725–746.

63. Hill JL, Gettes LS. Effects of acute coronary artery occlusion on local myocardial extracellular K$^+$ activity in swine. *Circulation* 1980; 61:768–778.

64. Hirche HJ, Franz C, Bos L, Bissig R, Lang R, Schramm M. Myocardial extracellular K$^+$ and H$^+$ increase and noradrenaline release as possible cause of early arrhythmias following acute coronary artery occlusion in pigs. *J Mol Cell Cardiol* 1980; 12:579–593.

65. Kleber AG. Resting membrane potential, extracellular potassium activity and intracellular sodium activity during acute global ischemia in isolated perfused guinea-pig hearts. *Circ Res* 1983; 52:442–450.

66. Dresdner KP, Kline R, Wit AL. Intracellular K$^+$ activity, intracellular Na activity and maximum diastolic potential of canine subendocardial Purkinje cells from one-day-old infarcts. *Circ Res* 1987; 60:122–132.

67. Dresdner KP, Kline RP, Wit AL. Cytoplasmic K$^+$ and N$^+$ activity in subendocardial canine Purkinje fibers from one day old infarcts using double-barrel ion sensitive electrodes. *Biophy J* 1985; 47:463.

68. Friedman PL, Stewart JR, Wit AL. Spontaneous and induced cardiac arrhythmias in subendocardial Purkinje fibers surviving extensive myocardial infarction in dogs. *Circ Res* 1973; 33:612–626.

69. Lazzara R, El-Sherif N, Scherlag BJ. Electrophysiological properties of canine Purkinje cells in one day old myocardial infarction. *Circ Res* 1973; 33:722–734.

70. Hordof AJ, Edie R, Malm JR, Hoffman BF, Rosen MR. Electrophysiological properties and response to pharmacological agents of fibers from diseased human atria. *Circulation* 1976; 54:774–779.

71. TenEick RE, Singer DH. Electrophysiological properties from diseased human atria: I. Low diastolic potential and altered cellular response to potassium. *Circ Res* 1979; 44:545–557.

72. Singer DH, Baumgarten CM, TenEick RE. Cellular electrophysiology of ventricular and other dysrhythmias: Studies on diseased and ischemic hearts. *Progr Cardiovasc Dis* 1981; 24:97–156.

73. Vassalle M. Electrogenic suppression of automaticity in sheep and dog Purkinje fibers. *Circ Res* 1970; 27:361–377.

74. Vassalle M. The relationship among cardiac pacemakers: Overdrive suppression. *Circ Res* 1977; 41:269–277.

75. Vassalle M. Cardiac pacemaker potentials at different extra- and intracellular K concentrations. *Am J Physiol* 1965; 208:770–775.

76. Vassalle M. Caress DL, Slovin AJ, Stuckey JH. On the cause of ventricular asystole during vagal stimulation. *Circ Res* 1967; 20:228–241.

77. Randall WC, Rinkema LE, Jones SB, Moran JF, Brynjolfsson G. Overdrive suppression of atrial pacemaker tissues in the alert, awake dog before and chronically after excision of the sinoatrial node. *Am J Cardiol* 1982; 49:1166–1175.

78. Glitsch HG. Characteristics of active Na transport in intact cardiac cells. *Am J Physiol* 1979; 236:H189–H199.

79. Gadsby DC, Cranefield PF. Electrogenic sodium extrusion in cardiac Purkinje fibers. *J Gen Physiol* 1979; 73:819–837.

80. Jordan JL, Yamaguchi I, Mandel WJ, McCullen AE. Comparative effects of overdrive on sinus and subsidiary pacemaker functions. *Am Heart J* 1977; 93:367–374.

81. Kodama I, Goto J, Ando A, Toyama I, Yamada K. Effects of rapid stimulation on the transmembrane action potentials of rabbit sinus node pacemaker cells. *Circ Res* 1980; 46:90–99.

82. Greenberg YJ, Vassalle M. On the mechanism of overdrive suppression in the guinea pig sino-atrial node. *J Electrocardiol* 1990; 37:53–67.

83. Gang ES, Reiffel JA, Livelli FD Jr, Bigger JT Jr. Sinus node recovery times following the spontaneous termination of supraventricular tachycardia and following atrial overdrive pacing. A comparison. *Am Heart J* 1983; 105:210–215.

84. Breithardt G, Seipel L, Loogen F. Sinus node recovery time and calculated sinoatrial conduction time in normal subjects and patients with sinus node dysfunction. *Circulation* 1977; 56:43–50.

85. Carmeliet E. The slow inward current: Non-voltage clamp studies. In: Zipes DP, Bailey JC, Elharrar V (eds). *The Slow Inward Current and Cardiac Arrhythmias*. The Hague: Martinus Nijhoff; 1980:97–110.

86. Hoffman BF, Dangman KH. Are arrhythmias caused by automatic impulse generation? In: Paes de Carvalho A, Hoffman BF, Lieberman M (eds). *Normal and Abnormal Conduction in the Heart*. Mount Kisco, NY: Futura; 1982:429–448.

87. Dangman KH, Hoffman BF. Studies on overdrive stimulation of canine cardiac Purkinje fibers: Maximum diastolic potential as a determinant of the response. *J Am Coll Cardiol* 1983; 2:1183–1191.

88. Falk RT, Cohen IS. Membrane current following activity in canine cardiac Purkinje fibers. *J Gen Physiol* 1984; 83:771–799.

89. Van Capelle FJL, Durer D. Computer simulation of arrhythmias in a network of coupled excitable elements. *Circ Res* 1980; 47:454–466.

90. Wit AL, Cranefield PF. Mechanism of impulse initiation in the atrioventricular junction and the effect of acetylstrophantidin (abstr) *Am J Cardiol* 1982; 49:921.

91. Kirchhof CJ, Bonke FIM, Allessie MA. Evidence for the presence of electrotonic depression of pacemakers in the rabbit atrioventricular node: The effects of uncoupling from the surrounding myocardium. *Basic Res Cardiol* 1988; 83:190–201.

92. Opthof T, van Ginneken ACG, Bouman LN, Jongsma HJ. The intrinsic cycle length in small pieces isolated from the rabbit sinoatrial node. *J Mol Cell Cardiol* 1987; 19:923–934.

93. Janse MJ, Van Capelle FJL. Electrotonic interactions across an inexcitable region as a cause of ectopic activity in acute regional myocardial ischemia: A study in intact porcine and canine hearts and computer models. *Circ Res* 1982; 50:527–537.

94. Boineau JP, Schuessler RB, Mooney CR, Wylds AC, Miller CB, Hudson RD, et al. Multicentric origin of the atrial depolarization waves: The pacemaker complex: Relation to dynamics of atrial conduction, P wave changes and heart rate control. *Circulation* 1978; 58:1036–1048.

95. Toda N, West TC. Changes in sino-atrial node transmembrane potentials on vagal stimulation of the isolated rabbit atrium. *Nature* 1965; 205:808–809.

96. Ferrer MI: *The Sick Sinus Syndrome*. Mount Kisco, NY: Futura; 1974.

97. Katz LN, Pick A. *Clinical Electrocardiography. The Arrhythmias*. Philadelphia: Lea & Febiger; 1956.

98. Jalife J, Moe GK. Effect of electrotonic potentials on pacemaker activity of canine Purkinje fibers in relation to parasystole. *Circ Res* 1976; 39:801–808.

99. Jalife J, Moe GK. A biologic model of parasystole. *Am J Cardiol* 1979; 43:761–772.

100. Moe GK, Jalife J, Mueller WJ, Moe B. A mathematical model of parasystole and its application to clinical arrhythmias. *Circulation* 1977; 56:968–979.

101. Euler DE, Jones SB, Gunnar WP. Koeb JM, Murdock DK, Randall

WC. Cardiac arrhythmias in the conscious dog after excision of the sinus node and crista terminalis. *Circulation* 1979; 59:468–475.

102. Loeb JM, Euler DE, Randall WC, Moran JF, Brynjolfsson G. Cardiac arrhythmias after chronic embolization of the sinus node artery: Alterations in parasympathetic pacemaker control. *Circulation* 1980; 61:192–198.

103. Randall WC, Rinkema LE, Jones SB, Moran JF, Brynjolfsson G. Functional characteristics of atrial pacemaker activity. *Am J Physiol* 1982; 242:H98–H106.

104. Gillette PC, Kugler JD, Garson A Jr, Gutgesell HP, Duff DF, McNamara DG. Mechanisms of cardiac arrhythmias after the Mustard operation for transposition of the great arteries. *Am J Cardiol* 1980; 45:1225–1230.

105. Klein HO, Lebson R, Cranefield PF, Hoffman BF. Effect of extrasystoles on idioventricular rhythm: Clinical and electrophysiologic correlation. *Circulation* 1973; 47:758–764.

106. Webb SW, Adgey AAJ, Pantridge JF. Autonomic disturbance of onset of acute myocardial infarction. *Br Med J* 1972; 3:89–92.

107. Lie KI, Wellens HJJ, Schuilenburg RM. Mechanism and significance of widened QRS complexes during complete atrioventricular block in acute inferior myocardial infarction. *Am J Cardiol* 1974; 33:833–839.

108. Dahl G, Isenberg G. Decoupling of heart muscle cells: Correlation with increased cytoplasmic calcium activity and with changes of nexus ultrastructure. *J Membr Biol* 1980; 53:63–75.

109. Weingart R. The actions of ouabain on intercellular coupling and conduction velocity in mammalian ventricular muscle. *J Physiol* 1977; 264:341–365.

110. Ellis D. The effects of external cations and ouabain on the intracellular sodium activity of sheep heart Purkinje fibers. *J Physiol* 1977; 273:211–240.

111. Davis LD. Effects of autonomic neurohumors on transmembrane potentials of atrial plateau fibers. *Am J Physiol* 1975; 229:1351–1364.

112. Tsien RW. Effects of epinephrine on the pacemaker potassium current of cardiac Purkinje fibers. *J Gen Physiol* 1974; 64:293–319.

113. Pliam MB, Krellenstein DJ, Vassalle M, Brooks C McC. The influence of norepinephrine, reserpine and propranolol on overdrive suppression. *J Electrocardiol* 1975; 8:17–24.

114. Armour JA, Hageman GR, Randall WC. Arrhythmias induced by local cardiac nerve stimulation. *Am J Physiol* 1972; 223:1068–1075.

115. Katzung BG, Hondeghem LM, Grant AO. Cardiac ventricular automaticity induced by current of injury. *Pflugers Arch* 1975; 360:193–197.

116. Rosen MR, Gelband H, Hoffman BF. Correlation between the effects of ouabain on the canine electrocardiogram and transmembrane potentials of isolated Purkinje fibers. *Circulation* 1973; 47:65–72.

117. Rosen MR, Gelband H, Merker C, Hoffman BF. Mechanisms of digitalis toxicity: Effects of ouabain on phase four of canine Purkinje fiber transmembrane potentials. *Circulation* 1973; 47:681–689.

118. Deck KA. Aenderungen des Ruhepotentials und der Kabeleigenschaften von Purkinje-Faden bei der Dehnung. *Pflugers Arch* 1964; 280:131–140.

119. Dudel J, Trautwein W. Das Aktionspotential und Mechanogramm des Herzmuskels unter dem Einflusz der Dehnung. *Cardiologia* 1954; 25:344–362.

120. Kaufmann R, Theopile U. Automatie fördernde Dehnungseffekte am Purkinje Faden, Papillarmuskeln und Vorhoftrabekeln von Rhesusaffen. *Pflugers Arch* 1967; 291:174–189.

121. Hansen DE, Craig CS, Hondeghem LM. Stretch-induced arrhythmias in the isolated canine ventricle: Evidence for the importance of mechanoelectrical feedback. *Circulation* 1990; 81:1094–1105.

122. Ferrier GR, Rosenthal JE. Automaticity and entrance block induced by focal depolarization of mammalian ventricular tissues. *Circ Res* 1980; 47:238–248.

123. Imanishi S, Surawicz B. Automatic activity in depolarized guinea-pig ventricular myocardium. *Circ Res* 1976; 39:751–759.

124. Brown HF, Noble SJ. Membrane currents underlying delayed rectification and pacemaker activity in frog atrial muscle. *J Physiol* 1969; 204:717–736.

125. Hume J, Katzung BG. Physiological role of endogenous amines in the modulation of ventricular automaticity in the guinea pig. *J Physiol* 1980; 309:275–286.

126. Cranefield PF, Aronson RS. Initiation of sustained rhythmic activity by single propagated action potentials in canine cardiac Purkinje fibers exposed to sodium-free solution or to ouabain. *Circ Res* 1974; 34:477–481.

127. Cranefield PF. Action potentials, afterpotentials and arrhythmias. *Circ Res* 1977; 41:415–425.

128. Cranefield PF, Aronson RS. Cardiac arrhythmias: The role of triggered activity and other mechanisms. Mt Kisco, NY: Futura; 1988.

129. Cramer M, Siegal M, Bigger JT Jr, Hoffman BF. Characteristics of extracellular potentials recorded from the sinoatrial pacemaker of the rabbit. *Circ Res* 1977; 41:292–300.

130. Wit AL, Boyden PA, Gadsby CD, Cranefield PF. Triggered activity as a cause of atrial arrhythmias. In: Narula OS (ed). *Cardiac Arrhythmias: Electrophysiology, Diagnosis and Management.* Baltimore: Williams & Wilkins; 1979:14–31.

131. Olsson SB, Blomström-Lundqvist C, Wohlfart B. Endocardial monophasic action potentials: Correlations with intracellular electrical activity. *Ann NY Acad Sci* 1990; 601:119–127.

132. Harriman RJ, Holzman R, Gough WB, Mehra R, Gomes JAC, El-Sherif N. In vivo demonstration of delayed afterdepolarization as a cause of ventricular rhythms in one day old infarction. *J Am Coll Cardiol* 1984; 3:478.

133. Priori SG, Mantica M, Schwartz PJ. Delayed afterdepolarizations elicited in vivo by left stellate ganglion stimulation. *Circulation* 1988; 78:178–185.

134. Fabiato A, Fabiato F. Contraction induced by a calcium-triggered release of calcium from the sarcoplasmic reticulum of single skinned cardiac cells. *J Physiol* 1975; 249:469–495.

135. Aronson RS, Gelles JM, Hoffman BF. Effect of ouabain on the current underlying spontaneous diastolic depolarization in cardiac Purkinje fibers. *Nature New Biol* 1973; 245:118–120.

136. Lederer WJ, Tsien RW. Transient inward current underlying arrhythmogenic effect of cardiotonic steroids in Purkinje fibers. *J Physiol* 1976; 263:73–100.

137. Kass RS, Lederer WJ, Tsien RW, Weingart R. Role of calcium ions in transient inward currents and after contractions induced by strophantidin in cardiac Purkinje fibers. *J Physiol* 1978; 281:187–208.

138. Kass RS, Tsien RW, Weingart R. Ionic basis of transient inward current induced by strophantidin in cardiac Purkinje fibers. *J Physiol* 1978; 281:209–226.

139. Karagueuzian HS, Katzung BG. Voltage clamp studies of transient inward current and mechanical oscillations induced by ouabain in ferret papillary muscle. *J Physiol* 1982; 327:255–271.

140. Vassalle M, Mugelli A. An oscillatory current in sheep cardiac Purkinje fibers. *Circ Res* 1981; 48:618–631.

141. Lipsius SL, Gobbins WR. Membrane currents, contractions and aftercontractions in cardiac Purkinje fibers. *Am J Physiol* 1982; 243:H77–H86.

142. Eisner DA, Lederer WJ. Inotropic and arrhythmogenic effects of potassium-depleted solutions on mammalian cardiac muscle. *J Physiol* 1979; 294:255–277.

143. Baker PF, Blaustein MP, Hodgkin AL, Steinhardt RA. The influence of calcium on sodium efflux in squid axons. *J Physiol* 1969; 200:431–458.

144. Mullins LJ. The generation of electrical currents in cardiac fibers by Na/Ca exchange. *Am J Physiol* 1979; 236:C103–C110.

145. Eisner DA, Lederer WJ. Na-Ca exchange: Stoichiometry and electrogenicity. *Am J Physiol* 1985; 248:C189–C202.

146. David LD. Effect of changes in cycle length on diastolic depolarization produced by ouabain in canine Purkinje fibers. *Circ Res* 1973; 32:206–214.

147. Ferrier GR, Saunders JH, Mendez C. A cellular mechanism for the generation of ventricular arrhythmias by acetylstrophantidin. *Circ Res* 1973; 32:600–609.

148. Ferrier GR, Moe GK. Effect of calcium on acetylstrophantidin-induced transient depolarizations in canine Purkinje tissue. *Circ Res* 1973; 33:508–515.

149. Hashimoto K, and Moe GK. Transient depolarizations induced by acetylstrophantidin in specialized tissue of dog atrium and ventricle. *Circ Res* 1973; 32:618–624.

150. Hogan PM, Wittenberg SM, Kocke FJ. Relationship of stimulation frequency to automaticity in the canine Purkinje fiber during ouabain administration. *Circ Res* 1973; 32:377–384.

151. Aronson RS, Cranefield PF. The effect of resting potential on the electrical activity of canine cardiac Purkinje fibers exposed to Na-free solution or to ouabain. *Pflugers Arch* 1974; 347:101–116.

152. Zipes DP, Arbel E, Knope RF, Moe GK. Accelerated cardiac escape rhythms caused by ouabain intoxication. *Am J Cardiol* 1974; 33:248–253.

153. Lown B, Cannon RL, Rossi MA. Electrical stimulation and digitalis drugs: Repetitive response in diastole. *Proc Soc Exp Biol Med* 1967; 126:697–701.

154. Lown B. Electrical stimulation to estimate the degree of digitalization: II. Experimental studies. *Am J Cardiol* 1968; 22:251–259.

155. Castellanos A, Lemberg L, Centurion MJ, Berkovits BV. Concealed digitalis-induced arrhythmias unmasked by electrical stimulation of the heart. *Am Heart J* 1967; 73:484–490.

156. Deitmer JW, Ellis D. The intracellular sodium activity of cardiac Purkinje fibers during inhibition and re-activation of the Na-K pump. *J Physiol* 1978; 284:241–259.

157. Lee CO, Dagostino M. Effect of strophantidin on intracellular Na ion activity and twitch tension of constantly driven cardiac Purkinje fibers. *Biophys J* 1982; 40:185–198.

158. Lee CO, Kang DH, Sokol JH, Lee KS. Relation between intracellular Na ion activity and tension of sheep cardiac Purkinje fibers exposed to dihydro-ouabain. *Biophys J* 1980; 29:315–330.

159. Reuter h, Seitz N. The dependence of calcium efflux from cardiac muscle on temperature and external ion composition. *J Physiol* 1968; 195:451–470.

160. Mullins JL. *Ion Transport in Heart,* New York: Raven Press; 1981.

161. Wit A, Cranefield PF. Triggered activity in cardiac muscle fibers of the simian mitral valve. *Circ Res* 1976; 38:85–98.

162. Boyden PA, Tilley LP, Albala A, Liu SK, Fenoglio JJ Jr, Wit AL. Mechanisms for atrial arrhythmias associated with cardiomyopathy: A study of feline hearts with primary myocardial disease. *Circ Res* 1984; 69:1036–1047.

163. Malfatto G, Rosen TS, Rosen MR. The response to overdrive pacing of triggered atrial and ventricular arrhythmias in the canine heart. *Circulation* 1988; 77:1139–1148.

164. Belardinelli L, Isenberg G. Actions of adenosine and isoproterenol on isolated mammalian ventricular myocyte. *Circ Res* 1983; 53:287–297.

165. Lazzara R, Marchi S. Electrophysiological mechanisms for the generation of arrhythmias with adrenergic stimulation. In: Brachman J, Schomig A (eds). *Adrenergic System and Ventricular Arrhythmias in Myocardial Infarction.* Heidelberg: Springer Verlag; 1989: 231–238.

166. Lerman BB, Belardinelli L, West A, Berne RM, DiMarco JP. Adenosine-sensitive ventricular tachycardia: Evidence suggesting cyclic AMP-mediated triggered activity. *Circulation* 1986; 74:270–280.

167. El-Sherif N, Zeiler R, Gough WB. Effects of catecholamine, verapamil, and tetrodotoxin on triggered automaticity in canine ischemic Purkinje fibers (abstr). *Circulation* 1980; 62:III-281.

168. El-Sherif N, Gough WB, Zeiler RH, Mehra R. Triggered ventricular arrhythmias in one day old myocardial infarction in the dog. *Circ Res* 1983; 52:566–579.

169. Reuter H. Localization of beta adrenergic receptors and effects of noradrenaline and cyclic nucleotides on action potentials, ionic currents and tension in mammalian cardiac muscle. *J Physiol* 1974; 242:429–451.

170. Horn EM, Johnson NJ, Bilezikian JP, Rosen MR. Developmental changes in the electrophysiological properties and the beta-adrenergic receptor-effector complex in atrial fibers of the canine coronary sinus. *Circ Res* 1989; 65:325–333.

171. Morad M, Rolett E. Relaxing effect of catecholamine on mammalian heart. *J Physiol* 1972; 224:537–558.

172. Fabiato A. Calcium-induced release of calcium from the cardiac sarcoplasmic reticulum. *Am J Physiol* 1983; 245:C1–C14.

173. Saito T, Otoguro M, Matsubara T. Electrophysiological studies on the mechanism of electrically induced sustained rhythmic activity in the rabbit right atrium. *Circ Res* 1978; 42:199–206.

174. Mary-Rabine L, Hordof AJ, Danilo P, Malm JR, Rosen MR. Mechanisms for impulse initiation in isolated human atrial fibers. *Circ Res* 1980; 47:267–277.

175. Aronson RS. Afterpotentials and triggered activity in hypertrophied myocardium from rats with renal hypertension. *Circ Res* 1981; 48:720–727.

176. Nordin C, Gilat E, Aronson RS. Delayed afterdepolarizations and triggered activity in ventricular muscle from rats with streptozotocin-induced diabetes. *Circ Res* 1985; 57:28–34.

177. Arlock P, Katzung BG. Effects of sodium substitutes on transient inward current and tension in guinea-pig and ferret papillary muscle. *J Physiol* 1985; 360:105–120.

178. Ferrier G. Effects of transmembrane potential on oscillatory afterpotentials induced by acetylstrophantidin in canine ventricular tissues. *J Pharmacol Exp Ther* 1981; 215:332–341.

179. Wasserstrom JA, Ferrier GR. Voltage dependence of digitalis afterpotentials, aftercontractions, and inotropy. *Am J Physiol* 1981; 241:H646–H653.

180. Henning B, Wit AL. Action potential characteristics control afterdepolarization amplitude and triggered activity in canine coronary sinus. *Circulation* 1981; 64:IV-50.

181. LeMarec H, Dangman KH, Danilo P, Rosen MR. An evaluation of automaticity and triggered activity in the canine heart one to four days after myocardial infraction. *Circulation* 1985; 71:1224–1236.

182. Gough WB, El-Sherif N. Dependence of delayed afterdepolarizations on diastolic potentials in ischemic Purkinje fibers. *Am J Physiol* 1989; 257:H770–H777.

183. Wit AL, Tseng G-N, Henning B, Hanna MS. Arrhythmogenic effects of quinidine on catecholamine-induced delayed afterdepolarizations in canine atrial fibers. *J Cardiovasc Electrophysiol* 1990; 1:15–30.

184. Sheu SS, Lederer WJ. Lidocaine's negative inotropic and antiarrhythmic actions: Dependence on shortening of action potential duration and reduction of intracellular sodium activity. *Circ Res* 1985; 57:578–590.

185. Aronson RS. Characteristics of action potentials of hypertrophied myocardium from rats with renal hypertension. *Circ Res* 1980; 47:443–454.

186. Moak JP, Rosen MF. Induction and termination of triggered activity by pacing in isolated canine Purkinje fibers. *Circulation* 1984; 69:149–162.

187. Wit AL, Gadsby DC, Cranefield PF. Electrogenic sodium extrusion can stop triggered activity in the canine coronary sinus. *Circ Res* 1981; 49:1029–1042.

188. Johnson N, Danilo P, Wit A, Rosen MR. Response to pacing of triggered activity occurring in catecholamine-treated canine coronary sinus. *Circulation* 1986; 741:1168–1179.

189. Gadsby DC, Cranefield PF. Direct measurement of changes in sodium pump current in canine cardiac Purkinje fibers. *Proc Natl Acad Sci USA* 1979; 76:1783–1787.

190. Johnson N, Rosen MR. The distinction between triggered activity and other cardiac arrhythmias. In: Brugada P, Wellens HJJ (eds). *Cardiac Arrhythmias: Where to Go from Here.* Mt Kisco, NY: Futura; 1987:129–145.

191. Dangman KH, Hoffman BF. The effects of single premature stimuli on automatic and triggered rhythms in isolated canine Purkinje fibers. *Circulation* 1985; 71:813–822.

192. Trautwein W: Mechanisms of tachyarrhythmias and extrasystoles. In: Sandoe E, Flenstad-Jenson E, Olesen K (eds). *Symposium on Cardiac Arrhythmias.* Sodertalje, Sweden: AB Astra; 1970:53–66.

193. January CT, Shorofsky S. Early afterdepolarizations: Newer insights into cellular mechanisms. *J Cardiovasc Electrophysiol* 1990; 1:161–169.

194. Mendez C, Delmar M. Triggered activity: Its possible role in cardiac arrhythmias. In: Zipes DP, Jalife J (eds). *Cardiac Electrophysiology and Arrhythmias.* Orlando, FL: Grune & Stratton, 1985:311–313.

195. Kupersmith J, Hoff P. Occurrence and transmission of localized repolarization abnormalities in vitro. *J Am Coll Cardiol* 1985; 6:152–160.

196. Wit AL, Wiggins JR, Cranefield PF. Some effects of electrical stimulation on impulse initiation in cardiac fibers: Its relevance for the determination of the mechanisms of clinical cardiac arrhythmias. In: Wellens JH, Lie KI, Janse MJ (eds). *The Conduction System of the Heart.* Philadelphia: Lea & Febiger; 1976:163–181.

197. Antzelevitch C, Sicouri S. Clinical relevance of cardiac arrhythmias generated by afterdepolarizations: Role of M cells in the generation of U waves, triggered activity and torsade de pointes. *J Am Coll Cardiol* 1994; 23:259–277.

198. BP, Rosen MR. Effects of pacing on triggered activity induced by early afterdepolarizations. *Circulation* 1984; 69:1013–1025.

199. Brachmann J, Scherlag BJ, Rosenshtraukh LV, Lazzara R. Bradycardia dependent triggered activity: Relevance to drug-induced multiform ventricular tachycardia. *Circulation* 1983; 68:846–856.

200. Kay GN, Plumb VJ, Arciniegas JG, Henthorn RW, Waldo AL. Torsade de pointes: The long-short initiating sequence and other clinical features: Observations in 32 patients. *J Am Coll Cardiol* 1983; 2:806–817.

201. Ben David J, Zipes DP. Differential response to right and left ansae subclaviae stimulation of early afterdepolarizations and ventricular tachycardia induced by cesium in dogs. *Circulation* 1988; 78:1241–1250.

202. Levine JH, Spear JF, Guarnieri T, Weisfeldt M, de Langen CDJ, Becker LC, et al. Cesium chloride-induced long QT syndrome: Demonstration of afterdepolarizations and triggered activity in vivo. *Circulation* 1985; 72:1092–1104.

203. Strauss HC, Bigger JT Jr, Hoffman BF. Electrophysiological and beta-blocking effects of MJ 1999 on dog and rabbit cardiac tissue. *Circ Res* 1970; 26:661–678.

204. Carmeliet E. Electrophysiologic and voltage clamp analyses of the effects of sotalol on isolated cardiac muscle and Purkinje fibers. *J Pharmacol Exp Ther* 1985; 232:817–825.

205. Dangman KH, Hoffman BF. In vivo and in vitro antiarrhythmic and arrhythmogenic effects of N-acetylprocainamide. *J Pharmacol Exp Ther* 1981; 217:851–862.

206. Roden DM, Hoffman BF. Action potential prolongation and induction of abnormal automaticity by low quinidine concentrations in canine Purkinje fibers: Relationship to potassium and cycle length. *Circ Res* 1985; 56:857–867.

207. Davidenko JM, Cohen L, Goodrow R, Antzelevitch C. Quinidine-induced action potential prolongation, early afterdepolarizations, and triggered activity in canine Purkinje fibers: Effects of stimulation rate, potassium, and magnesium. *Circulation* 1989; 79:674–686.

208. Colatsky T. Mechanisms of action of lidocaine and quinidine on action potential duration in rabbit cardiac Purkinje fibers: An effect on steady-state sodium currents. *Circ Res* 1982; 50:17–27.

209. Selzer A, Wray HW. Quinidine syncope: Paroxysmal ventricular fibrillation occurring during treatment of chronic atrial arrhythmias. *Circulation* 1964; 30:17–26.

210. Smith WM, Gallagher JJ. "Les torsades de pointes": An unusual ventricular arrhythmia. *Ann Intern Med* 1980; 93:578–584.

211. Olshansky B, Martins J, Hunt S. N-acetyl procainamide causing torsades de pointes. *Am J Cardiol* 1982; 50:1439–1441.

212. Kuck KH, Kunze DP, Roewer N, Bleifield W. Sotalol-induced torsade de pointes. *Am Heart J* 1984; 107:179–180.

213. Bailie DS, Inoue H, Kaseda S, Ben-David J, Zipes DP. Magnesium suppression of early afterdepolarizations and ventricular tachyarrhythmias induced by cesium in dogs. *Circulation* 1988; 77:1395–1402.

214. Tzivoni D, Keren A, Cohen AM, Loebel H, Zahavi I, Chenzbraun A, et al. Magnesium therapy for torsade de pointes. *Am J Cardiol* 1984; 53:528–530.

215. Perticone F, Adinolfi L, Bonaduce D. Efficacy of magnesium sulfate in the treatment of torsade de pointes. *Am Heart J* 1986; 112:847–849.

216. Lewis T. *The Mechanism and Graphic Registration of the Heart Beat*, 3d ed. London: Shaw Sons; 1925.

217. Smeets JLRM, Allessie MA, Lammers WJEP, Bonke FIM, Hollen J. The wavelength of cardiac impulse and reentrant arrhythmias in isolated rabbit atrium: The role of heart rate, autonomic transmitters, temperature, and potassium. *Circ Res* 1986; 58:96–108.

218. Garrey W. The nature of fibrillary contraction of the heart: Its relation to tissue mass and form. *Am J Physiol* 1914; 33:397–414.

219. El Sherif N, Carel EB, Yin H, Restivo M. The electrophysiological mechanism of ventricular arrhythmias in the long Q-T syndrome: Tridimensional mapping of activation and recovery patterns. *Circ Res* 1996; 79:474–492.

220. Coumel P, Cabrol C, Fabiato A, Gourgon R, Slama R. Tachycardie permanente par rhythme reciproque. *Arch Mal Coeur* 1967; 60:1830–1864.

221. Critelli G, Gallagher JJ, Monda V, Coltorti F, Scherillo M, Rossi L. Anatomic and electrohysiologic substrate of the permanent form of junctional reciprocating tachycardia. *J Am Coll Cardiol* 1984; 4:601–610.

222. Wit AL, Cranefield PF, Hoffman BF. Slow conduction and reentry in the ventricular conducting system: II. Single and sustained circus movement in networks of canine and bovine Purkinje fibers. *Circ Res* 1972; 30:11–22.

223. Boyden PA. Activation sequence during atrial flutter in dogs with surgically induced right atrial enlargement: I. Observations during sustained rhythms. *Circ Res* 1988; 62:596–608.

224. Shimizu A, Nozaki A, Rudy Y, Waldo AL. Onset of induced atrial flutter in the canine pericarditis model. *J Am Coll Cardiol* 1991; 17:1223–1234.

225. Waldo AL, Cooper TB. Spontaneous onset of type I atrial flutter. *J Am Coll Cardiol* 1996; 28:707–712.

226. Olshansky B, Okumura K, Hess PG, Waldo AL. Demonstration of an area of slow conduction in human atrial flutter. *J Am Coll Cardiol* 1990; 16:1639–1648.

227. Klein H, Karp RB, Kouchoukos NT, Zorn GL Jr, James TN, Waldo AL. Intraoperative electrophysiological mapping of the ventricles during sinus rhythm in patients with a previous myocardial infarction:

228. Fozzard HA. Conduction of the action potential. In: Berne RM (ed): *The Cardiovascular System*. Bethesda, MD: The American Physiological Society; 1979:335–356.

229. Weidmann S. The effect of the cardiac membrane potential on the rapid availability of the sodium carrying system. *J Physiol* 1955; 127:213–224.

230. Gettes LS, Reuter H. Slow recovery from inactivation of inward currents in mammalian myocardial fibers. *J Physiol* 1974; 240:703–724.

231. Dodge FA, Cranefield PF. Nonuniform conduction in cardiac Purkinje fibers. In: Paes de Carvalho A, Hoffman BF, Lieberman M (eds). *Normal and Abnormal Conduction in the Heart*. Mt Kisco, NY: Futura; 1982:379–395.

232. Tisen RW. Calcium channels in excitable cell membranes. *Annu Rev Physiol* 1983; 45:341–358.

233. Zipes DP, Mendez C. Action of manganese ions and tetrodotoxin on atrioventricular nodal transmembrane potentials in isolated rabbit hearts. *Circ Res* 1973; 32:447–454.

234. Spach MS, Miller WT, Geselowitz DB, Barr RC, Kootsey JM, Johnson EA. The discontinuous nature of propagation in normal canine cardiac muscle: Evidence for recurrent discontinuities of intracellular resistance that effect membrane currents. *Circ Res* 1981; 48:39–54.

235. Spach MS, Miller WT, Dolber PC, Kootsey JM, Sommer JR, Mosher EC. The functional role of structural complexities in the propagation of depolarization in the atrium of the dog: Cardiac conduction disturbances due to discontinuities of effective axial resistivity. *Circ Res* 1982; 50:175–191.

236. Sommer JR, Dolber PC, Cardiac muscle: The ultrastructure of its cells and bundles. In: Hoffman BF, Lieberman M, Paes de Carvalho A (eds). *Normal and Abnormal Conduction of the Heart Beat*. Mt Kisco, NY: Futura; 1982:1–27.

237. Hoyt RH, Cohen ML, Saffitz JE. Distribution and three-dimensional structure of intercellular junctions in canine myocardium. *Circ Res* 1989; 64:563–574.

238. Roberts DE, Hersh LT, Scher AM. Influence of cardiac fiber orientation on wavefront voltage, conduction velocity and tissue resistivity in the dog. *Circ Res* 1979; 44:701–712.

239. Clerc L. Directional differences of impulse spread in trabecular muscle from mammalian heart. *J Physiol* 1976; 255:335–346.

240. Saffitz JE, Kanter HL, Green KG, Tolley TK, Beyer EC. Tissue-specific determinants of anisotropic conduction velocity in canine atrial and ventricular myocardium. *Circ Res* 1994; 74:1065–1070.

241. Spach MS, Dolber PC. Relating extracellular potentials and their derivatives to anisotropic propagation at a microscopic level in human cardiac muscle: Evidence for uncoupling of side-to-side fiber connections with increasing age. *Circ Res* 1986; 58:356–371.

242. Spach MS, Dolber PC, Heidlage JF. Influence of the passive anisotropic properties on directional differences in propagation following modification of the sodium conductance in human atrial muscle: A model of reentry based on anisotropic discontinuous propagation. *Circ Res* 1988; 62:811–832.

243. Hunter PJ, McNaughten PA, Noble D. Analytical models of propagation in excitable cells. *Prog Biophys Mol Biol* 1975; 30:99–144.

244. Dominguez C, Fozzard HA. Influence of extracellular K^+ concentration on cable properties and excitability of sheep cardiac Purkinje fibers. *Circ Res* 1970; 26:565–574.

245. Spach MS, Miller WT, Miller-Jones E, Warren RB, Barr RC. Extracellular potentials related to intracellular action potentials during impulse conduction in anisotropic canine cardiac muscle. *Circ Res* 1979; 45:188–204.

246. Rudy Y, Quan W. A model study of the effects of the discrete cellular structure on electrical propagation in cardiac tissue. *Circ Res* 1987; 61:815–823.

247. Quan W, Rudy Y. Unidirectional block and reentry of cardiac excitation: A model study. *Circ Res* 1990; 60:367–382.

248. DeMello WC. Effect of intracellular injection of calcium and strontium in cell communication in heart. *J Physiol* 1975; 250:231–245.

249. Hess SP, Weingart R. Intracellular free calcium modified by pH_i in sheep cardiac Purkinje fibres. *J Physiol* 1980; 307:60P–61P.

250. Van Dam RTh: Experimenteel onderzoek naar het prikkelbaarheidsverloop van de hartspier. Thesis. Amsterdam: University of Amsterdam, Klein Offsetdrukkerij Poortpers; 1960.

251. Rensma PL, Allessie MA, Lammers WJEP, Bonke FIM, Schalij MJ.

Length of excitation wave and susceptibility to reentrant atrial arrhythmias in normal conscious dogs. *Circ Res* 1988; 62:395–410.

252. Allessie MA, Bonke FIM, Schopman FJG. Circus movement in rabbit atrial muscle as a mechanism of tachycardia: 2. The role of nonuniform recovery of excitability in the occurrence of unidirectional block as studied with multiple microelectrodes. *Circ Res* 1976; 39:168–177.

253. Han J, Moe GK. Nonuniform recovery of excitability of ventricular muscle. *Circ Res* 1964; 14:44–60.

254. Janse MJ. The effects of changes in heart rate on the refractory period of the heart. Thesis. Amsterdam: University of Amsterdam, Mondeel-Offsetdrukkerij; 1971.

255. Wallace AG, Mignone RS. Physiologic evidence concerning the reentry hypothesis for ectopic beats. *Am Heart J* 1966; 72:60–70.

256. Kuo C-S, Munakata K, Reddy CP, Surawicz B. Characteristics and possible mechanisms of ventricular arrhythmia dependent on the dispersion of action potential durations. *Circulation* 1983; 67:1356–1367.

257. Cranefield PK, Klein HO, Hoffman BF. Conduction of the cardiac impulse: 1. Delay, block and one-way block in the pressed Purkinje fibers. *Circ Res* 1971; 28:199–219.

258. Joyner RW, Overholt ED, Ramza B, Veenstra RD. Propagation through electrically coupled cells: Two inhomogeneously coupled cardiac tissue layers. *Am J Physiol* 1984; 247:H596–H609.

259. Goldstein SS, Rall W. Changes in action potential shape and velocity for changing core conductor geometry. *Biophys J* 1974; 14:731–757.

260. Overholt ED, Joyner RW, Veenstra RD, Rawling D, Wiedmann R. Unidirectional block between Purkinje and ventricular layers of papillary muscles. *Am J Physiol* 1984; 247:H584–H595.

261. Janse MJ, Wilms-Schopman F, Wilensky RJ, Tranum-Jensen J. Role of the subendocardium in arrhythmogenesis during acute ischemia. In: Zipes DP, Jalife J (eds). *Cardiac Electrophysiology and Arrhythmias,* Orlando, FL: Grune & Stratton, 1985:353–362.

262. Gilmour RF, Evans JJ, Zipes DP. Purkinje-muscle coupling and endocardial response to hyperkalemia, hypoxia, and acidosis. *Am J Physiol* 1984; 247:H303–H311.

263. Gilmour RF, Evans JJ, Zipes DP. Preferential interruption of impulse transmission across Purkinje-muscle junctions by interventions that depress conduction. In: Zipes DP, Jalife J (eds). *Cardiac Electrophysiology and Arrhythmias,* Orlando, FL: Grune Stratton; 1985:287–300.

264. Delmar M, Michaels DC, Johnson T, Jalife J. Effects of increasing intercellular resistance on transverse and longitudinal propagation in sheep epicardial muscle. *Circ Res* 1987; 60:780–785.

265. Delgado C, Steinhaus B, Delmar M, Chialvo DR, Jalife J. Directional differences in excitability and margin of safety for propagation in sheep ventricular epicardial muscle. *Circ Res* 1990; 67:97–110.

266. Frame LH, Page RL, Boyden PA, Fenoglio JJ Jr, Hoffman BF. Circus movement in the canine atrium around the tricuspid ring during experimental atrial flutter and during reentry in vitro. *Circulation* 1987; 76:1155–1175.

267. Moe GK. On the multiple wavelet hypothesis of atrial fibrillation. *Arch Int Pharmacodyn* 1962; 140:180–188.

268. Moe GK, Rheinboldt WC, Abildskov JA. A computer model of atrial fibrillation. *Am Heart J* 1964; 67:200–220.

269. Coumel P. Role of the autonomic nervous system in paroxysmal atrial fibrillation. In: Touboul P, Waldo AL (eds). *Atrial Arrhythmias.* St Louis: Mosby–Year Book; 1990:248–261.

270. Allessie MA, Lammers WJEP, Bonke FIM, Hollen J. Experimental evaluation of Moe's multiple wavelet hypothesis of atrial fibrillation. In: Zipes DP, Jalife J (eds). *Cardiac Electrophysiology and Arrhythmias.* New York: Grune & Stratton, 1985:265–275.

271. Waldo AL. Mechanisms of atrial fibrillation, atrial flutter, and ectopic atrial tachycardia—A brief review. *Circulation* 1987; 75-III:37–40.

272. Allessie MA, Bonke FIM, Schopman FJG. Circus movement in rabbit atrial muscle as a mechanism of tachycardia: 3. The "leading circle" concept—A new model of circus movement in cardiac tissue without the involvement of an anatomical obstacle. *Circ Res* 1977; 41:9–18.

273. Allessie MA, Lammers WJEP, Bonke FIM, Hollen J. Intra-atrial reentry as a mechanism for atrial flutter by acetylcholine and rapid pacing in the dog. *Circulation* 1984; 70:123–135.

274. Okumura K, Plumb VJ, Pagé PL, Waldo AL. Atrial activation sequence during atrial flutter in the canine pericarditis model and its effects on the polarity of the flutter wave in the electrocardiogram. *J Am Coll Cardiol* 1991; 17:509–518.

275. Cosío FG: Endocardial mapping of atrial flutter. In: Touboul P, Waldo AL (eds). *Atrial Arrhythmias—Current Concepts and Management.* St Louis: Mosby–Year Book; 1990:229–240.

276. Spinelli W, Hoffman BF. Mechanisms of termination of reentrant atrial arrhythmias by class I and class III antiarrhythmic agents. *Circ Res* 1989; 65:1565–1579.

277. Wit AL, Dillon SM. Anisotropic reentry. In: Zipes DP, Jalife J (eds). *Cardiac Electrophysiology—From Cell to Bedside.* Philadelphia: Saunders; 1990:353–364.

278. Allessie MA, Bonke FIM, Schopman FJG. Circus movement in rabbit atrial muscle as a mechanism of tachycardia. *Circ Res* 1973; 32:54–62.

279. Dillon S, Allessie MA, Ursell PC, Wit AL: Influence of anisotropic tissue structure on reentrant circuits and the sub-epicardial border zone of subacute canine infarcts. *Circ Res* 1988; 63:182–206.

280. Schalij MJ: Anisotropic conduction and ventricular tachycardia. PhD thesis. Maastricht, The Netherlands: University of Limburg; 1988.

281. Peters NS, Coromilas J, Costeas CA, DeRuyter B, Wit AL. Variation of the excitable gap permits preexcitation without reset of reentrant ventricular tachycardia circuits. *Circulation* 1993; 88 (Part 4, #2):I–117.

282. Winfree AT. Electrical instability in cardiac muscle: Phase singularities and rotors. *J Theor Biol* 1989; 138:353–405.

283. Winfree AT. Ventricular reentry in three dimensions. In: Zipes DP, Jalife J (eds). *Cardiac Electrophysiology: From Cell to Bedside.* Philadelphia: Saunders; 1990:224–234.

284. Courtemanche M, Winfree AT. Re-entrant rotating waves in a Beeler-Reuter based model of two-dimensional cardiac electrical activity. *Int J Bifurc Chaos* 1991; 1:431–444.

285. Davidenko JM, Kent PF, Chialvo DR, Michaels DC, Jalife J. Sustained vortex-like waves in normal isolated ventricular muscle. *Proc Natl Acad Sci USA* 1990; 87:8785–8789.

286. Jalife J, Davidenko J, Michaels DC. A new perspective on the mechanisms of arrhythmias and sudden cardiac death: Spiral waves of excitation in heart muscle. *J Cardiovasc Electrophysiol* 1991; 2(suppl 3):S133–S152.

287. Winfree AT. Vortex action potentials in normal ventricular muscle. In: Jalife J (ed). Mathematical Approaches to Cardiac Arrhythmias. *Ann NY Acad Sci* 1990; 591:190–207.

288. Shibata N, Chen P-S, Dixon EG, Wolf PD, Danieley ND, Smith WM, et al. Influence of shock strength and timing on induction of ventricular arrhythmias in dogs. *Am J Physiol* 1988; 225:H891–H901.

289. Chen P-S, Wolf PD, Dixon EG, Danieley ND, Frazier DW, Smith WM, Ideker RE. Mechanism of ventricular vulnerability to single premature stimuli in open-chest dogs. *Circ Res* 1988; 62:1191–1209.

290. Mayer AG: Rhythmical pulsation in Scyphomedusae: II. *Pap Tortugas Lab Carnegie Inst Wash* 1908; 1:113–131.

291. Mines GR. On circulating excitation in heart muscles and their possible relations to tachycardia and fibrillation. *Trans R Soc Can* 1914; 8(ser III, sec IV):43–52.

292. Goldreyer BN, Gallagher JJ, Damato AN. The electrophysiologic demonstration of atrial ectopic tachycardia in man. *Am Heart J* 1973; 85:205–215.

293. Scheinman MM, Basu D, Holenberg M. Electrophysiologic studies in patients with persistent atrial tachycardia. *Circulation* 1974; 50:266–273.

294. Strauss HC, Saroff AL, Bigger JT Jr, Giardina GV. Premature atrial stimulation as a key to the understanding of sinoatrial conduction in man: Presentation of data and critical review of the literature. *Circulation* 1973; 47:86–93.

295. Gillette PC, Garson A Jr. Electrophysiologic and pharmacologic characteristics of automatic ectopic atrial tachycardia. *Circulation* 1977; 56:571–575.

296. Klein HO, Cranefield PF, Hoffman BF. Effect of extrasystoles on idioventricular rhythm. *Circ Res* 1972; 30:651–665.

297. Palileo EV, Ashley WW, Swiryn S, Bauernfeind RA, Strasberg B, Petropoulis AT, et al. Exercise provokable right ventricular outflow tract tachycardia. *Am Heart J* 1982; 104:185–193.

298. Sung RJ, Shen EN, Morady F, Scheinman MM, Hess D, Botvinick CH. Electrophysiologic mechanism of exercise-induced sustained ventricular tachycardia. *Am J Cardiol* 1983; 51:525–530.

299. Wellens HJJ. Value and limitations of programmed electrical stimulation of the heart in the study and treatment of tachycardias. *Circulation* 1978; 57:845–853.

300. Goldreyer BN, Bigger JT Jr. Site of reentry in paroxysmal supraventricular tachycardia in man. *Circulation* 1971; 43:15–26.

301. Bigger JT Jr, Goldreyer BN. The mechanism of supraventricular tachycardia. *Circulation* 1970; 42:673–688.

302. Waldo AL. Cardiac pacing: Role in diagnosis and treatment of disorders of cardiac rhythm and conduction. In: Rosen MRR, Hoffman BF (eds). *Cardiac Therapy.* Boston: Martinus Nijhoff; 1983:299–336.

303. Waldo AL, MacLean WAH, Karp RB, Kouchoukos NT, James TN. Entrainment and interruption of atrial flutter with atrial pacing: Studies in man following open heart surgery. *Circulation* 1977; 56:737–744.

304. Waldo AL, Plumb VJ, Henthorn RW. Observations on the mechanism of atrial flutter. In: Surawicz B, Reddy CP, Prystowsky EN (eds). *Tachycardias.* The Hague: Martinus Nijhoff; 1984:213–229.

305. Olshansky B, Okumura K, Henthorn RW, Waldo AL. Characterization of double potentials in human atrial flutter: Studies during transient entrainment. *J Am Coll Cardiol* 1990; 15:833–841.

306. Waldo AL. Some observations concerning atrial flutter in man. *PACE* 1983; 6:1181–1189.

307. MacLean WAH, Plumb VJ, Waldo AL. Transient entrainment and interruption of ventricular tachycardia. *PACE* 1981; 4:358–366.

308. Waldo AL, Henthorn RW, Plumb VJ, MacLean WAH. Demonstration of the mechanism of transient entrainment and interruption of ventricular tachycardia with rapid atrial pacing. *J Am Coll Cardiol* 1984; 3:422–430.

309. Okumura K, Olshansky B, Henthorn RW, Epstein AE, Plumb VJ, Waldo AL. Demonstration of the presence of slow conduction during sustained ventricular tachycardia in man. *Circulation* 1987; 75:369–378.

310. Waldo AL, Plumb VJ, Arciniegas JG, MacLean WAH, Cooper TB, Priest MF, et al. Transient entrainment and interruption of AV bypass pathway type paroxysmal atrial tachycardia: A model for understanding and identifying reentrant arrhythmias in man. *Circulation* 1982; 67:73–83.

311. Okumura K, Henthorn RW, Epstein AE, Plumb VJ, Waldo AL. Further observations on transient entrainment: Importance of pacing site and properties of the components of the reentry circuit. *Circulation* 1985; 72:1293–1307.

312. Brugada P, Waldo AL, Wellens HJJ. Transient entrainment and interruption of atrioventricular tachycardia. *J Am Coll Cardiol* 1987; 9:769–775.

313. Henthron RW, Okumura K, Olshansky B, Waldo AL. A fourth criterion for transient entrainment: The electrogram equivalent of progressive fusion. *Circulation* 1988; 77:1003–1012.

314. Chen P-S, Lowe JE, German LD, Vidaillet HJ Jr, Greer GS, Smith WM, et al. Mapping ventricular fusion beats during entrainment. *Circulation* 1986; 74-II:484.

315. El-Sherif N, Gough WB, Restivo M. Reentrant ventricular arrhythmias in the late myocardial infarction period: 14. Mechanisms of resetting, entrainment, acceleration, or termination of reentrant tachycardia by programmed electrical stimulation. *PACE* 1987; 10:341–371.

316. Waldecker B, Coromilas J, Saltman AE, Dillon SM, Wit AL. Overdrive stimulation of functional reentrant circuits causing ventricular tachycardia in the infarcted canine heart—Resetting and entrainment. *Circulation* 1993; 87:1286–1305.

317. Boyden PA, Frame LH, Hoffman BF. Activation mapping of reentry around an anatomic barrier in the canine atrium. *Circulation* 1989; 79:406–416.

318. Shimizu A, Nozaki A, Rudy Y, Waldo AL. Multiplexing studies of effects of rapid atrial pacing on the area of slow conduction during atrial flutter in canine pericarditis model. *Circulation* 1991; 83:983–994.

319. Frank R, Tonet JL, Kounde S, Farenq G, Fontaine G. Localization of the area of slow conduction during ventricular tachycardia. In: Brugada P, Wellen HJJ (eds). *Cardiac Arrhythmias: Where to Go From Here?* Mount Kisco, NY: Futura; 1987:191–208.

320. Morady F, Frank R, Kou WH, Tonet JL, Nelson SD, Kounde S, et al. Identification and catheter ablation of a zone of slow conduction in the reentrant circuit of ventricular tachycardia in humans. *J Am Coll Cardiol* 1988; 11:775–782.

321. Stevenson WG, Weiss JN, Wiener I, Nademanee K, Wohlgelernter D, Yeatman L, et al. Resetting of ventricular tachycardia: Implications for localizing the area of slow conduction. *J Am Coll Cardiol* 1988; 11:522–529.

322. Almendral JM, Rosenthal ME, Stamato NJ, Marchlinski FE, Buxton AE, Frame LH, et al. Analysis of the resetting phenomenon in sustained uniform ventricular tachycardia: Incidence and relation to termination. *J Am Coll Cardiol* 1986; 8:294–300.

323. Almendral JM, Stamato NJ, Rosenthal ME, Marchlinski FE, Miller JM, Josephson ME. Resetting response patterns during sustained ventricular tachycardia: Relationship to the excitable gap. *Circulation* 1986; 74:722–730.

324. Stamato NJ, Rosenthal ME, Almendral JM, Josephson ME. The resetting response ventricular tachycardia to single and double extrastimuli: Implications for an excitable gap. *Am J Cardiol* 1987; 60:596–601.

325. Bernstein RC, Frame LH. Ventricular reentry around a fixed barrier: Resetting with advancement in an in vitro model. *Circulation* 1990; 81:267–280.

326. Frame LH, Page RL, Hoffman BF. Atrial reentry around an anatomic barrier with a partially refractory excitable gap. *Circ Res* 1986; 58:495–511.

327. Rosen MR, Fisch C, Hoffman BF, Danilo P, Lovace DE, Knoebel SB. Can accelerated atrioventricular junctional escape rhythms be explained by delayed afterdepolarizations? *Am J Cardiol* 1980; 45:1272–1284.

328. Rosen MR, Reder RF. Does triggered activity have a role in the genesis of cardiac arrhythmias? *Ann Intern Med* 1981; 94:794–801.

329. Gorgels APM, Beekman HDM, Brugada P, Dassen WRM, Richards DAB, Wellens HJJ. Extrastimulus-related shortening of the first post pacing interval in digitalis-induced ventricular tachycardia: Observations during programmed electrical stimulation in the conscious dog. *J Am Coll Cardiol* 1983; 1:840–857.

330. Wit AL, Rosen MR. Afterdepolarizations and triggered activity. In: Fozzard HA, Jennings RB, Haber E, et al (eds). *The Heart and Cardiovascular System: Scientific Foundations.* New York: Raven Press; 1986:1449–1490.

331. Akhtar M. Supraventricular tachycardias: Electrophysiologic mechanisms, diagnosis, and pharmacologic therapy. In: Josephson ME, Wellens HJJ (eds). *Tachycardias: Mechanisms, Diagnosis, Treatment.* Philadelphia: Lea & Febiger; 1984:137–169.

332. Josephson ME, Marchlinski FE, Buxton AE, Waxman HL, Doherty JU, Kienzle MG, et al. Electrophysiologic basis for sustained ventricular tachycardia—Role of reentry. In: Josephson ME, Wellens HJJ (eds). *Tachycardias: Mechanisms, Diagnosis, Treatment.* Philadelphia: Lea & Febiger; 1984:305–323.

333. Vos MA, Gorgels APM, Leunisse JDM, Brugada P, Wellens HJJ. The effect of an entrainment protocol on ouabain-induced ventricular tachycardia. *PACE* 1989; 12:1485–1493.

334. Brugada P, Wellens HJJ. Programmed electrical stimulation of the human heart: General principles. In: Josephson ME, Wellens HJJ (eds). *Tachycardias: Mechanisms, Diagnosis, Treatment.* Philadelphia: Lea & Febiger; 1984:61–89.

335. Jackman WM, Clark M, Friday KJ, Aliot EM, Anderson J, Lazzara R. Ventricular tachyarrhythmias in the long QT syndromes. *Med Clin North Am* 1984; 68:1079–1109.

336. Schecter E, Freeman CC, Lazzara R. Afterdepolarizations as a mechanism for the long QT syndrome. Electrophysiologic studies of a case. *J Am Coll Cardiol* 1984; 3:1556–1561.

337. Coumel P, LeClercq J, Dessertenne F. Torsades de pointes. In: Josephson ME, Wellens HJJ (eds). *Tachycardia: Mechanisms, Diagnosis, Treatment.* Philadelphia: Lea & Febiger; 1984:325–351.

RECOGNITION, CLINICAL ASSESSMENT, AND MANAGEMENT OF ARRHYTHMIAS AND CONDUCTION DISTURBANCES

Robert J. Myerburg / Kenneth M. Kessler / Agustin Castellanos

The diagnosis and management of cardiac arrhythmias and conduction disturbances can be structured in an algorithm consisting of three interacting components: (1) electrocardiographic analysis of the rhythm disturbance, (2) assessment of the clinical setting, and (3) identification of an endpoint and method of therapy.[1]

Electrocardiographic recognition of arrhythmias requires an organized system of analysis of atrial and ventricular myocardial activation and deduction of atrioventricular (AV) conduction patterns. Forms of arrhythmias are separated into those ambient events that cause only limited symptoms, but may be triggering arrhythmias under appropriate conditions,[2] (e.g., premature atrial or ventricular impulses), and those that are sustained symptomatic and/or potentially fatal arrhythmias [e.g., supraventricular tachycardias (SVTs), ventricular tachycardias (VTs), ventricular fibrillation (VF) or bradycardias] (Table 27-1).

Clinical settings are broadly divided into those that cause acute or transient electrophysiologic abnormalities, such as acute ischemia, the acute phase of myocardial infarction, electrolyte disturbances, or proarrhythmic effects of antiarrhythmic drugs, and those that are chronic and provide the substrate for persistent or recurrent arrhythmias. Commonly, the latter include chronic ischemic heart disease, cardiomyopathies, and the anatomic and physiologic substrate for the various paroxysmal supraventricular tachyarrhythmias.[3] Analogous to the concept of "triggering" and "sustained" arrhythmias, transient ischemia or hemodynamic disturbances may be viewed as *triggering events* and chronic ischemic heart disease, or the hypertrophied or myopathic heart, as sustaining *substrates*.

The goals, or endpoints, of therapy of cardiac arrhythmias are dependent on the forms, clinical settings, and mechanisms of arrhythmia. Broadly, goals of treatment may be antiarrhythmic (targeted to the suppression of ambient or triggering arrhythmias or events) or antitachycardiac, antifibrillatory, or heart-rate supporting (in which the goal is prevention or reversion of sustained arrhythmias), whether the arrhythmias are well tolerated, symptomatic, or life-threatening.

TABLE 27-1

ASSESSMENT OF CARDIAC ARRHYTHMIAS

Forms of cardiac arrhythmias
  Ambient or triggering arrhythmias (e.g., premature atrial or ventricular impulses)
  Sustained or potentially lethal arrhythmias (e.g., supraventricular or ventricular tachycardias, ventricular fibrillation, sustained bradyarrhythmias)
Clinical settings in which arrhythmias occur
  Acute, transient (e.g., acute ischemic events, metabolic disturbances)
  Chronic, persistent, recurrent (e.g., chronic ischemic heart disease, cardiomyopathy, anatomic/physiologic substrate for paroxysmal supraventricular tachycardia, chronic conducting system disease)
Endpoints of management
  Antiarrhythmia (suppress ambient/triggering arrhythmias)
  Antitachycardia/antifibrillatory (prevent or revert tachycardias or fibrillation)
  Heart rate support (prevent symptomatic bradycardias)

Source: Modified from Myerburg et al.,[1] with permission of the American Heart Journal.

PRINCIPLES OF CARDIAC RHYTHM ANALYSIS

The Standard Electrocardiogram

The standard 12-lead electrocardiogram (ECG) and rhythm strips provide a direct and easily accessible method for diagnosing disturbances of cardiac rhythm. The simultaneous 3-lead rhythm strip accompanying the 12-lead ECG on modern ECG machines, plus the option of recording a longer 1-lead rhythm strip, will yield sufficient information for a prompt and accurate diagnosis of most cardiac rhythms.

For many arrhythmias, analysis requires only the recognition of P-wave and QRS morphology, their relative timing, and their vectors. Simple inspection of the tracing may be sufficient, but the analysis of more complex arrhythmias is facilitated by the use of ladder diagrams. First used extensively by Sir Thomas Lewis, they are also referred to as *Lewis lines*. The ladders are usually constructed with three tiers—A, AV, and V (Fig. 27-1A)—but additional tiers may be helpful in depicting events related to sinoatrial (SA) conduction (Fig. 27-1B) or ventricular ectopic rhythms (Fig. 27-1C).

The A and V tiers are used to depict activation of atrial (A) and ventricular (V) muscle, respectively. The middle tier (AV) is used to infer conduction characteristics in the AV junction. Since atrial and ventricular activation are the only direct registrations of cardiac electrical activity on the standard

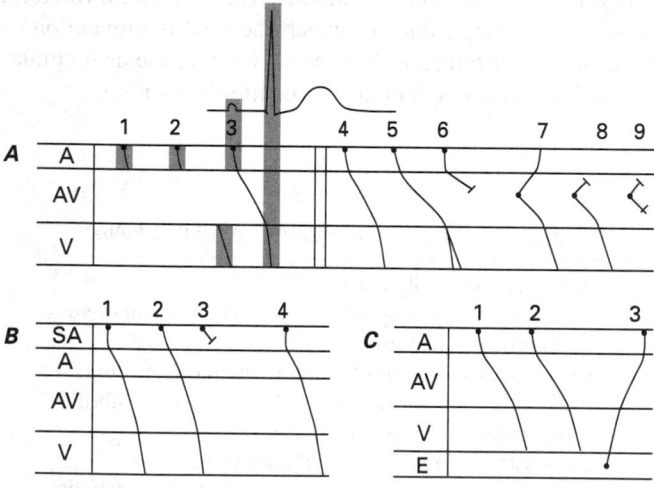

FIGURE 27-1

Ladder diagrams for analysis of cardiac arrhythmias. *A.* Charting of P wave and QRS complexes and deduction of conduction relationships for a normal sinus impulse are demonstrated in A1 to A3. The diversion of lines shown in the V level in A5 is used to indicate aberrant intraventricular conduction, and the incomplete cross-hatched line in the AV level in A6 represents an impulse blocked in the AV junction. The AV junctional impulses with retrograde and antegrade conduction (A7), retrograde block and antegrade conduction (A8), and block in both directions resulting in a concealed extrasystole (A9) are shown next. *B.* Diagram used to analyze sinoatrial conduction is demonstrated. A sinus impulse that fails to conduct to the atrium is indicated as in B3. *C.* Ventricular ectopic activity (E) is depicted as shown in C3, which represents a premature ventricular contraction with retrograde conduction to the atrium.

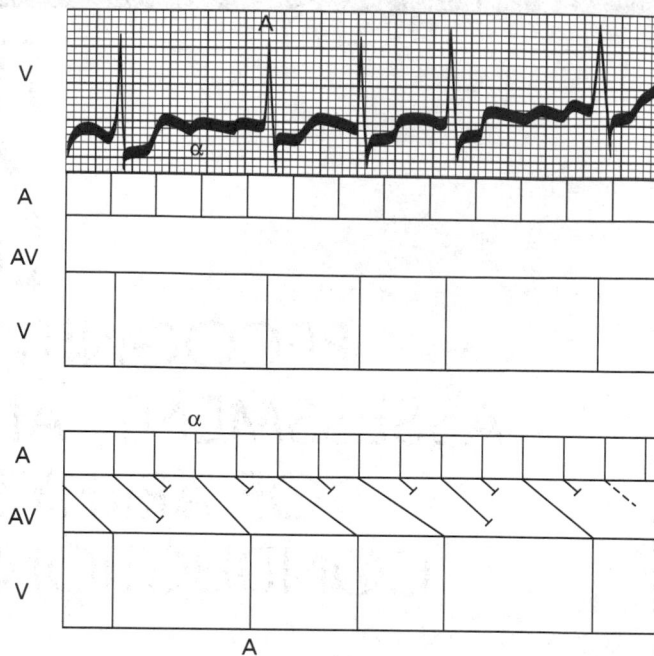

FIGURE 27-2

Construction of ladder diagrams for analyzing specific arrhythmias. *Stage 1:* Draw lines to represent atrial activity (seen and inferred by measurement) and ventricular complexes. *Stage 2:* Since in flutter the FR interval usually ranges between 0.26 and 0.45 s, start by connecting the F wave *a* to the QRS *A* in this example. As successive impulses are diagrammed, it becomes apparent that there is a basic 2:1 AV conduction with a Wenckebach period of the alternate cycles. (From Marriott HJL. Armchair arrhythmias. Tampa Tracings, 1966. Reproduced with permission.)

ECG, they are diagrammed first. The "A" line is drawn from the beginning of the P wave, and the "V" line from the beginning of the QRS. Time is indicated by the slope of the line, and the site within a tier in which impulse propagation begins (upper, middle, or lower) shows the direction the impulse is traveling. The site of origin may be represented by a black dot. A blocked impulse is indicated by a short bar at a right angle to the line indicating direction of conduction, and aberrant intraventricular conduction is shown as a pair of slightly divergent lines. A variety of such examples are shown in Fig. 27-1.

In using the diagram, particularly for complex arrhythmias, the first caution is to draw only what can be seen or inferred with certainty. Subsequently, the AV tier can be used to diagram proposed mechanisms of conduction (Fig. 27-2).

Special Leads

When the standard ECG does not provide sufficient information to establish a diagnosis, usually due to inability to identify P waves, special lead systems may be used. A bipolar esophageal lead can record left atrial activity, and an intraatrial electrode catheter can record atrial activity from within the right atrium. For both techniques, it is necessary to have at least one standard surface ECG lead recorded simultaneously with the special lead.

Continuous Monitor Recordings

Continuous monitoring of cardiac rhythm may be performed in hospital in special care units or in the ambulatory patient using various types of portable recording devices. Both types of systems now provide the capability for simultaneous two-lead recordings that improve diagnostic yield considerably. Long-term storage capabilities for inpatient monitoring permit off-line analysis of complex rhythm disturbances if the physician is not available at the time the arrhythmia occurs. The two most popular leads for use in bedside monitoring are lead II and MCL-I, the latter providing a pattern similar to V_1. For infrequently occurring arrhythmias, a number of "event recorders" are now available. They allow the patient to activate the device when an event occurs, providing internal storage that can be transmitted by telephone to a central station for later review. Transtelephonic transmitters also can be used in real time for more persistent or frequent events.

Exercise Testing for Cardiac Arrhythmias

Treadmill stress testing may be used to initiate an evanescent arrhythmia, document an exercise relationship to its onset, and evaluate both efficacy of therapy and adverse responses in some circumstances. The standard treadmill is used, and thallium or echocardiographic imaging is not necessary unless an ischemic basis correlating with the onset of arrhythmia is suspected. The procedure is especially useful for eliciting and evaluating therapy of exercise-induced ventricular arrhythmias [either premature ventricular contractions (PVCs) or VT], for distinguishing between autonomic and structural disease mechanisms for sinus or AV node dysfunction, and for evaluating adverse effects of drug therapy, such as rate-dependent proarrhythmic effects (see below). It may also provide some general insight into the refractory periods of accessory pathways in the Wolff-Parkinson-White (WPW) syndrome.

Signal-Averaged Electrocardiography; Heart Rate Variability; Baroreceptor Sensitivity

These three techniques provide information on the probability of life-threatening arrhythmias, whether used separately or combined with other estimates of risk [e.g., PVCs and nonsustained VT on 24-h ambulatory monitoring, ejection fraction (EF) measurements]. They have been applied most intensively after myocardial infarction.

Signal-averaged electrocardiography employs amplification of low-amplitude signals occurring after the termination of the standard electrocardiographic QRS complex, as recorded by high-amplification techniques. The low-amplitude signals are repetitive electrical events caused by a delayed activation sequence of part(s) of the ventricular muscle mass. Their repetitive timing allows them to be amplified during signal averaging, while random noise is being canceled out. The resultant signal is a high-gain, high-frequency QRS complex, followed by low-amplitude signals representing the late

potentials. The terminal delayed activation pattern represents a pathophysiologic marker for susceptibility to ventricular arrhythmias. It results from fragmented activation in an area of delayed conduction, which is a well-established substrate for reentrant arrhythmias.

Although no one set of standard definitions is universally accepted, the general characteristics of an abnormal signal-averaged ECG include: (1) a prolonged filtered QRS complex ($\geq$115 ms) with a normal duration of the standard QRS complex; (2) the terminal portion of the filtered QRS complex <40 μV for $\geq$39 ms; and (3) less than 20 μV of amplitude during the last 40 ms of the filtered QRS complex.[4] At least two of the three criteria must be abnormal to consider the tracing abnormal, and many would require all three to be abnormal (Fig. 27-3). Residual high-frequency noise content must be <1 μV with a 25-Hz high-pass cut-off (<0.7 μV with a 40-Hz high-pass cut-off).

Signal-averaged electrocardiography is most useful for demonstrating presence and absence of risk for ventricular arrhythmias and sudden death after myocardial infarction.[5] It is most powerful as a negative predictor of risk, in that a normal signal-averaged ECG after healing of myocardial infarction identifies a >97 percent probability of remaining free of ventricular arrhythmias. The positive predictive accuracy is less powerful and is heavily influenced by other variables, such as EF and ambient ventricular arrhythmias. Signal-averaged electrocardiography alone has a positive predictive value in the range of 20 percent, and combined with a low EF and ambient arrhythmias, the risk may be as high as 50 percent in some subgroups (see "Ventricular Arrhythmias," below).

Heart rate variability studies provide estimates of sympathetic and parasympathetic balance.[6] The normal patterns of variability of sinus rate over time are blunted in subgroups of myocardial infarction and cardiac arrest survivors who appear to be at increased risk for recurrent events.[6,7] As is the case for signal-averaged electrocardiography, the test is used primarily for prognostic information rather than as a therapeutic guide.

Baroreceptor sensitivity estimates the relationship between phenylephrine-induced blood pressure increase and concomitant fall in heart rate, as an indication of parasympathetic responsiveness to the pure α-adrenergic stimulus.[8] Following a myocardial infarction, a *blunted* baroreceptor sensitivity predicts an increased risk of VT and death. A recent large study also demonstrated its power for predicting adverse outcome following a myocardial infarction, which was further enhanced when combined with other risk variables, such as low EF and ambient arrhythmias.[9]

Intracardiac Electrocardiography and Electrophysiologic Studies

These procedures, which are described in detail in Chap. 29, can be used to diagnose many disturbances in rhythm and conduction for which surface electrocardiography is insufficient. Intracardiac electrophysiologic studies are also used

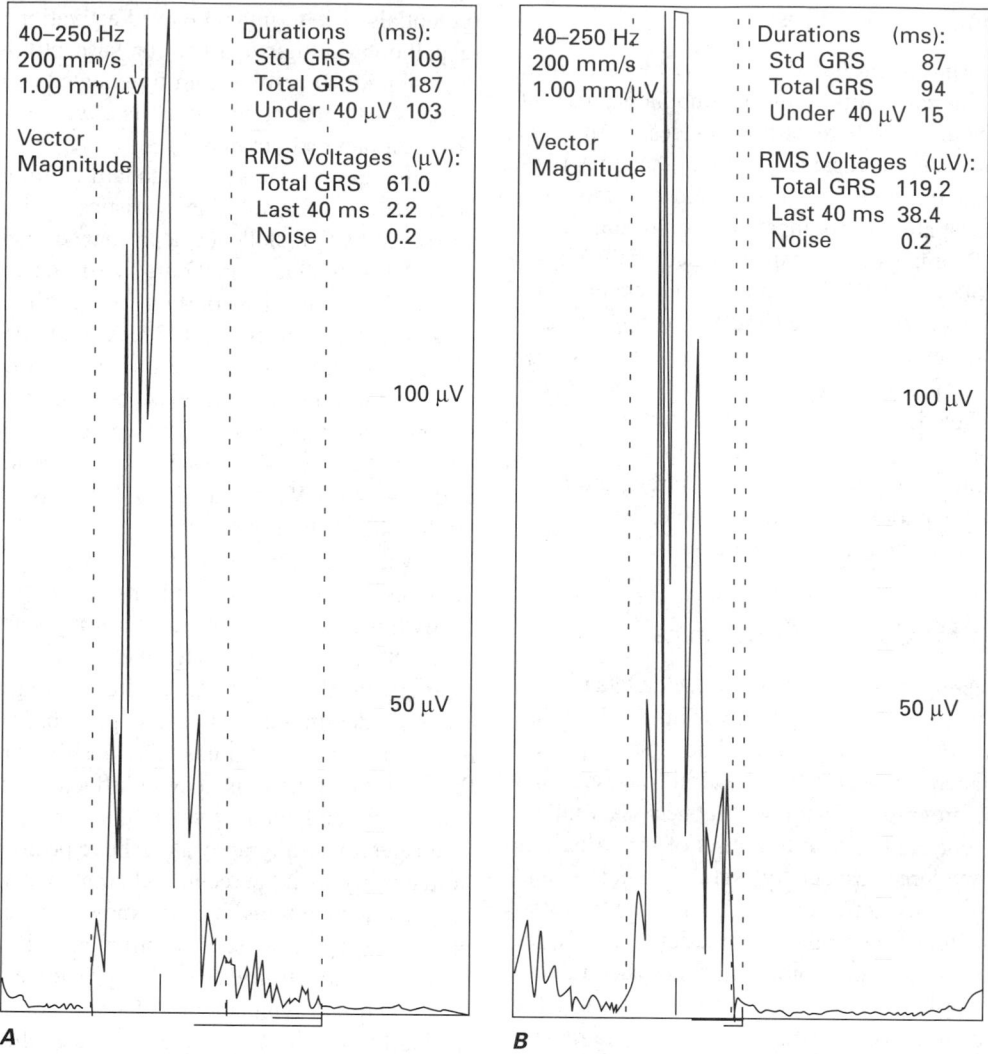

FIGURE 27-3

A. Normal signal-averaged vector complex. *B.* Abnormal signal-averaged vector complex. All three signal-averaged measurements are abnormal. The signal-averaged QRS duration is 187 ms, low-amplitude signals are 103 ms in duration, and the root-mean-square voltage is 2.2 μV. (Courtesy of Paul F. Walter, M.D.)

to define appropriate therapy and to test the results of therapy for various forms of supraventricular and ventricular arrhythmias. The use of multicatheter electrode systems, providing simultaneous recordings from many intracardiac sites (Fig. 27-4), allows mapping of the sequence of excitation in the atria, AV junction, and ventricle. Intracardiac mapping procedures permit the identification of sites of accessory pathways, mechanisms of ventricular tachyarrhythmias, and the reentrant pathways or sites of origin of supraventricular tachyarrhythmias. Such techniques provide the basis for electrocardiographically guided therapy such as radiofrequency (RF) ablation. In addition, the distinction between AV block above and below the level of the bundle of His, and between true AV block and pseudo-AV block caused by concealed extrasystoles, is also possible. Specific clinical applications are provided in the appropriate sections below and in Chap. 29.

Intraoperative Multiarray Epicardial Mapping and Endocardial Catheter Mapping

Mapping of pathways and sites of origin for both ventricular and supraventricular tachyarrhythmias has greatly improved both surgical results and the use of catheter techniques for nonsurgical ablation procedures. Multiple electrode arrays allow simultaneous recordings from many points during the same cardiac cycle, generating maps of activation during a surgical procedure. This technology allows the clinical electrophysiologist and surgeon to identify target areas for surgical ablation. Figure 27-5, Plate 48, provides an example of a computer-generated epicardial activation map from a multielectrode array, demonstrating the sequence of activation in

FIGURE 27-5

See color Plate 48.

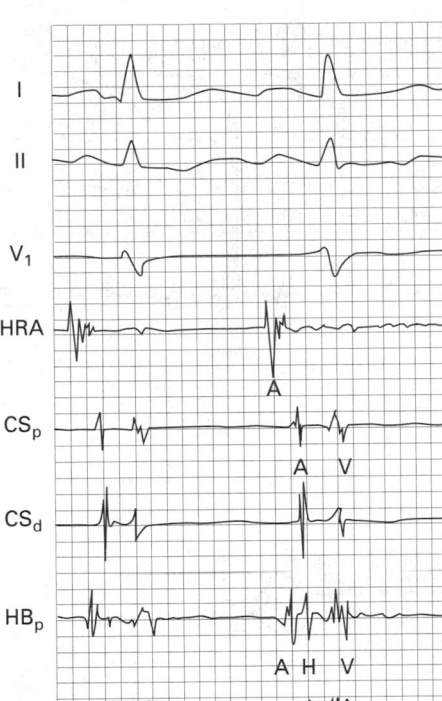

FIGURE 27-4

Intracardiac recordings during electrophysiologic testing. Recordings during sinus rhythm in a multicatheter study are illustrated. The comprehensive intracardiac study includes the recording of atrial activity (A), the His bundle deflection (H), and ventricular activity (V) used to determine the timing and sequences of activation at various intracardiac sites. A-activity is recorded from the high right atrium (HRA), and both A and V activity are recorded from a proximal (HB$_p$) and distal (HB$_d$) site in the His bundle region and from proximal (CS$_p$) and distal (CS$_d$) sites within the coronary sinus. The CS sites record atrial and ventricular activity from the posterior/posteroseptal and posterolateral/lateral areas, respectively. V-activity is also recorded from the right ventricle (RV), either the apex or outflow tract, depending upon the positioning of the catheter in the right ventricle. For more detailed mapping procedures, more sites in the coronary sinus or sites around the tricuspid ring can be recorded, or the left ventricle can be mapped by a retrograde recording catheter from the femoral artery. Less extensive studies using fewer catheters and recording sites can be used for different clinical purposes. The configuration shown is standard for studies of supraventricular tachycardias. For ventricular tachycardia studies, three catheters can be used (HRA, HB, RV) for the diagnostic study.

a patient with VT undergoing surgery for the arrhythmia. Although quite successful in prior years, intraoperative mapping for WPW syndrome has been largely displaced by catheter mapping and ablation techniques, except for a few specific clinical circumstances (see below). The technique of left ventricular (LV) endocardial catheter mapping for identification of sites appropriate for catheter ablation of VT is demonstrated in Fig. 27-6.

OVERVIEW OF MANAGEMENT STRATEGIES

Management strategies for cardiac arrhythmias have become far more complex in recent years compared to the limited pharmacologic approaches of the past. There is better understanding of the underlying systemic and cardiac factors that can be modified to influence predisposition to arrhythmias, the range of indications for pharmacologic therapy has contracted, and nonpharmacologic interventions have been expanded (Table 27-2). Many patients now are managed with multiple interventions, with one therapeutic mode complementary to another.

TABLE 27-2

SUMMARY OF APPROACHES TO ARRHYTHMIA MANAGEMENT

General systemic interventions
  Respiratory support
  Hemodynamic support
  Metabolic and electrolyte control
  Neurophysiologic control
Electropharmacologic therapy
  Control triggering events
    Suppress triggering arrhythmias
    Prevent/reverse arrhythmogenic factors (e.g., antiischemic therapy, electrolyte replacement)
  Control sustained arrhythmias
    Acute interventions
    Chronic prevention
  Control ventricular rate
Catheter ablation procedures
  Paroxysmal supraventricular tachycardia
    AV nodal reentry
    WPW syndrome
    AV node modification in atrial fibrillation
    Atrial flutter
  Atrial, sinus node, and AV junctional tachycardias
  Ventricular tachycardias
Surgical intervention
  Antiarrhythmic surgery
    Anomalous pathways[a]
    Aneurysmectomy, endocardial resection
    Cryoablation
  Antiischemic surgery
  Structural heart disease surgery
Electronic devices
  Acute applications
    Cardioversion
    Defibrillation
    Temporary pacemakers
  Long-term applications
    Permanent pacemakers
    Implantable cardioverter defibrillators

[a] Limited clinical application at the time of this writing.

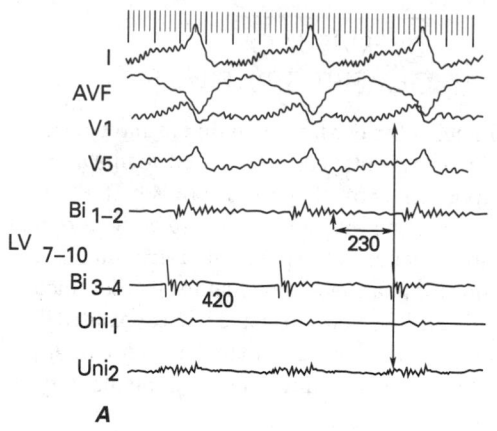

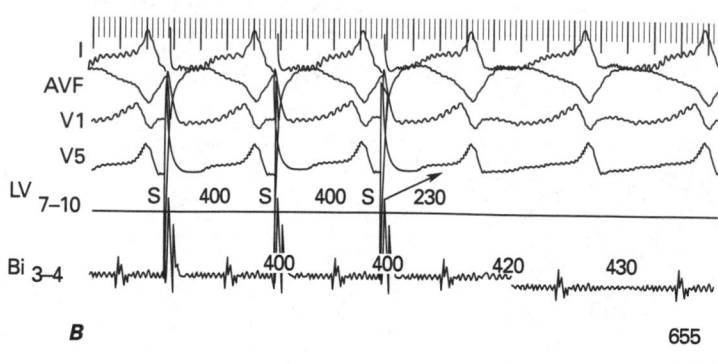

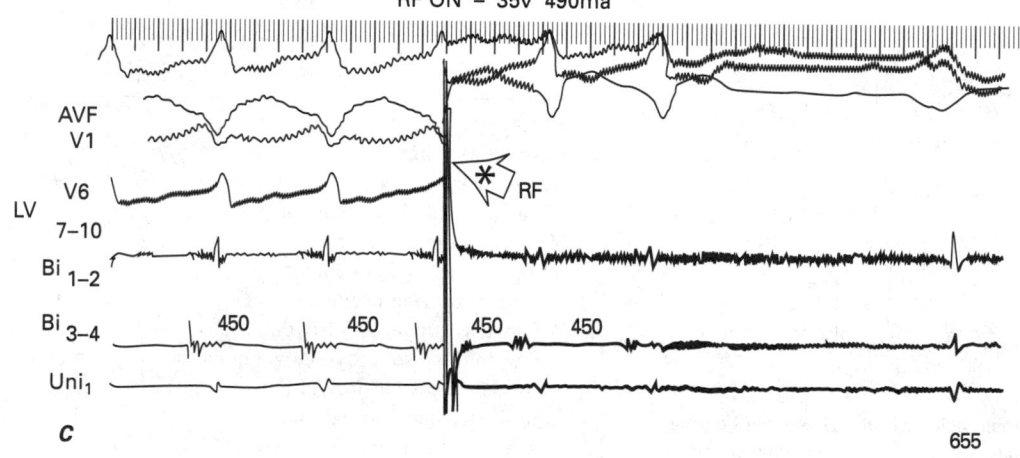

FIGURE 27-6

Left ventricular endocardial catheter mapping and radiofrequency ablation of ventricular tachycardia (VT) *A*. Bipolar (Bi) and Unipolar (Uni) recordings from an LV mapping site. The sustained ventricular tachycardia has a cycle length ranging from 420 to 450 ms. Onset of the VT QRS is indicated by the vertical line. Fractionated electrical activity is recorded from the distal bipolar electrode pair (Bi 1-2). A small potential immediately precedes the QRS onset, and fractionated signals extend 210 ms after the onset. *B*. The tachycardia is entrained during pacing and a cycle length of 400 ms [note the identical morphology of the complexes following pacing stimuli (concealed entrainment, entrainment with concealed fusion)], and a return to the spontaneous (unpaced) VT cycle length after cessation of pacing. The interval between the pacing stimulus and the onset of the responding QRS complex is the same as the interval between the end of the fractionated electrogram in *A* and the onset of the following QRS complex. *C*. Radiofrequency energy applied through a catheter positioned at the same location results in prompt termination of the tachycardia, loss of fractionated electrograms, and return to sinus rhythm. (From Stevenson WG, et al. Identification of reentry circuit sites during catheter mapping and radiofrequency ablation of ventricular tachycardia late after myocardial infarction. *Circulation* 1993; 88[part 1]:1647–1670. Reproduced with permission of the American Heart Association.)

A complete management plan for any arrhythmia must consider and distinguish between (1) an underlying structural etiology (coronary heart disease, cardiomyopathy, WPW syndrome, etc.) and (2) transient functional factors that interact with the underlying structural abnormality (e.g., hemodynamic, electrolyte, metabolic, and respiratory abnormalities) (see Table 27-3).[3,10] The identification of contributing factors, which interact with underlying etiology as the proximate cause of an arrhythmia, is inherent to any treatment plan. Contributing factors may be systemic or cardiac. The major systemic abnormalities include hemodynamic dysfunction, hypoxia, acidosis, electrolyte disturbances, toxic or proarrhythmic drug effects, and endocrine abnormalities. Central nervous system factors, including fluctuations in autonomic tone, may cause or aggravate specific arrhythmias. Prompt reversal of serious arrhythmias may follow control of these disturbances.

Primary and secondary arrhythmias must be distinguished for both management and prognosis. An arrhythmia that results from an electrophysiologic disturbance caused by a disease process, independent of a significant change in hemodynamic function, is defined as a *primary* arrhythmia; an arrhythmia that results from an electrical disturbance initiated by hemodynamic deterioration or metabolic abnormalities is a *secondary* arrhythmia (Fig. 27-7). In the former, antiarrhythmic drugs may be used prior to the development of a clinically manifest electrophysiologic disturbance (e.g., the use of lidocaine in patients with PVCs during acute myocardial infarction) or after an electrophysiologic abnormality has developed in order to prevent or revert a sustained primary arrhythmia. In secondary arrhythmias, the use of hemodynamically active drugs to support the failing circulation may prevent electrical disturbances; but once electrical disturbances develop, antiarrhythmic and hemodynamically active drugs have complementary roles.

Direct cardiac interventions for control of arrhythmias include pharmacologic approaches, ablation of specific foci involved in arrhythmogenesis, antiarrhythmic surgical approaches, and implantable devices designed to control tachyarrhythmic events or to prevent symptomatic bradyarrhythmias (Table 27-2). The antiarrhythmic drugs may be classified into groups using the modified Vaughn Williams system, which categorizes them on the basis of electropharmacologic and electrophysiologic properties (see Table 27-4). This classification is useful and practical for the clinician but has increasingly evident shortcomings. These include difficulty categorizing new drugs, exclusion of some drugs with obvious antiarrhythmic properties (e.g., adenosine), and inability to

TABLE 27-3
CAUSES OF CARDIAC ARRHYTHMIAS: STRUCTURE AND FUNCTION

Structural Abnormalities	Functional Factors
Coronary heart disease	Transient alterations of coronary blood flow
Acute myocardial infarction	Vasomotor dynamics
Chronic ischemic heart disease	Acute ischemia
Ventricular hypertrophy	Reperfusion after ischemia
Secondary left ventricular hypertrophy	Systemic factors
Hypertrophic cardiomyopathy	Hemodynamic fluctuations
Obstructive	Hypoxia, acidosis
Nonobstructive	Electrolyte imbalance
Myopathic ventricles	Neurophysiologic alterations
Dilated cardiomyopathy	Central nervous system influences
Pericarditis, myocarditis	Receptor function
Noninfectious inflammatory diseases	Neurotransmitters
Infiltrative diseases	Toxic substances
Structural electrophysiology abnormalities	Proarrhythmic drugs
Sinus node, AV node, and His-	Idiosyncratic
Purkinje disease	Dose-dependent
Accessory pathways	Cardiotoxic substances

Source: Modified from Myerburg et al.,[3] with permission of the American Journal of Cardiology.

correlate drug class with specific effects as antiarrhythmic agents. A new classification system, the Sicilian gambit,[11] has been developed for the purpose of providing deeper insight into drug effects, therapeutic targets, mechanisms of action, and responses (Fig. 27-8).

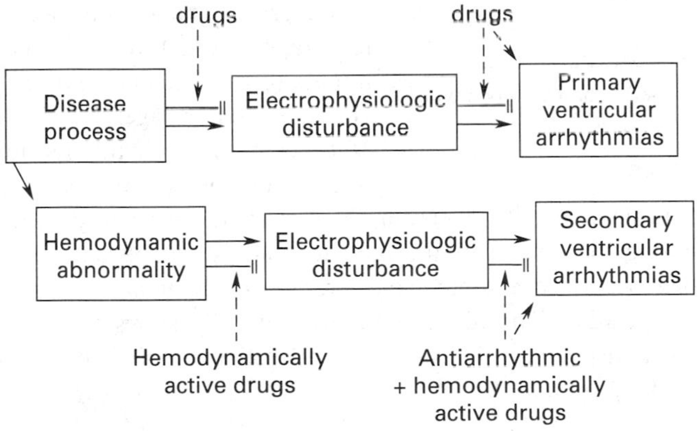

The usual dosages and routes of administration for the antiarrhythmic agents approved by the U.S. Food and Drug Administration at the time of writing are listed in Table 27-5. A number of other drugs are presently at various stages of study for ventricular and supraventricular arrhythmia indications.

SUPRAVENTRICULAR ARRHYTHMIAS

Sinus Rhythms and Sinus Tachycardia

The range of rates defining normal sinus rhythm is between 60 and 100 impulses per minute. The rhythm is usually regular, but when the variation between the longest and shortest cycle on a resting tracing exceeds 0.12 s, sinus arrhythmia is present (Fig. 27-9A). This normal variant is most common in children and decreases with advancing age. It is defined as *phasic sinus arrhythmia* if the cycle lengths shorten with inspiration and lengthens with expiration. If unrelated to the respiratory cycle, it is referred to as *nonphasic sinus arrhythmia.*

A sinus rhythm at a rate below 60 impulses per minute is defined as *sinus bradycardia* (Fig. 27-9C); its significance is much more dependent upon clinical circumstance than absolute rate (see "Sinus Bradycardia," below). It may be normal, even at rates in the mid-to-low 30s, in highly trained young athletes at rest, while it is generally considered abnormal even at rates in the high 40s in the elderly.

FIGURE 27-7

Primary and secondary arrhythmias. When a disease process directly initiates an electrophysiologic disturbance, the resulting arrhythmia is referred to as *primary.* In contrast, when the disease process produces a hemodynamic abnormality that in turn initiates the electrophysiologic disturbance, a resulting arrhythmia is referred to as *secondary.* Antiarrhythmic drugs may be used to prevent the electrophysiologic disturbance, prevent the electrophysiologically unstable heart from developing a manifest arrhythmia, or reverse a primary arrhythmia. In secondary arrhythmias, hemodynamically active drugs are used to prevent or reverse secondary electrophysiologic disturbances, usually in conjunction with antiarrhythmic drugs. Antiarrhythmic drugs alone are less likely to be effective for secondary arrhythmias. (Modified from Myerburg et al.[1] Reproduced with permission from the publisher.)

TABLE 27-4

MODIFIED VAUGN WILLIAMS CLASSIFICATION OF DRUGS APPROVED FOR ANTIARRHYTHMIC USES

Examples	Depolarization	Repolarization
Class I: Membrane-active drugs		
IA Quinidine (Quinaglute, Quinidex, Cardioquin)	Moderate depression of Na$^+$ current; intermediate kinetics	Prolonged
Procainamide (Pronestyl, Procan-SR)		
Disopyramide (Norpace)		
Moricizine (Ethmozine)		
IB Lidocaine (Xylocaine)	Limited depression of Na$^+$ current; rapid kinetics	No effect or shortened
Tocainide (Tonocard)		
Mexiletine (Mexitil)		
Phenytoin (Dilantin)		
IC Flecainide (Tambocor)	Marked depression of Na$^+$ current; slow kinetics	Minimal effect
Propafenone (Rhythmol)		
Class II: β-Adrenoceptor blocking drugs		
Propranolol (Inderal)		
Esmolol (Brevibloc)		
Acebutolol (Sectral)		
Class III: Drugs that prolong repolarization		
Amiodarone (Cordarone)		
Bretylium tosylate (Bretylol)		
Sotalol (Betapace)		
Ibutilide (Corvert)		
Class IV: Ca^{2+}-entry blocking drugs		
Verapamil (Isoptin, Calan)		
Diltiazem (Cardizem)		
Unclassified in this system		
Digoxin (Lanoxin)		
Adenosine (Adenocard)		

Note: Drugs identified by name are limited to those approved for antiarrhythmic use by the U.S. Food and Drug Administration at the time of this writing.

A sinus rate above 100 impulses per minute is defined as *sinus tachycardia*. Sinus rates in excess of 100 per minute are normal in infants and children under 2 years of age. Occasional normal adults will have resting sinus rates slightly in excess of 100 per minute. Faster and persistent inappropriate sinus tachycardia, probably mediated by autonomic factors, may cause disturbing or disabling symptoms.[12] If fast enough and persisting for months, it may precipitate a reversible form of tachycardia-induced heart failure.[13]

The category of physiologic sinus tachycardias includes the normal sinus rate responses to exercise, excitement, anxiety, and other emotional stresses. Pharmacologic sinus tachycardias result from medications such as epinephrine, ephedrine, amyl nitrate, isoproterenol, and atropine and may occur upon exposure to alcohol, nicotine, or caffeine. The heart rate responses are a result of the pharmacologic properties of these drugs. Pathologic sinus tachycardia may be secondary to noncardiac systemic factors or due to specific cardiac abnormali-

ties. Among the secondary causes are fever, hypoxemia, hemorrhage, hypotension, thyrotoxicosis, and anemia. Cardiovascular causes include congestive heart failure, myocardial infarction, and pulmonary embolism.

ELECTROCARDIOGRAPIC FEATURES

The ECG in sinus tachycardia reveals a rate in excess of 100 per minute accompanied by a normal PR relationship and a normal P-wave vector (Fig. 27-9*B*). The upper rate range of sinus tachycardia varies according to the patient's clinical status and factors responsible for the tachycardia. For instance, in the physiologic tachycardia group, the upper limit in the normal adult during exercise testing may range from 160 to 190 per minute, whereas the highly trained athlete may attain a rate of at least 200 per minute under maximal effort. In contrast, the pharmacologic tachycardias do not commonly induce a rate exceeding 130 per minute, whereas the rate that is secondary to pathologic causes may range from 120 to 140 per minute (e.g., hypotension, hypovolemia, hemorrhage, fever) to 160 per minute (hyperthyroidism, severe heart failure). In a persistent sinus tachycardia, the rate characteristically varies during the course of the day, in contrast to the fixed rate that occurs in ectopic tachycardias or AV nodal reentrant tachycardia. Carotid sinus massage usually slows the sinus rate transiently, with a return to the baseline rate after cessation of the procedure.

MANAGEMENT OF SINUS TACHYCARDIA

Sinus tachycardia, except when it is an appropriate response to acute physical or emotional stress, is usually categorized as persistent and is easily recognized. Its management almost always depends on control of exogenous or endogenous systemic factors or of an underlying cardiac disease. Its differentiation from other SVTs at rates of 150 or more a minute may be achieved with carotid sinus massage, which typically produces a gradual slowing followed by a gradual return to the baseline rate. Specific therapy is rarely required; when it is, β-adrenergic blockade will often achieve at least partial

DRUG	CHANNELS: NA Fast	NA Med	NA Slow	Ca	K	μ	RECEPTORS: α	β	M_2	P	PUMPS: Na-K ATPase	CLINICAL EFFECTS: Left ventricular function	Sinus Rate	Extra-cardiac	ECG EFFECTS: PR interval	QRS width	JT interval
Lidocaine	Low											→	→	Moderate			↓
Mexiletine	Low											→	→	Moderate			↓
Tocainide	Low											→	→	High			↓
Moricizine	High (I)											↓	→	Low		↑	
Procainamide		High (A)			Moderate							↓	→	High	↑	↑	↑
Disopyramide		High (A)			Moderate				Low			↓	→	Moderate	↑↓	↑	↑
Quinidine		High (A)			Moderate		Low		Low			→	↑	Moderate	↑↓	↑	↑
Propafenone		High (A)						Moderate				↓	↓	Low	↑	↑	
Flecainide			High (A)		Low							↓	→	Low	↑	↑	
Encainide			High (A)									↓	→	Low	↑	↑	
Bepridil	Low			High	Moderate							?	↓	Low			↑
Verapamil	Low			High			Moderate					↓	↓	Low	↑		
Diltiazem				Moderate								↓	↓	Low	↑		
Bretylium					High		Agonist/Antagonist	Agonist/Antagonist				→	↓	Low			↑
Sotalol					High			High				↓	↓	Low	↑		↑
Amiodarone	Low			Low	High		Moderate	Moderate				→	↓	Low	↑		↑
Alinidine					Moderate	High						?	↓	High			
Nadolol								High				↓	↓	Low	↑		
Propranolol	Low							High				↓	↓	Low	↑		
Atropine									High			→	↑	Moderate	↓		
Adenosine										Agonist		?	↓	Low	↑		
Digoxin									Agonist		High	↑	↓	High	↑		↓

Relative potency of block: ○ Low ⊜ Moderate ● High A = Activated state blocker
□ = Agonist ◪ = Agonist/Antagonist I = Inactivated state blocker

FIGURE 27-8
The Sicilian gambit approach to antiarrhythmic drugs. This figure summarizes the important actions of drugs on membrane channels, receptors, and ion pumps in the heart, as well as on the ECG, sinus rate, and left ventricular function. Because clinical and ECG effects are diverse, the table unavoidably includes some degree of subjectivity. Accordingly, the shading of the symbols and the direction of the arrows should not be taken as absolute. Moreover, the clinical information presented refers to the patient who does not have importantly compromised left ventricular function prior to the drug administration.

For the section on channels, receptors, and pumps, the actions of drugs on the sodium (Na^+), calcium (Ca^{2+}), potassium channels (I_K and I_f) are indicated. Sodium channel blockade is subdivided into three groups of actions characterized by fast (tau $<$ 300 ms), medium (tau = 200–1500 ms), and slow (tau $>$ 1500 ms) time constants for recovery from block. This parameter is a measure of use dependence and predicts the likelihood that a drug will decrease conduction velocity of normal Na^+-dependent tissues in the heart and perhaps the propensity of a drug for causing bundle branch block or proarrhythmia. The rate constant for onset of block might be even more clinically relevant. Blockade in the inactivated (I) or activated (A) state is indicated.

Drug interaction with receptors (α-adrenergic, β-adrenergic, muscarinic subtype 2 [M_2], and A_1 purinergic [P]), and drug effects on the sodium/potassium pump [Na^+, K^+-ATPase], are indicated. Filled triangles indicate antagonist or inhibitory actions; unfilled triangles indicate direct- or indirect-acting agonists or stimulators. The intensity of the action is indicated by the various shadings.

The absence of a symbol indicates lack of effect. The use of a question mark (?) indicates uncertainty concerning effect. The arrows in the clinical effect and ECG section indicate direction; no quantitative differentiation has been made between weak and strong effects. The effects listed for ECG, left ventricular function, sinus rate, and "extracardiac" are those that may be seen at therapeutic plasma levels. Deleterious effects that may appear with concentrations above the therapeutic range are not listed.

Antiarrhythmic drug actions. LVFX, left ventricular function. [From Schwartz PJ, Zaga A. The Sicilian Gambit revisited. *Eur Heart J* 1992; 13 (suppl F):23–29. Reproduced with permission.]

TABLE 27-5

ANTIARRHYTHMIC DRUGS: DOSAGE AND KINETICS

Drug	Usual Dosing Range[a]	Half-Life, h	Therapeutic Range, μg/mL	Plasma Protein Binding, %	Major Route of Excretion
Class IA					
Quinidine	Oral sulfate: 200–600 mg q 6 h	5–7	2.3–5	80	H
	Oral long acting: 330–660 mg, q 8 h or q 6 h				
Procainamide	Oral: 250–750 mg, q 4 h or q 6 h	3–5	4–10	15	R[b]
	Oral long-acting: 500–1500 mg, q 8 h or q 6 h				
	IV: 10–15 mg/kg at 25 mg/min, then 1–6 mg/min				
Disopyramide	Oral: 100–200 mg q 8 h or q 6 h	8–9	2–5	35–95	H/R
Moricizine[c]	Oral: 150–300 mg q 12 h to q 8 h	6–13	—	95	H
Class IB					
Lidocaine	IV:1–3 mg/kg at 20–50 mg/min, then 1–4 mg/min	1–2	1–5	60	H
Tocainide	Oral: 400–600 mg q 8–12 h	15	4–10	10	H
Mexiletine	Oral: 200–400 mg q 8 h	10–12	0.5–2.0	55	H
Class IC					
Flecainide	Oral: 100–200 mg q 12 h	20	0.4–1.0	40	H
Propafenone[d]	Oral: 150–300 mg q 8 h	2–10	0.5–1.5[e]	95	H
Class II					
Propanolol	Oral: 10–100 mg q 6 h	4–6	0.04–0.10	95	H
	IV: 0.1 mg/kg in divided 1-mg doses				
Esmolol	IV: 500 mg/kg per min × 1 min followed by 50 mg/kg per min × 4 min, repeat with 50-mg increments to maintenance dose to 200 mg/kg per min	9 min	—	55	H
Acebutolol	Oral: 200–600 mg b.i.d.	3–4	—	26	H/R
Class III					
Amiodarone	Oral: 600–1600 mg/day × 1–3 weeks, then 200–400 mg/day	50 days	1–2.5	96	H
	IV: 15 mg/min × 10 min, then 1 mg/min × 6 h, then maintenance at 0.5 mg/min	?	?		
Bretylium	IV: 5–10 mg/kg at 1–2 mg/kg, then 0.5–2.0 mg/min	8–14	0.5–1.5	—	R
Sotalol[d]	Oral: 80–320-mg q 12 h	10–15	—	0	R
Ibutilide	IV: (for >60 kg) 1 mg over 10 min; may repeat × 1 10 min after completion of initial dose[f]	2–12	—	40	H
Class IV					
Verapamil	Oral: 80–32 mg q 6–8 h	3–8	0.1–0.15	90	H
	IV: 5–10 mg in 1–2 min				
Diltiazem	IV: 0.25 mg/kg body wt over 2 min; if response inadequate, wait 15 min, then 0.35 mg/kg over 2 min; maintenance 10–15 mg/h	3.5–5.0	0.1–3.0	70–80	H
Other					
Digoxin	Oral: 1.25–1.5 mg in divided doses over 24 h followed by 0.125–0.375 mg/day	36	0.8–1.4 ng/mL	30	R
	IV: Approximately 70% of oral dose				
Adenosine	IV: 6 mg rapidly; if unsuccessful within 1–2 min, 12 mg rapidly	10 s	—	—	—

[a] All dosing should follow FDA-approved guidelines as outlined in package insert or *Physicians' Desk Reference*. See also Chap. 30. Does not include pediatric use in infants and young children.)

[b] Parent compound metabolized to active metabolite (NAPA) in liver; both active metabolite and unmetabolized parent compound excreted by kidneys.

[c] Shares classes IB, IC activities.

[d] Shares class II activity.

[e] Active metabolite limits significance of these measurements.

[f] D/C upon arrhythmia conversion or for ventricular tachycardia or prolongation of QT or QT_c.

Note: H, hepatic; R, renal.

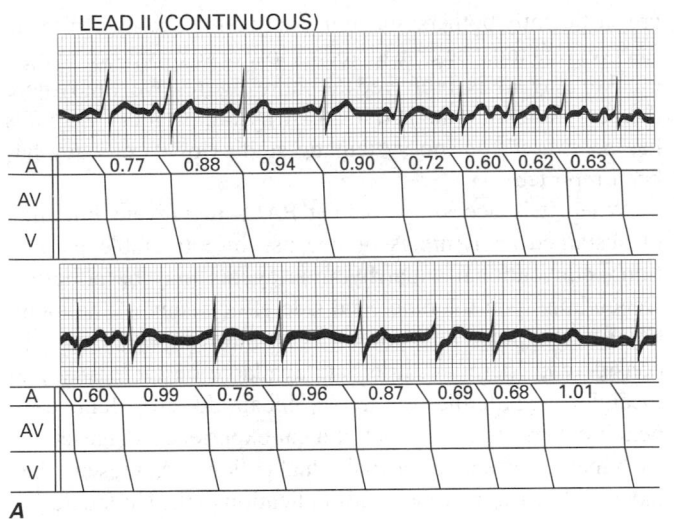

LEAD II (CONTINUOUS)

A

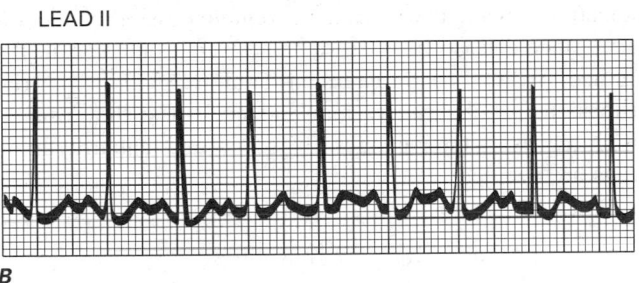

LEAD II

B

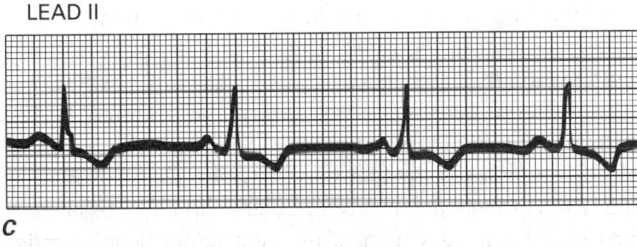

LEAD II

C

FIGURE 27-9

A. Sinus arrhythmia. The sinus cycles are indicated in seconds in the atrial (A) tier; they range from 0.60 to 1.01 s. Note that the P-wave amplitude increases as the sinus pacemaker accelerates. *B.* Sinus tachycardia. Note normally shaped and directed P waves, normal PR interval, and a rate of almost 150 per minute. *C.* Sinus bradycardia. Note normally directed (but abnormally wide) P waves, normal PR interval, and a rate of slightly more than 50 per minute.

control of the sinus rate. In uncomplicated acute myocardial infarction, the sinus rate may be controlled with small doses of propranolol (10 to 20 mg every 6 h). Persistent sinus tachycardia occurs in thyrotoxicosis, and higher doses of propranolol may be required for its control. Persistent sinus tachycardia during heart failure or hypovolemic states will respond promptly to an improving hemodynamic status as the primary problem is corrected. The chronic form of nonparoxysmal sinus tachycardia, symptomatic or associated with heart failure, may require RF energy modification or ablation of the sinus node area[14] if it is not controllable by drug therapy.

Premature Atrial Impulses

Atrial extrasystoles or premature atrial contractions (PACs) are extremely common and may occur in normal individuals or in the presence of systemic or cardiac abnormalities. They occur at any age, including infancy, and were observed in 0.4 percent of 122,000 asymptomatic healthy males, 16 to 50 years of age, in the U.S. Air Force.[15] Because of the cross-sectional nature of this data base and the limited electrocardiographic sample size per individual, the actual prevalence is likely to be considerably higher. Both endogenous (febrile illnesses, thyrotoxicosis, emotional stress, etc.) and exogenous (alcohol, tobacco, or caffeine consumption) systemic factors may initiate or worsen atrial extrasystolic activity. Among cardiac causes, myopericarditis, ischemia, heart failure, and digitalis intoxication are all precipitating or contributing factors.

ELECTROCARDIOGRAPHIC FEATURES

The PAC is characterized by (1) a P wave that occurs before the next expected sinus impulse, and (2) a change in the vector of the early P wave. The PR interval of the conducted PAC is usually normal or minimally prolonged (see Fig. 27-10). Much more marked prolongation of the PR interval occurs occasionally and may indicate the presence of dual AV nodal pathway physiology. More subtle electrocardiographic patterns include (1) superimposition of the premature P wave on the T wave of the preceding sinus impulse, and (2) an unexpected pause due to failure of conduction of a PAC to the ventricles. In both instances, careful inspection of the T wave of the sinus impulse before the PAC will reveal a distortion of the T wave, sometimes minimal, indicating the presence of the PAC. When the coupling interval of the PAC to the previous sinus P wave is short, aberrant intraventricular conduction makes the diagnosis dependent upon recognition of the P wave distorting the previous T wave (Fig. 27-10*B*). The hallmark of timing of PACs is the less than fully compensatory pause. Since the premature P wave commonly resets the sinus cycle, the PAC is bracketed by a cycle terminated by the early P wave and a return cycle close to the underlying sinus cycle length (Fig. 27-10*A*). The sum of the two cycles will be less than fully compensatory. Occasionally, fully compensatory pauses or longer than compensatory pauses occur because of failure to invade and reset the sinus node cycle or delay of its return because of overdrive suppression.

MANAGEMENT OF PREMATURE ATRIAL CONTRACTIONS

PACs usually do not require treatment, especially when they occur in normal individuals or when due to systemic influences or minor cardiac abnormalities such as mitral valve prolapse and acute viral pericarditis. When PACs may be triggering events[2] for sustained arrhythmias, their management may become important. Generally, SVT due to AV nodal reentry or the WPW syndrome, paroxysmal atrial fibrillation, or the rare instances of induction of sustained ventricular arrhythmia by supraventricular impulses are best managed by therapy tar-

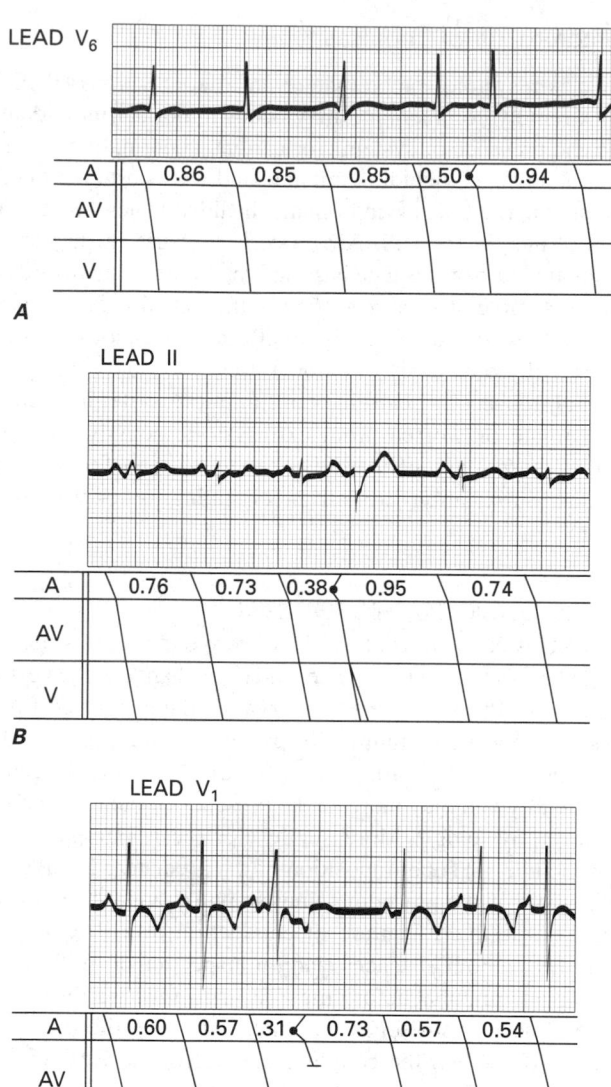

FIGURE 27-10

A. The fifth impulse is an atrial premature beat; there is a premature P wave (usually labelled P′) followed by a normal QRS-T complex, and the postextrasystolic pause is longer than the sinus cycle but less than compensatory. *B.* The fourth impulse is an atrial premature beat with aberrant intraventricular conduction; there is a premature P wave followed by an anomalous QRS-T complex; the postextrasystolic pause is less than compensatory. *C.* Nonconducted atrial premature beat. Following the third ventricular complex, a P′ wave negatively deforms the ST segment and is not followed by a ventricular response.

geted to the prevention of the sustained arrhythmias. But occasionally suppression of triggering PACs is helpful.

Annoying palpitations are a common symptom of PACs in patients who have either no underlying heart disease or mitral valve prolapse. Reassuring the patient of the benign nature of the arrhythmia may suffice, and no therapy is necessary other than removal of inciting factors such as cigarettes, coffee, alcohol, and excessive fatigue. When the palpitations

are sufficiently bothersome to impact on the quality of life, an intervention must be considered. A low dose of a β-adrenergic blocking agent is preferred to more aggressive (and more dangerous) membrane-active antiarrhythmic agents. Digitalis has been tried, but no systematic studies of its efficacy has been reported.

When it is necessary to treat PACs to prevent initiation of sustained arrhythmias or because of intolerable palpitations, conventional antiarrhythmic agents may be effective. Depending upon tolerance and side effects, any of the membrane-active drugs or β-adrenoceptor blocking agents may be considered. There are little data available on the efficacy of tocainide, mexiletine, flecainide, encainide, propafenone, or beta blockers for PACs, but clinical experience suggests that each may be effective for individual patients. At present, they have not been approved for this indication in the United States. Class IC (see Table 27-4) drugs should be avoided for this indication in patients with even the remote possibility of coronary artery disease because of the adverse outcome in the Cardiac Arrhythmia Suppression Trial (CAST).[16,17] Atrial distension in heart failure may induce PACs; they usually disappear as hemodynamics improve, and antiarrhythmic drugs are avoided.

Supraventricular Tachyarrhythmias

This category includes all tachyarrhythmias that originate above the bifurcation of the bundle of His or incorporate tissues proximal to the bifurcation of the bundle of His in a reentrant circuit. The diagnosis requires an atrial chamber rate of 100 or more per minute; the ventricular rate may be less when AV conduction is incomplete. SVTs usually have narrow QRS complexes, but they may be wide because of aberrant conduction through the intraventricular conducting tissue, participation of a bypass tract in the ventricular depolarization pattern, or in the presence of coexisting bundle branch block.

SVTs may be separated into three groups based on duration: brief paroxysms, persistent, and chronic. Arrhythmias that are paroxysmal in onset and offset [e.g., paroxysmal SVT (PSVT) due to AV nodal reentry or WPW syndrome, paroxysmal atrial fibrillation, paroxysmal atrial flutter] tend to be recurrent and of short duration—i.e., seconds to hours. Persistent tachycardias [e.g., sinus tachycardia, ectopic atrial tachycardia (nonparoxysmal), multifocal atrial tachycardia, longer episodes of PSVT or atrial flutter of fibrillation] may last for days or weeks and may be associated with a specific contributing pathophysiologic factor such as decompensated chronic obstructive pulmonary disease, pulmonary emboli, electrolyte disturbances, or drug toxicity. They tend to be recurrent when an underlying structural cause such as atrial disease or mitral valve disease is the dominant pathophysiologic factor. When a transient functional abnormality dominates, such as hypoxemia, heart failure, or an electrolyte abnormality, they may be isolated clinical events, reappearing only if or when the inciting event occurs. Longstanding or chronic SVTs (chronic atrial flutter, chronic atrial fibrillation) do not revert if untreated, often fail to revert even with attempted treatment, and if reverted will frequently recur despite therapy.

The management of an SVT is dictated by its mechanism and whether it is expressed as brief paroxysms, persistent tachycardias or chronic arrhythmias. Table 27-6 provides an overview of the methods available for management of acute and recurrent PSVTs.

THE REENTRANT PAROXYSMAL SUPRAVENTRICULAR TACHYCARDIAS

PSVT may be due to AV nodal reentry, the WPW syndrome, or intraatrial or sinus node reentry. Most of the interventions for SVT listed in Table 27-6 are applicable to these arrhythmias.

PSVT Due to AV Nodal Reentry

This is the most common form of PSVT. The underlying pathophysiologic disturbance in AV nodal reentry is the presence of dual pathways in the region of the AV node. Previously thought to be restricted to the compact anatomic AV node itself, it is now recognized that dual-pathway physiology behaves as though there are two types of conduction pathways in the *region* of the AV node; one pathway is capable of faster conduction, which usually has a longer refractory period, and the other is more slowly conducting and has a shorter refractory period. Both the slow and fast pathways have components in the low atrial approaches to the AV node (Fig. 27-11).

In the presence of dual AV nodal physiology, a premature atrial impulse with a sufficiently short coupling interval may block in the fast pathway, allowing conduction to proceed through the slow pathway (Fig. 27-11*B*). This results in slower-than-normal conduction through the AV node, prolonging the PR interval abruptly. The slowly propagating impulse may then reenter the fast pathway in the retrograde direction and arrive at the proximal end after it has recovered excitability. When this occurs, a circuit is completed and the impulse may then reenter the slow pathway if it too has regained excitability (Fig. 27-11*C*). Once established, this reentrant pattern will continue until the relationship between conduction velocities and refractory periods in the two pathways is disturbed so as to interrupt the cycle. The circulating impulse progresses through the His-Purkinje system to ventricular muscle each time it passes the distal end of the reentrant loop and provides retrograde atrial activation each time it passes the proximal end. Because antegrade conduction is slow and retrograde conduction

rapid, atrial activity begins soon after the onset of ventricular activation, creating an inability to identify P waves on the standard ECG during AV nodal reentrant tachycardia (Fig. 27-12), because it is within the QRS complex. The characteristic alignment of electrograms recorded during AV nodal reentrant tachycardia is shown in Fig. 27-13*A*. In a much less common form of AV nodal reentry, the circulating wavefront proceeds antegradely down the fast pathway and retrogardely up the slow pathway, creating a sequence of excitation of atria that is delayed relative to ventricular activation because of slow retrograde conduction. This form of AV nodal reentrant tachycardia is characterized by a long RP interval and a short PR interval, with a clearly visible inverted P wave in II, III, and aV_F. The electrophysiologic findings in the common and uncommon forms of AV nodal reentry are compared in Figs. 27-13*A* and -13*B* (see also Chap. 26).

Electrocardiographic Features PSVT due to AV nodal reentry is characterized by an abrupt onset and offset and usually has a narrow QRS complex without clearly discernable P waves. The rate is commonly in the range of 160 to 190 per minute but may be as slow as 120 to 130 per minute and occasionally faster than 200 per minute. When preexisting bundle branch block is present, the tachycardia will reflect the preexisting wide QRS complex, and functional bundle branch block due to tachycardia may also occur, making a distinction from ventricular tachyarrhythmias difficult (Fig. 27-14). Functional bundle branch block may have either a left or a right bundle pattern.

Management of PSVT Due to AV Nodal Reentry PSVT due to AV nodal reentry is a benign disturbance, requiring intervention primarily for the patient's comfort and sense of well-being. When it coexists with other disease processes in which the tachyarrhythmia is poorly tolerated, such as ischemic heart disease or mitral stenosis, it may have more serious implications. Occasionally, the rate is rapid enough to cause

TABLE 27-6

MANAGEMENT OF PAROXYSMAL SUPRAVENTRICULAR TACHYCARDIAS

	Acute	Long-Term
Physiologic interventions	Rest, sedation Valsalva maneuver Carotid sinus massage	Self-administered Valsalva maneuver, carotid sinus massage Avoid inciting factors
Pharmacologic therapy	Drugs with direct effect on AV nodal or accessory pathway Drugs that control ventricular rate	Drugs that alter properties of AV node or accessory pathways Drugs that control ventricular rate
Catheter ablation and surgical techniques	—	Ablation of reentrant pathway Modification of AV node
Electronic devices	Temporary pacing Cardioversion	Permanent pacemaker

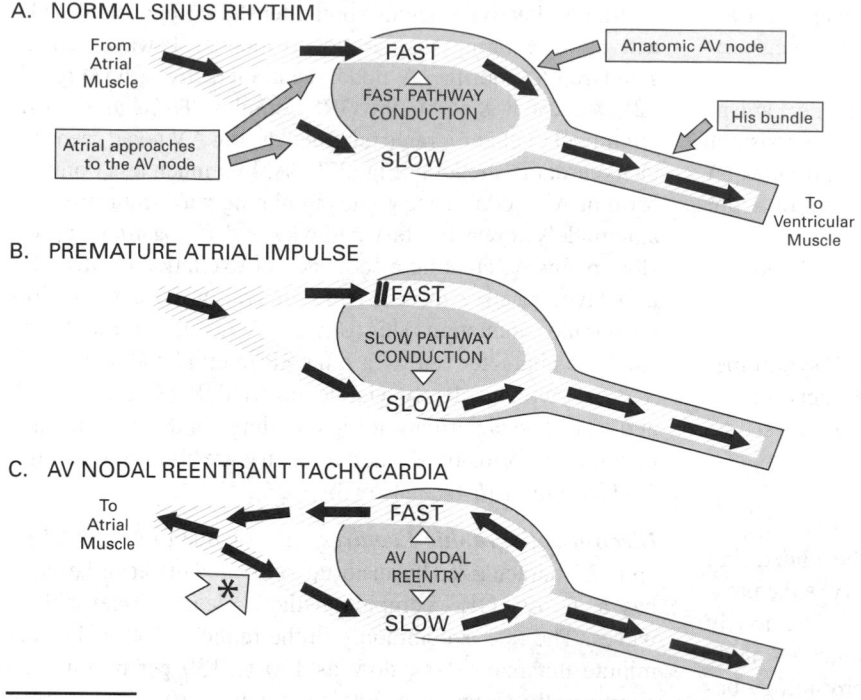

A. NORMAL SINUS RHYTHM

B. PREMATURE ATRIAL IMPULSE

C. AV NODAL REENTRANT TACHYCARDIA

FIGURE 27-11

Mechanism of paroxysmal supraventricular tachycardia due to AV nodal reentry. PSVT due to AV nodal reentry is due to the presence of dual AV nodal pathways with different conduction properties and refractory periods. Although the fast and slow pathways were previously thought to be within the anatomic AV node, the pathways are now viewed as having critical components in the atrial approaches to the AV node. Nonetheless, the dual-pathway physiology concept is valid. *A.* During sinus rhythm in the presence of dual AV nodal pathway, the fast pathway (which generally has a longer refractory period) is primarily responsible for AV transmission because of slower propagation in the other pathway. *B.* A premature atrial impulse blocks in the fast pathway because of its longer refractory period and propagates down the slow pathway, prolonging the PR interval and allowing retrograde invasion of the fast pathway because its tissue remains polarized because of block of the descending impulse. *C.* Echo beats or AV nodal reentrant tachycardia will occur when the time relationships between slow pathway conduction and recovery of excitability at the site of block in the fast pathway allow the impulse to reenter the slow pathway after retrograde fast pathway transmission. The atria are also activated retrogradely. In a much less common form of AV nodal reentry, a shorter refractory period in the fast pathway reverses the loop, with antegrade conduction down the fast pathway and retrograde conduction up the slow pathway (see Fig. 27-13 for examples). Radiofrequency energy for slow pathway ablation therapy is applied at the site indicated by the asterisk (*).

near-syncope or syncope in otherwise normal individuals, although such rates are more common in PSVT due to WPW (see below).

Rest, sedation, and vagotonic maneuvers are simple means for reverting acute episodes, and patients can be taught self-administered vagotonic maneuvers for recurrences. Patients should be advised to avoid inciting factors such as smoking, alcohol, extreme fatigue, and stress. Many of the effective pharmacologic interventions for acute episodes used in the past have given way to new drug therapy. Infusions of sympathomimetic (phenylephrine, methoxamine) and parasympathomimetic drugs (edrophonium, neostigmine) have been supplanted by intravenous adenosine, Ca^{2+}-entry blockers, digoxin, or β-adrenergic blockers for managing the acute episodes. Adenosine, 6 mg given intravenously (see Fig. 27-12), followed by one or two 12-mg boluses if necessary, is effective and safe[18] for acute treatment. Because of its very

short duration of action and lack of the negative inotropic effects of Ca^{2+}-entry blockers, it is now preferred to other acute pharmacologic therapies, especially when managing a patient with concomitant structural heart disease. A 5-mg bolus of verapamil, followed by one or two additional 5-mg boluses 10 min apart if the initial dose does not convert the arrhythmia, has been an effective regimen in up to 90 percent of patients with PSVT due to AV node reentry.[19,20] However, it must not be used for an unknown wide QRS tachycardia because of risk of adverse effects when used in patients who have VT.[21] Intravenous diltiazem is also effective.[22,23] Initial treatment consists of a bolus of 0.25 mg/kg body weight administered over 2 min. If the response is inadequate, a repeat bolus of 0.35 mg/kg over 2 min is administered 15 min later. Intravenous digoxin, 0.5 mg infused over 10 min and repeated if necessary, may convert the arrhythmia. An additional 0.25 mg every 4 h to a maximum dose of 1.5 mg in 24 h may be used. A slow infusion of propranolol may be used[24]; 1 mg/min is given to a total dose of 5 to 10 mg or a significant fall in blood pressure. The class IA antiarrhythmic agents, which appear to depress conduction in the fast pathway, may be tried if other drugs fail.[25]

Several special points must be remembered. When the QRS complex is wide and VT is mistakenly diagnosed as SVT with aberrant conduction, intravenous verapamil frequently causes a clinically significant fall in blood pressure and potentially lethal events.[21] Unless it is absolutely known that a wide QRS tachycardia is due to aberrant intraventricular conduction or preexisting bundle branch block, verapamil should not be used. Similarly, in patients with coexisting hemodynamically significant underlying heart disease, intravenous propranolol must be used with caution, if at all. For those few patients in whom the clinical setting demands an immediate return to a normal sinus mechanism, DC cardioversion can be employed. A low-energy shock (10 to 50 W·s) may be sufficient; larger energies are used if necessary. If DC cardioversion should be avoided, pacing the right atrium or ventricle via a temporary pacing catheter is usually successful[26] (see Chap. 34).

Long-term control of recurrent PSVT due to AV nodal reentry may be achieved with pharmacologic therapy or catheter ablation. Surgical techniques and electronic devices have been used in the past but are now virtually obsolete. Patients who have infrequent, well-tolerated episodes that are short-lived and/or respond to self-administered physiologic maneuvers (Table 27-6) may require no chronic interventions. In many others, pharmacologic therapy is sufficient. Most patients will have reduced numbers and severity of attacks with simple medications such as digoxin in standard maintenance doses, propranolol, or verapamil. These drugs act by altering conduction velocities and refractory periods in the AV nodal pathways, disrupting the delicate balance required for initiation or maintenance of sustained arrhythmias. Membrane-active antiarrhythmic drugs may prevent recurrences, both by suppressing triggering premature impulses and by depressing conduction in the retrograde (fast) pathway of the AV nodal reentrant circuit.[25] However, the risk of potentially serious proarrhythmic responses, combined with other troublesome side effects, limits their use for these arryhthmis, since other options are available.

Invasive electrophysiologic studies to guide therapy[27] have been used for difficult cases, but recent experience with RF catheter ablation techniques[28] has demonstrated that the procedure is safe and very effective for PSVT due to AV nodal reentrant tachycardia.[29,30] It has, therefore, emerged as the treatment of choice for patients with frequent arrhythmic episodes and/or poor tolerance of drugs (see also Chap. 31). It is also the preferred option for pharmacologically controllable AV nodal reentrant tachycardia by patients who want to avoid pharmacologic side effects. Curative surgical techniques that preserve AV node conduction[31] are available, as are antitachycardia pacing devices,[32] but they are rarely used anymore.

PSVT Due to Accessory Pathways (the Wolff-Parkinson-White Syndrome)

WPW syndrome appears to be the second most common cause of PSVT. Since it also occurs in a concealed form, in which the standard ECG is normal during sinus rhythm because of inability of the accessory pathway to conduct in the antegrade direction, the total number of PSVTs that are due to accessory pathways may be considerably higher than previous estimates. As in AV nodal reentry, the pathophysiology of reentrant tachyarrhythmias in WPW syndrome relates to the presence of two pathways between the atria and the ventricles that have different conduction properties and refractory periods. In the majority of patients, the effective refractory period of the accessory pathway exceeds that of the normal AV nodal–His-Purkinje pathway. Therefore, a premature atrial impulse may block at the accessory pathway and conduct antegradely down the normal pathway, ultimately entering the accessory pathway in the retrograde direction and reentering the atrium to establish a circus movement tachycardia referred to as *orthodromic* (see Fig. 27-15A). Because the normal pathway is used for ventricular activation and the accessory pathway for return to the atria, the delta wave is absent, causing the

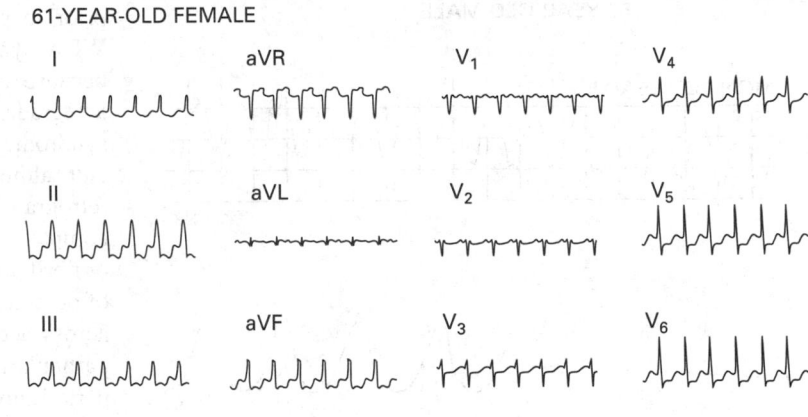

61-YEAR-OLD FEMALE

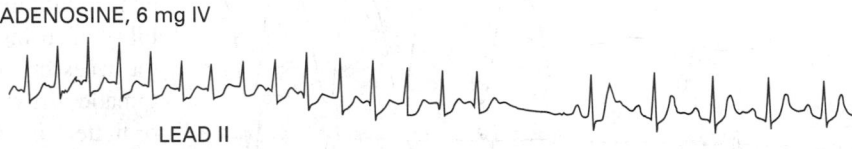

ADENOSINE, 6 mg IV

LEAD II

FIGURE 27-12

Paroxysmal supraventricular tachycardia due to AV nodal reentry. Narrow QRS complexes with ST-segment depression are seen (*upper panel*). *Lower panel:* adenosine, 6 mg intravenously, abruptly alters AV nodal properties and terminates the tachycardia. The ST-T wave pattern immediately returns to normal.

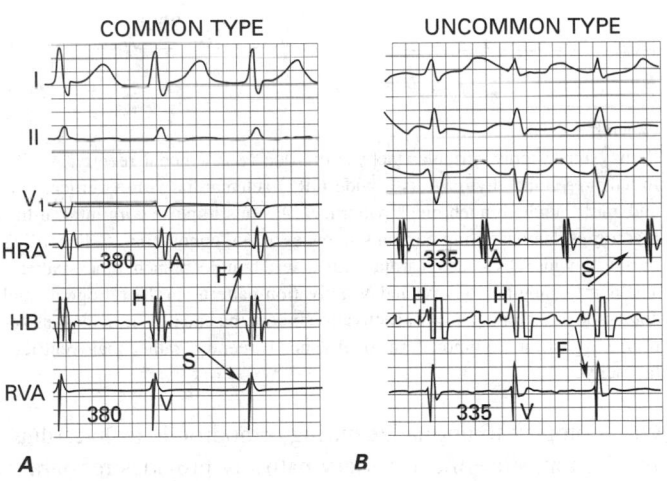

FIGURE 27-13

Common and uncommon forms of AV nodal reentrant tachycardia recorded during electrophysiologic studies. *A.* The common type of AV nodal reentrant tachycardia, antegrade conduction in the slow pathway and retrograde in the fast pathway, results in atrial (A) and ventricular (V) activation that are close to one another in time. Characteristically, intracardiac recordings demonstrate a "lining up" of atrial and ventricular electrograms, indicating that the atria are activated before completion of ventricular activation. *B.* In the uncommon type of AV nodal reentrant tachycardia, antegrade fast pathway and retrograde slow pathway conduction change the relative timing pattern so that atrial activation is delayed relative to ventricular activation, and the electrograms are not in line. In this form of PSVT, the RP interval is longer than the PR interval on the ECG, which results in inscription of the retrograde P wave *after* the ST-T wave of the related ventricular impulse. The uncommon type of AV nodal reentrant tachycardia may be difficult to distinguish from other arrhythmias such as ectopic atrial tachyarrhythmias or concealed Wolff-Parkinson-White syndrome (see text).

68-YEAR-OLD MALE

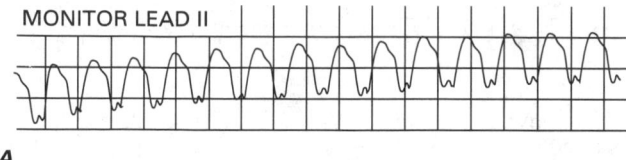

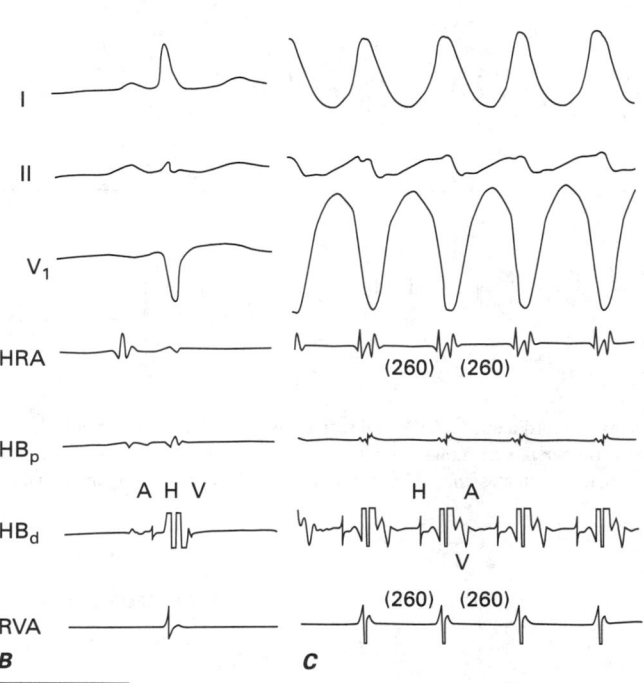

FIGURE 27-14

Paroxysmal supraventricular tachycardia due to AV nodal reentry. *A*. The initial presenting rhythm was a wide QRS tachycardia with a vertical axis and a left bundle branch block pattern. *B*. A sinus impulse with intracardiac recordings demonstrating normal sequences of AV conduction. *C*. Recording during a wide QRS tachycardia with a left bundle branch block pattern. The nearly simultaneous A- and V-activation patterns in the retrograde and antegrade directions (i.e., atrial activation before the end of ventricular activation) suggest the common form of AV nodal reentry, rather than ventricular tachycardia.

QRS complex to normalize during orthodromic tachycardias. In addition, since the accessory pathway provides retrograde conduction to the atria, P waves, if seen, are usually inverted in the inferior and lateral leads. The stability of the reentrant circuit depends upon the conduction properties and refractory periods of the two pathways. In a much less common form of PSVT, a shorter refractory period in the anomalous pathway results in block of an initiating premature atrial impulse in the normal pathway, with antegrade conduction down the anomalous pathway and then retrograde invasion of the normal AV nodal pathway to establish an *antidromic* tachycardia. The QRS complex is wide, having the characteristics of a ventricular complex originating near the insertion site of the anomalous pathway (Fig. 27-15*B*). These wide QRS tachycardias may be difficult to distinguish from ventricular tachyarrhythmias if the existence of WPW syndrome was not known

prior to presentation with a tachyarrhythmia. In concealed WPW syndrome,[33] only orthodromic tachycardias can occur because of inability of the bypass tract to conduct in the antegrade direction. Distinction between concealed WPW syndrome and AV nodal reentrant tachycardia may be difficult, although a faster rate (>200 per minute) and a visible retrograde P wave after, rather than lost within, the QRS complex favor concealed WPW syndrome. When atrial flutter or fibrillation occurs in patients with WPW syndrome, the risk of potentially lethal arrhythmias due to very rapid conduction across accessory pathways must be considered. The risk is particularly treacherous in patients with short-refractory-period anomalous pathways since atrial fibrillation may induce ventricular fibrillation.

PSVT in WPW syndrome may begin in childhood or not appear until middle age. In asymptomatic patients, the probability of losing the capacity for antegrade conduction across the accessory pathway increases with advancing age.[34] Symptomatic arrhythmias may be due to PSVT, atrial fibrillation or flutter, or both in individual patients. In a series of 212 patients with tachyarrhythmias and WPW, PSVT alone occurred in 64 percent, atrial fibrillation alone in 20 percent, and both in 16 percent.[35] Since the reentrant tachyarrhythmias tend to be more rapid than those in patients with AV nodal reentry, they may be more symptomatic. Light-headedness, near-syncope, and syncope appear to occur more commonly in WPW with PSVT or atrial fibrillation than in AV nodal reentry.

A risk of sudden death in patients with WPW has been emphasized, but the magnitude of the risk is unknown, even in those with short refractory periods. Other factors that appear to influence risk are the presence of multiple bypass tracts and a family history of premature sudden death.[36]

Electrocardiographic Features   The most common patterns recorded during PSVT due to WPW syndrome are narrow QRS tachycardias at rates ranging from 160 to 240 per minute. Rates may occasionally be faster or somewhat slower. When the tachycardia is antidromic, the QRS complexes are wide and have characteristics similar to fully preexcited impulses during sinus rhythm or PACs (see Fig. 27-15*B*). In atrial fibrillation with WPW syndrome, if the accessory pathway has a refractory period longer than the normal pathway, the delta wave will disappear and patterns typical of atrial fibrillation with narrow QRS complexes will be recorded. In contrast, when the refractory period of the accessory pathway is shorter, wide QRS complexes dominate the tracing (Fig. 27-16). Multiple bypass tracts are suggested by multiple wide QRS complex morphologies during atrial fibrillation with preexcited conduction (Fig. 27-16*B*). The grossly irregular rhythm, wide QRS complexes, and a mean ventricular rate in excess of 200 per minute are clues supporting WPW with atrial fibrillation in the differential diagnosis of a wide QRS complex tachycardia. Another form of wide QRS tachycardia in WPW is orthodromic tachycardia with functional bundle branch block. When a patient with left lateral bypass tract abruptly develops a wide QRS complex with a left bundle branch block pattern

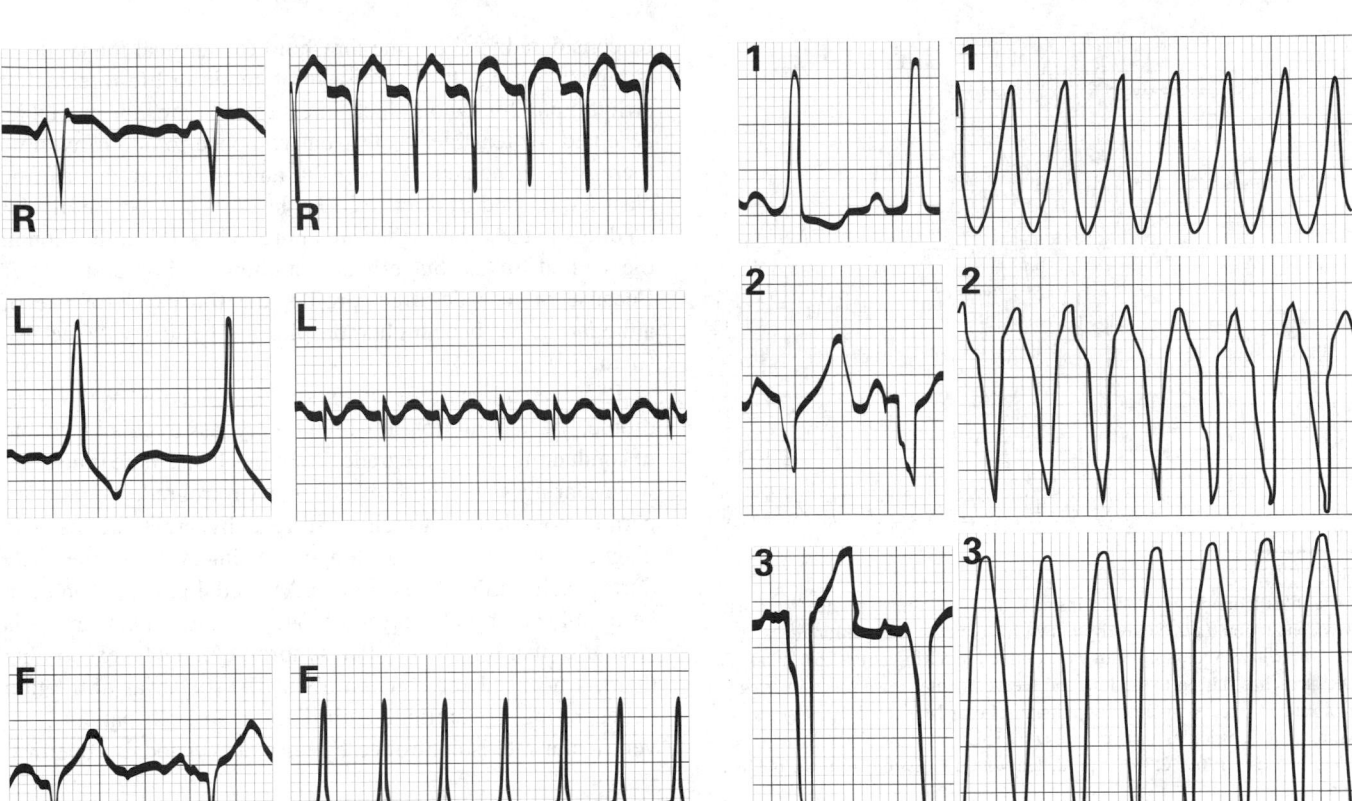

FIGURE 27-15
Wolff-Parkinson-White syndrome with reciprocating tachycardia. *A.* Before and during an "orthodromic" tachycardia. *B.* From another patient, before and during an "antidromic" tachycardia.

during orthodromic tachycardia, the diagnosis of SVT with aberrancy is strongly suspected when the cycle length of the tachycardia *lengthens*. Functional left bundle branch block delays arrival of the circulating impulse at the distal end of a left-sided accessory pathway, thereby lengthening the tachycardia cycle. Under most other conditions, appearance of functional left bundle branch block correlates with *shortening* of the tachycardia cycle length, because the accelerating tachycardia rate encroaches on the refractory period of the left bundle branch (see also Chap. 26).

Management of PSVT Due to WPW Syndrome This form of reentrant SVT is amenable to a broad range of interventions. Careful attention to the details of therapy is required because a subgroup of patients is at risk for potentially lethal arrhythmias due to very rapid conduction across the accessory pathway during atrial flutter or fibrillation. This concern influences the pharmacologic approaches to PSVT in the WPW syndrome, since drugs have different effects on accessory pathways and the AV node, and because reciprocating PSVT may convert to atrial flutter or fibrillation.[37]

Physiologic interventions and vagomimetic drugs can be used safely during acute episodes of reciprocating tachycardia.

In addition, adenosine, verapamil diltiazem, propranolol, and membrane-active antiarrhythmic agents such as procainamide, quinidine, or disopyramide may be used to convert acute reentrant tachycardias. Verapamil[38,39] and lidocaine[40] may accelerate the ventricular rate during atrial flutter or fibrillation in the WPW syndrome, however, and should be avoided if atrial fibrillation is present or if the patient has previously demonstrated alternation between atrial fibrillation and reciprocating tachycardia. Digoxin must be avoided in patients with WPW because it may shorten the refractory period of the accessory pathway[41] as well as atrial muscle. Should this occur in the presence of unrecognized atrial flutter or fibrillation or with the conversion of a reciprocating tachycardia to atrial fibrillation, the patient could develop a life-threatening tachyarrhythmia due to rapid accessory pathway conduction.[42] Whenever there is doubt, therapy should be limited to those drugs that will depress conduction in the accessory pathway or prolong its refractory period, such as the membrane-active antiarrhythmic agents (e.g., intravenous procainamide), or to agents such as adenosine that usually have no effect on an accessory pathway. Electrical cardioversion should be used if other means have failed or as initial therapy if the patient has extremely rapid rates causing hemodynamic intolerance of the tachycardia.

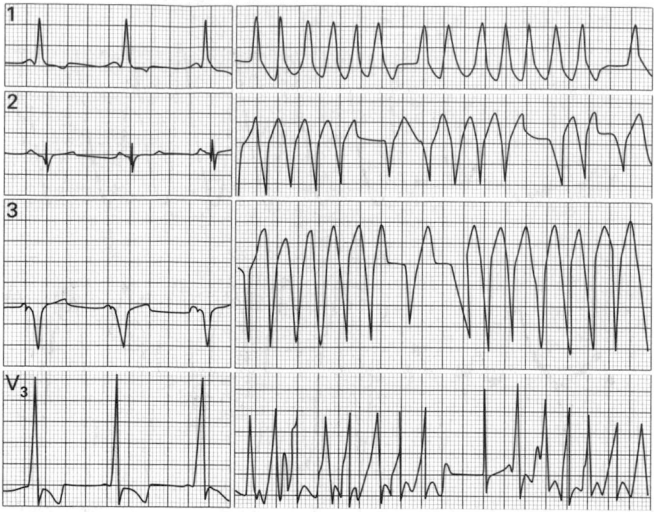

FIGURE 27-16

Atrial fibrillation in Wolff-Parkinson-White syndrome with accessory pathway conduction. *Left:* Sinus rhythm with a typical preexcitation (delta wave) pattern. *Right:* Accessory pathway conduction during atrial fibrillation. The QRS axis has shifted to the left, and the ventricular rhythm is now irregular at a rate in excess of 200 per minute. (From Marriott HJL, Rogers HM. Mimics of ventricular tachycardia associated with the WPW syndrome. *J Electrocardiol* 1969; 2:77. Reproduced with permission from the publisher and author.)

The approach to long-term management of patients with WPW syndrome is determined by the physiologic characteristics of the bypass tract and the frequency, duration, and symptoms of arrhythmias. Three approaches to therapy are available: drugs, surgery, and catheter ablation. The latter, using an RF energy source (Fig. 27-17), is now the preferred method for treatment of patients with tachycardias symptomatic enough to limit their quality of life (e.g., near-syncope, syncope) or with symptomatic life-threatening arrhythmias in WPW (e.g, atrial fibrillation with short refractory period bypass tracts)[31,32,43] (see Chap. 31). Surgery is reserved for the occasional cases not amenable to catheter ablation and for some who require surgery for other causes as well.[44] Intracardiac electrophysiologic studies provide information on drug efficacy and pharmacologic effects on the bypass tract,[45] but this invasive procedure is not required for all patients.[46] Patients who demonstrate a good clinical response to therapy, measured in terms of reduced frequency or rate of tachyarrhythmic episodes, can be managed noninvasively; patients with intermittent delta wave and no clinical arrhythmia need no therapy. On the other hand, patients who have frequent or poorly tolerated tachyarrhythmias, those who are prone to episodes of atrial flutter or fibrillation[47] (particularly if they develop wide QRS complexes during their tachyarrhythmias, suggesting bypass tract conduction), or those who have a family history of WPW and sudden death[36,48] should be evaluated by electrophysiologic testing. In such patients, catheter ablation using RF energy has emerged as the intervention of choice when available in an experienced laboratory and accepted by the patient.[30,43,49] In the event of failure of the technique to interrupt the tract(s), surgical interventions may

be considered,[50,51] but the threshold for surgical intervention is higher. Among those with symptomatic or life-threatening arrhythmias for whom such interventions are not available, accepted, or feasible, a clear-cut response to antiarrhythmic therapy is mandated. Among the antiarrhythmic agents, the class IA, IC, and III drugs (see Table 27-4) may be useful. Not all drugs in these categories are approved for this indication in the United States, but efficacy studies are impressive.[52–56] Because of its side-effect profile, the threshold for use of amiodarone has been higher, despite good efficacy[54] (see also Chap. 30).

PSVT also occurs in patients with *concealed* WPW syndrome,[33,57] a condition in which the bypass tract is incapable of conducting in the antegrade direction. Thus, there is no delta wave during sinus rhythm, but intact retrograde conduction permits completion of reciprocating tachycardia circuits. The diagnosis is suggested by longer RP intervals on the ECG during tachycardia than occur in AV nodal reentry[33] and can be established by electrophysiologic testing. Management is similar to that for other WPW syndrome patients, except that there is no need for concern about risk of atrial fibrillation degenerating to ventricular fibrillation. In such patients, the ventricular rate is controlled by normal AV nodal properties,

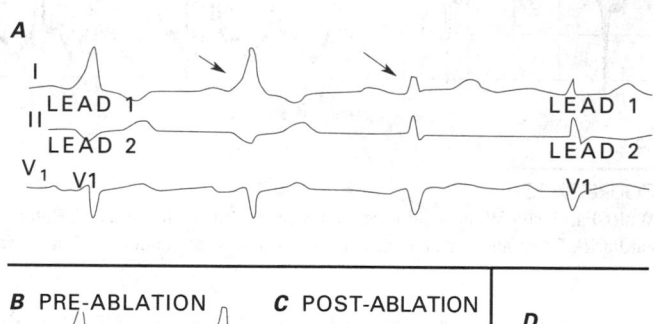

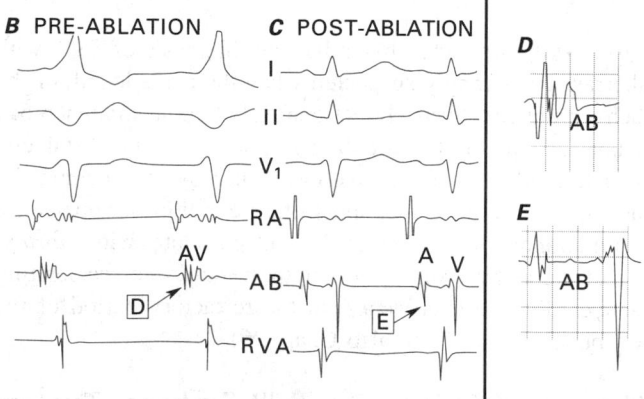

FIGURE 27-17

Radiofrequency ablation in Wolff-Parkinson-White (WPW) syndrome in a 52-year-old female. The patient had frequent recurrent supraventricular tachycardias due to WPW syndrome. *A.* Standard leads I, II, and V₁ demonstrate disappearance of the delta wave from one impulse to the next, 5 s after beginning the application of radiofrequency energy (compare successive QRS complexes indicated by arrows). *B.* Prior to ventricular ablation, the interval between atrial (A) and (V) activation at the site of the ablation catheter is less than 50 ms, and the sharp spike between A and V likely represents activity in the bypass tract. *C.* Immediately after ablation, the AV interval at the site of the ablation catheter (AB) is lengthened to 150 ms, and the accessory pathway spike has disappeared. *D* and *E.* Enlargements of *D* and *E* from panels *B* and *C*, respectively. (RA, right atrium, AB, ablation catheter, RVA, right ventricular apex.)

since the accessory pathway cannot provide antegrade conduction.

OTHER PAROXYSMAL REENTRANT SVTs

The other reentrant SVTs are far less common than PSVT due to AV node reentry or WPW syndrome. The PSVT due to sinus node reentry[58,59] may be difficult to distinguish clinically and by ECG from sinus tachycardia, except for its paroxysmal onset and offset. P-wave morphology is similar to that in sinus tachycardia. Intraatrial reentry[59,60] may be difficult to distinguish from certain forms of automatic ectopic atrial tachycardia. Intraatrial or sinus node reentry are distinguished from PSVT due to AV node reentry or WPW on a standard ECG because P waves precede narrow QRS complexes during these tachycardias. Atriofascicular and nodoventricular pathways (Mahaim tracts)[61] may cause PSVT with wide QRS complexes having a left bundle branch block pattern. Intracardiac electrophysiologic studies are usually very helpful in distinguishing between these various PSVTs.

There is no generally accepted and predictably effective approach to therapy. Intraatrial reentrant tachycardia may be treated with conventional membrane-active antiarrhythmic agents, β-adrenergic blocking agents, or perhaps Ca^{2+}-entry blockers. Sinus node reentry may respond to digoxin, propranolol, diltiazem, or verapamil. Surgical interventions[62] are only rarely considered for these arrhythmias because of their usually benign nature, but catheter ablation with RF energy may prove to be useful for many (see also Chap. 31).

ECTOPIC ATRIAL TACHYCARDIAS

These arrhythmias are usually persistent, are commonly referred to as "nonparoxysmal," and may be associated with specific inciting factors. There are experimental and clinical reasons to suspect that ectopic atrial tachycardia could be due to mechanisms of reentry[63] or automaticity (enhanced spontaneous phase 4 depolarization)[64] or could be a clinical expression of triggered activity.[65] An underlying toxic or metabolic cause is commonly identified as the factor responsible for ectopic atrial tachycardia, but some are persistent or recurrent, likely due to focal atrial disease. When an ectopic atrial rate is in the range of 160 to over 200 per minute and associated with 2:1 conduction or variable block in a patient receiving digitalis, a digitalis-toxic rhythm must be suspected strongly. Decompensated chronic lung disease, metabolic abnormalities (including acute alcohol abuse), electrolyte disturbances, and hypoxemia should be considered when digitalis toxicity has been excluded. Various forms of cardiac disease, including acute myocardial infarction, also may cause ectopic atrial tachycardia. Such diseases occasionally originate from atrial suture lines, such as in patients who have previously had complex congenital heart disease surgery with a major atrial component.

Electrocardiographic Features

P waves are usually normal to small in amplitude and may be difficult to identify when the ventricular rate is rapid (Fig. 27-18). Atrial activity does not slow during carotid sinus massage, but AV conduction is usually impeded, making P

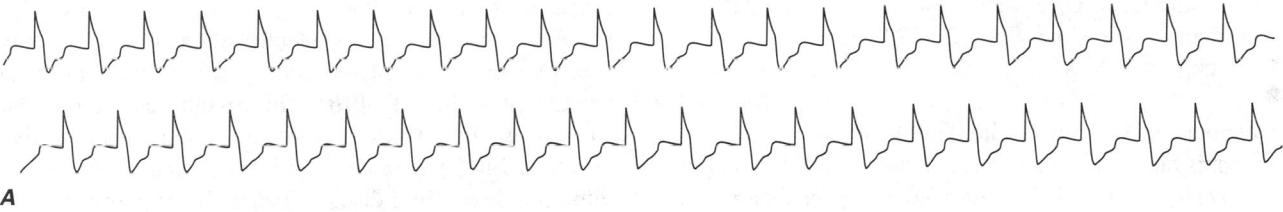

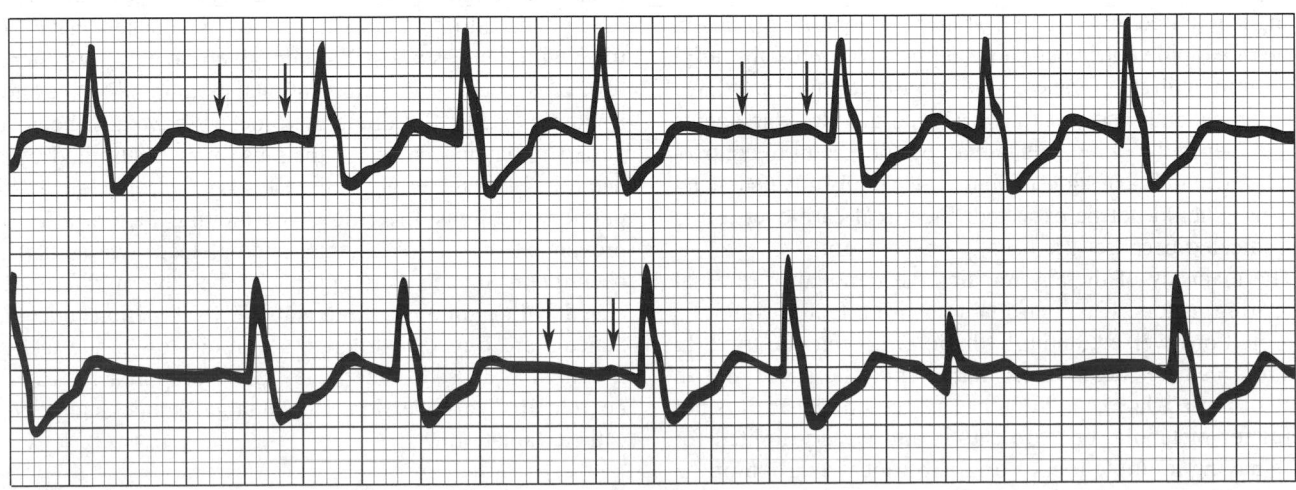

FIGURE 27-18

Ectopic atrial tachycardia. *A.* A 20-s continuous recording demonstrates a regular tachycardia at a ventricular rate of approximately 140 per minute. *B.* During carotid sinus massage, ventricular conduction becomes irregular and diminutive P waves at twice the basic ventricular rate are evident. Impaired AV conduction with little or no effect on atrial activity is characteristic of the response of an ectopic atrial tachycardia to carotid sinus massage.

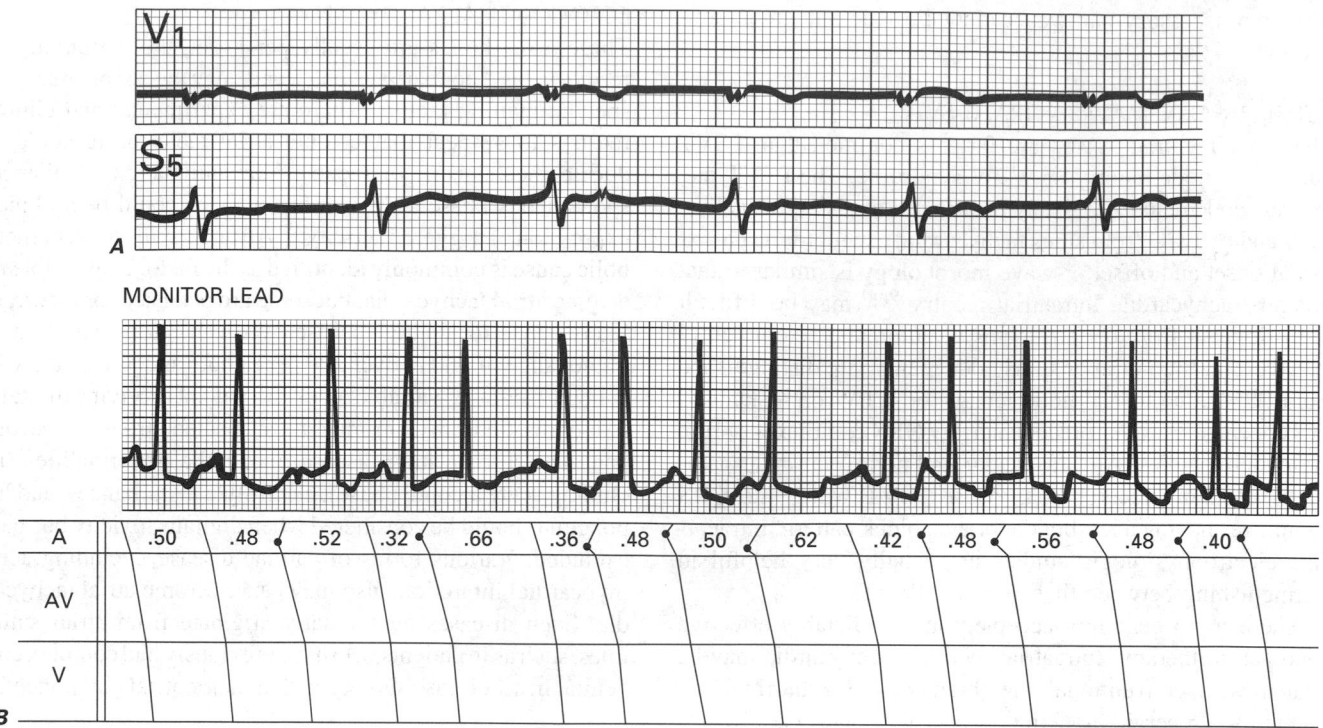

FIGURE 27-19

A. Atrial tachycardia with 2:1 AV block due to digitalis intoxication. Note the diminutive P waves, barely visible even in V_1. *B.* Multifocal (chaotic) atrial tachycardia. Note the constantly changing form of the ectopic P waves

and the irregular rhythm at a mean rate of 122 per minute. Three or more distinct P-wave morphologies are required to make the diagnosis.

waves more evident. When ectopic atrial tachycardia is due to digitalis intoxication, P waves may be "diminutive" and the ventricular rate slow (Fig. 27-19*A*) because of high-grade block.

Management of Ectopic Atrial Tachycardias

Treatment is dictated by identification and reversal of inciting factors, by ablation of a defined focal source when identifiable, and by control of the heart rate when necessary. Temporary pacing is required infrequently. More commonly, the problem is one of a rapid ventricular rate. Attempts to control the atrial arrhythmia with membrane-active antiarrhythmic drugs have not been generally successful. β-Adrenergic blocking agents or Ca^{2+}-entry blocking agents may be successful in controlling the arrhythmia in some patients, but a uniformly beneficial response should not be expected. Electrical cardioversion is not indicated because it is usually unsuccessful.

The mainstay of therapy remains the removal or reversal of inciting factors. If a controllable inciting factor cannot be identified or reversed, antiarrhythmic drugs may be tried. In addition, catheter ablation techniques may be successful in some of those whose condition has a structural basis. It is not useful for metabolic or toxic causes and is very limited for those having multiple foci of origin. Surgical excision of the site of origin of a chronic ectopic atrial tachycardia can be achieved with intraoperative mapping.[66] It should be used only under very extraordinary circumstances, however, since atrial disease is commonly multifocal.

MULTIFOCAL ATRIAL TACHYCARDIA; CHAOTIC ATRIAL RHYTHM

The diagnosis requires the identification of P waves having three or more different morphologies that occur at different cycle lengths (Fig. 27-19*B*). The rhythm, as the name indicates, is usually chaotic, but the rate is not usually excessive (less than 140 per minute).[67] It is most commonly associated with underlying lung disease, metabolic abnormalities, electrolyte disturbances, and in rare instances toxic causes such as digitalis intoxication. Calcium-entry blockers have been tried with some success[68] when given acutely, but there is little or no success with conventional membrane-active antiarrhythmic agents. β-Adrenergic blockers have also been suggested,[69] but feasibility of their use may be limited by the nature of the underlying disease (e.g., chronic obstructive pulmonary disease). Removal of inciting factors (e.g., improvement of P_{O_2}, P_{CO_2}, pH, and/or electrolyte status) has been the most successful approach when the rhythm is associated with pulmonary or metabolic dysfunction, but many patients are forced to tolerate a chronic low-grade tachyarrhythmia because of inefficacy of any approach. There is no role for cardioversion, implantable devices, surgery, or catheter ablation.

ATRIAL FLUTTER

Atrial flutter is a rapid regular atrial tachyarrhythmia that is less common than the PSVTs or atrial fibrillation. It is observed infrequently in normal individuals,[70] but may occur at any age in the presence of underlying atrial abnormalities such as those secondary to mitral valve disease, congenital heart disease, cardiomyopathies, and, less frequently, coronary artery disease. Subgroups at particularly high risk for developing atrial flutter are children, adolescents, and young adults who have undergone corrective surgery for complex congenital heart diseases, most notably transposition of the great vessels, tetralogy of Fallot, or atrial septal defects.[71]

Atrial flutter has been separated into two types, classic, or type I, and type II.[72] The distinction is based upon (1) the ability to entrain and interrupt classic (type I) flutter with atrial pacing techniques, and (2) a faster atrial rate in type II flutter. Untreated type I flutter usually has atrial rates between 280 and 320 per minute, commonly very close to 300 per minute. Type I, however, may occur infrequently at rates as low as 240 to 250 and as high as 340 per minute. In type II flutter, the atrial rate is commonly at least 340 to 350 per minute and occasionally may be as fast as 450 per minute. The ventricular rate in atrial flutter is usually a defined fraction of the atrial rate—2:1 conduction in type I flutter generating a ventricular rate of 150 per minute and 4:1 conduction at 75 per minute. Group beating may occur, often reflecting two levels of block in the AV junction with a Wenckebach phenomenon influencing the impulses conducting below the site of 2:1 block[73] (see also Chap. 26).

Clinically, atrial flutter may occur in brief, persistent, or chronic forms, and therapeutic approaches are influenced by the clinical pattern.

Electrocardiographic Features

Atrial flutter generates a defined pattern of atrial activity in the ECG. Classically, a sawtooth pattern is identifiable in leads II, III, and aV_F (Fig. 27-20). The electrical activity appears continuous in these leads, without a defined isoelectric baseline between flutter waves. The exception is in slow atrial flutter, as may occur in the presence of antiarrhythmic drugs, in which a discernible isoelectric line may appear in these leads. In contrast to leads II, III, and aV_F, other leads (most notably lead V_1) generally have discrete flutter waves inscribed with an isoelectric line between them (Fig. 27-20). The pattern in leads II, III, and aV_F likely reflects continuous electrical activity in the reentrant pathway in the low right atrium, while the pattern in lead V_1 reflects discrete wavefronts of activation approaching an area remote from the reentrant loop. Leads I and V_6 may generate intermediate patterns. In type II flutter, the electrocardiographic patterns are similar, except for the faster rate.

The most common AV conduction ratios in atrial flutter are 2:1 and 4:1, generating a ventricular rate of approximately 150 and 75 per minute, respectively. In young children and

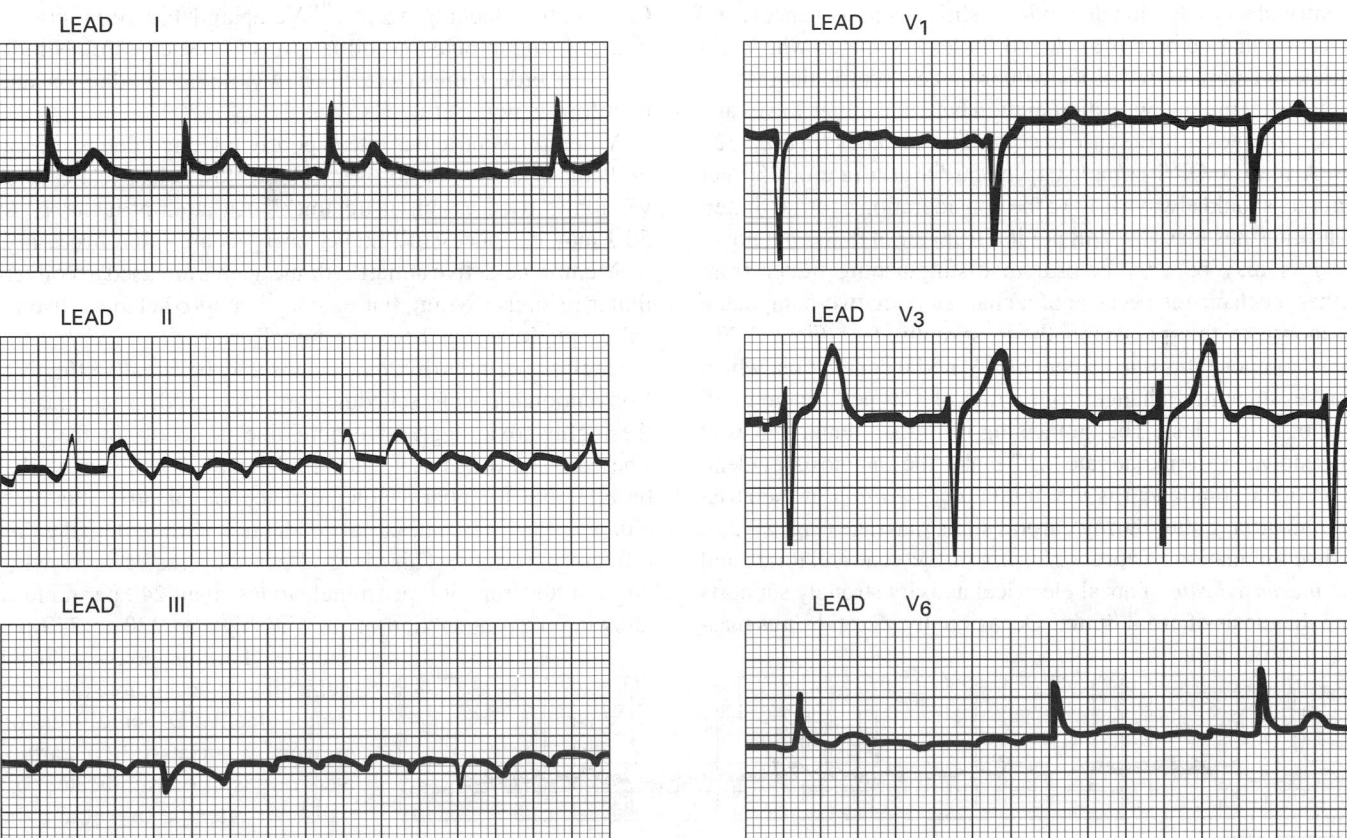

FIGURE 27-20
Atrial flutter. Note the "sawtooth" pattern in leads II and III, discrete atrial waves in V_1, and poorly registered atrial activity in leads I and V_6.

MONITOR LEAD II

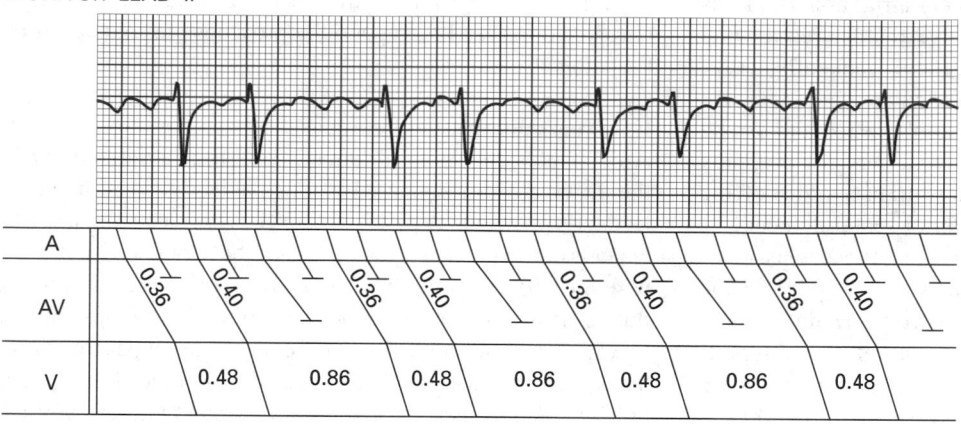

FIGURE 27-21

Atrial flutter with alternating 4:1 and 2:1 conduction. This common cause of bigeminal rhythm is almost always due to 2:1 AV conduction high in the AV junction and 3:2 Wenckebach periods at a lower level, as diagrammed.

rarely in adults, 1:1 AV conduction may occur, resulting in a ventricular rate of 300 per minute. Continuous 3:1 and 5:1 ratios are very rare, but alternating 2:1 and 4:1 ratios are common, generating a bigeminal pattern. Such patterns commonly contain Wenckebach periods at the lower level of block (Fig. 27-21). Occasionally, the second impulse of the bigeminal pattern is aberrantly conducted in the ventricles, requiring a distinction between the Ashman phenomenon (aberrant intraventricular conduction due to long-short cycle sequences) and a ventricular ectopic beat. Atrial flutter associated with high-grade or complete AV block will produce a ventricular rate below 60 per minute, with dissociation between flutter waves and QRS complexes in the case of complete AV block (Fig. 27-22).

A narrow QRS complex tachycardia at a rate of 150 per minute should always lead to the consideration of atrial flutter. Carotid sinus massage will not interrupt atrial flutter but nonetheless may be very helpful in distinguishing flutter from other mechanisms because of a characteristic two-component response to this parasympathetic stimulus (see Fig. 27-23). One component is impairment of AV nodal conduction, which causes an abrupt change from a rate of 150 per minute to 75 per minute or less. The unmasking of hidden flutter waves at the slower ventricular rate will make the diagnosis evident. The other component is the unique *acceleration* of the atrial rate in atrial flutter during carotid sinus massage (Fig. 27-23). The combination of abrupt *slowing* of the ventricular rate and an *increased rate* of atrial electrical activity strongly supports the diagnosis of atrial flutter. Occasionally, carotid sinus mas-

sage will cause atrial flutter to convert to atrial fibrillation.

Management of Paroxysmal Atrial Flutter

Treatment of acute paroxysmal atrial flutter differs from the treatment of PSVT due to AV nodal reentry or AV reciprocating mechanisms. Carotid sinus massage will not interrupt atrial flutter but transiently slows the ventricular rate by impairing AV nodal conduction (Fig. 27-23). The pharmacologic treatment of atrial flutter may be directed to reversion to a sinus mechanism or to control of the ventricular rate. The usual ventricular rate of 150 impulses per minute (± 10 impulses per minute) may be well tolerated in the absence of myocardial dysfunction, symptomatic coronary artery disease, or mitral stenosis. The ventricular rate should be slowed with digitalis before antiarrhythmics are instituted to convert the atrial arrhythmia to avoid very rapid rates associated with drug-induced 1:1 AV conduction.[74] Control of the heart rate during the paroxysm may also be achieved with Ca^{2+}-entry blocking agents.[20] Verapamil has been studied in detail, and intravenous diltiazem is also successful. Nifedipine has little clinical effect on AV nodal conduction and therefore is not useful.

When the ventricular rate is poorly tolerated due to effects on hemodynamics or coronary blood flow, electrical cardioversion is used as initial treatment. An attempt using 10 to 50 J may be successful; higher energies are often necessary.

Membrane-active antiarrhythmic agents are used to convert flutter to sinus rhythm, but efficacy is unpredictable. Historically, quinidine has been the initial drug of choice, but the other class IA antiarrhythmic agents may be equally effective. Conventional dosing schedules are now used, in contrast to the highly toxic aggressive quinidine protocols of the past. The class IC drugs (e.g., flecainide, propafenone) may also be effective for pharmacologic reversion of atrial flutter,[52] although they slow intraatrial conduction without lengthening refractory periods. This drug effect may result in slowing atrial flutter from 300 per minute to less than 240 per minute, allowing 1:1 conduction at rates as high as 220 to 240 per minute. Failing conversion or achieving an acceptable rate with drugs, elective DC cardioversion is usually successful. If cardioversion is contraindicated or fails, an attempt to entrain the atrium with rapid atrial pacing may result in conversion to sinus rhythm[75,76] (see Chap. 34).

Pharmacologic management

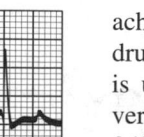

FIGURE 27-22

Atrial flutter (type II) with complete AV block. The atrial rate is 366 per minute, and the ventricular rate is 40 per minute. The ventricular rhythm remains regular, while the relationship between atrial and ventricular complexes varies.

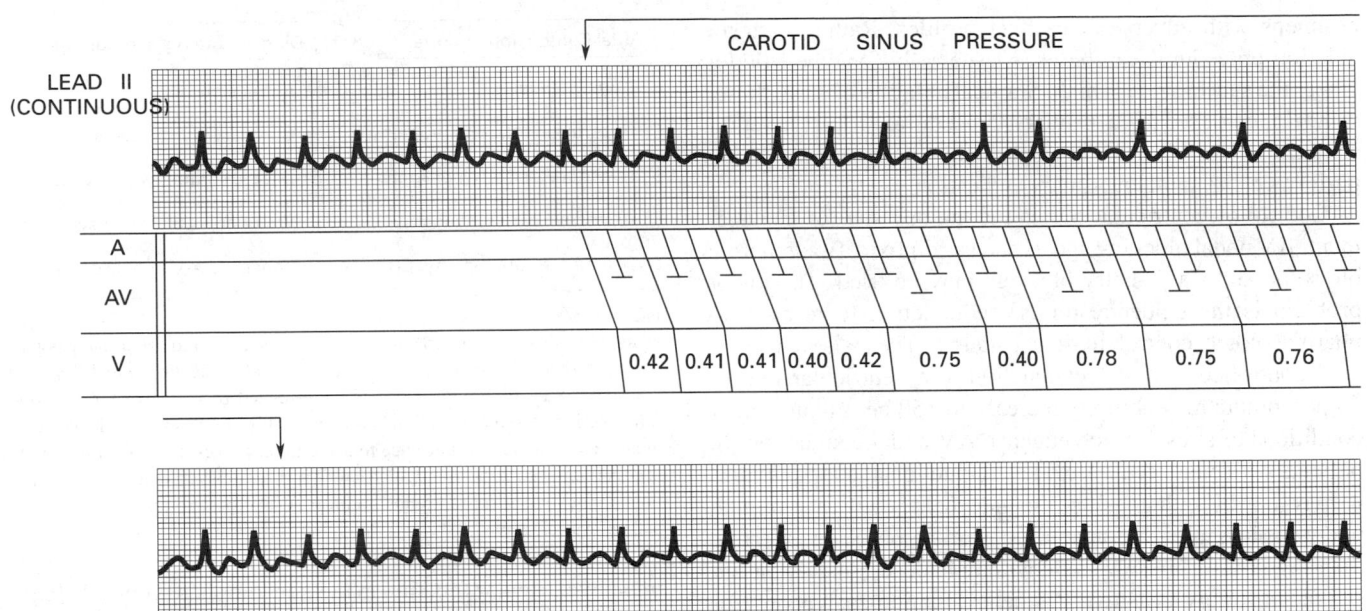

FIGURE 27-23

Atrial flutter and carotid sinus massage. At the beginning of the strip, AV conduction is occurring at the common 2:1 ratio, and flutter waves can be suspected but not proved; however, during carotid sinus massage, the conduction ratio increases to 4:1 and the flutter waves are easily recognized. Note the tendency of the atrial (flutter) rate to increase slightly during the parasympathetic stimulus.

for recurrences of the paroxysmal form of atrial flutter include long-term use of antiarrhythmic therapy to prevent the arrhythmia and the use of AV nodal blocking agents to control heart rate during recurrences. For the former, the class IA antiarrhythmic agents, especially quinidine, have been used with variable success. Other class I drugs (classes IB and IC) and class III drugs are potentially useful, but the concern with the action of class IC drugs in atrial flutter cited above limits their use. Control of ventricular rate is best achieved with digitalis because of safety and efficacy considerations. Long-term oral use of verapamil for control of rate in recurrent atrial flutter is less predictably effective than intravenous use to slow the rate during a paroxysm.[19] Beta-adrenergic blocking agents have been used, and if the drugs are well tolerated, the dose can be titrated to clinical β-blocking efficacy by heart rate and blood pressure criteria. Subsequent observations of ventricular rates during recurrences will establish efficacy. There is little or no excess incidence of embolic events during paroxysmal atrial flutter or during its reversion. Anticoagulants are not used before, during, or after reversion. In recent years, RF catheter ablation procedures have been used with increasing frequency for patients with atrial flutter, especially for patients with frequent symptomatic episodes of atrial flutter or those resistant to drug therapy. RF ablation permanently interrupts the reentrant pathway responsible for type I flutter with a high probability of success[77,78] and avoids the need for long-term pharmacologic therapy among these patients.

Management of Persistent Atrial Flutter

Atrial flutter may occur in a persistent form secondary to noncardiac factors such as thyrotoxicosis or pulmonary embolism, although it is most common in the presence of chronic heart disease. Persistent or chronic atrial flutter occurs, but not commonly, in otherwise normal persons. Patients subject to recurrent episodes of persistent atrial flutter can be maintained on long-term antiarrhythmic therapy, usually one of the class IA drugs. Class IC and class III drugs may also be effective in some. However, RF ablation has emerged as the therapy of choice for symptomatic patients in this category.[71] If RF ablation fails or is not desired by the patient, therapeutic approaches during recurrences include additional antiarrhythmic agents for reverting atrial flutter and agents that will control the ventricular rate. Acute antiarrhythmic therapy may include intravenous procainamide or ibutilide[79] or orally administered drugs that prolong refractoriness (e.g., sotolol). Electrical reversion, however, may still be required. Surgical approaches are feasible[56] but have largely yielded to catheter ablation techniques.

Management of Chronic Atrial Flutter

Some patients will remain in chronic atrial flutter despite aggressive antiarrhythmic therapy, and flutter may recur predictably shortly after DC cardioversion. This usually occurs in the setting of advanced heart disease; may occur as the forerunner of chronic atrial fibrillation; and appears to be more frequent with the variants of flutter, such as type II atrial flutter. It may occur rarely in otherwise normal persons[70] and more commonly in association with other SVTs, such as WPW and AV nodal reentry.[80] If the ventricular rate is adequately controlled and the patient is asymptomatic, chronic atrial flutter need not be treated aggressively. In these cases, there is little justification for the use of complex antiarrhythmic drug regimens with adverse side-effect profiles. Rather, catheter ablation procedures can be used, especially for type I flutter where the success rate is high. Surgical ablation of atrial flutter is no longer used as a primary procedure. In rare circumstances, it can be used in conjunction with surgery being performed for another primary indication.

Control of ventricular rate is the major issue for management. AV nodal blocking agents such as digoxin, β-adrenergic blockers, and Ca^{2+}-entry blockers may be tried. The major problem is the tendency for AV conduction to respond to pharmacologic control in step patterns. The patient who is well controlled with 4:1 conduction at a ventricular rate of 75 per minute may abruptly increase to 150 per minute under conditions of stress, which enhance AV nodal conduction. In patients with enhanced AV nodal conduction and atrial flutter, it may be difficult to slow the rate below 150 per minute pharmacologically. Verapamil appears to be more effective than digoxin for the AV node with enhanced conduction but is not uniformly effective. Catheter ablation techniques for AV node modification or interruption is indicated for heart rate control in patients who are resistant to, or intolerant of, AV nodal blocking drugs and who have failed ablation attempts to interrupt the flutter pathway. It is almost always successful but requires pacemaker implantation to manage heart rate subsequent to the procedure. Surgery solely for interruption of the AV junction is no longer performed.[62] Long-term anticoagulation is not generally used for chronic atrial flutter, although the potential risk of embolism in atrial flutter is being reevaluated.[81]

ATRIAL FIBRILLATION

The prevalence, presentation, clinical significance, and long-term implications of atrial fibrillation depend heavily upon the clinical circumstances in which it occurs. Among the cross-sectional studies of prevalence, there is a large gradient across age categories, ranging from less than 0.5 percent in young adults to the range of 1 to 5 percent through the decades from 40 to 70 years and reaching rates in excess of 10 percent in some beyond age 70.[82] At each age, however, prevalence is powerfully influenced by the presence of disease, especially (but not exclusively) mitral valve disease. The high prevalence in rheumatic mitral valve disease has been emphasized in the past, but it is likely that risk with any cause of mitral valve disease of equivalent severity is just as high. The clinical presentation ranges from minimally symptomatic or asymptomatic incidental findings to acute pulmonary edema in patients with advanced mitral or aortic stenosis. Between these extremes, atrial fibrillation may herald the presence of noncardiac disorders (e.g., thyrotoxicosis), alert to the significance of another cardiac disorder (e.g., WPW syndrome), constitute a transient complicating factor of another cardiac disorder (e.g., acute myocardial infarction or systemic arterial hypertension), or occur as an isolated event having no inherent significance (e.g., lone paroxysmal atrial fibrillation in healthy young adults). The hemodynamic consequences of atrial fibrillation are due to two factors: (1) the loss of atrial systole may

Atrial Contraction Important	Diastolic Intervals Important
▷ Aortic stenosis	▷ Mitral stenosis
▷ Hypertrophic cardiomyopathy	▷ Coronary artery disease
▷ Hypertension/LV hypertrophy	▷ Dilated cardiomyopathy; CHF
▷ Restrictive cardiomyopathy	▷ Wolf-Parkinson-White syndrome
▷ Dilated cardiomyopathy; CHF	▷ Enhanced A-V nodal conduction

FIGURE 27-24

Hemodynamic factors in atrial fibrillation. Atrial fibrillation creates the potential for two hemodynamic defects: (1) loss of atrial contraction, which provides the presystolic atrial "kick"; and (2) rate-related reduction of the diastolic filling period. Atrial contraction is important to ventricles with reduced compliance and low-output states due to myocardial factors. Diastolic filling time is important in conditions in which a longer diastolic is beneficial to impaired flow states, such as mitral stenosis, coronary atherosclerosis, and some myopathic ventricles.

impair ventricular function in the noncompliant ventricle [e.g., aortic stenosis, left ventricular hypertrophy (LVH)] or the dilated ventricle with systolic dysfunction, and (2) a rapid ventricular rate will encroach upon the diastolic filling period of the left ventricle and the diastolic flow time of the coronary arteries (Fig. 27-24). The risk of embolism and stroke is a long-term concern of special importance (see below). Atrial fibrillation may occur in paroxysmal, persistent, and chronic patterns (Fig. 27-25).

Electrocardiographic Features

Atrial fibrillation is characterized electrocardiographically by grossly disorganized atrial electrical activity that is irregular in respect to both rate and rhythm. There is no visually discernible timing pattern to the atrial electrical activity on the surface ECG or to electrogram sequences recorded by catheter electrodes. Specific patterns of AV conduction sequences (ventricular responses) have been proposed as a result of sophisticated analytic techniques[83]; this provides some physiologic insight but does not yet have practical clinical value. Atrial fibrillatory waves are best seen in standard lead V_1 and are usually clearly evident in II, III, and aV_F as well. They may be quite large and coarse or almost imperceptible (compare panels A and B in Fig. 27-26). In the absence of discernible atrial electrical activity, a grossly irregular ventricular rhythm still suggests

Definition	Duration
¥ Paroxysmal	Minutes/hours
- Short-lasting	Seconds → <1 hour
- Long-lasting	≥1 hour; → ≤48 hours
¥ Persistent	Two days → weeks
¥ Chronic	Months / years

FIGURE 27-25

Clinical expression of atrial fibrillation. Atrial fibrillation may occur in brief paroxysms, a more persistent form lasting from days to weeks, or chronically. Approaches to therapy are dictated by these patterns in conjunction with the hemodynamic considerations shown in Fig. 27-24.

LEAD V₁

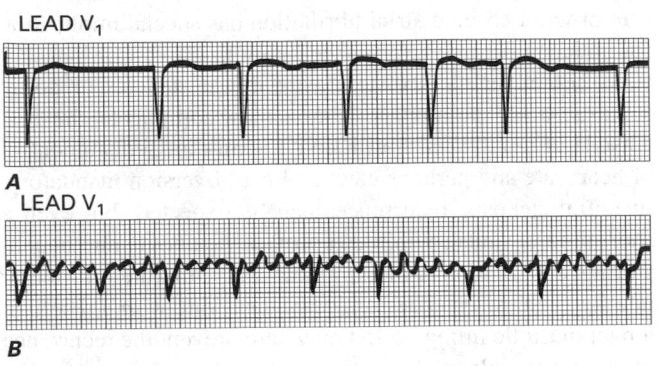

A

LEAD V₁

FIGURE 27-26

A. Fine atrial fibrillation, leaving virtually no imprint on the baseline ("straight-line" fibrillation). *B.* Coarse atrial fibrillation; the fibrillatory waves are the size of respectable flutter waves but are irregular.

LEAD V₁

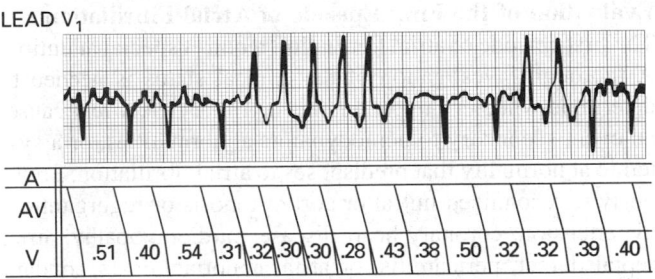

A	
AV	
V	.51 .40 .54 .31 .32 .30 .30 .28 .43 .38 .50 .32 .32 .39 .40

FIGURE 27-28

Atrial fibrillation with repetitive aberrant ventricular conduction. The impulses that end the shortest ventricular cycles (0.28 to 0.32 s) are anomalous, widened complexes. Note that the cycle preceding the onset of the salvos of anomalous beats is *relatively* long in comparison with the anomalous complexes (0.54 and 0.50 s), in accordance with Ashman's phenomenon. Thus, these almost certainly represent a right bundle branch block type of ventricular aberration rather than ventricular ectopy.

the presence of atrial fibrillation. Coarse atrial fibrillation is occasionally difficult to distinguish from atrial flutter waves, but the irregular ventricular response, in the absence of a repetitive pattern, is again helpful in making the distinction. In contrast, obvious coarse fibrillatory waves with a regular ventricular response, especially when slow, suggests the coexistence of high-grade AV block with atrial fibrillation.

One of the more challenging exercises in clinical electrocardiography is the distinction between aberrant intraventricular conduction and ventricular ectopy in the presence of atrial fibrillation. Aberrant conduction tends to occur when a long ventricular cycle is followed by a short cycle. This long-short cycle sequence, with the short cycle terminated by an aberrantly conducted beat, is referred to as the *Ashman phenomenon*.[84] It is important to recognize that "long" and "short" cycles are relative terms and carry no implications of absolute value (compare Figs. 27-27 and 27-28). A series of short cycles, if short enough, may generate runs of consecutively aberrant beats imitating VT (Fig. 27-28). Thus, additional criteria for distinction between aberrancy and ectopy are re-

quired. In general, an initial QRS vector similar or identical to that of narrow QRS complexes and a typical right bundle branch block pattern, in association with a long-short cycle sequence, strongly favor aberrancy over ectopy.[85] Left bundle branch block aberrancy also occurs but is far less common. It is more likely when aberrant conduction is persistent (i.e., functional bundle branch block during a sustained SVT) (Fig. 27-14), while it is unusual in single-cycle aberrancy (Fig. 27-27). Atrial fibrillation alters intraventricular conduction only through the following mechanisms: (1) functional bundle branch block or aberrancy (Fig. 27-29), (2) loss of delta waves in WPW syndrome with normal pathway conduction during atrial fibrillation, or (3) totally preexcited QRS complexes during atrial fibrillation in WPW syndrome (Fig. 27-16). The QRS complex during atrial fibrillation will be similar to that recorded during sinus rhythm under all other circumstances. In patients with preexisting bundle branch block who develop atrial fibrillation with rapid ventricular responses, the distinction from VT may be difficult.

LEAD V₁

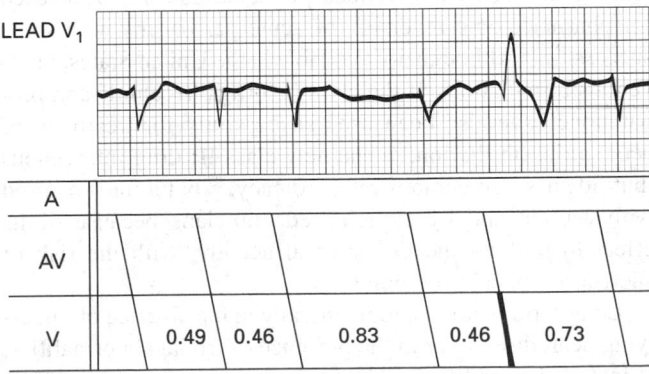

A	
AV	
V	0.49 0.46 0.83 0.46 0.73

FIGURE 27-27

Ashman's phenomenon. During atrial fibrillation, the impulse ending a short cycle preceded by a relatively long cycle manifests aberrant intraventricular conduction. In this example, the aberrant impulse shows typical right bundle branch block type aberration in lead V₁, with an rSR′ pattern and the initial deflection identical with that of the preceding and following normally conducted impulses.

MCL–1 MONITOR LEAD (CONTINUOUS)

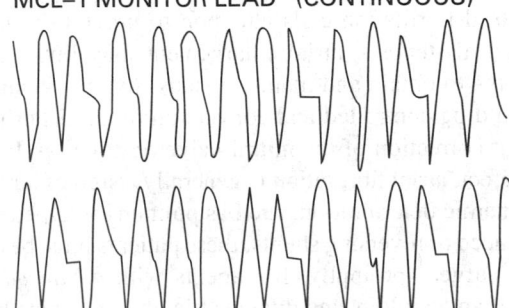

FIGURE 27-29

Irregular wide QRS tachycardia. A rapid irregular rhythm with wide QRS complexes having a left bundle branch block pattern is recorded. The rhythm is atrial fibrillation with abnormal intraventricular conduction. Irregular, wide QRS tachycardias also occur in Wolff-Parkinson-White syndrome with atrial fibrillation and conduction down the accessory pathway or in rare cases of irregular ventricular tachycardia.

Evaluation of the First Episode of Atrial Fibrillation

The first episode of atrial fibrillation requires special attention. A thorough investigation of the clinical status is needed to determine whether the patient has a primary electrical cause, an event secondary to hemodynamic abnormalities, or a systemic abnormality that predisposes to atrial fibrillation. Previously unrecognized mitral or aortic stenosis or regurgitation, hypertension, coronary heart disease, cardiomyopathy, atrial septal defect, pericarditis, or atrial abnormalities secondary to left or right ventricular overload are among cardiac causes that must be excluded. Pulmonary emboli and metabolic abnormalities such as thyrotoxicosis also must be considered. The identification of associated factors at the time of the first episode of atrial fibrillation may dictate future management. In the absence of an identifiable cause, so-called lone atrial fibrillation carries a good prognosis,[86] especially if it is a single event or intermittently recurrent. Chronic lone atrial fibrillation may indicate a higher risk,[87] although conflicting data[86] question the validity of this conclusion. In a young, healthy individual in whom there is no evidence of structural heart disease, paroxysmal episodes of lone atrial fibrillation may occur under conditions of exogenous precipitating factors, such as excessive cigarette, alcohol, and/or coffee consumption; stress or fatigue; and, rarely, upon cessation of extreme exercise.

In the absence of organic heart disease or coexistent WPW syndrome, long-term management after the first episode need include no more than avoidance or removal of precipitating factors and following the patient over time to estimate the frequency of recurrences. In the presence of treatable cardiac or noncardiac causes, management must include attention to precipitating and predisposing factors. For instance, in atrial fibrillation occurring during the acute phase of myocardial infarction, which has been observed in up to 18 percent of monitored patients, spontaneous reversion is very common and rate control is the only therapy needed. In the setting of thyrotoxicosis, there is no rationale for trying to convert atrial fibrillation until the thyrotoxic state is controlled; in the interim, the ventricular rate may be slowed with propranolol. When atrial fibrillation calls attention to previously undiagnosed mitral stenosis, atrial enlargement may limit success of attempts to obtain and maintain sinus rhythm. Ventricular rate should be controlled and conversion of atrial fibrillation can await correction of the mitral valve obstruction. In atrial septal defect, atrial fibrillation is generally a sign of advanced hemodynamic deterioration, such as pulmonary hypertension and balanced or reversing shunts; these patients must be evaluated for surgery promptly. In patients with *advanced* heart disease of any etiology and dilated atria, the first episode may herald a chronic fibrillatory state. An attempt to revert the rhythm, either pharmacologically or electrically, the latter usually with a concomitant pharmacologic agent, may be an appropriate option; but the recurrence rate is very high.[88-90] If the patient will benefit from the hemodynamic advantage provided by an atrial contraction, the attempt at reversion is warranted despite the high probability of recurrence. The re-

cent onset of chronic atrial fibrillation has special implication for anticoagulation therapy (see below).

In hemodynamically significant mitral stenosis or aortic stenosis, acute pulmonary edema may complicate the first episode of rapid atrial fibrillation, making immediate control of heart rate and perhaps electrical cardioversion mandatory. In mitral stenosis, recurrences can be expected; but even a short time in sinus rhythm can provide hemodynamic benefit and allow institution of therapy that will control the ventricular rate for the next episode. A slower heart rate with a resultant longer diastolic filling period may help prevent the recurrence of pulmonary edema. In aortic stenosis, dependence upon the atrial kick for optimal hemodynamic function of the noncompliant hypertrophied left ventricle, rather than encroachment on the diastolic filling period, is the major concern. In some patients, multiple cardioversions may be necessary while preparing for surgery.

Management of Short-Duration Paroxysmal Atrial Fibrillation

Paroxysms of atrial fibrillation lasting less than 48 h in the absence of underlying heart disease are usually managed conservatively. Rest, mild sedation with 5 to 10 mg of diazepam, and digitalis for control of the ventricular rate is an accepted approach. After the first episode, patients who have lone atrial fibrillation can be reassured in respect to the absence of underlying organic heart disease and guided to avoid precipitating factors. In the presence of heart disease, particularly when the hemodynamic circumstances require either the mechanical benefit of atrial systole or a slow ventricular rate for adequate diastolic filling (Fig. 27-24), immediate reversion to sinus rhythm or slowing of the ventricular rate may be mandatory. The presence of clinical signs of heart failure may require immediate cardioversion to achieve either or both of these goals. If the patient is clinically stable, pharmacologic approaches to control the rate (digitalis or intravenous verapamil or diltiazem) may be attempted, as may antiarrhythmic agents. Among the latter, intravenous procainamide has been used for pharmacologic reversion of acute paroxysms with some success.[91,92] Although not available in the United States, intravenous formulations of the class IC drugs flecainide and propafenone have also been used successfully for treatment of acute atrial fibrillation.[93] The new class III drug intravenous ibutilide has also demonstrated efficacy,[79] but it must be used with caution and by experienced clinicians because of its effect to prolong the QT interval acutely, with the risk of short-term torsades de pointes.

Long-term pharmacologic therapy in the absence of underlying heart disease, or in the presence of trivial abnormalities, is intended to reduce or eliminate recurrent episodes and to control ventricular rate during recurrences, should they occur. Digitalis, β-adrenergic blockers, or Ca^{2+}-entry blockers are used for rate control as described for atrial flutter. Digitalis controls ventricular rate at rest, although it appears less effective for limiting effort-induced increases in ventricular rate during atrial fibrillation.[94]

Prevention of episodes of atrial fibrillation may be achieved with class IA, IC, or III antiarrhythmic drugs. If episodes are clinically benign and infrequent, the threshold for such treatment is higher than if they are symptomatic. Efficacy is uneven, and proarrhythmic or toxic side effects are of concern. During short paroxysms of atrial fibrillation ($\leq$48 to 72 h), anticoagulation is not required prior to reversion; long-term anticoagulation is not necessary for patients subject to brief paroxysmal attacks[95] (Fig. 27-25; Table 27-7).

Management of Persistent Atrial Fibrillation

The decision to intervene in longer episodes of atrial fibrillation is based on the balance between hemodynamic tolerance and the likelihood of being able to control future episodes. More recently, consideration of the effects of "electrical remodeling" of atrial myocytes during persistent atrial fibrillation,[96] favoring persistence of the arrhythmia and resistance to reversion, has begun to lead to a more aggressive approach to early reversion.[97]

Many patients with organic heart disease have intermittent episodes of persistent atrial fibrillation prior to establishing

---

TABLE 27-7

ANTICOAGULATION OF PATIENTS WITH ATRIAL FIBRILLATION

Indications
  Rheumatic mitral valve disease with recurrent or chronic atrial fibrillation
  Dilated cardiomyopathy with recurrent persistent or chronic atrial fibrillation
  Prosthetic valves
  Prior to ($\geq$3 weeks) elective cardioversion of persistent or chronic atrial fibrillation
  Coronary heart disease or hypertensive heart disease with recurrent persistent or chronic atrial fibrillation
  Atrial fibrillation in thyrotoxicosis (while awaiting long-term control; elective cardioversion)
  Chronic or persistent lone atrial fibrillation, age $\geq$60 years
Controversial; or limited data
  Coronary or hypertensive heart disease with normal left atrial size, after first episode of paroxysmal atrial fibrillation
  Elective cardioversion of atrial fibrillation of short duration (2–3 days) with normal left atrial size
  Chronic or persistent lone atrial fibrillation, age <60 years
Not indicated
  Lone atrial fibrillation, short paroxysms (<48 h)
  Most clinical settings associated with short paroxysms (minutes to hours)
Relative contraindications
  Difficulty controlling prothrombin times
  Dementia
  Malignancies, especially associated with bleeding risk
  Prior major bleeding events
  Uncontrolled hypertension

---

chronic atrial fibrillation.[98] These are the most difficult patients for management since antiarrhythmic efficacy for control of recurrences is unpredictable. Prediction of the ability to control ventricular rate by AV nodal blocking agents is better but still imperfect. After treating the first episode of persistent atrial fibrillation, many clinicians avoid repeated electrical cardioversions for recurrences of a persistent pattern in patients with advanced organic heart disease if they are well tolerated hemodynamically. If elective cardioversion is to be attempted, 3 weeks of anticoagulation should precede the procedure to reduce embolic risk. If cardioversion is not attempted and the patient has recurrent episodes of atrial fibrillation lasting $\geq$48 to 72 h, long-term anticoagulant with warfarin is indicated. If the patient is without structural disease, is aged $\leq$60 years, and has a normal echocardiogram and no prior history of embolism, cardioversion may be carried out earlier and long-term warfarin therapy is unnecessary.

In the presence of cardiac disease, atrial fibrillation is likely to revert and recur intermittently until the condition evolves into chronic atrial fibrillation. When this occurs, the best therapeutic approach may be control of ventricular rate during recurrences. Membrane-active antiarrhythmic agents are often used in an attempt to limit the number of recurrences, but efficacy is unpredictable and risk of side effects is high. The flecainide data suggest efficacy,[56,99] especially for patients with good LV function and those free of underlying coronary artery disease.[14,15] Class III antiarrhythmic drugs also appear effective.[92] Despite these considerations, the long-term benefit of prevention of atrial fibrillation by drug therapy versus control of heart rate remains uncertain. A large multicenter study is currently in progress to answer this question.

Management of Chronic Atrial Fibrillation

The ventricular rate in chronic atrial fibrillation is usually more predictably controlled than in recurrent episodes of paroxysmal or persistent atrial fibrillation. Pharmacologic or electrical cardioversion in patients with advanced heart disease and atrial enlargement is attempted in the hope of achieving a hemodynamic benefit, but the short- and long-term success rates are low.[88–90] Until more data are available, the choice between restoration of sinus rhythm and heart rate control in atrial fibrillation is a matter for individual clinical judgment; but most agree that no more than one attempt at electrical cardioversion is warranted in the presence of adequate levels of a membrane-active antiarrhythmic agent. Among patients with diverse diseases who have been electrically cardioverted, approximately one-third will revert to atrial fibrillation within 1 week and two-thirds within 12 months.[88,90] If the rhythm reverts to chronic atrial fibrillation shortly after cardioversion, the probability of long-term maintenance of sinus rhythm by pharmacologic approaches is nearly nil. The ventricular rate is then controlled as outlined above.

Pharmacologic control of ventricular rate may be problematic in recurrent episodes of both persistent and chronic atrial fibrillation. Under both circumstances, catheter modification of the AV junction or complete interruption (catheter ablation) of the AV junction with permanent pacing may provide heart rate control.[100] Other nonpharmacologic strategies for control of atrial fibrillation include surgical procedures designed to establish sinus node control of the ventricular rate and rhythm. The "corridor" procedure[101] establishes a pathway from sinus node to AV node, while the MAZE procedure[102] interrupts pathways necessary for maintaining fibrillation and reestablishes both rate control and mechanical function. A newly conceived device, the implantable atrial defibrillator,[103] and catheter ablation techniques for preventing atrial fibrillation (i.e., catheter-based MAZE procedure)[104] are both currently under evaluation. The ultimate role for each of these approaches in the management of patients with recurrent or chronic atrial fibrillation remains to be determined.

Anticoagulation of Patients with Atrial Fibrillation

This is an important component in the management of patients with persistent or chronic atrial fibrillation. Patients with atrial fibrillation have a greater than fivefold increase in risk of stroke, compared to control populations without atrial fibrillation.[105–108] In addition, there are specific high-risk subgroups. Among patients with rheumatic heart disease, the risk exceeds by up to 17 times that of a control group.[106,107] Other subgroups at high risk include patients with dilated cardiomyopathy, dilated left atrium of any cause, atrial fibrillation of recent onset, and a history of prior embolism. Patients with atrial fibrillation and LV hypertrophy are also at increased risk, as are thyrotoxic patients.[109] In one study, the chronic form of lone atrial fibrillation has been reported to be associated with a relative increase in risk of embolic stroke,[110] although other studies have not identified an increased risk. It is generally agreed, however, that patients older than 60 years with lone atrial fibrillation are at risk and should be anticoagulated with warfarin.[111] As a group, the nonrheumatic disease states associated with atrial fibrillation tend to have excess risks in the range of five- to sixfold among various studies.[82] Absolute risks differ little between the various rheumatic and nonrheumatic etiologies, however, with event rates in the range of 4 to 6 percent for each, except for lone atrial fibrillation, which has a considerably lower rate.[82,86,110] The risk of embolic events tends to cluster around changes in rhythm—the highest incidence occurring within the first year after onset of chronic atrial fibrillation[106] and a concentrated 1 to 2 percent risk occurring in the first days after conversion to sinus rhythm.[112–114]

The issue of anticoagulation in atrial fibrillation hinges on a balance between efficacy of preventing embolic events and risk of bleeding (Table 27-7). Until recently, most of the data on efficacy of anticoagulation for reducing incidence of embolic events in atrial fibrillation were from poorly controlled or uncontrolled studies, and there was no consensus based on the available data.[105] The available combination of risk data and retrospective or uncontrolled efficacy data[89,94,105] tended to result in the practice of using long-term anticoagulation for patients with a rheumatic etiology

and for those with advanced structural diseases associated with atrial fibrillation. Such patients included those with coronary artery disease and a prior embolism, idiopathic dilated cardiomyopathy, and prosthetic cardiac valves. Several recent placebo-controlled studies have now provided clarification of the role and methods for anticoagulation in patients with nonrheumatic atrial fibrillation. In one multicenter randomized trial, the Stroke Prevention in Atrial Fibrillation (SPAF) Study, aspirin, 325 mg/day, and warfarin, with prolongation of prothrombin times to 1.3 to 1.8 times control, were each compared to placebo among a population of 1330 patients.[115] During a mean follow-up of 1.3 years, ischemic stroke or systemic embolization occurred at a rate of 6.3 percent per year in the placebo group, compared to 3.6 percent per year in the aspirin-treated group, a 42 percent reduction in the treated group ($p < .02$). Among the patients eligible for warfarin, the event rate in the untreated group was 7.4 percent compared to 2.3 percent in the treated group, a 67 percent reduction ($p < .01$). Primary embolic events and deaths combined were reduced by 58 percent in the warfarin group and 32 percent in the aspirin group. Thus both warfarin and aspirin were effective, but the design of the study prevented comparison of the two treatments. Although both chronic atrial fibrillation and intermittent atrial fibrillation were included in the study, the data reported do not permit a determination of any difference in risk or benefit for the two patterns. In another study, the Canadian Atrial Fibrillation Anticoagulation (CAFA) Study, the placebo group experienced a 5.2 percent embolism/stroke rate compared to 3.5 percent in a warfarin-treated group, a relative reduction of 37 percent with treatment.[116] The differences did not reach statistical significance since the study was prematurely terminated because of outcome data from other large studies suggesting benefit. Among two other studies, the Copenhagen AFASK Study[117] and the Boston Area Anticoagulation Trial in Atrial Fibrillation,[118] warfarin again demonstrated significant reductions in risk (82 and 87 percent, respectively), while aspirin demonstrated only a 14 percent reduction in the Copenhagen study (nonsignificant),[117] even though it was associated with a 42 percent reduction in the SPAF study.[115] Collectively, these studies demonstrate a significant benefit for reduction of embolism and stroke in nonrheumatic atrial fibrillation patients with the use of warfarin and likely with aspirin as a less-effective alternative (see Chap. 99). More recent data have reaffirmed that warfarin is superior to aspirin and provided additional insight into effective warfarin dose ranges.[119] In patients at high risk for embolic events, fixed low-dose warfarin [0.5 to 3.0 mg/day; international normalized ratio (INR) = 1.2 to 1.5] plus aspirin (325 mg/day) was inferior to conventional dose-adjusted warfarin (INR target = 2.0 to 3.0).

Indications for anticoagulation prior to elective cardioversion have not undergone the same scrutiny for efficacy as has now been provided for intermittent and chronic atrial fibrillation. Nonetheless, there is enough information available to warrant the routine use of anticoagulation prior to elective cardioversion of recent onset (>48 to 72 h), persistent atrial fibrillation or chronic atrial fibrillation, particularly when associated with an enlarged left atrium or other structural diseases regardless of etiology. Anticoagulation with warfarin is started 3 to 4 weeks before elective cardioversion and is maintained for 3 to 4 weeks subsequently. Anticoagulation may be used less uniformly prior to elective cardioversion of atrial fibrillation of short duration (<48 to 72 h), particularly if it is lone atrial fibrillation or associated with minimal structural disease and normal atrial dimensions. The risk-benefit data are less clear under these conditions.

The potential efficacy of anticoagulation must be weighed against its risk. Patients receiving anticoagulants retain a risk of embolization ranging from 1 to greater than 3 percent per year,[82,89,114–118] depending upon disease states. Furthermore, there is a significant incidence of major bleeding events requiring transfusion or life-threatening events among patients on long-term anticoagulation. In one report,[120] the incidence was 4.3 percent per treatment year. In the SPAF study,[115] however, bleeding risk hovered around 1.5 percent and did not differ among aspirin-treated, warfarin-treated, and placebo groups. Lower warfarin dosing than used previously, titrated to an INR of 2.0 to 3.0,[121] may be one reason for the reduction of bleeding risk with warfarin use. Since the risk of bleeding is increased significantly with prothrombin times greater than 2.5 times control and INR ≥ 5.0, the inability to control the prothrombin time, including the inability of the patient to comply with the prescribed dosages, must be considered relative contraindications. Intracranial bleeds are considered among the major complications and may have an incidence of 1 to 2 percent per treatment year.[122] Table 27-7 lists indications and relative contraindications for anticoagulation in patients with atrial fibrillation. The physician must balance accepted indications and risks in judging whether or not to use anticoagulation in individual patients. In most circumstances now, however, one should err on the side of use rather than avoidance if risk/benefit is not clear, assuming the INR is assiduously maintained between 2.0 and 3.0 in candidates at higher risk for bleeding complications.

ATRIOVENTRICULAR JUNCTIONAL AND ACCELERATED VENTRICULAR RHYTHMS

Rhythm disturbances that originate in the AV junction include premature AV junctional impulses, accelerated junctional rhythms, and AV junctional tachycardias that may be automatic or reentrant. Those arrhythmias that incorporate the AV junction as part of a larger reentrant pathway (i.e., various tachycardias or echo beats incorporating accessory pathways) and PSVT due to AV nodal reentry are discussed elsewhere. Junctional escape rhythms at rates of 40 to 60 per minute during sinus bradycardia or AV block are normal physiologic back-up phenomena, which are usually hemodynamically stable; failure of normal junctional escape mechanisms resulting in significant bradycardia will be discussed later.

The normal inherent rate of AV junctional automatic activity is 40 to 60 per minute, and those of subordinate pacemakers

at the fascicular or ventricular level are 20 to 40 per minute. Faster rates from either of these levels are considered "accelerated" rhythms up to 100 impulses per minute, at which point they take on the general definition of a tachycardia. Accelerated junctional and ventricular rhythms and most nonparoxysmal AV junctional tachycardias are thought to be due to enhanced automatic activity.[123,124] Clinical and experimental observations suggest that the mechanism of acceleration is enhanced phase 4 depolarization, although other forms of abnormal automaticity, including triggered activity initiated by afterdepolarizations, may also originate in the AV junction[125,126] (see also Chap. 26).

AV Junctional Premature Beats

These occur much less frequently than premature atrial or ventricular complexes. The timing of P waves and QRS complexes is variable, however. The P waves may precede QRS complexes by 0.12 s or less, may be concealed within the QRS complexes, or may appear in the ST segment following the QRS complex (Fig. 27-30). The P waves are usually inverted in leads II, III, and aV_F; isoelectric to slightly negative in leads I and V_6; and upright in the right precordial leads. The QRS complexes are narrow except when aberrant intraventricular conduction is present. When the P waves precede the QRS complex, distinction from premature atrial complexes may be difficult, and when aberrant intraventricular conduction is present and the P wave is within or after the QRS complex, the distinction from premature ventricular complexes may be impossible without intracardiac recordings.

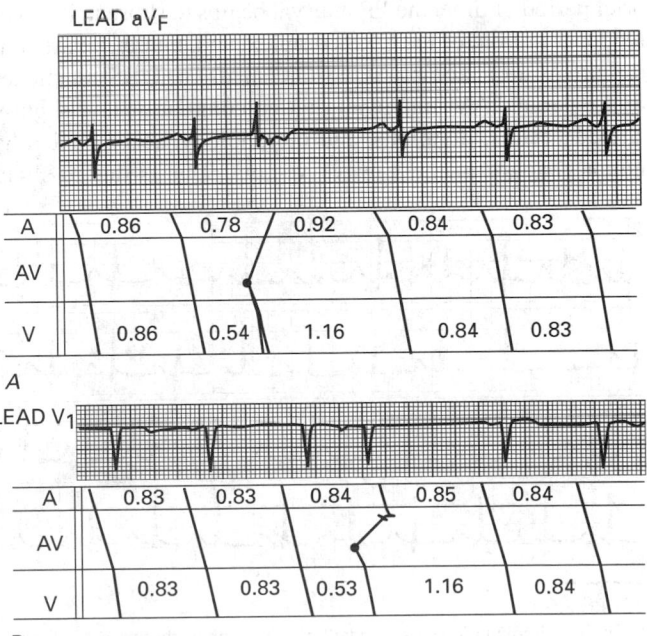

FIGURE 27-30

A. AV junctional extrasystole. The retrograde P wave follows the premature QRS complex, which shows some degree of ventricular aberration. *B.* The fourth complex is an AV premature impulse without retroconduction to the atria, leaving the sinus rhythm undisturbed.

There are no special aspects to the management of AV junctional premature beats. They generally require no treatment; when treated, however, they are approached using the same principles applied to the treatment of premature ventricular complexes (see below).

Accelerated Junctional and Accelerated Ventricular Rhythms

Accelerated rhythms derive from subordinate pacemakers and emerge when the sinus rate is less than the normally suppressed focus. Sinus bradycardia combined with enhanced automaticity of the subordinate site is the common pathophysiology. Ischemia (especially inferior wall myocardial ischemia or infarction), digitalis intoxication, electrolyte disturbances (especially hypokalemia), and hypoxemia may enhance phase 4 depolarization in the AV junction or intraventricular specialized conducting system, accelerating the rate of impulse formation of the subordinate pacemakers located at these sites. Digitalis intoxication, various degrees of AV block, and sinus node depression may accompany AV junctional acceleration producing complex ECG patterns. In inferior wall ischemia, subordinate pacemaker acceleration is commonly associated with sinus node depression, the latter permitting escape and usurpation of pacemaker function even with only modest AV junctional acceleration (e.g., 60 to 70 impulses per minute). These rhythms are almost always hemodynamically stable.

The typical electrocardiographic pattern is apparent shortening of the PR interval as the PP intervals prolong, leading to emergence of the subordinate QRS complexes as they assume the pacemaker function (Fig. 27-31). After a usually brief period of time, the PP interval begins to shorten, P waves reappear in front of the QRS complex, and, finally, ventricular capture by atrial activity is reestablished. The QRS complexes of accelerated AV junctional rhythm commonly have slightly altered vectors, durations, and morphology, accompanied by minor changes in the T-wave vectors. This is due to slight

changes in conduction patterns resulting from the altered origin of the propagatory wavefront in the ventricles, and these changes are diagnostically useful in uncertain instances.

Accelerated AV junctional and ventricular rhythms generally require no specific antiarrhythmic therapy. In ischemia, they are usually self-limiting in duration and of no major consequence hemodynamically; when associated with digitalis intoxication or electrolyte disturbances, they promptly reverse with control of these toxic or metabolic influences. In fact, specific antiarrhythmic drugs might suppress a subordinate pacemaker that is needed to maintain cardiac output in the presence of dysfunction of normal sinus node pacemakers. If a faster ventricular rate or AV sequencing is desirable for hemodynamic benefits, attempts to enhance cardiac rates may be achieved pharmacologically or by pacing. Atropine, 0.6 to 1.2 mg intravenously, may increase sinus rate and allow the sinus to resume its normal pacemaking function if AV conduction is intact. Atropine will have little or no influence on the rate of the accelerated AV junction focus. Temporary atrial or ventricular pacing may be used to support the heart rate if it is slow enough to impair hemodynamics, but it is rarely necessary.

AV Junctional Tachycardia

Enhanced AV junctional rhythm may occasionally double its rate abruptly to a true tachycardic range.[127] This likely represents an automatic focus firing at the faster rate with 2:1 exit block, which abruptly changes to 1:1 exit. In acute ischemic events, it may be desirable to reduce the rate with antiarrhythmic agents. These incidents are commonly self-limited, however, and will usually cease spontaneously or revert to 2:1 exit block.

Ectopic or persistent nonparoxysmal AV junctional tachycardia may occur intermittently in patients with chronic heart disease and appears to be more frequent and more important in children, particularly after surgical correction of congenital defects.[128,129] The response to treatment is unpredictable, and the rhythm may be resistant to conventional antiarrhythmic drugs. Catheter ablation has been suggested for some patients, however.[129]

An arrhythmia referred to as *permanent junctional reciprocating tachycardia* is characterized by a long RP–short PR reentry pattern and may be due to a very slowly conducting retrograde accessory pathway.[130–132] It is persistent, though not truly incessant; tends to occur in children; and is difficult to treat pharmacologically. Some success with class IC antiarrhythmic agents has been reported in children,[133] and catheter ablation has been used successfully.

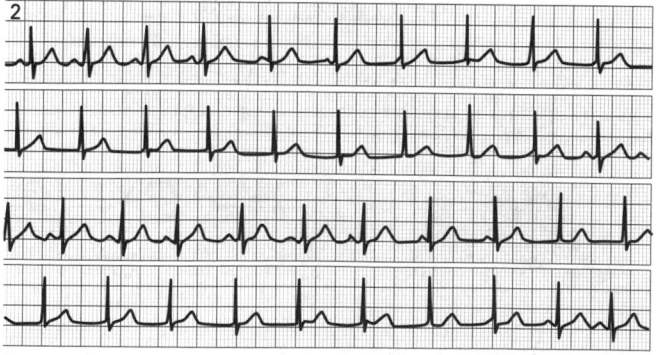

FIGURE 27-31
Accelerated idiojunctional (idionodal?) rhythm with isorhythmic AV dissociation. After four sinus beats, the sinus rate slows slightly, enabling an accelerated junctional pacemaker to escape at a rate of 94 per minute. After several seconds the sinus pacemaker accelerates and recaptures the ventricles. The same sequence is then repeated (the strips are continuous). (From Marriott HJL. Workshop in electrocardiography. Tampa Tracings, 1972. Reproduced with permission from the publisher and author.)

VENTRICULAR ARRHYTHMIAS

Attitudes and approaches to the evaluation and management of ventricular arrhythmias have undergone dramatic changes in recent years. New insight into the risk implied by ventricular arrhythmias in various clinical settings, some clarification of the risk-benefit ratio of antiarrhythmic drug treatment, and the refinement of nonpharmacologic methods of treatment all have developed in parallel in recent years. The equilibrium between the risk implied by an arrhythmia and the proarrhythmic risk of a drug[134–137] has been dramatically emphasized by the results of the CAST Study.[16,17] The implications of that study have resulted in major changes in indications and methods for treatment of some ventricular arrhythmias. The *urge* to treat, based upon limited scientific support in the past, has yielded to indications based upon the *need* to treat, with indications for treatment now modulated by a better definition of the risk of treatment. Clinical approaches to the patient with ventricular arrhythmias require a clear analysis of the interrelationships between electrocardiographic forms of arrhythmias, the specific clinical setting in which it occurs, and realistic goals of therapy (Tables 27-1 and 27-2).

Definitions, Classification of Risk, and Endpoints of Therapy

When the approach to cardiac arrhythmias shown in Table 27-1 is applied to ventricular arrhythmias, "forms" may be separated into the various patterns of ambient PVCs and of sustained arrhythmias such as sustained VT or VF (Fig. 27-32). The former are present continuously and intermittently over time and identify risk in presence of structural heart disease. They may also serve a triggering function for hemodynamically significant or life-threatening arrhythmias (VT or VF) under appropriate conditions. This distinction, however,

TABLE 27-8

SPECIFIC FORMS OF VENTRICULAR TACHYCARDIA

Duration	ECG Pattern
Salvo (3–5 impulses)	Uniform morphology VT[a]
Nonsustained VT (6 impulses, 29 s)	Polymorphic VT; torsades de pointes
Sustained VT (≥30 s)	Right ventricular outflow pattern
	Bidirectional tachycardia

[a] VT, ventricular tachycardia.

is an oversimplification because of the lack of a uniformly accepted classification system to estimate risk and the complexity of the interaction between chronic PVCs, the stability of underlying disease, and the severity of LV dysfunction.

The conventional definition of VT, which is three or more consecutive ventricular ectopic impulses at a rate of 120 or greater, is too broad to apply to current evaluation and management strategies. A distinction between bursts of nonsustained VT lasting for up to 30 s and sustained VT lasting 30 s or more (Table 27-8) may be more useful for the proper evaluation of bedside clinical information, ambulatory monitoring data, the results of invasive electrophysiologic testing, and responses to therapy. In addition to defining VT by its duration, useful information is contained in the definition of VT from its ECG pattern. Slow, monomorphic patterns of nonsustained VT are less symptomatic and may denote lower risk than faster, polymorphic VT patterns.

Estimates of risk of chronic PVCs are based upon frequency and/or forms of PVCs[138] in conjunction with the underlying state of the heart. Data on the risk predicted by PVCs after convalescence from myocardial infarction have been analyzed relative to both frequency and forms.[138–143] Based upon the frequency in Fig. 27-33, most studies demonstrate increased risk with frequencies of 10 or more ectopic impulses per hour, and one major study demonstrated a sharp increase in risk moving across the range of 1 to 9 impulses per hour.[143] Similarly, in the hierarchy of forms, couplets indicate only a small increase in risk compared to uniform or multiform single PVCs,[143] and salvos indicate a significantly higher risk.[142,143] There are insufficient data to determine whether longer runs (i.e., nonsustained VTs ≥6 consecutive impulses) constitute an even higher risk. Within the hierarchy of forms, unifocal, multiform, couplets, and salvos are considered among the triggering PVCs, and sustained VT and VF are the potentially lethal forms. Nonsustained VT may be an intermediate or transitional form[1] (Fig. 27-32); pathophysiologically, it may be either a self-terminating expression of sustained VT or an intense trigger. Patterns such as bigeminy and trigeminy are simply an expression of frequency and contain no inherent information concerning risk beyond frequency.

In evaluating or managing any form of ventricular arrhythmia, an approach based upon clinical information beyond the

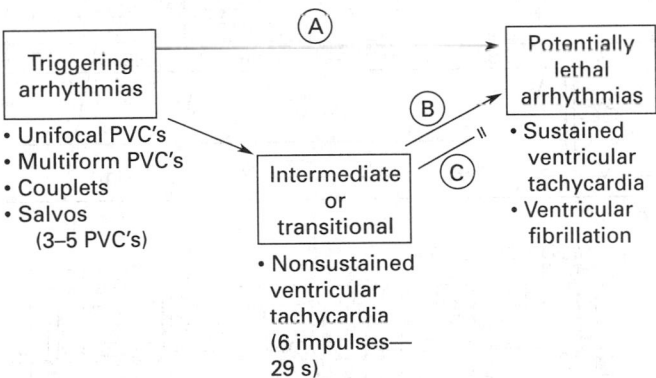

FIGURE 27-32

Forms of ventricular arrhythmias; triggering versus potentially lethal arrhythmias. Chronic, subacute, or acute premature ventricular contractions (PVCs) may function as triggering events to initiate potentially lethal arrhythmias at a time when the ventricular myocardium is susceptible to sustained ventricular tachycardia (VT) or ventricular fibrillation (VF) (arrows A and B). Unifocal and multiform PVCs, couplets, salvos (3 to 5 PVCs), and sustained VT are included among the triggering forms, while sustained VT or VF are the potentially lethal sustained arrhythmias. Nonsustained VT may be considered an intermediate or transitional form, functioning as an intense trigger to initiate potentially lethal arrhythmias (B) or as an "incomplete" form of VT (C). Approaches to therapy may be targeted to suppression of triggering events or prevention of initiation of lethal arrhythmias by stabilizing the myocardial mass. (Modified from Myerburg et al.[1] Reproduced with permission from the publisher.)

HIERARCHY OF FREQUENCIES	HIERARCHY OF FORMS
CLASS 0 – NIL	CLASS A – UNIFORM MORPHOLOGY, UNIFOCAL
CLASS I – RARE < 1 ectopic impulse/hour	CLASS B – MULTIFORM, MULTIFOCAL
CLASS II – INFREQUENT 1 to 9 ectopic impulses/hour	CLASS C – REPETITIVE FORMS • COUPLETS • SALVOS, REPETITIVE RESPONSES (3–5 consecutive inpulses)
CLASS III – INTERMEDIATE 10 to 29 ectopic impulses/hour	CLASS D – NON-SUSTAINED VENTRICULAR TACHYCARDIA (from 6 consecutive ectopic impulses to runs lasting up to 30 seconds)
CLASS IV – FREQUENT ≥ 30 ectopic impulses/hour	CLASS E – SUSTAINED VENTRICULAR TACHYCARDIA (runs of ectopic activity ≥ 30 seconds)

FIGURE 27-33

Classification of ventricular arrhythmias based on hierarchies of frequency and forms. Hierarchical schemes for estimating risk of ventricular arrhythmias have been developed based on frequency and forms of ventricular arrhythmias. In some clinical settings, frequencies in the range of 1 to 9 ectopic impulses per hour become significant, and in most settings of clinically significant heart disease, risk based on frequency plateaus in the range of 10 to 30 ectopic impulse per hour. Among forms of ventricular arrhythmias, the repetitive forms, particularly salvos or nonsustained ventricular tachycardia, indicate higher risk in most clinical settings. (Modified from Myerburg et al.[138] Reproduced with permission from the publisher.)

pattern of the arrhythmia itself must be developed. Very high frequencies and/or advanced forms connote little or no increased risk in the absence of structural heart disease, except for certain polymorphic nonsustained VTs. Risk begins to increase with the presence of organic heart disease and becomes prominent with falling EFs.[142,143] A simplified but useful clinically based classification incorporates both form and frequency along with clinical disease information. Bigger[144] suggested classifying ventricular arrhythmias as "benign," "potentially malignant," and "malignant" based on these considerations. As an extension of this concept, frequency, forms, severity of cardiac disease, and LV function (EF) can be integrated into a clinical classification of benign (no independent increase in risk), significant (independent increase in risk), and potentially lethal (untreated, can lead to proximate fatality). While these clinically based approaches have not been quantitated, they do provide a conceptual framework for classifying arrhythmias.

Management of PVCs must be further analyzed in regard to specific etiology [e.g., low-risk mitral valve prolapse (MVP) versus high-risk idiopathic dilated cardiomyopathy], and PVCs in acute or subacute clinical settings must be distinguished from those occurring in chronic settings. Finally, endpoints of therapy that are based upon suppression of underlying ectopy (i.e., background PVCs) are separated from endpoints based upon prevention of potentially lethal arrhythmias (i.e., sustained VT or VF) (see Table 27-1).

Premature Ventricular Contractions

ELECTROCARDIOGRAPHIC RECOGNITION OF PVCS

Ventricular arrhythmias originate in the specialized conducting tissue distal to the bifurcation of the bundle of His or in true ventricular myocardium. Accordingly, they are characterized by a prolonged ventricular depolarization (i.e., wide QRS complex), an alteration in the sequence of ventricular activation (i.e., a change in the QRS vector), and alterations in the timing sequence of consecutive QRS complexes (prematurity, escape rhythms). No one of these criteria or set of criteria are totally sensitive and specific for ectopic impulses of ventricular origin. On occasion, PVCs demonstrate narrow QRS complexes, have a vector very similar to the normal QRS vector, or have timing little changed from the normal sinus sequence. Nonetheless, the majority of impulses originating in the ventricles have QRS complexes of at least 0.12 s and a shift in the QRS vector, and most single PVCs or initiating beats for runs of ventricular ectopic activity are premature. PVCs may fail to conduct to the atria or may demonstrate retrograde atrial activation. In either case, the sinus cycle is usually not interrupted, resulting in a *fully compensatory pause* (Fig. 27-34). The pause is characterized by an interval between the P wave of the sinus impulse immediately before the PVC and the first

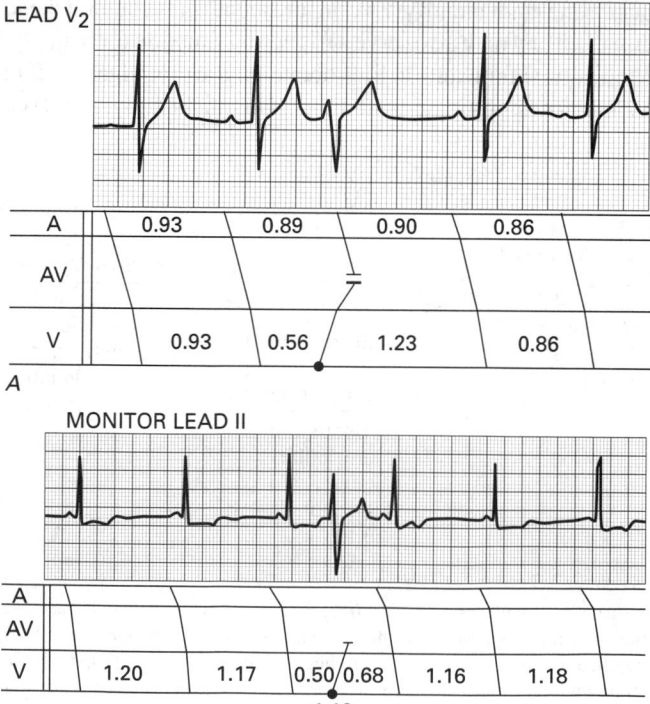

FIGURE 27-34

Ventricular premature contractions. *A*. The third impulse is wide and bizarre, and since the sinus rhythm is undisturbed (next sinus P wave indicated by arrow), the postextrasystolic pause is compensatory. *B*. The fourth impulse is an interpolated ventricular premature contraction; it is sandwiched between two consecutive conducted sinus beats.

sinus P wave after the PVC equal to twice the sinus cycle length (Fig. 27-34*A*). If the sinus rate is relatively slow, PVCs may be interpolated between two sinus beats with no alteration of the sinus cycle length (Fig. 27-34*B*). Exceptions to the compensatory pause rule do occur (Fig. 27-35) and occasionally complicate diagnostic criteria. PVCs that presumably originate in the fascicles of the specialized conducting system may have more narrow QRS complexes with only slight alterations in the QRS vector.

PVCs are usually coupled to the preceding sinus beat by a fixed coupling interval. This generalization has exceptions, in that PVCs having different QRS morphologies may have different coupling intervals,[145] and PVCs having the same morphology in a given patient may have different coupling intervals as pathophysiologic conditions change. The pattern of fixed coupling has led to a concept of a physiologic relationship between the sinus beat and the PVC and is used as an argument in favor of reentrant or triggered-activity mechanisms for common PVCs. In contrast, parasystolic rhythms refer to an independent ectopic rhythm, with the focus of origin being protected in the sense that descending impulses cannot enter and reset the parasystolic focus but can create a field of refractoriness around it, limiting the rate and timing of impulses that exit the focus. Thus, the parasystolic focus, automatic in nature, can deliver impulses to the myocardium but cannot be reset by impulses originating elsewhere. Accordingly, the ECG reflects the presence of competing pacemakers, the sinus node, and a protected automatic ectopic ventricular focus, creating the classic triad of (1) variable coupling between sinus beats and ectopic QRS complexes, (2) fusion beats, and (3) a fixed common denominator of interectopic intervals between manifest parasystolic extrasystoles (Fig. 27-36). In recent years, however, classic concepts of parasystole have been altered by the discovery that parasystole

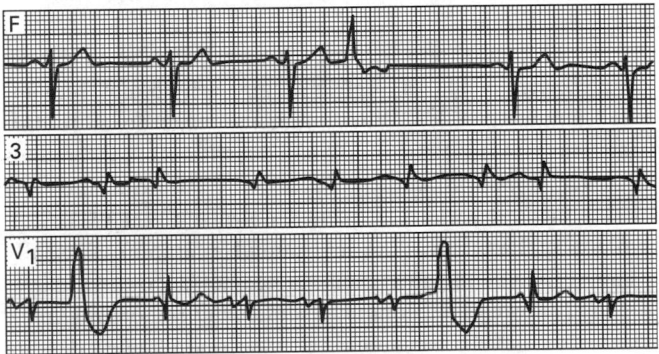

FIGURE 27-35

Exceptions to the rules for compensatory pauses. *Top.* Ventricular extrasystole with less than compensatory pause. Retrograde conduction to the atria (retrograde P wave deforms first part of ST segment) discharges the sinus pacemaker early and thus shortens the postextrasystolic cycle. *Middle.* Atrial premature contraction followed by fully compensatory pause. The third and eighth beats are atrial extrasystoles, but presumably because they suppress the sinus pacemaker, they are followed by compensatory pauses. *Bottom.* Ventricular extrasystoles with less than compensatory pauses. Each postextrasystolic cycle ends in an escape beat and so is slightly less than compensatory.

may be modulated by relationships between the parasystolic focus and impulses originating in the sinus node. Sinus impulses occurring early in the parasystolic cycle tend to shorten the cycle length of the parasystolic focus, whereas those arriving in the latter half of the cycle tend to lengthen the cycle length of the parasystolic focus.[146] Parasystolic patterns may also occur with atrial extrasystolic activity.

MANAGEMENT OF PREMATURE VENTRICULAR CONTRACTIONS

Management of PVCs in the Absence of Significant Structural Heart Disease

PVCs occur in many healthy individuals. In the absence of heart disease, there is little or no increased risk,[147] and the risk-benefit ratio of antiarrhythmic therapy does not support a need for routine treatment. For the patient who complains of disturbing palpitations due to PVCs, however, the clinician may have to attempt to relieve the symptom (Fig. 27-37). Reassurance and avoidance of potentially aggravating factors (e.g., tobacco, coffee, caffeine-containing soft drinks, environmental stress, stimulants) should be tried before specific pharmacologic therapy. For the latter, mild anxiolytic drugs or β-adrenergic blockers (which may sedate, reduce PVC frequency, and decrease the strength of postextrasystolic impulses causing the perception of palpitations) are preferred. When used for this purpose, low doses of β-adrenergic blockers are often sufficient—e.g., 5 to 20 mg of propranolol qid or an equivalent dose of other preparations. The endpoint, relief of symptoms, may not necessarily be accompanied by significantly reduced PVC frequency. The frequency of PVCs may be modulated by underlying heart rate,[148] and thus manipulations of sympathetic and parasympathetic balance may be useful. Because of their side-effect profiles, class I antiarrhythmic agents are rarely indicated in this clinical setting, and the class III agent amiodarone is unnecessarily potent. PVCs are often more prominent with pregnancy and premenstrually and increase in frequency with age.[149]

There may be an urge to be more aggressive in the management of patients who have advanced forms of PVCs (i.e., salvos, nonsustained VT) or a high frequency of PVCs (30 or more PVCs per hour) in the absence of structural disease. Kennedy et al.,[147] however, reported no increased risk of death in a cohort of such persons followed for a mean of over 6 years. Some specific forms of nonsustained VT may predict some increase in risk—e.g., polymorphic runs (see below).

The occurrence of PVCs in patients with MVP has gained special attention for three reasons: (1) the high prevalence of MVP, (2) the prevalence of PVCs in patients with MVP, and (3) the very small risk of sustained VT or VF. Annoying palpitations are a common complaint, but the arrhythmia does not require treatment in the vast majority. There are limited data suggesting that the patients at highest risk for serious ventricular arrhythmias can be subgrouped by the presence of nonspecific ST-T wave changes in leads II, III, and

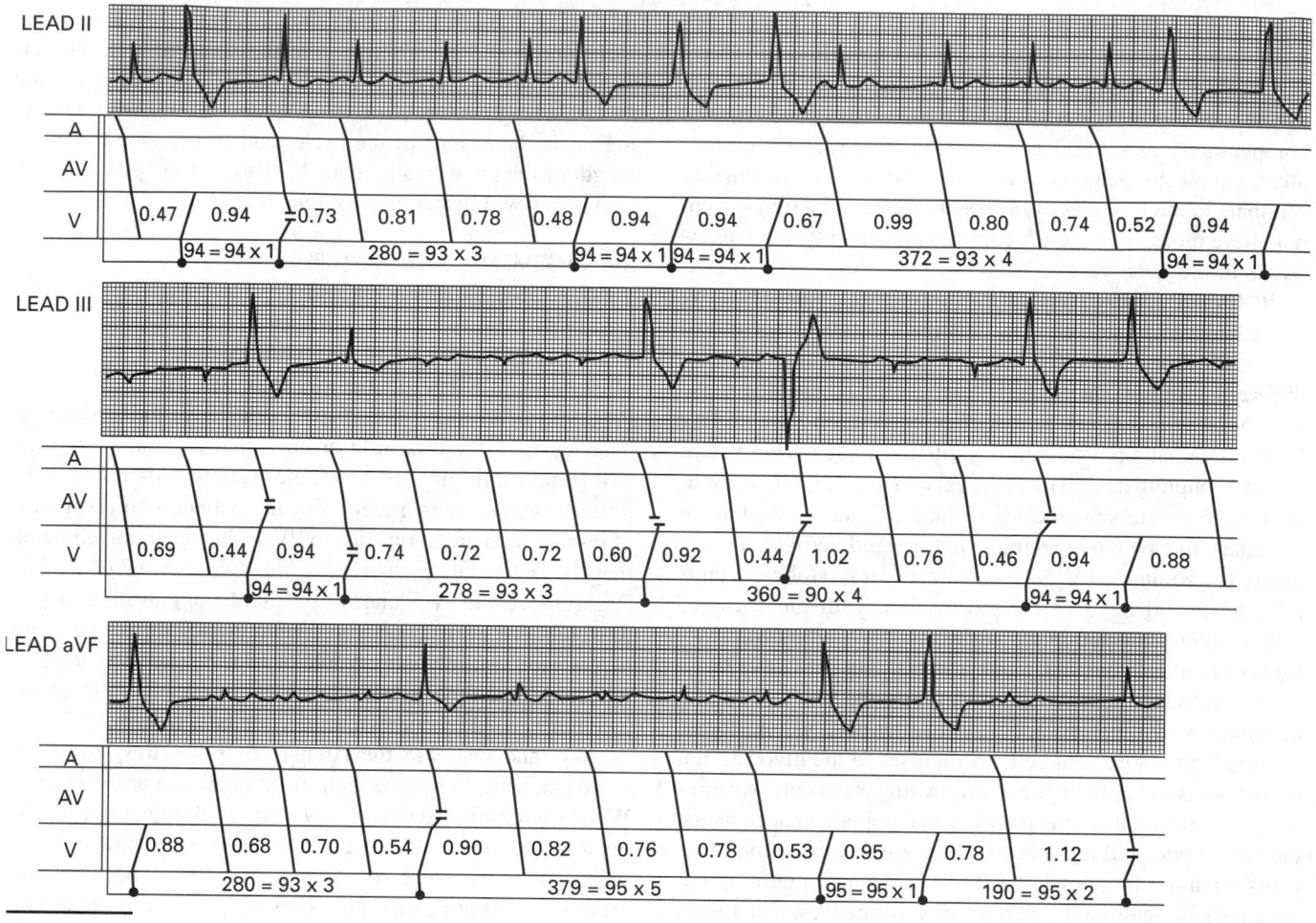

FIGURE 27-36

Ventricular parasystole. The strips are continuous. Note that (1) the interval between an ectopic beat and the preceding sinus beat varies; (2) the interectopic intervals all have a common denominator of 0.90 to 0.95 s; and (3) there are occasional fusion beats (third beat in top strip; fourth beat in second strip; last beat in bottom strip). (From Hurst JW, Myerburg R. *Introduction to Electrocardiography*. New York: McGraw-Hill; 1973. Reproduced with permission from the publisher and authors.)

aV$_F$[150,151] in conjunction with advanced grades of ventricular arrhythmias and redundancy of the mitral valve echocardiographically.[152] The approach to treatment of patients with benign forms of PVCs in MVP should be no different than that outlined for individuals with no structural abnormalities. β-Adrenergic blocking agents are often sufficient to control the symptoms, and membrane-active antiarrhythmic drugs should be avoided. Patients at risk for more serious arrhythmias, as outlined above, may require more aggressive treatment; membrane-active drugs are considered for use in this special situation for patients with salvos or nonsustained VT. The rare MVP patient who has had sustained VT or survived after VF is managed by the approaches generally used for these potentially lethal arrhythmias in other clinical settings (see below) (see also Chap. 64).

Management of PVCs in Acute Syndromes

PVCs are nearly ubiquitous in acute myocardial infarction, but the threshold for treatment remains unsettled. The original concept of "warning arrhythmias" published by Lown et al.[153]

remains an indication for aggressive treatment, even though the predictive value of such warning arrhythmias remains unsubstantiated.[154,155] Other opinions range from routine treatment with lidocaine of all patients with acute infarctions to prevent PVCs as well as VT or VF[156,157] to a threshold for treatment at various frequencies of manifest PVCs. Suppression of PVCs in acute myocardial infarction is usually accomplished with intravenous lidocaine (a bolus of 50 to 100 mg followed by a continuous infusion of 2 to 4 mg/min), with intravenous procainamide as a second choice (100 mg every 5 min to a total dose of 500 to 750 mg, followed by an infusion of 1 to 4 mg/min). Both drugs have significant side effects, especially with improper dosing. Furthermore, although their "routine" use is supported by practice, these drugs have not been shown to change hospital mortality in patients for whom prompt medical attention and electrical defibrillation are available. Lidocaine levels and binding both increase during the course of acute myocardial infarction,[158] theoretically rendering free drug levels stable. The practice of tapering the lidocaine infusion to avoid toxicity[159] is not appropriate if free drug concentration represents active drug and does not rise. Caution is warranted until these points are confirmed (see also Chap. 47).

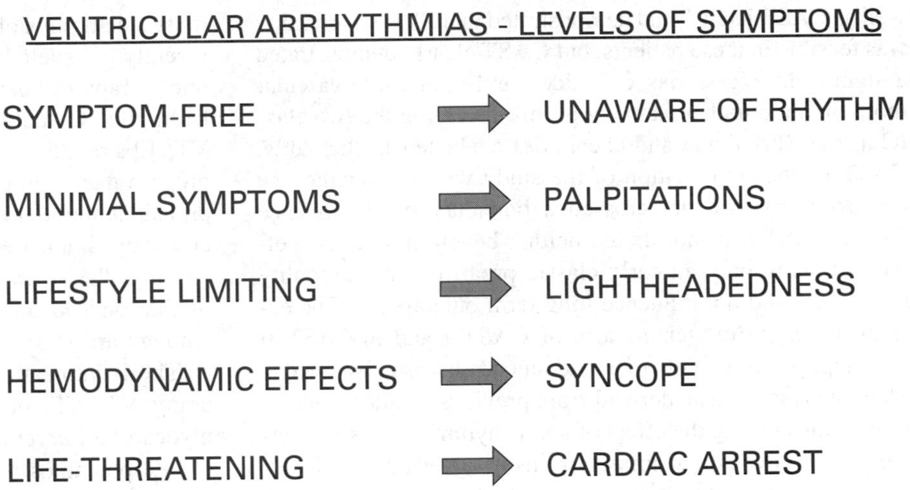

A number of other acute cardiac states are associated with the emergence of PVCs. Transient ischemic events have a high incidence of PVCs during and immediately after ischemia and are accompanied by a risk for sustained VT or VF.[160–162] The primary intervention for controlling PVCs in these settings is the reversal of ischemia.[160] On first contact, however, intravenous lidocaine or procainamide should be administered to suppress the arrhythmias. Clinical circumstances characterized by myocardial reperfusion—e.g., Prinzmetal's angina, thrombolysis in acute myocardial infarction, balloon deflation during percutaneous transluminal coronary angioplasty (PTCA)—may cause reperfusion-induced arrhythmias. The arrhythmias generated include PVCs and accelerated ventricular rhythms (e.g., postthrombolysis or PTCA) or nonsustained VT (often polymorphic) after reversal of coronary spasm.[162] These arrhythmias are usually transient and self-limiting but may evolve into sustained VT or VF.[161,162] Although there are theoretical and experimental reasons to suspect that Ca^{2+}-mediated electrophysiologic disturbances occur during reperfusion,[163,164] intravenous lidocaine is currently used to treat reperfusion-induced arrhythmias. It is used in the same dose and with the same infusion techniques as in acute myocardial infarction. Severe heart failure and acute pulmonary edema are commonly accompanied by frequent and advanced forms of PVCs[165,166]; as in acute myocardial infarction with low-output states, the PVCs are considered secondary to the hemodynamic abnormality (Fig. 27-1). The use of antiarrhythmic agents while the hemodynamic status is being stabilized is appropriate but may have only limited success until adequate hemodynamic control is achieved.

Acute and subacute myocarditis and pericarditis are commonly accompanied by PVCs, and sustained VT or VF may occur infrequently,[167] even in the absence of heart failure. Frequent PVCs and salvos or nonsustained VT are usually treated until the carditis has resolved. In those patients who have not had sustained VT or VF, conventional antiarrhythmic agents are given orally and titrated to suppression of the PVCs if possible, or at least to achieve suppression of repetitive forms. Antiarrhythmic therapy is continued for a minimum of 2 months, and then the patient is taken off antiarrhythmic drugs while still being monitored. If advanced forms do not reappear, the drug is not restarted; if they do reappear, treatment is continued for another 2 to 3 months, after which the

VENTRICULAR ARRHYTHMIAS - LEVELS OF SYMPTOMS

SYMPTOM-FREE	⟹ UNAWARE OF RHYTHM
MINIMAL SYMPTOMS	⟹ PALPITATIONS
LIFESTYLE LIMITING	⟹ LIGHTHEADEDNESS
HEMODYNAMIC EFFECTS	⟹ SYNCOPE
LIFE-THREATENING	⟹ CARDIAC ARREST

FIGURE 27-37

Approaches to management of ventricular arrhythmias. Treatment of ventricular arrhythmias is dictated by symptoms and clinical risk. Asymptomatic premature ventricular contractions (PVCs) in the absence of disease usually need not be treated. Ventricular arrhythmias in the presence of advanced and/or acute disease states commonly indicate high risk, although therapy is not necessarily targeted to the PVCs themselves. A range of considerations of risk versus quality of life exists between these two extremes (see text for details).

same procedure is carried out. Myocarditis that has not evolved into a cardiomyopathic state is only rarely followed by frequent or complex forms of PVCs beyond 6 months. Virtually all other acute cardiac syndromes and many acute systemic disorders may be associated with PVCs that will abate with resolution of the initiating abnormality. In most systemic disorders, PVCs do not require antiarrhythmic therapy.

Management of Chronic PVCs in the Presence of Cardiac Disease

Chronic PVCs carry a different connotation in patients with established heart disease than in those free of disease. Sudden and total death rates are increased in patients who have frequent or repetitive PVCs in the major categories of chronic cardiac disease in the United States, including chronic ischemic heart disease,[139–143] hypertensive heart disease, and the cardiomyopathies.[1,165,166,168,169] When frequent PVCs and/or salvos or runs of nonsustained VT are accompanied by a reduced EF, both the arrhythmia and the EF contribute to risk, and the rate of sudden death is increased.[142,143] Bigger et al.[143] observed a 2-year mortality of 42 percent for postinfarction patients with salvos or nonsustained VT and an EF of less than 30 percent, compared to a 2-year mortality of 12 percent for patients with salvos or nonsustained VT and an EF of 50 percent or more. The 2-year rate fell to 7 percent for patients with only single PVCs and an EF of 50 percent or more. Use of beta blockers after infarction should reduce this risk substantially in the higher risk subgroup.

Attitudes and approaches to the management of frequent and repetitive forms of chronic PVCs after myocardial infarction have changed dramatically since the results of the CAST study were published.[16,170] Previous studies[171,172] as well as CAST itself[16] had demonstrated that PVC suppression was feasible in these patients, but CAST clearly demonstrated a significant excess risk of sudden and total cardiovascular mortality among the treatment groups receiving the two class IC agents (flecainide and encainide) evaluated in the study. CAST II, the continuation of the study with moricizine, the one drug that had not crossed a boundary of significance during CAST I, demonstrated neither benefit nor adverse effect, showing only an early classic proarrhythmic mortality risk, which did not influence long-term outcome.[170] The enrollment in the moricizine arm of CAST I and in CAST II was a population with more advanced disease, by design. Meta-analyses of data derived from previous smaller randomized studies testing the effect of antiarrhythmic drugs on mortality after myocardial infarction also suggested an adverse effect of most antiarrhythmic drugs when used in postmyocardial infarction patients.[173] Accordingly, the drugs used in CAST are now contraindicated following myocardial infarction in patients with asymptomatic or mildly symptomatic PVCs, and there is a trend away from the use of any membrane-active antiarrhythmic agent in such patients. Recent randomized, placebo-controlled trials testing the possible benefit of amiodarone in postmyocardial infarction patients demonstrated no benefit on total mortality,[174,175] although one trial demonstrated benefit relative to sudden death (the primary endpoint in the study).[175] Beta-adrenoceptor blocking agents, however, have a substantial beneficial effect on long-term outcome in the postmyocardial infarction patient.[176,177] In addition, they are effective in suppressing repetitive forms of PVCs in many patients.[178] Beta blockers, therefore, have evolved as the drugs of choice following myocardial infarction in patients with mildly symptomatic PVCs. While no properly randomized study directed to a sudden and total death outcome as a result of PVC suppression using beta-adrenoceptor blocking agents has been reported, the existing randomized data on mortality in patients following myocardial infarction in general demonstrates beneficial effects.[176,177]

Management becomes more difficult following myocardial infarction in patients with *symptomatic* repetitive forms of PVCs, especially when accompanied by a low EF. Such patients have a higher risk of sudden death, and it is not known whether or not the CAST data should be extrapolated to this population as well. Because of the CAST study, class IC agents are generally avoided in these patients, but clinicians may use other antiarrhythmic drugs if they are well tolerated and no adverse effects are observed soon after initiation of therapy. Regardless of the depression of EF, β-adrenergic blocking agents should be tried initially; if they are effective and well tolerated, they are the preferred treatment, even in this category. Another approach is the use of antiarrhythmic therapy guided by the results of programmed electrical stimulation in patients who have coronary heart disease, low EFs, nonsustained VT clinically, and induced VT during invasive electrophysiologic testing.[179] The reported results appear beneficial, but the interpretation is limited by the absence of concurrent placebo-controlled observations, as is the case in most electrophysiologically guided data for such patients. A recently completed trial comparing conventional antiarrhythmic therapy (80 percent amiodarone) to implantable defibrillators in a population of such patients who had nonsustained VT, EFs ≤ 35 percent, inducible sustained VT, and failed programmed stimulation-guided therapy with intravenous procainamide, demonstrated a major benefit in favor of the automatic implanted defibrillator.[180] While the benefit was striking, the study population represents a small subgroup of the total postmyocardial infarction population who have ambient arrhythmias.

The identification of patients at increased risk of developing VT, VF, or sudden cardiac death after surviving a myocardial infarction may be enhanced by the identification of late potentials by signal-averaged electrocardiography or abnormal heart rate variability. The combination of a low EF (<35 percent), advanced PVC forms, and either a positive signal-averaged ECG[181] or abnormal heart rate variability[182] has identified subgroups with a 1-year mortality risk as high as 30 to 40 percent and 2½-year mortality up to 50 percent.

Chronic PVCs are very common in patients with advanced idiopathic dilated cardiomyopathy and in patients with hypertrophic cardiomyopathy, and both groups have a major risk of arrhythmic sudden death. In some reports, more than 90 percent of patients with dilated cardiomyopathy have frequent PVCs and over 50 percent have salvos or nonsustained VT.[165,166] Efficacy of antiarrhythmic therapy for both suppression of chronic PVCs and prevention of VT and VF is unclear and perhaps is quite limited in these patients. Nonetheless, treatment remains customary even though it is not known whether or not the CAST data can be extrapolated to this group. When treatment is prescribed, the patient should be hospitalized for initiation of antiarrhythmic therapy because of proarrhythmic risk in cardiomyopathy.[183] Secondary ventricular arrhythmias in patients who have chronic heart failure (Fig. 27-1) may respond to control of heart failure. In one carefully designed study, treatment with an angiotensin-converting enzyme inhibitor had a very favorable effect on both parameters of heart failure and ventricular ectopy.[184]

When antiarrhythmic drugs are to be used, the selection of a drug or a combination of drugs for high-risk patients with chronic PVCs is complex. The class IA drugs are moderately effective but have a high incidence of allergic reactions (e.g., procainamide) and poorly tolerated side effects (e.g., quinidine). They may also produce significant further myocardial depression in patients with an already reduced EF (e.g., disopyramide). Moricizine appears to be better tolerated, but all have significant risks of proarrhythmic effects, although many of these events are not life-threatening.[185] Among the class IB agents (e.g., tocainide, mexiletine), efficacy might be good in some patients and the proarrhythmic incidence is lower, but there is a high incidence of uncomfortable side effects. The currently available IC agents (flecainide, propafenone) are very effective for reducing ventricular ectopy and are well tolerated in patients with normal or only minimally depressed LV function. Their use is not indicated for patients with ischemic heart disease because of the adverse outcome observed in CAST[16] and is limited more generally by the fact that the incidence of proarrhythmic effects and myocardial depression is highest in the subgroup at greatest need for the intervention—i.e., those with repetitive forms and impaired LV function. It is not yet known, however, whether the higher absolute risk of adverse effects in patients with abnormal LV function is balanced by a benefit in this higher risk group.[186] Specifically, the long-term effects of the class I agents on death rates in patient groups other than the lower risk category enrolled in CAST are unknown at present. In regard to proarrhythmic risk, there are differences among the various drug groups. Class IA drugs are predominantly associated with classical proarrhythmia (torsades de pointes), which usually appears shortly after initiation of therapy.[187] Class III drugs have the same pattern of proarrhythmia, perhaps with a lower incidence of torsades de pointes for amiodarone. Sotolol demonstrates a dose-dependent incidence of torsades, in contrast to the idiosyncratic pattern for the class IA drugs. The common denominator between class IA and class III drugs, which likely contributes to this concordant proarrhythmic pattern, is moderate-to-marked prolongation of repolarization as reflected in QT interval prolongation. In contrast, the class IC drugs, which have minimal effect on repolarization, have a low rate of classic proarrhythmia—i.e., torsades de pointes. They may, however, worsen clinical arrhythmias or generate a new rapid sinusoidal sustained VT[188] (Fig. 27-38). In addition, the excess death rate in CAST, attributed to proarrhythmia, extended over the entire period of drug exposure rather than close in time to the start of treatment. A possible explanation for this pattern is a tendency for the class IC drugs to interact with sporadic intercurrent events, such as transient ischemia or LV dysfunction.[17] Such an explanation is consistent with disturbed conduction patterns (depolarization) contributing to proarrhythmia rather than repolarization abnormalities[11] (see also Chap. 30). It is also consistent with the observation in CAST that increased risk of mortality in the flecainide and encainide arms was accompanied by a decreased incidence of nonfatal ischemic events compared to their placebo groups.

Combining drug classes has been found to be effective by some, although carefully controlled studies are limited[189];

combinations such as a class IA and a class IB drug may be tried. The class II drugs, β-adrenergic blocking agents, have been mentioned earlier, and many consider them the first choice of therapy even if the EF is reduced. They may be used in combination with class I drugs in some patients. Class III drugs have been approved only for use in life-threatening arrhythmias, although amiodarone and sotolol are both appropriate for selected patients with symptomatic runs of nonsustained VT and advanced LV dysfunction. The available data on amiodarone is promising for patients with life-threatening arrhythmias,[190,191] but the specific benefit for patients with PVCs and nonsustained VT in the presence of advanced heart disease is unclear. In the CHF-STAT study, which randomized ischemic and nonischemic myopathies and PVCs to amiodarone and placebo, no mortality benefit was observed.[192] Another study, GESICA, which randomized cardiomyopathic patients to the same drug versus placebo, however, showed a survival benefit for the amiodarone-treated group.[193] PVC stratification was not carried out in the latter. In both studies, amiodarone-treated patients with nonischemic cardiomyopathies tended to respond more favorably to the drug than those with ischemic cardiomyopathies. The class IV drugs, Ca^{2+}-entry blockers, have no role in the treatment of chronic PVCs.

With any of these drugs or drug combinations, attention to underlying heart disease and systemic factors is necessary.

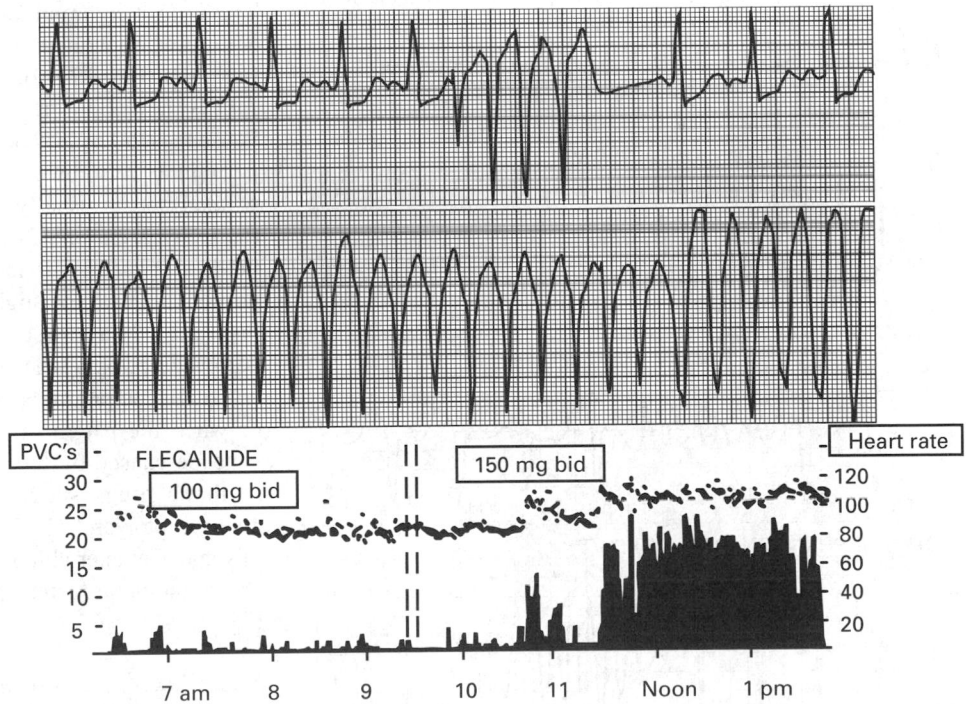

FIGURE 27-38

Proarrhythmic response to flecainide acetate in a 62-year-old male. The trend recording demonstrates heart rate variations (dots) and frequency of premature ventricular contractions (PVC) (bars). While the patient received flecainide acetate, 100 mg every 12 h, ventricular ectopic impulses occurred at a mean frequency of 1.2 PCVs per minute and the mean heart rate was 98 per minute. After the dose was increased to 150 mg q 12 h, there was a marked increase in total PVC frequency, including the generation of salvos (*top tracing*) and the emergence of runs of spontaneous sustained ventricular tachycardia (*lower tracing*) that had not previously been present. (From Myerburg et al.[188] Reproduced with permission of the publisher.)

Treatment for limiting the frequency of episodes of transient ischemia, maximizing LV function, maintaining electrolyte balance, and controlling blood pressure all may act in concert with antiarrhythmic agents to limit the risk of cardiac morbidity and mortality in patients with chronic PVCs.

The endpoint of treatment (see Table 27-1) of patients who have structural heart disease and high-risk forms and frequency of chronic PVCs is not at all clear. The pharmacodynamics of PVC suppression differ from those of VT prevention,[194] and quantitative PVC suppression is difficult to achieve. Suppression of advanced forms of PVCs (couplets, salvos, nonsustained VT) appears to be an acceptable and achievable endpoint for high-risk patients with these forms on baseline ambulatory monitoring,[195] even if quantitative PVC suppression cannot be achieved. General guidelines include suppression of 70 to 80 percent of total PVCs on a 24-h ambulatory monitor[196] and complete (or nearly complete) suppression of salvos or nonsustained VT.[197]

Nonsustained Ventricular Tachycardia

Nonsustained runs of VT (salvos of three to five consecutive impulses or nonsustained VT of six impulses to 30 s) (Fig.

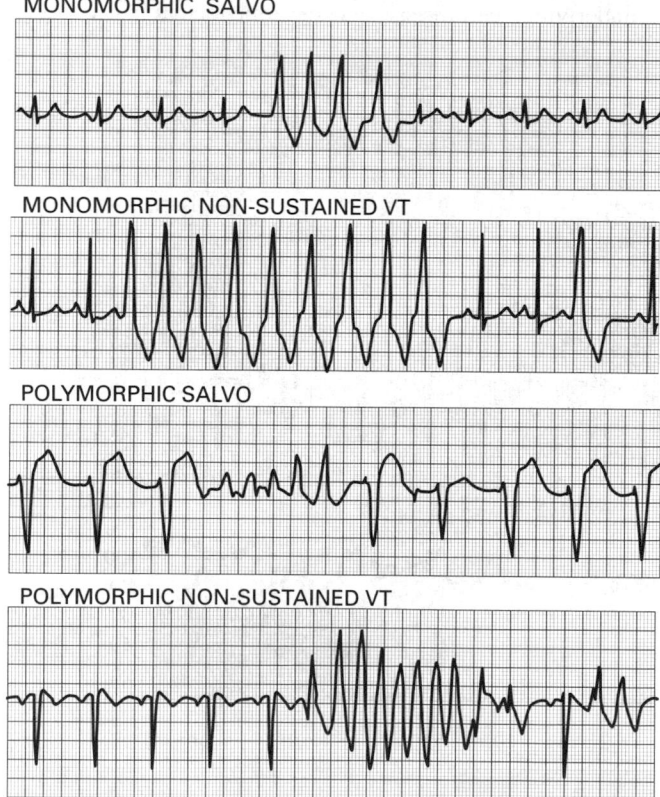

MONOMORPHIC SALVO

MONOMORPHIC NON-SUSTAINED VT

POLYMORPHIC SALVO

POLYMORPHIC NON-SUSTAINED VT

FIGURE 27-39

Nonsustained forms of ventricular tachycardia (VT). Runs of repetitive ventricular impulses (rates ≥ 100/minute) lasting <30 s are subgrouped into salvos of three to five consecutive impulses and nonsustained VT of six or more impulses in duration. Both forms may be further defined according to morphology as monomorphic or polymorphic.

27-39) are considered indicators of high risk for potentially fatal arrhythmias (sustained VT or VF) in most clinical settings. There are important exceptions, however. Patients who have no organic disease or limited cardiac abnormalities do not appear to have increased risk, although some patients who have very rapid polymorphic VT may be at increased risk. Even in the absence of an increased mortality risk, severe symptoms such as transient light-headedness, near-syncope, or syncope, require therapy (Fig. 27-37). At the other extreme, cardiomyopathy patients and those who have advanced coronary artery disease with a poor EF are among the highest risk groups. Conceptually, nonsustained VT may be viewed as self-terminating VT or as an intense triggering event in a susceptible myocardium (Fig. 27-32).[1] Treatment is generally similar to that outlined for other patterns of PVCs, although it is suggested that patients with prior myocardial infarction who have nonsustained VT, low EFs, and are inducible into VT in the clinical electrophysiology laboratory are at higher risk.[179] It has been suggested, but not proven, that these patients benefit from therapy guided by electrophysiologic testing. Implantable cardioverter defibrillator (ICD) therapy has demonstrated decreased mortality than best conventional therapy in one randomized trial of such patients.[180]

Repetitive Monomorphic Ventricular Tachycardia

This is an uncommon form of repetitive salvos or nonsustained VT, often separated from one another by only a few sinus impulses (Fig. 27-40).[198] Occasionally, it is continuous and fulfills the definition for sustained VT. The tachycardia rate is usually 150 or less per minute but may be greater than 200 per minute in some cases. The syndrome is more common in women and is usually benign.[198–200] The QRS patterns of the tachycardia on 12-lead ECGs suggest a right ventricular outflow tract origin (left bundle branch block pattern with normal, vertical, or slightly rightward axis), and the mechanism is likely a form of enhanced automaticity.[201] Treatment is considered only when structural heart disease is also present, when the palpitations are poorly tolerated by the patient, or when the patient has light-headedness, near-syncope, or syncope caused by the arrhythmia. Membrane-active antiarrhythmic drugs should be avoided if possible, and beta-adrenoceptor and Ca^{2+}-entry blocking agents are effective in some. Catheter ablation is an option for the more sustained or symptomatic forms and has a high rate of success[202] (see Fig. 27-41).

Sustained Ventricular Tachycardia

Sustained VT may originate in the specialized conducting system distal to the bundle of His, in ventricular myocardium, or by an interaction between the two. By definition, it occurs at a heart rate of 100 per minute or more and lasts for 30 s or more. An abnormally rapid ventricular rhythm not meeting the strict definition of "tachycardia" (faster than 40 to 50 impulses per minute but slower than 100 per minute) is referred to as an *accelerated ventricular rhythm*. Runs of VT less than 30 s in duration that impair hemodynamics enough to cause symptoms of reduced peripheral or central nervous system blood flow are considered the functional equivalent of a sustained ventricular tachyarrhythmia. Although generally considered to be included among the life-threatening cardiac arrhythmias, benign forms of sustained VT do exist. They occur in persons without apparent structural heart disease, and a functional basis can be identified in some instances (see below).

The etiology of VT will determine its mechanism and clinical presentation. For example, in the patient with prior myocardial infarction and a defined ventricular aneurysm, sustained monomorphic VT occurs at rates ranging from 140 to 200 per minute, most commonly in the range of 150 to 180 per minute (Fig. 27-42*A*).

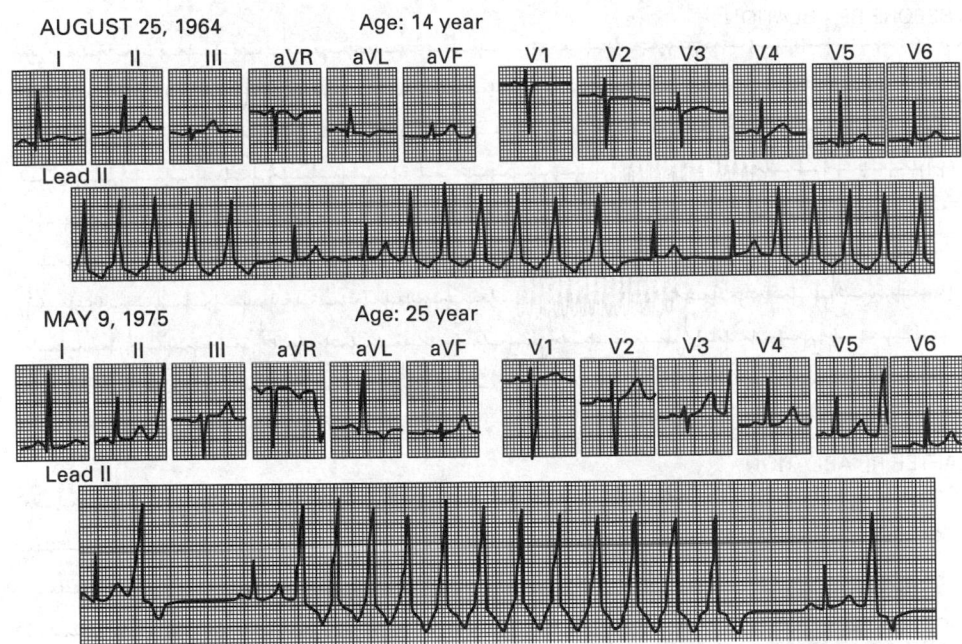

FIGURE 27-40

Repetitive monomorphic ventricular tachycardia (RMVT). RMVT is commonly benign but may be symptomatic in some patients. The most benign form (Gallavardin tachycardia; Parkinson-Papp syndrome) is characterized by runs of nonsustained VT, commonly separated by only a few sinus beats. It is occasionally sustained and usually suppresses with exercise. It is more comon in women and has a QRS morphology suggesting a right ventricular outflow tract origin. In this example, an 11-year follow-up shows persistence of the arrhythmia, with no other significant ECG abnormalities, in a patient who has remained asymptomatic without therapy.

This arrhythmia usually employs stable reentrant pathways and may be hemodynamically well tolerated. In contrast, patients with transient myocardial ischemia often have more rapid ventricular tachyarrhythmias (in excess of 200 per minute) that may be polymorphic or sinusoidal (Fig. 27-42*B*). The mechanism is not clearly defined but likely may be either reentrant or automatic, including the possibility of triggered activity. These forms of VT tend to be hemodynamically and electrically unstable, with a higher risk of degenerating to VF than chronic recurrent monomorphic VT. They tend not to persist for long periods of time, in contrast to the sustained monomorphic VTs, which may persist for hours in some patients. These forms of VT either degenerate to VF, convert to a stable monomorphic VT, or spontaneously revert to sinus rhythm (see also Chap. 26).

Some patients will tolerate sustained monomorphic VT remarkably well, although the risk that sustained VT will degenerate into VF must always be kept in mind. When the hemodynamic status is stable and there is no evidence of myocardial ischemia, acute infarction, or poor central nervous system perfusion, electrical cardioversion can await a therapeutic trial of intravenous drug. With acute myocardial infarction, falling blood pressure, or evidence of ischemia, immediate cardioversion is indicated. In patients who are already receiving antiarrhythmic agents because of prior sustained VT or for treatment of other ventricular arrhythmias, recurrent sustained VT presents a challenging therapeutic problem. If it

is known that the patient has not complied with antiarrhythmic regimens, standard intravenous regimens may be tried, but more commonly this is not the case. Plasma concentrations of the prescribed antiarrhythmics should be ordered at the time of presentation, even though the information may not be available for initial management. The distinction between recurrence of the previous VT or proarrhythmic effects caused by antiarrhythmic agents is a major dilemma. Proarrhythmia should be suspected if the VT morphology is different from the previously identified clinical VT morphology, if antiarrhythmic agents have been recently prescribed or changed, if there is marked prolongation of the QT interval, or if the VT has a polymorphic or torsades de pointes configuration. If there are repeated recurrences after cardioversion, the possibility of proarrhythmia should be seriously entertained and temporary pacing may be useful. Other causes of repeated recurrence include ischemia, heart failure, autonomic surges, or electrolyte disturbances.

ELECTROCARDIOGRAPHIC RECOGNITION OF SUSTAINED VT

Having met the rate and duration criteria for a sustained tachyarrhythmia, the distinction between sustained ventricular tachyarrhythmias and supraventricular tachyarrhythmias with abnormal intraventricular conduction patterns is based upon a complex set of electrocardiographic criteria. The evaluation of the patient's general clinical status is only of limited value

BEFORE RF ABLATION

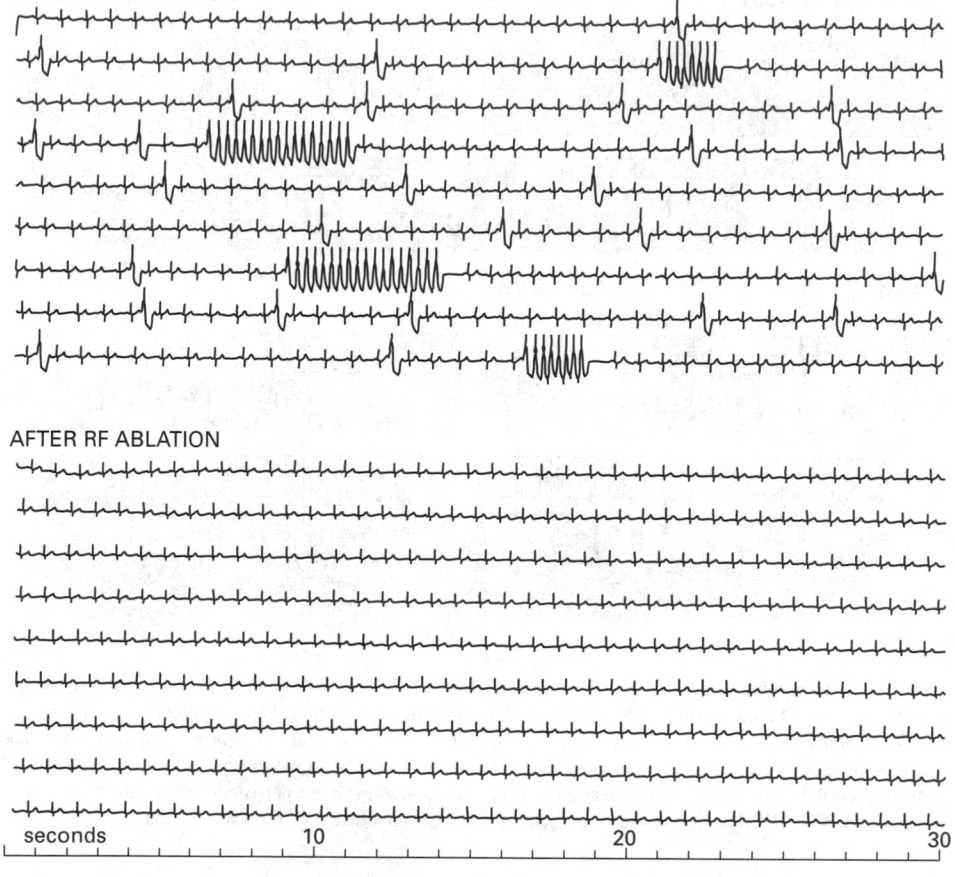

AFTER RF ABLATION

seconds   10   20   30

FIGURE 27-41

Symptomatic repetitive monomorphic ventricular tachycardia (RMVT). In this example of RMVT, the patient presented with a 6-month history of palpitations, episodic lightheadedness, and a few episodes of syncope. RMVT was observed on ambulatory monitoring (*upper tracing*); radiofrequency ablation of a focus in the right ventricular outflow tract was curative (*lower tracing*).

A QRS duration greater than 0.14 s favors VT as the cause of a wide QRS complex tachyarrhythmia. It is nonspecific, however, and is commonly observed in patients with SVT in the presence of a preexisting bundle branch block. SVT with QRS complexes greater than 0.14 s occurs only rarely as a consequence of aberrant intraventricular conduction when QRS complexes are normal during sinus rhythm. In addition, antidromic tachycardias in WPW syndrome usually have QRS complexes longer than 0.14 s in duration and therefore may mimic VT. The mean QRS axis is also of limited help in distinguishing between SVT with aberration and VT. Abnormal left-axis deviation ($-30°$ or beyond) favors VT but does not exclude SVT with preexisting bundle branch block or various supraventricular arrhythmias associated with accessory pathways. Some unusual VTs are associated with a left bundle branch block pattern and right-axis deviation.

QRS configurations have been carefully studied in both VT and SVT with aberrant intraventricular conduction and are of considerable help in distinguishing between the two. Generally, concordantly positive or negative QRS complexes across the precordium from V_1 to V_6 strongly favor VT over aberrant intraventricular conduction (Fig. 27-45). In addition, patterns in specific leads may be helpful. In V_1, a right bundle branch block configuration that is monophasic (R) or biphasic (qR) suggests VT, while a triphasic pattern (rSR) strongly favors aberrant intraventricular conduction.[203] R-wave amplitude in V_1 during the tachycardia that exceeds that during sinus rhythm favors VT, and an initial R wave during the tachycardia of 30 ms duration or longer also favors VT. In V_1 and V_2, a notched downslope on an S wave suggests VT, as does an interval of 70 ms or more from onset of the QRS to the negative peak of the S wave. In lead V_6, a deep S wave with an R:S ratio below 1 and a qR or QS pattern both favor VT.[204,205] Each of these criteria may be altered or modified in individual cases by the presence of preexisting intraventricular conduction abnormalities.

Several additional features of tachyarrhythmias may be helpful. Polymorphic tachyarrhythmias are almost exclusively ventricular in origin but must be carefully distinguished from atrial fibrillation in patients with WPW syndrome who have

for distinguishing very rapid SVTs or VTs as the cause of hypotension or syncope. Nonetheless, the distinction between SVTs and VTs at the bedside is important because of its clinical and therapeutic implications.

Electrocardiographic criteria derive from atrial/ventricular timing relationships and from QRS durations, configurations, and axes. The presence of ventriculoatrial dissociation, with clearly discernible P waves, independent of a regular QRS rhythm, is strongly suggestive of VT (Fig. 27-43A), as is the presence of P waves associated with alternate QRS complexes (see Fig. 27-44). The latter, best identified in lead V_1, is due to 2:1 retrograde block because of the rate of the tachycardia. The presence of a 1:1 relationship between P waves and QRS complexes, with a short RP interval (as in Fig. 27-43B), is also considered supportive evidence for VT. A variety of SVTs with aberrant intraventricular conduction may mimic this pattern, however, and therefore it is not conclusive. Finally, in the presence of ventriculoatrial dissociation, a fortuitously timed sinus impulse may fuse with the wide QRS complex due to VT and produce a single cycle of an altered (usually narrowed) QRS complex (Fig. 27-43C). Such fusion beats are helpful when present but are not common.

multiple bypass tracts.[206] A tachycardia characterized by a wide QRS pattern with a left bundle branch configuration in the precordial leads and right-axis deviation in the frontal plane leads is also usually ventricular in origin. A regular rhythm with alternating QRS axes (a bidirectional pattern) alteration is likely to be ventricular in origin, while paired group beating with bidirectional alteration is likely to be due to aberrant conduction terminating the shorter cycles. Finally, VTs, presumably originating in proximal bundle branches or fascicles, may inscribe relatively or absolutely narrow QRS complexes (Fig. 27-46).

The cycle length of tachyarrhythmias is of little additional value in distinguishing between VTs and SVTs. Although monomorphic VT associated with coronary heart disease and LV aneurysms tend to have rates below 220 per minute, ventricular arrhythmias due to ischemia and/or reperfusion may be considerably faster, in some instances approaching 250 to 280 per minute (Fig. 27-42B). SVTs, particularly those associated with WPW syndrome, may approach similar rates and may be difficult to distinguish from VTs. Antiarrhythmic drugs may also alter electrocardiographic patterns. An example is the slowing of atrial flutter by class IA or class IC antiarrhythmic agents to atrial rates of 240 per minute or less, allowing 1:1 conduction. Particularly for the class IC agents, slowed intraventricular conduction at these rates widens the QRS complexes, resulting in patterns that may be difficult to distinguish from rapid sustained *ventricular* tachyarrhythmias.

ACUTE MANAGEMENT OF SUSTAINED MONOMORPHIC VT

This form of VT may occur in acute or chronic ischemic heart disease syndromes, idiopathic dilated or hypertrophic cardiomyopathy, and less frequently in inflammatory or infiltrative disease states or as a primary electrical disturbance. Management depends upon the clinical setting and the clinical characteristics of the tachycardia.

In acute myocardial infarction, sustained VT occurs most commonly within 24 h of the onset. It carries a risk of degenerating into VF and must be treated aggressively. If the patient

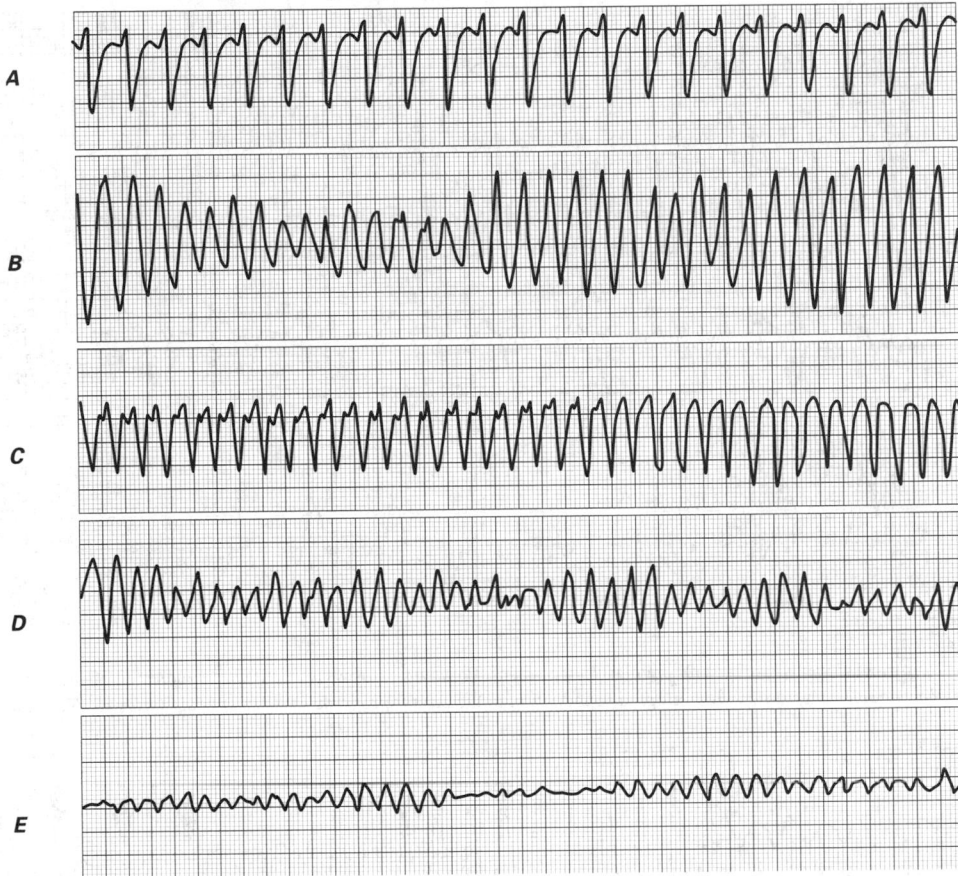

FIGURE 27-42

Different forms of sustained potentially fatal ventricular tachycardias (VTs). *A.* Sustained monomorphic VT recorded from a patient with a left ventricular aneurysm. *B.* Sustained polymorphic VT in a patient with myocardial ischemia. *C.* Ventricular flutter: a sine wave configuration at a cycle length of 200 to 220 ms. *D.* Coarse ventricular fibrillation (VF). *E.* Fine VF. A careful distinction between the different morphologies and rates of tachyarrhythmia contains important information for prognosis and management.

is clinically stable and the arrhythmia electrically stable, a 75- to 100-mg bolus of intravenous lidocaine, followed by a continuous infusion of 1 to 4 mg/min may be tried. The infusion dose depends upon the patient's age, size, and general clinical status.[207] In heart failure and low-output states, the dose should be reduced. If the VT does not revert immediately or if the patient is hypotensive, immediate DC cardioversion is required. Following cardioversion, intravenous lidocaine is continued to prevent recurrences. If VT recurs with lidocaine, 100-mg boluses of procainamide are infused at 5-min intervals to a total loading dose of 500 to 1000 mg, followed by a constant infusion of 2 to 4 mg/min.[208] If breakthroughs occur on both drugs, the next drug of choice is bretylium tosylate[209] or intravenous amiodarone.[210] Bretylium is administered as a loading dose of 5 mg/kg intravenously infused over 15 min, repeated if necessary, and followed by a 0.5- to 2.0-mg/min infusion. Total dose should not exceed 25 mg/kg per 24 h. Amiodarone is administered intravenously with a loading dose of 150 mg infused over 10 min, followed by a continuous infusion of 1 mg/min for 6 h, and then a maintenance infusion at a rate of 0.5 mg/min. Antiarrhythmic therapy may be

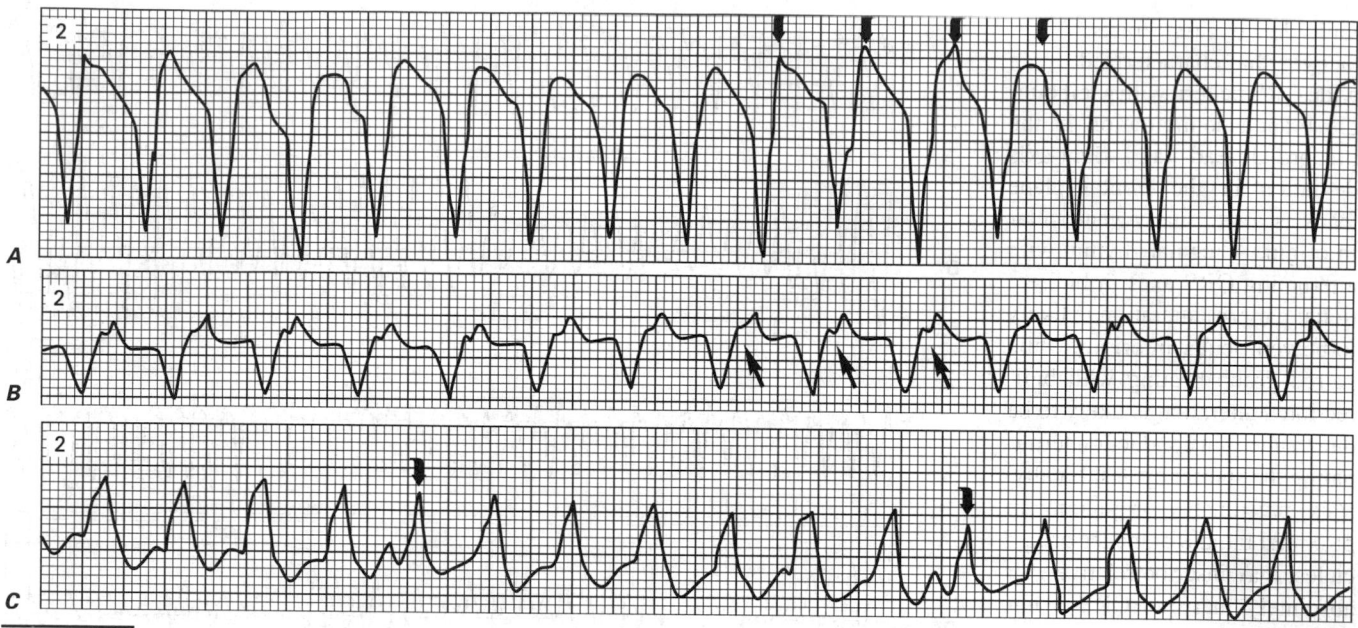

FIGURE 27-43

A. Ventricular tachycardia with regular independent P waves (arrows).
B. Ventricular tachycardia with retrograde conduction to the atria (retrograde

P waves indicated by arrows.) *C.* Ventricular tachycardia with fusion (Dressler's) beats (arrows). Note the sinus P wave preceding each fusion beat.

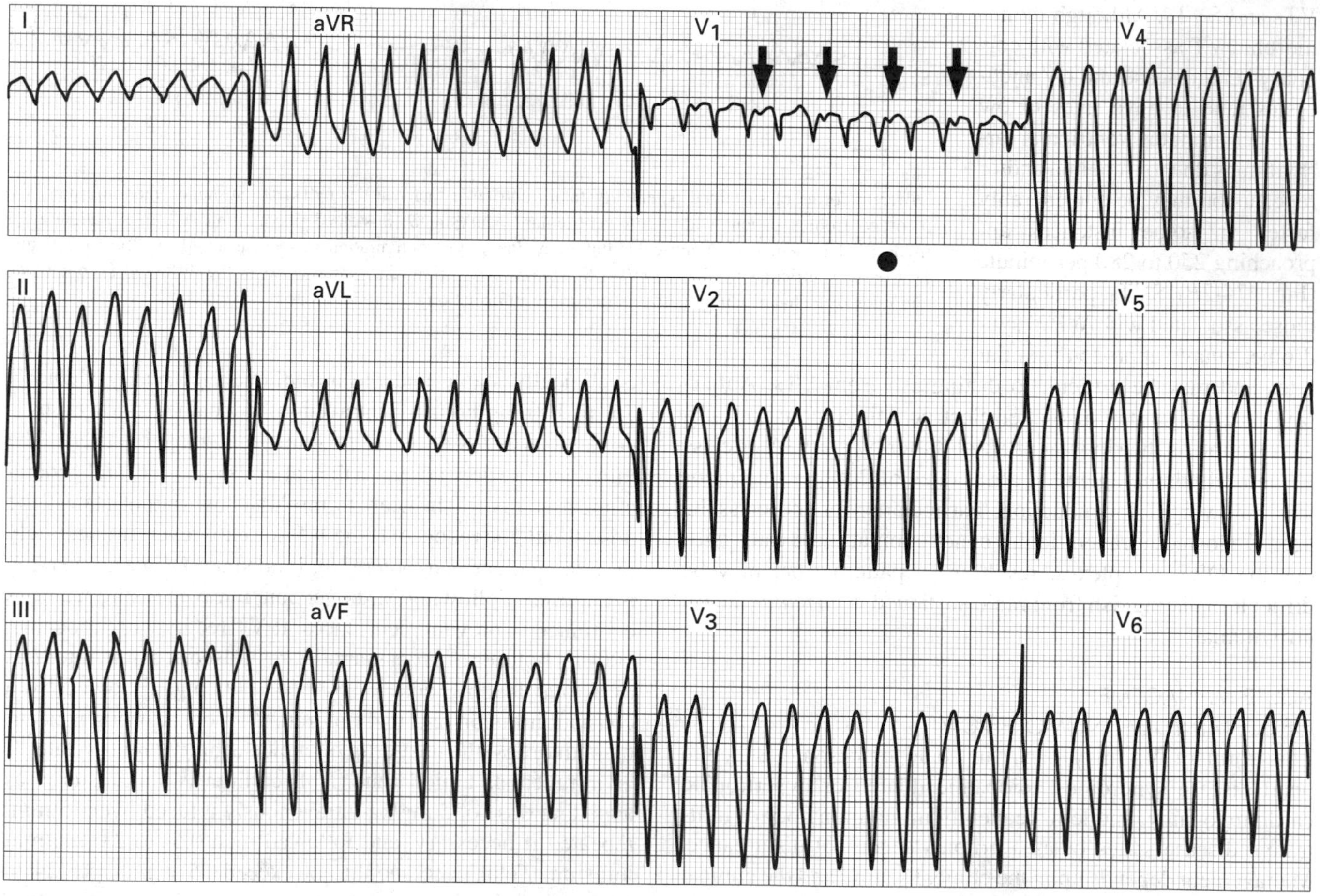

FIGURE 27-44

A rapid wide QRS tachycardia in a 22-year-old female with a history of prior chest wall trauma and a left ventricular aneurysm. Ventricular tachycardia is suggested by the history and QRS pattern (see text), but useful confirmatory information is present in the form of 2:1 retrograde conduction, resulting in

P waves following alternate QRS complexes, most clearly seen in lead V_1 (arrows). In difficult cases, the presence of a 2:1 VA conduction pattern is strongly supportive of ventricular tachycardia.

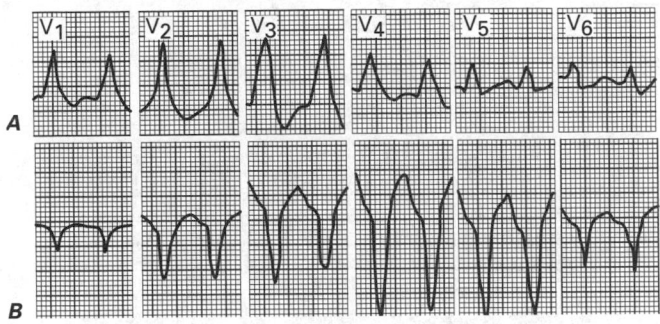

FIGURE 27-45
Ventricular tachycardia with concordant QRS complexes across precordium. *A.* All upright. *B.* All inverted.

stopped after 48 to 72 h, since the risk of recurrence is small at that point. Sustained VT during the acute phase of transmural myocardial infarction is due to transient factors and does not predict later recurrent arrhythmias (see also Chap. 47).

A second clinical category of sustained VT related to acute myocardial infarction is that which occurs during the convalescent period.[211] It is unrelated pathophysiologically to the VT that occurs early and has much more serious long-term implications. It is most common in patients with large anterior wall myocardial infarction. Management of the acute event requires intravenous antiarrhythmic drugs and/or cardioversion, using an algorithm similar to that described for acute-phase VT. There is, however, a very high death rate during follow-up of these patients, in part related to the size of the infarct. One report cited an 83 percent death rate during a mean follow-up of 7 months using empiric antiarrhythmic therapy.[212] Others have reported a somewhat better outcome when such patients undergo electrophysiologic testing for evaluation of drug therapy and/or surgical interventions,[213] although mortality is still high—approximately 25 percent total mortality during a mean follow-up of 16 months. Sustained VT in patients beyond the convalescent phase of myocardial infarction (6 to 8 weeks) has a somewhat less ominous prognosis than convalescent phase VT but is still

considered life-threatening and requires special interventions (see below).[212]

Sustained VT may complicate other acute or transient cardiac syndromes, including ischemia/reperfusion sequences associated with coronary spasm or thrombolysis early after the onset of myocardial infarction, heart failure,[214] acute myocarditis,[167] and almost any toxic or metabolic disturbance of sufficient severity. Therapeutic approaches include both conventional arrhythmia treatment, as described above for sustained VT in acute myocardial infarction, and careful attention to underlying predisposing factors.

LONG-TERM MANAGEMENT OF VT
IN CHRONIC ISCHEMIC HEART DISEASE
The long-term management of recurrent VT in patients with chronic ischemic heart disease has evolved into a complex clinical exercise. Prevention of recurrences is related to successful management of the underlying precipitating factors, such as ischemia and hemodynamic status, as well as to specific antiarrhythmic approaches.

Four general approaches to antiarrhythmic therapy are available: (1) antiarrhythmic therapy guided by invasive electrophysiologic testing or by ambulatory monitoring or exercise testing; (2) surgical procedures designed to excise or cryoablate reentrant pathways or automatic foci; (3) catheter ablation procedures; and (4) ICDs (see Table 27-9). The relative proportion of patients managed by each of these four techniques has been changing in recent years, with fewer but more selective surgical approaches, fewer antiarrhythmic drug trials after one or two drug failures, and broader use of ICD therapy. The use of catheter ablation techniques for VT in chronic ischemic heart disease is largely palliative,[215] often employed as adjunctive therapy with other primary approaches. As technology improves, however, it may develop broader applications (see below).

Pharmacologic Management
Invasive electrophysiologic testing to guide pharmacologic therapy has become a standard part of treatment for patients with recurrent monomorphic sustained VT in ischemic heart disease. An initial study free of antiarrhythmic drugs is required to demonstrate inducibility of the clinical VT and its characteristics at baseline, with a few exceptions, before evaluating medical or surgical interventions. Baseline studies may be avoided in patients with left main coronary artery disease or unstable angina pectoris.

Although there have been controversies about the validity of different protocols for programmed electrical stimulation in patients who have clinical sustained ventricular arrhythmias,[216] up to 95 percent of inducible sustained monomorphic VTs can be induced by right ventricular stimulation, using up to two drive cycle lengths between 600 and 400 ms, from two right ventricular locations (apex and outflow tract), with up to three extrastimuli (see also Chap. 29). In at least 80 percent of patients with chronic ischemic heart disease and recurrent monomorphic sustained VT, the clinical tachyarrhythmias can be induced at a baseline study free of antiar-

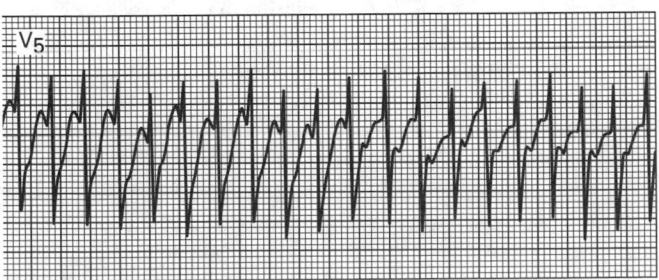

FIGURE 27-46
Ventricular tachycardia (VT) with narrow QRS complexes. The tracings were recorded from a 39-year-old male with ischemic cardiomyopathy and recurrent VT. Multiple VT morphologies were recorded, one of which was this narrow QRS morphology. These may be recognized by their onset if the latter is available but often may be very difficult to distinguish from supraventricular tachycardia with altered repolarization patterns. The diagnosis of the narrow QRS VT shown was confirmed by invasive electrophysiologic studies.

TABLE 27-9

THERAPEUTIC OPTIONS FOR VENTRICULAR ARRHYTHMIAS, CARDIAC ARREST, OR UNEXPLAINED SYNCOPE IN PATIENTS WITH CHRONIC ISCHEMIC HEART DISEASE

Clinical Event	Laboratory-Induced Arrhythmia	Drug Therapy	Surgery; Angioplasty	Implantable Devices	Catheter Ablation
Sustained monomorphic ventricular tachycardia (VT): Hemodynamically stable	Single morphology VT	Membrane active	Antiarrhythmic surgery ± Antiischemic	Tiered therapy	Yes
	Multiple morphology VTs	Membrane active (lower success rate)	Antiischemic, if substrate identified	Tiered therapy	Very low success rate
Hemodynamically unstable	Single morphology VT	Membrane active; β-adrenergic blockers	Antiischemic, if substrate identified	Defibrillation mode (? tiered therapy)	No
	Multiple morphology VTs	Membrane active (lower success rate); β-adrenergic blockers	Antiischemic, if substrate identified	Defibrillation mode (? tiered therapy)	No
Polymorphic ventricular tachycardia	Sustained or nonsustained VT	β-adrenergic blockers; ? amiodarone	Antiischemic, if substrate identified	Defibrillation mode	No
Ventricular fibrillation (VF)	Sustained monomorphic VT	Membrane active		Tiered therapy	Low success rate
	Polymorphic VT; nonsustained VT	β-adrenergic blockers; ? amiodarone	Antiischemic, if substrate identified	Defibrillation mode	No
	Ventricular fibrillation	? β-adrenergic blockers; ? amiodarone		Defibrillation mode	No
Cardiac arrest: mechanism unknown; suspected ventricular arrhythmia	Noninducible	β-adrenergic blockers or amiodarone (uncertain efficacy)	Antiischemic, if substrate identified	Defibrillation mode	No
Unexplained syncope: suspected ventricular arrhythmia	Inducible VT	Membrane active; β-adrenergic blockers; amiodarone		Tiered therapy or defibrillation mode	Low success rate
	Noninducible or inducible VF	? β-adrenergic blockers; ? amiodarone (unknown efficacy)	Antiischemic, if substrate identified	Defibrillation mode	No

Note: Modes of therapy are not mutually exclusive. Combination therapy, with an ancillary second therapy, is a commonly used strategy (see text).

rhythmic agents. The subsequent identification of a drug regimen that will prevent reinduction into the same sustained monomorphic VT is associated with a reduction of risk of recurrent VT at 1 year of follow-up. The risk appears to decrease from 30 to 40 percent if VT remains inducible on therapy to 10 to 15 percent if therapy results in noninducibility.[217] The results of acute intravenous testing of a drug should

not be extrapolated to long-term oral therapy without retesting on the oral regimen, because intravenous regimens do not predict responses on oral drug.[218] In addition, a drug capable of preventing induction of a VT previously induced during baseline testing can be identified in only a minority of patients (~20 to 35 percent in various studies). Moreover, the success rate for membrane-active drugs is considerably lower if multiple monomorphic VTs are induced at baseline.[219] Left ventricular EF strongly influences probability of recurrence. Among cardiac arrest survivors, an EF $\leq$ 30 percent predicts a mortality rate approximately twice as high as patients in the same category with EFs > 30 percent.[220] A similar relationship likely exists for patients who present clinically with sustained VT. Unfortunately, all statements about the potential benefit of therapy guided by programmed electrical stimulation are based upon comparisons of groups who did (responders) or did not (nonresponders) convert from an inducible status to a noninducible status as a result of the therapy. Randomized, placebo-controlled studies of patients who convert to a noninducible status on therapy, with a similar strategy for patients with VT that remains inducible, are still lacking. Such studies would determine whether it is the therapy or simply the ability to change inducibility status that is determining outcome. In one study of patients who had had VT or VF and met criteria for both the invasive electrophysiologic approach (i.e., inducibility at baseline) and the ambulatory monitoring approach (30 or more PVCs per hour), a randomized comparison revealed a significantly lower arrhythmia recurrence rate with therapy guided by the invasive testing technique[221]—20 percent recurrence rate of symptomatic VT at 24 months with invasive procedures versus 50 percent with noninvasive procedures. The study, however, did not identify a difference in death rate, possibly because of the small number of patients randomized. In another study, a drug or drug combination that did not prevent inducibility during invasive electrophysiologic study, but did prolong the cycle length of induced VT by more than 100 ms with stable hemodynamics, predicted a favorable mortality outcome, even though the incidence of recurrent VT was not different from in those who failed to show any measure of a successful response.[222] Patients who have a partial response to a drug regimen (i.e., induced runs of 6 or more, but fewer than 15 impulses) also appear to have a lower risk of recurrent VT.[223] Many electrophysiologists currently will accept induced runs of less than 10 impulses on therapy as a satisfactory endpoint, and almost all will accept less than 6. Any change in therapy established by invasive electrophysiologic testing because of drug intolerance or clinical failure should be evaluated by repeat testing.[217,224]

Noninvasive management strategies for VT require identification of frequent (i.e., $\geq$10 to $\geq$30 PVCs per hour in various studies) and/or repetitive PVC forms (i.e., salvos, nonsustained VT) at baseline monitoring or VT induced during exercise testing. Reduction of PVC frequency (80 percent or more suppression) and abolition of complex forms is the usual endpoint for a successful response. This approach has been reported to be successful in some studies,[195,225] even among patients who have failed to achieve a successful endpoint by invasive electrophysiologic testing.[225] Unfortunately, it is not yet clear which patients who fail invasive electrophysiologic testing require surgical or implantable device management, even when noninvasive methods are successful,[226] and many clinicians now use surgical treatment or implantable devices for such patients.

A large multicenter randomized trial, entitled Electrophysiological Study Versus Electrocardiographic Monitoring (ESVEM), was designed to compare programmed electrical stimulation with ambulatory monitoring techniques for guiding therapy in patients who had sustained VT, survived cardiac arrest, or syncope presumed due to a ventricular arrhythmia.[227,228] The data showed no difference between the two methods for prediction of efficacy or mortality benefit, although there was a small trend favoring programmed stimulation during early follow-up in the coronary disease subgroup (see Chap. 33). Failure by both invasive and noninvasive criteria connotes a poor prognosis and requires other considerations for therapy—i.e., surgery or implantable devices.

Surgical Therapy

Patients who have recurrent sustained monomorphic VT, associated with prior myocardial infarction and inducibility into a hemodynamically stable tachycardia, should be considered for antiarrhythmic surgery. The indication is reinforced by the presence of discrete ventricular aneurysms and bypassable coronary artery lesions. Surgery is recommended, in the absence of contraindications, for such patients who fail electrophysiologic testing with antiarrhythmic drugs.[217,229,230] It may also be recommended in lieu of successful drug therapy by electrophysiologic criteria if the patient has exceptionally good surgical anatomy and/or requires revascularization. Patients without discrete aneurysms who have large dyskinetic areas may have sites of origin of VT mapped in the cardiac electrophysiology laboratory and operating room if they are inducible into stable monomorphic tachycardias. Mapping allows the identification of areas that may be attacked by endocardial resection or surgical cryoablation.[231] Map-guided surgical procedures employing resection, cryoablation, and revascularization have markedly improved the clinical outcome of surgically treated patients[232] (Fig. 27-47). Overall surgical results have also benefited from the preferred use of ICDs in patients previously referred for surgery out of desperation (see Chap. 33). Coronary bypass surgery may be used as primary therapy for patients who have recurrent VT initiated by transient ischemic episodes.[233] It is also a valuable adjunct to antiarrhythmic surgery (see Table 27-9).

Catheter Ablation Techniques

The combination of LV endocardial mapping by catheter techniques and RF energy delivery systems provides the capability for catheter ablation therapy of sustained, hemodynamically stable VTs.[215,234,235] These techniques are currently limited to only a small fraction of patients as primary therapy,[235] however, but are useful as an adjunct to ICD therapy (see Fig. 27-48). Future improvements of mapping techniques and energy delivery systems may enhance the use of catheter ablation as primary therapy in the future.

Implantable Defibrillators

The role of ICD therapy for patients with ventricular tachyarrhythmias has expanded dramatically in recent years

77-YEAR-OLD MALE

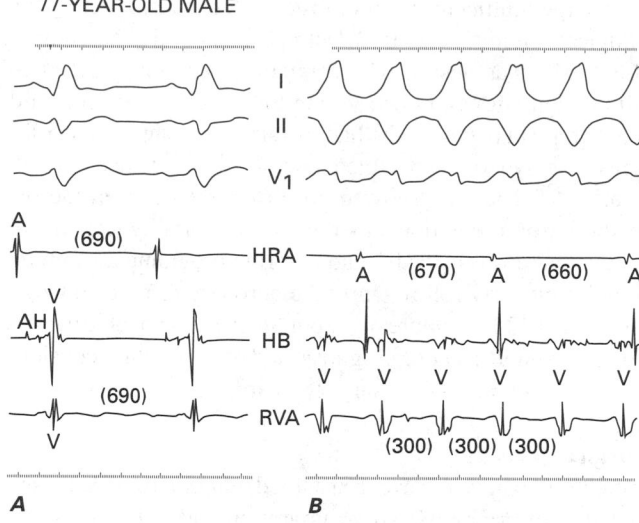

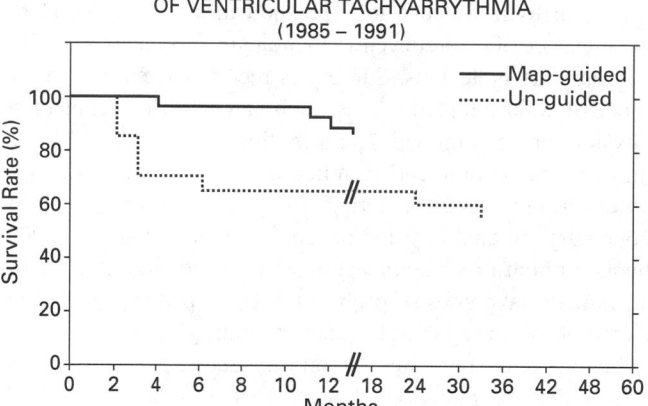

FIGURE 27-47

Benefit of map-guided antiarrhythmic surgery on outcome. *A* and *B*. Normal sinus rhythm and induced, hemodynamically stable ventricular tachycardia (VT) in a patient with the same VT clinically. The ability to induce and sustain the clinical VT by programmed stimulation makes the patient a favorable surgical candidate if the appropriate surgical anatomy is present (see text). *C*. Actuarial curves show outcome of patients who had surgery for recurrent sustained VT, comparing outcome after map-guided surgery with intraoperative ablation procedures to the subgroup of patients who could not be mapped at the time of surgery. Primary surgical success rate and survival are improved by intraoperative mapping.

(see Table 27-9). It is no longer necessary or desirable to test a long sequence of antiarrhythmic drugs. Rather, failure of no more than one or two drugs during electrophysiologic study is generally considered an indication for ICD therapy. Their use is amplified by enrichments such as antitachycardia pacing, low-energy conversion, and defibrillation, using programmable tiered-therapy algorithms, back-up bradyarrhythmia pacing, and electrogram storage for retrieving and analyzing events.

Patients who present with clinical VT and have inducible, hemodynamically *unstable* VT associated with ischemia be-

fore surgery should receive an ICD after revascularization surgery if they remain inducible into VT. Surgical placement of epicardial patches at the time of surgery for possible use later is obsolete in view of the demonstrated efficacy of transvenous endocardial defibrillation lead systems.[236] The routine use of an ICD after antiarrhythmic surgery, even if successful by postsurgical programmed stimulation study, has been advocated[237] but has gained only limited acceptance. ICDs are indicated for patients with recurrent or unstable VT whose arrhythmias have not been (or cannot be) controlled surgically and do not respond to medical therapy[238,239] and may be considered for some patients with EF below 30 percent, even if they do respond to drug therapy. ICDs with antitachycardia pacing capabilities and programmable tiered therapy have expanded the scope of device therapy for recurrent sustained VT. The availability of antitachycardia pacing obviates the need for antiarrhythmic surgery in at least some (perhaps many) patients who have been considered surgical candidates on the basis of anatomy and physiology in the recent past (Fig. 27-49) (see also Chap. 33).

LONG-TERM MANAGEMENT OF VT IN NONISCHEMIC HEART DISEASE

Sustained VT in patients with idiopathic dilated cardiomyopathy, dilated cardiomyopathies due to specific etiologies, or hypertrophic cardiomyopathies carries a poor prognosis. Management approaches differ from those used for patients with ischemic heart disease (see Table 27-10).

Invasive electrophysiologically guided therapy is applicable in the small fraction of patients with dilated cardiomyopathy who have clinical sustained monomorphic VT,[240,241] although it is not clear that the long-term outcome is altered by drug therapy. In a subgroup of these patients, sustained VT is due to bundle branch reentry,[242] which can be cured by catheter ablation of the right bundle branch. Electrophysiologically guided management does not appear useful in idiopathic dilated cardiomyopathy patients who have survived out-of-hospital VF or have clinical nonsustained VT.[243] There is almost no role for surgical therapy in these patients at present, but the ICD is an appropriate means of management. The device appears effective for reverting potentially fatal arrhythmias in patients who have cardiomyopathy,[244] but the long-term outcome may be dominated by LV function. The evaluation of ICD therapy in these patients has been confounded by the observation that, in some (perhaps a substantial fraction) of these patients, sudden death is caused by the bradyarrhythmic/asystole/pulseless-electrical-activity complex, which would not benefit from any form of antiarrhythmic therapy.[245] The availability of ICD with electrogram storage capability should begin to clarify the magnitude of this problem. Ultimately, identification of groups at risk for specific mechanisms will help define the best therapy, but such data are currently lacking.

Sustained VT is also a late consequence and poor prognostic sign in patients with hypertrophic cardiomyopathy.[246–248]

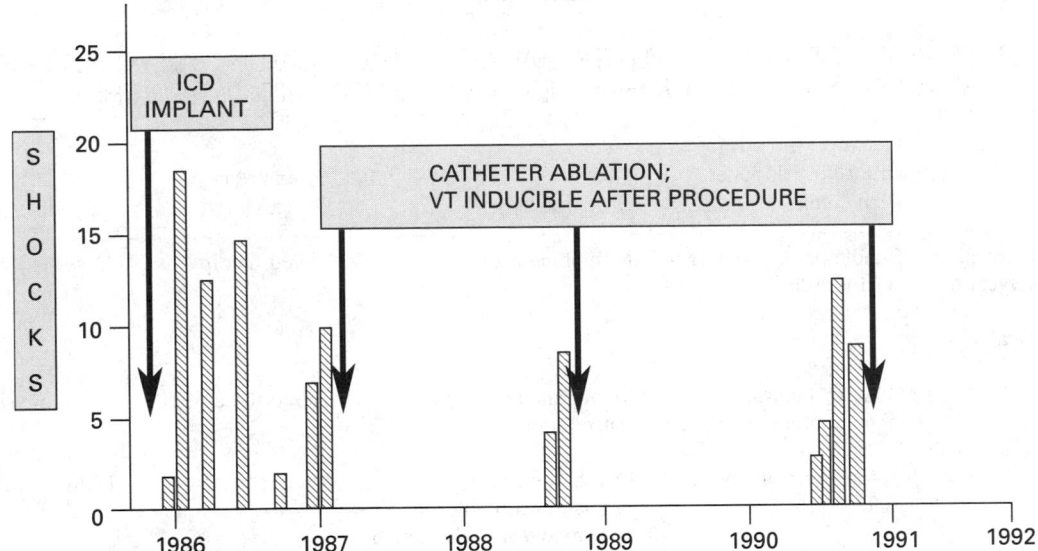

FIGURE 27-48

Catheter ablation for ventricular tachycardia (VT) as an adjunct to an implantable cardioverter defibrillator. A 57-year-old male with recurrent life-threatening episodes of sustained VT who received an implantable cardioverter defibrillator (ICD) had multiple shocks for arrhythmias that were resistant to all antiarrhythmic agents attempted. Left ventricular mapping and catheter ablation in a VT reentrant pathway in 1987 provided freedom from recurrent ICD discharges for approximately 19 months, after which the multiple ICD discharges recurred. Additional ablation procedures 18 or more months apart provided relief from the recurrent discharges, despite the fact that VT remained inducible. While of limited value as primary therapy for life-threatening ventricular arrhythmias in patients with coronary heart disease or cardiomyopathy because of risk of recurrence (see text), this procedure can provide benefit as an adjunct to other primary forms of therapy by avoiding frequent discharges and improving the quality of life.

In this setting, the use of electrophysiologic testing has been limited because of unvalidated concerns about the ability to cardiovert the severely hypertrophied and obstructed ventricle,[248,249] and there is no uniform opinion regarding the best approach to management of these patients, other than the accepted need for therapy. In this entity, again the trend in recent years has been toward ICD therapy rather than pharmacologic therapy, particularly among higher risk subgroups. Preoperative electrophysiologic testing is also avoided in patients with severe aortic stenosis who have survived sustained VT or VF.

Less Common Clinical Causes of Sustained Monomorphic VT

CATECHOLAMINE/METABOLICALLY MEDIATED VT

There are a limited number of patients in whom sustained VT appears mediated by catecholamines or other neurophysiologic influences.[250,251] Sustained VT in these patients is commonly induced by physical or emotional stress. Isoproterenol infusions may be used to initiate the VT, which may then be suppressed and subsequently prevented by β-adrenergic blocking agents (Fig. 27-50). Another small group of patients have sus-

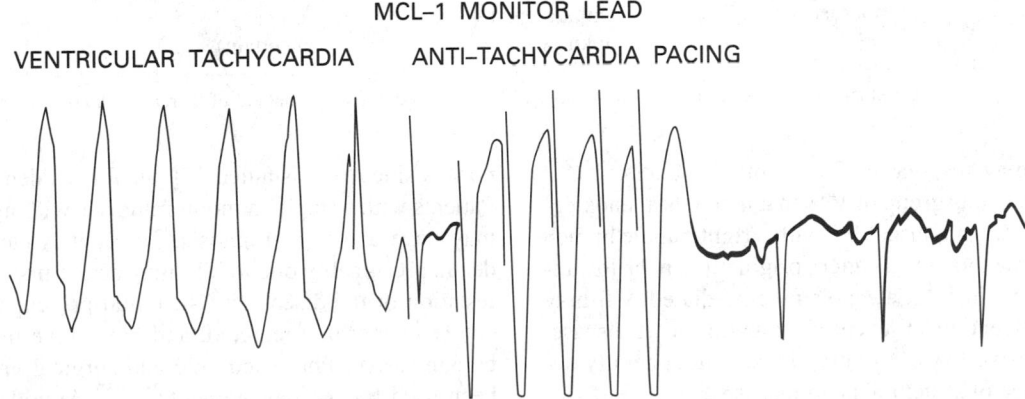

FIGURE 27-49

Implantable cardioverter defibrillator with antitachycardia pacing. The figure demonstrates the end of a run of induced sustained ventricular tachycardia (*left*) followed by antitachycardia pacing that converts the rhythm back to normal sinus (*right*). The device will revert to a defibrillator mode if programmed pacing sequences fail to convert the rhythm.

TABLE 27-10

LONG-TERM THERAPEUTIC OPTIONS FOR VENTRICULAR ARRHYTHMIAS, CARDIAC ARREST, OR UNEXPLAINED SYNCOPE IN PATIENTS WITH NONISCHEMIC DILATED CARDIOMYOPATHIES

Clinical Event	Electrophysiology Laboratory–Induced Arrhythmia	Drug Therapy	Implantable Devices	Catheter Ablation
Sustained monomorphic ventricular tachycardia (VT): Hemodynamically stable	Bundle branch reentrant tachycardia	Membrane active	Tiered therapy	Yes
	Other or multiple monomorphic reentrant VTs	Membrane active (low success rate)	Tiered therapy	Very low success rate
	Automatic monomorphic VT	Membrane active; ? β-adrenergic blockers; ? hemodynamically active drugs	No	Unlikely to be effective
Hemodynamically unstable	Single morphology VT	Membrane active; β-adrenergic blockers	Defibrillation mode (? tiered therapy)	Yes, if bundle branch reentry
	Multiple morphology VTs	Membrane active (very low success rate); β-adrenergic blockers	Defibrillation mode (? tiered therapy)	No
Polymorphic ventricular tachycardia	Sustained or nonsustained	Membrane active; β-adrenergic blockers or amiodarone (efficacy unknown)	Defibrillation mode	No
Ventricular fibrillation (VF)	Ventricular tachycardia	? β-adrenergic blockers; ? amiodarone	Tiered therapy	For bundle branch reentry; ? success rate
	Ventricular fibrillation	? β-adrenergic blockers; ? amiodarone (efficacy uncertain)	Defibrillation mode	No
Cardiac arrest: Mechanism unknown; suspected ventricular arrhythmia	Noninducible	β-adrenergic blockers or amiodarone (efficacy unknown)	Defibrillation mode	No
Unexplained syncope: Suspected ventricular arrhythmia	Sustained ventricular tachycardia	Membrane active: β-adrenergic blockers; amiodarone	Tiered therapy or defibrillation mode	For bundle branch reentry; ? success rate
	Noninducible; inducible nonsustained VT or VF	β-adrenergic blockers; amiodarone (efficacy unknown)	Defibrillation mode (efficacy uncertain)	No

Note: Modes of therapy are not mutually exclusive. Combination therapy, with an adjunctive second method of therapy, is a common strategy (see text).

tained VT that may respond to Ca^{2+}-entry blockers.[252–254] This is a heterogeneous group of VTs that includes adenosine-sensitive VT[252] and an unusual VT with a right bundle branch block/left-axis deviation QRS pattern originating in the low interventricular septum.[254] Catecholamine-mediated VT may occur in the presence or absence of structural heart disease; when it is responsive to Ca^{2+}-entry blockers, it generally occurs in the absence of structural heart disease.

RIGHT VENTRICULAR DYSPLASIA AND VENTRICULAR ARRHYTHMIAS

Arrhythmogenic right ventricular dysplasia (ARVD) or right ventricular cardiomyopathy (RVCM) may be associated with nonsustained or sustained VT and/or sudden cardiac death. Patients with a stable monomorphic VT without near-syncope may have a better prognosis,[255] but it is clear that sudden death, presumably due to VF, may be the first and only manifestation of the disease.[256] At initial presentation, the future course cannot be predicted, and preventive measures should be aggressive. Pharmacologic and surgical approaches have been used for its management.[255,257] Amiodarone and class IC drugs have been suggested to be effective for ARVD patients with symptomatic arrhythmias. The term *isolated right ventricular cardiomyopathy*[256,258] has been used as an alternative for ARVD, and more recently it is being viewed as an ARVD/RVCM complex.[259] The entity may occur spo-

Isoproterenol Infusion.

42 y.o. female   4 µg/min   Propranolol

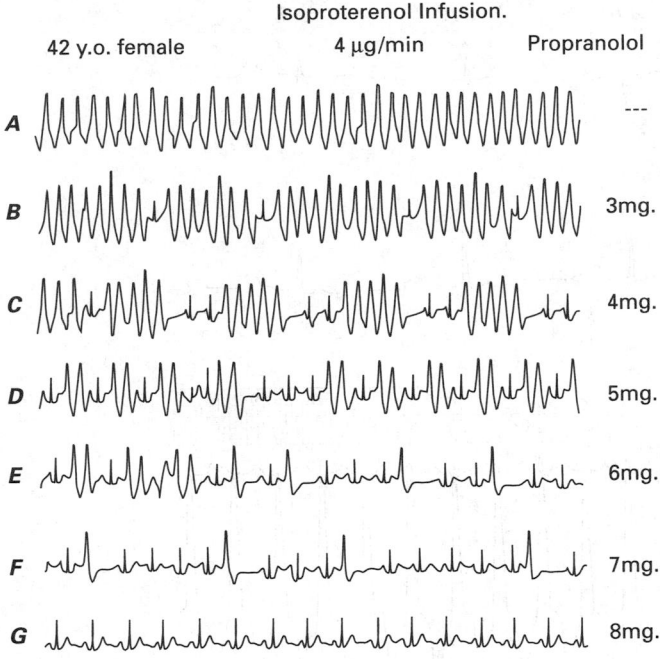

FIGURE 27-50

Catecholamine-mediated ventricular tachycardia (VT) in an otherwise healthy female. Psychologic stress or isoproterenol infusion could initiate the arrhythmia in this patient. During this sequence, a 4-µg/min isoproterenol infusion initiated the VT (A), and the patient was treated with intravenous propranolol. After the first 3 mg of propranolol (B), occasional sinus beats interrupted the tachycardia. On a milligram-by-milligram basis up to a total dose of 8 mg of propranolol, there was further suppression of VT to the point of salvos (C, D, E), frequent premature ventricular contractions (F), and complete suppression of ectopic activity (G).

radically or in familial clusters, although the inheritance pattern is unknown.

The 12-lead electrocardiographic pattern of the patient with ARVD is helpful. In sinus rhythm, anterior precordial T-wave inversions are commonly present (Fig. 27-51), sometimes with notching in the ST segment of V_1 and V_2 as well. The monomorphic tachycardia has a left bundle branch block morphology, reflecting its origin from the right ventricle.

VENTRICULAR TACHYCARDIA AFTER CONGENITAL HEART DISEASE SURGERY

Sustained VT or VF may appear years after repair of complex congenital heart defects,[260] especially tetralogy of Fallot and transposition of the great vessels. The arrhythmias are potentially lethal and must be treated pharmacologically,[261] surgically,[262] or with ICDs in selected cases.

BIDIRECTIONAL VENTRICULAR TACHYCARDIA

This arrhythmia (Fig. 27-52) is usually a manifestation of digitalis intoxication and responds to standard measures.

Polymorphic Ventricular Tachycardia; Torsades de Pointes

The polymorphic VTs, including the specific variant referred to as torsades de pointes, is a tachycardia pattern with im-

portant clinical implications. As a group, the polymorphic tachycardias tend to be more unstable electrically than the monomorphic tachycardias, occur at faster rates, have a higher likelihood of producing transient central nervous system symptoms (syncope, near-syncope) due to reduced cardiac output, and establish a higher risk for spontaneous degeneration to VF. The polymorphic tachycardias do not generally persist as long as the monomorphic tachycardias, either spontaneously reverting to a normal rhythm, degenerating to VF, or triggering a monomorphic tachycardia in susceptible patients.

The specific variant of polymorphic tachycardia characterized by QRS peaks that seem to twist around the baseline (Fig. 27-53) is referred to as *torsades de pointes*. The orthodox definition of torsades de pointes includes the predisposing electrocardiographic pattern, namely a prolonged QT interval.[263] The same electrocardiographic pattern, however, may occur in the absence of QT prolongation.[264] Torsades de pointes may occur as a consequence of congenital prolongation of the QT interval or may be associated with acquired QT prolongations due to any of a group of diverse factors (see below). Less specific patterns of polymorphic VT may also occur in a number of other acquired disease settings, often not associated with prolonged QT intervals or with transient prolongations.

CONGENITAL LONG QT INTERVAL SYNDROME

The congenital long QT interval syndrome, which is present persistently from childhood, is characterized by the presence of long QT intervals and/or prominent U waves on the standard 12-lead ECG (Fig. 27-54). The affected patients are prone to episodes of torsades de pointes, which may cause transient light headedness or syncope or sudden cardiac death. Arrhythmias may occur at rest, under emotional stress, or with exercise (Fig. 27-55).

The two general patterns of the syndrome are the Romano-Ward syndrome,[265,266] which has an autosomal dominant inheritance pattern, and the Jervell–Lange-Nielson syndrome,[267] which has an autosomal recessive inheritance pattern and is associated with congenital deafness. The Romano-Ward pattern of inheritance is far more common than the Jervell–Lange-Nielson pattern.

For many years, congenital long QT interval syndrome has been viewed as being a consequence of abnormal patterns of cardiac autonomic neural innervation, based in part upon the fact that the entity could be treated with β-adrenergic blocking agents or surgical ablation of the left stellate ganglion.[268] Recent progress in the molecular genetics of the syndrome, however, has clearly demonstrated that inherited defects in membrane ion channel molecular structure and function underlie the disease. To date, multiple variations of specific genetic abnormalities have been identified on five chromosomes (Fig. 27-56), and the specific gene products and their physiologic dysfunctions are being studied for each. The first abnormality identified is on chromosome 11[269]; linkage analysis had suggested an association with the Harvey-*ras* gene, but subsequent observations have demonstrated that the affected locus encodes a potassium channel, likely I_{KS} (the slowly

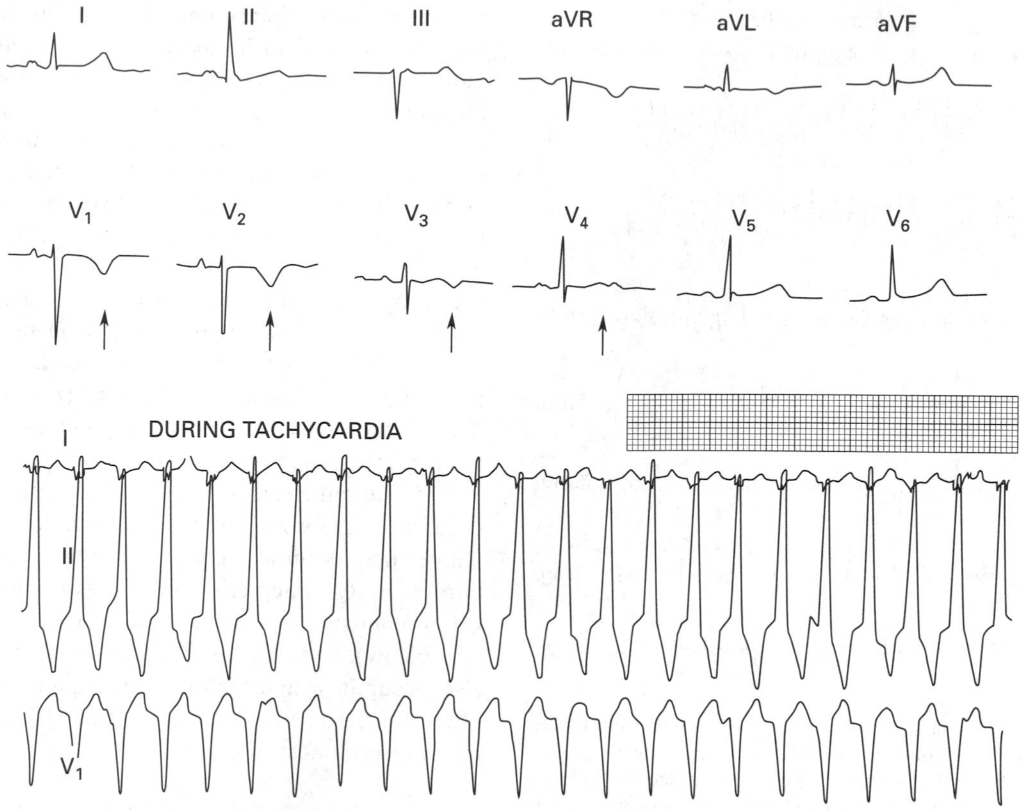

FIGURE 27-51

Right ventricular dysplasia with ventricular tachycardia. Episodic wide QRS tachycardia, with near-syncope, in a 33-year-old man. The left bundle branch block pattern of the tachycardia suggests a right ventricular origin, and the inverted T waves in V_1 to V_3 are characteristic of right ventricular dysplasia.

activating delayed rectifier channel). This channel also appears to be affected in at least one variety of the Jervell–Lange-Neilsen syndrome. Subsequently, two other genetic patterns have been found among multiple families. An abnormality has been mapped to a locus on chromosome 7, identifying a gene which appears to encode HERG,[270] a repolarizing potassium channel that is, or is similar to, the rapidly activating delayed rectifier channel (I_{KR}). Another locus, identified on chromosome 3, encodes SCN5A, the human cardiac sodium channel gene.[271] One defective pattern on the latter gene encodes a 3-amino acid deletion, which results in failure of the channel to close properly after activation. The depolarizing leak of Na^+ current competes with and delays repolarization by the normal potassium channel. Drugs that block the sodium channel, such as mexiletine, have been suggested as a possible

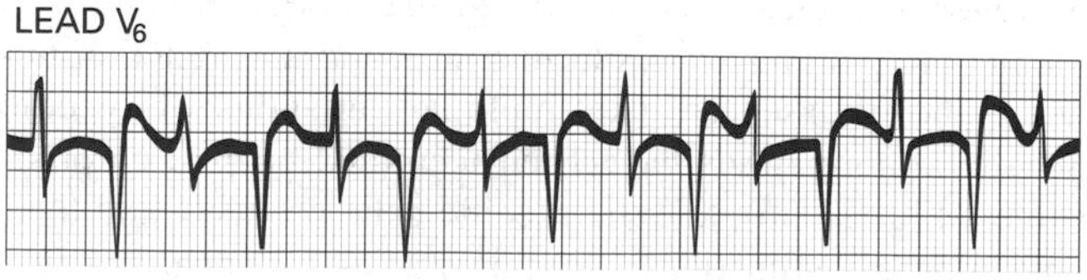

pharmacologic therapy for this specific variant of the syndrome.[272] A fourth genetic abnormality on chromosome 4 has been identified in a single family and may be a unique mutant in that family.[273] Finally, the fifth chromosome affected is chromosome with the new information on genetically based ion-channel abnormalities as the underlying mechanisms in the congenital long QT interval syndromes, the role of the autonomic nervous system is being reevaluated. It is likely, but unproven, that the ion-channel abnormalities provide structural substrates at a molecular level, predisposing to long QT intervals, and that the autonomic nervous system is involved in triggering the actual arrhythmias. For the other general variety of congenital long QT interval syndromes, the Jervell–Lange-Nielson syndrome, specific genetic patterns are not yet defined.

A recently reported syndrome of torsades de pointes with normal QT intervals[264] may also have a congenital basis, although cases are infrequent and adequate studies have not yet occurred. Another pattern is the complex of right bundle branch block, persistent ST-segment elevation in the anterior leads, and sudden death.[274] The reported patients have spontaneous and inducible polymorphic VT, whether sustained or nonsustained, with normal QT intervals. As yet it is unclear whether these two syndromes should be classified with abnormalities of repolarization.

LEAD V_6

FIGURE 27-52

Bidirectional tachycardia. The tachycardia is regular at a rate of 160, but the vector of the QRS-T complexes alternates.

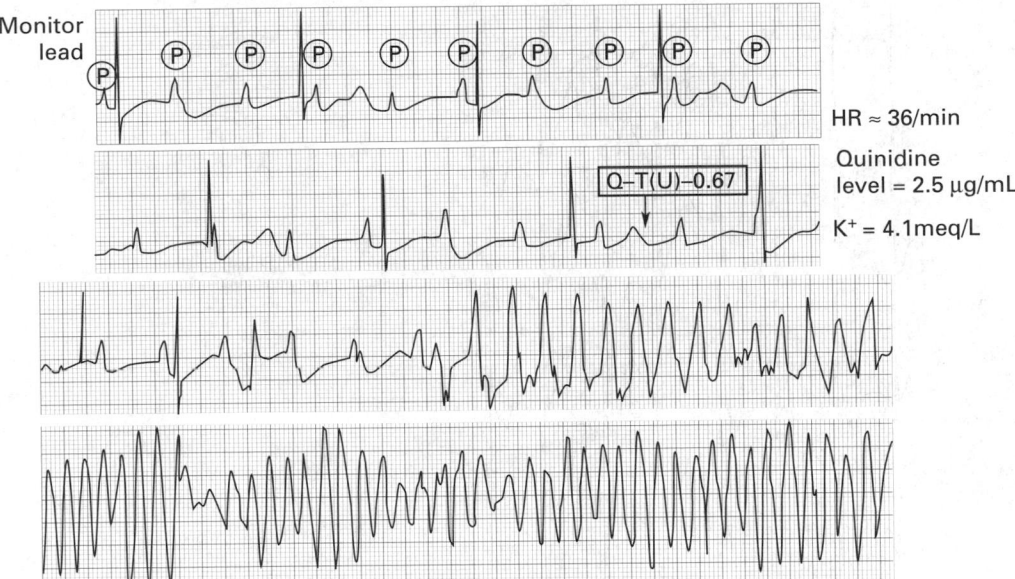

FIGURE 27-53

Torsades de pointes. The patient, a 49-year-old female, has complete heart block and was receiving quinidine sulfate for a ventricular arrhythmia. The rhythm shown in the bottom two strips occurred shortly after institution of therapy. Note the prolonged QT(U) interval (0.67 s) and the onset of classical torsades de pointes.

ACQUIRED LONG QT INTERVAL SYNDROME

The most common causes for acquired long QT interval syndromes are the antiarrhythmic drugs, classically quinidine but also other class IA agents and class III agents, with prolongation of the QT interval preceding the arrhythmia.[275] Bradycardia, hypokalemia, and hypomagnesemia contribute to the risk.[276–278] QT prolongation induced by class IA agents appears to be idiosyncratic in most cases and occurs among a small subsegment of the population exposed to the drugs. This suggests specific individual susceptibility, which might be inherited, but no inheritance pattern has as yet been identified. The class III drugs, particularly sotolol, prolong the QT interval in

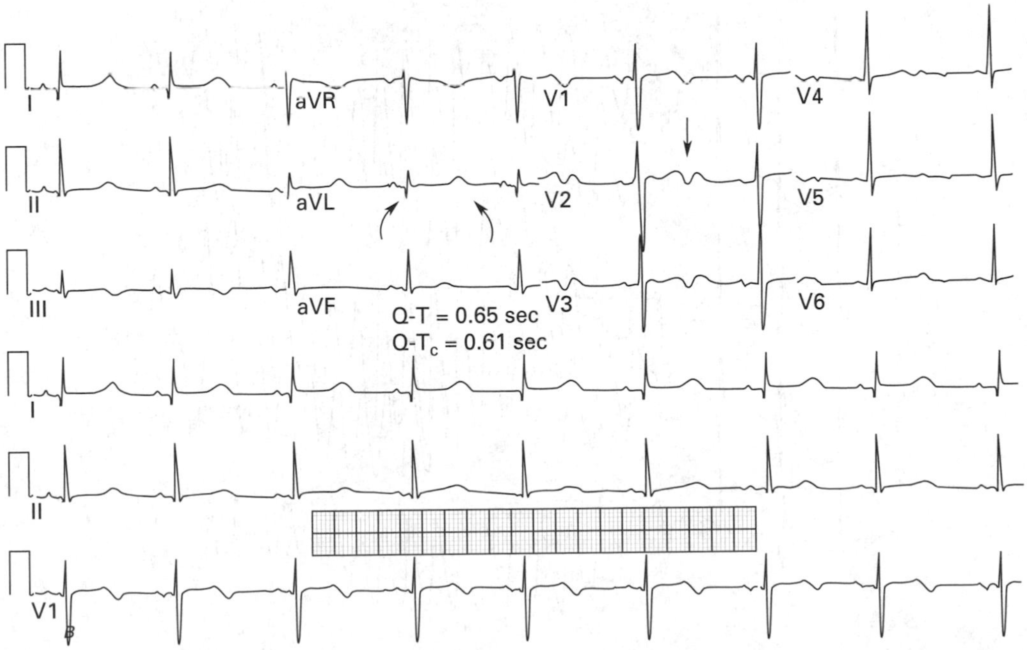

FIGURE 27-54

Congenital long QT interval syndrome. A 12-lead ECG was recorded in a 25-year-old female with congenital deafness and a history of recurrent syncope throughout her life (Jervell–Lange-Nielson syndrome). Many episodes of syncope occurred during or immediately after exercise and were commonly preceded by palpitations. She had never been treated. The tracing reveals a corrected QT interval of 610 ms with marked notching of the TU waves in the anterior precordial leads.

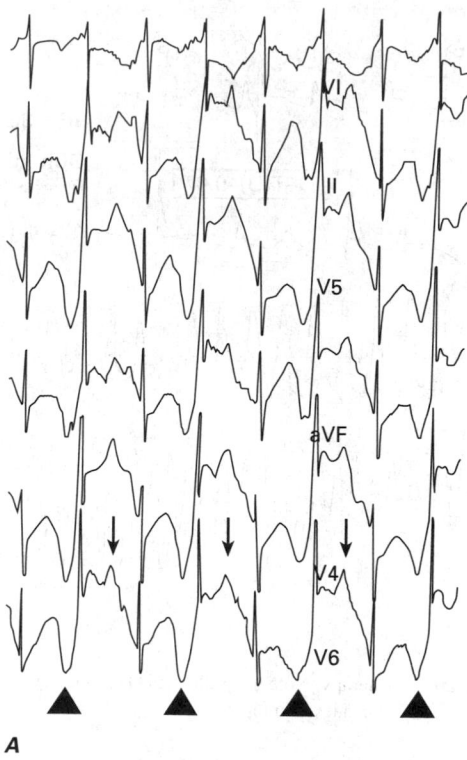

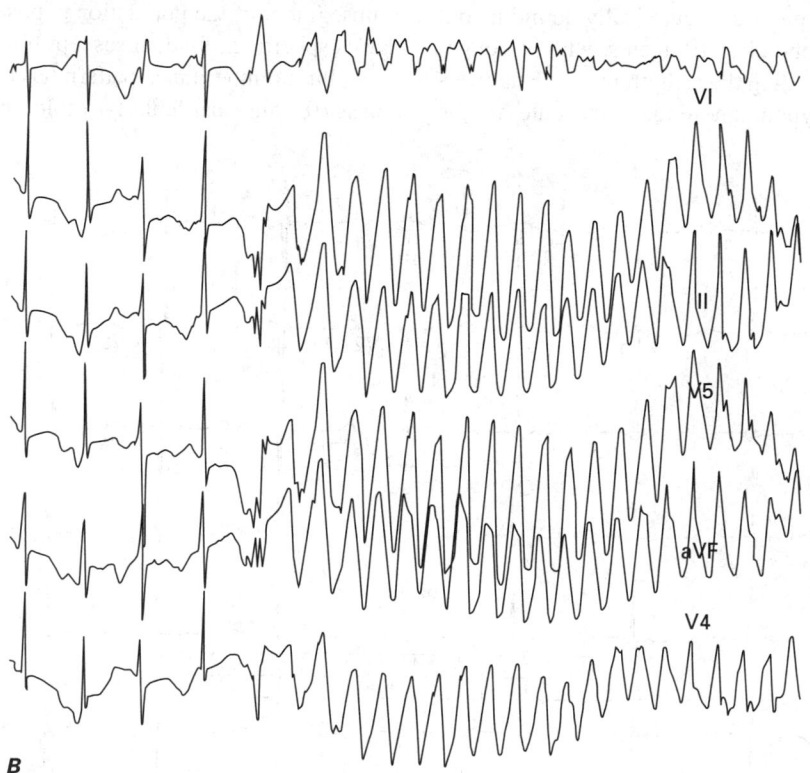

FIGURE 27-55

Congenital long QT interval syndrome. Treadmill stress testing was carried out in the patient shown in Fig. 27-54. *A*. At 4 min and 2 s into a Bruce protocol, ST-T alternans was observed, followed shortly by torsades de pointes (*B*).

a dose-dependent pattern, consistent with its major pharmacologic effect of blocking the delayed rectifier channel and thus prolonging the QT interval. This has implications for monitoring adverse drug effects at the initiation of therapy.

There is a growing list of other drugs that may also block repolarizing currents, prolong the QT interval, and establish susceptibility to torsades de pointes. These include the phenothiazines, certain antibiotics, pentamidine (Nebupent), cocaine, and terfenadine (Seldane), among others. The mechanisms of terfenadine-induced torsades de pointes is particularly instructive.[279] The parent compound, in addition to antihistamine effects, also blocks the delayed rectifier current, which can result in prolongation of the QT interval. Under normal conditions after oral ingestion, however, the parent compound is converted by a P450 enzyme in the liver to a metabolite that is an effective antihistamine but does not block the delayed rectifier current. Concomitant use of drugs that block specific enzymes in the hepatic P450 enzyme system, however [e.g., ketoconazole (Nizoral)], allows the parent compound to be absorbed and to circulate, creating the propensity to torsades de pointes in a small group of patients. Sudden deaths have been reported with this combination therapy.[280] Other causes of acquired long QT interval syndrome with torsades de pointes include acute ischemia and reperfusion, acute central nervous system injury, liquid protein diets, and various other drugs.[277,281,282]

ELECTROCARDIOGRAPHIC FEATURES

Torsades de pointes is characterized by sequential beat-to-beat variations in mean QRS axis, causing the QRS complexes to appear to twist about the baseline (Figs. 27-53 and 27-55). Characteristically, the tachycardia rate varies between 150 and 300 per minute, and the QT interval is prolonged during sinus rhythm. Episodes of tachycardia may be nonsustained or sustained, preceded by a long-short cycle sequence initiated by late PVCs, and may degenerate into VF. Torsades de pointes is a classic proarrhythmic manifestation of class IA antiarrhythmic agents. Class IC antiarrhythmic agents may express proarrhythmia in the form of an incessant monomorphic VT that is sinusoidal in pattern and often at slower rates (see Fig. 27-38) (see also Chap. 26).

MANAGEMENT OF CONGENITAL LONG QT INTERVAL SYNDROME

The clinical expression of arrhythmias in congenital long QT interval syndrome is episodic and transient, ranging from

GENETICS OF CONGENITAL LONG Q-T SYNDROME

Syndrome	Inheritance	Chromosome	Gene	Product
Romano-Ward				
LQT-1	Dominant	11p 15.5	KVLQT1	K^+ channel (I_{Ks})
LQT-2	Dominant	7q35-36	HERG	K^+ channel (I_{Kr})
LQT-3	Dominant	3p21-24	SCN5A	Na^+ channel
LQT-4	Dominant	4q25-27	?	(?)
LQT-5	Dominant	21q22.1	mink	K^+ channel
.		-22.2		[compnent, co-assembly unit?]
.				
.				
LQT-n (?)		(?)	(?)	(?)
—	Recessive	11p 15.5	KVLQT1	K^+ channel
Jervell, Lange-Nielson				

FIGURE 27-56

Genetic basis for congenital long QT interval syndromes. Abnormalities have been linked to five chromosomes among families with the Romano-Ward form of congenital long QT interval syndromes. At present, specific genetic abnormality and gene products are identified, at least in part, for four of the five. Multiple mutations or deletions are possible at each locus. The genetic asis for the Jervell–Lange-Nielson (autosomal recessive form of the syndrome) may be similar to LQT-1 in some families, but other loci are likely as well.

palpitations to syncope to sudden death. Ambient arrhythmias are not usually sustained enough to make acute management a common clinical need. When required, however, intravenous β-adrenergic blockade, intravenous Mg^{2+}, pacing, and/or lidocaine are appropriaste, depending on the genetic variant and pattern of the arrhythmia. A new category of drugs, the K^+-channel openers, may ultimately prove useful as well.

Because of the continuing risk of transition of torsades de pointes to VF in patients with congenital long QT interval syndrome throughout life, careful long-term management is important from the time of diagnosis. A 12-lead ECG should be recorded in anyone with *unexplained* near-syncope, syncope, and/or symptomatic palpitations, especially with repetitive beats. In selected patients, stress testing and ambulatory monitoring may help clarify uncertain findings. Genetic testing should be generally available in the near future.

Long-term therapy includes β-adrenergic blockade and/or left cardiac sympathetic denervation.[268,283] Placement of an ICD should be considered for patients with resistant arrhythmias. The present information on a variety of genetically controlled ion-channel dysfunctions may lead to new therapeutic approaches in the near future. For instance, mexiletine may be a specific therapy for the variant associated with the SCN5A gene on chromosome 3, which encodes the cardiac Na^+ channel.[272] It is anticipated that other channel-specific therapies will be identified in the future.

MANAGEMENT OF ACQUIRED LONG QT INTERVAL SYNDROME

Treatment is directed at the underlying cause(s), with careful attention to electrolyte and metabolic disturbances and to identifying and reversing or removing iatrogenic factors. Although electrical cardioversion may interrupt torsades de pointes, the arrhythmia frequently recurs as long as the offending influence is present. In addition, many runs are nonsustained. Intravenous magnesium sulfate is often effective, especially when torsades de pointes is due to quinidine. It may be given in a dose of 2 g over 2 min followed by an infusion of 2 to 20 mg/min. Overdrive atrial or ventricular pacing to induce rate-related QT shortening may also be required. Acceleration of the underlying heart rate with isoproterenol infusion to shorten the acquired QT interval prolongation may be effective but should be avoided in patients with symptomatic ischemic heart disease, if possible. Lidocaine also may be beneficial, as may other class IB drugs. These drugs tend to shorten the QT interval in normal myocardium. Class IA and class III antiarrhythmic agents should be avoided, since they prolong the QT interval.

Ventricular Fibrillation and Flutter

Ventricular fibrillation is a terminal arrhythmia, uniformly requiring rapid initiation of emergency measures. Ventricular flutter with loss of consciousness and rapid unstable VT may be clinically and hemodynamically equivalent to VF and is treated identically when accompanied by the clinical picture of cardiac arrest. VF occurs commonly in the setting of acute ischemia or unpredictably in advanced chronic ischemic heart disease. Moreover, it is the apparent mode of death in 25 to 50 percent of cardiac fatalities. Among patients with nonischemic cardiomyopathies,[284,285] cardiac arrest is the mode of death in up to 50 percent of all fatalities. In the past, it has been assumed that VF is the mechanism of most of these events, but it is clear now that a substantial proportion of these events are due to bradyarrhythmias and asystole[285] and, importantly, to acute hemodynamic dysfunction.

VF may also develop during hypoxia, atrial fibrillation with rapid ventricular responses in WPW syndrome, R-on-T pacing or asynchronized cardioversion, or electrical accidents due to improper grounding of electrical devices or as proarrhythmic effects of antiarrhythmic drugs. A particularly high-risk setting for VF is acute myocardial infarction with right or left bundle branch block. VF may occur de novo, but among patients with out-of-hospital cardiac arrest, VT commonly precedes the onset of VF (see also Chap. 26).

ELECTROCARDIOGRAPHIC FEATURES

The electrocardiographic pattern of VF is described by gross disorganization without identifiable repetitive waveforms or intervals (Fig. 27-42*D* and *E*). At the onset, VF may be "coarse" in pattern, but over time, it loses its amplitude and becomes "fine" (<0.2 mV). Successful defibrillation and survival rates are decreased in patients with the fine pattern of VF. In ventricular flutter (Fig. 27-42*C*), a sine wave configuration is present, having a cycle length in the range of 200 to 240 ms. Rapid polymorphic VTs may be difficult to distinguish from VF electrocardiographically, but maintained con-

sciousness suggests VT rather than VF, the latter defined by loss of effective mechanical function. Hemodynamic findings may be initially stable in ventricular flutter or very rapid polymorphic VT, but hypotension, loss of consciousness, and degeneration to VF are common.

MANAGEMENT OF VENTRICULAR FLUTTER AND VENTRICULAR FIBRILLATION

There are two major goals of therapy: (1) immediate life support and resuscitation, and (2) long-term prevention of recurrences. Basic life support with standard cardiopulmonary resuscitation (Chap. 37) is used until emergency defibrillation at 200 or more J can be carried out (see Chap. 32). After three unsuccessful shocks at energies up to 360 J, 1 mg of epinephrine should be administered by intravenous push and defibrillation attempted again.

Early defibrillation is essential to survival.[286] Resistance of defibrillation may occur due to patient size, improper paddle placement, improper use of conducting media, acidosis, hypoxemia, or electrolyte disturbances.[287] Some antiarrhythmic drugs may raise the defibrillation threshold. Energy thresholds for defibrillation may be decreased by administration of bretylium, lidocaine, or epinephrine, the latter especially when the fibrillatory waveform is fine. Immediate steps to improve metabolic and electrolyte disturbances are required, paramount of which is to establish an airway, followed by techniques to support ventilation.[288] In rare instances, "spontaneous" reversion of VF[289] or "medical" defibrillation with bretylium[209] has been reported. A physiologic or pharmacologic increase in catecholamines has been postulated as the underlying mechanism.

After successful defibrillation, careful attention to the total clinical status of the patient and prophylactic antiarrhythmic drugs are required. Intravenous therapy with lidocaine, procainamide, or, in resistant cases, amiodarone or bretylium may be useful. In addition to oxygenation and improving the metabolic milieu, aggressive steps to identify and treat or prevent recurrent ischemia or heart failure are necessary, since they may act as pathophysiologic triggers for recurrences.[4,214]

In the in-hospital setting, early recognition and aggressive treatment of VT may prevent VF. In the patient with acute myocardial infarction, early VF (≤48 h), as with early VT, is not associated with an independent influence on posthospital mortality risk and does not justify long-term antiarrhythmic therapy.[290–292] When VF occurs as a convalescent-phase complication of acute myocardial infarction, however, aggressive long-term antiarrhythmic management is indicated (see above).[293,294] The vast majority of patients who have VT or VF in the convalescent phase after acute myocardial infarction (3 days to 8 weeks) will have inducible ventricular arrhythmias at baseline electrophysiologic study.[213]

Among survivors of out-of-hospital VF not caused by acute myocardial infarction, control of ischemia and heart failure is essential. The clinical context[295,296] is evaluated in terms of the interaction between structural abnormalities (coronary heart disease, myopathy, hypertrophy, anatomic electrical abnormalities) and functional states (ischemia/reperfusion, systemic factors including congestive heart failure, metabolic and electrolyte disturbances, neurophysiologic interactions, and toxic effects). For long-term management of the risk of arrhythmia, results of invasive electrophysiologic testing of pharmacological efficacy is one accepted approach.[297] Only about 33 to 40 percent of survivors, however, will be inducible into a reproducibly inducible ventricular tachyarrhythmia at baseline.[296,297] A similar fraction will be inducible into nonsustained VT or VF (Fig. 27-57), and 20 to 30 percent are noninducible. The subgroup whose unexpected VF is related to transient ischemia, in contrast to an underlying structural basis, is less likely to be inducible at baseline.[298] With high-risk forms of arrhythmias on ambulatory monitoring or exercise testing, but without inducible arrhythmia at baseline by invasive testing, drug therapy can be guided by suppression of these spontaneous arrhythmias by noninvasive techniques[195,225,226] as long as the EF is greater than 40 percent. For such patients with lower EFs, the use of ICDs is emerging as the preferred treatment.

Usefulness of long-term drug therapy is limited by the fact that no more than 20 to 30 percent of the patients with inducible arrhythmias will have a drug identified that will prevent inducibility. In one randomized study without placebo control (ESVEM), a class III antiarrhythmic agent with beta-blocking effect, sotolol, appeared more effective than other drugs for survivors of VT and VF.[228] Whether amiodarone will have equivalent (or greater) benefit remains to be determined. Patients who have recurrences despite drug therapy predicted to be effective during testing, those in whom an endpoint of therapy cannot be established, or those in whom the risk of recurrence remains high because underlying precipitating factors cannot be adequately controlled should receive ICDs.[296] The development of programmable devices with diagnostic electrogram storage capability and transvenous lead systems is expanding the set of circumstances in which ICDs are preferred therapy (see Chap. 33). The relative benefit of ICDs versus empiric amiodarone (or other drugs), in terms of total mortality during follow-up, however, is not established for the overall population of survivors of a cardiac arrest.

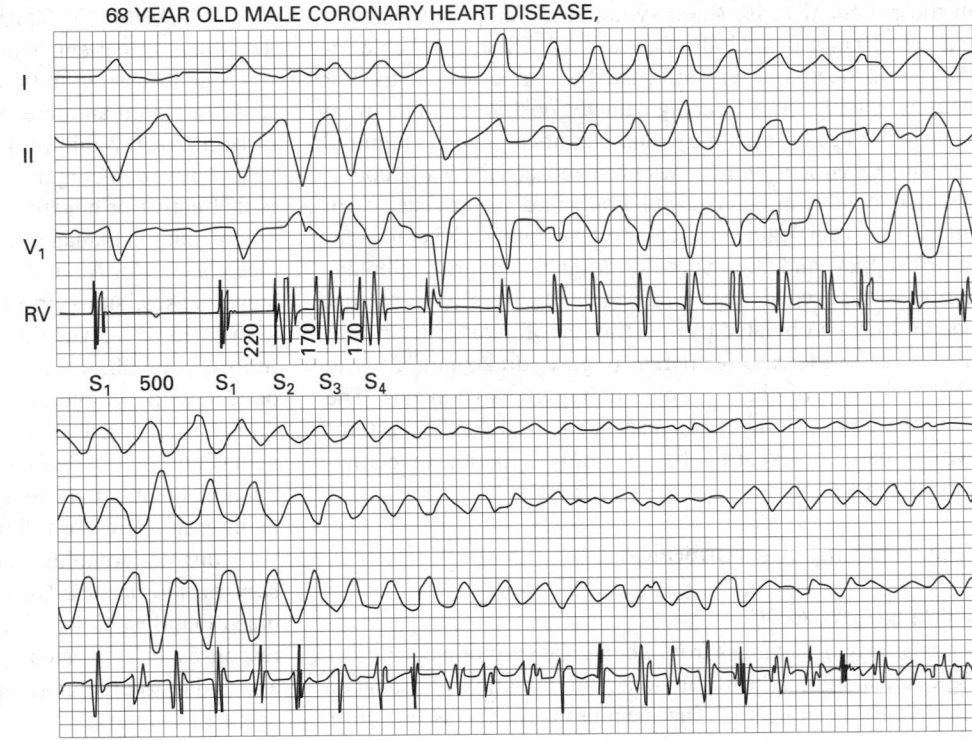

68 YEAR OLD MALE CORONARY HEART DISEASE,

FIGURE 27-57

Programmed electrical stimulation study in a survivor of out-of-hospital cardiac arrest. The patient had ischemic heart disease, and polymorphic ventricular tachycardia degenerating to ventricular fibrillation was reproducibly induced prior to bypass surgery. After surgery, the tachycardia was no longer inducible

BRADYARRHYTHMIAS

Bradyarrhythmias may be due to depression or failure of impulse formation or to failure of AV conduction. They are often asymptomatic, but when symptoms of hypoperfusion occur, resulting from inadequate cerebral or coronary blood flow or worsening of congestive heart failure at rest or during exercise, treatment is required. Symptoms are almost always due to inadequate heart rate, although under some circumstances, such as with aortic stenosis or hypertrophic cardiomyopathy, loss of synchronized atrial contraction may contribute to symptoms. Bradyarrhythmias may be due solely to cardiac factors but are often caused or aggravated by noncardiac factors such as drugs, autonomic imbalance, hypothyroidism, hypothermia, or hyperkalemia.[299] Furthermore, the hypoperfusion associated with bradycardia may be multifactorial, such as may occur in acute inferior wall infarction, in which bradycardia and LV dysfunction may be additive. In all cases, careful evaluation of both cardiac and noncardiac factors is necessary. If the patient is symptomatic, the first step in management is to increase the heart rate, which is readily accomplished by parasympatholytic drugs (e.g., atropine) or sympathomimetic drugs (e.g., isoproterenol). Underdosing with atropine (e.g., ≤0.3 mg) may cause a centrally mediated bradycardia and should be avoided. In addition, sympathomimetics must be used cautiously in all patients and avoided in the patient with ischemic symptoms. Temporary external pacing offers a logical alternative.[300,301] Stable, reliable increases in heart rate are afforded by temporary ventricular demand pacing from a pacing catheter positioned in the right ventricular apex. Temporary dual-chamber pacing is required for those cases in which synchronized atrial contraction is deemed beneficial, such as in bradycardia associated with inferior wall and right ventricular infarction.[302] General circulatory support and elimination of drugs that aggravate bradycardia is the second step in management. Rarely, permanent pacing may be obviated by substitution of a vasodilator drug that tends to increase heart rate (e.g., hydralazine)[303,304] in place of negative chronotropic antihypertensive agents. The administration of ephedrine has been used in the past for symptomatic bradycardia but is rarely superior to permanent pacing.

Failure of Impulse Formation

SINUS BRADYCARDIA

Sinus bradycardia ranges from a benign asymptomatic physiologic adjustment in heart rate to a symptomatic expression of sinus node dysfunction. The asymptomatic forms are most often benign and related to physiologic (e.g., training effect) or pathologic (e.g., inferior wall infarction) excesses in vagal tone.[305–309] Although most commonly due to impaired impulse formation, it may also be caused by SA block.

ELECTROCARDIOGRAPHIC FEATURES OF SINUS BRADYCARDIA AND SINOATRIAL BLOCK

Sinus bradycardia is defined as a rate less than 60 impulses per minute, with the pacemaker impulse originating in the sinus node, resulting in P waves of normal amplitude and vector. It is rarely considered outside of the physiologic range until rates are under 50 per minute. In well-trained athletes and during sleep, rates of 40 per minute or less may occur normally. Sinus bradycardia is commonly accompanied by some degree of sinus arrhythmia.

SA block, referring to abnormal conduction of a sinus impulse from the SA node to the atrial muscle, is categorized as first-degree (delayed conduction), second-degree (intermittent), or third-degree (complete) block. Vagal stimulation, digitalis, and ischemia are the most common predisposing factors in these otherwise rare conduction disorders. SA block may be recognized by the absence of expected P waves and the subsequent QRS complex. First- and third-degree SA blocks cannot be recognized on the standard clinical ECG, but second-degree SA block may be identified because of its intermittent pattern. Characteristically, in SA Wenckebach, the PP and RR intervals will progressively shorten together before a dropped P-QRS complex results in a pause; a recurrent pattern may be identified (Fig. 27-58B). Sinoatrial Wenckebach periods are frequently overlooked and mislabeled as sinus arrhythmia. Intermittent 2:1 block may also be deduced from standard rhythm strips (Fig. 27-59), but persistent 2:1 SA block is indistinguishable from sinus bradycardia.

MANAGEMENT OF SINUS BRADYARRHYTHMIAS

Treatment of patients who have asymptomatic bradycardia is often unnecessary and may even be detrimental, such as in those in whom an increase in rate may aggravate myocardial ischemia or LV failure. In the symptomatic patient, elimination of reversible aggravating factors is essential. When this is ineffective or negative chronotropic agents are essential to overall patient management, permanent pacing may be needed (see Chap. 34). A similar approach is taken for patients with sinus pauses, sinus arrest, or SA exit block, which may be associated with myocardial infarction, myocarditis, sinus node fibrosis, digitalis excess, or excess vagal tone.[310,311] In the patient with symptomatic hypersensitive carotid sinus syndrome,[312,313] medical treatment is usually inadequate. Permanent ventricular or dual-chamber pacing[314] is usually effective but occasionally may not relieve symptoms because of a coexisting vasodepressor reflex.[315]

A distinct complex, referred to as *neurocardiogenic syncope* or *neurally mediated vasodepressor syncope*, has combined manifestations of sinus bradycardia and vasodepressor responses. It is revealed by the response to head-up tilt testing and is due to an abnormal reflex, the afferent limb of which originates in the LV wall.[316] The efferent limb is parasympathetic, causing both peripheral decreases in vascular tone, leading to hypotension, and sinus node depression, leading to sinus bradycardia. In the majority of patients, the vasodepressor component dominates, limiting the effectiveness of pacing therapy.[317] Among pharmacologic agents, β-adrenergic blockers have been most useful, presumably by the mechanism of blocking the sympathetically mediated afferent limb of the reflex[318] (see Chap. 35).

Sick-Sinus Syndrome

Sick-sinus syndrome[319–321] is a generalized abnormality of cardiac impulse formation and intraatrial and AV conduction abnormalities[305,322,323] that may be manifested by variable combinations of brady- and tachyarrhythmias.[324] Treatment, therefore, must be individualized to each patient's manifestations of the syndrome.[325] Often the patient is asymptomatic, or the symptoms are mild and nonspecific. Negative chronotropic agents are avoided or discontinued,[321,326] and permanent pacing may be delayed until the patient is more clearly symptomatic.[327,328] In the clearly symptomatic patient, treatment may include a combination of antiarrhythmic agents and permanent pacing for intrinsic and drug-induced bradycardias. Ironically, the eventual development of atrial fibrillation in patients with sick-sinus syndrome may alleviate symptoms, since heart rate control in atrial fibrillation can be more consistently achieved. Dual-chamber pacing is preferred to avoid pacemaker syndrome (see Chap. 34), and DDD pacing with rate-responsive functions is preferred for patients with intermittent or persistent sinus bradyarrhythmias. Automatic mode-switching function is useful for patients with intermittent tachyarrhythmic components. For patients with chronic atrial fibrillation, rate-responsive VVI pacing is preferred.[329] Digitalis is used with

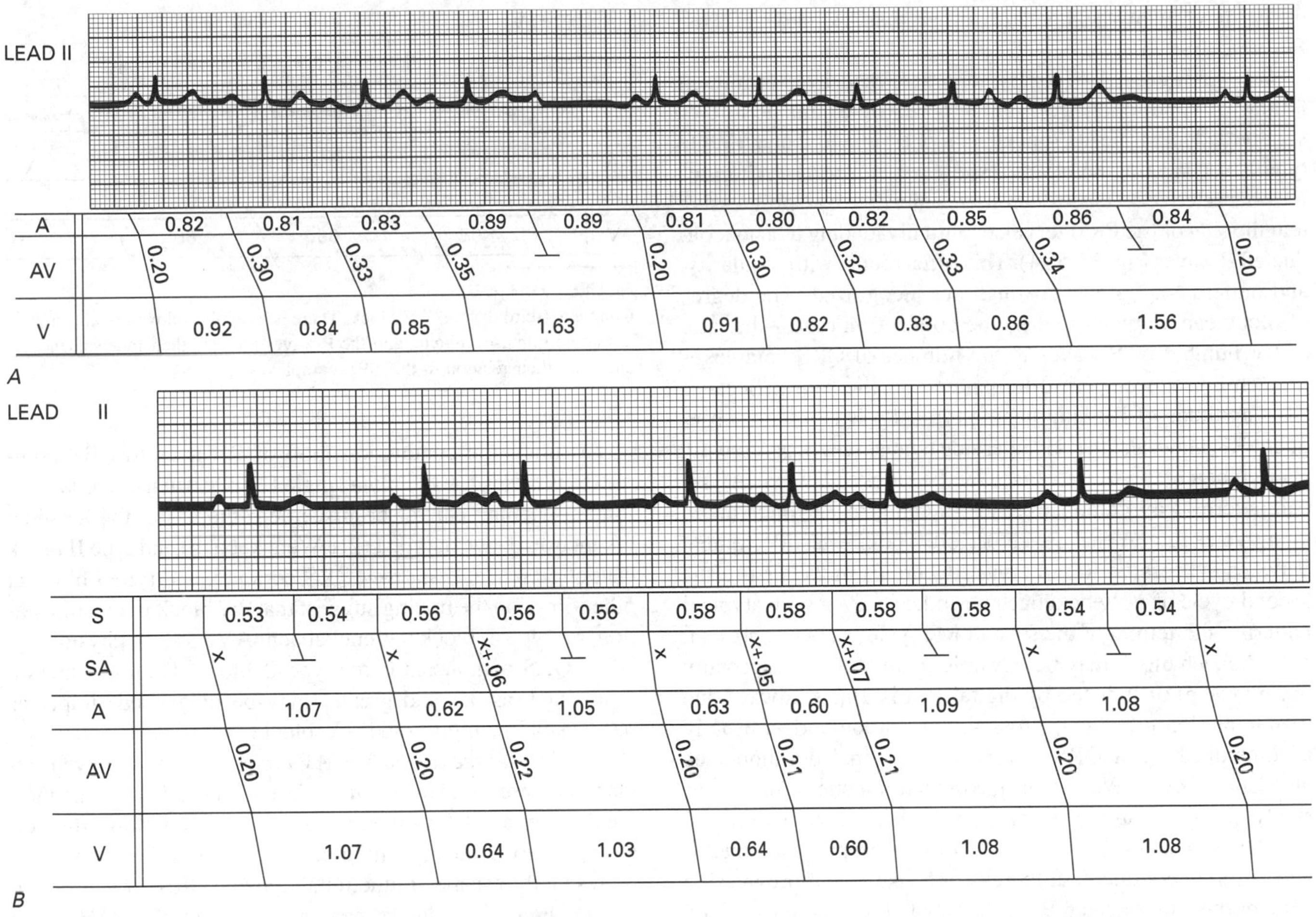

LEAD II

A	0.82	0.81	0.83	0.89	0.89	0.81	0.80	0.82	0.85	0.86	0.84
AV	0.20	0.30	0.33	0.35		0.20	0.30	0.32	0.33	0.34	0.20
V	0.92	0.84	0.85	1.63		0.91	0.82	0.83	0.86	1.56	

A

LEAD II

S	0.53	0.54	0.56	0.56	0.56	0.58	0.58	0.58	0.58	0.54	0.54
SA	x		x	x+.06		x	x+.05	x+.07		x	x
A	1.07		0.62		1.05		0.63	0.60	1.09		1.08
AV	0.20		0.20	0.22		0.20	0.21	0.21		0.20	0.20
V	1.07		0.64		1.03		0.64	0.60	1.08		1.08

B

FIGURE 27-58

Wenckebach phenomenon. *A.* A 5:4 and 6:5 AV Wenckebach period. Note that the PR interval progressively lengthens, but by a decreasing increment; therefore the ventricular cycle tends to shorten (at least for the first two cycles following the dropped beat). *B.* A 3:2 and 4:3 sinoatrial Wenckebach period with 2:1 sinoatrial block at beginning and end of strip. (From Hurst JW, Myerburg R. *Introduction to Electrocardiography.* New York: McGraw-Hill; 1973. Reproduced with permission from the publisher and authors.)

caution[326] and, when needed, is easier to titrate once the patient is permanently paced. When such patients require therapy with antiarrhythmic drugs that slow sinus rates and/ or impair AV conduction (e.g., beta blockers, amiodarone), management of drug therapy may be facilitated by pacemaker back-up.

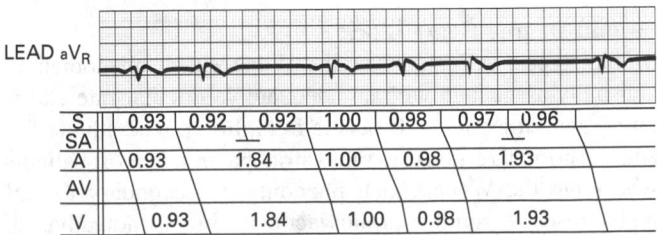

LEAD aV_R

S	0.93	0.92	0.92	1.00	0.98	0.97	0.96
SA							
A	0.93	1.84		1.00	0.98	1.93	
AV							
V	0.93	1.84		1.00	0.98	1.93	

FIGURE 27-59

Sinoatrial (SA) block. In each pause the entire P-QRS-T sequence is missing, and the long cycle is approximately equal to two of the sinus cycles. The pattern is the equivalent of a Möbitz type II block at the level of the AV junction.

AV Conduction Abnormalities

Heart block refers to abnormalities of impulse conduction that may result from normal physiologic variations (e.g., vagal tone) or pathologic influences.[330] Management is determined by assessing the degree of block, symptoms, and clinical setting. Recurrent episodes of the Wenckebach phenomenon (type I, second-degree AV block) may be asymptomatic and require no therapy in the well-conditioned individual or athlete, while transient complete AV block accompanying an acute anterior wall myocardial infarction is a high-risk marker that may indicate permanent pacing, whether or not symptoms of AV block have occurred.

ELECTROCARDIOGRAPHIC PATTERNS

First-degree AV block is defined as a PR interval in excess of 0.2 s at normal heart rates. When the QRS complexes are of normal duration and configuration, it is usually due to prolonged conduction at the level of the AV node. If bundle branch or fascicular block is present, the conduction delay may be at the level of either the AV node or His-Purkinje system.

Second-degree AV block is characterized by intermittent failure of conduction from atria to ventricles and is further subdivided into type I (Wenckebach phenomenon) and Möbitz type II second-degree block. *Type I second-degree AV block* is characterized electrocardiographically by progressive lengthening of the PR interval, eventually leading to a nonconducted P wave (Fig. 27-58A). This often recurs with regularity, and patterns of "group beating" are recognized. The degree of block can be quantified by the conduction ratio—the ratio of the number of P waves to the number of QRS complexes in each episode or period terminated by the pause. Because the magnitude of PR lengthening typically is less with subsequent RR intervals, the RR intervals themselves progressively shorten before the pause caused by the blocked P wave. Atypical patterns may demonstrate lengthening of RR intervals in later cycles of a Wenckebach period. The greatest decrement between successive RR intervals occurs from the first to the second cycle of a Wenckebach period, and even with atypical patterns, shortening of the second RR cycle is always present. Wenckebach block may be physiologic in athletes (especially during sleep) or induced by digitalis. It is almost always due to impaired conduction across the AV node and is usually accompanied by a QRS complex of normal duration (see also Chap. 34). A Wenckebach conduction pattern may occur rarely across an area of disease in the His-Purkinje system.

In *type II second-degree AV block,* appropriately timed P waves fail to conduct, but there is not a pattern of progressive PR lengthening. Isolated P waves may fail to conduct, or fixed patterns (e.g., 2:1 at rates which are expected to conduct 1:1 under normal physiologic conditions) may occur. Infranodal block is the rule, and QRS complexes tend to be widened due to disease in the His bundle or intraventricular conducting system. Type II block is most often associated with organic cardiac disease and is frequently progressive. When the QRS complex is narrow with Möbitz type II block, block in the His bundle is likely (Fig. 27-60); when it is widened, block below the His bundle is the rule.

LEAD aVF

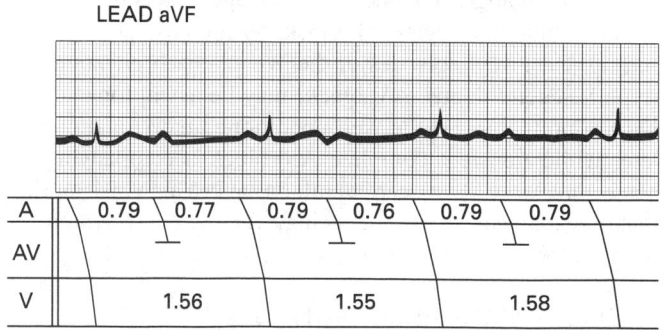

FIGURE 27-60

A form of second-degree AV block. There are two P waves to each QRS 2:1 AV block (alternate sinus impulses are blocked). This pattern can be caused by block in the AV node (Wenckebach), intra-Hisian block, or distal block (see text).

LEAD V₂

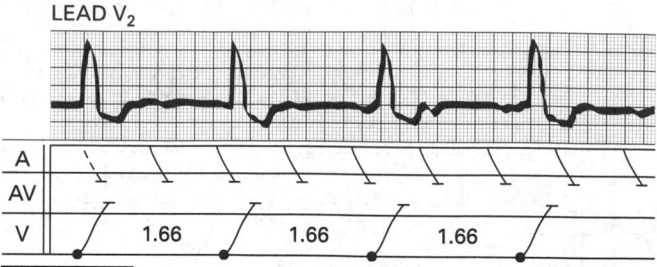

FIGURE 27-61

Complete (third degree) AV block. There is a regular idioventricular rhythm at rate 36 impulses/minute, and the P waves indicate their independence by changing their relation to the QRS complexes.

At times, the conduction ratio of P waves to QRS complexes is fixed at 2:1. Only a single PR interval is recorded and PR lengthening cannot be discerned; therefore, the absolute distinction between type I (2:1 Wenckebach) and type II block cannot be made. A narrow QRS complex and type I block at other times on the tracing suggest that 2:1 block is a manifestation of type I block (Wenckebach–AV nodal) physiology. Wide QRS complexes favor type II block. High conduction ratios such as 3:1 and greater may be diagnosed simply as paroxysmal or high-grade AV block.

In *third-degree (complete) AV block*, the atrial and ventricular rates are regular but dissociated (Fig. 27-61). At times, the P waves and QRS rates are so similar (isorhythmic dissociation) as to make this judgment difficult. QRS complexes represent the escape of junctional (narrow QRS) or ventricular (wide QRS) subordinate pacemakers. Complete AV block may be preceded by years of varying and/or progressive lower grades of block as well as by bundle branch and fascicular blocks. It is common to observe long rhythm strips that demonstrate not-quite-complete AV block. Occasional capture beats interrupt a regular escape rhythm. The conducted P waves are critically timed within a narrow range. The clinical implication of this pattern is the same as complete heart block.

MANAGEMENT OF AV BLOCK

First-Degree Heart Block
Isolated first-degree AV block is never symptomatic and is not an indication for temporary or permanent pacing.[331]

Second-Degree Heart Block
Möbitz type I AV block, or the Wenckebach phenomenon, is usually associated with an adequate ventricular rate and is rarely symptomatic.[332] It occurs in highly trained athletes[333] and is a normal response to rapid atrial pacing. In most patients who have the Wenckebach phenomenon secondary to AV nodal disease, routine prophylactic pacing is not advised, as it is minimally symptomatic (if at all) and tends not to progress.[334] Rarely, the effective ventricular rate is slow and patients are symptomatic, requiring pacing if vagolytic maneuvers are ineffective. The prognosis in patients who have underlying organic heart disease is determined by the extent of the

underlying disease, not the Möbitz type I block.[334] It is common in the acute phase of inferior wall myocardial infarction and rarely requires temporary pacing in this setting. Reversion is usually prompt—measured in hours to days.

Möbitz type II block is less common but implies more significant disease in the conduction system. The site of block is almost always below the AV node and usually below the bundle of His. Therefore, slower escape rhythms and risk of progression to complete heart block are of concern. It is almost always associated with a defined disease process. Permanent pacing is indicated,[331] except where Möbitz type II block is induced by rapid artificial pacing.[335,336] The purpose of pacing is primarily to protect against symptomatic events such as syncope and thus to protect the patient from injury to him- or herself, or to others. Available data do not suggest that pacemakers will prolong the life of patients with Möbitz type II block. The selection among specific designs of pacing devices is discussed in Chap. 34.

A special circumstance involves 2:1 AV block, in which the underlying mechanism and site of block remain obscure. The decision to treat is inferred from the clinical setting. Wide QRS complexes, sudden onset of periods of block, and inadequate escape rates favor type II block, whereas narrow complexes and coincident episodes of typical type I block favor Wenckebach block.

Another variant pattern is multilevel block in the AV junction. This commonly occurs during atrial tachycardias and may be functional, pharmacologic, or pathologic. The pattern of multilevel block during atrial tachycardia may be deceiving. In this pattern, a basic 2:1 pattern, with Wenckebach conduction patterns of the impulses that conduct through the area of 2:1, produces group beating of the ventricles. This may result in relatively slow ventricular rates, but the primary problem is the atrial arrhythmias with physiologic or insignificant pathologic responses at the level of the AV node. His bundle electrograms may be diagnostic, but such invasive studies are indicated only when needed for a therapeutic decision.[337–339]

Paroxysmal AV Block

Runs of consecutive atrial impulses that fail to conduct to the ventricles may last for up to 10 to 20 s and may be associated with syncope. Unless a clearly defined reversible cause is identified, permanent pacing is required.

Complete AV Block

Complete heart block may be acute in onset or chronic; it may produce abrupt significant symptoms or may be asymptomatic and discovered incidentally. When acute and symptomatic, evaluation and rate support are urgently needed. Pharmacologic intervention with atropine or isoproterenol is usually most readily available. The latter should be avoided in the ischemic setting, and external pacing instituted if needed.[300,301] Reliable rate control is achieved by ventricular or dual-chamber temporary cardiac pacing. Permanent pacing is indicated unless those factors responsible for the heart block

are reversible or when transient complete block complicates an acute inferior wall infarction.[331]

Although commonly asymptomatic or minimally symptomatic, patients with congenital AV block usually are managed with permanent pacemakers. The choice between ventricular and dual-chamber pacing, and considerations for rate-responsive pacing in various clinical conditions, are discussed in Chap. 34.

AV Dissociation

This diagnosis is not synonymous with AV block but occurs in conjunction with block as well as in its absence. It implies an abnormality of intrinsic pacemaker activity that may be slowing of normal pacemaker activity (*default*), acceleration of a normally subordinate or latent pacemaker (*usurpation*), AV block, or a combination of these.

ELECTROCARDIOGRAPHIC FINDINGS

AV dissociation implies that the atria and ventricles each have manifest independent pacemakers. In the setting of AV block, a junctional or ventricular pacemaker emerges as an escape rhythm; if it fails or if the escape is too slow, AV block will become a symptomatic or terminal rhythm. The atria and ventricles may beat independently if a normally subordinate junctional or ventricular pacemaker discharges faster than the sinus or atrial pacemaker and 1:1 retrograde conduction is absent. Since AV block is not necessarily present, ventricular capture by impulses of sinus origin commonly occur as a result of fortuitous timing relationships between sinus node activity and ventricular refractoriness. At times, capture beats and junctional or ventricular beats coincide and generate fusion beats (Fig. 27-62).

MANAGEMENT

Treatment, when needed, is directed to the underlying cause. It is important to evaluate whether symptoms are present and whether they are due to a rapid or slow rate. Suppression of tachyarrhythmias, such as AV dissociation in VT, is the primary goal when symptoms are related primarily to the tachyarrhythmia and an intact intrinsic or artificial pacemaker is present. Intermittent ventricular ectopy may be an escape phenomenon in an otherwise asymptomatic patient who has an underlying persistent bradycardia. In such a case, rate support with pacing is indicated and will often relieve the symptoms and ventricular ectopy. If initial therapy is mistakenly targeted to tachycardia, the underlying bradycardia may worsen due to drug suppression of lower intrinsic pacemaker sites.[340]

Indications for Pacing

Pacing is indicated for symptomatic bradyarrhythmias that have no identifiable reversible cardiac or noncardiac cause.[341,342] Prophylactic pacing to prevent mortality or the onset of life-threatening symptoms is controversial, since

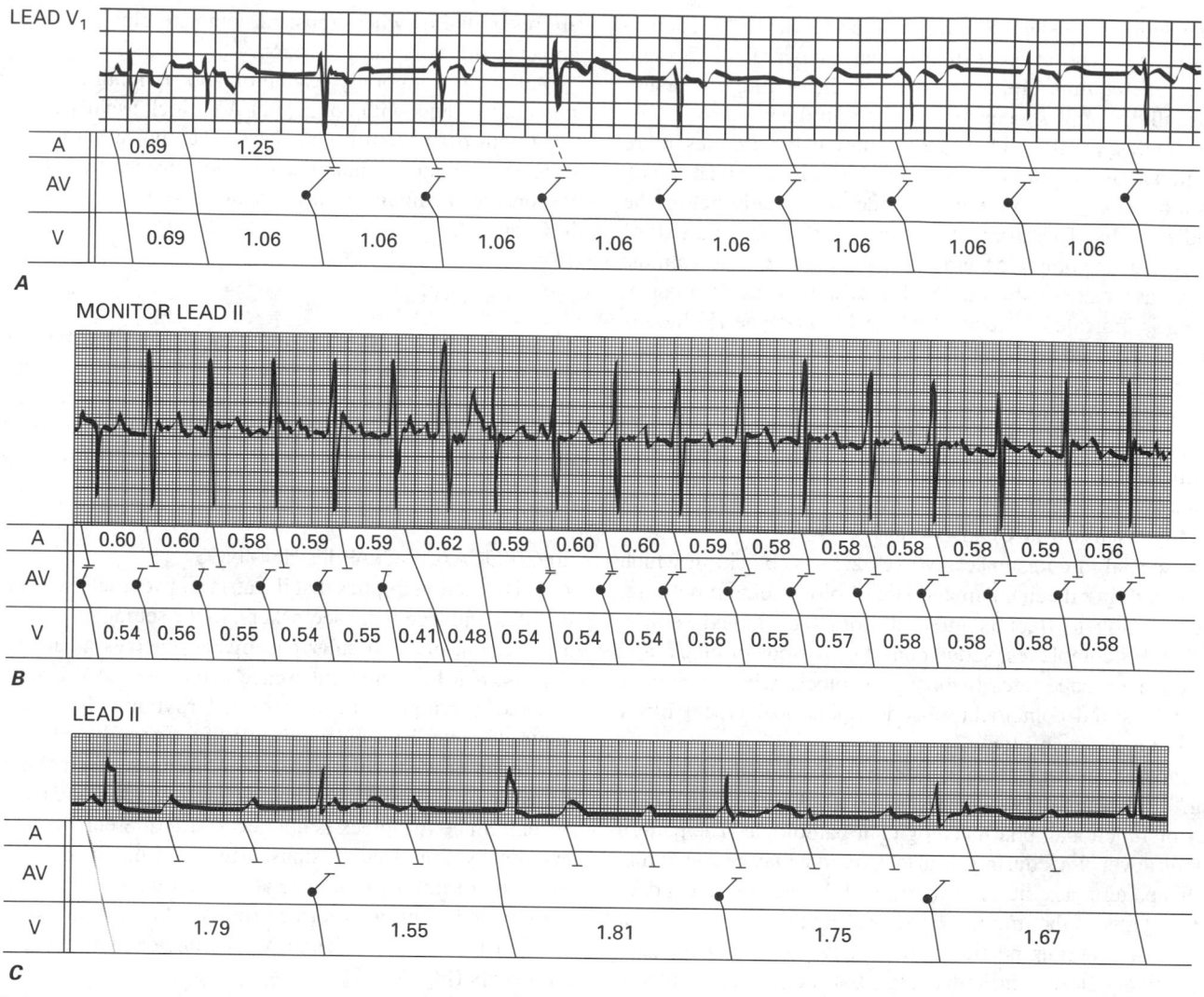

FIGURE 27-62

Atrioventricular dissociation *A.* Sinus arrhythmia: The bradycardic phase enables the AV node to escape, with resulting dissociation. *B.* Atrioventricular tachycardia: The tachycardia enables the AV pacemaker to usurp control of the ventricles, with resulting dissociation; the seventh and eighth beats are ventricular captures, the seventh, ending the shorter cycle, showing ventricular aberration. *C.* High-grade AV block permits the AV node to escape (second, fourth, and fifth beats) with resulting dissociation.

increased risk of death is more likely related to the severity of underlying organic heart disease. The benefits of pacing, though theoretically sound, often lack rigorous proof of effectiveness. Less controversial is the use of permanent pacing to reduce symptomatic bradyarrhythmic events[341,342] (see also Chap. 34).

Temporary pacing is indicated for AV block associated with acute anterior wall infarction if the heart rate is excessively slow and/or associated with rate-dependent hypotension and is advanced in some newly acquired left or right bundle branch block accompanied by hemiblock.[343] The availability of external pacing techniques[300,301] has tended to relax the sense of urgency for prophylactic pacing catheters in these settings. New left bundle branch block or preexisting right or left bundle branch block does not require pacing. Permanent pacing is often recommended for those with acute anterior

wall infarction who have had transient complete heart block.[344] The change in long-term survival, however, is not well documented.[345] Temporary pacing can often be avoided in AV block associated with inferior infarction since block is often related to ischemia or parasympathetic reflexes, is often asymptomatic, and reverses with time.[346] If hypotension occurs in inferior infarction that is not due to hypovolemia or right ventricular infarct, temporary pacing for severe sinus bradycardia or higher grades of AV block is often used. Permanent pacing after AV block in inferior infarction is required only very rarely.

Permanent prophylactic pacing in bifascicular block is not routinely recommended.[347,348] In patients at high risk for complete heart block (e.g., Kearns-Sayre syndrome) or recurrent neurologic symptoms associated with advanced HV prolongation (e.g., HV longer than 70 to 80 ms), however, prophylactic pacing may be of benefit.[349] Guidelines for permanent cardiac pacemaker implantation have been published[331] and are further discussed in Chap. 34.

Pacemaker-Associated Arrhythmias

As pacemakers have become more sophisticated, there has been an increasing need to identify normal and abnormal pacemaker rhythms as well as difficulty in identifying them. The baseline pacing pattern is dependent on the pacemaker design and the interaction with the patient's intrinsic rhythm. These aspects, as well as pacemaker testing, are reviewed in detail in Chap. 34. Apparent pacemaker malfunctions are frequently due to observer inexperience and lack of knowledge of pacemaker electronics. Unusually rapid or slow rates may connote pacemaker malfunction, but programming changes, magnet activation, and over- and undersensing must be excluded. Fusion beats, pseudofusion, and ventricular-triggered pacing may cause confusion. Fusion beats occur when there is overlap in the timing of paced and normal beats and the morphology of the fused complex is midway between the normal and paced QRS complexes. Ventricular-triggered pacing becomes confusing when a PVC occurs and is thought to be triggered by the pacemaker because of the width of the complex and the presence of a pacemaker artifact. The pacing artifact occurs slightly after the initiation of the PVC, providing a clue to ventricular ectopy. Inappropriate bradycardias may be induced by oversensing by the pacemaker or by normal sensing of extracardiac stimuli such as myopotentials (skeletal muscle activity) or extracorporeal inhibition by electromagnetic or RF waves. "Cross talk" can result in arrhythmias, for instance, when the ventricular lead senses atrial activity.

Dual-chamber pacing may lead to a variety of arrhythmias that are actually an undesirable byproduct of normal pacemaker function. Arrhythmias may be initiated by asynchronous ventricular or atrial stimulation (DVI pacemakers), interruption of ventricular sensing during ventricular blanking (all dual-chamber pacemakers), or asynchronous atrial or ventricular stimulation in the magnet mode (all dual-chamber pacemakers). Furthermore, dual-chamber units create an artificial bypass tract that may become operative in the presence of ventriculoatrial conduction. When a ventricular event, either paced or spontaneous, results in retrograde atrial activation, the latter may be sensed by the atrial electrode returning to the ventricle after an appropriate AV delay. A paced ventricular response follows, and the process repeats itself. This artificial arrhythmia has been called an "endless loop" tachycardia[350] (Fig. 27-63). Spontaneous termination of the reentry tachycardia may occur by fatigue or block in the retrograde limb. Treatment includes reprogramming of pacemaker parameters, including extension of the atrial refractory period of the pacemaker or avoidance of the DDD or VDD mode (at the extreme,

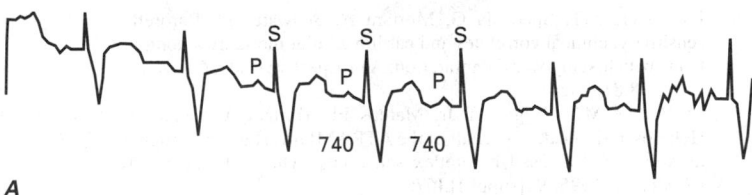

FIGURE 27-63

Pacemaker-mediated (endless-loop) tachycardia. The patient had a DDD pacemaker and presented with episodes of sustained rapid heart action. The tracing (lead II) demonstrates (*A*) atrial tracking with ventricular pacing at a cycle length of 740 ms and (*B*) ventricular pacing with retrograde atrial activation. The retrograde P waves (P') following each paced QRS are sensed by the atrial sensing lead and trigger a ventricular pacing spike (S) followed by the paced QRS with repeated retrograde atrial activation.

the VVI mode is used). In order to guard against rapid ventricular pacing and response to sudden increases in atrial rate, physiologic pacemakers tend to have an upper rate limit control. Earlier models suddenly drop to 2:1 pacing rates. Recent models often induce a gradual Wenckebach-type response. The pacemaker electronically creates a Wenckebach phenomenon with a gradually increasing number of dropped QRS complexes (see Chap. 34).

REFERENCES

1. Myerburg RJ, Kessler KM, Zaman L, Fernandez P, De Marchena E, Castellanos A. Pharmacologic approaches to management of arrhythmias in patients with cardiomyopathy and heart failure. *Am Heart J* 1987; 114:1273–1279.

2. Castellanos A, Aranda J, Befeler B, Myerburg RJ. Intraventricular reentrant tachycardias. In: Schlant RC, Hurst JW, eds. *Advances in Electrocardiography.* New York: Grune & Stratton; 1976: 131–142.

3. Myerburg RJ, Kessler KM, Bassett AL, Castellanos A. A biological approach to sudden cardiac death: Structure, function and cause. *Am J Cardiol* 1989; 63:1512–1516.

4. Breithardt G, Cain ME, El-Sherif N, Flowers NC, Hombach V, Janse M, et al. Standards for analysis of ventricular late potentials using high-resolution or signal-averaged electrocardiography: A statement by a task force committee of the European Study of Cardiology, the American Heart Association, and the American College of Cardiology. *J Am Coll Cardiol* 1991; 17:999–1006.

5. Kuchar DL, Thorburn CW, Sammel NL. Prediction of serious arrhythmic events after myocardial infarction. Signal-averaged electrocardiogram, Holter monitoring, and radionuclide ventriculography. *J Am Coll Cardiol* 1987; 9:531–538.

6. Kleiger RE, Miller JP, Bigger JT, Moss AJ. Decreased heart rate variability and its association with increased mortality after acute myocardial infarction. *Am J Cardiol* 1987; 59:256–262.

7. Huikuri HV, Valkama JO, Airaksinen KE, Seppanen T, Kessler KM, Takkunen JT, et al. Frequency domains measures of heart rate variability before the onset of nonsustained and sustained ventricular tachycardia in patients with coronary artery disease. *Circulation* 1993; 87:1220–1228.

8. La Rovere MT, Specchia G, Mortara A, Schwartz PJ. Baroreflex sensitivity, clinical correlates and cardiovascular mortality among patients with first myocardial infarction: A prospective study. *Circulation* 1988; 78:816–824.

9. La Rovere MT, Bigger JT Jr, Marcus FI, Mortara A, Camm AJ, Hohnloser SH, et al., on behalf of the ATRAMI investigators. Prognostic value of depressed baroreflex sensitivity: The ATRAMI Study. *Circulation* 1995; 92[suppl I]:I676.

10. Myerburg RJ, Kessler KM, Castellanos A. Pathophysiology of sudden cardiac death. *Pacing Clin Electrophysiol* 1991; 23:127–135.

11. Task Force of the Working Group on Arrhythmias of the European Society of Cardiology. The Sicilian gambit: A new approach to the classification of antiarrhythmic drugs based on their actions on antiarrhythmogenic mechanisms. *Circulation* 1991; 84:1831–1851.

12. Bauernfeind RA, Amat-y-Leon F, Dhingra RC, Kehoe R, Wyndham C, Rosen KM. Chronic nonparoxysmal sinus tachycardia in otherwise healthy persons. *Ann Intern Med* 1979; 91:702–710.

13. Packer DL, Bardy GH, Worley SJ, Smith MP, Cobb FR, Coleman RE, et al. Tachycardia-induced cardiomyopathy: A reversible form of left ventricular dysfunction. *Am J Cardiol* 1986; 57:563–570.

14. Lee RJ, Kalman JM, Fitzpatrick AP, Epstein LM, Fisher WG, Olgin JE, et al. Radiofrequency catheter modification of the sinus node for "inappropriate" sinus tachycardia. *Circulation* 1995; 92:2919–2928.

15. Hiss RG, Lamb LE. Electrocardiographic findings in 122,043 individuals. *Circulation* 1962; 25:947–961.

16. Echt DS, Liebson PR, Mitchell B, Peters RW, Obias-Manno D, Barker AH, et al. Mortality and morbidity in patients receiving encainide, flecainide, or placebo. The Cardiac Arrhythmia Suppression Trial. *N Engl J Med* 1991; 324:781–788.

17. Akhtar M, Breithardt G, Camm AJ, Coumel P, Janse MJ, Lazzara R, et al. CAST and beyond: Implications of the Cardiac Arrhythmia Suppression Trial. *Circulation* 1990; 81:1123–1127.

18. DiMarco JP, Sellers TD, Lerman BB, Greenberg ML, Berne RM, Belardinelli L. Diagnostic and therapeutic use of adenosine in patients with supraventricular tachyarrhythmias. *J Am Coll Cardiol* 1985; 6:417–425.

19. Rinkenberger RL, Prystowsky EN, Heger JJ, Troup PJ, Jackman WM, Zipes DP. Effects of intravenous and chronic oral verapamil administration in patients with supraventricular tachyarrhythmias. *Circulation* 1980; 62:996–1010.

20. Waxman HL, Myerburg RJ, Appel R, Sung RJ. Verapamil for control of ventricular rate in paroxysmal supraventricular tachycardia and atrial fibrillation or flutter: A double-blind randomized cross-over study. *Ann Intern Med* 1981; 94:16.

21. Stewart RB, Bardy GH, Greene LH. Wide complex tachycardia: Misdiagnosis and outcome after emergent therapy. *Ann Intern Med* 1986; 104:766–771.

22. Rozanski JJ, Zaman L, Castellanos A. Electrophysiologic effects of diltiazem hydrochloride in supraventricular tachycardia. *Am J Cardiol* 1982; 49:621–628.

23. Betriu A, Chaitman BR, Bourassa MG, Brevers G, Scholl J, Bruneau P, et al. Beneficial effect of intravenous diltiazem in the acute management of paroxysmal supraventricular tachyarrhythmias. *Circulation* 1983; 67:88–94.

24. Wu D, Denes P, Dhingra R, Khan A, Rosen KM. The effects of propranolol on induction of A-V nodal reentrant paroxysmal tachycardia. *Circulation* 1974; 50:665–677.

25. Wu D, Hung JS, Kuo CT, Hsu KS, Shieh WB. Effects of quinidine on atrioventricular nodal reentrant paroxysmal tachycardia. *Circulation* 1981; 64:823–831.

26. Batchelder J, Zipes DP. Treatment of tachyarrhythmias by pacing. *Arch Intern Med* 1975; 135:1115–1124.

27. Bauernfeind RA, Wyndham CR, Dhingra RC, Swiryn SP, Palileo E, Strasberg B, et al. Serial electrophysiologic testing of multiple drugs in patients with atrioventricular nodal reentrant paroxysmal tachycardia. *Circulation* 1980; 62:1341–1349.

28. Gallagher J, Svenson R, Kasell J, German L, Bardy G, Broughton A, et al. Catheter technique for closed-chest ablation of the atrioventricular conduction system: A therapeutic alternative for treatment of refractory supraventricular tachycardia. *N Engl J Med* 1982; 306:194–200.

29. Lee MA, Morady F, Kadish A, Schamp DJ, Chin MC, Scheinman MM, et al. Catheter modification of the atrioventricular junction with radiofrequency energy for control of atrioventricular nodal reentry tachycardia. *Circulation* 1991; 83:827–835.

30. Calkins H, Sousa J, El-Atassi R, Rosenheck S, deBuitleir M, Kou WH, et al. Diagnosis and cure of the Wolff-Parkinson-White syndrome or paroxysmal supraventricular tachycardias during a single electrophysiologic test. *N Engl J Med* 1991; 324:1612–1618.

31. Ross DL, Johnson DC, Denniss AR, Cooper MJ, Richards DA, Uther JB. Curative surgery for atrioventricular junctional ("A-V nodal") reentrant tachycardia. *J Am Coll Cardiol* 1985; 6:1383–1392.

32. den Dulk K, Bertholet M, Brugada P, Bar FW, Richards D, Dennoulin JC, et al. Clinical experience with implantable devices for control of tachyarrhythmias. *Pacing Clin Electrophysiol* 1984; 7:548–556.

33. Sung RJ, Castellanos A, Gelband H, Myerburg RJ. Mechanisms of reciprocating tachycardia initiated during sinus rhythm in concealed Wolff-Parkinson-White syndrome. *Circulation* 1976; 54:338–344.

34. Klein GT, Yee R, Sharma AD. Longitudinal electrophysiologic assessment of asymptomatic patients with the Wolff-Parkinson-White electrocardiographic pattern. *N Engl J Med* 1989; 320:1229–1233.

35. Wellens HJJ. Wolff-Parkinson-White syndrome: I. Diagnosis, arrhythmias and identification of the high risk patient. *Mod Concepts Cardiovasc Dis* 1983; 52:53–56.

36. Vidaillet HJ Jr, Pressley JC, Henke E, Harrell FE Jr, German LD. Familial occurrence of accessory A-V pathways (preexcitation syndrome). *N Engl J Med* 1987; 317:65–69.

37. Sung RJ, Castellanos A, Mallon SM, Bloom MG, Gelband H, Myerburg RJ. Mechanisms of spontaneous alteration between reciprocating tachycardia and atrial flutter-fibrillation in the Wolff-Parkinson-White syndrome. *Circulation* 1977; 56:409–415.

38. Gulamhusein S, Ko P, Carruthers SG, Klein GJ. Acceleration of the ventricular response during atrial fibrillation in the Wolff-Parkinson-White syndrome after verapamil. *Circulation* 1982; 65:348–354.

39. McGovern B, Garan H, Ruskin JN. Precipitation of cardiac arrest by verapamil in patients with Wolff-Parkinson-White syndrome. *Ann Intern Med* 1986; 104:791–794.

40. Akhtar M, Gilbert CJ, Shenasa M. Effect of lidocaine on atrioventricular response via the accessory pathway in patients with Wolff-Parkinson-White syndrome. *Circulation* 1981; 63:435–441.

41. Wellens HJJ, Durrer D. Effect of digitalis on atrioventricular conduction and circus movement tachycardias in patients with Wolff-Parkinson-White syndrome. *Circulation* 1973; 47:1229–1233.

42. Sellers TD, Bashore TM, Gallagher JJ. Digitalis in the preexcitation syndrome: Analysis during atrial fibrillation. *Circulation* 1977; 56:260–267.

43. Jackman WM, Wang X, Friday KJ, Roman CA, Moulton KR, Beckman KJ, et al. Catheter ablation of accessory atrioventricular pathways (Wolff-Parkinson-White syndrome) by radiofrequency current. *N Engl J Med* 1991; 324:1605–1611.

44. Guiraudon GM, Guiraudon CM, Klein GJ, Yee R, Thakur RK. Operation for the Wolff-Parkinson-White syndrome in the catheter ablation era. *Ann Thorac Surg* 1994; 57:1084–1088.

45. Wellens HJJ, Brugada P. Value of programmed stimulation of the heart in patients with the Wolff-Parkinson-White syndrome. In: Josephson ME, Wellens HJJ, eds. *Tachycardias: Mechanisms, Diagnosis, Treatment.* Philadelphia: Lea & Febiger; 1984: 199–221.

46. Prystowsky EN. Indications for intracardiac electrophysiologic studies in patients with supraventricular tachycardia. *Circulation* 1987; 75(suppl III):III119–III122.

47. Klein GJ, Bashore TM, Sellers TD, Pritchett ELC, Smith WM, Gallagher JJ. Ventricular fibrillation in the Wolff-Parkinson-White syndrome. *N Engl J Med* 1979; 301:1080–1085.

48. Castellanos A, Myerburg RJ. Changing perspectives in the preexcitation syndromes. *N Engl J Med* 1987; 317:109–111.

49. Scheinman MM. Catheter ablation for patients with ventricular preexcitation syndromes. In: Benditt DG, Benson DW, eds. *Cardiac Preexcitation Syndromes.* Boston: Martinus Nijhoff; 1986:493–506.

50. Cox JL, Cain ME. Surgery for preexcitation syndromes. In: Benditt DG, Benson DW, eds. *Cardiac Preexcitation Syndromes.* Boston: Martinus Nijhoff; 1986:527–534.

51. Guiraudon GM, Klein GJ, Sharma AD, Jones DL, McLellan DG. Surgery for Wolff-Parkinson-White syndrome: Further experience with an epicardial approach. *Circulation* 1986; 74:525–529.

52. Camm J, Hellestrand KJ, Nathan AW, Bexton RS. Clinical usefulness of flecainide acetate in the treatment of paroxysmal supraventricular arrhythmias. *Drugs* 1985; 29:713.

53. Prystowsky EN, Klein G, Rinkenberger RL, Heger JJ, Naccarelli GV, Zipes DP. Clinical efficacy and electrophysiologic effects of encainide

in patients with Wolff-Parkinson-White syndrome. *Circulation* 1984; 69:278–287.

54. Fogoros RN, Anderson KP, Winkle RA, Swerdlow CD, Mason JW. Amiodarone: Clinical efficacy and toxicity in 96 patients with recurrent drug refractory arrhythmias. *Circulation* 1983; 68:88–94.

55. Breithardt G, Borggrefe M, Wiebringhaus E, Seipel L. Effect of propafenone in the Wolff-Parkinson-White syndrome: Electrophysiologic findings and long term follow-up. *Am J Cardiol* 1984; 54:29D–39D.

56. Pritchett EL, DaTorre SD, Platt ML, McCarville SE, Hougham AJ. Flecainide acetate treatment of paroxysmal supraventricular tachycardia and paroxysmal atrial fibrillation: Dose-response studies. *J Am Coll Cardiol* 1991; 17:297–303.

57. Neuss H, Schlepper M, Thormann J. Analysis of reentry mechanisms in the three patients with concealed Wolff-Parkinson-White syndrome. *Circulation* 1975; 51:75–81.

58. Wu D, Amat-y-Leon F, Denes P, Dhingra RC, Pietras RJ, Rosen KM. Demonstration of sustained sinus and atrial reentry as a mechanism of paroxysmal supraventricular tachycardia. *Circulation* 1975; 51:234–243.

59. Wu D, Denes P, Amat-y-Leon, Dhingra RC, Wyndham CRC, Bauernfeind R, et al. Clinical electrocardiographic and electrophysiologic observations in patients with paroxysmal supraventricular tachycardia. *Am J Cardiol* 1978; 41:1045–1051.

60. Coumel P, Flammang D, Attuel P, Leclercq JF. Sustained intra-atrial reentrant tachycardia: Electrophysiologic study of 20 cases. *Clin Cardiol* 1979; 2:167–178.

61. Gallagher JJ, Smith WM, Kassell JH, Benson DW, Sterba R, Grant RO. Role of Mahaim fibers in cardiac arrhythmias in man. *Circulation* 1981; 64:176–189.

62. Cox JL. The status of surgery for cardiac arrhythmias. *Circulation* 1985; 71:413–417.

63. Allessie MA, Bonke FIM, Schopman FJG. Circus movement in rabbit atrial muscle as a mechanism of tachycardia. III. The "leading circle" concept: A new model of circus movement in cardiac tissue without the involvement of an anatomical obstacle. *Circ Res* 1977; 41:9–18.

64. Gelband H, Bush HL, Rosen MR, Myerburg RJ, Hoffman BF. Electrophysiologic properties of isolated preparations of human atrial myocardium. *Circ Res* 1972; 30:290–300.

65. Mary-Rabine L, Hordof AJ, Danilo P Jr, Malm JR, Rosen MR. Mechanisms for impulse initiation in isolated human atrial fibers. *Circ Res* 1980; 47:267–277.

66. Josephson ME, Spear JF, Harken AH, Horowitz LN, Dorio RJ. Surgical excision of automatic atrial tachycardia: Anatomic and electrophysiologic correlates. *Am Heart J* 1982; 104:1076–1085.

67. Shine KI, Kastor JA, Yurchak PM. Multifocal atrial tachycardia. Clinical and electrocardiographic features in 32 patients. *N Engl J Med* 1968; 279:344–349.

68. Salerno DM, Anderson B, Sharkey PJ, Iber C. Intravenous verapamil for treatment of multifocal atrial tachycardia with and without calcium pretreatment. *Ann Intern Med* 1987; 107:623–628.

69. Wang K, Goldfarb JL, Gobel F, Richman HG. Multifocal atrial tachycardia. *Arch Intern Med* 1977; 137:161–164.

70. Fosmoe RJ, Averill KH, Lamb LE. Electrocardiographic findings in 67,375 asymptomatic subjects. II: Supraventricular arrhythmias. *Am J Cardiol* 1960; 6:84–95.

71. Garson A, Bink-Boelkens M, Hesslein PS, Hordof AJ, Keane JF, Neches WH, et al. Atrial flutter in the young: A collaborative study of 380 cases. *J Am Coll Cardiol* 1985; 6:871–878.

72. Waldo AL, Henthorn RW, Plumb VJ. Atrial flutter: Recent observations in man: In: Josephson ME, Wellens HJJ, eds. *Tachycardias: Mechanisms, Diagnosis, Treatment.* Philadelphia: Lea & Febiger; 1982:113–135.

73. Slama R, Leclercq JF, Rosengarten M, Coumel PH, Bouvrain Y. Multilevel block in the atrioventricular node during atrial tachycardia and flutter alternating with Wenckebach phenomenon. *Br Heart J* 1979; 42:463–470.

74. Robertson CE, Miller HC. Extreme tachycardia complicating the use of disopyramide in atrial flutter. *Br Heart J* 1980; 44:602–603.

75. Waldo AL, MacLean WH, Karp RP, Kouchoukos NT, James TN. Entrainment and interruption of atrial flutter with atrial pacing. Studies in man following open heart surgery. *Circulation* 1977; 56:737–745.

76. Camm J, Ward D, Spurrell R. Response of atrial flutter to overdrive atrial pacing and intravenous disopyramide phosphate, singly and in combination. *Br Heart J* 1980; 44:240–247.

77. Touboul P, Saoudi N, Georges A, Kirkorian G. Electrophysiological basis of catheter ablation in atrial flutter. *Am J Cardiol* 1989; 64:79J–82J.

78. Waldo AL, Touboul P, eds. *Atrial Flutter: Advances in Mechanisms and Management.* Armonk, NY: Futura Publishing; 1996.

79. Ellenbogen KA, Stambler BS, Wood MA, Sager PT, Wesley RC Jr, Meissner MD, et al., for the Ibutelide Investigators. Efficacy of intravenous ibutelide for rapid termination of atrial fibrillation and atrial flutter: A dose-response study. *J Am Coll Cardiol* 1996; 28:130–136.

80. Benditt DG, Pritchett EL, Gallagher JJ. Spectrum of regular tachycardias with wide QRS complexes in patients with accessory atrioventricular pathways. *Am J Cardiol* 1978; 42:828–838.

81. Waldo AL. Atrial flutter: Mechanisms, clinical features, and management. In: Zipes DP, Jalife J, eds. *Cardiac Electrophysiology: From Cell to Bedside,* 2d ed. Philadelphia: Saunders; 1995:666–681.

82. Cairns JA, Connolly ST. Nonrheumatic atrial fibrillation: Risk of stroke and role of antithrombotic therapy. *Circulation* 1991; 84:469–481.

83. Shrier A, Dubarsky H, Rosengarten M, Guevara MR, Nattal S, Glass L. Prediction of complex atrioventricular conduction rhythms in humans with use of the atrioventricular nodal recovery curve. *Circulation* 1987; 76:1196–1205.

84. Gouaux JL, Ashman R. Auricular fibrillation with aberration simulating ventricular paroxysmal tachycardia. *Am Heart J* 1947; 34:366–373.

85. Marriott HJL, Sandler LA. Criteria, old and new, for differentiating between ectopic ventricular beats and aberrant ventricular conduction in the presence of atrial fibrillation. *Prog Cardiovasc Dis* 1966; 9:18–28.

86. Kopecky SL, Gersh BJ, McGoon MD, Whisnant JP, Holmes DR, Ilstrup DM, et al. The natural history of lone atrial fibrillation: A population-based study over three decades. *N Engl J Med* 1987; 317:669–674.

87. Gajewski J, Singer RB. Mortality in an insured population with atrial fibrillation. *JAMA* 1981; 245:1540–1544.

88. Morris JM, Peter RH, Mcintosh HD. Electrical conversion of atrial fibrillation: Immediate and long-term results and selection of patients. *Ann Intern Med* 1966; 65:216–231.

89. Mancini GBJ, Goldberger AL. Cardioversion of atrial fibrillation: Consideration of embolization, anticoagulation, prophylactic pacemaker and long-term success. *Am Heart J* 1982; 104:617–621.

90. Van Gelder IC, Crijns HJ, Van Gilst WH, Verwer R, Lie KI. Prediction of uneventful cardioversion and maintenance of sinus rhythm from direct-current electrical cardioversion of chronic atrial fibrillation and flutter. *Am J Cardiol* 1991; 68:41–46.

91. Fenster PE, Comess KA, Marsh R, Katenberg C, Hager WD. Conversion of atrial fibrillation to sinus rhythm by acute intravenous procainamide infusion. *Am Heart J* 1983; 106:501–504.

92. Prystowsky EN, Benson DW Jr, Fuster V, Hart RG, Kay GN, Myerburg RJ, et al. Management of patients with atrial fibrillation: A statement for health care professionals from the subcommittee on electrocardiography and electrophysiology of the American Heart Association. *Circulation* 1996; 93:1262–1277.

93. Suttorp MJ, Kingma JH, Jessurun ER, Lie-A-Huen L, van Hemel NM, Lie KI. The value of class IC antiarrhythmic drugs for acute conversion of paroxysmal atrial fibrillation or flutter to sinus rhythm. *J Am Coll Cardiol* 1990; 16:1722–1727.

94. Klein HO, Kaplinsky E. Verapamil and digoxin: Their respective effects on atrial fibrillation and their interaction. *Am J Cardiol* 1982; 50:894–902.

95. Dunn M, Alexandre J, DeSilva R, Hildner F. Antithrombotic therapy in atrial fibrillation. *Chest* 1986; 89:68s–73s.

96. Wijffels MCEF, Kirchhof CJHJ, Dorland R, Allessie MA. Atrial fibrillation begets atrial fibrillation: A study in awake chronically instrumented goats. *Circulation* 1995; 92:1954–1968.

97. Allessie MA, Konings K, Kirchhof CJHJ, Wijffels M. Electrophysiologic mechanisms of perpetuation of atrial fibrillation. *Am J Cardiol* 1996; 77:10A–23A.

98. Takahashi N, Seki A, Imataka K, Fuji J. Clinical features of paroxysmal atrial fibrillation: An observation of 94 patients. *Jpn Heart J* 1981; 22:143–149.

99. Berns E, Rinkenberger RL, Jeang MK, Dougherty AH, Jenkins M, Naccarelli GV. Efficacy and safety of flecainide acetate for atrial tachycardia or fibrillation. *Am J Cardiol* 1987; 59:1337–1341.

100. Morady E, Calkins H, Langberg JJ, Armstrong WF, de Buitleir M, El-Atassi R, et al. A prospective randomized comparison of direct

current and radiofrequency ablation of the atrioventricular junction. *J Am Coll Cardiol* 1993; 21:102–109.

101. Leitch JM, Klein G, Yee R, Guiraudon G. Sinus node-atrioventricular node isolation: Long-term results with the "corridor" operation for atrial fibrillation. *J Am Coll Cardiol* 1991; 17:970–975.

102. Cox JL, Boineau JP, Schuessler RB, Ferguson TB Jr, Cain ME, Lindsay BD, et al. Successful surgical treatment of atrial fibrillation: Review and clinical update. *JAMA* 1991; 266:1976–1980.

103. Hillsley RE, Wharton JM. Implantable atrial defibrillator. *J Cardiovasc Electrophysiol* 1995; 6:634–648.

104. Swartz JF, Pellersels G, Silvers J, Patten L, Cervantez D. A catheter-based curative approach to atrial fibrillation in humans (abstr). *Circulation* 1994; 90(suppl I):I-335.

105. Olshansky B, Waldo AL. Atrial fibrillation: Update on mechanism, diagnosis, and management. *Mod Concepts Cardiovasc Dis* 1987; 56:23–27.

106. Wolf PA, Dawber TR, Thomas HE. Epidemiologic assessment of chronic atrial fibrillation and risk of stroke: The Framingham study. *Neurology* 1978; 28:973–977.

107. Wolf PA, Kannel WB, McGee DL, Meeks SL, Bharucha NE, McNamara PM. Duration of atrial fibrillation and imminence of stroke: The Framingham study. *Stroke* 1983; 14:664–667.

108. Kannel WB, Abbott RD, Savage DD, McNamara PM. Epidemiologic features of chronic atrial fibrillation. *N Engl J Med* 1982; 306:1018–1022.

109. Staffurth JS, Gibberd MC. Arterial embolism in thyrotoxicosis with atrial fibrillation. *Br Med J* 1977; 2:688–690.

110. Brand FN, Abbott RD, Kannel WB, Wolf PA. Characteristics and prognosis of lone atrial fibrillation. *JAMA* 1985; 254:3449–3453.

111. Wolf PA, Abbott RD, Kannel WB. Atrial fibrillation: A major contributor to stroke in the elderly: The Framingham study. *Arch Intern Med* 1987; 147:1561–1564.

112. Lown B. Electrical reversion of cardiac arrhythmias. *Br Heart J* 1967; 29:469–489.

113. Resenkov L, McDonald L. Complications in 220 patients with cardiac dysrhythmias treated by phased direct current shock and indications for electrocardioversion. *Br Heart J* 1967; 29:926–936.

114. Bjerkelund CJ, Orning OM. The efficacy of anticoagulant therapy in preventing embolism related to DC electrical conversion of atrial fibrillation. *Am J Cardiol* 1969; 23:208–216.

115. Stroke Prevention in Atrial Fibrillation Investigators. Stroke prevention in atrial fibrillation study: Final results. *Circulation* 1991; 84:527–539.

116. Connolly SJ, Laupacis A, Gent M, Roberts RS, Cairns JA, Joyner C, for the CAFA Study Co-investigators. Canadian atrial fibrillation anticoagulation (CAFA) study. *J Am Coll Cardiol* 1991; 18:349–355.

117. Peterson P, Boysen G, Godtfredsen J, Andersen ED, Andersen B. Placebo-controlled, randomized trial of warfarin and aspirin for prevention of thromboembolic complications in chronic atrial fibrillation: The Copenhagen AFASAK study. *Lancet* 1989; 1:175–179.

118. Boston Area Anticoagulation Trial in Atrial Fibrillation Investigators. The effect of low-dose warfarin on the risk of stroke in patients with non-rheumatic atrial fibrillation. *N Engl J Med* 1990; 323:1505–1511.

119. Stroke Prevention in Atrial Fibrillation Investigators. Adjusted-dose warfarin versus low-intensity, fixed-dose warfarin plus aspirin for high-risk patients with atrial fibrillation: Stroke Prevention and Atrial Fibrillation III randomized clinical trial. *Lancet* 1996; 348:633–638.

120. Forfar JC. A 7-year analysis of haemorrhage in patients on long-term anticoagulant treatment. *Br Heart J* 1979; 42:128–132.

121. European Atrial Fibrillation Trial Study Group. Optimal oral anticoagulant therapy in patients with nonrheumatic atrial fibrillation and recent cerebral ischemia. *N Engl J Med* 1995; 33:5–10.

122. Whisnant JP, Cartlidge NEF, Elveback LR. Carotid and vertibral-basilar transient ischemic attacks: Effect of anticoagulants, hypertension, and cardiac disorders on survival and stroke occurrence—a population study. *Ann Neurol* 1978; 3:107–115.

123. Hoffman BF, Rosen MR. Cellular mechanisms for cardiac arrhythmias. *Circ Res* 1981; 43:115.

124. Friedman PL, Stewart JR, Wit AL. Spontaneous and induced cardiac arrhythmias in subendocardial Purkinje fibers surviving extensive myocardial infarction in dogs. *Circ Res* 1973; 33:612–626.

125. Rosen MR, Fisch C, Hoffman BF, Danilo P Jr, Lovelace DE, Knoebel SB. Can accelerated atrioventricular junctional escape rhythms be explained by delayed afterdepolarizations? *Am J Cardiol* 1980; 45:1272–1284.

126. Sclarowsky S, Strasberg B, Fuchs J, Lewin RF, Arditi A, Klainman E, et al. Multiform accelerated idioventricular rhythm in acute myocardial infarction: Electrocardiographic characteristics and response to verapamil. *Am J Cardiol* 1983; 52:43–47.

127. deSoyza N, Bissett JK, Kane JJ, Murphy ML, Doherthy JE. Association of accelerated idioventricular rhythm and paroxysmal ventricular tachycardia in acute myocardial infarction. *Am J Cardiol* 1974; 34:667–670.

128. Garson A, Gillette PC. Junctional ectopic tachycardia in children: Electrocardiography, electrophysiology and pharmacologic response. *Am J Cardiol* 1979; 44:298–302.

129. Gillette PC, Garson A, Porter J, Ott D, McVey P, Zinner A, et al. Junctional automatic ectopic tachycardia: New proposed treatment of transcatheter His bundle ablation. *Am Heart J* 1983; 106:619–623.

130. Green M, Heddle B, Dassen W, Wehr M, V Abdollah H, Brugada P, et al. Value of QRS alternation in determining the site of origin of narrow QRS supraventricular tachycardia. *Circulation* 1983; 68:368–373.

131. Brugada P, Bar FWHM, Vanagt EJ, Friedman PR, Wellens HJJ. Observations in patients showing A-V junctional echoes with a shorter P-R than R-P interval: Distinction between intranodal reentry and reentry using an accessory pathway with a long conduction time. *Am J Cardiol* 1981; 48:611–622.

132. Brugada P, Farre H, Green M, Heddle B, Roy D, Wellens HJJ. Observations in patients with supraventricular tachycardia having a P-R interval shorter than the R-P interval: Differentiation between atrial tachycardia and reciprocating atrioventricular tachycardia using an accessory pathway with long conduction times. *Am Heart J* 1984; 107:556–570.

133. Perry JC, McQuinn RL, Smith RT, Gothing C, Fredell P, Garson A. Flecainide acetate for resistant arrhythmias in the young: Efficacy and pharmacokinetics. *J Am Coll Cardiol* 1989; 14:185–191.

134. Velebit V, Podrid P, Lown B, Cohen BH, Graboys TB. Aggravation and provocation of ventricular arrhythmia by antiarrhythmic drugs. *Circulation* 1982; 65:886–894.

135. Ruskin JN, McGovern B, Garan H, DeMarco JP, Kelly E. Antiarrhythmic drugs: A possible cause of out-of-hospital cardiac arrest. *N Engl J Med* 1983; 309:1302–1306.

136. Myerburg RJ, Kessler KM, Prineas RJ. The cardiac arrhythmia suppression trial (letter). *N Engl J Med* 1989; 321:1754.

137. Starmer CF, Lastra AA, Nesterenko VV, Grant AO. Proarrhythmic response to sodium channel blockade: Theoretical model and numerical experiments. *Circulation* 1991; 84:1364–1377.

138. Myersburg RJ, Kessler KM, Luceri RFM, Zaman L, Trohman RG, Estes D, et al. Classification of ventricular arrhythmias based on parallel hierarchies of frequency and form. *Am J Cardiol* 1984; 54:1355–1358.

139. Moss AJ, Schnitzler R, Green R, DeCamilla J. Ventricular arrhythmias 3 weeks after acute myocardial infarction. *Ann Intern Med* 1971; 75:837–841.

140. Vismara LA, Amsterdam BA, Mason DT. Relation of ventricular arrhythmias in the late-hospital phase of acute myocardial infarction to sudden death after hospital discharge. *Am J Med* 1975; 59:6–12.

141. Ruberman W, Weinblatt E, Goldberg JD, Frank CW, Chaudhary BS, Shapiro S. Ventricular premature complexes and sudden death after myocardial infarction. *Circulation* 1981; 64:297–305.

142. Schulze RA, Strauss HW, Pitt B. Sudden death in the year following myocardial infarction: Relationship of ventricular premature contractions in the late hospital phase and left ventricular ejection fraction. *Am J Med* 1977; 62:192–199.

143. Bigger JT, Fleiss JL, Kleiger R, Miller JP, Rolnitzky LM, and the Multicenter Postinfarction Research Group. The relationships among ventricular arrhythmias, left ventricular dysfunction, and mortality in the 2 years after myocardial infarction. *Circulation* 1984; 69:250–258.

144. Bigger JT Jr. Current approaches to drug treatment of ventricular arrhythmias. *Am J Cardiol* 1987; 60:10F–20F.

145. Kessler KM, McAuliff D, Chakko S, Castellanos A, Myerburg RJ. Multiform ventricular complexes: A transitional arrhythmia form? *Am Heart J* 1989; 118:441–444.

146. Castellanos A, Luceri RM, Moleiro F, Kayden DA, Trohman RG, Zaman L, et al. Annihilation, entrainment and modulation of ventricular parasystolic rhythms. *Am J Cardiol* 1984; 54:17–322.

147. Kennedy HL, Whitlock JA, Sprague MK, Kennedy LJ, Buckingham TA, Goldberg RJ. Long-term follow-up of asymptomatic healthy subjects with frequent and complex ventricular ectopy. *N Engl J Med* 1985; 313:193–197.

148. Winkle RA. The relationship between ventricular ectopic beat frequency and heart rate. *Circulation* 1982; 66:439–446.

149. Kostis JB, McCrone K, Moreyra AE, Gotzoyannis S, Aglitz NM, Natarajan N, et al. Premature ventricular complexes in the absence of identifiable heart disease. *Circulation* 1981; 63:1351–1356.

150. Campbell RWF, Godman MG, Fiddler GI, Marquis RM, Julian DG. Ventricular arrhythmias in the syndrome of balloon deformity of mitral valve: Definition of possible high risk group. *Br Heart J* 1976; 38:1053–1057.

151. Pocock WA, Bosman CK, Chesler E, Barlow JE, Edwards JE. Sudden death in primary mitral valve prolapse. *Am Heart J* 1984; 107:378–382.

152. Nishimura RA, McGoon MD, Shub C, Miller FA, Ilstrup DM, Tajik AJ. Echocardiographically documented mitral valve prolapse: Long-term follow-up of 237 patients. *N Engl J Med* 1985; 313:1305–1309.

153. Lown B, Fakhro AM, Hood WB, Thorn GW. The coronary care unit: New perspectives and directions. *JAMA* 1967; 199:156–166.

154. El-Sherif N, Myerburg RJ, Scherlag BJ, Befeler B, Aranda JM, Castellanos A, et al. Electrocardiographic antecedents of primary ventricular fibrillation. Value of the R-on-T phenomenon in myocardial infarction. *Br Heart J* 1976; 38:415–422.

155. DeSozya N, Meacham D, Murphy ML, Kane JJ, Doherty JE, Bissett JK. Evaluation of warning arrhythmias before paroxysmal ventricular tachycardia during acute myocardial infarction in man. *Circulation* 1979; 60:814–818.

156. Wyman MG, Hammersmith L. Comprehensive treatment plan for the prevention of primary ventricular fibrillation in acute myocardial infarction. *Am J Cardiol* 1974; 33:661–667.

157. Lie KI, Wellens HJJ, Van Capelli FJ. Lidocaine in the prevention of primary ventricular fibrillation. A double-blind randomized study of 212 consecutive patients. *N Engl J Med* 1974; 291:1324–1326.

158. Routledge PA, Stargel WW, Wagner GS, Shand DG. Increased alpha-1-acid glycoprotein and lidocaine distribution in myocardial infarction. *Ann Intern Med* 1980; 293:701–704.

159. LeLorier J, Genon D, Latour Y. Pharmacokinetics of lidocaine after prolonged intravenous infusions in uncomplicated myocardial infarction. *Ann Intern Med* 1977; 87:700–702.

160. Maseri A, Severi S, Marzulio P. Role of coronary arterial spasm in sudden coronary ischemic death. *Ann NY Acad Sci* 1982; 382:204–217.

161. Tzivoni D, Keren A, Granot H, Gottlieb S, Benhorin J, Stern S. Ventricular fibrillation caused by myocardial reperfusion in Prinzmetal's angina. *Am Heart J* 1983; 105:323–325.

162. Myerburg RJ, Kessler KM, Mallon SM, Cox MM, de Marchena E, Interian A Jr, et al. Life-threatening ventricular arrhythmias in patients with silent myocardial ischemia due to coronary artery spasm. *N Engl J Med* 1992; 326:1451–1455.

163. Kimura S, Bassett AL, Saoudi NC, Cameron JS, Kozlovskis PL, Myerburg RJ. Cellular electrophysiologic changes and "arrhythmias" during experimental ischemia and reperfusion in isolated cat ventricular myocardium. *J Am Coll Cardiol* 1986; 7:833–841.

164. Furukawa T, Bassett AL, Furukawa N, Kimura S, Myerburg RJ. The ionic mechanism of reperfusion-induced early afterdepolarizations in feline left ventricular hypertrophy. *J Clin Invest* 1993; 91:1521–1531.

165. Maskin CS, Siskin SJ, LeJemtal TH. High prevalence of nonsustained ventricular tachycardia in severe congestive heart failure. *Am Heart J* 1983; 207:896–901.

166. Chakko CS, Gheorghiade M. Ventricular arrhythmias in severe heart failure: Incidence, significance, and effectiveness of antiarrhythmic therapy. *Am Heart J* 1985; 109:497–504.

167. Vignola PA, Aonuma K, Swaye PS, Rozanski JJ, Blankstein RL, Benson J, et al. Lymphocytic myocarditis presenting as unexplained ventricular arrhythmias: Diagnosis with endomyocardial biopsy and response to immunosuppression. *J Am Coll Cardiol* 1984; 4:812–819.

168. Meinertz T, Hofmann T, Kasper W, Treese N, Bechtold H, Stienen U, et al. Significance of ventricular arrhythmias in idiopathic dilated cardiomyopathy. *Am J Cardiol* 1984; 53:902–907.

169. Holmes J, Kubo SH, Cody RJ, Kligfield P. Arrhythmias in ischemic and nonischemic dilated cardiomyopathy: Prediction of mortality by ambulatory electrocardiography. *Am J Cardiol* 1985; 55:146–151.

170. The Cardiac Arrhythmia Suppression Trial II Investigators. Effect of the antiarrhythmic agent moricizine in survival after myocardial infarction. *N Engl J Med* 1992; 327:227–233.

171. Bigger JT. Methodology for clinical trials with antiarrhythmic drugs to prevent cardiac deaths: U.S. experience. *Cardiology* 1987; 74(suppl 2):40–56.

172. The Cardiac Arrhythmia Pilot Study (CAPS) Investigators. Effects of encainide, flecainide, imipramine, and moricizine on ventricular arrhythmias during the year after acute myocardial infarction: The CAPS study. *Am J Cardiol* 1988; 61:501–509.

173. Hine LK, Laird NM, Hewitt P, Chalmers TC. Meta-analysis of empirical long-term antiarrhythmic therapy after myocardial infarction. *JAMA* 1989; 262:3037–3040.

174. Julian DG, Camm AJ, Frangin G, Janse MJ, Munoz A, Schwartz PJ, Simon P, for the European Myocardial Infarct Amiodarone Trial Investigators. Radomised trial of effect of amiodarone on mortality in patients with left-ventricular dysfunction after recent myocardial infarction: EMIAT. *Lancet* 1997; 349:667–674.

175. Cairns JA, Connolly SJ, Roberts R, Gent M, the Canadian Amiodarone Myocardial Infarction Arrhythmia Trial Investigators. Randomised trial of outcome after myocardial infarction in patients with frequent or repetitive ventricular premature depolarisations: CAMIAT *Lancet* 1997; 349:675–682.

176. Beta-Blocker Heart Attack Research Group. A randomized trial of propranolol in patients with acute myocardial infarction. 1. Mortality results. *JAMA* 1982; 247:1707–1714.

177. Pederson TR and the Norwegian Multicenter Study Group. Six-year follow-up of the Norwegian multicenter study on timolol after acute myocardial infarction. *N Engl J Med* 1985; 313:1055–1058.

178. Woosley RL, Kornhauser D, Smith R, Reele S, Higgins SB, Nics RS, et al. Suppression of chronic ventricular arrhythmias with propranolol. *Circulation* 1979; 60:819–827.

179. Gomes JA, Harriman RI, Kaing P, El-Sherif N, Chowdhry I, Lyons J. Programmed electrical stimulation in patients with high-grade ventricular ectopy: Electrophysiologic findings and prognosis for survival. *Circulation* 1984; 70:43–51.

180. Moss AM, Hall WJ, Cannom DS, Daubert JP, Higgins SL, Klein H, et al, for the Multicenter Automatic Defibrillator Implantation Trial Investigators. Improved survival with an implanted defibrillator in patients with coronary disease at high risk for ventricular arrhythmia. *N Engl J Med* 1996; 335:1933–1940.

181. Gomes JA, Winters SL, Stewart D, Horowitz S, Milner M, Barreca P. A new noninvasive index to predict sustained ventricular tachycardia and sudden death in the first year after myocardial infarction: Based on signal-averaged electrocardiogram, radionucleotide ejection fraction, and Holter monitoring. *J Am Coll Cardiol* 1987; 10:349–357.

182. Bigger JT, Fleiss JL, Steinman RC, Rolintsky LM, Kleiger RS, Rottman JN. Frequency domain measures of heart period variability and mortality after myocardial infarction. *Circulation* 1992; 85:164–171.

183. Morganroth J, Anderson JL, Gentzkow CD. Classification by type of arrhythmia predicts frequency of adverse cardiac events from flecainide. *J Am Coll Cardiol* 1986; 8:607–615.

184. Webster MWI, Fitzpatrick MA, Nicholis MG, Ikram H, Wells JE. Effect of enalapril on ventricular arrhythmias in congestive heart failure. *Am J Cardiol* 1985; 56:566–569.

185. Myerburg RJ, Kessler KM, Chakko S, Cox MM, Fernandez P, Interian A Jr, et al. Future evaluation of antiarrhythmic therapy. *Am Heart J* 1994; 127:1111–1118.

186. Myerburg RJ, Kessler KM, Castellanos A. Sudden cardiac death: Epidemiology, transient risk, and intervention assessment. *Ann Intern Med* 1993; 119:1187–1197.

187. Minardo JD, Heger JJ, Miles WM, Zipes DP, Prystowsky EN. Clinical characteristics of patients with ventricular fibrillation during antiarrhythmic drug therapy. *N Engl J Med* 1988; 319:257–262.

188. Myerburg RJ, Kessler KM, Cox MM, Huikuri H, Terracall E, Interian A, et al. Reversal of proarrhythmic effects of flecainide acetate and encainide hydrochloride by propranolol. *Circulation* 1989; 80:1571–1579.

189. Anderson JL. Rationale of combination antiarrhythmic drug therapy. *Cardiovasc Clin* 1985; 16:307–327.

190. Herre JM, Sauve MJ, Malone P, Griffin JC, Helmy I, Laneberg JJ, et al. Long-term results of amiodarone therapy in patients with recurrent sustained ventricular tachycardia or ventricular fibrillation. *J Am Coll Cardiol* 1989; 13:442–449.

191. The CASCADE Investigators. Randomized antiarrhythmic drug therapy in survivors of cardiac arrest (the CASCADE Study). *Am J Cardiol* 1993; 72:280–288.

192. Singh SN, Fletcher RD, Fisher SB, Singh BN, Lewis HD, Deedwania PC, et al, for the Survival Trial of Antiarrhythmic Therapy in Congestive Heart Failure. Amiodarone in patients with congestive heart failure and asymptomatic ventricular arrhythmia. *N Engl J Med* 1995; 333:77–82.

193. Doval HC, Nul DR, Grancelli HO, Perrone SV, Bortman GR, Curiel R, for Grupo de Estudio de la Sobrevida en la Insuficiencia Cardiaca en Argentina (GESICA). Randomised trial of low-dose amiodarone in severe congestive heart failure. *Lancet* 1994; 344:493–498.

194. Myerburg RJ, Kessler KM, Kiem I, Pefkaros KC, Conde CA, Cooper D, et al. The relationship between plasma levels of procainamide, suppression of premature ventricular contractions, and prevention of recurrent ventricular tachycardia. *Circulation* 1981; 64:280–290.

195. Graboys TB, Lown B, Podrid PJ, DeSilva R. Long-term survival of patients with malignant ventricular arrhythmias treated with antiarrhythmic drugs. *Am J Cardiol* 1982; 50:437–443.

196. Morganroth J, Michelson EL, Horowitz LN, Josephson ME, Pearlman AS, Dankman WB. Limitations of routine long-term electrocardiographic monitoring to assess ventricular ectopic frequency. *Circulation* 1978; 58:408–414.

197. Vlay SC, Kallman CH, Reid RP. Prognostic assessment of survivors of ventricular tachycardia and ventricular fibrillation with ambulatory monitoring. *Am J Cardiol* 1984; 54:87–90.

198. Gallavardin L, Veil P. Deux nouveaux cas d'extrasystolic-ventriculaire avec salves tachycardiques. *Arch Mal Coeur* 1929; 22:738–741.

199. Buxton AE, Marchlinski FE, Doherty JU, Cassidy DM, Vassalo JA, Flores BT, et al. Repetitive monomorphic ventricular tachycardia: Clinical and electrophysiologic characteristics in patients with and without organ heart disease. *Am J Cardiol* 1984; 54:997–1002.

200. Coumel P, Leclercq JF, Attuel P, Rosengarten M, Milosevic D, Slama P, et al. Tachycardies ventriculaires en salves: Etude electrophysiologique et therapeutique. *Arch Mal Coeur* 1980; 73:155–164.

201. Rahilly GT, Prystowsky EN, Zipes DP, Naccerelli GV, Jackson WM, Heger JJ. Clinical and electrophysiologic findings in patients with otherwise normal electrocardiograms. *Am J Cardiol* 1982; 50:459–468.

202. Klein LS, Shih H-T, Hackett FK, Zipes DP, Miles WM. Radiofrequency catheter ablation of ventricular tachycardia in patients without structural heart disease. *Circulation* 1992; 85:1666–1674.

203. Marriott HJL. Differential diagnosis of supraventricular and ventricular tachycardia. *Cardiology* 1990; 77:209–220.

204. Wellens HJJ, Bar FRWM, Lie KI. The value of the electrocardiogram in the differential diagnosis of a tachycardia with a widened QRS complex. *Am J Med* 1978; 64:27–33.

205. Wellens HJJ, Bar FRHM, Vanagt EJDM, Brugada P. Medical treatment of ventricular tachycardia: Considerations in the selection of patients for surgical treatment. *Am J Cardiol* 1982; 49:187–193.

206. Colavita PG, Packer DL, Pressley JC, Ellenbogen KA, O'Callaghan WG, Gilbert MR, et al. Frequency, diagnoses, and clinical characteristics of patients with multiple atrioventricular pathways. *Am J Cardiol* 1987; 59:601–606.

207. Thompson PD, Melmon KL, Richardson JA, Cohn K, Cudihee R, Steinbrunn W, et al. Lidocaine pharmacokinetics in advanced heart failure, liver disease and renal failure in humans. *Ann Intern Med* 1973; 78:499–508.

208. Giardina EG, Heissenbuttel RH, Bigger JT. Intermittent intravenous procainamide to treat ventricular arrhythmias. Correlation of plasma concentration with effect on arrhythmia, electrocardiogram, and blood pressure. *Ann Intern Med* 1973; 78:183–193.

209. Holder DA, Sniderman AD, Fraser G, Fallen EL. Experience with bretylium tosylate by a hospital cardiac arrest team. *Circulation* 1977; 55:541–544.

210. Scheinman MM, Levine JH, Cannom DS, Friehling T, Kopelman HA, Chilson DA, et al. Dose-ranging study of intravenous amiodarone in patients with life-threatening ventricular tachyarrhythmias. *Circulation* 1995; 92:3264–3272.

211. Myerburg RJ, Zaman L, Luceri R, Kessler KM, Kayden D, Castellanos A. Antiarrhythmic drug therapy after myocardial infarction. In: Kulbertus HE, Wellens HJJ, eds. *The First Year after a Myocardial Infarction*. Mt. Kisco, NY: Futura: 1983; 321–339.

212. Wellens HJJ, Bar FWH, Vanagt EJDM, Brugada P. Medical treatment for ventricular tachycardia: Considerations in the selection of patients for surgical therapy. *Am J Cardiol* 1982; 49:186–193.

213. DiMarco JP, Lerman BB, Kron IL, Sellers TD. Sustained ventricular tachyarrhythmias within 2 months of acute myocardial infarction: Results of medical and surgical therapy in patients resuscitated from the initial episode. *J Am Coll Cardiol* 1985; 6:759–768.

214. Packer M. Sudden unexpected death in patients with congestive heart failure. A second frontier. *Circulation* 1985; 72:681–685.

215. Garan H, Kuchar D, Freeman C, Finkelstein D, Ruskin JN. Early assessment of the effect of map-guided transcatheter intracardiac electric shock on sustained ventricular tachycardia secondary to coronary artery disease. *Am J Cardiol* 1988; 61:1018–1023.

216. Wellens HJJ, Brugada P, Stevenson WG. Programmed electrical stimulation of the heart in patients with life-threatening ventricular arrhythmias: What is the significance of induced arrhythmias and what is the correct stimulation protocol? *Circulation* 1985; 72:1–7.

217. Swerdlow CD, Winkle RA, Mason JW. Determinant of survival in patients with ventricular tachycardias. *N Engl J Med* 1983; 308:1436–1442.

218. Interian A Jr, Zaman L, Velez-Robinson E, Kozlovskis P, Castellanos A, Myerburg RJ. Paired comparisons of efficacy of intravenous and oral procainamide in patients with inducible sustained ventricular tachyarrhythmias. *J Am Coll Cardiol* 1991; 17:1581–1586.

219. Mitrani RD, Biblo LA, Carlson M, Gatzoylas KA, Henthorn RW, Waldo AL. Multiple monomorphic ventricular tachycardia configurations predict failure of antiarrhythmic drug therapy guided by electrophysiologic study. *J Am Coll Cardiol* 1993; 22:1117–1122.

220. Wilbur DJ, Garan H, Finkelstein D, Kelly E, Newell J, McGovern B, et al. Out-of-hospital cardiac arrest: Use of electrophysiologic testing in the prediction of long-term outcome. *N Engl J Med* 1988; 318:19–24.

221. Mitchell LB, Duff HJ, Manyari DE, Wyse DG. A randomized clinical trial of the noninvasive and invasive approaches to drug therapy of ventricular tachycardia. *N Engl J Med* 1987; 317:1681–1687.

222. Waller TJ, Kay HR, Spielman SR, Kutalek SP, Greenspan AM, Horowitz LN. Reduction in sudden death and total mortality by antiarrhythmic therapy evaluated by electrophysiologic drug testing: Criteria of efficacy in patients with sustained ventricular tachycardia. *J Am Coll Cardiol* 1987; 10:83–89.

223. Rae AP, Greenspan AM, Spielman SR, Sokoloff NM, Webb CR, Kay HR, et al. Antiarrhythmic drug efficacy for ventricular tachyarrhythmias associated with coronary artery disease as assessed by electrophysiologic studies. *Am J Cardiol* 1985; 55:1494–1499.

224. Myerburg RJ, Kessler KM, Estes D, Conde CA, Luceri RM, Zaman L, et al. Long-term survival after pre-hospital cardiac arrest: Analysis of outcome during an 8-year study. *Circulation* 1984; 70:538–546.

225. Kim SG, Seiden SW, Felder SD, Waspe LE, Fisher JD. Is programmed stimulation of value in predicting the long-term success of antiarrhythmic therapy for ventricular tachycardias? *N Engl J Med* 1986; 315:356–362.

226. Kim SG. The management of patients with life-threatening ventricular tachyarrhythmias: Programmed stimulation or Holter monitoring (either or both)? *Circulation* 1987; 76:1–5.

227. The ESVEM Investigators. Determinants of predicted efficacy of antiarrhythmic drugs in the Electrophysiologic Study Versus Electrocardiographic Monitoring Trial. *Circulation* 1993; 87:323–329.

228. Mason JW, for the Electrophysiologic Study Versus Electrocardiographic Monitoring Investigators. A comparison of electrophysiologic testing with Holter monitoring to predict antiarrhythmic-drug efficacy for ventricular tachyarrhythmias. *N Engl J Med* 1993; 329:445–451.

229. Weiner I, Mindich B, Pitchon R. Determinant of ventricular tachycardia in patients with ventricular aneurysms: Results of intraoperative epicardial and endocardial mapping. *Circulation* 1982; 65:856–861.

230. Josephson ME, Harken AH, Horowitz LN. Endocardial excision. A new surgical technique for the treatment of recurrent ventricular tachycardia. *Circulation* 1979; 60:1430–1439.

231. Gallagher JJ, Anderson RW, Kasell JH, Rice JR, Pritchett ELC, Gault JH, et al. Cryoablation of drug resistant ventricular tachycardia in a patient with a variant of scleroderma. *Circulation* 1978; 57:190–197.

232. Cox JL. Ventricular tachycardia surgery: A review of the first decade and a suggested contemporary approach. *Semin Thorac Cardiovasc Surg* 1989; 1:97–103.

233. Condini MA, Sommerfeldt I, Eybel CE, DeLaria GA, Messer JV. Efficacy of coronary bypass grafting in exercise-induced ventricular tachycardia. *J Thorac Cardiovasc Surg* 1981; 81:502–506.

234. Fontaine G, Lechat PH, Cansell A, Guiraudon G, Linares-Cruz E, Koulibal M, et al. Advances in the treatment of cardiac arrhythmias in the last decade: Definition and role of ablative techniques. In: Fontaine G, Scheinman MM, eds. *Ablation in Cardiac Arrhythmias*. Mt. Kisco, NY: Futura; 1987:5–20.

235. Stevenson WG. Ventricular tachycardia after myocardial infarction: From arrhythmia surgery to catheter ablation. *J Cardiovasc Electrophysiol* 1995; 6:942–950.

236. Kleman JM, Castle LW, Kidwell GA, Maloney JD, Morant VA, Trohman RG, et al. Non-thoracotomy-versus-thoracotomy-implantable defibrillators: Intentions-to-treat comparison of clinical outcomes. *Circulation* 1994; 90:2833–2842.

237. Platia EV, Griffith LSC, Watkins L, Mower MM, Guarnieri T, Mirowski M, et al. Treatment of malignant ventricular arrhythmias with endocardial resection and implantation of the automatic cardioverter-defibrillator. *N Engl J Med* 1986; 314:213–216.

238. Mirowski M, Reid PR, Winkle RA, Mower MM, Watkins L, Stinson GB, et al. Mortality in patients with implanted automatic defibrillators. *Ann Intern Med* 1983; 98:585–588.

239. Echt DS, Armstrong K, Schmidt P, Oyer PE, Stinson EB, Winkle RA. Clinical experience, complications, and survival in 70 patients with the automatic implantable cardioverter/defibrillator. *Circulation* 1985; 7:289–296.

240. Poll DS, Marchinski FE, Buxton AE, Josephson ME. Usefulness of programmed stimulation in idiopathic dilated cardiomyopathy. *Am J Cardiol* 1986; 58:992–997.

241. Rae AP, Spielman SC, Kutalek SP, Kay HR, Horowitz LN. Electrophysiologic assessment of antiarrhythmic drug efficacy for ventricular tachyarrhythmias associated with dilated cardiomyopathy. *Am J Cardiol* 1987; 59:291–295.

242. Caceres J, Jazayeri M, McKinnie J, Avitall B, Denker ST, Tchou P, et al. Sustained bundle branch reentry mechanism of clinical tachycardia. *Circulation* 1989; 79:256–270.

243. Das SK, Morady F, DiCarlo L, Baerman J, Krol R, DeBultleir M, et al. Prognostic usefulness of programmed ventricular stimulation in idiopathic dilated cardiomyopathy without symptomatic ventricular arrhythmias. *Am J Cardiol* 1986; 58:998–1000.

244. Myerburg RJ, Luceri RM, Thurer R, Cooper DK, Zaman L, Interian A, et al. Time to first shock and clinical outcome in patients receiving automatic implantable cardioverter defibrillators. *J Am Coll Cardiol* 1989; 14:508–514.

245. Myerburg RJ, Estes D, Zaman L, Luceri RM, Kessler KM, Trohman RG, et al. Outcome of resuscitation from bradyarrhythmic or asystolic prehospital cardiac arrest. *J Am Coll Cardiol* 1984; 4:1118–1122.

246. Anderson KP. Sudden death, hypertension, and hypertrophy. *J Cardiovasc Pharm* 1984; 6:(suppl III):S498–S503.

247. Goodwin JF, Krikler DM. Arrhythmia as a cause of sudden death in hypertrophic cardiomyopathy. *Lancet* 1976; 2:937–940.

248. Kowey PR, Eisenberg R, Engel TR. Sustained arrhythmias in hypertrophic obstructive cardiomyopathy. *N Engl J Med* 1984; 310:1566–1569.

249. Anderson KP, Stinson EB, Derby GC, Oyer PE, Mason JW. Vulnerability of patients with obstructive hypertrophic cardiomyopathy to ventricular arrhythmia induction in the operating room. *Am J Cardiol* 1983; 51:811–816.

250. Coumel P, Rosengarten MD, Leciereq JF, Attuel P. Role of sympathetic nervous system in non-ischemic ventricular arrhythmias. *Br Heart J* 1982; 47:137–147.

251. Sung RJ, Shapiro WA, Shen EN, Morady F, Davis J. Effects of verapamil on ventricular tachycardias possibly caused by reentry, automaticity, and triggered activity. *J Clin Invest* 1983; 72:350–360.

252. Lerman BB, Belardinelli L, West A, Berne RM, DiMarco JP. Adenosine-sensitive ventricular tachycardia: Evidence suggesting cyclic AMP–mediated triggered activity. *Circulation* 1986; 74:270–280.

253. Ward DE, Nathan AW, Camm AJ. Fascicular tachycardia sensitive to calcium antagonists. *Eur Heart J* 1984; 5:896–905.

254. Ohe T, Shimomura S, Aihara N, Kamakura S, Matsuhisa M, Sato I, et al. Idiopathic sustained left ventricular tachycardia: Clinical and electrophysiologic characteristics. *Circulation* 1988; 77:560–568.

255. Marcus FI, Fontaine GH, Guiraudon G, Frank R, Laurenceau JL, Malergue C, et al. Right ventricular dysplasia; A report of 24 adult cases. *Circulation* 1982; 65:384–398.

256. Thiene G, Nava A, Corrado D, Rossi L, Pinnelli N. Right ventricular cardiomyopathy and sudden death in young people. *N Engl J Med* 1988; 318:129–133.

257. Guiraudon GM, Klein GJ, Guiamhusein SS, Painvin GA, DelCampo C, Gonzales JC, et al. Total disconnection of the right ventricular free wall: Surgical treatment of right ventricular tachycardia associated with right ventricular dysplasia. *Circulation* 1983; 67:463–470.

258. Fitchett DH, Sugrue DD, MacArthur CG, Oakley CM. Right ventricular dilated cardiomyopathy. *Br Heart J* 1984; 51:25–29.

259. Fortaine G, Fontaliran F, Rosas Andrade F, Velasquez E, Tonet J, Jouven X, et al. The arrhythmogenic right ventricle: Dysplasia versus cardiomyopathy. *Heart Vessels* 1995; 10:227–235.

260. Dunnigan A, Pritzker MR, Benditt DG, Benson DW. Life-threatening ventricular tachycardias in late survivors of surgically corrected tetralogy of Fallot. *Br Heart J* 1984; 52:198–206.

261. Garson A, Randall DC, Gillette PC, Smith RT, Moak JP, McVey P, et al. Prevention of sudden death after repair of tetralogy of Fallot: Treatment of ventricular arrhythmias. *J Am Coll Cardiol* 1985; 6:221–227.

262. Harken AH, Horowitz LN, Josephson ME. Surgical correction of recurrent sustained ventricular tachycardia on complete repair of tetralogy of Fallot. *J Thorac Cardiovasc Surg* 1980; 80:779–781.

263. Fontaine G, Frank R, Grosgogeat Y. Torsades de pointes: Definition and management. *Mod Concepts Cardiovasc Dis* 1982; 51:103–108.

264. Leenhardt L, Glaser E, Burguera M, Nürnberg M, Maison-Blanche P, Coumel P. Short-coupled variant of torsade de pointes: A new electrocardiographic entity in the spectrum of idiopathic ventricular tachyarrhythmias. *Circulation* 1994; 89:206–215.

265. Ward OC. A new familial cardiac syndrome in children. *J Irish Med Assoc* 1964; 54:103–106.

266. Romano C. Congenital cardiac arrhythmia. *Lancet* 1965; 1:658–659.

267. Jervell A, Lange-Nielsen F. Congenital deaf mutism, functional heart disease with prolongation of the Q-T interval, and sudden death. *Am Heart J* 1957; 54:59–78.

268. Schwartz PJ, Locati EH, Moss AJ, Crampton RS, Trazzi R, Ruberti U. Left cardiac sympathetic denervation in the therapy of congenital long QT syndrome: A worldwide report. *Circulation* 1991; 84:503–511.

269. Keating MT, Atkinson D, Dunn C, Timothy K, Vincent GM, Leppert M. Linkage of a cardiac arrhythmia, the long Q-T syndrome, and the Harvey *ras*-1 gene. *Science* 1991; 252:704–706.

270. Curran ME, Splawski I, Timothy KW, Vincent GM, Green ED, Keating MT. A molecular basis for cardiac arrhythmia: HERG mutations cause long QT syndrome. *Cell* 1995; 80:795–803.

271. Wang Q, Shen J, Splawski I, Atkinson D, Li Z, Robinson JL, et al. SCN5A mutations associated with an inherited cardiac arrhythmia, long Q-T syndrome. *Cell* 1995; 80:805–811.

272. Schwartz PJ, Priori SG, Locati EH, Napolitano C, Cantù F, Towbin JA, et al. Long Q-T syndrome patients with mutations of the SCN5A and HERG genes have differential responses to Na$^+$-channel blockade and to increases in heart rate: Implications for gene-specific therapy. *Circulation* 1995; 92:3381–3386.

273. Schott JJ, Charpentier F, Peltier S, Folley P, Drouin E, Bonhour JB, et al. Mapping of a gene for long Q-T syndrome to chromosome 4q25-27. *Am J Hum Genet* 1995; 57:1114–1122.

274. Brugada P, Brugada J. Right bundle branch block, persistent ST segment elevation, and sudden cardiac death: A distinct clinical and electrocardiographic syndrome—a multicenter report. *J Am Coll Cardiol* 1992; 20:1391–1396.

275. Denes P, Gabster A, Huang SK. Clinical, electrocardiographic and follow-up observations in patients having ventricular fibrillation during Holter monitoring. *Am J Cardiol* 1981; 48:9–27.

276. Krikler DM, Curry PVL. Torsades de pointes, an atypical ventricular tachycardia. *Br Heart J* 1976; 38:117–120.

277. Smith WM, Gallagher JJ. "Les torsades de pointes": An unusual ventricular arrhythmia. *Ann Intern Med* 1980; 93:578–584.

278. Keren A, Tzivoni D, Gavish D, Levi J, Gottlieb S, Benhorin J, et al. Etiology, warning signs and therapy of torsades de pointes—a study of ten patients. *Circulation* 1981; 64:1167–1174.

279. Monahan BP, Ferguson CL, Killeavy ES, Lloyd BK, Troy J, Cantilgna LR, Jr. et al. Torsade de pointes occurring in association with terfenadine use. *JAMA* 1990; 264:2788–2790.

280. Woosley RL, Chen Y, Freiman JP, Gillis RA. Mechanism of the cardiotoxic actions of terfenadine. *JAMA* 1993; 269:1532–1536.

281. Bhandari AK, Scheinman M. The long Q-T syndrome. *Mod Concepts Cardiovasc Dis* 1985; 54:45–50.

282. Stratmann HG, Kennedy HL. Torsades de pointes associated with drugs and toxins: Recognition and management. *Am Heart J* 1987; 113:1470–1482.

283. Schwartz PJ, Locati EH, Moss AJ, Crampton RS, Trazzi R, Ruberti U. Left cardiac sympathetic denervation in the therapy of congenital long QT syndrome: A worldwide report. *Circulation* 1991; 84:503–511.

284. Packer M. Sudden unexpected death in patients with congestive heart failure. A second frontier. *Circulation* 1985; 72:681–685.

285. Luu M, Stevenson WG, Stevenson LW, Baron K, Walden J. Diverse

mechanisms of unexpected cardiac arrest in advanced heart failure. *Circulation* 1991; 80:1675–1680.

286. Cummins RO, Ornato JP, Thies WH, Pepe P. Improving survival from sudden cardiac arrest: The "chain of survival" concept. *Circulation* 1991; 83:1832–1847.

287. Creed JD, Packard JM, Lambrew CT, Lewis AJ. Defibrillation and synchronized cardioversion. In: McIntyre KM, Lewis AJ, eds. *Textbook of Advanced Cardiac Life Support*. Dallas: American Heart Association; 1983:89–96.

288. Emergency Cardiac Care Committee and Subcommittees, American Heart Association. Guidelines for cardiopulmonary resuscitation and emergency cardiac care. *JAMA* 1992; 268:2172–2275.

289. Interian A, Trohman RG, Castellanos A, Cox M, Zaman L, Myerburg RJ. Spontaneous conversion of ventricular fibrillation in cardiogenic shock for acute myocardial infarction. *Am J Cardiol* 1987; 50:1200–1201.

290. Behar S, Goldbourt U, Reicher-Reiss H, Kaplinsky E, The Principal Investigators of the SPRINT Study. Prognosis of acute myocardial infarction complicated by primary ventricular fibrillation. *Am J Cardiol* 1990; 66:1208–1211.

291. Volpi A, Cavalli A, Franzosi MG, Maggioni A, Mauri F, Santoro G, et al. One-year prognosis of primary ventricular fibrillation complicating acute myocardial infarction. *Am J Cardiol* 1989; 63:1174–1178.

292. Nicod P, Gilpin E, Nicod P, Gilpin C, Dittrich H, Wright M, et al. Late clinical outcome in patients with early ventricular fibrillation after myocardial infarction. *J Am Coll Cardiol* 1988; 11:464–470.

293. Lie KI, Leim KL, Schullenberg RM, David GK, Durrer D. Early identification of patients developing late in-hospital ventricular fibrillation after discharge from the coronary care unit. *Am J Cardiol* 1978; 41:674–677.

294. Hauer RNW, Lie KI, Liem KL, Durrer D. Long-term prognosis in patients with bundle branch block complicating acute anteroseptal infarction. *Am J Cardiol* 1982; 49:1581–1585.

295. Myerburg RJ, Kessler KM, Castellanos A. Sudden cardiac death: Structure, function and time-dependence of risk. *Circulation* 1992; 85(suppl I):I2–I10.

296. Myerburg RJ, Kessler KM. Management of patients who survive cardiac arrest. *Mod Concepts Cardiovasc Dis* 1986; 55:61–66.

297. Wilber DJ, Garan H, Finkelstein D, Kelly E, Newell J, McGovern B, et al. Out-of-hospital cardiac arrest: Use of electrophysiologic testing in the prediction of long-term outcome. *N Engl J Med* 1988; 318:19–24.

298. Morady F, DiCarlo L, Winston S, Davis JC, Scheinman MM. Clinical features and prognosis of patients with out-of-hospital cardiac arrest and a normal electrophysiologic study. *J Am Coll Cardiol* 1984; 4:39–44.

299. Kunis RL, Garfein OB, Pepe AJ, Dwyer EM. Deglutition syncope and atrioventricular block selectively induced by hot food and liquid. *Am J Cardiol* 1985; 55:613.

300. Falk RH, Zoll PM, Zoll RH. Safety and efficiency of non-invasive cardiac pacing. A preliminary report. *N Engl J Med* 1983; 309:1166–1168.

301. Zoll PM, Zoll RH, Falk RH, Clinton JE, Eitel DR. External non-invasive temporary cardiac pacing: Clinical trials. *Circulation* 1985; 71:937–944.

302. Love JC, Haffajee MD, Gore MD, Alpert JS. Reversibility of hypotension and shock by atrial or atrioventricular sequential pacing in patients with right ventricular infarction. *Am Heart J* 1984; 108:5–13.

303. Weiss AT, Rod JL, Gotsman MD, Lewis BS. Hydralazine in the management of symptomatic sinus bradycardia. *Eur J Cardiol* 1981; 12:261–270.

304. Lewis BS, Rozenman Y, Mardler A, Rodeanu ME, Shefer A, Halon DA. Chronotropic effect of hydralazine and its mechanism in symptomatic sinus bradycardia. *Am J Cardiol* 1987; 59:93–96.

305. Kang PS, Gomes JA, Kelen G, El-Sherif N. Role of autonomic regulatory mechanism in sinoatrial conduction and sinus nodal automaticity in sick sinus syndrome. *Circulation* 1981; 64:832–838.

306. Yabek SM, Swensson RE, Jarmakani JM. Electrocardiographic recognition of sinus node dysfunction in children and young adults. *Circulation* 1977; 56:235–239.

307. Mackintosh AF. Sinoatrial disease in young people. *Br Heart J* 1981; 45:62–66.

308. Rasmussen V, Haunso S, Skagen K. Cerebral attacks due to excessive vagal tone in heavily trained persons. A clinical and electrophysiologic study. *Acta Med Scand* 1978; 204:401–405.

309. Bharati S, Nordenberg A, Bauernfeind R, Varghese JP, Carvalho AG, Rosen KM, et al. The anatomic substrate for the sick sinus syndrome in adolescents. *Am J Cardiol* 1980; 46:156–172.

310. DeMoulin JC, Kulbertus HE. Histopathological correlates of sinoatrial disease. *Br Heart J* 1978; 40:1384–1389.

311. Thery C, Gosselin B, Lekieffre J, Warrenbourg H. Pathology of the sinoatrial node. Correlation with electrocardiographic findings in 111 patients. *Am Heart J* 1977; 93:735–740.

312. Walter PF, Crawley IS, Dorney ER. Carotid sinus hypersensitivity and syncope. *Am J Cardiol* 1978; 42:396–403.

313. Davies AB, Stephens MR, Davies AG. Carotid sinus hypersensitivity in patients presenting with syncope. *Br Heart J* 1979; 42:583–586.

314. Madigan NP, Fiaker GC, Curtis JJ, Reid J, Mueller KJ, Murphy BS. Carotid sinus hypersensitivity: Beneficial effects of dual-chamber pacing. *Am J Cardiol* 1984; 53:1034–1040.

315. Wenger TL, Dohrmann ML, Strauss HC, Conley MJ, Wechsler AD, Wagner GS. Hypersensitive carotid sinus syndrome manifested as cough syncope. *Pacing Clin Electrophysiol* 1980; 3:332–339.

316. Sra JS, Anderson AJ, Sheikh SH, Avitall B, Tchou PJ, Troup PJ, et al. Unexplained syncope evaluated by electrophysiologic studies and head-up tilt testing. *Ann Intern Med* 1991; 114:1013–1019.

317. Sra JS, Jazayeri MR, Avitall B, Dhala A, Deshpande S, Blanck Z, et al. Comparison of cardiac pacing with drug therapy in the treatment of neurocardiogenic (vasovagal) syncope with bradycardia or asystole. *N Engl J Med* 1993; 328:1085–1090.

318. Cox MM, Pearlman BA, Mayor MR, Silberstein TA, Levin E, Pringle L, et al. Acute and long-term beta-adrenergic blockade for neurocardiogenic syncope. *J Am Coll Cardiol* 1995; 26:1293–1298.

319. Bigger JT Jr, Reiffel JA. Sick sinus syndrome. *Annu Rev Med* 1979; 30:91–118.

320. Chung EK. Sick sinus syndrome: Current views. *Mod Concepts Cardiovasc Dis* 1980; 49:61–66.

321. Crossen KJ, Cain ME. Assessment and management of sinus node dysfunction. *Mod Concepts Cardiovasc Dis* 1986; 55:43–48.

322. Narula OS. Atrioventricular conduction disturbances in patients with sinus bradycardia. *Circulation* 1971; 44:1096–1110.

323. Jordan JA, Yamaguchi L, Mandel WJ. Studies on the mechanisms of sinus node dysfunction in a sick sinus syndrome. *Circulation* 1978; 57:217–223.

324. Rosenqvist M, Vallin H, Edhag O. Clinical electrophysiologic course of sinus node diseases: Five-year follow-up study. *Am Heart J* 1985; 109:513–522.

325. Benditt DG, Benson DW, Kreitt J, Dunnigan A, Pritzker MR, Crouse L, et al. Electrophysiologic effects of theophylline in young patients with symptomatic bradyarrhythmias. *Am J Cardiol* 1983; 52:1223–1229.

326. Gomes JA, Kang PS, El-Sherif N. Effects of digitalis on the human sick sinus node after pharmacologic autonomic blockade. *Am J Cardiol* 1981; 48:783–788.

327. Dhingra RC, Amat-y-Leon F, Wyndham C, Deedwania PC, Wu; D, Denes P, et al. Clinical significance of prolonged sinoatrial conduction time. *Circulation* 1977; 55:8–15.

328. Gann D, Tolentino A, Samet P. Electrophysiologic evaluation of elderly patients with sinus bradycardia: A long-term follow-up study. *Ann Intern Med* 1979; 90:24–29.

329. Rosenqvist M, Brandt J, Schuller H. Atrial versus ventricular pacing in sinus node disease: A treatment comparison study. *Am Heart J* 1986; 111:292–297.

330. Denes P. Atrioventricular and intraventricular block. *Circulation* 1987; 75(suppl III):III19–III25.

331. Dreifus LS, Fisch C, Griffin JC, Gillette P, Mason JW, Parsonnet V. Guidelines for implantation of cardiac pacemakers and antiarrhythmic devices. *J Am Coll Cardiol* 1991; 18:1–13.

332. Zipes DP. Current topics. Second degree atrioventricular block. *Circulation* 1979; 60:465–472.

333. Zeppilli P, Feniel R, Sassara M, Pisrami MM, Casell G. Wenckebach second degree A-V block in top-ranking athletes: An old problem revisited. *Am Heart J* 1980; 100:281–294.

334. Strasberg B, Amat-y-Leon F, Dhingra RC, Palileo E, Swiryn S, Barenerfeind R, et al. Natural history of chronic second degree atrioventricular nodal block. *Circulation* 1981; 63:1043–1049.

335. Damato AN, Varghese PJH, Caracta AR, Akhtar M, Lau SH. Functional 2:1 A-V block within the His Purkinje system. Simulation of type II A-V block. *Circulation* 1973; 47:534–542.

336. Woelfel A, Simpson RJ Jr, Foster JR. Functional "type I-like" distal atrioventricular block induced by atrial pacing. *Am J Cardiol* 1984; 54:1363–1364.

337. Zipes DP, Dimarco JP, Gillette PC, Jackman WM, Myerburg RJ, Rahimtoola SH. Guidelines for clinical intracardiac electrophysiological and catheter ablation procedures: A report of the American College Cardiology/American Heart Association Task Force on Practice Guidelines (Committee on Clinical Intracardiac Electrophysiologic and Catheter Ablation Procedures), developed in collaboration with the North American Society of Pacing and Electrophysiology. *Circulation* 1995; 92:673–691.

338. Gallastregui J, Hariman RJ. Indications for intracardiac electrophysiologic studies in patients with atrioventricular and intraventricular blocks not associated with acute myocardial infarction. *Circulation* 1987; 75(suppl III):III103–III106.

339. Bhandari AK, Rahimtoola SH. Intracardiac electrophysiologic studies in patients with atrioventricular and intraventricular blocks not associated with acute myocardial infarction. Discussion. *Circulation* 1987; 75(suppl III):III107–III109.

340. Tenczer J, Littmann L, Rohia N, Fenyvesi T. The effects of overdrive pacing and lidocaine on atrioventricular junctional rhythm in man: The role of abnormal automaticity. *Circulation* 1985; 72:480–486.

341. Mond HG. The bradyarrhythmias: Current indications for permanent pacing (Part I). *Pacing Clin Electrophysiol* 1981; 4:432–442.

342. Mond GH. The bradyarrhythmias: Current indications for permanent pacing (Part II). *Pacing Clin Electrophysiol* 1981; 4:538–547.

343. Gunnar RM, Bourdillon PVD, Dixon DW, Fuster V, Karp RB, Kennedy JW, et al. ACC/AHA guidelines for the early management of patients with acute myocardial infarction. *Circulation* 1990; 82:664–707.

344. Hindman MC, Wagner GS, Jaro M. The clinical significance of bundle branch block complicating acute myocardial infarction. 2. Indications for temporary and permanent pacemaker insertion. *Circulation* 1978; 58:689–699.

345. Watson RDS, Glober DR, Page AJF, Littier WA, Davies P, DeGiovanni J, et al. The Birmingham trial of permanent pacing in patients with intraventricular conduction disorders after acute myocardial infarction. *Am Heart J* 1984; 108:496–501.

346. Kastor JA. Atrioventricular block. *N Engl J Med* 1975; 292:462–465.

347. Dhingra RC, Palileo E, Strasberg B, Swiryn S, Bauerfeind RA, Wyndham C, et al. Significance of the HV interval in 517 patients with chronic bifascicular block. *Circulation* 1982; 64:1265–1271.

348. McAnulty JH, Rahimtoola DH, Murphy ES, Kauffman S, Ritzmann LW, Kanarek P, et al. A prospective study of sudden death in high risk bundle branch block. *N Engl J Med* 1978; 299:209–215.

349. Scheinman MM, Peters RW, Modin G, Brennan M, Mies C, O'Young J. Prognostic value of infranodal conduction time in patients with chronic bundle branch block. *Circulation* 1977; 56:240–244.

350. Furman S, Fischer JD. Endless loop tachycardia in the A-V universal (DDD) pacemaker. *Pacing Clin Electrophysiol* 1982; 5:486–489.

28

LONG-TERM CONTINUOUS ELECTROCARDIOGRAPHIC RECORDING

R. Joe Noble / Douglas P. Zipes

Long-term electrocardiographic recording is a method of recording the electrocardiogram (ECG) over extended time periods; the recording is subsequently analyzed for rhythm and ST-segment and T-wave alterations.[1-3] Technological advances in the past few years have provided a diversity of recording, transmitting, and analysis systems.

INDICATIONS

Ambulatory ECG recording may be helpful in recognizing, characterizing, and, less frequently, quantitating arrhythmias in patients with symptoms potentially related to an arrhythmia; the recording of a rhythm disturbance simultaneous with a patient's symptoms may be the only means of diagnosis, particularly when the symptoms and arrhythmia are relatively infrequent. Importantly, the recording of a normal rhythm when the patient is symptomatic may prove equally valuable in excluding a rhythm disturbance as the cause for the patient's symptoms. Not only is it important to correlate an abnormal rate and rhythm with the symptom complex but, from the ambulatory record, also to determine the precise mechanism of arrhythmia. Some concept of the frequency of the arrhythmia, as demonstrated by the ambulatory record, is clinically helpful, but precise quantitation of the frequency of premature ventricular complexes, for instance, is rarely required.

Ambulatory ECG recordings are indicated in certain patients to assess risk for future cardiac events—specifically in those patients with idiopathic hypertrophic cardiomyopathy, patients who have survived myocardial infarction with substantial left ventricular dysfunction, patients with long QT intervals, those with dilated cardiomyopathy and symptoms consistent with arrhythmia, and in some patients with the Wolff-Parkinson-White syndrome.[4]

Patients who undergo treatment for complex arrhythmias, such as sustained supraventricular tachyarrhythmias or ventricular tachycardia, may benefit from ambulatory ECG recordings in order to assess the efficacy of therapy. Similarly, patients in whom pacemakers have been implanted who have symptoms consistent with pacemaker malfunction or who require evaluation of their rate-responsive physiologic pacing function may require long-term ECG recording.

Heart rate variability may be accurately measured by long-term ambulatory ECG recordings and may be helpful in patients with sleep apnea or those with coronary disease in whom further prognostic information is sought.[4]

The recording of the ECG pattern (as opposed to the rhythm) may be helpful in the detection of myocardial ischemia. Long-term ambulatory ECG recording is indicated for patients suspected of Prinzmetal's variant angina, in whom the simultaneous recording of ST-segment elevation with symptoms should confirm the diagnosis. Also, long-term recording may be of diagnostic help in patients with symptomatic angina who are unable to undergo exercise testing. Silent myocardial ischemia—i.e., ST-segment depression on the ECG in the absence of symptoms—may be detected by ambulatory monitoring. Clear indications for ambulatory recording in this setting have not as yet been established, but such recordings may be indicated for postinfarction patients with ventricular ectopy or in patients with chronic angina to establish the efficacy of their antiischemic therapy.[4]

The reader is referred to *Guidelines for Ambulatory Electrocardiography*, published jointly by the American College of Cardiology and American Heart Association, for a more complete consideration of clinical indications for ambulatory ECG recordings.[4]

RECORDING TECHNIQUES

Three general types of instruments for acquiring data are currently available: continuous recorders, intermittent or "event" recorders, and instruments for real-time recording and transmission of electrocardiograms (Table 28-1).

Continuous Recorders

The ECG can be recorded continuously on tape (either reel-to-reel or cassette) or digitally in solid-state memory. The tape recorder is a battery-powered, miniaturized device with very slow tape speed and is small enough to be suspended by a strap over the shoulder or around the waist.

All digital recording systems amplify, digitize, and store the ECG in solid-state memory. Two types of digital recorders

TABLE 28-1

TYPES OF ELECTROCARDIOGRAPHIC RECORDING INSTRUMENTS

Type	Recording	Scanning	Transmitting
"Holter"			
Analog	All ECG complexes "Full Disclosure"	Technician with computer assistance, templating, area determination and superimposition	None
Digital—continuous recording	All ECG complexes "Full Disclosure"	Technician with computer assistance, templating, area determination and superimposition	Transtelephonic
Digital—real-time analysis	Computer analysis of ECG and selected ECG printouts	Real time by microprocessor with retrospective technician editing	None
"Event Recorder"			
"Postevent," nonlooping, without memory			
Hand-held (including credit card size) wristwatch–type	ECG, selected by patient activation	Direct visualization	Transtelephonic
Automatic electronic sensor, in DDD pacemaker	ECG, when activated automatically by sensor	Direct visualization of analysis or ECG	Direct telemetry
"Pre-event," looping, with memory			
Wristwatch type monitor worn with attached electrodes	ECG, selected by patient activation, with memory of pre-event	Direct visualization	Transtelephonic
Subcutaneous, implanted digital recorder	ECG, selected by patient activation with memory of pre-event	Direct visualization	Direct telemetry
Automatic electronic sensor, in ICD or pacemaker	ECG, when activated by firing of ICD or recognized by sensor in pacemaker, with memory	Direct visualization of analysis or ECG	Direct telemetry
"Real Time"			
Real-time transtelephonic monitoring	ECG at central monitoring station—no recording at device	Direct visualization	Transtelephonic

are available. In the first, each QRS complex is recorded, similar in this sense to the continuous tape recording. Some of these recorders have been miniaturized to the size of a credit card. With the second, microcomputers and microelectronic circuits sample the cardiac rhythm in real time as it is being recorded, convert the analog signal into a digital signal, and analyze the data in terms of maximal and minimal rates, RR intervals, and change in RR intervals. Within minutes of the instrument's disconnection from the patient, the information can be retrieved in the form of a histogram covering the entire recording period and a printout of selected segments in real time can be obtained. This instrument is different from those used to make continuous tape or digital recordings in that the actual ECG has not been recorded on tape; only the histogram has been stored; however, selected brief segments of the patient's ECG, e.g., 6- to 10-s intervals, can also be stored. Microcomputers that can analyze electronic data over prolonged periods, even several days, have been developed.

Most current systems provide channels sufficient to record at least three ECG leads, which are essential to differentiate between ventricular arrhythmias and supraventricular arrhythmias with aberrancy and also to assess ST-T segments. The frequency response of current systems should conform to accepted ECG standards[5,6] and digital records should eliminate distortion of low-frequency signals; consequently, accurate ST-T configurations should generally be recorded.[7,8] Most current recorders are equipped with an event marker, consisting of a button the patient pushes to note the time of a symptom. Activation of the event recorder marks the tape or digital record so that the symptom and recording can be correlated during analysis. The patient carries a diary in which are entered any symptoms experienced during the recording period, the patient's activities, and the time at which the symptoms occurred.

The lead systems on recorders vary from one manufacturer to another. At least two leads should be simultaneously recorded, either V_1 and V_5 or bipolar limb and unipolar chest leads. Meticulous attention must be paid to placing the electrodes on the patient's chest, since poor electrode contact will produce technically inadequate recordings (Fig. 28-1).

Event Recorders

An alternative method records not continuously but only when the patient senses symptoms, or an event. Of the numerous event recorders available, there are two basic types, which are differentiated on the basis of memory.

In the *postevent recorder*, without memory, the unit may continuously monitor the ECG via attached leads. The patient wears the recorder continuously, activating it when symptoms appear; this device does not record the ECG until it is activated. Alternatively, the patient may carry a miniature solid-state recorder (sufficiently small to fit into a pocket or purse) with which the rhythm can be recorded whenever the symptoms appear, simply by placing the unit on the precordium. Some newer devices are the size of a credit card, to be carried in a wallet or worn as a necklace. The recorded data are stored in memory until the patient submits the information either directly or transtelephonically to an ECG receiver, where it is recorded. When a tape is employed, the tape is then erased, and subsequent data can be recorded and transmitted to facilitate the recording of rhythm or pattern during several symptomatic episodes. When digital acquisition devices are used, a prolonged, continuous event can be recorded and stored or the device can be programmed to acquire multiple events.

With a *preevent recorder*, employing a memory loop, the rhythm is monitored continuously via leads either at the

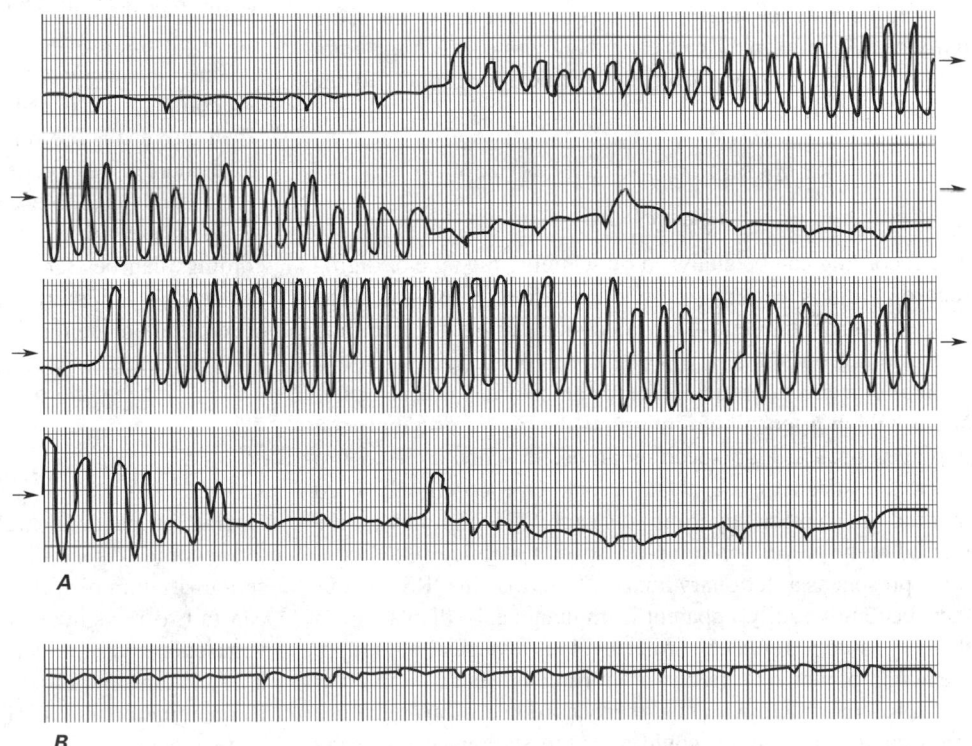

FIGURE 28-1

Artifact recorded on Holter monitor. *A*. A loose electrode was responsible for the artifactual tracing mimicking ventricular flutter-fibrillation recorded by the monitor. *B*. A simultaneous ECG confirmed continuous sinus rhythm, and the patient remained asymptomatic.

extremities or over the precordium and a recorder resembling a wristwatch or a miniaturized device worn as a necklace or on a belt. Patients activate the unit when they experience symptoms, so that an abnormal rhythm or an ECG synchronous with the symptoms can be recorded. The loop recorder is capable of recording information several seconds or minutes before or after a recognized event; the number of events that can be recorded and the allotment of recording time prior to and after activation of the unit are programmable.

A miniaturized *event recorder* has been developed, which can be implanted subcutaneously to be mechanically activated by the patient to record an ECG when the patient suffers serious symptoms (such as syncope) at widely spaced intervals.[9] Incorporating a memory loop, the preevent ECG is recorded, and the resultant recording is transmitted by telemetry to a receiver for analysis.

Event recording is also provided by some newer-generation DDD pacemakers and implantable automatic defibrillators. These instruments automatically recognize abnormal rhythms, such as tachycardia, and provide, via telemetric transmission, either actual ECG records or an analysis of the number, rate, and duration of recognized arrhythmias.

Real-Time Monitoring

As another variation, the device that acquires data can transmit the ECG information directly and transtelephonically, in real time, and without recording the data in the unit. With such a device, for instance, the patient can transmit his or her ECG daily or even multiple times each day, with or without symptoms, at some distance from the medical institution to the recording station.

SCANNING AND ANALYSIS TECHNIQUES

The recording can be analyzed by scanning the tape or digital record at high speed, by printing it out directly, or—as in the case of microcomputers—by processing during the recording and printing out the analysis at the end of sampling.

Scanning techniques include technician-dependent analysis, in which a technician interprets the cardiac rhythm as it is played back at high speed on an oscilloscope at 30 to 120 times the speed of the actual event. One commonly used method of scanning superimposes each QRS complex on the immediately preceding complex, so that identical QRS contours present as a stationary image. Variations in QRS contour then become readily apparent. Simultaneously displayed on the oscilloscope for each cardiac cycle is a vertical bar graph, the height of which is directly proportional to each RR interval and QRS morphology. Thus, the occurrence of a premature ventricular extrasystole would alter the stationary image by producing a variation in the QRS contour, alter the pitch and sound of the audio signal, and shorten the vertical bar reflecting cycle lengths. When such an abnormal event is noted, the tape can be played at a normal rate of speed for analysis on a standard ECG machine.

To minimize the human factor and provide accurate quantitative data, the tape can be analyzed by a semiautomated electronic analyzer, which quantitates the number of abnormalities it recognizes. The accuracy of the system depends on the system's ability to distinguish abnormal from normal.

A computer can be interfaced with the scanner to quantitate the data even more accurately. The playback analysis can occur at up to 240 times the normal rate. Electronic analyzers and computers, as well as the scanner, can be programmed to recognize the patient's own QRS complex template and then to recognize any deviation from the normal. The computer program can provide summaries of heart rates, heart rate variability, frequency of premature atrial or ventricular extrasystoles, coupling intervals, runs of tachycardia or other arrhythmias, and variations in QRS, ST, QT, or T pattern during any time period. Hard copies can be printed out for verification. When arrhythmias or pattern changes are detected, an automatic ECG printout can be triggered by the event marker or by the computer.

Scanning services are available and can generally provide reasonably accurate analysis at less cost than can small institutions or offices with smaller volumes of long-term ECG recordings. Recorders can be purchased, leased, or rented.

An alternative to scanning is the *direct printout* of the entire record. Prolonged ECG records are compressed to reduce the amount of paper that the physician must examine; when brief events are recorded, compression is not necessary. By directly writing out the entire ECG, the need for a trained technician and scanners may be obviated.

Since *microcomputers* assess the ECG in real time, as it is recorded, there is no need for a scanner or expert technician when the results are printed out. The physician evaluates the trend chart or any recorded rhythm strip.

As noted in Table 28-1, all of the event recordings, the real-time recording, as well as some of the continuous recordings can be transmitted transtelephonically to receivers for analysis and interpretation. Those recordings of implanted pacemakers or defibrillators are available by telemetry.

COMPARISON OF TECHNIQUES FOR PROLONGED ELECTROCARDIOGRAPHIC RECORDING

Operator-dependent, high-speed audiovisual analysis of the tape, without direct printout or electronic analysis, recognizes serious rhythm disturbances. On the other hand, the operator can fail to recognize as many as one-third to two-thirds of ventricular and supraventricular arrhythmias. Operator-dependent systems are affected by the capabilities of the operator. If quantitation is unimportant, this system of analysis is quite adequate.

Electronic analysis systems improve upon the sensitivity and specificity of interpretation of long-term ECG recordings. Computer analysis systems are said to be 90 to 95 percent accurate in quantitating ectopic complexes.[10–12] Current computer-based systems that permit operator editing are even more sensitive and accurate, but both electronic and computer analysis systems increase cost. One reason for the stated accuracy of computer interpretations is that ventricular ectopy is responsible for most broad, complex beats. Supraventricular ectopy with aberrancy or intermittent preexcitation is not accurately diagnosed by computer, but the relatively low frequency of these complexes does not statistically alter sensitivity calculations. Both electronic and computer analysis systems increase cost.

"Full disclosure"—i.e., hard-copy printout of the entire record—provides a visual analysis of the record to identify immediately complex disturbances such as ventricular tachycardia or prolonged asystolic intervals. In addition, it is often useful to have hard-copy ECG data available (as opposed to those derived from analysis of the ECG data) with which to compare subsequent records. The direct printout does not quantitate the actual number of events. Assuming care in interpretation, the direct printout may be more sensitive than high-speed, operator-dependent, and semiautomated systems with operator editing in identifying pairs or triplets of consecutive ectopic complexes.

An event recorder does not require a scanner or an experienced technician; however, the continuously recording event recorder itself is more expensive than a continuously recording tape recorder. The postevent recorder, without memory, which the patient applies only when symptoms appear, is less expensive. Both types of event recorders provide an ECG record more quickly than a system that requires scanning,[13] but neither creates a long-term record of the ECG during asymptomatic intervals. The automatic event recorders incorporated in pacemakers and implantable defibrillators are limited by the accuracy and sensitivity of the algorithm used to detect abnormalities. Any event recorder clearly allows correlation between the patient's symptoms and the rhythm. The only technique currently available to record rhythm events leading up to and following infrequently occurring symptoms is the memory-loop event recorder.

When more rapid identification of a rhythm abnormality in an outpatient is essential, as in the patient with a potentially dangerous rhythm disturbance, real-time transmitters permit frequent and even automatic transtelephonic transmission of the ambulatory record to a hospital or clinic telemetry receiver. The monitor technician can then quickly identify a serious rhythm abnormality and arrange for the patient's proper management.

Those microcomputers that analyze the rhythm in real time, simultaneous with the recording, should prove at least as accurate as other high-speed playback analysis systems. More importantly, longer periods can be monitored than are practical for other systems. The cost of the analysis is independent of the duration of recording, so that patient cost should be less for prolonged periods of monitoring. Finally, the analysis of the entire recording and the actual printout of the specific ECG segment are available within minutes of the recording. On the other hand, only limited segments of actual ECG records are generally available, and the accuracy of abnormal rhythm or pattern recognition remains dependent upon the computer algorithm; this recognition is far from perfect, since many problems in the computer analysis of complex rhythm disturbances remain unsolved.

Whichever system is employed, the ultimate accuracy of ECG interpretation depends on the technician and overreading physician; scanners and computers cannot differentiate complex patterns (supraventricular arrhythmias with aberrancy as opposed to ventricular arrhythmias or preexcitation) or even artifact. The clinical application of the data is solely the function of the responsible physician. No data-acquisition system or scanner, no computer, and no technician can substitute for the well-trained physician in determining the significance of any recorded data and their clinical utility.

Selection of Device

The ultimate selection of a long-term ECG recording system depends on individual patient needs. If a precise count of ectopy is required, a continuous recorder with computer-based analysis is essential. On the other hand, if the purpose of the recording is to detect ventricular tachycardia or asystole, an event recorder, a microcomputer, or direct printout of the entire record would be an excellent choice. Either a microcomputer or an event recorder provides an opportunity to monitor over prolonged periods of time, and either is of benefit to the patient whose rhythm disturbance occurs infrequently. When the goal is to correlate the patient's rhythm or ECG pattern with symptoms that are very infrequent (at weekly intervals or less), the patient-applied and patient-activated event recorder is the optimal choice. However, if the patient's symptoms are of such brief duration (seconds) or severity (frank syncope) to preclude capture by such a unit, then a loop event recorder is required. This and the direct printout are less expensive for an individual physician's or small clinic's use, and both are more cost-effective than prolonged ambulatory (Holter) recordings, whether indicated for assessment of palpitations[14] or such serious symptoms as syncope.[15] The implantable event recorder with memory may prove optimal for those patients with syncopal events so widely spaced (weeks or months) as to render other devices impractical.[9]

Except with large scanning services, it is impractical for an individual physician to have available all the monitoring techniques for each individual patient's needs. Hence, the physician's selection of a system is based upon his or her own patient population, the frequency of using this test, the availability of dependable scanning services, and the associated cost analysis. The physician would do well to realize that any or all of the systems described above are available alone or in combination. The more detailed and precisely quantitated the final report, generally the more expensive the equipment and personnel required. All systems recognize ventricular tachycardia or marked bradycardia and, qualitatively at least, detect ectopy. For clinical purposes, this amount of information is usually sufficient. The practicing physician does not really require precise quantitation, since the therapeutic and prognostic significance of such quantitation is not yet known. In short, technology exceeds clinical assimilation of the results at the present time.

DURATION OF RECORDING

A standard resting ECG, which records less than 1 min of cardiac rhythm, detects ventricular premature systoles in about 8 percent of patients with known coronary artery disease; this frequency doubles if the recording period is extended to 12 h.[16] A 48-h ECG recording period detects additional and more complex ventricular arrhythmias and supraventricular tachyarrhythmias; it also displays the character and frequency of rhythm disturbances during sleep as well as during awake periods.

Arrhythmias are often evanescent, occurring only rarely. In such patients, 24-h ECG recordings are unlikely to detect the abnormal rhythm. Even when arrhythmias are frequent, marked variation in the frequency and complexity of the rhythm disturbance is expected, with variations occurring during and between days. Spontaneous reduction in the frequency of ventricular ectopy of 50 to 90 percent is common.[17,18] For screening purposes, 24-h ECG tape recording seems an optimal compromise between the practical limits of recording and the point of diminishing return.[16,19,20]

If a reduction in total number of premature ventricular complexes is the goal of antiarrhythmic therapy, then more than one control 24-h ECG recording and several recordings while the patient is receiving therapy are required to prove efficacy.[19,20] The total number of premature ventricular complexes must be reduced by about 80 percent.[17,18,21] On the other hand, since it has not yet been demonstrated that reducing the total number of premature ventricular complexes necessarily implies the elimination of more dire ventricular rhythm disturbances or sudden death, this is often not the physician's goal. Instead, simply preventing sustained, symptomatic ventricular tachycardia may be the therapeutic goal,[22] in which case multiple 24-h recordings are less essential.

The ideal duration of recording varies from patient to patient, depending on the physician's goals. If the objective is to correlate the cardiac rhythm or pattern with a symptom such as syncope, palpitations, or chest pain, then the *monitoring period* must be extended sufficiently to incorporate a symptomatic period, whether these intervals occur with a frequency of hours or months. The *actual recording period*, however, may be only seconds.

RECORDINGS OF ST SEGMENTS AND T WAVES

For several reasons, both technical and physiologic, long-term ECG recording devices do not provide the same degree of reliability in the interpretation of the pattern of the ST segment and T wave as in the detection of rhythm disturbances. Technical limitations have included unsatisfactory low-frequency responses, which have precluded accurate display of the very low frequency ST segment and T waves.[7,8] Another limitation has been the use of a one-lead system. Just as a single lead on a standard ECG might not record "ischemic" ST-segment and T-wave changes during myocardial ischemia, so a single lead is inadequate for this purpose with prolonged recording. Technical improvements in more recently developed models, including the expansion of the lower-limit frequency response and the use of two leads, have enhanced the reliability of QRS-ST-T pattern interpretation with long-term recording. Despite these improvements, most manufacturers have not assured that the appropriate specifications for recording apply not only to the amplifier but also to the recorder, playback system, and printout device.[23]

Even more important than these technical considerations, however, are certain physiologic limitations. For instance, standing, hyperventilation, eating, anxiety, use of drugs, and change in heart rate are all daily events that may result in depression of the ST segment or inversion of the T wave to simulate ischemic changes. Striking ST-segment elevation has been recorded during prolonged recording in patients without organic heart disease.[24]

Despite these limitations, preliminary evaluations of the technique of prolonged ECG recording to detect ischemic heart disease have indicated in some instances (1) that patients who display ischemic ST segment–T wave changes are more likely to develop overt manifestations of ischemic heart disease subsequently than those who do not display such alterations and (2) that a similar ECG pattern during recording correlates with angiographic evidence of coronary artery disease.[25-27] The sensitivity and specificity of the technique, however, remain to be determined.

Long-term ECG recording proves superior to exercise testing in detecting angina at rest (Chap. 46) accompanied by ST-segment elevation, which cannot be reproduced with exercise (Prinzmetal's variant angina) (Fig. 28-2). Another potential use of prolonged ECG recording is to correlate symptoms that occur during normal daily activity with ECG evidence of ischemia. In this setting, the demonstration of significant ST segment–T wave alterations that cannot be reproduced by hyperventilation or change in position, particularly when reinforced by documentation in the patient's diary of simultaneous symptoms of angina, prove highly suggestive of ischemic heart disease. In still other patients, in whom exercise testing is precluded by physical disability, ambulatory recording may be helpful. Also, in patients in whom exercise testing produces negative results yet symptoms highly suggestive of myocardial ischemia continue with other specific activities, prolonged ECG recording provides useful information.

ARTIFACTS AND ERRORS

Artifacts registered during prolonged ECG recording have mimicked virtually every variety of supraventricular and ventricular bradycardia and tachycardia and have led to misdiagnosis.[28,29]

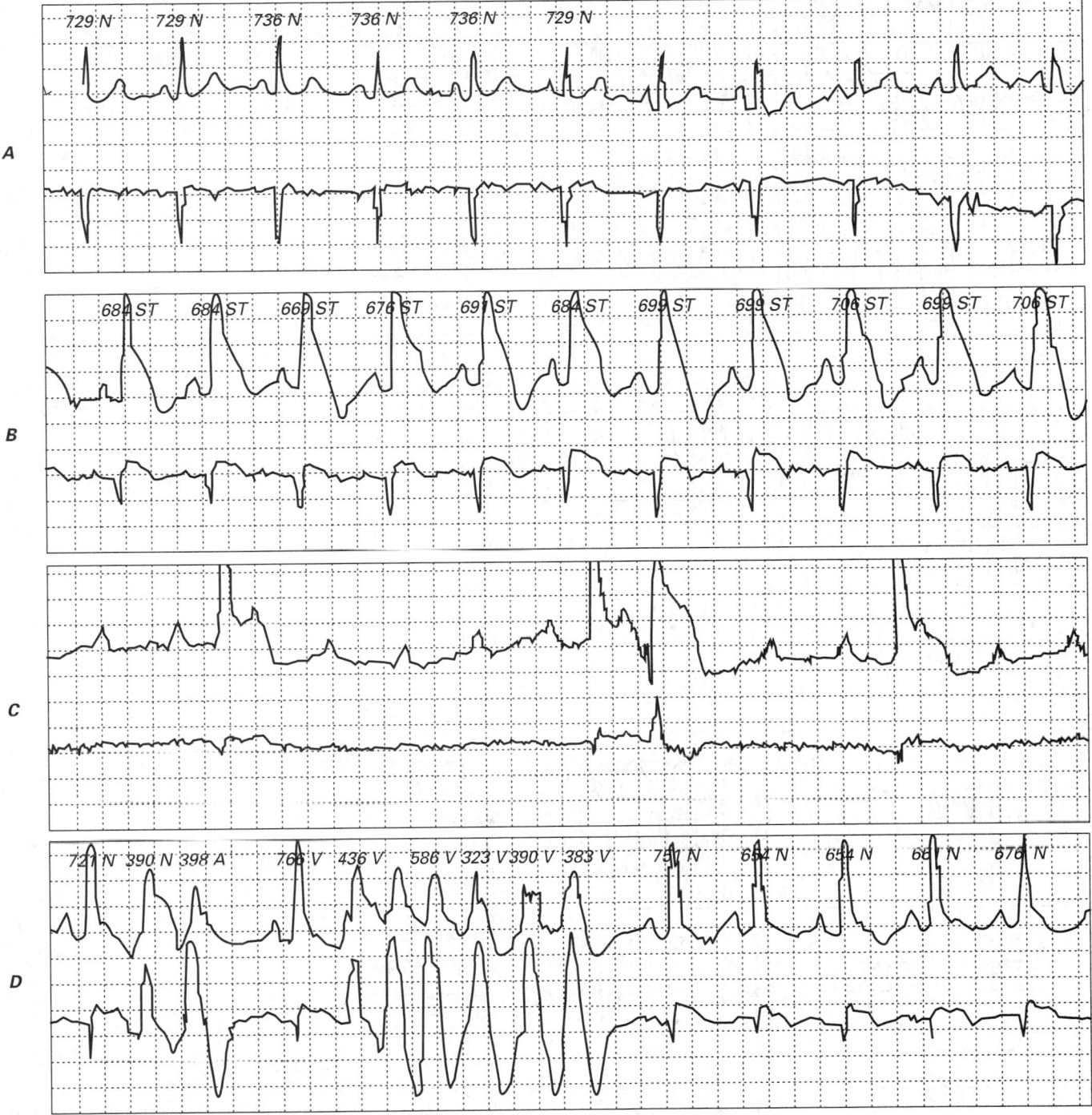

FIGURE 28-2

Ambulatory ECG recording in Prinzmetal's variant angina. *A.* Control. Lead II (*top*), precordial lead (*bottom*). *B.* Marked ST-segment elevation (resembling monophasic action potential), associated with mild angina. *C.* High-grade AV block and continued ST-segment elevation, associated with near syncope. *D.* Nonsustained ventricular tachycardia with continued ST-segment elevation associated with palpitations and light-headedness.

Most of these artifacts are identical to those plaguing the standard 12-lead ECG but are simply detected more frequently due to the length of the recording; however, many are unique to extended recording by virtue of the magnetic tape recorder.

Probably the most common artifact is that resulting from a loose electrode (Fig. 28-1) or mechanical "stimulation" of the electrode. In Fig. 28-3, ventricular tachycardia is simulated by the patient "scratching" the electrodes. Failure of either the battery or the motor of the recorder generally results in a slowing of the tape speed as the ECG is recorded. When played back, the heart rate will appear fast; i.e., it will mimic a tachycardia (Fig. 28-4). The interpreter may be alerted to the artifact by the concomitant shortening of all ECG intervals (PR, QRS, QT, and RR) and decrease in QRS voltage. Con-

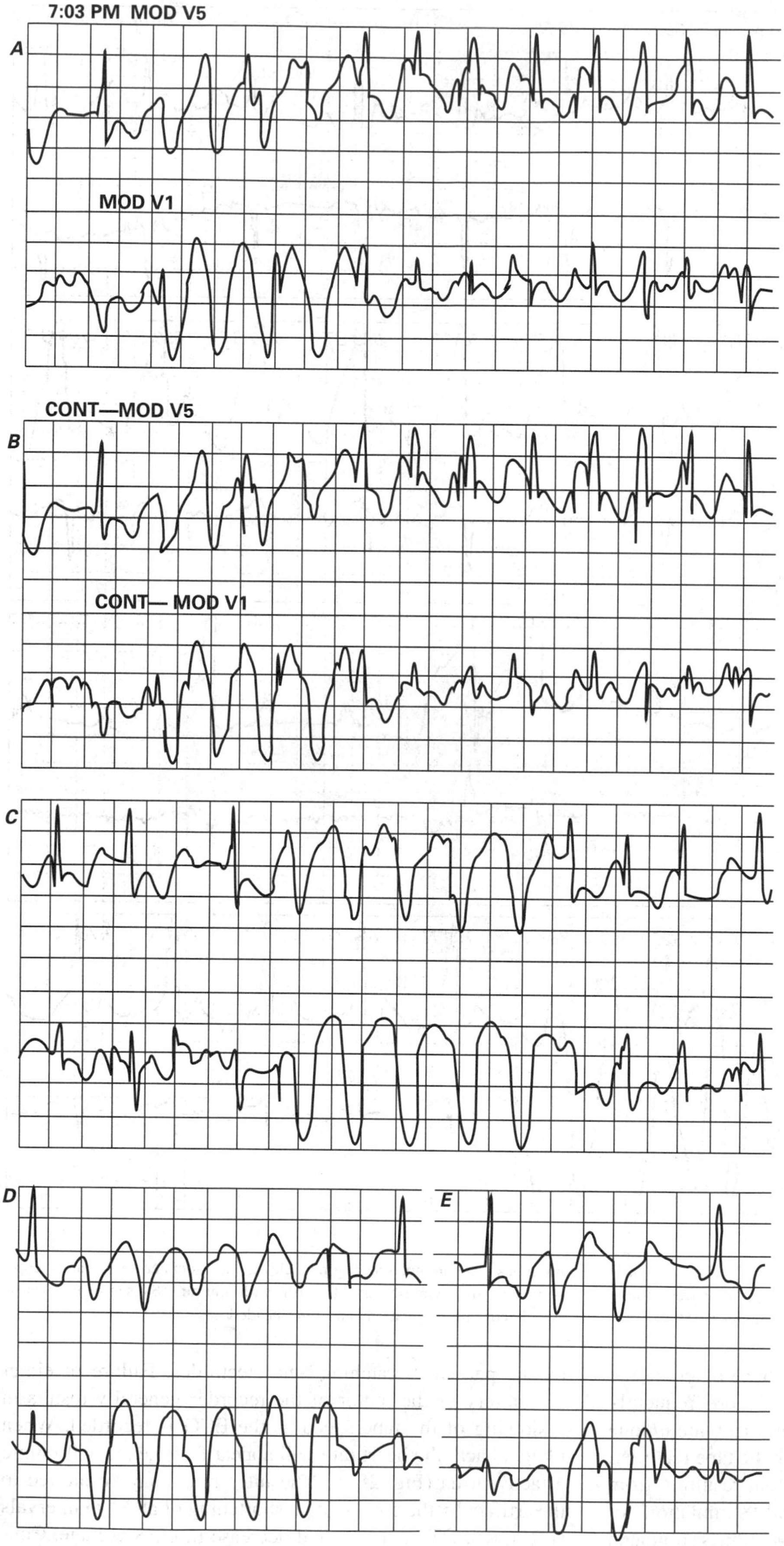

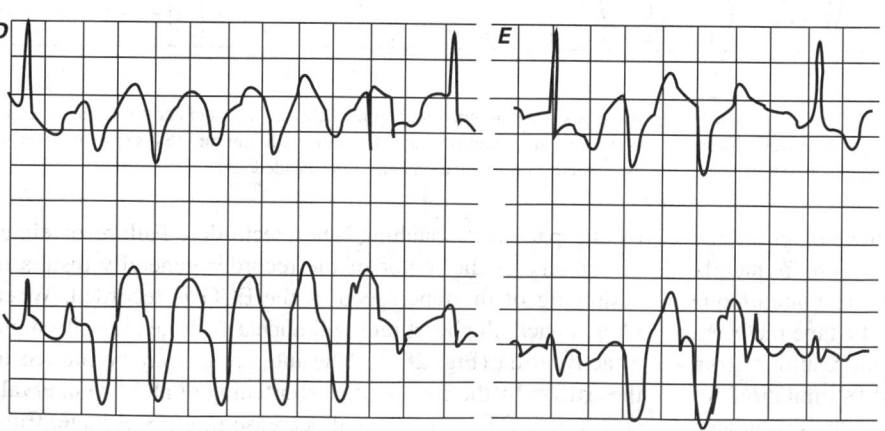

7:03 PM MOD V5

A

MOD V1

CONT—MOD V5

B

CONT— MOD V1

C

D

E

FIGURE 28-3

Mechanical stimulation of electrodes mimicking ventricular tachycardia. Regular, rapid (160 per minute) broad QRS complexes were repeatedly recorded in both leads V_1 and V_5 and interpreted as ventricular tachycardia (*A* through *D*) or pairs of premature ventricular complexes (PVCs) (*E*). Antiarrhythmic therapy was administered. However, the clue to the artifactual recording is the normal QRS "marching through" the "ventricular tachycardia" and the fact that the coupling interval between the last normal complex preceding the "tachycardia" and the first complex following it are often so short as to be unphysiologic. Intense pruritus from the electrodes elicited scratching, which explained the artifacts.

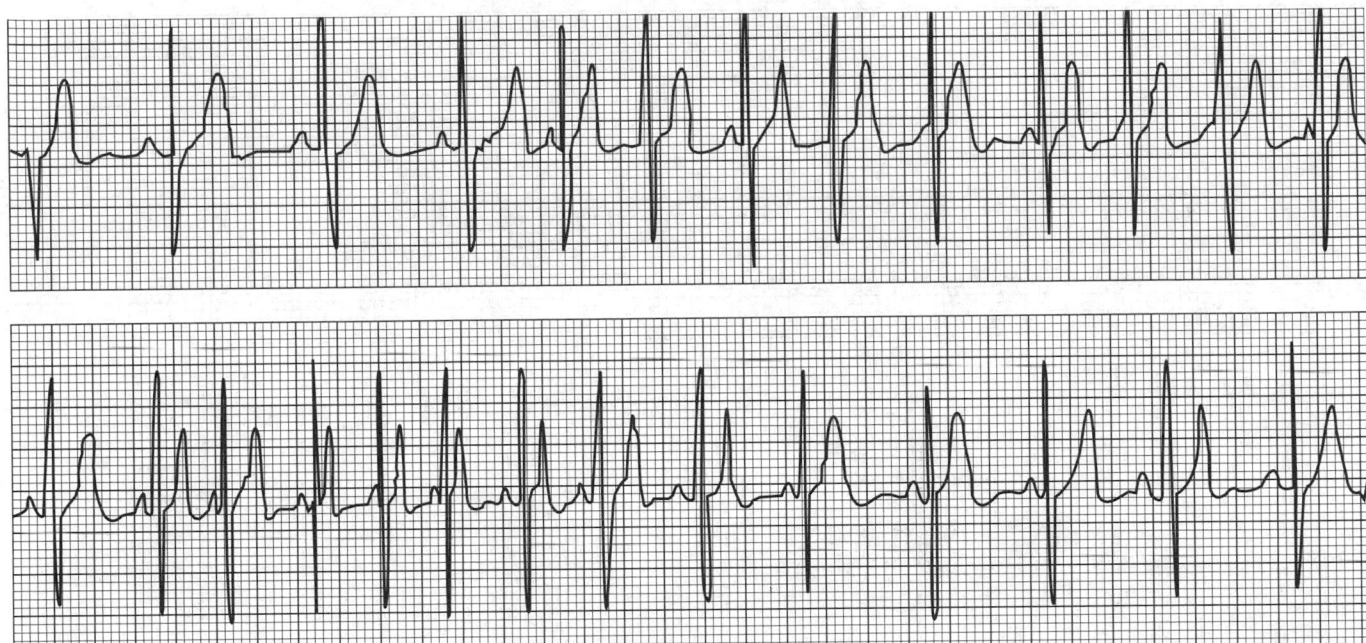

FIGURE 28-4

Deceleration of tape during recording. Supraventricular tachycardia is simulated toward the end of the top and beginning of the second trace, as the tape, which transiently slowed as a result of battery failure during recording, was played back on recording paper at proper speed. Note the foreshortening of the duration of the P wave, PR interval, QRS complex, and QT interval.

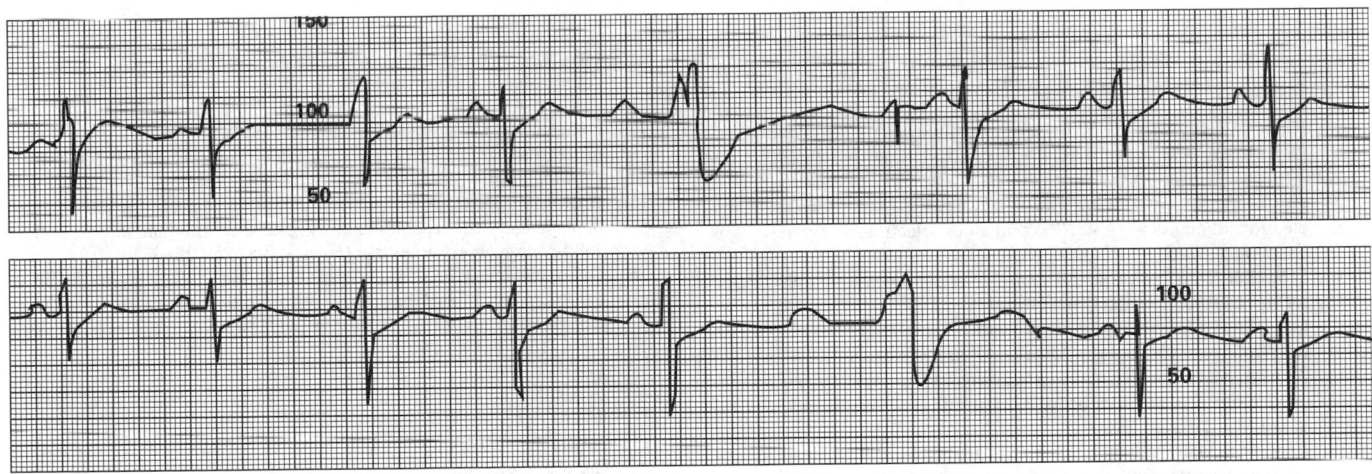

FIGURE 28-5

Deceleration of tape during playback. Slowing or sticking of the tape during playback spreads out the P wave, PR interval, and QRS complex to resemble sinus deceleration, or transient atrioventricular or intraventricular conduction delay. (Fifth complex in top trace; sixth complex in bottom trace.)

versely, transient slowing or sticking of the tape during playback will suggest bradycardia or atrioventricular (AV) or intraventricular conduction disturbances (Fig. 28-5). Recording an ECG on a previously used tape that is incompletely erased results in the simultaneous registration of two ECGs and potentially the misinterpretation of a "parasystolic" ectopic rhythm (Fig. 28-6). Digital recording in solid-state memory eliminates these various mechanical failures of tape recordings.

The technician and/or physician who interprets prolonged ECG recordings must have a working knowledge of these and other potential artifacts in order to interpret the records properly.

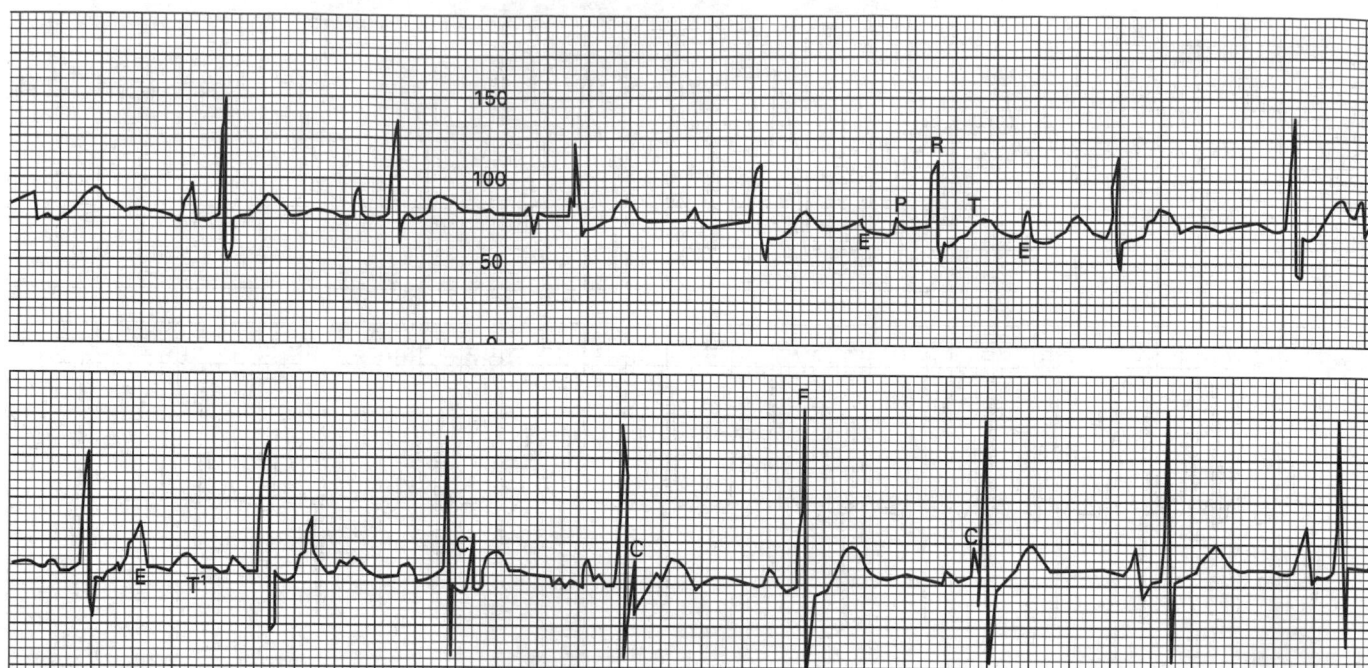

FIGURE 28-6

Incomplete erasure of tape. Two independent ventricular rhythms are identified: a larger QRS, labeled R, whose P wave and T wave are also labeled, and a smaller QRS, considered "ectopic," and labeled E; its T wave is labeled T'. The sequence could be recorded with a piggyback heart transplant, or in Siamese twins. Alternatively, ectopic complex E might be misinterpreted to represent a parasystolic rhythm even fusing with complex R at F. The very short coupling intervals (C) preclude this possibility and indicate that the ECG record of one patient is superimposed on that of another.

REFERENCES

1. Holter NJ. New method for heart studies: Continuous electrocardiography of active subjects over long periods is now practical. *Science* 1961; 134:1214–1220.
2. Gilson JS, Holter NJ, Glassock WR. Clinical observations using this electrocardiocorder—AVSEP continuous electrocardiographic system. *Am J Cardiol* 1964; 14:204–217.
3. Schneller SJ. State-of-the-art ambulatory electrocardiographic monitoring. *Cardiol Trends* 1990; 10:1–4.
4. Guidelines for Ambulatory Electrocardiography. A report of the American College of Cardiology/American Heart Association Task Force on Assessment of Diagnostic and Therapeutic Cardiovascular Procedures (Subcommittee on Ambulatory Electrocardiography). *J Am Coll Cardiol* 1989; 13:249–258.
5. Report of Committee on Electrocardiography, American Heart Association. Recommendations for standardization of leads and of specifications for instruments in electrocardiography and vectorcardiography. *Circulation* 1967; 35:583–602.
6. Sheffield LT, Berson A, Bragg-Remschel D, Gillette PC, Hermes RE, Hinkle L, et al. Recommendations for standards of instrumentation and practice in the use of ambulatory electrocardiography. *Circulation* 1985; 71:626A–636A.
7. Hinkle LE Jr, Meyer J, Stevens M, Carver ST. Recordings of the ECG of active men. *Circulation* 1967; 36:752–765.
8. Crawford MH, Mendoza CA, O'Rourke RA, White DH, Boucher CA, Gorwit J. Limitations of continuous ambulatory electrocardiogram monitoring for detecting coronary artery disease. *Ann Intern Med* 1978; 89:1–5.
9. Krahn AD, Klein GJ, Norris C, Yee R. The etiology of syncope in patients with negative tilt table and electrophysiological testing. *Circulation* 1995; 92:1819–1824.
10. Stein IM, Plunkett J, Troy M. Comparison of techniques for examining long-term ECG recordings. *Med Instrum* 1980; 14:69–72.
11. Fitzgerald JW, Spitz AL, Winkle RA, Harrison DC. Quantitation of ambulatory electrocardiograms (abstr). *Circulation* 1977; 56(suppl 3):178.
12. Knoebel SB, Lovelace DE, Rasmussen S, Wash SE. Computer detection of premature ventricular complexes: A modified approach. *Am J Cardiol* 1976; 38:440–447.
13. Brown AP, Dawkins KD, Davies JG. Detection of arrhythmias: Use of a patient-activated ambulatory electrocardiogram device with a solid-state memory loop. *Br Heart J* 1987; 58:251–253.
14. Kinlay S, Leitch J, Neil A, Chapman B, Hardy D, Fletcher P. Event recorders yield more diagnoses and are more cost-effective than 48-hour Holter monitoring in patients with palpitations. *Ann Intern Med* 1996; 124 (1,pt 1):16–20.
15. Fogel R, Evans J, Prystowsky E. Utility and cost of event recorders in the diagnosis of palpitations, presyncope and syncope. *Am J Cardiol* 1997; 79:207–208.
16. Lown B, Wolf M. Approaches to sudden death from coronary heart disease. *Circulation* 1971; 14:130–142.
17. Winkle RA. Antiarrhythmic drug effect mimicked by spontaneous variability of ventricular ectopy. *Circulation* 1978; 57:1116–1121.
18. Morganroth J, Michelson EL, Horowitz LN, Josephson ME, Pearlman AS, Dunkman WB. Limitations of routine long-term ambulatory electrocardiographic monitoring to assess ventricular ectopic frequency. *Circulation* 1978; 58:408–414.
19. Lopes MG, Runge P, Harrison DC, Schroeder JS. Comparison of 24 versus 12 hours of ambulatory ECG monitoring. *Chest* 1975; 67:269–273.
20. Kennedy HL, Chandra V, Sayther KL, Caralis DG. Effectiveness of increasing hours of continuous ambulatory electrocardiography in detecting maximal ventricular ectopy. *Am J Cardiol* 1978; 42:925–930.
21. Sami M, Kraemer H, Harrison DC, Houston N, Shimasaki C, DeBusk RF. A new method for evaluating antiarrhythmic drug efficacy. *Circulation* 1980; 62:1172–1179.
22. Winkle RA, Alderman EL, Fitzgerald JW, Harrison DC. Treatment of recurrent symptomatic ventricular tachycardia. *Ann Intern Med* 1976; 85:1–7.

23. Berman DA, Rozanski AL, Knoebel SB. The detection of silent ischemia: Cautions and precautions. *Circulation* 1987; 75:101–105.

24. Golding B, Wolf E, Tzivoni D, Stern S. Transient S-T elevation detected by 24-hour ECG monitoring during normal daily activity. *Am Heart J* 1973; 86:501–507.

25. Stern S, Tzivoni D. Early detection of silent ischaemic heart disease by 24-hour electrocardiographic monitoring of active subjects. *Br Heart J* 1974; 36:481–486.

26. Wolf E, Tzivoni D, Stern S. Comparison of exercise tests and 24-hour ambulatory electrocardiographic monitoring in detection of ST-T changes. *Br Heart J* 1974; 36:90–95.

27. Stern S, Tzivoni D. Dynamic changes in the ST-T segment during sleep in ischemic heart disease. *Am J Cardiol* 1973; 32:17–20.

28. Krasnow AZ, Bloomfield DK. Artifacts in portable electrocardiographic monitoring. *Am Heart J* 1976; 91:349–357.

29. Malek J, Glushien A. To the editor: Artifacts in portable ECG monitoring. *Ann Intern Med* 1972; 77:1004.

29

TECHNIQUES OF ELECTROPHYSIOLOGIC TESTING

Masood Akhtar

The recording of intracavitary electrocardiographic signals and various forms of pacing programs have experienced enormous growth during the past three decades. Recordings of intracardiac signals from the region of the His bundle, initially made by Scherlag et al.,[1] were rapidly applied to clinical problems including atrioventricular (AV) blocks and supraventricular and ventricular tachyarrhythmias.[1-10] Such recordings were then complemented by pacing to unmask sinus node dysfunction and AV conduction abnormalities as well as to initiate supraventricular tachycardias (SVTs).[3,8] Intracardiac electrophysiologic studies (EPSs) now find utility in a variety of cardiac arrhythmias, including sinus node dysfunction, intraventricular and AV conduction disturbances, SVTs, ventricular tachycardias (VTs), preexcitation syndromes, and ventricular fibrillation (VF). Such studies are now also employed as a prelude to correction of various arrhythmias and conduction defects. This chapter addresses recording and pacing techniques and their clinical utility.[9,10]

TECHNIQUES OF INTRACARDIAC ELECTROPHYSIOLOGIC STUDIES[11]

The exact type of electric signal recordings, specific equipment used, and pacing protocol depend upon the nature of the clinical problem, the type of electrophysiologic assessment, and the anticipated course of action. Routine cardiac EPSs are performed in a nonsedated postabsorptive state. Although some degree of sedation is advisable in apprehensive patients, drugs that may alter the properties of the cardiac conduction system should be avoided. Antiarrhythmic drugs are usually stopped prior to these studies. In selected cases, antiarrhythmic drugs may be continued if a clinical event occurred while the patient was on a specific agent. Customarily, other cardioactive drugs that are necessary for nonar-rhythmic cardiovascular problems such as hypertension, angina, and heart failure are continued.

The typical electrode catheters used for both recording and cardiac stimulation are multipolar (sizes varying from 4 to 8 F). Catheters can be inserted via peripheral veins such as the antecubital or femoral veins and, at times, the subclavian and internal jugular veins may be used. When a catheter is intended to be left in place for several days, subclavian and internal jugular veins are preferable. After using local anesthesia, a guidewire is inserted percutaneously through a needle and a sheath is advanced over the guidewire. A catheter is then guided fluoroscopically through the sheath to position in the appropriate cardiac chamber. For most electrophysiologic testing, the catheter is placed in the high right atrium, at the His bundle, or at the right bundle branch region across the tricuspid valve and right ventricular apex or outflow. For accessory pathways or AV junctional tachycardias, a catheter is placed in the region of the coronary sinus. Heparinization is recommended by continuous infusion of approximately 1000 units per hour. For EPSs, good contact between the electrodes and the walls of the various chambers is critical. For His bundle and right bundle branch recording, the catheter is introduced via the femoral vein, advanced across the tricuspid valve, and gradually withdrawn until an appropriate recording from the right bundle and/or the His bundle is obtained (Fig. 29-1). Placement of a coronary sinus catheter can be accomplished via an arm, internal jugular, or subclavian vein. If necessary, coronary sinus catheterization can also be accomplished via a femoral approach. For a routine study, left-sided heart catheterization is seldom necessary. In patients with VT and/or left-sided accessory pathways, however, this is performed for diagnostic or therapeutic purposes. Continuous heparinization is desirable for left heart catheterization to avoid thromboembolic complications.

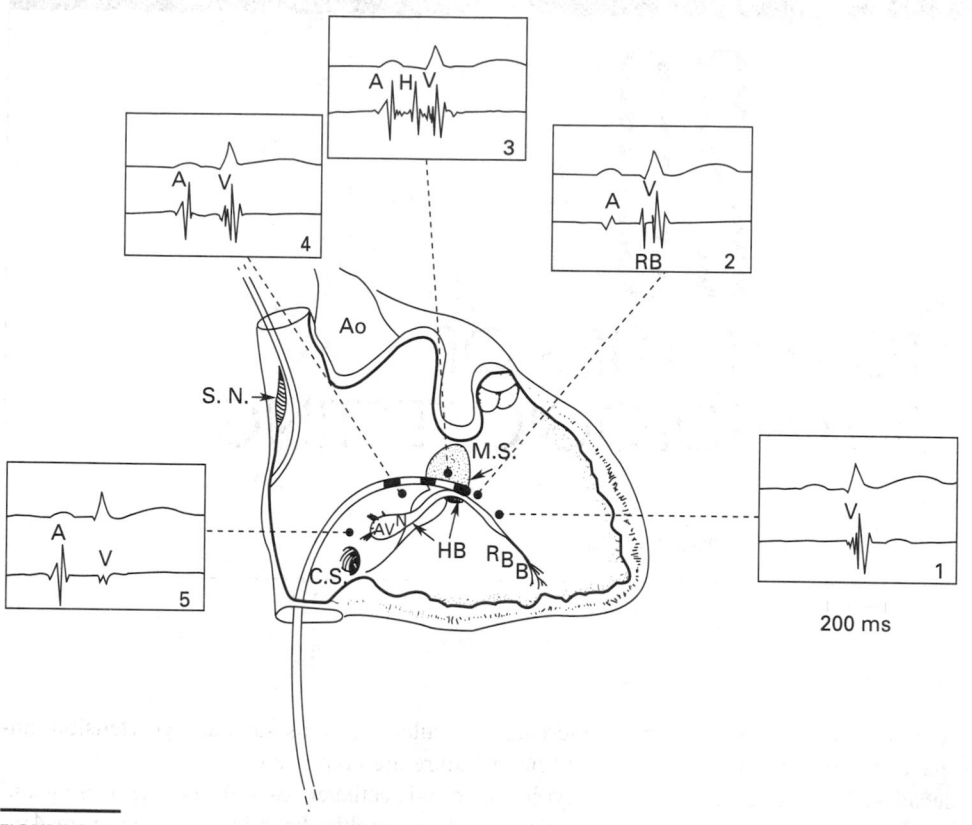

200 ms

FIGURE 29-1

Intracardiac recordings from the specialized conduction system in the AV junction. The recording of various electrograms along the right side of the interventricular septum with gradual withdrawal of the catheter across the tricuspid valve is shown. The intracardiac recordings are labeled. Numbers 1 through 5 refer to intracardiac location of catheters along with corresponding electrogram. (CS, coronary sinus; SN, sinus node; Ao, aorta; MS, membranous septum; AVN, atrioventricular node; HB, His bundle; RBB, right bundle branch; A, atrial deflection; H and RB, His and right bundle potentials; V, ventricular deflection.) (From Gallagher JJ, Damato AN. Technique of recording His bundle activity in man. In: Grossman W, ed. *Cardiac Catheterization and Angiography*. Philadelphia: Lea & Febiger; 1980:283–301. Reproduced with permission from the publisher and authors.)

Electrophysiologic Recordings

Once the electrode catheters are placed appropriately, the connections are made via a junction box and isolation units to prevent excess current in the event of random electrical surges. All of the electrograms are displayed simultaneously on a multichannel oscilloscopic recorder. In addition to the intracardiac signals, several unfiltered surface electrocardiographic leads, i.e., X, Y, Z or leads I, II, or aV_F and V_1, are recorded. To reduce the noise generated with the low-frequency signals, the usual filtering frequency for intracardiac signals is between 30 and 40 Hz for the high-pass and 500 Hz for the low-pass filters. Although appropriately placed electrode catheters will record appropriate signals at any filtering frequency, filter settings between 30 to 40 and 500 Hz are best suited for sharp intracardiac signals such as those from the His bundle and accessory pathways (Fig. 29-2). Undesirable low-frequency signals can be reduced by a high-pass filter setting of more than 50 to 100 Hz. On the other hand, 60-cycle interference can be eliminated with a low-pass filter setting at 50 Hz. Alteration in the high-bandpass filter

for surface electrocardiography can markedly alter the scalar electrocardiographic morphology. Amplification is frequently necessary to identify desirable signals from the specialized conduction system. This can lead to superimposition of the larger myocardial signals on various electrocardiographic tracings. In most recording equipment, however, there are limiting filters that allow the adjustment of amplitude limits.

The main value of intracardiac/electrocardiographic tracings is timing of electric events. To acquire true local electrical activity, a bipolar electrogram with an interelectrode distance of less than 1 cm is desirable. When unipolar electrograms are obtained, a rapid intrinsic deflection will identify a point of local activation. For routine intracardiac electrocardiographic studies, unipolar electrograms provide relatively limited advantage over bipolar signals, and therefore, the latter are more often utilized. The above description relates to the routine diagnostic invasive EPSs. In other clinical situations, different types of diagnostic methods are employed. For example, during intraoperative mapping, direct placement of electrodes over the epicardium or endocardium is necessary to get appropriate signals for identifying the origin and route of impulse propagation.[12] These electrodes can be in the form of either hand-held probes or plaques that can be placed or sutured over the myocardium. Socks and balloons incorporating several electrodes can also be used for epicardial and endocardial mapping techniques, respectively.[13,14] All electrical signals can be recorded on either a disk or frequency-modulated tape for permanent storage.

Programmed Electrical Stimulation

After satisfactory placement of the electrode catheters, patches, or other forms of recording equipment, programmed stimulation is initiated. The usual site of pacing is the right atrium or left atrium via the coronary sinus. For ventricular stimulation, the pacing sites are the right ventricular apex, outflow tract, and rarely some other right ventricular site. A variety of pacing programs can be utilized, depending upon the nature of the underlying arrhythmic problem under investi-

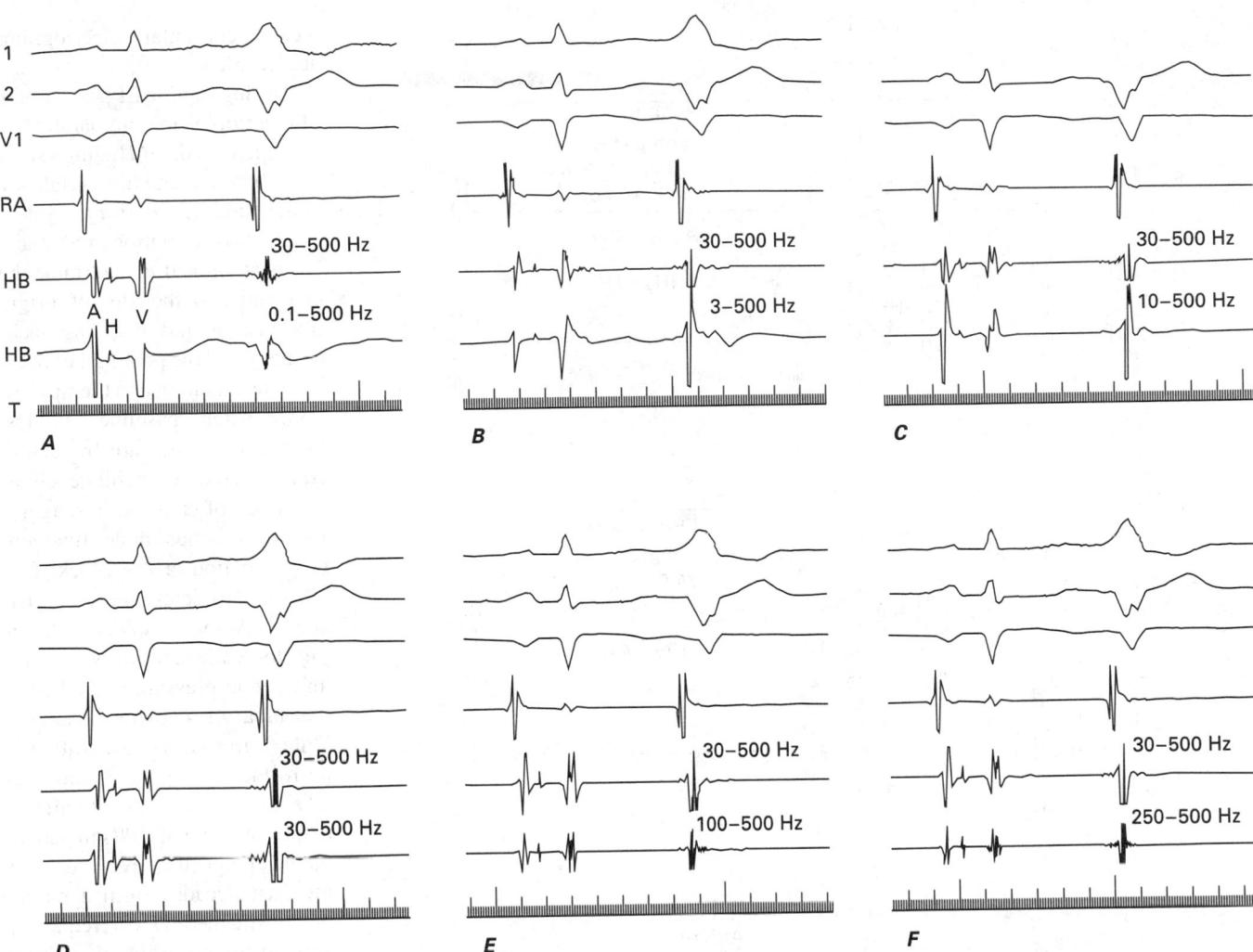

FIGURE 29-2

Effects of various filtering frequencies on the morphologic appearance of intracardiac electrograms *A* through *F*. The tracings from top to bottom are ECG leads I, II, V$_1$, right atrial (RA), two His bundle (HB) electrograms, and time (T) line. Similar abbreviations are used in subsequent figures and tracings. In each panel, the first beat is of sinus origin and is followed by a spontaneous ventricular premature beat. The top HB, RA, and RV are filtered at 30 to 500 Hz (i.e., the usual filtering frequencies). The bottom HB tracing shows the effect of various filtering frequencies on the appearance. The low-frequency signals are mostly eliminated at high-bandpass filter frequency settings above 10 Hz (*C*). The low-bandpass filter settings above 500 Hz generally do not have a significant effect on the intracardiac electrogram appearance. It should be pointed out that the high-bandpass setting reduces the overall magnitude of the electrogram, necessitating an increase in amplification. It should also be noted that at all frequencies depicted, the HB deflection can be clearly identified. (From Akhtar.[11] Reproduced with permission from the publisher and authors.)

gation. At least two formats of pacing protocol are common. The first format is incremental pacing, which is pacing at a constant cycle length with gradual shortening until the occurrence of a desirable event, such as induction of a tachycardia and production of AV block. Otherwise the incremental atrial pacing is continued until the onset of AV nodal Wenckebach phenomenon: a physiologic response at faster pacing rates. Fixed cycle length pacing is also used for the induction of supraventricular tachyarrhythmias and study of ventriculo-atrial conduction. Bursts of pacing at a constant cycle length are occasionally used to induce SVT, VT, or VF or for study of sinus node function and integrity of subsidiary pacemakers.

The second pacing format is premature (or extra) stimulation from atrial or ventricular sites. For the study of a physio-logic phenomenon, refractory periods, and conduction characteristics, a single extra stimulus is usually applied after a series of beats with a constant cycle length (Fig. 29-3). The scanning is initiated late during electrical diastole, and the coupling interval is progressively decreased until the atrial and/or ventricular muscle is refractory. For induction of SVTs, single, two, or more extra stimuli are delivered (Fig. 29-4). For the induction of VT, up to three ventricular extra stimuli are employed. The sensitivity of pacing protocols seems to be directly related to the number of extra stimuli utilized.[15] This occurs, however, at the expense of specificity when poly-morphic VT/VF can be induced at very short coupling intervals using multiple extra stimuli. Regardless of the pacing protocol, the induction of sustained monomorphic VT consti-

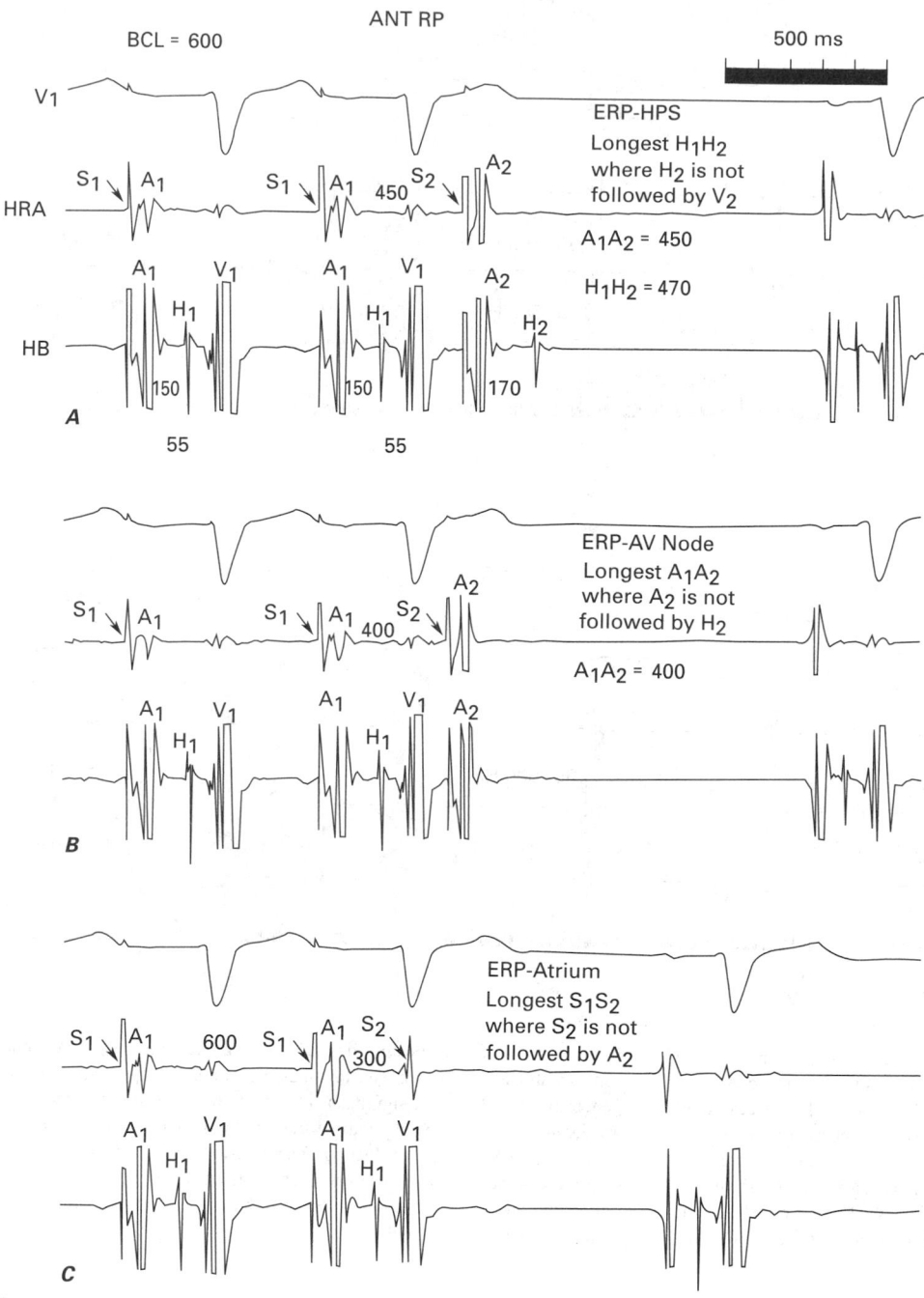

FIGURE 29-3

Determination of cardiac refractory periods during atrial pacing (*A* through *C*). During a basic cycle length pacing at 600 ms (S_1S_1 or A_1A_1), atrial premature stimulation (S_2 or A_2) at progressively shorter coupling intervals (S_1S_2 or A_1A_2) is depicted. The definition of the effective refractory period (ERP) of the His-Purkinje system (HPS), AV node, and atrium are labeled. (ANT RP, antegrade refractory period.) (From Akhtar.[11] Reproduced with permission from the publisher and authors.)

local ventricular electrograms are avoided.[16]

During routine EPSs, a variety of electrophysiologic parameters are measured, including sinus node function and intraatrial, AV nodal, and His-Purkinje system conduction. Initiation of SVT and VT is attempted to determine the mechanisms, the site of origin (by pacing and mapping techniques), and the potential of overdrive termination as a therapy option. After baseline studies, intravenous drugs are frequently administered to facilitate either induction of tachycardias, aggravation of sinus node function, or production of AV block (Fig. 29-5), or to determine drug efficacy.[17] At the completion of testing, the catheters are withdrawn and gentle pressure is applied at the area of catheter insertion. Unless arterial catheterization is performed, the patients are usually allowed to ambulate after 4 to 6 h. The role of EPSs in patient management has evolved over the past decades from a purely diagnostic method to a frequently applied therapeutic tool. A brief outline of the value of clinical EPSs in various arrhythmia settings is outlined separately under diagnostic and therapeutic categories.

INVASIVE ELECTROPHYSIOLOGIC STUDIES FOR DIAGNOSIS

Sinus Node Dysfunction[3,4]

Electrophysiologic studies are generally performed to detect suspected sinus node dysfunction in patients with dizziness, presyncope, syncope, etc., in whom the diagnosis cannot be made noninvasively. EPSs are not indicated with sinus node dysfunction or with obvious sinus node dysfunction demonstrable from the surface electrocardiogram. The most frequently performed test is that of sinus node suppression using overdrive atrial pacing. After pacing at several basic cycle lengths for a period of approximately 30 s or longer, the pacing is interrupted. The resultant escape

tutes a specific response and is seldom induced in patients not prone to such arrhythmias clinically. In contrast, the induction of polymorphic VT/VF with three extra stimuli can be nonspecific and does not provide a reliable guide for serial testing. Both polymorphic VT and VF can be avoided to a great extent if short coupling intervals (<200 ms) and the induction of latency between the stimulus artifact and the

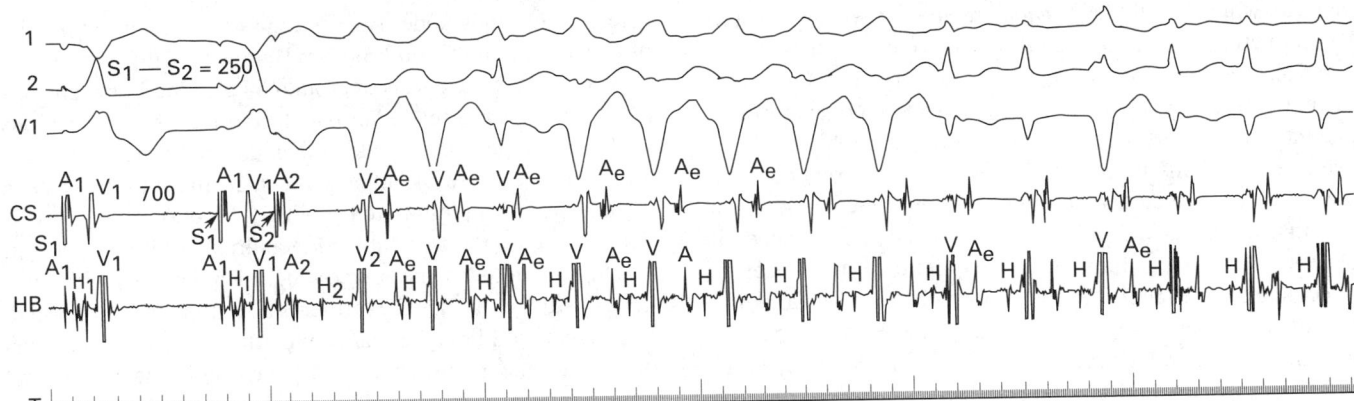

FIGURE 29-4

Induction of supraventricular tachycardia (SVT) in Wolff-Parkinson-White syndrome. The tracings are labeled. Atrial pacing from coronary sinus (CS) is done at 700 ms basic cycle. During the basic drive pacing, left free wall accessory pathway conduction to the ventricle produces ventricular preexcitation. A single premature beat (S_2) blocks in the accessory pathway (AP) and conducts over the normal pathway with a left bundle branch block morphology, and the SVT is initiated. Note the intermittent normalization of the QRS complex during this SVT. (From Jazayeri M, Caceres J, Tchou P, Mahmud R, Denker S, Akhtar M. Electrophysiologic characteristics of sudden QRS axis deviation during orthodromic tachycardia. *J Clin Invest* 1989; 83(3):952–959. Reproduced with permission from the publisher and authors).

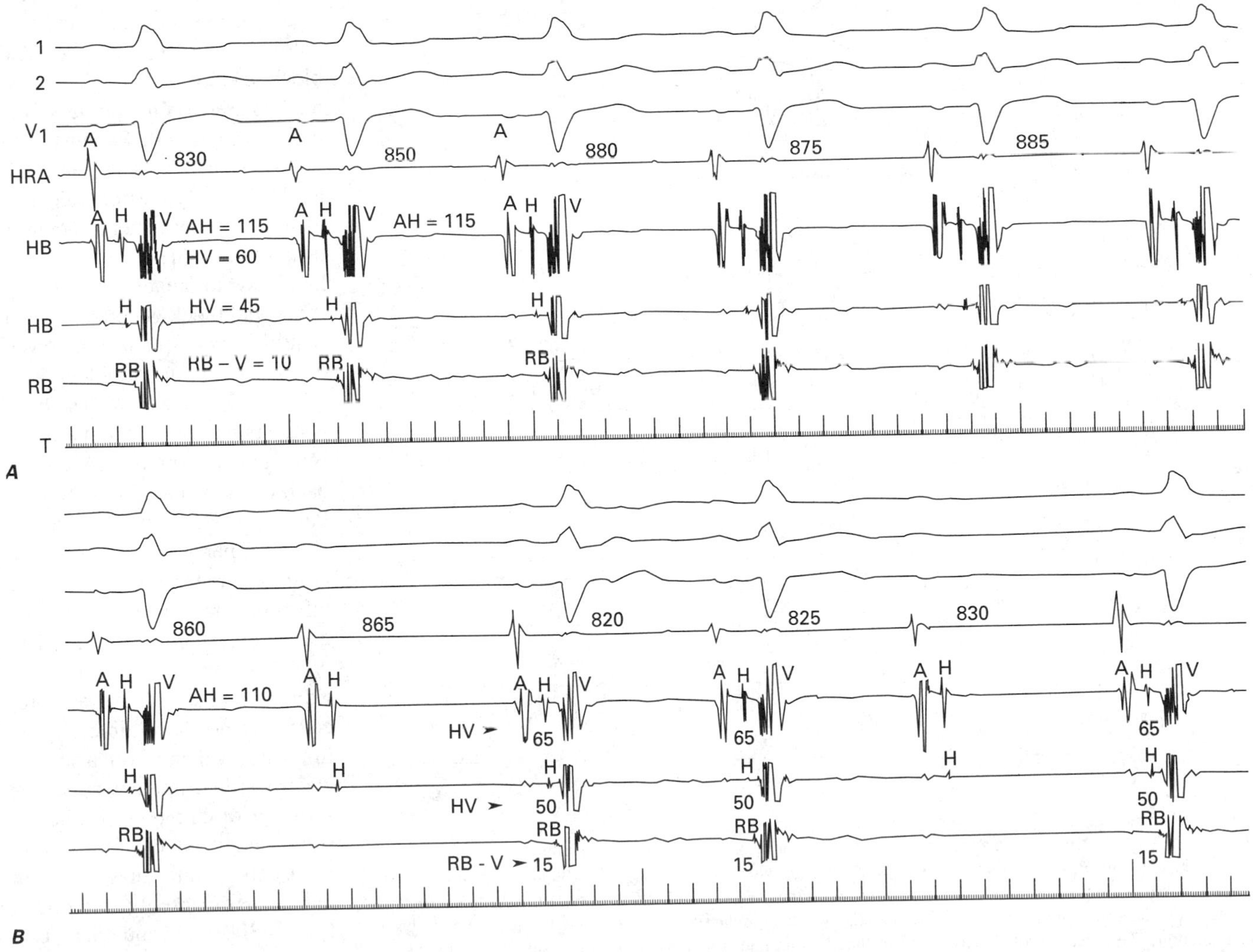

FIGURE 29-5

Atrioventricular block in the His-Purkinje system (HPS). *A.* Control. 1:1 AV conduction is depicted in a patient with unexplained syncope. Following 150 mg of intravenous procainamide (*B*), a second-degree AV block in the HPS is noted (i.e., His bundle potential is not followed by a QRS complex), an abnormal response to a small dose of procainamide suggesting AV block in the HPS as a potential cause of syncope.

interval, which is called *sinus node recovery time*, is measured. By deducting the predominant sinus cycle length from this interval, one can obtain the so-called corrected sinus node recovery time. In one study, sinus node recovery time in patients with sinus node disease averaged 3087 ms,[3] and averaged 1073 ms in normal individuals. In another series,[6] the value for corrected sinus node recovery time was less than 525 ms in normal individuals and exceeded those values in patients with overt sinus node dysfunction. More recently, direct sinus node recordings have been obtained by amplification of recording from catheters placed in close proximity to the sinus node,[18,19] where both the sinus node automaticity and sinoatrial conduction can be determined more accurately.

In the vast majority of patients with true sinus node disease, sinoatrial conduction abnormalities are the predominant reason for sinus node dysfunction. The sinoatrial conduction time in the absence of obvious sinus node disease is less than 100 ms. The sensitivity of sinus node recovery time for the detection of sinus node dysfunction is 54 percent while that of sinoatrial conduction time is 51 percent, with a combined sensitivity of the two tests of around 64 percent. Poor sensitivity of such testing relates in part to the fact that in previous studies documented episodes of sinus bradycardia or sinus arrest due to neurocardiogenic mechanisms may have been included as examples of sinus node dysfunction.[20] The specificity of the two tests combined is approximately 88 percent. It is important to test the AV conduction in patients with sinus node dysfunction since the former is also frequently abnormal. In patients with bradycardia/tachycardia syndrome, tachycardias are frequent, particularly those arising in the atrium, and testing may also be necessary for the proper diagnosis and therapy of the concomitant tachyarrhythmia.

Atrioventricular Block

In asymptomatic patients with first-degree AV block (prolonged PR interval), electrophysiologic assessment is unnecessary, regardless of the QRS morphology of the conducted beats. In asymptomatic individuals with second-degree AV block, electrophysiologic assessment is used to find the site of the block (Fig. 29-6). Patients with intra-Hisian or infra-Hisian block tend to have a more unpredictable course, and permanent pacing is usually desirable.[21] On the other hand, asymptomatic patients with AV nodal block generally do not require permanent pacing. Even though the intranodal block usually presents as Wenckebach phenomenon or Mobitz type I, it is not uncommon to see Wenckebach phenomena within the His-Purkinje system or within the His bundle. There is no difference in prognosis regardless of how the infra- or intra-Hisian second-degree block manifests itself, i.e., type I versus type II. On occasion, intranodal blocks are preceded by no discernible change in PR interval and from a surface electrocardiogram may appear as forms of Mobitz type II. The absolute length of the PR interval is usually quite diagnostic in that it is markedly prolonged (i.e., >300 ms), and there is a PR shortening exceeding 100 ms following the block beat. In symptomatic patients with second-degree AV block, the role

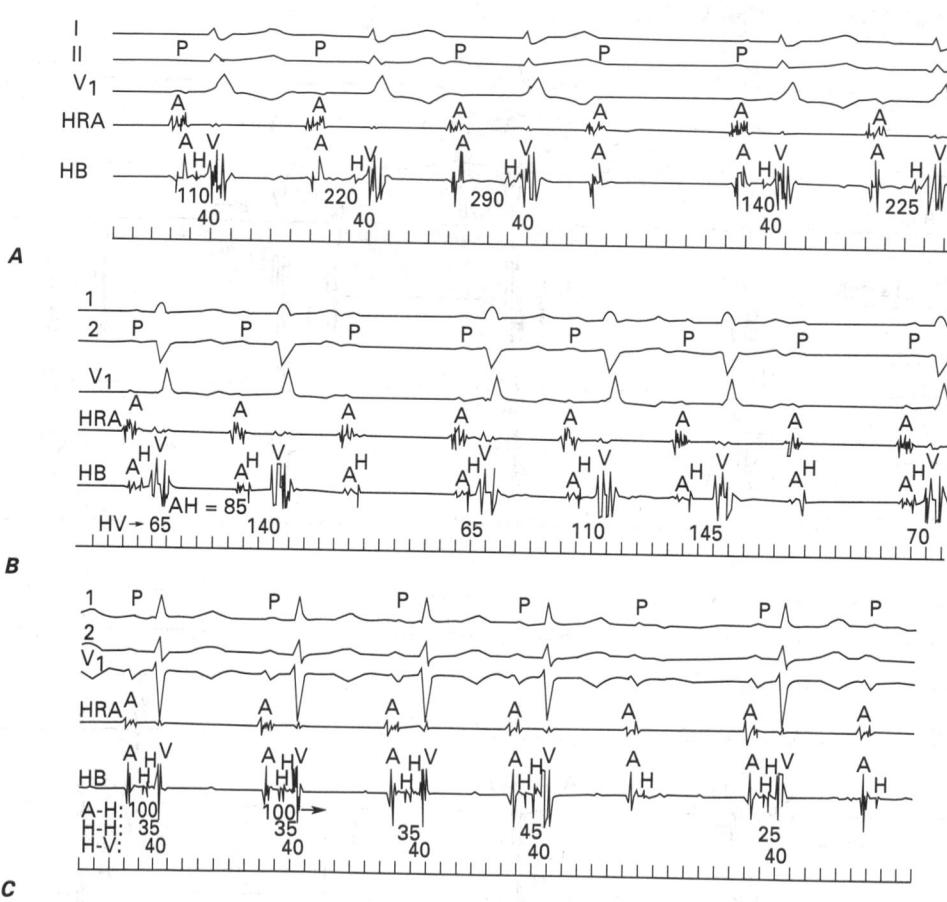

FIGURE 29-6

His bundle (HB) electrograms in AV block. The tracings are from three different patients with second-degree AV block. In *A* and *B*, the conducted QRS complexes are wide and associated with bundle branch block. In *A*, the block is within the AV node (i.e., the A wave on the HB is not followed by an HB deflection). In *B*, it can be appreciated that the block is distal to the HB even though the surface ECG demonstrates a Wenckebach phenomenon. The latter can obviously occur in the His-Purkinje system as well, as depicted in this figure. *C*. Site of block is within the HB. This is suggested by split HB potentials (labeled H and H′), and the block is distal to the H but proximal to the H′. Intra-His block is difficult to diagnose from the surface ECG but can be suspected when a Mobitz type II occurs in association with a normal PR interval and a narrow QRS complex. (From Akhtar.[17] Reproduced with permission from the publisher and author.)

of EPS is limited because permanent pacing is the appropriate intervention. On the other hand, if the patient's symptoms cannot be explained on the basis of AV block and may be related to another arrhythmia, such as VT, EPSs should be considered. In patients with third-degree or complete AV block, EPSs are seldom required and permanent pacing is the obvious option in symptomatic patients.

For EPSs to determine the site of AV block, it is critical to have the catheter across the AV junction that records the His bundle. A discernible His bundle recording allows one to determine the exact site of AV conduction abnormality, i.e., proximal to, within, or distal to the His bundle region. This, in combination with surface electrocardiographic morphology of conducted beats, allows one to identify precisely the location of conduction abnormality. The normal atrial to His bundle activation time (A-H) is approximately 50 to 140 ms, while the His to ventricular myocardial depolarization interval (H-V) measures 35 to 55 ms.

If 1:1 AV conduction is noted during EPSs in patients suspected of intermittent AV block, incremental atrial pacing should be done to see if AV block could be reproduced. AV block in the His-Purkinje system is abnormal during incremental atrial pacing but is a physiologic response during atrial extrastimulation (see Fig. 29-3A) or with abrupt acceleration of atrial pacing rate. First- and second-degree block in the AV node are considered physiologic responses during incremental atrial pacing or atrial extrastimulation (see Fig. 29-3B).

Wide QRS Tachycardia

Wide QRS tachycardia occurs due to a variety of electrophysiologic mechanisms, both from supraventricular and ventricular mechanisms in the presence and absence of accessory pathways (Fig. 29-7).[22] The underlying nature of the wide QRS tachycardia is critical for both prognosis and therapy. EPSs have proven invaluable in distinguishing the various etiologies (Fig. 29-8). With few exceptions, when the nature of the arrhythmic problem is not well known and the direction of therapy is not clear, patients with wide QRS tachycardia should undergo EPS. This is particularly true in situations where non-pharmacologic therapy is the desired goal.

Unexplained Syncope

Unexplained syncope is predominantly due to cardiovascular mechanisms. The two most common reasons for cardiovascular syncope are cardiac arrhythmias and neuro-cardiogenic dysfunction, often referred to as *vasodepressor syncope*.[23–28] Electro-

physiologic evaluation constitutes an integral part of the evaluation of patients with unexplained syncope. During such studies, all arrhythmic possibilities such as sinus node dysfunction, AV conduction abnormalities, SVT, and VT should be excluded. Neurocardiogenic mechanisms constitute the most common causes of syncope in patients without structural heart disease, and incomplete assessment in these patients may lead to inappropriate therapy (Fig. 29-9).[20,23] The possibility of neurocardiogenic dysfunction should always be considered in younger patients (<50 years) with syncope and documented bradycardia (sinus arrest or AV block) and can be unmasked on a tilt table. The triage of patients towards one or the other, i.e., electrophysiologic testing versus head-up tilt, is fairly simple and predicted by clinical history and the presence or absence of structural heart disease.[23] Patients with underlying structural heart disease, such as old myocardial infarction, primary myocardial disease, or poor left ventricular function, generally have underlying VT to explain the symptoms of syncope (Fig. 29-10). When arrhythmias occur in patients without overt structural heart disease, sinus node dysfunction, AV block (particularly intra-Hisian block), or SVTs are likely. On rare occasion, VT can occur in the absence of an overt structural heart disease.

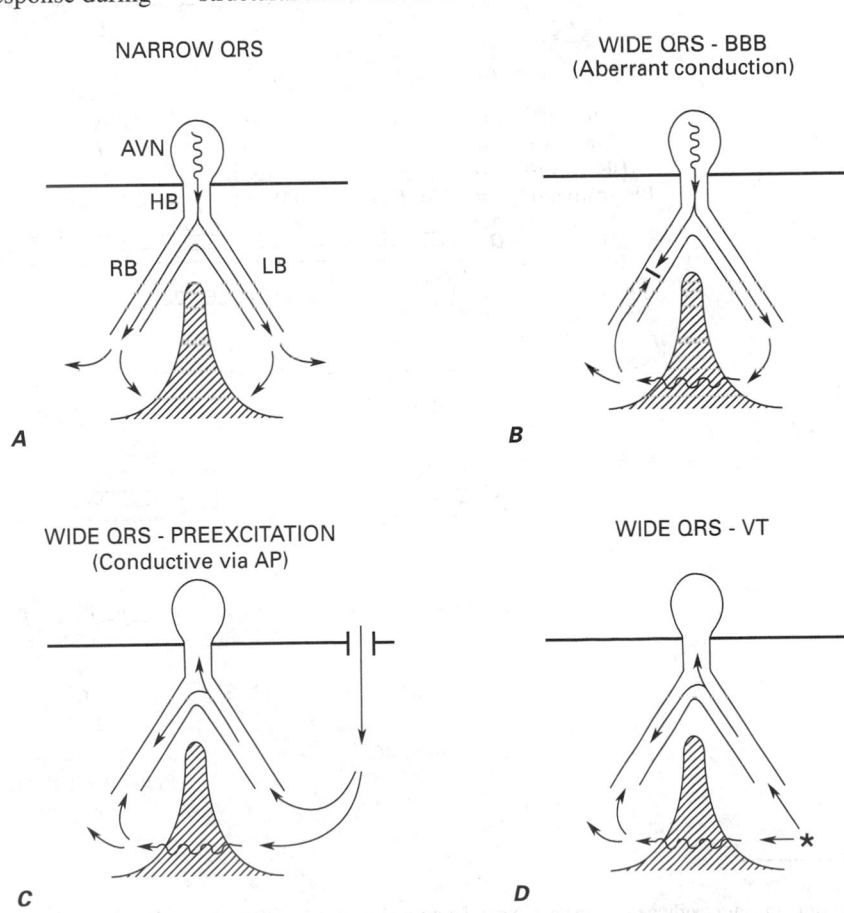

FIGURE 29-7
Wide QRS tachycardia. Routes of impulse propagation during a wide QRS tachycardia in various settings are depicted. It should be noted that only in *A* and *B* is His bundle activation expected to precede ventricular activation. This helps the delineation from other causes of wide QRS tachycardia shown in *C* and *D*.

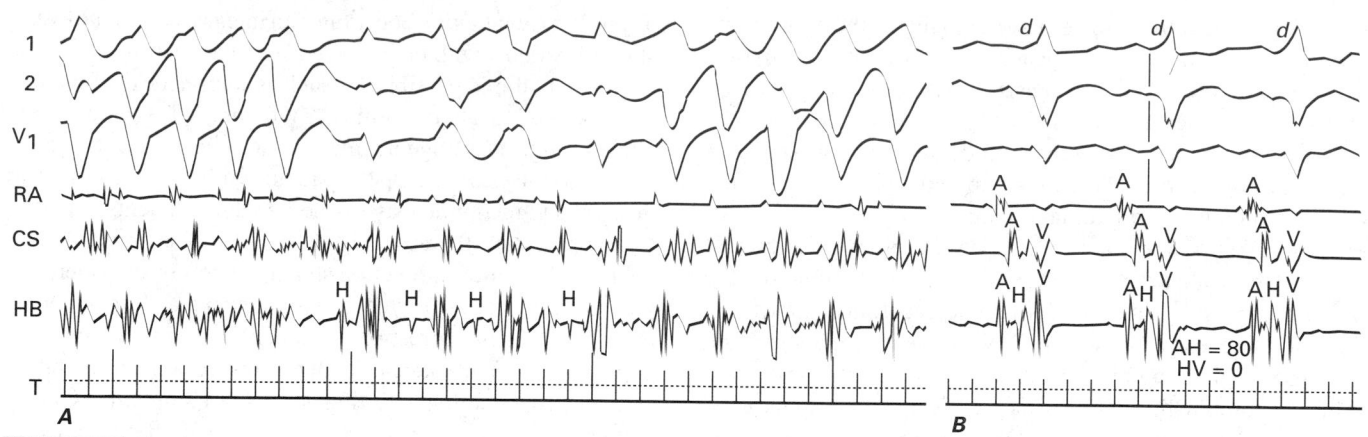

FIGURE 29-8

Wide QRS tachycardia. *A.* Wide QRS complexes of at least two varieties are seen. Those showing a left bundle branch block pattern are due to conduction over an accessory pathway, while those with a right bundle branch pattern are aberrant in nature. Note the His bundle activation prior to both narrow and aberrant complexes but not before preexcited complexes. A right posteroseptal preexcitation can be appreciated in *B*, with a short PR, a delta wave (*d*), an HV of zero, and negative delta wave in lead V_1.

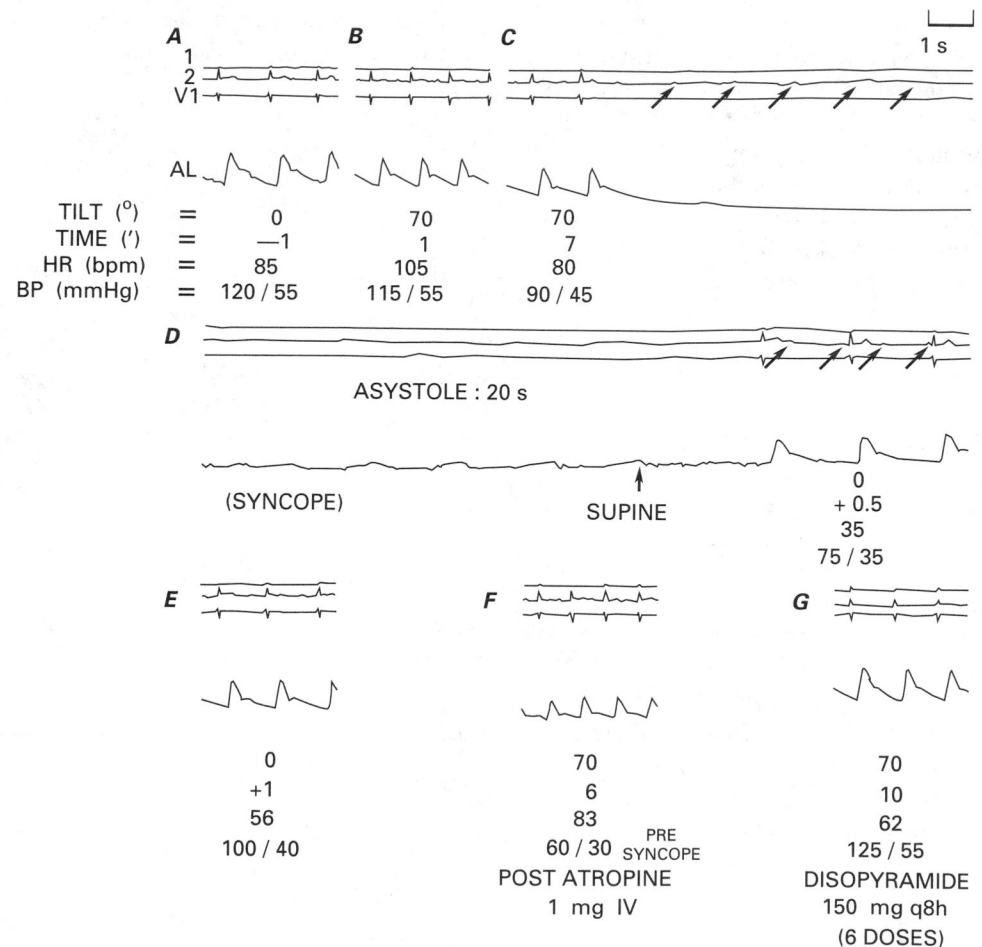

FIGURE 29-9

Asystole in neurocardiogenic syncope. Note the normal heart rate (HR) and blood pressure (BP) in supine position. At the beginning of head-up tilt at 70° (*B*), some degree of tachycardia is noted. Seven minutes after the onset of tilt (*C*), an episode of AV block occurs and is followed by sinus arrest and a total asystole of 20 s. Syncopal episodes follow. Presyncope is still present when asystole is prevented by atropine (*F*). Findings in panel *C* might tempt one to prescribe permanent pacing, an inappropriate choice of therapy. In this patient with neurocardiogenic syncope, disopyramide (*G*) prevented hypotension and syncope without the need for a permanent pacemaker. This patient has remained asymptomatic on this therapy for more than 6 years now. (From Sra et al.[23] Reproduced with permission from the publisher and authors.)

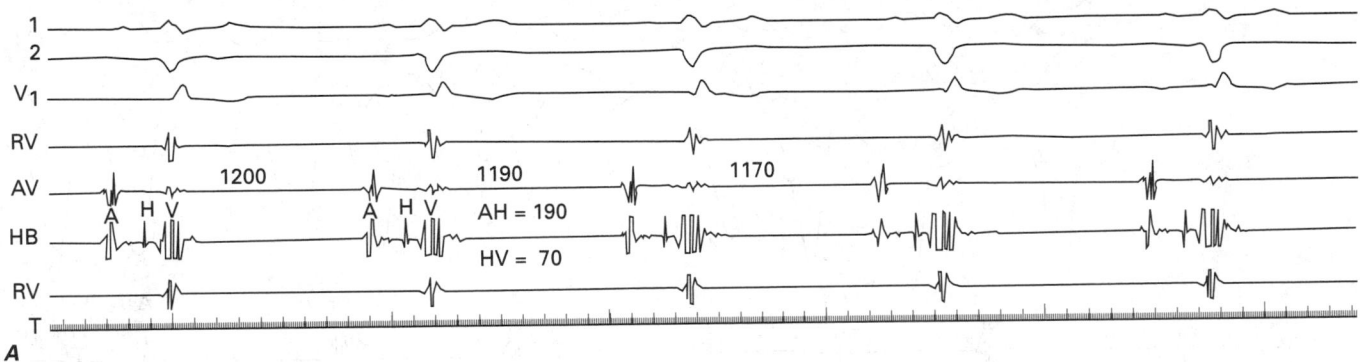

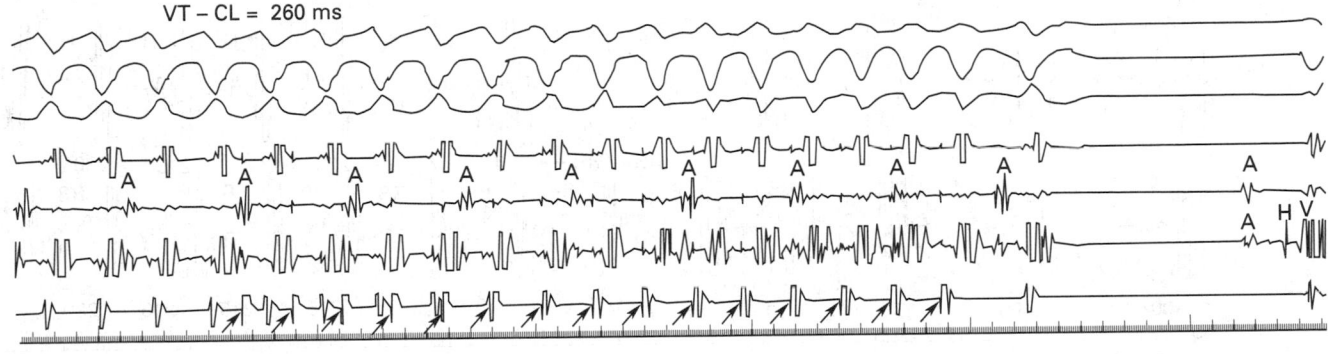

FIGURE 29-10

Arrhythmic causes of syncope. *A.* Sinus rhythm in a patient with unexplained syncope. Sinus bradycardia, bifascicular block, and a long PR interval from surface ECG suggest possible bradycardia etiology. In this patient, however, ventricular tachycardia (*B*) was inducible with ventricular extrastimulation and was the actual cause of syncope. Control of ventricular tachycardia (VT) without a pacemaker was sufficient to prevent syncope in this patient. Termination of tachycardia and restoration of sinus rhythm is shown in *B*.

Survivors of Sudden Cardiac Death

In most patients with documented episodes of cardiac arrest from the onset, VF can be documented. Patients dying suddenly generally have underlying structural heart disease (usually coronary artery disease or primary myocardial disease) and are prone to VT/VF due to electrical instability. It seems prudent to investigate both the nature and extent of organic heart disease and also to assess vulnerability to recurrent VT/VF. At the present time, EPS is considered a routine part of the overall patient assessment in this group of individuals.[29–31]

EPSs in survivors of VT/VF are desirable for a variety of reasons. Some are listed below.

1. Not infrequently, the underlying VT leading to cardiac arrest is bundle branch reentry (Fig. 29-11). This arrhythmia is preferably managed with bundle branch ablation, which is curative, rather than with an implantable cardioverter defibrillator (ICD).

2. Several VT morphologies or other types of tachycardia may be induced in addition to VT. Lack of awareness of such arrhythmias may complicate patient management. For example, the presence of rapid SVT may require separate attention to prevent unnecessary ICD shocks.

3. In some cases, supraventricular arrhythmia may trigger VT/VF. This may happen in patients with severe coronary artery disease, congestive heart failure, Wolff-Parkinson-White syndrome, etc. The elimination of the underlying causes constitutes more rational therapy and should be considered at the outset.

4. Patients with VT/VF often have underlying sick sinus syndrome or AV block, which can be further aggravated with antiarrhythmic drugs and may require permanent pacing. Considering that the current ICDs do not provide dual-chamber pacing, a separate pacing system may have to be implanted. Assessment for this eventuality should be done during the conduct of an EPS.

INVASIVE CARDIAC ELECTROPHYSIOLOGIC STUDIES FOR THERAPEUTIC INTERVENTION

Because of the episodic nature of most cardiac arrhythmias, it is difficult to assess the efficacy of any therapeutic intervention unless the arrhythmia in question can be replicated. Diagnostic EPS provides that opportunity, and it seems logical to use the same tool to assess therapeutic interventions.[32–34] This method to assess efficacy can be applied for both pharmacologic and nonpharmacologic therapy.

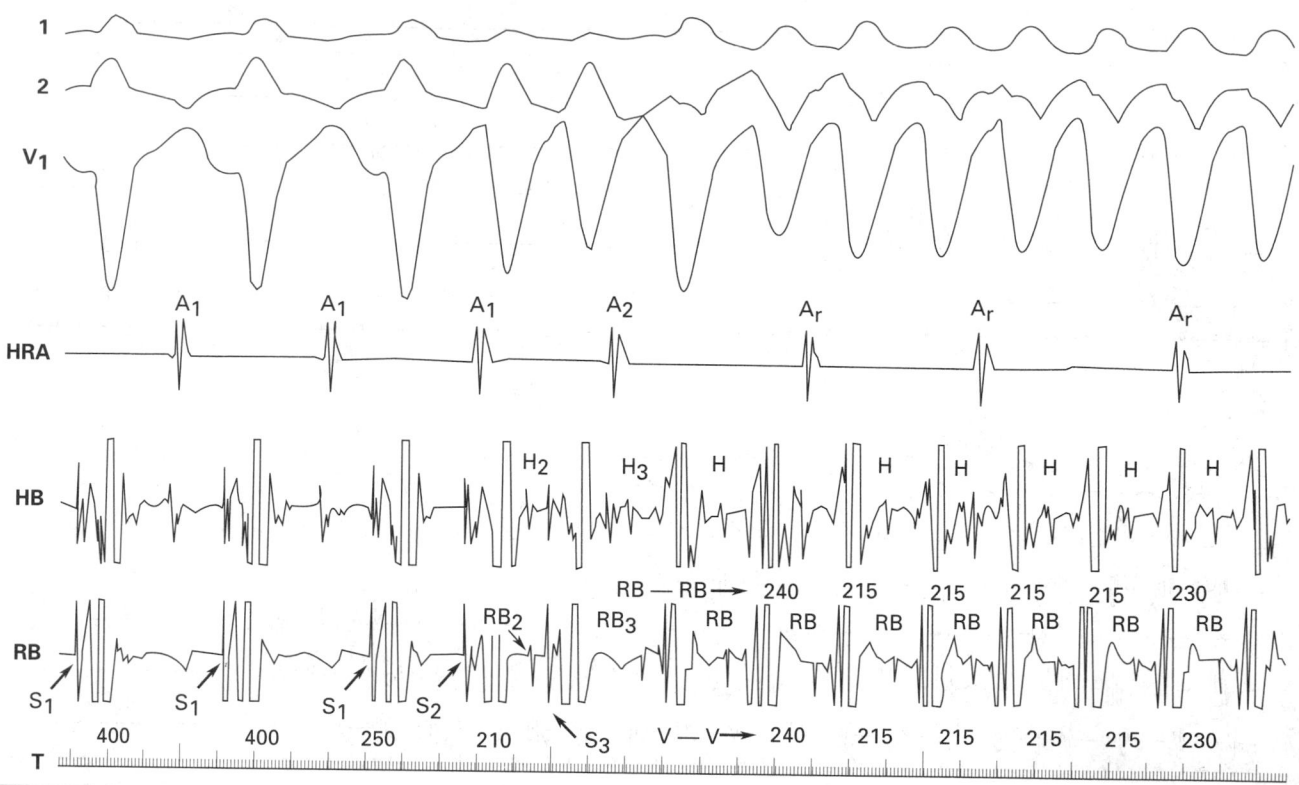

FIGURE 29-11

Induction of sustained VT due to bundle branch reentry (BBR). The surface ECG and intracardiac tracings are labeled. Basic cycle length (S_1S_1) is 400 ms during ventricular pacing. Sustained BBR is induced with two extra stimuli (S_2S_3). Note that the His bundle and RB deflections precede the QRS, suggesting supraventricular tachycardia with aberrant conduction. However, there is 2:1 VA block, indicating the ventricular nature of this tachycardia.

Without HB/RB recordings, the diagnosis can be difficult and, consequently, the likelihood of inappropriate therapy will be high. RB-RB and V-V intervals are labeled. (From Jazayeri M, Sra J, Akhtar M. Wide QRS complexes: Electrophysiologic basis of a common electrocardiographic diagnosis. *J Cardiovasc Electrophysiol* 1992; 3:36–39. Reproduced with permission from the publisher and authors.)

Pharmacologic Therapy

It is arguable whether or not the assessment of pharmacologic intervention is essential in patients with relatively benign cardiac arrhythmias. The clinical course can be observed to determine if control has been achieved. With life-threatening tachycardias, such as VT/VF, or with severe manifestations of cardiac arrhythmias, such as syncope or presyncope, it is desirable to assess efficacy of pharmacologic intervention. (Fig. 29-12).[33,34] The technique of drug testing has been developed whereby the elimination of inducibility of a given tachycardia is assessed following a drug administration. Both the drug efficacy and its lack can be evaluated using this method. When drug therapy does eliminate induction of a previously inducible tachycardia, the addition of isoproterenol will frequently demonstrate reversal of therapeutic drug effect.[35,36] This is helpful in considering additional beta-blocker therapy. The latter can be accomplished with ease in patients with good left ventricular function, whereas the addition of beta blockers may pose a problem in patients with VT and poor left ventricular function. Failure of serial drug testing is associated with a significant recurrence rate and a strong indication for nonpharmacologic intervention.

Recently, some controversy has arisen regarding the value of EPS for prediction of drug efficacy in comparison to ambulatory monitoring.[37] However, because of the infrequency of spontaneous VT/VF in most patients with life-threatening ventricular arrhythmias, ambulatory monitoring is an impractical method. EPS, when conducted appropriately, i.e., using aggressive and complete pacing protocols, remains the most effective means of directing patients into pharmacologic versus nonpharmacologic management strategies.

Nonpharmacologic Therapy

Nonpharmacologic intervention has become an integral part of patient management in cardiac arrhythmias. With documented cardiac arrest from VF, implantation of an automatic ICD is fairly common, and electrophysiologic assessment for such therapy is important, as was outlined above. Additional indications for study include documented VF or hypotensive VT and no inducible VT/VF, where no other forms of therapy can be rationally prescribed and implantation of an ICD is the obvious choice.[38] Subsequent to the implantation of an ICD, postoperative testing for the efficacy of detection and termination of VT or VF by the device also requires electrophysiologic assessment. With newer devices, antitachycardia function, low-energy cardioversion, and cardiac defibrillation

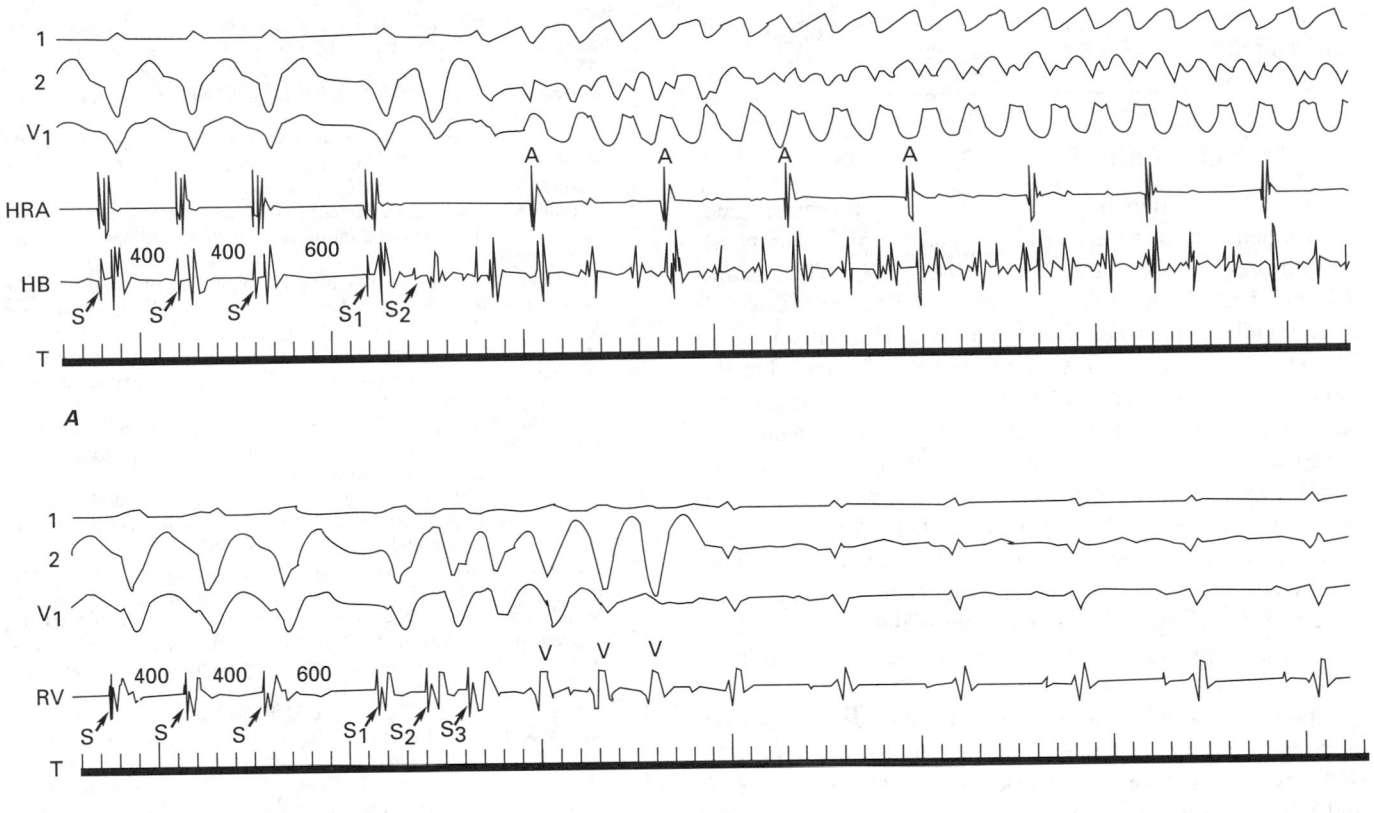

FIGURE 29-12

A. Control. B. Post PA + mexiletine. Initiation of sustained monomorphic VT of myocardial origin is shown in A. After oral procainamide and mexiletine, the sustained VT could not be induced despite using a more aggressive pacing protocol.

can be programmed. When problems are encountered following discharge of a patient with an ICD, electrophysiologic reassessment is frequently necessary both for reprogramming and for the detection of any unexplained events. Most of the newer devices permit a noninvasive initiation and termination of VT/VF and reprogramming. For assessment of other electrophysiologic parameters (e.g., AV conduction, SVTs), however, transvenous catheterization may be necessary.

Patients with coronary artery disease and mappable VT are also candidates for VT surgery.[39–41] Preoperative EPS assessment for this possibility is important if coronary artery bypass surgery, aneurysm resection, or both are being contemplated. Surgery for VT in the form of endocardial resection or cryoablation can be performed very effectively and relatively safely in patients with a left ventricular ejection fraction greater than 20 percent. This curative procedure will provide effective control in approximately 75 percent of the patients who have monomorphic VT that can be appropriately mapped.

Surgery for SVT has gone through a significant evolution. The introduction of catheter ablative techniques has made it rare for patients to undergo surgery for Wolff-Parkinson-White syndrome and/or AV nodal reentrant tachycardia. Some individuals with resistant atrial fibrillation and flutter and those

who fail catheter ablative therapy may still be considered candidates for such a procedure, but this is now becoming exceedingly rare.

CATHETER ABLATION TECHNIQUES[42–46]

The realization that many sites of origin of VT and SVT can be effectively mapped has made the catheter ablative technique a rational approach. The radiofrequency form of energy delivered through a catheter has permitted controlled trauma to cardiac tissue to abolish or modify reentrant circuits. This is true for both SVT and VT. Unifocal atrial tachycardia, AV nodal reentry of all varieties, and accessory pathways including atriofascicular fibers can be cured in over 90 percent of patients with radiofrequency catheter ablation. Among the VTs, bundle branch reentrant tachycardia seen in association with dilated cardiomyopathy (both ischemic and nonischemic) is an ideal substrate for catheter ablation. Patients with monomorphic VT associated with myocardial scarring or other substrates can also be considered candidates, particularly when they are not suitable for VT surgery and have failed drug therapy. Additionally, in patients with incessant VT or frequency VT with inadequate control despite ICD therapy,

VT ablation should be considered. In all of these patient subsets, initial EPS evaluation is crucial.

IATROGENIC PROBLEMS ENCOUNTERED DURING EPS

Mechanical irritation from catheters during placement and even when not being manipulated can cause a variety of arrhythmias and conduction disturbances.[38] These include induction of atrial, junctional, and ventricular ectopic beats and right bundle branch block and thus AV block in the His-Purkinje system in patients with preexisting left bundle branch block during right ventricular catheterization.[47] Obviously, AV block in the His-Purkinje system can occur in patients with preexisting right bundle branch block during left ventricular catheterization. Ventricular stimulation can also occur from physical movement of the ventricular catheter coincident with atrial contraction, producing electrocardiographic patterns of ventricular preexcitation. Recognition of all these iatrogenic patterns is important for avoiding misinterpretation of electrophysiologic phenomena and the significance of findings in the laboratory.

Certain types of arrhythmias must be avoided at all costs, such as atrial and ventricular fibrillation. Atrial fibrillation will obviously not permit study of any other form of SVT, and VF will require prompt cardioversion, making it difficult to continue the EPS. If atrial fibrillation must be initiated for diagnostic purposes (i.e., to assess ventricular response over the accessory pathway in Wolff-Parkinson-White syndrome), it should be done at the end of the study. Patients with a prior history of atrial fibrillation are more prone to the occurrence of sustained atrial fibrillation in the laboratory. Frequently, this will occur during initial placement of catheters, and excessive manipulation of catheters in the atria should therefore be avoided.

Risks and Complications

The complication rate is relatively low when only right heart catheterization is done, with almost negligible mortality.[48,49] Other complications include deep venous thrombosis, pulmonary embolism, infection at catheter sites, systemic infection, pneumothorax, and perforation of a cardiac chamber or coronary sinus. The occurrence of potentially lethal arrhythmias such as rapid VT or VF is common in the laboratory. These are not necessarily counted as complications, however, but are often expected and anticipated events. Nonetheless, the common occurrence of these events makes the electrophysiology laboratory a place for only highly trained personnel equipped to handle such problems.

REFERENCES

1. Scherlag BJ, Lau SH, Helfant RH, Berkowitz WD, Stein E, Damato AN. Catheter technique for recording His bundle activity in man. *Circulation* 1969; 39:13–18.
2. Goldreyer BN, Bigger JT. Spontaneous and induced reentrant tachycardia. *Ann Intern Med* 1969; 70:87–98.
3. Mandel WJ, Hayakawa H, Danzig R, Marcus HS. Evaluation of sino-atrial node function in man by overdrive suppression. *Circulation* 1971; 44:59–66.
4. Narula OS, Samet P, Javier RP. Significance of the sinus node recovery time. *Circulation* 1972; 45:140–158.
5. Damato AN, Lau SH, Helfant RH, Stein E, Patton RD, Scherlag BJ, et al. A study of heart block in man using His bundle recordings. *Circulation* 1969; 39:297–305.
6. Narula OS, Scherlag BJ, Samet P, Javier RP. Atrioventricular block: Localization and classification by His bundle recordings. *Am J Med* 1971; 50:146–165.
7. Goldreyer BN, Damato AN. The essential role of atrioventricular conduction delay in the initiation of paroxysmal supraventricular tachycardia. *Circulation* 1971; 43:679–687.
8. Wellens HJJ, Schuilenberg RM, Durrer D. Electrical stimulation of the heart in patients with the Wolff-Parkinson-White syndrome type A. *Circulation* 1971; 43:99–114.
9. Mason JW, Winkel RA. Electrode catheter arrhythmia induction in the selection and assessment of antiarrhythmic drug therapy for recurrent ventricular tachycardia. *Circulation* 1978; 58:971–985.
10. Ruskin JN, DiMarco JP, Garan H. Out of hospital cardiac arrest: Electrophysiologic observations in selection of long-term antiarrhythmic therapy. *N Engl J Med* 1980; 303:607–613.
11. Akhtar M. Invasive cardiac electrophysiologic studies: An introduction. In: Parmley WW, Chatterjee K, eds. *Cardiology*, vol 1: *Physiology, Pharmacology, Diagnosis*. Philadelphia: Lippincott; 1991:1–17.
12. Josephson ME, Harken PH, Horowitz LN. Endocardial excision: A new surgical technique for the treatment of recurrent ventricular tachycardia. *Circulation* 1979; 60:1430–1439.
13. Fann JI, Loeb JM, LoCicero J III, et al. Endocardial activation mapping and endocardial pace-mapping using a balloon apparatus. *Am J Cardiol* 1985; 55:1076.
14. Mickleborough LL, Harris L, Downar E, et al. A new intraoperative approach for endocardial mapping of ventricular tachycardia. *J Thorac Cardiovasc Surg* 1988; 95:271.
15. Brugada P, Green M, Abdollah H, Wellens HJ. Significance of ventricular arrhythmias initiated by programmed ventricular stimulation: The importance of the type of ventricular arrhythmia induced and the number of premature stimuli required. *Circulation* 1984; 69:87–92.
16. Avitall B, McKinnie J, Jazayeri M, Akhtar M, Tchou P. Induction of ventricular fibrillation versus monomorphic ventricular tachycardia during programmed stimulation: Role of premature beat conduction delay. *Circulation* 1992; 85:1271–1278.
17. Akhtar M. Clinical application of electrophysiologic studies in the management of patients requiring pacemaker therapy. In: Barold S, ed. *Modern Cardiac Pacing*. Mount Kisco, NY: Futura; 1985:3–17.
18. Hariman RJ, Krongrad E, Boxer RA, Weiss MB, Steeg CN, Hoffman BF. Method for recording electrical activity of the sinoatrial node and automatic atrial foci during cardiac catheterization in human subjects. *Am J Cardiol* 1980; 45:775–781.
19. Gomes JA. The sick sinus syndrome and evaluation of the patient with sinus node disorders. In: Parmley WW, Chatterjee K, eds. *Cardiology*, vol 1: *Physiology, Pharmacology, Diagnosis*. Philadelphia: Lippincott; 1991:1–15.
20. Sra JS, Jazayeri MR, Avitall B, Dhala A, Deshpande S, Blanck Z, et al. Comparison of cardiac pacing with drug therapy in the treatment of neurocardiogenic (vasovagal) syncope with bradycardia or asystole. *N Engl J Med* 1993; 328:1085–1090.
21. Dhingra RC, Wyndham CRC, Bauernfiend R, Swiryn S, Deedwania PC, Smith T, et al. Significance of block distal to the His bundle induced by atrial pacing in patients with chronic bifascicular block. *Circulation* 1979; 60:1455–1464.
22. Akhtar M, Jazayeri M, Avitall B, McKinnie J, Tchou P. Electrophysiologic spectrum of wide QRS complex tachycardia. In: Zipes DP, Jalife J, eds. *Cardiac Electrophysiology: From Cell to Bedside*. Orlando, FL: Saunders; 1990:635–646.
23. Sra J, Anderson A, Sheikh S, Avitall B, Tchou P, Troup P, et al. Unexplained syncope evaluated by electrophysiologic studies and head-up tilt testing. *Ann Intern Med* 1991; 114:1013–1019.
24. DiMarco JP, Garan H, Ruskin JN. Cardiac electrophysiologic techniques in recurrent syncope of unknown cause. *Ann Intern Med* 1981; 95:542–548.
25. Akhtar M, Shenasa M, Denker S, Gilbert CJ, Rizwi N. Role of cardiac electrophysiologic studies in patients with unexplained recurrent syncope. *Pacing Clin Electrophysiol* 1983; 6:192–201.

26. Morady F, Scheinman MM. The role and limitations of electrophysiologic testing in patients with unexplained syncope. *Int J Cardiol* 1983; 4:229–234.

27. Teichman SL, Felder DS, Matos JA, Kim SG, Waspe LE, Fisher, JD. The value of electrophysiologic studies in syncope of undetermined origin: Report of 150 cases. *Am Heart J* 1985; 110:469–479.

28. Moazez F, Peter T, Simonson J, Mandel WJ, Vaughn C, Gang E. Syncope of unknown origin: Clinical noninvasive and electrophysiologic determinants of arrhythmia induction and symptom recurrence during longterm follow-up. *AHJ* 1991; 121:81 88.

29. Akhtar M, Garan H, Lehmann MH, Troup PJ. Sudden cardiac death: Management of high-risk patients. *Ann Intern Med* 1991; 114:499–512.

30. Ruskin JN, DiMarco JP, Garan H. Out-of-hospital cardiac arrest: Electrophysiologic observations and selection of long-term antiarrhythmic therapy. *N Engl J Med* 1980; 303:607–612.

31. Morady F, Scheinman MM, Hess DS, Sung RJ, Shen E, Shapiro W. Electrophysiologic testing in the management of survivors of out-of-hospital arrest. *Am J Cardiol* 1983; 51:85–89.

32. Wu D, Wyndham CR, Denes P, Amat-y-Leon F, Miller RH, Dhingra RC, et al. Chronic electrophysiological study in patients with recurrent paroxysmal tachycardia: A new method for developing successful oral antiarrhythmic therapy. In: Kulbertus HE, ed. *Reentrant Arrhythmias*. Baltimore: University Park Press; 1976:294.

33. Horowitz LN, Josephson ME, Farshidi A, Spielman SR, Michelson EL, Greenspan AM. Recurrent sustained ventricular tachycardia: Role of the electrophysiologic study in selection of antiarrhythmic regimens. *Circulation* 1978; 58:986–997.

34. Mason JW, Winkle RA. Accuracy of ventricular tachycardia induction study for predicting long term efficacy and inefficacy of antiarrhythmic drugs. *N Engl J Med* 1980; 303:1073–1077.

35. Niazi I, Naccarelli G, Dougherty A, Rinkenberger R, Tchou P, Akhtar M. Treatment of atrioventricular node reentrant tachycardia with encainide: Reversal of drug effect with isoproterenol. *J Am Coll Cardiol* 1989; 13:904–910.

36. Jazayeri M, Van Wyhe G, Avitall B, McKinnie J, Tchou P, Akhtar M. Isoproterenol reversal of antiarrhythmic effects in patients with inducible sustained ventricular tachyarrhythmias. *J Am Coll Cardiol* 1989; 14:705–711.

37. Mason JW. A comparison of electrophysiologic testing with Holter monitoring to predict antiarrhythmic-drug efficacy for ventricular tachyarrhythmias. *N Engl J Med* 1993; 329:445–451.

38. Akhtar M, Avitall B, Jazayeri M, Tchou P, Troup P, Sra J, et al. Role of implantable cardioverter defibrillator therapy in the management of high risk patients. *Circulation* 1992; 85(suppl I):I131–I139.

39. Josephson ME, Harken AH, Horowitz LN. Long-term results of endocardial resection from sustained ventricular tachycardia in coronary disease patients. *Am Heart J* 1982; 104:51–57.

40. Caceres J, Werner P, Jazayeri M, Akhtar M, Tchou P. Efficacy of cryosurgery alone for refractory monomorphic sustained ventricular tachycardia due to inferior wall infarct. *J Am Coll Cardiol* 1988; 11:1254–1259.

41. Caceres J, Akhtar M, Werner P, Jazayeri M, McKinnie J, Avitall B, et al. Cryoablation of refractory sustained ventricular tachycardia due to coronary artery disease. *Am J Cardiol* 1989; 63:296–300.

42. Jackman WM, Wang X, Friday KJ, Roman CA, Moulton KP, Beckman KJ, et al. Catheter ablation of accessory atrioventricular pathways (Wolff-Parkinson-White syndrome) by radiofrequency current. *N Engl J Med* 1991; 324:1605–1611.

43. Calkins H, Sousa J, El-Atassi R, Rosenheck S, de Buitleir M, Kou WH, et al. Diagnosis and cure of the Wolff-Parkinson-White syndrome or paroxysmal supraventricular tachycardias during a single electrophysiologic test. *N Engl J Med* 1991; 324:1612–1618.

44. Jazayeri M, Hempe SL, Sra JS, Dhala AA, Blanck Z, Deshpande SS, et al. Selective transcatheter ablation of the fast and slow pathways using radiofrequency energy in patients with atrioventricular nodal reentrant tachycardia. *Circulation* 1992; 85:1318–1328.

45. Saoudi N, Atallah G, Kirkorian G, Touboul P. Catheter ablation of the atrial myocardium in human type I atrial flutter. *Circulation* 1990; 81:762–771.

46. Klein LS, Shih HT, Hackett FK, Zipes DP, Miles WM. Radiofrequency catheter ablation of ventricular tachycardia in patients without structural heart disease. *Circulation* 1992; 85:1666–1674.

47. Akhtar M, Damato AN, Gilbert-Leeds CJ, Batsford WP, Reddy CP, Gomes JA, et al. Induction of iatrogenic electrocardiographic patterns during electrophysiologic studies. *Circulation* 1977; 56:60–65.

48. Di Marco JP, Garan H, Ruskin JN. Complications in patients undergoing cardiac electrophysiologic procedures. *Ann Intern Med* 1982; 97:490–493.

49. Horowitz L. Risks and complications of clinical cardiac electrophysiologic studies: A prospective analysis of 1000 consecutive patients. *J Am Coll Cardiol* 1987; 9:1261–1268.

30

ANTIARRHYTHMIC DRUGS

Raymond L. Woosley

Antiarrhythmic drugs have been developed with the expectation that they would extend and improve life for many patients with cardiovascular disease and those with a history of life-threatening arrhythmias. Their usefulness, however, has been limited by ineffectiveness and/or toxicity. In mortality trials, benefit has not been seen and worsened mortality has been observed with some drugs. Care must be taken, therefore, in deciding the mode of treatment, or in fact whether or not to treat at all. Many antiarrhythmic agents are available today or under development; however, the need for so many is an indication that no agent is completely effective for all patients and that every agent has the potential for inducing serious adverse effects. In fact, drug selection is often empiric; however, the side-effect profiles of the available drugs are very different and are often the determining factor in drug selection. Known side effects may completely eliminate the use of certain classes of drugs for a specific patient. Because of the narrow margin between effective and potentially toxic dosages, it is essential that physicians be thoroughly familiar with the pharmacology, dosage, and adverse effects of any of these agents.

The use of antiarrhythmic drugs has been dramatically altered by the findings of the Cardiac Arrhythmia Suppression Trial (CAST).[1] This study was designed to test the hypothesis that suppression of asymptomatic ventricular arrhythmias in patients with recent myocardial infarction would reduce mortality from cardiac arrest and/or arrhythmic sudden death. Prior to the CAST, antiarrhythmic drugs were prescribed for these patients to suppress asymptomatic arrhythmias and thus improve mortality. Based on the results of a feasibility and planning trial of the Cardiac Arrhythmia Pilot Study (CAPS), the CAST evaluated encainide, flecainide, and moricizine because they were all tolerated and had reasonable ability to suppress symptomatic ventricular arrhythmias. In April 1989, the CAST was interrupted by the Data Safety and Monitoring Committee, and encainide and flecainide were removed because they had been found to increase mortality two- to three-fold. The CAST II continued to evaluate the remaining drug,

moricizine. However, the CAST II was also terminated prematurely in August 1991 when it became apparent that moricizine was producing a similar trend toward harm and there was no reasonable chance that a beneficial effect on mortality could be detected.[2] These results shocked the medical community but have influenced thinking in this and many other areas of medicine. Hine et al.[3] reported a meta-analysis of the CAST and similar studies with sodium channel blocking antiarrhythmic drugs and found overall support for the conclusion of the CAST. The CAST has also led to recommendations by the Food and Drug Administration (FDA) for more restrictive labeling for all sodium channel blocking antiarrhythmic drugs. In 1991, these drugs were given class labeling with indications for the treatment of documented ventricular arrhythmias that, in the judgment of the physician, are life threatening. Exceptions are quinidine and flecainide, both of which have an indication for supraventricular arrhythmias.

Because of discouraging results with sodium channel blocking drugs, drugs that prolong the action potential (often termed class III) have been studied. Developers had been encouraged since one drug with this action, amiodarone, may improve mortality in patients with prior myocardial infarction.[4] Dofetilide, ibutilide, and the *d*-isomer of sotalol all prolong the action potential duration and were developed in the hope that they would have the efficacy of amiodarone but lack its propensity to cause serious side effects. But, the first of these drugs to be evaluated in a mortality trial, *d*-sotalol, has been found to increase mortality after myocardial infarction.[5] Clearly these are the most complex drugs in clinical use today and require care in their use.

CLASSIFICATION OF ANTIARRHYTHMIC DRUGS

Antiarrhythmic drugs are often classified according to their electrophysiologic effects.[6] The scheme most often described was originally proposed by Vaughan Williams as a classification of drug actions that should be antiarrhythmic, not a classification of drugs.[6] This is a subtle but important distinction that is made for the following reasons:

- Most antiarrhythmic drugs have multiple actions, hence their pharmacology is more complex than indicated by a simple drug classification scheme.
- The actions of a given drug differ in different cardiac tissues.
- Many antiarrhythmic agents have pharmacologically active metabolites whose activity may be quite different from and in a class other than that of the parent compound.
- The relative amounts of these metabolites produced is genetically determined for several of these drugs and often varies extensively within the population.

Drugs having class I action possess "local anesthetic," or "membrane-stabilizing," activity. Their predominant action is to block the fast inward sodium channel. This produces a decrease in the maximum depolarization rate, V_{max}, of the action potential (phase 0) and slows intracardiac conduction. These agents have been further subclassified as belonging to class IA, IB, or IC on the basis of their effects on specific aspects of intracardiac conduction and refractoriness.[7] Drugs having class IA action include quinidine, procainamide, and disopyramide. These agents also produce measurable increases in ventricular refractoriness and prolongation of the QT interval. Lidocaine, mexiletine, and tocainide have actions belonging to class IB. Their potency for blocking sodium channels is only moderate, and in isolated tissues, they shorten the action potential duration (APD) and refractoriness. They generally exert little effect on PR, QRS, or QT intervals. Drugs with class IC actions are the newer, more potent agents: flecainide and propafenone. Because these are potent sodium channel inhibitors, slowing conduction velocity while having little effect on repolarization, they increase the PR and QRS intervals but cause little change in QT.

Class II action refers to beta-adrenergic antagonism, possessed by agents such as propranolol, timolol, and metoprolol. While these drugs are effective for treatment of supraventricular arrhythmias and tachyarrhythmias secondary to excessive sympathetic activity, they are not very effective in the treatment of severe arrhythmias, such as recurrent ventricular tachycardia. Although the mechanism is unknown, they are the only drugs found effective in preventing sudden cardiac death in patients with prior myocardial infarction.

Drugs whose predominant effect is to prolong the duration of the cardiac action potential and refractoriness have class III action, e.g., amiodarone, sotalol, bretylium, ibutilide, and N-acetylprocainamide (NAPA), the major metabolite of procainamide.

Class IV action is calcium channel antagonism. Drugs with this action include verapamil, bepridil, diltiazem, and nifedipine.

Because of the many limitations of the Vaughan Williams classification of antiarrhythmic drugs, a new approach has been proposed,[8] termed the *Sicilian gambit*. This classification system is based on the differential effects of antiarrhythmic drugs on (1) channels, (2) receptors, and (3) transmembrane pumps. The grouping is based primarily on the predominant action of drugs but also considers the other ancillary actions that may be clinically relevant. As shown in Fig. 30-1, because of the sequence of drugs listed, the symbols for these primary actions are aligned diagonally. For example, in this system quinidine is a sodium channel antagonist (moderate time constant for recovery from block) with potassium channel- and alpha-blocking activity. This provides a more complete and accurate description of the pharmacologic actions of the drugs than simply "class IA." When combined with an understanding of the electrophysiologic role of these actions, one can predict the effects likely to occur in vivo. In this case one would expect conduction slowing, increased APD (and refractoriness), and vasodilation to result from these three actions of quinidine.

The Sicilian gambit also creates a framework in which newly discovered actions of drugs can be readily added. While it emphasizes the multiple actions of drugs and the subtle differences and similarities that exist, it is more complete than the simple grouping in the Vaughan Williams classification. At present, our understanding of the pharmacology of these drugs has progressed to the point that the Vaughan Williams "shorthand" is an oversimplification that can be misleading. The increased detail of the new system reflects the current state of our knowledge at a level necessary for optimal use of these drugs.

Due to the low efficacy of any one agent, the treatment of acute or chronic ventricular arrhythmias frequently necessitates the use of multiple drugs, sequentially or in combination. One may produce increased sodium channel blockade and, hopefully, increase drug efficacy by using combinations of drugs with different kinetics of interaction with the sodium channel. Basic to these considerations is an understanding of the regulation of sodium channel function. Hodgkin and Huxley[9] proposed that sodium channels exist in three distinct states: open, closed, and inactivated. According to the modulated receptor theory of cardiac sodium channel regulation proposed by Hille and by Hondeghem and Katzung,[10] sodium channels in each of these states have differing affinities for a given local anesthetic drug (Fig. 30-2).

The theory also provides a potential explanation for the phenomenon of "frequency," or "use," dependence. Use dependence is the increase in conduction block observed at an increasing rate of stimulation in response to sodium channel blocking antiarrhythmic agents. Since an increase in the rate of stimulation increases the number of sodium channels in the open and inactivated states, antiarrhythmic agents having greater affinity for activated (open) or inactivated channels (as opposed to rested channels) would have a greater opportunity to bind to the receptor and slow conduction. Therefore, greater block will occur during tachycardia, leaving less drug action at normal heart rates. Also, antiarrhythmic drugs have different affinities for the states of the sodium channel, and this is manifested as different rates for onset or recovery from block. Drugs that slowly associate with the receptor will cause block to accumulate over the first few cardiac cycles, such

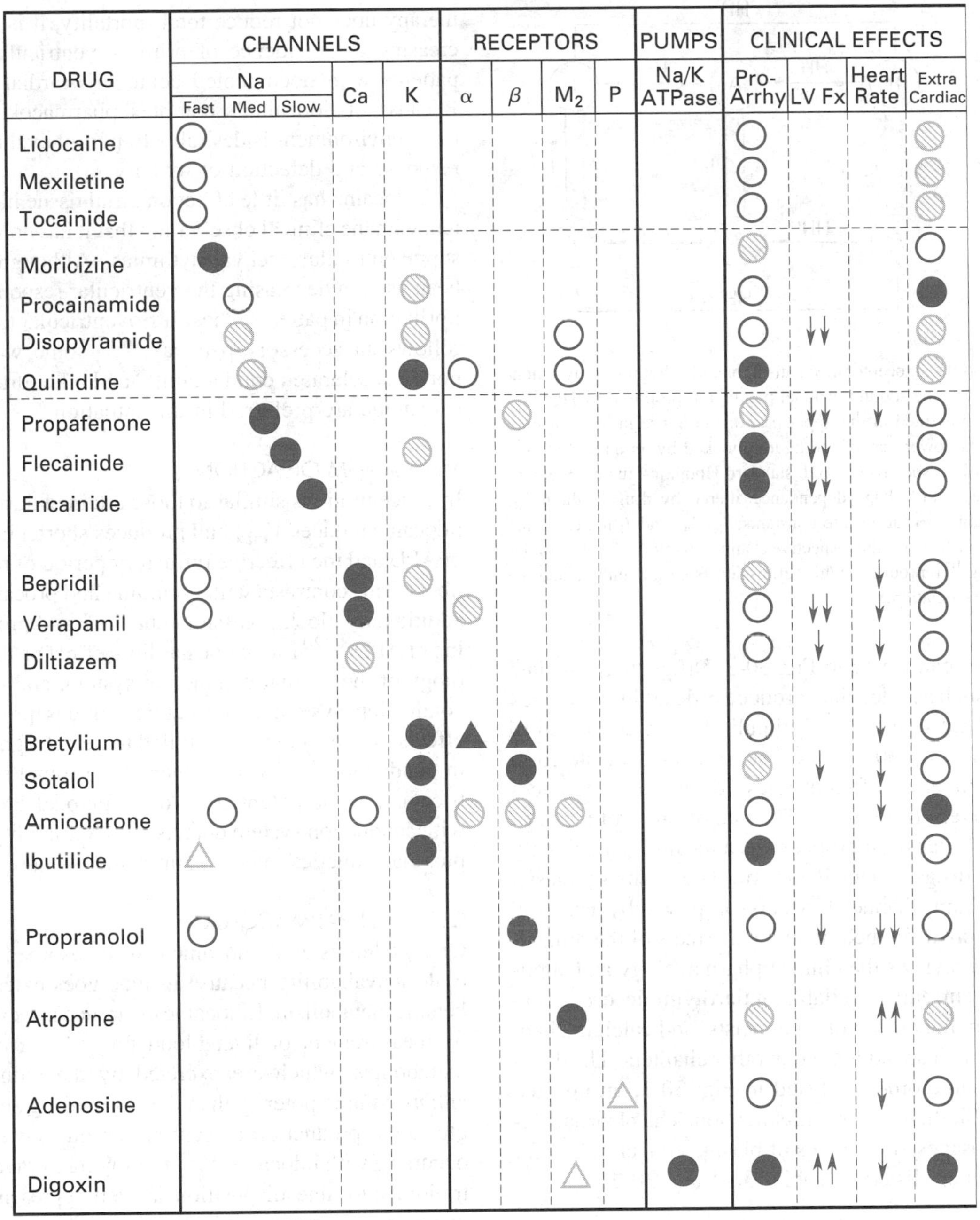

DRUG	CHANNELS — Na Fast	CHANNELS — Na Med	CHANNELS — Na Slow	CHANNELS — Ca	CHANNELS — K	RECEPTORS — α	RECEPTORS — β	RECEPTORS — M₂	RECEPTORS — P	PUMPS — Na/K ATPase	CLINICAL EFFECTS — Pro-Arrhy	CLINICAL EFFECTS — LV Fx	CLINICAL EFFECTS — Heart Rate	CLINICAL EFFECTS — Extra Cardiac
Lidocaine	○ low										○			▨
Mexiletine	○ low										○			▨
Tocainide	○ low										○			▨
Moricizine	● high										▨			○
Procainamide		○			▨						○			●
Disopyramide		▨			▨			○			○	↓↓		
Quinidine		▨			●	○		○			●			▨
Propafenone			●		▨		▨				▨	↓↓	↓	○
Flecainide			●		▨						●	↓↓		○
Encainide			●								●	↓↓		○
Bepridil	○			●	▨						▨		↓	○
Verapamil	○			●		▨					○	↓↓	↓	○
Diltiazem				▨							○		↓	○
Bretylium					●	▲	▲				▨		↓	○
Sotalol					●		●				▨	↓	↓	○
Amiodarone		○		○	●		▨	▨			○		↓	●
Ibutilide	△				●						●			○
Propranolol	○						●				○	↓	↓↓	○
Atropine								●			▨		↑↑	▨
Adenosine									△		○		↓	○
Digoxin								△		●	●	↑↑	↓	●

Symbol legend: ○ = low; ▨ = moderate; ● = high; △ = agonist; ▲ = agonist/antagonist.

FIGURE 30-1

Summary of the potentially most important actions of drugs on membrane channels, receptors, and ionic pumps in the heart. Listed are drugs used to modify cardiac rhythm. Most are marketed as antiarrhythmic agents. The drugs (rows) are ordered in a fashion similar to the columns so that generally the symbols for their predominant action(s) form a diagonal. Drugs with multiple actions (e.g., amiodarone) depart strikingly from the diagonal trend. The actions of drugs on the sodium, calcium, and potassium channels are indicated. Sodium channel blockade is subdivided into three groups of actions characterized by fast ($\leq$300 ms), medium (Med) (300–1500 ms), and slow ($\geq$1500 ms) time constants for recovery from block. This parameter is a measure of use dependence and predicts the likelihood that a drug will decrease conduction velocity of normal sodium-dependent tissues in the heart and perhaps the propensity of a drug for causing bundle branch block or proarrhythmia. Drug interaction with receptors α, β, M₂, and P (alpha- and beta-adrenergic, muscarinic subtype, and A₁ purinergic) and drug effects on the sodium-potassium pump (Na/K ATPase) are indicated. Filled circles indicate antagonist or inhibitory actions; open circles indicate direct or indirect acting agonists or stimulators. The darkness of the symbol increases with the intensity of the action. Filled triangles for bretylium indicate its biphasic action to initially stimulate α and β receptors by release of norepinephrine followed by subsequent block of norepinephrine release and indirect antagonism of these receptors. (Antagonist relative potency: ○, low; ▨, moderate; ●, high; △ = agonist; ▲ = agonist/antagonist.) (Adapted from the Task Force of the Working Group on Arrhythmias of the European Society of Cardiology,[8] with permission.)

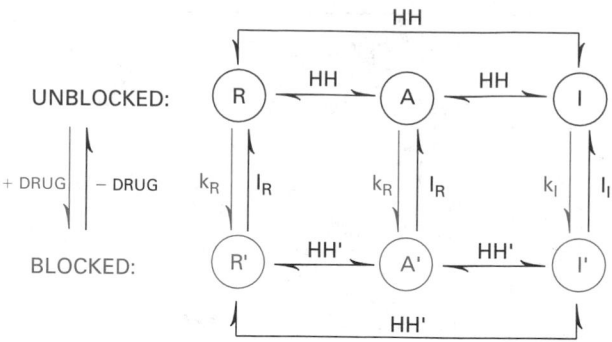

FIGURE 30-2

Diagram of the modulated receptor mechanism for antiarrhythmic drug action. The three fractions of the sodium channel population proposed by Hodgkin and Huxley are represented in the upper part of the figure in the drug-free condition and in the lower part of the figure, blocked by an antiarrhythmic agent (R', A', and I', respectively). HH, standard Hodgkin-Huxley rate constants; HH', same, with voltage dependence altered by drug binding; k_R, k_A, and k_I represent association rate constants; I_R, I_A, and I_I represent the dissociation rate constants for the respective channel fractions. (From Hondeghem and Katzung,[10] reproduced with permission from the authors and the American Heart Association.)

as shown for procainamide in Fig. 30-3. Drugs that associate more rapidly, such as lidocaine, produce little additional block after the first beat in a train of stimuli. This is compared to procainamide in Fig. 30-3. Likewise, drugs dissociate from the sodium channel at different rates, leading to differences in rates of recovery from block. The rate of onset of block of sodium channels has been proposed as a means to subclassify antiarrhythmic drugs.[11] This is the correlate of the subclassification of sodium channel blockers proposed by Harrison that was based on differences in clinical effects of the drugs.[7]

This chapter reviews the clinical pharmacology and applications of the currently available antiarrhythmic drugs, excluding digoxin, beta receptor antagonists, and calcium channel blockers, which are addressed in other chapters. The drugs appear in the same order as listed in Fig. 30-1, an updated revision of the Sicilian gambit classification. The pharmacokinetics, usual dosages, and ranges of plasma concentration for the major drugs are listed in Tables 30-1 and 30-2.

DRUGS

Lidocaine (Xylocaine)

CLINICAL APPLICATIONS

Lidocaine, introduced as a local anesthetic, was first used as an antiarrhythmic agent in the 1950s for the treatment of arrhythmias arising during cardiac catheterization.[12] It is the most widely used intravenous antiarrhythmic drug. Since extensive first-pass metabolism makes it unsatisfactory for oral use, congeners were developed that would possess similar sodium channel blocking actions and be active when taken orally.

Lidocaine is very often the drug of first choice for the acute suppression of ventricular arrhythmias. Although such

therapy does not reduce total mortality, it is effective in decreasing the incidence of primary ventricular fibrillation in patients with documented acute myocardial infarction.[13,14] Because of lidocaine's complex pharmacokinetics, a monitored environment is desirable to permit evaluation of patient response and detection of toxicity.

Lidocaine has little effect on atrial tissue in vitro,[15] consistent with the clinical observation that it has no value in treating supraventricular tachyarrhythmias. Although lidocaine has been used in decreasing the ventricular response during atrial fibrillation in patients whose atrioventricular (AV) conduction follows an accessory pathway,[16,17] some workers have reported accelerated conduction,[18] and other drugs such as procainamide are preferred in this situation.

MECHANISM OF ACTION

In concentrations similar to those attained during clinical use, lidocaine reduces $\dot{V}_{max}$ and produces shortening or no change in APD and the effective refractory period of normal Purkinje fibers. This contrasts with quinidine and procainamide, which additionally block potassium channels and produce lengthening of APD.[19,20] Lidocaine has little effect on the electrophysiology of the normal conduction system, and in patients with conduction system abnormalities, it has produced variable effects. Some studies have failed to detect significant changes in conduction,[21,22] while others have found slowing of ventricular rate or potentiation of infranodal block in patients with conduction system defects.[23,24] Variability in dosage and pharmacokinetics may explain some of these discrepancies.

CLINICAL PHARMACOLOGY

Orally administered lidocaine is well absorbed, but it has poor oral bioavailability because it undergoes extensive first-pass hepatic metabolism. Lidocaine clearance is well approximated by measurement of liver blood flow.[25,26] The two desethyl metabolites, which are excreted by the kidneys, have less antiarrhythmic potency than the parent drug and may contribute to the production of central nervous system side effects occurring with lidocaine.[27,28] Following intravenous administration, lidocaine disposition is well represented by a two-compartment pharmacokinetic model.[29] Since antiarrhythmic activity is correlated with lidocaine's concentration in the central compartment and the half-life of distribution out of this compartment is rapid (8 min), regimens employing a series of multiple loading doses and a maintenance infusion should be used to achieve and then maintain a therapeutic plasma and myocardial lidocaine concentration.

Regardless of the loading regimen employed, the lidocaine concentration eventually reaches steady state dependent only on drug infusion rate and its clearance. The time required to reach steady-state conditions is approximately 8 to 10 h in normal individuals and up to 20 to 24 h in some patients with heart failure and/or liver disease. This is longer than often anticipated because of the failure to recognize the relatively long elimination half-life (1.5 to 2 h in normal subjects and longer in patients with heart failure or hepatic disease).

DOSAGE
AND ADMINISTRATION

Lidocaine's primary use is for acute rapid suppression of ventricular arrhythmias. Single intravenous boluses will achieve only transient therapeutic effects because the drug is rapidly distributed out of the plasma and myocardium; therefore, multiple loading doses should be used in order to achieve more sustained therapeutic plasma levels of lidocaine rapidly. Based on pharmacokinetic models validated in clinical studies, several regimens have been designed to maintain a relatively constant therapeutic level. For a stable patient, a total loading dose of lidocaine should be approximately 3 to 4 mg per kilogram of body weight administered over 20 to 30 min. After injection of an initial dose of 1 mg/kg over 2 min, a series of three loading "boluses" can be administered slowly (50 mg each over 2 min) 8 to 10 min apart, while the patient is continuously observed for the development of side effects. Loading should be stopped should the usually transient, mild central nervous system side effects persist or serious unwanted effects occur.

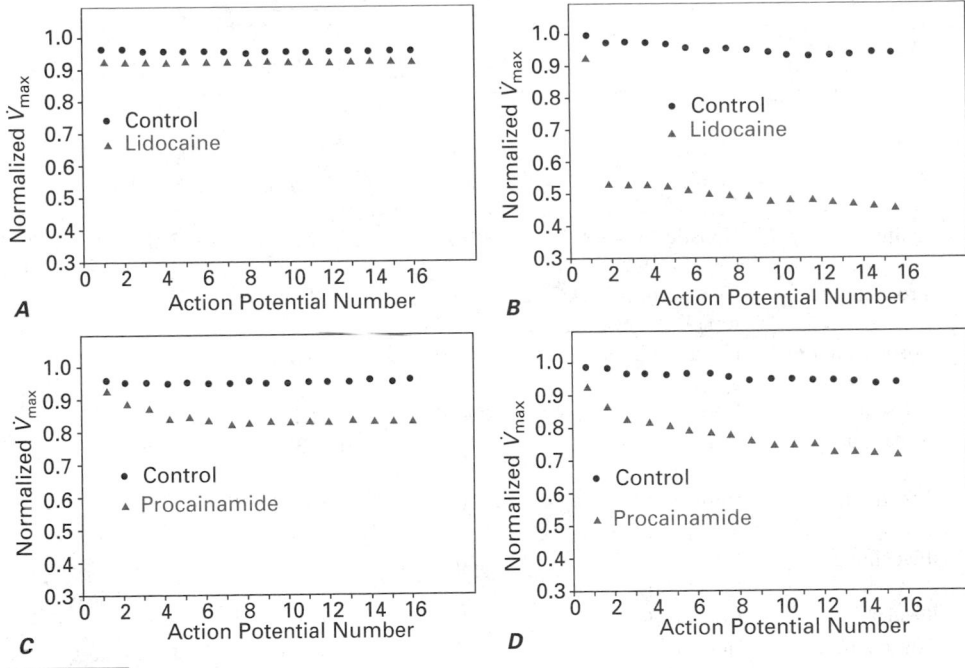

FIGURE 30-3

Rate- (interval-) dependent depression of $\dot{V}_{max}$ by lidocaine and procainamide. Following a 20-s rest period, a train of 16 action potentials was elicited using interstimulus intervals (ISIs) of 1 s or 200 ms, in the presence (triangles) or absence (squares) of lidocaine or procainamide. For the duration of the train, $\dot{V}_{max}$ was relatively constant when measured at either ISI in the absence of drug. In the presence of lidocaine (22 μM), stimulation at an ISI of 1 s (A) produced no use-dependent block. However, stimulation at 200 ms (B) produced a 50 percent reduction in $\dot{V}_{max}$ from baseline, which was first observed for the second action potential and was constant thereafter. A different pattern is seen in the presence of 276 μM procainamide, which produced a significant depression of $\dot{V}_{max}$ at an ISI of 1 s (C). This depression was more pronounced when the ISI was shortened to 200 ms (D). Unlike the case for lidocaine, the use-dependent depression of $\dot{V}_{max}$ due to procainamide required multiple action potentials to approach steady-state values. (From Ehring BR, Moyer JW, Hondeghem LM. Quantitative structure activity studies of antiarrhythmic properties in a series of lidocaine and procainamide derivatives. *J Pharmacol Exp Ther* 1989; 244:479–492. Reproduced with permission from the authors and publisher.)

Another effective and well-tolerated loading regimen was outlined by Wyman et al.[30] For a 75-kg person, an initial bolus of 75 mg was given, followed by 50 mg every 5 min to a total dose of 225 mg. This regimen usually achieves and maintains plasma concentrations within usual therapeutic guidelines (1.5 to 5 μg/mL). A priming dose of 75 mg followed by a loading infusion of 150 mg over 18 min has also been used successfully.[31] At the time of initiation of the loading regimen, a maintenance infusion, designed to replace ongoing losses due to drug elimination, should be started. This may be calculated as the product of the desired plasma concentration (about 3 μg/mL) and the expected clearance. This usually yields a dosage in the range of 20 to 60 μg per kilogram of body weight per minute.

Even in normal individuals, there is great variability in the peak plasma concentration and, consequently, in the calculated size of the central compartment for lidocaine. Therefore, during loading, the patient's electrocardiogram (ECG), blood pressure, and mental status should be monitored; the process should be stopped at the first sign of lidocaine excess. When symptomatic arrhythmias persist in the presence of documented adequate

dosage, defined by side effects or plasma concentration in excess of 5 to 7 μg/mL, another agent should be used.

If the maintenance infusion has reached steady state but the concentration is below the level needed to prevent recurrence and the arrhythmia reappears while side effects are absent, the appropriate actions are as follows: (1) obtain a plasma sample for measurement of lidocaine concentration for future reference, (2) administer a small bolus of lidocaine (25 to 50 mg), and (3) increase the maintenance infusion rate proportionally. The plasma concentration can be used to estimate clearance for calculation of the final maintenance infusion (i.e., clearance equals infusion rate divided by plasma concentration at steady state). Little therapeutic effect is evident at lidocaine plasma concentrations below 1.5 μg/mL, whereas the risk of toxicity increases above 5 μg/mL. In some patients, however, concentrations in the range of 5 to 9 μg/mL may be required for arrhythmia suppression and can safely be achieved with cautious drug administration.[32]

Once steady-state conditions have been achieved, simply terminating a lidocaine infusion will result in a gradual decline in plasma levels over the next 8 to 10 h as elimination occurs. Not only is there no reason to taper lidocaine infusions, but

TABLE 30-1

PHARMACOKINETICS OF ANTIARRHYTHMIC DRUGS

Agent	Inactivation or Elimination,[a] %	Protein Binding, %	V_D, L/kg	Elimination Half-life, h	Bioavailability, %	Apparent Oral Clearance, mL/min
Quinidine	Hepatic (50–90) Renal (10–30)	80–90	2.5	3–19	70	200–400
Procainamide	Hepatic (40–70)[b] Renal (30–60)	15	2	2–4	100	400–700
Disopyramide	Hepatic (20–30) Renal (40–50)	20–50	0.6	6–8	80–90	90
Lidocaine	Hepatic (90)	40–70	1.1	1.5–4	35[c]	700–1000[c]
Tocainide	Hepatic (30–40) Renal (40)	10	1.5–3	8–20	90	150–200
Mexiletine	Hepatic (85–90)[b] Renal (10–15)	70	5.5–9.5	8–20	90	400–700
Flecainide	Hepatic (70)[b] Renal (30)	40	7–10	7–26	90–95	200–800
Propafenone	Hepatic (99)[b]	90	3–4	2–24[b]	10–50[b]	800–5000[b]
Amiodarone	Hepatic (99)	95	20–200	13–103 days	20–80	6500–11,000
Bretylium	Renal (90)	Low	3–4	4–16	25[c]	1300

[a] Renal—elimination of unchanged drug.

[b] Dependent on metabolic phenotype (see text).

[c] Not recommended for oral administration.

TABLE 30-2

DOSAGE AND PLASMA CONCENTRATION RANGES FOR ANTIARRHYTHMIC AGENTS[a]

Agent	Usual Initial Dosage[b]	Modification of Dosage in Disease[c]	Dosage Range	Maximum Single Dose	Therapeutic Range,[d] µg/mL
Quinidine (sulfate)	200 mg q 6 h	None	800–2400 mg/day	600	0.7–5.5
Procainamide (sustained release)	500 mg q 6 h	↓ CHF ↓ RI	2000–6000 mg/day	1500	4–8
Disopyramide	100 mg q 6 h	↓ CHF ↓ HI ↓ RI	300–1200 mg/day	300	2–5
Lidocaine	See text	↓ CHF ↓ HI	1–4 mg/min IV	—	1.5–5
Tocainide	400 mg q 8 h	↓ HI ↓ RI	1200–2400 mg/day	800	4–10
Mexiletine	200 mg q 8 h	↓ CHF ↓ HI?	600–1200 mg/day	400	0.7–2
Flecainide	100 mg q 12 h	↓ CHF ↓ RI ↓ HI?	200–400 mg/day	200	0.2–1
Propafenone	150 mg q 8 h	See text	300–900 mg/day	300	0.5–3?
Amiodarone	600–1400 mg/day (load)	None	200–600 mg/day	600	1–2
Bretylium	See text	↓ RI	1–4 mg/min IV	—	—

[a] These are general guidelines only. Dosage should be determined for each patient based on clinical presentation, disease states, clinical response, and tolerance to the drug.

[b] Dosage usually recommended in absence of significant cardiac, renal, or hepatic failure.

[c] CHF, congestive heart failure; HI, hepatic insufficiency; RI, renal insufficiency. See text for details.

[d] The range of therapeutic plasma concentrations is a statistical range that should be considered only a guideline to therapy.

it may be dangerous if oral antiarrhythmic therapy is initiated since unpredictable additive effects may occur between lidocaine and newly started oral therapy. If a patient has reached steady-state equilibrium, it is possible to estimate when the plasma lidocaine concentration will fall below usually therapeutic levels. The plasma lidocaine concentration should be determined at the time the infusion is terminated, and the number of half-lives needed for that level to reach approximately 1.5 μg/mL are estimated from the following equation:

$t_{1/2}$ = plasma concentration $\times$ V_D $\times$ 0.693/infusion rate,

where V_D is the volume of distribution.

Plasma concentration and infusion are known components of the equation. V_D is usually 1.1 L/kg but may be reduced by half in heart failure.

MODIFICATION OF DOSAGE IN DISEASE STATES

Initial loading regimens require no adjustment in patients with renal or liver disease[29]; however, maintenance infusions must be decreased in liver disease and heart failure to compensate for decreased clearance. Since clearance alone is altered in liver disease with little change in the volume of distribution, the half-life of elimination is prolonged greatly (to almost 5 h) and steady-state conditions will not be achieved until 20 to 25 h following the institution of an intravenous infusion. Despite the fact that lidocaine metabolites are excreted by the kidneys, renal disease has not been reported to exert any significant effect on lidocaine dosing regimens. With mechanical ventilation, there is a decrease in cardiac output and hepatic blood flow and a decrease in lidocaine dosage is required.[33] Patients with congestive heart failure achieve lidocaine levels that are almost double those in normal individuals given the same dose.[29] Since the central volume of distribution is generally halved, loading doses should be reduced by 50 percent; since clearance is approximately halved, maintenance doses should be reduced proportionately from an infusion rate of 30 μg/mL per kilogram of body weight per minute used for normal patients to about half that figure. The time required to achieve steady-state conditions following the institution of a maintenance infusion is still 8 to 10 h in many patients because of concomitant changes in V_D and clearance, resulting in a half-life similar to that seen in patients without heart failure.

In summary, general recommendations for initial lidocaine dosage selection should be adjusted for each patient based on clinical presentation, clinical response, and the results of plasma level monitoring. Some patients with congestive heart failure may experience toxicity when given an infusion of 0.5 mg/mL, so that blood level monitoring is essential for proper dosage adjustment.

In postmyocardial infarction patients receiving lidocaine infusions for more than 24 h, plasma lidocaine levels can increase and the elimination phase half-life can increase up to 50 percent.[34] This increase is due, in part, to changes occurring in protein binding of lidocaine during the first few days of therapy. Assays for plasma lidocaine measure the sum of both protein-bound and free lidocaine as total lidocaine and thus do not give a true picture of the amount of free drug

available. An increase in plasma lidocaine occurring at this time often reflects an elevation in plasma levels of alpha-1-acid glycoprotein (AAG), to which it binds,[35] and does not always indicate an increase in free, active drug. In this case, the lidocaine dosage should not be reduced to compensate for the higher total plasma concentration as long as the patient displays no adverse effects. Subsequent decreases in AAG concentrations will result in an apparent decrease in plasma lidocaine, which may reflect a drop in only that fraction bound to AAG.

ADVERSE REACTIONS

Central nervous system symptoms are the most frequent side effects of lidocaine administration. A rapid bolus can induce seizures. With more gradual attainment of excessive levels, drowsiness, dysarthria, and dysesthesia may occur. Excessive lidocaine can also cause coma, which is a consideration in postcardiac arrest, and can depress cardiac function, decrease lidocaine clearance, and produce an even greater increase in lidocaine concentrations. Advanced degrees of sinus node dysfunction have been reported in isolated instances.[36,37] In patients with conduction abnormalities below the AV node, lidocaine should be administered cautiously, if at all, unless a temporary pacemaker is readily available.

DRUG INTERACTIONS

An additive or synergistic depression of myocardial function or conduction may occur during combined therapy using lidocaine with other antiarrhythmic agents,[38] especially during conversion from lidocaine to another antiarrhythmic agent. A pharmacokinetic drug interaction between propranolol and lidocaine has been described experimentally and in humans in which beta-adrenergic blockade caused a decrease in cardiac output and liver blood flow with a resultant decreased lidocaine clearance.[39,40] Cimetidine has been reported to decrease lidocaine's volume of distribution, decrease splanchnic (and hence liver) blood flow, and inhibit the enzymes responsible for lidocaine metabolism. This may raise lidocaine plasma concentrations, and both loading and maintenance dosages may require downward adjustment in patients receiving cimetidine.[41]

Mexiletine (Mexitil)

CLINICAL APPLICATIONS

Mexiletine is used in the treatment of ventricular arrhythmias and has, on occasion, been effective in treating arrhythmias that were refractory to several other agents. Success rates vary between 6 and 60 percent, and more than half of the studies suggest limited efficacy (less than 20 percent).[42] Mexiletine does not prolong the QT interval and, therefore, can be useful with a history of torsades de pointes or long QT syndrome when quinidine, sotalol, procainamide, or disopyramide are contraindicated. While the rate of response to mexiletine when used alone is low, it has been combined successfully with quinidine,[42] propranolol,[43] or procainamide.[44] This mode of therapy takes advantage of the additive, and perhaps synergistic, antiarrhythmic response produced by the combination of these agents. Lower than usual dosages of both agents can be used so that dosage-related adverse effects are reduced concomitantly.

DESCRIPTION

Mexiletine is an orally active lidocaine congener with class IB sodium channel blocking activity and structural similarity to tocainide. It was originally developed as an anorexiant and anticonvulsant agent, and its antiarrhythmic properties were only later recognized. Mexiletine exerts minimal effects on both hemodynamics and myocardial contractility, even in patients with severe congestive heart failure.[45]

MECHANISM OF ACTION

Mexiletine has class IB action and blocks fast sodium channels, decreasing $\dot{V}_{max}$ and shortening the repolarization phase of ventricular myocardium.[46,47]

CLINICAL PHARMACOLOGY

Mexiletine's systemic bioavailability approximates 90 percent,[48] with a large volume of distribution (5.5 to 9.5 L/kg), reflecting extensive tissue uptake. About 1 percent of total body content of mexiletine is in the plasma compartment, with approximately 70 percent of this bound to serum proteins. Mexiletine has little first-pass metabolism but is eliminated primarily by hepatic metabolism, with only 10 to 15 percent being excreted unchanged in the urine.[49,50] Its half-life of elimination is between 8 and 20 h (9 and 12 h for healthy subjects), with the time needed to reach steady state ranging between 1 and 3 days.[51] Mexiletine undergoes extensive hepatic metabolism by CYP2D6[49,52] and, consequently, clearance is extremely variable (see below).

DOSAGE AND ADMINISTRATION

Mexiletine therapy should be initiated with a low dosage, which is increased at 2- to 3-day intervals until efficacy or intolerable side effects such as tremor or other central nervous system symptoms develop. With normal renal function, the recommended initial oral mexiletine dosage is 200 mg every 8 h. As with most drugs having extensive liver metabolism, clearance will be widely variable within the population. This is especially true for mexiletine because CYP2D6, responsible for its metabolism, is missing in 7 percent of the Caucasian population. Also, consideration of dosage adjustment to compensate for the action of agents (discussed below) that induce or inhibit hepatic mexiletine metabolism is required.

MODIFICATION OF DOSAGE IN DISEASE STATES

Patients with renal failure who also inherit a deficiency of hepatic CYP2D6 are likely to have extremely slow elimination for mexiletine,[53] and for this reason, all renal failure patients should be given low initial doses. Elimination half-life and clearance may be prolonged by overt congestive heart failure[54] and hepatic failure,[55] and dosage reduction is required.

ADVERSE REACTIONS

Adverse reactions to mexiletine are dose-related and neurologic and include tremor, visual blurring, dizziness, dysphoria, and nausea. Thrombocytopenia has been reported to occur infrequently with mexiletine therapy,[56,57] and a positive antinuclear antibody test occurs rarely. Severe bradycardia and abnormal prolongation of sinus node recovery time have been reported in patients with the sick-sinus syndrome,[58] and at high concentrations, worsening of heart block has been reported.[59] Oral mexiletine does not depress ventricular function or induce increased heart failure,[60,61] although intravenous mexiletine, which is not available in the United States, has been noted to increase congestive heart failure.[62]

DRUG INTERACTIONS

Mexiletine's hepatic metabolism can be increased by phenobarbital, phenytoin (Dilantin), or rifampicin, which will reduce the half-life of mexiletine, possibly reducing an effective dose to an ineffective one.[51,63,64] Conversely, if treatment with an inducing agent is stopped, an effective dose may become toxic.

In one study, mexiletine decreased the clearance and increased the plasma concentrations of theophylline.[65] Quinidine inhibits the CYP2D6 enzyme partially responsible for mexiletine clearance, and plasma concentration of mexiletine may increase in those individuals who have the enzyme (93 percent of Caucasians).

Procainamide (Pronestyl-SR, Procan-SR)

CLINICAL APPLICATIONS

Procainamide, like quinidine, is effective against both supraventricular and ventricular arrhythmias.[66,67] Although the two drugs have similar electrophysiologic effects, they are clinically different, and one agent may be effective for a patient when the other is not. Procainamide is useful in acute management of patients with reentrant supraventricular tachycardia and atrial fibrillation and flutter associated with Wolff-Parkinson-White syndrome.[68–71]

Although lidocaine is more often used, procainamide is also used intravenously to suppress ventricular arrhythmias occurring immediately following myocardial infarction or to convert sustained ventricular tachycardia. Since it takes approximately 20 min to administer a loading dose of procainamide safely, its use is limited to those situations where adequate time is available. Its advantage over lidocaine is the potential for conversion to oral therapy using the same agent. Lidocaine is usually used, however, because the initial loading dose can be given within a 2- to 5-min period.

The active metabolite of procainamide, *N*-acetylprocainamide (acecainide, NAPA), was investigated as an antiarrhythmic drug. It has been shown to be effective in the treatment of ventricular arrhythmias, but its use is limited by a narrow therapeutic index.[70,71]

DESCRIPTION

The development of procainamide as an antiarrhythmic agent resulted from a systematic search for a useful congener of procaine, whose use was precluded by adverse reactions.[72] NAPA, the major metabolite of procainamide, produces antiarrhythmic activity in some patients, although not always those who respond to procainamide.[70] This is most likely due to the drug's very different electrophysiologic actions.[73] Since procainamide is an effective agent but is not without adverse effects, it has served as a prototype for development of several of the newer antiarrhythmic agents.

MECHANISM OF ACTION

Like other agents demonstrating class I activity, procainamide slows conduction and decreases automaticity and excitability of atrial and ventricular myocardium and Purkinje fibers.[74] Because of its effect on potassium channels, it also prolongs APD and refractoriness. Compared to quinidine, procainamide has very little vagolytic activity and does not prolong the QT interval to as great an extent.[66] NAPA has predominantly class III antiarrhythmic activity; it prolongs APD and refractoriness in both atrial and ventricular myocardium and prolongs the QT interval.[69,75] It has little or no effect on $\dot{V}_{max}$, in either Purkinje fibers or ventricular cells, and does not alter His-Purkinje conduction velocity because of its very low potency as a sodium channel antagonist.

CLINICAL PHARMACOLOGY

Procainamide is rapidly absorbed and 100 percent orally bioavailable. About 15 percent of procainamide is bound to serum proteins. Procainamide's short half-life of elimination of 2 to 4 h in patients with normal renal function necessitates dosing every 3 to 6 h. Dosing every 6 to 8 h is possible with sustained-release preparations.

Slightly more than half of the general population are phenotypic rapid acetylators of procainamide and quickly convert it to NAPA, a metabolite with very pure class III antiarrhythmic action.[70] As would be expected, however, the response to one agent does not predict response to the other. When each is given as the sole agent, the usually effective plasma concentration is 4 to 8 μg/mL for procainamide and 7 to 15 μg/mL for NAPA.[70] During oral procainamide therapy, both agents are present in variable amounts, and there is no way to determine the contribution of NAPA to arrhythmia suppression under these conditions. Consequently, the utility of measuring plasma levels of procainamide during chronic therapy is limited because of this variable hepatic conversion to NAPA. Monitoring plasma concentrations for determination of compliance or prevention of toxicity is feasible and recommended (see below).

DOSAGE AND ADMINISTRATION

Procainamide is available for either intravenous or oral use. With normal renal and cardiac function, the initial recommended oral maintenance dose is 50 mg/kg per day. Frequent administration is required for oral procainamide, which is inconvenient and makes compliance difficult. A sustained-release form of procainamide is available, which permits dosing every 6 to 8 h. During chronic therapy, levels of NAPA

may accumulate to effective or toxic levels in some individuals, resulting in achievement of maximum pharmacologic effect long after the time procainamide itself reaches steady state.[70,76] Therefore, the elimination half-life for procainamide may be misleading as a predictor of time to the occurrence of stable pharmacologic action. Thus, dosage should be initiated at conservative levels, and the patient should be monitored carefully until both procainamide and its metabolite reach steady state. The plasma concentration of procainamide usually associated with an antiarrhythmic effect is from 4 to 8 μg/mL.[70] Patients with ventricular tachycardia may need higher levels for prevention of induction by programmed stimulation,[77] although such dosage frequently leads to adverse effects. Since the electrophysiological effects of procainamide and NAPA are quite different, monitoring of patients receiving procainamide should at some point include measurement of plasma concentrations of both agents to determine their relative concentrations. Patients who are rapid acetylators or who have impaired renal function have plasma concentrations of NAPA higher than procainamide. These individuals should be monitored for excessive accumulation of NAPA during dose titration to maintain plasma levels below 20 μg/mL. The practice of using the sum of the plasma concentration of procainamide and NAPA is not recommended (see above).

When administered intravenously, procainamide can be given as a constant 25-min loading infusion of 275 μg/min per kilogram of body weight or by a series of doses ($\leq$100 mg delivered over 3 min) given every 5 min, up to a total dose of 1 g.[78,79] If the loading infusion is well tolerated with no hypotension and less than 25 percent QRS or QT widening, a maintenance intravenous infusion of 20 to 60 μg/kg per minute can then be given. Larger and more rapid loading infusions of 1 g over 15 to 20 min have been given in the electrophysiology laboratory to prevent induction of ventricular tachycardia by programmed ventricular stimulation. A second loading infusion of 0.5 to 1 g has been given in some instances where an initial loading infusion was well tolerated but ineffective. These large dosages are accompanied by a higher incidence of hypotension and conduction disturbance and often result in attainment of unacceptably high plasma concentration.

MODIFICATION OF DOSAGE IN DISEASE STATES

With renal dysfunction or a low cardiac output, both procainamide and NAPA in usual doses may accumulate to potentially toxic levels and the dose should be reduced.[80]

Increased plasma levels of procainamide and/or NAPA may occur with congestive heart failure because of decreased urinary excretion and hydrolysis of procainamide.[81] On the other hand, one study of procainamide pharmacokinetics following a single intravenous bolus revealed no difference in volume of distribution, clearance, elimination half-life, unbound drug fraction, and peak procainamide concentrations between patients with congestive heart failure and normal individuals.[82] Although intravenous procainamide does depress myocardial contractility and lower blood pressure, worsening of heart failure is uncommon during oral therapy when the usual dosages and plasma concentrations are maintained.

ADVERSE REACTIONS

Side effects associated with long-term procainamide therapy limit its usefulness. Up to 40 percent of patients discontinue therapy in the first 6 months due to adverse reactions. The potential exists for arrhythmia aggravation, including the development of torsades de pointes due to procainamide or, more often, NAPA.[83,84] Therefore, just as with all agents possessing class IA activity, procainamide should not be used in patients with a long QT syndrome, a history of torsades de pointes, or hypokalemia.[85] In order to reduce the occurrence of proarrhythmia, potassium levels should be maintained above 4 meq/L when taking procainamide.

Between 15 and 20 percent of patients receiving procainamide develop a lupus-like syndrome, which is often difficult to recognize but regresses with discontinuation of treatment. The syndrome begins insidiously as mild arthralgia but usually progresses to frank arthritis, fever, malar erythematous rash, and pleural and/or pericardial effusions, with serum antibodies against nucleoprotein (histone) appearing as antinuclear antibodies with a "smooth" or "diffuse" pattern. These symptoms abate if procainamide is discontinued and generally resolve at a rate proportional to their duration.

Almost all patients treated chronically develop detectable antinuclear antibodies, but only 15 to 20 percent develop symptoms of the lupus syndrome. Therefore, it is unnecessary to discontinue therapy solely because of the positive antinuclear antibody titer. The patient should be fully informed of the symptoms, which should be reported, so therapy can be discontinued at the earliest symptoms or signs of the lupus syndrome. Continuing procainamide after the development of the early symptoms of the lupus syndrome is dangerous because of the above-noted possibility of pleural effusion and potentially lethal pericardial tamponade.[86]

More recently, procainamide therapy has been associated with the development of agranulocytosis. It has been suggested, but not proven, that the sustained-release form of the drug may be especially capable of inducing this toxicity.[87] The manufacturer recommends that a white blood count be obtained every 2 weeks for the first 3 months. Heart block and sinus node dysfunction can occur in patients with preexisting conduction system abnormalities.[88]

DRUG INTERACTIONS

Unlike quinidine, procainamide does not cause an increase in digoxin levels. There are few reports of interactions between procainamide and other drugs. Its clearance is reduced between 30 and 50 percent by cimetidine, which blocks the renal tubular secretion of procainamide.[89,90] A similar competition has been found between procainamide and its predominant metabolite, NAPA.[76] Ranitidine affects procainamide pharmacokinetics by reducing both its renal clearance and its absorption, the former by 14 to 23 percent and the latter by 10 to 24 percent, depending on the dose.[91]

Disopyramide (Norpace)

CLINICAL APPLICATIONS

Disopyramide is effective against a broad range of supraventricular and ventricular arrhythmias, its antiarrhythmic profile being similar to that of quinidine and procainamide.

DESCRIPTION

Disopyramide has class IA action and, in contrast to quinidine and procainamide, is better suited for long-term therapy, having relatively little associated chronic toxicity. While newer than quinidine or procainamide, disopyramide is still one of the older antiarrhythmic agents, having been in use in the United States since 1977. Its negative inotropic and anticholinergic actions occur frequently and limit its usefulness.

MECHANISMS OF ACTION

Disopyramide's antiarrhythmic effects are predominantly those associated with sodium and potassium channel blockade. Its effects are similar to those of quinidine and procainamide on automaticity, conduction, and refractoriness in atrial and ventricular tissue.[92–94]

CLINICAL PHARMACOLOGY

Disopyramide's oral bioavailability is 80 to 90 percent.[95] Its half-life of elimination, usually 6 to 8 h, is lengthened to as much as 15 h in cardiac patients.[96] About half of the compound is eliminated by the kidneys unchanged, and the remainder as an active metabolite, resulting from hepatic N-dealkylation.[97–99] Protein binding of disopyramide is complex, with between 20 and 50 percent of disopyramide being bound to plasma proteins. For most drugs, the percentage bound to plasma protein is a constant over the usual range of therapeutic concentrations. The saturation of disopyramide-binding sites on plasma proteins means that there are disproportionate increases in levels of free drug in plasma compared to the magnitude of dosage increment.[97,100]

DOSAGE AND ADMINISTRATION

Loading doses are not recommended with disopyramide. The usually effective dosage for disopyramide is 100 to 400 mg three to four times daily, to a maximal dose of 800 mg/day. Therapy should be very carefully titrated, beginning with low doses and allowing ample time for achievement of steady-state equilibrium.

While rapid fluctuations in plasma concentration are undesirable, they are difficult to avoid because of disopyramide's saturable protein binding. The controlled-release form of disopyramide may be useful in reducing adverse effects by decreasing fluctuations in the concentration of free disopyramide in plasma.[101] Because of saturable protein binding,[15] the generally accepted therapeutic range for total disopyramide in plasma of 2 to 5 μg/mL should not be strictly relied on. While monitoring the plasma concentrations of free disopyramide has been recommended,[102] the range of concentrations associated with arrhythmia suppression has not been clearly delineated and overlaps with that causing adverse effects.

MODIFICATION OF DOSAGE IN DISEASE STATES

Patient response to disopyramide should be monitored especially closely following acute myocardial infarction because both the absorption and elimination of disopyramide are decreased at this time.[103,104] In fact, in view of disopyramide's negative inotropic actions and changes in levels of binding proteins in plasma following a myocardial infarction, other antiarrhythmic agents should be considered first.

Disopyramide is contraindicated in patients with uncompensated heart failure because it can worsen failure.[105] The initial dosage of disopyramide should be reduced to 50 to 100 mg every 12 h in patients with renal insufficiency[96] or decreased hepatic function.[106]

ADVERSE REACTIONS

The predominant side effects of disopyramide include new or worsened congestive heart failure and symptoms resulting from dose-related anticholinergic actions, including urinary retention, constipation, dry mouth, and esophageal reflux.[107] Because of this anticholinergic action, patients with obstructive uropathy or glaucoma should not receive this agent.[107] For some patients, the anticholinergic side effects can be prevented or alleviated by concomitant use of cholinesterase inhibitors such as physostigmine and neostigmine without reduction in antiarrhythmic efficacy.[108] As with all agents that prolong repolarization, disopyramide should not be used in patients with long QT syndrome, hypokalemia, or a history of torsades de pointes[109] because of the potential for arrhythmia aggravation. Direct actions of disopyramide on the sinus node can lead to excessive bradycardia in patients with sinus nodal dysfunction,[110] and this may contribute to development of torsades de pointes in patients with hypokalemia.[111]

DRUG INTERACTIONS

Disopyramide does not increase digoxin levels,[112] and the effects of warfarin are not potentiated by disopyramide.[113] Phenytoin, rifampicin, and phenobarbital induce hepatic metabolism of disopyramide, thus increasing its elimination and potentially leading to loss of antiarrhythmic effect.[114–116] Significant depression of myocardial contractility may result from the combined administration of disopyramide with beta-adrenergic or calcium channel antagonists and should be avoided in patients with severe impairment of ventricular function.[117]

Quinidine

CLINICAL APPLICATIONS

Quinidine has been used successfully for a variety of supraventricular and ventricular arrhythmias, including conversion of atrial fibrillation or flutter,[118,119] supraventricular tachycardia,[66,120] ventricular extrasystoles,[121–123] and ventricular tachycardia and fibrillation.[124,125] On the other hand, a

grouped analysis of six small placebo-controlled trials in patients with atrial fibrillation showed a statistically significant increase in mortality for the patients treated with quinidine.[126] Because of the similarity to the results in the CAST and CAST II, one must assume that the results of this meta-analysis are valid until a definitive prospective study is available.

DESCRIPTION

Quinidine is one of the most widely used antiarrhythmic agents in the United States, being effective in the treatment of a variety of supraventricular and ventricular arrhythmias. A great deal of controversy exists over its use and whether or not it should ever be initially prescribed to outpatients. This concern is reflected in the current labeling for quinidine products and all other antiarrhythmic drugs in which initiation of therapy in the hospital is recommended.

MECHANISM OF ACTION

Quinidine has multiple actions, but the action thought by many to be primarily responsible for its efficacy is block of the rapid inward sodium channel. This results in a decrease in V_{max} of the action potential upstroke and slowed conduction, more marked in the His-Purkinje system than in the atria. Quinidine's effects on sodium channels are greatest at increased heart rate and less negative membrane potential, i.e., they are pH-, rate-, and voltage-dependent. Dose-related changes in the ECG are increases in PR, QRS, and QT_c intervals, which reflect quinidine's multiple actions.[127]

CLINICAL PHARMACOLOGY

Quinidine's effective dosage varies among individuals because of several factors. Although quinidine sulfate is usually administered every 6 h, there is wide variation in its elimination half-life of 3 to 19 h.[128] Plasma protein binding also varies widely, ranging from 50 to 95 percent.[128] Oral bioavailability is approximately 70 percent, and oral clearance ranges from 200 to 400 mL/min. Quinidine is inactivated or eliminated by both hepatic metabolism (50 to 90 percent) and renal elimination (10 to 30 percent). Several potentially active metabolites are formed in amounts that vary among individuals,[129] but for most, their clinical role has not been determined. One of quinidine's metabolites, 3-hydroxyquinidine, has been shown to possess antiarrhythmic activity when given to humans.[129] Experimental data indicate some contribution by metabolites of quinidine to its antiarrhythmic action.[130–132]

DOSAGE AND ADMINISTRATION

Quinidine therapy (as the sulfate) is usually initiated with an oral dosage of 200 mg every 6 h, and the dosage is carefully titrated every 3 or more days. Elderly patients often require lower dosages of quinidine because of both reduced clearance and volume of distribution. Quinidine is available commercially in at least three different forms: quinidine sulfate, gluconate, and polygalacturonate. Since the quinidine content varies among these at 83, 62, and 60 percent, respectively, the need for dosage adjustment should be considered if one form is substituted for another. The usually effective dosage of quinidine sulfate ranges from 800 to 2400 mg/day, with the maximum recommended single dose being 600 mg. Because the half-life varies from 3 to 19 h, one should wait 2 to 4 days between dosage increases to prevent unexpected drug accumulation. The range of therapeutic plasma concentrations measured using assays that differentiate quinidine from its metabolites is 0.7 to 5.5 μg/mL.[133,134] Rapid escalation in quinidine dosage has been used to convert atrial fibrillation, but this therapy is no longer recommended because of unnecessary toxicity.

Intravenous therapy with quinidine is usually avoided if alternatives are feasible. Vasodilation and hypotension result from quinidine-induced alpha-adrenergic blockade. If quinidine is given intravenously (as quinidine gluconate), the patient should be carefully monitored and the infusion rate should be no greater than 16 mg/min. This should be discontinued if hypotension is observed or the QRS is prolonged by more than 30 percent.

MODIFICATION OF DOSAGE IN DISEASE STATES

No adjustment in initial dosage is usually needed for patients with renal or hepatic disease,[135,136] although due to decreased protein binding in patients with hepatic failure, lower than usual total plasma concentration can produce toxicity.[137] Slower dose titration is advisable to permit attainment of steady state and accumulation of active metabolites; however, because the usual range of effective dosages is wide, dosage for these patients is not markedly different. Patients with rapid quinidine elimination may require higher dosages (up to 600 mg every 6 h). This is often due to induction of hepatic metabolism caused by other drugs.

Patients with congenital long QT syndrome, hypokalemia, or a history of torsades de pointes[138] should not be given quinidine because of their increased risk for this form of proarrhythmic event. For patients with congestive heart failure, problems associated with use of quinidine are proarrhythmia and digitalis (either digitoxin or digoxin) toxicity. Prudent use of quinidine in these individuals requires the following: (1) that titration begin at a reduced dosage; (2) that dosage of any cardiac glycoside being administered concomitantly be reduced; and (3) that plasma electrolyte levels, especially potassium, be maintained above 4 meq/L.

Although quinidine does possess some direct negative inotropic effects, these are usually counteracted by its vasodilatory effect; therefore, oral quinidine appears to be well tolerated hemodynamically when given at dosages producing usual plasma concentrations, even in patients with reduced ventricular function.[139] In a study of over 650 patients, 35 percent of whom had congestive heart failure, quinidine therapy resulted in no induction or worsening of congestive heart failure.[140] On the other hand, a significant problem for patients with congestive heart failure receiving quinidine therapy is proarrhythmia, with quinidine-induced torsades de pointes being potentiated in the setting of bradycardia and low serum levels of magnesium or potassium.[111,141]

ADVERSE REACTIONS

Marked prolongation of the QT interval has been seen in some patients receiving low or usual dosages of quinidine, and the risk of torsades de pointes is markedly increased. This arrhythmia may be responsible for quinidine syncope, which occurs in as many as 5 to 10 percent of patients within the first days of quinidine treatment, and for quinidine-induced sudden death.[142] Torsades de pointes usually occurs in patients (females > males) with low serum concentrations of quinidine, hypokalemia, poor ventricular function, and bradycardia.[142,143] In a recent study by Drici et al., dihydrotestosterone reduced the sensitivity to quinidine's effects on the QT interval in animals.[144] This study indicated that sex hormones have direct effects on cardiac tissue that may be responsible for the difference in the incidence of torsades de pointes in men and women.[144]

For patients who develop torsades de pointes, treatment with pacing or isoproterenol is very effective. Magnesium sulfate injection has also been recommended as initial therapy for torsades de pointes, although controlled trials are not available. These measures should also include correction of hypokalemia. Clinically, it is essential to distinguish torsades de pointes from polymorphic ventricular tachycardia occurring in the setting of a normal QT interval, because the latter should be treated with local anesthetic antiarrhythmic drugs and may be worsened by the above treatment for torsades de pointes.

Since quinidine acts via alpha-adrenergic blockade to produce vasodilatation,[145] hypotension may occur, especially in patients concomitantly receiving nitrates or other vasodilators. Other adverse effects include a high incidence of diarrhea and vomiting, tinnitus at high plasma levels, rare thrombocytopenia,[146] and, in unusual cases, conduction block in patients with existing conduction system disease.[140] In patients treated with quinidine for atrial flutter without prior AV nodal blockade by digitalis,* there have been reports of sudden increases in AV conduction and rapid ventricular rates.[145] This results from a slight reduction of the flutter rate and enhanced AV nodal conduction due to quinidine's anticholinergic effects. This permits 1:1 conduction through the AV node, often at 200 to 250 beats per minute. This may be of particular concern for patients receiving other drugs that increase conduction through the AV node, such as beta-adrenergic agonists.

DRUG INTERACTIONS

Quinidine metabolism is inhibited by cimetidine[147] and induced by phenytoin, phenobarbital,[148] and rifampicin,[146] with the latter agents leading to reduced, often subtherapeutic, quinidine concentrations.

Clinical digoxin toxicity has been described in 20 to 40 percent of patients receiving quinidine and digoxin concurrently.[147] The magnitude of this interaction is dependent on quinidine dosage, and in some patients it may not appear until

---

* Digitalis is used in the treatment of atrial fibrillation, atrial flutter, and other arrhythmias. This important drug is discussed in Chap. 23.

the dosage is increased to higher levels.[149,150] The rise in digoxin levels appears with the first dose of quinidine; therefore, it is suggested that digoxin dosage be halved when quinidine therapy is initiated. A similar interaction has been reported for quinidine and digitoxin.

Quinidine is a potent inhibitor of the hepatic cytochrome P450 specific for debrisoquine metabolism (CYP2D6),[151–153] although it is not metabolized by this specific P450 isozyme.[154,155] Thus, it may interfere with the biotransformation and actions of pharmacologic agents dependent on this cytochrome for their metabolism, which include propafenone, mexiletine, flecainide, metoprolol, timolol, sparteine, and bufuralol.[156] Quinidine worsens neuromuscular blockade in patients with myasthenia gravis[157] and may prolong the effects of succinylcholine.[158]

Propafenone (Rythmol)

CLINICAL APPLICATIONS

Propafenone was developed in Germany, where it has been marketed since 1977. It is similar to other antiarrhythmic agents in overall efficacy and patient tolerance. It has a role in the treatment of many types of arrhythmias, including supraventricular arrhythmias.[159]

CLINICAL PHARMACOLOGY

Propafenone has been described as having class IC antiarrhythmic activity because of its potent ability to slow conduction velocity with little change in APD.[160,161] It has a marked structural similarity to propranolol, and studies have shown that propafenone can accumulate during continued administration to levels capable of producing clinically significant beta-adrenergic inhibition.[162,163]

Propafenone, like mexiletine and flecainide, is eliminated by a metabolic pathway that has a polymorphic pattern of inheritance. Patients deficient in CYP2D6 activity, which is responsible for the metabolism of debrisoquine, encainide, metoprolol, timolol, flecainide, mexiletine, sparteine, and many other drugs, have very slow elimination of propafenone and fail to form measurable quantities of the potentially active metabolite, 5-hydroxypropafenone.[164] The accumulation of high concentrations of propafenone leads to significant beta-receptor antagonism at both low and high dosages in poor metabolizers but only at high dosages in extensive metabolizers of propafenone.[165] Although metabolic phenotype does not seem to dramatically influence the antiarrhythmic response to propafenone,[164] it clearly influences the degree of beta blockade occurring during therapy.

DOSAGE AND ADMINISTRATION

Effective dosages range from 300 to 900 mg/day in two to four divided dosages. In order to prevent unexpected accumulation of pharmacologic action, propafenone dosage should not be changed more frequently than every 3 days; there is slow elimination of the parent drug in poor metabolizers, and

there is slow accumulation of the metabolite(s) in extensive metabolizers.

Patients with reduced ventricular function, especially those receiving propafenone, should be carefully monitored for deterioration in ventricular function, which may result from beta-adrenergic receptor antagonism and/or the direct negative inotropic effect.[166]

MODIFICATION OF DOSAGE IN DISEASE STATES

Dosage recommendations for patients with cardiac, renal, or hepatic dysfunction are not yet available.

DRUG INTERACTIONS

It is very likely that there will be drug interactions between propafenone and other agents that utilize or inhibit cytochrome CYP2D6 for their metabolism. Such an interaction has been documented already between propafenone and metoprolol[167] and should be expected with timolol, many antidepressants, many neuroleptics, and perhaps other agents. Quinidine, which inhibits this cytochrome, inhibits the formation of 5-hydroxypropafenone in extensive metabolizers[168]; however, the clinical consequence of such inhibition is unknown and difficult to predict. One would expect greater beta blockade to occur after combining quinidine with propafenone therapy because of the resulting higher propafenone concentrations.

Flecainide (Tambocor)

CLINICAL APPLICATIONS

Flecainide is very effective in suppressing a variety of ventricular and supraventricular tachycardias.[169,170] The finding of increased mortality when flecainide is given to patients with ischemic heart disease has led to restricted usage (see above); however, there has been no evidence to indicate that this increase in mortality is seen when flecainide is given to treat supraventricular arrhythmias in patients without known coronary artery disease.[171] Overall, the antiarrhythmic response to flecainide in patients with symptomatic life-threatening ventricular arrhythmias is not markedly better than with older agents such as quinidine or procainamide.[169,172] Although it is far better tolerated than older agents, its negative inotropic actions restrict its use to patients having moderately well-preserved ventricular function. Likewise, its potential to increase mortality in patients with ischemic heart disease limits its usefulness.

DESCRIPTION

Flecainide has sodium channel blocking activity and is considered to have class IC actions. It has also been found to block the delayed rectifier potassium channel in feline ventricular myocytes, and this action may be clinically relevant.[173]

Flecainide slows intraventricular conduction velocity more than it prolongs effective refractory periods.[174] It prolongs AH and HV intervals and measurably increases PR and QRS intervals on the surface ECG at therapeutic doses. The QT_c interval is slightly increased, primarily due to prolongation of the QRS, but its ability to block the delayed rectifier may contribute to QT changes.

CLINICAL PHARMACOLOGY

The systemic bioavailability of oral flecainide is 90 to 95 percent,[175] and most of flecainide is metabolized in the liver to compounds that are not pharmacologically active at the concentrations usually found in plasma.[169] Flecainide, like many other antiarrhythmic agents, is metabolized by CYP2D6.[176] Because flecainide is also eliminated by the kidneys to a considerable extent, the enzyme deficiency has little effect on the pharmacokinetics of flecainide. If, however, those patients without the enzyme develop renal insufficiency or if renal patients are given a drug that blocks the metabolism, extremely high plasma concentrations are likely to occur.[177] A potential advantage of flecainide is its very slow elimination, with half-life ranging from 7 to 23 h in normal individuals and tending to be even longer (14 to 26 h) in patients with cardiac disease, even in the absence of heart failure.[175,178]

DOSAGE AND ADMINISTRATION

The usual dosage of flecainide for ventricular arrhythmias is 100 to 150 mg every 12 h in patients without cardiac or renal failure. A total daily dosage of more than 400 mg may sometimes be used under close medical monitoring (see below). Patients with supraventricular tachycardia are recommended to receive 50 mg every 12 h as a starting dose. The range of therapeutic plasma concentrations of flecainide is reported to be between 200 and 1000 ng/mL, although adverse effects may occur in some patients at concentrations within this range,[179,180] and many patients tolerate concentrations well above this range. To reduce the incidence of adverse effects, flecainide therapy should start with a low dosage that is maintained until steady state has been reached (at least 4 days) and altered relative to clinical response.

MODIFICATION OF DOSAGE IN DISEASE STATES

With cardiac failure, the usual initial dose is 50 to 100 mg every 12 h. Since 7 percent of Caucasian patients with renal failure will not have the CYP2D6 enzyme and because flecainide is usually eliminated by both metabolism and renal excretion, all patients with renal failure should be given very low dosages and titrated very carefully. Plasma concentration monitoring will be essential in patients with renal disease or cardiac or hepatic dysfunction. Any significant reduction in ejection fraction should be expected to lengthen elimination half-life and hence the time needed to attain steady-state equilibrium, while reductions in clearance may occur in renal or hepatic dysfunction and lead to higher plasma concentrations at steady state.

ADVERSE REACTIONS

Although aggravation of arrhythmias seen in the early days of flecainide's evaluation was often due to excessive initial doses and frequent dose increments, flecainide has a potential to induce proarrhythmic events, even when prescribed as recommended. This is especially true in patients with severe heart disease and if flecainide is given in higher dosages.[181] Because of its negative inotropic effects at dosages necessary to suppress arrhythmias, flecainide produces a measurable decrease in left ventricular function in most patients.[182,183] The increased mortality seen in the CAST seems to be confined to patients with structural heart disease.[171] A retrospective study of five multiple-dose efficacy trials showed that of patients with a history of congestive heart failure, oral flecainide precipitated heart failure in 15 percent.[184] A dose-related depression of myocardial performance was found after rapid (1 to 2 mg/kg) intravenous injections.[185]

Other side effects of flecainide include depression of sinus node activity in patients with preexisting sinus node dysfunction[186] and prolongation of QRS and PR intervals on the surface ECG. If below 25 percent, these effects do not necessarily indicate excessive dosage.

Flecainide increases pacing thresholds by as much as 200 percent and should therefore be used with caution in patients dependent upon pacemakers.[187,188] It also increases the threshold for electrical defibrillation, so patients with implanted devices should be evaluated carefully.[189]

DRUG INTERACTIONS

Cimetidine reduces flecainide clearance and prolongs flecainide elimination half-life.[190] Studies in normal volunteers have demonstrated an increase in the plasma concentrations of digoxin and propranolol when flecainide is coadministered.[191,192] Not unexpectedly, propranolol and flecainide have been found to have additive negative inotropic effects. An interaction with amiodarone, resulting in elevation of plasma flecainide concentration and necessitating reduction of flecainide dosage, has been described.[193]

Calcium Channel Blockers

Some calcium channel blockers are also used as antiarrhythmic agents.[194,195] Verapamil and diltiazem are useful in the management of supraventricular tachycardia, where they are administered to slow the ventricular rate in patients with atrial fibrillation or flutter and to treat and prevent AV nodal reentrant tachycardia. Intravenous diltiazem is useful for the temporary control of rapid ventricular rate during atrial fibrillation and flutter. In controlled clinical trials, conversion to sinus rhythm occurred with diltiazem and placebo with equal frequency (see also Chap. 54).

Bretylium (Bretylol)

CLINICAL APPLICATIONS

Bretylium is effective for acute therapy of ventricular tachycardia and/or ventricular fibrillation. Because it produces complex indirect effects via the autonomic nervous system, it should be reserved for patients who have failed to respond to lidocaine.

DESCRIPTION

Because of its sympatholytic activity, bretylium tosylate was first evaluated in the 1950s for the treatment of hypertension; however, a very high incidence of orthostatic hypotension and unreliable oral absorption led to its disfavor for chronic therapy. After its antiarrhythmic activity was discovered in animals,[196] it was eventually marketed in the United States as intravenous therapy for life-threatening ventricular arrhythmias. Bretylium is usually employed only after patients have not responded to lidocaine.

MECHANISM OF ACTION

In addition to the indirect electrophysiologic changes caused by the drug's action on postganglionic autonomic neurons, bretylium has a direct class III action that causes an increase in APD and refractoriness in ventricular muscle and Purkinje fibers.[197] When clinically relevant concentrations of bretylium are studied in normal tissues, no changes are seen in V_{max}, maximum diastolic potential, or conduction velocity. Studies have found that bretylium reduces the degree of dispersion of repolarization across the boundary between normal and ischemic tissue by acting predominantly on normal tissue.[198] Transient increases in membrane potential and conduction velocity are seen early after bretylium administration and are presumed to be due to the local release of catecholamines.

When initially administered, bretylium causes the release of norepinephrine from postganglionic adrenergic neurons.[199] Bretylium is transported into the neuron by the norepinephrine pump, and extensive accumulation in the neuron is then associated with a blockade of further release or uptake of norepinephrine by the neuron. The blockade of uptake of circulating or infused catecholamines leads to supersensitivity that is functionally similar to a denervated state.

CLINICAL PHARMACOLOGY

Bretylium is poorly absorbed after oral administration, with bioavailability of approximately 25 percent, and is therefore available only for parenteral administration. It is eliminated almost entirely unchanged in the urine, and clearance correlates well with creatinine clearance.[200] It is probably actively secreted by the base transport system in the distal tubules of the kidney.

DOSAGE AND ADMINISTRATION

The usual intravenous dosage for bretylium is 5 mg/kg given at a rate dependent upon the clinical setting.[201] During cardiac emergencies, it should be given by rapid injection into a central intravenous line. In less acute situations, giving a loading infusion of the same dose but over 10 to 20 min will reduce the incidence of nausea and vomiting. The loading dose should be repeated after 20 min if the arrhythmia is still present. A total loading dose of 20 mg/kg may be required, and dosages up to 9 g in 24 h have been given without serious adverse effects. Maintenance infusions of 1 to 4 mg/min should be given, depending upon body size and renal function. Heart rhythm and blood pressure should be monitored care-

fully, especially during the first few hours of bretylium therapy.

MODIFICATION OF DOSAGE IN DISEASE STATES

In patients with renal insufficiency, bretylium clearance is reduced and half-life prolonged; therefore, the maintenance infusion for bretylium should be reduced to the lowest effective dosage. There are no data to guide dosage adjustment in cardiac or hepatic impairment, but it is unlikely that the dosage should be altered in these patients.

ADVERSE REACTIONS

When bretylium is given by rapid intravenous injection, many patients experience nausea and vomiting. The release of norepinephrine by bretylium has the potential to cause increased blood pressure, but severe hypertension has not been described. Increased frequency of ventricular arrhythmias is often seen at this time and can lead to the need for more frequent cardioversion. The reduction in peripheral vascular resistance can cause symptomatic hypotension in volume-depleted patients, but this can be readily corrected if recognized, although hypotension could prove dangerous in patients with fixed valvular obstruction. Bradycardia has been reported in some patients with abnormalities of the conduction system when given large intravenous dosages of bretylium.

In stable patients, either low or high dosages of bretylium can cause a transient increase in heart rate, blood pressure, contractility, peripheral vascular resistance, and arrhythmia frequency, followed by a fall in standing blood pressure and peripheral vascular resistance.[202] Orthostatic hypotension is almost uniformly seen in patients receiving bretylium and sometimes lasts for days after discontinuation of therapy. Dosages that are well below those required for antiarrhythmic efficacy are capable of causing orthostatic hypotension. When hypotension develops during bretylium therapy, it should be corrected with intravenous volume expansion, and adequate doses of bretylium should be given to suppress arrhythmias.

DRUG INTERACTIONS

Other than those with tricyclic antidepressants, no drug interactions have been reported. One would expect, however, that there might be competition for renal tubular secretion with procainamide, NAPA, cimetidine, and other organic bases.

Sotalol (Betapace)

CLINICAL APPLICATIONS

Sotalol has been used for up to 20 years in many countries for angina and hypertension, and it was in this setting that its value as an antiarrhythmic agent was first observed. Sotalol is unlike other beta-adrenergic antagonists in that it prolongs the action potential, producing a parallel increase in refractoriness of cardiac tissues.[203] This unique combination of properties makes sotalol effective in a variety of supraventricular and ventricular arrhythmias. It has been found to be effective in patients with sustained ventricular tachycardia evaluated by programmed ventricular stimulation. In a controlled comparison to procainamide, sotalol was effective in 30 percent of patients with inducible sustained ventricular tachycardia, whereas only 20 percent responded to procainamide ($p < .2$).[204] This is consistent with the response rate for sotalol (31 percent) in the ESVEM trial sponsored by the National Institutes of Health, which compared therapy guided by programmed electrical stimulation to therapy guided by ambulatory monitoring.[205] In this study, a mean of only 12 percent of patients responded to the other antiarrhythmic drugs evaluated.

MECHANISM OF ACTION

Sotalol has two main actions, each of which can contribute to its antiarrhythmic efficacy.[206] The drug was originally synthesized for its actions as a beta-adrenergic receptor antagonist. Unlike other beta-receptor antagonists, it markedly prolongs refractoriness in atrial and ventricular tissues, a class III antiarrhythmic action. These actions slow heart rate; decrease AV nodal conduction; and increase refractoriness of atrial, ventricular, AV nodal, and AV accessory pathways in both the anterograde and retrograde directions.[207] When given in dosages between 160 and 640 mg/day there are increases of 40 to 100 ms in the QT interval and 10 to 40 ms in QT_c.

CLINICAL PHARMACOLOGY

Oral bioavailability of sotalol is greater than 90 percent, and peak concentrations are seen 2.5 to 4 h after a dose. It is not bound to plasma proteins and is eliminated by the kidneys unchanged, with an elimination half-life of approximately 12 h. Because of the relatively long half-life and twice daily dosing regimen, it is recommended that testing for efficacy be conducted near the end of the dosing interval at steady state. Age, per se, does not influence the pharmacokinetics of sotalol other than that due to the natural decline in renal function that occurs with age. Dosage adjustment must be made for alterations in renal function (see below).

DOSAGE AND ADMINISTRATION

Sotalol is available only in the oral form in the United States. The recommended initial dose of sotalol is 80 mg every 12 h. In patients with relatively normal renal function, steady state will occur in 2 to 3 days. If evaluation at this dosage indicates a lack of response without evidence of excessive effects on repolarization (QT below 500 ms), the dosage may be increased to 160 mg twice daily and, if necessary, to 240 mg twice daily. Some patients with life-threatening arrhythmias have required dosages of 640 mg/day.

MODIFICATION OF DOSAGE IN DISEASE STATES

Because sotalol is mainly eliminated unchanged in the urine, the dosage must be adjusted for altered renal function. For patients with a creatinine clearance greater than 60 mL/min, the usual dosing interval is every 12 h. If the creatinine clearance (CL_{CR}) is between 30 and 60 mL/min, however, the recommended interval between doses is 24 h. For patients

with CL_{CR} between 10 and 30 mL/min, the interval should be every 36 to 48 h or the usual dose halved and given every 24 h. The dosage for patients with CL_{CR} below 10 mL/min should be individualized. Because of the increased risk of proarrhythmia and congestive heart failure, patients with reduced cardiac output should be given lower doses and monitored carefully.

ADVERSE REACTIONS

A major concern with sotalol treatment has been the occurrence of torsades de pointes. Reports of this syndrome have predominantly been cases of suicidal overdoses or in patients who were receiving concomitant diuretics and inadequate potassium replacement. Clearly, hypokalemia and bradycardia are predisposing factors for the development of this arrhythmia during sotalol therapy, as they are with quinidine, disopyramide, and procainamide. The manufacturer observed an overall incidence of torsades de pointes of 2 percent, broken down to 4 percent with sustained ventricular tachycardia and 1.5 percent with supraventricular arrhythmias. It is more common in females with congestive heart failure and with a history of sustained ventricular tachycardia (7 percent). The incidence of torsades de pointes should be minimized by careful screening for predisposing factors such as bradycardia, baseline prolongation of the QT interval, and electrolyte disturbances, (especially hypokalemia); careful dose escalation beginning at 160 mg/day; and limiting the maximum QT interval prolongation to less than 550 ms.

The incidence of new or worsened congestive heart failure is only about 3 percent. This is somewhat lower than expected for a drug with potent beta-blocking actions but may be attenuated because of the increased inotropy produced by its action to prolong repolarization. Other side effects typical of beta blockers are to be expected, including bronchospasm in asthmatic patients, masking the signs and symptoms of hypoglycemia in diabetic patients, and catecholamine hypersensitivity withdrawal syndrome[205] (see also Chap. 54).

DRUG INTERACTIONS

Concomitant use of sotalol with agents that prolong repolarization has the potential to increase the likelihood of torsades de pointes. No pharmacokinetic interactions have been seen with sotalol and/or warfarin, digoxin, cholestyramine, or hydrochlorothiazide. Because of the beta-blocking actions of sotalol, it is likely that there would be increased pharmacologic effect if the drug is combined with calcium channel blockers, antihypertensive agents, or antiarrhythmic agents.

Amiodarone (Cordarone)

CLINICAL APPLICATIONS

Although amiodarone has been reported to have efficacy in a wide range of arrhythmias, the U.S. FDA has recommended it only for life-threatening ventricular arrhythmias refractory to other available forms of therapy. Nevertheless, there are now numerous trials in the literature describing the efficacy of amiodarone in the conversion and slowing of atrial fibrillation, AV nodal reentrant tachycardia, and tachycardias associated with the Wolff-Parkinson-White syndrome.[208,209] The reasons for amiodarone's limited labeling are: (1) the documented potentially lethal complications of chronic amiodarone therapy, (2) the difficulties associated with its variable time for onset of action, and (3) multiple dangerous drug interactions.

After the results of CAST, antiarrhythmic drugs are examined for their effects on mortality. After several small or uncontrolled trials seemed to indicate that amiodarone could have a beneficial effect on mortality,[4,210] adequate trials were undertaken. The Veteran's Administration trial, Congestive Heart Failure Survival Trial of Antiarrhythmic Therapy (CHF STAT),[211] examined the effects of amiodarone on total mortality in patients with a history of congestive heart failure, more than 10 premature ventricular contractions per hour on ambulatory monitoring, and an ejection fraction below 40 percent. The study found no difference in the placebo- and amiodarone-treated arms. Two other major trials have evaluated amiodarone in patients with recent myocardial infarction. The Canadian Myocardial Infarction Amiodarone Trial (CAMIAT)[212] and the European Myocardial Infarction Amiodarone Trial (EMIAT)[213] were recently completed. The results of these trials are mixed in that neither found amiodarone to reduce overall mortality, but the Canadian trial reported a reduced incidence of ventricular fibrillation or arrhythmic death among survivors of myocardial infarction with ventricular ectopy. Importantly, there was no increase in mortality, as has been seen with other antiarrhythmic drugs.

In 1993, an intravenous formulation of amiodarone became available in the United States. Although it had been used extensively in most countries for many years, controlled trials only became available in recent years. Two recently completed controlled trials demonstrated the value of amiodarone in patients with recurrent life-threatening ventricular tachycardia or fibrillation. A comparison of three dosages found that the recurrence of arrhythmia decreased with increasing dosages of 125, 500, and 1000 mg per 24 h.[214] Hypotension was the major side effect seen, but it occurred equally in all groups, about 26 percent. The second study in a similar group of patients was a comparison of bretylium to two doses of amiodarone.[215] The arrhythmia event rate for the first 48 h of therapy was equivalent for the high dose of amiodarone and bretylium, and both were more effective than the low dose of amiodarone. Hypotension was common in all groups but significantly higher in the bretylium group. It appears that amiodarone is effective when given by the intravenous route.

DESCRIPTION

Amiodarone is an iodinated benzofuran that has structural similarity to thyroxine and procainamide and was originally developed as an antianginal agent. It was incidentally noted to suppress a wide variety of ventricular and supraventricular arrhythmias effectively. This efficacy has been assumed to be due to its prolongation of refractoriness and APD in myocardial tissue (Vaughan Williams class III antiarrhythmic activity), although amiodarone has been found to have many diverse pharmacologic actions (see Table 30-1); the one(s) responsible for its high degree of antiarrhythmic efficacy remain unidentified.

MECHANISM OF ACTION

In intracellular recordings of rabbit cardiac myocytes, amiodarone prolongs APD and increases refractoriness of both atrial and ventricular myocardium, Purkinje fibers, and sinus and AV nodal tissues. Amiodarone decreases phase 0 depolarization of myocardial cells, blocks sodium channels that are in the inactivated state, and slows phase 4 depolarization of the sinus node as well as conduction through the AV node.[216,217] The electrophysiologic actions of the major metabolite of amiodarone, desethylamiodarone (DEA), differ from those of amiodarone, with the metabolite having greater effects on conduction due to effects on sodium channels and, hence, upon conduction.[218] Intracoronary injection of amiodarone has shown little cardiac effect compared to DEA's ability to prolong cardiac refractoriness.[219]

Electrophysiologic changes in humans depend on the route of administration and the duration of therapy. Following acute intravenous amiodarone administration, prolongation of the AH interval and an increase in the refractory periods of the AV node and bypass tracts are seen, but this may be due to the presence of the solubilizing agent, polysorbate 80 (Tween 80), in the intravenous formulation. No acute changes occur in either sinus rate or atrial or ventricular refractoriness, whereas these are prolonged during chronic oral therapy. Chronic amiodarone therapy also prolongs the AH and HV intervals and the PR and QT intervals of the surface ECG. Data conflict on the time course of these changes and how they might relate to antiarrhythmic efficacy. Changes in APD and refractoriness are seen in hypothyroidism, similar to changes resulting from oral amiodarone therapy.[220] Since these changes can be prevented in animals by coadministration of thyroid hormone with amiodarone,[221] some have concluded that amiodarone's antiarrhythmic efficacy is due to production of "cardiac hypothyroidism." This is supported by the observation that amiodarone's major metabolite causes noncompetitive inhibition of thyroid hormone binding to nuclear receptors.[222] On the other hand, amiodarone also causes noncompetitive blockade of alpha and beta receptors[223] and muscarinic receptors,[224] and both calcium and sodium channel blockade—any combination of which may contribute to its antiarrhythmic efficacy.

CLINICAL PHARMACOLOGY

Amiodarone is a highly lipid-soluble compound with extremely variable and complex pharmacokinetics. It is slowly absorbed from the gastrointestinal tract, and bioavailability varies over a fourfold range.[225] Amiodarone is extensively metabolized to DEA, and little, if any, is excreted unchanged in the urine. Concentrations of DEA in plasma vary from 0.4 to 2.0 times that of amiodarone during chronic therapy.[226] This metabolite has antiarrhythmic potency equal to or greater than amiodarone in in vitro and animal models.[227] Amiodarone is rapidly concentrated in some tissues, including myocardium, but accumulates more slowly in others, such as adipose tissue. It redistributes out of myocardial tissue while still accumulating in adipose and other tissues.[226,228] Until all tissues are saturated, rapid redistribution out of the myocardium may be responsible for early recurrence of arrhythmias after discontinuation of therapy or rapid reduction of dosage. Because of drug accumulation in tissues, the volume of distribution for amiodarone is very large, 20 to 200 L/kg.[228] After intravenous administration, the measured half-life in plasma is from 4.8 to 68.2 h,[229] with tissue uptake being the primary factor responsible for the decline in plasma concentration. As tissues become saturated, however, the decline in plasma levels is slow, reflecting mainly elimination and slow redistribution of drug out of adipose and muscle tissues. This leads to slow and extremely variable elimination from plasma, with half-lives ranging from 13 to 103 days at steady state.[228] It is also possible that amiodarone inhibits its own elimination after chronic therapy, contributing to the differences between half-life early in therapy to that after prolonged therapy.

DOSAGE AND ADMINISTRATION

Without a loading dose, amiodarone requires several weeks to months before producing its antiarrhythmic action. Large intravenous dosages or oral loading dosages can hasten the onset of therapeutic effects. From small prospective studies, loading dosages have varied from 600 to 1400 mg/day for 2 to 21 days.[230] Recent large clinical trials have utilized a lower loading dose of 600 to 800 mg daily for 14 days.[211,231] Because of relatively rapid redistribution out of myocardial tissue, the dosage should be tapered over a period of several weeks. The usual maintenance dose varies from 200 to 600 mg/day, and because of the severe nature of adverse reactions, the lowest effective dosage should be prescribed. Patients with supraventricular arrhythmias may respond to lower dosages than those with ventricular arrhythmias, but there are many exceptions and no comparative trials are available. Because of the variable pharmacokinetics and oral bioavailability, generalizations such as this may be unreliable. Some patients with extensive absorption (~80 to 90 percent bioavailability) of even low doses may have the same drug exposure as a person with limited bioavailability given a high dose.

For intravenous administration, the manufacturer recommends a three-phase infusion over the first 24 h: 150 mg over 10 min, followed by 360 mg over the next 6 h, followed by 0.5 mg/min. The drug can be continued at this rate, but monitoring of plasma concentrations is recommended. An additional 150 mg can be infused over 10 min for those patients who continue to have recurrent ventricular tachycardia or fibrillation or whose arrhythmia recurs during downward titration of the infusion. Concentrations of drug greater than 3 mg/mL should be given through a central catheter to prevent phlebitis. Also, the surfactant properties of the drug alter the size of a drop, and pumps that count drops will give approximately 30 percent less drug than intended.

Amiodarone concentrations are usually between 1 and 2 μg/mL during effective oral therapy.[232,233] Similar concentrations of DEA accumulate during therapy and, although this is unproven, are likely to contribute to antiarrhythmic efficacy. Because of extensive overlap between the range of concentrations required for arrhythmia suppression and those associated with toxicity, monitoring of plasma concentrations is of limited value. Clearly, levels of amiodarone above 3 to 4 μg/mL for prolonged periods of time are associated with a higher incidence of adverse effects.[234]

MODIFICATION OF DOSAGE IN DISEASE STATES

Long-term oral therapy with amiodarone appears to be well tolerated hemodynamically in patients with congestive heart failure. In the Veteran's Administration trial discussed above, amiodarone failed to prolong life for congestive heart failure patients with arrhythmias but was associated with improved ventricular function.[211]

ADVERSE REACTIONS

Intravenous amiodarone at dosages greater than 5 mg/kg decreases contractility and peripheral vascular resistance, producing severe hypotension in some instances. Some of this effect, like the electrophysiologic effects described earlier, may be due to the effects of polysorbate 80 or benzyl alcohol, since oral administration at usual dosages improves myocardial contractility.

The safety of amiodarone is controversial. The early reports found it to be very well tolerated and described it as the "ideal antiarrhythmic drug." Some studies continue to find that it is safe and effective, even in the treatment of arrhythmias in children,[235] although the experience with amiodarone in the United States, with a very high incidence of intolerable and sometimes lethal reactions, differs from that in Europe. Determination of the incidence of adverse reactions is difficult because of highly variable dosages and durations of treatment.[216,236]

The most serious adverse reaction is lethal interstitial pneumonitis,[216,237] which may be more common in patients with preexisting lung disease. Monitoring is essential since the pneumonitis is reversible if detected early. A chest x-ray every 3 months may be useful, but serial pulmonary function tests are of little value for follow-up. Hyper- or hypothyroidism is seen in about 4 percent of patients.[220] Accumulation of corneal microdeposits is almost uniform during long-term therapy and in many cases can progress to the point of interfering with vision.[238] Some Caucasian patients notice a slate-gray or bluish discoloration of sun-exposed areas of the skin.[239] Many also complain of photosensitivity, which can sometimes be prevented or alleviated with sunscreens and garments. Thirty percent or more of patients have abnormally elevated serum hepatic enzyme levels, and progression to jaundice and cirrhosis has been reported.[240,241] Serial laboratory tests to screen for amiodarone toxicity can be costly and generally are of little value; however, it is wise to obtain a reliable assessment of baseline tests, including complete blood count, blood chemistry, tests of thyroid and pulmonary function, a slit-lamp examination, and measurement of blood levels of other drugs whenever possible.

DRUG INTERACTIONS

Amiodarone has been found to interfere with the clearance of many drugs. This may involve the formation of a metabolically inactive cytochrome P450 Fe(II)–metabolite complex, which has been described in animals treated with amiodarone,[242] and may explain the unexpected accumulation of warfarin,[243] quinidine, procainamide, disopyramide, mexiletine, and propafenone[244] and the resulting bleeding, heart block, or torsades de pointes. It does not, however, explain interaction with drugs eliminated predominantly by the kidneys, such as digoxin.[245] The elimination of other drugs may be impaired by amiodarone, and the lowest effective dosage should be sought.

Ibutilide (Corvert)

CLINICAL APPLICATIONS

Ibutilide is the first drug given FDA approval for the rapid conversion of recent-onset atrial fibrillation or flutter.[246,247] It has not been tested in other arrhythmias or in patients with atrial fibrillation or flutter of long duration (>90 days). It should not be given to patients who have hypokalemia, hypomagnesemia, or QT_c prolongation at baseline >440 ms. In placebo-controlled studies summarized in the manufacturer's labeling, the placebo conversion rate for atrial fibrillation or flutter was approximately 2 percent. Ibutilide terminated the arrhythmia in approximately 44 percent of patients treated with 1 mg followed by either 0.5 or 1 mg. Approximately 20 percent of patients responded to the first infusion, and approximately 25 percent of those not responding to the first infusion responded to the second infusion. Response usually occurred at 20 to 30 min, ranging from 5 to 88 min after infusion. The response in patients with atrial fibrillation and atrial flutter were not significantly different in the trials performed.

DESCRIPTION

Ibutilide is a remarkably potent methanesulfonamide analogue of sotalol that prolongs cardiac action potential duration and has class III action to prolong cardiac refractoriness and action potential duration.

MECHANISM OF ACTION

The mechanism of action of ibutilide is controversial. The manufacturer claims that the drug's class III action is due to a "unique" ability to increase an inward sodium current, as observed in guinea pig ventricular myocytes at $10^{-7}\ M$ concentrations. Higher concentrations ($10^{-5}\ M$) increase a potassium current to shorten action potential duration.[248] On the other hand, as has been seen with dofetilide, sotalol, and other methanesulfonamides, $10^{-8}\ M$ concentrations block the rapid component of the delayed rectifier potassium current, I_{Kr}, in mouse and human cardiac cells.[249]

CLINICAL PHARMACOLOGY

Ibutilide is only available at this time for intravenous administration. When given over 10 min, it distributes rapidly in a multiexponential fashion, with the relevant component having a half-life from 2 to 12 h (mean = 6 h). The plasma concentration and pharmacokinetics are highly variable, and dosing is recommended on the basis of weight. The drug is mainly eliminated by oxidative hepatic metabolism, and systemic clearance is rapid (about 29 mL/min per kilogram). Since formal drug interaction studies have not been performed, it is not possible to anticipate which enzymes are likely responsible for its elimination.

DOSAGE AND ADMINISTRATION

Ibutilide is given undiluted or diluted in saline as an infusion over 10 min. The recommended dose for a patient over 60 kg is 1 mg and for a patient under 60 kg is 0.01 mg/kg. For patients whose arrhythmias have not converted by 10 min after completion of the first dose, a second dose of equal size can be administered. Since conversion of the arrhythmias is usually associated with peak levels, slower infusion rates are not likely to be as effective.

It is essential that patients receiving ibutilide be treated in a carefully monitored environment during and at least 4 h subsequent to treatment. The FDA-approved labeling recommends that skilled personnel, facilities, and medication for defibrillation or resuscitation must be readily available.

MODIFICATION OF DOSAGE IN DISEASE STATES

Although specific studies with heart failure and renal or hepatic disease have not been conducted, current information does not indicate that any dosage adjustments should be necessary in these conditions. Patients with severe left ventricular dysfunction, however, have a higher risk of developing ventricular arrhythmias, including torsades de pointes. Since the duration of drug effect is determined by distribution, it is very possible that patients with severe congestive heart failure will have decreased volumes of distribution and hence an exaggerated and prolonged duration of effect.

ADVERSE REACTIONS

The most serious adverse reaction is torsades de pointes, which has been seen in 1.7 percent of patients. There were, however, only 586 patients participating in trials, and patients with a $QT_c > 440$ ms or potassium concentrations <4 meq/L were excluded. In spite of these precautions, the incidence of sustained polymorphic ventricular tachycardia requiring cardioversion was 1.7 percent. Another 2.7 percent developed nonsustained polymorphic ventricular tachycardia, 4.9 percent nonsustained monomorphic ventricular tachycardia, 1.5 percent AV block, and 1.9 percent bundle branch block. The risk of polymorphic ventricular tachycardia was highest in patients who were female and/or had evidence of reduced ventricular performance. The incidence of these adverse effects may well be higher in general clinical use where electrolyte disorders and concomitant therapies may be more common.

DRUG INTERACTIONS

No specific drug interaction studies have been performed. Concomitant beta receptor or calcium channel antagonists do not apparently interact, although data are limited.

Beta-Receptor Antagonists (See Chap. 54)

Adenosine (Adenocard)

CLINICAL APPLICATIONS

Adenosine is very effective for the acute conversion of paroxysmal supraventricular tachycardia (PSVT) due to reentry involving the AV node. Sixty percent of patients respond at a dose of 6 mg, and an additional 32 percent respond when given a higher dose of 12 mg. Some patients with PSVT associated with the Wolff-Parkinson-White syndrome have also been found to respond to adenosine. Because of the fleeting and relatively selective action of adenosine on the AV node, some have suggested that it be used as a diagnostic tool in patients with narrow and wide complex tachycardia.[250] It is preferable to make the correct diagnosis before giving any drugs, because of their risk of adverse effects.

DESCRIPTION

Adenosine is a nucleoside formed in the body by serial dephosphorylation of adenosine triphosphate (ATP), from cyclic adenosine monophosphate, or from hydrolysis of S-adenosylhomocysteine. It is formed both intra- and extracellularly, and its actions are rapidly terminated by transport into cells followed by metabolism. The actions of adenosine are highly dependent on the rate and route of administration. A rapid intravenous injection into a central venous line is thought to activate carotid body chemoreceptors and usually produces an initial increase in blood pressure of 10 to 15 mmHg, followed by a small and transient decrease. These reflexes are attenuated during surgery, and in this setting, adenosine decreases peripheral vascular resistance, increases cardiac output, and increases heart rate moderately. Bolus injections also produce biphasic effects on heart rate. Approximately 20 s after injection, sinus bradycardia occurs for 10 to 15 s, followed by sinus tachycardia thought to be due to chemoreceptor activation. Activation of the carotid chemoreceptors stimulates respiration and causes secondary activation of pulmonary stretch receptors. Adenosine has a direct effect of slowing AV nodal conduction, which can result in transient AV block. Although adenosine has no direct effect on the His-Purkinje system, it does attenuate the effects of catecholamine stimulation and, in patients with heart block, can block acceleration of the ventricular escape rate by isoproterenol. Adenosine usually has no effect on anterograde or retrograde accessory pathway conduction. Pathways that demonstrate decremental conduction often respond to adenosine, probably because they are partially depolarized and can be hyperpolarized by adenosine. Slow injections into a peripheral line often produce no clinical benefit or changes in blood pressure or heart rate.

MECHANISM OF ACTION

The development of synthetic agonists and antagonists of adenosine receptors has made possible the subclassification of A_1 and A_2 receptor subtypes. The A_1 receptors are present in myocardial cells and mediate the negative inotropic, dromotropic, and chronotropic actions of adenosine. The A_2 receptors are present in the endothelium and vascular smooth muscle cells and cause coronary vasodilatation, when activated.

The efficacy of adenosine in PSVT is most likely due to the following actions in atrial myocardium and the AV node: (1) hyperpolarization of sinoatrial nodal cells and slowing of rate of firing, (2) shortening of the action potential of atrial cells, and (3) depression of conduction velocity in the AV node. These actions are due to activation of A_1 adenosine receptor subtypes, which leads to activation of cyclic AMP–independent, acetylcholine/adenosine-regulated potassium current, $I_{ACh,Ado}$.

CLINICAL PHARMACOLOGY

After intravenous injection, adenosine is rapidly transported into red blood cells and endothelial cells. A half-life of elimination has been estimated as 1.5 to 10 s. The drug is rapidly metabolized in the plasma and in cells to form inosine and adenosine monophosphate. Maximal pharmacologic effects are seen within 30 s after injection into a peripheral intravenous line but occur within 10 to 20 s when given into a central line.

DOSAGE AND ADMINISTRATION

Adenosine should be injected intravenously into a proximal tubing site and flushed quickly with saline. For adults, the initial dose is 6 mg injected over 1 to 2 s. If the arrhythmia persists, a 12-mg dose can be injected 1 to 2 min later. This can be repeated, but doses larger than 12 mg are not recommended by the manufacturer. A dosage regimen based on body weight has been proposed, with an initial dose of 50 $\mu g/kg$ incremented by 50 $\mu g/kg$ until the PSVT is terminated or side effects become intolerable.[250] Higher doses may be required for patients who have received caffeine or theophylline because of their antagonistic effects at A_1 receptors. Lower doses are recommended if the patients are receiving dipyridamole or carbamazepine.

MODIFICATION OF DOSAGE IN DISEASE STATES

Although the pharmacokinetics of adenosine are unlikely to be altered in patients with renal or hepatic disease, these patients often have electrolyte imbalances that could alter the clinical response. Although patients with congestive heart failure have not been reported to respond abnormally, cardiac transplant patients appear to require one-third to one-fifth of the usual dose because of denervation hypersensitivity.[251]

ADVERSE REACTIONS

Adenosine is contraindicated in patients with sick-sinus syndrome or second- or third-degree heart block unless the patient has a functioning artificial pacemaker. Because of the rapid clearance of adenosine, side effects such as facial flushing, dyspnea, or chest pressure last less than 60 s. Although intrapulmonary administration of adenosine has precipitated bronchospasm in asthmatic patients, this has not been reported with intravenous administration. Other less frequent side effects include nausea, lightheadedness, headache, sweating, palpitations, hypotension, and blurred vision. Intravenous theophylline, which has been recommended to reverse the effects of adenosine, should be prepared and ready for injection.

DRUG INTERACTIONS

There are several proven interactions that can increase or decrease the activity of adenosine. Dipyridamole pretreatment increases the potency of adenosine, probably because it blocks cellular uptake of adenosine.[252] On the other hand, caffeine and theophylline antagonize the actions of adenosine.[253] The manufacturer cautions that carbamazepine may potentiate the actions of adenosine.

INVESTIGATIONAL DRUGS

There are only a few new antiarrhythmic agents under development in the United States at this time. Several of these, such as dofetilide or E-4031, are analogues of sotalol and/or NAPA, which have been selected for testing because they have class III activity but lack the other actions such as beta-adrenergic receptor inhibition or sodium channel blocking activity.[254,255] Some impetus for the development of these sotalol-like agents lies in the hope that they will have amiodarone's efficacy without its toxicity. Amiodarone is a very effective antiarrhythmic, and agents with the potential to have a similar degree of efficacy but to lack its toxicity are being tested.[256] Unfortunately, it seems unlikely that these new drugs will have markedly improved efficacy because of their electrophysiologic similarity to modest agents such as NAPA, clofilium, and d-sotalol.[75,254] The recent early termination of the SWORD trial (d-sotalol) certainly does not bode well for this group of drugs.[5]

REFERENCES

1. CAST investigators: Preliminary report. Effect of encainide and flecainide on mortality in a randomized trial of arrhythmia suppression after myocardial infarction. *N Engl J Med* 1989; 321:406–412.
2. CAST-II Investigators. Effect of the antiarrhythmic agent moricizine on survival after myocardial infarction (abstr). *N Engl J Med* 1992; 327:227–233.
3. Hine LK, Laird NM, Hewitt P, Chalmers TC. Meta-analysis of empirical long-term antiarrhythmic therapy after myocardial infarction. *JAMA* 1989; 262:(21):3037–3040.
4. Pfisterer ME, Kiowski W, Brunner H, Burckhardt D, Burkart F. Long-term benefit of 1-year amiodarone treatment for persistent complex ventricular arrhythmias after myocardial infarction. *Circulation* 1993; 87:309–311.
5. Waldo AL, Camm AJ, deRuyter H, Friedman PL, MacNiel DJ, Pauls JF, et al. Effect of d-sotalol on mortality in patients with left ventricular dysfunction after recent and remote myocardial infarction. *Lancet* 1996; 348:7–12.
6. Vaughan Williams EM. A classification of arrhythmic actions reassessed after a decade of new drugs. *J Clin Pharmacol* 1984; 24:129–147.
7. Harrison DC. Antiarrhythmic drug classification: New science and practical applications. *Am J Cardiol* 1985; 56:185–187.
8. Task Force of the Working Group on Arrhythmias of the European Society of Cardiology. The Sicilian gambit: A new approach to the classification of antiarrhythmic drugs based on their actions on arrhythmogenic mechanisms. *Circulation* 1991; 84(4):1831–1851.
9. Hodgkin AL, Huxley AF. A quantitative description of membrane current and its application to conduction and excitation in nerve. *J Physiol* 1952; 117:500–544.
10. Hondeghem LM, Katzung BG. Test of a model of antiarrhythmic drug action: Effects of quinidine and lidocaine on myocardial conduction. *Circulation* 1980; 61(6):1217–1224.
11. Campbell TJ. Kinetics of onset of rate-dependent effects of class I antiarrhythmic drugs are important in determining their effects on refractoriness in guinea-pig ventricle, and provide a theoretical basis for their subclassification. *Cardiovasc Res* 1983; 17:344–352.
12. Southworth JL, McKusick VA, Pierce EC II, Rawson FL Jr. Ventricular fibrillation precipitated by cardiac catheterization. *JAMA* 1950; 143:717–720.
13. Lie KI, Wellens HJ, van Capelle FJ, Durrer D. Lidocaine in the prevention of primary ventricular fibrillation. A double-blind, randomized study of 212 consecutive patients. *N Engl J Med* 1974; 291:1324–1326.
14. MacMahon S, Collins R, Peto R, Koster RW, Yusuf S. Effects of prophylactic lidocaine in suspected acute myocardial infarction. *JAMA* 1988; 260(13):1910–1916.
15. Pedersen LE, Bonde J, Graudal NA, Backer NV, Hansen JS, Kampmann JP. Quantitative and qualitative binding characteristics of disopyramide in serum from patients with decreased renal and hepatic function. *Br J Clin Pharmacol* 1987; 23:41–46.
16. Rosen KM, Barwolf C, Ehsani A, Rahimtoola SH. Effects of lidocaine and propranolol on the normal and anomalous pathways in patients with preexcitation. *Am J Cardiol* 1972; 30:801–809.
17. Josephson ME, Kastor JA, Kitchen JGI. Lidocaine in Wolff-Parkinson-White syndrome with atrial fibrillation. *Ann Intern Med* 1976; 84:44–45.
18. Akhtar M, Gilbert CJ, Shenasa M. Effect of lidocaine on atrioventricular response via the accessory pathway in patients with Wolff-Parkinson-White syndrome. *Circulation* 1981; 63:435–441.
19. Davis LD, Temte JV. Electrophysiological actions of lidocaine on canine ventricular muscle and Purkinje fibers. *Circ Res* 1969; 24:639–655.
20. Bigger JT Jr, Mandel WJ. Effect of lidocaine on the electrophysiological properties of ventricular muscle and Purkinje fibers. *J Clin Invest* 1970; 49:63–77.
21. Kunkel F, Rowland M, Scheinman MM. The electrophysiologic effects of lidocaine in patients with intraventricular conduction defects. *Circulation* 1974; 49:894–899.
22. Bekheit S, Murtagh JG, Morton P, Fletcher E. Effect of lignocaine on conducting system of human heart. *Br Heart J* 1973; 35:305–311.
23. Gupta PK, Lichstein E, Chadda KD. Lidocaine-induced heart block in patients with bundle branch block. *Am J Cardiol* 1974; 33:487–492.
24. Aravindakshan V, Kuo C, Gettes LS. Effect of lidocaine on escape rate in patients with complete atrioventricular block. A. Distal His block. *Am J Cardiol* 1977; 40:177–183.
25. Stenson RE, Constantino RT, Harrison DC. Interrelationships of hepatic blood flow, cardiac output, and blood levels of lidocaine in man. *Circulation* 1971; 43:205–211.
26. Zito RA, Reid PR. Lidocaine kinetics predicted by indocyanine green clearance. *N Engl J Med* 1978; 298:1160–1163.
27. Blumer J, Strong JM, Atkinson AJ Jr. The convulsant potency of lidocaine and its N-dealkylated metabolites. *J Pharmacol Exp Ther* 1973; 186:31–36.
28. Narang PK, Crouthamel WG, Carliner NH, Fisher ML. Lidocaine and its active metabolites. *Clin Pharmacol Ther* 1978; 24:654–662.
29. Thomson PD, Melmon KL, Richardson JA, Cohn K, Steinbrunn W, Cudihee R, et al. Lidocaine pharmacokinetics in advanced heart failure, liver disease and renal failure in humans. *Ann Intern Med* 1973; 78:499–508.
30. Wyman MG, Slaughter RL, Farolino DA, Gore S, Cannom DS, Goldreyer BN, et al. Multiple bolus technique for lidocaine administration in acute ischemic heart disease. II. Treatment of refractory ventricular arrhythmias and the pharmacokinetic significance of severe left ventricular failure. *J Am Coll Cardiol* 1983; 2:764–769.
31. Stargel WW, Shand DG, Routledge PA, Barchowsky A, Wagner GS.

Clinical comparison of rapid infusion and multiple injection methods for lidocaine loading. *Am Heart J* 1981; 102:872–876.

32. Alderman EL, Kerber RE, Harrison DC. Evaluation of lidocaine resistance in man using intermittent large-dose infusion techniques. *Am J Cardiol* 1974; 34:342–349.

33. Richard C, Berdeaux A, Delion F, Riou B, Rimailho A, Giudicelli JF, et al. Effect of mechanical ventilation on hepatic drug pharmacokinetics. *Chest* 1986; 90:837–841.

34. Kuhlkamp V, Meerhof J, Schmidt F, Mayer F, Ickrath O, Haasis R, et al. Electrophysiologic effects and efficacy of cibenzoline on stimulation-induced atrial fibrillation and flutter and implications for treatment of paroxysmal atrial fibrillation. *Am J Cardiol* 1990; 65:628–632.

35. Routledge PA, Shand DG, Barchowsky A, Wagner G, Stargel WW. Relationship between alpha 1-acid glycoprotein and lidocaine disposition in myocardial infarction. *Clin Pharmacol Ther* 1981; 30:154–157.

36. Cheng TO, Wadhwa K. Sinus standstill following intravenous lidocaine administration. *JAMA* 1973; 223:790–792.

37. Marriott HJL, Phillips K. Profound hypotension and bradycardia after a single bolus of lidocaine. *J Electrocardiol* 1974; 7:79–82.

38. Cote P, Harrison DC, Basile J, Schroeder JS. Hemodynamic interaction of procainamide and lidocaine after experimental myocardial infarction. *Am J Cardiol* 1973; 32:937–942.

39. Branch RA, Shand DG, Wilkinson GR, Nies AS. The reduction of lidocaine clearance by dl-propranolol: An example of hemodynamic drug interaction. *J Pharmacol Exp Ther* 1973; 184:515–519.

40. Ochs HR, Carstens G, Greenblatt DJ. Reduction in lidocaine clearance during continuous infusion and by coadministration of propranolol. *N Engl J Med* 1980; 303:373–377.

41. Feeley J, Wilkinson GR, McAllister CB, Wood AJJ. Increased toxicity and reduced clearance of lidocaine by cimetidine. *Ann Intern Med* 1982; 96:592–593.

42. Duff HJ, Primm PK, Roden D, Oates JA, Woosley RL. Mexiletine in the treatment of resistant ventricular arrhythmias: Enhancement of efficacy and reduction of dose-related side effects by combination with quinidine. *Circulation* 1983; 67:1124–1128.

43. Leahey EBJ, Heissenbuttel RH, Giardina EV, Bigger JT Jr. Combined mexiletine and propranolol treatment of refractory ventricular arrhythmia. *Br Med J* 1980; 281:357–358.

44. Ruskin JN, DiMarco JP, Garan H. Out-of-hospital cardiac arrest: Electrophysiologic observations and selection of long-term antiarrhythmic therapy. *N Engl J Med* 1980; 303:607–613.

45. Stein J, Podrid P, Lown B. Effects of oral mexiletine on left and right ventricular function. *Am J Cardiol* 1984; 54:575–578.

46. Yamaguchi I, Singh BN, Mandel WJ. Electrophysiological effects of mexiletine on isolated rabbit atria and canine ventricular muscle Purkinje fiber. *Cardiovasc Res* 1979; 13:288–296.

47. Weld FM, Bigger JT Jr, Swistel D, Bordiuk J, Lau YH. Electrophysiological effects of mexiletine (KO1173) on ovine cardiac Purkinje fibers. *J Pharmacol Exp Ther* 1979; 210:222–228.

48. Prescott LF, Clements JA, Pottage A. Absorption, distribution, and elimination of mexiletine. *Postgrad Med J* 1977; 53(suppl 1):50–55.

49. Beckett AH, Chidomere EC. The distribution, metabolism and excretion of mexiletine in man. *Postgrad Med J* 1977; 53(suppl 1):60–66.

50. Campbell NPS, Kelley JG, Adgey AAJ, Shanks RG. The clinical pharmacology of mexiletine. *Br J Clin Pharmacol* 1978; 6:103–108.

51. Woosley RL, Wang T, Stone W, Siddoway L, Thompson K, Duff HJ, et al. Pharmacology, electrophysiology, and pharmacokinetics of mexiletine. *Am Heart J* 1984; 107:1058–1065.

52. Brown JE, Shand DG. Therapeutic drug monitoring of antiarrhythmic agents. *Clin Pharmacokinet* 1982; 7:125–148.

53. el Allaf D, Henrard L, Crochelet L, Delapierre D, Carlier J, Dresse A. Pharmacokinetics of mexiletine in renal insufficiency. *Br J Clin Pharmacol* 1982; 14:431–435.

54. Leahey EBJ, Giardina EV, Bigger JT Jr. Effect of ventricular failure on steady state kinetics of mexiletine. *Clin Res* 1980; 26:239A.

55. Pentikainen PJ, Hietakorpi S, Halinen MO, Lampinen LM. Cirrhosis of the liver markedly impairs the elimination of mexiletine. *Eur J Clin Pharmacol* 1986; 30:83–88.

56. Fasola GP, D'Osualdo F, de Pangher V, Barducci E. Thrombocytopenia and mexiletine (letter). *Ann Intern Med* 1984; 100:162.

57. Girmann G, Pees H, Scheurlen PG. Pseudothrombocytopenia and mexiletine (letter). *Ann Intern Med* 1984; 100:767.

58. Roos JC, Paalman ACA, Dunning AJ. Electrophysiological effects of mexiletine in man. *Br Heart J* 1976; 38:1262–1271.

59. Campbell RWF, Dolder MA, Prescott LF, Talbot RG, Murray A, Julian DG. Comparison of procainamide and mexiletine in prevention of ventricular arrhythmias after acute myocardial infarction. *Lancet* 1975; 1:1257–1259.

60. Klein MD, Levine PA, Ryan TJ. Antiarrhythmic efficacy, pharmacokinetics and clinical safety of tocainide in convalescent myocardial infarction patients. *Chest* 1980; 77:726–730.

61. Stein J, Podrid PJ, Lampert S, Hirsowitz G, Lown B. Long-term mexiletine for ventricular arrhythmia. *Am Heart J* 1984; 107:1091–1098.

62. Saunamaki KI. Hemodynamic effects of a new anti-arrhythmic agent mexiletine (Ko 1173) in ischaemic heart disease. *Cardiovasc Res* 1975; 9:788–792.

63. Campbell RWF. Mexiletine. *N Engl J Med* 1987; 316:29–34.

64. Pentikainen PJ, Koivula IH, Hiltunen HA. Effect of rifampicin treatment on the kinetics of mexiletine. *Eur J Clin Pharmacol* 1982; 23:261–266.

65. Bigger JT Jr. The interaction of mexiletine with other cardiovascular drugs. *Am Heart J* 1984; 107:1079–1085.

66. Hoffman BF, Rosen MR, Wit AL. Electrophysiology and pharmacology of cardiac arrhythmias. VII. Cardiac effects of quinidine and procaine amide. *Am Heart J* 1975; 90:117–122.

67. Wellens HJJ, Durrer D. Effect of procaine amide, quinidine and ajmaline in the Wolff-Parkinson-White syndrome. *Circulation* 1974; 50:114–120.

68. Elson J, Strong JM, Lee W, Atkinson AJ Jr. Antiarrhythmic potency of N-acetylprocainamide. *Clin Pharmacol Ther* 1975; 17:134–140.

69. Dangman KH, Hoffman BF. In vivo and in vitro antiarrhythmic and arrhythmogenic effects of N-acetyl procainamide. *J Pharmacol Exp Ther* 1981; 217:851–862.

70. Roden DM, Reele SB, Higgins SB, Wilkinson GR, Smith RF, Oates JA, et al. Antiarrhythmic efficacy, pharmacokinetics and safety of N-acetylprocainamide in human subjects: Comparison with procainamide. *Am J Cardiol* 1980; 46:463–468.

71. Kluger J, Drayer DE, Reidenberg M, Ellis G, Lloyd V, Tyberg T, et al. The clinical pharmacology and antiarrhythmic efficacy of acetylprocainamide in patients with arrhythmias. *Am J Cardiol* 1980; 45:1250–1257.

72. Mark LC, Kayden HJ, Steele JM, Rovenstine EA, et al. The physiologic disposition and cardiac effects of procaine amide. *J Pharmacol Exp Ther* 1951; 102:5–15.

73. Jaillon P, Winkle RA. Electrophysiologic comparative study of procainamide and N-acetylprocainamide in anesthetized dogs: Concentration-response relationships. *Circulation* 1979; 60: 1385–1394.

74. Komeichi K, Tohse N, Nakaya H, Shimizu M, Zhu MY, Kanno M. Effects of N-acetylprocainamide and sotalol on ion currents in isolated guinea-pig ventricular myocytes. *Eur J Pharmacol* 1990; 187:313–322.

75. Jaillon P, Rubenson D, Peters F, Mason JW, Winkle RA. Electrophysiologic effects of N-acetylprocainamide in human beings. *Am J Cardiol* 1981; 47:1134–1140.

76. Funck-Brentano C, Jared LL, Roden DM, Woosley RL. Interaction of procainamide and N-acetylprocainamide in man. *Circulation* 1987; 76(suppl):IV-520.

77. Myerburg RJ, Kessler KM, Kiem I, Pefkanos KC, Conde CA, Cooper D, et al. Relationship between plasma levels of procainamide, suppression of premature ventricular complexes and prevention of recurrent ventricular tachycardia. *Circulation* 1981; 64:280–290.

78. Giardina EV, Heissenbuttel RH, Bigger JT Jr. Intermittent intravenous procainamide to treat ventricular arrhythmias. Correlation of plasma concentration with effect on arrhythmia, electrocardiogram and blood pressure. *Ann Intern Med* 1973; 78:183–193.

79. Lima JJ, Goldfarb AL, Conti DR, Golden LH, Bascomb BL, Benedetti GM, et al. Safety and efficacy of procainamide infusions. *Am J Cardiol* 1979; 43:98–105.

80. Karlsson E. Clinical pharmacokinetics of procainamide. *Clin Pharmacokinet* 1978; 3:97–107.

81. du Souich P, Erill S. Metabolism of procainamide in patients with chronic heart failure, chronic respiratory failure and chronic renal failure. *Eur J Clin Pharmacol* 1978; 14:21–27.

82. Kessler KM, Kayden DS, Estes DM, Koslovskis PL, Sequira R, Trohman RG, et al. Procainamide pharmacokinetics in patients with acute myocardial infarction or congestive heart failure. *J Am Coll Cardiol* 1986; 7:1131–1139.

83. Jackman WM, Clark M, Friday KJ, Aliot EM, Anderson JL, Lazzara R. Ventricular tachyarrhythmias in the long QT syndrome. *Med Clin North Am* 1984; 68:1079–1109.

84. Olshansky B, Martins J, Hunt S. *N*-acetyl procainamide causing torsades de pointes. *Am J Cardiol* 1982; 50:1439–1441.

85. Brachmann J, Scherlag BJ, Rosenshtraukh LV, Lazzara R. Bradycardia-dependent triggered activity: Relevance to drug-induced multiform ventricular tachycardia. *Circulation* 1983; 68:846–856.

86. Kosowsky BD, Taylor J, Lown B, Ritchie RF. Long-term use of procaine amide following acute myocardial infarction. *Circulation* 1973; 47:1204–1210.

87. Ellrodt AG, Murata GH, Riedinger MS, Stewart ME, Mochizuki C, Gray R. Severe neutropenia associated with sustained-release procainamide. *Ann Intern Med* 1984; 100:197–201.

88. Wyse DG, McAnulty JH, Rahimtoola SH. Influence of plasma drug level and the presence of conduction disease on the electrophysiologic effects of procainamide. *Am J Cardiol* 1979; 43:619–626.

89. Somogyi A, McLean A, Heinzow B. Cimetidine-procainamide pharmacokinetic interaction in man: Evidence of competition for tubular secretion of basic drugs. *Eur J Clin Pharmacol* 1983; 25:339–345.

90. Christian CDJ, Meredith CG, Speeg KV Jr. Cimetidine inhibits renal procainamide clearance. *Clin Pharmacol Ther* 1984; 36:221–227.

91. Somogyi A, Bochner F. Dose and concentration dependent effect of ranitidine on procainamide disposition and renal clearance in man. *Br J Clin Pharmacol* 1984; 18:175–181.

92. Danilo P Jr, Hordof AJ, Rosen MR. Effects of disopyramide on electrophysiologic properties of canine cardiac Purkinje fibers. *J Pharmacol Exp Ther* 1977; 201:701–710.

93. Mirro MJ, Watanabe AM, Bailey JC. Electrophysiological effects of disopyramide and quinidine on guinea pig atria and canine Purkinje fibers. *Circ Res* 1980; 46:660–668.

94. Befeler B, Castellanos A, Wells DE, Vagueiro MC, Yeh BK. Electrophysiologic effects of the antiarrhythmic agent disopyramide phosphate. *Am J Cardiol* 1975; 35:282–287.

95. Dubetz DK, Brown NN, Hooper WD, Eadie MJ, Tyrer JH. Disopyramide pharmacokinetics and bioavailability (letter). *Br J Clin Pharmacol* 1978; 6:279–281.

96. Johnston A, Henry JA, Warrington SJ, Hamer NAJ. Pharmacokinetics of oral disopyramide phosphate in patients with renal impairment. *Br J Clin Pharmacol* 1980; 10:245–248.

97. Rangno RE, Warnica W, Ogilvie RI, Kreeft JH, Bridger E. Correlation of disopyramide pharmacokinetics with efficacy in ventricular tachyarrhythmia. *J Int Med Res* 1976; 4(suppl 1):54–58.

98. Hinderling PH, Garrett ER. Pharmacokinetics of the antiarrhythmic disopyramide in healthy humans. *J Pharmacokinet Biopharm* 1976; 4:199–230.

99. Hinderling PH, Garrett ER. Pharmacodynamics of the antiarrhythmic disopyramide in healthy humans. Correlation of the kinetics of the drug and its effect. *J Pharmacokinet Biopharm* 1976; 4:231–242.

100. Meffin PJ, Robert EW, Winkle RA, Harapat S, Peters FA, Harrison DC. The role of concentration-dependent plasma protein binding in disopyramide disposition. *J Pharmacokinet Biopharm* 1979; 7:29–46.

101. Davies RF, Siddoway LA, Shaw L, Barbey JT, Roden DM, Woosley RL. Immediate- versus controlled-release disopyramide: Importance of saturable binding. *Clin Pharmacol Ther* 1993; 54:16–22.

102. Edvardsson N, Olsson SB. Clinical value of plasma concentrations of antiarrhythmic drugs. *Eur Heart J* 1987; 8(suppl A):83–89.

103. Kumana CR, Rambihar VS, Tanser PH, Cairns JA, Gupta RN, Wildeman RA, et al. A placebo-controlled study to determine the efficacy of oral disopyramide phosphate for the prophylaxis of ventricular dysrhythmias after acute myocardial infarction. *Br J Clin Pharmacol* 1982; 14:519–527.

104. Ilett KF, Madsen BW, Woods JD. Disopyramide kinetics in patients with acute myocardial infarction. *Clin Pharmacol Ther* 1979; 26:1–7.

105. Podrid PJ, Schoenberger A, Lown B. Congestive heart failure caused by oral disopyramide. *N Engl J Med* 1980; 302:614–617.

106. Bonde J, Gradual NA, Pedersen LE, Balslov S, Angelo HR, Svendsen TL, et al. Kinetics of disopyramide in decreased hepatic function. *Eur J Clin Pharmacol* 1986; 31:73–77.

107. Mokler CM, Hillman RA. Nature of the anticholinergic action of some antiarrhythmic drugs. *Pharmacol Res Commun* 1972; 4:171–178.

108. Teichman SL, Ferrick A, Kim SG, Matos JA, Waspe LE, Fisher JD. Disopyramide-pyridostigmine interaction: Selective reversal of anticholinergic symptoms with preservation of antiarrhythmic effect. *J Am Coll Cardiol* 1987; 10:633–641.

109. Schweitzer P, Mark H. Torsades de pointes caused by disopyramide and hypokalemia. *Mt Sinai J Med* 1982; 49:110–114.

110. LaBarre A, Strauss HC, Scheinman MM, Evans GT, Bashore T, Tiedman JS, et al. Electrophysiological effects of disopyramide phosphate on sinus node function in patients with sinus mode dysfunction. *Circulation* 1979; 59:226–235.

111. Roden DM, Hoffman BF. Action potential prolongation and induction of abnormal automaticity by low quinidine concentrations in canine Purkinje fibers. Relationship to potassium and cycle length. *Circ Res* 1985; 56:857–867.

112. Risler T, Burk M, Peters U, Grabensee B, Seipel L. On the interaction between digoxin and disopyramide. *Clin Pharmacol Ther* 1983; 34:176–180.

113. Sylven C, Anderson P. Evidence that disopyramide does not interact with warfarin. *Br Med J* 1983; 286:1181.

114. Kessler JM, Keys PW, Stattford RW. Disopyramide and phenytoin interaction. *Clin Pharm* 1982; 1:263–264.

115. Aitio M, Mansury L, Tala E, Haataja M, Aitio A. The effect of enzyme-induction on the metabolism of disopyramide in man. *Br J Clin Pharmacol* 1981; 11:279–285.

116. Aitio M, Vuorenmaa T. Enhanced metabolism and diminished efficacy of disopyramide by enzyme induction. *Br J Clin Pharmacol* 1980; 9:149–152.

117. Cumming AD, Robertson C. Interaction between disopyramide and practolol. *Br Med J* 1979; 2:1264.

118. Sodermark T, Edhag O, Sjogren A, Jönssen B, Olsson A, Oro L, et al. Effect of quinidine on maintaining sinus rhythm after conversion of atrial fibrillation or flutter: A multicenter study from Stockholm. *Br Heart J* 1975; 37:486–492.

119. Levi GF, Proto C. Combined treatment of atrial fibrillation with quinidine and beta-blockers. *Br Heart J* 1972; 34:911–914.

120. Wu D, Kou H, Hung J. Exercise-triggered paroxysmal ventricular tachycardia. *Ann Intern Med* 1981; 95:410–414.

121. Bloomfield SS, Romhilt DW, Chou T, Fowler NO. Natural history of cardiac arrhythmias and their prevention with quinidine in patients with acute coronary insufficiency. *Circulation* 1973; 47:967–973.

122. Yount EH, Rosenblum M, McMillan RL. Use of quinidine in treatment of chronic auricular fibrillation. *Arch Intern Med* 1952; 89:63–69.

123. Weisman SA. Do's and don'ts in the treatment of auricular fibrillation with quinidine. *Am J Cardiol* 1959; 3:333–335.

124. Carliner NH, Crouthamel WG, Fisher ML, Mugmon MA, Vassar DL, Narang PK, et al. Quinidine therapy in hospitalized patients with ventricular arrhythmias. *Am Heart J* 1979; 98:708–715.

125. Winkle RA, Gradman AH, Fitzgerald JW. Antiarrhythmic drug effect assessed from ventricular arrhythmia reduction in the ambulatory electrocardiogram and treadmill test: Comparison of propranolol, procainamide and quinidine. *Am J Cardiol* 1978; 42:473–480.

126. Coplen SE, Antman EM, Berlin JA, Hewitt P, Chalmers TC. Efficacy and safety of quinidine therapy for maintenance of sinus rhythm after cardioversion. A meta-analysis of randomized control trials. *Circulation* 1990; 82(4):1106–1114.

127. Woosley RL, Sale M. QT interval: A measure of drug action. *Am J Cardiol* 1993; 72:36B–43B.

128. Sokolow M, Edgar AL. Blood quinidine concentrations as a guide in the treatment of cardiac arrhythmias. *Circulation* 1950; 1:576–592.

129. Vozeh S, Oti-Amoako K, Uematsu T, Follath F. Antiarrhythmic activity of two quinidine metabolites in experimental reperfusion arrhythmia: Relative potency and pharmacodynamic interaction with the parent drug. *J Pharmacol Exp Ther* 1987; 43:297–301.

130. Vozeh S, Bindschedler M, Huy-Riem HA, Kaufmann G, Guentert TW, Follath F. Pharmacodynamics of 3-hydroxyquinidine alone and in combination with quinidine in healthy persons. *Am J Cardiol* 1987; 59:681–684.

131. Kavanagh KM, Wyse DG, Mitchell LB, Gilhooly T, Gillis AM, Duff HJ. Contribution of quinidine metabolites to electrophysiologic responses in human subjects. *Clin Pharmacol Ther* 1989; 46:352–358.

132. Thompson KA, Blair IA, Woosley RL, Roden DM. Comparative in vitro electrophysiology of quinidine, its major metabolites and dihydroxyquinidine. *J Pharmacol Exp Ther* 1987; 241:84–90.

133. Drayer DE, Lorenzo B, Reidenberg MM. Liquid chromatography and fluorescence spectroscopy compared with a homogeneous enzyme immunoassay technique for determining quinidine in serum. *Clin Chem* 1981; 27:308–310.

134. Lehmann CR, Boran KJ, Pierson WP, Melikian AP, Wright GJ. Quini-

dine assays: Enzyme immunoassay versus high performance liquid chromatography. *Ther Drug Monit* 1986; 8:336–339.

135. Drayer DE, Lowenthal DT, Restivo KM, Schwartz A, Cook CE, Reidenberg MM. Steady-state serum levels of quinidine and active metabolites in cardiac patients with varying degrees of renal function. *Clin Pharmacol Ther* 1978; 24:31–39.

136. Kessler KM, Humphries WC, Black M, Spann JF. Quinidine pharmacokinetics in patients with cirrhosis or receiving propranolol. *Am Heart J* 1978; 96:627–635.

137. Ochs HR, Greenblatt DJ, Woo E. Clinical pharmacokinetics of quinidine. *Clin Pharmacokinet* 1980; 5:150–168.

138. Kay GN, Plumb VJ, Arciniegas JG, Henthorn RW, Waldo AL. Torsades de pointes: The long-short initiating sequence and other clinical features. Observations in 32 patients. *J Am Coll Cardiol* 1983; 2:806–817.

139. Gottlieb SS, Weinberg M. Hemodynamic and neurohormonal effects of quinidine in patients with severe left ventricular dysfunction secondary to coronary artery disease or idiopathic dilated cardiomyopathy. *Am J Cardiol* 1991; 67:728–731.

140. Cohen IS, Jick H, Cohen SI. Adverse reactions to quinidine in hospitalized patients: Findings based on data from the Boston Collaborative Drug Surveillance Programs. *Prog Cardiovasc Dis* 1977; 20:151–163.

141. Dargie HJ, Cleland JGF, Leckie BJ, Inglis CG, East BW, Ford I. Relation of arrhythmias and electrolyte abnormalities to survival in patients with severe chronic heart failure. *Circulation* 1987; 75(suppl):IV-98–IV-107.

142. Roden D, Woosley R, Primm R. Incidence and clinical features of the quinidine-associated long-QT syndrome: Implications for patient care. *Am Heart J* 1986; 111:1088–1093.

143. Makkar RR, Fromm BS, Steinman RT, Meissner MD, Lehmann MH. Female gender as a risk factor for torsades de pointes associated with cardiovascular drugs. *JAMA* 1993; 270:2590–2597.

144. Drici MD, Burklow TR, Haridasse V, Glazer RI, Woosley RL. Sex hormones prolong the QT interval and down-regulate potassium channel expression in the rabbit heart. *Circulation* 1996; 94:1471–1474.

145. Schmid PG, Nelson LD, Mark AL, Heistad DD, Abboud FM. Inhibition of adrenergic vasoconstriction by quinidine. *J Pharmacol Exp Ther* 1974; 188:124–134.

146. Nair MR, Duvernoy WF, Leichtman DA. Severe leukopenia and thrombocytopenia secondary to quinidine. *Clin Cardiol* 1981; 4:247–257.

147. Polish LB, Branch RA, Fitzgerald GA. Digitoxin-quinidine interaction: Potentiation during administration of cimetidine. *South Med J* 1981; 74:633–634.

148. Data JL, Wilkinson GR, Nies AS. Interaction of quinidine with anticonvulsant drugs. *N Engl J Med* 1976; 294:699–702.

149. Leahey EBJ, Reiffel JA, Drusin RE, Heissenbuttel RH, Lovejoy WP, Bigger JT Jr. Interactions between quinidine and digoxin. *JAMA* 1978; 240:533–534.

150. Bussey HI. The influence of quinidine and other agents on digitalis glycosides. *Am Heart J* 1982; 104:289–302.

151. Brinn R, Brosen K, Gram LF, Haghfelt T, Otton SV. Spartine oxidation is practically abolished in quinidine-treated patients. *Br J Clin Pharmacol* 1986; 22:194–197.

152. Inaba T, Tyndale RE, Mahon WA. Quinidine: Potent inhibition of spartine and debrisoquine oxidation in vivo (letter). *Br J Clin Pharmacol* 1986; 22:199–200.

153. Spiers CJ, Murray S, Boobis AR, Seddon CE, Davies DS. Quinidine and the identification of drugs whose elimination is impaired in subjects classified as poor metabolizers of debrisoquine. *Br J Clin Pharmacol* 1986; 22:739–743.

154. Guengerich FP, Muller-Enoch D, Blair IA. Oxidation of quinidine by human liver cytochrome P-450. *Mol Pharmacol* 1986; 30:287–295.

155. Mikus G, Ha HR, Vozeh S, Zekorn C, Follath F, Eichelbaum M. Pharmacokinetics and metabolism of quinidine in extensive and poor metabolizers of spartine. *Eur J Clin Pharmacol* 1986; 31:69–72.

156. Brosen K, Gram LF, Haghfelt T, Bertilsson L. Extensive metabolizers of debrisoquin become poor metabolizers during quinidine treatment. *Pharmacol Toxicol* 1987; 60:312–314.

157. Kornfeld P, Horowitz SH, Genkins G, Papatestas AE. Myasthenia gravis unmasked by antiarrhythmic agents. *Mt Sinai J Med* 1976; 43:10–14.

158. Grogono AW. Anesthesia for atrial fibrillation. Effect of quinidine on muscle relaxation. *Lancet* 1963; 2:1039–1040.

159. Connolly SJ, Mulji AS, Hoffert DL, Davis CA, Schragge BW. Randomized placebo-controlled trial of propafenone for treatment of atrial tachyarrhythmias after cardiac surgery. *J Am Coll Cardiol* 1987; 10:1145–1148.

160. von Philipsborn G, Gries J, Hofmann HP, Krieskott H, Kretzschmar R, Muller CD, et al. Pharmacological studies on propafenone and its main metabolite 5-hydroxypropafenone. *Arzneimittelforschung* 1984; 34:1489–1497.

161. Valenzuela C, Delgado C, Tamargo J. Electrophysiological effects of 5-hydroxypropafenone on guinea pig ventricular muscle fibers. *J Cardiovasc Pharmacol* 1987; 10:523–529.

162. McLeod AA, Stiles GL, Shand DG. Demonstration of beta adrenoceptor blockade by propafenone hydrochloride: Clinical pharmacologic, radioligand binding, and adenylate cyclase activation studies. *J Pharmacol Exp Ther* 1984; 228:461–466.

163. Muller-Peltzer H, Greger G, Neugebauer G, Hollman M. Beta-blocking and electrophysiological effects of propafenone in volunteers. *Eur J Clin Pharmacol* 1983; 25:831–833.

164. Siddoway LA, Thompson KA, McAllister CB, Roden DM, Woosley RL. Polymorphism of propafenone metabolism and disposition in man: Clinical and pharmacokinetic consequences. *Circulation* 1987; 75:785–791.

165. Lee JT, Funck-Brentano C, Lineberry MD, Chaffin PL, Roden DM, Woosley RL. Beta receptor antagonism by propafenone in man: Influence of polymorphic metabolism (abstr). *Clin Res* 1988; 36:294A.

166. Baker BJ, Dinh H, Kroskey D, deSoyza NDB, Murphy ML, Franciosa JA. Effect of propafenone on left ventricular ejection fraction. *Am J Cardiol* 1984; 54(suppl):20D–22D.

167. Wagner F, Kalusche D, Trenk D, Jahnchen E, Roskamm H. Drug interaction between propafenone and metoprolol. *Br J Clin Pharmacol* 1987; 24:213–220.

168. Funck-Brentano C, Kroemer HK, Pavlou H, Woosley RL, Roden DM. Genetically-determined interaction between propafenone and low dose quinidine: Role of active metabolites in modulating net drug effect. *Br J Clin Pharmacol* 1989; 27:435–444.

169. Roden DM, Woosley RL. Flecainide. *N Engl J Med* 1986; 315:36–41.

170. Hellestrand KJ, Nathan AW, Bexton RS, Spurrell RAJ, Camm AJ. Cardiac electrophysiologic effects of flecainide acetate for paroxysmal reentrant junctional tachycardias. *Am J Cardiol* 1983; 51:770–776.

171. Pritchett EL, Wilkinson WE. Mortality in patients treated with flecainide and encainide for supraventricular arrhythmias. *Am J Cardiol* 1991; 67(11):976–980.

172. The Flecainide-Quinidine Research Group. Flecainide versus quinidine for treatment of chronic ventricular arrhythmias. A multicenter clinical trial. *Circulation* 1983; 67:1117–1123.

173. Follmer CH, Colatsky TJ. Block of delayed rectifier potassium current, I_K, by flecainide and E-4031 in cat ventricular myocytes. *Circulation* 1990; 82(1):289–293.

174. Estes NAM III, Garan H, Ruskin JN. Electrophysiological properties of flecainide acetate. *Am J Cardiol* 1984; 53(suppl):26B–29B.

175. Conrad GJ, Ober RE. Metabolism of flecainide. *Am J Cardiol* 1984; 53(suppl):41B–51B.

176. Haefeli W, Bargetzi M, Follath F, Meyer UA. Potent inhibition of cytochrome P450IID6 (debrisoquin 4-hydroxylase) by flecainide in vitro and in vivo. *J Cardiovasc Pharmacol* 1990; 15:776–779.

177. Johnston A, Warrington S, Turner P. Flecainide pharmacokinetics in healthy volunteers: The influence of urinary pH. *Br J Clin Pharmacol* 1985; 20:333–338.

178. Franciosa JA, Wilen M, Weeks CE, Tannenbaum R, Kvam DC, Miller AM. Pharmacokinetics and hemodynamic effects of flecainide in patients with chronic low output heart failure (abstr). *J Am Coll Cardiol* 1983; 1:699.

179. Winkelman BR, Leinberger H. Life-threatening flecainide toxicity. A pharmacodynamic approach. *Ann Intern Med* 1987; 106:807–814.

180. Salerno DM, Granrud GA, Sharkey P, Asinger RW. Pharmacodynamics and side effects of flecainide acetate. *Clin Pharmacol Ther* 1986; 40:101–107.

181. Morganroth J, Horowitz LN. Flecainide: Its proarrhythmic effect and expected changes on the surface electrocardiogram. *Am J Cardiol* 1984; 53(suppl):89B–94B.

182. Josephson MA, Kaul S, Hopkins J, Kvam DC, Singh BN. Hemodynamic effects of intravenous flecainide relative to the level of ventricular function in patients with coronary artery disease. *Am Heart J* 1985; 109:41–45.

183. Muhiddin KA, Turner P, Blackett A. Effect of flecainide on cardiac output. *Clin Pharmacol Ther* 1985; 37:260–263.

184. Rotmensch HH, Belhassen B, Ferguson RK. Amiodarone—benefits and risks in perspective. *Am Heart J* 1982; 104:1117–1119.

185. Josephson MA, Ikeda N, Singh BN. Effects of flecainide on ventricular function: Clinical and experimental correlations. *Am J Cardiol* 1984; 53(5):95B–100B.

186. Vik-Mo H, Ohm O, Lund-Johansen P. Electrophysiological effects of flecainide acetate in patients with sinus nodal dysfunction. *Am J Cardiol* 1982; 50:1090–1094.

187. Hellestrand KJ, Nathan AW, Bexton RS, Camm AJ. Electrophysiologic effects of flecainide acetate on sinus node function, anomalous atrioventricular connections and pacemaker thresholds. *Am J Cardiol* 1984; 53(suppl):30B–38B.

188. Hellestrand KJ, Burnett PJ, Milne JR, Bexton RS, Nathan AW, Camm AJ. The effect of the antiarrhythmic agent flecainide on acute and chronic pacing thresholds. *Pacing Clin Electrophysiol* 1983; 6:892–899.

189. Hernandez R, Mann DE, Breckinridge S, Williams GR, Reiter MJ. Effects of flecainide on defibrillation thresholds in the anesthetized dog. *J Am Coll Cardiol* 1989; 14:777–781.

190. Tjandra-Maga TB, van Hecken A, van Melle P, Verbesselt R, deSchepper PJ. Altered pharmacokinetics of oral flecainide by cimetidine. *Br J Clin Pharmacol* 1986; 22:108–110.

191. Weeks CE, Conard GJ, Kvam DC, Fox JM, Chang SF, Paone RP, et al. The effect of flecainide acetate, a new antiarrhythmic, on plasma digoxin levels. *J Clin Pharmacol* 1986; 26:27–31.

192. Lewis GP, Holtzman JL. Interaction of flecainide with digoxin and propranolol. *Am J Cardiol* 1984; 53(suppl):52B–57B.

193. Shea P, Lal R, Kim SS, Schechtman K, Ruffy R. Flecainide and amiodarone interaction. *J Am Coll Cardiol* 1986; 7:1127–1130.

194. Rowland E. Antiarrhythmic drugs—class IV. *Eur Heart J* 1987; 8(suppl A):61–63.

195. Singh BN, Nademanee K, Baky SH. Calcium antagonists. Clinical use in the treatment of arrhythmias. *Drugs* 1983; 25:125–153.

196. Bacaner MB. Treatment of ventricular fibrillation and other acute arrhythmias with bretylium tosylate. *Am J Cardiol* 1968; 21:530–543.

197. Bigger JT Jr, Jaffe CC. The effect of bretylium tosylate on the electrophysiologic properties of ventricular muscle and Purkinje fibers. *Am J Cardiol* 1971; 27:82–92.

198. Cardinale R, Sasyniuk BI. Electrophysiological effects of bretylium tosylate on subendocardial Purkinje fibers from infarcted canine hearts. *J Pharmacol Exp Ther* 1978; 204:159–174.

199. Nishimura M, Watanabe Y. Membrane action and catecholamine release action of bretylium tosylate in normoxic and hypoxic canine Purkinje fibers. *J Am Coll Cardiol* 1983; 2:287–295.

200. Narang PK, Adir J, Josselson J, Yacobi A. Pharmacokinetics of bretylium in man after intravenous administration. *J Pharmacokinet Biopharm* 1980; 8:363–372.

201. Chow MSS, Kluger J, DiPersio DM, Lawrence R, Fieldman A. Antifibrillatory effects of lidocaine and bretylium immediately postcardiopulmonary resuscitation. *Am Heart J* 1985; 110:938–943.

202. Duff HJ, Roden DM, Yacobi A, Robertson D, Wang T, Mattucci RJ, et al. Bretylium: Relations between plasma concentrations and pharmacologic actions in high-frequency ventricular arrhythmias. *Am J Cardiol* 1985; 55:395–401.

203. Singh BN, Nademanee K. Sotalol: A beta-blocker with unique antiarrhythmic properties. *Am Heart J* 1987; 114:121–139.

204. Singh BN, Kehoe R, Woosley RL, Scheinman M, Quart B. Multicenter trial of sotalol compared with procainamide in the suppression of inducible ventricular tachycardia: A double-blind, randomized parallel evaluation. Sotalol Multicenter Study Group. *Am Heart J* 1995; 129:87–97.

205. Mason JW, ESVEM Investigators. A comparison of seven antiarrhythmic drugs in patients with ventricular tachycardias. *N Engl J Med* 1993; 329:452–458.

206. Wang T, Bergstrand RH, Thompson KA, Siddoway L, Duff HJ, Woosley RL, et al. Concentration-dependent pharmacologic properties of sotalol. *Am J Cardiol* 1986; 57:1160–1165.

207. Kopleman HA, Woosley RL, Lee JT, Roden DM, Echt DS. Electrophysiologic effects of intravenous and oral sotalol for sustained ventricular tachycardia secondary to coronary artery disease. *Am J Cardiol* 1988; 61:1006–1011.

208. Graboys TB, Podrid PJ, Lown B. Efficacy of amiodarone for refractory supraventricular tachyarrhythmias. *Am Heart J* 1983; 106:870–876.

209. Horowitz LN, Spielman SR, Greenspan AM, Mintz GS, Morganroth J, Brown R, et al. Use of amiodarone in the treatment of persistent and paroxysmal atrial fibrillation resistant to quinidine therapy. *J Am Coll Cardiol* 1985; 6:1402–1407.

210. Peters RW, Fisher ML. Use of amiodarone. *Choices Cardiol* 1994; 8:57–60.

211. Singh SN, Fletcher RD, Gross-Fisher S, Singh BN, Lewis HD, Deedwania PC, et al. Amiodarone in patients with congestive heart failure and asymptomatic ventricular arrhythmia. *N Engl J Med* 1995; 333:77–82.

212. Cairns JA, Connolly SJ, Roberts R, Gent M, CAMIAT. Randomized trial of outcome after myocardial infarction in patients with frequent or repetitive premature depolarizations: CAMIAT (abstr). *Lancet* 1997; 349:675–682.

213. Julian DG, Camm AJ, Frangin G, Janse MJ, Munoz A, Schwartz PJ, et al. Randomized trial of effect of amiodarone on mortality in patients with left-ventricular dysfunction after recent myocardial infarction: EMIAT. *Lancet* 1997; 349:667–674.

214. Scheinman MM, Levine JH, Cannom DS, Friehling T, Kopelman HA, Chilson DA, et al. Dose-ranging study of intravenous amiodarone in patients with life-threatening ventricular tachyarrhythmias (abstr). *Circulation* 1995; 92:3264–3272.

215. Kowey PR, Levine JH, Herre JM, Pacifico A, Lindsay BD, Plumb VJ, et al. Randomized, double-blind comparison of intravenous amiodarone and bretylium in the treatment of patients with recurrent, hemodynamically destabilizing ventricular tachycardia or fibrillation (abstr). *Circulation* 1995; 92:3255–3263.

216. Mason JW. Amiodarone. *N Engl J Med* 1987; 316:455–466.

217. Mason JW, Hondeghem LM, Katzung BG. Amiodarone blocks inactivated cardiac sodium channels. *Pflugers Arch* 1983; 396:79–81.

218. Talajic M, DeRoode MR, Nattel S. Comparative electrophysiologic effects of intravenous amiodarone and desmethylamiodarone in dogs: Evidence for clinically relevant activity of the metabolite. *Circulation* 1987; 75:265–271.

219. Nanas JN, Mason JW. Pharmacokinetics and regional electrophysiological effects of intracoronary amiodarone administration. *Circulation* 1995; 91:451–461.

220. Albert SG, Alves LE, Rose EP. Thyroid dysfunction during chronic amiodarone therapy. *J Am Coll Cardiol* 1987; 9:175–183.

221. Singh BN, Nademanee K. Amiodarone and thyroid function: Clinical implications during antiarrhythmic therapy. *Am Heart J* 1983; 106:857–869.

222. Latham KR, Sellitti DF, Goldstein RE. Interaction of amiodarone and desethylamiodarone with solubilized nuclear thyroid hormone receptors. *J Am Coll Cardiol* 1987; 9:872–876.

223. Charlier R, Deltour G, Baudine A, Chaillet F. Pharmacology of amiodarone, an anti-anginal drug with a new biological profile. *Arzneimittelforschung* 1968; 18:1408–1417.

224. Cohen-Armon M, Schreiber G, Sokolovsky M. Interaction of the antiarrhythmic drug amiodarone with the muscarinic receptor in rat heart and brain. *J Cardiovasc Pharmacol* 1984; 6:1148–1155.

225. Pourbaix S, Berger Y, Desager J, Pacco M, Harvengt M. Absolute bioavailability of amiodarone in normal subjects. *Clin Pharmacol Ther* 1985; 37:118–123.

226. Adams PC, Holt DW, Storey GC, Morley AR, Callaghan J, Path MRC, et al. Amiodarone and its desethyl metabolite: Tissue distribution and morphologic changes during long-term therapy. *Circulation* 1985; 72:1064–1075.

227. Nattel S, Davies M, Quantz M. The antiarrhythmic efficacy of amiodarone and desethylamiodarone, alone and in combination, in dogs with acute myocardial infarction. *Circulation* 1988; 77:200–208.

228. Holt DW, Tucker GT, Jackson PR, McKenna WJ. Amiodarone pharmacokinetics. *Br J Clin Pract* 1986; 44(suppl):109–114.

229. Plomp TA, van Rossum JM, Robles de MEO, van Lier T, Maes RA. Pharmacokinetics and body distribution of amiodarone in man. *Arzneimittelforschung* 1984; 34:513–520.

230. Siddoway LA, McAllister CB, Wilkinson GR, Roden DM, Woosley RL. Amiodarone dosing: A proposal based on its pharmacokinetics. *Am Heart J* 1983; 106:951–956.

231. Cairns JA, Connolly SJ, Gent M, Roberts R. Post-myocardial infarction mortality in patients with ventricular premature depolarizations. *Circulation* 1991; 84:550–557.

232. Escoubet B, Coumel P, Poirier J, Maison-Blanche P, Jaillon P, LeClercq J-F, et al. Suppression of arrhythmias within hours after a

single oral dose of amiodarone and relation to plasma and myocardial concentrations. *Am J Cardiol* 1985; 55:696–702.

233. Mostow ND, Vrobel TR, Noon D, Rakita L. Rapid suppression of complex ventricular arrhythmias with high-dose oral amiodarone. *Circulation* 1986; 73:1231–1238.

234. Greenberg ML, Lerman BB, Shipe JR, Kaiser DL, DiMarco JP. Relation between amiodarone and desethylamiodarone plasma concentrations and electrophysiological effects, efficacy and toxicity. *J Am Coll Cardiol* 1987; 9:1148–1155.

235. Coumel P, Fidelle J. Amiodarone in the treatment of cardiac arrhythmias in children: One hundred thirty-five cases. *Am Heart J* 1980; 100:1063–1069.

236. Mason JW, the Amiodarone Study Group. Toxicity of amiodarone (abstr). *Circulation* 1985; 72(suppl):III–272.

237. Veltri EP, Reid PR. Amiodarone pulmonary toxicity: Early changes in pulmonary function test during amiodarone rechallenge. *J Am Coll Cardiol* 1985; 6:802–805.

238. Orlando RG, Dangel ME, Schaal SF. Clinical experience and grading of amiodarone keratopathy. *Ophthalmology* 1984; 91:1184–1187.

239. Zachary CB, Slater DN, Holt DW, Storey GCA, MacDonald DM. The pathogenesis of amiodarone-induced pigmentation and photosensitivity. *Br J Dermatol* 1984; 110:451–456.

240. Simon JB, Manley PN, Brien JF, Armstrong PW. Amiodarone hepatotoxicity simulating alcoholic liver disease. *N Engl J Med* 1984; 311:167–172.

241. Rigas B, Rosenfeld LE, Barwick KW, Enriquez R, Helzberg J, Batsford WP, et al. Amiodarone hepatotoxicity: A clinicopathologic study of five patients. *Ann Intern Med* 1986; 104:348–351.

242. Larrey D, Tinel M, Letteron P, Geneve J, Descatoire V, Pessayer D. Formation of an inactive cytochrome P-450 Fe(II)-metabolite complex after administration of amiodarone in rats, mice and hamsters. *Biochem Pharmacol* 1986; 35:2213–2220.

243. Almog S, Shafran N, Halkin H, Weiss P, Farfel Z, Martinowitz U, et al. Mechanism of warfarin potentiation by amiodarone: Dose- and concentration-dependent inhibition of warfarin elimination. *Eur J Clin Pharmacol* 1985; 28:257–261.

244. Marcus FI. Drug interactions with amiodarone. *Am Heart J* 1983; 106:924–930.

245. Fenster PE, White NWJ, Hanson CD. Pharmacokinetic evaluation of the digoxin-amiodarone interaction. *J Am Coll Cardiol* 1985; 5:108–112.

246. Stambler BS, Wood MA, Ellenbogen KA. Comparative efficacy of intravenous ibutilide versus procainamide for enhancing termination of atrial flutter by atrial overdrive pacing. *Am J Cardiol* 1996; 77:960–966.

247. Guo GB, Ellenbogen KA, Wood MA, Stambler BS. Conversion of atrial flutter by ibutilide is associated with increased atrial cycle length variability. *J Am Coll Cardiol* 1996; 27:1083–1089.

248. Lee KS. Ibutilide, a new compound with potent class III antiarrhythmic activity, activates a slow inward Na^+ current in guinea pig ventricular cells. *J Pharmacol Exp Ther* 1992; 262:99–108.

249. Yang T, Snyders DJ, Roden DM. Ibutilide, a methanesulfonanilide antiarrhythmic, is a potent blocker of the rapidly activating delayed rectifier K^+ current (IKr) in AT-1 cells. Concentration-, time-, voltage-, and use-dependent effects (see comments). *Circulation* 1995; 91:1799–1806.

250. Lerman BB, Belardinelli L. Cardiac electrophysiology of adenosine: Basic and clinical concepts. *Circulation* 1991; 83(5):1499–1509.

251. Ellenbogen K, Thames M, DiMarco JP, Sheehan H, Lerman BB. Electrophysiologic effects of adenosine in the transplanted human heart: Evidence for supersensitivity. *Circulation* 1990; 81:821–828.

252. Lerman BB, Wesley RC, Belardinelli L. Electrophysiologic effects of dipyridamole on atrioventricular nodal conduction and supraventricular tachycardia: Role of endogenous adenosine. *Circulation* 1989; 80:1536–1543.

253. DiMarco JP, Sellers TD, Lerman BB, Greenberg ML, Berne RM, Belardinelli L. Diagnostic and therapeutic use of adenosine in patients with supraventricular tachyarrhythmias. *J Am Coll Cardiol* 1985; 6:417–425.

254. Baskin EP, Serik CM, Wallace AA, Brookes LM, Selnick HG, Claremon DA, et al. Effects of new and potent methanesulfonanilide class III antiarrhythmic agents on myocardial refractoriness and contractility in isolated cardiac muscle. *J Cardiovasc Pharmacol* 1991; 18(3):406–414.

255. Wettwer E, Scholtysik G, Schaad A, Himmel H, Ravens U. Effects of the new class III antiarrhythmic drug E-4031 on myocardial contractility and electrophysiological parameters. *J Cardiovasc Pharmacol* 1991; 17:480–487.

256. Manning AS, Bruyninckx C, Ramboux J, Chatelain P. SR 33589, a new amiodarone-like agent: Effect on ischemia- and reperfusion-induced arrhythmias in anesthetized rats. *J Cardiovasc Pharmacol* 1995; 26:453–461.

31

TREATMENT OF CARDIAC ARRHYTHMIAS WITH CATHETER-ABLATIVE TECHNIQUES

Melvin M. Scheinman

Over the past several years various techniques have been introduced using catheter ablative procedures for patients with cardiac arrhythmias. Particularly impressive are some of the newer techniques utilizing radiofrequency energy sources for patients with supraventricular arrhythmias. This chapter reviews the techniques, results, and clinical indications for these procedures.

TECHNIQUES

Ablation of the Atrioventricular Junction

The technique of catheter ablation of the atrioventricular (AV) junction was first developed in canines[1] and subsequently applied for control of drug-refractory atrial arrhythmias in patients.[2,3] Multipolar electrode catheters are inserted by vein and positioned just across the tricuspid valve and against the apex of the right ventricle (Fig. 31-1). The catheter across the tricuspid valve is manipulated to allow the recording of the largest unipolar His bundle potential (Fig. 31-2).[2] Radiofrequency energy 350 to 500 kHz is applied between the distal electrode and a large back patch. After persistent AV block is observed, a permanent cardiac pacemaker is inserted (Fig. 31-3).

Atrioventricular Nodal Modification for Patients with Atrial Fibrillation

A more recent innovation has been use of AV nodal modification for achieving rate control in patients with atrial fibrillation.[4,5] This technique involves placement of radiofrequency lesions over the posterior or midseptum in order to achieve the desired reduction in rate during atrial fibrillation. The procedure entails a 20 percent risk of inducing complete AV

block, which usually occurs within the first 48 h after the ablation. In addition, late recurrence of rapid rate has been reported in approximately 10 percent of patients. The available data suggest that the bulk of suitably selected patients with

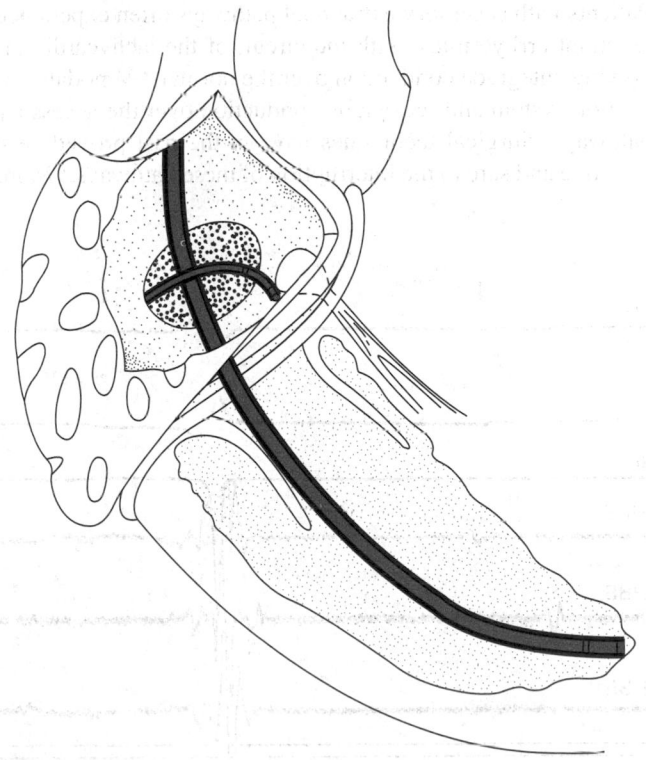

FIGURE 31-1

Catheter positions for patients undergoing AV junctional ablation. One catheter is placed over the region of the AV node, while a second catheter is placed against the apex of the right ventricle.

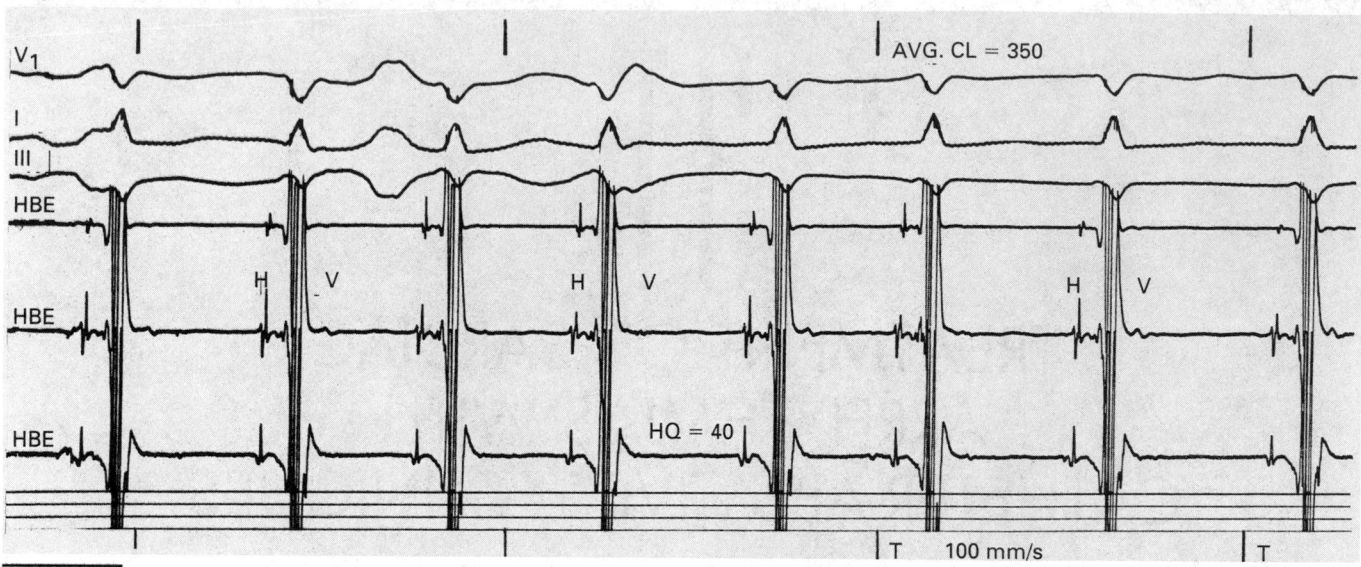

FIGURE 31-2

Atrial fibrillation with rapid ventricular response prior to ablation.

atrial fibrillation and rapid rate resistant to drug therapy will respond to AV nodal modification. This technique is of no value for relief of symptoms related to the irregular rhythm per se.

Ablation of Accessory Pathways

Patients with accessory extranodal pathways often experience reentrant arrhythmias, with the circuit of the tachycardia involving antegrade conduction over the normal AV-nodal conduction system and retrograde conduction over the accessory pathway.[6] Surgical techniques have in the past proved very effective and safe in the interruption of these pathways.[7] More

recently, a variety of catheter techniques have been introduced for catheter ablation of these pathways. Fisher et al.[8] were the first to use this technique for ablation of left free wall accessory pathways via the coronary sinus. Accessory AV pathways occur anywhere along the cardiac annulus or in the septum. The majority of pathways are found traversing the left AV groove. These pathways are currently approached by inserting a steerable multipolar electrode catheter into the femoral artery with retrograde catheterization of the left ventricle.[9] The catheter is then placed under the mitral annulus in the putative site of the accessory pathway (Fig. 31-4). An alternative technique involves use of transseptal catheteriza-

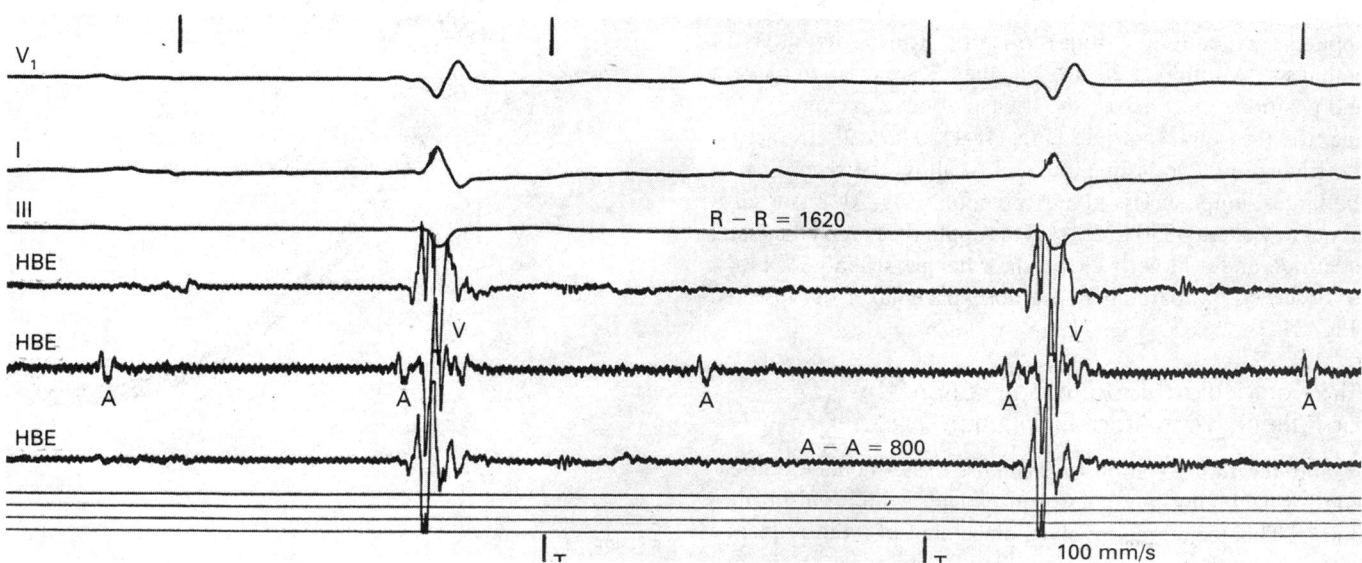

FIGURE 31-3

After completion of the ablation, complete AV block is achieved.

tion with placement of the catheter along the atrial margin of the mitral annulus.[10] One or more applications of radiofrequency energy are applied in order to ablate the pathways. In contrast, most septal and all right free wall pathways are approached by right-sided catheterization.

Modification of the Atrioventricular Node in Atrioventricular Nodal Reentrant Tachycardia

Patients with AV nodal reentrant tachycardia are thought to have two pathways within or in close proximity to the AV node. These pathways show fast and slow conducting properties and have different refractory periods. Techniques have been introduced that allow for selective ablation of either pathway. The fast pathway is approached by withdrawing the catheter to a more proximal location while recording the His bundle potential, which is associated with a large-amplitude atrial electrogram and a very small or absent His deflection.[11] Application of radiofrequency energy to this area results in abrupt prolongation of the PR, since ablation of the fast pathway forces conduction to occur over the slow pathway. An alternative technique for ablation of the slow pathway was introduced by Roman and associates,[12] where the radiofrequency energy is applied posteriorly between the os of the coronary sinus and the septal leaflet of the tricuspid valve. Successful application of the latter technique does not result in a change in the PR or AH. The approach described for slow-pathway ablation may be successfully accomplished either by using anatomic landmarks or searching for specific so-called slow-pathway potentials. This technique has proved to be more effective and safer than attempts at fast-pathway ablation.

Ablation of Atrial Flutter/Atrial Tachycardia

Very effective techniques have recently been introduced for ablation of atrial flutter. Patients with a "typical" flutter pattern have a reentrant circuit localized to the right atrium. The critical slow zone appears to reside in the isthmus between the inferior vena cava and the tricuspid annulus.[13] A catheter is used to apply serial lesions, creating a line of block across the isthmus, with initial results suggesting success in 85 to 90 percent of patients.[14]

Patients with atrial tachycardia may be treated with catheter-ablative techniques.[15] The catheter is manipulated to find the earliest endocardial atrial potential relative to the surface P wave (Fig. 31-5). Foci of atrial tachycardia are localized along the crista terminalis or atrial appendage in the right atrium. Left atrial foci occur around the superior pulmonary veins or left atrial appendage.[16] Once the earliest site is located, radiofrequency energy is applied in order to ablate the atrial focus (Fig. 31-6).

Modification of Sinus Node Function in Patients with Inappropriate Sinus Tachycardia

Patients with inappropriate sinus tachycardia have a resting tachycardia with abrupt increases in rate with mild exertion.[17]

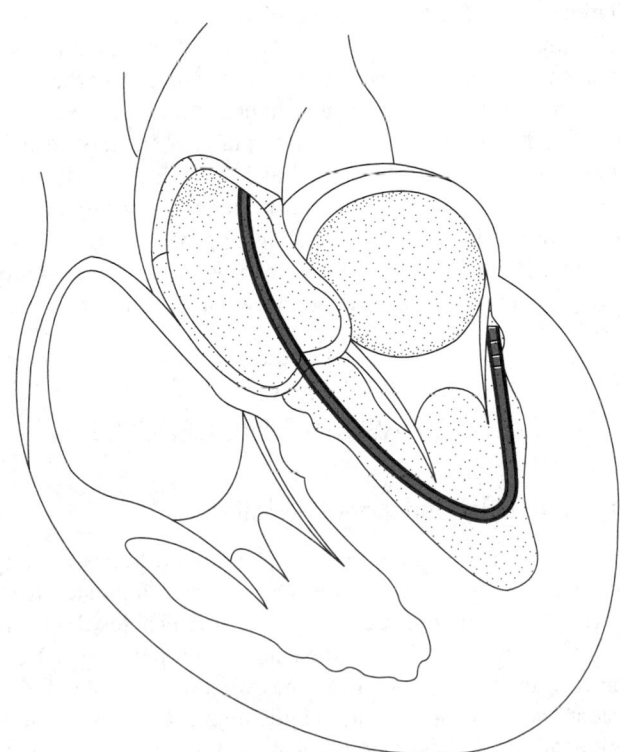

FIGURE 31-4
Schema depicting retrograde aortic technique for ablation of a left free wall accessory pathway. The catheter is passed across the aortic valve and placed under the mitral annulus.

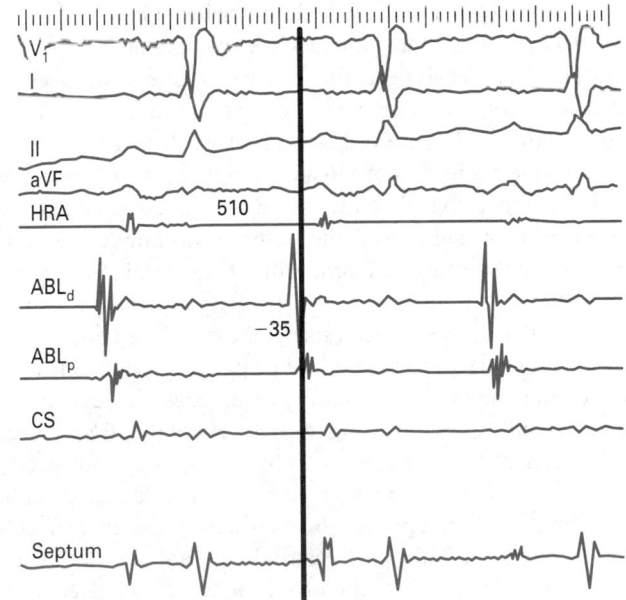

FIGURE 31-5
Simultaneous surface V_1, I, II, and intracardiac recordings from the high right atrium (HRA), distal (ABL_d) and proximal (ABL_P) electrodes from the ablating catheter, coronary sinus (CS), and low right atrial septum (Septum) in a patient with atrial tachycardia. The earliest atrial electrogram was 35 ms prior to the inscription of the surface P waves.

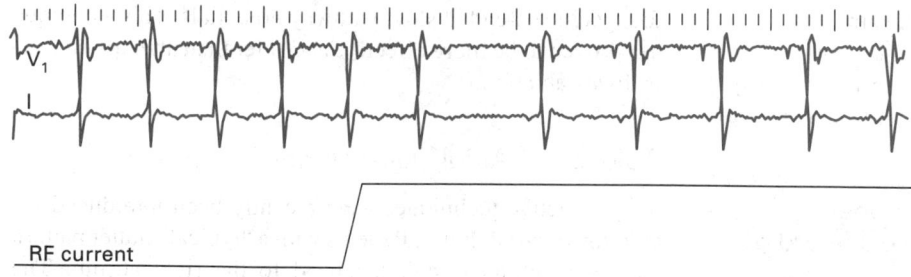

FIGURE 31-6

Same patient as in Fig. 31-5 showing application of radiofrequency energy with abrupt termination of the atrial tachycardia.

Typically, the arrhythmia shows diurnal variation with slowing to normal rates at night. These patients have an increased intrinsic heart rate and excessive response to exercise or catecholamines.[17] Catheter-ablative techniques have been introduced that allow for identification of the most rapid pacemaker region of the sinus node complex.[18] This is usually found over the superior crest of the crista terminalis. One or more radiofrequency lesions are placed in this area, producing dramatic decreases in the sinus rate.[19] In addition, when this procedure is successful, there is marked attenuation of the heart rate response to exercise or catecholamines.

Ablation of Ventricular Tachycardia Foci

The most demanding of the catheter-ablative techniques is attempted ablation of foci initiating ventricular tachycardia. For this procedure, multipolar electrode catheters are inserted into the right ventricle, coronary sinus, and left ventricle. Ventricular tachycardia is induced by using standard stimulation protocols, and the catheters are manipulated within the ventricles in order to determine the earliest ventricular endocardial electrogram (during ventricular tachycardia) in relation to at least three reference orthogonal surface leads.[20] Ventricular overdrive pacing is used in an attempt to entrain the tachycardia and to prove that the earliest endocardial potentials precede (rather than follow) the tachycardia complex. In addition, the putative focus of ventricular tachycardia is paced in an effort to determine whether the paced complexes are identical or similar to the induced tachycardia.[21] The latter procedure is known as pace mapping. For patients with ventricular tachycardia due to coronary artery disease, concealed entrainment is manifest by a prolonged paced spike to QRS, a paced QRS identical to spontaneous tachycardia, and a postpacing interval identical to the spontaneous ventricular tachycardia cycle length, which appears to best identify the critical slow zone for the ventricular tachycardia reentrant circuit.[22] Once the putative isthmus is found, one or more radiofrequency applications are delivered from the distal electrode near this endocardial site to a chest-wall patch.

A subset of patients with ventricular tachycardia and structural heart disease particularly amenable to catheter ablation are those with bundle branch reentrant arrhythmias. These patients are recognized by having a left intraventricular con-

duction delay or a frank pattern of left bundle branch block. The majority have an associated cardiomyopathy and all have prolonged infranodal conduction. In these patients, the tachycardia mechanism involves bundle-to-bundle conduction.[23] Catheter cure may be achieved by ablation of the right bundle branch. The right bundle is usually draped superficially over the right septal surface and the right bundle potential is usually easily located. The right bundle may be ablated either by direct current or preferably by radiofrequency discharges.[23] Even after successful ablation of the right bundle branch, further electrophysiologic testing is in order to exclude ventricular tachycardia emanating from myocardial sources.

Other forms of ventricular tachycardia that may be particularly amenable to catheter ablation are those occurring in patients without structural cardiac disease. These patients present with tachycardia emanating from either the right ventricular outflow tract[24] or from the inferior left septum.[25] Patients with tachycardia emanating from the right ventricular outflow show a pattern of left bundle branch block with an inferior axis. The arrhythmia is often exercise-induced and may respond to carotid massage or treatment with adenosine or beta blockers. This arrhythmia is thought to be a cyclic AMP-dependent triggered arrhythmia. The hallmark of proper ablation includes detection of early areas in the outflow tract and a precise correspondence between the paced map and spontaneous ventricular tachycardia. Another important site of ventricular tachycardia in normal hearts may emanate from the left apical septum. This arrhythmia is characterized by a pattern of right bundle branch block associated with a left superior axis. This arrhythmia most often responds to intravenous verapamil. Modes of ablative approaches include recording a Purkinje potential just in front of the QRS and/or a paced map that corresponds to the spontaneous tachycardia.

RESULTS OF CATHETER-ABLATIVE PROCEDURES

Atrioventricular Junctional Ablation

To date, the largest experience in the United States relating to the various ablative procedures has been accumulated from the voluntary ablation registry of NASPE (Tables 31-1 and 31-2).[26] At present, AV junctional ablation is performed using radiofrequency energy application, with a success rate of 97.3 percent and very infrequent complications. The most serious complication is postprocedure death, which occurred in 4 of 2142 patients undergoing ablation. One death was due to an acute myocardial infarction, three patients had postprocedure episodes of torsades de pointes, and two had pericarditis and tamponade.

TABLE 31-1

RESULTS OF ATRIOVENTRICULAR JUNCTIONAL ABLATION

	AV Junctional Ablation	Accessory Pathway Ablation			AVNRT		Atrial Flutter	Atrial Tachycardia
		LFW	RFW	Septal	Slow	Fast		
Total performed	2084	3096	885	1446	5092	331	570	569
Success, percent	97.3 (3° AV block achieved)	93	85	87	97	46	72	71
Significant complications, number (percent)	79 (3.7)		99 (1.8)		40 (0.7)		4 (0.7)	10 (1.7)
Procedure-related deaths	4	4						

Abbreviations: LFW = left free wall, RFW = right free wall, AVNRT = atrioventricular nodal reentrant tachycardia.

Source: Modified from Scheinman,[26] with permission.

Ablation of Accessory Pathways

In the NASPE voluntary registry,[26] ablation of accessory pathways was attempted in 5427 patients. The overall rate of successful ablation for left-sided pathways was 93 percent, as compared with a success rate of 85 percent for right free wall and 87 percent for septal accessory pathways. Significant complications, including four procedure-related deaths, occurred in 1.8 percent of patients. The most frequent major complication was pericarditis (10 patients) or frank tamponade (7 patients), complete AV block (9 patients), cerebrovascular accident (8 patients), and aortic (4 patients) or mitral valve damage (2 patients). Three patients had damage to the coronary arteries, including one patient with a left main occlusion requiring angioplasty.

Ablation for Patients with Atrioventricular Node Reentry

The largest reported series of patients undergoing catheter treatment of AV node reentry again comes from the NASPE

TABLE 31-2

RESULTS OF ABLATION FOR VENTRICULAR TACHYCARDIA

	Total	Success	Percent Successful
VT associated with coronary disease	257	170	66
VT associated with cardiomyopathy	124	84	68
VT in structurally normal heart	463	392	85
Significant complications	20		
Procedure-related deaths	0		

Abbreviations: VT = ventricular tachycardia.

Source: Modified from Scheinman,[26] with permission.

voluntary registry,[26] which included 5092 patients who underwent ablation of a slow pathway. The success rate was 97 percent in these patients, and the only significant complication was development of inadvertent complete AV block (0.7 percent). In contrast, attempted ablation of a fast pathway was much less successful (46 percent), with a higher incidence of AV block.

Ablation of Atrial Flutter/Atrial Tachycardia

A total of 570 patients underwent attempted flutter ablation in the NASPE registry. The reported success rate for flutter was 72 percent and for atrial tachycardia (569 patients) 71 percent. Reported complications included development of complete AV block (two patients), pericardial tamponade (one patient), and pulmonary embolus.

Ablation of Ventricular Tachycardia

Successful ablation was more frequent in those with ventricular tachycardia associated with no structural heart disease (85 percent), including those with right ventricular outflow tract tachycardia or left septal tachycardia, compared with ablation for ventricular tachycardia associated with coronary artery disease (66 percent) or idiopathic cardiomyopathy (68 percent).[26] Major complications included cardiac tamponade, systemic emboli, AV block, and femoral artery thrombosis. No procedure-related deaths were reported.

ADVANTAGES AND DISADVANTAGES OF CATHETER-ABLATIVE TECHNIQUES

Advantages

The use of catheter-ablative techniques has greatly affected our approach to the management of patients with supraventricular tachycardia. Catheter ablation of the AV junction has replaced the need for surgical ablation of the His bundle for patients with atrial arrhythmias refractory to drug therapy.

Furthermore, use of catheter procedures allows cure of patients with reentrant supraventricular arrhythmias. The initial reports suggest a cure rate of 90 to 100 percent with minimal serious adverse effects.[27,28] For selected patients with ventricular tachycardia, catheter-ablative procedures may obviate the need for surgical intervention. This is particularly true for patients with bundle branch reentry or for those with right ventricular outflow tract or left septal tachycardias.

Disadvantages

The chief disadvantage of atrioventricular junctional ablation is the need for chronic cardiac pacing after successful ablation. Another serious adverse effect is the reported 2 to 4 percent incidence of polymorphous ventricular tachycardia occurring in the postablative period.[28] This arrhythmia is more common in patients with severe myocardial disease, bradycardia, electrolyte abnormalities; it may be enhanced by use of class IA antiarrhythmic agents. The chief complication reported for patients undergoing AV modification procedures for AV-nodal reentry is the risk of complete AV block. Attempted ablation of the slow AV-nodal pathway promises to diminish or obviate this risk.

The risks of catheter ablation of accessory pathways appears to be related to the pathway site. Reported complications for left free wall pathways include the risk of systemic embolization, tamponade, or damage to the left circumflex coronary artery. Ablation of septal pathways carries the risk of causing inadvertent complete AV block. Fortunately, the risk of significant complications appears to be on the order of approximately 2 percent.

Major complications have been reported in the use of catheter ablation treatment of ventricular tachycardia. Such complications include the risk of cerebrovascular accidents, damage to the aortic valve, or tamponade.

CONCLUSION

The introduction of catheter-ablative techniques has completely revolutionized our approach to the management of patients with supraventricular tachycardia. These techniques have evolved to the point where curative ablative procedures are recommended as the treatment of choice for all symptomatic patients with tachycardias mediated by accessory pathways and for most patients with symptomatic AV-nodal reentrant tachycardia. Complete AV-junctional ablation is the procedure of choice for those with drug-refractory atrial arrhythmias, while selected patients with ventricular arrhythmias may benefit from catheter-ablative techniques; however, the vast majority of these patients are best managed by drugs, devices, or surgical therapy.

REFERENCES

1. Gonzalez R, Scheinman M, Margaretten W, Rubinstein M. Closed-chest electrode-catheter technique for His bundle ablation in dogs. *Am J Physiol* 1981; 241:H283–H287.

2. Scheinman MM, Morady F, Hess DS, Gonzalez R. Catheter-induced ablation of the atrioventricular junction to control refractory supraventricular arrhythmias. *JAMA* 1982; 248:851–855.

3. Gallagher JJ, Svenson RH, Kasell JH, et al. Catheter technique for closed-chest ablation of the atrioventricular conduction system: A therapeutic alternative for the treatment of refractory supraventricular tachycardia. *N Engl J Med* 1982; 306:194–200.

4. Williamson BD, Man KC, Daoud E, Niebauer M, Strickberger SA, Morady F. Radiofrequency catheter modification of atrioventricular conduction to control the ventricular rate during atrial fibrillation. *N Engl J Med* 1994; 331:910–917.

5. Della Bella P, Carbucicchio C, Tondo C, Riva S. Modulation of atrioventricular conduction by ablation of the "slow" atrioventricular node pathway in patients with drug-refractory atrial fibrillation or flutter. *J Am Coll Cardiol* 1995; 25:39–46.

6. Gallagher JJ, Gilbert M, Swenson RH, Sealy WC, Kasell J, Wallace AG. Wolff-Parkinson-White syndrome: The problem, evaluation, and surgical correction. *Circulation* 1975; 51:767–785.

7. Gallagher JJ, Sealy WC, Cox JL, Kasell JH. Results of surgery for preexcitation in 200 consecutive cases. In: Levy S, Scheinman MM, eds. *Cardiac Arrhythmias: From Diagnosis to Therapy.* Mt. Kisco, NY: Futura; 1984:323–340.

8. Fisher JD, Brodman R, Kim SG, Matos JA, Brodman E, Wallerson D. Attempted nonsurgical electrical ablation of accessory pathways via the coronary sinus in the Wolff-Parkinson-White syndrome. *J Am Coll Cardiol* 1984; 4:685–694.

9. Jackman WM, Wang XH, Friday KJ, Roman CA, Moulton KP, Beckman KJ. Catheter ablation of accessory atrioventricular pathways (Wolff-Parkinson-White syndrome) by radiofrequency current. *N Engl J Med* 1991; 324:1605–1611.

10. Lesh MD, Van Hare GF, Scheinman MM, Ports TA, Epstein LA. Comparison of the retrograde and transseptal methods for ablation of left free wall accessory pathways. *J Am Coll Cardiol* 1993; 22:542–549.

11. Lee MA, Morady F, Kadish A, Schamp DJ, Chin MC, Scheinman MM. Catheter modification of the atrioventricular junction with radiofrequency energy for control of atrioventricular nodal reentry tachycardia. *Circulation* 1991; 83:827–835.

12. Roman CA, Wang X, Friday KJ, Moulton KP, Margolis PD, Klonis D. Catheter technique for selective ablation of slow pathway in AV nodal reentrant tachycardia (abstr). *PACE* 1990; 13:498.

13. Olgin JE, Kalman JM, Fitzpatrick AP, Lesh MD. Role of right atrial endocardial structures as barriers to conduction during human type I atrial flutter: Activation and entrainment mapping guided by intracardiac echocardiography. *Circulation* 1995; 92:1839–1848.

14. Saxon LA, Kalman JM, Olgin JE, Scheinman MM, Lee RJ, Lesh MD. Results of catheter ablation for atrial flutter. *Am J Cardiol* 1995; 26:431–438.

15. Tracy CM, Swartz JF, Fletcher RD, et al. Radiofrequency catheter ablation of ectopic atrial tachycardia using paced activation sequence mapping. *J Am Coll Cardiol* 1993; 21:910–917.

16. Tang CW, Scheinman MM, Van Hare GF, Epstein LM, Fitzpatrick AP, Lee RJ, et al. Use of P wave configuration during atrial tachycardia to predict site of origin. *J Am Coll Cardiol* 1995; 26:1315–1324.

17. Morillo CA, Klein GJ, Thakur RK, Li H, Zardini M, Yee R. Mechanism of inappropriate sinus tachycardia: Role of sympathovagal balance. *Circulation* 1994; 90:873–877.

18. Kalman JM, Lee RJ, Fisher WG, Chin MC, Ursell P, Stillson CA, et al. Radiofrequency catheter modification of sinus pacemaker function guided by intracardiac echocardiography. *Circulation* 1995; 92:3070–3081.

19. Lee RJ, Kalman JM, Fitzpatrick AP, Epstein LM, Fisher WG, Olgin JE, et al. Radiofrequency catheter modification of the sinus node for "inappropriate" sinus tachycardia. *Circulation* 1995; 92:2919–2928.

20. Marchlinski FE, Almendrah JM, Cassidy DM, et al. Localization of endocardial site for catheter ablation of ventricular tachycardia. In: Fontaine G, Scheinman MM, eds. *Ablation in Cardiac Arrhythmias.* Mt. Kisco, NY: Futura; 1987:289–302.

21. Josephson ME, Waxman HL, Cain ME, Gardner MJ, Buxton AE. Ventricular activation during ventricular endocardial pacing: II. Role of pace mapping to localize origin of ventricular tachycardia. *Am J Cardiol* 1982; 50:11–22.

22. Stevenson WG, Weiss JN, Weiner I, et al. Resetting of ventricular tachycardia: Implications for localizing the area of slow conduction. *J Am Coll Cardiol* 1988; 11:522.

23. Tchou P, Jazayeri M, Denker S, Dongas J, Caceres J, Akhtar M. Transcatheter electrical ablation of right bundle branch: A method of treating macroreentrant ventricular tachycardia attributed to bundle branch reentry. *Circulation* 1988; 78:246–257.

24. Klein LS, Shih H-T, Hackett FK, et al. Radiofrequency catheter ablation of ventricular tachycardia in patients without structural heart disease. *Circulation* 1992; 85:1666.

25. Coggins DL, Lee RJ, Sweeney J, Chien WW, Van Hare G, Epstein L, et al. Radiofrequency catheter ablation as a cure for idiopathic tachycardia of both left and right ventricular origin. *J Am Coll Cardiol* 1994; 23:1333–1341.

26. Scheinman MM: NASPE survey on catheter ablation. *PACE* 1995; 18:1474–1478.

27. Calkins H, Sousa J, el-Atassi R, Rosenheck S, deBuitleir M, Kou WH. Diagnosis and cure of the Wolff-Parkinson-White syndrome or paroxysmal supraventricular tachycardias during a single electrophysiologic test. *N Engl J Med* 1991; 324:1612–1618.

28. Evans-Bell GT Jr, Scheinman MM, Bardy G, Borggrefe M, Brugada P, Fisher J, et al. Predictors of in-hospital mortality after DC catheter ablation of atrioventricular junction: Results of a prospective, international, multicenter study. *Circulation* 1991; 84:1924–1937.

CHAPTER 32

EXTERNAL CARDIOVERSION AND DEFIBRILLATION

Bernard Lown / Regis A. DeSilva

The external application of electrical current is standard treatment for termination of atrial and ventricular tachyarrhythmias, and the safe application of such treatment requires a thorough knowledge of the electrical principles involved and the proper procedures to be followed. *Cardioversion* is the discharge of electrical energy synchronized on the R wave, while *defibrillation* refers to unsynchronized discharge. The electrophysiologic basis for cardioversion is probably the closure of the "excitable gap" in a reentrant circuit. Abolition of the circuit for the arrhythmia may be accomplished with energy levels as low as 1 to 5 J, and this might account for the success in terminating reentrant arrhythmias such as atrial flutter and ventricular tachycardia. Defibrillation requires energy levels up to 360 J, and this may be due to the necessity for depolarizing a large number of multiple asynchronous reentrant circuits.

PROCEDURE

Elective cardioversion should preferably be done in the early morning with the patient in the fasting state. In urgent cases, meals should be withheld for as long as possible. Serum levels for electrolytes, digoxin, blood urea nitrogen, and creatinine should be obtained, and hypokalemia should be corrected before cardioversion is attempted. Digitalis glycosides should be withheld only on the day of cardioversion, but if digitalis toxicity is suspected, the procedure is postponed until the problem is resolved. An intravenous line is inserted, vital signs and the electrocardiogram (ECG) are monitored, and equipment for cardiopulmonary resuscitation (CPR) is made available. General anesthesia is administered, or intravenous diazepam or minazolam is used for sedation.

Synchronization with the tallest R wave on the ECG prevents accidental triggering of ventricular fibrillation, and this should be checked after each discharge. Improper synchronization may occur when there is bundle branch block with a tall R' wave, when the T wave is highly peaked, and with artifactual spikes from a malfunctioning pacemaker. Electrodes are placed in either an anterior-lateral position or an anterior-posterior position. The anterior electrode is placed parasternally in the right second and third intercostal spaces. The lateral electrode is positioned over the cardiac apex. If a flat posterior electrode is available, it is placed at the tip of the angle of the left scapula. The envelope of current flow in either configuration is along the long axis of the heart; it encompasses the bulk of cardiac tissue and minimizes travel through high-impedance bony tissue. Electrode paste, with firm pressure on the electrodes, should be used to provide adequate electrical contact and to reduce transthoracic impedance. Bridging of the electrodes by conductive paste should be avoided as this will reduce the amount of energy delivered to the heart. Prior to discharge, CPR should be stopped and an "All clear" signal should be given to avoid accidental shocking of attendants.

Energy titration reduces both energy use and complications. The initial setting may be as low as 10 J for atrial flutter and stable ventricular tachycardia, and the energy output is increased progressively to 25, 50, 100, 200, and 360 J for reversion of arrhythmias. Lead II of the ECG is monitored to determine whether sinus rhythm has been reestablished. *If ventricular arrhythmias emerge after a discharge, xylocaine is administered prophylactically before the next discharge and cardioversion cautiously continued*. Following cardioversion, a proper airway is maintained and adequate ventilation delivered until recovery from anesthesia occurs. Vital signs and cardiac rhythm are monitored continuously for at least 24 h to detect the late emergence of malignant arrhythmias, which may occur in patients with suspected digitalis or quinidine toxicity.

TREATMENT OF
SPECIFIC ARRHYTHMIAS

Atrial Fibrillation

Cardioversion should be attempted at least once if no contrain-dications exist and if there is a reasonable expectation that sinus rhythm can be maintained. Normal rhythm following cardioversion obviates the need for long-term anticoagulation, with a decrease in fatigue, increase in exercise capacity, and improvement in cerebral blood flow. Treatment with quinidine or disopyramide for 48 h before cardioversion may prevent early recurrence. Success of cardioversion in maintaining si-nus rhythm is dependent on factors such as the duration of arrhythmia, the size of the left atrium, underlying conduction system disease, presence of valvular heart disease, and the patient's age. Overall, the success may be over 90 percent using 200 J or less, and the mean energy level required being 87 J.[1] Recurrence of arrhythmia is predicted by a left atrial size of 45 mm or greater and a less than 10 percent increase in the A wave on Doppler echocardiography postcardioversion.[2] Successful cardioversion results in a decrease in both right and left atrial volumes.[3]

Higher energy levels may be required to terminate atrial fibrillation in congestive heart failure, and treatment of heart failure before cardioversion will increase the success rate. Acute myocardial infarction is not a contraindication to car-dioversion; in fact, prompt reversion would help prevent in-farct extension by decreasing the heart rate and reducing oxygen consumption. In patients with conduction system dis-ease, arrhythmias such as atrial ectopic activity, severe sinus bradycardia, sinus arrest, junctional rhythm, or multifocal atrial tachycardia may follow cardioversion, with only gradual restoration of sinus rhythm. In such cases, atropine or isopro-terenol treatment may be required. If conduction system dis-ease is suspected (e.g., a slow ventricular response in the absence of drug treatment), cardioversion should be avoided as asystole may result. Energy titration, as described earlier, anticipates this complication, and attempts at cardioversion are abandoned if the first few discharges evoke bradyarrhyth-mia. Other patients who may not benefit from cardioversion are those with severe mitral valve disease with a "giant" scarred atrium, those with mitral valve replacement, patients with chronic recurrent paroxysmal atrial tachyarrhythmias, and those with intolerance to antiarrhythmic drugs.

Thromboembolism may result from stasis and inadequate emptying of the left atrial appendage with low transmitral flow velocity. Anticoagulation reduces the incidence of emboli and is recommended in the absence of contraindications.[4,5] *Warfarin is started a minimum of 3 weeks before cardiover-sion to maintain a prothrombin time of 1.3 to 1.5 times the control value, or an international normalized ration (INR) of 2.0 to 3.0.* Treatment is maintained for 4 weeks after cardiover-sion because delayed embolism from residual clot may occur. Such embolism may result if there is delayed resumption of atrial activity due to "stunning" after successful cardioversion

in atrial fibrillation.[6] Doppler echocardiography is useful in documenting the presence of atrial contraction, as the absence of an atrial A wave suggests electromechanical dissociation.[2] Anticoagulation beyond 4 weeks is indicated in the presence of recurrent bouts of atrial fibrillation, prosthetic valves or cardiomyopathy or if there is a history of previous emboli-zation.

Anticoagulation for 3 weeks prior to cardioversion is prob-ably unnecessary if atrial fibrillation has been documented to have been present for less than 48 to 72 h (unless intraatrial clot has been demonstrated by echocardiography) and in emergency situations. In such cases, heparin is administered and simultaneous treatment with warfarin initiated prior to cardioversion. The absence of thrombus documented by trans-esophageal echocardiography is not an adequate reason to withhold anticoagulation as it does not protect the patient from the risk for thromboembolism.[7,8] Although transesophageal echocardiography has been used to guide the decision whether to cancel cardioversion, it should be remembered that 3 to 4 weeks of anticoagulation prior to cardioversion is inadequate for resolution of thrombus in some patients.[9,10] If warfarin is contraindicated, aspirin may be utilized, but there is no definitive evidence that treatment with this agent or dipyrami-dole protects against embolism. *In pure atrial flutter and in supraventricular tachycardia, anticoagulation is necessary only if atrial fibrillation is concomitantly present.*

Atrial Flutter

If drug treatment with an agent such as propafenone or sotalol is unsuccessful, cardioversion is the treatment of choice for this arrhythmia. In many cases, the arrhythmia does not recur and maintenance drug treatment may not be necessary. This arrhythmia is often benign unless there is 1:1 atrioventricular conduction, when syncope may occur. Low-energy shocks easily revert this arrhythmia, and the mean energy level re-quired is 25 J; 95 percent of cases require 50 J or less.

Supraventricular Tachycardia

Because this arrhythmia is often responsive to vagal maneu-vers and/or to several antiarrhythmic drugs, cardioversion is only rarely necessary for reversion. If such treatment fails, cardioversion with energy levels between 100 and 360 J are required. *In paroxysmal atrial tachycardia with block due to digitalis intoxication, cardioversion is extremely hazardous as ventricular fibrillation and death may result.* When digitalis toxicity is suspected, energy titration is cautiously attempted, with xylocaine pretreatment for ventricular arrhythmia if nec-essary. If low-energy discharges provoke high grades of ar-rhythmia or atrioventricular block, cardioversion is discon-tinued.

Ventricular Tachycardia

When a chest thump and intravenous xylocaine, bretylium tosylate, or procainamide fail to terminate ventricular tachy-cardia, cardioversion should be performed promptly. Unless the arrhythmia is clinically unstable, sedation is administered. Energy titration is performed in stable ventricular tachycardia, and as little as 1 to 5 J may succeed; in 90 percent of cases, 10 J or less is successful in terminating the arrhythmia. Only rarely is more than 100 J necessary. When ventricular tachycardia is rapid and the QRS complex and T wave indistinguishable, or if the patient becomes syncopal due to hemodynamic deterioration, an unsynchronized discharge of 100 J is delivered immediately. If this attempt fails, discharges of 200, 300, and 360 J should be administered consecutively until sinus rhythm is restored. Polymorphic ventricular tachycardia and torsades de pointes that is not self-terminating may be similarly treated.

Ventricular Fibrillation

External defibrillation is generally performed using a standard defibrillator or with an automatic external defibrillator (AED). Defibrillation, performed by using unsynchronized discharge, is utilized only for ventricular fibrillation and for pulseless ventricular tachycardia. This setting is also used for "blind defibrillation" in an unmonitored patient in cardiac arrest, and the electrode positions are similar to those used for cardioversion. The procedure for defibrillation is delivery of an initial shock of 200 J following institution of CPR, followed by a second 200- or 300-J shock and a third 360-J shock if ventricular fibrillation persists. If these attempts fail, 0.5 to 1.0 mg of intravenous epinephrine is given and defibrillation at 360 J attempted again. Prospective clinical studies show that 200 J or less is often sufficient for defibrillation of adults of normal weight, and there is little evidence that, even in heavier adults, discharges beyond 400 J are necessary. As a rule, for children, 1 to 2 J/kg is recommended, and in small children and infants, as little as 10 J might suffice. Following successful termination of ventricular fibrillation, the airway is kept clear of secretions and vomitus, adequate ventilation with supplemental oxygen is continued, and the patient monitored in an appropriate setting for further management. If defibrillation occurs outside of a medical facility, the patient is physically stabilized and transported to a hospital as soon as possible.

A variety of lightweight AEDs are now available, using either damped sinusoidal or monophasic truncated exponential waveforms with varying types of hardware and software.[11] These devices include features such as strip-chart recorders, screen displays, and voice-synthesizer messages for the operator and devices to record the ECG and the voices of the operators. These defibrillators are fitted with computed algorithms that recognize ventricular fibrillation or rapid ventricular tachycardia when presented with approximately 8 s of cardiac rhythm, permitting automatic firing of the device within 8 to 10 s. These devices are intended for use in the field, where highly-trained personnel are unavailable and therapeutic options are limited. Adhesive defibrillator pads are attached to the patient's chest in the positions recommended for standard defibrillation. Resuscitative maneuvers are stopped, and radio transmitters and receivers are switched off during initial signal recording to prevent interference. Signal recognition takes up to 15 s before the defibrillator fires; prior to firing, the device will automatically announce the imminent delivery of a shock by providing a printed message, a visual alarm, or a voice statement so that attendants are not accidentally shocked. Following delivery of the first shock, CPR is not reinstituted so that signal analysis may be accomplished by the device and additional shocks delivered if necessary. If defibrillation is successful, the device is turned off and the patient transported rapidly to the nearest emergency room.

The major determinant for success or failure of defibrillation is delay in delivery of the first shock. Failure to resuscitate may occur because of operator error or because of irreversibility of the underlying condition, when cardiac damage is very extensive or when ventricular fibrillation has been so prolonged that severe metabolic derangements have occurred. In refractory ventricular fibrillation, correction of hypoxia and acid-base imbalance and the administration of isoproterenol (to convert fine-grain fibrillation to coarse-grain fibrillation) all render successful defibrillation more likely. If this approach is unsuccessful, rapid serial delivery of two or three 360-J shocks may succeed due to successive reductions in transthoracic impedance and delivery of higher current levels. Rarely, fine-grain fibrillation may appear as asystole on a monitor, and defibrillation should be attempted. Newer defibrillators, which automatically measure transthoracic impedance before delivery of the shock, and current-based defibrillators (rather than an energy-based system) delivering 30 to 40 amperes per shock, offer promise in patients who are difficult to defibrillate because of high chest-wall impedance.[12,13] If all resuscitative efforts fail to revive the patient, a rapid and thorough assessment of the resuscitative and defibrillation procedures is necessary to check for errors such as electrode placement and the use of appropriate energy levels. With AEDs, it is essential to check for proper contact of the defibrillator pads and for proper signal analysis. If, however, no errors are detected and if the patient is not responsive, a decision about terminating resuscitation must be made.

COMPLICATIONS

Morphologic and functional cardiac damage may follow the use of high-energy shocks. Elevation of creatine kinase levels following electrical discharge is transient; it derives from skeletal muscle and usually does not mask the diagnosis of acute myocardial infarction. Intracellular potassium is also released by electrical trauma. This release is accentuated by digitalis toxicity, contributing to the emergence of ventricular arrhythmias. Electrocardiographic signs of hyperkalemia may be present after high-energy shocks. The occurrence of serious ventricular arrhythmias is related to the presence of hypokalemia, digitalis toxicity, severity of heart disease, improper synchronization, and the repeated use of high levels of energy. Asystole and cardiac arrest are rare and occur when there is severe conduction system disease. When ventricular fibrillation occurs several hours after cardioversion, it may be due to toxicity from digoxin, quinidine, or both.

Pulmonary edema following cardioversion occurs most often in the presence of mitral or aortic valvular disease or left ventricular dysfunction. These factors, in conjunction with electrically induced alterations in myocardial function, fluid overload, delayed return of atrial function, and pulmonary embolism, all contribute to pulmonary edema. The risk of systemic embolization has already been discussed. Unexplained hypotension sometimes occurs after cardioversion, and fluid treatment will correct this problem. Following cardioversion or defibrillation, pacing thresholds may increase due to myocardial burns caused by transmission of electrical energy to the paced site. Because the increase in threshold may increase gradually over weeks with subsequent loss of capture by the pacemaker, serial pacing threshold measurements for 2 months is recommended. Defibrillator electrodes should be placed at least 12 cm from the generator before discharge. In patients with implanted cardioverter-defibrillators who fail internal defibrillation, an external shock should be attempted.

Cardioversion has been safely performed during pregnancy, and fetal death has not been reported as a direct consequence of treatment. Nonetheless, fetal monitoring, with an obstetrician in consultation, should be available whenever possible. Despite the possible complications described with the use of electrical energy, cardioversion and defibrillation have been performed for several decades now with a high degree of safety whenever guidelines and precautions are adhered to.

REFERENCES

1. Lown B. Electrical reversion of cardiac arrhythmias. *Br Heart J* 1967; 29:469–489.

2. Dethy M, Chassat C, Roy D, Mercier LA. Doppler echocardiographic predictors of recurrence of atrial fibrillation. *Am J Cardiol* 1988; 62:723–726.

3. Gosselink AT, Crijns HJ, Hamer HP. Changes in left and right atrial size after cardioversion of atrial fibrillation: Role of mitral valve disease. *J Am Coll Cardiol* 1993; 22:1666–1672.

4. Dunn M, Alexander J, DeSilva R, Hildner F. Antithrombotic therapy in atrial fibrillation. *Chest* 1989; 95(suppl):18S–127S.

5. Prystowsky EN, Benson DW, Fuster V, Hart RG, Kay GN, Myerburg RJ, et al. Management of patients with atrial fibrillation. *Circulation* 1996; 93:1262–1277.

6. Grimm RA, Stewart WJ, Maloney JD, Cohen GI. Impact of electrical cardioversion for atrial fibrillation on left atrial appendage function and spontaneous echo contrast: Characterization by simultaneous transesophageal echocardiography. *J Am Coll Cardiol* 1993; 22:359–366.

7. Moreyra E, Finklehor RS. Limitations of transesophageal echocardiography in the risk assessment of patients before nonanticoagulated cardioversion from atrial fibrillation and flutter: An analysis of pooled trials. *Am Heart J* 1995; 129:71–75.

8. Black IW, Fatkin D, Sagar KB, Khandheria BK, Leung DY, Galloway JM. Exclusion of atrial thrombus by transesophageal echocardiography does not preclude embolism after cardioversion of atrial fibrillation. A multicenter study. *Circulation* 1994; 89:2509–2513.

9. Stoddard MF, Dawkins PR. Transesophageal echocardiographic guidance of cardioversion in patients with atrial fibrillation. *Am Heart J* 1995; 129:1204–1215.

10. Fatkin D, Kuchar DI. Transesophageal echocardiography before and during direct current cardioversion of atrial fibrillation: Evidence for "atrial stunning" as a mechanism of thromboembolic complications. *J Am Coll of Cardiol* 1994; 23:307–316.

11. Weisfeldt ML, Kerber RE, McGoldrick P, Moss AJ, Nichol G, Ornato JP, et al. American Heart Association Report on the Public Access Defibrillation Conference, December 8–10, 1994. *Circulation* 1995; 92:2740–2747.

12. Kerber RE, Martins JB, Kienzle MG, Constantin L, Olshansky B, Hopson R, et al. Energy, current and success in defibrillation and cardioversion: Clinical studies using an automated impedance-based method of energy adjustment. *Circulation* 1988; 77:1038–1046.

13. Lerman BB, DiMarco JP, Haines DE. Current-based versus energy-based ventricular defibrillation: A prospective study. *J Am Coll Cardiol* 1988; 12:1259–1264.

33

THE IMPLANTABLE CARDIOVERTER DEFIBRILLATOR

Peter A. O'Callaghan / Jeremy N. Ruskin

HISTORICAL PERSPECTIVE

Sudden cardiac death is estimated to claim 350,000 lives annually or 25 lives per million people per week in the United States.[1] The principal cause of sudden cardiac death remained unclear until in-field electrocardiogram (ECG) monitoring demonstrated a high prevalence of ventricular fibrillation (VF) in victims of out-of-hospital cardiac arrest.[2] In more than 80 percent of cases, sudden death is caused by the abrupt onset of ventricular tachycardia (VT) that either persists or more commonly progresses to VF.[3] *Since self-termination of VF is exceedingly rare, the single most important factor determining survival in victims is the time between the onset of collapse and the first defibrillation attempt.*[4] Overall mortality associated with out-of-hospital cardiac arrest remains above 75 percent, mainly because of the delay in providing effective therapy to afflicted individuals.[5]

As originally conceived by Mirowski,[6] the implantable defibrillator was designed to circumvent the delay in providing definitive therapy to ambulatory individuals with life-threatening ventricular tachyarrhythmias by the use of intrathoracic electrical countershock. The first experimental model of the implantable defibrillator was built at Sinai Hospital in Baltimore and successfully tested in 1969 in a dog.[7] After 10 years of research and development, Mirowski and coworkers[8] performed the first automatic defibrillator implantation in a human at the Johns Hopkins University Medical Center on February 4, 1980. The internal defibrillator responds by delivering an electrical shock between intrathoracic electrodes within 10 to 20 s of arrhythmia onset, a time frame in which the potential for arrhythmia reversal approaches 100 percent. As these devices are capable of responding immediately to spontaneous ventricular tachyarrhythmias, the implantable cardioverter-defibrillator (ICD) has proved to be a reliable and effective means of preventing sudden cardiac death in survivors of out-of-hospital cardiac arrest.

SYSTEM COMPONENTS AND FUNCTION

The ICD system consists of two basic components: a pulse generator and lead electrodes for arrhythmia detection and for therapy delivery. In addition to internal defibrillation, all of today's manufactured devices also provide synchronized cardioversion and bradycardia pacing. The pulse generator contains a battery, energy-storing electrolytic capacitors, and electronic components. The outer covering of the pulse generator is made of titanium with a header of epoxy. The header has two to four electrode receptacles to receive the rate sensing/pacing and shocking leads. The characteristics of some of the currently available ICDs are outlined in Table 33-1.

Sensing and Detection

Reliable sensing and detection of ventricular tachyarrhythmias are essential for proper functioning of the ICD. In brief, an endocardial lead senses ventricular depolarization, either by true bipolar sensing between a distal tip electrode and a proximal ring electrode (e.g., Transvene, Medtronic) or by integrated bipolar sensing between a distal tip electrode and the right ventricular (RV) shocking electrode (e.g., Endotak, CPI). During sensing, the sense amplifier amplifies, filters, and rectifies the incoming signals. It then compares them to a sensing threshold and produces a set of RR intervals for the detection algorithm to use (Fig. 33-1). *Intracardiac electrogram amplitude can vary markedly between rhythms such as sinus rhythm, VT, and VF or even during the same rhythm (e.g., VF). Therefore all ICDs utilize some form of automatic adjusting signal amplifier.* Fixed gain and sensitivity as used in pacemaker technology would result in either undersensing or oversensing, depending on the settings chosen. Automatic gain control (Ventritex, CPI, and Intermedics) automatically and continuously varies the gain so that the amplitude of the processed

TABLE 33-1

FEATURES OF REPRESENTATIVE ICD DEVICES[a] IN USE OR UNDERGOING CLINICAL EVALUATION

Manufacturer	Model	Dimensions, mm	Volume, mL	Weight, g	Max Stored Energy, J	Max Delivered Energy, J	Active Can Available	Stored EGM	EGM Type	History Log, No. Events	Status
Biotronik	Phylax 06	76 × 63 × 17	69	109	30	30	Yes	3.5 mins	Near field	30	CE
CPI	Ventak Mini	85 × 57 × 17.5	73	136	33	29	Yes	5 mins	Far field	69	A
CPI	Ventak Mini II	75 × 57 × 17.5	64	125	30	27	Yes	5 mins	Far field	69	A
Medtronic	Jewel 7219	83.5 × 63 × 18	80	129	34	33	Yes	12 s	Far or near field	5	A
Medtronic	Micro Jewel	74.4 × 62 × 18.5	72	116	34	33	Yes	15 min	Far or near field	150	A
Intermedics	Res-Q Micron	88 × 60 × 16	69	123	32	30	Yes	5 mins	Far or near field	59	CE
Telectronics	Sentry 4310	83 × 57 × 18	78	142	41	30	Yes	100 s	Near field	250	CE
Ventritex	Cadet V-115	72 × 65 × 17	73	129	42	37	No	8 min	Near field	60	A
Ventritex	Contour V-145	72.6 × 64.8 × 15.2	57	109	42	37	Yes	16 min	Near field	60	CE

[a]All devices listed feature biphasic defibrillation, cardioversion, antitachycardia pacing, and bradycardia pacing capabilities.

Note: A = approved for use in United States; CE = clinical evaluation in United States; CPI = Cardiac Pacemakers Incorporated; EGM = ventricular electrogram.

signal is constant. Autoadjusting sensitivity threshold (Medtronic, Telectronics) sets the sensitivity to a proportion of the amplitude of the last sensed event, and the sensitivity then gradually increases until the next event is sensed. The sensed R waves are then analyzed using an algorithm to detect a tachyarrhythmia that should be treated.

VENTRICULAR FIBRILLATION DETECTION

Devices employ rate criteria as the sole method of detecting VF. An *X/Y* detector triggers when *X* out of the previous *Y* sensed intervals (typical setting 8/12 intervals) are shorter than the VF detection interval. This approach is very good at ignoring the effect of a small number of undersensed events due to small-amplitude signals during VF. The utilization of rate detection in an *X/Y* detection algorithm results in maximal sensitivity at the expense of specificity. Any tachycardia with a cycle length less than the tachycardia detection interval will be detected as VF by the device, and VF therapy will be initiated. In most devices a reconfirmation algorithm must be fulfilled during or at the end of capacitor charging and prior to the delivery of therapy (noncommitted device). In one study, the ability of the device to continue tachycardia sensing during capacitor charging and to abort shock therapy for self-terminating events prevented unnecessary shocks in 37 percent of patients during a mean follow-up period of 10 months.[10]

VENTRICULAR TACHYCARDIA DETECTION

ICDs have at least two and frequently more tachyarrhythmia detection zones. The fastest tachyarrhythmia zone is the "VF detection" zone. Between this zone and sinus rhythm, "VT zone(s)" can be programmed. Although rate is the principal detection criterion, the detection algorithm is different from that in the VF zone. In contrast to VF detection, most VT detection algorithms require a programmable number of consecutive intervals shorter than the VT detection interval. An interval longer than the VT detection interval (e.g., due to RR variability in atrial fibrillation) would reset the counters. In addition, optional VT detection enhancements, including onset and stability criteria, are programmable to increase specificity. The onset criterion is intended to distinguish sinus tachycardia with a gradual rate increase from VT characterized by a sudden rate increase. The stability criterion is used to differentiate sustained monomorphic VT with a small variation in cycle length from atrial fibrillation with large cycle length variability. In practice there is considerable overlap of both stability and onset values between VT and nonventricular tachycardias.[11] Although programming of these values improves specificity, it does so at the risk of prolonging detection times or even of failure to detect an episode and should be reserved for the detection of hemodynamically tolerated, sustained monomorphic VT. "Sustained rate duration" is a programmable safety feature intended to avoid excessive delay in therapy delivery due to either onset or stability criteria. In the event of a satisfied rate detection criterion and nonfulfilled enhancement detection parameters, the programmed therapy will be delivered after the sustained rate duration.

Ventricular Fibrillation Therapy

ICDs employ electrical defibrillation as the sole therapy option for the treatment of VF. In contrast to cardiac pacing, which requires depolarization during diastole of a small number of cells located very close to the electrode, defibrillation requires

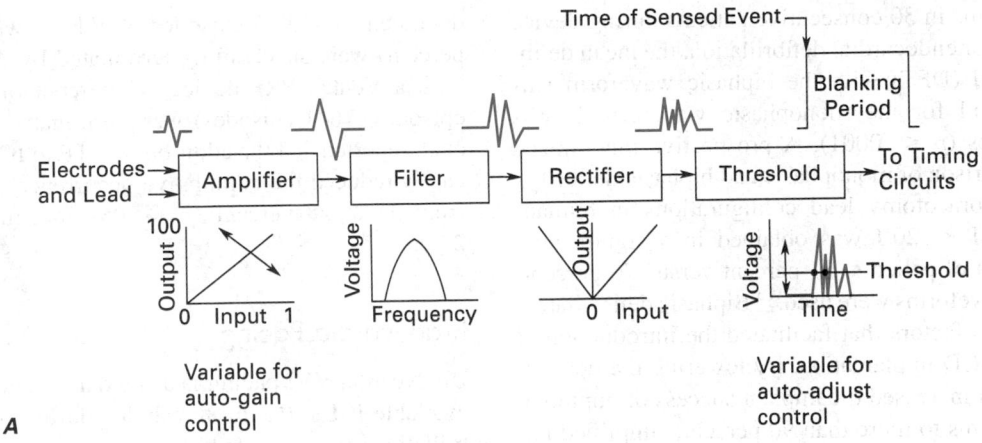

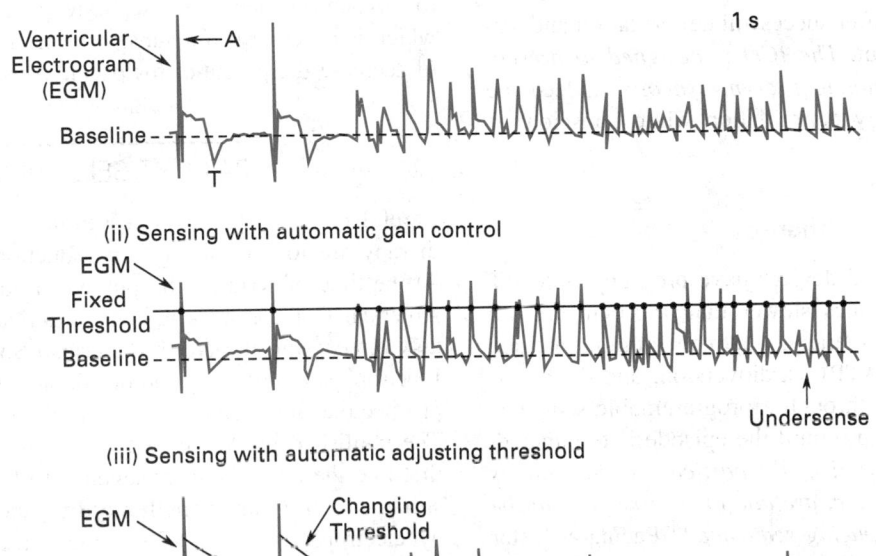

FIGURE 33-1

Sensing of electrogram signals by implantable cardioverter-defibrillators. *A.* A functional block diagram for an ICD sense amplifier consists of an amplifier that may be fixed or have automatic gain control, a bandpass filter to reject low-frequency T waves and high-frequency noise, a rectifier to eliminate polarity dependency, and a threshold detector that may be fixed or autoadjusting. The net result is a single pulse for each sensed event that is used by timing circuits to determine a series of cycle lengths. The effects of each block on a biphasic electrogram are shown above the blocks, and each functional operation is shown below each block. *B.* Sinus rhythm and

ventricular fibrillation signals are shown for the raw electrogram in panel (i), for automatic gain control in panel (ii), and for automatic adjusting threshold in panel (iii). For panel (ii), the small electrograms are amplified compared to panel (i), and sensing is shown by the dots where the signal crosses the fixed threshold. For panel (iii), the electrograms are the same as in panel (i), and the threshold varies according to the amplitude of the electrogram; sensing is again shown by the dots where the signal crosses the variable threshold. (From Olson WH,[9] reproduced with permission from the publisher and author.)

---

depolarization of the majority of ventricular myocardial cells, many of which are relatively refractory and can be up to 10 cm away. Successful defibrillation may require voltages up to 150 times greater than the voltage of the ICD battery (~6.4 V). A capacitor is used to store charge immediately prior to therapy delivery. This energy is then delivered be-

tween the high-voltage electrodes and depolarizes the intervening myocardium, thereby restoring baseline rhythm.

Reversing electrode polarity during capacitor discharge (biphasic waveform) lowers defibrillation energy requirements. Neuzner et al. performed a prospective randomized comparison of the defibrillation efficacy of monophasic and biphasic waveforms in 30 consecutive patients during device implantation.[12] For endocardial defibrillation, the mean defibrillation threshold (DFT) with the biphasic waveform was 12.5 ± 4.9 J, and for the monophasic waveform it was 22.2 ± 5.6 Joules ($p < .0001$). A prospective randomized cross-over comparison of monophasic and biphasic defibrillation using nonthoracotomy lead configurations in humans found that a DFT < 20 J was obtained in a significantly greater proportion of patients (91 percent versus 76 percent) when biphasic waveforms were used.[13] Biphasic defibrillation is one of the main factors that facilitated the introduction of nonthoracotomy ICD implantation. By lowering the defibrillation threshold, it increased the implant success of nonthoracotomy lead systems to more than 90 percent, simplified implant testing, and resulted in the development of smaller, lower energy output devices. The time interval between VF onset and delivery of defibrillation energy is usually 10 to 20 s. During this time the subject commonly loses consciousness, which is regained after successful defibrillation and restoration of cardiac output. *The ICD is designed to prevent sudden cardiac death, not to prevent syncope.* Indeed the delivery of a high-energy defibrillation while conscious is painful for patients.

Ventricular Tachycardia Therapy

All currently manufactured devices have programmable VT zone(s) for tachycardia rates slower than those in the VF zone. In contrast to VF therapy, treatment options include antitachycardia pacing (ATP), cardioversion, and defibrillation. Therapy progresses through a programmable sequence of responses (tiered therapy) until the episode is terminated. *Most sustained monomorphic VTs, particularly in patients with coronary artery disease, are due to reentry and can be terminated by a critical pacing sequence.*[14] Pacing at faster rates increases the probability of VT termination but also increases the risk of tachycardia acceleration. ATP, with backup defibrillation if acceleration occurs, is an attractive, well-tolerated treatment that avoids high-energy shock therapy, which is painful and diminishes battery life. Pacing usually commences as a percentage of the sensed tachycardia cycle length (adaptive pacing) rather than at a fixed cycle length. Repeated and more aggressive pacing trains can be administered. This results in either termination of the tachycardia or progression to the next treatment modality (cardioversion or defibrillation).

Cardioversion, in contrast to defibrillation, is a synchronized shock usually of low energy (see Chap. 32). Compared to high-energy defibrillation, low-energy cardioversion reduces the time to therapy and conserves battery life. Efficacy rates and acceleration rates are similar for these two treatment modalities.[15] ATP successfully terminates 65 to 90 percent and accelerates 3 to 21 percent of induced VTs.[16] ATP success rates in terminating spontaneous VT have been higher, probably due to longer tachycardia cycle lengths and selection bias. Follow-up of 1221 patients with a Medtronic PCD device

documented 15,985 episodes of VT, of which 14,301 (89.4 percent) were successfully terminated by ATP[17]; in patients with a Ventak PRx device, 91 percent of spontaneous VT episodes (1641 episodes) were terminated by ATP.[18] Gross et al. reported that the addition of ATP to ICD therapy significantly reduced the cumulative occurrence of first ICD shock from 36 to 28 percent ($p < .05$) at a mean follow-up of 2 years.[19]

Bradycardia Pacing

Bradycardia VVI pacing is a standard feature of all currently available ICDs. Pacing thresholds during VT and after defibrillation are frequently higher than those needed for bradycardia pacing, and in some devices the pacing output for these various conditions are separately programmable. In the near future, devices will have dual-chamber pacing capability, both to obviate the need for separate pacemaker implantation, which is necessary in a substantial minority of patients, and to decrease the potential for pacemaker-ICD interactions.

PATIENT SELECTION

Careful patient selection is essential if the benefits of ICD therapy are to translate into a reduction in total mortality. At the time of writing, the published guidelines of both the American College of Cardiology/American Heart Association task force[20] and the North American Society of Pacing and Electrophysiology[21] are outdated, and the results of most prospective multicenter clinical trials are not yet available. The published guidelines are based on the assumption that first-line therapy in the management of VF or symptomatic sustained VT is antiarrhythmic drug therapy, guided either by electrophysiologic (EP) studies or electrocardiographic monitoring, and that ICD therapy is reserved either for those who are not adequately suppressed or who cannot be assessed by these techniques. There are many reasons why ICD implantation should be considered as first-line therapy in patients with life-threatening ventricular tachyarrhythmias. First, up to 30 percent of cardiac arrest survivors and patients with symptomatic sustained VT have no inducible arrhythmia at baseline EP study, and therefore efficacy of drug therapy cannot be assessed.[22] Second, induced VT/VF in cardiac arrest survivors and in patients with symptomatic sustained VT is suppressed by EP-guided drug therapy in only 20 to 50 percent of cases.[23] Therefore, in the majority of patients, ventricular tachyarrhythmia is either noninducible at baseline or is nonsuppressed by drug therapy. Third, in patients with poor left ventricular ejection fraction (EF < 30 percent)[22] or with substrates other than chronic coronary atherosclerosis,[24,25] EP-guided therapy predicts efficacy poorly. Finally, and most importantly, the sudden death rate seems to be higher even in patients whose ventricular tachyarrhythmia is suppressed by EP-guided drug therapy compared to those who undergo primary ICD implantation.[26–31]

Current guidelines employed at our institution are listed in Table 33-2. Although ICD therapy is, or may be, indicated according to these guidelines, it may not be the only reasonable option. Until the results of studies comparing the best available ICDs with the best available drug therapy are known (Table 33-3), we consider, and discuss with our patients, the risks and benefits of ICD therapy, amiodarone therapy, and, in select cases, EP-guided sotalol therapy. Although the role of EP study in assessing the efficacy of amiodarone is unclear, it is our clinical practice to perform an EP study after oral loading with 10 g of amiodarone. If a hemodynamically significant ventricular tachyarrhythmia is induced or if the clinical arrhythmia is more easily induced, amiodarone therapy is unlikely to be effective and an ICD is advised. Usually EP-guided sotalol therapy is considered only in those patients with underlying ischemic heart disease who are inducible at

baseline EP testing and whose EF is > 30 percent. Candidates for ICD therapy generally fall into one of four categories: (1) cardiac arrest survivors, (2) those with symptomatic sustained VT, (3) those with syncope of unknown origin with inducible VT, and (4) asymptomatic patients at high risk for future life-threatening arrhythmic events.

Cardiac Arrest Survivors

Aborted sudden cardiac death is caused by ventricular tachyarrhythmia, asystole, or electromechanical dissociation (see Chap. 36). The most common underlying pathology is severe chronic coronary atherosclerosis in 56 to 78 percent of patients in all published series. The remaining patients have other structural heart diseases including cardiomyopathy, myocardial hypertrophy, and valvular heart disease. A small proportion of patients have structurally normal hearts, and in this group sudden cardiac death may be due to congenital long QT syndrome, ventricular preexcitation, or idiopathic ventricular fibrillation (see Chap. 36).

Survivors of cardiac arrest, in the absence of an acute myocardial infarction within 48 h, are at high risk of future recurrence. Data from Seattle in the 1970s showed a 30 to 40 percent 1-year mortality rate in untreated patients following an episode of out-of-hospital ventricular fibrillation.[39] Workup of cardiac arrest survivors usually includes an assessment of left ventricular EF, cardiac catheterization, and invasive EP testing. Left ventricular dysfunction is a powerful independent predictor of risk for recurrent cardiac arrest and sudden cardiac death. A left ventricular EF ≤ 30 percent was associated with a relative risk of 2.6 for recurrent cardiac arrest in survivors of out-of-hospital cardiac arrest.[22] Cardiac catheterization identifies those survivors of sudden cardiac death who have critical obstructive coronary artery disease. It is our practice to revascularize these patients whenever feasible, as this has been shown to improve long-term outcome.[40] We routinely perform invasive EP testing prior to and following revascularization, except in the presence of left main coronary artery disease, and advise ICD implantation in those with inducible VF or hemodynamically significant VT. *Those patients with preserved left ventricular function who are inducible at baseline EP study and noninducible following revascularization are a low-risk group whose treatment usually consists of beta blockade.* We routinely perform EP studies in cardiac arrest survivors. This provides baseline data on sinus node dysfunction and conduction system disease as well as inducibility of both VF and sustained monomorphic VT. Occasionally, it uncovers a readily treatable cause of cardiac arrest such as bundle branch reentry or preexcitation. Although ICD implantation without a baseline EP study is reported,[41] we do not at present support this practice.

TABLE 33-2

GUIDELINES FOR ICD IMPLANTATION

I. **ICD indicated**
   A. Cardiac arrest not due to acute ischemia or infarction[a] or reversible causes
   B. Documented sustained VT with hemodynamic compromise
   C. Syncope of unknown origin in structural heart disease patients with inducible sustained VT.

II. **ICD may be indicated**
   A. Inducible nonclinically documented VT following ablative or surgical therapy in high-risk patients
   B. Asymptomatic nonsustained VT + prior MI + left ventricular EF < 0.35 + inducible sustained VT that remains inducible despite IV procainamide
   C. Highly symptomatic long QT interval despite optimal medical therapy
   D. Cardiac arrest in the setting of acute ischemia plus inducible VF or hemodynamically significant VT despite optimal revascularization
   E. Hemodynamically stable sustained monomorphic VT

III. **ICD Contraindicated**
   A. Sustained VT or VF due to reversible causes (acute infarction, ischemia, electrolyte abnormalities, or drug proarrhythmia)
   B. Syncope of unknown origin and noninducible on EP testing
   C. Incessant or very frequent VF or VT
   D. Cardiac (NYHA class IV) or other comorbid illnesses that severely limit life expectancy (<6 months).
   E. Psychiatric contraindications.
   F. VF due to AF in WPW syndrome which is amenable to RFA surgery.

[a]Acute infarction is within 48 h of the time of onset of infarction.
Note: AF = atrial fibrillation; EP = electrophysiologic; MI = myocardial infarction; RFA = radiofrequency ablation; WPW = Wolff-Parkinson-White.

Symptomatic Sustained Ventricular Tachycardia

Another subset of patients in whom the ICD is being used with increasing frequency comprises those with spontaneous

TABLE 33-3
PROSPECTIVE MULTICENTER ICD TRIALS

Trial	Type	Study Population	Treatment Groups	Endpoints	Start Date	Status
CASH (Cardiac Arrest Study Hamburg)[32]	Secondary prophylaxis	Cardiac arrest survivors and inducible VT or VF	ICD vs. amiodarone vs. metoprolol vs. propafenone	Total mortality Cardiac arrest or ventricular tachyarrhythmia recurrence	1987	Ongoing Propafenone limb terminated due to excess mortality
CIDS (Canadian Implantable Defibrillator study)[33]	Secondary prophylaxis	(i) Cardiac arrest survivors, or (ii) syncopal VT or (iii) symptomatic VT + EF < 35%	ICD vs. amiodarone	Total mortality Quality of life Costs	1990	Ongoing
AVID (Antiarrhythmics Versus Implantable Defibrillators[34]	Secondary prophylaxis	(i) cardiac arrest survivors, or (ii) VT with either syncope or hypotension + EF < 40%	ICD vs. amiodarone or guided sotalol therapy	Total morality Quality of life Costs	1993	Ongoing
MADIT (Multicenter automatic Defibrillator Implantation Trial)[35]	Primary prophylaxis	Prior MI with EF < 35%, nonsustained VT and inducible, nonsuppressible VT or VF	ICD vs. conventional medical therapy	Total mortality First cardiac event Quality of life	1990	Terminated by Safety Monitoring Committee due to significantly fewer deaths in ICD group
CABG patch (Coronary artery Bypass Graft Patch) Trial[36]	Primary prophylaxis	CABG with EF < 36% and positive SAECG	ICD + CABG vs. CABG only	Total mortality	1990	Ongoing
CAT (Cardiomyopathy Trial)[37]	Primary prophylaxis	Dilated cardiomyopathy with EF < 30% and no symptomatic ventricular arrhythmias	ICD vs. control group	Total mortality Sudden death	1991	Ongoing
MUSTT (Multicenter Unsustained Tachycardia Trial)[38]	Primary prophylaxis	CAD with EF < 40%, nonsustained VT and inducible VT or VF	ICD in nonsuppressible group vs. antiarrhythmic drug in suppressible group vs. no treatment	Sudden arrhythmic death or spontaneous sustained VT	1992	Ongoing
SCD HeFT (Sudden Cardiac Death in Heart Failure Trial)	Primary prophylaxis	Ischemic cardiomyopathy or nonischemic dilated cardiomyopathy with CHF(NYHA II–III) and EF < 35%	ICD vs. amiodarone vs. placebo	Total mortality Arrhythmic mortality Quality of life Costs	1996	Starting

Note: CAD = coronary artery disease; CHF = congestive heart failure; MI = myocardial infarction; SAECG = signal averaged electrocardiogram.

and induced sustained monomorphic VT. In this subset of patients, potential therapeutic options are more numerous, including EP-guided antiarrhythmic drug therapy, guided or empiric amiodarone therapy, surgical aneurysmectomy with map-guided subendocardial resection, transcatheter radiofrequency ablation (see Chap. 31), or an ICD with antitachycardia pacing capabilities. The limitations of EP-guided antiarrhythmic drug therapy are discussed above. Long-term amiodarone therapy is limited by drug intolerance and organ toxicity. Combined aneurysmectomy and intraoperative map-guided subendocardial resection yields a low rate of arrhythmia recurrence but is only indicated in selected patients with drug-

refractory VT secondary to ischemic heart disease who have a discrete left ventricular aneurysm. Transcatheter radiofrequency ablation is suitable in only about 10 percent of patients with spontaneous sustained VT screened at our institution.[42] Transcatheter radiofrequency ablation is rarely employed as sole therapy in patients with underlying structural heart disease; however, it may be curative in patients with bundle branch reentry or idiopathic VT.

In patients with left ventricular dysfunction and rapid VTs, particularly when associated with hemodynamic compromise, the ICD is increasingly seen as first-line therapy. Antitachycardia pacing is highly effective in a majority of patients with recurrent monomorphic VT and is usually imperceptible to the patient, a feature that enhances patient acceptance of these devices. The various therapeutic options available should be considered as complementary, rather than competing, therapies. In managing individual patients, more than one therapy or even all therapies may be employed over a period of time.

Syncope of Unknown Origin

Syncope is a common, usually benign condition (see Chap. 35). When associated with structural heart disease and inducible VT at EP study, however, it carries a high risk of sudden cardiac death. One study reported a sudden death rate of 48 percent at 3 years in patients with syncope of unknown origin and inducible sustained VT, compared to 9 percent in patients with a negative EP study.[43] In patients at high risk of sudden cardiac death, such as those with structural heart disease, poor left ventricular function, and/or inducible sustained VT, ICD implantation, amiodarone, or guided sotalol therapy are all reasonable options.

Asymptomatic High-Risk Patients

A majority of patients at high risk for sudden cardiac death have not previously experienced a sustained ventricular tachyarrhythmia. Since current mortality rates associated with out-of-hospital cardiac arrest are in the range of 70 to 85 percent, it is evident that primary prevention strategies will have the greatest impact on reducing mortality from sudden cardiac death.[44] Prophylactic ICD implantation involves placing the device in a patient who is considered at high risk but has never had a spontaneous episode of sustained VT or VF, with the aim of treating the first episode effectively and thereby preventing sudden death. Defining populations of patients who are at sufficiently high risk that prophylactic ICD implantation would be medically justified is difficult and is the focus of several prospective clinical trials (Table 33-3). These trials test the hypothesis that prophylactic ICD implantation reduces not only sudden cardiac death but also total mortality. Included are select patients with left ventricular dysfunction and nonsustained VT [Multicenter Automatic Defibrillator Implantation Trial (MADIT) and Multicenter Unsustained Tachycardia Trial], patients with dilated cardiomyopathy (Cardiomyopathy Trial), and high-risk patients following coronary artery bypass graft (Coronary Artery Bypass Graft Patch Trial).

Nonsustained VT in the setting of a previous myocardial infarction and left ventricular dysfunction is associated with a 2-year mortality rate of approximately 30 percent. MADIT was designed to determine if prophylactic implantation of a cardioverter-defibrillator in high-risk coronary patients with asymptomatic nonsustained VT would improve survival compared to conventional medical therapy.[35] Over 5 years, 196 patients from 32 centers in the United States and Europe were enrolled: requirements included prior myocardial infarction, EF < 35 percent, New York Heart Association (NYHA) class I to III, a documented episode of nonsustained VT, and inducible, nonsuppressible sustained VT they were random-

ized to either ICD ($n = 95$) or conventional medical therapy ($n = 101$). MADIT was terminated early by the Safety Monitoring Committee because of significantly improved survival in the ICD arm.[35] One month after randomization, amiodarone therapy was used in 2 percent of the ICD group and 80 percent of the conventional therapy group. There were 15 (15.8 percent) deaths in the ICD group and 39 (38.6 percent) deaths in the conventional group (hazard ratio 0.46; 95 percent confidence interval = 0.26 to 0.82; $p < .009$). This study has major implications as it suggests not only that prophylactic ICD therapy can save lives in a group of patients frequently seen in clinical practice but also that ICD therapy saves lives compared to amiodarone therapy. The results of the above ongoing clinical trials and cost-benefit analyses will determine the role of prophylactic ICD implantation in the future.

IMPLANTATION AND TESTING

Patches to Pectoral Implants

An ICD system includes the pulse generator, rate sensing/pacing, and shocking leads. Although the feasibility of transvenous catheter defibrillation systems was demonstrated in the early 1970s,[45,46] there were practical problems with the use of this approach. These included the sensitive dependence of the catheter's position within the right ventricle for proper functioning and high defibrillation energy requirements, which approached the maximum energy output of the ICD device. Animal experiments indicated that the lowest, most consistent, and most stable energy requirements for successful defibrillation were achieved with patch electrodes placed directly on the epicardium.[47] The earliest ICD systems consisted of epicardial patches surgically placed by means of a thoracotomy, with either epicardial screw-in leads or an endocardial lead for rate sensing (Fig. 33-2). The pulse generator was placed in an abdominal pocket. Transthoracic approaches developed for the implantation of epicardial patches include the anterolateral thoracotomy, subcostal thoracotomy, the subxiphoid approach, and the median sternotomy.[49] The patch electrodes can be placed either intrapericardially or extrapericardially. Extrapericardial patch placement is preferred to avoid injury to epicardial vessels and to facilitate future cardiac operations. The need for thoracotomy limited the use of ICDs in some high-risk patients and was responsible for most of the morbidity and mortality associated with ICD implantation.

Two separate developments made transvenous nonthoracotomy systems feasible. First, the development of reliable integrated lead systems, which incorporate both shocking and sensing/pacing elements, and second, biphasic defibrillation waveforms. Initial defibrillation circuits consisted of RV and superior vena cava (SVC) coils inserted either as two separate leads (e.g., Transvene, Medtronic) or as a single lead (e.g., Endotak, CPI). A patch electrode was implanted subcutaneously over the left chest wall, if needed to achieve an adequate DFT. Biphasic defibrillation waveforms lowered DFTs sig-

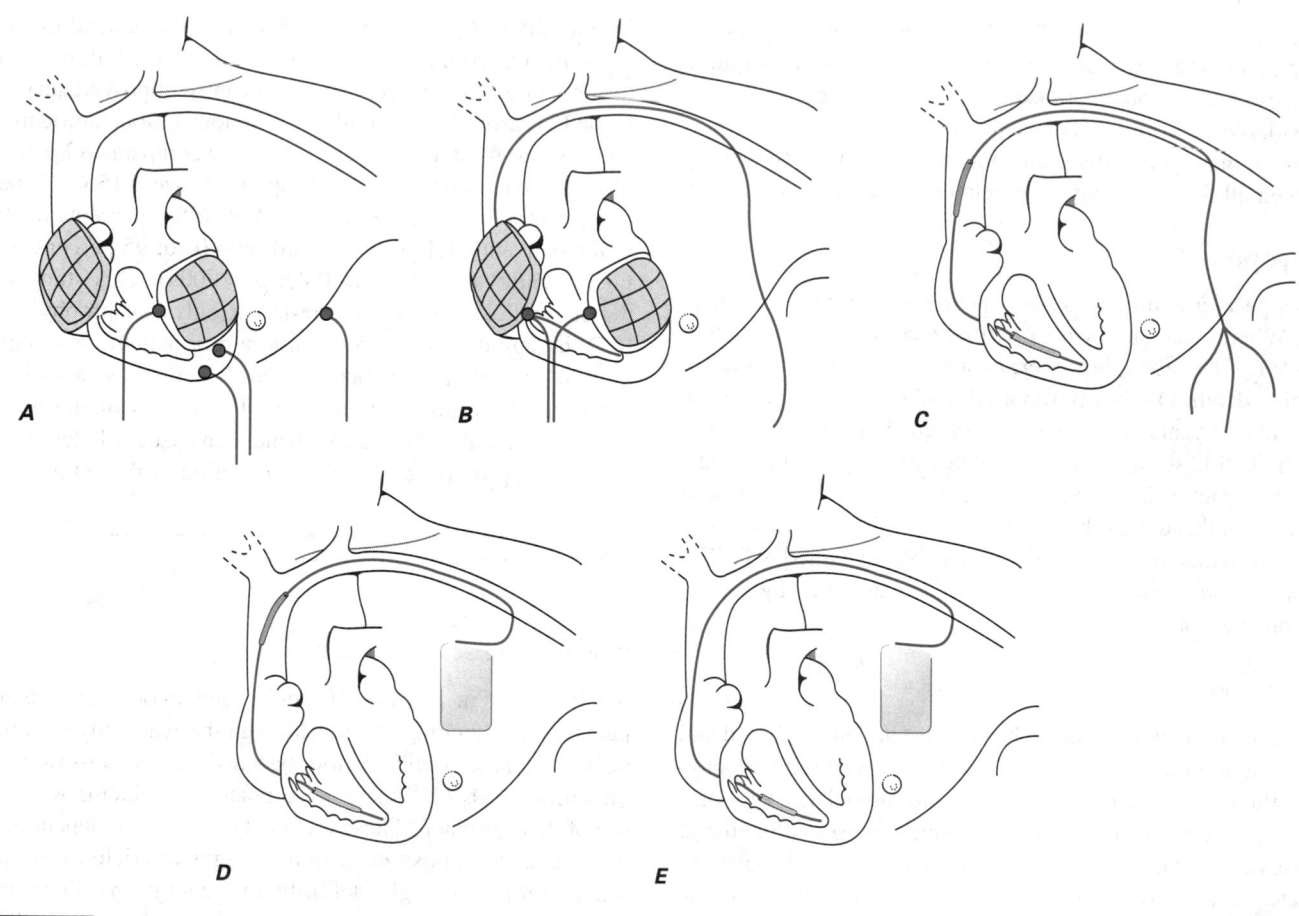

FIGURE 33-2

Schematic representation of defibrillation lead systems. RV = right ventricle; SVC = superior vena cava; SQ = subcutaneous.

Implant Technique	Sensing Circuit	Defibrillation Circuit	Pulse Generator Site
A. Thoracotomy	Epicardial rate sensing leads	Epicardial patch to patch	Abdominal
B. Thoracotomy	Endocardial rate sensing lead	Epicardial patch to patch	Abdominal
C. Nonthoracotomy	Endocardial rate sensing lead	Endocardial RV to SVC coil ± SQ patch (left chest wall)	Abdominal
D. Nonthoracotomy	Endocardial rate sensing lead	Endocardial RV to SVC coil ± SQ patch (left infraclavicular)	Pectoral
E. Nonthoracotomy	Endocardial rate sensing lead	Unipolar RV coil to "active can" ± SVC coil	Pectoral

(*Adapted from Gold MR, Shorofsky SR,*[48]) with permission.

nificantly compared to monophasic waveforms and resulted in a greater proportion of successful implants using a coil-to-coil configuration. Transvenous ICD systems resulted in lower perioperative mortality and morbidity, shorter hospital stay, lower cost, and comparable long-term efficacy.[50,51] Transve-nous ICD implantation with satisfactory DFTs was accomplished in over 90 percent of patients.[52]

With technological advances, pulse generator size decreased to the extent that pectoral implantation became feasible (Table 33-1). The defibrillation pathway in the initial pectoral implants used an RV-to-SVC coil configuration and, if necessary to achieve adequate DFTs, a patch electrode was placed under the device.[53] This rapidly led to unipolar defibrillation systems, the titanium case of the pulse generator acting as a large surface area defibrillation patch electrode ("active can").[54] The defibrillation pathway in pectoral active-can implants is RV coil to active can. An SVC coil may be included in the defibrillation pathway to lower DFTs. Although prospective randomized trials are lacking, simple unipolar transvenous defibrillation results in DFTs comparable to those reported with epicardial lead systems.[55] Today, pectoral implantation of an active can is the technique of first choice in most institutions. Despite major advances in lead technology and defibrillation waveforms, a small proportion of individuals still require thoracotomy and epicardial patch placement to achieve adequate DFTs.

Implantation Testing

The ability to defibrillate VF reproducibly is fundamental to the success of ICD therapy in preventing sudden cardiac death. Accomplishing this goal requires meticulous device testing at the time of implantation. Implantation testing may be considered a three-step process: lead testing, defibrillation testing, and ICD system testing.

LEAD TESTING
Correct positioning of an integrated lead usually involves advancing its tip as close to the apex of the right ventricle as possible. During sinus rhythm, R-wave amplitude, rate of change of the signal voltage (slew rate), pacing threshold, and pacing lead impedance are assessed. The larger the signal amplitude and the greater the slew rate during sinus rhythm, the more likely it is that the signals during VT and VF will be detected easily. The minimum acceptable R-wave amplitude is >5 mV, to ensure satisfactory sensing during both sinus rhythm and VF. If necessary the lead is repositioned until satisfactory results are obtained. In addition to testing sensing and pacing functions, a low-energy R-wave synchronized shock is given between the defibrillation electrodes to determine the high-voltage lead impedance prior to initiating VF.

DEFIBRILLATION TESTING
Defibrillation testing requires the repeated induction of VF and repeated attempts at defibrillation. VF is induced either by a critically timed T-wave shock, very rapid burst pacing, or occasion-

ally alternating current. As defibrillation energy requirements increase with time, testing is standardized by maintaining VF for 10 s prior to attempting defibrillation. If attempts at defibrillation using an implant support system and the test lead configuration fail, a 360-J external defibrillation is performed. A 5-min interval is allowed between successive tests. The concept of a DFT implies that at a certain energy level defibrillation success changes abruptly from 0 to 100 percent. Unfortunately, there is no clear-cut distinction between successful and unsuccessful energy levels. Rather, the relationship between defibrillation energy and success is best described as a sigmoidal dose-response curve, the probability of success increasing steadily with each increase in energy until a 100 percent success plateau is reached (Fig. 33-3). The DFT is defined as the minumum energy producing defibrillation success and may be significantly lower than the lowest energy required for 100 percent success (E_{100}). To ensure efficacy of the implanted device in the future and to allow for rising defibrillation energy requirements due to such factors as altering substrate or addition of certain antiarrhythmic drugs, defibrillation shock intensities must be programmed so that the ICD output is 10 to 15 J above E_{100}. Full characterization of the dose-response curve would require more shocks than are compatible with patient safety. In clinical practice, two types of testing methods are performed—one aims to verify that the ICD can be programmed with an adequate safety margin between maximum output and the shock intensities tested at implant (margin verification protocol), and the other aims to define the minimum energy producing defibrillation success (DFT testing protocol).[57] At our institution, the minimum acceptable testing to proceed with implantation using a given defibrillation configuration is at least three successful conversion attempts and no failure at

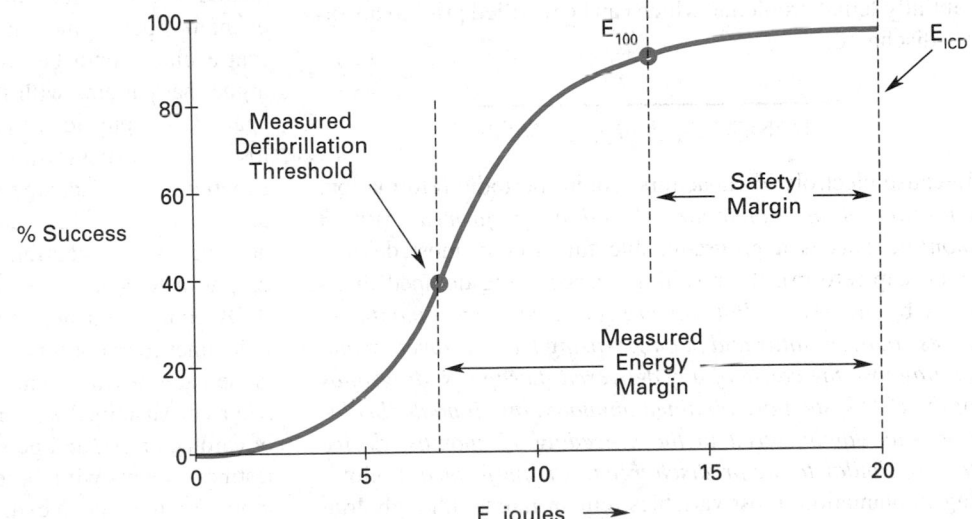

FIGURE 33-3
Percent probability for successful defibrillation versus shock energy. The measured ICD energy margin is the energy difference between the lowest conversion success [defibrillation threshold (DFT)] and the programmed ICD energy: energy margin = E_{ICD} − DFT. The ICD safety margin is the energy difference between the lowest energy required for 100 percent success at implant (E_{100}) and the programmed ICD energy: safety margin = E_{ICD} − E_{100}. (Adapted from Singler I, Lang D,[56] with permission.)

an energy level 10 J and preferably 15 J below the maximum energy output of the device. In patients who are tolerating the fibrillation-defibrillation episodes, a step-down method is employed to assess the defibrillation threshold. If an adequate safety margin cannot be demonstrated, testing is repeated with reverse polarity, different lead configurations, or after the addition of an extra electrode. If unsuccessful, we leave a long endocardial integrated rate-sensing/shocking lead in place and a cardiac surgeon performs epicardial patch(es) placement. After adequate safety margins are demonstrated, the leads are tunnelled to the abdomen and connected to a pulse generator.

ICD TESTING

ICD testing involves intraoperative testing of the entire system to ensure satisfactory sensing, acceptable pacing threshold, and lead impedances and to demonstrate that the final system detects and defibrillates VF appropriately. Only after all these criteria are fulfilled is the system deemed to be successfully implanted and adequately tested.

Predischarge Testing

Prior to discharge, a chest x-ray is reviewed to rule out lead dislodgement and the patient is subjected to a further device test. Noninvasive programmed stimulation (NIPS) is performed using the device programmer. VF is induced noninvasively, either by a critically timed T-wave shock or by burst pacing. Appropriate sensing of induced VF and the ability to defibrillate with an adequate safety margin are confirmed. Sustained monomorphic VT may be induced by NIPS with up to three extrastimuli and ATP algorithms tested. Predischarge testing occasionally uncovers otherwise unsuspected and potentially lethal problems, which can be rectified prior to hospital discharge.

LONG-TERM FOLLOW-UP

Because electrolytic capacitors require periodic reformation, *charging of the capacitors should be performed every 3 months.* This is a programmable function in most devices (auto-cap reform), the resulting charge being dumped internally by the device. *Patients are reviewed every 3 months to assess battery status and pacing/sensing lead parameters and to diagnose the cause of any delivered therapy. Radiographs of the ICD system are obtained annually, and if no defibrillation was administered in the preceding 12 months, device testing similar to the predischarge test is performed.* Following implantation, most variables remain fixed, although drug therapy may change and underlying disease processes may worsen. Long-term oral amiodarone can increase defibrillation thresholds.[58,59] Repeat testing of the ICD is recommended in these individuals to confirm adequate function, especially in those with minimal safety margins established at the time of intraoperative DFT testing.

Elective Replacement

Almost all patients with an ICD should be considered for pulse generator replacement when there is evidence of battery depletion, since late shocks occurring many years after primary implantation appear to define a continuing need for this therapy in many patients.[60] The decision to replace the device in patients without previous shocks must be individualized and depends on factors such as the presenting arrhythmia, the circumstances of its occurrence, the nature and severity of underlying heart disease, the results of EP testing, and the presence of other comorbid factors. Patients requiring generator replacement are admitted electively and have the same generator or an upgraded model implanted. Lead electrodes are not routinely changed at the time of generator replacement unless a problem is identified. Confirmation of previously established rate-sensing lead electrogram amplitude is performed as well as defibrillation testing, followed by testing of the new pulse generator. Several studies have confirmed the stability over time of DFTs in most patients.[61,62] In occasional patients, however, defibrillation energy requirements may be unexpectedly elevated at the time of generator replacement, supporting the practice of routine defibrillation testing.[63]

Psychosocial Issues

The ICD is generally well accepted in the vast majority of patients for whom this therapy is recommended.[64,65] Before implantation, the implications of having an ICD must be thoroughly discussed. The issue causing the greatest ambivalence among patients is the potential restriction of lifestyle related to driving. Because of the potential risk of an arrhythmia recurrence and the delivery of high-energy shocks, most physicians who implant ICDs agree that some restriction on driving should be considered. Since the risk of a recurrent arrhythmic event may persist indefinitely and because the timing of recurrent events cannot be predicted accurately, some physicians argue that patients with ICDs should not be allowed to drive again. Other physicians permit driving in patients who do not lose consciousness with their arrhythmias or who have not experienced a discharge after an arbitrary length of follow-up, usually 6 to 12 months. This approach is problematic, however, since recurrent arrhythmic events may still occur despite a long initial shock-free interval. Patients receiving ICDs comprise a heterogeneous population, and one set of guidelines may not serve all cases. At one end of the spectrum is the patient with impaired ventricular function, documented recurrent sustained ventricular arrhythmias causing syncope or cardiac arrest, and persistent inducibility at the time of EP testing. Patients with these characteristics are likely to receive more frequent device discharges. At the other end of the spectrum are asymptomatic high-risk patients. A more restrictive approach to the issue of driving seems appropriate for the former group of patients but is inappropriate for the latter and may make patients unwilling to accept ICD therapy. At present, few states in the United States have specific laws for patients with life-threatening arrhythmias, and no state makes any distinction between patients managed with an ICD versus those managed medically.[66] Therefore there is no legal consensus to guide physicians in advising patients with ICDs. At present, a conservative approach seems prudent, particularly for patients with a history of previous sustained arrhythmias who are deemed at high risk for recurrent arrhythmic events. Many implanting centers have ICD support groups that meet several times a year to discuss issues relating to their devices. These groups provide a forum for patients with ICDs to discuss issues with one another and with implanting physicians and nurses. Support groups of this nature provide an invaluable service to patients with these devices.

COMPLICATIONS AND TROUBLESHOOTING

ICD therapy is associated with well-known risks (Table 33-4) that must be weighed against the potential benefits of automatic ventricular tachyarrhythmia therapy. Lead-related problems can result in failure to sense, failure to pace, and either inappropriate defibrillation shocks or inability to defibrillate ventricular tachyarrhythmias. Pacing and sensing problems are more common with epicardial leads; lead dislodgement is more common with endocardial leads.[17,50] A lead fracture or insulation defect may present as a medical emergency due to frequent inappropriate shocks or a potentially fatal lead problem may remain undetected. Fortunately, careful regular follow-up, including assessment of pacing/sensing characteristics, impedance measurements, and radiographs of the ICD system, will identify the majority of asymptomatic problems.[67]

One of the most devastating complications is infection of the

TABLE 33-4
ICD COMPLICATIONS

PROCEDURE-RELATED

Short-term
Proarrhythmia (atrial fibrillation, ventricular tachyarrhythmia storm)
Respiratory (atelectasis, aspiration, pulmonary embolism, pneumonia, ARDS, pleural effusion)
Pericardial (pericarditis, effusion)
Myocardial infarction
Cerebrovascular accident
Hematoma (pulse generator pocket or subcutaneous patch)
Seroma (pulse generator pocket or subcutaneous patch)
Subclavian stick complications (pneumothorax, air embolism, subclavian artery puncture)
Venous thromboembolism
Phrenic nerve stimulation

Long-term
Infection
Erosion
Migration
Venous thromboembolism
Constrictive pericarditis
Patch-related vessel erosion
Endocarditis

SYSTEM-RELATED

Lead dislodgement (Gross dislodgment, microdislodgment, Twiddler's syndrome)
Lead conductor fracture
Lead insulation defect
Lead perforation (± diaphragmatic pacing)
Lead malposition
Loose set screw
Loose adaptor
Exit block
Patch crinkling
Premature battery depletion

THERAPY-RELATED

Inappropriate treatment
Overdetection
Noise (e.g., sensing artifact due to lead defect; electromagnetic interference)
Double-counting (e.g., T waves, R waves, pacing spikes)
Misdiagnosis of atrial fibrillation or sinus tachycardia
Detection failure
Undersensing
"Drop-out" (prolonged detection time)
Total failure to detect episode
Redetection failure
Proarrhythmia
Acceleration or degeneration of hemodynamically tolerated ventricular tachycardia
Inappropriate treatment triggering ventricular tachyarrhythmia
Appropriate treatment triggering atrial fibrillation

infection resemble those observed with permanent pacemaker implantation but occur more frequently. In the PCD multicenter trial of 1221 patients, of whom approximately half received an epicardial system via a thoracotomy approach and half an endocardial system with tunnelling to an abdominal device, the infection rate was higher in the endocardial system recipients than the epicardial system recipients (4.8 percent versus 2.3 percent; $p = .028$).[17] Direct intraoperative contamination is thought to be the source of most infections. However, due to the low virulence of some organisms (e.g., *Staphylococcus epidermis*), infections may not become obvious for a considerable time after implantation. In general, explantation of the entire ICD system, sometimes requiring open heart surgery, is mandatory. After a regimen of intense antibiotic therapy, usually for 6 weeks, and if all clinical evidence of infection is resolved, reimplantation at a different site may be performed, but the risk of reinfection is higher than for a primary implant. The necessity for surgical revision of the ICD system, including lead repositioning, insertion of a new lead, or explantation of the device, reflects the frequency of serious ICD complications. Between 5.5 and 9.8 percent of patients with epicardial systems required surgical revision during follow-up, compared with 7.1 to 16.4 percent of patients with endocardial systems.[17,51,68,69]

The long-term complication rate for pectoral implants is less well known at present. With abdominal implantation of endocardial lead systems, lead fractures frequently occur at the lower costal margin and in the abdominal pocket, and extensive subcutaneous tunnelling is thought to increase the risk of infection. Pectoral implantation should potentially result in fewer long-term complications. A multicenter pectoral implant trial (active can) of 473 patients had an overall complication rate of 6 percent and complications requiring system revision in 4.2 percent of patients.[70] Of note was the complete absence of device infections. Further studies and longer follow-up are required to assess the complication rate of pectoral implantation fully as it is possible that other complications, such as device migration or erosion, may increase in frequency.

Troubleshooting

The management of a patient who has received an ICD discharge is a challenging problem. Symptoms preceding an ICD discharge are difficult to interpret, as ventricular tachyarrhythmias may cause minimal or no symptoms. Over the years, ICDs have advanced from therapeutic devices providing basic diagnostic data, such as event counters or RR interval information, to sophisticated electrocardiographic monitoring units (Table 33-1). Analysis of stored intracardiac electrograms results in a confident diagnosis of most ICD discharges. The recordings are either from the sensing electrode (near-field) or from the high-voltage defibrillation coils (far-field) during the time interval preceding, during, and following ICD therapy; during aborted therapy; or during sinus rhythm. In addi-

tion, there are marker channels that annotate each sensed event. In general, changes in electrogram morphology compared to sinus rhythm are consistent with ventricular tachyarrhythmias, whereas an identical electrogram morphology is consistent with supraventricular arrhythmias. Atrial activity can often be identified with far-field electrograms. Approximately 25 percent of ICD discharges are inappropriate (Table 33-4), most commonly due to atrial fibrillation or sinus tachycardia resulting in a ventricular rate above the tachycardia detection rate.[71] Other less frequent problems include overdetection (noise, double counting), undersensing, redetection failure, or ICD-induced proarrhythmia and are usually apparent on careful analysis of stored electrogram data. Accurate interpretation is needed to institute the appropriate action, which may include device reprogramming, alteration of antiarrhythmic therapy, or surgical revision of the ICD system.

EFFICACY AND ECONOMICS

Sudden Cardiac Death

As a therapeutic modality, the ICD is unequalled in its ability to prevent sudden cardiac death. Combining the results of large single-center and multicenter studies in over 4000 patients, the sudden death rate is <2 percent per year up to 5 years postimplantation.[72] Although the ICD provides a highly effective therapy for reducing mortality from sudden cardiac death in high-risk patients, a small incidence of sudden death remains in patients with these devices.[73] Device failures are extremely rare (below 1 percent) and may be attributed to factors such as lead fracture or migration, premature battery depletion, and generator malfunction.[74] Deaths in the setting of documented refractory VF and normal device function are also described.[73] The factors accounting for the resistance to defibrillation in these cases are incompletely understood and may, in some cases, result from severe ischemia and/or end-stage pump failure. High DFTs at the time of implantation or a rise in the DFT postimplant as well as asystole and electromechanical dissociation may account for other instances of sudden death.[75,76]

The sudden death rates reported in ICD patients compare favorably with patients treated either with amiodarone[26,29,30] or EP-guided sotalol or type I antiarrhythmic therapy.[22,27,31]

Perioperative Mortality

ICD implantation by thoracotomy exposes the patient to a nontrivial initial risk. Published perioperative mortality ranges from 1 to 6 percent.[72] This has been reduced substantially to between 0 and 1.4 percent by the use of nonthoracotomy lead systems and should remain low as the procedure is simplified by pectoral implantation. Although no randomized prospective trial has compared epicardial with endocardial implantation, during a multicenter study of 1221 implants, approximately half were implanted using thoracotomy and epicardial patches and half using a nonthoracotomy approach and endocardial lead electrodes in a nonrandomized manner.[17] Perioperative 3-day mortality was 0.8 percent in endocardial implant recipients and 4.2 percent in epicardial implant recipients ($p <.001$).

Total Mortality

Although all published studies have uniformly reported low sudden death rates, some investigators have argued that total mortality is not reduced with ICDs compared to the best available conventional antiarrhythmic therapy. Although sudden death is markedly reduced, overall mortality in ICD recipients can be up to 20 percent at 2 years.[72] Early ICD pioneers proved that the ICD reliably terminated life-threatening ventricular arrhythmias. Once the ability of the ICD to prevent sudden death became established, it became extremely difficult to design prospective randomized trials in high-risk patients.[77] In the absence of prospective trial data, several indirect approaches have been employed in an attempt to confirm the benefit of ICD therapy in reducing overall mortality. Comparisons with historical controls,[78,79] case-control studies,[26,80,81] and projected survival from time of appropriate ICD discharge[82–88] and comparison between those using and not using their devices[89,90] have all suggested that ICD therapy improves overall survival. Each one of these analyses is flawed. Survival today is improved compared to historical controls because of aspirin, beta blockers, angiotensin-converting enzyme inhibitors as well as more aggressive reperfusion and revascularization. Case control studies either compare ICDs with outmoded forms of medical therapy such as type I antiarrhythmics or are criticized for differences in clinical characteristics between groups. Determining whether an arrhythmia resulting in an ICD discharge would have been fatal had the ICD not been implanted is difficult and susceptible to marked overestimation of efficacy. While none of these studies is above criticism, assessing the evidence accumulated by all these studies combined, *one can reasonably conclude that the ICD prolongs survival in certain subsets of patients with life-threatening ventricular tachyarrhythmias.*

It is now recognized that the primary endpoint to assess the benefit of ICD therapy should be total mortality, which would include deaths during the waiting period prior to ICD implantation, perioperative mortality, and all-cause mortality during follow-up. At present, several ongoing prospective multicenter trials are addressing the efficacy of ICD therapy in reducing total mortality (Table 33-3). The ability of the ICD to impact on total mortality, however, depends on the proportion of overall mortality that is accounted for by sudden cardiac death in a given population of patients. Based on reasonable assumptions that sudden deaths constitute one-half of postarrest cardiac deaths and that 80 percent of sudden deaths are due to ventricular tachyarrhythmias, a 90 percent reduction in sudden tachyarrhythmic deaths can only yield a 36 percent reduction in total cardiac mortality.[91] In patients with preserved left ventricular function (EF > 40 percent)

and mild or no symptoms of congestive heart failure (NYHA class I to II), the survival benefit of the ICD relative to drug therapy is likely to be late and may not be demonstrated for years after implantation. In patients with moderately depressed left ventricular function (EF 30 to 40 percent) and moderate symptoms of congestive heart failure (NYHA class II to III), the relative survival benefit of the ICD is likely to be early but may not be sustained due to conversion of sudden to nonsudden cardiac deaths in patients with advancing heart failure. In patients with severely impaired left ventricular function (EF > 30 percent) and severe symptomatic congestive heart failure (NYHA class IV), there is unlikely to be a significant improvement in overall mortality despite a low sudden death rate.[91] Optimizing patient selection to ensure that a low sudden death rate will translate into a significant reduction in long-term survival is the challenge for the future.

Cost Effectiveness

The cost of the ICD with leads ranges between $20,000 and $28,000. Hospital costs associated with the evaluation of patients with life-threatening arrhythmias and subsequent ICD implantation may exceed these figures. The cost effectiveness of the implantable defibrillator is well within the range of currently accepted life-saving technology.[92] Moreover, as this technology evolves, it is likely to become more cost effective. Noninvasive programmed stimulation capabilities and sophisticated diagnostic features permit outpatient evaluation and device reprogramming and reduce the need for ambulatory or in-hospital ECG monitoring in many patients. Antitachycardia pacing therapy may reduce the frequency of rehospitalization in patients with recurrent VT. Earlier decision-making and the use of pectoral implants should reduce the length of hospital stay and costs associated with initial implantation of these devices substantially. Wever et al. compared two treatment strategies in postinfarct sudden death survivors.[28,93] Patients were randomly assigned either to early ICD implantation as first-line therapy ($n = 29$) or to a conventional therapeutic strategy of starting with EP-guided drug therapy and proceeding to map-guided VT surgery and/or ICD implantation in those who remained inducible ($n = 31$). In the conventional group, 20 patients failed EP-guided antiarrhythmic therapy and subsequently underwent map-guided VT surgery (6 patients) or ICD implantation (14 patients). Total mortality was 14 percent in the early ICD group and 35 percent in the conventional group after 24 months. Of the 11 patients who remained on antiarrhythmics as sole therapy, two died in the hospital prior to retesting, five died after discharge, and one survived a recurrent cardiac arrest followed by ICD implantation. Median total costs were similar for both strategies ($47,000 versus $47,500, 1992 costs). Median total costs per patient in the early ICD group were higher only during the first 3 months of follow-up; after that, the EP-guided strategy was more costly. Cost-effectiveness ratio was estimated as the median of total costs per patient per day alive. The cost-effectiveness ratios were $63 and $94 for the early ICD and

EP-guided strategy groups, respectively, per patient per day alive. Patients discharged with antiarrhythmic drugs as sole therapy had the lowest total costs ($23,500 per patient) but the highest mortality, resulting in the worst cost-effectiveness ratio ($196 per patient per day alive). Although the results can be criticized due to the use of type I antiarrhythmics in patients with ischemic heart disease, it is the first prospective randomized trial comparing the efficacy and cost effectiveness of two different treatment strategies.

FUTURE DIRECTIONS

ICD technology is evolving rapidly. More efficient defibrillation waveforms, improved lead systems, and advances in battery and capacitor technology will hopefully enable the ICD of the future to approach more closely the size of today's permanent pacemakers, thereby facilitating pectoral implantation. Multiple intracardiac electrogram sources (e.g., near-field, far-field, or atrial), annotated marker channels, and expanded memory for event storage and Holter functions should substantially facilitate the management of patients following device discharges and provide new insights into the pathophysiology of sudden cardiac death. Devices incorporating an atrial electrode resulting in "DDD-ICDs" will help differentiate ventricular from supraventricular tachycardias and permit antitachycardia atrial pacing in response to supraventricular arrhythmias. In addition, these units will obviate the need for separate permanent pacemaker implantation and reduce the risk of pacemaker-ICD interactions. The incorporation of a reliable hemodynamic sensor to differentiate hemodynamically stable from hemodynamically compromising tachyarrhythmias would help identify the most appropriate therapy for each arrhythmia. Technological advances, simplification of the implantation procedure, and employment of the ICD as first-line therapy should result in fewer complications, less morbidity, and shorter hospital length of stay.

More important than technological advances in the next few years will be a clearer understanding of the role of ICD therapy in the secondary and primary prophylaxis of sudden cardiac death. Careful patient selection to reduce overall mortality as well as sudden cardiac death will ensure that both patients and society benefit.

DEDICATION

This chapter is dedicated to the memory of Ross Brooks, colleague and coauthor of "The Implantable Cardioverter-Defibrillator" in the 8th edition of this text.

REFERENCES

1. Gillum RF. Sudden coronary death in the United States. *Circulation* 1989; 79:756–765.
2. Kerber RE, Jensen SR, Gascho JA, Grayzel J, Hoyt R, Kennedy J. Determinants of defibrillation: A prospective analysis of 183 patients. *Am J Cardiol* 1983; 52:739–745.
3. DeLuna AB, Coumel P, Leclercq JF. Ambulatory sudden cardiac death: Mechanisms of production of fatal arrhythmias on the basis of 157 cases. *Am Heart J* 1989; 117:151–159.
4. Pionkowski RS, Thompson BM, Gruchow HW, Aprahamian CV, Darin JC. Resuscitation time in ventricular fibrillation—a prognosis indicator. *Ann Emerg Med* 1983; 12:733–738.
5. Weaver WD, Cobb LA, Hallstrom AP, Fahrenbruch C, Copass MK, Ray R. Factors influencing survival after out-of-hospital cardiac arrest. *J Am Coll Cardiol* 1986; 7:752–757.
6. Mirowski M. The automatic implantable cardioverter/defibrillator: An overview. *J Am Coll Cardiol* 1985; 6:461–466.
7. Mirowski M, Mower MM, Langer A, Hellman MS, Schreibman J. A chronically implanted system for automatic defibrillation in active conscious dogs. Experimental model for treatment of sudden death from ventricular fibrillation. *Circulation* 1978; 58:90–93.
8. Mirowski M, Reid PR, Mower MM, Watkins L, Gott VL, Schauble JF, et al. Termination of malignant ventricular arrhythmias with an implanted automatic defibrillator in human beings. *N Engl J Med* 1980; 303:322–324.
9. Olson WH. Tachyarrhythmia sensing and detection. In: Singler I, ed. *Implantable Cardioverter Defibrillator*. New York: Futura; 1994:71–107.
10. Hurwitz JL, Hook BG, Flores BT, Marchlinski FE. Importance of abortive shock capability with electrogram storage in cardioverter-defibrillator devices. *J Am Coll Cardiol* 1993; 21:895–900.
11. Neuzner J, Pitschner HF, Schlepper M. Programmable VT detection enhancements in implantable cardioverter defibrillator therapy. *Pacing Clin Electrophysiol* 1995; 18(pt II):539–547.
12. Neuzner J, Pitschner HF, Huth C, Schlepper M. Effects of biphasic waveform pulse on endocardial defibrillation efficacy in humans. *Pacing Clin Electrophysiol* 1994; 17:207–212.
13. Block M, Hammel D, Bocker D, Borggrefe M, Budde T, Isbruch F, et al. A prospective randomised cross-over comparison of mono- and biphasic defibrillation using nonthoracotomy lead configurations in humans. *J Cardiovasc Electrophysiol* 1994; 5(7):581–590.
14. Almendral J, Arenal A, Villacastin JP, San Roman D, Bueno H, Alday JM, et al. The importance of antitachycardia pacing for patients presenting with ventricular tachycardia. *Pacing Clin Electrophysiol* 1993; 16(II):535–539.
15. Brady GH, Poole JE, Kudenchuk PJ, Dolack GL, Kelso D, Mitchell R. A prospective randomised repeat-crossover comparison of anti-tachycardia pacing with low-energy cardioversion. *Circulation* 1993; 87:1889–1896.
16. Rosenqvist M. Pacing techniques to terminate ventricular tachycardia. *Pacing Clin Electrophysiol* 1995; 18(II): 592–598.
17. The PCD Investigator Group. Clinical outcome of patients with malignant ventricular tachyarrhythmias and a multiprogrammable implantable cardioverter-defibrillator implanted with or without thoracotomy: An international multicenter study. *J Am Coll Cardiol* 1994; 23:1521–1530.
18. Porterfield JG, Porterfield LM, Smith BA, Bray L, Voshage L, Martinez A, and the Ventak PRx Phase I Investigators. Conversion rates of induced versus spontaneous ventricular tachycardia by a third generation cardioverter defibrillator. *Pacing Clin Electrophysiol* 1993; 16(II):170–178.
19. Gross JN, Sackstein RD, Song SL, Chang CJ, Kawinishi DT, Furman S. The antitachycardia pacing ICD: Impact on patient selection and outcome. *Pacing Clin Electrophysiol* 1993; 16(II):165–169.
20. Dreifus LS, Fisch C, Griffin JC, Gillette PC, Mason JW, Parsonnet V. Guidelines for implantation of cardiac pacemakers and antiarrhythmic devices: A report of the American College of Cardiology/American Heart Association Task Force on Assessment of Diagnostic and Therapeutic Cardiovascular Procedures (Committee on Pacemaker Implantation). *J Am Coll Cardiol* 1991; 18:1–13.
21. Lehman MH, Saksena S for the NASPE Policy Conference Committee. Implantable cardioverter defibrillators in cardiovascular practice: Report of the Policy Conference of the North American Society of Pacing and Electrophysiology. NASPE Policy Conference Committee. *Pacing Clin Electrophysiol* 1991; 14:969–979.
22. Wilber DJ, Garan H, Finkelstein D, Kelly E, Newell J, McGovern B, et al. Out-of-hospital cardiac arrest. Use of electrophysiologic testing in the prediction of long-term outcome. *N Engl J Med* 1988; 318:19–24.
23. Trouton TG, Powell AC, Garan H, Ruskin JN. Risk identification for sudden cardiac death—implications for implantable cardioverter-defibrillator use. *Prog Cardiovasc Dis* 1993; 36(3):195–208.

24. Fananapazir L, Epstein SE. Hemodynamic and electrophysiologic evaluation of patients with hypertrophic cardiomyopathy surviving cardiac arrest. *Am J Cardiol* 1991; 67:280–287.

25. Poll DS, Marchlinsky FE, Buxton AE, Doherty JU, Waxman HL, Josephson ME. Sustained ventricular tachycardia in patients with idiopathic dilated cardiomyopathy: Electrophysiologic testing and lack of response to antiarrhythmic drug therapy. *Circulation* 1984; 70:451–456.

26. Fogoros RN, Fiedler SB, Elson JJ. The automatic implantable cardioverter-defibrillator in drug-refractory ventricular tachyarrhythmias. *Ann Intern Med* 1987; 107:635–641.

27. Mason JW for the Electrophysiologic Study versus Electrocardiographic Monitoring Investigators. Comparison of seven antiarrhythmic drugs in patients with ventricular tachyarrhythmias. *N Engl J Med* 1993; 329:452–458.

28. Wever EF, Hauer RN, Van Capelle FL, Tijssen JG, Crijns HJ, Algra A, et al. Randomised study of implantable defibrillator as first-choice therapy versus conventional strategy in postinfarct sudden death survivors. *Circulation* 1995; 91(8):2195–2203.

29. Herr JM, Sauve MJ, Malone P, Griffin JC, Helmy I, Langberg JJ, et al. Long-term results of amiodarone therapy in patients with recurrent sustained ventricular tachycardia or ventricular fibrillation. *J Am Coll Cardiol* 1989; 13:442–449.

30. The CASCADE Investigators: Randomized antiarrhythmic drug therapy in survivors of cardiac arrest (the CASCADE Study). *Am J Cardiol* 1993; 72:280–287.

31. Fogoros RN, Elson JJ, Bonnet CA, Fiedler SB, Chenarides JG. Long-term outcome of survivors of cardiac arrest whose therapy is guided by electrophysiologic testing. *J Am Coll Cardiol* 1992; 19:780–788.

32. Siebels J, Kuck KH, and The CASH Investigators. Implantable cardioverter defibrillator compared with antiarrhythmic drug treatment in cardiac arrest survivors (the Cardiac Arrest Study Hamburg). *Am Heart J* 1994; 127:1139–1144.

33. Connolly SJ, Gent M, Roberts RS, Dorian P, Green MS, Klein GJ, et al. Canadian implantable defibrillator study (CIDS): Study design and organization. *Am J Cardiol* 1993; 72(F):103–108.

34. The AVID Investigators. Antiarrhythmics versus implantable defibrillators (AVID)—rationale, design, and methods. *Am J Cardiol* 1995; 75:470–475.

35. Moss AJ, Hall WJ, Cannom DS, Daubert JP, Higgins SL, Klein H, et al. Improved survival with an implanted defibrillator in patients with coronary disease at high risk for ventricular arrhythmias. *N Engl J Med* 1996; 335:1933–1940.

36. Brachman J, Freigang K, Saggau W. Coronary artery bypass graft trial. *Pacing Clin Electrophysiol* 1993; 16(II):571–575.

37. The German Dilated Cardiomyopathy Study Investigators. Prospective studies assessing prophylactic therapy in high risk patients: The German Dilated Cardiomyopathy Study (GDCMS)—study design. *Pacing Clin Electrophysiol* 1992; 15(III):697–700.

38. Buxton AE, Fisher JD, Josephson ME, Lee KL, Pryor DB, Prystowsky EN, et al. Prevention of sudden death in patients with coronary artery disease: The Multicenter Unsustained Tachycardia Trial (MUSTT). *Prog Cardiovasc Dis* 1993; 36(3):215–226.

39. Cobb LA, Baum RS, Alvarez H, Schaffer WA. Resuscitation from an out-of-hospital ventricular fibrillation: Four years follow-up. *Circulation* 1975; 52:223–228.

40. Kelly P, Ruskin JN, Vlahakes GJ, Buckley MJ, Freeman CS, Garan H. Surgical coronary revascularisation in survivors of prehospital cardiac arrest: Its effect on inducible ventricular arrhythmias and long-term survival. *J Am Coll Cardiol* 1990; 15:267–273.

41. Dolack GL, Poole JE, Kudenchuk PJ, Raitt MH, Gelva MJ, Anderson J, et al. Management of ventricular fibrillation with transvenous defibrillators without baseline electrophysiologic testing or antiarrhythmic drugs. *J Cardiovasc Electrophysiol* 1996; 7:197–202.

42. Kim YH, Sosa-Suarez G, Trouton TG, O'Nunain SS, Osswald S, McGovern BA, et al. Treatment of ventricular tachycardia by transcatheter radiofrequency ablation in patients with ischemic heart disease. *Circulation* 1994; 89:1094–1102.

43. Bass EB, Elson JJ, Fogoros RN, Peterson J, Arena VC, Kapoor WN. Long-term prognosis of patients undergoing electrophysiologic studies for syncope of unknown origin. *Am J Cardiol* 1988; 62:1186–1191.

44. Eisenberg MS, Hallstrom A, Bergner L. Long-term survival after out-of-hospital cardiac arrest. *N Engl J Med* 1982; 306:1340–1343.

45. Mirowski M, Mower MM, Staewen WS, Denniston RH, Mendelhoff AI. The development of the transvenous automatic defibrillator. *Arch Intern Med* 1972; 129:773–779.

46. Schuder JC, Stoeckle H, Gold JH, West JA, Keskar PY. Experimental ventricular defibrillation with an automatic and completely implanted system. *Trans Am Soc Artif Intern Org* 1970; 16:207–214.

47. Mower MM. In the beginning: From dogs to humans. *Pacing Clin Electrophysiol* 1995; 18(11):506–511.

48. Gold MR, Shorofsky SR. Transvenous defibrillation lead systems. *J Cardiovasc Electrophysiol* 1996; 570–580.

49. Mahomed Yousuf. Surgical techniques for implantation of the implantable cardioverter-defibrillator. In: Zipes DP, Jalife J, eds. *Cardiac Electrophysiology: From Cell to Bedside*, 2d ed. Philadelphia: Saunders; 1995; 1412–1425.

50. Zipes DP, Roberts D. Results of the international study of the implantable pacemaker cardioverter-defibrillator. A comparison of epicardial and endocardial lead systems. The Pacemaker-Cardioverter-Defibrillator Investigators. *Circulation* 1995; 92(1):59–65.

51. Hauser RG, Kurschinski DT, McVeigh K, Thomas A, Mower MM. Clinical results with nonthoracotomy ICD systems. *Pacing Clin Electrophysiol* 1993; 16(pt II):141–148.

52. Raviele A, Gasparini G for the Italian Endotak Investigator Group. Italian multicenter clinical experience with endocardial defibrillation: Acute and long-term results in 307 patients. *Pacing Clin Electrophysiol* 1995; 18(pt II):599–608.

53. Markewitz A, Kaulbach H, Mattke S, Dorwarth U, Weinhold C, Hoffman E, et al. One incision approach for insertion of implantable cardioverter defibrillators. *Ann Thorac Surg* 1994; 58(6):1609–1613.

54. Bardy GH, Johnson G, Poole JE, Dolack GL, Kudenchuk PJ, Kelso D, et al. A simplified, single-lead unipolar transvenous cardioversion-defibrillation system. *Circulation* 1993; 88:543–547.

55. Poole JE, Bardy GH, Kudenchuk PJ, Dolack GL, Raitt MH, Mehra R, et al. Prospective randomised comparison of biphasic waveform tilt using a unipolar defibrillation system. *Pacing Clin Electrophysiol* 1995; 18:1369–1373.

56. Singer I, Lang D. Defibrillation threshold: Clinical utility and therapeutic implications. *Pacing Clin Electrophysiol* 1992; 15(6):932–949.

57. Lang JL, KenKnight BH. Implant support devices. In: Singer I, ed. *Implantable Cardioverter Defibrillator*. New York: Futura; 1994; 223–252.

58. Guarnieri T, Levine JH, Veltri E, Griffith LSC, Watkins L, Juanteguy J, et al. Success of chronic defibrillation and the role of antiarrhythmic drugs with automatic implantable cardioverter/defibrillator. *Am J Cardiol* 1987; 60:1061–1064.

59. Kelly PA, Cannom DS, Garan H, Mirabal GS, Harthorne JW, Hurtivz RJ, et al. The automatic implantable cardioverter-defibrillator. Efficacy, complications, and survival in patients with malignant ventricular arrhythmias. *J Am Coll Cardiol* 1988; 11:1278–1286.

60. Grimm W, Marchlinski FE. Shock occurrence in patients with an implantable cardioverter-defibrillator without spontaneous shocks before first generator replacement for battery depletion. *Am J Cardiol* 1994; 73(13):969–970.

61. Wetherbee JN, Chapman PD, Troup PJ, Veneth-Rogers, Thakur RK, Hossein TG, et al. Long-term internal cardiac defibrillation threshold stability. *Pacing Clin Electrophysiol* 1989; 12:443.

62. Joachim-Trappe H, Klein H, Frank G, Wenzlaff P. Do the defibrillation thresholds of an automatic defibrillator remain acceptable with time? (Abstract). *Pacing Clin Electrophysiol* 1989; 12:664.

63. Vlay SC. Defibrillation testing. Necessary but evil. *Am Heart J* 1989; 117:499–504.

64. Luderitz B, Jung W, Deister A, Manz M. Patient acceptance of implantable cardioverter defibrillator devices: Changing attitudes. *Am Heart J* 1994; 127(2):1179–1184.

65. May CD, Smith PR, Murdock CJ, Davis MJ. The impact of the implantable cardioverter defibrillator on quality-of-life. *Pacing Clin Electrophysiol* 1995; 18:1411–1418.

66. Strickberger SA, Cantillon CO, Friedman PL. When should patients with lethal ventricular arrhythmias resume driving? An analysis of state regulations and physician practices. *Ann Intern Med* 1991; 115:560–563.

67. Drucker EA, Brooks R, Garan H, Sweeney MO, Ruskin JN, McGovern BA, et al. Malfunction of implantable cardioverter defibrillators placed by a nonthoracotomy approach: Frequency of malfunction and value of chest radiography in determining cause. *Am J Roentgenol* 1995; 165(2):275–279.

68. Saksena S, Poczobutt-Johanos M, Castle LW, Fogoros RN, Alpert BL, Kron J, et al, for the Guardian Multicenter Investigators Group. Long-term multicenter experience with a second-generation implantable pacemaker-defibrillator in patients with malignant ventricular tachyarrhythmias. *J Am Coll Cardiol* 1992; 19:490–499.

69. Korte K, Jung W, Spehl S, Wolpert C, Moosdorf R, Manz M, et al. Incidence of ICD lead related complications during long-term follow-up. *Pacing Clin Electrophysiol* 1995; 18:2053–2061.

70. Bardy GH, Yee R, Jung W, for the Active Can Investigators. Multicenter experience with a pectoral unipolar implantable cardioverter-defibrillator. *J Am Coll Cardiol* 1996; 28:400–410.

71. Marchlinski FE, Callans DJ, Gottlieb CD, Schwartzman D, Preminger M. Benefit and lessons learned from stored electrogram information in implantable defibrillators. *J Cardiovasc Electrophysiol* 1995; 6:832–851.

72. Block M, Breithardt G. Long-term follow-up and clinical results of implantable cardioverter-defibrillators. In: Zipes DP, Jalife J, eds. *Cardiac Electrophysiology: From Cell to Bedside,* 2d ed. Philadelphia: Saunders; 1995; 1412–1425.

73. Steinman RT, Thomas AC, Schuger C, Lehmann MH. Clinical findings in monitored cases of sudden cardiac death in patients with an automatic implantable defibrillator (abstract). *Pacing Clin Electrophysiol* 1989; 12:646.

74. Vlay S, Olson LC, Burger L. Internal cardioverter defibrillator component failure. *Pacing Clin Electrophysiol* 1990; 13:1086–1087.

75. Luu M, Stevenson WG, Stevenson LW, Baron K, Walden J. Diverse mechanisms of unexpected cardiac arrest in advanced heart failure. *Circulation* 1989; 80:1675–1680.

76. Kempf FC, Josephson ME. Cardiac arrest recorded on ambulatory electrograms. *Am J Cardiol* 1984; 53:1577–1582.

77. Fogoros RN. The effect of the implantable cardioverter defibrillator on sudden death and on total survival. *Pacing Clin Electrophysiol* 1993; 16(II):506–510.

78. Liberthson RR, Nagel EL, Hirschman JC, Nussenfeld SR. Prehospital ventricular fibrillation: Prognosis and follow-up course. *N Engl J Med* 1974; 291:317–321.

79. Goldberg RJ, Gore JM, Haffajee CI, Alpert JS, Dalen JE. Outcome after cardiac arrest during myocardial infarction. *Am J Cardiol* 1987; 59:251–255.

80. Newman D, Sauve MJ, Herr J, Langberg JJ, Lee MA, Titus C, et al. Survival after implantation of the cardioverter defibrillator. *Am J Cardiol* 1992; 69:899–903.

81. Powell AC, Fuchs T, Finkelstein DM, Garan H, Cannom DS, McGovern BA, et al. Influence of implantable cardioverter-defibrillators on the long-term prognosis of survivors of out-of-hospital cardiac arrest. *Circulation* 1993; 88;1083–1092.

82. Fogoros RN, Elson JJ, Bonnet CA, Fiedler SB, Burkholder JA. Efficacy of the automatic implantable cardioverter-defibrillator in prolonging survival in patients with severe underlying cardiac disease. *J Am Coll Cardiol* 1990; 16:381–386.

83. Levine JH, Mellits ED, Baumgardner RA, Veltri EP, Mower M, Grunwald L, et al. Predictors of first discharge and subsequent survival in patients with automatic implantable cardioverter-defibrillators. *Circulation* 1991; 84:556–558.

84. Bocker D, Block M, Isbruch F, Wietholt D, Hammel D, Borggrefe M, et al. Do patients with implantable defibrillators live longer? *J Am Coll Cardiol* 1993; 21:1638–1644.

85. Mirowski M, Reid PR, Winkle RA, Mower MM, Watkins L, Stinson EB, et al. Mortality in patients with implanted automatic defibrillators. *Ann Intern Med* 1983; 98:585–588.

86. Akhtar M, Avitall B, Jazayeri M, Tchou P, Troup P, Sra J, et al. Role of implantable cardioverter-defibrillator therapy in the management of high risk patients. *Circulation* 1992; 85(suppl I):I,131–I,139.

87. de Marchena E, Chakko S, Fernandez P, Villa A, Cooper D, Wozniak P, et al. Usefulness of the automatic implantable cardioverter defibrillator in improving survival of patients with severely depressed left ventricular function associated with coronary artery disease. *Am J Cardiol* 1991; 67:812–816.

88. Tchou PJ, Kadri N, Anderson J, Caceras JA, Jazayeri M, Akhtar M. Automatic implantable cardioverter defibrillators and survival in patients with left ventricular dysfunction and malignant ventricular arrhythmias. *Ann Intern Med* 1988; 109:529–534.

89. Myerburg RJ, Luceri RM, Thurer R, Copper DK, Zaman L, Interian A, et al. Time to first shock and clinical outcome in patients receiving an automatic implantable cardioverter-defibrillator. *J Am Coll Cardiol* 1989; 14:508–514.

90. Fogoros RN, Elson JJ, Bonnet CA. Survival of patients who have received appropriate shocks from their implantable defibrillators. *Pacing Clin Electrophysiol* 1991; 14:1842–1845.

91. Sweeney MO, Ruskin JN. Mortality benefits and the implantable cardioverter-defibrillator. *Circulation* 1994; 89:1851–1858.

92. Kuppermann M, Luce BR, McGovern B, Podrid PJ, Bigger JT, Ruskin JN. An analysis of the cost effectiveness of the implantable defibrillator. *Circulation* 1990; 81:91–100.

93. Wever EF, Hauer RN, Schrijvers G, van Capelle FJ, Tijssen JG, Crijns HJ, et al. Cost-effectiveness of implantable defibrillators as first-choice therapy versus electrophysiologically guided, tiered strategy in postinfarct sudden death survivors. A randomised study. *Circulation* 1996; 93:489–496.

34

CARDIAC PACEMAKERS

Raul D. Mitrani / Robert J. Myerburg / Agustin Castellanos

The concept of pacemakers for bradycardia originated in the 1950s. Initial units were bulky, required frequent battery changes, and had no programmability. Over the past three decades, cardiac pacing has undergone tremendous growth. The modern pacemaker generator weighs 25 to 35 g, is fully programmable for dual-chamber pacing, provides rate response to activity or metabolic changes, has telemetry of battery function, incorporates algorithms to respond to changes in intrinsic rhythms, and can store a history of the patient's arrhythmic events. The quantity of varied and different features continues to increase. A number of current and comprehensive reviews are available,[1–4] and the reader is referred to these for more detailed discussion of selected topics.

The basic pacemaker system consists of a pulse generator connected to one or two leads attached to the heart. Almost all modern pacemakers use a lithium-iodide battery. Pacing is accomplished by sending current pulses through the lead to a distal electrode (cathode), which initiates depolarization of the myocardium. The electrical circuit is completed by current returning through the anode. In unipolar pacing systems, the anode is incorporated into the pacemaker generator shell, whereas in bipolar systems, the anode consists of a separate electrode proximal to the electrode tip within the same lead.

CODES
FOR CARDIAC PACING

Pacemakers are coded by a specific abbreviation, according to the type of pacemaker and mode of pacing. In common usage, the first three or four letters are used, but a total of five letters has been defined by the North American Society of Pacing and Electrophysiology (NASPE) and the British Pacing and Electrophysiology Group (BPEG)[5] (Table 34-1).

The first three letters refer to the type of pacemaker or pacing mode that is being employed. The first letter refers to

the chamber(s) being paced, and the second letter refers to the chamber(s) being sensed. The letter A indicates atrial pacing or sensing, and V refers to ventricular pacing or sensing. If A and V are both being paced and/or sensed, the designation D, dual-chamber pacing or sensing, is used. The third letter refers to the response to a sensed event, whether it is a normal complex, a premature complex, or a sensing artifact. The pacemaker can either inhibit (I) pacing output from one or both of its leads, or it can trigger (T) pacing at a programmable interval after the sensed event. The detailed description of and indications for different pacing modes will be described.

The fourth letter designation represents either the type of programmability or whether the pacemaker is capable of providing rate-responsive pacing. In common usage, only the rate responsiveness of the pacemaker is noted. For the past several years, most implanted pacemakers in the United States have been fully programmable and capable of telemetry. Therefore, it is rare to note the type of programmability of the pacing unit.

Finally, the fifth letter represents cardiac devices that are capable of treating atrial or ventricular tachyarrhythmias. It is possible to describe implantable defibrillators by the NASPE/ BPEG code, but in clinical practice, this code is rarely used for defibrillators because of the increased complexity inherent in implantable defibrillators. In contrast, there are occasional patients with atrial pacemakers with antitachycardia pacing function, and these pacemakers may be described by the NASPE/BPEG designation.

TEMPORARY
PACING

Temporary pacing is a modality required to provide patients with heart rate support when they experience intermittent or persistent hemodynamically relevant bradyarrhythmias or to provide standby pacing for patients at increased risk for sud-

TABLE 34-1

THE NASPE/BPEG PACEMAKER CODE

Chamber Paced	Chamber Sensed	Response to Sensed Event	Programmability/Rate Response
O (none)	O	O	O
A (atrium)	A	I (inhibit)	R (rate responsive)
V (ventricle)	V	T (triggered)	P (simple programmable)
D (dual)	D	D (I + T)	M (multiprogrammable)
S (single chamber—A or V)	S		C (communicating)

den and complete heart block. Occasionally, temporary pacing is used to control sustained atrial or ventricular tachyarrhythmias. The endpoint for temporary pacing is either resolution of a temporary indication for pacing or implantation of a permanent pacemaker for a continuing indication. Assessment of the risk-benefit ratio is required prior to placing a temporary pacemaker. Furthermore, the clinician must decide whether to insert a temporary transvenous pacemaker or to rely on a noninvasive external unit.[6,7]

Indications

The indications for temporary pacing are listed in Table 34-2. In general, indications for temporary pacing may include patients who are at high risk for developing complete heart block, as is the case in patients with acute myocardial infarction and alternating bundle branch blocks. Other indications for temporary pacing include those indications for permanent pacing when patients are symptomatic and cannot wait for the permanent pacemaker. In general, it would be advisable to place the permanent pacemaker as soon as possible to avoid the separate procedure of a temporary pacemaker.

Temporary pacing is also indicated when a patient has bradycardia causing symptomatic or hemodynamic compromise. Temporary pacing at rates of 80 to 100 beats per minute can be used to prevent bradycardia-dependent ventricular arrhythmias or those associated with a long QT interval and torsades de pointes. Temporary atrial pacing is occasionally used to restore atrioventricular (AV) synchrony in patients with temporary sinus arrest who have intact AV conduction. Toxic drug effects, such as digitalis toxicity, or metabolic abnormalities, such as hyperkalemia, may produce a temporary symptomatic bradycardia requiring temporary pacing.[8] Transient or permanent damage to the AV junction during electrophysiologic studies with radiofrequency ablation may be another indication for temporary pacing.

Lyme disease is a specific cause of carditis that has been associated with various degrees of AV block in some patients.[8-11] In the presence of high-degree or complete AV block (see Chap. 26), the escape rhythm consists of a slow, wide QRS complex or asystole. Temporary cardiac pacing is

necessary in the more advanced cases, but implantation of a permanent pacemaker is generally not necessary for patients with Lyme disease since the AV block almost always resolves.

Prophylactic temporary pacing is often used during cardiac catheterization and occasionally before permanent pacemaker implantation or pacemaker generator change. It is unusual, however, to implant a temporary pacemaker before other surgical procedures in patients who do not otherwise have standard indications for temporary or permanent pacing.

Occasionally, temporary pacing is used for management of tachyarrhythmias for overdrive pacing of atrial or ventricular arrhythmias. The most common clinical setting is generally in the postoperative period after major cardiac surgery, when atrial flutter may be pace-terminated into sinus rhythm.[12]

TABLE 34-2

INDICATIONS FOR TEMPORARY (TRANSVENOUS) PACING

I. Symptomatic sinus nodal dysfunction/bradyarrhythmias
  A. Drug- or electrolyte-induced
II. Symptomatic high- or third-degree AV block
  A. Acquired or congenital heart block with symptoms
  B. Postoperative after cardiac surgery
  C. After radiofrequency ablation of the AV junction
III. Acute myocardial infarction
  A. Class I indications[a]
    1. Third-degree AV block
    2. New bifascicular block with first-degree AV block
    3. Alternating bundle branch block
    4. Symptomatic bradycardia with hypotension from any etiology
    5. Mobitz type II second-degree AV block
  B. Class II indications[a]
    1. New or indeterminate RBBB with LAHB or LPHB or first-degree AV block
    2. New or indeterminate LBBB
    3. Recurrent sinus pauses not responsive to atropine
IV. Prior to pacemaker generator change in patients who are pacemaker-dependent
V. Bradycardia-dependent tachyarrhythmias/long QT syndrome with torsades de pointes

[a] See Table 34-3 for definition of class I or class II indications.
Note: AV = atrioventricular; LAHB = left anterior hemiblock; LBBB = left bundle branch block; LPHB = left posterior hemiblock; RBBB = right bundle branch block.

Acute Myocardial Infarction

The use of temporary pacing in acute myocardial infarction can be accomplished by transcutaneous systems in those patients without active need for pacing and in those patients at low or moderate risk for developing complete heart block. Because transcutaneous systems are uncomfortable during active pacing for prolonged periods of time, transvenous pacing may be placed in patients requiring active pacing or in those patients at increased risk for developing complete heart block[13] (Table 34-2).

Conduction abnormalities in the setting of acute anterior infarction are usually due to infranodal conduction disturbances. This is manifested by bundle branch block, high-grade AV block, or complete AV block. Escape rhythms tend to have a wide QRS complex and are slow, thereby causing hemodynamic symptoms. The presence of severe conduction system disturbances generally indicates extensive damage; therefore, the prognosis for patients with anterior infarction who require temporary pacing is very poor.

In patients with inferior infarction, any conduction disturbance is likely to be proximal to the His bundle. These are manifested on the electrocardiogram (ECG) by narrow QRS complex escape rhythms at rates between 40 and 60 beats per minute, with generally stable hemodynamic courses. Since the extent of damage is less, the prognosis is better. Therefore, in the presence of inferior infarction, there is less of a role for temporary cardiac pacing. It should be limited to those patients with symptoms (angina, hypotension, etc.) associated with the bradycardia or possibly to persistence of rates less than 40 beats per minute.

Although patients with inferior myocardial infarction are less likely to require temporary pacing, the recent guidelines on the use of temporary pacing in patients with acute infarction do not differentiate between anterior and inferior infarction.[13] Temporary pacing is indicated in the presence of high-degree (Mobitz type II second-degree AV block) or complete AV block because of the likelihood that these patients will be hemodynamically unstable with their bradyarrhythmia. Any symptomatic bradycardia with hypotension is also an indication for temporary pacing. Additionally, the presence of new bifascicular block generally places patients at increased risk for complete AV block, especially with associated first-degree AV block; therefore, temporary pacing would be reasonable. Specifically, a new right bundle branch block with right or left axis deviation, new left bundle branch block with first-degree AV block, and alternating bundle branch block place patients at increased risk for complete heart block. It is unclear whether patients with new left bundle branch block with normal PR interval or with new right bundle branch block (with normal axis) require temporary pacing.

Selected patients with right ventricular infarction or other patients who require AV synchrony may require dual-chamber AV pacing. Most patients who need temporary transvenous pacing, however, receive a single ventricular lead because of its ease of use.

Techniques

The techniques and clinical competence required to implant temporary pacemakers have been described elsewhere.[1,14,15] Catheters are generally placed into the right heart by percutaneous sheaths placed into the internal jugular, subclavian, brachial, or femoral vein. If the expected duration for temporary pacing is long, then it is preferable not to use the femoral vein in order to prevent infection. For temporary VVI pacing, the catheter is advanced under fluoroscopic guidance into the right ventricle. If fluoroscopy is not available, the pacing catheter can be advanced into the right ventricle using intracardiac electrograms to position the lead. For atrial pacing leads, it is generally preferable to use a temporary "J" lead and place it into the right atrial appendage in order to obtain maximum lead stability and prevent dislodgment.

Transcutaneous pacing is a common method for noninvasively pacing patients who require a prophylactic temporary pacer or emergent pacing.[6,7,16] For patients at risk for developing complete heart block, it serves as a backup VVI pacemaker. It can be activated quickly in situations in which emergency ventricular pacing is required. The unit incorporates two large pads placed in an anterior and posterior position. The main drawback is the high energy requirements (50 to 100 mA at 20 to 40 ms), which cause skeletal muscle stimulation and pain.

INDICATIONS FOR PERMANENT PACEMAKERS

A complete list of cardiac pacemakers and details for their indications, including some controversies regarding these indications, have been reviewed elsewhere.[3,17-20] Indications for pacemakers can be subdivided into three classifications (Table 34-3). The indications for permanent pacemakers are listed in Table 34-4 according to the most recent recommendations published by a joint task force of the American College of Cardiology and American Heart Association in 1991.[17] These recommendations serve as guidelines, and there are other factors in clinical situations that may affect the decision factor. Many indications for pacemaker implantation are predicated by the presence of symptoms. Many symptoms such as fatigue or subtle symptoms of congestive heart failure,

TABLE 34-3

CLASSIFICATION OF INDICATIONS FOR PACEMAKERS

Class I	Conditions for which there is general agreement that permanent pacemakers should be implanted
Class II	Conditions for which permanent pacemakers are frequently used, but there is divergence of opinion with respect to the necessity of their insertion
Class III	Conditions for which there is general agreement that devices are unnecessary

TABLE 34-4

GUIDELINES FOR IMPLANTATION OF PACEMAKERS

	Class I	Class II	Class III
Acquired AV block	Permanent or intermittent AV block with: Syncope or presyncope Congestive heart failure Mental confusion (that improves with temporary pacing) Symptomatic ventricular ectopy or tachycardia related to the lack of adequate escape rhythm Escape rhythm <40 bpm or documented asystole >3 s Chronotropic incompetence of escape pacemaker associated with symptoms Atrial fibrillation, flutter, or other SVT, with complete or advanced AV block associated with any condition listed above Second-degree AV block, permanent or intermittent, with symptomatic bradycardia Persistent complete or advanced second-degree AV block	Asymptomatic complete AV block with ventricular rate <40 bpm Asymptomatic type II second-degree AV block (permanent or intermittent) Asymptomatic type I second-degree AV block at or below the bundle of His	First-degree AV block Asymptomatic type I second-degree AV block above the level of the bundle of His
After myocardial infarction	Persistent complete or advanced second-degree AV block Transient advanced AV block and associated BBB Symptomatic AV block at any level	Persistent advanced AV block at the AV node level	Transient AV conduction disturbances without intraventricular conduction defects or with isolated left anterior fascicular block Acquired left anterior fascicular block Persistent first-degree AV block in the presence of old or age-indeterminate BBB
Bifascicular or trifascicular block	Bifascicular block with intermittent complete heart block associated with symptoms Bifascicular block with intermittent type II second-degree AV block with symptoms	Bifascicular block with intermittent type II second-degree AV block without symptoms Bifascicular or trifascicular block with syncope not proven to be due to AV block but other causes of syncope not identifiable HV interval >100 ms or pacing-induced infra-His block	Fascicular block without AV block or symptoms Fascicular block with first-degree AV block without symptoms
Sinus node dysfunction	Sinus node dysfunction with documented symptomatic bradycardia (in some patients, this will occur as a result of long-term essential drug therapy of a type and dose for which there is no acceptable alternative)	Sinus node dysfunction, occurring spontaneously or as a result of necessary drug therapy, with heart rates <40 bpm without clear association between significant symptoms and bradycardia	Sinus node dysfunction in asymptomatic patients, including those in whom substantial sinus bradycardia is a consequence of long-term drug treatment Sinus node dysfunction in patients in whom symptoms suggestive of bradycardia are clearly documented not to be associated with a slow heart rate
Hypersensitive carotid sinus and neurovascular syndromes	Recurrent syncope associated with clear, spontaneous events provoked by carotid sinus stimulation; minimal carotid sinus pressure induces asystole of >3 s duration in the absence of any medication that depresses the sinus node or AV conduction	Recurrent syncope without clear, provocative events and with a hypersensitive cardioinhibitory response Syncope with associated bradycardia reproduced by head-up tilt (with or without provocative maneuvers or isoproterenol) in which a temporary pacemaker and second head-up tilt test can establish the likely benefits of a permanent pacemaker	A hyperactive cardioinhibitory response to carotid sinus stimulation in the absence of symptoms Vague symptoms (dizziness or lightheadedness) with a hyperactive cardioinhibitory response to carotid sinus stimulation Recurrent syncope, lightheadedness, or dizziness in the absence of a cardioinhibitory response

Note: BBB = bundle branch block; bpm = beats per minute; HV interval = conduction time from bundle of His to earliest ventricular activation; SVT = supraventricular tachycardia.

however, may be recognized only in retrospect, after placement of a permanent pacemaker.

Specific Causes and Patterns of AV Block

It is generally agreed that complete heart block, permanent or intermittent, at any anatomic level and associated with symptoms such as dizziness, lightheadedness, congestive heart failure, or confusion is a class I indication for a permanent pacemaker. In asymptomatic patients, a ventricular rate <40 beats per minute or pauses >3.0 s are also generally considered indications for pacemaker implantation.

In the setting of an acute myocardial infarction, pacemakers are indicated for high-grade or complete block in the His-Purkinje system. In the setting of inferior infarction, AV block typically occurs at the level of the AV node; it may be due to reversible injury and/or autonomic tone and usually subsides in days to weeks.

In the presence of bifascicular or trifascicular block, intermittent third-degree or type II second-degree AV block usually indicates the need for a permanent pacemaker. When these patients present with syncope, a pacemaker may be required. But an electrophysiology study may be required to rule out other causes of syncope (i.e., ventricular tachycardia), particularly if structural heart disease is present. Additionally, during electrophysiology study, a finding of a markedly prolonged HV interval (> 80 ms),[21] pacing, or drug-induced infra-His block[22] suggests an indication for permanent pacing (see Chapter 29).

In asymptomatic patients with second-degree AV block, type I or type II, cardiac pacing may be required if the level of block is infranodal because the prognosis for complete heart block in patients with infranodal block appears to be the same whether the AV block is type I or type II. Furthermore, with 2:1 AV block, the level of block may be difficult to determine. In the presence of a bundle branch block and 2:1 AV block, the level of block is usually, but not always, infranodal and, therefore, may be a class II indication for cardiac pacing.

In asymptomatic and otherwise healthy patients, the presence of intermittent second-degree type I AV block may be considered a manifestation of enhanced vagal tone.[20,23,24] In asymptomatic elderly patients with type I second-degree AV block and structural heart disease, however, there is some divergence of opinion as to whether permanent pacing should[20,25,26] or should not[17,24] be considered. Many patients may become symptomatic during clinical follow-up.[20,27] Electrophysiologic testing to determine the level of block may be helpful.

Classically, first-degree AV block has not been considered an indication for permanent pacing (class III).[17] Recent studies, however, have reported a benefit of DDD pacing in symptomatic patients with first-degree AV block.[19,28] With marked PR interval prolongation, atrial systole occurs after ventricular systole, which may produce symptoms such as the pacemaker syndrome (see below). Additionally, because there is not an appropriately timed ventricular systole occurring at the end of atrial systole, end-diastolic mitral regurgitation develops, which may be of clinical significance in patients with left ventricular systolic dysfunction.[19,29] For this reason, dual-chamber pacing may play a role in selected patients with decreased systolic function and prolonged PR interval by optimizing the AV interval and improving hemodynamics.[29,30] Long-term studies have not been performed, however.

Congenital AV Block

The site of AV block in congenital heart block is usually at the level of the AV node. Patients typically have narrow QRS complex rhythms and tend to be asymptomatic, but congenital AV block is associated with serious and possibly fatal complications, including syncope and sudden death.[31-35] In one study,[33] a mean daytime heart rate <50 beats per minute was associated with sudden death or need for pacemaker. Exercise testing is useful to assess heart rate response at rest and exercise.[33] Other indicators of poor outcome include prolonged QT interval (corrected for heart rate), cardiomegaly, atrial enlargement, and decreased left ventricular systolic function.

Cardiac pacing is thus indicated in all symptomatic patients with congenital AV block. In asymptomatic patients with congenital AV block, the indications for pacing are summarized in Table 34-5. These indications are consistent with either an insufficient junctional escape rate to meet the patient's hemodynamic and metabolic needs, an unstable junctional escape rhythm, possible proarrhythmia resulting from persistent bradyarrhythmia, or coexistence of other congenital cardiac defects.

Sinus Nodal Dysfunction

Sinus nodal dysfunction has become the most common indication for pacing in the United States. The guidelines (Table 34-4) stress the importance of correlating symptoms with bradyarrhythmias. Often, it is difficult to correlate ECG findings with symptoms. Furthermore, symptoms may be nebulous. For instance, the presence of fatigue and dyspnea may be due to a bradyarrhythmia but may also be due to lack of conditioning or other cardiac dysfunction.

TABLE 34-5

INDICATIONS FOR PERMANENT PACING IN PATIENTS WITH ASYMPTOMATIC CONGENITAL AV BLOCK

Mean daytime heart rate less than 50 beats per minute
Chronotropic incompetence on exercise
Sudden prolongation of RR interval during sleep consistent with high AV block
Cardiomegaly or decreased left ventricular systolic function
Atrial chamber enlargement
Prolonged QT interval (corrected for heart rate) or ventricular ectopy

The presence of the tachycardia/bradycardia syndrome is especially common in patients with paroxysmal atrial arrhythmias. The bradyarrhythmia often occurs at the termination of tachycardia (Fig. 34-1) and can lead to pauses of several seconds. Drugs used to suppress such tachyarrhythmias may lead to symptomatic bradycardia, in which case a bradycardia pacemaker would be required.

Patients with asymptomatic bradyarrhythmias should be evaluated carefully prior to placing a pacemaker. Athletes commonly have physiologic bradycardia, even with heart rates <40 beats per minute, due to enhanced vagal tone. Asymptomatic bradyarrhythmias, particularly nocturnal, may be a marker of sleep apnea in patients without obvious signs and symptoms of sleep apnea.[36]

Carotid Sinus Syndrome

The diagnosis of carotid sinus syndrome (CSS) is typically made by demonstrating asystolic pauses of >3 s with carotid sinus massage or a vasodepressor response of >50 mmHg associated with clear symptoms provoked by carotid sinus stimulation, such as wearing a tight shirt or turning one's head. Vague symptoms such as dizziness associated with a hyperactive cardioinhibitory response to carotid sinus stimulation are generally not an indication for permanent pacing.

Improvement of symptoms and suppression of syncope have been demonstrated by treating patients with cardiac pacing,[37–41] particularly dual-chamber pacing.[41–43] Single-chamber atrial pacing is contraindicated because of the increased risk of transient AV block. Some studies suggest that hemodynamic evaluation of patients may enable them to be stratified into groups to select those for whom VVI pacing would be sufficient. VVI pacing has been effective in selected patients with predominantly cardioinhibitory CSS if there is no evidence of hypotension induced by ventricular pacing. However, DDD pacing is probably better in patients with CSS associated with vasodepressor as well as cardioinhibitory components.

Neurocardiogenic Syncope

Patients with neurocardiogenic syncope tend to be younger than patients with CSS. Furthermore, neurocardiogenic syncope is often associated with peripheral vasodilatation, and medication is generally effective for prevention of the reflex that causes the vagal efferent responses. Cardiac pacing has been shown to prevent the bradycardia and AV block associated with neurocardiogenic syncope, but patients still typically experience hypotension, vasodilatation, and other associated symptoms.[44] For these reasons, cardiac pacing plays little role for most patients with neurocardiogenic syncope.[45,46] Other studies, however, suggest that even though pacemakers do not prevent the vasovagal reflexes associated with neurocardiogenic syncope, pacing may prevent syncope and convert a vasovagal episode to an episode of dizziness and presyncope.[47,48]

Hypertrophic Cardiomyopathy

In patients with hypertrophic cardiomyopathy (HCM) and left ventricular outflow tract (LVOT) gradients, traditional therapies have included beta-adrenergic blockers, calcium channel blockers, left ventricular septal myectomy, or mitral valve replacement (see Chaps. 69 and 74). Recent studies have shown that DDD pacing with a programmed short AV interval reduces LVOT gradients and improves symptoms in patients with obstructive HCM.[49–54] With ventricular pacing at short AV interval, the right ventricular apex is preexcited by the pacemaker, causing altered left ventricular depolarization and paradoxical septal motion. This causes the septum to move away from the posterior left ventricular wall in systole, thereby widening the LVOT during systole. The gradient is reduced, and less contractility is required to maintain cardiac output. The reduction in LVOT gradient in patients with chronic pacemakers is maintained in sinus rhythm even if the pacemaker is inactivated[51,53]; this suggests that the reduction of the LVOT gradient reduces stimuli for maintenance of the hypertrophic left ventricle. Furthermore, there is evidence that the benefit of DDD pacing is maintained over the long term.[54]

With dual-chamber pacing and short AV interval, the left

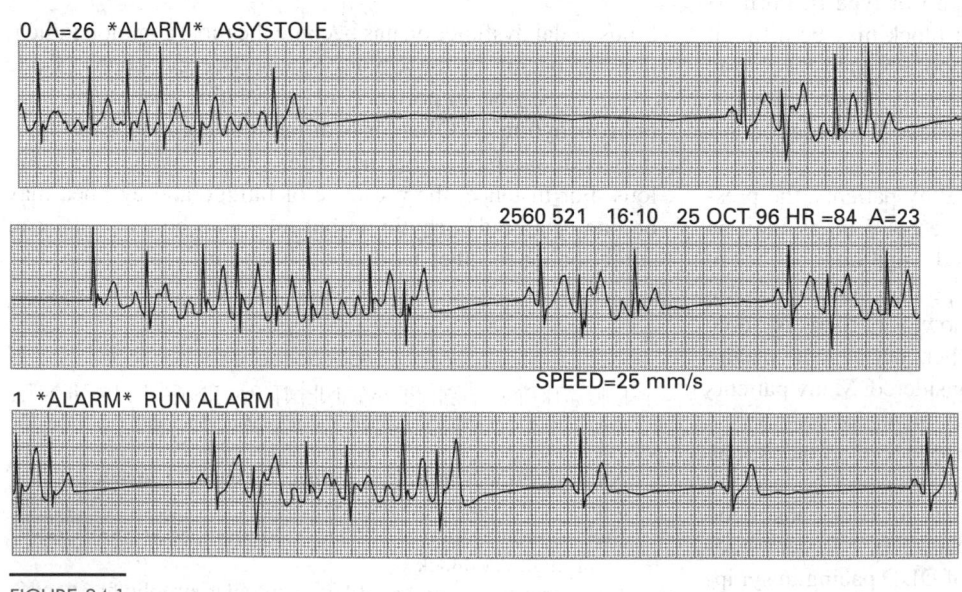

0 A=26 *ALARM* ASYSTOLE

2560 521 16:10 25 OCT 96 HR =84 A=23

SPEED=25 mm/s

1 *ALARM* RUN ALARM

FIGURE 34-1

This is a continuous electrocardiographic tracing from a patient with sick sinus syndrome who complained of palpitations and near-syncope. The patient was mostly symptomatic from the pauses following abrupt termination of his atrial fibrillation. Note the frequent abrupt terminations, followed by pauses up to 6 s before resumption of atrial fibrillation.

ventricular apex empties early in systole before septal contraction, which may also play a role in the favorable hemodynamic response. However, acute hemodynamic measurements during pacing with very short AV intervals have demonstrated a decrease in cardiac output, increase in left atrial pressure, and a prolongation of relaxation indices[55] consistent with a deterioration of diastolic function. Therefore, the AV interval should be programmed to the longest interval that still allows for left ventricular preexcitation, which would decrease but not eliminate the deleterious effects of pacing with short AV intervals.[55] Occasionally, radiofrequency ablation of the AV node may be required to allow for ventricular preexcitation of the left ventricle.[54]

Patients with preexisting left bundle branch block also have altered left ventricular depolarization. Patients with drug-refractory, symptomatic obstructive HCM who have preexisting left bundle branch block, however, still derive relief of symptoms and reduction in LVOT gradient when a DDD pacemaker is placed.[54–56]

In contrast to obstructive HCM, patients with nonobstructive symptomatic HCM experience limited symptomatic improvement and no objective evidence of hemodynamic benefit with DDD pacing and short AV interval.[57] These patients frequently require reinstitution of medical therapy. Therefore, permanent cardiac pacing cannot be recommended for patients with symptomatic nonobstructive HCM.

Dilated Cardiomyopathy

There were some initial reports indicating that dual-chamber pacemakers programmed with a short AV interval might be beneficial to patients with dilated cardiomyopathy and heart failure who did not have any other indications for cardiac pacing,[29,58,59] and that the patients with first-degree AV block derived the most hemodynamic benefit. However, as opposed to earlier reports, which were not randomized, a double-blind randomized study in 12 patients with chronic congestive heart failure showed no hemodynamic or clinical benefit from dual-chamber pacing.[60] Therefore, the use of dual-chamber pacemakers in patients with chronic congestive heart failure cannot be routinely recommended but may occasionally be beneficial to patients with first-degree heart block.[29]

PACEMAKER HARDWARE AND METHODS OF IMPLANT

Pacemaker implant was initially a major surgical procedure requiring thoracotomy and was performed in the operating suite. Currently, nearly all pacemakers are implanted through a transvenous approach, and the implants are performed by either cardiologists or surgeons. The choice of using an operating room or a catheterization laboratory for the implant procedure probably plays little role in procedural-related complications,[61,62] but a cardiac catheterization laboratory involves lower hospital costs.[62]

A full description of the surgery has been reviewed elsewhere.[1,63] Venous access for lead placement generally is through a subclavian venipuncture or a cephalic vein cutdown. The use of subclavian venipuncture is technically easier, and this vein can almost always accommodate two leads. With the subclavian venipuncture, there exists the risk of puncturing the subclavian artery or the apex of the lung, causing a pneumothorax. Furthermore, if pacing leads are placed medially, there is the additional long-term risk of lead insulation breaks or fractures (Fig. 34-2) because the leads may be gradually "crushed" by the clavicle and first rib. Lateral puncture of the subclavian or axillary vein may be associated with increased risk of pneumothorax. Using intravenous contrast in the ipsilateral arm during venipuncture, however, may allow for safe lateral subclavian venous puncture.[64]

Cephalic venous cutdown requires more expertise and avoids the risk of pneumothorax.[65] It is believed that there is less risk for the crush syndrome with long-term placement of leads, but it is not always possible to perform a cephalic vein cutdown. With the use of bipolar leads, it is less likely that two leads can be introduced into this vein; therefore, at least one subclavian venous puncture is usually required.

Hardware

The pulse generator generally weighs between 25 and 40 g. Selection is based upon the physical requirements of the patient in addition to the pacing modes required, special pacing features needed, and battery capacity. It would be unusual for one pacemaker generator model to be the optimal and most cost-effective model for all patients. An algorithm for choosing a pacemaker system and pacing mode is presented in Fig. 34-3.

Pacemaker leads can be unipolar or bipolar (Figs. 34-4 and 34-5). Unipolar leads use a distal electrode in the catheter as the cathode and the shell of the pacemaker generator as the anode. Therefore, the myocardium and adjacent tissue complete the circuit. A bipolar lead consists of two separate conductors and electrodes within the lead. Since the electrodes for sensing in a bipolar lead are much closer together, bipolar signals are sharper, with less extraneous noise (Fig. 34-6).

Unipolar leads are simpler to design, smaller in diameter, and, because of their simplicity, less likely to fracture or develop insulation problems. Because of their small size, it is easier to pass two unipolar leads through a cephalic venous approach. There are, however, several disadvantages to unipolar lead systems. Because the unipolar lead uses body tissue to complete the circuit, there is the possibility of causing muscle stimulation. Most pacemakers avoid this by placing the stimulating surface of the pacemaker anterior so that it interfaces with subcutaneous tissue and not the pectoralis muscle. Unipolar sensing is far more likely to pick up extracardiac signals, including myopotentials (Fig. 34-6), far-field sensing of remote cardiac potentials (far-field sensing), and electromagnetic interference. Finally, unipolar pacing is generally contraindicated in patients who have a concomitant implantable defibrillator. Therefore, most leads implanted today are bipolar.

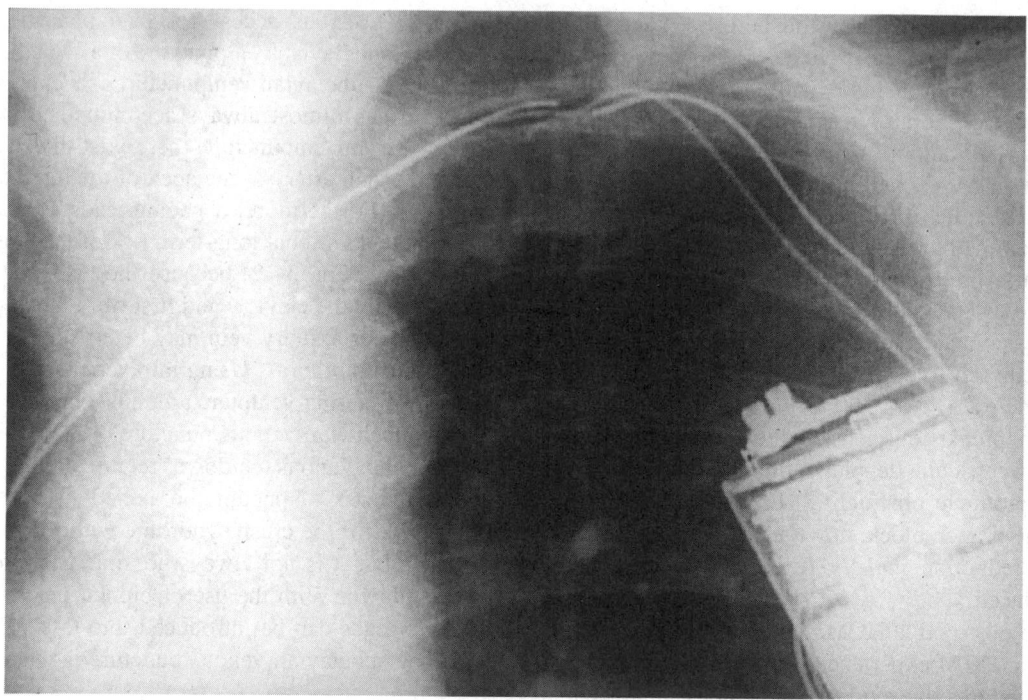

FIGURE 34-2
Close-up of a chest x-ray of a patient with a dual-chamber pacemaker. Note complete fracture of both leads at the costoclavicular junction, causing complete pacemaker malfunction.

Leads are attached to the heart by active or passive fixation. Active fixation involves the use of some type of exposed or retractable screw within the lead system that fixes the lead to the heart (Fig. 34-5). Passive fixation involves the use of tines, which are short protuberances that extend proximal to the distal electrode and interact with myocardial tissue to hold the lead in place. The use of either type of lead system depends on the preference of the implanting physician. Active fixation leads are used more in the atrium and allow fixation of the leads almost anywhere within the right atrium or ventricle.

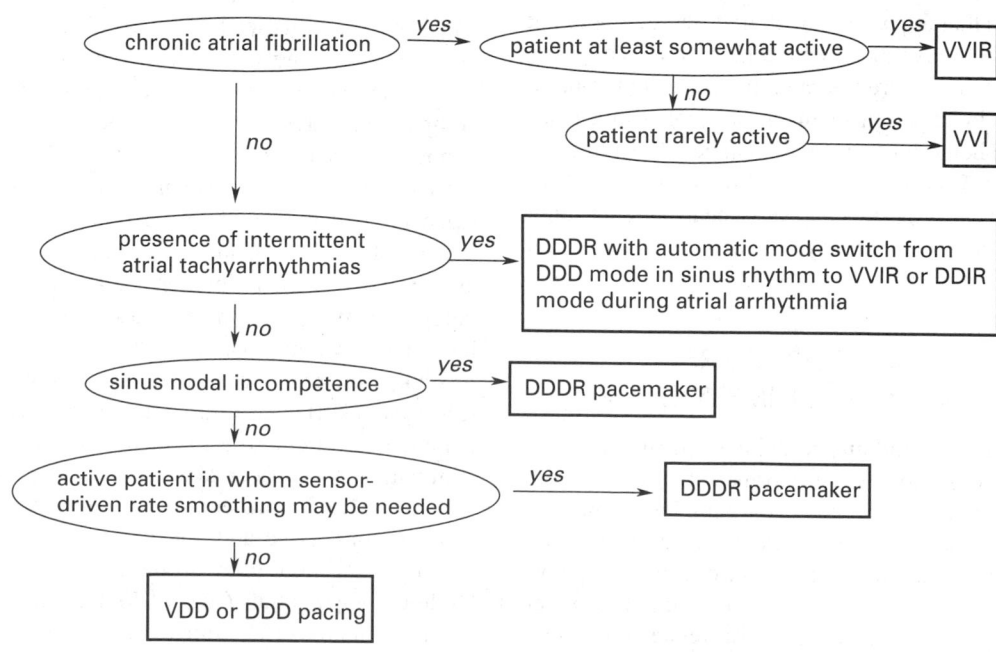

FIGURE 34-3
An algorithm for choosing a pacemaker model and pacemaker mode in patients with intermittent or fixed AV block. See text for details.

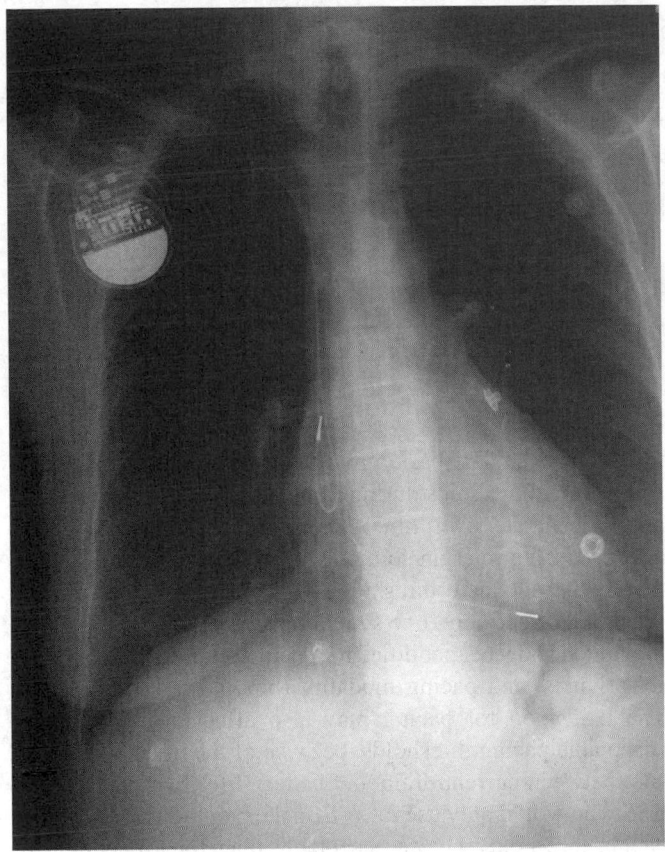

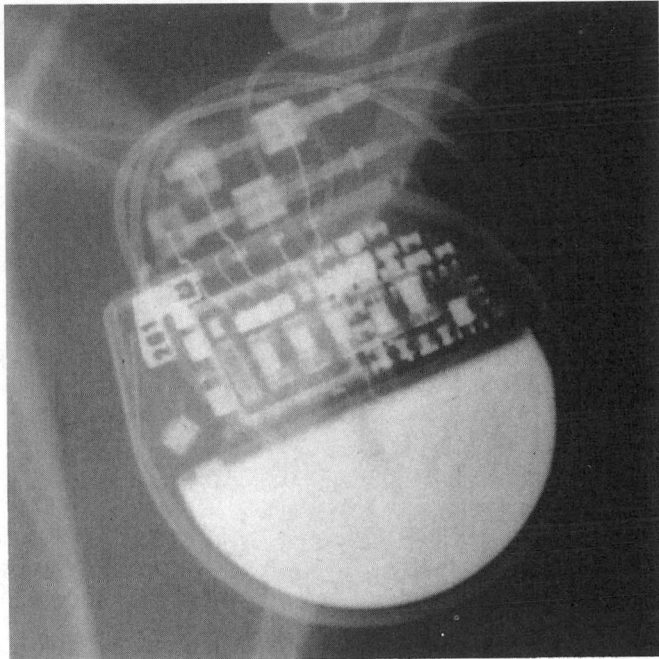

B

A

FIGURE 34-4

A. Chest x-ray of a patient with a dual-chamber unipolar pacemaker. The leads are placed in the right atrial appendage and in the right ventricular apex, respectively. Note only one electrode at the distal tip of each lead. *B.* Close inspection of the pacemaker generator shows that the ventricular lead has pulled out of the header with very minimal contact between the ventricular electrodes and the metal contacts in the pacemaker header. This caused intermittent failure to sense and pace in this patient.

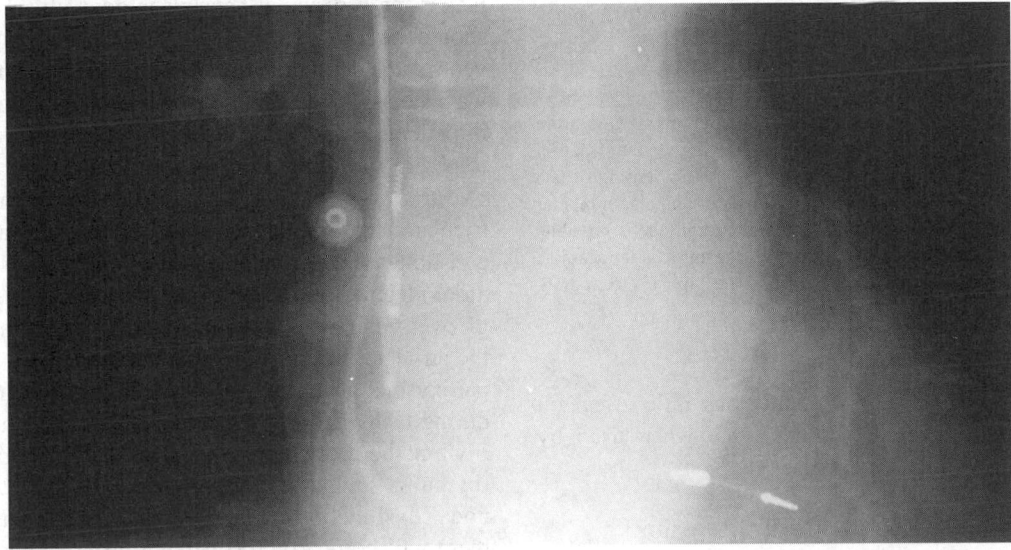

FIGURE 34-5

Chest x-ray from a patient with a bipolar dual-chamber pacing system. The atrial lead is attached to the right atrial appendage by active fixation (screw-in lead), and the screw is visible on the chest x-ray. The ventricular lead is attached to the ventricle by passive fixation.

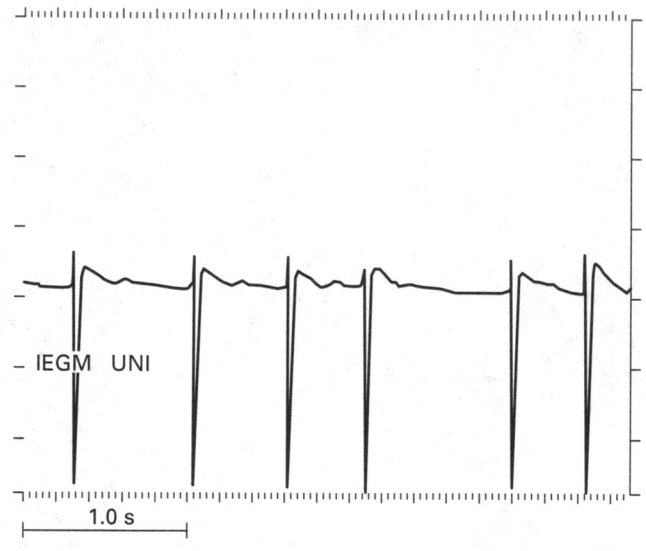

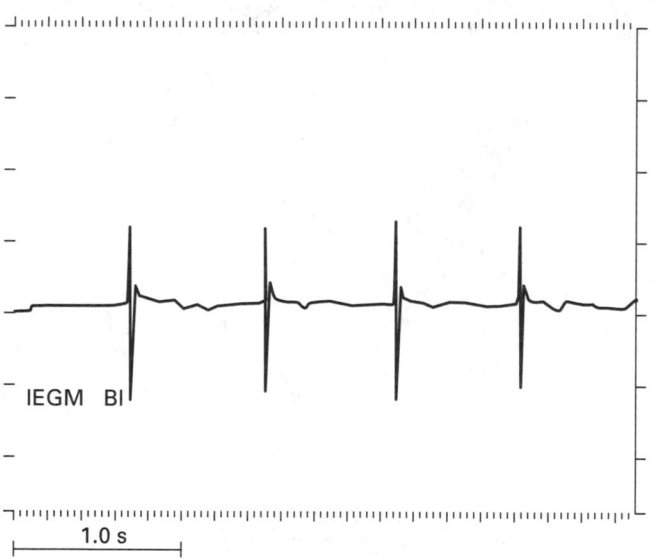

FIGURE 34-6

Unipolar (*top*) and bipolar (*bottom*) intracardiac electrograms (IEGM) from a patient with a ventricular pacemaker whose underlying rhythm is atrial fibrillation. Note that the bipolar signal is sharper, with less sensing of far-field ventricular electrical activity or T waves. With either unipolar or bipolar electrograms, direct measurement of the electrogram amplitude is possible. Each division on the left represents 1 mV. Therefore, the unipolar intracardiac electrogram is 2 to 3 mV from baseline to peak. The bipolar electrogram would be expected to be approximately 2 mV.

The use of either type of lead probably has little effect on complication rate or lead dislodgment rate when used by experienced operators.

Lead Placement and Acute Threshold Testing

Atrial and ventricular leads are placed into the appropriate chambers after ensuring adequate pacing and sensing thresholds (Table 34-6). Most pacemaker units are capable of pacing

TABLE 34-6

ACCEPTABLE PACING AND SENSING THRESHOLDS DURING IMPLANT

	Atrial	Ventricular
Pacing threshold at 0.5 ms	<1.2 V	<1.0 V
Sensing threshold (bipolar)	>1.5–2 mV	>5 mV
Sensing threshold (unipolar)	>2–2.5 V	>5 mV
Impedance[a]	300–1400 Ω	300–1400 Ω

[a] New high-impedance leads result in less current drain and improved longevity.

to at least 5 V. The basic premise in obtaining acute pacing and sensing thresholds during implant is that these thresholds may degenerate over time. Therefore, there should be an adequate safety margin so that even if thresholds degenerate, there exist adequate thresholds to perform safe pacing and sensing. Furthermore, one should be aware of the type of unit implanted and its capabilities for pacing outputs, programmed sensitivities, and pacing modality (bipolar versus unipolar). The indication for pacing may also affect decisions about acceptable pacing thresholds, because of the inverse relationship between current drain and battery life. In a patient with CSS who would only use the pacemaker sporadically, a higher pacing threshold may be acceptable than for a patient with complete heart block in whom it is expected that there will be 100 percent ventricular pacing. Therefore, ventricular pacing threshold should be less than 1 V at 0.5 ms; however, in patients who are pacemaker-dependent, the best threshold should be obtained.

For sensing functions, ventricular electrograms should measure at least 5 mV and frequently measure in excess of 10 to 20 mV. Since the programmed sensitivity of the pacemaker for ventricular sensing is generally 2 to 3 mV, there should be an adequate safety margin for sensing intrinsic ventricular depolarization without the risk of oversensing T waves or other artifacts. During implantation of pacemakers in patients with complete heart block, it may not be possible to obtain the ventricular sensing threshold.

Atrial electrograms are generally much smaller than ventricular electrograms, and many factors play a role as to what constitutes acceptable thresholds. In unipolar systems, a larger atrial electrogram is important because of the increased risk of oversensing myopotentials or other artifactual signals if the atrial sensitivity is programmed too low. In patients with paroxysmal atrial fibrillation or flutter, the atrial electrogram during tachycardia might be much smaller than during sinus rhythm; therefore, the maximal atrial electrogram during sinus rhythm is sought. Conversely, in patients with marked sinus nodal dysfunction or bradycardia, where it is expected that there will be nearly 100 percent atrial pacing, atrial sensing thresholds may not be as important.

Atrial pacing thresholds should also be related to the expected need for atrial pacing. Although ideal thresholds may be less than 1 V, it is reasonable to accept higher pacing thresholds in patients with AV block and preserved sinus nodal function in whom it is more important to obtain adequate atrial sensing thresholds.

Many extraneous factors may affect atrial or ventricular pacing and sensing thresholds. There is some variation to these thresholds, depending on the autonomic tone or the electrolyte status. There is an expected rise in acute thresholds within 1 to 4 weeks following implant due to acute inflammation, and this rise appears to be more exaggerated with active fixation lead systems. Many drugs, particularly antiarrhythmic medications, may affect pacing thresholds. The presence of new myocardial infarction around the leads would be expected to lead to deterioration of pacing and/or sensing thresholds. Some leads that are steroid-eluting generally limit the acute rise in pacing threshold. Long-term lead thresholds appear to stabilize some time after 3 to 6 months.[66]

PACEMAKER FOLLOW-UP

The goal for pacemaker follow-up should be to perform a systematic long-term evaluation of the pacemaker as it relates to and functions with the patient and his or her individual needs. These goals are outlined in Table 34-7. Complete guidelines for pacemaker follow-up have been described.[67]

It is desirable to perform a direct evaluation to check pacemaker and lead function and to optimize pacemaker programming at least once per year. With the increasing sophistication of pacemakers, more visits may be required to optimize features such as rate responsiveness or other special features as described below. In patients with dual-chamber pacemakers and patients with single-chamber pacemakers who are pacemaker-dependent, more frequent direct evaluations may be warranted. Similarly, in patients with pacemaker generators or leads that are under alert, more intensive follow-up may be needed.

In most pacers, there is a stable period of pacer function starting 6 to 12 months following implant until the expected time for battery depletion. In patients with single-chamber pacers with hardware that is not under alert and in whom reprogramming may not be expected or needed, follow-up periods may be prolonged up to 1-year intervals or longer, providing the patients can easily be seen when problems present.[68]

Transtelephonic Monitoring

Technology is available for simple devices to be used by patients to transmit their ECG by telephone to a receiving station so that their ECG rhythm may be analyzed to detect normal or abnormal pacemaker function.[67,69] In this way, a spontaneous pacing rhythm can be assessed for normal or abnormal pacing function. More importantly, by applying a magnet to the pacemaker and observing the "magnet rate" during the transtelephonic monitoring (TTM), evaluation of adequate battery function is possible. During TTM, changes in pacing rate or loss of output can always be detected. Ventricular oversensing or atrial pace/sense problems can sometimes be detected during TTM.[67]

Follow-up using TTM should probably be individualized according to the type of pacemaker, whether the patient is pacemaker-dependent, the age of the pulse generator and its expected longevity, the presence of any pacemaker component under advisory or warning, and patient clinical factors. As stated above, during the expected stable period it is reasonable to have only intermittent TTM follow-ups. Finally, TTM should not replace periodic direct evaluation of pacer function because of the very limited capabilities of TTM to provide detailed information. The maximal allowable TTM follow-up schedule using Medicare guidelines is presented in Table 34-8.

Components for Direct Evaluation of Pacemaker Systems

CHECKING PACING THRESHOLDS AND PROGRAMMING PACING OUTPUTS

Pacemakers should always be programmed for maximal safety, particularly in patients who are pacemaker-dependent. In order to understand how to program pacemakers safely and efficiently, some basic principles will be reviewed.

Current Drain

Ultimately, the longevity of the battery will be a function of the current drain versus battery capacity. There is nominal current drain for running pacemaker circuitry and sensing intracardiac electrograms; however, most current drain is a result of pacing output. The current delivered per pacing pulse is a function of the voltage divided by the lead impedance ($I = V/R$; Ohm's law). Therefore, it is desirable to be able to implant leads with low pacing voltage thresholds and high impedance. Many manufacturers now offer "high impedance" pacing leads in order to prolong the longevity of pacemakers.

TABLE 34-7

GOALS OF PACEMAKER FOLLOW-UP

Monitor pacemaker generator and lead function

Maximize longevity of generator by programming suitable pacing outputs

Optimize pacing parameters to meet patient needs during rest and exercise

Minimize problems and pacemaker-related complications by adequate programming of parameters

Anticipate need for pacemaker generator replacement

Educate the patient

Maintain accurate patient address and telephone number to contact patient as device or lead advisories occur

Maintain adequate and separate pacemaker charts

Source: Adapted from Bernstein et al.,[67] with permission.

TABLE 34-8

1994 MEDICARE GUIDELINES FOR CARDIAC PACEMAKER FOLLOW-UP USING TRANSTELEPHONIC MONITORING (TTM)

Pacemaker Type	Months after Implant	Scheduled Frequency of TTM, Weeks
Newer pacer with increased longevity[a]		
Single chamber	<1	2
	2–48	12
	49–72	8
	>73	4
Dual chamber	<1	2
	2–30	12
	31–48	8
	>49	4
Older pacer with decreased longevity[a]		
Single chamber	<1	2
	2–36	8
	>37	4
Dual chamber	<1	2
	2–6	4
	7–36	8
	>37	4

[a] Newer pacers or those with increased longevity include those that demonstrate better than 90% longevity at 5 years, whose output voltage decreases <50% over at least 3 months, and whose magnet mode (asynchronous) rate decreases <20% or 5 pulses per minute over the same period.
Source: Adapted from Bernstein et al.,[67] with permission.

The Strength-Duration Curve (Fig. 34-7)

The strength-duration curve relates voltage and pulse width. This curve is dynamic during the first 2 to 3 months following implant. With an acute rise in threshold, the curve is expected to shift upwards by two to four times and then subsequently shift back downwards to a level greater than the initially obtained values. At pulse widths less than 0.2 ms, the curve is steep; at pulse widths exceeding 1.0 ms, the curve is flat. With this kind of relationship, programming pulse widths greater than 1 ms generally does not add a safety margin to the pacing output but does increase battery current drain substantially. Similarly, programming pacing pulse widths less than 0.2 ms may not allow a sufficient safety margin at even high-voltage amplitudes.

Energy Expenditure

The total energy expenditure of the pacemaker is defined as follows: Energy equals the square of the voltage times the pulse width divided by the impedance:

$$\left(E = \frac{V^2 \cdot \text{pulse width}}{\text{impedance}} \right)$$

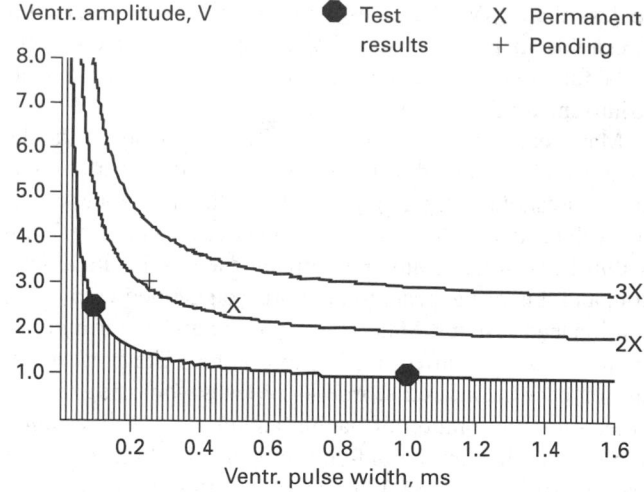

FIGURE 34-7

A sample of a strength-duration curve. The voltage threshold at 2.5 V was 0.1 ms, and the pulse width threshold at 1.0 ms was 1.0 V. Sample curves are shown providing for two and three times the safety margin for programming voltage and pulse width. Ventr. = ventricular.

According to this relationship, energy expenditure is more dependent on voltage output than on pulse width. Therefore, it is preferable to reduce voltage output rather than pulse width to conserve battery life.

Pacing Threshold

At implant, it is standard to fix the pulse width at 0.5 ms and to reduce the voltage to the lowest setting that maintains consistent pacing—which is the pacing threshold (Fig. 34-8). One can fix the pulse width at any value, however (usually between 0.3 and 1.0 ms), and calculate a voltage threshold. Similarly, one can fix the voltage at a certain value and reduce the pulse width to the lowest value that maintains consistent pacing, which would also define the pacing threshold. Either method is acceptable to define a pacing threshold during long-term follow-up.

Safety Margin

The safety margin for pacing outputs can be calculated by multiples of either the pulse width or voltage threshold. For example, if the threshold at 0.5 ms is 1.5 V, then a pacing output of 0.5 ms and 3.0 V would yield an energy safety margin of fourfold, given the relationship between energy and voltage. Similarly, if the pulse width threshold at 3.0 V is 0.15 ms, then a pacing output of 3.0 V and 0.6 ms would provide a fourfold energy safety margin.

Acute Pacing Outputs

Because the extent of the acute rise in pacing thresholds may be difficult to predict, it is better to program high pacing outputs (i.e., 5.0 V/0.5 ms) at implant and during the first 6 to 24 weeks after implant. Usually, a pacemaker is initially programmed with at least a four- to sixfold safety margin in

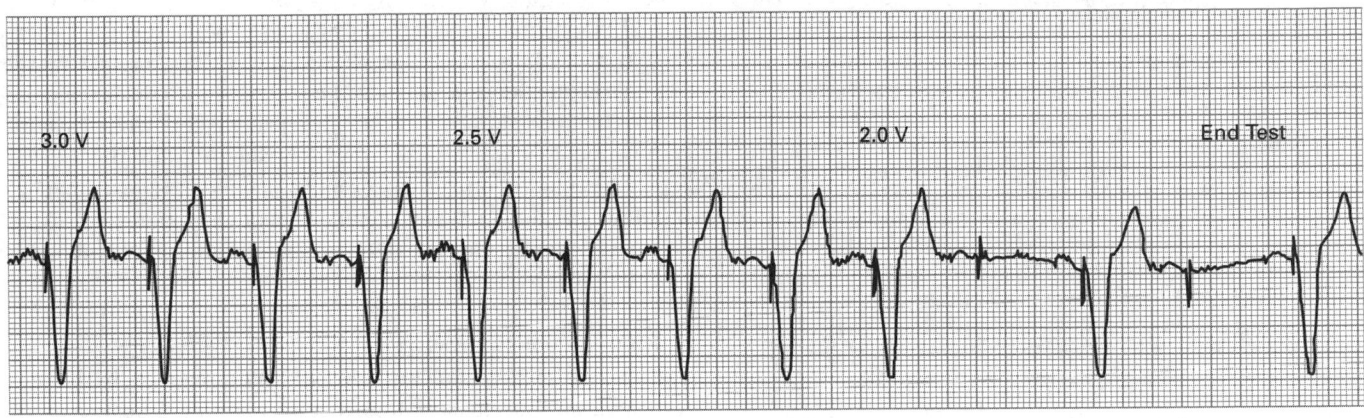

FIGURE 34-8

Ventricular pacing threshold in a patient can be calculated by holding the pulse width constant and automatically decreasing the voltage in 0.5-V decrements every four complexes. As shown, ventricular pacing was maintained at

2.5 V but was inconsistent at 2.0 V. Therefore, the voltage threshold in this patient was 2.5 V at 0.5 ms.

pacing outputs. A greater safety margin may be desired in patients who are pacemaker-dependent. Typically, greater safety margins are also desired in ventricular leads than in atrial leads. Steroid-eluting leads generally result in blunting of the acute rise in threshold,[70–73] which may allow for lower pacing outputs early after implant.

Chronic Pacing Outputs

In the time frame of 2 to 6 months, the pacing thresholds tend to stabilize. There may still be variability in pacing thresholds due to electrolyte shifts, hyperkalemia, ischemia, infarction, changes in autonomic tone, and various drugs. Therefore, at that point, chronic pacing outputs may be programmed (Table 34-9). There are other factors to consider. For patients in whom a pacemaker serves as a backup unit and will likely pace only rarely (i.e., pacing for CSS), the outputs may be programmed higher than recommended because longevity will not be greatly affected by pacing.

Almost all pacing batteries consist of lithium-iodine systems, which generate 2.8 V. It is most efficient to pace at the voltage of the battery (2.5 to 2.8 V). Therefore, the longevity

of pacemakers can be improved if pacing outputs are reduced to 2.5 V with pulse widths programmed two to four times the pulse width thresholds.

OTHER FEATURES

Sensing

Evaluation of sensing of atrial and ventricular intracardiac electrograms can be performed by different algorithms. In order to test atrial sensing, the pacemaker needs to be programmed temporarily at a programmed atrial rate less than the intrinsic sinus rate. In order to test ventricular sensing, there are various options, depending on whether there is intact AV conduction and whether the pacemaker unit is single or dual chamber. In patients with intact AV conduction, ventricular sensing can be assessed in the VVI mode if the programmed ventricular rate is less than the intrinsic heart rate. Alternatively, with intact AV conduction, the AV delay can be increased to allow AV conduction and thereby allow for ventricular sensing in the DDD mode. Sensing can be performed by increasing the programmed sensitivity until the intrinsic P or R wave is no longer sensed (Fig. 34-9). Alternatively, in some units, telemetry of atrial or ventricular electrograms allows for direct measurement of the electrogram amplitude (Fig. 34-6). Lastly, in some pacemakers, there are automated sensing algorithms whereby atrial or ventricular electrograms are automatically measured by the pacemaker.

Lead Function

Lead function is assessed by checking pacing and sensing function. Additionally, telemetry of the lead impedances provides additional information on lead integrity. Although there is wide variability of normal lead impedances, chronic lead impedances should not vary widely between outpatient follow-up visits. A lead with a fractured conductor may exhibit a markedly elevated lead impedance. Insulation breaks manifest by reduced lead impedances. Lead fractures or insulation

TABLE 34-9

RECOMMENDATIONS FOR PACING OUTPUTS

	Atrial Leads	Ventricular Leads
Pacemaker dependent	2–3 times PW threshold	4 times PW threshold
	1.5–1.8 times V threshold	2 times V threshold
Not pacemaker dependent	2 times PW threshold	2–3 times PW threshold
	1.5 times V threshold	1.5–1.8 times V threshold

Note: PW = pulse width; V = voltage.

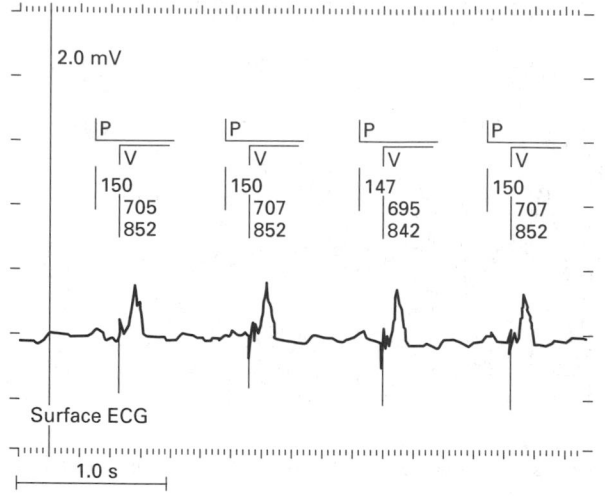

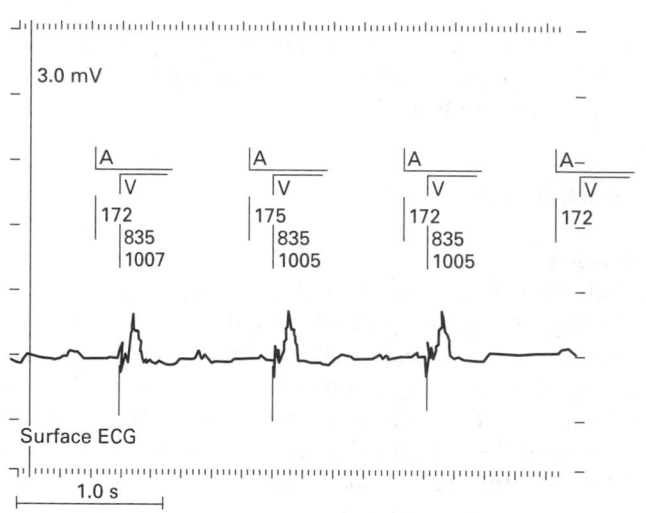

FIGURE 34-9

Top. P-wave synchronous ventricular pacing, with marker channels "P" indicating sensed P waves and "V" indicating paced ventricular complex. At 2 mV there was appropriate P-wave sensing. *Bottom.* "A" indicates that the pacemaker is pacing the atrium. At the programmed sensitivity of 3 mV, there was undersensing of the P wave and therefore atrial pacing occurred. Hence, the sensed P-wave amplitude is between 2 and 3 mV.

breaks often are intermittent problems. Therefore, normal lead impedances and pacing and sensing thresholds do not rule out these problems. The leads can be stressed by having the patient change position and do various arm movements, and these provocative maneuvers sometimes facilitate diagnosis of lead-related problems that are not otherwise observed.

Battery Function

Almost all pacemakers use lithium-iodide batteries, which have an initial battery voltage of 2.8 V. Battery voltages can be measured directly, and at a certain level [elective replacement index (ERI)], the pacemaker unit requires elective generator change. At a lower battery voltage [end of life (EOL)], there is potential loss of pacemaker function; therefore, immediate generator change is mandated.

Battery function can also be assessed without formal interrogation. Many pacemakers reset to a VVI mode at a preset pacing rate, or the pacing rate decreases to less than the programmed lower rate of the pacemaker when battery function reaches the ERI or EOL stage. Additionally, the magnet mode causes asynchronous pacing at a preset magnet rate for each particular pacemaker model. Some pacemakers have separate magnet rates for EOL and/or ERI battery voltages.

Rate Responsiveness

Many patients with chronotropic incompetence have rate-responsive pacemakers that require periodic adjustments of the rate-responsive features to optimize clinical responsiveness. The programmable variables include a rate-responsive upper pacing rate, which may be a programmable variable separate from the upper tracking rate. With certain rate-response sensors, such as activity, a threshold for detecting activity is programmed so that below that threshold, rate responsiveness is inactive. Finally, some type of rate-response slope may be programmed in order to determine the pacing rate at a certain activity level. During outpatient follow-up, the appropriateness of rate responsiveness can be assessed. Some pacemakers store data with respect to the use of rate responsiveness over a certain period of time. Otherwise, one can simply have the patient walk briskly for 2 to 3 min and assess the heart rate to determine if it is appropriate, given the patient's age and clinical status. Some pacemakers offer algorithms whereby the physician chooses the appropriate heart rate for "brisk walking," and the pacemaker automatically calculates the optimal rate-responsive programming.

Data Recall

One of the most recent advances in pacemaker follow-up is the ability of the pacemaker to store certain information with respect to pacer function. For instance, it is possible with certain pacers to interrogate the breakdown of pacing versus sensing. In dual-chamber pacing, this information provides useful information with respect to how much atrial or ventricular sensing or pacing was done. For instance, in a patient with complete heart block, it is expected that there would be nearly 100 percent ventricular pacing, but if that patient has adequate chronotropic function, there would be predominantly atrial sensing.

Some pacers can be programmed to store certain events, such as when a patient had an episode of atrial or ventricular tachyarrhythmia, and store intracardiac electrograms associated with these events.

Chest Radiograph (Posteroanterior and Lateral)

A standard chest x-ray (Figs. 34-4 and 34-5) is recommended as part of the predischarge evaluation performed within 1 week of implant. This is to ensure appropriate placement of leads and to rule out lead migration. This chest x-ray would also serve as a baseline for future studies should problems develop.

ECG Rhythm Strips, with and without Magnet

These are used to evaluate the patient's underlying rhythm and interactions with any arrhythmias present.

Myopotential Oversensing

In patients with unipolar pacing systems, the patient undergoes a series of arm movements to rule out myopotential oversensing.

PACEMAKER FUNCTION AND MODES

Magnet Mode

Virtually all pacemakers are designed to pace in an asynchronous mode when they come into contact with a magnetic field. The response to a magnet varies according to manufacturer, pacemaker model, and sometimes even the mode in which a pacer is programmed. Single-chamber pacers respond to magnets by asynchronous pacing at either the programmed rate or a special magnet rate (Fig. 34-10). This allows a simple noninvasive method to assess pacing at the bedside, in the office, or even at home. In patients who are pacemaker-dependent and experiencing oversensing, thereby inhibiting pacemaker output, a magnet is a convenient short-term method to ensure pacing. Furthermore, pacemakers usually have one

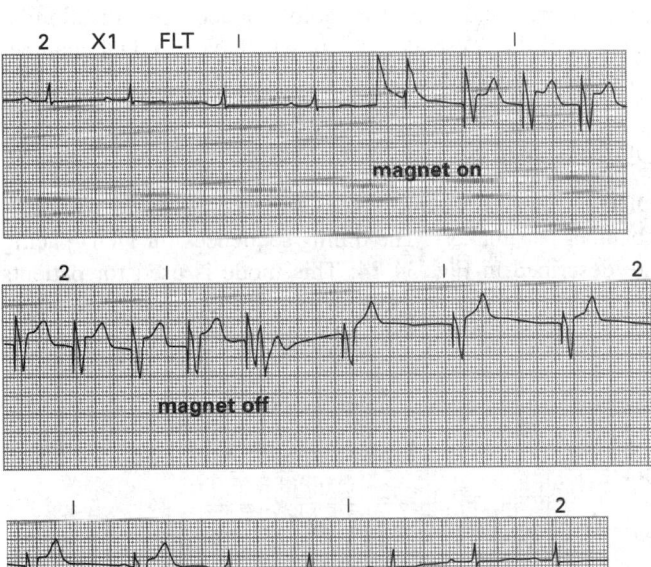

FIGURE 34-10

An electrocardiogram of a patient with sinus nodal dysfunction and first-degree AV block who has an implanted VVI pacemaker. Note that application of a magnet causes VVI pacing in the asynchronous mode at a rate of approximately 95 beats per minute. After the magnet is removed, the pacemaker reverts to VVI at 50 beats per minute until the patient's sinus rhythm inhibits pacemaker function.

magnet rate for a battery that is intact and another one for a battery that is at the ERI or EOL stage. If these rates are known, applying a magnet to a pacemaker is an easy noninvasive method to assess battery status. It also causes continuous pacing output, allowing for analysis of pacing capture function.

VVI Mode

In the VVI mode, a pacemaker operates as shown in Fig. 34-11. The lower rate is converted to an interval (milliseconds). After a paced or sensed ventricular event, a programmable refractory period for sensing prevents inappropriate sensing of T waves. After the pacemaker ventricular refractory period, there is an interval extending to the escape interval during which time the pacemaker may sense a ventricular event, if one occurs before the end of the interval; otherwise, there is ventricular pacing output.

Hysteresis is a programmable function in which the ventricular escape interval is longer after a sensed ventricular event than after a paced ventricular event. This feature is intended to conserve battery life and maintain an intrinsic rhythm, because the effective rate at which a pacer begins to pace is lower than the actual rate of the pacemaker (Fig. 34-12). For example, in a patient with intact AV conduction, if the pacemaker is programmed to a lower rate of 70 pulses per minute and the hysteresis rate is 50 beats per minute, the patient's intrinsic rhythm would have to decrease to less than 50 beats per minute for one cycle in order to establish pacing at 70 pulses per minute. The intrinsic rate would have to exceed the lower rate of the pacemaker (70 beats per minute) in order to inhibit pacemaker output once pacing is established.

Hysteresis is a function that originated with VVI pacers in patients with sinus nodal dysfunction in order to preserve AV synchrony and battery function. It is more hemodynamically beneficial to have sinus rhythm at a rate slightly lower than the lower rate of the pacemaker rather than initiating ventricular pacing. With hysteresis, ventricular pacing would not occur until the sinus rate is substantially lower than the lower rate.

AAI Pacing

AAI pacing is similar to VVI pacing, except that the pacemaker is stimulating the atrium. This mode of pacing and type of pacemaker are more common in Europe than in the United States. AAIR is an excellent mode of pacing in a patient with sinus node dysfunction and normal AV nodal and His-Purkinje function.[74–76] The timing sequences are the same for AAI as for VVI pacing. Atrial sensitivities are programmed to much lower values (increased sensitivity) in order to sense intrinsic P waves safely. This frequently leads to oversensing of far-field ventricular electrograms (Fig. 34-13). A longer atrial sensing refractory period needs to be programmed to avoid this problem.

Patients with sinus nodal dysfunction may develop AV block, which may be a source of concern when using AAI

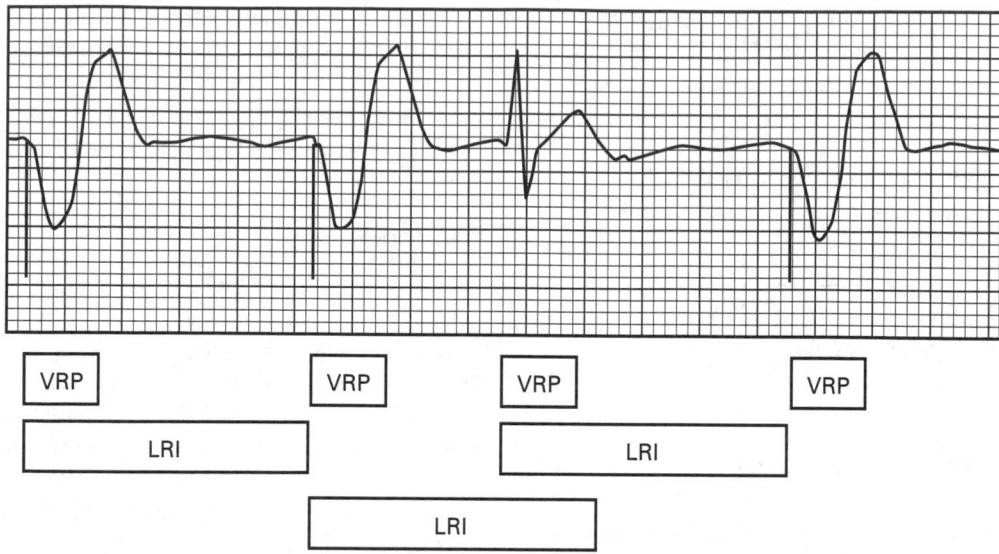

FIGURE 34-11

Schematic diagram of the pacemaker timing cycles during VVI pacing. After a ventricular paced or ventricular sensed event, the pacemaker begins a ventricular refractory period (VRP). This is a programmable value usually between 250 and 400 ms. During this time, a sensed ventricular event will not initiate a new timing interval and will not reset the pacemaker. The lower rate interval (LRI) of the pacemaker corresponds to the programmed lower rate. If this interval expires and there is no sensed ventricular event following the end of the ventricular refractory period, the pacemaker stimulates the ventricle (second and fourth complex) and the VRP and LRI begin anew. If there is an intrinsic ventricular depolarization between the end of the VRP and during the LRI, then ventricular output is inhibited and the VRP and LRI begin anew.

pacing. However, with careful selection of patients,[74–76] including those with relatively normal PR intervals and absence of bundle branch block, an atrial pacemaker can usually be implanted with low risk for complete heart block developing. It is usually desirable to assess AV nodal function further by demonstrating 1:1 AV conduction with atrial pacing at rates exceeding 130 to 140 beats per minute during implant of an AAI pacer.

If there are concomitant atrial arrhythmias, therapy to suppress atrial tachyarrhythmias may lead to prolongation of intrinsic AV conduction. In this case, it is reasonable to implant a dual-chamber pacemaker. Furthermore, many of these patients are candidates for radiofrequency modification or ablation of the AV node,[77–79] in which case, a dual-chamber pacemaker is required.

DDD Pacing

DDD pacing is the most common pacing mode for dual-chamber pacemakers. The timing sequences for DDD pacing are described in Fig. 34-14. This mode is used for patients with AV node and/or sinus node dysfunction.

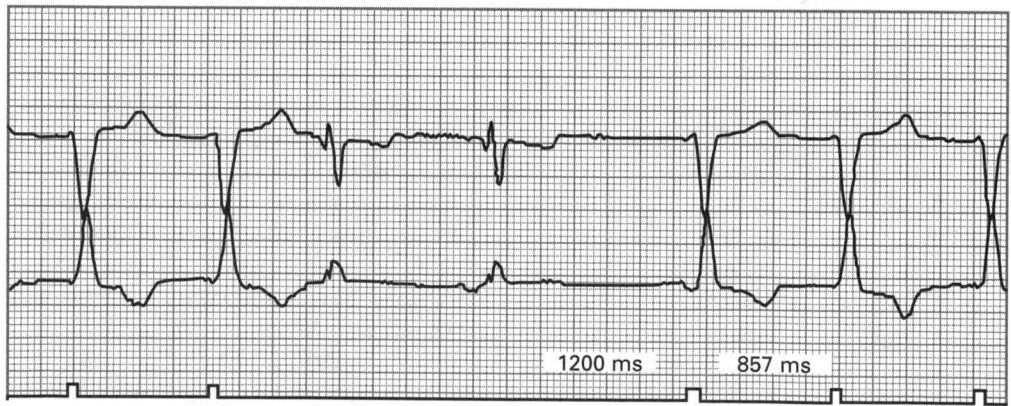

FIGURE 34-12

A patient with atrial fibrillation and the VVI pacemaker with lower rate of 70 pulses per minute (857 ms) and hysteresis rate of 50 beats per minute (1200 ms). The square pulses in the bottom line represent pacing output. This tracing (two leads recorded simultaneously) represents normal hysteresis function. See text for discussion.

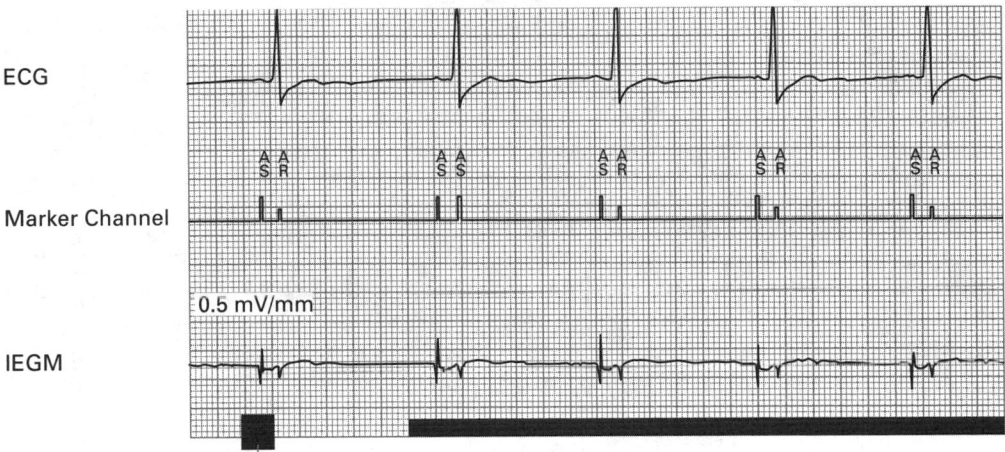

FIGURE 34-13

Surface electrocardiogram, marker channel, and intracardiac electrogram of a patient with an atrial pacemaker and normal sinus rhythm. Note the atrial electrograms corresponding to the P waves of approximately 2 mV and a far-field ECG corresponding to the QRS complex of approximately 1 mV. Therefore, with a programmed sensitivity of 0.5 mV, there is far-field sensing of the ventricular depolarization. In an AAI pacemaker, this could lead to inappropriate sensing and pacing at less than the lower rate. To avoid sensing of these far-field electrograms (AS), the atrial refractory period may be extended so that the electrograms fall within the refractory period (AR). When the far-field electrogram falls within the refractory period, the lower rate interval is not reset.

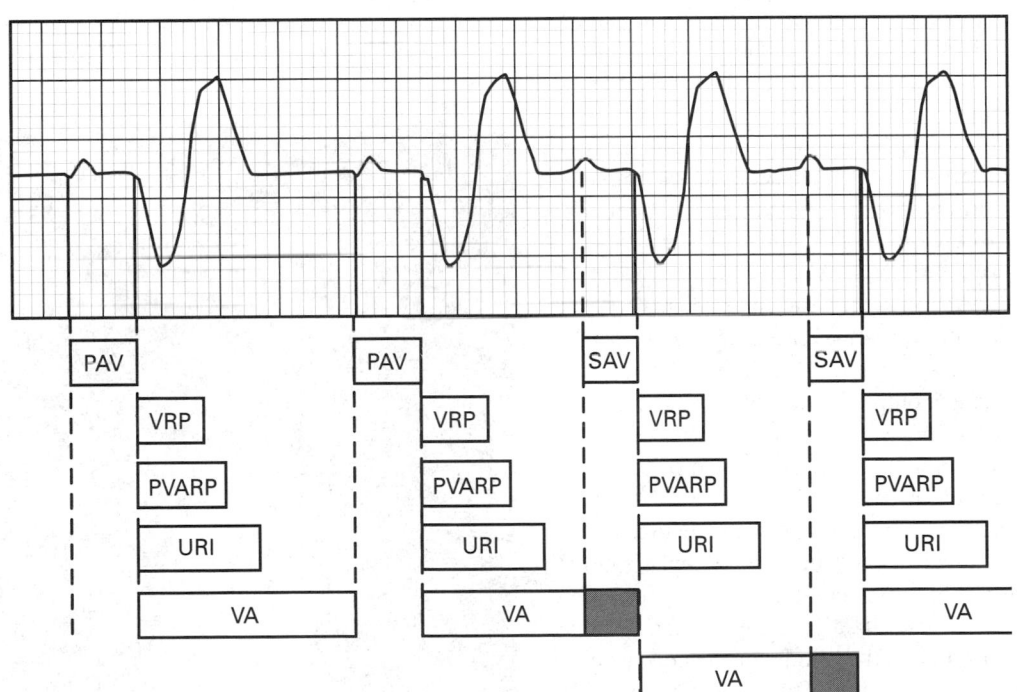

FIGURE 34-14

Schematic diagram of DDD pacing with selected timing cycles and refractory periods. After a paced atrial complex, the paced AV interval (PAV) begins. If there is no ventricular depolarization before this interval expires, the pacemaker response is to output a ventricular impulse. After a paced ventricular output, several refractory periods and timing cycles are initiated. The ventricular refractory period (VRP) is the time during which a ventricular event will not reset the timing intervals. The postventricular refractory period (PVARP) represents the time during which an atrial event will not be sensed or will not reset the timing intervals. The upper rate interval represents the shortest interval (maximum rate) that a pacemaker will ventricular pace corresponding to the programmed upper tracking rate. The ventricular-atrial escape interval (VA) represents the time during which, if there is no sensed atrial electrogram, atrial pacing occurs. The programmed lower rate corresponds to the AV interval and the VA interval. During the first two complexes, there were no sensed atrial complexes; therefore, the VA interval expired and atrial pacing occurred. During the third and fourth complexes, there were sensed atrial electrograms following the PVARP and before the VA interval expired (shaded area in the VA bar). Note that atrial sensing usually occurs after the start of the P wave, representing the atrial conduction time to the atrial electrodes. The programmed AV interval following a sensed atrial complex (SAV) may be programmed at a value lower than the PAV to obtain equivalent PR intervals.

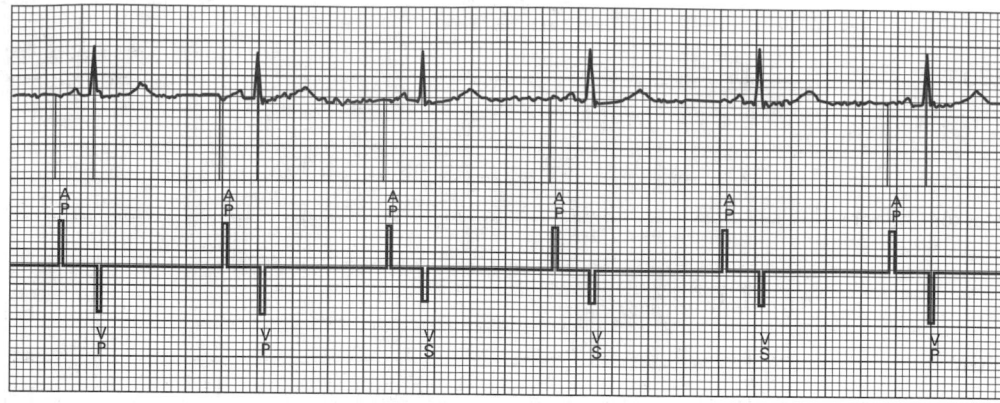

FIGURE 34-15

Surface electrocardiogram with marker channels of a patient with a dual-chamber pacemaker in the DDD mode. Note atrial pacing of all complexes. The first, second, and last complexes have paced ventricular outputs in the middle of the QRS complex. Compared to the third, fourth, and fifth complexes, which do not have these ventricular pacing spikes, there is no change in the QRS complex. This is consistent with "pseudofusion" of the QRS complex. This is due to the fact that the ventricular depolarization is not sensed by the pacemaker until the middle or end of the QRS complex in this particular patient. Subtle variations in the conducted PR interval account for the fact that some of the complexes have a paced ventricular complex and some do not.

DDD PACING IN PATIENTS WITH SINUS NODE DYSFUNCTION

Patients with sinus node dysfunction may have intermittent or chronic sinus bradycardia requiring intermittent or continuous atrial pacing. If patients have intact AV conduction, the pacemaker functions as an AAI pacer. Due to the fact that patients with sinus node dysfunction frequently have AV nodal or His-Purkinje disease, however, patients with DDD pacemakers frequently demonstrate fused ventricular complexes originating from ventricular stimulation and through the natural AV conduction system. The degree of fusion of the ventricular complex between pacing from a right ventricular lead and conduction down the AV nodal–His-Purkinje system depends in large part on the difference between the programmed AV interval and the intrinsic AV conduction time.

In order for ventricular output to be inhibited in patients with DDD pacemakers, the conduction time between the sensed or paced atrial complex to the right ventricular lead must be less than the programmed sensed or paced AV interval. Therefore, it is not uncommon that pacemakers sense the ventricular electrogram late during ventricular depolarization, especially with right ventricular conduction delay or right bundle branch block. In these situations, the pacemaker may pace in the ventricular mode in the middle or towards the end of the QRS complex (Fig. 34-15). This is consistent with normal pacemaker function and is termed *pseudofusion*. One strategy to avoid fusion or pseudofusion is to program a long AV interval; however, if the AV interval is too long, then the benefits of AV synchrony are lost during those times when AV pacing occurs.

PATIENTS WITH AV BLOCK AND NORMAL SINUS NODE FUNCTION

In the DDD mode, if the lower rate of the pacer is programmed at a sufficiently low value to permit atrial tracking, the pacemaker stimulates the ventricle synchronously with intrinsic P waves. If a patient does not require atrial pacing, it may be reasonable to implant a dual-chamber pacer with a single tripolar or quadripolar lead that allows atrial sensing and ventricular pacing and sensing (Fig. 34-16). These VDD pac-

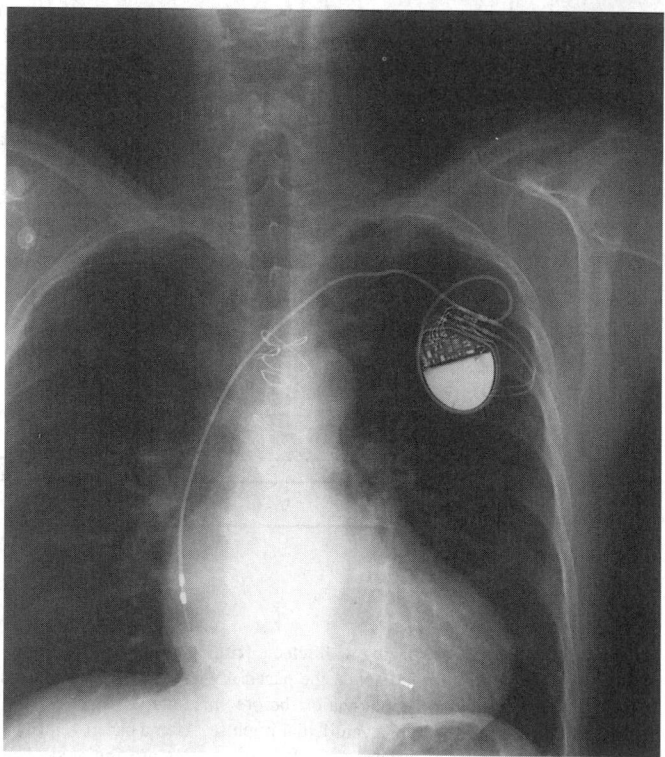

FIGURE 34-16

Chest x-ray showing a single lead in the heart. Note the bipolar electrodes in the atrium and the single electrode in the ventricle. This pacemaker system is capable of VDD pacing. Therefore, it senses atrial depolarizations and can pace or sense in the ventricle.

ing systems allow for ease of implant and for bipolar atrial sensing. Atrial sensing may not be as reliable with a fixed atrial lead, since the atrial electrodes are not attached to the atrial wall in these systems. The amplitude of atrial electrograms may change with body position, leading to occasional atrial undersensing.[80–82]

PATIENTS WITH A TACHYCARDIA-BRADYCARDIA PATTERN OF SICK SINUS SYNDROME

In these patients, the pacer may be used for intermittent atrial and/or AV pacing. During atrial tachyarrhythmias, however, the DDD mode would be disadvantageous because of tracking of atrial tachyarrhythmias. One useful mode would be the DDI mode. This is particularly useful for patients who have intact AV conduction. When patients are in sinus rhythm or experiencing episodes of atrial tachyarrhythmia, the pacer is inhibited. During episodes of bradyarrhythmia, the pacer functions in an atrial or AV pacing mode. In general, the DDI pacing mode is inappropriate for patients with permanent or intermittent AV block because of lack of AV synchrony if a patient has a sinus rate higher than the programmed lower rate of the pacemaker.

PACEMAKER TIMING INTERVALS AND UPPER RATE BEHAVIOR

AV Interval

The AV interval is divided into three zones. The first 20 to 40 ms of this interval is the atrial blanking period. The ventricular channel is blanked during this period to prevent inappropriate sensing of atrial output (cross talk). Cross talk is a greater problem in unipolar than in bipolar systems. The next part of the AV interval occurs from the end of the blanking period to approximately 100 to 120 ms after the atrial pacing output. If a ventricular sensed event occurred at this point, it would be nonphysiologic because of the short elapsed AV interval. The pacemaker responds with a ventricular output at a short AV interval (100 to 120 ms), which is a safety feature (ventricular safety pacing—Fig. 34-17). Ventricular safety pacing is a feature that ensures ventricular pacing in case the sensed event was not a ventricular depolarization; instead, pacing occurs at a short interval so that the pacing output falls before the T wave. Finally, if there is a sensed event in the latter part of the AV interval, the pacemaker response is to inhibit ventricular pacing output.

Upper Rate Behavior

The total atrial refractory period (ARP) consists of the AV interval and the postventricular ARP. The total ARP is a programmable value that can be calculated in milliseconds. Ventricular tracking of atrial events cannot exceed a frequency shorter than the total ARP. By dividing 60,000 ms/min by the total ARP, a rate can be calculated that is the upper rate at which a pacemaker can track atrial events at a 1:1 ratio.

At atrial rates exceeding this value, every other atrial event will fall within the pacemaker refractory period (postventricular ARP) and there will be 2:1 pacemaker AV block. Therefore, the rate corresponding to the total ARP corresponds to the pacemaker 2:1 rate.

The upper tracking rate is a separate programmable value. The upper tracking rate is generally programmed at a rate less than that corresponding to the total ARP rate. This leads to pacemaker Wenckebach behavior when the patient's atrial rate exceeds the programmed upper rate (Fig. 34-18). The Wenckebach interval is defined as the difference between the programmed upper rate and the rate corresponding to the total ARP.

Therefore, when a patient has a sinus or other atrial tachycardia, the pacemaker can track the P waves in a 1:1 fashion up to either the upper programmed rate of the pacer or the pacemaker 2:1 rate, whichever is lower. If the 2:1 pacemaker rate is lower, there may be deleterious hemodynamic consequences for an exercising patient in whom the ventricular response would abruptly drop by nearly half. For this reason, a Wenckebach interval is preferred by programming the total ARP to a sufficiently short interval or the upper rate of the pacemaker to a rate that is less than the 2:1 AV block rate.

There are various strategies available for active patients with DDD pacemakers who require physiologic upper rates. Many pacemakers offer autoadjusting AV intervals that shorten with increasing rates. By shortening the AV interval, the total ARP decreases, which allows greater upper tracking rates before reaching the rate of 2:1 AV block. Another strategy involves sensor driven rate smoothing. The rate-responsive features are activated, and a separate upper sensor-driven rate, different from the upper atrial tracking rate, may be programmed. This allows maintenance of increased ventricular pacing rates driven by the sensor when the atrial rate exceeds the upper tracking rate or the 2:1 rate, and prevents AV Wenckebach or 2:1 AV block. Therefore, this is a form of sensor-driven rate smoothing.[83] When sensor-driven ventricular pacing occurs, there may be loss of AV synchrony, but AV synchrony appears to be less important at faster rates than at rates less than 100.[83–86]

USE OF PACEMAKERS IN DIFFERENT CLINICAL SITUATIONS

Paroxysmal Atrial Fibrillation, Flutter, and Other Tachyarrhythmias

Dual-chamber pacing with atrial tracking presents unique problems when the atrial rhythm is a pathologic atrial tachyarrhythmia rather than a physiologic sinus tachycardia. During atrial fibrillation, there are so many sensed atrial events occurring at rapid rates that a DDD pacemaker responds with an attempt to track these electrograms up to but not exceeding the upper rate (Figs. 34-19 and 34-20). The ECG hallmark is an irregularly irregular ventricular paced rhythm at a mean rate just below the upper rate. Of course, if the patient has

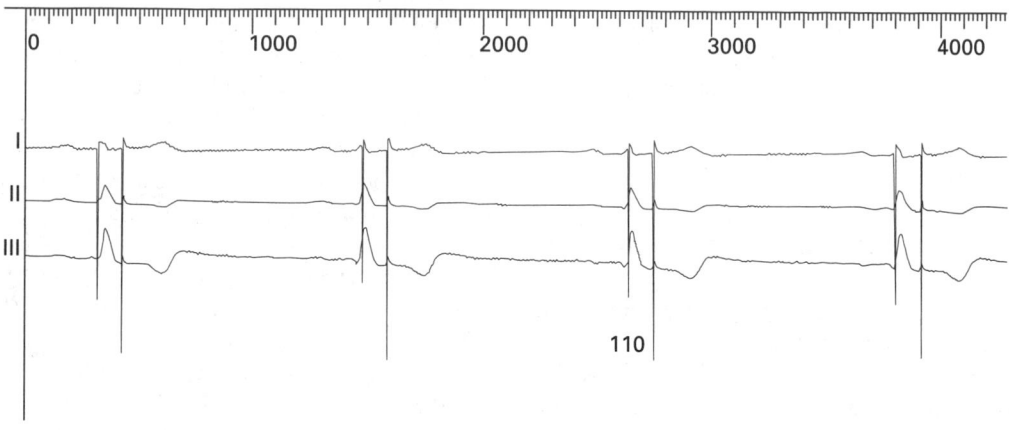

FIGURE 34-17

Surface leads I, II, and III are shown at paper speed of 50 mm/s. Note that there is complete undersensing of the P wave. The pacemaker therefore tends to pace at the lower rate interval, which corresponds with an intrinsic QRS complex. This QRS complex is sensed within the ventricular safety period, triggering ventricular safety pacing. For this particular pacemaker, ventricular safety pacing occurs at 110 ms after atrial pacing in order to avoid ventricular pacing during the T wave.

intrinsic AV conduction, the patient's ventricular rate is not controlled by the pacemaker but rather by the intrinsic AV nodal conduction.

There are various strategies for preventing inappropriate upper tracking behavior during atrial tachyarrhythmias. In a patient with intact AV conduction and paroxysmal atrial tachyarrhythmias, DDI or DDIR modes may be appropriate (Fig. 34-19). In this mode of pacing, there is no tracking of atrial events. If there is a sinus or other atrial sensed electro-gram, the pacer will inhibit atrial pacing output. Ventricular pacing occurs only at the lower rate interval. For patients

with sick sinus syndrome, the clinical problem necessitating a pacemaker is either the bradycardia resulting from intrinsic sinus node dysfunction or the bradyarrhythmias resulting from therapy to suppress the tachyarrhythmias. Therefore, DDIR is very effective therapy for patients with sick sinus syndrome who have intrinsic AV conduction.

A new feature available in some pacemakers for avoiding upper rate tracking during atrial arrhythmias is automatic mode switching (Fig. 34-20). Depending on the pacer model, the basic principle involves automatically switching pacer modes from DDD[R] to VVI[R] or DDI[R] when the atrial

5268-2   TM197 21:42   15 FEB 94 III MON HR = 87 A = 3

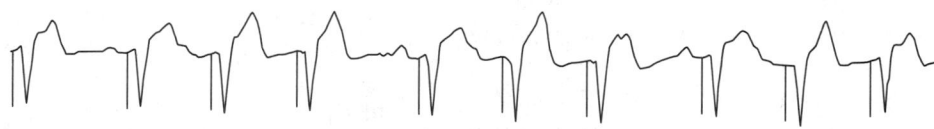

SPEED = 25 mm/s

ICK 5268-2   TM197 17:57   16 FEB 94 II MON HR = 92 A = 0

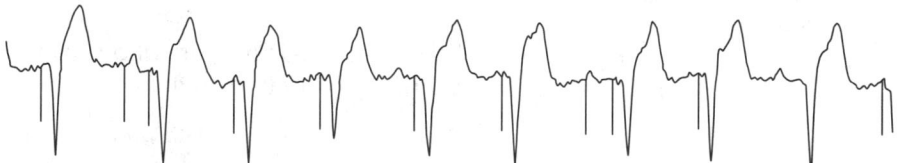

D = 25 mm/s

FIGURE 34-18

Top. Sinus tachycardia in a patient with AV block and a DDD pacemaker with a programmed upper rate of 100 beats per minute, which is less than the intrinsic sinus rate. Note that the interval between the sensed P wave and the paced ventricular complex lengthens progressively, until there is a P wave (within the T wave) following the first, fourth, and seventh paced ventricular complexes without subsequent ventricular pacing, consistent with pacemaker Wenckebach. *Bottom.* The pacemaker is programmed in the DDDR mode with upper rate of 100 beats per minute. The presence of rate response, during activity, acts to smooth the upper rate, preventing the longer pauses during pacemaker Wenckebach.

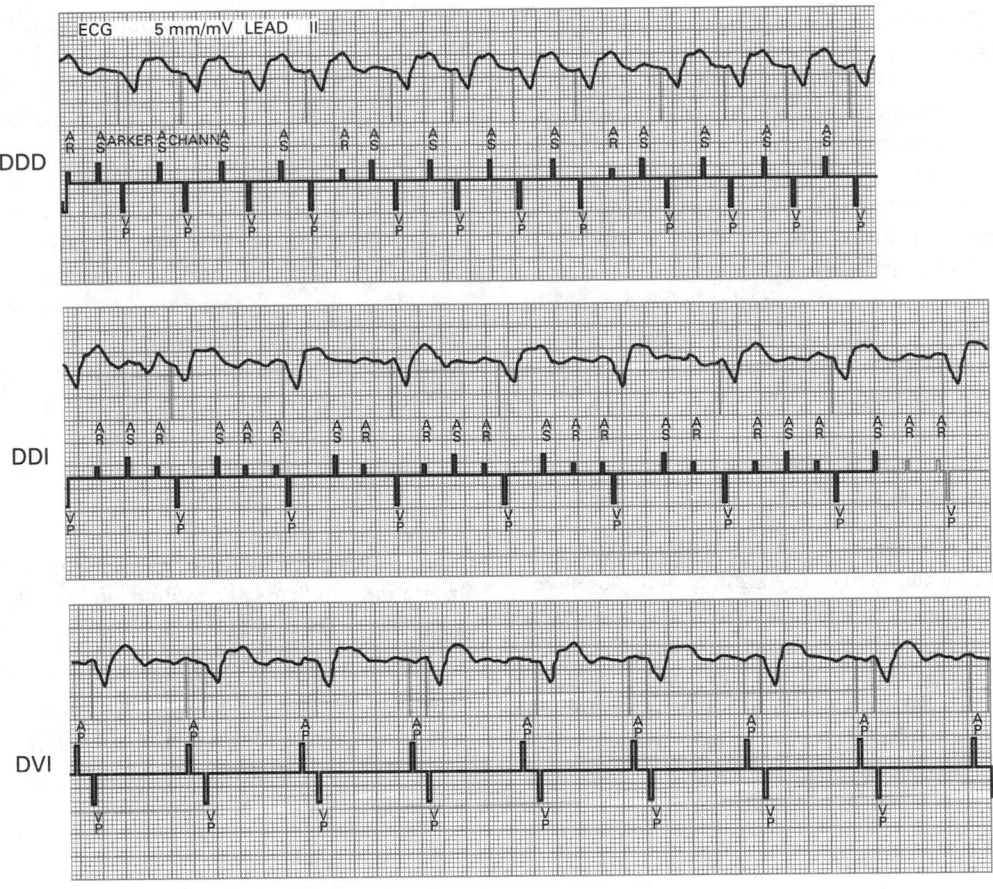

FIGURE 34-19
Tracings of a patient with a dual-chamber pacemaker who has underlying atrial fibrillation. Electrocardiograms and corresponding marker channels are shown for pacing modes DDD, DDI, and DVI, respectively. Note that during DDD, the pacemaker rhythm is an irregularly irregular paced ventricular rhythm at, but not exceeding, the upper rate of the pacemaker. In the DDI mode, there is no tracking of the atrial fibrillation; therefore, it functions effectively as a VVI pacemaker so long as the patient is in atrial fibrillation. In the last tracing, the mode is DVI; therefore, there is no sensing of atrial electrograms, which accounts for the AV sequential pacing pattern. This mode is generally not used when the DDI mode is available. AR = sensed atrial electrogram in the pacemaker refractory period; AS = sensed atrial electrogram; VP = ventricular paced complex.

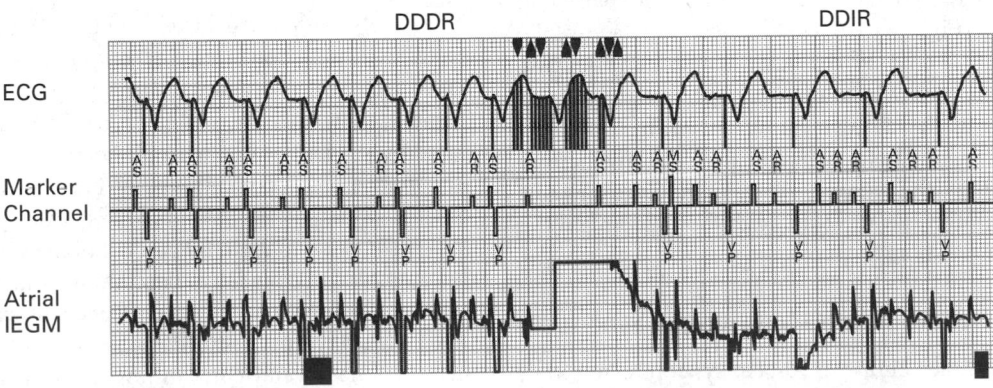

FIGURE 34-20
Electrocardiogram, marker channels, and intracardiac atrial electrograms (IEGMs) are shown for a patient with atrial fibrillation. At the left-hand part of the tracing, there is upper track pacing at an irregular rate due to the atrial fibrillation. Automatic mode switch was programmed on (indicated by the triangles), and the pacemaker automatically mode switched (MS) to the DDIR mode. Note the prolonging of ventricular cycle lengths after mode switch was activated.

rhythm changes from sinus rhythm to an atrial fibrillation or flutter or other tachycardia. The automatic mode switch may occur at the upper rate of the pacemaker or at a separate programmable mode switch rate. It may occur with a single or multiple sequential premature atrial complexes, depending on the pacemaker model.

In the future, there may be novel pacing strategies to prevent or reduce the occurrence of atrial tachyarrhythmias. Recently, it has been reported that multisite pacing in the atrium may reduce the occurrence of episodes of atrial fibrillation.[87,88] Other pacing strategies for reducing episodes of atrial fibrillation include algorithms for increasing the pacing rate following premature atrial complexes.

Chronic Atrial Fibrillation or Other Atrial Tachyarrhythmia

It is generally agreed that any patient with chronic atrial fibrillation or other atrial tachyarrhythmia should not have a dual-chamber pacemaker. Patients with chronic atrial tachyarrhythmia and high-degree or complete AV block generally benefit from a VVIR pacemaker unless their functional status is limited, in which case a VVI pacemaker would suffice. In patients with chronic atrial fibrillation or other atrial tachyarrhythmia and tachycardia-bradycardia syndrome, a VVI or VVIR pacemaker may be appropriate. Depending on the mean ventricular response and functional capabilities of the patient, the VVI mode with hysteresis would be appropriate if the patient requires a backup pacemaker.

Complete or Intermittent Third-Degree AV Block

Patients with complete or intermittent third-degree AV block generally receive a DDD pacemaker (Fig. 34-3). If the sinus nodal function is intact, the ventricle is generally paced synchronously with the P wave after a programmed AV delay. Because some of these patients would not require atrial pacing, some manufacturers offer a single tripolar or quadripolar lead that utilizes a bipole in the atrial cavity for atrial sensing and a unipole or bipole attached to the right ventricle for ventricular pacing or sensing (Fig. 34-16). This mode of pacing (VDD) facilitates implant since only one lead is required. Because the atrial lead is not attached to the atrium, however, there is marked variation in the atrial electrogram with respiratory and positional changes. This problem is alleviated by increasing atrial sensitivities, but atrial sensing may not be as reliable as with a fixed atrial lead. Currently, with these floating atrial leads, atrial pacing is not reliable.

Carotid Sinus Syndrome and Vasovagal Syncope

Patients with one of the neurally mediated syncope syndromes generally have intact sinus and AV nodal function. They are frequently controlled medically (e.g., neurocardiogenic syncope, see Chap. 35) but may require episodic pacing in some cases. Because of combined vasodepressor and cardioin-hibitory responses, patients may benefit from dual-chamber pacing.[37–48] Additionally, they would benefit from a pacing rate exceeding the rate that would normally be programmed as a lower rate. For instance, if a patient with vasovagal syncope experiences an episode with bradycardia and hypotension and has a dual-chamber pacemaker programmed to a lower rate of 50 pulses per minute, the pacemaker response would be to pace at 50 when the patient's intrinsic rate fell below 50. During one of these episodes, however, the patient would benefit more from a pacing rate of 75 to 100 pulses per minute, which may further alleviate the symptoms from the hypotension. With standard DDD pacing, the only way to pace at lower rates of 75 to 100 beats per minute would be to always pace at these rates, which would be inappropriate in otherwise healthy patients with intact sinus and AV nodal function. Certain pacemakers now offer features that allow for pacing at an intervention rate for a short period of time, possibly triggered by a precipitous drop in a patient's intrinsic heart rate, which may be more beneficial from a hemodynamic standpoint. These features are known as *scanning hysteresis* or *rate drop response.*

HEMODYNAMICS OF CARDIAC PACING

In theory, a multiprogrammable DDD pacemaker will optimize and maintain AV synchrony and heart rate in order to allow cardiac output to meet the metabolic needs of the patient, whether resting, sleeping, or exercising. Cardiac output is a function of heart rate and stroke volume. There are many variables involved in determining cardiac output through an effect on stroke volume, such as the autonomic tone, physical condition of the patient, left ventricular diastolic and systolic function, and peripheral vascular resistance. As seen in Table 34-10, there are many variables in pacing systems that can affect cardiac hemodynamic function.

AV Synchrony

In patients with fixed stroke volume (i.e., left ventricular systolic dysfunction), cardiac output is determined almost exclusively by heart rate.[89] In younger patients, however, particularly well-trained athletes, cardiac output is controlled more by stroke volume than by heart rate. Nevertheless, the importance of AV synchrony has been recognized in several clinical situations. In patients at rest, AV synchrony appears to contribute up to 20 to 30 percent of the cardiac output.[89–92] In patients with congestive heart failure due to left ventricular systolic dysfunction, the dependence of cardiac output on AV synchrony appears to decrease secondary to the already increased left ventricular filling pressures. Any improvement in cardiac output with restoration of AV synchrony, however, may be clinically significant and possibly improve survival.[93] Additionally, in patients with left ventricular hypertrophy or diastolic dysfunction due to other etiologies, AV

TABLE 34-10

EFFECTS OF CARDIAC PACING VARIABLES ON CARDIAC HEMODYNAMIC FUNCTION

Variable	Comment
AV synchrony	More important in patients with diastolic dysfunction and during resting heart rates
	Required for most patients with one of the neurally mediated syncope syndromes
	Prevents AV valve regurgitation that is observed with ventricular contraction against open AV valves
	Prevents increase in pulmonary venous or central venous pressure seen when atria contract against closed AV valves
AV interval	Short AV interval in patients with hypertrophic cardiomyopathy
	AV interval in most clinical situations is between 120 and 200 ms
	Shorter AV interval after sensed P wave than during AV sequential pacing to have equivalent PR intervals
Rate responsiveness	Useful in patients with chronotropic incompetence
	Rate responsiveness as complementary and not alternative feature to AV synchrony
	Useful as a rate smoothing feature during upper tracking rate behavior in DDD patients to prevent deleterious effects of pacemaker AV Wenckebach or 2:1 AV block
Pacing site	Right ventricular apex is preferred in patients with hypertrophic cardiomyopathy to have left ventricular apical pre-excitation preceding septal activation
	??Usefulness of high septal ventricular pacing to pace His bundle and have normal ventricular activation sequence
	??Multisite pacing in atrium to prevent atrial fibrillation or further optimize cardiac hemodynamic function

synchrony plays an even greater role in maintaining cardiac output.

There have been several acute and long-term hemodynamic studies demonstrating the advantage of atrial-based pacing (AAI or DDD) compared to VVI pacing.[89–98] Additionally, many studies have shown that maintenance of AV synchrony improves quality of life, particularly at rest.[96,97] In fact, many patients who have VVI pacers may not recognize the extent of their symptoms until they have an upgrade to a DDD system. This advantage of dual-chamber pacing is observed in patients with AV block and sick sinus syndrome.

Morbidity of VVI Pacing Compared to Atrial-Based Pacing

There have been several retrospective studies examining the morbidity and mortality of patients with DDD or AAI pacing versus VVI pacing. Many retrospective studies have demonstrated that atrial-based pacing (DDD) is associated with decreased clinical events, including atrial fibrillation, congestive heart failure, stroke, and death,[98–111] mainly in patients with sick sinus syndrome but also in patients with AV block. There were many limitations with these retrospective studies,[112] however, and randomized prospective studies are currently under way.

With VVI pacing, in the absence of AV synchrony and in the presence of retrograde VA conduction, the atrium contracts against closed AV valves, causing atrial distention. This is probably the mechanism causing the reported increased incidence of atrial fibrillation, which in turn can be associated with the higher stroke rate. Even in the absence of retrograde conduction, during VVI pacing with VA dissociation, depending on the atrial and ventricular rates, most atrial systoles will be ineffective or contract against closed AV valves, producing a similar deleterious effect on atrial size and function.

Pacemaker Syndrome

The pacemaker syndrome is a constellation of signs and symptoms representing adverse reaction to VVI pacing.[113–117] Most of the symptoms relate to loss of AV synchrony and to retrograde conduction. The symptoms include orthostatic hypotension, near syncope, fatigue, exercise intolerance, malaise, weakness, cough, awareness of heart beat, chest fullness, neck fullness, headache, chest pain, and other symptoms that may be nonspecific. On examination, these patients may have intermittent or persistent cannon A waves and possible liver pulsation. The ECG demonstrates VVI pacing present at the time of their symptoms.

The basis for pacemaker syndrome is not only the loss of AV synchrony but also the presence of ventricular-atrial conduction. Atrial contraction against closed AV valves leads to increases in jugular and pulmonary venous pressure, causing cough and malaise in patients with intact cardiac function and congestive heart failure in other patients with structural heart disease. As mentioned before, atrial distention may lead to atrial fibrillation and the associated sequelae. Furthermore, distended atria can lead to reflex vasodepressor effects mediated by the autonomic nervous system and diuresis mediated by elevated levels of atrial natriuretic peptide.[118,119] The presence of increased atrial natriuretic peptide may be a marker for and not necessarily a contributor to the pacemaker syndrome.[120] Therefore, if patients have decreased cardiac output and arterial pressure secondary to VVI pacing, autonomic and humoral reflexes can lead to further hypotension and hemodynamic deterioration.

Other pacing modalities may produce the pacemaker syndrome if AV synchrony is not present. If a patient with AV block has a pacemaker programmed in the DDI mode and the sinus rate exceeds the lower rate, AV dissociation may produce symptoms compatible with the pacemaker syndrome. Some patients with severe intraatrial conduction delay may experience inappropriate timing between left atrial systole and left ventricular contraction, leading to retrograde atrial flow.[121] This may necessitate the addition of a coronary sinus pacing lead to advance left atrial systole.[88,122]

The management of pacemaker syndrome in patients with sick sinus syndrome usually requires restoration of AV synchrony. In many patients, an upgrade to a dual-chamber pacer is indicated. In some patients with intact sinus and AV conduction, lowering the pacing rate in VVI mode and using the hysteresis mode may promote more sinus rhythm, lessening the symptoms associated with sick sinus syndrome. Using the VVIR mode by itself will not prevent or reduce symptoms from the pacemaker syndrome. It is important to note that many patients may experience mild symptoms of the pacemaker syndrome and learn to live with these symptoms. It is not unusual for patients to recognize the symptoms of pacemaker syndrome only after an upgrade to a dual-chamber pacemaker, when they feel much better.[123] Most patients prefer DDD pacing to VVI pacing in various clinical and hemodynamic studies.[117,123–125]

AV Interval

The role of the AV interval and the optimal AV interval for improving hemodynamic function have been studied.[126–132] In general, for most patients, the optimal AV interval corresponds to the physiologic range for normal PR intervals; that is, an AV interval of approximately 150 ± 50 ms. In clinical practice, however, most patients' quality of life is not significantly different with AV intervals that are "optimized by noninvasive assessment" or with AV intervals that are "suboptimal."[132]

There are other considerations when programming AV intervals. With AV sequential pacing, the start of the P wave corresponds to the start of the AV interval, whereas with P-wave synchronous ventricular pacing, the start of the P wave begins approximately 20 to 70 ms prior to the start of the AV interval, depending on the conduction time from the sinus node to the atrial electrodes. The optimal AV interval for P-wave synchronous ventricular pacing would be shorter than the optimal AV interval for AV sequential pacing.[133] Therefore, in order to achieve similar hemodynamic effects from ventricular pacing following a sensed or paced P wave, the sensed AV interval should be programmed approximately 40 to 50 ms shorter than the paced AV interval. Additionally, left ventricular cardiac function is more dependent on left atrial to left ventricular relationships rather than right atrial to right ventricular AV interval. For this reason, there is much variability between patients with respect to programming AV intervals.

Lastly, the PR interval in normal patients shortens as the heart rate increases during exercise.[134,135] Therefore, many

pacers now offer programmable rate-adaptive AV delays that automatically shorten the AV delay with increasing heart rates.

RATE-RESPONSIVE PACEMAKERS

The ability of a pacemaker to increase the lower rate in response to a physical or physiologic stimulus is termed *rate-responsive*, *rate-adaptive*, or *sensor-driven* pacing. This is indicated by the letter R in the fourth position of the NASPE/BPEG pacing code. Rate-responsive pacing is based upon signals generated by sensor systems that respond to parameters or activities that correlate with physiologic need for increased cardiac pacing rate. Depending on the programmable features available, this sensor can increase the lower rate of the pacer to meet a patient's metabolic needs during physical exertion.

Sensors were first used in single-chamber pacemakers in the early 1960s[136] but did not become popular until the 1980s.[136–147] Numerous sensors have been developed with the goal of providing sensor input into the pacemaker, which can then be used to provide rate-adaptive pacing.

Hemodynamic Evaluation of Rate-Adaptive Pacing

Cardiac output is a function of ventricular rate and stroke volume, modified by variables such as AV synchrony, ventricular preload, ventricular afterload, and autonomic state. In normal individuals at rest, a pacing-induced increase in ventricular rate usually results in a transient increase in cardiac output followed by decrease in stroke volume, returning cardiac output toward normal. When there is a physiologic need for increased cardiac output, however, such as during exercise, stroke volume is maintained during increased ventricular pacing rate.

The role of the atrium and the need for AV synchrony remain less certain during faster rates compared with heart rates under 100 beats per minute. In patients with fixed AV and retrograde ventricular-atrial block, pacing in the VDD mode compared with VVI pacing matched to the atrial rate (without AV synchrony) appears to provide similar cardiac output.[84–86] Multiple studies have shown that the change in work capacity correlates with ventricular rate during exercise, whether the ventricular rate is triggered by spontaneous atrial activity or by a pacemaker sensor. This is why there has been controversy as to whether VVIR pacing may be an alternative to DDD pacing. Patients spend most of their time during rest at heart rates less than 100 beats per minute, however. As discussed, AV synchrony at rest plays a great role in optimizing cardiac output as well as improving the general sense of well-being and quality of life. Therefore, VVIR pacemakers should not usually be considered as an alternative to DDD pacing in patients who would otherwise benefit from AV synchrony.

If a patient has a VVI pacemaker and ventriculo-atrial conduction, or a DDD pacemaker programmed with long AV intervals so that the P wave is closer to the preceding R wave, deleterious hemodynamic consequences may result. In either circumstance, there would be a decrease in cardiac output since the atrium would consistently pace against closed AV valves, producing increases in the pulmonary and jugular venous pressures. This would also produce symptoms of the pacemaker syndrome. Dual-chamber pacemakers currently available often have options of rate-adaptive AV intervals. Such an option provides the advantage of maintaining normal AV relationships during exercise and preventing retrograde atrial contraction.

RATE-ADAPTIVE SENSORS

There are multiple rate-adaptive sensors, either available or under development.[136–150] Actively based sensors are used most commonly. These are piezoelectric crystal systems that are very sensitive to detection of vibration, particularly that induced by up-down motion (activity) or acceleration (forward-backward motion).

The drawback of activity-based pacers is that they do not provide feedback that is proportional to physiologic need. For instance, climbing up stairs requires more work than going down stairs; however, going down stairs is usually faster and would activate the sensor more than climbing up stairs. This leads to faster-paced rates while going down stairs. Similarly, other activity with little body vibrations may produce ineffective rate adaptation from the pacemaker. Therefore, true physiologic sensors are desirable for rate-responsive pacing. The role of physiologic sensors is to provide some measurable index of activity, exercise, or catecholamine state that can provide a more accurate input to the pacemaker for rate-adaptive pacing. The QT interval is affected by heart rate but also independently by catecholamines. Therefore, pacers can measure the interval from the ventricular stimulus to the end of the sensed T wave and modulate the heart rate based on this measurement. The drawback of this technique is that the patient has to be ventricular paced in order to measure the QT, or stimulus-T, interval.

Since there exists a close relationship between respiratory rate or minute ventilation and heart rate, various sensors incorporate measurements of respiratory effort. These systems are based upon measurement of transthoracic impedance between the pacemaker lead and the pulse generator. The impedance increases with inspiration and decreases with expiration; the amplitude of the impedance changes is proportional to the tidal volume. Minute ventilation is the product of the tidal volume and respiratory rate. Thus, minute ventilation can provide an accurate physiologic estimate of metabolic needs. One of the disadvantages of this system is that energy is required to measure impedance, which increases the current drain from the pacemaker generator.

There are a number of other sensor systems available or under development. Many use physiologic parameters, such as pH, oxygen saturation, stroke volume, or temperature. The premise behind all of these is that the measured parameters can provide an accurate measure of a patient's metabolic needs, which can be used to guide rate responsiveness. There are various benefits and drawbacks to the different methods, and at this time there is no consensus as to which sensor is best.

DUAL SENSORS

Some sensor systems provide the advantage of more physiologic pacing during steady state but have a slow response time during initiation of exercise. Other sensors, particularly piezoelectric (activity) sensors, have fast response times at initiation of activity but may not produce physiologic responses during peak or steady-state activity. Some single- and dual-chamber pacers have dual-sensor technology. These systems use a piezoelectric sensor to provide fast responses during the start of exercise to augment the heart rate and a more physiologic sensor (QT, minute ventilation) to provide more proportional heart rate response during exercise.[151–153]

Programming Rate-Adaptive Parameters

The parameters for programming rate responsiveness include the lower and upper activity rates. In many pacers, a separate programmable upper activity and atrial tracking rate is possible. With activity-based sensors, a programmable value for threshold of detection of activity is often required. In elderly patients with slower movements, a lower threshold for detection of activity may be required to optimize rate-responsive features. Once the threshold for detection is achieved, then a slope may be programmed according to the frequency of the activity to match this to a pacing rate. A treadmill test may be required to optimize pacemaker programming. In practice, it is often sufficient to have the patient walk for a few minutes and program the rate-responsive features to achieve what would be expected to be a physiologic pacing rate for that patient. Many pacers now have algorithms that record beat-by-beat heart rates or sample heart rates every few seconds in order to provide immediate feedback during an office or clinic visit as to the paced rate achieved with a few minutes of walking. Some pacers will calculate what the optimal rate-responsive programming should be, based on the activity of the patient during a brief walk and the heart rate desired for that level of activity.

PACEMAKER COMPLICATIONS

Pacemaker complications can occur at the time of implantation, with injury to the heart, lung, or blood vessels. Other complications can occur early or late after implantation and can be due to any of the causes listed in Table 34-11. A complete review of pacemaker complications has been given elsewhere.[1]

Complications of Pacemaker Implant

There are many potential complications of surgical implantation of a pacemaker. Some of these complications relate to the subclavian venous puncture and include subclavian arterial puncture, pneumothorax, hemothorax, or air embolus. Rarely,

TABLE 34-11

PACEMAKER COMPLICATIONS

Early Complications— Surgical	Early Complications— Other	Late Complications
Pneumothorax	Lead dislodgment	High thresholds
Hematoma	Pacemaker	Lead failure
Cardiac	syndrome	Pacemaker failure
perforation	Loose setscrew	Loose setscrew
Subclavian	High thresholds	Diaphragmatic
artery puncture	Diaphragmatic	stimulation
Brachial plexus	stimulation	Infection
injury		Skin erosion
Wound		Battery depletion
dehiscence		Venous thrombosis
Infection		Pacemaker
Pain		syndrome
		Pain

a lead may be introduced into the left ventricle through an inadvertent subclavian arterial puncture or through an unrecognized atrial or ventricular septal defect.[154,155]

Cardiac perforation is a potentially serious and often unrecognized complication of pacemaker lead insertion. This may be recognized at the time of lead insertion by fluoroscopic confirmation of the position of the lead, diaphragmatic stimulation, or hypotension resulting from cardiac tamponade. In the absence of anticoagulation, perforation usually does not lead to tamponade if the lead is withdrawn and repositioned. The presence of a right bundle branch block pattern with pacing is sometimes a sign of perforation.

After implantation, cardiac perforation may be recognized by pericardial pain, friction rub, increasing ventricular pacing threshold, diaphragmatic stimulation, or pericardial effusion. The presence of these signs is not diagnostic of cardiac perforation, and echocardiograms should be performed to examine the lead position. If perforation is suspected and the patient is hemodynamically stable, clinical observation is often the prudent course.

Infections related to pacemaker implantation are rare. The use of prophylactic antibiotics is a common practice, and the irrigation of the pacemaker pocket with an antibiotic solution may help prevent infection. Early infections may be caused by *Staphylococcus aureus* and can be aggressive. Late infections are commonly related to *S. epidermidis* and may have a more indolent course. Occasionally, pacemaker infections are misdiagnosed as pacemaker allergy. Other signs of infection include local inflammation and abscess formation, erosion of the pacer, and fever with positive blood culture without an identifiable focus of infection. Transesophageal echocardiography may help determine whether vegetations are present on the pacemaker lead.[156,157] If the pacemaker is infected, removal of the pacemaker leads and generator is usually required.[158]

Complications related to venous leads include venous occlusion with resulting superior vena cava syndrome or thrombosis of the subclavian vein with ipsilateral arm edema.[159–163] Acute thrombosis may be treated with heparin and warfarin and managed conservatively if the patient responds to anticoagulation. Invasive and surgical interventions, including venoplasty and stent placement, have been described.[159,163] Most occlusions, partial or complete, may occur over time and tend to be asymptomatic because of the formation of venous collaterals.

Mechanical Complications

During implant, the leads are connected to the pulse generator by a setscrew mechanism. If the setscrew is loose (Fig. 34-4), pacemaker malfunction may occur, manifested by increased impedance and intermittent or complete failure to capture.

The pacemaker leads are subject to long-term complications. The insulation of the leads may break, leading to problems with oversensing (due to electrical noise), undersensing, and failure to capture (due to current leak). This problem often manifests intermittently and may be difficult to detect during a routine pacer check. The patient may complain of pectoral muscle stimulation due to current leak around an insulation break.[164] An abnormally low impedance with demonstrable lead malfunction is usually diagnostic for insulation break. It is often useful to have the patient perform provocative maneuvers while monitoring an ECG (and marker channels) and/or measuring impedances in order to detect these insulation breaks. In the past, polyurethane insulation appeared to have more problems with long-term insulation break than silicone insulation.

Leads may also fracture over time (Fig. 34-2). Early lead fractures lead to increased impedances associated with failure to capture, oversensing, and undersensing. Some leads use retention wires to preform an atrial lead so that it is more likely to attach and remain within the atrial appendage. Fracture of a retention wire does not cause any pacemaker malfunction; however, it can lead to serious complications, including cardiac perforation and death, when it penetrates through the insulation into the atrial cavity.[165]

Twiddler's syndrome is a term applied to patients who intentionally or unintentionally manipulate their pulse generator, causing twisting of the entire pacemaker system. This leads to lead dislodgment or fracture. This may also result from an excessively large pacemaker pocket allowing rotation of the pacemaker.

Electromagnetic Interference with Pacemaker Function

In general, electromagnetic interference (EMI) can originate from a variety of sources that have the potential to adversely affect pacemaker function. In Table 34-12, some of the more common sources of EMI are listed with their potential effects on pacemakers.

TABLE 34-12

SOURCES OF ELECTROMAGNETIC INTERFERENCE AND POTENTIAL EFFECTS

	Possible Pacemaker Response		
Type of Interference	Damage to Pacemaker	Total Inhibition	Rate Increase
Magnetic resonance imaging	Y	N	Y
Cellular phones (digital)	N	Y	Y
Electrocautery	U	Y	Y
Defibrillation (external or internal)	U	N	N
Extracorporeal shock wave lithotripsy	U	Y	U
Therapeutic radiation	Y	U	U
Radiofrequency ablation	U	Y	U
Electroshock therapy	U	U	U

Note: N = no; Y = yes; U = unlikely, but possible.

Unipolar pacemakers are usually more susceptible to EMI than bipolar pacemakers because the sensing circuit encompasses a larger area compared to bipolar sensing. Factors that affect EMI have to do with the source of the interference and the proximity to the pacemaker generator. Many of these sources are located in a hospital environment or in specialized places such as construction sites. Sources of EMI at home and the office usually do not pose a problem for patients.

The effects of EMI vary according to its source and the type of pacemaker. Inhibition of pacing output can potentially be life-threatening for patients who are pacemaker-dependent. If the EMI is interpreted as atrial events by the pacemaker, then inappropriate ventricular pacing may occur in patients with DDD pacemakers, since these pacemakers attempt to "track" these events, which are interpreted as atrial. EMI often causes electrical noise that causes the pacemaker to function in a "noise reversion mode." The actual function of this mode differs among the different pacemakers; but this mode involves switching to an asynchronous pacing mode. After elimination of this interference, pacers generally revert to the previously programmed mode; however, it is possible for EMI to cause pacemakers to revert to a backup pacing mode. Backup pacing in some models is unipolar VVI pacing at a preset rate.

Occasionally, EMI causes permanent damage to the pulse generator. Therapeutic radiation can damage the complementary metal oxide semiconductors that are part of most modern pacemakers. Generally doses in excess of 5000 rads, but as little as 1000 rads, may induce pacemaker circuitry damage, which in turn can cause pacemaker failure or even induce a runaway pacemaker. If the pacemaker cannot be shielded from the field of radiation, then consideration should be given to reimplanting the pacemaker at a distant site.

In studies examining interactions between pacemakers and cellular telephones,[166–170] it was noted that digital telephones may cause intermittent pacemaker dysfunction. These adverse effects observed included pacemaker inhibition, inappropriate ventricular tracking (in VDD or DDD pacemakers), or resetting the pacemaker to a backup asynchronous mode. Such interference was noted to be more likely in patients with unipolar rather than bipolar systems. Furthermore, interference was generally noted when the phones were within 10 cm of the pacemaker generator, ipsilateral to the generator implant site and held closely to it. Other factors associated with such interference include increased energy output by the cellular phone and maximal sensitivity by the pacemaker. Because of the diversity of cellular phones and pacemakers that have different shielding capabilities against EMI, it is difficult to draw firm conclusions on the use of digital cellular telephones.[168] No consistent problems have been detected with analogue telephones. In guidelines issued by the U.S. Food and Drug Administration in November 1995, no special precautions were recommended for analogue cellular telephones.[169] It is advisable for patients to use analogue cellular telephones or to keep digital cellular (with power outputs <3 W) phones 20 cm away from their pacemaker generator. Therefore, the use of digital cellular telephones over the ear poses little if any clinically significant health risk.[170] In special circumstances, patients' ECGs may be monitored during use of their cellular telephones.

PACEMAKER MALFUNCTION

Pacemaker malfunction can be categorized as abnormal pacing rate, loss of capture, oversensing, undersensing, or other erratic behavior. The approach to diagnosing pacemaker malfunction is to inspect the ECG carefully, interrogate the pacemaker; check pacing and sensing thresholds, lead impedances, and battery voltage/magnet rate; and perform a chest x-ray. Many instances of pacemaker malfunction actually represent normal function of the pacemaker (Table 34-13). Usually, causes of pacer malfunction may be diagnosed noninvasively, but occasionally, surgery is required to diagnose problems.

Abnormal Pacing Rates

Abnormal pacing rates can be due to normal or abnormal pacing function (see Table 34-13). Failure of the pacemaker to produce output is usually due to oversensing. Occasionally, there is pacemaker output that is not visible because of bipolar pacing producing very low amplitude pacing artifacts (artifacts from digital ECG recording are commonly difficult to visualize). Conversely, absence of pacing stimuli may be due to interruption of current flow from a lead fracture, insulation break, or a loose setscrew.

TABLE 34-13
CAUSES OF ABNORMAL PACING RATES

Normal Pacer Function	Abnormal Pacer Function
Hysteresis	Oversensing or under-sensing
Different sleep rate/lower rate	Battery depletion causing fixed slow rate
Scanning hysteresis/rate drop response causing an increased "intervention" pacing rate for vasovagal episodes	Component failure
Magnet mode	Pacemaker reset due to electromagnetic interference

Abnormally fast pacing rates are usually due to normal pacing function. They may be in response to rate-adaptive sensors. In DDD pacemakers, upper rate pacing may be due to sinus tachycardia, atrial tachyarrhythmias, or pacemaker-mediated tachycardia (Table 34-14). In either case, the pacemaker function is normal and is responding either to a rapid atrial rate or to retrograde atrial activity. Rarely, very rapid ventricular pacing ("runaway pacemakers") can cause life-threatening problems requiring disconnection of the pacemaker. Occasionally, abnormal pacing rates can be due to an

TABLE 34-14
CAUSES OF UPPER RATE BEHAVIOR
IN DDD PACEMAKERS (AND AV BLOCK)

	ECG Characteristics	Response to Magnet
Sinus tachycardia	1:1 AV pacing, pacemaker Wenckebach or 2:1 block depending on the PVARP, upper rate, and sinus rate	No change in paced rhythm after magnet removed
Atrial fibrillation	Irregularly irregular paced ventricular rhythm up to but not exceeding the upper rate	No change in paced rhythm after magnet removed
Pacemaker-mediated tachycardia	Regular paced ventricular rhythm equal to or less than upper rate	Termination of tachycardia

Note: PVARP = postventricular atrial refractory period.

unstable lead position where the lead is swinging between heart chambers.

Loss of Capture

The loss of pacemaker capture occurs when there is a visible pacing stimulus and no atrial or ventricular depolarization. This may be intermittent or persistent. Most problems occur at the pacemaker lead/tissue interface. For instance, lead dislodgment can cause obvious failure to capture. An increase in the pacing threshold above the pacing output can occur as part of the rise above initial threshold within a few weeks following lead placement (Fig. 34-21), or because of drug therapy, electrolytes, myocardial infarction, or ischemia. Fracture of the lead, insulation breaks, and loose setscrews are mechanical problems that can cause failure to capture. Lastly, battery depletion may cause the pacing output to decline sufficiently so that pacing failure occurs.

Loss of capture requires a check of pacing threshold, pacing lead impedance, and a chest x-ray. For instance, if the problem is an elevated pacing threshold, pacing outputs must be increased. Abnormal lead impedances may confirm a lead failure and the need for lead replacement.

Oversensing

This is a problem that leads to abnormal pacing rates with pacemaker pauses. Generally, unipolar lead systems are more susceptible to oversensing. The sources for oversensing can be intracardiac, extracardiac, or due to EMI. Analysis of the ECG, especially with pacemaker interrogation and pacemaker marker channels, may help to determine the cause. If the oversensing is regular, analysis of the pauses may suggest T-wave or P-wave oversensing. T-wave oversensing can usually be eliminated by decreasing the sensitivity (increasing the millivoltage required to sense electrical activity) or increasing the ventricular refractory period.

Oversensing due to lead fracture, insulation break, or other electrode problems will usually be random and erratic (Fig. 34-22). With early lead problems, the malfunction is intermittent and may be exacerbated by certain body positions or motions. In later stages, the combination of oversensing, undersensing, and failure to capture is almost always diagnostic of a lead-related problem. Programming to an asynchronous mode may temporarily control this problem while awaiting a lead replacement, which should be carried out as promptly as possible.

Cross talk inhibition is a phenomenon usually seen in unipolar pacers. It is due to ventricular sensing of atrial output. This is currently a rare problem because of blanking periods and ventricular safety pacing.

Myopotential oversensing is usually a problem in unipolar but not bipolar systems. These skeletal myopotentials generate interference, which tends to correspond to certain activity. The optimal solution is reprogramming the sensitivity to a level high enough to avoid myopotential sensing, while pre-

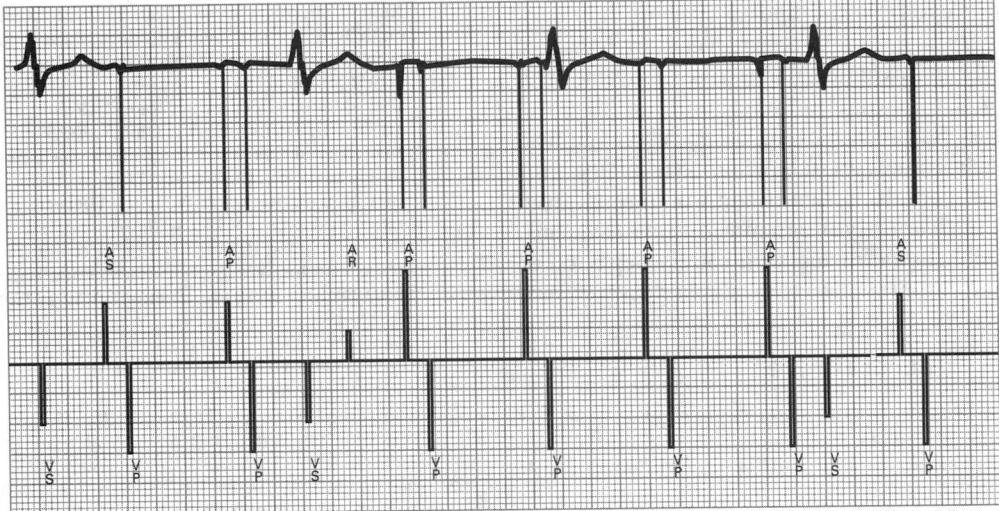

FIGURE 34-21

Electrocardiogram marker channels of a patient with a dual-chamber pace-maker. Note that the atrial pacing outputs (AP) are capturing the atrium, and there is appropriate P-wave sensing (AS or AR). However, none of the ventricular outputs are capturing the ventricle. This is a tracing of a patient who had a pacemaker placed 3 weeks prior to acquisition of this ECG, and the pacing threshold had exceeded the tracing output.

serving an adequate safety margin to sense intrinsic cardiac depolarizations.

Undersensing

An inadequate intracardiac signal can lead to undersensing (Fig. 34-17). The intracardiac electrograms can deteriorate due to inflammation or scar formation at the tissue/lead interface. Additionally, certain drugs, electrolyte abnormalities, infarction, ischemia, lead fracture, or insulation breaks can lead to undersensing. Cardioversion or defibrillation can also cause attenuation of intracardiac electrograms. Usually, undersensing is a greater problem in the atrium than in the ventricle. The optimal solution is to program an enhanced sensitivity

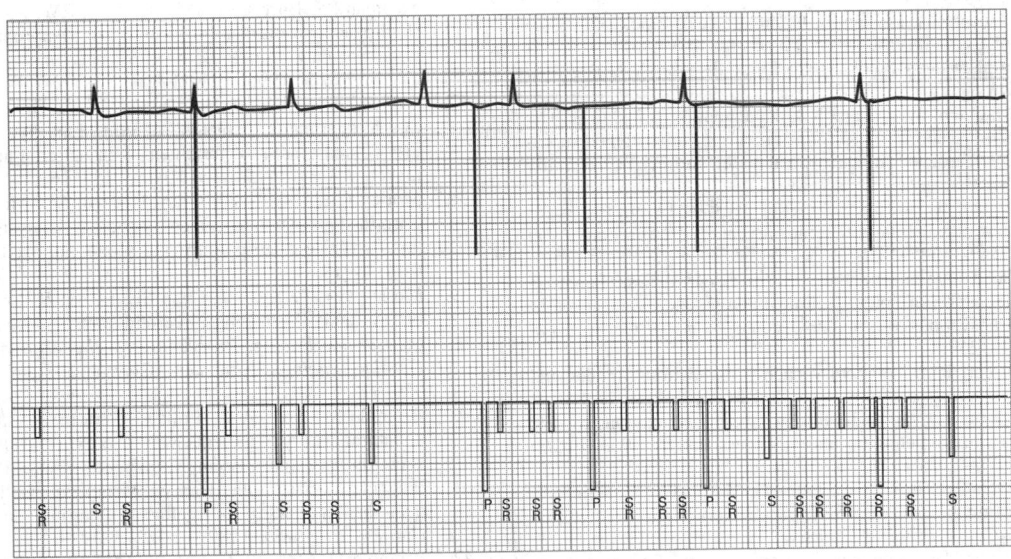

FIGURE 34-22

Electrocardiogram and marker channels are shown for a patient with a ventricular lead impedance break. Note that based on the ECG, there is failure to sense, as manifested by the second and fourth pacing outputs coming very shortly after the QRS complex. There is failure to capture, demonstrated by the second and third pacing outputs, which should capture the ventricle. There is also evidence of oversensing, as demonstrated by the long pause between the fourth and fifth pacing outputs during a diastolic period that exceeds the interval between the previous two pacing outputs. In general, when there is evidence of oversensing, undersensing, and failure to capture, then the likely etiology is either a lead insulation break, lead fracture, or other mechanical problem. The marker channels confirm the above ECG findings. There are sensed ventricular events (S or SR) that do not correspond to surface QRS complexes, consistent with oversensing. Additionally, the erratic pattern of sensed ventricular events is consistent with electrical noise. There are also lack-of-sense markers corresponding to QRS complexes; finally, there are ventricular pace markers (P) that fail to capture the ventricle.

(decrease sensing level). With bipolar systems, the programmed sensitivity can usually be reduced to levels of 0.25 mV in the atrium, avoiding undue risk of oversensing extraneous potentials.

Other etiologies for undersensing occur when intrinsic atrial or ventricular complexes fall within one of the programmed refractory periods. Undersensing would result from a pacer that was inadvertently programmed to an asynchronous mode (occasionally occurring with battery depletion or pacemaker generator reset).

REFERENCES

1. Furman S, Hayes DL, Holmes DR. *A Practice of Cardiac Pacing*, 3d ed. Mount Kisco, NY: Futura; 1993.

2. Barold SS, Mugica J. *New Perspectives in Cardiac Pacing*, 3d ed. Mount Kisco, NY: Futura; 1992.

3. Kusumoto FM, Goldschlager N. Cardiac pacing. *N Engl J Med* 1996; 334:89–98.

4. Ellenberger KA, Kay GN, Wilkoff BL, eds. *Clinical Cardiac Pacing.* Philadelphia: Saunders; 1995.

5. Bernstein AD, Camm AJ, Fletcher R, et al. The NASPE/BPEG generic pacemaker code for antibradyarrhythmia and adaptive rate pacing and antitachyarrhythmia devices. *Pacing Clin Electrophysiol* 1987; 10:794–799.

6. Zoll PM, Zoll RH, Falk RH, Clinton JE, Eitel DR, Antman EM. External noninvasive temporary cardiac pacing: Clinical trials. *Circulation* 1985; 71:937–944.

7. Zoll PM. Noninvasive temporary cardiac pacing. *J Electrophysiol* 1987; 1:156.

8. McAllister HF, Klementowicz PT, Andrews C, et al. Lyme carditis: An important cause of reversible heart block. *Ann Intern Med* 1989; 110:339.

9. Rubin DA, Sorbera C, Baum S, et al. Acute reversible diffuse conduction system disease due to Lyme disease. *Pacing Clin Electrophysiol* 1990; 13:1367–1373.

10. Kimball SA, Janson PA, LaRaia PJ. Complete heart block as the sole presentation of Lyme disease. *Arch Intern Med* 1989; 149:1897.

11. Vlay SC. Complete heart block due to Lyme disease. *N Engl J Med* 1984; 315:1418.

12. Waldo AL, MacLean WA, Karp RB, Kouchoukos NT, James TN. Continuous rapid atrial pacing to control recurrent or sustained supraventricular tachycardias following open heart surgery. *Circulation* 1976; 54:245–250.

13. Ryan TJ, Anderson JL, Antman EM, et al. ACC/AHA guidelines for the management of patients with acute myocardial infarction. *J Am Coll Cardiol* 1996; 1328–1419.

14. Francis GS (lead author) and the ACP/ACC/AHA Task Force on Clinical Privileges in Cardiology. Clinical competence in insertion of a temporary transvenous ventricular pacemaker. *J Am Coll Cardiol* 1994; 23:1254–1257.

15. Hauser RG, Vicari RM. Temporary pacing: Indications, modes and techniques. *Med Clin North Am* 1986; 70:813–827.

16. Trigano JA, Birkui PJ, Mujica J. Noninvasive transcutaneous cardiac pacing: Modern instrumentation and new perspectives. *Pacing Clin Electrophysiol* 1992; 15:1937.

17. Dreifus LS, Fisch C, Griffin JC, Gillette PC, Mason JW, Parsonnet V. Guidelines for implantation of cardiac pacemakers and antiarrhythmia devices. *J Am Coll Cardiol* 1991; 18:1–13.

18. Barold SS. ACC/AHA guidelines for implantation of cardiac pacemakers: How accurate are the definitions of atrioventricular and intraventricular conduction blocks? *Pacing Clin Electrophysiol* 1993; 16:1221–1226.

19. Barold SS. Indications for permanent cardiac pacing in first-degree AV block: Class I, II, or III? *Pacing Clin Electrophysiol* 1996; 19:747–751.

20. Connelly DT, Steinhaus DM. Mobitz type I atrioventricular block: An indication for permanent pacing? *Pacing Clin Electrophysiol* 1996; 19:261–264.

21. Scheinman MM, Peters RW, Sauve MJ, Desai J, Abbott JA, Cogan J, et al. Value of HQ interval in patients with bundle branch block and the role of prophylactic permanent pacing. *Am J Cardiol* 1982; 50:1316–1322.

22. Dhingra RC, Wyndham C, Bauernfeind R, Swiryn S, Deedwania PC, Smith T, et al. Significance of block distal to the His-bundle induced by atrial pacing in patients with chronic bifascicular block. *Circulation* 1979; 60:1455–1464.

23. Zipes D. Second degree AV block. *Circulation* 1979; 60:465–472.

24. Strasberg B, Amat-Y-Leon F, Dhingra RC, Palileo E, Swiryn S, Bauernfeind R, et al. Natural history of chronic second-degree AV block. *Circulation* 1981; 63:1043–1049.

25. Shaw DB, Kekwick CA, Veale D, Gowers J, Whistance T. Survival in second degree AV block. *Br Heart J* 1985; 53:587–593.

26. Clarke M, Sutton R, Ward D, et al. Recommendations for pacemaker prescription for symptomatic bradycardia. Report of a working party of the British Pacing and Electrophysiology Group. *Br Heart J* 1991; 66:185–191.

27. Dhingra RC, Denes P, Wu D, Chuquimia R, Rosen KM. The significance of second degree AV block and bundle branch block. *Circulation* 1974; 49:638–646.

28. Kim YH, O'Nunain S, Trouton T, et al. Pseudo-pacemaker syndrome following inadvertent fast pathway ablation for AV nodal reentrant tachycardia. *J Cardiovasc Electrophysiol* 1993; 4:178–182.

29. Nishimura RA, Hayes DL, Holmes DR, Tajik AJ. Mechanism of hemodynamic improvement by dual-chamber pacing for severe left ventricular dysfunction: An acute Doppler and catheterization hemodynamic study. *J Am Coll Cardiol* 1995; 25:281–288.

30. Auricchio A, Sommariva L, Salo RW, Scafuri A, Chiariello L. Improvement of cardiac function in patients with severe congestive failure and coronary artery disease by dual-chamber pacing with shortened AV delay. *Pacing Clin Electrophysiol* 1993; 16:2034–2043.

31. McHenry MM. Factors influencing longevity in adults with congenital heart block. *Am J Cardiol* 1972; 29:416.

32. Dewey RC, Capeless MA, Levy AM. Use of ambulatory electrocardiographic monitoring to identify high risk patients with congenital complete heart block. *N Engl J Med* 1987; 316:835.

33. Reybrouck T, Vanden Eynde BB, Cumoulin M, Van der Hauwaert LG. Cardiorespiratory response to exercise in congenital complete AV block. *Am J Cardiol* 1989; 64:896.

34. Cobe SM. Congenital complete heart block. *Br Med J* 1983; 286:1769.

35. Sholler GF, Walsh EP. Congenital complete heart block in patients without anatomic cardiac defects. *Am Heart J* 1989; 118:1193.

36. Stegman SS, Burroughs JM, Henthorn RW. Asymptomatic bradyarrhythmias as a marker for sleep apnea: Appropriate recognition and treatment may reduce the need for pacemaker therapy. *Pacing Clin Electrophysiol* 1996; 19:899–904.

37. Sugrue DD, Gersh BJ, Holmes DR, Wood DL, Osborn MJ, Hammill SC. Symptomatic "isolated" carotid sinus hypersensitivity: Natural history and results of treatment with anticholinergic drugs or pacemaker. *J Am Coll Cardiol* 1986; 7:158–162.

38. Morley CA, Perrins EJ, Grant C, Chan SL, McBrien DJ, Sutton R. Carotid sinus syncope treated by pacing. Analysis of persistent symptoms and role of atrioventricular sequential pacing. *Br Heart J* 1982; 47:411–418.

39. Morley CA, Perrins EJ, Chan SL, Sutton R. Long-term comparison of DVI and VVI pacing in carotid sinus syndrome. In: Steinback K, ed. *Cardiac Pacing. Proceedings of the VIIth World Symposium on Cardiac Pacing.* Darmstadt, Germany: Steinkopff Verlag; 1983: 929–935.

40. Brignole M, Nemzzi C, Lolli G, Sartore B, Barra M. Natural and unnatural history of patients with severe carotid sinus hypersensitivity: A preliminary study. *Pacing Clin Electrophysiol* 1988; 11:1628–1635.

41. Brignole M, Sartore B, Barra M, Menozzi C, Lolli G. Ventricular and dual-chamber pacing for treatment of carotid sinus syndrome. *Pacing Clin Electrophysiol* 1989; 12:582–590.

42. Brignole M, Menozzi C, Lolli G, Oddone D, Gianfranchi L, Bertulla A. Pacing for carotid sinus syndrome and sick sinus syndrome. *Pacing Clin Electrophysiol* 1990; 13:2071–2075.

43. Brignole M, Menozzi C, Lolli G, Oddone D, Gianfranchi L, Bertulla A. Validation of a method for choice of pacing mode in carotid sinus syndrome with or without sinus bradycardia. *Pacing Clin Electrophysiol* 1991; 14:196–203.

44. El-Bedawi KM, Wahbha MMAE, Hainsworth R. Cardiac pacing does not improve orthostatic tolerance in patients with vasovagal syncope. *Clin Autonom Res* 1994; 4:233–237.

45. Maloney JD, Jaeger FJ, Rizo-Patron C, Zhu DW. The role of pacing for the management of neurally mediated syncope: Carotid sinus syndrome and vasovagal syncope. *Am Heart J* 1994; 127:1030–1037.

46. Sra JS, Jazayeri MR, Avitall B, Dhala A, Deshpande S, Blanck Z, et al. Comparison of cardiac pacing with drug therapy in the treatment of neurocardiogenic (vasovagal) syncope with bradycardia or asystole. *N Engl J Med* 1993; 328:1085–1090.

47. Petersen MEV, Chamberlain-Webber R, Fitzpatrick AP, Ingram A, Williams T, Sutton R. Permanent pacing for cardioinhibitory malignant vasovagal syndrome. *Br Heart J* 1994; 71:274–281.

48. Fitzpatrick A, Theodorakis G, Ahmed R, Williams T, Sutton R. Dual-chamber pacing aborts vasovagal syncope induced by head-up 60 degree tilt. *Pacing Clin Electrophysiol* 1991; 14:13–19.

49. Johnson AD, Daily PO. Hypertrophic subaortic stenosis complicated by high degree heart block: Successful treatment with atrial synchronous ventricular pacemaker. *Chest* 1975; 67:491–494.

50. McDonald K, McWilliams E, O'Keeffe B, Maurer B. Functional assessment of patients treated with permanent dual-chamber pacing as a primary treatment for hypertrophic cardiomyopathy. *Eur Heart J* 1988; 9:893–898.

51. Fananapazir L, Cannon RO, Tripodi D, Panza JA. Impact of dual-chamber permanent pacing in patients with obstructive hypertrophic cardiomyopathy with symptoms refractory to verapamil and beta-adrenergic blocker therapy. *Circulation* 1992; 85:2149–2161.

52. Nishimura RA, Trusty JM, Hayes DL, Ilstrup DM, Larson DR, Hayes SN, et al. Dual-chamber pacing for hypertrophic cardiomyopathy: A randomized, double-blind, crossover trial. *J Am Coll Cardiol* 1997; 29:435–441.

53. Jeanrenaud X, Goy JJ, Kappenberger L. Effects of dual-chamber pacing in hypertrophic obstructive cardiomyopathy. *Lancet* 1992; 339:1318–1323.

54. Fananapazir L, Epstein ND, Curiel RV, Panza JA, Tripodi D, McAreavey D. Long term results of dual-chamber (DDD) pacing in obstructive hypertrophic cardiomyopathy. Evidence for progressive symptomatic and hemodynamic improvement and reduction of left ventricular hypertrophy. *Circulation* 1994; 90:2731–2742.

55. Nishimura RA, Hayes DL, Ilstrup DM, Holmes DR, Tajik M. Effect of dual-chamber pacing on systolic and diastolic function in patients with hypertrophic cardiomyopathy. Acute doppler echocardiographic and catheterization hemodynamic study. *J Am Coll Cardiol* 1996; 27:421–430.

56. McAreavey D, Tripodi D, Epstein N, Fananapazir L. Dual-chamber pacing relieves outflow tract obstruction in hypertrophic cardiomyopathy despite pre-existing left bundle branch block. *J Am Coll Cardiol* 1993; 21:123A.

57. Cannon RO, Tripodi D, Dilsizian V, Panza JA, Fananapazir L. Results of permanent dual-chamber pacing in symptomatic nonobstructive hypertrophic cardiomyopathy. *Am J Cardiol* 1994; 73:571–576.

58. Brecker SJD, Xiao HB, Sparrow J, Gibson DG. Effects of dual-chamber pacing with short atrioventricular delay in dilated cardiomyopathy. *Lancet* 1992; 340:1308–1312.

59. Auricchio A, Sommariva L, Salo RW, Scafuri A, Chiariello L. Improvement of cardiac function in patients with severe congestive heart failure and coronary artery disease by dual-chamber pacing with shortened AV delay. *Pacing Clin Electrophysiol* 1993; 16:2034–2043.

60. Gold MR, Feliciano Z, Gottlieb SS, Fisher ML. Dual-chamber pacing with a short atrioventricular delay in congestive heart failure: A randomized study. *J Am Coll Cardiol* 1995; 26:967–973.

61. Miller GB, Leman RB, Kratz JM, Gillette PC. Comparison of lead dislodgment and pocket infection rates after pacemaker implantation in the operating room versus the catheterization laboratory. *Am Heart J* 1988; 115:1048–1051.

62. Stamato NJ, O'Toole MF, Enger EL. Permanent pacemaker implantation in the cardiac catheterization laboratory versus the operating room: An analysis of hospital charges and complications. *Pacing Clin Electrophysiol* 1992; 15:2236–2239.

63. Smyth NPD. Pacemaker implantation: Surgical techniques. *Cardiovasc Clin* 1983; 14:31–44.

64. Higano ST, Hayes DL, Spittell PC. Facilitation of the subclavian-introducer technique with contrast venography. *Pacing Clin Electrophysiol* 1990; 13:681–684.

65. Furman S. Venous cutdown for pacemaker implantation. *Ann Thorac Surg* 1986; 41:438–439.

66. Gumbrielle TP, Bourke JP, Sinkovic M, Tynan M, Kittpawong P, Gold RG. Long-term thresholds of nonsteroidal permanent pacing leads: A 5-year study. *Pacing Clin Electrophysiol* 1996; 19:829–835.

67. Bernstein AD, Irwin ME, Parsonnet V, Wilkoff BL, Black WR, Buckingham TA, et al. Report of the NASPE policy conference on anti-bradycardia pacemaker follow-up: Effectiveness, needs and resources. *Pacing Clin Electrophysiol* 1994; 17(pt 1):1714–1729.

68. Grendahl H. Pacemaker follow-up with prolonged intervals in the stable period 1 to 5 years postimplant. *Pacing Clin Electrophysiol* 1996; 19:1219–1224.

69. Sweesy W, Erickson SL, Crago JA, Castor KN, Batey RL, Forney RC. Analysis of the effectiveness of in office and transtelephonic follow-up in terms of pacemaker system complications. *Pacing Clin Electrophysiol* 1994; 17:2001–2003.

70. Rhoden WE, Llewellyn MJ, Schofield SW, Bennett DH. Acute and chronic performance of a steroid-eluting electrode for ventricular pacing. *Int J Cardiol* 1992; 37:209.

71. Mond H, Stokes KB, Helland J, Griff L, Kertes P, Pate B, et al. The porous titanium steroid-eluting electrode: A double-blind study assessing the stimulation threshold effects of steroid. *Pacing Clin Electrophysiol* 1988; 11:214–219.

72. Mond H, Stokes KB. The electrode-tissue interface: The revolutionary role of steroid elution. *Pacing Clin Electrophysiol* 1992; 15:95–107.

73. Mond HG, Stokes KB. The steroid eluting electrode: A 10-year experience. *Pacing Clin Electrophysiol* 1996; 19:1016–1020.

74. Brandt J, Anderson H, Fahraens T, Schuller H. Natural history of sinus node disease treated with atrial pacing in 213 patients—implications for selection of stimulation mode. *J Am Coll Cardiol* 1992; 20:633.

75. Brandt J, Schuller H. Pacing for sinus node disease: A therapeutic rationale. *Clin Cardiol* 1994; 17:495.

76. Katritsis D, Camm M. AAI pacing mode: When is it indicated and how can it be achieved? *Clin Cardiol* 1993; 16:339.

77. Feld GK, Fleck RP, Fujimura O, Prothro DL, Bahnson TD, Ibarra M. Control of rapid ventricular response by radiofrequency catheter modification of the atrioventricular node in patients with medically refractory atrial fibrillation. *Circulation* 1994; 90:2299–2307.

78. Williamson BD, Man KC, Daoud E, Niebauer M, Strickberger SA, Morady F. Radiofrequency catheter modification of atrioventricular conduction to control the ventricular rate during atrial fibrillation. *N Engl J Med* 1994; 331:910.

79. Rodriguez LM, Smeets JL, Xie B, de Chillou C, Cheriex E, Pieters F, et al. Improvement in left ventricular function by ablation of atrioventricular nodal conduction in selected patients with lone atrial fibrillation. *Am J Cardiol* 1993; 72:1137–1140.

80. Toivonen L, Lommi J. Dependence of atrial sensing function on posture in a single-lead atrial triggered ventricular (VDD) pacemaker. *Pacing Clin Electrophysiol* 1996; 19:309–313.

81. Crick JCP. European multicenter prospective follow-up study of 1002 implants of a single lead VDD pacing system. *Pacing Clin Electrophysiol* 1991; 14:1724–1744.

82. Naegeli B, Osswald S, Pfisterer M, Burkart F. VDDR pacing: Short- and long-term stability of atrial sensing with a single lead system. *Pacing Clin Electrophysiol* 1996; 19(pt 1):455–464.

83. Higano ST, Hayes DL, Eisinger G. Sensor driven rate smoothing in a DDDR pacemaker. *Pacing Clin Electrophysiol* 1989; 12:922–929.

84. Wirtzfeld A, Schmidt G, Himmier FC, Stangl K. Physiological pacing. Present status and future developments. *Pacing Clin Electrophysiol* 1987; 10:41–56.

85. Fananapazir L, Bennett DH, Monks P. Atrial synchronized ventricular pacing. Contribution of the chronotropic response to improved exercise performance. *Pacing Clin Electrophysiol* 1983; 6:601–608.

86. Nordlander R, Hedman A, Pehrsson SK. Rate responsive pacing and exercise capacity—a comment. *Pacing Clin Electrophysiol* 1989; 12:749–751.

87. Saksena S, Praiash A, Hill M, Krol RB, Munsif AN, Mathew PP, et al. Prevention of recurrent atrial fibrillation with chronic dual-site right atrial pacing. *J Am Coll Cardiol* 1996; 28:687–694.

88. Daubert C, Mabo P, Berder V. Arrhythmia prevention by permanent atrial resynchronization in advanced interatrial block. *Eur Heart J* 1990; 11:237–242.

89. Oldroyd KG, Rae A, Carter R, Wingate C, Cobbe SM. Double-blind crossover comparison of the effects of dual-chamber pacing (DDD) and ventricular adaptive (VVIR) pacing on neuroendocrine variables, exercise performance and symptoms in complete heart block. *Br Heart J* 1991; 65:188–193.

90. Kruse I, Annian K, Conradson TB, Ryden L. A comparison of the acute and long-term hemodynamic effects of ventricular inhibited and atrial synchronous ventricular inhibited pacing. *Circulation* 1982; 56:846–855.

91. Karlof I. Hemodynamic effect of atrial triggered versus fixed rate pacing at rest and during exercise in complete heart block. *Acta Med Scand* 1975; 197:195–206.

92. Nitsch J, Seiderer M, Bull U, Luderitz B. Evaluation of left ventricular performance by radionuclide ventriculography in patients with AV versus ventricular demand pacemakers. *Am Heart J* 1984; 107:906–911.

93. Stewart WJ, Dicola VC, Harthorne JW, Gillam LD, Weyman AE. Doppler ultrasound measurement of cardiac output in patients with physiologic pacemakers. *Am J Cardiol* 1984; 54:308–312.

94. Alpert MA, Curtis JJ, Sanfelippo W, Flaker GC, Walls JT, Makerji V, et al. Comparative survival following permanent ventricular and dual-chamber pacing for patients with chronic symptomatic sinus node dysfunction with and without congestive heart failure. *Am Heart J* 1987; 13:958–965.

95. Hartzler GO, Maloney JD, Curtiss JJ, Barnhorst DA. Hemodynamic benefits of AV sequential pacing after cardiac surgery. *Am J Cardiol* 1977; 40:234.

96. Lukl J, Doupal V, Heinc P. Quality-of-life during DDD and dual sensor VVIR pacing. *Pacing Clin Electrophysiol* 1994; 17:1844.

97. Lau CP, Tai YT, Lee PWE, Cheung B, Tang MO, Lam WK. Quality-of-life in DDDR pacing: AV synchrony or rate adaptation? *Pacing Clin Electrophysiol* 1994; 17:1838–1843.

98. Rosenqvist NI, Brandi J, Schuller H. Atrial versus ventricular pacing in sinus node disease: A treatment comparison study. *Am Heart J* 1986; 111:292–297.

99. Feuer N, Shandling AH, Messenger JC, Castellanet CD, Thomas LA. Influence of cardiac pacing mode on the long-term development of atrial fibrillation. *Am J Cardiol* 1989; 64:1376–1379.

100. Grimm W, Langefeld H, Bernhard M, Clisiek K. Symptoms, cardiovascular risk profile and spontaneous ECG in paced patients: A five-year follow-up study. *Pacing Clin Electrophysiol* 1990; 13:2086–2090.

101. Markewitz A, Schad N, Hemmer W, Beiniheim C, Ciavolella M, Weinhold C. What is the most appropriate stimulation mode in patients with sinus node dysfunction. *Pacing Clin Electrophysiol* 1986; 9:1115–1120.

102. Hesselson AB, Parsormet V, Bernstein AD, Bonavita GJ. Deleterious effects of long-term single-chamber ventricular pacing in patients with sick sinus syndrome: The hidden benefits of dual-chamber pacing. *J Am Coll Cardiol* 1992; 19:1542–1549.

103. Rosenqvist M, Brandt J, Schuller H. Long-term pacing in sinus node disease: Effects of stimulation mode on cardiovascular morbidity and mortality. *Am Heart J* 1988; 116:16–22.

104. Santini M, Alexidou G, Arisalone G, Cacciatore G, Cini R, Turrito G. Relation of prognosis in sick sinus syndrome to age, conduction defects and modes of permanent cardiac pacing. *Am J Cardiol* 1990; 65:729–735.

105. Sasaki Y, Furihata A, Suyama K, Furihata Y, Koike S, Kobayashi T, et al. Comparison between ventricular inhibited pacing and physiologic pacing in sick sinus syndrome. *Am J Cardiol* 1991; 67:771–774.

106. Sgarbossa EB, Pinski SL, Maloney JD. The role of pacing modalities in long-term survival in the sick sinus syndrome. *Ann Intern Med* 1993; 119:359–365.

107. Sgarbossa EB, Pinski SL, Maloney JD, Simmons TW, Wilkoff BL, Castle LW, et al. Chronic atrial fibrillation and stroke in paced patients with sick sinus syndrome: Relevance of clinical characteristics and pacing modalities. *Circulation* 1993; 88:1045–1053.

108. Stangl K, Wirtzfeld A, Alt E, Blomer H. Difference between atrial single chamber pacing (AAI) and ventricular single chamber pacing (VVI) with respect to prognosis and antiarrhythmic effect in patients with sick sinus syndrome. *Pacing Clin Electrophysiol* 1990; 13:2080–2085.

109. Camm J, Katritsis D. Ventricular pacing for sick sinus syndrome—a risky business? *Pacing Clin Electrophysiol* 1990; 13:695–699.

110. Alpert MA, Curtiss JJ, Sanfellippo JF, Flaker GC, Walls JT, Mukerji V, et al. Comparative survival after permanent ventricular and dual-chamber pacing for patients with chronic high degree atrioventricular block with and without preexistent congestive heart failure. *J Am Coll Cardiol* 1986; 7:925–932.

111. Linde-Edelstam C, Gullberg B, Nordlander R, Pehrsson SK, Rosenqvist M, Ryden L. Longevity in patients with high degree AV block paced in the atrial synchronous or the fixed rate ventricular inhibited mode. *Pacing Clin Electrophysiol* 1992; 14:304–313.

112. Lamas GA, Estes NM III, Schneller S, Glaker OC. Does dual-chamber or atrial pacing prevent atrial fibrillation? The need for a randomized controlled trial. *Pacing Clin Electrophysiol* 1992; 15:1109–1113.

113. Furman S. Pacemaker syndrome. *Pacing Clin Electrophysiol* 1994; 17:14.

114. Schuller H, Brandt J. The pacemaker syndrome: Old and new causes. *Clin Cardiol* 1991; 14:336–340.

115. Travill CM, Sutton R. Pacemaker syndrome: An iatrogenic condition. *Br Heart J* 1992; 68:163.

116. Ausubel K, Furman S. The pacemaker syndrome. *Ann Intern Med* 1985; 103:420–429.

117. Heldman D, Mulvihill D, Nguyen H, et al. True incidence of pacemaker syndrome. *Pacing Clin Electrophysiol* 1990; 13:1742–1750.

118. Stangl K, Weil J, Seitz K, Laule M, Gerzer R. Influence of AV synchrony on the plasma levels of atrial natriuretic peptide (ANP) in patients with total AV block. *Pacing Clin Electrophysiol* 1988; 11:1176–1181.

119. Noll B, Krappe J, Goke B, Maisch B. Influence of pacing mode and rate on peripheral levels of atrial natriuretic peptide (ANP). *Pacing Clin Electrophysiol* 1989; 12:1763–1769.

120. Clemo HF, Baumgarten CM, Stambler BS, Wood MA, Ellenbogen KA. Atrial natriuretic factor. Implications of cardiac pacing and electrophysiology. *Pacing Clin Electrophysiol* 1994; 17:70.

121. Grant SCD, Bennet DH. Atrial latency in a dual-chamber pacing system causing inappropriate sequence of cardiac chamber activation. *Pacing Clin Electrophysiol* 1992; 15:116.

122. Daubert C, Mabo P, Berder V, et al. Atrial tachyarrhythmias associated with high degree interatrial conduction block: Prevention by permanent atrial resynchronisation. *Eur J Pacing Electrophysiol* 1994; 3:35.

123. Sulke N, Drisas A, Bostock J, Wells A, Morris R, Sowton E. "Subclinical" pacemaker syndrome: A randomized study of symptom-free patients with ventricular demand (VVI) pacemakers upgraded to dual-chamber devices. *Br Heart J* 1992; 67:57.

124. Rediker DE, Eagle KA, Homma S, Gillam LD, Harthorne JW. Clinical and hemodynamic comparison of VVI versus DDD pacing in patients with DDD pacemakers. *Am J Cardiol* 1988; 61:323–329.

125. Sulke N, Chambers J, Dritsas A, Sowton E. A randomized double-blind crossover comparison of four rate-responsive pacing models. *J Am Coll Cardiol* 1991; 17:696.

126. Haskell RJ, French WJ. Optimum AV interval in dual-chamber pacemakers. *Pacing Clin Electrophysiol* 1986; 9:670–675.

127. Janosik DL, Pearson AC, Buckingham TA, Labovitz AJ, Redd RM. The hemodynamic benefit of differential atrioventricular delay intervals for sensed and paced atrial events during physiologic pacing. *J Am Coll Cardiol* 1989; 14:499–507.

128. Mehta D, Gilmore S, Ward D, Camm AJ. Optimal AV delay at rest and during exercise in patients with dual-chamber pacemakers: A non-invasive assessment by continuous wave Doppler. *Br Heart J* 1989; 61:161–166.

129. Pearson AC, Janosik DL, Redd RR, Buckingham TA, Blum RI, Labovitz AJ. Doppler echocardiographic assessment of the effect of varying atrioventricular delay and pacemaker mode on left ventricular filling. *Am Heart J* 1988; 115:611–621.

130. Leman RB, Kratz JM. Radionuclide evaluation of dual-chamber pacing: Comparison between variable AV intervals and ventricular pacing. *Pacing Clin Electrophysiol* 1985; 8:408–414.

131. Videen JS, Huang SK, Bazgan ID, Mechling E, Patton DD. Hemodynamic comparison of ventricular pacing, atrioventricular sequential pacing and atrial synchronous ventricular pacing using radionuclide ventriculography. *Am J Cardiol* 1986; 57:1305–1308.

132. Frielingsdor J, Deseo T, Gerber AE, Bertel O. A comparison of quality-of-life in patients with dual-chamber pacemakers and individually programmed atrioventricular delays. *Pacing Clin Electrophysiol* 1996; 19:1147–1154.

133. Janosik DL, Pearson AC, Buckingham TA, Labovitz M, Redd RM. The hemodynamic benefit of differential AV delay intervals for sensed and paced atrial events during physiologic pacing. *J Am Coll Cardiol* 1989; 14:499–507.

134. Rees M, Haennel RG, Black WR, Kappagoda T. Effect of rate-adapting AV delay on stroke volume and cardiac output during atrial synchronous pacing. *Can J Cardiol* 1990; 6:445–452.

135. Ryden L, Karisson O, Kristensson BE. The importance of different AV intervals for exercise capacity. *Pacing Clin Electrophysiol* 1988; 11:1051–1052.

136. Cammili L, Alcidi L, Papeschi G, Wiechmaim V, Padeletti L, Grassi

G. Preliminary experience with the pH-triggered pacemaker. *Pacing Clin Electrophysiol* 1978; 1:448–457.

137. Rickards AF, Donaldson RM, Thalen HJ. The use of QT interval to determine pacing rate. Early clinical experience. *Pacing Clin Electrophysiol* 1983; 6:346–354.

138. Alt E, Hirgstetter C, Heinz M, Blomer H. Rate control of physiologic pacemakers by central venous blood temperature. *Circulation* 1986; 73:1206–1212.

139. Benditt DG, Mianulli M, Fetter J, Benson DW Jr, Dunnigan A, Molina E, et al. Single-chamber cardiac pacing with activity initiated chronotropic response. Evaluation by cardiopulmonary exercise testing. *Circulation* 1987; 75:184–189.

140. Benditt DG, Milstein S, Buetikofer J, Gornick CC, Mianulli M, Fetter J. Sensor-triggered, rate variable cardiac pacing. Current technologies and clinical implications. *Ann Intern Med* 1987; 107:714–724.

141. Bennett T, Sharma A, Sutton R. Development of a rate adaptive pacemaker based on the maximum rate-of-rise of right ventricular pressure (RV dP/dt max). *Pacing Clin Electrophysiol* 1992; 15:219–234.

142. Bloomfield P, Macareavey D, Kerr F, Fananapazir L. Long-term follow-up of patients with the QT rate adaptive pacemaker. *Pacing Clin Electrophysiol* 1989; 12:1114.

143. den Dulk K, Bouwels L, Lindemans F, Rankin I, Brugada P, Wellens HJ. The Activitrax rate-responsive pacemaker system. *Am J Cardiol* 1988; 61:107–112.

144. Fearnot NE, Jolgren DL, Tacker WA, Nelson JP, Geddes LA. Increasing cardiac rate by measurement of right ventricular temperature. *Pacing Clin Electrophysiol* 1984; 7:1240–1245.

145. Lau DP, Antoniou A, Ward DE, Camm AJ. Initial clinical experience with a minute ventilation sensing rate modulated pacemaker. Improvements in exercise capacity and symptomatology. *Pacing Clin Electrophysiol* 1988; 11:1815–1822.

146. Lau DP. The range of sensors and algorithms used in rate adaptive cardiac pacing. *Pacing Clin Electrophysiol* 1992; 15:1177–1211.

147. Lau CO, Tai Y, Fong P. Clinical experience with an activity sensing DDDR pacemaker using an accelerometer sensor. *Pacing Clin Electrophysiol* 1992; 15:334–343.

148. Lipkin DP, Buller N, Frenneaux M, Ludgate I, Lowe T, Webb SC, et al. Randomized crossover trial of rate responsive Activitrax and conventional fixed rate ventricular pacing. *Br Heart J* 1987; 58:613–616.

149. Mond H, Strathinore N, Kertes P, Hunt D, Baker G. Rate responsive pacing using a minute ventilation sensor. *Pacing Clin Electrophysiol* 1988; 11:1866–1874.

150. Ruiter J, Heemels J, Kee D, van Mechelen R. Adaptive rate pacing controlled by the right ventricular preejection interval. Clinical experience with a physiological pacing system. *Pacing Clin Electrophysiol* 1992; 15:886–894.

151. Celiker A, Alehan D, Tokel NK, Lenk MK, Ozome S. Experience with dual-sensor rate-responsive pacemakers in children. *Eur Heart J* 1996; 17:1251–1255.

152. Provenier F, Van Acker R, Backers J, Van Wassenhove E, De Meyer V, Jordaens L. Clinical observations with a dual-sensor rate-adaptive single chamber pacemaker. *Pacing Clin Electrophysiol* 1992; 15:1821–1825.

153. Cowell R, Morris-Thurgood J, Paul V, Ilsley C, Carum M. Are we being driven to two sensors? Clinical benefits of sensor cross-checking. *Pacing Clin Electrophysiol* 1993; 16:1441–1444.

154. Mazzetti H, Cussaut A, Tentori C, Dussaut E, Lazzari JO. Transarterial permanent pacing of the left ventricle. *Pacing Clin Electrophysiol* 1990; 13:588–592.

155. Winner SJ, Boon NA. Transvenous pacemaker electrodes placed unintentionally in the left ventricle: Three cases. *Postgrad Med J* 1989; 65:98–102.

156. Vilacosta I, Zamorano J, Camino A, San Roman JA, Rollan MJ, Pinto A. Infected transvenous permanent pacemakers: Role of transesophageal echocardiography. *Am Heart J* 1993; 125:904–906.

157. Vilacosta I, Sarria C, San Roman JA, Jimenez J, Castillo JA, Iturralde E, et al. Usefulness of transesophageal echocardiography for diagnosis of infected transvenous permanent pacemakers. *Circulation* 1994; 89:2684–2687.

158. Smith HJ, Fernot NE, Byrd CL, Wilkoff BL, Love CJ, Sellers TD. Five-years experience with intravascular lead extraction. *Pacing Clin Electrophysiol* 1994; 17:2016.

159. Spittell PC, Vlietstra RE, Hayes DL, Higano ST. Venous obstruction due to permanent transvenous pacemaker electrodes: Treatment with percutaneous transluminal balloon venoplasty. *Pacing Clin Electrophysiol* 1990; 13:2714.

160. Spittell PC, Hayes DL. Venous complications after insertion of a transvenous pacemaker. *Mayo Clin Proc* 1992; 67:258–265.

161. Antonelli D, Turgeman Y, Kaveh Z, Artoul S, Rosenfeld T. Short-term thrombosis after transvenous permanent pacemaker insertion. *Pacing Clin Electrophysiol* 1989; 12:280–282.

162. Mazzetti H, Dussaut A, Tentori C, Dussaut E, Lazzari JO. Superior vena cava occlusion and/or syndrome related to pacemaker leads. *Am Heart J* 1993; 125:831–837.

163. Lindsay HS, Chennells PM, Perrins EJ. Successful treatment by balloon venoplasty and stent insertion of obstruction of the superior vena cava by an endocardial pacemaker lead. *Br Heart J* 1994; 71:363–365.

164. Chauvin M, Brecheumacher C. Muscle stimulation caused by a pacemaker current leakage: The role of the insulation failure of a polyurethane coating. *J Electrophysiol* 1987; 1:326–329.

165. Kawanish D, Brinken J, Kay GN, Love C, Mutter M, Pioger G, et al. Prevalence of fracture of an atrial pacemaker lead J-shape retention wire in a multicenter study. *Circulation* 1995; 92:I150.

166. Naegeli B, Osswald S, Deola N, Burkart F. Intermittent pacemaker dysfunction caused by digital mobile telephones. *J Am Coll Cardiol* 1996; 27:1471–1477.

167. Barbaro V, Barolini P, Donato A, Militello C, Altamura G, Ammirati F, et al. Do European GSM mobile phones pose a potential risk to pacemaker patients? *Pacing Clin Electrophysiol* 1995; 18:1218–1224.

168. Ellenbogen FC, Wood MA. Cellular telephones and pacemakers: Urgent call or wrong number? (editorial). *J Am Coll Cardiol* 1996; 27:1478–1479.

169. Hayes DL, VonFeldt LK, Neubauer SA, Rasmussen MJ, Christiansen JR. Does cellular phone technology cause pacemaker or defibrillator interference? (abstr). *Pacing Clin Electrophysiol* 1995; 18:842.

170. Hayes DL, Wang PJ, Reynolds DN, Estes M III, Griffith JL, Steffens RA, et al. Interference with cardiac pacemakers by cellular telephones. *N Engl J Med* 1997; 336:1473–1479.

SYNCOPE, SUDDEN DEATH, AND CARDIOPULMONARY RESUSCITATION

35

DIAGNOSIS AND MANAGEMENT OF SYNCOPE

Harisios Boudoulas / Steven D. Nelson / Stephen F. Schaal / Richard P. Lewis

Syncope is a sudden and transient loss of consciousness. The occurrence of syncope in the general population, as reflected in the 26-year surveillance of the Framingham Study, is 3.0 percent in men and 3.5 percent in women in the general population. As a general rule, the incidence of syncope increases with the age.[1]

As an initial presentation, syncope denotes a diversity of disorders ranging from a benign episode to sudden death. Studies in recent years have documented the multiple causes and the widely divergent mortality risks associated with an episode of syncope. On the basis of these studies, patients with a transient episode of altered consciousness (presyncope) and those with complete loss of consciousness (syncope) can be classified into three broad categories[2,3] (Table 35-1): *cardiac syncope, noncardiac syncope,* and *syncope of undetermined cause.* The relative incidence of these categories varies with the clinical site from which the patients are selected. In the emergency room, noncardiac syncope is most common. For patients admitted to the hospital, cardiac syncope is the most common diagnosis. Among all patients in whom syncope or presyncope is the presenting symptom, an etiologic diagnosis cannot be readily established in approximately one-third.[4-7]

Clearly, the highest mortality occurs among those with cardiac syncope. Among all patients with syncope associated with cardiac disease, sudden death is inordinately frequent.

TABLE 35-1
CLASSIFICATION OF SYNCOPE

I. Noncardiac
II. Cardiac
III. Undetermined cause

NONCARDIAC SYNCOPE (Table 35-2)

Sudden transient loss or impairment of consciousness occurs under a wide variety of circumstances. The pathophysiologic mechanisms, diagnostic features, and therapy for these disorders will be discussed below.

Neurocardiogenic Syncope

The syndrome of neurocardiogenic syncope, the common faint (also referred to as neurally mediated hypotension, vasovagal syncope, vasodepressor syncope), is one of the most common causes of syncope.[8-10] This disorder is considered to be an abnormality in the complex neurocardiovascular interactions responsible for maintaining systemic and cerebral perfusion (Fig. 35-1).

TABLE 35-2
CLASSIFICATION OF NONCARDIAC SYNCOPE

Neurocardiogenic	Metabolic, drugs
Orthostatic	Hypoxia
Cerebrovascular	Hypoglycemia
Seizure disorders	Hyperventilation, panic
Carotid sinus hypersensitivity	attacks
Situational	Ethanol, other drugs
Cough	Other forms of syncope or
Swallowing	conditions mimicking
Valsalva	syncope
Micturition	Vertigo
Defecation	Migraine
Diver's	Psychiatric
Postprandial	

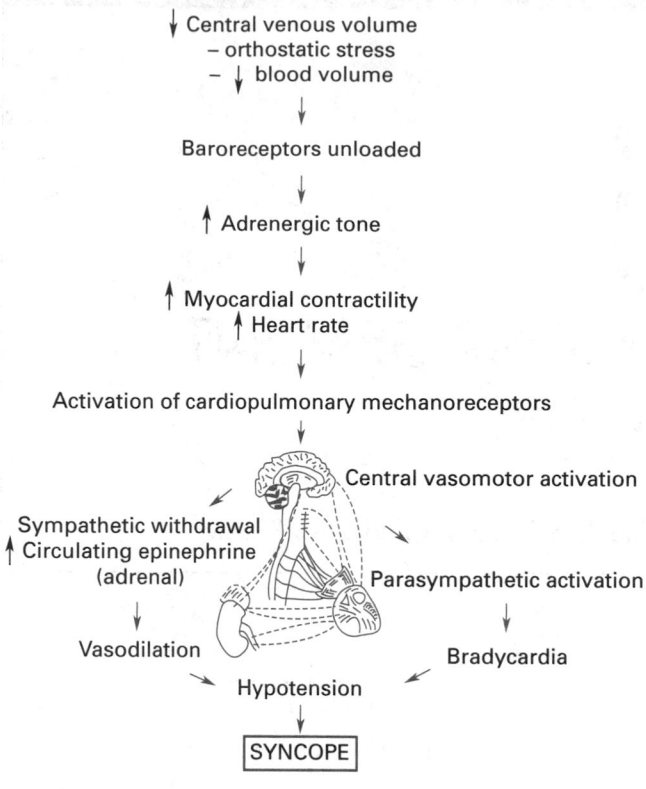

FIGURE 35-1

Presumed mechanism of neurocardiogenic syncope. Schematic presentation. ↑ = increase; ↓ = decrease.

PATHOPHYSIOLOGY

The pathophysiology of neurocardiogenic syncope is quite complex and incompletely understood.[11–15] Under normal circumstances, upright posture causes venous pooling and a transient decrease in arterial pressure, resulting in an unloading of baroreceptors. Reflex augmentation of sympathetic activity and parasympathetic withdrawal result in peripheral arterial vasoconstriction, venoconstriction, and an increase in heart rate and contractility. These adaptive mechanisms serve to maintain normal systemic and cerebral perfusion. Neuroendocrine systems (e.g., renin-angiotensin and vasopressin) may be important modulators of homeostasis during prolonged periods of orthostatic stress.[10]

Individuals susceptible to neurocardiogenic syncope are unable to maintain the adaptive neurocardiovascular responses to upright posture for prolonged periods of time. These patients tend to have a modest reduction in central blood volume, which is aggravated by upright posture.[16] Increases in circulating catecholamines and cardiac adrenergic tone in response to orthostatic stress result in increased myocardial contractility.[17] Studies in animal models suggest that, under these conditions, cardiopulmonary mechanoreceptors are activated, resulting in increased neural traffic across afferent C fibers leading to the central nervous system vasomotor center; this in turn results in reflex paradoxical vasodilation (vasodepressor response) and bradycardia (cardioinhibitory response).[18,19] The final result is hypotension, cerebral hypoperfusion, cere-

bral anoxia, and syncope. This paradoxical reflex is believed to be a variant of the Bezold-Jarisch reflex and has also been documented during nitrate therapy for acute myocardial ischemia, and during acute hemorrhagic syndromes.[19–22] In addition, central vasomotor center activation is believed to cause several of the prodromal symptoms of diaphoresis, nausea, vomiting, and dyspnea that frequently accompany neurocardiogenic syncope. Recent evidence from patients with denervated hearts (i.e., cardiac transplantation patients) and those with neurocardiogenic syncope raises the possibility that other neurohumoral mechanisms, primarily involving the peripheral circulation, may play an important role.[23]

The mechanism of paradoxical vasodilation observed during neurocardiogenic syncope is incompletely understood. Clinical studies have shown that serum epinephrine concentrations surge prior to the syncopal event with resultant intense β_2 activation, which may cause inappropriate vasodilation and syncope.[24,25] Withdrawal of peripheral sympathetic neural activity at the time of neurocardiogenic syncope has also been demonstrated by direct recordings of sympathetic neural activity.[26]

The paradoxical bradycardia (cardioinhibitory response) during neurocardiogenic syncope is due to a surge in cardiac parasympathetic tone and usually lags vasodilation by several seconds.[27] The cardioinhibitory response is highly variable, ranging from a relative bradycardia with heart rates in the 40 to 60 beats per minute range to profound periods of asystole (Fig. 35-2). Variable degrees of atrioventricular (AV) block and junctional escape rhythms are observed as well. *Bradycardia aggravates but is not the principal cause of hypotension during neurocardiogenic syncope.* Maintaining heart rate with atropine or cardiac pacing will often reduce, but not prevent, symptomatic hypotension during neurocardiogenic syncope. Elderly patients with neurocardiogenic syncope are likely to have a predominant vasodepressor response without a significant cardioinhibitory component.

CLINICAL CHARACTERISTICS

Predisposition to neurocardiogenic syncope occurs under a wide variety of clinical circumstances. Indeed, the neurocardiogenic reaction per se may be the ultimate cause of most types of syncope. Neurocardiogenic syncope is often noted in individuals receiving sympathetic blocking agents and vasodilator drugs for hypertension, in elderly individuals receiving tranquilizers, in patients with acute or chronic anemia, and in those with transient reductions in blood volume, such as occur following a brisk diuresis or blood donation. Neurocardiogenic syncope complicates acute febrile infections and occurs with prolonged recumbency in chronic illness. Normal individuals at prolonged bed rest have a propensity for fainting, particularly when they arise abruptly from a sitting or recumbent position. Neurocardiogenic syncope is probably the most frequent cause of cardiovascular collapse during dental manipulations (dental syncope).[28] Neurocardiogenic syncope has been noted to follow strenuous exercise and may also occur during rapid acceleration in air flight, particularly

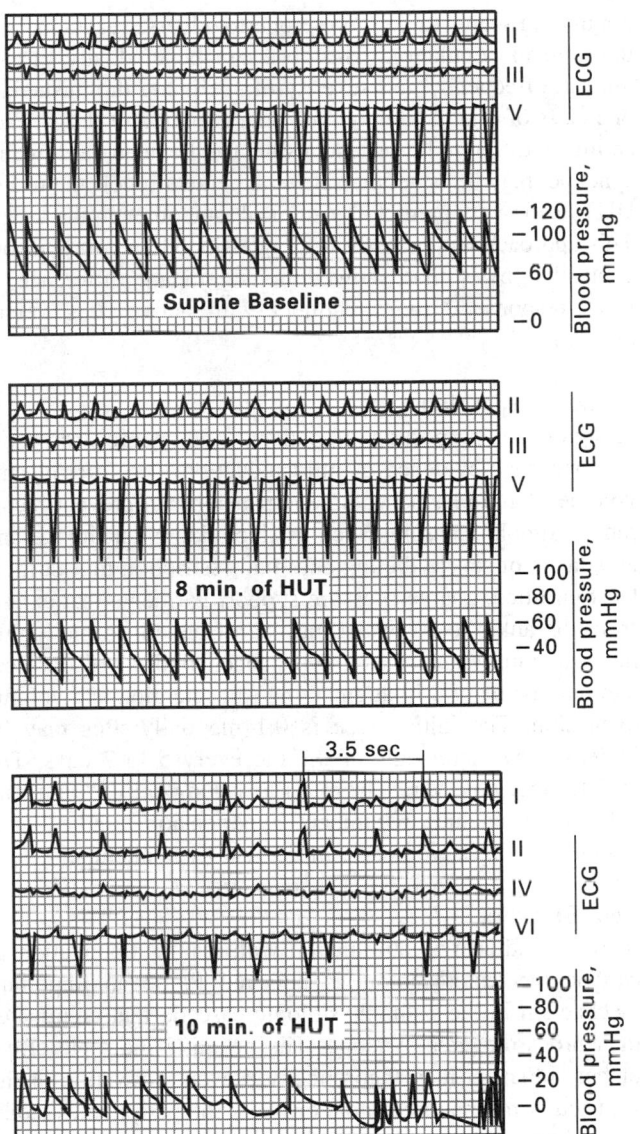

FIGURE 35-2

Heart rate and blood pressure response to 60° head-up tilt in patients with syncope of undefined origin. *Top.* Baseline recordings with blood pressure of approximately 130/70 mmHg and heart rate of 75 beats per minute. *Middle.* After 8 min of tilt, heart rate falls gradually to 45 beats per minute with progressive decrease in blood pressure. *Bottom.* Syncope occurs with profound hypotension and 3.5-s asystolic period. (From Schaal et al.,[3] with permission.)

when centrifugal force is applied in the head-to-foot position.[2,3] Neurocardiogenic syncope of an unusual type may occur in pregnancy, being precipitated when the patient is supine and reversed when the patient assumes a lateral decubitus or upright posture (see also Chap. 92).

The identification of aggravating factors ("triggers") is important not only for the diagnosis but also for the prevention of syncope. Situations that decrease central venous volume or increase cardiovascular adrenergic tone are particularly important in the aggravation of neurocardiogenic syncope. The postprandial state, exertion in warm environments, prolonged upright posture, sodium restriction or diuretic use,

and emotional or stressful situations are but a few important triggers to consider. Recent evidence suggests a relationship between chronic fatigue syndrome and neurocardiogenic syncope.[29]

The classic syncopal spell is often preceded by a constellation of prodromal symptoms occurring several seconds prior to the syncopal event. The prodrome may include symptoms of nausea, headache, diaphoresis, dizziness, chest pain, palpitations, dyspnea, and paresthesia. These symptoms may also persist for several minutes to several hours after the syncopal episode has resolved. Patients with sudden loss of consciousness may not report prodromal symptoms. Usually the spell occurs when the patient is upright and is less likely while seated. *Syncope while supine should prompt the search for etiologies other than neurocardiogenic syncope.*

During the syncopal episode, patients typically appear pale and diaphoretic, with a slow, diminished pulse. Occasionally, seizure-like activity may occur during asystolic periods. The syncopal spell classically resolves spontaneously once the patient is in the supine position but may recur if the patient stands or sits upright soon after the initial spell. The observations of a bystander are particularly helpful. *If the patient experiences a prolonged period of confusion after the syncopal event or is incontinent, etiologies other than neurocardiogenic syncope should be considered.*

Natural History

The frequency and clinical significance of neurocardiogenic syncope are highly variable. Neurocardiogenic syncope may occur as a single isolated event or as a cluster of spells over weeks to months, or it may be a recurrent lifetime problem. The overall prognosis in patients with neurocardiogenic syncope is quite favorable compared to arrhythmic or left ventricular outflow obstructive forms of cardiac syncope. A very small subset of patients has been described as having "malignant" neurocardiogenic syncope.[29–33] This form of syncope is characterized by profound periods of asystole with sudden loss of consciousness, potentially leading to severe trauma and a theoretically increased risk of ischemia-mediated ventricular tachyarrhythmias. This risk is greatest in patients with underlying structural heart disease.

DIAGNOSTIC EVALUATION

Head-up tilt (HUT) testing has become a useful diagnostic study for the identification of patients with neurocardiogenic syncope.[34–38] The sensitivity, specificity, and reproducibility of HUT testing depend on the patient population studied and the HUT protocol employed.[34–46] HUT at an angle of 60° to 90° for a time period of 20 to 60 min has been found to yield a sensitivity ranging from 20 to 74 percent. Longer durations of HUT (45 to 60 min) lead to improved sensitivity without a significant increase in false-positive responses.[38–40] Recent studies suggest that the optimal HUT angle should be between 60° and 80°. Tilt angles less than 45° sacrifice sensitivity, while angles greater than 80° can result in more false-positive studies.[38,44] An average of 63 percent of patients studied with

HUT after a negative electrophysiologic study were found to have a positive HUT response, suggesting that a significant proportion of patients with unexplained syncope have neurocardiogenic syncope.[40] The specificity of HUT testing is typically greater than 90 percent, while the reproducibility is reportedly greater than 70 percent.[44,45] Isoproterenol infusion during HUT testing has been shown to improve sensitivity.[37] Low-dose isoproterenol infusion (<2 µg/min) has been shown to nearly double the number of positive responses compared to baseline (short-duration HUT), with an acceptable specificity of 93 percent and reproducibility of 83 percent.[42] High doses of isoproterenol, especially at HUT angles of greater than 80°, markedly increase the incidence of false-positive responses.[44]

MANAGEMENT

Immediate therapy for the common faint consists of placing the patient in a recumbent position with the head down. With profound and persistent bradycardia, intravenously administered atropine may be required. Vasopressor therapy is rarely needed to reverse hypotension.

The management of recurrent neurocardiogenic syncope is challenging and sometimes unsatisfactory. The choice of therapy should be based on an understanding of the neurocardiovascular cascade that eventually culminates in neurocardiogenic syncope. First-line therapy includes counseling the patient to avoid dehydration, prolonged periods of standing motionless, and situations known to trigger syncope. Increased salt intake may be beneficial, if not contraindicated. Patients should be educated to recognize premonitory symptoms and, if they are present, to assume a recumbent position and cough in order to maintain cerebral perfusion.

The severity and frequency of recurrence of neurocardiogenic syncope are highly variable.[47] As a result, its pharmacologic management must be highly individualized and is not necessarily lifelong in duration. Patients with infrequent, near-syncopal spells may respond to conservative measures alone. Frequent syncopal spells, especially if trauma occurs, usually necessitate pharmacologic interventions (Table 35-3).

Therapeutic options include volume expansion, beta-adrenergic receptor blockade, anticholinergic agents, methylxanthines, serotonin reuptake inhibitors, and, rarely, artificial cardiac pacing. A stepped approach to pharmacologic therapy is advisable, starting with low initial doses, as this patient

TABLE 35-3

THERAPEUTIC OPTIONS FOR NEUROCARDIOGENIC SYNCOPE

Counseling
Volume expansion
Beta blockers
Anticholinergic agents
Serotonin reuptake inhibitors
Methylxanthines
Cardiac pacing

population seems to be more prone to adverse reactions than the general population. The dose can be gradually titrated until the frequency and severity of spells are diminished. If one class of drug is ineffective, a combination of drugs, each acting on different limbs responsible for the neurocardiogenic syncope, may be beneficial. Several centers report the use of HUT testing to predict the clinical outcome of therapy.[35] This approach has recently been questioned by two placebo-controlled trials that showed no significant difference in HUT response during treatment with active drug versus placebo.[48,49]

Volume Expansion

A significant proportion of patients with neurocardiogenic syncope have evidence of mild reduction in central plasma volume,[16] and plasma volume expansion can prevent recurrence. Simple measures such as liberalizing salt intake and avoidance of severe dieting and fluid restriction may suffice. Custom-fitted, counterpressure support garments that extend from the ankle to the waist may be of benefit in the highly motivated individual. In some instances, fludrocortisone acetate may be helpful in augmenting salt retention and volume expansion. The initial dose is 0.1 mg daily; this may be increased by increments of 0.1 mg every 5 to 7 days. The maintenance dose varies from 0.1 to 1.0 mg daily.[50] Potential side effects include recumbent hypertension, marked fluid retention, congestive heart failure, and hypokalemia.

Beta Blockers

Increased adrenergic stimulation with resultant activation of cardiac mechanoreceptors is believed to be an important mechanism in the pathophysiologic cascade that culminates in neurocardiogenic syncope. The negative inotropic effect of beta blockers may theoretically prevent activation of the ventricular mechanoreceptors or block the peripheral vasodilator effects of beta-adrenergic receptor stimulation. Oral metoprolol has been shown to prevent symptom recurrence in patients with neurocardiogenic syncope. In addition, intravenous metoprolol can blunt the hypotension and bradycardia during HUT testing.[51] Recent studies suggest that patients who require isoproterenol infusion during tilt to elicit neurocardiogenic syncope are more likely to respond to beta blockers than are patients who are tilt-positive without isoproterenol provocation.[52]

Anticholinergic Agents

During neurocardiogenic syncope, certain subsets of patients experience profound bradycardia that can aggravate the hypotension associated with vasodilation. This subset is believed to have a sudden surge in vagal activity because the bradyarrhythmia, but not the vasodilation, can be prevented by intravenous atropine. The profound bradyarrhythmias are primarily observed in the young and presumably healthy age group. Despite the unimpressive response of neurocardiogenic syncope to atropine, certain other anticholinergic drugs may be of benefit, if tolerated.[53]

Transdermal scopolamine has been shown to be a useful preventive agent in certain subsets of patients with recurrent neurocardiogenic syncope.[16,54] Its mechanism of action is poorly understood. Certainly, the anticholinergic actions of scopolamine may be important in preventing the hypotension that is due to bradycardia. More important, however, may be the scopolamine-induced depressant effect on the central nervous system transmission to the autonomic nervous system. These central actions of scopolamine are believed to be important for the prevention of the nausea of motion sickness, which may incidentally involve neuropathways common to the vasovagal pathways.[55]

The class 1A antiarrhythmic drug, disopyramide, has known anticholinergic and negative inotropic properties. These properties, which are considered undesirable effects of disopyramide in the therapy of tachyarrhythmias, may prevent the activation of cardiopulmonary mechanoreceptors and the neurogenic reflex observed in neurocardiogenic syncope. Disopyramide has been shown to prevent tilt-induced syncope and to prevent spontaneous syncopal spells.[56] Antiarrhythmic drugs such as disopyramide, however, must be used with caution because of their potential for proarrhythmia. In addition, the noncardiovascular anticholinergic side effects of disopyramide may be intolerable for some patients. Recent data have raised questions concerning the efficacy of disopyramide as compared to placebo control in a small number of patients with neurocardiogenic syncope.[56]

Serotonin Reuptake Inhibitors

Recent data have led to the suggestion that serotonin may be an important mediator of inappropriate vasodilation and bradycardia in animal models of hemorrhagic shock. Blockade of serotonin receptors with methysergide can block this event. Recent clinical studies, somewhat paradoxically, suggest that the serotonin reuptake inhibitors fluoxetine hydrochloride (Prozac) and sertraline hydrochloride (Zoloft) may both be beneficial in the prevention of neurocardiogenic syncope after 4 to 6 weeks of therapy in approximately 55 percent of patients with severe, recurrent neurocardiogenic syncope.[57,58]

Methylxanthines

Theophylline appears to reduce the frequency of neurocardiogenic syncope in patients who can tolerate this drug. Two separate clinical studies have shown that theophylline can prevent recurrences in greater than 70 percent of patients.[59,60] Even low doses of theophylline (6 to 12 mg/kg per day) appear to have benefit in those patients who cannot tolerate higher doses. Unfortunately, side effects such as nervousness, anxiety, and gastrointestinal abnormalities limit the usefulness of theophylline in this setting. Methylxanthines, such as theophylline, appear to have three different pharmacologic effects that may be beneficial therapeutically. In low concentrations, methylxanthines are potent adenosine receptor antagonists. Recent evidence suggests that adenosine phosphates can provoke syncope in susceptible patients.[61] At "therapeutic" serum concentrations, theophylline acts as a phosphodiesterase inhibitor and as a calcium transport inhibitor, both of which may be important in maintaining peripheral vascular tone.[62]

Cardiac Pacing

The role of artificial cardiac pacing for the management of neurocardiogenic syncope is controversial.[63,64] Similar to the use of anticholinergics, pacing is valuable in preventing the component of hypotension that is due to bradycardia; however, peripheral vasodilation may still occur despite heart rate control as noted. *Cardiac pacing should be reserved for those patients who have documented episodes of prolonged bradycardia associated with the syncopal spell.* Pacing may be especially beneficial in those rare patients with malignant neurocardiogenic syncope due to cardiac asystole.[30] Temporary pacing during HUT-provoked syncope can be used to identify the patient who may benefit from permanent pacing. These patients typically require pharmacologic therapy in addition to cardiac pacing to prevent the vasodepressor component. Dual-chamber pacing is the preferred mode of pacing in order to maintain AV synchrony.[64]

Orthostatic Syncope (Orthostatic Hypotension)

Orthostatic hypotension is a disorder in which assumption of the upright posture is associated with a fall in arterial pressure associated with light-headedness, blurring of vision, and a sense of weakness and unsteadiness.[2,3,65–69] Hypotension is progressive over a period of seconds to minutes, depending upon the degree of loss in reflex adaptation. If the fall in perfusion pressure to the brain is profound, syncope occurs. If the individual assumes the recumbent posture, arterial pressure rapidly normalizes and consciousness is restored.

From the diagnostic viewpoint, orthostatic hypotension is conveniently classified under three major causes[2,3]: *venous pooling and/or blood volume depletion, pharmacologic agents,* and *neurogenic causes* (Table 35-4). In certain cases, circulating endogenous vasodilators may result in orthostatic hypotension and syncope.

VENOUS POOLING AND/OR BLOOD VOLUME DEPLETION

Excessive venous pooling accounts for the postural hypotension accompanying sustained bed rest, prolonged standing, pregnancy, and marked venous varicosities. Tall, asthenic individuals with poorly developed musculature are particularly prone to this form of postural hypotension.[68–74] Deconditioning of normal autonomic reflex vasoconstriction may contribute to the orthostatic hypotension associated with prolonged bed rest and following extended periods of weightlessness in astronauts.[2,3] Blood volume depletion accounts for the orthostatic hypotension associated with dehydration, excessive diuresis, anemia, hemorrhage, excessive gastrointestinal fluid loss, third-space sequestration, prolonged fever, renal dialysis, excessive perspiration, adrenal insufficiency, pheochromocytoma, and diabetes insipidus.[74–79]

TABLE 35-4

CAUSES OF ORTHOSTATIC SYNCOPE

Venous pooling or volume depletion	Neurogenic causes
Prolonged bed rest	Diabetes mellitus
Prolonged standing	Alcoholic neuropathy
Pregnancy	Spinal cord disease
Venous varicosities	Amyloidosis
Blood loss	Multiple sclerosis
Dehydration	Multiple cerebral infarcts
Pharmacologic agents	Parkinsonism
Antihypertensive drugs	Tabes dorsalis
Sympathetic blocking agents	Syringomyelia
Calcium channel blockers	Idiopathic orthostatic hypotension
Converting enzyme inhibitors	Shy-Drager syndrome (multiple system atrophy)
Nitrates	Circulating endogenous vasodilators
Diuretics	Hyperbradykinism
Antidepressants, antipsychotic drugs	Mastocytosis
Phenothiazides	Carcinoid syndrome
Tranquilizers	
Antiparkinsonian drugs	
Central nervous system depressants	

PHARMACOLOGIC AGENTS

Pharmacologically induced postural hypotension is a complicating side effect in the administration of several classes of drugs, including antihypertensives, sympathetic blocking agents, diuretics, nitrates, calcium channel blockers, converting enzyme inhibitors, antidepressants, phenothiazines, tranquilizers, antipsychotic drugs, antiparkinsonian drugs, and central nervous system depressants.[74,80]

NEUROGENIC CAUSES

Neurogenic postural hypotension has been observed in a wide variety of diseases affecting the autonomic nervous system. Specific entities include diabetes mellitus, alcoholic neuropathy, spinal cord injury, idiopathic orthostatic hypotension, and Shy-Drager syndrome[75-79] (see Table 35-4). Administration of adrenergic blocking drugs and vasodilators may accentuate the predisposition to orthostatic hypotension in patients with primary neurogenic postural hypotension.[80]

In the idiopathic form of orthostatic hypotension, postural hypotension is accompanied by relatively fixed heart rate, heat intolerance, anhidrosis, nocturnal polyuria, urinary and anal sphincter dysfunction, and impotency.[77,78] In the Shy-Drager syndrome, orthostatic hypotension is accompanied by multiple central nervous system manifestations and is referred as *multiple system atrophy*.[75,79] The central nervous system manifestations in multiple system atrophy may be indistinguishable from those of idiopathic Parkinson's disease and may precede or follow the onset of orthostatic hypotension.

The prognosis appears to be worse in patients with multiple system atrophy than in those with idiopathic orthostatic hypotension, with death often resulting from general debilitation and its complications. Severe supine hypertension may complicate the presence of orthostatic hypotension.

When the total or central blood volume is depleted in the presence of an intact autonomic nervous system, pallor, coldness of the extremities, tachycardia, and sweating are evident. Relative bradycardia may occur at the time of syncope, and the clinical presentation may be identical to that of neurocardiogenic syncope. When orthostatic hypotension is due to loss or severe impairment of autonomic reflexes, the syncope is associated with little or no change in heart rate, and there is an absence of the pallor, sweating, and other manifestations observed in patients with intact autonomic reflexes.

THERAPY

Effective therapy in postural hypotension is closely linked to an accurate diagnosis. Primary emphasis must be based on treatable causes, in particular, pharmacologically induced postural hypotension, blood volume loss, venous pooling, and reversible disease entities. A summary of treatment modalities currently applied among patients with chronic orthostatic hypotension is presented[2,3] in Table 35-5. The wide variety of recommended approaches reflects the frequently disappointing therapeutic response to each of these modalities. Commonly, multiple maneuvers are necessary to achieve optimum control of postural hypotension. Of singular importance is the need to have the patient avoid experiences, such as dehydration, that accentuate postural hypotension and to restrict the use of pharmacologic agents that induce blood volume depletion, vasodilation, and sympathetic blockade.[80] *Patients should be instructed about simple adaptive maneuvers, in-*

TABLE 35-5

TREATMENT OF CHRONIC ORTHOSTATIC HYPOTENSION

I. Evaluation for reversible and accentuating disease entities
II. Specific modalities for irreversible orthostatic hypotension
  A. Mechanical measures
    1. Head-up position of bed
    2. Lower body compression garment
    3. Slow motion and calf muscle flexing on arising
  B. Volume expansion
    1. High-salt diet
    2. Fludrocortisone acetate
  C. Pharmacologic agents
    1. Sympathomimetics
    2. Vasoconstrictors
    3. Beta-receptor blockers
    4. Alpha$_2$-receptor agonists
  D. Atrial pacing

cluding slow rising from a recumbent or sitting position, flexing of the calf muscles during assumption of the upright posture, and avoidance of prolonged immobility during standing. The use of erythropoietin to expand red blood cell mass and blood volume has been used to maintain pressure in the upright posture in certain cases of orthostatic hypotension.[81]

Cerebrovascular Syncope

In patients with extensive occlusive disease of the origins of the brachiocephalic vessels, such as pulseless disease (e.g., aortic arch syndrome and Takayasu's arteritis), syncope is not uncommon.[2,3,82] With lesser degrees of cerebral occlusive disease, as with atherosclerotic narrowing, transient lowering of arterial pressure such as that immediately following assumption of the upright posture may be followed by vague symptoms suggesting impaired cerebral blood flow. In patients with cerebrovascular occlusive disease, a transient decrease in cardiac output and arterial pressure may provoke syncope at levels of arterial pressure that would otherwise be tolerated (see also Chap. 99).

Impairment or loss of consciousness in relation to changing positions of the head, particularly hyperextension and lateral rotation, has been attributed to mechanical narrowing of the vertebral arteries by skeletal deformities of the cervical spine. Such symptoms have been observed in patients with Klippel-Feil deformity, cervical spondylosis, and severe cervical osteoarthritis. Altered consciousness is often preceded by vestibular symptoms. When vertigo is a predominant symptom, the syndrome of benign postural vertigo must be considered.[2,3]

Among patients with major occlusive disease of the carotid-vertebrobasilar arterial system, manual compression of the carotid artery as a test for carotid sinus hypersensitivity may induce syncope, at times associated with focal neurologic signs. The occurrence of syncope under such circumstances may be misdiagnosed as carotid sinus syndrome. The occurrence of a cerebrovascular accident following manual compression of the carotid sinus has been reported in patients with carotid disease, and *carotid sinus massage should be avoided in patients with symptomatic or suspected occlusive carotid vascular disease.*

Syncope in the *subclavian steal syndrome* is caused by major occlusive disease of the subclavian artery proximal to the origin of the vertebral artery. During upper extremity exercise, blood flow is shunted retrograde, by the circle of Willis, to the distal subclavian artery. The consequent decrease in cerebral circulation induces cerebral ischemia.[2,3,82] This syndrome is suggested by the findings of diminished brachial arterial pressure on the affected side, a bruit that is maximal over the supraclavicular area adjacent to the origin of the vertebral artery, and the induction of symptoms by exercise of the involved extremity.

While focal neurologic symptoms and signs are the usual neurologic manifestations of cerebral emboli, transient loss of consciousness can be a primary presenting symptom. *Syncopal episodes are more likely to occur when atherosclerotic* occlusive disease involves the vertebrobasilar system, with compromised perfusion to the medullary arousal center. In vertebrobasilar vascular insufficiency, syncope or presyncope is nearly always preceded by symptoms of vertigo, diplopia, dysarthria, and ataxia. The episodes are generally attributed to microemboli arising from an atherosclerotic plaque, although vasospasm or postural hypotension may contribute (see also Chap. 99).

THERAPY

The treatment of recurrent syncope in cerebrovascular disease is predicated on an accurate diagnosis. In this regard, it is essential to segregate the potential contribution of cardiac and vascular factors and their interplay. Anticoagulants and/or platelet antiaggregant agents are recommended for the prevention of embolic disease from the heart or central vessels (see Chap. 52). Surgical endarterectomy should be considered in carotid arterial occlusive disease.

Seizure Disorders

Differentiation of the various forms of syncope from the loss of consciousness during a generalized convulsive seizure is often made on the basis of history alone.[83] Grand mal epilepsy as a cause of sudden loss of consciousness is suggested by the dramatic nature of the onset of the attack, which is often preceded by an aura. Other observations that aid in distinguishing epilepsy are the absence of hypotension and cardiac arrhythmia (other than sinus tachycardia); the presence of sustained tonic-clonic convulsive movements with upturning of the eyes; prolonged unconsciousness; urinary incontinence; and postictal drowsiness, headache, and confusion. While any of these findings occasionally occur in episodes of syncope, the frequent association of these several events generally allows differentiation of epilepsy as its cause. In fact, it is common for patients with true syncope to be incorrectly diagnosed as having a seizure disorder (see also Chap. 99). Akinetic seizures and absence (petite mal) seizures may be difficult to differentiate from syncope. The occurrence in childhood, a past history of recurrent episodes, and the absence of pallor in witnessed episodes are helpful diagnostic findings. *Temporal lobe seizures are the most likely form of epilepsy to masquerade as syncope.*

An abnormal electroencephalogram (EEG) between episodes of altered consciousness can aid in distinguishing a seizure disorder when clinical observations are not definitive, and in some instances continuous EEG and electrocardiogram (ECG) monitoring are required.

Carotid Sinus Hypersensitivity

Compression of the carotid sinus in normal persons is often associated with transient slowing of the heart and mild hypotension. In some patients, such stimulation is followed by a profound slowing of heart rate and/or a marked diminution of arterial pressure. This disorder is referred to as *carotid sinus hypersensitivity.*

There are three forms of carotid sinus syncope, as originally described by Weiss and Baker:[84] cardioinhibitory, vasodepressor, and mixed type.

CARDIOINHIBITORY TYPE

The *cardioinhibitory type of carotid sinus syncope* is the most common. It is associated with slowing of the heart rate secondary to marked sinus bradycardia, sinoatrial block, and/ or high-degree AV block. Syncope in this instance is related to the prolonged asystole rather than to a fall in peripheral vascular resistance.

VASODEPRESSOR TYPE

The *vasodepressor type of carotid sinus syncope* is that form of the syndrome in which syncope occurs as a result of a primary decrease in arterial pressure in the absence of profound bradycardia. Presyncopal signs, such as nausea, sweating, and pallor, are usually not observed, and the fall in arterial pressure may be precipitous.

MIXED FORM

In the *mixed form of carotid sinus syncope* with bradycardia and hypotension, the vasodepressor component may not be evident until after atropine blockade or during cardiac pacing. Under such circumstances, carotid sinus massage uncovers the hypotension in the absence of bradycardia.

Carotid sinus syncope and presyncope are commonly found in elderly patients in whom symptoms of light-headedness and impaired consciousness may be initiated by relatively minor stimulation of the carotid sinus.[2,3] Carotid sinus hypersensitivity in the elderly is often associated with generalized atherosclerosis.

The frequency of a hypersensitive response to manual carotid sinus compression in elderly persons enjoins caution whenever this maneuver is attempted. Digital carotid massage should first be attempted with a very gentle and brief (2 to 4 s) compression, always when the patient is supine and with monitoring of the heart rate and blood pressure.[85–88] *The presence of carotid artery bruits is a relative contraindication to carotid massage.*

Carotid sinus syncope has been observed in patients with neoplasms, inflammatory masses, and lymph nodes in the neck adjacent to the carotid sinus.[89] Carotid sinus syncope is well established as a complication of carotid body and parotid tumors. In certain patients, carotid sinus hypersensitivity may be documented only when carotid sinus massage is performed in the upright position or during HUT studies.

THERAPY

Thorough patient education concerning avoidance of carotid sinus pressure may be effective in preventing syncopal episodes. Anticholinergic and sympathomimetic agents may be tried, but inadequacy of drug therapy and the occurrence of side effects may necessitate pacemaker therapy. AV sequential pacing appears to minimize the hypotensive effect of cardiac pacing and, hence, is the preferred form of pacemaker therapy

in the mixed form of carotid sinus syncope. It is important that pacemaker effectiveness be verified objectively through observation of the effect of carotid sinus stimulation on cardiac rhythm and arterial pressure following pacemaker insertion.[2,3]

Situational Syncope

The term *situational syncope* has been applied to a group of syndromes that is defined by the circumstances that precipitate the event. In the past the syncope in these disorders has been attributed mainly to mechanical factors. Recent observations suggest that, at least in part, neurocardiogenic factors contribute to the syncope.

COUGH SYNCOPE

Also called laryngeal vertigo, tussive syncope and posttussive syncope, cough syncope is associated with loss of consciousness following a paroxysm of vigorous coughing. It is often seen in robust men and children but rarely in women. Cerebral blood flow is impaired by the marked increase in cerebrospinal fluid pressure during coughing, which increases cerebrovascular resistance. There is also a "concussive effect" transmitted via the cerebrospinal fluid. Reflex-induced sinus bradycardia, sinus arrest, and AV block have been observed in patients with cough syncope.[90,91]

In the treatment of cough syncope, the patient should be informed of the deleterious effects of vigorous coughing. Cessation of smoking and initiation of bronchodilator and anti-inflammatory therapy for associated bronchitis are mandatory for the prevention of cough-induced syncope.

SWALLOWING, OR DEGLUTITION, SYNCOPE

Deglutition syncope has been reported in association with tumor, diverticulum, achalasia, stricture, and spasm of the esophagus. In some patients no abnormality can be identified radiologically or endoscopically. Syncope is usually associated with sinus bradycardia, sinus arrest, or high-degree AV block.[92]

Similar mechanisms have been implicated in syncope following distension of the viscera, glossopharyngeal neuralgia, fainting associated with irritation of the pleura or peritoneum, and cardiac asystole associated with esophagoscopy or bronchoscopy.[93]

VALSALVA SYNCOPE

Valsalva syncope is related to prolonged increases in intrathoracic pressure that may be observed during a sustained Valsalva maneuver. With prolonged exhalation against a closed glottis, there is a progressive fall in venous return, arterial pressure, and cardiac output.[2,3] These hemodynamic changes may be sufficient to impair cerebral circulation. An episode of Valsalva syncope may be the first indication of the presence of a disorder predisposing to syncope (e.g., cerebrovascular occlusive disease or sick sinus syndrome). Instruction to the patient regarding avoidance of sustained Valsalva maneuvers is essential in preventing recurring episodes.

MICTURITION SYNCOPE

Micturition syncope is often seen in adult men with nocturia. During or immediately following voiding there is a loss of consciousness, often without premonitory symptoms. The ingestion of large quantities of alcoholic beverages before retiring is common.[2,3,94] A similar type of syncope may be observed following drainage of the distended bladder or after removal of large quantities of ascitic fluid. The loss of consciousness in these circumstances may be related to bradycardia and a sudden reflex decrease in peripheral arterial resistance induced by the precipitous fall of intraabdominal volume. The loss of consciousness of typical micturition syncope is precipitated by such factors as the Valsalva maneuver in the upright posture and the peripheral vasodilation associated with a warm bed and recent alcohol consumption.

DEFECATION SYNCOPE

Defecation syncope occurs most commonly in the elderly, usually after arising from bed at night or during manual disimpaction of the rectum.[2,3,95] It has been attributed to sudden decompression of the rectum. Valsalva-related syncope could also explain some instances of this form of syncope. Many patients with defecation syncope have underlying gastrointestinal or cardiovascular disease.

DIVER'S SYNCOPE

Diver's syncope is an unusual and poorly understood form of loss of consciousness or even sudden death that may occur in underwater diving. Some instances may be forms of neurocardiogenic syncope. Hypoxia and bradycardia of the diving reflex may be contributing factors.[2,3]

POSTPRANDIAL SYNCOPE

Hypotension postprandially may result in presyncope and/or syncope and is most common in the elderly. The mechanisms of postprandial hypotension and syncope are not fully understood. Possible contributing factors include inadequate sympathetic nervous system compensation for meal-induced splanchnic blood pooling, impairments in baroreflex function, inadequate postprandial increase in cardiac output, impairment of peripheral vasoconstriction, and release of gastrointestinal peptides.[96,97]

TREATMENT

Therapy of situational syncope should be individualized and should be addressed to the specific circumstance associated with it. Episodes of syncope may be prevented by anticholinergic drugs such as atropine if they are administered prior to a procedure. Other measures include avoidance of vasodilators before meals and/or resting in a supine position after meals for patients with postprandial hypotension and sitting while urinating for men with micturition syncope. Octreotide, a somatostatin analog, has been shown to be effective in patients with postprandial hypotension, but it is expensive and must be given parenterally.[96,97]

Metabolic Syncope

HYPOXIA-RELATED SYNCOPE

Hypoxia may induce syncope that is related directly to a lack of oxygen or to an episode of neurocardiogenic syncope initiated during a period of oxygen lack.[96] In the presence of cardiovascular disease, pulmonary insufficiency, and anemia, symptoms of hypoxia occur at lesser levels of oxygen deprivation. The impairment of consciousness due to hypoxia is accompanied by sinus tachycardia, while arterial pressure is usually normal. Short-term exposure to moderate altitude may be related to otherwise unexplained syncope in healthy, young adults. The environmental setting in which impaired consciousness due to hypoxia occurs usually leaves little difficulty in its differentiation from other forms of syncope.

HYPOGLYCEMIA-RELATED SYNCOPE

This form of syncope may be associated with weakness, sweating, a sensation of hunger, confusion, and altered consciousness. The symptoms are unrelated to posture and usually respond promptly to food ingestion or intravenous glucose administration. Impaired consciousness is usually associated with sinus tachycardia and is rarely accompanied by hypotension. In contrast to syncope of circulatory origin, it is gradual in onset. Recently, hypoglycemia has been implicated as a possible factor that may trigger neurocardiogenic syncope.[2,3]

HYPERVENTILATION, PANIC ATTACKS, AND SYNCOPE

In normal persons, anxiety is accompanied by varying degrees of hyperventilation. In the hyperventilation syndrome or in a panic episode, anxiety is associated with an inordinate degree of hyperventilation[99] (see Chap. 90). Symptoms of hypocapnia and alkalosis may dominate the clinical picture. During the episode, the patient may complain of a tightness in the chest and a feeling of suffocation. These symptoms may be followed by confusion, a sense of unreality, bewilderment, light-headedness, and a feeling of panic. Symptoms of palpitation, precordial oppression, and dyspnea may suggest an acute cardiac or pulmonary catastrophe. Digital and circumoral paresthesias may develop and, in severe cases, may be accompanied by carpopedal spasm, which is probably related to alkalosis-induced decreases in serum ionized calcium. The symptoms may be protracted and persist while the subject is sitting or in recumbency. During hyperventilation, there is slight hypotension but no profound fall in arterial pressure, while the heart rate is rapid. Although mentation is impaired, complete loss of consciousness rarely occurs. Typical neurocardiogenic syncope may be superimposed, making identification of the syndrome more difficult. *The induction of a typical episode by voluntary hyperventilation is helpful in distinguishing this syndrome and aids in educating the patient regarding the prevention and control of attacks.*

Other Forms of Syncope or Conditions Mimicking Syncope

VERTIGO

Although recurrent episodes of vertigo may first be described by the patient as a loss or impairment of consciousness, careful attention to the history will usually reveal the true nature of this symptom. In true vertigo there is a keen sense of movement, either of the environment or of the patient. Falling may be abrupt; it is not due to weakness of postural tone but to a loss of balance. The lack of true loss or impairment of consciousness, the increased distress with head movement, the associated nystagmus, and the findings of normal arterial pressure and pulse during an attack help differentiate vertigo from syncope.[2,3]

MIGRAINE-RELATED SYNCOPE

Symptoms suggesting syncope are unusual in ordinary types of migraine. In rare instances in which the basilar arterial system is involved (as opposed to the more usually affected carotid system), the premonitory aura of migraine terminates in a period of unconsciousness of several minutes' duration. The unconsciousness is slow in onset and may be preceded by a dreamlike state. When the patient awakens, there is severe headache, typically in the occipital area. This form of migraine usually afflicts young women and has a strong menstrual association. The symptoms in syncopal migraine may suggest hyperventilation and/or hysterical syncope.

HYSTERICAL SYNCOPE

Altered consciousness of circulator origin may be mimicked by hysteria. Hysterical episodes occur most frequently in young adults, often with severe emotional illness, and generally in the presence of an audience. The individual slumps gently, even gracefully, to the floor or in a convenient chair or sofa, typically without injury or awkwardness. The patient may be motionless or may exhibit symbolic restrictive movements. Episodes are of varying duration and may last an hour or more. Although the patient is unresponsive to verbal stimulation, there is evidence, such as eyelid movement, that consciousness is well preserved, and no abnormalities in pulse, arterial pressure, or skin color are evident.

CARDIAC SYNCOPE

Either severe obstruction of cardiac output or disturbances of cardiac rhythm can produce syncope of cardiac origin.[2,3,100–112] Obstructive lesions and arrhythmias frequently coexist; indeed, one abnormality may accentuate the other. Common disorders associated with cardiac syncope are listed in Table 35-6.

TABLE 35-6

COMMON DISORDERS ASSOCIATED WITH CARDIAC SYNCOPE

I. Obstruction of cardiac output
  A. Left heart
    1. Aortic stenosis
    2. Hypertrophic cardiomyopathy
    3. Prosthetic valve malfunction
    4. Mitral stenosis
    5. Left atrial myxoma (rare)
  B. Right heart
    1. Eisenmenger syndrome
    2. Tetralogy of Fallot
    3. Pulmonary embolism
    4. Pulmonary stenosis
    5. Primary pulmonary hypertension
    6. Cardiac tamponade
II. Cardiac arrhythmia
  A. Sinoatrial disease
  B. Atrioventricular block
  C. Supraventricular tachycardia
  D. Ventricular tachycardia/fibrillation
  E. Pacemaker related
    1. Pacemaker syndrome
    2. Pacemaker malfunction
    3. Pacemaker-induced tachycardia

Syncope Related to Obstruction of Cardiac Output

Obstruction to cardiac output sufficient to cause syncope may occur on the left or right side of the heart. Syncope, particularly that occurring with effort, is a major symptom of aortic stenosis and is often the initial presentation.[2,3] The mechanisms are unclear, but studies suggest a reflex fall in peripheral vascular resistance as the usual cause. Failure of cardiac output to increase adequately during exercise, while peripheral resistance decreases, may play a role (see also Chap. 63). Transient arrhythmias can also induce syncope in aortic stenosis. Syncope associated with effort (often occurring immediately after effort) is observed in patients with hypertrophic cardiomyopathy as well. Nonexertional syncope related to acute decreases in preload or afterload, to inotropic stimulation, or to transient arrhythmias may also occur in hypertrophic cardiomyopathy (see also Chap. 74). Left-sided heart prosthetic valve malfunction can produce transient and at times profound obstruction to blood flow with syncope (see also Chap. 67). A left atrial myxoma may obstruct left ventricular filling, leading to low cardiac output and syncope. The obstruction of left ventricular inflow in atrial myxoma may be posturally induced (see also Chap. 86). Mitral stenosis can produce cardiac syncope but usually does so only when tachycardia or other arrhythmias supervene (see also Chap. 64).

Primary pulmonary hypertension and pulmonary hypertension secondary to congenital heart disease may both be complicated by syncope, particularly effort-related syncope. In these conditions limitation of right ventricular outflow markedly inhibits the cardiac output during increased peripheral demand. The fall in peripheral resistance in the presence of an inability to increase cardiac output may result in profound hypotension. A reflex fall in peripheral resistance similar to that which occurs with aortic stenosis may play a role. In a young patient without a cardiac murmur who presents with syncope during or shortly after exertion, primary pulmonary hypertension should be considered (see also Chap. 59). In pulmonary stenosis and pulmonary embolism, similar mechanisms may account for syncope. Pulmonary embolism as a cause of syncope should also be suspected in paraplegic patients.[113] In tetralogy of Fallot, the magnitude of flow through the right-to-left shunt increases when systemic resistance falls with effort, since the right ventricular outflow obstruction is usually fixed.[2,3] This shunting results in marked arterial hypoxia, which may precipitate a syncopal episode (see also Chap. 70).

Cardiac tamponade, which affects both the right and the left side of the heart, can produce syncope, but this is extremely rare. The likelihood of syncope is increased by concomitant arrhythmias.

Syncope Related to Cardiac Arrhythmia

Arrhythmias are a common cause of syncope and must be considered in any patient, particularly when cardiac disease is present. Either extreme of ventricular rate—bradycardia or tachycardia—can depress cardiac output to the point of critical hypotension with cerebral hypoperfusion and syncope. As noted earlier for other forms of syncope, a neurocardiogenic reaction may be precipitated by the hemodynamic effects of arrhythmias[114] (see also Chaps. 26 and 27). The most common arrhythmias producing syncope or presyncope are profound sinus bradycardia, sinoatrial exit block or sinus pause, high-grade AV block, supraventricular tachycardia, ventricular tachycardia/fibrillation, and the pacemaker syndrome. Although arrhythmias occur in the absence of demonstrable underlying cardiac disease, they are usually secondary to such disorders as ischemic heart disease, cardiomyopathy, valvular heart disease (including mitral valve prolapse), and primary conduction system disease.

Primary degenerative disease of the sinus node and the specialized conduction tissue is the most common cause of sinoatrial disease (*sick sinus syndrome*; see Chap. 27). The sick sinus syndrome may be manifested by persistent or episodic sinus bradycardia or sinoatrial exit block with impaired junctional escape rhythm and frequently supraventricular tachycardias. The appearance of alternating sinus bradycardia with paroxysmal supraventricular tachycardia of diverse types is quite common and is referred to as the *bradycardia-tachycardia syndrome. Syncope often occurs with asystole or bradycardia at the termination of tachycardia, when overdrive suppression of the sinoatrial or junctional pacemakers is present.*[2,3] A high incidence of associated AV and intraventricular conduction defects occurs in the sick sinus syndrome. Thus, AV block, impaired junctional escape rhythm, or ventricular arrhythmias may actually be responsible for syncope in the setting of sick sinus syndrome.

High-grade AV block may be due to disease of either the AV node or the His-Purkinje system. Disease of the AV node is associated with a functional junctional pacemaker and a normal QRS complex, while AV block due to disease of the His-Purkinje system is usually associated with a wide complex idioventricular escape rhythm, which may be quite slow and unreliable. Bifascicular block associated with a prolonged PR interval is associated with a substantial risk of developing high-grade AV block and syncope. Progression to high-grade AV block in patients with bifascicular block and a normal PR interval is less common. Ventricular tachycardia can cause syncope in patients with AV block or other bradycardic rhythms, since torsades de pointes is usually pause dependent (see Chap. 27).

Sinus bradycardia, AV block, or cardiac asystole may be mediated by reflex vagal mechanisms and have been observed in a variety of disease states or during diagnostic procedures (see above). Ventricular asystole (usually sinus arrest, although AV block can occasionally be noted) is most commonly due to neurocardiogenic syncope. Paroxysmal sinus bradycardia or AV block can also occur in apparently healthy young individuals; certain of these patients may have mitral valve prolapse.[109] Paroxysmal supraventricular tachycardias usually do not produce syncope in young individuals. Syncope, however, may occur in individuals who have accessory AV pathways due to the Wolff-Parkinson-White (WPW) syndrome, wherein supraventricular tachycardia is associated with a very rapid ventricular response. Studies have shown, however, that syncope during supraventricular tachycardia may be related to vasomotor factors and not be due solely to heart rate (Fig. 35-3).[114–116] Atrioventricular node reentry, atrial fibrillation, or atrial flutter may be associated with a rapid ventricular rate in the setting of baseline short PR interval, or tachycardia occurring during or postexercise may cause syncope. Patients with cardiac disease, particularly obstructive outflow disorders, and older individuals may more commonly have hypotension significant enough to cause cerebral hypoperfusion and syncope.

Paroxysmal ventricular tachycardia may produce syncope at any age and can occur as a manifestation of most types of cardiac disease in which there are structural abnormalities and/or ischemia. Ventricular tachycardia is the most common arrhythmic cause of syncope in most series. In some patients, ventricular and supraventricular tachycardia coexist[2,3] (see Chap. 27).

Syncope may occur with ventricular tachycardia in the setting of the long QT syndrome. The long QT interval syndrome may be congenital or acquired[110] (see also Chaps. 12 and 27). The recognition of the long QT syndromes depends on demonstration of QT prolongation and of recurrent syn-

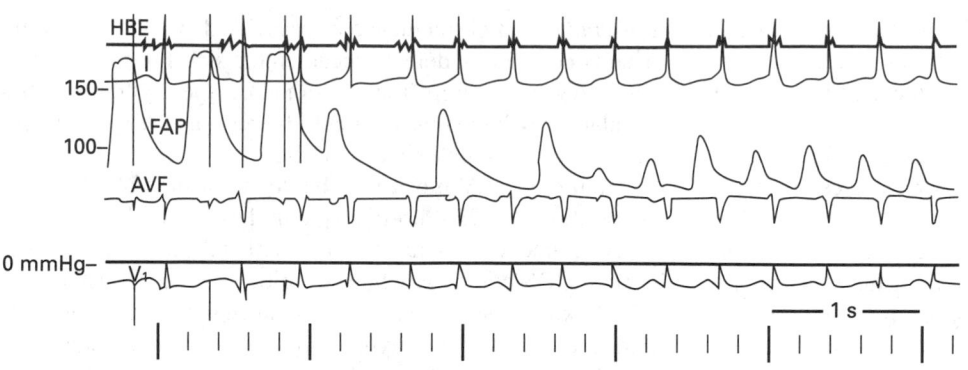

FIGURE 35-3
Atrial premature depolarization induction of supraventricular tachycardia in patient with tachycardia and syncope. Tachycardia rate was 170/min but associated with moderate hypotension in supine state. HBE = His bundle electrocardiogram; FAP = femoral artery pressure; I, AVF, V_1 = electrocardiographic leads. (From Schaal et al.,[3] with permission.)

cope, which is almost always due to ventricular arrhythmia. The ventricular arrhythmia is usually torsades de pointes. Ventricular tachycardia in the long QT syndromes is often triggered by exercise or stress reaction. A pause (usually after ventricular ectopy) is most common since the early afterdepolarizations thought responsible for torsades are bradycardia-dependent.[110,111]

It is particularly important to recognize the polymorphic ventricular tachycardia associated with acquired long QT syndromes, because it is an uncommon phenomenon and is a potentially life-threatening side effect of many drugs and metabolic abnormalities. The most frequent causes of acquired long QT syndromes are antiarrhythmic drugs and electrolyte disorders (hypokalemia and hypomagnesemia).

A variety of other drugs may produce arrhythmias or arrhythmia aggravation, resulting in syncope or presyncope. Beta-blocking drugs, calcium channel blocking agents, sotalol, and amiodarone are some of the more common agents that may cause significant sinus bradycardia or atrioventricular block. Digitalis may occasionally cause sinoatrial exit block or atrioventricular block, particularly in patients with sinoatrial or atrioventricular node disease. Supraventricular and ventricular tachycardias can be a result of digitalis therapy, particularly in patients with organic heart disease and hypokalemia. Theophylline and beta agonists, used for therapy of chronic obstructive pulmonary disease, may precipitate ventricular or supraventricular arrhythmias. Therapy with diuretics often causes hypokalemia and hypomagnesemia, which predispose to supraventricular and ventricular arrhythmias. Both caffeine and alcohol may precipitate either atrial or ventricular tachycardia.

In patients with an artificial ventricular pacemaker, syncope may be secondary to pacemaker malfunction or to the pacemaker syndrome (see Chap. 34). Dual-chamber pacemakers can produce pacemaker-mediated tachycardias when there is retrograde conduction of the ventricular impulse to the atria. Improvements in technology have reduced the incidence of this complication.[117]

DIAGNOSTIC EVALUATION OF SYNCOPE ASSOCIATED WITH CARDIAC DISEASE

While the history and physical examination often establish the diagnosis of obstructive cardiac syncope, laboratory studies are usually required for the determination of the severity of the disorder.[2,3] Cardiac catheterization is required when corrective cardiac surgery is contemplated.

By far the most challenging diagnostic evaluation occurs when arrhythmic cardiac syncope is suspected. Such patients often have evidence of underlying cardiovascular disease, which, when present, portends a poor prognosis. Thus, diagnostic studies directed to the nature and severity of the underlying cardiac disease must be pursued in addition to the arrhythmia evaluation.

The various diagnostic tests used for the evaluation of arrhythmic syncope are listed in Fig. 35-4. Because of the transient nature of most arrhythmias, the routine ECG is generally of limited value. It is, however, very useful in identifying patients with abnormalities that may predispose to syncope, such as prior infarction, WPW pattern, and AV or bundle branch block.[2,3]

The technique of signal-averaged ECG for detecting late potentials can be used as a noninvasive screening test for detecting a high-risk subset of patients prone to lethal ventricular arrhythmias. The accuracy of the signal-averaged ECG in predicting the induction of sustained monomorphic ventricular tachycardia in high-risk patients with coronary artery disease who undergo electrophysiologic studies is good.[118–124]

Exercise testing can directly provoke arrhythmias in patients with a history suggesting exercise-induced arrhythmias. It should be performed when exertional arrhythmias are suspected but not documented by ambulatory monitoring or when ischemia is suspected (see also Chap. 15).[125,126]

Continuous ECG monitoring is a widely used screening test for suspected arrhythmic syncope. It has low yield in unselected patients. *It is important to recognize that one 24-h monitoring period may not be sufficient for detecting transient rhythm disturbances. The diagnostic yield, moreover, increases only slightly with more prolonged monitoring*[125–128] (see also Chap. 28).

When ambulatory monitoring does not document an arrhythmia, a patient-activated electrocardiographic device (event recorder) may prove efficacious. This type of monitoring is effective in documenting infrequent arrhythmia. It should not be used in patients with suspected life-threatening arrhythmias.[129–132]

When noninvasive testing is inconclusive for the diagnosis of suspected arrhythmic syncope, an electrophysiologic study should be performed on high-risk patients (i.e., those with underlying heart disease, suspicious arrhythmia by ECG monitoring, or recurrent syncope). The patient without identifiable heart disease is less likely to have the cause of syncope identified by electrophysiologic study.[133–141] The cause of syncope most commonly identified by electrophysiologic study is ventricular tachycardia.

Electrophysiologic studies are useful in stratifying risk among symptomatic patients with bundle branch block or patients with bifascicular block. Patients with normal electrophysiologic study results have a favorable prognosis even without treatment.[142,143] Patients undergoing permanent pacing on the basis of electrophysiologic testing also have a favorable prognosis, with a low rate of symptom recurrence.[144–147]

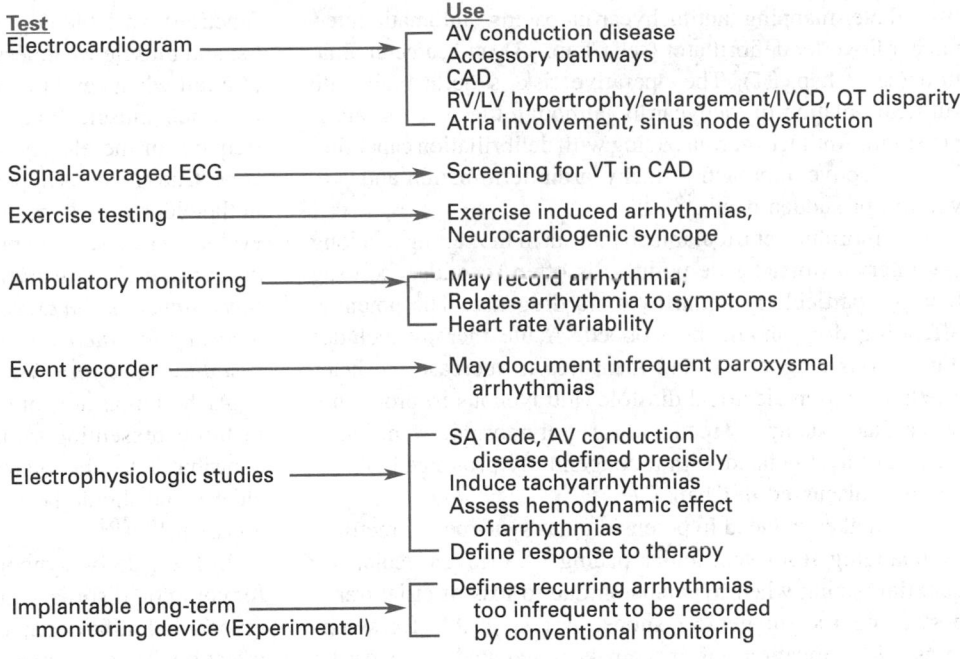

FIGURE 35-4

Diagnostic tests that can be used for the evaluation of arrhythmic syncope. AV = atrioventricular; CAD = coronary artery disease; RV/LV = right ventricular/left ventricular; IVCD = intraventricular conduction defect; VT = ventricular tachycardia; SA = sinoatrial.

The prognosis in patients with syncope due to supraventricular tachycardia is usually good, since therapeutic approaches are available (i.e., drugs and radiofrequency ablation). The prognosis in patients with inducible ventricular tachycardia is less favorable but is improved when specific therapy can be demonstrated to inhibit the inducibility of ventricular tachycardia or with the use of an implantable cardioverter defibrillator.

TREATMENT OF CARDIAC SYNCOPE

Obstructive Heart Disease

For the patient with syncope caused by obstructive heart disease, cardiac surgery is often the treatment of choice.[2,3,148] Patients with hypertrophic cardiomyopathy and syncope may respond well to pharmacologic therapy. Recent studies have suggested that an AV sequential pacemaker might control symptoms in certain patients with hypertrophic cardiomyopathy.[148] In rare cases with severe obstruction and persistent symptoms, surgery must be considered (see Chap. 74). Among all patients with obstructive heart disease and recurrent syncope, the diagnosis of fixed pulmonary hypertension is most difficult to treat because effective therapeutic options are limited (see Chap. 59).

Arrhythmic Syncope

A detailed discussion of therapy for cardiac arrhythmias is presented in Chap. 27. Some general principles of arrhythmia management as they apply to patients with syncope will be summarized here. Treatment of arrhythmic syncope requires

accurate definition of the arrhythmia associated with syncope or presyncope.[2,3]

The bradycardic rhythm disturbances responsible for syncope, primarily AV and sinoatrial pauses or exit block, usually require the implantation of a pacemaker. Patients receiving drugs that cause or contribute to the bradyarrhythmia, however, may benefit from withdrawal or substitution of the offending agent. The patient with bradycardia-tachycardia syndrome usually requires pacemaker therapy, because the antiarrhythmic agents required for control of the tachycardia will often further suppress sinoatrial function.

Implicit in the approach to the tachycardias causing syncope is the accurate diagnosis of a specific tachycardia. The definition of the tachycardia and the response to antiarrhythmic therapy are often best achieved in the electrophysiologic laboratory.[2,3] Patients with syncope due to supraventricular tachycardia associated with an accessory pathway are most often approached with catheter ablation of the accessory pathway. Catheter ablation is also a successful mode of therapy in the patient with AV nodal reentry supraventricular tachycardia associated with a rapid heart rate[149,150] (see Chap. 31).

Therapy of paroxysmal ventricular tachycardia responsible for syncope is best guided by pharmacologic testing in the electrophysiologic laboratory.[2,3] Predictive accuracy of therapeutic effectiveness due to antiarrhythmic agents is higher with electrophysiologic testing than with ambulatory monitoring or exercise testing. Empiric drug therapy, except for amiodarone, for ventricular tachycardia causing syncope appears to offer no benefit. Other modalities of therapy for ventricular tachyarrhythmias include surgical ablative techniques guided by catheter mapping, antitachycardia pacing, automatic internal cardioverter defibrillator (see Chap. 33), and catheter ablation (see Chap. 31). The operative risk is quite high with surgical ablation of tachycardia, although the success rate is also high. Antitachycardia pacing with defibrillation capability is an effective approach to tachycardia termination and prevention of sudden death.[151-155]

Polymorphic ventricular tachycardia in the setting of a long QT interval (torsades de pointes) is often secondary to drug therapy, particularly antiarrhythmic drug use. The potential offending drug should be stopped. Acute therapy includes intravenous magnesium and measures to increase the heart rate and shorten electrical diastole (intravenous isoproterenol or cardiac pacing). Treatment of polymorphic ventricular tachycardia associated with a congenitally prolonged QT interval is discussed in Chap. 27.

Pacemaker-induced hypotension and syncope are rectified by changing from ventricular pacing to atrioventricular sequential pacing when hypotension due to loss of atrial transport or neurocardiogenic response is responsible for symptoms. Identification of pacemaker-mediated tachycardia usually requires only pacemaker programming changes. Pacemaker malfunction or myopotential inhibition requires a change in programming or replacement of the defective part of the system.

SYNCOPE OF UNDETERMINED CAUSE

Despite careful diagnostic evaluation, the cause of syncope often cannot be defined. Unexplained syncope probably has a broad spectrum of etiologies. The varying mortality in patients with syncope of undetermined cause probably reflects the varying incidence of undetected cardiac syncope. A certain number of these patients probably have experienced syncope of multiple causes.

SPECIAL PROBLEMS IN SYNCOPE

Syncope in the Elderly

Elderly persons are particularly prone to develop syncope or presyncope. The aging process can result in diminished cerebral oxygen delivery by a variety of physiologic mechanisms, including decreased cerebral blood flow from low cardiac output, cerebral vascular disease, decreased hemoglobin, and lower arterial P_{O_2}. In addition, cerebral arteriolar sclerosis may be present and may necessitate a normal arterial perfusion pressure. Thus, many older patients have only marginal cerebral oxygen delivery at rest.[156-161] Physiologic defenses against a fall in blood pressure may also be impaired as discussed above.

The aged may also suffer from multiple sensory deficits (e.g., in vision, vestibular function, peripheral sensory nerve function), variable degrees of dementia, bradykinesis, arthritis, and muscle weakness, all of which enhance the likelihood of a fall when cerebral perfusion is marginal. "Drop" attacks, in which muscle tone in the lower extremities is lost, are frequent in the elderly and must be distinguished from syncope. Carotid sinus hypersensitivity also is relatively common in the elderly, as is postprandial syncope, and they should be evaluated as discussed previously. *The elderly frequently have multisystem disease and are likely to be taking several medications, sometimes in excessive amounts, that may aggravate the tendency to syncope (e.g., antihypertensive drugs, diuretics, vasodilators, antiarrhythmic drugs, or psychoactive drugs).*

Arrhythmias are common in elderly individuals, especially in those presenting with syncope. Syncope is a significant contributor to unexplained automobile accidents among the elderly and should be suspected when external causes are not apparent.[162,163]

In the elderly, syncope may be the presenting complaint for common disorders such as pneumonia, viral illness, acute myocardial infarction, occult hemorrhage, or urinary tract infection. Thus, the management of syncope in the aged often requires initial management of underlying diseases, with subsequent evaluation to determine if such therapy controls syncope.

Multifactorial Syncope

In many instances, syncope requires that a constellation of events occurs, either simultaneously or in sequence. Without the full complex the patient may note only light-headedness or perhaps no definable symptoms. A careful history is required to elucidate such complex presentations.

Transient abnormalities such as fever, fatigue, hypoglycemia, or drug ingestion may increase the likelihood of syncope. Coexisting diseases may decrease the patient's physiologic defenses for maintaining adequate cerebral perfusion to sustain consciousness. A cardiac arrhythmia that ordinarily would not produce syncope may become a contributory factor when other predisposing factors are present (Fig. 35-5). With respect to combined causes of syncope, it is notable that in the original description of Adams-Stokes syncope, the patients exhibited a permanently slow pulse rate accompanied by aortic stenosis.[164,165]

The development of the neurocardiogenic reaction may determine whether a given stimulus initiates syncope. This relationship has been shown in such diverse causes of syncope as aortic stenosis, vasodilator drug therapy, volume loss, pulmonary embolism, tachyarrhythmias, pacemaker syndrome, postprandial state in the elderly, and postexercise. A common pathophysiologic mechanism that may trigger neurocardiogenic syncope is diminished venous return to the right side of the heart.[166]

Syncope and Sudden Death

Sudden death is common in those with known cardiac syncope (both obstructive and arrhythmic), but occasionally sudden

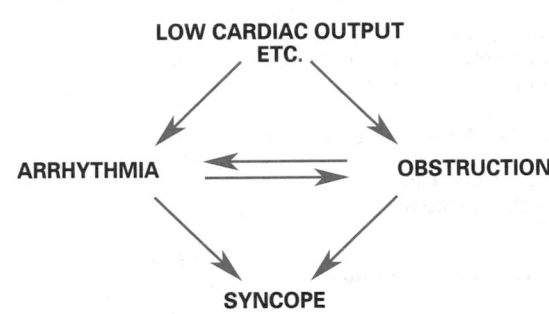

FIGURE 35-5

Frequently, multiple factors must be present simultaneously or in sequence for syncope to occur as a result of an arrhythmia or obstruction to cardiac output. (From Boudoulas and Lewis,[178] with permission.)

death may also occur in presumptive noncardiac syncope and syncope of unknown cause. It would appear, therefore, that in some patients, syncope is a harbinger of sudden death. Patients with advanced heart failure and syncope are at especially high risk for sudden death regardless of the etiology.[167] Syncope is also associated with high mortality in patients with hypertrophic cardiomyopathy. It is not always clear to what extent the occurrence of syncope per se is a risk factor for sudden death or whether the risk is more related to the underlying disease.

Recurrent Syncope

In up to one-third of all patients with syncope, it is a recurring event. It is interesting that for most patients the persistence of syncope increases morbidity from trauma but does not increase mortality. Such recurrences most often reflect a lack of effective therapy and/or a failure to establish the correct diagnosis.[2,3] Unexplained syncope in patients with negative preliminary investigations has a broad spectrum of etiologies, the most common of which is bradycardia. An implantable long-term monitoring device is useful for establishing a diagnosis when symptoms are recurrent but too

infrequent for conventional monitoring techniques.[168] Recurrent syncope is particularly common in a subset of patients with mitral valve prolapse in whom dysautonomia, arrhythmia, and hypovolemia all play a role.[109] In certain patients with unexplained recurrent syncope, especially in individuals with multiple physical symptoms, screening for psychiatric disorder may be necessary.[99] In patients with recurrent syncope, advice regarding the avoidance of certain activities, such as working with dangerous equipment, is needed and, in some cases in which public safety is involved, a change in jobs is required (e.g., pilots or bus drivers).

Exercise and Syncope

Individuals with a history of syncope associated with activity and who participate in physical activities or competitive athletics constitute a special problem. Since exercise syncope may be a manifestation of serious underlying cardiac disease, complete evaluation is indicated to define the cause of syncope prior to recommendation for participation in sports. *Identification of myocardial abnormalities by physical examination and echocardiogram is paramount to the prevention of potential sudden cardiac death.*[169–176]

Syncope may occur during or immediately after exercise. The most common causes of exercise-induced syncope are shown in Fig. 35-6. Neurocardiogenic syncope is not uncommon in highly trained individuals with high resting vagal tone, but caution should be used in making this diagnosis without first excluding underlying structural myocardial abnormality. HUT studies can be used to assess patients at risk for neurocardiogenic syncope, but this test lacks sensitivity and specificity in highly trained individuals. Exercise testing is useful, especially if the syncope is exercise-induced. Exercise-induced ventricular ectopy, sustained ventricular tachycardia, or rapid supraventricular tachycardia requires electrophysiologic evaluation and general cardiologic evaluation.

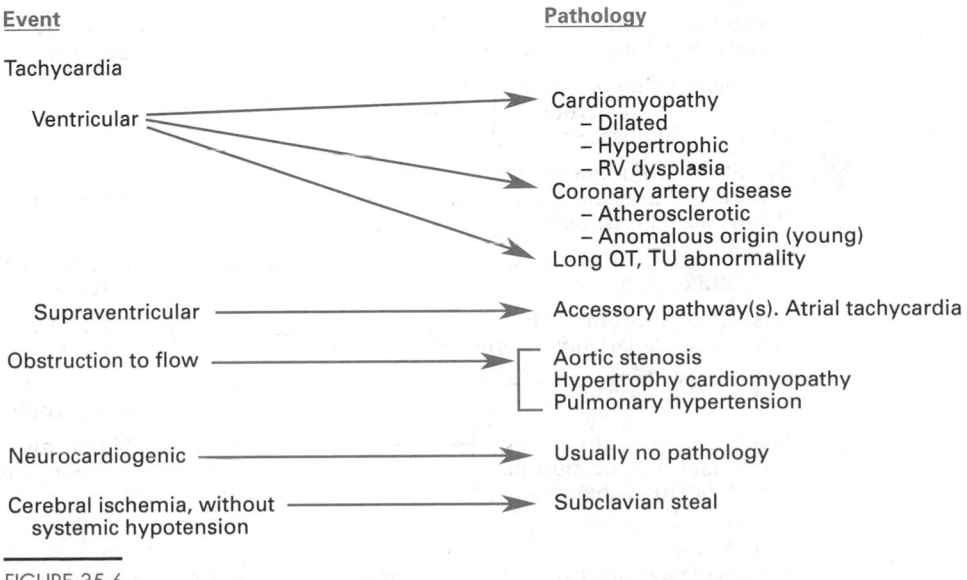

FIGURE 35-6

Exercise-induced syncope. Events and underlying pathology. RV = right ventricular.

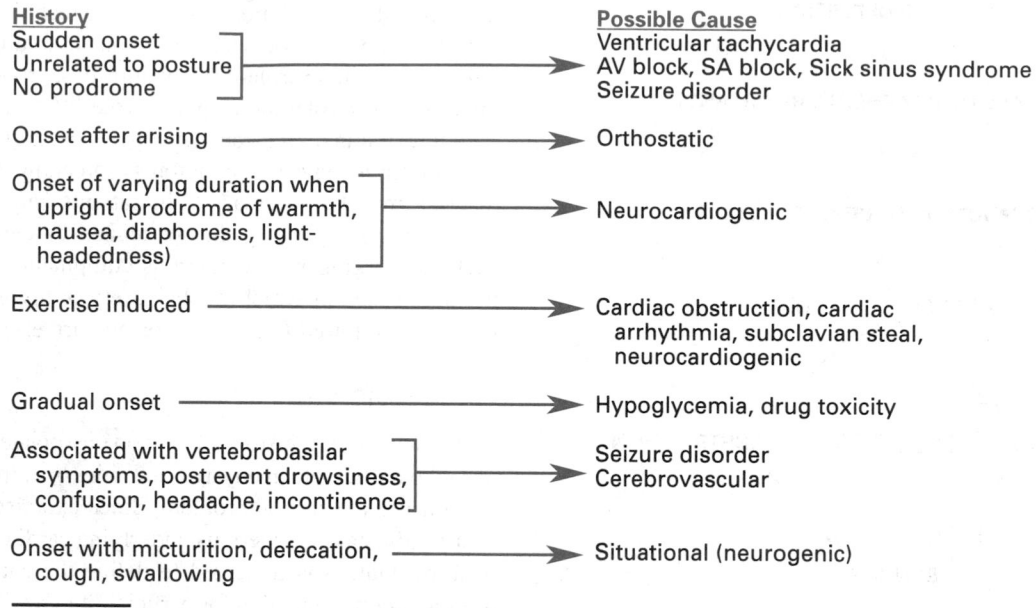

FIGURE 35-7
Differential diagnosis of syncope based on history. AV = atrioventricular; SA = sinoatrial.

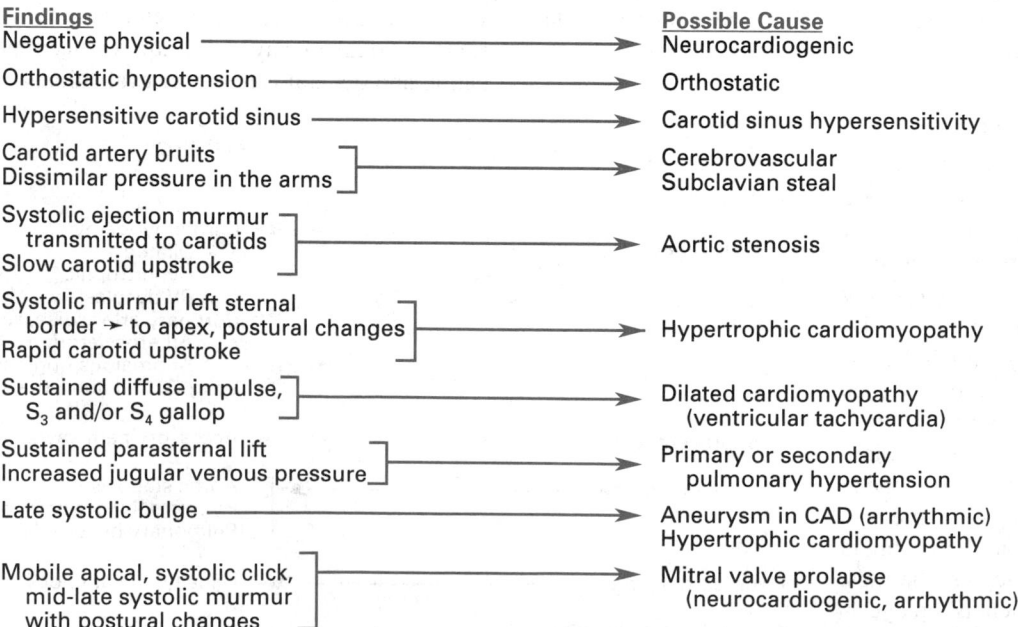

FIGURE 35-8
Differential diagnosis of syncope based on physical examination. CAD = coronary artery disease.

Final recommendation and advice to participate in sports with high, moderate, or low intensity should be individualized. Recommendations should be balanced between restricting activity unduly and reducing chance of death or injury from the participation in sports.

DIAGNOSTIC EVALUATION OF SYNCOPE: AN OVERVIEW

In the initial approach to the diagnosis of syncope, it is essential to distinguish the underlying cause in terms of the three basic categories outlined in Table 35-1.[2,3] This differentiation is accomplished in a majority of patients by a history (Fig. 35-7), physical examination (Fig. 35-8), and ECG (Fig. 35-9) and is supplemented by routine laboratory studies, including echocardiography (Fig. 35-10). Further, Figs. 35-6 and 35-11 provide a useful framework for initiating a diagnostic evaluation of syncope based on age and in cases where syncope is induced with physical activities.[177–184]

The extent of evaluation should initially be predicated on the estimation of mortality and morbidity risk, which is high in cardiac syncope or syncope associated with cardiac disease and low in syncope without structural heart disease. While cost effectiveness in diagnostic testing should be practiced, the need for an assiduous search should not be dismissed when lethal disease is suspected.

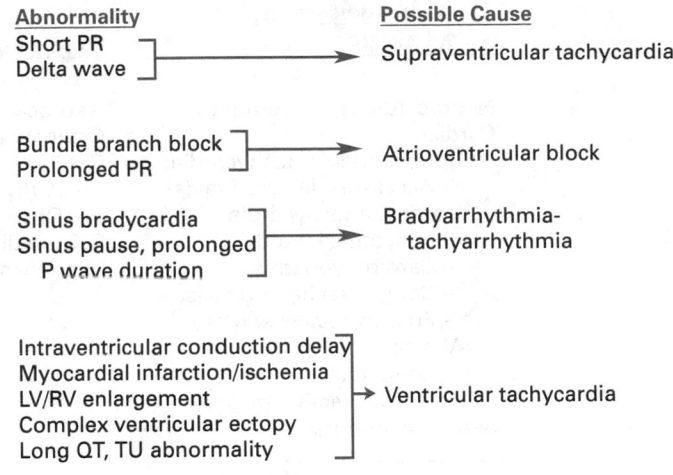

FIGURE 35-9

Differential diagnosis of syncope based on the electrocardiogram. LV/RV = left ventricular/right ventricular.

Hospitalization for more complete evaluation of syncope is often required for the elderly and for patients with suspected arrhythmic syncope (Fig. 35-12). When patients in such a selected group undergo a thorough evaluation, including an electrophysiologic study, an arrhythmic basis for syncope can be found in the majority of patients. *Negative results are often*

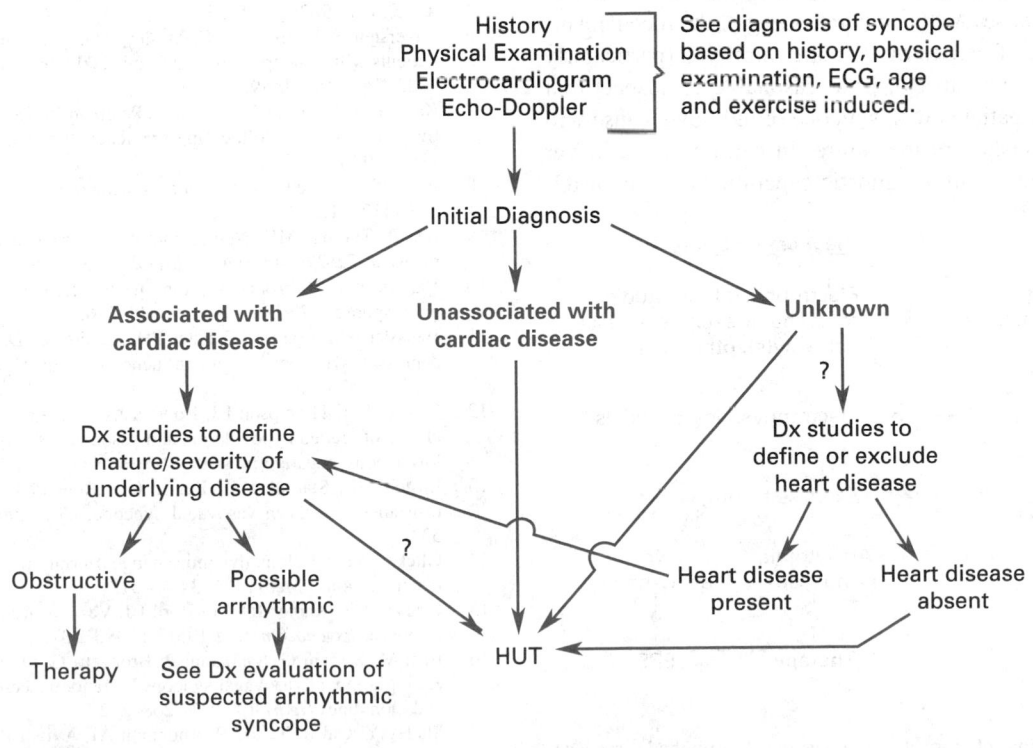

FIGURE 35-10

Basic schema for diagnostic evaluation of syncope. ECG = electrocardiogram; Dx = diagnostic; HUT = head-up tilt.

Children, Adolescents, Young Adults	Middle Age	Elderly
Neurocardiogenic (common)	Neurocardiogenic	Cardiac
Cardiac	Orthostatic	– Arrhythmic
Supraventricular tachycardia	Cardiac	– Obstructive
– Accessory AV pathway(s)	– Arrhythmic	Orthostatic
Ventricular tachycardia	– Obstructive	Neurocardiogenic
– Idiopathic long QT	Seizure disorders	Drug induced
– Cardiomyopathy	Pharmacologic agents	Cerebrovascular
– Congenital heart disease		Carotid sinus hypersensitivity
– Post corrective surgery		Seizure disorders
AV block		Combined causes
– Congenital		
– Post corrective surgery		
Seizure disorders		

FIGURE 35-11

Common causes of syncope by age. AV = atrioventricular.

as important as actual identification of an arrhythmia, since the negative evaluation usually denotes a favorable long-term prognosis. Long-term follow-up suggests that a reduction in both morbidity and mortality can be achieved by therapy guided by electrophysiologic study results. Unfortunately, no controlled studies exist (or are likely to be done) to establish these benefits conclusively.

The diagnostic evaluation of the patient with syncope of unknown cause presents a perplexing problem, particularly when syncope occurs repeatedly and because it may be a harbinger of sudden death, especially when undetected cardiac syncope is the cause. As the understanding of the mechanisms and the breadth of causes of syncope improves (particularly the role of multiple causes), it is reasonable to suspect that the incidence of patients with syncope of unknown cause will be further diminished in the future. In certain cases, newer pacemaker devices with diagnostic capabilities can be used.

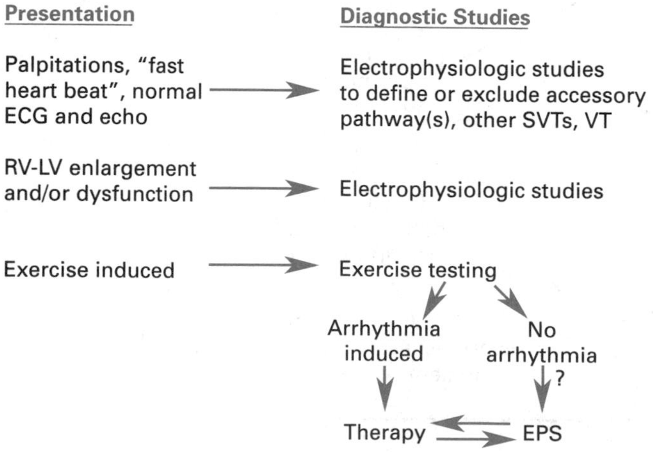

Presentation	Diagnostic Studies
Palpitations, "fast heart beat", normal ECG and echo ⟶	Electrophysiologic studies to define or exclude accessory pathway(s), other SVTs, VT
RV-LV enlargement and/or dysfunction ⟶	Electrophysiologic studies
Exercise induced ⟶	Exercise testing

Arrhythmia induced   No arrhythmia

Therapy ⟷ EPS

FIGURE 35-12

Diagnostic evaluation of patients with suspected arrhythmic syncope. RV/LV = right ventricular/left ventricular; SVT = supraventricular tachycardia; VT = ventricular tachycardia; ECG = electrocardiogram; Echo = echocardiogram; EPS = electrophysiologic studies; SAECG = signal-averaged electrocardiogram.

REFERENCES

1. Savage DD, Corwin L, McGee DL, Kannel WB, Wolf PA. Epidemiologic features of isolated syncope: The Framingham Study. *Stroke* 1985; 16:626–629.
2. Boudoulas H, Weissler AM, Lewis RP, Warren JV. The clinical diagnosis of syncope. *Curr Probl Cardiol* 1982; 7:6–40.
3. Schaal SF, Nelson SD, Boudoulas H, Lewis RP. Syncope. *Curr Probl Cardiol* 1992; 17:211–264.
4. Martin GJ, Adams SL, Martin HG, Mathews J, Zull D, Scanlon PJ. Prospective evaluation of syncope. *Ann Emerg Med* 1984; 13:499–504.
5. Day SC, Cook EF, Funkenstein H, Goldman L. Evaluation and outcome of emergency room patients with transient loss of consciousness. *Am J Med* 1982; 73:15–23.
6. Silverstein MD, Singer DE, Mulley AG, Thibault GE, Barnett GO. Patients with syncope admitted to medical intensive care units. *JAMA* 1982; 248:1185–1189.
7. Kapoor WN, Karpf M, Wieland S, Peterson JR, Levey GS. A prospective evaluation and follow-up of patients with syncope. *N Engl J Med* 1983; 309:197–204.
8. Abbond F. Neurocardiogenic syncope. *N Engl J Med* 1993; 328:1117–1120.
9. Rea R, Thomas MD. Neural control and vasovagal syncope mechanisms. *J Cardiovasc Electrophysiol* 1993; 4:587–595.
10. Van Lieshout JJ, Wouter W, Karemaker JM, Eckberg DL. The vasovagal response. *Clin Sci* 1991; 81:575–586.
11. Weissler AM, Warren JV, Estes EH, McIntosh HD, Leonard JJ. Vasodepressor syncope. Factors influencing cardiac output. *Circulation* 1957; 15:875–883.
12. Murray RH, Thompson LJ, Bowers JA, Albright CD. Hemodynamic effects of graded hypovolemia and vasodepressor syncope induced by lower body negative pressure. *Am Heart J* 1968; 76:799–811.
13. Epstein SE, Stampfer M, Beiser GD. Role of the capacitance and resistance vessels in vasovagal syncope. *Circulation* 1968; 37:524–533.
14. Glick G, Yu PN. Hemodynamic changes during spontaneous vasovagal reactions. *Am J Med* 1963; 34:42–51.
15. Graham DT, Kabler JD, Lunsford LJ. Vasovagal fainting: A diphasic response. *Psychosom Med* 1961; 23:493–507.
16. Biffi M, Boriani G, Sabbatani P, Bronzetti G, Frabetti L, Zannoli R, et al. Malignant vasovagal syncope: A randomised trial of metoprolol and clonidine. *Heart* 1997; 77:268–272.
17. Shalev Y, Gal R, Tchou P, Anderson AJ, Avitall B, Akhtar M, et al. Echocardiographic demonstration of decreased left ventricular dimension and vigorous myocardial contraction during syncope induced by head-up tilt. *J Am Coll Cardiol* 1991; 18:748–751.
18. Thoren P. Role of cardiac vagal C-fibers in cardiovascular control. *Rev Physiol Biochem Pharmacol* 1979; 86:1–94.

19. Oberg B, Thoren P. Increased activity in left ventricular receptors during hemorrhage or occlusion of caval veins in the cat: A possible cause of the vasovagal reaction. *Acta Physiol Scand* 1972; 85:164–173.

20. Mark A. The Bezold-Jarisch reflex revisited: Clinical implications of inhibitory reflexes originating in the heart. *J Am Coll Cardiol* 1983; 1:90–102.

21. Come PC, Pitt B. Nitroglycerin-induced severe hypotension and bradycardia in patients with acute myocardial infarction. *Circulation* 1976; 54:624–628.

22. Rosoff MH, Cohen MV. Profound bradycardia after amyl nitrate in patients with a tendency to vasovagal episodes. *Br Heart J* 1986; 55:97–100.

23. Fitzpatrick AP, Banner N, Cheng A, Yacoub M, Sutton R. Vasovagal reactions may occur after orthotopic heart transplantation. *J Am Coll Cardiol* 1993; 21:1132–1137.

24. Sra JS, Murthy V, Natale A, Jazayeri MR, Dhala A, Deshpande S, et al. Circulatory and catecholamine changes during head-up tilt testing in neurocardiogenic (vasovagal) syncope. *Am J Cardiol* 1994; 73:33–37.

25. Chosy JJ, Graham DT. Catecholamines in vasovagal fainting. *J Psychosom Med* 1984; 46:94–103.

26. Wallin BG, Sundlof G. Sympathetic outflow in muscles during vasovagal syncope. *J Auton Nerv Syst* 1982; 6:287–291.

27. Chen MY, Goldenberg IF, Milstein S, Buetikofer J, Almquist A, Benditt DG. Cardiac electrophysiologic and hemodynamic correlates of neurally mediated syncope. *Am J Cardiol* 1989; 63:66–72.

28. Boorin MR. Anxiety. Its manifestation and role in the dental patient. *Dent Clin North Am* 1995; 39:523–539.

29. Bou-Holagah I, Rowe PC, Kan J, Calkins H. The relationship between neurally mediated hypotension and the chronic fatigue syndrome. *JAMA* 1995; 274:961–967.

30. Milstein S, Buetikofer J, Lesser J, Goldenberg IF, Benditt DG, Gornick C, et al. Cardiac asystole: A manifestation of neurally mediated hypotension-bradycardia. *J Am Coll Cardiol* 1989; 14:1626–1632.

31. Maloney JD, Jaeger FJ, Fouad-Tarazi FM, Morris HH. Malignant vasovagal syncope: Prolonged asystole provoked by head-up tilt. *Cleve Clin J Med* 1988; 55:542–548.

32. Tizes R. Cardiac arrest following routine venipuncture. *JAMA* 1976; 236:1846–1847.

33. Folino AF, Buja GF, Martini B, Miorelli M, Nava A. Prolonged cardiac arrest and complete AV block during upright tilt test in young patients with syncope of unknown origin—prognostic and therapeutic implications. *Eur Heart J* 1992; 13:1416–1421.

34. Benditt DG, Remole S, Bailin S, Dunnigan A, Asso A, Milstein S. Tilt table testing for evaluation of neurally mediated (cardioneurogenic) syncope: Rationale and proposed protocols. *Pacing Clin Electrophysiol* 1991; 14:1528–1537.

35. Kosinski D, Grubb BP. Neurally mediated syncope with an update on indications and usefulness of head-up tilt table testing and pharmacologic therapy. *Curr Opin Cardiol* 1994; 9:53–64.

36. Milstein S, Reyes WJ, Benditt DG. Upright body tilt for evaluation of patients with recurrent, unexplained syncope. *Pacing Clin Electrophysiol* 1989; 12:117–124.

37. Almquist A, Goldenberg IF, Milstein S, Chen MY, Chen X, Hansen R, et al. Provocation of bradycardia and hypotension by isoproterenol and upright posture in patients with unexplained syncope. *N Engl J Med* 1989; 320:346–351.

38. Fitzpatrick AP, Theodorakis G, Vardas P, Sutton R. Methodology of head-up tilt testing in patients with unexplained syncope. *J Am Coll Cardiol* 1991; 17:125–130.

39. Sneddon JF, Slade A, Seo H, Camm AJ, McKenna WJ. Assessment of the diagnostic value of head-up tilt testing in the evaluation of syncope in hypertrophic cardiomyopathy. *Am J Cardiol* 1994; 73:601–604.

40. Raviele A, Gasparini G, DiRode F. Usefulness of head-up tilt in evaluating patients with syncope of unknown origin and negative electrophysiology study. *Am J Cardiol* 1990; 65:1322–1327.

41. Kenny RA, Bayliss J, Ingram A, Sutton R. Head-up tilt: A useful test for investigating unexplained syncope. *Lancet* 1986; 1:1352–1355.

42. Morello CA, Klein GJ, Zandri S, Yee R. Diagnostic accuracy of a low-dose isoproterenol head-up tilt protocol. *Am Heart J* 1995; 129:901–906.

43. Waxman MB, Yao L, Cameron DA, Wald RW, Roseman J. Isoproterenol induction of vasodepressor type reaction in vasodepressor-prone persons. *Am J Cardiol* 1989; 63:58–65.

44. Natale A, Akhtar M, Jazayeri M, Dhala A, Blanck Z, Deshpande S, et al. Provocation of hypotension during head-up tilt testing in subjects with no history of syncope or presyncope. *Circulation* 1995; 92:54–58.

45. Grubb BP, Wolfe D, Temesy-Armos P, Hahn H, Elliott L. Reproducibility of head-up tilt table test in patients with syncope. *Pacing Clin Electrophysiol* 1992; 15:1477–1488.

46. Sheldon R, Rose S, Flanagan P, Koshman ML, Killam S. Risk factors for syncope recurrence after a positive tilt-table test in patients with syncope. *Circulation* 1996; 93:973–981.

47. Ruiz GA, Peralta A, Gonzalez-Zuelgaray J, Duce E. Evolution of patients with clinical neurocardiogenic (vasovagal) syncope not subjected to specific treatment. *Am Heart J* 1995; 130:345–350.

48. Morillo CA, Leitch JW, Yee R, Klein GJ. A placebo-controlled trial of intravenous and oral disopyramide for prevention of neurally mediated syncope induced by head-up tilt. *J Am Coll Cardiol* 1993; 22:1843–1848.

49. Moya A, Permanyer-Miralda G, Sagrista-Sauleda J, Carne X, Rius T, Mont L, et al. Limitations of head-up tilt test for evaluating the efficacy of therapeutic interventions in patients with vasovagal syncope: Results of a controlled study of etilefrine versus placebo. *J Am Coll Cardiol* 1995; 25:65–69.

50. Schatz IJ. Management of orthostatic hypotension. In: Schatz IJ, ed. *Orthostatic Hypotension.* Philadelphia: FA Davis; 1986; pp 98–100.

51. Goldenberg IF, Almquist A, Dunbar DN, Milstein S, Pritzker MR, Benditt DG. Prevention of neurally mediated syncope by selective β-1 adrenoreceptor blockade (abstract). *Circulation* 1987; 76(suppl IV): IV-133.

52. Lippman N, Stein KM, Lerman BB. Differential therapeutic responses of patients with isoproterenol-dependent and isoproterenol-independent vasodepressor syncope. *Am Heart J* 1994; 128:1110–1116.

53. McLaran CJ, Gersch BJ, Osborn MJ. Increased vagal tone as an isolated finding in patients undergoing electrophysiologic testing for recurrent syncope: Response to long-term anticholinergic agents. *Br Heart J* 1986; 55:53–57.

54. Jaeger FJ, Fouad-Tarazi FM, Abi-Samra FM, Cruse RF, Castle LW, Maloney JD. Transdermal scopolamine for the treatment of vasovagal syncope (abstract). *Clin Res* 1987; 35:832A.

55. Kosinski D, Grubb BP, Temesy-Armos P. Pathophysiological aspects of neurocardiogenic syncope: Current concepts and new perspectives. *Pacing Clin Electrophysiol* 1995; 18:716–724.

56. Milstein S, Buetikofer J, Dunnigan A, Benditt DG, Gormick C, Reyes WJ. Usefulness of disopyramide for prevention of upright tilt-induced hypotension-bradycardia. *Am J Cardiol* 1990; 65:1339–1344.

57. Grubb BP, Wolfe DA, Samoil D, Temesy-Armos P, Hahn H, Elliott L. Usefulness of fluoxetine hydrochloride for prevention of resistant upright tilt induced syncope. *Pacing Clin Electrophysiol* 1993; 16:458–464.

58. Grubb BP, Samoil D, Kosinski D, Kip K, Brewster P. Use of sertraline hydrochloride in the treatment of refractory neurocardiogenic syncope in children and adolescents. *J Am Coll Cardiol* 1994; 24:490–495.

59. Benditt DG, Benson W, Kreitt J, Dunnigan A, Pritzker MR, Crouse L, et al. Electrophysiologic effects of theophylline in young patients with recurrent symptomatic bradyarrhythmias. *Am J Cardiol* 1983; 52:1223–1229.

60. Nelson SD, Stanley M, Love CJ, Coyne KS, Schaal SF. The autonomic and hemodynamic effects of oral theophylline in patients with vasodepressor syncope. *Arch Intern Med* 1991; 151:2425–2429.

61. Flammang D, Luizy J, Waynberger M. Re-initiation and quantification of the vasovagal syndrome by the adenosine 5′ triphosphate (ATP) test: Assessment of the best therapy (abstract). *Pacing Clin Electrophysiol* 1990; 13:539.

62. Rall TW. Evolution of the mechanisms of action of methylxanthines from calcium mobilizers to antagonists of adenosine receptors. *Pharmacologist* 1982; 24:277–287.

63. Sra JS, Jazayeri MR, Avitall B, Dhala A, Deshpande S, Blanck Z, et al. Comparison of cardiac pacing with drug therapy in the treatment of neurocardiogenic (vasovagal) syncope with bradycardia or asystole. *N Engl J Med* 1993; 328:1085–1090.

64. Fitzpatrick A, Tagodorekis G, Williams T, Ahmed R, Sutton R. Dual-chamber pacing aborts vasovagal syncope induced by 60° head-up tilt. *Pacing Clin Electrophysiol* 1991; 14:13–19.

65. Schatz IJ. Orthostatic hypotension. Functional and neurogenic causes. *Arch Intern Med* 1984; 144:773–777.

66. Thomas JE, Schirger A, Fealey RD, Sheps SG. Orthostatic hypotension. *Mayo Clin Proc* 1981; 156:117–125.

67. Johnson RH. Orthostatic hypotension in neurological disease. *Cardiology* 1976; 61(suppl 1):150–152.

68. Ziegler MG. Postural hypotension. *Annu Rev Med* 1980; 31:239–245.

69. Levine BD, Giller CA, Lane LD, Buckey JC, Blomqvist G. Cerebral versus systemic hemodynamics during graded orthostatic stress in humans. *Circulation* 1994; 90:298–306.

70. Hilsted J, Parving HH, Christensen NJ, Galbo H. Hemodynamics in diabetic orthostatic hypotension. *J Clin Invest* 1981; 68:1427–1434.

71. Page MM, Watkins PJ. Provocation of postural hypotension by insulin in diabetic autonomic neuropathy. *Diabetes* 1976; 25:90–95.

72. Polinsky RJ, Taylor IL, Chew P, Weise V, Kopin IJ. Pancreatic polypeptide responses to hypoglycemia in chronic autonomic failure. *J Clin Endocrinol Metab* 1982; 54:48–52.

73. Cryer PE, Silverberg AB, Santiago JV, Shah SD. Plasma catecholamines in diabetes: The syndromes of hypoadrenergic and hyperadrenergic postural hypotension. *Am J Med* 1978; 64:407–416.

74. Leier CV, Boudoulas H. *Cardiorenal Disorders and Diseases*, 2d ed. Mount Kisco, NY: Futura Publishing; 1992.

75. Shy GM, Drager GA. A neurologic syndrome associated with orthostatic hypotension. *Arch Neurol* 1960; 2:511–527.

76. Kontos HA, Richardson DW, Norvell JE. Norepinephrine depletion in idiopathic orthostatic hypotension. *Ann Intern Med* 1975; 82:336–341.

77. Ziegler MG, Lake CR, Kopin IJ. The sympathetic nervous system defect in primary orthostatic hypotension. *N Engl J Med* 1977; 296:293–297.

78. Kopin IJ, Polinsky RJ, Oliver JA, Oddershede IR, Eberj MH. Urinary catecholamine metabolites distinguish different types of sympathetic neuronal dysfunction in patients with orthostatic hypotension. *J Clin Endocrinol Metab* 1983; 57:632–637.

79. Khurana RK, Nelson E, Azzarelli B, Garcia JH. Shy-Drager syndrome: Diagnosis and treatment of cholinergic dysfunction. *Neurology* 1980; 30:805–809.

80. Low PA, Gilden JL, Freeman R, Sheng K, McElligott MA. Efficacy of midodrine vs placebo in neurogenic orthostatic hypotension. A randomized, double blind multicenter study. *JAMA* 1997; 277:1046–1051.

81. Hoeldtke RD, Streeten DHP. Treatment of orthostatic hypotension with erythropoietin. *N Engl J Med* 1993; 329:611–615.

82. Bousser MG, Dubois B, Castaigne P. Transient loss of consciousness in ischemic cerebral events: A study of 557 ischemic strokes and transient ischemic attacks. *Ann Intern Med* 1980; 132:300–307.

83. Benbadis SR, Wolgamuth BR, Goren H, Brener S, Fouad-Tarazi F. Value of tongue biting in the diagnosis of seizures. *Arch Intern Med* 1995; 155:2346–2349.

84. Weiss S, Baker JP. The carotid sinus reflex in health and disease: Its role in the causation of fainting and convulsions. *Medicine* 1933; 12:297–354.

85. Graux P, Carlioz R, Guyomar Y, Lemaire N, Rihani R, Cornaert P, et al. Characteristics and influence of different clinical forms on the development and prognosis of carotid sinus syndrome. *Arch Mal Coeur Vaiss* 1995; 88:999–1006.

86. El-Sayed H, Hainsworth R. Relationship between plasma volume, carotid baroreceptor sensitivity and orthostatic tolerance. *Clin Sci* 1995; 88:463–470.

87. Nishizaki M, Arita M, Sakurada H, Ohta T, Yamawake N, Numano F, et al. Long-term follow-up of the reproducibility of carotid sinus hypersensitivity in patients with carotid sinus syndrome. *Jpn Circ J* 1995; 59:33–39.

88. Tea SH, Mansourati J, L'Heveder G, Mabin D, Blanc JJ. New insights into the pathophysiology of carotid sinus syndrome. *Circulation* 1996; 93:1411–1418.

89. Blanc J, Heveder GL, Mansourati J, Tea SH, Guillo P, Mabin D. Assessment of a newly recognized association. Carotid sinus hypersensitivity and denervation of sternocleidomastoid muscles. *Circulation* 1997; 95:2548–2551.

90. Hart G, Oldershaw PJ, Cull RE, Humphrey P, Ward D. Syncope caused by cough-induced complete atrioventricular block. *Pacing Clin Electrophysiol* 1982; 5:564–566.

91. Mattle HP, Nirkko AC, Baumgartner RW, Sturzenegger M. Transient cerebral circulatory arrest coincides with fainting in cough syncope. *Neurology* 1995; 45:498–501.

92. Bortolotti M, Cirignotta F, Labo G. Atrioventricular block induced by swallowing in a patient with diffuse esophageal spasm. *JAMA* 1982; 248:2297–2299.

93. Ferrante L, Artico M, Nardacci B, Fraioli B, Cosentino F, Fortuna A. Glossopharyngeal neuralgia with cardiac syncope. *Neurosurgery* 1995; 36:58–63.

94. Godec CJ, Cass AS. Micturition syncope. *J Urol* 1981; 126:551–556.

95. Kapoor WN, Peterson J, Karpf M. Defecation syncope: A symptom with multiple etiologies. *Arch Intern Med* 1986; 146:2377–2382.

96. Jansen RW, Connelly CM, Kelley-Cagnon M, Parker JA, Lipsitz LA. Postprandial hypotension in elderly patients with unexplained syncope. *Arch Intern Med* 1995; 155:945–952.

97. Jansen RWMM, Lipsitz LA. Postprandial hypotension: Epidemiology, pathophysiology, and clinical management. *Ann Intern Med* 1995; 122:286–295.

98. Nicholas R, O'Meara PD, Calonge N. Is syncope related to moderate altitude exposure? *JAMA* 1992; 268:904–906.

99. Kapoor WN, Fortunato M, Hanusa BH, Schulberg HC. Psychiatric illnesses in patients with syncope. *Am J Med* 1995; 99:505–512.

100. Aminoff MJ, Scheinman MM, Griffin JC, Herre JM. Electrocerebral accompaniments of syncope associated with malignant ventricular arrhythmias. *Ann Intern Med* 1988; 108:791–796.

101. Constantin L, Martins JB, Fincham RW, Dagli RD. Bradycardia and syncope as manifestations of partial epilepsy. *J Am Coll Cardiol* 1990; 15:900–905.

102. Grech ED, Ramsdale DR. Exertional syncope in aortic stenosis: Evidence to support inappropriate left ventricular baroreceptor response. *Am Heart J* 1991; 121:603–606.

103. Schwartz LS, Goldfisher J, Sprague GJ, Schwartz SP. Syncope and sudden death in aortic stenosis. *Am J Cardiol* 1969; 23:647–658.

104. Nienaber CA, Hiller S, Speilmann RP, Geiger M, Kuck KH. Syncope in hypertrophic cardiomyopathy: Multivariate analysis of prognostic determinants. *J Am Coll Cardiol* 1990; 15:948–955.

105. Dressler W. Effort syncope as an early manifestation of primary pulmonary hypertension. *Am J Med Sci* 1952; 223:131–143.

106. Scarpa WJ. The sick sinus syndrome. *Am Heart J* 1983; 92:648–651.

107. Talwar KK, Edvardsson N, Varnauskas E. Paroxysmal vagally mediated AV block with recurrent syncope. *Clin Cardiol* 1985; 8:337–340.

108. Beder SD, Cohen MH, Riemenschneider TA. Occult arrhythmias as the etiology of unexplained syncope in children with structurally normal hearts. *Am Heart J* 1985; 109:309–313.

109. Boudoulas H, Wooley CF. *Mitral Valve Prolapse and the Mitral Valve Prolapse Syndrome.* Mount Kisco, NY: Futura Publishing; 1988.

110. Moss AJ, Schwartz PJ, Crampton RS, Tzivoni D, Locati EH, MacCluer J, et al. The long QT syndrome: Prospective longitudinal study of 328 families. *Circulation* 1991; 84:1136–1144.

111. Soffer J, Dreifus LS, Michelson EL. Polymorphous ventricular tachycardia associated with normal and long QT intervals. *Am J Cardiol* 1982; 138:30–35.

112. Krikler DM, Curry PV. Torsade de pointes: An atypical ventricular tachycardia. *Br Heart J* 1976; 38:117–120.

113. Chen SY, Wang YH, Hwang JJ, Huang TS, Lai JS, Lien IN. Pulmonary embolism presenting as syncope in paraplegia: A case report. *Arch Phys Med Rehabil* 1995; 76:387–390.

114. Brignole M, Gianfranchi L, Menozzi C, Raviele A, Oddone D, Lolli G, et al. Role of autonomic reflexes in syncope associated with paroxysmal atrial fibrillation. *J Am Coll Cardiol* 1993; 22:1123–1129.

115. Alicandri C, Fouad FM, Tarazi RC, Castle L, Morant V. Three cases of hypotension and syncope with ventricular pacing: Possible role of atrial reflexes. *Am J Cardiol* 1978; 42:137–142.

116. Leitch JW, Klein GJ, Yee R, Leather RA, Kim YH. Syncope associated with supraventricular tachycardia. *Circulation* 1992; 85:1064–1071.

117. Ausubel K, Boal BH, Furmen S. Pacemaker syndrome: Definition and evaluation. *Cardiol Clin* 1985; 3:587–589.

118. Kuchar DL, Thorburn CW, Sammel NL. Signal-averaged electrocardiogram for evaluation of recurrent syncope. *Am J Cardiol* 1986; 58:949–953.

119. Gang ES, Peter T, Rosenthal ME, Oseran D, Mandel WJ, Deng ZW, et al. Detection of late potentials on the surface electrocardiogram in unexplained syncope. *Am J Cardiol* 1986; 58:1014–1020.

120. Winters SL, Stewart D, Gomes JA. Signal averaging of the surface QRS complex predicts inducibility of ventricular tachycardia in patients with syncope of unknown origin: A prospective study. *J Am Coll Cardiol* 1987; 10:775–781.

121. Nalos PC, Gang ES, Mandel WJ, Laddenheim ML, Lass Y, Peter T. The signal-averaged electrocardiogram as a screening test for inducibility of sustained ventricular tachycardia in high risk patients: A prospective study. *J Am Coll Cardiol* 1987; 9:539–548.

122. Cain ME, Anderson JL, Arnsdorf MF, Mason JW, Scheinman MM, Waldo AL. ACC Expert Consensus Document. Signal-averaged electrocardiography. *J Am Coll Cardiol* 1996; 27:238–249.

123. Englund A, Rosenqvist M, Bergfeldt L. Use of signal-averaged electrocardiography for predicting inducible sustained monomorphic ventricular tachycardia in patients with bundle branch block with and without a history of syncope. *Am Heart J* 1995; 130:481–488.

124. Steinberg JS, Prystowsky E, Freedman RA, Moreno F, Katz R, Kron J, et al. Use of the signal-averaged electrocardiogram for predicting inducible ventricular tachycardia in patients with unexplained syncope: Relation to clinical variables in a multivariate analysis. *J Am Coll Cardiol* 1994; 23:99–106.

125. Boudoulas H, Schaal SF, Lewis RP, Robinson JL. Superiority of 24-hour outpatient monitoring over multi-stage exercise testing for the evaluation of syncope. *J Electrocardiol* 1979; 12:103–108.

126. Boudoulas H, Geleris P, Schaal SF, Leier CV, Lewis RP. Comparison between electrophysiologic studies and ambulatory monitoring in patients with syncope. *J Electrocardiol* 1983; 16:91–96.

127. Dewey RC, Capeless MA, Levy AM. Use of ambulatory electrocardiographic monitoring to identify high risk patients with congenital complete heart block. *N Engl J Med* 1987; 316:835–839.

128. Gibson TC, Heitzman MR. Diagnostic efficacy of 24-hour electrocardiographic monitoring for syncope. *Am J Cardiol* 1984; 53:1013–1017.

129. Linzer M, Prystowsky EN, Brunetti LL, Varia IM, German LD. Recurrent syncope of unknown origin diagnosed by ambulatory continuous loop ECG recording. *Am Heart J* 1988; 116:1632–1634.

130. Shen WK, Holmes DR Jr, Hammill SC. Transtelephonic monitoring: Documentation of transient cardiac rhythm disturbances. *Mayo Clin Proc* 1987; 63:109–112.

131. Fetter JG, Stanton MS, Benditt DG, Trusty J, Collins J. Transtelephonic monitoring and transmission of stored arrhythmia detection and therapy data from an implantable cardioverter defibrillator. *Pacing Clin Electrophysiol* 1995; 18:1531–1539.

132. Kinlay S, Leitch JW, Neil A, Chapman BL, Hardy DB, Fletcher PJ. Cardiac event recorders yield more diagnoses and are more cost-effective than 48-hour Holter monitoring in patients with palpitations. *Ann Intern Med* 1996; 124:16–20.

133. DiMarco JP, Garan H, Harthorne JW, Ruskin JN. Intracardiac electrophysiologic techniques in recurrent syncope of unknown cause. *Ann Intern Med* 1981; 95:542–548.

134. Bhandari AK, Shapiro WA, Shen EN, Morady F, Mason J, Scheinman MM. Electrophysiologic testing in patients with the long QT syndrome. *Circulation* 1985; 71;63–71.

135. Olshansky B, Mazuz M, Martins JB. Significance of inducible tachycardia in patients with syncope of unknown origin: A long-term follow-up. *J Am Coll Cardiol* 1985; 5:216–223.

136. Click RL, Gersh BJ, Sugrue DD, Holmes DR Jr, Wood KL, Osburn MJ, et al. Role of invasive electrophysiologic testing in patients with symptomatic bundle branch block. *Am J Cardiol* 1987; 59:817–823.

137. Krol RB, Morady F, Flaker G, DiCarlo LA Jr, Baerman JM, Hewett J, et al. Electrophysiologic testing in patients with unexplained syncope: Clinical and noninvasive predictors of outcome. *J Am Coll Cardiol* 1987; 10:358–363.

138. Doherty JU, Pembrook-Rogers D, Grogan EW, Falcone R, Buxton AE, Marchlinski FE, et al. Electrophysiologic evaluation and follow-up characteristics of patients with recurrent unexplained syncope and presyncope. *Am J Cardiol* 1985; 55:703–708.

139. Kushner JA, Kou WH, Kadish AM, Moran F. Natural history of patients with unexplained syncope and a nondiagnostic electrophysiologic study. *J Am Coll Cardiol* 1989; 74:391–396.

140. Boudoulas H, Schaal SF, Lewis RP. Electrophysiologic risk factors in syncope. *J Electrocardiol* 1978; 11:339–342.

141. Englund A, Bergfeldt L, Rehnqvist N, Astrom H, Rosenqvist M. Diagnostic value of programmed ventricular stimulation in patients with bifascicular block: A prospective study of patients with and without syncope. *J Am Coll Cardiol* 1995; 26:1508–1515.

142. Mitchell LB, Duff HJ, Manyari DE, Wyse DG. A randomized clinical trial of the noninvasive and invasive approaches to drug therapy of ventricular tachycardia. *N Engl J Med* 1987; 317:1681–1687.

143. Morady F, Shen E, Schwartz A. Long-term follow-up of patients with recurrent unexplained syncope evaluated by electrophysiologic testing. *J Am Coll Cardiol* 1983; 2:1053–1059.

144. Baedeker W, Stein H, Theiss W, Goedel-Meinen L, Schmidt G, Blomer H. Syncopes of unclear etiology: Diagnosis, follow-up observations and pacemaker therapy. *Dtsch Med Wochenschr* 1987; 112:128–134.

145. Bellinder G, Nordlander R, Pehrsson SK, Astrom H. Atrial pacing in the management of sick sinus syndrome: Long-term observation for conduction disturbances and supraventricular tachyarrhythmias. *Eur Heart J* 1986; 7:105–109.

146. Langenfeld H, Grimm W, Marsch B, Dochsiek K. Course of symptoms and spontaneous ECG in pacemaker patients: A 5-year follow-up study. *Pacing Clin Electrophysiol* 1988; 11:2198–2206.

147. Moss AJ, Liu JE, Gottlieb S, Locati EH, Schwartz PJ, Robinson JL. Efficacy of permanent pacing in the management of high-risk patients with long QT syndrome. *Circulation* 1991; 84:1524–1529.

148. Nishimura RA, Giuliani ER, Brandenburg RO, Danielson GK. Hypertrophic cardiomyopathy. In: Giuliani ER, Gersh BJ, McGoon MD, Hayes DL, Schaff HV, eds. *Mayo Clinic Practice of Cardiology,* 3d ed. Chicago: Mosby-Year Book; 1996:689–711.

149. Jackman WM, Xunzhang W, Friday K, Roman C, Moulton KP, Beckman KJ, et al. Catheter ablation of accessory atrioventricular pathways (Wolff-Parkinson-White syndrome) by radio-frequency current. *N Engl J Med* 1991; 324:1605–1611.

150. Calkins H, Sousa J, El-Atassi R, Rosensheck S, de Buitleir H, Kou WH, et al. Diagnosis and cure of the Wolff-White-Parkinson syndrome or paroxysmal supraventricular tachycardia during a single electrophysiologic test. *N Engl J Med* 1991; 324:1612–1618.

151. Weiner DA, Levine SR, Klein MD. Ventricular arrhythmias during exercise testing: Mechanism, response to coronary bypass surgery and prognostic significance. *Am J Cardiol* 1984; 53:1553–1559.

152. Echt DS, Armstrong K, Schmidt P, Dyer PE, Stinson EB, Winkle RA. Clinical experience, complications, and survival in 70 patients with the automatic implantable cardioverter/defibrillator. *Circulation* 1985; 71:289–296.

153. Scheinman MM. Nonpharmacologic treatment of life-threatening cardiac arrhythmias. *Am Heart J* 1987; 114:1291–1298.

154. Manolis AS, Rastegar H, Estes NA. Automatic implantable cardioverter defibrillator: Current status. *JAMA* 1989; 262:1362–1368.

155. Mirowski M, Reid PR, Mower MM, Watkins L, Gott VL, Schauble JF, et al. Termination of malignant ventricular arrhythmias with an implanted automatic defibrillator in human beings. *N Engl J Med* 1980; 330:322–324.

156. Lipsitz LA. Syncope in the elderly. *Ann Intern Med* 1983; 99:92–105.

157. Lipsitz LA, Marks ER, Koestner J, Jonsson PV, Wei JY. Reduced susceptibility to syncope during postural tilt in old age: Is beta-blockade protective? *Arch Intern Med* 1989; 149:2709–2712.

158. Jonsson PV, Lipsitz LA, Kelley M, Koestner J. Hypotensive responses to common daily activities in institutionalized elderly. *Arch Intern Med* 1990; 150:1518–1524.

159. Lipsitz LA, Nyquist RP Jr, Wei JY, Rowe JW. Postprandial reduction in blood pressure in the elderly. *N Engl J Med* 1983; 309:81–83.

160. O'Mahony D. Pathophysiology of carotid sinus hypersensitivity in elderly patients. *Lancet* 1995; 346:950–952.

161. Ooi WL, Barrett S, Hossain M, Kelley-Gagnon M, Lipsitz LA. Patterns of orthostatic blood pressure change and their clinical correlates in a frail, elderly population. *JAMA* 1997; 277:1299–1304.

162. Rehm CG, Ross SE. Syncope as etiology of road crashes involving elderly drivers. *Am Surg* 1995; 61:1006–1008.

163. Rehm CG, Ross SE. Elderly drivers involved in road crashes: A profile. *Am Surg* 1995; 61:435–437.

164. Adams R. Cases of diseases of the heart, accompanied with pathological observations. *Dublin Hosp Rep* 1827; 4:353–453.

165. Stokes W. Observations on some permanently slow pulse. *Dublin Q J Clin Med Sci* 1846; 2:73–85.

166. Bondar RL, Kassam MS, Stein F, Dunphy PT, Fortney S, Riedesel ML. Simultaneous cerebrovascular and cardiovascular responses during presyncope. *Stroke* 1995; 26:1794–1800.

167. Middlekauff HR, Stevenson WG, Stevenson LW, Saxon LA. Syncope in advanced heart failure: High risk of sudden death regardless of origin of syncope. *J Am Coll Cardiol* 1993; 21:110–116.

168. Lascault G, Barnay C, Cazeau S, Frank R, Medvedowsky JL. Etude preliminaire d'un stimulateur double chambre a fonction diagnostique. *Arch Mal Coeur Vaiss* 1995; 88:451–457.

169. Leenhardt A, Lucet V, Denjoy I, Grau F, Ngoc DD, Coumel P. Catecholaminergic polymorphic ventricular tachycardia in children. A 7-year follow-up of 21 patients. *Circulation* 1995; 91:1512–1519.

170. Salim MA, DiSessa TG. QT interval response to exercise in children with syncope. *Am J Cardiol* 1994; 73:976–978.

171. Noh CI, Song JY, Kim HS, Choi JY, Yun YS. Ventricular tachycardia and exercise-related syncope in children with structurally normal hearts: Emphasis on repolarization abnormality. *Br Heart J* 1995; 73:544–547.

172. Sinkovec M, Rakovec P, Zorman D, Antolic G, Grad A. Exertional syncope in a patient with aortic stenosis and right coronary artery disease. *Eur Heart J* 1995; 16:276–278.

173. Williams CC, Bernhardt DT. Syncope in athletes. *Sports Med* 1995; 19:223–234.

174. Thomson HL, Atherton JJ, Khafagi FA, Frenneaux MP. Failure of reflex venoconstriction during exercise in patients with vasovagal syncope. *Circulation* 1996; 93:953–959.

175. Balaji S, Oslizlok PC, Allen MC, McKay CA, Gillette PC. Neurocardiogenic syncope in children with a normal heart. *J Am Coll Cardiol* 1994; 23:779–785.

176. Liberthson RR. Sudden death from cardiac causes in children and young adults. *N Engl J Med* 1996; 334:1039–1044.

177. Kapoor WN, Peterson J, Wieand HS, Karpf M. Diagnostic and prognostic implications of recurrences in patients with syncope. *Am J Med* 1987; 83:700–708.

178. Boudoulas H, Lewis RP. Cardiac syncope: Diagnosis, mechanism, and management. In: Hurst JW, et al, eds. *The Heart,* 6th ed. New York: McGraw-Hill; 1986: 321–329.

179. Calkins H, Shyr Y, Frumin H, Schork A, Morady F. The value of the clinical history in the differentiation of syncope due to ventricular tachycardia, atrioventricular block, and neurocardiogenic syncope. *Am J Med* 1995; 98:365–373.

180. Linzer M, Yang EH, Estes NA, Wang P, Vorperian VR, Kapoor WN. Diagnosing syncope. Part 1: Value of history, physical examination, and electrocardiography. *Ann Intern Med* 1997; 126:989–996.

181. Gilman JK. Syncope in the emergency department. *Emerg Med Clin North Am* 1995; 13:955–971.

182. Manolis AS. Evaluation of patients with syncope: Focus on age-related differences. Parts I and II. *ACC Current Journal Review* 1994:13–18.

183. Kroenke K, Lucas CA, Rosenberg ML, Scherokman B, Herbers JE, Wehrie PA, et al. Causes of persistent dizziness. A prospective study of 100 patients in ambulatory care. *Ann Intern Med* 1992; 117:898–904.

184. Krahn AD, Klein GJ, Norris C, Yee R. The etiology of syncope in patients with negative tilt table and electrophysiological testing. *Circulation* 1995; 92:1819–1824.

36

SUDDEN CARDIAC DEATH

Erica D. Engelstein / Douglas P. Zipes

DEFINITION OF SUDDEN CARDIAC DEATH

Sudden cardiac death describes the unexpected natural death due to a cardiac cause within a short time period from the onset of symptoms in a person without any prior condition that would appear fatal. The definition of sudden cardiac death should include the time interval from onset of the symptoms leading to collapse and then to death (which can usually be established only in the presence of a witness), the unexpected nature of the event, prior disease, and specific cause of death. Lack of all this information has led to many inconsistencies in the definition of sudden cardiac death (Table 36-1).[1–11] More recent definitions have focused on time intervals of 1 h or less, which normally identify sudden cardiac death populations having a high proportion (up to 91 percent) of arrhythmic death.[12,13] An inconsistency related to the definition of sudden cardiac death is inherent in the term itself. Death is an absolute and irreversible event. Because of improvements in emergency medical systems and community-based resuscitation, however, patients may survive the sudden death episode, which is a contradiction in terms. Ultimately though, the distinction between sudden cardiac death, non–sudden cardiac death and non–cardiac death is relevant more from a historical perspective, and total mortality is a more definitive end point in assessing the efficacy of an intervention aimed at improving survival.

EPIDEMIOLOGY

Incidence

Sudden cardiac death accounts for approximately 300,000 to 400,000 deaths yearly in the United States, depending on the definition used (Table 36-1).[1–11] When its definition is restricted to death less than 2 h from onset of symptoms,

12 percent of all natural deaths were sudden and 88 percent of these were due to cardiac disease. In autopsy-based studies, a cardiac etiology of sudden death has been reported in 60 to 70 percent of sudden death victims.[14,15] Sudden cardiac death is the most common, and often the first, manifestation of coronary heart disease (CHD) and is responsible for half the mortality from cardiovascular disease, which remains the main cause of death in this country. In the Framingham Study,[1–3] a 26-year survey of 5128 subjects (age 30 to 62) without evidence of cardiac disease at entry, 13 percent of all natural deaths were sudden, accounting for 50 percent of the mortality from CHD. Fifty percent of sudden cardiac deaths in men and 64 percent in women occurred in people without known CHD. The proportion of sudden cardiac death was lower (20 to 34 percent) in patients with known coronary heart disease. Sudden cardiac death was the first symptom of CHD in 10 percent of all coronary events in men and 8 percent of those in women.

The overall annual incidence of sudden cardiac death in the United States is probably best estimated with data derived from the National Center for Health Statistics.[10] This database from 40 states represents 71 percent of the U.S. population. Based on a combination of the place of death (out of hospital or emergency room) and diagnosis of CHD as an estimate of sudden cardiac death, the sudden cardiac death incidence in 1985 was 1.9 in men and 0.6 in women, resulting in 223,864 deaths of a total of 399,324 deaths from ischemic heart disease. Sudden cardiac death rates in developed countries outside the United States are comparable to those in the United States. Using methods similar to those of the National Center for Health Statistics study,[10] the World Health Organization reported an annual incidence of sudden cardiac death of 1.9 in men and 0.6 in women, again accounting for nearly half the deaths from CHD in a surveillance study of 3.5 million men and women aged 20 to 64 years.[16] Sudden cardiac death rates in developing countries are considerably lower, paralleling

TABLE 36-1

INCIDENCE OF SUDDEN CARDIAC DEATH IN SELECTED REGIONAL POPULATION STUDIES

Study	Patient Population	Definition of Sudden Cardiac Death	SCD (CHD Deaths)	Annual Incidence of SCD (per 1000 population)	Known CHD, %	Proportion of CHD Deaths, %	Comments
Framingham,[1–3] 1948–1974	5128 M + F 30–62 years; no prior CHD	<1 h	M:160(350) F: 73(196)	*Age: 45–54 55–64 65–74* M: 1.1 2.7 2.6 F: 0.3 0.4 1.2	M: 50 F: 36	M: 46 F: 35	18% M (24% F) had SCD as first symptom of CHD
Tecumseh,[4] 1959–1965	M + F ≥30 years	<1 h		2.0	40	46	
Baltimore,[5,6] 1964–1965	M + F 40–64 years	<24 h, witnessed	661 (1098)	*<2 h 2–24 h* M: 2.02 1.14 F: 0.39 0.34	51	60	
Allegheny,[7] 1970–1981	White M 35–44 years	<24 h, OOH, no disability	433		43	78	50% decline in CHD mortality, 77% due to decrease in SCD mortality
Worcester,[8] 1975–1988	M + F ≥25 years	OOH + ER		*1975 1978 1981 1984* 2.65 1.74 1.70 1.48			
Minnesota,[9] 1970–1980	M + F 30–74 years	OOH + ER		*Year: 1970 1980* M: 3.11 2.44 F: 0.96 0.7	M: 26[a] F: 16	M: 67 F: 60	
40 U.S. states,[10] 1980–1985	M + F 35–74 years	OOH + ER	223,864 (399,324)	M: 1.91[b] F: 0.57	56	M: 60 F: 50	
Denmark,[11] 1982	M + F ≥25 years	<24 h	166	*Age: 25–50 50–69 ≥70* M: 1.1 2.7 2.6 F: 0.3 0.4 1.2	75	13% of all deaths (1309)	19% had no prodrome or known heart disease

[a] Acute myocardial infarction only.
[b] White population only.

Abbreviations: CHD = coronary heart disease; ER = emergency room deaths; F = female; M = male; OOH = out-of-hospital deaths; SCD = sudden cardiac death.

the rates of ischemic heart disease as a whole (Fig. 36-1). In the United States, several populations-based studies have documented a decline (15 to 19 percent) in the incidence of sudden cardiac deaths caused by CHD since the early 1980s.[7,17]

Influence of Age, Race, and Gender

Since up to 80 percent of individuals suffering sudden cardiac death have CHD, its epidemiology parallels to a great extent that of CHD.

AGE

The incidence of sudden cardiac death increases with age, in both men and women as well as whites and nonwhites because of the higher prevalence of ischemic heart disease at older age (Fig. 36-2).[3] Among patients with CHD, however, the proportion of coronary deaths that are sudden decreases with age.[1,3]

RACIAL DIFFERENCES

An analysis of cardiac death rates from 40 U.S. states between 1980 and 1985 showed that the rate of sudden coronary death is higher in blacks than in whites (men, 66 versus 61 percent; women, 56 versus 50 percent).[10] The annual age-adjusted incidence of sudden cardiac death in a cohort of 860 white and 117 black cardiac arrest victims in Seattle between 1984 and 1986 was also higher in blacks than in whites: 3.4 percent versus 1.6 percent per 1000 population ($p < .001$).[18] A similar difference was reported in an analysis of 6451 cardiac arrest victims in Chicago.[19] Not only was the sudden cardiac death rate higher but the overall survival was also lower in blacks than in whites (10.2 percent versus 16.7 percent, $p < .07$, in Seattle, and 0.8 percent versus 2.6 percent, $p < .001$, in Chicago). In both studies, blacks were less likely to receive bystander cardiopulmonary resuscitation (CPR) and were less often found to have ventricular fibrillation as the presenting rhythm. The differences in outcome could not be accounted for by differences in emergency medical team response time or administration of advanced cardiac life support. It is more likely that the higher incidence of sudden cardiac death and poorer outcome in blacks is due to differences in health and socioeconomic status.

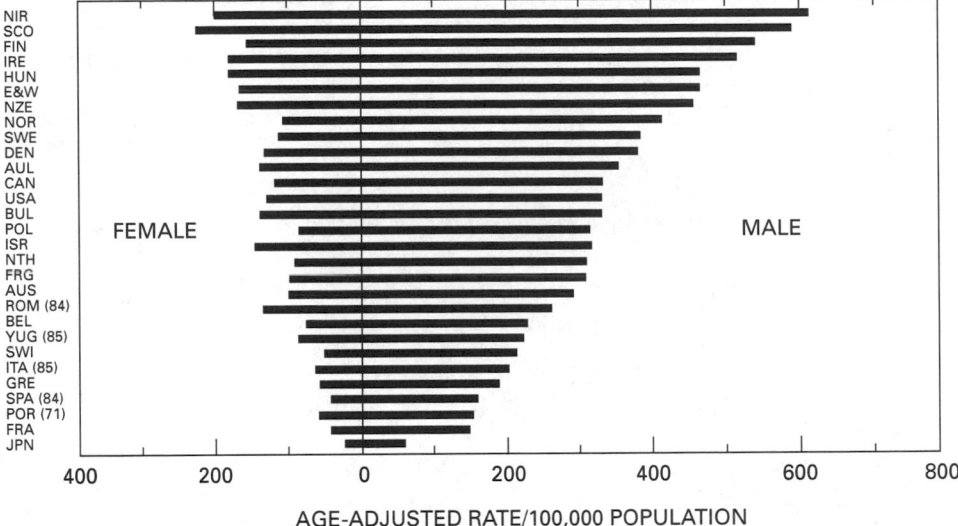

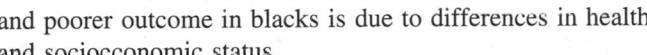

FIGURE 36-1

Sudden cardiac death rates by sex and country, ages 35 to 74 years, compiled from death certificates by the World Health Organization, Geneva, 1986. (Reprinted with permission from Manolio TA, Furberg CD. Epidemiology of sudden cardiac death. In: Akhtar M, Myerburg RJ, Ruskin JN, eds. *Sudden Cardiac Death.* Baltimore: Williams & Wilkins; 1994:3–20.)

GENDER

Sudden cardiac death has a much higher incidence in men than in women, reflecting gender differences in the incidence of CHD.[1–3] Between 70 and 89 percent of sudden cardiac deaths occur in men, and the annual incidence of sudden cardiac death in men is overall three to four times higher than in women. A higher percentage (64 percent) of sudden cardiac death in women than in men (50 percent) occurs in patients without prior evidence of coronary heart disease.[3] Among survivors of cardiac arrest, women are more likely than men to have other forms of structural heart disease (valvular heart disease, 13 percent versus 5 percent; idiopathic dilated cardiomyopathy, 19 percent versus 10 percent) or a "normal" heart (10 percent versus 3 percent), and only 45 percent of women as opposed to 80 percent of men have underlying CHD.[20]

Sudden Cardiac Death in the Young

Sudden cardiac death accounts for 19 percent of sudden deaths in children between 1 and 13 years of age and 30 percent between 14 and 21 years.[21] The overall incidence is low, 600 cases per year as compared with approximately 300,000 per year in the adult population. Structural cardiac abnormalities can be identified in over 90 percent of young victims of sudden cardiac death (Table 36-2).[21–33] About 40 percent of sudden cardiac deaths in the pediatric population occur in patients with surgically treated congenital cardiac abnormalities; in the majority of young victims, however, sudden cardiac death is often the first manifestation of underlying cardiac disease in otherwise healthy-appearing individuals.[34] The most common

causes of sudden cardiac death in the first three decades of life are myocarditis, hypertrophic cardiomyopathy, congenital coronary artery anomalies, atherosclerotic coronary heart disease, conduction system abnormalities, mitral valve prolapse, and aortic dissection. Among young people with known cardiac disease, aortic stenosis, and primary or secondary pulmo-

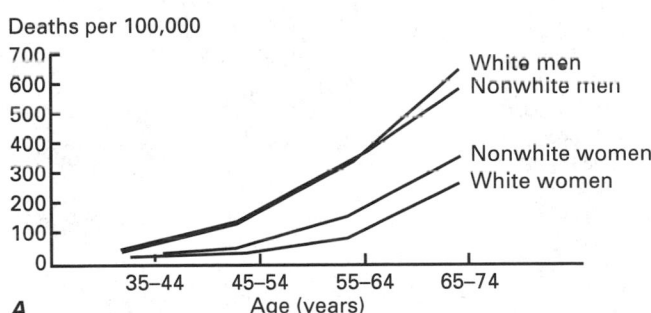

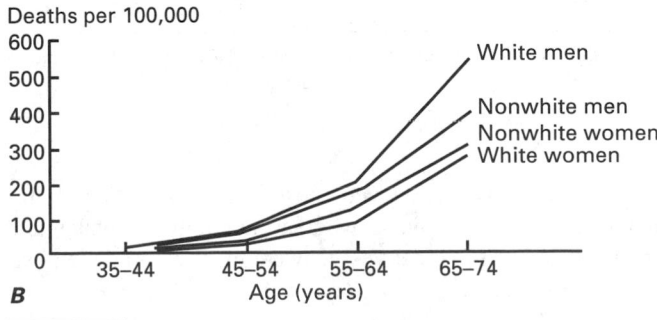

FIGURE 36-2

Plots of mortality rates (deaths per 100,000) for ischemic heart disease occurring (*A*) out of hospital or in emergency room (an estimate for sudden cardiac death rate) and (*B*) occurring in the hospital, by age, sex, and race in 40 states during 1985. (From the National Center for Health Statistics. Reprinted with permission from Gillum.[10])

TABLE 36-2

CAUSES OF SUDDEN CARDIAC DEATH IN YOUNG PERSONS

Study	N	Age, Years	Male, %	Myocarditis, %	CHD, %	HCM, %	RVCM, %	DCM, %	Congenital, %	Primary Arrhythmia or Conduction Abnormality, %	MVP, %	Preceding Symptoms	Exertion-Related, %
Burke,[23] Maryland, 1981–1988	690	14–40	77	5	48	10			2	3			5
Kennedy,[24] St. Louis C., 1981–1982	27	1–29			19	11			22				8
Drory,[25] Israel, 1976–1985	118	9–39	83	25	58	13				4		Dizziness, chest pain, syncope (54%)	23
Driscoll,[26] Olmstead C., 1950–1982	7	1–22	66	20		20			40	20		Syncope (25%)	17
Neuspiel,[21] Allegheny C., 1972–1980	51	1–21	58	27		10		24		12		Prior heart disease (41%)	22
Topaz,[27] St. Paul, 1960–1983	50	7–35	58	24	4	12			6		24	Family history (16%)	16
Phillips,[28] U.S. Air Force, 1965–1985	19	17–28	90	42	25	20					10		79
Kramer,[29] Israeli soldiers, 1974–1986	24	17–30	100	29	17	25		4		4	13	Syncope, fever, chest pain, (61%)	14
Thiene,[30] Northern Italy, 1979–1993	163	18–35		7	35	6	12	5	5	10	10		
Mollander,[31] Sweden, 1974–1979	9	1–20	56	44		22			33				33
Keeling,[32] Oxford, UK, 1965–1984	42	2–20		14	2	12		7	64				
Shen,[33] Olmstead C., 1960–1984	31	20–40	65	10	46	5	8		10	5			3

Abbreviations: CHD = coronary heart disease; DCM = dilated cardiomyopathy; HCM = hypertrophic cardiomyopathy; MVP = mitral valve prolapse; RVCM = right ventricular cardiomyopathy.

nary vascular obstruction were most common in patients without prior cardiac surgery, whereas tetralogy of Fallot and transposition of the great vessels were more common in postoperative patients.[34,35]

Risk Factors for Sudden Cardiac Death

Since a majority of sudden cardiac deaths in the adult population occur in patients with CHD, risk factors for sudden car-

diac death are similar to those of CHD, making a high-risk profile for CHD (Chap. 41) a high-risk profile for sudden cardiac death. In the Framingham Study—a multivariate prediction model based on known coronary risk factors such as *age, systolic blood pressure, left ventricular hypertrophy, intraventricular block or nonspecific abnormalities on the electrocardiogram (ECG), elevated serum cholesterol, glucose intolerance, decreased vital capacity, smoking, relative weight, and heart rate*—identified in the upper decile of multivariate risk 53 percent of men and 42 percent of women at risk for sudden cardiac death (Fig. 36-3).[1–3] Despite the fact that numerous population-based epidemiologic studies have shown a strong relationship of cardiovascular risk factors to the incidence of coronary heart disease and that of sudden cardiac death, none of them has identified a single set of risk factors specific for sudden cardiac death (Table 36-3).[1,2,36–39] The only coronary risk factors that seem to carry a disproportionate high risk for sudden cardiac death are those related to life style and psychosocial factors.[1,2,40–46]

CIGARETTE SMOKING

In the Framingham Study, the annual incidence of sudden cardiac deaths increased from 13 per 1000 in nonsmokers to 31 per 1000 in those smoking more than 20 cigarettes per day.[1,2,40] *People who stopped smoking had a prompt reduction in CHD mortality compared with those who continued to smoke irrespective of the duration of prior smoking habits.*[40,41] Smoking has been shown to act as a trigger for sudden cardiac death in predisposed patients by a variety of mechanisms, such as increase in platelet adhesiveness, decrease in ventricular fibrillation threshold, acceleration of heart rate, increase in blood pressure, induction of coronary

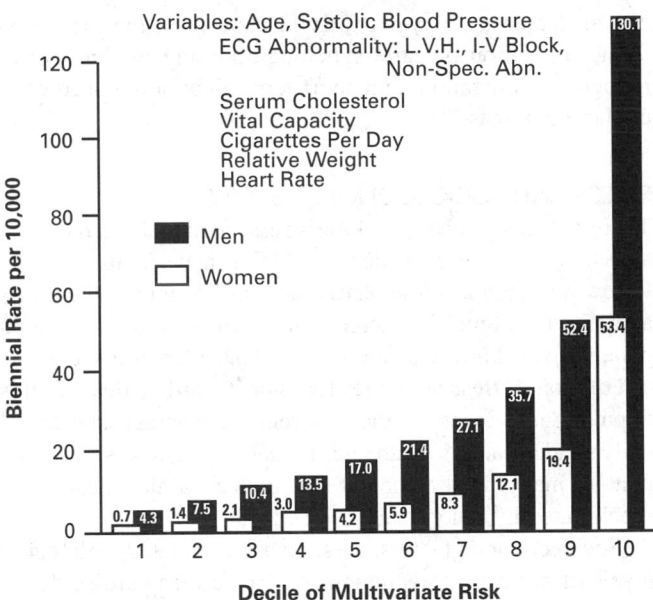

FIGURE 36-3

Risk of sudden cardiac death by decile of multivariate risk: 26-year follow-up, the Framingham Study. Abbreviations: ECG = electrocardiographic; I-V = intraventricular; LVH = left ventricular hypertrophy; Non-Spec. Abn. = nonspecific abnormality. (Reprinted with permission from Kannel and Schatzkin.[2])

TABLE 36-3

RISK FACTORS FOR SUDDEN CARDIAC DEATH IN POPULATION-BASED STUDIES

Study	Study Population	Risk Factors for SCD	
Kannel et al.[1,2] (Framingham Study)	5128 men and women, age 30–62, no CHD at entry: 546 CHD deaths over 26 years, 46% (men) and 35% (women) SCD	Men: LVH (by ECG) Cholesterol Systolic BP Relative body weight Cigarette smoking	Women: Vital capacity Cholesterol Hematocrit Serum glucose
Hinkle et al.[36]	269,755 men, age 20–65: 1839 CHD deaths over 5 years, 60% SCD	Hypertension Cigarette smoking Alcohol History of CHD LVH (by ECG) Enlarged heart (CXR) CHF PVCs	
Demirovic[37] (Yugoslavia Cardiovascular Disease study)	6614 men, age 35–62, no CHD at entry: 143 CHD deaths over 15 years, 75% SCD	Age Blood pressure Cigarette smoking	
Beaglehole et al.,[38] Aukland, New Zealand	300 cases of SCD, age <70	Cigarette smoking Low-level HDL	
Kagan et al.,[39] Hawaii	7591 middle-aged Japanese men living in Hawaii	Blood pressure Cholesterol Cigarette smoking Positive family history LVH (by ECG)	

Abbreviations: CHD = coronary heart disease; CHF = congestive heart failure; CXR = chest x-ray; HDL = high-density lipoproteins; LVH = left ventricular hypertrophy; PVC = premature ventricular contractions; SCD = sudden cardiac death.

spasm, decrease in oxygen-carrying capacity of the circulation by accumulation of carboxyhemoglobin and impairment of myoglobin utilization, and short-term nicotine-induced catecholamine release.[40]

STRESS AND SOCIOECONOMIC STATUS

There are many reports linking stress, particularly emotional stress, to sudden cardiac death.[42,43] For instance, in the hours following the Northridge earthquake in California, there was a more than fourfold increase in sudden cardiac death in patients with known or unknown CHD, illustrating the role of emotional stress as trigger for sudden cardiac death in this population.[44] Based on the difference of average and actual daily sudden cardiac death rates in that period, it was estimated that as many as 40 percent of sudden cardiac deaths are precipitated by emotional stress.

Socioeconomic factors, presumably associated with higher levels of stress, can also contribute to sudden cardiac death. For instance, a more than threefold increase of sudden cardiac death following myocardial infarction was reported in men with low levels of education and complex ventricular ectopy compared with better-educated men with the same arrhythmias.[45] In a study of sudden cardiac death in women, those who died suddenly were less often married, had fewer children, and had greater educational discrepancies with their spouses compared to age-matched controls in the same neighborhood.[46]

PHYSICAL ACTIVITY

There is increasing evidence that regular physical activity may help prevent CHD and its complications.[2,47–50] On the other hand, the value of vigorous exercise in patients with known CHD is controversial, and several studies have reported triggering of sudden cardiac death and acute myocardial infarction by vigorous exercise.[51,52] Emergency medical records show that in adults, 11 to 17 percent of cardiac arrest victims collapsed during or immediately after exertion, although the amount of exertion is rarely quantified.[48] The increased risk of cardiac arrest due to ventricular fibrillation during or after exercise is also evident in cardiac rehabilitation programs and exercise stress testing in patients with heart disease. In these situations, cardiac arrests rates of 1 in 12,000 to 15,000 (rehabilitation) and 1 per 2000 (stress testing) have been reported, which is at least six times higher than the general incidence of sudden cardiac death for patients known to have heart disease.[48] Because of immediate and successful defibrillation in most cases, these reported cases of cardiac arrest have rarely been fatal. These observations, however, do support the concept that vigorous physical activity can trigger cardiac arrest due to ventricular fibrillation. On the other hand, there is increasing experimental evidence that regular exercise may prevent ischemia-induced ventricular fibrillation and death by altering autonomic function, specifically by increasing vagal reflexes.[53] Thus, it appears that the beneficial effects of regular exercise on cardiovascular

morbidity and mortality are partially offset by (vigorous) exertion-induced sudden cardiac death in patients with underlying heart disease.

Sudden Cardiac Death in Competitive Athletes

Sudden cardiac death in competitive athletes is an extremely rare event. Between 10 and 25 sports-related sudden deaths from cardiac causes occur annually in the United States.[22] The annual incidence of sudden cardiac death during exercise is 1 per 200,000 among Air Force recruits who have been prescreened by general physical examination[28] and 1 per 250,000 among unscreened young runners.[54] Collapse usually occurs during or shortly after exercise, either in training or during competition. Although, unfortunately, sudden cardiac death is often the first manifestation of their disease, the majority of sudden cardiac deaths in athletes occur in persons with underlying cardiac disease.[23,55–57] Age has been shown to be the most useful variable in predicting the underlying cardiac disease[55] (Fig. 36-4). In athletes below 35 years of age, the vast majority of sudden cardiac deaths arise from a variety of congenital cardiovascular diseases, most commonly hypertrophic cardiomyopathy, congenital coronary artery anomalies, and aortic rupture associated with Marfan's syndrome. Atherosclerotic coronary artery disease (CAD) is found in only about 10 percent of athletes in this younger age group, compared with 80 percent in those older than 35 years.[55]

Screening programs for identifying relatively rare cardiac abnormalities in a large population of asymptomatic athletes are often costly and inefficient.[58] Guidelines for such screening have therefore been published; they are based mainly on detailed personal and family history, physical examination, and ECG, with echocardiography and other noninvasive tests reserved for those with any positive finding during the initial evaluation.[59] Guidelines have also been published outlining which athletes with cardiac arrhythmias can participate in competitive athletics[59] (see also Chap. 95).

MECHANISM OF SUDDEN CARDIAC DEATH

The Relationship between Structure and Function in Sudden Cardiac Death

A vast majority of patients who have experienced sudden cardiac death have had cardiac structural abnormalities. In the adult population, these consist predominantly of coronary heart disease, cardiomyopathies, valvular heart disease, and abnormalities of the conduction system. These structural changes provide the substrate for ventricular tachyarrhythmias, which represent the cause of sudden cardiac death in most cases. It is important to recognize the role of triggering factors, such as fluctuations in the autonomic nervous system, electrolyte abnormalities, and proarrhythmic effects of drugs

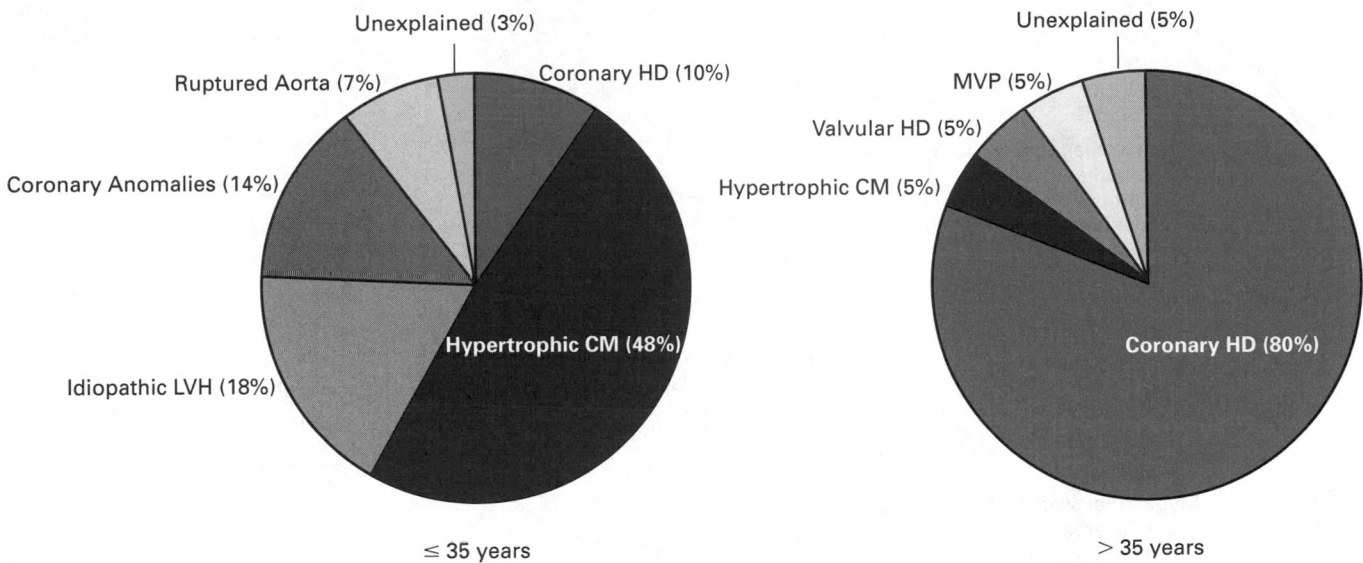

FIGURE 36-4

Causes of sudden cardiac death in competitive athletes by age group. There is evidence for structural heart disease in nearly all athletes who die suddenly of cardiac causes. In athletes younger than 35 years, hypertrophic cardiomyopathy is more prevalent, whereas in those older than 35 years, coronary heart disease is the most frequent cause. CM = cardiomyopathy; HD = heart disease; LVH = left ventricular hypertrophy; MVP = mitral valve prolapse. (Reprinted with permission from Maron et al.[55])

in the initiation of ventricular arrhythmias resulting in sudden cardiac death (Fig. 36-5).[60,61] Strategies aimed at eliminating or reducing the triggers of arrhythmias may prove to be efficient short- and midterm solutions, since many of the structural abnormalities cannot be cured or require long-term risk-factor modification to prevent their development.

Tachyarrhythmias versus Bradyarrhythmias in Sudden Cardiac Death

Ventricular fibrillation is the first recorded rhythm in approximately 70 percent of patients who have cardiac arrest.[62,63] Sustained ventricular tachycardia is only rarely (<2 percent) documented as the initial rhythm, but it is unknown how often it precedes and precipitates ventricular fibrillation. In a series of 157 patients who were wearing an ambulatory ECG monitor at the time of their cardiac arrest, primary ventricular fibrillation was documented in 8 percent, ventricular tachycardia degenerating into ventricular fibrillation in 62 percent, and torsades de pointes in 13 percent.[64]

Electromechanical dissociation and asystole are found in about 30 percent of patients experiencing cardiac arrest, and this finding is usually related to the time interval from collapse to first monitoring of the rhythm, suggesting that it is a later manifestation of cardiac arrest.[62,63] The incidence of bradycardia as the first documented rhythm varies according to the population studied. In patients who have died suddenly while wearing an ambulatory ECG monitor, bradyarrhythmias as the initial rhythm were documented in 17 percent (26 of 231).[65] In a group of 21 patients with severe congestive heart failure awaiting cardiac transplantation, bradycardia or electromechanical dissociation accounted for 62 percent of sudden

cardiac deaths.[66] Ambulatory ECG recordings demonstrated that even in patients with atrioventricular or intraventricular conduction defects, ventricular tachyarrhythmias are most often the mode of recurrent cardiac arrest.[64,67] A sudden slowing of the heart rate may also trigger ventricular tachyarrhythmias in normal hearts, potentially by greatly prolonging ventricular refractoriness.[68] Therefore, treatment of bradycardia may prevent the onset of tachyarrhythmias and is an important consideration in the prevention of sudden cardiac death.

Since ventricular fibrillation is the most frequent cause of sudden cardiac death, understanding the mechanisms responsible for this arrhythmia is essential in its prevention and treatment. A complete discussion is beyond the scope of this chapter (see Chaps. 26 and 27). Fundamentally, electrical inhomogeneity is most likely the basis of fibrillation, setting the stage for unidirectional block and reentrant excitation.[69] Experimental and theoretical evidence suggests that myocardial reentry caused by spiral waves of excitation may be important.[70]

Role of Ischemia

The electrophysiologic effects of acute ischemia include a decrease in amplitude and upstroke velocity of the cardiac action potential, depolarization of the resting membrane potential and shortening of action potential duration.[69] The changes in refractoriness during ischemia occur inhomogenously, largely caused by local abnormalities in extracellular K^+ and acidosis. Refractory periods in the ischemic myocardium shorten after the first 2 min of coronary occlusion along with the shortening of the action potential duration. Partially

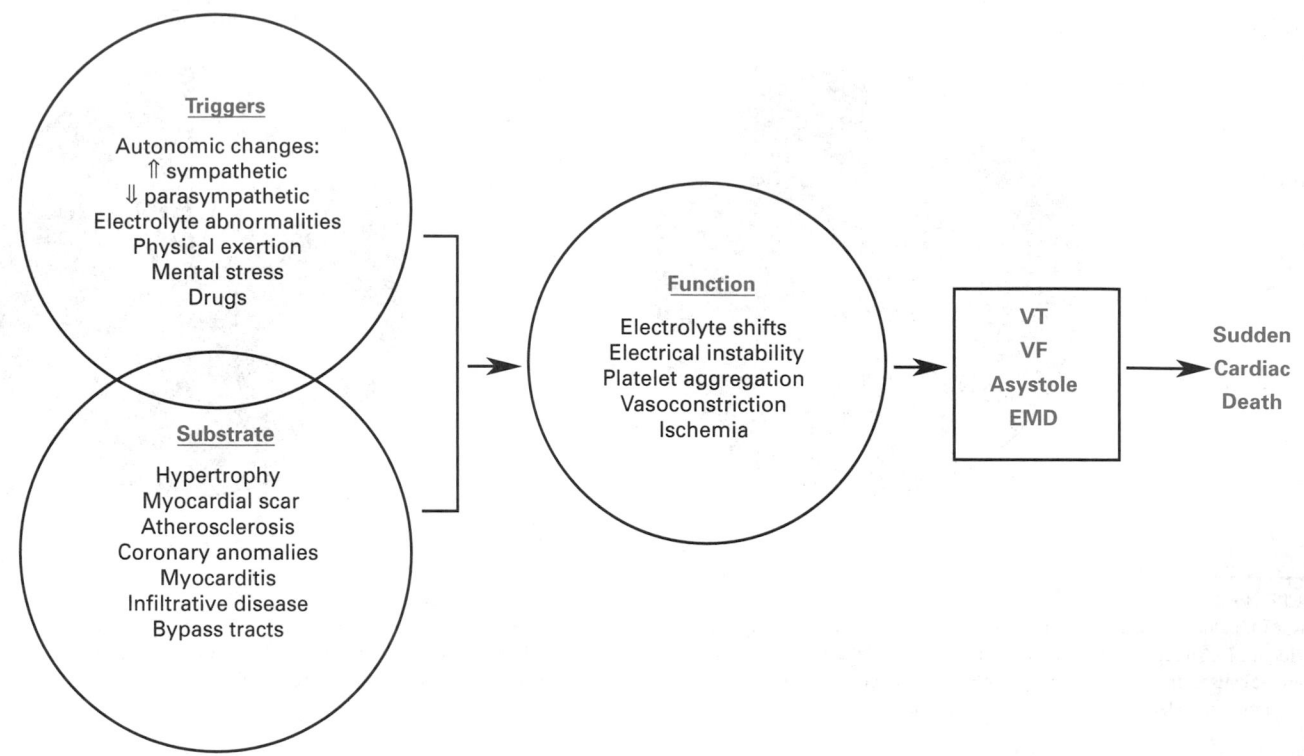

FIGURE 36-5

Interaction between structural cardiac abnormalities, functional changes, and triggering factors in the pathophysiology of sudden cardiac death. The role of triggering factors, such as changes in autonomic tone or reflexes, is increasingly being recognized. EMD = electromechanical dissociation; VF = ventricular fibrillation; VT = ventricular tachycardia.

depolarized fibers, however, may remain inexcitable even after completion of repolarization, eventually prolonging refractoriness despite shortening of the action potential duration. This postrepolarization refractoriness may further contribute to inhomogeneities in electrophysiologic properties within and around the ischemic zone, causing significant conduction delays, unidirectional block, and reentrant arrhythmias. In addition, cellular uncoupling occurs after 20 to 25 min of ischemia, causing conduction to become slow and discontinuous.[71]

Ventricular arrhythmias during experimental acute ischemia occur in two peaks, one between 2 and 10 min following coronary occlusion and the second at 15 to 20 min. Rapid polymorphic ventricular tachycardias and ventricular fibrillation are the characteristic arrhythmias during the early stages of ischemia and are the cause of sudden cardiac death.[72] Activation mapping during ventricular fibrillation has demonstrated that the initial arrhythmias are due to reentry, which is facilitated by the inhomogeneous conduction velocities and refractory periods in and around the ischemic zone. The second peak of ventricular arrhythmias coincides with a peak in catecholamine release, and other mechanisms such as abnormal automaticity or triggered activity have been invoked. Ventricular tachyarrhythmias also occur frequently during reperfusion of the infarct zone, as seen after administration of thrombolytic agents.[73]

In the subacute phase of myocardial infarction (within the first 3 days), sudden cardiac death may occur due to ventricular fibrillation in the setting of frequent premature ventricular complexes (PVCs). These ventricular arrhythmias have been shown to be predominantly due to abnormal impulse initiation consistent with abnormal automaticity and are clinically manifest as accelerated idioventricular rhythm or idioventricular tachycardia. These arrhythmias appear to arise for the most part from surviving Purkinje fibers in the subendocardial border zone of a transmural infarction. These arrhythmias usually subside after 2 to 3 days in parallel with the normalization of the resting membrane potential and action potential duration of Purkinje fibers and have no prognostic significance for development of late arrhythmias.[69]

In the late phases following myocardial infarction, when the infarction is healed, reentrant excitation appears to be the principal mechanism of ventricular arrhythmias. Critical areas of the reentrant circuit are formed by surviving myocardial cells in the epicardial and endocardial border zone of a healed infarction, as well as surviving intramural fibers within the infarct zone[72] (see also Chap. 26).

Mechanoelectrical Feedback

Left ventricular dysfunction has been identified as the strongest independent predictor of sudden cardiac death. Despite the clinical recognition that acute heart failure can precipitate ventricular tachyarrhythmias, the mechanism by which this occurs is incompletely understood. Beside mechanisms related to acute and chronic ischemia, it has been shown that acute changes in the mechanical state of the heart related to altered preload and contractility can have direct electrophysiologic effects that may precipitate arrhythmias; this relationship is usually referred to as *mechanoelectrical feedback*.[74] An increase in both left ventricular preload and contractility has been shown to shorten action potential duration in the canine ventricle.[74] An increase in right ventricular pressure has been shown to shorten action potential duration in humans.[75] The cellular mechanism by which this occurs is unknown, but there is some evidence that these changes might be mediated by fluctuation of intracellular calcium.[74]

Role of the Autonomic Nervous System in the Genesis of Arrhythmias

There is increasing evidence that cardiac abnormalities associated with a high risk of sudden cardiac death are accompanied by changes in autonomic innervation of the heart. Myocardial infarction, for instance, has been shown to cause regional cardiac sympathetic and parasympathetic denervation not only in the infarcted area but also in the region apical to the infarct because of interruption of afferent and efferent nerve fibers transversing the infarct zone.[76] The denervated areas show supersensitivity to catecholamine infusion, with disproportionate shortening of action potential duration and refractoriness.[77] This autonomic heterogeneity may predispose to arrhythmia development by creating dispersion of refractoriness and/or conduction. Studies with metaiodobenzylguanidine (MIBG) scintigraphy in humans have demonstrated evidence of sympathetic denervation in 10 of 12 patients with spontaneous ventricular tachyarrhythmias after myocardial infarction and 2 of 7 postinfarction patients without ventricular arrhythmias.[78] Preconditioning ischemia, which may reduce fatal arrhythmias during acute coronary occlusion, has been shown to preserve the efferent sympathetic and parasympathetic response during the early period after coronary artery occlusion in the dog.[79]

Whereas sympathetic activation favors the onset of life-threatening cardiac arrhythmias, vagal activation has been shown to have a protective effect in the presence of tonic sympathetic stimulation.[80] This is thought to be due, at least in part, to the antiadrenergic effects of vagal stimulation via reduction of norepinephrine release and inhibition of adenylate cyclase via inhibitory G proteins. Because it is difficult to study the effects of vagal activity on ventricular electrophysiological properties directly, the behavior of the sinus node has been used as a surrogate by measuring indices of heart rate variability (reflecting primarily tonic vagal activity) and evaluating baroreflex sensitivity (a measure of reflex vagal activity). Susceptibility to ventricular fibrillation and sudden cardiac death provoked by ischemia in a chronic (4-week) infarct model has been associated with decreased baroreflex

sensitivity in dogs.[53] The risk of sudden cardiac death in this model increased from 20 percent for a baroreflex sensitivity >15 ms/mmHg to 91 percent for a slope of <9 ms/mmHg. Myocardial infarction reduced baroreflex sensitivity 4 weeks after myocardial infarction in 73 percent of animals studied compared to control. A transient (<3 months) decrease in baroreflex sensitivity following myocardial infarction has also been demonstrated in humans.[81] The prognostic value of baroreflex sensitivity in humans has been suggested in several studies.[82,83] Modulation of vagal tone may offer a new approach to prevention of sudden cardiac death. Prevention of ischemia-induced ventricular fibrillation was achieved in dogs, in which heart rate variability (by 74 percent) and baroreflex sensitivity (by 69 percent) were increased by daily exercise training.[84]

CARDIAC DISEASES ASSOCIATED WITH SUDDEN CARDIAC DEATH (TABLE 36-4)

Ischemic Heart Disease

CORONARY ATHEROSCLEROSIS

In survivors of cardiac arrest, CHD is found in 40 to 86 percent of patients, depending on age and gender of the population studied.[85] In most pathologic studies, a greater than 75 percent cross-sectional stenosis in at least one major coronary artery is used to distinguish coronary from noncoronary heart disease as the presumed etiology for sudden cardiac death. Although the majority of patients who suffer sudden cardiac death have severe multivessel CAD, fewer than half of the patients resuscitated from ventricular fibrillation evolve evidence of myocardial infarction by elevated cardiac enzymes, and less than a quarter have Q-wave myocardial infarction.[62] Despite the lack of clinical evidence for myocardial infarction in the majority of patients resuscitated from sudden cardiac death, a recent occlusive coronary thrombus has been reported in 15 to 64 percent of victims of sudden death caused by ischemic heart disease,[86] and several detailed pathologic studies have documented the presence of acute coronary arterial lesions (plaque fissure, plaque hemorrhage and thrombosis) in 38 to 95 percent of patients dying suddenly.[87–89] Healed infarctions are present in 44 to 82 percent of hearts of sudden cardiac death victims at autopsy and in 38 to 91 percent of survivors of cardiac arrest.[90] Studies demonstrating the sudden occlusion of previously only minimally stenosed coronary arteries, which are presumably a weaker stimulus for development of collaterals than high-grade lesions, suggest an important role of coronary collateralization in the presentation of coronary artery disease as sudden cardiac death.[91] This mitigating effect of coronary collateralization is further supported by a study of exercise testing in 894 healthy men followed for a mean of 12.7 years. In this study, the initial coronary event was acute myocardial infarction or sudden cardiac death in 73 percent of those with a normal stress test, as opposed to 20

TABLE 36-4

CARDIAC ABNORMALITIES ASSOCIATED WITH SUDDEN CARDIAC DEATH

Ischemic heart disease
  Coronary atherosclerosis
    Acute myocardial infarction
    Chronic ischemic cardiomyopathy
  Anomalous origin of coronary arteries
  Hypoplastic coronary artery
  Coronary artery spasm
  Coronary artery dissection
  Coronary arteritis
  Small vessel disease
Nonischemic heart disease
  Cardiomyopathies
    Idiopathic dilated cardiomyopathy
    Hypertrophic cardiomyopathy
    Hypertensive cardiomyopathy
    Right ventricular cardiomyopathy
  Infiltrative and inflammatory heart disease
    Sarcoidosis
    Amyloidosis
    Hemochromatosis
    Myocarditis
  Valvular heart disease
    Aortic stenosis
    Aortic regurgitation
    Mitral valve prolapse
    Infective endocarditis
  Congenital heart disease
    Tetralogy of Fallot
    Transposition of the great vessels (post-Mustang/
      Senning)
    Ebstein's anomaly
    Pulmonary vascular obstructive disease
    Congenital aortic stenosis
  Primarily electrical abnormalities
    Long QT syndrome
    Wolff-Parkinson-White syndrome
    Congenital heart block
    Idiopathic ventricular fibrillation
      Syndrome of RBBB, ST-elevation, and sudden
        death (Brugada syndrome)
      Nocturnal sudden death in Southeast Asian men
        (Pokkuri syndrome)
Drug-induced and other toxic agents
  Antiarrhythmic drugs (classes Ia, Ic, III)
  Erythromycin
  Terfenadine
  Pentamidine
  Psychotropic drugs (tricyclic antidepressants,
    chlorpromazine)
  Cocaine
  Alcohol
  Phosphodiesterase inhibitors
Electrolyte abnormalities
  Hypokalemia
  Hypomagnesemia
  Hypercalcemia
  Anorexia nervosa and bulimia
  Liquid protein dieting
  Diuretics

percent of those with an abnormal stress test.[92] It has been hypothesized that chronic ischemia may be a stimulus for development of coronary collaterals, which in turn could have a protective effect during acute coronary occlusion. Of note, patients with silent ischemia during exercise testing have the same likelihood of developing an acute myocardial infarction or sudden cardiac death as do symptomatic patients.[93]

Since coronary artery disease is the major substrate of sudden cardiac death, risk stratification following myocardial infarction is an important step in the prevention of sudden cardiac death. Few variables, mainly frequent PVCs (>10/h), reduced left ventricular ejection fraction (<40 percent), and use of digitalis are independent risk factors for sudden versus nonsudden cardiac death following myocardial infarction.[94–97] The incidence of sudden cardiac death in the first 2 years after myocardial infarction ranged from 11 to 18 percent in these studies. The variables identified to predict sudden cardiac death following myocardial infarction in these studies are better in selecting a low-risk population for sudden cardiac death than predicting who will die suddenly. In the absence of frequent PVCs and with a normal left ventricular ejection fraction following myocardial infarction, the risk of sudden cardiac death is low (less than 2 percent in the first year).[98] On the other hand, even when all clinical risk factors for sudden cardiac death are present following myocardial infarction, the reported risk varies between 10 and 40 percent and generally does not warrant prophylactic antiarrhythmic therapy. Hopefully, risk-stratification models incorporating other methods (heart rate variability, baroreflex sensitivity, nonlinear dynamics, T-wave alternans, imaging of the cardiac autonomic innervation) assessing triggers of sudden cardiac death such as autonomic fluctuations and electrical instability will enhance their positive predictive value (see also Chap. 47).

NONATHEROSCLEROTIC DISEASE OF THE CORONARY ARTERIES

Several nonatherosclerotic diseases of the coronary arteries are associated with increased risk of sudden cardiac death precipitated by cardiac ischemia. *Congenital coronary artery anomalies*, found in approximately 1 percent of all patients undergoing angiography and in 0.3 percent of patients undergoing autopsy, *have been complicated by sudden cardiac death in up to about 30 percent of patients, often exercise-related.*[99] Origin of the left main coronary artery from the right aortic sinus or origin of the right coronary artery from the left coronary sinus were most frequently the cause. It has been postulated that acute ischemia is due to compression of the anomalous coronary artery between the pulmonary artery and aorta during exercise-induced expansion of these vessels and to diminished coronary flow reserve due to the slitlike orifice and acute takeoff angle of the anomalous vessel.[99]

Life-threatening ventricular arrhythmias and sudden cardiac death have been described in patients with *coronary artery spasm* (Prinzmetal's anginal, variant angina). In a series of 81 patients with coronary artery spasm, 13 patients

(16 percent) had at least one episode of cardiac arrest due to ventricular fibrillation.[100,101] Significant arrhythmias during attacks of variant angina were documented in 41 percent of these patients and appeared to be associated with a higher risk of sudden cardiac death. Calcium-channel blockers are effective in many patients in preventing coronary spasm and appear also to protect from malignant ventricular arrhythmias if the attacks can be completely abolished.[100,101]

Sudden cardiac death has been described as a rare complication of *coronary artery dissection* in Marfan's syndrome, after labor and delivery, secondary to trauma or coronary catheterization, as a consequence of syphilitic aortitis, or as an extension of aortic dissection. *Myocardial bridges* have been reported in association with sudden cardiac death during exercise, but they are also an incidental finding at autopsy in up to 20 percent of patients dying of other causes.

Cardiomyopathies

IDIOPATHIC DILATED CARDIOMYOPATHY

Idiopathic dilated cardiomyopathy is the substrate for approximately 10 percent of sudden cardiac deaths in the adult population. Mortality rates in idiopathic dilated cardiomyopathy are high, reaching 10 to 50 percent annually, depending on the severity of disease.[102] In an overview of 14 studies including 1432 patients with idiopathic dilated cardiomyopathy, the mean mortality rate after a follow-up of 4 years was 42 percent, with 28 percent of deaths classified as sudden.[102] Sudden cardiac death in idiopathic dilated cardiomyopathy is usually attributed to ventricular tachyarrhythmias on the basis of the high frequency of complex ventricular ectopy found in these patients.[103] The terminal event can, however, also be asystole or electromechanical dissociation, especially in patients with advanced left ventricular dysfunction.[66] Factors potentially contributing to the generation of arrhythmias in idiopathic dilated cardiomyopathy are mechanoelectrical feedback, electrolyte depletion due to chronic diuretic therapy, excessive activation of the sympathetic nervous and renin-angiotensin systems, and proarrhythmic effects.[104]

Risk stratification of patients with idiopathic dilated cardiomyopathy is difficult because there are few clinical predictors specific for sudden cardiac death.[105] Patients with idiopathic dilated cardiomyopathy have a very high incidence of ventricular ectopy, with simple PVCs, complex PVCs, and non-sustained ventricular tachycardia present in 94 percent, 76 percent, and 40 percent, respectively, thus limiting their prognostic value by a low specificity.[103] The prognostic value of intraventricular conduction delays on ECG, which are associated with decreased survival, is again not specific for sudden cardiac death, whereas late potentials, recorded by signal-averaged ECGs, can be detected only in a minority of patients with idiopathic dilated cardiomyopathy.[106] Although mortality is higher in patients with advanced heart failure, the proportion of sudden cardiac deaths is not increased.[107] The only clinical variable that identifies patients with a higher risk of sudden cardiac death in this population is syncope.[102] The value of electrophysiologic testing in patients with idiopathic dilated cardiomyopathy is limited, since it frequently results in the initiation of polymorphic ventricular tachycardia or ventricular fibrillation, which appear to be nonspecific findings, and the absence of inducible ventricular tachyarrhythmias in this population does not accurately predict a low risk for sudden cardiac death[108] (see Chap. 73).

HYPERTROPHIC CARDIOMYOPATHY

The incidence of sudden cardiac death in patients with hypertrophic cardiomyopathy (HCM) is 2 to 4 percent per year in adults, and a 4 to 6 percent per year in children and adolescents.[109] A review of 78 patients with HCM who died suddenly or survived a cardiac arrest episode showed that 71 percent were younger than 30 years of age, 54 percent were without functional limitation, and 61 percent were performing sedentary or minimal physical activity at the time of cardiac arrest.[110] The mechanism of sudden cardiac death in HCM is not clear. Primary arrhythmias, hemodynamic events with diminished stroke volume, and/or ischemia have been implicated.[109,111] Assessment of autonomic function in patients with HCM revealed abnormal responses of heart rate and blood pressure to exercise in two-thirds, which was associated with a more malignant clinical course, suggesting that autonomic imbalance may be important in the genesis of sudden cardiac death in these patients.[112]

There are few predictors of sudden cardiac death in patients with HCM. A clinical history of aborted sudden cardiac death or sudden death in family members indicates a worse prognosis, as does onset of symptoms in childhood.[110] Hemodynamic and echocardiographic variables such as left ventricular wall thickness or the presence of outflow tract obstruction are not useful in identifying patients at high risk for sudden cardiac death. Ambulatory ECG monitoring has been reported to be of some value in identifying patients with HCM at risk for sudden cardiac death.[113] Sustained ventricular tachyarrhythmias, predominantly rapid polymorphic ventricular tachycardia, have been induced in 27 to 43 percent of patients with HCM at electrophysiologic study, but their prognostic significance is controversial.[113,114] Absence of inducible sustained ventricular tachyarrhythmias at electrophysiologic study, absence of nonsustained ventricular tachycardia on ambulatory ECG, and no history of "impaired consciousness" (i.e., cardiac arrest or syncope) identified a subset (22 percent) of patients with HCM with a low (<1 percent) risk for sudden cardiac death.[114] In approximately 50 percent of families with HCM, different missense mutations in the β-cardiac myosin heavy-chain gene have been identified, and the location of the mutation appeared to influence survival[115] (see Chaps. 69 and 74).

HYPERTENSIVE CARDIOMYOPATHY

Left ventricular hypertrophy as detected by electrocardiography is a strong independent risk factor for cardiovascular deaths and, in particular, sudden cardiac death in patients who also have a history of hypertension.[117,118] In the Framingham Study, ECG evidence of left ventricular hypertrophy doubled the risk of sudden cardiac death.[116] Echocardiographic studies showed an incremental risk for cardiovascular deaths of 1.73 in men and 2.12 in women for each 50 g increment in the index of left ventricular mass.[116] The proposed mechanism for this increased mortality in patients with left ventricular hypertrophy is ventricular tachyarrhythmias,[117] potentially triggered by transient myocardial ischemia.[118] Transient ischemia might be favored by increased oxygen demand of the hypertrophied muscle and reduced blood supply due to microcirculatory disturbance. Long-term, repeated transient ischemic episodes could lead to increased interstitial fibrosis, forming the substrate for ventricular arrhythmias.[119] Other potential contributing factors to the increased risk of sudden cardiac death in hypertensive cardiomyopathy are electrolyte disturbances associated with therapy of hypertension with diuretics.[120,121] Whether or not therapy for hypertension will reduce the increased risk of sudden cardiac death is unclear at this time. A metaanalysis of 12 antihypertensive trials involving more than 50,000 hypertensive patients treated with placebo or active medication showed no effect on sudden cardiac death events[122] (see also Chap. 58).

ARRHYTHMOGENIC RIGHT VENTRICULAR DYSPLASIA

A predominantly right ventricular cardiomyopathy characterized by fatty or fibromatous replacement of myocardium and recurrent ventricular tachycardia with multiple left bundle branch block morphologies, arrhythmogenic right ventricular dysplasia (ARVD) is a rare cause of sudden cardiac death except in a few endemic regions.[123] In patients with ARVD, ventricular tachycardia is often precipitated by exercise and its induction is usually catecholamine-sensitive at electrophysiologic study.[123,124] The course and prognosis of ARVD is highly variable and difficult to predict. The annual incidence of sudden cardiac death in ARVD has been estimated to be about 2 percent despite various treatments[125,126] (see Chap. 27).

Valvular Heart Disease

The risk of sudden cardiac death in asymptomatic patients with aortic stenosis or regurgitation appears to be low.[127,128] In contrast, in the presurgical era, sudden cardiac death was one of the three most common types of death in symptomatic patients with aortic stenosis, the other two being bacterial endocarditis and congestive heart failure.[129] There appears to be an increased risk of sudden cardiac death following aortic valve replacement for aortic stenosis or regurgitation.[130,131] In 831 patients receiving a Bjork-Shiley prosthesis in the aortic (341 patients), mitral (345 patients), or double-valve (145 patients) position, the incidence of sudden cardiac death in the subgroups was 1.8 percent, 3.5 percent, and 4 percent, respectively, over a follow-up of 7 years.[131] Malignant tachyarrhythmias have been suggested as the cause of sudden cardiac mortality in these patients, given the more frequent presence of PVCs in patients who died suddenly compared with those who died of other causes. Transient complete heart block is relatively common following both aortic (17.6 percent) and mitral (13 percent) valve replacement, pointing to bradyarrhythmias as the potential precipitating factor for sudden cardiac death[132] (see also Chap. 63).

MITRAL VALVE PROLAPSE

Whether or not mitral valve prolapse (MVP) is a cause of sudden cardiac death is controversial. The prevalence of MVP is so high (4 to 5 percent of the general population and up to 17 percent of young women) that its presence may just be a coincidental finding in victims of sudden cardiac death and not causally related.[133,134] The overall 8-year probability of survival in a group of 237 asymptomatic or minimally symptomatic patients with echocardiographically documented MVP who were prospectively followed was not significantly different from that for a matched control population.[134] On the other hand, MVP may not always be benign, since in a significant number of victims of sudden cardiac death, especially in the young female population, MVP is the only structural cardiac disease found.[27,135] Naturally, they may have had a primary electrical disease unrelated to mitral valve prolapse.[136] Patients with MVP associated with mitral regurgitation and left ventricular dysfunction are clearly at higher risk for complications such as infective endocarditis, cerebroembolic events and sudden cardiac death.[137,138] Some victims of sudden cardiac death with MVP, mild mitral regurgitation, and normal left ventricular function had been treated with antiarrhythmic agents, raising the possibility of proarrhythmia as the cause of death.

The proposed cause of sudden cardiac death in patients with MVP is a ventricular tachyarrhythmia based on finding increased incidence of complex ventricular ectopy on ambulatory ECG in patients with mitral valve prolapse who experienced sudden cardiac death.[136,140] A prolonged QTc interval and changes in autonomic tone have also been related to sudden cardiac death in patients with MVP.[139] Several risk factors for sudden cardiac death have been identified in asymptomatic or mildly symptomatic MVP patients without significant mitral regurgitation, including mitral valve annular circumference, thickness of the anterior and posterior mitral valve leaflets, presence and extent of endocardial plaque, and the presence or absence of redundant mitral valve leaflets on M-mode echocardiography[134,139] (see Chap. 65).

Inflammatory and Infiltrative Myocardial Disease

Any inflammatory disease can cause sudden cardiac death due to either ventricular tachyarrhythmias or complete heart block. Histologic findings suggestive of *myocarditis* have been reported in 10 to 44 percent of young victims of sudden cardiac death (Table 36-2).[22] In adults, the diagnosis of myocarditis is made much less frequently, perhaps because of concurrent structural heart disease or because the late manifestations of the disease are indistinguishable from idiopathic dilated cardiomyopathy (see Chap. 76). In South America, however, myocarditis due to specific pathogens such as *Chagas' disease,* is the most frequent cause of cardiomyopathy and related sudden cardiac death.[140] Patients with infective endocarditis may also be at risk for sudden cardiac death due to acute coronary emboli from valvular vegetations. More often, sudden cardiac death during or following infective endocarditis is caused by acute hemodynamic deterioration due to valvular failure. An intramyocardial abscess can also be causing ventricular tachycardia leading to sudden cardiac death.

Infiltrative cardiomyopathies such as primary or secondary *amyloidosis, hemochromatosis,* or *sarcoidosis* have been associated with predominantly cardiac conduction defects but also ventricular tachyarrhythmias and sudden cardiac death. Ventricular tachycardia is sometimes the mode of presentation of sarcoidosis, can usually be reproduced by programmed electrical stimulation, and is associated with a high rate of recurrent arrhythmia and sudden cardiac death.[141]

Congenital Heart Disease

An increased risk of sudden cardiac death due to an arrhythmia has been found predominantly in four congenital conditions: tetralogy of Fallot, transposition of the great vessels, aortic stenosis, and pulmonary vascular obstruction.[34] Patients who have undergone reparative surgery for *tetralogy of Fallot* have a reported risk of sudden cardiac death of 6 percent before age 20.[142,143] A QRS duration $\geq$180 ms was found to be the most sensitive predictor of sudden cardiac death and ventricular tachyarrhythmias in 178 adults after repair of tetralogy of Fallot and correlated with other parameters of right ventricular volume overload.[143] *Transposition of the great vessels (post-Mustard/Senning)* is associated with a 2 to 8 percent rate of late sudden cardiac death, which is due in some cases to sinus node dysfunction and in others to ventricular tachyarrhythmias (Chap. 70). Sudden cardiac death is often (45 to 60 percent) the mode of death in patients with *primary* or *secondary pulmonary hypertension* (Chap. 59). Death is often precipi-

tated by general anesthesia, dehydration, exertion, or pregnancy. Any manipulation that decreases systemic vascular resistance, increases right to left shunting, and decreases pulmonary flow, leading to peripheral desaturation may trigger lethal arrhythmias and sudden cardiac death.[144] The sudden cardiac death risk in *congenital aortic stenosis* is estimated to be 1 percent, and occurs predominantly in symptomatic patients with severe left ventricular hypertrophy. *Ebstein's anomaly* is frequently (up to 25 percent) associated with the presence of accessory pathways and Wolff-Parkinson-White syndrome, which carries a small risk of sudden cardiac death. *Congenital heart block* without associated structural heart disease occurs in 1 of 20,000 infants, and a moderate decrease in heart rate is usually well tolerated. A maternal risk factor is systemic lupus erythematosus. Patients with severe bradycardia, however, have a tendency to develop ventricular arrhythmias. Pacemaker therapy has virtually eliminated the risk of sudden cardiac death in this population.[144]

Primary Electrical Abnormalities

LONG-QT SYNDROME

Sudden cardiac death is one of the hallmarks of the idiopathic long-QT syndrome (LQTS).[145–147] The prolonged QT interval reflects abnormal prolongation of repolarization. Other characteristics of this disorder, in addition to prolonged (>460 ms) QT interval, include abnormal T-wave contours, relative sinus bradycardia, a family history of early sudden death, and a propensity for recurrent syncope and sudden cardiac death due to polymorphic ventricular tachycardia (torsades de pointes) and ventricular fibrillation. Over 90 percent of the congenital forms of LQTS have been linked to four specific chromosomal defects, resulting in a genetically based classification (LQTS 1 through 4, Table 36-5) with important functional and prognostic implications.[147] Several mutations have been identified in each gene, and this locus heterogeneity

TABLE 36-5

CLASSIFICATION OF THE LONG-QT SYNDROME (LQTS) BASED ON THE GENETIC ABNORMALITY

Syndrome	Chromosomal Location	Defective Gene	Affected Currents	Characteristic T-Wave Shape	Comments
LQTS 1	11 (11p15.5)	*KVLQT1*	Potassium (I_K)	Broad	
LQTS 2	7 (7q35-36)	*HERG*	Potassium, delayed rectifier (I_{Kr})	Low amplitude	Current improves with increased extracellular potassium concentration
LQTS 3	3 (3p21-24)	*SCN5A*	Sodium (I_{Na})	Delayed onset	QTc interval shortens with tachycardia
LQTS 4 Jervell and Lange-Nielsen	4 (4q25-27) Not identified	Not identified	? Chloride		

appears to be important prognostically. Defects in outward currents (potassium) or impaired inactivation of inward currents (sodium) can cause abnormal prolongation of the action potential repolarization, enhancing the propensity to develop early afterdepolarizations (EADs) that may initiate arrhythmias[147] (see Chaps. 26 and 27).

Carriers of the LQT gene have been reported to have a 5 percent incidence of aborted sudden cardiac death and a 63 percent incidence of recurrent syncope.[146] The mean age at presentation was 24 years and the annual incidence of sudden cardiac death and recurrent syncope was 1.3 percent and 8.6 percent, respectively, in a series of 196 patients enrolled in an international registry.[145] Multivariate analysis in the registry population identified female gender, congenital deafness, history of syncope, and a documented episode of torsades de pointes or ventricular fibrillation as independent risk factors for postenrollment syncope or sudden cardiac death.[145] Echocardiography has also been reported to reveal specific wall motion abnormalities associated with an increased risk (relative risk, 2.75) of syncope and sudden cardiac death.[148] Genetic typing in the future may facilitate risk stratification, providing valuable information not only about the underlying abnormality but also about the expected severity of the disease and preferred therapy.[147]

WOLFF-PARKINSON-WHITE SYNDROME

The risk of sudden cardiac death in patients with Wolff-Parkinson-White (WPW) syndrome is less than 1 per 1000 patient-years of follow-up.[149] Although a rare event, it is an important one to consider, since it usually occurs in otherwise healthy individuals, and, in the era of catheter ablation of accessory pathways, is a curable cause of sudden cardiac death.[150] Almost all survivors of sudden cardiac death with WPW have had symptomatic arrhythmias prior to the event, but up to 10 percent had sudden cardiac death as their first manifestation of the disease.[151-155] The mechanism of sudden cardiac death in most patients with the WPW syndrome is presumably the development of atrial fibrillation with rapid ventricular rates due to conduction over an accessory pathway and subsequent degeneration into ventricular fibrillation. The best predictor for development of ventricular fibrillation is a rapid ventricular response over the accessory pathway during atrial fibrillation, with the shortest interval between preexcited ventricular beats (i.e., those conducted over the accessory pathway) being ≤250 ms.[151-155] Although this short RR interval is a highly sensitive marker, identifying virtually 100 percent of patients at high risk for ventricular fibrillation, its specificity is low, since this finding is present in approximately 20 percent of asymptomatic patients with WPW syndrome[151] and 50 percent of those with mild to moderate symptoms due to atrioventricular reentrant tachycardia.[152] An electrophysiologic study offers the opportunity to assess conduction properties of the accessory pathways, the propensity to develop tachyarrhythmias, and the possibility of curing the patient with catheter ablation at minimal risk.

IDIOPATHIC VENTRICULAR FIBRILLATION

Although the list of potential causes of sudden cardiac death continues to grow, a definite cause of sudden cardiac death cannot be established in approximately 1 percent of patients dying suddenly or after successful resuscitation from cardiac arrest.[156] These instances of sudden cardiac death without evident cause are presumed to be due to idiopathic ventricular fibrillation. The incidence of idiopathic ventricular fibrillation is higher in selected populations such as younger patients (up to 14 percent in patients below 40 years of age who had sudden cardiac death[157]) or female survivors of sudden cardiac death unrelated to myocardial infarction (10 percent[20]). The risk of recurrent ventricular fibrillation in this young and otherwise healthy patient population ranges between 22 and 37 percent at 2 to 4 years.[156,158,159] In survivors of cardiac arrest due to idiopathic ventricular fibrillation, the diagnosis is made by exclusion if extensive cardiac workup (including physical examination, laboratory tests for acute myocardial infarction and electrolyte abnormalities, ECG, exercise test, echocardiography, cardiac catheterization, and electrophysiologic study to exclude significant conduction system abnormalities or accessory pathways) reveals no abnormality that is thought to account for the ventricular fibrillation episode. In a review of 54 published cases with presumed idiopathic ventricular fibrillation, patients were younger (mean age 36 ± 16 years) than those who had sudden cardiac death associated with structural heart disease, and there was a relatively higher proportion of women.[156] Noninvasive evaluation including exercise testing and ambulatory ECG monitoring may help confirm the diagnosis of idiopathic ventricular fibrillation in selected patients in whom rapid, nonsustained runs of polymorphic ventricular tachycardia can be documented. Unfortunately, such markers are present in less than half the patients with this disorder.[156,160] The prognostic role of electrophysiologic evaluation in these patients is controversial: sustained rapid polymorphic ventricular tachycardia or ventricular fibrillation is inducible in 38 to 75 percent of patients studied[156,159-161]; however, these arrhythmias are generally considered a nonspecific finding,[162,163] and noninducibility of ventricular fibrillation in this patient population did not predict a more favorable outcome.[159]

Several distinct clinical or electrophysiologic patterns in patients with idiopathic ventricular fibrillation have been described. They include a syndrome of "nocturnal sudden cardiac death in Southeast Asian men" among previously healthy refugees from Southeast Asia,[164] a similar entity in young Japanese men (Pokkuri disease),[165] and a putative "syndrome of right bundle branch block, persistent ST segment elevation and sudden cardiac death due to ventricular fibrillation" (or Brugada syndrome).[166] At this time it is unclear whether these entities represent a different pathophysiologic condition or whether they are forms of previously described arrhythmogenic cardiac diseases.[167]

In any case, it should be kept in mind that the diagnosis of "idiopathic" ventricular fibrillation is made by exclusion and therefore depends on the sensitivity of the diagnostic tests used. With the development and validation of new diagnostic tools, including autonomic imaging and genetic testing, many forms of "idiopathic" sudden cardiac death in "structurally normal" hearts may have to be reclassified.[78]

Drugs and Other Toxic Agents

PROARRHYTHMIA

The apparent paradox that antiarrhythmic agents can cause arrhythmias has been recognized since introduction of quinidine in 1918.[168] The results of the Cardiac Arrhythmia Suppression Trial (CAST) showed an increased mortality in postinfarction patients treated with encainide, flecainide, and moricizine as compared with placebo, despite effective antiarrhythmic efficacy as documented by the suppression of PVCs.[169] Besides antiarrhythmic drugs, many other agents with diverse actions have been implicated in the induction of tachyarrhythmias.[170] Among commonly used drugs associated with the risk of producing ventricular arrhythmias leading to sudden cardiac death are erythromycin, terfenadine, hismanal, pentamidine, and certain psychotropic drugs, such as tricyclic antidepressants and chlorpromazine, which generally affect repolarization. Phosphodiesterase inhibitors and other positive inotropic agents that increase intracellular calcium loading have also been shown to be proarrhythmic and to increase the risk of sudden cardiac death, despite their beneficial effects on hemodynamic parameters.[171] Suggested proarrhythmia mechanisms of classes Ia and III antiarrhythmic drugs—as well as psychotrophic drugs, erythromycin, and pentamidine—include increased prolongation of refractoriness (QT interval of the ECG) and development of early afterdepolarizations.[172] The initiation of the arrhythmia is often triggered by bradycardia or a characteristic "long-short" coupling interval that initiates a pause-dependent prolongation of the QT interval. The ventricular tachycardia in this setting has commonly a typical torsades de pointes morphology. This form of proarrhythmia may be facilitated by electrolyte abnormalities such as hypokalemia or hypomagnesemia. It is usually an early event during drug therapy (within 3 days) and concomitant therapy with digitalis and diuretic agents may predispose patients to this complication.[173] Since it is not possible to predict who will develop proarrhythmic effects, initiation of antiarrhythmic therapy in a telemetry unit is recommended (see Chaps. 26, 27, and 30).

A second mechanism of proarrhythmia, observed predominantly with class Ic antiarrhythmic drugs such as flecainide and propafenone, appears to be associated with acute ischemic events and occurs more frequently in patients with ischemic cardiomyopathy.[174] It is believed that the antiarrhythmic drug exacerbates ischemia-induced myocardial conduction delays, in an inhomogenous fashion, and promotes reentrant ventricular tachycardias.[174]

COCAINE AND ALCOHOL

The increasingly widespread use of cocaine in the United States has led to the realization that this drug can precipitate life-threatening cardiac events, including sudden cardiac death. In a series of 41 survivors of cardiac arrest due to ventricular fibrillation in patients 18 to 35 years of age, one-third had ingested alcohol or drugs (cocaine, heroin, or tricyclic agents).[175] The combination of alcohol and cocaine is especially dangerous due to the generation of a unique metabolite, cocaethylene, that has enhanced cardiotoxicity.[176] Cocaine causes coronary vasoconstriction, increases cardiac sympathetic effects, and precipitates cardiac arrhythmias irrespective of the amount ingested, prior use, or whether or not there is an underlying cardiac abnormality.[177] The combination of increased oxygen demand due to sympathetic stimulation and diminished coronary flow due to vasoconstriction may precipitate ischemia-induced arrhythmias and sudden cardiac death (see Chap. 80).

Electrolyte Abnormalities

Hypokalemia is often found in patients during and following resuscitation from a cardiac arrest. Although it is often a secondary phenomenon due to catecholamine-induced potassium shift into the cells, primary hypokalemia can also be arrhythmogenic. There is an almost linear inverse relationship between serum potassium concentration and the probability of ventricular tachycardia in patients with acute myocardial infarction.[178] A decrease in extracellular potassium hypopolarizes the resting membrane potential, shortens the plateau duration, prolongs the phase of rapid repolarization in ventricular fibers, and causes an increase in pacemaker activity in Purkinje cells, triggering ventricular arrhythmias.[179] These changes in repolarization may increase the dispersion of the recovery of excitability and facilitate reentrant ventricular arrhythmias.[179] Many of the electrophysiologic effects of hypokalemia are similar to those caused by digitalis and catecholamine stimulation, explaining the high risk of ventricular arrhythmias when a combination of these factors is present.

An association between *magnesium deficiency* and sudden cardiac death has been reported in humans, especially as a cofactor in drug-induced torsades de pointes.[180] Hypomagnesemia in humans is generally associated with congestive heart failure, digitalis use, chronic diuretic use, hypokalemia, and hypocalcemia, making it difficult to establish whether the hypomagnesemia alone caused the sudden cardiac death. Acute administration of magnesium has been successfully used in the treatment of drug-induced torsades de pointes, although hypomagnesemia is not usually documented in this situation.

Changes in intracellular concentration of calcium may also be arrhythmogenic.[179] An *increase in intracellular calcium* concentration causes oscillatory release of calcium from the sarcoplasmic reticulum and gives rise to delayed afterdepolarizations, which may lead subsequently to ventricular arrhythmias due to triggered activity. Increases in intracellular calcium are believed to play a significant role in arrhythmias associated with digitalis glycosides, catecholamine-induced ventricular tachycardia, reperfusion arrhythmias, and the proarrhythmic effect seen with phosphodiesterase inhibitors and other positive inotropic agents.

Several studies in patients with hypertension who received treatment with diuretics suggested an increased risk of sudden cardiac death due to therapy with *non–potassium-sparing diuretics.*[181] Drug-induced potassium or magnesium depletion leading to cardiac arrhythmias has been suggested as the underlying mechanism (see also Chap. 26).

Electrolyte abnormalities are thought to be the cause of sudden cardiac death in patients with severe eating disorders, such as *anorexia nervosa, bulimia,* or who are on *liquid protein diets.* Sudden cardiac death due to ventricular tachycardia related to prolongation of the QT interval has been reported in a few patients with anorexia nervosa and bulimia.[182] It is thought to account partially for the high fatality rate of this eating disorder.

CLINICAL PRESENTATION AND MANAGEMENT OF THE PATIENT WITH CARDIAC ARREST

Out-of-Hospital Cardiac Arrest

Cardiac arrest is characterized by abrupt loss of consciousness, which would uniformly lead to death in the absence of an acute intervention, although spontaneous reversions rarely occur. Prodromal symptoms such as chest pain, dyspnea, fatigue, and palpitations may be present in up to half of patients presenting with cardiac arrest but are generally nonspecific and lead to medical evaluation in only a minority of patients.[11,186] About 75 percent of cardiac arrests occur at home and about two-thirds are witnessed.[183,184] Individuals who live alone and women appear more likely to have unwitnessed deaths.[185] The average age of cardiac arrest victims is around 65 years and 70 to 80 percent are men.[184]

As discussed above, the most common mechanisms of cardiac arrest are ventricular tachyarrhythmias, followed by bradyarrhythmias or asystole. The most important determinant of successful resuscitation is the time interval from cardiovascular collapse to initial intervention. Since most patients are found in ventricular fibrillation, time to successful defibrillation is a key element in the acute management of the cardiac arrest victim (Fig. 36-6). *The importance of early intervention is reflected in the "chain of survival" concept of emergency*

cardiac care systems: early access, early CPR, early defibrillation, and early advanced cardiac life support.[186] This concept has led to the development of tiered medical emergency systems in most urban areas. Following activation of the emergency call (911) system, the first response consists of emergency medical technicians or fire departments from the nearest location, who are trained to provide basic CPR and defibrillation. The second response is by paramedics who are trained in advanced cardiac life support, including endotracheal intubation, intravenous medications, and additional defibrillation if necessary.

Initiation of bystander CPR by people trained in basic cardiac life support is another important element of early intervention and improves the chances of successful resuscitation. In an overview of 17 controlled studies of survival from out-of-hospital cardiac arrest, bystander CPR was associated with a greater than twofold odds ratio of survival (28 ± 16 percent of 5565 patients receiving bystander CPR versus 12 ± 11 percent of 8329 patients who did not).[186] The association between early CPR and improved survival appears to be related to the beneficial effects of CPR on ventricular fibrillation. The earlier CPR is performed, the greater the proportion of patients who are found in ventricular fibrillation as opposed to bradycardia or asystole.[63] Further, successful defibrillation is more likely when early CPR is performed. Community-based CPR training programs, such as those implemented in Seattle and Minneapolis, resulted in training of 20 to 25 percent of the adult population and have led to a higher likelihood of bystander CPR being administered in out-of-hospital cardiac arrest. The percentage of patients receiving

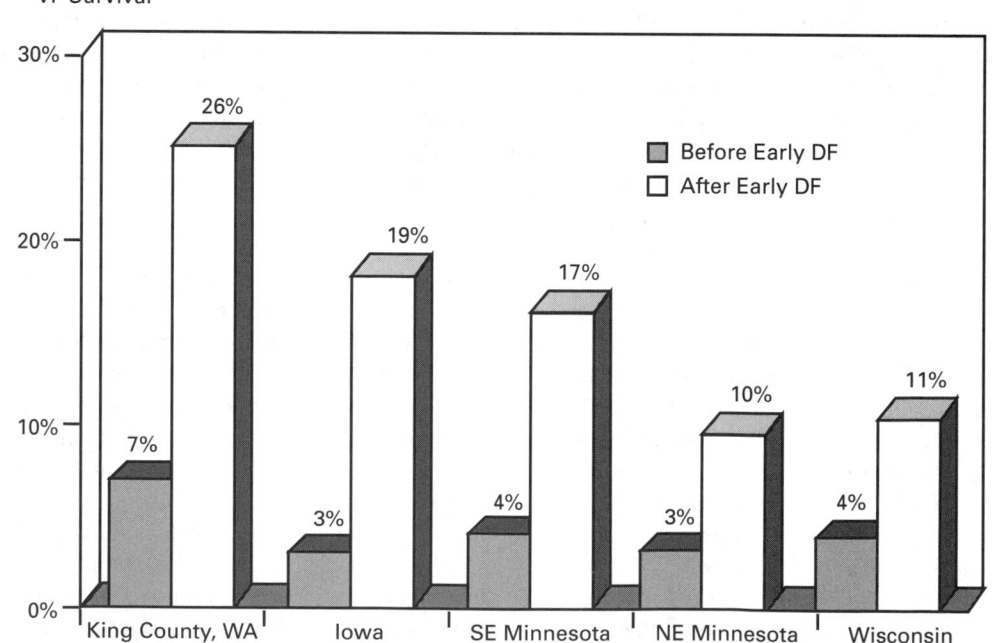

FIGURE 36-6

Survival before (*open boxes*) and after (*shaded boxes*) implementation of early defibrillation programs by EMT. (Reproduced with permission from Ornato JP et al. Community experience in treating out-of-hospital cardiac arrest. In: Akhtar M, Myerburg RJ, Ruskin JN, eds. *Sudden Cardiac Death.* Baltimore: Williams & Wilkins; 1994:450–462.)

bystander CPR varies in the communities studied between 8 and 54 percent, with an average around 30 percent.[184] Another, perhaps more efficient approach is targeted CPR training for persons who have an increased likelihood of having to perform CPR. It has been suggested that learning CPR be a mandatory course in high school, much like learning how to drive a car.[187]

In order to improve the time to initial defibrillation, early defibrillation by nonmedical personnel, such as firefighters, has been advocated. The widespread use of *automatic external defibrillators has the potential to improve significantly the availability of early defibrillation.*[186,188] These are relatively simple and inexpensive devices that have an automatic detection and treatment algorithm for ventricular tachyarrhythmias. The addition of interposed abdominal compression to standard CPR techniques has been reported to improve the outcome, particularly in patients found in asystole or electromechanical dissociation.[189]

Although its duration is the most important determinant of successful ventricular defibrillation, other factors should be kept in mind. It has been estimated that in humans only about 4 percent of the transthoracic current actually traverses the heart, the rest being shunted by the thoracic cage and lungs.[190] The transthoracic impedance is inversely proportional to the size of defibrillator patches and the force applied on the paddles. It also depends on the location of the paddles and the paddle-skin coupling material, and it decreases with the number of shocks applied.[191] To improve defibrillation efficacy, especially in individuals with large chests and expected high transthoracic impedance, the operator should use a gel/cream or saline-soaked gauze between the paddles and the skin and press firmly on the largest hand-held paddles available; several successive shocks may be necessary.[192] Recent experimental evidence suggests that ischemia-triggered release of endogenous adenosine may have deleterious effects on the success of defibrillation.[193] Development of specific adenosine antagonists and their administration during CPR in patients found in ventricular fibrillation might further improve defibrillation success.

Survival and Prognosis after Cardiac Arrest

Survival to hospital discharge after cardiac arrest varies from 1.4 to 28 percent.[62,63,184,194,195] Marked differences in survival following out-of-hospital cardiac arrest have been reported in different communities, being lowest in large cities such as New York (1.4 percent) and Chicago (4 percent)[195] and highest (28 percent) in Seattle, a midsized urban community where many of the early intervention concepts have been pioneered.[196] The in-hospital mortality following successful resuscitation outside the hospital remains high, in the range of 30 to 50 percent[62,63,197] (Fig. 36-7). The most important factors associated with increased in-hospital mortality after out-of-hospital cardiac arrest are cardiogenic shock after defibrillation, age ≥60 years, requirement of four or more shocks for defibrillation, absence of an acute myocardial infarction, and coma on admission to the hospital.[62,197]

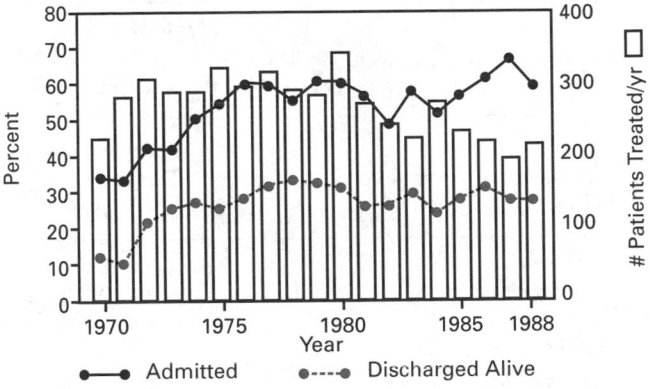

FIGURE 36-7

Percentage of out-of-hospital cardiac arrest victims admitted to the hospital by emergency medical service personnel and subsequently discharged alive during the period from 1970 to 1988. (Reproduced with permission from Cobb LA et al. Community-based interventions for sudden cardiac death: Impact, limitations, and changes. *Circulation* 1992; 85:I98–I102.)

Survival depends largely on the initial recorded rhythm.[62,63,184,194,195] Some 40 to 60 percent of patients who are found in ventricular fibrillation are successfully resuscitated, but only about one-fourth of patients survive to be discharged from the hospital. The outcome is much better in the small (<7 percent) group of patients in whom ventricular tachycardia is the initial documented rhythm: 88 percent survive to the hospital and 76 percent are discharged alive. Bradycardias and electromechanical dissociation as the presenting rhythms are associated with the worst prognosis, and very few (<5 percent) of these patients survive to discharge from the hospital.[63] Other factors associated with improved survival are a low "comorbidity index," reflecting chronic conditions such as history of heart failure, diabetes, hypertension, gastrointestinal disorders, as well as recent symptoms prior to the event.[198]

An important consideration in the treatment of the cardiac arrest victim is the appropriateness of CPR and the use of life-sustaining therapies in patients with a low likelihood of survival, such as chronically ill people found in asystole or electromechanical dissociation. Their chances to survive until hospital discharge are less than 1 percent. Further, many older people prefer to die suddenly rather than experience chronic suffering.[199] Advance directives, when available, and consultation with family members and personal physicians might aid in the difficult decision process of when to administer supportive care rather than aggressive management.

MANAGEMENT OF CARDIAC ARREST SURVIVORS AND RISK STRATIFICATION FOR SUDDEN CARDIAC DEATH

Establishing the Underlying Cardiac Pathology

The initial management following successful resuscitation from cardiac arrest consists of allowing a period of hemody-

TABLE 36-6

DIFFERENCES IN CLINICAL STATUS IMMEDIATELY BEFORE DEATH IN PATIENTS DYING PRIMARILY OF ARRHYTHMIA VERSUS CIRCULATORY FAILURE

Clinical Status Immediately before Death	Arrhythmic Deaths, %, N = 82	Circulatory Failure Deaths, %, N = 59
Comatose	0/82 (0%)	56/59 (95%)
Standing or actively moving	39/82 (48%)	0/59 (0%)
Terminal arrhythmia		
Ventricular fibrillation	15/18 (83%)	3/9 (33%)
Asystole	3/18 (17%)	6/9 (67%)
Duration of terminal illness		
<1 h	53/82 (65%)	4/59 (7%)
>24 h	17/82 (21%)	48/59 (81%)
Nature of terminal illness		
Acute cardiac events	80/82 (98%)	8/59 (14%)
Noncardiac events	1/82 (1%)	51/59 (86%)

Source: Modified with permission from Hinkle et al.[13]

namic and respiratory stabilization, after which every effort should be made to establish the cause of cardiac arrest. For this, the underlying cardiac disease should first be determined. History and physical examination may provide the first clues. Myocardial infarction has to be excluded by serial enzymes and ECG changes. Echocardiography can help in evaluating left ventricular function, regional wall motion abnormalities, valvular heart disease, or other cardiomyopathies. Stress-imaging studies can demonstrate inducible ischemia. Cardiac catheterization is often recommended to evaluate the coronary anatomy and right and left ventricular hemodynamic parameters. Other tests such as radionuclide studies, magnetic resonance imaging, or cardiac biopsy may be necessary in selected patients. As discussed above, an underlying cardiac disease can be found in nearly all patients.

Primary versus Secondary Cardiac Arrest

One of the important questions following cardiac arrest is whether it was primarily due to acute circulatory or respiratory failure or to an arrhythmia. Although all these events are usually present during the arrest, it is important to distinguish whether the arrhythmia preceded or followed the hemodynamic collapse. While several clinical and historical clues help to answer this question (Table 36-6), the distinction sometimes cannot be made with certainty. Separating primary from secondary cardiac arrest has important prognostic and therapeutic consequences. In 142 survivors of cardiac arrest with coronary artery disease, the 1-year survival was 89 percent, 80 percent, and 71 percent in the patients classified as having had cardiac arrest secondary to acute myocardial infarction (44 percent of patients), secondary to an ischemic event (34 percent), or due to a primary arrhythmic event (22 percent), respectively.[85] Patients who present with cardiac

arrest secondary (and within 48 h) to an acute transmural myocardial infarction have a similar prognosis as those who have an acute myocardial infarction without an arrhythmia.[62] Specific antiarrhythmic therapy is therefore usually not recommended if cardiac arrest occurs during or within 2 days of an acute Q-wave myocardial infarction. In contrast, if the arrhythmia is the primary event and myocardial infarction developed secondary to the acute hemodynamic deterioration during the arrhythmia, then antiarrhythmic therapy with a drug or device is recommended unless a transient or reversible cause is identified.[85]

Every effort should be made to exclude potentially reversible causes of sudden cardiac death (Table 36-7), including transient ischemic episodes in patients who are candidates for complete revascularization and in whom the onset of the arrhythmia is clearly preceded by ischemic ECG changes or symptoms.

Other reversible etiologies for cardiac arrest include transient severe electrolyte disturbances and proarrhythmic effects of antiarrhythmic drugs and other pharmacologic agents. It can be difficult to establish a causal relationship between the proarrhythmic agent and the malignant ventricular arrhythmia as opposed to its being a coincidental finding. A pathologic prolongation of the QTc interval preceding initiation of arrhythmia and return of the QTc interval to normal following discontinuation of the presumed proarrhythmic agent is strongly suggestive of a cause-effect relationship. Occasionally, especially when type Ia agents are implicated in the cardiac arrest event, electrophysiologic evaluation with programmed stimulation after washout and following reexposure to these agents is necessary to confirm proarrhythmia as the sole cause of the episode of cardiac arrest. Another setting in

TABLE 36-7

POTENTIALLY REVERSIBLE CAUSES OF CARDIAC ARREST DUE TO VENTRICULAR FIBRILLATION

Myocardial ischemia
Prinzmetal's angina
Proarrhythmia
  Antiarrhythmic agents
  Other drugs
Electrolyte abnormalities
Hypoxia
Acute congestive heart failure

which a reversible etiology for cardiac arrest is often present is the hemodynamically unstable patient in the early postoperative period following cardiac surgery. Infusion of positive inotropic agents, electrolyte imbalances, and hypoxia are often precipitating factors.

Risk Stratification for Sudden Cardiac Death

Several clinical, noninvasive, and invasive strategies can aid in the risk stratification of patients for sudden cardiac death. The choice of the appropriate test is largely determined by the underlying cardiac disease.

Clinical History

Four independent prognostic variables for sudden cardiac death related to *clinical history* were identified in a study of 200 patients who suffered from ventricular fibrillation or sustained ventricular tachycardia following myocardial infarction: (1) cardiac arrest at the time of the first documented episode of arrhythmia, (2) New York Heart Association (NYHA) class III or IV, (3) ventricular fibrillation or ventricular tachycardia occurring early after myocardial infarction (3 days to 2 months), and (4) history of multiple previous myocardial infarctions.[200] Risk stratification for sudden cardiac death using these four variables can identify subgroups with a sudden cardiac death incidence ranging from 0 to 28 percent. Of note, patients without hemodynamic collapse at the time of the arrhythmia and with ventricular tachycardia occurring more than 2 months after myocardial infarction, a subgroup that constituted 40 percent of the study population, were reported to have a 0 percent incidence of sudden cardiac death at 26 months. Syncope in patients with a left ventricular ejection fraction below 30 percent is associated with increased risk of sudden cardiac death (about 50 percent at 3 years) irrespective of finding an arrhythmic cause.[201]

Left Ventricular Function

Left ventricular dysfunction is a major independent predictor of total and sudden cardiac mortality in patients with ischemic as well as nonischemic cardiomyopathy.[202–205] In survivors of cardiac arrest who have a left ventricular ejection fraction below 30 percent, the risk of sudden cardiac death exceeds 30 percent over 1 to 3 years if the patients do not have inducible ventricular tachycardia; it ranges between 15 and 50 percent in those who have inducible ventricular tachyarrhythmias despite therapy with drugs that suppressed the inducible arrhythmias or with empiric amiodarone.[206–208] *Assessment of left ventricular function by clinical history (e.g., a history of congestive heart failure) and by other noninvasive methods (echocardiography, radionuclide studies) or invasive means (angiography) is therefore essential in the evaluation of a patient at risk for sudden cardiac death.*[203] Unfortunately, detection of severe left ventricular dysfunction serves to predict total cardiac mortality but does not distinguish patients who will die suddenly from those who will die of progressive congestive heart failure.[107,203,204]

Electrocardiographic Abnormalities

In survivors of out-of-hospital cardiac arrest, the presence of atrioventricular block or intraventricular conduction defects on ambulatory ECG (72 h) is associated with a higher recurrence rate of cardiac arrest (10 of 14 patients versus 1 of 28 patients without).[63] Other ECG parameters that have been reported to be associated independently with an increased risk of sudden cardiac death are prolongation of the QT interval (in the absence of inherited or acquired long-QT syndrome),[209] increased dispersion of the QT interval,[210,211] and an increase of resting heart rate above 90, particularly in men without a history of coronary artery disease.[212]

Detection of nonsustained ventricular arrhythmias by ambulatory ECG monitoring has been reported to be of value in the risk stratification of patients for sudden cardiac death.[202,213–216] The incidence of sudden cardiac death in the 2 years following myocardial infarction in 766 patients enrolled in the Multicenter Post-Infarction Research Group increased with the frequency of PVCs detected during 24-h ECG monitoring from 3 percent for <1/h to 14 percent for >30/h; similarly, patients with nonsustained ventricular tachycardia runs had a higher (17 percent) incidence of sudden cardiac death than those with single PVCs (6 percent).[202] The prognostic value of ambulatory ECG monitoring in patients with congestive heart failure is limited by the high incidence of these arrhythmias (up to 88 percent) in this population, resulting in a low specificity of this parameter.[217]

Baroreflex Sensitivity

Reduced *baroreflex sensitivity*, reflecting mainly an impairment in the vagal efferent component of the baroreceptor reflex, may help to predict cardiovascular mortality and arrhythmic events in particular in patients following myocardial infarction. In two prospective studies including a total of 200 patients following myocardial infarction, baroreflex sensitivity was significantly reduced in the 14 patients with sudden cardiac death or life-threatening arrhythmias compared to those without (<3 ms/mmHg versus 8 ms/mmHg).[83,84] The prognostic significance of baroreflex sensitivity was not diminished in patients with reduced left ventricular function and carried the highest relative risk for arrhythmic events, superior to that of other prognostic variables including left ventricular function.

Heart Rate Variability

Another noninvasive measure of sympathovagal balance is *heart rate variability*, beat-to-beat variations of RR intervals and their mathematically derived parameter. Several measures of heart rate variability have been reported to be associated with an increased risk of sudden and total cardiac death following myocardial infarction, underscoring the importance of the autonomic nervous system in the evolution of life-threatening arrhythmias.[216,218–220] In a study of 808 survivors of myocardial infarction, heart rate variability of <50 ms carried a 5.3 relative risk of mortality compared with the group with a heart rate variability of >100 ms.[218] In a prospective study of 6693 nonselected and consecutive patients who underwent 24-h AECG monitoring, those with a heart rate variability of <25 ms had a fourfold higher risk of sudden cardiac death than patients with higher variability.[220] The sensitivity, specificity, positive predictive value, and relative risk in the prediction of arrhythmic events following myocardial infarction have been reported to be 60, 94, 55, and 10.4 for reduced heart rate variability [standard deviation of RR intervals (SDNN), <50 ms] and 80, 91, 44, and 23.1, respectively, for decreased baroreflex sensitivity (<3.0 ms/mmHg).[221] A prospective international study is in progress to assess the prognostic significance of diminished baroreflex sensitivity and heart rate variability 20 days after myocardial infarction in a large population.[222]

Nonlinear Dynamics

According to the chaos theory, apparently irregularly irregular events such as ventricular ectopy are nonrandomly distributed in time and their clustering can be quantified by fractal geometric analysis.[223] Fractal clustering of ventricular ectopy has been associated with sudden cardiac death in patients with mitral regurgitation and has also been demonstrated in other patients with life-threatening ventricular arrhythmias.[223] The physiologic correlate for a low fractal dimension appears to be transient increases in cardiac sympathetic tone.[224]

T-Wave Alternans

Macroscopic T-wave changes with an alternating pattern have been observed in patients with long-QT syndrome prior to onset of ventricular fibrillation as well as in the setting of mechanical alternans, as is sometimes present during cardiac tamponade. Recent studies have indicated that T-wave alternans that is discernible only by computer averaging techniques may be a more ubiquitous phenomenon that can identify patients at risk for ventricular arrhythmias.[225] Techniques for computer-assisted analysis of T-wave alternans are being developed and may provide a quantitative, noninvasive method for assessing susceptibility to ventricular fibrillation. T-wave alternans assessed by computer analysis has been shown to predict arrhythmia-free survival over 20 months with a nearly 90 percent sensitivity and specificity in a small cohort of 66 patients[226] (see Chaps. 26, 27, and 47).

Late Potentials

Late potentials, microvolt waveforms extending the duration of a filtered QRS complex detected by *signal-averaging electrocardiography* (SAECG), have been shown to be helpful in the risk stratification of patients following myocardial infarction. The prognostic significance of late potentials has been demonstrated in several studies, which reported a 17 to 29 percent incidence of sudden cardiac death, ventricular fibrillation, or sustained ventricular tachycardia in patients with an abnormal SAECG, in contrast to 0.8 to 3.5 percent in those without.[227] Although the negative predictive value of a normal SAECG is good, the application of SAECG in risk stratification for sudden cardiac death is limited by a low positive predictive value in patients following myocardial infarction as well as by its low sensitivity in patients with nonischemic cardiomyopathies[106,228,229] (see also Chap. 27).

Electrophysiologic Studies

Electrophysiologic studies have advanced our understanding of life-threatening ventricular arrhythmias and facilitated the development of new therapies for their prevention and treatment. *Induction of sustained monomorphic ventricular tachycardia is the generally accepted end point for programmed stimulation, whereas induction of nonsustained ventricular arrhythmias, polymorphic ventricular tachycardia, or ventricular fibrillation may be a nonspecific finding depending on the aggressiveness of the stimulation protocol.*[163,230] Information obtained during the electrophysiologic study—such as ventricular tachycardia rate, morphology, origin, mechanism, and hemodynamic stability—is crucial to determine whether the patient is a candidate for serial drug testing, catheter ablation therapy, surgical therapy, or an implantable defibrillator. In patients who present with sustained monomorphic ventricular tachycardia, ventricular tachycardia is reproducibly inducible in the vast majority, especially in those with coronary artery disease.[230] Another group in whom electrophysiologic testing is useful includes those patients with structural heart disease presenting with unexplained syncope. Ventricular tachycardia is the most common abnormal finding in these patients, but demonstration of His-Purkinje conduction disease or hemodynamically unstable supraventricular tachycardia can also be important. *In patients with CHD, reduced left ventricular function, and documented nonsustained ventricular tachycardia, electrophysiologic studies can help select patients who would benefit from antiarrhythmic therapy.* In survivors of cardiac arrest due to ventricular fibrillation, the prognostic value of electrophysiologic testing is less clear. Since sustained ventricular tachycardia or ventricular fibrillation is inducible in less than half the patients, suppression of induction of ventricular fibrillation by antiarrhythmic therapy is an unreliable end point, and even patients with no inducible ventricular arrhythmias remain at a high risk for recurrent cardiac arrest.[231,232] Nevertheless, in survivors of cardiac arrest, electrophysiologic study may reveal the mechanism of arrest, have prognostic significance, and help select an appropriate therapy.[233,234] The routine use of electrophysiologic testing following myocardial infarction in patients with nonischemic cardiomyopathy is controversial, and the appropriate end points are unclear[231,235] (see Chap. 29).

TREATMENT OPTIONS FOR PATIENTS AT RISK FOR SUDDEN CARDIAC DEATH

General Considerations

There are few direct and randomized comparisons of various treatment strategies to prevent sudden cardiac death. Since reduction of sudden cardiac death rates does not necessarily parallel total mortality, reduction in total mortality is a more appropriate end point in assessing antiarrhythmic efficacy. Patient selection affects the outcome of different treatment strategies. For example, in patients at low risk of sudden cardiac death, proarrhythmia or surgical mortality might outweigh the benefits achieved with an antiarrhythmic intervention. On the other hand, in patients at high risk for recurrent cardiac arrest, the risk-benefit profile of antiarrhythmic treatment strategies may be more favorable. Selection of therapy is further limited by the patient's baseline characteristics. For instance, *only patients with inducible sustained ventricular arrhythmias are good candidates for electrophysiologically guided antiarrhythmic drug therapy, and radiofrequency ablation of ventricular tachycardia is an option only in patients with hemodynamically stable monomorphic ventricular tachycardia or bundle branch reentry.* In an era of limited health care resources, the cost-effectiveness of different treatment strategies is another element to be considered in choosing therapy. Last but not least, quality of life is an important aspect in the selection of the most appropriate therapy.

Pharmacologic Therapy

BETA BLOCKERS

Of all the therapies currently available for the prevention of sudden cardiac death, none are more established or more effective in patients with coronary heart disease than beta blockers.[236,237] Although beta blockers are less effective in suppressing spontaneous or induced ventricular ectopy when compared with other membrane-active antiarrhythmic agents, both nonselective beta blockers (timolol, propranolol) and cardioselective agents such as metoprolol have been shown in placebo-controlled randomized trials to reduce total mortality by 20 to 36 percent, in large part because of a reduction of sudden cardiac death.[237–240] In a review of 19,000 post–myocardial infarction patients who were randomized to beta blockers or placebo, active treatment was associated with a decrease in total mortality of 20 percent, of sudden cardiac death rate of 30 percent, and of reinfarction by 35 to 40 percent.[241] Beta blockers are effective in the setting of ventricular arrhythmias provoked by a high sympathetic tone, as in patients with congenital long-QT syndrome,[145] arrhythmogenic right ventricular dysplasia,[127] or congestive heart failure.[242] Importantly, the beneficial effects of beta blockers on cardiac mortality are most pronounced in patients who are at higher risk for sudden cardiac death, such as patients with congestive heart failure, atrial and ventricular arrhythmias post–myocardial infarction, and diabetes[236] (see also Chaps. 27 and 54).

ANGIOTENSIN-CONVERTING ENZYME INHIBITORS

Vasodilator therapy is an effective treatment in patients with congestive heart failure and has been shown to reduce mortality by up to 40 percent in the first year.[243–245] Despite the beneficial effect on total mortality, the effects of angiotensin-converting enzyme (ACE) inhibitors on sudden cardiac death are conflicting. In a study comparing isosorbide dinitrate/hydralazine with enalapril in 804 men with moderate heart failure, the reduction in mortality in the enalapril group (25 percent at 2 years) was due to a lower incidence of sudden cardiac death, raising the question whether or not ACE inhibitors have an added antiarrhythmic effect.[243] In two other large, randomized trials of enalapril versus placebo in patients with severe[244] and moderate[245] heart failure, however, sudden cardiac death rates were similar in the treatment and control groups despite a total mortality reduction of 30 percent at 1 year.

CLASS I ANTIARRHYTHMIC DRUGS

The role of antiarrhythmic drug therapy in the prevention of sudden cardiac death has changed considerably since placebo controlled trials such as CAST demonstrated that suppression of spontaneous nonsustained ventricular arrhythmias with certain drugs does not necessarily result in improved survival.[169] In CAST, type Ic antiarrhythmic drugs such as encainide, flecainide, and moricizine were associated with excess mortality from arrhythmias in asymptomatic postinfarct patients with frequent ventricular ectopy despite effective suppression of spontaneous ventricular ectopy.[169] These results were interpreted as being due to an excessive proarrhythmic effect, which outweighed the lower mortality risk of these patients. Whether the risk-benefit ratio between pro- and antiarrhythmic effect of antiarrhythmic drugs is different in other patient populations or with other antiarrhythmic drugs is not clear, since there are very few placebo-controlled randomized trials with total mortality as an end point.

There is no evidence that other class I antiarrhythmic drugs can prolong survival in any patient group studied, and they may even be harmful. Results of a metaanalysis of empiric long-term antiarrhythmic therapy after myocardial infarction with mostly class I antiarrhythmic agents (mexiletine, phenytoin, tocainide, flecainide, encainide, procainamide, aprindine, imipramine, and moricizine) showed either no beneficial effects or detrimental effects on mortality despite effective reduction of PVCs.[246,247] A metaanalysis of lidocaine in acute myocardial infarction suggested an increase in in-hospital mortality despite a reduction in the prevalence of ventricular fibrillation.[248] Empiric use of these drugs in patients with sustained ventricular arrhythmias has been associated with a very high rate of sudden cardiac death, between 30 and 70 percent at 2 years.[249] In a randomized trial between electrophysiologically guided conventional (i.e., class I drugs) therapy versus empiric amiodarone in survivors of cardiac arrest (CASCADE), overall survival was lower in the conventional arm (78, 62, and 32 percent at 2, 4, and 6 years, respectively; Fig. 36-8).[250] The propafenone arm was stopped early in the Cardiac Arrest Study Hamburg (CASH) because of excess mortality in cardiac arrest survivors compared with amiodarone, beta blockers, and implantable defibrillators[251] (see also Chaps. 27 and 47).

SOTALOL

Sotalol, in the currently marketed form of a racemic mixture of the *d*- and *l*-stereoisomers, is a potent class III antiarrhythmic agent with nonselective beta-blocking effects.[252] Sotalol has been reported to suppress inducible ventricular tachycardia in 30 to 40 percent of patients who present with sustained ventricular arrhythmias. In a randomized trial of sotalol and other antiarrhythmic agents in patients with sustained ventricular tachycardia, the arrhythmia recurrence rate (21 percent at 1 year) and the arrhythmic death rate (12 percent at 4 years) was half of that achieved with class I agents.[253] The beta-blocking effect of sotalol seems to be essential for its benefit, since a trial of the *d*-isomer (class III antiarrhythmic effect only, devoid of beta-blocking effect) in patients with prior myocardial infarction was associated with increased mortality.[254] The most serious side effect encountered with sotalol is proarrhythmia (mostly torsades de pointes), which has been reported to occur in up to 8 percent of treated patients.[252] In survivors of cardiac arrest, sotalol therapy was less effective than implantable cardioverter defibrillators.[255,255a]

AMIODARONE

Amiodarone is widely considered the most effective antiarrhythmic agent for therapy of supraventricular and ventricular arrhythmias. It is a class III antiarrhythmic agent with additional class I, II and IV properties and has unusual pharmacokinetics with a delayed onset of action and an elimination half-life of up to 53 days after chronic therapy[256] (see Chap. 30). In contrast to that of other antiarrhythmic agents, the long-term clinical efficacy of amiodarone is poorly predicted by the results of electrophysiologic evaluation.[207,208] Uncontrolled trials in patients with sustained ventricular tachycardia or ventricular fibrillation demonstrated a relatively low incidence of sudden cardiac death in patients treated with amiodarone, despite a high recurrence rate of ventricular arrhythmias. The sudden cardiac death rate at 1, 3, and 5 years in two series of 462 and 589 patients with mostly sustained ventricular arrhythmias was 9 percent, 15 to 16 percent, and 21 to 22 percent, respectively, whereas the arrhythmia recurrence rate was approximately 20 percent, 30 percent, and 40 percent during the same time period.[207,208] Again, the most important predictor of sudden cardiac death in patients treated with amiodarone for sustained ventricular tachycardia or ventricular fibrillation is left ventricular ejection fraction. In a series of 122 such patients with mostly coronary artery disease, the actuarial probability of sudden cardiac death at 5 years was 5 percent when the ejection fraction was $\geq$40 percent and 49 percent when the ejection fraction was <40 percent.[257]

Amiodarone has been shown to reduce significantly sudden cardiac death rates following myocardial infarction in several placebo-controlled randomized studies, but its effects on total mortality are inconsistent.[258] The Basel Antiarrhythmic Study of Infarct Survival (BASIS), a prospective randomized trial of empiric amiodarone, ambulatory ECG-guided conventional antiarrhythmic therapy, or placebo in 312 patients with complex ventricular ectopy following myocardial infarction, showed that amiodarone significantly reduced total mortality at 1 year from 13 percent in the placebo group to 5 percent

in amiodarone-treated patients ($p < .05$).[259] On the other hand, amiodarone therapy did not reduce total mortality compared with placebo in nearly 2700 post–myocardial infarction patients enrolled in the Canadian Amiodarone Myocardial Infarction Arrhythmia Trial (CAMIAT)[260] and the European Myocardial Infarction Amiodarone Trial (EMIAT),[261] despite a 50 percent risk reduction in the arrhythmic mortality.

In patients with congestive heart failure, who are at high risk for sudden cardiac death, prophylactic therapy with amiodarone has been shown to decrease mortality (by 28 percent) in the Argentinean Grupo de Estudio de la Sobrevida en la Insuficiencia Cardiaca en Argentina (GESICA) trial,[262] but not in the Veterans Administration heart failure study.[263] Comparison of the two patient populations and subgroup analysis suggested that prophylactic amiodarone might be more beneficial in patients with nonischemic cardiomyopathy, found in greater number in the GESICA study.

In patients who survived cardiac arrest not associated with myocardial infarction, empiric amiodarone therapy has been shown to be superior to electrophysiologically guided conventional therapy.[250] Survival free of cardiac death, resuscitated cardiac arrest, and defibrillator shocks associated with syncope at 1, 3, and 5 years was 91 percent, 76 percent, and 63 percent, respectively, in the amiodarone-treated patients, compared with 77 percent, 56 percent, and 46 percent in the conventionally treated patients (Fig. 36-8). The efficacy of amiodarone in reducing total mortality in patients with ventricular fibrillation or hemodynamically unstable ventricular tachycardia compared to implantable cardioverter (ICD) treatment has been evaluated prospectively in the randomized Amiodarone Versus Implantable Defibrillator (AVID) study, which re-

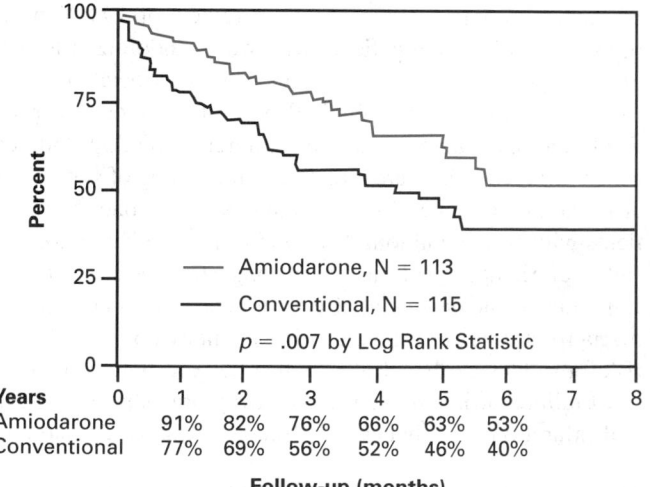

Years	0	1	2	3	4	5
Amiodarone	91%	82%	76%	66%	63%	53%
Conventional	77%	69%	56%	52%	46%	40%

Follow-up (months)

FIGURE 36-8

Cumulative "cardiac survival" for all patients in a randomized trial between electrophysiologically guided conventional (i.e., class I drugs) therapy (*black line*) versus empiric amiodarone (*green line*) in survivors of cardiac arrest (CASCADE Trial). End points included total cardiac mortality, resuscitated cardiac arrest, and syncopal implanted cardioverter/defibrillator shocks. Survival in the conventional therapy arm was lower than in the amiodarone arm. (Reprinted with permission from the CASCADE Investigators.[250])

ported a survival benefit in the patients randomized to ICD therapy.[255a] Prospective, randomized trials addressing a similar question in cardiac arrest survivors are the ongoing Canadian Implantable Defibrillator Study (CIDS)[264] and Cardiac Arrest Study Hamburg (CASH).[251] These studies will help to define the role of amiodarone treatment in patients at risk for sudden cardiac death.

Intravenous Amiodarone

The recent approval of intravenous amiodarone in the United States has added a powerful parenteral drug for the acute treatment of patients with life-threatening ventricular arrhythmias.[265] The efficacy of intravenous amiodarone in patients with recurrent, hemodynamically unstable ventricular tachycardia refractory to lidocaine, procainamide, and bretylium is approximately 40 percent in prospective studies, and about 80 percent of the arrhythmias are suppressed within the first 48 h. A loading dose of 5 mg/kg over the first 30 min and a total dose of 1000 mg in the first 24 h is recommended. Additional boluses of 150 mg may be necessary for arrhythmia control.[266] Compared with bretylium, intravenous amiodarone was at least as effective and caused significantly less hypotension than did bretylium in 302 patients with recurrent or incessant ventricular arrhythmias refractory to lidocaine and procainamide[267] (see also Chaps. 27 and 30).

Device Therapy

AUTOMATIC IMPLANTABLE CARDIOVERTER-DEFIBRILLATOR

The ICD was initially developed to recognize ventricular fibrillation or rapid ventricular tachycardia and terminate it automatically by delivering one or more high-energy shocks.[268] Newer-generation defibrillators have the additional ability to deliver low-energy cardioversion, antitachycardia pacing for ventricular tachycardia, and antibradycardia pacing. In addition, the extended storage capabilities of new defibrillator systems permit retrospective analysis of the stored electrograms during arrhythmia detection, allowing more accurate conclusions about the type of arrhythmia recognized by the device (supraventricular or ventricular), their mode of initiation, and effects of additional antiarrhythmic therapy. The first generation of epicardial defibrillators required a thoracotomy to place the sensing and defibrillator leads epicardially and the generator size mandated implantation of the device in an abdominal pocket. The development of biphasic waveforms, "active cans" (the generator case itself serves as a defibrillator electrode), and more efficient capacitors has made it possible to reduce the size of the defibrillators, which can now be implanted subpectorally with a transvenous endocardial lead system that integrates both pace/sense and high-voltage defibrillation abilities. Endocardial placement has reduced the perioperative mortality associated with defibrillator implants from 4 to 5 to less than 1.0 percent.[269]

Implantable cardioverter defibrillators are very effective in terminating ventricular tachyarrhythmias (Table 36-8). In a large data base of 2834 epicardial and endocardial defibrilla-

tors implanted in 2807 patients between 1989 and 1993, 98.8 percent of 7470 ventricular fibrillation episodes were detected and 97.9 percent of 42,132 ventricular tachycardia episodes were successfully terminated by the device.[269] The long-term outcome of patients with implantable defibrillators is also favorable, considering that virtually all patients receiving such devices are at high risk for sudden cardiac death, since they had either cardiac arrest or recurrent ventricular tachycardia refractory to medical therapy prior to implantation of the device. Defibrillator therapy has been shown to effectively reduce the annual incidence of sudden cardiac death in patients with severe underlying cardiac disease (less than 5 percent)[270,271] as well as in patients without significant structural heart disease (0 percent).[272] Despite effective reduction of the mortality from sudden cardiac death, however, long-term survival in patients with severely depressed left ventricular function is still poor despite defibrillatory therapy, and their overall cardiac mortality does not appear to be reduced in direct proportion to the reduction in sudden cardiac death.[273] Compared to the best currently available antiarrhythmic drug therapy, ICDs have recently been shown to improve survival in patients with a history of ventricular fibrillation or ventricular tachycardia. In the multicenter, prospective, and randomized AVID trial, which enrolled 1016 such patients, the ICD group had a 38 and 25 percent reduction in overall mortality at one and three years, respectively, compared to the group of patients taking amiodarone or solatol.[255a] Despite the undisputed efficacy of implantable defibrillators in preventing sudden (cardiac) death, there are several major questions that remain to be answered: (1) Which patients will benefit most from defibrillator therapy? (2) Do ICDs improve quality of life? (3) Are ICDs cost-effective compared with antiarrhythmic drug therapy and (4) Will adjunctive antiarrhythmic drug therapy add to the efficacy of ICDs?

The prophylactic (before the initial cardiac arrest event) use of defibrillators in high-risk populations is currently under investigation in patients with a left ventricular ejection fraction ≤30 percent; patients with impaired left ventricular ejection fraction and positive signal-averaged ECG who are undergoing operative revascularization; and patients with nonsustained ventricular tachycardia, coronary artery disease, and reduced left ventricular function.[274] A recently completed study (Multicenter Automatic Defibrillator Implantation Trial, MADIT)[275] demonstrated a survival benefit of defibrillator therapy compared with conventional therapy in patients with nonsustained ventricular tachycardia, post–myocardial infarction, and inducible sustained ventricular tachycardia not suppressed by procainamide; it has led to the approval of prophylactic implantation of defibrillators in this narrowly defined patient population.

The number of patients who could benefit from an ICD implant is increasingly larger due to the lower mortality and morbidity associated with the implantation of newer endocardial devices, which can be implanted with techniques similar to those of bradycardia pacemaker insertion. ICDs can effectively protect against both tachycardic and bradycardic sudden

TABLE 36-8

SURVIVAL IN PATIENTS WITH IMPLANTABLE CARDIOVERTER DEFIBRILLATORS

Study	No. of Patients	Clinical Characteristics	Follow-up, Years	Sudden Death, %	Cardiac Mortality, %	Total Mortality, %
Zipes et al.[269]		61±13 years, 83% M, CHD 76%, LVEF 34%			5.7	8.3
	2807		1	1.8		
Winkle et al.[271]	270	58±12 years, 80% M, CHD 78%, LVEF 34%	1	0.9	7.0	7.7
			5	4.4	23.8	26.2
Powell et al.[273]	150	57±13 years, 73% M, CHD 62%	2	3.3	13.3	19.3
		EF≥40%	1			4.5
			5			4.5
		EF<40%	1			6.1
			5			35.7
Fogoros et al.[270]	119	62 + 9 years, 76% M, CHD 82%	2			
		EF<30%	1			6
			3			33
		EF≥30%	1			1
			3			4
Meissner et al.[272]	28	42±14 years, 54% M LVEF>50%, no significant structural heart disease	3	0ᵃ	0	7

[a] Four patients (14%) had appropriate shocks.

Abbreviations: CHD = coronary heart disease; EF = ejection fraction; F = female; LV = left ventricular; M = male; SCD = sudden cardiac death.

cardiac death regardless of the underlying heart disease or various triggers of arrhythmias. Since their mode of action is therapeutic rather than preventive, ICD therapy might effectively be combined with other antiarrhythmic strategies such as drugs or catheter ablation to prevent frequent recurrences of tachyarrhythmias. Selection of patients who will most likely benefit from ICDs and timing of implantation are two of the many questions remaining to be determined (see also Chap. 33).

PERMANENT PACEMAKER

Permanent pacing appears to have a beneficial effect on survival in patients with congenital long-QT syndrome.[276,277] The beneficial effects of permanent pacing may be related to prevention of bradycardia and pauses, potentially contributing to a more homogeneous repolarization, as well as rate-dependent shortening of the QTc interval in patients with mutation in the sodium-channel gene (*SCN5A*)[147] (see Chap. 27).

Patients with obstructive hypertrophic cardiomyopathy at increased risk for sudden cardiac death may also benefit from pacemaker implantation. In a series of 84 patients with this condition who had severe, drug-refractory symptoms and a history of syncope in half the patients, only two sudden cardiac deaths occurred during the 2.5-year follow-up period after pacemaker implantation.[278] This approximately 1 percent annual mortality compares favorably with the annual incidence of sudden cardiac death in hypertrophic cardiomyopathy of 2 to 4 percent per year in adults and 4 to 6 percent per year in children and adolescents[110] in previous studies. While most studies have shown a decrease in left ventricular outflow tract gradient, however, pacing may have deleterious effects on other hemodynamic parameters, and there are no controlled trials demonstrating improved survival[278,279] (see Chap. 74).

Role of Surgery

REVASCULARIZATION

There is a reduced prevalence of sudden cardiac death after coronary artery bypass grafting (CABG).[280,281] Among the 13,476 patients in the Coronary Artery Surgical Study (CASS) registry, all of whom had significant coronary artery disease, operable vessels, and no significant valvular disease, the mean incidence of sudden cardiac death during the 4.6-year average follow-up was 5.2 percent in patients treated medically and 1.8 percent in those treated surgically.[280] The beneficial effect of CABG was even more pronounced in the subgroup of patients with reduced left ventricular ejection fraction and multivessel disease, where survival free from sudden cardiac death at 5 years was 91 percent for the surgical group versus 69 percent in the medical group. CABG also seems to be beneficial in patients with cardiac arrest prior to hospitalization. In an uncontrolled study of 265 survivors of cardiac arrest, 32 percent underwent CABG and 68 percent were treated medically.[282] After adjusting for differences in baseline variables between the two treatment groups, the use of CABG was associated with a significant risk reduction in recurrent cardiac arrest (risk ratio 0.48, CI 0.24 to 0.97). The protective effect of CABG from recurrent cardiac arrest appears to be best in patients with reversible ischemia as their major pathophysiologic factor in sudden cardiac death. These patients are characterized by critical coronary artery disease, significant regions of myocardium at risk for ischemia, and no inducible monomorphic ventricular arrhythmias at electrophysiologic study.[206,282] Despite the encouraging results of CABG in survivors of cardiac arrest, it should be noted that only a minority of these patients are candidates for operative revascularization and that monomorphic ventricular tachycardia, which is often associated with ventricular scars from healed myocardial infarctions, is usually not controlled by myocardial revascularization alone.[283]

ANTIARRHYTHMIA SURGERY

Electrophysiologically guided subendocardial resection and cryoablation are potentially curative surgical options in patients with recurrent monomorphic ventricular tachycardia, in whom areas of slow conduction around myocardial scars are critical for sustaining ventricular tachycardia. Long-term follow-up of this operative technique has yielded a clinical success rate of nearly 90 percent in eliminating the presenting ventricular tachycardia in patients who survive surgery. The technique is limited, however, by the high surgical mortality of 10 to 15 percent.[284] The best candidates for electrophysiologically guided subendocardial resection are patients who require coronary revascularization and have a well-defined left ventricular aneurysm.

Another surgical technique aimed at reducing sudden cardiac death rates in high-risk patients is left cardiac sympathetic denervation in the therapy of congenital long-QT syndrome.[285] The goal of this surgery is selective partial sympathetic denervation of the heart. In a review of 85 long-QT patients who continued to have recurrent syncope and cardiac arrest despite beta-blocker therapy and subsequently underwent left sympathectomy, the cardiac event rate was reduced from 22 ± 32 to 1 ± 3 per patient and the number of patients with cardiac events decreased from 99 to 45 percent.[285] The rate of sudden cardiac death over a follow-up period of nearly 6 years was 8 percent (see also Chap. 27).

Catheter Ablation Therapy

Catheter ablation of arrhythmias has emerged as a curative approach for many supraventricular arrhythmias and a few specific forms of ventricular tachycardias.[150] The role of catheter ablation in the prevention of sudden cardiac death is less well established, but this therapy form has been successfully employed in selected cases. Rarely, supraventricular tachycardias with a rapid ventricular response may degenerate into fatal ventricular tachyarrhythmias and cardiac arrest.[286]

Radiofrequency catheter ablation can eliminate the risk of a rapid ventricular response by abolishing conduction over an accessory pathway in patients with WPW syndrome, or it can slow or completely block conduction over the atrioventricular node in patients with atrial arrhythmias and rapid, medically uncontrolled atrioventricular conduction.

Radiofrequency catheter ablation can potentially prevent sudden cardiac death in patients with documented and inducible bundle branch reentrant ventricular tachycardia as the only mechanism for cardiac arrest.[287] The role of catheter ablation in other forms of ventricular tachycardia is less well established. Catheter ablation of ventricular tachycardia in patients with structural heart disease is currently feasible in only a small subset of patients who present with a hemodynamically relatively well tolerated monomorphic ventricular tachycardia.[288] Although the acute success rate in eliminating the index arrhythmia in a few specialized centers is near 60 percent, these patients often have extensive coronary heart disease, and other ventricular tachycardia morphologies recur frequently during follow-up, necessitating additional therapies.[289] Improved mapping techniques of the ventricular tachycardia circuit, better catheters, and perhaps other energy sources may help improve the efficacy of catheter ablation for ventricular tachycardia and potentially expand its role in the prevention of sudden cardiac death (see also Chap. 31).

SUMMARY

Sudden cardiac death affects more than 300,000 individuals in the United States annually and accounts for half the mortality from coronary heart disease. The vast majority of people who have experienced sudden cardiac death have underlying structural heart disease, which in the adult population is most frequently coronary heart disease, but a variety of other cardiac disorders can cause sudden cardiac death as well. Ventricular tachycardia/fibrillation and less often bradycardia/asystole are responsible for sudden cardiac death. Autonomic changes such as increased sympathetic and decreased parasympathetic reflexes appear to be important in triggering or predisposing to sudden cardiac death. Long-term survival following a cardiac arrest episode is still poor (<30 percent). The time delay to defibrillation and/or bystander administration of CPR directly influences survival. Use of an automatic implantable cardioverter/defibrillator and amiodarone are effective therapeutic options to treat survivors of cardiac arrest, but with the exception of beta blockers, prophylactic choices to prevent sudden cardiac death are inadequate. Several reasons explain the difficulty to prevent sudden cardiac death. First, sudden cardiac death often occurs in people without previously known heart disease. Second, we cannot identify with acceptable sensitivity and specificity a large percentage of the individuals who experience sudden cardiac death. Third, the mechanisms that precipitate arrhythmias causing sudden cardiac death are diverse and for the most part not known. Short-term efforts to improve the survival of sudden cardiac death victims should be directed toward delivering CPR and electrical therapy as soon as possible after the onset of an arrest.[187] Long-term goals should be focused on the prevention of sudden cardiac death and encompass basically four interrelated, stepwise objectives[187]: (1) more accurate and specific identification of the patients at risk, (2) identification and characterization of mechanisms responsible for ventricular tachycardia/ventricular fibrillation and bradycardia/asystole, (3) identification of interventions that prevent these arrhythmias, and (4) testing of these interventions in the individuals at risk.

REFERENCES

1. Kannel WB, Thomas HE Jr. Sudden coronary death: The Framingham Study. *Ann NY Acad Sci* 1982; 382:3–20.
2. Kannel WB, Schatzkin A. Sudden death: Lessons from subsets in population studies. *J Am Coll Cardiol* 1985; 5(suppl):141B–149B.
3. Kannel WB, Cupples LA, D'Agostino RB. Sudden death risk in overt coronary heart disease: The Framingham study. *Am Heart J* 1987; 113:799–804.
4. Chiang BN, Perlman LV, Fulton M, Ostrander LD, Epstein FH. Predisposing factors in sudden cardiac death in Tecumseh, Michigan. *Circulation* 1970; 41:31–37.
5. Kuller L, Lilienfeld A, Fischer R. Epidemiological study of sudden and unexpected deaths due to arteriosclerotic heart disease. *Circulation* 1966; 34:1056–1068.
6. Kuller L, Lilienfeld A, Fischer R. An epidemiological study of sudden and unexpected death in adults. *Medicine* 1967; 46:341–361.
7. Kuller KH, Perper JA, Dai WS, Rutan G, Traven N. Sudden death and the decline in coronary heart disease mortality. *J Chronic Dis* 1986; 39:1001–1019.
8. Goldberg RJ, Gore JM, Alpert JS, Dalen JE. Incidence and acute fatality rates of acute myocardial infarction (1975–1988): The Worcester Heart Attack Study. *Am Heart J* 1988; 115:751–767.
9. Gillum RF, Folsom A, Luepker RV, Jacobs DR Jr, Kottke TE, Gomez-Marin O, et al. Sudden death and acute myocardial infarction in a metropolitan area, 1970–1980: The Minnesota Heart Survey. *N Engl J Med* 1983; 309:1353–1358.
10. Gillum RF. Sudden coronary death in the United States: 1980–1985. *Circulation* 1989; 79:756–765.
11. Madsen AK. Ischemic heart disease and prodromes of sudden death. *Br Heart J* 1985; 54:27–32.
12. Goldstein S. The necessity of a uniform definition of sudden coronary death: Witnessed death within 1 hour of the onset of acute symptoms. *Am Heart J* 1982; 103:156–159.
13. Hinkle LE, Thaler HT. Clinical classification of cardiac deaths. *Circulation* 1982; 65:457–464.
14. Leach IH, Blundell JW, Rowley JM, Turner DR. Acute ischemic lesions in death due to ischemic heart disease: An autopsy study of 333 cases of out-of-hospital death. *Eur Heart J* 1995; 16:1181–1185.
15. Matoba R, Shikata I, Iwai K, Onishi S, Fujitani M, Yoshida K, et al. An epidemiologic and histopathological study of sudden cardiac death in Osaka Medical Examiner's office. *Jpn Circ J* 1989; 53:1581–1588.
16. Myocardial Infarction Community Registers. *Public Health in Europe 5.* Copenhagen: Regional Office for Europe, World Health Organization; 1976.
17. Goldberg RJ. Declining out-of-hospital sudden coronary death rates: Additional pieces of the epidemiologic puzzle. *Circulation* 1989; 79:1369–1373.
18. Cowie MR, Fahrenbuch CE, Cobb LA, Hallstrom AP. Out-of-hospital cardiac arrest: Racial differences in outcome in Seattle. *Am J Public Health* 1993; 83:955–959.
19. Becker LB, Han BH, Meyer PM, Wright FA, Rhodes KV, Smith DW, et al. Racial differences in the incidence of cardiac arrest and subsequent survival. *N Engl J Med* 1993; 329:600–606.
20. Albert CM, McGovern BA, Newell JB, Ruskin JN. Sex differences in cardiac arrest survivors. *Circulation* 1996; 93:1170–1176.
21. Neuspiel DR, Kuller LH. Sudden and unexpected natural death in childhood and adolescence. *JAMA* 1985; 254:1321–1325.
22. Liberthson RR. Sudden death from cardiac causes in children and young adults. *N Engl J Med* 1996; 334:1039–1044.
23. Burke AP, Farb A, Virmani R, Goodin J, Smialck JE. Sports-related sudden cardiac death in young adults. *Am Heart J* 1991; 121:568–575.
24. Kennedy HL, Whitlock JA, Buckingham TA. Cardiovascular sudden death in young persons (abstr). *J Am Coll Cardiol* 1984; 3:485.
25. Drory Y, Turetz Y, Hiss Y, Lev B, Fisman EZ, Pines A, et al. Sudden unexpected deaths in persons less than 40 years of age. *Am J Cardiol* 1991; 68:1388–1392.
26. Driscoll DJ, Edwards WD. Sudden unexpected death in children and adolescents. *J Am Coll Cardiol* 1985; 5(Suppl):118B–121B.
27. Topaz O, Edwards JE. Pathologic features of sudden death in children, adolescents and young adults. *Chest* 1985; 87:476–482.
28. Philips M, Robinowitz M, Higgins JR, Boran KJ, Reed T, Virmnai R. Sudden cardiac death in Air Force recruits: A 20-year review. *JAMA* 1986; 256:2696–2699.
29. Kramer MR, Drory Y, Lev B. Sudden death in young Israeli soldiers: Analysis of 83 cases. *Isr J Med Sci* 1989; 25:620–624.
30. Thiene G, Nava A, Corrado D, Rossi L, Pennelli N. Right ventricular cardiomyopathy and sudden death in young people. *N Engl J Med* 1988; 318:129–133.
31. Molander N. Sudden natural death in later childhood and adolescence. *Arch Dis Child* 1982; 57:572–576.
32. Keeling JW, Knowles SAS. Sudden death in childhood and adolescence. *J Pathol* 1989; 159:221–224.
33. Shen WK, Edwards WD, Hammill SC, Bailey KR, Ballard DJ, Gersh BJ. Sudden unexpected nontraumatic death in 54 young adults: A 30-year population-based study. *Am J Cardiol* 1995; 76:148–152.
34. Garson A Jr, McNamara DG. Sudden death in a pediatric cardiology population, 1958–1983: Relation to prior arrhythmias. *J Am Coll Cardiol* 1985; 5(Suppl):134B–137B.
35. Lambert EC, Menon VA, Wagner HR, Vlad P. Sudden unexpected death from cardiovascular disease in children: A cooperative international study. *Am J Cardiol* 1974; 34:89–96.
36. Hinkle LE. Short-term risk factors for sudden death. *Ann NY Acad Sci* 1982; 382:22–37.
37. Demirovic J. Risk factors in the incidence of sudden cardiac death and possibilities for its prevention. Doctoral thesis. Belgrade, Yugoslavia: University of Belgrade Press; 1985.
38. Beaglehole R, Stewart AW, Bonita R, Jackson RT, Sharpe DN. Myocardial infarction and sudden death in Auckland. *NZ Med J* 1984; 97:715–718.
39. Kagan A, Yano K, Reed DM, MacLean CJ. Predictors of sudden cardiac death among Hawaiian-Japanese men. *Am J Epidemiol* 1989; 130:268–277.
40. Kannel WB. Update on the role of cigarette smoking in coronary heart disease. *Am Heart J* 1981; 101:310–326.
41. Hallstrom AP, Cobb LA, Ray R. Smoking as a risk factor for recurrence of sudden cardiac arrest. *N Engl J Med* 1986; 314:271–274.
42. Lown B. Sudden cardiac death: Biobehavioral perspective. *Circulation* 1987; 76:1181–1196.
43. Engel GL. Sudden and rapid death during psychologic stress: Folk lore or folk wisdom? *Ann Intern Med* 1971; 74:771–782.
44. Leor J, Poole WK, Kloner RA. Sudden cardiac death triggered by an earthquake. *N Engl J Med* 1996; 334:413–419.
45. Weinblatt E, Ruberman W, Goldberg JD, Frank CW, Shapiro S, Chaudhary BS. Relation of education to sudden death after myocardial infarction. *N Engl J Med* 1978; 299:60–65.
46. Talbott E, Kuller LH, Petre K, Perper J. Biologic and psychosocial risk factors of sudden death from coronary disease in white women. *Am J Cardiol* 1977; 39:858–864.
47. Lakka TA, Venalainen JM, Rauramaa R, Salonen R, Tuomilehto J, Salonen JT. Relation of leisure-time physical activity and cardiorespiratory fitness to the risk of acute myocardial infarction in men. *N Engl J Med* 1994; 330:1549–1554.
48. Cobb LA, Weaver WD. Exercise: A risk factor for sudden death in patients with coronary heart disease. *J Am Coll Cardiol* 1986; 7:215–219.
49. Williams PT. Physical activity and public health. *JAMA* 1995; 274:533–534.
50. Brownell KD, Bachorik PS, Ayerle RS. Changes in plasma lipid and lipoprotein levels in men and women after a program of moderate exercise. *Circulation* 1982; 65:477–484.
51. Mittleman MA, Maclure M, Toffer GH, Sherwood JB, Goldberg RJ, Muller JE. Triggering of acute myocardial infarction by heavy physical exertion—Protection against triggering by regular exertion. *N Engl J Med* 1993; 329:1677–1683.

52. Thompson PD, Stern MP, Williams P, Duncan K, Haskell WL, Wood PD. Deaths during jogging or running: A study of 18 cases. *JAMA* 1979; 242:1265–1267.

53. Schwartz PJ, Vanili E, Stramba-Badiale M, de Ferrari GM, Billman GE, Foreman RD. Autonomic mechanisms and sudden death: New insights from the analysis of baroreceptor reflexes in conscious dogs with and without a myocardial infarction. *Circulation* 1988; 78:969–979.

54. Koplan JP. Cardiovascular deaths while running. *JAMA* 1979; 242:2578–2579.

55. Maron BJ, Epstein SE, Roberts WC. Causes of sudden death in competitive athletes. *J Am Coll Cardiol* 1986; 7:204–214.

56. Maron BJ, Roberts WC, McAllister HA, Rosing DR, Epstein SE. Sudden death in young athletes. *Circulation* 1980; 62:218–229.

57. Jensen-Urstad M. Sudden death and physical activity in athletes and nonathletes. *Scand J Med Sci Sports* 1995; 5:279–284.

58. Maron BJ, Bodison S, Wesley Y, Tucker E, Green KJ. Results of screening a large population of intercollegiate athletes for cardiovascular disease. *J Am Coll Cardiol* 1987; 10:1214–1222.

59. Maron BJ, Mitchell JH. 26th Bethesda Conference: Recommendations for determining eligibility for competition in athletes with cardiovascular abnormalities. *J Am Coll Cardiol* 1994; 24:845–899.

60. Myerburg R, Kessler KM, Bassett AL, Castellanos A. A biological approach to sudden cardiac death: Structure, function and cause. *Am J Cardiol* 1989; 63:1512–1516.

61. Willich SN, Maclure M, Mittleman M, Arntz HR, Muller JE. Sudden cardiac death: Support for a role of triggering in causation. *Circulation* 1993; 87:1442–1450.

62. Green HL. Sudden arrhythmic cardiac death: Mechanisms, resuscitation and classification: The Seattle Perspective. *Am J Cardiol* 1990; 65:4B–12B.

63. Myerberg RJ, Conde CA, Sung RJ, Castellanos A. Clinical, electrophysiologic, and hemodynamic profile of patients resuscitated from prehospital cardiac arrest. *Am J Med* 1980; 68:568–576.

64. Bayes de Luna A, Coumel P, Leclercq J. Ambulatory sudden cardiac death: Mechanism of production of fatal arrhythmia on the basis of data from 157 cases. *Am Heart J* 1989; 117:151–159.

65. Bayes deLuna AB, Coumel P, Leclercq JF. Ambulatory sudden cardiac death: Mechanisms of production of fatal arrhythmia. *Am Heart J* 1989; 117:151–159.

66. Luu M, Stevenson WG, Stevenson LW, Baron K, Walden L. Diverse mechanisms of unexpected cardiac arrest in advanced heart failure. *Circulation* 1989; 80:1675–1680.

67. Nikolic G, Bishop RL, Singh JB. Sudden death during Holter monitoring. *Circulation* 1982; 66:218–225.

68. Satoh T, Zipes DP. Rapid rates during bradycardia prolong ventricular refractoriness and facilitate ventricular tachycardia induction with cesium in dogs. *Circulation* 1996; 94:217–227.

69. Janse MJ, Wit AL. Electrophysiologic mechanisms of ventricular arrhythmias resulting from myocardial ischemia and infarction. *Physiol Rev* 1989; 69:1049–1154.

70. Jalife J, Davidenko JM, Michaels DC. A new perspective in the mechanism of arrhythmias and sudden cardiac death: Spiral waves of excitation in heart muscle. *J Cardiovasc Electrophysiol* 1991; 2:S133–S152.

71. Dillon SM, Allessie MA, Ursell PC, Wit AL. Influence of anisotropic tissue structure on reentrant circuits in the epicardial border zone of subacute canine infarcts. *Circ Res* 1988; 63:182–206.

72. Pogwizd SM, Corr PB. Mechanisms underlying the development of ventricular fibrillation during early myocardial ischemia. *Circ Res* 1990; 66:672–695.

73. Balke CW, Kaplinsky E, Michelson EL, Naito M, Dreifus LS. Reperfusion ventricular tachyarrhythmias: Correlation with antecedent coronary artery occlusion tachyarrhythmias and duration of myocardial ischemia. *Am Heart J* 1981; 101:449–456.

74. Lerman BB, Burkhoff D, Yue DT, Franz MR, Sagawa K. Mechanoelectrical feedback: Independent role of preload and contractility in modulation of canine ventricular excitability. *J Clin Invest* 1985; 76:1843–1850.

75. Levine JH, Guarnieri T, Kadish AH, White RI, Calkins H, Kan JS. Changes in myocardial repolarization in patients undergoing balloon valvuloplasty for congenital pulmonary stenosis: Evidence for contraction-excitation feedback in humans. *Circulation* 1988; 77:70–77.

76. Barber MJ, Mueller TM, Henry DP, Felten SY, Zipes DP. Transmural myocardial infarction in the dog produces sympathectomy in noninfarcted myocardium. *Circulation* 1983; 67:787–796.

77. Inoue H, Zipes DP. Results of sympathetic denervation in the canine heart: Supersensitivity that may be arrhythmogenic. *Circulation* 1987; 75:877–887.

78. Stanton MS, Tuli MM, Radtke NL, Heger JJ, Miles WM, Mock BH, et al. Regional sympathetic denervation after myocardial infarction in humans detected noninvasively using I-123-metaiodobenzylguanidine. *J Am Coll Cardiol* 1989; 14:1519–1526.

79. Miyazaki T, Zipes DP. Protection against autonomic denervation following acute myocardial infarction by preconditioning ischemia. *Circ Res* 1989; 64:437–448.

80. Takahashi N, Zipes DP. Vagal modulation of adrenergic effects on canine sinus and atrioventricular nodes. *Am J Physiol* 1983; 244:H775–H781.

81. Schwartz PJ, Zaza A, Pala M, Locati E, Beria G, Zanchetti A. Baroreflex sensitivity and its evolution during the first year after myocardial infarction. *J Am Coll Cardiol* 1988; 12:629–636.

82. La Rovere MT, Specchia G, Mortara A, Schwartz PJ. Baroreflex sensitivity, clinical correlates and cardiovascular mortality among patients with a first myocardial infarction: A prospective study. *Circulation* 1988; 78:816–824.

83. Farrell TG, Odemuyiwa O, Bashir Y, Paul V, Camm A. Prognostic value of baroreflex sensitivity after acute myocardial infarction. *Br Heart J* 1992; 66:129–137.

84. Hull SJJ, Vanoli E, Adamson PB, Verrier RL, Foreman RD, Schwartz PJ. Exercise training confers anticipatory protection from sudden death during myocardial ischemia. *Circulation* 1994; 89:548–552.

85. Goldstein S, Landis J, Leighton R, Ritten G, Vasu CM, Lantis A, et al. Characteristics of the resuscitated out-of-hospital cardiac arrest victim with coronary heart disease. *Circulation* 1981; 64:977–984.

86. Davies M. Pathological view of sudden cardiac death. *Br Heart J* 1981; 45:88–96.

87. Davies MJ, Thomas A. Thrombosis and acute coronary artery lesions in sudden cardiac ischemic death. *N Engl J Med* 1984; 310:1137–1140.

88. Van Dantzig J, Becker A. Sudden cardiac death and acute pathology of coronary arteries. *Eur Heart J* 1986; 7:987–991.

89. Roberts WC, Kragel AH, Gertz D, Roberts LS. Coronary arteries in unstable pectoris, acute myocardial infarction and sudden coronary death. *Am Heart J* 1994; 127:1588–1593.

90. Meissner MD, Ahktar M, Lehman MH. Nonischemic sudden tachyarrhythmic death in atherosclerotic heart disease. *Circulation* 1991; 84:904–912.

91. Ambrose JA, Tannenbaum MA, Alexopoulos D, Hjemdahl-Monsen CE, Leavy J, Weiss M, et al. Angiographic progression of coronary artery disease in the development of myocardial infarction. *J Am Coll Cardiol* 1988; 12:56–62.

92. McHenry PL, O'Donnell J, Morris SN, Jordan JJ. The abnormal exercise electrocardiogram in apparently healthy men: A predictor of angina pectoris as an initial coronary event during long-term follow-up. *Circulation* 1984; 70:547–551.

93. Weiner DA, Ryan TJ, McCabe CH, Chaitman BR, Sheffield LT, Tristani FE, et al. Risk of developing an acute myocardial infarction or sudden death in patients with exercise-induced silent myocardial ischemia: A report from the Coronary Artery Surgery Study (CASS) registry. *Am J Cardiol* 1988; 62:1155–1158.

94. Goldstein S, Friedman L, Hutchinson R, and the Aspirin Myocardial Infarction Study Group. Timing, mechanism and clinical setting of witnessed deaths in postmyocardial infarction patients. *J Am Coll Cardiol* 1984; 3:1111–1117.

95. Marcus FI, Cobb LA, Edwards JE, and the Multicenter Post-infarction Research Group. Mechanism of death and prevalence of myocardial ischemic symptoms in the terminal event after acute myocardial infarction. *Am J Cardiol* 1988; 61:8–15.

96. Holmes DR Jr, Davis K, Gersh BJ, Mock MB, Pettinger MB, and Participants in the Coronary Artery Surgery Study (CASS). Risk factor profiles of patients with sudden cardiac death and death from other cardiac causes: A report from the Coronary Artery Surgery Study (CASS). *J Am Coll Cardiol* 1989; 13:524–530.

97. Muharji J, Rude R, Poole K, Gustafson N, Thomas TJ, Strauss HW, et al. Risk factors for sudden death after acute myocardial infarction: Two year follow-up. *Am J Cardiol* 1994; 54:31–56.

98. Middlekauff HR, Stevenson WG, Tilliseh JH. Prevention of sudden death in survivors of myocardial infarction: A decision analysis approach. *Am Heart J* 1992; 123:475–480.

99. Taylor AJ, Rogan KM, Virmani R. Sudden cardiac death associated with isolated congenital coronary artery anomalies. *J Am Coll Cardiol* 1992; 20:640–647.

100. McAlpin RN. Cardiac arrest and sudden unexpected death in variant angina: Complications of coronary spasm that can occur in the absence of severe organic coronary stenosis. *Am Heart J* 1993; 125:1101–1017.

101. Myerburg RJ, Kessler KM, Mallon SM, Cox MM, DeMarchena E, Interian A Jr, et al. Life threatening ventricular tachycardia in patients with silent myocardial ischemia due to coronary artery spasm. *N Engl J Med* 1992; 326:1451–1455.

102. Tamburro P, Wilber D. Sudden death in idiopathic dilated cardiomyopathy. *Am Heart J* 1992; 124:1035–1045.

103. Larsen L, Markham J, Haffajee CI. Sudden death in idiopathic dilated cardiomyopathy: Role of ventricular arrhythmias. *Pacing Clin Electrophysiol* 1993; 16:1051–1059.

104. Tomaselli GF, Beuckelman DJ, Calkins HG, Berger RD, Kessler PD, Lawrence JH, et al. Sudden cardiac death in heart failure: The role of abnormal repolarization. *Circulation* 1994; 90:2434–2539.

105. Hofmann T, Meinertz T, Kasper W, Geibel A, Zehender M, Hohnloser S, et al. Mode of death in idiopathic dilated cardiomyopathy: A multivariate analysis of prognostic determinants. *Am Heart J* 1988; 116:1455–1463.

106. Middlekauff HR, Stevenson WG, Woo MA, Moser DK, Stevenson LW. Comparison of frequency of late potentials in idiopathic dilated cardiomyopathy and ischemic cardiomyopathy with advanced congestive heart failure and their usefulness in predicting sudden death. *Am J Cardiol* 1990; 66:1113–1117.

107. Packer M. Lack of correlation between ventricular arrhythmias and sudden death in patients with chronic heart failure. *Circulation* 1992; 85(suppl I):I-50–I-56.

108. Naccarelli GV, Prystowski EN, Jackmann WM, Heger J, Rahilly GT, Zipes DP. Role of electrophysiologic testing in managing patients who have ventricular tachycardia unrelated to coronary artery disease. *Am J Cardiol* 1982; 50:165–171.

109. McKenna WJ, Camm AJ. Sudden death in hypertrophic cardiomyopathy. *Circulation* 1989; 80:1489–1492.

110. Maron BJ, Roberts WC, Epstein SE. Sudden death in hypertrophic cardiomyopathy: A profile of 78 patients. *Circulation* 1992; 65:1388–1394.

111. Dilsizian V, Bonow RO, Epstein SE, Fananapazir L. Myocardial ischemia detected by thallium scintigraphy is frequently related to cardiac arrest and syncope in young patients with hypertrophic cardiomyopathy. *J Am Coll Cardiol* 1993; 22:796–804.

112. Counihan PJ, Fei L, Bashir Y, Farrell TG, Haywood GA, McKenna WJ. Assessment of heart rate variability in hypertrophic cardiomyopathy: Association with clinical and prognostic features. *Circulation* 1993; 88:1682–1690.

113. Fananapazir L, Chang AC, Epstein SE, McAreavey D. Prognostic determinants in hypertrophic cardiomyopathy: Prospective evaluation of a therapeutic strategy based on clinical, Holter, hemodynamic, and electrophysiologic findings. *Circulation* 1992; 86:730–740.

114. Fananapazir L, Tracy CM, Leon MB, Winkler JB, Cannon RO, Bonow RO, et al. Electrophysiologic abnormalities in patients with hypertrophic cardiomyopathy: A consecutive analysis of 155 patients. *Circulation* 1989; 80:1259–1268.

115. Watkins H, Rosenzweig A, Hwang DS, Levi T, McKenna W, Seidman CE, et al. Characteristics and prognostic implications of myosin missense mutations in familial hypertrophic cardiomyopathy. *N Engl J Med* 1992; 326:1108–1114.

116. Levy D, Garrison RJ, Savage DD, Kannel WB, Castelli WP. Prognostic implications of echocardiographically determined left ventricular mass in the Framingham Heart Study. *N Engl J Med* 1990; 322:1561–1566.

117. Zehender M, Faber T, Koscheck U, Meinertz T, Just H. Ventricular tachyarrhythmias, myocardial ischemia, and sudden cardiac death in patients with hypertensive heart disease. *Clin Cardiol* 1995; 18:377–383.

118. Scheler S, Motz W, Strauer BE. Transiente Myokardischämie bei Hypertonikern. *Z Kardiol* 1989; 78:197–203.

119. Tanaka M, Fujiwara H, Onodera T. Quantitative analysis of myocardial fibrosis in normals, hypertensive hearts and hypertrophic cardiomyopathy. *Br Heart J* 1986;55:575–581.

120. Siskovick DS, Raghunathan TE, Psaty BM, Koepsell TD, Wicklund KG, Lin X, et al. Diuretic therapy for hypertension and the risk of primary cardiac arrest. *N Engl J Med* 1994; 330:1899–1900.

121. Hoes AW, Grobbee DE, Lubsen J, Man in't Veld AJ, van der Does E, Hofman A. Diuretics, beta-blockers, and the risk for sudden cardiac death in hypertensive patients. *Ann Intern Med* 1995; 123:481–487.

122. Szlachcic J, Tubau JF, Massie BM, O'Kelly BF. Coronary morbidity and mortality, preexisting silent coronary artery disease and mild hypertension. *Ann Intern Med* 1989; 110:1017–1026.

123. Thiene G, Nava A, Corrado D, Rossi L, Pennelli N. Right ventricular cardiomyopathy and sudden death in young people. *N Engl J Med* 1988; 318:129–133.

124. Haissaguerre M, Le Metayer P, D'Ivernois C, Barat JL, Montserrat P, Warin JF. Distinctive response of arrhythmogenic right ventricular disease to high dose isoproterenol. *PACE* 1990; 13:2119–2126.

125. Marcus FI, Fontaine G, Frank R, Gallagher JJ, Reiter JM. Long term follow-up in patients with arrhythmogenic right ventricular disease. *Eur Heart J* 1989; 10(suppl D):68–73.

126. Lenery R, Brugada P, Janssen J, Cheriex E, Dugernier T, Wellens HJJ. Nonischemic sustained ventricular tachycardia: Clinical outcome in 12 patients with arrhythmogenic right ventricular dysplasia. *J Am Coll Cardiol* 1989; 14:96–105.

127. Pellikka PA, Nishimura RA, Bailey KR, Tajik AJ. The natural history of adults with asymptomatic, hemodynamically significant aortic stenosis. *J Am Coll Cardiol* 1990; 15:1012–1017.

128. Bonow RO, Lakatos E, Maron BJ, Epstein SE. Serial long-term assessment of the natural history of asymptomatic patients with chronic regurgitation and normal left ventricular systolic function. *Circulation* 1991; 84:1625–1635.

129. Braunwald E. On the natural history of severe aortic stenosis. *J Am Coll Cardiol* 1990; 15:1018–1020.

130. Foppl M, Hoffmann A, Amann FW, Roth J, Stulz P, Hasse J, et al. Sudden cardiac death after aortic valve surgery. *Clin Cardiol* 1989; 12:202–207.

131. Alvarez L, Escudero C, Figuera D, Castillo-Olivares JL. Late sudden cardiac death in the follow-up of patients having a heart valve prosthesis. *J Thorac Cardiovasc Surg* 1992; 104:502–510.

132. Keefe DL, Griffin JC, Harrison DC, Stinson EB. Atrioventricular conduction abnormalities in patients undergoing isolated aortic or mitral valve replacement. *PACE* 1985; 8:393–398.

133. Farb A, Tang AL, Atkinson JB, McCarty WF, Virmani R. Comparison of cardiac findings in patients with mitral prolapse who die suddenly to those who have congestive heart failure from mitral regurgitation and to those with fatal noncardiac conditions. *Am J Cardiol* 1992; 70:234–239.

134. Nishimura RA, McGoon MD, Shub C, Miller FA Jr, Ilstrup DM, Tajik AJ. Echocardiography documented mitral valve prolapse: Long term follow-up of 238 patients. *N Engl J Med* 1985; 313:1305–1309.

135. Vohra J, Sathe S, Warren R, Tatouis J, Hunt D. Malignant ventricular arrhythmias in patients with mitral valve prolapse and mitral regurgitation. *PACE* 1993; 16:387–393.

136. Martini B, Basso C, Thiene G. Sudden death in mitral valve prolapse with Holter monitoring–documented ventricular fibrillation: Evidence of coexisting arrhythmogenic right ventricular cardiomyopathy. *Int J Cardiol* 1995; 49:274–278.

137. Marks AR, Choong CY, Sanfilippo AJ, Ferre M, Weyman AE. Identification of high-risk and low-risk subgroups of patients with mitral-valve prolapse. *N Engl J Med* 1989; 320:1031–1036.

138. Devereux RB. Diagnosis and prognosis of mitral valve prolapse. *N Engl J Med* 1989; 320:1077–1079.

139. Puddu PE, Pasternac A, Tubau JF, Krol R, Farey L, deChamplain J. QT interval prolongation and increased plasma catecholamine levels in patients with mitral valve prolapse. *Am Heart J* 1983; 105:422–428.

140. Ramos SG, Matturi L, Rossi L, Rossi MA. Lesions of mediastinal paraganglia in chronic chagasic cardiomyopathy: Cause of sudden death? *Am Heart J* 1996; 131:417–420.

141. Winter SL, Cohen M, Greenberg S, Stein B, Curwin J, Pe E, et al. Sustained ventricular tachycardia associated with sarcoidosis: Assessment of the underlying cardiac anatomy and the prospective utility of programmed ventricular stimulation, drug therapy and implantable antitachycardia device. *J Am Coll Cardiol* 1991; 18:937–943.

142. Cullen S, Celermajer DS, Franklin RCG, Hallidie-Smith KA, Deanfield JE. Prognostic significance of ventricular arrhythmias after repair of tetralogy of Fallot: A 12-year prospective study. *J Am Coll Cardiol* 1994; 23:1151–1155.

143. Gatzoulis MA, Till JA, Somerville J, Redington AN. Mechanoelectrical interaction in Tetralogy of Fallot: QRS prolongation relates to right

ventricular size and predicts malignant ventricular arrhythmias and sudden death. *Circulation* 1995; 92:231–237.

144. Moss AJ, Adams FH. Sudden cardiac death. In: Moss AJ, Adams FH eds, *Heart Disease in Infants, Children and Adolescents Including the Fetus and Young Adult II,* 5th ed. Baltimore: Williams & Wilkins; 1995:1610–1619.

145. Moss AJ, Schwartz PJ, Crampton RS, Locati E, Carleen E. The long QT syndrome: A prospective international study. *Circulation* 1985; 71:17–24.

146. Vincent GM, Timothy KW, Leppert M, Keating M. The spectrum of symptoms and QT intervals in carriers of the gene for the long-QT syndrome. *N Engl J Med* 1992; 327:846–852.

147. Roden DM, Lazzara R, Rosen M, Schwartz PJ, Towbin J, Vincent JM. Multiple mechanisms in the long QT syndrome: Current knowledge, gaps, and future directions. The SADS Foundation Task Force on LQTS. *Circulation* 1996; 94: 1996–2012.

148. Nador F, Beria G, De Ferrari GM, Stramba-Badiale M, Locati EH, Lotto A, et al. Unsuspected echocardiographic abnormality in the long QT syndrome: Diagnostic, prognostic and pathogenetic implications. *Circulation* 1991; 84:1530–1542.

149. Munger TM, Packer DL, Hammill SC, Feldman SC, Bailey KR, Ballard DJ, et al. A population study of the natural history of Wolff-Parkinson-White syndrome in Olmsted County, Minnesota, 1953–1989. *Circulation* 1993; 87:866–873.

150. Jackman WM, Wang XZ, Friday KJ, Roman CA, Moulton KP, Beckman KJ, et al. Catheter ablation of accessory atrioventricular pathways (Wolff-Parkinson-White syndrome) by radiofrequency current. *N Engl J Med* 1991; 324:1605–1611.

151. Leitch JW, Klein GJ, Yee R, Murdock C. Prognostic value of electrophysiologic testing in asymptomatic patients with Wolff-Parkinson-White pattern. *Circulation* 1990; 82:1718–1723.

152. Zardini M, Yee R, Thakur RK, Klein GJ. Risk of sudden arrhythmic death in the Wolff-Parkinson-White syndrome: current perspectives. *Pacing Clin Electrophysiol* 1994; 17:966–975.

153. Klein GJ, Bashore TM, Sellers TD, Pritchett EL, Smith WM, Gallagher JJ. Ventricular fibrillation in the Wolff-Parkinson syndrome. *N Engl J Med* 1979; 301:1080–1085.

154. Chen SA, Chiang CE, Tai CT, Lee SH, Chiou CW, Ueng KC, et al. Longitudinal clinical and electrophysiological assessment of patients with symptomatic Wolff-Parkinson-White syndrome and atrioventricular node reentrant tachycardia. *Circulation* 1996; 93:2023–2032.

155. Bromberg BI, Lindsay BD, Cain ME, Cox JL. Impact of clinical history and electrophysiologic characterization of accessory pathways on management strategies to reduce sudden death among children with Wolff-Parkinson-White syndrome. *J Am Coll Cardiol* 1996; 27:690–695.

156. Viskin S, Belhassen B. Idiopathic ventricular fibrillation. *Am Heart J* 1990; 120:661–671.

157. Morady F, Scheinman MM, Hess DS, Chen R, Stanger P. Clinical characteristics and results of electrophysiologic testing in young adults with ventricular tachycardia or ventricular fibrillation. *Am Heart J* 1983; 106:1306–1314.

158. Siebels J, Schneider MAE, Geiger M, Kuck KH. Unexpected recurrences in survivors of cardiac arrest without organic heart disease (abstr). *Eur Heart J* 1991; 12(suppl):86.

159. Wever EPD, Hauer RNW, Oomen A, Peters RHJ, Bakker PFA, Robles de Medina EO. Unfavorable outcome in patients with primary electrical disease who survived an episode of ventricular fibrillation. *Circulation* 1993; 88:1021–1029.

160. Wellens HJJ, Lemery R, Smeets JL, Brugada O, Gorgels AP, Cheriex EC, et al. Sudden death without overt heart disease. *Circulation* 1992; 85(suppl I):92–97.

161. Aizawa Y, Naitoh N, Washizuka T, Takahashi K, Uchiyama H, Shiba M, et al. Electrophysiological findings in idiopathic recurrent ventricular fibrillation: Special reference to mode of induction, drug testing, and long-term outcomes. *PACE* 1996; 19:929–939.

162. Brugada P, Abdollah H, Heddle B, Wellens HJJ. Results of a ventricular stimulation protocol using a maximum of 4 premature extrastimuli in patients without documented or sustained ventricular arrhythmias. *Am J Cardiol* 1983; 52:1214–1218.

163. DiCarlo LA Jr, Morady F, Schwartz AB, Shen EN, Baerman JM, Krol RB, et al. Clinical significance of ventricular fibrillation-flutter induced by programmed ventricular stimulation. *Am Heart J* 1985; 109: 959–963.

164. Kirschner JW, Eckner FAO, Baron RC. The cardiac pathology of sudden, unexplained nocturnal death in Southeast Asian refugees. *JAMA* 1986; 256:2700–2705.

165. Gotoh K. A histopathological study of the conduction system in so-called "Pokkuri disease" (sudden unexpected cardiac death of unknown origin in Japan). *Jpn Circ J* 1976; 40:753–768.

166. Brugada P, Brugada J. Right bundle branch block, persistent ST segment elevation and sudden cardiac death, a distinct clinical and electrocardiographic syndrome. *J Am Coll Cardiol* 1992; 20:1391–1396.

167. Corrado D, Nava A, Buja G, Martini B, Fasoli G, Oselladore L, et al. Familial cardiomyopathy underlies syndrome of right bundle branch block, ST segment elevation and sudden death. *J Am Coll Cardiol* 1996; 27:443–448.

168. Frey W. Weitere Erfahrungen mit Chinidin bei absoluter Herzunregelmäßigkeit. *Wien Klin Wochenschr* 1918; 55:849–853.

169. Echt DS, Liebson PR, Mitchell B, Peters RW, Oblas-Manno D, Barken AH, et al. Mortality and morbidity in patients receiving encainide, flecainide, or placebo: The Cardiac Arrhythmia Suppression Trial. *N Engl J Med* 1991; 324:781–788.

170. Podrid PJ. Aggravation of arrhythmia: A complication of antiarrhythmic drugs. *J Cardiovasc Electrophysiol* 1993; 4:311–319.

171. Packer M, Medina N, Yushak M. Hemodynamic and clinical limitations of long term inotropic therapy with amrinone in patients with severe congestive heart failure. *Circulation* 1984; 70:1038–1047.

172. Patterson E, Szabo B, Scherlag BJ, Lazzara R. Arrhythmogenic effects of antiarrhythmic drugs. In: Zipes DP, Jalife J, eds. *Cardiac Electrophysiology: From Cell to Bedside.* Philadelphia: Saunders; 1995: 496–511.

173. Minardo JD, Heger JJ, Miles WM, Zipes DP, Prystowsky EN. Clinical characteristics of patients with ventricular fibrillation during antiarrhythmic drug therapy. *N Engl J Med* 1988; 319:257–262.

174. Nattel S, Pederson DH, Zipes DP. Alteration in regional myocardial distribution and arrhythmogenic effects of aprindine produced by coronary artery occlusion in the dog. *Cardiovasc Res* 1981; 15:80–85.

175. Raymond JR, van den Berg EK Jr, Knapp MJ. Nontraumatic prehospital death in young adults. *Arch Intern Med* 1988; 148:303–308.

176. Hearn WL, Flynn DD, Hine GW, Rose S, Cofino JC, Mantero-Atienza C, et al. Cocaethylene: A unique cocaine metabolite displays high affinity for the dopamine transporter. *J Neurochem* 1991; 56:698–701.

177. Isner JM, Estes M III, Thompson PD, Costanzo-Nordin MR, Subramanian R, Miller G, et al. Acute events temporally related to cocaine abuse. *N Engl J Med* 1986; 315:1438–1443.

178. Nordrehaug JE, Johannessen KA, van der Lippe G. Serum potassium concentrations as a risk factor of ventricular arrhythmias early in acute myocardial infarction. *Circulation* 1985; 71:645–649.

179. Gettes LS. Electrolyte abnormalities underlying lethal ventricular arrhythmias. *Circulation* 1992; 85(suppl I):I70–I76.

180. Eisenberg MJ. Magnesium deficiency and sudden death. *Am Heart J* 1992; 124:544–549.

181. Hoes AW, Grobbe DE, Peet TM, Lubsen J. Do non-potassium-sparing diuretics increase the risk of sudden cardiac death in hypertensive patients? Recent evidence. *Drugs* 1994; 47:711–733.

182. Isner JM, Roberts WC, Heymsfield SB, Yager J. Anorexia nervosa and sudden death. *Ann Intern Med* 1985; 102:49–52.

183. Litwin PE, Eisenberg MS, Hallstrom AP, Cummins RO. The location of collapse and its effect on survival from cardiac arrest. *Ann Emerg Med* 1987; 16:787–791.

184. Eisenberg MS, Horwood BT, Cummins RO, Reynolds-Haertie R, Hearne TR. Cardiac arrest and resuscitation: A tale of 29 cities. *Ann Emerg Med* 1990; 19:179–186.

185. Kuller LH, Perper JA, Cooper MC. Sudden and unexpected death due to atherosclerotic heart disease. *Mod Trends Cardiol* 1974; 3:292–332.

186. Cummins RO, Ornato JP, Thies WH, Pepe PE. Improving survival from sudden cardiac arrest: The "chain of survival" concept. *Circulation* 1991; 83:1832–1847.

187. Zipes DP. Sudden cardiac death. Future approaches. *Circulation* 1992; 85(suppl I):I-160–I-166.

188. Weaver WD, Cobb LA, Fahrenbruch CE, Hill DL, Copass MK, Hallstrom AP. Use of the automatic external defibrillator in the management of out-of-hospital cardiac arrest. *N Engl J Med* 1988; 319:661–666.

189. Sack JB, Kesselbrenner MB, Jarrad A. Interposed abdominal compression CPR and resuscitation outcome during asystole and electromechanical dissociation. *Circulation* 1992; 86:1692–1700.

190. Lerman BB, Deale OC. Relation between transcardiac and transthoracic current during defibrillation in humans. *Circ Res* 1990; 67:1420–1426.

191. Kerber RE, Grayzel J, Hoyt R, Marcus M, Kennedy J. Transthoracic resistance in human defibrillation: Influence of body weight, chest size, serial shocks, paddle size and paddle contact pressure. *Circulation* 1981; 63:676–682.

192. Emergency Cardiac Care Committee and Subcommittees, American Heart Association. Guidelines for cardiopulmonary resuscitation and emergency cardiac care. *JAMA* 1992; 268:2172–2295.

193. Lerman BB, Engelstein ED. Metabolic determinants of defibrillation: Role of adenosine. *Circulation* 1995; 91:838–844.

194. Becker LB, Ostrander MP, Barrett J, Xondos GT. Outcome of CPR in a large metropolitan area: Where are the survivors? *Ann Emerg Med* 1991; 20:355–361.

195. Lombardi G, Gallagher EJ, Gennis P. Outcome of out-of-hospital cardiac arrest in New York City: The pre-hospital arrest survival evaluation. (PHASE) study. *JAMA* 1994; 271:678–683.

196. Cobb LA, Hallstrom AP. Community-based cardiopulmonary resuscitation: What have we learned? *Ann NY Acad Sci* 1982; 382:330–342.

197. Dickey W, Adgey J. Mortality within hospital after resuscitation from ventricular fibrillation outside hospital. *Br Heart J* 1992; 67:334–338.

198. Hallstrom AP, Cobb LA, Yu BH. Influence of comorbidity on the outcome of patients treated for ventricular fibrillation. *Circulation* 1996; 93:2019–2022.

199. Longstretch WT, Cobb LA, Fahrenbruch CE, Copass MK. Does age affect outcomes of out-of-hospital cardiopulmonary resuscitation? *JAMA* 190; 264:2104–2100.

200. Brugada P, Talajic M, Smeets J, Mulleneers R, Wellens HJJ. The value of the clinical history to assess prognosis of patients with ventricular tachycardia or ventricular fibrillation after myocardial infarction. *Eur Heart J* 1989; 10:747–752.

201. Middlekauff HR, Stevenson WG, Saxon LA. Prognosis after syncope: Impact of left ventricular function. *Am Heart J* 1993; 125:121–127.

202. Bigger JT, Fleiss JL, Kleiger R, Miller JP, Rolnitzky LM, the Multicenter Post-Infarction Research Group. The relationship among ventricular arrhythmias, left ventricular dysfunction, and mortality in the 2 years after myocardial infarction. *Circulation* 1983; 69:250–258.

203. Greenberg H, McMaster P, Dwyer EM Jr, and the Multicenter Postinfarction Research Group. Left ventricular dysfunction after acute myocardial infarction: Results of a prospective multicenter study. *J Am Coll Cardiol* 1984; 4:867–874.

204. Wilson JR, Schwartz J, Sutton M, Ferraro N, Horowitz LW, Reichek N, et al. Prognosis in severe heart failure: Relation to hemodynamic measurements and ventricular ectopic activity. *J Am Coll Cardiol* 1983; 2:403–410.

205. Stevenson WG, Stevenson LW, Middlekauf HR, Saxon LA. Sudden death prevention in patients with advanced ventricular dysfunction. *Circulation* 1993; 88:2953–2961.

206. Wilber DJ, Garan H, Finkelstein D, Kelly E, Wewll J, McGovern B, Ruskin JN. Out-of-hospital cardiac arrest: Use of electrophysiologic testing in the prediction of long-term outcome. *N Engl J Med* 1988; 318:19–24.

207. Herre JM, Sauve MJ, Malone P, Griffin JC, Helmy I, Langberg J, et al. Long term results of amiodarone therapy in patients with recurrent sustained ventricular tachycardia or ventricular fibrillation. *J Am Coll Cardiol* 1989; 13:442–449.

208. Weinberg BA, Miles WM, Klein LS, Bolander JE, Dusman RE, Stanton MS, et al. Five-year follow-up of 589 patients treated with amiodarone. *Am Heart J* 1993; 125:109–120.

209. Algra A, Tijssen JGP, Roelandt JRTC, Pool J, Lubsen J. QTc prolongation measured by standard 12-lead electrocardiography is an independent risk factor for sudden death due to cardiac arrest. *Circulation* 1991; 83:1884–1894.

210. Day CP, McComb JM, Campbell RWF. QT dispersion, an indication of arrhythmia risk in patients with long QT intervals. *Br Heart J* 1990; 63:342–344.

211. Barr CS, Naas A, Freeman M, Lang CC, Struthers AD. QT dispersion and sudden unexpected death in chronic heart failure. *Lancet* 1994; 343:327–329.

212. Shaper AG, Wannamethee G, Macfarlane PW, Walker M. Heart rate in ischemic heart disease and sudden cardiac death in middle-aged British men. *Br Heart J* 1993; 70:49–55.

213. Holmes J, Kubo SH, Cody RJ, Kligfield P. Arrhythmias in ischemic and nonischemic dilated cardiomyopathy: Prediction of mortality by ambulatory electrocardiography. *Am J Cardiol* 1985; 55:146–151.

214. Gomes JA, Winters SL, Stewart D, Horowitz SL, Milner M, Barreca P. A new noninvasive index to predict ventricular tachycardia and sudden death in the first year after myocardial infarction: Based on signal averaged electrocardiogram, radionuclide ejection fraction and Holter monitoring. *J Am Coll Cardiol* 1987; 10:349–357.

215. Kuchar DL, Thornburn CW, Sammel NL. Prediction of serious arrhythmic events after myocardial infarction: Signal averaged electrocardiogram, Holter monitoring and radionuclide ventriculography. *J Am Coll Cardiol* 1987; 9:531–538.

216. Farrell TG, Bashir Y, Cripps T, Malik M, Poloniecki J, Bennett ED, et al. Risk stratification for arrhythmic events in post-infarction patients based on heart rate variability, ambulatory electrocardiographic variables and the signal-averaged electrocardiogram. *J Am Coll Cardiol* 1991; 18:687–697.

217. Chakko CS, Cheorghiade M. Ventricular arrhythmias in severe heart failure: Incidence, significance, and effectiveness of antiarrhythmic therapy. *Am Heart J* 1985; 109:497–504.

218. Kleiger RE, Miller JP, Bigger JT, Moss AJ, the Multicenter Post-Infarction Research Group. Decreased heart rate variability and its association with increased mortality after acute myocardial infarction. *Am J Cardiol* 1987; 59:256–262.

219. Bigger JT Jr, Fleiss JL, Steinman RC, Roinitsky LM, Kleiger RE, Rottman JN. Frequency domain measures of heart period variability and mortality after myocardial infarction. *Circulation* 1992; 85:164–171.

220. Algra A, Tijssen JPG, Roelandt JRTC, Pool J, Ludsen J. Heart rate variability from 24 hour electrocardiography and the 2-year risk for sudden death. *Circulation* 1993; 88:180–185.

221. Barron HV, Lesh MD. Autonomic nervous system and sudden cardiac death. *J Am Coll Cardiol* 1996; 27:1053–1060.

222. Schwartz PJ, La Rovere MT, Vanoli E. Autonomic nervous system and sudden cardiac death: Experimental basis and clinical observations for post-myocardial infarction risk stratification. *Circulation* 1992; 85(suppl I):I-77–I-91.

223. Stein KM, Borer JS, Hochreiter C, Kliegfield P. Fractal clustering of ventricular ectopy and sudden death in mitral regurgitation. *J Electrocardiol* 1992; 25:S178–S181.

224. Stein KM, Karagounis LA, Anderson JL, Kliegfield P, Lerman BB. Fractal clustering of ventricular ectopy correlates with sympathetic tone preceding ectopic beats. *Circulation* 1995; 91:722–727.

225. Rosenbaum DS, He B, Cohen RJ. New approaches for evaluating cardiac electrical activity: Repolarization alternans and body surface imaging. In: Zipes DP, Jalife J, eds. *Cardiac Electrophysiology: From Cell to Bedside.* Philadelphia: Saunders; 1995:1187–1197.

226. Rosenbaum DS, Jackson LE, Smith JM, Garan H, Ruskin JN, Cohen RJ. Electrical alternans and vulnerability to ventricular arrhythmias. *N Engl J Med* 1994; 330:235–241.

227. Simson MB. Noninvasive identification of patients at high risk for sudden cardiac death: Signal-averaged electrocardiography. *Circulation* 1992; 85(suppl I):I-145–I-151.

228. Mancini DM, Wong SL, Simson MB. Prognostic value of an abnormal signal-averaged electrocardiogram in patients with nonischemic congestive cardiomyopathy. *Circulation* 1993; 87:1083–1092.

229. Gomes JA, Winters SL, Ergin A, Machae J, Estioko M, Alexopoulos D, et al. The clinical and electrophysiological determinants, treatment and survival of patients with sustained malignant ventricular tachyarrhythmias late postmyocardial infarction. *J Am Coll Cardiol* 1990; 17:320–326.

230. Ruskin JN. Role of invasive electrophysiologic testing in the evaluation of and treatment of patients at high risk for sudden cardiac death. *Circulation* 1992; 85(suppl I):I-152–I-159.

231. Andresen D, Steinbeck G, Bruggeman T, Haberl R, Fink L, Schröder R. Prognosis of patients with sustained ventricular tachycardia and of survivors of cardiac arrest not inducible by programmed stimulation. *Am J Cardiol* 1992; 70:1250–1254.

232. Poole JE, Mathisen TL, Kudenchuck PJ, McAnulty JH, Swerdlow CD, Bardy GH, et al. Long-term outcome in patients who survived out-of-hospital ventricular fibrillation and who undergo electrophysiologic studies: Evaluation by electrophysiologic subgroups. *J Am Coll Cardiol* 1990; 16:657–665.

233. Benditt DG, Benson DW Jr, Klein GJ, Pritzker MR, Kriett JM, Anderson RW. Prevention of recurrent sudden cardiac arrest: Role of pro-

vocative electropharmacologic testing. *J Am Coll Cardiol* 1983; 2:418–425.

234. Waller TJ, Kay HR, Spielman SR, Kutalek SP, Greenspan AM, Horowitz LN. Reduction in sudden death and total mortality by antiarrhythmic therapy evaluated by electrophysiologic drug testing: Criteria of efficacy in patients with sustained ventricular tachyarrhythmia. *J Am Coll Cardiol* 1987; 10:83–89.

235. Bourke JP, Richards DAB, Ross DL, Wallace EM, McGuire MA, Uther JB. Routine programmed electrical stimulation in survivors of acute myocardial infarction for prediction of spontaneous ventricular tachyarrhythmias during follow-up: Results, optimal stimulation protocol and cost-effective screening. *J Am Coll Cardiol* 1991; 18:780–788.

236. Kendall MJ, Lynch KP, Hjalmarson A, Kjekshus J. β-blockers and sudden cardiac death. *Ann Intern Med* 1995; 123:358–367.

237. Yusuf S, Peto R, Lewis J, Collins R, Sleight P. Beta blockade during and after myocardial infarction: An overview of the randomized trials. *Prog Cardiovasc Dis* 1985; 27:335–371.

238. Beta-Blocker Heart Attack Research Group. A randomized trial of propranolol in patients with acute myocardial infarction: I. Mortality results. *JAMA* 1982; 247:1707–1714.

239. Schwartz PJ, Motolese M, Pollavini G, Ruberti U, Trazzi R, et al. Prevention of sudden cardiac death after a first myocardial infarction by pharmacological or surgical antiadrenergic interventions. *J Cardiovasc Electrophysiol* 1992; 3:2–16.

240. Norwegian Multicenter Study Group. Timolol-induced reduction in mortality and reinfarction in patients surviving myocardial infarction. *N Engl J Med* 1981; 304:801–807.

241. Singh BN. Advantages of beta-blockers versus antiarrhythmic agents and calcium-antagonists in secondary prevention after myocardial infarction. *Am J Cardiol* 1990; 66:9C–20C.

242. Furberg C, Hawkins C, Lichstein E. Effect of propranolol in postinfarction patients with mechanical or electrical complications. *Circulation* 1984; 69:761–765.

243. Cohn JN, Johnson G, Ziesche S, Cobb F, Francis G, Tristani F, et al. A comparison of enalapril with hydralazine-isosorbide dinitrate in the treatment of congestive heart failure. *N Engl J Med* 1991; 325:303–310.

244. CONSENSUS Trial Study Group. Effects of enalapril on mortality in severe congestive heart failure: Results of the Cooperative North Scandinavian Enalapril Survival Study (CONSENSUS). *N Engl J Med* 1987; 316:1429–1435.

245. SOLVD Investigators. Effect of enalapril on survival in patients with reduced left ventricular ejection fractions and congestive heart failure. *N Engl J Med* 1991; 325:293–302.

246. Hine L, Laird N, Hewitt P, Chalmers TC. Metaanalysis of empirical long-term antiarrhythmic therapy after myocardial infarction. *JAMA* 1989; 262:3037–3040.

247. Teo KK, Yusuf S, Furberg CD. Effects of prophylactic antiarrhythmic drug therapy in acute myocardial infarction. *JAMA* 1993; 270:1589–1595.

248. Hine LK, Laird N, Hewitt P, Chalmers TC. Meta-analysis evidence against prophylactic use of lidocaine in acute myocardial infarction. *Arch Intern Med* 1989; 149:2694–2698.

249. Moosvi AR, Goldstein S, Medendorp SV, Landis JR, Wolfe RA, Leighton R, et al. Effect of empiric antiarrhythmic therapy in resuscitated out-of-hospital cardiac arrest: Victims with coronary artery disease. *Am J Cardiol* 1990; 65:1192–1197.

250. The CASCADE Investigators. Randomized antiarrhythmic drug therapy in survivors of cardiac arrest (the CASCADE study). *Am J Cardiol* 1993; 72:280–287.

251. Siebels J, Kuck KH. Implantable cardioverter defibrillator compared with antiarrhythmic drug treatment in cardiac arrest survivors [The Cardiac Arrest Study Hamburg (CASH)]. *Am Heart J* 1994; 127:1139–1144.

252. Hohnloser SH, Woosley RL. Drug therapy: Sotalol. *N Engl J Med* 1994; 331:31–38.

253. Mason JW. A randomized comparison of electrophysiologic study to electrocardiographic monitoring for prediction of antiarrhythmic drug efficacy in patients with ventricular tachyarrhythmias. *N Engl J Med* 1993; 329:445–451.

254. Waldo AL, Camm AJ, deRuyter H, Friedman PL, MacNeil DJ, Pauls JF, et al. Effect of d-sotalol on mortality in patients with left ventricular dysfunction after recent and remote myocardial infarction: The SWORD Investigators. (Survival With Oral d-Sotalol). *Lancet* 1996; 348:7–12.

255. AVID Investigators. Antiarrhythmics Versus Implantable Defibrillators (AVID)—Rationale, design and methods. *Am J Cardiol* 1995; 75:470–475.

255a. NIH News Release: NHLBI stops arrhythmia study–Implantable cardiac defibrillators reduce deaths. NHLBI Communication 1997; 301:496–497.

256. Zipes DP, Prystowsky EN, Heger JJ. Amiodarone: Electrophysiologic actions, pharmacokinetics and clinical effects. *J Am Coll Cardiol* 1984; 3:1059–1071.

257. Olson PJ, Woelfel A, Simpson RJ Jr, Foster JR. Stratification of sudden death risk in patients receiving long-term amiodarone treatment for sustained ventricular tachycardia or ventricular fibrillation. *Am J Cardiol* 1993; 71:823–826.

258. Nademanee K, Singh BN, Stevenson WG, Weiss JN. Amiodarone and post MI patients. *Circulation* 1993; 88:764–774.

259. Burkart F, Pfisterer M, Kioski W, Follath F, Burchhardt D, Jordi H. Effect of antiarrhythmic therapy on mortality in survivors of myocardial infarction with asymptomatic complex ventricular arrhythmias: Basel Antiarrhythmic Study of Infarct Survival (BASIS). *J Am Coll Cardiol* 1990; 16:1711–1718.

260. Cairns JA, Connolly SJ, Roberts R, Gent M. Randomized trial of outcome after myocardial infarction in patients with frequent or repetitive ventricular premature depolarizations: CAMIAT. Canadian Amiodarone Myocardial Infarction Trial Investigators. *Lancet* 1997; 349:675–682.

261. Julian DJ, Camm AJ, Frangin G, Janse MJ, Munoz A, Schwartz PJ, et al. Randomized trial of effect of amiodarone on mortality in patients with left-ventricular dysfunction after recent myocardial infarction. EMIAT, European Myocardial Infarction Amiodarone Trial Investigators. *Lancet* 1997; 349:667–674.

262. Doval HC, Nul DR, Grancelli HO, Perrone SV, Bortman GR, Curie R, et al. Randomised trial of low-dose amiodarone in severe congestive heart failure. Grupo de Estudio de la Sobrevida en la Insuficiencia Cardiaca en Argentina (GESICA). *Lancet* 1994; 344:493–498.

263. Singh SN, Fletcher RD, Fisher SG, Singh BN, Lewis HD, Deedwania PC, et al. Amiodarone in patients with congestive heart failure and asymptomatic ventricular arrhythmia. *N Engl J Med* 1995; 13:333;121–122.

264. Connolly SJ, Gent M, Roberts RS, Dorian P, Green MS, Kein GJ, et al. Canadian Implantation Defibrillator Study (CIDS): Study design and organization. *Am J Cardiol* 1993; 72:103F–108F.

265. Scheinman MM. Parenteral antiarrhythmic drug therapy in ventricular tachycardia/ventricular fibrillation: Evolving role of class III agents—Focus on amiodarone. *J Cardiovasc Electrophysiol* 1995; 6:914–919.

266. Levine JH, Massumi A, Scheinman MM, Winkle RA, Platia EV, Chilson DA, et al. Intravenous amiodarone for recurrent sustained hypotensive ventricular tachyarrhythmias. *J Am Coll Cardiol* 1996; 27:67–75.

267. Kowey PR, Levine JH, Herre JM, Pacifico A, Lindsay BD, Plumb VJ, et al. Randomized, double-blind comparison of intravenous amiodarone and bretylium in the treatment of patients with recurrent, hemodynamically destabilizing ventricular tachycardia or fibrillation. *Circulation* 1995; 92:3255–3263.

268. Mirowski M, Reid PR, Mower MM, Watkins L, Gott VL, Schauble JF, et al. Termination of malignant ventricular arrhythmias with an implanted automatic defibrillator in human beings. *N Engl J Med* 1980; 303:322–324.

269. Zipes DP, Roberts D, for the Pacemaker-Cardioverter-Defibrillator Investigators. Results of the International Study of the implantable pacemaker cardioverter-defibrillator: A comparison of epicardial and endocardial lead systems. *Circulation* 1995; 92:59–62.

270. Fogoros RN, Elson JJ, Bonnet CA, Fiedler GB, Burkholder JA. Efficacy of the automatic implantable cardioverter-defibrillator in prolonging survival in patients with severe underlying cardiac disease. *J Am Coll Cardiol* 1990; 16:381–386.

271. Winkle RA, Mead RH, Ruder MA, Gaudiani VA, Smith WA, Buch WS, et al. Long-term outcome with the automatic implantable cardioverter-defibrillator. *J Am Coll Cardiol* 1989; 13:1353–1361.

272. Meissner MD, Lehmann MH, Steinman RT, Mosteller RD, Akhtar M, Calkins H, et al. Ventricular fibrillation in patients without significant structural heart disease: A multicenter experience with implantable cardioverter defibrillator therapy. *J Am Coll Cardiol* 1993; 21:1406–1412.

273. Powell AC, Fuchs T, Finkelstein DM, Garan H, Cannon DS, McGovern

BA, et al. Influence of implantable cardioverter defibrillators on the long term prognosis of survivors of out of hospital cardiac arrest. *Circulation* 1993; 88:1083–1092.

274. Kuck KH. Value of prophylactic implantable cardioverter defibrillator therapy. *PACE* 1994; 17:514–516.

275. Moss AJ, Hall WJ, Cannom DS, Daubert JP, Higgins SL, Klein H, et al. Improved survival with an implanted defibrillator in patients with coronary disease at high risk for ventricular arrhythmia. *N Engl J Med* 1996; 335:1933–1940.

276. Moss AJ, Liu JE, Gottlieb S, Locati EH, Schwartz PJ, Robinson JL. Efficacy of permanent pacing in the management of high-risk patients with long QT syndrome. *Circulation* 1991; 84:1524–1529.

277. Eldar M, Griffin JC, VanHare GF, Witherell C, Bhandari A, Benditt D, et al. Combined use of beta-adrenergic blocking agents and long-term cardiac pacing for patients with long QT syndrome. *J Am Coll Cardiol* 1992; 20:830–837.

278. Fananapazir L, Epstein ND, Curiel RV, Panza JA, Tripodi D, McAreavey D. Long-term results of dual chamber (DDD) pacing in obstructive hypertrophic cardiomyopathy: Evidence for progressive symptomatic and hemodynamic improvement and reduction of left ventricular hypertrophy. *Circulation* 1994; 90:2731–2742.

279. Nishimura RA, Hayes DL, Ilstrup DM, Holmes DR, Tajik AJ. Effect of dual-chamber pacing on systolic and diastolic function in patients with hypertrophic cardiomyopathy: Acute Doppler echocardiographic and catheterization hemodynamic study. *J Am Coll Cardiol* 1996; 27:421–430.

280. Holmes DR Jr, Davis KB, Mock MB, Fisher LD, Gersh BJ, Killip T, et al. The effect of medical and surgical treatment in patients with coronary artery disease: A report from the Coronary Artery Surgery Study. *Circulation* 1986; 73:1254–1263.

281. Varnauskas E, and the European Coronary Surgery Study Group. Survival, myocardial infarction and employment status in a prospective randomized study of coronary bypass surgery. *Circulation* 1985; 72(suppl V):V-90–V-101.

282. Every NR, Fahrenbruch CE, Hallstrom AP, Weaver WD, Cobb LA. Influence of coronary bypass surgery on subsequent outcome of patients resuscitated from out of hospital cardiac arrest. *J Am Coll Cardiol* 1992; 19:1435–1439.

283. Kelly P, Ruskin JN, Vlahakes GJ, Buckley MJ, Freeman CS, Garan H. Surgical coronary revascularization in survivors of prehospital cardiac arrest: Its effect on inducible ventricular arrhythmias and long-term survival. *J Am Coll Cardiol* 1990; 15:267–273.

284. Hargrove WC, Josephson ME, Marchlinski FE, Miller JM. Surgical decisions in the management of sudden cardiac death and malignant ventricular arrhythmias: Subendocardial resection, the automatic internal defibrillator, or both. *J Thorac Cardiovasc Surg* 1989; 97:923–928.

285. Schwartz PJ, Locati EH, Moss AJ. Left cardiac sympathetic denervation in the therapy of congenital long QT syndrome: a world-wide report. *Circulation* 1991; 84:503–511.

286. Wang YS, Scheinmann MM, Chien WW, Cohen TJ, Lesh MD, Griffin JC. Patients with supraventricular tachycardia presenting with aborted sudden death: Incidence, mechanism and long-term follow-up. *J Am Coll Cardiol* 1991; 18:1711–1719.

287. Langberg JJ, Desai J, Dullet N, Scheinman MM. Treatment of macroreentrant ventricular tachycardia with radiofrequency ablation of the right bundle branch. *Am J Cardiol* 1989; 63:1010–1013.

288. Stevenson WG, Khan H, Sager P, Saxon LA, Middlekauff HR, Natterson PD, et al. Identification of reentry circuit sites during catheter mapping and radiofrequency ablation of ventricular tachycardia late after myocardial infarction. *Circulation* 1993; 88:1647–1670.

289. Gonska BD, Cao K, Schaumann A, Dorszewski A, von zur Muhlen F, Kreuzer H. Catheter ablation of ventricular tachycardia in 136 patients with coronary artery disease: Results and long-term follow-up. *J Am Coll Cardiol* 1994; 24:1506–1514.

CARDIOPULMONARY RESUSCITATION AND THE SUBSEQUENT MANAGEMENT OF THE PATIENT

Nisha Chibber Chandra / Myron L. Weisfeldt

HISTORICAL ISSUES

Since biblical times, humans have attempted to restore life to the dead or nearly dead individual. In the eighteenth century, bellows were used to inflate the lungs. One technique that gained broad use in this century was the Schafer prone pressure method of artificial respiration, in which the lower back was pressed cyclically, thus forcing air from the lungs.[1] At the time, all these methods were viewed as a means primarily for providing lung ventilation. Since these techniques almost certainly provided repeated fluctuation of intrathoracic pressure, as discussed below, they also likely provided some circulation of blood as well. In 1954, Elam and colleagues showed that mouth-to-mouth or mouth-to-nose resuscitation was superior to the Schafer method in terms of efficacy of ventilation.[2] The importance of the circulation of blood was also recognized, and direct or internal cardiac massage became an accepted technique as early as 1916. Despite proven efficacy, internal massage remains fraught with complications and is rarely employed even by trained personnel.[3,4]

In the 1930s, Wiggers pioneered the study of the mechanisms and treatment of ventricular fibrillation.[5] Only recently has the importance of prompt defibrillation taken a primary position in improving survival from sudden cardiac death. This follows on the success of implanted defibrillators and development of less expensive semiautomatic defibrillators for first-responder use. In 1960, Kouwenhoven and coworkers developed the present technique of external chest compression in the supine position and coupled this with artificial respiration.[6] These investigators proposed that during chest compression in the arrested state, the heart was squeezed or massaged between the sternum and vertebral column, resulting in the forward flow of blood. This technique of cardiopulmonary resuscitation (CPR) gained rapid popularity and was shown to be effective.[7] Subsequent studies in large populations have confirmed that survival from prehospital cardiac arrest is dependent upon both prompt CPR and prompt defibrillation.

MECHANISMS OF MOVEMENT OF BLOOD DURING CARDIOPULMONARY RESUSCITATION

The original hypothesis, as mentioned above, suggested that blood flow to the periphery during external chest compression resulted from direct compression of the heart between the sternum and the vertebral column.[6] According to this concept, chest compression ("systole"), similar to internal cardiac massage, resulted in blood being squeezed from both ventricles into the great arteries as the pulmonary and aortic valves opened. Retrograde flow of blood was prevented by closure of the mitral and tricuspid valves. During the release phase of chest compression ("diastole"), the ventricles recoiled to their original shape and filled by a suction effect while elevated arterial pressure was thought to close both the pulmonic and aortic valves.

This widely held concept is not, however, consistent with a number of observations in animal models[8] and humans[9] that suggest a correlation between the rise in intrathoracic pressure during chest compression and the apparent magnitude of carotid flow and pressure. The importance of fluctuations in intrathoracic pressure as a means for generating blood flow is further supported by the observations of Criley et al. that, by the continuous and early initiation of coughing, patients in ventricular fibrillation can maintain consciousness as long as cough is continued.[10] The critical ingredient of the cough is clearly a rise in intrathoracic pressure, probably with no cardiac compression. Criley's observations strongly suggest that following cardiac arrest, a rise in intrathoracic pressure is a potent mechanism for the movement of blood to the brain in humans.[10]

EXPERIMENTAL OBSERVATIONS

For brain blood flow to occur during CPR, a carotid arterial-to-jugular pressure gradient must be present during chest compression. In large animals, chest compression during CPR results in an essentially equal rise in central venous, right atrial, pulmonary artery, aortic, esophageal, and lateral pleural space pressures with no transcardiac gradient being developed (Fig. 37-1).[11]

In large animals, aortic pressure is transmitted directly to the carotid arteries, but retrograde transmission of intrathoracic venous pressure into the jugular veins is prevented by valves at the thoracic inlet. Thus, during chest compression ("systole"), a peripheral arteriovenous pressure gradient appears, and blood flow occurs consequent to this gradient. During compression, there is no pressure gradient across the heart; therefore, the heart cannot be the pump responsible for generating blood flow during CPR. In fact, the heart functions merely as a passive conduit. When chest compression is released ("diastole"), intrathoracic pressures fall toward zero, and venous flow into the right side of the heart and lungs

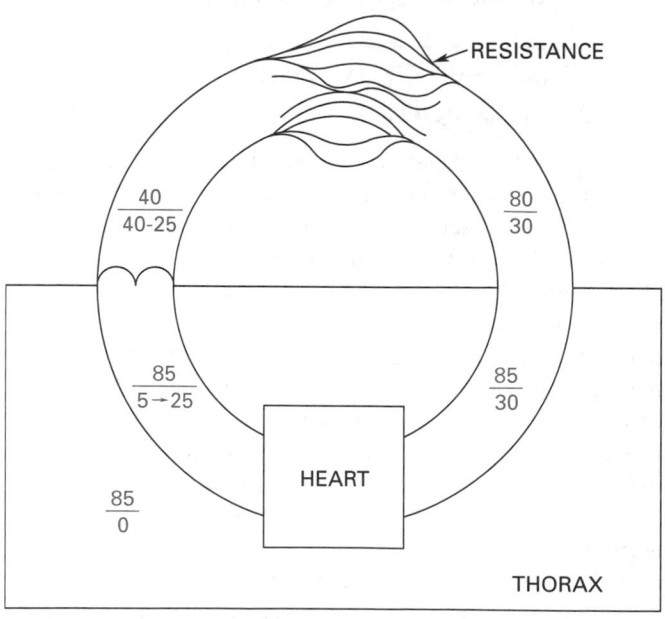

FIGURE 37-1

Representative pressures recorded during conventional cardiopulmonary resuscitation with forward carotid flow. Pressures are those recorded during compression. Intrathoracic pressures were indexed from esophageal pressures. There is no significant pressure gradient across the heart. The extrathoracic arterial pressure is similar to the intrathoracic aortic pressure. The extrathoracic venous pressure is markedly lower than the intrathoracic venous (right atrial) pressure. There is an extrathoracic arteriovenous pressure gradient that results in forward flow.

occurs. During "diastole," a modest gradient also develops between the intrathoracic aorta and the right atrium and determines myocardial flow. Limited retrograde flow occurs into the aorta from extrathoracic arteries, raising aortic diastolic pressure and increasing coronary flow. The rise in intrathoracic pressure during chest compression is likely a consequence of airway collapse, which occurs at the level of the small bronchioles and results in air trapping. With the release of chest compression, this airway collapse is relieved.[11,12]

Unlike the hemodynamic pattern described above, in some animals intrathoracic vascular pressures during vigorous chest compression are much higher than pleural pressure.[13] In such animals, the rise in vascular pressures probably result from compression of the heart during chest compression, and the classic mechanism of direct cardiac compression is probably operating in these animls. Even during cardiac compression, however, venous valves at the thoracic inlet remain essential for establishing a peripheral arteriovenous pressure gradient, which facilitates peripheral flow. It is likely that flow produced by the two mechanisms operating simultaneously can occur, and in such situations the resultant flow is additive.

The position of the mitral valve during chest compression came to be regarded as a "marker" for the mechanism of blood flow during CPR, with mitral valve closure suggesting direct cardiac compression.[14] Some investigators, using transesophageal echocardiography, have demonstrated mitral valve closure during CPR in humans.[15] Others have reported that the mitral valve remains open during chest compression.[16] Recent animal studies have demonstrated that mitral valve closure or position cannot be used to identify the primary mechanism for blood flow during CPR.[17]

Studies of the perfusion of vital organs indicate that during CPR (irrespective of the primary mechanism for blood flow), cerebral flow is dependent on the gradient between the carotid artery and the intracranial pressure during "systole," with myocardial flow being dependent on the gradient between the aorta and right atrium during "diastole."[18]

Building on these concepts, several experimental maneuvers and techniques have been developed to increase arterial pressure during chest compression; these are undergoing clinical evaluation. Some of these techniques require special equipment, whereas others can be performed by unequipped health care providers.

EXPERIMENTAL TECHNIQUES OF CARDIOPULMONARY RESUSCITATION

The technique of perithoracic high-pressure vest inflation without airway manipulation (vest CPR) allows cyclical increments in intrathoracic pressure to 100 to 150 mmHg during external chest compression by the vest and has been shown to significantly increase cerebral and myocardial blood flow during CPR in animals.[19] This technique employs a special computer-controlled pneumatic vest device positioned around the chest. Initial human data confirm higher vascular pressures during vest CPR as compared with conventional resuscitation.[20] A multicenter, randomized, in-hospital trial is presently ongoing to test whether or not the rapid initiation of vest CPR improves survival.

Active compression-decompression CPR (ACD-CPR) requires a special suction-cup plunger-type device that can be readily deployed by first responders. It incorporates a negative pressure "pull" on the thorax during the release phase of chest compression and slightly improves vascular pressures and air exchange during CPR.[21] The mechanism of benefit from this technique of resuscitation may relate to improved venous return and/or increased intrathoracic pressure during chest compression as a consequence of changes in the bony thorax. Although initially small clinical reports appeared favorable, recent larger in-hospital and out-of-hospital studies in cardiac arrest patients have shown no survival benefit of ACD-CPR.[22]

In cardiac arrest in animals, aortic infusion during CPR via catheters placed retrograde has been shown to improve coronary flow and survival. Human experience with this technique is, however, limited. Emergency cardiopulmonary bypass during cardiac arrest is also undergoing clinical evaluation following promising animal studies.

"High-impulse CPR" requires no special equipment and has been shown to improve vascular pressures.[13] Clinical experience with this technique is limited. Interposed abdominal compression (IAC) CPR can be performed by one or two unequipped health care providers. It increases carotid flow and improves survival in animals. Clinical trials with in-hospital CPR in humans have also shown improved survival as compared with conventional CPR.[23] In this technique, the upper abdomen is compressed when the chest is released. The mechanism of benefit with IAC-CPR in humans is unclear but may relate to improved venous return, decreased arterial runoff, or greater rise in intrathoracic pressure (with the diaphragm pushed up before chest compression).

Recently, the technique of phased chest and abdominal compression-decompression has also undergone animal and clinical testing. This technique is a mechanized IAC-CPR in which the rescuer uses a special chest-abdomen manual compression device (the Lifestick Resuscitator); the chest and abdomen are thus compressed alternately. The originators of this technique suggest that it, though similar to IAC-CPR, is safer and more effective. Clinical studies are presently ongoing. In summary, despite extensive evaluation, none of the experimental techniques of resuscitation have shown benefit in large human populations studied by independent investigators.

Although such experimental techniques do not lend themselves to routine clinical use, their study has resulted in a better understanding of physiology that, in turn, allows several aspects of external chest compression to be manipulated in order to optimize vital-organ perfusion pressures.[24] First, greater sternal force augments myocardial and cerebral perfusion but can also result in greater tissue injury. Second, adequate duration of compression during each chest compression–release cycle is critical for maintaining maximal myocardial and cerebral blood flow during resuscitation. At higher rates of chest compression, an optimal chest compres-

sion duration of 50 percent of cycle time is more easily achieved. Based on these data, changes in the American Heart Association (AHA) recommendations regarding chest compression rate evolved.[25] The 1986 standards recommend an increase in the rate of chest compression from the historical 60 beats per minute to 80 to 100 beats per minute.

OBSERVATIONS IN HUMANS

Unfortunately, at this point we can draw no final conclusion as to the frequency or importance of the two mechanisms (cardiac compression or generalized increase in intrathoracic pressure) during conventional cardiopulmonary resuscitation in humans. Published studies, however, suggest that manipulation of intrathoracic pressure is probably the dominant mechanism.[26] In a number of patients, comparable arterial and right atrial pressures have been observed as well as the presence of a pressure gradient at the thoracic inlet upon withdrawing an intravascular catheter from the superior vena cava to the extrathoracic internal jugular vein.[11,27,28] This hemodynamic pattern favors the concept of forward flow of blood through manipulation of intrathoracic pressure. This concept is further strengthened by the observation that maneuvers designed to increase intrathoracic pressure during chest compression— such as prolonged compression or vest CPR—are rewarded by a significant increase in peripheral arterial pressure.[20] Perhaps the strongest evidence supporting the theory of manipulation of intrathoracic pressure as a mechanism for blood flow in humans is found in the documented efficacy of "cough CPR."[10] In some patients, who are usually thin chested with cardiomegaly, extremely high arterial pressures are generated with conventional CPR. In a few of these patients, central venous pressure was found to be lower than arterial pressure. This hemodynamic picture suggests cardiac compression. In other patients, however, this higher arterial pressure may reflect higher generalized intrathoracic pressure during chest compression. This may be a result of functional airway obstruction due to airway collapse, pulmonary congestion, and/or bronchospasm.[12] In the majority of the patients in whom radial artery pressure has been measured during CPR, the arterial pressure has been relatively low and similar to that seen in the dog during conventional CPR.[26,27]

In human beings (and also in animals), it is not essential to think about the mechanisms of blood flow during CPR in an exclusive fashion. As the force of chest compression changes or as chest wall anatomy and chest compliance change during prolonged resuscitation, the dominant mechanism for blood flow (during resuscitation) may also change.

DIAGNOSIS AND IDENTIFICATION OF CARDIAC ARREST

Cardiac arrest is defined as the sudden cessation of effective cardiac pumping function as a result of either ventricular asystole (electrical or mechanical) or ventricular fibrillation.

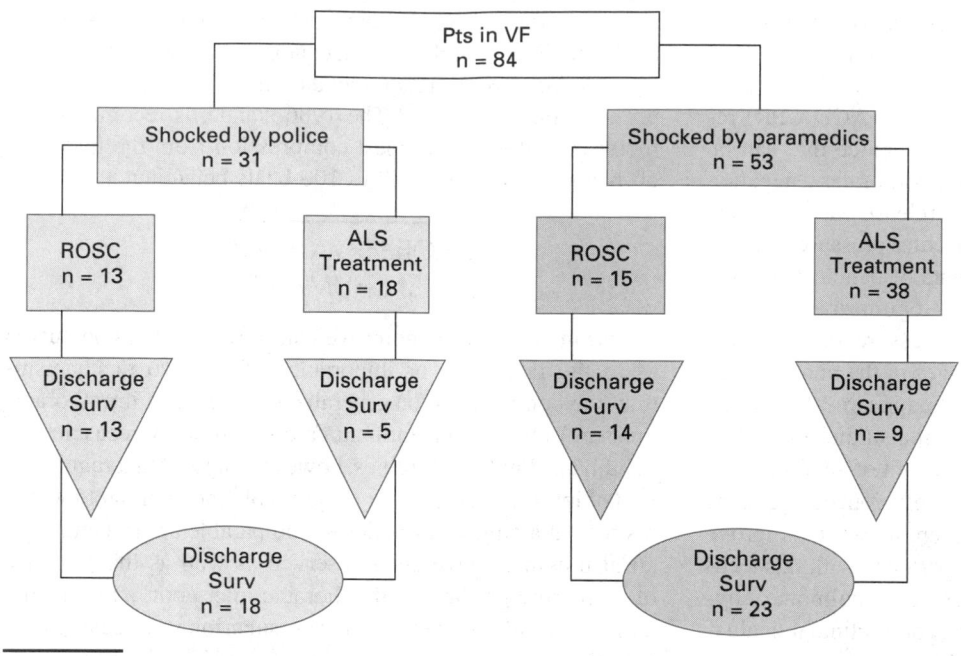

FIGURE 37-2

Police and paramedical treatment groups and patient outcome. VF-ventricular fibrillation; ROSC-restoration of spontaneous circulation; ALS-advanced life support. (From White et al.,[31] with permission.)

Rapid diagnosis and treatment are essential because (1) more than a few minutes of total cardiac arrest result in permanent cerebral anoxic damage and (2) the success of resuscitative measures is related to the rapidity with which they are instituted following arrest. Based on these and other observations, the concept of early activation of Emergency Medical Systems (EMS) has evolved for victims of out-of-hospital cardiac arrest[29] (see also Chap. 36).

Preliminary Patient Evaluation and Triage

Cardiac arrest should be considered in the differential diagnosis of sudden collapse in any patient. It can be clinically confirmed by pulseless major vessels and absent heart sounds. Although respirations (agonal respirations) may continue for a minute or two, the patient with cardiac arrest rapidly becomes cyanotic and unconscious.

Once the diagnosis of cardiac arrest is made and no trauma is suspected, the unconscious patient should be positioned supine on a firm surface and the airway opened using the head tilt–chin lift technique or alternative strategies, as described below (in the discussion of ventilation during CPR). The patient should immediately receive rescue breathing either with a bag-valve mask device or with mouth-to-mouth breathing. Simple airway barrier devices, which are easily deployed, can be used to minimize direct patient contact and are preceived as being more hygienic during mouth-to-mouth resuscitation. Following airway opening and rescue breathing, chest compressions should be promptly initiated at approximately 80 to 100 per minute. Recent animal data suggests

that ventilation can be deferred for several minutes in witnessed cardiac arrest without changing survival if chest compressions are initiated promptly. Confirmation of these observations in humans is needed before such practice is recommended.

If available, an electrocardiogram (ECG) can confirm the diagnosis and identify asystole, ventricular fibrillation, or electromechanical dissociation as the mechanism of arrest. Cardiopulmonary resuscitation (CPR), however, should be initiated immediately, as described above, once the clinical diagnosis is made without delaying to obtain this information. If a defibrillator but not an ECG is immediately available, a 200-J countershock should be administered without delay. Prehospital CPR studies in several patients have confirmed that the mechanism of cardiac arrest is usually ventricular fibrillation and that survival is critically dependent on the time to defibrillation.[30] Most hospitals and paramedics are now equipped with defibrillators with "quick look" paddles that simultaneously allow the ECG rhythm to be analyzed. On the basis of the rhythm, an etiology for the arrest can then be explored in a more focused way and appropriate therapy initiated.

AUTOMATIC EXTERNAL DEFIBRILLATORS

Based on these observations, automatic external defibrillators (AEDs) were developed for use by first (minimally trained) responders, and were shown to dramatically improve survival after prehospital arrest.[31,32] AEDs have been successfully used by nontraditional health care professionals (airline crews and police) with dramatic improvement in patient survival. All these programs have included strict physician-guided training and supervision. Perhaps the most compelling results of this strategy of emergency care were reported recently by White et al. in Rochester, Minnesota, where police initiated AED defibrillation and resuscitation resulted in a survival to hospital discharge of approximately 50 percent (Fig. 37-2).[31] AEDs have an approximately 90 percent sensitivity and specificity for successfully recognized ventricular fibrillation. They are designed for use by first responders or persons with little medical training (e.g., fire fighters, EMS technicians). These devices have varying degrees of automation and can deliver several successive defibrillatory shocks by two self-adhesive electrodes that are placed by the user on the left anterior chest.

It is highly recommended that all first responder units be equipped with AEDs. The use of AEDs by nontraditional health care professionals and possibly by trained lay persons is currently the focus of intense research.

RESPIRATORY ARREST

Respiratory arrest is the cessation of effective respiratory effort. It can result from airway obstruction (due to a foreign body or other causes), drowning, smoke inhalation, drug overdose, head trauma, cerebrovascular accident, or suffocation. When respiratory arrest occurs suddenly (as with foreign-body obstruction), the patient rapidly becomes cyanotic, though a palpable pulse with blood pressure, consciousness, and ineffective respiratory efforts may be maintained for several minutes. Opening the airway and/or rescue breathing may be all that is necessary to resuscitate such a patient.

The Heimlich maneuver is recommended for relieving foreign-body airway obstruction. It is implemented by standing behind the victim and delivering a series of sharp thrusts to the upper abdomen with a closed fist.[33] Abdominal thrusts can also be used directly in the unconscious, supine patient to help dislodge a foreign body mechanically. The Heimlich maneuver can also be self-administered by placing the fist between the naval and xiphoid process and delivering a series of quick upward thrusts. If incorrectly administered, this maneuver can lead to visceral damage.[34] When properly used, however, the technique is both safe and effective. Manual removal of a foreign body should be used only in the unconscious victim. This can be achieved by opening the victim's mouth and attempting to dislodge any obvious foreign body with a finger. As a single method, back blows may not be as effective as the Heimlich maneuver in adults. For this reason, the Heimlich maneuver is considered the technique of choice.

VENTILATION DURING CARDIOPULMONARY RESUSCITATION

Clearing the airway is of the utmost importance. Foreign bodies, loose dentures, or any other oral obstruction should be removed. Next, the head tilt–chin lift technique, which causes the tongue to move anteriorly, is used to open the airway. The chin is lifted forward with the fingers of one hand supporting the jaw and the head is tilted back by the other hand on the forehead of the patient.[35] The head tilt–neck lift method of opening the airway is also commonly employed and is an acceptable technique for use by the skilled rescuer. Here, the head is tilted back with one hand on the forehead; the other hand is placed behind the neck, lifting it upward to open the airway. If no spontaneous respirations are present, mouth-to-mouth (or mouth-to-nose) ventilation is immediately initiated, with adequacy being judged by the rise and fall of the patient's chest with each breath. To minimize gastric distention, it is necessary to deliver slow (1- to 2-s) ventilatory breaths.

Equipped rescuers will use a barrier device or a bag-mask technique of ventilation together with a small plastic oral "airway," which moves the tongue anteriorly. Adequate ventilation is difficult with the bag-mask technique, since a single rescuer often has difficulty maintaining an adequate seal on the face, and rapid bag deflation commonly results in gastric distention and aspiration. Slow (1- to 2-s) ventilation must be employed if the bag-mask technique is used.

Several invasive airway adjuncts have also been developed for use by nonphysician health care providers in prehospital situations.[36] The esophageal obturator airway (EOA), esophageal gastric tube airway (EGTA), the Combitube, and the pharyngotracheal lumen airway are among those that have been used in the prehospital setting. Considerable training and skill are needed in placing and using these devices properly. Serious, life-threatening complications have been reported following the use of the EOA or EGTA; after successful resuscitation, if an EOA was used, balloon deflation frequently results in the regurgitation of gastric contents.[36] As a consequence, the recent trend in most EMS systems has been to train paramedics in endotracheal intubation, which can be successfully implemented in the field.

Endotracheal intubation remains the ideal technique for ensuring adequate ventilation during CPR. It can be implemented rapidly, but much valuable time can be wasted by repeated unskilled attempts at intubation. If this technique is used, CPR should be discontinued for no more than 20 to 30 s while the tube is being passed into the airway. If more than 20 to 30 s elapse without successful intubation, the laryngoscope should be withdrawn and CPR reinstituted. Whenever possible, a nasogastric tube should be inserted to drain the stomach and thus decrease the chances of aspiration.

The optimal requirements for ventilation during CPR in human beings remain unknown. No study has clearly identified the optimal timing, sequence in relation to chest compression, or tidal volume needed during CPR. The American Heart Association (AHA) recommendations advise 10 to 12 slow ventilatory breaths per minute with a tidal volume of 800 to 1200 mL per breath.[29] During the first few minutes of cardiac arrest without prior hypoxia, as noted above, animal studies suggest that ventilation is less important relative to chest compression and defibrillation. Airflow from chest compression alone and air in the lungs at the time of arrest may be sufficient initially.[37,38] Human confirmation of these observations is necessary before changes in clinical recommendations can be made.

CHEST COMPRESSION DURING CARDIOPULMONARY RESUSCITATION

The AHA has published *Standards for Cardiopulmonary Resuscitation and Emergency Cardiac Care*.[29] In reference to external chest compression, they advise (1) 80 to 100 sternal compressions per minute, (2) 50 percent of each compression-relaxation cycle to be compression, and (3) one slow (1- to 2-s) ventilation for every five compressions if two trained rescuers are performing CPR, and two slow (1- to 2-s) ventilatory breaths every 15 chest compressions if lay rescuers or one trained person is performing CPR. As mentioned earlier, at such faster rates of chest compression, a prolongation of chest compression is more easily achieved by most individuals. In addition to these recommendations, it is critical in performing chest compression to use sufficient force to depress the sternum by approximately 2 in. (5 to 6 cm). As this is usually difficult to gauge, sufficient chest compression force should be used to generate a palpable femoral or carotid arterial pulse.

Airway, breathing, chest compression, "ABC," is the specific sequence used to initiate CPR in the United States and many other countries.[29] However, in the Netherlands, "CAB" is the common technique for CPR implementation, with resuscitation outcomes similar to those reported for "ABC" in the United States. No human studies have compared the "ABC" technique of resuscitation with "CAB." Both techniques are effective. "ABC" CPR remains the dominant technique for CPR implementation in the United States with survival rates as high as 35 percent in cities with advanced EMS systems[30,32] (see Chap. 36).

Despite its proven efficacy, the recently perceived risk of infectious disease transmission during CPR has reduced the willingness of both lay and medical personnel to initiate mouth-to-mouth ventilation and CPR in unknown victims of cardiac arrest. In an effort to respond to these concerns and encourage layman CPR, some cities have mandated the public availability and use of barrier devices during mouth-to-mouth ventilation. The effectiveness of such barrier devices is, however, unknown. To overcome this limitation, potential rescuers who are reluctant to initiate CPR because of the perceived risk of infection should be encouraged to activate the EMS system immediately, open the victim's airway, and then initiate and continue chest compressions only until paramedics arrive. The paramedics can then initiate ventilation with the necessary protective equipment.

DEFINITIVE THERAPY

The AHA's 1992 *Guidelines for Cardiopulmonary Resuscitation and Emergency Cardiac Care* have adopted a new classification for therapeutic recommendations.[29] This classification allows a relative therapeutic value to be assigned to a given strategy of treatment.

Class I   :   Definitely helpful
Class IIA: Acceptable, probably helpful
Class IIB: Acceptable, possibly helpful, probably not harmful
Class III: Not indicated, may be harmful

In the following text, these specific therapeutic classifications will be mentioned when appropriate.

During cardiac arrest, the ECG will usually show rapid ventricular tachycardia or fibrillation, asystole, or heart block—or it may be near normal.

Ventricular Tachycardia or Fibrillation

With ventricular fibrillation, an attempt at electrical defibrillation should be made as quickly as possible. Successful defibrillation is accomplished by the passage of adequate electrical current (amperes) through the heart (see also Chap. 32). Current flow is dependent on the energy chosen (joules) and the transthoracic impedance (ohms), or resistance to current flow. Factors that affect transthoracic impedance include the energy selected, electrode size, skin-paddle coupling material, the number and time interval of previous shocks, the distance between the electrodes (size of the chest), phase of ventilation, and paddle electrode pressure.[39] Human transthoracic impedance ranges from 15 to 150 ohms, with the average adult impedance being 70 to 80 ohms. If transthoracic impedance is high, low-energy shocks are ineffective in generating enough current to achieve successful defibrillation. Transthoracic impedance can be reduced by firm pressure on hand-held electrode paddles and a gel/cream, or saline-soaked gauze pads, between the electrode and the skin.[39] In addition, proper electrode/paddle placement is essential; one electrode should be placed to the right of the upper sternum below the clavicle and the other to the left of the nipple, with the center of the electrode in the midaxillary line. An acceptable alternative is one electrode anteriorly over the left precordium and the other posteriorly behind the heart in the right infrascapular location. The latter positioning is best achieved by using preadhesive rather than hand-held electrodes. In female patients with large breasts, the electrodes are best placed to the right of the upper sternum and either under or lateral to the left breast. Direct current is employed during defibrillation. The paddles, coated with low-resistance gel, are applied firmly to the chest and then discharged with 200 J, which is repeated at 200 to 300 J if the first shock is unsuccessful. The current AHA standards suggest that a third 360-J shock be delivered if ventricular fibrillation persists.[30] These three shocks should be delivered in rapid succession. Prospective studies by Adgey and others have shown 85 to 90 percent successful defibrillation using only 200 J in patients weighing up to 90 kg.[40,41] Some advocate higher-energy defibrillation, but few currently use more than 400 J.[42] High-energy defibrillation may cause more cardiac injury, and there is no clear evidence that it increases the frequency of successful resuscitation.[43] The importance of transthoracic impedance as a determinant of successful defibrillation has led to the concept of "current-based" defibrillation. Here, the operator selects electrical current (amperes) instead of energy (joules). Such an approach avoids the problem of an inappropriately low energy selection in patients with high impedance (with consequent low current flow and failure to defibrillate), or selection of high energy in patients with low impedance, which could result in excessive current flow, myocardial injury, and failure to defibrillate. Recent advances in defibrillator design have made such an approach feasible by displaying an instantaneous measurement of transthoracic impedance. Clinical studies with this technique support its effectiveness.[44]

When the ECG shows "fine" fibrillation waves, defibrillation efforts are often unsuccessful. The administration of epinephrine (5 to 10 mL of 1:10,000) intravenously (IV) results in a more vigorous and coarse fibrillation that is more responsive to defibrillation. This effect is likely due to improved coronary flow following epinephrine administration (see below) and perhaps direct myocardial effects on the electrical properties for defibrillation. If defibrillation fails, it is likely that marked acidosis or hypoxemia is present. Emphasis should be on hyperventilation with supplemental oxygen to correct both hypoxemia and metabolic acidosis.[45] Sodium bicarbonate might then be administered (1 meq/kg) to aid in the management of acidosis, and defibrillation should be repeated with 320 to 400 J. By using instantaneous Fourier transformation analysis, Brown et al. have demonstrated that the coarseness of the waveform of ventricular fibrillation may be highly predictive of subsequent survival and appears to correlate with coronary flow.[46] Animal data suggest that techniques or drugs that increase the "coarseness" of the ventricular fibrillation waveform may increase the likelihood of successful defibrillation. Preliminary human data to confirm these observations is encouraging, though the technique of instantaneous waveform analysis is still undergoing clinical testing.[46]

For recurrent ventricular fibrillation, the administration of 75 to 100 mg IV of lidocaine followed by repeat defibrillation may increase the likelihood of returning to a stable rhythm. Lidocaine is an effective antiarrhythmic agent for recurrent ventricular fibrillation. Amiodarone (a bolus of 150 to 300 mg over 10 min, 1.0 to 2.0 mg/min for 6 h, then 0.5 to 1.0 mg/min for 6 to 24 h) intravenously has recently been shown to be of modest benefit for recurrent ventricular fibrillation in patients failing treatment with lidocaine alone. Procainamide or bretylium can additionally be used in patients failing lidocaine, but both can cause considerable hypotension.[29,47,48] For recurrent ventricular fibrillation in the setting of ischemia, intravenous propranolol or other intravenous beta blockers are remarkably effective drugs. Beta blockers seem particularly helpful in the setting of primary ventricular fibrillation complicating acute myocardial infarction.

Hyperkalemia is a readily treated condition that can cause atrioventricular (AV) block, impaired intraatrial and intraventricular conduction, and occasionally ventricular fibrillation or, less commonly, asystole. It can be recognized by the development of tall, peaked T waves with a normal QT interval and sine wave–like ventricular tachycardia. Life-threatening hyperkalemia responds most readily to calcium infusion; 10 to 30 mL of 10% calcium gluconate is infused intravenously over 1 to 5 min under constant ECG monitoring. Calcium counteracts the adverse effects of potassium on the neuromuscular membranes but does not alter plasma potassium. Its effect, though immediate, is transient. Hyperkalemia should subsequently be treated by glucose-insulin or ion-exchange resins (see also Chap. 27). Sodium bicarbonate is also used as an agent to lower potassium.

With ventricular tachycardia, cough may reverse the arrhythmia without defibrillation, and repeated cough may maintain the conscious state as a result of the rise in intrathoracic pressure.[10,49] The efficacy of the precordial thump (precordial chest blows) has been variably reported in patients with ventricular tachycardia. A thump is generally ineffective for terminating prehospital ventricular fibrillation or asystole. Hence, it should never be used in the patient with ventricular tachycardia and a pulse unless a defibrillator is immediately available.

Asystole or Heart Block

For patients with prehospital cardiac arrest, asystole has been shown to be an ominous rhythm with a very low likelihood of successful resuscitation.[30] On the other hand, asystole due to vagal stimulation is the commonest cause of cardiac arrest associated with anesthesia induction and surgical procedures. Asystole also occurs as a result of heart block or sinus node disease (see Chap. 27). Atropine (0.5 mg) given intravenously and repeated in 5 min can be used acutely to prevent or reverse severe bradycardia in many of these settings.

If asystole is witnessed or of short duration, vigorous blows to the precordium may sometimes restart the heart. Rhythmic chest blows may maintain limited perfusion and can be continued if needed while palpating the femoral or carotid pulse until other treatment is available. If the chest blow fails, cardiopulmonary resuscitation should be initiated and intravenous epinephrine (5 to 10 mL of 1:10,000) administered. Possible treatable causes of asystole—such as acidosis, hypoxemia, hyper- or hypokalemia, and hypothermia—should be considered and treated appropriately if suspected. If an overdose of calcium channel blocker is suspected, calcium chloride, 1 g given as an intravenous bolus may be very effective (class IIA recommendation). Resuscitation measures may result in the return of a slow ventricular rhythm, which can subsequently be supported with atropine (1 to 2 mg IV) until a temporary pacemaker is placed. Temporary pacing is the optimal treatment for true asystole or profound bradycardia. Obviously, considerable skill and training are required for temporary transvenous pacemaker placement (see Chap. 34). Transcutaneous pacing has been developed as a noninvasive and simple technique that can be implemented rapidly. It uses external surface electrodes with a high-voltage pacing source. Higher voltages are required to overcome transthoracic resistance, but they are painful and are therefore used mainly on unconscious patients. The energy delivered to the heart by this technique is variable, as is its efficacy. Recently, pacing sources with longer pacing stimulus duration have been developed and may offer less painful and more effective pacing. Prehospital studies of transcutaneous pacing for asystole have not confirmed an improvement in survival.[50] It may, however, be of some benefit for patients early in asystole (class IIB intervention). Clinical evidence does not support its routine use in all patients with asystole.

In rare instances, very fine ventricular fibrillation may result in an almost straight line on a single-lead ECG and thus be mistaken for "asystole." In such cases, where the diagnosis of asystole is in question, it is suggested that a perpendicular ECG lead be viewed. Rotation of "quick look" ECG paddles by 90° easily achieves this. If ventricular fibrillation is present, the perpendicular ECG lead will demonstrate a typical fibrillation pattern, whereas in true asystole, a straight line will be seen in all ECG leads. If ventricular fibrillation is diagnosed, the initial treatment should be according to the outline above—i.e, three successive countershocks. There is little value in defibrillating true asystole.

Electromechanical Dissociation

In electromechanical dissociation (EMD), there is evidence of organized electrical activity on the ECG at a reasonable rate but failure of effective perfusion (no pulse or blood pressure). The most treatable causes of this condition are hypovolemia due to severe hemorrhage, pericardial tamponade, tension pneumothorax, hypoxia, hypothermia, acidosis, hyperkalemia, and massive pulmonary embolism. Signs of these problems should be sought and definitive therapy undertaken with fluids and/or blood replacement, pericardiocentesis, placement of a pleural needle or tube, endotracheal intubation, and other maneuvers as deemed necessary. These conditions should also be strongly considered if CPR results in no palpable pulse or evidence of perfusion. Unfortunately, many patients with electromechanical dissociation have primary myocardial failure. Following diagnosis, ventilation should be optimized and epinephrine administered. Calcium chloride was used for EMD, but prospective studies have not shown it to improve survival.[51] In acute myocardial infarction, sudden electromechanical dissociation is a sign of myocardial rupture. In such cases, pericardiocentesis and surgical repair can rarely result in survival.

ESTABLISHMENT OF AN INTRAVENOUS ROUTE

While external chest compression and artificial ventilation are continued, a plastic catheter should be inserted into a large peripheral vein. Drug administration during CPR should be accomplished only from a source above the diaphragm, since there is little cephalad flow from veins below the diaphragm. If a peripheral vein cannot be cannulated, a cutdown should be attempted or a central venous line placed by a percutaneous route. If CPR is properly performed, drugs administered through a peripheral line will often reach the arterial circulation within 15 to 30 s.[45] Recent data suggest that a 20-mL fluid bolus significantly improves peripheral drug delivery to the central compartment. Intracardiac injections are unnecessary except when there is no intravenous access. If an intravenous route is unavailable, epinephrine (1 to 2 mg in 10 mL of sterile distilled water) and lidocaine (50 to 100 mg in 10 mL of sterile distilled water) can be administered by way of the endotracheal tube into the bronchial tree. The drug should be injected through a long catheter passed beyond the tip of the endotracheal tube. Cardiac compression should be withheld, and several insufflations with an Ambu bag should immediately follow drug administration to aid drug absorption through aerosolization.

MAJOR DRUGS USED DURING CARDIOPULMONARY RESUSCITATION

Drugs that are used for the treatment of various arrhythmias are mentioned above. Catecholamines are used in cardiac arrest to (1) increase arterial and coronary perfusion during and following CPR, (2) stimulate spontaneous contraction during asystole, (3) make fine ventricular fibrillation more responsive to defibrillation, and (4) act as an inotropic agent.

Epinephrine is effective in achieving all these goals. Recent studies have extensively evaluated the hemodynamic effects of epinephrine during resuscitation and have clearly shown it to be the singularly most important drug for common use during CPR. Animal studies show that during conventional CPR, cerebral and myocardial perfusion pressures are low. Epinephrine increases brain and heart flow by two mechanisms: (1) It prevents carotid artery collapse and raises arterial pressure during both chest compression and the release phase of chest compression (i.e., "systole" and "diastole," respectively). This results in higher carotid arterial "systolic" and aortic "diastolic" pressures, which, in turn, are reflected in higher cerebral perfusion and myocardial perfusion pressures and flow. (2) It preferentially reduces blood flow to the external carotid, renal, and splanchnic beds, thereby redirecting flow toward the brain and heart.[52,53]

Arterial collapse at the thoracic inlet has been shown to be the critical limiting factor for cerebral perfusion pressure and flow during prolonged CPR. Arterial collapse results from high extravascular intrathoracic pressures, low intravascular volumes, and loss of arterial tone. Collapse results in a precipitous fall in carotid arterial and hence cerebral perfusion pressure. Epinephrine during CPR can not only reverse arterial collapse but also prevent it from developing. With the administration of epinephrine during conventional manual CPR in the dog, cerebral blood flow can be maintained at approximately 15 percent and myocardial flow at approximately 5 percent of prearrest values for 20 min.

These data strongly support the early and frequent use of epinephrine during CPR in an effort to optimize the perfusion of vital organs. Hence, once the diagnosis of cardiac arrest is established and CPR initiated, epinephrine should be administered as soon as possible. The recommended dose is 0.5 to 1 mg IV, and this dose should be repeated at approximately 3- to 5-min intervals unless effective cardiac activity is restored. Although promising in the animal model, large clinical trials failed to demonstrate improved survival with high-dose epinephrine.[54,55] Hence, most experts would use 1 mg IV uniformly. Higher doses may be used for the second and third dose (3 and 5 mg) if the initial dose, CPR, and defibrillation fail.[29] If an intravenous route is not available, epinephrine can be administered down the endotracheal tube; 10 mL of a 1:10,000 solution should be used, and this can also be repeated every 3 to 5 min.

The benefits of epinephrine are principally due to the alpha vasoconstriction induced by this agent. The inotropic effects of the drug may not be helpful, since these effects increase myocardial oxygen demand, even during ventricular fibrillation, when supply or blood flow is limited.[56] Consequently, there is some interest in using a pure vasoconstrictor during CPR rather than epinephrine. Animal studies of vital organ perfusion and human survival studies comparing epinephrine and phenylepinephrine (a pure alpha vasoconstrictor) have yielded similar results. With asystole, the chronotropic effects of epinephrine may be useful.

The recommended dose of epinephrine (1 mg IV every 3 to 5 min) is comparable to a 0.007 to 0.014 mg/kg dose in a 70-kg person. This dose has been questioned, since animal studies using higher doses of epinephrine have shown improved blood flow to vital organs and improved survival.[53] Other studies of higher doses of epinephrine, however, have shown increased myocardial oxygen demand despite this improved blood flow.[56] Higher than recommended doses of epinephrine have been reported to increase arterial pressure and coronary perfusion pressure in a small number of human studies. These studies spawned an intense interest in the use of higher doses of epinephrine during CPR. Results from several prospective randomized out-of-hospital clinical trials of more than 2400 adult cardiac arrest victims, however, have shown no statistically significant improvement in survival to hospital admission or discharge when higher doses of epinephrine (0.1 to 0.2 mg/kg) were compared with standard doses.[54,55] On the other hand, these trials did not demonstrate any obvious deleterious effect of the higher doses of epinephrine. Hence, higher-dose epinephrine should be considered a class IIB recommendation.

Norepinephrine is a potent vasoconstrictor and generally produces a rise in blood pressure; it is also an inotropic agent. Its disadvantage is renal and mesenteric vasoconstriction, and it should not be used in the initial phase of resuscitation. This agent is most useful where severe hypotension is present but where the chronotropic effects of epinephrine are not desirable (as in acute myocardial infarction or severe ischemia). This agent should be administered cautiously, since severe tissue injury results from extravasation around an intravenous site. A large prehospital trial failed to identify any differences in survival following treatments with norepinephrine, high-dose epinephrine, or standard epinephrine.[54]

Similarly, dopamine (a chemical precursor of norepinephrine) and dobutamine (a synthetic catecholamine) are preferred for use as inotropic agents because of their lesser chronotropic effect. Recent animal data suggests that dobutamine may be particularly effective in reducing postresuscitation left ventricular dysfunction. Isoproterenol (a synthetic catecholamine) is a pure adrenergic agonist and effective vasodilator. Therefore, its use during CPR is contraindicated since it can significantly decrease vital organ perfusion pressures. In patients with a palpable pulse, however, it is useful for treatment of bradycardia due to heart block or asystole until a temporary pacemaker is placed (see also Chap. 34).

Sodium Bicarbonate

The recent AHA recommendations deemphasize the role of sodium bicarbonate and suggest that much less sodium bicar-

bonate should be used than previously advocated for acid-base control during cardiac arrest. As with other types of metabolic acidosis, if adequate alveolar ventilation is achieved, the metabolic acidosis of arrest is partially corrected through P_{CO_2} excretion.[45] Recent clinical trials failed to demonstrate improved outcome from cardiac arrest with buffer therapy.[57] Rather, several deleterious effects of bicarbonate administration including metabolic acidosis, hypernatremia, and hyperosmolality have been reported. Ideally, sodium bicarbonate should be given according to the results of measurement of arterial blood pH, P_{CO_2} determination, and calculation of the base deficit. Bicarbonate should be used, if at all, only after more established interventions such as defibrillation, ventilation with endotracheal intubation, and pharmacologic therapies (epinephrine and antiarrhythmic drugs) have been tried.[29] If needed, 1 meq/kg of sodium bicarbonate should be administered; then no more than half this dose may be repeated every 15 min. Excessive use of sodium bicarbonate can result in metabolic alkalosis, hypernatremia, and hyperosmolality. On the other hand, bicarbonate may be most useful during the immediate postresuscitation period, when a profound metabolic acidosis occurs. In most instances during CPR, its use should be considered as a class IIB recommendation.[30]

Calcium chloride (5 to 7 mg/kg) enhances the contractile state of the heart and is indicated in treating severe hypotension due to an overdose of calcium channel blocker or hyperkalemia. It is no longer recommended for use in asystole or electromechanical dissociation.[29,51]

TERMINATION OF CARDIOPULMONARY RESUSCITATION

Despite resuscitative efforts, the patient in cardiac arrest may not regain spontaneous circulation. The decision to end (or even initiate) CPR should be based on a physician's assessment of the patient's prior advance directives (if known) and the cerebral, cardiovascular, and general status of the patient.[58,59] Failure is likely if there is absence of organized ventricular ECG activity and/or peripheral perfusion after 10 to 15 min of adequate CPR and appropriate therapy. Recent studies have demonstrated that continued in-hospital CPR efforts (in patients failing prehospital advanced cardiac life support) are not only expensive but also unsuccessful.[66] Persistent deep unconsciousness and absence of respiration, reflex response, or pupillary reaction suggest cerebral death, and resuscitative efforts are usually unproductive. These guidelines, however, should be altered in patients with hypothermia, barbiturate overdose, and perhaps following electrocution, where recovery has been seen even after hours of resuscitation.[60]

POSTARREST CARE

Patients who have been successfully resuscitated usually require monitoring in an intensive care setting. These patients are prone to develop cardiac arrhythmias, hemodynamic and ventilatory instability, and ischemic encephalopathy. Ventilatory support with a respirator may well be necessary initially. Serial arterial blood-gas determinations should be made to identify hypoxemia and assess the rapidly changing acid-base status.

Several therapeutic strategies have been employed in animal models to help reduce hypoxic encephalopathy after cardiac arrest. None (including emergency cardiopulmonary bypass, which is currently undergoing clinical testing) have clearly been shown to be beneficial in humans. The treatment of encephalopathy after cardiac arrest involves the prevention of further hypoxia and hypotension. For cerebral edema after cardiac arrest, methylprednisolone (60 to 100 mg) or dexamethasone sodium phosphate (12 to 20 mg IV every 6 h) has been recommended, but there is no conclusive evidence that these agents are beneficial. High-dose barbiturates or lidoflazine have also been shown to reduce postarrest brain injury in animal studies; the value of this therapy in human beings is negligible. The prognosis of the patient with anoxic encephalopathy is related to the depth and continued duration of cerebral dysfunction (see also Chap. 99). Failure to exhibit neurologic improvement 72 h following resuscitation is usually an ominous sign. Clinical and laboratory evaluations (electroencephalography, sensory evoked potentials) are often employed to help define prognosis and thus guide further care in such individuals.

Other potential life-threatening problems in the postarrest period include acute renal failure, bowel infarction, infection, adult respiratory distress syndrome, and sepsis. Patients regaining consciousness may have postarrest amnesia or may develop psychotic behavior.

OUTCOME OF RESUSCITATION

In their initial study, Kouwenhoven and colleagues reported a 24 percent successful resuscitation and discharge rate from the hospital. Recent studies have shown that with a paramedical response system, a near 40 percent successful out-of-hospital resuscitation rate can be achieved.[30,61] Many of these patients die in hospital, however, with the dominant cause of death being anoxic encephalopathy. Recent data suggest that somatosensory evoked potentials may be useful and highly predictive in identifying patients who are likely to have irreversible brain injury.[62] The critical factors for successful out-of-hospital resuscitation include approximately 7 min total duration of CPR, approximately 4 min from collapse to the initiation of CPR, and approximately 10 min to successful delivery of first countershock. It is important to point out, however, that the quality of life for patients surviving to hospital discharge is often quite good, with most discharged patients being able to return to gainful employment.

CHAIN OF SURVIVAL

The concept of a "chain of survival" has been adopted by several agencies and underscores the importance of an inte-

grated public education and health care system if outcome from prehospital cardiac arrest is to be optimized.[29] Early access (to EMS systems), early CPR (to include bystander CPR), early defibrillation (to include the use of AEDs), and early advanced cardiac life support (ACLS) care are the major "links" in the chain, and any one "weak" link weakens the whole "chain of survival."

This is best exemplified in two recent publications that reported on prehospital cardiac arrest outcomes in New York and Chicago, where survival rates were only 1 to 2 percent. Despite a mature EMS system and considerable public training in CPR, delayed defibrillation—due to traffic, elevators, and other factors—contributed significantly to the poor outcome in these studies.[63,64] Other cities, where prompt defibrillation has been possible, have reported a 20 to 30 percent survival rate.[65] To overcome this tragic limitation, AEDs were developed and have been shown to facilitate prompt defibrillation and thereby improve survival. Hence, the American Heart Association/American College of Cardiology have jointly recommended that all professional first-responder units (especially in rural areas where long transport times are common) be equipped with AEDs. The safety and usefulness of this lifesaving technology in the hands of non-traditional first responders has been recently tested. Qantas Airlines cabin crews were AED-equipped and have successfully resuscitated victims in midair. Extending the concept of training the nontraditional but often first responder, the City of Rochester police force was trained in the use of AEDs. All police cars were AED equipped, and the appropriate and prompt use of defibrillation dramatically reduced mortality.[31] Cheaper, self instructing AEDs have been developed. The American Heart Association is pioneering the "public access defibrillation" program to examine the feasibility of such devices being used by trained "lay first responders" and possibly also in the homes of high risk patients or in public areas.

If mortality from out-of-hospital arrest is to be reduced, public education programs to increase awareness of the warning signs of a heart attack and teach CPR are critical. Such programs are presently being tested. Despite similar efforts by other training agencies, however, the incidence of bystander CPR nationwide remains low.[63,64] This may have several explanations, including a lack of training in high-risk populations, poor performance or lack of retention despite training, unnecessarily complex training programs, or a fear of communicable disease during mouth-to-mouth resuscitation. This last issue has become particularly significant in the 1990s. Individuals should be reassured that the likelihood of disease transmission is minimal, 70 percent of arrest victims collapse at home, and if an individual is still unwilling to do mouth-to-mouth CPR, he or she should be taught to at least activate EMS ("call") and start chest compressions ("pump"). Ventilation ("blow") could then be started by suitably equipped trained EMS rescuers. Present data indicate that a refocusing of basic life support (BLS) training programs is essential, with efforts being targeted at simplification of training, with specific education and training penetration into high-risk patient groups (older patients and minority groups). The CPR message must be kept simple (for example, "call-pump-blow"). These goals must be achieved if the first two links in the chain of survival (early access and early CPR) are to be strengthened. Universal 911 would facilitate early and easy access and should be encouraged in all communities. Minimal standards of performance and excellence for EMS systems should be established and monitored. Dispatcher-assisted CPR teaches CPR on the telephone to the person who is calling to report the arrest (while professional help is in transit) and has been shown to be effective. The Seattle–King County EMS system is proof that such efforts directly improve outcome.[65] On the other hand, the Chicago–New York experience is a chilling reminder of the consequence of one weak link in the chain of survival. The outcome from prehospital arrest can be improved only if each community strives to optimize its own chain of survival.

REFERENCES

1. Comroe JH. Retrospectroscope: In comes the good air. *Am Rev Respir Dis* 1979; 119:803–809.
2. Elam JO, Brown ES, Elder JD. Artificial respiration by mouth-to-mask method. *N Engl J Med* 1954; 250:749–754.
3. Sanders AB, Kern KB, Ewy GA. Open chest massage for resuscitation from cardiac arrest. *Resuscitation* 1988; 16:153–154.
4. Eldor J, Frankel DZN, Davidson JT. Open chest cardiac massage: A review. *Resuscitation* 1988; 16:155–162.
5. Wiggers CJ. The physiologic basis for cardiac resuscitation from ventricular fibrillation method of serial defibrillation. *Am Heart J* 1940; 20:413–422.
6. Kouwenhoven WB, Jude JR, Knickerbocker GG. Closed chest cardiac massage. *JAMA* 1960; 173:1064–1067.
7. Jude JR, Kouwenhoven WB, Knickerbocker GG. Cardiac arrest: Report of application of external cardiac massage on 118 patients. *JAMA* 1961; 178:1063–1071.
8. Weale FE, Rothwell-Jackson RL. The efficiency of cardiac massage. *Lancet* 1962; 1:990–992.
9. MacKenzie GJ, Taylor SH, McDonald AH, Donald KW. Hemodynamic effects of external cardiac compression. *Lancet* 1964; 1:1342–1345.
10. Criley JM, Blaufuss AN, Kissel GL. Cough-induced cardiac compression. *JAMA* 1976; 236:1246–1250.
11. Rudikoff MT, Maughan WL, Effron M, Freund P, Weisfeldt ML. Mechanisms of flow during cardiopulmonary resuscitation. *Circulation* 1980; 61:345–351.
12. Halperin H, Brower R, Weisfeldt ML, Tsitlik J, Chandra N, Cristiano L, et al. Air trapping in the lungs during cardiopulmonary resuscitation in dogs: A mechanism for generating changes in intrathoracic pressure. *Circ Res* 1989; 65:946–954.
13. Maier GW, Tyson GS, Olsen CO, Kerstein KH, Davis JW, Conn EH, et al. The physiology of external cardiac massage: High impulse cardiopulmonary resuscitation. *Circulation* 1984; 70:86–101.
14. Feneley MP, Maier GW, Gaynor JW, Gall SA, Kisslo JA, Davis JW, et al. Sequence of mitral valve motion and transmitral blood flow during manual cardiopulmonary resuscitation in dogs. *Circulation* 1987; 76:363–375.
15. Deshmukh HG, Weil MH, Gudipati CV, Trevino RP, Bisera J, Rackow EC. Mechanism of blood flow generated by precordial compression during CPR:I. Studies on closed chest precordial compression. *Chest* 1989; 95:1092–1099.
16. Werner JA, Greene HL, Janko CL, Cobb LA. Visualization of cardiac valve motion in man during external chest compression using two-dimensional echocardiography: Implications regarding the mechanism of blood flow. *Circulation* 1981; 63:1417–1421.
17. Halperin HR, Weiss JL, Guerci AD, Chandra N, Tsitlik JE, Brower R, et al. Cyclic elevation of intrathoracic pressure can close the mitral valve during cardiac arrest in dogs. *Circulation* 1988; 78:754–760.

18. Koehler RC, Chandra N, Guerci AD, Tsitlik J, Traytsman RJ, Rogers MC, et al. Augmentation of cerebral perfusion by simultaneous chest compression and lung inflation with abdominal binding following cardiac arrest in dogs. *Circulation* 1983; 67:266–275.
19. Halperin HR, Guerci AD, Chandra N, Herskowitz A, Tsitlik JE, Niskanen RA, et al. Vest inflation without simultaneous ventilation during cardiac arrest in dogs: Improved survival from prolonged cardiopulmonary resuscitation. *Circulation* 1986; 74:1407–1415.
20. Halperin HR, Tsitlik JE, Gelfand N, Weisfeldt ML, Gruben KG, Levin HR, et al. A preliminary study of cardiopulmonary resuscitation with circumferential compression of the chest with use of a pneumatic vest. *N Engl J Med* 1993; 329:762–768.
21. Cohen TJ, Tucker KJ, Lurie KG, Redberg RF, Dutton JP, Dwyer KA, et al. Active compression-decompression resuscitation: A new method of cardiopulmonary resuscitation. *JAMA* 1992; 267:2916–2923.
22. Stiell IG, Hébert PC, Wells GA, Laupacis A, Vandemheen K, Dreyer JF, et al. The Ontario trial of active compression-decompression cardiopulmonary resuscitation for in-hospital and prehospital cardiac arrest. *JAMA* 1996; 275:1417–1423.
23. Sack J, Kesselbrenner M, Bergman D. Survival from in-hospital arrest with interposed abdominal counterpulsation during cardiopulmonary resuscitation. *JAMA* 1992; 276:379–385.
24. Halperin HR, Tsitlik JE, Guerci AD, Levin HR, Shi AY, Chandra N, et al. Determinants of blood flow to vital organs during cardiopulmonary resuscitation in dogs. *Circulation* 1986; 73:539–551.
25. Standards and guidelines for cardiopulmonary resuscitation (CPR) and emergency cardiac care (ECC). *JAMA* 1986; 255:2905–2989.
26. Swenson RD, Weaver WD, Nisaken RA, Martin J, Dahlberg S. Hemodynamics in humans during conventional and experimental methods of cardiopulmonary resuscitation. *Circulation* 1988; 78:630–639.
27. Chandra NC, Tsitlik JE, Halperin HR, Guerci AD, Weisfeldt ML. Observations of hemodynamics during cardiopulmonary resuscitation. *Crit Care Med* 1990; 18:929–934.
28. Paradis N, Martin G, Goetting M, Rosenberg J, Rivers E, Appleton T, et al. Simultaneous aortic, jugular bulb, and right atrial pressures during cardiopulmonary resuscitation in humans: Insights into mechanisms. *Circulation* 1989; 80:361–368.
29. Emergency Cardiac Care Committee and Subcommittees, American Heart Association: Guidelines for cardiopulmonary resuscitation and emergency cardiac care. *JAMA* 1992; 268:2171–2302.
30. Eisenberg MS, Horwood BT, Cummins RO, et al. Cardiac arrest after resuscitation: A tale of 29 cities. *Ann Emerg Med* 1990; 19:179–186.
31. White RD, Asplin BR, Bugliosi TF, Hankins DG. High release survival from out-of-hospital ventricular fibrillation with rapid defibrillation by both police and paramedics. *Acad Emerg Med* 1996; 3.422.
32. Weaver WD, Hill D, Fahrenbruch CE, Copass MK, Martin JS, Cobb LA, et al. Use of the automatic external defibrillation in the management of out-of-hospital cardiac arrest. *N Engl J Med* 1988; 319:661–666.
33. Heimlich HJ. A life saving maneuver to prevent from choking. *JAMA* 1975; 234:398–401.
34. Visintine RE, Baick CH. Ruptured stomach after Heimlich maneuver. *JAMA* 1975; 234:415.
35. Greene DG, Elam JO, Dobkin AB, Studley CL. Cine-fluorographic study of hypertension of the neck and upper airway patency. *JAMA* 1961; 176:570–573.
36. Pepe PE, Zacharich BS, Chandra NC. Update on invasive airway techniques in resuscitation. *Ann Emerg Med* 1993; 22:393–403.
37. Chandra NC, Gruben KG, Tsitlik JE, Brower R, Guerci AD, Halperin HR, et al. Observations of ventilation during resuscitation of a canine model. *Circulation* 1994; 90:3070–3075.
38. Locke CJ, Berg RA, Sanders AB, Davis MF, Milander MM, Kern KB, et al. Bystander cardiopulmonary resuscitation: Concerns about mouth to mouth contact. *Arch Intern Med* 1995; 155:938–943.
39. Sirna SJ, Fergusson DW, Charbonnier F, Kerber RE. Electrical cardioversion in humans: Factors affecting transthoracic impedance. *Am J Cardiol* 1988; 62:1048–1052.
40. Adgey AAJ, Patton JN, Campbell NPS, Webb SW. Ventricular defibrillation: Appropriate energy levels. *Circulation* 1979; 60:219–223.
41. Gascho JA, Crampton RS, Cherwek ML, Sipes JM, Hunter FP, O'Brien WM. Determinants of ventricular defibrillation in adults. *Circulation* 1979; 60:231–240.
42. Tacker WA, Ewy GA. Emergency defibrillation dose, recommendation and rationale. *Circulation* 1979; 60:223–225.

43. Weaver WD, Cobb LA, Copass MK, Hallstrom AP. Ventricular defibrillation: A comparative trial using 175-J and 320-J shocks. *N Engl J Med* 1982; 307:1101–1106.

44. Lerman BB, DiMarco JP, Haines D. Current-based versus energy-based ventricular defibrillation: A prospective study. *J Am Coll Cardiol* 1988; 12:1259–1264.

45. Bishop RL, Weisfeldt ML. Sodium bicarbonate administration during cardiac arrest: Effect of arterial pH, P_{CO_2} and osmolality. *JAMA* 1976; 235:506–509.

46. Brown CG, Dzwoncyk R, Martin DR. Physiologic measurement of the ventricular fibrillation ECG signal: Estimating the duration of ventricular fibrillation. *Circulation* 1993; 22:70–74.

47. Kowey PR, Levine JH, Herre JM, Pacifico A, Lindsay BD, Plumb VJ, et al. Randomized, double-blind comparison of intravenous amiodarone and bretylium in the treatment of patients with recurrent, hemodynamically destabilizing ventricular tachycardia and fibrillation. *Circulation* 1995; 92:3255–3263.

48. Haynes RE, Copass MK, Chinn TL, Cobb LA. Comparison of bretylium tosylate and lidocaine in management of out-of-hospital ventricular fibrillation: A randomized clinical trial. *Am J Cardiol* 1981; 48:353–356.

49. Wei JY, Greene HL, Weisfeldt ML. Cough-facilitated conversion of ventricular tachycardia. *Am J Cardiol* 1980; 45:174–176.

50. Cummins RO, Grave JR, Larsen MP, Hallstrom AP, Hearne TR, Cilerti J, et al. Out-of-hospital transcutaneous pacing by emergency medical technicians in patients with asystolic cardiac arrest. *N Engl J Med* 1993; 328:1377–1382.

51. Stueven HA, Thompson BM, Aprahamian C, Tonsfeldt DJ. Calcium chloride: Reassessment of use in asystole. *Ann Emerg Med* 1984; 13:820–822.

52. Michael JR, Guerci AD, Koehler RC, Shi AY, Tsitlik J, Chandra N, et al. Mechanisms by which epinephrine augments cerebral and myocardial perfusion during cardiopulmonary resuscitation in dogs. *Circulation* 1984; 69:822–835.

53. Brown CG, Wermn HA, Davis EA, Hobson J, Hamlin RL. The effects of graded doses of epinephrine on regional myocardial blood flow during cardiopulmonary resuscitation in swine. *Circulation* 1987; 75:491–497.

54. Callaham M, Madsen CD, Barton CW, Saunders CE, Pointer J. A randomized clinical trial of high-dose epinephrine and norepinephrine vs standard dose epinephrine in prehospital cardiac arrest. *JAMA* 1992; 268:2667–2672.

55. Brown CG, Martin DR, Pepe PE, Steuven H, Cummins RO, Gonzalez E, et al. A comparison of standard-dose and high-dose epinephrine in cardiac arrest outside the hospital. *N Engl J Med* 1992; 327:1051–1055.

56. Ditchey RV, Lindenfeld J. Failure of epinephrine to improve the balance between myocardial oxygen supply and demand during closed chest resuscitation in dogs. *Circulation* 1988; 78:382–389.

57. Dybvik T, Strand T, Steen PA. Buffer therapy during out-of-hospital cardiopulmonary resuscitation. *Resuscitation* 1995; 29:89–95.

58. Luce JM, Raffin TA. Withholding and withdrawal of life support from critically ill patients. *Chest* 1988; 94:621–626.

59. Niemann JT. Cardiopulmonary resuscitation. *N Engl J Med* 1992; 327:1075–1080.

60. Ravitch MM, Lane R, Safar P, Steichen FM, Knowles P. Lightning stroke: Report of a case with recovery after cardiac massage and prolonged artificial respiration. *N Engl J Med* 1961; 264:36–38.

61. Eisenberg MS, Hallstrom A, Bergner L. Long-term survival after out-of-hospital cardiac arrest. *N Engl J Med* 1982; 306:1340–1343.

62. Berek K, Lechleitner P, Luef G, Felber S, Saltuari L, Schinnerl A, et al. Early determination of neurological outcome after prehospital cardiopulmonary resuscitation. *Stroke* 1995; 26:543–549.

63. Lombardi G, Gallagher J, Gennis P. Outcome of out-of-hospital cardiac arrest in New York City: The pre-hospital arrest survival evaluation (PHASE) study. *JAMA* 1994; 271:678–683.

64. Becker LB, Ostrander MP, Barrett J, Kondos GT. Outcome of CPR in a large metropolitan area—Where are the survivors? *Ann Emerg Med* 1991; 20:355–361.

65. Cummins RO. From concept to standard-of-care? Review of the clinical experience with automated external defibrillators. *Ann Emerg Med* 1989; 12:1269–1275.

66. Gray WA, Capone RJ, Most AS: Unsuccessful emergency medical resuscitation—Are continued efforts in the emergency department justified? *N Engl J Med* 1991; 325:1393–1398.

COLOR PLATES*

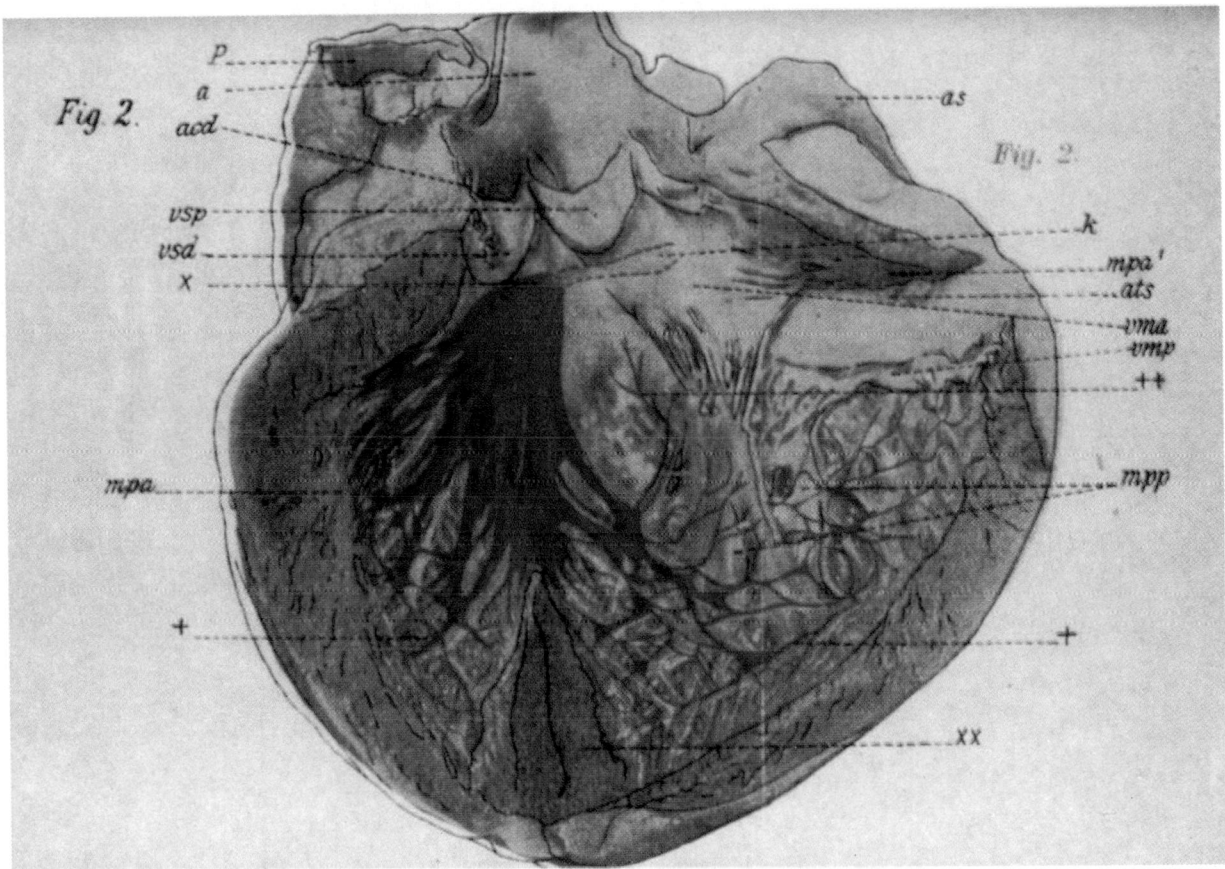

Plate 1 (Fig. 2-77) This diagram is taken from the monograph of Tawara (1906), which established and elucidated the significance of the atrioventricular conducton axis. It shows the fanlike arrangement of the left bundle branch. The clinical value of the so-called concept of hemiblocks should not be extended to presume that the left bundle branch is arranged anatomically in bifascicular fashion. As shown here, it is arranged as a fan, and if it divides at all, it forms three rather than two divisions. [From Tawara (see Ref. 143 in Chap. 2). Figure provided from Anderson RH, Wilcox BR, Becker AE: Anatomy of the normal heart. In: Hurst JW, editor in chief. *Atlas of the Heart.* New York, Gower Medical Publishing, 1988, p. 1.115. Used with permission from the publisher.]

---

* The figures in each Plate have been double-numbered in order to indicate the chapter in which they are cited and the order of their citation therein.

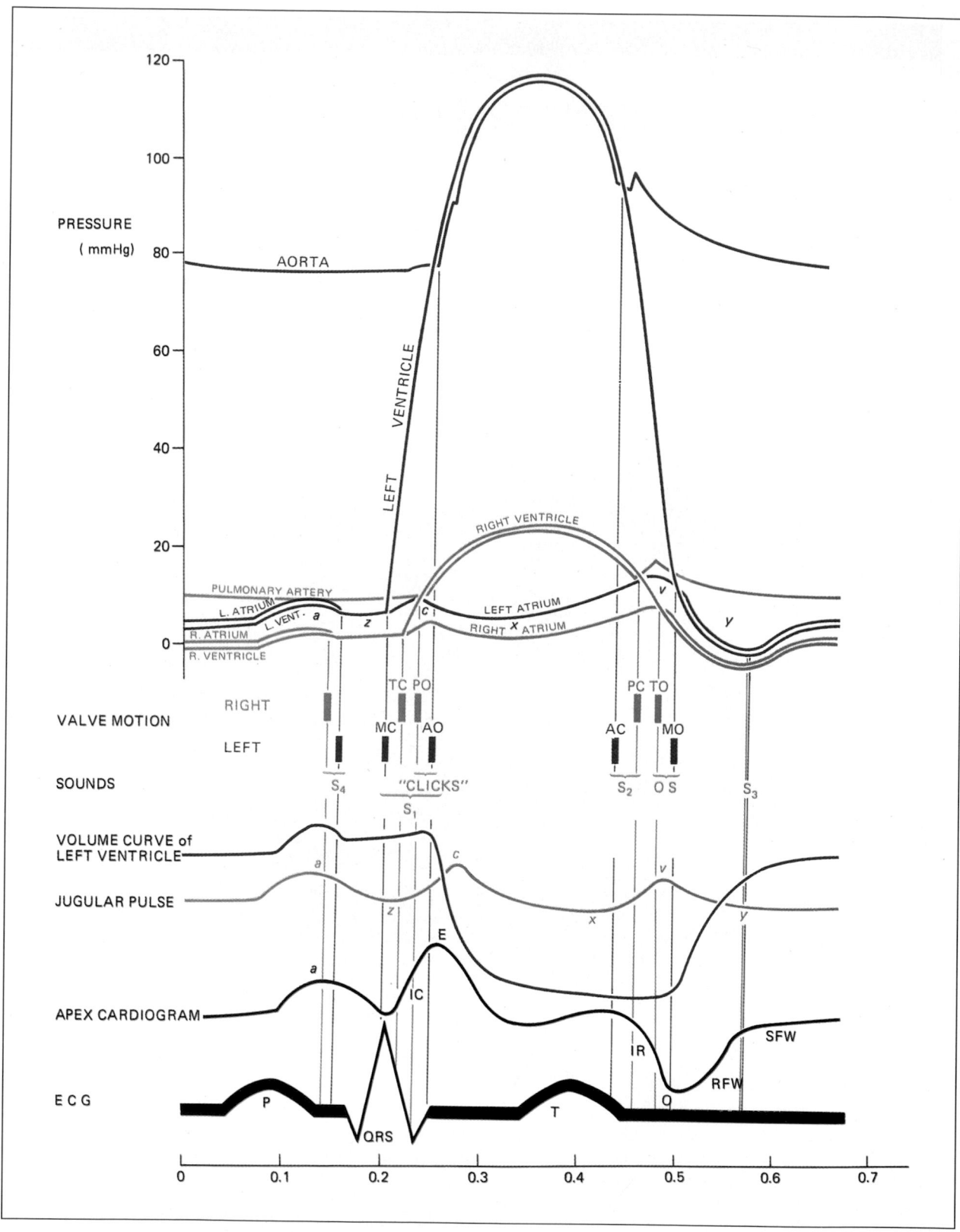

Plate 2 (Fig. 3-31) Diagram of the cardiac cycle, showing the pressure curves of the great vessels and cardiac chambers, valvular events and heart sounds, left ventricular volume curve, jugular pulse wave, apex cardiogram (Sanborn piezo crystal), and the electrocardiogram. For illustrative purposes, the time intervals between the valvular events have been modified and the z point has been prolonged. Valve motion: MC = mitral component of the first heart sound; MO = mitral valve opening; TC = tricuspid component of the first heart sound; TO = tricuspid valve opening; AC = aortic component of the second heart sound; AO = aortic valve opening; PC = pulmonic valve component of the second heart sound; PO = pulmonic valve opening; OS = opening snap of atrioventricular valves. Apex cardiogram: IC = isovolumic or isovolumetric (isochoric) contraction wave; IR = isovolumic or isovolumetric (isochoric) relaxation wave; O = opening of mitral valve; RFW = rapid-filling wave; SFW = slow-filling wave.

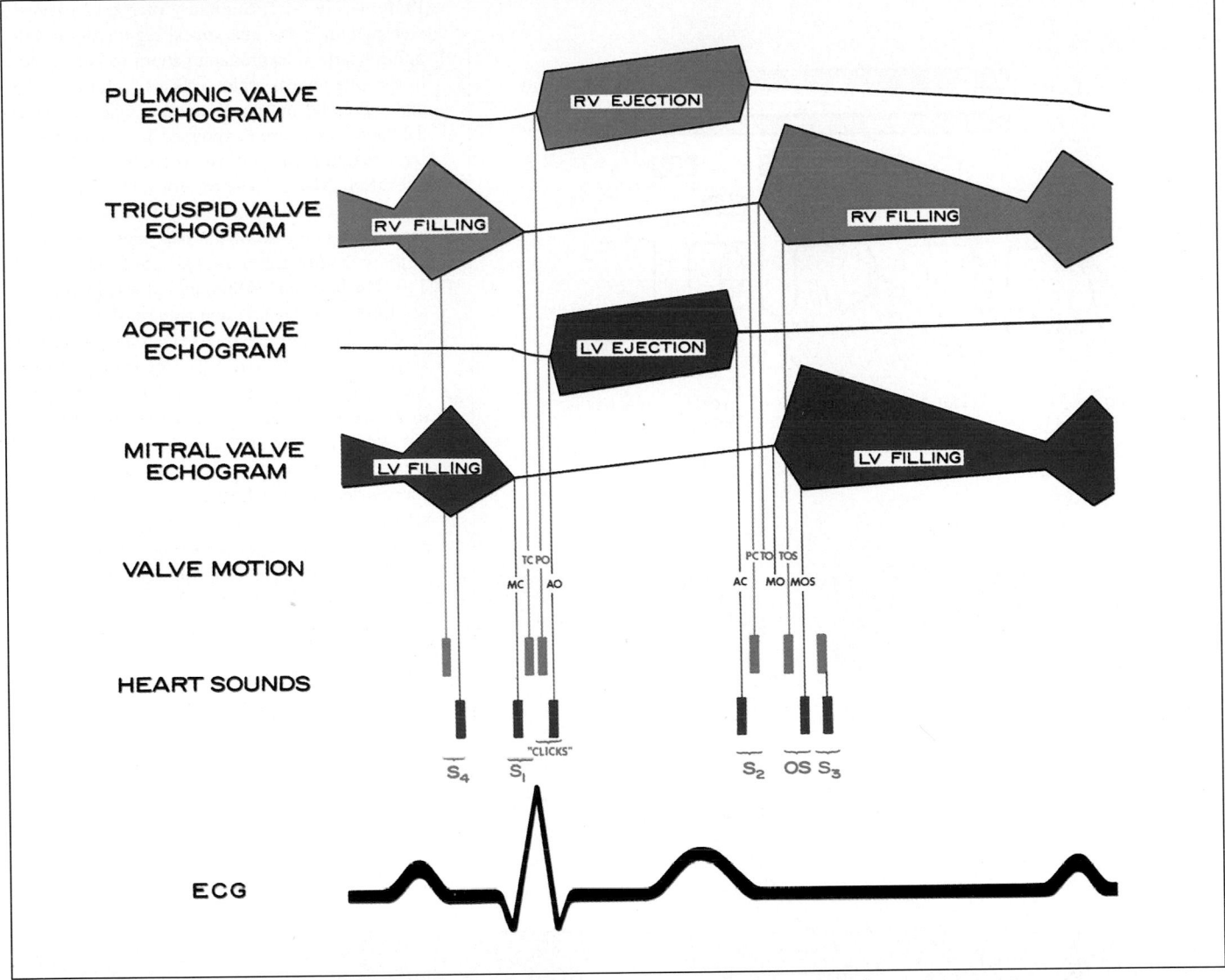

Plate 3 (Fig. 3-32) Schematic presentation of the relationships between electrical and mechanical events and heart sounds during the cardiac cycle. The sequences of ejection from, and of filling of, the right ventricle are indicated by the schematic echograms of the pulmonic valve and the tricuspid valve. The corresponding phases of the left ventricle are indicated by the schematic echograms of the aortic valve and the mitral valve. The isovolumic contraction phase for each ventricle occurs in the short phase between the end of filling and the onset of ejection, whereas isovolumic filling occurs in the brief phase between the end of ejection and the onset of filling.

The right atrium starts contracting before the left atrium; on the other hand, the left ventricle starts contracting prior to the contraction of the right ventricle. Because of the relatively higher pressure in the aorta than in the pulmonary artery, the phases of isovolumic contraction and isovolumic relaxation of the left ventricle are much longer than for the right ventricle. As a result, although left ventricular contraction begins first, right ventricular ejection begins prior to left ventricular ejection and also ends after that of left ventricular ejection. Thus, the phase of active ejection for the right ventricle is longer than that of the left ventricle. On the other hand, the total duration of systole, including isovolumic contraction and relaxation, is normally longer for the left ventricle.

The normal sequence of the heart sounds and valve motion is schematically depicted: MC = the mitral component of the first heart sound (S_1); TC = the tricuspid component of the first sound (S_1); PO = pulmonic valve opening; AO = aortic valve opening; AC = aortic component of the second heart sound (S_2); PC = pulmonic component of the second heart sound (S_2); TO = tricuspid valve opening; TOS = tricuspid opening snap; and MOS = mitral valve opening snap. Normally, the sound produced by the opening of the cardiac valves is not audible; however, in disease states the opening of the mitral or tricuspid valve may produce an "opening snap," which usually occurs about the moment when the respective valve leaflets just reach maximal opening. Similarly, very vigorous tensing and opening of the aortic and pulmonic valves can produce ejection or opening "clicks" or sounds analogous to the opening snaps of the AV valves. An aortic and pulmonic valve opening click or sound may occur anywhere between the onset of valve opening, as illustrated, and the point of maximal opening of the respective valve, where it more commonly occurs. The sound occurring at the end of the rapid-filling phase of the ventricle is referred to as a *third heart sound* (S_3), *ventricular filling sound,* or *ventricular gallop.* The sound that occurs during or shortly after the P wave on the electrocardiogram and that is associated with an atrial contribution to ventricular filling is referred to as the *fourth heart sound* (S_4). Both third (S_3) and fourth (S_4) heart sounds may originate from either ventricle. The motion of the valve leaflets is depicted schematically in the valve echograms; for illustrative purposes, not all time intervals are depicted proportionately.

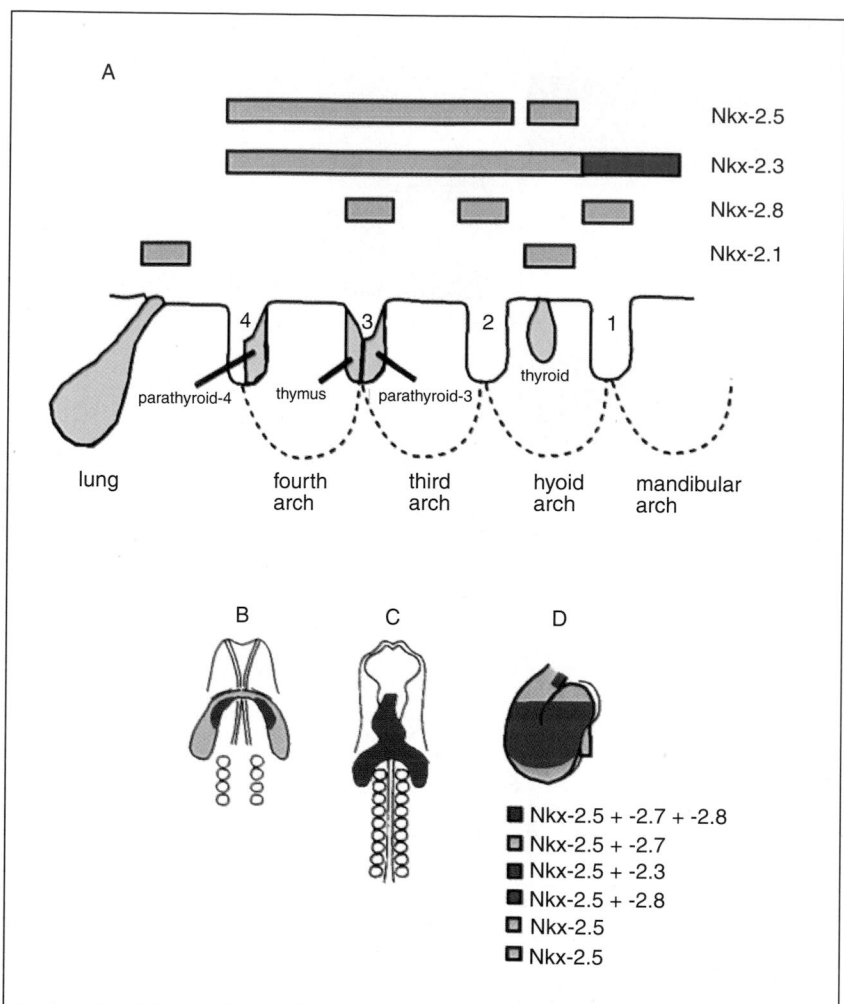

Plate 4 (Fig.7-22) Summary of Nkx-2 expression pattern in the pharyngeal region and developing heart. *A.* Expression pattern of Nkx genes in the pharyngeal region. Nkx-2.3 and Nkx-2.5 are expressed in broad patterns, whereas Nkx-2.1 and Nkx-2.8 are expressed in a more localized manner. In contrast to chicken Nkx-2.3, zebrafish Nkx-2.3 expression extended more anteriorly, which is indicated by the deep purple box. Only one side of the pharyngeal region is depicted, with the branchial clefts numbered 1–4. The branchial arches are indicated with dotted lines. *B–D.* Expression pattern of Nkx genes in the developing heart. *B.* HH stage 7. *C.* HH stage 10. *D.* Late stage. The genes that correspond to a given color are indicated at the base of *D.* Zebrafish Nkx-2.7 expression pattern is not known at late stages of development. Early Nkx-2.3 expression is not indicated because of species-species variation. References for expression domains are as follows: mouse Nkx-2.1[120]; *Xenopus,* chicken, and zebrafish Nkx-2.3[121–123]; mouse, chicken, *Xenopus,* and zebrafish Nkx-2.5[87, 90, 91, 123]; zebrafish Nkx-2.7.[123]

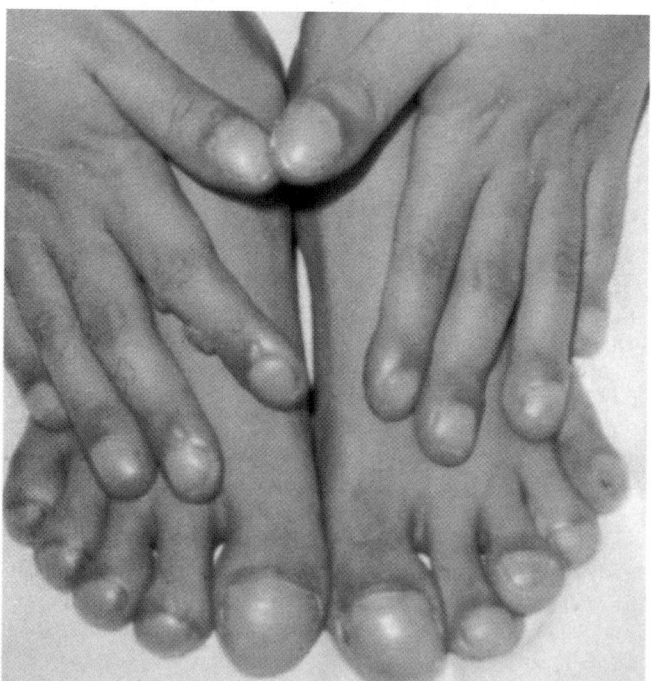

Plate 5 (Fig. 10-12) Symmetric cyanosis. Equal cyanosis and clubbing of hands and feet due to transposition of great vessels and a ventricular septal defect *without* patent ductus arteriosus.

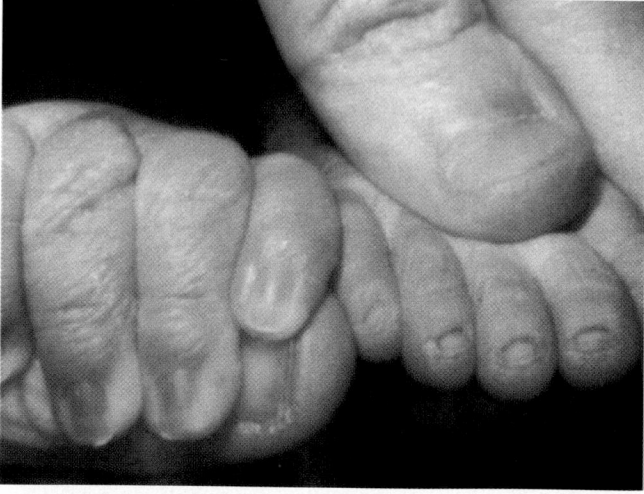

Plate 6 (Fig. 10-13) Differential cyanosis. Cyanosis of fingers (*left*) greater than that of toes due to transposition of great vessels *with* patent ductus arteriosus.

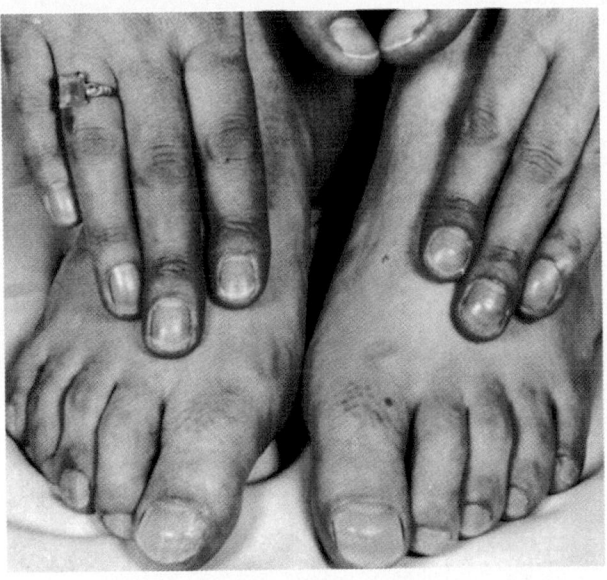

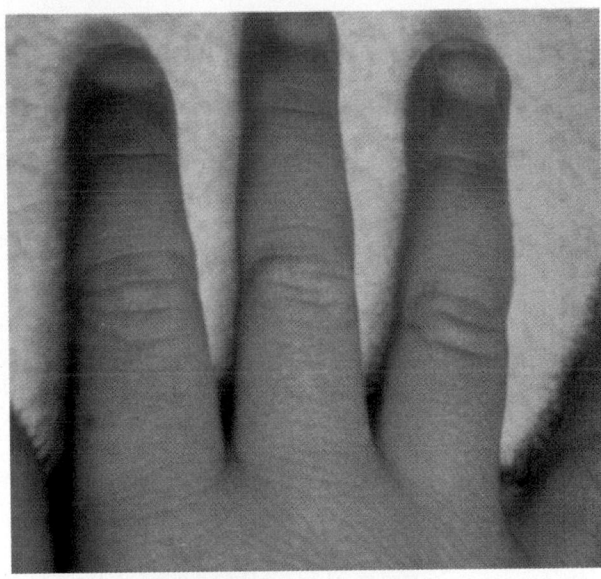

Plate 7 (Fig. 10-14) Differential cyanosis. Clubbing of left hand (compare thumbs) and cyanosis of left hand and all toes due to patent ductus arteriosus with pulmonary hypertension and normally related great vessels. (Courtesy of Dr. Joseph K. Perloff, University of California, Los Angeles.)

Plate 8 (Fig. 10-15) Tuft erythema. Erythema of fingertips due to small right-to-left shunt from AV canal defect.

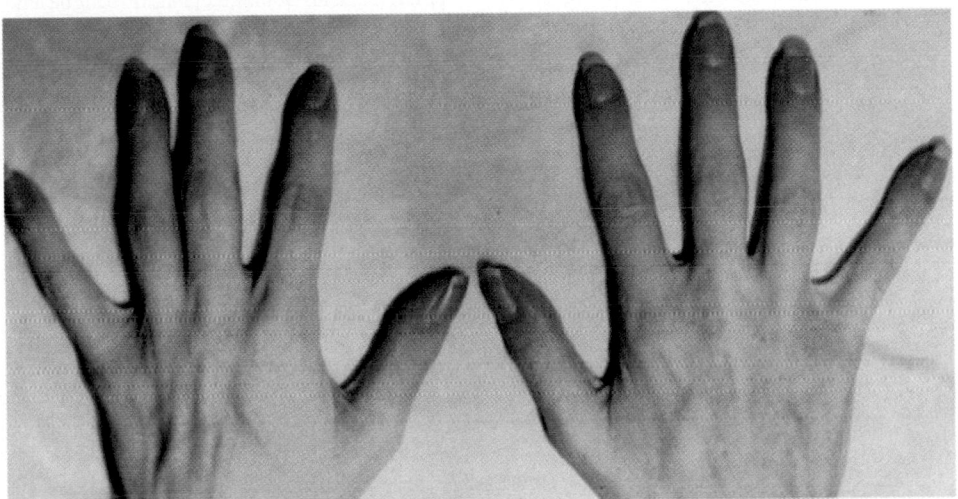

Plate 9 (Fig. 10-16) Clubbing due to bacterial endocarditis.

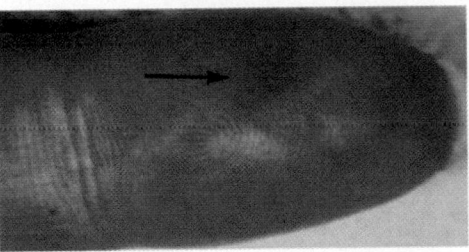

Plate 10 (Fig. 10-18) Osler's node (*arrow*).

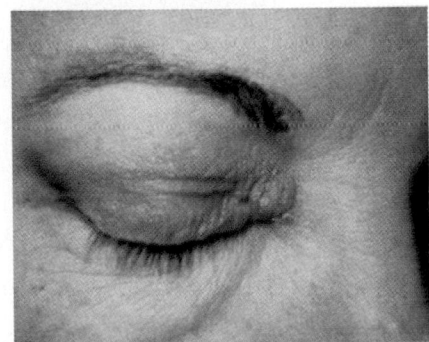

Plate 11 (Fig. 10-30) Dermatomyositis. A violaceous hue and edema of upper eyelid may be associated with myocardial disease.

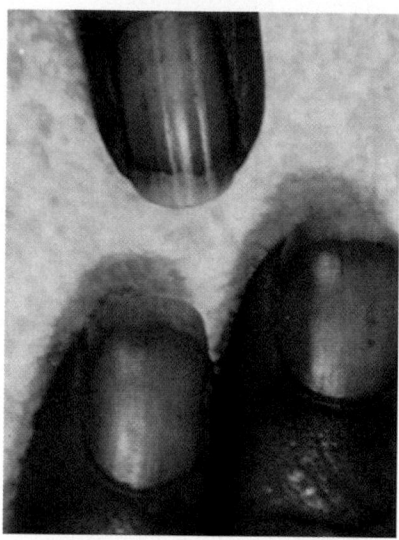

Plate 12 (Fig. 10-35) Hereditary hemorrhagic telangiectasia. Telangiectasia under nails. (From Silverman ME, Hurst JW. The hand and the heart. *AM J Cardiol* 1968; 22:609. With permission from the publisher.)

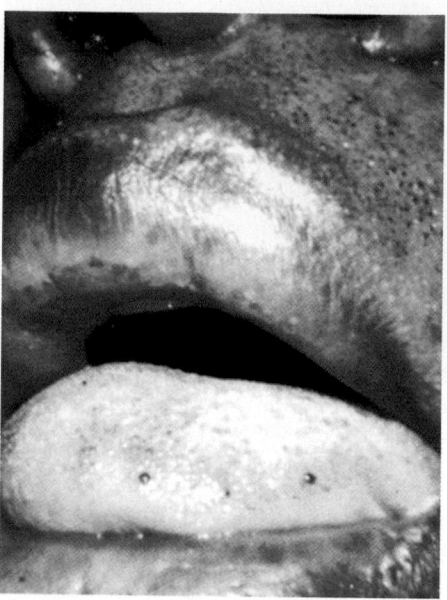

Plate 13 (Fig. 10-36) Hereditary hemorrhagic telangiectasia. Telangiectasia of tongue and lips may be associated with a pulmonary arteriovenous fistula.

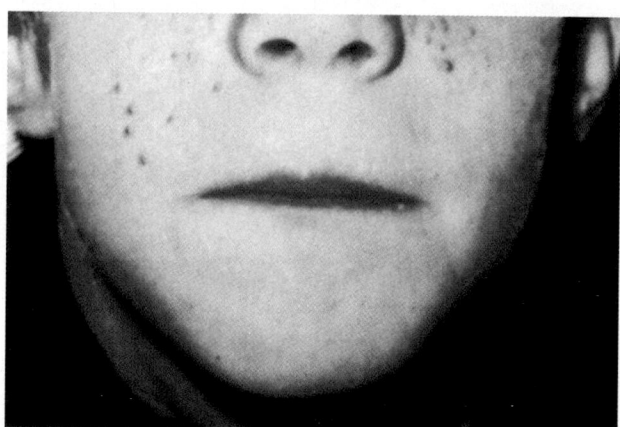

Plate 14 (Fig. 10-37) Tuberous sclerosis. Adenoma sebaceum may be associated with rhabdomyomas of the myocardium.

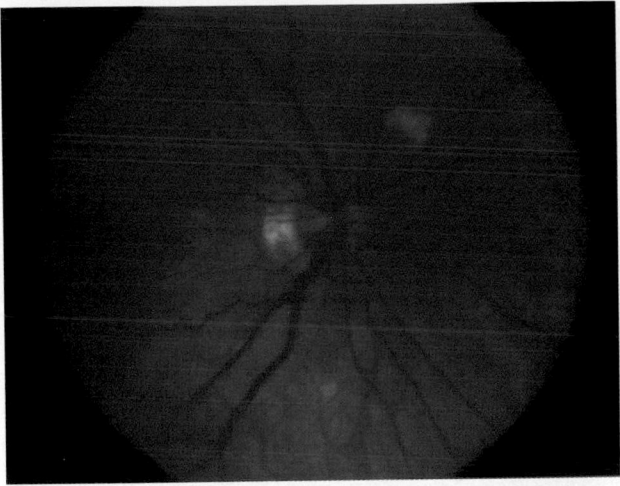

Plate 15 (Fig. 11-1) Retinal cotton-wool spot. Cotton-wool spots are most frequently found close to the optic disk. Although they occur in acute uncontrolled systemic hypertension, the more common cause now, in younger patients, is infection with the human immunodeficiency virus (HIV).This normotensive 37-year-old man had no visual symptoms and no other retinopathy. There is a myopic crescent at the temporal disk edge, which is not abnormal. He died of complications related to the acquired immunodeficiency syndrome (AIDS) 2 years later.

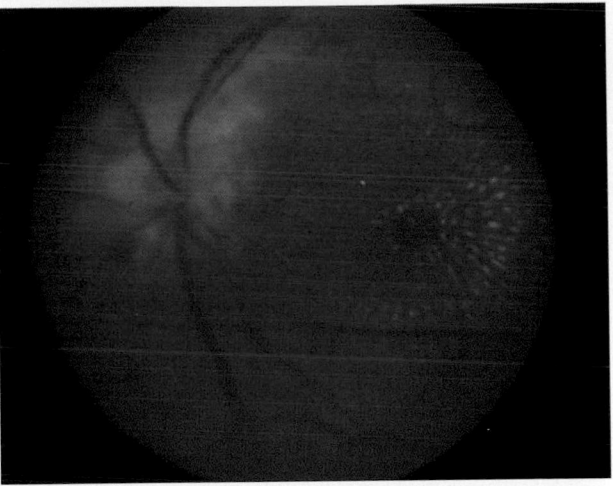

Plate 16 (Fig. 11-2) Disk swelling and hard exudate in a macular "star" pattern. In this hypertensive patient with periarteritis nodosa, vascular leakage has led to the deposit of hard exudates around the fovea. Radial perifoveal connective tissue results in the star pattern of the exudate. Note also that the optic disk is edematous, with blurred margins, secondary to hypertension.

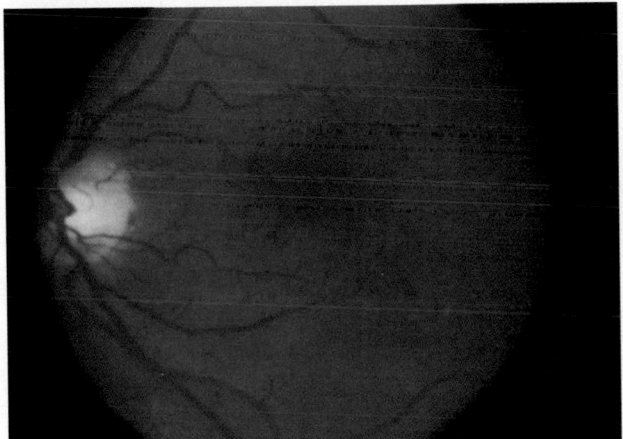

Plate 17 (Fig. 11-3) Background diabetic retinopathy. Retinal microaneurysms, dot-and-blot hemorrhages, and a few fine upper temporal hard exudates are diagnostic of early diabetic retinopathy. The patient had no visual symptoms, but retinopathy of this magnitude can often be seen in patients with insulin-requiring diabetes of 15 or more years' duration.

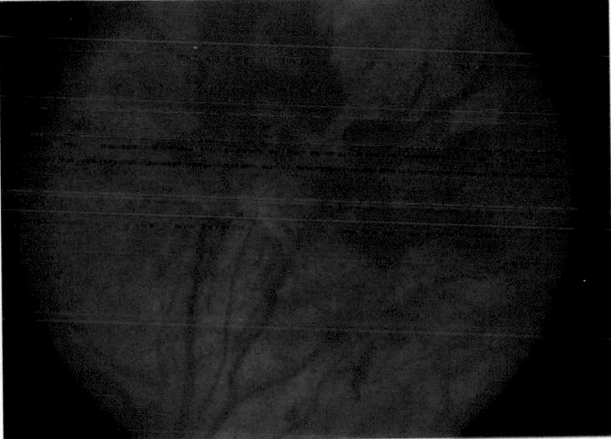

Plate 18 (Fig. 11-4) Proliferative diabetic retinopathy with preretinal hemorrhage. When neovascularization develops, preretinal and vitreous hemorrhages are much more likely to occur. Easily visible neovascularization either in the periphery of the retina, as in this diabetic patient, or at the disk is an indication for immediate panretinal laser photocoagulation.

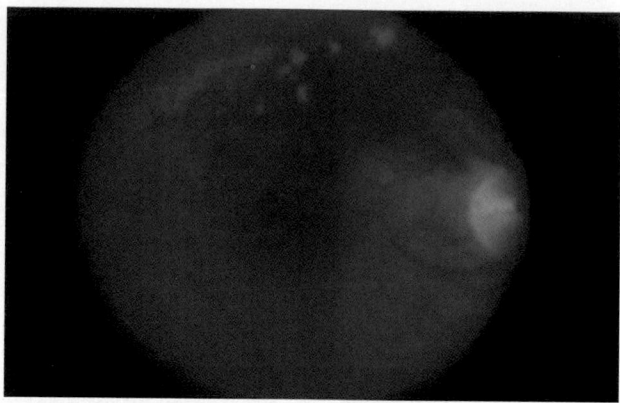

Plate 19 (Fig. 11-6) Branch retinal vein obstruction. Thickening of the retinal arterial wall in diabetes and hypertension may compromise the lumen of the vein, where they share a common adventitial sheath at an arteriovenous crossing. The resulting obstruction produces hemorrhagic retinopathy in the drainage area of the affected vein. Note here how the flame-shaped pattern of blood outlines the arcuate pattern of the nerve fibers as they run toward the optic disk.

A   *B*

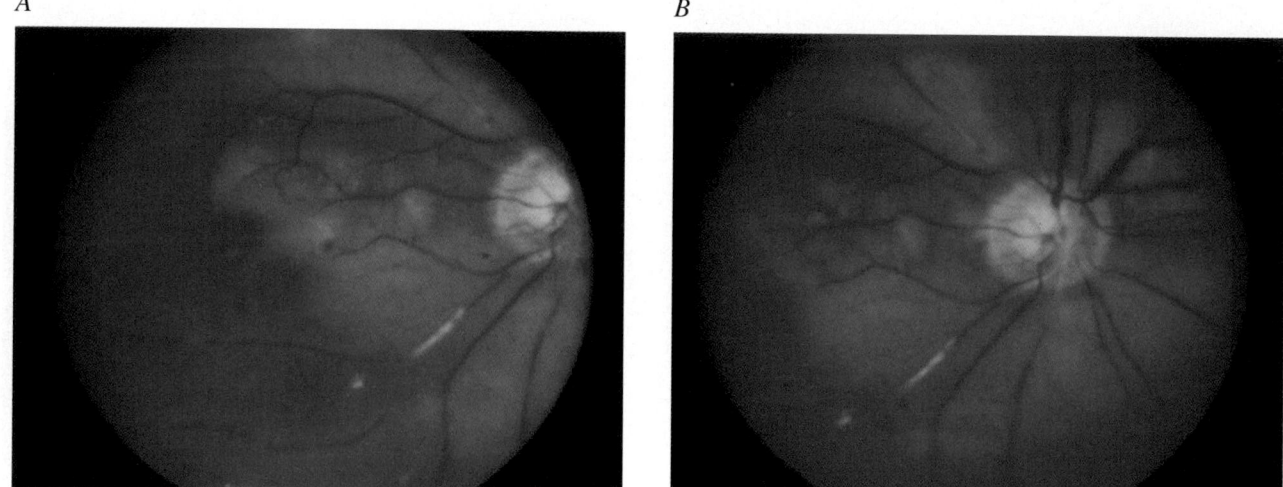

Plate 20 (Fig. 11-7) Embolic retinal arterial obstruction (*A* and *B*). Cholesterol crystals may dislodge from the walls of the heart, aortic arch, or carotids. Carried into the retinal circulation as Hollenhorst plaques, they seldom obstruct the arterioles completely. Although amaurosis fugax is more common, the embolic burden may occasionally be so large as to produce retinal infarction. Note in the photograph of the macular area (*A*) that this patient's fovea remains red, while there is a pale, cloudy swelling nasal to it. This has produced a half "cherry-red" spot. With complete central retinal artery occlusion, the red foveal area is completely surrounded by pale swollen retina. Hollenhorst cholesterol plaques can be seen in both the upper and lower temporal retinal arteries. In *A*, the inferior temporal arteriole demonstrates "boxcar" segmentation of the blood column, indicative of very slow flow.

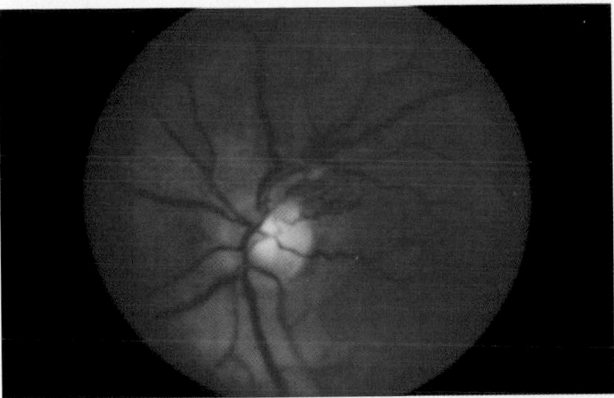

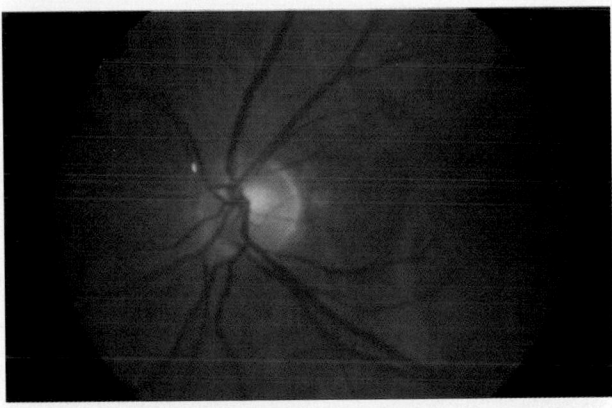

Plate 21 (Fig. 11-8) Neovascularization after branch retinal vein obstruction. New vessels may develop late after obstruction of a branch of the central retinal vein. These most often serve to shunt flow around the obstructed vessel site and are thus not as exuberantly proliferative as those seen in diabetic retinopathy.

Plate 22 (Fig. 11-10) Calcific retinal embolus associated with aortic valvular disease. Calcific aortic valvular disease and valve replacement surgery may result in retinal emboli. Like cholesterol emboli, these calcific flecks lodge at arterial bifurcations but seldom obstruct flow completely. They are white and glitter in the ophthalmoscope beam. Somewhat similar emboli may be seen after the intravenous injection of illicit drugs expanded with talc.

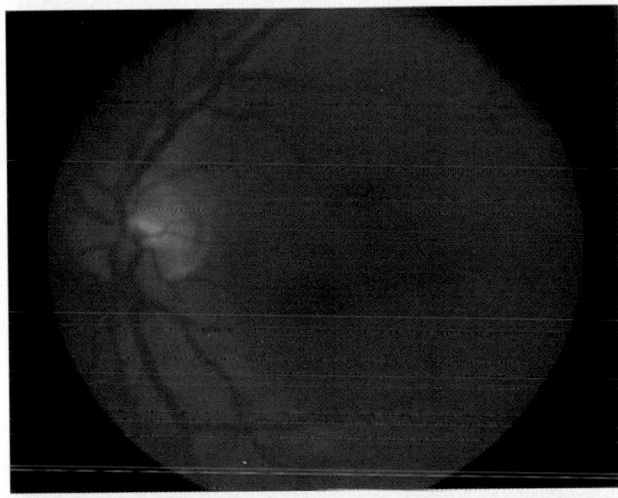

Plate 23 (Fig. 11-11) Retinal hemorrhages after cardiac catheterization. Following cardiac catheterization, symptomatic and asymptomatic retinal hemorrhages may occur. The latter are more common. Presumably, these are the result of embolic events. Note, in this recently catheterized patient, the two oval hemorrhages and a small area of cloudy swelling just inferiorœand temporal to the fovea.

A

B

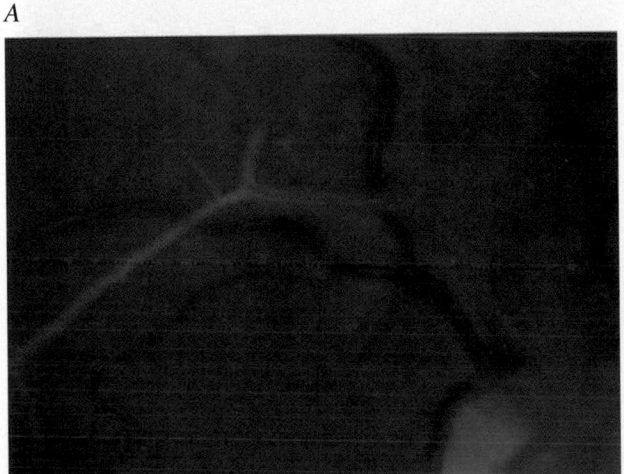

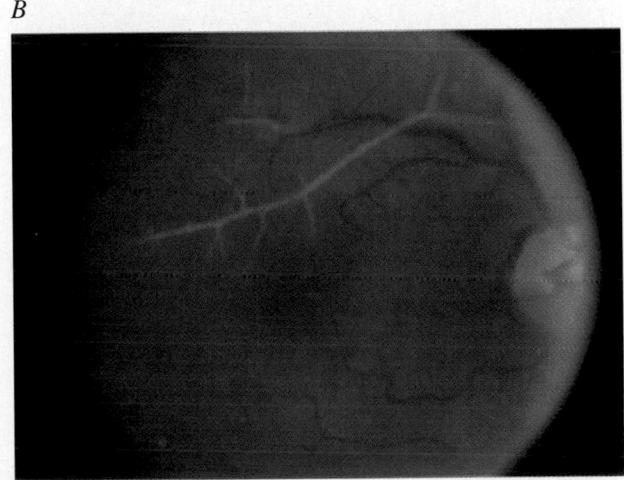

Plate 24 (Fig. 11-13) *A*. Retinal arteriosclerosis. This 75-year-old hypertensive woman has marked arteriosclerosis of the upper temporal retinal arteriole and its branches. When the narrowed blood column can no longer be seen, the thickened wall produces the "silver-wire" appearance seen here. Where the arteriole crosses its associated vein, the course of the vein is altered, and its blood column cannot be seen. This venous "nicking" and "banking" is associated with impairment of outflow, and the affected veins become darker, larger, and more tortuous. *B*. Low-power view showing the silver-wire arteriole.

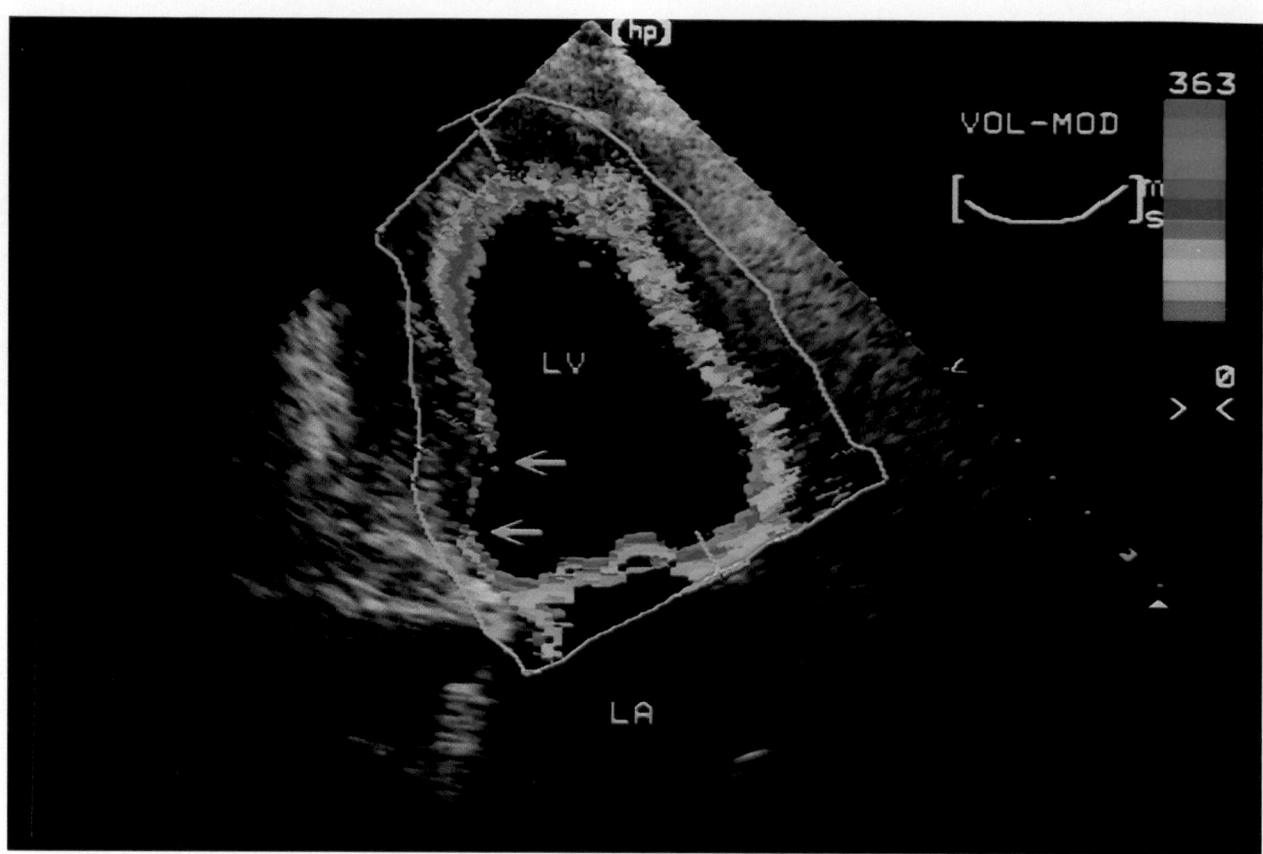

Plate 25 (Fig. 14-23) Color kinesis image (apical 2-chamber view) from a patient with an inferobasal infarction. Systolic motion in this area (*arrows*) is markedly diminished.

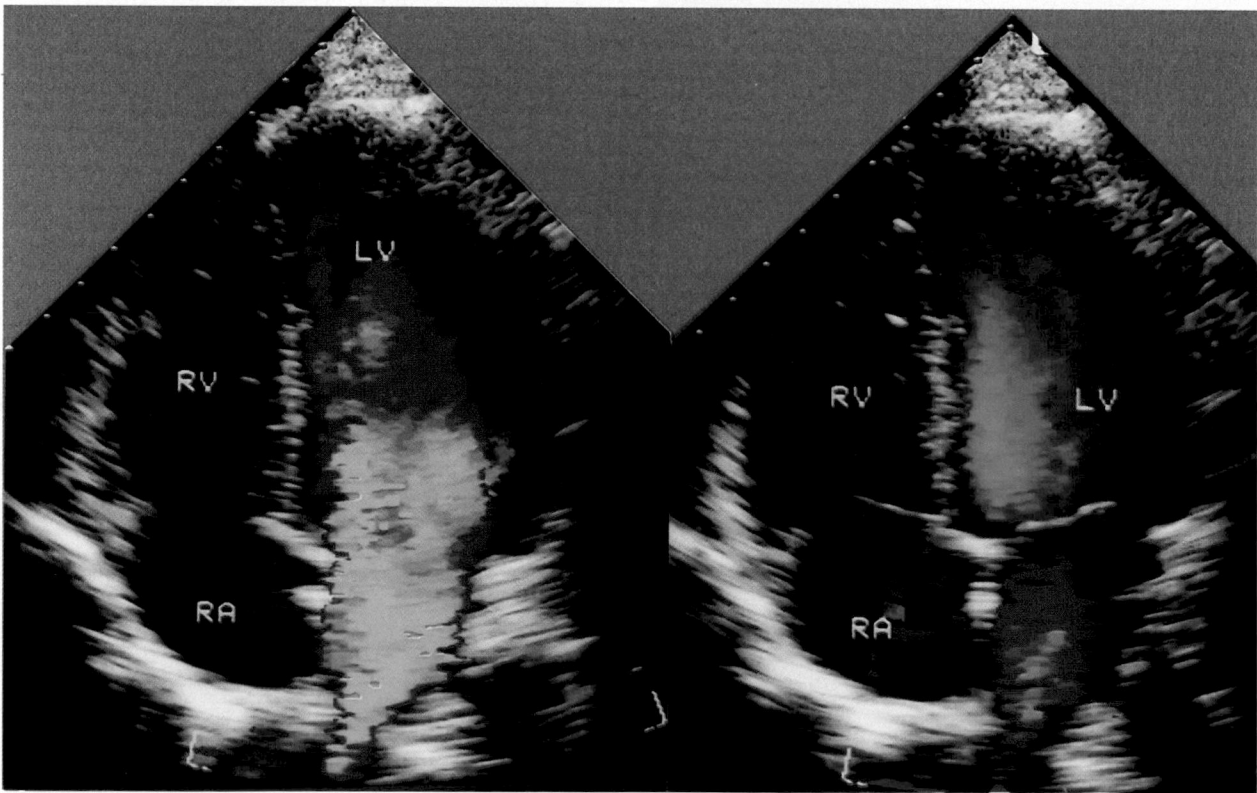

Plate 26 (Fig 14-30) Apical four-chamber images with color-flow Doppler during diastole and systole. Red flow indicates movement toward the transducer (diastolic filling); blue flow indicates movement away from the transducer (systolic ejection).

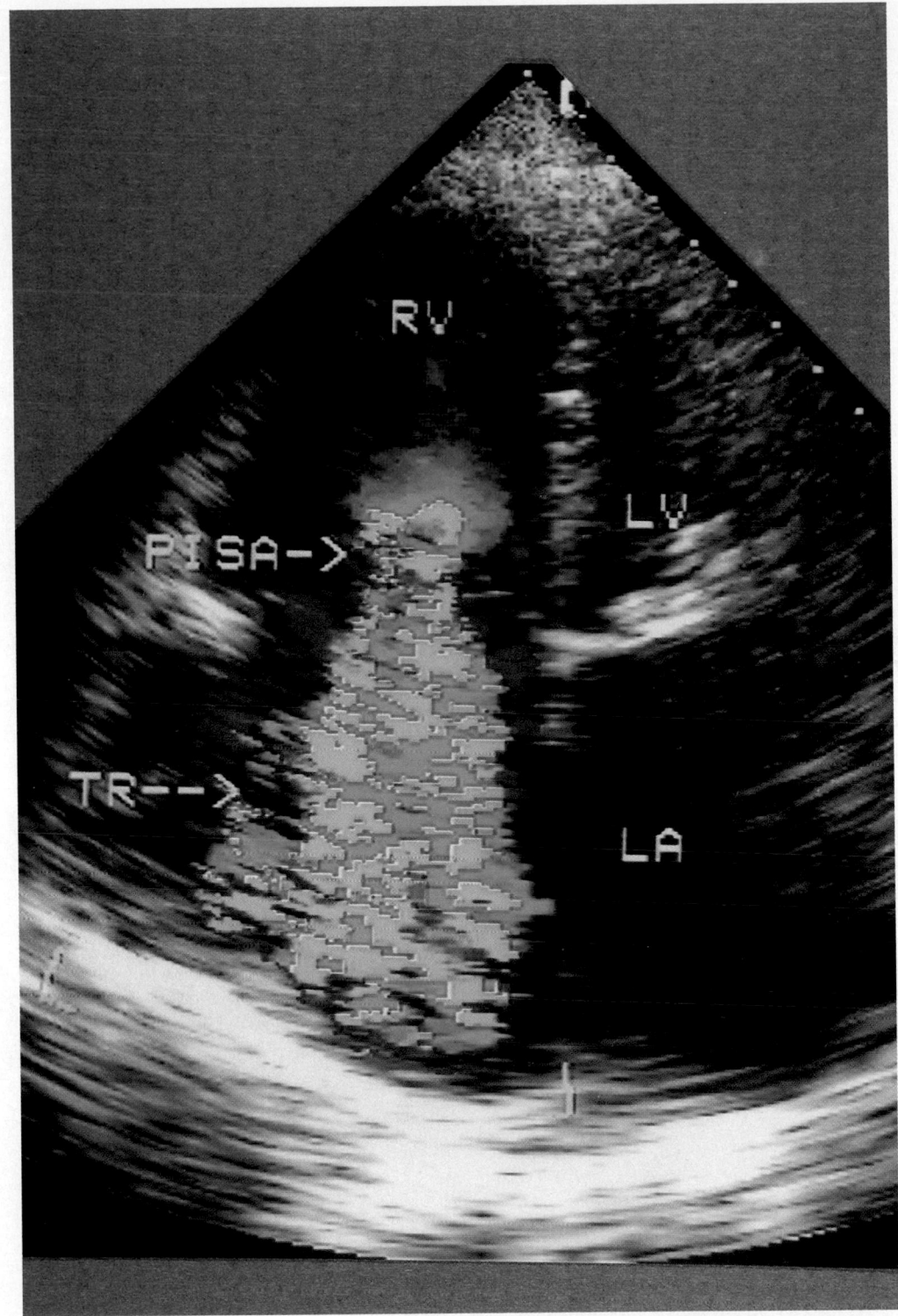

Plate 27 (Fig. 14-31) Apical four-chamber view of severe tricuspid regurgitation. The Doppler color jet fills the right atrium. PISA = proximal isovelocity surface area; LV = left ventricle; LA = left atrium; RV = right ventricle.

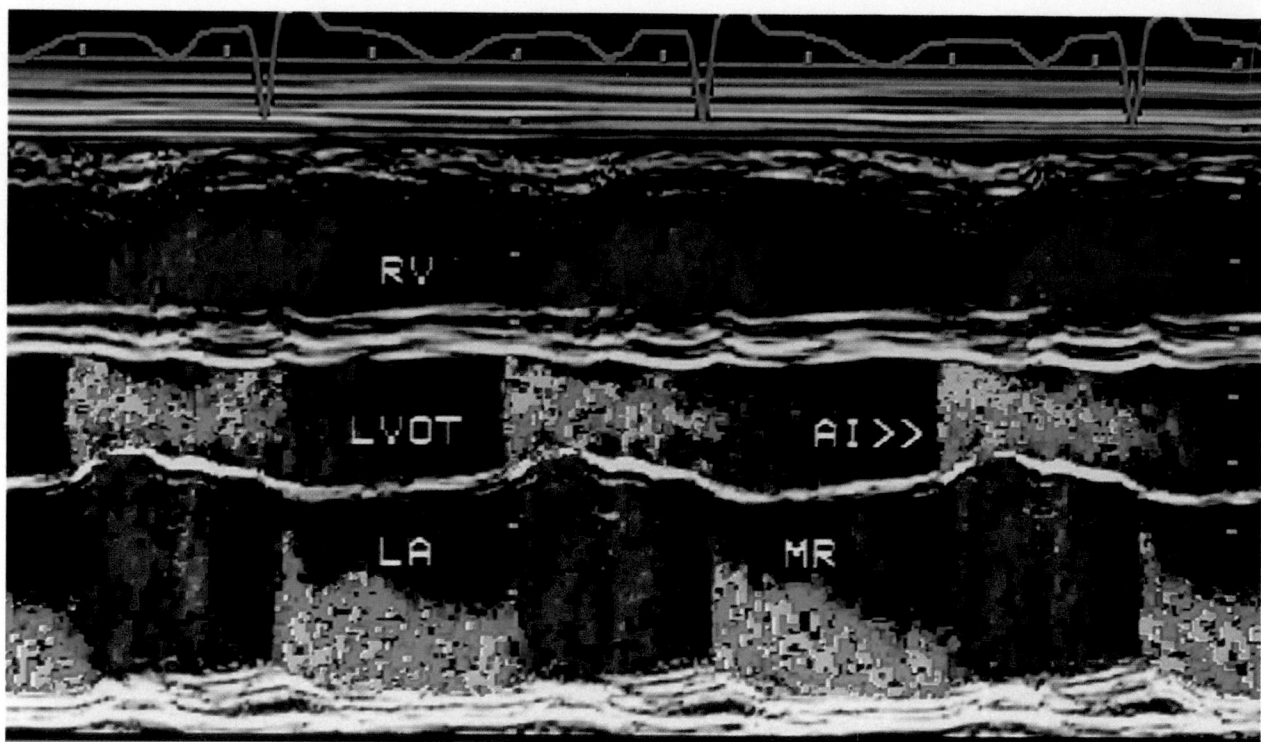

Plate 28 (Fig. 14-32) Color-flow Doppler superimposed on an M-mode image. The transducer is in parasternal position, and the cursor is directed through the left ventricular outflow tract (LVOT) and left atrium (LA). The patient under study has both aortic insufficiency (AI) and mitral regurgitation (MR). RV = right ventricle.

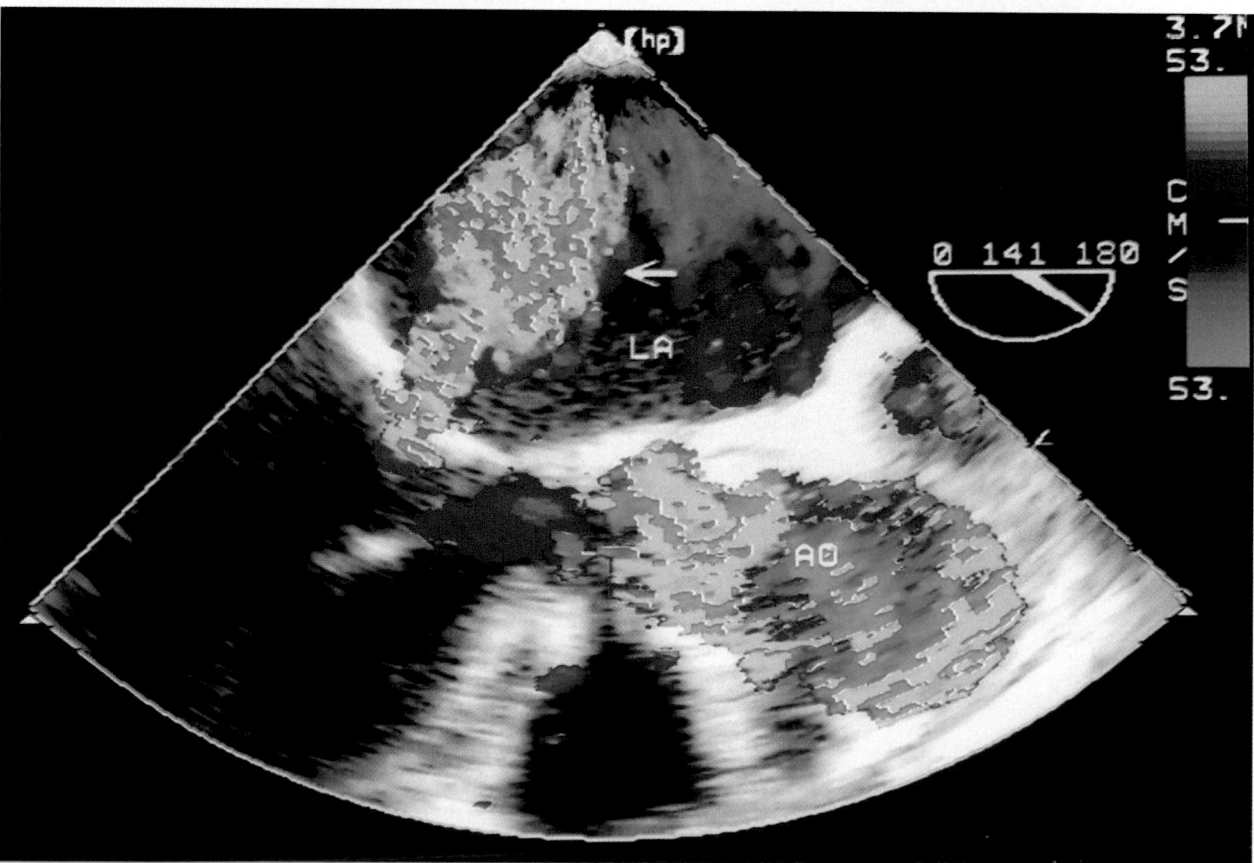

Plate 29 (Fig. 14-49) Transesophageal echocardiography image ("three-chamber" plane) demonstrating a jet of mitral regurgitation (*arrow*) in the left atrium (LA). AO = aorta; LV = left ventricle.

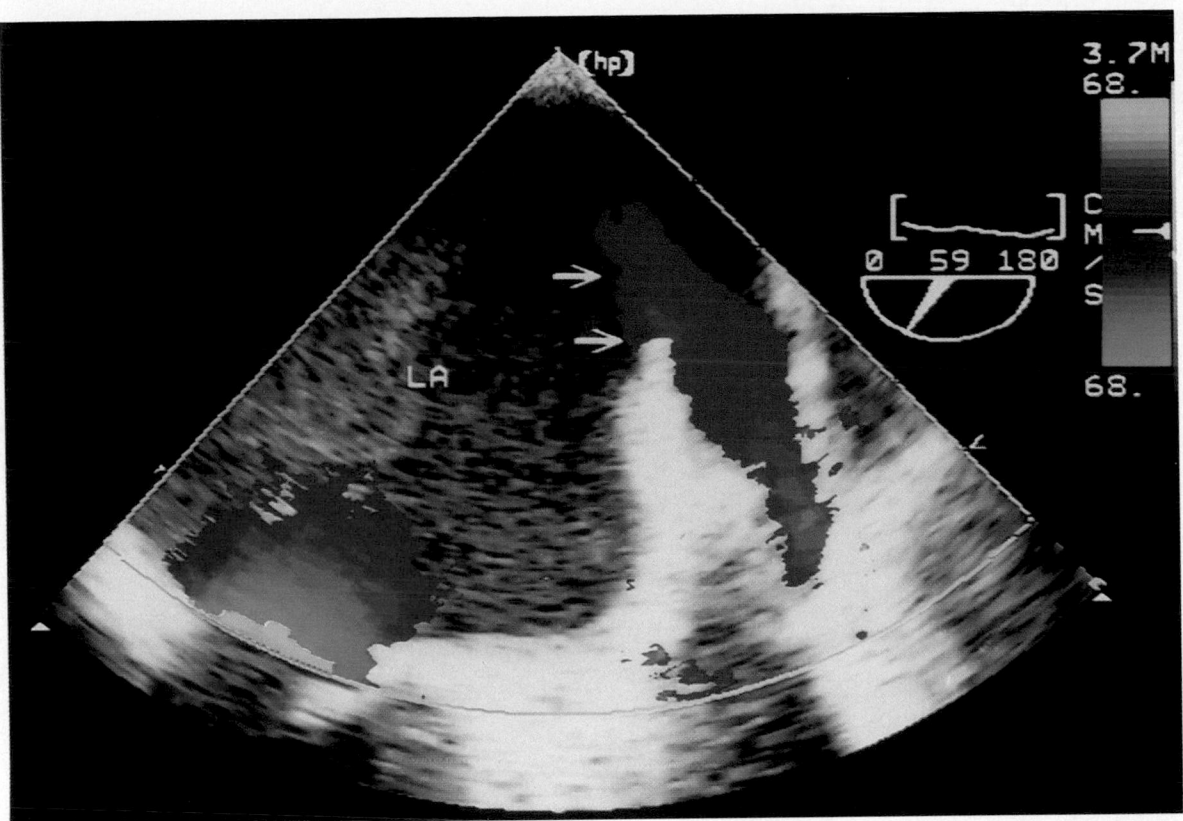

Plate 30 (Fig. 14-50) Transesophageal echocardiography image of pulmonary venous flow (*arrows*) entering the left atrium (LA) during diastole.

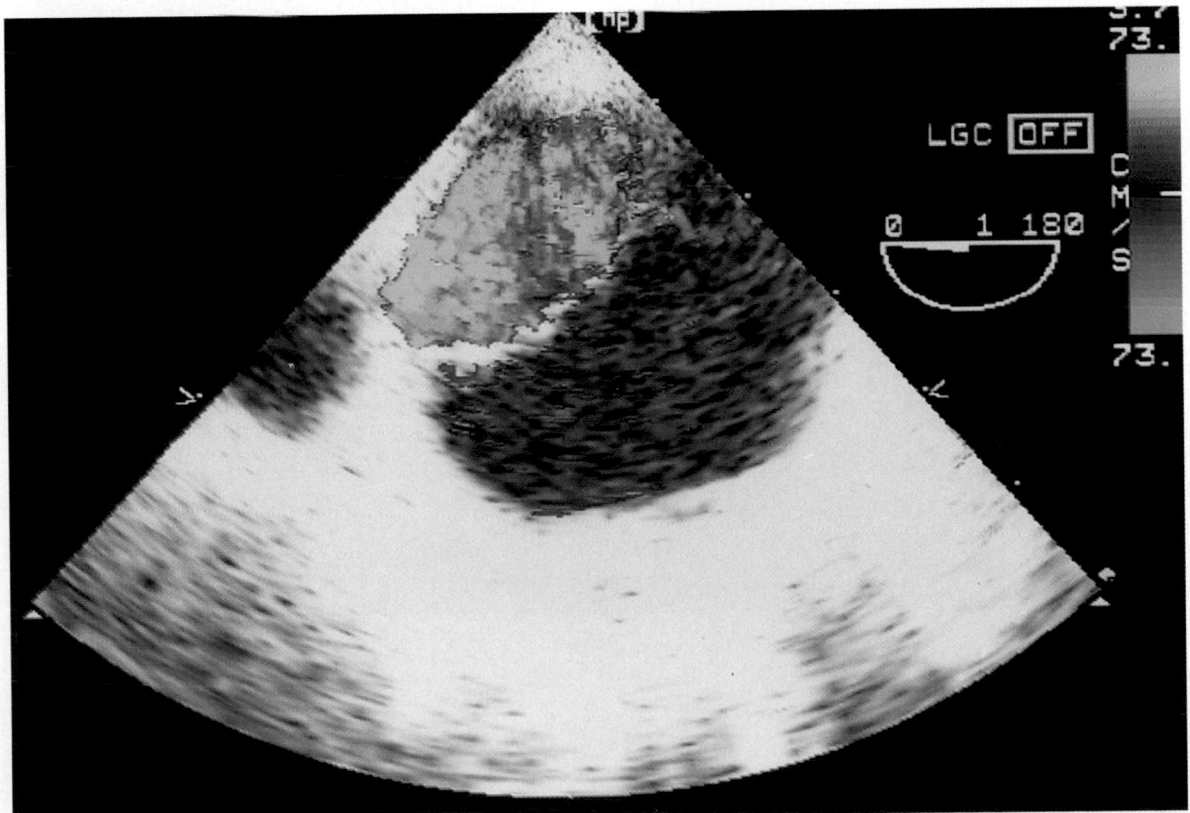

Plate 31 (Fig. 14-51) Transverse TEE image of a descending aortic dissection. The true lumen is color-coded orange. The false lumen is mostly devoid of flow, but a small blue jet of communication between the two channels is present.

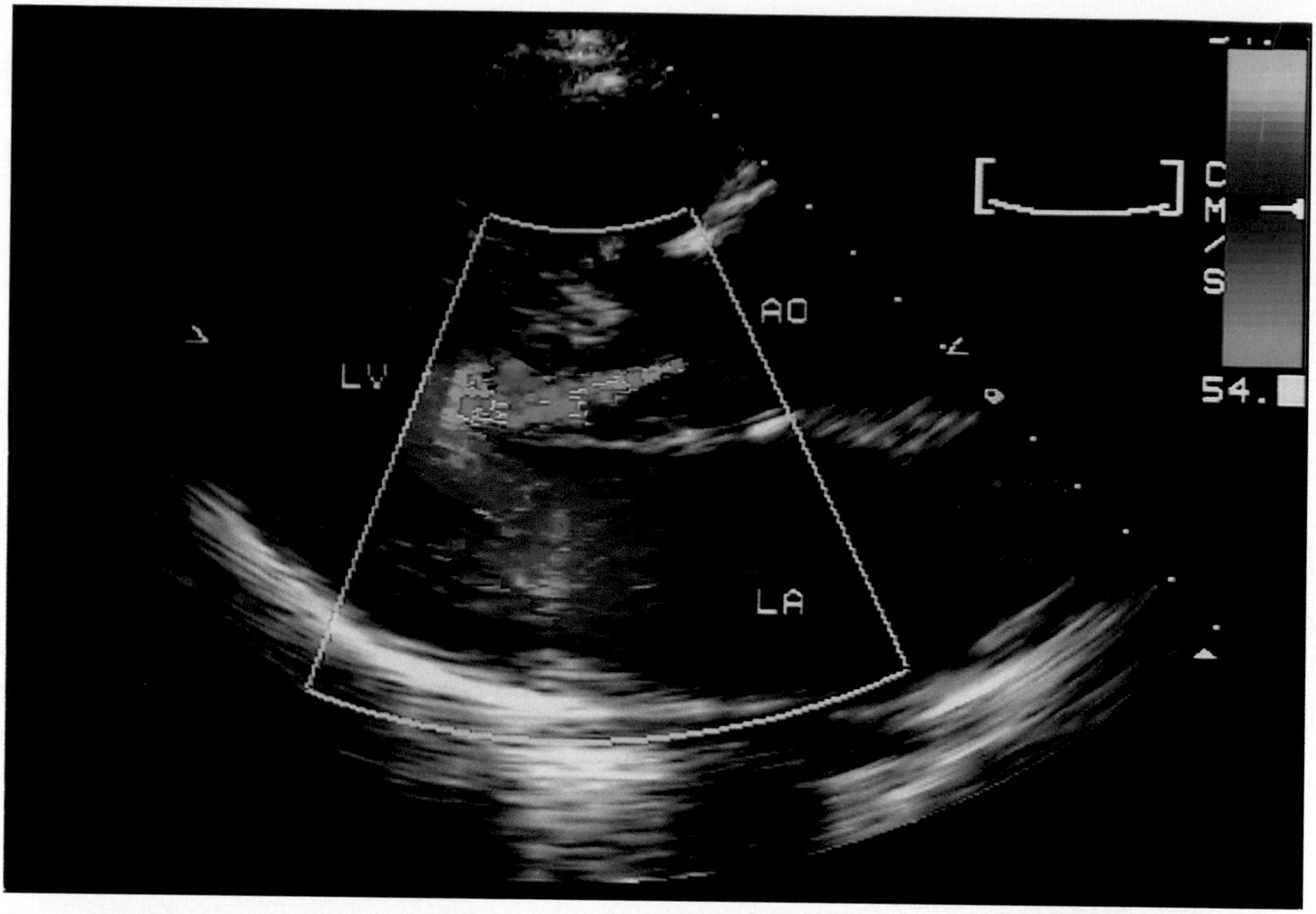

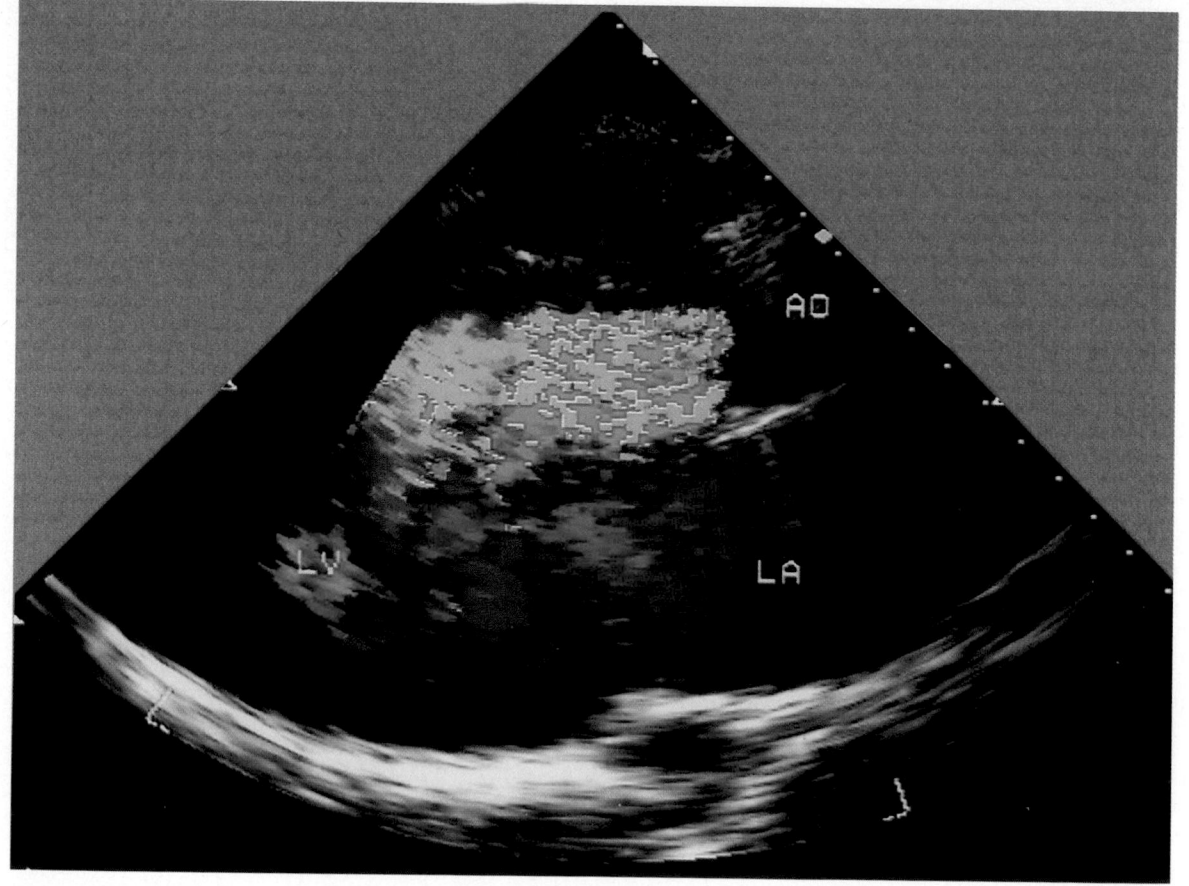

A

B

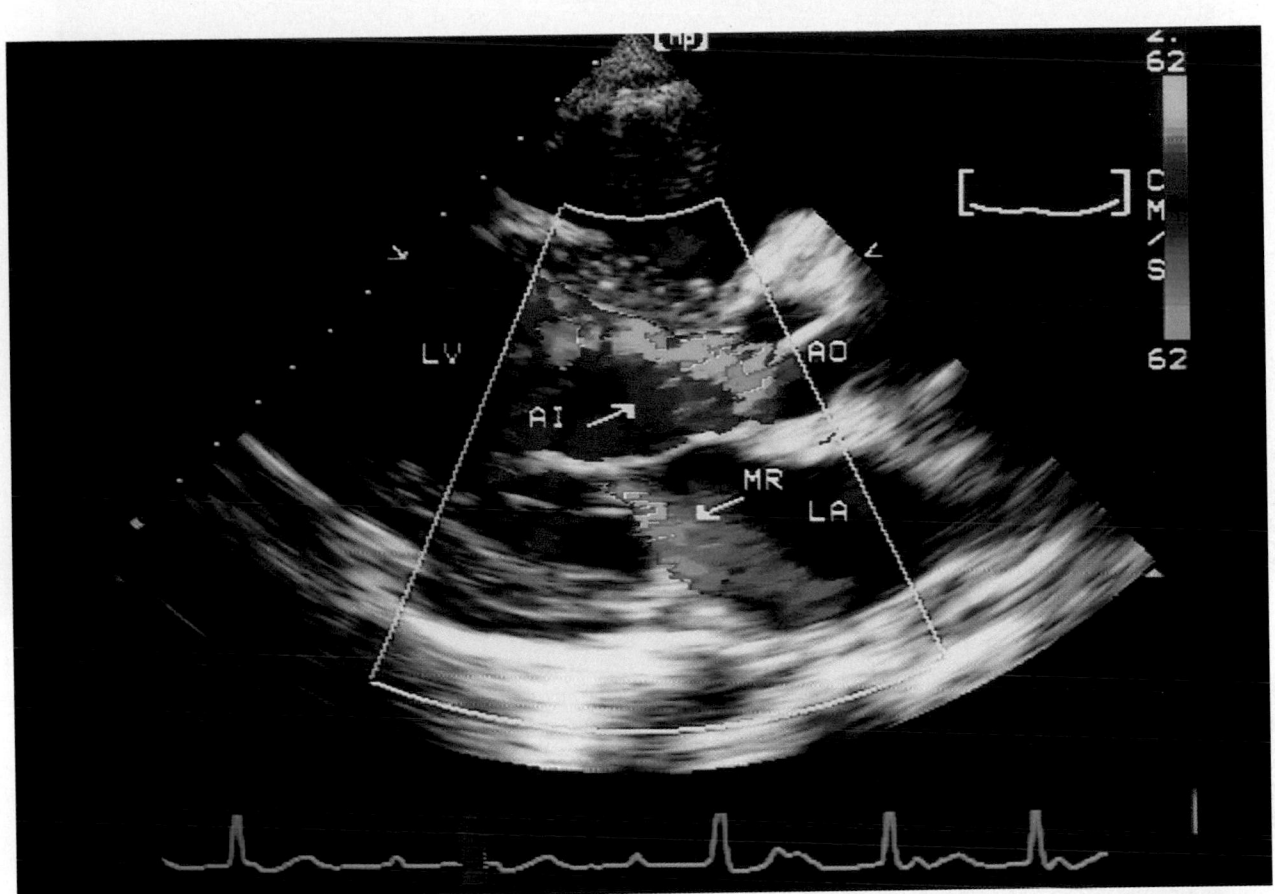

C

Plate 32 (Fig. 14-64) *A*. Parasternal long-axis plane showing a multicolor jet (indicating turbulent flow) of aortic regurgitation in the left ventricular outflow tract. The jet is narrow in width, suggesting mild regurgitation. AO = aorta; LA = left atrium; LV = left ventricle. *B*. Parasternal long-axis plane with color-flow Doppler imaging. The aortic regurgitant (AR) color jet is as wide as the left ventricular outflow tract, suggesting severe AR. AO = aorta; LA = left atrium; LV = left ventricle. *C*. Parasternal long-axis image of acute severe aortic insufficiency (AI). The accompanying marked elevation of left ventricular (LV) diastolic pressure causes diastolic mitral regurgitation (MR). AO = aorta; LA = left atrium.

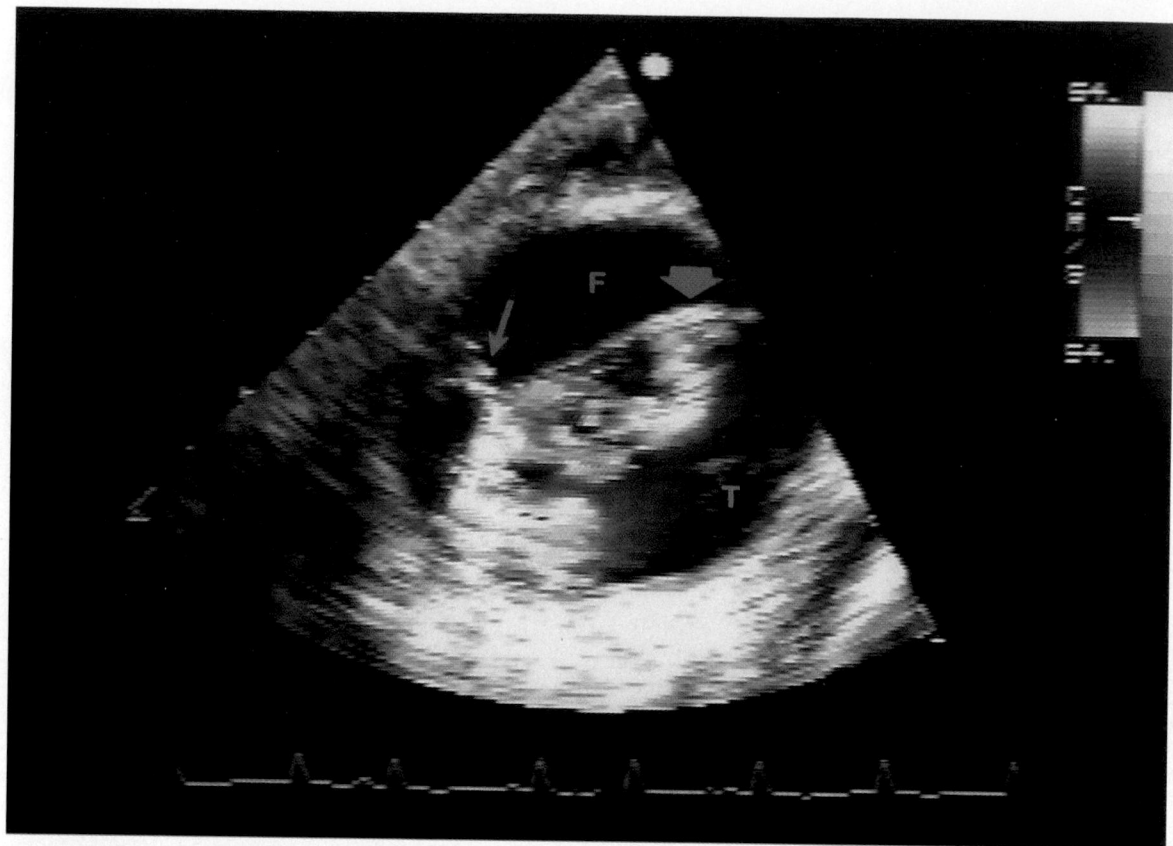

Plate 33 (Fig. 14-69) Transverse TEE view of an aortic dissection. The false (F) and true (T) lumens are separated by an intimal flap (*large arrow*). The communication between the two channels is visible (*small arrow*).

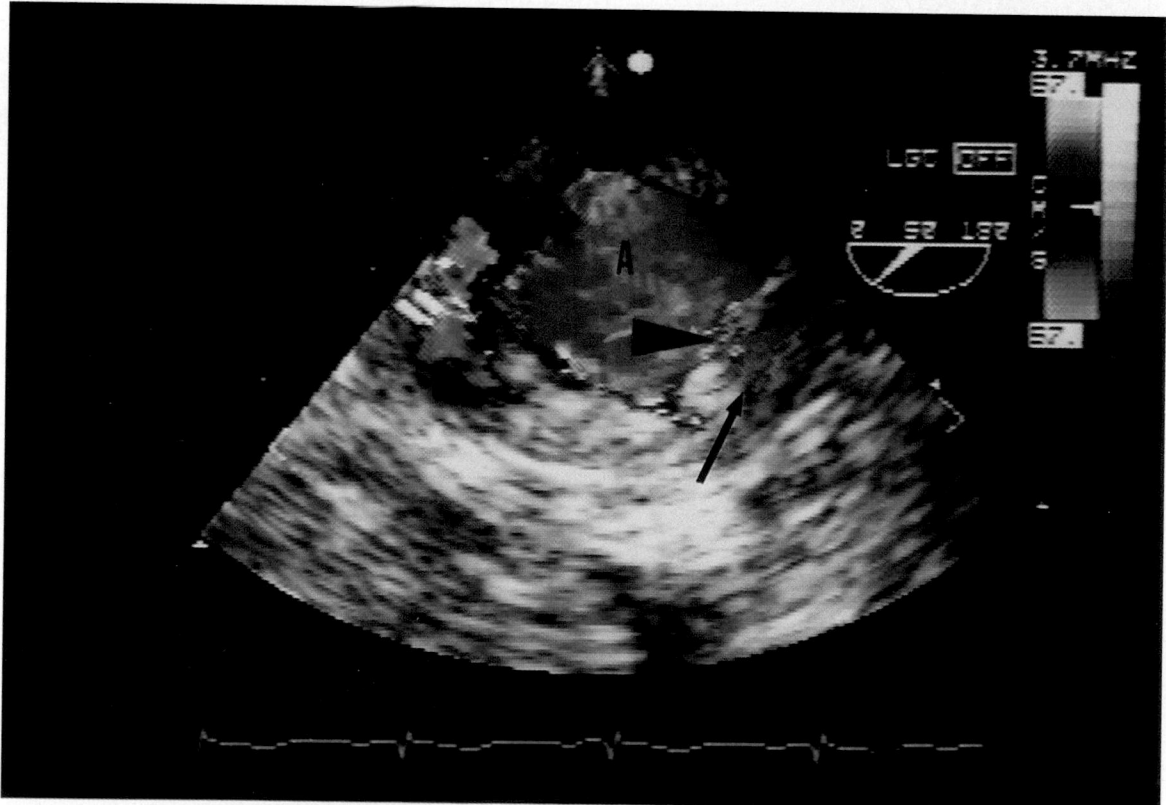

Plate 34 (Fig. 14-71) Transverse TEE view of penetrating ulceration in the proximal portion of the descending aorta (A). The mouth of the ulcer crater is visible (*large arrowhead*), as is blood flow within the atheroma (*arrow*).

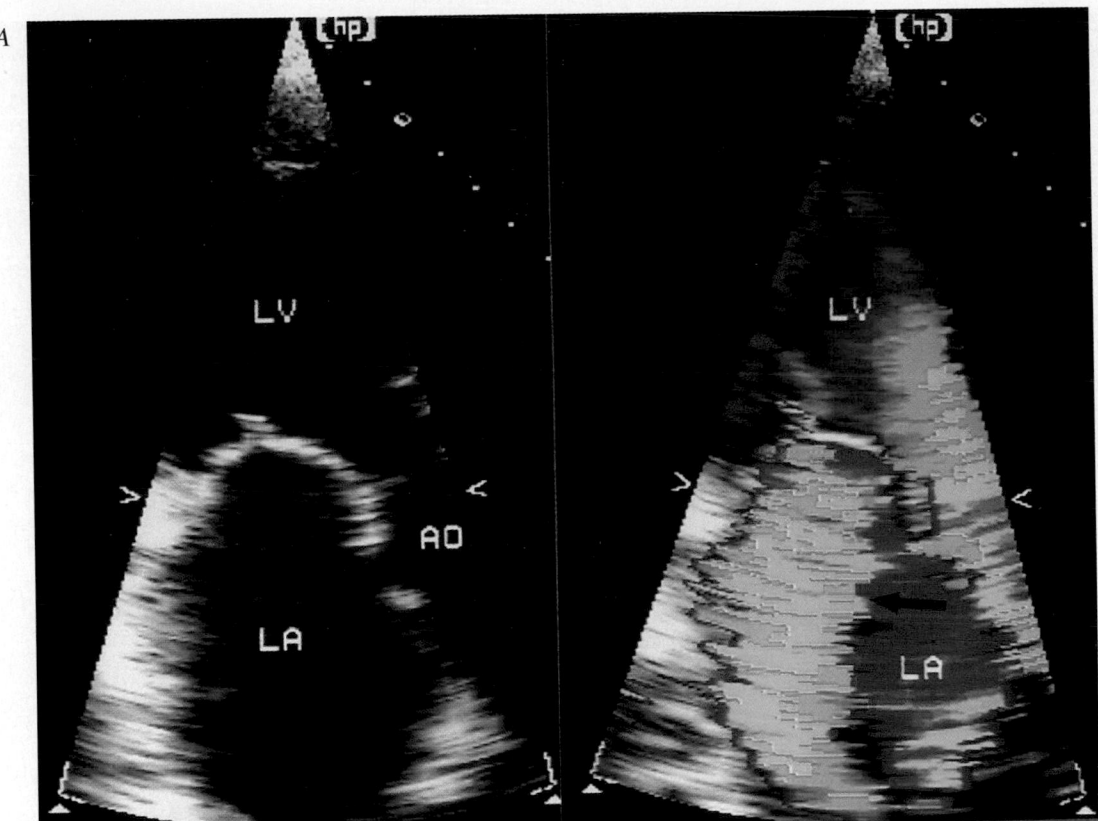

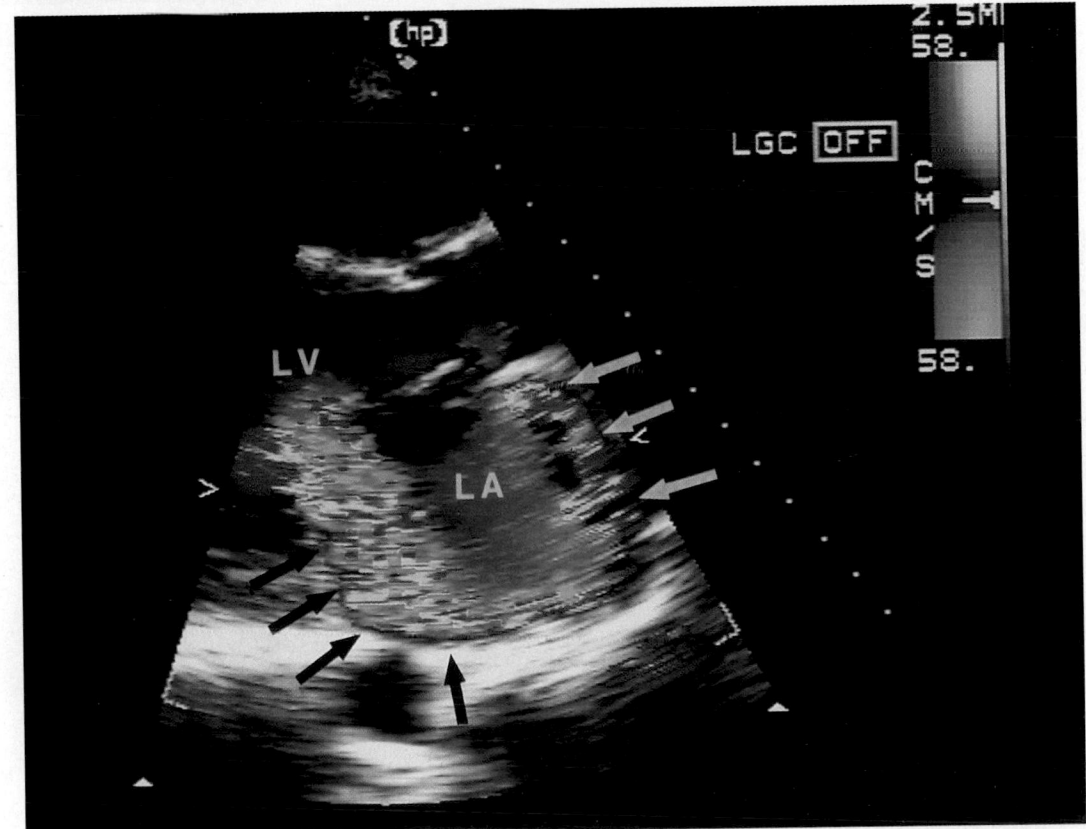

Plate 35 (Fig. 14-77) *A*. Mitral regurgitation. *Left*: apical 3-chamber plane. *Right*: same plane with color Doppler imaging. A large jet of mitral regurgitation (*arrow*) is present. AO = aorta; LA = left atrium; LV = left ventricle. *B*. Parasternal long-axis view from a patient with angiographically proved severe mitral regurgitation. The color Doppler jet in this case is directed posteriorly and eccentric (*black arrows*). The jet "hugs" the wall of the left atrium (LA) and wraps around all the way to the aortic root (*white arrows*). LV = left ventricle.

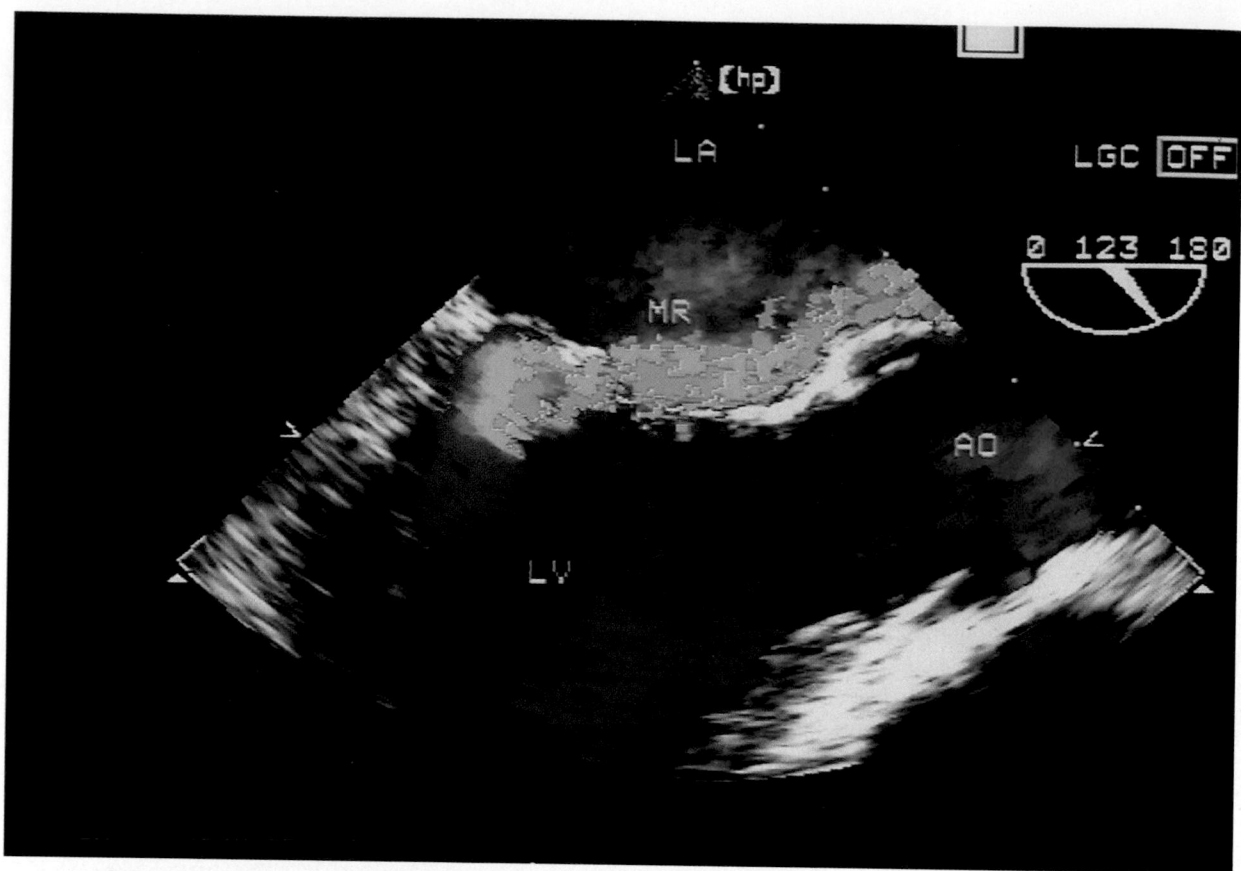

Plate 36 (Fig. 14-78*B*) Color Doppler imaging demonstrates an eccentric jet of MR directed anteriorly toward the aortic root (AO). LA = left atrium; LV = left ventricle.

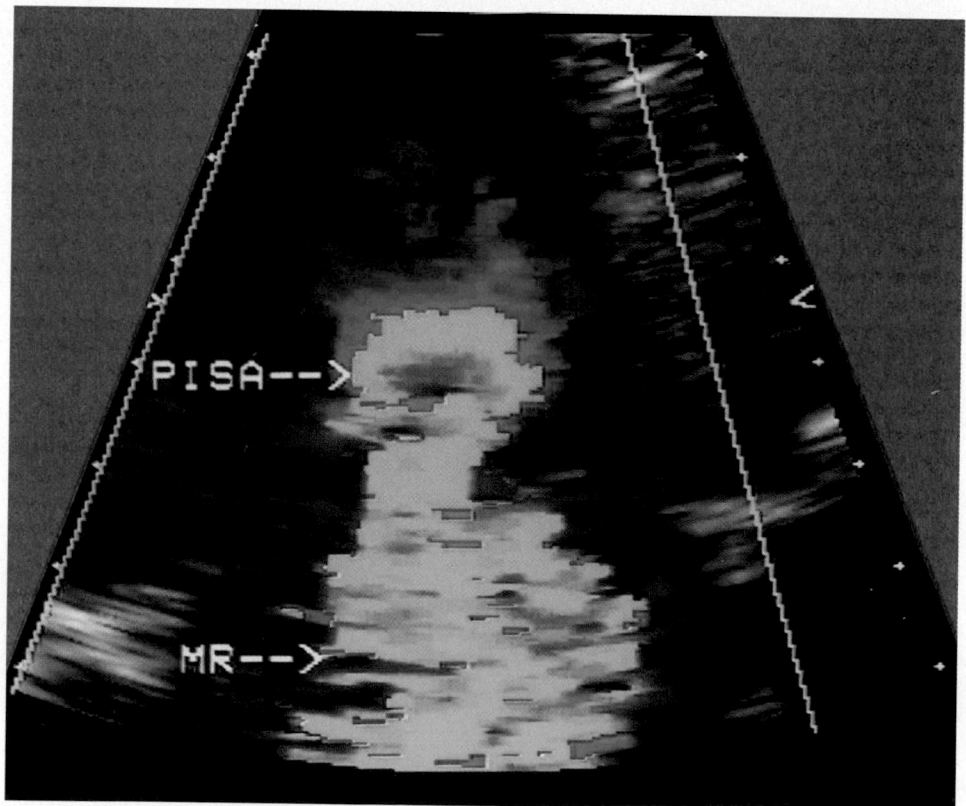

Plate 37 (Fig. 14-80*B*) Magnified view (from the apical 4-chamber plane) of mitral regurgitation (MR) demonstrating color Doppler flow convergence proximal to the mitral valve (PISA).

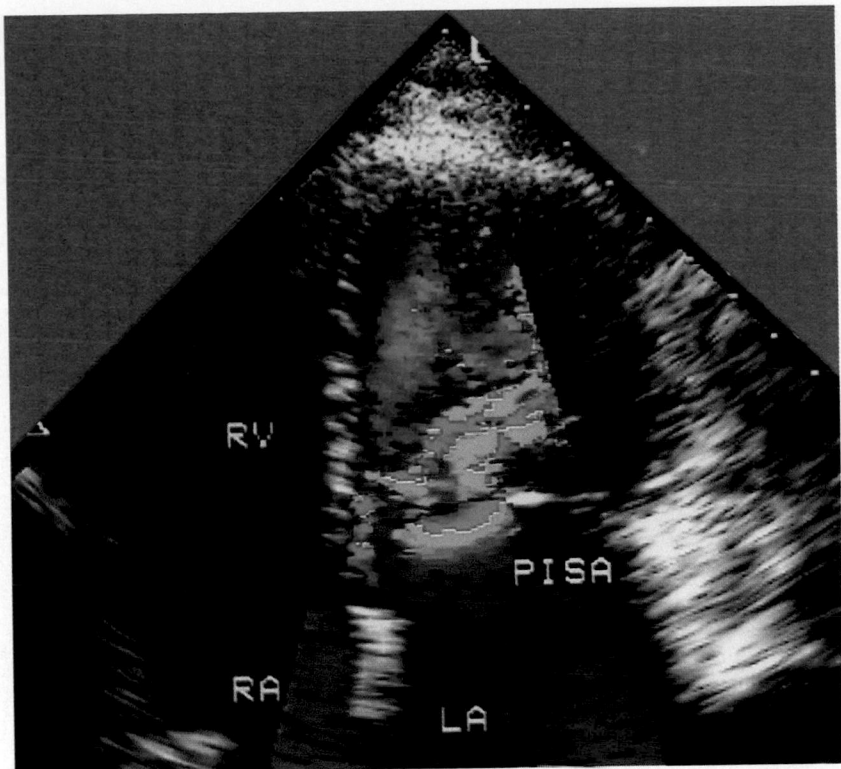

Plate 38 (Fig. 14-81) Apical four-chamber plane in mitral stenosis. Color flow imaging in the mitral valve region shows flow convergence (PISA) proximal to the valve during diastole. LA = left atrium; RA = right atrium; RV = right ventricle.

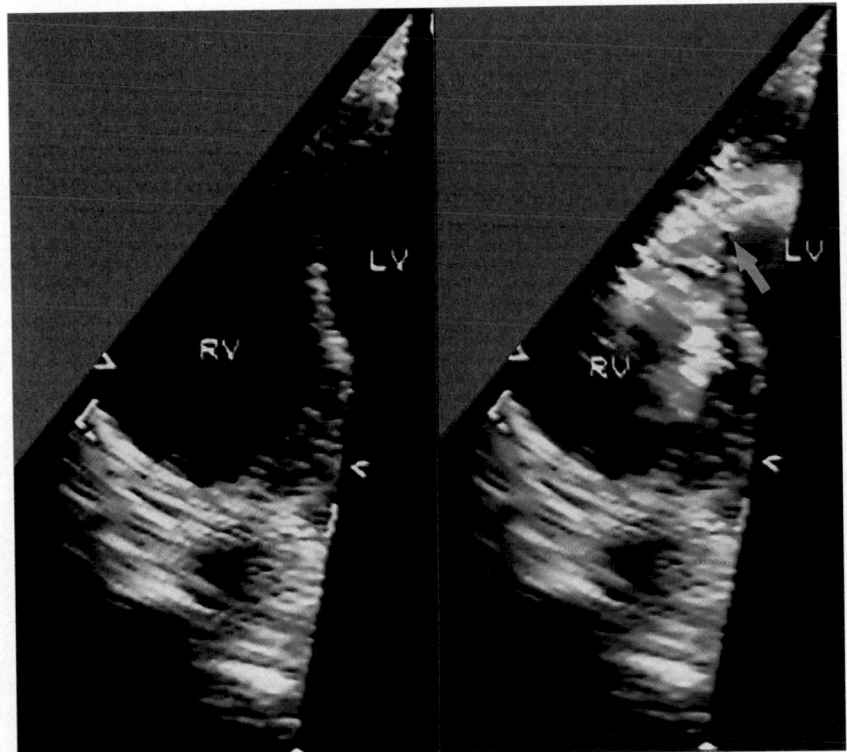

Plate 39 (Fig. 14-102) Modified apical four-chamber image of a distal septal ventricular septal rupture. With 2D imaging (*left*), the distal septum is incompletely visualized. With color Doppler imaging, however, a high-velocity aliased color jet is seen in the right ventricle (RV). In addition, an area of flow convergence is seen on the left ventricular (LV) side of the rupture (*arrow*).

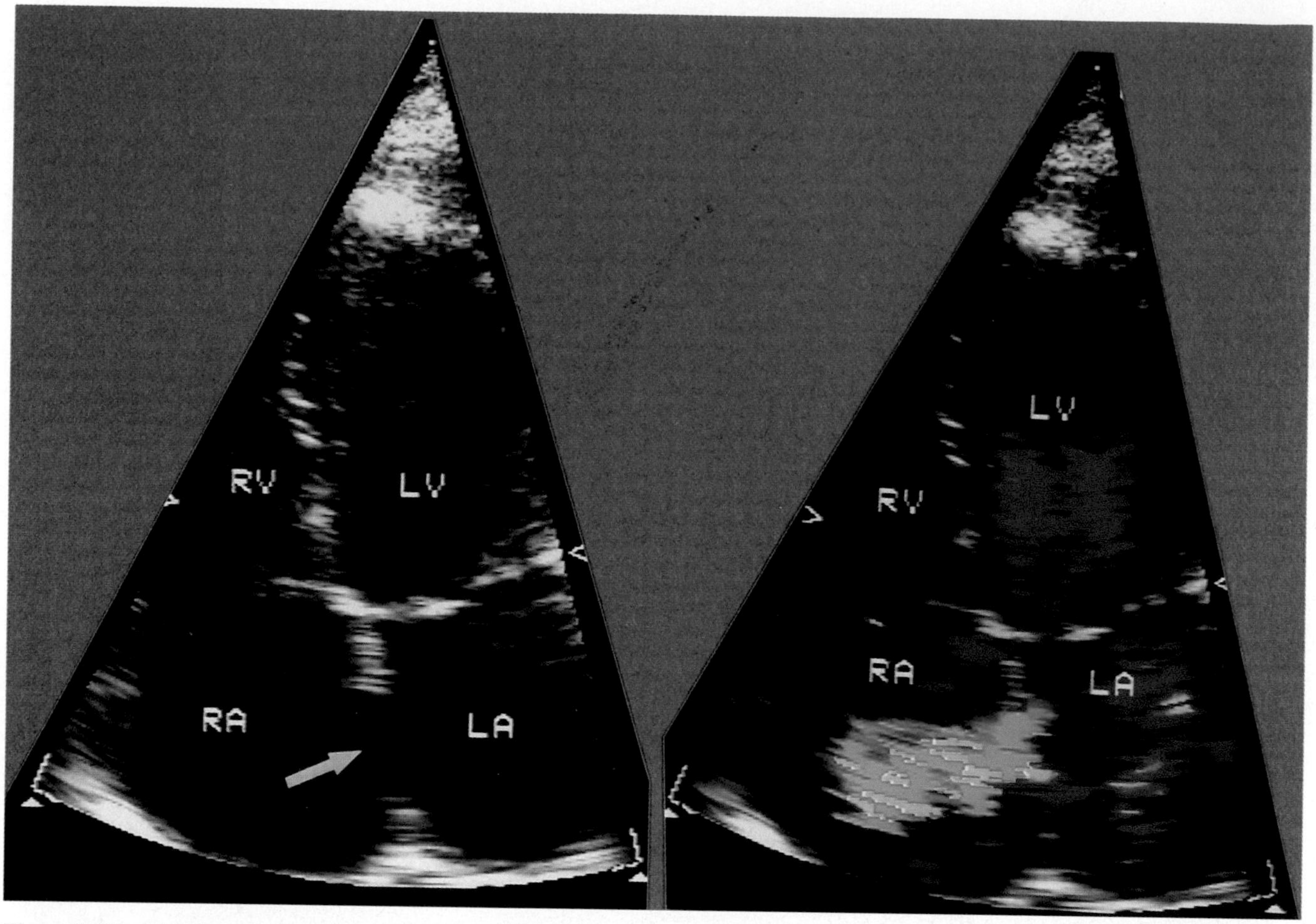

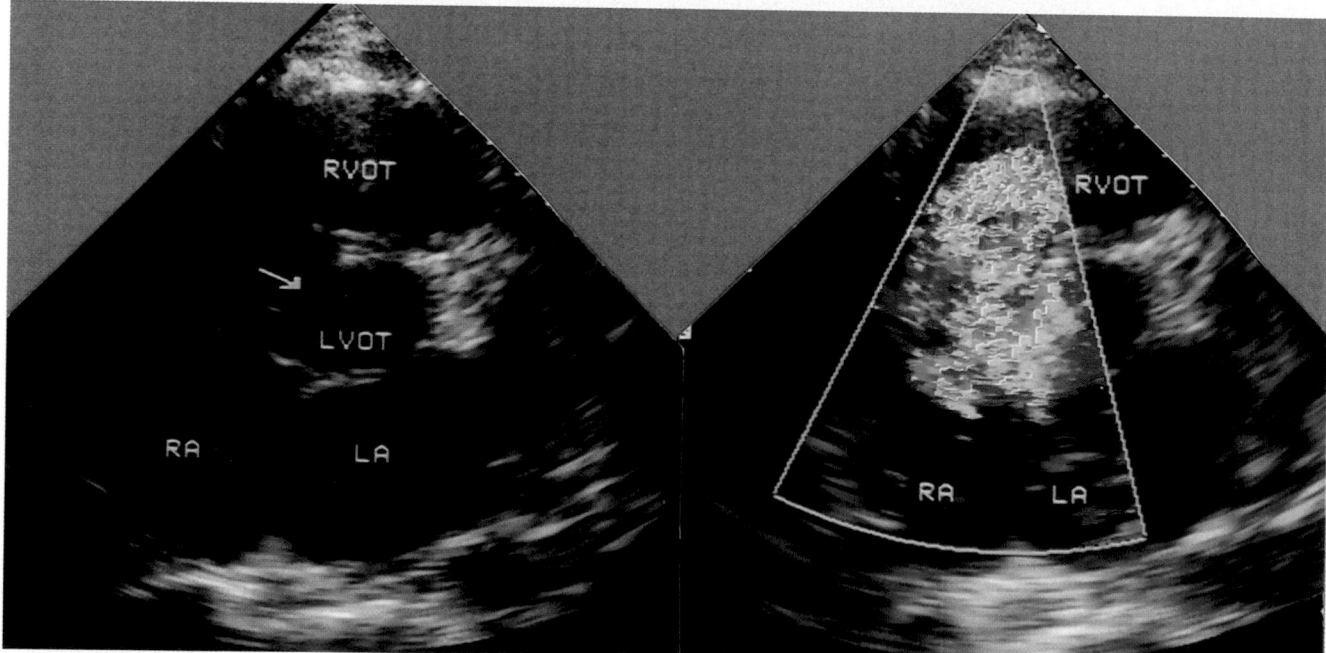

Plate 40 (Fig.14-110*A*) Apical four-chamber view of an ostium secundum atrial septal defect (ASD). On the left, a defect in the mid atrial septum is apparent (*arrow*). On the right, there is color flow through the shunt. RV = right ventricle; RA = right atrium; LA = left atrium; LV = left ventricle.

Plate 41 (Fig. 14-114) Parasternal short-axis images of a large perimembranous ventricular septal defect (VSD) (*arrow*) without (*left*) and with (*right*) superimposed color flow Doppler. A large, turbulent color jet crosses the VSD during systole (*right*). RVOT = right ventricular outflow tract; RA = right atrium; LA = left atrium; LVOT = left ventricular outflow tract.

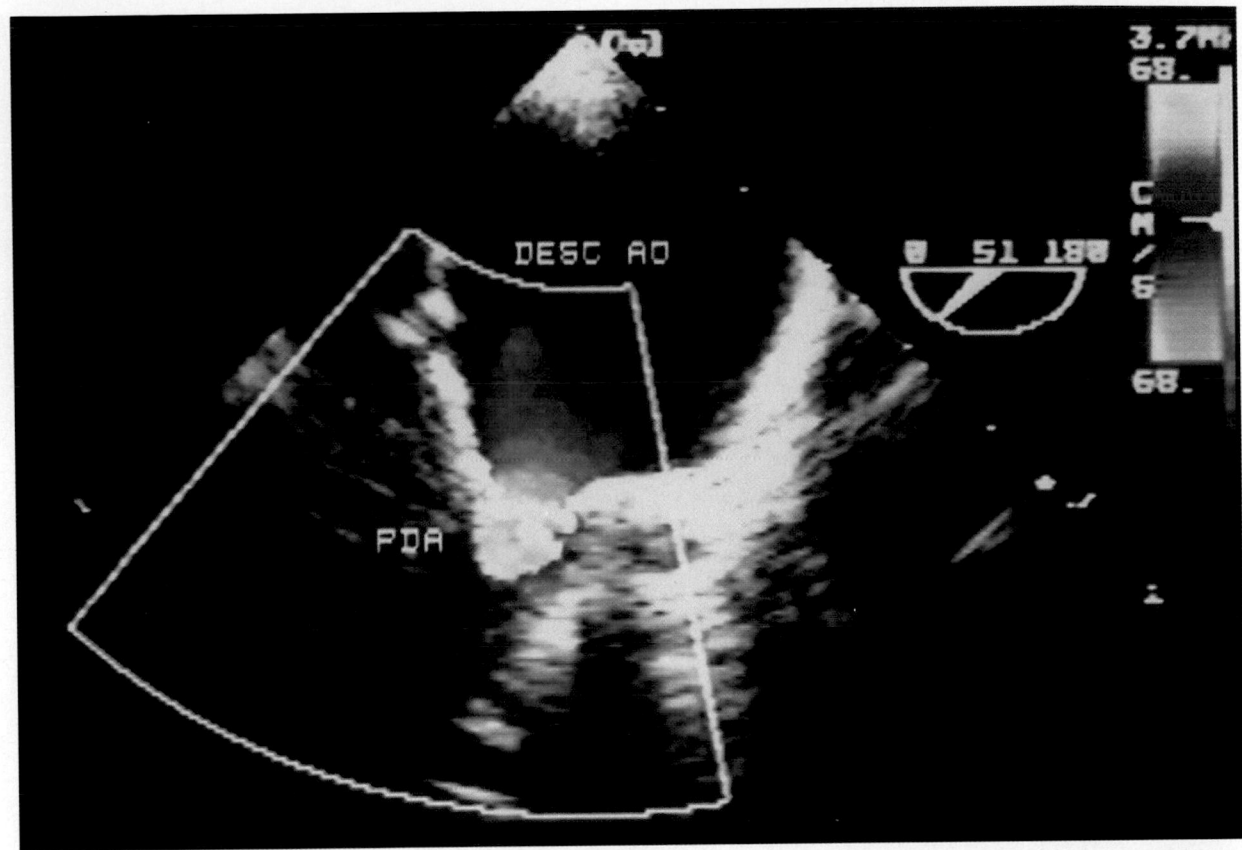

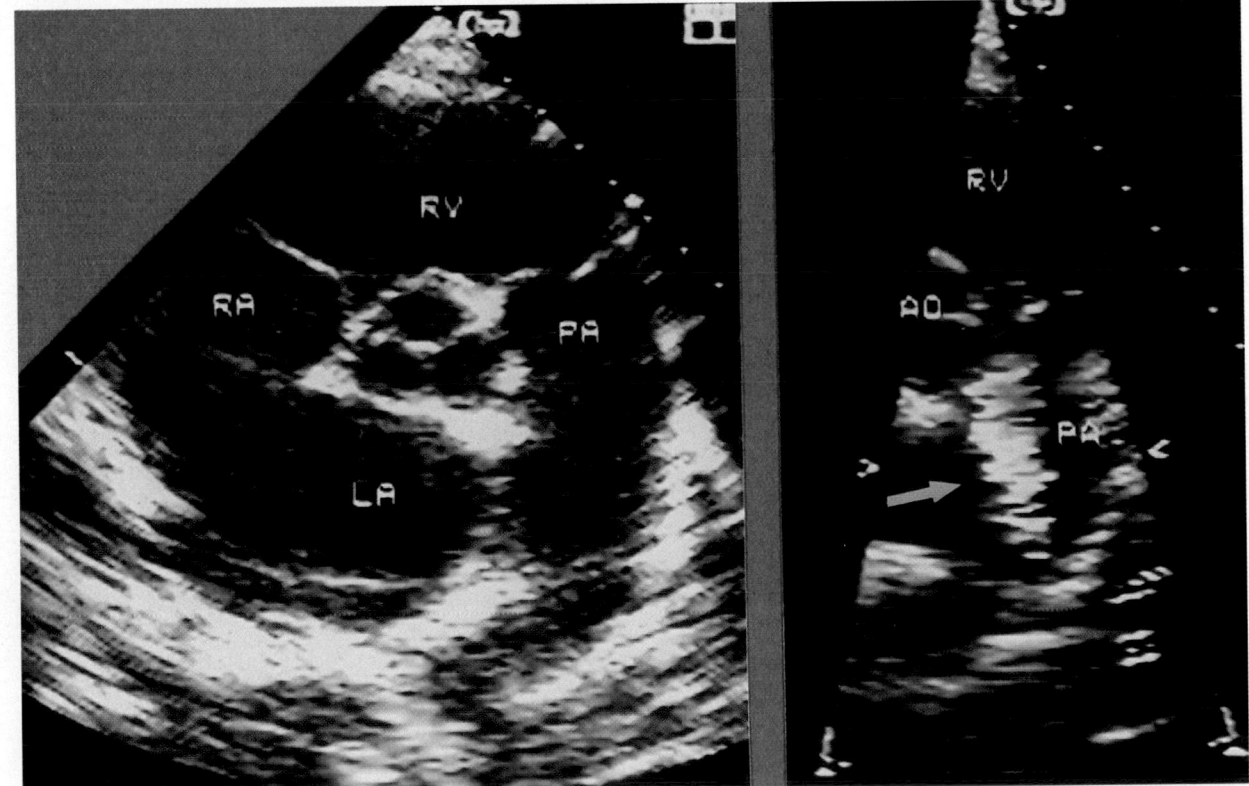

Plate 42 (Fig. 14-115) *A.* Transesophageal image of a patent ductus arteriosus (PDA). Color Doppler imaging shows flow from the descending aorta (DESC AO) into the PDA. (Courtesy of Bruce J. Kimura, M.D.) *B.* Parasternal short-axis images at the aortic valve level. On the left, the pulmonary artery (PA) is somewhat enlarged. On the right, color imaging reveals diastolic flow within the PA, consistent with a patent ductus arteriosus. RV = right ventricle; RA = right atrium; LA = left atrium; AO = aorta.

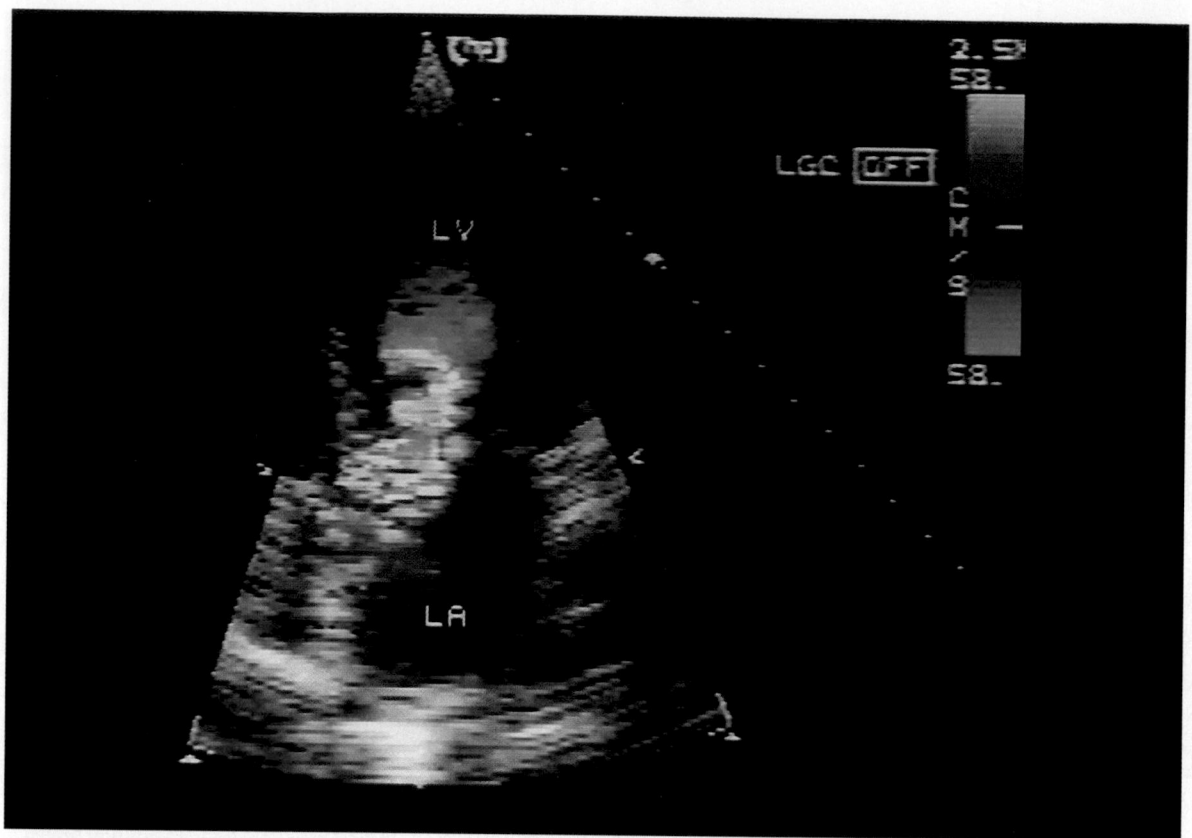

Plate 43 (Fig. 14-122*B*) Apical five-chamber view of discrete subaortic stenosis with color flow Doppler, demonstrating aliasing and proximal flow convergence in the left ventricular outflow tract. LV = left ventricle; LA = left atrium.

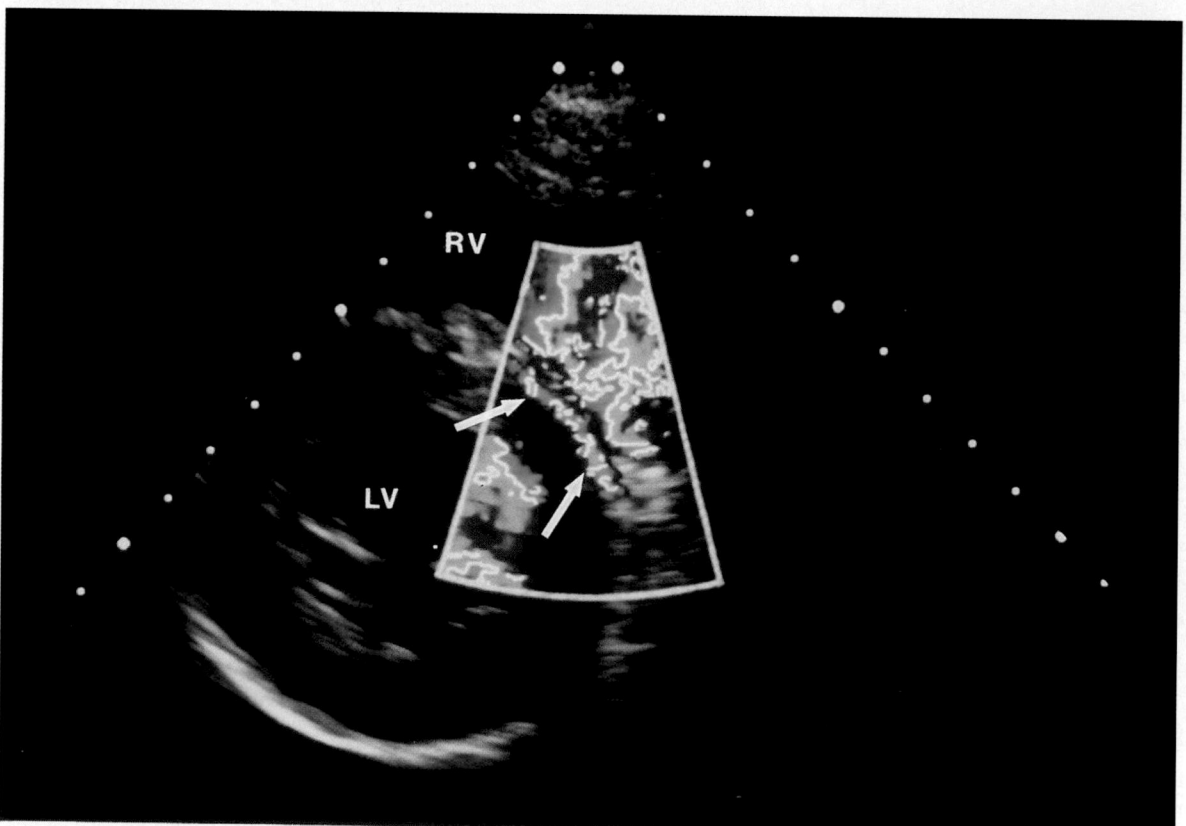

Plate 44 (Fig. 14-141) Transthoracic short-axis image of a coronary artery within the interventricular septum (*arrows*). LA = left ventricle; RV = right ventricle.

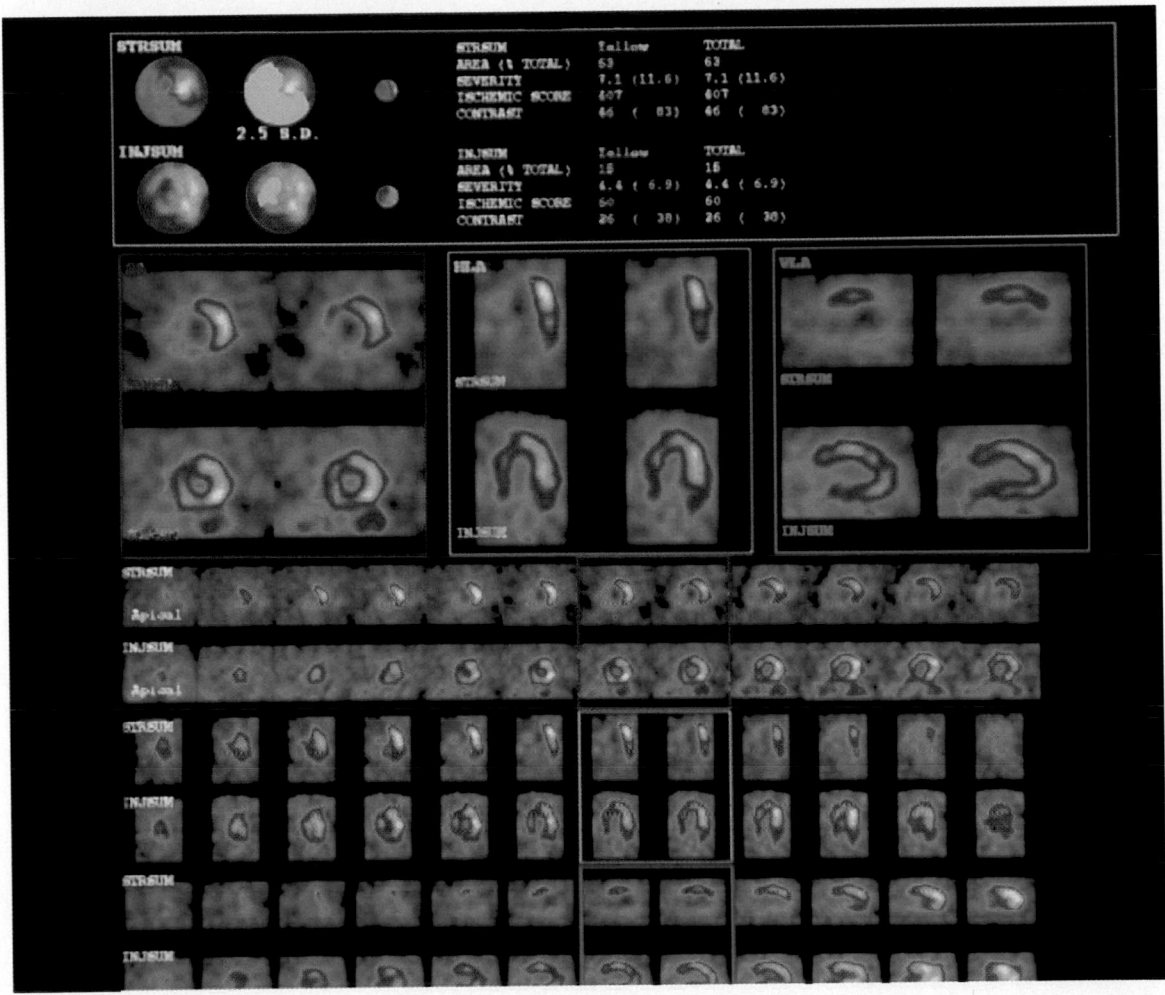

Plate 45 (Fig. 17-8) This patient is a 47-year-old man with a previous history of coronary artery disease (CAD) and myocardial infarction (MI). He exercised for 7 METS (metabolic equivalents of exercise) on the Bruce protocol to 76 percent of age-predicted maximum heart rate with no chest discomfort, but he had an abnormal ECG-ST. Gated planar Tl[201] images acquired simultaneously in the 45° LAO and 45° RAO projections showed abnormal wall motion of the septum. Quantitative bull's-eye images include the normal file (*left column*), the patient data (*second column from left*), the standard deviation map (*second from right*), and the patient data with abnormal area indicated by the blackened area (at 2.5 SD below the normal file). Row 1 shows the stress data; row 2 shows the reinjection images; and row 3 shows the reversibility maps. The graphic overlay (*right*) relates the defect region to the approximate distributions of coronary arteries.

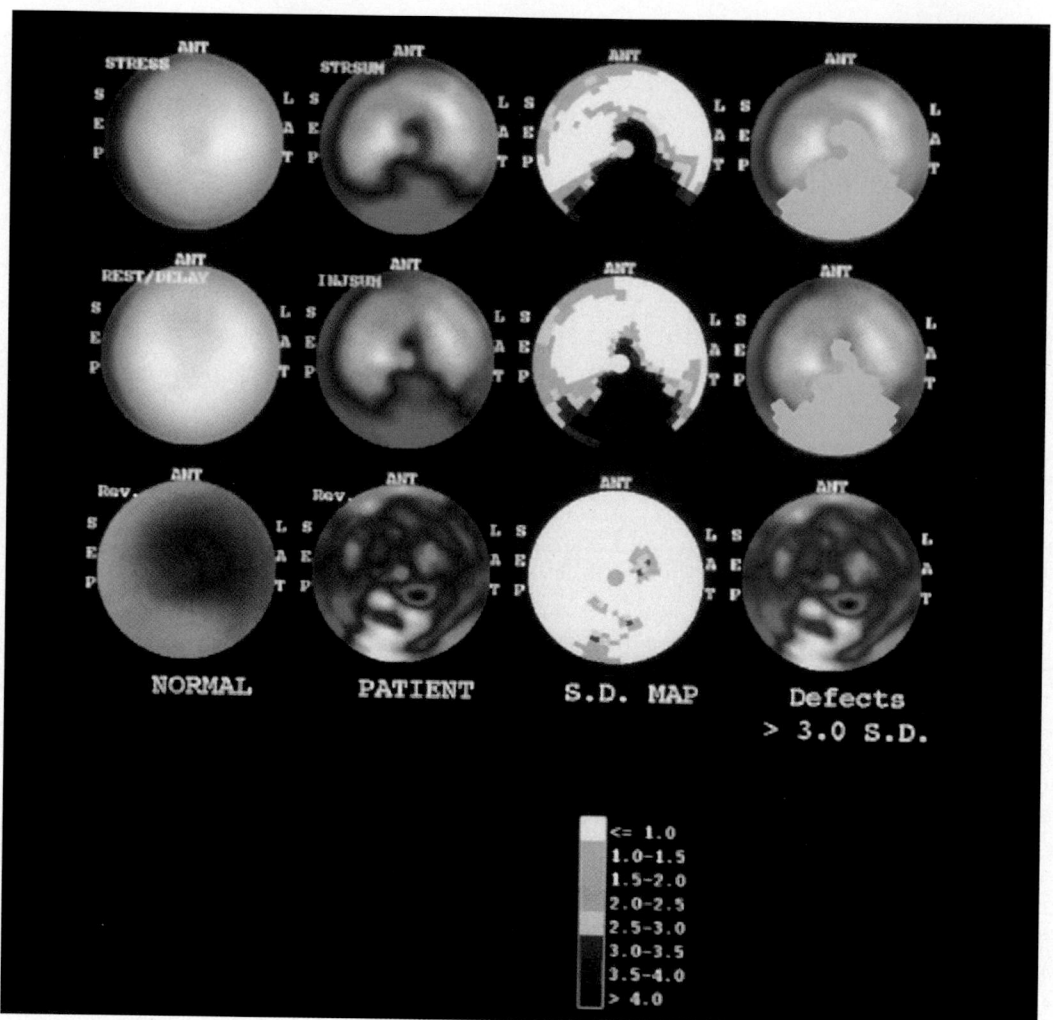

Plate 46 (Fig. 17-9) For the patient shown in the previous figure, the summary review screen from the INSPECT program for quantitative analysis and display of SPECT Tl^{201} myocardial perfusion imaging. Bull's-eye displays are shown (*top left*) along with quantitative information on extent and severity of defects (*top right*). Short-axis, vertical long-axis, and horizontal long-axis slices are displayed in subsequent rows, with stress images on top and reinjection images on the bottom. Quantitative analysis shows a large defect (63 percent of the left ventricle); the anteroseptal and apical portions of the defect are fixed, and the inferoseptal and inferolateral defects are reversible on rest/reinjection images. Consistent with the SPECT images, cardiac catheterization revealed an anterior wall dyskinetic region, 100-percent occlusion of the left anterior descending cornonary artery, and a 70-percent stenosis of the right coronary artery.

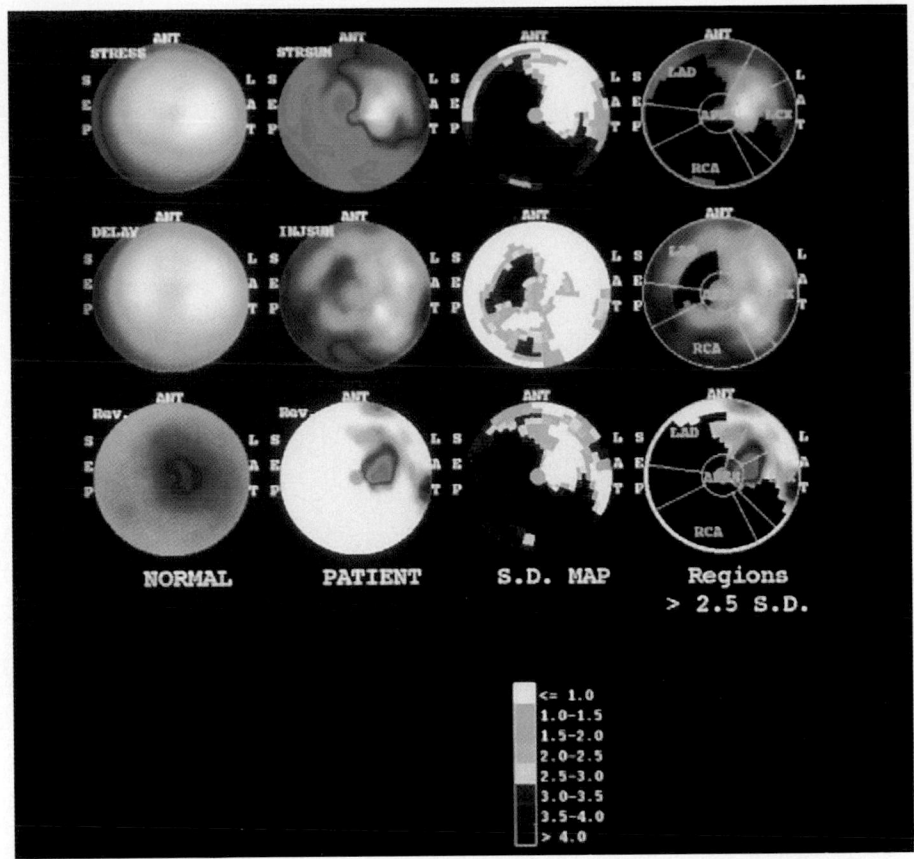

Plate 47 (Fig. 17-10) This patient is a 75-year-old woman with a previous myocardial infarction. She exercised to 4 METS on the Bruce protocol to 122 percent of maximum predicted heart rate with equivocal ECG-ST and no chest discomfort. Gated planar Tl^{201} images acquired simultaneously in the 45° LAO and 45° RAO projections showed abnormal wall motion of the inferolateral wall. SPECT Tl^{201} images (*top row*) showed a large defect on stress (41 percent of left ventricle) with no change on reinjection images (*second row*).

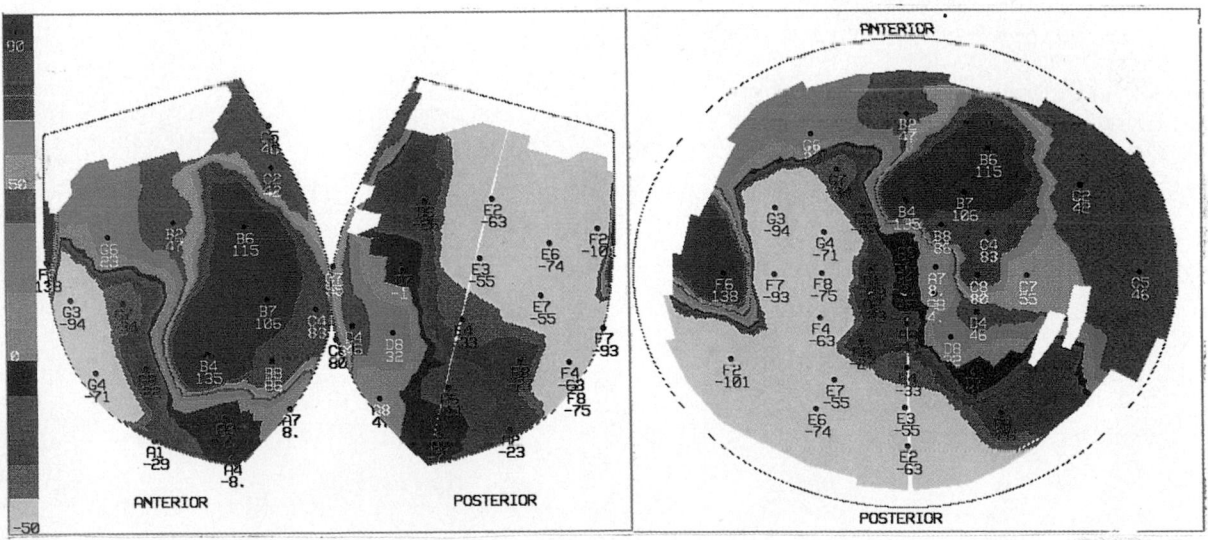

Plate 48 (Fig. 27-5) Computerized epicardial activation map recorded with a multielectrode array during a surgical procedure for sustained monomorphic ventricular tachycardia. Ventricular tachycardia has been induced, and the sites of activation are expressed (numbers in milliseconds) with respect to a reference site of activation located on the free wall of the right ventricle. The earliest activation with respect to the reference site is shown in light teal (e.g., A8 = 4 ms after reference site activation). The activation times preceding activation of the reference site are shown in yellow (earliest), orange, and red (closest to activation of the reference site). Activation sites that follow the reference site are shown in dark green, blue, and purple. The map provides the sequence of activation during VT. Times are in milliseconds.

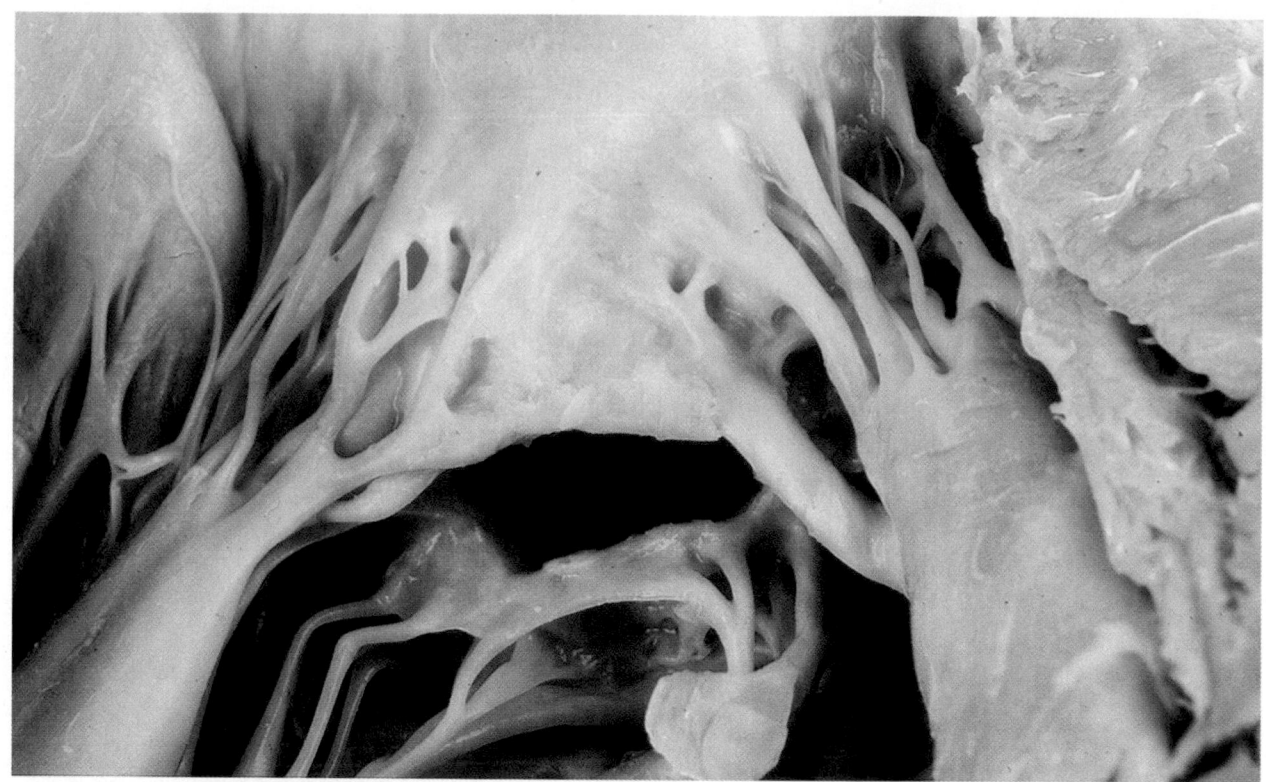

Plate 49 (Fig. 64-7) Anatomic example of rheumatic MR. Note the thickening of the leaflet and chordae and the retraction of the mitral tissue. (Courtesy of Dr. W. D. Edwards.)

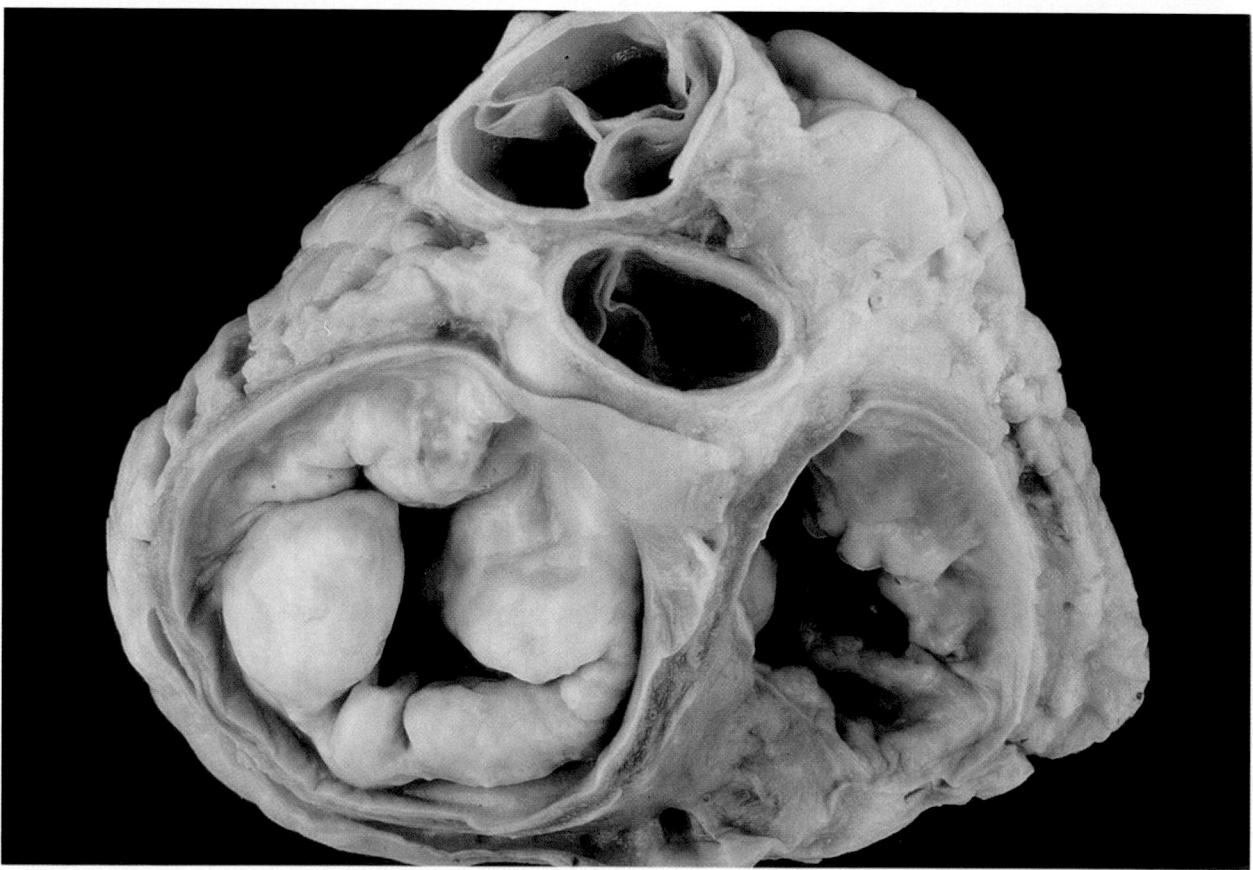

Plate 50 (Fig.64-8) Anatomic example of MR due to mitral valve prolapse seen from the atrial view (*the mitral orifice is on the left of picture*). Note the redundancy of the leaflets with excess tissue. (Courtesy of Dr. W. D. Edwards.)

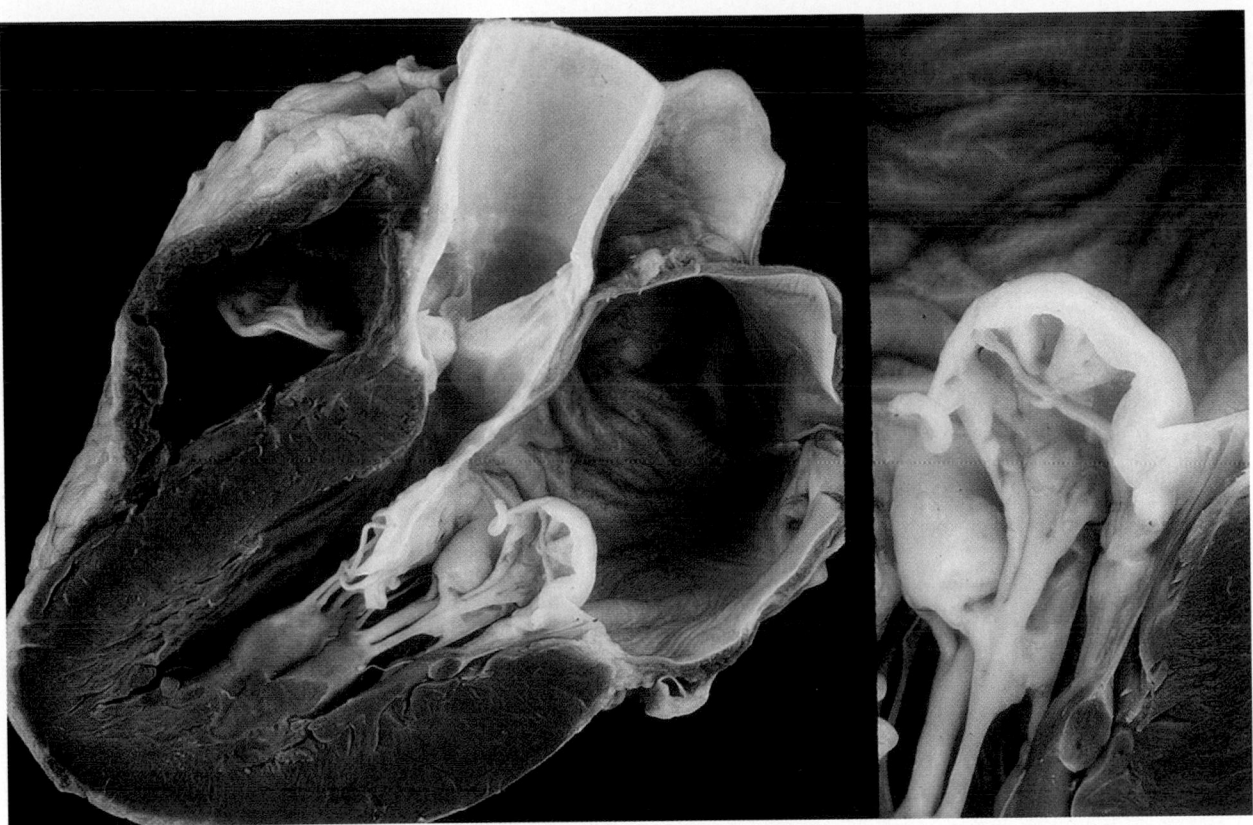

Plate 51 (Fig. 64-9) Anatomic example of a flail posterior leaflet with ruptured chord. On the right of the picture, close-up view of the ruptured chord. Otherwise the left atrium is enlarged, and the valvular tissue normal. (Courtesy of Dr. W. D. Edwards.)

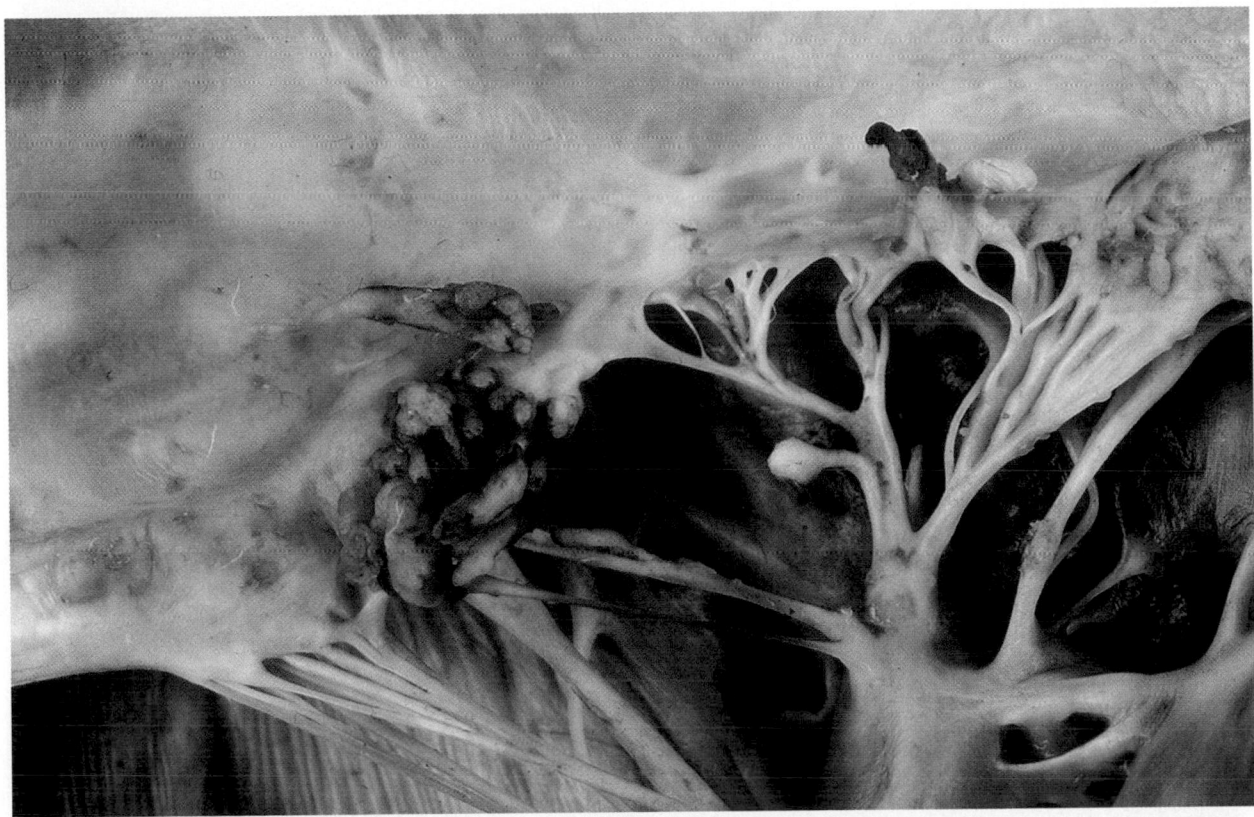

Plate 52 (Fig. 64-10) Anatomic example of MR due to endocarditis. Note the vegetations of the anterior leaflet and the ruptured chords. (Courtesy of Dr. W. D. Edwards.)

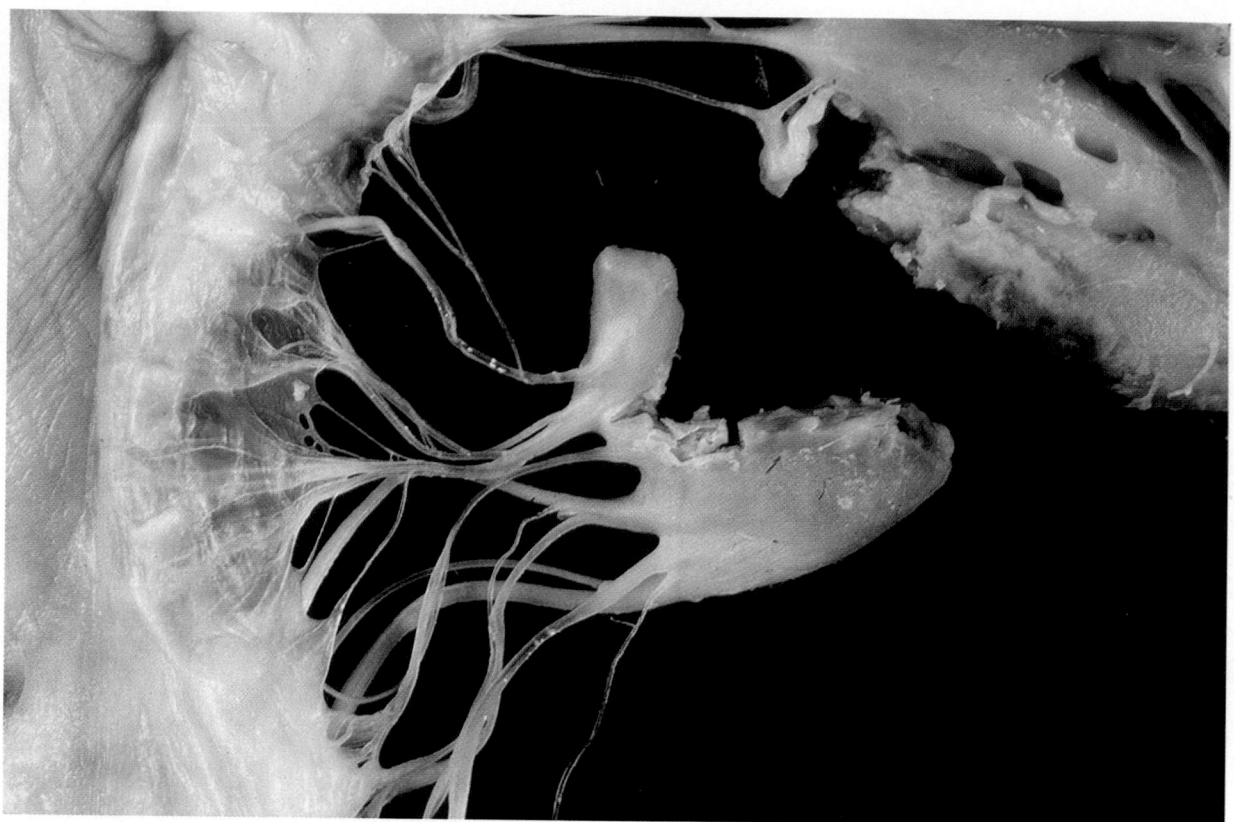

Plate 53 (Fig. 64-11) Anatomic example of a ruptured posterior papillary muscle. Note the normal valvular tissue otherwise. (Courtesy of Dr. W. D. Edwards.)

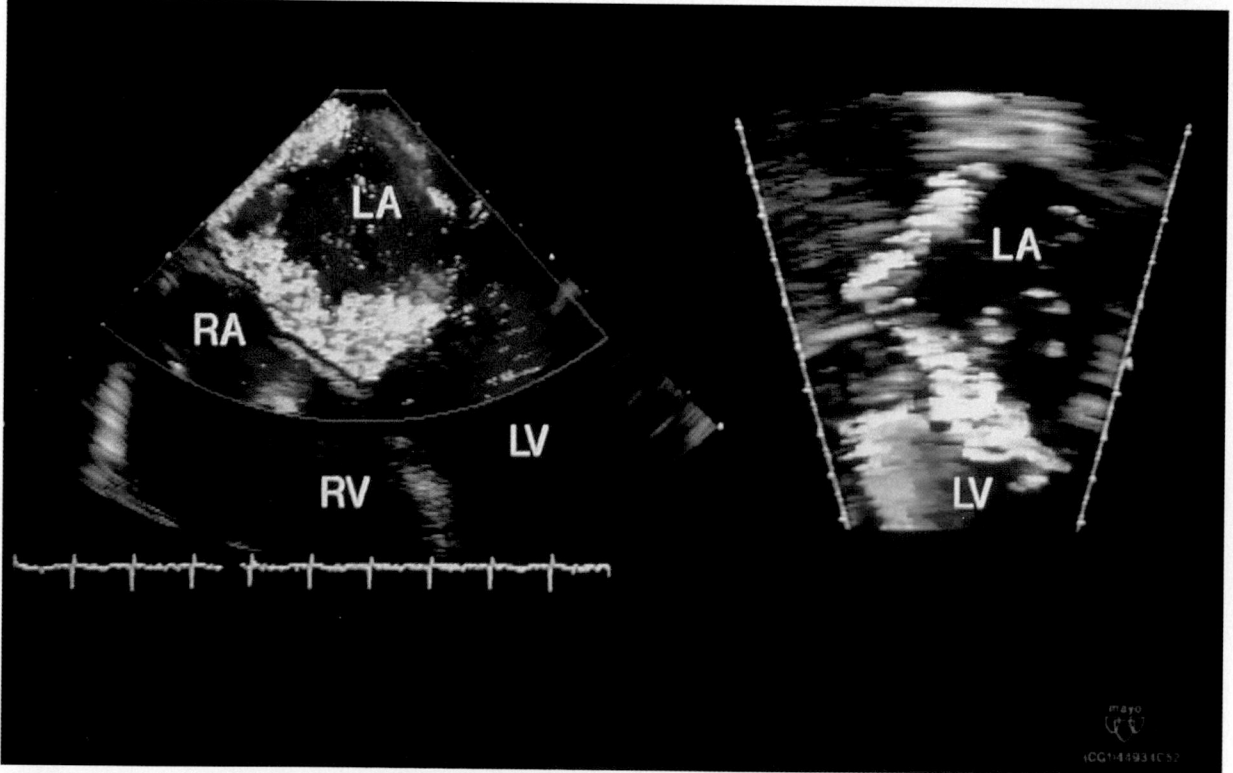

Plate 54 (Fig. 64-19) Color flow imaging of an eccentric jet (*flail posterior leaflet*). *Left:* Transesophageal (*horizontal plane*) echocardiography. *Right:* Transthoracic echocardiography. Note that with both modalities the jet is thinned, impinging on the atrial wall and tending to underestimate this severe regurgitation.

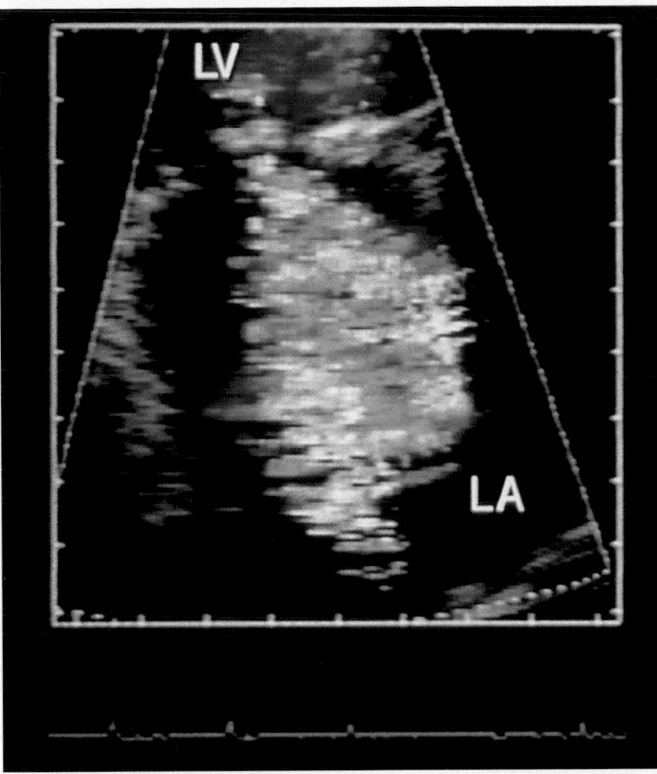

Plate 55 (Fig. 64-20) Color flow imaging of a central jet of a functional mitral regurgitation by transthoracic echocardiography. Note that the jet is free, expands in the left atrium, and tends to overestimate this moderate regurgitation.

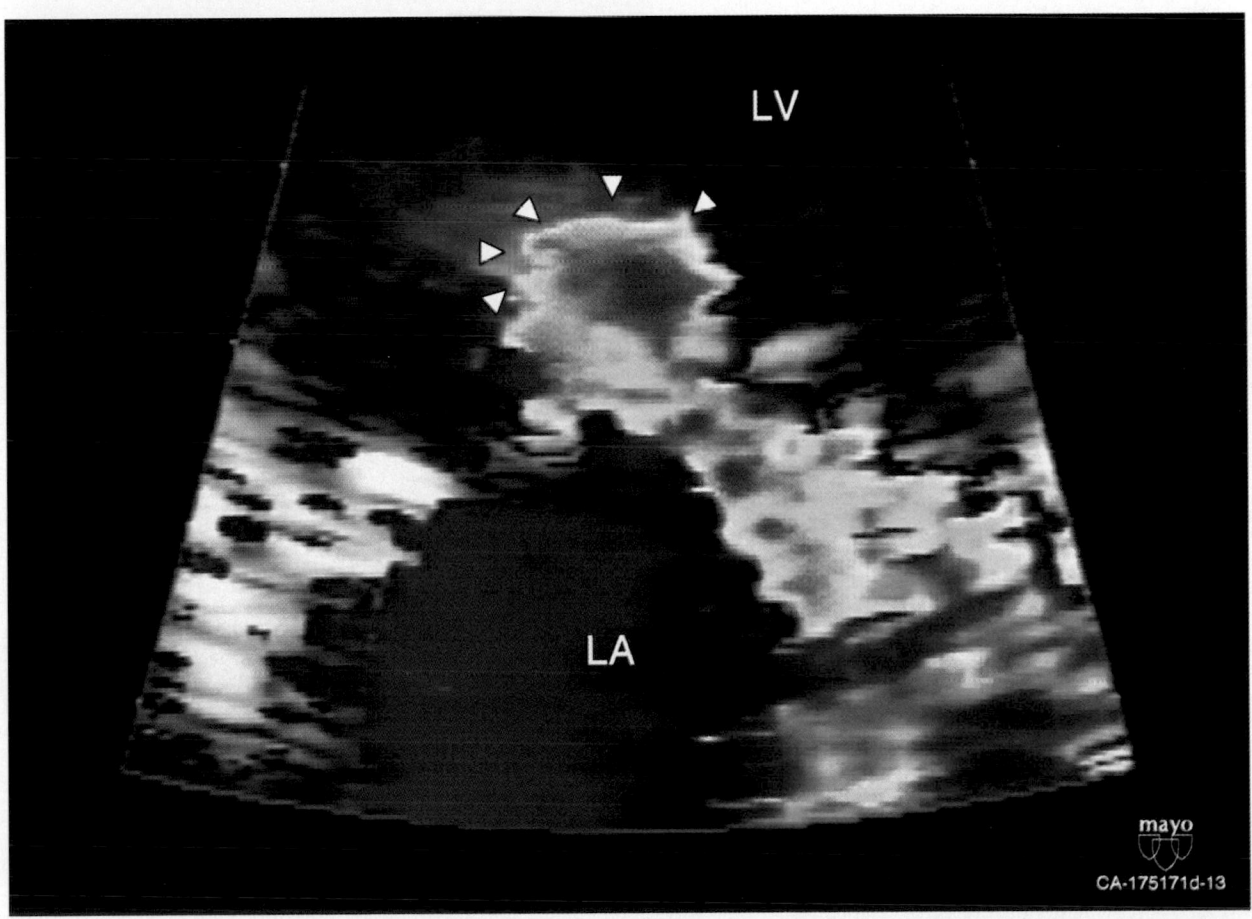

Plate 56 (Fig. 64-22) Color flow imaging of the proximal flow convergence of a mitral regurgitation due to a flail posterior leaflet (by transthoracic echocardiography). The downward baseline shift of the color flow scale enlarges the size of the flow convergence, which is easily measurable.

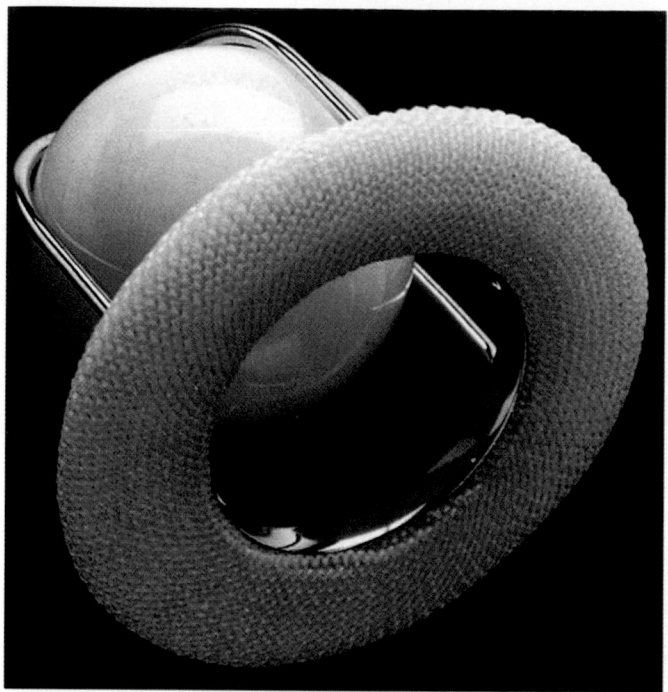

Plate 57 (Fig. 67-1) Starr-Edwards ball valve—aortic. The aortic valve has three struts, and the mitral valve has four struts. The sewing ring is thickly upholstered to improve coaptation with irregular tissue beds.

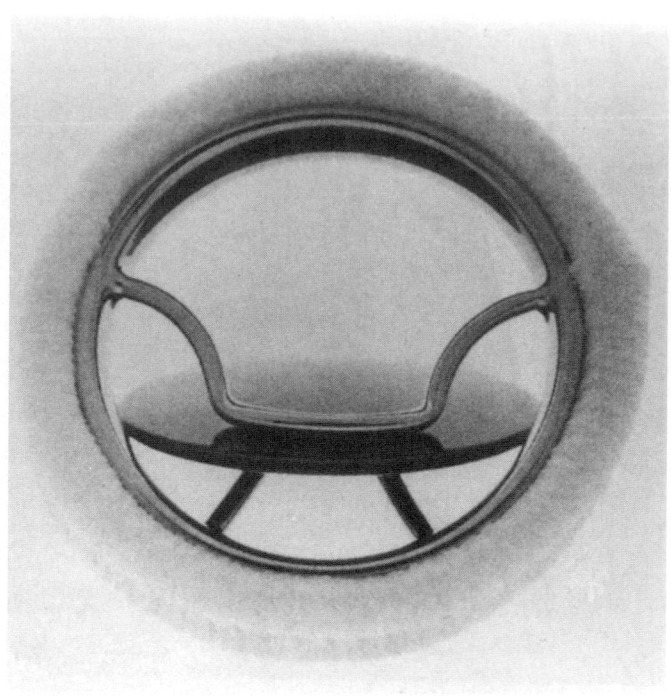

Plate 58 (Fig. 67-2) Björk-Shiley tilting valve-spherical disk model. This is *not* the valve that had strut fracture problem.

A

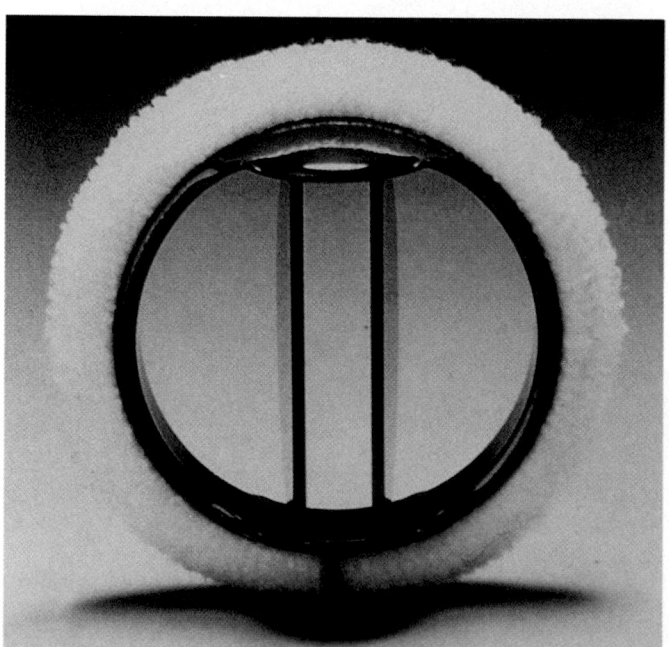

B

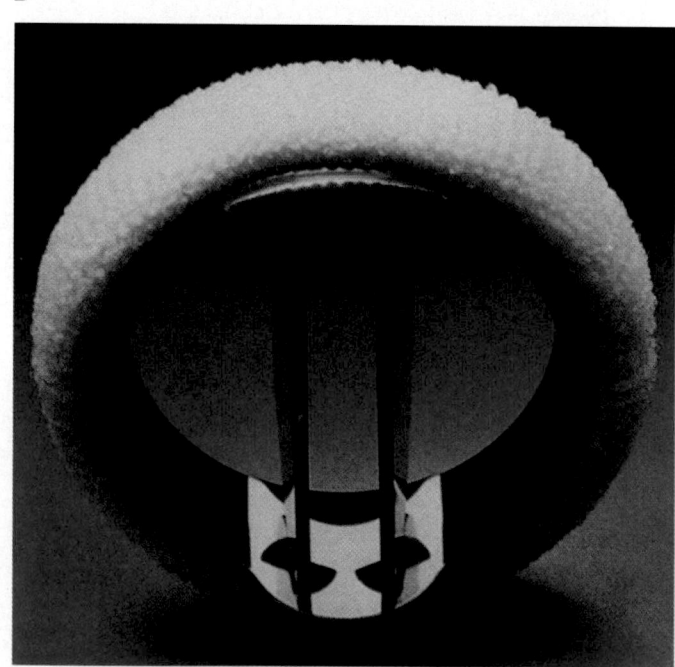

Plate 59 (Fig. 67-3) St. Jude bileaflet valve. The housing of the valve is a cylindrically shaped piece of pyrolitic carbon with two rounded tabs, called *pivot guards,* which project up from the inflow side. The inside surfaces of these tabs are flat and contain two butterfly-shaped indentations that retain the leaflets. Small "ears" at the end of each diameter of the thin hemispherical leaflet fit into these indentations, which secure the leaflets in the housing and define their limits of travel.

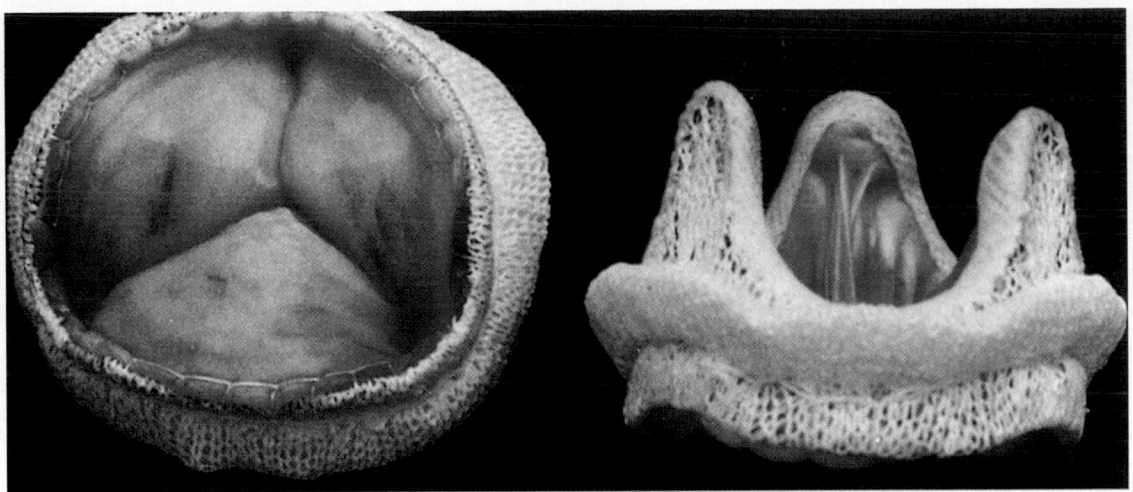

Plate 60 (Fig. 67-4) Carpentier-Edwards porcine bioprosthesis. (From Grunkemeier G et al[85]. Reproduced by permission)

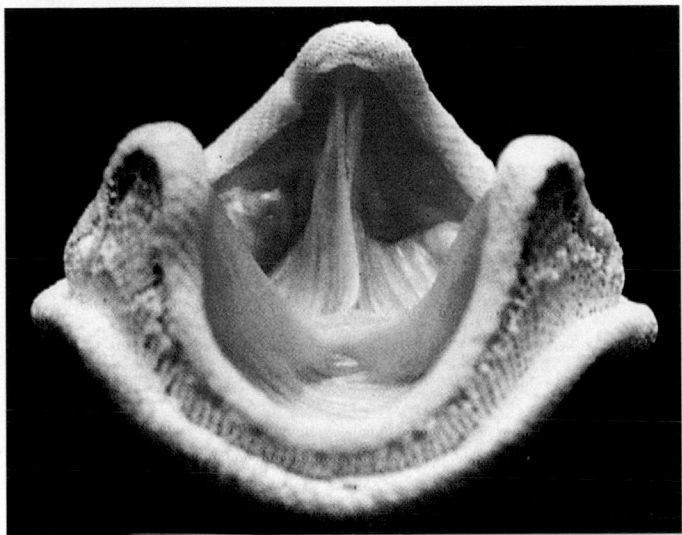

Plate 61 (Fig. 67-5) Carpentier-Edwards SupraAnnular aortic porcine bioprosthesis. (From Grunkemeier G et al[85]. Reproduced by permission)

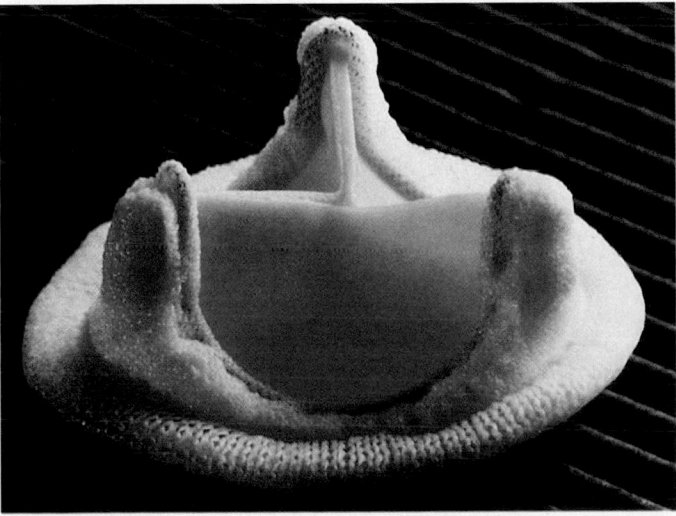

Plate 62 (Fig. 67-6) Carpentier-Edwards bovine pericardial bioprosthesis. (From Grunkemeier G et al[85]. Reproduced by permission)

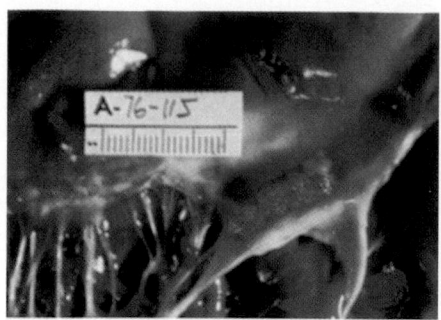

Plate 63 (Fig. 82-3) Typical vegetation of nonbacterial thrombotic endocarditis, found at necropsy in a cachectic patient who died with disseminated lung cancer.

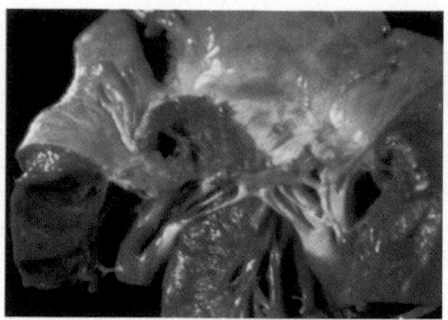

Plate 64 (Fig. 82-5) Typical vegetation of bacterial endocarditis, complicated by perforation of the anterior mitral valve leaflet. Note that the valve shows preexisting chronic rheumatic disease, with thickening, deformity, and fusion of chordae tendineae.

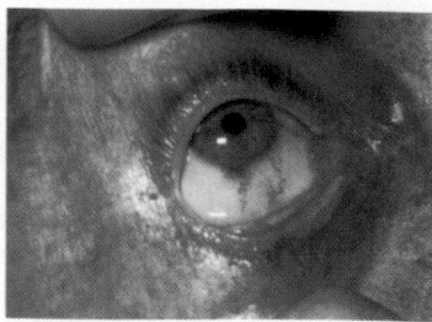

Plate 65 (Fig. 82-7) Typical conjunctival petechia in a patient with SBE due to *Streptococcus sanguis*.

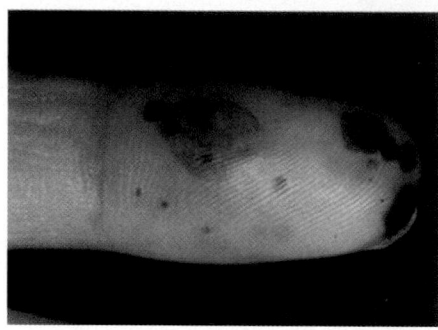

Plate 66 (Fig. 82-8) Ischemic, hemorrhagic, and pustular lesions on the extremities in acute *Staphylococcus aureus* endocarditis.

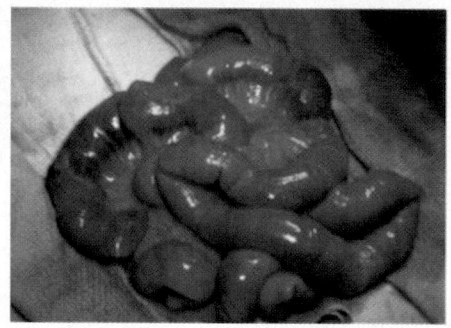

Plate 67 (Fig. 82-9) Segmental ischemia and necrosis in the gut, presenting as acute abdomen.

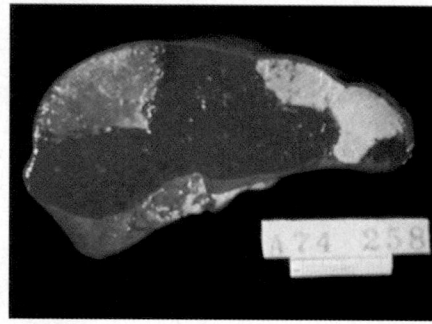

Plate 68 (Fig. 82-10) Infarctions in the spleen.

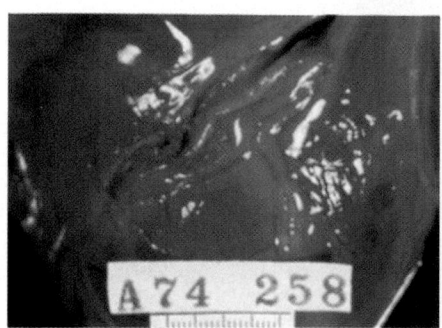

Plate 69 (Fig 82-11) An infected embolus in a coronary artery.

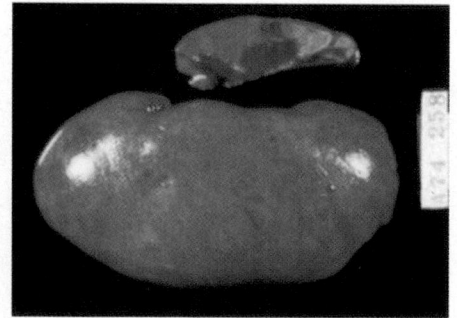

Plate 70 (Fig. 82-12) Kidney from a case of subacute bacterial endocarditis, showing two abnormalities: (1) typical ischemic infarctions due to emboli and (2) swelling and petechiae ("flea-bitten kidney") due to immune-complex glomerulonephritis.

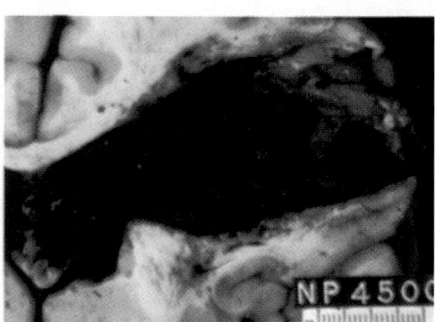

Plate 71 (Fig. 82-13) Massive cerebral hemorrhage with intraventricular extension due to rupture of a small, peripheral mycotic aneurysm. The patient had been *bacteriologically* cured of *Staphylococcus epidermidis* endocarditis several weeks previously. Cultures of the blood, valve, and aneurysm taken at necropsy were negative.

CORONARY
HEART DISEASE

38

THE NATURAL HISTORY OF ATHEROSCLEROTIC CORONARY HEART DISEASE: A HISTORICAL PERSPECTIVE

Gottlieb C. Friesinger II / J. Willis Hurst

DEFINITIONS

The description of the clinical events caused by a disease in *untreated* patients is referred to as the *natural history* of the disease. Patients may experience no clinical signs or symptoms while the disease progresses, signs and symptoms that are characteristic of the disease, or a sudden or gradual death. The condition itself may last for minutes, hours, days, months, or years—and the patient may die of a noncardiac cause or causes.

Obviously, it is not possible to determine the value of medical or surgical treatment unless the natural history of the disease is known. Accordingly, this is an extremely important aspect of medical knowledge.

The simple presence of atherosclerosis of the coronary arteries is not the subject of this chapter. This chapter deals with the natural history of atherosclerotic coronary heart disease. The addition of the words *heart disease* to the descriptive term implies that the atheromatous process has progressed to the point that it interferes with coronary artery blood flow. When this occurs, the myocardium becomes ischemic or necrotic.

The characteristics of the clinical syndromes caused by atherosclerotic coronary heart disease must also be defined, because the natural history of each syndrome is different. From a clinical point of view, it is useful to divide atherosclerotic coronary heart disease into stable and unstable subsets. All subsets may have silent manifestations of ischemia, arrhythmias, or ventricular dysfunction with or without concomitant symptomatic episodes.

The most common stable syndrome is *stable angina pectoris*. This subset is defined as angina pectoris in which there has been no change in the precipitating events, the duration of attacks, or the frequency of the episodes during the previous 60 days (see Chap. 45).

The unstable syndromes consist of unstable angina pectoris, myocardial infarction with and without complications, and sudden death. *Unstable angina pectoris* is defined as angina pectoris occurring for the first time, angina pectoris that has appeared during the last 60 days, stable angina that has accelerated in frequency, and prolonged episodes of angina pectoris that last longer than formerly or that are precipitated by less effort (see Chap. 46). *Myocardial infarction* can be diagnosed in patients who have chest discomfort that is characteristic of myocardial ischemia but who exhibit objective evidence of myocardial necrosis (see Chap. 47). *Sudden and unexpected death* is defined as instantaneous death with or without previous evidence of atherosclerotic coronary heart disease; it may result from acute ischemia or be the result of past necrosis with scarring (see Chaps. 27, 36, and 47).

"Silent" or painless myocardial ischemia may occur in patients who are completely asymptomatic and have never been symptomatic, have had a previous myocardial infarction, or have angina pectoris but also have episodes of painless myocardial ischemia (see Chap. 45). Similarly, arrhythmias and ventricular dysfunction may be completely asymptomatic.

These definitions must be kept in mind as one analyzes the reports that deal with the natural history of the various syndromes.

DIFFICULTIES IN STUDYING THE NATURAL HISTORY OF ATHEROSCLEROTIC CORONARY HEART DISEASE

Atherosclerotic coronary heart disease is a chronic condition. Once present, it remains with the patient for life. The disease may be active and then become quiescent and later become active again.

Until the 1950s, *no treatment* was available for atherosclerotic coronary heart disease and its complications except nitroglycerin, oxygen, digitalis, quinidine, the advice to avoid the effort that caused angina, and the prescription of a long period of rest in bed when a "heart attack" occurred. Because treatment was limited, it would seem that an analysis of the reports about the disease published prior to the 1950s should enable one to establish the natural history of the disease. The problem prior to the 1950s was that *the diagnosis of the disease was not always correct.* Undoubtedly, many patients who were thought to have angina pectoris due to coronary atherosclerosis did not have it. This occurred because diagnostic methods were limited to an analysis of the patient's symptoms, interpretation of the electrocardiogram during exercise, and examination of the coronary arteries at autopsy. Myocardial infarction was both underdiagnosed and overdiagnosed. This was the case because the recognition of myocardial infarction depended on the results of the physical examination, the interpretation of the electrocardiogram, the temperature curve, the white blood count, the sedimentation rate, and the results of autopsy.

After the 1950s, *diagnostic methods improved* and valuable objective information became available. Cardiac enzymes could be measured, electrocardiographic interpretation improved, and the electrocardiographic exercise stress test was used more frequently. About the same time, however, *treatment also improved:* longer-acting nitrates were utilized, procainamide was used, new pressor agents became available, anticoagulants were used, coronary care units were developed, coronary arteriography was commonly performed, and nuclear techniques were beginning to be used. Still later, beta blockers, calcium antagonists, new antiarrhythmic drugs, coronary bypass surgery, coronary angioplasty and other catheter-based treatment interventions, thrombolytic therapy, cardiac pacemakers, external and internal defibrillators, and cardiac transplantation became fully developed, and diagnostic methods, including coronary arteriography and nuclear studies, became more refined. *Accordingly, the advances made in diagnostic methods were paralleled by advances made in effective treatment.* Because of this, it was not possible to study the natural history of the disease; clinical trials were designed to compare the results of a new therapy with the "best therapy of the day." For example, clinical trials were designed to compare the results of coronary bypass surgery with the results of the best medical therapy of the era. All patients in the clinical trials received what was believed to be the best treatment of the day. While this masked the natural history of the disease,

it was considered to be good news, because both the medical and surgical treatment of the disease improved dramatically after the 1950s. In addition, even when the trials included large numbers of patients, they represented a selected (biased) population in reference to natural history, and generalization may be problematic. This is particularly true for the elderly and women, who are regularly underrepresented in studies.

THE RESULTS OF OBSERVATIONS MADE PRIOR TO THE FIFTIES

William Heberden first used the term *angina pectoris* in a lecture before the Royal College of Physicians in 1768. His classic article on the subject appeared in 1772 and should be reread at least annually.[1] Although he does not categorize the patients into the subsets of disease we currently recognize, one can identify the patients with stable angina pectoris, unstable angina pectoris, myocardial infarction, and sudden death in his report. He stated in his 1772 report that he had seen at least 20 men and 1 woman with the condition, and all of them were above the age of 50 years. Of his 21 patients, 6 died suddenly.

After Heberden died, his son published Heberden's manuscript, in which he described the clinical features of "nearly a hundred people with this disorder, out of which number there have been three women."[2]

Heberden recognized the seriousness of the symptoms because more than one-third of his original 21 patients died. It is also highly likely that some of his patients did not have atherosclerotic coronary heart disease. This question will, of course, never be answered, because when Heberden made his observations, he had no idea that the symptoms he described were due to atherosclerotic coronary heart disease. This giant step in understanding was made by Jenner in 1772, when he concluded that angina pectoris was caused by disease of the coronary arteries. Jenner wrote about his observation in a letter to Parry; Parry later credited Jenner in his own publication in 1799.[3]

Little else was written about the disease until J. B. Herrick described "Clinical Features of *Sudden Obstruction of the Coronary Arteries*" (emphasis added) in 1912.[4] Herrick pointed out the following:

> Obstruction of a coronary artery or any of its large branches has long been regarded as a serious accident. Several events contributed toward the prevalence of the view that this condition was almost always suddenly fatal.... But there are reasons for believing that even large branches of the coronary arteries may be occluded—at times acutely occluded—without resulting in death, at least without death in the immediate future....[4]

Herrick's description of the clinical features associated with coronary thrombosis and the events prior to and after the attack should accompany one's annual reading of Heberden's description of angina pectoris.

Although physicians in general ignored Herrick's message, a few scholars did heed his advice. Among them were Drs. Paul White of Boston and Paul Wood of London. Their books on heart disease offer not only the results of their own meticulous observations but also their descriptions of others, observations that influenced their views about the natural history of atherosclerotic coronary heart disease.[5,6]

In 1951, Paul White emphasized that

The condition, unsuspected in life, may be discovered only on postmortem examination after a noncardiac death in ripe old age; or symptoms and signs may be marked and obvious in a fulminating acute catastrophe of severe coronary occlusion, cutting off the blood supply to a large mass of heart muscle, that may kill in a few hours or a few days. The prognosis depends not only on the degree and speed of involvement of the myocardium but also on the treatment, the reserve strength of the heart, and complications.[7]

The definitions of stable and unstable syndromes, and silent myocardial ischemia offered earlier in this chapter, were not used in the long follow-up of symptomatic patients who were observed during the first half of the twentieth century. This, of course, makes it impossible to use the data to establish an accurate natural history for each of the subsets of the disease. Despite this limitation, it is useful to review the observations of White, Wood, and others.

In 1943, White, Bland, and Miskall reported that the average life expectancy from the onset of *angina pectoris* is 9 to 10 years. About 10 percent of the patients lived almost 20 years.[8]

In 1947 Montgomery et al. reported the results of a 10-year follow-up of 3440 patients with *angina pectoris* and discovered that 405 of these patients were alive at the end of the follow-up period.[9]

In 1952, Block et al. reported the 5- to 23-year follow-up of 6882 patients with *angina pectoris* and found that 15 percent of these patients died in the first year and about 9 percent each year thereafter.[10] The investigators emphasized that the resting electrocardiogram added powerful predictive information.

In 1946, Parker et al. reported that women had a better prognosis than men and that patients over the age of 40 years fared better than patients under that age.[11] These observations have not been supported by data that have became available during the last two decades (see discussion below).

In 1937, Harold Feil wrote a short, classic article entitled "Preliminary Pain in Coronary Thrombosis."[12] He observed 15 patients with coronary thrombosis; 14 of them had evidence of myocardial infarction. The patients had mild attacks of substernal pain preceding the clinical picture of coronary thrombosis by hours or days—usually from 12 to 48 h. This syndrome of *preliminary pain* was later called *coronary insufficiency*.

In 1956, Paul Wood commented on *acute coronary insufficiency*.[13] By then, the term was used to designate patients with new-onset angina pectoris or those with prolonged episodes of chest discomfort due to myocardial ischemia who had no objective signs of myocardial infarction. The term *preinfarction angina pectoris* was also used to designate this group of patients. Today, this subset of patients is commonly labeled as having *unstable angina pectoris*. Wood pointed out that the results of long-term follow-up studies had not been completed on such patients.[14] It was well known, as Feil had pointed out earlier, that such patients commonly had a myocardial infarction within hours, days, or weeks following the onset of unstable symptoms and that the mortality of patients with acute coronary insufficiency was greater than in patients with stable angina pectoris.[12]

In 1956, Wood described the natural history of *myocardial infarction* as follows.[14] He quoted Yater et al., who, in 1948, reported the follow-up of 866 relatively young patients who had myocardial infarction. Some 16 percent of the patients died instantly and another 10 percent died within 15 min.[15] Wood concluded that at least one-third of all patients with acute coronary artery occlusion died of ventricular fibrillation or cardiac asystole.[14] Such patients do not live long enough to be admitted to the hospital.

Wood pointed out that *arrhythmias* also occurred in hospitalized patients with myocardial infarction and that many of the arrhythmias jeopardized the patient's life. He reported that ventricular tachycardia occurred in 2 percent of patients, ventricular fibrillation in 10 percent, and complete heart block in 1 percent.[14,16]

Wood estimated that *cardiogenic shock* occurred in 10 to 15 percent of patients with myocardial infarction; he quoted Selzer's study indicating that the condition was fatal in two-thirds to three-fourths of the patients.[14,17]

Wood reported that *congestive heart failure* occurred during the 28 days following a myocardial infarction in 10 to 15 percent of patients and that it was the cause of death in 3 to 5 percent. Little was written about the heart failure caused by ischemic cardiomyopathy.

Thromboembolic lesions were reported to occur with alarming frequency. Hellerstein and Martin reported that thromboembolic episodes were clinically recognized in 20 percent of patients with myocardial infarction and that 45 percent of autopsied patients had emboli.[18] Some 23.5 percent of the emboli were to the lungs, 14.4 percent to the kidneys, 8.8 percent to the spleen, 7.7 percent to the brain, 5.5 percent to the peripheral arteries, 1.9 percent to the mesenteric arteries, and 0.5 percent to the carotid artery or aorta.[18]

Cardiac rupture occurred in 1.5 to 3 percent of patients with myocardial infarction according to Oblath et al.[19]

Rupture of the papillary muscle was considered to be rare and, when present, caused the death of the patient.[19]

Wood reported that *rupture of the interventricular septum* occurred "occasionally" and that more than half of the patients died.[20]

Wartman and Hellerstein reported that *left ventricular aneurysm* developed in 22 percent of fatal cases of myocardial infarction but was clinically recognized in less than half of the patients.[21]

Wood reported that 10 percent of patients with myocardial infarction had a *pericardial friction rub*.[22]

As pointed out above, in 1956, Paul Wood concluded from his own observations and the work of others that about one-quarter of patients with an *acute coronary event died suddenly*.

The condition referred to as *silent myocardial ischemia* was not discussed to any degree prior to the last two decades.

Electrocardiographic abnormalities were used to predict the future of patients with symptomatic atherosclerotic coronary heart disease. In 1952, Block et al. reported on 6882 patients with symptomatic atherosclerotic coronary heart disease. They found the following 10-year mortalities: 47 percent in patients with normal electrocardiograms; 75 percent in patients with atherosclerotic coronary heart disease with abnormal Q waves or disease related T-wave abnormalities; 75 percent in patients with inferior myocardial ischemia; and 90 percent in patients with anterior or lateral myocardial ischemia.[10] These observations presaged the development of the concept that left ventricular dysfunction is a powerful predictive factor—the electrocardiographic abnormalities being markers for past infarction and scarring.

In later years, studies were reported describing the use of abnormalities found in the stress electrocardiogram to predict the natural history of the disease.

RESULTS OF OBSERVATIONS MADE AFTER THE 1950s

Sones performed the first coronary arteriogram in October 1958. Although the initial procedure was performed inadvertently, Sones's prepared mind sensed its potential value immediately. The work was reported in *Modern Concepts of Cardiovascular Disease* in 1962.[23] This diagnostic procedure enabled physicians to identify the location and extent of the atherosclerotic plaques in the coronary arteries, and left ventricular angiography made it possible to determine the ejection fraction of the left ventricle. These two measurements were then used to study the natural history of the disease. This was a giant step forward in diagnostic work in that very useful objective data could be obtained in a living human being. A great lesson was learned: physicians soon discovered that they were not always correct in their prearteriographic diagnoses of the presence of absence of atherosclerotic coronary heart disease based on the interpretation of clinical data.

Coronary arteriography and left ventriculography revolutionized the clinician's approach to diagnosis. Clinicians moved from considering primarily subjective data (complaints such as angina and dyspnea) to semiquantitative objective data that, in turn, broadened the context of the natural history. Physicians also learned that objective data may be more powerful than subjective data in the evaluation of a patient and that the *total* evidence should be considered when diagnosis, prognosis, and natural history are contemplated. In day-to-day practice, physicians moved from asking the local expert diagnostician to see those of their patients with chest pain that they had difficulty

in diagnosing to ordering a coronary arteriogram and left ventriculogram or performing a functional test.

As pointed out in the initial part of this chapter, medical treatment also improved after the 1950s. Accordingly, randomized clinical trials never included a group of patients who received none of the new, effective medications; all patients in the trials received the best of modern therapy. Therefore, a new procedure being studied was randomly assigned to a group of patients who also received medical treatment. The result was then compared to the results found in a group of patients who received only the medical treatment. Analysis of the data became even more difficult when the "best" medical treatment changed during the period of the trial, as new information revealed the value of another medication.

Some Important General Considerations

The influence of age, gender, and socioeconomic factors was studied more extensively in the decades following the 1950s.

AGE

The majority of patients with atherosclerotic coronary heart disease are more than 65 years old; older patients have higher mortality and more complications. Acute myocardial infarction dramatically illustrates this problem.[24,25] Mortality under the age of 60 is low, but it increases steadily with age and increases dramatically after the age of 70. Comorbidity is often cited as a reason for the high rates of mortality and complications. While this is undoubtedly true, the excellent study of Maggioni et al.—of the age-related mortality among patients with first myocardial infarction treated with thrombolysis—revealed that age was a powerful independent predictor of in-hospital and postdischarge mortality rates.[26]

Age-related changes in the cardiovascular system and other organs make it reasonable to assume that aging per se constitutes a major reason for the increased morbidity and mortality in older persons. These age-related changes include diastolic dysfunction, degenerative changes in the conduction system, reduced responses to catecholamine and sympathetic stimuli, and major alterations in the pharmacokinetics and pharmacodynamics of drugs. Such age-related changes have major implications for the response of older patients to the disease and its treatment.

The presentation of symptoms due to atherosclerotic coronary heart disease is often different in older patients than in younger ones. Silent infarction[27] (estimated to be 40 percent of all cases in patients above age 65) and painless presentations such as dyspnea, worsening heart failure, and central nervous system symptoms are much more frequent in older patients (see Chap. 47). These features must be taken into account in interpreting reports of natural history in older patients. In general, not only do more typical presentations provide for easier diagnosis, but they also portend more favorable prognosis in elderly patients.

Noninvasive tests of ventricular function, because of age-related diastolic dysfunction, and induced ischemia must also be interpreted differently in the elderly. Available data indicate that the ability to exercise to a reasonable level is a favorable prognostic feature, and such patients have substantially lower mortality than those not able to perform exercise tests. Noncardiac reasons for inability to exercise seem equally important to cardiac limitations. Changes in the ST segment of the electrocardiogram are much less predictive of events in older patients than in younger ones. Systematic unbiased data derived from echocardiographic and nuclear medicine tests are not available, so their incremental value is not known.

FEMALE GENDER

Cardiovascular disease is the most common cause of death in women in the United States. The relation of female gender to the development and prognosis of atherosclerotic coronary heart disease is complicated.[28] The powerful protective effect of the premenopausal state in preventing and postponing the condition is fully appreciated; women tend to develop atherosclerotic coronary heart disease approximately 10 years later than men.

Women are less vulnerable than men to sudden cardiac death and less likely to have myocardial infarcts as the first manifestation of atherosclerotic coronary heart disease. Typical and atypical symptoms of angina pectoris are less likely to be associated with significant epicardial coronary atherosclerosis in women, especially in those under the age of 60 or 65.[28,29] Functional tests[30-36] are associated with much higher false-positive rates in women than in men. Multiple studies have found the exercise-induced ST-segment shift to be falsely positive in women 40 to 60 percent of the time. The expected increase in exercise-induced ejection fraction occurs less often in normal women than in normal men. Although thallium perfusion studies are more sensitive and specific than exercise-induced ST-segment shifts, they are not as sensitive or predictive in women as in men, perhaps because of attenuation artifacts related to the breast and diaphragm.[30] Hence, the problems in diagnosing atherosclerotic coronary heart disease in women are substantial, making it critical that the accuracy of diagnosis be a part of any report discussing the natural history of this condition in women.

Complications are fewer in women after the onset of angina, but they may be more frequent after myocardial infarction.[37,38] However, since the disease occurs an average 10 years later in women and because women have a higher incidence of other risk factors and comorbid features—particularly hypertension, diabetes, and obesity—it is difficult to assess the effect of female gender per se. Acute myocardial infarction has been studied most extensively and estimates of the relative risk of women as opposed to men have varied from unity to as high as 1.5.[39-46]

There are multiple reports indicating a gender bias in reference to the use of diagnostic and therapeutic procedures, but interpretation is complicated by the possibility of overuse and overtreatment in low-risk men.[47-52] *The point has been clearly made, however; atherosclerotic coronary heart disease manifest as angina, infarct, and sudden death is as common in women after age 60 as it is in men.*

Socioeconomic Factors

There are abundant data indicating that the increase in death rate from any cause in both genders and in white and black Americans is related to a variety of socioeconomic features, particularly education and income. There has been the perception that conventional risk factors cluster in the lower socioeconomic groups and that this phenomenon can explain the increased incidence of atherosclerotic coronary heart disease.[53] However, only about 50 percent of atherosclerotic coronary heart disease can be explained by known risk factors. The socioeconomic status proved to be independent predictors in patients with established atherosclerotic coronary heart disease.[54] Adjusting for other variables, stable and postmyocardial infarction patients of higher socioeconomic status have a more favorable clinical course. Studies of longer duration, with adjustment for multiple known risk factors, demonstrate an increased relative risk for study participants of lower socioeconomic status.[55] Other studies have been conducted in the United States and Europe, and the results are similar.[56-60] An instructive study involves 17,530 British civil servants who were initially evaluated in 1968. This well-done study demonstrated a coronary mortality rate 3.6 times higher in the group with the lowest socioeconomic status. Kaplan and Keil[53] review the published data and make a convincing case for the role played by socioeconomic status in the natural history of atherosclerotic coronary heart disease. Although no simple relationship between socioeconomic status, risk for cardiovascular disease, and long-term outcome for manifest atherosclerotic coronary heart disease can be devised, the evidence is consistent and persuasive that lower socioeconomic status is an independent and significant determinant of long-term outcome.

Stable Angina Pectoris

The key pathophysiologic feature in patients with chronic stable angina pectoris is the predictable development of myocardial ischemia due to an increase in oxygen demand in the presence of fixed atherosclerotic lesions in the coronary arteries. Apparent variability in the ischemic threshold may be due to a combination of myocardial oxygen-consumption determinants operating simultaneously (e.g., walking after a heavy meal or experiencing anxiety during physical effort) or alterations in coronary artery tone.

The "total ischemic burden," which includes the symptomatic plus the silent episodes, is a useful concept in estimating prognosis, but its actual clinical use is not practical. A close inverse relationship between the time of occurrence of ST-segment depression on the treadmill and the number of silent ischemic episodes and/or the total time of ischemia found by 24-h ambulatory monitoring has been demonstrated.[61] Hence, the time of occurrence of exercise-induced ST-segment depression was better than the occurrence of angina in assessing total ischemic burden; this emphasizes the importance of objective data.

The "average" annual mortality of medically treated patients with a history of stable angina pectoris and angiographically proven coronary atherosclerosis but without left main coronary artery obstruction is 2 to 4 percent, but the spectrum of prognosis is very broad. This estimate is derived from data collected in the 1960s and 1970s.[62–68]

It is not surprising that the severity and frequency of symptoms are of limited value in assessing prognosis in stable angina pectoris. Many patients can prevent or minimize their symptoms by using nitroglycerin prophylactically and by avoiding activities that provoke angina pectoris; this complicates the interpretation of symptoms in assessing prognosis. Instructive observations have been reported by Califf et al.[66] Angina pectoris was classified on a scale of 0 to 3, class 0 being truly stable angina and class 3 being unstable or variant angina; classes 1 and 2 comprised intermediate symptoms. In this sophisticated retrospective analysis of 5886 patients, 44 percent had class 0 angina, and the number of daily episodes did not have independent prognostic significance. Left ventricular function (ejection fraction) was the most important prognostic factor. In angina pectoris groups 1 to 3—the less predictable forms of angina—the number of daily episodes did provide prognostic information that contributed to the other independent variables, such as left ventricular function and the extent of coronary arteriosclerosis.

Easily obtained clinical variables have prognostic importance in patients with stable angina pectoris. The presence of hypertension and abnormalities on the resting electrocardiogram, such as nonspecific ST-T wave changes and Q waves, worsen the prognosis. If neither hypertension nor electrocardiographic abnormality is present, the mortality rate is as low as 2 percent per year. If both are present, the mortality is substantially higher, probably at least 5 percent annually.[65] These features continue to have adverse effects on prognosis even in patients who have undergone coronary bypass surgery.[69,70]

Ambient ventricular ectopy as a separate prognostic factor is controversial because it tends to be associated with ventricular dysfunction and may be reduced by ischemia, but certain types of complex ventricular ectopy worsen prognosis.[67]

A wide variety of objective functional tests are available, but simple exercise testing has provided the most overall valuable information on the prognosis of stable angina pectoris.[71–75] The single most important prognostic determinant with exercise testing is exercise tolerance, but blood pressure, ST-segment shifts, and the occurrence of angina are important features in assessing prognosis (see Chap. 45).

THE INFLUENCE OF THE SITE
OF CORONARY ARTERY OBSTRUCTION
ON THE NATURAL HISTORY
OF THE DISEASE

In the early seventies, the Veterans Administration began a randomized trial in order to study the value of coronary artery bypass surgery in the treatment of symptomatic atherosclerotic coronary heart disease. The study, reported in 1975, revealed that male patients with stable angina pectoris for 6 months who had left main coronary artery disease and were treated medically had a 3-year survival of about 60 percent, whereas those who were treated surgically with coronary artery bypass surgery had a 3-year survival of nearly 85 percent.[76] The investigators described the medical treatment as follows: "Medically randomized patients received conventional medical treatment, including short- and long-acting coronary vasodilators, diuretics, digitalis, and beta-blocking agents as indicated."[76]

Once these observations had been made, patients with left main coronary artery obstruction were no longer randomized; they were subjected to coronary artery bypass surgery.

Another Veterans Administration trial revealed, in a $4\frac{1}{2}$ year follow-up of medically treated male patients with stable angina pectoris who had triple-vessel coronary disease, that their survival was between 75 and 80 percent.[77]

The medical treatment consisted of "Nitrates, beta-blocking agents, antihypertension medication, antiarrhythmic drugs, diuretics, digitalis, and dietary regulation."[77]

Bruschke et al., working at the Cleveland Clinic, provided the profession with valuable information in 1977.[78] They found a 10-year survival of about 70 to 75 percent in patients with angina pectoris who had single-vessel coronary artery disease; 50 to 55 percent in patients with double-vessel coronary artery disease; and 25 percent in patients with disease of the left main coronary artery. This retrospective study was valuable because the investigation followed patients who had arteriograms in whom bypass surgery could have been performed had it been fully developed at the time. Bruschke et al. did not characterize the angina pectoris into stable and unstable subsets, and some patients who were followed had heart failure. The medical treatment used in these patients was not discussed.

Because of these studies, physicians began to determine the natural hsitory of individual patients according to the number of coronary arteries that were obstructed, the location of the obstruction in the coronary arteries, and the physical characteristics of the obstructing lesions.

THE INFLUENCE OF THE EJECTION FRACTION
ON THE NATURAL HISTORY OF THE DISEASE

In 1979, Hammermeister et al. emphasized the importance of using the ejection fraction to determine the natural history of patients with suspected atherosclerotic coronary heart disease.[79] The concluded that "For the 733 medically treated patients, the Cox's regression analysis showed that the left ventricular ejection fraction was the most predictive of survival, followed by age, number of vessels with stenosis(es), and ventricular arrhythmias on the resting electrocardiogram."[79]

The details of the medical treatment were not discussed.

In 1982 Mock et al. reported on 20,088 medically treated patients listed in the CASS registry.[80] The conclusions of their work is presented here with permission:

The cumulative 4-year survival of medically managed patients was analyzed to determine the survival of specific subsets of patients with obstructive coronary disease. The vital status of 99.8% of the patients was known. The 4-year survival of medically treated patients with no significant obstructive disease was 97%, in contrast to 92%, 84%, and 68% in patients with one-, two-, and three-vessel disease, respectively. The presence of left main coronary artery disease decreased survival significantly. The 4-year survival decreased from 70% to 60% in patients with three-vessel disease when significant obstruction of the left main coronary artery was also present. Patients with significant coronary artery disease who had an ejection fraction $\geqq 50\%$, 35–49%, and 0–34% had a 4-year survival of 92%, 83%, and 58%, respectively. The systolic contraction pattern was assessed in five selected segments and given a score of 1–6, with a score of 1 for normal function, increasing to 6 if an aneurysm was present. In a patient with normal LV contraction in all five segments of the LV ventricular angiogram, the LV score would equal 5. Patients with an LV score of 5–11, 12–16, and 17–30 had 4-year survivals of 90%, 71%, and 53%, respectively. Patients with good LV function (a score of 5–11) had a 4-year survival of 94%, 91%, and 79% for one-, two-, and three-vessel disease, respectively. Patients with poor left ventricular function (score of 17–30) had a 4-year survival rate of 67%, 61%, and 42% in one-, two-, and three-vessel disease, respectively. Thus, LV function is a more important predictor of survival than the number of diseased vessels.[80]

The details of medical treatment were not presented. The patients undoubtedly received nitrates, beta blockers, and calcium antagonists. The study reveals how the number of obstructed coronary arteries and the ejection fraction, or altered systolic contraction pattern, conspire to determine the mortality of patients with atherosclerotic coronary heart disease. These and many similar studies emphasize the importance of including multiple clinical, laboratory, and angiographic variables (including exercise tolerance, discussed below) in order to get the best estimate of prognosis and to understand natural history.

Unstable Angina Pectoris

In 1973, Gazes et al. reported on the 10-year follow-up of 140 patients who were hospitalized because of unstable angina pectoris.[81] They found an 18 percent 1-year mortality in patients who had preexisting stable angina pectors who continued to have episodes of angina pectoris accompanied by ST-segment displacement while in the hospital. The medical treat-

ment used in these patients included "Period of rest, nitrates (long-acting and sublingual nitroglycerin), sedatives, analgesia, and low calorie–low fat diet. The beta blockers were not available until the latter part of the study. Ninety-one patients received warfarin and/or heparin."

The National Cooperative Study of unstable angina pectoris excluded patients with left main coronary artery obstruction.[82] This study, completed in 1978, again revealed the seriousness of the problem. The patients assigned to medical treatment had a 10 percent mortality rate and a 19 percent infarction rate; 36 percent had to have bypass surgery during the 30 months of follow-up. Vigorous medical management included "Bed rest in the coronary care unit and administration of oxygen, beta adrenergic blocking drugs used to maximal therapeutic doses, long-acting nitrates as often as every 2 to 3 hours, nitroglycerin as required, sedative drugs, digitalis and diuretic therapy when indicated and control of blood pressure as needed. Anticoagulant therapy is used at the discretion of the physician."

Note again that these figures do not reveal the true natural history of the condition. The data simply reveal that intense medical management of unstable angina pectoris is not satisfactory.

As mentioned above, physicians began to use subjective *and* objective data to identify specific subsets of patients. The objective information that is germane to the current discussion of unstable angina pectoris includes the physical appearance of the obstructive lesion seen on the coronary arteriogram and the occurrence of ST-segment shifts in the electrocardiogram during ischemic episodes (silent or symptomatic). The arteriographic features of the unstable plaque located in the coronary artery that is responsible for the unstable syndromes has been described by several investigators.[83–85] This advance in knowledge enables physicians to predict the likelihood and seriousness of additional future coronary events.

Variant Angina Pectoris

Patients with variant angina pectoris have coronary artery spasm. Almost all patients have some degree of atherosclerosis of the coronary arteries. Waters et al. pointed out that 18 percent of patients either die or have a myocardial infarction within 3 months after symptoms begin.[86] The medical treatment used in their study included the following:

Before hospitalization 79 of the 132 patients were being treated with topical or long-acting oral nitrates, 73 with beta receptor blocking agents and one with a calcium antagonist drug. In the hospital, beta receptor blocking therapy was discontinued in all cases. Treatment during hospitalization was not uniform but varied according to several factors including the availability of calcium antagonist drugs and shifts in our opinion about optimal management of this condition. Perhexiline maleate was the only calcium antagonist drug available to treat the first 27 patients; thereafter, nifedipine, diltiazem, or verapamil, alone or in combination, was used in nearly all patients.[86]

Silent Myocardial Ischemia

Silent ischemia can be subdivided into group 1 (patients who have no symptoms and have never had symptoms but have signs of ischemia in the electrocardiogram or thallium scan); group 2 (episodes of myocardial ischemia on the electrocardiogram or thallium scan after remote myocardial infarction); and group 3 (patients with angina pectoris who also have signs of episodic painless myocardial ischemia on the electrocardiogram or thallium scan).[87] Peter Cohn's excellent book, entitled *Silent Myocardial Ischemia and Infarction,* is a rich source of information on this subject.[88]

Although studies of patients in group 1 are few, all data indicate a favorable prognosis, with angina pectoris being the most likely first symptom.

Gottlieb et al. studied patients with unstable angina pectoris who exhibited episodes of painless ischemia on continuous electrocardiographic monitoring.[89] Sixteen percent of their patients with silent ischemia had a myocardial infarction within 1 month, compared with 3 percent of patients who did not.

Silent or painless myocardial ischemia is now appreciated by most physicians. Less appreciated is the detrimental effect of silent ventricular dysfunction (no dyspnea) and silent arrhythmias (no palpitation, dizziness, syncope, etc.) on the natural history of the disease.

Myocardial Infarction

About 25 percent of myocardial infarcts are "silent." Patients with diabetes mellitus or those who are elderly are even more likely to have painless infarcts.

The overall mortality of patients with myocardial infarction who reach the hospital ranges from 12 to 20 percent (see Chap. 47). The natural history of myocardial infarction cannot be ascertained, because modern treatments for arrhythmias, heart failure, and shock are instituted immediately. More recently, thrombolytic therapy, angioplasty, bypass surgery, and aortic balloon pumps have also been introduced.

Patients with myocardial infarction who are above age 70 have a poorer prognosis than those who are below that age. Women do not fare as well as men. Multiple studies show that the *first* myocardial infarct in older patients has less enzyme leak (indicating less myocardial necrosis), despite the dramatic increase in mortality and more complications related to left ventricular dysfunction. This paradox must be attributable to cardiovascular and other age-related changes, making the older patient less able to tolerate the stress of myocardial infarction. In addition, the more favorable outcome of inferior infarction as opposed to an anterior location is not seen in older patients, perhaps because they have a higher incidence of right ventricular myocardial infarction and/or merely because of age-related cardiac and pulmonary changes.

Patients with large infarcts, determined by extensive changes in the electrocardiogram or marked elevation of serum creatine phosphate (CK), have a poorer prognosis than those with minor changes in the electrocardiogram and only a small rise in serum CK. A note of caution—the electrocardiograms of patients with previous infarcts are commonly abnormal. The more abnormal the preinfarct tracings are, the less likely it is that new infarcts will show new changes. A new but small infarct that creates little change in the new tracing may be very serious, because the amount of newly destroyed myocardium is added to the amount of previously damaged muscle to create an even larger area of damage. The same reasoning holds for the level of serum CK. Second and third infarcts may not cause the serum enzymes to become more than slightly elevated, signifying a small area of myocardial necrosis. But when a small infarct occurs in a patient who has had previous infarcts, the new, small area of infarction may be very serious because the new damage is added to the area of previous myocardial damage. Although the new infarct may be small, it may be more serious than the patient's original larger infarct.

In general, patients with an anterior myocardial infarction have a higher mortality than patients with an inferior myocardial infarction. Patients with a Q-wave infarcts have a higher mortality than patients with non-Q-wave infarcts. Patients who have right ventricular infarcts in addition to inferior infarcts have a much higher mortality than patients with inferior infarcts alone (see Chap. 47). Patients with acute heart failure due to myocardial infarction probably have a mortality in the range of 50 percent. Patients with cardiogenic shock probably have a mortality of about 90 percent.

Ischemic Cardiomyopathy

Ischemic cardiomyopathy was not discussed in the literature prior to the 1950s. Today, there is an increasing number of such patients because the patients treated earlier with bypass surgery, angioplasty, and modern medical therapy are living to develop cardiomyopathy (see Chap. 73). In clinical trials, the majority, as many as 80 percent of recruited patients, have ischemic cardiomyopathy. Such patients may undergo cardiac transplantation after a period of modern treatment for heart failure has failed. The natural history of such patients is not known because all of them are treated vigorously, but it is obviously dismal. Within the context of a dismal outcome, some patients live longer than others. The more severe the symptoms, the lower the ejection fraction, and the older the patients, the worse the prognosis.[90] Annual mortality varies from less than 5 percent to 50 percent, depending on the combination of attributes present.

Sudden Cardiac Death

Sudden and unexpected death, with or without previous symptoms, is still common and occurs in about 30 percent of patients with atherosclerotic coronary heart disease (see Chaps. 27, 36, and 47).

A majority of sudden cardiac deaths occur outside the hospital; valuable information on this subject has been provided by an extensive communitywide program of resuscitation in Seattle, Washington.[91–94] Most patients who suffered sudden cardiac death outside the hospital and were resuscitated did not have diagnosable myocardial infarction. Twenty-six percent of patients without myocardial necrosis suffered recurrent sudden cardiac death within 1 year. In contrast, when acute myocardial infarction was diagnosed, survivors of out-of-hospital sudden cardiac death had a 1-year mortality of 4 percent. This important statistic indicates that so-called primary ventricular fibrillation, occurring early in the course of acute myocardial infarction and unaccompanied by other complications of ventricular dysfunction, does not carry an ominous long-term prognosis when treated promptly. The high incidence of recurrent ventricular fibrillation in the year following resuscitation in noninfarct patients is almost certainly associated with chronic advanced ventricular dysfunction with the propensity for recurrent ischemia or reentrant mechanisms involving scars that produce recurrent ventricular tachycardia or ventricular fibrillation.

Electrocardiographic Stress Test

Whereas the result of an electrocardiogram exercise stress test has diagnostic value, its use to determine the prognosis of patients with stable angina pectoris became widespread only during the last two decades. Patients who can achieve a heart rate of 160 or who can reach stage 4 of the Bruce protocol without developing angina, undue dyspnea, or ST-segment abnormalities on the electrocardiogram have an annual mortality of about 1 or 2 percent. Patients who are unable to reach stage 2 because of angina, dyspnea, or ST-segment displacement on the electrocardiogram have an annual mortality of about 6 to 10 percent.

A total of 4083 patients from the Coronary Artery Surgical Study Registry had 30 clinical and exercise variables analyzed.[74] Exercise duration was confirmed as the important exercise test variable, but ST-segment response also proved to have independent (incremental) prognostic value. The overall mortality, with a minimum of 3 years follow-up, was 5 percent. On the basis of only two exercise variables, a high-risk subset (492 patients) with an annual mortality of more than 5 percent had 1 mm or greater ST-segment depression at a low level of exercise (Bruce stage 1 or less). A low-risk subset (1302 patients) with an annual mortality of less than 1 percent had less than 1 mm ST-segment depression in the final exercise of stage 3 or higher. Hence, in this very large sample, nearly 50 percent of the patients could be divided into high- and low-risk subsets on the basis of these two simply obtained exercise variables. In 572 patients with three-vessel disease and good ventricular function, a wide spectrum of 4-year survival was seen. A small group of this subset achieved stage 5 on the Bruce protocol and had no mortality, while only 53 percent of the patients who were unable to achieve stage 1 survived 4 years. This study demonstrates that left ventricular function, exercise duration, and ST shifts are more predictive than the extent of coronary atherosclerosis. Mark et al. studies 2842 patients and developed and validated a clinical rule requiring only three variables—exercise time, degree of ST-segment shift, and the occurrence and severity of angina. Their study emphasized that symptoms have additive predictive value when other features are equal.[75]

The earlier the ST segment becomes displaced during the exercise test and the longer it remains displaced after the test is discontinued, the worse the prognosis (see Chap. 45).

Radionuclide and Echocardiograms

The use of radionuclide studies and the echocardiogram as diagnostic and prognostic tools are discussed in Chaps. 14 and 17. Overall, these techniques have provided limited insights into prognosis natural history, since their development has coincided with the evolution of drug and interventional therapies. A positive finding on these imaging tests virtually always results in additional diagnostic and/or therapeutic maneuvers that minimize the possibility of studying the predictive value of the finding. Patients in whom interventions are not pursued represent highly selected cases.

HOW DOES ONE REACT TO THE INFORMATION?

An analysis of the available information regarding the natural history of atherosclerotic coronary heart disease leads one to have the following reactions:

The natural history of atherosclerotic coronary heart disease reported and discussed by Drs. Paul White, Paul Wood, and others in the 1950s continues to be useful. Although limited by the lack of diagnostic tools, their conclusions about the natural history of the disease were less influenced by effective treatment than is the case today.

There are no recent studies that reveal the natural history of atherosclerotic coronary heart disease because modern clinical trials are designed to determine if a new treatment, such as coronary bypass surgery, is superior to modern medical treatment in altering the course of the disease. It is no longer possible to study the natural history of the disease because modern effective treatment cannot be withheld from the patients enrolled in a clinical trial. *However, the current view is that the natural history of the disease may be different now than it was formerly, because many Americans are smoking less, eating less fat, and exercising more than they did 50 years ago.* Certain events obviously occur with less frequency today than they did formerly. For example, emboli associated with myocardial infarction occur less often today than reported by Hellerstein and Martin in 1947.[18]

The interaction between the knowledge of the natural history and treatment of atherosclerotic coronary heart disease is a critical part of every clinician's decision-making process. Today, unlike the attempts made prior to the 1950s to establish the natural history and prognosis of the disease that were determined mainly by subjective data, the natural history and prognosis are currently determined by the subjective *and* objective data available on the majority of patients we treat. In current practice, it is tempting to focus on a single feature, symptom, abnormality in the electrocardiogram, arteriographic finding, or abnormality on a functional test as the determinant of prognosis and allow it to dictate clinical decision making. It is the total evidence that must be considered in determining the natural history and prognosis of the disease.

The natural history of this disease remains unpredictable in individual patients. Surprises are in store for any physician who takes care of a number of patients with this malady. Witness the surprise that is expressed, even by physicians, when someone in the neighborhood dies suddenly and unexpectedly because he or she had no former symptoms and had been "checked" recently by a doctor. Also, note the surprise, even among physicians, that accompanies the survival of a patient with inoperable three-vessel atherosclerotic coronary heart disease who has lived 10 years beyond the time he or she should have died (according to statistical data).

How should we react to the statistics that accompany the discussion of the natural history of atherosclerotic coronary heart disease? At first glance, many of the figures please us. It is good to know that only 5 percent of a certain subset of patients will die in a 5-year follow-up period when the figure could have been 20 percent. If, however, the patients are only 35 years old when they are diagnosed, the fact that 5 in 100 of these "young" patients will die before age 40 should be viewed with alarm and deemed unacceptable.

On the other hand, Dr. Paul White wrote the following sentences about the patients who had symptoms and signs of the disease at an "advanced age."[95] It is interesting to note that these sentences were the last lines in the fourth edition of his book *Heart Disease,* the final edition of the book, which changed the course of cardiology.

> In closing this chapter and the book itself may I suggest that after all neither a high, even 100 percent, mortality from cardiovascular disease nor sudden death itself are to be regretted, provided they take place at an advanced age after a healthy and happy and useful life right up to the last minute. In fact this is actually an ideal goal toward which man may strive, for it means the eradication not only of other diseases, such as the infections of the past, and the cancers, accidents, and the wars of the present, but also the control of the serious cardiovascular threats (such as hypertension and coronary atherosclerosis). . . .[95]

As one reviews the great advances that have been made in the treatment of this disease, one cannot escape feeling that much has been accomplished but that even the greatest therapeutic triumph will fade into obscurity when it is possible to prevent the disease. *This is true because the current treatment of the disease, great as it is, does not alter the natural history of the disease to a satisfactory degree.* Consider the sudden deaths and myocardial infarcts that still occur, as well as the cost and suffering that accompany bypass surgery, angioplasty, certain medications, and even a single day in a coronary care unit.

REFERENCES

1. Heberden W. Some account of a disorder of the breast. *Med Trans Coll Physicians* 1772; 2:59–67.
2. Heberden W. *Commentaries on the History and Care of Disease.* London: Payne; 1802.
3. Parry CH. *An Inquiry into the Symptoms and Causes of the Syncope Anginosa, Commonly Called Angina Pectoris.* Bath, England; Crutwell; 1799.
4. Herrick JB. Clinical features of sudden obstruction of the coronary arteries. *JAMA* 1912; 59:2015–2020.
5. White PD. *Heart Disease,* 4th ed. New York: Macmillan; 1951:555–556.
6. Wood P. *Diseases of the Heart and Circulation,* 2d ed. Philadelphia: Lippincott; 1956:716, 723, 725, 739, 740, 750.
7. White PD. *Heart Disease,* 4th ed. New York: Macmillan; 1951:555.
8. White PD, Bland EF, Miskall EW. The prognosis of angina pectoris: A long time follow-up of 497 cases, including a note on 75 additional cases of angina pectoris decubitus. *JAMA* 1943; 123:801–804.
9. Montgomery GE Jr, Dry TJ, Gage RP. Further observations on the prognosis in angina pectoris due to coronary sclerosis: A study of 405 patients who survived 10 or more years. *Minn Med* 1947; 30:162–165.
10. Block WJ Jr, Crumpacker EL, Dry TJ, Gage RP. Prognosis of angina pectoris: Observations in 6,882 cases. *JAMA* 1952; 150:259–264.
11. Parker RL, Dry TJ, Willius FA, Gage RP. Life expectancy in angina pectoris. *JAMA* 1946; 131:95–100.
12. Feil H. Preliminary pain in coronary thrombosis. *Am J Med* 1937; 193:42–48.
13. Wood P. *Diseases of the Heart and Circulation,* 2d ed. Philadelphia: Lippincott; 1956:725.
14. Wood P. *Diseases of the Heart and Circulation,* 2d ed. Philadelphia: Lippincott; 1956:740.
15. Yater WM, Traum AH, Brown WG, Fitzgerald RP, Geisler MA, Wilcox BB. Coronary artery disease in men eighteen to thirty-nine years of age. *Am Heart J* 1948; 36:334–372, 481–526, 683–722.
16. Mintz SS, Katz LN. Recent myocardial infarction: An analysis of five hundred and seventy-two cases. *Arch Intern Med* 1947; 80:205–236.
17. Selzer A. The immediate sequelae of myocardial infarction: The relation to the prognosis. *Am J Med Sci* 1948; 216:172–178.
18. Hellerstein HK, Martin JW. Incidence of thrombo-embolic lesions accompanying myocardial infarction. *Am Heart J* 1947; 33:443–452.
19. Oblath RW, Levinson DC, Griffith GC. Factors influencing rupture of heart after myocardial infarction. *JAMA* 1952; 149:1276–1281.
20. Wood P. *Diseases of the Heart and Circulation,* 2d ed. Philadelphia: Lippincott; 1956:743.
21. Wartman WB, Hellerstein HK. The incidence of heart disease in 2,000 consecutive autopsies. *Ann Intern Med* 1948; 28:41–65.
22. Wood P. *Diseases of the Heart and Circulation,* 2d ed. Philadelphia: Lippincott, 1956:745.
23. Sones FM Jr, Shirey EK. Cine coronary arteriography. *Mod Concepts Cardiovasc Dis* 1962; 31:735–738.
24. Solomon CG, Lee TH, Cook EF, Weisberg MC, Brad DA, Rouan GW, et al. Comparison of clinical presentation of acute myocardial infarction in patients older than 65 years of age to younger patients: Multicenter chest pain study experience. *Am J Cardiol* 1989; 63:772–776.
25. Goldberg RJ, Gore JM, Gurwitz JHA, Alpert JS, Brady P. Strohsnitter W, et al. The impact of age on the incidence and prognosis of initial acute myocardial infarction: The Worcester Heart Attack Study. *Am Heart J* 1989; 117:543–549.

26. Maggioni AP, Maseri A, Fresco C, Franzosi MG, Mauri F, Santoro E, et al. Age-related increase in mortality among patients with first myocardial infarctions treated with thrombolysis. *N Engl J Med* 1993; 329:1442–1448.

27. Nadelmann J, Frishman WH, Ooi WL, Tepper D, Greenberg S, Guzik H, et al. Prevalence, incidence and prognosis of recognized and unrecognized myocardial infarction in persons aged 75 years or older: The Bronx Aging Study. *Am J Cardiol* 1990; 66:533–537.

28. Wenger NK, Speroff L, Packard B (eds). *Cardiovascular Health and Disease in Women.* Greenwich, CT: LeJacq Communications; 1993.

29. McGovern PG, Pankow JS, Shahar E, Doliszny KM, Folsom AR, Blackburn H, et al. Recent trends in acute coronary heart disease: Mortality, morbidity, medical care, and risk factors. *N Engl J Med* 1996; 334:884–890.

30. Gibbons RJ. Exercise ECG testing with and without radionuclide studies. In: Wenger NK, Speroff L, Packard B, eds. *Cardiovascular Health and Disease in Women.* Greenwich, CT: LeJacq Communications; 1993; 73–80.

31. Sketch MM, Mohiuddin SM, Lynch JD, Zencka AE, Runco V. Significant sex differences in the correlation of electrocardiographic exercise testing and coronary arteriograms. *Am J Cardiol* 1975; 36:169–173.

32. Guiteras P, Chaitman BR, Waters DD, Bourassa MG, Scholl JM, Ferguson RJ, et al. Diagnostic accuracy of exercise ECG lead systems in clinical subsets of women. *Circulation* 1982; 65:1465–1474.

33. Barolsky SM, Gilbert CA, Faruqui A, Nutter DO, Schlant RC. Differences in electrocardiographic response to exercise of women and men: A non-Bayesian factor. *Circulation* 1979; 60:1021–1027.

34. Gibbons RJ, Lee KL, Cobb F, Jones RH. Ejection fraction response to exercise in patients with chest pain and normal coronary arteriograms. *Circulation* 1981; 64:952–957.

35. Higginbotham MB, Morris KG, Coleman RE, Cobb FR. Sex-related differences in the normal cardiac response to upright exercise. *Circulation* 1984; 70:357–366.

36. Hanley PC, Zinsmeister AR, Clements IP, Bove AA, Brown ML, Gibbons RJ. Gender-related differences in cardiac response to supine exercise assessed by radionuclide angiography. *J Am Coll Cardiol* 1989; 13:624–629.

37. Murabito JM, Evans JC, Larson MG, Levy D. Prognosis after the onset of coronary heart disease: An investigation of differences in outcome between the sexes according to initial coronary disease presentation. *Circulation* 1993; 88:2548–2555.

38. Weintraub WS, Wenger NK, Jones EL, Craver JM, Guyton RA. Changing clinical characteristics of coronary surgery patients: Differences between men and women. *Circulation* 1993; 88:(suppl II)79–86.

39. Orencia A, Bailey K, Yawn BP, Kottke TE. Effect of gender on long-term outcome between the sexes according to initial coronary disease presentation. *JAMA* 1993; 269:2392–2397.

40. Vaccarino V, Krumholz HM, Berkman LF, Horwitz RI. Sex differences in mortality after myocardia infarction: Is there evidence for an increased risk for women? *Circulation* 1995; 91:1861–1871.

41. Tofler GH, Stone PH, Muller JE, Willich SN, Davis VG, Poole WK, et al. Effects of gender and race on prognosis after myocardial infarction: Adverse prognosis for women, particularly black women. *J Am Coll Cardiol* 1987; 9:473–482.

42. Dittrich H, Gilpin E, Nicod P, Cali G, Henning H, Ross J Jr. Acute myocardial infarction in women: Influence of gender on mortality and prognostic variables. *Am J Cardiol* 1988; 62:1–7.

43. Fiebach NH, Viscoli CM, Horwitz RI. Differences between women and men in survival after myocardial infarction: Biology or methodology? *JAMA* 1990; 263:1092–1096.

44. Bueno H, Vidan MT, Almazan A, Lopez-Sendon JL, Delcan JL. Influence of sex on the short-term outcome of elderly patients with a first acute myocardial infarction. *Circulation* 1995; 92:1133–1140.

45. Jenkins JS, Flaker GC, Nolte B, Price LA, Morris D, Kurz J, et al. Causes of higher in-hospital mortality in women than in men after acute myocardial infarction. *Am J Cardiol* 1994; 73:319–322.

46. Maynard C, Litwin PE, Martin JS, Weaver WD. Gender differences in the treatment and outcome of acute myocardial infarction: Results from the Myocardial Infarction Triage and Intervention Registry. *Arch Intern Med* 1992; 152:972–976.

47. Chiriboga DE, Yarzebski J, Goldberg JR, Chen Z, Gurwitz J, Gore JM, et al. A community-wide perspective of gender differences and temporal trends in the use of diagnostic and revascularization procedures for acute myocardial infarction. *Am J Cardiol* 1993; 71:268–273.

48. Steingart RM, Packer M, Hamm P, Coglianese ME, Gersh B, Geltman EM, et al. Sex differences in the management of coronary artery disease. *N Engl J Med* 1991; 325:226–230.

49. Krumholz HM, Douglas PS, Lauer MS, Pasternak RC. Selection of patients for coronary angiography and coronary angiography and coronary revascularization early after myocardial infarction: Is there evidence for a gender bias? *Ann Intern Med* 1992; 116:785–790.

50. Funk M, Griffey KA. Relation of gender to the use of cardiac procedures in acute myocardial infarction. *Am J Cardiol* 1994; 74:1170–1173.

51. Ayanian JZ, Epstein AM. Differences in the use of procedures between women and men hospitalized for coronary heart disease. *N Engl J Med* 1991; 325:221–225.

52. Bearden D, Allman R, McDonald R, Miller S, Pressel S, Petrovitch H. Age, race, and gender variation in the utilization of coronary artery bypass surgery and angioplasty in SHEP: SHEP Cooperative Research Group—Systolic Hypertension in the Elderly Program. *J Am Geriatr Soc* 1994; 42:1143–1149.

53. Kaplan GA, Keil JE. Socioeconomic factors and cardiovascular disease: A review of the literature. *Circulation* 1993; 88(4:I):1973–1998.

54. Williams RB, Barefoot JC, Califf RM, Haney TL, Saunders WB, Pryor DB, et al. Prognostic importance of social and economic resources among medically treated patients with angiographically documented coronary artery disease. *JAMA* 1992; 267:520–524.

55. Liu K, Cedres LB, Stamler J, Dyer A, Stamler R, Nanas S, et al. Relationship of education to major risk factors and death from coronary heart disease, cardiovascular diseases, and all causes: Findings of three Chicago epidemiologic studies. *Circulation* 1982; 66:1308–1314.

56. Holme I, Helgeland A, Hjermann I, Leren P. Socio-economic status as a coronary risk factor: The Oslo study. *Acta Med Scand Suppl* 1982; 660:147–151.

57. Doornbos G, Kromhout D. Educational level and mortality in a 32-year follow-up study of 18-year-old men in the Netherlands. *Int J Epidemiol* 1990; 19:374–379.

58. Salonen JT. Socioeconomic status and risk of cancer, cerebral stroke, and death due to coronary heart disease and any disease: A longitudinal study in eastern Finland. *J Epidemiol Community Health* 1982; 36:294–297.

59. Marmot MG, Kogevinas M, Elston MA. Social/economic status and disease. *Annu Rev Public Health* 1987; 8:111–135.

60. Rose G, Marmot MG. Social class and coronary heart disease. *Br Heart J* 1981; 45:13–19.

61. Rocco MB, Barry J, Campbell S, Nabel E, Cook EF, Goldman L, et al. Circadian variation of transient myocardial ischemia in patients with coronary artery disease. *Circulation* 1987; 75:395–400.

62. European Coronary Surgery Study Group. Prospective randomized study of coronary artery bypass surgery in stable angina pectoris: Second interim report. *Lancet* 1980; 2:491–495.

63. Murphy ML, Hultgren HN, Detre K, Thomsen J, Takaro T. Treatment of chronic stable angina: A preliminary report of survival data of the randomized Veterans Administration Cooperative Study. *N Engl J Med* 1977; 297:621–627.

64. Proudfit WJ, Bruschke AV, MacMillan JP, Williams GW, Sones FM Jr. Fifteen-year survival study of patients with obstructive coronary artery disease. *Circulation* 1983; 68:986–997.

65. Frank CW, Weinblatt E, Shapiro S. Angina pectoris in men: Prognostic significance of selected medical factors. *Circulation* 1973; 47:509–517.

66. Califf RM, Mark DB, Harrell FE Jr, Hlatky MA, Lee KL, Rosati RA, et al. Importance of clinical measures of ischemia in the prognosis of patients with documented coronary artery disease. *J Am Coll Cardiol* 1988; 11:20–26.

67. Ruberman W, Weinblatt E, Goldberg JD, Frank CW, Shapiro S, Chaudhary BS. Ventricular premature complexes in prognosis of angina. *Circulation* 1980; 61:1172–1178.

68. Friesinger GC, Page EE, Ross RS. Prognostic significance of coronary arteriography. *Trans Assoc Am Phys* 1970; 49:489–497.

69. Yusuf S, Zucker D, Peduzzi P, Fisher LD, Takaro T, Kennedy JW. Effect of coronary artery bypass graft surgery on survival: Overview of 10-year results from randomised trials by the Coronary Artery Bypass Graft Surgery Trialists Collaboration. *Lancet* 1994 344:563–570.

70. Lytle BW, Loop FD, Cosgrove DM, Taylor PC, Goormastic M, Peper W, et al. Fifteen hundred cornary reoperations: Results and determi-

nants of early and late survival. *J Thorac Cardiovasc Surg* 1987; 93:847–859.

71. McNeer JF, Margolis JR, Lee KL, Kisslo JA, Peter RH, Kong Y, et al. The role of the exercise test in the evaluation of patients for ischemic heart disease. *Circulation* 1978; 57:64–70.

72. Dagenais GR, Rouleau JR, Christen A, Fabia J. Survival of patients with a strongly positive exercise electrocardiogram. *Circulation* 1982; 65:452–456.

73. Gohlke H, Samek L, Betz P, Roskamm H. Exercise testing provides additional prognostic information in angiographically defined subgroups of patients with coronary artery disease. *Circulation* 1983; 68:979–985.

74. Weiner DA, Ryan TJ, McCabe CH, Chaitman BR, Sheffield T, Ferguson JC, et al. Prognostic importance of a clinical profile and exercise test in medically treated patients with coronary artery disease. *J Am Coll Cardiol* 1984; 3:772–779.

75. Mark DB, Hlatky MA, Harrell FE, Lee KL, Califf RM, Pryor DB. Exercise treadmill score for predicting prognosis in coronary artery disease. *Ann Intern Med* 1987; 106:793–800.

76. Takaro T, Hultgren HN, Lipton MJ, Detre KM, and Participants in the Study Group. The VA Cooperative Randomized Study of Surgery for Coronary Arterial Occlusive Disease: II. Subgroup with significant left main lesions. *Circulation* 1975; 54(suppl 3):107–116.

77. Read RC, Murphy ML, Hultgren HN, Takaro T. Survival of men treated for chronic stable angina pectoris: A cooperative randomized study. *J Thorac Cardiovasc Surg* 1978; 75:1–12.

78. Bruschke AVG, Proudfit WL, Sones FM Jr. Progress study of 590 consecutive nonsurgical cases of coronary disease followed 5–9 years: I. Arteriographic correlations. *Circulation* 1973; 47:1147–1153.

79. Hammermeister KE, DeRouen TA, Dodge HT. Variables predictive of survival in patients with coronary disease: Selection by univariate and multivariate analyses from the clinical, electrocardiographic, exercise, arteriographic, and quantitative angiographic evaluations. *Circulation* 1979; 59:421–430.

80. Mock MB, Ringqvist I, Fisher LD, Davis KB, Chaitman BR, Kouchoukos NT, et al. Survival of medically treated patients in the coronary artery surgery study (CASS) registry. *Circulation* 1982; 66:562–568.

81. Gazes PC, Mobley EM Jr, Faris HM Jr, Duncan RC, Humphries GB. Preinfarctional (unstable) angina—A prospective study—Ten-year follow-up. *Circulation* 1973; 48:331–337.

82. National Cooperative Study group to compare medical and surgical therapy. Unstable angina pectoris: I. Report of protocol and patient population. *Am J Cardiol* 1976; 37:896–902.

83. Fuster V, Badimon L, Baimon JJ, Chesebro JH. The pathogenesis of coronary artery disease and the acute coronary syndromes (first of two parts). *N Engl J Med* 1992; 236:242–318.

84. Ambrose JA, Winters SL, Arora RR, Eng A, Riccio A, Gorlin R, et al. Angiographic evolution of coronary artery morphology in unstable angina. *J Am Coll Cardiol* 1986; 7:472–478.

85. Davies MJ, Thomas AC, Knapman PA, Hangartner JR. Intramyocardial platelet aggregation in patients with unstable angina suffering sudden ischemic cardiac death. *Circulation* 1986; 73:418–427.

86. Waters DD, Szlachcic J, Miller DD, Theroux P. Clinical characteristics of patients with variant angina complicated by myocardial infarction or death within one month. *Am J Cardiol* 1982; 49:658–664.

87. Cohn PF: Asymptomatic coronary artery disease: Pathophysiology, diagnosis, management. *Mod Concepts Cardiovasc Dis* 1981; 50:55–60.

88. Cohn PF. *Silent Myocardial Ischemia and Infarction.* New York: Marcel Dekker; 1993:8–18, 87–97.

89. Gottlieb SO, Weisfeldt ML, Ouyang P, Mellitus ED, Gerstenblith G. Silent ischemia as a marker for early unfavorable outcomes in patients with unstable angina. *N Engl J Med* 1986; 314:1214–1219.

90. The SOLVD Investigators: Effect of enalapril on survival in patients with reduced left ventricular ejection fractions and congestive heart failure. *N Engl J Med* 1991; 325:293–302.

91. Cobb LA, Conn RD, Samson WE. Prehospital coronary care: The role of rapid response mobile intensive coronary care system. *Circulation* 1971; 43:II-139. (See also *JAMA* 1985.)

92. Cobb LA, Baum RS, Alvarez HA III, Schaffer WA. Resuscitation from out-of-hospital ventricular fibrillation: 4 years follow-up. *Circulation* 1985; 52:III-223–III-235. (See also *JAMA* 1985.)

93. Schaffer WA, Cobb LA. Recurrent ventricular fibrillation and modes of death in survivors of out-of-hospital ventricular fibrillation. *N Engl J Med* 1975; 293:259–262.

94. Weaver DW, Lorch GS, Alvarez HA III, Cobb LA. Angiographic findings and prognostic indicators. *Circulation* 1976; 54:895–900.

95. White PD: *Heart Disease,* 4th ed. New York: Macmillan; 1951:956.

39

FACTORS INFLUENCING ATHEROGENESIS

Russell Ross

THE LESIONS OF ATHEROSCLEROSIS

Atherosclerosis is not a single disease entity. In fact, the lesions of atherosclerosis represent a common response of the artery to numerous, potentially different forms of insult. The lesions of atherosclerosis take different forms depending upon their anatomic site; the age, genetic constitution, and physiologic status of the affected individual; and the risk factors to which each individual has been exposed. Examination of the lesions of atherosclerosis reveals that each lesion contains the elements of an inflammatory response together with varying levels of fibroproliferative response.[1-5] If it is an early lesion (fatty streak, see below), it consists largely of monocyte-derived macrophages and T lymphocytes. Thus, it is a pure, highly specialized inflammatory response. The intermediate and advanced lesions also contain these elements, together with smooth muscle cells, which migrate, proliferate, and lay down extracellular matrix, presumably as part of a healing response to the insult and inflammation. Hyperlipidemia is commonly associated with the process of atherogenesis. Thus, together with the inflammatory-fibroproliferative response, both intracellular and extracellular lipid accumulation can be found in association with many of the lesions. In each instance, the relative degree to which each of the cells responds to different atherogenic stimuli determines the unique combination that defines the type and extent of the resulting lesion.[6,7]

The lesions of atherosclerosis occur principally within the innermost layer of the artery wall, the intima. They include the fatty streak, the fibrous plaque, and the so-called complicated lesions[1-3] (see Chap. 40). Secondary changes have been noted in the media of the artery underlying the lesion, principally in association with the more advanced lesions of atherosclerosis (Fig. 39-1).

The Fatty Streak

The process of atherogenesis begins in childhood with the development of fat, lipid-rich lesions called fatty streaks (see Chap. 40). Studies using monoclonal antibodies specific for macrophages, T cells, and smooth muscle cells have shown that early fatty streaks appear to consist of macrophages together with variable numbers of T lymphocytes. As the lesions expand, they contain smooth muscle cells that have migrated into the intima as well. As a consequence, these lesions become mixed macrophage–T lymphocyte–smooth muscle lesions in which both macrophages and smooth muscle are lipid-laden. Each of these cell types contains deposits of cholesterol and cholesterol oleate. Fatty streaks can be found in the aorta shortly after birth and appear in increasing numbers between the ages of 8 and 18 years. Fatty streaks appear in the coronary arteries at about age 15 and continue to increase in amount in these vessels through the third decade of life.[5,8]

The lesions are yellowish and sessile in appearance and cause little or no obstruction of the affected artery and no clinical sequelae. The fatty streak is ubiquitous in young people, even in those populations that do not appear to develop severe atherosclerosis. This observation suggests that lipid deposition does not inevitably lead to the advanced lesions of atherosclerosis but that a number of other factors are associated with the progression of the lesions and with the development of the more complex form of atherosclerosis, the fibrous plaque.

The Fibrous Plaque

More advanced lesions begin to develop around the age of 25 in those populations in which there is a high incidence of atherosclerosis and its clinical sequelae. The fibrous plaque is grossly white in appearance and becomes elevated, so that

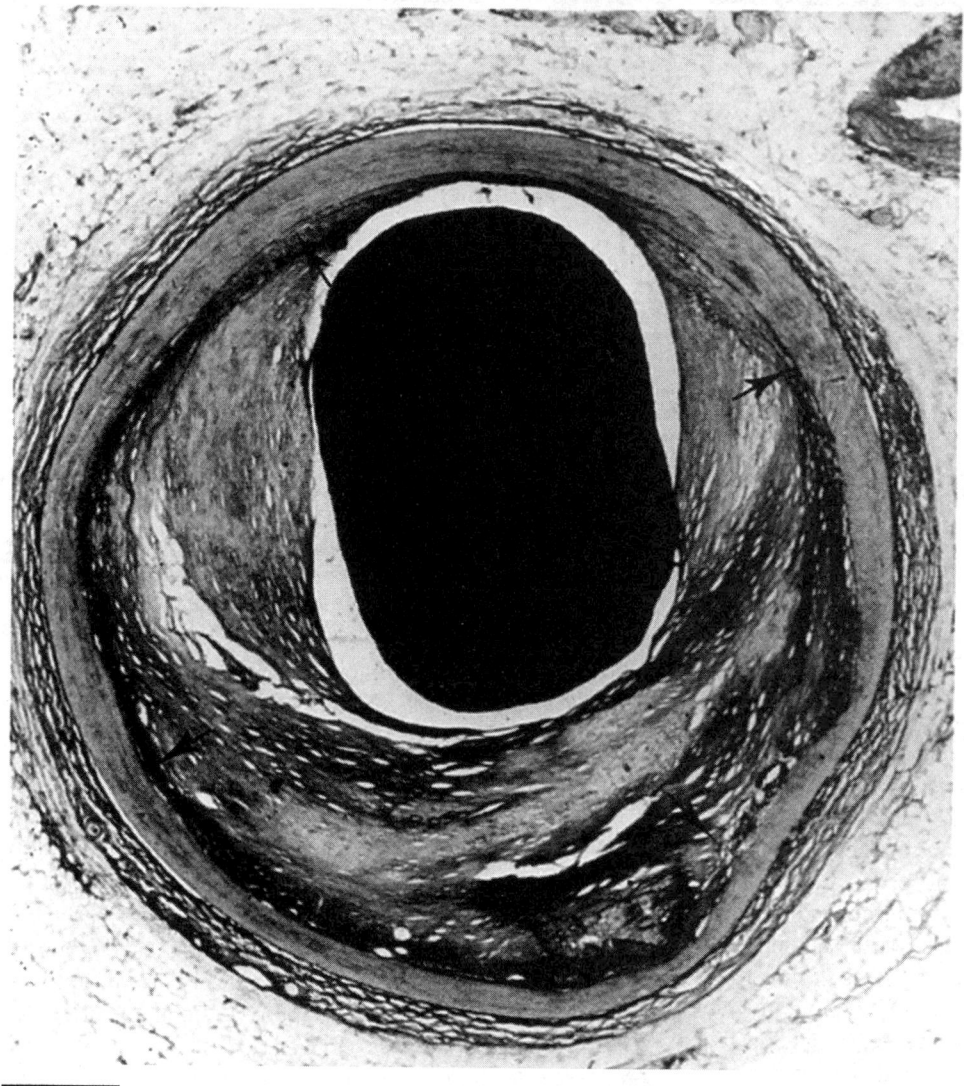

FIGURE 39-1

Classical light micrograph of a cross section of a coronary artery that contains a large atherosclerotic lesion. The lumen of the artery is relatively small. The original lumen is indicated by the arrows. In this preparation, it is virtually impossible to see cellular detail and, in particular, to determine the type of cells involved in the formation of the lesion.

proved but has been questioned because, although fatty streaks in young individuals are often found in the same anatomic location in the coronary and extracranial cerebral arteries as fibrous plaques in older individuals, fatty streaks also occur in anatomic sites that are different from those in which fibrous plaques appear. The reasons for these differences are not understood. It has been suggested that in those instances where their location is different, the fatty streaks may simply have regressed and disappeared, whereas in the instances where the anatomic location is the same, lesion progression has occurred.[9] There is a lesion that is generally accepted as a forerunner of the fibrous plaque. This is known as fibromusculoelastic or intermediate lesion of the intima, which consists of proliferated smooth muscle cells surrounded by connective tissue and contains little to no lipid.[1,5,6]

Immunohistochemical examination of fibrous plaques with cell-specific monoclonal antibodies has shown that the fibrous cap of the lesion consists of numerous smooth muscle cells surrounded by a dense connective tissue matrix, often intermixed with numerous macrophages. This cap covers a deeper layer of macrophages (many of which are filled with lipid in hypercholesterolemic individuals) that are often intermixed with variable numbers of T lymphocytes. Deeper in the lesion there may be necrotic debris and extracellular lipid, and deeper still, there may be numerous proliferated smooth muscle cells. *The presence of T lymphocytes in lesions raises the possibility that an immune response may be important in lesion genesis or progression and that some lesions may represent an autoimmune response.*

The Advanced (Complicated) Lesion— Plaque Disruption and Sudden Death

The complicated lesions of atherosclerosis (see Chap. 40) occur in increasing frequency with advancing age. The fibrous plaque can become vascularized both from the luminal as well as the medial aspects. In the complicated lesion the

it may protrude into the lumen of the artery (see Chap. 40). If this lesion progresses sufficiently, it can occlude the lumen and compromise the vascular supply of the involved tissue. The principal change that occurs within the arterial intima during the development of the fibrous plaque consists of migration and proliferation of smooth muscle cells. These cells usually form a fibrous cap owing to the deposition by the cells of new connective tissue matrix and to the accumulation of intracellular and extracellular lipids. This fibrous cap covers a deeper deposit of varying amounts of extracellular lipid and cell debris[4] (Fig. 39-2).

It has been suggested that fibrous plaques are derived from fatty streaks that continue the process of cell proliferation, lipid accumulation, and connective tissue formation and that the deep core of lipid and cell debris results from inadequate blood supply and cell necrosis. Such a relation has not been

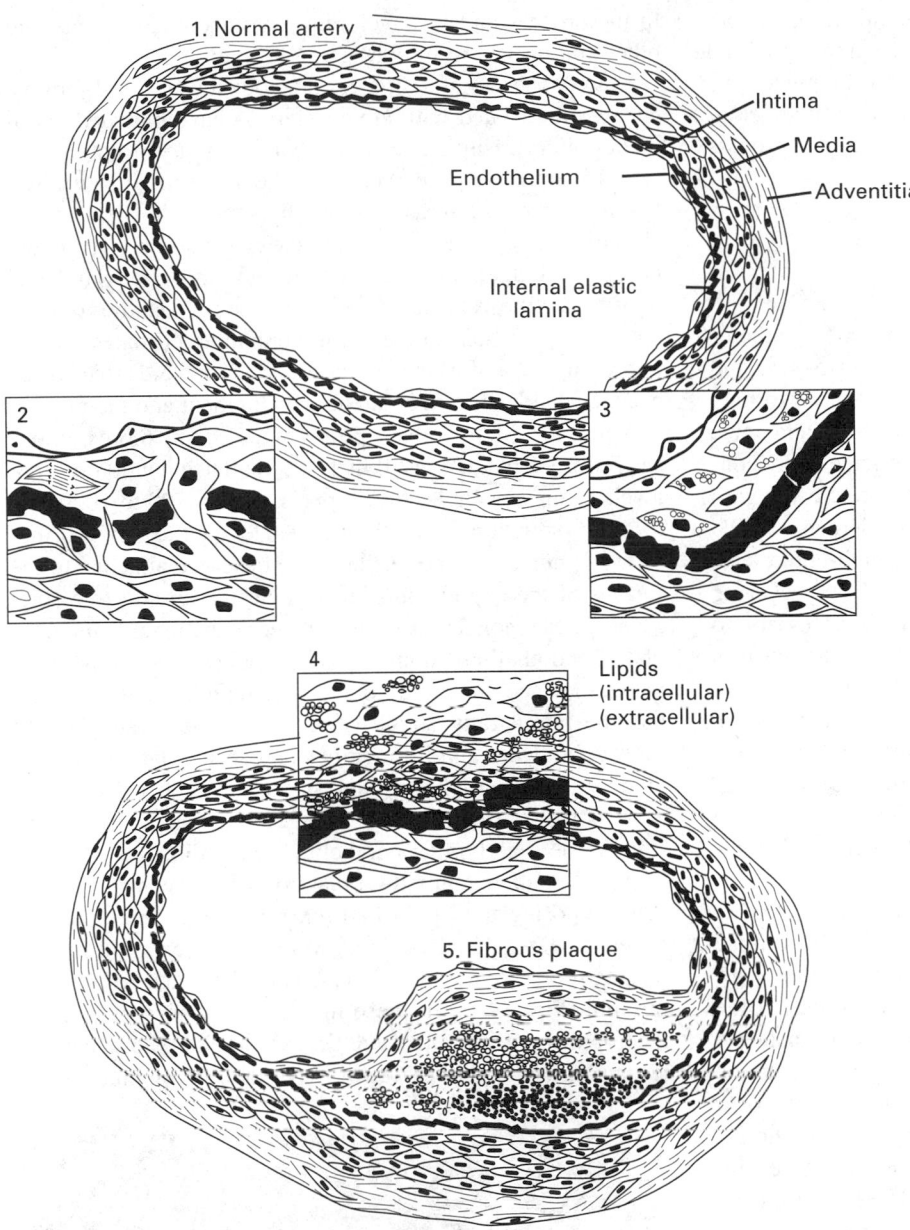

FIGURE 39-2
A series of possible stages in the development of the various lesions of atherosclerosis. (1) The appearance of a normal muscular artery and its component layers; the intima bounded by endothelium and internal elastic lamina, the media, and adventitia. In children and young adults, the intima is thin and contains only an occasional smooth muscle cell; with age, it slowly and uniformly increases in thickness and cell content. It is important to note that there are no fibroblasts present in either the intima or the media of mammalian arteries. Fibroblasts are found only in the adventitia. (2) The first phase of a developing lesion in atherosclerosis; a focal thickening of the intima consists of an increase in smooth muscle cells and extracellular matrix. Smooth muscle cells are shown proliferating within the intima; two are in the process of migrating through fenestrae of the internal elastic lamina. Subsequent to or possibly concomitant with internal smooth-muscle proliferation, accumulation of intercellular lipid deposits (3) or extracellular lipid (4) or both occurs, resulting in a fatty streak. A fibrous plaque (5) may result from a continued accumulation of a connective tissue cap covering increased numbers of smooth muscle cells laden with lipids, extracellular lipid, and cell debris overlying a deeper extracellular pool of lipid. A complicated lesion may form as a result of continuing cell degeneration, ingress of blood constituents, and calcification superimposed upon the elements present in the fibrous plaque. Observations made at necropsy and experiments such as those described in the text suggest that this may represent the sequence of events that occurs in humans. (Reprinted with permission from Glomset JA, Ross R. Atherosclerosis and the arterial smooth muscle cell. *Science* 1973; 180:1332. Copyright © 1973 by the American Association for the Advancement of Science.)

necrotic "lipid-rich core" increases in size and often becomes calcified. The lesions may become increasingly complex as a result of hemorrhage and calcification, and the intimal surface may develop fissures or cracks, may disintegrate and ulcerate, and may become involved with thrombotic episodes that can lead to occlusive disease. Such thrombi may then organize and further increase the thickness of the plaque while progressively reducing the size of the arterial lumen. It is not uncommon that as the intimal lesions progress, the number of smooth muscle cells in the underlying media decreases and the media undergoes atrophy, which can sometimes result in aneurysmal changes rather than lead to thrombotic occlusion of the artery.

There is quite a range of variability in the degree of severity of the lesions of atherosclerosis in different arteries. Individual lesions of atherosclerosis can vary greatly in their composition and organization. The typical advanced, complicated lesion contains a large, necrotic core. The artery "attempts to protect" the core by covering it with a fibrous cap, which can vary greatly in density and consistency.[4] Plaques that contain large, atheromatous cores may rupture, particularly when the lesion is located at sites of irregular flow and where the fibrous cap is thin and poorly developed. Plaque disruption may account for many of the thrombi that are responsible for acute coronary syndromes.[10,11] The site of fibrous cap rupture usually occurs where there are collections of macrophages, which can form numerous proteolytic enzymes, including metalloproteases.[12–15] Thus, the site of rupture of the fibrous cap may be at the shoulder of the lesion where the cap is thinnest and where the concentration of macrophages, often present as foam cells, is the greatest. Various forms of stress may be placed on the fibrous cap, due to alterations in the structure of the artery by the lesion itself and by its location at branches and bifurcations.

Recognition that the components of inflammation, smooth muscle proliferation, connective tissue formation, and lipid accumulation represent the key elements of developing lesions of atherosclerosis has led to the utilization of a number of models of experimentally induced disease to study this process in different animal species.

EXPERIMENTALLY INDUCED ATHEROSCLEROSIS

At least five species have been widely used in studying atherogenesis: rabbits, chickens, swine, nonhuman primates, and genetically modified mice. Most early work was performed in rabbits; however, swine, nonhuman primates, and mice homozygous for apolipoprotein E (ApoE) deficiency are considered to develop lesions that correspond more closely with those that occur in human beings. Atherosclerosis can be induced in most animal models by a high-fat, high-cholesterol diet. A principal shortcoming of this approach, however, is that to produce more advanced lesions, it is necessary to maintain animals on such diets for years. Even though it is possible to induce the lesions in a relatively short period (1 to 3 years in the monkey), it is not clear that the lesions produced in this manner actually simulate those that may require 20 to 30 years to form in human beings. On the other hand, the rate at which lesions form in humans is not entirely clear, since some may progress more rapidly than had heretofore been considered to be possible.[16]

A major, recent development in the field of atherosclerosis research has been the evolution of genetically modified mice that develop lesions of atherosclerosis similar to those observed in humans.[17] Not only are the lesions similar but the cellular events that precede lesion formation and the anatomic sites where the lesions form also have been shown to be similar in at least one of these strains of mice. Mice of a particular inbred strain (C57BL/6), when fed a high-cholesterol, high-fat diet containing cholic acid, show marked increases in plasma cholesterol levels and develop extensive fatty lesions at the root of the aorta.[18] Using gene knockout technology, two laboratories have generated mice deficient in ApoE, a cholesterol-carrying lipoprotein made principally in the liver, which participates in the recognition and clearance of low-density lipoprotein (LDL) by lipoprotein receptors in the liver. When fed a chow diet, these mice develop cholesterol levels of 400 to 600 mg/dL and, over time, lesions of atherosclerosis.[18–20] Other mouse models that have been studied include mice deficient in the LDL receptor gene[21] and transgenic mice with the human ApoB or lipoprotein (a) gene.[22,23]

In the homozygous ApoE-deficient mice, fatty streaks form after monocyte and lymphocyte adhesion, which then progress to intermediate and advanced lesions over time. In these mice the atherogenic stimuli appear to be chylomicron and very low density lipoprotein (VLDL) remnants. These mice and several other mouse models of atherogenesis should prove to be valuable tools in exploring the cells and molecules involved

in the process and in developing pharmacologic agents and other approaches to inhibit lesion formation.

Approaches to studying the smooth muscle proliferative changes associated with atherosclerosis have included endothelial injury resulting from mechanical injury from varying types of intraarterial catheters,[24] chemically induced injury (from sources such as chronic hypercholesterolemia[25] or chronic homocystinemia),[26] immune-type injuries[27] (from exposure to antigen-antibody complexes), and virally induced injury in entities such as Marek's disease.[28] In studies of diet-induced hypercholesterolemia in nonhuman primates, Faggiotto et al[29,30] and Masuda and Ross[31,32] have described the changes that lead to fatty streak development and the manner in which some fatty streaks progress to become more complicated fibrous plaques. Within 12 days after induction of high levels of plasma cholesterol (approximately 700 to 1000 mg/dL)[29,30] or within 1 month at lower levels (200 to 400 mg/dL),[31,32] numerous monocytes were observed attached to the surface of the endothelium throughout the arterial tree (Fig. 39-3). These monocytes probe between junctional complexes of the endothelium, migrate, and localize subendothelially, where they accumulate lipid and become foam cells to establish the initial fatty streak (Fig. 39-4). These fatty streaks form at branches and bifurcations and accumulate increasing numbers of macrophages and smooth muscle cells; in the process they create a markedly uneven surface contour and stretch the overlying endothelium exceedingly thin (Fig. 39-5). After about 5 months, breaks occur between endothelial cells, exposing the lipid-filled macrophages, some of which appear to enter the circulation. Many of the exposed macrophages serve as sites where platelets adhere and form mural thrombi (Fig. 39-6). In these monkeys, the sites of platelet-macrophage interactions were first observed in the iliac arteries, and after longer periods of hypercholesterolemia, similar

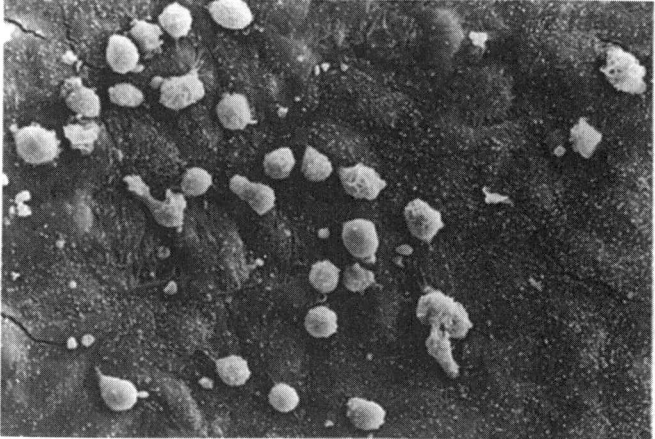

FIGURE 39-3

Scanning electron micrograph demonstrating the adherence of leukocytes (monocytes and T lymphocytes) to the endothelium in a segment of the aorta from a nonhuman primate that had been hypercholesterolemic (250 mg/dL) for 1 month. Most of the cells are rounded; however, a few of them have begun to spread on the surface over which they migrate prior to entry into the artery wall between the endothelial cells.

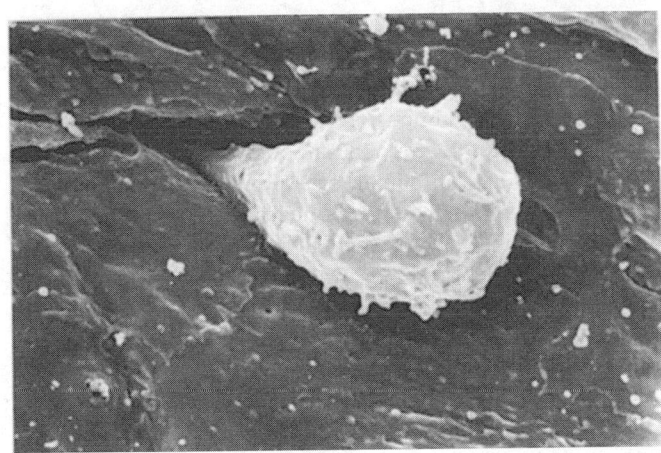

FIGURE 39-4

Scanning electron micrograph demonstrating a leukocyte that has found a port of entry between endothelial cells after having adhered to the surface of the endothelium. This cell is in the process of chemotaxis into the subendothelium, where it will participate in the formation of a fatty streak.

changes occurred at higher levels in the abdominal and thoracic aorta. Interestingly, the anatomic sites that were previously involved with platelet-macrophage interactions are the same sites that 1 to 2 months later contain proliferative smooth muscle lesions of atherosclerosis (Fig. 39-7). Similar studies of chronic hypercholesterolemia have been described in Watanabe heritable hyperlipemic rabbits (WHHL)[33,34] and in ApoE-deficient mice.[19,20] The same cellular interactions and process of lesion progression from fatty streak to intermediate lesion to fibrous plaque were observed in these two different animal models as those observed in the nonhuman primates. They also show the same increase in lesion progression in a cephalad direction that was observed in the earlier studies, suggesting a relationship between the early fatty streak and the ultimate advanced lesion, or fibrous plaque.

These studies, together with more recent observations in humans and numerous other experimental animals, further support observations that endothelial alterations, or "injury," cause cell-surface changes that induce leukocyte adhesion and the development of a specialized inflammatory response that

results in fatty streaks. It is probable that most fibrous plaques derive from fatty streaks through their continued expansion and by the induction of a fibroproliferative or healing response. Furthermore, both activated endothelial cells and macrophages can produce growth factors, including platelet-derived growth factor (PDGF), colony stimulating factor (CSF), transforming growth factor β (TGF-β), and numerous others are shown by Northern analysis for messenger ribonucleic acid (mRNA), and by histochemical demonstration of the presence of many of these proteins within the lesions of atherosclerosis. These factors can have profound effects by inducing endothelial activation, smooth muscle migration and proliferation, connective tissue formation, and macrophage replication.

Despite the fact that each of the animal models that has been studied has its shortcomings, the models have provided new and supportive information that relate to observations in human lesions and correlate with in vitro models that principally use cell culture techniques. The latter have permitted in-depth studies of endothelium, smooth muscle, macrophages, T cells, and platelets and have provided insight into the interrelationships among these cells, which are discussed later in this chapter. For example, on the basis of in vitro studies demonstrating the importance of oxidation mechanisms in vascular cell inflammatory responses, studies with antioxidants in animal models utilizing the antioxidant probucol, and more recently other antioxidants such as vitamin E have demonstrated

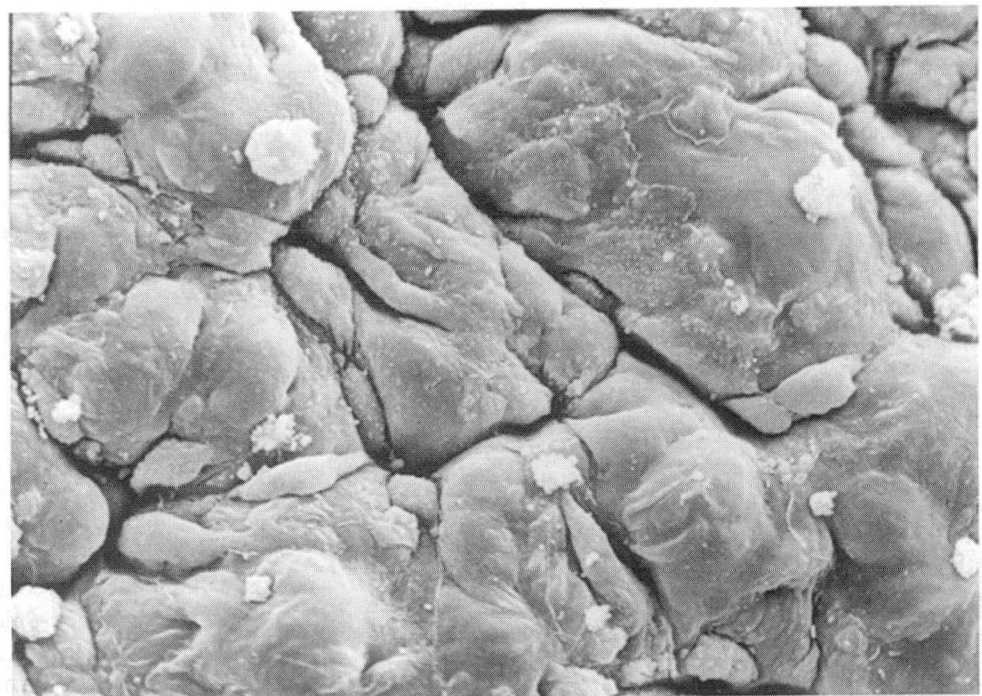

FIGURE 39-5

Scanning electron micrograph demonstrating the uneven appearance of the surface of a fatty streak in a hypercholesterolemic nonhuman primate. The domelike configurations and deep folds between these elevated regions represent accumulations of lipid-filled macrophages (foam cells) and T lymphocytes beneath the endothelial cells. Additional adherent leukocytes can be seen on the surface of the fatty streak that may potentially participate in the expansion of the lesion. Thus, the endothelium covering the surface of the fatty streak is altered and induces additional leukocyte adhesion, chemotaxis, and foam cell formation, so that the fatty streak can expand.

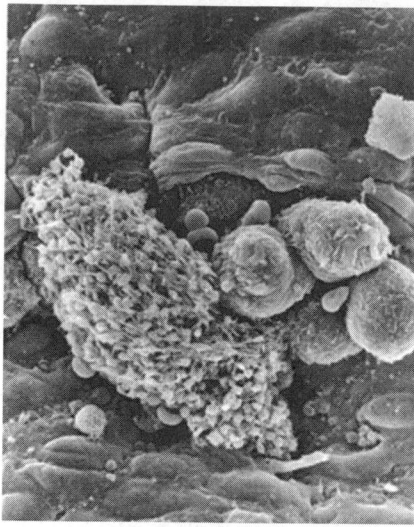

FIGURE 39-6

Scanning electron micrograph of a portion of a fatty streak that has become exposed due to separation between endothelial cells at their junctional attachment sites. The expanding lesion appears somehow to induce this separation, leading to exposure of the underlying lipid-filled macrophages, several of which have become a site for thrombus formation. The mural platelet thrombus that has formed on the left side of the micrograph demonstrates that many of these macrophages can become thrombogenic sites and potentially represent sites where the platelets may release their products, including several growth-regulatory molecules.

further that lesions of atherosclerosis can be markedly inhibited in the WHHL rabbit (model of familial homozygous hypercholesterolemia). Furthermore, antioxidants can inhibit fatty streak formation in hypercholesterolemic nonhuman primates. The latter studies were carried out for only 11 months

and thus were not of sufficient duration to have an impact on the formation of advanced lesions. Nevertheless, the data are striking; antioxidant therapy has the potential of being both preventive and, if administered for a sufficiently long time, may induce lesion regression, although the latter has not yet been demonstrated in human or experimental animals.

The cellular responses described in hypercholesterolemic nonhuman primates, rabbits, and the ApoE-deficient mouse have been verified in humans. Davies et al.[35] examined a series of hearts that contained advanced coronary atherosclerosis that were removed for transplant purposes. The hearts were perfusion-fixed as rapidly as possible after their removal and were examined by light and by scanning and transmission electron microscopy. Virtually the same cellular responses—including increased adherence and transendothelial migration of monocytes and T lymphocytes and localization in the intima to form the early fatty streaks—were observed. Further, sites of endothelial separation over expanding fatty streaks were observed to be covered by platelet mural thrombi, similar to the mural thrombi that formed on the exposed migrating macrophages in the nonhuman primates and rabbits. Ultimately, the cellular makeup of the advanced lesions of atherosclerosis in the human lesions are essentially identical to those observed in the experimental animals. In essence these observations represent the hallmarks of marked, chronic inflammation associated with a subsequent fibroproliferative process. Due to the excessive nature of both the inflammation and the fibroproliferative processes, the incursion of the lesion into the lumen of the artery, and secondary changes that lead to thrombosis and organization of the thrombi, these lesions continue to expand. When there is no compensatory arterial dilation, they will encroach upon the lumen and lead to clinical sequelae. Thus, *atherosclerosis represents an excessive, chronic inflammatory-fibroproliferative response that begins as a protective response but in its excess becomes the disease process.*

HYPOTHESIS OF ATHEROGENESIS

Historical View of Atherogenesis

Atherosclerosis has been recognized in humans for thousands of years. Lesions of atherosclerosis were identified in Egyptian mummies dating from as early as the fifteenth century B.C. Long has discussed the development of clinical-pathologic correlations that evolved during the era when autopsy examination permitted the formulation of a hypothesis relating the degree of atherosclerosis to the incidence of myocardial infarction and stroke.[36] In the mid–nineteenth century, Virchow proposed the idea that some form of injury to the artery wall associated with an inflammatory response resulted in what was then considered to be the degenerative lesion of atherosclerosis.[37] This idea was subsequently modified by Antischkow[38] and further included the role of platelets and thrombogenesis in atherosclerosis, as expanded by Duguid[39] in 1948. Many of the modern views of atherosclerosis stem from the

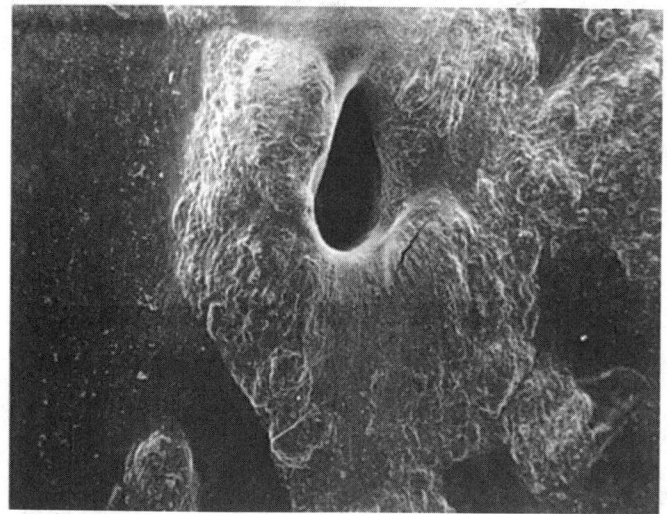

FIGURE 39-7

Low-power scanning electron micrograph of an intermediate or fibrofatty lesion that has formed at the inflow track of one of the intercostal arteries in the thoracic aorta of a chronically hypercholesterolemic nonhuman primate. The elevation due to the fibroproliferative response and continuing accumulation of macrophages in this lesion can be seen at this site. This may potentially go on to become a fibrous plaque.

work of John French,[40] who noted that the structural integrity of the endothelial lining of the artery represented a key element in the maintenance of normal arterial function and that alterations in endothelial integrity might precede a sequence of events that would lead to the various forms of the lesions of atherosclerosis. Thus, over the years, numerous theories concerning the etiology and pathogenesis of atherosclerosis have been developed.

The Response-to-Injury Hypothesis

One basis for the response-to-injury hypothesis of atherosclerosis[1,6,7,41] lies in the marked similarity observed by many investigators between the ubiquitous fibromusculoelastic lesions noted at autopsy and a similar lesion that can be induced in a number of animal species, including nonhuman primates, rabbits, ApoE-deficient mice, and swine after different forms of arterial endothelial injury.

The hypothesis (Fig. 39-8) posits that some form of "injury" to the endothelium results in structural and/or functional alterations in the endothelial cells. Factors such as chronic hypercholesterolemia[25]; altered shear stress from the flow of blood over the endothelial cells, which may occur at branch points or bifurcations in arteries in hypertension[42]; and dysfunction induced by toxins,[1] viruses,[28,43,44] bacteria, chlamydia,[45] genetic factors such as elevated homocysteine,[26] or other injurious agents may lead to changes in the nature of the protective barrier established by the endothelial cells. In the normal artery, the endothelial cells form a continuous monolayer that regulates the passage of substances from the plasma to the underlying artery wall.[46-48]

Injury to the endothelial cells may alter their permeability characteristics and change endothelial cell-cell or endothelial cell–connective tissue relations, permitting hemodynamic forces to induce focal endothelial cell dysfunction and thus permit interactions to occur between elements from the blood and the wall of the artery (see also Chap. 4).

Endothelial cells not only play an important role as a permeability barrier, but also form a thromboresistant surface that promotes the continuous flow of blood throughout the vascular tree. The thromboresistant character of the endothelium appears to be due principally to at least three factors produced by the cells. These factors have been identified, but some of their physiologic roles are relatively poorly understood. They are the cell-surface glycoproteins and proteoglycans that form the surface coat of the endothelial cells; a prostaglandin derivative, prostacyclin (PGI$_2$)[49]; and perhaps the most potent agent, nitric oxide (NO).[50] Prostacyclin and NO are potent vasodilatory agents and potent inhibitors of platelet aggregation. Both endothelial cells and smooth muscle cells are capable of synthesizing prostacyclin and NO (discussed in greater detail below).

Injury to the endothelium that results in alterations in function would permit plasma constituents such as lipoproteins to have more ready access to the artery wall. Injury and other factors that affect endothelial function may not result in any changes in the morphology of the endothelial monolayer that

lines the artery. Endothelial dysfunction could alter the thromboresistant character of the lumen of the artery, so that platelets could interact directly at sites of endothelial injury. If the injury were sufficiently severe, the endothelial cells might desquamate and be lost into the bloodstream, leading to exposure of the underlying connective tissue to platelets and to other elements in the circulation. The response-to-injury hypothesis suggests that the interaction between constituents in the plasma, platelets and monocyte/macrophages, T cells and the endothelium or the connective tissue could result in activation of a number of cells, including platelets, with release of contents normally stored within the granules of the platelets, and with release from activated macrophages or foam cells, from activated T cells, or even from endothelium of proinflammatory agents and growth factors. In most cases, the advanced lesions probably form due to macrophage–smooth muscle interactions. The early fatty streak contains principally macrophages and variable numbers of T cells. Platelet interactions may be relatively rare unless thrombosis occurs. Direct progression of fatty streaks to fibrous plaques probably represents the most common course of atherogenesis in hypercholesterolemia. The exposure of the artery wall at sites of injury to factors derived from platelets and/or macrophages, together with components from the plasma such as lipoproteins and hormones, would then lead to focal proliferation of arterial smooth muscle cells. According to the hypothesis, this smooth muscle proliferation would be derived from two sources: preexisting intimal smooth muscle cells and medial smooth muscle cells that are attracted to and migrate and proliferate within the intima at sites of "injury." Such a local stimulus could also lead to the formation of new connective tissue matrix constituents by the proliferating smooth muscle cells and to the deposition of lipids both within and around the proliferated cells.

According to this hypothesis, if the injury to the endothelium were a self-limited event and if endothelial function were restored, the proliferative lesions might be capable of regressing. If this were the case, the lesions would be reversible and, if they had not reached a critical size, would be clinically silent. There is evidence both in experimental animals and in human beings that the lesions of atherosclerosis can, under intensive lipid-lowering therapy, regress.[51-53]

On the other hand, if the injury at focal sites in the artery wall is either of long standing or chronically repeated over periods of many years, the lesions could continue to progress, become increasingly complex in terms of their composition, and eventually lead to the principal clinical sequelae of atherosclerosis—myocardial infarction and cerebral infarction. The capacity of the endothelium to regenerate and restore endothelial integrity at sites of injury may be critical in determining whether the lesions of atherosclerosis enlarge, remain relatively constant in size, or regress. The superimposition of risk factors that might possibly affect this balance by providing a chronic source of injury or by somehow altering the normal tissue response to injury might change the balance so that lesions would be slowly progressive. As an example, the

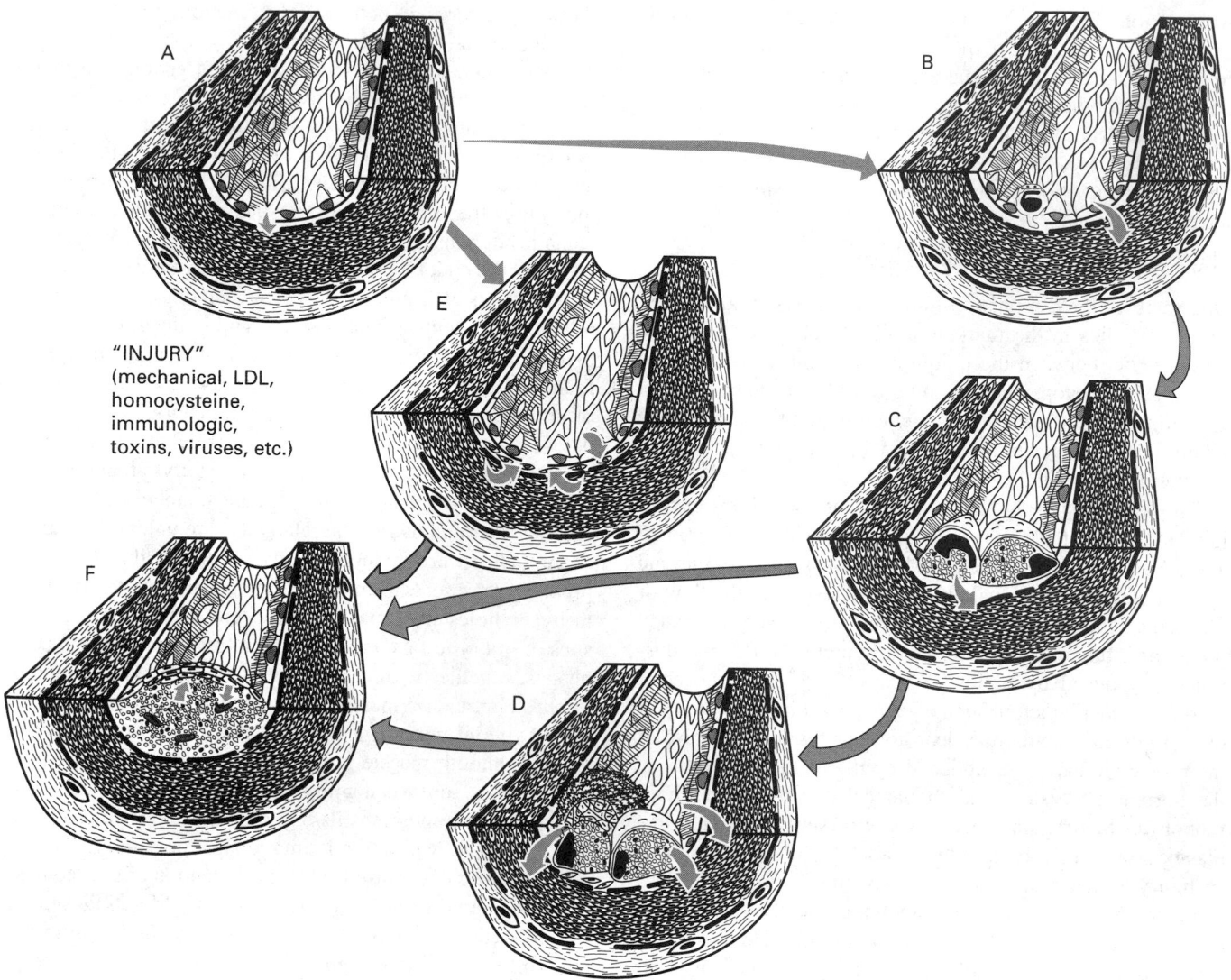

"INJURY"
(mechanical, LDL,
homocysteine,
immunologic,
toxins, viruses, etc.)

FIGURE 39-8

Revised response-to-injury hypothesis. Advanced intimal proliferative lesions of atherosclerosis may occur by at least two pathways. the pathway demonstrated by the clockwise (long) arrows to the right has been observed in experimentally induced hypercholesterolemia. Injury to the endothelium (A) may induce growth factor secretion (*short arrow*). Monocytes attach to endothelium (B), which may continue to secrete growth factors (*short arrow*). Subendothelial migration of monocytes (C) may lead to fatty-streak formation and release of growth factors such as PDGF (*short arrow*). fatty streaks may become directly converted to fibrous plaques (*long arrow from C to F*) through release of growth factors from macrophages or endothelial cells or both. Macrophages may also stimulate or injure the overlying endothelium. In some cases, macrophages may lose their endothelial cover and platelet attachment may occur (D), providing three possible sources of growth factors—platelets, macrophages, and endothelium (*short arrows*). Some of the smooth muscle cells in the proliferative lesion itself (F) may form and secrete growth factors such as PDGFs (*short arrows*). An alternative pathway for development of advanced lesions of atherosclerosis is shown by the arrows from A to E to F. In this case, the endothelium may be injured but remain intact. Increased endothelial turnover may result in growth factor formation by endothelial cells (A). This may stimulate migration of smooth muscle cells from the media into the intima, accompanied by endogenous production of PDGF by smooth muscle as well as growth factor secretion from the "injured" endothelial cells (E). These interactions could then lead to fibrous plaque formation and further lesion progression (F). (Reprinted by permission of The New England Journal of Medicine. Ross R. the pathogenesis of atherosclerosis: An update. *N Engl J Med* 1986; 314:488. Copyright 1986. Massachusetts Medical Society. All right reserved.)

increased levels of plasma low-density lipoprotein (LDL) associated with hypercholesterolemia may provide a source of injury to the endothelial cells and may also convert what might otherwise be a limited tissue response to injury to frank, progressive lesions of atherosclerosis.[1]

This hypothesis has stimulated a great deal of experimental work, leading to an improved understanding of factors that determine the capacity of the endothelial cells to maintain themselves as an integral continuous cell layer and to studies of those factors that control the growth of endothelium. Of equal importance, many studies have elucidated the factors that modify the capacity of arterial smooth muscle cells to form connective tissue proteins, to synthesize and metabolize lipids and lipoproteins, and to proliferate in response to different mitogenic factors. One of the more important observations resulting from examination of this hypothesis is the discovery that platelets, macrophages, and smooth muscle cells can release several potent mitogens, among them PDGF.[54] It has been suggested that this factor may play an important role in inducing the intimal smooth muscle proliferative response seen in experimentally induced atherosclerosis and in atherosclerosis in human beings (discussed in greater detail below).

A number of important questions have arisen concerning the factors that promote proliferation of smooth muscle and endothelial cells and the mechanisms whereby lesions of atherosclerosis may regress. More is becoming known concerning the factors such as metalloproteases, that are responsible for the turnover of connective tissue matrix within the artery wall, and that may be responsible for removing the matrix from lesions. The response-to-injury hypothesis has provided explanations for some of these phenomena. Much has been learned regarding the capacity of endothelial cells, macrophages, and smooth muscle cells to bind and metabolize lipoprotein and to make growth factors and their inhibitors as well as other modifiers of cell function and connective tissue metabolism.

Thus, in essence, *the response-to-injury hypothesis of atherosclerosis suggests that the "injury" to the endothelial cells lead to alterations in the endothelium that induce a long-standing chronic, inflammatory response.*[1,55,56] Because this injury and response occur intermittently or continuously over a prolonged period of time, the inflammation may become excessive. Both the excessive inflammatory response, involving both macrophages and T lymphocytes, and the resulting fibroliferative response in their excess become a disease process in themselves. It is not uncommon for such fibroliferative responses, when they are excessive, to become disease entities. This is probably the case not only in atherosclerosis but also in rheumatoid arthritis, pulmonary fibrosis, and hypertrophic scars. This excessive inflammatory, fibroliferative process thus lies at the heart of the response-to-injury hypothesis of atherosclerosis.[1]

The Role of Lipids

Both lesion initiation and lesion progression in atherosclerosis appear to be associated in many individuals with markedly increased elevations of plasma LDL. The accumulation of lipid within proliferated smooth muscle cells, within macrophages in the lesions, and within the extracellular connective tissue matrix is a common finding, particularly in the lesions of atherosclerosis.[3,4,57] The presence of elevated levels of LDL suggests that cholesterol internalization and esterification by cells may be accelerated to such a degree that proliferated smooth muscle cells within lesions become filled with cholesterol oleate. Many of the cells may go on to become necrotic and may release their lipid into the extracellular spaces. In the presence of excess plasma LDL, which is relatively rich in cholesterol linoleate, the debris may be a mixture of both types of cholesterol esters.

Many studies have demonstrated that modified or oxidized lipoproteins play a key role in the process of atherogenesis, particularly in hyperlipidemic individuals. This role was first appreciated when it was shown that antioxidant therapy, using the lipid-lowering drug probucol, could diminish lesion formation in genetically hyperlipidemic rabbits[58,59] and that subsequently a similar approach could inhibit the inflammatory response, or fatty streak formation, in hyperlipidemic nonhuman primates as well.[60,61] Oxidized and otherwise modified LDL can be taken up by scavenger receptors on monocyte-derived macrophages, can be chemotactic for these cells, can be toxic to endothelium, and may induce apoptosis in macrophages and possibly in other cell types. Furthermore, modified lipoproteins may induce the development of metalloproteinases and other enzymes that participate in connective tissue matrix degradation and in further modification of the lesions.[10]

Although a recent clinical trial of probucol in humans was not shown to produce definitive results by angiographic examination in patients on the antioxidant for 2 years, this trial does not necessarily prove the inefficacy of this approach. The observation of Sasahara et al.[60] and Chang et al.[61] that probucol therapy could statistically significantly decrease fatty streak formation and thus prevent initiation of lesion formation, provide clues about the role of oxidized or modified LDL in this process. It is possible that for antioxidants to have an effect on humans who have well-established, advanced lesions of atherosclerosis, a much longer period of treatment may be required, possibly for 5 to 10 years, before decreases in advanced lesions occur or prevention of lesion progression can be documented.[62,63]

The roles of lipids in atherogenesis have been amply demonstrated, initially by individuals with familial, homozygous hypercholesterolemia who lack functional LDL receptors and also by WHHL rabbits, which possess a similar molecular lesion. Two genetically modified mice, the ApoE-deficient mouse and the fat-led LDL receptor–deficient mouse, also develop extensive lesions of atherosclerosis.[19–21] Recommendations have been made in the United States for ideal levels of plasma cholesterol and plasma LDL cholesterol. In addition, approaches to diet and/or therapy, including lipid-lowering drugs, have been recommended to attain these goals (see Chap. 53).[64–66] Studies such as the Scandinavian Simvastatin Survival Study (4S)[67] and the West of Scotland Study (WOSCOPS)[68] demonstrate the clinical benefits of lipid lowering. It must also be recognized, however, that there are other factors besides lipids in this multifactorial disease. Many individuals who are not hyperlipidemic by conventional standards develop clinical sequelae of atherosclerosis. The interactions among lipids and other factors and the means of induction are discussed below.

The Role of Risk Factors

A number of risk factors for atherosclerosis have become reasonably well established on the basis of their relation, in epidemiologic studies, to the incidence of clinically manifest disease (Chap. 41). Unfortunately, there is no basis for comparison between risk factors and the severity or extent of the lesions of atherosclerosis. Among many factors that have been shown to be important are hyperlipidemia, hypertension, cigarette smoking, male sex, and diabetes mellitus. These have, in general, been associated with an increased incidence of fibrous plaques and their sequelae. The associations are relatively strong when they are made on a group comparison basis, although all of the studies have demonstrated a high degree of variability among individuals within even the most homogeneous of groups.[69]

HYPERLIPIDEMIA

Hyperlipidemia, endogenous (genetic) and diet-induced, is considered to be among the most important agents responsible for severe atherosclerosis and for high frequency of atherosclerotic disease in industrially developed parts of the world. Saturated fats became implicated in the increased incidence of atherosclerosis when it was found that they elevated the concentration of plasma cholesterol; however, the specific contributions of cholesterol, saturated fats, polyunsaturated fats, and total fats in atherosclerosis are still unclear. It has become possible to demonstrate an unequivocal association between ingestion of dietary cholesterol and plasma cholesterol levels and the incidence and prevalence of coronary disease within population groups. The results of the Lipid Research Clinics Trial[70,71] demonstrated a direct association between the plasma lipoprotein profile, cholesterol levels, and morbidity and mortality from coronary atherosclerosis. As noted above, at least three large clinical trials have demonstrated the efficacy of lipid lowering with hydroxymethylglutarylcoenzyme A (HMG-CoA) reductase inhibitors, or statins, together with dietary approaches and other cholesterol lowering agents, to reduce the clinical sequelae of atherosclerosis (see Chap. 53). The 4S trial[67] demonstrated an approximately 40 percent reduction in the incidence of myocardial infarction as well as a further reduction in the need for procedural intervention in hyperlipidemic individuals. The dramatic results in this study pointed to the benefits of reducing plasma LDL cholesterol and elevating high-density lipoprotein (HDL) cholesterol. Subsequently, the efficacy of this approach was shown in WOSCOPS in which hyperlipidemic patients with no personal history of clinical events but with a strong family history of cardiac events were enrolled.[68] This study suggests that there will be clinical benefits in using both dietary and pharmacologic approaches to lower plasma cholesterol.

Brown et al.[72] have demonstrated that some semiocclusive lesions of atherosclerosis, followed in individuals by angiography, can be induced to regress and decrease in size during a sufficient period of reduced plasma cholesterol levels. Those studies provided an unequivocal demonstration that some lesions of atherosclerosis can regress under appropriate conditions. Guidelines have been issued by the National Institutes of Health related to plasma cholesterol and lipoproteins. All individuals should have these measured as a routine part of their physical examination. Cholesterol levels below 200 mg/ dL are considered normal, levels of 200 to 240 mg/dL are considered borderline and should be treated by diet modification, and levels greater than 240 mg/dL should be treated with drug therapy. Similarly, LDL levels less than or equal to 130 mg/dL are considered normal, levels of 130 to 159 borderline, and levels greater than 160 mg/dL require therapy[65] (see Chap. 53).

There is a great deal of variation from individual to individual in terms of dietary intake of fats and of plasma cholesterol levels. There is also intrinsic variation in plasma cholesterol levels among individuals who consume the same diet but respond differently to it. There is little question that dietary cholesterol directly affects the levels of plasma cholesterol.[73] Dietary cholesterol may also affect the incidence of atherosclerosis by altering the profile of plasma lipoproteins and possibly by changing the structural or functional properties of these lipoproteins.[74] Increased dietary cholesterol generally results in an increase in LDL cholesterol, with a lesser increase in HDL cholesterol. Low density lipoprotein leads to increased uptake of lipid in cells, whereas HDL plays a role in removing lipid from cells and is thus protective (see Chaps. 41 and 53).

HYPERTENSION

Hypertension has been established unequivocally as an associated risk factor in that individuals with elevated blood pressure show accelerated atherogenesis, an increased incidence of coronary heart disease, and in particular, an increased incidence of cerebrovascular disease. The effects of hypertension appear to be independent of other risk factors in an epidemiologic sense; however, it does not appear to be a primary cause of advanced atherosclerosis in those populations in which the incidence of clinically manifest atherosclerosis is less than average.

The means by which hypertension induces atherogenesis are not clear, although there are many humoral mediators of blood pressure that may participate in this process. For example, renin, angiotensin, β-adrenergic substances, and other hypertensive agents may induce cellular changes that lead to atherogenesis. Fry,[42] as well as others have suggested that altered flow characteristics, including the eddy currents and backflow of blood, particularly in hypertensive individuals, at selected anatomic sites within the arterial tree may result in focally altered endothelium and in the development of atherosclerotic lesions very much as suggested in the response-to-injury hypothesis discussed earlier.

An important component in hypertension is the renin/angiotensin system, which plays a critical role in circulatory and fluid electrolyte homeostasis. Angiotensin II is the ultimate end product of the cleavage of its precursors, angiotensinogen, and angiotensin I, by renin and angiotensin converting enzyme, respectively, and is both the systemic and tissue-derived hormone that activates target organs including arteries, the kidneys, adrenal glands, and the heart. Locally, angiotensin II exerts autocrine-paracrine effects on arteries as well as the heart, and it can play an important role in the development of atherosclerosis. Angiotensin II is a potent vasoconstrictor, binds to receptors on smooth muscle cells that lead to the activation of phospholipases, and activates receptor-operated calcium channels, leading to calcium influx and increased smooth muscle contractility. Angiotensin II also induces secondary gene expression for growth factors such as TGF-β, PDGF, and fibroblast growth factor (FGF). Through these complex interactions, the hormonal influences that result in hypertension can lead to the development of lesions of atherosclerosis, particularly when they interact with other risk factors such as elevated plasma lipids.[75,76]

CIGARETTE SMOKING

Cigarette smoking provides perhaps the strongest and most consistent correlation with the increased incidence of atherosclerotic disease and appears to be a major contributor to increased risk of disease, generally in combination with other risk factors. Unfortunately, there is relatively little information concerning the means by which cigarette smoking exerts an impact at the cellular level. Early studies suggested that carbon monoxide might be a causative agent; however, these have not been confirmed. Becker et al.[77] identified agents derived from cigarette smoke that may be injurious to the artery wall. It has also been suggested that inhalation of cigarette smoke may result in the exposure of arterial cells to free radicals or other mutagens that transform the smooth muscle cells and result in the stimulation of their proliferation.[78] Apparently, cessation of cigarette smoking decreases the risk for development of the clinical sequelae of atherosclerosis and possibly may augment regression of lesions. Further research is clearly required to identify the factors in cigarette smoke that are responsible for its cardiovascular effects and to determine the mechanisms by which these factors alter cellular metabolism (see also Chap. 41).

GENDER

Perhaps one of the best documented and most consistent risk factors for coronary atherosclerosis is male sex. This gender-dependent differential risk is accentuated in nonwhite populations, and it has been suggested that females have a decreased incidence because of a protective function exerted by estrogens. Paradoxically, large doses of estrogenic hormones appear to increase cardiovascular mortality in men who have had one myocardial infarction and among those under treatment for prostatic cancer. Recently, a study of estrogens and their effects on smooth muscle cells and other elements of atherogenesis showed that estrogens can have an antiproliferative effect on smooth muscle and can be protective to the endothelium in relation to stimulation by growth factors, cytokines, and other agents.

The protective effects of estrogen in preventing atherosclerosis have been clearly demonstrated in epidemiologic studies.[79,80] Estrogen is not only antiproliferative[81] for smooth muscle but also has been shown to be capable of modulating acetylcholine-mediated dilation of atherosclerotic coronary arteries in premenopausal female nonhuman primates.[82] Thus the possibility of diminishing the effects of this disease by

hormonal treatment in postmenopausal women is under intensive investigation.

DIABETES

Another risk factor known to be associated with an increased incidence of atherosclerosis and myocardial infarction is diabetes mellitus. The mechanisms involved are poorly understood. There is, unfortunately, no consistency in the evidence related to whether elevated concentrations of plasma cholesterol and lipoproteins occur in diabetics whose concentrations of blood and urine glucose are carefully regulated. There does appear to be some evidence suggesting a decreased concentration of HDL cholesterol in diabetics and a high prevalence of hypertension associated with hyperglycemia.[83] The basic mechanisms associated with the proliferation of smooth muscle–type cells in the magnesium of the kidney in renal complications of diabetes and in increased thickness of capillary basement membrane in diabetics with microvascular disease may bear some similarity to smooth muscle proliferation in atherogenesis. In general, the alterations in the arterial tree in diabetics that precede the lesions of atherogenesis are not well documented and are poorly understood (see also Chaps. 41 and 78).

HOMOCYSTEINE

Elevated levels of plasma homocysteine (hyperhomocysteinemia) may be important in the population at large not only as a risk factor for atherosclerosis but also as a direct cause of the disease. Consistent observations from many studies with over 2000 subjects, including the Framingham Study, have shown that hyperhomocysteinemia together with low concentrations of folates and vitamin B$_6$ in the plasma, based upon their role in homocysteine metabolism, are associated with an increased risk of extracranial carotid artery stenosis, particularly in elderly individuals.[84]

Levels of homocysteine in the plasma above 14 μm/L appear to be associated with an increased incidence of atherosclerosis.[85,86] These increased levels of plasma homocysteine can occur from the genetic absence of the rate-limiting enzymes in homocysteine metabolism as well as from decreased levels of the vitamins noted above that play a role in this system. Elevated homocysteine appears to be toxic to the endothelium, depresses the capacity of endothelium to make nitric oxide, and induces endothelial dysfunction. As noted above, alterations in endothelial functions induced by agents including homocysteine may play a role in the process of atherogenesis. Once clinical trials have been completed to determine the appropriate levels of homocysteine for the population at large, it should be possible for the vast majority of patients to adjust their levels of plasma homocysteine by adjusting the level of folic acid in their diets.

Although a great deal of new information, discussed below, has evolved concerning our understanding of endothelial cells, smooth muscle cells, macrophages, and platelets and the interactions among these cells, the specific role of each of the risk factors that is associated with increased incidence of atherosclerosis on an epidemiologic basis remains, for the most part, to be investigated and elucidated. This information will be critical if we are to proceed with the development of improved means of diagnosis, prevention, and intervention in this disease process (see also Chap. 44).

CELLULAR MODULATIONS IN ATHEROSCLEROSIS

Endothelium

THE BARRIER ROLE
Endothelial cells provide a selective permeability barrier, a blood-compatible interface, and a thromboresistant lining to the artery wall, and they are metabolically active. Many studies of endothelial permeability using various tracer molecules have demonstrated the presence of pinocytotic vesicles, transendothelial channels, and intracellular clefts in different kinds of endothelium. The junctional complexes between endothelial cells and the artery wall appear to be functionally dynamic structures that can respond to stimuli such as changes in blood pressure and pharmacologic agents. The surface components, at the molecular level, of the endothelial cells appear to influence the selective permeability of the endothelium.[87,88] Endothelial cells have been shown by the Steins[89] to be capable of transporting plasma lipoproteins of given sizes into the artery wall via vesicles. Thus, molecules like HDL would be transported, but larger lipoproteins the size of VLDL or chylomicrons would have difficulty in crossing the endothelial barrier without some kind of alteration of these lipid-rich particles (see also Chap. 4).

Endothelium normally prevents leukocyte and platelet adhesion by forming PGI_2 and NO.[47] The disruption of this barrier has been shown in a number of experimental animals to result in opportunities that permit interactions between platelets and the artery wall at sites of endothelial injury, resulting in the formation of an intimal smooth muscle proliferative response. If endothelial cells are removed by abrasion with an intraarterial catheter, sites of exposure of the subendothelial connective tissue are quickly coated with a "carpet" of degranulated platelets (Fig. 39-9). The interaction of products released from the platelets and plasma constituents at such sites of endothelial injury precedes a sequence of events that begins with focal smooth muscle migration and proliferation and eventually leads to the development of a fibromusculoelastic lesion. If this mechanical injury is mod-

ified by the addition of a high-fat, high-cholesterol diet to the experiment, the hyperlipemic animals whose endothelium has been mechanically injured develop intimal proliferative lesions essentially identical to fibrous plaques. In the normocholesterolemic animals, such endothelial injury leads to a fibromusculoelastic proliferative lesion that, over a period of 6 months, may undergo regression, whereas in hypercholesterolemic animals, the lesions become slowly progressive and show no signs of regression (Figs. 39-10 and 39-11).

Ross and Harker observed that monkeys that received no mechanical injury but that were only fed a high-fat, high-cholesterol diet for a year or longer showed signs of endothelial injury as determined morphologically and by measurements of endothelial cell turnover at selected sites in the arterial tree.[25]

Faggiotto et al.[29,30] and Masuda and Ross[31,32] have observed a sequence of events in chronic hypercholesterolemic monkeys that culminates in dysjunction of endothelium overlying foam cells in fatty streaks derived from blood monocytes. Exposure of the foam cells leads to platelet interactions with both the macrophages and the exposed connective tissues. These interactions occur at the same anatomic sites that 1 to 2 months later are occupied be extensive smooth muscle proliferative lesions of atherosclerosis. Virtually identical observations also have been made in hypercholesterolemic rabbits[33,34] and in human coronary arteries with lesions of atherosclerosis.

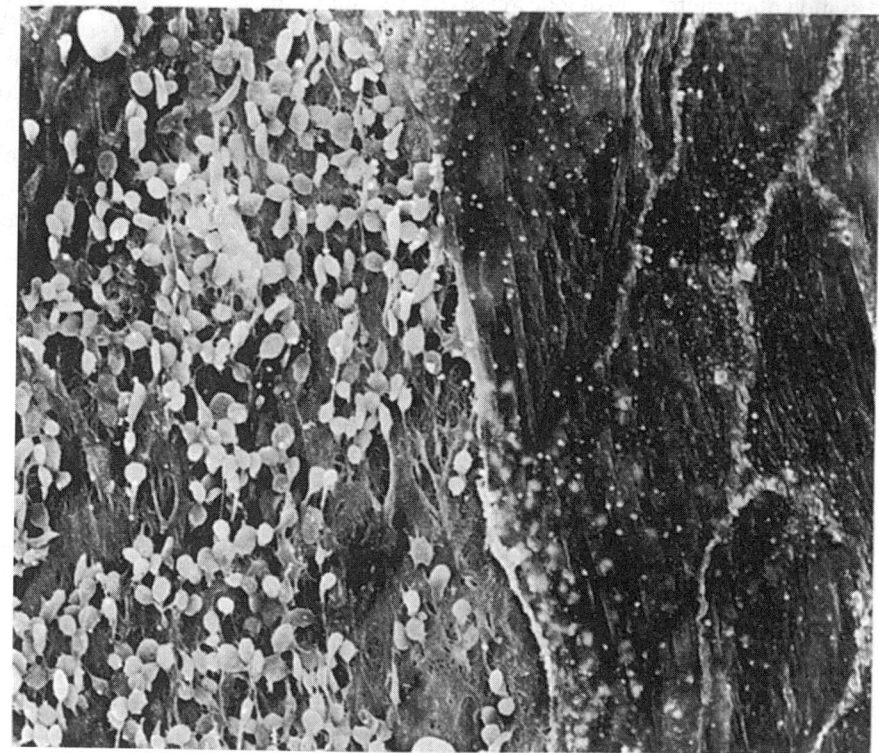

FIGURE 39-9

Scanning electron micrograph presenting a surface view of an artery in which the endothelial cells shown on the right have been removed with a catheter in the left portion of the micrograph. Demonstrates platelets, seen as the small ovoid bodies attached to the subendothelial connective tissue that was exposed upon injury to the endothelium. These platelets tend to adhere to the exposed connective tissue and to one another. In the process of doing so, they release their intracellular contents.

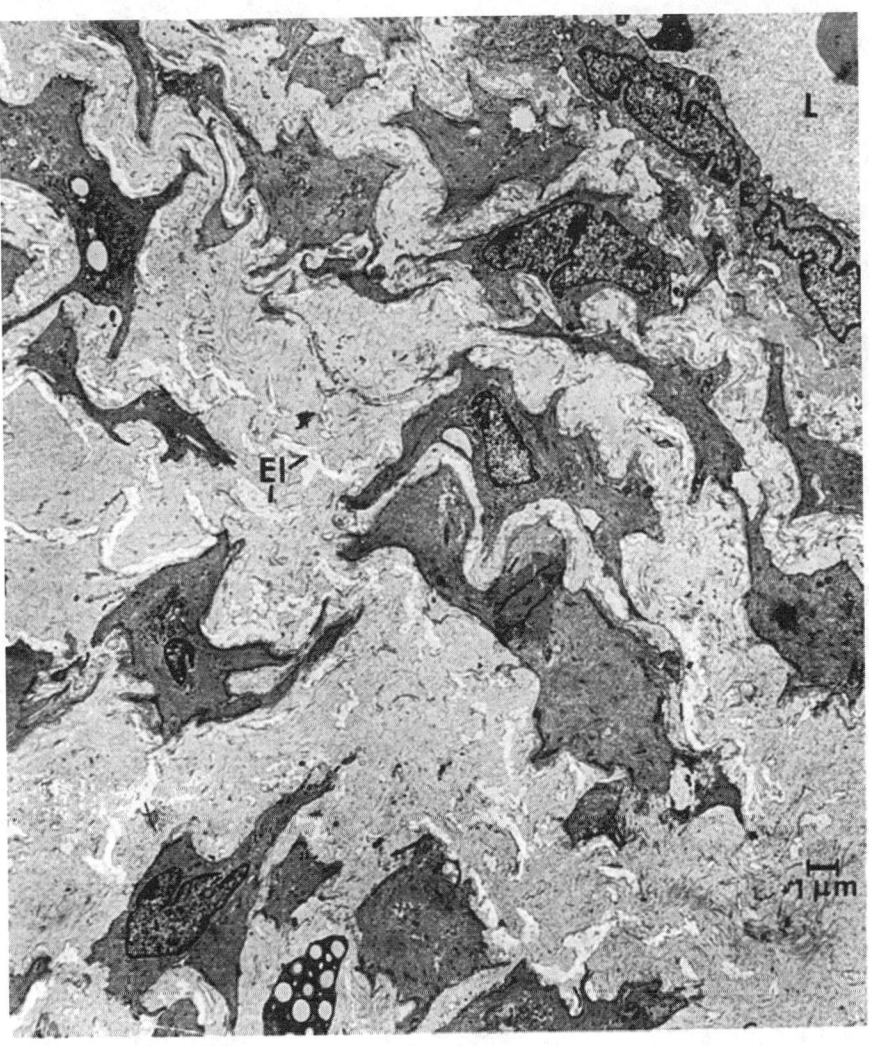

FIGURE 39-10

Electron micrograph of part of the intima from the right iliac artery of a macaque 3 months after the endothelium was removed with an intravascular balloon catheter. the lumen (L) is to the upper right. Endothelial cells cover the markedly thickened intima, which contains large numbers of smooth muscle cells surrounded by a matrix of small elastic fibers (El), collagen, and proteoglycan.

(ICAM-1). ICAM-1 is induced by altered shear and turbulent forces on the endothelial cells and is present at sites of slow flow and decreased shear, particularly opposite flow dividers. VCAM-1 has been shown to be upregulated in endothelium in animals that have elevated LDL cholesterol. Both of these molecules play a key role and perhaps act synergistically to cause the leukocytes to adhere and to spread. Another molecule formed by endothelium, pericellular adhesion molecule (PeCAM), has been shown to participate in interendothelial migration by the adherent leukocytes into the subendothelial space or intima of the artery. Thus, *the earliest phase of the chronic, inflammatory response that has become recognized to be the hallmark of atherogenesis is represented by leukocyte adhesion due to the formation of these attachment and adherence molecules on the surfaces of the endothelium and the leukocytes.*[91–93]

A second factor is transmigration of these adherent leukocytes between endothelial cells to localize in the subendothelial matrix, where they establish the first lesion of atherosclerosis, the fatty streak (Fig. 39-4). This transmigration of leukocytes is mediated by PeCAM and by chemotactic factors that can be generated both by the endothelial cells and by the underlying smooth muscle cells. Oxidized LDL, referred to above, can act as one of these chemotactic reagents and can also induce the endothelial cells and the underlying smooth muscle cells to form a second potent chemotactic factor, monocyte chemotactic protein 1 (MCP-1), which may also actively participate in this inflammatory process.

In addition to leukocyte adhesion, the intimal smooth muscle proliferation seen to accompany functional alteration of the endothelial cell barrier has been shown to be associated with the interactions between platelets and the exposed subendothelium at such sites of injury (discussed below).

ENDOTHELIAL CELL CULTURE

Arterial endothelial cells have been successfully cultured from a number of species, including the cow, rabbit, swine, nonhuman primate, and human being.[94,95] Endothelial cells from each of these species demonstrate a number of common characteristics. They grow, as they do in vivo, in a unique, continuous monolayer and, unlike cells such as smooth muscle or fibroblasts, appear to be truly "contact-inhibited." That is, the cells become quiescent when they remain in contact and become confluent. If the monolayer is disrupted—for exam-

It is now recognized that one of the earliest, principal changes that occurs in the endothelium after hyperlipidemia or in hypertensive individuals is increased adherence of leukocytes, specifically monocytes and T lymphocytes, to the endothelial cells at particular sites in the artery wall. These adherent leukocytes occur in clusters and appear to do so due to the formation of increased amounts of specific cell-surface adhesion molecules that are responsible for the leukocyte adhesion (Fig. 39-3).[1,90] Several of the cell-surface glycoproteins that form on both the leukocytes and the endothelial cells have been identified, isolated, and purified. These molecules include a class of adhesion factors called *selectins* (E, L, and P selectins) that appear to play a role in inducing rolling and attachment of monocytes and T lymphocytes to endothelium. These act together with the *immunoglobulin* family of cell adhesion molecules that includes vascular cell adhesion molecule 1 (VCAM-1) and intercellular adhesion molecule 1

ple, by wounding—the cells are stimulated to synthesize new deoxyribonucleic acid (DNA) synthesis and proliferation, whereas those in the monolayer at a distance from the wound appear to remain relatively quiescent. This peculiar characteristic of the growth of endothelium is so strikingly different from that of smooth muscle cells that it has been suggested that these two different cell types are under different sets of controls of their growth and that somehow cell-cell contact appears to be important in determining the state of quiescence of endothelial cells. Endothelial cells grown in culture have been shown to be capable of forming a number of connective tissue matrix macromolecules, including particular types of collagen,[96] transporting lipids, synthesizing prostacyclin,[49] factor VIII,[97] angiotensin-converting enzyme,[98] and, of particular importance, NO.[50] They are also able to maintain many aspects of their differentiated phenotype through several passages (see also Chap. 4).

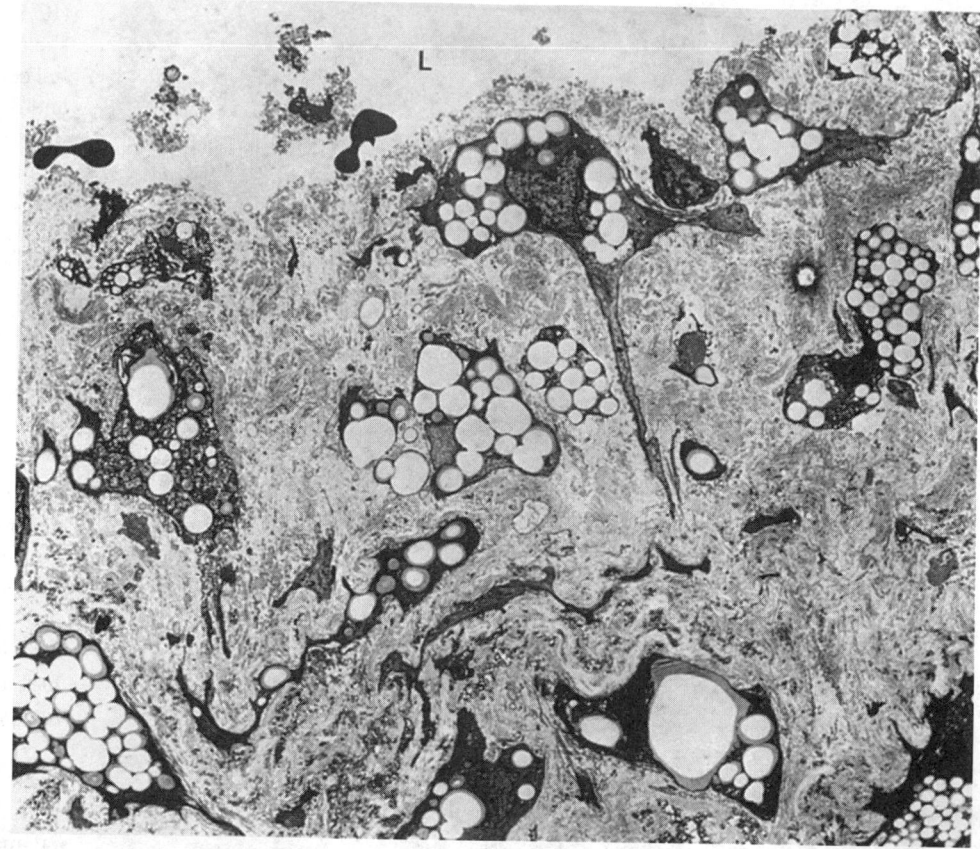

FIGURE 39-11

Electron micrograph of a portion of an intimal lesion in the iliac artery of a monkey on a hyperlipidemic diet 6 months after balloon injury. Most of the smooth muscle cells in the lesion contain large lipid deposits. The cells are surrounded by small, globular, membranous deposits in the connective tissue. An endothelial cover is lacking at the luminal surface (L) at the crest of the lesion.

ENDOTHELIUM-DERIVED GROWTH FACTORS

Endothelial cells have been shown to be capable of forming growth factors in culture. One of these substances is a form of PDGF capable of stimulating cells such as fibroblasts and smooth muscle to proliferate.[99] Endothelial cells in culture release PDGF into the medium after they have been exposed to plasma or to serum-free medium.[100] It is not yet known whether or not it is formed by endothelial cells in vivo, although in situ hybridization techniques have demonstrated the presence of mRNA for both chains of PDGF in arterial endothelium.[101] This observation could have potential importance in atherogenesis, because PDGF formation could induce lesion progression,

Upon exposure to appropriate angiogenic factors such as vascular endothelial growth factor (VEGF) and FGF, the endothelium may form microvascular channels that are derived either from adventitial capillaries or from the endothelium lining the lesions of atherosclerosis. These microvascular channels may result in a highly vascularized advanced atherosclerosis and could ultimately play a role in the intralesion hemorrhage and thrombosis that may occur in later stages of the disease.

Smooth Muscle

SMOOTH MUSCLE PROLIFERATION

Smooth muscle cells have long been recognized to possess a number of features important to normal arterial function, including their capacity to contract, maintain arterial tonus, and synthesize connective tissue proteins. Perhaps the most important phenomena associated with the smooth muscle cell are the processes of cell migration, proliferation, and matrix synthesis in atherogenesis. Since intimal smooth muscle proliferation is an important early feature in atherogenesis, the factors responsible for this proliferative response are under intensive investigation in vivo and in vitro. It is well known that serum provides all of the factors necessary for smooth muscle proliferation in cell culture. Arterial smooth muscle cells from a large number of species can be grown in culture and are able to maintain their differentiated phenotype under these conditions.[102,103]

Ross and coworkers,[54] as well as several other laboratories,[104,105] have demonstrated that the principal mitogenic component present in whole blood serum but missing in cell-free, plasma-derived serum and that is responsible for the proliferation of arterial smooth muscle cells in culture is a mitogen derived from the platelet, the PDGF. The observation that smooth muscle proliferation in culture is stimulated principally by this mitogen led to a series of studies to examine the role of platelets in smooth muscle proliferation induced in vivo. Since that time, several other smooth muscle cell mitogens, including FGF and heparin-binding epidermal growth factor-like growth factor (HB-EGF) have also been shown potentially to be involved in atherogenesis.

As described above, several forms of endothelial injury result in adherence of platelets at sites of injury. Platelet adherence is followed by activation, degranulation, and release into the artery wall of material stored in the platelet granules. Together with plasma constituents, these platelet products can have far-reaching effects upon the smooth muscle cells of the artery wall.

Harker et al. demonstrated that in homocystinuria, a genetic disease of childhood commonly associated with markedly increased incidence of atherosclerosis (discussed above), platelets appear to interact at sites where the endothelium has somehow been injured by increased levels of plasma homocysteine.[26] They demonstrated this association by measuring the survival of autologous platelets labeled with chromium 51 in homocystinuric children and observed that the greater the levels of plasma homocysteine, the greater the decrease in platelet survival. As a result of these observations, they developed an animal model of homocystinuria by chronically infusing homocysteine in baboons. In this model, they showed a similar correlation between elevated levels of plasma homocysteine and decreased levels of platelet survival (or increased platelet utilization). When they maintained the baboons on a homocystinemic regimen for 3 months, they observed an increased incidence of missing endothelial cells by morphometric examination of whole-mount preparations of the aorta. Their studies established a correlation between the amounts of injured endothelium, the decrease in platelet survival, and the formation of proliferative smooth muscle atherosclerotic lesions at the sites of endothelial injury.

Harker and colleagues went on to demonstrate that if they administered to the homocystinemic baboons one of two pharmacologic agents that could inhibit platelet interactions with the injured artery wall, they could prevent the intimal smooth muscle proliferative lesions that otherwise developed.[26] One of these agents, dipyridamole, returned platelet survival to normal levels and is known to inhibit both platelet phosphodiesterase activity and platelet adherence. The other agent, sulfinpyrazone, appeared to somehow protect the endothelial cells, since the sulfinpyrazone-treated homocystinemic baboons demonstrated fewer areas of endothelial injury. In both approaches, platelet survival levels were normalized and the proliferative lesions of atherosclerosis were prevented. These were the first data to correlate a requirement for platelet function with experimentally induced atherosclerosis.

Other approaches to examining these same phenomena were taken by Moore et al.[106] and by Friedman et al.[107] In both of their studies, atherosclerosis was induced in rabbits by injuring the endothelium with an intraarterial catheter. In each case the investigators induced a thrombocytopenia by administration of a specific antiplatelet antiserum. The animals made thrombocytopenic in this manner had no proliferative atherosclerosis lesions, whereas the control animals had extensive lesions.

Using a different approach, Fuster and colleagues[108] examined the incidence of atherosclerosis in the aortas of swine fed a high-fat, high-cholesterol diet. They were able to study the role of platelets by trying to induce atherosclerosis with a high-cholesterol diet in a group of swine that were homozygous for von Willebrand's disease as compared with a group of normal swine. The swine with severe von Willebrand's disease had essentially no factor VIII—von Willebrand's factor—in their plasma. Normally this factor is required for platelet adherence and release. The control animals on the high-lipid diet developed intimal infiltrates of lipid but no smooth muscle proliferative lesions. In the absence of von Willebrand's factor, platelet interactions may be somewhat inhibited in the hypercholesterolemic swine with von Willebrand's disease. All of these studies point to the importance of platelet interactions at sites of endothelial alterations that precede the formation of experimentally induced proliferative lesions of atherosclerosis (see Chap. 44).

Recent studies at the cellular and molecular levels in smooth muscle and endothelial cells have elucidated the intracellular signaling pathways that are activated when cells are induced to migrate chemotactically or to multiply after exposure to growth factors such as PDGF. Clearly separable intracellular signaling pathways for migration versus proliferation have been identified in human arterial smooth muscle cells after PDGF binds to its appropriate receptor and induces one or the other of these two phenomena.[109,110] Based upon the tyrosine molecules in the C-terminal portion of the PDGF receptor that are phosphorylated after binding to PDGF, phosphorylation leads to activation of specific elements in the cytosol, such as phospholipases, or to intermediate molecules, such as ras, raf, and the mitogen-activated protein (MAP) kinase cascade in the cells that ultimately lead to actin polymerization (in the case of smooth muscle chemotaxis) or to cell cycle traverse (in the case of smooth muscle proliferation) due to the activation of the appropriate intracellular signaling pathway. The migration signal pathway can be inhibited without affecting the proliferation signal pathway and vice versa.[109,110] The expansion of our understanding of the intracellular molecules and pathways that are required for these activities may someday lead to the development of pharmaceutical agents that can alter these pathways and thus control activities that are critical to the development of the lesions of atherosclerosis. Not only cell migration and proliferation are important in atherogenesis but also control of cell turnover, which includes programmed cell death, or apoptosis; that is important in cell accumulation and lesion size. Factors that regulate apoptosis in both smooth muscle and endothelium, as well as macrophages (see below) are beginning to be understood.[10] Those elements that control these activities may be crucial in understanding how to proceed in controlling progression or regression of the lesions of atherosclerosis.

LIPID METABOLISM

Since lipids are essential components of all cells, it is not surprising that they are involved in a number of cell functions and metabolic processes, as they represent the principal constituents of all cell membranes. Both the plasma membrane and the internal membranous compartments of all cells, including smooth muscle, are composed of phospholipids, proteins, and cholesterol, principally unesterified cholesterol. Esterified cholesterol is found in smooth muscle only under abnormal conditions. Accumulations of cholesterol ester in smooth muscle cells and macrophages lead to the development of foam cells found in the lesions of atherosclerosis. Some experiments have shown that smooth muscle cells can acquire cholesterol both by de novo synthesis[111] and from an exogenous source of cholesterol-carrying lipoproteins.[112] Such a dual mechanism may help the cell to protect itself against possible deficits in cholesterol.

Smooth muscle cells and many other cells can also protect themselves against excess cholesterol. The mechanism that has evolved for this purpose is the surface-located, high-affinity LDL receptor.[113,114] These receptors bind LDL, and the cell then internalizes the bound LDL by the process of endocytosis and transports it to lysosomes, where the LDL is degraded and free cholesterol is liberated for use by the cell that inhibits the synthesis of LDL receptors. In addition, the presence within the cell of excess cholesterol provides a signal that inhibits cholesterol synthesis by the rate-limiting intracellular enzyme HMG-CoA reductase (see Chap. 53).

Under normal circumstances, sterol balance in the cell maintains a given receptor level for LDL at the cell surface. In this way the requirements for extracellular cholesterol are met by concentrations of plasma LDL that are not atherogenic. Increased concentrations of plasma LDL may alter the endothelial barrier and bring large amounts of LDL in direct contact with the smooth muscle cell, which may ingest much of the LDL by bulk-phase endocytosis, bypassing the high-affinity receptor mechanism and leading to increased esterification and storage of cholesterol esters and the development of foam cells (see also Chap. 44).

As discussed above, several studies[58–62] have observed that antioxidant drugs protect hyperlipidemic rabbits and nonhuman primates by decreasing lesion formation due to decrease in oxidation of LDL. In hypercholesterolemia, the oxidized LDL may act primarily as the injurious agent to endothelium and is taken up by macrophages via their scavenger receptors. *Oxidized LDL is not only toxic to the endothelium and the surrounding cells in the intima but also chemotactic for monocytes and can activate monocyte-derived macrophages to produce growth factors and cytokines. It may be the principal culprit in advancing the lesions of atherosclerosis in hyperlipidemic individuals.*

Evidence is accumulating in favor of the notion that HDL, in contrast to LDL, is a negative factor in the development of atherosclerosis. Two mechanisms have been proposed to explain how HDL might be a deterrent against atherosclerosis. The first suggests that HDL augments the removal of cholesterol from cells such as smooth muscle. The second mechanism involves the apparent ability of HDL to influence the binding and absorption of LDL by cells such as smooth muscle. Neither of these mechanisms, however, has been shown to be responsible for control of cellular cholesterol.

In addition to metabolizing and responding to growth regulatory molecules, it has now been shown that smooth muscle cells themselves can form PDGF A chain. Smooth muscle cells can be induced to form PDGF-AA by other growth-regulatory molecules, such as TGF-β, or by the cytokines, interleukin-1 (IL-1) and tumor necrosis factor (TNF). In each case, the cells proliferate in culture due to autocrine stimulation by the PDGF-AA that the smooth muscle cells themselves form. Thus, under appropriate stimulation, it is entirely possible that smooth muscle cells may continue to proliferate in the artery wall if they are exposed to agents that appropriately induce them to stimulate themselves in an autocrine fashion.

The Macrophage

Macrophages are commonly found in early lesions of atherosclerosis as well as in advanced lesions like the fibrous plaque. They are probably the principal cell responsible for advanced lesion formation. In their studies of hypercholesterolemia in nonhuman primates, Faggiotto et al.[29,30] and Masuda and Ross[31,31] found that monocyte-derived macrophages were the major component of the fatty streaks in these animals and were found in abundance in fibrous plaques as well. A new observation made in those studies was the separation of endothelium over advancing lesions, leading to exposure of subendothelial, lipid-laden macrophages (foam cells) that sometimes became the foci for platelet adherence and formation of mural thrombi. Such cellular interactions were often found at anatomic sites (branches and bifurcations) that 1 to 2 months later were sites of advanced, proliferative smooth muscle lesions, The expansion of the macrophage-rich fatty streaks appeared possibly to predispose to rupture of endothelial junctions of overlying, thinly stretched endothelium. This junctional rupture established the conditions for macrophage exposure and for macrophage-platelet interactions. Macrophages could conceivably play several roles in lesion progression and possibly in regression as well. In tissue culture, macrophages have been shown to release mitogens as potent as those derived from platelets into the culture medium.[115] It has recently been shown that the mitogens formed by appropriately activated macrophages include both forms of PDGF (that is, dimers of both the A and B chains of the molecule),[116] TGF-α,[117] TGF-β,[118] IL-1, and possibly FGF. Since the macrophage is the principal cell of fatty streak and is located throughout the fibrous plaque, it would appear that it may, in fact, be the principal source of growth factors responsible for the progression of fatty streaks to fibrous plaques.

This concept is further supported by the recent observations that macrophages in all stages of atherogenesis contain reasonably large amounts of PDGF B-chain protein.[119] This discovery was made using a monoclonal antibody specific for PDGF B-chain, which, when used for immunohistochemistry, demonstrates the presence of this protein in a Golgi, rough endoplasmic reticulum–type distribution within the cells. Furthermore, using complementary DNA probes for PDGF B-chain and in situ hybridization, mRNA for PDGF-B (presumably PDGF-BB) can be shown to be present in these cells as well. Furthermore, there is increased expression of genes for PDGF in circulating monocytes in hypercholesterolemic patients.[120] Thus, the fact that both the message and the protein are present in these cells and that they have the capacity to secrete PDGF-BB in culture supports the notion that the macrophages are a principal source of mitogens, platelet interactions may occur only under certain circumstances, whereas macrophages are always present. Thus the majority of lesions may progress due to macrophage activation. This could occur through direct secretion of growth factors by the macrophages themselves or by macrophage secretion of cytokines such as TNF-α and IL-1. TNF-α has been shown to affect profoundly endothelial cells and to induce them to make PDGF.[121] IL-1 induces smooth muscle cells also to make PDGF. Macrophage activation and endothelial or smooth muscle interactions such as those that could occur in the fatty streak may lead to oxidation of lipid (which in turn could injure endothelium) and to formation and release of cytokines that result, directly or indirectly, in smooth muscle proliferation. Thus PDGF may play a principal role in the process of lesion progression.

Macrophages are not only potentially responsible for smooth muscle and endothelial proliferation but they also represent one of the principal replicating cells in the process of atherogenesis. It is now accepted that macrophage proliferation in the lesions can be as prominent as smooth muscle proliferation and that replication of these cells is important in lesion formation and progression. Macrophages appear to multiply in the lateral margins of advanced lesions of atherosclerosis and are responsible for the majority of foam cells that make up not only the fatty streak but the other lesions of atherosclerosis as well.

It has been recognized that unstable advanced lesions of atherosclerosis, which often have thin fibrous caps, may be the principal basis for sudden death and thus myocardial infarctions and stroke[10,11,122] (see Chap. 40). Sites where the fibrous caps have ruptured have been shown to be related to loci of activated macrophages, which can produce numerous hydrolytic enzymes such as metalloproteases that can degrade fibrin, collagen, elastic fibers, and proteoglycans. Thus the monocytes/macrophages are not only critical components in the normal host-defense mechanisms, but they play critical roles in lesion formation and progression by forming growth factors and cytokines and in lesion disruption by forming degradative enzymes that have profound effects in this inflammatory, fibroproliferative response.

T Lymphocytes

As noted above, T lymphocytes are ubiquitous in all phases of atherogenesis, as determined by the use of antibodies that recognize the different types of T cells. Some 10 to 20 percent of the lymphocytes in the lesions express antigens such as CD3. Approximately 60 percent of these express the CD4 antigen and 30 percent the CD8 antigen. T cells presumably enter the lesion by mechanisms similar to those used by monocytes, namely, via adhesion molecules on the surface of the endothelium. Many of these T cells have IL-2 receptors and HLA-DR on their surfaces. Both activated macrophages and T cells are present in the lesions and proliferate.[123] The antigens that bring the T cells in may include viruses, oxidized or modified LDL,[124] and possibly heat shock proteins. Thus the potential for macrophage–T cell interactions in the lesions of atherosclerosis is reasonably good, although the specific antigens that elicit this cellular, immune response remain to be identified.

Platelets

Aggregates of platelets, or mural thrombi, are commonly observed in every phase of lesion formation during atherogenesis in nonhuman primates. Similar aggregates have been observed in human lesions, as described above. Because platelets can provide a number of growth-regulatory molecules and cytokines to the tissues upon their activation and release, the presence of platelet aggregates may be important in lesion progression. This is particularly the case in the special type of neointimal smooth muscle proliferative response that forms after balloon catheter angioplasty and also may be critical in progression of advanced lesions of atherosclerosis, which characteristically develop fissures, cracks, or ulcerations, which can serve as sites for mural thrombosis. If the mural thrombus is not occlusive, it could serve as a rapid means of increase in lesion size due to the organization of the thrombus by smooth muscle cells that migrate from the lesion adjacent to the thrombus into the thrombus due to the presence of numerous chemotactic growth-regulatory molecules, in particular PDGF (see also Chaps. 40 and 52).

GROWTH REGULATORY MOLECULES, CYTOKINES, AND OTHER LOW MOLECULAR WEIGHT SUBSTANCES

A number of cytokines and other growth-regulatory molecules have been shown to be capable of either directly or indirectly influencing smooth muscle cell replication and connective tissue formation. For example, TGF-β is a potent inhibitor of cell replication. It also will induce secondary gene expression of PDGF A-chain in smooth muscle cells, PDGF-AA secretion, and smooth muscle proliferation at low doses. At high doses, it is a potent inhibitor of smooth muscle replication. At the same time, TGF-β is probably the most potent molecule known to induce the synthesis of connective tissue molecules, such as collagen, proteoglycans, and elastic fiber proteins.

Like TGF-β, the cytokines IL-1 and TNF-α also induce secondary gene expression for PDGF in smooth muscle cells and endothelium, respectively, as noted previously. These two molecules can also have profound effects on cells. Since they represent principal products of activated macrophages, they could play critical roles in lesion progression or regression. Finally, many cells appear to contain FGF, which can be released during cell injury. This is true for endothelium, smooth muscle, and macrophages. Thus, injury sufficient to induce increased cell permeability or, if severe enough, cell lysis and release of FGF could also be important in furthering proliferation of both the smooth muscle cells and potentially even endothelial cells, should this occur within the tissues. Additionally, other molecules have been discovered, the function of which in atherosclerosis is not clear but may be important. An example is HB-EGF. This molecule is as potent a mitogen for smooth muscle as is PDGF, binds to the EGF receptor, and can be formed by smooth muscle cells or activated macrophages. Northern analysis of human atherosclerotic lesions has demonstrated the presence of this molecule. Its potential role in atherogenesis is under active investigation.

Platelet-Derived Growth Factor

PDGF is a mitogen that is stored in the alpha granule of the platelets and consists of two highly homologous chains (A and B) of 16,000 and 14,000 molecular weight, has a molecular weight of approximately 32,000, and is highly cationic (pI 9.8), stable, disulfide-bonded protein. This growth factor is extremely potent, as it will cause proliferation of all susceptible cells in culture at a level of 5 ng/mL of culture medium (equivalent to addition of 5 percent whole blood serum). As discussed earlier in this chapter, PDGF is the principal mitogen in whole blood serum to which cells characteristically respond by cell proliferation. Exposure of smooth muscle to this factor results in a sequence of events that includes binding of the molecules to receptors on the surface of the cells. This then induces intracellular signals that stimulate the cell to traverse the cell cycle, leading to DNA synthesis and cell multiplication.

PDGF stimulates a number of phenomena in addition to DNA synthesis upon exposure to smooth muscle cells. It causes increases in pinocytosis, protein synthesis, RNA synthesis, and lipid metabolism. Chait et al.[112] observed that exposure of arterial smooth muscle cells to this growth factor results in increased binding of LDL to the cells due to formation of an increased number of high-affinity receptors for LDL at the cell surface. This increased binding of LDL permits the cells to utilize exogenous sources of cholesterol for cell multiplication more effectively. Habenicht et al.[111] demonstrated that this mitogen also stimulates increased cholesterol synthesis by cells if an exogenous source of cholesterol is not available to them. Davies and Ross[125] observed that smooth muscle cells exposed to PDGF undergo a marked increase in

the rate of endocytosis of tracer molecules. In other words, exposure to this mitogen results in an increase in a number of cellular activities, many of which are associated with cell proliferation and with new protein synthesis and therefore with connective tissue formation.[126] Thus, exposure to this factor could potentially provide the trigger that results in the inhibition of all the components of a proliferative lesion PDGF is clearly operative in cell culture and has recently been shown to be formed by endothelium, macrophages, and even appropriately activated smooth muscle cells. Thus most of the cells involved in lesion development are probably involved in PDGF generation during the process of atherogenesis.[127] Formation of this growth factor, together with others elaborated by the cells, is probably dependent upon particular cellular interactions. The role of functional platelets and macrophages in inducing experimental atherosclerosis in vivo is unquestioned. The role of PDGF in stimulating mitogens in cell culture is clear and is rapidly becoming clarified in vivo, particularly in view of its presence in macrophages in the lesions, as noted above (see also Chaps. 4 and 7).

Nitric Oxide and Prostaglandins

A great deal has been learned about nitric oxide (NO) and the prostaglandins, all of which may play critical roles in the metabolism of endothelium, smooth muscle, and platelets in atherogenesis.[49,50,128,129] All three of these cell types are capable of converting the fatty acid arachidonic acid into prostaglandin endoperoxides that can lead to the formation of two important end products, thromboxin A_2 (TXA$_2$), formed by platelets, and prostacyclin (PGI$_2$), formed by endothelium and smooth muscle. Arachidonic acid is derived either from diet or from linoleic acid, a fatty acid in the membrane of cells. TXA$_2$ is a powerful vasoconstrictor and capable of stimulating smooth muscle contraction and platelet aggregation. It has a short half-life and breaks down spontaneously into a stable substance, thromboxane B_2. A number of inhibitors of thromboxane synthesis markedly reduce platelet aggregation, including aspirin and indomethacin. PGI$_2$ is the principal product of cyclooxygenase activity in the walls of arteries and veins and is synthesized by both endothelium and smooth muscle from arachidonic acid. PGI$_2$ is also unstable and is a potent vasodilator as well as an inhibitor of platelet aggregation. The balance between these two substances may be important in determining whether arteries undergo vasoconstriction or dilation as well as platelet adhesion, aggregation, and thrombosis (see also Chap. 3).

Perhaps the most important vasoactive substance that plays critical roles in hypertension and in atherosclerosis is NO. This molecule was first called endothelial-derived relaxing factor and may circulate primarily as a nitrosothiol adduct after combining with sulfhydryl groups, proteins, or possibly free amino acids.[130,131] NO can be produced by several enzymes including a constitutive NO synthase made by endothelium, which can be stimulated by a variety of hormones such as acetylcholine, bradykinin, histamine, or endothelin[132,133] and by mechanical factors resulting from alterations in flow. NO synthesis can be inhibited by certain arginine derivatives. NO can diffuse across cell membranes and bind to the heme in soluble guanylate cyclase resulting in increased production of cyclic guanosine monophosphate (GMP), which can have many effects including increased permeability and decreased phosphorylation of myosin light chain, leading directly to muscle relaxation. NO inhibits platelet aggregation and production of endothelin (another potent vasoconstrictor molecule made by endothelial cells). NO plays a major role in maintaining normal tonus in the artery. Decreases in NO can lead to vasoconstriction, whereas increases can lead to vasodilation. Individuals who are hyperlipidemic and have extensive atherosclerosis appear to have impaired vasodilation, suggesting either impairment in NO synthase or excessive degradation of NO, likely by oxygen free radicals. NO may also have arterial protective effects, since mice lacking the gene for endothelial NO synthase become hypertensive.[134] Thus the induction of increased levels of NO in individuals who are atherogenic poses an interesting area for future study (see also Chaps. 4 and 44).

REFERENCES

1. Ross R. The pathogenesis of atherosclerosis: A perspective for the 1990s. *Nature* 1993; 362:801–809.
2. Stary HC. Macrophages, macrophage foam cells, and eccentric intimal thickening in the coronary arteries of young children. *Atherosclerosis* 1987; 64:91–108.
3. Stary HC, Chandler AB, Glagov S, Guyton JR, Insull W Jr, Rosenfeld ME, et al. A definition of initial, fatty streak, and intermediate lesions of atherosclerosis. *Circulation* 1994; 89:2462–2478.
4. Stary HC, Chandler AB, Dinsmore RE, Fuster V, Glagov S, Insull W, et al. A definition of advanced types of atherosclerotic lesions and a histological classification of atherosclerosis. *Circulation* 1995; 92:1355–1374.
5. Wissler RW, Hiltscher L, Oinuma T, PDAY Research Group. The lesions of atherosclerosis in the young: From fatty streaks to intermediate lesions. In: Fuster V, Ross R, Topol EJ, eds. *Atherosclerosis and Coronary Artery Disease*. Philadelphia: Lippincott-Raven; 1996: 475–489.
6. Ross R, Glomset JA. The pathogenesis of atherosclerosis. *N Engl J Med* 1976; 295:420–425.
7. Ross R. The pathogenesis of atherosclerosis—an update. *N Engl J Med* 1986; 314:488–500.
8. U. S. Department of Health, Education and Welfare. *Arteriosclerosis: A Report by the National Heart and Lung Institute Task Force on Arteriosclerosis, II.* DHEW pub. (NIH) 72-219. 1971:1 365.
9. McGill HC Jr. Atherosclerosis: Problems in pathogenesis. *Atheroscler Rev* 1977; 2:27–65.
10. Libby P. Molecular bases of the acute coronary syndromes. *Circulation* 1995; 91:2844–2850.
11. Falk E, Shah PK, Fuster V. Coronary plaque disruption. *Circulation* 1995; 92:657–671.
12. Moreno PR, Falk E, Palacios IF, Newell JB, Fuster V, Fallon JT. Macrophage infiltration in acute coronary syndromes: Implications for plaque rupture. *Circulation* 1994; 90:775–778.
13. Galis ZS, Sukhova GK, Lark MW, Libby P. Increased expression of matrix metalloproteinases and matrix degrading activity in vulnerable regions of human atherosclerotic plaques. *J Clin Invest* 1994; 94:2493–2503.
14. Nikkari ST, O'Brien KD, Ferguson M, Hatsukami T, Welgus HG, Alpers CE, et al. Interstitial collagenase (MMP-1) expression in human carotid atherosclerosis. *Circulation* 1995; 92:1393–1398.
15. Brown DL, Hibbs MS, Kearney M, Loushin C, Isner JM. Identification of 92-kD gelatinase in human coronary atherosclerotic lesions: Associ-

ation of active enzyme synthesis with unstable angina. *Circulation* 1995; 91:2125–2131.
16. DeBakey ME. Patterns of atherosclerosis and rates of progression. *Atheroscler Rev* 1976; 3:1–56.
17. Breslow JL. Mouse models of atherosclerosis. *Science* 1996; 272:685–688.
18. Zhang SH, Reddick RL, Burkey B, Maeda N. Diet-induced atherosclerosis in mice heterozygous and homozygous for apolipoprotein E gene disruption. *J Clin Invest* 1994; 94:937–945.
19. Reddick RL, Zhang SH, Maeda N. Atherosclerosis in mice lacking ApoE: Evaluation of lesional development and progression. *Arterioscler Thromb* 1994; 14:141–147.
20. Nakashima Y, Plump AS, Raines EW, Breslow JL, Ross R. ApoE-deficient mice develop lesions of all phases of atherosclerosis throughout the arterial tree. *Arterioscler Thromb* 1994; 14:133–140.
21. Ishibashi S, Goldstein JL, Brown MS, Herz J, Burns DK. Massive xanthomatosis and atherosclerosis in cholesterol-fed low density lipoprotein receptor-negative mice. *J Clin Invest* 1994; 93:1885–1893.
22. Callow MJ, Verstuyft J, Tangirala R, Palinski W, Rubin EM. Atherogenesis in transgenic mice with human apolipoprotein B and lipoprotein (a). *J Clin Invest* 1995; 96:1639–1646.
23. Mancini FP, Newland DL, Mooser V, Murata J, Marcovina S, Young SG, et al. Relative contribution of apolipoprotein (a) and apolipoprotein-B to the development of fatty lesions in the proximal aorta of mice. *Arterioscler Thromb Vasc Biol* 1995; 15:1911–1916.
24. Bjorkerud S, Bondjers G. Arterial repair and atherosclerosis after mechanical injury: I. Permeability and light microscopic characteristics of endothelium in non-atherosclerotic and atherosclerotic lesions. *Atherosclerosis* 1971; 13:355–363.
25. Ross R, Harker LA. Hyperlipidemia and atherosclerosis. *Science* 1976; 193:1094–1100.
26. Harker LA, Ross R, Slichter SJ, Scott CR. Homocystine-induced arteriosclerosis: The role of endothelial cell injury and platelet response in its genesis. *J Clin Invest* 1976; 58:731–741.
27. Minick CR, Murphy GE. Experimental induction of atheroarteriosclerosis by the synergy of allergic injury to arteries and lipid-rich diet: II. Effect of repeated injections of horse serum in rabbits fed a lipid-rich, cholesterol-poor diet. *Am J Pathol* 1973; 73:265–300.
28. Fabricant CG, Fabricant J, Litrenta MM, Minick CR. Virus induced atherosclerosis. *J Exp Med* 1978; 48:335–340.
29. Faggiotto A, Ross R, Harker L. Studies of hypercholesterolemia in the nonhuman primate: I. Changes that lead to fatty streak formation. *Arteriosclerosis* 1984; 4:323–340.
30. Faggiotto A, Ross R. Studies of hypercholesterolemia in the nonhuman primate: II. Fatty streak conversion to fibrous plaque. *Arteriosclerosis* 1984; 4:341–356.
31. Masuda J, Ross R. Atherogenesis during low-level hypercholesterolemia in the nonhuman primate: I. Fatty streak formation. *Arteriosclerosis* 1990; 10:164–177.
32. Masuda J, Ross R. Atherogenesis during low-level hypercholesterolemia in the nonhuman primate: II. Fatty streak conversion to fibrous plaque. *Arteriosclerosis* 1990; 10:178–187.
33. Rosenfeld ME, Tsukada T, Gown AM, Ross R. Fatty streak initiation in Watanabe heritable hyperlipemic and comparably hypercholesterolemic fat-fed rabbits. *Arteriosclerosis* 1987; 7:9–23.
34. Rosenfeld ME, Tsukada T, Chait A, Bierman EL, Gown AM, Ross R. Fatty streak expansion and maturation in Watanabe heritable hyperlipemic and comparably hypercholesterolemic fat-fed rabbits. *Arteriosclerosis* 1987; 7:24–34.
35. Davies MJ, Woolf N, Rowles PM, Pepper J. Morphology of the endothelium over atherosclerotic plaques in human coronary arteries. *Br Heart J* 1988; 60:459–464.
36. Long ER. The development of our knowledge of arteriosclerosis. In: Cowdry EV, ed. *Arteriosclerosis: A Survey of the Problem*. New York: Macmillan; 1933:19–52.
37. Virchow R. *Gesammelte Adhandlungen zur Wissenschaftlichen Medicin*. Frankfurt-am-Main: Meidinger Sohn; 1856:458–636.
38. Anitschkow NN. A history of experimentation on arterial atherosclerosis in animals. In: Blumenthal HT, ed. *Cowdry's Arteriosclerosis*, 2d ed. Springfield, IL: Charles C Thomas; 1967:21–44.
39. Duguid JB. Thrombosis as a factor in the pathogenesis of coronary atherosclerosis. *J Pathol Bacteriol* 1946; 58:207–212.
40. French JE. Atherosclerosis in relation to the structire and function of the arterial intima, with special reference to the endothelium. *Int Rev Exp Pathol* 1966; 5:253–353.

41. Ross R, Glomset JA. Atherosclerosis and the arterial smooth muscle cell. *Science* 1973; 180:1332–1339.

42. Fry DL. Hemodynamic forces in atherogenesis. In: Scheinberg P, ed. *Cerebrovascular Diseases.* Tenth Princeton Conference. New York: Raven Press; 1976:77–95.

43. Hajjar DP, Fabricant CG, Minick CR, Fabricant J. Virus-induced atherosclerosis: Herpesvirus infection alters arterial cholesterol metabolism and accumulation. *Am J Pathol* 1986; 122:62–70.

44. Hajjar DP. Viral pathogenesis of atherosclerosis: Impact of molecular mimicry and viral genes. *Am J Pathol* 1991; 139:1195–1211.

45. Grayston JT, Kuo C, Coulson AS, Campbell LA, Lawrence RD, Lee MJ, et al. *Chlamydia pneumoniae* (TWAR) in atherosclerosis of the carotid artery. *Circulation* 1995; 92:3397–3400.

46. Gimbrone MA Jr. Vascular endothelium in health and disease. In: Haber E, ed. *Molecular Cardiovascular Medicine.* New York: Scientific American Medicine; 1995:49–61.

47. DiCorleto PE, Gimbrone MA Jr. Vascular endothelium. In: Fuster V, Ross R, Topol EJ, eds. *Atherosclerosis and Coronary Artery Disease.* Philadelphia: Lippincott-Raven; 1996:387–399.

48. Griendling KK, Alexander RW. Endothelial control of the cardiovascular system: Recent advances. *FASEB J* 1996; 10:283–292

49. Moncada S, Higgs EA, Vane JR. Human arterial and venous tissue generate prostacyclin (prostaglandin x), a potent inhibitor of platelet aggregation. *Lancet* 1977; 2:18–20.

50. Snyder SH. No endothelial NO. *Nature* 1995; 377:196–197.

51. Wissler RW, Vesselinovitch D. Studies of regression of advanced atherosclerosis in experimental animals and man. *Ann NY Acad Sci* 1976; 275:363–378.

52. Blankenhorn DH, Nessim SA, Johnson RL, Sanmarco ME, Azen SP, Cashin-Hemphill L. Beneficial effects of combined colestipol-niacin therapy on coronary atherosclerosis and coronary venous bypass grafts. *JAMA* 1987; 257:3233–3240.

53. Superko HR, Krauss RM. Coronary artery disease regression: Convincing evidence for the benefit of aggressive lipoprotein management. *Circulation* 1994; 90:1056–1069.

54. Ross R, Glomset JA, Kariya B, Harker L. A platelet-dependent serum factor that stimulates the proliferation of arterial smooth muscle cells in vitro. *Proc Natl Acad Sci USA* 1974; 71:1207–1210.

55. Munro JM, Cotran R. The pathogenesis of atherosclerosis: Atherogenesis and inflammation. *Lab Invest* 1988; 58:249–261.

56. Hajjar DP, Nicholson AC. Atherosclerosis: An understanding of the cellular and molecular basis of the disease promises new approaches for its treatment in the near future. *Am Sci* 1995; 83:460–467.

57. Geer JC, McGill HC Jr, Strong JP. The fine structure of human atherosclerotic lesions. *Am J Pathol* 1961; 38:263–287.

58. Kita T, Nagano Y, Yokode M, Ishii K, Kume H, Ooshima A, et al. Probucol prevents the progression of atherosclerosis in Watanabe heritable hyperlipidemic rabbit, an animal model for familial hypercholesterolemia. *Proc Natl Acad Sci USA* 1987; 84:5928–5931.

59. Carew TE, Schwenke DC, Steinberg D. Antiatherogenic effect of probucol unrelated to its hypocholesterolemic effect: Evidence that antioxidants in vivo can selectively inhibit low density lipoprotein degradation in macrophage-rich fatty streaks and slow the progression of atherosclerosis in the Watanabe heritable hyperlipidemic rabbit. *Proc Natl Acad Sci USA* 1987; 84:7725–7729.

60. Sasahara M, Raines EW, Chait A, Carew TE, Steinberg D, Wahl PW, et al. Inhibition of hypercholesterolemia-induced atherosclerosis in the nonhuman primate by probucol: I. Is the extent of atherosclerosis related to resistance of LDL to oxidation? *J Clin Invest* 1994; 94:155–164.

61. Chang MY, Sasahara M, Chait A, Raines EW, Ross R. Inhibition of hypercholesterolemia-induced atherosclerosis in the nonhuman primate by probucol: II. Cellular composition and proliferation. *Arterioscler Thromb Vasc Biol* 1995; 15:1631–1640.

62. Steinberg D. Antioxidants and atherosclerosis: A current assessment. *Circulation* 1991; 84:1420–1425.

63. Greenberg ER, Sporn MB. Antioxidant vitamins, cancer, and cardiovascular disease. *N Engl J Med* 1996; 334:1189–1190.

64. Pedersen TR. Lowering cholesterol with drugs and diet. *N Engl J Med* 1995; 333:1350–1351.

65. National Cholesterol Education Program. Second report of the Expert Panel on Detection, Evaluation, and Treatment of High Blood Cholesterol in Adults (Adult Treatment Panel II). *Circulation* 1994; 89:1333–1445.

66. Pyörälä K, De Backer G, Graham I, Poole-Wilson P, Wood D. Prevention of coronary heart disease in clinical practice: Recommendation of the Task Force of the European Society of Cardiology, European Atherosclerosis Society and European Society of Hypertension. *Eur Heart J* 1994; 15:1300–1331.

67. Scandinavian Simvastatin Survival Study Group. Randomised trial of cholesterol lowering in 4444 patients with coronary heart disease: The Scandanavian Simvastatin Survival Study (4S). *Lancet* 1994; 344:1383–1389.

68. Shepherd J, Cobbe SM, Ford I, Isles CG, Lorimer AR, MacFarlane PW, et al. Prevention of coronary heart disease with pravastatin in men with hypercholesterolemia. *N Engl J Med* 1995; 333:1301–1307.

69. McGill HC Jr. Risk factors for atherosclerosis. *Adv Exp Med Biol* 1978; 104:273–280.

70. Lipid Research Clinics Program, Lipid Metabolism-Atherogenesis Branch, National Heart, Lung, and Blood Institute. The lipid research clinics coronary primary prevention trial results: I. Reduction in incidence of coronary heart disease. *JAMA* 1984; 251:351–364.

71. Lipid Research Clinics Program, Lipid Metabolism-Atherogenesis Branch, National Heart, Lung, and Blood Institute. The lipid research clinics coronary primary prevention trial results: II. The relationship of reduction in incidence of coronary heart disease to cholesterol lowering. *JAMA* 1984; 251:365–374.

72. Brown BG, Albers JJ, Fisher LD, Schaefer FM, Lin J-T, Kaplan C, et al. Regression of coronary artery disease as a result of intensive lipid-lowering therapy in men with high levels of apolipoprotein B. *N Engl J Med* 1990; 323:1289–1298.

73. Grundy SM. Dietary fats and sterols. In: Levy R, Rifkind B, Dennis B, Ernst N, eds. *Nutrition, Lipids, and Coronary Heart Disease.* New York: Raven Press, 1979:89–118.

74. McGill HC Jr. The relationship of dietary cholesterol to serum cholesterol concentration and to atherosclerosis in man. *Am J Clin Nutr* 1979; 32(suppl):2664–2702.

75. Dzau VJ, Chobanian AV. Renin-angiotensin system and atherosclerotic vascular disease. In: Fuster V, Ross R, Topol EJ, eds. *Atherosclerosis and Coronary Artery Disease.* Philadelphia: Lippincott-Raven; 1996:237–242.

76. Paul M, Bachmann J, Ganten D. The tissue renin-angiotensin system in cardiovascular disease. *Trends Cardiovasc Med* 1992; 2:94–99.

77. Becker CG, Dubin T, Wiedemann HP. Hypersensitivity to tobacco antigen. *Proc Natl Acad Sci USA* 1976; 73:1712–1716.

78. Stafford RS, Becker CG. Cigarette smoking and atherosclerosis. In: Fuster V, Ross R, Topol EJ, eds. *Atherosclerosis and Coronary Artery Disease.* Philadelphia: Lippincott-Raven; 1996:303–325.

79. Wenger NK, Speroff L, Packard B. Cardiovascular health and disease in women. *N Engl J Med* 1993; 329:247–256.

80. Stampfer MJ, Colditz GA, Willett WC, Manson JE, Rosner B, Speizer FE, et al. Postmenopausal estrogen therapy and cardiovascular disease. *N Engl J Med* 1991; 325:756–762.

81. Sullivan TR, Karas RH, Aronovitz M, Faller GT, Ziar JP, Smith JJ, et al. Estrogen inhibits the response-to-injury in a mouse carotid artery model. *J Clin Invest* 1995; 96:2482–2488.

82. Williams JK, Shively CA, Clarkson TB. Determinants of coronary artery reactivity in premenopausal female cynomolgus monkeys with diet-induced atherosclerosis. *Circulation* 1994; 90:983–987.

83. Aronson D, Rayfield EJ. Diabetes and obesity. In: Fuster V, Ross R, Topol EJ, eds. *Atherosclerosis and Coronary Artery Disease.* Philadelphia: Lippincott-Raven; 1996:327–359.

84. Selhub J, Jacques PF, Bostom AG, D'Agostino RB, Wilson PWF, Belanger AJ, et al. Association between plasma homocysteine concentrations and extracranial carotid-artery stenosis. *N Engl J Med* 1995; 332:286–291.

85. Robinson K, Mayer EL, Miller DP, Green R, van Lente F, Gupta A, et al. Hyperhomocysteinemia and low pyridoxal phosphate: Common and independent reversible risk factors for coronary artery disease. *Circulation* 1995; 92:2825–2830.

86. Hopkins PN, Wu LL, Wu J, Hunt SC, James BC, Vincent GM, et al. Higher plasma homocyst(e)ine and increased susceptibility to adverse effects of low folate in early familial coronary artery disease. *Arterioscler Thromb Vasc Biol* 1995; 15:1314–1320.

87. Simionescu N, Simionescu M, Palade GE. Permeability of muscle capillaries to small heme-peptides: Evidence for the existence of patent transendothelial channels. *J Cell Biol* 1975; 64:586–607.

88. Renkin EM. Multiple pathways of capillary permeability. *Circ Res* 1977; 41:735–743.

89. Stein Y, Stein O. Interaction between serum lipoproteins and cellular components of the arterial wall. *Biochem Atheroscler* 1979; 7:313–344.

90. Springer TA, Cybulsky MI. Traffic signals on endothelium for leukocytes in health, inflammation, and atherosclerosis. In: Fuster V, Ross R, Topol EJ, eds. *Atherosclerosis and Coronary Artery Disease.* Philadelphia: Lippincott-Raven, 1996:511–537.

91. Springer TA. Traffic signals for lymphocyte recirculation and leukocyte emigration: The multistep paradigm. *Cell* 1994; 76:201–314.

92. Carlos TM, Harlan JM. Leukocyte-endothelial adhesion molecules. *Blood* 1994; 84:2068–2101.

93. Bevilacqua MP. Endothelial-leukocyte adhesion molecules. *Annu Rev Immunol* 1993; 11:767–804.

94. Gimbrone MA Jr. Culture of vascular endothelium. *Prog Hemost Thromb* 1976; 3:1–28.

95. Jaffe EA, Nachman RL, Becker CG, Minick CR. Culture of human endothelial cells derived from umbilical veins: Identification by morphologic and immunologic criteria. *J Clin Invest* 1973; 52:2745–2756.

96. Jaffe EA, Minick CR, Adelman B. Synthesis of basement membrane by cultured human endothelial cells. *Circulation* 1975; 51(suppl 1):11.

97. Jaffe EA, Hoyer LW, Nachman RL. Synthesis of antihemophilic factor antigens by cultured human endothelial cells. *J Clin Invest* 1973; 52:2757–2764.

98. Gimbrone MA Jr, Alexander RW. Angiotensin II stimulation of prostaglandin production in cultured human vascular endothelium. *Science* 1975; 189:219–220.

99. Gajdusek C, DiCorleto P, Ross R, Schwartz SM. An endothelial cell derived growth factor. *J Cell Biol* 1980; 85:467–472.

100. DiCorleto PE, Bowen-Pope DF. Cultured endothelial cells produce a platelet-derived growth factor-like protein. *Proc Natl Acad Sci USA* 1983; 80:1919–1923.

101. Wilcox JN, Smith KM, Williams LT, Schwartz SM, Gordon D. Platelet-derived growth factor mRNA detection in human atherosclerotic plaques by in situ hybridization. *J Clin Invest* 1988; 82:1134–1143.

102. Ross R, Kariya B. Morphogenesis of vascular smooth muscle in atherosclerosis and cell culture. In: Bohr DF, Somlyo AP, Sparks HV, eds. *Handbook of Physiology—The Cardiovascular System II: Circulation, Vascular Smooth Muscle.* Bethesda, MD: American Physiological Society; 1980:69–91.

103. Chamley-Campbell J, Campbell GR, Ross R. The smooth muscle cell in culture. *Physiol Rev* 1979; 59:1–61.

104. Kohler N, Lipton A. Platelets as a source of fibroblast growth-promoting activity. *Exp Cell Res* 1974; 87:297–301.

105. Heldin C-H, Wasteson A, Westermark B. Partial purification and characterization of platelet factors stimulating the multiplication of normal human glial cells. *Exp Cell Res* 1977; 109:429–437.

106. Moore S, Friedman RJ, Singal DP, Gauldie MA, Blajchman MA, Roberts RS. Inhibition of injury induced thromboatherosclerotic lesions by anti-platelet serum in rabbits. *Thromb Haemost* 1976; 35:70–81.

107. Friedman RJ, Stemerman MB, Wenz B, Moore S, Gauldie J, Gent M. The effect of thrombocytopenia on experimental atherosclerotic lesion formation in rabbits: Smooth muscle cell proliferation and re-endothelialization. *J Clin Invest* 1977; 60:1191–1201.

108. Fuster V, Bowie EJW, Lewis JC, Fass DN, Owen CA Jr, Brown AL. Resistance to arteriosclerosis in pigs with von Willebrand's disease: Spontaneous and high cholesterol diet–induced arteriosclerosis. *J Clin Invest* 1978; 61:722–730.

109. Bornfeldt KE, Raines EW, Nakano T, Graves LM, Krebs EG, Ross R. Insulin-like growth factor-I and platelet-derived growth factor-BB induce directed migration of human arterial smooth muscle cells via signaling pathways that are distinct from those of proliferation. *J Clin Invest* 1994; 93:1266–1274.

110. Bornfeldt KE. Intracellular signaling in arterial smooth muscle migration versus proliferation. *Trends Cardiovasc Med* 1996; 6:143–151.

111. Habenicht AJR, Glomset JA, Ross R. Relation of cholesterol and mevalonic acid to the cell cycle in smooth muscle and Swiss 3T3 cells stimulated to divide by platelet-derived growth factor. *J Biol Chem* 1980; 255:5134–5140.

112. Chait A, Ross R, Albers JJ, Bierman EL. Platelet-derived growth factor stimulates activity of low density lipoprotein receptors. *Proc Natl Acad Sci USA* 1980; 77:4084–4088.

113. Brown MS, Faust JR, Goldstein JL. Role of the low density lipoprotein receptor in regulating the content of free and esterified cholesterol in human fibroblasts. *J Clin Invest* 1975; 55:783–793.

114. Goldstein JL, Brown MS. The low-density lipoprotein pathway and its relation to atherosclerosis. *Annu Rev Biochem* 1977; 46:897–930.

115. Leibovich SJ, Ross R. A macrophage-dependent factor that stimulates the proliferation of fibroblasts in vitro. *Am J Pathol* 1976; 84:501–513.

116. Shimokado K, Raines EW, Madtes DK, Barrett TB, Benditt EP, Ross R. A significant part of macrophage-derived growth factor consists of at least two forms of PDGF. *Cell* 1985; 43:277–286.

117. Madtes DK, Raines EW, Sakariassen KS, Assoian RK, Sporn MB, Bell GI, et al. Induction of transforming growth factor-alpha in activated human alveolar macrophages. *Cell* 1988; 53:285–293.

118. Assoian RK, Fleurdelys BE, Stevenson HC, Miller PJ, Madtes DK, Raines EW, et al. Expression and secretion of type beta transforming growth factor by activated human macrophages. *Proc Natl Acad Sci USA* 1987; 84:6020–6024.

119. Ross R, Masuda J, Raines EW, Gown AM, Katsuda S, Sasahara M. Localization of PDGF-B protein in macrophages in all phases of atherogenesis. *Science* 1990; 248:1009–1012.

120. Billett MA, Adbeish IS, Alrokayan SAH, Bennett AJ, Marenah CB, White DA. Increased expression of genes for platelet-derived growth factor in circulating mononuclear cells of hypercholesterolemic patients. *Arterioscler Thromb Vasc Biol* 1996; 16:399–406.

121. Hajjar KA, Hajjar DP, Silverstein RL, Nachman RL. Tumor necrosis factor-mediated release of platelet-derived growth factor from cultured endothelial cells. *J Exp Med* 1987; 166:235–245.

122. Falk E, Shah PK, Fuster V. Pathogenesis of plaque disruption. In: Fuster V, Ross R, Topol EJ, eds. *Atherosclerosis and Coronary Artery Disease.* Philadelphia: Lippincott-Raven; 1996:491–507.

123. Rekhter MD, Gordon D. Active proliferation of different cell types, including lymphocytes, in human atherosclerotic plaques. *Am J Pathol* 1995; 147:668–677.

124. Stemme S, Faber B, Holm J, Wiklund O, Witztum JL, Hansson GK. T lymphocytes from human atherosclerotic plaques recognize oxidized low density lipoprotein. *Proc Natl Acad Sci USA* 1995; 92:3893–3897.

125. Davies PF, Ross R. Mediation of pinocytosis in cultured arterial smooth muscle and endothelial cells by platelet-derived growth factor. *J Cell Biol* 1978; 79:663–671.

126. Burke JM, Ross R. Synthesis of connective tissue macromolecules by smooth muscle. *Int Rev Connect Tissue Res* 1979; 8:119–157.

127. Ross R. Platelet-derived growth factor. *Annu Rev Med* 1987; 38:71–79.

128. Moncada S, Vane JR. Arachidonic acid metabolites and the interactions between platelets and blood-vessel walls. *N Engl J Med* 1979; 300:1142–1147.

129. Moncada S, Vane JR. Mode of action of aspirin-like drugs. *Adv Intern Med* 1979; 24:1–22.

130. Furchgott RF, Zawadzki JV. The obligatory role of endothelial cells in the relaxation of arterial smooth muscle by acetylcholine. *Nature* 1980; 288:373–379.

131. Dinerman JL, Lowenstein CJ, Snyder SH. Molecular mechanisms of nitric oxide regulation: Potential relevance to cardiovascular disease. *Circ Res* 1993; 73:217–222.

132. Masaki T, Yanagisawa M, Goto K, Kimura S. Role of endothelin in mechanisms of local blood pressure control. *J Hypertens* 1990; 8(suppl 7):S107–S112.

133. Lerman A, Holmes DR Jr, Bell MR, Garratt KN, Nishimura RA, Burnett JC Jr. Endothelin in coronary endothelial dysfunction and early atherosclerosis in humans. *Circulation* 1995; 92:2426–2431.

134. Huang PL, Huang Z, Mashimo H, Bloch KD, Moskowitz MA, Bevan JA, et al. Hypertension in mice lacking the gene for endothelial nitric oxide synthase. *Nature* 1995; 377:239–242.

40

PATHOLOGY OF CORONARY ATHEROSCLEROSIS

Michael J. Davies

THE PROCESS OF ATHEROSCLEROSIS

Atherosclerosis is an intimal disease of arteries ranging in size from the aorta to the epicardial coronary artery that is characterized by discrete intimal plaques, although at an advanced stage the lesions may coalesce. Each plaque has combinations of extracellular lipid, lipid contained within cells that have foamy cytoplasm, and connective tissue matrix proteins, such as collagen, produced by smooth muscle cells. The majority of the foam cells are derived from monocytes, which enter the plaque from the arterial lumen.

Lipid is a fundamental component of the atherosclerotic plaque, which is essentially an inflammatory/repair response in the vessel wall invoked by lipid.[1] Lesions that consist entirely of proliferating smooth muscle cells, such as the response to endothelial denudation in animal models or after angioplasty in humans, are a pure repair response to mechanical injury and are not atherosclerosis.

Intimal thickening that consists solely of connective tissue and smooth muscle cells is an adaptive response of the vessel wall to flow and is not atherosclerosis.[2,3] Such intimal thickening occurs at branching points in human coronary arteries from a young age. Concentric intimal thickening also develops in coronary arteries distal to chronic high-grade stenosis or occlusion. Adaptive intimal thickening, while it often occurs in the same arterial sites as coronary atherosclerosis, is not an initiating factor for plaque formation.[2,3]

Morphological Forms of Atherosclerotic Plaques

The intimal surface of an opened human coronary artery reveals several types of plaque. Some are flat yellow dots or lines (fatty streaks), and others are raised above the surface as oval humps, which range in color from white to yellow (raised fibrolipid plaques).

Observations made on human necropsies allow a developmental sequence to be proposed for plaques based on cohorts of individuals dying at different ages from noncardiac disease.[2] In children from 5 to 10 years of age, fatty streaks are often present in the coronary arteries, suggesting that they are the initial point in a sequence of plaque development.[4] Raised plaques appear later in life, and, by 20 years of age, are present in areas such as the proximal left anterior descending coronary artery, where fatty streaks are most prevalent in earlier life.[4] *By middle age, most subjects will have coronary plaques of all types, suggesting that plaque initiation continues throughout life.*

The American Heart Association has recommended a nomenclature for the types of plaques and has suggested ways in which they may evolve.[5]

Plaque Evolution

The initial lesion (type I) develops when monocytes migrate from the lumen of the artery across the intact endothelium to accumulate in the intima. The type II lesion is the fatty streak, which consists of a focal accumulation of lipid-filled foam cells immediately beneath the intact endothelium. The type III lesion also contains small pools of extracellular lipid. These first three stages of plaque development are predictable, but from this point on, a wide range of possible evolutionary paths exist. While stage I to stage III plaques are the precursors of more advanced lesions, they do not cause clinical symptoms.

Stage IV is characterized by two additional features. Smooth muscle cells appear within the lesion beneath the endothelium, and the pools of extracellular lipid coalesce to form a lipid core. Stage V shows significant connective tissue deposition and the formation of a fibrous capsule containing the lipid core. The portion of this capsule separating the core from the lumen is the plaque cap. The lipid core is often bright yellow due to the presence of carotenoid pigment.

Plaques with a lipid core and a fibrous cap are designated as type Va (Figs. 40-1 and 40-2). *Type VI plaques are those complicated by thrombosis, which predominantly develops in Va plaques.* Another developmental attribute of plaques is heavy calcification (type Vb). Another form of advanced plaque (type Vc) is almost entirely composed of collagen and smooth muscle cells, with a trivial lipid component.

Basic Mechanisms in Plaque Formation

FOAM CELL FORMATION

In experimental models and human disease, the first morphologic phenomenon observed in plaque formation is adhesion of monocytes to an intact endothelial surface.[1,6] This adhesion is followed by monocyte migration into the intima. In the intima, monocytes are activated, converted to macrophages, and may divide.[7] Lipid uptake by macrophages then leads to the formation of the foam cell. These observations have created a paradox in that, although plasma low-density lipoprotein (LDL) freely enters the intima, it should not be taken up by macrophages, which lack the appropriate receptor. The apparent paradox can now be explained in the context of the chemical changes that LDL undergoes as it is modified by the cells in the arterial wall. The first minor modifications of the LDL molecule occur close to the endothelial surface.[8] This initial change produces a proinflammatory molecule called *minimally modified low-density lipoprotein* (MMLDL),[9] which contributes to the endothelial expression of molecules mediating monocyte adhesion, such as *vascular cell adhesion molecule* (VCAM).[10] Other inflammatory mediators such as *intercellular adhesion molecule* (ICAM), *monocyte chemotac-*

tic protein (MCP-1),[11] and *macrophage colony stimulating factor* (MCSF)[12] are also induced (see also Chaps. 4 and 44). These factors act in concert to cause monocyte migration and to allow the incoming monocytes to establish themselves and divide in the intima. Further changes in the LDL molecule lead to an oxidized form (oxidized LDL), which is recognized by the *macrophage scavenger receptor*. The scavenger receptor does not down-regulate, as does the receptor for native LDL, and the cell becomes laden with lipid because of continued unregulated uptake. The macrophage foam cells that result produce a range of inflammatory cytokines including tumor necrosis factor alpha (TNF-α)[13] and metalloproteinases[14] as well as the procoagulant tissue factor.[15] This sequence of lipid oxidation and lipid uptake by macrophages forms a credible explanation for the formation of foam cells, and oxidized LDL has been shown within macrophages in both human and rabbit atherosclerosis[16] (see also Chap. 39).

The endothelial surface is intact in the initial phase of coronary atherosclerosis. There is no exposure of the subendothelial connective tissue matrix and therefore no adhesion of platelets to the vessel wall.

LIPID CORE FORMATION

Extracellular lipid is derived from two possible sources. Some may be derived directly from LDL bound to proteoglycans within the intima,[17] but much of the cholesterol and esters in the lipid core is released from the cytoplasm of dying foam cells. Macrophages may be killed by lipid peroxides formed by LDL oxidation, but there is now evidence that cell death is by apoptosis.[18] Deprivation of growth factors such as MCSF-1 may induce apoptosis, particularly in association with the TNF-α present in large amounts in cellular plaques.

Lipid cores are potential spaces in the connective tissue matrix of the intima that are filled with cellular debris and cholesterol. Active plaques contain numerous macrophages clustered at the edge of the core with the expression of a range of metalloproteinases[14] that likely are engaged in the active destruction of the collagen matrix.

SMOOTH MUSCLE PROLIFERATION AND CAP FORMATION

The caps of plaques with a lipid core consist of a lattice of collagen within which are lacunae containing smooth muscle cells that produce the connective tissue matrix. Smooth muscle cell migration and proliferation as well as collagen deposition are

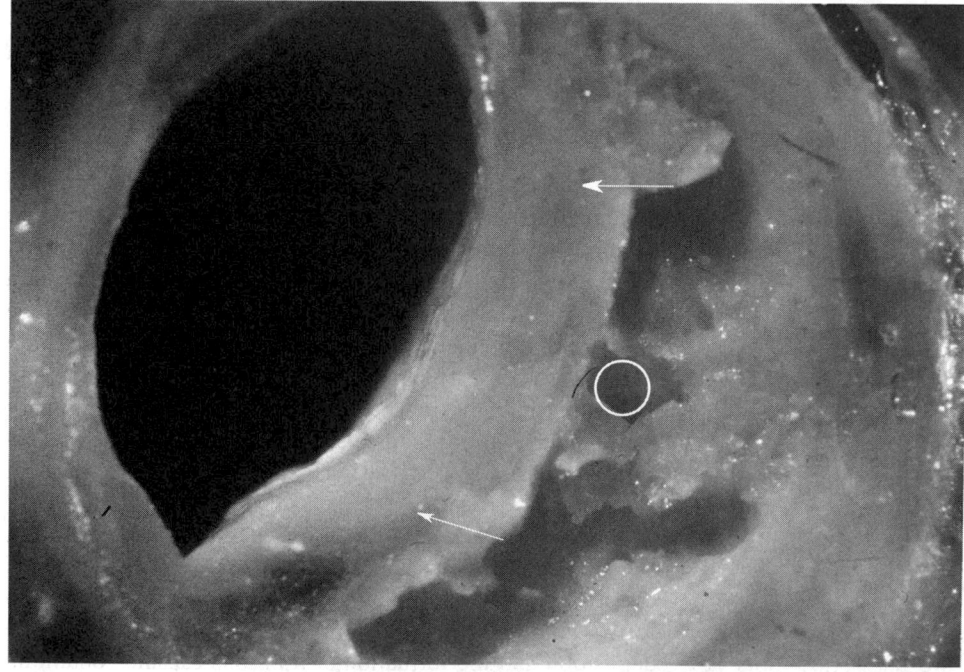

FIGURE 40-1

Human coronary artery in which there is a large lipid-rich plaque with a core (○) and a thick cap (*arrows*). This lesion would be designated as a type Va plaque.

driven by growth factors produced by virtually every cell type, including smooth muscle cells themselves.[19] Platelets, fibrin, and thrombin can also stimulate smooth muscle proliferation if deposited on the vessel wall,[20] and there is increasing recognition that fibrinogen passes into the intima and can be converted to fibrin. Such fibrin is usually removed by plasminogen activation. Any residual fibrin/thrombin complexes are potent stimulators of smooth muscle proliferation. The plaque cap is now recognized as a dynamic structure in which there is deposition of collagen[21] balanced by degradation of the connective tissue matrix by a range of proteases. Numerous cytokines control this balance.[21]

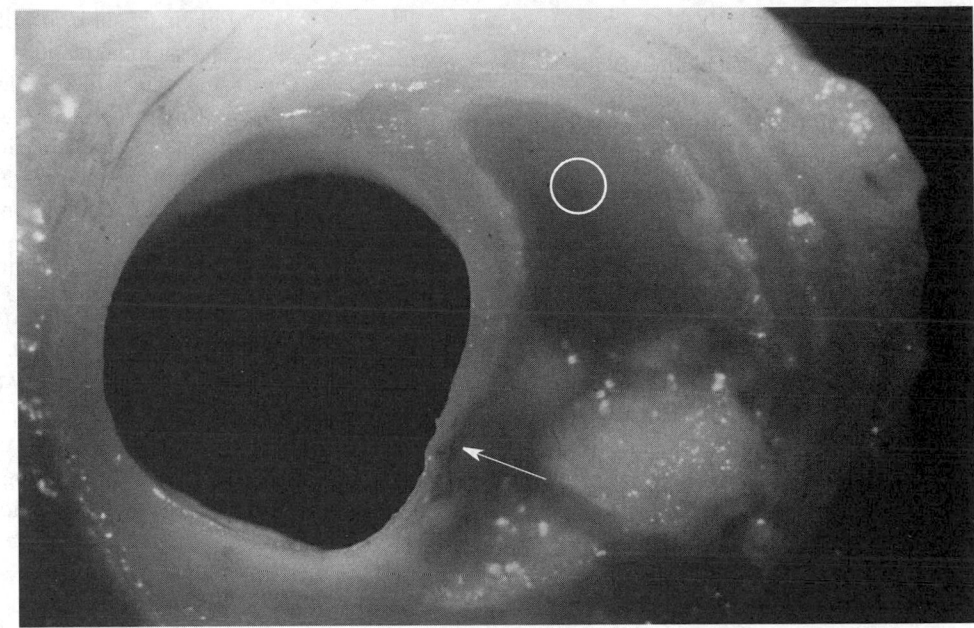

FIGURE 40-2

Human coronary artery in which there is a large lipid-rich plaque with a core (○), but in contrast to Fig. 40-1, the cap (*arrow*) is thin. This lesion is also a type Va plaque.

IMMUNE MECHANISMS IN PLAQUE FORMATION

Plaques contain T lymphocytes,[22] the function of which may be, in part, to modify smooth muscle proliferation via the production of interferon-γ. B lymphocytes are absent from the plaque itself but are present, often in large numbers, in the adjacent adventitia. Oxidized LDL is strongly antigenic, and the B lymphocytes produce autoantibodies that can be measured in the plasma and may provide a marker of the activity or extent of the atherosclerotic process.[23]

PLAQUE VASCULARIZATION

The normal media is avascular, but once intimal thickening occurs, new vessels grow in from the adventitia and reach the base of the plaque. Neovascularization may be visible on angiography in life.[24] The vessels that lie close to the base of the core are thin-walled, and extravasation of red cells is very common. When the core contains platelets, however, a direct continuity with the lumen is found via a cap tear (see below). Transmedial vessels strongly express adhesion molecules such as VCAM and may be another route by which monocytes enter the plaque.[25]

CLINICAL SYMPTOMS
AND PLAQUE TYPES

The presence of advanced plaques of types IV and Va allows clinical symptoms to develop. Atherosclerosis is a biphasic disease; in the first stage, advanced plaques are generated but the patient is asymptomatic; in the second stage, symptoms develop. Plaques are ubiquitous in Western

populations, but not everyone develops ischemic heart disease. Large scale epidemiologic studies—including the International Geographic Survey,[26] the Pathological Determinants of Atherosclerosis in Youth (PDAY) study,[4] and the Bogalusa Heart Study[27]—have produced consistent confirmation.

In all geographic populations, the mean number of coronary plaques present in a large number of autopsied patients who die from all causes predicts the incidence of ischemic heart disease in that population. The risk factors for large numbers of subjects developing ischemic heart disease depend on how many advanced plaques are present. Smokers will, on average, have more plaques than nonsmokers. Similar data exist for hyperlipidemia, hypertension, and diabetes (see Chap. 41). Thus risk factors operate in part by increasing the number of plaques that can potentially progress to cause symptoms. Such epidemiologic studies, however, do not mean that an individual cannot die of a single, strategically placed plaque.

The majority of types IV and Va advanced plaques are clinically silent and angiographically invisible because they do not encroach upon the lumen of the coronary artery.[3,28] Two mechanisms are responsible for this phenomenon. First, the media behind an atherosclerotic plaque undergoes thinning and atrophy, which allows the plaque to bulge outward rather than inward. Second, *the development of an intimal plaque causes remodeling of the arterial wall, increasing the external diameter and allowing the plaque to be accommodated without altering the lumen dimensions.* Intravascular ultrasound confirms that coronary angiography is very insensitive for the detection of plaques[29] (see also Chap. 49).

Plaque Heterogeneity

Common to all type Va plaques is the presence of a fibromuscular cap, but, even so, there is considerable heterogeneity (Figs. 40-1 and 40-2). The cap may be relatively thick and uniform, or it may vary in thickness with interspersed thin areas. Thick caps have high numbers of smooth muscle cells, while relatively thin caps often have fewer smooth muscle cells and contain appreciable numbers of macrophages. The lipid core may occupy over 70 percent of the overall volume of the plaque or as little as 10 percent. Core margins may be surrounded by macrophages, or there may be no macrophages. *Plaque heterogeneity therefore involves both the micromorphology of the lesion (core size, cap thickness) and the degree of inflammatory activity.* A plaque in inflammatory terms can be "hot" or burnt out. There is no readily discernible relation between plaque size and any of the variables that contribute to plaque heterogeneity.

Mechanisms of Induction of Symptoms

Three major mechanisms lead to clinical symptoms (see also Chap. 39). First, thrombosis leads to acute decreases in flow in a coronary artery. Second, a plaque grows without the clinically apparent involvement of thrombosis to the point that the lumen size is reduced to a degree that causes flow limitation during exercise.

Finally, in subjects with coronary atherosclerosis, coronary vasomotor tonal responses are abnormal. This disordered control of tone, which reflects in part endothelial dysfunction (see also Chaps. 4 and 44) may take the form of local spasm at the site of an eccentric plaque in which there is a residual segment of normal vessel wall or vasospasm may be a more generalized phenomenon.

Acute Ischemic Syndromes

The major factor initiating acute ischemia in the crescendo form of unstable angina, acute myocardial infarction, and in a high proportion of sudden ischemic deaths is a thrombus of sufficient size to protrude into the arterial lumen. This assertion does not imply that thrombosis is the only factor, but necropsy studies, angiography, and angioscopy as well as the success of fibrinolytic therapy in restoring arterial patency in infarct-related arteries all indicate a dominant role for thrombosis.

FACTORS INDUCING PLAQUE THROMBOSIS
Postmortem study of human coronary thrombi causing death has shown the involvement of two distinct processes.[30]

Endothelial Erosion
The endothelial surface over many plaques of types IV and Va has been shown to develop small foci of endothelial cell loss,[31,32] which expose the subendothelial connective tissue and lead to local platelet adhesion. The initial response involves interaction of von Willebrand's factor, collagen, and fibronectin with the Ia/Ib platelet receptors. Further thrombus growth is dependent upon the platelet IIb/IIIa receptor and its reaction with fibrinogen. These small thrombi do not cause symptoms, usually because they consist of only a monolayer of platelets and are demonstrable only by ultramicroscopic methods (Fig. 40-3). They indicate that *the endothelium overlying an active lesion is in a state of constant regeneration and may therefore be functionally abnormal.* Larger areas of endothelial denudation or erosion may, however, initiate thrombi capable of causing symptoms. The characteristic of these thrombi is that they are adherent to the luminal surface of the plaque and there is no intraplaque thrombosis (Fig. 40-4). Endothelial erosion is associated with the

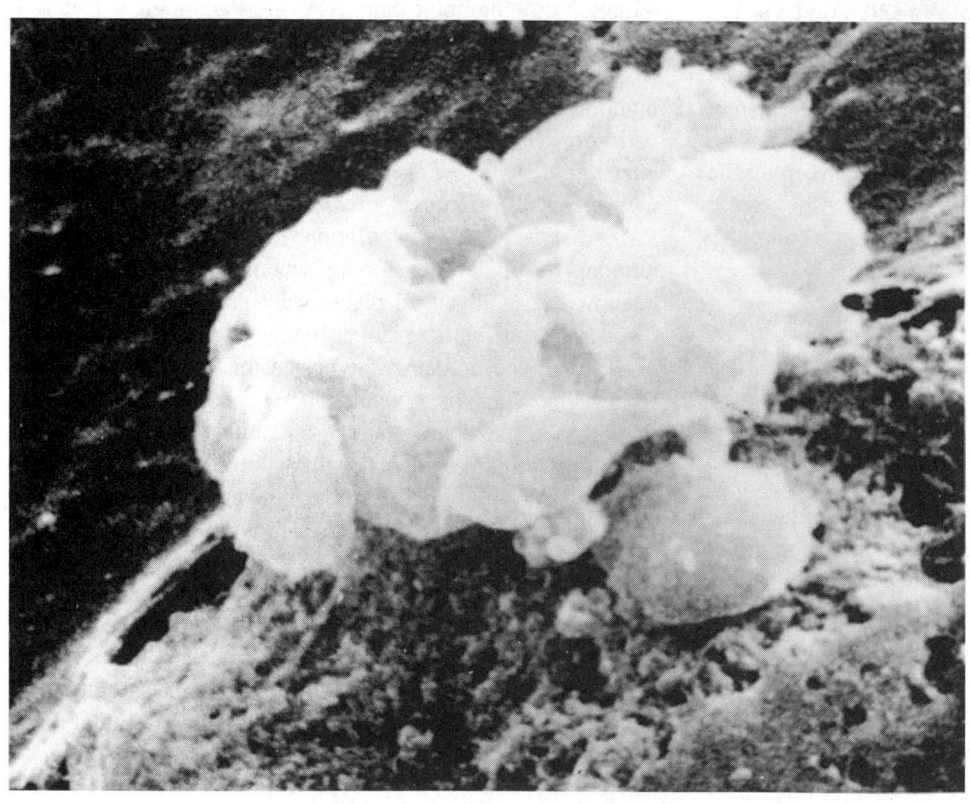

FIGURE 40-3
Scanning electron micrograph of human coronary artery. A single endothelial cell has undergone denudation. Over the exposed subendothelial tissue, a small clump of platelets has formed. No platelets adhere to adjacent intact endothelial cells.

presence of activated macrophages and of T lymphocytes in association with class II major histocompatibility complex (MHC) expression on adjacent smooth muscle cells, indicating an intense local inflammatory/immune reaction.[33] *Superficial thrombosis causes at least one-quarter of significant coronary thrombi[30] but has been reported in some series to be more frequent.[34]* In 50 cases of sudden ischemic death, 22 were associated with thrombus due to erosion of the endothelial surface of a plaque that was rich in proteoglycans rather than lipid. This study showed this form of superficial plaque thrombosis was relatively more common in women.[34]

Plaque Disruption

Up to three-quarters of major coronary thrombi are caused by plaque disruption (also known as plaque cracking, fissuring, rupture, or ulceration). In disruption, the cap of a plaque with a lipid-rich core will tear; blood from the lumen of the artery then enters the lipid core, where the presence of tissue factor and collagen induces platelet adhesion, aggregation, and activation.[35] Thrombus formation within the core itself expands

and distorts the plaque, while the torn cap may project into the lumen (Fig. 40-5). Necropsy study of disrupted coronary and aortic plaques compared with intact plaques in the same individuals shows that plaques with a large lipid core occupying more than 50 percent of overall plaque volume and having a high macrophage density, a thin cap, and low smooth muscle cell density are the most vulnerable to rupture.[36–38] Of interest, core size and cap thickness, which are two major determinants of plaque vulnerability, are not statistically related and neither is related to absolute plaque size or to the degree of stenosis.[38]

Postdisruption Events

The events that follow an episode of plaque cap disruption are dynamic and occur in stages

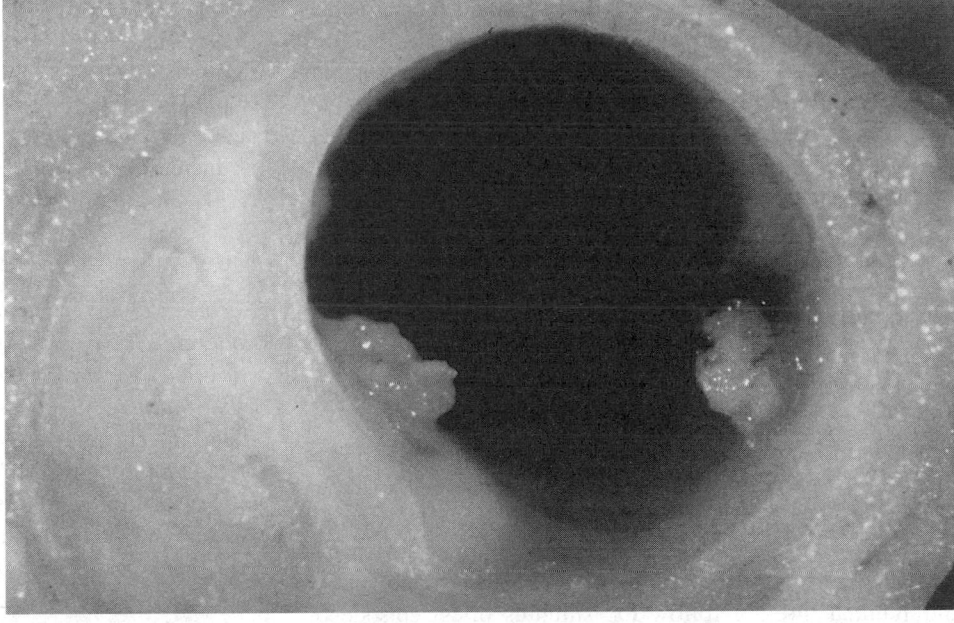

FIGURE 40-4

Two small thrombi due to endothelial erosion over a plaque. The thrombi are stuck onto the surface of the plaque—there is no intraplaque component of thrombus.

(Fig. 40-6). Progression can be halted at any stage. The initial stage has, in the past, often been referred to as *plaque* or *intimal hemorrhage*,[39] *intraplaque hematoma*, and *hemorrhagic dissection*.[40] These names imply that the intraplaque component is predominantly composed of red cells. A large component, however, is composed of platelets and fibrin, justifying the name *intraplaque thrombus*. Within the area of

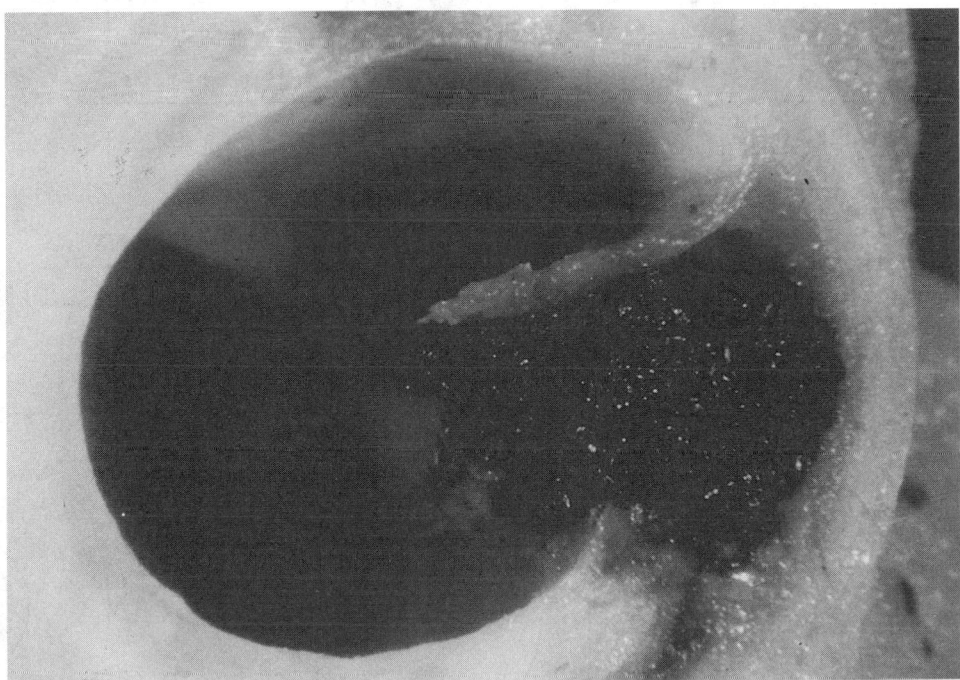

FIGURE 40-5

Plaque disruption in which the torn cap of a plaque projects into the lumen. The original site of the lipid core is filled with thrombus, which protrudes into but does not occlude the lumen.

the torn cap at the interface with the lumen, the thrombus composition is predominantly densely packed fibrin. From this transition zone mural thrombus may project out into lumen without totally preventing antegrade flow. In the final stage, thrombus is predominantly made up of a loose network of fibrin-containing, enmeshed red blood cells and totally occludes the arterial lumen.

Plaque disruption is a stimulus to the formation of thrombosis within the lumen. Many factors control whether or not thrombosis occurs. The magnitude of the tear varies; at one extreme it may be a narrow fissure running from the lumen to the core, at the other extreme the whole cap may be lost with extrusion of core material into the lumen. Another important factor is the local blood flow. Reduction of flow, either due to spasm or because of a large expansion of the plaque by thrombus within the core, increases the likelihood of major thrombosis within the lumen. The systemic balance of prothrombotic and natural fibrinolytic mechanisms is another factor influencing whether or not major intraluminal thrombi follow the stimulus of an episode of plaque disruption.

Plaque Healing

Plaque disruption is followed by a healing response. Natural fibrinolysis will remove a variable amount of the thrombus,

which is followed by smooth muscle proliferation and deposition of new collagen. This healing process is analogous to that which follows angioplasty. The end stage of an episode of plaque disruption can range from a trivial increase in plaque size[41] through more significant increases in size, resulting in an increase in stenosis severity or to chronic total occlusion (Fig. 40-6).

Mechanism of Intimal Tears

Reconstruction of human atherosclerotic plaques that have undergone disruption shows that the majority have a large core of extracellular cholesterol occupying over 50 percent of the plaque by volume.[42] Computer models of plaques using finite element analysis have been used to show the distribution of circumferential wall stress in systole.[42,43] Normally, systolic circumferential stress is evenly distributed. Lipid cores are soft and cannot sustain stress, which has to be distributed elsewhere. The displaced stress is redistributed to the plaque cap. Focal points of maximal stress may be up to 10 times greater than that experienced by the rest of the arterial wall. Studies of coronary plaques show that the site of tearing coincides with the calculated point of maximal stress.[43] Concentration of stress on the plaque cap is also particularly enhanced in thin caps of plaques, causing minimal stenosis.[44] All of these studies emphasize the concept that plaques with

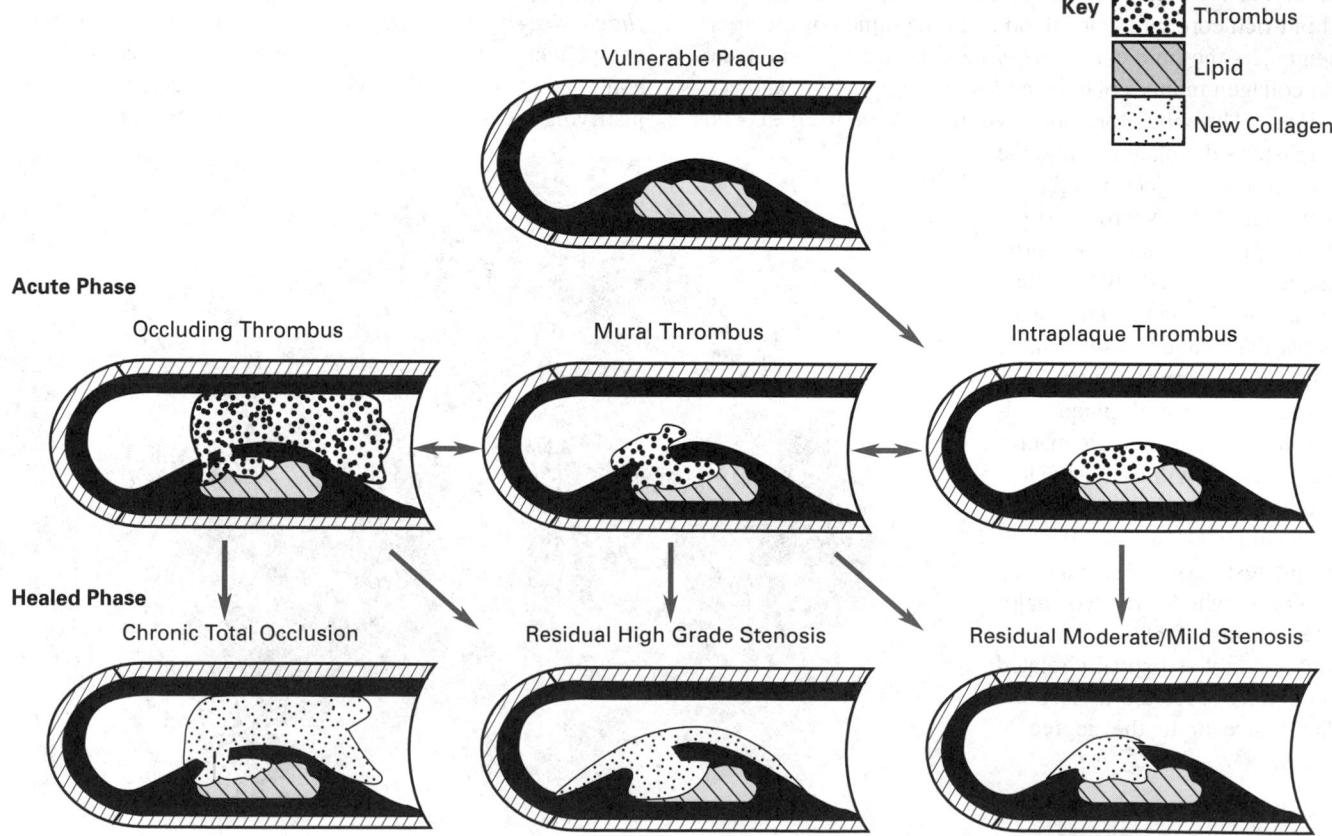

FIGURE 40-6

Diagram of the dynamic state of the acute thrombotic response with different stages—intraplaque, mural nonocclusive, and occlusive thrombus. The end result, after healing by smooth muscle proliferation, ranges from chronic total occlusion to mild increase in stenosis.

lipid cores and thin caps are mechanically inefficient, with stresses impinging excessively upon the cap.

Another important aspect of plaque disruption is the innate mechanical strength of the cap tissue. Mechanical testing in vitro of cap tissue shows that a reduction in collagen and glycosoaminoglycans and an increase in the number of lipid-filled macrophages interact to reduce the amount of stress needed to fracture the tissue even after correction for the cross-sectional area of the test sample.[45] Collagen types and elastin content do not alter absolute tissue strength. These results lead to consideration of whether or not the cap is undergoing active destruction by proteases. Macrophages have the capacity when activated by the cytokines TNF-α and interleukin-1 (IL-1) to secrete inactive *metalloproteinases* (MMP).[14] These connective tissue-degrading enzymes include interstitial collagenase (MMP1), gelatinase B (MMP9), stromelysins 1, 2, and 3 (MMP 3, 10, and 11), and a membrane type (MTMPP). When activated by plasmin or by inactivation of intrinsic inhibitors in the tissue, these metalloproteinases can degrade the connective tissue matrix. Both metalloproteinase mRNA and protein have been found in large amounts in the cap and core area,[46] but their activity may be neutralized by tissue inhibitors (TIMPS). Sections of plaques laid on a gelatin substrate in vitro, however, show that lysis occurs in focal areas, indicating that active degradation of collagen is occurring.[47] *Plaque cap tears can therefore be seen as resulting from a destructive process initiated by macrophages that gains ascendancy over the repair process of collagen deposition by smooth muscle cells.*

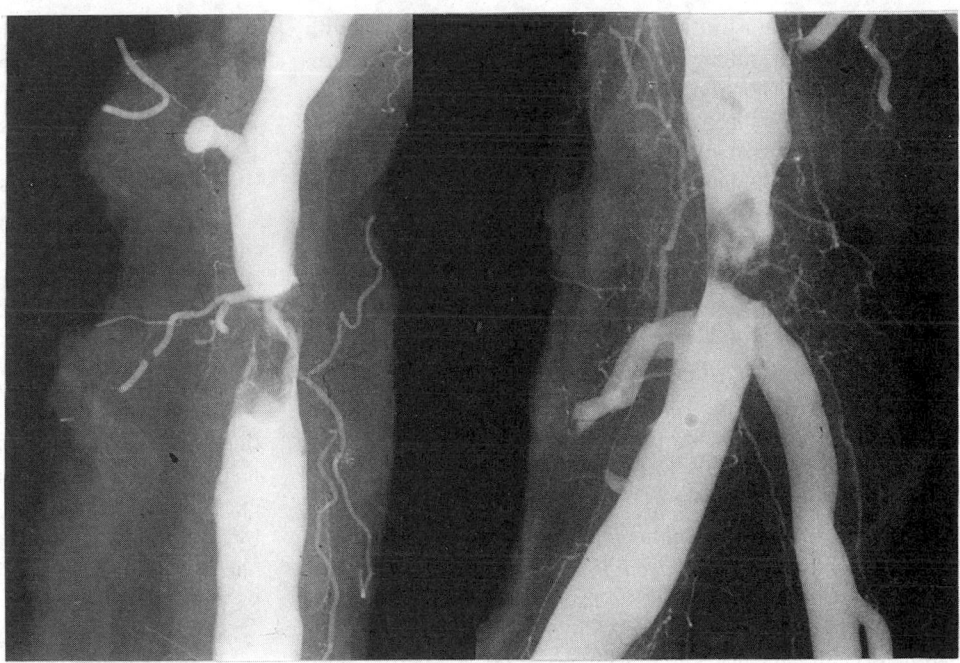

FIGURE 40-7

Postmortem angiograms of two patients who died suddenly after a prodrome of intermittent resting chest pain. Both had disrupted plaques. The angiograms show the typical eccentric stenoses with ragged edges. Both have related intraluminal thrombi—proximal in one (*left*) and distal in the other (*right*).

farction, emphasize the presence of eccentric stenoses with ragged outlines, designated as type II, and of intraluminal filling defects.[48] Necropsy studies (Fig. 40-7) confirm that these angiographic appearances are due to nonocclusive thrombi developing over a disrupted plaque.[37] *A major cause of unstable angina is, therefore, a culprit plaque over which thrombus is arrested at an intermediate stage in which it is neither occlusive nor resolved sufficiently to allow the plaque to reseal and heal.*

Necropsy studies of unstable angina are biased toward the worst-case scenario. To an extent, this limitation can be overcome by studies of plaque material retrieved by atherectomy of the culprit lesion. Such studies confirm that macrophage infiltration is a feature of unstable plaques.[49] A number of atherectomy studies have shown that thrombotic material is recovered from a far higher proportion of plaques causing unstable as compared to stable angina but that this correlation is not 100 percent.[50,51] A far smaller proportion of apparently stable plaques also shows thrombotic material. Haft and colleagues,[52] for example, found thrombus in atherectomy material in 49 of 57 cases of unstable angina (86 percent) and in 7 of 24 cases of stable angina (29 percent). Material removed from unstable angina–related plaques shows an increased number of lipid-filled macrophages,[49] increased expression of tissue factor,[15] and increased gelatinase B content.[53] Atherectomy removes a random portion of the plaque, and this may explain the absence of thrombus in some cases of unstable angina. Timing is also important. Atherectomy samples that show accelerated growth with storiform smooth muscle cell proliferation[54] can be explained by the sample's having been

DETAILED PATHOLOGY OF CLINICAL SYNDROMES IN ISCHEMIC HEART DISEASE

Unstable Angina

Intermittent ischemia occurring at rest is the hallmark of unstable angina and is related to "dynamic" stenosis, i.e., the obstruction to flow varies rather than being fixed (see Chap. 46). Two main mechanisms, mural thrombosis at the site of a culprit plaque and varying vasomotor tone, have been proposed. Neither process is exclusive and both may operate contemporaneously.

Angiographic studies in unstable angina of the crescendo form, in which there is a clear risk of subsequent acute in-taken after healing is initiated. This pattern is associated with plaques that cause angina at rest without a crescendo pattern. Angioscopy is probably more sensitive than angiography in identifying plaque thrombosis. A recent study[55] shows 70 out of 95 (73.7 percent) of patients with unstable angina had plaque thrombus. Four out of 27 patients (14.8 percent) who had only exercise-related pain showed thrombus.

Pathologic studies show platelet emboli into the distal myocardium lead to small foci of acute myocardial necrosis in subjects dying suddenly after unstable angina.[56,57] These small platelet emboli within the myocardium show intense expression of the IIb/IIIa receptor (Fig. 40-8).

The arterial pathology of unstable angina differs from that of acute myocardial infarction only in that the artery remains open and some antegrade flow is retained while in the latter antegrade flow ceases for at least a period of time, usually some hours. Unstable angina of the crescendo type, non-Q wave, or nontransmural infarction, and transmural infarction are different points in a continuous spectrum. It is therefore not surprising that sensitive methods of detecting myocardial necrosis, such as measuring plasma troponin-T levels, can be used to detect subjects with the clinical diagnosis of unstable angina who are at high risk of death or further infarction.[58]

The essence of the arterial pathology of unstable angina is that the process of thrombosis is arrested at the point of exposed mural thrombus. This arrest represents a balance between many active forces and does not imply that the thrombotic surface has become inert. The risk of thrombotic occlusion developing at the site remains increased for at least 6

to 12 weeks and systemic hypercoagulative activity is also elevated for several months.[59] Residual thrombotic material continues to be highly thrombogenic until it is completely replaced by smooth muscle cells and new connective tissue.[60] Lymphocyte activation during unstable angina,[61] increased plasma neutrophil and monocyte adhesion molecule levels,[62] and elevated C-reactive protein levels[63] all indicate continuing inflammatory activity following an episode of unstable angina.

Vasomotor Tonal Abnormalities in Unstable Angina

There is now abundant evidence in humans and in animals that atherosclerotic arteries have inappropriate vasoconstrictor responses. Vasoconstriction, which has been induced both by exercise and intracoronary infusion of acetylcholine, is caused by a failure of normal vasodilatory responses, due, at least in part, to diminished nitric oxide release by the endothelium (see Chaps. 4 and 44).

Some cases of unstable angina have localized dynamic vasoconstriction, either at a site of eccentric stenosis or in a segment with minimal or no angiographic narrowing.[64–66] It is uncertain why one such lesion should acquire vasomotor excitability. Increased endothelin-1 production within plaques may be a contributing factor.[67] In one case, small amounts of thrombus, too small to be detected angiographically, were found on the endothelial surface at surgery.[68] The local release of vasoactive substances by platelets is one possible cause of spasm, and this possibility is supported by experimental models of coronary injury in pigs.[69] Another postulated cause is related to the heavy adventitial inflammation; mast cells may release pharmacologically active substances that directly act on adventitial nerve tissue.[70,71] The Prinzmetal variant form of angina frequently occurs in arteries that have some angiographic evidence of atherosclerosis but without an element of high-grade fixed stenosis[72,73] (see also Chap. 46).

Acute Myocardial Infarction

The blood supply of the mammalian myocardium is regional; each major branch of the coronary arteries supplies a specific segment of myocardium. There is considerable interspecies variation in the degree of innate cross-flow between adjacent epicardial arteries; humans and pigs

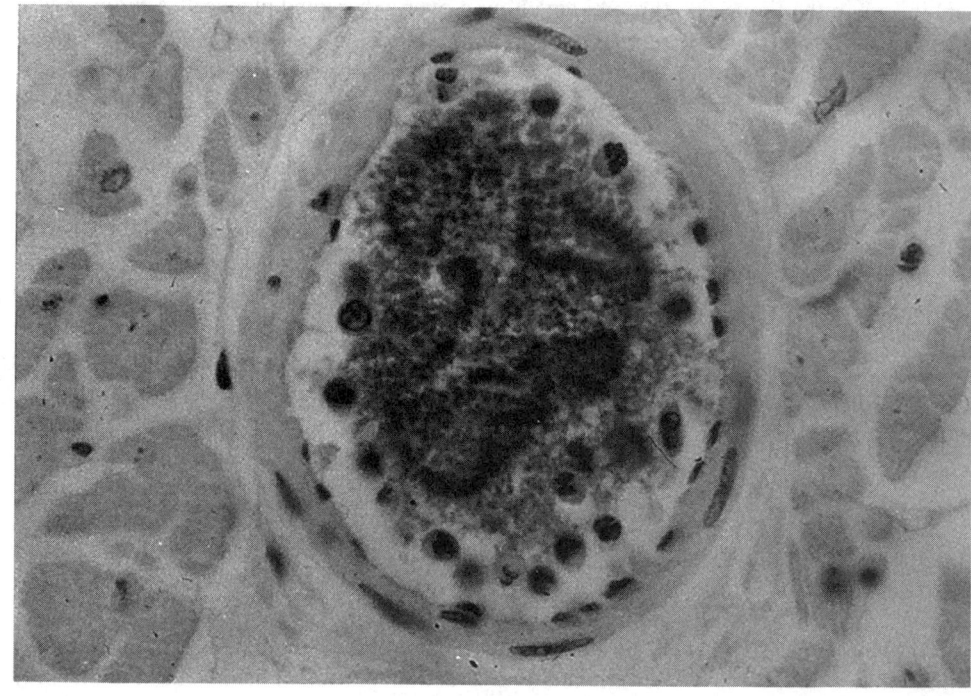

FIGURE 40-8

An intramyocardial artery distal to a disrupted plaque in a major epicardial artery is occluded by a mass of platelets and white blood cells. The platelets are expressing the IIb/IIIa receptor (immunohistochemical staining with IIb/IIIa antibody).

share the property of having little natural collateral development.

In experimental animal models, the only way to produce regional infarction is to occlude the coronary artery supplying a given area. Clinical studies of regional myocardial infarction in humans confirm the importance of occlusion of the subtending ("infarct-related") artery. Angiography during the early hours of infarction shows the subtending artery to the region to be occluded.[74] The frequency with which occlusion is detected after a myocardial infarction diminishes with the passage of time; as antegrade flow returns (because of spontaneous lysis of thrombus), filling defects are seen within the lumen over a type II stenosis. Fibrinolytic therapy increases the speed with which the subtending artery reopens. These data suggest that a dynamic thrombotic process is occurring. Necropsy studies show a higher frequency of total thrombotic occlusion than equivalent angiographic studies of survivors of acute infarction. These findings suggest that persistent occlusion has an adverse influence on survival, probably by being linked to larger infarct size.[75]

Reconstruction of the microanatomy of occlusive coronary thrombi shows the majority to be due to plaque rupture in which there is both an intraplaque and an intraluminal component (Fig. 40-9). The thrombus found at autopsy varies in age in different areas of the clot, suggesting that it is formed by an intermittent process taking place over some days. The intraplaque component of the thrombus consists predominantly of platelets; the thrombus within the fissure site is formed of densely packed fibrin. Much of the intraluminal thrombus, particularly that distal to the fissured plaque, is "venous" in type, suggesting that it has formed in a static column of blood. At least part of the intraluminal thrombus may thus be a late phenomenon. In vivo radiolabeling studies in subjects who subsequently died of acute infarction show that both fibrinogen and platelets given after the onset of the infarction can be incorporated into the coronary thrombus. Detailed studies, however, showed that the thrombus within the fissured plaque is not labeled, i.e., predates infarction, while a proportion of thrombus in the lumen is labeled, i.e., postdates infarction.[40]

INTERRELATION OF INFARCT MORPHOLOGY AND ARTERIAL THROMBI

Human regional infarcts may be formed of transmural necrosis of uniform age. Such infarcts are closely analogous to experimental infarction in the dog and represent the consequences of thrombus occurring suddenly and progressing to occlusion over a very short time in a vessel in which there was minimal or no preexisting stenosis. There may, however, be preexisting high-grade stenosis that has invoked collateral formation.[76-78] In such arteries thrombosis may occur without causing any infarction. Thrombosis may be mural and associated with distal embolization of platelet masses or intermittently occlusive prior to the final occlusive episode.[79] Antegrade flow may or may not be restored spontaneously within a period of hours. These more complex developmental patterns of thrombosis are associated with regional infarcts that are built up by the coalescence of small, often microscopic areas of necrosis of different ages. Retention of areas of viable myocardium mixed with necrotic areas is common. Infarcts that are regional but confined to the subendocardial zone (nontransmural) are almost always of this type. In humans, nontransmural infarction, as compared with transmural infarction, has a higher frequency of previously established collateral flow and/or restoration of antegrade flow over the culprit plaque.[80,81] The sinister complications of infarct expansion, infarct rupture, and cardiogenic shock are virtually confined to transmural infarcts and are associated with persistent total occlusion of long segments of coronary artery.

Coronary Artery Pathology in Stable Exertional Angina

Angiographic and necropsy studies[82] show that the basis of stable angina is segments of coronary artery in which the

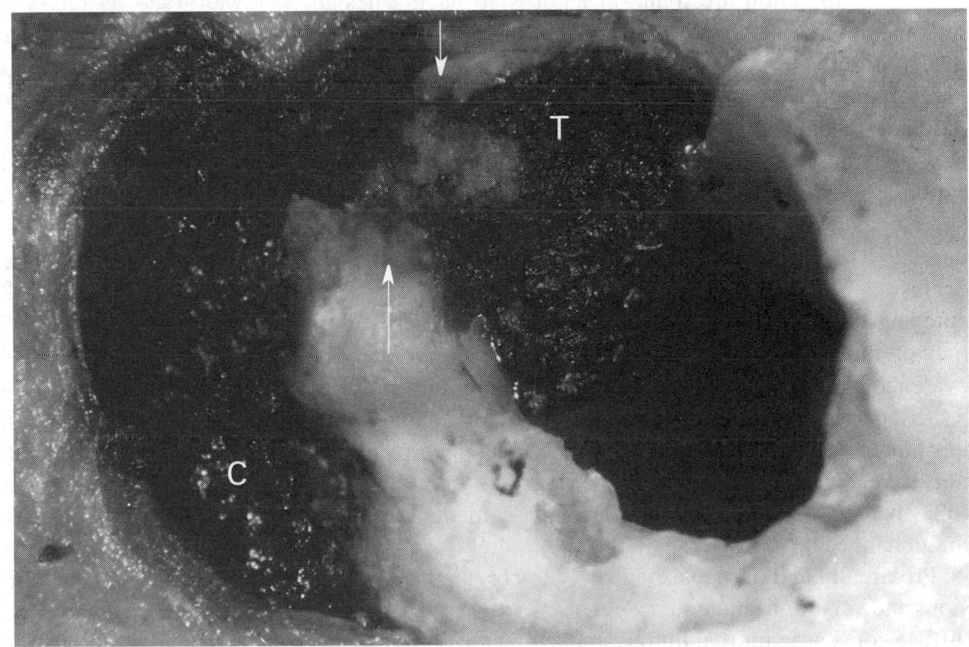

FIGURE 40-9
Plaque disruption related to an acute regional infarct. There is a mass of thrombus within the lipid core (C), which is continuous with thrombus (T) in the lumen via a discrete fissure (*arrows*) in the cap. The thrombus is not occlusive, presumably due to natural lysis.

lumen is reduced in diameter by at least 50 percent (75 percent cross-sectional area) compared to the adjacent normal artery. Such stenoses are potentially flow-limiting on exertion. The number of arteries involved and the number of stenotic segments vary widely from case to case, with autopsy studies inevitably showing the more severe end of the spectrum. The morphology of lesions causing chronic high-grade stenosis can best be appreciated in coronary arteries that have been fixed after autopsy by perfusion with formalin at systolic pressures. In such preparations the lumen is nearly circular in outline, indicating that the slitlike lumen shape shown in many pathology studies is an artifact. Segments of high-grade stenosis may be eccentric; that is, there is an arc of vessel wall that has retained its normal media opposite the plaque (Fig. 40-2).[83] Alterations in vascular tone in this residual segment of normal media may alter the cross-sectional area of the lumen. Stenoses may, however, be concentric, surrounding the lumen and limiting variation in lumen size.

The constituents of the plaques that cause high-grade stenosis vary in the relative amounts of lipid and collagen that are present. Plaques causing high-grade stenosis can either be relatively simple and have a lipid core (type Va) or be solid and fibrous (type Vc). Many are complex and have heavy calcification, or they consist of plaques formed on top of another or of plaques that have coalesced (Vb). In general, the higher the grade of angiographic stenosis, the more the plaque tends to be rich in collagen.[84] Such group data, however, hide the fact that even at high grades of stenosis, a plaque with a large lipid core can be present.

Many patients with stable angina but without a clinical history of infarction are found at autopsy to have a healed regional infarct. Arteries that supply such regions may be totally occluded by fibrous tissue, have high-grade stenosis due to complex type Vb plaques, or have many new, small vascular channels contained within the original lumen. This last appearance is pathognomonic of recanalization by organization of previous occlusive thrombus. In subjects with stable angina, such recanalized segments may also be present and unrelated to old scars, illustrating the fact that thrombotic occlusion is not inevitably followed by infarction. In one autopsy study of 54 men with stable angina who died within 6 h of the onset of symptoms, 38 cases had microscopic evidence of previous healed myocardial infarction; of these, 33 (87 percent) had one or more arterial segments in which the lumen was multichanneled. In the 16 patients who did not have microscopic evidence of an old infarction, 10 (62.5 percent) had one or more arterial segments that were multichanneled.[82]

Proximally and particularly distally to chronic total occlusions and very high-grade stenoses (<75 percent by diameter), diffuse concentric intimal fibrous thickening develops and the lumen is markedly reduced in size. This change may hinder attempts at angioplasty to restore normal flow and is probably a hemodynamic response rather than the result of atherosclerosis per se.[3]

CORONARY ANASTOMOSES (COLLATERALS)

Anastomotic flow is impossible to demonstrate in life or at necropsy without angiography. Anastomoses occur at several different levels. Local adventitial vessels open and provide very localized anastomoses at sites of short segments of high-grade or total chronic occlusion. While such periarterial vessels may show up strikingly in angiograms, the caliber of individual vessels is small and useful flow may not be achieved. Similar-sized vessels develop within the arterial lumen, passing through an old organized thrombus. Larger anastomoses develop between adjacent arteries on the epicardial surface. These may be as much as 1000 μm in diameter and are probably preexisting smaller arteries altered by flow-induced pressure differentials between different coronary beds. These anastomoses at the epicardial surface are probably the most important functionally and develop a characteristic corkscrew configuration in angiograms. In areas of nontransmural scarring within the myocardium, a plexus of large subendocardial vessels appears that has a structure resembling that of venous sinusoids. In very diffusely scarred ventricles, these channels fill throughout the ventricle from injection into one coronary artery.

MECHANISMS OF PROGRESSION AND REGRESSION

Any morphologic explanation of disease progression must take into account a number of clinical observations.[85–87] Sequential clinical angiographic studies show that progression is phasic and unpredictable in any particular arterial segment. High-grade lesions do not necessarily appear at sites where lower-grade lesions were previously present. New lesions causing luminal stenosis over 50 percent in diameter can appear between two angiographic examinations in apparently normal segments of artery. The sites of future acute occlusions causing infarction cannot be predicted. The progression of separate lesions in an individual is unrelated, and the progression of lesions in "normal" segments is often greater than in areas recognized to have an irregular outline. Thus individual plaques can enter an accelerated growth phase that is unrelated to their degree of stenosis. Despite this unpredictable behavior, high-grade stenoses (>70 percent by diameter) do tend to progress, particularly if the segment is long. Chronic total occlusions follow such high-grade lesions three times more frequently than in the case of less severe lesions[89] but frequently do not invoke infarction because of collateral development. Sequential coronary angiograms show that increases in the overall extent of disease also predict the risk of acute ischemic events in the future.[90,91]

Episodes of plaque disruption were initially regarded as events that inevitably caused thrombosis within the arterial lumen and were therefore usually manifest as episodes of acute myocardial ischemia. Several pathology studies have altered this concept. In a significant proportion of patients who had coronary atherosclerosis but who died of noncardiac causes such as accidents, small, recent plaque disruptions were found at autopsy. Up to 16 percent of such individuals who have diabetes and/or hypertension have these lesions.[92] In three studies of patients who died of acute myocardial ischemia, many were found at necropsy to have had two or three separate areas of disruption, although one was usually larger and regarded as the culprit lesion causing death.[93–95] Such data suggest that *episodes of plaque disruption are a characteristic feature of the progression of atherosclerosis and that many are clinically silent.*

An episode of plaque disruption heals by smooth muscle proliferation, replacing residual thrombus. The repair process is identical to that which follows plaque disruption produced by angioplasty. The final outcome of an episode of plaque disruption can range from chronic total occlusion at one extreme to a mild increase in stenosis at the other extreme (Fig. 40-6). It is apparent that one mode of generating new high-grade stenotic lesions is the healing of an episode of disruption that has not been clinically expressed as acute ischemia.

Lipid lowering trials have shown that disease progression can be slowed but that the degree of reduction in narrowing is minimal. Two trials designed to study the risk of acute events after lipid lowering by drugs demonstrated a 30 percent drop in acute ischemic events and a fall in all-cause mortality. The effect becomes apparent after 18 months of therapy[96,97] (see also Chap. 53).

The nature of the plaque is an important component of determining both the risk of acute ischemic events and progression to high-grade stenosis (see also Chap. 39). *Vulnerable plaques, which have large lipid cores and high macrophage activity, either undergo disruption to cause an acute clinical event or remain silent with an increased degree of stenosis in the healing phase.* Vulnerable plaques are distributed across the full range of stenosis, but—because of the absence of collateral flow—major disruptions occurring in arteries without prior high-grade stenosis are more likely to cause infarction than are highly stenotic lesions. *Thus, the risk of any subject having an acute ischemic event is determined by the absolute numbers of vulnerable plaques present. A current challenge is that there is no current clinical method to determine the number and site of these plaques.*

The mechanism(s) by which lowering levels of plasma lipids reduces plaque vulnerability (increases stability) is unclear. The plaque may lose some lipid from the core and smooth muscle proliferation may allow new collagen formation, solidifying the plaque and restoring its mechanical efficiency. Regression studies in primates[98,99] suggest that this can occur; in Watanabe rabbits, it was found that a reduction of monocyte/macrophage density follows lipid lowering.[100] Lipid lowering may, however, act by simply reducing the numbers and activity of macrophages within the plaque.

REFERENCES

1. Ross R. The pathogenesis of atherosclerosis—A perspective for the 1990s. *Nature* 1993; 362:801–809.

2. Stary HC. Evolution and progression of atherosclerotic lesions in coronary arteries of children and young adults. *Arteriosclerosis* 1989; 9:1–19.

3. Glagov S, Bassiouny HS, Giddens DP, Zarins CK. Intimal thickening: Morphogenesis, functional significance and detection. *J Vasc Invest* 1995; 1:2–14.

4. Wissler RW. An overview of the quantitative influence of several risk factors on progression of atherosclerosis in young people in the United States. *Am J Med Sci* 1995; 310:S29–S36.

5. Stary HC, Chandler AB, Dinsmore RE, Fuster V, Glagov S, Insull W, et al. A definition of advanced types of atherosclerotic lesions and a histological classification of atherosclerosis: A report from the Committee on Vascular Lesions of the Council on Atherosclerosis, American Heart Association. *Circulation* 1995; 92:1355–1374.

6. Faggiotto A, Ross R, Harker L. Studies of hypercholesterolemia in the non-human primate: I. Changes that lead to fatty streak formation. *Arteriosclerosis* 1984; 4:323–340.

7. Gordon D, Reidy MA, Benditt EP, Schwartz SM. Cell proliferation in human coronary arteries. *Proc Natl Acad Sci USA* 1990; 87:4600–4604.

8. Steinberg D, Witztum JL. Lipoproteins and atherogenesis. *JAMA* 1990; 264:3047–3052.

9. Berliner JA, Territo MC, Sevanian A. Minimally modified low density lipoprotein stimulates monocyte endothelial interactions. *J Clin Invest* 1990; 85:1260–1266.

10. O'Brien KD, Allen MD, McDonald TO, Chait A, Harlan JM, Fishbein D, et al. Vascular cell adhesion molecule-1 is expressed in human coronary atherosclerotic plaques: Implications for the mode of progression of advanced coronary atherosclerosis. *J Clin Invest* 1993; 92:945–951.

11. Nelken NA, Coughlin SR, Gordon D, Wilcox JN. Monocyte chemoattractant protein-1 in human atheromatous plaques. *J Clin Invest* 1991; 88:1121–1127.

12. Rosenfeld ME, Yla-Herttuala S, Lipton BA, Ord VA, Witztum JL, Steinberg D. Macrophage colony-stimulation factor mRNA and protein in atherosclerotic lesions of rabbits and man. *Am J Pathol* 1992; 140:291–300.

13. Barath P, Fishbein MC, Cao J, Berenson J, Helfant RH, Forrester JS. Tumor necrosis factor gene expression in human vascular intimal smooth muscle cells detected by in situ hybridization. *Am J Pathol* 1990; 137:503–509.

14. Dollery CM, McEwan JR, Henney A. Matrix metalloproteinases and cardiovascular disease. *Circ Res* 1995; 77:863–868.

15. Annex BH, Denning SM, Channon KM, Sketch MH, Stack RS, Morrissey JH, et al. Differential expression of tissue factor protein in directional atherectomy specimens from patients with stable and unstable coronary syndrome. *Circulation* 1995; 91:619–622.

16. Yla-Herttuala S, Palinski W, Rosenfeld ME, Parthasarathy S, Carew T, Butler S, et al. Evidence for the presence of oxidatively modified low density lipoprotein in atherosclerotic lesions of rabbit and man. *J Clin Invest* 1989; 84:1086–1095.

17. Guyton JR, Klemp KF. Development of the atherosclerotic core region: Chemical and ultrastructural analysis of microdissected atherosclerotic lesions from human aorta. *Arterioscler Thromb* 1994; 14:1305–1314.

18. Ball RY, Stower EC, Burton JH, Cary NR. Evidence that the death of macrophage foam cells contributes to the lipid core of atheroma. *Atherosclerosis* 1995; 114:45–54.

19. Raines EW, Ross R. Smooth muscle cells and the pathogenesis of the lesions of atherosclerosis. *Br Heart J* 1993; 69:S30–S37.

20. Bini A, Fenoglio JJ, Mesa-Tejada R, Kudryk B, Kaplan KL. Identification and distribution of fibrinogen, fibrin and fibrin(ogen) degradation products in atherosclerosis: Use of monoclonal antibodies. *Arteriosclerosis* 1989; 9:109–121.

21. Libby P. Molecular bases of the acute coronary syndromes. *Circulation* 1995; 91:2844–2850.

22. Libby P, Hansson GK. Involvement of the immune system in human atherogenesis: Current knowledge and unanswered questions. *Lab Invest* 1991; 64:5–15.

23. Salonen JT, Yla-Herttuala S, Yamamoto R, Butler S, Korpela H, Salonen R, et al. Auto-antibody against oxidised LDL and progression of carotid atherosclerosis. *Lancet* 1992; 339:883–887.

24. Barger AC III, Beeuwkes R. Rupture of coronary vasa vasorum as a trigger of acute myocardial infarction. *Am J Cardiol* 1990; 66:41G–43G.

25. O'Brien KD, McDonald TO, Chait A, Allen M, Alpers C. Neovascular expression of E-selectin, intercellular adhesion molecule-1, and vascular cell adhesion molecule-1 in human atherosclerosis and their relation to intimal leukocyte content. *Circulation* 1996; 93:672–682.

26. McGill HC. *The Geographic Pathology of Atherosclerosis*. Baltimore: Williams & Wilkins; 1968:38–77.

27. Tracy RE, Newman WP, Wattigney WA, Berenson GS. Risk factors and atherosclerosis in youth: Autopsy findings of the Bogalusa Heart Study. *Am J Med Sci* 1995; 310:S37–S41.

28. Glagov S, Weisenberd E, Zarins CK, Stankunavicius R, Kolettis GJ. Compensatory enlargement of human atherosclerotic coronary arteries. *N Engl J Med* 1987; 316:1371–1375.

29. Tuzcu EM, Hobbs RE, Rincon G, Bott-Silverman C, De Franco AC, Robinson K, et al. Occult and frequent transmission of atherosclerotic coronary disease with cardiac transplantation: Insights from intravascular ultrasound. *Circulation* 1995; 91:1706–1713.

30. Davies MJ. A macroscopic and microscopic view of coronary thrombi. *Circulation* 1990; 82:1138–1146.

31. Davies MJ, Woolf N, Rowles PM, Pepper J. Morphology of the endothelium over atherosclerotic plaques in human coronary arteries. *Br Heart J* 1988; 60:459–464.

32. Burrig KF. The endothelium of advanced arteriosclerotic plaques in humans. *Arterioscler Thromb* 1991; 11:1678–1689.

33. van der Wal AC, Becker AE, van der Loos CM, Das PK. Site of intimal rupture or erosion of thrombosed coronary atherosclerotic plaques is characterized by an inflammatory process irrespective of the dominant plaque morphology. *Circulation* 1994; 89:6–44.

34. Farb A, Burke AP, Tang AL, Liang Y, Mannan P, Smialek J, et al. Coronary plaque erosion without rupture into a lipid core: A frequent cause of coronary thrombosis in sudden coronary death. *Circulation* 1996; 93:1354–1363.

35. Fernandez-Ortiz A, Badimon JJ, Falk E, Fuster V, Meyer B, Mailhac C, et al. Characterization of the relative thrombogenicity of atherosclerotic plaque components: Implication for consequences of plaque rupture. *J Am Coll Cardiol* 1994; 23:1562–1569.

36. Davies MJ, Richardson PD, Woolf N, Katz DR, Mann J. Risk of thrombosis in human atherosclerotic plaques: Role of extracellular lipid, macrophage, and smooth muscle cell content. *Br Heart J* 1993; 69:377–381.

37. Davies MJ, Thomas AC. Plaque fissuring—The cause of acute myocardial infarction, sudden ischaemic death and crescendo angina. *Br Heart J* 1985; 53:363–373.

38. Mann JM, Davies MJ. Vulnerable plaque: Relation of characteristics to degree of stenosis in human coronary arteries. *Circulation* 1996; 94:928–931.

39. Falk E. Plaque rupture with severe pre-existing stenosis precipitating coronary thrombosis: Characteristics of coronary atherosclerotic plaque underlying fatal occlusive thrombi. *Br Heart J* 1983; 50:127–134.

40. Fulton WFM. Pathological concepts in acute coronary thrombosis: Relevance to treatment. *Br Heart J* 1993; 70:403–408.

41. Marshall JC, Waxman HL, Sauerwein A, Gilchrist I, Kurnik PB. Frequency of low-grade residual coronary stenosis after thrombolysis during acute myocardial infarction. *Am J Cardiol* 1990; 66:773–778.

42. Richardson PD, Davies MJ, Born GVR. Influence of plaque configuration and stress distribution on fissuring of coronary atherosclerotic plaques. *Lancet* 1989; 2:941–944.

43. Cheng GC, Loree HM, Kamm RD, Fishbein MC, Lee RT. Distribution of circumferential stress in ruptured and stable atherosclerotic lesions: A structural analysis with histopathological correlation. *Circulation* 1993; 87:1179–1187.

44. Loree HM, Kamm RD, Stringfellow RG, Lee RT. Effects of fibrous cap thickness on peak circumferential stress in model atherosclerotic vessels. *Circ Res* 1992; 71:850–858.

45. Lendon CL, Davies MJ, Born GVR, Richardson PD. Atherosclerotic plaque caps are locally weakened when macrophages density is increased. *Atherosclerosis* 1991; 87:87–90.

46. Henney AM, Wakeley PR, Davies MJ, Foster K, Hembry R, Murphy G, et al. Localization of stromelysin gene expression in atherosclerotic plaques by in situ hybridization. *Proc Natl Acad Sci USA* 1991; 88:8154–8158.

47. Galis ZS, Sukhova GK, Lark MW, Libby P. Increased expression of matrix metalloproteinases and matrix degrading activity in vulnerable regions of human atherosclerotic plaques. *J Clin Invest* 1994; 94:2493–2503.

48. Ambrose JA, Winters SL, Arora RR. Angiographic evolution of coronary artery morphology in unstable angina. *J Am Coll Cardiol* 1986; 7:472–478.

49. Moreno PR, Falk E, Palacios IF, Newell JB, Fuster V, Fallon JT. Macrophage infiltration in acute coronary syndromes: Implications for plaque rupture. *Circulation* 1994; 90:775–778.

50. Escaned J, van Suylen RJ, MacLeod DC, Ulmans VA, de Jong M, Bosman FT, et al. Histologic characteristics of tissue excised during directional coronary atherectomy in stable and unstable angina pectoris. *Am J Cardiol* 1993; 71:1442–1447.

51. Rosenschein U, Ellis SG, Haudenschild CC, Yakbov SJ, Muller DW, Dick RJ, et al. Comparison of histopathologic coronary lesions obtained from directional atherectomy in stable angina versus acute coronary syndromes. *Am J Cardiol* 1994; 73:508–510.

52. Haft JI, Christou CP, Goldstein JE, Carnes RE. Atherectomy and complex coronary lesions. In: Ambrose JA, ed. *Complex Coronary Lesions in Acute Coronary Syndromes*. Armonk, NY: Futura; 1996:73–85.

53. Brown DL, Hibbs MS, Kearney M, Loushin C, Isner JM. Identification of 92-kD gelatinase in human coronary atherosclerotic lesions: Association of active enzyme synthesis with unstable angina. *Circulation* 1995; 91:2125–2131.

54. Flugelman MY, Virmani R, Correa R, Yu ZX, Farb A, Leon MB, et al. Smooth muscle cell abundance and fibroblast growth factors in coronary lesions of patients with nonfatal unstable angina: A clue to the mechanism of transformation from the stable to the unstable clinical state. *Circulation* 1993; 88:2493–2500.

55. White CJ, Ramee SR, Collins TJ, Escobar AE, Karsan A, Shaw D, et al. Coronary thrombi increase PTCA risk: Angioscopy as a clinical tool. *Circulation* 1996; 93:253–258.

56. Davies MJ, Thomas AC, Knapman PA, Hangartner R. Intramyocardial platelet aggregation in patients with unstable angina suffering sudden ischaemic cardiac death. *Circulation* 1986; 73:418–427.

57. Falk E. Unstable angina with fatal outcome: Dynamic coronary thrombosis leading to infarction and/or sudden death. *Circulation* 1985; 71:699–708.

58. Lindahl B, Venge P, Wallentin L, FRISC Study Group. Relation between troponin T and the risk of subsequent cardiac events in unstable coronary artery disease. *Circulation* 1996; 93:1651–1657.

59. Hoffmeister HM, Jur M, Wendel HP, Heller W, Seiper L. Alterations of coagulation and fibrinolytic and kallikrein-kinin systems in the acute and postacute phases in patients with unstable angina. *Circulation* 1995; 91:2520–2527.

60. Badimon L, Chesebro JH, Badimon JJ. Thrombus formation on ruptured atherosclerotic plaques and rethrombosis on evolving thrombi. *Circulation* 1992; 86:III74–85.

61. Neri Serneri GG, Anbbate R, Gori AM, Attanasio M, Martini F, Giusti B, et al. Transient intermittent lymphocyte activation is responsible for the instability of angina. *Circulation* 1992; 86:790–797.

62. Mazzone A, De Servi S, Ricevuti G, Mazzucchelli I, Fossati G, Pasotti D. Increased expression of neutrophil and monocyte adhesion molecules in unstable coronary artery disease. *Circulation* 1993; 88:358–363.

63. Dinerman JL, Mehta JL, Saldeen IGP, Emerson S, Wallin R, Darda R. Increased neutrophil elastase release in unstable angina pectoris and acute myocardial infarction. *J Am Coll Cardiol* 1990; 15:1559–1563.

64. Reddy KG, Nair RN, Sheehan HM, Hodgson JM. Evidence that selective endothelial dysfunction may occur in the absence of angiographic or ultrasound atherosclerosis in patients with risk factors for atherosclerosis. *J Am Coll Cardiol* 1994; 23:833–843.

65. Bugiardini R, Pozzati A, Ottani F, Morgagni GL, Puddu P. Vasotonic angina: A spectrum of ischemic syndromes involving functional abnormalities of the epicardial and microvascular coronary circulation. *J Am Coll Cardiol* 1993; 22:417–425.

66. Yamagishi M, Miyatake K, Tamai J, Nakatani SM, Koyma J, Nissen SE. Intravascular ultrasound detection of atherosclerosis at the site of focal vasospasm in angiographically normal or minimally narrowed coronary segments. *J Am Coll Cardiol* 1994; 23:352–357.

67. Zeiher AM, Goebel H, Schachinger V, Ihling C. Tissue endothelin-1 immunoreactivity in the active coronary atherosclerotic plaque: A clue to the mechanism of increased vasoreactivity of the culprit lesion in unstable angina. *Circulation* 1995; 91:941–947.

68. Brown B, Bolson EL, Dodge HT. Dynamic mechanisms in human coronary stenosis. *Circulation* 1984; 70:917–922.

69. Lam JY, Chesebro JH, Steele PM, Badimon L, Fuster V. Is vasospasm related to platelet deposition: Relationship in a porcine preparation of arterial injury in vivo. *Circulation* 1987; 76:243–248.

70. Forman MB, Oates JA, Robertson D. Increased adventitial mast cells in a patient with coronary spasm. *N Engl J Med* 1985; 313:1138–1141.

71. Kohchi K, Takebayashi S, Hiroki T, Nobuyoshi M. Significance of adventitial inflammation of the coronary artery in patients with unstable angina: Results at autopsy. *Circulation* 1995; 71:709–716.

72. Rizzon P, Rossi L, Calabrese P, Franchini G, DiBase M. Angiographic and pathologic correlations in Prinzmetal variant angina. *Angiology* 1978; 29:486–490.

73. Roberts WC, Curry RC, Isner JM. Sudden death in Prinzmetal's angina with coronary spasm documented by arteriography: Analysis of three necropsy cases. *Am J Cardiol* 1982; 50:203–210.

74. Stadius ML, Maynard C, Fritz JK. Coronary anatomy and left ventricular function in the first 12 hours of acute myocardial infarction: The Western Washington randomized intracoronary streptokinase trial. *Circulation* 1985; 72:292–301.

75. Davies MJ, Woolf N, Robertson WB. Pathology of acute myocardial infarction with particular reference to occlusive coronary thrombi. *Br Heart J* 1976; 38:659–664.

76. Cohen M, Sherman W, Rentrop KP, Gorlin R. Determinants of collateral filling observed during sudden controlled coronary occlusion in human subjects. *J Am Coll Cardiol* 1989; 13:297–303.

77. Habib GB, Heibig J, Forman SA, Brown BG, Roberts R, Terrin ML, et al. Influence of coronary collateral vessels on myocardial infarct size in humans. *Circulation* 1991; 83:739–746.

78. Fuster V, Frye RL, Kennedy MA, Connolly DC, Mankin HT. The role of collateral circulation in the various coronary syndromes. *Circulation* 1979; 59:1137–1144.

79. Hackett D, Davies G, Chierchia S, Maseri A. Intermittent coronary occlusion in acute myocardial infarction. Value of thrombolytic and vasodilator therapy. *N Engl J Med* 1987; 317:1055–1059.

80. DeWood MA, Sifter WF, Simpson CS. Coronary arteriographic findings soon after non-Q-wave myocardial infarction. *N Engl J Med* 1986; 315:417–423.

81. Piek JJ, Becker AE. Collateral blood supply to the myocardium at risk in human myocardial infarction: A quantitative post-mortem assessment. *J Am Coll Cardiol* 1988; 11:1290–1296.

82. Hangartner JRW, Charleston AJ, Davies MJ, Thomas AC. Morphological characteristics of clinically significant coronary artery stenosis in stable angina. *Br Heart J* 1986; 56:501–508.

83. Waller BF. The eccentric coronary atherosclerotic plaque: Morphologic observations and clinical relevance. *Clin Cardiol* 1989; 12:14–20.

84. Kragel AH, Reddy SG, Wittes JT, Roberts WC. Morphometric analysis of the composition of atherosclerotic plaques in the four major epicardial coronary arteries in acute myocardial infarction and in sudden coronary death. *Circulation* 1989; 80:1747–1756.

85. Moise A, Lesperance J, Theroux P, Taeymans Y, Goulet C, Bourassa MG. Clinical and angiographic predictors of new total coronary occlusion in coronary artery disease: Analysis of 313 non-operated patients. *Am J Cardiol* 1984; 54:1176–1181.

86. Ambrose JA, Tannenbaum MA, Alexopoulos D, Hjemdahl CE, Borrico S, Gorlin R, et al. Angiographic progression of coronary artery disease and the development of myocardial infarction. *J Am Coll Cardiol* 1988; 12:56–62.

87. Little WC, Constantinescu M, Applegate RJ. Can coronary angiography predict the site of a subsequent myocardial infarction in patients with mild-to-moderate artery disease? *Circulation* 1988; 78:1157–1166.

88. Giroud D, Li JM, Urban P, Meier B, Rutishauser W. Relation of the site of acute myocardial infarction to the most severe coronary arterial stenosis at prior angiography. *Am J Cardiol* 1992; 69:729–732.

89. Petursson KK, Jonmundsson EH, Brekkan A, Hardarson T. Angiographic predictors of new coronary occlusions. 1995; 129:515–520.

90. Waters D, Craven TE, Lesperance J. Prognostic significance of progression of coronary atherosclerosis. *Circulation* 1993; 87:1067–1075.

91. Azen SP, Mack WJ, Cashin-Hemphill L, LaBree L, Shircore AM, Selzer RH, et al. Progression of coronary artery disease predicts clinical coronary events: Long-term follow-up from the cholesterol lowering atherosclerosis study. *Circulation* 1996; 93:34–41.

92. Davies MJ, Bland JM, Hangartner JWR, Angelini A, Thomas AC. Factors influencing the presence or absence of acute coronary artery thrombi in sudden ischaemic death. *Eur Heart J* 1989; 10:203–208.

93. Davies MJ, Thomas AC. Thrombosis and acute coronary artery lesions in sudden cardiac ischaemic death. *N Engl J Med* 1984; 310:1137–1140.

94. Falk E. Plaque rupture with severe pre-existing stenosis precipitating coronary thrombosis: Characteristics of coronary atherosclerotic plaque underlying fatal occlusive thrombi. *Br Heart J* 1983; 50:127–131.

95. Frink RJ. Chronic ulcerated plaques: New insights into the pathogenesis of acute coronary disease. *J Invas Cardiol* 1994; 6:173–185.

96. 4S Group. Randomised trial of cholesterol lowering in 4444 patients with coronary heart disease: The Scandinavian Simvastatin Survival Study (4S). *Lancet* 1994; 344:1383–1389.

97. Shepherd J, Cobbe SM, Ford I, Isles CG, Lorimer AR, MacFarlane PW, et al. Prevention of coronary heart disease with pravastatin in men with hypercholesterolemia. *N Engl J Med* 1995; 333:1301–1307.

98. Small DM, Bond MG, Waugh D, Prack M, Sawyer JK. Physicochemical and histological changes in the arterial wall of non-human primates during progression and regression of atherosclerosis. *J Clin Invest* 1984; 73:1590–1605.

99. Kaplan JR, Manuck SB, Adams MR, Williams JK, Register TC, Clarkson TB. Plaque changes and arterial enlargement in atherosclerotic monkeys after manipulation of diet and social environment. *Arterioscler Thromb* 1993; 13:254–263.

100. Shiomi M, Ito T, Tsukada T, Yata T, Watanabe Y, Tsujita Y, et al. Reduction of serum cholesterol levels alters lesional composition of atherosclerotic plaques: Effect of pravastatin sodium on atherosclerosis in mature WHHL rabbits. *Arterioscler Thromb Vasc Biol* 1995; 15:1938–1944.

RISK FACTORS AND THE PREVENTION OF CORONARY HEART DISEASE

David J. Maron / Paul M. Ridker / Thomas A. Pearson

Epidemiologic research has identified risk factors that increase the likelihood of coronary heart disease (CHD) events. Basic and clinical studies have revealed plausible biological links between many of the risk factors and atherosclerosis and have demonstrated that management of risk factors can improve coronary endothelial function, stop the progression of atherosclerosis, prevent disruption and thrombosis of vulnerable atherosclerotic plaque, and reduce CHD morbidity and mortality (see Chap. 44). When risk factors coexist, they multiply the risk of CHD severalfold[1] (Fig. 41-1).

Identification and management of risk factors are essential in preventing CHD in high-risk asymptomatic individuals (*primary prevention*) and in preventing recurrent events in patients with established disease (*secondary prevention*). *Risk factor management should be thought of as prevention or treatment of the atherosclerotic disease process itself and, as such, should be included as an integral part of any management plan for the many acute or chronic manifestations of this disease.* Risk factors may be conceptualized as modifiable versus unmodifiable, proatherogenic versus prothrombotic, and chronic versus acute. The intensity of risk factor intervention should correspond to the patient's level of risk. The presence of unmodifiable risk factors may necessitate more intense management of modifiable risk factors. A recent Bethesda Conference proposed a classification scheme according to the strength of evidence that risk factor intervention favorably affects outcome.[2] This chapter is organized to reflect that classification scheme (Table 41-1) and reviews CHD risk factors, discusses the efficacy and cost-effectiveness of managing risk factors, and provides practical recommendations for preventive cardiology practice.

RISK FACTORS FOR WHICH INTERVENTIONS HAVE PROVED TO LOWER RISK OF CORONARY HEART DISEASE

Cigarette Smoking

Strong dose-responsive relationships between cigarette smoking and CHD have been observed in both sexes, in the young and the elderly, and in all racial groups.[3] Cigarette smoking increases risk two- to threefold and interacts with other risk factors to multiply risk (Fig. 41-1). There is no evidence that filters or other modifications of the cigarette reduce risk.[4] Passive smoking also increases CHD risk.[5,6] Pipe smoking and cigar smoking, when not inhaled, as well as oral tobacco use, whether chewing tobacco or snuff, carry rather small risks but are related to later resumption of cigarette smoking. Clearly, cigarette smoking remains a leading preventable cause of mortality, much of it due to cardiovascular disease.

Pathophysiologic studies have identified a panoply of mechanisms through which cigarette smoking may cause CHD. Smokers have increased levels of oxidation products, including oxidized low-density lipoproteins (LDL).[7] Cigarette smoking also lowers the cardioprotective levels of high-density lipoproteins (HDL). These effects, along with direct effects of carbon monoxide and nicotine, produce endothelial damage. Possibly through these mechanisms, smokers have increased vascular reactivity.[8] Cigarette smoking is also related to increased levels of fibrinogen[9] and increased platelet aggregability.[10]

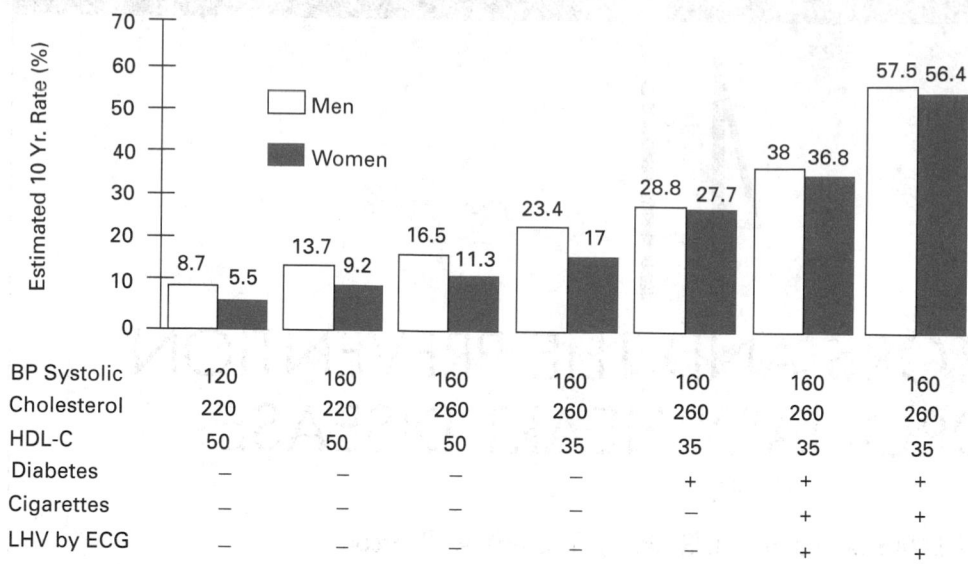

BP Systolic	120	160	160	160	160	160	160
Cholesterol	220	220	260	260	260	260	260
HDL-C	50	50	50	35	35	35	35
Diabetes	–	–	–	–	+	+	+
Cigarettes	–	–	–	–	–	+	+
LHV by ECG	–	–	–	–	–	+	+

FIGURE 41-1

Estimated 10-year risk of coronary heart disease in hypothetical 55-year-old men and women according to levels of various risk factors. Based on Framingham Heart Study data. Lipid units are milligrams per deciliter. (From Wilson.[1] Reprinted by permission of Elsevier Science Inc. from Wilson PWF: Established risk factors and coronary artery disease: The Framingham Study. *Am J Hypertens*, 1994; 7:7S–12S. Copyright 1994 by American Journal of Hypertension, Inc.)

PRIMARY PREVENTION

Cessation of smoking is associated with a precipitous fall in CHD events. *In a previous smoker, the relative risk declines nearly to that of a nonsmoker in a year or less.*[11] It is estimated that a 35-year-old who quits smoking extends survival by 3 to 5 years,[12] with much of the improved life expectancy caused by a reduction of CHD deaths.

SECONDARY PREVENTION

The risk of a recurrent event in the patient surviving a myocardial infarction (MI) is strikingly reduced by smoking cessation. Compared with the patient who continues to smoke, most studies suggest that the risk of recurrence can be reduced by 50 percent.[13,14] *The benefits of achieving complete abstinence from smoking in the patient with CHD compare favorably with the health benefits of any intervention in modern cardiology.*

COST-EFFECTIVENESS

Cost-effectiveness analysis is used to consider both the effectiveness of an intervention and its cost and is commonly expressed as a ratio of cost in dollars per quality-adjusted years of life gained.[2] The validity of the assumptions used to determine direct and indirect costs is critical to computing an accurate ratio. By convention, less than $20,000 per year of life saved is considered highly cost-effective, $20,000 to $40,000 is relatively cost-effective, and greater than $60,000 is considered expensive. Interventions to achieve smoking cessation are among the most cost-effective in either primary or secondary prevention, with or without the use of nicotine replacement therapy.[15,16] Physician counseling of middle-

aged patients without vascular disease is estimated to cost only $1000 to $1400 per year in men and $1700 to $3000 per year in women.[17] The use of nicotine gum by these patients increases the cost to up to $9000 per year in men and $13,500 per year in women.[18] In contrast, counseling to achieve smoking cessation in MI patients is exceptionally cost-effective, costing only $250 per year of life saved.[19]

PRACTICE RECOMMENDATIONS

Nothing less than complete cessation of smoking and other tobacco use should be acceptable in patients with cardiovascular disease. The cardiovascular specialist often has unique opportunities to influence a patient's behavior. After an acute event, the patient and family members may be especially receptive to a smoking cessation intervention. Key elements of a successful smoking cessation program are outlined in Table 41-2.[20]

Lipids and Lipoproteins

See Chap. 53 for a complete discussion of lipid metabolism and the diagnosis and treatment of lipid disorders.

TOTAL AND LDL CHOLESTEROL AS RISK FACTORS FOR ATHEROSCLEROSIS

Elevated LDL cholesterol is considered a major cause of CHD. Numerous prospective epidemiologic studies have identified a continuous, graded, direct relationship between serum total cholesterol level and CHD incidence[21] (see Chap. 38). This relationship has been confirmed in numerous countries, in women, in the elderly, and in middle-aged adults.[22] Cholesterol levels obtained in young adulthood predict coronary disease decades later.[23] The level of total and LDL-cholesterol interacts with other risk factors to multiply risk[1] (Fig. 41-1). Elevated LDL-cholesterol levels have been related to recurrent events and CHD death in patients with established CHD.[24] Elevated LDL-cholesterol levels appear to be involved with all stages of atherogenesis: endothelial dysfunction, plaque formation and growth, and plaque instability and disruption. Elevated LDL-cholesterol levels in the plasma lead to increased retention of LDL particles in the arterial wall, their oxidation, and the secretion of various inflammatory mediators and chemoattractants[25] (see Chap. 39). One sequela of this is the disruption of endothelial cell functions by the oxidized LDL,[26] with subsequent loss of production of endothelial-

TABLE 41-1

CARDIOVASCULAR RISK FACTORS: THE EVIDENCE SUPPORTING THEIR ASSOCIATION WITH DISEASE, THE USEFULNESS OF MEASURING THEM, AND THEIR RESPONSIVENESS TO INTERVENTION

Risk Factor	Evidence for Association with CVD		Clinical Measurement Useful?	Response to	
	Epidemiologic	Clinical Trials		Nonpharmacologic Therapy	Pharmacologic Therapy
Category I (risk factors for which interventions have been proved to lower CVD risk)					
Cigarette smoking	+ + +	+ +	+ + +	+ + +	+ +
LDL cholesterol	+ + +	+ + +	+ + +	+ +	+ + +
High fat/cholesterol diet	+ + +	+ +	+ +	+ +	–
Hypertension	+ + +	+ + + (stroke)	+ + +	+	+ + +
Left ventricular hypertrophy	+ + +	+	+ +	–	+ +
Thrombogenic factors	+ + + (fibrinogen)	+ + + (aspirin, warfarin)	+ (fibrinogen)	+	+ + + (aspirin, warfarin)
Category II (risk factors for which interventions are likely to lower CVD risk)					
Diabetes mellitus	+ + +	+	+ + +	+ +	+ + +
Physical inactivity	+ + +	+ +	+ +	+ +	–
HDL cholesterol	+ + +	+	+ + +	+ +	+
Triglycerides; small, dense LDL	+ +	+ +	+ + +	+ +	+ + +
Obesity	+ + +	–	+ + +	+ +	+
Postmenopausal status (women)	+ + +	–	+ + +	–	+ + +
Category III (risk factors associated with increased CVD risk that, if modified, might lower risk)					
Psychosocial factors	+ +	+	+ + +	+	–
Lipoprotein(a)	+	–	+	–	+
Homocysteine	+ +	–	+	+ +	+ +
Oxidative stress	+	–	–	+	+ +
No alcohol consumption	+ + +	–	+ +	+ +	–
Category IV (risk factors associated with increased CVD risk but which cannot be modified)					
Age	+ + +	–	+ + +	–	–
Male gender	+ + +	–	+ + +	–	–
Low socioeconomic status	+ + +	–	+ + +	–	–
Family history of early-onset CVD	+ + +	–	+ + +	–	–

Note: CVD, cardiovascular disease; HDL, high-density lipoprotein; LDL, low-density lipoprotein; +, weak, somewhat consistent evidence; + +, moderately strong, rather consistent evidence; + + +, very strong, consistent evidence; –, evidence poor or nonexistent.
Source: From Fuster and Pearson.[2] Reprinted with permission from the American College of Cardiology (*J Am Coll Cardiol* 1996; 27:957–1047).

derived relaxing factors. Treatment of elevated LDL-cholesterol levels has been shown to reestablish normal coronary vasodilatory response to acetylcholine.[27,28] LDL is also a potent mitogen for smooth muscle cells; progressive growth of atherosclerotic plaques can be halted by the lowering of LDL-cholesterol levels. Atherosclerotic plaques with a large lipid core and numerous lipid-filled macrophages are prone to rupture[29] (see Chap. 40). Thus, the epidemiologic and biologic evidence strongly supports LDL-cholesterol's role in atherosclerosis.

LOW HDL CHOLESTEROL AS A RISK FACTOR FOR ATHEROSCLEROSIS

Numerous prospective epidemiologic studies have demonstrated a continuous, inverse relationship between HDL-cholesterol levels and the incidence of CHD.[30] The relationship

TABLE 41-2

SUCCESSFUL ELEMENTS OF A SMOKING CESSATION PROGRAM

I. Obtain a complete smoking history, including assessment of nicotine addiction and environmental exposures.
II. Give advice to quit smoking.
   A. Express concern.
   B. Review benefits of quitting.
   C. Review risks of continuing.
III. Determine the patient's willingness to quit smoking; if unwilling, the patient should identify reasons for unwillingness.
IV. In the patient willing to quit, initiate a smoking cessation program with combination of both behavioral and pharmacologic interventions.
   A. Provide behavioral interventions, including smoking cessation pamphlets, self-monitoring with a diary of cigarette use, setting a quit date, identifying a support person, and removing all cues from the home and work environment.
   B. In the addicted smoker, consider replacement therapy with nicotine gum or transdermal patch.
V. Arrange for follow-up.
   A. Provide reminder on quit date.
   B. See patient shortly after quit date to assess success.
   C. If unsuccessful, identify barriers and work to remove them.

Note: Modified from Pearson.[20]

has been observed in men and women, including the elderly,[31] and appears independent of total or LDL-cholesterol levels. The total cholesterol to HDL-cholesterol ratio is a better predictor of CHD than the HDL-cholesterol level alone.[30] Since interventions focus on individual lipid subfractions, however, the National Cholesterol Education Program has elected to treat the individual lipoproteins rather than the ratio. *Two important mechanisms by which HDL is thought to play a protective role against atherosclerosis are reverse cholesterol transport and inhibition of LDL oxidation.*

TRIGLYCERIDES AND SMALL, DENSE LDL PARTICLES AS RISK FACTORS FOR ATHEROSCLEROSIS

The relationship between triglycerides and CHD has been less clear. In men, univariate analyses have consistently demonstrated a direct dose-response relationship. This relationship usually disappears after adjustment for other risk factors such as HDL cholesterol, obesity, and diabetes.[32] *Hypertriglyceridemia, however, has been found to be an independent risk factor in women.*[33] Thus, triglyceride-rich lipoproteins and/or their remnants may impart some risk for atherosclerosis. Several mechanisms have been proposed to explain the triglyceride-CHD association. First, several familial syndromes associated with early CHD are characterized by elevated LDL-cholesterol and triglyceride levels. Second, some patients with hypertriglyceridemia have a predominance of small, dense

LDL particles. Small, dense LDLs are felt to be particularly atherogenic[34] and may require interventions different from those targeting elevated LDL cholesterol. (A high level of plasma apoprotein B in the presence of normal LDL cholesterol may be presumptive evidence of this pattern.) Third, fasting hypertriglyceridemia may be a marker of exaggerated postprandial hyperlipidemia, which may promote the uptake of atherogenic triglyceride-rich lipoprotein remnants by endothelial cells.[35] Finally, serum triglyceride levels are strongly related to fibrinogen and factor VII in numerous epidemiologic studies.[36] Therefore, a number of mechanisms, direct and indirect, may link serum triglycerides and CHD.

PRIMARY PREVENTION

A number of trials to lower elevated LDL-cholesterol levels have been conducted over the past three decades. Early studies using diets, bile acid–binding resins, and fibric acid derivatives generally were able to demonstrate reductions in CHD endpoints, including both fatal and nonfatal events.[37] These interventions resulted in modest reductions in LDL cholesterol (generally 9 to 11 percent versus control groups). In some of these trials, reductions in CHD deaths in the treatment groups were counterbalanced by excess deaths due to noncardiac causes. (For a discussion of this issue, please refer to Chap. 53.)

More recently, the West of Scotland Coronary Prevention Study examined the effects of an HMG-CoA reductase inhibitor ("statin"), pravastatin (40 mg/day), in hypercholesterolemic Scottish men free of MI.[38] The randomized, placebo-controlled trial demonstrated a significant 31 percent reduction in nonfatal MI and CHD deaths ($p = .001$) and a 22 percent reduction in total mortality ($p = .051$) at the end of 6 years. Unlike previous trials, there was no excess of non-CHD deaths in the intervention group. The benefits of intervention appeared within 6 months after initiation of treatment. Large reductions in the need for revascularization and hospitalization were also observed. Therefore, with statins available, prevention of CHD in relatively high-risk patients appears feasible. Demonstration of benefit in groups at lower risk, such as women, those with few risk factors, and younger men, has not been attempted.

SECONDARY PREVENTION

Numerous studies have proven the worth of lowering LDL cholesterol in patients with evidence of atherosclerosis. Again, early studies in CHD patients demonstrated the ability of older agents, such as bile acid–binding resins and niacin, to reduce CHD events. More recently, a large number of studies have used serial angiograpic endpoints to test the cholesterol hypothesis.[39] These studies tested a variety of interventions, some of them nonpharmacologic, with nonintervention controls. Despite small but significant changes in the rate of progression of coronary atherosclerosis, the reduction in the rate of coronary events was surprisingly large, ranging from 22 to 89 percent. This supports the notion that although the bulk of atherosclerotic plaque is changed minimally by LDL-cholesterol reduction, the composition of the plaque is altered favorably (see Chap. 44). Large secondary prevention trials using statins have been reported recently[40,41] (see Chap. 53). In general, these studies demonstrated large reductions in CHD events similar to those shown in the serial angiographic trials. Not only did these studies reduce revascularization procedures, MI, and cardiac death but they also extended their benefits to reductions in stroke, congestive heart failure, and total mortality.

Low HDL-cholesterol levels are related to recurrent CHD events, even in the absence of elevated total cholesterol levels.[24,42] No trials have been completed in which HDL-cholesterol levels were raised in patients with otherwise normal or near-normal LDL-cholesterol levels.

COST-EFFECTIVENESS

Studies of the cost-effectiveness of cholesterol-lowering have demonstrated the importance of effective therapies in patients at highest risk. Studies of LDL-cholesterol reduction with statins have demonstrated cost-effectiveness in CHD patients. Estimates of cost per year of life range from $22,900 in asymptomatic 55- to 64-year-old men with total cholesterol < 250 mg/dL to actual cost savings in hypercholesterolemic, male CHD patients 45 to 54 years old.[43] In a direct cost analysis of the Scandinavian Simvastatin Survival Study, cost of simvastatin therapy ranged from $3800 for 70-year-old men with a cholesterol level of 309 mg/dL to $27,400 for 35-year-old women with a cholesterol level of 213 mg/dL.[44] When indirect costs were considered, the results ranged from a savings in the youngest patient to a cost of $13,300 per year of life gained in older patients. In contrast, the use of less effective agents, such as bile acid–binding resins, in low-risk, asymptomatic patients does not appear to be cost-effective.[45]

PRACTICE RECOMMENDATIONS

Please refer to Chap. 53 for a complete discussion of the treatment of lipid disorders for primary and secondary prevention according to the National Cholesterol Education Program guidelines.[46]

Hypertension

Several major prospective epidemiologic studies have found that both systolic and diastolic hypertension have a strong, positive, and graded relationship to CHD without evidence of a threshold risk level of blood pressure.[47–49] The risk imposed by hypertension is heightened substantially when other risk factors are present (see Fig. 41-1). Hypertension clusters with insulin resistance, hyperinsulinemia, glucose intolerance, dyslipidemia, left ventricular hypertrophy (LVH), and obesity and occurs in isolation in fewer than 20 percent of individuals.[50] The potential mechanisms by which hypertension may cause CHD include impaired endothelial function, increased endothelial permeability to lipoproteins, increased adherence of leukocytes, increased oxidative stress, and hemodynamic stress that may trigger acute plaque rupture.

PRIMARY PREVENTION

A meta-analysis of 17 randomized trials of antihypertensive drugs in over 47,000 men and women with mild to moderate hypertension found that stroke was reduced by 38 percent and CHD was reduced by 16 percent.[48] The mean difference in diastolic blood pressure over 5 years between treatment and control groups was 5 to 6 mmHg. An important subset in whom events were reduced were elderly patients with isolated systolic hypertension (systolic blood pressure ≥ 160 mmHg, diastolic blood pressure ≤ 90 mmHg).

For a prolonged 5- to 6-mmHg difference, observational studies predict reductions of 35 to 40 percent in stroke risk and 20 to 25 percent in CHD risk. Although clinical trials indicate that antihypertensive therapy achieves the reduction in stroke expected from observational studies, the reduction in CHD is not as great as expected. Potential explanations for this are as follows: (1) the shortfall was due to chance; (2) the duration of observation was too short, and the full benefit was not seen; (3) the treatment benefits were partially offset by metabolic side effects of medications; (4) excessive reduction in diastolic blood pressure led to excess CHD events; or (5) metabolic disturbances associated with hypertension that potentiate CHD were not corrected by the antihypertensive therapy used in the studies (see "Insulin Resistance Syndrome," below). Most of these trials were based on diuretic therapy, with or without beta blockers, leading some experts to propose that adverse metabolic consequences of diuretics were responsible for the less-than-expected benefits of antihypertensive treatment. Nevertheless, diuretics and beta blockers are the only classes of antihypertensives extensively tested to date that have been shown to reduce CHD morbidity and mortality in primary prevention. The efficacy of newer antihypertensives in reducing initial coronary events is currently being tested.[51] Blood pressure can be lowered by weight loss, exercise, salt restriction, and avoidance of alcohol,[49] but the long-term utility of these measures to prevent CHD in hypertensive individuals has not been tested in randomized controlled studies (see also Chap. 58).

SECONDARY PREVENTION

Clinical trials to test the effect of blood pressure lowering per se in CHD patients have not been performed.

COST-EFFECTIVENESS

Treatment of hypertension for primary prevention is highly cost-effective, with an estimated cost per year of life saved of about $23,000 (in 1993 dollars) for moderate to severe hypertension and twice as much for mild hypertension.[2] Estimates (in 1993 dollars) vary depending on the choice of medication, ranging from $14,000 per year of life saved for propranolol, $20,000 for hydrochlorothiazide, and up to $90,000 for newer medications. The cost-effectiveness of blood pressure lowering for secondary prevention is unknown.

PRACTICE RECOMMENDATIONS

The authors agree with the goal of the Joint National Committee on Detection, Evaluation, and Treatment of High Blood

Pressure of achieving a blood pressure < 140/90 mmHg.[49] (See Chap. 58 for a complete discussion of the treatment of hypertension.)

Left Ventricular Hypertrophy

Left ventricular hypertrophy, defined either by electrocardiography or by echocardiography, is a potent independent risk factor for CHD. LVH often begins as an adaptive mechanism to compensate for excess hemodynamic load, including increased afterload from systemic arterial hypertension (see Chap. 56). In addition to hypertension, LVH is associated with obesity, salt intake, alcohol consumption, advanced age, and genetic predisposition.[52] Progressive LVH may lead to decreased left ventricular compliance, decreased coronary reserve, ventricular ectopy, and ultimately, impaired systolic function. Many antihypertensive drugs can reduce LVH, although not all drugs are equally effective in this regard despite their equipotent blood pressure lowering capabilities. Angiotensin-converting enzyme (ACE) inhibitors are the most effective in regression of LVH,[53] but it is possible to achieve LVH regression with calcium channel blockers, beta blockers, and diuretics. The Framingham Heart Study observed that electrocardiographic evidence of LVH regression was associated with a reduction in cardiovascular disease morbidity and mortality.[54] Randomized clinical trials have not yet tested whether regression of LVH lowers CHD risk, but the observational data merit its classification as a risk factor that should be modified.[2]

Thrombogenic Factors   (See "Antiplatelet and Anticoagulant Therapy," below.)

RISK FACTORS FOR WHICH INTERVENTIONS ARE LIKELY TO LOWER RISK OF CORONARY HEART DISEASE

Insulin Resistance Syndrome: The Basis of Multiple Risk Factors

Reaven[55,56] has hypothesized that *resistance to insulin-stimulated glucose uptake and compensatory hyperinsulinemia are the common metabolic bases for a cluster of coronary risk factors, particularly hypertension, diabetes, hypertriglyceridemia, low HDL, predominance of small, dense LDL, and an increased plasminogen activator inhibitor (PAI) concentration.* A number of observations have supported this hypothesis. Hypertensive individuals, both treated and untreated, obese and nonobese, are hyperinsulinemic compared with a matched group of normotensive individuals. Although not a necessary condition for the expression of the insulin resistance syndrome, obesity, particularly when located centrally (in the abdomen), exacerbates insulin resistance, and weight loss improves insulin sensitivity. Resistance to insulin and compensatory hyperinsulinemia are found in type II diabetes and enhance hepatic very low density lipoprotein triglyceride secretion and hypertriglyceridemia with associated low HDL cholesterol. Hyperinsulinemia may raise blood pressure through sympathetic nerve stimulation and/or renal sodium retention. Insulin sensitivity is associated with endothelial nitric oxide production in healthy persons, providing a clue as to how insulin resistance may promote CHD directly.[57] Furthermore, hyperinsulinemia has been found in a prospective study to be an independent risk factor for CHD in nondiabetic men after adjusting for body weight, blood pressure, and dyslipidemia.[58]

A comprehensive lifestyle approach is required to address the cluster of risk factors related to insulin resistance. Weight loss and physical activity are clear goals because they counteract insulin resistance. Although a high-carbohydrate, low-fat diet is clearly beneficial for hypercholesterolemia, it might be detrimental in insulin-resistant, hypertriglyceridemic patients.[56]

Diabetes Mellitus

Diabetes mellitus is an independent risk factor for CHD, increasing risk by two to three times for men and three to five times for women.[59] CHD is the leading cause of death in diabetic patients, and approximately 25 percent of MI survivors have diabetes.[46] *The CHD risk for a premenopausal diabetic woman is similar to the risk of a nondiabetic man; hence, diabetes abolishes the usual protective effect of being a premenopausal female.*[60] Diabetic women have twice the risk of recurrent MI compared with diabetic men.[61] The greater risk of CHD in diabetic women compared to diabetic men may be explained in part by the greater adverse effect of diabetes on lipoproteins in women.[62] Potential mechanisms by which diabetes may cause atherosclerosis include low HDL, high triglycerides/increased lipoprotein remnant particles, increased small, dense LDL, elevated lipoprotein(a) [Lp(a)] concentration, enhanced lipoprotein oxidation, glycation of LDL, increased fibrinogen, increased platelet aggregability, increased PAI-1, impaired fibrinolysis, increased von Willebrand factor, hyperinsulinemia, and impaired endothelial function.

PRIMARY AND SECONDARY PREVENTION

Despite overwhelming observational data that diabetes increases the risk of CHD, there are few data available to determine if glycemic control reduces risk. The University Group Diabetes Program was the only large-scale randomized clinical trial able to study cardiovascular endpoints in patients with non-insulin-dependent diabetes mellitus, and treatment with sulfonylurea therapy was associated with *increased* cardiovascular mortality.[63] The Diabetes Control and Complications Trial studied the effect of intensive insulin therapy in insulin-dependent diabetes mellitus patients.[64] Intensive therapy reduced microvascular endpoints, but the study was not of sufficient size to examine CHD endpoints.

COST-EFFECTIVENESS

The cost-effectiveness of treating diabetes for primary and secondary prevention of CHD has not been established.

PRACTICE RECOMMENDATIONS

Weight loss and exercise are key therapeutic interventions because they improve the constellation of metabolic abnormalities that accompany diabetes. Although the optimal proportion of dietary fat and carbohydrate is controversial, calorie restriction for obesity and avoidance of sugar and saturated fat are definitely recommended. *Beta blockers should not be withheld from diabetic patients following MI unless strong contraindications exist, because diabetic MI survivors have fewer deaths if treated with a beta blocker.*[65] The National Cholesterol Education Program guidelines recommend a more aggressive LDL goal (<100 mg/dL) in primary prevention of CHD in diabetic patients[46] (see Chap. 78).

Physical Inactivity

Physical inactivity roughly doubles the risk of CHD. Data linking sedentary lifestyle with CHD derive from numerous lines of evidence including animal studies, observational studies, and clinical trials examining the effect of exercise on risk factors and clinical endpoints. Moderate-intensity exercise reduces coronary atherosclerosis and widens coronary arteries in monkeys fed an atherogenic diet compared with monkeys fed the same diet but forced to be sedentary.[66] Physical activity slows progression of angiographically defined coronary atherosclerosis in humans.[67] Over 50 observational studies, primarily of men, have established that physical fitness, on-the-job physical activity, and leisure-time physical activity reduce the risk of CHD.[68] Higher levels of physical fitness and leisure-time physical activity are associated with lower rates of all-cause mortality, independent of other risk factors.[68] These studies of physical activity are subject to important potential biases including self-selection and unmeasured confounding variables. The risk of MI and sudden cardiac death is greatest during exercise, leading some to question the benefits of exercise. The overall risk of MI and sudden cardiac death, however, is reduced among those who exercise regularly.[69] The greatest reduction in risk is between sedentary individuals and those who do regular moderate-intensity activity. Smaller gains are achieved by participating in high-intensity as compared with moderate-intensity activity. In addition to decreasing myocardial oxygen demand and increasing myocardial efficiency and electrical stability, other potential mechanisms by which physical activity may reduce CHD risk include increasing HDL, reducing blood pressure, reducing obesity, improving insulin sensitivity, decreasing platelet aggregation, and increasing fibrinolysis.[68]

PRIMARY PREVENTION

A randomized, controlled trial of physical activity for primary prevention of CHD is not likely to be conducted because of cost and compliance.

SECONDARY PREVENTION   (See Chap. 55 on cardiac rehabilitation.)

Metaanalyses of randomized trials of cardiac rehabilitation with exercise in over 4000 MI survivors demonstrated a 20 to 25 percent reduction in cardiovascular mortality, although there were no significant differences in nonfatal reinfarction.[70,71] Most of the studies combined exercise training with other risk factor modification. The small number of trials with exercise as the only intervention does not permit definitive conclusions. The benefit of physical activity in female CHD patients is also unknown.

COST-EFFECTIVENESS

The cost-effectiveness of physical activity for primary prevention is not established. Given the low monetary cost of physical activity and its numerous favorable effects on other risk factors, exercise for primary prevention may prove to be highly cost-effective. The cost-effectiveness of cardiac rehabilitation has been estimated (in 1993 dollars) at less than $8000 per quality-adjusted year of life gained.[2]

PRACTICE RECOMMENDATIONS

The American College of Sports Medicine and the Centers for Disease Control and Prevention recommend that every adult should accumulate 30 min or more of moderate-intensity physical activity on most, preferably all, days.[72] Only about 20 percent of U.S. adults meet this goal. The American Heart Association recommends a minimal goal of 30 min of moderate-intensity activity three to four times a week for patients with CHD.[73] Large-scale studies indicate that high-intensity physical activity is *not* required to achieve a mortality benefit, and that 200 kcal expended daily in moderate-intensity physical activity will confer the majority of CHD risk reduction that exercise can provide. To accomplish this requires about 30 min of brisk walking; however, intermittent activity also provides substantial benefit.[72] Therefore, the minimal goal of 30 min can be accumulated in short bouts of typical daily activities like walking, walking up stairs, housework, and gardening. Apparently healthy men over 40 and women over 50 who are sedentary should undergo treadmill testing before starting a vigorous physical activity program (intensity > 60 percent of individual maximum oxygen consumption).[74] For secondary prevention, exercise testing is recommended to guide exercise prescription, and high-risk patients should exercise in a medically supervised setting.[73] Structured exercise programs, whether on-site or at home, help compliance with an exercise prescription[75] (see also Chap. 15).

Obesity

Approximately one-third of the U.S. adult population is obese, and the prevalence is increasing.[76] Obesity promotes insulin resistance, hyperinsulinemia, hypertension, hypertriglyceridemia, low HDL cholesterol, and LVH.[77,78] Many observational studies have found that *obesity strongly and positively correlates with the risk of CHD in univariate analysis.* In multivariate analysis, when controlling statistically for risk factors such as hypertension, diabetes, and dyslipidemia, obesity is usually not found to be an independent risk factor. This should not be construed to mean that obesity is not an important risk factor. Rather, it reflects that much of the adverse consequences of obesity are mediated through resultant metabolic risk factors acting as pathogenetic links in the causal pathway. Nevertheless, some large prospective observational studies of long duration indicate that obesity is an independent risk factor for coronary and cardiovascular mortality in men and women.[79–81] In general, the greater the degree of overweight, the higher the risk of coronary mortality. The central distribution of body fat (typical male pattern abdominal obesity) predicts CHD in men independently of body-mass index and other major risk factors.[82] Weight loss improves insulin sensitivity and glucose disposal; reduces blood pressure, triglycerides, and LVH; and increases HDL cholesterol.[77,78]

PRIMARY AND SECONDARY PREVENTION

Although weight loss leads to a number of favorable short-term changes in metabolism, it is unknown if long-term weight loss results in reduced CHD events. No primary or secondary prevention trials of weight loss have been conducted.

COST-EFFECTIVENESS

The cost-effectiveness of weight loss is unknown. Given the favorable effect of weight loss on other risk factors, it may prove to be highly cost-effective.

PRACTICE RECOMMENDATIONS

Weight reduction to ideal body weight should be recommended to persons whose weight is ≥120 percent of ideal and for patients with lesser degrees of overweight but who have non-insulin-dependent diabetes mellitus, elevated triglycerides, low HDL levels, or hypertension.[73] Attainment of ideal body weight and its maintenance can be accomplished by control of caloric intake and by increased physical activity. Nevertheless, successful long-term weight loss is extremely difficult to achieve. Since obesity increases with age, prevention of initial weight gain in young people is the ideal goal. Smoking cessation is associated with weight gain, on average 4.4 kg for men and 5.0 kg for women.[83] The health hazards of smoking exceed the risks of moderate obesity; therefore, cigarette smokers should be given the clear message that smoking cessation is of the highest priority even if it results in weight gain. Weight reduction with pharmacologic agents is not recommended; the role of newer agents such as fenfluramine in CHD prevention is undefined.

Postmenopausal Status

CHD is relatively uncommon in premenopausal women. There is a dramatic rise in CHD incidence in women after age 55, coinciding with increasing age and a decline in endogenous estrogen levels. Early menopause (natural or surgical) is associated with increased CHD risk.[84] These observations are consistent with the notion that estrogen deficiency permits or promotes CHD and that estrogen reduces risk. Numerous observational studies show that postmenopausal users of estrogen replacement therapy (ERT) have a 50 percent lower risk of initial CHD events compared with nonusers.[84] Because of their observational design, these studies have been subject to selection bias and uncontrolled or unknown confounding variables. In most of these studies, ERT has been unopposed by concomitant progestin therapy. Estrogen may reduce CHD by raising HDL, lowering LDL, lowering small, dense LDL, inhibiting LDL oxidation, lowering Lp(a), lowering fibrinogen levels, and enhancing endothelium-dependent and independent coronary vasodilation. In women with CHD, sublingual estrogen increases time to ST depression on treadmill testing,[85] and intracoronary estrogen corrects endothelium-dependent vasodilation.[86]

Unopposed ERT increases the risk of endometrial carcinoma, but the addition of a progestin erases that risk.[84] Estrogen with or without progestin may increase the risk of breast cancer slightly, particularly among older women who have taken hormones for 5 or more years.[84,87] For women aged 65 to 74 years, the absolute risk of dying from CHD over the next 10 years is 15 times that of dying from endometrial cancer and 6 times that of dying from breast cancer.[88] The Postmenopausal Estrogen/Progestin Interventions Trial assessed differences between placebo, unopposed estrogen, and three estrogen/progestin combinations over 3 years on selected CHD risk factors in healthy postmenopausal women.[89] Compared with placebo, estrogen alone or in combination with a progestin raised HDL cholesterol and produced significantly lower fibrinogen levels. The best regimen for raising HDL cholesterol was unopposed estrogen, but in women with an intact uterus this caused a high rate of atypical or adenomatous endometrial hyperplasia.

PRIMARY AND SECONDARY PREVENTION

Two large clinical trials are currently in progress to assess the efficacy of hormone replacement for primary and secondary prevention of CHD. Until the results of these trials become available, clinical decisions must be based on observational and short-term clinical trials.

COST-EFFECTIVENESS

The cost-effectiveness of ERT for prevention of CHD is undefined.

PRACTICE RECOMMENDATIONS

Although evidence from a clinical trial is still lacking, ERT is recommended in postmenopausal women with CHD or at high risk for CHD unless they have a personal history of breast cancer or a metabolic contraindication (e.g., serum triglycerides > 400 mg/dL). If the patient has an intact uterus, combination therapy with a progestin is strongly recommended. Oral (versus transdermal) administration of estrogen is recommended because this results in a greater magnitude of benefit on lipoproteins.[90] ERT appears to decrease the risk of cardiovascular disease among postmenopausal women who smoke,[91] hence we do not view smoking as a contraindication to ERT.

RISK FACTORS FOR WHICH INTERVENTIONS MIGHT LOWER RISK OF CORONARY HEART DISEASE

Psychosocial Factors

The role of personality, environment, social support, social contact, stress and lack of control at work, and depression have all been associated with increased risk for CHD. See Chap. 89 for a discussion of these topics.

Acute emotional reactions have been implicated as triggers of acute coronary syndromes. In the absence of atherosclerosis, mental stress causes vasodilation or no change in the diameter of epicardial coronary arteries. In the presence of atherosclerosis, mental stress induces silent myocardial ischemia[92] and coronary vasoconstriction.[93] An episode of anger is capable of triggering acute MI.[94] There was a fivefold increase in the number of sudden cardiac deaths related to atherosclerosis on the day of one of the strongest earthquakes ever recorded in North America.[95] Most of these deaths did not occur in association with heavy physical exertion and were presumably related to major emotional stress. In most cases, the length of time between the earthquake and sudden death was less than 1 h. Potential mechanisms by which acute emotional stress could trigger coronary events are release of catecholamines, leading to an increase in heart rate, blood pressure, myocardial oxygen demand, vasoconstriction, platelet aggregability, and coagulation with an inhibition of fibrinolysis. These factors could contribute to the rupture of a vulnerable plaque with subsequent thrombosis or to the precipitation of ventricular arrhythmias.

PRACTICE RECOMMENDATIONS
Optimal comprehensive secondary prevention should include attempts to identify and treat depression and anxiety in patients with CHD. Group support and stress management can be provided in formal cardiac rehabilitation programs.

Lipoprotein(a)

Lp(a) consists of an LDL particle linked via a disulfide bond to an apo(a) polypeptide chain. Because of homology between apo(a) and plasminogen, Lp(a) has been hypothesized to serve as a competitive inhibitor for plasminogen binding and thus may inhibit endogenous fibrinolysis.[96] Lp(a) is largely genetically determined, and distributions differ between men and women as well as between races.

Several retrospective case-control studies support the view that Lp(a) is an independent risk factor for future thromboembolic disease. However, results of the major prospective studies evaluating baseline Lp(a) concentration and future risks of MI and stroke have been inconsistent.[97–101] One possibility to explain these divergent results may relate to the fact that Lp(a) appears to be a greater marker of risk among patients with hypercholesterolemia.[98,102]

PRIMARY AND SECONDARY PREVENTION
While nicotinic acid and estrogen appear to reduce Lp(a) levels in some patients, no data are available that indicate that reducing plasma levels results in reduced risk.

PRACTICE RECOMMENDATIONS
It is not yet clear whether Lp(a) provides information independent of the baseline lipid profile, and no recommendation for screening can be made. If elevated levels prove clearly to increase risk among hypercholesterolemic individuals, however, it may be prudent to lower LDL-cholesterol levels even more aggressively in such individuals than current guidelines dictate. Knowledge of Lp(a) levels may also be useful in the selection of LDL-lowering drugs (e.g., niacin and estrogen) and may identify a possible treatable cause in the occasional patient with CHD and none of the major risk factors.

Total Plasma Homocysteine Level

Total plasma homocysteine level reflects the sum of homocysteine and homocysteinyl moieties of oxidized disulfides, homocystine, and cysteine-homocysteine. Together, these amino acid derivatives appear to have direct toxic effects on the vascular endothelium and can result in the oxidation of LDL, both important steps in atherogenesis. While there are genetic determinants of total homocysteine level (see Chap. 69), the most important factor affecting plasma concentration is dietary intake of folate and vitamins B_6 and B_{12}.[103]

A series of cross-sectional and case control studies strongly supports an independent association between total plasma homocysteine level and atherosclerotic risk[104] (Fig. 41-2). In addition, prospective studies have found increased risk of MI[105,106] and stroke[107] among patients with moderate hyperhomocysteinemia. When pooled, these data suggest that as much as 10 percent of the population risk of CHD may be attributable to homocysteine level.[104]

PRIMARY AND SECONDARY PREVENTION
While folate and vitamins B_6 and B_{12} reduce homocysteine concentration, no randomized trial data are available that indicate that reducing plasma levels results in reduced risk.

PRACTICE RECOMMENDATIONS
Measurement of homocysteine may be useful in patients with CHD in the absence of major risk factors or with a history of recurrent arterial thromboses. Within the United States, folate fortification is being considered because of clinical trial evidence that this intervention reduces incidence of first trimester neural tube defects. Folic acid, 1 to 2 mg/day, reduces homocysteine levels at low cost and without side effects.

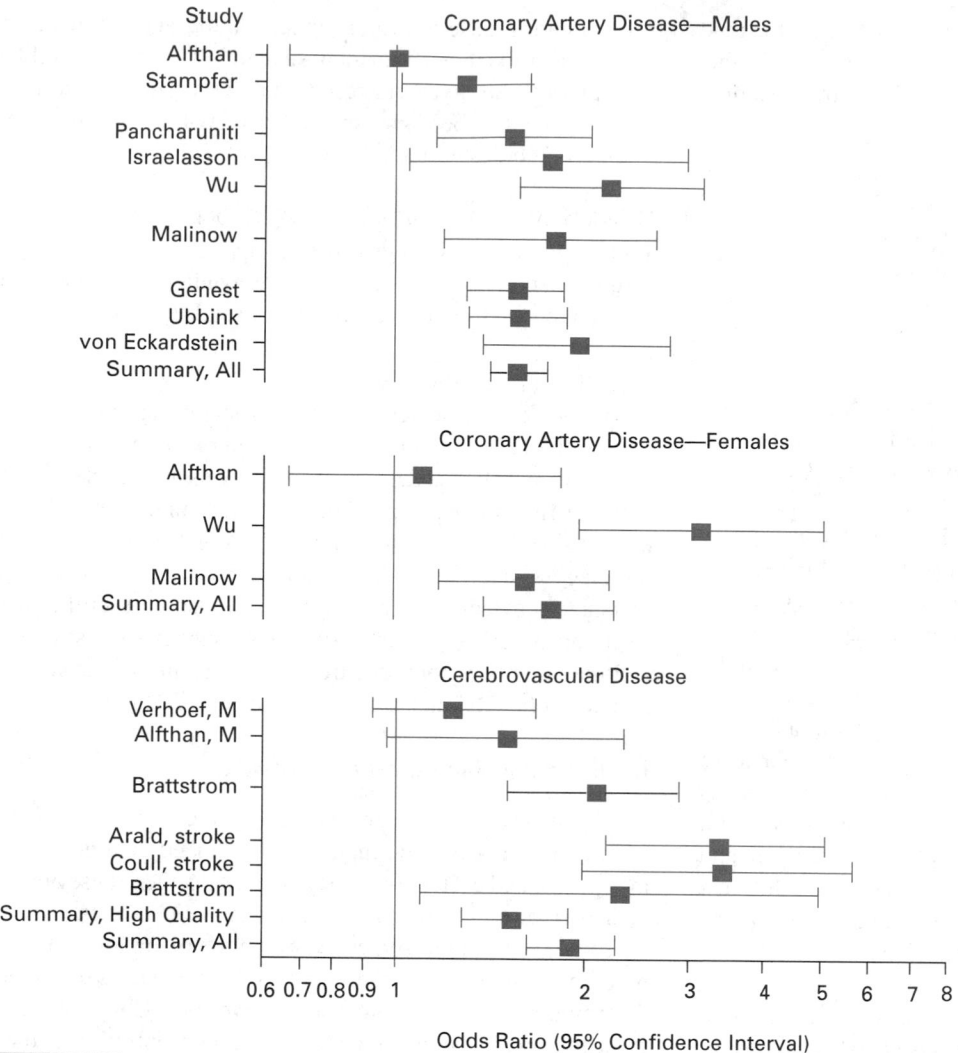

FIGURE 41-2

Quantitative analysis of studies of total homocysteine and vascular disease presented as odds ratios with 95% confidence intervals on a log scale based on a 5-μmol/L increase in total homocysteine. An odds ratio greater than 1.0 indicates that elevated total homocysteine levels increase the risk for vascular disease. For each study, the odds ratio estimate was calculated from the mean levels of total homocysteine in cases and controls by the linear discriminant function method. Unless indicated, odds ratios are for both males (M) and females. The "Summary, All" included all studies in each figure, and the "Summary, High Quality" included only those studies classified as high quality. (From Boushey et al.,[104] *JAMA* 1995; 274:1049–1057. Copyright 1995, American Medical Association.)

Oxidative Stress

Oxidative modification of LDL has been hypothesized to play a major role in the initiation and progression of atherosclerosis.[25] Because naturally occurring antioxidants such as vitamins E, C, and beta-carotene may slow this process, there has been substantial interest in these compounds as agents for both primary and secondary prevention. A series of observational epidemiologic studies supports the hypothesis that increased dietary intake of antioxidants is associated with reduced cardiovascular risk, with the strongest evidence for vitamin E[108–111] (Fig. 41-3). Unfortunately, it is impossible to conclude from observational studies that a given vitamin supplement is responsible for observed vascular risk reduc-tion, since individuals who take vitamins are also likely to employ other preventive lifestyle and dietary measures. This issue can only be resolved through large-scale, randomized clinical trials.

PRIMARY PREVENTION

In the Alpha-Tocopherol, Beta-Carotene Cancer Prevention Study, which enrolled 29,133 male smokers,[112] there was no evidence that vitamin E (given as 50 mg of alpha-tocopherol daily) reduced the subsequent risk of CHD or stroke, and a small increase in rates of cerebral hemorrhage was reported. In the same trial, beta-carotene was associated with a small increase in lung cancer and deaths due to CHD. In the Carotene and Retinol Efficacy Trial conducted among 18,314 smokers, former smokers, and asbestos-exposed workers,[113] the combined use of 30 mg/day of beta-carotene plus 25,000 IU of retinol was associated with a small but statistically significant increase in lung cancer and all-cause mortality as well as a non-significant increase in cardiovascular mortality. In contrast, among 22,071 men participating in the Physicians' Health Study who were randomly allocated to 50 mg of beta-carotene on alternate days for a period of 12 years, supplementation resulted in no evidence of benefit or harm in terms of the incidence of cardiovascular disease or cancer.[114]

SECONDARY PREVENTION

In the Cambridge Heart Antioxidant Study,[115] higher doses of vitamin E were found to reduce rates of nonfatal MI substantially among a group of patients with known CHD. Specifically, in this high-risk secondary prevention trial, the use of 400 to 800 IU of alpha-tocopherol daily over an average period of only 17 months was associated with a statistically significant 47 percent risk reduction in cardiovascular death and nonfatal infarction.

PRACTICE RECOMMENDATIONS

Based upon these randomized trial data, it is impossible to make recommendations for or against supplementation with vitamins E or C to prevent CHD, although beta-carotene appears to carry no benefit. However, given observational evidence suggesting benefit for diets high in fruits and vegetables, it is prudent to continue such diets, since vitamins E and C are only two of the several hundred micronutrients that may have chemopreventive properties.

No Alcohol Consumption

Heavy alcohol intake is associated with increased risks of death from several causes and is a major public health concern. However, cross-sectional, case-control, and prospective cohort studies indicate that mild to moderate alcohol consumption is associated with reduced rates of CHD compared with abstainers.[116–118] These studies suggest a J-shaped relationship between level of alcohol consumption and total mortality such that a protective effect is apparent at low levels of consumption (one to two beverages daily), while there is substantial hazard among heavy consumers.[119] In large part, this dose-dependent balance reflects summation of three effects: (1) a positive association between alcohol use and cancer; (2) a U-shaped relationship between alcohol use and total cardiovascular disease due to increased risks of cardiomyopathy, sudden death, and hemorrhagic stroke among heavy drinkers; and (3) a well-established L-shaped protective effect for coronary disease.[119,120]

Several mechanisms are important in the cardioprotective effect of moderate alcohol use. Alcohol intake increases total HDL-cholesterol levels as well as HDL2 and HDL3 cholesterol.[121–124] Alcohol consumption also has potentially beneficial effects on fibrinolytic function[125,126] and on platelet aggregation.[127,128]

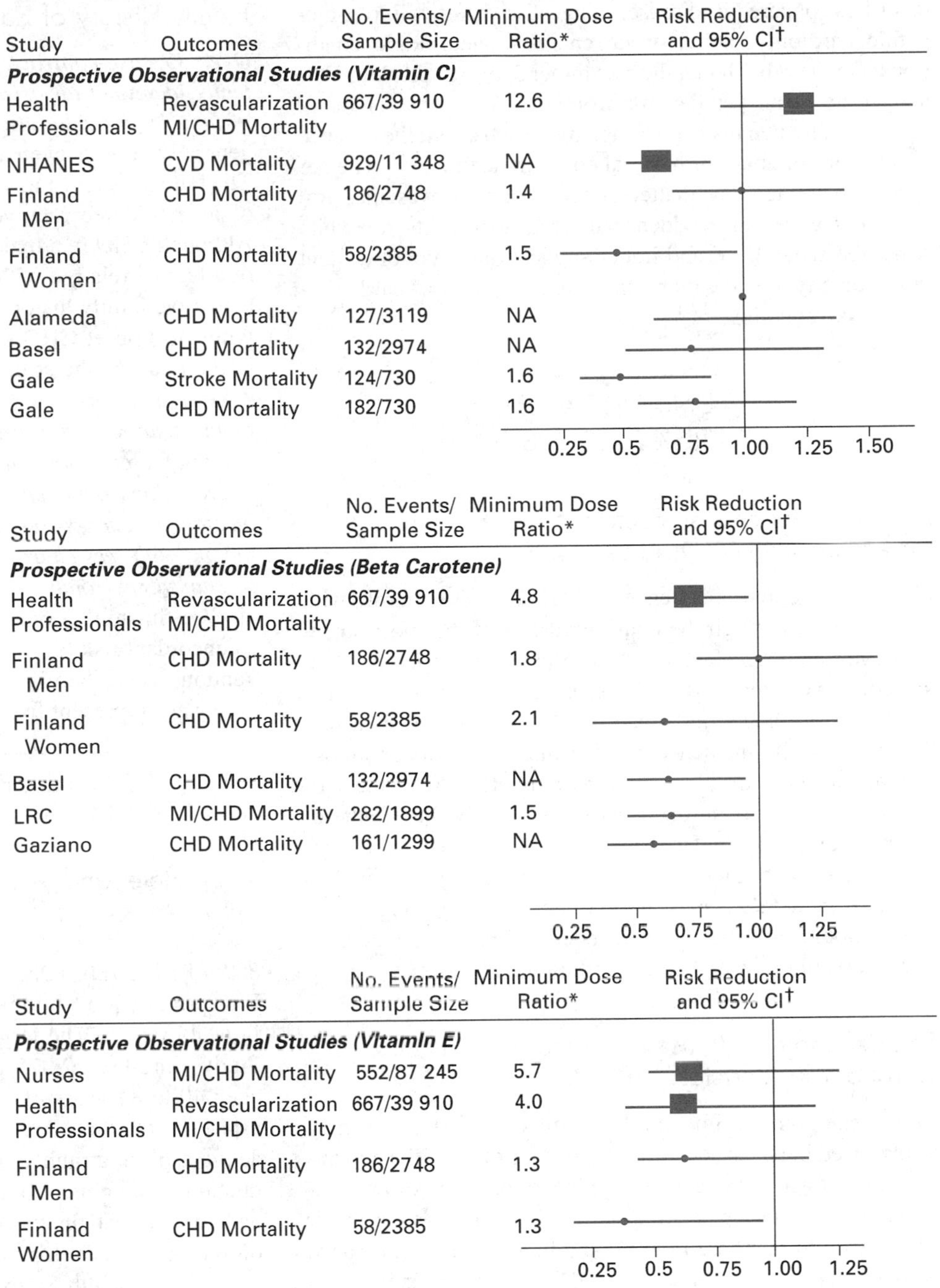

PRIMARY AND SECONDARY PREVENTION

There have been no randomized trials of alcohol use for primary or secondary prevention.

FIGURE 41-3

Prospective observational studies of effects of vitamin C (*top panel*), beta carotene (*middle panel*), and vitamin E (*bottom panel*) on cardiovascular endpoints. The horizontal bars represent 95% confidence intervals. The size of the square showing the reduction is approximately proportional to the square root of the overall sample size multiplied by the number of events. MI, myocardial infarction; NHANES, National Health and Nutrition Examination Survey; LRC, Lipid Research Clinic. *The minimum dose ratio refers to the minimum relative differences in intake levels or antioxidant vitamin doses between comparison groups. †Risk reduction is the relative reduction in the odds ratio, standardized mortality ratio, or relative risk. (From Jha et al.,[111] with permission from the publisher and authors.)

PRACTICE RECOMMENDATIONS

How best to advise patients concerning the potential use of alcohol for cardiovascular protection is a complex process, because of this agent's potential for abuse.[129] Abstinence is advised for patients who are pregnant or who have hepatic disorders, pancreatic disease, congestive heart failure, idiopathic cardiomyopathy, or degenerative neurologic conditions. On the other hand, the recommendation to drink moderately (one drink per day for women, two drinks for men), may be safe when made on a case-by-case basis in the absence of a history of abuse or medical contraindication.[129] Whether specific beverage type matters in terms of cardiovascular protection is uncertain. Evidence indicating benefits for white wine, red wine, beer, and liquor suggest that alcohol content rather than type is the more important predictor of cardiovascular risk reduction.[117,118]

UNMODIFIABLE RISK FACTORS

Age and Sex as Risk Factors for Atherosclerotic Disease

The incidence and prevalence of CHD increase sharply with age, so that age might be considered one of the most potent cardiovascular risk factors. Atherosclerotic involvement of the coronary arteries is well established in men by young adulthood, as shown in Korean war and Vietnam war casualties.[130,131] CHD incidence rates in men are similar to those in women 10 years older.[132] Approximately 52 percent of women and 46 percent of men will eventually die of atherosclerotic diseases.[133] The increased risk of men and older persons should trigger more intense management of modifiable risk factors. Persons at very advanced age (e.g., 75+ years) should have the risks and benefits of preventive cardiology interventions weighed on an individual basis.

Socioeconomic Status: An Unmodifiable Coronary Risk Factor?

At any one point in time, markedly different CHD rates may be observed between socioeconomic subgroups of the population, as defined by occupation, education, income, or other measures. As a group becomes affluent, its members use their new wealth to purchase high-fat and high-salt foods, tobacco products, and automobiles. Less affluent groups lag behind this development, achieving access to these deleterious behaviors later. Affluent groups then learn about and adopt healthful lifestyles, reducing deleterious behaviors. Again, less affluent and less educated groups lag behind, eventually exceeding the rates of CHD in those educated groups whose CHD rates have begun to fall.

Currently, persons with low socioeconomic status are at high risk for CHD. A number of mechanisms may explain this.[134] First, risk factors for atherosclerosis, such as smoking, hypertension, obesity, and sedentary lifestyle, are higher in persons with low socioeconomic status. Second, some of these risk factors, as well as psychosocial responses to stressors, may increase exposure to CHD triggers in these groups. Finally, these groups may have less access to care.

Family History of Early-Onset CHD

Over 35 case-control and prospective studies have consistently identified an association between CHD and a history of first-degree relatives with early onset CHD.[135] This risk generally persists even after adjustment for other risk factors. The family history most predictive of coronary disease is that of a first-degree relative developing CHD at an early age. Although CHD in a male relative with onset at age 55 or less or a female relative with onset at age 65 or less is defined as a positive family history,[46] the larger the number of relatives with early-onset CHD or the younger the age of CHD onset in the relative, the stronger the predictive value.[136,137]

Although considered a nonmodifiable risk factor, a positive family history should result in the careful screening of individual risk factors known to aggregate in families. Such familial aggregations may represent monogenic factors with known phenotypic expressions and inheritance patterns, polygenic factors with less clear modes of expression and inheritance, or shared environments. In early CHD families, Williams et al.[137] *estimate that only 10 percent of families will not have a concordant risk factor, most of which are amenable to intervention. Thus, family members of patients with CHD at a young age represent fruitful targets for risk factor assessment.*

OTHER PHARMACOLOGIC THERAPY

Antiplatelet and Anticoagulant Therapy (See also Chap. 52.)

PRIMARY PREVENTION

Two primary prevention trials of aspirin have been completed in healthy men. The largest of these, the Physicians' Health Study, enrolled 22,071 apparently healthy male physicians aged 40 to 84 years of age and randomized them to 325 mg aspirin on alternate days or to placebo.[138] Among those given active aspirin, a highly statistically significant 44 percent reduction in nonfatal MI was observed. In this study, aspirin had little effect on the clinical characteristics of MI[139] or on the rate of development of angina pectoris.[140] When the Physicians' Health Study data are combined with those of a similar trial among British men,[141] an overall 32 percent reduction in risk of first nonfatal MI appears to be associated with chronic aspirin prophylaxis.[142] These trials have also demonstrated the efficacy of low-dose aspirin in the prevention of MI among patients with stable angina pectoris.[143] At this time, no data on primary prevention with warfarin are available, although a large-scale trial evaluating low-dose warfarin and aspirin among high-risk individuals is nearing completion.[144]

SECONDARY PREVENTION

At least 25 trials have been completed in the study of antiplatelet therapy for secondary prevention.[145] Overall, among patients with known clinical manifestations of atherosclerotic disease, antiplatelet therapy is associated with a 32 percent reduction in subsequent MI, 27 percent reduction in subsequent nonfatal stroke, and 15 percent reduction in vascular mortality.[146]

Few studies of anticoagulant therapy in the secondary prevention of coronary disease are available. In the Dutch Sixty Plus Study,[147] patients over 60 years of age who had been taking anticoagulants following infarction were randomly assigned to continue or discontinue warfarin. Patients continuing anticoagulant therapy had a 26 percent lower mortality rate and a 51 percent lower reinfarction rate.

The utility of warfarin initiated soon after infarction has also been demonstrated.[148] In a trial of 1214 patients with acute or subacute MI, the randomized use of warfarin with a target INR between 2.8 and 4.8 was associated with a 24 percent reduction in mortality, a 34 percent reduction in nonfatal reinfarction, and a 55 percent reduction in stroke over a mean period of 37 months. These reductions were achieved with acceptably low bleeding rates for those assigned to warfarin.

COST-EFFECTIVENESS

For primary prevention, aspirin is likely to be extremely cost-effective because of its low cost and high efficacy for preventing MI. Following MI, both aspirin and anticoagulant therapy have been shown to be cost saving.[149]

PRACTICE RECOMMENDATIONS

The United States Preventive Services Task Force has recommended that low-dose aspirin be considered in men age 40 and over who are at high risk for MI and lack contraindications.[150] While observational data generally support the use of aspirin in women,[151] the risk-to-benefit ratio in women may differ from that of men since the average age at first infarction is higher. For secondary prevention, 80 to 325 mg of aspirin daily is recommended, with treatment continued indefinitely. If aspirin is contraindicated, warfarin is recommended for secondary prevention, with an INR goal of 2 to 3.5.[73]

FIBRINOGEN

Plasma fibrinogen level has been shown in several studies to predict the future risk of MI and stroke.[152-155] When pooled, these studies indicate that individuals with fibrinogen concentrations in the upper third of the control distribution have a relative risk of future cardiovascular disease 2.0 to 2.5 times that of individuals with lower levels[156] (Fig. 41-4). High fibrinogen levels result in increased whole blood viscosity and may play a direct role in atherogenesis and platelet aggregation. While fibrinogen levels increase with

smoking, age, oral contraceptive use, and diabetes, fibrinogen is poorly correlated with the lipid profile and therefore may provide additional risk information beyond lipid and lipoprotein measurement.

ENDOGENOUS FIBRINOLYSIS: TISSUE PLASMINOGEN ACTIVATOR, PAI-1, AND D-DIMER

The activity of the endogenous fibrinolytic system reflects a balance between plasma concentration of tissue-type plasminogen activator (tPA) and its primary inhibitor, PAI-1. Prospective studies of initially healthy individuals[157] as well as patients with known CHD[155,158] indicate that elevated antigen levels of both enzymes are associated with increased risk of future MI. Further, prospective data also indicate that tPA antigen level is a potent marker of risk for stroke.[159]

Because both tPA and PAI-1 contribute to the net fibrinolytic balance, it has been hypothesized that individuals at risk for future vascular occlusive events suffer from a net inhibition of fibrinolytic function, a finding supported in at least one prospective study.[160] Other data, however, indicate that elevations of D-dimer are also associated with increased risk of future MI[161] and peripheral vascular disease.[162] Since plasma D-dimer levels increase with fibrinogen turnover, these data raise the possibility that the endogenous fibrinolytic system is activated among individuals at risk.

Evidence is not available to support fibrinogen reduction as a measure to prevent CHD, although smoking cessation, physical activity, and hormone replacement therapy[89,163] all favorably affect fibrinogen levels. Other fibrinogen-reducing agents such

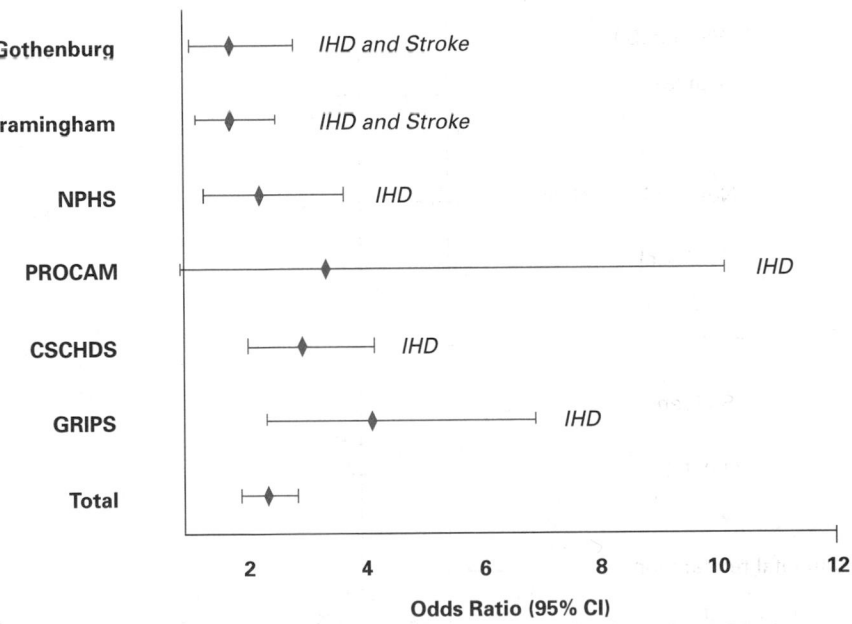

FIGURE 41-4

Odds ratios for cardiovascular events in persons with fibrinogen levels in the upper tertile compared to the lower tertile. Odds ratios and 95% confidence intervals in prospective epidemiologic studies. IHD, ischemic heart disease; CSCHDS, The Caerphilly and Speedwell Collaborative Heart Disease Studies; GRIPS, The Göttingen Risk, Incidence, and Prevalence Study; NPHS, Northwick Park Heart Study; PROCAM, Prospective Cardiovascular Münster Study. (From Ernst and Resch,[156] with permission from the publisher and authors.)

as bezafibrate are also under investigation in ongoing clinical trials.[164] Many factors affect endogenous fibrinolytic activity including obesity, estrogen status, and exercise. In addition, pharmacologic interventions may soon be available that can favorably shift fibrinolytic function in an attempt to reduce vascular risk. To date, aspirin therapy, alcohol use, and ACE inhibitors have all shown promise in this regard.

Beta-Adrenergic Blocking Agents

Beta-adrenergic blocking agents reduce heart rate, systemic blood pressure, and ventricular contractility, all factors that decrease myocardial oxygen consumption (see Chap. 54). Beta blockers further have antiarrhythmic properties and appear to increase thresholds for ventricular fibrillation.[165]

PRIMARY PREVENTION

Little clinical trial data are available that directly test beta-blocking agents in the primary prevention of MI. The use of this class of agents in the treatment of hypertension, however, has been shown to be efficacious for CHD prevention,[166] and in general the beta blockers have few long-term side effects.

SECONDARY PREVENTION

The utility of beta-blocking agents in the acute, subacute, and chronic phases following MI has been demonstrated in many clinical trials (Fig. 41-5). Overview analyses indicate that therapy with beta blockers reduces mortality approximately 20 percent compared to placebo.[167,168] The mortality effect of long-term beta blockade results primarily from prevention of sudden death (pooled relative risk = 0.68), presumably due to a reduction in the incidence and complexity of ventricular arrhythmias. Beta blockers have also proven effective in reducing rates of nonfatal reinfarction (pooled relative risk = 0.74), an effect more likely to result from chronic reductions in heart rate, contractility, and vascular stress.

COST-EFFECTIVENESS

Estimates of the cost of beta blockers after MI range from $3600 per year of life saved when used in high-risk patients to $23,400 per year of life saved when used in low-risk patients.[169] This is cost-effective as compared with other accepted CHD interventions.

PRACTICE RECOMMENDATIONS

For primary prevention, beta blockers are recommended as first-line therapy for hypertension.[49] For secondary prevention, beta blockers are recommended in post-MI patients with arrhythmias, left ventricular dysfunction, and inducible ischemia.[73] Although specific studies of beta-blocker cessation are not available, it is commonly recommended that beta-blocker therapy be continued indefinitely as long as side effects are not present.[165]

Angiotensin-Converting Enzyme Inhibitors

PRIMARY PREVENTION

Although ACE inhibitors are used widely as first-line therapy for hypertension, no data on primary prevention with this class of drugs are available. A large-scale trial is in progress.[51]

SECONDARY PREVENTION

ACE inhibitors reduce mortality in patients with congestive heart failure and reduced left ventricular ejection fraction.[170–172] More recently, this class of agents has been recognized as important adjunctive therapy following acute MI.[173] The primary rationale for using these agents in this setting is based upon the experimental observation that ACE inhibition slows the process of ventricular remodeling.[174,175] This effect appears time-dependent in that the use of ACE inhibition after

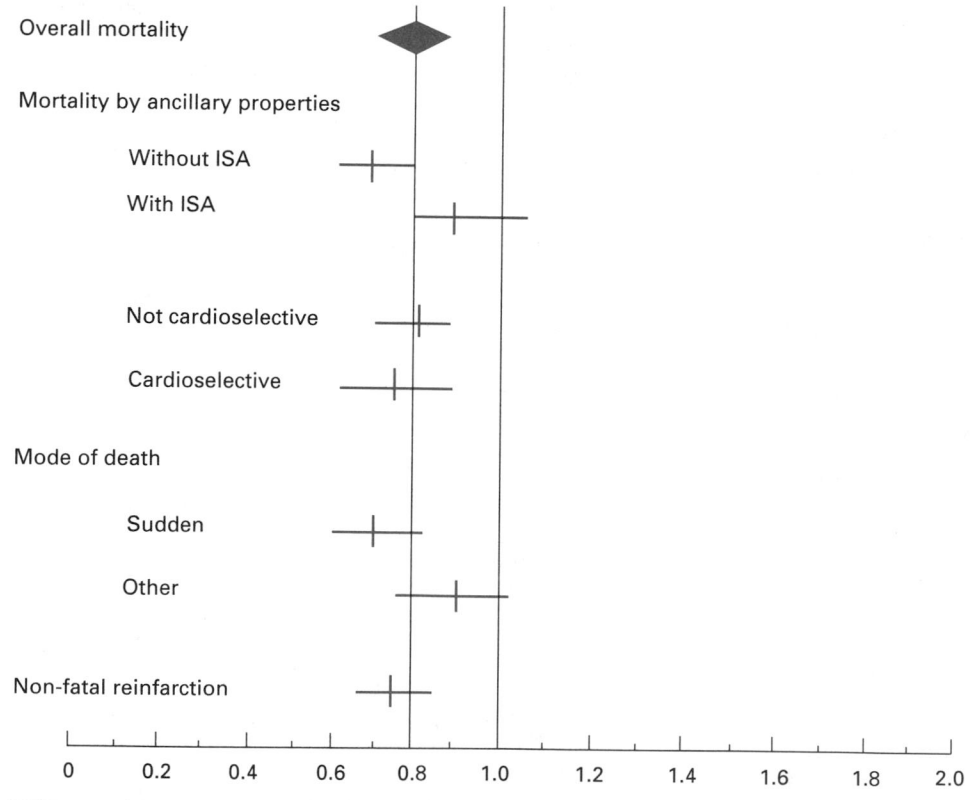

FIGURE 41-5

Meta-analysis of effects of long-term beta-blocker therapy in survivors of myocardial infarction according to total mortality, mortality by ancillary properties of agent tested, mode of death, and nonfatal reinfarction. ISA, intrinsic sympathomimetic activity. Data presented as odds ratios (active:control) with horizontal bars representing approximate 95% confidence intervals. (From Yusuf et al.,[167] with permission from the publisher and authors.)

MI requires a sufficient length of therapy to result in detectable changes in ventricular volumes and size. The observation in several trials that rates of recurrent MI may also be reduced with ACE inhibition[173,176,177] raises the possibility that these agents also result in enhanced endogenous fibrinolysis.[178]

COST-EFFECTIVENESS

The cost-effectiveness of ACE inhibitor therapy after MI in patients with left ventricular ejection fraction ≤ 0.40 compares favorably with other commonly accepted therapies for patients with CHD. Depending on the age of the patient and the assumptions used, estimates for the cost-effectiveness of captopril range from $3600 to $60,800 per quality-adjusted life-year.[179]

PRACTICE RECOMMENDATIONS

No data are available to recommend ACE inhibitors for primary prevention. For secondary prevention, ACE inhibitors should be considered among patients with congestive heart failure, reduced left ventricular function, and prior MI. Whether ACE inhibitors should be used in broader populations of patients at risk is under investigation.

THE PRACTICE OF PREVENTIVE CARDIOLOGY

Despite overwhelming evidence regarding the efficacy of risk factor intervention and the presence of clear guidelines for secondary prevention[73] (see Table 41-3), the levels of risk factor management in patients with established CHD are disappointingly low. Among MI survivors, only 40 percent receive beta blockers, 60 percent of patients with reduced left ventricular ejection fraction take ACE inhibitors, and 70 percent take aspirin.[180] Following MI, only 20 percent of smokers receive smoking cessation counseling,[180] and only 20 to 30 percent of patients receive cholesterol-lowering diet or drug regimens.[181] Fewer than 40 percent of CHD patients participate in formal cardiac rehabilitation programs.[182]

Barriers to Implementation of Preventive Cardiology Services

A number of barriers to the implementation of preventive services have been identified.[183,184] These barriers occur at the level of the patient, the physician, the health care setting, and the community and society[185–187] (see Table 41-4).

Strategies to Improve Preventive Cardiology Services

IMPROVING PATIENT COMPLIANCE

Understanding of the process of behavior change provides an important basis for designing behavioral interventions. The "readiness for change" model proposed by Prochaska and DiClemente[188] proposes that patients do not make decisions to change their behavior radically; rather, they go through a series of smaller decisions, leading up to the actual behavior change. The following approach is suggested to improve adherence[187]: (1) secure the patient's understanding and acceptance of treatment; (2) establish specific behavioral goals to be achieved and a schedule to achieve them; (3) write out specific treatment recommendations; (4) anticipate and address common concerns and misconceptions; (5) tailor treatment to the patient's daily circumstances, and elicit family or peer understanding and support, if possible; (6) teach the patient self-monitoring skills to provide performance feedback; (7) review performance and reinforce positive behavior during subsequent visits; and (8) refer selected patients to special programs.

IMPROVING PHYSICIAN PERFORMANCE

Cardiovascular specialists should receive training in risk factor assessment and management. American Heart Association/American College of Cardiology guidelines provide unambiguous goals for the physician[73] (Table 41-3). However, guidelines alone, without incentives or other means to facilitate them, are by no means an assurance of implementation.[189]

Organization of Preventive Cardiology Services

Hospitals, health care organizations, and practices have a number of organizational resources available to implement improvements in preventive cardiology services. Central laboratories can be used to identify and prompt the care of patients, such as those with hypercholesterolemia. Computer-based reminder systems have led to increased attention to preventive interventions.[190] Nurse case-management has enjoyed increasing popularity in the treatment of hypertension, diabetes, smoking, and hypercholesterolemia. A recent randomized trial demonstrated significant reductions in smoking and LDL cholesterol in MI survivors referred to a nurse case-manager.[191] Another study, the Stanford Coronary Risk Intervention Project, used a nurse case-manager and multiple risk factor intervention and demonstrated significant reductions in the rate of progression of coronary atherosclerosis and clinical cardiac events.[192] Such a program improves patient adherence and compliance, patient self-monitoring of progress, and the early identification of treatment failure and/or increasing CHD symptoms. The development of preventive cardiology specialty clinics offers a centralization of physician specialists and nonphysician experts in nursing, nutrition, exercise physiology, smoking cessation, and psychology. Finally, hospitals and health systems can implement quality assurance programs, using risk factor management services as a quality-of-care indicator. These performance reports can provide feedback to the physician, practice, or health system to guide further improvement.[193] The organization of preventive cardiology services should facilitate both improved efficiency and the allocation of resources and reimbursements needed to allow widespread implementation of preventive cardiology practice.

TABLE 41-3

GUIDE TO COMPREHENSIVE RISK REDUCTION FOR PATIENTS WITH CORONARY AND OTHER VASCULAR DISEASE

Risk Intervention	Recommendations

Smoking
  Goal: complete
  cessation
	Strongly encourage patient and family to stop smoking.
	Provide counseling, nicotine replacement, and formal cessation programs as appropriate.

Lipid management
  Primary goal:
  LDL < 100 mg/dL
  Secondary goals:
  HDL > 35 mg/dL;
  TG < 200 mg/dL
	Start AHA Step II Diet in all patients: ≤30% fat, <7% saturated fat, <200 mg/day cholesterol.
	Assess fasting lipid profile. In post-MI patients, lipid profile may take 4 to 6 weeks to stabilize. Add drug therapy according to the following guide:

LDL < 100 mg/dL	LDL 100 to 130 mg/dL	LDL > 130 mg/dL	HDL < 35 mg/dL
No drug therapy	Consider adding drug therapy to diet:	Add drug therapy to diet:	Emphasize weight management and physical activity. Advise smoking cessation.

TG < 200 mg/dL	TG 200 to 400 mg/dL	TG > 400 mg/dL	
Statin Resin Niacin	Statin Niacin	Consider combined drug therapy (niacin, fibrate, statin)	If needed to achieve LDL goals, consider niacin, statin, fibrate.

If LDL goal not achieved, consider combination therapy.

Risk Intervention	Recommendations

Physical activity
  Minimum goal: 30 min
  3 to 4 times per week
	Assess risk, preferably with exercise test, to guide prescription.
	Encourage minimum of 30 to 60 min of moderate-intensity activity 3 or 4 times weekly (walking, jogging, cycling, or other aerobic activity) supplemented by an increase in daily lifestyle activities (e.g., walking breaks at work, using stairs, gardening, household work). Maximum benefit 5 to 6 h a week.
	Advise medically supervised programs for moderate- to high-risk patients.

Weight management	Start intensive diet and appropriate physical activity intervention, as outlined above, in patients >120% of ideal weight for height. Particularly emphasize need for weight loss in patients with hypertension, elevated triglycerides, or elevated glucose levels.
Antiplatelet agents/ anticoagulants	Start aspirin 80 to 325 mg/day if not contraindicated. Manage warfarin to international normalized ratio = 2 to 3.5 for post-MI patients not able to take aspirin.
ACE inhibitors post-MI	Start early post-MI in stable high-risk patients [anterior MI, previous MI, Killip class II (S_3 gallop, rales, radiographic CHF)]. Continue indefinitely for all with LV dysfunction (ejection fraction ≤ 40%) or symptoms of failure. Use as needed to manage blood pressure or symptoms in all other patients.
Beta blockers	Start in high-risk post-MI patients (arrhythmia, LV dysfunction, inducible ischemia) at 5 to 28 days. Continue 6 months minimum. Observe usual contraindications. Use as needed to manage angina rhythm or blood pressure in all other patients.
Estrogens	Consider estrogen replacement in all postmenopausal women. Individualize recommendation consistent with other health risks.
Blood pressure control Goal: ≤140/90 mmHg	Initiate lifestyle modification—weight control, physical activity, alcohol moderation, and moderate sodium restriction—in all patients with blood pressure >140 mmHg systolic or 90 mmHg diastolic. Add blood pressure medication, individualized to other patient requirements and characteristics (i.e., age, race, need for drugs with specific benefits) if blood pressure is not less than 140 mmHg systolic or 90 mmHg diastolic in 3 months or if *initial* blood pressure is >160 mmHg systolic or 100 mmHg diastolic.

Note: ACE, angiotensin-converting enzyme; CHF, congestive heart failure; HDL, high-density lipoprotein; LDL, low-density lipoprotein; LV, left ventricular; MI, myocardial infarction; TG, triglycerides.

Source: From Smith et al.,[73] with permission from the authors and publisher.

TABLE 41-4

BARRIERS TO IMPLEMENTATION OF PREVENTIVE SERVICES

Patient
  Lack of knowledge and motivation
  Lack of access to care
  Cultural factors
  Social factors
Physician
  Problem-based focus
  Feedback on prevention is negative or neutral
  Time constraints
  Lack of incentives, including reimbursement
  Lack of training
    Poor knowledge of benefits
    Perceived ineffectiveness
    Lack of skills
  Lack of specialist-generalist communication
  Lack of perceived legitimacy
Health care settings (hospitals, practices, etc.)
  Acute care priority
  Lack of resources and facilities
  Lack of systems for preventive services
  Time and economic constraints
  Poor communication between specialty and primary care providers
  Lack of policies and standards
Community/society
  Lack of policies and standards
  Lack of reimbursement

Source: From Pearson et al,[185] with permission.

REFERENCES

1. Wilson PWF. Established risk factors and coronary artery disease: The Framingham Study. *Am J Hypertens* 1994; 7:7S–12S.
2. Fuster V, Pearson TA. 27th Bethesda Conference: Matching the intensity of risk factor management with the hazard for coronary heart disease events. *J Am Coll Cardiol* 1996; 27:957–1047.
3. Department of Health and Human Services. *The Health Consequences of Smoking: Cardiovascular Disease: A Report of the Surgeon General.* DHHS publication (PHS) 84-50204. Washington, DC, Office on Smoking and Health, US Government Printing Office, 1983.
4. Castelli WP, Garrison RJ, Dawber TR, McNamara PM, Feinlieb M, Kannel WB. The filter cigarette and coronary heart disease: The Framingham Study. *Lancet* 1981; 2:109–113.
5. Fielding JE, Phenow KJ. Health effects of involuntary smoking. *New Engl J Med* 1988; 319:1452–1460.
6. Glantz SA, Parmley WW. Passive smoking and heart disease. Mechanisms and risks. *JAMA* 1995; 273:1047–1053.
7. Frei B, Forte TM, Ames BN, Cross CE. Gas phase oxidants of cigarette smoke induce lipid peroxidation and changes in lipoprotein properties in human blood plasma. Protective effects of ascorbic acid. *Biochem J* 1991; 277:133–138.
8. Celermajer DS, Sorensen KE, Georgakopoulos D, Bull C, Thomas O, Robinson J, et al. Cigarette smoking is associated with dose-related and potentially reversible improvement of endothelium-dependent dilation in healthy young adults. *Circulation* 1993; 88:2149–2155.
9. Folsom AR, Wu KK, Davis CE, Conlan MG, Sorlie PD, Szklo M. Population correlates of plasma fibrinogen and factor VII, protective cardiovascular risk factors. *Atherosclerosis* 1991; 91:191–205.
10. Rival J, Riddle JM, Stein PD. Effects of chronic smoking on platelet function. *Thromb Res* 1987; 45:75–85.
11. Gordon T, Kannel WB, McGee D, Dawber TR. Death and coronary attacks in men after giving up cigarette smoking. A report from the Framingham Study. *Lancet* 1974; 2:1345–1348.
12. Tsevat J, Weinstein MC, Williams LW, Tosteson AN, Goldman L. Expected gains in life expectancy from various coronary heart disease risk factor modifications. *Circulation* 1991; 83:1194–1201.
13. Wilhelmsson C, Vedin JA, Elmfeldt D, Tibblin G, Wilhelmsen L. Smoking and myocardial infarction. *Lancet* 1975; 1:415–419.
14. Hermanson B, Omenn GS, Kronmal RA, Gersh BJ. Beneficial six-year outcome of smoking cessation in older men and women with coronary heart disease. Results from the CASS registry. *N Engl J Med* 1988; 319:1365–1369.
15. Tsevat J. Impact and cost-effectiveness of smoking interventions. *Am J Med* 1992; 93:43S–47S.
16. Goldman L, Garber AM, Grover SA, Hlatky MA. Cost-effectiveness of assessment and management of risk factors. *J Am Coll Cardiol* 1996; 27:1020–1030.
17. Cummings SR, Rubin SM, Oster G. The cost-effectiveness of counseling smokers to quit. *JAMA* 1989; 261:75–79.
18. Oster G, Huse DM, Delea TE, Colditz GA. Cost-effectiveness of nicotine gum as an adjuvant to physicians' advice against cigarette smoking. *JAMA* 1986; 256:315–318.
19. Krumholz HM, Cohen BJ, Tsevat J, Pasternack RC, Weinstein MC. Cost-effectiveness of a smoking cessation program after myocardial infarction. *J Am Coll Cardiol* 1993; 22:1697–1702.
20. Pearson TA. Smoking cessation: Clinical evaluation and management of the cigarette smoker. In: Kelly WN, ed. *Textbook of Internal Medicine.* Philadelphia: Lippincott; 1992:1870–1874.
21. Stamler J, Wentworth D, Neaton JD. Is relationship between serum cholesterol and risk of premature death from coronary heart disease continuous and graded? *JAMA* 1986; 256:2823–2828.
22. Law MR, Wald NJ, Thompson SG. By how much and how quickly does reduction in serum cholesterol concentration lower risk of ischemic heart disease? *Br Med J* 1994; 308:367–372.
23. Klag MJ, Ford DE, Mead LA, He J, Whelton PK, Liang K-Y, et al. Serum cholesterol in young men and subsequent cardiovascular disease. *N Engl J Med* 1993; 328:313–318.
24. Pekkanen J, Linn S, Heiss G, Suchindran CM, Leon A, Rifkind BM, et al. Ten-year mortality from cardiovascular disease in relation to cholesterol level among men with and without preexisting cardiovascular disease. *N Engl J Med* 1990; 322:1700–1707.
25. Steinberg D, Parthasarathy S, Carew TE, Khoo JC, Witztum JC. Beyond cholesterol. Modifications of low-density lipoproteins that increase its atherogenicity. *N Engl J Med* 1989; 320:915–924.
26. Flavahan NA. Atherosclerosis or lipid induced endothelial dysfunction. Potential mechanisms underlying reduction in EDRF/nitric oxide activity. *Circulation* 1992; 85:1927–1938.
27. Treasure CB, Klein JL, Weintraub WS, Talley J, Stillabauer ME, Kosinski AS, et al. Beneficial effects of cholesterol-lowering therapy on the coronary endothelium in patients with coronary artery disease. *N Engl J Med* 1995; 332:481–487.
28. Anderson TJ, Meredith IT, Yeung AC, Frei B, Selwyn AP, Ganz P. The effect of cholesterol-lowering and antioxidant therapy on endothelium-dependent coronary vasomotion. *N Engl J Med* 1995; 332:488–493.
29. Falk E, Shah PK, Fuster V. Coronary plaque disruption. *Circulation* 1995; 92:657–671.
30. Gordon DJ, Probstfield JL, Garrison RJ, Neaton JD, Castelli WP, Knoke JD, et al. High-density lipoprotein cholesterol and cardiovascular disease. Four prospective American studies. *Circulation* 1989; 79:8–15.
31. Manolio T, Pearson TA, Wenger NK, Barrett-Connor E, Payne GH, Harlan WR. Cholesterol and heart disease in older persons and women. *Ann Epidemiol* 1992; 2:161–176.
32. Hulley SB, Rosenman RH, Bawol RD, Brand RJ. Epidemiology as a guide to clinical decisions. The association between triglyceride and coronary heart disease. *N Engl J Med* 1980; 302:1383–1389.
33. Castelli WP. The triglyceride issue: A view from Framingham. *Am Heart J* 1986; 112:432–437.
34. Austin MA, Breslow JL, Hennekens CH, Buring JE, Willett WC, Krauss RM. Low-density lipoprotein subclass patterns and risk of myocardial infarction. *JAMA* 260:1917–1921.
35. Zilversmit DB. Atherosclerosis: A postprandial phenomenon. *Circulation* 1979; 60:473–485.
36. Folsom AR, Wu KK, Davis CE, Conlan MG, Sorlie PD, Szklo M.

Population correlates of plasma fibrinogen and factor VII, putative cardiovascular risk factors. *Atherosclerosis* 1991; 91:191–205.

37. Rossouw JE. Secondary prevention of coronary heart disease. In: Rifkind BM, ed. *Lowering Cholesterol in High-Risk Individuals and Populations.* New York: Marcel Dekker; 1995:46–67.

38. Shepherd J, Cobbe SM, Ford I, Isles CG, Lorimer AR, MacFarlane PW, et al. Prevention of coronary heart disease with pravastatin in men with hypercholesterolemia. *N Engl J Med* 1995; 333:1301–1307.

39. Brown BG, Zhao X-Q, Sacco DE, Albers JJ. Lipid lowering and plaque regression. New insights into prevention of plaque disruption and clinical events in coronary disease. *Circulation* 1993; 87:1781–1791.

40. Scandinavian Simvastatin Survival Study Group. Randomized trial of cholesterol lowering in 4444 patients with coronary heart disease: The Scandinavian Simvastatin Survival Study (4S). *Lancet* 1994; 344:1383–1389.

41. Sacks FM, Pfeffer MA, Moye LA, Rouleau JL, Rutherford JD, Cole TG, et al. The effect of pravastatin on coronary events after myocardial infarction in patients with average cholesterol levels. *N Engl J Med* 1996; 335:1001–1009.

42. Miller M, Seidler A, Kwiterovich PO, Pearson TA. Long-term predictors of subsequent cardiovascular events with coronary artery disease and "desirable" levels of plasma total cholesterol. *Circulation* 1992; 86:1165–1170.

43. Goldman L, Weinstein MC, Goldman PA, Williams LW. Cost-effectiveness of HMG-CoA reductase inhibition for primary and secondary prevention of coronary heart disease. *JAMA* 1991; 265:1145–1151.

44. Johannesson M, Jönsson B, Kjekshus J, Olsson AG, Pedersen TR, Wedel H. Cost-effectiveness of simvastatin treatment to lower cholesterol levels in patients with coronary heart disease. *N Engl J Med* 1997; 336:332–336.

45. Cohen DJ, Goldman L, Weinstein C. The cost-effectiveness of programs to lower serum cholesterol. In: Rifkind BM, ed. *Lowering Cholesterol in High-Risk Individuals and Populations.* New York: Marcel Dekker; 1995:311–336.

46. Expert Panel on Detection, Evaluation, and Treatment of High Blood Cholesterol in Adults (Adult Treatment Panel II). *Circulation* 1994; 89:1329–1445.

47. MacMahon S, Peto R, Cutler J, Collins R, Sorlie P, Neaton J, et al. Blood pressure, stroke, and coronary heart disease. Part I. Prolonged differences in blood pressure: Prospective observational studies for the regression dilution bias. *Lancet* 1990; 335:765–774.

48. Collins R, MacMahon S. Blood pressure, antihypertensive drug treatment and the risks of stroke and of coronary heart disease. *Br Med Bull* 1994; 50:272–298.

49. Members of the Joint National Committee on Detection, Evaluation, and Treatment of High Blood Pressure. The fifth report of the Joint National Committee on detection, evaluation, and treatment of high blood pressure (JNC V). *Arch Intern Med* 1993; 153:154–183.

50. Kannel WB. Blood pressure as a cardiovascular risk factor: Prevention and treatment. *JAMA* 1996; 275:1571–1576.

51. Davis BR, Cutler JA, Gordon DJ, Furberg CD, Wright JT Jr., Cushman WC, et al. Rationale and design for the Antihypertensive and Lipid Lowering Treatment to Prevent Heart Attack Trial (ALLHAT). *Am J Hypertens* 1996; 9(4 pt 1):342–360.

52. Messerli FH, Soria F. Ventricular dysrhythmias, left ventricular hypertrophy, and sudden death. *Cardiovasc Drugs Ther* 1994; 8(suppl 3):557–563.

53. Dahlof B, Pennert K, Hansson L. Reversal of left ventricular hypertrophy in hypertensive patients: A metaanalysis of 109 treatment studies. *Am J Hypertens* 1992; 5:95–110.

54. Levy D, Salomon M, D'Agostino RB, Belanger AJ, Kannel WB. Prognostic implications of baseline electrocardiographic features and their serial changes in subjects with left ventricular hypertrophy. *Circulation* 1994; 90:1786–1793.

55. Reaven GM. Role of insulin resistance in human disease. *Diabetes* 1988; 37:1595–1607.

56. Reaven GM. Syndrome X: 6 years later. *J Intern Med* 1994; 236(suppl 736):13–22.

57. Petrie JR, Ueda S, Webb DJ, Elliott HL, Connell JMC. Endothelial nitric oxide production and insulin sensitivity: A physiologic link with implications for pathogenesis of cardiovascular disease. *Circulation* 1996; 93:1331–1333.

58. Després J-P, Lamarche B, Mauriège P, Cantin B, Dagenais GR, Moorjani S, et al. Hyperinsulinemia as an independent risk factor for ischemic heart disease. *N Engl J Med* 1996; 334:952–957.

59. Krolewski AS, Warram JH, Valsania P, Martin BC, Laffel LMB, Christlieb R. Evolving natural history of coronary artery disease in diabetes mellitus. *Am J Med* 1991; 90(suppl 2A)56S–61S.

60. Bierman E. George Lyman Duff Memorial Lecture. Atherogenesis in diabetes. *Arterioscler Thromb* 1992; 12:647–656.

61. Abbott RD, Donahue RP, Kannel WB, Wilson PWF. The impact of diabetes on survival following myocardial infarction in men vs. women: The Framingham Study. *JAMA* 1988; 260:3456–3460.

62. Walden CE, Knopp RH, Wahl PW, Beach KW, Strandness E Jr. Sex differences in the effect of diabetes mellitus on lipoprotein triglyceride and cholesterol concentrations. *N Engl J Med* 1984; 311:953–959.

63. The University Group Diabetes Program. A study of the effects of hypoglycemic agents on vascular complications in patients with adult-onset diabetes. II. Mortality results. *Diabetes* 1970; 19(suppl 2):787–830.

64. The Diabetes Control and Complications Trial Research Group. The effect of intensive treatment of diabetes on the development and progression of long-term complications in insulin-dependent diabetes mellitus. *N Engl J Med* 1993; 329:977–986.

65. Gundersen T, Kjekshus J. Timolol treatment after myocardial infarction in diabetic patients. *Diabetes Care* 1983; 6:285–290.

66. Kramsch DM, Aspen AJ, Abramowitz BM, Kreimendahl T, Hood WB. Reduction of coronary atherosclerosis by moderate conditioning exercise in monkeys on an atherogenic diet. *N Engl J Med* 1981; 305:1483–1489.

67. Hambrecht R, Niebauer J, Marburger C, Grunze M, Kälberer B, Hauer K, et al. Various intensities of leisure time physical activity in patients with coronary artery disease: Effects on cardiorespiratory fitness and progression of coronary atherosclerotic lesions. *J Am Coll Cardiol* 1993; 22:468–477.

68. Haskell WL. Sedentary lifestyle as a risk factor for coronary heart disease. In: Pearson TA, Criqui MH, Luepker RV, Oberman A, Winston M, eds. *Primer in Preventive Cardiology.* Dallas: American Heart Association; 1994:173–187.

69. Siscovick DS, Weiss NS, Fletcher RH, Lasky T. The incidence of primary cardiac arrest during vigorous exercise. *N Engl J Med* 1984; 311:874–877.

70. Oldridge NB, Guyatt GH, Fischer ME, Rimm AA. Cardiac rehabilitation after myocardial infarction: Combined experience of randomized clinical trials. *JAMA* 1988; 260:945–950.

71. O'Connor GT, Buring JE, Yusuf S, Goldhaber SZ, Olmstead EM, Paffenbarger RS, et al. An overview of randomized trials of rehabilitation with exercise after myocardial infarction. *Circulation* 1989; 80:234–244.

72. Pate RR, Pratt M, Blair SN, Haskell WL, Macera CA, Bouchard C, et al. Physical activity and public health: A recommendation from the Centers for Disease Control and Prevention and the American College of Sports Medicine. *JAMA* 1995; 273:402–407.

73. Smith SC Jr, Blair SN, Criqui MH, Fletcher GF, Fuster V, Gersh BJ, et al. Preventing heart attack and death in patients with coronary disease. AHA Consensus Panel Statement. *Circulation* 1995; 92:2–4.

74. American College of Sports Medicine. *Guidelines for Exercise Testing and Prescription,* 4th ed. Philadelphia: Lea & Febiger; 1991.

75. King AC, Haskell WL, Taylor CB, Kraemer HC, DeBusk RF. Group-vs home-based exercise training in healthy older men and women: A community-based clinical trial. *JAMA* 1991; 266:1535–1542.

76. Kuczmarski RJ, Flegal KM, Campbell SM, Hohnson CL. Increasing prevalence of overweight among U.S. adults: The National Health and Nutrition Examination Surveys, 1960 to 1991. *JAMA* 1994; 272:205–211.

77. Pi-Sunyer FX. Short-term medical benefits and adverse effects of weight loss. *Ann Intern Med* 1993; 119(7 pt 2):722–726.

78. MacMahon SW, Wilcken DEL, Macdonald GJ. The effect of weight reduction on left ventricular mass: A randomized controlled trial in young, overweight hypertensive patients. *N Engl J Med* 1986; 314:334–339.

79. Hubert HB, Feinleib M, McNamara PM, Castelli WB. Obesity as an independent risk factor for cardiovascular disease: A 26-year follow-up of participants in the Framingham Heart Study. *Circulation* 1983; 67:968–977.

80. Manson JE, Willett WC, Stampfer MJ, Colditz GA, Hunter DJ, Hankinson SE, et al. Body weight and mortality among women. *N Engl J Med* 1995; 333:677–685.

81. Jousilahti P, Tuomilehto J, Vartiainen E, Pekkanen J, Puska P. Body weight, cardiovascular risk factors, and coronary mortality: 15-year follow-up of middle-aged men and women in eastern Finland. *Circulation* 1996; 93:1372–1379.

82. Larsson B. Regional obesity as a health hazard in men: Prospective studies. *Acta Med Scand Suppl* 1988; 723:45–51.

83. Flegal KM, Troiano RP, Pamuk ER, Kuczmarski RJ, Campbell SM. The influence of smoking cessation on the prevalence of overweight in the United States. *N Engl J Med* 1995; 333:1165–1170.

84. Belchetz PE. Hormonal treatment of postmenopausal women. *N Engl J Med* 1994; 330:1062–1071.

85. Rosano GMC, Sarrel PM, Poole-Wilson PA, Collins P. Beneficial effect of oestrogen on exercise-induced myocardial ischaemia in women with coronary artery disease. *Lancet* 1993; 342:133–136.

86. Collins P, Rosano GMC, Sarrel PM, Ulrich L, Adamopoulos S, Beale CM, et al. 17 β-estradiol attenuates acetylcholine-induced coronary arterial constriction in women but not men with coronary heart disease. *Circulation* 1995; 92:24–30.

87. Colditz GA, Hankinson SE, Hunter DJ, Willett WC, Manson JE, Stampfer MJ, et al. The use of estrogens and progestins and the risk of breast cancer in postmenopausal women. *N Engl J Med* 1995; 332:1589–1593.

88. Goldman L, Tosteson ANA. Uncertainty about postmenopausal estrogen: Time for action, not debate. *N Engl J Med* 1991; 325:800–802.

89. The Writing Group for the PEPI Trial. Effects of estrogen or estrogen/progestin regimens on heart disease risk factors in postmenopausal women: The postmenopausal estrogen/progestin interventions (PEPI) trial. *JAMA* 1995; 273:199–208.

90. Walsh BW, Schiff I, Rosner B, Greenberg L, Ravnikar V, Sacks FM. Effects of postmenopausal estrogen replacement on the concentrations and metabolism of plasma lipoproteins. *N Engl J Med* 1991; 325:1196–1204.

91. Stampfer MJ, Colditz GA, Willett WC, Manson JE, Rosner B, Speizer FE, et al. Postmenopausal estrogen therapy and cardiovascular disease: Ten-year follow-up from the Nurses' Health Study. *N Engl J Med* 1991; 325:756–762.

92. Rozanski A, Bairey CN, Krantz DS, Friedman J, Resser KJ, Morell M, et al. Mental stress and the induction of silent myocardial ischemia in patients with coronary artery disease. *N Engl J Med* 1988; 318:1005–1012.

93. Yeung AC, Vekshtein VI, Krantz DS, Vita JA, Ryan TJ Jr, Ganz P, et al. The effect of atherosclerosis on the vasomotor response of coronary arteries to mental stress. *N Engl J Med* 1991; 325:1551–1556.

94. Mittleman MA, Maclure M, Sherwood JB, Mulry RP, Tofler GH, Jacobs SC, et al. Triggering of acute myocardial infarction onset by episodes of anger. *Circulation* 1995; 92:1720–1725.

95. Leor J, Poole WK, Kloner RA. Sudden cardiac death triggered by an earthquake. *N Engl J Med* 1996; 334:413–419.

96. Scanu AM. Lipoprotein(a): A genetic risk factor for premature coronary heart disease. *JAMA* 1992; 267:3326–3329.

97. Ridker PM, Hennekens CH, Stampfer MJ. A prospective study of lipoprotein(a) and the risk of myocardial infarction. *JAMA* 1993; 270:2195–2199.

98. Schaefer EJ, Lamon-Fava S, Jenner JL, McNamara JR, Ordovas JM, Davis CE, et al. Lipoprotein(a) levels and risk of coronary heart disease in men. The Lipid Research Clinics Coronary Primary Prevention Trial. *JAMA* 1994; 271:999–1003.

99. Cremer P, Nagel D, Labrot B, Mann H, Muche R, Elster H, et al. Lipoprotein Lp(a) as predictor of myocardial infarction in comparison to fibrinogen, LDL cholesterol and other risk factors: Results from the prospective Gottingen Risk Incidence and Prevalence Study (GRIPS). *Eur J Clin Inv* 1994; 24:444–453.

100. Wald NJ, Law M, Watt HC, Wu T, Bailey A, Johnson AM, et al. Apolipoproteins and ischaemic heart disease: Implications for screening. *Lancet* 1994; 343:75–79.

101. Ridker PM, Stampfer MJ, Hennekens CH. Plasma concentration of lipoprotein(a) and the risk of future stroke. *JAMA* 1995; 273:1269–1273.

102. Maher VMG, Brown BG, Marcovina SM, Hillger LA, Zhao X-Q, Albers JJ. Effects of lowering elevated LDL cholesterol on the cardiovascular risk of lipoprotein(a). *JAMA* 1995; 274:1771–1774.

103. Selhub J, Jacques PF, Wilson PWF, Rush D, Rosenberg IH. Vitamin status and intake as primary determinants of homocysteinemia in an elderly population. *JAMA* 1993; 270:2693–2698.

104. Boushey CJ, Beresford SAA, Omenn GS, Motulsky AG. A quantitative assessment of plasma homocysteine as a risk factor for vascular disease: Probable benefits of increasing folic acid intakes. *JAMA* 1995; 274:1049–1057.

105. Stampfer MJ, Malinow MR, Willett WC, Newcomer LM, Upson B, Ullmann D, et al. A prospective study of plasma homocyst(e)ine and risk of myocardial infarction in US physicians. *JAMA* 1992; 268:877–881.

106. Arnesen E, Refsum H, Bonaa KH, Ueland PM, Forde OH, Nordrehaug JE. Serum total homocysteine and coronary heart disease. *Int J Epidemiol* 1995; 24:704–709.

107. Perry IJ, Refsum H, Morris RW, Ebrahim SB, Ueland PM, Shaper AG. Prospective study of serum total homocysteine concentration and risk of stroke in middle-aged British men. *Lancet* 1995; 346:1395–1398.

108. Stampfer MJ, Hennekens CH, Manson JE, Colditz GA, Rosner B, Willett WC. Vitamin E consumption and the risk of coronary disease in women. *N Engl J Med* 1993; 328:1444–1449.

109. Rimm ER, Stampfer MJ, Ascherio A, Giovannucci E, Colditz GA, Willett WC. Vitamin E consumption and the risk of coronary disease in men. *N Engl J Med* 1993; 328:1450–1456.

110. Greenberg ER, Baron JA, Karagas MR, Stukel TA, Nierenberg DW, Stevens MM, et al. Mortality associated with low plasma concentration of beta carotene and the effect of oral supplementation. *JAMA* 1996; 275:699–703.

111. Jha P, Flather M, Lonn E, Farkouh M, Yusuf S. The antioxidant vitamins and cardiovascular disease. A critical review of epidemiologic and clinical trial data. *Ann Intern Med* 1995; 123:860–872.

112. Alpha-Tocopherol, Beta-Carotene Cancer Prevention Study Group. The effect of vitamin E and beta carotene on the incidence of lung cancer and other cancers in male smokers. *N Engl J Med* 1994; 330:1029–1035.

113. Omenn GS, Goodman GE, Thornquist MD, Balmes J, Cullen MR, Glass A, et al. Effects of the combination of beta-carotene and vitamin A on lung cancer incidence, total mortality, and cardiovascular mortality in smokers and asbestos-exposed workers. *N Engl J Med* 1996; 334:1150–1155.

114. Hennekens CH, Buring JE, Manson JE, Stampfer MJ, Rosner B, Cook NR, et al. Lack of effect of long-term supplementation with beta-carotene on the incidence of malignant neoplasms and cardiovascular disease. *N Engl J Med* 1996; 334:1145–1149.

115. Stephens NG, Parsons A, Schofiled PM, Kelly F, Cheeseman K, Mitchinson MJ. Randomized controlled trial of vitamin E in patients with coronary disease: Cambridge Heart Antioxidant Study (CHAOS). *Lancet* 1996; 347:781–786.

116. Moore RD, Pearson TA. Moderate alcohol consumption and coronary artery disease: A review. *Medicine (Baltimore)* 1986; 65:242–267.

117. Stampfer MJ, Colditz GA, Willett WC, Speizer FE, Hennekens CH. A prospective study of moderate alcohol consumption and the risk of coronary disease and stroke in women. *N Engl J Med* 1988; 319:267–273.

118. Rimm EB, Giovannucci EL, Willett WC, Colditz GA, Ascherio A, Rosner B, et al. Prospective study of alcohol consumption and risk of coronary disease in men. *Lancet* 1991; 338:464–468.

119. Gaziano JM. Alcohol and coronary heart disease. Biological Effects of Low Level Exposure 1995; 4:1–5 (newsletter).

120. Maclure M. Demonstration of deductive meta-analysis: Ethanol intake and risk of myocardial infarction. *Epidemiol Rev* 1993; 15:1–24.

121. Langer RD, Criqui MH, Reed DM. Lipoproteins and blood pressure as biological pathways for effect of moderate alcohol consumption on coronary heart disease. *Circulation* 1992; 85:910–915.

122. Suh I, Shaten BJ, Cutler JA, Kuller LH. Alcohol use and mortality from coronary heart disease: The role of high-density lipoprotein cholesterol: The Multiple Risk Factor Intervention Trial Research Group. *Ann Intern Med* 1992; 116:881–887.

123. Haskell WL, Camargo C Jr, Williams PT, Vranizan KM, Krauss RM, Lindgren FT, et al. The effect of cessation and resumption of moderate alcohol intake on serum high-density-lipoprotein subfractions. *N Engl J Med* 1984; 310:805–810.

124. Gaziano JM, Buring JE, Breslow JL, Goldhaber SZ, Rosner B, VanDenburgh M, et al. Moderate alcohol intake, increased levels of high-density lipoprotein and its subfractions, and decreased risk of myocardial infarction (see comments). *N Engl J Med* 1993; 329:1829–1834.

125. Ridker PM, Vaughan DE, Stampfer MJ, Glynn RJ, Hennekens CH.

Association of moderate alcohol consumption and plasma concentration of endogenous tissue plasminogen activator. *JAMA* 1994; 272:929–933.

126. Hendriks HFJ, Veenstra J, Velthuis-te Wierik EJM, Schaafsma G, Kluft C. Effects of moderate dose of alcohol with evening meal on fibrinolytic factors. *BMJ* 1994; 308:1003–1006.

127. Deykin D, Janson P, McMahon L. Ethanol potentiation of aspirin-induced prolongation of the bleeding time. *N Engl J Med* 1982; 306:852–854.

128. Elmer O, Goransson G, Zoucas E. Impairment of primary hemostasis and platelet function after alcohol ingestion in man. *Haemostasis* 1984; 14:223–228.

129. Pearson TA. What to advise patients about drinking alcohol: The clinician's conundrum. *JAMA* 1994; 272:967–968.

130. Enos WF Jr, Beyer JC, Holmes RH. Pathogenesis of coronary disease in American soldiers killed in Korea. *JAMA* 1955; 58:912–914.

131. McNamara JJ, Molot MA, Stremple JF, Cutting RT. Coronary artery disease in combat casualties in Vietnam. *JAMA* 1971; 216:1185–1187.

132. Castelli WP. Epidemiology of coronary heart disease: The Framingham study. *Am J Med* 1984; 76(2A):4–12.

133. Thom TJ. Cardiovascular disease mortality among United States women. In: Eaker ED, Packard B, Wenger NK, Clarkson TB, Tyroler HA, eds. *Coronary Heart Disease in Women.* New York: Haymarket Doyma; 1987.

134. Kaplan GA, Keil JE. Socioeconomic factors and cardiovascular disease: A review of the literature. *Circulation* 1993; 88:1973–1998.

135. Hopkins PN, Williams RR. Human genetics and coronary heart disease: A public health perspective. *Annu Rev Nutr* 1989; 9:303–345.

136. Rissanen AM. Familial occurrence of coronary heart disease: Effect of age at diagnosis. *Am J Cardiol* 1979; 44:60–66.

137. Williams RR, Hopkins PN, Wu LL, Schumacher C, Hunt SC. Evaluating family history to prevent early coronary heart disease. In: Pearson TA, Criqui MH, Luepker RV, Oberman A, Winston M, eds. *Primer in Preventive Cardiology.* Dallas: American Heart Association; 1994:93–106.

138. Steering Committee of the Physician's Health Study Research Group. Final report on the aspirin component of the ongoing Physician's Health Study. *N Engl J Med* 1989; 321:129–135.

139. Ridker PM, Manson JE, Buring JE, Goldhaber SZ, Hennekens CH. Clinical characteristics of nonfatal myocardial infarction among individuals on prophylactic low-dose aspirin therapy. *Circulation* 1991; 84:708–711.

140. Manson JE, Grobbee DE, Stampfer MJ, Taylor JO, Goldhaber SZ, Gaziano JM, et al. Aspirin in the primary prevention of angina pectoris in a randomized trial of physicians. *Am J Med* 1990; 89:772–776.

141. Peto R, Gray R, Collins R, Wheatley K, Hennekens C, Jamrozik K, et al. Randomised trial of prophylactic daily aspirin in British male doctors. *Br Med J* 1988; 296:313–316.

142. Hennekens CH, Peto R, Hutchison GB, Doll R. An overview of the British and American aspirin studies. *N Engl J Med* 1988; 318:923–924.

143. Ridker PM, Manson JE, Gaziano MJ, Buring JE, Hennekens CH. Low dose aspirin therapy for chronic stable angina: A randomized clinical trial. *Ann Intern Med* 1991; 114:835–839.

144. Meade TW, Wilkes HC, Stirling Y, Brennan PJ, Kelleher C, Browne W. Randomized controlled trial of low dose warfarin in the primary prevention of ischemic heart disease in men at high risk: Design and pilot study. *Eur Heart J* 1988; 9:836–843.

145. Hennekens CH, Buring JE, Sandercock P, Collins R, Peto R. Aspirin and other antiplatelet agents in the secondary and primary prevention of cardiovascular disease. *Circulation* 1989; 80:749–756.

146. Antiplatelet Trialists Collaboration. Collaborative overview of randomized trials of antiplatelet treatment. Part I: Prevention of vascular death, myocardial infarction, and stroke by prolonged antiplatelet therapy in different categories of patients. *Br J Med* 1994; 308:81–106.

147. Sixty Plus Reinfarction Study Research Group. A double-blind trial to assess long-term anticoagulant therapy in elderly patients after myocardial infarction. *Lancet* 1980; 2:989–993.

148. Smith P, Arnesen H, Holme I. The effect of warfarin on mortality and reinfarction after myocardial infarction. *N Engl J Med* 1990; 323:147–152.

149. Cairns JA, Markham BA. Economics and efficacy in choosing oral anticoagulants or aspirin after myocardial infarction. *JAMA* 1995; 273:965–967.

150. US Preventive Services Task Force. Aspirin prophylaxis. In: *Guide to Clinical Preventive Services: Report of the US Preventive Services Task Force.* Baltimore: Williams & Wilkins; 1989.

151. Manson JE, Stampfer MJ, Colditz GA, Willett WC, Rosner B, Speizer FE, et al. A prospective study of aspirin use and primary prevention of cardiovascular disease in women. *JAMA* 1991; 266:521–527.

152. Meade TW, Mellows S, Brozovic M, Miller GJ, Chakrabarti RR, North WR, et al. Haemostatic function and ischemic heart disease: Principal results of the Northwick Park Heart Study. *Lancet* 1986; 2:533–537.

153. Wilhelmsen L, Svärdsudd K, Korsan-Bengtsen K, Larsson B, Welin L, Tibblin G. Fibrinogen as a risk factor for stroke and myocardial infarction. *N Engl J Med* 1984; 311:501–505.

154. Kannel WB, Wolf PA, Castelli WP, D'Agostino RB. Fibrinogen and risk of cardiovascular disease. The Framingham Study. *JAMA* 1987; 258:1183–1186.

155. Thompson SG, Kienast J, Pyke SDM, Haverkate F, van de Loo JC. Hemostatic factors and the risk of myocardial infarction or sudden death in patients with angina pectoris. *N Engl J Med* 1995; 332:635–641.

156. Ernst E, Resch KL. Fibrinogen as a cardiovascular risk factor: A meta-analysis and review of the literature. *Ann Intern Med* 1993; 118:956–963.

157. Ridker PM, Vaughan DE, Stampfer MJ, Manson JE, Hennekens CH. Endogenous tissue-type plasminogen activator and risk of myocardial infarction. *Lancet* 1993; 341:1165–1168.

158. Hamsten A, Walldius G, Szamosi A, Blomback M, DeFaire U, Dahlén G, et al. Plasminogen activator inhibitor in plasma: Risk factor for recurrent myocardial infarction. *Lancet* 1987; 2:3–9.

159. Ridker PM, Hennekens CH, Stampfer MJ, Manson JE, Vaughan DE. Prospective study of endogenous tissue plasminogen activator and risk of stroke. *Lancet* 1994; 343:940–943.

160. Meade TW, Ruddock V, Stirling Y, Charkrabarti R, Miller GJ. Fibrinolytic activity, clotting factors, and long-term incidence of ischaemic heart disease in the Northwick Park Heart Study. *Lancet* 1993; 342:1076–1079.

161. Ridker PM, Hennekens CH, Cerskus A, Stampfer MJ. Plasma concentration of cross-linked fibrin degradation product (D-dimer) and the risk of future myocardial infarction among apparently healthy men. *Circulation* 1994; 90:2236–2240.

162. Fowkes FGR, Lowe GDO, Housley E, Rattray A, Rumley A, Elton RA, et al. Cross-linked fibrin degradation products, progression of peripheral arterial disease, and risk of coronary heart disease. *Lancet* 1993; 342:84–86.

163. Nabulsi AA, Folsom AR, White A, Patsch W, Heiss G, Wu KK, et al, for the Atherosclerosis Risk in Communities Study Investigators. Association of hormone replacement therapy with various cardiovascular risk factors in postmenopausal women. *N Engl J Med* 1993; 328:1069–1075.

164. Goldbourt U, Behar S, Reicher-Reiss H, Agmon J, Kaplinsky E, Graff E, et al. Rationale and design of a secondary prevention trial of increasing serum HDL cholesterol and reducing triglycerides after myocardial infarction in patients with clinically manifest atherosclerotic heart disease (the Bezafibrate Infarction Prevention Study). *Am J Cardiol* 1993; 71:909–915.

165. Stone PH, Sacks FM. Strategies for secondary prevention. In: Manson JE, Ridker PM, Gaziano JM, Hennekens CH, eds. *Primary Prevention of Myocardial Infarction.* London: Oxford University Press; 1996.

166. Wikstrand J, Warnold I, Olsson G, Tuomilehto J, Elmfeldt D, Berglund G. Primary prevention with metoprolol in patients with hypertension: Mortality results from the MAPHY Study. *JAMA* 1988; 259:1976–1982.

167. Yusuf S, Peto R, Lewis J, Collins R, Sleight P. Beta blockade during and after myocardial infarction: An overview of the randomized trials. *Prog Cardiovasc Dis* 1985; 27:335–371.

168. Lau J, Antman EM, Jimenez-Silva J, Kupelnick B, Mosteller F, Chalmers T. Cumulative meta-analysis of the therapeutic trials for myocardial infarction. *N Engl J Med* 1992; 327:248–254.

169. Goldman L, Sia STB, Cook EF, Rutherford JD, Weinstein MC. Costs and effectiveness of routine therapy with long-term beta-adrenergic antagonists after acute myocardial infarction. *N Engl J Med* 1988; 319:152–157.

170. The Consensus Clinical Trial Study Group. Effects of enalapril on mortality in severe congestive heart failure: Results of the Cooperative

North Scandinavian Enalapril Survival Study (CONSENSUS). *N Engl J Med* 1987; 316:1429–1435.

171. The SOLVD Investigators. Effect of enalapril on survival in patients with reduced left ventricular ejection fractions and congestive heart failure. *N Engl J Med* 1991; 325:293–302.

172. The SOLVD Investigators. Effect of enalapril on mortality and the development of heart failure in asymptomatic patients with reduced left ventricular ejection fractions. *N Engl J Med* 1992; 327:685–691.

173. Pfeffer JM, Fischer TA, Pfeffer MA. Angiotensin-converting enzyme inhibition and ventricular remodeling after myocardial infarction. *Annu Rev Physiol* 1995; 57:805–826.

174. Pfeffer MA, Lamas GA, Vaughan DE, Parisi AF, Braunwald E. Effect of captopril on progressive ventricular dilatation after anterior myocardial infarction. *N Engl J Med* 1988; 319:80–86.

175. Sharpe N, Smith H, Murphy J, Hannan S. Treatment of patients with symptomless left ventricular dysfunction after myocardial infarction. *Lancet* 1988; 1:255–259.

176. Pfeffer MA, Braunwald E, Moye LA, Basta L, Brown EJ Jr, Cuddy TE, et al. Effect of captopril on mortality and morbidity in patients with left ventricular dysfunction after myocardial infarction. Results of the Survival and Ventricular Enlargement Trial. *N Engl J Med* 1992; 327:669–677.

177. Yusuf S, Pepine CJ, Garces C, Pouleur H, Salem D, Kostis J, et al. Effects of enalapril on myocardial infarction and unstable angina in patients with low ejection fractions. *Lancet* 1992; 340:1173–1178.

178. Ridker PM, Gaboury CL, Conlin PR, Seely EW, Williams GH, Vaughan DE. Stimulation of plasminogen activator inhibitor in vivo by infusion of angiotensin II: Evidence of a potential interaction between the renin angiotensin system and fibrinolytic function. *Circulation* 1993; 87:1969–1973.

179. Tsevat J, Duke D, Goldman J, Pfeffer MA, Gervasio AL, Soukup JR, et al. Cost-effectiveness of captopril therapy after myocardial infarction. *J Am Coll Cardiol* 1995; 26:914–919.

180. Vogel RA. Risk factor intervention and coronary artery disease: Clinical strategies. *Coron Artery Dis* 1995; 6:466–471.

181. Pearson TA. Personal communication, 1995.

182. Cardiac Rehabilitation Guideline Panel. *Cardiac Rehabilitation: Clinical Practice Guideline.* Department of Health and Human Services, Public Health Service, Agency for Health Care Policy and Research. DHHS publication No. AHCPR 96-0672, Oct 1995.

183. Kottke TE, Blackburn H, Brekke MC, Solberg LI. The systematic practice of preventive cardiology. *Am J Cardiol* 1987; 59:690–694.

184. Davis JE, McBride PE, Bobula JA. Improving prevention in primary care: Physicians, patients, and process (editorial; comment). *J Fam Pract* 1992; 35:385–387.

185. Pearson TA, McBride PE, Houston Miller N, Smith SC. Organization of preventive cardiology service. *J Am Coll Cardiol* 1996; 27:1039–1047.

186. Haynes RB. Determinants of compliance: The disease and mechanisms of treatment. In: Haynes RB, Taylor DW, Schlant DL, eds. *Compliance in Health Care.* Baltimore: Johns Hopkins University Press; 1979.

187. Levine DM. Behavioral and psychosocial factors, processes, and strategies. In: Pearson TA, Criqui MH, Luepker RV, Oberman A, Winston M, eds. *Primer in Preventive Cardiology.* Dallas: American Heart Association; 1994:217–226.

188. Prochaska JO, DiClemente CC. Stages and processes of self-change of smoking: Toward an integrative model of change. *J Consult Clin Psychol* 1983; 51:390–395.

189. Lomas J, Anderson GM, Domnick-Pierre K, Vayda E, Enkin MW, Hannah WJ. Do practice guidelines guide practice? The effect of a consensus statement on the practice of physicians. *N Engl J Med* 1989; 321:1306–1311.

190. Harris RP, O'Malley MS, Fletcher SW, Knight BP. Prompting physicians for preventive procedures: A five-year study of manual and computer reminders. *Am J Prev Med* 1990; 6:145–152.

191. DeBusk RF, Miller NH, Superko HR, Dennis CA, Thomas RJ, Lew HT, et al. A case-management system for coronary risk factor modification after acute myocardial infarction. *Ann Intern Med* 1994; 120:721–729.

192. Haskell WL, Alderman EL, Fair JM, Maron DJ, Mackey SF, Superko HR, et al. Effects of intensive multiple risk factor reduction on coronary atherosclerosis and clinical cardiac events in men and women with coronary artery disease: The Stanford Coronary Risk Intervention Project (SCRIP). *Circulation* 1994; 89:975–990.

193. Epstein A. Performance reports on quality: Prototypes, problems, and prospects. *N Engl J Med* 1995; 333:57–61.

42

NONATHEROSCLEROTIC CORONARY HEART DISEASE

Bruce F. Waller

Although atherosclerotic disease of the coronary arteries is the most common cause of luminal narrowing and coronary heart disease, there are multiple nonatherosclerotic (congenital and acquired) causes of severe luminal narrowing and subsequent clinical coronary events (angina pectoris, acute myocardial infarction, and sudden death) (Table 42-1).

Various nonatherosclerotic coronary artery diseases can reduce or interrupt coronary blood flow by various mechanisms: (1) fixed luminal obstructions (internal narrowing), (2) encroachment of the lumen by disease of the arterial wall or adjacent tissues (external narrowing), or (3) both.[1] Reduction in coronary arterial blood flow may also result from dynamic changes in the walls of an otherwise normal artery (spasm) or from a disproportion of myocardial oxygen supply and demand. In view of current trends toward rapid coronary artery reperfusion to salvage jeopardized myocardium during evolving acute myocardial infarction, the various nonatherosclerotic etiologies of coronary artery disease must be kept in mind.

FREQUENCY OF NONATHEROSCLEROTIC CORONARY NARROWING PRODUCING FATAL MYOCARDIAL INFARCTION

Approximately 4 to 7 percent of all patients with acute myocardial infarction and nearly four times this percentage for patients under age 35 do not have atherosclerotic coronary artery disease (CAD) as demonstrated by coronary arteriography, at necropsy, or both.[1–5] In view of the fact that coronary angiography simply represents an image of one lumen, the specificity for etiology of the coronary luminal narrowing is extremely low. Review of necropsy studies[1,3,4] suggests that approximately 95 percent of patients with fatal acute myocar-

dial infarction have at least one major epicardial coronary artery with severe luminal narrowing or total occlusion (Fig. 42-1). The remaining 5 percent of patients apparently have normal major epicardial coronary arteries. Of the 95 percent of patients with severe coronary luminal narrowing, 95 percent have typical atherosclerotic plaque with a superimposed thrombus in 85 percent of these.

The remaining 5 percent of the patients with severe coronary luminal narrowing have a host of etiologies (Table 42-1), including coronary arteritis, trauma, systemic metabolic disorders, intimal fibrous proliferation, and coronary emboli. Medical centers with large populations of cardiac transplant patients will exceed the 5 percent nonatherosclerotic approximation owing to the high frequency of intimal fibrous proliferation in the coronary arteries late after transplantation. Of the 5 percent of patients seen at necropsy after fatal acute myocardial infarction with normal or nearly normal epicardial coronary arteries, perhaps 50 to 60 percent represent clinical coronary spasm, but the remaining 40 to 50 percent represent a combination of congenital coronary artery anomalies, spontaneous recanalization, and mismatches of coronary supply and myocardial demand (see also Chap. 40).

CONGENITAL CORONARY ARTERY ANOMALIES

Variation in the origin, course, or distribution of the epicardial coronary arteries are found in 1 to 2 percent of the population (Table 42-2; Fig. 42-2).[1,6–14] Certain types of these anomalies—including ostial lesions, passage of a major artery between the walls of the pulmonary trunk, a major coronary artery originating from the pulmonary trunk, or perhaps myo-

TABLE 42-1

NONATHEROSCLEROTIC CAUSES OF CORONARY ARTERY DISEASE (CORONARY HEART DISEASE)

Congenital anomalies
  Anomalous origin from the aorta
  Right-from-left sinus of Valsalva
  Left-from-right sinus of Valsalva
  Single coronary artery
  Atresia of coronary ostium
  High-takeoff coronary ostium
  Ostial ridges
  Anomalous origin from the pulmonary trunk
  Fistula
  Myocardial bridges ("tunneled" epicardial artery)
Embolus
  Natural
  Thrombus
  Tumor
  Calcium
  Vegetation (infective, noninfective)
  Iatrogenic
  Cardiac surgery
  Cardiac catheterization
  Coronary angioplasty
  Prosthetic valves
  Paradoxical
Dissection
  Coronary artery
  Aortic
Spasm
Trauma
  Nonpenetrating
  Penetrating
  Surgery
  Catheterization
Arteritis
  Takayasu's disease
  Polyarteritis nodosa
  Systemic lupus erythematosus
  Kawasaki's syndrome (mucocutaneous lymph node
    syndrome)
  Syphilis
  Other infections (infective endocarditis, *Salmonella*,
    parasites)
  Burger's disease
  Giant-cell arteritis

Metabolic disorders
  Mucopolysaccharidoses (Hurler, Hunter)
  Homocystinuria
  Fabry's disease
  Amyloid
Intimal proliferation
  Irradiation therapy
  Cardiac transplantation
  Fibromuscular hyperplasia (methysergide therapy)
  Ostial cannulation
  Transluminal balloon angioplasty
  Idiopathic infantile arterial calcification (juvenile internal
    sclerosis)
  Cocaine
External compression
  Aortic aneurysm
  Tumor metastases
  Muscle bridges
Thrombosis without underlying atherosclerotic plaque
  Polycythemia
  Thrombocytosis
  Hypercoagulability
Substance abuse
  Cocaine
  Amphetamines
Myocardial oxygen demand-supply disproportion
  Aortic stenosis
  Systemic hypotension
  Carbon monoxide poisoning
  Increased myocardial function (thyrotoxicosis)
Intramural coronary artery disease (small vessel disease)
  Hypertrophic cardiomyopathy
  Amyloid
  Cardiac transplantation
  Neuromuscular
  Diabetes mellitus
Normal coronary arteries

Sources: Adapted from Waller,[1] Alpert and Braunwald,[2] Cheitlin et al.,[4] and Baim and Harrison.[5]

cardial "bridges"—may produce ischemia with subsequent myocardial infarction[8] (see also Chaps. 16 and 70).

ORIGIN OF BOTH RIGHT AND LEFT CORONARY ARTERIES FROM THE SAME SINUS OF VALSALVA

When either the right or left coronary artery arises from the left or right sinus of Valsalva, respectively, the anomalous

vessel transverses the base of the heart in a course anterior to the pulmonary trunk, posterior to the aorta, or between the aorta and pulmonary trunk (Figs. 42-3 and 42-4). At least 43 cases have been reported with necropsy where the origin of the left main coronary artery is from the right sinus with passage between the aorta and pulmonary trunk.[7] In 79 percent of these patients,[34] death was related to the anomaly with sudden death or an acute myocardial infarction. At necropsy, 5 of 26 patients age less than 20 years old had myocardial infarcts.[7] When the right coronary artery originates from the

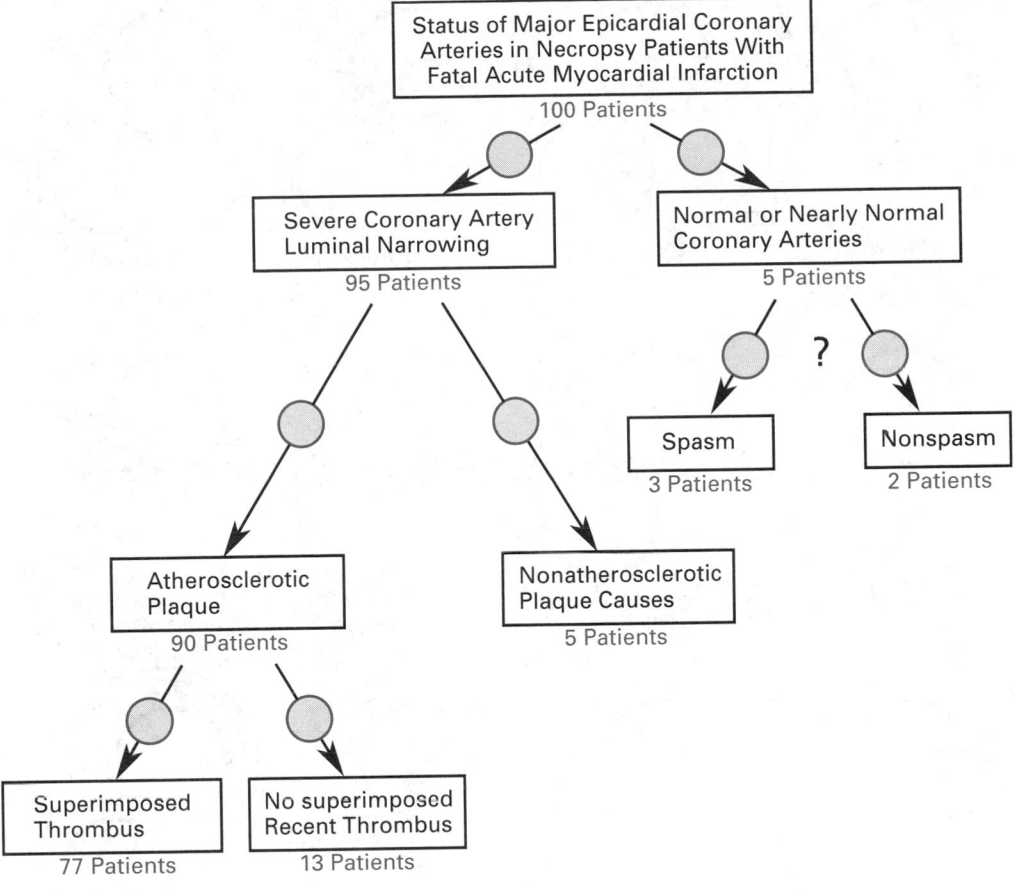

FIGURE 42-1
Diagram displaying the approximate breakdown of status of major epicardial coronary arteries in necropsy patients with fatal acute myocardial infarction. (From Waller.[10] Reproduced with permission from the publisher, editor, and author.)

TABLE 42-2

CERTAIN CORONARY ARTERIAL ANOMALIES ASSOCIATED WITH CLINICAL CORONARY EVENTS OR CORONARY ARTERY NARROWING

Anomalous origin of one or more coronary arteries from the aorta	High-takeoff coronary ostia
Origin of both right (R) and left (L) from same sinus of Valsalva	Ostial narrowing
R + LM (left main) from right sinus	Syphilis
R + LM (left main) from left sinus	Takayasu's disease (pulseless disease)
Single coronary artery	Fibromuscular hyperplasia (drug-induced)
Arising from right sinus	Aortic valve surgery
Arising from left sinus	Fibrous ridges
Arising from posterior sinus	Protruding masses
Anomalous origin of one or more coronary arteries from pulmonary trunk (PT)	Calcific nodules
Origin of R from PT	Supravalvular aortic stenosis
Origin of LM from PT	Aortic dissection
Origin of left anterior descending from PT	Adhesion of aortic cusp to sinus wall
Origin of left circumflex from PT	Embolism
Coronary artery atresia	Fibroelastosis
Atresia of R	Coronary artery fistula
Atresia of LM	Myocardial bridges

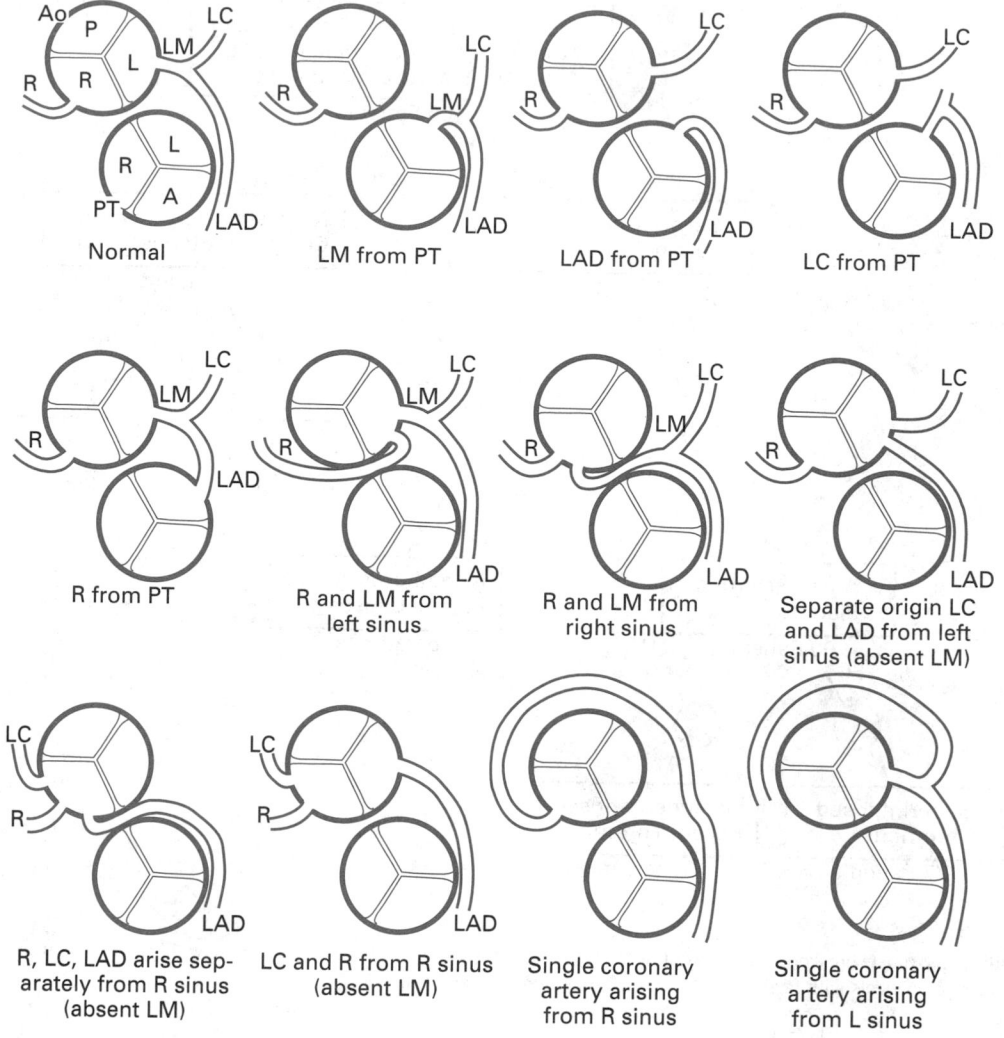

FIGURE 42-2

Diagram showing various congenital coronary artery anomalies which have been associated with clinical symptomatic heart disease. A = anterior cusp; Ao = aorta; L = left cusp; LAD = left anterior descending; LC = left circumflex; LM = left main; P = posterior cusp; PT = pulmonary trunk; R = right cusp or right coronary artery.

left sinus of Valsalva and passes between the aorta and pulmonary trunk, symptoms of myocardial ischemia, infarction, or sudden death may occur.[7] Of 12 patients with this anomaly,[9] 3 died suddenly, and 2 had angina or syncope. At necropsy, transmural ventricular scars (healed infarction) were seen in two.

The mechanism of ischemia, infarction, and/or sudden death in this coronary anomaly appears related to the shape of the coronary ostium of the anomalous vessel (Fig. 42-4). Normally, the coronary ostia are round to oval in shape, but in this anomaly, the coronary artery has an acute angle of takeoff that makes the ostium slitlike in shape. With increased cardiac output, the aorta dilates with stretching of the aortic wall, so that this slitlike ostium may become severely narrowed (Figs. 42-3 to 42-6). It is unlikely that there is "compression" of the anomalous coronary artery by the aorta and pulmonary trunk, in view of the marked differ-ences in diastolic pressures. At best, there would be an anterior shift of the anomalous vessel rather than a viselike compression.

SINGLE CORONARY ARTERY

Origin of the entire coronary circulation from a single aortic ostium has been termed *single coronary*. This anomaly is rare in the absence of other associated anomalies of the heart (Fig. 42-1). One or more branches of the single artery may cross the base of the heart in a fashion described above and thus may be exposed to the risks of ischemia owing to acute angulation.[5] Angina pectoris and myocardial lactate production have been demonstrated in patients with single coronary arteries where coronary atherosclerosis or an anomalous coronary artery passage was absent[13] (see also Chap. 70).

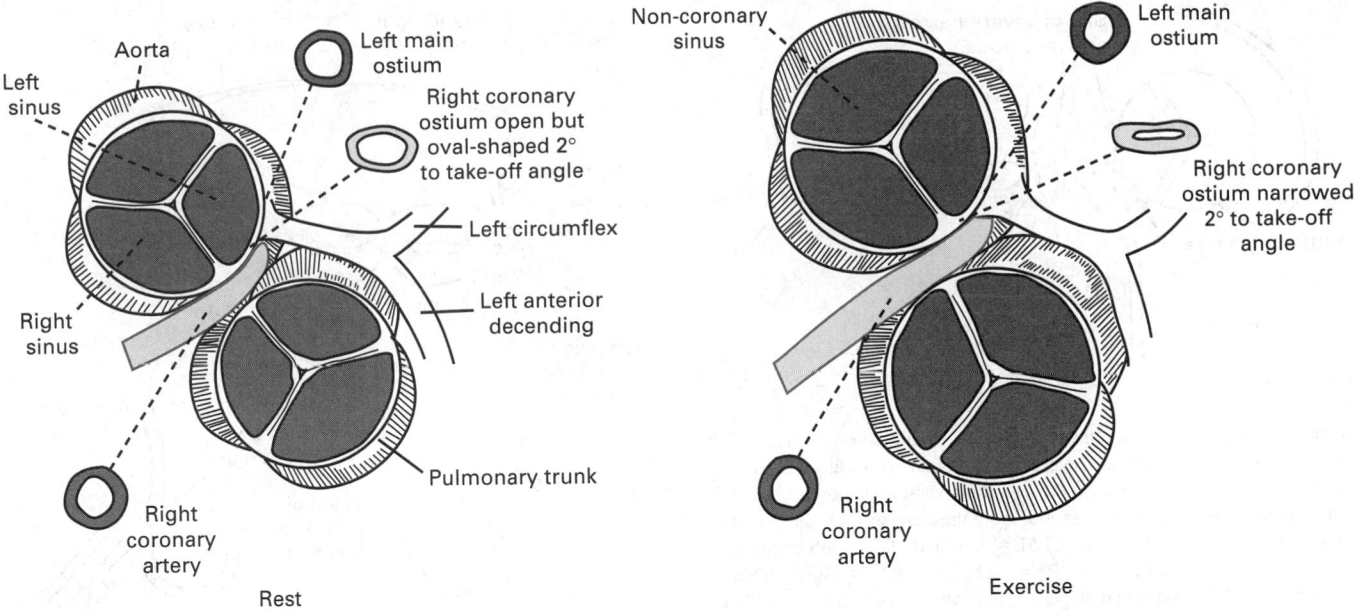

FIGURE 42-3

Diagram showing the proposed mechanism of myocardial ischemia produced by anomalous origin of the right coronary artery from the left sinus of Valsalva. With exercise, the aorta and pulmonary trunk dilate, thereby reducing the already narrowed coronary ostium of the anomalous right coronary. (From Waller.[10] Reproduced with permission from the publisher, editor, and author.)

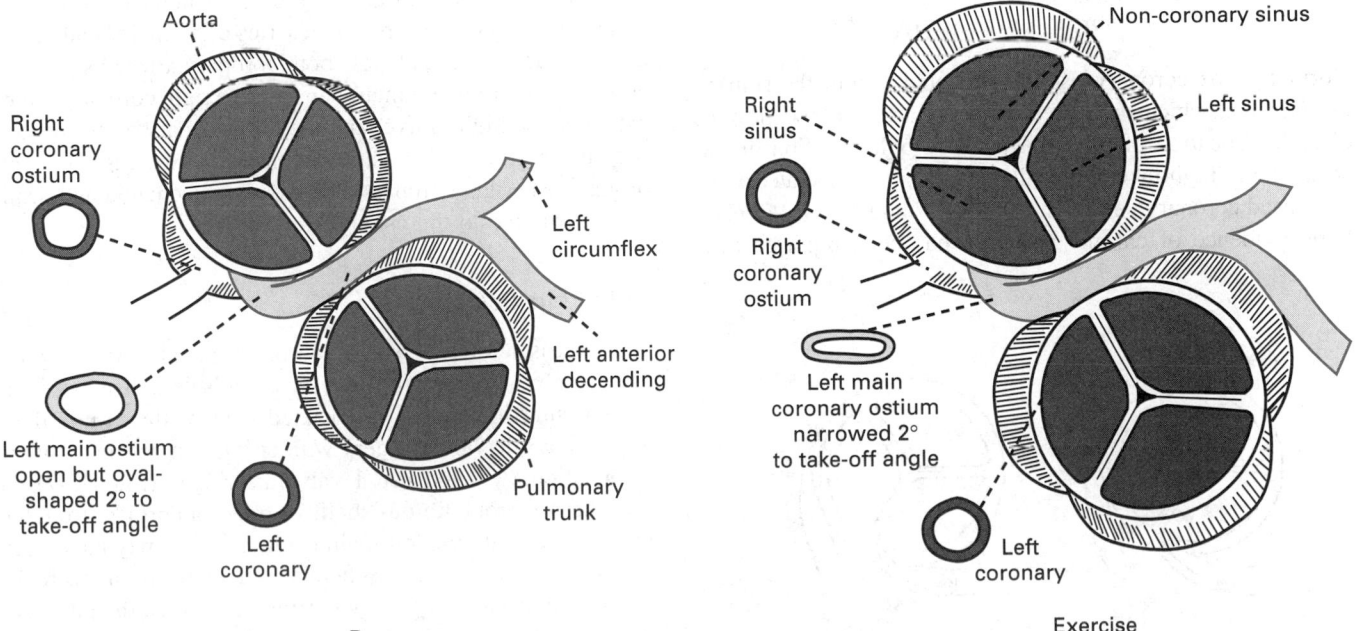

FIGURE 42-4

Diagram showing the proposed mechanism of myocardial ischemia produced by anomalous origin of the left coronary artery from the right sinus of Valsalva. With exercise, the aorta and pulmonary trunk dilate, thereby reducing the already narrowed coronary ostium of the anomalous left coronary. (From Waller.[10] Reproduced with permission from the publisher, editor, and author.)

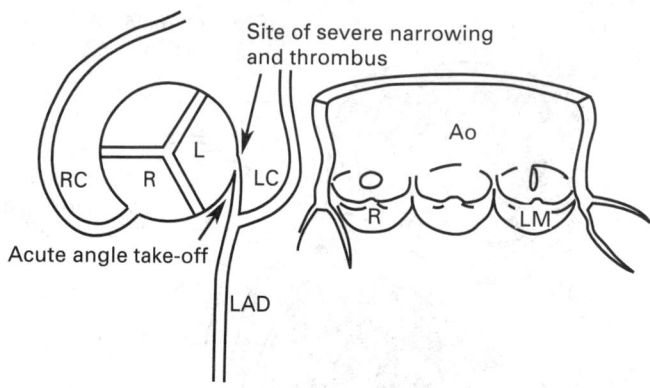

FIGURE 42-5

Diagram showing acute angle takeoff of the left main coronary artery with ostial ridge and slitlike orifice. The proximal left main is occluded by atherosclerotic plaque and thrombus, but the remaining vessels are normal. Accelerated coronary atherosclerosis may result from the acute angle takeoff malformation. Ao = aorta; L = left cusp; LM = left main; LC = left circumflex; LAD = left anterior descending; R = right cusp; RC = right coronary. (From Menke.[11] Reproduced with permission from the publisher and author.)

CORONARY ARTERY ATRESIA

Atresia of one of the two main coronary ostia may be associated with myocardial ischemia and infarction in infancy or childhood.[5] The involved vessel becomes dependent on collateral coronary blood flow from the contralateral coronary artery.

HIGH-TAKEOFF CORONARY OSTIA

Normally, the coronary ostia are located within the sinuses of Valsalva, which optimizes coronary artery blood flow in diastole. Location of the ostia in the tubular portion of the aorta (i.e., "high-takeoff" position) may be associated with decreased coronary perfusion (Figs. 42-7 and 42-8). Morphologic evidence of chronic ischemia has been reported in a

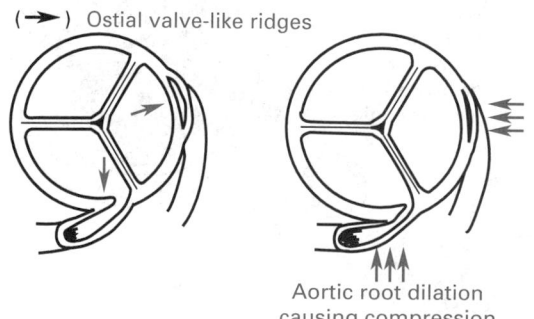

FIGURE 42-6

Diagram illustrating ostial valvelike ridges and the proposed mechanism of ostial compression with aortic root dilation. (From Virmani et al.[12] Reproduced with permission from the publisher and author.)

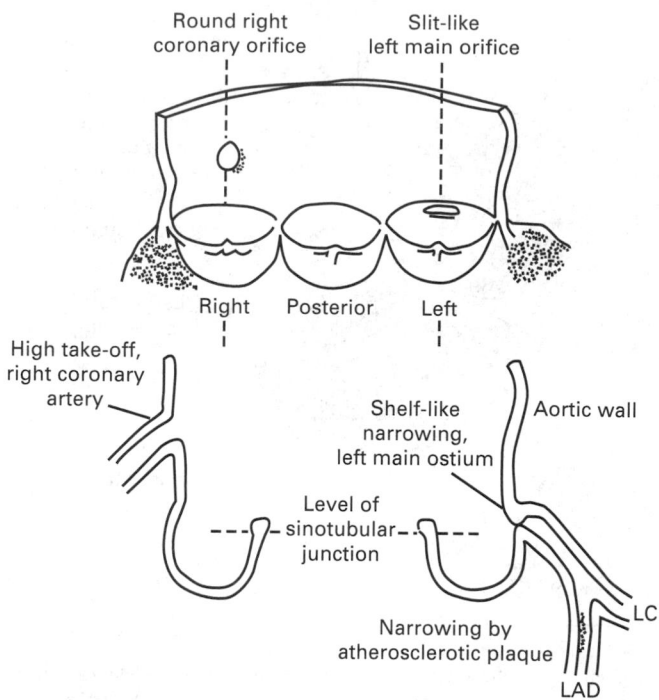

FIGURE 42-7

Diagram showing high takeoff position of the right coronary artery and the nonatherosclerotic fibrous ridge occluding the left main coronary ostium. LAD = left anterior descending; LC = left circumflex. (From Foster et al.[14] Reproduced with permission from the publisher and author.)

patient with a high-takeoff right coronary artery who had right and left ventricular wall scarring.[14,15] High-takeoff position of the coronary ostium also has been postulated as a cause of sudden coronary death.[16] In a series of 54 major and minor coronary artery anomalies,[17] both coronary artery ostia arose above the sinotubular junction in two, the right coronary artery ostium arose high in five, and the left coronary artery ostium was in a high-takeoff position in three. In two cases of high origin of the right coronary artery ostium, ischemia and death were attributed to the ostial lesion in one.[18]

Ostial Fibrous Ridges

Nonatherosclerotic causes of coronary ostial narrowing include syphilis,[19] Takayasu's disease (pulseless disease),[20] fibromuscular hyperplasia associated with methysergide therapy,[21,22] aortic valve surgery with or without coronary artery cannulation,[14,23] and ostial valvelike ridges (Fig. 42-7). A nonatherosclerotic fibrous shelflike ridge can project from the wall of aorta into the left main ostium.[14,15] It may have been responsible for chronic ischemia and myocardial necrosis. Other rare diseases that may narrow or occlude the coronary ostia have been summarized by Baroldi[24]: (1) a nonatheromatous, calcific protrusion from the sinotubular junction into the right or left ostium; (2) saccular aneurysm of the aorta; (3) aortic dissection extending into the coronary ostium—the right ostium involved more commonly than the left; (4) supravalvular aortic stenosis with severe intimal thickening; (5) obliteration of the ostium due to adhesion of the free edge of an aortic cusp to the aortic wall above the coronary ostium; (6) occlusion by embolus (see below); and (7) occlusive fibroelastosis.

ANOMALOUS ORIGIN OF ONE OR TWO CORONARY ARTERIES FROM THE PULMONARY TRUNK

Anomalous origin of a coronary artery from the pulmonary trunk (Figs. 42-9 and 42-10) may be responsible for myocardial ischemia and infarction in infants and children. In more than 90 percent of cases,[5,7] the left main is the anomalous artery; thus the anteroseptal and anterolateral left ventricular myocardium may be at jeopardy for injury. Asymptomatic older patients with this coronary anomaly are usually found when they present with an abnormal electrocardiogram (ECG), a systolic murmur, or sudden death.[7] The murmur and abnormal ECG are the result of papillary muscle and/or anteroseptal myocardial wall damage (see Chap. 47).

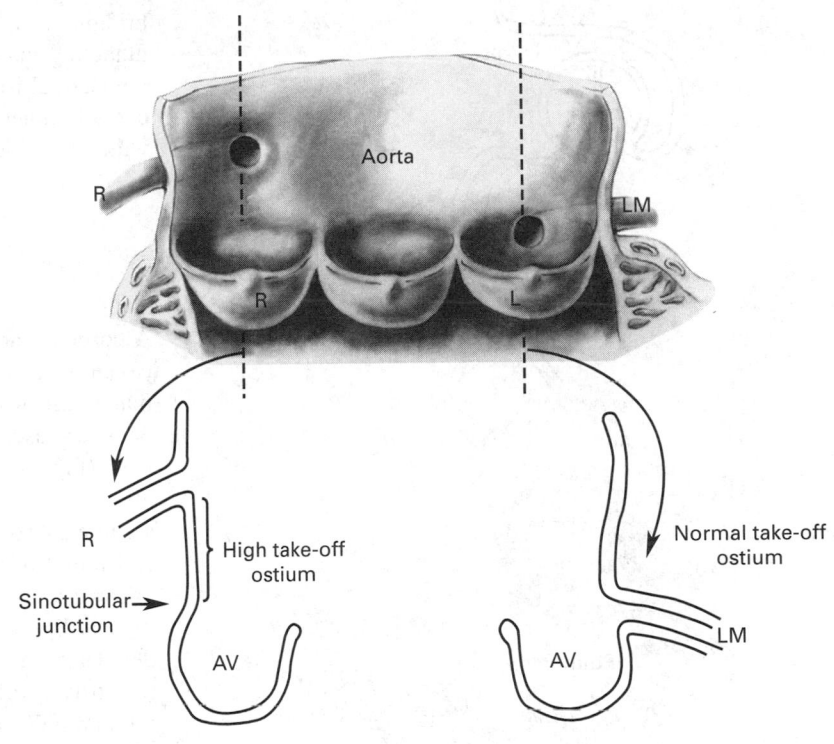

FIGURE 42-8

Diagram showing origin of right coronary ostium above the sinotubular junction—"high-takeoff position." AV = aortic valve; L = left cusp; LM = left main; R = right cusp or right coronary artery.

MYOCARDIAL BRIDGES ("TUNNELED" EPICARDIAL CORONARY ARTERY)

The coronary arteries may dip into the myocardium for varying lengths and then reappear on the heart's surface (Figs. 42-11 to 42-18). The muscle overlying the intramyocardial segment of the epicardial coronary artery is termed a *myocardial bridge*, and the artery coursing within the myocardium is called a *tunneled artery* (see Figs. 42-11 to 42-13).[25–63] Tunneled coronary arteries have long been recognized anatomically,[25] but suggested associations between myocardial ischemia and myocardial bridges have heightened their clinical relevance.[26,27]

Tunneled coronary arteries have been presumed congenital in origin.[28] At least three factors have been postulated to account for differences between the high frequency of tunneled major coronary arteries observed at necropsy (5[29] to 86 percent[30,57]) and the lower frequency of tunneled coronary arteries observed

angiographically (0.5[26] to 12 percent[31,32,58–60]) or associated with symptoms of myocardial ischemia (18 percent[32]): (1) length of the tunneled coronary segment, (2) degree of systolic compression, and (3) heart rate. Longer tunneled segments of coronary arteries,[27] more severe systolic diameter narrowing of the tunneled segment,[27] and tachycardia[33] may contribute to the production of myocardial ischemia with myocardial

CORONARY ARTERIES ARISING FROM PULMONARY TRUNK ASSOCIATED WITH MYOCARDIAL INFARCTION

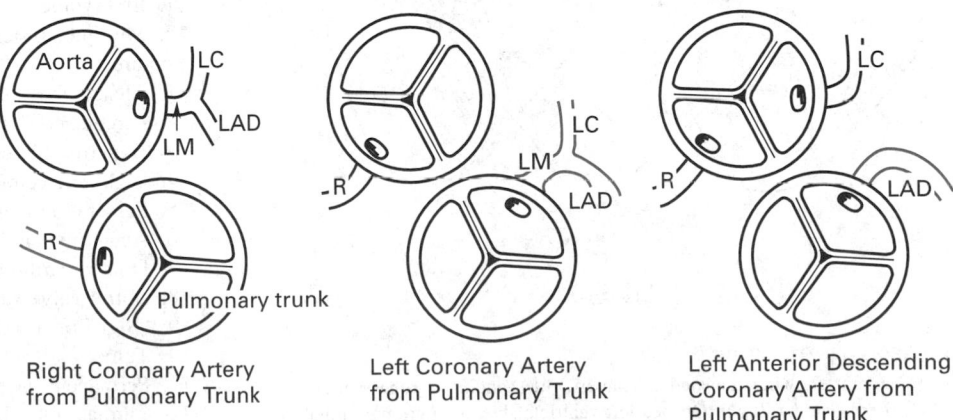

Right Coronary Artery from Pulmonary Trunk

Left Coronary Artery from Pulmonary Trunk

Left Anterior Descending Coronary Artery from Pulmonary Trunk

FIGURE 42-9

Anomalous origin of one or two major epicardial coronary arteries from the pulmonary trunk. (From Waller.[1] Reproduced with permission from the publisher, editor, and author.) For abbreviations, see Fig. 42-2.

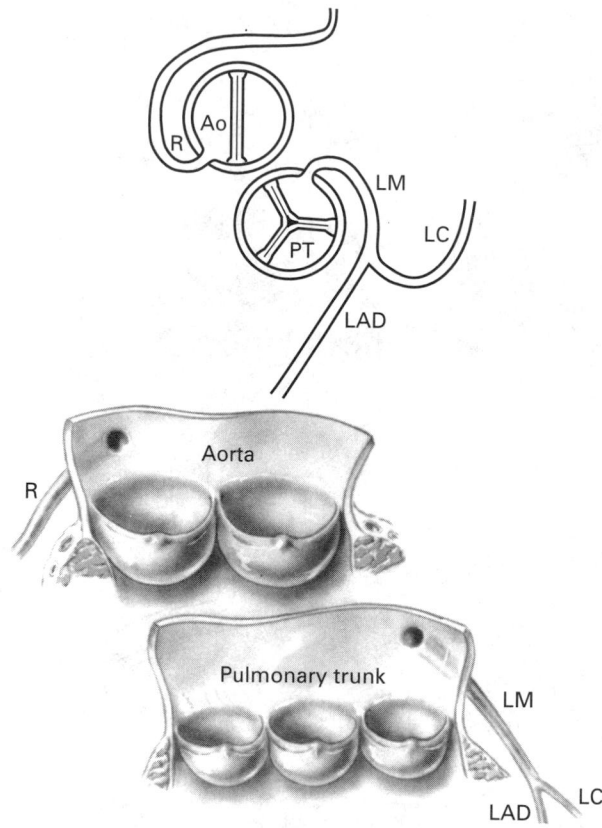

FIGURE 42-10

Anomalous origin of the main (LM) coronary artery from the pulmonary trunk causing acute myocardial infarction in an infant. Of interest is both the anomalous LM and normal right coronary arteries arise in high-takeoff positions from the pulmonary trunk and aorta (Ao) respectively. LAD = left anterior descending; LC = left circumflex.

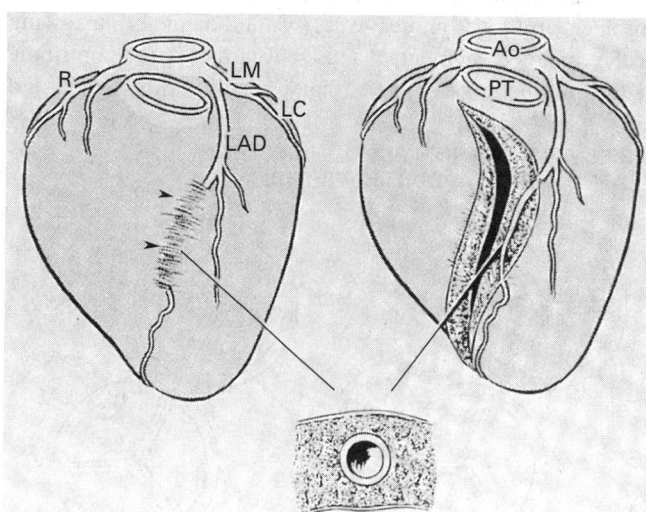

FIGURE 42-11

Left: Diagram showing tunneled left anterior descending coronary artery (LAD) (*arrowheads*). *Right:* Opened left ventricle showing intramyocardial segment. *Below:* Transverse section of left ventricular wall showing tunneled coronary artery surrounded by myocardium. (From Waller.[1] Reproduced with permission from the publisher, editor, and author.)

bridging (see Figs. 42-17 and 42-18). The length of coronary tunneling may not always be an important factor in causing myocardial ischemia, as three cases with left main intramyocardial tunneling of greater than 40 mm have been described without evidence of myocardial ischemia[34,35] (see Fig. 42-19).

CORONARY ARTERY FISTULA

A coronary artery fistula is an abnormal communication between an epicardial coronary artery and a cardiac chamber, major vessel (vena cava, submonary veins, pulmonary artery), or other vascular structure (mediastinal vessels, coronary sinus) (Fig. 42-20).[5,64–113] This infrequent abnormality can affect any age and is the most important hemodynamically significant coronary artery anomaly.[5,64–113] Many are small and found incidentally during coronary arteriography, while others are identified as the cause of a continuous murmur, myocardial ischemia angina, acute myocardial infarction, sudden death coronary steal, congestive heart failure, endocarditis, stroke, arrhythmias, coronary aneurysm formation (rupture, emboli), or superior vena cava syndrome.[64–76] Of over 33,000 patients undergoing coronary arteriography,[34] coronary artery fistula occurred in 0.1 percent,[76] whether due to congenital[77–85] or acquired causes[76–113] (Table 42-3). Fistulas from the right coronary artery are more common than from the left[64–113] and over 90 percent of the fistulas drain into the venous circulation.[64–113] Most fistulas are single communications, but multiple fistulas have been identified.[106] The natural history of coronary artery fistulas is variable, with

TABLE 42-3

CAUSES AND ASSOCIATIONS
OF CORONARY ARTERY FISTULA

I. Congenital[77–85]
  1. Embryonic
  2. Multiple; systemic hemangioma
II. Acquired
  1. Closed-chest ablation of accessory pathway[86]
  2. Percutaneous coronary balloon angioplasty[87–89]
  3. Hypertrophic cardiomyopathy[90]
  4. Right/left ventricular septal myectomy[101]
  5. Penetrating and nonpenetrating trauma[102–104]
  6. Acute myocardial infarction[91,93]
  7. Dilated cardiomyopathy[94]
  8. Mitral valve surgery[95]
  9. "Sign" of mural thrombus[96]
  10. Tumor[100]
  11. Permanent pacemaker placement[99]
  12. Cardiac transplant[92]
  13. Endomyocardial biopsy[97,98]
  14. Coronary artery bypass grafting[105]

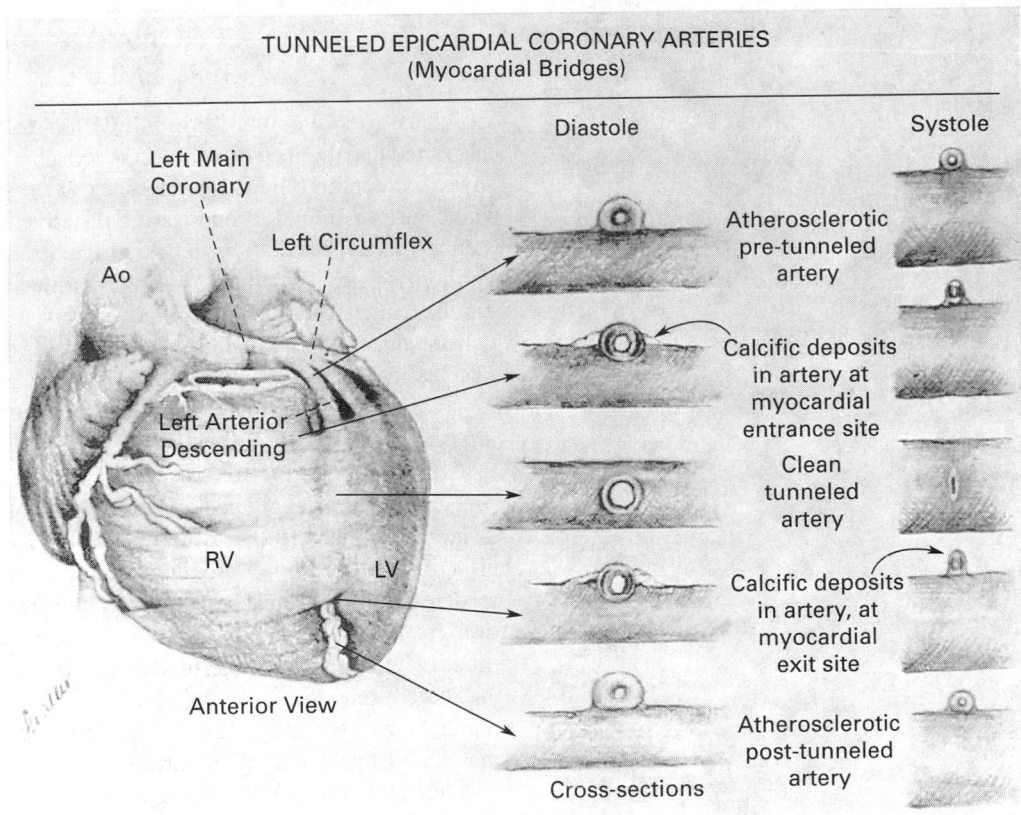

TUNNELED EPICARDIAL CORONARY ARTERIES
(Myocardial Bridges)

Diastole   Systole

Left Main Coronary

Left Circumflex

Ao

Left Arterior Descending

Atherosclerotic pre-tunneled artery

Calcific deposits in artery at myocardial entrance site

Clean tunneled artery

RV   LV

Calcific deposits in artery, at myocardial exit site

Anterior View

Atherosclerotic post-tunneled artery

Cross-sections

FIGURE 42-12
Diagram showing segments of tunneled and nontunneled epicardial coronary artery with changes during ventricular systole and diastole. Ao = aorta; LV = left ventricle; RV = right ventricle. (From Waller.[10] Reproduced with permission from the publisher, editor, and author.)

long periods of stability in some and sudden onset or gradual progression of symptoms in others. Spontaneous closure is uncommon.[106–108] Surgical repair of the fistula is recommended for symptomatic patients and for those asymptomatic patients at risk for future complications (coronary steals, aneurysms, large shunts).[109–112] Transcatheter embolization of fistulas has been reported.[113] Direct connection between a major epicardial coronary artery and a cardiac chamber or major vessel (vena cava, coronary sinus, pulmonary artery) is the most common hemodynamically significant coronary artery anomaly (Fig. 42-19).[5] Fistulas from the right coronary artery are more common than from the left. Over 90 percent of the fistulas drain into the venous circulation.[5] Myocardial ischemia has been documented in some patients with coronary artery fistulas who have no evidence of coronary atherosclerosis.[5]

Treatment of symptomatic, clinically recognized myocardial bridges has involved beta and calcium channel blockers (control of tachycardia and antispasmodic effects) and surgery. Several cases have now been reported[61–63] in which "supraarterial myotomy" (release of myocardial bridge, excision of myocardial bridge) has resulted in relief of symptoms and improvement in previously abnormal nuclear imaging tests. High-frequency intraoperative echocardiography has been used to image the intramyocardial coronary artery before and after surgical release.[61]

CORONARY ANEURYSMS

Aneurysm formation of the coronary arteries may result from congenital or acquired conditions. Congenital coronary artery aneurysms are found most commonly in the right coronary artery.[114] Abnormal flow patterns within the aneurysm may lead to thrombus formation, with subsequent vessel occlusion, distal thromboembolization, and myocardial infarction.[115] In general, angina pectoris or acute myocardial infarction present in patients less than 20 years of age should prompt suspicion of a congenital coronary artery anomaly or a congenital coronary artery aneurysm.[114] Coronary artery aneurysms are found in about 1.5 percent of patients studied at necropsy or by coronary arteriography.[37] Coronary artery aneurysms, which may be multiple, can be congenital or the result of atherosclerosis, trauma, angioplasty, atherectomy, laser procedures, arteritis (including syphilis), mycotic emboli, mucocutaneous lymph node syndrome (Kawasaki's disease), systemic lupus erythematosus,[116] or dissection (spontaneous or secondary) (Table 42-4). Atherosclerosis-induced aneurysms are thought to result from primary thinning and/or destruction of the media and may represent up to 50 percent of the causes (Table 42-4). Angioplasty, atherectomy, vasculitis, and arteritis may also damage the arterial wall (media) and lead to coronary aneurysms.

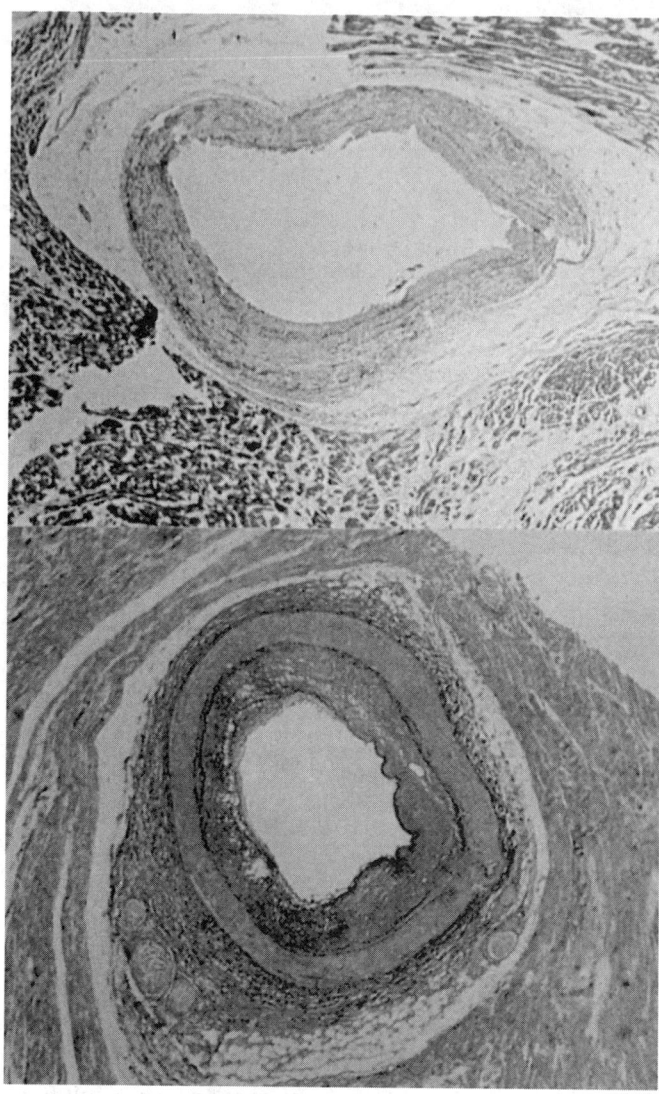

FIGURE 42-13
Tunneled epicardial coronary arteries. Two examples of tunneled left anterior descending coronary arteries. Each artery is surrounded by myocardium. (From Waller.[1] Reproduced with permission from the publisher, editor, and author.)

TABLE 42-4
CAUSES OF CORONARY ARTERIAL ANEURYSMS

Atherosclerosis (destruction of coronary media)
Trauma
Angioplasty
Atherectomy
Laser
Arteritis (including syphilis, lupus erythematosus)
Mycotic emboli
Mucocutaneous lymph node syndrome (Kawasaki's disease)
Congenital
Dissection
Neoplasm
Connective tissue disorders (Ehlers-Danlos, Marfan's)

CORONARY ARTERY EMBOLI

Coronary arterial emboli (Figs. 42-21 to 42-25) are clinically suspected in patients who develop severe chest pain with acute myocardial infarction in the presence of a prosthetic left-sided valve, active infective endocarditis, native left-sided valve stenosis, atrial fibrillation, left ventricular aneurysm, dilated cardiomyopathy (Fig. 42-22), known cardiac tumor, or during cardiac catheterization or cardiac surgery. Coronary emboli can be due to natural, iatrogenic, or "paradoxical" causes (Table 42-5) (Figs. 42-21 to 42-25). Coronary embolism most often involves the left anterior descending coronary artery.[36]

Coronary embolism is suspected as the cause of acute myocardial infarction when, at necropsy, the zone of necrosis is large but discrete (since there was little time to develop effective collaterals). Embolic coronary artery lesions can resolve completely and spontaneously and provide an explanation for angiographically normal coronary arteries several months following an acute myocardial infarction.[36]

The consequences of coronary embolism depend on two major factors (see Fig. 42-25): the size of the embolus and the size of the lumen of the artery in which it becomes impacted.[139,140] The smaller the embolus, the greater the chance that it will travel distally to a small coronary arterial segment and the less the likelihood of myocardial infarction or fatal arrhythmia.[139] An embolus so small that it travels distally and impacts in a single intramural vessel is probably clinically silent and observed only at necropsy.[139,140] The status of the coronary lumen before the embolus appears also determines the subsequent myocardial consequences. An embolus to a previously normal coronary artery is likely to migrate distally and result in localized myocardial infarction because of absence of collaterals. An embolus traveling to a previously diseased coronary artery is more likely to impact proximally. Emboli to the left main coronary arteries are rare but usually fatal (see Fig. 42-24).[140]

CORONARY ARTERY DISSECTION

Separation of the media by hemorrhage with or without an associated intimal tear is termed *coronary artery dissection*. The medial separation forces the intimal-medial layer (wall of true channel) toward the true coronary lumen and produces distal myocardial ischemia/infarction (Figs. 42-26 and 42-27). Coronary artery dissections may be primary or secondary (Table 42-6).[141–168] Secondary coronary artery dissections are more frequent, especially those associated as an extension from aortic root dissection (8 percent).[5] Primary coronary artery dissections may occur spontaneously or as a consequence of coronary angioplasty or angiography, cardiac surgery, or chest trauma (0.3 percent).[158] Most spontaneous coronary artery dissections occur in women who are most

TABLE 42-5

ETIOLOGY OF CORONARY ARTERY EMBOLI

Natural
  Vegetation
  Active infective endocarditis (native valve)
  Active infective endocarditis (prosthetic valve)
  Mural endocarditis
  Noninfective (marantic) endocarditis
  Calcific deposit
  Aortic valve stenosis
  Mitral valve stenosis
  Intracardiac thrombus
  Left ventricle (myocardial infarction, cardiomyopathy,
    fibroelastosis with mural thrombus, ventricular
    aneurysm)
  Left atrium—appendage (low-cardiac-output states)
  Left atrium—body (mitral stenosis, native or prosthetic)
  Pulmonary veins (mitral stenosis)
  Intracardiac tumor
  Primary (myxoma)
  Secondary (extension from pulmonary veins, lymphatic
    extension, direct extension)
  Coronary artery
  Plaque rupture (cholesterol)
  Thrombus dislodgment

Iatrogenic
  Cardiac surgery (ostial cannulization, prosthetic valve,
    patch repair)
  Cardiac catheterization and angiography (catheter
    thrombus, catheter fragments)
  Coronary angioplasty, other interventions, catheter
    balloon valvuloplasty and thrombolysis
  Prosthetic valves (thrombus, vegetation, occluders,
    leaflets, cloth covering, struts)
  Cardioversion (left atrial thrombus, left ventricular
    thrombus)
  Cardiac resuscitation (thrombus)
  Trauma—blunt penetrating, nonpenetrating, foreign body
    (bullet)
  "Paradoxical"
  Congenital heart disease (atrial septal defect, ventricular
    septal defect)
  Probe patent foramen ovale defect (thrombophlebitis,
    right atrial catheters)
  Pulmonary hypertension (acquired atrial septal defect)
  Interatrial flap valve (fossa ovale aneurysm)

Source: Waller.[1] Reproduced with permission from the author, editor, and publisher.

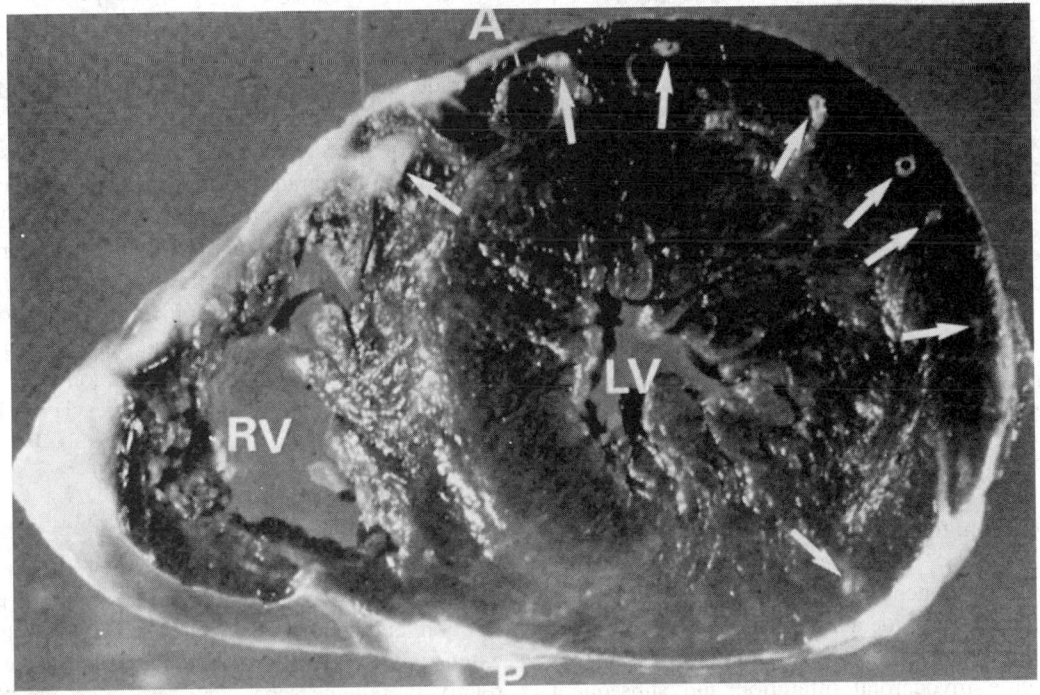

FIGURE 42-14

Transverse section of ventricular myocardium showing the "arcade" of tunneled epicardial coronary arteries (*arrows*). A = anterior; LV = left ventricle; RV = right ventricle; P = posterior. (From Waller.[1] Reproduced with permission from the publisher, editor, and author.)

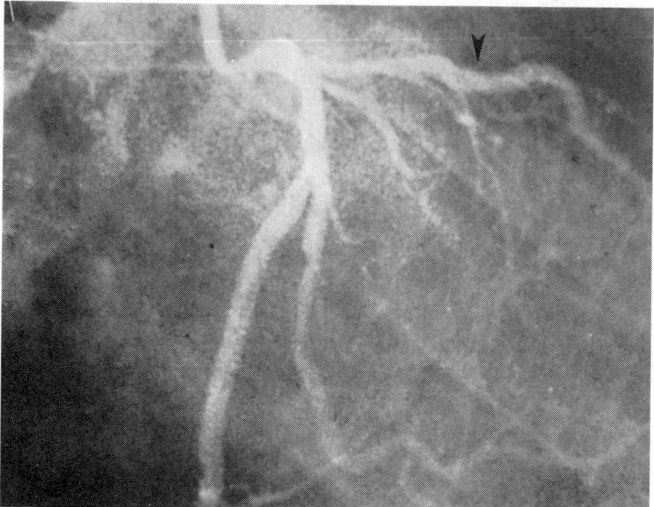

A

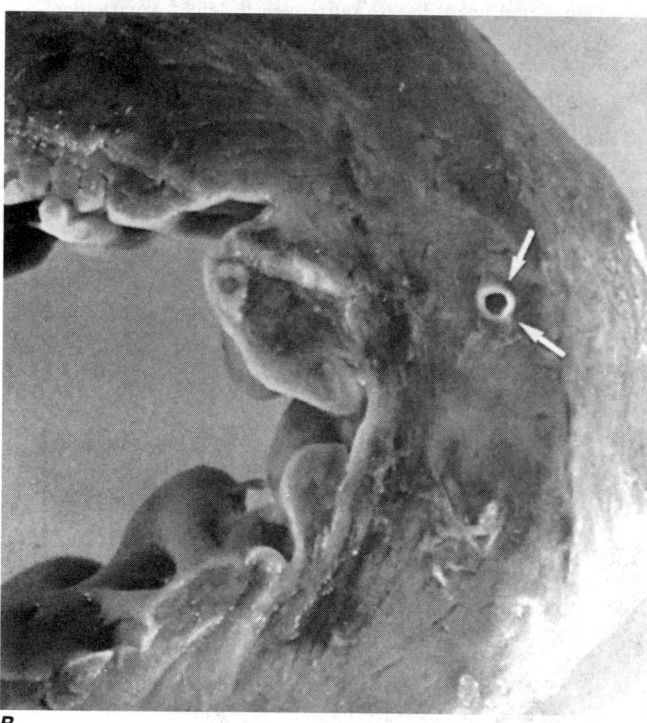

B

FIGURE 42-15

Tunneled epicardial coronary artery. *A.* Coronary angiogram showing tunneled segment of epicardial coronary artery. *B.* Corresponding segment of tunneled left circumflex coronary artery (*arrow*). (From Waller.[1] Reproduced with permission from the publisher, editor, and author.)

commonly postpartum; they may be associated with coronary artery wall eosinophils.[141–165] The left anterior descending artery is the one most frequently involved. Systemic hypertension does not appear to provide a significant factor of risk.[114]

Spontaneous coronary artery dissection may result in sudden death or acute myocardial infarction and subsequent death. Parenthetically, localized and limited coronary artery dissection (i.e., intimal-media tear) appears necessary for a clinically successful coronary artery balloon angioplasty procedure[143,144] (see also Chap. 48).

TABLE 42-6

CAUSES OF CORONARY ARTERY DISSECTIONS[141–168]

I. Spontaneous
  A. Post- or peripartum[142,146,148,156,160,161,163,164,166,167]
  B. With or without eosinophilia[142,156,161,163]
  C. Idiopathic[145,150–152,154,158,159,162,163,165]
  D. Systemic hypertension[155]
  E. Coronary spasm
  F. Aortic root dissection[163] (hypertension, medial degeneration)
  G. Arteritis[162]
  H. Fibromuscular hyperplasia
II. Trauma
  A. Post- or peripartum[146,148,160,164,167]
  B. Blunt chest[157] (penetrating, nonpenetrating)
  C. Coronary angiography[153]
  D. Coronary interventions[147,168] (angioplasty, atherectomy, laser, stenting, rotablade)
  E. Cardiac surgery (coronary bypass, coronary ostial cannulation, endarterectomy)
  F. Aortic root dissection[149] (surgery, nonpenetrating, penetrating)

Coronary angioplasty dissections viewed in short- or long-axis tomographic images help distinguish dissections that are *therapeutic* (mechanism) from those which are *complications of angioplasty* (complications).[168] In the short-axis image, dissection involving more than 50 percent of the coronary media circumference has been considered a complication. Similarly, in the long-axis image, dissections (antegrade, retrograde, or both) longer than 1 cm in length have also been defined as a complication of angioplasty (Fig. 42-28). A combination of dissection >50 percent of short-axis circumference and >1 cm antegrade or retrograde of long-axis length may result in "intussusception" of intimal-medial tissue. Spiral dissections ("the ugly") are among the most serious dissection injuries after balloon angioplasty (Fig. 42-29). The spiral dissection as reviewed angiographically appears to alternate from side to side, extending antegrade and retrograde (Fig. 42-29A), or it has an unaltered dissection course but appears alternating from limited angiographic views (Fig. 42-29B).

CORONARY ARTERY SPASM

Coronary artery luminal narrowing produced by spasm has been associated with angina pectoris, acute myocardial infarction, and sudden death[141,169–195] (Chap. 46). Despite the extensive clinical information about coronary artery spasm, relatively few necropsy data are available.[169–181] Smooth muscle cells in the coronary artery wall may contract in response to various neurologic and pharmacologic stimuli and temporarily reduce the vessel lumen. Specific pathogenesis of this disorder is unknown[180] (see also Chap. 44). Enhanced

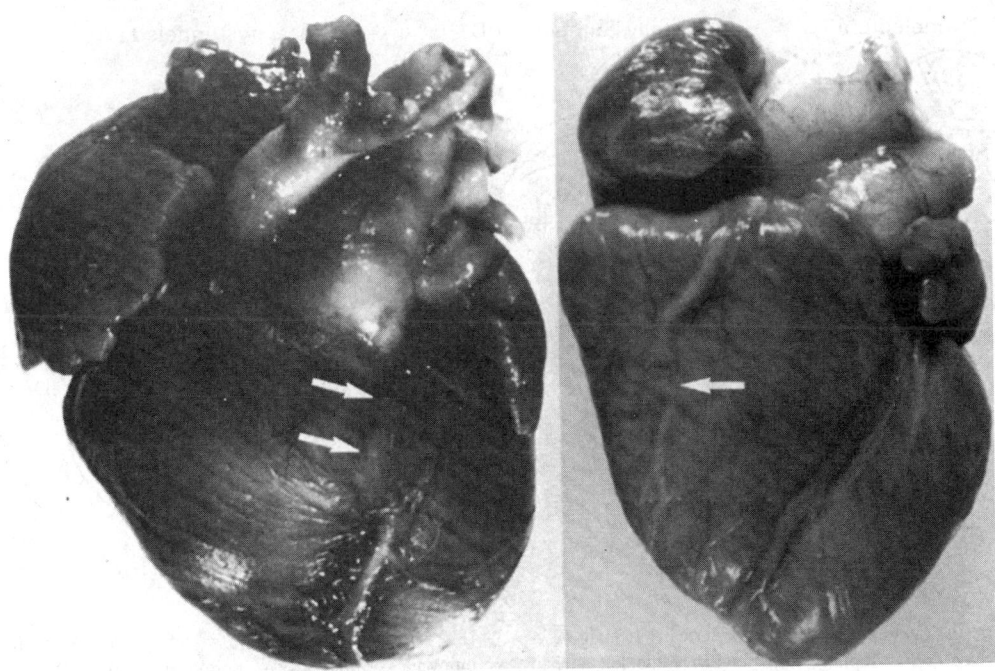

FIGURE 42-16

Tunneled left anterior epicardial coronary arteries from two newborn infants. *Left:* Tunneled left anterior descending. *Right:* Tunneled marginal branch of right coronary artery. (From Waller.[1] Reproduced with permission from the publisher, editor, and author.)

alpha-adrenergic tone[191] and various vasoactive substances—such as histamine, catecholamines, prostaglandins, thromboxane[189–192]—are presently thought to be relevant factors. Necropsy findings have been reviewed in 13 previously reported cases and in 3 new cases[141,180,195] (Figs. 42-30 and 42-31).

Most of the 13 previous patients with clinical evidence of spasm had significant fixed coronary luminal narrowing due to atherosclerotic plaque, although coronary angiograms during life did not recognize these lesions found at necropsy.[141,195] In one of the original patients described by Prinzmetal and colleagues,[169] both major epicardial coronary arteries were "markedly sclerotic," and the "posterior coronary artery" was 80 percent narrowed. Of the subsequent 12 necropsy patients, 10 had at least one major artery severely narrowed by atherosclerotic plaque at necropsy.[169–181] The three necropsy patients with clinical spasm[141,180] all had se-

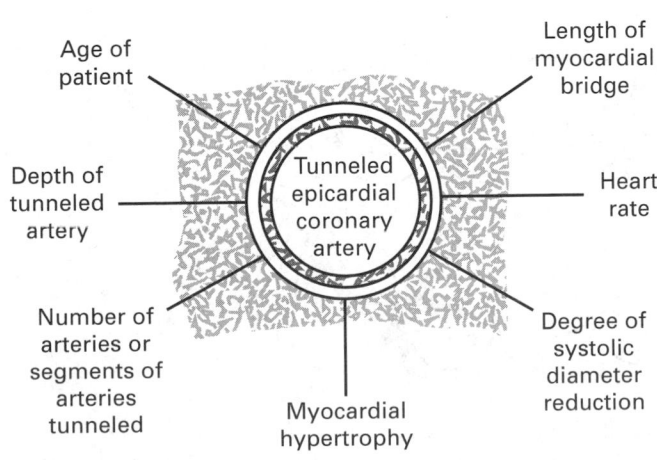

FIGURE 42-17

Diagram showing some of the clinical and anatomic factors in a tunneled epicardial coronary artery. (From Waller.[1] Reproduced with permission from the publisher, editor, and author.)

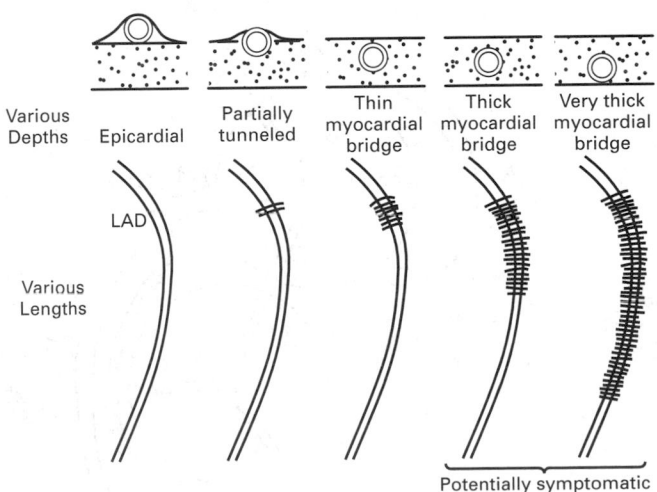

FIGURE 42-18

Diagram showing morphologic variations in tunneling (length of tunneled segment, depth of tunneled segment). (From Waller.[1] Reproduced with permission from the publisher, editor, and author.)

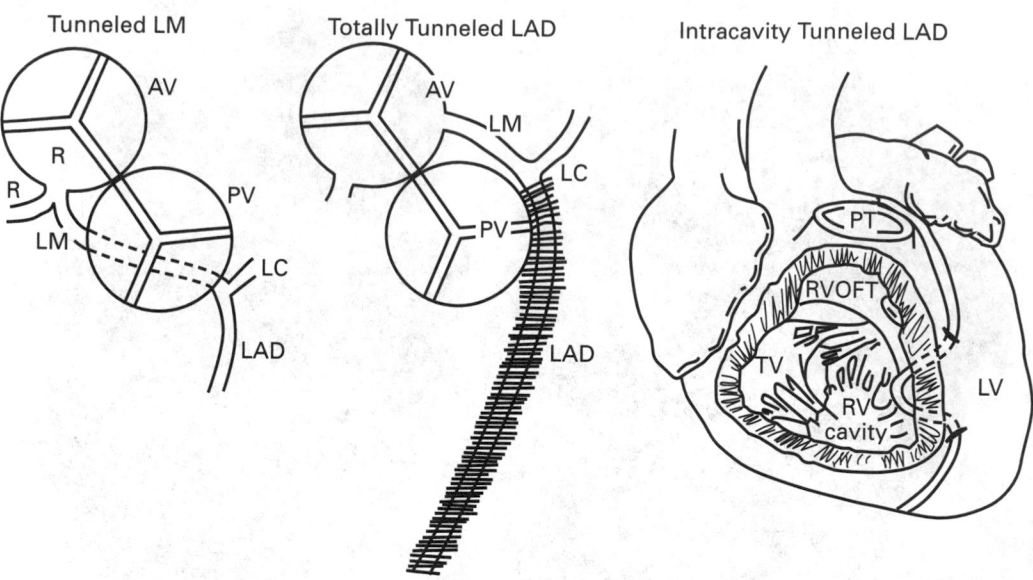

FIGURE 42-19

Diagram showing extremes of tunneled coronary arteries: left main (LM) tunneled through the ventricular septum, total length of the left anterior descending (LAD) located within the myocardium, tunneled segment of LAD becoming intracavitary. AV = aortic valve; LAD = left anterior descending; LC = left circumflex; LM = left main; LV = left ventricular; PT = pulmonary trunk; PV = pulmonary valve; RVOFT = right ventricular outflow tract; RV = right ventricle; TV = tricuspid valve. (From Waller.[1] Reproduced with permission from the publisher, editor, and author.)

vere luminal coronary narrowing by atherosclerotic plaque at least in the artery in which spasm had been demonstrated during life (see Figs. 42-30 and 42-31). In general, histologic sections of the left anterior descending artery at the site of spasm disclosed luminal concentric plaque that had a predominance of smooth muscle cells, suggesting that the lesion may have been responsive to pharmacologic and neurologic stimuli compared with "garden-variety" fibrotic and calcified athero-

sclerotic plaque (Fig. 42-31). In a patient with normal angiograms and documented myocardial infarction, "intimal ridges" were observed on postmortem angiography; these were interpreted as evidence of spasm.[194] Similar ridges have been noted at necropsy in a patient with coronary artery spasm.[195] Histology of the ridges disclosed typical atherosclerotic plaque,[196] suggesting that varying degrees of dynamic muscular contraction may be superimposed upon fixed atheroscle-

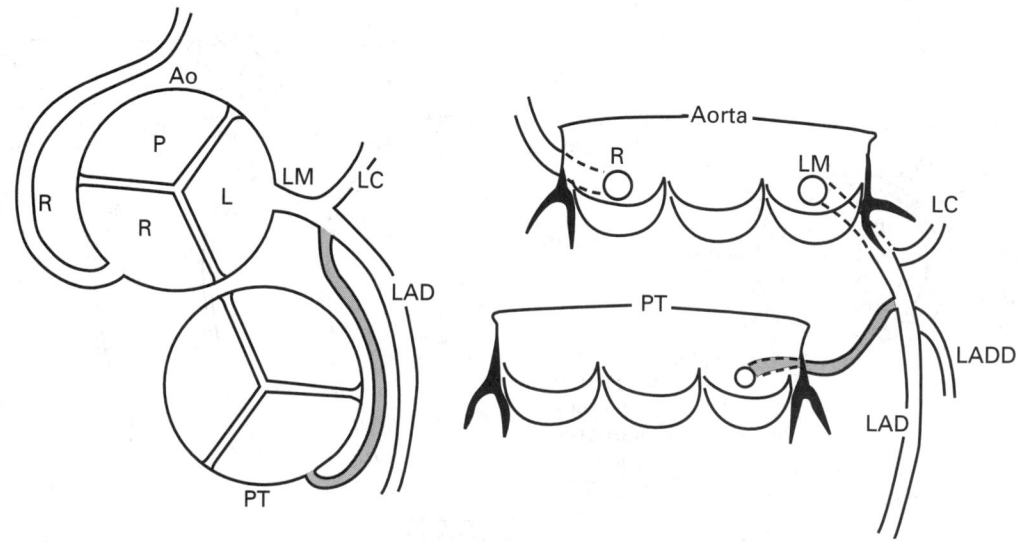

FIGURE 42-20

Diagram showing coronary artery fistula connecting pulmonary trunk and left anterior descending (LAD) artery. It originally was misdiagnosed as an anomalous coronary artery. LADD = diagonal branch of LAD: LC = left circumflex; LM = left main; R = right.

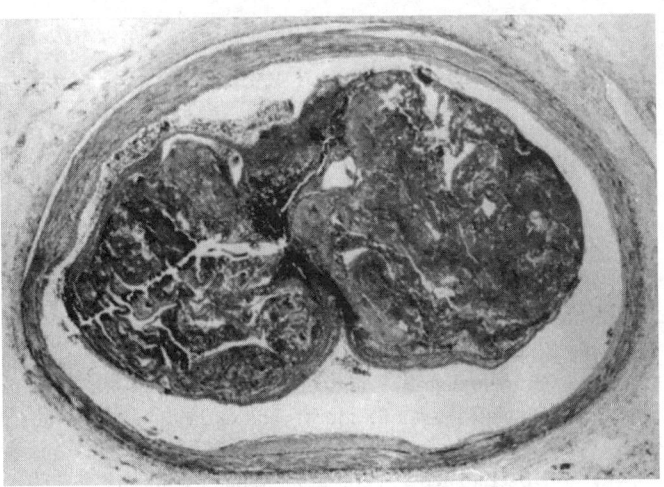

FIGURE 42-21

Coronary artery embolus. Fibrin-platelet thrombus occluding the left anterior descending coronary artery. The source of the embolus was not established, but the patient recently underwent cardiac surgery. (From Waller.[1] Reproduced with permission from the publisher, editor, and author.)

rotic lesions, presumably related to the amount of smooth muscle present.[141] Coronary artery smooth muscle depletion ("medial attenuation"), which accompanies advanced degrees of luminal narrowing by atherosclerotic plaque, suggests diminished potential for coronary wall spasm.[196] It has recently been suggested that medial "contraction" bands may represent a morphologic-histologic marker for arteries that have spasm during life[197] (see also Chap. 46).

Eccentric atherosclerotic plaques have a segment of disease-free wall with preserved media which presumably has the potential for spasm[198] (see also Chap. 44). In patients with clinical coronary spasm, unstable and stable angina pectoris, and episodes of silent myocardial ischemia, where 448 segments were narrowed by more than 75 percent in cross-sectional area by plaques, 15 percent of these segments had a variable arc of disease-free wall with normal media. Other studies have found a similar 15 to 20 percent of the coronary wall normal in 70 percent of cases studied.[200–205] This disease-free coronary segment represents a site of "vasospastic potential" and could convert a hemodynamically insignificant lesion of less than 50 percent cross-sectional area into a hemodynamically significant one of more than 75 percent narrowing.

Three newly recognized associations and/or causes of coronary spasm include general anesthesia,[184] "allergic angina" (histamine-induced),[185] and postpartum bromocriptine usage.[186] Acute ST segment elevation has been noted following induction of general anesthesia in some patients with angiographically normal coronary arteries.[184] In postpartum women receiving bromocriptine in the presence of pregnancy-induced hypertension acute myocardial infarction has occurred.[186] Coronary spasm also occurs with balloon angioplasty and coronary interventional procedures,[187] catheter-related angiography, and neurofibromatosis.[188]

Endothelial cell dysfunction has been proposed to explain coronary vasospasm.[189] In response to increases in shear stress, platelet products and other agonists, normal endothelial cells release endothelium-derived relaxing factor (nitric oxide), resulting in vasodilation.[189] When endothelium is damaged, as occurs with hypertension, elevated cholesterol, smoking, or use of cocaine, endothelial nitric oxide is reduced or lost. Thus, when platelets aggregate at such sites with release of vasospastic substances such as serotonin (5HT) and thromboxane A_2, arterial smooth muscle cells contract, causing spasm.[190]

CORONARY ARTERY TRAUMA

Coronary artery trauma may produce myocardial ischemia and/or acute myocardial infarction. Traumatic injury may result from a nonpenetrating blunt chest wall injury such as a steering-wheel injury, penetration trauma such as a laceration from a stab wound or bullet, coronary bypass surgery as from inadvertent ligation, laceration, or intimal dissection, or after coronary angiography or angioplasty resulting in dissection, rupture, or embolus. Nonpenetrating trauma may produce coronary injury and subsequent myocardial infarction due to coronary dissection, contusion and thrombosis, fistula formation, and/or coronary artery aneurysm formation.[5] Extensive coronary artery dissections occur more commonly as the result of catheter or cannula injury in normal or nearly normal arteries as opposed to coronary arteries with severe atherosclerotic plaque (see also Chap. 87).

CORONARY ARTERY ARTERITIS (VASCULITIS)

Epicardial coronary arteritis (vasculitis) is a rare event but has been reported in several conditions (Table 42-7). The resulting coronary injury may lead to myocardial ischemia/infarction with or without associated coronary artery thrombosis. This type of coronary artery damage has been classified by route(s) of entry[24]: *direct extension* from adjacent organ or tissue infections, e.g., epicardial or myocardial abscess from aortic valve endocarditis, pericardial infections such as tuberculosis; *hematogenous spread* through the coronary lumen or vasa vasorum; and *unknown* route of entry. In the direct extension route of entry, the adventitial layer of the artery is initially involved, whereas in the hematogenous route the coronary intimal layer is initially involved. Evidence of coronary arteritis has included[24] the following: (1) focal artery necrosis with or without calcification; (2) acute coronary artery thrombosis or recanalized thrombus associated with underlying atherosclerotic plaque; (3) rupture of the vessel wall unassociated with trauma or an interventional procedure; (4) coronary artery wall thickening with secondary luminal narrowing; or (5) wall thickening with aneurysm formation.[204] Specific coronary lesions may also be seen with systemic diseases such as tuberculosis or polyarteritis periarteritis.

TABLE 42-7

SOME CONDITIONS ASSOCIATED WITH CORONARY ARTERY ARTERITIS (VASCULITIS)

Tuberculosis[24,238,239]
Polyarteritis nodosa[24,205,310–324]
Giant–cell arteritis[205,226–228,266–277]
Systemic lupus erythematosus[205,358–362]
Burger's disease (thromboangiitis obliterans)[205,303–307]
Wegener's granulomatosis[205,342–355]
Salmonella[4,340]
Leprosy[4]
Mucocutaneous lymph node syndrome[326–339]
Takayasu's disease[208,247–265]
Typhus[232]
Infective endocarditis[341]
Rheumatic diseases[205,276–297]
Ankylosing spondylitis[293]
Syphilis[5,114,205,233–237]
Malaria[241]
Schistosoma haematobium[242]
Rickettsial infections[205,242–244]
Viruses[205,245,246]

Source: Waller.[1] Reproduced with permission from the author, editor, and publisher.

A more recent classification of coronary vasculitides has been based upon known and unknown causes and involvement of size of vessel (medium-sized, small-sized) (Table 42-8).[205] With the exception of infectious angiitis resulting from syphilitic, mycobacterial or rickettsial infection, the causes and pathogenesis of most coronary vasculitides are either unknown or incompletely understood. Vasculitic syndromes may be caused by deposition of immune complex in the vessel walls.[209–214] The specific antigen has been identified in only a few cases, such as hepatitis B. Circulating immune complexes associated with hepatitis B infection may cause more than one type of vasculitic syndrome,[205] producing periarteritis nodosa in arteries of muscles and hypersensitivity angiitis in venules while eliciting the production of anti-immunoglobulin antibodies, leading to cryoglobulinemia. Thus, a classification of vasculitides *based solely* on immunological studies is incomplete[205] (see also Chap. 85).

GENERAL CONCEPTS

The earliest vasculitic syndrome was named *periarteritis nodosa*[215] because of the nodules along the course of small arteries.[205] Because the inflammatory changes are not only periarterial, *polyarteritis* may be a better term.[216] Periarteritis nodosa has become a "wastebasket designation" of any vasculitis whose cause was unknown.[205] The term *necrotizing angiitis*[217] has been used to designate arterial and venous lesions; there are five types[217,218]: (1) hypersensitivity angiitis, (2) allergic granulomatous angiitis, (3) rheumatoid arteri-

TABLE 42-8

CLASSIFICATION OF VASCULITIDES

1. Infectious angiitis

Syphilitic	Rickettsial
Mycobacterial	Viral
Pyogenic bacteria or fungal	Whipple bacillus

2. Noninfectious angiitis
   A. Involving large, medium-sized, and small blood vessels

   Takayasu's arteritis

   Granulomatous (giant-cell) arteritis

   Cranial (temporal) arteritis and extracranial giant-cell arteritis

   Disseminated visceral granulomatous angiitis

   Granulomatous angiitis of the central nervous system

   Arteritis of rheumatic-rheumatoid disease and spondyloarthropathies

   B. Involving predominantly medium-sized and small blood vessels

   Thromboangiitis obliterans (Buerger's disease)

   Polyarteritis (periarteritis)

Polyarteritis nodosa	Infantile polyarteritis
Microscopic polyarteritis	Kawasaki's disease

   Pathergic-allergic granulomatosis and angiitis

   Wegener's granulomatosis

   Churg-Strauss syndrome

   Necrotizing sarcoid granulomatosis

   Vasculitis of collagen-vascular disease

Rheumatic fever	Relapsing polychondritis
Rheumatoid arthritis	Systemic sclerosis
Seronegative arthropathies	Sjögren's syndrome
Systemic lupus erythematosus	Behçet's syndrome
Dermatomyositis/polymyositis	Cogan's syndrome

   C. Involving predominantly small blood vessels

   Hypersensitivity angiitis (synonym: leukocytoclastic or allergic vasculitis)

Serum sickness	Mixed cryoglobulinemia
Schönlein-Henoch purpura	Hypocomplementemia
Drug-induced angiitis	Inflammatory bowel disease
Malignancy-associated vasculitis	Primary biliary cirrhosis
Retroperitoneal fibrosis	Goodpasture's syndrome

Source: Lie.[208] Reproduced with permission from the author, editor, and publisher.

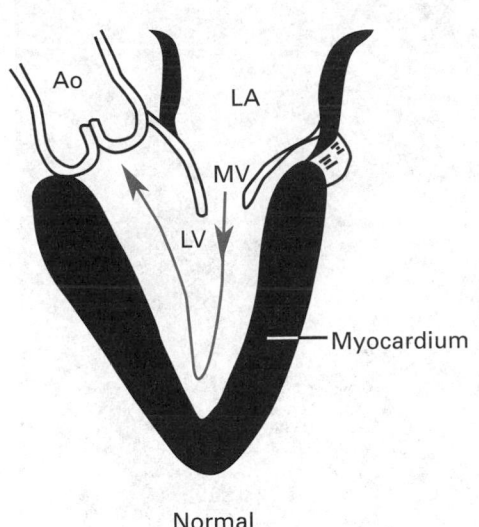

Normal

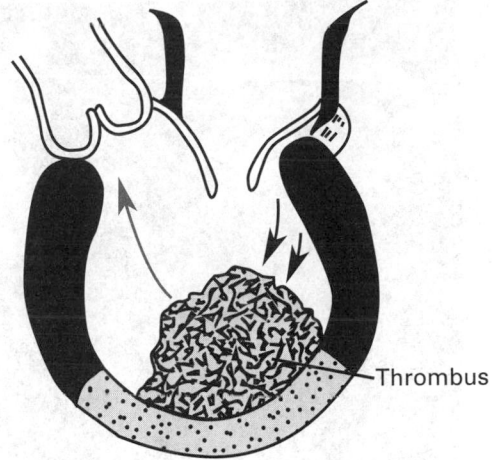

Idiopathic Dilated
Cardiomyopathy

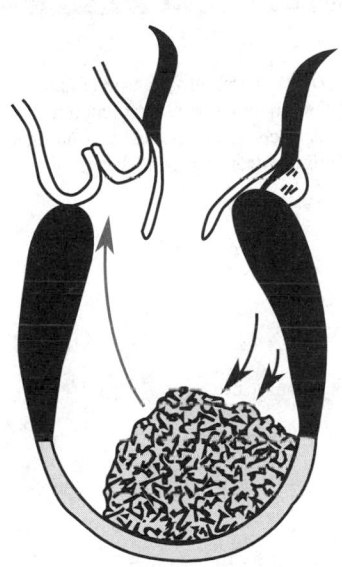

Coronary Dilated
Cardiomyopathy

("Ischemic Cardiomyopathy")

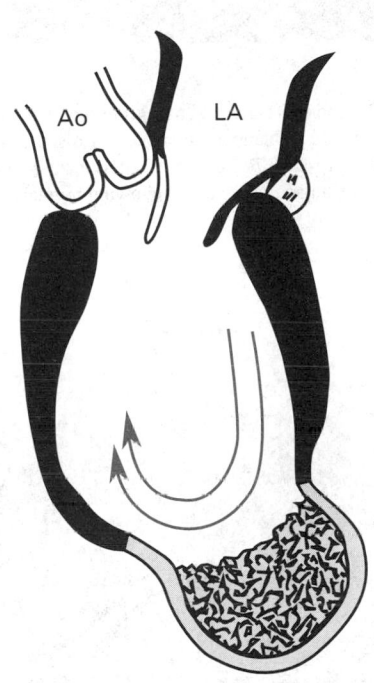

Left Ventricular Aneurysm

FIGURE 42-22

Diagram showing factors associated with emboli from left ventricular (LV) thrombus in three conditions: (1) idiopathic dilated cardiomyopathy (IDC); (2) coronary dilated cardiomyopathy (CDC); (3) left ventricular aneurysm. Thrombus protruding into the LV cavity (IDC, CDC) is more likely to embolize than thrombus protected within the sac of an LV aneurysm. Underlying myocardial contraction is more likely to propel thrombus out the LV outflow tract than paradoxical motion of LV aneurysm. Ao = aorta; LA = left atrium; MV = mitral valve. (From Cabin and Robins.[138] Reproduced with permission from the publisher, editor, and author.)

tis, (4) periarteritis nodosa, and (5) temporal arteritis. The term *hypersensitivity angiitis* has been considered synonymous with small-vessel vasculitis and is used to imply that the angiitis is due to an allergic response to proteins, drugs, vaccines, or infections.[205] Allergic *granulomatous angiitis* (Churg-Strauss syndrome) is a variant of polyarteritis charac-terized by necrotizing vasculitis with extravascular granulomas and eosinophilia associated with asthma or allergic rhinitis.[205,219–221] *Rheumatic arteritis*[222] describes vascular lesions in rheumatic diseases with both rheumatic and necro-tizing vascular lesions. *Temporal arteritis* (giant-cell arteritis) involves large and small extracranial arteries, including the

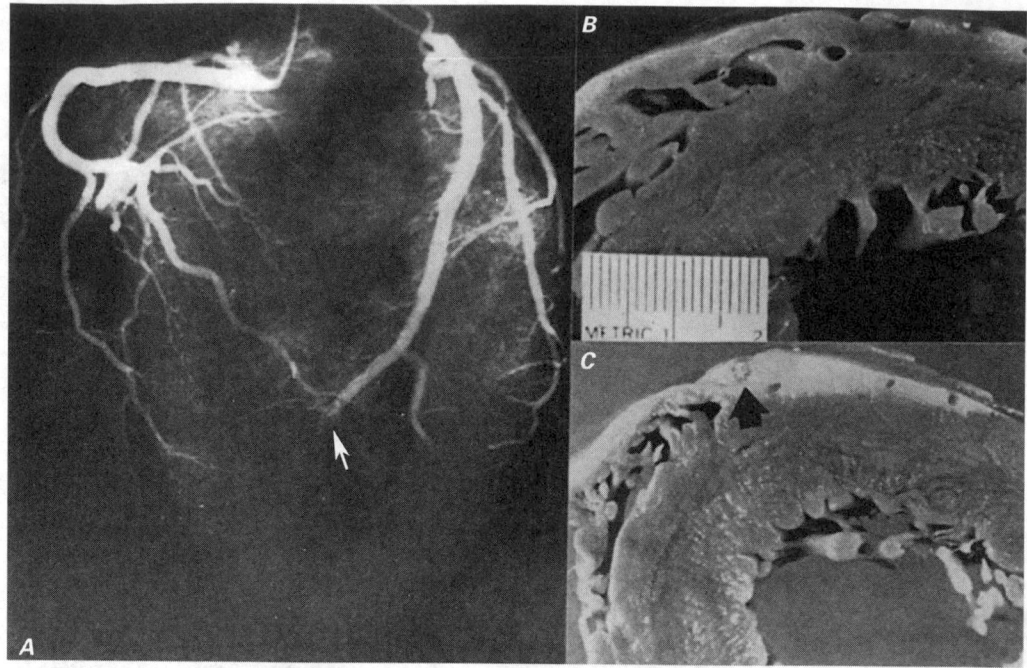

FIGURE 42-23

Coronary artery embolus *A.* Postmortem coronary angiogram showing normal epicardial coronary arteries except for sudden cutoff of the distal third of the left anterior coronary artery *(arrow). B.* Portion of anterior left ventricle and proximal left anterior descending coronary artery showing normal artery.

C. Site *(arrow)* of embolic occlusion of the left anterior descending coronary artery. The remaining distal left anterior descending, right, left circumflex and left main coronary arteries were normal. (From Waller.[1] Reproduced with permission from the publisher, editor, and author.)

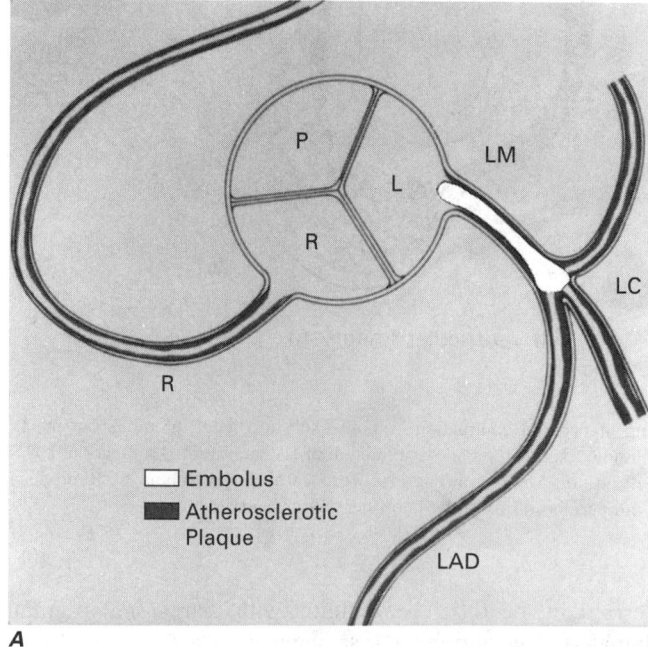

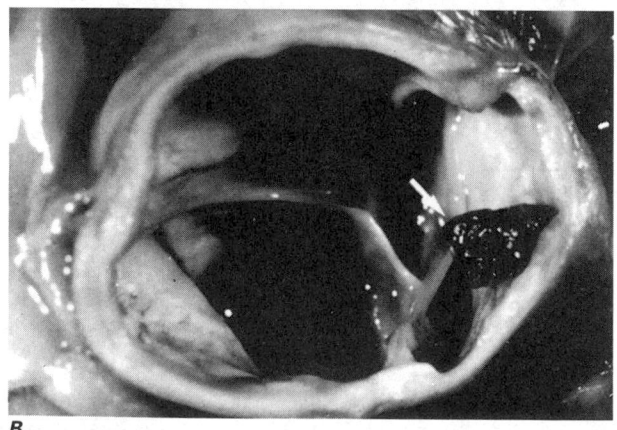

FIGURE 42-24

Coronary artery embolism. *A.* Diagram showing location and extent of occlusion of the left main (LM) coronary artery by an embolus. *B.* Photograph of aortic root showing embolus protruding from the LM coronary ostium

(arrow). LAD = left anterior descending; LC = left circumflex; R = right. (From Waller et al.[140] Reproduced with permission from the publisher, editor, and author.)

CORONARY ARTERIAL EMBOLI

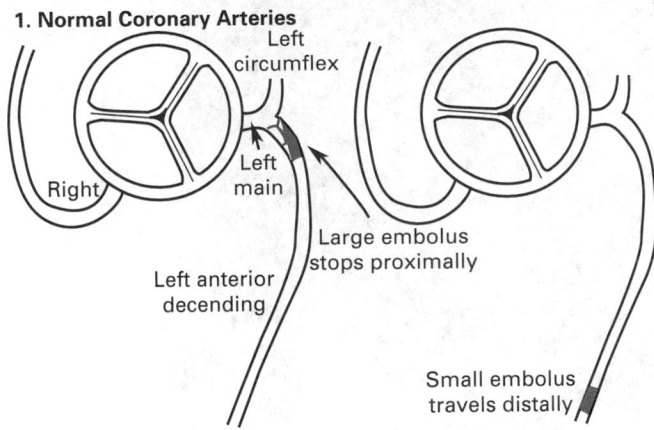

1. **Normal Coronary Arteries**

Left circumflex

Left main

Right

Left anterior decending

Large embolus stops proximally

Small embolus travels distally

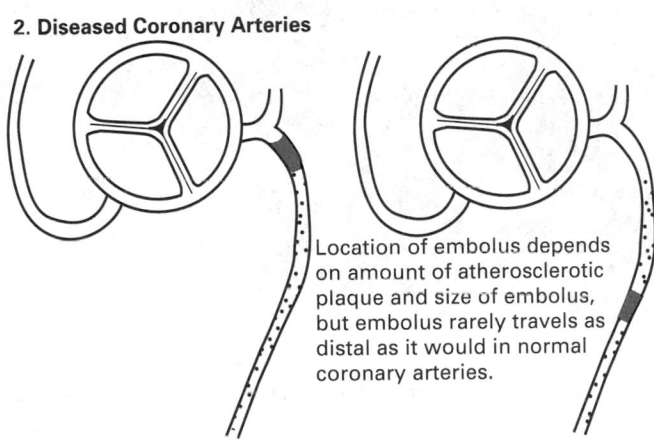

2. **Diseased Coronary Arteries**

Location of embolus depends on amount of atherosclerotic plaque and size of embolus, but embolus rarely travels as distal as it would in normal coronary arteries.

FIGURE 42-25
Coronary emboli in normal and diseased coronary arteries. (From Waller,[1] Reproduced with permission from the publisher, editor, and author.)

coronary arteries, and blindness may be a serious complication.[205,223–228] Despite its limitations, this classification[217,218] remains a basis for the diagnosis of vasculitides. The classification of coronary vasculitis is closely tied to that of vasculitides in general[205] and relates to the predominant type and size of vessels affected (Table 42-8)[229,230] (see also Chap. 85).

INFECTIOUS ANGIITIS

Various microorganisms may cause vasculitis in vessels of any size and involve the vessel by extension of the acute or chronic infective process from an adjacent tissue or organ[24] or from the lumen by hematogenous spread (Table 42-8). The inflammatory response produces variable reactions including suppurative inflammation bacteria, proliferative response (typhoid[232]), hemorrhagic (anthrax) and histiocytic and granulomatous response (leprosy, syphilis, tuberculosis).[4,205] The most important angiitic infections affecting the coronary arteries include syphilis, tuberculosis, and syphilitic arteritis. All

three stages of syphilis show arteritic features. The most important vascular lesion of tertiary syphilis, coronary ostial stenosis, seen in up to 4 percent of patients with tertiary syphilis,[5,233–235,236] can occur independent of aortic involvement.[205,235] Syphilitic arteritis is characterized by a chronic inflammation with adventitial fibrosis and patchy destruction of media with a lymphoplasmacytic infiltrate. Gummas can be found in 20 percent of cases,[237] but spirochetes are rarely detected.[205] The first 3 to 4 mm of the left and right coronary arteries may be involved with an obliterative arteritis[114]; angina and acute myocardial infarction may result from syphilitic involvement.[236]

TUBERCULOUS ARTERITIS

Tuberculous coronary arteritis occurs mainly in patients with pericardial and myocardial tuberculosis.[238,239] Granuloma may involve the adventitia, intima, or the entire wall[24,239] and result from several infectious angiitic agents. Endocarditis and septicemia are the most common underlying causes of infectious angiitis and mycotic aneurysm formation.[205,240] Any type of gram-positive or gram-negative organism may be involved. Myocarditis with abscesses and pericarditis frequently accompany infectious coronary angiitis. Mucormycosis, aspergillosis, and *Candida* (Fig. 42-32) are examples of fungi and systemic yeast infections associated with coronary angiitis. Malarial parasites and parasitized red blood cells also may plug larger coronary arteries.[241] *Schistosoma haematobium* has been found in a major epicardial coronary artery associated with myocardial infarction.[242] Rickettsial infections may produce angiitis in small vessels of the heart[205,243]; these infections consist of a lymphomononuclear infiltrate with or without thrombosis. A direct toxic effect from rickettsiae may produce angiitis.[244] Viruses have also been implicated in vasculitis by direct invasion of immunologic mechanisms.[205] Virus-induced vasculitides in humans are represented by polyarteritis associated with hepatitis-B antigenemia[205,245,246] and herpes zoster.[205]

NONINFECTIOUS ANGIITIS

Various noninfectious causes of angiitis involve large- to medium-sized (predominately medium- and small-sized) blood vessels (Table 42-8).[205]

Takayasu's Arteritis

Takayasu's disease (pulseless disease) is one of the coronary vasculitides associated with aortitis; others are temporal arteritides and rheumatic disease. Takayasu's disease is a chronic, occlusive inflammatory disease of unknown etiology[205,247–256] with a worldwide distribution and greater incidence in young to middle-aged female Asians.[249–250] Involvement of the coronary arteries occurs 15 to 25 percent of cases

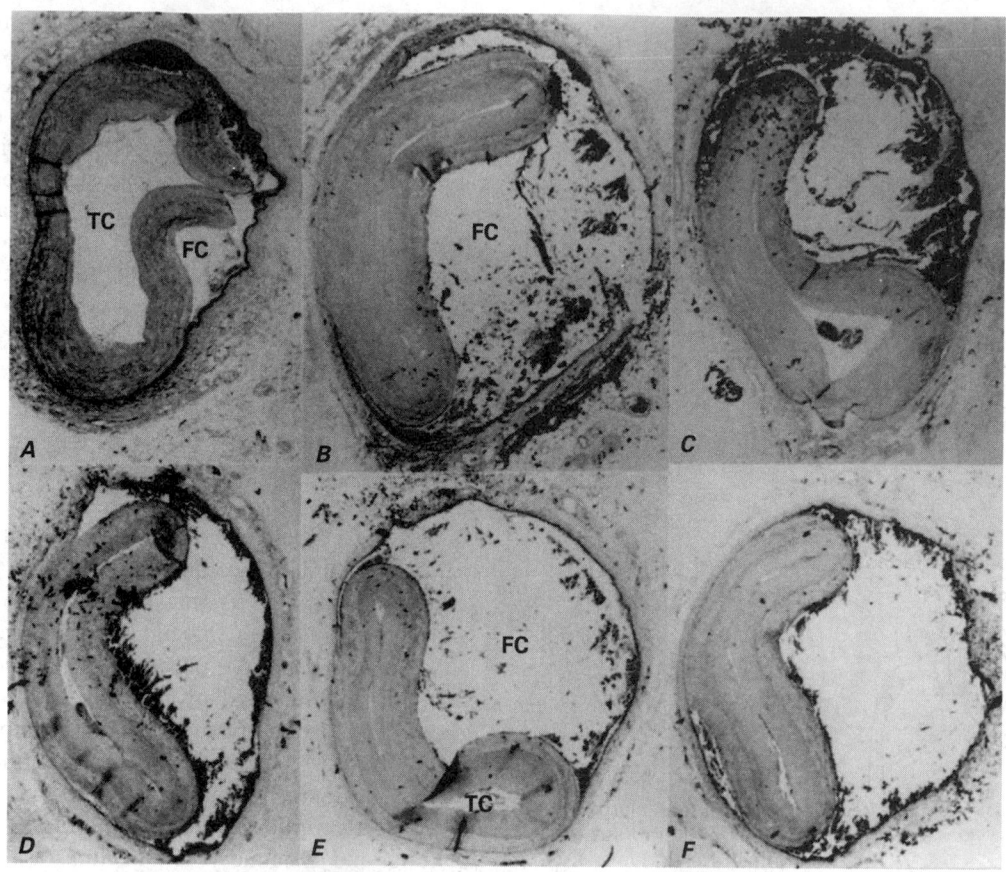

FIGURE 42-26

Coronary artery dissection. Serial cross-section (A-F) showing dissection of the left anterior descending coronary artery. The true channel (TL) is severely compromised by external compression from the false channel (FC) ("dissec-tion channel"). (From Waller.[1] Reproduced with permission from the publisher, editor, and author.)

and may be the lethal complication (Fig. 42-33),[248,250–255,257] commonly involving the coronary ostium[248,257,258–263] with segmental involvement of distal coronary arteries.[252–255,264] Rarely, diffuse coronary arteritis is produced by Takayasu's disease.[265]

Granulomatous Giant-Cell Arteritis (Temporal Arteritis)

Granulomatous giant-cell arteritis may occur independently or, more commonly, may be associated with temporal arteritis in 10 to 15 percent of patients.[205,226–228,266–277] Histologically proven giant-cell coronary arteritis is rare, and cases leading to fatal myocardial infarction are even rarer (Fig. 42-34).[205,266,269–272,274] The arterial wall lesion is a granulomatous inflammation with giant cells found along degenerative internal elastic membrane.[274] The intima becomes greatly thickened, and ultimately the vessel is converted into a fibrous cord. Luminal thrombosis may also be present in 16 cases of temporal arteritis reported by Harrison[275]; only 1 case involved the epicardial coronary arteries. Giant-cell arteritis of the intramural (intramyocardial) coronary arteries (Fig. 42-35) may also occur in association with temporal arteritis and giant-cell arteries[266] (see also Chap. 85).

Arteritis of Rheumatic Disease

Rheumatic diseases commonly affect the aorta and are morphologically indistinguishable from granulomatous aortitis.[205,276–293] Coronary arteritis at necropsy has been detected in up to 20 percent of patients with rheumatoid arthritis, usually involving small intramural vessels.[276–297] The small-vessel arteritis may also involve conduction system vessels leading to various forms of heart block.[291–293] Rheumatoid coronary vasculitis producing myocardial infarction is rare.[282–285,296,297] Histologically, extraaortic rheumatoid vasculitis (coronary artery vasculitis) is usually a polyarteritis type of necrotizing angiitis[205,281,286–290] and not a giant-cell arteritis (Fig. 42-36). Small myocardial vessels may also be severely narrowed in ankylosing spondylosis. Occlusion of the left main ostium has been described.[293]

Thromboangiitis Obliterans (Buerger's Disease)

Thromboangiitis obliterans (Buerger's disease), which is very rare (Fig. 42-37),[205,303–307] is a nonatherosclerotic, occlusive, inflammatory vascular disease of unknown cause occurring mainly in young males who are heavy smokers of cigarettes.[205] In a few patients, the coronary arteries have shown focal polymorphonuclear infiltrates, histiocytes, and giant

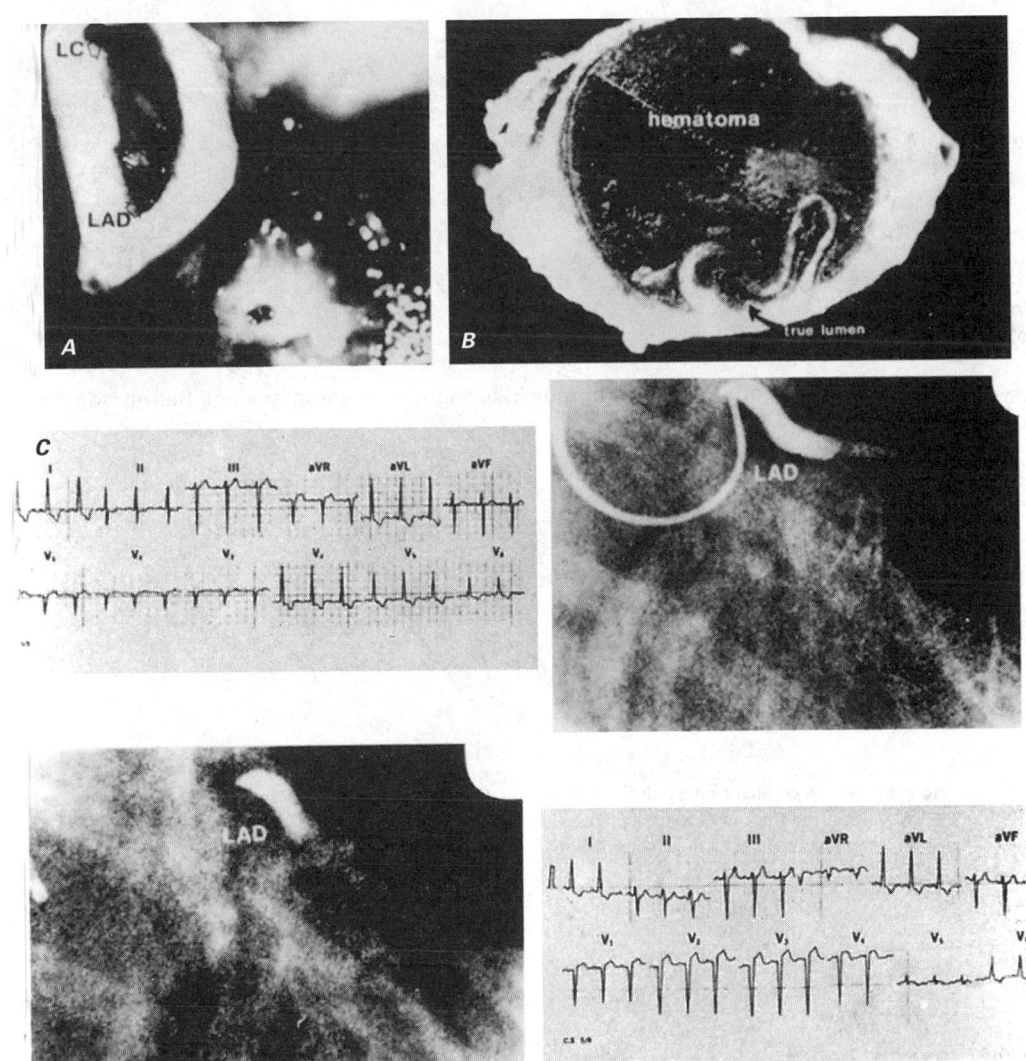

FIGURE 42-27

Coronary artery dissection. Occlusion of the left anterior descending (LAD) artery due to dissection. *A.* The LAD and left circumflex (LC) are seen through the left main artery. *B.* Cross section shows hematoma in false channel severely narrows native (true channel) unobstructed lumen. *C.* Sequential electrocardiographic and angiographic findings. (From Isner and Donaldson.[141] Reproduced with permission from the publisher, editor, and author.)

cells with or without coronary artery thrombosis.[304] Coronary involvement is rare,[304] although coronary thrombosis may be seen.[308] Buerger's disease involving a saphenous vein bypass graft has also been documented.[309]

POLYARTERITIS GROUP OF NECROTIZING ANGIITIS

Classic Polyarteritis Nodosa

Classic polyarteritis nodosa is a chronic systemic disease manifest by infarction or hemorrhage in various target organs as the result of necrotizing vasculitis.[215] Male patients are affected twice as often as female, with a mean age of 45 years.[205,310–314] It is probably the most common cause of coronary angiitis with both epicardial and intramural coronary arteries being affected (Fig. 42-38).[24,310–320] In a review of

66 necropsy cases,[315] 41 (62 percent) had involvement of the epicardial coronary arteries, including 25 cases (61 percent) with involvement of both the epicardial and intramural coronary arteries, while 16 cases (39 percent) had only involvement of the intramural arteries. Frequently, various stages of acute disease and healing are seen in the same arterial segment. The acute phase has an acute cellular reaction with destruction of the media and internal elastic membrane.[316] The healing stage results in fibrous internal proliferation. Coronary arteries may dilate to form small berry-like aneurysms (becoming occluded by thrombus), rupture, or produce fatal myocardial infarction,[315,317,318–320] pericardial tamponade, or sudden death (see also Chap. 85).

Infantile Polyarteritis

Polyarteritis nodosa occurring in infants under 2 years of age (infantile polyarteritis) differs from the clinical pathologic

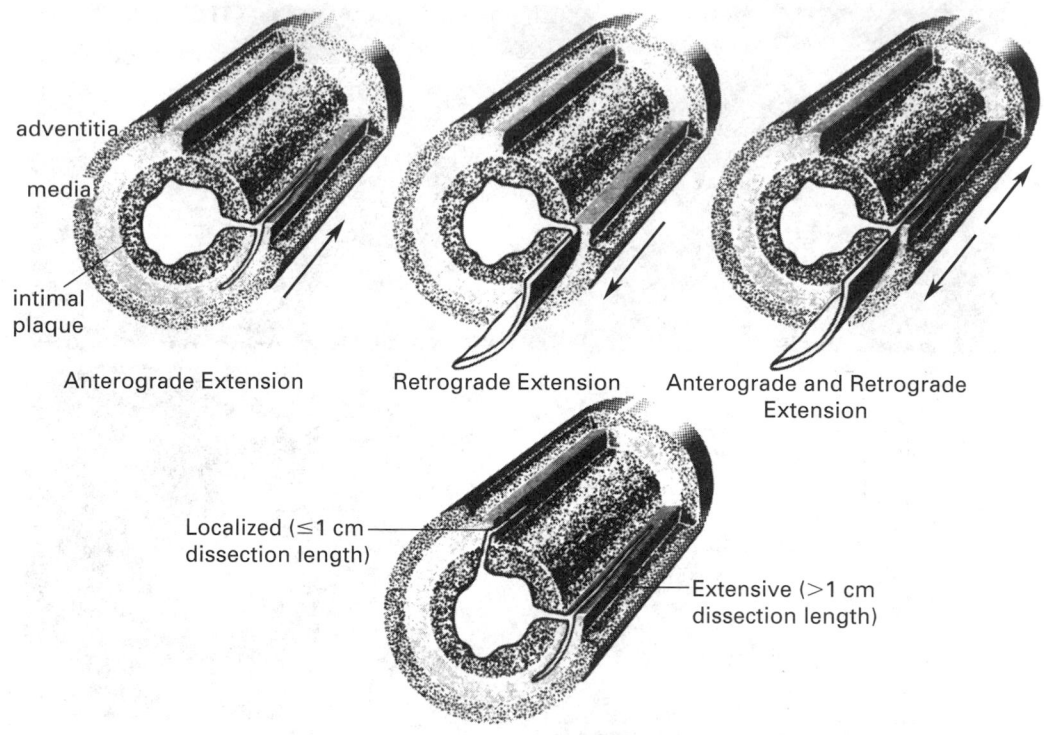

FIGURE 42-28

Diagram showing morphologic definition of coronary artery dissections in balloon angioplasty (long-axis plane): localized (mechanism) (≤1 cm in total dissection length) and extension (complications) (≥1 cm in total length).

(From Waller et al.[168] Reproduced with permission from the author, editor, and publisher.)

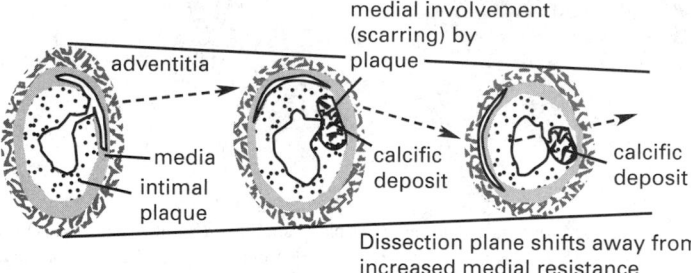

A

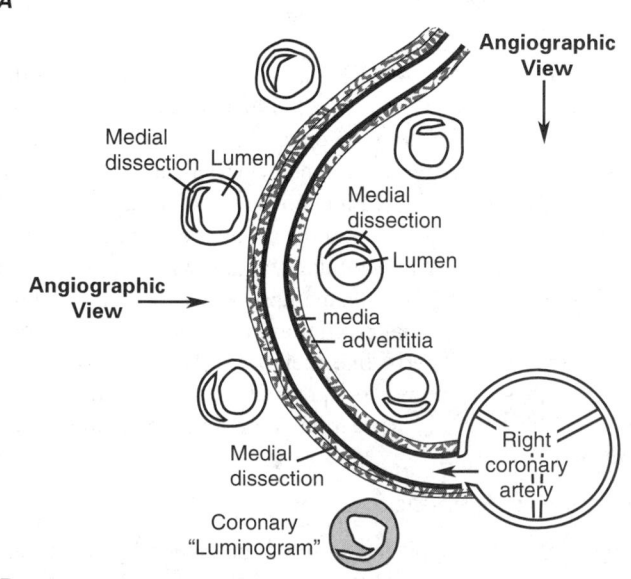

B

FIGURE 42-29

Diagram showing pathologic change accounting for angiographic appearance of coronary artery "spiral" dissection. *A.* Alteration in course of dissection. *B.* Angiographic appearance of unaltered course of dissection. (From Waller et al.[168] Reproduced with permission from the author, editor, and publisher.)

features of classical polyarteritis no-dosa.[205,321–324] Infantile disease involves a higher frequency (79 percent) of coronary vasculitis and aneurysmal disease of the coronary arteries with sparing of vessels in other locations (Fig. 42-39).[205,321–324] Kawasaki's disease may involve children up to 8 or 10 years of age[205] rather than being confined to patients under 2 as in infantile polyarteritis.[325]

Kawasaki's Disease (Mucocutaneous Lymph Node Syndrome)

Kawasaki's disease, or mucocutaneous lymph node syndrome, is an acute febrile exanthematous illness of children first de-scribed in the Japanese literature in 1967 and reported in the English literature in 1974.[326] It has subsequently been reported in children worldwide and in all racial groups.[327] In about 20 percent of children with the acute illness, a vasculitis of the coronary vasa vasorum leads to coronary arterial aneurysm formation, thrombosis, acute myocardial infarction, and sudden death.[326–339] Estimates of death from acute infarction or ventricular analytic range from 1 to 2 percent.[332–334] Late pre-sentation with myocardial infarction sec-ondary to dislodged aneurysmal thrombo-sis may also occur (Figs. 42-40 and 42-41).[332,333,335,337] Pathologically, the acute phase shows a necrotizing angiitis involving media and adventitial layers. Some children have survived into adult-hood, with coronary artery aneurysms identified later in life (Figs. 42-40 and 42-41).[339] The differential diagnosis of coronary artery aneurysms in adults in-cludes previously undiagnosed Kawa-saki's disease presumably occurring dur-ing childhood. Coronary arteriography results in 1100 children ages 4 months to 13 years identified 262 (24 percent) patients with the disease. In these, coronary occlusion was present in 76 percent; segmental stenosis in 5.7 percent; localized steno-sis in 23.7 percent; aneurysms in 35.5 percent; and dilatation in 27.5 percent.[338] The incidence of both occlusion and seg-mental stenosis was lowest in the group studied shortly after the onset of the illness, whereas the prevalence of coronary aneurysm was highest in this early group.

Allergic Granulomatosis and Angiitis: Wegener's Granulomatosis and Churg-Strauss Syndrome

Wegener's granulomatosis is a necrotizing vasculitis of un-known cause classically involving the upper and lower respira-

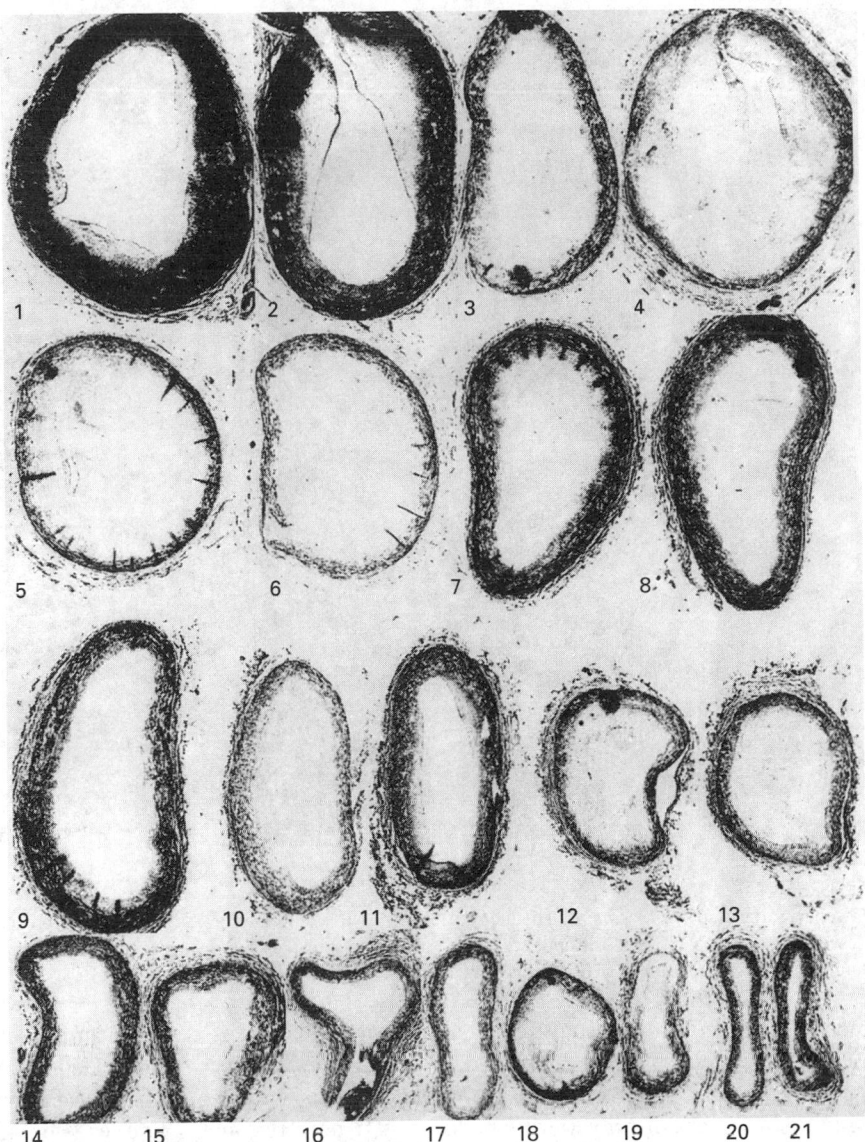

FIGURE 42-30
Coronary artery spasm. Composite of coronary artery cross sections of a patient with coronary spasm during life. Clinical spasm involved segments 3 to 7. Severe atherosclerotic plaque is seen in 8 of the 21 segments. (From Roberts et al.[180] Reproduced with permission from the author, editor, and publisher.)

tory tracts and the kidneys.[205,342–355] Cardiovascular involve-ment in Wegener's granulomatosis was described in one of three cases reported in 1936.[345] About 30 additional necropsy cases have been described subsequently, 14 of these (48 per-cent) showed small-vessel necrotizing coronary vasculitis (Fig. 42-42).[205,353,354] Fibrinoid necrosis of the small and medium-sized coronary arteries[342] and occlusion of larger epicardial coronary arteries with myocardial infarction[343] have been reported. In a large clinical series of patients with Wegeners granulomatosis, 12 percent had cardiac involve-ment largely manifest by pericarditis and coronary arteritis.[355] Some patients with this disease develop unusual cardiac com-plications such as pericardial tamponade and later constrictive pericarditis, high-grade atrioventricular block, and atrial

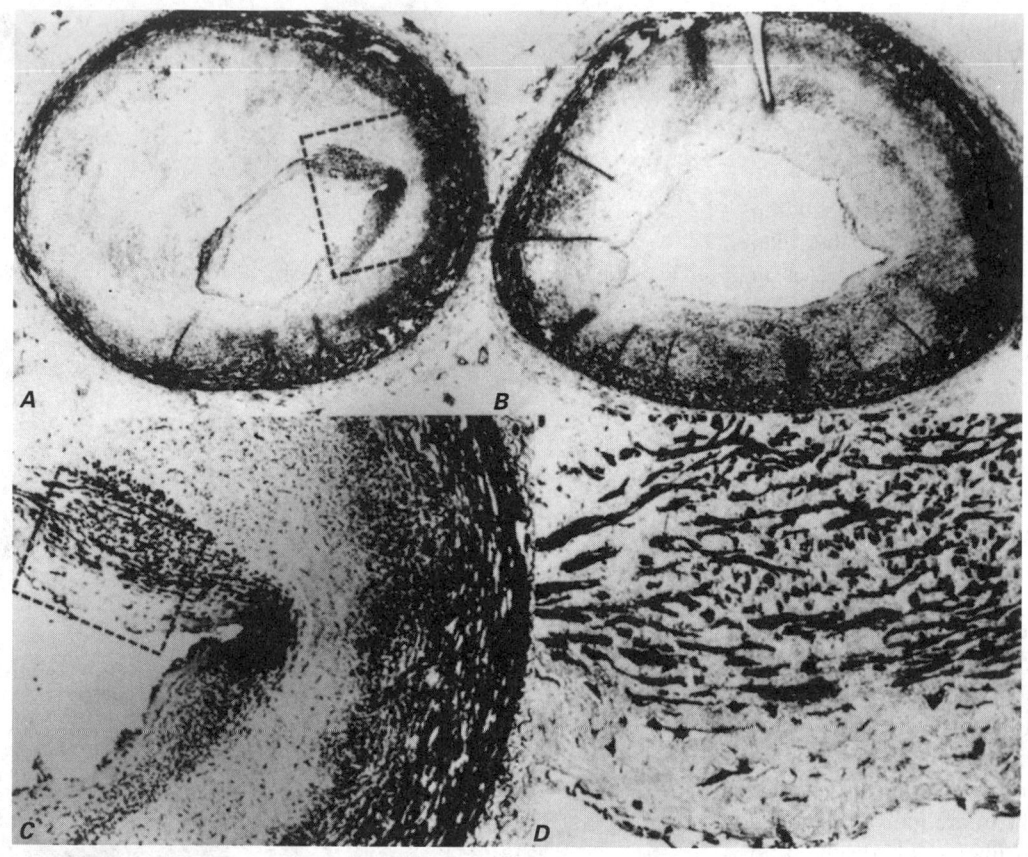

FIGURE 42-31
Coronary artery spasm. *A and B*. Histology sections of the left anterior descending coronary artery at the approximate site of spasm showing severe luminal narrowing. *C and D*. Higher magnifications of the internal plaque

showing the predominance of smooth muscle cells. (From Roberts et al.[180] Reproduced with permission from the author, editor, and publisher.)

tachycardia resistant to usual treatment measures. In this series,[355] all patients improved with cyclophosphamide therapy.

Churg-Strauss syndrome (allergic granulomatosis and angiitis) is a variant of polyarteritis nodosa[205,219] occurring in patients with asthma or an allergy history.[219–221,356] It is

characterized by necrotizing angiitis with extravascular granulomas and eosinophilia. The heart is commonly involved with this disease, with granulomatous vasculitis of the coronary arteries (Fig. 42-42). Granulomatous myocarditis may occur with or without the coronary angiitis[357] (see also Chap. 85).

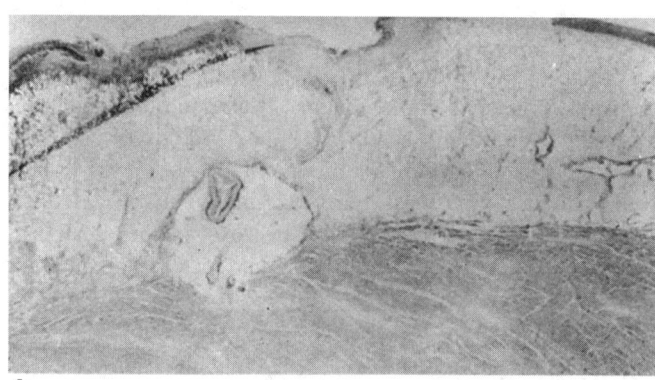

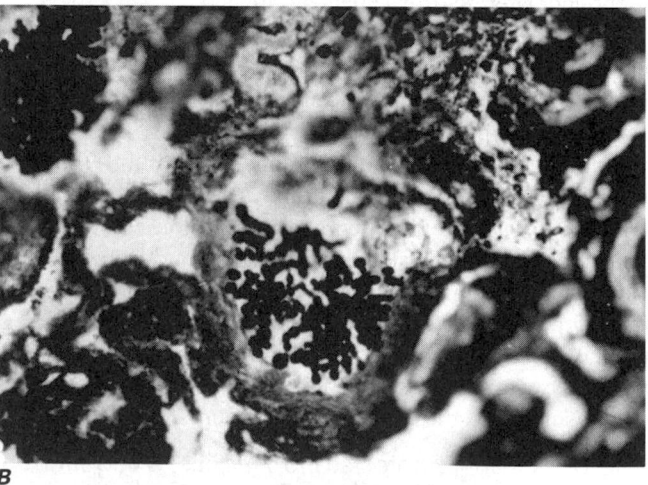

FIGURE 42-32
Coronary arteritis. *A*. Extensive yeast (*Candida*) pericarditis, which involves the adventitial layer of a branch of a major subepicardial coronary artery.

B. Closeup shows the budding yeast organisms (GMS stain). (From Waller.[1] Reproduced with permission from the author, editor, and publisher.)

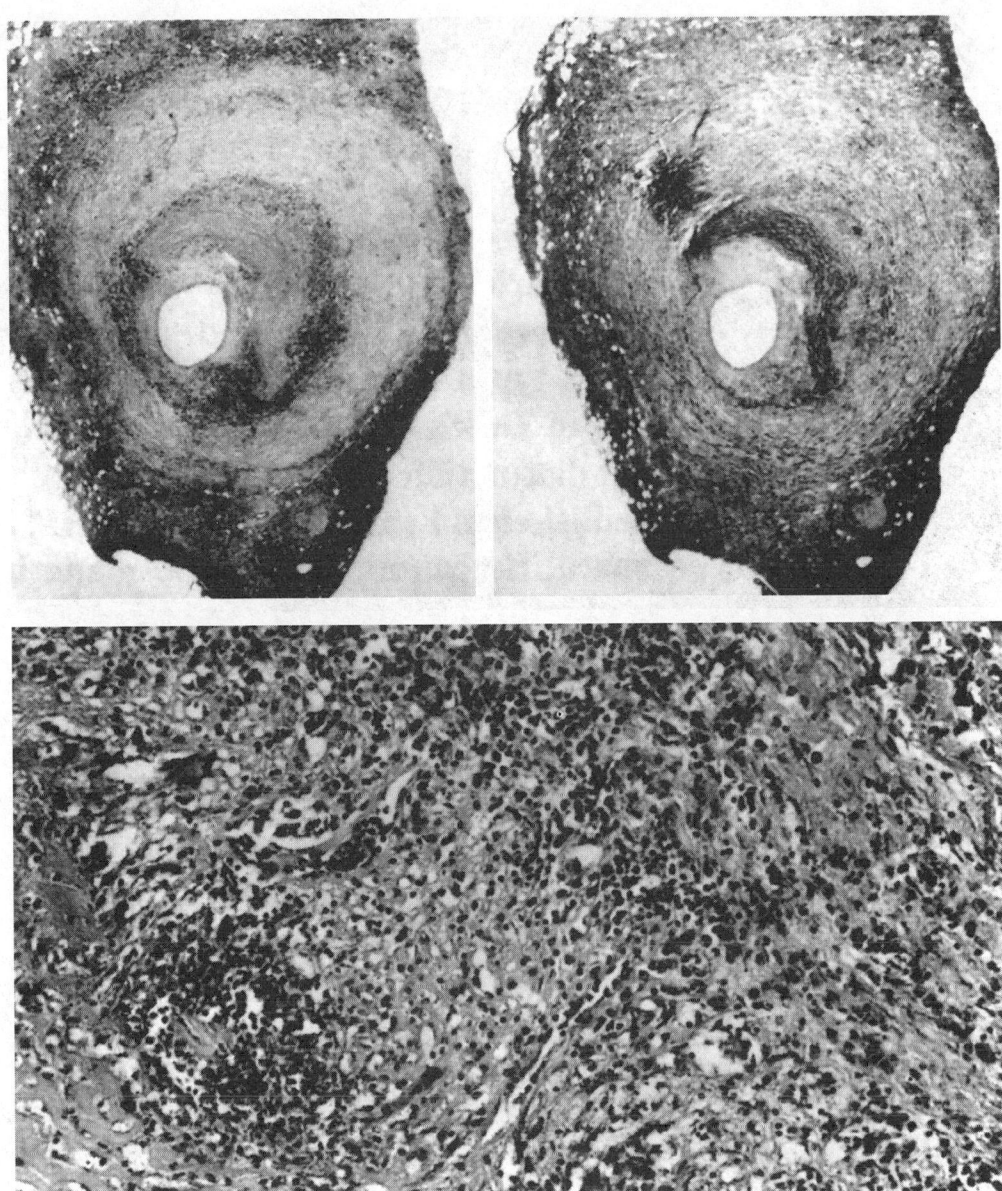

FIGURE 42-33

Top: Matching hematoxylin-eosin (*left*) and elastic stain (*right*) sections of coronary artery in Takayasu's arteritis. Note transmural fibrosis and inflammatory infiltrate in media of artery (×16). *Bottom:* Closeup view of lymph-oplasmacytic infiltrate with giant cells in media of coronary artery (×160). (From Lie.[205] Reproduced with permission from the author, editor, and publisher.)

COLLAGEN VASCULAR DISEASE VASCULITIS

Collagen vascular diseases generally involve arthritis, myositis, carditis, dermatitis, and inflammatory vascular changes to varying degrees.[358] They include systemic lupus erythematosus, rheumatoid vasculitis, systemic sclerosis, and polymyositis. Rheumatoid vasculitis is discussed above. One of the most common conditions with coronary vasculitis is systemic lupus erythematosus (Fig. 42-43). Several young patients with this disease and absent coronary atherosclerosis have suffered acute myocardial infarction[359–362] (see also Chap. 85). At necropsy, the coronary arteries in these patients have shown internal fibrous proliferation, possibly representing healed arteritis. Necrotizing vasculitis frequently leads to fatal coronary thrombosis and myocardial infarction,[205,360] rarely associated with thrombotic occlusion of all three major arteries.[360] Smaller intramural coronary arteries are also involved frequently with fibrinoid necrosis and subsequent fibrosis.[114] Recently myocardial infarction has been seen with a proximal right coronary artery aneurysm at necropsy. It was postulated that the coronary aneurysm represented a sequela of systemic lupus erythematosus arteritis similar to Kawasaki's disease.[362] Necrotizing vasculitis occurs less commonly in other entities

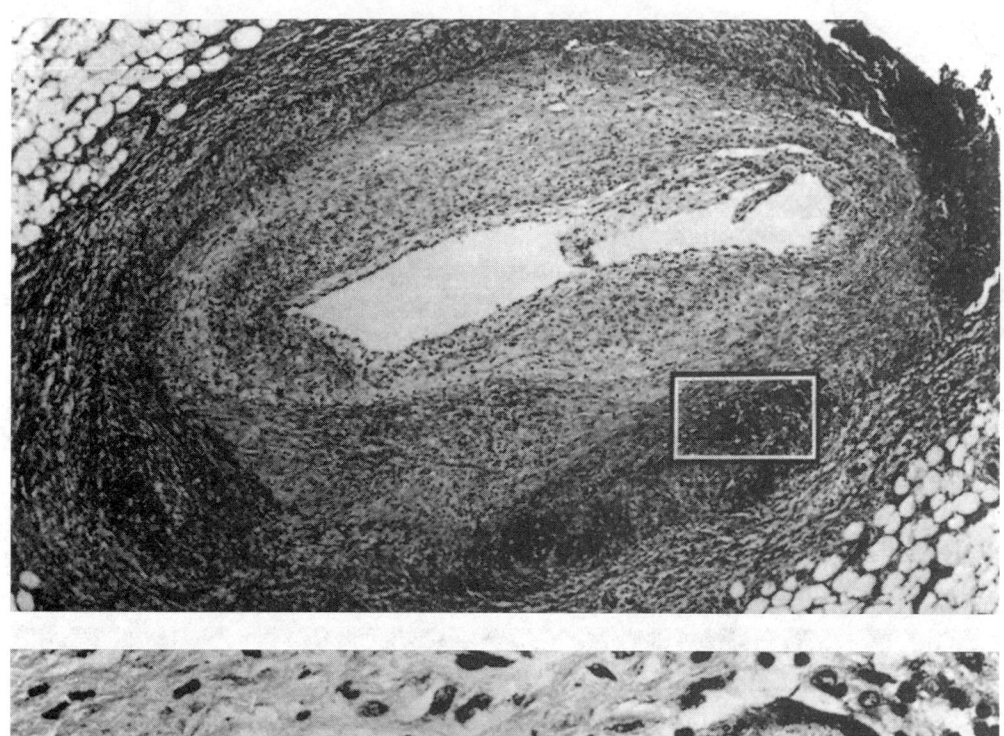

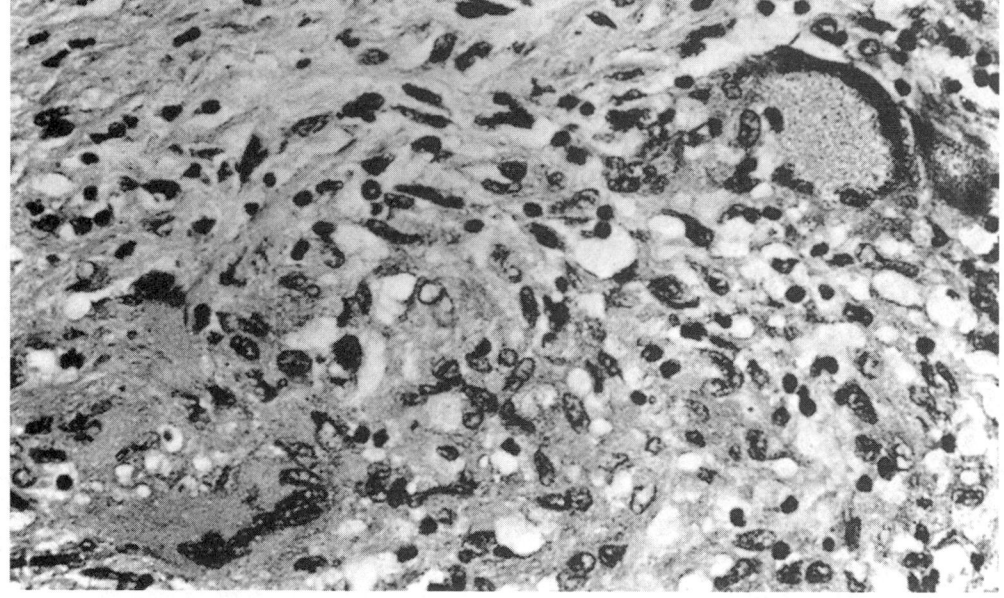

FIGURE 42-34

Top: Low-power view of granulomatous coronary arteritis associated with giant-cell aortitis (hematoxylin-eosin, ×40). *Bottom:* Closeup view of boxed area (hematoxylin-eosin ×400). (From Lie.[205] Reproduced with permission from the author, editor, and publisher.)

of collagen vascular disease such as dermatopolymyositis,[363] systemic sclerosis,[364] Behçet's syndrome,[365] and Cogan's syndrome.[205,366]

HYPERSENSITIVITY ANGIITIS (ALLERGIC VASCULITIS)

Hypersensitivity angiitis describes a miscellaneous group of necrotizing vasculitides that involve both epicardial and intramural coronary arteries.[205] This includes drug-induced vasculitis,[367] which, when generalized, may involve the heart. Histologically, drug-induced vasculitis cannot be separated from primary vasculitis or from hypersensitivity angiitis associated with a known underlying disease or malignancy such as serum sickness, mixed cryoglobulinemia, or Schönlein-Henoch purpura, etc. (Table 42-8).[205] Correct diagnosis cannot be made without clinical information about drug usage. Organ-transplantation arteritis[205,368] is also in this category representing a form of immune-mediated vascular injury (see Chap. 25).

METABOLIC DISORDERS NARROWING CORONARY ARTERIES

Specific metabolic substances may accumulate in the walls of large and small coronary arteries as a result of inborn errors of metabolism. The deposition of this material may severely

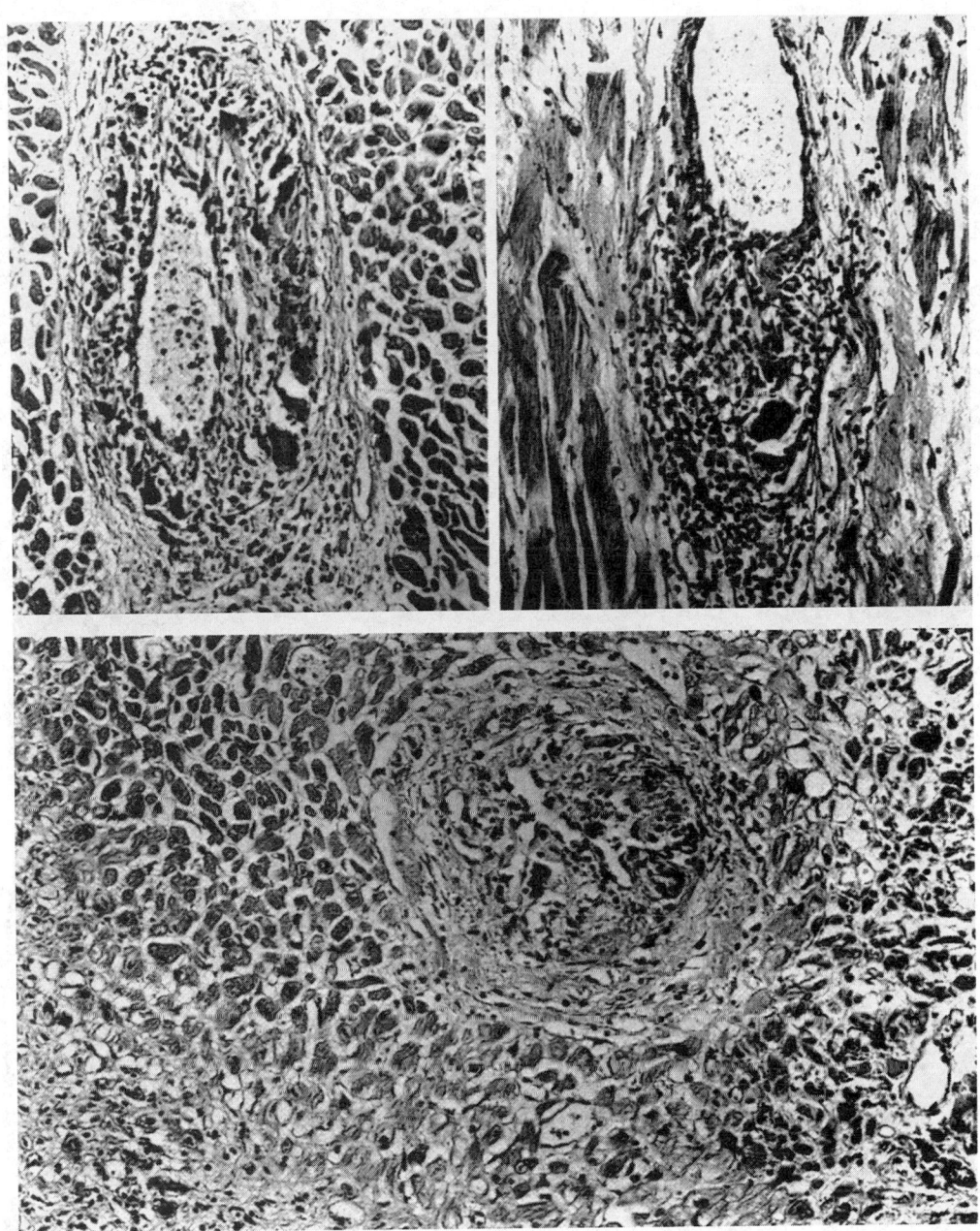

FIGURE 42-35

Top left and right: Giant cell arteritis of intramural coronary arteries associated with temporal arteritis and giant cell arteritis (hematoxylin-eosin, ×160). *Bottom:* Granulomatous coronary arteritis in disseminated visceral giant cell angiitis (hematoxylin-eosin, ×160). (From Lie.[205] Reproduced with permission from the author, editor, and publisher.)

narrow the coronary artery lumen and produce acute myocardial infarction.[5] Inherited inborn errors of metabolism that are known to affect major epicardial coronary arteries include Hunter's and Hurler's diseases (mucopolysaccharidoses).[293,369–371] The involvement of the coronary arteries in these disorders may be so severe as to occlude totally the vessel and to produce myocardial ischemia/infarction. Other disorders of metabolism such as primary oxalosis,[372] Fabry's disease,[114] Sandhoff's disease (gangliosidoses),[373] and homocystinuria may affect smaller coronary vessels by severe intimal proliferation[374] (see also Chap. 69).

INTIMAL PROLIFERATION

Fibrous hyperplasia and smooth muscle proliferation in the coronary arteries may severely narrow the lumen and produce myocardial ischemia/infarction. The process may be associated with mediastinal irradiation,[375] fibromuscular hyperplasia of the renal arteries,[5] the use of methysergide,[22,376] ostial cannulation during cardiac surgery, aortic valve replacement,[23] and unknown causes.[377, 378–380] Up to 50 percent of patients undergoing cardiac transplantation develop signifi-

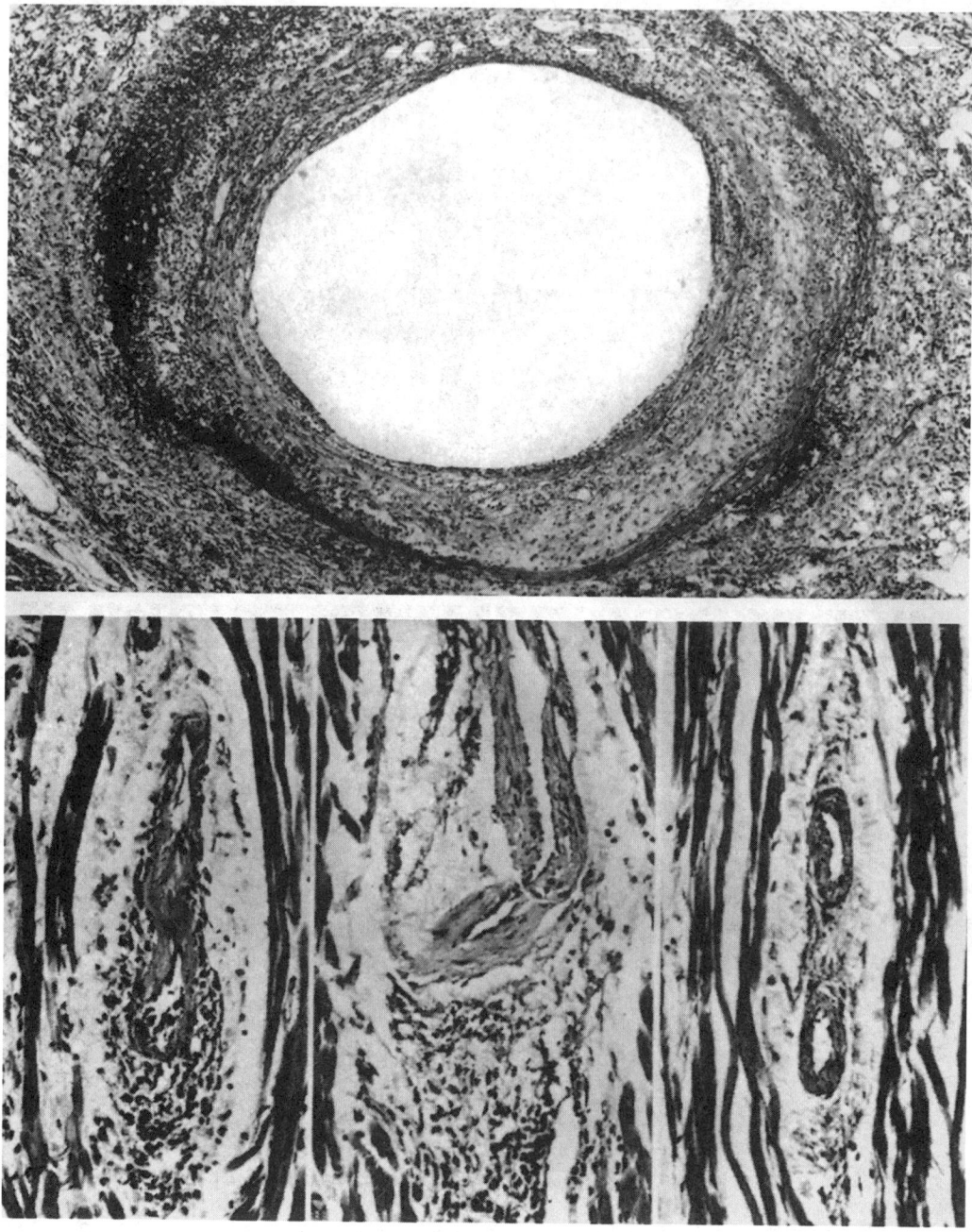

FIGURE 42-36

Top: Polyarteritis type necrotizing angiitis of epicardial coronary artery in rheumatoid arthritis (hematoxylin-eosin, ×160). *Bottom:* Variations of small vessel coronary arteritis in rheumatic fever (hematoxylin-eosin, ×160).

(From Lie.[205] Reproduced with permission from the author, editor, and publisher.)

cant narrowing of epicardial coronary arteries or total occlusion by intimal fibrous proliferation within 3 to 5 years after transplantation.[381] Myocardial infarction and sudden death may result from this "chronic rejection" process. Fibrosis of the intramural vessels may also occur. Intimal damage from immunologic rejection is believed to be the basis for the accelerated intimal fibrous hyperplasia involving the coronary arteries (see also Chap. 25). A morphologic assessment of 61 human cardiac allografts of short- and long-term survival has been provided.[382] Allographs were divided into two groups: fibrous lesions confined to the proximal regional of epicardial arteries and those with diffuse necrotizing vasculitis of the entire system. Disease in the proximal region begins as concentric fibrous thickening. Diffuse disease (necrotizing vasculitis) was invariably associated with acute myocardial rejection with severe intimal lesions of large and small epicardial

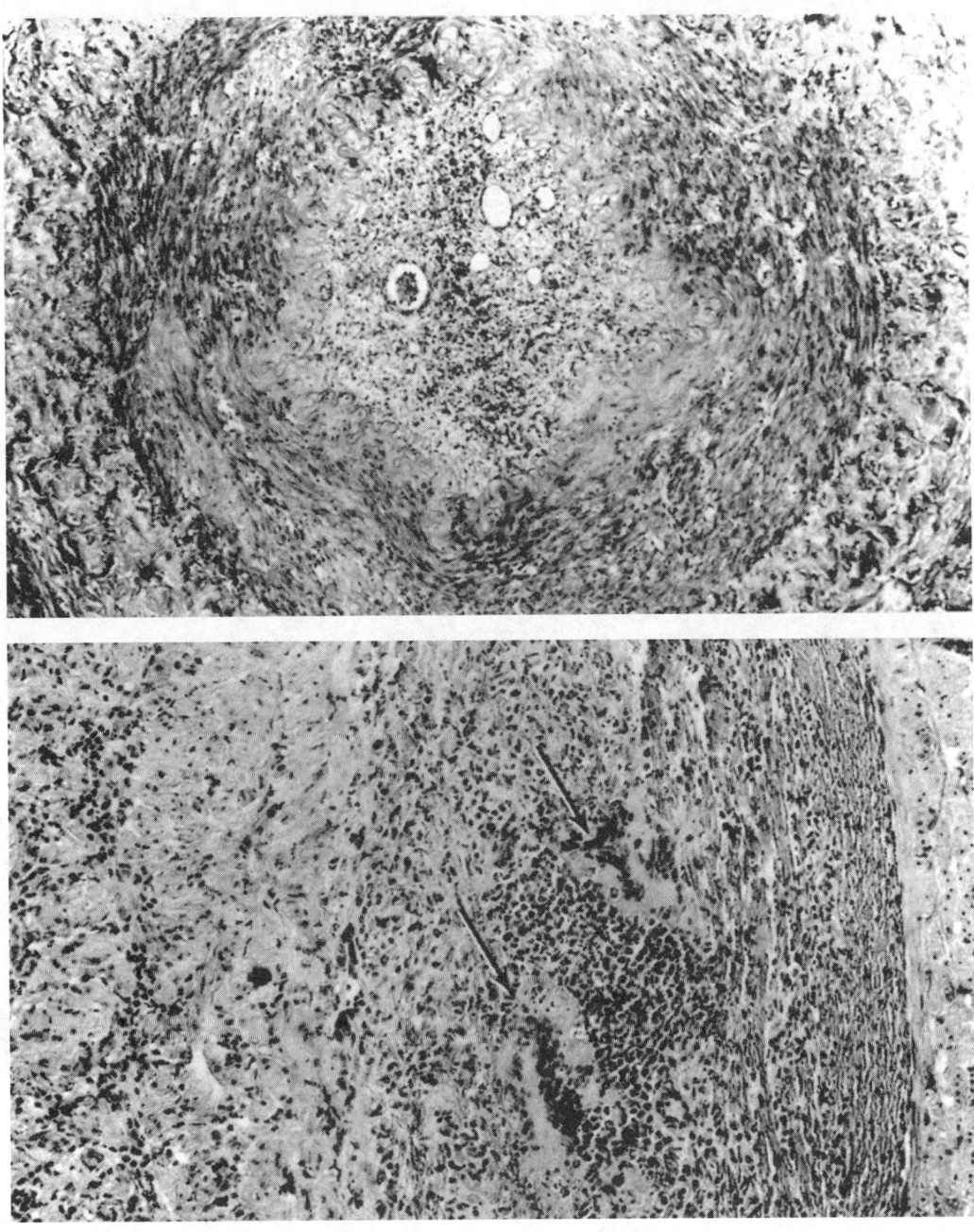

FIGURE 42-37

Top: Subacute stage of Buerger's disease of coronary artery with organizing thrombus (hematoxylin-eosin, ×160). *Bottom:* Involvement of coronary vein in Buerger's disease with typical intraluminal microabscesses and giant cells (*arrows*) (hematoxylin-eosin, ×160). (From Lie.[205] Reproduced with permission from the author, editor, and publisher.)

and intramural arteries.[382] These authors and others[383] have postulated that disease results from healing of a necrotizing vasculitis. Intravascular ultrasound[384] has shown intimal hyperplasia which was easily detected; its severity predicted the development of cardiac events including myocardial infarction, unstable angina, or sudden death, despite the presence of a normal coronary arteriogram.

A similar histologic picture of intimal fibrous proliferation is seen in epicardial coronary arteries late after undergoing percutaneous balloon angioplasty (Fig. 42-44).[143,144] Intimal fibrous proliferation of the left main coronary artery has been reported late after balloon angioplasty of a lesion in the proximal left anterior descending coronary artery.[385] This may be due to intimal reaction from balloon rubbing of the intimal surface and/or extension of the fibrous process from the angioplasty dilation site (see also Chap. 48).

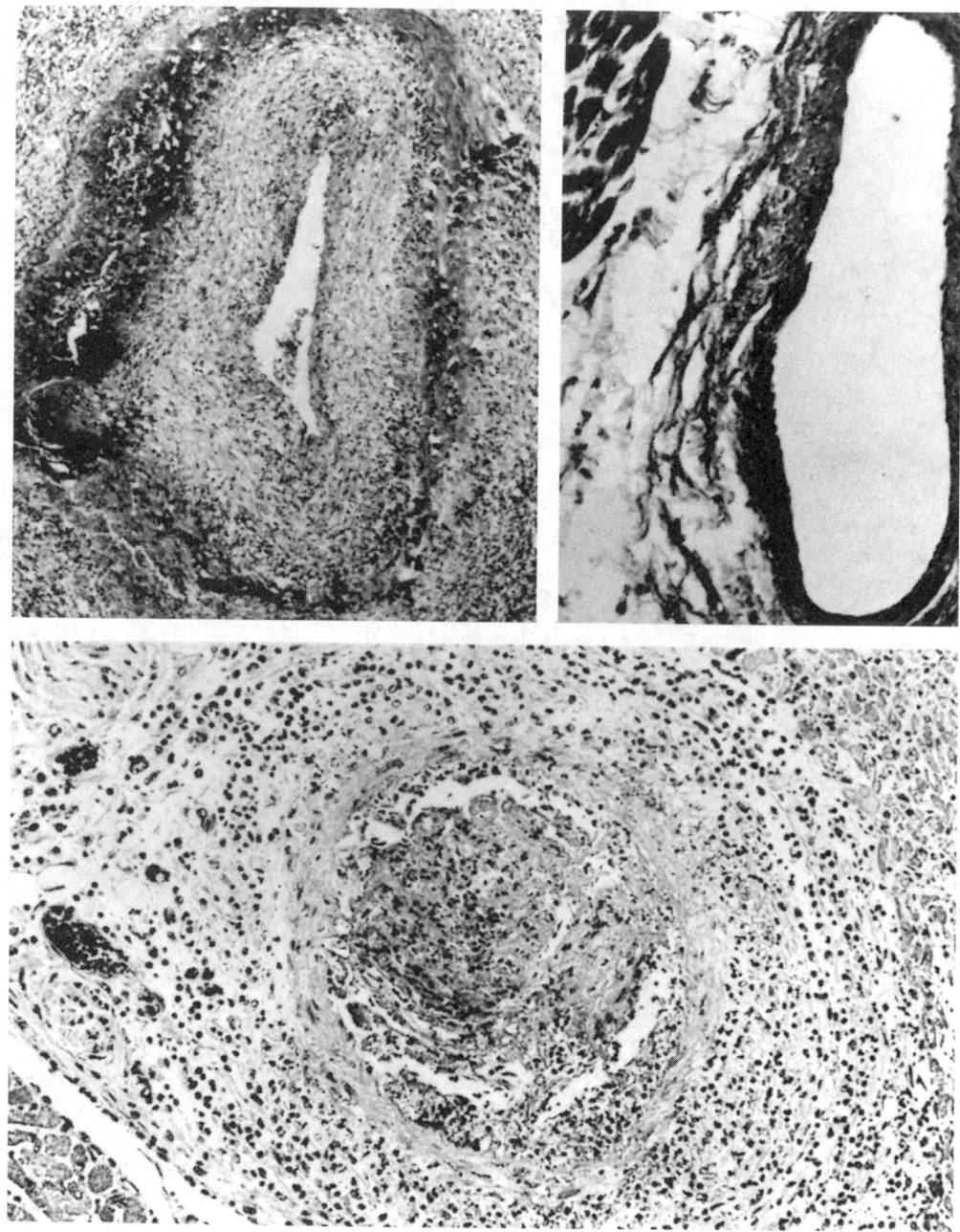

FIGURE 42-38

Top: Necrotizing angiitis (*left*) and histologically normal (*right*) segments of epicardial coronary arteries in classic polyarteritis nodosa (hematoxylin-eosin, ×16). *Bottom:* Necrotizing angiitis with fibrinoid necrosis of intramu-ral coronary artery (hematoxylin-eosin, ×160). (From Lie.[205] Reproduced with permission from the author, editor, and publisher.)

EXTERNAL COMPRESSION

External compression of the epicardial coronary arteries may result in severe luminal narrowing and progressive myocardial ischemia. External compression of a major epicardial coronary artery has been reported in patients with sinus of Valsalva aneurysms, chronic aortic dissection,[386] and epicardial tumor metastases.[387,388] Myocardial bridging (external muscle compression during ventricular systole) has been reviewed earlier.

METASTATIC IMPLANTS

Myocardial metastatic lesions from various tumors—including carcinomas, sarcomas, and lymphomas—may mimic a healed myocardial infarct at necropsy (Fig. 42-45). The discrete location or locations of these metastatic deposits generally are unrelated to specific coronary arterial supply zones, and the lesions are usually surrounded by normal myocardium. These two gross observations suggest the lesions are meta-

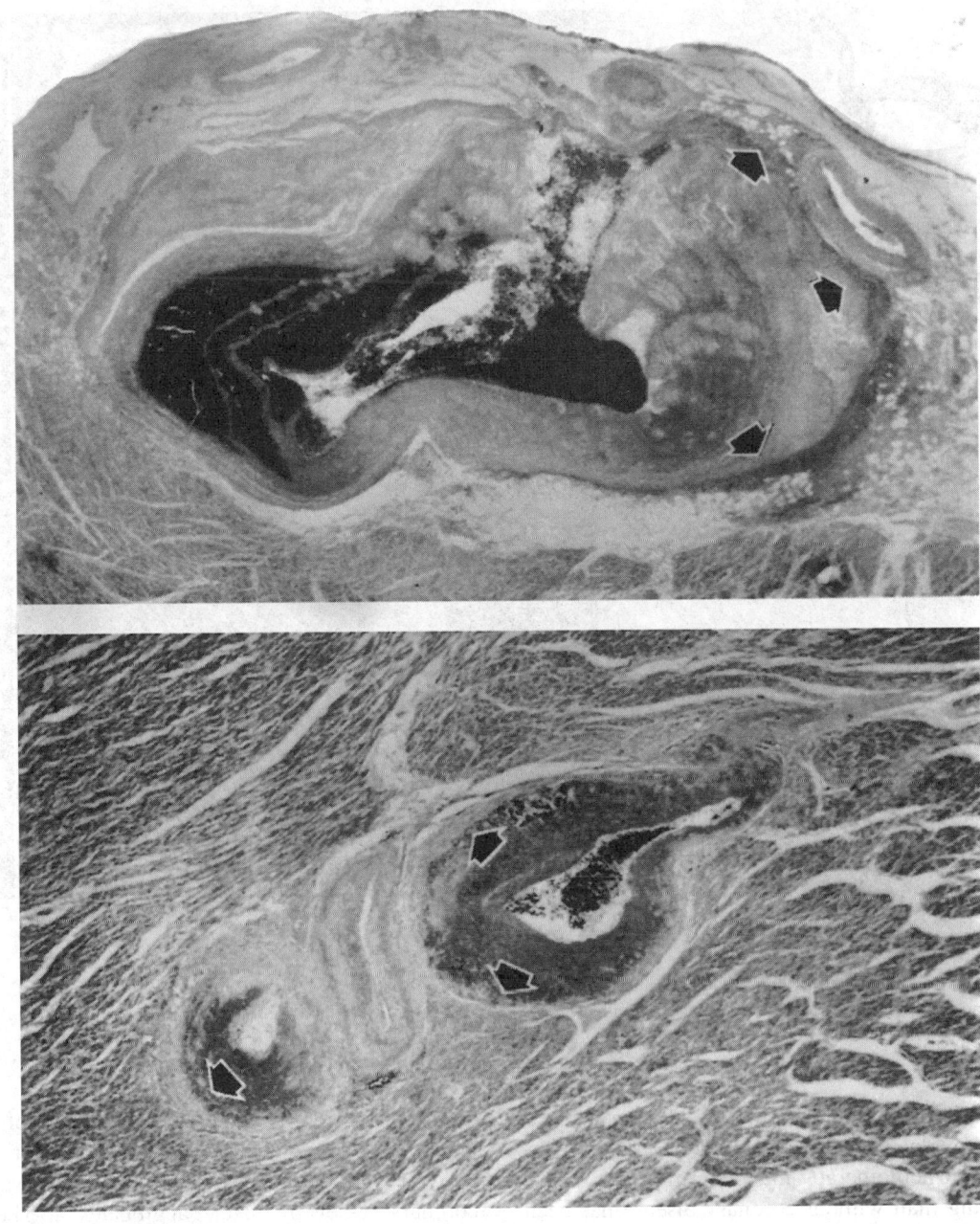

FIGURE 42-39

Necrotizing angiitis with aneurysmal disruption of epicardial (*arrows, top*) and intramural (*arrows, bottom*) coronary arteries in infantile polyarteritis nodosa (hematoxylin-eosin, ×160). (From Lie.[205] Reproduced with permission from the author, editor, and publisher.)

static tumor implants rather than healed myocardial infarcts (see also Chap. 86).

RADIATION-INDUCED CORONARY DISEASE

Intimal proliferation of epicardial coronary arteries involving the ostium, main segment, or both is well known and increasingly reported.[375,389–400] "Accelerated" or "premature" coronary atherosclerosis has been noted in young individuals undergoing previous mediastinal irradiation for various types of malignancies.[401–404] Internal proliferation following mediastinal radiation 5 to 10 years earlier is described as "intimal thickening *without* medial abnormalities." The intimal lesions (ostial or main segment of artery) consists of fibrous tissue *without* extra cellular lipid deposits.[375,399] Coronary ostial stenosis has an incidence of 0.13 to 2.7 percent of patients undergoing mediastinal irradiation treatment.[375,399] A few patients have developed acute myocardial infarction or unstable angina as a result of the radiation-induced lesions treated by myocardial revascularization[394,398] or angioplasty (see also Chap. 80).[398]

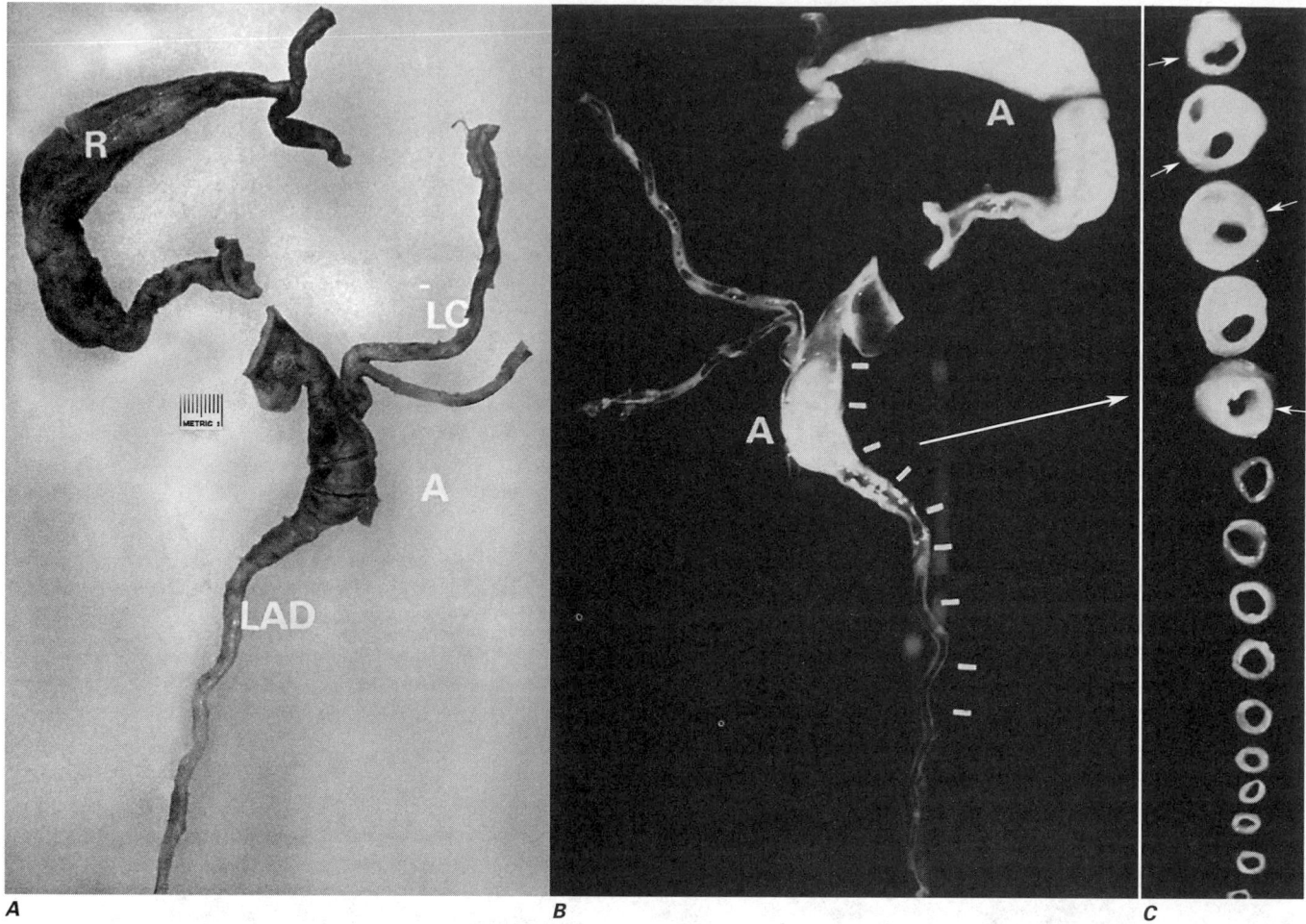

FIGURE 42-40

A. Epicardial coronary artery aneurysm involving the proximal left anterior descending (LAD) and right coronary artery (A) from an adult with probable Kawasaki's disease as a child. LC = left circumflex. *B.* Radiograph of coronary arterial tree in *A* showing calcific deposits. Cross section of the aneurysm (*A*) is shown in (*C*). Arrows indicate calcific deposits.

Because of their fibrous nature, many radiation-induced lesions do not provide the best substrate for dilation techniques.[143,144,385] Chemotherapy-induced myocardial infarction in a young man without coronary disease has been reported.[405] Cardiac invasion by tumor, hypercoagulable states, and coronary artery spasm are possible etiologies.[405] Vascular toxicity, including myocardial infarction has been reported following antineoplastic regimens containing Vinca alkaloids.[405]

CORONARY ARTERY THROMBOSIS WITHOUT UNDERLYING ATHEROSCLEROTIC PLAQUE (THROMBOSIS IN SITU)

Thrombotic occlusion of the coronary system unassociated with underlying atherosclerotic plaque may be seen with several hematologic diseases: thrombocytopenic purpura,[35] leukemia,[406] polycythemia vera,[407] sickle cell anemia,[114] and primary thrombocytosis.[408] Occasionally, acute myocardial infarction may be the initial manifestation of these hematologic disorders. A main factor responsible for the myocardial ischemia in these conditions is blockage of small intramural coronary vessels by platelet aggregates.[409] These platelet aggregates initially may form in the major coronary arteries, then embolize distally.

SUBSTANCE ABUSE (COCAINE)

Cocaine abuse is now a major health hazard; more than 22 million Americans have tried cocaine at least once, and 5 million are current users.[410] Recent reports have documented that cocaine abuse can result in myocardial ischemia and infarction in the absence of coronary artery disease,[410–420] and cocaine-induced coronary artery vasoconstriction has been reported in patients following the intranasal administration of cocaine[415,421–424] (see also Chap. 80).

Several instances of coronary artery thrombosis and spasm have been reported in patients who abuse cocaine. Acute

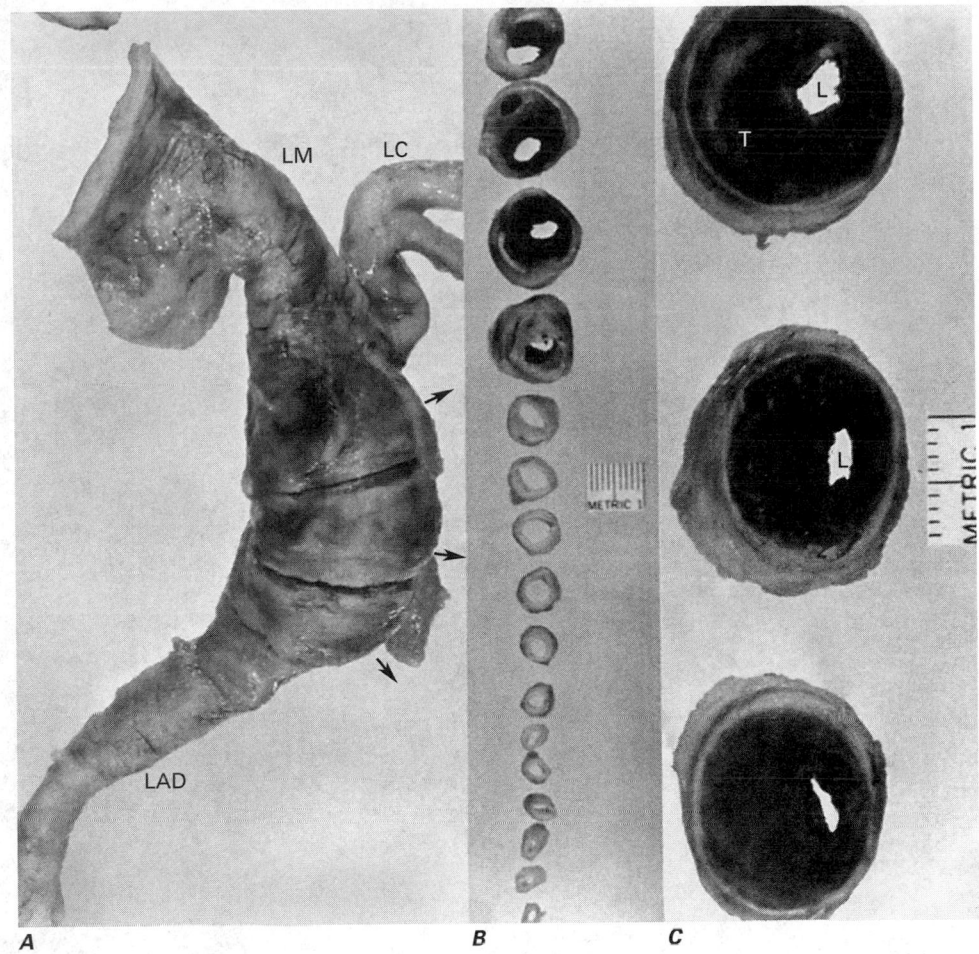

FIGURE 42-41

A. Close-up of left anterior descending (LAD) coronary aneurysm from Fig. 42-40 with cross-sections displayed in B. Note the intraaneurysmal thrombus.

C. Close-up of three transverse sections of coronary aneurysm shown in *A* and *B.* LM = left main; LC = left circumflex.

coronary thrombosis in association with cardiac events—including angina, acute myocardial infarction, and sudden death—has been reported.[410,413,422–424] In some instances, there is underlying atherosclerotic plaque; in others, the coronary arteries are normal. Coronary thrombosis occurring in coronary arteries free of atherosclerotic plaque suggests the role of cocaine-induced spasm, massive norepinephrine release in the heart, or possible primary thrombogenicity of cocaine or its metabolites.[421] Coronary spasm has been associated with cocaine usage and has been postulated as a mechanism of myocardial infarction in cocaine users with clean coronary arteries.[410, 425–431] In such cases, fibrointimal proliferation with coronary narrowing was attributed to underlying coronary artery spasm that caused focal vessel endothelial injury, platelet adherence, and aggregation. Platelets liberate platelet-derived growth factor (PDGF), which can induce intimal proliferative lesions. In patients with underlying coronary plaque, cocaine-induced spasm also may produce endothelial disruption at the surface of the plaque and promote platelet aggregation and further vasoconstriction from the release of platelet prostaglandins[432] (see also Chap. 80).

Recently, two drugs have been the center of debate over their potential for abuse versus use as psychotherapeutic agents and their complication in induction of arrhythmias.[433] Use of MDMA ("Ecstasy") (3,4-methylenedioxymethamphetamine) and MDEA ("Eve") (3,4-methylenedioxymethamphetamine) have been associated with five sudden deaths.[433] In three of these, Eve and Ecstasy may have induced fatal arrhythmias.

MYOCARDIAL OXYGEN DEMAND-SUPPLY DISPROPORTION

In this category are disease states in which there is failure to deliver adequate oxygen to the myocardium over a prolonged period or increased myocardial wall tension requiring increased oxygen supply. The classic example of the first situation is carbon monoxide poisoning,[4] which has been associated with extensive nontransmural infarction in the presence of normal epicardial coronary arteries. Prolonged shock from any cause can also result in extensive nontransmural necrosis and is frequently associated with transmural necrosis of the

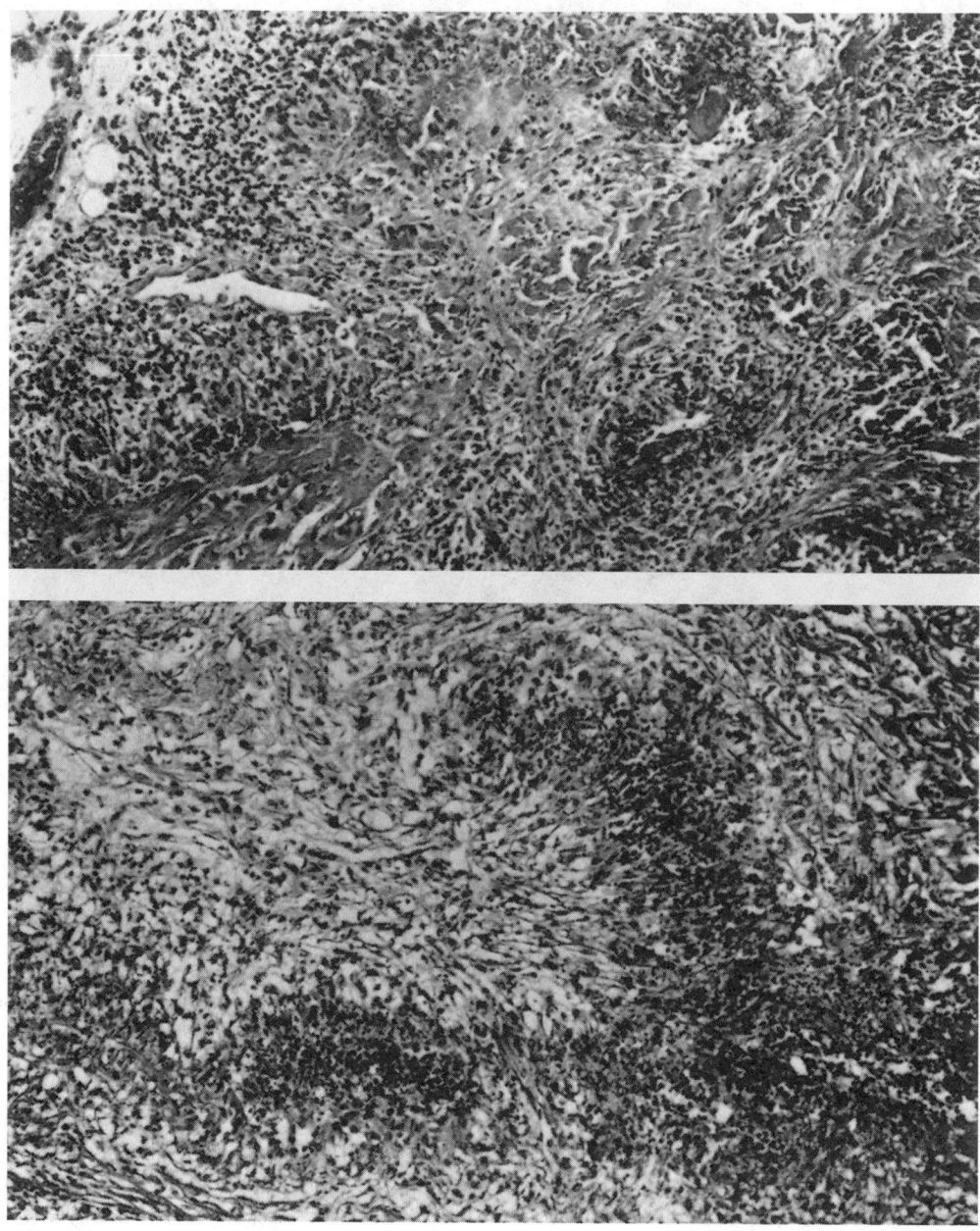

FIGURE 42-42
Granulomatous necrotizing angiitis of coronary arteries in Wegener's granulomatosis (*top*) and Churg-Strauss syndrome (*bottom*) (hematoxylin-eosin, ×160). (From Lie.[205] Reproduced with permission from the author, editor, and publisher.)

papillary muscles. One example of increased myocardial wall tension requiring increased coronary oxygen supply is aortic valve stenosis[4] (Chap. 63). In the face of increased oxygen demand with increased muscle mass, coronary blood supply may be limited by poor perfusion resulting from the lower coronary arterial pressure. In addition, poor perfusion results from the high coronary resistance caused by increased wall pressure on the intramural coronary arteries and the high left ventricular end-diastolic pressure from a stiff ventricle, with further limitation of the time in diastole for coronary blood flow occasioned by tachycardia.[4] Excessive myocardial oxygen demand exceeding supply and resulting in myocardial ischemia/infarction may also be seen in thyrotoxicosis,[434] which reflects increased metabolic rates and the adverse affects of tachycardia.

INTRAMURAL CORONARY ARTERY DISEASE (SMALL-VESSEL DISEASE)

Acute myocardial infarction may result from abnormally thickened or totally occluded intramural coronary arteries in the presence of normal extramural (epicardial) coronary arter-

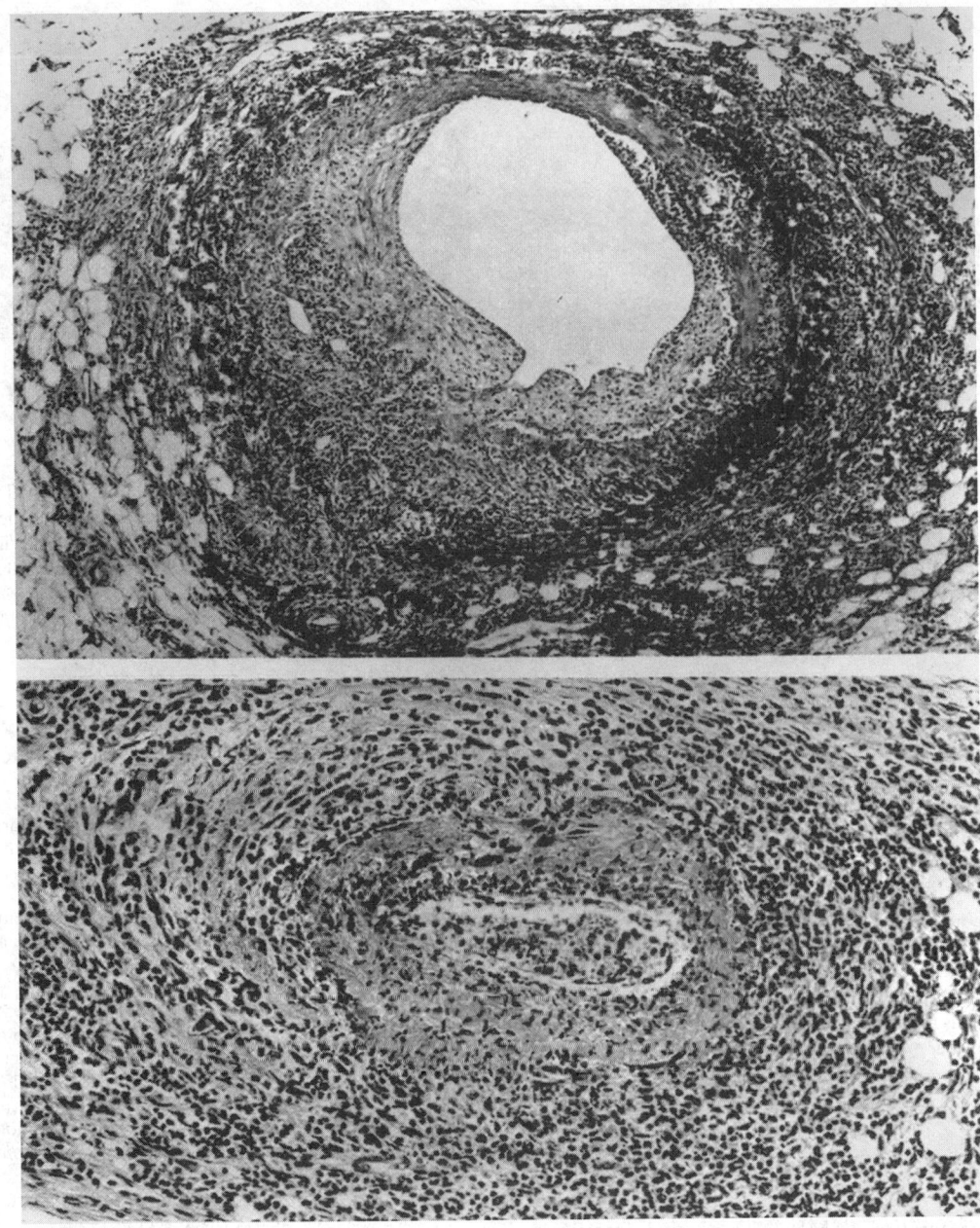

FIGURE 42-43

Necrotizing angiitis of epicardial (*top*) and intramural (*bottom*) coronary arteries in systemic lupus erythematosus (hematoxylin-eosin, ×160).

ies. A few of the conditions in this category include (1) hypertrophic cardiomyopathy, (2) diabetes mellitus, (3) amyloid heart disease,[434] (4) neuromuscular disorders (Friedreich's ataxia, progressive muscular dystrophy), (5) cardiac transplantation, (6) rheumatoid arthritis, (7) collagen-vascular disorders (scleroderma, systemic lupus erythematosus), (8) metabolism abnormalities (mucopolysaccharidoses, gangliosidoses), and (9) polyarteritis nodosa.[435–439]

Histologic abnormalities of small vessel coronary arteries have been reported in individuals who have died from toxic oil syndrome involving napeseed oil adulterated with aniline.[440]

Many of those who later died had scleroderma-like illnesses. Dense fibrosis of the sinus node, resembling scleroderma, was found with cystic degeneration of the sinus node (resembling lupus erythematosus) and fibromuscular dysplasia of small coronary vessels.

NORMAL EPICARDIAL CORONARY ARTERIES

There have been relatively few necropsy reports of patients with acute myocardial infarction who had angiographically

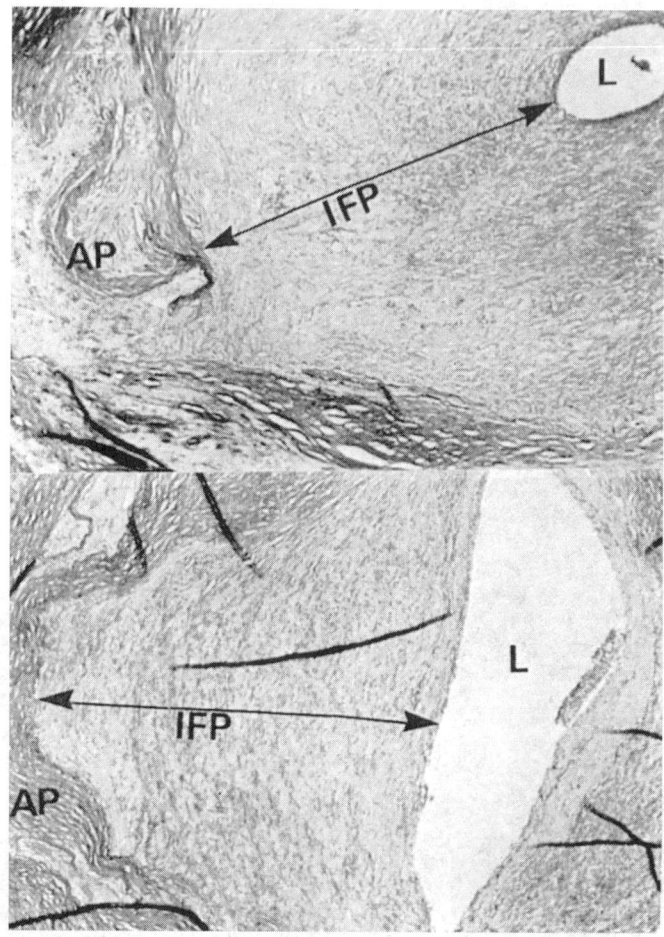

FIGURE 42-44

Intimal fibrous proliferation. Severe luminal narrowing of the left anterior descending coronary artery by intimal fibrous proliferation (IFP) several months after percutaneous balloon angioplasty. The IFP superimposes underlying atherosclerotic plaque (AP). L = lumen. (From Waller.[1] Reproduced with permission from the author, editor, and publisher.)

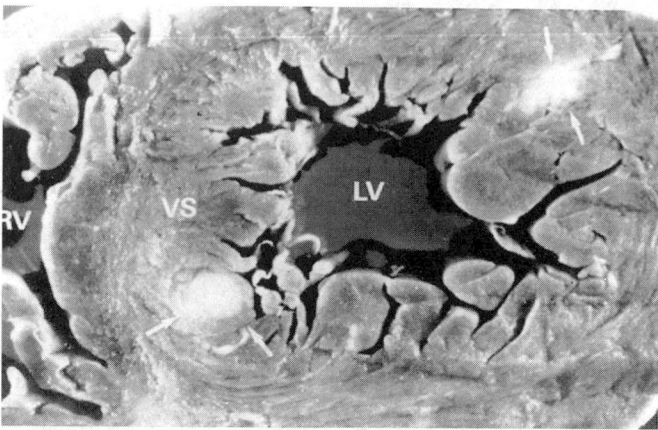

FIGURE 42-45

Metastatic deposits mimicking myocardial infarction. Transverse section of cardiac ventricle showing two discrete myocardial metastatic deposits of lymphoma. These whitish deposits may be mistakenly interpreted as healed myocardial infarctions in a patient with clean epicardial coronary arteries. LV = left ventricle; RV = right ventricle; VS = ventricular septum. (From Waller.[1] Reproduced with permission from the author, editor, and publisher.)

normal coronary arteries and normal coronary arteries at necropsy.[3,4,434,441,442] Of 100 consecutive necropsy cases of acute myocardial infarction (AMI),[3] 7 percent had infarcts without evidence of coronary luminal narrowing. In 10 patients with a typical picture of AMI who died within 25 days of onset of symptoms, the coronary arterial systems showed minimal or no luminal narrowing by atherosclerosis. No thrombotic material was observed in the coronary arteries despite the fact that the AMI was 2 days old in five patients and 3 to 4 days old in three. Possible explanations for this have included coronary artery spasm, coronary artery disease in vessels too small to be visualized angiographically, or coronary artery thrombosis or embolus with subsequent clot lysis. Myocardial infarction in postpartum women with normal epicardial coronary arteries has included two additional causes for possible spasm in these patients: bromocriptine utilized for suppression of lactation[186] and antiphospholipid syndrome with elevated anticardiolipin antibody levels, false-positive syphilis serology, and a history of deep venous thrombosis.[443]

REFERENCES

1. Waller BF. Atherosclerotic and nonatherosclerotic coronary artery factors in acute myocardial infarction. In: Pepine CJ (ed). *Acute Myocardial Infarction*. Philadelphia, Davis, 1989:29–104.
2. Alpert JS, Braunwald E. Acute myocardial infarction: Pathological, pathophysiological and clinical manifestations. In: Braunwald E (ed). *Heart Disease: A Textbook of Cardiovascular Medicine*. Philadelphia, Saunders, 1984:1262–1300.
3. Eliot RS, Baroldi G. Necropsy studies in myocardial infarction with minimal or no coronary luminal reduction due to atherosclerosis. *Circulation* 1974; 49:1127–1131.
4. Cheitlin MD, McAllister HA, deCastro CM. Myocardial infarction without atherosclerosis. *JAMA* 1975; 231:951–959.
5. Baim DS, Harrison DC. Nonatherosclerotic coronary heart disease (including coronary artery spasm). In: Hurst JW, et al (eds). *The Heart*, 5th ed. New York, McGraw-Hill, 1982:1158–1170.
6. Engel HJ, Torres C, Page HL. Major variations in anatomical origin of the coronary arteries: Angiographic observations in 4,250 patients without associated congenital heart disease. *Cathet Cardiovasc Diag* 1975; 1:157–161.
7. Roberts WC. Major anomalies of coronary arterial origin seen in adulthood. *Am Heart J* 1986; 111:941–963.
8. Levin DC, Fellows KE, Abrams HL. Hemodynamically significant primary anomalies of the coronary arteries. Angiographic aspects. *Circulation* 1978; 58:25–34.
9. Roberts WC, Siegel RJ, Zipes DP. Origin of the right coronary artery from the left sinus of Valsalva and its functional consequences: Analysis of 10 necropsy patients. *Am J Cardiol* 1982; 49:863–868.
10. Waller BF. Exercise related sudden death in young (age <30 years) and old (age >30 years) conditioned athletes. In: Wenger NK (ed). *Exercise and the Heart*, 2d ed. Cardiovascular Clinics. Philadelphia, Davis, 1985:9–73.
11. Menke DM, Jordan MD, Sut CH, Aust CH, Waller BF. Isolated and severe left main coronary atherosclerosis and thrombosis: A complication of acute angle takeoff of the left main coronary artery. *Am Heart J* 1986; 112:1319–1320.
12. Virmani R, Chun PKC, Goldstein RE, Rabinowitz M, McAllister HA. Acute takeoffs of the coronary arteries along the aortic wall and congenital coronary ostial valve-like ridges: Association with sudden death. *J Am Coll Cardiol* 1984; 3:766–771.
13. Joswig BF, Warren SE, Vieweg, WV, Hagan AD. Transmural myocardial infarction in the absence of coronary arterial luminal narrowing in a young man with single coronary arterial anomaly. *Cathet Cardiovasc Diag* 1978; 4:297–301.

14. Foster L, Waller BF, Pless JE. Hypoplastic coronary arteries and high takeoff position of the right coronary artery. *Chest* 1985; 88:299–301.

15. Foster L, Waller BF. Nonatherosclerotic fibrous ridges: A previously unrecognized cause of ostial left main stenosis. *J Indiana Med Assoc* 1983; 76:682–683.

16. Vlodaver Z, Amplatz K, Burchell HB, Edwards JE. *Coronary Heart Disease: Clinical, Angiographic and Pathologic Profiles.* New York, Springer-Verlag, 1976.

17. Alexander RW, Griffith GC. Anomalies of the coronary arteries and their clinical significance. *Circulation* 1956; 14:800–805.

18. Burth HC. Hoher und trichterformiger Ursprung der Herz Kanzarterien. *Beitr Pathol Anal* 1963; 128:139–148.

19. Holt S. Syphilitic ostial occlusion. *Br Heart J* 1977; 39:469–470.

20. Young JA, Sengupta A, Khaja FU. Coronary arterial stenosis, angina pectoris and atypical coarctation of the aorta due to nonspecific arteritis: Treatment, with aortocoronary bypass graft. *Am J Cardiol* 1973; 32:356–361.

21. Rozavi M. Unusual forms of coronary artery disease. In: D Vedt (ed). *Cleveland Clinic Cardiovascular Consultations.* Philadelphia, Davis, 1975:25.

22. Hudgson P, Foster JB, Walton JN. Methysergide and coronary artery disease. *Am Heart J* 1967; 74:854–855.

23. Yates JD, Kirsh MM, Sodeman TM, Walton JA, Brymer JF. Coronary ostial stenosis: A complication of aortic valve replacement. *Circulation* 1974; 49:530–534.

24. Baroldi G. Diseases of the coronary arteries. In: Silver MD (ed). *Cardiovascular Pathology.* New York, Churchhill Livingstone, 1983:341.

25. Reyman HC. Disertatis de vasis cordis propiis. *Bibl Anat* 1737; 2:366–373.

26. Noble J, Bourassa MG, Petitclerc R, Dyrda I. Myocardial bridging and milking effect of the left anterior descending coronary artery: Normal variant or obstruction? *Am J Cardiol* 1976; 37:993–999.

27. Faruqui AM, Maloy WC, Felner JM, Schlant RC, Logan WD, Symbas P. Symptomatic myocardial bridging of the coronary artery. *Am J Cardiol* 1978; 41:1305–1310.

28. Visscher DW, Mildes BM, Waller BF. Tunneled ("bridged") left anterior descending coronary artery in a newborn without clinical or morphological evidence of myocardial ischemia. *Cath Cardiovasc Diag* 1983; 9:493–498.

29. Edwards JC, Burnsides C, Swarm RL, Lansing AJ. Arteriosclerosis and extramural portions of coronary arteries in the human heart. *Circulation* 1956; 13:235–241.

30. Polacek P. Relation of myocardial bridges and loops in the coronary arteries to coronary occlusions. *Am Heart J* 1961; 61:44–52.

31. Levin DC, Fellows KE, Abrams HL. Hemodynamically significant primary anomalies of the coronary arteries. Angiographic aspects. *Circulation* 1978; 58:25–34.

32. Kramer JR, Kitazume H, Proudin WI, Sones IM. Clinical significance of isolated coronary bridges: Benign and frequent condition involving the left anterior descending artery. *Am Heart J* 1982; 103:283–288.

33. Ishimori T, Raizner AE, Chahine RA, Awdeh M, Luchi RJ. Myocardial bridges in man: Clinical correlations and angiographic accentuation with nitroglycerin. *Cathet Cardiovas Diag* 1977; 3:59–65.

34. Roberts WC, Dicicco BS, Waller BF, Kishel JC, McManus BM, Dawson SL. Origin of the left main from the right coronary artery or from the right aortic sinus with intramyocardial tunneling to the left side of the heart via the ventricular septum: The case against clinical significance of myocardial bridge or coronary tunnel. *Am Heart J* 1982; 104:303–305.

35. Schulte MA, Waller BF, Hull MT, Pless JE. Origin of the left anterior descending artery from the right aortic sinus with intramyocardial tunneling to the left side of the heart via the ventricular septum: A case against clinical and morphologic significance of myocardial bridging. *Am Heart J* 1985; 110:499–501.

36. Angelini P, Trivellato M, Donis J, Leachman RD. Myocardial bridges: A review. *Prog Cardiovasc Dis* 1983; 26:75–88.

37. Isner JM, Donaldson RF. Coronary angiographic and morphologic correlation. *Cardiol Clin* 1984; 2:571–92.

38. Nakajima K, Taki J, Bunko H, Tonami N, Tada A, Nanbu I, et al. Demonstration of therapeutic effect in a patient with myocardial bridge by exercise-myocardial SPECT imaging. *Clin Nucl Med* 1985; 10:116–117.

39. Kramer JR, Kitazume H, Krauthamer D, Raju NV, Loop FD, Proudfit WL. The prevalence of myocardial bridging and septal squeeze in patients with significant aortic stenosis. *Cleve Q* 1984; 51:35–38.

40. Carvalho VB, Macruz R, Decort LV, Arie S, Manrique R, Mello SC, et al. Hemodynamic determinants of coronary constriction in human myocardial bridges. *Am Heart J* 1984; 108:73–80.

41. Kitazume H, Kramer JR, Krauthamer D, Tobgi S, Proudfit WL, Sones FM. Myocardial bridges in obstructive hypertrophic cardiomyopathy. *Am Heart J* 1983; 106:131–135.

42. Pichard AD, Casanegra P, Marchant E, Rodriguez JA. Abnormal regional myocardial flow in myocardial bridging of the left anterior descending coronary artery. *Am J Cardiol* 1981; 47:978–982.

43. Chee TP, Jensen DP, Padnick MB, Cornell WP, Desser KB. Myocardial bridging of the left anterior descending coronary artery resulting in subendocardial infarction. *Arch Int Med* 1981; 141:1703–1704.

44. Traube C, Rafii S, Greenfield DH, Levine RS, Fox P. Progression of the milking effect of the coronary artery. *Chest* 1981; 79:475–476.

45. Greenspan M, Iskandrian AS, Catherwood E, Kimbiris D, Bemis CE, Segal BL. Myocardial bridging of the left anterior descending artery: Evaluation using exercise thallium-201 myocardial scintigraphy. *Cathet Cardiovasc Diagn* 1980; 6:173–180.

46. Kuhn FE, Reagan K, Mohler ER III, Satler LF, Lu DY, Rackley CE. Evidence for endothelial dysfunction and enhanced vasoconstriction in myocardial bridges. *Am Heart J* 1991; 122:1764–1766.

47. Voelker W, Euchner U, Dittmann H, Karsch KR. Long-term clinical course of patients with angina and angiographically normal coronary arteries. *Clin Cardiol* 1991; 14:307–311.

48. Feld H, Guadanino V, Hollander G, Greengart A, Lichstein E, Shani J. Exercise-induced ventricular tachycardia in association with a myocardial bridge. *Chest* 1991; 1295–1296.

49. Furniss SS, Williams DO, McGregor CG. Systolic coronary occlusion due to myocardial bridging—A rare cause of ischemia. *Int J Cardiol* 1990; 26:116–117.

50. Somanath HS, Reddy KN, Gupta SK, Murthy JS, Rao AS, Abraham KA. Myocardial bridge (MB): An angiographic curiosity? *Indian Heart J* 1989; 41:296–300.

51. Vasan RS, Bahl VK, Rajani M. Myocardial infarction associated with a myocardial bridge. *Int J Cardiol* 1989; 25:240–241.

52. Theron HD, Kleynhans PH, Marx JD, Jordaan PJ. Myocardial bridging as a cause of myocardial infarction: A case report. *S Afr Med J* 1988; 74:243–244.

53. Bennett JM, Bomerus P. Thallium-201 scintigraphy perfusion defect with dipyridamole in a patient with a myocardial bridge. *Clin Cardiol* 1988; 11:268–270.

54. Kracoff OH, Ovsyshcher I, Gueron M. Malignant course of a benign anomaly: Myocardial bridging. *Chest* 1987; 92:1113–1115.

55. Bestetti RB, Finzi LA, Amaral FT, Secches AL, Oliveira JS. Myocardial bridging of coronary arteries associated with an impending acute myocardial infarction. *Clin Cardiol* 1987; 10:129–131.

56. Bestetti RB, Costa RS, Zucolotto S, Oliveira JS. Fatal outcome associated with autopsy proven myocardial bridging of the left anterior descending coronary artery. *Europ Heart J* 1989; 10:573–576.

57. Ferreira AG Jr, Trotter SE, Konig B Jr, Decourt LV, Fox K, Olsen EG. Myocardial bridges: Morphological and functional aspects. *Br Heart J* 1991; 66:364–367.

58. Irvin RG. The angiographic prevalence of myocardial bridging in man. *Chest* 1982; 81:198–202.

59. Channer KS, Bukis E, Hartnell G, Rees JR. Myocardial bridging of the coronary arteries. *Clin Radiol* 1989; 40:355–359.

60. Wymore P, Yedlicka JW, Garcia-Medina V, Olivari MT, Hunter DW, Castaneda-Zuniga WR, et al. The incidence of myocardial bridges in heart transplants. *Cardiovasc Int Radiol* 1989; 12:202–206.

61. Watanabe G, Ohhira M, Takemura H, Tanaka N, Iwa T. Surgical treatment for myocardial bridge using intraoperative echocardiography. *J Cardiovasc Surg* 1989; 30:1009–1012.

62. Betriu A, Tubau J, Sanz G, Magrina J, Navarro-Lopez F. Relief of angina by periarterial muscle resection of myocardial bridges. *Am Heart J* 1980; 100:223–226.

63. Pey J, de Dios RM, Epeldegui A. Myocardial bridging and hypertrophic cardiomyopathy: Relief of ischemia by surgery. *Int J Cardiol* 1985; 8:327–330.

64. Gupta NC, Beauvais J. Physiologic assessment of coronary artery fistula. *Clin Nucl Med* 1991; 16:40–42.

65. Theman TE, Crosby DR. Coronary artery steal secondary to coronary arteriovenous fistula. *Can J Surg* 1981; 24:231–233, 236.

66. Nakashima M, Takashima S, Hashimoto K, Shiraishi M. Association of stroke and myocardial infarction in children. *Neuropediatrics* 1982; 13:47–49.

67. Macri R, Capulzini A, Fazzini L, Cornali M, Verunelli F, Reginato E. Congenital coronary artery fistula: Report of five patients, diagnostic problems and principles of management. *Thorac Cardiovasc Surg* 1982; 30:167–171.

68. Sethia B, Pollock JC. Coronary artery fistula following rupture of aneurysm of the sinus node artery into the right atrium. *Thorac Cardiovasc Surg* 1985; 33:191–192.

69. Zalman F, Andia AM, Wu KT, Moores WY, Hoit B, Maisel AS. Atherosclerotic coronary artery aneurysm progressing to coronary artery fistula: Presentation as myocardial infarction with continuous murmur. *Am Heart J* 1987; 114:427–429.

70. Fyfe DA, Edwards WD, Driscoll DJ. Myocardial ischemia in patients with pulmonary atresia and intact ventricular septum. *J Am Coll Cardiol* 1986; 8:402–406.

71. Lau G. Sudden death arising from a congenital coronary artery fistula. *Forens Sci Int* 1995; 73:125–130.

72. Takahashi M, Sekiguchi H, Fujikawa H, Mizuno O, Akazawa H, Kuroki S, et al. Multiple saccular aneurysm formation in a patient with bilateral coronary artery fistula: A case report and review of the literature. *Cardiology* 1995; 86:174–176.

73. Takahashi M, Sekiguchi H, Fujikawa H, Mito H, Eto M, Hojo Y, et al. Multicystic aneurysmal dilatation of bilateral coronary artery fistula. *Cathet Cardiol Diagn* 1994; 31:290–292.

74. Cason BA, Gordon HJ. Coronary steal caused by a coronary artery fistula. *J Cardiothorac Vasc Anesth* 1992; 6:65–67.

75. Rein AJ, Yatsiv I, Simcha A. Intracardiac causes of superior vena cava obstruction. *Eur J Pediatr* 1988; 148:98–100.

76. Vavuranakis M, Bush CA, Boudoulas H. Coronary artery fistulas in adults: Incidence, angiographic characteristics, natural history. *Cathet Cardiovasc Diagn* 1995; 35:116–120.

77. Aydogan U, Onursal E, Cantez T, Barlas C, Tanman B, Gurgan L. Giant congenital coronary artery fistula to left superior vena cava and right atrium with compression of left pulmonary vein simulating cor triatriatum—Diagnostic value of magnetic resonance imaging. *Eur J Cardiovasc Surg* 1994; 8:97–99.

78. Vigneswaran WT, Pollock JC. Pulmonary atresia with ventricular septal defect and coronary artery fistula: A late presentation. *Br Heart J* 1988; 59:387–388.

79. Shizukuda Y, Yonekura S, Tsuchihashi K, Tanaka S, Komatsu S, Iimura O. A case of a right coronary artery to left ventricle fistula observed over twenty years. *Jpn J Med* 1989; 28:510–514.

80. Wilde P, Watt I. Congenital coronary artery fistulae: Six new cases with a collective review. *Clin Radiol* 1980; 31:301–311.

81. Mori K, Onoe T, Ooka T. Three main coronary arteries to pulmonary artery fistula. *Jpn Circ J* 1981; 45:209–212.

82. Schneeweiss A, Rath S, Neufeld HN. Bilateral congenital coronary artery fistula. *Thorax* 1981; 36:697–698.

83. Adams P, Morris L, Ross I. Congenital left coronary artery–right ventricular fistula. *Austr Pediatr J* 1983; 19:47–50.

84. Nakashima T, Tsuji T, Miyanaga H, Imanishi H, Suto Y, Takeda S, et al. A case of blue rubber bleb nevus syndrome with coronary artery fistula to left ventricle. *Gastroenterol Jpn* 1983; 18:255–259.

85. Liu PR, Leong KH, Lee PC, Chen YT. Congenital coronary artery-cardiac chamber fistulae: A study of fourteen cases. *Chung Hua i Hsueh Tsa Chih* 1994; 54:160–5.

86. Mabo P, Le Breton H, De Place C, Daubert C. Asymptomatic pseudo-aneurysm of the left ventricle and coronary artery fistula after closed-chest ablation of an accessory pathway. *Am Heart J* 1992; 124:1637–1639.

87. Bata IR, MacDonald RG, O'Neill BJ. Coronary artery fistula as a complication of percutaneous transluminal coronary angioplasty. *Can J Cardiol* 1993; 9:331–335.

88. Iannone LA, Iannone DP. Iatrogenic left coronary artery fistula-to-left ventricle following PTCA: A previously unreported complication with nonsurgical management. *Am Heart J* 1990; 120:1215–1217.

89. Cheng TO. Coronary artery fistula related to dilatation of totally occluded vessel. *Clin Cardiol* 1994; 17:166.

90. Geist M, Rozenman Y, Hasin Y, Gotsman MS. Coronary artery–pulmonary artery fistula associated with hypertrophic cardiomyopathy. *Clin Cardiol* 1994; 17:93–94.

91. Shirai K, Ogawa M, Kawaguchi H, Kawano T, Nakashima Y, Arakawa K. Acute myocardial infarction due to thrombus formation in congenital coronary artery fistula. *Eur Heart J* 1994; 15:577–579.

92. Uchida N, Baudet E, Roques X, Laborde N, Billes MA. Surgical experience of coronary artery–right ventricular fistula in a heart transplant patient. *Eur J Cardiothorac Surg* 1995; 9:106–108.

93. Uy R, Sharma B, Franciosa JA. Acquired coronary artery fistula to the left ventricle after acute myocardial infarction. *Am J Cardiol* 1986; 58:557–558.

94. Doi YL, Takata J, Hamashige N, Yonezawa Y, Odawara H, Ozawa T. Congenital coronary arteriovenous fistula associated with dilated cardiomyopathy. *Chest* 1987; 91:464–466.

95. Lee RT, Mudge GH, Colucci WS. Coronary artery fistula after mitral valve surgery. *Am Heart J* 1988; 115:1128–1130.

96. Lucca MJ, Tomlinson GC. Acquired coronary artery fistula: a sign of mural thrombus. *Cathet Cardiovasc Diagn* 1988; 15:273–276.

97. Sandhu JS, Uretsky BF, Zerbe TR, Goldsmith AS, Reddy PS, Kormos RL, et al. Coronary artery fistula in the heart transplant patient: A potential complication of endomyocardial biopsy. *Circulation* 1989; 79:350–356.

98. Henzlova MJ, Nath H, Bucy RP, Bourge RC, Kirklin JK, Rogers WJ. Coronary artery to right ventricle fistula in heart transplant recipients: A complication of endomyocardial biopsy. *J Am Coll Cardiol* 1989; 14:258–261.

99. Saeian K, Vellinga T, Troup P, Wetherbee J. Coronary artery fistula formation secondary to permanent pacemaker placement. *Chest* 1991; 99:780–781.

100. Sherman D, Smith C, Marboe C, Mosca R, Weinberger J, Di Tullio M, et al. Right atrial angiosarcoma causing a coronary artery fistula: Diagnosis by transesophageal echocardiography. *Am Heart J* 1993; 126:254–256.

101. Gildein HP, Kleinert S, Layangool T, Wilkinson JL. Acquired coronary artery fistula in children after ventricular septal myectomy of the right or left ventricular outflow tract. *Am Heart J* 1995; 130:1124–1126.

102. Lowe JE, Adams DH, Cummings RG, Wesly RL, Phillips HR. The natural history and recommended management of patients with traumatic coronary artery fistulas. *Ann Thorac Surg* 1983; 36:295–305.

103. Haas GE, Parr GV, Trout RG, Hargrove WC III. Traumatic coronary artery fistula. *J Trauma* 1986; 26:854–857.

104. Kwan T, Salciccioli L, Elsakr A, Burack J, Feit A. Coronary artery fistula coexisting with a ventricular septal defect due to a penetrating gunshot wound. *Cathet Cardiovasc Diagn* 1995; 34:235–239.

105. Tami LF. Coronary artery-right ventricular fistula after coronary artery bypass grafting. *Clin Cardiol* 1993; 16:155–157.

106. Sapin P, Frantz E, Jain A, Nichols TC, Dehmer GJ. Coronary artery fistula: An abnormality affecting all age groups. *Medicine* 1990; 69:101–113.

107. Hackett D, Hallidie-Smith KA. Spontaneous closure of coronary artery fistula. *Brit Heart J* 1984; 52:477–479.

108. Griffiths SP, Ellis K, Hordof AJ, Martin E, Levine OR, Gersony WM. Spontaneous complete closure of a congenital coronary artery fistula. *J Am Coll Cardiol* 1983; 2:1169–1173.

109. John S, Perianayagam WJ, Muralidharan S, Nandakumar V, Mansfield R, Krishnaswamy S, et al. Surgical treatment of congenital coronary artery fistula. *Thorax* 1981; 36:350–354.

110. Rim RS, Yang YJ, Chiu IS, Lin FY, Chu SH, Hung CR. Surgical management of congenital coronary artery fistula. *J Formos Med Assoc* 1985; 84:683–692.

111. Wellens F, Deuvaert F, Leclerc JL, Primo G. Coronary artery fistula: An absolute surgical indication. *Acta Chirurg Belg* 1984; 84:339–344.

112. Kostis JB, Burns JJ, Moreyra AE, Pichard AD. Recurrent coronary artery fistula. *Clin Cardiol* 1984; 7:307–313.

113. Reidy JF, Anjos RT, Qureshi SA, Baker EJ, Tynan MJ. Transcatheter embolization in the treatment of coronary artery fistulas. *J Am Coll Cardiol* 1991; 18:187–192.

114. Wenger NK. Nonatherosclerotic causes of myocardial ischemia and necrosis. In: Hurst JW, et al. (eds). *The Heart*, 4th ed. New York, McGraw-Hill, 1978:1345–1362.

115. Glickel SZ, Maggs PR, Ellis FH. Coronary artery aneurysm. *Ann Thorac Surg* 1978; 25:372–376.

116. Sumino H, Kanda T, Sasaki T, Kanazawa N, Takeuchi H. Myocardial infarction secondary to coronary aneurysm in systemic lupus erythematosus: An autopsy case. *Angiology* 1995; 46:527–530.

117. Teja K, Crampton RS. Intramural coronary arteritis from cholesterol emboli: A rare case of unstable angina preceding sudden death. *Am Heart J* 1985; 110:168–170.

118. Choy DS, Stertzer S, Loubeau JM, Kessler H, Quilici P, Rotterdam H, et al. Embolization and vessel wall perforation in argon laser recanalization. *Lasers Surg Med* 1985; 5:297–308.

119. Arvan S. Mural thrombi in coronary artery disease: Recent advances in pathogenesis, diagnosis, and approaches to treatment. *Arch Intern Med* 1984; 144:113–116.

120. Charles RG, Epstein EJ. Diagnosis of coronary embolism: A review. *J R Soc Med* 1983; 76:863–869.

121. Hartman RB, Harrison EE, Pupello DF, Vijayanagar R, Sbar SS. Characteristics of left ventricular thrombus resulting in perioperative embolism: A complication of coronary artery bypass grafting. *J Thorac Cardiovasc Surg* 1983; 86:706–709.

122. Rath S, Har-Zahav Y, Battler A, Agranat O, Neufeld HN. Coronary arterial embolus from left atrial myxoma. *Am J Cardiol* 1984; 54:1392–1393.

123. Tubbs RR, Picha GC, Levin HS, Groves L, Barenberg S. Cotton emboli of the coronary arteris. *Hum Pathol* 1980; 11:76–80.

124. Keon WJ, Heggtveit HA, Leduc J. Perioperative myocardial infarction caused by atheroembolism. *J Thorac Cardiovasc Surg* 1982; 84:849–855.

125. Charles RG, Epstein EJ, Holt S, Coulshed N. Coronary embolism in valvular heart disease. *Q J Med* 1982; 51:147–161.

126. Camann WR, Sacks GM, Schools AG, Heggeness ST, Reilly DT, Concepcion, M. Nearly fatal cardiovascular collapse during total hip replacement: Probable coronary arterial embolism. *Anesth Analg* 1991; 72:245–248.

127. Wiegand V, Tebbe U, Helmchen U, Kreuzer H. Coronary arterial embolism due to valvular debris after percutaneous valvuloplasty of calcific mitral stenosis. *Clin Cardiol* 1988; 11:793–796.

128. Goulah RD, Rose MR, Strober M, Haft JI. Coronary dissection following chest trauma with systemic emboli. *Chest* 1988; 93:887–888.

129. Mercereau D, Klinke WP. Paradoxical coronary embolism associated with an unusual interatrial flap valve. *Can J Cardiol* 1988; 4:140–143.

130. Saenz CB, Harrell RR, Sawyer JA, Hood WP. Acute percutaneous transluminal coronary angioplasty complicated by embolism to a coronary artery remote from the site of infarction. *Cathet Cardiovasc Diagn* 1987; 13:266–268.

131. Lifschultz BD, Donoghue ER, Leestma JE, Boade WA. Embolization of cotton pledgets following insertion of porcine cardiac valve bioprostheses. *J Foren Sci* 1987; 32:1796–1800.

132. Johnson D, Gonzalez-Lavin L. Myocardial infarction secondary to calcific embolism: An unusual complication of bioprosthetic valve degeneration. *Ann Thorac Surg* 1986; 42:102–103.

133. Cina SJ, Raso DS, Crymes LW, Upshur JK. Fatal suture embolism to the left anterior descending coronary artery: A case report and review of the literature. *Am J Forens Med Pathol* 1994; 15:142–145.

134. Saber RS, Edwards WD, Bailey KR, McGovern TW, Schwartz RS, Holmes DR. Coronary embolization after balloon angioplasty or thrombolytic therapy: An autopsy study of 32 cases. *J Am Coll Cardiol* 1993; 22:1283–1288.

135. Hopkins HR, Pecirep DP. Bullet embolization to a coronary artery. *Ann Thorac Surg* 1993; 56:370–372.

136. Nagaoka H, Funakoshi N, Innami R, Fujiwara A, Watanabe M. Left ventricular aneurysm, normal coronary arteries and embolization in a patient with systemic lupus erythematosus. *Chest* 1993; 103:287–288.

137. Yutani C, Imakita M, Ueda-Ishibashi H, Katsuragi M, Fujita H. Coronary artery embolism with special reference to invasive procedures as the source. *Mod Pathol* 1992; 5:244–249.

138. Cabin HS, Roberts WC. Left ventricular aneurysm, intraaneurysmal thrombus and systemic embolus in coronary heart disease. *Chest* 1980; 77:586–590.

139. Roberts WC. Coronary embolism: A review of causes, consequences and diagnostic considerations. *Cardiovasc Med* 1978; 3:699–709.

140. Waller BF, Dixon DS, Kem RW, Roberts WC. Embolus to the left main coronary artery. *Am J Cardiol* 1982; 50:658–660.

141. Isner JM, Donaldson RF. Coronary angiographic and morphologic correlation. In: Waller BF (ed). *Cardiac Morphology*. Cardiology Clinics. Philadelphia: Saunders; 1984:571–592.

142. Rabinowitz M, Virmani R, McAllister HA. Spontaneous coronary artery dissection and eosinophilic infiltration: A cause-and-effect relationship? *Am J Med* 1982; 72:923–928.

143. Waller BR. Pathology of transluminal balloon angioplasty used in the treatment of coronary heart disease. *Hum Pathol* 1987; 18:476–484.

144. Waller BF. Crackers, breakers, stretchers, drillers, scrapers, shavers, burners, welders and melters: The future of atherosclerotic coronary

145. Antoniucci D, Magi Diligenti L. Spontaneous dissection of the three major coronary arteries. *Eur Heart J* 1990; 11:1130–1134.

146. Mather PJ, Hansen CL, Goldman B, Inniss S, Pina I, Norris R, et al. Postpartum multivessel coronary dissection. *J Heart Lung Transpl* 1994; 13:533–537.

147. Wasserman L, Wolf P, Podolin R, Bloor CM. Dissecting aneurysm of a coronary artery due to percutaneous transluminal balloon angioplasty. *Am J Cardiovasc Pathol* 1990; 3:271–274.

148. Ehya H, Weitzner S. Postpartum dissecting aneurysm of coronary arteries in a patient with sarcoidosis. *South Med J* 1980; 73:87–88.

149. Lantos G, Sos TA, Sniderman KW, Saddekni S, Hilton S. Dissecting hematoma of the thoracic aorta extending into a coronary artery: Angiographic demonstration. *Radiology* 1980; 135:329–330.

150. Molloy PJ, Ablett MB, Anderson KR. Left main stem coronary artery dissection. *Br Heart J* 1980; 43:705–708.

151. Shin P, Minamino T, Onishi S, Kitamura H. Dissecting aneurysms of the coronary arteries. *Acta Pathol Japon* 1982; 32:713–724.

152. van der Bel-Kahn J. Recurrent primary coronary artery dissecting aneurysm. *Am J Clin Pathol* 1982; 78:394–398.

153. Morise AP, Hardin NJ, Bovill EG, Gundel WD. Coronary artery dissection secondary to coronary arteriography: Presentation of three cases and review of the literature. *Cathet Cardiovasc Diagn* 1981; 7:283–296.

154. Gibson WG, Reimer KA. Multiple coronary artery dissections in old age: A unique case. *Arch Pathol Lab Med* 1980; 104:419–421.

155. Paidipaty BB, Husain M, Puri VK. Right coronary artery occlusion after acute proximal dissection. *Crit Care Med* 1983; 11:574–575.

156. Virmani R, Forman MB, Robinowitz M, McAllister HA. Coronary artery dissections. *Cardiol Clin* 1984; 2:633–646.

157. Boland J, Limet R, Trotteur G, Legrand V, Kulbertus H. Left main coronary dissection after mild chest trauma: Favorable evolution with fibrinolytic and surgical therapies. *Chest* 1988; 93:213–214.

158. Nishikawa H, Nakanishi S, Nishiyama S, Nishimura S, Kato K, Yanagishita Y, et al. Primary coronary artery dissection: Its incidence, mode of the onset and prognostic evaluation. *J Cardiol* 1988; 18:307–317.

159. Wisecarver J, Jones J, Goaley T, McManus B. Spontaneous coronary artery dissection: The challenge of detection, the enigma of cause. *Am J Forens Med Pathol* 1989; 10:60–62.

160. Movsesian MA, Wray RB. Postpartum myocardial infarction. *Br Heart J* 1989; 62:154–156.

161. Burkey D, Love J, Fanning J, Lambrew C. Multiple spontaneous coronary artery dissections in a middle aged woman: Support for an underlying eosinophilic arteritis predisposing to intimal disruption. *Cathet Cardiovasc Diagn* 1993; 30:303–305.

162. Siegel RJ, Koponen M. Spontaneous coronary artery dissection causing sudden death: Mechanical arterial failure or primary vasculitis. *Arch Pathol Lab Med* 1994; 118:196–198.

163. Bateman AC, Gallagher PJ, Vincenti AC. Sudden death from coronary artery dissection. *J Clin Pathol* 1995; 48:781–784.

164. Sage MD, Koelmeyer TD, Smeeton WM. Fatal postpartum coronary artery dissection: A light- and electron-microscope study. *Am J Forens Med Pathol* 1986; 7:107–111.

165. Thayer Jo, Healy RW, Maggs PR. Spontaneous coronary artery dissection. *Ann Thorac Surg* 1987; 44:97–102.

166. Emori T, Goto Y, Maeda T, Chiba Y, Haze K. Multiple coronary artery dissections diagnosed in vivo in a pregnant woman. *Chest* 1993; 104:289–290.

167. Shaver PJ, Carrig TF, Baker WP. Postpartum coronary artery dissection. *Br Heart J* 1978; 40:83–86.

168. Waller BF, Orr CM, Pinkerton CA, Van Tassel J, Peters T, Slack JD. Coronary balloon angioplasty dissections: The good, the bad, and the ugly. *J Am Coll Cardiol* 1992; 20:701–706.

169. Prinzmetal M, Kennamer R, Merliss R, Wada T. Angina pectoris: I. A variant form of angina pectoris. Preliminary report. *Am J Med* 1959; 27:375–388.

170. Peretz DI. Variant angina pectoris of Prinzmetal. *Can Med Assoc J* 1961; 85:1101–1102.

171. Gianelly R, Mugler F, Harrison DC. Prinzmetal's variant of angina pectoris with only slight coronary atherosclerosis. *Calif Med* 1968; 108:129–132.

172. Silvermann ME, Flamm MD. Variant angina pectoris: Anatomic findings and prognostic implications. *Ann Intern Med* 1971; 75:339–343.

173. Dhurandhar RW, Watt DL, Silver MD, Trimble AS, Adelman AS.

artery disease? A clinical-morphologic assessment. *J Am Coll Cardiol* 1989; 13:969–987.

Prinzmetal's variant form of angina with arteriographic evidence of coronary arterial spasm. *Am J Cardiol* 1972; 30:902–905.

174. Cosby RS, Giddins JA, See JR, Mayo M. Variant angina: Case reports and critique. *Am J Med* 1972; 53:739–742.

175. Cheng TO, Bashour T, Kelser GA, Weiss L, Baos J. Variant angina of Prinzmetal with normal coronary arteriograms: A variant of the variant. *Circulation* 1973; 47:476–485.

176. Donsky MS, Harris MD, Curry GC, Blomquest CG, Willerson JT, Mullins CB. Variant angina pectoris: A clinical and coronary arteriographic spectrum. *Am Heart J* 1975; 89:571–578.

177. Wiener L, Kasparian H, Duca PR, Walinsky P, Gottlieb RS, Henckel F, et al. Spectrum of coronary arterial spasm: Clinical, angiographic and myocardial metabolic experience in 29 cases. *Am J Cardiol* 1976; 38:945–955.

178. Bharati S, Dhingra RC, Lev M, Towne WD, Rahimtoolah SH, Rosen KM. Conduction system in a patient with Prinzmetal's angina and transient atrioventricular block. *Am J Cardiol* 1977; 39:120–125.

179. Maseri A, L'Abbate A, Baroldi G, Chierchia S, Marzilli M, Ballestra AM, et al. Coronary vasospasm as a possible cause of myocardial infarction: A conclusion derived from the study of "preinfarction" angina. *N Engl J Med* 1978; 299:1271–1277.

180. Roberts WC, Curry RC, Isner JM, Waller BF, McManue BM, Constantine MR, et al. Sudden death in Prinzmetal's angina with coronary spasm documented by angiography: Analysis of 3 necropsy patients. *Am J Cardiol* 1982; 50:203–210.

181. Brown BF. Coronary vasospasm: Observations linking the clinical spectrum of ischemic heart disease to the dynamic pathology of coronary, atherosclerosis. *Arch Intern Med* 1981; 141:716–722.

182. Conti CR. Large vessel coronary vasospasm: Diagnosis, natural history and treatment. *Am J Cardiol* 1985; 55:41B–49B.

183. Lambert CR, Pepine CJ. Coronary artery spasm and acute myocardial infarction. *Cardiovasc Clin* 1989; 20:131–140.

184. Zainea M, Duvernoy WF, Chauhan A, David S, Soto E, Small D. Acute myocardial infarction in angiographically normal coronary arteries following induction of general anesthesia. *Arch Intern Med* 1994; 154:2495–2498.

185. Kounis NG, Zavras GM. Histamin induced coronary artery spasm: The concept of allergic angina. *Br J Clin Prac* 1991; 45:121–128.

186. Ruch A, Duhring JL. Postpartum myocardial infarction in a patient receiving bromocriptine. *Obstet Gynecol* 1989; 74:448–451.

187. Fischell TA. Coronary artery spasm after percutaneous transluminal coronary angioplasty: Pathophysiology and clinical consequences. *Cathet Cardiovasc Diagn* 1990; 19:1–3.

188. Halper J, Factor SM. Coronary lesions in neurofibromatosis associated with vasospasm and myocardial infarction. *Am Heart J* 1984; 108:420–422.

189. Shepherd JT, Katusic ZS, Vedernikov Y, Vanhoutte PM. Mechanisms of coronary vasospasm: Role of endothelium. *J Mol Cell Cardiol* 1991; 23(suppl 1):125–131.

190. Kalsner S. Coronary artery spasm: Multiple causes and multiple roles in heart disease. *Biochem Pharmacol* 1995; 49:859–871.

191. Hillis LD, Braunwald E. Coronary artery spasm. *N Engl J Med* 1978; 299:695–702.

192. Ginsburg R, Birstow MR, Harrison DC, Stinson EB. Studies with isolated human coronary arteries: Some general observations, potential mediators of spasm, role of calcium antagonists. *Chest* 1980; 78:180–186.

193. Maseri A, Severi S, De Nes M, L'Abbate A, Chierchia S, Marzilli M, et al. "Variant" angina: One aspect of a continuous spectrum of vasospastic myocardial ischemia. *Am J Cardiol* 1978; 42:1019–1035.

194. El-Maraghi NRH, Sealey BJ. Recurrent myocardial infarction in a young man with coronary arterial spasm, demonstrated at autopsy. *Circulation* 1980; 61:199–207.

195. Isner JM, Donaldson RF, Katsas GC. Spasm at autopsy: A prospective study (abstr). *Circulation* 1983; 68:III–1028.

196. Isner JM, Fortin AH, Fortin RV. Depletion of smooth muscle from the media of atherosclerotic coronary arteries: A potential factor in the pathogenesis of myocardial ischemia and the variable response to anti-anginal therapy (abstr). *Clin Res* 1983; 31:193A.

197. Factor SM, Cho S. Smooth muscle contraction bands in the media of coronary arteries: A postmortem marker of antemortem coronary spasm? *J Am Coll Cardiol* 1985; 6:1329–1337.

198. Waller BF. The eccentric coronary atherosclerotic plaque: Morphologic observations and clinical relevance. *Clin Cardiol* 1988; 12:14–20.

199. Hangartner JRW, Charleston AJ, Davies MJ, Thomas AC. Morphologic characteristics of clinically significant coronary artery stenosis in stable angina. *Br Heart J* 1986; 56:501–508.

200. Quyyumi AA, Al-Rufaii HK, Olsen EGJ, Fox KM. Coronary anatomy in patients with various manifestations of three vessel coronary artery disease. *Br Heart J* 1985; 54:362–366.

201. Hort W, Moosdorf R, Kalbfleisch H, Kohler F, Milzner-Schwarz U, Frenzel H. Postmortale Untersuchungen uber Lokalisation und Form der starksten Stenosen in den Koronararterien und ihre Beziehung zu den Risikofaktoren. *Z Kardiol* 1977; 66:333–340.

202. Freudenberg H, Lichtlen PR. Das Normale Wandsegment bei Koronarstenosen—ein postmortale Studie. *Z Kardiol* 1981; 70:863–869.

203. Saner HE, Gobel FL, Salomonowitz E, Erlich DA, Edwards JE. The disease-free wall in coronary atherosclerosis: Its relation to degree of obstruction. *J Am Coll Cardiol* 1985; 6:1096–1099.

204. Manion WC. Infectious angiitis. In, Orbison JL, Smith DE (eds): *The Peripheral Blood Vessels*. Baltimore: Williams & Wilkins; 1963:221.

205. Lie JT. Coronary vasculitis: A review in the current scheme of classification of vasculitis. *Arch Pathol Lab Med* 1987; 111:224–233.

206. Parillo JE, Fauci AS. Coronary vasculitis. In Ansell BM, Simkin PA (eds). *The Heart and Rheumatic Disease*. Woburn, MA, Butterworth, 1984:213–233.

207. Manion WC. Infectious angiitis. In Orbison JL, Smith DE (eds). *The Peripheral Blood Vessels*. Baltimore, Williams and Wilkins, 1963:221–231.

208. DeShazo RD. The spectrum of systemic vasculitis. A classification to aid diagnosis. *Postgrad Med* 1975; 58:78–82.

209. Paronetto F. Systemic nonsuppurative necrotizing angiitis. In: Miescher PA, Muller-Eberhard HJ, eds. *Textbook of Immunopathology*, 2d ed. New York: Grune & Stratton, 1976; 1012–1024.

210. Christian CL, Sergent JS. Vasculitis syndromes: Clinical and experimental models. *Am J Med* 1976; 61:385–392.

211. Conn DL, McDuffie FC, Holley KE, Schroeter AL. Immunologic mechanisms in systemic vasculitis. *Mayo Clin Proc* 1976; 51:511–518.

212. Fauci AS, Hayne BF, Katz P. The spectrum of vasculitis: Clinical, pathogenic, immunologic, and therapeutic considerations. *Ann Intern Med* 1978; 89:660–676.

213. Soter NA, Austen KF. Pathogenetic mechanisms in necrotizing vasculitides. *Clin Rheum Dis* 1980; 6:233–253.

214. McCluskey RT, Fienberg R. Vasculitis in primary vasculitides, granulomatoses, and connective tissue diseases. *Hum Pathol* 1983; 14:305–315.

215. Kussmaul A, Maier R. Uber eine bisher nicht beschriebene eigenthumliche Arterienerkrankung (periarteritis nodosa), die mit Morbus Brightii und rapid fortschreitender allgemeiner Muskellahmung einhergeht. *Disch Arch Klin Med* 1866; 1:484–518.

216. Dickson WE. Polyarteritis acuta nodosa and periarterits nodosa. *J Pathol Bacteriol* 1908; 12:31–57.

217. Zeek PM. Periarteritis nodosa: A critical review. *Am J Clin Pathol* 1952; 22:777–790.

218. Zeek PM. Periarteritis and other forms of necrotizing angiitis. *N Engl J Med* 1953; 248:764–772.

219. Churg J, Strauss L. Allergic granulomatosis, allergic angiitis, and periarteritis nodosa. *Am J Pathol* 1951; 27:277–294.

220. Churg J. Allergic granulomatosis and granulomatous vascular syndromes. *Ann Allergy* 1963; 21:619–628.

221. Lanham JG, Elkon KB, Pusey CD, Hughes GF. Systemic vasculitis with asthma and eosinophilia: A clinical approach to the Churg-Strauss syndrome. *Medicine* 1984; 63:65–81.

222. Von Glahn WC, Pappenheimer AM. Specific lesions of peripheral blood vessels in rheumatism. *Am J Pathol* 1926; 2:235–250.

223. Huthinson J. Diseases of the arteries: On a peculiar form of thrombotic arteritis of the aged which is sometimes productive of gangrene. *Arch Surg London* 1890; 1:323–329.

224. Horton BT, Magath TB, Brown GE. An underscribed form of arteritis of the temporal vessels. *Mayo Clin Proc* 1932; 7:700–701.

225. Horton BT, Magath TB, Brown GE. Arteritis of the temporal vessels. *Arch Intern Med* 1934; 53:400–410.

226. Cooke WT, Cloake PC, Govan AD, Colbeck JC. Temporal arteritis: A generalized vascular disease. *Q J Med* 1946; 15:47–75.

227. Hamilton CR, Shelley WM, Tumulty PA. Giant cell arteritis: Including temporal arteritis and polymyalgia rheumatica. *Medicine* 1971; 50:1–27.

228. Ostberg G. On arteritis: With special reference to polymyalgia arteritica. *Acta Pathol Microbiol Immunol Scand A* 1973; 237:1–59.

229. Somer T. Thrombo-embolic and vascular complications in vasculitis syndromes. *Eur Heart J* 1993; 14(suppl K):24–29.

230. Kawai S, Fukuda Y, Okada R. Atherosclerosis of the coronary arteries in collagen disease and allied disorders with special reference to vasculitis as a preceding lesion of coronary atherosclerosis. *Jpn Circ J* 1982; 46:1208–1221.

231. Karsner HT. *Acute Inflammations of Arteries.* Springfield, IL, Charles C Thomas, 1947.

232. Allen AC, Spitz S. A comparative study of the pathology of scrub typhus (Tsutsugamushi disease) and other rickettsial diseases. *Am J Pathol* 1945; 21:603–682.

233. Moritz AR. Syphilitic coronary arteritis. *Arch Pathol Lab Med* 1931; 11:44–59.

234. Bruenn HG. Syphilitic disease of the coronary arteries. *Am Heart J* 1934; 9:421–436.

235. Scharfman WB, Wallach JB, Angrist A. Myocardial infarction due to syphilitic coronary ostial stenosis. *Am Heart J* 1950; 40:603–613.

236. Holt S. Syphilitic ostial occlusion. *Br Heart J* 1977; 39:469–470.

237. Heggtveit HA. Syphilitic aortitis: A clinicopathologic study of 100 cases, 1950 to 1960. *Circulation* 1964; 29:346–355.

238. Rose AG. Cardiac tuberculosis. A study of 19 patients. *Arch Pathol Lab Med* 1987; 111:422–426.

239. Gouley BA, Bellet S, McMillan TM. Tuberculosis of the myocardium: Report of six cases with observations on involvement of coronary arteries. *Arch Intern Med* 1933; 51:244–263.

240. Manion WC. Infectious angiitis. In: Orbison JL, Smith DE (eds). *The Peripheral Blood Vessels.* Baltimore: Williams & Wilkins; 1963; 221–231.

241. Merkel WC. Plasmodium falciparum malaria: The coronary and myocardial lesions observed in autopsy in two cases of acute fulminating *P. falciparum* infection. *Arch Pathol* 1946; 41:290–298.

242. Gazayerli M. Unusual site of a schistosome worm in the circumflex branch of the left coronary artery. *J Egypt Med Assoc* 1939; 22:34–39.

243. Allen AC, Spitz S. A comparative study of the pathology of scrub typhus (Tsutsugamuschi's disease) and other rickettsial diseases. *Am J Pathol* 1945; 21:603–681.

244. Moe JB, Mosher DF, Kenyon RH, White JD, Stookey JL, Bagley LR. Functional and morphological changes during experimental Rocky Mountain spotted fever in guinea pigs. *Lab Invest* 1976; 35:235–245.

245. Sergent JS. Vasculitides associated with viral infections. *Clin Rheum Dis* 1980; 6:339–350.

246. Sergent JS, Lockshin MD, Christian CL, Gocke DJ. Vasculitis with hepatitis B antigenemia: Long-term observations in nine patients. *Medicine* 1976; 55:1–18.

247. Heibel RH, O'Toole JD, Curtiss EI, Medsger TA, Reddy SP, Shaver JA. Coronary arteritis in systemic lupus erythematosus. *Chest* 1976; 69:700–703.

248. Cipriano PR, Silverman JF, Perlroth MG, Grupp RB, Wexler L. Coronary arterial narrowing in Takayasu's aortitis. *Am J Cardiol* 1977; 39:744–750.

249. Judge RD, Currier RD, Gracie WA, Figley MM. Takayasu's arteritis and the aortic arch syndrome. *Am J Med* 1962; 32:379–392.

250. Strachan RW. The natural history of Takayasu's arteriopathy. *Q J Med* 1964; 33:57–69.

251. Ueda H. Clinical and pathological studies of aortitis syndrome: Committee report. *Jpn Heart J* 1968; 9:76–87.

252. Hachiya J. Current concepts of Takayasu's arteritis. *Semin Roentgenol* 1970; 5:245–259.

253. Lupi-Herrera E, Sanchez-Torres G, Marcus-Hamer J, Mispireta J, Horowitz S, Vela JE. Takayasu's arteritis: Clinical study of 107 cases. *Am Heart J* 1977; 93:94–103.

254. Ischikawa K. Natural history and classification of occlusive thromboarteriopathy (Takayasu's disease). *Circulation* 1978; 57:27–35.

255. Rose AG, Sinclair-Smith CC. Takayasu's arteritis: A study of 16 cases. *Arch Pathol Lab Med* 1980; 104:231–237.

256. Hall S, Barr W, Lie JT, Stanson AW, Kazmier FJ, Hunder GG. Takayasu arteritis: A study of 32 North American patients. *Medicine* 1985; 64:89–99.

257. Aufderheide AC, Henke BW, Parker EH. Granulomatous coronary arteritis (Takayasu's disease). *Arch Pathol Lab Med* 1981; 105:647–649.

258. Hashimoto Y, Numano F, Maruyama Y, Oniki T, Kasuya K, Kakuta T, et al. Thallium 201 stress scintigraphy in Takayasu arteritis. *Am J Cardiol* 1991; 67:879–882.

259. Kinare SG. Cardiac lesions in nonspecific aortoarteritis: An autopsy study. *Indian Heart J* 1994; 46:65–69.

260. Takei M, Sasaki Y, Suyama K, Furihata A, Chino C, Midorikana T, et al. Surgically treated case of complete obstruction of the left main coronary artery caused by Takayasu's arteritis. *Am Heart J* 1993; 126:458–459.

261. Tanaka M, Abe T, Takeuchi E, Watanabe T, Tamaki S. Revascularization for coronary ostial stenosis in Takayasu's disease with calcified aorta. *Ann Thorac Surg* 1992; 53:894–895.

262. Nakano S, Shimazaki Y, Keneko M, Kaneko M, Taniguchi K, Miyamoto Y, et al. Transaortic patch angioplasty for left coronary ostial stenosis in a patient with Takayasu's aortitis. *Ann Thorac Surg* 1992; 53:694–696.

263. Aufderheide AC, Henke BW, Parker EH. Granulomatous coronary arteritis. *Arch Pathol Lab Med* 1981; 105:647–649.

264. Rosen H, Gaton E. Takayasu's arteritis of coronary arteries. *Arch Pathol Lab Med* 1972; 94:225–229.

265. Case 46-1967. Case records of the Massachusetts General Hospital: Weekly clinicopathological exercise. *N Engl J Med* 1967; 277:1025–1033.

266. Lie JT, Failoni DD, Davis DC. Temporal arteritis with giant cell aortitis, coronary arteritis, and myocardial infarction. *Arch Pathol Lab Med* 1986; 110:857–860.

267. Klein RG, Hunder GG, Stanson AW, Sheps SG. Large vessel involvement in giant cell (temporal) arteritis. *Ann Intern Med* 1975; 83:806–812.

268. Harris M. Dissecting aneurysm of the aorta due to giant cell arteritis. *Br Heart J* 1968; 30:840–844.

269. Morrison AN, Abitbol M. Granulomatous arteritis with myocardial infarction: A case report with autopsy findings. *Ann Intern Med* 1955; 42:691–700.

270. Crompton MR. The visual changes in temporal (giant cell) arteritis: Report of a case with autopsy findings. *Brain* 1959; 82:377–390.

271. Martin JF, Kittas C, Triger DR. Giant cell arteritis of coronary arteries causing myocardial infarction. *Br Heart J* 1980; 43:487–489.

272. Save-Soderbergh J, Malmvall BE, Andersson R, Bengtsson RA. Giant cell arteritis as a cause of death: Report of nine cases. *JAMA* 1985; 255:493–496.

273. Lie JT. Disseminated visceral giant cell arteritis: Histopathologic description and differentiation from other granulomatous vasculitides. *Am J Clin Pathol* 1978; 69:299–305.

274. Ainsworth RW, Gresham GA, Balmforth GV. Pathologic changes in temporal arteries removed from unselected cadavers. *J Clin Pathol* 1961; 14:115–119.

275. Harrison CV. Giant-cell or temporal arteritis: A review. *J Clin Pathol* 1948; 1:197–211.

276. Paulley JW. Coronary ischemia and occlusion in giant cell (temporal) arteritis. *Acta Medica Scand* 1980; 208:257–263.

277. Zvaifler NJ, Weintraub AM. Aortitis and aortic insufficiency in chronic rheumatic disorders: A reappraisal. *Arthritis Rheum* 1963; 6:241–245.

278. Heggtveit HA, Hennigar GR, Morrione TG. Panaortitis. *Am J Pathol* 1963; 42:151–172.

279. Reimer KA, Rodgers RF, Oyasu R. Rheumatoid arthritis with rheumatoid heart disease and granulomatous aortitis. *JAMA* 1976; 235:2510–2512.

280. Sokoloff L. Cardiac involvement in rheumatoid arthritis and allied disorders: current concepts. *Mod Concept Cardiovasc Dis* 1964; 33:847–850.

281. Lie JT. Rheumatoid arthritis and heart disease. *Prim Cardiol* 1982; 8:137–152.

282. Swezey RL. Myocardial infarction due to rheumatoid arthritis. *JAMA* 1967; 199:855–857.

283. Karten I. Arteritis, myocardial infarction, and rheumatoid arthritis. *JAMA* 1969; 210:1717–1720.

284. Voyles WF, Searles RP, Bankhurst AD. Myocardial infarction caused by rheumatoid vasculitis. *Arthritis Rheum* 1980; 23:860–883.

285. Morris PB, Imber MJ, Heinsimer JA, Hlatky MH, Reimer KA. Rheumatoid arthritis and coronary arteritis. *Am J Cardiol* 1986; 57:689–690.

286. Pagel W. Polyarteritis nodosa and the rheumatic diseases. *J Clin Pathol* 1951; 4:137.

287. Cruickshank B. The arteritis of rheumatoid arthritis. *Ann Rheum Dis* 1954; 13:136–145.

288. Schmid FR, Cooper NS, Ziff M, McEwen C. Arteritis in rheumatoid arthritis. *Am J Med* 1961; 30:56–83.

289. Glass D, Soter NA, Schur PH. Rheumatoid vasculitis. *Arthritis Rheum* 1976; 19:950–952.

290. Scott DG, Bacon PA, Tribe CR. Systemic rheumatoid vasculitis: A clinical and laboratory study of 50 cases. *Medicine* 1981; 60:288–297.

291. James TN. De Subitaneis Mortibus: XXIII. Rheumatoid arthritis and ankylosing spondylitis. *Circulation* 1977; 55:669–677.

292. Hoffman FG, Leight L. Complete atrioventricular block associated with rheumatoid disease. *Am J Cardiol* 1965; 16:585–592.

293. Grismer JT, Anderson WR, Weiss L. Chronic occlusive rheumatic coronary vasculitis and myocardial dysfunction. *Am J Cardiol* 1976; 20:739–745.

294. Kawai S, Okada R, Sugimoto H, Okada M, Fukuda Y. An autopsied case of a two month old infant with granulomatous pancarditis having severe vasculitis and valvulitis. *Jpn Circ J* 1983; 47:1325–1330.

295. Bely M, Apathy A, Beke Martos E. Cardiac changes in rheumatoid arthritis. *Acta Morphol Hung* 1992; 40:149–186.

296. Voyles WF, Searles RP, Bankhurst AD. Myocardial infarction caused by rheumatoid vasculitis. *Arthritis Rheum* 1980; 23:860–863.

297. Fujita M, Abe M, Itoh T, Saitoh K, Noguchi M, Sano K, et al. Nonarthritic rheumatoid valvulitis with coronary arteritis causing myocardial infarction. *Virchows Arch* 1992; 420:109–112.

298. Buerger L. Thromboangiitis obliterans: A study of the vascular lesions leading to presenile spontaneous gangrene. *Am J Med Sci* 1908; 136:567–580.

299. McKusick VA, Harris WS, Otteson OE, Goodman RM, Sheiley WM, Bloudwell K. Buerger's disease: A distinct clinical and pathologic entity. *JAMA* 1962; 181:5–12.

300. Wessler S. Buerger's disease revisited. *Surg Clin North Am* 1969; 49:703–713.

301. Williams G. Recent views on Buerger's disease. *J Clin Pathol* 1969; 22:573–578.

302. Vink M. Symposium on Buerger's disease. *J Cardiovasc Surg* 1973; 14:1–51.

303. Gilkes R, Dow J. Aortic involvement in Buerger's disease. *Br J Med* 1973; 46:110–114.

304. Saphir O. Thromboangiitis obliterans of the coronary arteries and its relation to arteriosclerosis. *Am Heart J* 1936; 12:521–535.

305. Gore I, Burrows S. A reconsideration of the pathogenesis of Buerger's disease. *Am J Clin Pathol* 1958; 29:319–330.

306. Ohno H, Matsuda Y, Takashiba K, Hamada Y, Ebihara H, Hyakuna E. Acute myocardial infarction in Buerger's disease. *Am J Cardiol* 1986; 57:690–691.

307. Mautner GC, Mautner SL, Lin F, Roggin GM, Roberts WC. Amounts of coronary arterial luminal narrowing and composition of the material causing the narrowing in Buerger's disease. *Am J Cardiol* 1993; 71:486–490.

308. Averbuck SH, Silbert S. Thromboangiitis obliterans: Cause of death. *Arch Intern Med* 1934; 54:436–465.

309. Lie JT. Thromboangiitis obliterans (Buerger's disease) in a saphenous vein arterial graft. *Hum Pathol*. In press.

310. Fronert PP, Sheps SG. Long-term follow-up study of polyarteritis nodosa. *Am J Med* 1967; 43:8–14.

311. Sack M, Cassidy JT, Bole GG. Prognostic factors in polyarteritis. *J Rheumatol* 1975; 2:411–420.

312. Leib ES, Restivo C, Paulus HE. Immunosuppressive and corticosteroid therapy of polyarteritis nodosa. *Am J Med* 1979; 67:941–947.

313. Cohen RD, Conn DL, Ilstrup DM. Clinical features, prognosis, and response to treatment in polyarteritis. *Mayo Clin Proc* 1980; 55:146–155.

314. Scott DG, Becon PA, Elliott PJ, Tribe CK, Wallington TB. Systemic vasculitis in a district general hospital 1972–1980: Clinical and laboratory classification and prognosis in 80 cases. *Q J Med* 1982; 51:292–311.

315. Holsinger DR, Osmondson PJ, Edwards JE. The heart in polyarteritis nodosa. *Circulation* 1962; 25:610–617.

316. Arkin A. A clinical and pathological study of periarteritis nodosa. *Am J Pathol* 1930; 6:401–426.

317. Sinclair W, Nitsch E. Polyarteritis nodosa of the coronary arteries: Report of a case with rupture of an aneurysm and intrapericardial hemorrhage. *Am Heart J* 1949; 38:898–904.

318. Przybojewski JZ. Polyarteritis nodosa in the adult: Report of a case with repeated myocardial infarction and a review of cardiac involvement. *S Afr Med J* 1981; 60:512–518.

319. Swalwell CI, Reddy SK, Rao VJ. Sudden death due to unsuspected coronary vasculitis. *Am J Forens Med Pathol* 1991; 12:306–312.

320. Sugihara N, Genda A, Shimizu M, Suematsu T, Kita Y, Shimizu K, et al. Intramural coronary angiitis of periarteritis nodosa proved by endomyocardial biopsy. *Am Heart J* 1990; 119:1414–1416.

321. Ettinger RE, Nelson AM, Buske EC, Lie JT. Polyarteritis nodosa in childhood: A clinical pathologic study. *Arthritis Rheum* 1979; 22:820–825.

322. Petty RE, Maligilavy DB, Cassidy JT, Sullivan DB. Polyarteritis in childhood: A clinical description of eight cases. *Arthritis Rheum* 1977; 20:392–394.

323. Roberts FB, Fetterman GH. Polyarteritis nodosa in infancy. *J Pediatr* 1963; 63:519–529.

324. Munro-Faure H. Necrotizing arteritis of the coronary vessels in infancy: Case report and review of the literature. *Pediatrics* 1959; 23:914–926.

325. Tanaka N, Naoe S, Masuda H, Ueno T. Pathological study of sequelae of Kawasaki disease (MCLS): With special reference to the heart and coronary arterial lesions. *Acta Pathol Japon* 1986; 36:1513–1527.

326. Kawasaki T, Kosaki F, Okawa S, Shigematsu I, Yanagawa H. A new infantile acute febrile mucocutaneous lymph node syndrome (MLNS) prevailing in Japan. *Pediatrics* 1974; 54:271–276.

327. Melish ME. Kawasaki syndrome (the mucocutaneous lymph node syndrome). *Annu Rev Med* 1982; 33:569–585.

328. Tanaka N. Kawasaki disease (acute febrile infantile mucocutaneous lymph node syndrome) in Japan: Relationship with infantile polyarteritis nodosa. *Pathol Microbiol* 1975; 43:204–218.

329. Langing BH, Larson EJ. Are infantile periarteritis nodosa with coronary artery involvement and fatal mucocutaneous lymph node syndrome the same? Comparison of 20 patients from North America with patients from Hawaii and Japan. *Pediatrics* 1977; 59:651–662.

330. Amano S, Hozama F, Hamashima Y. Pathology of Kawasaki disease: I. Pathology and morphology of the vascular changes. *Jpn Circ J* 1979; 43:633–643.

331. Amano S, Hozama F, Hamashima Y. Pathology of Kawasaki disease: II. distribution and incidence of the vascular lesions. *Jpn Circ J* 1979; 43:741–748.

332. Fukushige J, Nihill MR, McNamara DG. Spectrum of cardiovascular lesions in mucocutaneous lymph node syndrome. *Am J Cardiol* 1980; 45:98–107.

333. Kitamura S, Kawashima Y, Fujita T, Mori T, Oyama C, Fujino M. Aortocoronary bypass grafting in a child with coronary artery obstruction due to mucocutaneous lymph node syndrome: Report of a case. *Circulation* 1976; 53:1035–1040.

334. Kato H, Koike S, Yamamoto M, Ito Y, Yano E. Coronary aneurysms in infants and young children with acute febrile mucocutaneous lymph node syndrome. *J Pediatr* 1975; 86:892–898.

335. Tanimoto T, Kamiya T, Misawa H, Manabe H, Go S, Yutani C. An autopsied case of an elementary school boy with sudden death four years after Kawasaki disease: On the problem of present method of cardiac mass screening of school children. *Jpn Circ J* 1981; 45:1438–1442.

336. Kitamura S, Kawachi K, Harima R, Sakakihara T, Hiruse H, Kawashima Y. Surgery for coronary heart disease due to mucocutaneous lymph node syndrome: Report of 6 patients. *Am J Cardiol* 1983; 51:444–448.

337. Quam JP, Edwards WD, Bambara JF, Luzier TL. Sudden death in an adolescent four years after recovery from mucocutaneous lymph node syndrome. *J Forens Sci* 1986; 31:1135–1141.

338. Suzuki A, Kamiya T, Kuwahara N, Ono Y, Kohata T, Takahashi O, et al. Coronary arterial lesions of Kawasaki disease: Cardiac catheterization findings of 1100 cases. *Pediatr Cardiol* 1986; 7:3–9.

339. Sakai Y, Takayanagi K, Inoue T, Yamaguchi H, Hayashi T, Moruoka S, et al. Coronary artery aneurysms and congestive heart failure: Possible long term course of Kawasaki disease in an adult. A case report. *Angiology* 1988; 39:625–630.

340. Hennigar GR, Thabet R, Bundy WE, Sutton LE. Salmonellosis complicated by pancarditis: Report of a case with autopsy findings. *J Pediatr* 1953; 43:524–531.

341. Saphir O, Katz LN, Gore I. The myocardium in subacute bacterial endocarditis. *Circulation* 1950; 1:1155–1167.

342. Parrillo JE, Fauci AS. Necrotizing vasculitis, coronary angiitis and the cardiologist. *Am Heart J* 1980; 99:547–554.

343. Gatenby PA, Lytton DG, Bulteau VG, O'Reilly B, Basten A. Myocardial infarction in Wegener's granulomatosis. *Aust NZ J Med* 1976; 6:336–340.

344. Klinger H. Grenzformen der periarteritis nodosa. *Frankfurt Z Pathol* 1931; 42:455–480.

345. Wegener F. Uber generalisierte, septische Gefasserkrankugen. *Verh Dtsch Ges Pathol* 1936; 29:202–210.

346. Wegener F. Uber eine eigenartige rhinogene Granulomatose mit besonderer Beteiligung des Arteriensystems und der Nieren. *Beitr Pathol Anat* 1939; 102:36–68.

347. Fahey J, Leonard E, Churg J, Godman G. Wegener's granulomatosis. *Am J Med* 1954; 17:168–179.

348. Godman G, Churg J. Wegener's granulomatosis: Pathology and review of the literature. *Arch Pathol Lab Med* 1954; 58:533–553.

349. Fienberg R. Pathergic granulomatosis. *Am J Med* 1955; 19:829–831.

350. Walton EW. Giant cell granuloma of the respiratory tract (Wegener's granulomatosis). *Br Med J* 1958; 2:265–270.

351. Fauci AS, Wolff SM. Wegener's granulomatosis: Studies in 18 patients and a review of the literature. *Medicine* 1973; 52.535–561.

352. Pambakian H, Tighe JR. Breast involvement in Wegener's granulomatosis. *J Clin Pathol* 1971; 24:343–347.

353. Forstot JZ, Overlie PA, Neufeld GK, Harmon CE, Forstut SL. Cardiac complications of Wegener granulomatosis: A case report of complete heart block and review of the literature. *Semin Arthritis Rheum* 1980; 10:148–154.

354. Allen DC, Doherty CC, O'Reilly DP. Pathology of the heart and the cardiac conduction system in Wegener's granulomatosis. *Br Heart J* 1964; 52:674–678.

355. Schiavone WA, Ahmad M, Ockner SA. Unusual cardiac complications of Wegener's granulomatosis. *Chest* 1985; 88:745–748.

356. Lie JT. Classification of vasculitis and a reappraisal of allergic granulomatosis and angiitis. *Mt Sinai J Med* 1986; 53:429–439.

357. Cupps TR, Fauci AS. *The Vasculitides*. Philadelphia, Saunders, 1981:211.

358. Rich AR. Hypersensitivity in disease, with special reference to periarteritis nodosa, rheumatic fever, disseminated lupus erythematosus, and rheumatoid arthritis. *Harvey Lect* 1947; 42:106 147.

359. Meller J, Conde CA, Deppisch LM, Donoso E, Dact S. Myocardial infarction due to coronary atherosclerosis in three young adults with systemic lupus erythematosus. *Am J Cardiol* 1975; 35:309–314.

360. Bonfiglio TA, Botti RE, Hagstrom JWC. Coronary arteritis, occlusion and myocardial infarction due to lupus erythematosus. *Am Heart J* 1972; 83:153–158.

361. Benisch BM, Pervez N. Coronary artery vasculitis and myocardial infarction with systemic lupus erythematosus. *NY State J Med* 1974; 74:873 874.

362. Sumino H, Kanda T, Sasaki T, Kanazawa N, Takeuch H. Myocardial infarction secondary to coronary aneurysm in systemic lupus erythematosus: An autopsy case. *Angiology* 1995; 46:527–530.

363. Denbow CE, Lie JT, Tancredi RG, Bunch TW. Cardiac involvement in polymyositis: A clinicopathologic study of 20 autopsied patients. *Arthritis Rheum* 1979; 22:1088–1092.

364. Follansbee WP. The cardiovascular manifestations of systemic sclerosis. *Curr Probl Cardiol* 1986; 11:245–297.

365. Schimizu T, Ehrlich GE, Inaba G, Hayashi K. Behçet disease. *Semin Arthritis Rheum* 1979; 8:223–260.

366. Haynes BF, Kaiser-Kupfer MI, Mason P, Fauci AS. Cogan syndrome: Studies in 13 patients, long term follow-up and a review of the literature. *Medicine* 1980; 59:426–441.

367. Mullick FG, McAllister HA, Wagner BM, Fenoglio JJ Jr. Drug related vasculitis: Clinicopathologic correlation in 30 patients. *Hum Pathol* 1979; 10:313–325.

368. Uys CJ, Rose AG. Pathologic findings in long term cardiac transplants. *Arch Pathol Lab Med* 1984; 108:112–116.

369. Brosius FC, Roberts WC. Coronary artery disease in the Hurler syndrome. *Am J Cardiol* 1981; 47:649–653.

370. Renteria VG, Ferrans VJ, Roberts WC. The heart in the Hurler syndrome: Gross histologic and ultrastructural observations in five necropsy cases. *Am J Cardiol* 1976; 38:487–501.

371. Lindsay S. The cardiovascular system in gargoylism. *Br Heart J* 1950; 12:17–32.

372. Stauffer M. Oxalosis: Report of a case with a review of the literature and discussion on pathogenesis. *N Engl J Med* 1960; 263:386–390.

373. Blieden LC, Desnick RJ, Carter JB, Krivit W, Moller JH, Sharp HL. Cardiac involvement in Sandhoff's disease: An inborn error of glycosphingolipid metabolism. *Am J Cardiol* 1974; 34:83–88.

374. Blieden LC, Moller JH. Cardiac involvement in inherited disorders of metabolism. *Prog Cardiovasc Dis* 1974; 16:615 631.

375. Brosius FC III, Waller BF, Roberts WC. Radiation heart disease: Analysis of 16 young (aged 15 to 33 years) necropsy patients who received over 3500 rads to the heart. *Am J Med* 1981; 70:519–530.

376. Brill IC, Brodeur MTH, Oyama AA. Myocardial infarction in two sisters less than 20 years old. *JAMA* 1971; 217:1345–1348.

377. Trimble AS, Bigelow WG, Wigle ED. Coronary ostial stenosis: A late complication of coronary perfusion in open-heart surgery. *J Thorac Cardiovasc Surg* 1969; 57:792–795.

378. Lie JT, Berg KK. Isolated fibromuscular dysplasia of the coronary arteries with spontaneous dissection and myocardial infarction. *Hum Pathol* 1987; 18:654–656.

379. Przybojewski JZ, Rossouw J. Severe isolated left mainstem coronary artery stenosis: A case report. *S Afr Med J* 1986; 69:133–136.

380. Dominguez FE, Tate LG, Robinson MJ. Familial fibromuscular dysplasia presenting as sudden death. *Am J Cardiovasc Pathol* 1988; 2:269–272.

381. Billingham M. Personal communication, 1988.

382. Johnson DE, Gao SZ, Schroeder JS, DeCampl WM, Billingham ME. The spectrum of coronary artery pathologic findings in human cardiac allografts. *J Heart Transpl* 1989; 8:349–359.

383. Gravanis MB. Allograft heart accelerated atherosclerosis: Evidence for cell mediated immunity in pathogenesis. *Mod Pathol* 1989; 2:495–505.

384. Mehra MR, Ventura HO, Stapleton DD, Smart FW, Collins TC, Ramee SR. Presence of severe intimal thickening by intravascular ultrasonography predicts cardiac events in cardiac allograft vasculopathy. *J Heart Lung Transpl* 1995; 14:632–639.

385. Waller BF, Pinkerton CA, Foster LN. Morphologic evidence of accelerated left main coronary artery stenosis: A late complication of percutaneous transluminal angioplasty of the proximal left anterior descending coronary artery. *J Am Coll Cardiol* 1987; 9:1019–1023.

386. Giritsky AS, Ricci MT, Reitz BA, Shumway NE. Extrinsic coronary artery obstruction by chronic aortic dissection. *Ann Thorac Surg* 1981; 32:289–293.

387. Gardia Rinaldi R, Von Koch L, Howell JP. Aneurysm of the sinus of Valsalva producing obstruction of the left main coronary artery. *J Thorac Cardiovascular Surg* 1976; 72:123–126.

388. Kopelson G, Herwig KJ. The etiologies of coronary artery disease in cancer patients. *Int J Radiat Oncol Biol Phys* 1978; 4:895–906.

389. Applefeld MM, Wiernik PH. Cardiac disease after radiation therapy for Hodgkin's disease: Analysis of 48 patients. *Am J Cardiol* 1983; 51:1679–1681.

390. SebagMontefiore D, Hope Stone H. Radiation induced coronary heart disease. *Br Heart J* 1993; 69:481–482.

391. Radwaner BA, Geringer R, Goldmann AM, Schwartz MJ, Kemp HG Jr. Left main coronary artery stenosis following mediastinal irradiation. *Am J Med* 1987; 82:1017–1020.

392. Schulman HE, Korr KS, Myers TJ. Left internal thoracic artery graft occlusion following mediastinal radiation therapy. *Chest* 1994; 105:1881–1882.

393. Benoff LJ, Schweitzer P. Radiation therapy induced cardiac injury. *Am Heart J* 1995; 129:1193–1196.

394. Reber D, Birnbaum DE, Tollenaere P. Heart diseases following mediastinal irradiation: Surgical management. *Eur J Cardiothor Surg* 1995; 9:202–205.

395. Raviprasad GS, Salem BI, Gowda S, Leidenfrost R. Radiation induced mitral and tricuspid regurgitation with severe ostial coronary artery disease: A case report with successful surgical treatment. *Cathet Cardiovasc Diagn* 1995; 35:146–148.

396. Simon EB, Ling J, Mendizabal RC, Midwall J. Radiation induced coronary artery disease. *Am Heart J* 1984; 108:1032–1034.

397. Chen MF, Yang CY, Wu CC, Chen WJ, Liau CS, Hou SW, et al. Heart diseases following radiotherapy. *J Formos Med Assoc* 1991; 90:398–402.

398. Handler CE, Livesey S, Lawton PA. Coronary ostial stenosis after radiotherapy: Angioplasty or coronary artery surgery? *Br Heart J* 1989; 61:208–211.

399. Grollier G, Commeau P, Mercier V, Lognone T, Gofard M, Scanu P, et al. Post radiotherapeutic left main coronary ostial stenosis: Clinical and histological study. *Eur Heart J* 1988; 9:567–570.

400. Tenet W, Missri J, Hager D. Radiation induced stenosis of the left main coronary artery. *Cathet Cardiovasc Diagn* 1986; 12:169–171.

401. McEniery PT, Dorosti K, Schiavone WA, Pedrick TJ, Sheldon WC. Clinical and angiographic features of coronary artery disease after chest irradiation. *Am J Cardiol* 1987; 60:1020–1024.

402. Mittal B, Deutsch M, Thompson M, Dameshek HL. Radiation induced accelerated coronary arteriosclerosis. *Am J Med* 1986; 81:183–184.

403. Om A, Ellahham S, Vetrovec GW. Radiation induced coronary artery disease. *Am Heart J* 1992; 124:1598–1602.

404. Orzan F, Brusca A, Conte MR, Presbitero P, Figliomeni MC. Severe coronary artery disease after radiation therapy of the chest and mediastinum: Clinical presentation and treatment. *Br Heart J* 1993; 69:496–500.

405. House KW, Simon SR, Pugh RP. Chemotherapy induced myocardial infarction in a young man with Hodgkin's disease. *Clin Cardiol* 1992; 15:122–125.

406. Fomina LG. A case of myocardial infarct in acute leukemia. *Sov Med* 1960; 24:141–143.

407. Wirth L. Myocardial infarction as the initial manifestation of polycythemia vera. *Mil Med* 1960; 125:544–548.

408. Spach MS, Howell DA, Harris JS. Myocardial infarction and multiple thrombosis in a child with primary thrombocytosis. *Pediatrics* 1963; 31:268–276.

409. James TN. Pathology of the small coronary arteries. *Am J Cardiol* 1963; 20:679–691.

410. Isner JM, Estes NAM III, Thompson PD, Costanzo-Nordin MR, Subramanian R, Miller G, et al. Acute cardiac events temporally related to cocaine abuse. *N Engl J Med* 1968; 315:1438–1443.

411. Simpson RW, Edwards WD. Pathogenesis of cocaine-induced ischemic heart disease. *Arch Pathol Lab Med* 1986; 110:479–484.

412. Zimmerman FH, Gustafson GM, Kemp HG. Recurrent myocardial infarction associated with cocaine abuse in a young man with normal coronary arteries: Evidence for coronary artery spasm culminating in thrombosis. *J Am Coll Cardiol* 1987; 9:964–968.

413. Smith HWB, Liberman HA, Brody SL, Battey LL, Donohue BC, Morris DC. Acute myocardial infarction temporally related to cocaine use: Clinical angiographic and pathophysiologic observations. *Ann Intern Med* 1987; 107:13–18.

414. Patel R, Haider B, Ahmed S, Regan TJ. Cocaine-related myocardial infarction: High prevalence of occlusive coronary thrombi without significant obstructive atherosclerosis (abstr). *Circulation* 1988; 78(suppl II):II-436.

415. Lange RA, Cigarroa RG, Yancy CW, Willard JE, Popma JJ, Sills MN, et al. Cocaine-induced coronary artery vasoconstriction. *N Engl J Med* 1989; 321:1557–1562.

416. Waller BF. Cocaine and the heart. *Indiana Med* 1988; 81:956–959.

417. Inoue H, Zipes DP. Cocaine induced supersensitivity and arrhythmogenesis. *J Am Coll Cardiol* 1988; 11:867–874.

418. Pallasch TJ, McCarty FM, Jastak JT. Cocaine and sudden cardiac death. *J Oral Maxillofac Surg* 1989; 47:1188–1191.

419. Perreault CL, Hauge NL, Morgan KG, Allen PD, Morgan JP. Negative inotropic and relaxant effects of cocaine on myopathic human ventricular myocardium and epicardial coronary arteries in vitro. *Cardiovasc Res* 1993; 27:262–268.

420. Virmani R, Robinowitz M, Smialek JE, Smyth DF. Cardiovascular effects of cocaine: An autopsy study of 40 patients. *Am Heart J* 1988; 115:1068–1076.

421. Lam D, Goldschlager N. Myocardial injury associated with polysubstance abuse. *Am Heart J* 1988; 115:675–680.

422. Rod JL, Zucker RD. Acute myocardial infarction shortly after cocaine inhalation. *Am J Cardiol* 1987; 59:161.

423. Kossowsky WA, Lyon AF. Cocaine and myocardial infarction: A probable connection. *Chest* 1984; 86:729–731.

424. Hollander JE, Hoffman RS. Cocaine-induced myocardial infarction: An analysis and review of the literature. *J Emerg Med* 1992; 10:169–177.

425. Miller GW. The cocaine habit. *Am Fam Physician* 1985; 31:173–176.

426. Wetli CV, Wright RK. Death caused by recreational cocaine use. *JAMA* 1979; 241:2519–2522.

427. Benchimol A, Bartall H, Desser KB. Acceleration of ventricular rhythm and cocaine abuse. *Ann Intern Med* 1978; 88:519–520.

428. Nanji AA, Filipenko JD. Asystole and ventricular fibrillation associated with cocaine intoxication. *Chest* 1984; 85:132–133.

429. Schachne JS, Roberts BH, Thompson PD. Coronary artery spasm and myocardial infarction associated with cocaine use. *N Engl J Med* 1984; 310:1665–1666.

430. Howard RE, Hueter DC, Davis GJ. Acute myocardial infarction following cocaine abuse in a young woman with normal coronary arteries. *JAMA* 1985; 254:95–96.

431. Simpson RW, Edwards WD. Pathogenesis of cocaine-induced ischemic heart disease: Autopsy finding in a 21-year-old man. *Arch Pathol Lab Med* 1986; 110:479–484.

432. Virmani R, Robinowitz M, Smialek JE, Smyth DF. Cardiovascular effects of cocaine: An autopsy study of 40 patients. *Am Heart J* 1988; 115:1068–1076.

433. Dowling GP, McDonough ET, Bost RO. Eve and ecstasy: A report of five deaths associated with the use of MDEA and MDMA. *J Am Coll Cardiol* 1987; 257:1615–1617.

434. Barbour DJ, Roberts WC. Frequency of acute and healed myocardial infarcts in fatal cardiac amyloidosis. *Am J Cardiol* 1988; 62:1134–1135.

435. Nichols GR, Davis GJ, Lefkowitz JB. Sudden death due to fibromuscular dysplasia of the sinoatrial nodal artery. *J Kentucky Med Assoc* 1989; 87:504–505.

436. James TN. Morphologic characteristics and functional significance of focal fibromuscular dysplasia of small coronary arteries. *Am J Cardiol* 1990; 65:12G–22G.

437. Mosseri M, Yarom R, Gotsman MS, Hasin Y. Histologic evidence for small vessel coronary artery disease in patients with angina pectoris and patent large coronary arteries. *Circulation* 1986; 74:964–972.

438. Oberai B, Adams CW, High OB. Myocardial and renal arteriolar thickening in cigarette smokers. *Atherosclerosis* 1984; 52:185–190.

439. Arey JB, Segal R. Fibromuscular dysplasia of intramyocardial coronary arteries. *Pediatr Pathol* 1987; 7:97–103.

440. James TN, Posada de la Paz M, Abaitua Borda I, Gomez-Sanchez MA, Martinez-Tello FJ, Soldevilla LB. Histologic abnormalities of large and small coronary arteries, neural structures, and the conduction system of the heart found in postmortem studies of individuals dying from the toxic oil syndrome. *Am Heart J* 1991; 121:803–815.

441. Friedberg CK, Horn H. Acute myocardial infarction not due to coronary artery occlusion. *JAMA* 1939; 112:1675–1679.

442. Baroldi G, Scomazzoni X. *Coronary Circulation in the Normal and Pathologic Heart.* Washington, DC: American Registry of Pathology, Armed Forces Institute of Washington DC, U.S. Government Printing Office 1967:1–80.

443. Thorp JM, Chescheir NC, Fann B. Postpartum myocardial infarction in a patient with antiphospholipid syndrome. *Am J Perinatol* 1994; 11:1–3.

43

PATHOPHYSIOLOGY OF MYOCARDIAL ISCHEMIA

Stephen M. Factor / Robert J. Bache

The heart functions almost exclusively as an aerobic organ with little capacity for anaerobic metabolism. Even during resting conditions, 70 to 80 percent of the oxygen in the blood perfusing the coronary arteries is extracted by the myocardium.[1] Because of the limited ability to increase oxygen availability by further increasing oxygen extraction, increases of myocardial demand during exercise or other stress must be met by equivalent increases of coronary blood flow. Myocardial ischemia results when the arterial blood supply fails to meet the needs of the heart muscle for oxygen and metabolic substrate. Since direct measurements of myocardial blood flow are not generally available in the clinical setting, myocardial ischemia is recognized by the consequences that it produces. Even mild ischemia can be evident as the result of anginal pain, electrocardiographic changes, and the cessation of regional cardiac contractile function, while severe sustained ischemia is likely to result in myocardial infarction. Persistent systolic dysfunction resulting from cumulative and recurrent ischemia can result in left ventricular failure.

PRIMARY CAUSES OF MYOCARDIAL ISCHEMIA

Under normal circumstances, coronary blood flow closely parallels myocardial metabolic demands despite wide fluctuations in oxygen consumption by the heart.[1] Cardiac metabolism appears unable to outstrip its blood supply in normal individuals, even at extreme limits of activity, so that excessive demand is never a primary cause of ischemia.[2,3] The myocardial oxygen supply can be approximated by the product of myocardial blood flow and arterial oxygen content. Precise evaluation of the sufficiency of the myocardial oxygen supply, however, must be made at the level of the mitochondria. As oxygen diffuses from the capillaries into the myocardial myocytes, ischemia occurs when the partial pressure of oxy-

gen (P_{O_2}) available at the mitochondria falls below the level required to rephosphorylate the ATP being utilized for myocardial work.[4] In vitro experiments have shown that the critical level of P_{O_2} for the mitochondria is below 1 mmHg and thus far less than in coronary venous blood, where values of P_{O_2} seldom fall below 15 mmHg. The difference between the critical level of mitochondrial P_{O_2} and the coronary venous P_{O_2} suggests that diffusion of oxygen from the capillary bed to the mitochondria has an important role in determining the myocardial oxygen supply.[5]

Anatomic evidence of closed precapillary sphincters in the beating heart indicates that myocardial capillaries are not all functional at all times.[6] These findings are supported by physiologic evidence of variability of blood flow to different regions of the heart (*spatial heterogeneity*) and, in any given region, variability of blood flow with time (*temporal heterogeneity*).[7,8] Analysis of these findings in terms of a diffusion model for oxygen suggests that changes in the number of open capillaries can exert an important influence on local myocardial P_{O_2}.[5] During ischemia, all of the myocardial capillaries are likely to be recruited, so that diffusion of oxygen is limited by the anatomic capillary density. Myocardial capillaries parallel myocytes with a ratio of approximately one capillary for each myocardial cell, which places each cell in contact with three to four capillaries.[9] This ratio of one capillary per myocyte remains constant in adults and is unchanged with cardiac hypertrophy.[9] It is likely that the resultant decrease in capillary density contributes to the increased vulnerability to ischemia in the hypertrophied heart[10] (Table 43-1). Other factors that limit exchange between myocardium and blood, such as myocardial edema, fibrosis, capillary obstruction by microemboli, or precapillary vasoconstriction, could also contribute to the development of ischemia. Decreases in arterial oxygen content, such as with anemia, hypoxia, or abnormal hemoglobins, reduce the myocardial oxygen supply and would also precipi-

TABLE 43-1

CAUSES OF INCREASED VULNERABILITY
TO ISCHEMIA IN THE PRESSURE OVERLOADED
HYPERTROPHIED LEFT VENTRICLE

Insufficient growth of coronary vessels
  Impaired minimum coronary vascular resistance
    Decreased coronary vasodilator reserve
  Increased intercapillary perfusion distance for O_2 and metabolic substrate
Increased extravascular compressive forces
  Increased left ventricular filling pressure
  Prolonged duration of systole with reduced diastolic coronary perfusion

tate ischemia if not compensated for by an increase in blood flow.

The most frequently recognized cause of myocardial ischemia is occlusive coronary atherosclerosis, which either causes direct arterial narrowing or produces coronary obstruction by inducing thrombus formation. Coronary narrowing can also occur secondary to stenosis of the coronary ostia produced by primary disease of the aorta, coronary embolism, or inflammatory disease of the coronary arteries. Coronary artery spasm, either in an angiographically normal coronary artery or at the site of an atherosclerotic plaque, can transiently interrupt blood flow and produce severe transmural myocardial ischemia.[11] In occasional individuals, coronary small-vessel constriction can limit myocardial blood flow and lead to ischemia during exercise or other stress.[12] Regardless of the precise cause, a limited arterial blood supply is common to both mild or incipient ischemia and to severe ischemia, so that factors that determine blood flow are a pervasive aspect in the consideration of myocardial ischemia. Consequently, it is appropriate to review the mechanisms responsible for normal regulation of coronary blood flow.

Coronary Autoregulation

A fundamental property of the normal coronary circulation is the almost complete independence of blood flow from changes in perfusion pressure. If cardiac function and the composition of the arterial blood remain constant, steady-state values of coronary blood flow are remarkably constant.[13] Coronary perfusion pressure is normally identical to aortic pressure and is maintained within narrow limits by arterial baroreceptor activity. When an atheroma causes coronary artery narrowing, pressure distal to the obstruction is reduced by the resistance caused by the obstruction, but ische-

mia is avoided by a compensatory decrease in resistance in the distal arteriolar bed.[14] This autoregulatory response is a fundamental mechanism for maintaining myocardial perfusion in the presence of occlusive coronary artery disease.

The mechanism that allows coronary flow to be independent of perfusion pressure (*autoregulation*) is likely identical to the mechanism that adjusts the tone of the coronary vessels in response to changing metabolic needs of the myocardium. Recent evidence indicates that hyperpolarization of the vascular smooth muscle cell membrane caused by opening of ATP-sensitive potassium channels (K^+_{ATP}) contributes to both autoregulation and metabolic vasoregulation of coronary blood flow.[15] Thus, progressively more K^+_{ATP} channels become activated as coronary pressure is decreased, so that essentially all K^+_{ATP} channels are opened when coronary perfusion pressure reaches the lower limit of autoregulation.[16] Furthermore, blockade of vascular smooth muscle K^+_{ATP} channels causes a decrease of coronary blood flow, which results in contractile dysfunction both under resting conditions and during exercise.[17] The mechanism by which K^+_{ATP} channels are opened in response to increasing myocardial metabolic demands or decreased coronary perfusion pressure is unclear, but it could result from direct sensing of tissue oxygen tension or from a metabolite released by the myocardium. As shown in Fig. 43-1, adenosine produced by myocardial myocytes can contribute to metabolic coronary vasodilation. When coronary blood flow is insufficient to meet myocardial metabolic demands, ATP consumption exceeds production, with a resultant increase in myocardial ADP content. Within the myocyte, two molecules of ADP are acted upon by the enzyme myokinase to produce one molecule each of ATP and AMP. The ectoenzyme 5′-nucleotidase can then act on the increased pool of AMP to produce adenosine, which diffuses into the interstitial fluid. Since adenosine is a potent

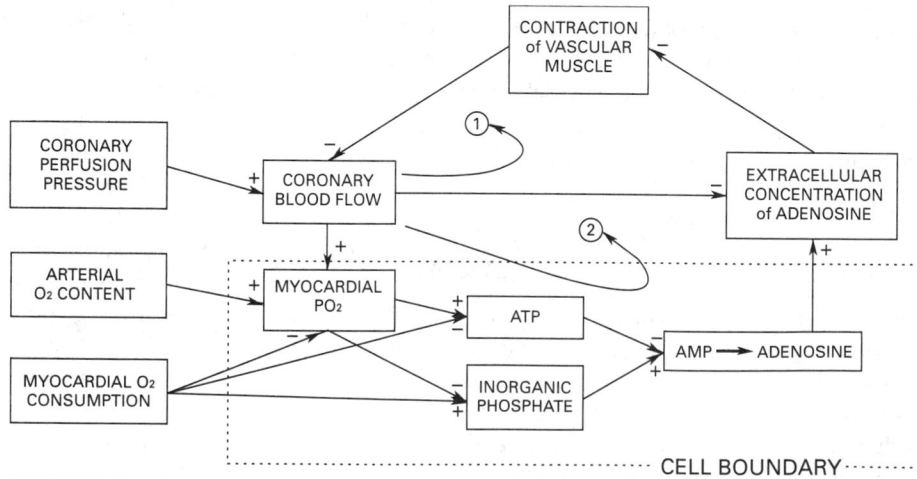

FIGURE 43-1

Diagram of feedback mechanism of regulation of coronary blood flow by adenosine.[1] Each variable is characterized as to its effect, that is, whether it increases ($+$) or decreases ($-$) the variable it acts on. In this type of diagram, negative feedback is characterized by having an odd number of negative signs in the feedback loop. Two negative-feedback loops involving coronary blood flow are indicated: involving (1) only extracellular variables, and (2) intracellular variables. In this diagram, the balance between supply and demand is represented in terms of delivery and utilization of oxygen.[1]

vasodilator of coronary resistance vessels, the increase in interstitial fluid adenosine augments coronary blood flow and acts to restore the balance between energy supply and demand.[18] In addition to adenosine there are numerous endogenous vasoactive substances, including those derived from the vascular endothelium such as nitric oxide and prostaglandins, platelet products such as thromboxane A_2 and serotonin, and agonists originating from autonomic neurons such as norepinephrine. It is likely that regulation of myocardial blood flow in the face of changes in coronary perfusion pressure and alterations of myocardial metabolic demand involves multiple redundant mechanisms. Furthermore, the mechanisms that control vasomotor tone may be different in diseased than in normal coronary vessels.

Effect of Myocardial Contraction on Coronary Blood Flow

Unlike other organs, in which blood flow varies directly with arterial driving pressure so that highest flow rates occur in systole when arterial pressure is highest, in the heart systolic contraction throttles blood flow, so that coronary flow normally occurs predominantly during diastole.[19] Impedance to coronary blood flow produced by the contracting myocardium is not uniform across the left ventricular wall. Thus, when coronary inflow is limited to systole, a steep transmural gradient of perfusion occurs, with selective reduction of flow to the subendocardium.[20,21] Impedance to blood flow produced by the contracting myocardium results in part from shearing forces within the left ventricular wall, which tend to pinch off intramural vessels within the left ventricular wall. These shearing forces, however, have been found to account for only a small fraction of total systolic impedance to coronary flow.[22] Furthermore, the effects of shearing forces on coronary flow are uniform transmurally and cannot explain the progressively increasing impedance to blood flow from epicardium to endocardium produced by cardiac contraction.[22]

During systole, the left ventricular endocardium is exposed to intracavitary pressure, while the epicardium is exposed to intrathoracic pressure. Myocardial perfusion during systole reflects this pressure difference across the left ventricular wall. Although the magnitude and pattern of the gradient of intramyocardial pressure across the left ventricular wall are uncertain, it is clear that effective intramyocardial pressure is highest in the subendocardium and falls progressively in the more superficial myocardial layers.[23] The blood vessels within the left ventricular wall act as collapsible tubes, and flow in collapsible tubes is inhibited in proportion to the magnitude of the external forces compressing the vessels. This phenomenon is termed the *vascular waterfall* and explains the increasing impedance to blood flow during systole in proportion to the depth of the muscle layer.[24] Impedance to blood flow produced by the vascular waterfall is additive to vasomotor tone in the coronary resistance vessels, but even during maximal coronary vasodilation, the extravascular component of coronary resistance in the beating heart accounts for 25 to 35 percent of total coronary resistance.[24] With maximal coronary vasodilation, extravascular compressive forces become the principal determinant of the transmural distribution of blood flow.

Systole does not normally inhibit the blood supply to the right ventricle, since right ventricular intracavitary pressure (and thus effective tissue pressure within the right ventricular wall) remains well below coronary perfusion pressure throughout the cardiac cycle.[25] In pulmonary hypertension, however, the increase in right ventricular systolic pressure can impede blood flow in a manner similar to that in the left ventricle.[26] During acute severe elevation of right ventricular systolic pressure secondary to acute pulmonary artery obstruction, systolic impairment of right ventricular myocardial blood flow can contribute to the development of right ventricular failure by limiting right ventricular perfusion and contributing to the development of ischemia.[26,27]

Subendocardial Ischemia

In the normal heart, blood flow to the subendocardium is maintained slightly greater than subepicardial flow, reflecting greater systolic stress development and higher oxygen consumption in the deeper myocardial layers.[28] Maintenance of adequate blood flow despite systolic underperfusion requires a perfusion gradient favoring flow to the subendocardium during diastole. This diastolic gradient of blood flow favoring the subendocardium requires that the resistance vessels maintain a greater state of vasodilation in the subendocardium than in the subepicardium. Because of the need for greater vasodilation of the subendocardial resistance vessels during basal conditions, the vasodilator reserve available to increase blood flow during periods of stress is least in this region.[29]

In response to a proximal arterial stenosis, the coronary resistance vessels undergo vasodilation to compensate for the resistance offered by the stenosis in an attempt to maintain adequate myocardial blood flow.[14] This compensatory vasodilation of the resistance vessels compromises the capacity for additional vasodilation during subsequent increases of myocardial oxygen demands. The degree of coronary artery stenosis that elicits maximal metabolic vasodilation of the resistance vessels is termed a *critical stenosis*, since any further reduction of luminal area will cause a decrease in coronary blood flow. Furthermore, in the presence of a critical stenosis, an increase of myocardial oxygen demands will result in myocardial ischemia, since the resistance vessels have no further capacity for metabolic vasodilation.

When blood flow is limited by a proximal stenosis rather than by the coronary resistance vessels, myocardial hypoperfusion and ischemia occur preferentially in the subendocardium. Redistribution of blood flow away from the subendocardium is the result of several interrelated mechanisms that occur when arterial inflow is insufficient to meet myocardial demands. First, since vasodilator reserve is least in the subendocardium, maximal vasodilation occurs first in this region, so that further reductions of perfusion pressure distal to the stenosis cannot be met by further vasodilation.[29] In contrast, residual vasodilator reserve may still exist in the subepicardium, allowing further vasodilation in this region to maintain blood flow. Second, a flow-limiting arterial stenosis alters the phasic pattern of coronary blood flow. Since the stenosis limits maximum flow rates through the proximal artery, and since maximal coronary flow rates occur in diastole, the influence of the stenosis is to decrease flow preferentially in diastole so that a greater fraction of flow occurs in systole.[30] Because cardiac contraction selectively impedes blood flow to the subendocardium, the increased systolic component of flow is delivered preferentially to the subepicardium. Finally, at the low levels of perfusion pressure that can exist distal to a flow-limiting coronary stenosis, extravascular forces can influence the transmural distribution of blood flow during diastole.[31] Since diastolic extravascular pressure is highest in the subendocardium, interaction between this compressive force and the low intravascular distending pressure distal to a flow-limiting coronary stenosis preferentially impedes perfusion of the subendocardium.[31] This effect is augmented with the onset of ischemia, because of the ischemia-induced increase in diastolic intracavitary pressure secondary to decreased myocardial compliance. The subendocardium is especially susceptible to ischemia, not only because this region is most vulnerable to hypoperfusion but also because oxygen requirements are highest in the subendocardium owing to the greater systolic tension development in this region.[28]

Coronary Vasomotion

In the normal heart, the proximal coronary arteries contribute only a small fraction of total vascular resistance so that normal spontaneous changes in vasomotor tone can occur without significantly affecting blood flow. With the development of atheromatous disease, however, a significant fraction of resistance to blood flow can reside in the proximal coronary artery. Approximately 70 percent of coronary atheromata are eccentric in location, leaving the uninvolved portion of the arterial wall able to undergo vasomotor changes.[32] In this situation, even modest degrees of coronary vasomotion can markedly influence stenosis severity. Thus, coronary vasoconstriction produced by alpha-adrenergic activity or circulating vasoactive peptides, which would be benign in a normal coronary artery, could significantly impair blood flow when the lumen is nearly obstructed by disease.[33] In addition to this modest vasoconstrictor activity, in occasional susceptible individuals coronary artery spasm can occur in either an angiographically normal or an atheromatous coronary artery to produce the severe primary reduction of coronary blood supply characteristic of Prinzmetal's variant angina.[11]

In patients with a compliant coronary artery stenosis, quantitative coronary angiographic studies have demonstrated that supine bicycle exercise results in worsening of stenosis severity.[34] This can result from passive collapse of the stenosis as well as from active vasoconstriction (Table 43-2). Passive worsening of stenosis severity occurs as metabolic vasodila-

TABLE 43-2

MECHANISMS FOR WORSENING OF SEVERITY OF A COMPLIANT CORONARY ARTERY STENOSIS DURING EXERCISE

Passive collapse
   Decrease in stenosis distending pressure secondary to metabolic vasodilation of coronary resistance vessels
Active vasoconstriction
   Exercise-induced activation of the alpha-adrenergic nervous system

tion of the resistance vessels causes an increased pressure loss across the stenosis with a decrease in distal coronary artery pressure. The distal coronary artery pressure represents the distending pressure for the stenosis.[35] In response to the decrease in distal coronary artery pressure during exercise, a compliant stenosis tends to collapse, resulting in an increase in stenosis severity.[36] In addition to this passive effect, sympathetic nervous system activation during exercise can result in active vasoconstriction at sites of eccentric stenoses, thereby further contributing to worsening of stenosis severity. Coronary artery vasoconstriction is especially marked during isometric exercise, since sympathetic nervous system activation is more prominent than during dynamic exercise.[37] Worsening of stenosis severity during exercise can be prevented by nitroglycerin, which causes dilation of compliant coronary stenoses.[34] Calcium channel blockers also prevent constriction of a compliant stenosis during exercise, although these agents cause less epicardial artery vasodilation than nitroglycerin.[38] Beta-adrenergic blockers can inhibit worsening of stenosis severity during dynamic exercise; this beneficial effect appears to result from blunting of resistance vessel dilation by limiting the increase of oxygen demands during exercise, thereby avoiding the marked decrease in distal coronary artery pressure that results in passive collapse of the stenosis.[39]

The vascular endothelium contributes importantly to modulation of vasomotor tone in the coronary arterial system. Furchgott and Zawadski[40] demonstrated that acetylcholine caused relaxation of isolated coronary artery rings when the endothelium was intact but contraction when the endothelium was removed. Subsequent studies have demonstrated that a number of agents, including acetylcholine, bradykinin, and histamine, cause coronary vasodilation indirectly by engaging specific receptors on the endothelium, which then cause release of an endogenous vasodilator termed *endothelium-derived relaxing factor* (EDRF).[41] EDRF appears to be nitric oxide or a closely related compound with a very short half-life produced by the constitutive endothelial cell enzyme nitric oxide synthase. Nitric oxide synthase acts on the amino acid arginine to produce nitric oxide, which diffuses to the underlying vascular smooth muscle to cause vasodilation.[42] The shearing force of the flowing blood modulates nitric oxide production, providing a mechanism by which the proximal coronary arteries undergo vasodilation in response to the increased blood flow during exercise or other stress.[43] Endothelium-dependent nitric oxide–mediated vasodilation is impaired or lost in atherosclerotic coronary arteries.[44] This has been demonstrated by the finding that the vasodilator response to intraarterial acetylcholine, which is observed in patients with angiographically normal coronary arteries, is converted to vasoconstriction in patients with atherosclerotic coronary artery disease.[45] In addition to vasodilator factors, the endothelium produces vasoconstrictor peptides called *endothelins*.[46] Although circulating endothelin levels are increased in myocardial infarction and shock, the role of these agents in control of the coronary circulation is at present unclear. Nevertheless, it is likely that endothelial dysfunction contributes to abnormal vasoconstrictor activity in some patients with coronary atherosclerosis.

It has generally been assumed that during ischemia local metabolic influences would cause maximal vasodilation of the coronary resistance vessels. Studies in experimental animals, however, have demonstrated that vasomotor tone can exist even in the presence of a coronary artery stenosis sufficiently severe to cause myocardial hypoperfusion, lactate production, and depression of contractile function.[47] Failure of ischemia to cause maximal vasodilation of coronary resistance vessels occurs because a substantial fraction of microvascular resistance resides in vessels that are not under metabolic control. Metabolic vasodilation and autoregulation occur predominantly in arterioles <100 μm in diameter.[48] Approximately 40 percent of total coronary resistance, however, resides in small arteries between 100 and 400 μm in diameter, which are not under metabolic control.[49] Thus, ischemia would cause metabolic vasodilation of microvessels <100 μm in diameter but would not cause vasodilation of vessels >100 μm in diameter, which represent nearly half of total coronary resistance. In the normal heart, the increase in blood flow produced by metabolic arteriolar vasodilation would likely result in flow-mediated nitric oxide–dependent vasodilation of arterial microvessels >100 μm in diameter. In patients with endothelial dysfunction secondary to atherosclerosis, hyperlipidemia, or hypertension, however, flow-mediated nitric oxide–dependent vasodilation of the larger resistance vessels is likely to be impaired or absent. Furthermore, sympathetic activation during exercise can cause alpha-adrenergic receptor–mediated coronary vasoconstriction, which opposes metabolic vasodilation.[50] Coronary resistance vessels in regions of ischemic myocardium are also responsive to other vasoconstrictors including thromboxane A$_2$.[51] Thus, it is possible that sympathetic activation during exercise or vasoconstrictors released in the proximal coronary artery by activated platelets could worsen myocardial hypoperfusion by causing vasoconstriction of the coronary resistance vessels.

Coronary Collateral Blood Flow

Total occlusion of a major coronary artery will result in ischemia or infarction of the dependent myocardium unless alternative arterial pathways exist. Although the normal human heart has preexisting connections between distal coronary artery branches, these native collateral vessels are usually insufficient to prevent infarction. In response to gradual obstruction of a coronary artery, however, collateral vessels can undergo sufficient growth to restore an adequate blood supply to the dependent myocardium. Transformation of the native rudimentary intercoronary anastomotic channels into mature collateral vessels involves a complex sequence of vessel injury, inflammation, and cellular proliferation.[52] Within the first 2 to 3 days after coronary occlusion, the small preexisting collateral vessels show extensive damage, with rupture of the internal elastic lamina, and appear as thin-walled, overstretched arterioles. This period of early transformation is marked by extensive perivascular inflammation with infiltration of monocytes and macrophages.[53] Mitotic activity is seen in endothelial and smooth muscle cells, with prominent intimal proliferation and subintimal hyperplasia.[50] As cellular proliferation continues and inflammation subsides, the collateral channels take on an organized smooth muscle coat, so that within 6 to 12 months after coronary occlusion they are similar in appearance to small arteries of comparable size.[52] As would be inferred from their appearance, these mature collateral channels do not function as passive conduits but have considerable vasomotor capability. Thus, developed collateral channels undergo vasoconstriction in response to the vasoactive amines angiotensin II and vasopressin and vasodilation in response to nitroglycerin and atrial natriuretic peptide.[54] In addition, collateral vessels undergo vasoconstriction in response to serotonin and thromboxane A$_2$, suggesting that these platelet products would be capable of impairing perfusion of collateral-dependent myocardium.[55]

There is considerable evidence that a functioning coronary collateral system can provide protection against myocardial ischemia in humans. Pathologic studies have shown that approximately 20 percent of all chronic total coronary artery occlusions found at autopsy are not associated with infarction of the dependent myocardium.[56] Presumably, in these patients coronary occlusion proceeded gradually, allowing sufficient time for an effective collateral circulation to develop before total occlusion occurred. In both experimental animals and in patients, even acute coronary occlusion frequently does not result in infarction of all of the dependent myocardium. Preservation of myocardium in the ischemic region is quantitatively related to the degree of coronary collateral inflow.[57] In patients undergoing coronary angioplasty, the presence of well-developed collateral vessels can minimize or prevent the development of a regional left ventricular wall motion abnormality during occlusion of the coronary artery with the angioplasty balloon.[58] Similarly, in patients undergoing thrombolytic therapy to interrupt the course of acute myocardial infarction, an effective coronary collateral system has been shown to delay the progression of ischemic injury, thereby extending the time period during which reperfusion can result in salvage of ischemic myocardium.[59]

The usual stimulus for development of an effective coronary collateral circulation is the presence of high-grade occlusive coronary artery disease. Cohen et al.[60] demonstrated that angiographically well-developed collateral vessels are regularly found only in patients with greater than 80 percent stenosis of a major coronary artery. Although the rate of development of collateral vessels in response to a high-grade coronary artery stenosis is not known, approximately three-quarters of patients suffering acute myocardial infarction develop angiographically well-functioning collaterals within 2 to 5 weeks after acute coronary occlusion.[61] The rate of collateral vessel development in response to stenotic lesions that do not produce total coronary occlusion may proceed at a slower rate. McHenry et al.[62] have provided evidence that antecedent exercise-induced myocardial ischemia can modify the syndrome that occurs in response to total coronary occlusion. Thus, when apparently healthy individuals with a previously positive exercise stress test experienced a coronary event, they were likely to suffer the onset of new or unstable angina, whereas similar individuals with a previously normal stress test were more likely to suffer myocardial infarction or sudden death. This finding suggests that the presence of a coronary stenosis sufficient to result in an ischemic response during exercise was also sufficient to cause development of coronary collateral vessels, which then exerted a protective influence when the coronary stenosis proceeded to total occlusion. These observations indicate that development of a functioning collateral circulation can be an effective long-term adaptation to occlusive coronary artery disease.

Although well-developed coronary collateral vessels can provide an alternative arterial blood supply to maintain perfusion of the dependent myocardium during resting conditions, patients with viable but collateral-dependent myocardium commonly have evidence of stress-induced myocardial ischemia. Collateral perfusion can be further compromised by disease in the coronary artery supplying the collateral vessels. When collateral channels are unable to increase blood flow adequately to the dependent myocardium during exercise, the distribution of blood flow will be similar to that observed when perfusion is limited by an arterial stenosis, with ischemia occurring preferentially in the subendocardium.[63] The maximum capacity for blood flow through collateral channels is not fixed but may be increased in response to collateral vasodilators such as nitroglycerin, while exercise capacity can be decreased following administration of collateral vasoconstrictors such as vasopressin or ergonovine.[64,65]

Coronary Steal

Under certain conditions, an increase in blood flow in one region of the heart can cause a decreased flow in another region as the result of *coronary steal*. The conditions necessary for coronary steal include (1) a common coronary artery having some resistance to blood flow, which supplies two myocardial regions in parallel; and (2) a stenosis in one of the two recipient arteries, which results in preexisting resistance vessel dilatation in that perfusion region.[66] The key to interpreting coronary steal is the pressure at the point where the common

vessel branches into the two parallel circulations. A decrease in pressure at this point will cause a decrease in flow in the already vasodilated circulation. This occurs when blood flow increases through the common vessel as a result of vasodilation in the active circulation.

The resistance of the common supply vessel is a critical determinant of the potential for development of coronary steal.[67] If the proximal artery has minimal resistance, large increases in flow will cause only minor decreases in pressure at the branch point. Conversely, if resistance in the proximal artery is markedly increased by occlusive atherosclerotic disease, autoregulation will recruit increasing portions of the vasodilator reserve in both distal branches and diminish the potential for steal.[14] Thus, the ability to develop steal is dependent upon an optimal degree of partial obstruction of the common coronary artery proximal to the bifurcation. Although vasodilation in one of two parallel regions is often used as evidence of coronary steal, small concomitant decreases in resistance in the common vessel or in the other parallel vascular bed could completely offset the tendency for a flow reduction. This possibility may be difficult to exclude whenever a coronary steal mechanism is considered to result from a coronary vasodilator drug. Drugs such as nitroglycerin elicit selective vasodilation in larger coronary vessels and therefore tend to prevent coronary steal. Drugs such as dipyridamole that override the normal autoregulatory mechanisms and cause vasodilation of the resistance vessels have potential for eliciting coronary steal.[68]

The conditions governing collateral blood flow are frequently conducive to the development of coronary steal. Collateral blood flow always occurs in parallel with flow to an adjacent normally perfused region, and often the adjacent region has a large vasodilator reserve. In fact, steal of collateral blood can be ruled out following a stimulus for small-vessel vasodilatation only if both regions are ischemic or if the collateral vessels are so well developed that no ischemia occurs. On the other hand, with a critical level of collateral blood flow resulting in a region balanced on the verge of ischemia, changes in demand are more likely to cause myocardial ischemia than are changes in supply caused by a steal mechanism.

Left Ventricular Hypertrophy

Left ventricular hypertrophy confers an increased risk for the development of myocardial ischemia. In hypertensive patients, left ventricular hypertrophy detected echocardiographically is associated with a substantially increased incidence of angina pectoris, myocardial infarction, and sudden death.[69] In dogs with left ventricular hypertrophy secondary to renovascular hypertension, acute coronary artery occlusion results in larger infarcts and a greater incidence of sudden death than in normal animals.[70] A coronary stenosis that results in similar reductions of distal pressure produces more severe subendocardial ischemia during exercise in animals with left ventricular hypertrophy than in normal animals.[71]

Increased vulnerability to ischemia results from both structural and functional abnormalities in the hypertrophied heart. Although both epicardial arteries and intramural vessels increase in size during hypertrophy, this vascular growth is less than would be expected from the increase in myocardial mass.[70] In agreement with this, studies in both human subjects and experimental animals with chronic pressure overload have demonstrated impaired coronary vasodilator reserve in the hypertrophied left ventricle.[72] The capillary:myocyte ratio remains near unity during hypertrophy, so that intercapillary diffusion distances for oxygen are increased in proportion to the increased myocyte diameter.[9] In addition to these structural alterations, functional abnormalities result in subendocardial ischemia during exercise.[73] Methods that measure only total coronary inflow may fail to detect this abnormality, since normal or supernormal subepicardial blood flow can exist in parallel with an underperfused subendocardium, resulting in a normal value for mean blood flow. Transmural redistribution of blood flow away from the subendocardium during exercise or other stress appears to be the consequence of abnormally increased extravascular forces resulting from the decreased compliance and increased cavitary pressure in the hypertrophied left ventricle.[73] These structural and functional abnormalities in the pressure-overloaded hypertrophied left ventricle cause increased sensitivity to the effects of occlusive coronary artery disease and, if sufficiently severe (as in critical aortic stenosis), can result in exercise-induced myocardial ischemia even in the absence of coronary disease.

Determinants of Myocardial Oxygen Consumption

Although the primary cause of myocardial ischemia is an impaired arterial blood supply, ischemia does not occur until the tissue demand for oxygen to support energy generation outstrips the supply. Accordingly, the determinants of myocardial oxygen consumption play a decisive role in setting the threshold for ischemia. The normal heart is dependent on aerobic metabolism for contractile function; therefore oxygen consumption closely parallels energy production. Although the exact relationship between myocardial mitochondrial respiration and cardiac pump function is difficult to define, good correlations exist between myocardial oxygen consumption and indexes based on pressure and volume measurements.[74,75] Three factors have been identified that have important, and possibly independent, effects on myocardial oxygen consumption. A discussion of each follows.

SYSTOLIC WALL TENSION

Systolic wall tension is directly proportional to ventricular systolic pressure and, according to the Laplace relationship, is also directly proportional to the ventricular diameter. Since systolic wall tension cannot be measured directly, systolic arterial pressure is used as a surrogate for wall tension. Since the effect of the ventricular diameter is neglected, the relationship with absolute oxygen consumption is imprecise. Nevertheless, changes in systolic arterial pressure do reflect changes in systolic wall tension. Wall tension is inversely proportional to wall thickness and consequently decreases with increased wall thickness. With compensated hypertrophy secondary to pressure overload, wall thickness is increased in proportion to the increase in systolic pressure, so that systolic wall stress (force per unit area) is generally normal during resting conditions.

MYOCARDIAL CONTRACTILITY

Myocardial contractility describes the contraction velocity and rate of force development independent of loading conditions. Increases in myocardial contractility result in increased energy expenditure and increased oxygen consumption. The maximum rate of rise of ventricular pressure during isovolumic contraction (dP/dt_{max}) has been widely used to estimate changes in myocardial oxygen consumption produced by alterations of contractility. This measurement changes in parallel with myocardial contractility but can also be influenced by both left ventricular preload and afterload.

HEART RATE

Heart rate serves as a summing factor for systolic wall tension and contractility, which are expressed on a per beat basis. For this reason, heart rate bears a strong relationship to the rate of myocardial energy utilization. In addition, increases of heart rate directly result in increased myocardial contractility, which contributes to increased myocardial metabolic demands.

RATE-PRESSURE PRODUCT

The product of heart rate and systolic arterial pressure (rate-pressure product) is useful for estimating changes in myocardial oxygen consumption. It should be kept in mind, however, that in the setting of coronary artery disease it may be difficult to balance the factors determining myocardial blood flow quantitatively against the factors that predict demand. Furthermore, with the onset of ischemia, myocardial aerobic metabolism rapidly decreases and contractile failure ensues. Under these conditions, the determinants of energy demand in the ischemic region are likely to be unrelated to global indices, which principally reflect mechanical function in the normal myocardium.

SUPPLY AND DEMAND CONSIDERATIONS IN THE THERAPY OF CORONARY ARTERY DISEASE

The mechanisms that apply at the onset of myocardial ischemia are summarized diagrammatically in Fig. 43-2. This diagram is a model that can be used to assess the effect of an intervention on the balance of myocardial supply and demand. The three underlying conditions of the model are that (1) the availability of blood flow to the myocardium determines the adequacy of supply, (2) the resistance vessels in the ischemic myocardium are vasodilated as the result of autoregulation, and (3) the critical regions to analyze are the subendocardial layers in segments of the heart supplied by occluded arteries. In the model, the effect of each of the

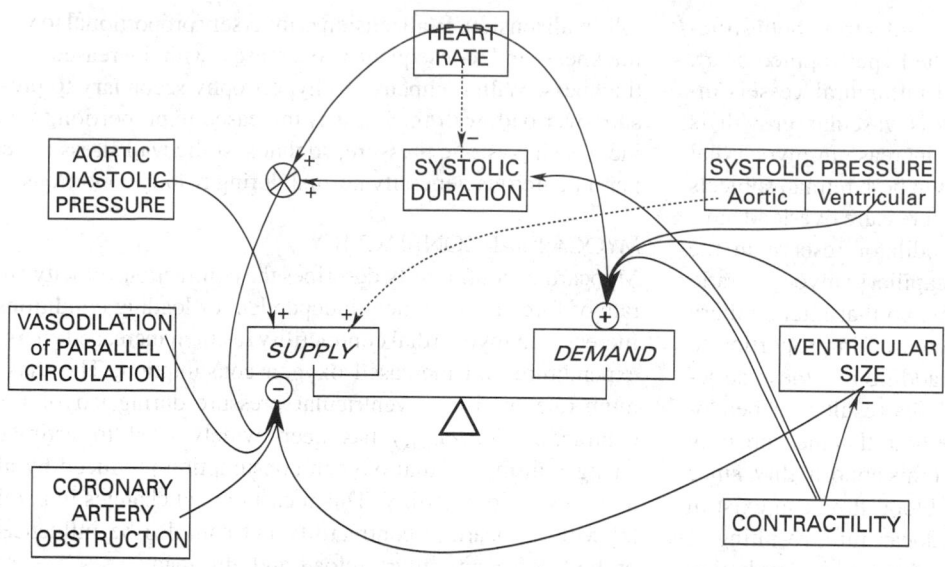

FIGURE 43-2

Diagram summarizing the factors in the balance of oxygen supply and demand in ischemic subendocardium. An increase in each variable is characterized as to its effect in increasing ($+$) or decreasing ($-$) the variables it acts on. The product ($\times$) of heart rate and systolic duration decreases the relative diastolic time and thereby decreases supply. Interactions of secondary importance are shown by dotted lines. Some interactions have direct effects on the balance of oxygen supply and demand (e.g., effect of aortic diastolic pressure on supply), while other interactions have a secondary effect on supply or demand (e.g., contractility effect on ventricular size).

factors on the balance of oxygen supply and demand in the ischemic subendocardium is shown by arrows. An increase in each variable is characterized as to whether it causes an increase ($+$) or a decrease ($-$) in the variable(s) it acts upon, which (depending on the side of the equation affected) either raises or lowers the balance in favor of oxygen supply. Several factors, such as aortic pressure and coronary artery occlusion, act only on one side of the balance and therefore have predictable effects on myocardial ischemia. Other variables affect both supply and demand and tend to shift the balance in an additive manner, e.g., ventricular size and heart rate. Contractility has the most complex interaction with the factors determining supply and demand. Although contractility causes an increase in myocardial oxygen consumption, the end result of a positive inotropic intervention on oxygen demand could be offset by a reduction of ventricular size and, consequently, systolic wall tension. In addition, increased contractility tends to increase the blood supply by (1) reducing diastolic compression of the subendocardial layers, (2) shortening systole with a resultant increase in the diastolic perfusion interval, and (3) decreasing ventricular volume. The model is helpful in understanding the complexity of the balance between oxygen supply and demand and to caution against oversimplified interpretations of the effect of an intervention.

PATHOLOGY OF MYOCARDIAL ISCHEMIA

Coronary ischemia that develops rapidly and then persists for a sufficient period leads to the evolution of cardiac tissue

necrosis known as *myocardial infarction*. A myocardial infarction is both a spatial and temporal event, the size and histopathology of which are dependent on the availability of coronary collateral blood supply and the metabolic demands of the tissue. As discussed above, the primary determinant of myocardial necrosis is blood flow; a diminution of coronary supply below a critical but often not predictable threshold leads to cell death. It is clear from studies on brief transient coronary artery occlusion[76] as well as from observations in animals and patients subjected to complete cessation of coronary flow during open heart surgery, however, that myocardial necrosis is not inevitable if blood flow is restored within a finite period of time. The complex pathophysiologic interrelationships between the coronary anatomy, the development of transient or permanent coronary occlusion leading to myocellular necrosis, and the identification and evolution of the infarction process will be explored in the succeeding sections.

Coronary Artery Anatomy and Pathology

Sudden obstruction of any coronary artery or a smaller branch vessel theoretically would not cause myocardial ischemia or necrosis if the coronary circulation was *diffusely* interconnected at all levels and if flow was homogeneous across the collateralized vascular bed. Even if myocardial infarction did develop because of inadequate collateralization of inhomogeneous flow, the pattern of tissue necrosis would likely be irregular and patchy, with indistinct borders possibly representing ischemic but surviving myocardium. Although larger collateral vessels can be demonstrated in the epicardial and subepicardial layers, the critical determinant of adequate blood supply to the myocardium is at the microcirculatory level where capillaries provide oxygen and nutrients to myocytes. If capillaries were diffusely interconnected and were derived from both patent and occluded stem vessels, myocardial cells might be maintained in an ischemic but viable state despite coronary artery occlusion. Two such hypothetical patterns are illustrated in Fig. 43-3, either of which could account for ischemic and surviving myocells at the lateral border of an infarct, e.g., a lateral border zone. If capillaries were organized in this way, there might be gradual and progressive diminution of blood flow toward the center of the perfusion field of a coronary artery, thereby leading to a "bullseye" pattern of infarction.

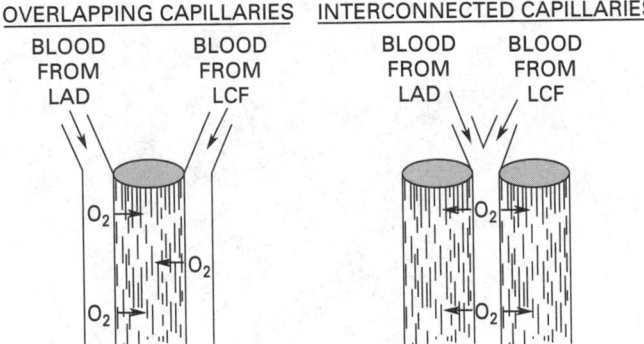

FIGURE 43-3

Two hypothetical capillary anatomic patterns that could explain the existence of surviving but ischemic myocardium at the lateral border of an acute myocardial infarction. On the left, each myocardial cell is intimately associated with interdigitating or overlapping capillaries derived from separate large coronary arteries. Occlusion of one main vessel would allow the cell to be supplied by oxygenated blood from the patent artery in diminished amounts as compared with normal. On the right, capillaries derived from two major vessels are interconnected, so that occlusion of one coronary artery would allow cells to be partially supplied by the patent vessel. With both patterns, enough substrate might be provided from the nonoccluded vascular bed to keep the myocardial cells viable, though ischemic. LAD, left anterior descending coronary artery; LCF, left circumflex artery. (From Factor et al.[86] Reproduced with permission from the American Heart Association, Inc., and the authors.)

Even though blood flow measurements with microspheres apparently do display a gradual falloff toward the center of an infarction, however,[77] there are alternative explanations for intermediate levels of coronary flow: if tissue at the border of an infarct is discretely necrotic and normal, it could be so interdigitated that it cannot be separated by rather gross methods. Accordingly, intermediate levels of flow or other markers of tissue damage [e.g., creatine kinase (CK)], simply represent averages of two distinct cell populations.

In fact, a number of sensitive techniques have shown that there is a sharp transition between normal and ischemic myocardium.[78–83] Additionally, serial section of completed infarcts with three-dimensional reconstruction has revealed that infarcts are remarkable complex along their lateral borders, with numerous interdigitating peninsulas of histologically normal and necrotic myocardium[84] (Fig. 43-4). Standard two-dimensional histology of infarctions gives a false impression of the spatial characteristics of the tissue, in that the discrete peninsulas are seen as "islands" separated from homologous tissue. These islands were previously viewed as histologic markers of ischemic but surviving tissue supplied by intermediate levels of blood flow. Reconstruction demonstrates a markedly interdigitated border with a sharp distinction between normal and necrotic myocardium. The explanation for this sharp border, not surprisingly, reflects the anatomy of the microcirculation. Perfusion studies of dog[85] and human[86] hearts reveals that there are no microvascular connections at the boundaries between regions perfused by separate large coronary arteries. The discrete blood supply is illustrated in Fig. 43-5, where two microcirculatory territories abut but do not anastomose. Termi-

nal homologous capillaries form loops rather than interconnecting with heterologous capillaries. Thus, the coronary circulation is a functional end-artery system, in which significant interconnections are present in the subepicardial layers. The theoretical patterns suggested in Fig. 43-3 do not represent the reality of the cardiac microcirculation.

One important consequence of the end-artery circulation in the heart is that the region of myocardium at risk following obstruction of a coronary artery is sharply delineated by the anatomic territory of the capillary bed supplied by that artery. Tissue outside the artery bed is not ischemic, nor is it jeopard-

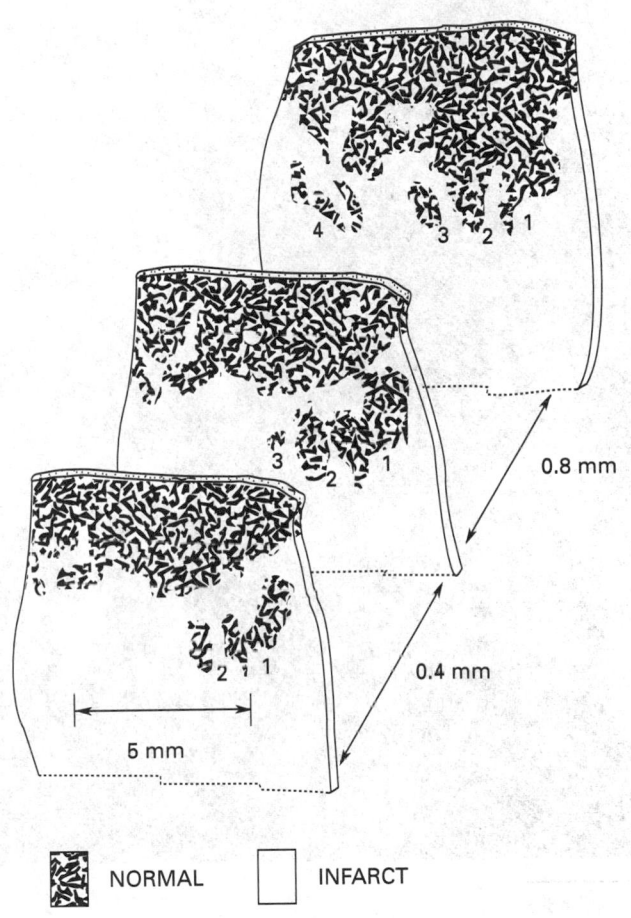

FIGURE 43-4

Composite illustration, based on original drawings of three myocardial sections. Intervening sections have been omitted for clarity. Preserved subepicardial normal myocardium (shaded area) can be seen at the top of each section. In the foreground, two islands of normal tissue (1 and 2) are completely separated from the subepicardial normal zone. Two sections deeper within the block, island 2 is still isolated. At the same level, a new island (3) becomes apparent. The last drawing, four sections away, shows complete continuity between islands 1 and 2 and the overlying subepicardial myocardium. Island 3 is larger at this level and becomes attached in subsequent sections. Several islands on the left (4) progressively enlarge and eventually become peninsulas. Additionally, the islands of necrotic tissue (unshaded) within the subepicardial zone demonstrate continuity with the infarct region at various levels and therefore are also peninsulas. The reconstruction illustrates that the border region consists of numerous interdigitated peninsulas that may appear as islands of normal or necrotic tissue when any one section is viewed. (From Factor et al.[84] Reproduced with permission from the publisher and authors.)

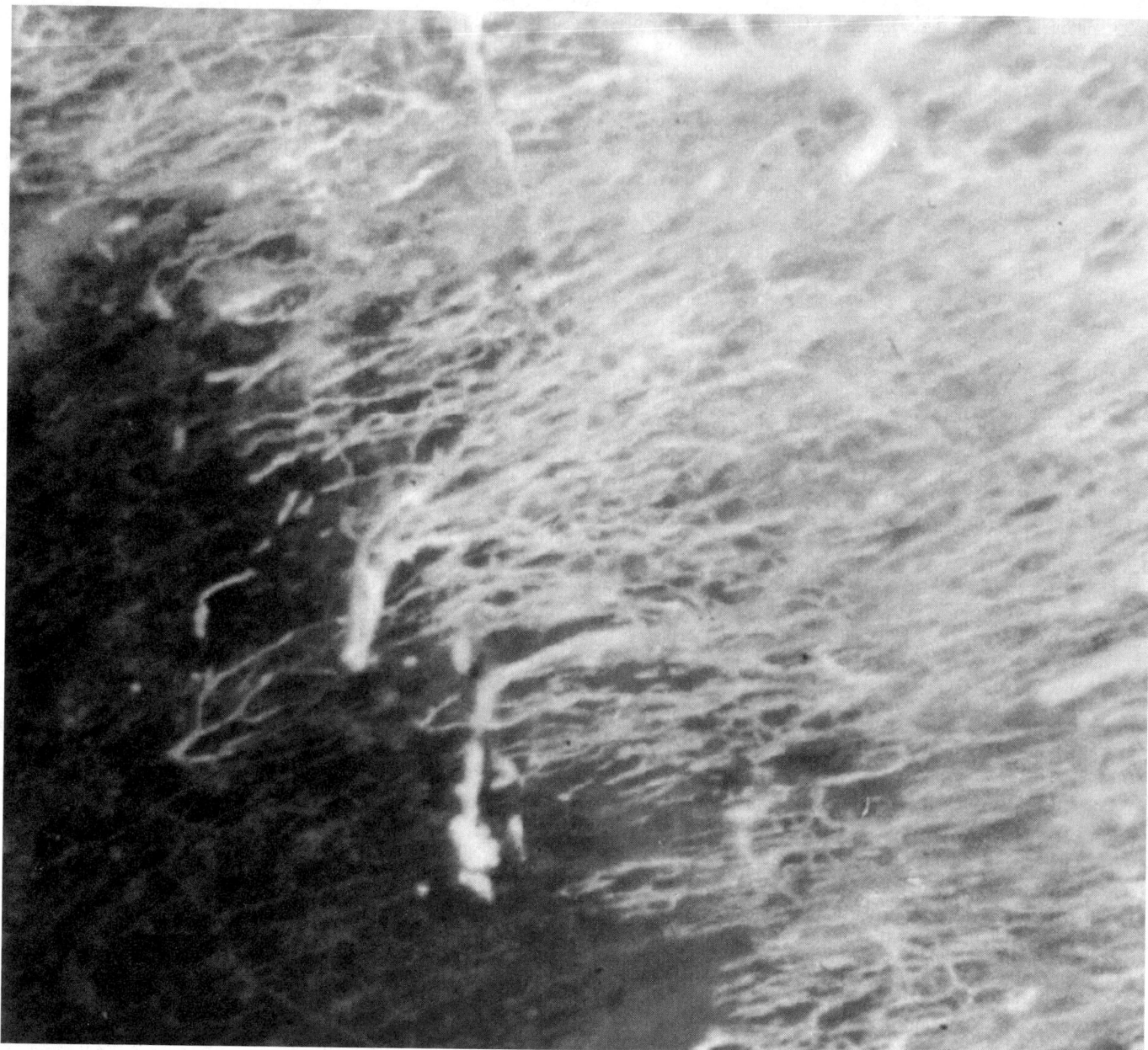

FIGURE 43-5

Multiple capillaries filled with white silicone rubber (Microfil) via injection of one coronary artery approach a zone perfused by an adjacent artery that is filled with red silicone rubber (reproduced here as gray). Where the white- and red-filled capillaries abut, they loop back on themselves, forming sharp hairpin turns. Some loops appear incomplete because they extend out of the section or out of the plane of focus. No anastomoses with capillaries perfused with different colors are noted, nor is there a complex alternation of red- and white-filled capillaries in this border region.

ized unless there is a coronary steal (see above). The concept of a region at risk determined by the arterial anatomy is emphasized by finding a close correlation between the size of an infarct and the size of the occluded artery bed.[87,88] When the cellular histology of infarcted or normal myocardium is compared with the microvascular supply, there is an extremely close relationship between the microcirculation derived from the occluded artery and the necrotic tissue.[89] Such analysis demonstrates that the highly complex, interdigitated histologic border results from an equally complex, interdigitated (but discrete) microvascular supply.

One can conclude from these observations that the coronary anatomy organized into an end-vessel system determines the area at risk of infarction if the supply vessel becomes occluded. Although preformed collaterals may mitigate the consequences of coronary occlusion, they are predominantly epicardial vessels, which, as previously discussed, are affected by intraventricular and intramural pressures that limit their perfusion of the subendocardium. In addition, since they are located proximal to the terminal capillary loops, their distal affects may be attenuated where they are most required to keep tissue viable. The anatomy of the coronary circulation leads to numerous areas at risk, progressing from the subendo-cardium to the subepicardium and potentially involving the tissue supplied by a single arteriolar-capillary unit up to the largest stem coronary vessel.

Coronary Artery Occlusion

Previous sections have emphasized that the primary determinant of myocardial viability is blood flow, although metabolic phenomena may modify the temporal and spatial characteristics of the process (see "Ischemic Preconditioning," below). The degree of ischemia is also a function of the extent of preformed collaterals. In the normally collateralized dog, abrupt coronary occlusion leads to a transmural gradient of flow in the myocardium, with the lowest flows in the subendocardium and relatively higher flows in the subepicardium. In the sheep without significant collaterals, coronary occlusion leads to dense ischemia throughout the risk region. In humans, the situation is more complex; collaterals may or may not be present, multiple coronary arteries may have partial or complete occlusion, and the arteries supplying the collaterals may themselves be diseased. Thus, the risk region may be more difficult to ascertain, and the beneficial effects of collaterals may not be predictable.

In experimental animals, myocardial infarcts generally are produced by a *sudden* occlusion of an anatomically normal coronary artery. In humans, the time course of total or complete coronary obstruction is often difficult to determine, but it appears to occur over a relatively brief interval of minutes to hours. Although human coronary arteries at postmortem generally reveal complete luminal occlusion with thrombi correlated with transmural infarction, recent observation suggests that subtotal occlusions may be seen in some individuals, along with infarcted tissue in different stages of organization. Additionally, the use of directional coronary atherectomy (DCA) devices in living patients who are undergoing acute coronary syndromes has provided a histopathologic "window" into events that may precede acute myocardial infarction. In patients with incipient or early infarction, coronary arteries may have intramural plaque thrombosis or plaque rupture prior to complete thrombotic occlusion of the lumen (Fig. 43-6). This, together with incomplete thrombotic occlusions, suggests that human infarcts may occur in a stepwise and progressive, or "stuttering," pattern, rather than

with the abrupt onset characteristic of myocardial infarctions seen in animal models.

As a rule, the coronary vessel supplying the area at risk in most patients reveals atherosclerosis with luminal narrowing.[90] Yet atherosclerosis is a chronic disease that takes months or years to evolve. Since atherosclerosis and myocardial infarction occur over different time frames, their frequent association is not reasonable proof of causation. Postmortem studies and more recent observations of DCA tissue removed from patients with acute coronary syndromes, however, emphasize that the atherosclerotic plaque as the underlying substrate for most coronary occlusive lesions must be modified by acute superimposed processes. These will be discussed in the following sections.

Coronary Thrombosis

There has been considerable controversy about the role played by coronary thrombosis in the etiology of acute myocardial infarction,[91] with a number of studies suggesting that thrombi were secondary to the infarction.[92–94] Currently, however, there is general agreement that in fatal acute transmural infarction more than 90 percent have associated coronary thrombosis, whereas significantly fewer cases of subendocardial infarction or sudden death have coronary thrombi, thus suggesting different pathophysiologic mechanisms for these latter two events.[95] Coronary angiography performed during the early stages of infarct development has provided the evidence required to settle this issue. DeWood et al.[96] evaluated patients in the first 4 h and found 87 percent with thrombotic occlusion,

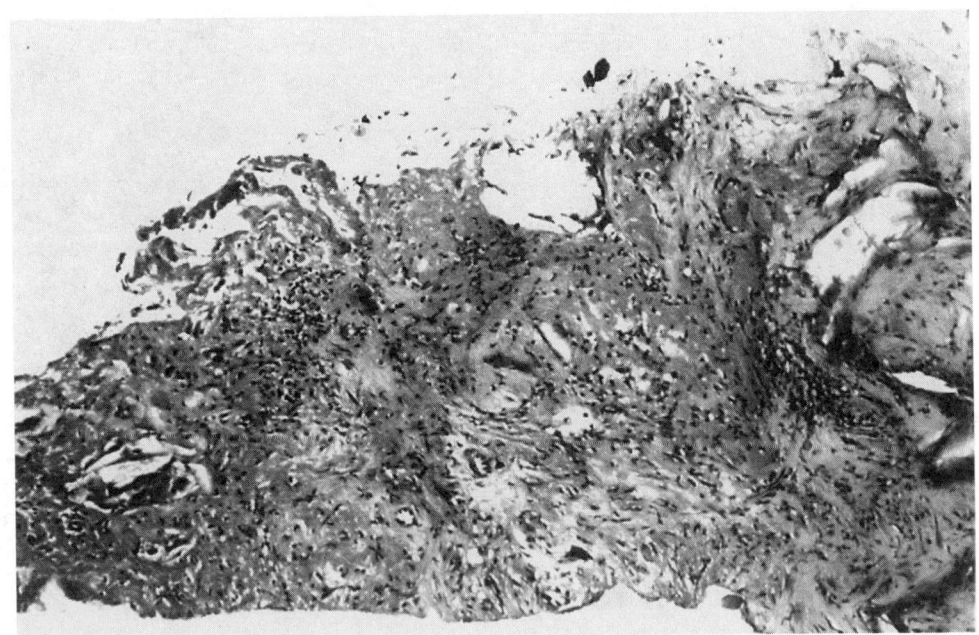

FIGURE 43-6

Coronary artery plaque material obtained with a directional coronary atherectomy device. The patient had unstable angina at the time of the procedure. The complex plaque material includes cholesterol, inflammatory cells, calcium, and platelet-fibrin thrombus. The presence of intraplaque hemorrhage, thrombosis, and inflammation is correlated with acute exacerbation (e.g., unstable angina) in patients with chronic atherosclerotic lesions. ($\times 150$)

with the percentage falling to 65 percent when patients were studied 12 to 24 h after onset. The decreased frequency of thrombi over time is probably explained by spontaneous thrombolysis, fragmentation, and distal embolization with infarct evolution. The efficacy of thrombolytic agents such as streptokinase and tissue plasminogen activator, demonstrated in numerous studies,[97] serves as further verification that coronary thrombosis is a critical event in infarct development. The ability to reestablish coronary flow with these agents, or by employing mechanical interventions such as percutaneous transluminal coronary angioplasty or DCA, is predicated on the concept that the coronary occlusion is due to an intraluminal thrombus and/or an unstable atherosclerotic plaque (see below). Improvement of left ventricular function and in-hospital mortality[98] supports the efficacy of these procedures and suggests that reperfusion occurred by thrombolysis.

Even if it is accepted that coronary thrombosis is a primary cause of sudden coronary obstruction, it is also clear that thrombi occur most often in diseased vessels with subtotal atherosclerotic luminal compromise.[90] Although alterations of blood flow with increased turbulence and shear stress, along with direct atherosclerotic damage to the vessel intima, may induce platelet adherence to underlying collagen with initiation of the coagulation cascade, other dynamic mechanisms are now known to be involved. It is beyond the scope of this chapter to review the complex interrelationships between the cellular, humoral, cytokine, and coagulability parameters that are involved. However, two specific events, plaque disruption and coronary artery spasm, are critical processes that have attained prominence based on in vivo and postmortem studies, and they require discussion.

Atherosclerotic Plaque Rupture

The human coronary atherosclerotic plaque is a complex structure composed of connective tissue, calcium, lipid, and inflammatory cells in differing proportions from patient to patient. Thin-walled vessels may enter the plaque and be potential sources of mural hemorrhage. Plaques may be *eccentric* (localized primarily along one segment of the wall) or *concentric* (localized circumferentially); regardless of their orientation, some intact smooth muscle is usually present in the residual medial layer, which may be a source of vessel vasomotion or vascular spasm under the appropriate stimulus. The consistency of plaques depends on the proportion of their component elements: A heavily calcified and fibrotic plaque is hard, while the plaque composed predominantly of cholesterol ester and lipid-containing macrophages is soft. Not infrequently, the soft lipid core of a plaque may be covered by a relatively thin cap of fibrous connective tissue separating the plaque material from the luminal blood flow (Fig. 43-7).

A number of studies have associated acute coronary thrombosis with rupture or cracks of the thin fibrous cap and release of the plaque material into the vascular lumen. Carefully performed studies have found between 78 and 93 percent[99–101] of acute coronary thrombi at postmortem can be identified as secondary to plaque rupture, confirming earlier work of Friedman and Van den Bovenkamp,[102] who found 98 percent concordance between thrombi and plaque rupture. Plaque rupture may induce thrombosis by any one or a combination of several mechanisms: (1) contact of platelets with exposed collagen, leading to thrombocyte adherence and the buildup of a platelet plug; (2) release of tissue thromboplastin from the plaque material, inducing the initiation of the clotting cascade; and (3) mechanical obstruction of the vessel lumen by the plaque components. What causes the thin-walled fibrous cap to crack or rupture leading to release of the plaque debris is still unknown. Among potential mechanisms, recent postmortem evidence suggests that coronary spasm may play a role.[103] In addition, it is known that plaques contain T cells and macrophages, which may release

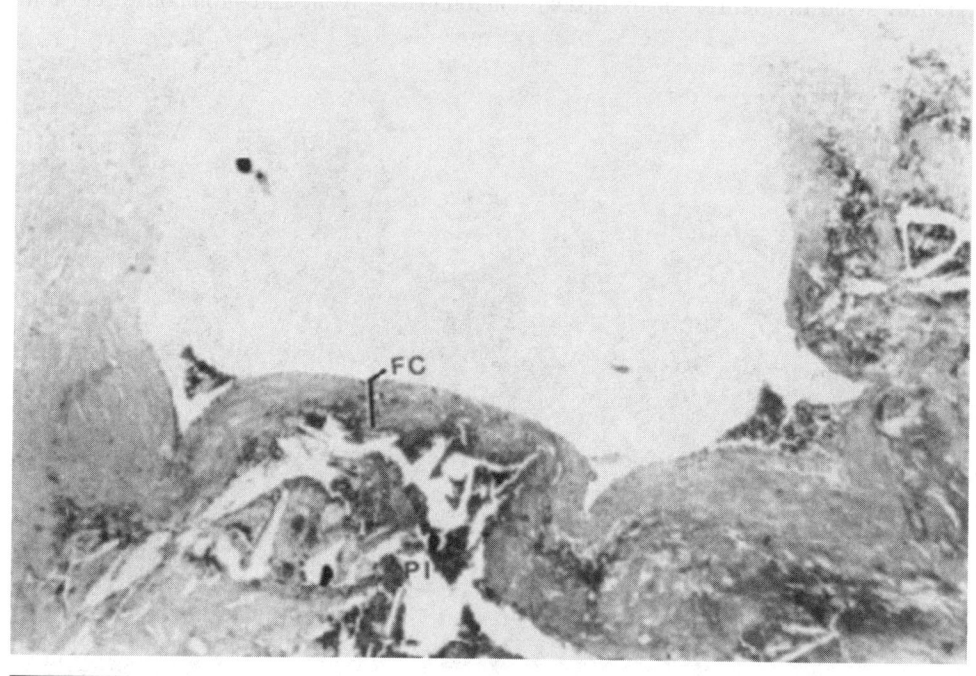

FIGURE 43-7
Segment of right coronary artery from a patient with an acute transmural myocardial infarction in the distribution of this vessel, associated with recent coronary thrombosis. The vessel was serially sectioned. At this level, there is a thin fibrous cap (FC) overlying a bulging atherosclerotic plaque (Pl) composed of cholesterol crystals (empty spaces), hemorrhage, and debris. A subsequent section revealed complete rupture of the plaque into the lumen with occlusive thrombus admixed with the plaque material. (×60)

collagenases or cytokines that may affect plaque integrity; mechanical disruption of the surface fibrous cap may also be a factor.[104,105]

Coronary Artery Spasm

The knowledge that coronary thrombosis is linked to the pathogenesis of acute myocardial infarction has developed in parallel with evidence that ischemic syndromes can be produced by coronary artery spasm, an old idea originally proposed by Latham[106] over a century ago and subsequently elaborated on by Sir William Osler[107] in 1910. There are now firm data that coronary artery spasm plays a major role in classical and variant angina pectoris as well as in acute myocardial infarction.[108–110] Angiographic studies performed in patients with clinical symptomatology or during provoked attacks have provided direct evidence that vasospasm can cause partial or complete coronary obstruction. Led by the pioneering efforts of Maseri et al.[111] in Europe and Oliva and Breckenridge[112] in the United States, there is now general acceptance for this view. What induces the vasospasm in most instances remains unknown;[110] however, preventive therapy with calcium channel blocking agents and nitrates has now entered the standard armamentarium for the treatment and prevention of the ischemic syndromes. It is also not known whether or not spasm due to a pathologic contraction of medial smooth muscle in one or several segments of a vessel and lasting for a brief or indeterminate period is solely responsible for dynamic coronary obstruction.

Recent observations have altered the emphasis on medial smooth muscle in the pathogenesis of coronary artery spasm and have focused attention on the critical role of endothelial cells in the maintenance of vascular homeostasis. Endothelial cells not only play a role in the adhesion of platelets and inflammatory cells to the luminal surface but also serve to elaborate a number of mediators that can relax (prostacyclin and nitric oxide) or constrict (endothelins) vessels.[113] These mediators provide exquisite control of vascular tone in normal blood vessels, but with derangements of endothelial integrity induced by trauma, toxins, or atherosclerosis among others, the balance may be upset, leading to loss of vasodilatory capacity.[114,115] Since endothelial integrity is also critical for the prevention of atherosclerosis and its alteration may initiate atherosclerosis through elaboration of multiple inflammatory cytokines and cell surface adhesion molecules,[116] it can be seen that two of the major pathologic processes affecting coronary artery patency (e.g., atherosclerosis and spasm) are interrelated, with the common pathway being the endothelial cell.

Although coronary artery spasm may occlude a vessel without any other associated vascular pathology, most often the spasm occurs in the setting of coronary atherosclerosis. If the occlusion is of sufficient duration (see below), tissue injury or necrosis may supervene before vascular relaxation restores blood flow. There is also evidence that coronary vasospasm is often the initiating event in the development of an acute thrombus.[117] Support for this concept comes from experimental studies demonstrating that arterial constriction induced with norepinephrine[118] or nonocclusive ligation[119] can lead to vessel wall damage, including endothelial injury and subsequent thrombosis. Cocaine, also, as an inhibitor of the reuptake of norepinephrine at the neuromuscular junction, causes a sustained local elevation of norepinephrine, thereby accounting for the well-known association of this illicit agent with vasospasm, acute coronary thrombosis, and myocardial infarction. Chronically, cocaine use may lead to coronary artery plaque formation, even in individuals devoid of systemic atherosclerosis. As suggested above, coronary vasospasm may also be implicated in the frequent plaque ruptures associated with thrombi. Thus, endothelial integrity, vasospasm, atherosclerosis, and coronary thrombosis are all related phenomena and can act together to enhance the occurrence of any single event leading to coronary artery occlusion. It is the interplay of complex static and dynamic events in the coronary vessel that produces obstructive vascular changes intimately associated with the pathogenesis and pathophysiology of myocardial ischemia.

Patterns of Acute Myocardial Infarction

The onset of abrupt coronary obstruction, induced by several of the mechanisms discussed in the previous sections, leads to the development of transmural ischemia within the area at risk determined by the coronary anatomy. At least partially because collateral flow increases from the deepest subendocardial layers to the subepicardium, the jeopardized myocardium within the risk region dies in a transmural pattern beginning in the subendocardium. This progression of necrosis has been termed a *wavefront* based on several classic studies by Jennings and coworkers.[120,121] They demonstrated in experimental animals that, with coronary occlusions ranging from 40 min up to 3 to 4 h followed by 2 to 4 days of reperfusion, progressively more tissue undergoes necrosis in a wavelike pattern from the subendocardium to the subepicardium, whereas 6-h reperfused infarcts did not differ from a 24-h infarct produced by permanent occlusions. These observations have been confirmed by several laboratories,[122,123] strongly indicating that this temporal and spatial progression of necrosis across the ventricular wall represents a fundamental pathophysiologic phenomenon. This phenomenon also appears to be applicable to human infarcts. A comparative study of human subendocardial infarct extension following permanent coronary artery occlusion revealed an identical pattern to that seen in dogs with 40-min subendocardial infarcts and subsequent transmural extension.[123]

There are several important implications that can be drawn from this work. Most significant is the conclusion that jeopardized myocardium undergoes necrosis in a sequential fashion, beginning in the subendocardium and extending toward the epicardium. The salvage of tissue in the epicardial layers is dependent on either the restoration of blood flow to this zone through the transiently occluded coronary artery or the presence of sufficient collateral supply to this area to prevent necrosis. By inference, then, *subendocardial infarctions in humans are likely to be secondary to intermittent coronary artery occlusions.* These may occur due to coronary artery spasm with spontaneous or drug-induced relaxation or to luminal thrombosis with spontaneous or iatrogenic clot lysis; in either case, the restoration of blood flow most likely must occur within a narrow time frame of several hours. Despite the evidence favoring blood flow–mediated transmural extension of myocardial necrosis, a recent study showed that the subendocardium was more vulnerable to damage than the subepicardium, even in the absence of all blood flow in the tissue.[124] This suggests that subendocardial vulnerability may be due to metabolic or other unknown factors.

Because of the complexity of atherosclerotic coronary disease in humans and the unpredictability of collateral supply, it is difficult to know whether or not the relatively short time course available for reperfusion and salvage of subepicardial myocardium demonstrated experimentally also applies to actual patients. If transmural necrosis is essentially completed within 3 to 6 h, there is little time available for institution of measures that will restore blood flow to the area at risk. Early reperfusion in animals has been shown to salvage myocardial function[125] and to have positive effects on survival, even when infarct size did not significantly differ from that produced by permanent coronary occlusion.[126] In contrast, early reperfusion may lead to preservation of increased numbers of myocytes in the immediate subendocardial zone[123]; it has been suggested that these cells may be responsible for ventricular arrhythmias that may have adverse consequences in the postinfarction period.[127,128] Thus, although it seems logical to believe that reperfusion is invariably beneficial, the preservation of jeopardized tissue otherwise destined to die may have unanticipated adverse results. This subject has also become more complex recently with evidence that previously ischemic myocardium may be less susceptible to subsequent ischemic events due to preconditioning (see below). Thus, patients with classic or atypical angina may develop some degree of protection that may prolong the survival of myocardium beyond the time course suggested by the wavefront studies.

Morphologic Effects of Reperfusion

Myocardial infarction secondary to complete obstruction of a coronary artery is not entirely devoid of blood flow if collateral vessels are present, but the flows are below the threshold required to maintain viability. Despite this insufficient circulation, an infarct in which minimal reperfusion occurs evolves into a relatively pale, yellow-white zone of necrotic muscle over several days, with demarcation from the normal muscle by a rim of hyperemia. Mottling and hemorrhage may be present focally, but they are only due to residual flow and stasis. In contrast, a reperfused infarct is hemorrhagic (Fig. 43-8), with the hemorrhage localized within the necrotic tissue in the subendocardium; the hemorrhage is due to microvascular injury. There has been considerable debate over whether

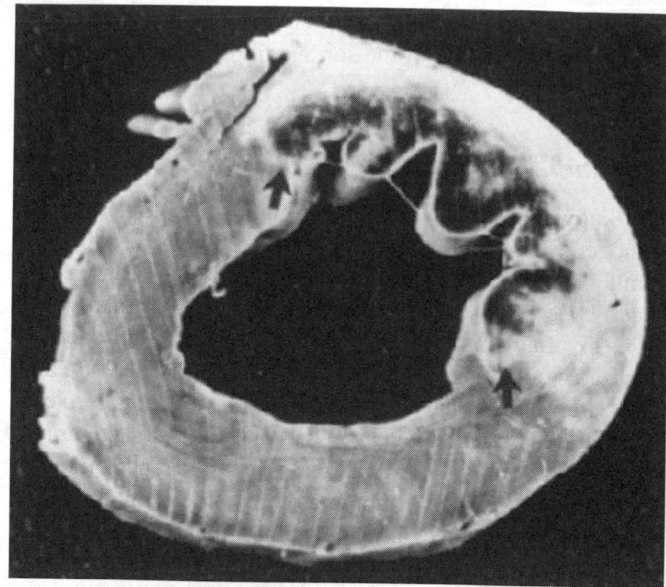

FIGURE 43-8
Left ventricle of a dog following a 40-min occlusion of the left anterior descending coronary artery (LAD) with 24 h of reperfusion. The region of risk has been delineated by perfusing the LAD with white silicone rubber. Note the dark subendocardial hemorrhage, which was histologically verified to be within the necrotic zone. Laterally, the hemorrhage and necrosis closely approach the lateral extent of the risk region (arrows).

reperfusion and the elicited intramyocardial hemorrhage have immediate or more chronic adverse consequences. The weight of evidence now strongly supports the view that reperfusion does not affect the ultimate evolution and healing of the infarct. This point is of considerable practical importance because of the clinical application of techniques to reestablish blood flow to infarcting myocardium during the active phase of necrosis. Reperfusion has a number of other consequences that may be related primarily to cell membrane damage.[129] The pathogenesis of the membrane damage remains in dispute, although the involvement of free oxygen radicals following reoxygenation of ischemic tissue has been promoted actively over the past decade. Whether or not oxygen and/or hydroxyl free radicals are generated during ischemia-reperfusion and whether or not they are deleterious to cells that would otherwise be viable are still areas of considerable debate and practical importance. Several recent commentaries have reviewed the salient issues on both sides.[130,131] Regardless of the cause, reperfusion leads to development of myocardial cell swelling,[132] accumulation of calcium in mitochondria,[133] accelerated washout of cellular enzymes,[134] and the presence of characteristic contraction bands.[135,136] These contraction bands are the morphologic marker of reperfusion injury, indicating that myocardial cells were ischemically damaged and then subsequently supplied with oxygenated blood. For example, they are seen in acute subendocardial infarction throughout the necrotic zone, and they have been described following coronary bypass grafting of patients with acute myocardial ischemia, where they are secondary to surgical reperfusion.[131] They may also be observed along the periphery of transmural infarctions, often associated with focal mitochondrial calcification (Fig. 43-9). In this location, they are probably related to diffusion of oxygenated substrate from the normally perfused tissue.

Morphology of Nonreperfused Infarcts

There are several characteristic features of predominantly nonreperfused infarctions that permit histologic identification and approximate dating. These features were outlined by Mallory et al.[137] in a classic paper in 1939, and they were verified more recently by Fishbein and colleagues.[138] The major limitation of histology is the insensitivity of light microscopy in early infarctions; morphologic alterations are not clearly defined in the first 6 to 12 h of infarct development, although experienced observers may see subtle signs of necrosis even in the first several hours. A variety of histochemical and ultrastructural methods have been employed to circumvent these problems, but light microscopy with hematoxylin-eosin staining still remains the "gold standard" for infarcts older than 12 to 24 h. The primary advantage of histology, particularly when compared with ultrastructure, is the ability to examine large regions of myocardium and to correlate the changes with vascular markers that can identify the area at risk. For definitive diagnosis of early infarcts of less than 6 h duration, however, other methods are required.

The most significant histologic marker of infarction is the presence of increased sarcoplasmic eosinophilia, or hypereosinophilia, characteristic of coagulation necrosis, which can be appreciated within the first 24 h (Fig. 43-9). Myocytes at this stage may also be attenuated and aligned in parallel bundles of wavy fibers,[139] but this is not a constant finding. The waviness is related to stretching of the necrotic tissue by the surrounding viable myocardium, with subsequent relaxation postmortem. Because of stretching, cross-striations are less prominent but are still present with increased sarcomeric spacing. Nonreperfused infarcts may have congested vessels and interstitial edema, but prominent intercellular hemorrhage is usually absent. Even without reperfusion, however, some blood flow is usually present in the infarct zone unless collaterals are absent; because of this, some viable myocytes may be seen surrounding vessels deep

within the necrotic tissue. Focal contraction bands and myocytolytic changes typical of reperfusion are usually seen along the periphery of the infarction. Whether this is related to reperfusion through collaterals, diffusion from the noninfarcted zone, or is due to the effects of catecholamines is not known. As previously noted, this is also the region where focal cellular calcification can be identified.

Cellular and reparative phenomena are somewhat variable from patient to patient. They are dependent on the underlying host inflammatory response, residual blood flow within the infarct zone, and blood flow within the myocardium surrounding the infarct. General observations reveal the following schema and are summarized in Table 43-3. Within the first 12 h, polymorphonuclear leukocytes (PMNs) marginate in vessels and begin to migrate into the interstitial spaces; this PMN response is most likely mediated by cytokine release from the ischemically injured tissues, and it plays a role in further damage to the myocardium.[140] By 24 to 48 h, all infarcts have infiltrates of PMNs at variable depths within the necrotic tissue, moving from the periphery toward the center. The variability probably reflects the extent of local blood flow, which may not be sufficient to keep the myocardium viable but may be capable of bringing inflammatory cells into the area. Lymphatic and venous drainage from the infarct zone carry away cellular proteins and enzymes that leak through damaged membranes and that may be measured systemically

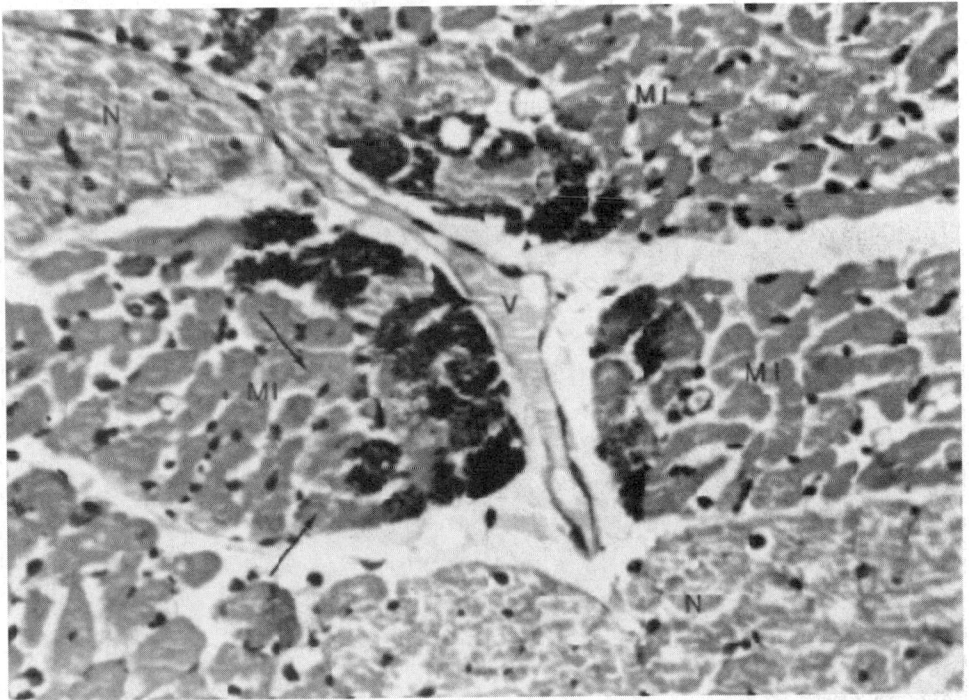

FIGURE 43-9
Histologic border of the 24-h canine transmural infarction. The darker, hypereosinophilic necrotic myocardial cells (MI) are sharply delimited from peninsulas of normal myocardium (N). In the region surrounding a thin-walled patent vessel (V), the necrotic cells contain finely granular calcium precipitate (black in this photomicrograph), which extends two to three cells away from the vessel. A few contraction bands are observed in the same area (arrows). The spatial orientation of the calcification and contraction bands suggests that they were secondary to diffusion of substrate from the noninfarcted zone or the patent vessel. (×150)

TABLE 43-3

HEALING OF MYOCARDIAL INFARCTION[a]

	0–6 h	6–12 h	12–24 h	1–2 days	2–4 days	4–7 days	7–14 days	>14 days
Hypereosinophilia	+/−	++/−	++	++	++	+	−	−
Wavy myocardium	+	++	++	++	+/−	−	−	−
PMNs	+/−	++/−	++	+++	+++	++	+	−
Cell lysis	−	−	+/−	+	++	+++	++	−
Macrophages	−	−	+/−	+	++	++	+++	++
Fibroblasts	−	−	−	+/−	+	++	+++	+++
Endothelial cells	−	−	−	−	+/−	++	+++	+++
Collagen	−	−	−	−	−	+/−	++	+++

[a] Progression and intensity of various histologic and cellular parameters involved in the organization and healing of myocardial infarctions from onset (0–6 h) beyond 14 days

as markers of necrosis, such as CK. Serial sectioning of acute infarcts demonstrates that the PMN collections are not homogeneous but discontinuous.[84] Absent blood flow related to microcirculatory damage (no-reflow phenomenon),[141] vascular thrombi within the infarct region, or inadequate collaterals may account for this discontinuity.

By 2 to 4 days, the degree of PMN inflammation has increased and inflammatory cells begin to undergo necrosis and fragmentation. Centripetal degeneration of necrotic myocytes is observed, and the peripheral infarct begins to demonstrate admixtures of mononuclear inflammatory cells including lymphocytes, mast cells, and macrophages. The latter often contain lipofuscin pigment from the breakdown of myocytes. Eosinophils are an inconstant feature, but they may be observed in this early period.

Within the first 4 to 7 days, although PMNs are still present, chronic inflammatory infiltration increases. At the periphery of the infarct, progressing toward the central zone, fibroblasts and new capillaries can be identified. By 1 week, this granulation tissue is well defined and loose collagen is being deposited in the interstitium. This process of scar formation progresses for weeks until a densely collagenized healed infarct is present. In very large infarctions, presumably where there is complete absence of blood flow in the center of the risk region, mummified necrotic myocytes surrounded by scar may be seen months or years after healing is complete. For most infarctions, scarring is generally completed within 6 to 8 weeks.

Alterations in Postinfarct Period

Although the authors have stressed that myocyte necrosis secondary to ischemia is a temporal event that takes a minimum of several hours for completion across the ventricular wall, it is equally true that once the infarct has developed fully, there may be associated remodeling changes with time in the immediate and distant regions of the ventricle that have adverse consequences for the heart. There has been recent popularization of this concept in descriptions of infarct expansion and extension.[142] *Expansion* refers to the dilatation and thinning of the infarct without superimposed new myocyte necrosis. In one study,[143] infarct expansion was identified in 59 percent of 76 consecutive acute transmural myocardial infarcts, with severe expansion occurring in infarcts greater than 5 days old. The authors have observed marked infarct thinning within the first 3 days (Fig. 43-10) and even as early as 1 day after onset, particularly if the infarct results in ventricular rupture. The pathogenesis of this pronounced thinning is unknown. Although it may be related to attenuation and disruption of

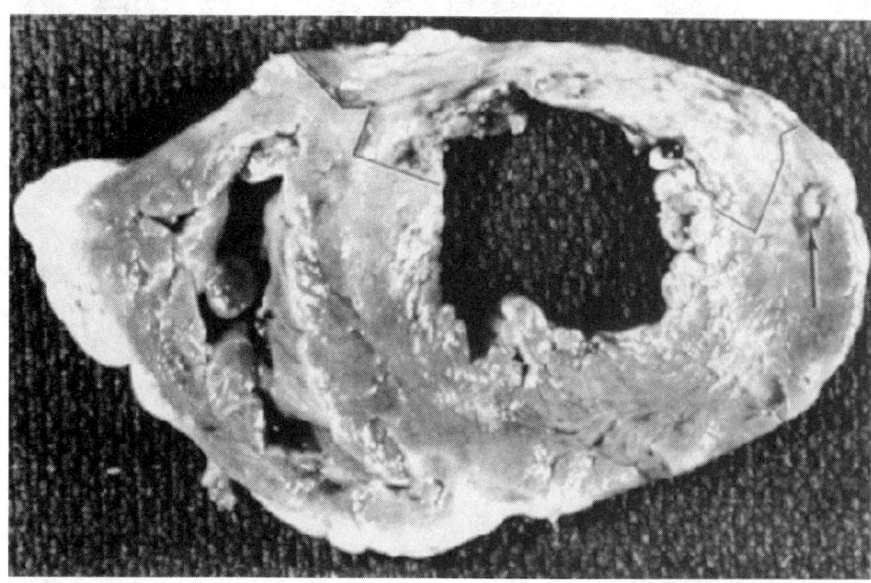

FIGURE 43-10
There is marked thinning of the posterior free wall secondary to a transmural acute myocardial infarction (approximately 72 h old). There was ventricular rupture present at another level. The infarct is demarcated at its gross lateral borders; a region of acute necrosis (arrow) is present peripheral to the main infarct.

myocardial fibers, recent observations suggest that it may be secondary to disruption or destruction of the interstitial connective tissue matrix of the heart. Myocardial cells are surrounded by a complex connective tissue skeleton that serves to attach myocytes to each other and to other structures in the heart.[144] It appears that even in very early infarction, there is loss or damage to this matrix, suggesting profound alterations in its composition and integrity (Fig. 43-11). Disruption of the matrix holding myocardial cells to each other may account for their slippage during infarction, leading to expansion and wall thinning, ventricular aneurysm formation, or myocardial rupture.[145] Thus, collagen degradation is an active part of myocardial necrosis,[146] and it occurs approximately concurrent with collagen synthesis in the infarct zone and even in the normal myocardium.[147] Both processes contribute to ventricular remodeling following infarction. Recent evidence suggests there may be a benefit for late perfusion in infarcts beyond the time in which myocardium can be salvaged, based on an enhancement of the reparative processes.[148]

In contrast to infarct thinning without new necrosis, *extension* refers to the development of additional myocardial necrosis adjacent to the initial infarct.[142] In the study reported by Hutchins and Bulkley, they described relatively small zones of contraction band necrosis in 17 percent of 76 acute infarctions and ascribed its occurrence to transient hypoperfusion.[143] Because of the small volume of myocardium involved, they believed that this process was probably hemodynamically insignificant. A clinical study by Fraker et al.,[149] however, identified acute extension in 13 percent of 458 patients with acute infarction and observed a fourfold increase in in-hospital mortality and decreased 1-year survival. Although the mechanism for extension is unknown, experimental infarcts in which the risk region is precisely defined reveal that extension can occur in the normal nonrisk zone.[150] The contraction band morphology of the necrosis and its localization suggest that catecholamines and/or microvascular spasm may be implicated.

Identification of the vascular area at risk with histologic infarct extension into the normal region links this phenomenon to the development of new necrosis at a distance from the initial infarct. This necrosis may represent a second myocardial infarction due to transient or complete obstruction of a main coronary artery with

features of a non-Q-wave or Q-wave infarction. Not infrequently, however, new necrosis is identified with contraction band or myocytolytic morphology in the epicardium or midventricular wall, and this is not in the vascular distribution expected with main coronary artery occlusion. The pathogenesis of this necrosis is unknown, but it may be similar to that proposed for acute extension.

Ischemic Myocardial Dysfunction without Necrosis (Stunned Myocardium)

There has been increasing recent interest in the phenomenon of *stunned myocardium*—the development of persistent me-

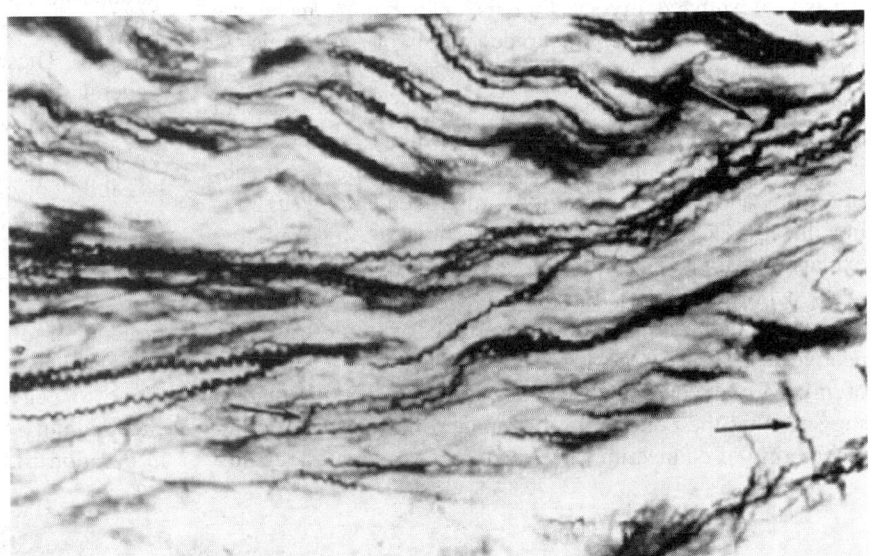

A

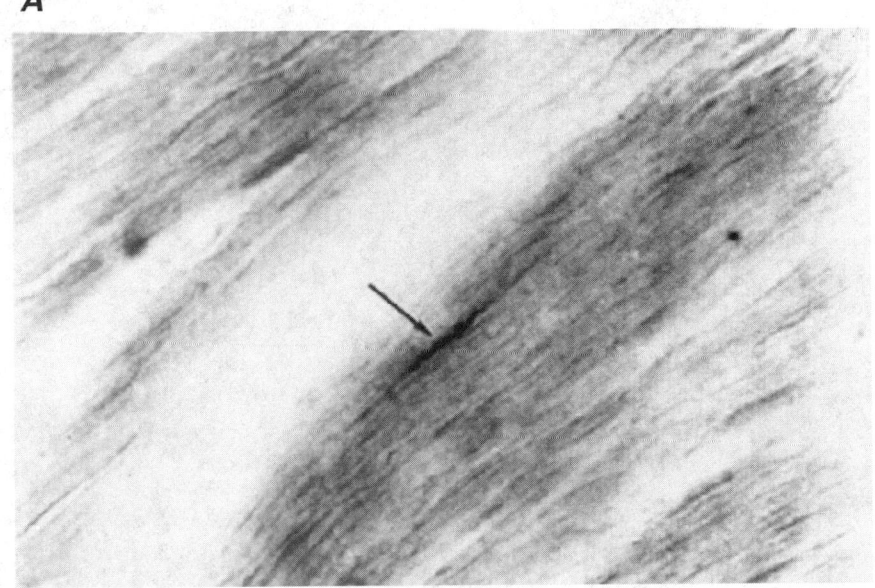

B

FIGURE 43-11

A. Section of normal myocardium from a patient with a 27-h-old ruptured infarct has been reacted with the del Rio Hortega silver stain to demonstrate the extent of the extracellular skeletal framework in this specimen.[145] Note the dark silver-positive collagen fibers in the extracellular space, some of which (arrows) act as struts between myocardial cells. (×150) *B.* Section from the same heart taken from the myocardial rupture site. With the exception of a single silver-positive fiber (arrow), none of the skeletal framework is apparent in this area. (×150)

chanical dysfunction of the ventricle with ischemic insults insufficient to produce necrosis.[151] The dysfunctional stunned myocardium has contractile abnormalities with systolic bulging and wall thinning. Although originally described in experimental animals, stunning may have important clinical implications. Patients may develop transient or persistent dysfunction secondary to intermittent coronary occlusions with angina pectoris or incipient infarction interrupted by coronary thrombolysis or percutaneous transluminal coronary angioplasty. Global ventricular dysfunction following cardiac surgery with cardiopulmonary bypass may also be a form of stunning. Regardless of the underlying precipitating event, the pathogenesis of stunned myocardium is unknown. A metabolic cause has been suggested due to depression of ATP levels.[152] Other postulated mechanisms include damage due to oxygen free radicals or abnormal sarcoplasmic reticulum calcium transport.[153,154] Against a primary metabolic defect, however, is the fact that inotropic stimulation with dopamine or epinephrine can lead to marked functional improvement,[155] suggesting that the contractile machinery is intact. An alternative explanation for this paradox has been proposed by Zhao et al.,[156] who demonstrated striking alterations of intercellular connective tissue in stunned canine myocardium. Focal connective tissue fibers were destroyed or absent without evidence of myocardial cell damage (Fig. 43-12). This observation suggests that the contractile dysfunction may result from an untethering of connections between viable myocytes, leading

to cell and mural layer slippage. The implication of these observations is that active collagenolysis is provoked by ischemia, even without necrosis or inflammation.

Myocardial Hibernation

As an extension of the more acute phenomenon of stunned myocardium, chronically ischemic but viable myocardium has been described as *hibernating*. This tissue, in contrast to stunned myocytes, does have profound myocellular structural changes in addition to *increased* interstitial matrix.[157] The loss of contractile elements, nuclear changes, depletion of sarcoplasmic reticulum, and mitochondrial alterations have been interpreted as evidence of de-differentiation of myocytes.[157] These changes are often observed in chronically ischemic subendocardial tissue. Although immediate functional recovery does not usually occur after restoration of adequate blood flow, the viability of the tissue does give some possibility of improvement in function following revascularization procedures.

Ischemic Preconditioning

In addition to causing myocardial stunning, a transient coronary occlusion insufficient to produce infarction has been found to convey a protective effect against subsequent ischemic injury.[158] Thus, coronary occlusions as brief as 5 min in duration followed by a short period of reperfusion cause a marked reduction in infarct size during a subsequent, more prolonged coronary occlusion.[158] This protective effect, termed *ischemic preconditioning* is relatively short-lived, lasting no more than 1 to 2 h after the initial brief period of ischemia.[159] The preconditioning effect is distinct from stunning, since stunning can persist long after preconditioning has disappeared.[160] Furthermore, interventions that prevent or attenuate stunning do not necessarily interfere with the preconditioning effect. The mechanism for preconditioning is not completely elucidated but may be dependent on a reduction of myocardial metabolic demands; this is supported by a decreased rate of ATP utilization and slowed anaerobic glycolysis during ischemia in the preconditioned heart.[161] This protective effect appears to be mediated through adenosine, since preconditioning can be blocked with adenosine receptor inhibitors, while specific

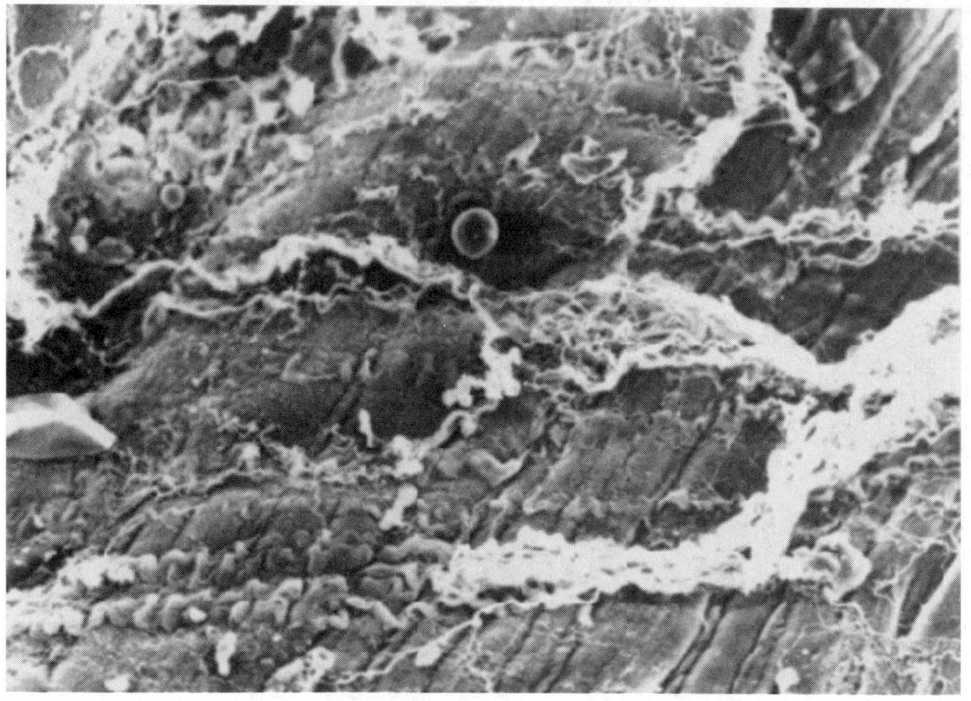

FIGURE 43-12

Scanning electron micrograph from the stunned region of canine myocardium following 12 episodes of transient 5 min ischemia with 10 min of reperfusion after each occlusion. The myocardium is viable; however, there is severe degeneration and unraveling of the surface connective tissue fibers. This degradation of collagen may account for the marked increase of compliance in the stunned region. [From Zhao et al.[156] Reprinted with permission from the American College of Cardiology (*J Am Coll Cardiol* 1987; 10:1322–1344.)]

adenosine receptor agonists are capable of mimicking the preconditioning effect.[162] Adenosine production is dependent on the ectoenzyme 5'-nucleotidase associated with the myocardial cell membrane; recent evidence indicates that this enzyme is activated during the initial ischemic episode, resulting in increased adenosine production and preconditioning.[163] Although the clinical importance of the preconditioning phenomenon is as yet unclear, it is possible that the transient ischemia that may precede total coronary occlusion can modify the subsequent course of myocardial infarction. Recent analysis of the Thrombolysis in Myocardial Infarction (TIMI)-4 Study data demonstrated significant improvement in multiple clinical parameters of outcome in patients who had experienced angina pectoris prior to myocardial infarction compared to those who were free of angina.[164]

REFERENCES

1. Berne RM, Rubio R. Coronary circulation. In: Berne RM, Sperelakis S, eds. *Handbook of Physiology*. sec. 2: *The Cardiovascular System* vol. 1: *The Heart*. Bethesda, MD: American Physiological Society; 1979:873.
2. Hastings AB, White FC, Sanders TM, Bloor CM. Comparative physiological responses to exercise stress. *J Appl Physiol* 1982; 52:1077–1083.
3. Laughlin MH, Korthuis RJ, Duncker DJ, Bache RJ. Control of blood flow to cardiac and skeletal muscle during exercise. In: Rowell LB, Shepherd JT, eds. *Regulation and Integration of Multiple Systems*. American Physiological Society Handbook Section 12, New York: Oxford University Press; 1996:770–838.
4. Chance B. Pyridine nucleotide as an indicator of the oxygen requirements for energy-linked functions of mitochondria. *Circ Res* 1976; 38(suppl 1):31–38.
5. Popel AS. Theory of oxygen transport to tissue. *Crit Rev Biomed Eng* 1989; 17:257–321.
6. Rose CP, Goresky CA, Belanger P, Chen MJ. Effect of vasodilation and flow rate on capillary permeability surface product and interstitial space size in the coronary circulation. *Circ Res* 1980; 47:312–328.
7. Austin RE, Aldea GS, Coggins DL, Flynn AE, Hoffman JIE. Profound spatial heterogeneity of coronary reserve. *Circ Res* 1990; 67:319–331.
8. Sestier FJ, Mildenberger RR, Klassen GA. Role of autoregulation in spatial and temporal perfusion heterogeneity of canine myocardium. *Am J Physiol* 1978; 235:H64–H71.
9. Rakusan K, Moravec J, Hatt PY. Regional capillary supply in the normal and hypertrophied rat heart. *Microvasc Res* 1980; 20:319–326.
10. Turek Z, Rakusan K. Log normal distribution of intercapillary distance in normal and hypertrophic rat heart as estimated by the method of concentric circles. Its effect on tissue oxygenation. *Pflugers Arch* 1981; 391:17–21.
11. Lanza GA, Pedrotti P, Pasceri V, Lucente M, Crea F, Maseri A. Autonomic changes associated with spontaneous coronary spasm in patients with variant angina. *J Am Coll Cardiol* 1996; 28:1249–1256.
12. Cannon RO, Schenke WH, Quyyumi A, Bonow RO, Epstein SE. Comparison of exercise testing with studies of coronary flow reserve in patients with microvascular angina. *Circulation* 1991; 83:III77–III81.
13. Defily DV, Chilian WM. Coronary microcirculation: Autoregulation and metabolic control. *Basic Res Cardiol* 1995; 90:112–118.
14. Gould KL, Lipscomb K, Calvert C. Compensatory changes of the distal coronary vascular bed during progressive coronary constriction. *Circulation* 1975; 51:1085–1094.
15. Nelson MT, Quayle JM. Physiological roles and properties of potassium channels in arterial smooth muscle. *Am J Physiol* 1995; 268 (*Cell Physiol* 37):C799–C822.
16. Komaru T, Lamping KG, Eastham CL, Dellsperger KC. Role of ATP-sensitive potassium channels in coronary microvascular autoregulatory responses. *Circ Res* 1991; 69:1146–1151.
17. Duncker DJ, Van Zon NS, Altman JD, Pavek TJ, Bache RJ. Role of K^+_{ATP} channels in coronary vasodilation during exercise. *Circulation* 1993; 88:1245–1253.
18. Berne RM. The role of adenosine in the regulation of coronary blood flow. *Circ Res* 1980; 47:807–813.
19. Sabiston DC, Gregg DE. Effects of cardiac contraction on coronary blood flow. *Circulation* 1957; 15:14–20.
20. Downey JM, Kirk ES. Inhibition of coronary blood flow by a vascular waterfall mechanism. *Circ Res* 1975; 36:753–760.
21. Hess DS, Bache RJ. Transmural distribution of myocardial blood flow during systole in the awake dog. *Circ Res* 1976; 38:5–15.
22. Downey JM, Downey HF, Kirk ES. Effect of myocardial strains on coronary blood flow. *Circ Res* 1974; 34:286–292.
23. Brandi G, MacGregor M. Intramural pressure in the left ventricle of the dog. *Cardiovasc Res* 1969; 3:472–475.
24. Permutt S, Riley RL. Hemodynamics of collapsible vessels with tone: The vascular waterfall. *J Appl Physiol* 1963; 18:924–932.
25. Hess DS, Bache RJ. Transmural right ventricular myocardial blood flow during systole in the awake dog. *Circ Res* 1979; 45:88–94.
26. Gold FL, Bache RJ. Transmural right ventricular blood flow during acute pulmonary artery hypertension in the sedated dog: Evidence for subendocardial ischemia despite residual vasodilator reserve. *Circ Res* 1982; 51:196–204.
27. Schwartz GG, Steinman S, Garcia J, Greyson C, Massie B, Weiner MW. Energetics of acute pressure overload of the porcine right ventricle. In vivo ^{31}P nuclear magnetic resonance. *J Clin Invest* 1992; 89:909–918.
28. Weiss HH, Neubauer JD, Lipp JD, Sinha AK. Quantitative determination of regional oxygen consumption in the dog heart. *Circ Res* 1978; 42:394–401.
29. Hoffman JIE. Determinants and prediction of transmural myocardial perfusion. *Circulation* 1978; 58:381–391.
30. Bache RJ, McHale PA, Greenfield JC Jr. Transmural myocardial perfusion during restricted coronary inflow in the awake dog. *Am J Physiol* 1977; 232:H645–H651.
31. Domenech RJ. Regional diastolic coronary blood flow during diastolic ventricular hypertension. *Cardiovasc Res* 1978; 12:639–645.
32. Freudenberg H, Lichtlen PR. The normal wall segment in coronary stenosis—a postmortem study. *Z Kardiol* 1981; 70:863–870.
33. Hossack KF, Brown BG, Stewart DK, Dodge HT. Diltiazem-induced blockade of sympathetically mediated constriction of normal and diseased coronary arteries: Lack of epicardial coronary dilatory effect in humans. *Circulation* 1984; 70:465–471.
34. Gage JE, Hess OM, Murakami T, Ritter M, Grimm J, Krayenbuchl HP. Vasoconstriction of stenotic coronary arteries during exercise in patients with classic angina pectoris: Reversibility by nitroglycerin. *Circulation* 1996; 73:865–876.
35. Schwartz JS, Bache RJ. Effect of arteriolar dilution on coronary artery diameter distal to coronary stenoses. *Am J Physiol* 1985; 249(*Heart Circ Physiol* 18):H981–H988.
36. Schwartz JS, Tockman B, Cohn JN, Bache RJ. Exercise-induced fall in flow through stenotic coronary arteries in the dog. *Am J Cardiol* 1982; 50:1409–1443.
37. Brown BG, Lee AB, Bolson EL, Dodge HT. Reflex constriction of significant coronary stenosis as a mechanism contributing to ischemic left ventricular dysfunction during isometric exercise. *Circulation* 1984; 70:18–24.
38. Frielingsdorf J, Seiler C, Kaufmann P, Vassalli G, Suter T, Hess OM. Normalization of abnormal coronary vasomotion by calcium antagonists in patients with hypertension. *Circulation* 1996; 93:1380–1387.
39. Bortone AS, Hess OM, Gaglione A, Suter T, Nonogi H, Grimm J, et al. Effect of intravenous propranolol on coronary vasomotion at rest and during dynamic exercise in patients with coronary artery disease. *Circulation* 1990; 81(4):1225–1235.
40. Furchgott RF, Zawadski JV. The obligatory role of endothelial cells in the relaxation of arterial smooth muscle by acetylcholine. *Nature* 1980; 288:373–376.
41. Furchgott RF, Vanhoutte PM. Endothelium-derived relaxing and contracting factors. *FASEB J* 1989; 3:2007–2018.
42. Ignarro LJ, Byrns RE, Buga GM, Wood KS. Endothelium-derived relaxing factor from pulmonary artery and vein possesses pharmacologic and chemical properties identical to those of nitric oxide radical. *Circ Res* 1987; 61:866–879.
43. Noris M, Morigi M, Donadelli R, Aiello S, Foppolo M, Todeschini M, et al. Nitric oxide synthesis by cultured endothelial cells is modulated by flow conditions. *Circ Res* 1995; 76:536–543.

44. Friedman PC, Mitchell GC, Heistad DD, Armstrong ML, Harrison DO. Atherosclerosis impairs endothelium-dependent vascular relaxation to acetylcholine and thrombin in primates. *Circ Res* 1988; 58:783–789.

45. Ludmer PL, Selwyn AP, Shook TL, Wayne RR, Mudge GH, Alexander RW, et al. Paradoxical vasoconstriction induced by acetylcholine in atherosclerotic coronary arteries. *N Engl J Med* 1986; 315:1046–1051.

46. Omland T, Bonarjee VV, Lie RT, Caidahl K. Neurohumoral measurements as indicators of long-term prognosis after acute myocardial infarction. *Am J Cardiol* 1995; 76:230–235.

47. Aversano T, Becker LC. Persistence of coronary vasodilator reserve despite functionally significant flow reduction. *Am J Physiol* 1985; 248:H403–H411.

48. Chilian WM, Layne SM. Coronary microvascular responses to reductions in perfusion pressure. *Circ Res* 1990; 66:1227–1238.

49. Chilian WM, Eastham CL, Marcus ML. Microvascular distribution of coronary vascular resistance in beating left ventricle. *Am J Physiol* 1986; 25 (*Heart Circ Physiol* 20):H779–H788.

50. Laxson DD, Dai X, Homans DC, Bache RJ. The role of alpha$_1$- and alpha$_2$-adrenergic receptors in mediating coronary vasoconstriction in hypoperfused ischemic myocardium during exercise. *Circ Res* 1989; 65:1688–1697.

51. Bache RJ, Dai X. The thromboxane A$_2$ mimetic, U46619, worsens myocardial hypoperfusion during exercise in the presence of a coronary stenosis. *Cardiovasc Res* 1992; 26:351–356.

52. Schaper W. *The Collateral Circulation of the Heart.* Amsterdam: Elsevier North-Holland; 1971.

53. Schaper J, Konig R, Franz D, Schaper W. The endothelial surface of growing coronary collateral arteries. Intimal margination and diapedesis of monocytes. A combined SEM and TEM study. *Virchows Arch A* 1976; 370:193–205.

54. Hautamaa PV, Dai X, Homans DC, Bache RJ. Vasomotor activity of the moderately well-developed canine coronary collateral circulation. *Am J Physiol* 1989; 256(*Heart Circ Physiol* 25):H890–H897.

55. Wright L, Homans DC, Laxson DD, Dai X, Bache RJ. Effect of serotonin and thromboxane A$_2$ on blood flow through moderately well-developed coronary collateral vessels. *J Am Coll Cardiol* 1992; 19:687–693.

56. Baroldi G, Scomazzoni G. *Coronary Circulation in the Normal and the Pathologic Heart.* Washington, DC: Department of the Army; 1967:217–228.

57. Rivas F, Cobb FR, Bache RJ, Greenfield JC Jr. Relationship between blood flow to ischemic regions and extent of myocardial infarction. *Circ Res* 1976; 38:439–447.

58. Cohen M, Rentrop KP. Limitation of myocardial ischemia by collateral circulation during sudden controlled coronary artery occlusion in human subjects: A prospective study. *Circulation* 1986; 74:469–476.

59. Rentrop KP, Feit F, Sherman W, Stecy P, Hosat S, Cohen M, et al. Late thrombolytic therapy preserves left ventricular function in patients with collateralized total coronary occlusion: Primary endpoint findings of the second Mount Sinai–New York University reperfusion trial. *J Am Coll Cardiol* 1989; 14:58–64.

60. Cohen M, Sherman W, Rentrop KP, Gorlin R. Determinants of collateral filling observed during sudden controlled coronary artery occlusion in human subjects. *J Am Coll Cardiol* 1989; 13:297–303.

61. Schwartz H, Leiboff RH, Bren GB, Wasserman AG, Katz RJ, Varghese PJ, et al. Temporal evolution of the human coronary collateral circulation after myocardial infarction. *J Am Coll Cardiol* 1984; 4:1008–1093.

62. McHenry PL, O'Donnell J, Morris SN, Jordan JJ. The abnormal exercise electrocardiogram in apparently healthy men: A predictor of angina pectoris as an initial coronary event during long-term follow-up. *Circulation* 1984; 70:547–551.

63. Bache RJ, Schwartz JS. Myocardial blood flow during exercise after gradual coronary occlusion in the dog. *Am J Physiol* 1983; 245(*Heart Circ Physiol* 14):131–138.

64. Foreman BW, Dai X, Bache RJ. Vasoconstriction of canine coronary collateral vessels with vasopressin limits blood flow to collateral dependent myocardium during exercise. *Circ Res* 1991; 69:657–664.

65. Pupita G, Maseri A, Kaski JC, Galassi AR, Gavrielides S, Davies G, et al. Myocardial ischemia caused by distal coronary-artery constriction in stable angina pectoris. *N Engl J Med* 1990; 323:514–520.

66. Bache RJ, Duncker DJ. Coronary steal. *Am Coll Cardiol Curr J Rev* 1994; 3:9–12.

67. Demer LL, Gould KL, Goldstei RA, Kirkeeide RL. Noninvasive assessment of coronary collaterals in man by PET perfusion imaging. *J Nucl Med* 1990; 31:259–270.

68. Picano E, Pogliani M, Lattanzi F, Disante A, L'Abbate A. Exercise capacity after acute aminophylline administration in angina pectoris. *Am J Cardiol* 1988; 63:14–16.

69. Koren MJ, Devereux RB, Casale PN, Savage DD, Laragh JH. Relation of left ventricular mass and geometry to morbidity and mortality in uncomplicated essential hypertension. *Ann Intern Med* 1991; 114:345–352.

70. Mueller TM, Tomanek RJ, Kerber RE, Marcus ML. Myocardial infarction in dogs with chronic hypertension and left ventricular hypertrophy. *Am J Physiol* 1980; 239:H731–H735.

71. Bache RJ, Wright L, Laxson DL, Dai X. Effect of a coronary stenosis on myocardial blood flow during exercise in the chronically pressure overloaded hypertrophied left ventricle. *Circulation* 1990; 81:1967–1973.

72. Bache RJ. Effects of hypertrophy on the coronary circulation. *Prog Cardiovasc Dis* 1988; 31:403–440.

73. Duncker DJ, Van Zon NS, Crampton M, Herrlinger S, Homans DC, Bache RJ. *Am J Physiol* 1994; 266 (*Heart Circ Physiol* 35):H795–H810.

74. Sarnoff SJ, Braunwald E, Welch GH Jr, Case RB, Stainsby WN, Marcruz R. Hemodynamic determinants of oxygen consumption of the heart with special reference to the tension time index. *Am J Physiol* 1958; 192:148–156.

75. Rook GA, Feigl EO. Work as a correlate of canine left ventricular oxygen consumption, and the problem of catecholamine wasting. *Circ Res* 1982; 50:273–286.

76. Jennings RB, Sommers HM, Smyth GA, Flack HA, Linn H. Myocardial necrosis induced by temporary occlusion of a coronary artery in the dog. *Arch Pathol* 1960; 70:68–78.

77. Hirzel HO, Sonneblick EH, Kirk ES. Absence of a lateral border zone of intermediate creatine phosphokinase depletion surrounding a central infarct 24 hours after acute coronary occlusion in the dog. *Circ Res* 1977; 673–683.

78. Marcus ML, Kerber RE, Ehrhardt J, Abboud FM. Three-dimensional geometry of acutely ischemic myocardium. *Circulation* 1975; 52:254–263.

79. Barlow CH, Chance B. Ischemic areas in perfused rat hearts: Measurement by NADH Fluorescence photography. *Science* 1976; 193:909–910.

80. Harken AH, Barlow CH, Harden WR 3d, Chance B. Two- and three-dimensional display of myocardial ischemic "border zone" in dog. *Am J Cardiol* 1978; 42:954–959.

81. Janse MJ, Cinca J, Morena H, Fiolet JWT, Kleber AG, DeVries GP, et al. The "border zone" in myocardial ischemia. An electrophysiological, metabolic, and histochemical correlation in the pig heart. *Circ Res* 1979; 44:576–588.

82. Harken AH, Simson MB, Haselgrove J, Wetstein L, Harden WR III, Barlow CH. Early ischemia after complete coronary ligation in the rabbit, dog, pig, and monkey. *Am J Physiol* 1981; 241:H202–H210.

83. Yellon DM, Hearse DJ, Crome R, Grannel J, Wyse RKH. Characterization of the lateral interface between normal and ischemic tissue in the canine heart during evolving myocardial infarction. *Am J Cardiol* 1981; 47:1233–1239.

84. Factor SM, Sonnenblick EH, Kirk ES. The histologic border zone of acute myocardial infarction: Islands or peninsulas? *Am J Physiol* 1978; 92:111–124.

85. Okun EM, Factor SM, Kirk ES. End-capillary loops in the heart: An explanation for discrete myocardial infarctions without border zones. *Science* 1979; 206:565–567.

86. Factor SM, Okun EM, Minase T, Kirk ES. The microcirculation of the human heart: End-capillary loops with discrete perfusion fields. *Circulation* 1982; 66:1241–1248.

87. Lowe JE, Reimer KA, Jennings RB. Experimental infarct size as a function of the amount of myocardium at risk. *Am J Pathol* 1978; 90:363–378.

88. Lee JT, Ideker RE, Reimer KA. Myocardial infarct size and location in relation to the coronary vascular bed at risk in man. *Circulation* 1981; 64:526–534.

89. Factor SM, Okun EM, Kirk ES. The histologic border of acute canine myocardial infarction: A function of microcirculation. *Circ Res* 1981; 48:640–649.

90. Brosius FC III, Roberts WC. Significance of coronary arterial thrombus in transmural acute myocardial infarction. A study of 54 necropsy patients. *Circulation* 1981; 63:810–816.

91. Muller JE. Coronary artery thrombosis: Historical aspects. *J Am Coll Cardiol* 1983; 1:893–896.

92. Erhlich JC, Shinohara Y. Low incidence of coronary thrombosis in myocardial infarction. A restudy by serial block technique. *Arch Pathol* 1964; 78:432–445.

93. Roberts EC, Buja M. The frequency and significance of coronary arterial thrombi and other observations in fatal acute myocardial infarction: A study of 107 necropsy patients. *Am J Med* 1972; 52:425–443.

94. Silver MD, Baroldi G, Mariani F. The relationship between acute occlusive coronary thrombi and myocardial infarction studies in 100 consecutive patients. *Circulation* 1980; 61:219–227.

95. Buja LM, Willerson JT. The role of coronary artery lesions in ischemic heart disease. *Hum Pathol* 1987; 18:451–461.

96. DeWood MA, Spores J, Notske R, Mouser LT, Burroughs R, Golden MS, et al. Prevalence of total coronary occlusion during the early hours of transmural myocardial infarction. *N Engl J Med* 1980; 303:897–902.

97. Rapaport E. Thrombolytic agents in acute myocardial infarction. *N Engl J Med* 1989; 320:861–864.

98. White HD, Norris RM, Brown MA, Takayama M, Maslowski A, Bass NM, et al. Effect of intravenous streptokinase on left ventricular function and early survival after acute myocardial infarction. *N Engl J Med* 1987; 317:850–855.

99. Ridolfi RL, Hutchins GM. The relationship between coronary artery lesions and myocardial infarcts: Ulceration of atherosclerotic plaques precipitating coronary thrombosis. *Am Heart J* 1977; 93:468–486.

100. Horie T, Sekiguchi M, Hirosawa K. Coronary thrombosis in pathogenesis of acute myocardial infarction. *Br Heart J* 1978; 40:153–161.

101. Falk E. Plaque rupture with severe pre-existing stenosis precipitating coronary thrombosis. Characteristics of coronary atherosclerosis plaques underlying fatal occlusive thrombi. *Br Heart J* 1983; 50:127–134.

102. Friedman M, Van den Bovenkamp GJ. The pathogenesis of coronary thrombus. *Am J Pathol* 1966; 48:19–45.

103. Factor SM, Cho S. Smooth muscle contraction bands in the media of coronary arteries: A post-mortem marker of ante-mortem spasm? *J Am Coll Cardiol* 1985; 6:1329–1337.

104. van der Wal AC, Becker AE, van der Loos CM, Das PK. Site of intimal rupture or erosion of thrombosed coronary atherosclerotic plaques is characterized by an inflammatory process irrespective of the dominant plaque morphology. *Circulation* 1994; 89,36–44.

105. Farb A, Burke AP, Tang AL, Liang Y, Mannan P, Smialek J, et al. Coronary plaque erosion without rupture into a lipid core. A frequent cause of coronary thrombosis in sudden coronary death. *Circulation* 1996; 93:1354–1363.

106. Latham PM. Lecture 37. In: *Collected Works*. London: New Sydenham Society; 1886:1:445.

107. Osler W. Lumleian lectures on angina pectoris. *Lancet* 1910; 1:839.

108. Buja LM, Hillis LD, Petty CS, Willerson JT. The role of coronary arterial spasm in ischemic heart disease. *Arch Pathol Lab Med* 1981; 105:221–226.

109. Gorlin R. Role of coronary vasospasm in the pathogenesis of myocardial ischemia and angina pectoris. *Am Heart J* 1982; 103:598–603.

110. Yasue H, Omote S, Takizawa A, Nagao M. Coronary arterial spasm in ischemic heart disease and its pathogenesis. A review. *Circ Res* 1983; 52(suppl 1):147–152.

111. Maseri A, L'Abbate A, Baroldi G, Chierchia S, Marzilli M, Ballestra AM, et al. Coronary vasospasm as a possible cause of myocardial infarction. A conclusion derived from the study of "preinfarction" angina. *N Engl J Med* 1978; 299:1271–1277.

112. Oliva JPB, Breckenridge JC. Arteriographic evidence of coronary arterial spasm in acute myocardial infarction. *Circulation* 1977; 56:366–374.

113. Rubanyi GM, Botelho LHP. Endothelins. *FASEB J* 1991; 5:2713–2720.

114. Forstermann U, Mugge A, Alheid U, Haverich A, Frolich JC. Selective attenuation of endothelium-mediated vasodilation in atherosclerotic human coronary arteries. *Circ Res* 1988; 62:185–190.

115. Harrison DG. From isolated vessels to the catheterization laboratory. Studies of endothelial function in the coronary circulation of humans. *Circulation* 1989; 80:703–706.

116. Berman JW, Calderon TM. The role of endothelial adhesion molecules in the development of atherosclerosis. *Cardiovasc Pathol* 1992; 1:17–28.

117. Dalen JE, Ockene IS, Alpert JS. Coronary spasm, coronary thrombosis, and myocardial infarction: A hypothesis concerning the pathophysiology of acute myocardial infarction. *Am Heart J* 1982; 104:1119–1124.

118. Joris I, Majno G. Endothelial changes induced by arterial spasm. *Am J Pathol* 1981; 102:346–358.

119. Gertz SD, Uretsky G, Wajnberg RS, Navot N, Gotsman MS. Endothelial cell damage and thrombus formation after partial arterial constriction: Relevance to the role of coronary artery spasm in the pathogenesis of myocardial infarction. *Circulation* 1981; 63:476–486.

120. Reimer KA, Lowe JE, Rasmussen MM, Jennings RB. The wavefront phenomenon of ischemic cell death. I. Myocardial infarct size vs. duration of coronary occlusion in dogs. *Circulation* 1977; 56:786–794.

121. Reimer KA, Jennings RB. The "Wavefront Phenomenon" of myocardial ischemic cell death. II. Transmural progression of necrosis within the framework of ischemic bed size (myocardium at risk) and collateral flow. *Lab Invest* 1979; 40:633–664.

122. Schaper W, Frenzel H, Hort W, Winkler B. Experimental coronary artery occlusion. II. Spatial and temporal evolution of infarcts in the dog heart. *Basic Res Cardiol* 1979; 74:233–239.

123. Forman R, Cho S, Factor SM, Kirk ES. Acute myocardial infarct extension into a previously preserved subendocardial region at risk in dogs and patients. *Circulation* 1983; 67:117–183.

124. Eng C, Cho S, Factor SM, Kirk S. A non-flow basis for the vulnerability of the subendocardium. *J Am Coll Cardiol* 1987; 9:374–379.

125. Lavellee M, Cox D, Patrick TA, Vatner SF. Salvage of myocardial function by coronary artery reperfusion 1, 2, and 4 hours after occlusion in conscious dogs. *Circ Res* 1983; 53:235–247.

126. Baughman KL, Maroko PR, Vatner SF. Effects of coronary artery reperfusion on myocardial infarct size and survival in conscious dogs. *Circulation* 1981; 63:317–322.

127. Fenoglio JJ, Karagueuzian HS, Friedman PL, Albala A, Wit AL. Time course of infarct growth toward the endocardial surface during the first 24 hours after coronary occlusion. *Am J Physiol* 1979; 236:H356–H370.

128. Karagueuzian HS, Fenoglio JJ, Weiss MB, Wit AL. Coronary occlusion and reperfusion: Effects on subendocardial cardiac fibers. *Am J Physiol* 1980; 236:H581–H593.

129. Frame LK, Lopez JA, Khaw BA, Fallon JT, Haber E, Powell WJ Jr. Early membrane damage during coronary reperfusion in dogs. Detection by radiolabeled anticardiac myosin. *J Clin Invest* 1983; 72:535–544.

130. Kloner RA, Przyklenk K, Whittaker P. Deleterious effects of oxygen radicals in ischemia/reperfusion. Resolved and unresolved issues. *Circulation* 1989; 80:1115–1127.

131. Kehrer JP. Concepts related to the study of reactive oxygen and cardiac reperfusion injury. *Free Radic Res Commun* 1989; 5:305–314.

132. Whalen DA, Hamilton DG, Ganote CE, Jennings RB. Effect of a transient period of ischemia on myocardial cells. Effects on cell volume regulation. *Am J Pathol* 1974; 74:381–398.

133. Shen AC, Jennings RB. Myocardial calcium and magnesium in acute ischemic injury. *Am J Pathol* 1972; 67:414–440.

134. Hearse DJ. Reperfusion of the ischemic myocardium. *J Mol Cell Cardiol* 1977; 9:605–616.

135. Sommers HM, Jennings RB. Experimental acute myocardial infarction, histologic and histochemical studies of early myocardial infarcts induced by temporary or permanent occlusion of a coronary artery. *Lab Invest* 1964; 13:1491–1503.

136. Bulkley BH, Hutchins GM. Myocardial consequences of coronary artery bypass graft surgery: The paradox of necrosis in areas of revascularization. *Circulation* 1977; 56:906–913.

137. Mallory GK, White PD, Salcedo-Salgar J. The speed of healing of myocardial infarction: A study of the pathologic anatomy in 72 cases. *Am Heart J* 1939; 18:647–671.

138. Fishbein MC, MacLean D, Maroko PR. The histopathologic evolution of myocardial infarction. *Chest* 1978; 73:843–849.

139. Bouchardy B, Majno G. Histopathology of early myocardial infarcts: A new approach. *Am J Pathol* 1974; 74:301–330.

140. Weiss SJ. Tissue destruction by neutrophils. *N Engl J Med* 1989; 320:365–376.

141. Kloner RA, Ganote CE, Jenning RB. The "no-reflow" phenomenon after temporary coronary occlusion in the dog. *J Clin Invest* 1974; 54:1496–1508.

142. Weisman HF, Healy B. Myocardial infarct expansion, infarct extension, and re-infarction: Pathophysiologic concepts. *Prog Cardiovasc Dis* 1987; 30.73–110.

143. Hutchins GM, Bulkley BH. Infarct expansion versus extension: Two different complications of acute myocardial infarction. *Am J Cardiol* 1978; 41:1127–1132.

144. Robinson TF, Cohen-Gould L, Factor SM. Skeletal framework of mammalian heart muscle. Arrangement of inter- and pericellular connective tissue structures. *Lab Invest* 1983; 49:482–498.

145. Factor SM, Robinson TF, Dominitz R, Cho S. Alterations of the myocardial skeletal framework in acute myocardial infarction with and without ventricular rupture. *Am J Cardiovasc Pathol* 1987; 1:91–98.

146. Takahashi S, Barry AC, Factor SM. Collagen degradation in ischemic rat hearts. *Biochem J* 1990; 265:233–241.

147. Cleutjens JPM, Verluyten MJA, Smits JFM, Daemen MJAP. Collagen remodeling after myocardial infarction in the rat heart. *Am J Pathol* 1995; 147:325–338.

148. Richard V, Murry CE, Reimer KA. Healing of myocardial infarcts in dogs. Effects of late reperfusion. *Circulation* 1995; 92:1991–2001.

149. Fraker TD Jr, Wagner GS, Rosati RA. Extension of myocardial infarction: Incidence and prognosis. *Circulation* 1979; 60:1127–1129.

150. Factor SM, Okun EM, Kirk ES. Microextension of acute myocardial necrosis into the normal zone of 7 day canine infarcts. *Circulation* 1979; 60(suppl 2):114.

151. Braunwald E, Kloner RA. The stunned myocardium: Prolonged, postischemic ventricular dysfunction. *Circulation* 1982; 66:1146–1149.

152. DeBoer LWV, Ingwall JS, Kloner RA, Braunwald E. Prolonged derangements of canine myocardial purine metabolism after a brief coronary artery occlusion not associated with anatomic evidence of necrosis. *Proc Natl Acad Sci USA* 1980; 77:5471–5475.

153. Przyklenk K, Kloner RA. Superoxide dismutase plus catalase improve contractile function in the canine model of the "stunned myocardium." *Circ Res* 1986; 58:148–156.

154. Ellis SG, Wynne J, Braunwald E, Henschke CI, Sandor T, Kloner RA. Response of reperfusion salvaged, stunned myocardium to inotropic stimulation. *Am Heart J* 1984; 107:13–19.

155. Becker LC, Levine JH, DiPaula AF, Guarnieri T, Aversano T. Reversal of dysfunction in postischemic stunned myocardium by epinephrine and postextrasystolic potentiation. *J Am Coll Cardiol* 1986; 7:580–589.

156. Zhao M, Hong Z, Robinson TF, Factor SM, Sonnenblick EH, Eng C. Profound structural alterations of the extracellular collagen matrix in postischemic dysfunctional ("stunned") but viable myocardium. *J Am Coll Cardiol* 1987; 10:1322–1334.

157. Ausma J, Cleutjens J, Thone F, Flameng W, Ramaekers F, Borgers M. Chronic hibernating myocardium: Interstitial changes. *Mol Cell Biochem* 1995; 147:35–42.

158. Murry CE, Jennings RB, Reimer KA. Preconditioning with ischemia: A delay of lethal cell injury in ischemic myocardium. *Circulation* 1986; 74:1124–1136.

159. Murry CE, Richard VJ, Reimer KA, Jennings RB. Ischemic preconditioning slows energy metabolism and delays ultrastructural damage during a sustained ischemic episode. *Circ Res* 1990; 66:913–931.

160. Murry CE, Richard VJ, Jennings RB, Reimer KA. Myocardial protection is lost before contractile function recovers from ischemic preconditioning. *Am J Physiol* (*Heart Circ Physiol*) 1991; 260:H796–H804.

161. Vuorinen K, Ylitalo K, Peuhkurinen K, Raatikainen P, Ala-Rami A, Hassinen IE. Mechanisms of ischemic preconditioning in rat myocardium. Roles of adenosine, cellular energy state, and mitochondrial FlFo-ATPase. *Circulation* 1995; 91:2810–2818.

162. Lui GS, Thornton J, Van Winkle DM, Stanley AWH, Olsson RA, Downey JM. Protection against infarction afforded by preconditioning is mediated by A1 adenosine receptors in rabbit heart. *Circulation* 1991; 84:350–356.

163. Kitakaze M, Hori M, Takashima S, Sato H, Inoue M, Kamada T. Ischemic preconditioning increases adenosine release and 5' nucleotidase activity during myocardial ischemia and reperfusion in dogs. *Circulation* 1993; 87:208–215.

164. Kloner RA, Shook T, Przyklenk K, Davis VG, Junio L, Mathews RV, et al. Previous angina alters in-hospital outcome in TIMI 4. A clinical correlate to preconditioning? *Circulation* 1995; 91:37–45.

44

THE CORONARY ISCHEMIC SYNDROMES: RELATIONSHIP TO THE BIOLOGY OF ATHEROSCLEROSIS

R. Wayne Alexander / Kathy K. Griendling

INTRODUCTION

The coronary ischemic syndromes, which include stable angina, unstable angina, and myocardial infarction, have been extensively studied and characterized. Their pathophysiologic basis may be related to increased oxygen demand in the setting of a flow-limiting lesion or, especially in unstable angina or myocardial infarction, there may be primary decreases in blood flow caused by vasospasm and thrombosis. Although the clinical syndromes are almost exclusively associated with atherosclerosis of the epicardial coronaries, efforts have been made only in recent years to relate the syndromes of coronary ischemia to the biology of atherosclerosis. There has been increasing interest in explaining the clinical syndromes in terms of the biology of the underlying disease for two major reasons. First, the clinical cardiologist has a need to understand the episodic nature of the unstable ischemic syndromes, in particular, while at the same time appreciating that there is a dynamism to even the so-called stable anginal syndromes. Second, the extraordinary progress in understanding the basic pathobiology of atherosclerosis has now made the attempts to reconcile the clinical cardiologist's observations with those of the experimental and clinical pathologist worthwhile. The pathologist and cardiologist traditionally have had very different views of atherosclerosis. The pathologist views the disease as chronic and frequently considers that there is a linear growth in lesion size and luminal encroachment. The cardiologist, on the other hand, sees the disease in its late stages as an episodic event frequently presenting with acute myocardial infarction or the subacute development of unstable angina pectoris. Although both of these clinical entities may be superimposed upon stable angina, their cyclic and episodic nature is still one of the most prominent manifestations of chronic coronary

atherosclerosis. One of the most intriguing conundrums in cardiovascular medicine involves the problem of understanding the cellular mechanisms by which a chronic stable atherosclerotic lesion is transformed to a state in which it fissures or ruptures and supports clot formation—the substrate for the development of unstable angina or myocardial infarction. The process in the lesion leading to unstable angina or infarction has been referred to generically as *activation,* and the lesion has been called *active.* This chapter will provide a mechanistic framework that will permit conceptualization of the process in cell biological terms. It will also provide an explanation for the spectrum of the ischemic coronary syndromes in the context of the rapidly expanding body of knowledge concerning the cell biology of atherosclerosis.

BIOLOGY OF ATHEROSCLEROSIS

The fundamental features of atherosclerosis are discussed in detail in Chaps. 39 and 40. The atherosclerotic lesion occurs almost exclusively in the large conduit and conduction vessels of the arterial system. The distribution is nonrandom. It occurs predominantly at flow dividers in areas of low shear stress. The lesion is characterized by the proliferation of medial smooth muscle cells that have been changed into a growth phenotype referred to as the *modulated state.*[1] Smooth muscle cells migrate into the intima and contribute to intimal thickening. Another major feature of an atherosclerotic lesion is the presence of blood monocytes that have adhered to the endothelium and migrated into the intima. These monocytes are transformed into tissue macrophage-like cells. These cells are the major source of the typical lipid-laden foam cells of the atherosclerotic lesion. The foam cells are caused primarily by the uptake of modified or oxidized low-density lipoprotein (LDL). Macrophages express the so-called scavenger receptor, which is a receptor that recognizes modified, but not native, LDL. More recently, it has been appreciated that atherosclerotic lesions have T cells as important constituents.[2] Furthermore, these are frequently memory T cells that express late activation antigens, suggesting that they have been immunologically activated.[3] An additional significant characteristic of an atherosclerotic lesion is neovascularization that is developed from new capillary vessel growth from the adventitial surface.[4] Thus, the atherosclerotic lesion has many features typical of inflammation.

The evolving concept that atherosclerosis is an inflammatory response to injury has led to considerable progress in the understanding of the basic pathogenesis of the disease.[5] As will be developed, this concept is also particularly relevant to the understanding of the episodic nature of clinical coronary disease. The artery exhibits a rather limited repertoire of responses to multiple injuries, all manifesting as an atherosclerotic lesion. The major injuries constitute the well-recognized risk factors. There is the metabolic injury of hyperlipidemia and the injury of physical forces induced by hypertension. As alluded to, physical forces—both shear and pressure—are thought to play a major role in the nonrandom distribution in the arterial system. The vessel may also respond to injury from smoking or to immune injury, as in transplant atherosclerosis. In addition, it may respond to the direct physical insult of balloon angioplasty.

As noted, viewing the lesion as an inflammatory response provides an important basis for considering the episodic nature of clinical coronary disease. An atherosclerotic lesion may be viewed as a chronic inflammatory nidus that may be quiescent or subject to periodic activation.

One of the most provocative new discoveries about the fundamental nature of atherosclerosis has come from work initiated by Steinberg and his colleagues.[6] Initially they observed that native LDL was not taken up readily by monocytes/macrophages in vitro, but that LDL modified by endothelial cells was readily taken up and foam cells were formed.[7] It

was found subsequently that one of the mechanisms involved in modification of LDL that would alter its handling by monocytes was oxidation of the particle with a marked increase in the content of lysophosphatidylcholine (LPC).[8] Modified LDL and LPC elicit a number of responses that are important in the pathogenesis of atherosclerosis, including stimulation of endothelial monocyte and lymphocyte adhesion molecules[9] and monocyte chemotactic protein expression.[10] These compounds will also stimulate growth factor production by the endothelium.[11] The central importance of enhanced oxidation mechanisms in atherosclerosis is emphasized by animal studies in which antioxidants, such as probucol, inhibit atherosclerotic lesion formation.[12]

ENDOTHELIUM

The endothelium plays the central role in controlling the biology of the vessel wall. It has been one of the main tenets in the study of atherosclerosis that a healthy endothelium is crucial to the prevention of disease development. This view evolved from early studies that demonstrated that mechanical removal of the endothelium facilitated lesion development in hypercholesterolemic monkeys. For a period of time, it was assumed that lesion development, in most instances, was associated with endothelial cell detachment exposing the subendothelial surface and permitting platelet adherence and clot formation with the release of growth factors.[13]

The concept of "dysfunction" of the endothelium developed when it became apparent that the endothelium, over most lesions, was intact morphologically.[14] Endothelial dysfunction implies that the normal functions of the endothelium may be modified or modulated to a maladaptive phenotypic state. This concept is central to the major, current views of the pathogenesis of the disease. The normal functions of the endothelium and the consequences of the development of dysfunction are summarized in Table 44-1.

Endothelial-Dependent Vasodilation

The endothelium has a number of critical functions. One of the most important of these is endothelial-dependent vasodilation (see Chap. 4). In 1980, Furchgott and Zawadzki demonstrated the existence of an endothelial-derived humoral factor, which they termed *endothelial-derived relaxing factor* (EDRF), that caused the dilatation of blood vessels by diffusing to the underlying smooth muscle cells and increasing cGMP.[15] Agents such as the muscarinic cholinergic agonist, acetylcholine, caused dilatation with an intact endothelium and contraction when the endothelium was removed (Fig. 44-1).

TABLE 44-1

NORMAL AND DYSFUNCTIONAL ARTERIAL ENDOTHELIUM

Normal Function	Dysfunction in Atherosclerosis	Cause(s) of Dysfunction
Antithrombotic	Potentially prothrombotic	Inflammatory cytokines Oxygen free radical production
Vasodilator	Decreased vasodilation ? Constrictor	Oxygen free radicals—degradation of NO causing decreased vasodilator activity
Growth inhibition	Growth promotion Loss of inhibition	Increased growth factor release; ? decreased inhibitor release
Anti-inflammatory	Proinflammatory—supports monocyte and T-cell localization into lesion	Increased leukocyte adhesion molecule and chemotactic protein expression

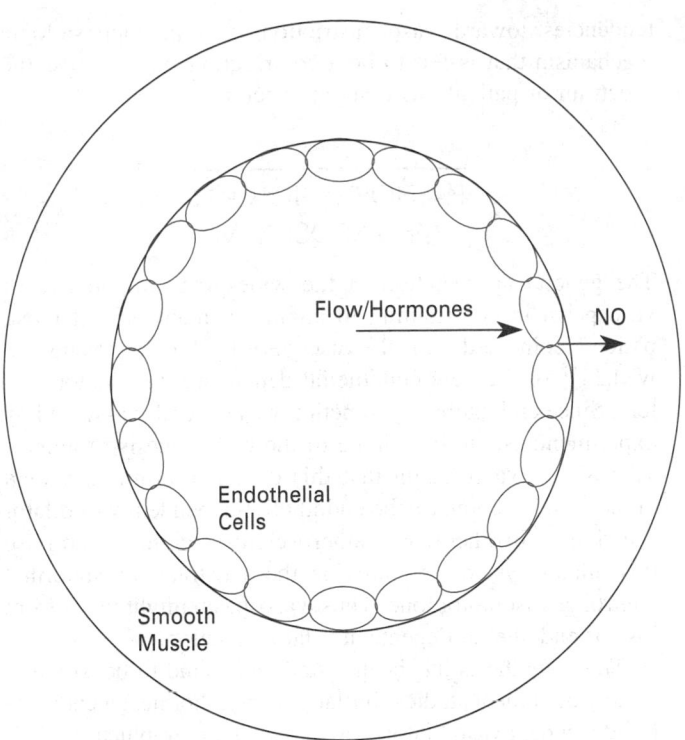

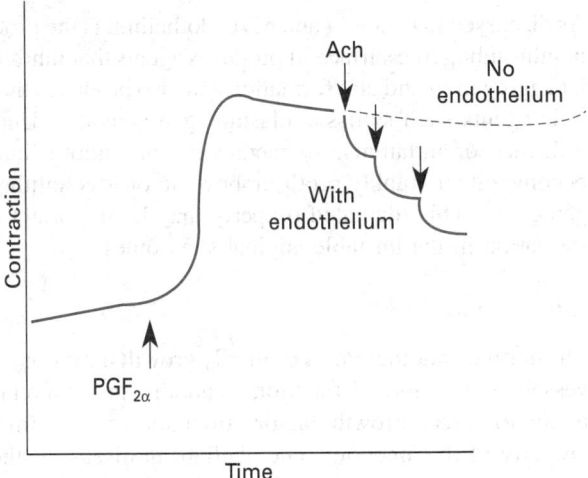

FIGURE 44-1

Endothelial-dependent dilatation. *Left:* An artery with stimuli acting upon the endothelium to cause the release of endothelial-derived relaxing factor or nitric oxide. This diffuses to the underlying smooth muscle to increase cGMP and cause relaxation. *Right:* The effects of the endothelial-dependent vasodilator acetylcholine (Ach) on an artery precontracted with PGF$_{2\alpha}$. In the presence of an intact endothelium, acetylcholine results in a dose-dependent relaxation. When endothelium is removed, acetylcholine no longer induces relaxation. PGF$_{2\alpha}$, platelet-derived growth factor.

Many, if not most, vasodilators, including serotonin, thrombin, flow, substance P, and adenine nucleotides, act through this mechanism.

Early work characterizing EDRF suggested similarities to nitric oxide (NO).[16] Nitric oxide has proven to be the most important of the endothelial-derived vasodilator substances. One of the characteristics of EDRF that was known to be shared with NO was its ease of degradation by oxygen free radicals.[17] The susceptibility of this important endogenous vasodilator to degradation by an oxidative environment is central to the understanding of disordered control of vasomotor tone clinically.

Support in humans for the concept that oxidative stress impairs endothelial function derives from the studies of Levine et al.,[18] who showed that the antioxidant ascorbic acid reverses impaired endothelium-dependent relaxation in brachial arteries of patients with coronary artery disease. Ting et al.[19] made similar observations in patients with diabetes mellitus. Furthermore, when lipid-lowering therapy (lovastatin) is combined with antioxidant therapy (probucol), a greater improvement in endothelium-dependent vasomotion is seen than with lovastatin alone.[20,21] These studies emphasize that excessive production of oxygen radicals may be a general metabolic feature of atherosclerotic arteries that may explain, in part, the abnormal vasomotor control and tendency toward vasospasm.

Inflammation

The endothelium also has a central role in controlling the development of inflammation by controlling the localization of circulating leukocytes. For example, localization of monocytes and lymphocytes to atherosclerotic lesion–prone areas is controlled by endothelial expression of leukocyte adhesion molecules, such as vascular cell adhesion molecule 1 (VCAM-1) (see Chap. 4).[22] In response to metabolic stress such as hyperlipidemia, the endothelium may also express chemotactic proteins such as monocyte chemotactic protein 1.[23] Inflammatory cytokines, such as tumor necrosis factor (TNF), interleukin-1 (IL-1), and interferon gamma, may be produced in the injured vessel and target the endothelium, potentially stimulating expression of adhesion molecules and chemotactic proteins.[24] Thus, the inflammatory response in, for example, an atherosclerotic lesion, may be self-perpetuating during active phases of the disease and may result in recruitment of additional inflammatory cells by cells resident cells in the lesion. Expression of certain adhesion molecules and chemotactic molecules also appears to be regulated by oxidation-sensitive mechanisms.[25,26] Thus, both the vasospastic and inflammatory manifestations of atherosclerosis that ultimately become important clinically may be related to excessive free radical production.

Thrombosis

As discussed in Chaps. 4 and 52, endothelium is the prototypic nonthrombogenic surface. It produces agents that inhibit platelet aggregation and clot formation and also produces thrombolytic agents such as tissue plasminogen activator. Under the influence of inflammatory mediators, the endothelium may become either frankly prothrombogenic or less antithrombogenic.[27,28] This regulated property may be important in clot formation in the unstable anginal syndromes.

Growth Control

The normal endothelium is primarily growth inhibitory. Blood vessels with a normal functional endothelium respond minimally to direct growth factor stimulation.[29] An important property of dysfunctional endothelium in disease is the shift from an antigrowth mode to a mode that promotes growth, in particular, of vascular smooth muscle in the vessel wall. The growth-inhibitory properties are not well understood. It is likely that the growth-promoting properties of the endothelium reflect stimulated production of growth factors such as platelet-derived growth factor B, insulin-like growth factor-1, and fibroblast growth factor.

STABLE
ANGINA PECTORIS

Stable angina is characterized by a consistent pain pattern that does not change over 6 to 8 weeks in either threshold, duration, or the setting in which it occurs (see Chap. 45). Pain characteristically occurs with exertion, emotional upset, or other stimuli that increase myocardial oxygen consumption. The threshold for pain is characteristically not absolutely fixed but is somewhat variable; that is, a stimulus that causes angina on one occasion may not on another, although a consistent pattern can usually be determined. Furthermore, when assessed by ambulatory monitoring, ischemia may be noted to occur at different heart rates.[30]

Hemodynamically significant obstructive disease of the coronary artery contributes to angina in situations where myocardial oxygen consumption is increased. Such obstructions account for the relatively reproducible time to onset of ischemia on treadmill exercise testing. A variability in angina threshold and the setting in which pain occurs is common, however, in everyday living. For example, a person may experience angina or ischemia at heart rates lower than those that cause ischemia on treadmill exercise testing and at rates that are somewhat inconstant.[30] This inconsistency in angina threshold in daily life is likely due to alterations in blood flow delivery—a result of changes in vasomotor tone rather than to unperceived changes in oxygen demand. Vasospasm causing ischemia was first demonstrated directly by angiography by Maseri and his colleagues in 1978.[31] They showed spontaneous occlusive coronary vasospasm in patients with unstable angina pectoris. Disordered control of vasomotor tone with tendencies toward vasoconstriction is a pathophysiologic mechanism that is felt to be a contributing factor across the spectrum of patients with angina pectoris.[32]

PATHOPHYSIOLOGY
OF VASOSPASM

The general appreciation of the widespread importance of vasospasm in contributing to angina in many, if not most, patients coincided with the discovery by Furchgott and Zawadzki[15] of the new endothelial-dependent vasodilator system. Since endothelial dysfunction was generally assumed by experimentalists to contribute to the pathogenesis of atherosclerosis, it was thought that this dysfunction might extend broadly and encompass the endothelial-dependent vasodilator functions.[33] In other words, atherosclerosis might compromise this dilator system and provide the substrate for abnormal control of vasomotor tone. Thus, vasospasm might result from loss of endothelial-dependent dilator function.

This hypothesis has been tested and found to be true in a variety of clinical studies. Initially, acetylcholine, an endothelial-dependent vasodilator, was shown angiographically to dilate normal coronary arteries and to constrict both minimal and advanced stenoses.[33] The pathophysiologic importance of these observations was emphasized by the findings that exercise[34] and cold pressor testing[35] dilated normal coronary arteries but constricted both minimally and advanced stenotic lesions (Figs. 44-2 and 44-3). Endothelial abnormalities were inferred in the exercise studies since acetylcholine and exercise had qualitatively identical effects on segments that dilated or constricted. Furthermore, endothelial-dependent relaxation of coronary arteries becomes defective with the presence of increasing numbers of risk factors, such as smoking and a family history for coronary artery disease, even before disease is angiographically apparent.[36] Recent preliminary studies using B-mode scanning of brachial arteries of young people with hypercholesterolemia indicated that flow-mediated dilatation, which is endothelial-dependent, is impaired, even at an early age.[37] This endothelial dysfunction is likely the substrate upon which more advanced coronary disease develops. Thus, endothelial-dependent dilation, probably the single most important intrinsic vasodilator system, is defective in atherosclerosis and undoubtedly contributes to the increased vasoconstriction and disordered vasomotor control in the disease.

Enhanced vasoconstrictor tone due to either increased local concentration of vasoconstrictor agonist or increased sensitivity of coronary vascular smooth muscle to vasoconstrictors might also contribute to vasospasm.[38] These possibilities have been somewhat more difficult to prove. The enhanced sensitivity to nonspecific vasoconstrictors, such as ergonovine, and the therapeutic efficacy in angina pectoris of vasodilators, such as calcium entry blockers, are consistent with the possibility that contraction-mediating mechanisms are augmented in atherosclerosis.

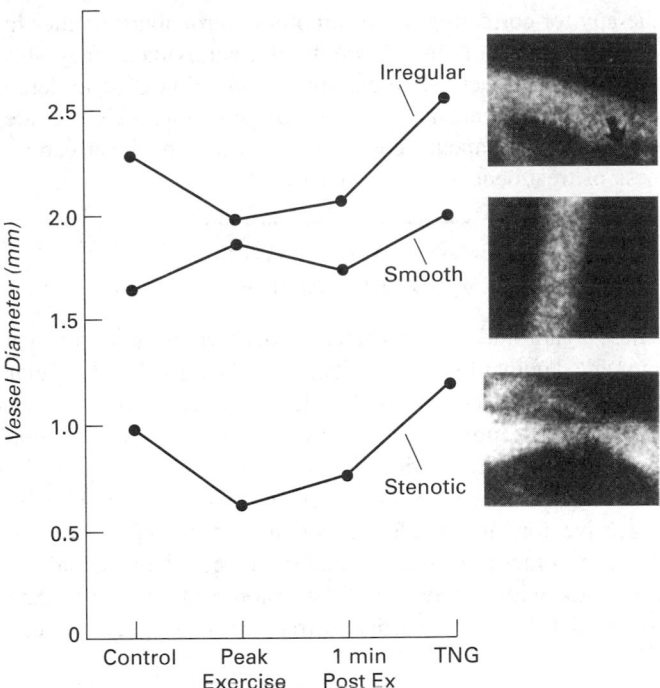

FIGURE 44-2

Exercise-induced changes in vasomotion in diseased and normal coronary arteries. The effects of exercise and nitroglycerin on vessel diameter as determined by quantitative coronary arteriography in a normal coronary segment and in segments with minimal obstruction and advanced stenosis are shown. Exercise induced on the catheterization table caused constriction of both the irregular segment (*upper panel*) and the segment with the high-grade stenosis (*lower panel*). In contrast, the segment that is angiographically smooth (*middle panel*) dilated in response to exercise. Endothelial dysfunction was implicated in these responses since simultaneous studies showed that segments constricting with exercise also constricted in response to acetylcholine, an endothelial-dependent vasodilator. In contrast, segments dilating to exercise dilated in response to acetylcholine. Beta blockade only partially attenuated the vasodilator response to exercise, thus invoking other mechanisms—presumably endothelial-dependent dilatation stimulated by flow. Note that all three segments dilate in response to nitroglycerin, an NO donor, which bypasses the defective endothelial control mechanism and dilates the smooth muscle directly. (From Gordon et al.[34] Reproduced with permission of the publisher and the authors.)

Cellular Mechanisms of Vasospasm

Both the clinical data already cited and data from hypercholesterolemic animals indicate that there is decreased activity of EDRF (NO) released by the endothelium. There are two possible explanations for this: (1) there is a decrease in production of NO, or (2) there is normal or increased production of NO by the endothelial cell with increased degradation to inactive metabolites before it can produce its effect on smooth muscle. There are data in experimental animals showing reversal of the endothelial-dependent vasodilator defect with administration of the NO precursor, the amino acid arginine.[39,40] Other evidence, however, favors the proposition that there is normal, or even increased, production of NO with enhanced degradation leading to decreased vasodilator activity.[41] In hypercholesterolemic rabbits, increased levels of NO metabolites were

measured in a setting of decreased EDRF dilator activity. Hypercholesterolemic rabbits have been shown to exhibit a dramatic increase in oxygen free radical production after only 1 month of cholesterol feeding.[42] The idea that free radical degradation of NO contributes to the contractile abnormality in atherosclerosis receives support from experiments on cholesterol-fed rabbits in which the defect in endothelial-dependent relaxation was largely reversed by superoxide dismutase, which scavenges the free radicals.[43] In the context of the previously reviewed data indicating that an abnormal redox state with enhanced oxidation in the atherosclerotic artery is central to the molecular mechanisms involved in the pathogenesis of atherosclerosis, the data on contraction are consistent with the presence of enhanced production of oxygen free radicals. Recent in situ hybridization and immunohistochemistry studies of human atherosclerotic lesions indicate increased, not decreased, expression of NO synthase in diseased arteries relative to normal arteries.[44] These clinical and experi-

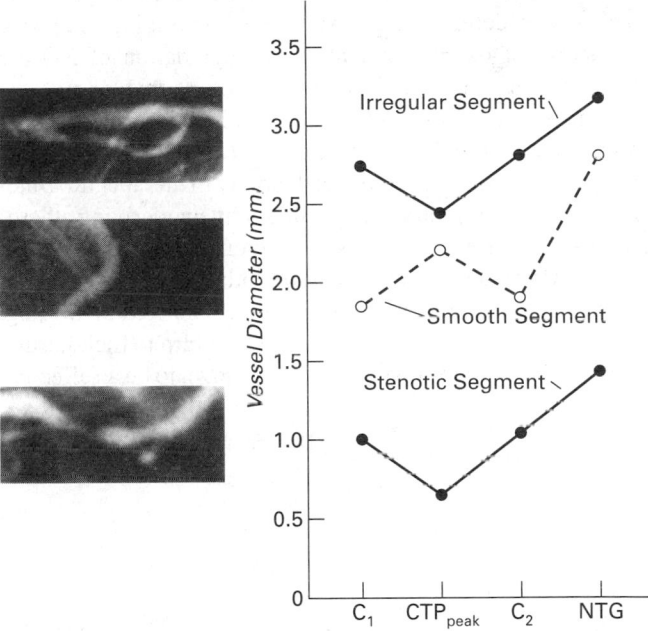

FIGURE 44-3

Effects of stimulation of the sympathetic nervous system by cold pressor testing of coronary artery diameter. At catheterization, the sympathetic nervous system was stimulated by the immersion of a hand in an ice slurry for 90 s. The *middle panel* shows a normal adaptive response to increase diameter at a time when myocardial oxygen consumption is increased, thus contributing to increased flow. This response in a perfectly smooth segment is contrasted with the response in a minimally diseased segment (*upper panel*) and a segment with advanced stenosis (*lower panel*). In both of these instances, there was constriction of the artery. In the case of the stenotic segment, this extent of constriction contributed importantly to a decrease in blood flow and might precipitate ischemia. The mechanisms mediating the dilator response undoubtedly include endothelial-dependent stimulation to dilatation caused by an increase in blood flow. The constrictor responses reflect, at least in part, the loss of endothelial-dependent dilatation. As in the case of exercise depicted in Fig. 44-2, nitroglycerin dilates both diseased and normal vessels by delivering nitric oxide directly to the smooth muscle. (From Nabel et al.[35] Reproduced with permission of the publisher and the authors.)

mental data confirm the existence of a fundamental defect in endothelial-dependent vasodilatation in atherosclerosis. A likely mechanism for this defect is increased degradation of NO by oxygen free radical production that is probably a fundamental characteristic of the disease.

The possibility of increased sensitivity of vascular smooth muscle constrictors as a contributor to vasospasm has been noted. The efficacy of calcium entry blockers in decreasing vasospasm suggests that there may be abnormal expression of voltage-dependent calcium channels that could enhance contractility. Mechanisms potentially contributing to vasospasm are summarized in Fig. 44-4.

Clinical Implications of Vasospasm

Abnormal control of vasomotor tone with a predominance of vasoconstrictor activity is present in virtually all patients with coronary artery disease, and this enhanced vasoconstrictor tone probably accounts for the efficacy of vasodilators, such as nitrates and calcium entry blockers, in treating angina. The mechanisms defined in animal models involving excessive production of oxygen radicals with degradation of NO are in agreement with the developing concept that one of the fundamental metabolic defects in the atherosclerotic artery is an enhanced oxidative state. Increased understanding of the biology of vasospasm should lead rapidly to therapeutic strategies to treat the primary abnormality of the underlying atherosclerosis. Experience in monkeys demonstrates that the defect in endothelial-dependent relaxation induced by hypercholesterolemia can be reversed by stopping cholesterol feeding, which forces serum cholesterol levels to return to their normal values.[45] Thus, lipid-lowering may be shown to be an effective

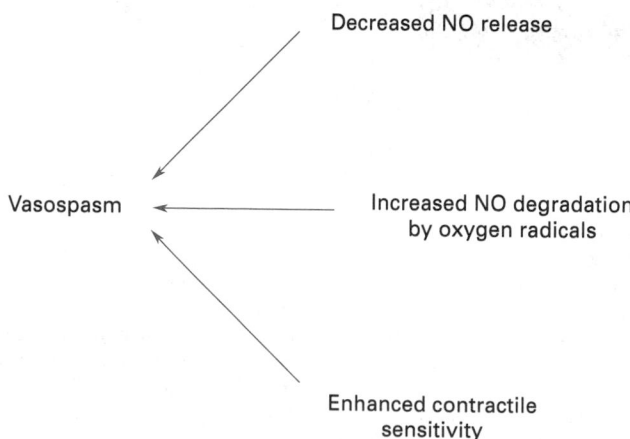

FIGURE 44-4

Mechanisms accounting for vasospasm. Decreased endothelial-dependent vasodilator function is a major contributor to the vasomotor abnormality in most patients with coronary artery disease. This may be associated with decreased nitric oxide release. A considerable amount of data suggests that the endothelium may produce normal, or even increased, amounts of nitric oxide. The vasodilator activity, however, is lost by enhanced degradation by the abnormal redox environment of the diseased artery with increased production of oxygen radicals. There may also be enhanced direct contractile sensitivity of vascular smooth muscle cells in diseased arteries. Increased local concentration of vasoconstrictor agents is possible.

therapy for correcting the vasomotor control abnormalities in coronary artery disease. In the future, antioxidants may also prove to be effective. Importantly, correction of disordered endothelial-dependent vasomotor abnormalities may provide eventually a therapeutic end-point for evaluating the effectiveness of treatment of atherosclerosis.

UNSTABLE ANGINA AND MYOCARDIAL INFARCTION

These syndromes are considered together because, from a biological point of view, it is likely that the underlying cellular mechanisms in the atherosclerotic plaque are similar, if not identical. The presence of mural thrombus is the common pathologic feature uniting the two syndromes.[46] It may be partially or transiently occlusive in unstable angina and totally occlusive for an extended period in myocardial infarction. The syndromes also share the underlying cellular mechanisms associated with conversion of the lesion from the stable state to one that has a propensity to fracture or rupture (see also Chap. 40).

Unstable angina and myocardial infarction are episodic events that are frequently superimposed upon a chronic stable angina pattern and are manifested by changing pain patterns. There may be a markedly lower exercise threshold for inducing pain, which may be of longer duration than usual. The pain may also occur at rest. A primary reduction of blood flow likely accounts for the rest pain and for the change in threshold. Unstable angina is frequently antecedent to myocardial infarction. This relationship between these two syndromes provides evidence, on clinical grounds alone, that the pathophysiologic mechanisms and the cellular basis must be similar.

Thrombosis superimposed on a fissured or ruptured complex plaque is present in most patients with acute myocardial infarction and is present in a high proportion of patients with advanced stages of unstable angina.[46] The development of mural thrombus with the associated decrease in lumen diameter probably accounts for the decrease in exertional threshold for angina or rest pain. In this context, the only fundamental difference between an atherosclerotic plaque causing either unstable angina or myocardial infarction is whether or not the thrombus is occlusive for a sufficient time to cause tissue death downstream. The thrombus most commonly occurs with disruption of the plaque or desquamation of endothelial cells[47] to expose thrombogenic surfaces and tissue thromboplastins. Clot could theoretically occur with intact endothelium since inflammatory mediators such as IL-1 and TNF, which are expressed in active, inflammatory lesions, can stimulate expression of the procoagulant tissue factor in human endothelial cells in culture.[27] Such a mechanism has not been demonstrated definitively in diseased arteries. Other products of inflammatory cells may contribute to the breakdown of the connective tissue skeleton of the plaque, compromising its structural integrity and predisposing it to fracture and fissuring.

Vasospasm also plays an important role in unstable angina, as already discussed.[31] The constrictor predominance present in stable angina may be enhanced in the unstable state by increased sensitivity to vasoconstrictors. Furthermore, the presence of clot with thrombin and platelet products such as 5-HT and thromboxane A_2 also may provide increased vasoconstrictor stimuli.[48]

Cellular Mechanisms of Unstable Angina and Myocardial Infarction

One of the more intriguing issues in cardiovascular medicine is why a chronic atherosclerotic lesion is converted to an active state, leading to enhanced vasoconstriction and thrombus formation with the resultant unstable angina and/or myocardial infarction. There is a compelling body of evidence that is consistent with enhanced inflammatory activity in these unstable states. In 1958, Pomerance showed increased numbers of inflammatory cells in the adventitia of the infarct-related arteries of patients who had died suddenly, thus minimizing the possibility that inflammatory response was secondary to the infarct.[49] The implication was that the inflammatory cells might, in fact, be a contributing factor. Increased subendothelial infiltration of the coronary arteries with monocytes and macrophages and also increased adventitial inflammatory cell numbers have been observed at autopsy in patients who had unstable angina.[50,51] A recent study showed that pultaceous plaques were frequent at sites of thrombosis and ulceration, and T cells and macrophages were prominent in other areas.[52] TNFα and IL-2 were expressed in these plaques.

Altered Plaque Structural Integrity

The increased numbers of inflammatory cells and their activation may be related directly to plaque instability, fracture or fissuring, and thrombus formation. Indeed, van der Wal et al.[53] showed that, regardless of dominant plaque morphology, the immediate site of plaque rupture or erosion is always marked by an inflammatory process. Macrophages may have protean effects on the vessel wall, the understanding of which may provide mechanistic insights into the relationship between the activation of the inflammatory response and development of the unstable coronary syndromes. Interactions between macrophages and lymphocytes are likely to be particularly important. As noted, there are resident macrophages and T cells in most atherosclerotic lesions.[2] Activation of the inflammatory response may precipitate expression of factors that recruit the additional leukocytes into the lesion in unstable angina.[50,51] For example, release of IL-1 or TNF by lymphocytes or macrophages (or endothelium) could increase expression of endothelial adhesion molecules to cause attachment to the overlying endothelium, resulting in movement of additional mononuclear cells into the intima. Similarly, production of chemotactic factors, such as monocyte chemotactic protein 1, which may be stimulated by cytokines, may also contribute to monocyte recruitment.[23]

Activation of lymphocytes and macrophages results in release of a number of additional substances that could be directly related to the pathogenesis of the unstable coronary syndromes. The release of oxygen free radicals and formation of H_2O_2, together with the secretion of degradative enzymes such as collagenase and haluronidase, can degrade connective tissue and compromise the structural integrity of the plaque, which, in the stable state with a dense connective tissue skeleton, may be quite resistant to rupture or fissuring. Rajagopalan et al.[54] showed that macrophage-derived foam cells from hypercholesterolemic rabbits do in fact produce $\cdot O_2^-$ and H_2O_2, and that these reactive oxygen species regulate the activity of smooth muscle–derived matrix metalloproteinases (MMP)-2 and MMP-9 (see Chap. 4). These enzymes degrade the extracellular matrix and thus permit cell migration and remodeling of the vessel wall. The cytokines produced by monocytes and macrophages also stimulate MMP expression in vascular wall cells. Indeed, increased levels of activated MMP-9, MMP-3, and MMP-1 have been found in the shoulder of atherosclerotic plaques and in regions of foam cell accumulation.[55] These observations provide support for the suggestion of Richardson and colleagues that macrophages may be degrading collagen and consequently compromising the structural integrity of the plaque. They described the fissuring of plaque at sites in the cap where there was an increased concentration of macrophages/foam cells.[56]

When the plaque does fracture because of compromise of its connective tissue skeletal framework or for other reasons, the clotting factors derived from macrophages and from the lipid core in the vessel wall contribute to luminal clot formation. As detailed previously, thrombus theoretically might also occur on a morphologically intact endothelium because of the capacity of cytokines to induce tissue factor production by endothelial cells in vitro.[27] Finally the neovascularization of the plaque with thin-walled vessels penetrating from the adventitial surface can lead to rupture, resulting in intramural hemorrhage and thrombus formation with disruption of plaque structure. The cellular events postulated to occur in an "active" atherosclerotic lesion are summarized in Fig. 44-5.

Episodic Thrombosis

Studies by Falk[57] have provided compelling evidence that clot formation in unstable angina is episodic, hence suggesting a potential explanation for the cyclic nature of the clinical manifestations of the disease. Autopsies of patients with a history of one or more episodes of unstable angina before dying of their ischemic heart disease showed a layering of thrombi of different ages in the epicardial infarct-related artery. Furthermore, downstream from the epicardial lesion, pathologic changes were observed, ranging from fibrotic areas of healed microinfarctions to recent platelet-rich isoemboli in the microvasculature. *These pathologic data viewed in the context of the evidence of episodic disease activation clinically suggest that the cyclic nature of the clinical presentation reflects recurrent changes in the biological state of the atherosclerotic lesion leading to recurrent thrombosis.*

According to the above synthesis, plaque rupture, and thus the propensity for infarction, would be a function of the bio-

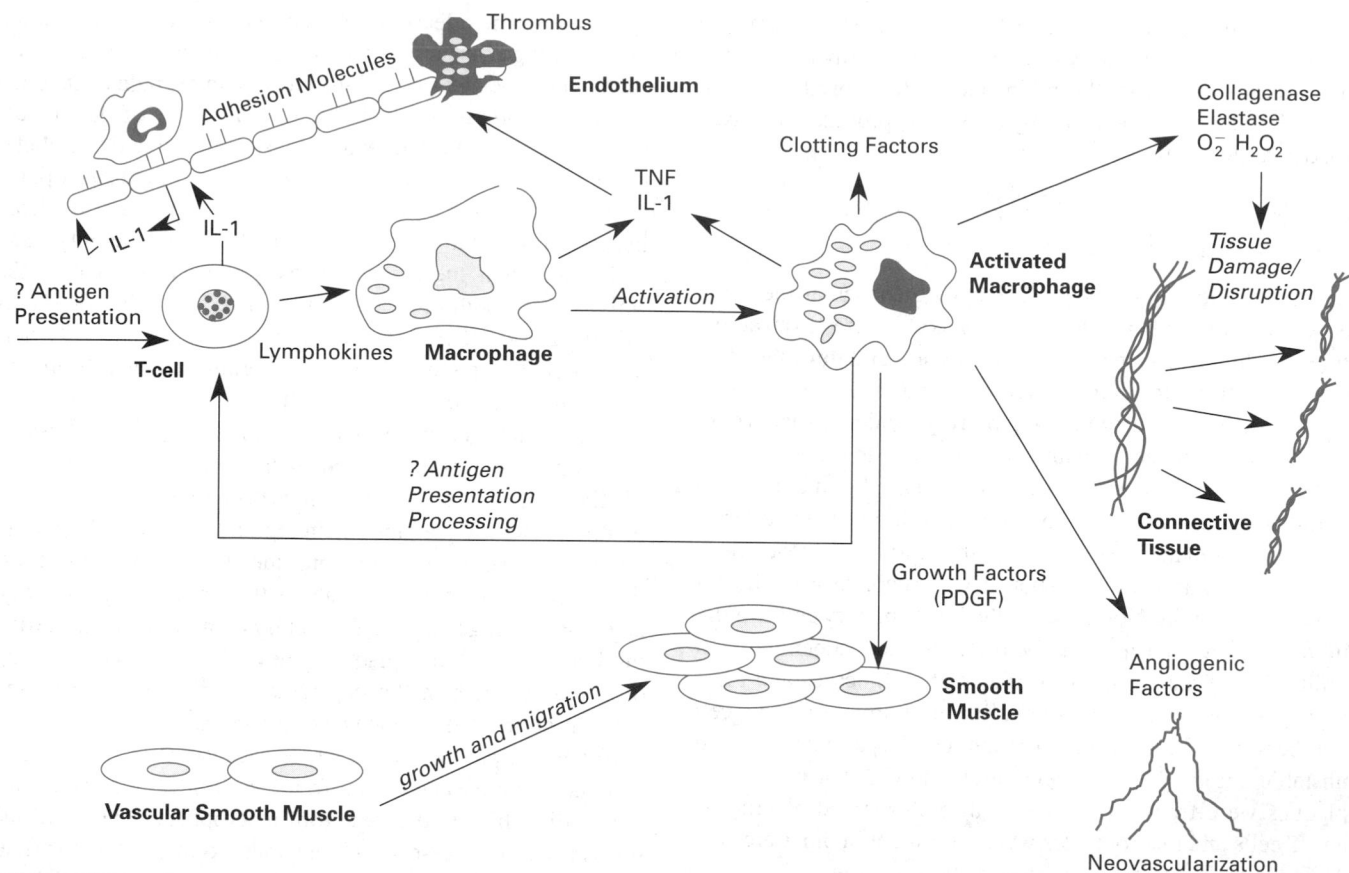

FIGURE 44-5

Postulated cellular mechanism in an "active" atherosclerotic lesion leading to mononuclear cell recruitment, lesion disruption, and clot formation. Activation of the lesion is thought to be associated with enhanced production of growth factors contributing to lesion growth through smooth muscle cell migration and proliferation. It is very likely that there is interaction between resident T cells and macrophages, and this may perhaps involve antigen presentation and/or processing that contributes to activation of the cells. Cytokine production will result in increased adhesion molecule expression and further recruitment of mononuclear cells and lymphocytes. The activated macrophage will produce procoagulant factors and growth factors. Impor-

tantly, the activated macrophage is likely to produce proteolytic agents, such as collagenase, elastase, and free radicals, that will lead to tissue damage and disruption. Fracture of the connective tissue can interfere with structural integrity of the plaque, leading to plaque fissuring and mural thrombus formation. The macrophages may also contribute angiogenic factors that increase the neovascularization of the plaque. This may be a source of intramural hemorrhage that can also compromise the structural integrity of the plaque. Decreasing inflammatory response in the plaque will, in the future, be a therapeutic objective, and possibly is a major contributor to the decrease in cardiac event rates that have been reported in lipid-lowering trials.

logical (inflammatory) state of the lesion rather than being closely related to the extent of stenosis. This concept has important clinical implications as discussed below.

Clinical Implications

The suggestion of an inflammatory cause of the unstable coronary syndromes is based upon the premise that conversion of a stable coronary atherosclerotic lesion to an unstable one may be caused by an activation of the resident and newly recruited monocytes/macrophages and T cells to cause an enhanced inflammatory response. *Thus, the recurrent nature of the unstable coronary syndromes may be related to the cyclic activation of a chronic inflammatory focus in a manner that might be analogous to the episodic activation of other chronic inflammatory diseases such as rheumatoid arthritis.* While the initiating factors for this episodic activation are

unknown, and details need to be confirmed, the proposed scenario is consistent with the available evidence about the pathogenesis of atherosclerosis and provides a synthesis and reconciliation with clinical observations.

PRECIPITATING EVENTS FOR LESION ACTIVATION

The mechanisms underlying lesion activation remain obscure. Clearly, the view of the process as having an inflammatory basis provides a conceptual framework for a better understanding. There are several possibilities. First, local mechanisms that are currently not known could initiate inflammatory cell activation and recruitment. Another consideration is the possibility that there is an antigen generated within the lesion that is presented by macrophages to T cells, leading to activation of the inflammatory response (Fig. 44-5). Although there is no firm basis for speculating about any specific antigen, it is interesting to note that oxidized LDL is a potent immunogen[58] and that some patients with atherosclerosis have circulating antibodies against the molecule.[59] At present, oxidized or modified LDL must be considered only a potential candidate antigen for stimulating local inflammation. It is also possible that modified lipids may generate an immune response within an atherosclerotic lesion. Cytokines produced during this activation could markedly affect growth and differentiation of vascular cells and mediate the response to injury.

There are data that raise intriguing questions concerning the possibility of systemic triggers of lesion activation. Spodick has called attention to the frequency with which patients who have had a myocardial infarction have a history of an antecedent febrile illness.[60] More recently, there have been reports that patients suffering acute cardiac events have a statistically significant increase in antibody titers to *Chlamydia pneumoniae* relative to controls.[61] Moreover, other analyses have suggested that chronic infection with *C. pneumoniae* may be a risk factor for coronary artery disease.[62] It is difficult to conceive, at present, of a mechanistic relationship between infection with this particular organism and lesion activation. Precipitation by infectious illness of acute episodes of other inflammatory diseases, such as rheumatoid arthritis, is a well-known phenomenon. In some cases of the unstable coronary syndromes, activation of the resident inflammatory cells in a previously quiescent coronary lesion by an infection triggering systemic inflammatory responses may occur.[63] There is some direct evidence of systemic activation of inflammatory responses during unstable angina. The acute-phase reactant, C-reactive protein, has been reported to be elevated in this circumstance.[64] In fact, a recent study suggested that C-reactive protein has some prognostic value for coronary events in patients with stable or unstable angina.[65] Furthermore, incubation of lymphocytes and mononuclear cells from patients with unstable angina is associated with production of tissue factor–like activity.[66] Tissue factor production was not observed 6 weeks later when the instability had resolved. Whether or not this evidence of systemic inflammatory response bears a cause-and-effect relationship to unstable angina remains to be determined. Nonetheless, these data also support the concept that the active coronary syndromes have an inflammatory component.

OVERVIEW

Two major propositions emerge from the synthesis of the clinical and experimental data reviewed here: (1) The manifestly episodic nature of the ischemic coronary syndromes and, in particular, the unstable syndromes reflects cyclic changes in the cell biology of the atherosclerotic plaque (Fig. 44-6); and (2) fundamentally, this cell biology is an inflammatory response to metabolic and/or physical injury to the endothelium initially. It follows, then, that the state of inflammatory activity of the lesion is critically important in determining the clinical course, and that the extent of stenosis of a lesion may

be of secondary importance as to whether or not a lesion is life-threatening. This view is consistent with the observations that the residual infarct-related lesion after thrombolysis is sometimes minimally stenotic[67,68] and that assessment of location and severity of stenosis angiographically does not permit reliable prediction of the location of subsequent myocardial infarction.[69] This formulation is also consistent with the observations in angiographic coronary regression trials with aggressive lipid-lowering regimens. For example, in the Familial Atherosclerosis Treatment Study (FATS), rather modest improvement (2 to 3 percent) in luminal diameter and/or lack of progression was associated with very substantial (~75 percent) reduction in cardiac event rates for death, myocardial infarction, or requirement for percutaneous transluminal coronary angioplasty (PTCA) or coronary artery bypass grafting.[70] Similarly, in the St. Thomas Atherosclerosis Regression Study (STARS), lowering cholesterol with diet, or diet plus cholestyramine, was associated with about a 75 percent reduction in cardiovascular events over 3 years while showing only modest improvement in lesion diameter or lack of progression.[71] Thus, lipid-lowering may favorably affect the biology of coronary lesions, making them less prone to activation and more resistant to structural breakdown and thrombus formation. This interpretation is consistent with the view that *the biological state, or activity, of an atherosclerotic lesion is a more important determinant of clinical course than is the extent of stenosis.*

These observations have considerable clinical significance. If, in fact, the life history of an atherosclerotic plaque is not one of continuous linear growth and luminal narrowing but, as the evidence suggests, consists of cyclic periods of growth associated with inflammatory activation and enhanced potential for catastrophic clinical events, then therapeutic objectives in the future may focus less exclusively on the hemodynamic consequences of a lesion and more on the prevention of lesion activation and on inactivation of an unstable lesion. An inactive lesion would be one with a minimal number of inflammatory cells in a quiescent state with an intact connective tissue framework and a relatively healthy overlying endothelium. This description applies to the coronary artery lesions of monkeys approximately 1 year after cessation of a high-cholesterol diet; during the hypercholesterolemic stage, these lesions had been highly cellular with marked impairment of endothelial vasodilator function.[72] Viewed in this context, a stenotic but inactive coronary artery lesion could have clinical consequences, such as exertional angina, but would have minimal devastating potential for plaque rupture or fissuring. Such an interpretation, as noted, might explain the marked reduction of clinical events in the FATS and other regression trials where angiographic improvements were modest.[70] This point of view would call into question any assertion that patients with coronary lesions that are neither highly stenotic or unstable should have PTCA or surgical revascularization.

The evidence available provides a rationale for active treatment of atherosclerosis by modification of known risk factors, such as smoking and hyperlipidemia, in most patients with

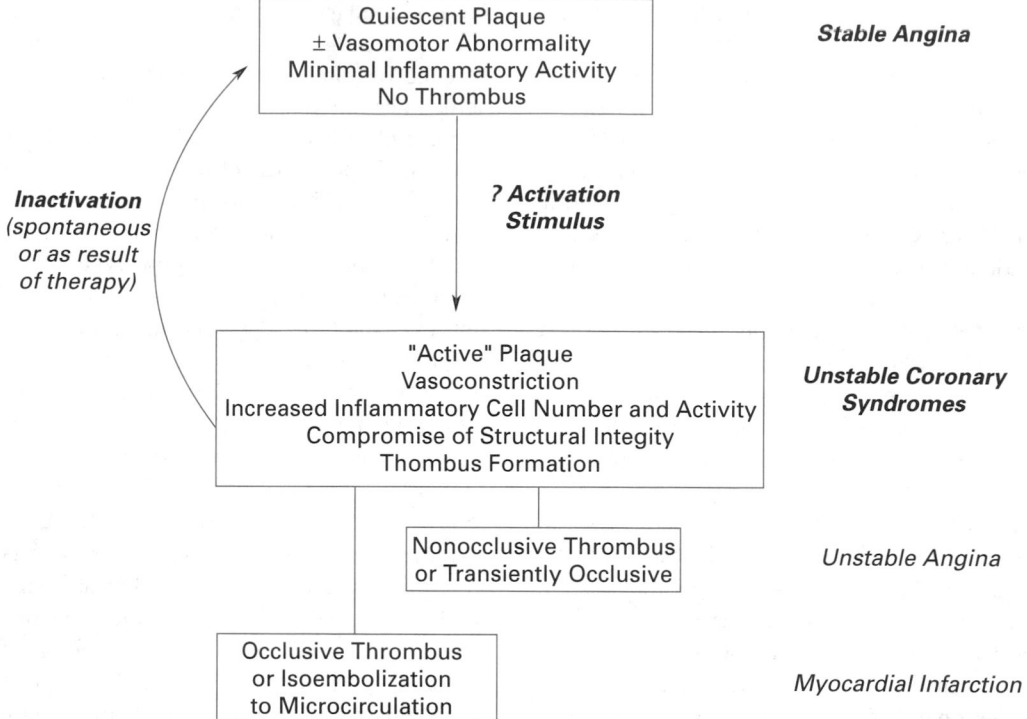

FIGURE 44-6

Cyclic nature of the coronary ischemic syndromes. Stable angina is associated with a plaque that has intact structural integrity and probably minimal inflammatory activity. Resident inflammatory cells are not in an active state. Effort angina is a result of the hemodynamic consequences of luminal narrowing as well as the loss of endothelial-dependent vasodilator mechanisms that may be chronic. An activation stimulus, the nature of which is not yet understood, likely causes increased inflammatory activity. There is increased recruitment of inflammatory cells, and there is activation of these cells. As a result of the activation, the tendencies for enhanced vasoconstriction become even more prominent. Because of the inflammatory response, there may be compromise of the structural integrity of the plaque that may be associated with fissuring or fracture with thrombus formation. A mural nonocclusive thrombus (or one that is only transiently occlusive) would be associated with unstable angina, whereas prolonged occlusion, or isoembolization, and microvascular occlusion would manifest as myocardial infarction. Inactivation of the plaque inflammatory activity would result in termination of the unstable state. The mechanisms for termination of lesion activity are also unknown but may be analogous to spontaneous inactivation, or quiescence, of inflammatory responses elsewhere. Plaque inactivation may account for the dramatic lowering of cardiac event rates in lipid-lowering regression trials.

clinical evidence of vascular disease at any stage of life or disease progression. With the rapid evolution of knowledge about the pathogenesis of atherosclerosis, one can anticipate even more effective and specific therapeutic approaches to the disease. If technology is developed that permits the reliable premorbid diagnosis of atherosclerosis itself, as opposed to the hemodynamic consequences of the disease, the implementation of effective therapy should make catastrophic coronary events much less common.

REFERENCES

1. Ross R, Masuda J, Raines EW. Cellular interactions, growth factors, and smooth muscle proliferation in atherogenesis. *Ann NY Acad Sci* 1990; 598:102–112.
2. Hansson GK, Jonasson L, Seifert PS, Stemme S. Immune mechanisms in atherosclerosis. *Arteriosclerosis* 1989; 9:567–578.
3. Stemme S, Holm J, Hansson GK. T lymphocytes in human atherosclerotic plaques are memory cells expressing CD45RO and the integrin VLA-1. *Arterioscler Thromb* 1992; 12:206–211.
4. Kamat BR, Galli SJ, Barger AC, Lainey LL, Silverman KJ. Neovascularization and coronary atherosclerotic plaque: Cinematographic localization and quantitative histologic analysis. *Hum Pathol* 1987; 18:1036–1042.
5. Munro JM, Cotran RS. The pathogenesis of atherosclerosis: Atherogenesis and inflammation. *Lab Invest* 1988; 58:249–261.
6. Steinberg D, Parthasarathy S, Carew TE, Khoo JC, Witztum JL. Beyond cholesterol. Modifications of low-density lipoprotein that increase its atherogenicity. *N Engl J Med* 1989; 320:915–924.
7. Henriksen T, Mahoney EM, Steinberg D. Enhanced macrophage degradation of low density lipoprotein previously incubated with cultured endothelial cells: Recognition by receptor for acetylated low density lipoprotein. *Proc Natl Acad Sci USA* 1981; 78:6499–6503.
8. Steinbrecher UP, Parthasarathy S, Leake DS, Witztum JL, Steinberg D. Modification of low density lipoprotein by endothelial cells involves lipid peroxidation and degradation of low density lipoprotein phospholipids. *Proc Natl Acad Sci USA* 1984; 81:3883–3887.
9. Fostegard J, Haegerstrand A, Gidlund M, Nilsson J. Biologically modified LDL increases the adhesive properties of endothelial cells. *Atherosclerosis* 1991; 90:112–126.
10. Cushing SD, Berliner JA, Valente AJ, Territo MC, Naval M, Parhami F, et al. Minimally modified low density lipoprotein induces monocyte chemotactic protein-1 in human endothelial cells and smooth muscle cells. *Proc Natl Acad Sci USA* 1990; 85:5134–5138.
11. Rajavashirth TB, Andalibi A, Territo MC, Berliner JA, Navab M, Fogelman AM, et al. Induction of endothelial cell expression of granulocyte and macrophage colony stimulating factors by modified low-density lipoproteins. *Nature* 1990; 344:254–257.
12. Carew TE, Schwenke DC, Steinberg D. Antiatherogenic effect of probucol unrelated to its hypocholesterolemic effect; evidence that antioxidants in vivo can selectively inhibit low density lipoprotein degradation in macrophage-rich fatty streaks and slow the progression

of atherosclerosis in the Watanabe heritable hyperlipidemic rabbit. *Proc Natl Acad Sci USA* 1987; 84:7725–7729.

13. Ross R, Glomset J, Harker L. Response to injury and atherogenesis. *Am J Pathol* 1977; 86:675–684.

14. Gimbrone MA Jr. Endothelial dysfunction and the pathogenesis of atherosclerosis. In: Gotto A, Smith LC, Allen B, eds. *Atherosclerosis-V. Proceedings of the Vth International Symposium on Atherosclerosis.* New York: Springer-Verlag; 1980:415–425.

15. Furchgott RF, Jawadzki JV. The obligatory role of endothelial cells in the relaxation of arterial smooth muscle by acetylcholine. *Nature* 1980; 288:373–376.

16. Palmer RM, Ferrige AG, Moncada S. Nitric oxide release accounts for the biological activity of endothelium-derived relaxing factor. *Nature* 1987; 327:524–526.

17. Gryglewski RJ, Palmer RM, Moncada S. Superoxide anion is involved in the breakdown of endothelium-derived vascular relaxing factor. *Nature* 1986; 320:454–456.

18. Levine GN, Frei B, Koulouris SN, Gernard MD, Keaney JF Jr, Vita JA. Ascorbic acid reverses endothelial vasomotor dysfunction in patients with coronary artery disease. *Circulation* 1996; 6:1107–1113.

19. Ting HH, Timimi FK, Boles KS, Creager SJ, Ganz P, Creager MA. Vitamin C improves endothelium-dependent vasodilation in patients with non-insulin-dependent diabetes mellitus. *J Clin Invest* 1997; 1:22–28.

20. Anderson TJ, Meredith IT, Yeung AC, Frei B, Selwyn AP, Ganz P. The effect of cholesterol-lowering and antioxidant therapy on endothelium-dependent coronary vasomotion. *N Engl J Med* 1995; 332:488–493.

21. Treasure CB, Klein JL, Weintraub WS, Talley JD, Stillabower ME, Kosinski AS, et al. Beneficial effects of cholesterol-lowering therapy on the coronary endothelium in patients with coronary artery disease. *N Engl J Med* 1995; 332:481–487.

22. Kume N, Cybulsky MI, Gimbrone MA Jr. Lysophosphatidylcholine, a component of atherogenic lipoproteins, induces mononuclear leukocyte adhesion molecules in cultured human and rabbit arterial endothelial cells. *J Clin Invest* 1992; 90:1138–1144.

23. Cushing SD, Berliner JA, Valente AJ, Territo MC, Navab M, Parhami F, et al. Minimally modified low density lipoprotein induces monocyte chemotactic protein-1 in human endothelial cells and smooth muscle cells. *Proc Natl Acad Sci USA* 1990; 87:5134–5138.

24. Libby P, Hansson GK. Involvement of the immune system in human atherogenesis: Current knowledge and unanswered questions. *Lab Invest* 1991; 64:5–15.

25. Capers Q IV, Alexander RW, Lou P, deLeon H, Wilcox JN, Ishizaka N, et al. Monocyte chemoattractant protein-1 expression in aortic tissues of hypertensive rats. *Circulation*, in press.

26. Marui N, Offerman M, Swerlick R, Kunsch C, Roxen CA, Ahmad M, et al. Vascular cell-adhesion molecule-1 (VCAM-1) gene-transcription and expression are regulated through an antioxidant sensitive mechanism in human vascular endothelial cells. *J Clin Invest* 1993; 92:1866–1874.

27. Bevilacqua MP, Gimbrone MA Jr. Inducible endothelial functions in inflammation and coagulation. *Semin Thromb Hemost* 1987; 13:425–433.

28. Bevilacqua MP, Schleff RR, Gimbrone MA Jr, Loskutoff DJ. Regulation of the fibrinolytic system of cultured human vascular endothelium by interleukin 1. *J Clin Invest* 1986; 78:587–591.

29. Edelman ER, Nugent MA, Smith LT, Karnovsky MJ. Basic fibroblast growth factor enhances the coupling of intimal hyperplasia and proliferation of vaso vasorum in injured rat arteries. *J Clin Invest* 1992; 89:465–473.

30. Deanfield JE, Maseri A, Selwyn AP, Ribeiro P, Chierchia S, Kirkler S, et al. Myocardial ischaemia during daily life in patients with stable angina: Its relation to symptoms and heart rate changes. *Lancet* 1983; 2:753–758.

31. Maseri A, Labbate A, Baroldi G, Chierchia S, Marzilli M, Ballestra AM, et al. Coronary vasospasm as a possible cause of myocardial infarction. A conclusion derived from the study of preinfarction angina. *N Engl J Med* 1978; 299:1271–1277.

32. Antman E, Muller J, Goldberg S, MacAlpin R, Rubenfire M, Tabatznik B, et al. Nifedipine therapy for coronary artery spasm. *N Engl J Med* 1980; 302:1269–1273.

33. Ludmer PL, Selwyn AP, Shook TL, Wayne RR, Mudge GH, Alexander RW, et al. Paradoxical vasoconstriction induced by acetylcholine in atherosclerotic coronary arteries. *N Engl J Med* 1986; 315:1046–1051.

34. Gordon JB, Ganz P, Nabel EG, Fish RD, Zebede J, Mudge GH, et al. Atherosclerosis influences the vasomotor response of epicardial coronary arteries to exercise. *J Clin Invest* 1989; 83:1946–1952.

35. Nabel EG, Ganz P, Gordon JB, Alexander RW, Selwyn AP. Dilation of normal and constriction of atherosclerotic coronary arteries caused by the cold pressor test. *Circulation* 1988; 77:43–52.

36. Vita JA, Treasure CB, Nabel EG, McLenachan JM, Fish RD, Yeung AC, et al. Coronary vasomotor response to acetylcholine relates to risk factors for coronary artery disease. *Circulation* 1990; 81:491–497.

37. Celermajer DS, Sorensen KE, Gooch VM, Spiegelhalter DJ, Miller OI, Sullivan ID, et al. Non-invasive detection of endothelial dysfunction in children and adults at risk of atherosclerosis. *Lancet* 1992; 340:1111–1115.

38. Ganz P, Alexander RW. New insights into the cellular mechanisms of vasospasm. *Am J Cardiol* 1985; 56:11E–15E.

39. Cooke JP, Singer AH, Tsao P, Zera P, Rowan RA, Billingham ME. Antiatherogenic effects of L-arginine in the hypercholesterolemic rabbit. *J Clin Invest* 1992; 90:1168–1172.

40. Rossitch E Jr, Alexander E 3d, Black PM, Cooke JP. L-Arginine normalizes endothelial function in cerebral vessels from hypercholesterolemic rabbits. *J Clin Invest* 1991; 87:1295–1299.

41. Minor RL Jr, Myers P, Guerra R Jr, Bates JN, Harrison DG. Diet-induced atherosclerosis increases the release of nitrogen oxides from rabbit aorta. *J Clin Invest* 1990; 86:2109–2116.

42. Ohara Y, Peterson TE, Harrison DG. Hypercholesterolemia increases endothelial superoxide anion production. *J Clin Invest* 1993; 91:2546–2551.

43. Mugge A, Elwell JH, Peterson TE, Hofmeyer TG, Heistad DD, Harrison DG. Chronic treatment with polyethylene-glycolated superoxide dismutase partially restores endothelium-dependent vascular relaxations in cholesterol-fed rabbits. *Circ Res* 1991; 69:1293–1300.

44. Sundell CL, Marsden PA, Subramanian RR, Pollock JS, Harrison DG, Wilcox JN. Nitric oxide synthase is expressed by endothelial cells overlying human atherosclerotic plaques. *Circulation* 1992; 86:I-473.

45. Freiman PC, Mitchell GG, Heistad DD, Armstrong ML, Harrison DG. Atherosclerosis impairs endothelium-dependent vascular relaxation to acetylcholine and thrombin in primates. *Circ Res* 1986; 58:783–789.

46. Mizuno K, Stomura K, Miyamoto A, Arakawa K, Shibuya T, Arai T, et al. Angioscopic evaluation of coronary-artery thrombi in acute coronary syndromes. *N Engl J Med* 1992; 326:287–291.

47. Sherman CT, Litvack F, Grundfest W, Lee M, Hickey A, Chaux A, et al. Coronary angioscopy in patients with unstable angina pectoris. *N Engl J Med* 1986; 315:913–919.

48. Willerson JT, Yao SK, McNatt J, Benedict CR, Anderson HV, Golino P, et al. Frequency and severity of cyclic flow alternations and platelet aggregation predict the severity of neointimal proliferation following experimental coronary stenosis and endothelial injury. *Proc Natl Acad Sci USA* 1991; 88:10624–10628.

49. Pomerance A. Periarterial mast cells in coronary atheroma and thrombosis. *J Pathol Bacteriol* 1958; 76:55–70.

50. Sato T, Takebayashi S, Kohchi K. Increased subendothelial infiltration of the coronary arteries with monocytes/macrophages in patients with unstable angina. *Atherosclerosis* 1987; 68:191–197.

51. Kohchi K, Takebayashi S, Hiroki T, Nobuyoshi M. Significance of adventitial inflammation of the coronary artery in patients with unstable angina: Results at autopsy. *Circulation* 1985; 71:709–716.

52. Arbustini E, Grasso M, Diegoli M, Pucci A, Bramerio M, Ardissino D, et al. Coronary atherosclerotic plaques with and without thrombus in ischemic heart syndromes: A morphologic, immunohistochemical, and biochemical study. *Am J Cardiol* 1991; 68:36B–50B.

53. van der Wal AC, Becker AE, van der Loos CM, Das PK. Site of intimal rupture or erosion of thrombosed coronary atherosclerotic plaques is characterized by an inflammatory process irrespective of the dominant plaque morphology. *Circulation* 1994; 89(1):36–44.

54. Rajagopalan S, Meng XP, Ramasamy S, Harrison DG, Galis ZS. Reactive oxygen species produced by macrophage-derived foam cells regulate the activity of vascular matrix metalloproteinases in vitro. *J Clin Invest* 1996; 98:2572–2579.

55. Galis ZS, Sukhova GK, Lark MW, Libby P. Increased expression of matrix metalloproteinases and matrix degrading activity in vulnerable regions of human atherosclerotic plaques. *J Clin Invest* 1994; 94:2493–2503.

56. Richardson PD, Davies MJ, Born GV. Influence of plaque configuration and stress distribution of fissuring of coronary atherosclerotic plaques. *Lancet* 1989; 2:941–944.

57. Falk E. Unstable angina with fatal outcome: Dynamic coronary thrombosis leading to infarction and/or sudden death. Autopsy evidence of recurrent mural thrombosis with peripheral embolization culminating in total vascular occlusion. *Circulation* 1985; 71:699–708.

58. Palinski W, Yla-Herttuala S, Rosenfeld ME, Butler SW, Socher SA, Parthasarathy S, et al. Antisera and monoclonal antibodies specific for epitopes generated during oxidative modification of low density lipoprotein. *Arteriosclerosis* 1990; 10:325–335.

59. Salonen JT Yla-Herttuala S, Yamamoto R, Butler S, Korpela H, Salonen R, et al. Autoantibody against oxidised LDL and progression of carotid atherosclerosis. *Lancet* 1992; 339:883–887.

60. Spodick DH. Infection and infarction. Acute viral (and other) infection in the onset, pathogenesis and mimicry of acute myocardial infarction. *Am J Med* 1986; 81:661–668.

61. Saikku P, Leinonen M, Tenkanen L, Linnanmaki E, Ekman MR, Manninen V, et al. Chronic *Chlamydia pneumoniae* infections as a risk factor for coronary heart disease in the Helsinki Heart Study. *Ann Intern Med* 1992; 116:273–278.

62. Thom DH, Wang SP, Grayston JT, Siscovick DS, Stewart DK, Kronmal RA, et al. *Chlamydia pneumoniae* strain TWAR antibody and angiographically demonstrated coronary heart disease. *Arterioscler Thromb* 1991; 11:547–551.

63. Valtonen VV. Infection as a risk factor for infarction and atherosclerosis. *Ann Med* 1991; 23:539–543.

64. Berk BC, Weintraub WS, Alexander RW. Elevation of C-reactive protein in active coronary artery disease. *Am J Cardiol* 1990; 65:168–172.

65. Haverkate F, Thompson SG, Pyke SD. Gallimore JR, Pepys MB. Production of C-reactive protein and risk of coronary events in stable and unstable angina. European Concerted Action on Thrombosis and Disabilities Angina Pectoris Study Group. *Lancet* 1997; 349:462–466.

66. Serveri GG, Abbate R, Gori AM, Attanasio M, Martini F, Giusti B, et al. Transient intermittent lymphocyte activation is responsible for the instability of angina. *Circulation* 1992; 86:790–797.

67. Ganz W, Buchbinder N, Marcus H, Mondkar A, Maddahi J, Charuzi Y, et al. Intracoronary thrombolysis in evolving myocardial infarction. *Am Heart J* 1981; 101:4–13.

68. Hackett D, Davies G, Maseri A. Pre-existing coronary stenoses in patients with first myocardial infarction are not necessarily severe. *Eur Heart J* 1988; 9:1317–1323.

69. Little WC, Constantinescu M, Applegate RJ, Kutcher MA, Burrows MT, Kahl FR, et al. Can coronary angiography predict the site of a subsequent myocardial infarction in patients with mild to moderate coronary artery disease? *Circulation* 1988; 78:1157–1166.

70. Brown G, Albers JJ, Fisher LD, Schaefer SM, Lin JT, Kaplan C, et al. Regression of coronary artery disease as a result of intensive lipid-lowering therapy in men with high levels of apolipoprotein B. *N Engl J Med* 1990; 323:1289–1298.

71. Watts GF, Lewis B, Brunt JNH, Lewis ES, Coltart DJ, Smith LDR, et al. Effect on coronary artery disease of lipid-lowering diet, or diet plus cholestyramine, in the St. Thomas Atherosclerosis Regression Study (STARS). *Lancet* 1992; 339:563–569.

72. Harrison DG, Armstrong ML, Freiman PC, Heistad DD. Restoration of endothelium-dependent relaxation by dietary treatment of atherosclerosis. *J Clin Invest* 1987; 80:1808–1811.

45

DIAGNOSIS AND MANAGEMENT OF PATIENTS WITH CHRONIC ISCHEMIC HEART DISEASE

Robert C. Schlant / R. Wayne Alexander

Angina pectoris (literally "strangling" in the chest) is a recurrent symptom complex of discomfort in the chest or related areas associated with myocardial ischemia and dysfunction but without myocardial necrosis. Characteristically, the discomfort is produced by exertion and is promptly relieved by rest or nitroglycerin.

HISTORICAL PERSPECTIVE

There were references to what would be recognized today as angina pectoris, myocardial infarction, and sudden death in ancient Egyptian, Greek, Biblical, and Talmudic sources. In 1768 William Heberden presented his classic description of angina pectoris in a lecture before the Royal College of Physicians and it was published in 1772.[1]

This classic description was again published with additions and minor changes in a chapter entitled "Pectoris Dolor" in his *Commentaries on the History and Cure of Diseases,* which was translated from the Latin and published by his son, also called William Heberden, in 1802, a year after Heberden's death.[2] The following quotation is from his original lecture:

> There is a disorder of the breast, marked with strong and peculiar symptoms, considerable for the kind of danger belonging to it, and extremely rare, of which I do not recollect any mention among medical authors. The seat of it, and sense of strangling and anxiety with which it is attended, may make it not improperly be called angina pectoris. Those who are afflicted with it are seized, while they are walking, and more particularly when they walk soon after eating, with a painful and most disagreeable sensation in the breast, which seems as if it would take their life away, if it were to increase or to continue: the moment they stand still all this uneasiness vanishes. In all other respects the patients are at the beginning of this disorder perfectly well, and in particular have no shortness of breath, from which it is totally different.
>
> After it has continued some months, it will not cease so instantaneously upon standing still; and it will come on, not only when the persons are walking, but when they are lying down, and oblige them to rise up from their beds every night for many months together; and in one or two very inveterate cases it has been brought on by the motion of a horse or a carriage, and even by swallowing, coughing, going to stool or speaking, or by any disturbance of mind. I have heard once, and only one person, say that he had known it to attack him when he was up and standing still or sitting.
>
> But most, whom I have seen, have been perfectly unaffected with riding in any manner, with speaking, swallowing, laughing, sneezing, or vomiting. One has told me that his complaint was greatest in winter; another, that it was aggravated by warm weather; in the rest the seasons were not suspected of making any difference.
>
> I have observed something like this affection of the breast in one woman who was paralytic, and have heard one or two young men complain of it in a slight degree; but all the rest, whom I have seen, who are at least twenty, were men, and almost all above 50 years old, and most of them with a short neck, and inclining to be fat. When a fit of this sort

comes on by walking, its duration is very short, as it goes off almost immediately upon stopping. If it comes on in the night, it will last an hour or two; and I have met with one, in whom it once continued for several days, during all which time the patient seemed to be in imminent danger of death.

When I first took notice of this distemper, and could find no satisfaction from books, I consulted an able physician of long experience, who told me that he had known several ill of it, and that all of them had died suddenly. This observation I have reason to think is generally true of such patients; having known six of those, for whom I have been consulted, die in this manner; and more perhaps may have experienced the same death, which I had no opportunity of knowing.

But the natural tendency of this illness be to kill the patients suddenly, yet unless it have a power of preserving a person from all other ails, it will easily be believed that some of those, who are afflicted with it, may die in a different manner, since this disorder will last, as I have known it more than once, near twenty years, and most usually attacks only those who are above fifty years of age. I have accordingly observed one, who sunk under a lingering illness of a different nature.

The os sterni is usually pointed to as the seat of this malady, but it seems sometimes as if it was under the lower part of it, and at other times under the middle or upper part, but always inclining more to the left side, and sometimes there is with it a pain about the middle of the left arm. What the particular mischief is, which is referred to these different parts of the sternum, it is not easy to guess, and I have had no opportunity of knowing with certainty. It may be a strong cramp, or an ulcer, or possibly both.

For the interested reader, Leibowitz has published an excellent history of coronary heart disease.[3] The syndrome of angina pectoris was described as rare in textbooks of medicine in 1866 (Austin Flint) and 1892 (William Osler). P.D. White wrote that "(angina pectoris) was still uncommon in my early professional years. But when the automobile came in the 1920s and the population at large became more prosperous and over nourished, the current epidemic of coronary heart disease, as shown prevailingly by the symptom angina pectoris, began and incidentally involved younger and younger men."[4]

In the United States, the peak mortality rate from coronary heart disease (CHD) occurred about 1962 to 1965, since when it has been steadily decreasing.[5]

ETIOLOGY

Angina pectoris is caused by coronary atherosclerosis in the vast majority of patients (see Chaps. 39 to 44, 53). Many nonatherosclerotic causes of coronary artery disease (CAD)

(Tables 42-1 and 42-2) can also produce angina pectoris or myocardial infarction; these are discussed in Chap. 42. Other conditions particularly associated with angina pectoris include congenital coronary artery abnormalities (Chaps. 42 and 70), aortic stenosis (Chap. 63), mitral stenosis that produces severe right ventricular hypertension (Chap. 64), hypertrophic cardiomyopathy (Chap. 74), and systemic arterial hypertension (Chaps. 56 and 57).

Conditions in which angina occurs less often include aortic regurgitation (Chap. 63), idiopathic dilated cardiomyopathy and specific forms of heart muscle disease (Chaps. 73 and 76), and syphilitic heart disease. Mitral valve prolapse (Chap. 65) is rarely a cause of true angina pectoris. Many conditions may alter the myocardial oxygen supply-demand relationship and worsen angina pectoris, including severe anemia, tachycardia, fever, hyperthyroidism, hypothyroidism, and Paget's disease of bone. Many of these are associated with a high cardiac output.

CLASSIFICATION

The Canadian Cardiovascular Society Grading Scale (Table 10-2) is currently widely used to classify the severity of angina pectoris.[6]

DIAGNOSIS

Symptoms

Angina pectoris is classified as stable when its characteristics (frequency, severity, duration, time of appearance, and precipitating factors) have not changed for the previous 60 days. Angina pectoris ("angina") may be described by the patient using a variety of descriptors (Table 45-1). The discomfort is often not painful. The wide variety of terms used to describe the discomfort at times reflects the patients' cultural background and life experience.

Certain descriptors of discomfort suggest that the discomfort is not angina pectoris (Table 45-2).[7] Other important characteristics of angina pectoris include its precipitating factors, location, mode of onset and duration, and disappearance (see Chap. 10).

Classically, the discomfort of chronic stable angina pectoris is precipitated by physical activity, emotions, eating, or cold

---

TABLE 45-1

COMMON TERMS USED TO DESCRIBE ANGINA PECTORIS

Pressure	Uncomfortable	Ache
Tightness	Swelling	Weight
Heaviness	Burning	Heartburn
Constricting	Dull	Soreness
Compressing	Searing	Bursting
Fullness	Hard	Like a toothache
Choking	Strangling	Like a vise
Discomfort	Indigestion	

TABLE 45-2

DESCRIPTORS OF DISCOMFORT NOT LIKELY TO BE ANGINA PECTORIS

Needlelike	Shooting	Pricking
Sticking	Jabbing	Cutting
Stabbing	Twitching	Like an ice pick
Knifelike	Itching	
Stinging	Tingling	

weather. Some patients are able to describe fairly precisely the amount of exercise (length of walking or number of stairs) at which they reproducibly experience their discomfort. In some patients the amount of exertion that produces angina is much less in the morning soon after arising. Upper extremity exertion may induce angina, at times more readily than walking.

Angina may be precipitated by cold temperatures or cold wind, which may also be associated with a decrease in the duration of exercise before the onset of discomfort. Angina may also occur after meals (prandial or postprandial angina) due to the increase in cardiac output.[8,9]

Many patients with angina will have symptoms if they walk up a hill after a large meal with a cold wind blowing in their face. Emotions, particularly anger, excitation, and frustration, may also precipitate angina in patients with significant coronary atherosclerosis. Cigarette smoking can also precipitate or lower the exertion threshold for angina pectoris in some patients.[10,11]

In most patients, a combination of factors is present, and the amount of exertion associated with discomfort frequently varies. Very often, an episode occurs after performing a certain amount of a particular activity at a certain time of the day, but not while performing even more strenuous activity at another time of day (see below).

In most instances, stable angina pectoris develops and increases to a plateau over 10 to 30 s and usually disappears after several minutes if the exertion is discontinued. Occasionally, the angina will disappear despite physical activity, so-called walk-through angina. Most patients have discomfort that lasts a few minutes or up to 10 to 15 min and, rarely, up to 30 min. When discomfort is documented to last more than 15 min, one should have a strong suspicion that there may have been necrosis of at least a few myocytes, which may be too few to be diagnosed as myocardial infarction (see Chaps. 46 and 47).

Discomfort that is sharp and stabbing, like an ice pick, and that has a sudden onset and lasts a few seconds is usually not due to myocardial ischemia (Table 45-2).

The discomfort of angina is most often located substernally or just to the left of the sternum. Some patients clench their fist over their sternum (Levine's sign) as they describe their discomfort. This sign has a high diagnostic accuracy. Less often, angina is located over the precordium. It is unusual for the discomfort to be located only at the apex of the heart. It can be located anywhere from the epigastrium to the neck, and rarely it may be located only in the neck, throat, arm, or back. Some patients state that they have a "funny" or "different" feeling that they cannot describe further. It is very rare that angina pectoris is located only below the costal margin.

The discomfort of angina pectoris often radiates down the arms or to the neck, jaw, teeth, shoulders, or back. Radiation to the left side is more common than to the right, but both sides can be involved. The radiation is characteristically down the ulnar aspect of the arm; frequently, the radiation is described as a numbness. Increased heat or humidity may also lower the exertional threshold at which angina occurs.

Amphetamines and across-the-counter cold remedies, which may increase the arterial blood pressure and heart rate, may precipitate angina, as can cocaine, which can also increase heart rate and blood pressure and produce coronary artery vasoconstriction or thrombosis (see Chap. 80). Nocturnal angina is the occurrence of angina at night. In some patients it may be related to an increase in blood volume and cardiac output as the result of assuming the recumbent position. Other possible causes include dreaming, unrecognized tachycardia, or a marked decrease in systemic arterial blood pressure. Some patients who have nocturnal angina as a consequence of the increase in blood volume respond to therapy with digoxin and diuretics. In general, both nocturnal and rest angina are strongly suggestive of unstable angina pectoris, which usually requires a prompt and thorough evaluation (see Chap. 46).

Conditions that increase myocardial oxygen requirements may exacerbate the occurrence of angina pectoris and, occasionally, may be associated with angina in the absence of significant CAD on routine coronary arteriography.

Angina Equivalents

As noted below, patients with stable angina have many episodes of myocardial ischemia that are asymptomatic or silent. In addition, patients may have episodes of myocardial ischemia that result in symptoms from either systolic or diastolic left ventricular dysfunction but that are not associated with chest discomfort or symptoms characteristic of angina pectoris. Like other types of angina, "angina equivalent" symptoms usually are associated with exertion and are relieved by rest and nitroglycerin. The most common symptoms are: (1) exertional dyspnea, which is probably related to alterations in diastolic relaxation and compliance due to myocardial ischemia; and (2) exertional fatigue or exhaustion, which is probably related to an acute decrease in cardiac output related to decreased systolic left ventricular function and/or associated mitral regurgitation from transient papillary muscle dysfunction.

Myocardial ischemia results in a slowing of the isovolumic relaxation rate and an upward shift of the left ventricular diastolic pressure-volume relation, together with a variable degree of depression of systolic function and changes in end-systolic volume.[12–18]

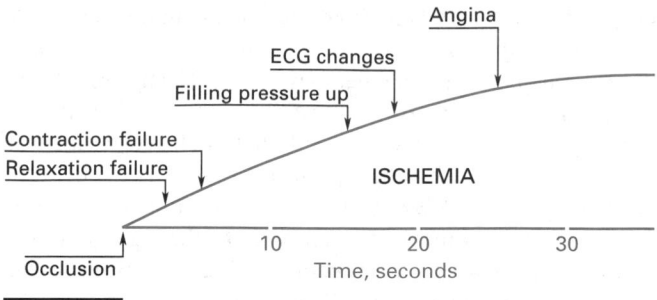

FIGURE 45-1

Appearance of events during transient coronary occlusion. (From Sigwart et al.[124] Reproduced with permission from the publisher and authors.)

In general, when myocardial ischemia is produced, diastolic dysfunction occurs before systolic dysfunction, which in turn often occurs prior to electrocardiographic (ECG) changes and before the symptom of angina pectoris (Fig. 45-1).

Patients with angina pectoris due to atherosclerosis have an increased frequency of the usual risk factors for atherosclerosis, including hypercholesterolemia, cigarette smoking, systemic arterial hypertension, diabetes mellitus, physical inactivity, and a family history of CAD in a parent or close relative before the age of 55. In women, the use of oral birth control pills and the postmenopausal state without estrogen replacement may contribute to the development and progression of atherosclerosis. These and other factors are discussed in Chaps. 41 and 53.

Physical Examination

During an attack of angina pectoris, many patients appear somewhat pale and quiet. They are frequently sweating. The heart rate and blood pressure are both often slightly elevated, and occasionally there are atrial or ventricular premature contractions. Abnormal systolic bulges may be present at the apex or at ectopic precordial areas.

A new gallop, usually an S_4 and occasionally an S_3, may be transiently present as well as an apical systolic murmur of mitral regurgitation from papillary muscle dysfunction.[19] Rarely, the second heart sound may demonstrate reversed splitting.[20,21]

A useful test to confirm the diagnosis in a patient experiencing discomfort is to perform carotid sinus massage for a few seconds while listening to the heart. If the patient experiences significant cardiac slowing, the physician should discontinue the massage and ask the patient whether the massage made the discomfort worse. If the patient replies "no" and adds that the massage made the discomfort go away, the diagnosis of angina pectoris is virtually established. On the other hand, if no slowing of the heart rate occurs, the test is indeterminate. Carotid sinus massage should not be performed until one has examined both carotid arteries for evidence of disease. In some patients, angina pectoris is relieved by performing a Valsalva maneuver, presumably by a decrease in myocardial oxygen requirements due to the decrease in left ventricular volume and wall stress produced by the decreased venous return. Patients with angina pectoris may have physical signs associated with hyperlipidemia, including arcus senilis, xanthelasma, and eruptive, tendon, and tuberous xanthomata (see Chap. 10).

Special Tests

INTRODUCTION

Most special tests in patients with suspected stable angina pectoris are performed either to establish the diagnosis or to obtain prognostic information.[22,23] In general, men with a history of classic angina pectoris have a higher probability of having significant CAD on coronary arteriography than do women.[24,25] The gender difference is even greater for patients with atypical angina pectoris. Table 45-3 and Fig. 45-2 provide

TABLE 45-3

PRETEST LIKELIHOOD OF CORONARY DISEASE ACCORDING TO AGE, SEX, AND SYMPTOMS[a,b]

Age, Years	Asymptomatic		Nonanginal Chest Pain		Atypical Angina		Typical Angina	
	Men	Women	Men	Women	Men	Women	Men	Women
35–45	0.037	0.007	0.105	0.027	0.428	0.155	0.809	0.454
	±0.024	±0.006	±0.063	±0.024	±0.144	±0.111	±0.104	±0.186
45–55	0.077	0.021	0.206	0.069	0.601	0.317	0.907	0.677
	±0.040	±0.018	±0.090	±0.051	±0.129	±0.160	±0.049	±0.167
55–65	0.111	0.054	0.282	0.127	0.690	0.465	0.939	0.839
	±0.049	±0.042	±0.100	±0.080	±0.106	±0.174	±0.029	±0.108
65–75	0.113	0.115	0.282	0.171	0.700	0.541	0.943	0.947
	±0.050	±0.078	±0.100	±0.097	±0.103	±0.169	±0.026	±0.057

[a] Each value represents the percentage ± standard error of the percentage.

[b] Assessment of anginal symptoms: (1) Is chest pain substernal? (2) Is it precipitated by exertion? (3) Is it relieved within 10 min by rest or nitroglycerin? Answers to three of three questions "yes" = typical angina. Answers to two of three questions "yes" = atypical angina. Answers to one of three questions "yes" = nonanginal chest pain. No complaints of chest discomfort above the diaphragm = asymptomatic.

Source: Adapted from Diamond GA: A clinically relevant classification of chest discomfort. *J Am Coll Cardiol* 1983; 1:574. Reproduced with permission from the author and the American College of Cardiology.

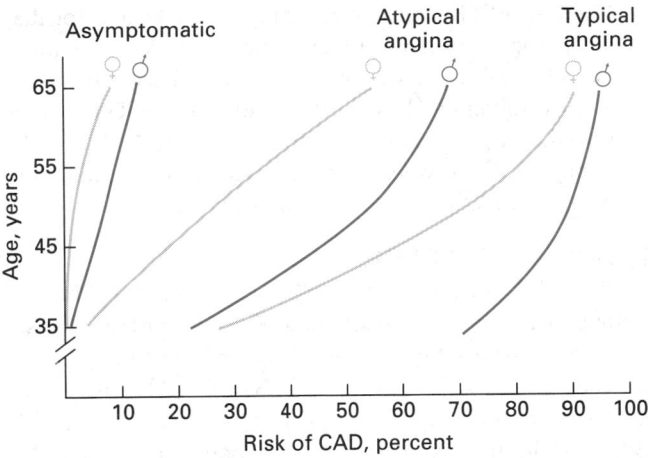

FIGURE 45-2

Influence of age, sex, and symptoms of coronary artery disease (CAD) derived from data of Diamond and Forrester.[24] (From Epstein SE. Implications of probability analysis on the strategy used for noninvasive detection of coronary artery disease. *Am J Cardiol* 1980; 46:491–499. Reproduced with permission from the publisher and author.)

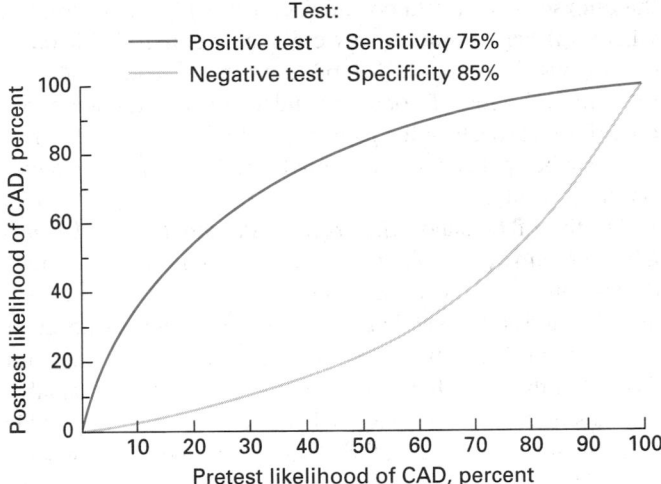

FIGURE 45-3

Influence of pretest likelihood of coronary artery disease (CAD) on the posttest likelihood of coronary artery disease. (From Epstein SE. Implications of probability analysis on the strategy used for noninvasive detection of coronary artery disease. *Am J Cardiol* 1980; 46:491–499. Reproduced with permission from the publisher and author.)

the likelihood for each gender by age and characteristics of the chest discomfort. They also illustrate one reason why women have more false-positive responses to ECG exercise testing than do men (see also Chap. 15). Table 45-4 provides a glossary of terms useful in the evaluation and selection of diagnostic tests. Bayes' theorem states that the pretest disease prevalence influences the posttest likelihood of significant CAD. This is illustrated in Fig. 45-3. In this figure, the posttest likelihood of CAD is plotted as a function of the pretest likelihood of disease, assuming that the test has a sensitivity

of 75 percent and a specificity of 85 percent, which are reasonable figures for ECG exercise testing. In many patients with known CAD, exercise testing is performed not for diagnostic but rather for prognostic purposes. Figure 45-4 illustrates the impact of Bayes' theorem when evaluating several diagnostic tests for coronary artery disease.

If one were to perform an exercise ECG test on a 55-year-old woman with atypical chest pain, with a pretest likelihood for coronary disease of 0.46, a positive test response would indicate her posttest likelihood to be 0.86. If she had a positive

TABLE 45-4

GLOSSARY OF TERMS

True positive (TP): Positive result in patient with disease
True negative (TN): Negative result in patient without disease
False positive (FP): Positive result in patient without disease
False negative (FN): Negative result in patient with disease

Sensitivity: $\dfrac{TP}{TP + FN}$

Specificity: $\dfrac{TN}{TN + FP}$

Predictive value of a positive test: $\dfrac{TP}{TP + FP}$

Predictive value of a negative test: $\dfrac{TN}{TN + FN}$

Bayes' theorem:

Probability of disease presence with a positive test =

$$\frac{\text{sensitivity} \times \text{prevalence}}{(\text{sensitivity} \times \text{prevalence}) + [(1 - \text{specificity}) \times (1 - \text{prevalence})]}$$

Probability of disease presence with a negative test =

$$\frac{(1 - \text{sensitivity}) \times \text{prevalence}}{[(1 - \text{sensitivity}) \times \text{prevalence}] + [\text{specificity} \times (1 - \text{prevalence})]}$$

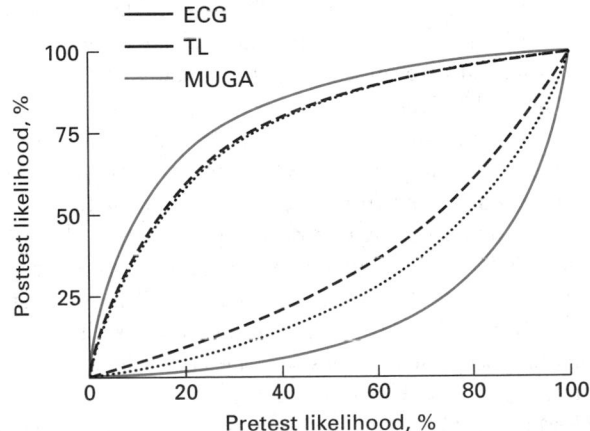

FIGURE 45-4

The use of Bayes' theorem in the diagnosis of coronary artery disease (ECG and radionuclide testing). The impact of exercise ECG, thallium (Tl), and ventriculographic (MUGA) test results as a function of pretest disease likelihood is shown. The curves above the line of identity represent positive test results. See text for additional discussion. (Adapted from Epstein SE: Implications of probability analysis on the strategy used for noninvasive detection of coronary artery disease. *Am J Cardiol* 1980; 46:491. Reproduced with permission from the publisher and author.)

thallium scan, her likelihood of disease would increase to 0.98, whereas if her thallium scan were negative, her likelihood of disease would decrease to 0.63. As long as additional tests meet the criterion of condition independence and are based on different aspects of the pathophysiologic process, this principle can be applied with additional tests to establish a diagnosis more firmly.

On the other hand, *diagnostic tests should only be performed to answer a specific clinical question.* From the above discussion, it should be apparent that a diagnostic test may be of limited additional diagnostic value in patients with either a very high (>0.80) or very (<0.20) low pretest risk for CAD. On the other hand, an exercise test may give valuable prognostic information, and nuclear scintigraphy may provide valuable information about the functional aspects of the coronary circulation.

EXERCISE-STRESS ELECTROCARDIOGRAPHY

Exercise-stress electrocardiography is the most widely applied test used to obtain objective evidence of myocardial ischemia and significant CAD. It is also employed to obtain prognostic data regarding ventricular performance in patients with known CAD.[26] See Chap. 15 for a more thorough discussion of exercise treadmill testing.

The sensitivity and specificity of exercise ECG testing have been stated to be 55 to 70 percent and 85 to 90 percent.[27] On the other hand, an extensive meta-analysis of 147 consecutive reports comparing exercise-induced ST depression with coronary arteriography in 24,074 patients found a wide variability in both sensitivity and specificity. The mean sensitivity was 68 percent [range, 23 to 100 percent; standard deviation (SD), 16 percent], and the mean specificity was 77 percent (range 17 to 100 percent; SD, 17 percent).[28,29]

Efforts to improve the clinical usefulness of exercise ECG testing in the diagnosis of CAD include development of a treadmill score[30,31] and a prognostic score and predicted 5-year survival determined from the amount of ST-segment depression, the degree of angina during exercise, and the duration of exercise (or equivalent).[32] Other techniques include the *ST/HR* slope (*ST* = ST-segment depression; *HR* = heart rate) calculated from linear regression of ST-segment depression against heart rate during peak exercise[33] and the simple *ST/HR* index in which additional ST-segment depression is divided by the overall change in *HR* throughout the exercise period.[34–36] To date none of these promising techniques has been clearly shown to be cost effective in daily practice.

Exercise ECG testing is of greatest diagnostic value in the evaluation of middle-aged men with atypical angina and a pretest probability of significant disease of 30 to 70 percent. Exercise ECG testing for diagnosis is somewhat more controversial when performed in women with typical or atypical angina; in men with atypical chest pain and complete right bundle branch block; in apparently healthy men more than 40 years old in special occupations (e.g., pilot, police officer, fire fighter, traffic controller); and in asymptomatic men with two or more major risk factors for coronary disease.

Exercise ECG testing is generally not indicated for diagnostic purposes in asymptomatic men and women who are apparently healthy or who have marginal chest pain.[37]

The overall clinical usefulness of exercise ECG testing for diagnostic purposes has been well reviewed.[24–26,28,29,38–41] It is relatively safe when performed using established guidelines and precautions[37,42] (see also Chap. 15).

RADIONUCLIDE SCINTIGRAPHY

Radionuclide techniques are discussed in detail in Chap. 17. Although it is more expensive, stress myocardial perfusion imaging provides higher sensitivity and specificity for the diagnosis of CAD than exercise ECG testing.[43–49] It may also be less dependent upon the level of exercise achieved.[50,51] Some of the findings that indicate a poor prognosis include an increased lung thallium 201 uptake, extensive perfusion defects, and postexercise transient left ventricular dilatation.[52–54] In general, a normal thallium-201 perfusion scan indicates that the likelihood of the patient experiencing a cardiac event is similar to the likelihood of the general population, even if the patient has known CAD.[51,55,56]

Pharmacologic stress testing, usually using dipyridamole, dobutamine, or adenosine, and thallium 201 can be employed in patients unable to exercise because of peripheral vascular disease, poor exercise tolerance, arthritis, neurologic disorders, or other contraindications. Stress perfusion scintigraphy is useful in the study of selected patients with chronic stable angina, patients with suspected CAD prior to noncardiac surgery (Chap. 83), or patients following myocardial infarction.[57–62] The use of technetium 99m sestamibi and other new agents may significantly improve imaging capabilities, particularly if they are used in combination with thallium 201[63] (see Chap. 17).

POSITRON EMISSION TOMOGRAPHY

Positron emission tomography (PET) promises to be even more accurate than standard thallium 201 single-photon emission computed tomography (SPECT) for the detection of CAD. It may also provide an estimate of coronary blood flow and coronary flow reserve as well as myocardial viability[64–66] (see Chap. 20).

Patients with stable angina may have persistent defects on 3-h redistribution imaging with thallium-201. About 30 to 40 percent of such patients may show improved perfusion and function after revascularization.[67] Viability can also be assessed using technetium 99m methoxyisobutyl isonitrile (99m Tc sestamibi) or PET with fluorine-18, 2-deoxyglucose.[68]

RADIONUCLIDE ANGIOGRAPHY

Radionuclide angiography, with the determination of peak exercise ejection fraction, is also useful for the diagnosis of CAD, although the presence of irregular heart rhythms, left bundle branch block, or marked left ventricular dysfunction limits its diagnostic value[69] (see also Chap. 17).

ECHOCARDIOGRAPHY

Transthoracic, Doppler, transesophageal, and stress echocardiography (Chap. 14) and intravascular ultrasound (Chap. 49) are all useful in the assessment of one or more subsets of patients with CAD. Routine echocardiography provides a good estimate of ventricular size and of regional and generalized left ventricular wall motion. This can be performed at rest, during exercise, or immediately afterwards.[70] Either routine or Doppler echocardiography can also be performed during or following pharmacologic stress with dobutamine, dipyridamole, or adenosine.[71–76] If adequate images can be obtained, exercise echocardiography has been reported to be comparable to radionuclide testing for the evaluation of CAD[66] (see Chap. 14).

CORONARY ARTERIOGRAPHY

It is controversial whether or not all patients with stable angina pectoris should undergo coronary arteriography. Some physicians routinely have cardiac catheterization and coronary arteriography performed to obtain an estimate of left ventricular regional and generalized wall motion and an evaluation of the extent and location of CAD. Other physicians are more selective and obtain coronary arteriography only if the diagnosis is in doubt or if revascularization by coronary artery bypass surgery (CABS) or coronary angioplasty is contemplated.

In general, patients whose symptoms are well controlled by medications and who have a good exercise tolerance are less likely to benefit significantly from revascularization. The authors tend toward earlier cardiac catheterization in many patients since exercise ECG, radionuclide, and echocardiographic testing may not always properly identify patients who are good candidates for revascularization.

DIFFERENTIAL DIAGNOSIS

Table 45-5 lists the differential diagnosis of angina pectoris. In most instances, the distinction is clear if one is able to obtain an accurate history and perform a complete physical examination.

TABLE 45-5

DIFFERENTIAL DIAGNOSIS OF ANGINA PECTORIS

Cardiovascular
  Myocardial ischemia
    Coronary atherosclerosis
    Coronary vasospasm
    Congenital coronary artery disease
      Anomalous origin
      Aberrant coronary artery
      Coronary arteriovenous fistula
    Kawasaki's disease
    Small vessel disease
    Microvascular angina (syndrome X)
    Systemic arterial hypertension
    Hypertrophic cardiomyopathy
    Idiopathic dilated cardiomyopathy
    Aortic valve disease
    Coronary artery dissection
      (Marfan's syndrome)
    Pulmonary hypertension
    Right ventricular hypertension
    Chronic obstructive pulmonary
      disease
    Syphilitic aortitis, coronary ostial
      disease
    Collagen-vascular disease
      Periarteritis nodosa
      Systemic lupus erythematosus
      Rheumatoid arthritis
    Cardiac amyloid
    Cardiac tumors
    Hereditary connective tissue
      disorders
      Pseudoxanthoma elasticum
      Cystic medial necrosis
      Homocystinuria
      Gargoylism

    Severe anemia, hypoxia
    High-dose x-irradiation
    Withdrawal from chronic
      nitroglycerin exposure
  Nonmyocardial ischemia
    Aortic dissection
    Discrete thoracic aortic aneurysm
    Mitral valve prolapse
    Tachycardia, bradycardia
    Palpitations
    Pericarditis
Thoracic-respiratory
  Pulmonary embolism, infarction
  Pneumothorax
  Pneumomediastinum (mediastinal
    emphysema)
  Pleuritis
  Epidemic pleurodynia (Bornholm's
    disease)
  Mediastinitis
  Intrathoracic malignancy
  Café Coronary
Gastrointestinal
  Gastroesophageal reflux, esophagitis
  Esophageal spasm
  Esophageal rupture (Mallory-Weiss
    syndrome; Boerhaave's syndrome)
  Esophageal impaction
  Hiatal hernia
  Cholecystitis, gallstones
  Gastritis
  Peptic ulcer disease
  Pancreatitis
  Splenic infarction
  Splenic flexure syndrome
Neuromuscular/skeletal

Chest wall pain
Costochondritis (Tietze's syndrome)
Cervical or thoracic degenerative
  arthritis, nerve compression,
  radiculopathy
    Cervical vertebral disk
    Intercostal neuralgia
Thoracic outlet (scalenus anticus)
  syndrome
Shoulder arthropathies
    Shoulder hand syndrome
Fibromyalgia (myofascial pain
  syndrome; fibromyositis)
    Pectoral, intercostal, serratus anterior
    Precordial catch syndrome
Cardiac causalgia
Bursitis
Superficial thrombophlebitis of thoracic
  veins (Mondor's syndrome)
Xiphoidalgia
Diaphragmatic flutter
Neurocutaneous
  Herpes zoster
Breast
  Pendulous breast syndrome
  Brassiere syndrome
Psychologic
  Anxiety
  Hyperventilation
  Panic attacks
  Depression
  Self-gain
  Munchhausen syndrome

Patients with hypertensive or valvular heart disease may have chest pain that is located at the apex rather than substernally and that is often associated with hyperesthesia of the left breast or precordium. Some patients with functional heart disease have apical pain that often occurs at rest. Chest wall pain, cervical arthritis, and subdeltoid bursitis can occur with exertion and be relieved by rest. It should be emphasized that not infrequently patients will have more than one type of chest discomfort. See Chap. 10 for a discussion of the differential diagnosis of chest pain.

PATHOPHYSIOLOGY

In patients with stable angina pectoris due to atherosclerotic CAD, there is little correlation between the severity and extent of the atherosclerosis and the severity of angina symptoms. There is also no apparent correlation between the location of the angina discomfort and the location of the myocardial ischemia. Women have angina as the initial manifestation of CHD more often than men, who commonly have acute myocardial infarction. The pathology of coronary atherosclerosis is discussed in detail in Chap. 40. The nonatherosclerotic causes of CHD are discussed in Chap. 42.

The fundamental feature of ischemic heart disease is the imbalance between the supply of coronary blood flow and the metabolic demands of the myocardium. This imbalance may be manifested episodically as angina pectoris or arrhythmias or chronically as congestive heart failure. The clinical evidence of ischemia is exhibited when myocardial demand exceeds the capacity of the coronary arteries to deliver an adequate supply of oxygen. In normal hearts there is excess capacity on the supply side so that ischemia does not occur even with very vigorous exercise.[77]

The presence of disease in either the epicardial coronary arteries or in the coronary microvasculature may result in imbalance between supply and demand at even modest levels of exercise. Understanding the determinants of coronary blood supply and myocardial metabolic demand is important in the management of chronic ischemic heart disease.

Myocardial Oxygen Demand

The major, clinically relevant determinants of oxygen demand are heart rate, contractility, and systolic wall tension (Table 3-2 and Fig. 45-5). A detailed discussion of the major and minor determinants of demand is presented in Chap. 3. Heart rate is one of the most important determinants of myocardial oxygen consumption $(M\dot{V}_{O_2})$[78] and is the one that is most easily manipulated pharmacologically in most patients.

Myocardial contractility, which is reflected in the rate of change of pressure (dP/dt), is a major determinant of oxygen consumption that is ordinarily not an important direct target for therapeutic manipulation. On the other hand, systolic wall tension is frequently an important factor in therapeutic considerations.

Systolic wall tension is directly related to the left ventricular systolic pressure and radius and inversely related to wall thickness. It follows that oxygen consumption can be decreased by decreasing systolic pressure and afterload. Reduction of preload through venodilation and thus of left ventricular distension and oxygen consumption is one of the important mechanisms for the therapeutic efficacy of nitrates in angina pectoris (see below). Positive inotropic agents may actually decrease oxygen consumption in patients with enlarged ventricles because the effects of decreasing radius may outweigh those of increasing contractility.

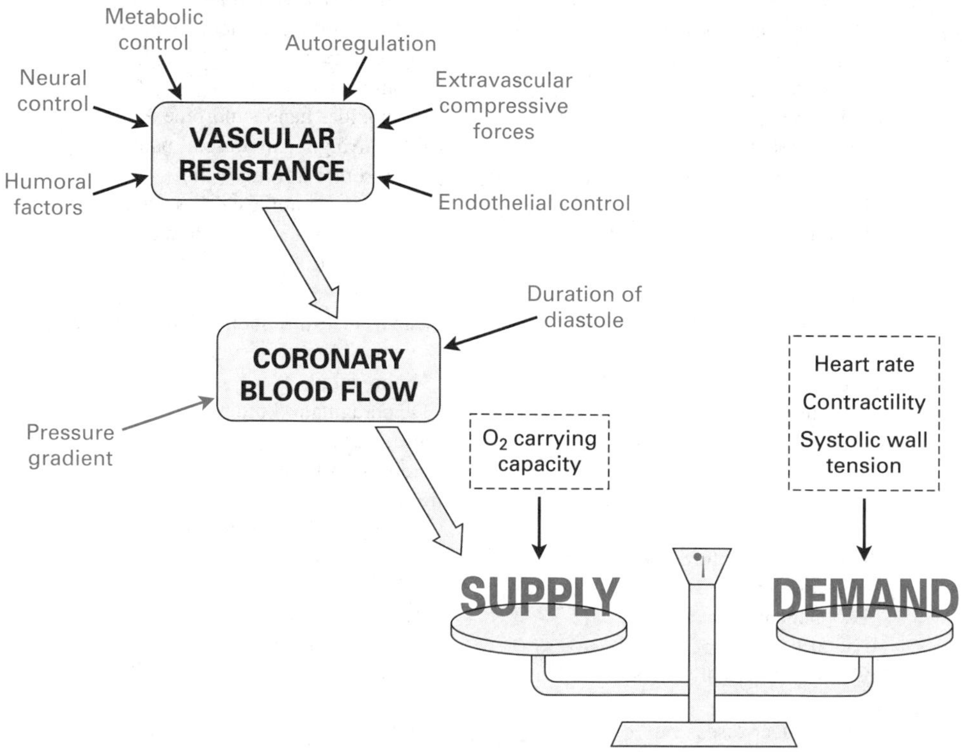

Myocardial Oxygen Supply

Oxygen supply to the myocardium is dependent upon the oxygen-carrying capacity of the blood and on blood flow. Decreased oxygen-carrying capacity may contribute to the development or exacerbation of myocardial ischemia in severe

FIGURE 45-5
Factors controlling myocardial oxygen supply and demand. (From Ardehali and Ports.[83] Modified with permission from the author and publisher.)

anemia. Most commonly, however, ischemia related to oxygen supply results from compromised coronary blood flow.

Normally the arteriolar resistance vessels are the primary regulators of myocardial blood flow since the epicardial arteries are low-resistance conduits. Narrowing of the large coronary arteries transiently by vasospasm or permanently by structural changes, as in atherosclerosis, may cause the development of resistance that is high enough to restrict blood flow. Until relatively recently, consideration of the factors limiting blood supply in ischemic heart disease has focused on the epicardial coronaries.

There has been increasing appreciation in ischemic disease of a pathophysiologic role of the microvasculature,[79,80] either concomitantly with atherosclerotic narrowing of the large-conduit arteries or predominantly, in anginal syndromes with normal epicardial arteries (syndrome X—discussed subsequently).[81,82]

The determinants of myocardial blood flow are relatively complex[83] and include: (1) metabolic control, (2) autoregulation, (3) extravascular compressive forces, (4) duration of diastole, (5) humoral agents composed of both circulating hormones and autocrine and paracrine factors produced within the arterial wall and in particular by the endothelium, (6) neural control, and (7) the pressure difference between aortic diastolic pressure and right atrial pressure. The factors controlling myocardial blood flow are depicted in Fig. 45-5. For a more complete discussion see Chaps. 3 and 43.

Myocardial blood flow is matched closely with myocardial work and metabolism.[78] The molecular mechanisms involved have not been completely defined but likely include adenosine, a degradation product of ATP that is released into the interstitium and is a potent dilator of microvessels[84,85] (see also Chaps. 3 and 43).

Myocardial blood flow is relatively constant (autoregulated) over a range of perfusion pressures between 60 and 160 mmHg.[86] Below a perfusion pressure of about 60 mmHg, vasodilator reserve is consumed and blood flow is directly related to perfusion pressure. Experimentally, loss of vasodilator reserve occurs distal to lesions with an 85 percent decrease in diameter.[87] A decrease in coronary blood flow, presumably due to vasoconstriction and loss of vasodilator reserve, has been observed in spite of an increase in blood pressure in response to cold pressor stimulation in patients with significant CAD.[88]

Extravascular compressive forces, including intrapericardial, intramyocardial, and intraventricular pressures, are important in the control of coronary blood flow and account for 30 to 50 percent of vascular resistance.[89] Since the intramyocardial and intraventricular pressures are maximal during systole and are exerted maximally on the subendocardium, the effects on blood flow are greatest on subendocardial vessels. Left ventricular subendocardial blood flow ceases during systole.[90] *Thus, the subendocardial blood flow is most vulnerable in any circumstance in which total blood flow is decreased or in which metabolic demands are increased and blood flow is limited.* Because of the systolic compressive forces, the subendocardium is also critically dependent on the duration of diastole for its blood flow (see also Chap. 3).

The coronary circulation is regulated by systemic hormonal influences and by neural control mechanisms that are not dissimilar from those in other vascular beds. Angiotensin II is a vasoconstrictor, and β-adrenergic agonists dilate and α-adrenergic agonists constrict coronary arteries, although there are some regional differences in distribution of receptors in vessels of different sizes. Very importantly, however, the integrated vasomotor response to the various vasoactive stimuli impinging upon a coronary artery or arteriole appears to be determined to a great extent by the functional state of the endothelium (see also Chaps. 4 and 44).

Endothelial Function and Coronary Vasomotor Control

The phenomenon of endothelial-dependent relaxation[91] and the identification of endothelial-derived relaxing factor as nitric oxide[92] are discussed in detail in Chap 4. The defect in endothelial-dependent dilatation in atherosclerotic epicardial coronary arteries with either advanced or minimally stenotic lesions that vasoconstrict in response to stimuli that are normally vasodilatory, such as acetylcholine, exercise, or cold pressure testing, is discussed in Chap. 44, as is the role of dysfunctional endothelium in both the stable and unstable coronary syndromes.

The prevailing view is that in nondiseased epicardial coronary arteries endothelial-dependent vasodilator mechanisms are predominant. Thus, interventions such as exercise,[93–97] mental stress,[98–100] cold pressor testing,[101,102] or even pacing-induced tachycardia,[103] which normally induce increases in $M\dot{V}_{O_2}$ and flow, are associated with epicardial dilatation that is, at least in part, endothelial-dependent. The presence of even nonocclusive, early atherosclerosis as well as of more advanced stenoses appears to attenuate this vasodilator mechanism and to result in the predominance of constrictor forces.

In illustration of this point, local infusion of the α-adrenergic agonist phenylephrine does not constrict normal coronary arteries of patients with intact endothelial-dependent dilatation.[104] In patients with even minimally diseased coronary arteries, however, constriction occurs at low concentrations of phenylephrine. Thus, in CAD there appears to be not only loss of endothelial-dependent dilatation but also enhanced vasoconstrictor sensitivity to catecholamines. This disordered vasomotor control is almost certainly an important contributor to the variability in anginal threshold that is seen commonly in many patients; it has been called *mixed angina* because it is felt to involve both high-grade stenoses and variable vasoconstrictor activity.[105] (It is discussed in more detail subsequently.)

Moderate vasoconstriction of a minimal stenosis may have little hemodynamic importance, whereas the same degree of vasoconstriction on a higher grade stenosis may markedly decrease blood flow and induce ischemia.

The Microvasculature and Coronary Ischemia

The realization of the potential importance of the coronary microvascular resistance vessels in the pathogenesis of angina pectoris developed from studies of patients with angina-like chest pain and angiographically normal epicardial coronary arteries.[106–114]

The coronary etiology of the chest pain was reenforced by the observations that a number of these patients had evidence of ischemia upon provocative exercise testing.[115] Many of these patients were eventually found to have abnormal vasodilator reserve.[116] Recent observations have implicated endothelial abnormalities in the disordered microvascular responses. Thus, in patients with angina and angiographically normal coronary arteries, endothelial-dependent vasodilatation of the resistance arteries, as reflected in the responses of blood flow to infusion of the endothelial-dependent vasodilator acetylcholine, was diminished relative to controls.[117]

In contrast, the flow responses to the nonendothelial-dependent dilators isosorbide dinitrate and papaverine were not different between patients and controls, suggesting that the intrinsic vasodilator capacity of the resistance arteries was not defective. Similar defects in endothelial-dependent increases in coronary flow have been observed in cardiac hypertrophy associated with hypertension, another condition that may be associated with angina pectoris but with angiographically normal epicardial coronaries.[118]

Morphologic data derived from analysis of biopsy specimens from patients with normal epicardial coronaries but with anginal syndromes are consistent with structural changes in the microvasculature that may reflect the observed functional abnormalities. In these patients there was capillary narrowing, with swollen endothelium encroaching on the lumen as well as decreased capillary density.[119]

Taken together, these data are consistent with the notion that the coronary microvasculature can develop dysfunction of vasomotor control mechanisms and, in particular, of endothelial-dependent vasodilatation that may become clinically significant in the setting of increased demand or $M\dot{V}_{O_2}$. In this case, loss of vasodilator reserve and/or the actual constriction of resistance arterioles might induce ischemia and chest pain.

Spectrum of Pathophysiologic Mechanisms Associated with the Stable Coronary Ischemic Syndromes

Symptomatic coronary ischemia associated with predominantly microvascular abnormalities in control of tone likely represents, pathophysiologically, one end of the spectrum of the anginal syndromes. Again pectoris or anginal equivalents, with a rather constant threshold for inducing symptoms that likely results from a fixed stenosis of an epicardial coronary, can be viewed as the other end of the spectrum. In between lie most patients who have a threshold for inducing angina that is somewhat variable from day to day or even at different times of the day, as discussed subsequently.

For example, the same activity that produces angina in the early morning may not do so in the afternoon or evening. These same patients may have a reproducible exercise level for inducing ischemia on formal exercise testing because of the increased myocardial oxygen consumption resulting from increases in heart rate, contractility, and blood pressure, which is associated with an increase in wall tension. This apparent paradox is explained by the presence of flow-limiting epicardial stenosis or stenoses and the concomitant association of episodic vasoconstriction.

This clinical scenario has been termed *mixed angina* by Maseri et al.[105] These patients have ischemia induced by both an increase in demand and a decrease in flow. The site(s) of vasoconstriction may be at an epicardial stenosis, in the microvasculature, or at both locations.[120] The concept of a variable flow reserve that interacts with differing metabolic demands to produce intermittent ischemia is depicted in Fig. 45-6. Variability of the flow reserve is undoubtedly a major contributor to a phenomenon such as the precipitation of angina by an activity that, even when repeated soon thereafter, subsequently does not cause angina.

A classic example is of the golfer who develops angina on the first or second hole and later, after resolution of the episode, can complete the round free of pain. Although loss or attenuation of endothelial-dependent vasodilator mechanisms is undoubtedly an important substrate permitting expression of vasoconstrictor stimuli, the predominant vasoconstrictors have not been identified.

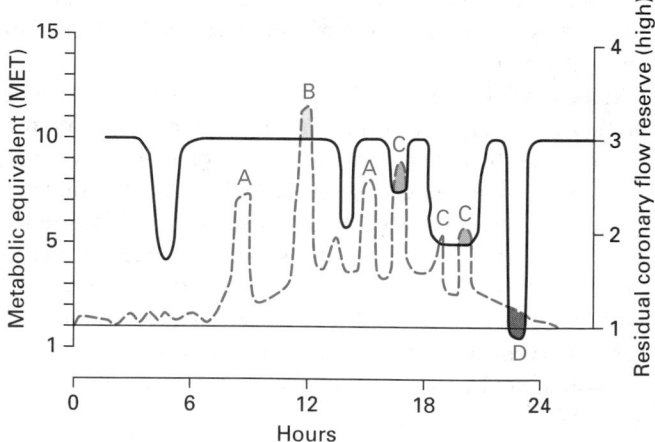

FIGURE 45-6

Concept of variable coronary flow reserve in presence of variable atherosclerotic obstruction. A: Episodes not associated with ischemia; B: ischemic episode occurring at levels of exercise exceeding threshold of residual coronary flow reserve; C: ischemic episodes occurring at lower levels of exercise when residual coronary flow is reduced; D: ischemic episodes occurring at rest in presence of maximal reduction in residual coronary flow reserve; (—) residual coronary flow reserve; (- - -) variable atherosclerotic obstruction, as measured by MET. (From Cohn PF. Mechanisms of myocardial ischemia. *Am J Cardiol* 1992; 70:14G–18G. Adapted from Maseri A. Role of coronary artery spasm in symptomatic and silent myocardial ischemia. *J Am Coll Cardiol* 1987; 9:249–262. Reproduced with permission from the authors and publishers.)

In the stable anginal syndromes these are likely neural and hormonal, whereas in the unstable syndromes platelet and coagulation products and inflammatory mediators are thought to be additional contributors. Patients with predominantly vasoconstrictor pathophysiology in an epicardial vessel have been classified as having vasospastic angina. Many of these patients may have unstable angina or Prinzmetal's variant angina (see Chap. 46).

Cellular Bases for the Clinical Manifestations of Ischemia

The cellular effects of myocardial ischemia are discussed in detail in Chaps. 43 and 47. The rapid decreases in systolic function and diastolic compliance that are associated with creatine phosphate depletion and ionic shifts will increase end-diastolic pressure. This pressure increase may be reflected in the pulmonary vascular pressures and may ultimately stimulate mechanoreceptors mediating dyspneic responses. Dyspnea may be an associated symptom with angina or may be present as an anginal equivalent in patients who do not develop pain.

The metabolic abnormalities induced by ischemia lead to cellular depolarization and the flow of electrical currents between normal and ischemic areas that are reflected on the ECG. ST-segment depression reflecting subendocardial hypoperfusion is the most common ECG manifestation of ischemia in chronic, stable angina during ambulatory monitoring or exercise testing.[121] Somewhat surprisingly, the electrical inhomogeneity inferred by ST-segment depression observed during exercise testing or ambulatory monitoring is not commonly associated with ventricular arrhythmias, especially of the complex or life-threatening type.[122]

Exercise-induced ventricular ectopic activity is not a reliable predictor of cardiac events in asymptomatic persons.[123]

Sequence of Events during Coronary Ischemia

Studies in which hemodynamic and ECG monitoring have been performed during spontaneous episodes of ischemia, usually in unstable patients or during balloon inflation at angioplasty, have provided insights into the sequential responses evoked at the onset of ischemia.

After balloon inflation, as implied above, relaxation failure or a decrease in compliance is the earliest event, occurring within seconds, and is followed by contractile dysfunction with a decrease in ejection fraction of up to one-third within 10 s.[124] ECG changes occur at about 20 s, and angina, if it occurs, does so beyond 25 s. These sequential events are depicted in Fig. 45-1.

It is implicit from considering this sequence that there are likely to be ischemic episodes that do not progress to angina. Since there are many patients who do not perceive coronary ischemic pain or have high pain thresholds, it follows that there is likely to be a substantial frequency of asymptomatic (silent) ischemia in the population with CAD. This, in fact, is the case, as will be discussed subsequently.

The various studies of patients with spontaneous or exercise-induced ischemia that have included hemodynamic and ECG monitoring have provided insights into and confirmed assumptions about the physiologic basis for a number of classic clinical observations about angina.

For example, as noted above, an anginal attack may be associated with new physical findings, including the development of an atrial gallop, systolic bulging of the precordium, mitral regurgitation due to papillary muscle dysfunction, and paradoxical splitting of the second sound. The atrial gallop reflects diastolic dysfunction and decreased compliance, while the remaining features reflect systolic dysfunction, including prolonged left ventricular ejection time accounting for the paradoxical splitting.

In addition, the crescendo-decrescendo nature of anginal pain, which is one of its most important differentiating characteristics, is reflected in the crescendo-decrescendo pattern of the development and resolution of ischemic ST-segment changes and elevations of left ventricular filling pressure during exercise-induced angina.

Circadian Rhythm of Coronary Ischemia

The incidence of myocardial infarction is highest in the morning in the first few hours after awakening.[125] Similarly, as many clinicians have observed, the threshold for precipitating anginal attacks in patients with stable angina appears to be lowest in the morning. Patients are more likely to develop ST-segment depression and angina at lower thresholds during exercise testing in the morning than in the afternoon.[126]

Studies with ambulatory ECG monitoring have confirmed that the incidence of both painful and painless episodes of ST-segment depression is highest in the morning[127] (Fig. 45-7) and, in particular, in the first few hours after awakening (Fig. 45-8).

The diurnal variation in ischemic threshold is likely related to endogenous rhythms of catecholamine secretion, which are highest in the morning, and to sensitivity to coronary vasoconstrictors, which appears to be highest in the morning since the dilating response to nitroglycerin is highest in patients at this time of day.[128] The increase in sympathetic nervous system activity is associated with increases in heart rate, blood pressure, and contractility. Taken together with the myocardial demands associated with activities of daily living, these various factors may converge to cause the morning increase in ischemic episodes.[129,130]

The lowered morning anginal threshold has important therapeutic implications. A decrease in the frequency of ischemia can be achieved by blunting of the morning surge of β-adrenergic stimulation with beta blockers chosen and administered in a manner to provide adequate pharmacologic effects in the morning. Furthermore, in patients with rather predictable morning angina, the use of nitroglycerin (TNG) soon after awakening may be useful in preventing angina in many instances.

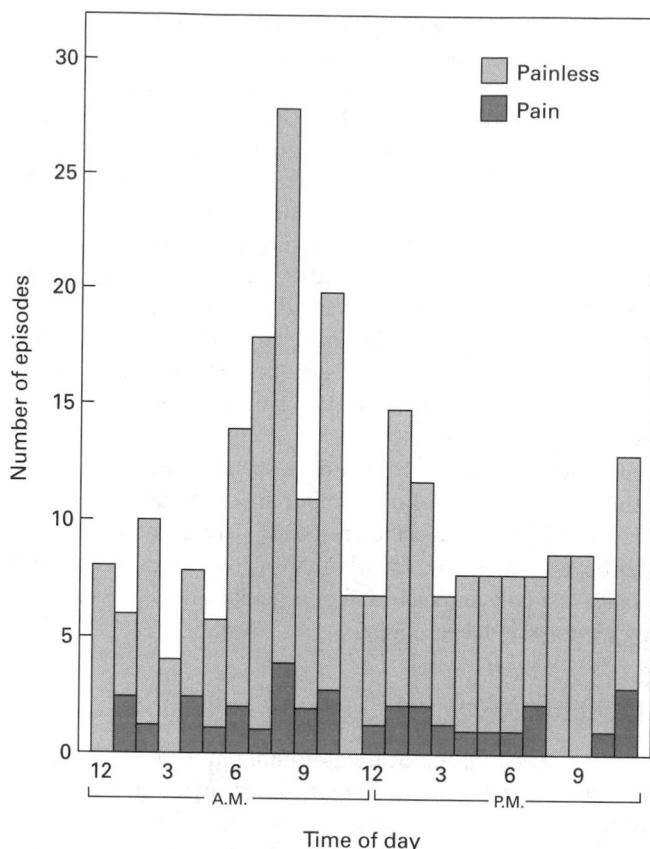

FIGURE 45-7

The hourly frequency of episodes of ischemic ST-segment depression in 24 patients with coronary disease monitored off therapy is greatest at 8 A.M. (From Rocco et al.[127] Reproduced with permission from the publisher and authors.)

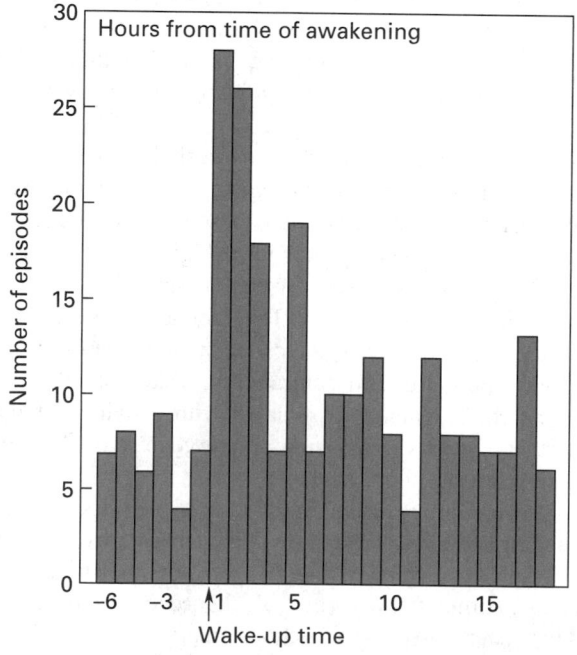

FIGURE 45-8

When the frequency of episodes is displayed hourly from the time of awakening, the peak activity occurs in the first and second hour after arising. (From Rocco et al.[127] Reproduced with permission from the publisher and authors.)

Mechanisms of Anginal Pain

Anginal pain may be a very useful warning system, although it is frequently insufficiently sensitive. Pain stimuli arise within the myocardium and most likely stimulate free nerve endings in the vicinity of small coronary vessels.[127] Impulses travel in afferent unmyelinated or small myelinated cardiac sympathetic nerves through the upper five thoracic sympathetic ganglia to dorsal horn cells and through the spinothalamic tract to the thalamus and then to the cortex.[131]

There is thought to be integration and modulation of these impulses at several levels including the cerebral cortex. This modulation may also contribute importantly to the variability in anginal threshold alluded to previously. At the cortical level, psychosocial and cultural factors may modulate the perception of pain.

The radiation patterns of angina are determined by the levels of the thoracic spinal cord that share the sensory inputs from the heart and from somatic structures. It was proposed that radiation of angina to the neck and jaw might be via vagal afferents, since this radiation pattern became more prominent after thoracic sympathectomy when this procedure was used to treat refractory angina.[132] This supposition has been challenged.[116]

The nature of the stimuli causing angina has been difficult to delineate. The causes are almost certainly chemical, and a number of candidate molecules including kinins, serotonin, hydrogen ions, and inflammatory mediators have been proposed. The usual lack of an association of, for example, inflammatory myocarditis either with pain in general or with anginal type pain specifically has directed attention away from inflammatory mediators. Substance P has been implicated as a potential cause of angina but does not provoke chest pain when infused into humans.[133]

On the other hand adenosine, which is increased during ischemia, has been shown to cause anginal type pain during intravenous infusion in normal volunteers.[134] The definitive nature of the stimuli causing anginal pain remains to be determined.

ASYMPTOMATIC (SILENT) ISCHEMIA IN STABLE CORONARY ARTERY DISEASE

The presence of clinically silent ischemic heart disease has intrigued physicians for decades, and the presence of unrecognized myocardial infarction was commented upon by Herrick in 1912.[135] The presence of extensive coronary disease and myocardial infarction at autopsy of apparently asymptomatic persons was emphasized subsequently.[136] Direct evidence of asymptomatic silent ischemia during exercise testing[137,138] or during ambulatory monitoring[139] heightened interest in the subject.[140,141]

Prevalence

Asymptomatic ischemic episodes may be present in patients across the spectrum of the ischemic coronary syndromes from stable to unstable angina or after myocardial infarction and may be observed in patients who are totally asymptomatic or are symptomatic with some episodes of ischemia but not with others.[142] Evidence suggests that silent ischemic episodes are present in virtually all patients with active unstable angina and in 36 to 38 percent of patients with stable, effort angina or in those with a remote (greater than 4 weeks previously) history of instability.[143] Cohn has estimated the prevalence in an adult population of asymptomatic CAD of an extent capable of inducing ischemia at approximately 5 percent.[144] ST-segment depression on ambulatory monitoring is rare in patients with proven absence of CAD[145] but has been reported to be more common in a general population, raising questions about the use of ambulatory monitoring as a screening mechanism.[141,146]

A prospective study of 68-year-old men with a 9.9 percent and a 6.6 percent prevalence of a history of angina pectoris or myocardial infarction, respectively, reported that 25 percent exhibited ST-segment depression on ambulatory ECG monitoring.[147] Ninety two percent of the "ischemic" episodes were asymptomatic. ST-segment depression was associated with increased cardiovascular risk, as discussed subsequently.

The true prevalence of silent ischemia is difficult to discern in the population and will obviously depend on age and the presence and activity of CAD. In the presence of CAD, however, it is apparent that episodes of asymptomatic ischemia are often more common than are painful episodes.[148]

Pathophysiology

Imbalance between coronary blood supply and myocardial oxygen demand in silent ischemia likely has the same fundamental causes as in stable angina, as discussed previously. There are unique aspects that must be considered. Why are some episodes of ischemia appreciated as pain (approximately 25 percent)[149] whereas others are asymptomatic? Why do some patients not experience pain with ischemia at all? Are the causes and functional consequences of silent ischemia the same as for painful ischemia, or is there something unique about this portion of the spectrum of ischemic manifestations?

An obvious possible explanation for painful as opposed to asymptomatic ischemia is that the ischemia, and thus the noxious stimulus, is more severe in the former than in the latter. There is, however, no strong correlation between the duration and severity of an ischemic episode and the development of anginal pain in chronic stable angina.[149] Symptomatic episodes lasted slightly longer and had a slightly higher frequency of severe ST-segment depression than did painless ones, but there was considerable overlap.

Chierchia et al. have assessed painful and asymptomatic ischemic episodes as follows: (1) ischemic episodes of less than 3 min duration that are associated with less than a 7-mmHg rise in end-diastolic pressure are usually painless; (2) episodes that are more severe and perhaps much more severe and/or longer may be painless or painful in the same patient.[150] Thus, the intensity of the ischemic stimulus does not appear

to account for the variability of the perception of pain in angina.[116]

An alternative explanation for lack of pain with myocardial ischemia is neurologic.[116] Neuropathy with defective sensory efferent nerves likely occurs in some patients and will be discussed subsequently in the context of diabetes. Modulation or extinction of pain stimuli in the central nervous system may contribute importantly to the variable expression of ischemic pain, as alluded to previously. This modulation may occur in spinal centers since transcutaneous nerve,[151] esophagal,[152] and dorsal column stimulation[153] can increase anginal threshold.

There is some evidence that modulation of pain-mediating efferent messages may also occur at supraspinal centers.[116] Psychological or cultural factors may affect pain perception. Subsets of patients with predominantly painless ischemia tend to have a higher threshold and tolerance for painful stimuli than do those who experience pain.[154–156] Thus, processing of pain signals in the central nervous system likely contributes to the variability of anginal threshold or to the absence of pain.

Diabetic patients have an increased incidence of painless myocardial infarction that is likely due, in part, to cardiac autonomic neuropathy.[157,158] They have an increased prevalence, relative to nondiabetic patients, of silent ischemia on exercise testing and ambulatory ECG monitoring.[159,160]

Causes and Functional Consequences of Asymptomatic Ischemia

Ischemia caused by the increased demand associated with exercise testing may be silent.[161] Ambulatory ECG monitoring has provided insights into potential mechanisms of many episodes of ischemia—painless or painful—during daily living. The heart rate at the onset of ischemia is generally lower with ambulatory than with exercise testing.[149,161] These observations suggest that increased vascular tone likely contributes to many episodes of ischemia.

The consequences for myocardial perfusion appear to be similar whether or not the ischemia is associated with chest pain and whether it is provoked or spontaneous. Thus, perfusion measured by rubidium 82 PET was decreased to a similar extent by exercise, cold pressor testing, and mental arithmetic or during spontaneous ischemia.[149,162]

Clinical Implications

The available data indicate that silent ischemia is a common, almost ubiquitous, component of the whole spectrum of the coronary syndromes. It thus appears to have no special implications but, in terms of predicting adverse events, has approximately the same significance as symptomatic ischemia.[163,164] The fundamental issues appear to be the extent and severity of ischemia, regardless of how it is detected or manifested, whether the disease is in a stable or unstable phase, and whether or not monitoring for silent ischemia and changing therapy to decrease or eliminate it decreases morbidity and mortality in a cost-effective manner. Unstable angina is discussed in Chap. 46.

Evidence of high-risk ischemia detected by exercise tolerance testing, with or without thallium or left ventricular blood pool imaging, and implications for treatment will be discussed subsequently. It seems prudent to attempt to reduce high-risk ischemia whether manifest with or without pain. Persistent severe ischemia in spite of medical therapy should lead to consideration of revascularization.

The role of ambulatory ECG monitoring to detect asymptomatic ischemia in routine patient care remains to be defined. At present there appears to be no obligatory, noninvestigational indication for its use.[141]

Treatment of Silent Ischemia

Most medical or interventional strategies that reduce symptomatic ischemia will also reduce asymptomatic ischemia.[165–168] The available data from early clinical trials of treatment of the asymptomatic (silent) ischemia in stable coronary disease have been summarized by Bertolet et al.[164] TNG is highly effective, and beta blockers appear to be somewhat more effective than calcium-entry blockers. Calcium antagonists may be most effective in preventing ischemia that occurs at lower heart rates when vasoconstriction may be a predominant factor, as discussed previously.

There has been a considerable evolution conceptually in the approaches to stable ischemic coronary disease with the appreciation that the total ischemic burden, and not just symptoms, may be the appropriate therapeutic target. While this concept is still being tested, other current developments are likely to revolutionize the approach to ischemic coronary disease.

The fundamental interrelationship between the biology of the atherosclerotic lesion and the coronary ischemic syndromes has been alluded to previously in the context of the contribution of endothelial dysfunction to disordered control of vasomotor tone and, in detail, in the broader scope in Chap. 44. Aggressive lipid lowering in coronary regression trials has shown dramatic lowering of subsequent cardiac event rates and improvement in endothelial function in some patients, even in the context of modest angiographic improvements.[169–181]

These observations suggest that the biology of atherosclerotic lesions is being favorably influenced and that ischemia can be diminished by marked lifestyle changes.[182,183] As discussed below, the treatment of atherosclerosis through risk factor modification should become a fundamental component of the treatment regimen for stable coronary disease with or without painful manifestations (see Chap. 41).

MEDICAL THERAPY

General

All patients with stable angina pectoris should have an evaluation of risk factors for coronary heart disease (see Chap. 41). Whenever possible, risk factors should be corrected. Of particular importance is the cessation of tobacco smoking or exposure to tobacco products in any other form, such as snuff, chewing tobacco, or passive smoking. Achievement of ideal body weight and optimal control of diabetes mellitus and of systemic arterial hypertension (Chap. 58) are very important.

In a randomized clinical trial of 333 male physicians with angina pectoris, low-dose aspirin (325 mg every other day) decreased the incidence of a first myocardial infarction by 87 percent.[184]

In the Swedish Angina Pectoris Aspirin Trial (SAPAT), a double-blind trial involving 2035 men and women, optimal symptom control was first obtained in all patients with sotalol (median dose, 160 mg/day), following which the patients were randomized to aspirin (75 mg/day) or placebo. The median duration of follow-up was 50 months. Compared to the placebo plus sotalol group, the aspirin plus sotalol group had a 34 percent reduction in primary outcome events (myocardial infarction and sudden death).[185]

Accordingly, patients with stable angina pectoris should be given aspirin in the absence of contraindications. The daily dose of aspirin should be individualized. A reasonable dose is 160 to 325 mg/day[186,187] (see also Chap. 52).

The Second Adult Treatment Panel[188] has recommended that dietary and, if necessary, drug therapy be employed to lower the low-density lipoprotein (LDL) cholesterol to or below 100 mg/dL (2.6 mmol/L) in patients with documented CHD (see Chaps. 41 and 53). For many patients, drug therapy (Chap. 53) will be required to reach this goal.

In a randomized clinical trial of 113 male patients with stable angina pectoris, 56 men assigned to a program of low-fat diet and intensive physical exercise had significantly slower progression of their coronary artery disease than 57 patients in the control group on usual care.[189]

The Scandinavian Simvastatin Survival Study was a randomized, double-blind, placebo-controlled study of 4444 patients aged 35 to 70 years (mean, 58.9 years) with angina pectoris and/or previous myocardial infarction and serum cholesterol levels of 213 to 310 mg/dL (5.5 to 8.0 mmol/L) receiving a lipid-lowering diet.[190] They were randomly assigned to placebo or simvastatin, 20 to 40 mg once daily. The median follow-up period was 5.4 years (range in survivors, 4.9 to 6.2 years). The risk of death was reduced by 30 percent ($p = .0003$) in those taking simvastatin and the risk of coronary death was reduced by 42 percent ($p = .00001$).

The Cholesterol and Recurrent Events (CARE) study evaluated the use of either pravastatin, 40 mg/day, or placebo in 4159 patients (3583 men and 576 women) with myocardial infarction who had plasma total cholesterol levels below 240 mg/dL (mean 209 mg/dL) and LDL cholesterol levels of 115 to 174 mg/dL (mean, 139 mg/dL).[191] There was a 24 percent reduction ($p = .003$) in the risk of a fatal coronary event or a nonfatal myocardial infarction. These results clearly demonstrate the benefit of cholesterol-lowering therapy when extended to the majority of patients with CAD who have cholesterol levels that are not markedly elevated.

Lipid-lowering therapy for patients with known CAD is cost effective.[192–195] An active exercise program, either individually directed or as part of a formal rehabilitation program (Chap. 55), is very helpful in achieving ideal body weight, decreasing coronary risk factors, and possibly even decreasing the risk of recurrent myocardial infarction.[196] Exercise training also increases the functional capacity of patients with stable angina pectoris.[189,197–204]

Nitrates

The standard first-line therapy of patients with stable angina pectoris is TNG, which usually relieves the symptoms in about 1 to 5 min.[205–211] TNG may be self-administered in the form of a sublingual tablet (0.3 to 0.6 mg) or as an oral spray, each puff of which delivers approximately 0.4 mg. Sublingual TNG tablets lose their potency over time and may require prescription refills every 2 to 3 months. Although few formulations have a longer shelf life, it is appropriate to advise the patient to keep only a small supply of tablets with them and to keep the remainder in sealed small brown bottles in the refrigerator. The oral TNG spray, which provides over 200 aerosol doses of 0.4 mg TNG, has a shelf life of more than 2 years and does not require refrigeration.

If patients have angina pectoris no more often than once a week, the use of only a rapidly acting TNG compound may be satisfactory, although the concurrent use of a beta blocker or calcium channel blocker or antagonist is frequently appropriate for blood pressure control. If the patient experiences angina pectoris more frequently than once a week, the additional use of a long-acting nitrate, beta blocker, or calcium channel blocker should be considered. Whenever possible, the patient should be instructed to take TNG prophylactically before an exertion or event known to precipitate angina pectoris.

Nitrates can also be administered in many other formulations, including a slowly dissolving buccal capsule, transdermally as an ointment or a patch, and sublingually or orally in forms that are more slowly absorbed and metabolized. When chronic nitrate therapy is first initiated, the dosage should be low and progressively increased to near the point of tolerance as judged by headache, dizziness, or postural hypotension. Table 23-1 lists the commonly used nitrates and their dosages. The use of a long-acting nitrate compound decreases the frequency of angina attacks and increases the amount of effort before angina (or angina equivalent) occurs.

The development of tolerance is a major disadvantage to chronic nitrate therapy.[205,212] In general, decreased effectiveness of TNG is encountered whenever a nitrate compound is regularly given without a 10- to 12-h nitrate-free period. The rate of development of nitrate tolerance increases with higher and more continuous dosages of nitrate compounds. For most patients, a satisfactory nitrate-free period is from about 9 P.M. to about 7 A.M. If patients are taking an oral nitrate in a form that is slowly metabolized, it may be necessary to administer the last dosage in the early evening.

For example, isosorbide dinitrate (10 to 60 mg) may be taken in doses of 30 mg twice a day at 8 A.M. and 5 P.M. or three times a day (8 A.M., 1 P.M., and 5 P.M.).[213] Nitroglycerin ointment or patches should usually be removed about 8 P.M. to 9 P.M. The administration of 20 mg isosorbide-5-mononitrate, which is the most important metabolite of isosorbide dinitrate, at 7 A.M. and 2 P.M. appears to prevent the development of tolerance in most patients.

It is important to be sure that the patient is on other antianginal therapy, such as a beta blocker or calcium antagonist, during the 10- to 12-h nitrate-free period. In patients who experience more episodes of angina between 9 P.M. and 7 A.M. than at other times, the nitrate-free period should be scheduled during other hours, often from about noon to 10 P.M. The physician should determine the ideal nitrate-free period in each individual patient. The interval is 8 to 12 h in most patients.

Nitrate tolerance is thought to be related to oxidation or depletion of sulfhydryl groups. The results of clinical trials to prevent tolerance by administering sulfhydryl donors such as acetylcysteine or methionine are variable, with some reports suggesting benefit[214–217] and others finding none.[218–220] Other postulated mechanisms of nitrate tolerance include activation of neurohumoral vasoconstrictive mechanisms, expansion of intravascular volume, and desensitization of soluble guanylate cyclase. Hydralazine may decrease the development of nitrate tolerance.[221] The pharmacology of nitrates is discussed in more detail in Chap. 23.

Beta-Adrenergic Blocking Agents

β-Adrenergic blocking agents are very effective in the management of patients with angina pectoris, in whom they improve exercise tolerance and decrease episodes of both symptomatic and asymptomatic (silent) myocardial ischemia. They function primarily by reducing the heart rate and myocardial contractility both at rest and especially during the normal increases with exertion. They also block reflex tachycardia that may be induced by TNG or arterial vasodilators.[222] There are many β-adrenergic blocking agents available, all of which block β_1-receptors. The pharmacology of beta blockers is discussed in detail in Chap. 54.

Agents that block only β_1-receptors are cardioselective beta blockers, while those that block both β_1- and β_2-receptors are nonselective blockers. These terms are relative, however, and in higher doses or in some patients, the selective agents can also produce some side effects associated with β_2-blockade. Some newer agents both block β_1-receptors and dilate blood vessels directly and are "vasodilator" beta blockers.

Beta blockers also differ in whether or not they have some intrinsic sympathomimetic activity; agents with this activity tend to produce less slowing of the resting heart rate. Beta blockers vary in their lipid and water solubility, a quality that can affect their duration of action and perhaps side effects. The membrane-stabilizing (or local anesthetic or quinidine-like) effect, which is unrelated to beta blockade, does not appear to be of clinical significance (see also Chap. 54).

Adverse effects of beta blockers related to beta blockade include excess bradycardia, hypotension, ventricular dysfunction, bronchospasm, inhibition of metabolic and circulatory response to hypoglycemia, and cold extremities. Adverse effects that are apparently unrelated to beta blockade include impotence, lethargy, depression, confusion, hallucination, and constipation.

In general, all beta blockers are effective in the management of patients with stable angina pectoris. It is generally appropriate to select agents that have been shown to be effective in clinical trials and that have properties least likely to produce adverse effects in an individual patient. Thus, cardioselective agents are preferred in patients who have a history of bronchospastic disease, diabetes mellitus, or peripheral vascular disease. Even cardioselective beta blockers, however, can worsen bronchial constriction. Similarly, all beta blockers can worsen heart block and left ventricular function and can worsen heart failure in patients with severe left ventricular dysfunction (see also Chaps. 54 and 73).

Beta blockers are usually administered in a dosage to lower the resting heart rate to 50 to 60 per minute; in some patients, even lower resting heart rates can be tolerated without symptoms. When beta-blocker therapy is discontinued, the dosage should be tapered over 4 to 10 days to avoid a rebound worsening of angina pectoris and possible myocardial infarction. The characteristics and dosages of individual beta blockers are shown in Tables 54-1, 54-2, 54-3, 54-7, and 54-10. Additional discussion of the selection of different beta blockers is provided below (see also Chap. 54).

Calcium Channel Blockers

Calcium channel entry blockers (or calcium antagonists) are diverse compounds that impede the entry of calcium into myocytes and smooth muscle cells. In general, they decrease myocardial oxygen requirements by producing arterial dilatation and reducing arterial blood pressure and afterload and by reducing myocardial contractility. Some, such as diltiazem and verapamil, also end to reduce heart rate.

Many calcium channel blockers also produce coronary vasodilatation and prevent coronary artery spasm. Different calcium channel blockers appear to interact with different receptors; they also vary significantly in their relative effects upon different vascular beds and the myocardium. They may be classified into papaverine derivatives (verapamil), dihydropyridines (nifedipine, nicardipine), benzodiazepine derivatives (diltiazem), mixed calcium and sodium channel blockers (bepridil), and some antihistamines (flunarizine). The pharmacology and recommended dosages of the calcium antagonists are discussed in detail in Chap. 54 and summarized in Tables 54-1 to 54-4.

Adverse effects include ankle edema, headache, palpitations, flushing, hypotension, and aggravation of angina due to coronary steal, especially with dihydropyridine derivatives

(nifedipine, nicardipine, etc.). Atrioventricular nodal delay may occur with verapamil and diltiazem; rarely, higher degrees of heart block occur, particularly when these agents are used concurrently with a beta blocker. All currently available calcium antagonists can have a negative inotropic effect, particularly verapamil. Other side effects include constipation, particularly with the use of verapamil.

All classes of calcium antagonists are effective in the management of patients with stable angina pectoris. In general, they are as effective as beta blockers, with which they are frequently used concurrently. Calcium antagonists are of special value in patients who have conditions that may be made worse by beta blockers, such as asthma, chronic obstructive pulmonary disease (COPD), or peripheral vascular disease.

Elderly patients often tolerate calcium antagonists better than beta blockers. Verapamil, which has a stronger negative inotropic effect, is useful in the management of patients with angina pectoris due to hypertrophic obstructive cardiomyopathy (see Chap. 74).

Combination Drug Therapy for Stable Angina Pectoris

Patients with infrequent episodes of angina can be managed effectively with short-acting nitrates. In patients with more frequent episodes of angina who may require a combination of a short- and a long-acting nitrate, the use of a long-acting beta blocker or a calcium channel blocker is advisable during a nitrate-free period initiated to prevent the development of nitrate tolerance. The use of a beta blocker or either diltiazem or verapamil tends to block the reflex tachycardia that is produced by nitrates in some patients.

In general, the combination of nitrates and nifedipine is more likely to be associated with reflex tachycardia or even supraventricular tachycardias than the combination of nitrates with other calcium channel blockers. Table 54-6 presents the rationale for combining nitrates and calcium channel blockers in the therapy of patients with angina pectoris.

The combination of beta blocker and calcium antagonist therapy is widely employed in the management of patients with stable angina pectoris. Table 54-5 presents the hemodynamic effects of beta blockers, calcium channel blockers, and combination treatment.

The combination of a beta blocker with verapamil is particularly likely to worsen heart failure and should be used with special caution in patients with left ventricular dysfunction. Similarly, the combination of a beta blocker and verapamil can produce heart block in some patients, particularly the elderly. The combination of a beta blocker and diltiazem is usually well tolerated, although it too can produce heart failure and heart block.

Triple therapy of patients with severe stable angina pectoris is relatively frequent, although often it is no more effective than double therapy. The physician should be especially cautious whenever employing triple therapy because of the increased likelihood of adverse side effects. The selection of the particular beta blocker and calcium channel blocker should be individualized, and the determination of the optimal combination often requires a series of therapeutic trials with various combinations.

Digitalis

Although digitalis is an inotrope and therefore would be expected to increase myocardial contractility and myocardial oxygen requirements, it may actually decrease myocardial oxygen requirements if it results in a decrease in left ventricular end-diastolic volume. This occurs because of the Laplace relationship (Chap. 3), wherein systolic wall tension is directly related to mean ventricular diameter. In addition, the perfusion of the subendocardium of the left ventricle may be improved if the digoxin decreases the left ventricular diastolic pressure.

Revascularization

Patients with stable angina pectoris may be appropriate candidates for revascularization either by CABS (Chap. 50) or percutaneous transluminal coronary angioplasty (coronary angioplasty) (Chap. 48). In general, this is an individual decision to be made by the patient with knowledge of the advantages and disadvantages either of medical therapy alone or of revascularization with either CABS or coronary angioplasty. While there are guidelines for indications for performing each of these procedures,[223,224] the guidelines are necessarily broad and do not include the many important variables for an individual patient. The indications for surgical revascularization are classified as shown in Table 45-6.

There are two general indications for a revascularization procedure: (1) the presence of symptoms that are not acceptable to the patient either because of restriction of physical activity and lifestyle or because of restrictions or side effects from medications, or (2) the presence of findings that indicate clearly that the patient would have a better prognosis with revascularization than with medical therapy. For some patients, the occurrence of angina may be so incapacitating despite optimal double or triple drug therapy that revascularization is desired. In other patients, the side effects from the medications necessary to control symptoms may be such that the patient prefers surgery. Anatomic considerations for revascularization are based upon an assessment of the grade or class of angina experienced by the patient, the presence and severity of evidence of myocardial ischemia on noninvasive stress testing, the degree of left ventricular function, and the distribution and severity of CAD. The indications for surgical revascularization and the results of such surgery are discussed in detail in Chap. 50.

Tables 45-7 and 45-8 show the guidelines for CABS in patients with stable angina pectoris recommended by the joint American College of Cardiology/American Heart Association Task Force in 1991.[223]

A review of randomized trials and registry studies revealed a trend for CABS to prolong survival in patients at high risk on the basis of clinical, functional, and anatomic characteristics in

TABLE 45-6

CLASSIFICATION OF INDICATIONS FOR THE CORONARY ARTERY BYPASS GRAFT OPERATION

Treatment Class	Description
I	Conditions for which the operation is indicated on the basis of a demonstrated advantage over medical treatment in terms of longevity or relief of symptoms, or both.
II	Conditions for which the operation is acceptable treatment but for which its advantages over medical treatment have not yet been fully defined.
III	Conditions for which the operation is not generally considered to be indicated, because of lack of demonstrated advantage over medical treatment.

Source: Kirklin et al.[223] Reproduced with permission from the publisher.

a comparison with medical therapy alone.[223,225–235] The 18-year follow-up of the Veterans Affairs Cooperative Study of Coronary Artery Bypass Surgery for Stable Angina found that CABS resulted in increased survival for patients with left main coronary artery disease and that other patients had relief of angina and better exercise performance for 5 years but that there was no difference at 10 years, presumably due to graft closure. Low-risk patients derived no survival benefit with surgical therapy at any time during the 18 years of follow-up.[226]

Transmyocardial laser revascularization is currently being evaluated in a controlled, randomized trial, and this procedure may prove useful in selected patients.[236,237]

Coronary angioplasty (see Chap. 48) has produced excellent results in patients with stable angina pectoris. Initially, it was used primarily in patients with single-vessel disease, and it is still the preferred technique of revascularization in most patients with single-vessel disease other than left main. Subsequently, coronary angioplasty has been widely employed in patients with multivessel disease.[224] A number of studies have compared the results of coronary angioplasty and CABS in patients with CAD.[238–244] Overall freedom from myocardial infarction and mortality appear to be similar for the two treatment strategies.

Angioplasty is associated with a greater need for repeat revascularization procedures. Angioplasty costs less initially, but the cost savings are largely lost after repeat procedures are performed (see Chaps. 48 and 50). In general, patients with single-vessel disease are revascularized by coronary angioplasty. Table 45-9 lists clinical features and the results of testing that have been found to indicate an increased risk and mortality over the next several years in patients with CHD.[37,164,223,224,245–247] These features are useful in evaluating patients for coronary arteriography and possible coronary revascularization.

TABLE 45-7

TREATMENT CLASS OF THE CORONARY ARTERY BYPASS OPERATION IN PATIENTS WITH CHRONIC STABLE CLASS I OR II ANGINA

CAD	Indication Class Left Ventricular Dysfunction			
	None	Mild	Moderate	Severe (but EF >0.20)
NO OR MILD MYOCARDIAL ISCHEMIA WITH NONINVASIVE STRESS TESTING				
Left main	I	I	I	I
3 vessel	II[a]	II[a]	I	I
2 vessel	II[a]	II[a]	II[a]	II[a]
1 vessel	III[b]	III[b]	II[a]	II[a]
MODERATE OR SEVERE MYOCARDIAL ISCHEMIA WITH NONINVASIVE STRESS TESTING				
Left main	I	I	I	I
3 vessel	I	I	I	I
2 vessel	II[a]	II[a]	II[a]	II[a]
1 vessel	III[b]	III[b]	II[a]	II[a]

[a] Class I if there is severe proximal stenosis in a large left anterior descending coronary artery.
[b] Class II if there is severe proximal stenosis in a large left anterior descending coronary artery.
Notes: Angina classified by Canadian Cardiovascular Society grades (Campeau[6]). Noninvasive stress testing includes exercise ECG testing, radionuclide scintigraphy, and radionuclide ventriculography. CAD, coronary artery disease; EF, ejection fraction.
Source: Kirklin et al.[223] Reproduced with permission from the publisher.

TABLE 45-8

TREATMENT CLASS OF THE CORONARY ARTERY BYPASS OPERATION IN PATIENTS WITH CHRONIC STABLE CLASS III OR IV ANGINA

CAD	Indication Class Left Ventricular Dysfunction			
	None	Mild	Moderate	Severe (but EF >0.20)
NO OR MILD MYOCARDIAL ISCHEMIA WITH NONINVASIVE STRESS TESTING				
Left main	I	I	I	I
3 vessel	I	I	I	I
2 vessel	II[a]	II[a]	II[a]	II[a]
1 vessel	II[a]	II[a]	II[a]	II[a]
MODERATE OR SEVERE MYOCARDIAL ISCHEMIA WITH NONINVASIVE STRESS TESTING				
Left main	I	I	I	I
3 vessel	I	I	I	I
2 vessel	II[a]	II[a]	II[a]	II[a]
1 vessel	II[a]	II[a]	II[a]	II[a]

[a] Class I if there is severe proximal stenosis in a large left anterior descending coronary artery.
Notes: Angina classified by Canadian Cardiovascular Society grades (Campeau[6]). Noninvasive stress testing includes exercise ECG testing, radionuclide scintigraphy, and radionuclide ventriculography. CAD, coronary artery disease; EF, ejection fraction.
Source: Kirklin et al.[223] Reproduced with permission from the publisher.

External Counterpulsation

External counterpulsation has been used in China for the treatment of patients with angina pectoris with some success. A recent report described a clinical trial of 18 patients using a device employing air counterpulsation of balloons around the calves, thighs, and buttocks for 1 h daily for a total of 36 h. In 14 patients, thallium scintigraphy showed a decrease in myocardial ischemia and an increase in exercise duration on maximal stress testing.[248] This innovative technique needs much more study before it can be recommended.

Neurostimulation

In contrast, neurostimulation appears to be a viable option in patients with refractory angina pectoris who are not suitable for revascularization.[151–153,249] After its safety is sufficiently established, it may become a useful alternative in highly selected patients who are refractory to conventional therapy.

TABLE 45-9

MAJOR PROGNOSTIC VARIABLES IN PATIENTS WITH CHRONIC STABLE ANGINA

Clinical
  Congestive heart failure
  NYHA Functional class
  Prior myocardial infarction
  Diuretic use
  Digitalis use
  Cardiomegaly
  S_3 gallop
  Ventricular arrhythmias
  ST-segment depression on resting ECG
  Angina frequency
  Angina duration
Exercise ECG testing
  Inability to exercise
  Poor exercise capacity (<5 METS) or maximal work (<100 W)
  ≥2 mm of ischemic ST-segment depression at a low work load (≤stage 2 or ≤130 beats per min)
  Failure to increase blood pressure (>130 mmHg) or a fall in blood pressure during exercise
  Early onset (stage 1) or prolonged duration (>5 min) of ST-segment depression
  Multiple leads (≥5) with ST-segment depression
  ST-segment elevation
  Inability to attain target heart rate (off medication)
  Exercise-induced ventricular couplets or tachycardia at a low work load
  ST/HR Slope ≥ 6 V per beat per min
  Angina
Thallium 201 scintigraphy
  Multiple severe initial thallium defects
  Multiple areas showing thallium redistribution
  Increased lung/heart thallium ratio
  Transient left ventricular dilatation
Radionuclide left ventricular imaging
  Ejection fraction ≤ 35 percent
  Multiple regional wall motion abnormalities
  Exercise-induced reduction in ejection fraction ≥ 10 percent
  Failure to increase ejection fraction ≥ 5 percent during exercise if ≤70 years age
  Exercise-induced left ventricular cavity dilatation
Ambulatory ECG Monitoring
  Prolonged ST-segment depression (≥60 min per 24 h)
  Marked ST-segment depression (≥2 mm)
  Frequent transient ischemic episodes (>6 per 24 h)

Notes: NYHA, New York Heart Association; METS, metabolic equivalents; HR, heart rate.

Chelation Therapy

There is no good scientific evidence that intravenous or oral chelation therapy is of benefit to patients with angina pectoris or with other forms of cardiovascular disease.[250] This is also true for other forms of cardiovascular disease, except for the treatment of hemachromatosis.

MANAGEMENT OF SPECIAL CATEGORIES

Systemic Arterial Hypertension

Patients with systolic arterial hypertension (SAH) often have angina pectoris. In most such patients, significant coronary atherosclerosis of the epicardial blood vessels is present, but some patients with SAH may have angina pectoris or even fatal myocardial infarction without significant obstruction of the large epicardial vessels. In some patients this may be due to the marked increase in myocardial oxygen requirements that exceed the coronary blood flow reserve, whereas others may have microvascular angina ("syndrome X") and abnormalities of the small coronary blood vessels (see below).

In many patients, treatment of the SAH with a beta blocker, calcium antagonist, or angiotensin-converting enzyme (ACE) inhibitor will also decrease myocardial oxygen requirements and prevent the development of angina pectoris. In general, efforts should be made to control the blood pressure both at rest and during exertion (see also Chap. 58).

Chronic Obstructive Pulmonary Disease Asthma

In general, beta blockers should be avoided in this subset of patients, and preference should be given to the use of nitrates and calcium blockers. Since many of these patients receive medications for their pulmonary disease that may increase their heart rate or even produce supraventricular tachycardia, such as sinus tachycardia or multifocal atrial tachycardia, it is preferable to use a cardiac-slowing calcium channel blocker such as diltiazem or verapamil.

Tachycardia can markedly increase myocardial consumption and precipitate myocardial ischemia. Some patients with a history of only asthma or only mild COPD may be able to tolerate small dosages of cardioselective beta blockers. When beta blockers are used in such patients, however, special caution and careful patient monitoring are appropriate. At times, very small dosages can prevent much of the tachycardia induced by the medications given for asthma or COPD.

Elderly Patients

In general, elderly patients tolerate calcium channel blockers better than beta blockers. The presence of sinus tachycardia or atrial fibrillation is a relative contraindication to the selection of nifedipine; in such patients, diltiazem or verapamil or even a beta blocker would be preferable. On the other hand, beta blockers, verapamil, and diltiazem can exacerbate heart block, and verapamil may produce troublesome constipation in some elderly patients. Some elderly patients are very sensitive to postural hypotension from short-acting nitrates.

Peripheral Vascular Disease

Although satisfactory clinical trials are lacking, many physicians have noted that patients with peripheral vascular disease may have a worsening of their symptoms when treated with a nonselective beta blocker, which might allow unopposed alpha-induced vasoconstriction. Alternatively, the worsening symptoms may be due to the decrease in arterial perfusion pressure. In general, it is preferable to treat patients with chronic stable angina who have peripheral vascular disease with nitrates and a channel blocker.

Diabetes Mellitus

Patients with chronic stable angina pectoris who have diabetes mellitus and who take insulin should preferably be treated with nitrates. A calcium antagonist may be used as a second drug. If it is necessary to use a beta blocker, one should use a cardioselective agent, which would be less likely to impair recognition of and recovery from insulin-induced hypoglycemia (see also Chap. 78).

Chronic Renal Disease

While beta blockers and calcium antagonists can normally be used effectively in patients with chronic angina and chronic renal insufficiency, careful monitoring may be necessary since many beta blockers and calcium channel blockers (Chap. 54) are excreted primarily by the kidneys. In addition, the decrease in arterial blood pressure can sometimes lower renal blood flow and worsen renal function (see also Chap. 94).

OTHER MANIFESTATIONS OF CHRONIC ISCHEMIC HEART DISEASE

Heart Failure

Patients with severe CAD that produces a loss of left ventricular myocardium, usually at least more than approximately 20 percent, or that results in a ventricular septal defect or significant mitral regurgitation may have significant left ventricular failure. While there may be significant hypertrophy of the remaining myocytes and interstitium (Chap. 21), the ventricle is unable to compensate fully, and there is often a syndrome of heart failure with decreased stroke volume and elevated diastolic filling pressures in the left ventricle. This can produce a syndrome of heart failure (see Chaps. 21 and 23) that is clinically predominant and often more incapacitating than the symptom of angina pectoris. Extremely rarely, patients may present with a syndrome of heart failure than can even resemble constrictive pericarditis and have no history of angina or myocardial infarction. This is one manifestation of the syndrome of *ischemic cardiomyopathy* (see also Chap. 73).

Patients who have severe left ventricular dysfunction due to CAD have a poor prognosis (see Chap. 38). In most instances, it reflects permanent, irreversible loss of myocytes. In a small percentage of patients, severe chronic CAD is associated with persistently impaired myocardial and left ventricular function at rest due to reduced coronary blood flow that can be partially or completely restored to normal either by improving blood flow or by reducing oxygen demand. This has been referred to as "hibernating myocardium."[251-256] This concept is important because there can be a significant improvement following good left ventricular revascularization. While this does not occur routinely,[257-271] it is important to take it into account before concluding that the left ventricular function of an individual patient is too low to consider revascularization surgery or that the etiology of the heart failure is not CHD.

At times, the latent function and myocardial viability of the left ventricle can be detected following a premature ventricular contraction. Radionuclide techniques[272-274] (Chap. 17), magnetic resonance imaging[275] (Chap. 19), echocardiography[273,274,276-280] (Chap. 14), and PET[281] (Chap. 20) are useful in detecting myocardial viability.[282-285]

The therapy of patients with heart failure due to ischemic heart disease is the same as for most patients with combined systolic and diastolic left ventricular failure, i.e., triple therapy with one or more diuretics, an ACE inhibitor, and digoxin (see Chap. 23). Because these patients frequently have overt or latent renal insufficiency, it may be necessary to use a combination of a long-acting nitrate (such as isosorbide dinitrate) and oral hydralazine in place of the ACE inhibitor.

In addition, since the remaining left ventricular myocardium usually has significant areas that are chronically or intermittently ischemic, these patients tend to be more sensitive to electrolyte disturbances, particularly hypokalemia and hypomagnesemia. The ischemic myocardium may also be more susceptible than the normal myocardium to arrhythmias and conduction disturbances from digitalis. Nevertheless, it is useful and should be given with appropriate monitoring.

Therapy with a beta blocker should also be considered. Such therapy has been found to be efficacious in recent studies (see Chap. 23). The beta blocker must be started in extremely low dosage, and the dosage very slowly increased over several months. Such therapy should be administered with very great care because of the danger of precipitating severe heart failure (see Chap. 23).

Cardiac transplantation is also frequently performed for severe heart failure due to CAD. The indications for, exclusions from, and results of cardiac transplantation are discussed in Chap. 25.

A patient with heart failure who has a large ventricular aneurysm may benefit from aneurysmectomy if there is sufficient remaining functioning left ventricular tissue (see Chap. 50). Similarly, heart failure due to severe mitral regurgitation can sometimes be significantly improved by corrective mitral valve surgery, which is often combined with coronary revascularization. The operative mortality for this procedure can be high (see Chap. 50).

Cardiac Arrhythmias, Conduction Disturbances

Chronic ischemic heart disease is a cause of many cardiac arrhythmias, including atrial and ventricular premature contractions, atrial fibrillation, sustained and nonsustained ventricular tachycardia, and ventricular fibrillation. The basic management is discussed in Chap. 27. In general, beta blockers should be employed whenever there is no strong contraindication, and type IC agents (Chap. 30) should be avoided unless the patient is symptomatic (see Chap. 27). In patients with atrial fibrillation, the ventricular response rate should be controlled with digoxin.

Patients with chronic atrial fibrillation should also be maintained on warfarin (INR = 2 to 3) unless there is a contraindication, in which case aspirin (81 to 325 mg/day) should be used. Patients in heart failure who have atrial fibrillation may benefit from electrical cardioversion (Chap. 32), although a very high percentage revert in the next few months.

Nevertheless, cardioversion can sometimes significantly improve overall cardiac function, even though for a short time. Patients with recurrent symptomatic ventricular tachycardia or ventricular fibrillation can be treated with an automatic implantable cardioverter defibrillator.[286] The use of these devices is discussed in Chap. 33. Conduction abnormalities are generally managed as described in Chaps. 27 and 34.

Embolic Disease

Patients with ischemic heart disease are likely to have systemic emboli, particularly patients with a history of systemic embolus, chronic atrial fibrillation, ventricular aneurysm, a large dyskinetic or hypokinetic area of myocardium, or a severely depressed left ventricular ejection fraction. Such patients should be considered for chronic, long-term, low-dose warfarin therapy (INR = 2 to 3) (see Chap. 52).

CHEST PAIN WITH NORMAL CORONARY ARTERIES

The combination of chest pain with many of the features of angina pectoris, although frequently atypical, and normal epicardial coronary arteries at cardiac catheterization has attracted a great deal of attention since the entity was first noted in the 1960s.[106,107]

These early studies identified many of the characteristics of what was subsequently characterized as a syndrome: female predominance; the frequent presence of ischemic ST-segment changes on the exercise ECG; inconsistent relationship between ECG changes and metabolic or hemodynamic evidence of ischemia; and pain that could be very severe, prolonged, atypical in location and precipitating events, and unresponsive commonly to usual anti-ischemic therapy.

The term *syndrome X* was applied to this diagnostic conundrum in 1973[287]; it is usually used to describe patients with the common features of angina-like pain and normal epicardial coronaries, but the term is also used to categorize groups that undoubtedly are pathophysiologically heterogeneous.[82] The continued use of the term is thus unfortunate and has been discouraged,[288] especially since there is another syndrome X, characterized by insulin resistance, hyperinsulinemia, and diabetes, that is associated with dyslipidemia, hypertension, and abdominal obesity[289] (see Chap. 78).

There may be some overlap between the two syndromes because a group of patients has been reported who have hyperinsulinemia, dyslipidemia, angina with normal coronary arteriograms, and presumed microvasculopathy.[290] A more specific terminology such as *angina with normal coronary arteriography* is preferable.[288]

Clinical Presentation and Characteristics

The essential features of the clinical presentation of patients with chest pain and normal coronary arteriograms were described previously. Patients, about 70 percent of whom are women with an average age of approximately 50 years, complain of pain that is frequently consistent with, but not typical of, angina pectoris that is associated with epicardial CAD. It may be precipitated by exertion, although the threshold for precipitating pain is highly variable.[79] As noted, its duration may be uncharacteristically long, and it may be unusually severe and is not commonly associated with symptoms such as diaphoresis.

TNG frequently does not give the characteristic rapid relief seen in usual angina pectoris. Approximately one-third of patients have hypertension or a history of hypertension without evidence of left ventricular hypertrophy.[82] The presence of left ventricular hypertrophy would result in the classification of patients as having hypertensive heart disease, which can result in similar chest pain syndromes and which probably overlaps mechanistically with the syndrome of chest pain with normal coronary arteriograms.[291]

Evidence for Ischemia

Ischemic ST-segment depression on exercise testing in the absence of epicardial CAD has been one of the hallmarks of syndrome X and has frequently been one of the criteria for its diagnosis.[82] More than 50 percent of patients evaluated at the National Institutes of Health for chest pain and normal coronaries had an ischemic ST-segment response.[292] Ischemic ST-segment depression and chest pain have been observed in two-thirds of patients but in no controls during the infusion of the vasodilator papaverine.[117]

Thallium perfusion abnormalities have been observed commonly in patients with chest pain and normal arteriograms, but no consistent correlation could be made among the extent of the defect, the positivity of the exercise test, and exercise tolerance.[293] In such patients there is a relatively high frequency of abnormal ventricular responses (decreased ejection fraction or regional wall motion abnormality) to exercise.[292] Thus, in many of these patients there is compelling evidence of perfusion abnormalities and ischemia that inferentially are related to abnormalities in the microvasculature.[259–299]

Metabolic studies have been performed in patients with chest pain and normal coronaries to evaluate evidence of ischemia developing during stress. Results assessing lactate production have been inconsistent. Rapid atrial pacing has been reported not to increase lactate production in this setting[294] or to increase it in about one-third of patients, while intracoronary papaverine infusion consistently increased cardiac lactate production.[117]

The available metabolic data do not permit definitive conclusions about the presence of ischemia. The methodologies used, however, may be insufficiently sensitive to detect the metabolic manifestations of ischemia if they are limited to relatively small areas of myocardium.

Myocardial Dysfunction

There is a growing body of data that is consistent with the notion that the myocardium is not normal in many patients with the chest pain–normal coronary artery syndrome, and a cardiomyopathic component of the syndrome has been implicated.[285,299,300] Endocardial biopsy has been reported to show mitochondrial swelling in myocardial cells[295] or hypertrophy and patchy fibrosis.[82,300]

Although patients with the syndrome have been said to have consistently normal left ventricular response to exercise,[301] development of wall motion abnormalities or a decrease in ejection fraction in sizeable subsets of patients with angina and normal epicardial coronaries has been reported.[292,302] Those patients with abnormalities of flow reserve were most likely to have abnormal ventricular responses and, among these, two-thirds of those with left bundle branch block exhibited exercise-induced ventricular dysfunction. The presence of resting or exercise-induced left bundle branch block has been shown by others to identify a subgroup within the syndrome to be at particularly high risk for the chronic deterioration in left ventricular ejection fraction.[299–303]

Romeo et al. also noted the relatively high frequency with which hypertension developed in these patients,[299] an association noted by others and alluded to previously. In analyzing their population they confirmed the heterogeneity of the syndrome and considered that it encompasses three groups: patients with ischemia who remain relatively stable, with or without worsening of the chest pain; those with borderline hypertension; and those with early cardiomyopathy. This for-

mulation also implies that the long-term prognosis is not as favorable as generally thought in all subsets of the syndrome.

Disordered Pain Perception

The intensity of the chest pain in the syndrome associated with normal coronary arteries, especially relative to stimuli that may appear mild or are not apparent, has led to speculation that there may be enhanced pain perception in many of these patients.[120] Patients with the syndrome have a low threshold for pain induction by stimuli such as forearm ischemia, cold pressor testing, or skin electrical stimulation.[304] They also may exhibit abnormal sensitivity to catheter manipulation, injection of normal saline into the atrium, pacing at the right ventricular apex, or injection of contrast into the left coronary artery.[305–307]

It has been proposed that release of high concentrations of adenosine in ischemic areas may account for the pain in many cases.[120] Thus, it may be that with respect to the cause of chest pain, patients with angina and normal coronary arteries can be divided into two groups—those with microvascular dysfunction and ischemia and those with neither.[82] The release of adenosine and stimulation of pain receptors may be related to pain in the former case, whereas nociceptive hypersensitivity with triggers such as ectopic beats, changes in loading conditions, or changes in heart rhythm, rate, or contractility may be involved in the latter.[307]

Approach to the Patient

The ideal approach to these patients would be to assess abnormalities of flow reserve using Doppler catheters and endothelial-dependent and endothelial-independent dilators. This approach is not practical, however, in most clinical environments. Evidence of ischemia should be sought using exercise echocardiogram, nuclear angiography, or exercise perfusion thallium imaging.

Those with evidence of ischemia should be given a trial of anti-ischemic therapy, preferably including nitrates and calcium channel blockers. Such trials are arguably indicated in most of these patients because of the relative insensitivity in detecting what may be small areas of ischemia. Borderline hypertensive patients or patients who become hypertensive should be treated effectively to keep blood pressure well within the normal range.

For those without evidence of ischemia and/or who do not respond to anti-ischemic therapy, general supportive therapy and reassurance should be provided. Narcotics and repeat hospitalization should be avoided. Noncardiac causes of chest pain obviously should be rigorously sought early in the course.

POTENTIAL RISK FACTORS

A low-fat, low-cholesterol diet and pharmacologic lowering of plasma total and LDL cholesterol as part of a comprehensive risk factor modification program significantly lowers the morbidity and mortality of patients with CAD.[177–183,190,191–318] In addition, elevated total serum cholesterol levels are associated with increased mortality both in middle-aged men with myocardial infarction and angina pectoris and in older persons.[319,320]

The endothelial dysfunction associated with hypercholesterolemia and/or CAD[169] improves within months after lowering of serum lipids levels.[80,171–175,321] Conversely, forearm endothelial function can be transiently impaired for 2, 3, or 4 h following a single high-fat meal[323] and also by smoking a cigarette.[324]

In addition to the usual lipid risk factors, a number of patient characteristics or possible dietary deficiencies have been suggested as being additional risk factors for cardiovascular morbidity or mortality (Table 45-10).[325–398] Most of these potential risk factors need better documentation. Furthermore, there is a need for clinical trials to document whether or not an intervention to influence any of these potential risk factors is cost effective.

Currently, the evidence is good that postmenopausal hormone replacement therapy favorably influences cardiovascular morbidity and mortality. The evidence remains more controversial for the other potential risk factors; however, one must use individual judgment regarding any potential benefit to an individual patient.

TABLE 45-10

POTENTIAL RISK FACTORS FOR PATIENTS WITH CHRONIC ISCHEMIC HEART DISEASE

Patient characteristics
  Increased visceral fat[325–328]
  Estrogen deficiency[329–339]
  Insulin resistance[340–343]
  Elevated plasma triglycerides[344,345]
  Elevated plasma lipoprotein(a)[346–349]
  Abnormal hemostatic factors:[350–361]
    Fibrinogen, von Willebrand factor
    Antigen, tissue plasminogen activator antigen,
    Antithrombin III, viscosity,
    C-reactive protein
  Elevated plasma plasminogen[362] activator inhibitor type-1 (PAI-1)
  Elevated plasma homocyst(e)ine[363–365]
  Elevated plasma ceruloplasmin
  Chlamydia pneumoniae infection[366,367]
  Reduced heart rate variability[368,369]
  Signal-averaged ECG late potentials[370]
  Mental and physical stress[371,372]
Low dietary consumption
  Beta carotene, vitamins C, E[373–383]
  Fiber[384]
  Fish, omega-3, omega-6 fatty acids[385]
  n-3 polyunsaturated fatty acids
  Arginine, L-glutamine[386–390]
Either excess or very low consumption
  Alcohol, red wine[391–398]

REFERENCES

1. Heberden W. Some account of disorder of the breast. *Med Trans R Coll Physicians (London)* 1772; 2:59–67.
2. Heberden W. *Commentaries on the History and Care of Disease.* London: T. Payne; 1802.
3. Leibowitz JO. *The History of Coronary Heart Disease.* Berkeley: University of California Press; 1970: 1–227.
4. White PD. Angina pectoris: Historical background. In: Paul O, ed. *Angina Pectoris.* New York: Medcom Press; 1974:1–11.
5. *1993 Heart and Stroke Facts Statistics.* Dallas: American Heart Association; 1992.
6. Campeau L. Grading of angina pectoris (letter). *Circulation* 1976; 54:522–523.
7. Willis PW III. Diagnosing angina pectoris. In: Paul O, ed. *Angina Pectoris.* New York: Medcom Press; 1974:19–32.
8. Cowley AJ, Fullwood LJ, Stainer K, Harrison E, Muller AF, Hampton JR. Postprandial worsening of angina: All due to changes in cardiac output? *Br Heart J* 1991; 66:147–150.
9. Colles P, Juneau M, Gregoire J, Lariver L, Desideri A, Waters D. Effect of a standardized meal on the threshold of exercise-induced myocardial ischemia in patients with stable angina. *J Am Coll Cardiol* 1993; 21:1052–1057.
10. Winniford MD, Wheelan KR, Kremers MS, Ugolini V, van den Berg E, Niggemann EH, et al. Smoking-induced coronary vasoconstriction in patients with atherosclerotic coronary artery disease: Evidence for adrenergically mediated alterations in coronary artery tone. *Circulation* 1986; 73:662–667.
11. Winniford MD, Jansen DE, Reynolds GA, Apprill P, Black WH, Hillis LD. Cigarette smoking–induced coronary vasoconstriction in atherosclerotic coronary artery disease and prevention by calcium antagonists and nitroglycerin. *Am J Cardiol* 1987; 59:203–207.
12. Parker JO, Ledwich JR, West RO, Case RB. Reversible cardiac failure during angina pectoris: Hemodynamic effects of atrial pacing in coronary artery disease. *Circulation* 1969; 39:745–757.
13. McLaurin LP, Rolett EL, Grossman W. Impaired left ventricular relaxation during pacing-induced ischemia. *Am J Cardiol* 1973; 32:751–757.
14. Barry WH, Books JZ, Alderman EL, Harrison DC. Changes in diastolic stiffness and tone of the left ventricle during angina pectoris. *Circulation* 1974; 49:255–263.
15. Mann T, Brodie BR, Grossman W, McLaurin LP. Effect of angina on the left ventricular diastolic pressure-volume relationship. *Circulation* 1977; 55:761–766.
16. Bourdillon PD, Lorell BH, Mirsky I, Paulus WJ, Wynne J, Grossman W. Increased regional myocardial stiffness of the left ventricle during pacing-induced angina in man. *Circulation* 1983; 67:316–323.
17. Carroll JD, Hess OM, Hirzel HO, Krayenbuehl HP. Exercise-induced ischemia: The influence of altered relaxation on early diastolic pressures. *Circulation* 1983; 67:521–528.
18. Lorrell B. Significance of diastolic dysfunction of the heart. *Annu Rev Med* 1991; 42:411–436.
19. Kono T, Sabbah HN, Rosman H, Alam M, Jafri S, Stein PD, et al. Mechanism of functional mitral regurgitation during acute myocardial ischemia. *J Am Coll Cardiol* 1992; 19:1101–1105.
20. Fowler NO. Clinical diagnosis. *Circulation* 1972; 42:1079–1097.
21. Martin CE, Shaver JA, Leonard JJ. Physical signs, apex cardiography, phonocardiography, and systolic time intervals in angina pectoris. *Circulation* 1972; 46:1098–1114.
22. Shub C. Stable angina pectoris: 2. Cardiac evaluation and diagnostic testing. *Mayo Clin Proc* 1990; 65:243–255.
23. Task Force of the European Society of Cardiology. Management of stable angina pectoris. *Eur Heart J* 1997; 18:394–413.
24. Diamond GA, Forrester JS. Analysis of probability as an aid in the clinical diagnosis of coronary-artery disease. *N Engl J Med* 1979; 300:1350–1358.
25. Rifkin RD, Hood WB Jr. Bayesian analysis of electrocardiographic exercise stress testing. *N Engl J Med* 1977; 297:681–686.
26. Reeves TJ. Use of stress electrocardiography in practice. *Heart Dis Stroke* 1992:13–18.
27. Levinson JR, Guiney TE, Boucher CA. Functional tests for myocardial ischemia. *Annu Rev Med* 1991; 42:119–126.

28. Gianrossi R, Detrano R, Mulvihil D, Lehmann K, Dubach P, Colombo A, et al. Exercise-induced ST depression in the diagnosis of coronary artery disease: A meta-analysis. *Circulation* 1989; 80:87–98.

29. Detrano R, Gianrossi R, Froelicher V. The diagnostic accuracy of the exercise electrocardiogram: A meta-analysis of 22 years of research. *Prog Cardiovasc Dis* 1989; 32:173–206.

30. Hollenberg M, Budge WR, Wisneski JA, Gertz EW. Treadmill score quantifies electrocardiographic responses to exercise and improves test accuracy and reproducibility. *Circulation* 1980; 61:276–285.

31. Veragari J, Hakki AH, Heo J, Iskandrian AS. Merits and limitations of quantitative treadmill exercise score. *Am Heart J* 1987; 114:819–826.

32. Mark DB, Shaw L, Harrell FE, Hlatky MA, Lee KL, Bengtson JR, et al. Prognostic value of a treadmill exercise score in outpatients with suspected coronary artery disease. *N Engl J Med* 1991; 325:849–853.

33. Kligfield P, Ameisen O, Okin PM. Heart rate adjustment of ST segment depression for improved detection of coronary artery disease. *Circulation* 1989; 79:245–255.

34. Lachterman B, Lehmann KG, Detrano R, Neutel J, Froelicher VF. Comparison of the ST/heart rate index to standard ST criteria for analysis of the exercise electrocardiogram. *Circulation* 1990; 82:44–50.

35. Bobbio M, Detrano R, Schmid J-J, Janosi A, Righetti A, Pfisterer M, et al. Exercise-induced ST depression and ST/heart rate index to predict triple-vessel or left main coronary disease: A multicenter analysis. *J Am Coll Cardiol* 1992; 19:11–18.

36. Kligfield P, Okin PM, Goldberg HL. Value and limitations of heart rate-adjusted ST segment depression criteria for the identification of anatomically severe coronary obstruction: Test performance in relation to method of rate correction, definition of extent of disease, and beta-blockade. *Am Heart J* 1993; 125:1262–1268.

37. Gibbons RJ, Balady GJ, Beasley JW, Bricker JM, Duvernoy WF, Froelicher VF, et al. ACC/AHA Guidelines for exercise testing: A report of the American College of Cardiology/American Heart Association Task Force on Practice Guidelines (Committee on Exercise Testing). *J Am Coll Cardiol* 1997; 30:260–315.

38. Bartel AG, Behar VS, Peter RH, Orgain ES, Kong Y. Graded exercise stress tests in angiographically documented coronary artery disease. *Circulation* 1974; 49:348–356.

39. Goldschlager N, Selzer A, Cohn K. Treadmill stress tests as indicators of presence and severity of coronary artery disease. *Ann Intern Med* 1976; 85:277–286.

40. McNeer JF, Margolis JR, Lee KL, Kisslo JA, Peter RH, Kong Y, et al. The role of the exercise test in the evaluation of patients for ischemic heart disease. *Circulation* 1978; 57:64–70.

41. Froelicher VF. *Exercise and the Heart: Clinical Concepts.* Chicago: Yearbook Medical Publishers; 1987.

42. Gibbons L, Blair SN, Kohl HW, Cooper K. The safety of maximal exercise testing. *Circulation* 1989; 80:846–852.

43. Botvinick EH. Stress imaging. Current clinical options for the diagnosis, localization, and evaluation of coronary artery disease. *Med Clin North Am* 1995; 79:1025–1061.

44. Ladenheim ML, Pollack BH, Royanski A, Berman DS, Staniloff HM, Forrester JS, et al. Extent and severity of myocardial reperfusion as predictors of prognosis in patients with suspected coronary artery disease. *J Am Coll Cardiol* 1986; 7:464–471.

45. Kaul S. A look at 15 years of planar thallium-201. *Am Heart J* 1989; 118:581–601.

46. Lotler TS, Diamond GA. Exercise thallium-201 scintigraphy in the diagnosis and prognosis of coronary artery disease. *Ann Intern Med* 1990; 113:684–702.

47. Beller GA. Pharmacologic stress imaging. *JAMA* 1991; 265:633–638.

48. Zaret BL, Wackers FJ. Nuclear cardiology (two parts). *N Engl J Med* 1993; 329;775–783, 855–863.

49. American College of Cardiology/American Heart Association Task Force on assessment of diagnostic and therapeutic cardiovascular procedures. Guidelines for clinical use of cardiac radionuclide imaging. *J Am Coll Cardiol* 1995; 2:521–547.

50. Esquivel L, Pollock SG, Beller GA, Gibson RS, Watson DD, Kaul S. Effect of the degree of effort on the sensitivity of the exercise thallium-201 stress test in symptomatic coronary artery disease. *Am J Cardiol* 1989; 63:160–165.

51. Iskandrian AS, Hakki AH, Kane-Marsh S. Exercise thallium-201 scintigraphy in men with non-diagnostic exercise electrocardiograms: Prognostic implications. *Arch Intern Med* 1986; 146:2189–2193.

52. Boucher CA, Zin LM, Beller GA, Okada RD, McKusick KA, Strauss HW, et al. Increased lung uptake of thallium-201 during exercise myocardial imaging: Clinical, hemodynamic and angiographic implications in patients with coronary artery disease. *Am J Cardiol* 1980; 46:189–196.

53. Kaul S, Finkelstein DM, Homma S, Leavitt M, Okada RD, Bousher CA. Superiority of quantitative exercise thallium-201 variables in determining long-term prognosis in ambulatory patients with chest pain: A comparison with cardiac catheterization. *J Am Coll Cardiol* 1988; 12:25–34.

54. Brown K. Prognostic value of thallium-201 myocardial perfusion imaging: A diagnostic tool comes of age. *Circulation* 1991; 83:363–381.

55. Pamelia FX, Gibson RS, Watson DD, Craddock GB, Sirowatka J, Beller GA. Prognosis with chest pain and normal thallium-201 exercise scintigrams. *Am J Cardiol* 1985; 55:920–926.

56. Staniloff HM, Forrester JS, Berman DS, Swan HJC. Prediction of death, myocardial infarction, and worsening chest pain using thallium scintigraphy and exercise electrocardiography. *J Nucl Med* 1986; 27:1842–1848.

57. Gibson RS, Watson DD, Craddock GB, Crampton RS, Kaiser DL, Denny MJ, et al. Prediction of cardiac events after uncomplicated myocardial infarction: A prospective study comparing predischarge exercise thallium-201 scintigraphy and coronary angiography. *Circulation* 1983; 68:321–326.

58. Boucher CA, Brewster DC, Darling RC, Okada RC, Strauss HW, Pohost GM. Determination of cardiac risk by dipyridamole-thallium imaging before peripheral vascular surgery. *N Engl J Med* 1985; 312:389–394.

59. Leppo J, Plaja J, Goinet M, Tumolo J, Paraskos JA, Cutler BS. Noninvasive evaluation of cardiac risk before elective surgery. *J Am Coll Cardiol* 1987; 9:269–276.

60. Hays JT, Mahmarian JJ, Cochran AJ, Verani MS. Dobutamine thallium-201 tomography for evaluating patients with suspected coronary artery disease unable to undergo exercise or vasodilator pharmacologic stress testing. *J Am Coll Cardiol* 1993; 21:1583–1590.

61. Forster T, McNeil AJ, Salustri A, Reijs AEM, el-Said EM, Roelandt JRTC, et al. Simultaneous dobutamine stress echocardiography and technetium-99m isonitrile single-photon emission computed tomography in patients with suspected coronary artery disease. *J Am Coll Cardiol* 1993; 21:1591–1596.

62. O'Keefe JH Jr, Bateman TM, Barnhard CS. Adenosine thallium-201 is superior to exercise thallium-201 for detecting coronary artery disease in patients with left bundle branch block. *J Am Coll Cardiol* 1993; 21:1332–1338.

63. Berman DS, Kiat H, Friedman JD, Wang FP, van Train K, Matzer L, et al. Separate acquisition rest thallium-201/stress technetium-99m sestamibi dual-isotope myocardial perfusion single-photon emission computed tomography: A clinical validation study. *J Am Coll Cardiol* 1993; 22:1455–1464.

64. Hutchins GD, Schwaiger M, Rosenspire KC, Krivokapich J, Schelbert HR, Kuhl DE. Non-invasive quantification of regional blood flow in the human heart using N-13 ammonia and dynamic positron emission tomographic imaging. *J Am Coll Cardiol* 1990; 15:1031–1042.

65. Geltman EM, Hennes GC, Senneff MJ, Sobel BE, Bergmann SR. Increased myocardial perfusion at rest and diminished perfusion reserve in patients with angina and angiographically normal coronary arteries. *J Am Coll Cardiol* 1990; 16:586–595.

66. Quinones MA, Verani MS, Haichin RM, Mahmarian JJ, Suarez J, Zoghbi W. Exercise echocardiography versus ^{201}Tl single-photon emission computed tomography in evaluation of coronary artery disease: Analysis of 292 patients. *Circulation* 192; 85:1026–1031.

67. Beller GA. Evaluation of myocardial viability using thallium-201 imaging. *Cardiol Rev* 1993; 1:78–86.

68. Bonow RO, Dilsizian V, Cuocolo A, Bacharach SL. Identification of viable myocardium in patients with chronic coronary artery disease and left ventricular dysfunction: Comparison of thallium scintigraphy with reinjection and PET imaging with 18F-fluoro-dioxide glucose. *Circulation* 1991; 83:26–37.

69. Gibbons RJ. Rest and exercise radionuclide angiography for diagnosis in chronic ischemic heart disease. *Circulation* 1991; 84(suppl 1):I93–I99.

70. Marwick TH, Nemec JJ, Pashkow FJ, Stewart WJ, Salcedo EE. Accuracy and limitations of exercise echocardiography in a routine clinical setting. *J Am Coll Cardiol* 1992; 19:74–81.

71. Berthe C, Pierard LA, Hiernaux M, Trotteur G, Lempereur P, Carlier J, et al. Predicting the extent and location of coronary artery disease in acute myocardial infarction by echocardiography during dobutamine infusion. *Am J Cardiol* 1986; 58:1167–1172.

72. Harrison MR, Smith MD, Friedman BJ, DeMaria AN. Uses and limitations of exercise Doppler echocardiography in the diagnosis of ischemic heart disease. *J Am Coll Cardiol* 1987; 10:809–817.

73. Cohen JL, Greene TO, Ottenweller J, Binenvaum SZ, Wilchfort SD, Kim CS. Dobutamine digital echocardiography for detecting coronary artery disease. *Am J Cardiol* 1991; 67:1311–1318.

74. Mazeika P, Nihoyannopoulos P, Nadazdin A, Oakley CM. Pharmacological stress echocardiography in the evaluation of coronary artery disease. *Postgrad Med J* 1991; 67(suppl 1):S21–S35.

75. Mazeika PK, Nadazdin A, Oakley CM. Stress Doppler echocardiography using dobutamine in coronary patients with and without ischaemia induction. *Eur Heart J* 1992; 13:1020–1027.

76. Martin TW, Seaworth JF, Johns JP, Pupa LE, Condos WR. Comparison of adenosine, dipyridamole, and dobutamine in stress echocardiography. *Ann Intern Med* 1992; 116:190–196.

77. Barnard RJ, Duncan HW, Livesay JJ, Buckberg GD. Coronary vasodilator reserve and flow distribution during near-maximal exercise in dogs. *J Appl Physiol: Resp Environ Exercise Physiol* 1977; 43:988–992.

78. Boerth RC, Covell JW, Pool PE, Ross J Jr. Increased myocardial oxygen consumption and contractile state associated with increases in heart rate in dogs. *Circ Res* 1969; 24:725–734.

79. Pupita G, Maseri A, Kaski JC, Galassi AR, Gavrielides S, Davies G, et al. Myocardial ischemia caused by distal coronary artery constriction in stable angina pectoris. *N Engl J Med* 1990; 323:514–520.

80. McGorisk GM, Treasure CB. Endothelial dysfunction in coronary heart disease. *Curr Opin Cardiol* 1996; 11:341–350.

81. Egashira K, Inou T, Hirooka Y, Yamada A, Urabe Y, Takeshita A. Evidence of impaired endothelium-dependent coronary vasodilatation in patients with angina pectoris and normal coronary angiograms. *N Engl J Med* 1993; 328:1659–1664.

82. Cannon RO III, Camici PG, Epstein SE. Pathophysiological dilemma of syndrome X. *Circulation* 1992; 85:883–892.

83. Ardehali A, Ports TA. Myocardial oxygen supply and demand. *Chest* 1990; 98:699–705.

84. Mubagwa K, Mullane K, Flameng W. Role of adenosine in the heart and circulation. *Cardiovasc Res* 1996; 32:797–813.

85. Olsson RA, Bunger R, Spann JAE. Coronary circulation. In: Fozzard HA, Haber E, Jennings RB, Katz AM, Morgan HE, eds. *The Heart and Cardiovascular System: Scientific Foundations*, 2d ed. New York: Raven; 1991:1393–1425.

86. Dole WP. Autoregulation of the coronary circulation. *Prog Cardiovasc Dis* 1987; 29:369–387.

87. Gould KL, Lipscomb K, Calvert C. Compensatory changes of the distal coronary vascular bed during progressive coronary constriction. *Circulation* 1975; 51:1085–1094.

88. Mudge GH Jr, Grossman W, Mills RM Jr, Lesch M, Braunwald E. Reflex increase in coronary vascular resistance in patients with ischemic heart disease. *N Engl J Med* 1976; 295:1333–1337.

89. Sabiston DC, Gregg DE. Effects of cardiac contraction on coronary blood flow. *Circulation* 1957; 15:14–20.

90. Lewis FB, Coffmann JD, Gregg DE. Effect of heart rate and intracoronary isoproterenol, levarterenol, and epinephrine on coronary flow and resistance. *Circ Res* 1961; 9:89–95.

91. Furchgott RF, Zawadzski JV. The obligatory role of endothelial cells in the relaxation of arterial smooth muscle by acetylcholine. *Nature* 1980; 288:373–376.

92. Palmer RMJ, Ferrige AG, Moncada S. Nitric oxide release accounts for the biological activity of endothelium-derived relaxing factor. *Nature* 1987; 327:524–526.

93. Brown BG, Bolson EL, Dodge HT. Dynamic mechanisms in human coronary stenosis. *Circulation* 1984; 42:917–922.

94. Gage JE, Hess OM, Murakami T, Ritter M, Grimm J, Krayenbuehl P. Vasoconstriction of stenotic coronary arteries during dynamic exercise in patients with classic angina pectoris: Reversibility by nitroglycerin. *Circulation* 1986; 73865–876.

95. Gordon JB, Ganz P, Nabel EG, Fish RD, Zebede J, Mudge GH, et al. Atherosclerosis influences the vasomotor response of epicardial coronary arteries to exercise. *J Clin Invest* 1989; 83:1946–1952.

96. Bortone AS, Hess OM, Eberli FR. Abnormal coronary vasomotion during exercise in patients with normal coronary arteries and reduced coronary flow reserve. *Circulation* 1991; 83:26–37.

97. Hess OM, Buchi M, Kirkeeide R, Niederer P, Anliker M, Gould KL, et al. Potential role of coronary vasoconstriction in ischemic heart disease: Effect of exercise. *Eur Heart J* 1900; 11(suppl B):58–64.

98. Bassen M, Marcus H, Ganz W. The effect of mild to moderate mental stress on coronary hemodynamics in patients with coronary artery disease. *Circulation* 1980; 62:933–935.

99. Deanfield JE, Kensett M, Wilson RA, Shea M, Horlock P, deLandsheere CM, et al. Silent myocardial ischaemia due to mental stress. *Lancet* 1984; 2:1001–1005.

100. Yeung AC, Vekshtein VI, Krantz DS, Vita JA, Ryan TJ, Ganz P, et al. The effect of atherosclerosis on the vasomotor response of coronary arteries to mental stress. *N Engl J Med* 1991; 325:1551–1556.

101. Zeiher AM, Drexler H, Wollschlaeger H, Saubier B, Just H. Coronary vasomotion in response to sympathetic stimulation in humans: Importance of the functional integrity of the endothelium. *J Am Coll Cardiol* 1989; 14:1181–1190.

102. Nabel EG, Ganz P, Gordon JB, Alexander RW, Selwyn AP. Dilation of normal and constriction of atherosclerotic coronary arteries caused by the cold pressor testing. *Circulation* 1988; 77:43–52.

103. Nabel EG, Selwyn AP, Ganz P. Paradoxical narrowing of atherosclerotic coronary arteries induced by increases in heart rate. *Circulation* 1990; 81:850–859.

104. Vita JA, Treasure CB, Yeung AC, Vekshtein VI, Fantasia GM, Fish RD, et al. Patients with evidence of coronary endothelial dysfunction as assessed by acetylcholine infusion demonstrate marked increase in sensitivity to constrictor effects of catecholamines. *Circulation* 1992; 85:1390–1397.

105. Maseri A, Chierchia S, Kaski JC. Mixed angina pectoris. *Am J Cardiol* 1985; 56:30E–33E.

106. Likoff W, Segal BL, Kasparian H. Paradox of normal selective coronary arteriograms in patients considered to have unmistakable coronary heart disease. *N Engl J Med* 1967; 276:1063–1066.

107. Kemp HG, Elliott WC, Gorlin R. The anginal syndrome with normal coronary arteriography. *Trans Assoc Am Physicians* 1967; 80:59–70.

108. Maseri A, Crea F, Kaski JC. Mechanisms of angina pectoris in syndrome X. *J Am Coll Cardiol* 1991; 17:499–506.

109. Cannon RO III, Camici PG, Epstein SE. Pathophysiological dilemma of syndrome X. *Circulation* 1992; 85:883–892.

110. Fuh MM-T, Jeng C-Y, Young MM, Sheu WH, Chen YD, Reaven GM. Insulin resistance, glucose intolerance, and hyperinsulinemia in patients with microvascular angina. *Metabolism* 1993; 42:1090–1092.

111. Cannon RO III. Angina pectoris with normal coronary angiograms. *Cardiol Clin* 1991; 9:157–166.

112. Quyyumi AA, Cannon RO III, Panza JA, Diodati JG, Epstein SE. Endothelial dysfunction in patients with chest pain and normal coronary arteries. *Circulation* 1992; 86:1864–1871.

113. Bugiardini R, Pozzati A, Ottani F, Murgagni GL, Puddu P. Vasotonic angina: A spectrum of ischemic syndromes involving functional abnormalities of the epicardial and microvascular coronary circulation. *J Am Coll Cardiol* 1993; 22:417–425.

114. Opherk D, Schuler G, Wetterauer K, Mauthey J, Schwartz F, Kubler W. Four-year follow-up study in patients with angina pectoris and normal coronary arteriograms ("syndromes X"). *Circulation* 1989; 80:1610–1616.

115. Legrand V, Hodgson JM, Bates ER, Aueron FM, Mancini GBJ, Smith JS, et al. Abnormal coronary flow reserve and abnormal radionuclide exercise test results in patients with normal coronary angiograms. *J Am Coll Cardiol* 1985; 6:1245–1253.

116. Cannon RO III, Watson RM, Rosing DR, Epstein SE. Angina caused by reduced vasodilator reserve of the small coronary arteries. *J Am Coll Cardiol* 1983; 1:1359–1373.

117. Egashira K, Inou T, Hirooka Y, Yamada A, Urabe Y, Takeshita A. Evidence of impaired endothelium-dependent coronary vasodilatation in patients with angina pectoris and normal coronary angiograms. *N Engl J Med* 1993; 328:1659–1664.

118. Treasure CB, Klein JL, Vita JA, Manoukian SV, Renwick GH, Selwyn AP, et al. Hypertension and left ventricular hypertrophy are associated with impaired endothelium-mediated relaxation in human coronary resistance vessels. *Circulation* 1993; 87:86–93.

119. Mosseri M, Schaper J, Admon D, Hasin Y, Gotsman MS, Sapoznikov D, et al. Coronary capillaries in patients with congestive cardiomyopathy or angina pectoris with patent main coronary arteries. Ultrastructural morphometry of endomyocardial biopsy samples. *Circulation* 1991; 48:203–210.

120. Maseri A, Crea F, Kaski JC, Davies G. Mechanisms and significance of cardiac ischemic pain. *Prog Cardiovasc Dis* 1992; 35:1–18.

121. Deanfield JE. Characteristics of silent and symptomatic ischemia in chronic stable angina: Comparison with unstable and vasospastic angina. In: Singh BM, ed. *Silent Myocardial Ischemia and Angina. Prevalence, Prognostic, and Therapeutic Significance.* New York: Pergamon; 1988:104–111.

122. Stern S, Tzivoni D. Ventricular arrhythmias, sudden death, and silent myocardial ischemia. *Prog Cardiovasc Dis* 1992; 35:19–26.

123. Nair CK, Aronow MH, Sketch R, Pagano JD, Lynch AN, Moose D, et al. Diagnostic and prognostic significance of exercise-induced premature ventricular complexes in men and women: A four-year follow-up. *J Am Coll Cardiol* 1983; 1:1201–1206.

124. Sigwart U, Grbic M, Payot J, Goy A, Essinger A, Fischer A. Ischemic events during coronary artery balloon occlusion. In: Rutishauser W, Roskamm H, eds. *Silent Myocardial Ischemia.* Berlin: Springer-Verlag; 1984:29–36.

125. Muller JE, Stone PH, Turi ZG, Rutherford JD, Czeisler CA, Parker C, et al. Circadian variation in the frequency of onset of acute myocardial infarction. *N Engl J Med* 1985; 313:1315–1322.

126. Kenkels U, Blumchen G, Ebner F. Zur Probleme von Belastungsprofungen in aungigkeit von der Tageszeit bei Patienten mit Koronarinsuffizienz. *Herz Kreisal* 1977; 9:343–346.

127. Rocco MB, Barry J, Campbell S, Nabel E, Cook EF, Goldman L, et al. Circadian variation of transient myocardial ischemia in patients with coronary artery disease. *Circulation* 1987; 75:395–400.

128. Yasue H, Omote S, Takizawa A, Nagao M, Miwa K, Tanaka S. Circadian variation of exercise capacity in patients with Prinzmetal's variant angina: Role of exercise-induced coronary arterial spasm. *Circulation* 1979; 59:938–948.

129. Rocco MB, Selwyn AP. Circadian rhythms and ischemic heart disease with particular reference to transient myocardial ischemia. In: Singh B, ed. *Silent Myocardial Ischemia and Angina.* New York: Pergamon; 1988:70–81.

130. Deanfield JE. Characteristics of silent and symptomatic ischemia in chronic stable angina: Comparison with unstable and vasospastic angina. In: Singh BM, ed. *Silent Myocardial Ischemia and Angina.* New York: Pergamon; 1988:104–111.

131. Rosen SD, Paulesu E, Frith CD, Frackowiak RSJ, Davies GJ, Jones T, et al. Central nervous pathways mediating angina pectoris. *Lancet* 1994; 344:147–150.

132. Lindgren I, Olivecrona H. Surgical treatment of angina pectoris. *J Neurosurg* 1947; 4:19–39.

133. Crossman DC, Larkin SW, Fuller RW. Substance P dilates epicardial coronary arteries and increases coronary blood flow in humans. *Circulation* 1989; 80:475–484.

134. Sylven C, Beerman B, Jonzon B. Angina pectoris–like pain provoked by intravenous adenosine in healthy volunteers. *Br Med J* 1986; 293:227–230.

135. Herrick JB. Clinical features of sudden obstruction of the coronary arteries. *JAMA* 1912; 59:2015–2020.

136. Roseman MD. Painless myocardial infarction: A review of the literature and analysis of 220 cases. *Ann Intern Med* 1954; 41:1–8.

137. Master AM, Geller AM. The extent of completely asymptomatic coronary artery disease. *Am J Cardiol* 1969; 23:173–179.

138. Froelicher VF, Yanowitz FG, Thompson AJ. The correlation of coronary angiography and the electrocardiographic response to maximal treadmill testing in 76 asymptomatic men. *Circulation* 1973; 48:597–604.

139. Stern S, Tzivoni D. Early detection of silent ischaemic heart disease by 24-hour electrocardiographic monitoring of active subjects. *Br Heart J* 1974; 36:481–486.

140. Gettes LS. Painless myocardial ischemia. *Chest* 1974; 66:612–613.

141. Mulcahy D, Husain S, Zalos G, Rehman A, Andrews NP, Schenke WH, et al. Ischemia during ambulatory monitoring as a prognostic indicator in patients with stable coronary artery disease. *JAMA* 1997; 277:318–324.

142. Cohn PF. Asymptomatic coronary artery disease: Pathophysiology, diagnosis, management. *Mod Conc Cardiovasc Dis* 1981; 50:55–60.

143. Serneri GGN, Doddi M, Arata L, Rostagno C, Dabizzi P, Coppo M, et al. Silent ischemia in unstable angina is related to an altered cardiac norepinephrine handling. *Circulation* 1993; 87:1928–1937.

144. Cohn PF. Prevalence of silent myocardial ischemia. In: Cohn PF, ed. *Silent Myocardial Ischemia and Infarction.* New York: Marcel Dekker; 1986:71–80.

145. Deanfield JE, Ribiero P, Oakley K, Kirkler S, Selwyn AP. Analysis of ST-segment changes in normal subjects: Implications for ambulatory monitoring in angina pectoris. *Am J Cardiol* 1984; 54:1321–1325.

146. Armstrong WF, Jordan JW, Morris SN, McHenry PL. Prevalence and magnitude of ST segment and T wave abnormalities in normal men during continuous ambulatory echocardiography. *Am J Cardiol* 1982; 49:1639–1642.

147. Hedblad B, Juul-Moller S, Svensson K, Hanson BS, Isacsson SO, Janzon L, et al. Increased mortality in men with ST segment depression during 24 h ambulatory long-term ECG recording: Results from prospective population study 'Men born in 1914,' from Malmo, Sweden. *Eur Heart J* 1989; 10:149–158.

148. Pepine CJ, Coy K, Lambert C. Silent myocardial ischemia during daily activities in asymptomatic patients with positive treadmill tests. In: Singh B, ed. *Silent Myocardial Ischemia and Angina.* New York: Pergamon; 1988:93–103.

149. Deanfield JE, Maseri A, Selwyn AP, Ribeiro P, Chierchia S, Kirkler S, et al. Myocardial ischemia during daily life in patients with stable angina: Its relation to symptoms and heart rate changes. *Lancet* 1983; 3:753–758.

150. Chierchia S, Lazzari M, Freedman B, Brunelli C, Maseri A. Impairment of myocardial perfusion and function during painless myocardial ischemia. *J Am Coll Cardiol* 1983; 1:924–930.

151. Mannheimer C, Carlsson CA, Vedin A, Wilhelmsson C. Transcutaneous electrical nerve stimulation (TENS) in angina pectoris. *Pain* 1986; 26:291–300.

152. Davies HA, Page Z, Rush EM, Brown AL, Lewis MJ. Esophageal stimulation lowers exertional angina threshold. *Lancet* 1985; 1:1011–1014.

153. Murphy DF, Giles KE. Dorsal column stimulation for pain relief from intractable angina pectoris. *Pain* 1987; 28:365–368.

154. Droste C, Roskamm H. Experimental pain measurements in patients with asymptomatic myocardial ischemia. *J Am Coll Cardiol* 1983; 1:940–945.

155. Glazier JJ, Chierchia S, Brown MJ, Maseri A. Importance of generalized defective perception of painful stimuli as a cause of silent myocardial ischemia in chronic stable angina pectoris. *Am J Cardiol* 1986; 58:667–672.

156. Falcone C, Sconocchia R, Guasti L, Codega S, Montemartini C, Specchia G. Dental pain threshold and angina pectoris in patients with coronary artery disease. *J Am Coll Cardiol* 1988; 12:348–352.

157. Bradley RF, Partamian JO. Coronary heart disease in the diabetic patient. *Med Clin North Am* 1993; 78:1093–1104.

158. Fearman I, Faccio E, Melei J. Autonomic neuropathy and painless myocardial infarction in diabetic patients: Histologic evidence of their relationships. *Diabetes* 1977; 26:1147–1158.

159. Nesto RW, Phillips RT, Kett KG. Angina and exertional myocardial ischemia in diabetic and nondiabetic patients: Assessment by exercise thallium scintigraphy. *Ann Intern Med* 1988; 108:170–175.

160. Chiariello M, Indolfi C, Cotecchia MR. Asymptomatic transient ST changes during ambulatory ECG monitoring in diabetic patients. *Am Heart J* 1985; 110:529–534.

161. Coy KM, Imperi GA, Lambert CR, Pepine CJ. Silent myocardial ischemia during daily activities in asymptomatic men with positive exercise test responses. *Am J Cardiol* 1987; 59:45–49.

162. Deanfield JE, Kensett M, Wilson RA, Shea M, Horlock P, deLandsheere CM, et al. Silent myocardial ischaemia due to mental stress. *Lancet* 1984; 2:1001–1005.

163. Pepine CJ. Is silent ischemia a treatable risk factor in patients with angina pectoris? *Circulation* 1990; 82(suppl II):II135–II142.

164. Bertolet BD, Hill JA, Pepine CJ. Treatment strategies for daily life silent myocardial ischemia: A correlation with potential pathogenic mechanisms. *Prog Cardiovasc Dis* 1992; 35:97–118.

165. Rogers WJ, Bourassa MG, Andrews TC, Bertolet BD, Blumenthal RS, Chaitman BR, et al. Asymptomatic Cardiac Ischemia Pilot (ACIP) Study: Outcome at 1 year for patients with asymptomatic cardiac ischemia randomized to medical therapy or revascularization. *J Am Coll Cardiol* 1995; 26:594–605.

166. Stone PH, Chaitman BR, McMahon RP, Andrews TC, MacCallum G, Sharaf B, et al. Asymptomatic Cardiac Ischemia Pilot (ACIP) Study: Relationship between exercise-induced and ambulatory ischemia in patients with stable coronary disease. *Circulation* 1996; 94:1537–1544.

167. Pepine CJ, Sharaf B, Andrews TC, Forman S, Geller N, Knatterud G, et al. Relation between clinical, angiographic and ischemic findings at baseline and ischemia-related adverse outcomes at 1 year in Asymp-

tomatic Cardiac Ischemia Pilot Study. *J Am Coll Cardiol* 1997; 29:1483–1489.

168. Davies RF, Goldberg AD, Forman S, Pepine CJ, Knatterud GL, Geller N, et al. Asymptomatic Cardiac Ischemia Pilot (ACIP) Study Two-Year Follow-up: Outcomes of patients randomized to initial strategies of medical therapy versus revascularization. *Circulation* 1997; 95:2037–2043.

169. Zeiher AM, Drexler H, Wollschläger H, Just H. Modulation of coronary vasomotor tone in humans. Progressive endothelial dysfunction with different early stages of coronary arterosclerosis. *Circulation* 1991; 83:391–401.

170. Brown BG, Zhao XQ, Sacco DE, Albers JJ. Lipid lowering and plaque regression: New insights into prevention of plaque disruption and clinical events in coronary disease. *Circulation* 1993; 87:1781–1791.

171. Leung W-H, Lau C-P, Wong C-K. Beneficial effect of cholesterol-lowering therapy on coronary endothelium-dependent relaxation in hypercholesterolemic patients. *Lancet* 1993; 341:1496–1500.

172. Treasure CB, Klein JL, Weintraub WS, Talley JD, Stillabower ME, Kosinski AS, et al. Beneficial effects of cholesterol-lowering therapy on the coronary endothelium in patients with coronary artery disease. *N Engl J Med* 1995; 332:481–487.

173. Anderson TJ, Meredith IT, Yeung AC, Frei B, Selwyn AP, Ganz P. The effects of cholesterol-lowering and antioxidant therapy on endothelium-dependent coronary vasomotion. *N Engl J Med* 1995; 332:488–493.

174. Stroes ESG, Koomans HA, de Bruin TWA, Rabelink TJ. Vascular function in the forearm of hypercholesterolaemic patients off and on lipid-lowering medication. *Lancet* 1995; 346:467–471.

175. Kroon AA, Aengevaeren WRM, van der Werf T, Uijen GJH, Reiber JHC, Bruschke AVG, et al. LDL-Apheresis Atherosclerosis Regression Study (LAARS): Effect of aggressive versus conventional lipid lowering treatment on coronary atherosclerosis. *Circulation* 1996; 93:1826–1835.

176. Lüscher TF, Tanner FC, Noll G. Lipids and endothelial function: Effects of lipid-lowering and other therapeutic interventions. *Curr Opin Lipidol* 1996; 7:234–240.

177. Waters D. Review of cholesterol-lowering therapy: Coronary angiographic and events trials. *Am J Med* 1996; 101(suppl 4A):34S–39S.

178. O'Keefe JH, Conn RD, Lavie CJ Jr, Bateman TM. The new paradigm in coronary artery disease: Altering risk factors, atherosclerotic plaques, and clinical prognosis. *Mayo Clin Proc* 1996; 71:957–965.

179. Watts GF, Burke V. Lipid-lowering trials in the primary and secondary prevention of coronary heart disease: New evidence, implications and outstanding issues. *Curr Opin Lipidol* 1996; 7:341–355.

180. Kinlay S, Selwyn AP, Delangrange D, Creager MA, Libby P, Ganz P. Biological mechanisms for the clinical success of lipid-lowering in coronary artery disease and the use of surrogate endpoint. *Curr Opin Lipidol* 1996; 7:389–397.

181. Andrews TC, Raby K, Barry J, Naimi CL, Allred E, Ganz P, et al. Effect of cholesterol reduction on myocardial ischemia in patients with coronary disease. *Circulation* 1997; 95:324–328.

182. Steinberg D. Oxidative modification of LDL and atherogenesis. *Circulation* 1997; 95:1062–1071.

183. Ornish D, Brown SE, Scherwitz LW, Billings JH, Armstrong WT, Ports TA, et al. Can lifestyle changes reverse coronary heart disease? *Lancet* 1990; 336:129–133.

184. Ridker PM, Manson JE, Gaziano JM, Buring JE, Hennekens CH. Low-dose aspirin therapy for chronic stable angina: A randomized, placebo-controlled clinical trial. *Ann Intern Med* 1991; 114:835–839.

185. Juul-Moller S, Edvardsson N, Jahnmatz B, Rosen A, Sorenson S, Omblus R. Double-blind trial of aspirin in primary prevention of myocardial infarction in patients with stable chronic angina pectoris. *Lancet* 1992; 340:1421–1425.

186. Stein B, Fuster V. Anticoagulants and platelet inhibitors. *Curr Opin Cardiol* 1990; 5:461–474.

187. Willard JE, Lange RA, Hillis LD. The use of aspirin in ischemic heart disease. *N Engl J Med* 1992; 327:175–181.

188. Summary of the Second Report of National Cholesterol Education Program (NCEP) Expert Panel on Detection, Evaluation, and Treatment of High Blood Cholesterol in Adults (Adult Treatment Panel II). *JAMA* 1993; 269:3015–3023.

189. Schuler G, Hambrecht R, Schlierf G, Niebauer J, Hauer K, Neumann J, et al. Regular physical exercise and low-fat diet. Effects on progression of coronary artery disease. *Circulation* 1992; 86:1–11.

190. Scandinavian Simvastatin Survival Study Group. Randomized trial of cholesterol lowering in 4444 patients with coronary heart disease. The Scandinavian Simvastatin Survival Study (4S). *Lancet* 1994; 344:1383–1389.

191. Sacks FM, Pfeffer MA, Moye LA, Rouleau JL, Rutherford JD, Cole TG, et al. The effect of pravastatin on coronary events after myocardial infarction in patients with average cholesterol levels. *N Engl J Med* 1996; 335:1001–1009.

192. Penderson TR, Kjekshus J, Berg K, Olsson AG, Wilhelmsen L, Wedel H, et al. Cholesterol lowering and the use of healthcare resources. Results of the Scandinavian Simvastatin Survival Study. *Circulation* 1996; 93:1796–1802.

193. Yusuf S, Anand S. Cost of prevention. The case of lipid lowering. *Circulation* 1996; 93:1774–1776.

194. Jönsson B, Johannesson M, Kjekshus J, Olsson AG, Pedersen TR, Wedel H. Cost-effectiveness of cholesterol lowering. Results from the Scandinavian Simvastatin Survival Study (4S). *Eur Heart J* 1996; 17:1001–1007.

195. Johannesson M, Jönsson B, Kjekshus J, Olsson AG, Pederson TR, Wedel H. Cost-effectiveness of simvastatin to lower cholesterol levels in patients with coronary heart disease. *N Engl J Med* 1997; 336:332–336.

196. Fletcher GF, Blair SN, Blumenthal J, Caspersen C, Chaitman B, Epstein S, et al. Statement on exercise benefits and recommendations for physical activity programs for all Americans. A statement for health care professionals by the Committee on Exercise and Cardiac Rehabilitation of the Council on Clinical Cardiology. American Heart Association. *Circulation* 1992; 86:340–344.

197. Redwood DR, Rosing DR, Epstein SE. Circulatory and symptomatic effects of physical training in patients with coronary artery disease and angina pectoris. *N Engl J Med* 1972; 286:959–965.

198. Amsterdam EA, Hughes JL III, DeMaria AN. Indirect assessment of myocardial oxygen consumption in the evaluation of mechanisms and therapy of angina pectoris. *Am J Cardiol* 1974; 33:737–743.

199. Sim DN, Neill WA. Investigation of the physiological basis for increased exercise threshold for angina pectoris after physical conditioning. *J Clin Res* 1974; 54:763–770.

200. Clausen JP. Circulatory adjustments to dynamic exercise and the effect of physical training in normal subjects and in patients with coronary artery disease. *Prog Cardiovasc Dis* 1976; 18:495.

201. Kennedy CC, Spiekerman RE, Lindsay MI, Mankin HT, Frye RL, McCallister BD. One-year graduated exercise program for men with angina pectoris. *Mayo Clin Proc* 1976; 51.231–236.

202. Ehsani AA, Health GW, Hagberg JM, Sobel BE, Holoszy JO. Effects of 12 months intense exercise training on ischemic ST segment depression in patients with coronary artery disease. *Circulation* 1981; 64:1116–1124.

203. Froelicher V, Jensen D, Genter F, Sullivan M, McKirnan MD, Witztum K, et al. A randomized trial of exercise training in patients with coronary artery disease. *JAMA* 1984; 252:1291–1297.

204. Tzivoni D, Maybaum S. Attenuation of severity of myocardial ischemia during repeated daily ischemic episodes. *J Am Coll Cardiol* 1997; 30:119–124.

205. Parker JO. Nitrate therapy in stable angina pectoris. *N Engl J Med* 1987; 316:1635–1642.

206. Abrams J. A reappraisal of nitrate therapy. *JAMA* 1988; 259(3):396–401.

207. Abrams J. Transdermal nitroglycerin in angina pectoris. *Eur Heart J* 1989; 10(suppl A):11–19.

208. Abrams J. Use of nitrates in ischemic heart disease. *Curr Probl Cardiol* 1992; 17:487–542.

209. Abrams J, ed. A symposium: Third North American conference on nitroglycerin therapy. *Am J Cardiol* 1992; 70(suppl B):1B–103B.

210. Frishman W, ed. Optimizing anti-anginal therapy: A consensus conference. *Am J Cardiol* 1992; 70(suppl G):1G–76G.

211. Thadani U. Secondary preventive potential of nitrates in ischemic heart disease. *Eur Heart J* 1996; 17(suppl F):30–36.

212. Leier CV. Nitrate tolerance. *Am Heart J* 1985; 110:224–232.

213. Parker JO, Farrell B, Lahey K, Moe G. Effect of intervals between doses on the development of tolerance to isosorbide dinitrate. *N Engl J Med* 1987; 316:1440–1444.

214. Horowitz JD, Antman EM, Lorell BH, Barry WH, Smith TN. Potentiation of the cardiovascular effects of nitroglycerin by *N*-acetylcysteine. *Circulation* 1983; 68:1247–1253.

215. Torresi J, Horowitz JD, Dusting GJ. Prevention and reversal of tolerance to nitroglycerin with *N*-acetylcysteine. *J Cardiovasc Pharmacol* 1985; 7:777–783.

216. Packer M, Lee WH, Kessler PD, Gottlieb SS, Medina N, Yushak M. Prevention and reversal of nitrate tolerance in patients with congestive heart failure. *N Engl J Med* 1987; 17:799–804.

217. Levy WS, Katz RJ, Ruffalo RL, Leiboff RH, Wasserman AG. Potentiation of the hemodynamic effects of acutely administered nitroglycerin by methionine. *Circulation* 1988; 78:640–645.

218. Parker JO, Farrell B, Labey KA, Rose BF. Nitrate tolerance: The lack of effect of *N*-acetylcysteine. *Circulation* 1987; 76:572–576.

219. Munzel T, Holtz J, Mulsch A, Stewart DJ, Bassenge E. Nitrate tolerance in epicardial arteries or in the venous system is not reversed by *N*-acetylcysteine in vivo, but tolerance-independent interactions exist. *Circulation* 1989; 79:188–197.

220. Dupris J, Lalonde G, Lemieux R, Rouleau JL. Tolerance to intravenous nitroglycerin in patients with congestive heart failure. Role of increased volume, neurohumoral activation and lack of prevention with N-acetylcysteine. *J Am Cardiol* 1990; 16:932–934.

221. Münzel T, Kurz S, Rajagopalan S, Thoenes M, Berrington WR, Thompson JA, et al. Hydralazine prevents nitroglycerin tolerance by inhibiting activation of a membrane-bound NADH oxidase. A new action for an old drug. *J Clin Invest* 1996; 98:1465–1470.

222. Thadani U, Davidson C, Singleton W, Taylor SH. Comparison of the immediate effects of five beta-adrenoreceptor-blocking drugs with different ancillary properties in angina pectoris. *N Engl J Med* 1979; 300:750–755.

223. Kirklin JW, Atkins CW, Blackstone E, Booth DC, Califf RM, Cohen LS, et al. American College of Cardiology/American Heart Association Task Force on Assessment of Diagnostic and Therapeutic Cardiovascular Procedures: Guidelines and indications for coronary artery bypass graft surgery. *J Am Coll Cardiol* 1991; 17:543–584.

224. Ryan TJ, Bauman WB, Kennedy JW, Kereikes OJ, King SB III, McCallister BD, et al. Guidelines for percutaneous transluminal coronary angioplasty. A report of the American College of Cardiology/American Heart Association Task Force on Assessment of Diagnostic and Therapeutic Cardiovascular Procedures (Committee on Percutaneous Transluminal Coronary Angioplasty). *J Am Coll Cardiol* 1993; 22:2033–2054.

225. Varnauskas E and the European Coronary Surgery Study Group. Twelve-year follow-up of survival in the randomized European Coronary Surgery Study. *N Engl J Med* 1988; 319:332–337.

226. The VA Coronary Artery Bypass Surgery Cooperative Study Group. Eighteen-year follow-up in the Veterans Affairs Cooperative Study of Coronary Artery Bypass Surgery for Stable Angina. *Circulation* 1992; 86:121–130.

227. Gersh BJ, Califf RM, Loop FD, Atkins CW, Pryor DB, Takaro TC. Coronary bypass surgery in chronic stable angina. *Circulation* 1989; 79(suppl I):I46–I59.

228. Alderman EL, Bourassa MG, Cohen LS, Davis KB, Kaiser GG, Killip T, et al. Ten-year follow-up of survival and myocardial infarction in the randomized Coronary Artery Surgery Study. *Circulation* 1990; 82:1629–1646.

229. Rogers WJ, Coggin CJ, Gersh BJ, Fisher LD, Myers WO, Oberman A, et al. Ten-year follow-up of quality of life in patients randomized to receive medical therapy or coronary artery bypass graft surgery: The Coronary Artery Surgery Study. *Circulation* 1990; 82:1647–1658.

230. Hammermeister KE, Morrison DA. Coronary bypass surgery for stable and unstable angina pectoris. *Cardiol Clin* 1991; 9:135–155.

231. Nwasokwa ON, Koss JH, Friedman GH, Grunwald MA, Bodenheimer MM. Bypass surgery for chronic stable angina: Predictors of survival benefit and strategy for patient selection. *Ann Intern Med* 1991; 114:1035–1049.

232. Yusuf S, Zucker D, Peduzzi P, Fisher LD, Takaro T, Kennedy JW, et al. Effects of coronary artery bypass graft surgery on survival: Overview of 10-year results from randomized trials by the Coronary Artery Bypass Graft Surgery Trialists Collaboration. *Lancet* 1994; 344:563–570.

233. Hillis LD. Coronary artery bypass surgery: Risks and benefits, realistic and unrealistic expectations. *J Invest Med* 1995; 43:17–27.

234. Davis KB, Chaitman B, Ryan T, Bittner V, Kennedy JW. Comparison of 15-years survival for men and women after initial medical or surgical treatment for coronary artery disease: A CASS registry study. *J Am Coll Cardiol* 1995; 25:1000–1009.

235. Kanagasaby RR, Parker DJ. Long-term results of coronary artery bypass grafting. *Curr Opin Cardiol* 1996; 11:568–573.

236. Frazier OH, Kadipasaoglu K. Transmyocardial laser revascularization. *Curr Opin Cardiol* 1996; 11:564–567.

237. Gassler N, Wintzer H-O, Stubbe H-M, Wullbrand A, Helmchen U. Transmyocardial laser revascularization. Histological features in human nonresponder myocardium. *Circulation* 1997; 95:371–375.

238. RITA Trial Participants. Coronary angioplasty versus coronary artery bypass surgery: Treatment of Angina (RITA) Trial. *Lancet* 1993; 341:573–580.

239. Hamm CW, Reimers J, Ischinger T, Rupprecht HJ, Berger J, Bleifeld W, et al. A randomized study of coronary angioplasty compared with bypass surgery in patients with symptomatic multivessel coronary disease. *N Engl J Med* 1994; 331:1037–1043.

240. King SB, Lembo NJ, Weintraub WS, Kosinski AS, Barnhart HX, Kutner MH, et al. A randomized trial comparing coronary angioplasty with coronary bypass surgery. *N Engl J Med* 1994; 331:1044–1050.

241. Harris WO, Mock MB, Orszulak TA, Schaff HV, Holmes DR. Use of coronary artery bypass surgical procedure and coronary angioplasty in treatment of coronary artery disease: Changes during a 10-year period at Mayo Clinic, Rochester. *Mayo Clin Proc* 1996; 71:927–935.

242. Anderson WD, King SB III. A review of randomized trials comparing coronary angioplasty and bypass grafting. *Curr Opin Cardiol* 1996; 11:583–590.

243. Weintraub WS, Jones EI, Morris DC, King SB III, Guyton RA, Craver JM. Outcome of reoperative coronary bypass surgery versus coronary angioplasty after previous bypass surgery. *Circulation* 1997; 95:868–877.

244. The Writing Group for the Bypass Angioplasty Revascularization Investigation (BARI) Investigators. Five-year clinical and functional outcome comparing bypass surgery and angioplasty in patients with multivessel coronary disease. A multicenter randomized trial. *JAMA* 1997; 277:715–721.

245. Guidelines for coronary angiography. A report of the ACC/AHA Task Force on Assessment of Diagnostic and Therapeutic Cardiovascular Procedures. *J Am Coll Cardiol* 1987; 10:935–950.

246. Pryor DB, Bruce RA, Chaitman BR, Fisher L, Gajewski J, Hammermeister KE, et al. Task Force I: Determination of prognosis in patients with ischemic heart disease. *J Am Coll Cardiol* 1989; 14:1016–1025.

247. Weiner DA. Risk stratification in angina pectoris. *Cardiol Clin* 1991; 9:39–47.

248. Lawson WE, Hui JCK, Soroff HS, Zheng ZS, Kayden DS, Sasvary D, et al. Efficacy of enhanced external counterpulsation in the treatment of angina pectoris. *Am J Cardiol* 1992; 70:859–862.

249. Hautvast RWM, DeJongste MJL, Ter Horst GJ, Blanksma PK, Lie KI. Angina pectoris refractory for conventional therapy—is neurostimulation a possible alternative treatment? *Clin Cardiol* 1996; 19:531–535.

250. Lewin MR. Chelation therapy for cardiovascular disease. *Texas Heart Inst J* 1997; 24:81–89.

251. Diamond GA, Forrester JS, deLuz PL, Wyatt HL, Swan HJC. Postextrasystolic potentiation of ischemic myocardium by atrial stimulation. *Am Heart J* 1978; 95:204–209.

252. Rahimtoola SH. The hibernating myocardium. *Am Heart J* 1989; 117:211–221.

253. Braunwald E, Rutherford J. Reversible ischemic left ventricular dysfunction: Evidence for "Hibernating Myocardium." *J Am Coll Cardiol* 1986; 8:1467–1470.

254. Rahimtoola SH. Clinical aspects of hibernating myocardium. *J Mol Cell Cardiol* 1996; 28:2397–2401.

255. Heusch G, Schulz R. Hibernating myocardium: A review. *J Mol Cell Cardiol* 1996; 28:2359–2372.

256. Vanoverschelde J-L J, Wijns W, Borgers M, Heyndrick G, Depré C, Flameng W, et al. Chronic myocardial hibernation in humans. From bedside to bench. *Circulation* 1997; 95:1961–1971.

257. Passamani E, Davis KB, Gillespie MJ, Killip T, and the CASS Principal Investigators and Their Associates. A randomized trial of coronary artery bypass surgery. Survival of patients with a low ejection fraction. *N Engl J Med* 1985; 312:1665–1671.

258. Louie HW, Laks H, Milgalter E, Drinkwater DC Jr, Hamilton MA, Brunken RC, et al. Ischemic cardiomyopathy. Criteria for coronary revascularization and cardiac transplantation. *Circulation* 1991; 84(suppl III):III290–III295.

259. Elefteriades JA, Tolis G Jr, Levi E, Mills LK, Zaret BL. Coronary artery bypass grafting in severe left ventricular dysfunction: Excellent survival with improved ejection fraction and functional state. *J Am Coll Cardiol* 1993; 22:1411–1417.

260. Milano CA, White WD, Smith LR, Jones RH, Lowe JE, Smith PK, et al. Coronary artery bypass in patients with severely depressed ventricular function. *Ann Thorac Surg* 1993; 56:487–493.

261. Baker DW, Jones R, Hodges J, Massie BM, Konstam MA, Rose MA. Management of heart failure. The role of revascularization in the treatment of patients with moderate or severe left ventricular systolic dysfunction. *JAMA* 1994; 272:1528–1534.

262. Alfieri O. Coronary artery bypass grafting for left ventricular dysfunction. *Curr Opin Cardiol* 1994; 9:658–663.

263. Shapira I, Isakov A, Yakirevich V, Topilsky M. Long-term results of coronary artery bypass surgery in patients with severely depressed left ventricle function. *Chest* 1995; 108:1546–1550.

264. Langenburg SE, Buchanan SA, Blackbourne LH, Scheri RP, Sinclair KN, Martinez J, et al. Predicting survival after coronary revascularization for ischemic cardiomyopathy. *Ann Thorac Surg* 1995; 60:1193–1197.

265. Kay GL, Sun G-W, Aoki A, Prejean CA Jr. Influence of ejection fraction on hospital mortality, morbidity, and costs for CABG patients. *Ann Thorac Surg* 1995; 60:1640–1651.

266. Di Carli MF, Asgarzadie F, Schelbert HR, Brunken RC, Laks H, Phelps ME, et al. Quantitative relation between myocardial viability and improvement in heart failure symptoms after revascularization in patients with ischemic cardiomyopathy. *Circulation* 1995; 92:3436–3444.

267. Mickleborough LL, Maruyama H, Takagi Y, Mohamed S, Sun Z, Ebisuzaki L. Results of revascularization in patients with severe left ventricular dysfunction. *Circulation* 1995; 92(suppl II):II73–II79.

268. Chan RKM, Raman J, Lee KJ, Rosalion A, Hicks RJ, Pornvilawan S, et al. Prediction of outcome after revascularization in patients with poor left ventricular function. *Ann Thorac Surg* 1996; 61:1428–1434.

269. Kaul TK, Agnihotri AK, Fields BL, Riggins LS, Wyatt DA, Jones CR. Coronary artery bypass grafting in patients with an ejection fraction of twenty percent or less. *J Thorac Cardiovasc Surg* 1996; 111:1001–1012.

270. Blitz A, Laks H. The role of coronary revascularization in the management of heart failure: Identification of candidates and review of results. *Curr Opin Cardiol* 1996; 11:276–290.

271. Elefteriades JA, Morales DLS, Gradel C, Tollis G Jr, Levi E, Zaret BL. Results of coronary artery bypass grafting by a single surgeon in patients with left ventricular ejection fraction ≤30%. *Am J Cardiol* 1997; 79:1573–1578.

272. Dilsizian V, Arrighi JA, Diodati JG, Quyyumi AA, Alvi K, Bacharach SL, et al. Myocardial viability in patients with chronic coronary artery disease: Comparison of ^{99m}Tc-sestamibi with thallium reinjection and [^{18}F] fluorodeoxyglucose. *Circulation* 1994; 89:578–587.

273. Botvinick EH. Stress imaging. Current clinical options for the diagnosis, localization, and evaluation of coronary artery disease. *Med Clin North Am* 1995; 79:1025–1061.

274. Perrone-Filardi P, Pace L, Prastaro M, Squame F, Betocchi S, Soricelli A, et al. Assessment of myocardial viability in patients with chronic coronary artery disease. Rest–4-hour–24-hour ^{201}Tl tomography versus dobutamine echocardiography. *Circulation* 1996; 94:2712–2719.

275. Steffens JC, Sakuma H, Bourne MW, Higgins CB. Magnetic resonance imaging in ischemic heart disease. *Am Heart J* 1996; 132:156–173.

276. Perrone-Filardi P, Pace L, Prastaro M, Piscione F, Betocchi S, Squame F, et al. Dobutamine echocardiography predicts improvement of hypoperfused dysfunctional myocardium after revascularization in patients with coronary artery disease. *Circulation* 1995; 91:2556–2565.

277. deFilippi CR, Willett DL, Irani WN, Eichhorn EJ, Velasco CE, Grayburn PA. Comparison of myocardial contrast echocardiography and low-dose dobutamine stress echocardiography in predicting recovery of left ventricular function after coronary revascularization in chronic ischemic heart disease. *Circulation* 1995; 92:2863–2868.

278. Picano E, Ostojic M, Varga A, Sicari R, Djordjevic-Dikic A, Nedeljkovic I, et al. Combined low dose dipyridamole-dobutamine stress echocardiography to identify myocardial viability. *J Am Coll Cardiol* 1996; 27:1422–1428.

279. Qureshi U, Nagueh SF, Afridi I, Vaduganathan P, Blaustein A, Verani MS, et al. Dobutamine echocardiography and quantitative rest-redistribution ^{201}Tl tomography in myocardial hibernation: Relation to contractile reserve to ^{201}Tl uptake and comparative prediction of recovery of function. *Circulation* 1997; 95:626–635.

280. Sawada S, Elsner G, Segar DS, O'Shaughnessy M, Khouri S, Foltz J, et al. Evaluation of patterns of perfusion and metabolism in dobutamine-responsive myocardium. *J Am Coll Cardiol* 1997; 29:55–61.

281. Maddahi J, Blitz A, Phelps M, Laks H. The use of positron emission tomography imaging in the management of patients with ischemic cardiomyopathy. *Adv Cardiac Surg* 1991; 7:163–188.

282. Ragosta M, Beller GA. The noninvasive assessment of myocardial viability. *Clin Cardiol* 1993; 16:531–538.

283. DeNofrio D, Loh E. Myocardial viability in patients with coronary artery disease and left ventricular dysfunction: Transplantation or revascularization? *Curr Opin Cardiol* 1996; 11:394–402.

284. Hendel RC, Chaudhry FA, Bonow RO. Myocardial viability. *Curr Probl Cardiol* 1996; 21:145–221.

285. Iskandrian AS, Heo J, Schelbert HR. Myocardial viability: Methods of assessment and clinical relevance. *Am Heart J* 1996; 132:1226–1235.

286. Moss AJ, Hall WJ, Cannom DS, Daubert JP, Higgins SL, Klein H, et al. Improved survival with an implanted defibrillator in patients with coronary disease at high risk for ventricular arrhythmias. *N Engl J Med* 1996; 335:1933–1940.

287. Kemp GH. Left ventricular function in patients with the anginal syndrome and normal coronary arteriograms. *Am J Cardiol* 1973; 32:375–376.

288. Kaplan MN. Syndromes X: Two too many. *J Am Coll Cardiol* 1992; 69;1643–1644.

289. Reaven GM. Role of insulin resistance in human disease. *Diabetes* 1988; 37:1595–1607.

290. Dean JD, Jones CJH, Hutchison SJ, Peters JR, Henderson AH. Hyperinsulinaemia and microvascular angina ("syndrome X"). *Lancet* 1991; 337:456–457.

291. Brush JE, Cannon RO, Schenke WH, Bonow RO, Leon MB, Maron BJ, et al. Angina due to coronary microvascular disease in hypertensive patients without left ventricular hypertrophy. *N Engl J Med* 1988; 319:1302–1307.

292. Cannon RO. Microvascular angina: Cardiovascular investigation regarding pathophysiology and management. In: Richter JE, Cannon RO, Reitman B, eds. *Unexplained Chest Pain*. Philadelphia: Saunders; 1991:1097–1118.

293. Tweddel AC, Martin W, Hutton I. Thallium scans in syndrome X. *Br Heart J* 1992; 68:48–50.

294. Camici PG, Marraccini P, Lorenzoni R, Buzzigoli G, Pecori N, Perissinotto A, et al. Coronary hemodynamic and myocardial metabolism in patients with syndrome X. Response to pacing stress. *J Am Coll Cardiol* 1991; 17:1461–1470.

295. Opherk D, Zebe H, Weihe E, Mall G, Durr C, Graveit D, et al. Reduced coronary dilatory capacity and ultrastructural changes of the myocardium in patients with angina pectoris but normal coronary arteriograms. *Circulation* 1981; 63:817–825.

296. Cannon RO, Epstein SE. "Microvascular angina" as a cause of chest pain with angiographically normal coronary arteries. *Am J Cardiol* 1988; 61:1338–1343.

297. Epstein SE, Cannon RO. Site of increased resistance to coronary flow in patients with angina pectoris and normal epicardial coronary arteries. *J Am Coll Cardiol* 1986; 8:459–461.

298. Motz W, Vogt M, Rabenay O, Scheler S, Luckhoff A, Straver BE. Evidence of endothelial dysfunction in coronary resistance vessels in patients with angina pectoris and normal coronary angiograms. *Am J Cardiol* 1991; 68:996–1003.

299. Romeo F, Rosano G, Martuscelli E, Lombardo L, Valente A. Long-term follow-up of patients initially diagnosed with syndrome X. *Am J Cardiol* 1993; 71:669–673.

300. Cannon RO, Dilsizian V, Correa R, Epstein SE, Bonow RO. Chronic deterioration in left ventricular function in patients with microvascular angina (abstr). *J Am Coll Cardiol* 1991; 17:28A.

301. Nihoyannopoulos P, Kaski JC, Crake T, Maseri A. Absence of myocardial dysfunction during stress in patients with syndrome X. *J Am Coll Cardiol* 1991; 18:1463–1470.

302. Opherk D, Zebe H, Schuler G, Weihe E, Mall G, Kubler W. Reduced coronary reserve and abnormal exercise left ventricular reserve in patients with syndrome X. *Arch Mal Coeur* 1983; 76:231–235.

303. Opherk D, Schuler G, Wetterauer K, Manthey J, Schwarz F, Kubler W. Four-year follow-up in patients with angina pectoris and normal coronary arteriograms ("syndrome X"). *Circulation* 1989; 80:1610–1616.

304. Turiel M, Galassi AR, Glazier JJ, Kaski JC, Maseri A. Pain threshold and tolerance in women with syndrome X and women with stable angina pectoris. *Am J Cardiol* 1987; 60:503–508.

305. Shapiro LM, Crake T, Poole-Wilson PA. Is altered cardiac sensation responsible for chest pain in patients with normal coronary arteries? Clinical observation during catheterization. *Br Med J* 1988; 296:170–171.

306. Cannon RO, Quyyumi AA, Schenke WH, Fananapazir L, Tucker EE, Gaughan AM, et al. Abnormal cardiac sensitivity in patients with chest pain and normal coronary arteries. *J Am Coll Cardiol* 1990; 16:1359–1366.

307. Maseri A, Crea F, Kaski JC, Davies G. Mechanisms of angina pectoris in syndrome X. *J Am Coll Cardiol* 1991; 17:499–506.

308. Smith SC Jr, Blair SN, Criqui MH, Fletcher GF, Fuster V, Gersh BJ, et al. Preventing heart attack and death in patients with coronary disease. *Circulation* 1995; 92:2–4.

309. Waters D, Pedersen TR. Review of cholesterol-lowering therapy: Coronary angiographic and events trials. *Am J Med* 1996; 101:4A34S–4A38S.

310. O'Keefe JH, Conn RD, Lavie CJ Jr, Bateman TM. Subspecialty Clinics: Cardiology. The new paradigm for coronary artery disease: Altering risk factors, atherosclerotic plaques, and clinical prognosis. *Mayo Clin Proc* 1996; 71:957–965.

311. Rackley CE. Monotherapy with HMG-CoA reductase inhibitors and secondary prevention in coronary artery disease. *Clin Cardiol* 1996; 19:683–689.

312. Watts GF, Burke V. Lipid-lowering trials in the primary and secondary prevention of coronary heart disease: New evidence, implications and outstanding issues. *Curr Opin Lipidol* 1996; 7:341–355.

313. Kinlay S, Selwyn AP, Delagrange D, Creager MA, Libby P, Ganz P. Biological mechanisms for the clinical success of lipid-lowering in coronary artery disease and the use of surrogate endpoints. *Curr Opin Lipidol* 1996; 7:389–397.

314. Schell WD, Myers JN. Regression of atherosclerosis: A review. *Prog Cardiovasc Dis* 1997; 39:483–496.

315. Merz CNB, Forrester JS. The secondary prevention of coronary artery disease. *Am J Med* 1997; 102:572–581.

316. Grundy SM. Cholesterol and coronary heart disease. *Arch Intern Med* 1997; 157:1177–1184.

317. Selwyn AP, Kinlay S, Libby P, Ganz P. Atherogenic lipids, vascular dysfunction, and clinical signs of ischemic heart disease. *Circulation* 1997; 95:5–7.

318. Andrews TC, Raby K, Barry J, Naimi CL, Allred E, Ganz P, et al. Effect of cholesterol reduction on myocardial ischemia in patients with coronary disease. *Circulation* 1997; 95:324–328.

319. Rosengren A, Hagman M, Wedel H, Wilhelmsen L. Serum cholesterol and long-term prognosis in middle-aged men with myocardial infarction and angina pectoris. A 16-year follow-up of the Primary Prevention Study in Göteborg, Sweden. *Eur Heart J* 1997; 18:754–761.

320. Corti M-C, Guralnik JM, Salive ME, Harris T, Ferrucci L, Glynn RJ, et al. Clarifying the direct relation between total cholesterol levels and death from coronary heart disease in older persons. *Ann Intern Med* 1997; 126:753–760.

321. Harrison DG. Endothelial function in atherosclerosis. *Basic Res Cardiol* 1994; 89(suppl 1):87–102.

322. O'Driscoll G, Green D, Taylor RR. Simvastatin, an HMG-coenzyme A reductase inhibitor, improves endothelial function within 1 month. *Circulation* 1997; 95:1126–1131.

323. Vogel RA, Corretti MC, Plotnick GD. Effect of a single high-fat meal on endothelial function in healthy subjects. *Am J Cardiol* 1997; 79:350–354.

324. Lekakis J, Papamichael C, Vemmos C, Nanas J, Kontoyannis D, Stamatelopoulos S, et al. Effect of acute cigarette smoking on endothelium-dependent brachial artery dilatation in healthy individuals. *Am J Cardiol* 1997; 79:529–531.

325. Donahue RP, Abbott RD, Bloom E, Reed DM, Yano K. Central obesity and coronary heart disease in men. *Lancet* 1987; 822–824.

326. Després J-P, Moorjani S, Lupien PJ, Tremblay A, Nadeau A, Bouchard C. Regional distribution of body fat, plasma lipoproteins, and cardiovascular disease. *Arteriosclerosis* 1990; 10:497–511.

327. Kissebah AH, Krakower GR. Regional adiposity and morbidity. *Physiol Rev* 1994; 74:761–811.

328. Cigolini M, Targher C, Bergamo Andreis IA, Tonoli M, Agostino G, De Sandre G. Visceral fat accumulation and its relation to plasma hemostatic factors in healthy men. *Arterioscler Thromb Vasc Biol* 1996; 16:368–374.

329. Sullivan JM, Vander ZR, Lemp GF, Hughes JP, Maddock V, Kroetz FW, et al. Estrogen replacement and coronary artery disease effect on survival in postmenopausal women. *Arch Intern Med* 1990; 150:2557–2562.

330. Stampfer MJ, Colditz GA. Estrogen replacement therapy and coronary heart disease: A quantitative assessment of the epidemiologic evidence. *Prev Med* 1991; 20:47–63.

331. Gilligan DM, Quyyumi AA, Cannon RO III. Effects of physiological levels of estrogen on coronary vasomotor function in postmenopausal women. *Circulation* 1994; 89:2545–2551.

332. Shahar E, Folsom AR, Salomaa VV, Stinson VL, McGovern PG, Shimakawa T, et al. Relation of hormone-replacement therapy to measures of plasma fibrinolytic activity. Atherosclerosis Risk in Communities (ARIC) Study Investigators. *Circulation* 1996; 93:1970–1975.

333. Colditz GA, Hankinson SE, Hunter DJ, Willett WC, Manson JE, Stampfer MJ, et al. The use of estrogens and progestins and the risk of breast cancer in postmenopausal women. *N Engl J Med* 1995; 332:1589–1593.

334. Grodstein F. Postmenopausal estrogen and progestin use and the risk of cardiovascular disease. *N Engl J Med* 1996; 335:453–461.

335. Grodstein F, Stampfer M. The epidemiology of coronary heart disease and estrogen replacement in postmenopausal women. *Prog Cardiovasc Dis* 1995; 38:199–210.

336. Sullivan JM, Fowlkes LP. Estrogens, menopause and coronary artery disease. *Cardiol Clin* 1996; 14:105–110.

337. Grodstein F, Stampfer MJ, Manson JE, Colditz GA, Willett WC, Rosner B, et al. Postmenopausal estrogen and progestin and the risk of cardiovascular disease. *N Engl J Med* 1996; 335:453–461.

338. Rosano GM, Sarrel PM, Poole-Wilson PA, Collins P. Beneficial effect of oestrogen on exercise-induced myocardial ischaemia in women with coronary artery disease. *Lancet* 1993; 342:133–136.

339. Davidson MH, Testolin LM, Maki KC, von Duvillard S, Drennan KB. A comparison of estrogen replacement, pravastatin, and combined treatment for the management of hypercholesterolemia in postmenopausal women. *Arch Intern Med* 1997; 157:1186–1192.

340. Després J-P, Marette A. Relation of components of insulin resistance syndrome to coronary diseases risk. *Curr Opin Lipidol* 1994; 5:274–289.

341. Laakso M. Insulin resistance and coronary heart disease. *Curr Opin Lipidol* 1996; 7:217–226.

342. Howard G, O'Leary DH, Zaccaro D, Haffner S, Rewers M, Hamman R, et al. Insulin sensitivity and atherosclerosis. The Insulin Resistance Atherosclerosis Study Investigations (IRAS). *Circulation* 1996; 93:1809–1817.

343. Steinberg HO, Chaker H, Leaming R, Johnson A, Brechtel G, Baron AD. Obesity/insulin resistance is associated with endothelial dysfunction. Implications for the syndrome of insulin resistance. *J Clin Invest* 1996; 97:2601–2610.

344. International Committee for the Evaluation of Hypertriglyceridemia as a Vascular Risk Factor. The hypertriglyceridemias: Risk and management. *Am J Cardiol* 1991; 68(suppl):1A–42A.

345. NIH Consensus Development Panel. Triglyceride, high-density lipoprotein, and coronary heart disease. *JAMA* 1993; 269:505–510.

346. Loscalzo J. Lipoprotein(a): A unique risk factor for atherothrombotic disease. *Arteriosclerosis* 1990; 10:672–679.

347. Ridker PM, Hennekens CH, Stampfer MJ. A prospective study of lipoprotein(a) and the risk of myocardial infarction. *JAMA* 1993; 27:2195–2199.

348. Bostom AG, Cupples LA, Jenner JL, Ordovas JM, Seman LJ, Wilson PW, et al. Elevated plasma lipoprotein(a) and coronary heart disease in men aged 55 years and younger: A prospective study. *JAMA* 1996; 27:544–546.

349. Stein JH, Rosenson RS. Lipoprotein Lp(a) excess and coronary heart disease. *Arch Intern Med* 1997; 157:1170–1176.

350. Ernst E. Plasma fibrinogen-independent cardiovascular risk factor. *J Intern Med* 1990; 277:365–375.

351. Ernst E, Resch KL. Fibrinogen as a cardiovascular risk factor: A meta-analysis and review of the literature. *Ann Intern Med* 1993; 188:956–963.

352. Yarnell JWG, Baker IA, Sweetnam PM, Bainton D, O'Brien JR, Whitehead PJ, et al. Fibrinogen, viscosity, and white blood cell count are major risk factors for ischemic heart disease. *Circulation* 1991; 83:836–844.

353. Thompson SG, Kienast J, Pyke SDM, Haverkate F, van de Loo JCW. Hemostatic factors and the risk of myocardial infarction or sudden death in patients with angina pectoris. *N Engl J Med* 1995; 332:635–641.

354. Dobroski DR, Loscalzo J. Thrombotic risk factors for atherosclerosis. *Coron Artery Dis* 1996; 7:919–932.

355. Benderly M, Graff E, Reicher-Reiss H, Behar S, Brunner D, Goldbourt U, et al. Fibrinogen is a predictor of mortality in coronary heart disease patients. *Arterioscler Thromb Vasc Biol* 1996; 16:351–356.

356. Thompson SG, Fechtrup E, Squire E, Heyse U, Breithardt G, van de Loo JCW, et al. Antithrombin III and fibrinogen as predictors of cardiac events in patients with angina pectoris. *Arterioscler Thromb Vasc Biol* 1996; 16:357–362.

357. Sweetnam PM, Thomas HF, Yarnel JWG, Beswick AD, Baker IA, Elwood PC. Fibrinogen, viscosity and the 10-year incidence of ischaemic heart disease. The Caerphilly and Speedwell Studies. *Eur Heart J* 1996; 17:1814–1820.

358. Lip GY, Blann AD. von Willebrand factor and its relevance to cardiovascular disorders. *Br Heart J* 1995; 74:580–583.

359. Haverkate F, Thompson SG, Pyke SDM, Gallimore JR, Pepys MB. Production of C-reactive protein and risk of coronary events in stable and unstable angina. *Lancet* 1997; 349:462–466.

360. Rabbani LE, Loscalzo J. Recent observations on the role of hemostatic determinants in the development of atherothrombotic plaque. *Atherosclerosis* 1994; 105:1–7.

361. Ridker PM, Cushman M, Stampfer MJ, Tracy RP, Hennekens CH. Inflammation, aspirin, and the risk of cardiovascular disease in apparently healthy men. *N Engl J Med* 1997; 336:973–979.

362. Ridker PM, Vaughn DE, Stampfer MJ, Manson JE, Hennekens CH. Endogenous tissue-type plasminogen activator and risk of myocardial infarction. *Lancet* 1993; 341:1165–1168.

363. Mayer EL, Jacobsen DW, Robinson K. Homocysteine and coronary atherosclerosis. *J Am Coll Cardiol* 1996; 27:517–527.

364. Nygard O, Nordrehaug JE, Refsum H, Ueland SE, Farstad M, Vollset SE. Plasma homocysteine levels and mortality in patients with coronary artery disease. *N Engl J Med* 1997; 337:230–236.

365. Graham IM, Daly LE, Refsum HM, Robinson K, Brattström LE, Ueland PM, et al. Plasma homocysteine as a risk factor for vascular disease. The European Concerted Action Project. *JAMA* 1997; 277:1775–1781.

366. Linnanmäki E, Leinonen M, Mattila K, Nieminen MS, Valtonen V, Saikku P. *Chlamydia pneumoniae*–specific circulating immune complexes in patients with chronic coronary heart disease. *Circulation* 1993; 87:1130–1134.

367. Ramirez JA, *Chlamydia pneumoniae*/Atherosclerosis Study Group. Isolation of *Chlamydia pneumoniae* from the coronary artery of a patient with coronary atherosclerosis. *Ann Intern Med* 1996; 125:979–982.

368. Carney RM, Saunders RD, Freedland KE, Stein P, Rich MW, Jaffe AS. Association of depression with reduced heart rate variability in coronary artery disease. *Am J Cardiol* 1995; 76(8):562–564.

369. van Boven AJ, Jukema JW, Crijns HJ, Lie KI. Heart rate variability profiles in symptomatic coronary artery disease and preserved left ventricular function: Relation to ventricular tachycardia and transient myocardial ischemia. Regression Growth Evaluation Statin Study (REGRESS). *Am Heart J* 1995; 130:1020–1025.

370. Lenihan DJ, Coyne E, Feldman B, Black R, Collins G. Frequency of late potentials on signal-averaged electrocardiograms during thallium stress testing in coronary artery disease. *Am J Cardiol* 1992; 70:432–435.

371. Wallén NH, Held C, Rehnqvist N, Hjemdahl P. Effects of mental and physical stress on platelet function in patients with stable angina pectoris and healthy controls. *Eur Heart J* 1997; 18:807–815.

372. Gullette ECD, Blumenthal JA, Babyak M, Jiang W, Waugh RA, Frid DJ, et al. Effects of mental stress on myocardial ischemia during daily life. *JAMA* 1997; 277:1521–1526.

373. Stampfer MJ, Hennekens CH, Manson JE, Colditz GA, Rosner B, Willett WC. Vitamin E consumption and the risk of coronary disease in women. *N Engl J Med* 1993; 328:1444–1449.

374. Rimm EB, Stampfer MJ, Ascherio A, Giovannucci E, Colditz GA, Willett WC. Vitamin E consumption and the risk of coronary heart disease in men. *N Engl J Med* 1993; 328:1450–1456.

375. Hennekens CH, Buring JE, Peto R. Antioxidant vitamins—benefits not yet proved. *N Engl J Med* 1994; 330:1080–1081.

376. Jha P, Flather M, Lonn E, Farkouh M, Yusof S. The antioxidant vitamins and cardiovascular disease. *Ann Intern Med* 1995; 123:860–872.

377. Hennekens C, Buring J, Manson J, Stampfer M, Rosner B, Cook NR, et al. Lack of effect of long-term supplementation with beta carotene on the incidence of malignant neoplasms and cardiovascular disease. *N Engl J Med* 1996; 334:1145–1149.

378. Stephens N, Parsons A, Schofield P, Kelly F, Cheeseman K, Mitchinson MJ. Randomised controlled trial of vitamin E in patients with coronary disease: Cambridge Heart Oxidation Study (CHAOS). *Lancet* 1996; 347:781–786.

379. Rapola JM, Virtamo J, Haukka JK, Heinonen OP, Albanes D, Taylor PR, et al. Effect of vitamin E and beta carotene on the incidence of angina pectoris. A randomized, double-blind, controlled trial. *JAMA* 1996; 275:693–698.

380. Levine GN, Frei B, Koulouris SN, Gerhard MD, Keaney JF, Vita JA. Ascorbic acid reverses endothelial vasomotor dysfunction in patients with coronary artery disease. *Circulation* 1996; 93:1107–1113.

381. Olsson AG, Yuan XM. Antioxidants in the prevention of atherosclerosis. *Curr Opin Lipidol* 1996; 7:374–380.

382. Price JF, Fowkes FGR. Antioxidant vitamins in the prevention of cardiovascular disease. The epidemiological evidence. *Eur Heart J* 1997; 18:719–727.

383. Rimm EB, Stampfer MJ. The role of antioxidants in preventive cardiology. *Curr Opin Cardiol* 1997; 12:188–194.

384. Rimm EB, Ascherio A, Giovannucci E, Spiegelman D, Stampfer MJ, Willett WC. Vegetable, fruit, and cereal fiber intake and risk of coronary heart disease among men. *JAMA* 1996; 275:447–451.

385. Conner WE. The beneficial effects of omega-3 fatty acids: Cardiovascular disease and neurodevelopment. *Curr Opin Lipidol* 1997; 8:1–3.

386. Tsao PS, McEvoy LM, Drexler H, Butcher EC, Cooke JP. Enhanced endothelial adhesiveness in hypercholesterolemia is attenuated by L-arginine. *Circulation* 1994; 89:2176–2182.

387. Egashira K, Hirooka Y, Kuga T, Mohri M, Takeshita A. Effects of L-arginine supplementation on endothelium-dependent coronary vasodilation in patients with angina pectoris and normal coronary arteriograms. *Circulation* 1996; 94:130–134.

388. Aji W, Ravalli S, Szaboles M, Jiang X C, Sciacca RR, Michler RE, et al. L-Arginine prevents xanthoma development and inhibits atherosclerosis in LDL receptor knockout mice. *Circulation* 1997; 95:430–437.

389. Adams MR, Jessup W, Celermajer DS. Cigarette smoking is associated with increased human monocyte adhesion to endothelial cells: Reversibility with oral L-arginine but not vitamin C. *J Am Coll Cardiol* 1997; 29:491–497.

390. Wolf A, Zalpour C, Theilmeier G, Wang B-Y, Anderson B, Tsao PS, et al. Dietary L-arginine supplementation normalizes platelet aggregation in hypercholesterolemic humans. *J Am Coll Cardiol* 1997; 29:479–485.

391. Criqui MH, Ringle BL. The French paradox: Does diet or alcohol explain the difference. *Lancet* 1994; 344:1719–1723.

392. Gronbaek M, Deis A, Sorensen TIA, Becker U, Schnohr P, Jensen G. Mortality associated with moderate intakes of wine, beer, or spirits. *BMJ* 1995; 310:1165–1169.

393. Demrow HS, Slane PR, Folts JD. Administration of wine and grape juice inhibits in vivo platelet activity and thrombosis in stenosed canine coronary arteries. *Circulation* 1995; 91:1182–1188.

394. Shaper AG. Alcohol and coronary heart disease. *Eur Heart J* 1995; 16:1760–1764.

395. Gaziano JM, Godfried SL, Hennekens CH. Alcohol and coronary heart disease. *Trends Cardiovasc Med* 1996; 6:175–178.

396. Pearson TA. Alcohol and heart disease. *Circulation* 1996; 94:3023–3025.

397. Camargo CA Jr, Stampfer MJ, Glynn RJ, Grodstein F, Gaziano JM, Manson JAE, et al. Moderate alcohol consumption and risk for angina pectoris or myocardial infarction in U.S. male physicians. *Ann Intern Med* 1997; 126:372–375.

398. Camargo CA Jr, Stampfer MJ, Glynn RJ, Gaziano M, Manson JAE, Goldhaber SZ. Prospective study of moderate alcohol consumption and risk of peripheral arterial disease in U.S. male physicians. *Circulation* 1997; 95:577–580.

46

DIAGNOSIS AND MANAGEMENT OF PATIENTS WITH UNSTABLE ANGINA

Pierre Théroux / David Waters

At the end of the twentieth century, unstable angina remains a clinical diagnosis: it is recognized by rapidly aggravating symptoms of angina pectoris, marking the transition from a chronic to an acute manifestation of coronary artery disease (CAD) and from no or stable symptoms to acute myocardial infarction (MI). As the underlying pathophysiologic processes became better known, the syndrome was established as a well-defined entity. Markers of the disease process are now being recognized. Although prognosis remains serious, diagnosis of unstable angina allows application of specific interventions, guided by risk evaluation, that modify the natural course of the disease to prevent the development of irreversible myocardial cell damage and MI.

HISTORICAL PERSPECTIVE

The concept of unstable angina originated early in this century from clinical observations of a high frequency of prodromal symptoms preceding MI[1–3] followed in mid-century by prospective observations of frequent MI and death in patients presenting with a changing pattern of chest pain.[4] In the 1960s, the syndrome was in search of a name, with varying terminology addressing symptoms (crescendo angina, status anginosus, accelerated angina), pathophysiology (coronary failure, acute coronary insufficiency),[5,6] or prognosis (impending MI, preinfarction angina). The term *unstable angina* proposed by Fowler was eventually retained.[7] The natural history of the disease was subsequently defined by risk strata.[8–10] Rapid progress in the understanding of the pathophysiology followed in the late 1970s, prompted by recognition of the critical role of a primary decrease in myocardial oxygen delivery. The early emphasis on abnormal and inappropriate coronary vasoconstriction[11] shifted in the past two decades to the demonstration of the critical role of the culprit plaque, with loss of endothelial integrity and activation of its cellular components triggering the formation of an intravascular thrombus and myocardial ischemia.[12–14] The parallel joint efforts of clinicians and basic scientists, helped by a rapidly growing technology, have allowed accelerated progress in management.

PATHOPHYSIOLOGIC MECHANISMS

The concept of the culprit lesion forms the basis for the new approach to the diagnosis and treatment of acute coronary artery syndromes. Unstable angina, like MI, is an acute manifestation of myocardial ischemia, clearly related to a regional decrease in blood flow caused by acute focal coronary obstruction. Intracoronary thrombi are observed at angiography in the majority of patients with an acute coronary syndrome.[15] Examples are shown in Figs. 46-1 and 46-2. Thus, although angiography was performed relatively late in the Thrombolysis in Myocardial Ischemia (TIMI) trial, within 24 h after hospital admission, clear images of thrombus were identified in 35 percent of patients, and possible thrombus in an additional 40 percent.[16] Ambrose et al. have associated unstable angina with eccentric coronary artery lesions with a narrow neck or irregular borders as opposed to the concentric lesions or eccentric lesions with a broad neck and smooth borders in stable angina.[17] Such angiographic features likely reflect changes that had already occurred compromising the structural integrity of the plaque.

The coronary anatomy before the unstable angina episode may be important in defining the high-risk plaque. Plaque

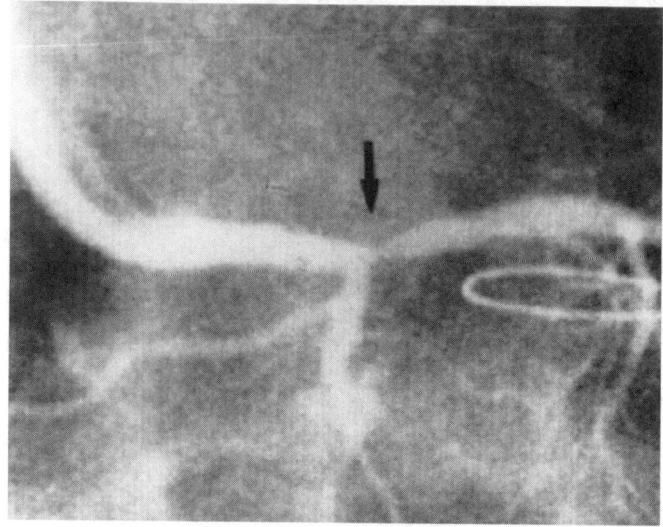

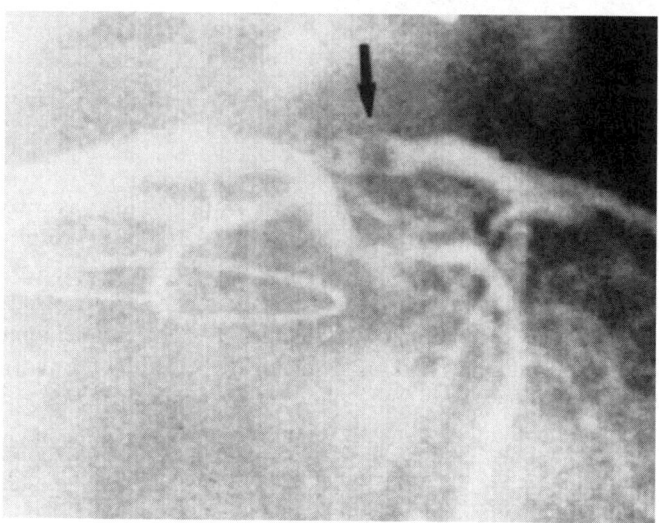

FIGURE 46-1

Left coronary dye injections obtained in a patient with stable angina who subsequently developed unstable angina. The injection during the stable state shows a 60 percent stenosis of the proximal left anterior descending coronary artery (*above*). One week later, the patient experienced a 30-min episode of chest pain at rest with transient ST-T changes in the anterior leads but no enzyme elevation. The angiogram obtained 2 h later displays an intraluminal globular radiotranslucent mass just distal to the previously described narrowing (*below*). This image represents a thrombus partially occluding the lumen that has acutely developed.

features favoring higher shear stress and flow separation over a narrow arterial segment, such as stenosis severity, acuteness of the outflow and inflow angles of the stenosis, and the presence of a nearby division branch, are associated with a higher risk of thrombosis.[18] The majority of lesions that occlude to produce acute syndromes are of only moderate severity, typically 45 to 60 percent lumen diameter reduction. The likelihood of a clinical event also increases with more numerous diseased coronary artery segments, possibly relating to a more active disease or by increasing the odds that one plaque ruptures.[19] If unstable angina is a marker of rapid, *acute* progression in the severity of segmental CAD, it is also a

harbinger of subsequent progression of *stenosis severity*. Follow-up angiographic studies performed after the acute phase have indeed documented that unstable angina is associated with a higher risk of subsequent progression of CAD, more specifically at the site of the active plaque but also at other sites.[20,21] Unstable angina is also associated with a high risk of recurrence.

The mechanisms for thrombotic occlusion are complex and require further elucidation of the close interdependence among the plaque, the endothelium, platelets, local coagulation and fibrinolytic factors, and inflammatory mediators (see Chap. 44). The interrelation is further influenced by hemodynamic and rheologic factors; the vasomotor response of the vessel; and systemic factors, including coagulation factors, epinephrine levels, plasma lipoprotein characteristics, and circadian and seasonal variations. A primary coagulation disorder is unusual in unstable angina; patients may, however, present with a so-called prethrombotic state, with elevated levels of various blood procoagulants. The formation of the thrombus, however, is generally conceived as a direct and physiologic response of the coagulation system to exposure of subendothelial thrombogenic substrate. The more fundamental causes of unstable angina are therefore within the plaque itself, with thrombus formation the triggering mechanism.

Patients dying suddenly have a high incidence of complicated atherosclerotic plaque, with plaque fissure and rupture covered by an intraluminal thrombus; these plaques are inflammatory and rich in extracellular lipid pool and are covered by a thin cap[12,13] (Fig. 46-3) (see also Chap. 40). The rupture within the plaque is often located at the junction of the cap with more normal tissue, where shear rate appears maximal.[22] The overlying thrombus comprises elements of various ages, indicating the cyclic nature of thrombosis in unstable angina,[23] which is compatible with the variability of symptoms and the tendency for recurrence. Plaques that undergo rupture frequently are relatively small, are relatively soft, and contain within the intima a deformable cavity filled with crystalline cholesterol and its ester.[24] The collagen exposed to the circulation after rupture triggers platelet deposition, the rate of which increases with higher shear rate.[25] The plaque is also rich in tissue factor, which forms a complex with factor VII to trigger formation of factor Xa and thrombin generation, further platelet aggregation, deposition of fibrin, and formation of an occlusive blood clot. Partial growth or regression of these intracoronary thrombi could explain some of the clinical features of unstable angina, including the intermittent clinical manifestations, the often unpredictable course, and the favorable response to antithrombotic therapy. Once initiated, the thrombotic process can perpetuate itself. The thrombus itself is a strongly thrombogenic surface, acting as a reservoir for the release of thrombin bound to fibrin leading to further thrombogenesis.[26,27]

Other mechanisms can also be operative in unstable angina and include the following: intraplaque hemorrhage by rupture of a vasa vasorum; distal coronary embolization of platelet aggregates; functional loss of the antithrombotic properties

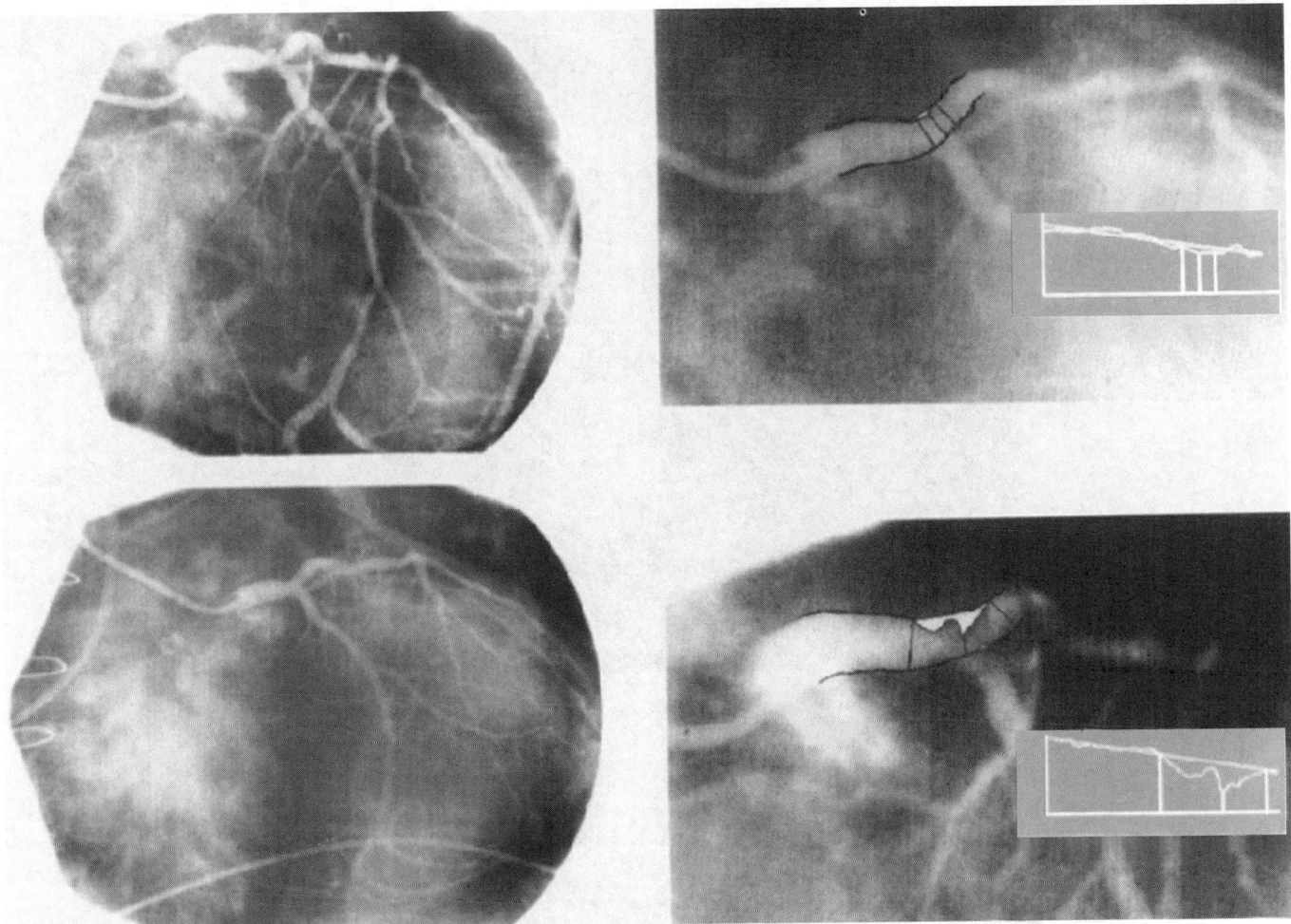

FIGURE 46-2

Computer-assisted analysis of two left coronary angiograms obtained at 1-year interval in the same patient. The angiogram at the top shows a minimal plaque in the distal left main vessel, well delineated by the computer analysis (*top right*). The second angiogram at the bottom was obtained after stabiliza-

tion of crescendo angina. The plaque has progressed to cause a 60 percent obstruction showing further the aspect of a complex, asymmetric, and ulcerated crater, representing a nidus for platelet aggregation and thrombus formation.

of the endothelium; and focal vasoconstriction precipitated by the release of local vasoactive agents, such as serotonin, thromboxane A₂, and endothelin.[28] The degree to which vasoconstriction contributes to the pathogenesis of unstable angina is likely variable. The abnormal vasoreactivity may persist after stabilization and contribute to recurrence; such a persisting abnormal response to exercise and to cold pressor test has been demonstrated at the site of the culprit lesion.[29]

Figure 46-4 schematically correlates the clinical manifestations with the pathophysiologic mechanisms.[27] The process can ultimately lead to complete coronary occlusion and MI. Its resolution may result in healing and a return to the clinical status existing before the unstable state. The release of platelet-derived growth factor and other mitogenic factors during healing may contribute not only to fibrotic organization of the intracoronary thrombi but also to rapid progression of CAD.[20,21,30] *Inherent to this perspective is the view that CAD is episodic and is associated with periodic plaque activation and growth that may be subclinical and lead to recurrence.*

The mechanisms that lead to plaque activation are important in understanding the disease process. Inflammation has a critical and fundamental role (Fig. 46-3). A low-grade chronic inflammatory disorder is present in atherosclerosis. The response-to-injury hypothesis of atherosclerosis proposes that endothelial dysfunction alters the proinflammatory properties of the endothelium to lead to adhesion and transmigration of monocytes into the subendothelium.[31] The monocytes become macrophages, and active scavengers of modified proteins and lipoproteins (such as oxidized low-density lipoprotein), release inflammatory mediators such as cytokines, secrete matrix degradation proteins, and generate immune responses, in concert with T cells, against foreign or neoantigens within the plaque. They also secrete factors leading to smooth muscle cell migration and proliferation. Pathologic studies of autopsy and of atherectomy specimens have shown abundant T lymphocytes, macrophages, and mast cells in the active plaque of unstable angina and MI,[32,33] and these are more at the erosion sites of the plaques than in unaffected

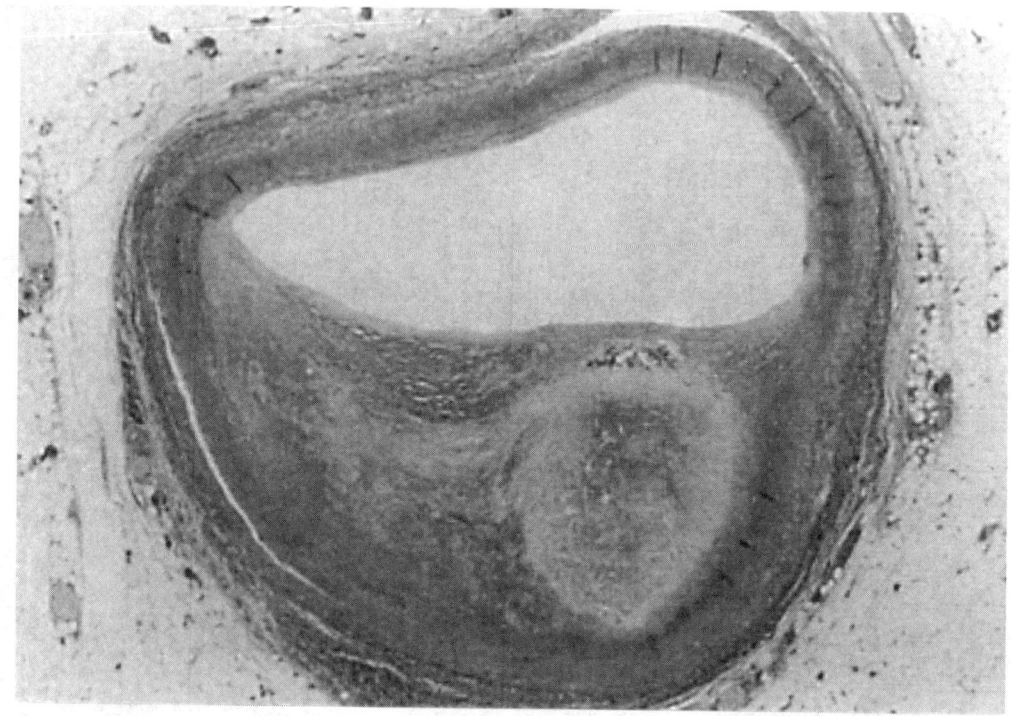

A

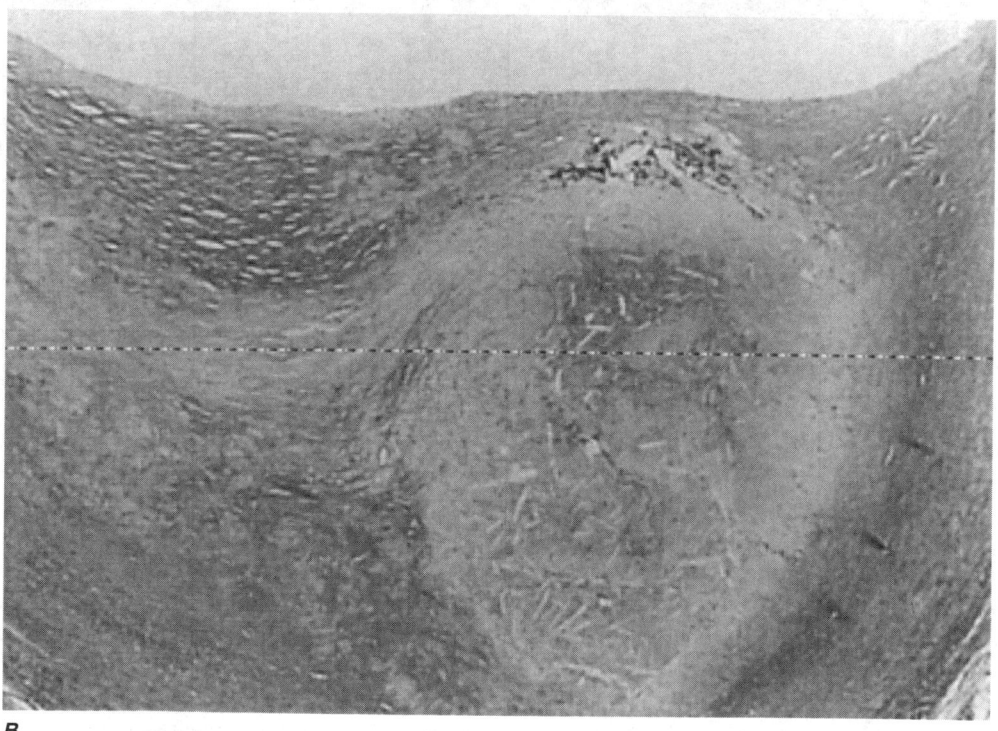

B

FIGURE 46-3

Photomicrographs illustrating composition and vulnerability of coronary artery plaques. *A.* The vulnerable plaque shown contains a core of soft, lipid-rich atheromatous gruel (devoid of blue-stained collagen) and a hard, collagen-rich sclerotic tissue. The fibrous tissue stabilizes the plaque and protects against disruption. *B.* The soft nucleus, as shown at high magnification, is infiltrated by foam cells and other inflammatory cells, indicating an active plaque, and is separated from the vascular lumen by a thin cap of fibrous tissue. It is highly vulnerable to rupture, exposing the highly thrombogenic gruel to flowing blood, leading to thrombosis. (From Falk et al.[30] Reproduced with permission of the American Heart Association and the author.)

areas (Table 46-1).[34] Cells are also activated; macrophages and lymphocytes express the HLA-DR antigens, and mast cells are degranulated with release of tryptase and chymase.[34] Metalloproteinases produced by macrophages and smooth muscle cells undermine and degrade the collagen in plaque matrix, and erode the fibrous cap. Macrophages enhance leukocyte recruitment and activation and secrete interleukin-1, tumor necrosis factor, tissue factor, and other chemotactic and procoagulant factors, which leads to more platelet deposition, platelet aggregation, and thrombus formation[35] (see Chaps. 4, 40, 43, 44, and 52). *The plaque causing unstable angina shares with atherosclerosis the same pathophysiologic mechanisms but with an exaggerated inflammatory reaction. The reasons for this extreme response remain to be investigated and may open new avenues for the control of atherosclerosis.* The inflammatory signals can be driven from continuous antigen stimulation. Candidate antigens are modified LDL-cholesterol molecules, toxins, and peptides derived from intracellular pathogens such as cytomegalovirus and *Chlamydia pneumoniae*.

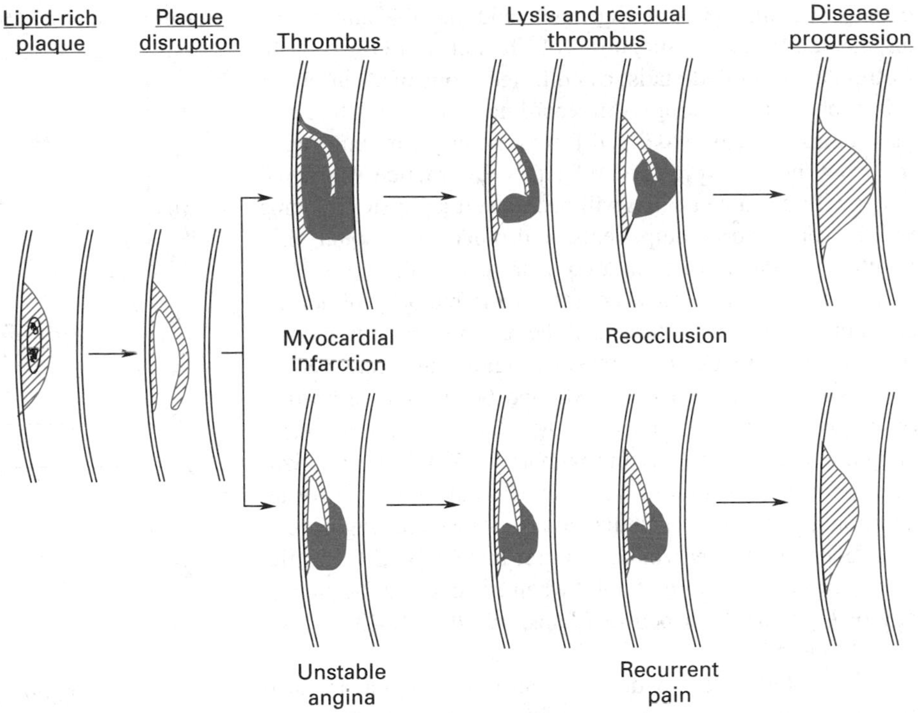

FIGURE 46-4

Schematic representation of plaque events leading to acute coronary syndromes. Plaque rupture is favored by high lipid content and by external forces applied. A deep fissure is a powerful stimulus for thrombus formation. A more superficial fissure leads to mural thrombus. The evolution is influenced by systemic factors and the balance between thrombogenic stimulation and plasma antithrombin and fibrinolytic activity. Complete prolonged lumen obstruction is associated with myocardial infarction; more transient occlusion or the presence of collateral circulation leads to one of the manifestations of unstable angina depending on the severity of ischemia. The healing process is associated with progression of atherosclerosis. (Adapted from Fuster et al.[27] Reproduced with permission of the authors and the publisher.)

DEFINITION AND INCIDENCE

Unstable angina encompasses a wide spectrum of symptomatic manifestations of CAD, intermediate between stable angina and MI. *Inherent to the definition is an evolving pattern of chest pain or discomfort that is new or that departs from the usual pattern of angina for a patient. It is extremely important to remember that patients often will not use the term pain to describe their symptoms.* Unstable angina can manifest as the first symptom of CAD or as an aggravation of preexisting symptoms. In either event, the symptoms suggest that pain is not triggered by an excessive workload but by a primary decrease in blood supply.

The exact incidence of unstable angina is difficult to assess because of the heterogeneity of the disease, the wide spectrum of clinical manifestations of variable severity, the variable threshold of tolerance to pain among patients influencing promptness in seeking medical consultation, the variability among physicians in their approach to management, and the relative lack of standardization in recording the hospital diagnosis. The ninth edition of the International Classification of Diseases of the World Health Organization, adopted by 46 different countries, uses a single

TABLE 46-1

DENSITIES OF INFLAMMATORY AND SMOOTH MUSCLE CELLS IN CORONARY INTIMAS FROM 20 PATIENTS WHO DIED OF MYOCARDIAL INFARCTION[a]

Intimal Areas	Mast Cells	Macrophages	T Lymphocytes	Smooth Muscle Cells
Erosion/rupture	28 (0–158)	217 (31–590)	31 (0–127)	191 (2–1300)
Adjacent areas	2 (0–20)	112 (4–460)	17 (0–39)	306 (7–1566)
Unaffected areas	1 (1–10)	49 (4–266)	9 (0–36)	813 (92–1700)

[a] Numbers of cell types (cells/mm^2, means and ranges) from three cross sections of intimal areas in which erosion and rupture were found in the autopsy specimens.

Source: From Kovanen et al.[34] Reproduced with permission of the American Heart Association and the authors.

code for the diagnosis of both stable and unstable angina and another code for the diagnosis of Q- and non-Q-wave MI. Computer-generated statistics collected from medical charts reflect physicians' accuracy in recording diagnoses. More precise diagnoses can be derived from coronary care unit registries, but their interpretation reflects local practice. Many patients with unstable angina will not consult a physician; some will be managed as outpatients, and others in-hospital, in a regular medical ward or in a coronary care unit.

Unstable angina now accounts for the majority of admissions in coronary care units, and the relative proportion compared with MI is steadily increasing, suggesting greater patient awareness of symptoms of CAD and better standardization of diagnosis by physicians. In the United States, unstable angina is responsible for approximately 750,000 hospitalizations per year and non-Q-wave myocardial infarction for an additional 250,000 hospitalizations.[36] Unstable angina can also recur many times in the natural history of CAD in the same patient, an important point when considering the pathology of CAD as described in Chaps. 39, 40, 41, 43, 44, 45, 47, 52, and 53.

The contemporary patterns of unstable angina are also evolving. The efficacy of the antithrombotic treatment has resulted in more standardized medical management; invasive procedures are now widely used within well-structured referral networks. Nevertheless, many differences exist between countries and between regions in the same country that must be considered in any prevalence and prognosis studies.

NATURAL HISTORY AND PROGNOSIS

Unstable angina carries a high risk of MI, death, and recurrent ischemia. Natural history studies have documented a 3-month incidence of MI ranging from 10 to 20 percent and a mortality rate between 4 and 10 percent.[37–39] Natural history studies can no longer be obtained since unstable angina is modified by antithrombotic therapy and more specifically by aspirin use in nearly all patients. Recent outcomes without antithrombotic therapy, however, can be obtained from the control groups in trials that have evaluated the efficacy of aspirin and/or heparin, and outcomes with antithrombotic therapy from ongoing trials evaluating newer antiplatelet and anticoagulant drugs against aspirin and heparin. In the Timi IIIB trial, with all patients administered aspirin, heparin, and antiischemic drugs, the overall rate of death or myocardial infarction at 42 days was 7.5 percent and at 12 months was 11.5 percent, as shown by the survival curves in Fig. 46-5.[40,41] The event rate, despite the frequent use of intervention procedures in this trial, remained high to stress the need for more effective treatment strategies.

CLASSIFICATION

The various classifications of unstable angina distinguish a primary and a secondary form. The former reflects primary

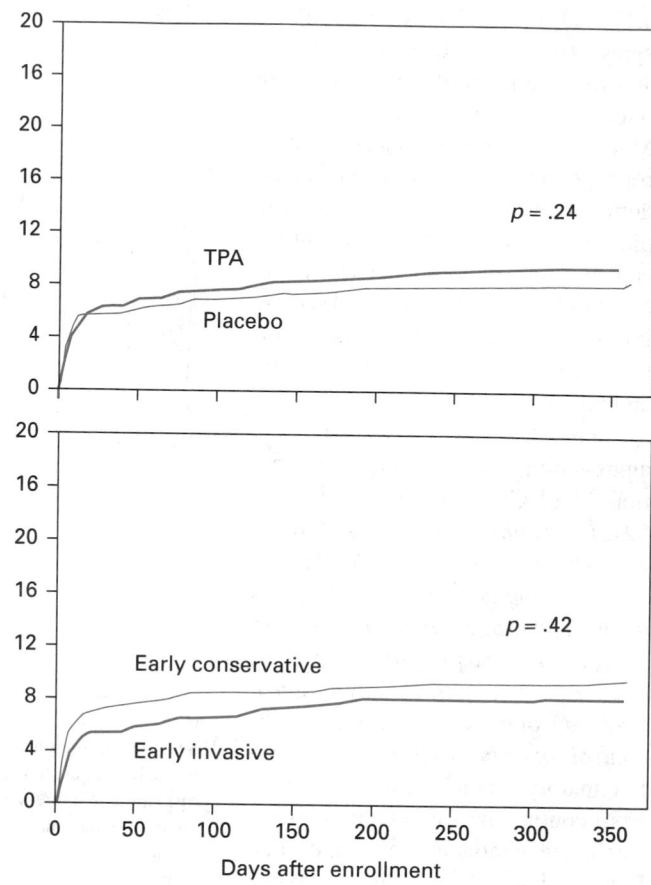

% cardiac death or MI

p = .24

TPA

Placebo

p = .42

Early conservative

Early invasive

Days after enrollment

FIGURE 46-5

One-year cumulative rates of death or myocardial infarction by randomized assignments in TIMI-IIIB. The 1473 patients enrolled were randomized in a 2 × 2 factorial design to tissue plasminogen activator or to placebo (*top*) and to an early invasive treatment strategy or early conservative strategy (*bottom*). No differences in the rates of death or myocardial infarction were seen at 6 weeks and at 1 year among the various treatment groups. Trends to more events were present with tissue-plasminogen activator and with the conservative strategy. (From Anderson et al.[41] Reproduced with permission of the author and publisher.)

pathologic changes at a plaque level, whereas the latter involves factors influencing myocardial oxygen demand, without a change in intrinsic plaque activity.

Secondary Unstable Angina

This form of unstable angina is partly a misnomer since it is provoked by different pathophysiologic mechanisms than those involved in primary unstable angina. *Any factor causing an increase in myocardial oxygen demand can lead to worsening of angina, usually in the presence of underlying CAD but also in its absence.* The major determinants of myocardial oxygen consumption are, in decreasing order of relative contribution, heart rate, the inotropic state of the myocardial fiber, and the afterload and preload conditions of the left ventricle. Typical conditions associated with a rapid heart rate are anemia, thyrotoxicosis, tachyarrhythmias, and fever. The inotropic state is increased by catecholamine stimulation, afterload by left ventricular outflow tract obstruction and severe hypertension, and preload by congestive heart failure and left ventricular dilatation. Other conditions impairing oxygen delivery such as low arterial P_{O_2}, anemia, polycythemia, and high blood viscosity may also be contributive. A more extensive listing of nonatherosclerotic aggravating conditions precipitating secondary unstable angina is provided in Table 46-2.

Primary Unstable Angina

Primary unstable angina implies that an underlying change in the biological state of the coronary circulation has developed. This change usually reflects activation and worsening of the inflammatory process associated with the underlying atherosclerosis. The active coronary lesion is prone not only to

structural disruption, as discussed above, but also to enhanced vasoconstriction because of impaired production of endothelium-derived relaxing factors (EDRF)[42] and possibly also by an increased production of endothelin.[43] The increased vasoconstriction can not only lead to a primary decrease in blood flow but can also contribute to endothelial disruption and plaque fracture, leading to platelet aggregation and thrombus formation. Exercise, cigarette smoking, and exposure to cold can provoke coronary vasoconstriction[44–46] and plaque disruption in a lesion, the structure of which has been weakened by an acute inflammatory response. Cocaine can induce intense vasoconstriction and intimal disruption, thrombosis, and MI in the absence or presence of severe atherosclerosis.[47–50]

CLASSIFICATION OF PRIMARY UNSTABLE ANGINA

Various classifications have been proposed for primary unstable angina. The classification of Gazes et al., based on clinical presentation, set the basis for subsequent classifications.[10] Three subgroups were defined: (1) initial onset of progressive, crescendo angina and pain at rest in a patient previously free of symptoms; (2) the same as (1) but occurring in a patient with known stable angina; and (3) episodes of chest pain at rest of more than 15 min duration not related to any obvious precipitating factor. More recently defined clinical presentations include postinfarction angina, variant angina, angina after coronary angioplasty, and angina after coronary artery bypass surgery (Table 46-3). Non-Q-wave MI is also now included in many clinical trials on unstable angina.

The classification proposed by Braunwald is now frequently used (Table 46-4).[51] This classification considers the clinical background and the severity of manifestations; and a subclassification, intensity of previous medical treatment and presence of ST-segment changes.

Maseri has introduced a prognostic classification of unstable angina that considers entry diagnosis and baseline and acute determinants of prognosis.[52] The classes are as follows: *de novo unstable angina*, with chest pain at rest and electrocardiographic changes; *destabilizing unstable angina*, with more

---

TABLE 46-2

PRECIPITATING FACTORS FOR SECONDARY UNSTABLE ANGINA UNRELATED TO THE BIOLOGY OF ATHEROSCLEROSIS

EXTRACORONARY FACTORS

Increase in myocardial oxygen demand
  Increase in heart rate
    Anemia
    Fever
    Tachyarrhythmias
    Thyrotoxicosis
  Increase in inotropic state
    High adrenergic state
    Use of sympathomimetic drugs
  Increase in afterload
    Aortic stenosis
    Obstructive hypertrophic cardiomyopathy
    Severe hypertension
  High preload
    Severe congestive heart failure
    High output states
  Interference with oxygen delivery
    Anemia
    Hypoxemia
    Polycythemia
    High blood viscosity

INTRINSIC CORONARY FACTORS[a]

Adrenergic stimulation
Cocaine or amphetamine intoxication
Thrombotic coronary artery disease (e.g., sickle cell anemia, polycythemia vera, thrombocytosis)
Coronary emboli (e.g., aortic and mitral valve disease, myxoma)
Coronary vasculitis (e.g., Takayasu's disease, cardiac allografts)
Trauma (e.g., coronary dissection, radiation)

[a] External factors interfering with coronary artery tone or reactivity, endothelial function, and/or intravascular coagulation.

TABLE 46-3

CLINICAL CLASSIFICATION OF UNSTABLE ANGINA[a]

I. Primary unstable angina pectoris
   A. Clinical presentation
      1. Onset of angina within 60 days
      2. Crescendo angina pectoris
      3. Angina pectoris at rest
   B. Clinical background
      1. Post–myocardial infarction angina pectoris
      2. Post–coronary angioplasty angina pectoris
      3. Post–bypass surgery angina pectoris
      4. Variant (Prinzmetal's) angina pectoris
II. Secondary unstable angina pectoris

[a] Patients with primary angina pectoris may have characteristics of more than one class.

TABLE 46-4

BRAUNWALD CLASSIFICATION OF UNSTABLE ANGINA (UA)[a]

Severity	Clinical Circumstances		
	A. Develops in Presence of Extracardiac Condition that Intensifies Myocardial Ischemia (Secondary UA)	B. Develops in Absence of Extracardiac Condition (Primary Unstable Angina)	C. Develops within 2 Weeks after Acute Myocardial Infarction (Postinfarction UA)
I. New onset of severe angina or accelerated angina; no rest pain	IA	IB	IC
II. Angina at rest within past month but not within preceding 48 h (angina at rest, subacute)	IIA	IIB	IIC
III. Angina at rest within 48 h (angina at rest, acute)	IIIA	IIIB	IIIC

[a] Patients with UA may be also divided into three groups: (1) absence of treatment for chronic stable angina, (2) treatment for chronic stable angina, or (3) maximal anti-ischemic therapy. They may also be divided into those with transient ST-T wave changes during pain.
Source: From Braunwald.[51] Reproduced with permission of the American Heart Association and the author.

severe angina in the previous 2 months in patients previously in a quiescent phase of the disease or with pervious stable angina; and *postinfarction angina*. Prognostic features present at baseline include the following: no previous myocardial infarction; a previous myocardial infarction without or with previous congestive heart failure or an ejection fraction below 40 percent; the total duration of ischemic episodes; and the input of other diagnostic tests, such as radionuclide imaging and biologic markers. Acute determinants of prognosis are: (1) *persisting instability*, defined as chest pain persisting during the last week; (2) *crescendo unstable angina*, with two episodes of pain, one lasting for more than 20 min or episodes with persisting electrocardiographic changes within the last 48 h; and (3) *refractory unstable angina*, with the same criteria for chest pain in the previous 48 h despite full medical treatment. The general concept of this definition is useful to evaluate prognosis and dictate treatment.

Rizik et al. have validated in a consecutive series of 1387 patients the prognostic value of a four-category classification: *acceleration of previously existing chronic stable angina* without new electrocardiographic changes (class IA) and with electrocardiographic changes (class IB); *exertional angina of new onset* without respect to electrocardiographic morphology (class 2); *new-onset resting angina* in previously asymptomatic patients or in patients with previously stable exertional angina (class 3); and *protracted chest pain of >20 min duration* with persistent abnormalities of subendocardial ischemia (class 4).[53]

Any classification can be expanded to include descriptors of unstable angina for a comprehensive approach to the patient, including anginal equivalents, medication used, severity, provocative factors, extent of coronary atherosclerosis, dynamics of the coronary artery obstructions, and left ventricular function (Table 46-5). The more exhaustive the classification,

the more it resembles an algorithm for risk evaluation and patient management.

DIAGNOSIS

The diagnosis of unstable angina integrates various steps that include the following: (1) symptoms recognition; (2) evaluation of the probability of coronary disease, including past medical history and signs of ischemia; (3) risk evaluation; and (4) treatment implementation.

TABLE 46-5

SUBCLASSIFICATION/DESCRIPTORS OF PRIMARY UNSTABLE ANGINA PECTORIS THAT INFLUENCE CLINICAL DECISION-MAKING

1. Presence or absence of a history of stable angina pectoris, myocardial infarction, or revascularization procedure
2. Duration of episodes of pain or of angina equivalents
3. Occurrence of symptoms or evidence of asymptomatic myocardial ischemia on or off pharmacologic therapy for angina pectoris and the characteristics of such therapy
4. Presence or absence of electrocardiographic changes at rest and/or during episodes of pain or angina equivalents
5. Objective evidence of asymptomatic, silent myocardial ischemia
6. Electrocardiographic and functional (echocardiographic, nuclear) response to exercise or to pharmacologic stress testing
7. Detailed characteristics of coronary artery atheromata and obstructions
8. Extent of coronary artery narrowing, coronary artery flow reserve, and response to vasoactive drugs such as nitroglycerin, acetylcholine, and ergonovine

Recognition of Symptoms

The term unstable angina *refers to a distinctive increase in the number, severity, or duration of anginal episodes within the previous 2 months.* It is important to recognize anginal equivalents; they can be, for example, inappropriate shortness of breath, undue fatigue, weakness or dizziness, nausea, or diaphoresis. The terms *angina* and *chest pain* are used interchangeably here but refer to the range of terms that patients may use to describe their discomfort arising from coronary ischemia. Examples include *soreness, burning, fullness, bursting.* Angina (or anginal equivalents) is present at a decreasing level of exercise, sometimes at minimal exercise. In its more typical form, angina occurs at rest. Angina may also occur at night. The episodes of chest pain, relative to the stable anginal state, may also be more severe, more prolonged, and less responsive to nitroglycerin, often with attacks recurring shortly after initial relief. They can also be unresponsive to nitroglycerin. An episode of chest pain that lasts a few hours can often be differentiated clinically from MI by its fluctuating character. The functional classification of the Canadian Cardiovascular Society, useful for documenting the clinical status of a patient before an episode of unstable angina, may be misleading during the acute phase of the disease with, at times, the paradoxical observation of symptoms occurring unpredictably at rest and not during physical activities (see Chaps. 10 and 45).

Clinical Presentation

Angina is said to be of new onset or *de novo* when developing in a previously asymptomatic patient and as *crescendo* or *accelerating* when symptoms of previous stable angina are getting more severe. The distinction between prolonged chest pain (30 min or more in duration) and non-Q-wave MI is made a posteriori when the results of cardiac enzyme measurements become available. Progress in the laboratory diagnosis with new markers of cell necrosis has increased the sensitivity and rapidity of diagnosis while narrowing the margins between the two clinical syndromes. *It is likely that the pathophysiologic basis of the two conditions is similar and that the differentiating feature of enzyme elevation merely reflects the extent and duration of compromised coronary blood flow* (see also Chap. 47). The therapeutic approach to non-Q-wave MI is now similar to that of unstable angina.

When evaluating symptoms, one needs to realize that "atypical" features are almost inherent in the definition of unstable angina. Indeed, features of the chest pain, such as prolonged duration and an unpredictable response to nitroglycerin, settings, such as at rest in a previously stable state, and variable threshold are atypical; yet these symptoms may assume diagnostic importance if they truly indicate unstable angina. The clinical features including site of pain, character, irradiation, provocative factors, and duration may be more atypical in women since the diagnostic criteria are largely derived from data generated in men. The initial manifestations of CAD are often less dramatic and more subtle in women.[54]

The various noninvasive tests are also, in general, less reliable indicators of the absence or presence of CAD in women.[55] On the other hand, the presence of risk factors, including a postmenopausal status, could be more predictive than in men.[55] Although the development of coronary disease in women occurs on average 10 years later than in men, unstable angina and MI are frequent in women and the prognosis may be worse,[56–58] dictating special attention. In the TIMI-III registry, women were less likely than men to receive intensive anti-ischemic therapy and less likely to undergo coronary angiography; they had less severe and less extensive coronary disease, yet had a similar risk of experiencing adverse events by 6 weeks.[57]

The diagnosis of vasospastic or Prinzmetal's variant angina is suggested by a peculiar pattern of chest pain occurring mainly in the early morning; the hallmark for diagnosis is transient ST-segment elevation during pain. Because of its very distinctive features compared to other forms of unstable angina, variant angina is discussed in a special section later in this chapter.

Clinical Background

Three specific clinical circumstances need to be recognized in unstable angina because they are associated with a distinct prognosis (see Table 46-3). *Early postinfarction ischemia* refers to patients with recurrent chest pain developing between 24 h and 1 month after an acute MI[59] (see Chap. 47). It complicates the clinical course of MI in 20 percent of patients with an incidence not significantly modified by thrombolysis.[60] Ischemia at a distance is defined by transient ST-T changes occurring in electrocardiographic leads away from the original infarct; it is more frequent in inferior infarcts and frequently is associated with two- or three-vessel disease.[61] Ischemia in the infarct zone occurs in the same electrocardiographic leads as the original infarct; it is usually associated with viable myocardium at jeopardy from a critical stenosis of the infarct-related artery and is most common in anterior MI.[61] *Unstable angina in patients with previous coronary bypass surgery* may account for as many as 20 percent of all patients admitted for unstable angina.[62] Although the early in-hospital course is similar in these patients as in patients without previous bypass surgery, the long-term prognosis is worse, with twice as many events. The numerous reasons are related to the extensive CAD in these patients, the frequent history of previous MI and left ventricular dysfunction, the rapid progression of disease in venous grafts, and reduced possibility for a new revascularization procedure.[63,64] The TIMI Registry prospective study enrolled 2048 patients, including 336 patients with previous bypass surgery.[64] Patients with previous surgery were most often men, white, and diabetic, with a history of angina or MI. Previous bypass surgery in this trial did not influence the duration of hospitalization and the likelihood of undergoing coronary angioplasty or bypass surgery. Death or MI occurred by day 10 in 4.5 percent of patients with previous surgery compared to 2.8 percent of those without previous surgery. At 1 year, 39.2 percent versus 30.2 percent had experienced death, MI, or recurrent ischemia ($p = .002$). The worse prognosis was not predicted independently by the previous surgery but was more related to the previously discussed baseline characteristics.[64]

On the other hand, *recurrent angina after coronary angioplasty* as opposed to bypass surgery has a better prognosis; it is encountered in approximately 20 to 30 percent of patients within the first 6 months after the procedure and is associated with angiographic restenosis.[65] Although the clinical presentation may resemble unstable angina, the pathophysiologic and prognostic implications are different. Myocardial infarctions are unusual in these patients because the stenosis reflects vascular smooth muscle proliferation and probably inappropriate vasoconstriction rather than thrombus formation on an unstable, active inflammatory lesion. Complications associated with a repeat coronary angioplasty are also infrequent. *When unstable angina occurs 6 months or more after the procedure, a new active lesion is likely present* (see also Chap. 48).

Likelihood of Coronary Artery Disease

The diagnosis of the unstable state can be difficult and somewhat imprecise if based mainly on symptoms. Thus, false-positive diagnoses occur commonly, and normal coronary angiograms can be found in as many as 10 to 20 percent of patients.[66] The less stringent the diagnostic criteria used, the more frequent is the likelihood of a false-positive diagnosis. Evaluation of the probability of CAD is, therefore, an essential step to diagnosis and to treatment. At times the diagnosis is obvious, but medical discrimination is often required as well as diagnostic aids. Here again, the initial approach is clinical. A previous MI or a previous coronary angiogram can be diagnostic of CAD. Age above 40 years with presence of risk factors substantially increases the likelihood of the disease; *risk factors have greater predictive value in women, and their presence correlates with the existence and extent of CAD in 55 percent of women but in only 39 percent of men.*[55] Signs of peripheral atherosclerosis are predictive of increased mortality rate in patients with CAD.[56] The physical examination is usually nonspecific but is essential to rule out a secondary cause of unstable angina. If performed at the time of chest pain, the examination may reveal signs of transient myocardial ischemia, such as a fourth heart sound, a mitral regurgitation murmur, or signs of left ventricular failure.

Diagnostic Aids

Routine diagnostic tests that help in diagnosis are first, the 12-lead electrocardiogram (ECG) and second, the plasma levels of protein markers of myocardial cell injury. Studies of regional myocardial function and of regional myocardial perfusion may sometimes be useful.

TWELVE-LEAD ELECTROCARDIOGRAM

The most frequent electrocardiographic abnormality in unstable angina and in non-Q-wave MI is ST-segment depres-

sion; it is observed in 30 percent of patients; T-wave inversions are reported in 20 percent of patients, and transient ST-segment elevation is seen in approximately 5 percent of patients.[10] Continuous ECG monitoring increases the yield for detecting transient ischemic changes (see Chap. 28).

ST-segment elevation reflects transient total occlusion of a major epicardial coronary artery segment without significant collateral flow, implying transmural myocardial ischemia. When rapidly reversible with nitroglycerin, it is one of the hallmarks of variant angina but can also be the result of a transient thrombotic occlusion. Tall upright T waves and pseudonormalization of previously negative T waves can also indicate transmural ischemia and are frequently encountered in variant angina and as early changes of acute MI. On the other hand, ST-segment depression and T-wave inversion indicate subendocardial ischemia. These changes tend to be more transient in unstable angina; in non-Q-wave MI, they are more sustained and may last for a few days or longer. The ECG changes carry more significance when they are evolving and are more sensitive and specific when observed during an episode of chest pain.[67]

Continuous ECG monitoring results in more frequent detection of myocardial ischemia and more specifically of clinically silent episodes. Such monitoring need not be performed routinely but can be useful in some patients to confirm control of disease and assess prognosis.

Some ECG patterns are useful for the diagnosis of specific coronary artery lesions (Fig. 46-6). Deeply negative T waves in the precordial leads, with the ST segment isoelectric or slightly elevated in leads V_2 and V_3 or depressed in leads V_4 or V_5, often indicate critical reduction of flow in the left anterior descending coronary artery, with proximal involvement when the changes include the anterolateral leads.[68] These patients are at high risk of a severe event. ST-segment depression in the right precordial leads in the setting of prolonged chest pain may represent true posterior wall infarction and should be managed according to the guidelines for the management of MI with ST-segment depression; recordings of dorsal leads V_7, V_8, and V_9 can reveal the ST-segment elevation in these patients. In general, the ECG leads showing the ST-T changes correspond well to the site of the culprit coronary lesion, especially when a previous MI is not present. Diffuse changes may indicate left main or three-vessel disease.

CARDIAC ENZYMES AND OTHER MARKERS OF MYOCARDIAL CELL NECROSIS

Elevation of the MB fraction of CK is currently the "gold standard" for the diagnosis of cell necrosis (see Chap. 47). An elevation is usually detected 6 to 12 h after the onset of a prolonged ischemic episode associated with cell necrosis. The measurements of mass activity based on immunoinhibition assays with monoclonal antibodies have improved the sensitivity and specificity of the diagnosis over previous assays measuring enzyme activity. More recently, other markers have been developed that have the potential of increasing rapidity, sensitivity, and specificity for the diagnosis of myocardial necrosis. Myoglobin is released very rapidly from the myocardial cell, and elevated levels can be detected in the plasma 3 h after the ischemic injury; the sensitivity of this marker is high, but specificity is low since myoglobin is also abundant in skeletal muscle. Troponin I and troponin T are very specific markers of myocardial cell injury, released in the plasma as early as CK. Troponin I or T elevations have a higher sensitivity for the detection of small amounts of myocardial necrosis but may also represent severe ischemia with leakage of the cytosolic content. Six percent of the cell pool of troponin T and 3 percent of the pool of troponin I are cytosolic. Numerous studies have now documented that elevated plasma levels of troponin T or troponin I are present in up to one-third of patients admitted for unstable angina, often in the presence of normal MB-CK values. Furthermore, an elevation is uniformly associated with an increased risk of a cardiac event during the acute phase and during the early follow-up period that is directly related to the amount of elevation.[69-71] Normal values do not rule out unstable angina but may indicate a better prognosis.

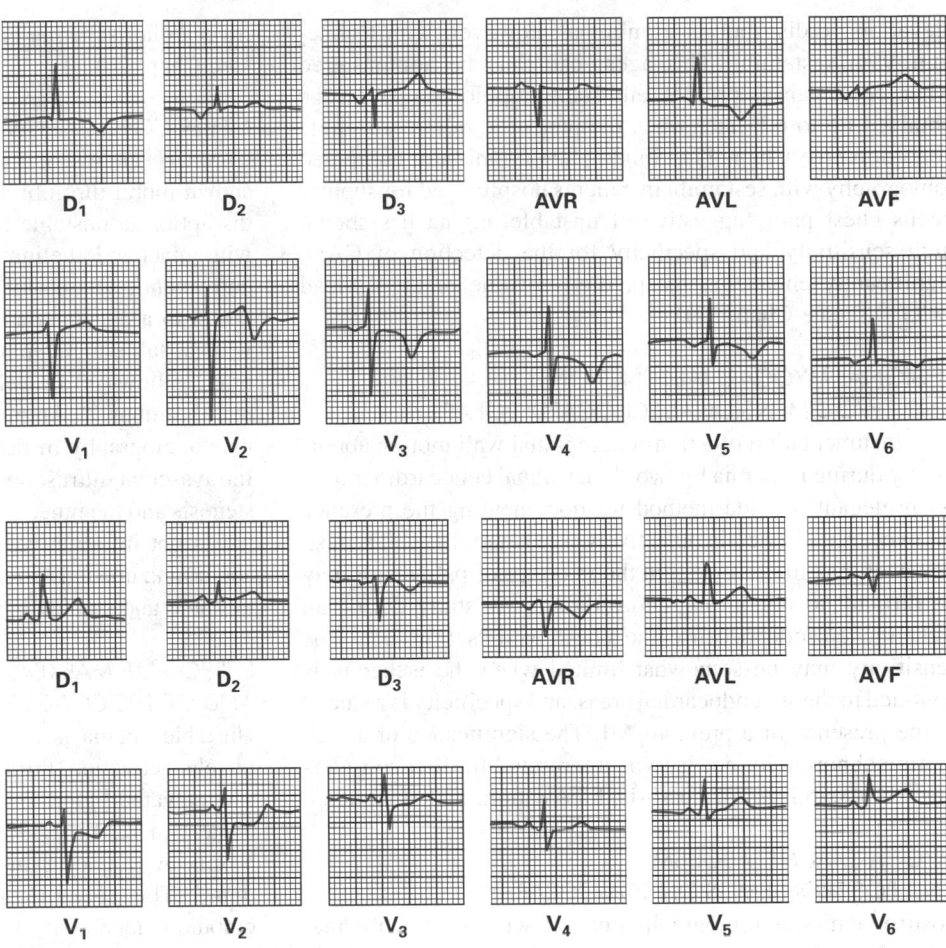

FIGURE 46-6

Specific ECG patterns in unstable angina. *Top.* The ECG shows deep T-wave inversion in the anterior lead extending to leads D_1 and AVL. It is strongly suggestive of a significant involvement of the proximal left anterior descending coronary artery and a large area of myocardium at risk. *Bottom.* The ST segment is depressed in leads V1 and V2. Closer inspection also revealed some ST elevation in the inferior leads. This ECG pattern in a patient with a prolonged chest pain indicates a true posterior wall infarct with an indication for fibrinolytic therapy.

CORONARY ANGIOGRAPHY

Coronary angiography provides unique information on the extent and severity of coronary artery stenotic lesions. Although not required for this purpose, it is nevertheless routinely performed in most centers in the majority of patients. *Coronary angiography should be obtained in higher risk patients to help select the best therapeutic approach.*

The traditional analysis of coronary angiograms in terms of severity and extent of CAD provides information only partly relevant to the diagnosis of unstable angina.[72] Indeed, the extent and severity of coronary lesions do not really help distinguish between patients with unstable angina, stable angina, or MI.[66] In the TIMI-IIIA angiographic study, 15 percent of patients had no stenosis of ≥60 percent and 4 percent had left main disease or left main equivalent; among the others, one-, two-, and three-vessel (≥60 percent stenosis) disease was found in 35, 39, and 26 percent of patients, respectively.[16] Some series have reported left main disease in as many as

10 percent of patients.[66] *Plaque morphology is more useful to characterize the culprit coronary lesion responsible for the ischemic state. These observations imply that the biologic characteristics of the plaque and not the severity of stenosis are critical determinants for the development of unstable angina* (see Chaps. 40 and 44).

MYOCARDIAL PERFUSION AND RADIONUCLIDE IMAGING

The diagnostic potential and the prognostic value of thallium-201 and technetium-99m sestamibi myocardial scintigraphy have been studied in patients with unstable angina (see Chap. 17). Thallium-201 injected during an episode of chest pain can document a perfusion defect with a high sensitivity. Injections during pain-free intervals documented defects in 40 to 60 percent of patients.[73] Washout abnormalities of thallium-201 have also been described.[74]

The rapid redistribution with thallium-201 necessitates immediate imaging, which may interfere with management of the unstable angina patient requiring immediate care and constant elevation. Redistribution is minimal, however, with technetium-99m sestamibi. This agent can thus be administered when chest pain is present, and scintigraphic images can be obtained up to 6 h later when the patient is in a more stable condition (see Chap. 17). Single-photon-emission computed tomography with sestamibi in patients hospitalized for spontaneous chest pain suggestive of unstable angina has shown high sensitivity and specificity for the detection of CAD, significantly enhancing the predictive value of the 12-lead ECG[67,75] (see Chap. 12).

REGIONAL MYOCARDIAL FUNCTION AND TWO-DIMENSIONAL ECHOCARDIOGRAPHY

The documentation of a transient regional wall motion abnormality during ischemia by two-dimensional echocardiography is an elegant bedside method for documenting the presence of myocardial ischemia objectively (see Chap. 14).[76] The test, however, has limited yield in the majority of patients. It may be difficult to obtain an echocardiographic study during an ischemic episode because the chest pain is transient. The sensitivity may be somewhat limited when the ischemia is confined to the subendocardial areas, and specificity is reduced in the presence of a previous MI. The significance of a wall motion abnormality needs to be interpreted further, considering the possibilities of necrosis, hibernation, and stunning.

MYOCARDIAL METABOLISM AND POSITRON EMISSION TOMOGRAPHY

Positron emission tomography imaging with the glucose analogue flourodeoxyglucose permits the detection of anaerobic metabolism. An increased uptake in regions of reduced perfusion indicates myocardial ischemia and reversibly injured myocardium and may be useful to distinguish between myocardial ischemia and infarction in certain circumstances (see Chap. 20).

OTHER CORONARY IMAGING TECHNIQUES

Coronary angioscopy performed in a few laboratories has shown mural thrombi and complex plaques with endothelial disruption in unstable angina, as opposed to smooth plaques with intact endothelium in stable angina. A gray-white lesion corresponds to fibrous plaque and a gray-yellow or yellow lesion to a degenerated fibrous plaque or atheroma. Patients with unstable angina have predominantly yellow lesions, more often yellow-red or yellow-pink.[77] MI is associated with a red thrombus.[78] Angioscopy is more sensitive andspecific than angiography in detecting the presence of a thrombus.[79] Intravascular ultrasound is useful to define the severity of stenosis and the inner core of the higher risk plaque accurately but is not informative about the presence of a thrombus or about fundamental differences in plaque composition between unstable and stable angina[79] (see Chap. 49).

SURROGATE MARKERS OF ACTIVATION OF PLATELETS AND OF THE COAGULATION SYSTEM

Unstable angina is accompanied by laboratory evidence of platelet activation, thrombin generation, and fibrin formation. The elevated blood levels of thromboxane B_2 and the urine content of 2,3-dinor thromboxane B_2, metabolites of thromboxane A_2 found in unstable angina, indicate platelet activation.[80] This elevation is frequently associated with angiographic evidence of thrombus formation and coincides with episodes of myocardial ischemia.[81] Thromboxane A_2, a potent stimulus to platelet aggregation and vasoconstriction, is released from activated platelets and also from activated leukocytes. Elevated levels of other platelet-specific proteins, such as beta-thromboglobulin and platelet factor 4, have been reported, but less consistently.[82] Flow cytometry provides a sensitive means to detect platelet activation; membrane P-selectin expression, fibrinogen binding to glycoprotein IIb/IIIa, and expression of activation epitotes (LIBS, ligand-induced binding sites) have been reported, but these measures are not highly predictive in individual patients because of considerable overlap between groups.[83,84]

Thrombin generation in vivo can be detected by various tests, some of which are shown in Fig. 46-7. The fragment of prothrombin 1 + 2 is released upon the conversion of prothrombin to thrombin. Two molecules of fibrinopeptide A are freed upon the

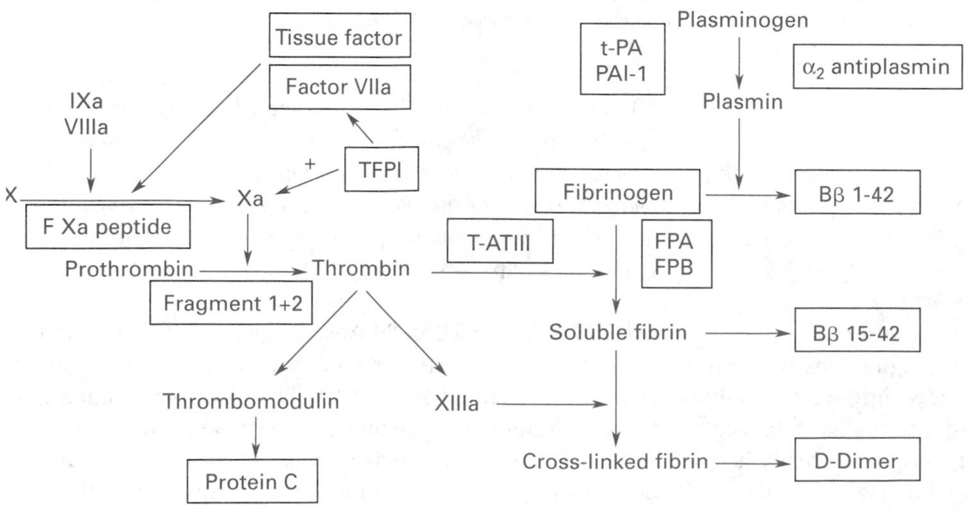

FIGURE 46-7
Diagram of the coagulation cascade showing some of the laboratory tests now available to evaluate the activity of the coagulation and fibrinolytic systems (the tests are within boxes). TFPI, tissue factor pathway inhibitor; T-ATIII, thrombin-antithrombin III complex; FPA, fibrinopeptide A; FPB, fibrinopeptide B; t-PA, tissue plasminogen activator; PAI-I, fast-acting inhibitor of tissue-type plasminogen activator; Bβ, polypeptide chain of fibrinogen.

catalytic transformation of one molecule of fibrinogen to fibrin by thrombin. Although the half-life of fibrinopeptide A is short, elevated levels can be detected in the blood and urine of patients with unstable angina.[85] Activation of the fibrinolytic system is also manifested by elevated levels of D-dimers, fibrin/fibrinogen degradation products, and of the fast inhibitor of tissue plasminogen activator.[86]

These surrogate markers are indicative of the thrombogenic etiology of unstable angina, and they have the potential of improving the diagnosis and of evaluating the response to treatment. The results of these tests may be affected by the technique of blood sampling and by other variables. They are at present a research tool (see also Chap. 52).

MARKERS OF INFLAMMATION

Systemic markers of the inflammatory process are increasingly recognized as being elevated in unstable angina. The acute phase reactants, fibrinogen, C-reactive protein, and amyloid A protein, are elevated in active disease.[87] In one series, for example, elevated levels of C-reactive protein and of serum amyloid A protein were detected in 65 percent of patients with an acute coronary syndrome.[88] Circulating leukocytes are activated,[89,90] and lymphocytes and monocytes may express a high procoagulant activity.[91,92] Interleukin 1 and interleukin 6 activity in the plasma may also be increased.[93,94] Interleukin-6 is responsible for the production of acute-phase reactant proteins by the liver and along with its main trigger, tumor necrosis factor, has intense proinflammatory and procoagulant activity. P-selectin, contained in the α granules of platelets and in the Weibel-Palade bodies of endothelial cells, is rapidly expressed at the cell surface following endothelial injury and platelet activation. Increased P-selectin plasma levels, as well as platelet-leukocyte aggregates, have been described in unstable angina.[95,96] P-selectin is the mediator for platelet binding to leukocytes and for leukocyte binding to the damaged endothelium. Elevation of plasma levels of leukocyte adhesion molecules has also been reported.[97] Additional research is needed to validate the value of these various markers as well as to determine the ones that will be most useful clinically to assess disease activity and disease control. The approach may be rewarding in facilitating understanding of the fundamental mechanisms of unstable angina and the reasons for a plaque to become unstable, forging the currently elusive link that exists between stable and unstable CAD.

RISK STRATIFICATION

Risk evaluation in unstable angina is a continuous process, initiated when diagnosis is suspected and updated during investigation and according to clinical evolution upon treatment. The early emphasis is focused on the acute disease process. Subsequently, it addresses the underlying atherosclerotic process and the determinants of long-term prognosis of CAD, keeping in mind that patients with unstable angina are at risk of recurrence and of rapid progression of atherosclerosis.

Prognosis in unstable angina, as in other manifestations of CAD, correlates strongly with the severity of the underlying CAD as assessed by the number of diseased vessels, the presence of left main disease or equivalents,[98,99] and with left ventricular function.[39,100,101] Some reports, however, provided conflicting interpretations,[39,102] emphasizing the specific nature of unstable angina and the importance of the anatomy and biology of the culprit lesion. Thus, complex lesions can be associated with a more severe prognosis than smooth lesions.[103] Yellow plaques with high lipid content, disrupted plaques, and the presence of a thrombus at the culprit lesion were associated in one angioscopic study with an eightfold increase in the risk of adverse outcome after balloon angioplasty.[104] Evaluation of the extent of myocardium at jeopardy is similarly important in risk evaluation.[98] Some of the features to consider in risk evaluation are summarized in Table 46-6.

TABLE 46-6

MARKERS OF RISK IN UNSTABLE ANGINA ASSOCIATED WITH AN ADVERSE OUTCOME[a]

	High Risk	Low Risk
Clinical presentation	Prolonged chest pain (>20 min)	De novo angina
	Repetitive pain	Effort angina
	Nocturnal pain	Little progression
	Hemodynamic instability	
Clinical background	Positive risk factors	Low probability of CAD
	Previous MI	
	Previous CABG	
ECG	ST-segment depression ≤ 1 mm	ECG normal or minimal changes
	Deeply inverted T waves	
Clinical evolution	Persistent instability on treatment	No recurrence of pain
Blood markers	Elevated CK values	Normal
	Elevated troponin T or I level	
	Inflammatory process	
Extent of CAD	Positive treadmill at low level	Negative treadmill or positive at high level
	Significant perfusion defects	

[a] Risk evaluation is performed at admission and updated as clinical status evolves.

Note: CABG, coronary artery bypass graft.

Prognosis During the Acute Phase

CLINICAL FEATURES

In general, *the more severe the clinical presentation, the worse the prognosis*. Thus, increasingly worse prognosis has been reported from new-onset angina to crescendo angina to angina at rest and to prolonged chest pain.[9,10,37] Recurrent chest pain on treatment is also associated with an adverse outcome. Prospective series, performed before modern treatment, have consistently described an unfavorable prognosis with chest pain persisting in-hospital. Its occurrence after 48 h in hospital was associated in one series with a 1-month mortality of 20 percent, in contrast to 2 percent without early in-hospital angina.[10] In another study, persisting pain after 12 h identified 86 percent of the patients with subsequent in-hospital MI.[9] In a multivariate analysis of clinical, electrocardiographic, and angiographic characteristics, recurrence of chest pain was the single most powerful predictor of prognosis in the acute phase. In a 12-month natural history study, angina that did not resolve early in the hospital course was the only predictor of subsequent cardiac events, which occurred during the early posthospital phase in 35 percent of patients with recurrent in-hospital angina as compared to 13 percent without.[39] Other important adverse prognostic features included previous cardiac history and, most importantly, left ventricular dysfunction.[105] The TIMI-III Prospective Registry examined in 3318 patients the influence of race, gender, and age on the incidence of death, MI, and recurrent ischemia at 42 days after entry.[57] Blacks were less likely than whites to undergo invasive procedures (odds 0.35, $p < .001$) and had a similar rate of death and MI but less recurrent ischemia; of those who underwent angiography, coronary stenoses were less extensive and less severe than in whites. Women were less likely than men to undergo angiography and revascularization and had less extensive stenotic disease, yet they had a similar risk of experiencing an adverse event. Striking differences were observed between patients older than 75 years and younger than 75 years. The elderly over 75 years received less aggressive medical treatment, were less likely to undergo angiography and an intervention, but had more extensive disease and a much higher event rate than those under 75 (relative risk 2.25, $p = .001$).

VALUE OF VARIOUS CLASSIFICATIONS

Classifications of unstable angina are aimed at defining prognosis. The classification proposed by Braunwald (Table 46-4) was partially validated in one study: The risk of recurrence of chest pain was highest in in-hospital patients in class III (angina within last 48 h), medium risk in class II (no angina within 48 h), and lowest in class I (no angina at rest); risk of recurrence was not influenced by the clinical situations A, B, and C (secondary, primary, postinfarction).[106] The severity class did not influence infarct-free survival at 6 months; patients with postinfarction angina, however, had a worse long-term prognosis. Prognosis was also less favorable when maximal medical therapy was required and when ECG

changes were present.[106] Rizik et al. have validated the in-hospital prognostic value of their classification.[53] The rate of occurrence of cardiac events, including refractory angina, MI, and death, was lowest in class IA (accelerating angina, no ECG changes), 2.7 percent; similar in class IB (accelerating angina, ECG changes) and II (new-onset exertional angina), 9.1 and 9.4 percent, respectively; higher in class III (new-onset rest angina), 20.1 percent; and highest in class IV (protracted angina), 42.8 percent. A prognostic grading system that takes into account the severity of recurrent angina is suggested in Table 46-7.

ELECTROCARDIOGRAPHIC CHANGES

The ECG is critically important in the evaluation of patients with chest pain. The presence of ischemic ST-T changes on the basal ECG carries important prognostic value.[53] Transient ST-T changes developing during chest pain provide further prognostic information.[10] In one study, the combination of ST-T fluctuation with ongoing symptoms of ischemia predicted a death rate of 42 percent at 1 year as compared with 5 percent at 2 years when absent.[107] In early postinfarction angina, the prognosis is also better when no ECG changes are present, rivaling the prognosis without early postinfarction angina.[108] The prognostic implications of ST-T changes are probably related to a high likelihood of extensive coronary disease, large ischemic zone, and possibly inadequate collaterals or collaterals jeopardized by multivessel disease. In contrast, the absence of ECG abnormalities is predictive of better prognosis.[109] *The absence of ECG abnormalities does not, however, rule out unstable angina.*

SILENT ISCHEMIA

Transient episodes of ST-segment depression on continuous ambulatory ECG recordings are reported in 10 to 66 percent of patients hospitalized for unstable angina.[110–113] The incidence is highest in patients with an abnormal baseline ECG or with an abnormal ECG during chest pain.[113] Silent ischemia, as is the case with symptomatic ischemia, is associated with severe CAD and a worse prognosis, with, in general, a twofold increase in the risk of MI and death as compared to the absence of silent ischemia. The discriminative power may be highest in patients with a duration of silent ischemia of 60 min or more over 24 h. In one study, the sensitivity of

TABLE 46-7

EVALUATION OF THE EARLY CLINICAL EVOLUTION

Class 0: No recurrent angina, no angina equivalents

Class 1: Occasional pain, not requiring modification of treatment

Class 2: Recurrent pain and/or ischemia controlled by intensification of medical treatment

Class 3: Recurrent angina, or ischemia, persisting despite intensive medical treatment

Class 4: Recurrent, severe ischemia, requiring urgent intervention

ST-segment depression on a 24-h ambulatory ECG recording to predict subsequent coronary events was similar to that of recurrence of chest pain (85 percent), but the specificity was higher, 75 percent versus 32 percent.[114] The enhanced predictive value in this study could have been related to the objective assessment of ischemia rather than relying on clinical endpoints.

BLOOD MARKERS

Elevation of the CK values denotes non-Q-wave MI and is associated with an adverse outcome that is directly proportional to the extent of elevation.[105] The newly developed markers of cell necrosis, such as troponin T and troponin I, add a new dimension to risk stratification. All studies, including recent large trials, have documented that an elevation in these proteins carries a three- to fourfold increase in the risk of death and of MI, both during hospitalization and during a follow-up extending to 6 months or more.[69–71,115–122] This prognostic information provided by troponin levels is independent of that of MB-CK.[69,121] In a sub-study by the investigators of GUSTO (Global Use of Strategies to Open Occluded Arteries), an elevation of troponin T above 0.1 μg/L was the strongest univariate predictor of an adverse outcome at 30 days.[121] The TIMI-IIIB report included 1404 patients with unstable angina or non-Q-wave MI.[122] The prognostic value of troponin I appears similar.[122] The cutoff values used to differentiate normal individuals from those with unstable angina and MI have varied between studies; in general, the higher the elevation of troponin I or T, the worse the prognosis (Fig. 46-8).

A new approach in risk stratification is now emerging with characterization of the blood proteins associated with inflammation. Levels of C-reactive protein $\geq$3 mg/L at hospital admission were associated with a poor response to medical therapy and a high risk of MI.[88] This prognostic value was present in patients with normal troponin T levels, suggesting that it marks a different aspect of the pathophysiology. High plasma levels of interleukin-6 were detected in 61 percent of patients with unstable angina and in 83 percent of patients with a complicated hospital course.[93] The prognostic value of the inflammation markers extends up to 1 year after hospital discharge[123] and also into the chronic phase of CAD.[124] The role of these markers of inflammation in clinical decision making has not yet been defined clearly. The Physicians' Health Study has shown that aspirin had more benefit in primary prevention in individuals with elevated levels of C-reactive protein at baseline.[125]

Late Prognosis

Risk stratification in unstable angina requires evaluation of the severity of CAD, directly by coronary angiography or by noninvasive means. Treadmill exercise testing can be performed safely *after stabilization* of unstable angina with medical treatment in many patients and is useful to predict long-term prognosis. In one study, cardiac events occurred at 1-year follow-up in 87 percent of patients with angina or ST-segment depression during the test compared to 29 percent of patients with a negative test.[126] In the RISC study, the number of leads with ST depression during exercise and a low maximal workload identified a high-risk group with death or MI at 1 year in 15.4 percent compared with 3.9 percent in a low-risk group.[127] In the Multicenter Myocardial Ischemia Research Group study, patients with an episode of unstable angina in the previous 6 months who had ST-segment depression $\geq$1 mm and an exercise duration less than 6 min showed a 3.4-fold increase in the risk of death, MI, or unstable angina.[128] *Exercise testing is not recommended as an early diagnostic procedure in patients with chest pain at rest; negative results may be misleading in the presence of a threatening thrombus associated with only a moderate degree of coronary*

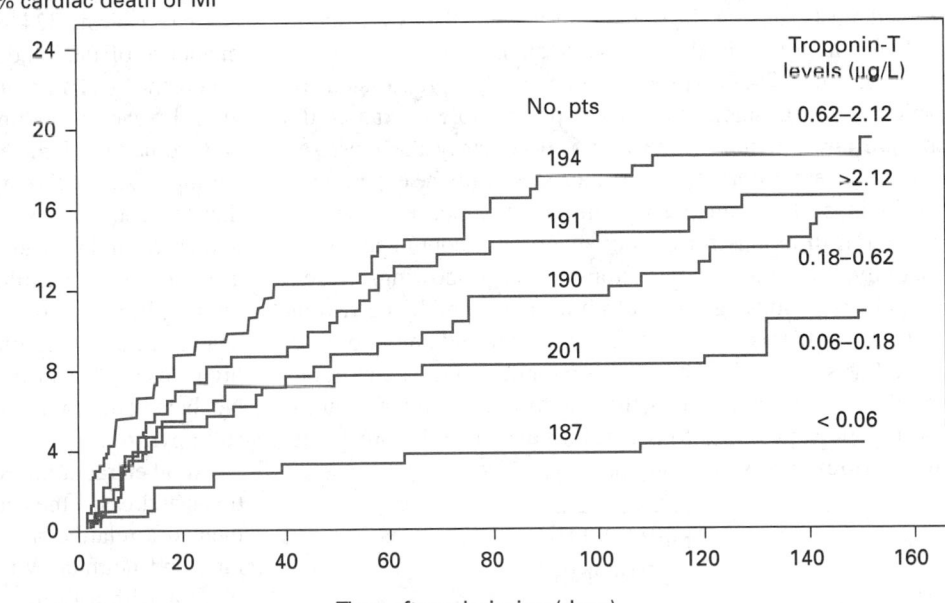

% cardiac death or MI

FIGURE 46-8

Cumulative risk of cardiac death or myocardial infarction based on maximal troponin T plasma levels obtained at admission for unstable angina and 12 and 24 h later. The number of patients in each group is shown. The risk increases from the lower to the higher quintiles. In the 217 patients with normal CK-MB mass values, the risk of a cardiac event was 13.0 percent with troponin T levels 0.06 to 0.18 μg/L and 4.6 percent with values below 0.06 μg/L. (From Lindahl et al.[120] Reproduced with permission of the author and the American Heart Association.)

occlusion at the time the test is performed. Exercise thallium-201 or technetium-99m sestamibi myocardial perfusion studies may provide additional diagnostic and prognostic information.[74,129,130] In a recent study of 126 consecutive patients treated medically, death and MI after 1 year occurred in only 2 percent of patients with a normal scan, compared with 14 percent of those with an abnormal scan and 25 percent with a reversible defect; counting rehospitalization as an event, incidences were respectively 12, 39, and 60 percent. The information provided by the diagnosis of a reversible defect was a strong independent predictor of prognosis, with a relative risk of 3.8 (95% confidence limits 1.6 to 8.6).[130] Dipyridamole perfusion scintigraphy is a useful alternative to treadmill exercise testing, as is stress echocardiography. The information derived from different testing modalities extends beyond detection of presence or absence of ischemia: it includes site(s), extent, and severity of ischemia, elements that can have prognostic value. The information can also orient treatment; for example, the selection of a lesion for angioplasty. Significant ischemia warrants invasive management and/or more intensive medical management.

Risk after an episode of unstable angina is further increased by an enhanced tendency to recurrence and to rapid progression of occlusive CAD. Angiographic progression in a series of 295 patients was twice as frequent after 8 ± 4 months in patients recatheterized after an episode of unstable angina as compared to patients recatheterized who had had stable angina; a complex morphology of the lesion was an additional predictor of progression.[131] Also, the accelerated progression in patients with a recurrent episode of unstable angina involved most often the site of the culprit lesion that was responsible for the first episode of unstable angina, marking a continuity in the disease process; conversely, progression in patients with unstable angina but prior stable angina could involve any previous stenosis, not necessarily the most severe.[132] These observations are consistent with the experimental findings of an enhanced proliferative response at the site of arterial thrombus formation[133] and with continued lesion "activity," as reflected by autopsy studies showing layered thrombi of various ages on culprit lesions[23] and by persisting elevation in the plasma levels of markers of inflammation and thrombosis.[124,125] The imputed role for thrombus in contributing to lesion progression is the scientific basis for new antithrombotic approaches to prevent accelerated atherosclerosis and also restenosis after angioplasty.[134,135]

THERAPEUTIC OPTIONS

Treatment of unstable angina can be divided into four broad categories: (1) antithrombotic therapy to control the underlying pathophysiologic process, (2) antianginal drugs to control and prevent symptoms and MI, (3) revascularization procedures directed against severely stenotic coronary lesions, and (4) risk factor modification and pharmacologic measures to slow or halt progression of atherosclerosis over the intermedi-

ate to long term. For discussion of this last category, see Chap. 41. Other therapies currently being investigated are target control of the inflammatory process and prevention of progression of cell ischemia to cell necrosis.

Cause-Specific Treatment: Antithrombotic Therapy

ANTIPLATELET THERAPY

Aspirin

Antiplatelet therapy, specifically aspirin, is now standard therapy for unstable angina, as it is for other manifestations of coronary disease (see Chap. 52). The Antiplatelet Trialists Group meta-analysis of more than 100,000 patients from 145 randomized controlled trials has shown homogeneous reduction in the risk of cardiovascular events with antiplatelet therapy in patients at all levels of risk, including acute and old MI, stroke, and stable and unstable angina.[136] The odds of infarction, stroke, or vascular death were reduced overall by more than 25 percent. In the 4000 patients with unstable angina, the risk reduction reached 35 percent after 6 months (9.1 percent versus 14 percent). Aspirin was used far more often than other antiplatelet drugs in these trials.

The benefits of aspirin in unstable angina are apparent during both the acute and follow-up phases. Four placebo-controlled trials have shown consistent benefits, despite differences in the populations studied, doses of aspirin used, time of initiation of treatment, and duration of follow-up.[137–140] In the Veterans Administration Cooperative Study involving 1266 men enrolled within 48 h after admission for unstable angina, aspirin, 324 mg daily, versus placebo reduced the incidence of fatal and nonfatal MI at 12 weeks from 10.1 to 5 percent.[137] The mortality rate remained 43 percent lower after 1 year follow-up. The second trial involved 555 men and women randomized to aspirin (325 mg four times daily), sulfinpyrazone (200 mg four times daily), both drugs, or neither.[138] The study was initiated within 8 days after hospital admission and was administered for an average of 18 months. The incidence of cardiac death and nonfatal MI was reduced with aspirin from 14.7 to 10.5 percent in the intention-to-treat analysis. Gastrointestinal side effects were frequent with these high doses of aspirin, occurring in 44 percent of patients. No benefit or favorable interaction of aspirin existed with sulfinpyrazone.

Another randomized placebo-controlled study of 479 patients addressed the acute phase of unstable angina and documented a relative risk reduction of 39 percent in the rate of fatal and nonfatal MI from 6.4 percent with placebo to 2.5 percent with aspirin.[139] The RISC study group tested a low aspirin dose of 75 mg daily in 945 men with unstable angina or non-Q-wave MI and confirmed a reduction in the rate of fatal and nonfatal MI at 5 days, from 5.7 to 2.5 percent, and at 90 days, from 17 to 6.5 percent.[140] The beneficial effects extended beyond 1 year (Fig. 46-9).[141]

Aspirin manifests numerous pharmacologic effects, many of which are only partly characterized. The primary mechanism accounting for the benefit in unstable angina is believed to be related to irreversible inhibition of the cyclooxygenase pathway in platelets, blocking formation of thromboxane A_2 and thromboxane A_2–induced platelet aggregation. This inhibition is complete with small doses of aspirin. The concomitant potential inhibition of prostacyclin generation by the endothelial cell does not seem to limit the protection afforded by aspirin significantly.

Ticlopidine

Ticlopidine, 250 mg twice a day, was compared in a randomized, open-label trial of 652 unstable angina patients of either sex to conventional antianginal therapy not including aspirin. After a follow-up of 6 months, ticlopidine reduced by 46 percent the rate of fatal and nonfatal MI, from 13.6 percent to 7.3 percent.[142] The benefit of ticlopidine in this study seemed to develop only after 2 weeks of treatment. This observation is compatible with the known delay of onset of action of this drug. Ticlopidine, unlike aspirin, does not block cyclooxygenase but interferes with the platelet activation mechanism mediated by adenosine diphosphate (ADP) and with transformation of the fibrinogen receptor, glycoprotein IIb/IIIa, into its high-affinity state (see also Chap. 52).

New Antiplatelet Agents

The benefits and limitations of aspirin have stimulated the development of many new therapies targeting various platelet functions, including adhesion and aggregation. Clopidogrel, a thienopyridine derivative closely related to ticlopidine, has been investigated in a large trial of 19,185 patients, the Clopidogrel versus Aspirin in Patients at Risk of Ischemic Events (CAPRIE) trial.[143] Patients with previous strokes, MI, and peripheral vascular disease were randomized to clopidogrel, 75 mg daily, or aspirin, 325 mg daily. An overall risk reduction of 8.7 percent was observed with clopidogrel compared to aspirin in the combined endpoint of stroke, MI, and vascular death. The benefits of clopidogrel were statistically significant in patients enrolled because of peripheral vascular disease but not in patients enrolled because of a previous MI. The side effect profile of clopidogrel was favorable, with no excess in total bleeding, gastrointestinal bleeding, thrombocytopenia, or neutropenia when compared with aspirin.

Selective inhibitors of thromboxane synthase and/or blockers of the thromboxane receptor have been investigated in

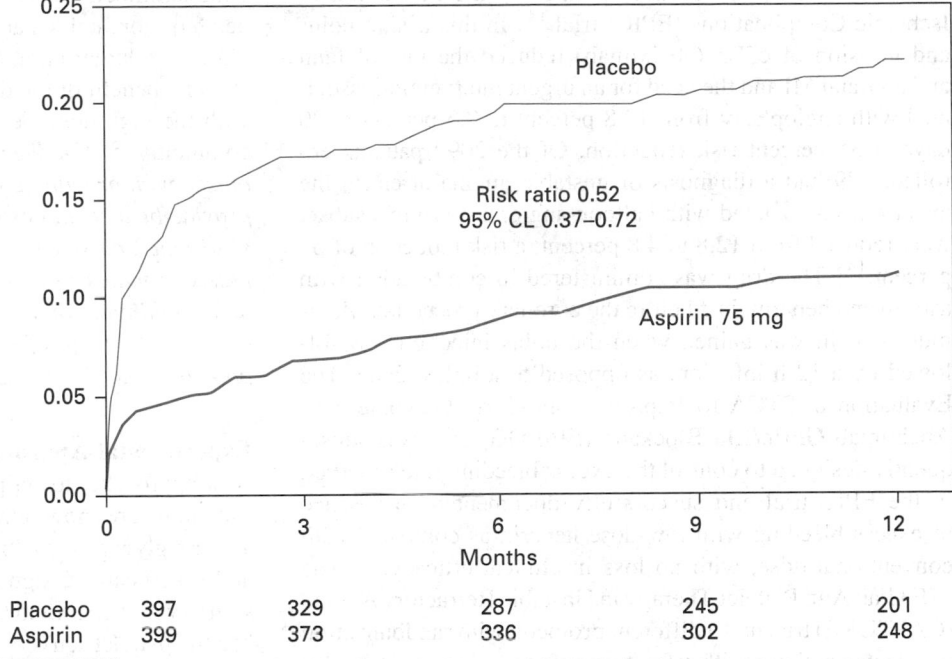

Probability of death or MI

Placebo	397	329	287	245	201
Aspirin	399	373	336	302	248

FIGURE 46-9

Risk of myocardial infarction or death during a 12-month follow-up after hospitalization for unstable angina, according to treatment assignment to aspirin (75 mg/day) or placebo. Severe angina requiring coronary angiography was also reduced from 29.2 to 20.8 percent (risk ratio, 0.71; 95% confidence limits, 0.56 to 0.91) (data not shown). (From Wallentin et al.[141] Reproduced with permission of the author and the editor.)

many trials without clear evidence of an advantage over aspirin, despite their potential of preserving prostacyclin formation.[144] Prostacyclin has not prevented complications in unstable angina patients.[145] Sulfinpyrazone and dipyridamole have also shown no benefit and are not recommended as antiplatelet agents.[138] Standard and low-molecular-weight heparin, the direct thrombin inhibitors, and the factor Xa inhibitors all inhibit platelet aggregation induced by thrombin and may thus counteract one of the most important pathways to platelet aggregation in acute coronary syndromes. These drugs are reviewed below, in "Anticoagulants," as well as in Chap. 52.

Glycoprotein IIb/IIIa Receptor Antagonists

The most promising new approach to inhibition of platelet aggregation in unstable angina and other acute coronary syndromes is inhibition of the platelet membrane integrin receptor glycoprotein IIb/IIIa. The glycoprotein IIb/IIIa integrin receptor is the final and obligatory pathway to platelet aggregation in response to all agonists. It can be inhibited in a dose-related manner by various drugs competing with the RGD (arginine-glycine–aspartic acid) sequence for fibrinogen binding to the receptor. The prototype of these inhibitors is c7E3, or abciximab, a monoclonal antibody.[146] Synthetic peptidic and nonpeptidic inhibitors mimicking the RGD (or KGD) sequence for fibrinogen binding and inhibiting the receptor highly specifically and reversibly have been synthesized. The monoclonal antibody is now approved for clinical use in high-risk coronary angioplasty following documentation of its protective effects in the Evaluation of 7E3 for the Prevention of Ischemic Complications (EPIC) trial.[147] In this trial, a bolus and infusion of c7E3 (abciximab) reduced the rate of fatal and nonfatal MI and the need for an urgent intervention associated with angioplasty from 12.8 percent to 8.3 percent at 30 days, a 35 percent risk reduction. Of the 2099 patients enrolled, 489 had a diagnosis of unstable angina at entry; the event rates associated with balloon angioplasty in this subset were reduced from 12.8 to 4.8 percent, a risk reduction of 62 percent.[148] The drug was administered in combination with aspirin and heparin, just before the coronary procedure. Maximum benefit was gained when the bolus injection was followed by a 12-h infusion, as opposed to a bolus alone. The Evaluation in PTCA to Improve Long-Term Outcome with Abciximab GPIIb/IIIa Blockade (EPILOG) trial was subsequently designed to control the excess bleeding rate observed in the EPIC trial and successfully documented an absence of excess bleeding with low-dose heparin as compared with conventional dose, with no loss in clinical efficacy.[149] The c7E3 Fab Anti Platelet Therapy in Unstable Refractory Angina (CAPTURE) trial had a different protocol, with randomization of selected patients with refractory angina and an angiographically documented culprit lesion suitable for angioplasty to c7E3 or to placebo.[150] Treatment was initiated 20 to 24 h before the angioplasty procedure and stopped 1 h after. Most events in this trial were related to the angioplasty procedure. The infusion of abciximab reduced the rate of MI during the infusion, before angioplasty, from 2.1 percent to 0.8 percent and the composite endpoint of death, MI, or need for an urgent intervention procedure at 1 month from 15.9 percent to 11.3 percent (risk ratio, 0.71; 95% confidence limits, 0.53 to 0.94; $p = .016$). The results of these trials with abciximab have documented an important benefit of the monoclonal antibody as an adjunct to percutaneous transluminal coronary angioplasty in high-risk cases.

The usefulness of glycoprotein IIb/IIIa antagonists to modify the course of unstable angina is presently being investigated in large trials. Integrelin, a synthetic peptidic glycoprotein IIb/IIIa inhibitor with the RGD sequence, is being studied in the Platelet IIb/IIIa in Unstable Angina: Receptor Suppression Using Integrelin Therapy (PURSUIT) trial. Two trials were just completed with tirofiban. The Platelet Receptor Inhibition for Ischemic Syndrome Management (PRISM) trial compared the clinical event rates occurring during a 48-h infusion of tirofiban or of heparin,[151] and the Platelet Receptor Inhibition for Ischemic Management in Patients Limited by Unstable Signs and Symptoms (PRISM-PLUS) trial evaluated the event rates at 1 week and 1 month following treatment with tirofiban, heparin, or the combination of tirofiban plus heparin.[152] Patients with high-risk unstable angina were enrolled in the latter trial. Previous pilot studies with integrelin, tirofiban, and lamifiban had suggested a benefit. In the Canadian lamifiban study involving 365 patients with unstable angina and non-Q-wave MI, the risk of death or nonfatal MI or the need for an urgent intervention procedure during a 72-

to 120-h infusion period decreased from 8.1 to 3.3 percent with lamifiban ($p = .04$); the highest doses also reduced death or nonfatal MI at 1 month from 8.1 to 2.5 percent ($p = .03$).[153] A larger pilot study with lamifiban, however, did not reveal a benefit of the drug, but an excess bleeding was noted with the high doses, especially when heparin was used concomitantly.[154] *Whether or not the glycoprotein IIb/IIIa antagonists, with or without concomitant aspirin and heparin, will provide benefits in unstable angina and other acute coronary syndromes, outside the context of adjunctive therapy to angioplasty, remains to be demonstrated in clinical trials. Orally active inhibitors of the glycoprotein IIb/IIIa receptor are now at an early stage of investigation. These drugs have much potential, but their risk/benefit ratios remain to be defined.*

Experimental Approach

New approaches to antiplatelet therapy targeting other platelet functions are now emerging. Thus, monoclonal antibody against glycoprotein Ib, inactive von Willebrand fragments, and specifically designed heparins can prevent platelet adhesion to von Willebrand factors. Inhibitors of selectins responsible for platelet-leukocyte interaction, of leukocyte integrins, and of platelet-derived growth factors are also under experimental investigation. The objective is to test the utility of attenuating the inflammatory reaction that leads to the active plaque and to cell proliferation.

ANTICOAGULANTS

Anticoagulants in unstable angina have been associated with marked early benefit but somewhat attenuated long-term results.

Standard Heparin

In a double-blind, randomized study of 479 unstable angina patients, intravenous heparin at therapeutic doses markedly reduced the incidence of fatal and nonfatal MI from 11.9 to 1.2 percent (risk ratio, 0.07; 95% confidence limits, 0.02 to 0.30; $p < .0001$) and of refractory angina from 22.9 to 9.6 percent (risk ratio, 0.48; 95% confidence limits, 0.25 to 0.70; $p < .0001$).[139] An extension of this trial directly comparing heparin with aspirin during the acute phase of unstable angina showed more benefit from heparin, with a risk difference in the incidence of death or MI of 2.9 percent ($p = .03$).[155] The early gains with heparin, however, were partly offset by an excess event rate after discontinuation of the drug. Death, MI, and recurrence of severe ischemia requiring an intervention occurred in 13 percent of patients clustered around a mean of 9.5 ± 5 h after discontinuation of heparin (Fig. 46-10).[156] Aspirin seemed partly effective in preventing this reactivation. The combination of heparin and aspirin was also the most effective therapeutic strategy in the RISC study at 5 days, with sustained benefits longer term when aspirin was administered concomitantly.[140] Another study has shown that the administration of an infusion of heparin reduced the incidence of severe refractory angina and of ambulatory ECG-detected ST-T segment shifts.[157] A study by Holdright et al. yielded different results, with no advantage of heparin over aspirin, but the event rate was unusually high, and MIs present before initiation of treatment were counted as events.[158]

Low-Molecular-Weight Heparins

The low-molecular-weight heparins exhibit better bioavailability than standard heparin. A small pilot study from Argentina suggested that they may have better efficacy than heparin as well.[159] Three larger randomized studies of approximately 1500 patients have recently been completed.[160–162] In the Fragmin during Instability in Coronary Artery Disease (FRISC) study of 1506 patients, dalteparin plus aspirin administered for 1 month, compared to placebo plus aspirin and no heparin, reduced the rate of death and MI at 6 days from 4.8 to 1.8 percent (risk ratio, 0.37; 95% confidence limits, 0.20 to 0.68) and the need for revascularization from 1.2 to 0.4 percent.[160] The reduction in the dose of dalteparin from twice a day to once a day after 6 days was associated with an increase in the event rate, documenting again the potential for reactivation of unstable angina. The overall difference was maintained at 6 weeks (Fig. 46-11). No differences were found in the rates for death, new MI, or revascularization procedures after 4 to 5 months. The FRIC study compared dalteparin to standard heparin to show no statistically significant differences between the two drug regimens; death or MI at day 6 had occurred in 9.3 percent of dalteparin patients and in 7.8 percent of standard heparin patients (NS).[161] A worrisome feature of this trial is that mortality was slightly higher, although of borderline statistical significance, in dalteparin-treated patients, 1.5 versus 0.4 percent (95 percent confidence limits, 0.09 to 0.99; $p = .057$). The Efficacy and Safety of Subcutaneous Enoxaparin in Non-Q Wave Coronary Events (Unstable Angina and Non-Q-Wave MI) (ESSENCE) trial, however, showed significantly better results with the low-molecular-weight heparin than with standard heparin. Enoxaparine at doses of 1 mg/kg subcutaneously twice a day was used in this trial for 3 to 8 days.[162] A total of 3171 patients were randomized. The composite endpoint of death, MI, or refractory angina was insignificantly reduced at 48 h from 7.4 percent with heparin to 6.2 percent with enoxaparine ($p = .176$), at 14 days from 19.8 to 16.6 percent ($p = .019$), and at 30 days from 23.3 to 19.8 percent ($p = .017$). A large

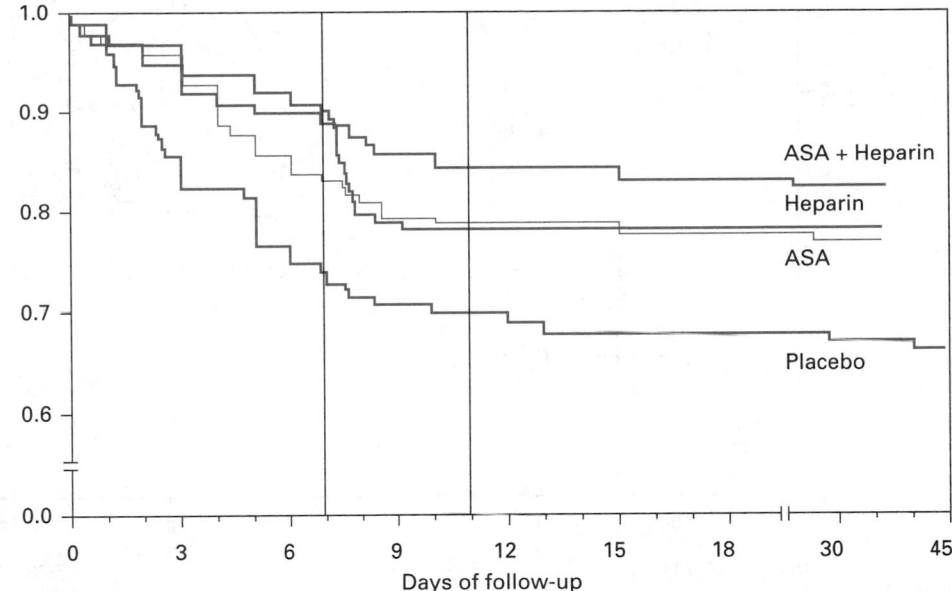

Probability of being free of an ischemic event

FIGURE 46-10

Kaplan Meier survival curves in patients randomized to aspirin (ASA), heparin, aspirin plus heparin, or placebo during the acute phase of unstable angina. The curves cover the study periods, including the double-blind administration of the study drugs, a 96-h period following drug discontinuation (indicated by the rectangle), and follow-up to 45 days. A cluster of ischemic events occurred at a mean of 9.5 ± 5 h following the discontinuation of heparin, showing rebound or reactivation of the disease following the discontinuation of heparin. (From Théroux P et al.[156] Reproduced with permission of the author and the editor.)

TIMI trial is now ongoing with enoxaparin. *The documentation of an equivalence between low- and standard-molecular-weight heparins would be useful findings because low-molecular-weight heparins can be administered subcutaneously with no monitoring required and because they cause fewer adverse effects. It is to be remembered that all low-molecular-weight heparins are not the same with regard to inhibition of factor X versus factor II and that the results obtained with various agents may differ.*

Direct Thrombin Inhibitors

The direct thrombin inhibitors do not require a cofactor for their effect and have no endogenous circulating inhibitors, resulting in a stable and reproducible anticoagulation (see Chap. 52). They effectively inhibit thrombin bound to fibrin within the blood clot and can therefore prevent further platelet activation and feedback reactivation of the coagulation process. Hirudin, the prototypical direct thrombin inhibitor, is now available as recombinant hirudin. Small peptides modeled after hirudin have been synthesized. Evaluated in pilot studies, they have provided encouraging results. Larger phase 3 trials, while confirming early benefit, have, however, been disappointing because the benefit was not well maintained after 1 and 6 months.

The GUSTO-II trials evaluated the safety and efficacy of r-hirudin in patients with acute chest pain with or without ST-segment evaluation.[163,164] The first phase of the trial, GUSTO-IIA, was stopped prematurely after enrollment of

Probability of cardiac death or MI

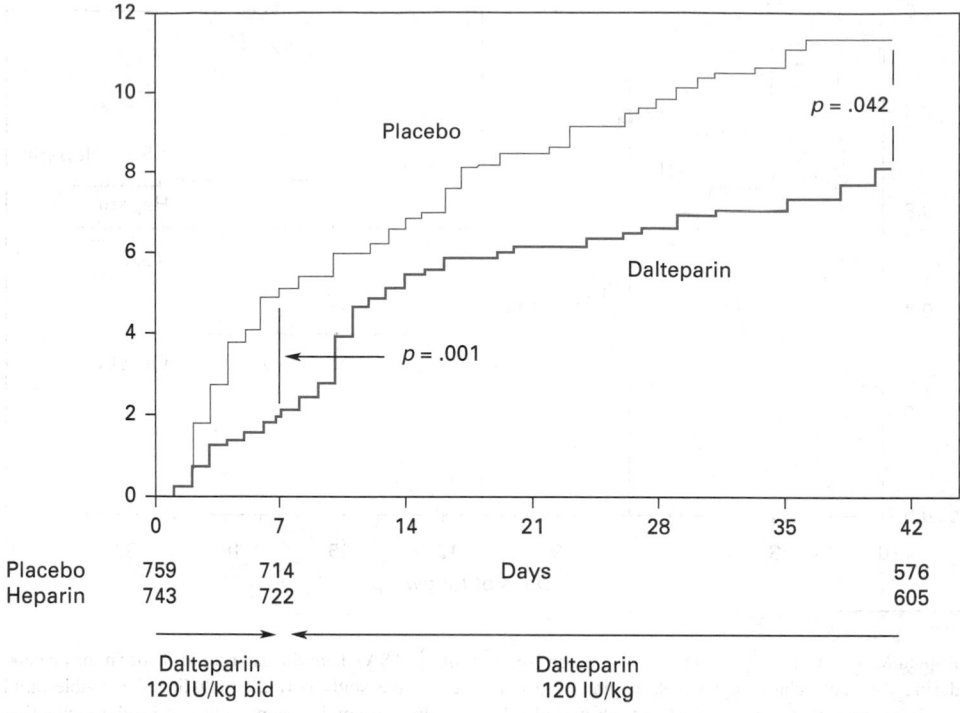

Placebo   759   714   576
Heparin   743   722   605

FIGURE 46-11

Kaplan Meier survival curves to 42 days after randomization showing the probability of death or myocardial infarction with dalteparin or placebo, all patients receiving aspirin. The curves show a bimodal distribution: they diverge early, favoring low-molecular-weight heparin; converge following reduction of the dose of dalteparin from twice daily to once daily at day 6; and diverge again later. The results document the efficacy of the low-molecular-weight heparin to prevent death, myocardial infarction, and severe angina in unstable angina. The drug did not prevent rebound, however, which became manifested with the dose reduction. (Reproduced with permission of the author and the editor, from Lars Wallentin: Low-molecular-weight heparin during instability in coronary artery disease. Fragmin during Instability in Coronary Artery Disease (FRISC) Study Group.[160] *Lancet* 1996; 347:561–568. © The Lancet Ltd., 1996.)

2564 patients because of excess bleeding with hirudin.[163] The dose subsequently was reduced to a 0.10-mg/kg bolus and a 0.1-mg/kg per hour infusion for the second phase. In GUSTO-IIB, the primary endpoint of death or nonfatal MI at 30 days occurred in 8.9 percent of patients with hirudin and 9.8 percent with heparin ($p = .06$). In the 4131 patients with ST-segment elevation, endpoints were reached in 9.9 and 11.3 percent of patients ($p = .13$), respectively, and in the 8011 patients without ST-segment elevation, in 8.3 and 9.1 percent ($p = .2$) (Fig. 46-12).[164] In contrast, the benefit of hirudin during the first 24 h was striking, a 1.3 percent event rate versus 2.1 percent with heparin, a risk reduction of 36 percent ($p = .001$), and at 48 h, 2.3 versus 3.1 percent (risk reduction, 25 percent; $p = .001$). In the Hirudin in a European Trial versus Heparin in the Prevention of Restenosis after PTCA (HELVETICA) trial, hirudin was administered to coronary angioplasty patients; the study also documented an early gain but no residual benefits after 6 months.[165] The Organization to Assess Strategies for Ischemic Syndromes (OASIS) pilot study used an intermediate dose of hirudin, 0.4-mg/kg bolus and 0.15-mg/kg per hour infusion, with dose titration to an activated partial thromboplastin time (aPTT) value between 60

and 100 s.[166] The rate of death, MI, and refractory angina at 7 days was reduced from 7.1 percent with heparin to 3.7 percent with the medium dose of hirudin ($p = .15$), and death, MI, and refractory or severe angina from 17.4 to 10.4 percent ($p = .05$). A large phase 3 trial to enroll 10,000 patients is ongoing.

Other synthetic direct thrombin inhibitors are available that interact differently with the thrombin molecule, have shorter half-life, and block thrombin effects differently. Inogatran and efegatran are small peptides. Argatoban is an arginine derivative. Aptamers inhibiting the thrombin active sites are also available. *Direct thrombin inhibitors do not currently provide a clear benefit over more standard therapy in unstable angina. Further research is required to define modalities for their application, such as optimal doses, and to maintain their early benefits for a longer term.*

New Anticoagulants

Many new anticoagulants are under development. Some act at more proximal and some at more distal levels of the coagulation cascade. The tissue factor–factor VIIa complex initiates both the intrinsic and extrinsic pathways of coagulation and can be blocked both by antibodies against the complex and by a recombinant form of the tissue factor pathway inhibitor. Direct inhibitors of factor Xa, such as the tick anticoagulant peptide and antistatin, can inhibit free factor Xa, as the heparins do, and also factor Xa at the platelet surface and within the prothrombinase complex. A recombinant form of activated protein C, a potent natural anticoagulant activated by the complex formed between thrombin and thrombomodulin at the endothelial level, is also being evaluated.

Oral Anticoagulants

No trials have adequately tested the value of oral anticoagulants for the longer term management of unstable angina, although some clinical observations have suggested that they could be of benefit.[5–8,167] The OASIS pilot study has suggested that coumadin could be useful in prolonging the early benefits of anticoagulants when used at therapeutic doses.[166] The strategy is now being tested in the large OASIS trial. In the Antithrombotic Therapy in Acute Coronary Syndromes

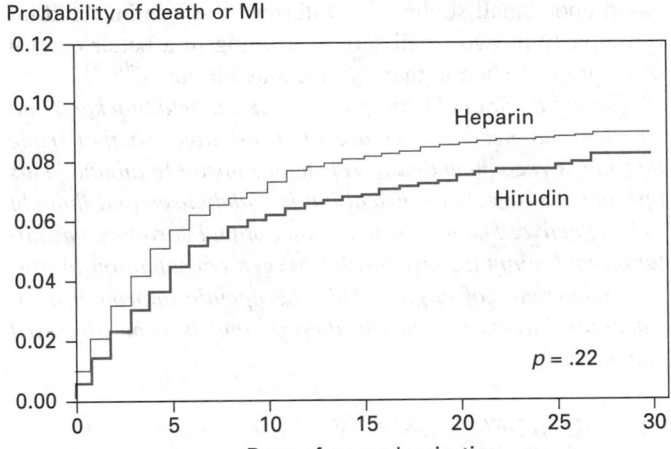

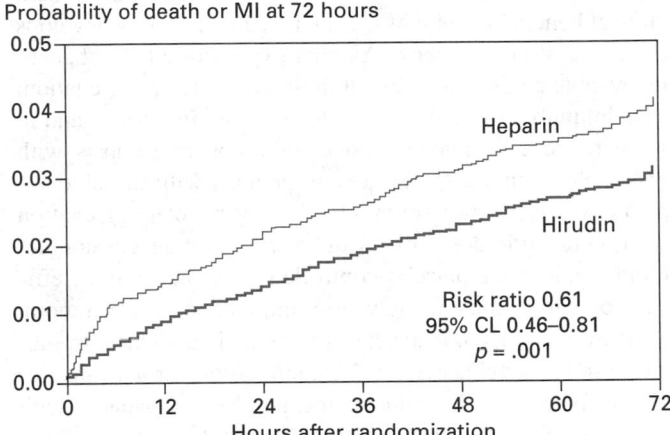

FIGURE 46-12

Kaplan Meier estimate of the probability of death, myocardial infarction, or reinfarction in patients with unstable angina or myocardial infarction without ST-segment elevation with treatment with intravenous heparin or intravenous recombinant hirudin (bolus of 0.1 mg/kg and infusion of 0.1 mg/kg per hour). The population includes 8011 of the 12,142 patients randomized in the Global

Use of Strategies to Open Occluded Coronary Arteries (GUSTO) IIb trial. Hirudin resulted in a statistically significant early risk reduction at 24 and 48 h (*left*), but this benefit was attenuated after 30 days (*right*). (From The GUSTO IIb Investigators.[164] Reproduced with permission of the author and the editor.)

(ATACS) study, 214 unstable angina patients not previously using aspirin were randomized 9.5 h after admission to aspirin alone or a combination of aspirin and heparin followed by coumadin for 12 weeks. The aspirin plus heparin combination resulted in reduction of ischemic events at 12 weeks from 27 to 10.5 percent; most benefit was present, however, early during treatment with heparin, and the benefit after 12 weeks was not statistically significant.[168] *Long-term oral anticoagulation following unstable angina is not recommended until additional results from clinical trials are available.*

FIBRINOLYTIC THERAPY

Clinical investigation has shown no benefits of thrombolysis in unstable angina and non-Q-wave MI.[169] In the Thrombolysis in Patients with Unstable Angina (UNASEM) study, recurrent angina was marginally more common in patients treated with thrombolytic therapy than in those who were not (27 versus 12 percent, *p* = .06), despite better restoration of coronary blood flow in the former group.[170] In the largest trial, TIMI-IIIB involving 1473 patients, death and MI occurred in 8.8 percent of patients treated with tissue plasminogen activator and in 6.2 percent of patients treated with placebo (*p* = NS) (see Fig. 46-5).[40] A trend toward a deleterious effect was also present with streptokinase compared to placebo in patients with unstable angina and venous bypass grafts.[171] Pooled data suggest that the risk of fatal or nonfatal MI in unstable angina patients treated with thrombolysis is significantly increased. Other studies have shown larger resting thallium-201 perfusion defects and longer duration of ST-segment shifts in patients treated with tissue plasminogen activator[172] and more frequent need for an urgent intervention because of recurrent ischemia.[173] *Thrombolysis is not indicated in patients with unstable angina, nor in patients with MI without ST-segment elevation, with the exception of patients present-*

ing with typical symptoms with left bundle branch block or true posterior infarction (see also Chap. 47).

Antianginal Therapy

The goal of antianginal therapy is to relieve myocardial ischemia by improving the ratio between oxygen supply and demand. This is accomplished by coronary vasodilation and by reducing the cardiac workload. Inappropriate vasoconstriction is often present in unstable angina, with secretion of potent vasoconstrictors and loss of the dilator properties of the endothelium. Coronary vasodilators may therefore induce striking improvement. Myocardial oxygen demand can be reduced effectively with beta blockers and, less consistently, with calcium channel blockers. The goal of treatment is to try to obtain favorable hemodynamic conditions within the range of patient comfort.

NITROGLYCERIN

Recommendations on the use of nitroglycerin are based on clinical experience more than on objective data derived from clinical trials. Indeed, the benefits of nitroglycerin for controlling chest pain and preventing clinical events have been examined in only a few small studies.[174–176] A decrease in angina episodes has been reported in 15 and 94 percent of patients with refractory angina treated with intravenous nitroglycerin for periods of 24 h to 3 weeks. Nitroglycerin reduces preload and afterload of the heart, produces coronary vasodilatation, and favors preferential flow to the ischemic zones. Nitroglycerin donates nitric oxide to the arterial wall and thus substitutes in part for reduced endothelium-derived nitric oxide production.[177] It acts by increasing the intracellular levels of cyclic guanosine monophosphate (cGMP). The precise mechanisms of benefit of nitroglycerin in unstable angina remain unclear.

Continuous infusions over several days are used with apparent clinical benefits in spite of the tolerance that rapidly develops to the use of nitroglycerin. Another explanation for its benefit in unstable angina could be inhibition of platelet aggregation. This inhibitory effect has been documented in vitro[178] and in vivo in the experimental model of coronary stenosis with endothelial damage.[179] Studies in patients with unstable angina have also shown some inhibition of platelet aggregation with therapeutic doses of nitroglycerin.[180] A recent double-blind, randomized placebo-controlled trial compared the efficacy of intravenous nitroglycerin, intravenous heparin, both, or neither to prevent recurrence of angina in patients hospitalized for rest angina within 6 months after coronary angioplasty. Nitroglycerin reduced the number of patients with recurrent rest angina from 70 to 43 percent (risk ratio, 0.61; 95% confidence limits, 0.47 to 0.79; $p = .0001$) and the number of patients requiring urgent intervention because of severe angina from 24 to 6.3 percent ($p = .0006$). Heparin was no better than placebo in the specific subset of unstable angina caused by restenosis.[181]

BETA-ADRENERGIC BLOCKERS

Beta blockers have become standard therapy in unstable angina despite the lack of data documenting a reduction in major cardiac events. They are used to prevent and control recurrent chest pain, based upon extrapolations from studies of other coronary syndromes and upon the results of small studies that have shown some efficacy.[182,183] They are most useful in patients with a high sympathetic tone manifest by sinus tachycardia and elevated blood pressure. They reduce myocardial oxygen demand and may also have additional protective effects. In a study of patients with chest pain suggestive of MI, beta blockers reduced the risk of developing MI by 13 percent.[183] Beta blockers may cause unopposed alpha-adrenergic vasoconstriction and, rarely, may exacerbate coronary spasm.[184] Beta blockers need individual titration. *The goal of treatment is to achieve a basal heart rate of 60 beats per minute or below.* Beta blockers can advantageously be administered intravenously when a rapid effect is needed, such as in a patient with evolving chest pain (see also Chap. 54).

CALCIUM CHANNEL BLOCKERS

Calcium channel blockers have been studied extensively in unstable angina.[185–191] Many trials have shown that verapamil, nifedipine, and diltiazem can efficiently control chest pain in unstable angina; the results in Prinzmetal's variant angina are most striking. *These trials, however, have failed to document a reduction in the rate of MI, death, and severe refractory angina.* In fact, an increased risk of MI has been reported with short-acting nifedipine used as monotherapy of unstable angina.[185,188] The combination of a beta blocker with nifedipine may, however, be safer and useful to prevent recurrent angina.[186,187] The newer dihydropyridines with longer half-lives have not been evaluated in unstable angina. Diltiazem and verapamil are as effective as propranolol in controlling recurrent ischemia and preventing cardiac events,

based upon small studies.[189] Diltiazem was administered intravenously in two small series, resulting in a better control of recurrent ischemia than intravenous nitrates.[190,191]

The antianginal effects of nitroglycerin, beta blockers, and calcium channel blockers are often additive, so that triple therapy is recommended in refractory unstable angina. This approach is largely empirical but is widely used and thought to be effective. The goal is to obtain optimal coronary vasodilation and minimize myocardial oxygen consumption to prevent recurrence of angina. This therapeutic approach is no substitute for antithrombotic therapy and is generally used concurrently.

INTRAAORTIC BALLOON PUMP

Intraaortic balloon counterpulsation can now be performed easily at the bedside using the transcutaneous approach. The augmented diastolic pressure favors diastolic flow through severe stenoses and may prevent complete occlusion by washing out thrombogenic material, while balloon deflation reduces cardiac work by systolic unloading. *The efficacy of the intraaortic balloon pump has not been evaluated in randomized studies, but clinical experience teaches that it is extremely efficacious in controlling recurrent ischemia and preventing complications in the patient at very high risk.* Indeed, patients will only rarely experience a cardiac complication while on counterpulsation. The technique can be associated with local complications in as many as 10 percent of cases and is not applicable in patients with obstructive aortic disease; it is contraindicated in patients with valvular aortic regurgitation. The local complications of lower limb ischemia are usually controlled by removing the catheter. Intraaortic balloon counterpulsation is most useful as a bridge to revascularization.[192] Used for a few days, it can help maintain patency at the site of a complicated coronary artery intervention procedure.[193] Intraaortic counterpulsation is used in 1 to 5 percent of patients to control severe recurrent ischemia, to stabilize hemodynamically unstable patients, and to prevent complications associated with coronary angiography, coronary angioplasty, and coronary bypass surgery.

Revascularization Procedures

Coronary artery bypass surgery has been applied to the management of unstable angina since the early 1970s, soon after its introduction in clinical practice. Coronary angioplasty was applied in the early 1980s, immediately after documentation of its feasibility in stable angina. These revascularization procedures are now widely used and are extremely useful in the management of unstable angina.

CORONARY ARTERY BYPASS SURGERY

Early reports have documented the feasibility of bypass vein graft surgery in unstable angina with a low operative mortality and with substantial relief of symptoms (see Chap. 50). The results, however, were offset by a perioperative infarction rate of 15 to 20 percent.[194,195] Comparative studies of a surgical versus a medical strategy for the management of unstable angina were initiated in the 1970s. In one series, the 23-month mortality was 21 percent in medically treated patients and 5.8 percent in surgical patients.[194] Five randomized trials, however, failed to demonstrate a benefit of surgery on survival. Mortality was the same in surgically and medically treated patients in the National Cooperative Study, performed in the 1970s.[101] In the larger and more recent Veterans Administration Cooperative Study involving 468 men, the rates of nonfatal MI at 2 years were 11.7 percent in patients treated surgically and 12.2 percent in patients treated medically ($p =$ NS).[196] Importantly, patients with left main disease and patients with a low ejection fraction were excluded from this study. Furthermore, subset analyses showed a favorable trend for surgery in patients with three-vessel disease and a significant benefit in patients with abnormal left ventricular function. The 5-year survival rates in patients with three-vessel disease were 89 percent with surgical and 75 percent with medical treatment. Prognosis was dependent upon ejection fraction in medically treated patients, but not in surgical patients, suggesting that the bad prognostic impact of impaired left ventricular function was attenuated by surgery (Fig. 46-13). Comparative mortalities were 27 and 14 percent in patients with ejection fractions between 30 and 49 percent ($p =$ .03).[196]

The randomized studies unanimously showed better long-term control of angina with surgical treatment and a high crossover rate of medical patients to surgery: 36 percent in the National Cooperative Study and 43 percent at 5 years in the Veterans Administration Cooperative Study. The latter study also reported a better quality of life in surgical patients.[197] Kaiser et al. reviewed 14 reports published from 1978 to 1988 involving 6136 patients with unstable angina

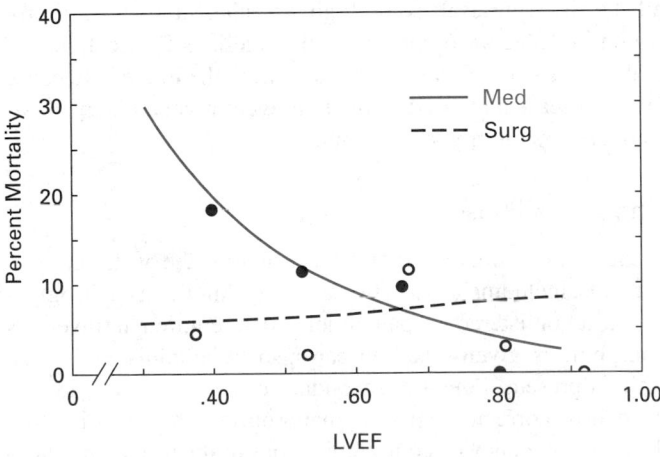

FIGURE 46-13

Results of the Veterans Administration study on the 2-year survival of patients with unstable angina randomized to medical or surgical treatment. No difference in survival rate existed between the two study groups. However, the ejection fraction influenced the results. The survival rate was poor in medically treated patients with a low ejection fraction. In surgically treated patients, survival was good and independent of a lower ejection fraction. (From Luchi et al.[196] Reproduced with permission of the author and the publisher.)

treated by coronary artery bypass grafting.[198] Patients with recent MI and patients operated on electively after stabilization with medical therapy were excluded. Mean operative mortality was 4.1 percent. The mean incidence of perioperative infarction was 9.9 percent, and the mean incidence of postoperative low cardiac output was 16 percent. The risk factors for morbidity and mortality were the same as for patients with stable angina, as were the results for angina relief and the long-term clinical course. After 7 to 10 years, 80 percent of patients were free of angina or had minimal symptoms; the annual rate of nonfatal MI was 3 to 4 percent; the survival rate at 10 years was 80 percent.

These results show that coronary bypass surgery can effectively control unstable angina and improve long-term survival in subsets of patients. It is often the only effective means of controlling symptoms in patients refractory to medical therapy. The perioperative MI rate has been reduced significantly, to 2 to 5 percent with better myocardial protective measures, although it can be as high as 20 percent in higher risk patients with previous bypass surgery, in patients with diabetes mellitus, and in patients with extensive CAD and impaired left ventricular function.[199–200] The shadow cast upon the late results of surgery by the high rate of venous graft occlusions has faded now that much higher late patency rates are achieved with one or more internal mammary artery conduits (see also Chap. 50).

CORONARY ANGIOPLASTY

Coronary angioplasty is an effective revascularization procedure, with long-term benefits comparable to bypass surgery in patients eligible for either intervention. Percutaneous procedures are not applicable to all patients: those with left main disease, left main equivalent, and severe three-vessel disease are generally referred to surgery. In the Bypass Angioplasty Revascularization Investigation (BARI) trial, diabetic patients with multivessel disease had a better 5-year survival when managed with surgery than with angioplasty.[201] A study from Brazil has also suggested that patients with proximal left anterior descending CAD could have better long-term outcome without MI and without the need for additional revascularization procedures when treated with bypass surgery.[202]

The primary success rate of coronary angioplasty in unstable angina is higher than 90 percent and very close to the success rates reported in stable angina. The risk of complications, including MI, emergency surgery, repeat angioplasty, and in-hospital mortality, may be higher, however[203–205]; it approaches 10 percent. The period of increased risk also extends through the follow-up period, when 31 percent of unstable angina patients experience an event at 12 months compared to 16 percent of patients with stable angina. The high complication rate appears partly related to the presence of an intracoronary thrombus[206] and may be higher when the intervention is performed earlier during the acute phase than when it is delayed. In one series, the incidence of Q-wave MI was 6.5 percent, of emergency surgery was 9.4 percent, and of follow-up mortality was 5.8 percent when the procedure was performed within 1 week after the onset of unstable angina, as opposed to 1.6, 4.8, and 1.7 percent, respectively, when delayed for 2 to 4 weeks.[206] Another series reported more major acute complications of angioplasty in unstable angina, 6 percent versus 0.5 percent in stable angina, and more restenosis during follow-up, 61 percent versus 43 percent.[207] In TIMI-IIIB, the procedure performed routinely 18 to 48 h after admission did not carry a higher risk than when performed later because of recurrent ischemia[40]; all patients, however had received a course of medical therapy. TIMI-IIIB was the single largest randomized trial comparing a routine invasive procedure to a routine conservative treatment in unstable angina and non-Q-wave MI. Early invasive management resulted in a higher rate of intervention, as dictated by protocol, but not as high as one could have expected, 61 percent versus 49 percent. The early invasive strategy, however, did not significantly influence the endpoints of death and MI at 6 weeks, 7.2 percent versus 7.8 percent with the conservative strategy ($p = .69$), and at 1 year, 10.8 percent versus 12.2 percent ($p = .42$) (see Fig. 46-5). Rehospitalization, residual ischemia, and the use of antianginal drugs were all more common in the conservative strategy group.

Recent progress in interventional cardiology may make these statistics obsolete. All trials recently performed with the blockers of the membrane receptor glycoprotein IIb/IIIa—abciximab in EPIC,[147] EPILOG,[149] and CAPTURE,[150] integrelin in the Integrelin to Minimize Platelet Aggregation and Prevent Coronary Thrombosis-2 (IMPACT-2) trial,[208] and tirofiban in the Randomized Efficacy Study of Tirofiban for Outcome and Restenosis (RESTORE) trial[209]—have shown a significant reduction reaching 50 percent in the complications associated with angioplasty procedures, including death, MI, and the need for stent implantation or an urgent procedure. Stent implantation, which has become more routinely used since these trials were completed, can also prevent complications of the procedures and effectively correct the acute complications. New trials are therefore warranted to compare more aggressive angioplasty to more aggressive medical management. Clearly, however, recurrence of significant ischemia is an indication for revascularization in unstable angina, to control angina, and possibly also to prevent MI.

Coronary angioplasty is therefore an option to consider in the management of patients with unstable angina when the coronary anatomy is suitable, preferably after initial medical stabilization, or more acutely in patients refractory to pharmacologic treatment. In very unstable patients with multivessel disease, angioplasty of the culprit lesion can be useful as an initial approach.[204] Nonrandomized studies have suggested that 3 to 6 days of heparin pretreatment may reduce the incidence of abrupt vessel closure from 10 percent to 2 percent.[210] Blockage of platelet aggregation with a glycoprotein IIb/IIIa antagonist is also recommended in addition to aspirin therapy. This approach should be preferred to intracoronary injection of fibrinolytic agents when a coronary thrombus is present or develops during the procedure.[146]

MANAGEMENT

Patients with active unstable angina should be hospitalized. Higher risk patients are best treated in a coronary care unit environment, while low-risk patients or patients with a doubtful diagnosis and a normal ECG can be rapidly managed in a chest pain unit or equivalent. Frequent evaluation of the characteristics of chest pain, of the 12-lead ECG, and the use of newer diagnostic techniques such as troponin T or troponin I measurements can lead to earlier and more accurate diagnosis.

Practice guidelines are useful for optimizing the screening of patients with chest pain, to diagnose MI, and to reduce length of hospital stay and hospital costs. Every year, acute MI is ruled out in nearly 2 million patients admitted in emergency rooms of U.S. hospitals.[211] The implementation of practice guidelines and physician education programs have resulted in significantly shorter hospital stays and reduced costs without compromising patient satisfaction and patient outcome after discharge.[212] The differences reported in treatment and outcome of patients treated by internists versus cardiologists favor the latter[213] and should be an incentive for better teaching programs, more standardized care, and periodic evaluation of the quality of care.

Practice guidelines on diagnosis, risk evaluation, and management of unstable angina have been published by a panel of experts convened by the Agency for Health Care Policy and Research and by the National Heart, Lung, and Blood Institute.[214] Patients are first evaluated for *likelihood of coronary disease*, based on previous history, characteristics of pain, and ECG changes, and for *immediate risk of the disease*, based on their history, characteristics of symptoms, momentum of symptoms, the ECG, and their hemodynamic condition. Figure 46-14, adapted from the guidelines, proposes a progression from noninvasive to invasive management on the basis of the risk appraisal; some high-risk characteristics are provided in Table 46-6, and general guidelines for treatment in Table 46-8. The initial measures address the immediate cause of the disease and of ischemia to prevent myocardial necrosis and irreversible myocardial damage.

The Acute Phase

General measures are indicated to assure the well-being of patients, including anxiolytics and stool emollients. Nitroglycerin is administered for pain relief and, if required, intravenous morphine is given. Oxygen can also be administered when pain is present. Potential secondary causes of angina are excluded or corrected, such as inappropriate tachycardia. Any bleeding tendency or contraindications to the use of antiplatelet drugs, anticoagulants, or fibrinolytic agents are assessed. Although attentive to patient need and comfort, the medical environment should not create an undue climate of fear or dependency.

A specific antithrombotic treatment is started at admission. Aspirin is administered to all patients with unstable angina

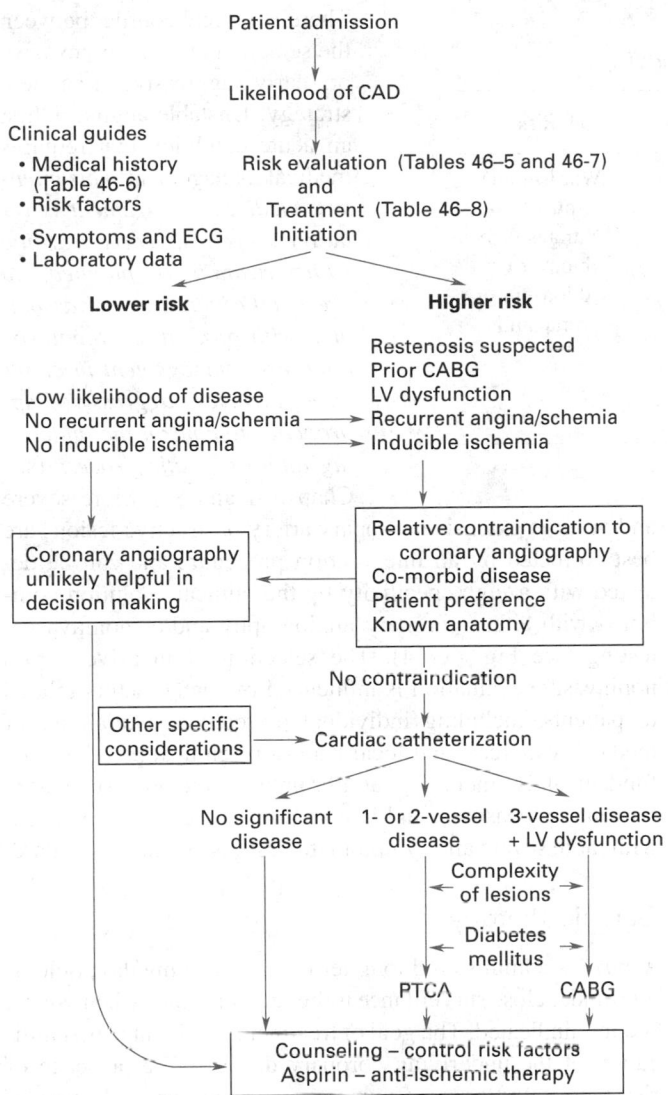

Patient admission

↓

Likelihood of CAD

↓

Risk evaluation (Tables 46–5 and 46–7)
and
Treatment (Table 46–8)
Initiation

Clinical guides
• Medical history
  (Table 46-6)
• Risk factors
• Symptoms and ECG
• Laboratory data

Lower risk   **Higher risk**

Restenosis suspected
Prior CABG
Low likelihood of disease   LV dysfunction
No recurrent angina/schemia → Recurrent angina/schemia
No inducible ischemia   → Inducible ischemia

Relative contraindication to
coronary angiography
Co-morbid disease
Patient preference
Known anatomy

Coronary angiography
unlikely helpful in
decision making

No contraindication

Other specific
considerations → Cardiac catheterization

No significant   1- or 2-vessel   3-vessel disease
disease   disease   + LV dysfunction
                                    Complexity
                                    of lesions
                                    Diabetes
                                    mellitus
                   PTCA   CABG

Counseling – control risk factors
Aspirin – anti-Ischemic therapy

FIGURE 46-14

Diagnosis, risk evaluation, and management of unstable angina based on the guidelines published by the U.S. Department of Health and Human Services, Public Health Service and Agency for Health Care Policy and Research (Clinical Practice Guideline, Number 10, AHCPR Publication No. 94-0602, Washington, DC, 1994). The clinical history and the ECG help establish the likelihood of disease, evaluate risk, and institute investigation and treatment appropriate to the individual patient. Progression from less to more invasive treatment is schematized. This global approach may result in optimal cost/ effectiveness and risk/benefit ratios in medical care.

and whenever a doubt exists on diagnosis. The initial loading dose of aspirin should be between 160 and 325 mg to achieve rapidly complete inhibition of thromboxane generation by platelets. Subsequent doses could be lower; 75 to 160 mg daily have been as effective as higher doses and associated with fewer side effects. Heparin is also indicated in all patients with any one of the high-risk features (Table 46-6); a bolus dose of 5000 units is first given, followed by an intravenous infusion titrated to an aPTT of 1.5 to 2.5 times normal. Ticlopidine, 250 mg twice per day, should be administered to patients who cannot tolerate aspirin. The delayed onset of action of

ticlopidine mandates the concomitant administration of heparin. Heparin alone, without aspirin, can be used in patients scheduled for early bypass surgery, to minimize subsequent blood loss. *In any case, antiplatelet therapy should be started before the discontinuation of heparin to prevent coronary events due to reactivation of the disease.* Antianginal therapy is also recommended, including intravenous nitroglycerin for initial treatment. Beta blockers are also indicated for angina control and, when prolonged pain is present, for their protective effect on ischemic myocardium. The dose is adjusted to maintain basal heart rate in the range of 50 to 60 beats per minute. Diltiazem or verapamil are good alternative choices if beta blockers are contraindicated; dihydropyridines alone are a poor choice. Triple therapy with nitroglycerin, a beta blocker, and a calcium antagonist is recommended in patients with recurrent angina. The decision to employ early conservative or early invasive therapy should be made rapidly so as not to prolong hospital stay.

Subsequent management is adjusted to the early clinical evolution and to the results of the clinical investigations. Recurrent ischemia, and especially during treatment and accompanied by ECG changes (see Table 46-6), is an indicator of ongoing active disease and of the need for more intensive medical treatment and of coronary angiography with a view to coronary revascularization, which mandates aggressive adjunctive therapy. These maneuvers in the more unstable patients may be performed under the protection of intraaortic balloon counterpulsation. Prompt fibrinolytic therapy is indicated if an acute MI with ST-segment elevation complicates the clinical course. Patients stable on medical therapy after 24 to 48 h are rapidly mobilized while treatment is adjusted from more acute to more long term. The duration of the acute phase of unstable angina is largely unknown. Clinical experience suggests that it may extend to 48 to 72 h past the last episode of pain, which probably reflects the time required for a plaque rupture to begin to heal. More recent data suggest that the underlying process may persist for weeks and months with a potential for reactivation.

The Subacute Phase

Potential residual latent ischemia or the severity of the underlying coronary lesions is evaluated at this stage using coronary angiography or some form of noninvasive test. Exercise testing or pharmacologic provocation with dipyridamole, thallium, or sestamibi scintigraphy (Chap. 17) or stress echocardiography (Chap. 14) are valid for risk stratification and permit the identification of patients with more severe obstructive lesions. Figure 49-14 identifies some of the many factors influencing the decision tree. Intravenous nitroglycerin is replaced by oral or transdermal treatment after 24 to 48 h, and heparin is discontinued when the patient is stable after 48 h on medical therapy or after an intervention procedure. *It is recommended to continue beta blockers for many months.* The patient is educated about the causes of the disease and on its modifiable clinical course before leaving the hospital;

TABLE 46-8

ACUTE MANAGEMENT OF UNSTABLE ANGINA

	High/Intermediate Risk	Low Risk
Treatment setting	Coronary care unit	Wards/home
Antithrombotic therapy	Aspirin + heparin	Aspirin
Anti-ischemic therapy	IV nitroglycerin + beta blocker and/or diltiazem or verapamil	Nitrates or beta blocker or diltiazem or verapamil
If persisting pain	Beta blockers + calcium antagonist Consider intraaortic counterpulsation Cardiac catheterization	

he or she is rapidly reintegrated to normal life, whenever possible. Counseling applies to all patients, whether an invasive intervention is performed or not. Unstable angina is associated in the following months with a high risk of recurrence and a high risk of rapid progression of CAD. Patients who have had a dilatation procedure performed are also at some risk of restenosis.

Early Invasive versus Early Conservative Strategies

Guidelines for management and for the respective merits of an early aggressive versus more conservative approach are provided by the TIMI-IIIB study. The 1473 patients enrolled received full medical therapy and were randomized to an early aggressive versus an early conservative treatment strategy.[40] The study was large enough to detect a 30 percent difference between the strategies. Coronary angiography was performed 18 to 48 h after randomization in the early invasive group, with angioplasty of culprit lesions with a suitable anatomy or bypass surgery if the patients were appropriate candidates. In the early conservative group, angiography was performed only when medical therapy failed, defined as one or more episodes of ischemic pain with ischemic ST-segment elevation or depression, ≥20 min duration of ST-segment shift on a 24-h ambulatory ECG recording, two or more perfusion defects on a thallium exercise scintigram, rest angina requiring readmission to hospital during the first 6 weeks, or Canadian Cardiovascular Society class III or IV angina with a positive exercise test. Coronary angiography had been performed at 6 weeks in 98 percent of patients in the early invasive arm and at 1 year in 99 percent, as compared with 64 and 73 percent, respectively, in the early conservative arm. Early revascularization did not significantly influence the endpoint of death and MI at 42 days, 7.2 versus 7.8 percent ($p = .69$), or at 12 months, 10.8 versus 12.2 percent ($p = .42$), as seen in Fig. 46-5. Repeat hospital admission, however, was less frequent with the early invasive strategy, 8 versus 14 percent at 6 weeks ($p < .001$) and 26 versus 33 percent at 1 year ($p < .005$). After 1 year, the use of antianginal therapy and the angina functional class were similar in the two strategies.

There is no real conflict between the selection of an early invasive or early aggressive treatment strategy. Unstable angina is first an acute condition that requires medical management. *This intensive medical management is required, even if early cardiac catheterization is planned, to prevent the increased risk associated with procedures. Similarly, long-term management in either case involves aggressive approaches to control the underlying atherosclerotic process* (see Chaps. 41 and 53). More severe and/or more extensive coronary artery obstructive lesions are best corrected by an intervention procedure and can be detected with a high specificity by the clinical evolution combined with either coronary angiography and/or noninvasive testing (see Fig. 46-14). The selection of invasive versus noninvasive evaluation is influenced by many factors related to patients, including individual preference, availability of medical resources, and local pattern of clinical practice. The fundamentals, including antithrombotic therapy, secondary preventive measures, and intervention procedures in patients with more severe and symptomatic lesions, are more standard.

Chronic Therapy

Aspirin is administered long term, 60 to 180 mg/day; ticlopidine under close surveillance is the second choice when aspirin is contraindicated. The goal of treatment at this stage is stabilization of the underlying coronary disease. The presence of risk factors and/or more numerous coronary artery lesions of any severity are associated with higher risk of progression and dictate a vigorous program for control of risk factors. This program includes control of blood cholesterol with prompt use of *lipid-lowering drugs*, particularly HMG CoA reductase inhibitors for their potential ability to alter plaque content and prevent plaque activation. *Beta-blocker therapy* helps to reduce the hemodynamic stress imposed on a fragile lesion, is antiarrhythmic, and is anti-ischemic. Smoking cessation and control of other risk factors have a major impact on the patient's long-term outcome. The clinical condition of the patient is reassessed after a few weeks to adjust therapy.

VARIANT ANGINA

In 1959, Prinzmetal et al.[215] described a syndrome characterized by angina at rest associated with transient ST-segment elevation. In most cases, exercise tolerance was well preserved and the attacks were cyclical in nature, often occurring in the early morning hours. The attacks did not last longer than ordinary anginal episodes, and the ST-segment elevation rapidly normalized as the chest pain receded. Ventricular arrhythmias and atrioventricular block sometimes occurred at the height of an attack, and both MI and sudden death were common complications.

With the advent of coronary arteriography, it soon became apparent that the syndrome was caused by transient coronary artery spasm, usually focal, and often at the site of coronary stenosis.[216] The underlying coronary disease can vary from a subtotal occlusion to a very mild stenosis, however, and in some cases, the coronary arteries are angiographically normal. Coronary spasm occurs in more than one artery in some patients,[217] and the site of spasm can sometimes fluctuate from one vessel to another.[218] Coronary artery spasm has been demonstrated to be the cause of MI in some patients who have only ST depression or pseudonormalization of abnormal T waves during episodes of angina.[219]

Pathophysiology

A central neural mechanism is unlikely to be involved since coronary spasm can occur in the denervated transplanted heart.[220] The frequency of attacks of variant angina is not reduced by alpha-adrenergic blockade,[221] blockade of serotonin receptors,[222] inhibition of thromboxane A_2 production,[223] or administration of prostacyclin.[224] Variant angina patients have been reported to have a higher prevalence of magnesium deficiency, as revealed by the magnesium loading test,[225] and hyperinsulinemia.[226]

Coronary spasm is usually localized to the site of an atherosclerotic lesion. *Even variant angina patients with normal-appearing arteries at angiography will invariably have atherosclerosis, demonstrable by intracoronary ultrasound, at the site of focal spasm.*[227] The response of other coronary segments to vasoconstrictive stimuli is normal, indicating that a generalized abnormality of coronary reactivity is not present.[228]

Normal endothelium modulates coronary tone by releasing EDRFs, the predominant one of which is nitric oxide (NO); this function is diminished at sites of early atherosclerosis and is impaired by hypercholesterolemia.[42] The EDRFs inhibit platelet aggregation; aggregating platelets release vasoconstricting substances that can act unopposed in the absence of EDRFs. Acetylcholine dilates arterial segments with normal endothelium by stimulating EDRF release but constricts segments with dysfunctional endothelium.[42] It is likely that loss of endothelial vasodilator function contributes to constriction in variant angina. Increased smooth muscle contractility also probably plays an important role (see also Chaps. 4, 43, and 44).

The pathophysiologic consequences of coronary spasm are well understood. Severe spasm rapidly induces transmural ischemia, resulting in regional dyskinesia and ST-segment elevation. If the ischemic zone is large, cardiac output and systemic arterial pressure will decrease. The risk of serious ventricular arrhythmias increases with the severity and extent of ischemia. Formation of a mural thrombus due to spasm

can generate local thrombotic activity that can be detected as increased circulating fibrinopeptide A levels.[229]

Clinical Features

Variant angina is uncommon, and the presenting symptoms are usually not remarkable enough to be distinguished immediately from unstable angina. Angina at rest occurs with a cyclical pattern and often with attacks occurring in the early morning hours. Exertional angina coexists in slightly more than half of the patients, but the ischemic threshold is extremely variable.[230] Variant angina can occur during the recovery phase of MI[231] or in patients who have had coronary bypass surgery[232] or recent angioplasty.[233]

Most patients with variant angina are heavy cigarette smokers, but their age, gender, and risk factor profiles are otherwise similar to other coronary patients.[234] Those with angiographically normal coronary arteries tend to be younger and more often women and often do not have more risk factors than noncoronary controls.[235] *One-quarter of variant angina patients have a history of migraine headaches, and one-quarter have symptoms of Raynaud's phenomenon.*[236] *Thus, variant angina in some cases may be part of a more generalized vasospastic diathesis.* Syncope, presumably due to ischemia-induced ventricular arrhythmia or to atrioventricular block, during rest angina is a useful diagnostic clue.

Cocaine causes coronary vasoconstriction[237] and can precipitate coronary spasm, sometimes with MI.[238] Neither coronary spasm nor myocardial infarction, however, can be documented in most patients presenting with chest pain after cocaine use.[238]

Physical examination of variant angina patients between attacks reveals no abnormalities. Routine laboratory tests, including cardiac enzymes, are likewise normal.

Variant angina can be most easily diagnosed by recording an ECG during an episode of rest angina. The ST-segment elevation that occurs during an attack will disappear promptly with the administration of nitroglycerin. As illustrated in Fig. 46-15, coronary spasm can induce ST elevation, ST depression, or pseudonormalization of abnormally negative T waves. Atrioventricular block may develop when the site of ST elevation is the inferior leads; ventricular arrhythmias, including ventricular fibrillation, can occur with ST elevation in any territory. The risk of these arrhythmias and conduction disturbances increases with the degree of ST-segment elevation.[236]

Diagnostic Procedures

The most important diagnostic procedure to obtain during an episode of pain at rest is a 12-lead ECG. When variant angina is suspected, ambulatory ECG monitoring can be useful to confirm the diagnosis. Exercise testing will provoke angina with ST elevation in approximately one-third of variant angina patients during an active phase of their disease.[239] The cold pressor test induces a variant angina attack in only 10 percent of patients.[239] Several different pharmacologic agents have been used to induce episodes of variant angina. Histamine[240]

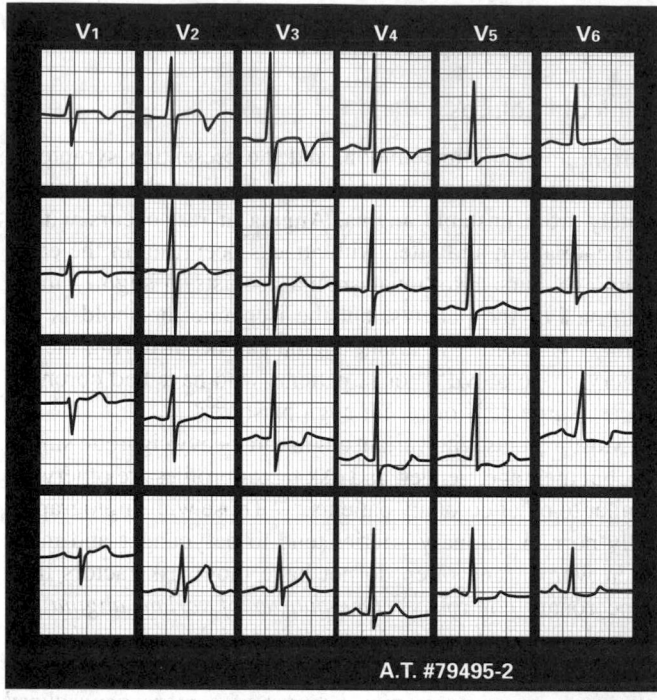

FIGURE 46-15
Electrocardiograms (leads V_1 to V_6) from a patient with active variant angina. Negative T waves are present in the control tracing (*top*). The other three tracings were recorded during separate episodes of rest angina and show (respectively) pseudonormalization of T waves, ST depression, and ST elevation.

and dopamine[241] provoke attacks in only one-quarter to one-half of variant angina patients. Intracoronary acetylcholine has a much higher sensitivity, 90 percent in one large series,[242] but should not be used without a temporary pacemaker if the right coronary (or dominant left coronary) artery is to be injected because of the high incidence of bradyarrhythmias and conduction disturbances from cholinergic effects in the atrioventricular node.

Ergonovine, an ergot alkaloid that constricts vascular smooth muscle by stimulating both alpha-adrenergic and serotoninergic receptors, is the agent most commonly used. When administered intravenously to patients with active variant angina at the time of coronary arteriography, more than 90 percent of patients will develop severe, focal coronary spasm.[243] Spontaneous and ergonovine-induced episodes of variant angina are very much similar. Examples of spontaneous and ergonovine-induced coronary spasm are illustrated in Fig. 46-16. Ergonovine causes physiologic coronary vasoconstriction and increases peripheral vascular resistance; these changes can induce myocardial ischemia with ST-segment depression if the underlying coronary stenoses are severe.[244] In a study in which ergonovine was administered to more than 1000 patients with various types of cardiac disease, coronary spasm was provoked in 38 percent of those with angina at rest, 14 percent of those with rest and effort angina, 4 percent of those with effort angina only, 20 percent of recent infarct

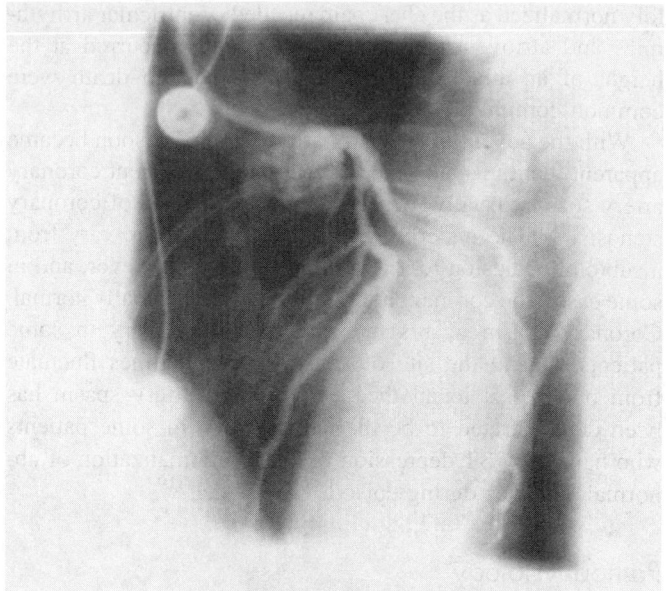

A

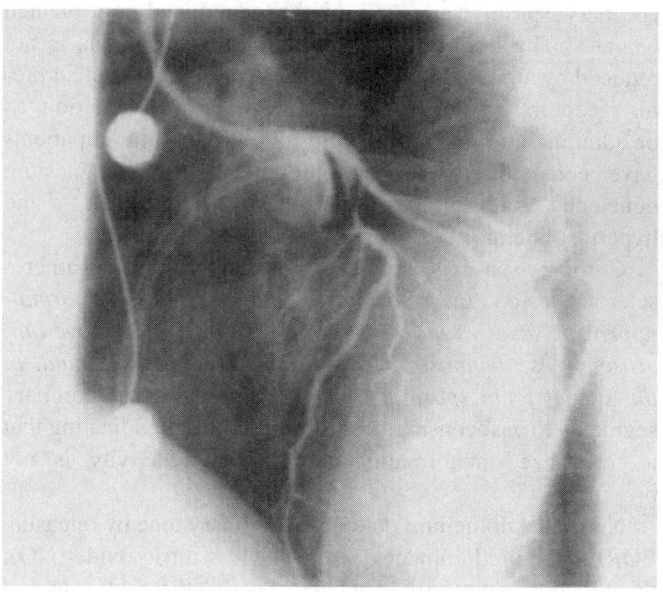

B

FIGURE 46-16
A. Left coronary arteriogram (45° LAD with 25° craniocaudal angulation) of a 47-year-old man with active variant angina. A 40 percent proximal LAD stenosis is present. The coronary arteries are otherwise normal angiographically. *B.* The control angina and ST elevation developed spontaneously during coronary arteriography. Repeat injections reveal severe focal spasm at the site of the lesion. The coronary spasm resolved immediately after nitroglycerin administration.

patients, 1 percent of those with atypical chest pain, and almost no patients without coronary disease.[245] A negative ergonovine test in the absence of coronary vasodilators in a patient with recent chest pain provides compelling evidence against coronary spasm as the cause.

Ergonovine testing has occasionally caused refractory coronary spasm resulting in death[246] and can induce multivessel

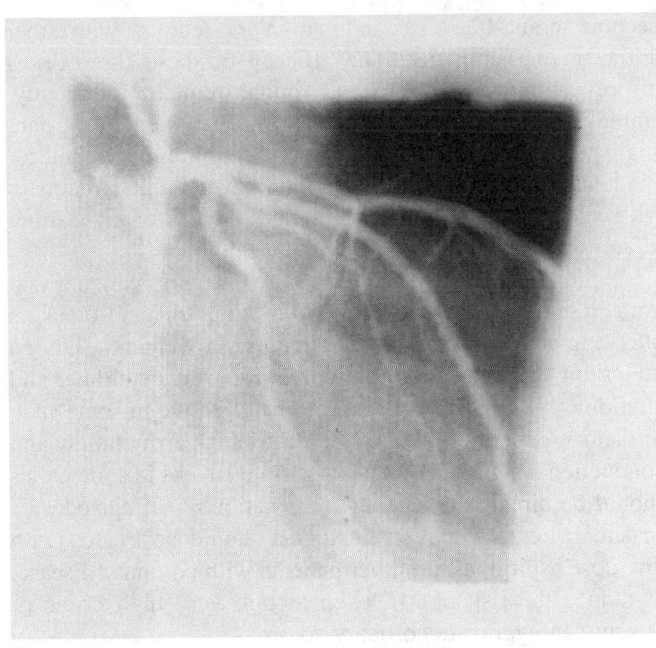

C

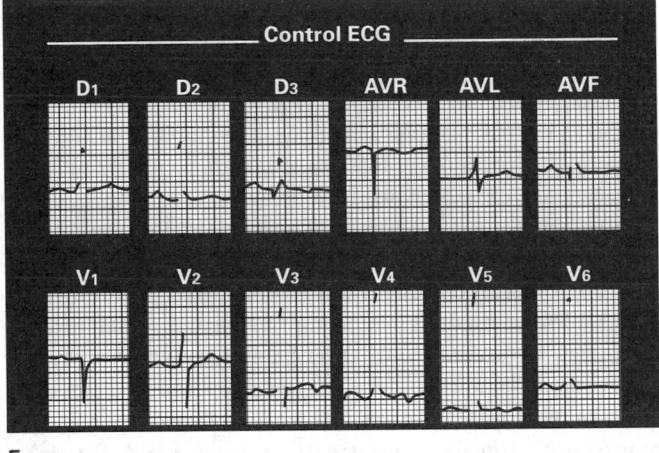

E

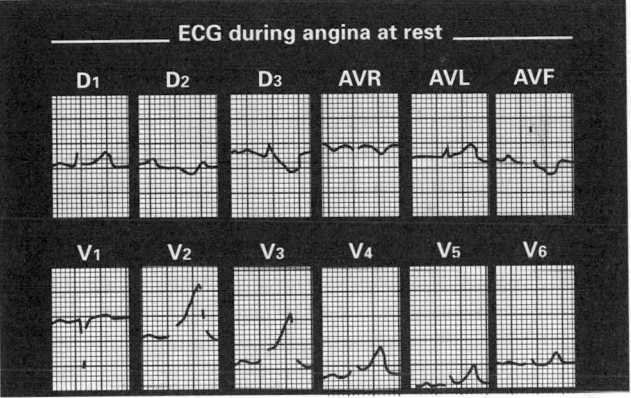

F

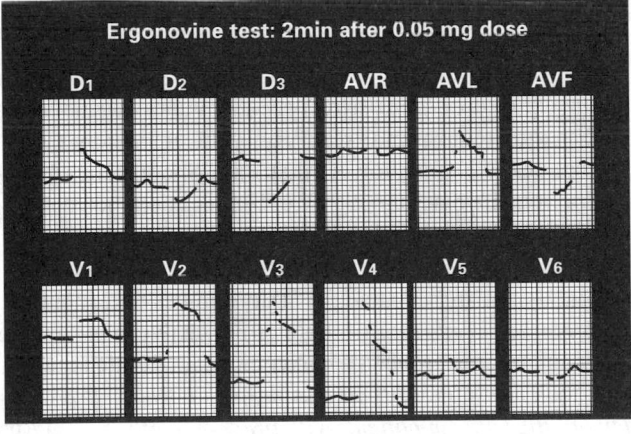

G

FIGURE 46-16 (continued)

C. Left coronary arteriogram in the RAO view after ergonovine administration. Severe coronary spasm is present both at the site of the LAD stenosis and distal to it. D. Resolution of ergonovine-induced spasm following nitroglycerin administration. E. Control electrocardiogram showing negative T waves in leads V_3 to V_6 with no other abnormalities. F. Electrocardiogram during a spontaneous attack of rest angina showing ST elevation in V_2 to V_5. These abnormalities disappeared 2 min after administration of sublingual nitroglycerin. G. Electrocardiogram following ergonovine administration. The ST segment is elevated in leads 1, AVL, and V_1 to V_5 with reciprocal ST depression in leads 2, 3, and AVF. Nitroglycerin rapidly reversed these abnormalities to normal. Ergonovine testing is unnecessary in patients with documented spontaneous attacks. (From Waters DD, Théroux P. The role of coronary artery spasm in Prinzmetal's angina. In: Chahine RA, ed. *Coronary Artery Spasm*, vol 6. Mount Kisco, NY: Futura; 1983:119–140. Reproduced with permission of the authors and the publisher.)

coronary spasm.[247] Selective intracoronary administration eliminates this risk and the systemic effects of the agents. The test should be stopped if significant vasoconstriction is observed on the angiogram, without waiting for development of chest pain or ST-segment changes. The cumulative intracoronary dose of ergonovine is 50 μg, compared to the cumulative intraarterial or intravenous dose of 0.3 to 1 mg.[217]

Contraindications to ergonovine testing include severe coronary disease, uncontrolled hypertension, pregnancy, severe left ventricular dysfunction, and recent stroke. A few investigators perform ergonovine testing outside the catheterization laboratory in patients with known coronary anatomy.[247,248] Under these conditions, the test can be used to assess the effect of therapy[249] or to detect the occurrence of spontaneous remission.[250] *The use of provocative testing outside the catheterization laboratory is controversial; most experts recommend that the test be performed only at the time of coronary arteriography so that nitroglycerin can be given by the intracoronary route if necessary. The test should never be performed on patients with unknown coronary anatomy.*

All patients with variant angina should undergo coronary arteriography unless an absolute contraindication is present. A provocative testing is performed most commonly when coronary arteriography reveals no organic stenoses severe enough to account for the patient's symptoms. Under these circumstances, positive responses are infrequent, particularly when symptoms are atypical. Provocative testing is often useful in patients with predominantly rest angina and a focal, proximal coronary stenosis because the response can influence the choice of therapy. For example, if spasm is not present, angioplasty might be the preferred therapy, whereas medical treatment might be a better choice if spasm is documented to be the cause of symptoms.

Treatment

Variant angina is difficult to treat because attacks occur unpredictably and frequently at rest. The goal of therapy should therefore be the elimination of all attacks. Spontaneous remission is a frequent outcome,[251,252] but MI is a common complication within the first 3 months after diagnosis, particularly in patients with underlying multivessel disease.[253] Nitroglycerin relieves variant angina attacks within minutes and should be used promptly. Long-acting nitrates are effective in preventing variant angina attacks, but the development of nitrate tolerance limits their usefulness. *Beta-adrenergic blocking drugs are often of little value in patients with predominantly vasospastic angina and may actually increase the duration of attacks.*[184,254]

The calcium channel blockers nifedipine,[255] diltiazem,[256] and verapamil[257] are very effective in preventing attacks of variant angina. More than half of the patients treated with one of these drugs become completely asymptomatic. The response is better at high doses; for example, nifedipine, 80 mg/day, diltiazem, 360 mg/day, or verapamil, 480 mg/day. Patients with an incomplete response to one drug often become angina-free on a combination of nifedipine with either diltiazem or verapamil. The efficacy of these three drugs in preventing variant angina is roughly equal.[249] Recently, amlodipine has been approved for the treatment of variant angina, but experience with it for this condition is limited.[258] Evidence from uncontrolled studies[259] suggests that treatment with calcium channel blockers reduces the risk of myocardial infarction (see also Chap. 54).

Approximately 20 percent of variant angina patients will not respond to treatment with two calcium channel blockers plus long-acting nitrates. Although not approved in the United States for this indication, amiodarone,[260] guanethidine, and clonidine[261] have been reported to be effective in some such refractory patients. Therapy for ventricular arrhythmias and conduction disturbances that complicate attacks in some cases should be directed toward the elimination of all episodes of spasm. Patients with variant angina should be treated with low-dose aspirin, as are other patients with coronary disease, to reduce the risk of MI, even though very high doses of aspirin can aggravate coronary spasm.[262]

Coronary bypass surgery should be considered in most patients with variant angina and significant multivessel atherosclerotic disease. Operative mortality and the perioperative infarction rate, however, are higher than for comparable patients without variant angina.[263,264] For example, in the Duke series three deaths and three nonfatal infarctions occurred perioperatively in 48 surgically treated patients.[263] Surgery almost invariably eliminates variant angina, and long-term outcome is excellent. Only one MI and no deaths were observed over 5 years of follow-up.

Bypass surgery will be successful when the anastomosis can be situated distal to the site of focal spasm but not when diffuse spasm involves the entire artery. Cardiac denervation by plexectomy in association with bypass surgery has yielded excellent results,[265] but this procedure has not been evaluated in a controlled study. The occurrence of spasm after cardiac transplantation or autotransplantation[266] argues against a beneficial effect from denervation. *Bypass surgery is not indicated for variant angina in the absence of significant organic stenoses.*

Many patients with variant angina have coronary lesions that are ideal for angioplasty. When such patients are pretreated with calcium channel blockers and given intravenous or intracoronary nitroglycerin during the procedure, the primary success rate is high.[233,267,268] Coronary spasm may persist or recur after successful angioplasty, however, and calcium channel blockers should therefore be continued. The restenosis rate is significantly higher than usual in patients with variant angina.[233,269] Coronary angioplasty is not indicated for patients with coronary spasm who have normal or nearly normal arteries on coronary arteriography.

Prognosis

The long-term prognosis of variant angina has been reported for several large series of patients from different coun-

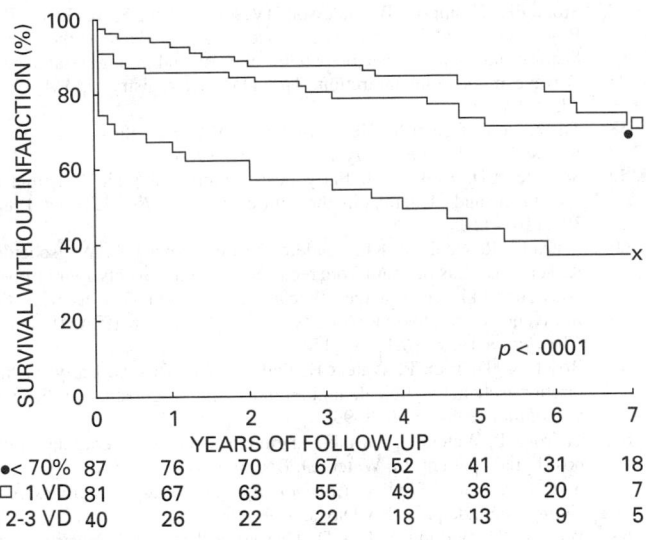

	0	1	2	3	4	5	6	7
● < 70%	87	76	70	67	52	41	31	18
□ 1 VD	81	67	63	55	49	36	20	7
× 2-3 VD	40	26	22	22	18	13	9	5

FIGURE 46-17

Survival without myocardial infarction in variant angina patients with no stenoses of 70 percent or more (●), those with one vessel disease (□), and those with multivessel disease (×). The outcome in the latter group of patients is much worse than in the other two groups. Events are clustered early in the follow-up period. (From Walling et al.[253] Reproduced with permission of the author and the American Heart Association.)

tries.[253,263,270–272] The extent and severity of the underlying coronary disease appear to be the most important factors influencing outcome. As illustrated in Fig. 46-17, survival without MI at 1 year in 217 consecutive patients was 93 percent for those without stenoses of 70 percent or more, 86 percent for patients with one-vessel disease, and 65 percent for those with multivessel disease.[248] At 5 years, the corresponding figures were 83, 74, and 44 percent, respectively. Other variables that correlate with a poor outcome include the presence of abnormal left ventricular function, ventricular arrhythmias during attacks, multivessel spasm, and the absence of treatment with calcium channel blockers. Patients who become angina-free may later experience recurrence of variant angina or may develop other manifestations of CAD.

REFERENCES

1. Osler W. The Lumleian lectures on angina pectoris. *Lancet* 1910; 1:697–701.
2. Sampson JJ, Eliaser M Jr. The diagnosis of impending acute coronary artery occlusion. *Am Heart J* 1937; 13:675–686.
3. Feil H. Preliminary pain in coronary thrombosis. *Am J Med Sci* 1937; 193:42–48.
4. Levy H. The natural history of changing pattern of angina pectoris. *Ann Intern Med* 1956; 44:1123–1135.
5. Vakil RJ. Intermediate coronary syndrome. *Circulation* 1961; 24:557–571.
6. Beamish RE, Storrie VM. Impending myocardial infarction. Recognition and management. *Circulation* 1960; 21:1107–1115.
7. Fowler NO. "Preinfarctional" angina: A need for an objective definition and for a controlled clinical trial of its management. *Circulation* 1971; 44:755–758.
8. Wood P. Acute and subacute coronary insufficiency. *Br Med J* 1961; 1:1779–1782.
9. Krauss KR, Hutter AM, De Sanctis RW. Acute coronary insufficiency course and follow-up. *Circulation* 1972; 45(suppl I):I66–I71.
10. Gazes PC, Mobly FM, Faris HM, Duncan RC, Humphries GB. Preinfarctional (unstable angina)—a prospective study—10 year follow-up. Prognostic significance of electrocardiographic changes. *Circulation* 1973; 48:331–337.
11. Maseri A, L'Abbate A, Baroldi G, Chierchia S, Marzilli M, Ballestra AM, et al. Coronary vasospasm as a possible cause of myocardial infarction: Conclusion derived from the study of "pre infarction angina." *N Engl J Med* 1978; 299:1271–1277.
12. Falk E. Plaque rupture with severe pre-existing stenosis precipitating coronary thrombosis: Characteristics of coronary atherosclerotic plaques underlying fatal occlusive thrombi. *Br Heart J* 1983; 50:127–134.
13. Davies MJ, Thomas AC. Plaque fissuring—The cause of acute myocardial infarction, sudden ischemic death, and crescendo angina. *Br Heart J* 1985; 53:363–373.
14. Willerson JT, Golino P, Eidt J, Campbell WB, Buja M. Specific platelet mediators and unstable coronary artery lesions. Experimental evidence and potential clinical implications. *Circulation* 1989; 80:198–205.
15. De Wood MA, Spores J, Notske R, Mouser LT, Burroughs R, Golden MS, et al. Prevalence of total coronary occlusion during the early hours of transmural myocardial infarction. *N Engl J Med* 1980; 303:897–902.
16. The TIMI IIIA Investigators. Early effects of tissue-type plasminogen activator added to conventional therapy on the culprit coronary lesion in patients presenting with ischemic cardiac pain at rest. Results of the Thrombolysis in Myocardial Ischemia (TIMI IIIA) Trial. *Circulation* 1993; 87:38–52.
17. Ambrose JA, Winters SL, Stern A, Eng A, Teichholtz LE, Gorlin R, et al. Angiographic morphology and the pathogenesis of unstable angina pectoris. *J Am Coll Cardiol* 1985; 5:609–616.
18. Taeymans Y, Théroux P, Lesperance J, Waters DD. Quantitative angiographic morphology of the coronary artery lesions at risk of thrombotic occlusion. *Circulation* 1992; 85:78–85.
19. Moise A, Lesperance J, Théroux P, Taeymans Y, Goulet C, Bourassa MG. Clinical and angiographic predictors of new total coronary occlusion in coronary artery disease: Analysis of 313 non-operated patients. *Am J Cardiol* 1984; 54:1176–1181.
20. Moise A, Théroux P, Taeymans Y, Descoings B, Lesperance J, Waters DD, et al. Unstable angina and progression of coronary atherosclerosis. *N Engl J Med* 1983; 309:685–689.
21. Ambrose JA, Winters SL, Arora RR, Eng A, Riccio A, Gorlin R, et al. Angiographic evolution of coronary artery morphology in unstable angina. *J Am Coll Cardiol* 1986; 7:472–478.
22. Richardson PD, Davies MJ, Born GVR. Influence of plaque configuration and stress distribution on fissuring of coronary atherosclerotic plaques. *Lancet* 1989; 2:941–944.
23. Falk E. Unstable angina with fatal outcome: Dynamic coronary thrombosis leading to infarction and/or sudden death. Autopsy evidence of recurrent mural thrombosis with peripheral embolization culminating in total vascular occlusion. *Circulation* 1985; 50:127–134.
24. Davies MJ, Woolf N, Rowles PM, Peper J. Morphology of the endothelium over atherosclerotic plaques in human coronary arteries. *Br Heart J* 1988; 60:459–464.
25. Badimon L, Badimon JJ, Turrito VT, Vallabhajosula S, Fuster V. Platelet thrombus formation on collagen type I: A model of deep vessel injury: Influence of blood rheology, von Willebrand factor and blood coagulation. *Circulation* 1988; 78:1431–1442.
26. Francis CW, Markham RE Jr, Barlow GH, Florack TM, Dobrzynski DM, Marder VJ. Thrombin activity of fibrin thrombi and soluble plasma derivatives. *J Lab Clin Med* 1983; 102:220–230.
27. Fuster V, Badimon L, Badimon JJ, Chesebro JH. Mechanisms of disease: The pathogenesis of coronary artery disease and the acute coronary syndromes. *N Engl J Med* 1992; 326:310–318.
28. Lam JYT, Chesebro JH, Steele PM, Badimon L, Fuster V. Is vasospasm related to platelet deposition? Relationship in a porcine preparation of arterial injury in vivo. *Circulation* 1987; 75:243–248.
29. Bogaty P, Hackett D, Davies G, Maseri A. Vasoreactivity of the culprit lesion in unstable angina. *Circulation* 1994; 90:5–11.
30. Falk E, Shah P, Fuster V. Coronary plaque disruption. *Circulation* 1995; 92:657–671.
31. Ross R. The pathogenesis of atherosclerosis: A perspective for the 1990s. *Nature* 1993; 362:801–809.
32. Sato T, Takebayashi S, Kohci K. Increased subendothelial infiltration of the coronary arteries with monocytes/macrophages in patients with unstable angina. *Atherosclerosis* 1987; 68:191–197.

33. Moreno PR, Falk E, Palacios IF, Newell JB, Fuster V, Fallon JT. Macrophage infiltration in acute coronary syndromes: Implications for plaque rupture. *Circulation* 1994; 90:775–778.

34. Kovanen PT, Kaartinen M, Paavonen T. Infiltrates of activated mast cells at the site of coronary atheromatous erosion or rupture in myocardial infarction. *Circulation* 1995; 92:1084–1088.

35. Bevilacqua MP. Endothelial-leukocyte adhesion molecules. *Ann Rev Immunol* 1993; 11:767–804.

36. National Center for Health Statistics. Vital and health statistics: Detailed diagnosis and procedures for patients discharged from short stay hospitals. Hyattsville, MD, U.S. Department of Health and Human Services, Public Health Service, Series 13, No. 90, 1987.

37. Bertolasi CA, Tronge JE, Riccitelli MA, Villamayor RM, Zuffardi E. Natural history of unstable angina with medical or surgical treatment. *Chest* 1976; 70:596–605.

38. Plotnic GD, Conti DR. Unstable angina: Angiography, short and long term morbidity, mortality, and symptomatic status of medically treated patients. *Am J Med* 1977; 63:870–873.

39. Mulcahy R, Daly L, Graham L, Hickey N, O'Donoghue S, Owens A, et al. Unstable angina: Natural history and determinants of prognosis. *Am J Cardiol* 1981; 48:525–528.

40. The TIMI IIIB Investigators. Effects of tissue plasminogen activator and a comparison of early invasive and early conservative strategies in unstable angina and non-Q-wave myocardial infarction: Results of the TIMI IIIB trial. *Circulation* 1994; 89:1545–1556.

41. Anderson HV, Cannon CP, Stone PH, Williams DO, McCabe CH, Knatterud GL, et al. One-year results of the Thrombolysis in Myocardial Infarction (TIMI) IIIB trial. *J Am Coll Cardiol* 1995; 26:1643–1650.

42. Vanhoutte PM, Shimokawa H. Endothelium-derived relaxing factor and coronary vasospasm. *Circulation* 1989; 80:1–9.

43. Lerman A, Edward BS, Hallett JW, Heublein DM, Sandberg SM, Burnett CJ Jr. Circulating and tissue endothelin immunoreactivity in advanced atherosclerosis. *N Engl J Med* 1991; 325:997–1001.

44. Brown BG, Lee AB, Bolson EL, Dodge HT. Reflex vasoconstriction of significant coronary artery stenosis as a mechanism contributing to ischemic left ventricular dysfunction during isometric exercise. *Circulation* 1984; 70:18–24.

45. Winniford MD, Wheelan KR, Kremers MS, Ugolini V, van den Berg E, Niggemann EH, et al. Smoking-induced coronary vasoconstriction in patients with atherosclerotic coronary artery disease: Evidence for adrenergically mediated alterations in coronary artery tone. *Circulation* 1986; 73:662–667.

46. Mudge GH, Grossman W, Mills RM, Braunwald E. Reflex increase in coronary vascular resistance in patients with ischemic heart disease. *N Engl J Med* 1976; 295:1333–1337.

47. Isner JM, Estes NAM III, Thompson PD, Costanzo-Nordin MR, Subramanian R, Miller G, et al. Acute cardiac events temporally related to cocaine abuse. *N Engl J Med* 1986; 315:1438–1443.

48. Hadjimihiades S, Covalesky V, Manno OV, Haaz WS, Mintz GS. Coronary arteriographic findings in cocaine abuse–induced myocardial infarction. *Cathet Cardiovasc Diagn* 1988; 14:33–36.

49. Flores ED, Lange RA, Cigarroa RG, Hillis LD. Effect of cocaine on coronary artery dimensions in atherosclerotic coronary artery disease: Enhanced vasoconstriction at sites of significant stenoses. *J Am Coll Cardiol* 1990; 16:74–79.

50. Togna G, Tempesta E, Togna AR, Dolci N, Cebo B, Caprino L. Platelet responsiveness and biosynthesis of thromboxane and prostacyclin in response to in vitro cocaine treatment. *Haemostasis* 1985; 15:100–107.

51. Braunwald E. Unstable angina. A classification. *Circulation* 1989; 80:410–414.

52. Maseri A. Unstable angina. In: Maseri A, ed. *Ischemic Heart Disease.* New York: Churchill Livingstone; 1995:533–557.

53. Rizik DG, Healy S, Margulis A, Vandam D, Bakalyar D, Timmis G, et al. A new clinical classification for hospital prognosis of unstable angina pectoris. *Am J Cardiol* 1995; 75:993–997.

54. Lerner DJ, Kannel WB. Patterns of coronary heart disease morbidity and mortality in the sexes: A 26-year follow-up of the Framingham population. *Am Heart J* 1986; 111:383–390.

55. Douglas PS, Ginsburg GS. The evaluation of chest pain in women. *N Engl J Med* 1996; 334:1311–1315.

56. Goldberg RJ, Gorak EJ, Yarzebski J, Hosmer DW, Dalen P, Gore JM, et al. A community-wide perspective of sex differences and temporal trends in the incidence and survival rates after acute myocardial infarction and out-of-hospital deaths caused by coronary heart disease. *Circulation* 1993; 87:1947–1953.

57. Stone PH, Thompson B, Anderson HV, Kronenberg MW, Gibson RS, Rogers WV, et al. The influence of race, gender, and age on the natural history and management of patients with unstable angina and non-Q-wave myocardial infarction. The TIMI III registry. *JAMA* 1996; 275:1104–1112.

58. The National Center for Health Statistics. Vital Statistics of the United States: 1981. Mortality. Hyattsville, MD, 1986.

59. Schuster EH, Bulkley B. Early post-infarction angina: Ischemia at a distance and ischemia in the infarct zone. *N Engl J Med* 1981; 305:1101–1105.

60. Schroder R, Neuhaus KL, Linderer T, Leizorovicz A, Wegscheider K, Tebbe U. Risk of death from recurrent ischemic events after intravenous streptokinase in acute myocardial infarction: Results from the Intravenous Streptokinase in Myocardial Infarction (ISAM) Study. *Circulation* 1987; 76:1144–1151.

61. Bosch X, Théroux P, Waters D, Pelletier GB, Roy D. Early postinfarction ischemia: Clinical, angiographic, and prognostic significance. *Circulation* 1987; 75:988–995.

62. Théroux P, Waters D. Unstable angina: Special considerations in the post-bypass patient. In: Waters D, Bourassa MG, Brest AN, eds. *Care of the Patient with Previous Coronary Bypass Surgery. Cardiovascular Clinics.* Philadelphia: FA Davis; 1991:169–191.

63. Waters DD, Walling A, Roy D, Théroux P. Previous coronary artery bypass grafting as an adverse prognostic factor in unstable angina pectoris. *Am J Cardiol* 1986; 58:465–469.

64. Kleiman NS, Anderson HV, Rogers WJ, Théroux P, Thompson B, Stone PH, for the TIMI Investigators. Comparison of outcome of patients with unstable angina and non-Q-wave acute myocardial infarction with and without prior coronary artery bypass grafting (Thrombolysis in Myocardial Ischemia III registry). *Am J Cardiol* 1996; 77:227–231.

65. Holmes DR Jr, Vliestra RE, Smith HV, Vetrovec GW, Kent KM, Cowley MJ, et al. Restenosis after percutaneous coronary angioplasty: A report from the PTCA registry of the National Heart, Lung, and Blood Institute. *Am J Cardiol* 1984; 53:77C–81C.

66. Rafflenbeul W, Russell RO, Lichtlen PR. Angiographic anatomy of coronary arteries in unstable angina pectoris. In: Rafflenbeul W, Lichtlen PR, Balcon R, eds. *Unstable Angina Pectoris.* New York: Thieme-Stratton, Inc; 1981:51–57.

67. Bilodeau L, Théroux P, Gregoire J, Gagnon D, Arsenault A. Technetium-99m sestamibi tomography in patients with spontaneous chest pain: Correlations with clinical, electrocardiographic and angiographic findings. *J Am Coll Cardiol* 1991; 18:1684–1691.

68. de Zwaan C, Baur FW, Janssen JHA, Cherier EC, Dassen WRM, Brugada P, et al. Angiographic and clinical characteristics of patients with unstable angina showing an ECG pattern indicating critical narrowing of the proximal LAD coronary artery. *Am Heart J* 1989; 117:657–664.

69. Hamm CW, Ravkilde J, Gerhardt, Jorgensen P, Peheim E, Ljungdahl L, et al. The prognostic value of serum troponin T in unstable angina. *N Engl J Med* 1992; 327:146–150.

70. Seino Y, Tomota Y, Takano T, Hayakama H. Early identification of cardiac events with serum troponin T in patients with unstable angina. *Lancet* 1993; 342:1236–1237.

71. Wu AHB, Abbas SA, Green S, Pearsal L, Dhakam S, Azar R, et al. Prognostic value of cardiac troponin T in unstable angina pectoris. *Am J Cardiol* 1995; 76:970–972.

72. Lesperance J, Théroux P, Hudon G, Waters D. A new look at coronary angiography: Plaque morphology as a help to diagnosis and to evaluate prognosis. *Int J Card Imaging* 1994; 10:75–94.

73. Brown KA, Okada RD, Boucher CA, Phillips HR, Strauss HW, Pohost GM. Serial thallium-201 imaging at rest in patients with unstable and stable angina pectoris: Relationship of myocardial perfusion at rest to presenting clinical syndrome. *Am Heart J* 1983; 106:70–77.

74. Freeman MR, Williams AE, Chisholm RJ, Patt NL, Greyson MD, Armstrong PW. Role of resting thallium-201 perfusion in predicting coronary anatomy, left ventricular wall motion, and hospital outcome in unstable angina pectoris. *Am Heart J* 1989; 117:306–314.

75. Hilton TC, Thompson RC, Williams HJ, Saylors R, Fulmer H, Stowers SA. Technetium-99m sestamibi myocardial perfusion imaging in the emergency room evaluation of chest pain. *J Am Coll Cardiol* 1994; 23:1016–1022.

76. Peels C, Visser CA, Funke Kupper AJF, Visser FC, Roos JP. Usefulness of two-dimensional echocardiography for immediate detection of myocardial ischemia in the emergency room. *Am J Cardiol* 1990; 65:687–691.

77. Thieme T, Wenecke KD, Meyer R, Brandenstein E, Hadebank D, Hinz A, et al. Angioscopic evaluation of atherosclerotic plaques: Validation by histomorphologic analysis and association with stable and unstable coronary syndromes. *J Am Coll Cardiol* 1996; 28:1–6.

78. Mizuno K, Satomura K, Miyamoto A, Arakawa K, Shibuya T, Arai T, et al. Angioscopic evaluation of coronary-artery thrombi in acute coronary syndromes. *N Engl J Med* 1992; 326:287–291.

79. De Feyter PJ, Ozaki Y, Baptista J, Escaned J, Mario CD, de Jaegere PPT, et al. Ischemia-related lesion characteristics in patients with stable and unstable angina. A study with intracoronary angioscopy and ultrasound. *Circulation* 1995; 92:1408–1413.

80. Fitzgerald DJ, Roy L, Catella F, Fitzgerald GA. Platelet activation in unstable coronary disease. *N Engl J Med* 1986; 315:983–989.

81. Hamm CW, Lorenz RL, Bleifeld W, Kupper W, Wober E, Weber PC. Biochemical evidence of platelet activation in patients with persistent unstable angina. *J Am Coll Cardiol* 1987; 10:998–1006.

82. Théroux P, Latour JG, De Lara J, Leger-Gauthier C. Fibrinopeptide A and platelet factor levels in unstable angina pectoris. *Circulation* 1987; 75:156–162.

83. Shattil SJ, Cunningham M, Hoxie JA. Detection of activated platelets in whole blood using activation-dependent antibodies and flow cytometry. *Blood* 1987; 70:307–315.

84. Warkentin TE, Powling MJ, Hardisty RM. Measurements of fibrinogen binding to platelets in whole blood by flow cytometry: A micromethod for the detection of platelet activation. *Br J Haematol* 1990; 76:387–394.

85. Merlini PA, Bauer KA, Oltrona L, Ardissino D, Cattaneo M, Belli C, et al. Persistent activation of coagulation mechanism in unstable angina and myocardial infarction. *Circulation* 1994; 90:61–68.

86. Hoffmeister HM, Jur M, Wendel HP, Heller W, Seipel J. Alterations of coagulation and fibrinolytic and kallikrein-kinin systems in the acute and postacute phases in patients with unstable angina pectoris. *Circulation* 1995; 91:2520–2527.

87. Berk BC, Weintraub WS, Alexander RW. Elevation of serum C-reactive protein in "active" coronary artery disease. *Am J Cardiol* 1990; 65:168–172.

88. Liuzzo G, Biasucci LM, Gallimore JR, Rebuzzi AG, Pepys MB, Maseri A. The prognostic value of C-reactive protein and serum amyloid A protein in severe unstable angina. *N Engl J Med* 1994; 331:417–424.

89. Biasucci L, D'onofrio G, Liuzzo G, Zini G, Monaco C, Caliguri G, et al. Intracellular neutrophil myeloperoxidase is reduced in unstable angina and acute myocardial infarction, but its reduction is not related to ischemia. *J Am Coll Cardiol* 1996; 27.611–616.

90. Carry M, Korley V, Willerson JT, Weigelt L, Ford-Hutchinson AW, Tagari P. Increased urinary leukotrienes excretion in patients with cardiac ischemia. *Circulation* 1992; 85:230–236.

91. Seneri GGN, Abbate R, Gori AN, Attanasio M, Martini F, Giusti B, et al. Transient intermittent lymphocyte activation is responsible for the instability of angina. *Circulation* 1992; 86:790–797.

92. Leatham EW, Bath PMW, Tooze JA, Camm AJ. Increased monocyte tissue factor expression in coronary disease. *Br Heart J* 1995; 73:10–13.

93. Biasucci LM, Vitelli A, Liuzzo G, Altamura S, Caligiuri G, Monaco C, et al. Elevated levels of interleukin-6 in unstable angina. *Circulation* 1996; 94:847–877.

94. Neumann FJ, Ott I, Gawaz M, Richardt G, Holzapfel H, Jochum M, et al. Cardiac release of cytokines and inflammatory responses in acute myocardial infarction. *Circulation* 1995; 92:748–755.

95. Ikeda H, Takajo Y, Ichiki K, Ueno T, Maki S, Noda T, et al. Increased soluble form of P-selectin in patients with unstable angina. *Circulation* 1995; 92:1693–1696.

96. Ito T, Nakai K, Ono M, Hiramori K. Can the risk for acute cardiac events in acute coronary syndrome be predicted by platelet membrane activation marker P-selectin? *Coron Artery Dis* 1995; 6:645–650.

97. Mazzone A, De Servi S, Ricevuti G, Mazzucchelli I, Fossat G, Pasotti G, et al. Increased expression of neutrophil and monocyte adhesion molecules in unstable coronary artery disease. *Circulation* 1993; 88:358–363.

98. Ouyang P, Brinker JA, Mellits ED, Weisfeldt ML, Gerstenblith G. Variables predictive of successful medical therapy in patients with unstable angina: Selection by multivariate analysis from clinical, electrocardiographic and angiographic evaluations. *Circulation* 1984; 70:367–376.

99. Alison HW, Russell RO, Mantle JA, Kouchoukos NT, Morashi RE, Rackley CE. Coronary anatomy and arteriography in patients with unstable angina pectoris. *Am J Cardiol* 1978; 41:204–209.

100. Scott SM, Luchi RJ, Deupree RH, Veterans Administration Unstable Angina Cooperative Study Group. Veterans Administration Cooperative Study Group for treatment of patients with unstable angina. Results in patients with abnormal left ventricular function. *Circulation* 1988; 78(suppl I):I113–I121.

101. Russell RO, Moraski RE, Kouchoukos N, Karp R, Mantle JA, Rogers WJ, et al. Unstable angina pectoris: National Cooperative Study Group to compare surgical and medical therapy. II. In-hospital experience and initial follow-up results in patients with one, two and three vessel disease. *Am J Cardiol* 1978; 42:839–848.

102. Castaner A, Roig E, Serra A, De Flores T, Magrina J, Azqueta M, et al. Risk stratification and prognosis of patients with recent onset angina. *Eur Heart J* 1990; 11:868–875.

103. Bugiardini R, Pozzati A, Borghi A, Morgagni GL, Ottani F, Muzi A, et al. Angiographic morphology in unstable angina and its relation to transient myocardial ischemia and hospital outcome. *Am J Cardiol* 1991; 67:460–464.

104. Waxman S, Sassower MA, Mittleman MA, Zarich S, Miyamoto A, Manzo KS, et al. Angioscopic predictors of early adverse outcome after coronary angioplasty in patients with unstable angina and non-Q-wave myocardial infarction. *Circulation* 1996; 93:2106–2113.

105. Murphy JJ, Connell PA, Hampton JR. Predictors of risk in patients with unstable angina admitted to a district general hospital. *Br Heart J* 1992; 67:395–401.

106. van Miltenburg-van Zijl AJM, Simoons ML, Veerhoek RJ. Incidence and follow-up of Braunwald subgroups in unstable angina pectoris. *J Am Coll Cardiol* 1995; 25:1286–1292.

107. Olson HG, Lyons KP, Aronow WS, Stinson PJ, Kuperus J, Waters HJ. The high risk angina patient. Identification by clinical features, hospital course, electrocardiography and technetium-99m stannous pyrophosphate scintigraphy. *Circulation* 1981; 64:674–684.

108. Bosch X, Théroux P, Pelletier GB, Waters D. Clinical and angiographic features and prognostic significance of early postinfarction angina with and without electrocardiographic signs of transient ischemia. *Am J Med* 1991; 91:493–501.

109. Severi S, Orsini E, Maraccini P, Michelessi C, L'Abbate A. The basal electrocardiogram and the exercise test in assessing prognosis in patients with unstable angina. *Eur Heart J* 1989; 9:441–446.

110. Gottlieb SO, Weisfeldt ML, Ouyang P, Mellitis ED, Gerstenblith G. Silent ischemia as a marker for early unfavorable outcomes in patients with unstable angina. *N Engl J Med* 1986; 314:1214–1219.

111. Nademanee K, Intarachot V, Josephson MA, Rieders D, Vaghaiwalla F, Singh BN. Prognostic significance of silent ischemia in patients with unstable angina. *J Am Coll Cardiol* 1987; 10:1 9.

112. Langer A, Freeman MR, Armstrong PW. ST segment shift in unstable angina. Pathophysiology and association with coronary anatomy and hospital outcome. *J Am Coll Cardiol* 1989; 13:1495–1502.

113. Wilcox I, Freedman SB, Kelly DT, Harris PJ. Clinical significance of silent ischemia in unstable angina pectoris. *Am J Cardiol* 1990; 65:1313–1316.

114. Bugiardini R, Borghi A, Pozzati A, Ruggeri A, Puddu P, Maseri A. Relation of severity of symptoms to transient myocardial ischemia and prognosis in unstable angina. *J Am Coll Cardiol* 1995; 25:597–604.

115. Ravkilde J, Horder H, Gerhardt L, Ljungdahl L, Petersson T, Tryding N, et al. Diagnostic performance and prognostic value of serum troponin T in suspected myocardial infarction. *Scand J Clin Lab Invest* 1993; 53:677–685.

116. Burlina A, Zaninotto M, Secchiero R, Rubin D, Accorsi F. Troponin T as a marker of ischemic myocardial injury. *Clin Biochem* 1994; 27:113–121.

117. Rebuzzi AG, Liuzzo G, Menini E, Grillo R, Biasucci L, Pala M, et al. Powerful prognostic value of troponin T and C-reactive protein in patients with unstable angina (abstr). *J Am Coll Cardiol* 1994; 23:77A.

118. Ravkilde J, Nissen H, Horder M, Thygensen K. Independent prognostic value of serum creatine kinase isoenzyme MB mass, cardiac troponin T and myosin light chain in suspected acute myocardial infarction. Analysis of 28 months of follow-up in 196 patients. *J Am Coll Cardiol* 1994; 23:574–578.

119. Murphy JJ, Ramesh P, Murphy JM, Hooper RJ. Troponin T risk assessment in patients with chest pain but without acute infarction (abstr). *Eur Heart J* 1996; 17(suppl):577.

120. Lindahl B, Venge P, Wallentin L, for the FRISC Study Group. Relation between troponin T and the risk of subsequent cardiac events in unstable coronary artery disease. *Circulation* 1996; 93:1651–1657.

121. Ohman EH, Armstrong PW, Christenson RH, Granger CB, Katus HA, Hamm CW, et al. Cardiac troponin T levels for risk stratification in acute myocardial ischemia. *N Engl J Med* 1996; 335:1333–1341.

122. Antman EM, Tanasijevic MJ, Thompson B, Schactman MS, McCabe CH, Cannon CP, et al. Cardiac-specific troponin I levels to predict the risk of mortality in patients with acute coronary syndromes. *N Engl J Med* 1996; 335:1342–1349.

123. Liuzzo G, Biasucci LM, Buffon A, Quaranta G, Caligiuri G, Monaco C, et al. Elevated C-reactive protein after waning of symptoms in unstable angina is associated with recurrence of instability during 12-month follow-up (abstr). *J Am Coll Cardiol* 1995; 25(Feb special):250A.

124. Thompson SG, Kienast J, Pyke SDM, Haverkate F, van de Loo JCW. Hemostatic factor and the risk of myocardial infarction or sudden death in patients with angina pectoris. *N Engl J Med* 1995; 332:635–641.

125. Ridker PM, Cushman M, Stampfer MJ, Tracy RP, Hennekens CH. Inflammation, aspirin, and the risk of cardiovascular disease in apparently healthy men. *N Engl J Med* 1997; 336:973–979.

126. Butman SM, Olson HG, Gardin JM, Piters KM, Hulett M, Butman LK. Submaximal exercise testing after stabilization of unstable angina pectoris. *J Am Coll Cardiol* 1984; 4:667–673.

127. Nyman I, Wallentin L, Areskog M, Areskog NH, Swahn E. Risk stratification by early exercise testing after an episode of unstable coronary disease. *Int J Cardiol* 1993; 39:131–142.

128. Moss AJ, Goldstein RE, Hall WJ, Bigger JT Jr, Fleiss JL, Greenberg H, et al. Detection and significance of myocardial ischemia in stable patients after recovery from an acute coronary event. Multicenter Myocardial Ischemia Research Group. *JAMA* 1993; 269:2379–2385.

129. Brown KA. Prognostic value of thallium-201 myocardial perfusion imaging in patients with unstable angina who respond to medical treatment. *J Am Coll Cardiol* 1991; 17:1053–1057.

130. Stratmann HG, Younis LT, Wittry MD, Amato M, Miller DD. Exercise technetium-99m myocardial tomography for the risk stratification of men with medically treated unstable angina pectoris. *Am J Cardiol* 1995; 76:236–240.

131. Chen L, Chester MR, Crook R, Kasi JC. Differential progression of complex culprit stenoses in patients with stable and unstable angina pectoris. *J Am Coll Cardiol* 1996; 28:597–603.

132. Chen L, Théroux P, Lesperance J, Hudon G. Differential pattern of progression of coronary artery disease in patients with unstable angina and previous stable or unstable angina. *Circulation*, submitted.

133. Willerson JT, Yao SK, McNatt J, Benedict CR, Anderson HV, Golino P, et al. Frequency and severity of cyclic flow alternations and platelet aggregation predict the severity of neointimal proliferation following experimental coronary stenosis and endothelial injury. *Proc Natl Acad Sci USA* 1991; 88:10624–10628.

134. Topol EJ, Califf RM, Weisman HF, Ellis SG, Tcheng JE, Worley S, et al. Randomized trial of coronary intervention with antibody against IIb/IIIa integrin for reduction of clinical restenosis: Results at six months. *Lancet* 1994; 343:881–886.

135. Maresta A, Balducelli M, Cantini L, Casari A, Chion R, Fabbri M, et al. Trapidil (triazolopyrimidine), a platelet-derived growth factor antagonist, reduces restenosis after percutaneous transluminal coronary angioplasty. Results of the randomized, double-blind STARC study. *Circulation* 1994; 90:2710–2715.

136. Antiplatelet Trialists' Collaboration. Collaborative overview of randomized trials of antiplatelet therapy—I: Prevention of death, myocardial infarction, and stroke by prolonged antiplatelet therapy in various categories of patients. *Br Med J* 1994; 308:81–106.

137. Lewis HD, Davis JW, Archibald DG, Steinke WE, Smitherman TC, Doherty JE, et al. Protective effects of aspirin against myocardial infarction and death in men with unstable angina. *N Engl J Med* 1983; 309:396–403.

138. Cairns JA, Gent M, Singer J, Finnie KJ, Frogatt GM, Holder DA, et al. Aspirin, sulfinpyrazone, or both in unstable angina. *N Engl J Med* 1985; 313:1369–1375.

139. Théroux P, Ouimet H, McCans J, Latour JG, Joly P, Levy G, et al. Aspirin, heparin, or both to treat acute unstable angina. *N Engl J Med* 1988; 319:1105–1111.

140. The RISC Group. Risk of myocardial infarction and death during treatment with low dose aspirin and intravenous heparin in men with unstable coronary disease. *Lancet* 1990; 336:827–830.

141. Wallentin LC, and the Research Group on Instability in Coronary Artery Disease in Southeast Sweden. Aspirin (75 mg/day) after an episode of unstable coronary disease: Long-term effects on the risk for myocardial infarction, occurrence of severe angina and the need for revascularization. *J Am Coll Cardiol* 1991; 18:1587–1593.

142. Balsano F, Rizzon P, Violi F, Scrutinio D, Cimminiello C, Aguglia F, et al. Antiplatelet treatment with ticlopidine in unstable angina. A controlled multicenter clinical trial. *Circulation* 1990; 82:17–26.

143. CAPRIE Steering Committee. A randomized, blinded trial of clopidogrel versus aspirin in patients at risk of ischaemic events (CAPRIE). *Lancet* 1996; 348:1329–1339.

144. Fiddler GI, Lumley P. Preliminary clinical studies with thromboxane synthase inhibitors and thromboxane receptor blockers. A review. *Circulation* 1990; 82(suppl 1):169–178.

145. Théroux P, Latour JG, Diodati J, Léger-Gauthier C, Morissette D, Bosch X, et al. Hemodynamic, platelet and clinical responses to prostacyclin in unstable angina pectoris. *Am J Cardiol* 1990; 65:1084–1089.

146. Coller BS. Blockade of platelet GPIIb/IIIa receptors as an antithrombotic strategy. *Circulation* 1995; 92:2373–2380.

147. The EPIC Investigators. Use of a monoclonal antibody directed against the platelet glycoprotein IIb/IIIa receptor in high-risk coronary angioplasty. *N Engl J Med* 1994; 330:949–955.

148. Lincoff AM, Califf RM, Anderson KA, Weisman HF, Aguirre FV, Kleiman NS, et al. Evidence for prevention of death and myocardial infarction with platelet membrane glycoprotein IIb/IIIa receptor blockade by c7E3 Fab (abciximab) among patients with unstable angina undergoing percutaneous coronary revascularization. *Circulation*: Submitted.

149. The EPILOG Investigators. Platelet glycoprotein IIb/IIa receptor blockade and low-dose heparin during percutaneous coronary revascularization. *N Engl J Med* 1997; 336:1689–1696.

150. The CAPTURE Investigators. Randomized placebo-controlled trial of abciximab before and during intervention in refractory unstable angina. *Lancet* 1997; 349:1429–1435.

151. The PRISM Investigators. Platelet receptor inhibition for ischemic syndrome management. Results presented at the Scientific Sessions, American College of Cardiology, Anaheim, CA, March 1997.

152. The PRISM-PLUS Investigators. Specific inhibition of platelet glycoprotein IIb/IIIa with tirofiban prevents acute coronary events in unstable angina and non-Q wave myocardial infarction. Submitted

153. Théroux P, Kouz S, Roy L, Knudtson M, Diodati JG, Marquis JF, et al. Platelet membrane receptor glycoprotein IIb/IIIa antagonism in unstable angina. The Canadian Lamifiban Study. *Circulation* 1996; 94:899–905.

154. PARAGON. Results presented at the American Heart Association meeting, New Orleans, LA, November, 1996.

155. Théroux P, Waters D, Qiu S, McCans J, de Guise P, Juneau M. Aspirin versus heparin to prevent myocardial infarction during the acute phase of unstable angina. *Circulation* 1993; 88:2045–2048.

156. Théroux P, Waters D, Lam J, Juneau M, McCans J. Reactivation of unstable angina after the discontinuation of heparin. *N Engl J Med* 1992; 327:141–145.

157. Neri-Serneri GG, Gensini GR, Poggesi L, Trotta F, Modesti PA, Boddi M, et al. Effect of heparin, aspirin or alteplase in reduction of myocardial ischemia in refractory unstable angina. *Lancet* 1990; 335:615–618.

158. Holdright D, Patel D, Cunningham D, Thomas R, Hubbard W, Hendry G, et al. Comparison of the effect of heparin and aspirin versus aspirin alone on transient myocardial ischemia and in-hospital prognosis in patients with unstable angina. *J Am Coll Cardiol* 1994; 24:39–45.

159. Gurfinkel EP, Manos EJ, Mejail RI, Cerda MA, Duronto EA, Garcia CN, et al. Low molecular weight heparin versus regular heparin or aspirin in the treatment of unstable angina and silent ischemia. *J Am Coll Cardiol* 1995; 26:313–318.

160. Fragmin during Instability in Coronary Artery Disease (FRISC) Study Group. Low-molecular-weight heparin during instability in coronary artery disease. *Lancet* 1996; 347:561–568.

161. FRIC Study Group. Low molecular weight heparin in the initial and prolonged treatment of unstable coronary disease—the fragmin in unstable coronary heart disease (abstr). *Eur Heart J* 1996; 17:306.

162. Cohen M, Demers C, Gurfinkel EP, Turpic AGG, et al. Low molecular weight heparin versus unfractionated heparin for unstable angina and non-Q wave myocardial infarction. (Presented at the American Heart Association Scientific Sessions, New Orleans, LA, November, 1996.) *N Engl J Med*, in press.

163. The Global Use of Strategies to Open Occluded Arteries (GUSTO) IIA Investigators. Randomized trial of intravenous heparin versus recombinant hirudin for acute coronary syndromes. *Circulation* 1994; 90:1631–1637.

164. The Global Use of Strategies to Open Occluded Coronary Arteries (GUSTO) IIB Investigators. A comparison of recombinant hirudin

with heparin for the treatment of acute coronary syndromes. *N Engl J Med* 1996; 335:775–782.

165. Serruys P, Herrman JPR, Simon R, Rutsch W, Bode C, Laarman GJ, et al. A comparison of hirudin with heparin in the prevention of restenosis after coronary angioplasty. *N Engl J Med* 1995; 333:757–763.

166. Organization to Assess Strategies for Ischemic Syndromes (OASIS) Investigators. Comparison of hirudin with heparin and warfarin with control for unstable angina and non-Q-wave MI in a randomized controlled trial (abstr). *Circulation* 1995; 52(suppl I):I416.

167. Williams DO, Kirby MG, McPherson K, Phear DM. Anticoagulant treatment in unstable angina. *Br J Clin Pract* 1986; 40:114–116.

168. Cohen M, Adams PC, Parry G, Xiong J, Chamberlain D, Wieczorek I, et al. Combination antithrombotic therapy in unstable rest angina and non-Q-wave infarction in non aspirin users. Primary endpoints analysis from the ATACS trial. *Circulation* 1994; 89:81–88.

169. Waters D, Lam JYT. Is thrombolytic therapy striking out in unstable angina? *Circulation* 1992; 86:1642–1644.

170. Bär FW, Vergheut FW, Col J, Materne P, Monassier JT, Geslin PG, et al. Thrombolysis in patients with unstable angina improves the angiographic but not the clinical outcome: Results of UNASEM, a multicenter, randomized, placebo-controlled clinical trial with anistreplase. *Circulation* 1992; 6:131–137.

171. Shabani F, Théroux P, de Guise P, Thibault B. A randomized, double-blind trial of streptokinase versus placebo for the management of unstable angina and non-Q-wave myocardial infarction in patients with previous coronary artery bypass surgery (abstr). *J Am Coll Cardiol* 1995:(special issue):421A.

172. Freeman MR, Langer A, Wilson RF, Morgan CD, Armstrong PW. Thrombolysis in unstable angina. Randomized double-blind trial of t-PA and placebo. *Circulation* 1992; 85:150–157.

173. Topol EJ, Nicklas JM, Kander NH, Walton JA, Ellis SG, Gorman L, et al. Coronary revascularization after intravenous tissue plasminogen activator for unstable angina pectoris: Results of a randomized, double-blind, placebo controlled trial. *Am J Cardiol* 1988; 62:368–371.

174. Dauwe F, Affaki G, Waters DD, Théroux P, Mizgala HF. Intravenous nitroglycerin in refractory unstable angina (abstr). *Am J Cardiol* 1979; 43:416.

175. Kaplan K, Davison R, Parker M, Przybylek J, Teagarden JR, Lesch M. Intravenous nitroglycerin for the treatment of angina at rest unresponsive to standard nitrate therapy. *Am J Cardiol* 1983; 51:694–698.

176. Curfman GD, Heinsimer JA, Lozner EC, Fung HL. Intravenous nitroglycerin in the treatment of spontaneous angina pectoris: A prospective randomized trial. *Circulation* 1983; 67:276–282.

177. Palmer RMJ, Ferrige AG, Moncada S. Nitric oxide release accounts for the biologic activity of endothelium-derived factor. *Nature* 1987; 327:524–526.

178. Schafer AI, Alexander RW, Handin RI. Inhibition of platelet function by organic nitrate vasodilators. *Blood* 1980; 55:649–654.

179. Folts JD, Stamler J, Loscalzo J. Intravenous nitroglycerin infusion inhibits cyclic blood flow responses caused by periodic platelet thrombus formation in stenosed coronary canine arteries. *Circulation* 1991; 83:2122–2127.

180. Diodati J, Théroux P, Latour JG, Lacoste L, Lam JYT, Waters D. Effects of nitroglycerin at therapeutic doses on platelet aggregation in unstable angina pectoris and acute myocardial infarction. *Am J Cardiol* 1990; 66:683–688.

181. Malekianpour M, Doucet S, Théroux P, Côté G, Bilodeau L, Tardif JC, et al. A randomized trial for treatment of unstable angina in patients with restenosis post coronary angioplasty (abstr). *J Am Coll Cardiol* 1997; 29:217A.

182. Yusuf S, Wittes J, Friedman L. Overview of results of randomized trials in heart disease. II. Unstable angina, heart failure, primary prevention with aspirin, and risk factor modification. *JAMA* 1988; 260:2259–2263.

183. Yusuf S, Ramsdale D, Peto R, Furse L, Bennett D, Bray C, et al. Early intravenous atenolol treatment in suspected acute myocardial infarction. *Lancet* 1980; 2:273–276.

184. Robertson RM, Wood AJJ, Vaughn WK, Robertson D. Exacerbation of vasotonic angina pectoris by propranolol. *Circulation* 1982; 65:281–285.

185. Muller JE, Turi ZG, Pearle DL, Schneider JF, Serfas DH, Morrison J. Nifedipine and conventional therapy for unstable angina pectoris: A randomized, double-blind comparison. *Circulation* 1984; 69:728–739.

186. Gerstenblith G, Ouyang P, Achuff SC, Bulkley BH, Becker LC, Mellits ED, et al. Nifedipine in unstable angina: A double-blind randomized trial. *N Engl J Med* 1982; 306:885–889.

187. Gottlieb SO, Weisfeldt ML, Ouyang P, Achuff SC, Baughman KL, Traill TA, et al. Effect of the addition of propranolol to therapy with nifedipine for unstable angina pectoris: A randomized, double-blind, placebo-controlled trial. *Circulation* 1986; 73:331–337.

188. Holland Interuniversity Nifedipine/Metoprolol Trial (HINT) Research Group. Early treatment of unstable angina in the coronary care unit: A randomized, double-blind, placebo-controlled comparison of recurrent ischemia in patients treated with nifedipine or metoprolol or both. *Br Heart J* 1986; 56:400–413.

189. Théroux P, Taeymans Y, Morissette D, Bosch X, Pelletier GB, Waters DD. A randomized study comparing propranolol and diltiazem in the treatment of unstable angina. *J Am Coll Cardiol* 1985; 5:717–722.

190. Fang ZY, Picart N, Abramowicz M, Unger P, Narraci P, Sobolski J, et al. Intravenous diltiazem versus nitroglycerin for silent and symptomatic myocardial ischemia in unstable angina pectoris. *Am J Cardiol* 1991; 68:42C–46C.

191. Göbel EJAM, Hautvast RWM, van Gilst WH, Spanjaard JN, Hillege HL, DeJongste MJL, et al. Randomized, double-blind trial of intravenous diltiazem versus glyceryl trinitrate for unstable angina pectoris. *Lancet* 1995; 346:1653–1657.

192. Weintraub RM, Aresty JM, Paulin S, Levine FH, Markis JE, LaRala PJ, et al. Medically refractory unstable angina. 1. Long-term follow-up of patients undergoing intra-aortic balloon counterpulsation and operation. *Am J Cardiol* 1979; 43:877–882.

193. Rankin JS, Newton JR Jr, Califf RM, Jones JR, Weschler AS, Oldham N, et al. Clinical characteristics and current management of medically refractory unstable angina. *Ann Surg* 1984; 200:457–465.

194. Hultgren HN, Pfeifer JF, Angel WW, Lipton MJ, Bilisoly J. Unstable angina: Comparison of medical and surgical patients. *Am J Cardiol* 1977; 39:734–740.

195. Selden R, Neill WA, Rizmann LW, Okies JE, Anderson RP. Medical versus surgical therapy for acute coronary insufficiency: A randomized study. *N Engl J Med* 1975; 293:1329–1333.

196. Luchi RJ, Scott SM, Deupree RH, Principal Investigators and their Associates of Veterans Administration Cooperative Study No. 28. Comparison of medical and surgical treatment for unstable angina pectoris. *N Engl J Med* 1987; 316:977–984.

197. Booth DC, Deupree RH, Hultgren HM, De Maria AN, Scott SM, Luchi RJ, et al. Quality of life after bypass surgery for unstable angina. 5-year follow-up results of a Veterans Affairs Cooperative Study. *Circulation* 1991; 83:87–95.

198. Kaiser GC, Schaff HV, Killip T. Myocardial revascularization for unstable angina pectoris. *Circulation* 1989; 79(suppl I):I60–I67.

199. Perrault L, Carrier M, Cartier R, Leclerc Y, Hebert Y, Diaz OS, et al. Morbidity and mortality of reoperation for coronary artery bypass grafting: Significance of atheromatous vein grafts. *Can J Cardiol* 1991; 7:427–430.

200. Craddock D, Iyer VS, Russell WJ. Factors influencing mortality and myocardial infarction after coronary artery bypass grafting. *Curr Opin Cardiol* 1994; 9:664–669.

201. The Bypass Angioplasty Revascularization Investigation (BARI) Investigators. Comparison of coronary bypass surgery with angioplasty in patients with multivessel disease. *N Engl J Med* 1996; 335:217–225.

202. Hueb WA, Bellotti G, de Oliveira SA, Arie S, de Albuquerque CP, Jatene AD, et al. The medicine, angioplasty or surgery study (MASS): A prospective, randomized trial of medical therapy, balloon angioplasty or bypass surgery for single proximal left anterior descending artery stenoses. *J Am Coll Cardiol* 1995; 26:1600–1605.

203. Dorros G, Cowley MJ, Simpson J, Bentivoglio LG, Block PC, Bourassa M, et al. Percutaneous transluminal coronary angioplasty: Report of complications from the National Heart, Lung, and Blood Institute PTCA Registry. *Circulation* 1983; 67:723–730.

204. de Feyter PJ, Serruys PW. Percutaneous transluminal coronary angioplasty for unstable angina. In: Topol EJ, ed. *Textbook of Interventional Cardiology*, 2d ed. Philadelphia: Saunders; 1994:274–291.

205. Rupprecht HJ, Brennecke R, Koitmeyer M, Bernhard G, Erbel R, Pop T, et al. Short- and long-term outcome after PTCA in patients with stable and unstable angina. *Eur Heart J* 1990; 11:964–973.

206. Myler RK, Shaw RE, Stertzer SH, Bashour TT, Ryan C, Hecht HS, et al. Unstable angina and coronary angioplasty. *Circulation* 1990; 82(suppl II):II88–II95.

207. Bauters C, Khanoyan P, McFadden EP, Quandaille P, Leblanche JM, Bertrand ME. Restenosis after delayed coronary angioplasty of the culprit vessel in patients with a recent myocardial infarction treated by thrombolysis. *Circulation* 1995; 91:1410–1418.

208. Schulman SP, Goldschmidt-Clermont PJ, Topol EJ, Califf RM, Navette FI, Willerson JT, et al. Effects of integrelin, a novel platelet glycoprotein antagonist, in unstable angina. A randomized multicenter trial. *Circulation* 1996; 94:2083–2089.

209. The RESTORE Investigators. The effects of glycoprotein IIb/IIIa blockade with tirofiban on adverse cardiac events in patients with unstable angina undergoing coronary angioplasty. *Circulation* 1997, in press.

210. Lukas MA, Deutsch E, Hirshfeld JW Jr, Kussmaul WG, Barnathan E, Laskey WK. Influence of heparin therapy on percutaneous transluminal coronary angioplasty outcome in patients with coronary arterial thrombus. *Am J Cardiol* 1990; 65:179–182.

211. Fineberg HV, Scadden D, Goldman L. Care of patients with a low probability of acute myocardial infarction. Cost effectiveness of alternatives to coronary-care-unit admission. *N Engl J Med* 1984; 310:1301–1307.

212. Weingarten SR, Riedenger MS, Conner L, Lee HL, Hoffman I, Johnson B, et al. Practice guidelines and reminders to reduce duration of hospital stay for patients with chest pain. *Ann Intern Med* 1994; 120:257–263.

213. Schreiber TL, Elkhatib A, Grines CL, O'Neill WW. Cardiologist versus internist management of patients with unstable angina: Treatment patterns and outcomes. *J Am Coll Cardiol* 1995; 26:577–582.

214. U.S. Department of Health and Human Services, Public Health Service. *Unstable Angina: Diagnosis and Management.* Clinical Practice Guideline, Number 10 (AHCPR Publication No. 94-0602). Washington, DC: 1994.

215. Prinzmetal M, Kennamer R, Merliss R, Wada T, Bor N. Angina pectoris. I. A variant form of angina pectoris. *Am J Med* 1959; 27:375–388.

216. MacAlpin RN, Kattus AA, Alvaro AB. Angina pectoris at rest with preservation of exercise capacity. Prinzmetal's variant angina. *Circulation* 1973; 47:946–958.

217. Onaka H, Hirota Y, Shimada S, Kita Y, Sakai Y, Kawakami Y, et al. Clinical observation of spontaneous anginal attacks and multivessel spasm in variant angina pectoris with normal coronary arteries: Evaluation by 24-hour 12-lead electrocardiography with computer analysis. *J Am Coll Cardiol* 1996; 27:38–44.

218. Ozaki Y, Keane D, Serruys P. Fluctuation of spastic location in patients with vasospastic angina: A quantitative angiographic study. *J Am Coll Cardiol* 1995; 26:1606–1614.

219. Maseri A, Severi S, De Nes M, L'Abbate A, Chierchia S, Marzilli M, et al. "Variant" angina: One aspect of a continuous spectrum of vasospastic myocardial ischemia. *Am J Cardiol* 1978; 42:1019–1035.

220. Kushwaha S, Mitchell AG, Yacoub MH. Coronary artery spasm after cardiac transplantation. *Am J Cardiol* 1990; 65:1515–1518.

221. Chierchia S, Davies G, Berkenboom G, Crea F, Crean P, Maseri A. α-Adrenergic receptors and coronary spasm: An elusive link. *Circulation* 1984; 69:8–14.

222. Freedman SB, Chierchia S, Rodriguez-Plaza L, Bugiardini R, Smith G, Maseri A. Ergonovine-induced myocardial ischemia: No role for serotonergic receptors? *Circulation* 1984; 70:178–183.

223. Robertson RM, Robertson D, Roberts LJ, Maas RL, FitzGerald GA, Friesinger GC, et al. Thromboxane A$_2$ in vasotonic angina pectoris. Evidence from direct measurements and inhibitor trials. *N Engl J Med* 1981; 304:998–1003.

224. Chierchia S, Patrono C, Crea F, Ciabattoni G, De Caterina R, Cinotti GA, et al. Effects of intravenous prostacyclin in variant angina. *Circulation* 1982; 65:470–477.

225. Goto K, Yasue H, Okumura K, Matsuyama K, Kugiyama K, Miyagi H, et al. Magnesium deficiency detected by intravenous loading test in variant angina pectoris. *Am J Cardiol* 1990; 65:709–712.

226. Shimabukuro M, Shinzato T, Higa S, Chibana T, Yoshida H, Nagamine F, et al. Enhanced insulin response relates to acetylcholine-induced vasoconstriction in vasospastic angina. *J Am Coll Cardiol* 1995; 25:356–361.

227. Yamagishi M, Miyatake K, Tamai J, Nakatani S, Koyama J, Nissen SE. Intravascular ultrasound detection of atherosclerosis at the site of focal vasospasm in angiographically normal or minimally narrowed coronary segments. *J Am Coll Cardiol* 1994; 23:352–357.

228. Kaski JC, Tousoulis D, Gavrielides S, McFadden E, Galassi AR, Crea F, et al. Comparison of epicardial coronary artery tone and reactivity in Prinzmetal's variant angina and chronic stable angina pectoris. *J Am Coll Cardiol* 1991; 17:1058–1062.

229. Irie T, Imaizumi T, Matuguchi T, Koyanagi S, Kanaide H, Takeshita A, et al. Increased fibrinopeptide A during anginal attacks in patients with variant angina. *J Am Coll Cardiol* 1989; 14:589–594.

230. Waters DD, Szlachcic J, Bourassa MG, Scholl JM, Théroux P. Exercise testing in patients with variant angina: Results, correlation with clinical and angiographic features and prognostic significance. *Circulation* 1982; 65:265–274.

231. Koiwaya Y, Torii S, Takeshita A, Nakagaki O, Nakamura M. Postinfarction angina caused by coronary arterial spasm. *Circulation* 1982; 65:275–280.

232. Waters DD, Théroux P, Crittin J, Dauwe F, Mizgala HF. Previously undiagnosed variant angina as a cause of chest pain after coronary artery bypass surgery. *Circulation* 1980; 61:1159–1164.

233. David PR, Waters DD, Scholl JM, Crépeau J, Szlachcic J, Lespérance J, et al. Percutaneous transluminal coronary angioplasty in patients with variant angina. *Circulation* 1982; 66:695–702.

234. Scholl JM, Benacerraf A, Ducimetiere P, Chabas D, Brau J, Chapelle J, et al. Comparison of risk factors in vasospastic angina without significant fixed coronary narrowing and no vasospastic angina. *Am J Cardiol* 1986; 57:199–202.

235. Miller D, Waters DD, Warnica W, Szlachcic J, Kreeft J, Théroux P. Is variant angina the coronary manifestation of a generalized vasospastic disorder? *N Engl J Med* 1981; 304:763–766.

236. Miller DD, Waters DD, Szlachcic J, Théroux P. Clinical characteristics associated with sudden death in patients with variant angina. *Circulation* 1982; 66:588–592.

237. Kloner RA, Hale S, Alker K, Rezkalla S. The effects of acute and chronic cocaine use on the heart. *Circulation* 1992; 85:407–419.

238. Gitter MJ, Goldsmith SR, Dunbar DN, Sharkey SW. Cocaine and chest pain: Clinical features and outcomes of patients hospitalized to rule out myocardial infarction. *Ann Intern Med* 1991; 115:277–282.

239. Waters DD, Szlachcic J, Bonan R, Miller DD, Dauwe F, Théroux P. Comparative sensitivity of exercise, cold pressor and ergonovine testing in provoking attacks of variant angina in patients with active disease. *Circulation* 1983; 67:310–315.

240. Okumura K, Yasue H, Matsuyama K, Morikami Y, Ogawa H, Obata K. Effect of H$_1$ receptor stimulation on coronary artery diameter in patients with variant angina: Comparison with effect of acetylcholine. *J Am Coll Cardiol* 1991; 17:338–345.

241. Crea F, Chierchia S, Kaski JC, Davies GJ, Margonato A, Miran DO, et al. Provocation of coronary spasm by dopamine in patients with active variant angina pectoris. *Circulation* 1986; 74:262–269.

242. Okumura K, Yasue H, Matsuyama K, Goto K, Miyagi H, Ogawa H, et al. Sensitivity and specificity of intracoronary injection of acetylcholine for the induction of coronary artery spasm. *J Am Coll Cardiol* 1988; 12:883–888.

243. Heupler FA Jr, Proudfit WL, Razavi M, Shirey EK, Greenstreet R, Sheldon WC. Ergonovine maleate provocative test for coronary arterial spasm. *Am J Cardiol* 1978; 41:631–640.

244. Crea F, Davies G, Romeo F, Chierchia S, Bugiardini R, Kaski JC, et al. Myocardial ischemia during ergonovine testing: Different susceptibility to coronary vasoconstriction in patients with exertional and variant angina. *Circulation* 1984; 69:690–695.

245. Bertrand ME, LaBlanche JM, Tilmant PY, Thieuleux FA, Delforge MR, Carre AG, et al. Frequency of provoked coronary arterial spasm in 1089 consecutive patients undergoing coronary arteriography. *Circulation* 1982; 65:1299–1306.

246. Buxton A, Goldberg S, Hirshfeld JW, Wilson J, Mann T, Williams DO, et al. Refractory ergonovine-induced coronary vasospasm: Importance of intracoronary nitroglycerin. *Am J Cardiol* 1980; 46:329–334.

247. Waters DD, Théroux P, Szlachcic J, Dauwe F, Crittin J, Bonan R, et al. Ergonovine testing in a coronary care unit. *Am J Cardiol* 1980; 46:922–930.

248. Ginsburg R, Lamb IH, Birstow MR, Harrison DC. Application and safety of outpatient ergonovine testing in accurately detecting coronary spasm in patients with possible variant angina. *Am Heart J* 1981; 102:698–702.

249. Waters DD, Théroux P, Szlachcic J, Dauwe F. Provocative testing with ergonovine to assess the efficacy of treatment with nifedipine, diltiazem and verapamil in variant angina. *Am J Cardiol* 1981; 48:123–130.

250. Waters DD, Szlachcic J, Théroux P, Dauwe F, Mizgala HF. Ergonovine testing to detect spontaneous remissions of variant angina during long-term treatment with calcium antagonist drugs. *Am J Cardiol* 1981; 47:179–184.

251. Waters DD, Bouchard A, Théroux P. Spontaneous remission is a frequent outcome of variant angina. *J Am Coll Cardiol* 1983; 2:195–199.

252. Previtali M, Panciroli C, Ardissino D, Chimienti M, Angoli L, Salerno JA. Spontaneous remission of variant angina documented by Holter monitoring and ergonovine testing in patients treated with calcium antagonists. *Am J Cardiol* 1987; 59:235–240.

253. Walling A, Waters DD, Miller DD, Roy D, Pelletier GB, Théroux P. Long-term prognosis of patients with variant angina. *Circulation* 1987; 76:990–997.

254. Tilmant PY, Lablanche JM, Thieuleux FA, Dupuis BA, Bertrand ME. Detrimental effect of propranolol in patients with coronary arterial spasm countered by combination with diltiazem. *Am J Cardiol* 1983; 52:230–233.

255. Morikami Y, Yasue H. Efficacy of slow-release nifedipine on myocardial ischemia episodes in variant angina pectoris. *Am J Cardiol* 1991; 68:580–584.

256. Pepine CJ, Feldman RL, Whittle J, Curry C, Conti CR. Effect of diltiazem in patients with variant angina: A randomized double-blind trial. *Am Heart J* 1981; 101:719–725.

257. Johnson SM, Mauritson DR, Willerson JT, Hillis LD. A controlled clinical trial of verapamil for Prinzmetal's variant angina. *N Engl J Med* 1981; 304:862–866.

258. Chahine RA, Feldman RL, Giles TD, Nicod P, Raizner AE, Weiss RJ, et al. Randomized placebo-controlled trial of amlodipine in vasospastic angina. *J Am Coll Cardiol* 1993; 21:1365–1370.

259. Yasue H, Takizawa A, Nagao M, Nishida S, Horie M, Kubota J, et al. Long-term prognosis for patients with variant angina and influential factors. *Circulation* 1988; 78:1–9.

260. Rutitzky B, Girotti AL, Rosenbaum MB. Efficacy of chronic amiodarone therapy in patients with variant angina pectoris and inhibition of ergonovine coronary constriction. *Am Heart J* 1982; 103:38–43.

261. Frenneaux M, Kaski JC, Brown M, Maseri A. Refractory variant angina relieved by guanethidine and clonidine. *Am J Cardiol* 1988; 62:832–833.

262. Miwa K, Kambara H, Kawai C. Exercise-induced angina provoked by aspirin administration in patients with variant angina. *Am J Cardiol* 1981; 47:1210–1214.

263. Mark DB, Califf RM, Morris KG, Harrell FE Jr, Pryor DB, Hlatky MA, et al. Clinical characteristics and long-term survival of patients with variant angina. *Circulation* 1984; 69:880–888.

264. Shubrooks SJ Jr, Bete JM, Hutter AM Jr, Block PC, Buckley MJ, Daggett WM, et al. Variant angina pectoris: Clinical and anatomic spectrum and results of coronary bypass surgery. *Am J Cardiol* 1975; 36:142–147.

265. Bertrand ME, Lablanche JM, Tilmant PY. Treatment of Prinzmetal's variant angina. Role of medical treatment with nifedipine and surgical coronary revascularization combined with plexectomy. *Am J Cardiol* 1981; 47:174–178.

266. Bertrand ME, Lablanche JM, Tilmant PY, Ducloux G, Warembourg H Jr, Soots G. Complete denervation of the heart (autotransplantation) for treatment of severe, refractory coronary spasm. *Am J Cardiol* 1981; 47:1375–1378.

267. Leisch F, Schützenberger W, Kerschner K, Herbinger W. Influence of a variant angina on the results of percutaneous transluminal coronary angioplasty. *Br Heart J* 1986; 56:341–345.

268. Bertrand ME, Lablanche JM, Thieuleux FA, Fourrier JL, Traisnel G, Asseman P. Comparative results of percutaneous transluminal coronary angioplasty in patients with dynamic versus fixed coronary stenosis. *J Am Coll Cardiol* 1986; 8:504–508.

269. Bertrand ME, Lablanche JM, Fourrier JL, Gommeaux A, Ruel M. Relation of restenosis after percutaneous transluminal coronary angioplasty to vasomotion of the dilated coronary arterial segment. *Am J Cardiol* 1989; 63:277–281.

270. Severi S, Davies G, Maseri A, Marzullo P, L'Abbate A. Long-term prognosis of "variant" angina with medical treatment. *Am J Cardiol* 1980; 46:226–232.

271. Nakamura M, Takeshita A, Nose Y. Clinical characteristics associated with myocardial infarction, arrhythmias, and sudden death in patients with vasospastic angina. *Circulation* 1987; 75:1110–1116.

272. Waters DD, Szlachcic J, Miller D, Théroux P. Clinical characteristics of patients with variant angina complicated by myocardial infarction or death within 1 month. *Am J Cardiol* 1982; 49:658–664.

47

DIAGNOSIS AND MANAGEMENT OF PATIENTS WITH ACUTE MYOCARDIAL INFARCTION

R. Wayne Alexander / Craig M. Pratt / Robert Roberts

Progress in the understanding of the pathogenesis of acute myocardial infarction (AMI) and of its treatment epitomizes scientific, evidence-based medicine at its best. Although myocardial infarction has long been a clinically recognized entity resulting from coronary artery atherosclerosis, its relative importance is a modern phenomenon. Its appearance as a modern epidemic reflects increasing longevity, permitting manifestation of chronic "degenerative" diseases such as atherosclerosis; the adoption of high-fat diets based on meats, permitted by increasing affluence; and decreased exercise, made possible by the increased mechanization of society. Osler devoted only a few pages in his textbook, published in 1892, to the discussion of AMI.[1]

The modern era can be said to have begun with the autopsy studies of Herrick, who concluded in 1912 that the clinical syndrome of myocardial infarction results from acute thrombotic occlusion of a coronary artery, with resulting downstream necrosis.[2] This conclusion was generally accepted for 60 years, and the term *coronary thrombosis* was not uncommonly used as the equivalent of *heart attack* or, more formally, *acute myocardial infarction*. The conventional wisdom was challenged in 1972, when it was suggested that the coronary artery thrombus may be the result rather than the cause of acute infarction, since autopsy studies—which were frequently performed several days after the acute event—did not uniformly show thrombus.[3] In retrospect, these findings can be explained by spontaneous lysis of a thrombus that had been occlusive for a sufficient amount of time to cause tissue necrosis. Definitive proof of the central role of thrombus formation in the pathogenesis of myocardial infarction came from angiographic studies performed during the first hours of the acute event,[4,5] a diagnostic strategy that had previously been thought to be contraindicated.[6]

The unequivocal demonstration of the role of the thrombus in AMI quickly led to the systematic testing of thrombolytic strategies to abort myocardial infarctions.[7–9] Analysis of data from several small trials of thrombolytic therapy with streptokinase suggested improved mortality in treated patients as early as 1982.[10] These early efforts were followed by a large number of major multicenter clinical trials on the treatment of acute myocardial infarction; these demonstrated in a rigorous fashion the efficacy of beta-adrenergic receptor blockers,[11] streptokinase versus no thrombolytic therapy,[12] and recombinant tissue plasminogen activator versus streptokinase[13] in reducing mortality. These and other major trials are discussed in detail further on. The major point to be made here is that large, adequately powered, randomized studies in the treatment of myocardial infarction have helped set a new standard and approach to the goal of enhancing the evidence-based practice of medicine while moving away from one based on previous practice patterns and intuitive extrapolations from pathophysiologic principles.

The availability of data from well-designed clinical trials has permitted the development, by panels of experts, of evidence-based practice guidelines for the treatment of myocardial infarction.[14,15] Furthermore, the confidence with which recommendations can be made for any particular diagnostic or therapeutic approach can be graded on the basis of judgments as to the strength of the supporting evidence. Thus, a committee convened by the American College of Cardiology/American Heart Association (ACC/AHA) Task Force on Practice Guidelines was charged with revising the ACC/AHA statement "Guidelines for the Early Management of Patients with Acute Myocardial Infarction," published in 1990.[14] The results of the deliberations of this committee, "Guidelines for the Management of Patients with Acute Myocardial Infarction," were published in late 1996.[15] The evidence and expert opinion supporting use of a therapy, intervention, or diagnostic procedure were weighed and expressed in ACC/AHA format as follows:

Class I: Conditions for which there is evidence and/or general agreement that a given procedure or treatment is beneficial, useful, and effective

Class II: Conditions for which there is conflicting evidence and/or a divergence of opinion about the usefulness/efficacy of a procedure or treatment

Class IIa: Weight of evidence/opinion is in favor of usefulness/efficacy

Class IIb: Usefulness/efficacy is less well established by evidence/opinion

Class III: Conditions for which there is evidence and/or general agreement that a procedure/treatment is not useful/effective and in some cases may be harmful[15]

In general, recommendations in this chapter are associated with a class I, II, or III designation to guide the reader in weighing diagnostic and therapeutic options.

The pathophysiologic bases and consequences of coronary artery disease and myocardial infarction are discussed elsewhere: natural history and prognosis (Chap. 38); pathogenesis of atherosclerosis (Chap. 39); pathology of coronary atherosclerosis (Chap. 40); risk factors and prevention (Chap. 41); nonatherosclerotic causes of coronary heart disease (spontaneous coronary artery dissection, aortic dissection, thrombosis associated with the use of birth-control pills, emboli, congenital coronary anomalies, metabolic abnormalities, blunt chest trauma, vasculitis, and drug abuse, especially cocaine) (Chap. 42); pathophysiology of myocardial ischemia (Chap. 43); pathophysiology of coronary artery disease as related to myocardial ischemic syndromes (Chap. 44); and thrombogenesis and antithrombotic therapy (Chap. 52).

The following are important general facts about myocardial infarction:

1. Approximately 900,000 persons in the United States experience acute myocardial infarction annually; of these, about 225,000 die. Of those who die, approximately one-half do so within 1 h of the onset of symptoms, before reaching a hospital.[15–17]

2. The majority of early deaths are the result of ventricular arrhythmias that can be readily aborted by defibrillation, either during prehospital care or in coronary care units (CCU) in the hospital.

3. The major cause of myocardial infarction is atherosclerotic disease of the epicardial coronary arteries, as noted. Although luminal narrowing resulting in hemodynamically significant obstruction of blood flow is the major cause of symptoms of coronary ischemia (Chap. 45), the majority of myocardial infarctions occur as a result of the disruption of arterial lesions that are not hemodynamically significant (<60 percent). This breakdown of the structural integrity of the arterial intima occurs because of weakening induced by proteolytic degrada-

tion of matrix proteins by products released from inflammatory leukocytes[18] and results in the exposure of blood to thrombogenic intimal material, causing obstructive clot formation. Local vasospasm may contribute to the obstruction. *These observations have led to the concept that the biological state of atherosclerotic lesions and not the extent of stenosis is the major determinant of whether or not plaque rupture and myocardial infarction occur.*

4. Myocardial infarction, or ischemia, is a segmental process limited to the distribution of the affected artery. Impaired contractility usually occurs within seconds of the cessation of blood flow. The process usually begins in the endocardium and spreads toward the epicardium. If flow is restored before cell death occurs, prolonged contractile impairment (stunning) may occur.

5. Episodes of ischemia preceding coronary occlusion enhance the survivability of myocardial cells (*ischemic preconditioning*).

6. Irreversible cardiac injury occurs if occlusion is complete for at least 15 to 20 min. Irreversible injury occurs maximally in the area at risk when occlusion is sustained for 4 to 6 h, but most of the damage occurs in the first 2 to 3 h. Thus, restoration of flow within the first 4 to 6 h is associated with salvage of the myocardium, but the salvage is exponentially greater if restoration occurs in 1 to 2 h.

7. Restoration of blood flow by thrombolysis results in myocardial salvage and improved mortality. The extent of the benefit is dependent upon restoration of near-normal blood flow (*open-artery hypothesis*), and is inversely related to the time between the onset of occlusion (symptoms) and the restoration of blood flow.

8. The percentage of tissue at risk that undergoes necrosis (infarct size) depends on existing collateral flow, which is highly variable and difficult to predict.

9. The major predictor of long-term outcome is infarct size, which is inversely related to the ejection fraction.

10. Q-wave infarction (usually presenting as ST-segment elevation) is a distinct clinical entity, as compared with non-Q-wave infarction (usually presenting with ST-segment depression). There are differential features in their clinical courses. (Q-wave infarction, untreated, has a relatively high in-hospital mortality rate that is very favorably influenced by thrombolysis, whereas non-Q-wave infarction has a lower in-hospital mortality and complication rate with a prolonged vulnerability to reinfarction. Thrombolysis may worsen the clinical outcome.) Although there is no close anatomic correlation between the presence and absence of Q waves and transmural and nontransmural myocardial infarction, the distinct clinical outcomes of patients presenting with ST-segment elevation and ST-segment depression have made this electrocardiographic feature a major initial decision point in assigning therapeutic strategies to patients presenting with symptoms compatible with AMI.

11. Because of their salutary effects on thrombus formation and ventricular arrhythmias, aspirin and beta-adrenergic blockers, respectively, have proven to be effective for secondary prevention in patients who have had a myocardial infarction. Aspirin has also been shown to be modestly effective for primary prevention in middle-aged males.

12. Lipid lowering and smoking cessation have both been shown to be effective in the primary and secondary prevention of myocardial infarction.

The enormous progress that has been made in understanding the pathogenesis and treatment of myocardial infarction has resulted in very substantial improvements in outcomes in recent years. Indeed, the "natural history" of treated patients has improved dramatically. The mortality rate in the pre-CCU era has been estimated to have been about 30 percent.[19] The mortality rate dropped dramatically, to about 15 percent, in the CCU era, which embraced the use of hemodynamic monitoring, defibrillation, and the use of beta blockers. The increased use of thrombolytics, coronary interventions, and aspirin has decreased the mortality of treated patients to 5 percent or less.[20] Nowadays, the major challenge is to bring the principles and lessons learned from the efforts of the past decade to everyday clinical practice.

CLINICAL ASPECTS

Predisposing Characteristics and Circumstances

The standard risk factors for the development of coronary artery disease (dyslipidemia, family history, age, male gender, cigarette smoking, diabetes mellitus, and hypertension) are well established and are discussed in Chap. 41. *Careful consideration of the probabilities of the presence of coronary artery disease is centrally important in the initial assessment and evaluation of testing results of any patient with chest pain.* The experienced clinician will calibrate his or her responses even within the context of algorithmic approaches to the evaluation of chest pain. For example, the 35-year-old male with atypical chest pain whose father died of coronary disease at less than age 50 and whose mother had a coronary bypass at age 55 would be viewed with a higher index of suspicion than if both his parents and grandparents were alive and well. This higher level of concern might translate into ordering diagnostic modalities with a higher level of sensitivity and specificity for detecting coronary artery disease in the former as opposed to the latter case.

As discussed in Chaps. 39, 40, and 44, atherosclerosis generally and including the disease in the coronary arteries is a chronic inflammation representing the response of the arterial wall to the stress imposed by various risk factors. Acute myocardial infarction has commonly been shown to occur as a result of the disruption of a coronary artery plaque at a site of a high density of inflammatory cells.[20] Thus, AMI can be thought of as resulting from the acute exacerbation of

a chronic inflammatory response. There is increasing clinical evidence supporting this view. Thus, unstable angina, a frequent antecedent of myocardial infarction,[21] has been shown to be associated with elevated plasma levels of the acute-phase reactant C-reactive protein.[22,23] Recent observations from the Physicians' Health Study, which showed that subjects with the highest levels of C-reactive protein have an increased long-term risk of cardiac events, is also supportive of the concept that inflammatory responses are important in the pathogenesis of acute myocardial infarction.[24] *Thus, events precipitating myocardial infarctions can be viewed as exacerbating the arterial inflammatory response and/or increasing the physical forces impinging on a coronary artery lesion weakened by inflammation, leading to rupture.*

Precipitating Events

There is little direct but intriguing indirect evidence that external factors might exacerbate the arterial inflammatory response. An association has been noted between acute myocardial infarction and antecedent mild respiratory syndromes.[24] It is possible that an infection, by activating systemic responses, could stimulate or activate previously quiescent atherosclerotic lesions. A more specific relationship between acute myocardial infarction and an infectious agent has been posited in the case of *Chlamydia pneumoniae*.[25–27] Increased antibody titers to *C. pneumoniae* in subsets of patients have been associated with increased risk for acute infarction, and acute infarction–associated increases in circulating immune complexes, followed by a subsequent increase in antibody titers, have been observed.[28] Evidence exists for the presence of chlamydiae in atherosclerotic coronary artery lesions.[29] Thus, it is possible that *C. pneumoniae* infection contributes to the inflammatory responses in atherosclerosis and that acute reinfection activates the inflammatory response, leading to myocardial infarction. This area requires further investigation.

There is considerable evidence associating AMI with emotional or environmental stresses. It is likely that the majority of these stresses involve activation of the sympathetic nervous system, with increases in locally released and circulating catecholamines. Increased sympathetic drive increases cardiac oxygen consumption by increasing contractility and rate. Sympathetic stimulation will also increase shear forces and stress on vascular atherosclerotic lesions by augmenting contraction and torque and elevating blood pressure. Superimposition of these forces on a vessel weakened by inflammation can lead to plaque rupture. Enhanced circulating catecholamine levels can increase the propensity for thrombus formation by activating platelets. Such a scenario likely explains the association (in about 4 to 7 percent of patients) between acute increases in physical exertion and the development of myocardial infarction, especially among those who do not exercise regularly.[30,31] Similarly, episodes of anger increase the risk of precipitating myocardial infarction in susceptible persons.[32] Distressing or changing life events reportedly occur with increased frequency in the months preceding a myocardial infarction.[33-35] A more recent well-controlled study found no correlation between the occurrence of acute infarction and the presence of unusual life events for up to 4 weeks prior to the event.[30]

It is apparent that any stressful event or intervention can precipitate AMI in a patient with "active," susceptible coronary atherosclerotic lesions. Anesthesia and surgery are well known to enhance the risk of myocardial infarction, and cardiac events are the leading cause of perioperative morbidity.[36] Perioperatively, stress can be induced by tachycardia and hypotension,[37] anemia,[38] and *hypothermia*.[39] A recent study in patients with coronary disease undergoing noncardiac surgery has shown that the usual perioperative hypothermia was associated with a relative risk of cardiac events of 2.2, as contrasted to a similar group in whom normothermia was maintained.[40] The salutary effects of maintaining normothermia were thought to be due to the prevention of cardiac stress imposed by activation of the sympathetic nervous system. By extension, many of the stressful events—such as pulmonary emboli, stroke, hypoxia, allergic responses, blood loss, etc.— that have been associated with the precipitation of acute myocardial infarction can likely be related to the effects of adrenergic stimulation by an excess of catecholamines.

Myocardial infarction can occur because of low perfusion pressure in shock of any etiology and can arise in severe aortic stenosis even in the absence of coronary artery disease because of excessive oxygen demands in a very hypertrophic ventricle with, for example, marked tachycardia. Other non-atherosclerotic causes of myocardial infarction, including trauma, embolism, and dissection, are discussed in Chap. 42. Vasospasm in the absence of angiographically demonstrable coronary artery disease has recently been reported to have caused acute myocardial infarction in several patients during general anesthesia.[41] Also, it is likely that vasospasm plays a central role in cocaine-induced myocardial infarction.[42]

Personality Types

It has been claimed that so-called coronary-prone individuals exhibit certain personality traits, such as compulsive hard work and being deadline-driven and excessively competitive. Categorizing people with such traits as "type A" and thus as being at increased risk for myocardial infarction was formerly widely discussed.[43] This concept is not widely accepted now,[44] and the psychological contributions to heart disease are generally considered to be more complex (see Chap. 89).

Circadian and Seasonal Variation

Results of the Multicenter Investigation of Limitation of Infarct Size (MILIS) study showed a marked circadian periodicity in the occurrence of myocardial infarction, with a peak prevalence between 6 A.M. and noon. The circadian rhythm was present whether the onset of the infarction was marked subjectively by the appearance of pain or objectively by plasma MB-CK levels. There was a threefold increase in the frequency of infarction at peak (9 A.M.) periods as compared

with trough (11 P.M.) periods.[45] As a corollary, sudden death attributed to ischemic heart disease has a similar circadian periodicity. Available data suggest that the rhythms both for the occurrence of myocardial infarction and for deaths from ischemic events are actually bimodal. These rhythms are characterized not only by the morning peak but also by a secondary, less pronounced late-afternoon or early-evening peak (6 to 8 P.M.).[46]

The mechanisms underlying this temporal distribution of ischemic events are not completely understood but are probably related to diurnal variations in thrombotic tendencies and to sympathetic nervous system activity. There is both an enhanced platelet aggregability[47] and a trough in intrinsic fibrinolytic activity during the morning hours.[48] A similar circadian variation is observed for cerebral infarction,[49] which further implicates an increased propensity for thrombosis in the morning hours. The blunting of the morning peak of myocardial infarction by both aspirin and beta-adrenergic blockers emphasizes the contributions of both the sympathetic nervous system and the coagulation pathways to the circadian rhythm of cardiovascular events.[50]

Other endogenous daily rhythms may be causally related. Ambulatory ST-segment changes in patients with coronary artery disease have demonstrated a close correlation between basal heart rate (which is higher in the morning) and the frequency of ischemic ST-segment changes.[51] These observations may be mechanistically related to the morning increase in tone noted in coronary artery segments with dysfunctional endothelium-dependent dilation in patients with chronic stable angina (see Chaps. 4 and 44).[52] Circadian variations in blood pressure[53] and plasma catecholamine levels[54] that parallel those of ischemic events have been observed. The morning increase in sympathetic activity not only increases the metabolic demand but may also cause coronary vasoconstriction that is unopposed by normal endothelial vasodilator mechanisms, as implied above.

There also appear to be exogenous rhythms that influence the development of acute myocardial infarction. In a working population, there is an increased risk for infarction on Mondays.[55] Seasonal variations have also been commented upon, with increases in the winter months of January through March.[56]

Symptoms

Prodromal symptoms antedating AMI are common and occur in at least 60 percent of patients.[57] Since at least 8 to 10 percent of AMIs are painless (not necessarily silent) and many ischemic episodes are silent,[58] it is apparent that the great majority of patients capable of sensing cardiac pain during periods of *unstable angina* do so in the hours, days, or sometimes weeks prior to the acute event. Most of these symptoms are anginal or angina-like, especially when assessed retrospectively in the context of the character of the pain of the acute infarct. The antecedent symptoms may also be anginal equivalents, such as paroxysmal dyspnea (see Chap. 45). The clinical features of unstable angina are discussed in Chap. 46. If one considers the general feeling of malaise and fatigue that many patients report having experienced prior to acute infarction, it is apparent that it is relatively unusual for the episode to be totally unheralded—a conclusion that is consistent with general clinical experience.

The *classic symptoms* of AMI involve chest discomfort that is commonly retrosternal or precordial in *location* and is described as pressure, aching, burning, crushing, squeezing, heavy, swelling, or bursting in *quality*.[59,60] The location of chest pain is usually of little help in differentiating ischemia/infarction from other causes of chest pain,[61] but severe chest pain (as opposed to vague discomfort) and the presence of associated symptoms (dyspnea, nausea, diaphoresis, etc.) are more commonly associated with AMI.[62] The discomfort often *radiates* over the anterior chest and frequently into the left arm or both arms (particularly the medial aspect), and/or into the neck or jaw. In unusual instances, the pain may be in the back, particularly between the scapulae. There may be skip areas with retrosternal pain—associated with jaw, antecubital fossa, or wrist pain—or no pain between the two sites. Moreover, the pain may appear only in the referral area. The *duration* of the pain of infarction is prolonged, lasting by definition longer than 15 min. While the intensity of the pain is usually steady following an initial crescendo, there is occasionally some waxing and waning. Sudden relief of pain may accompany reperfusion. *Associated symptoms* may include dyspnea, diaphoresis, nausea, and vomiting. Marked apprehension is common. Occasionally, presenting symptoms include syncope, acute confusion, agitation, stroke, or palpitations.

Approximately 23 percent of myocardial infarctions go unrecognized by patients because of the absence of symptoms or the lack of recognition of the significance of symptoms.[63] The common symptoms in this latter instance are nonclassic or atypical pain, dyspnea, nausea, vomiting, and/or epigastric pain. A myocardial infarction may also masquerade as the development or worsening of congestive heart failure, the appearance of an arrhythmia, an overwhelming sense of apprehension, profound weakness, acute indigestion, pericarditis, embolic stroke, or peripheral embolus.[64] Presentation with painless myocardial infarction is more common in the elderly than in the nonelderly, and this subgroup has an increased frequency of congestive heart failure as the initial presenting symptom.[65]

Physical Findings

GENERAL EXAMINATION

Features of the physical examination during AMI have been the subject of several reviews.[66,67] The patient is frequently sitting up because of a sense of suffocation or a feeling of shortness of breath. Most patients with cardiac pain or myocardial infarction have some sense of impending doom that is reflected in their facial expression. They may have a grayish appearance or one of panic or exhaustion. Diaphoresis is frequent. In severe cases, patients may be quite anxious, with an ashen or pale face beaded with perspiration.

The patient should be examined in both the supine and left lateral decubitus position. The major findings pertaining to the heart appear on palpation of the precordium in the left lateral position. It is important to rapidly ascertain the vital signs and the nature, character, and rhythm of the arterial pulse; to observe the jugular venous pulse; to check the peripheral pulses; to palpate the precordium; and to auscultate the chest and precordium. Examination of the extremities should include subjective assessment of the temperature and color of the feet. The presence of very cool feet, especially with acrocyanosis in the setting of tachycardia, suggests low cardiac output.

The heart rate and rhythm are very important indicators of cardiac function in the initial hours of myocardial infarction. *A normal rate usually indicates that the patient is not experiencing significant hemodynamic compromise.* In patients with inferior myocardial infarction, heart rates in the fifties and sixties are very common in the initial hours. Up to 60 percent of these patients initially have bradycardia, but the rate gradually increases over the next few hours. The bradycardia, which may be associated with secondary hypotension, results from the stimulation of myocardial receptors with vagal afferents. *Persistent sinus tachycardia beyond the initial 12 to 24 h is predictive of a very high mortality rate.* The pulse may be low in volume, reflecting decreased stroke volume. The blood pressure is usually normal but may be increased secondary to anxiety, or it may be decreased from cardiac failure. Blood pressure frequently normalizes temporarily with AMI in patients with hypertension. All peripheral pulses should be examined to observe their presence, and their status should be noted both to exclude current occlusion and to provide a baseline in case of future embolic events. The carotid pulse is most useful in assessing systolic upstroke time and stroke volume, which are decreased in the patient with a low-output state.

The rhythm of the pulse is very important because of the frequency of ectopic atrial and, in particular, ventricular beats in AMI. Observation of the jugular venous pulse is useful in determining whether ectopic beats are atrial or ventricular. A large A wave, indicating that the right atrium is contracting against a closed atrioventricular valve, suggests that the ectopic beat is ventricular.

The respiratory rate is usually within the normal range. However, patients who are extremely anxious often exhibit hyperventilation, and those with pulmonary edema and cardiac failure have an increased respiratory rate associated with shallow inspirations. Abnormal breathing patterns, such as Cheyne-Stokes respirations, are rare unless the patient is in cardiogenic shock.

Examination of the jugular venous pulse is important with AMI, especially in patients with an inferior infarction, because insights can be gained into possible involvement of the right ventricle. The right ventricle is commonly involved with inferior infarction, but right-sided failure is seen only with major right ventricular involvement. It may be manifest by an elevated jugular venous pressure. In addition, in many patients with right ventricular infarction, there is also a prominent A wave because of the decreased compliance of the right ventricle.[68] Kussmaul's sign, or an increase in the venous pressure on inspiration, may also be seen in right ventricular infarction because of decreased right ventricular compliance. Generally, right ventricular failure commonly reflects left ventricular failure, with secondary elevation in pulmonary and right ventricular pressures. This circumstance usually occurs with large anterior or anterolateral infarction.

EXAMINATION OF THE LUNGS

Basilar rales are frequently detected in AMI. Cardiac failure diagnosed on the basis of mild signs of pulmonary congestion occurs in 30 to 40 percent of patients with otherwise uncomplicated myocardial infarction. A clinical classification proposed by Killip provides some uniformity in terms of describing cardiac failure and pulmonary congestion. Class I patients do not have any pulmonary rales or a third heart sound. Class II patients have rales of a mild to moderate degree, involving less than 50 percent of the lung fields, and may or may not have an S3 gallop. Class III patients have rales more than halfway up the lung fields and an S3 gallop. Class IV patients are those in cardiogenic shock.

CARDIAC EXAMINATION

Palpation of the precordium may reveal evidence of regional wall motion abnormalities. Palpation should be performed with the patient initially lying in the supine position; this is often adequate to ascertain whether there is a localized normal apical impulse and also permits assessment for dyskinetic impulses (see Chap. 10). Frequently, one may not feel any precordial impulse with the patient in the supine position because of the decreased intensity of contraction and/or body habitus. With the patient in the left lateral decubitus position, one may palpate a diffuse rather than a localized apical impulse, akinesis, or a paradoxical bulging during late systole; in some patients, there is a palpable atrial contraction corresponding to an audible S4 gallop due to the decreased compliance of the left ventricle. One or more of these features of decreased contractility or lusitrophy and dyssynergy are frequently present in the early hours of AMI, particularly with extensive damage.

The first and second heart sounds are often very soft because of decreased contractility. The first heart sound may also be diminished because of a prolonged PR interval. If there is tachycardia, a shortened PR interval may result in a somewhat accentuated first heart sound. The second heart sound is usually normal; however, with extensive damage, there may be a single second sound. Rarely, paradoxical splitting may reflect severe left ventricular dysfunction. A fourth heart sound is often audible in patients with AMI. A third heart sound is heard in probably only about 15 to 20 percent of AMI patients. A pericardial friction rub is usually not heard until 48 to 72 h after the onset of myocardial infarction and

occurs in only about 10 percent of patients. The murmur of papillary muscle dysfunction is relatively common early in the course of infraction. This crescendo-decrescendo midsystolic murmur often reflects ischemia of the papillary muscles or the myocardial attachment rather than irreversible injury to these structures. This murmur usually disappears after the first 12 to 24 h if it is soft; however, if the murmur is moderate to loud in intensity, it may persist much longer, possibly throughout the patient's life. Mitral regurgitation is most commonly due to ischemia of the posteromedial papillary muscle (see also Chap. 10). Other findings on physical examination, such as the murmur of papillary muscle rupture or a ruptured ventricular septum, are described in appropriate sections under "Complications."

Diagnosis of Acute Myocardial Infarction

DIFFERENTIAL DIAGNOSIS

Myocardial infarction has typically been diagnosed on the basis of the triad of chest pain, electrocardiographic changes, and elevated plasma enzyme activity. Although AMI occurs without chest pain (20 to 25 percent of cases), chest pain remains the most common symptom and is usually responsible for the patient's seeking medical help. The differential diagnosis of prolonged chest pain is presented in Table 47-1. Chest pain, however, is not specific to cardiac disease, and it is often impossible on the basis of history alone to distinguish ischemia or infarction from other causes of chest pain. The differential diagnosis of chest pain is discussed in Chap. 45. Of patients presenting to the emergency department with chest pain, only about 14 percent are subsequently documented to have AMI.[69–72] Most patients at risk for myocardial infarction will be admitted to evaluate their chest pain unless definite noncardiac causes of chest pain—such as chest wall pain,

---

TABLE 47-1

DIFFERENTIAL DIAGNOSIS
OF PROLONGED CHEST PAIN

AMI
Aortic dissection
Pericarditis
Atypical anginal pain associated with hypertrophic cardiomyopathy
Esophageal, other upper gastrointestinal, or biliary tract disease
Pulmonary disease
Pleurisy: infectious, malignant, or immune disease–related
Embolus with or without infarction
Pneumothorax
Hyperventilation syndrome
Chest wall
Skeletal
Neuropathic
Psychogenic

hyperventilation, pleurisy, gastrointestinal pain, and so on—that are not imminently dangerous can be identified. In the CCU, only about 20 percent of patients admitted with chest pain have AMI.

ELECTROCARDIOGRAPHIC DIAGNOSIS

The electrocardiogram (ECG) is very sensitive for detecting myocardial ischemia and infarction but is frequently not powerful enough for differentiating ischemia from necrosis (see Chap. 12).[70,71,73] Serial ECGs during AMI will show some evolutionary changes in the majority of patients.[74] An ECG obtained during cardiac ischemic pain frequently but not always exhibits changes in repolarization. The absence of electrocardiographic changes during pain provides evidence but not proof that the pain is not ischemic in nature. The early electrocardiographic changes of T-wave inversion or ST-segment depression may reflect ischemia or infarction. ST-segment elevation is more specific for AMI and reflects the epicardial injury–associated total occlusion of an epicardial coronary artery. The hallmark of AMI is the development of abnormal Q waves,[75,76] which appear on the average 8 to 12 h from the onset of symptoms but may not develop for 24 to 48 h. Abnormal Q waves usually reflect tissue death and the development of an electrical dead zone. Since abnormal Q waves do not develop immediately, they are not very helpful for initial diagnostic management and therapeutic triage except to signify the presence or absence of prior myocardial infarction. The diagnostic serial electrocardiographic changes consist of ST-segment elevation with the development of T-wave inversion and the evolution of abnormal Q waves (Fig. 47-1).[744] The appearance of abnormal Q waves is very specific to AMI; however, they are present in less than 50 percent of patients with documented AMI.[77] Most of the other patients who have AMI will have electrocardiographic changes restricted to T-wave inversion or ST-segment depression or no change at all.[73] These patients represent the group with non-Q-wave infarction.[78]

The traditional concept that myocardial infarctions can be classified as transmural or nontransmural on the basis of the presence or absence of Q waves is misleading, since autopsy studies have demonstrated convincingly that pathologic Q waves may be associated with nontransmural infarction and may be absent with transmural infarction.[79–81] These misnomers have been replaced by the terms *Q-wave infarction* and *non-Q-wave infarction* for *transmural* and *nontransmural infarction*, respectively.[82] The evolution of a non-Q-wave infarction is characterized by a lack of development of an abnormal Q wave and by the appearance of reversible ST-T-wave changes with ST depression that usually return to normal over a few days, but are occasionally permanent. Differentiation between these two types of infarctions has become entrenched, since there are major differences in their pathogenesis, clinical manifestations, treatment, and prognosis (Table 47-2). The initiating events in the pathogenesis of Q-wave and non-Q-wave infarction are thought to be identical, namely, coronary occlusion induced by a thrombus superimposed on a plaque

together with vasoconstriction (see Chap. 40). There is considerable evidence, however, to indicate that in non-Q-wave infarction, early spontaneous reperfusion occurs, the mechanism of which remains uncertain. In contrast, in Q-wave infarction, the coronary occlusion is sustained at least for a long enough period to result in extensive necrosis.

One explanation for early spontaneous reperfusion is the lack of sustained vasoconstriction, which may contribute to occlusion.[83] The evidence supporting the existence of early spontaneous reperfusion in non-Q-wave infarction is as follows: (1) Coronary angiographic studies performed in the early hours after onset show that only about 20 to 30 percent of patients have complete coronary occlusion of infarct-related vessels; however, for Q-wave infarction, it is about 80 to 90 percent. (2) Infarct size is routinely much less than observed with Q-wave infarction, which is consistent with salvage by early reperfusion. (3) Peak plasma creatine kinase (CK) levels are reached on an average of 12 to 13 h after onset of symptoms, indicating early washout of the enzyme, as opposed to about 27 h after Q-wave infarction. (4) Reperfusion-induced contraction necrosis is extremely common, as it is in patients who undergo early reperfusion induced by thrombolytic therapy.[84] (5) Acute mortality rates are around 2 to 3 percent, compared with 10 percent for Q-wave infarction. (6) The complications are minimal compared with those after a Q-wave infarction. (7) Finally, the long-term prognosis is characterized by recurrent episodes of reinfarction, so that after about 2 years, survival is the same as that after Q-wave infarction.[78,85–88]

Traditional teaching has held that AMI could not be diagnosed electrocardiographically in the presence of a left bundle branch block because of the unpredictability of the depolarization and repolarization patterns. Recently, it has been suggested that marked ST-segment deviation, beyond what could be anticipated from the conduction abnormality, could be useful in the diagnosis of AMI in the setting of a left bundle branch block.[89]

The resting ECG is insensitive for detecting the presence of atherosclerotic coronary heart disease; it is normal in 50 percent of patients with angiographically significant coronary obstruction.[90] Nevertheless, an abnormally wide Q wave on a resting ECG has been the standard criterion for the diagnosis of a myocardial infarction for over 60 years.[91]

The electrocardiographic criteria for the diagnosis of AMI as outlined in the MILIS study are the presence, in the setting of chest pain, of any one of the following: (1) new or presumably new Q waves (at least 30 ms wide and 0.20 mV deep) in at least two leads from any of the following: (a) leads II, III, or aV_F; (b) leads V_1 through V_6; or (c) leads I and aV_L; (2) new or presumably new ST-T-segment elevation or depression (≥ 0.10 mV measured 0.02 s after the J point in two contiguous leads of the above-mentioned lead combination); or (3) a complete left bundle branch block in the appropriate clinical setting. An evaluation of these criteria in 1809 enzyme-confirmed infarctions found that 21 percent of the patients with an infarction had none of these changes.[92] Conversely, over

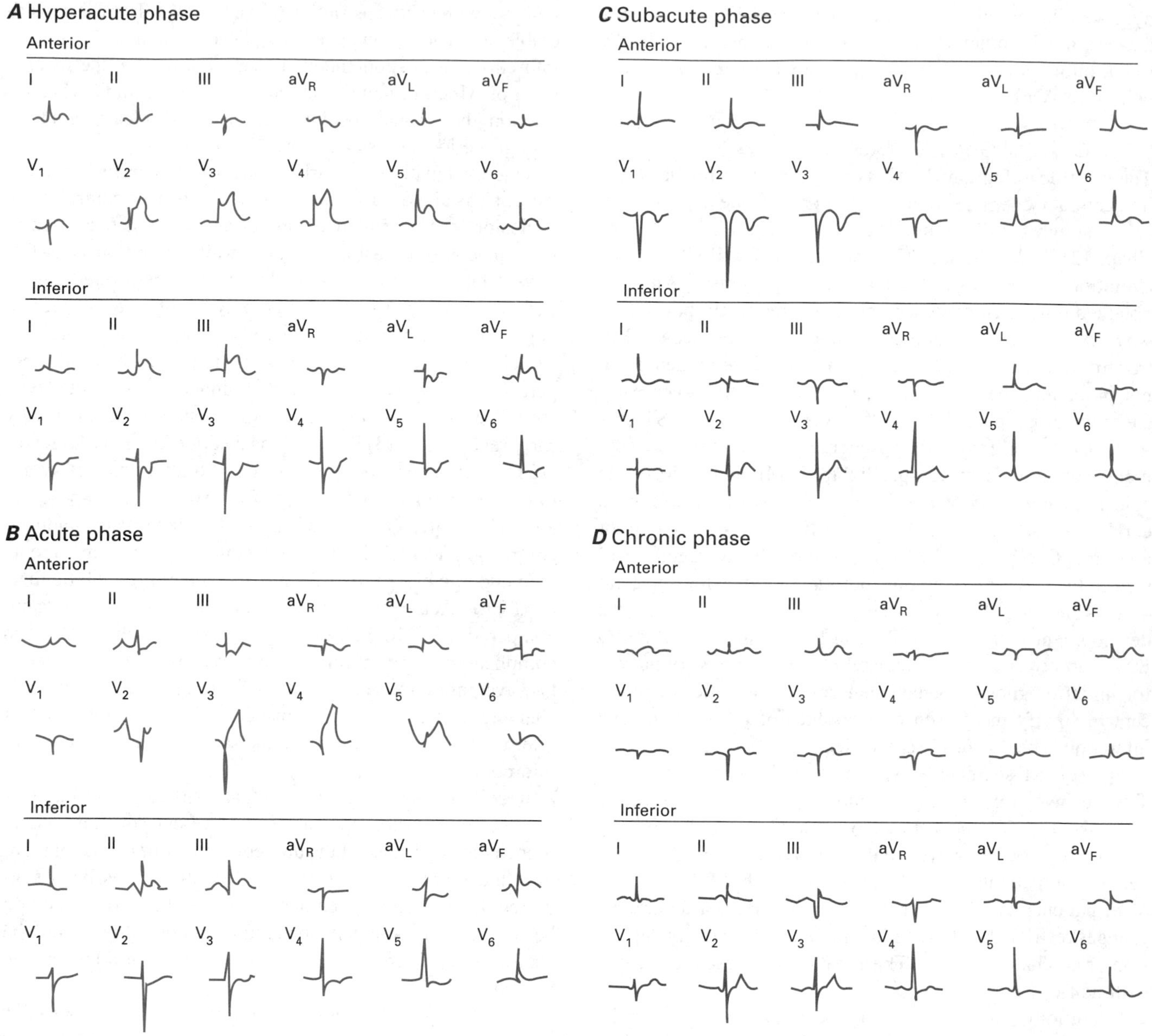

A Hyperacute phase

Anterior

I   II   III   aV_R   aV_L   aV_F

V_1   V_2   V_3   V_4   V_5   V_6

Inferior

I   II   III   aV_R   aV_L   aV_F

V_1   V_2   V_3   V_4   V_5   V_6

B Acute phase

Anterior

I   II   III   aV_R   aV_L   aV_F

V_1   V_2   V_3   V_4   V_5   V_6

Inferior

I   II   III   aV_R   aV_L   aV_F

V_1   V_2   V_3   V_4   V_5   V_6

C Subacute phase

Anterior

I   II   III   aV_R   aV_L   aV_F

V_1   V_2   V_3   V_4   V_5   V_6

Inferior

I   II   III   aV_R   aV_L   aV_F

V_1   V_2   V_3   V_4   V_5   V_6

D Chronic phase

Anterior

I   II   III   aV_R   aV_L   aV_F

V_1   V_2   V_3   V_4   V_5   V_6

Inferior

I   II   III   aV_R   aV_L   aV_F

V_1   V_2   V_3   V_4   V_5   V_6

FIGURE 47-1

Electrocardiographic evolution of acute anterior and inferior myocardial infarction. *A.* Hyperacute phase. There is marked ST-segment elevation in V_2 to V_5 in the anterior infarction and in II, III, and aV_f in the inferior infarction. In the inferior infarction, there are reciprocal changes or posterior involvement as reflected in the ST-segment depression in the precordial leads. There are no QRS changes in either case. *B.* Acute phase. Q waves indicating myocardial necrosis develop during this phase. There is some persistent ST-segment elevation and the T-wave vector generally points toward the infarct zone. *C.* Subacute phase. QRS changes are well developed and ST-segment elevation is still present. The T vector, or, more precisely, the terminal portion of the T vector, begins to point away from the infarct zone. *D.* Chronic phase. Minimal or no ST-segment elevation is present and the T wave is directed away from the infarct zone. (From Wagner et al.,[744] with permission.)

90 percent of patients who had ST-segment elevation of 0.1 mV, as described previously, were confirmed to have AMI. If the patients also had ST-segment depression in the so-called reciprocal leads, the infarction rate was 3 percent higher. Patients with a left branch bundle block or ST-segment depression without other abnormalities had a lower rate of infarction (46 and 52 to 56 percent, respectively). Furthermore, the presence of abnormal Q waves on the resting ECG accurately predicts the presence and location of left ventricular contraction abnormalities. In a study of 64 patients with abnormal Q waves on the ECG, all patients with abnormal Q waves in the anterior leads and 30 of 33 with abnormal Q waves in the inferior leads demonstrated contraction abnormalities in the corresponding left ventricular segments.[93] The evolution of a Q-wave myocardial infarction can be separated electrocardiographically into four phases: (1) hyperacute, (2) acute, (3) subacute, and (4) chronic stabilized (Fig. 47-1; see Chap. 12).

TABLE 47-2

DIFFERENCES BETWEEN PATIENTS WITH Q-WAVE AND NON-Q-WAVE MYOCARDIAL INFARCTION

Characteristic	Q-Wave	Non-Q-Wave
Prevalence	47%	53%
Incidence of coronary occlusion	80–90%	15–25%
ST-T segment elevation	80%	25%
ST-T segment depression	20%	75%
Postinfarction angina	15–25%	30–40%
Incidence of early reinfarction	5–8%	15–25%
1-Month mortality	10–15%	3–5%
2-Year mortality	30%	30%
Infarct size	Moderate to large 10–20%	Usually small
Residual ischemia		40–50%
Acute complication	Common	Uncommon
Therapy		
Thrombolysis	Indicated	Not indicated
Beta-adrenergic blockers	Indicated	Retrospective analysis shows ineffective
Calcium channel blockers		
Nifedepine	Possibly detrimental	Not determined
Diltiazem	Not indicated	Recommended
Verapamil	Beneficial	Possibly beneficial but not established

In the hyperacute phase (Fig 47-1), the earliest electrocardiographic manifestation of an acute infarction is usually a straightening of the normal upward concavity of the ST-T segment.[94] With further evolution, the straightened ST-T segment becomes elevated. The ST-T segment usually slopes upward, since the portion of the ST-T segment nearest the T wave is more elevated than the proximal portion. Also, the amplitude of the T wave is usually increased. Occasionally, the ST-T segment may be markedly elevated and yet retain its upward concavity. ST-T depressions in leads oriented toward the presumably noninfarcted myocardium were traditionally termed *reciprocal changes*. Recent studies have indicated that such ST-T depressions usually reflect more extensive infarction. In the subacute phase, the abnormal Q wave representing myocardial necrosis begins to appear, but the T-wave vector still points toward the infarct zone (Fig. 47-1). In the fully evolved phase, the ST-T segment begins to diminish in amplitude and becomes coved or convex upward. It blends into the now symmetrically inverted T waves (see Fig 47-1). The abnormal Q waves (>0.03 s in duration and more than 25 percent of the R-wave amplitude) appear

during this stage. During the chronic phase (Fig. 47-1), there is generally resolution of the ST- and T-wave changes, with the only residual change being an abnormal Q wave. Although the ST-T segments again become isoelectric, they are frequently horizontal, with a sharp-angled ST-T junction, rather than exhibiting the normal concavity. Occasionally, in small inferior infarctions, even the abnormal Q waves resolve.

Posterior myocardial infarction occurs in the posterior left ventricular wall. An isolated true posterior infarction is quite uncommon, since such an infarction is usually associated with an inferior or lateral infarction. Since there are no electrocardiographic leads oriented toward the posterior left ventricular wall, the electrocardiographic changes of a true posterior infarction are seen as mirror-image representations in leads V_1 to V_3. Perloff described the criteria for a true posterior infarction as follows: R waves of 0.04 s in lead V_1 and in contiguous right precordial leads with upright T waves, and, in the acute phase, ST-segment depression and an R/S ratio equal to or greater than 1 in leads V_1 and V_2.[94] Usually, there are associated changes of an inferior or lateral infarction. As the infarction evolves, the ST-segment depression decreases and the upright T-wave amplitude increases. It is helpful to turn the ECG upside down and look at it from the back while holding it to a strong light. The changes in leads V_1 and V_2, which might be overlooked on a direct glance, are seen as abnormal Q waves, ST-segment elevation, and T-wave inversion when viewed from this perspective.

Similarly, electrocardiographic diagnosis of right ventricular infarction offers special challenges. Since right ventricular infarction occurs in the presence of inferior left ventricular infarction, the resulting ST-segment elevation is usually overwhelmed in the conventional precordial leads overlying the right ventricle (V_2 and V_3) by the ST-segment elevation in the opposing left ventricular myocardium on the inferior surface. The right ventricular electrical forces might be manifest in this setting as a diminution of the usual reciprocal ST-segment depression seen in the right precordial leads in inferior infarction. If the injury to the inferior wall is minimal, ST-segment elevation will occasionally be seen in V_2 through V_4 in the presence of right ventricular infarction.[95] Otherwise, ST-segment elevation must be sought in the right chest leads, V_1, and V_3R through V_6R. ST-segment elevation in these leads provides reasonably strong evidence for the presence of right ventricular infarction.[96] A postmortem study has shown that a 25 percent or greater involvement of the right ventricle was necessary to produce ST-T-segment elevation.[97] Atrial infarction is usually reflected in PR-segment elevation or depression and P-wave abnormalities and is frequently associated with supraventricular arrhythmias, as discussed below.[98]

The phenomenon of "ischemia at a distance" reflects the occurrence, in AMI with ST-segment elevation, of ST-segment depression in other, frequently reciprocal leads, as alluded to in the discussion of right ventricular infarction. The question of whether these changes represent true reciprocal changes or subendocardial ischemia in the area has received considerable attention but usually cannot be resolved on an electrocardiographic basis alone.[99,100] Whether or not anterior ST-segment depression in the setting of inferior or lateral AMI represents reciprocal changes or anterior ischemia, the presence of the finding is associated with a less favorable prognosis than its absence.[101,102]

Criteria for electrocardiographic diagnosis of AMI in various areas of the heart are discussed more fully in Chap. 12. In view of a lack of sensitivity and specificity of the chest pain history or of the ECG, confirmation of the diagnosis of AMI is based on elevated plasma levels of cardiac-specific isoenzymes.

PLASMA DIAGNOSTIC MARKERS

Tissue Distribution of MB-CK, Troponin T, Troponin I, and Myoglobin

Myocardial necrosis is associated with the release of a variety of macromolecules, including enzymes, myoglobin, and contractile proteins that have been evaluated as potential diagnostic markers for AMI. The use of CK and MB-CK has become routine and is highly sensitive, specific, and cost-effective for diagnosing myocardial infarction.[103-105] The use of total CK alone without MB-CK yields a similar sensitivity, but specificity is markedly lower, in the range of 70 percent.[106] Creatine kinase consists of two monomers, each having a molecular weight of 43,000.[107] The isoenzymes of CK are formed by the association of two M monomers (MM-CK), which predominate in muscle (hence the name); or of two B monomers (BB-CK), which predominate in the brain and internal visceral organs; and a hybrid form (MB-CK), found in the heart, composed of one M subunit and one B subunit. The isoenzymes MM, MB, and BB are located in the cytoplasm of the cell. There are separate genes for each of the monomers, which have been isolated, cloned, and sequenced.[108,109] About 5 percent of cellular MM-CK activity is associated with the M line of the sarcomere in both heart and skeletal muscle,[110,111] and a significant amount is in the Z line in heart muscle.

Fifteen percent of the CK in the myocardium is in the form of MB-CK, which provides for its sensitivity and specificity as a diagnostic marker of acute myocardial infarction. Several investigators have found small amounts of MB-CK in normal adult skeletal muscle,[112,113] whereas others have failed to detect any cytosolic CK other than MM-CK.[114,115] MB-CK is alleged to increase (1 to 5 percent) in skeletal muscle following injury such as chronic exercise,[116,117] inflammation,[118] trauma,[119] and electrical injury.[120] In hereditary muscle diseases, such as Duchenne muscular dystrophy (DMD), there is also increased MB-CK in the range of 1 to 5 percent. During the first 6 weeks of life in utero, only BB-CK is synthesized, while at about the eighth week, M-CK synthesis is induced and rapidly supplants the B-CK in skeletal and cardiac muscle, such that by about the 12th week, MM-CK predominates.[121,122] It is believed that in DMD, the retained expression of the B-CK reflects the abnormal development

of these muscles. It is postulated that in the case of the reaction to muscle injury, undifferentiated skeletal muscle cells differentiate to form mature skeletal myocytes and thus repeat the developmental program of fetal skeletal muscle, but the expression of B-CK is transient.[123] In the adult human heart, 15 percent of total CK activity is MB-CK and the remainder is MM-CK, which is also the case in other primates.[124] Myoglobin, with a molecular weight of 17,000, is ubiquitously distributed throughout cardiac and skeletal muscles.[125]

Two new diagnostic cardiac markers have been introduced: troponin T[126] and troponin I,[127] which are part of the sarcomere complex. Troponin T has a molecular weight of 38,000, and troponin I, 23,000. There are three genes for each of the troponins that encode for slow and fast skeletal and cardiac muscle.[128] Cardiac troponin I has 31 amino acids, which are not present in the skeletal forms.[129] The recognition site of the antibody used in the assay is in the cardiac-specific region, which makes the test very specific as a marker for myocardial injury,[127] and since normal plasma levels of troponin I are near zero, it is also very sensitive. Furthermore, studies indicate that cardiac troponin I is not upregulated in skeletal muscle with hypertrophy or injury and the skeletal form is not upregulated in the heart with hypertrophy or injury.[130] Cardiac troponin T has 11 amino acids not present in the skeletal forms, which has permitted the development of a specific diagnostic test.[131,132] It has similar sensitivity to troponin I but somewhat less specificity in that the cardiac form may be upregulated in skeletal muscle with injury[133-135] and, while it is unlikely that the skeletal form is upregulated in the heart with hypertrophy or injury, this remains an unresolved issue.[136]

Temporal Profiles of MB-CK, Myoglobin, Troponin I, and Troponin T Released into Plasma

Plasma MB-CK activity following myocardial infarction is significantly elevated, such that reliable diagnostic sensitivity (>90 percent) is reached within 12 to 16 h of the onset of symptoms. Maximal levels of MB-CK are reached between 14 and 36 h, with a return to normal levels occurring after 48 to 72 h[137] (Fig. 47-2). In patients with minimal cardiac injury, such as occurs in non-Q-wave infarction or following effective early reperfusion, plasma MB-CK activity reaches maximal activity at about 12 to 15 h. In contrast, after Q-wave infarction with reperfusion, it reaches maximal activity at an average of 28 h. The plasma temporal profiles of troponin I and troponin T are very similar to those of total CK and MB-CK. Troponin I and troponin T are released into the plasma so that reliable diagnostic sensitivity (≥90 percent) is reached by 12 to 16 h and maximal activity is reached by 24 to 36 h. The levels return to normal within 10 to 12 days.[138] Plasma myoglobin is increased within 2 h of the onset of symptoms and remains increased for at least 7 to 12 h.[126]

Early Diagnosis (6 to 10 h of Onset): MB-CK Subforms and Myoglobin

In the United States, over five million patients with chest pain present annually to the emergency department but only about

10 percent with chest pain will subsequently be shown to have myocardial infarction.[139] About 50 percent of patients will have cardiac ischemia, 10 percent will have nonischemic cardiac pain, and about 30 percent will have pain of noncardiac origin.[140] It is important to have an early diagnosis to determine the initial therapeutic regimen and whether hospital admission is needed. In the United States, it is estimated that over $12 billion per year[141] is spent unnecessarily to exclude myocardial infarction in patients admitted to the hospital with chest pain without infarction. Thus, early, rapid diagnosis is required to triage patients, reduce costs, and select appropriate therapy in spite of the difficulty in distinguishing cardiac ischemia from infarction based on the patient's history,

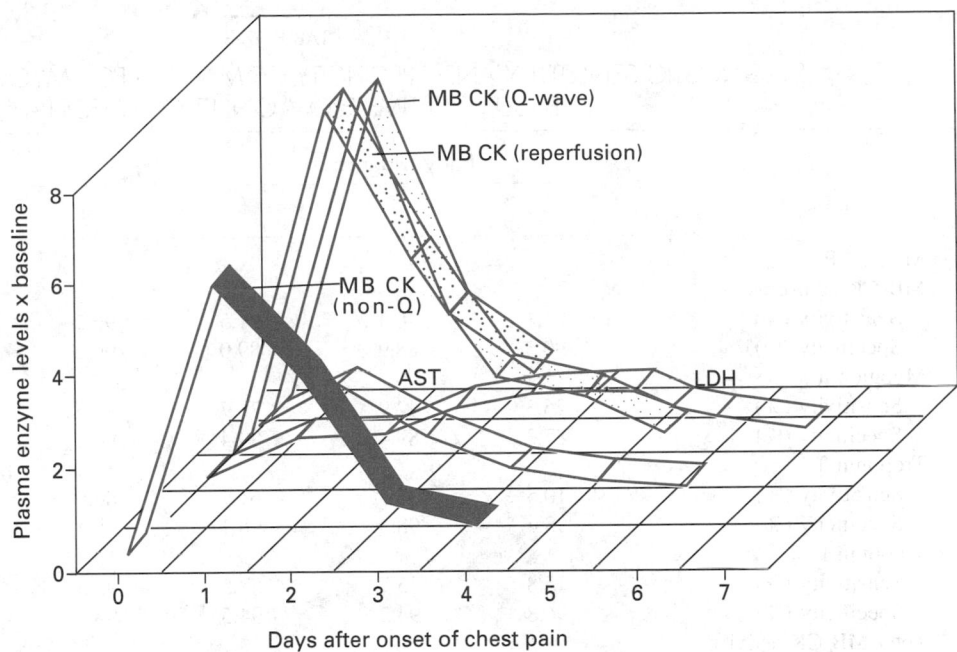

FIGURE 47-2
Typical plasma profiles for the MB isoenzyme of creatine kinase (MB-CK), aspartate amino transferase (AST), and lactate dehydrogenase (LDH) activities following onset of AMI.

physical examination, and the ECG, as noted. This difficulty is emphasized by the observation that over 50 percent of AMI patients in the United States[142] present with nonspecific ST-segment changes (non-Q-wave infarction) rather than ST-segment elevation (Q-wave infarction). The only specific electrocardiographic findings on admission for myocardial infarction are the recent development of ST-segment elevation or left bundle branch block. It is estimated that less than 50 percent of patients with AMI will have a diagnostic ECG, which represents only 5 percent of the total patients presenting with chest pain; thus, there is a need for an early objective marker (within 6 h of onset).[71] The ideal diagnostic test should have an assay performance time that is brief, and the marker must have a highly reliable negative predictive value, since only 10 percent of patients will have infarction, as noted. While a false-positive range of 5 to 10 percent is acceptable, a desirable false-negative range is 1 to 2 percent. Assessment of the plasma profile of the markers shows only two plausible candidates, namely, MB-CK subforms and myoglobin.

It was recognized for some time that MM and MB-CK, though present in tissue in single forms, exhibit different forms upon release into the circulation, as detected by electrophoresis.[143] In 1982, it was shown that upon release into the circulation, MM-CK is converted into three forms: MM-3, MM-2, and MM-1, and MB-CK is converted into MB-2 and MB-1, due to the proteolytic activity of carboxypeptidase-N, an enzyme present in the blood of all vertebrates.[144,145] Carboxypeptidase-N cleaves the terminal amino acid, lysine, from the M subunit of the MB-CK, which is positively charged, leaving the remaining molecule more negatively charged (MB-1). The more negative form (MB-1), upon elec-

trophoresis, separates from the parent tissue form (MB-2), giving rise to the two forms of MB-CK in plasma. A new technique utilizing 1400 V, which provides separation of the MB subforms within about 6 min,[146] is coupled with automated densitometric quantification; this produces a value for MB-2 activity, the plasma ratio of MB-2 to MB-1, and total MB-CK activity.[147,148] The current assay for the MB-CK subforms is completely automated and requires about 25 min. In the plasma, the MB-CK subforms are in equilibrium, with a ratio of MB-2 to MB-1 of 1 to 1. Normally, the baseline plasma MB-CK activity is in the range of 2 to 4 IU/L, or a protein concentration of 3 to 5 ng/L. Thus, for a reliable diagnosis of myocardial infarction based on total MB-CK activity, one requires an increase above 9 to 10 IU/L, or, for protein, above 7 to 9 ng/L. *When infarction occurs, MB-2, the tissue form, is initially released into the circulation in minute amounts so that total MB-CK remains within the normal range, but the ratio of MB-2 to MB-1 changes markedly and provides the basis for an early diagnosis of myocardial infarction.*

Previous studies[148] have shown that the assay for MB-CK subforms reliably diagnoses infarction within 6 h of the onset of symptoms. This was confirmed in a large, blinded, prospective study involving 1110 patients presenting consecutively with chest pain.[147] Similar studies with large sample sizes are not available for myoglobin, but smaller studies[126] suggest that myoglobin is a sensitive early diagnostic marker, and, if patients with conditions such as trauma are excluded, is also specific. The assay performance time required for any of the markers (CK, total MB-CK, MB-CK subforms, myoglobin, and troponins T and I) is only 20 to 25 min.

TABLE 47-3

DIAGNOSTIC SENSITIVITY AND SPECIFICITY OF MARKERS FOR MYOCARDIAL INFARCTION
BASED ON TIME FROM ONSET OF CHEST PAIN

Time, hours	Early Diagnosis			Late Diagnosis			
	2	4	6	10	14	18	22
MARKER							
MB-CK subforms							
Sensitivity (%)	21.1	46.4	91.5	96.2	90.6	80.9	53.1
Specificity (%)	90.5	88.9	89.0	90.2	90.0	89.9	92.2
Myoglobin							
Sensitivity (%)	26.3	42.9	78.7	86.5	62.3	57.5	42.9
Specificity (%)	87.3	89.4	89.4	90.2	88.3	88.8	91.3
Troponin T							
Sensitivity (%)	10.5	35.7	61.7	86.5	84.9	78.7	85.7
Specificity (%)	98.4	98.3	96.1	96.4	96.1	95.7	94.6
Troponin I							
Sensitivity (%)	15.8	35.7	57.5	92.3	90.6	95.7	89.8
Specificity (%)	96.8	94.2	94.3	94.6	92.2	93.4	94.2
Total MB-CK activity							
Sensitivity (%)	21.1	40.7	74.5	96.2	98.1	97.9	89.8
Specificity (%)	100.0	98.8	97.5	97.5	96.1	96.9	96.2
Total MB-CK mass							
Sensitivity (%)	15.8	39.3	66.0	90.4	90.5	95.7	95.7
Specificity (%)	99.2	98.8	100.0	99.6	98.9	99.6	99.1

The recent introduction of troponins T and I necessitates the need for diagnostic selection. In an attempt to provide comparative diagnostic sensitivity and specificity for all of the markers, a large, multicenter, prospective, double-blind study, the Diagnostic Marker Cooperative Study (DMCS), was performed, comprising 1004 patients admitted consecutively with chest pain.[140] A serial analysis of all markers was performed on a sample taken on admission, with another at 1 h, another every 2 h for up to 6 h from onset, and subsequently every 4 h for up to 24 h. Every effort was made to obtain the time of onset of symptoms. In keeping with previous observations, only 11 percent of the patients with chest pain were subsequently documented to have infarction ($n = 118$), of whom less than 47 percent had a diagnostic ECG (43 percent had ST-segment elevation and 4 percent had a left bundle branch block), with the remainder having nonspecific ST-T changes (non-Q-wave infarction). Cardiac ischemia accounted for 51 percent and nonischemic cardiac pain for another 9 percent, while in 29 percent the pain was of noncardiac origin. The diagnostic sensitivity and specificity of each of the markers are indicated in Table 47-3. MB-CK subforms afforded a sensitivity and specificity of 91 percent for the diagnosis of infarction within 6 h of the onset of symptoms. Myoglobin had a sensitivity of 83 percent during the same interval. The negative predictive value of MB-CK subforms within the initial 6 h of onset was 97 percent and that of myoglobin was 95 percent. *Thus, if a patient has a negative MB-CK subform test at 6 h after the onset of symptoms, one can reliably conclude that the patient does not have infarction.*

During the same interval of 6 h from onset, the total MB-CK (activity or mass assay) and troponins T and I afforded a sensitivity of only 65 percent. A major observation from this study—with significant diagnostic, therapeutic, and cost-saving implications—is the finding that MB-CK subforms correctly diagnosed 92 percent of the patients with myocardial infarction within 60 min of arriving in the emergency department. This was based on the results of the sample collected on admission to the emergency department and on a second sample collected 1 h later (Table 47-4). For the same two samples, however, myoglobin had a sensitivity of 83 percent. The mean time required to make the diagnosis of myocardial infarction using MB-CK subforms was 1.2 h ± 20 min from arrival in the emergency department, and a similar time was required to exclude those without infarction. It is evident from the data in Table 47-3 that total MB-CK, troponin T, and troponin I have high sensitivity and specificity for the diagnosis of myocardial infarction 12 to 16 h from the onset of

TABLE 47-4

DIAGNOSTIC SENSITIVITY OF MYOGLOBIN AND
MB-CK SUBFORMS ON ADMISSION AND 1 H LATER

Markers	Sample on Admission	Sample 1 h Later
MB-CK subform	67%	91%
Myoglobin	63%	78%

symptoms. It is noteworthy that the sensitivity of myoglobin decreases after about 7 or 8 h because of rapid renal clearance and thus may not be reliable after 10 to 12 h, particularly in patients with minimal injury.

SAMPLING INTERVALS AND THE DIAGNOSIS OF INFARCTION

In patients presenting within the first 10 h of the onset of myocardial infarction, the appropriate marker is either MB-CK subform or myoglobin, since other markers lack the necessary sensitivity. It is recommended that a blood sample be taken immediately on admission, 1 h later, then every 2 h until 6 h from the onset of symptoms, and then, if positive, every 6 h for 24 to 48 h. The MB-CK subform assay provides a diagnosis based on the first two samples (initial 1 h) in more than 90 percent of the patients with infarction. Once a sample is positive, one can sample every 6 h for 24 to 48 h. If the sample shows normal values for the MB-CK subforms, one must sample until 6 h from the onset of symptoms to reliably exclude infarction, at which time sampling can be discontinued. Sampling for 24 to 48 h in patients with positive MB-CK subforms is optional, but it is recommended for the following reasons: to obtain maximal total plasma MB-CK activity as a rough index of the extent of damage; to follow the decline in MB-CK subform activity as a baseline for subsequent procedures often performed, such as cardiac catheterization or percutaneous transluminal coronary angioplasty (PTCA); and to facilitate detection of early reinfarction, which accounts for 30 to 40 percent of in-hospital deaths in patients recovering from AMI. If the myoglobin is analyzed, a similar sampling algorithm is followed except that the interval required to exclude or include infarction with myoglobin may be longer, since with MB-CK subforms, 90 percent of patients with AMI are diagnosed within 60 min (two samples), whereas only 80 percent over the same interval will be diagnosed with myoglobin. Patients presenting 10 to 12 h or later after the onset of symptoms should have a sample taken on admission; if this is positive, it should be repeated every 6 h for 24 to 48 h. Total MB-CK, troponin T, or troponin I in this time frame will provide the desired diagnostic sensitivity and specificity. Normal total plasma MB-CK activity or protein concentrations at 12 to 16 h from the onset of symptoms excludes infarction with 95 to 100 percent reliability, as does a normal troponin T or I. Plasma myoglobin is not a reliable marker 8 to 10 h after the onset of symptoms. The upper level of normal for MB-2 is ≥ 2.6 IU/L, with a ratio of MB-2 to MB-1 of ≥ 1.7. The upper limit of normal for myoglobin is 85 ng/mL. The upper limit of total MB-CK activity is 9 IU/L, and for protein (mass) assays, 7 ng/mL. The upper limit of normal for troponin T is 0.1 ng/mL and for troponin I, 1.5 ng/mL. The guidelines below[78,149,150] are suggested as enzymatic criteria for the diagnosis of myocardial infarction (Table 47-5).

If there is a serial elevation in plasma MB-CK levels followed by a decrease to baseline, with a change of 25 percent or more between the two values or plasma MB-CK activity

TABLE 47-5

ENZYMATIC CRITERIA FOR DIAGNOSIS OF MYOCARDIAL INFARCTION

Serial increase, then decrease of plasma MB-CK, with a change >25% between any two values

MB-CK >10–13 U/L or >5% total CK activity

Increase in MB-CK activity >50% between any two samples, separated by at least 4 h

If only a single sample available, MB-CK elevation > twofold

Beyond 72 h, an elevation of troponin T or I or LDH-1 > LDH-2

increases 50 percent or more between two samples separated by at least 4 h and not more than 12 h:

1. Preferably, the diagnosis is made on the basis of no fewer than two samples in a 24-h period, separated by at least 4 h.

2. If only a single sample is present, the diagnosis must be made on the basis of an elevation above normal by at least twofold.

3. In patients admitted beyond 72 h from the onset of infarction, troponin T or I is preferred, since MB-CK levels may have returned to normal. The LDH isoenzymes would also be appropriate (see below).

These criteria have not been evaluated for troponin T or I but would probably serve as guidelines until further information is available. These principles are incorporated into the protocols for triaging patients in the emergency department, as illustrated in Fig. 47-3.

LIMITATIONS TO MYOGLOBIN, MB-CK, AND TROPONINS I AND T

Elevated plasma MB-CK as a diagnostic marker for myocardial infarction is associated with a very low incidence of false-negative results if samples are collected frequently and appropriately within 48 to 72 h of the onset of symptoms. However, false-positive results do occur, since trace amounts of MB-CK can be released from tissues other than the heart. Skeletal muscle injury may induce the synthesis of MB-CK, and has been documented after crush injury,[119] electrical injury,[120] dermatomyositis and polymyositis,[118] and DMD[151] as well as in professional athletes and marathon runners.[116,117] If one suspects that elevated plasma MB-CK activity is due to skeletal rather than cardiac muscle, the following should be considered: (1) The appropriate clinical setting, namely, skeletal muscle disease or trauma. (2) An atypical time course for the increase and decrease in plasma MB-CK activity, particularly if prolonged, as one might see in inflammatory disorders. (3) If MB-CK accounts for less than 5 percent of the total CK activity, then a skeletal muscle source should be suspected. Since tissues that contain MB-CK (other than the myocardium), such as skeletal muscle, contain only trace

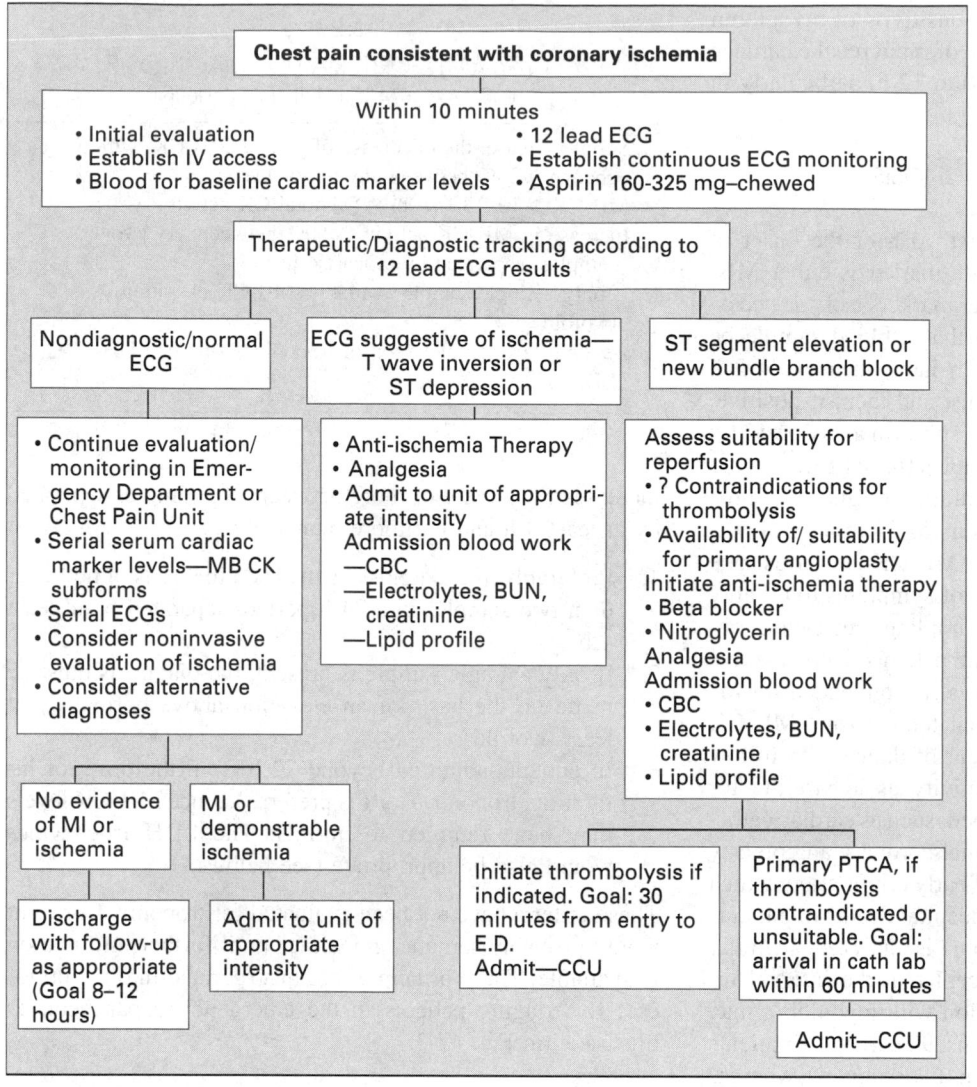

Chest pain consistent with coronary ischemia

Within 10 minutes
- Initial evaluation
- Establish IV access
- Blood for baseline cardiac marker levels
- 12 lead ECG
- Establish continuous ECG monitoring
- Aspirin 160-325 mg–chewed

Therapeutic/Diagnostic tracking according to 12 lead ECG results

Nondiagnostic/normal ECG

ECG suggestive of ischemia—T wave inversion or ST depression

ST segment elevation or new bundle branch block

- Continue evaluation/ monitoring in Emergency Department or Chest Pain Unit
- Serial serum cardiac marker levels—MB CK subforms
- Serial ECGs
- Consider noninvasive evaluation of ischemia
- Consider alternative diagnoses

- Anti-ischemia Therapy
- Analgesia
- Admit to unit of appropriate intensity
Admission blood work
—CBC
—Electrolytes, BUN, creatinine
—Lipid profile

Assess suitability for reperfusion
- ? Contraindications for thrombolysis
- Availability of/ suitability for primary angioplasty
Initiate anti-ischemia therapy
- Beta blocker
- Nitroglycerin
Analgesia
Admission blood work
- CBC
- Electrolytes, BUN, creatinine
- Lipid profile

No evidence of MI or ischemia

MI or demonstrable ischemia

Discharge with follow-up as appropriate (Goal 8–12 hours)

Admit to unit of appropriate intensity

Initiate thrombolysis if indicated. Goal: 30 minutes from entry to E.D. Admit—CCU

Primary PTCA, if thromboysis contraindicated or unsuitable. Goal: arrival in cath lab within 60 minutes

Admit—CCU

FIGURE 47-3

Algorithm for the initial assessment and evaluation of the patient with acute chest pain in the emergency department. The emergency department should be organized to facilitate the rapid triage of chest pain patients so that the initial evaluation, obtaining a 12-lead ECG, and establishing intravenous access and continuous monitoring are accomplished within 10 min. The path in the decision tree is determined by the results of the 12-lead ECG. The presence of ST-segment elevation diagnostic of AMI or of presumptively new BBB suggestive of this diagnosis should lead to the immediate consideration of the suitability of the patient for reperfusion therapy, which, if indicated, should be initiated within 30 min of the patient's arrival. The primary PTCA option is applicable only in those settings in which it is immediately available and can be performed by highly qualified interventional cardiologists. In general, patients should not be transferred for angioplasty if thrombolysis is an option. Thrombolysis is not indicated in patients with only ST-segment depression.

amounts (1 to 2 percent), elevated plasma MB-CK indicative of myocardial infarction should exceed 5 percent of total activity. At the time of peak plasma CK resulting from myocardial infarction, MB-CK levels usually make up 10 to 15 percent of the total activity. (4) A marked elevation of total CK activity of 20- to 30-fold suggests that the cause is more likely to be skeletal muscle injury. An elevated plasma MB-CK level may also be due to artifact. An analysis of samples for troponin I should determine whether the MB-CK is of cardiac origin. Those assays that do not differentiate the B from the M subunit may show elevations in MB-CK because

of detection of B-CK in the circulation resulting from injury to the prostate, uterus, gastrointestinal tract, or brain,[152–155] which are known to be rich in BB-CK. Similar artifactual elevations of plasma MB-CK may be seen in females following vaginal or cesarean delivery of a baby.[156] Release of BB-CK from the brain is seldom observed following cerebrovascular accidents,[157] but it may occur after trauma and infection or diffuse brain injury.[158] Finally, certain tumors, including those of the lung, brain and breast, may synthesize excessive amounts of BB-CK, which may be released into the circulation.[159] Hypothyroidism is associated with elevated levels of both total CK and MB-CK due to diminished clearance.[160] Occasionally, one sees what is referred to as macro CK-1, a complex of CK and macroglobulins, which migrates in the position of MB-CK upon electrophoresis[149,161] and results in a false-positive diagnosis of AMI. Macro CK-1 is more common in elderly women and in patients who are chronically ill, with an overall stated incidence of 1.6 percent in hospitalized patients.[161] This is not a problem for assays utilizing MB-CK monoclonal antibody, as is currently the case for most MB-CK assays. Electrocardioversion causes a significant elevation of total CK activity, but unless the procedure is repeated several times, it does not elevate plasma MB-CK. MB-CK is elevated in chronic renal failure[162]; however, it does not show any changes upon serial analysis and thus is not a significant diagnostic problem.

Troponin I has not been found to be elevated in patients with normal skeletal muscle, despite severe exercise or injury,[127] or in the blood of marathon runners.[163,164] Furthermore, in a recent study[165] involving 100 patients undergoing noncardiac surgery with extensive skeletal muscle injury, only 1 patient had a slight elevation of cardiac troponin I. Troponin I is not elevated in chronic renal failure.[127] *Troponin I would appear to be a more specific marker than MB-CK in patients with myocardial infarction and concomitant skeletal muscle injury, such as that following noncardiac surgery or severe muscle trauma.* However, the experience with troponin I is limited compared with the extensive experience with MB-CK; thus, the specificity may diminish as further studies are performed in clinical diseases affecting skeletal muscle or with various neoplasms. The specificity of troponin T with skeletal muscle injury has not yet been systematically determined.[166] An increase in troponin T has been reported in patients with polymyositis/dermatomyositis without cardiac involvement.[135] Wu et al.[167] recently documented that troponin T had lower specificity than MB-CK for myocardial damage. However, the antibody used in the assay for troponin T has been reported to have a 3.6 percent cross-reactivity with skeletal troponin T,[168] which may account for this lack of specificity. A recent assay with a more specific monoclonal antibody is now undergoing evaluation; it may offer greater diagnostic specificity. Troponin T, as in the case of MB-CK, has consistently been shown to be elevated in patients with chronic renal failure.[169]

RATIONALE FOR SELECTING A DIAGNOSTIC MARKER OR MARKERS

In view of the abundance of plasma markers and the increasing need to reliably triage patients with chest pain in a cost-effective manner, a careful choice must be made of which plasma marker or combination of markers will be utilized routinely. In selecting a marker for early diagnosis upon admission to the emergency department, there is essentially a choice between MB-CK subforms and myoglobin. MB-CK subforms, as compared with myoglobin, provide greater sensitivity as well as greater specificity overall for the early diagnosis of AMI. There has been extensive experience with the MB-CK subforms, while routine use of myoglobin for the diagnosis of infarction is minimal. Nevertheless, if patients with trauma are avoided, the specificity of myoglobin is quite acceptable, and it is the next best alternative for an early diagnosis, as indicated in Tables 47-3 and 47-4. Both assays are automated and simple to perform, requiring only about 25 min, and are identical in cost. For the diagnosis of patients presenting 10 h or later after the onset of symptoms, total MB-CK, which has been the standard for more than two decades, is extremely sensitive and specific, as would be troponin I or T. The time for performance of any of these latter three markers is also about 25 min, with identical costs. The choice of marker or markers used routinely may depend in part on the various tests with which the laboratory personnel are acquainted. However, there is little reason, based on diagnostic sensitivity and specificity, to assay all of these markers; in addition, the cost would be prohibitive. The single best assay for both early and late diagnosis is for the MB-CK subforms, from which total MB-CK can be derived as needed for late diagnosis. An assay of MB-CK subforms or myoglobin for early diagnosis, plus either troponin I or T for late diagnosis, is recommended. The available data for troponins I and T are somewhat limited compared with the extensive experience

with MB-CK; however, troponin I appears to be more specific than troponin T. In patients with renal failure, MB-CK[162] and troponin T[169] are artifactually elevated, while troponin I is not.[127] In most clinical situations where skeletal muscle involvement may be associated with elevated MB-CK, the extent of elevation is minimal and is less than 5 percent of total CK activity; it is usually not a diagnostic problem. Troponin I offers greater specificity and reliability in those clinical conditions. Whether troponin T offers enhanced specificity in clinical situations with skeletal muscle injury remains to be determined.[135] *The data from the DMCS indicate no advantage to simultaneously analyzing both MB-CK subforms and myoglobin for early diagnosis; similarly, for late diagnosis, there is little advantage to analyzing multiple markers.*

DIAGNOSIS OF ACUTE MYOCARDIAL INFARCTION IN PATIENTS 48 H OR MORE FROM THE ONSET OF SYMPTOMS

In patients admitted 48 to 72 h after the onset of symptoms, particularly when associated with minimal myocardial damage, plasma MB-CK may have returned to normal levels. In this situation, it has been traditional to utilize LDH isoenzymes, since LDH-1 activity peaks between 48 and 72 h and remains elevated for 10 to 14 days.[170] Recently, however, the preferred diagnostic marker has become troponin I or T. Both remain elevated for 10 to 14 days and offer greater sensitivity and specificity than LDH. The assays are also more rapid and convenient than those used for LDH isoenzymes. Patients presenting late should have blood samples analyzed for either troponin T or I. Late diagnosis, however, is probably required in less than 5 percent of patients.

ENZYMATIC ASSESSMENT IN PATIENTS UNDERGOING FIBRINOLYTIC THERAPY OR ANGIOPLASTY

Patients who receive fibrinolytic therapy or early angioplasty (within 4 to 6 h) should be assessed hourly for plasma MB-CK activity for the first 4 to 6 h, then every 6 to 8 hours for 36 h, with sampling reinitiated if chest pain or other features occur to suggest reinfarction. Following successful reperfusion, MB-CK is usually elevated within 30 to 60 min of the reperfusion and plasma activity reaches maximum levels within 10 to 15 h. Recent studies[171,172] have shown that 15 to 20 percent of patients undergoing elective PTCA have elevated plasma MB-CK, and these individuals have a worse prognosis over the subsequent 6 months.[173] It remains controversial whether routine sampling for MB-CK should be performed after elective PTCA, since changes in treatment based on increased MB-CK have not been assessed. In patients with triple-vessel disease or where complications are more likely, routine sampling with MB-CK subforms is recommended for 6 h; it should be discontinued if the results are normal. If they are positive, sampling should continue for at least 24 h, and the patient should be treated as having had myocardial damage.

DIAGNOSIS OF EARLY REINFARCTION

Diagnosis of early reinfarction (within 24 to 48 h) is difficult, since it represents an elevation superimposed on an already elevated plasma marker.[174,175] However, if MB-CK has returned to normal, then the diagnosis is relatively easy, since one sees a secondary increase in plasma MB-CK activity. Detection of early reinfarction with a secondary elevation in plasma MB-CK in patients who undergo successful thrombolysis is more appropriate, since MB-CK activity usually peaks within the first 10 to 15 h and returns to normal by 36 to 48 h. A secondary elevation of MB-CK activity 36 to 48 h after the onset of symptoms provides for a sensitive and specific diagnosis of reinfarction. In the latter situation, we define reinfarction as an increase of 50 percent or more in the plasma MB-CK activity above the preceding baseline (mean of the two preceding samples) in at least two samples separated by a minimum of 4 h within a 24-h interval, with an absolute value of ±9 IU/L or 7 ng/L in at least one sample.[137] If the MB-CK activity is on the downslope from the antecedent infarction, a 25 percent increase is considered diagnostic; however, this is always less reliable than a secondary elevation after the return of MB-CK activity to baseline. These criteria were found to be reliable in three large clinical trials: Nifedipine in Acute Myocardial Infarction, the Multicenter Investigation of Limitation and Infarct Size, and the Diltiazem Reinfarction Study.[78,149,150] Confirmation of reinfarction occurring early, however, is more appropriately diagnosed using the MB-CK subforms. The MB-2 is near normal by 18 to 24 h and usually peaks at 10 to 12 h, so a well-defined downslope is apparent after 12 to 16 h. The other markers, troponin T, tropo-

nin I and LDH, since they remain elevated for 10 to 14 days, lack the necessary sensitivity. Myoglobin, since it returns to normal early after onset, is also a sensitive marker, but because of venipuncture or other minor skeletal muscle trauma in the hospital setting, is often nonspecific.

PROGNOSTIC ROLE FOR BIOCHEMICAL MARKERS IN ASSESSMENT OF UNSTABLE ANGINA

Several studies have recently shown that patients presenting with the clinical diagnosis of unstable angina and minor elevations in MB-CK, troponin T, or troponin I have a more adverse outcome with respect to clinical events such as death, myocardial infarction, or the need for revascularization. In the GUSTO IIA trial,[176] of 835 patients with unstable angina, 36 percent had elevated troponin T and experienced increased mortality and other clinical events. Similarly, in the TIMI III trial,[177] of 1404 patients with non-Q-wave infarction and unstable angina, 41 percent had elevated troponin I and experienced increased mortality and other clinical events. In a study involving 593 patients with unstable angina, those with elevated MB-CK had increased mortality and other clinical events.[178]

It is now recommended that patients with unstable angina be assessed with one or more of these markers; however, treatment based on these indications and its long-term outcome have not been assessed. In the recent DMCS study,[140] there were 178 patients with unstable angina (rest pain of increased frequency or severity); the results of the various markers are shown in Fig. 47-4. This is the only study in which the sensitivity of all of the markers has been compared. There is a dilemma with respect to the interpretation of elevated plasma markers in patients with unstable angina. Does this mean that these proteins are released to ischemia (reversible injury) or that, in fact, limited infarction has occurred? Recent data[179] strongly indicate that the release of CK reflects irreversible injury. In a series of conscious animal studies, it was shown that 20 min of coronary artery occlusion is consistently associated with increased plasma CK activity and, on light and electron microscopy, myocardial necrosis. In contrast, animals undergoing 10 min of coronary occlusion who exhibited severe ischemia—as shown by ST-segment elevation, depletion of myocardial glycogen, and cell swelling—had no increase in

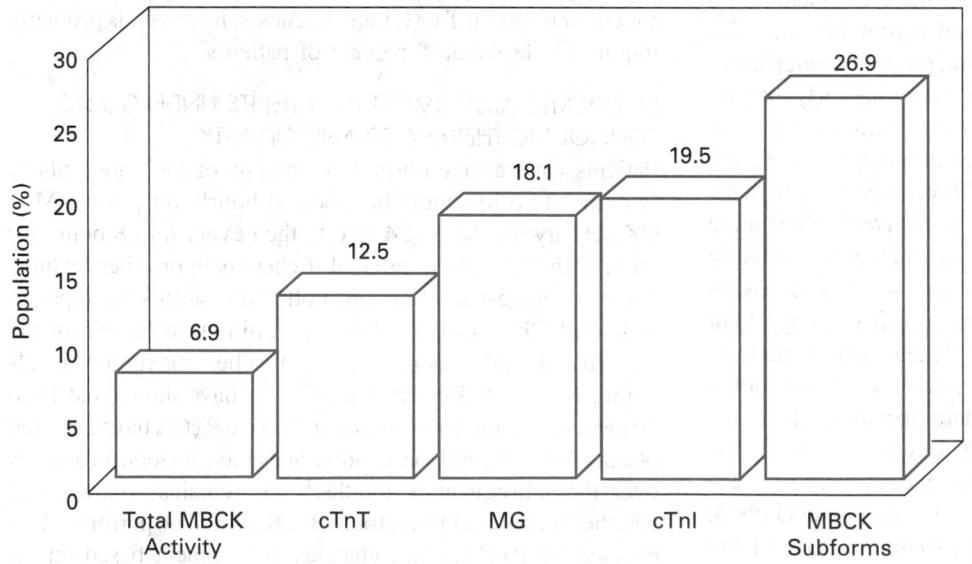

FIGURE 47-4

The above analysis is based on a prospective, multicenter, double-blind study involving the consecutive enrollment of 995 patients presenting to the emergency department. Diagnostic sensitivity and specificity for myocardial infarction of all markers [MB-CK subforms, myoglobin, total MB-CK (activity and mass), troponin T, and troponin I] were assessed serially every 1 to 2 h for 24 h. There were 119 (12.5 percent) patients with infarction and 203 (21 percent) with unstable angina. CK-MB subforms were most sensitive and specific (91 and 89 percent) within 6 h of onset versus myoglobin (78 and 89 percent). For late diagnosis, total MB-CK activity (derived from subforms) was the most sensitive and specific (96 and 98 percent) at 10 h from onset, followed by troponin I (96 and 93 percent), but not until 18 h, and troponin T (87 and 93 percent) at 10 h. In unstable angina, MB-CK subforms were increased in 29.5 percent, myoglobin in 23.7 percent, troponin I in 19.7 percent, and troponin T in 14.8 percent. (From Roberts et al.,[140] with permission.)

plasma CK. In the group of animals undergoing 15 min of coronary occlusion, only 30 percent had increased plasma CK activity, and each of these also showed microinfarction of the myocardium as detected by light and electron microscopy.[179] This finding—coupled with the observation that patients with proven obstructive coronary disease during exercise-induced ischemia, as documented by thallium scintigraphy, exhibited no increase in plasma MB-CK or MB-CK subforms—provides the basis for interpreting elevated plasma MB-CK levels as reflective of irreversible injury.[180] Fibrinolytic therapy has been shown to be detrimental[181] for the outcome in unstable angina; however, in non-Q-wave infarction, when given on an average of 9 h from onset, it showed no beneficial or detrimental effect. Early fibrinolytic, antithrombin, or antiplatelet therapy in patients with positive MB-CK subforms but ST-segment depression has yet to be evaluated. Similar studies have not been performed to determine whether increased troponin I or troponin T reflects cell death, although, since they are structural sarcomeric proteins, it is highly likely that their release does reflect cell necrosis. Since the molecular weight of troponin I is 23,000, however, and that of troponin T is 39,000, both of which are significantly less than that of MB-CK (82,000), the possibility of leakage with myocardial ischemia cannot be excluded.

DIAGNOSIS OF MYOCARDIAL INFARCTION AFTER SURGERY

Myocardial infarction after noncardiac surgery is also reliably determined from serial analysis of plasma MB-CK, MB-CK subforms, troponin T, or troponin I every 4 to 6 h.[106,182] There is a marked elevation of other enzymes due to tissue trauma, including total CK, but MB-CK, troponin T, and troponin I are highly specific to the myocardium. There is at least one study[165] showing that troponin I is more reliable than either total MB-CK or troponin T for the diagnosis of acute myocardial infarction in this setting. In the setting of cardiac surgery, however, MB-CK, like other cardiac enzymes, is almost always elevated due to manipulation and involvement of the myocardium and thus is not a reliable diagnostic index.[183,184] Nevertheless a severalfold elevation of MB-CK postoperatively is highly suggestive of periprocedural infarction, even in the absence of Q waves, although it lacks specificity as a sole criterion. Multifold elevations of troponin T or troponin I probably have the same implications postoperatively.

DIAGNOSIS OF PREVIOUS INFARCTION

Determining whether a patient has had a remote infarction to account for the subsequent development of cardiac failure or other clinical conditions can be difficult. Until recently, the only reliable means of diagnosis was the presence of Q waves on the ECG. Since less than 50 percent of infarctions develop Q waves and since a significant percentage of these Q waves disappear with time, the ECG can be nonspecific and unreliable in diagnosing remote infarction.[185,186] Thallium-201 (^{201}Tl) perfusion scanning or gated blood pool scanning with

technetium 99m (^{99m}Tc)–labeled red blood cells has been shown to be extremely reliable, sensitive, and specific in diagnosing remote infarction.[187] Studies were performed on patients at rest with thallium-201 imaging and radionuclide ventriculography on an average of 11 months (6 to 21 months) from the time of infarction. Perfusion defects were detected in 94 percent of the patients with infarction, and corresponding wall motion abnormalities were present in 78 percent. In 10 patients in whom the infarct size was less than 20 CK gram equivalents, wall motion abnormalities were found in only 50 percent. The ECG showed Q waves in only 56 percent. In the patients with persistent Q waves, infarct size was consistently greater than 20 CK gram equivalents, which was present in only 30 percent of the patients. Thus, these two techniques performed nearly 1 year after the event provided highly sensitive and specific assessments of infarction, with the thallium 201 being more sensitive than radionuclide ventriculography. Assessment by one or both of these techniques can be extremely valuable in determining the cause of a patient's symptoms when the ECG does not show Q waves or the patient has not had a previous history as well as in those patients in whom silent myocardial infarction has occurred.

OTHER BIOCHEMICAL ALTERATIONS

The stress of myocardial infarction elicits numerous hormonal and metabolic responses. For example, both catecholamines and growth hormones are elevated. It is noteworthy, however, that the serum cholesterol and lipoprotein fractions are relatively unchanged in the initial 1 to 2 days but decrease significantly over subsequent days and weeks. In establishing the baseline levels of these values for guiding future therapeutic interventions, measurements should be performed on admission or should be delayed for 6 to 8 weeks.[188,189] It should also be recognized that if myocardial infarction is occurring in individuals who have hypertension or for any reason are on medications such as diuretics, there may be significant electrolyte abnormalities that need to be treated, particularly in view of the increased propensity for arrhythmias, as with hypokalemia or alkalosis. The other abnormality seen on occasion is that of an increase in blood glucose following myocardial infarction, which, in some cases, particularly in patients with mild or moderate diabetes, may be associated with the development of significant ketoacidosis.[190,191] Not infrequently, it has also been shown that in the early days following myocardial infarction, the glucose tolerance curve is abnormal. It returns to normal after a few weeks. The white blood cell count is usually mildly to moderately elevated in 3 to 5 days.

Noninvasive Imaging in Acute Myocardial Infarction

CHEST ROENTGENOGRAM

The chest roentgenogram (x-ray) provides very important information in the evaluation of chest pain and contributes to an integrative assessment of the clinical situation. Its usefulness in the early stages of evaluation of a patient with chest pain is frequently compromised by the fact that one is usually dealing with a portable study performed in the emergency department or in the CCU. Nonetheless, the chest film may assist in excluding causes of chest pain such as pneumothorax, pulmonary infarction with effusion, aortic dissection, skeletal fractures, and so on. In the patient with acute infarction, the chest film can be useful in establishing the presence of pulmonary edema, in assessing heart size to assist in determining whether or not cardiomegaly is present, and in deciding whether heart failure or myocardial or valvular disease is acute or chronic. It must be emphasized that severe left ventricular failure can be present without manifesting pulmonary edema on the chest x-ray and that, conversely, improvement in the x-ray appearance can lag behind hemodynamic resolution of pulmonary congestion (see Chap. 13).

ECHOCARDIOGRAPHY

Because of the quality of the images provided, their wide availability, and the portability of these modalities, two-dimensional and Doppler echocardiography have become very useful tools in the assessment of the patient with suspected acute myocardial infarction[192–194] (see also Chap. 14). Echocardiography is particularly valuable in assessing the patient with a nondiagnostic ECG. The presence of a regional wall motion abnormality provides strong supportive evidence of acute coronary ischemia and is generally present in transmural or Q-wave myocardial infarction.[195–198] Wall motion abnormalities are less common in non-Q-wave infarction but are still present in the majority of cases. Nonetheless, small infarctions can be missed, and a wall motion abnormality may not necessarily be acute.[199] Echocardiography also provides an assessment of ventricular function; it is useful in predicting the prognosis[200] and in diagnosing right ventricular infarction.[201] It can also provide information concerning alternative diagnoses such as aortic dissection and, coupled with Doppler, can provide information on such complications as ruptured chordae tendineae with mitral regurgitation and ventricular septal defect[202] (see Chap. 14). It is useful in detecting ventricular thrombus and pericardial fluid. Thus, echocardiography is extremely useful in the initial assessment of AMI. General guidelines on its clinical use, including those for myocardial infarction, have been published recently.[203] Its usefulness in establishing the diagnosis of AMI per se, however, may diminish with the increased availability of rapid, sensitive, and specific blood markers.

The echocardiogram is also useful in the assessment of residual viable myocardium[204,205] and residual ischemia.[206]

MAGNETIC RESONANCE IMAGING

Magnetic resonance imaging (MRI) offers great promise in assessing AMI (see Chap. 19). Its major limitation is logistic, in that it requires transporting patients to the imaging facility—a major concern in the case of the acutely ill. It is potentially useful in the assessment of infarct size and viable myocardium and the extent of the ischemic insult as well as in estimating perfusion to ischemic and nonischemic areas.[207–209] Currently, MRI does not have a defined role in the routine management of AMI.

COMPUTED TOMOGRAPHY

Computed tomography (CT) is a powerful tool for cardiac imaging that gives high-resolution structural information (see Chap.18). Ventricular thickness and dimensions can be assessed.[210] Also, CT is highly sensitive for detecting a left ventricular thrombus.[211] It has the same logistic limitations as MRI in the management of AMI. It does not have a routine role in the management of infarction. Whether electron-beam CT, with its very rapid acquisition times, can have a role in routine management requires further investigation (see Chap. 18).

RADIONUCLIDE SCINTIGRAPHY

The radionuclide techniques available for the diagnosis of acute myocardial infarction are discussed in detail in Chap. 17, and are summarized in Table 47-6.[212] Guidelines for the use of cardiac radionuclide scanning have been published and suggest that the indications for its use in the diagnosis of acute infarction are limited to the unusual case in which history, electrocardiographic changes, and plasma markers are unreliable or unavailable.[212] There is no class I indication in the acute setting, and *routine* diagnostic use is not indicated (class III).[15,212]

If a patient presents more than 24 h after the onset of symptoms and there are no diagnostic electrocardiographic changes, ^{99m}Tc pyrophosphate, which is infarct-avid, has a moderate diagnostic sensitivity and specificity in this setting[213,214] (class IIa). Alternatively, infarct-avid antimyosin antibodies could be substituted for pyrophosphate in this circumstance, presumably with the same class IIa indication.[215,216] Another setting in which AMI might not be diagnosed by standard means is in the case of early presentation and successful reperfusion. In this case, serial rest perfusion imaging with ^{201}Tl or ^{99m}Tc sestamibi may show localized defects; ^{99m}Tc pyrophosphate may show local uptake,[15] but with relatively low sensitivity and specificity (class IIb).[212]

Radionuclide scintigraphy may have a diagnostic role in certain patients with right ventricular infarction by showing localized contractile abnormalities[217] or ^{99m}Tc pyrophosphate uptake (class IIa).[212]

Measurement of Myocardial Infarct Size

It has been established experimentally[218,219] and clinically,[220,221] as noted, that the major determinant of both an acute and a long-term prognosis following myocardial infarction is the extent of myocardial damage. In the early 1970s, there were major efforts to quantify infarct size through a variety of techniques, such as assessing the degree of ST-segment elevation on the ECG[222] and determining myocardial radioisotope uptake[223–225] and the kinetics of cardiac enzyme release into the circulation.[226]

TABLE 47-6

USES OF RADIONUCLIDE TESTING IN ACUTE MYOCARDIAL INFARCTION

| Indication | Diagnosis | | Indication | Risk Assessment | |
	Test	Class		Test	Class
1. RV infarction	Rest RNA	IIa	1. Residual ischemia	Stress (exercise/ pharmacological) thallium with redistribution	I
	^{99m}Tc pyrophosphate	IIa		Stress (exercise/ pharmacological) sestamibi with redistribution	
2. Infarction not diagnosed by standard means— early presentation with successful reperfusion	Rest myocardial perfusion imaging ^{99m}Tc pyrophosphate	IIb IIb	2. Myocardial infarct size	Tomographic thallium Tomographic sestamibi	IIa IIa
3. Infarction not diagnosed by standard means—late presentation	^{99m}Tc pyrophosphate	IIa	3. Hibernating myocardium	Early, late thallium	IIa
4. Routine diagnosis	Any technique	III	4. Ventricular function	RNA	I

Key: RV = right ventricular; RNA = radionuclide angiography; ^{99m}Tc = technetium 99m.
Source: The ACC/AHA task force,[212] with permission.

ENZYMATIC MEASUREMENT OF INFARCT SIZE

In the prereperfusion era, determination of the total amount of MB-CK released into the circulation was shown to provide a reasonable estimate of infarct size as correlated with postmortem studies.[227] With the advent of reperfusion as standard therapy, however, it was observed that there was a rapid washout of CK from the myocardium, and the ratio of CK released into the circulation to that depleted from the myocardium was altered, invalidating estimates of infarct size in this setting.[228]

ELECTROCARDIOGRAPHIC ESTIMATES OF INFARCT SIZE

The ECG has long been used to obtain a semiquantitative assessment of the extent of myocardial infarction. In general, it has been found, for example, that patients with anterior infarcts who develop Q waves in leads V_1 to V_6 usually have extensive damage and an unfavorable prognosis. Early studies demonstrated that the sum of ST-segment elevations measured in the precordial leads was useful in assessing the extent of myocardial injury in patients with anterior myocardial infarction.[229] The technique was limited, however, because it did not distinguish between reversible and irreversible ischemic changes and was dependent upon ventricular geometry.[230] More quantitative scoring systems were developed[231–233] but were not accurate enough to assess the effects of interventions.

For routine, practical clinical purposes, there are useful electrocardiographic indicators of infarct size that have prognostic significance. In an acute anterior infarction, the extent of jeopardized myocardium correlates with the number of precordial leads showing ST-segment elevation and QRS changes and with the extent of those changes.[234] In general, there is a direct relationship between the number of leads showing ST-segment elevation and mortality. ST-segment elevation in eight or nine leads is associated with a mortality of three to four times that of patients manifesting ST-segment elevation in only two or three leads.[235]

ASSESSMENT OF INFARCT SIZE BY IMAGING

As noted, infarct size can be assessed by echocardiography (see Chap. 14), computerized tomography (see Chap. 18), magnetic resonance imaging (see Chap. 19), positron emission tomography (see Chap. 20), or radionuclide scintigraphy (Table 47-6[212]) (see Chap. 17). For practical reasons, echocardiography is most commonly used in the acute evaluation. Ventricular function, as assessed after the acute episode by equilibrium-gated radionuclide angiography, correlates strongly with clinical outcomes in the absence[236,237] and presence of reperfusion therapy.[238,239] Recently, ^{99m}Tc sestamibi with tomographic imaging has been used to quantitate infarct size,[240,241] which was shown to be inversely related to the patient's outcome.[242,243] Thallium 201 can also be used to measure infarct size.[212]

Prehospital Care

Recommendations[15]:

Class I

1. Availability of 911 access
2. Availability of an emergency medical services (EMS) system staffed by persons trained to treat cardiac arrest with defibrillation, if indicated, and to triage patients with ischemic-type chest discomfort

Class IIa

1. Availability of a first-responder defibrillation program in a tiered response system
2. That health care providers educate patients/families about the signs and symptoms of AMI, about accessing EMS, and about medications

Class IIb

1. The use of 12-lead telemetry
2. Prehospital thrombolysis in special circumstances (e.g., transport time is greater than 90 min)

As mentioned previously, modern in-hospital care of the AMI patient has resulted in a substantial reduction in mortality. Some 40 to 65 percent of deaths from AMI, however, occur within an hour of the onset of symptoms and prior to arrival at a hospital.[244,245] Most of these deaths are attributable to ventricular fibrillation.[246] To achieve a further substantial decrease in the mortality rate, it will be necessary to reduce the incidence of deaths outside the hospital.[247] Since, as noted, the earlier thrombolytic therapy can be initiated in eligible patients, the better the outcome, it is also essential to bring patients with chest pain into the medical care system as soon as possible because of the need to shorten the time between the onset of symptoms and the initiation of thrombolytic therapy. To that end, in the United States, the National Heart, Lung and Blood Institute of the National Institutes of Health has instituted the National Heart Attack Alert Program as a coordinated plan to extend the ACC/AHA guidelines promoting rapid identification and treatment of patients with AMI.[248,249]

RECOGNITION AND MANAGEMENT

A further reduction in the mortality rate will require the combined efforts of the patient, bystanders, minimally trained "first responders" who are capable of applying defibrillation therapy, and/or paramedics as well as the patient's physician. It has been established that a prolonged delay time in responding to a patient's symptoms is the rate-limiting step in defining the prehospital phase of myocardial infarction. Mean delay time in such response is almost 3 h.[250] Most of this time is consumed in decision making, while failing to recognize or acknowledge the seriousness of the problem.[251] Additional components of the delay between the onset of symptoms and the initiation of definitive therapy involve prehospital evaluation, treatment, and transport time and the time involved with the diagnosis and initiation of treatment in the hospital. The National Registry of Myocardial Infarction found, in a review of 48,128 patients with confirmed AMI, that the average duration of the prehospital phase, defined as onset of chest pain to hospital presentation, was 5.1 h.

Strategies to Reduce Delay

Patient-specific issues for decreasing the delay in seeking assistance primarily involve education. The patient must perceive the symptoms, recognize their possible significance, and

conclude that medical help is appropriate. For some patients, the decision time is prolonged because of a lack of knowledge. It is interesting, however, that the length of time patients take to get help is not dependent on educational level, occupation, socioeconomic class, or past history of cardiac disease. In fact, patients with a past history of myocardial infarction or angina have an unexpectedly long decision time,[252] a situation that must be viewed, at least in part, as a failure by physicians to educate patients with established coronary artery disease as to the appropriate response to a change in or reappearance of their symptoms. In other cases, the decision time is prolonged by denial or by "diagnostic trials" with household remedies, patent medications, or previously prescribed drugs. It has been noted that only 10 percent of patients arriving at the hospital within 1 h of the onset of pain utilized nonprescription medications, while 41 percent of those arriving after 12 h did so.[245] The remainder of the delay time is consumed by "human factors," including the time a patient takes to modify existing social obligations and to prepare for going to the hospital. There is evidence that public education can reduce the time required for decision making.[251] *It follows that effective efforts by the physician and his or her staff in educating patients with coronary artery disease will have similar effects in inducing appropriate responses to ischemic coronary symptoms.* Prodromal symptoms occur in about two-thirds of patients with acute myocardial infarction, as discussed previously, and patients must be taught to recognize them.[247] Patients and their families must be given a specific plan of action after the recognition of symptoms that includes medications to be taken (nitroglycerin and possibly aspirin), mode of transportation to the hospital, and the location of the nearest hospital that offers emergency cardiac care. It is desirable that coronary patients have a copy of their resting ECG with them. They should be instructed not to delay by attempting to contact their physician and should be shown how to use the EMS system and how to contact it (911 in the United States). As opposed to personal transportation, utilizing EMS is desirable, because it permits the earliest possible access to expertise in defibrillation and resuscitation and facilitates evaluation in the field to prepare the hospital to receive the patient, as discussed below. The use of the EMS usually decreases the delay in initiating definitive care.[248] Since the capabilities of the EMS vary by locale, the physician must be familiar with the system in the patient's home area.

Instructions concerning medications to be taken at the onset of symptoms should be individualized. In general, patients are instructed to take nitroglycerin immediately at the onset of angina or a recognized anginal equivalent. If pain is not relieved, another nitroglycerin dose is taken at 5 min and a third at 10 min. If there is no relief by the third dose of nitroglycerin, the patient should be transported to the appropriate emergency facility. The physician should decide whether to incorporate the chewing of an aspirin tablet into this regimen when the decision is made to proceed to the hospital.

Bystanders/family members can play an important role in both shortening patient delay time and responding to an arrest.

It has been shown that a spouse's presence accelerated the hospital arrival time.[246] Furthermore, if basic life support is initiated by a bystander within 4 min of cardiac arrest and if defibrillation is accomplished within 8 min, 40 percent of patients will survive and be discharged from the hospital.[253]

EMERGENCY MEDICAL SERVICES

Many communities in the United States are served by a two-tier ambulance service consisting of basic and advanced life support units. Since these are usually more basic support units, the response time of these units is shorter and should ideally be less than 5 min.[15,254] The first responders may be any of a variety of public service employees who are trained in CPR and defibrillation and have been taught to have a sense of urgency in order to identify and treat the AMI patient rapidly. Automatic external defibrillators are safe and effective and can be used by even minimally trained first responders to analyze rhythms and deliver defibrillatory shocks to convert ventricular fibrillation.[15,255–259] Incorporation of automatic external defibrillators into emergency medical systems is highly desirable.[15] Minimally, it has been recommended that every ambulance transporting victims of cardiac arrest be equipped with a conventional defibrillator.[257]

The goal of any emergency medical system should be to include individuals who are trained in advanced life support techniques—including the use of antiarrhythmics as well as administration of intravenous fluids administration and analgesics—and who can reach the patient as soon as possible in a vehicle equipped as a CCU. Undirected EMS technicians can spend excessive amounts of time evaluating a patient with chest pain and actually delay the ultimate initiation of appropriate therapy.[15] The time elapsed between receiving a 911 call and the actual arrival in the hospital has been assessed, and, at over 46 min, was substantially longer than estimates (under 26 min) taken from the paramedics involved.[251] Most of this field time was consumed by the paramedic

on-scene time, which was not prolonged by acquisition of a 12-lead ECG. It has been demonstrated that, by the use of a standardized protocol (Table 47-7[15]), evaluation of the patient with chest pain by experienced emergency medical technicians, acquisition of a 12-lead ECG and initiation of therapy can be accomplished within 20 min.[15] The protocol should facilitate determination of the likelihood of AMI and the presence of comorbid conditions in which thrombolytic therapy would be dangerous. It should also identify those suspected AMI patients who are at high risk. Patients in this category include those with sinus tachycardia, hypotension, or pulmonary edema or those with signs of shock. It is ideal to be able to record 12-lead ECGs in the field to be transmitted to the hospital physician. The availability of these data facili-

---

TABLE 47-7

CHEST PAIN CHECKLIST FOR USE BY EMT/PARAMEDIC FOR DIAGNOSIS OF ACUTE MYOCARDIAL INFARCTION AND THROMBOLYTIC THERAPY SCREENING

Check each finding below. If all [yes] boxes are checked and ECG indicates ST elevation or new BBB, reperfusion therapy with thrombolysis or primary PTCA may be indicated. Thrombolysis is generally not indicated unless all [no] boxes are checked and BP ≤180/110 mmHg.

	Yes	No
Ongoing chest discomfort (≥20 min and <12 h)	☐	—
Oriented, can cooperate	☐	—
Age >35 y (>40 if female)	☐	—
History of stroke or TIA	—	☐
Known bleeding disorder	—	☐
Active internal bleeding in past 2 weeks	—	☐
Surgery or trauma in past 2 weeks	—	☐
Terminal illness	—	☐
Jaundice, hepatitis, kidney failure	—	☐
Use of anticoagulants	—	☐

Systolic/diastolic blood pressure
Right arm: ____/____
Left arm: ____/____

	Yes	No
ECG done	☐	—

*High-risk profile**	Yes	No
Heart rate ≥100 bpm	☐	—
BP ≤100 mmHg	☐	—
Pulmonary edema (rales greater than one half-way up)	☐	—
Shock	☐	—

*Transport to hospital capable of angiography and revascularization if needed.

Pain began	____	AM/PM
Arrival time	____	AM/PM
Begin transport	____	AM/PM
Hospital arrival	____	AM/PM

Key: EMT = emergency medical technician; ECG = electrocardiogram; BBB = bundle branch block; PTCA = percutaneous transluminal coronary angioplasty; BP = blood pressure; TIA = transient ischemic attack. Adapted from the Seattle/King County EMS Medical Record.
Source: Ryan et al.,[15] with permission.

tates establishing the diagnosis and allows for accelerating preparations to administer thrombolytic therapy.[260–262]

PREHOSPITAL THROMBOLYSIS

As mentioned above, there is unequivocal evidence that the earlier thrombolysis is administered to the AMI patient with ST-segment elevation, the more efficacious is the outcome[12,263,264]; in particular, the most favorable results are achieved when therapy is initiated within the first 1 to 2 h after the symptoms appear. It seems logical, therefore, that if thrombolysis could be initiated in appropriate patients during the prehospital phase by general practitioners or by EMS technicians guided by protocol, the 12-lead ECG, and communication with the emergency department physician, outcomes would be improved. Prehospital thrombolysis has been evaluated in several trials.[260,265–267] A metaanalysis of all of the trials showed a modest (17 percent) improvement in outcome, although none of the trials demonstrated significant improvement individually.[267] Prehospital thrombolysis, however, is fraught with a number of difficulties, beginning with the fact that only a small portion of chest pain patients (5 to 10 percent) have an AMI and are eligible to be treated with thrombolytics.[260,262,268,269] Thus, correctly selecting patients for thrombolytic therapy and avoiding its administration when not indicated or when contraindicated is difficult and has significant legal, medical, and economic implications. Because of these difficulties, prehospital thrombolysis should be emphasized primarily in those circumstances in which it can be administered 60 to 90 min before reaching the hospital (because of a long transport time) or when a physician is in the ambulance.[15] Generally, emphasis should be placed on rapid screening and diagnosis in the field to facilitate hospital triage and thrombolytic administration within 30 min of the patient's arrival.

EVALUATION AND MANAGEMENT OF CHEST PAIN PATIENT IN THE EMERGENCY DEPARTMENT

Recommendation[15]:

Class I

1. Emergency department AMI protocol that yields a targeted clinical examination, a 12-lead ECG within 10 min, and administration of thrombolytic therapy, as appropriate, within 30 min.

Background

In general, the goals of the emergency department with respect to chest pain patients are to rapidly identify those patients with acute myocardial infarction with both typical and atypical presentations so that appropriate therapy can be initiated; to recognize those patients with acute coronary syndromes (unstable angina) but without myocardial infarction and who,

thus, are at high risk; and to assess accurately those patients at low risk who are candidates for noninvasive evaluation and early discharge.[270]

As mentioned previously, the earlier reperfusion therapy is initiated in the subset of patients with diagnostic ST-segment elevation, the more favorable the clinical results (Fig. 47-5[263]).

An important objective, obviously, should be a triage system that minimizes the number of patients at high risk (AMI or unstable angina) who are inadvertently discharged from the emergency department while also minimizing the admission to high-intensity CCUs of low-risk patients without myocardial infarction—a goal of increasing urgency in this era of intense pressures for cost containment. Of patients admitted to a CCU, for example, less than 20 percent will have AMI, as noted.[271,272] In contrast, even in the current era of an enhanced appreciation for atypical presentations, an increased potential for litigation, and a decreased threshold for admission to exclude myocardial infarction, the missed diagnosis rate has still been about 4 percent,[147] a percentage that appears not to have changed substantially since the 1980s.[273–275]

The reasons for misdiagnosis of acute coronary syndromes in the emergency department have been studied extensively and have recently been reviewed.[270] The misinterpretation of ECGs has been reported to occur in approximately 20 to 40 percent of missed AMIs.[274,276,277] Equally disturbing are the reports, which are indictments of training or focus, that patients are discharged even though the physician has recognized ischemic symptoms or electrocardiographic changes.[273,276,277] A major contributing problem is that even experienced clinicians are imprecise in their clinical judgment as to the presence or absence of myocardial infarction in a given patient. Sensitivities of 80 to 90 percent and specificities of approximately 70 to 80 percent in diagnostic precision in determining the presence or absence of AMI based on clinical impressions have been reported.[70,274,278] The diagnostic problem, however, is not limited to the diagnosis of myocardial infarction but also applies to whether unstable angina is present (see also Chap. 46). Patients who are admitted to the hospital with chest pain and only transient ST-segment changes and without aggressive therapy have a 22 percent incidence of death and myocardial infarction after a 28-month follow-up,[279] a figure not dissimilar to that for patients with an initial confirmed infarction. These similarities in outcome of unstable angina and myocardial infarction are not surprising, since the fundamental underlying pathophysiologic mechanisms, disruption of the atherosclerotic plaque and thrombus formation, with or without vasospasm, are likely to be identical, the major difference being the extent of luminal compromise by the thrombus. *Thus, the clinical focus should not be simply to "rule out" acute myocardial infarction, but, taking a proactive approach, to "rule in" either acute infarction or unstable angina in an expeditious manner.[270] Once these urgent conditions have been excluded or ascertained to be of low probability, the next level of concern is determining the presence of other acute cardiovascular or cardiopulmonary*

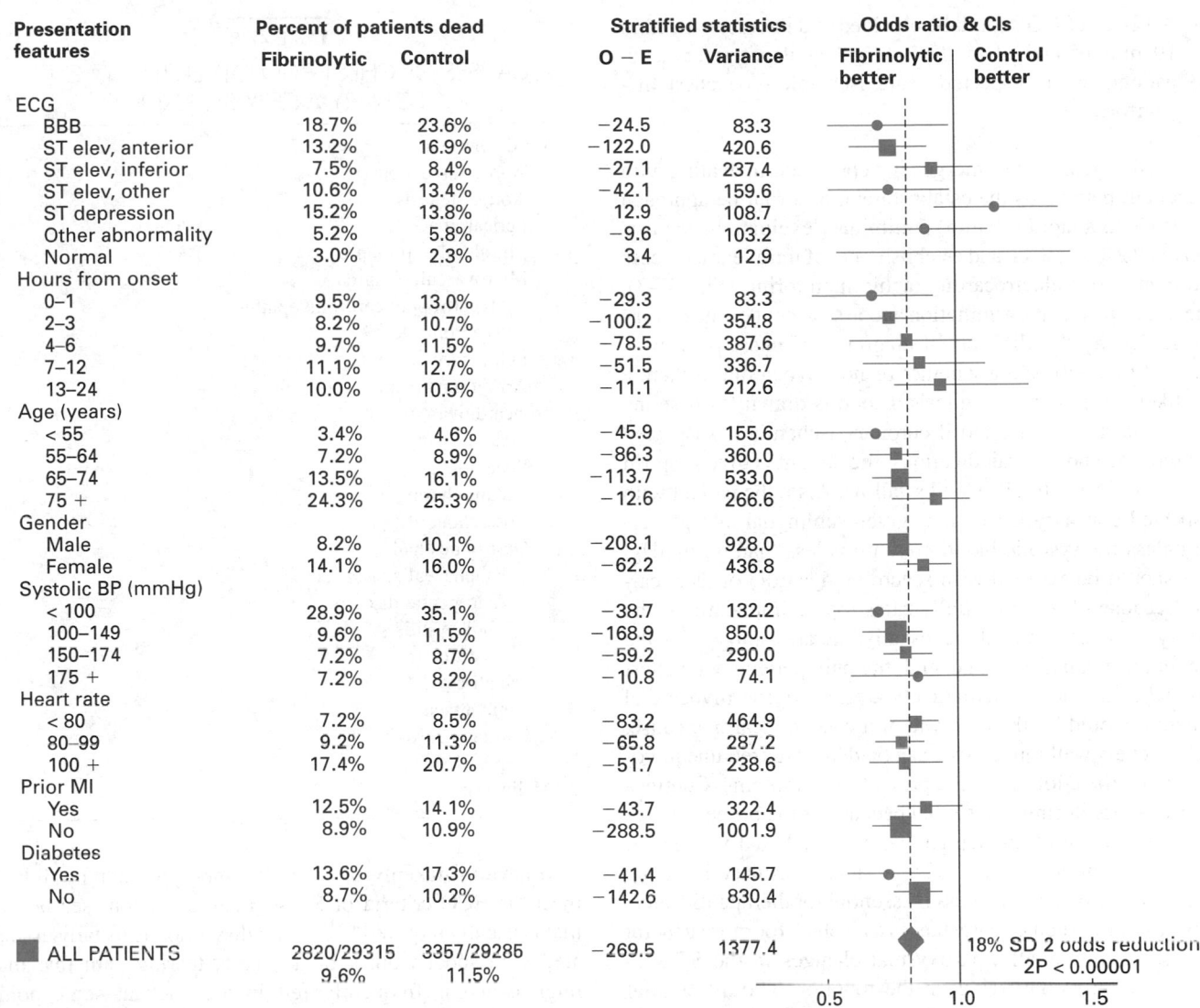

FIGURE 47-5

Proportional effects of fibrinolytic therapy on mortality during days 0 to 35 subdivided by presentation features. "Observed minus expected" (O-E) number of events among fibrinolytic-allocated patients (and its variance) is given for subdivisions of presentation features, stratified by trial. This is used to calculate odds ratios (ORs) of death among patients allocated to fibrinolytic therapy to that among those allocated control. The ORs (squares with areas proportional to the amount of "statistical information" contributed by the trials) are plotted with their 99 percent confidence intervals (CIs) (horizontal lines). Squares to the left of the solid vertical line indicate benefit (significant at $2p < .01$ only where the entire CI is to left of vertical line). Overall result and 95 percent CI represented by diamond, with overall proportion reduction in the odds of death and statistical significance given alongside. (From Fibrinolytic Therapy Trialists' Collaborative Group,[263] with permission.)

conditions, such as aortic dissection, pulmonary embolus, pericarditis, etc. The focus, subsequently, in a hierarchical fashion, is to establish whether or not stable coronary artery disease is present, to identify cardiovascular risk factors, and to consider noncardiac diagnoses, which, in nonurgent cases, can be evaluated further on an outpatient basis.

It has recently been suggested[270] that management of chest pain in the emergency department can be optimized by having the appropriate clinical focus, developing effective risk stratification approaches, and implementing systematic algorithmic protocols. There has been a great deal of interest in the development of actual or virtual chest pain units to facilitate the expeditious triage and management of chest pain patients, as discussed below.

Initial Approach, Detection, and Assessment of Risk

Recommendations[15]:

Class I

1. Supplemental oxygen, intravenous access, and continuous electrocardiographic monitoring should be established in all patients with acute ischemic-type chest discomfort.

2. A 12-lead ECG should be obtained and interpreted within 10 min of arrival in the emergency department in all patients with suspected acute ischemic-type chest discomfort.

A major goal of the emergency department in dealing with chest pain patients is the establishment of a routine approach that leads to a rapid (10 min) preliminary evaluation, acquisition of a 12-lead ECG, and establishment of intravenous access and continuous electrocardiographic monitoring (Fig. 47-3). The initial physical examination and assessment of the history are guided by the differential diagnosis of chest pain, with the goal of establishing whether or not myocardial ischemia is a likely or possible diagnosis. Blood is drawn for baseline cardiac marker levels, and if coronary ischemia is suspected and there are no contraindications, the patient is given aspirin of 160 to 325 mg to chew and swallow. Also, the patient with suspected coronary ischemia is given sublingual nitroglycerine unless the systolic blood pressure is less than 90 mmHg. This should be avoided with severe bradycardia or tachycardia. Because of the potentially catastrophic implications, the history of chest pain alone usually dictates entry into the system for evaluation. In general, the only patients with chest pain who are not systematically evaluated for myocardial ischemia would be those in whom a clear noncardiac cause, such as chest wall tenderness, can be demonstrated unequivocally to be the etiology of the presenting symptoms. Continuous ECG monitoring is essential because of the propensity for the development of sudden and potentially lethal ventricular arrhythmias in any patient with an acute coronary ischemic syndrome. Intravenous access is essential for therapeutic interventions under such circumstances as well as for more general purposes. Additionally, paroxysmal changes in the ST segment may be recognizable on the monitor. The differential diagnosis of chest pain and the clinical recognition of AMI were discussed previously. The causes of chest pain that are not the result of acute pathologic changes compromising the structural integrity of the large coronary arteries are listed in Table 47-8.

As a general rule, and as previously mentioned, one should begin the evaluation of the chest pain patient with the assumption that one is dealing with myocardial ischemia until proven otherwise. The three most serious and urgent alternative diagnoses that need to be considered specifically during the initial evaluation are *aortic dissection, acute pulmonary embolus,* and *acute pneumothorax. Acute pericarditis and myopericarditis* need to be considered as well.

Although relatively uncommon, aortic dissection must be considered and ruled in or out during the initial evaluation of the patient with chest pain, since specific intervention can decrease its high mortality. Furthermore, and not unexpectedly, administration of thrombolytic agents in the presence of aortic dissection is associated with high mortality.[280–282] Suspicion of dissection should be heightened especially in hypertensive patients or in those with marfanoid habitus (see also Chaps. 69 and 98). Most patients with aortic dissection

TABLE 47-8

CAUSES OF CHEST PAIN OTHER THAN ACUTE CORONARY ARTERY SYNDROMES

Cardiovascular
  Aortic dissection
  Aortic stenosis
  Pericarditis
  Mitral valve prolapse
  Microvascular angina
    Hypertrophic cardiomyopathy
    Syndrome X
  Pulmonary embolus
  Arrhythmia/palpitations
Noncardiovascular
  Pleurisy
  Pneumonia
  Pneumothorax
  Costochondritis
  Gastrointestinal
    Esophageal spasm/reflux
    Acid peptic disease
    Cholecystitis
    Gastritis
Psychiatric
  Panic attack
  Cardiac neurosis
  Depression
Malingering

who have mistakenly received thrombolytic therapy did not meet the ECG criteria of ST-segment elevation (see below) that is usually required.[281] Aortic dissection is usually associated with sudden onset of a severe, tearing pain that may migrate and is frequently felt in the back at some point. Differential blood pressures in the arms may be noted, and pulse differences in the carotids or arms may be observed. An echocardiogram and, in particular, transesophageal echocardiography can be very efficacious in the diagnosis of aortic dissection (see Chaps. 14 and 98).

Pulmonary embolus can be life-threatening and should be suspected in anyone with a sudden onset of shortness of breath and chest pressure or pain, especially if there is a history of being sedentary or immobilized and/or of deep venous thrombosis. There may be a pleural rub, and the chest roentgenogram is usually normal, although arterial hypoxia may be present (see Chap. 60). Similarly, pneumothorax may be associated with persistent chest pain, hypoxemia, and evidence of hypoventilation on physical examination.

Acute pericarditis may mimic acute myocardial infarction in that the pain can be substernal and persistent. Frequently, however, there will be a positional component as well as characteristics of pleurisy, with accentuation by deep breathing. Furthermore, the diffuse ST-segment elevation may lead to a misdiagnosis of myocardial infarction. The key differentiating features in pericarditis include PR depression, the diffuse nature of ST-segment elevation in most leads, and the absence of reciprocal changes (see Chaps. 12 and 81). The presence of a pericardial rub is a key diagnostic finding. Echocardiography, by demonstrating a pericardial effusion in the case of pericarditis or a wall motion abnormality in the case of acute ischemia, can be helpful in making the appropriate diagnosis. Hemorrhagic pericardial effusions have been reported in patients given thrombolytic therapy in the setting of acute pericarditis.[280,283]

Although usually not urgent, it should be kept in mind that esophageal disorders, as assessed retrospectively by motility studies, are very common in patients presenting with chest pain in whom cardiac ischemia is ruled out[284-287] (see also Chap. 45). In fact, among all patients presenting with chest pain, gastroesophageal disease has been observed to be the most common etiology (42 percent), whereas ischemic heart disease was present in 31 percent and chest wall syndromes were responsible in 28 percent.[288] Because of the high frequency of gastrointestinal disease in patients with chest pain, "GI cocktails" or antacids have been used as a diagnostic tool to guide triage and disposition. Only 25 percent of patients with esophageal pain, however, have been reported to obtain pain relief with antacids.[289] Furthermore, coincidental, spontaneous relief of ischemic chest pain at the time of administration of the GI cocktail could be misleading. Similarly, administration of nitroglycerin as a diagnostic strategy for ischemic disease could be misleading, because it can relieve esophageal spasm. Moreover, it has been found that pain relief after nitroglycerin did not predict unstable angina or AMI in the chest pain patient.[290] The use of these "response-to-treatment" strategies as major decision points in the evaluation of chest pain has been discouraged.[270] This reservation, however, applies primarily to those patients without diagnostic ECG changes, and does not preclude giving sublingual nitroglycerin to patients with chest pain and ST-segment elevation as a test of vasospasm or Printzmetal's angina.

DETECTION

The 12-Lead Electrocardiogram as a Guide to Management Strategy
The results of the 12-lead ECG guide the next level of decision making for the patient with chest pain thought to be compatible with myocardial ischemia (Fig. 47-3). The ECG interpretation is assigned to one of three categories: (1) ST-segment elevation in two or more leads or a presumptively new bundle branch block implicating acute coronary occlusion, usually thrombotic; (2) ST-segment depression and/or T-wave inversion implying subtotal occlusion and nontransmural ischemia; and (3) normal or nondiagnostic. The group with ST-segment elevation or a left bundle branch block is particularly important to define, as it is this group that has been shown to benefit from thrombolytic therapy. ST-segment elevation has a 46 percent sensitivity and a 91 percent specificity for the diagnosis of AMI.[92] There is no indication as yet of the benefit of thrombolytic therapy or primary angioplasty in those patients without ST-segment elevation or bundle branch block.

The ECG also serves as a basis for initial risk assessment. ST-segment elevation or a new left bundle branch block in the patient with chest pain defines a high-risk group, and in those with elevated ST segments, the mortality correlates positively with the number of leads with the ST changes.[235] The presence of ST-segment depression or T-wave inversion also defines a high-risk group. In patients with unstable angina or non-Q-wave myocardial infarction, ST-segment depression on the initial ECG of at least 1 mm in two leads during pain predicted major clinical events in the subsequent 3 months.[291] A nondiagnostic or normal ECG is associated with lower risk. For example, the incidence of myocardial infarction has been reported to be 10, 8, and 41 percent in patients who, at admission, had a normal, a nonspecific, or an abnormal ECG, respectively.[292] The incidence of complications paralleled the infarction rate—a predictable conclusion corroborated by other studies.[293,294]

As discussed previously, the initial ECG is diagnostic in less than 50 percent of patients with AMI,[295,296] and the measurement of serum markers of myocardial damage plays a major role in diagnosis. Measurement of CK-MB is the benchmark laboratory test, and the specificity and sensitivity of samples taken 2 h apart during serial sampling have been reported to be 91 and 94 percent, respectively.[297] The limitations of conventional CK-MB measurements and the role of myoglobin and the troponins have been discussed. The newly developed, rapid high-voltage method to separate $MB-CK_1$ and $MB-CK_2$ and to determine the ratio of the isoforms was described and may be particularly relevant to the initial evaluation in the emergency department, since it quickly provides information that not only facilitates establishing the appropriate diagnosis but also contributes to assigning a risk category to a patient.

As discussed previously, two-dimensional echocardiography can be useful as an adjunctive modality. It may be especially useful in detecting wall motion abnormalities in the presence of conduction abnormalities on the ECG.

RISK STRATIFICATION
Stratifying risk in the patient with AMI is an essential part of the management strategy during all phases of care. It permits not only the more precise calibration of treatment and diagnostic approaches with the level of risk but also, increasingly, facilitates the utilization of hospital resources appropriately. Traditional approaches to initial risk assessment have involved combinations of ECG changes and clinical manifestations. *High risk has been associated with age, ST-segment elevation or depression, T-wave inversions, and Q waves as well as prolonged chest pain, especially if it radiates to cardiac referral areas.*[70,274,298-300]

Quantitative assessments of risk have been developed to guide the management of chest pain patients in the emergency department.[294] *Predictors of an increased risk of complications included ECG evidence of ST-segment elevation or Q waves in two or more leads that are not known to have been present previously; ST-segment depression or T-wave inversions consistent with myocardial ischemia and not known to be present previously; pain worse than prior angina or the same as that experienced with prior myocardial infarction; systolic blood pressure of less than 100 mmHg; or rales bilaterally above the bases.* On the basis of these predictors, patients could be divided into four risk groups.[294] Furthermore, the risk could be updated if a complication occurred. This general approach can guide decisions concerning the level of intensity of the unit to which a patient is admitted and the length of observation required.

Blood levels of cardiac markers are prognostically important, as noted. *In particular, the levels of troponins (I and T) at presentation appear to be strong predictors of risk in patients with acute ischemic syndromes*[176,301] (See Chap. 46).

INITIAL MANAGEMENT

As discussed, one frequently does not have a definitive diagnosis of AMI in the chest pain patient in the emergency department, although this situation may ultimately be improved by the wider availability of the very rapid assays of blood cardiac markers, as discussed above. Nevertheless, the initial general treatment of the acute coronary syndromes is the same.

Routine General Measures

Oxygen Administration Recommendations for oxygen administration[15]:

Class I

1. Overt pulmonary congestion
2. Arterial oxygen desaturation (Sa_{O_2} less than 90 percent)

Class IIa

1. Routine administration of oxygen to all patients with uncomplicated myocardial infarction during the first 2 to 3 h

Class IIb

1. Routine administration of supplemental oxygen to patients with uncomplicated myocardial infarction beyond 3 to 6 h

Hypoxemia is not uncommon in patients with AMI, even with an uncomplicated course, and presumably because of ventilation-perfusion mismatch.[302] Oxygen administration has been reported to decrease ST-segment elevation in anterior myocardial infarction.[303] Thus, oxygen administration for up to several days has previously been routine. There is concern with this practice, however, since oxygen may increase vascular resistance, and there may not necessarily be increased delivery to tissues. Because of these concerns and because of the expense of prolonged oxygen administration, there appears to be little justification for extending its use in uncomplicated

myocardial infarction with an Sa_{O_2} of greater than 90 percent beyond 2 to 3 h.[15] Justification of its use in uncomplicated infarction can be based on its potential for limitating of ischemic injury and on the fact that nitroglycerin can induce ventilation-perfusion abnormalities due to its pulmonary vasodilator activity, thus contributing to hypoxia.

Oxygen administration should be continued in patients with pulmonary congestion and desaturation. In patients with complicated myocardial infarction, nasal oxygen or oxygen by face mask may be insufficient to maintain saturation, and positive-pressure breathing or intubation and mechanical ventilation may have to be considered. If necessary, they should be initiated promptly.

Analgesia The alleviation of pain and anxiety remains an essential element in the care of the patient with AMI. The pain and accompanying anxiety contribute to excessive activity of the autonomic nervous system and to restlessness. These factors, in turn, increase the metabolic demands of the myocardium. Physician reassurance from the beginning is an essential part of treatment and should be provided with compassion, patience, and confidence. Optimal care of the patient with AMI requires a team of experienced individuals who can help alleviate anxiety by their air of competence and caring.

It is a common clinical observation that reperfusion in acute myocardial infarction is associated with rapid relief of pain, suggesting that the pain is due to ongoing ischemia of the viable myocardium rather than to the effects of tissue necrosis. Thus, the approach to pain consists of the dual strategy of relieving ischemia and attacking the pain directly. Anti-ischemic therapy consists of reperfusion, beta blockers (if appropriate), nitrates, and oxygen administration, as discussed. Narcotics not only relieve pain directly but also indirectly by diminishing the sympathetic nervous system's drive and catecholamine secretion, which will increase blood pressure and drive cardiac chronotrophic and inotrophic responses to increase oxygen consumption and ischemia. The increased sympathetic drive will also enhance the propensity for serious ventricular arrhythmias. Morphine, in most instances, is the drug of choice, since it is well tolerated and offers analgesia without significant cardiac depression.[304] It also relieves anxiety and the feeling of doom commonly described. Morphine sulfate can be given at doses of 2 to 4 mg every 15 min until adequate relief has been obtained, which, in some patients, may require 25 to 30 mg.[305] The peak effect of intravenous morphine occurs within 15 to 20 min, thus requiring titration. Morphine has frequently been given in inadequate doses because of fear of respiratory depression or hypotension. Respiratory depression is less common in patients with myocardial infarction than generally, because of the anxiety and respiratory drive from hypoxia, and can be treated with intravenous naloxone should it occur.[15] Hypotension related to morphine is usually orthostatic and volume-dependent and is less common in supine patients.[306] In patients with severe ongoing pain, it may be prudent to avoid concomitant administration of substantial doses of morphine and vasodilators, such as nitroglycerin. In patients with an acute inferior myocardial infarction with bradycardia with or without hypotension, the vagolytic narcotic meperidine may be substituted for the parasympathomimetic morphine. If the patient's anxiety is not controlled by the administration of narcotics, mild sedation with a benzodiazepine is appropriate. Diazepam in doses of 5 mg orally every 8 to 12 h or alprazolam in doses of 0.25 mg every 8 h are most often used.

Nitroglycerin Recommendations for intravenous nitroglycerin[15]:

Class I

1. For the first 24 to 48 h in patients with AMI and congestive heart failure, large anterior infarction, persistent ischemia, or hypertension
2. Continued use (beyond 48 h) in patients with recurrent angina or persistent pulmonary congestion

Class IIa: None
Class IIb

1. For the first 24 to 48 h in all patients with AMI who do not have hypotension, bradycardia, or tachycardia
2. Continued use (beyond 48 h), perhaps in an oral or topical form, in patients with large or complicated infarction

Class III

1. Patients with systolic pressure less than 90 mmHg or severe bradycardia (less than 50 beats per minute)

Nitroglycerin has become very widely used in the treatment of AMI. It is an anti-ischemic agent not only by virtue of its actions to decrease preload and afterload, and thus to decrease oxygen demand, but also because of its vasodilator actions on epicardial coronary arteries and coronary collaterals. Consequently, and especially in patients with good collaterals, nitroglycerin is likely to increase flow into the ischemic regions.[307,308] Apart from relieving ischemia and pain, intravenous nitroglycerin, in early studies, appeared to reduce the likelihood of developing cardiac failure, infarct extension, or cardiac death. Both clinical data[309,310] and animal studies suggest that the early administration of nitroglycerin limits the extent of myocardial damage and favorably affects survival.[311] Long-term nitrates after reperfusion in animals favorably affect ventricular remodeling.[312]

Small, early trials before the widespread use of reperfusion suggested that the early administration of intravenous nitroglycerin was associated with improved morbidity and mortality. A metaanalysis of these trials suggested that the use of nitrates reduced the odds of mortality after AMI by greater than 30 percent.[313] The efficacy of nitrates in improving short-term mortality after AMI was tested prospectively in the GISSI-3 trial.[314] At 6 weeks, there was no significant difference between the nitrate and control groups. The power to

distinguish between the two, however, was diminished, because about one-half of the control group received nitrates during the first 2 days at the discretion of the attending physician. The angiotensin-converting enzyme (ACE) inhibitor lisinopril was tested in a similar fashion in GISSI-3. Mortality was decreased slightly at 6 weeks. The combined use of nitrates and lisinopril was associated with decreased mortality at both 6 weeks and 6 months compared with the no-nitrate group or with the group that received lisinopril alone. In another large trial, ISIS-4, which evaluated the effects of nitrates on mortality after myocardial infarction, no significant difference was noted at 35 days in comparison with the control group.[315] This trial was also compromised by the high frequency of discretionary nitrate use in the control group. A metaanalysis of all randomized, controlled trials involving the use of nitrates in AMI show a small, statistically significant reduction in mortality (about 5 percent).

The weight of the evidence does not justify the routine, long-term use of nitrates in uncomplicated AMI. The use of intravenous nitroglycerin early after acute infarction is justified because of its ease of titration, rapid onset, and ability to be quickly withdrawn in case of complications. Longer-term use of nitrates is appropriate in the case of recurrent ischemia, large infarction, congestive heart failure, or hypertension.

COMPLICATIONS AND LIMITATIONS The most serious complication of nitroglycerin is hypotension. The fall in blood pressure may cause reflex tachycardia, and, together with decreased perfusion pressure, may cause or worsen angina. Thus, nitroglycerin should be avoided with a systolic pressure of less than 90 mmHg. Caution should be exercised in the case of inferior wall infarction because of the possibility of right ventricular involvement. Nitroglycerin should be used only with extreme caution if at all in right ventricular infarction, because the right ventricle in this circumstance becomes extremely dependent upon preload, which can be diminished by the venodilating properties of the drug.[316] Similarly, nitroglycerin should be avoided in patients with severe bradycardia (heart rate less than 50 beats per minute), as hypotension may result.[317] If hypotension and bradycardia develop, nitroglycerin should be stopped, legs elevated, fluid administered, and atropine given if needed. Headache is a common side effect of nitrate administration.

Nitrate tolerance is common (see Chap. 91). With intravenous nitroglycerin, this may be recognized only as a diminution of clinical effect after 24 to 48 h. An increase in dose may be required.

DOSAGE OF NITROGLYCERIN Long-acting nitrates should generally not be used as initial therapy in acute myocardial infarction. Intravenous nitroglycerin is preferable, as noted, because of rapidity of onset, ease of titration, and ease of removal in case of complications. Dose titration can be assessed by frequent determinations of blood pressure and heart rate. Invasive monitoring is not essential but is probably prudent if high doses are required or if there is hemodynamic instability or uncertainty about the adequacy of ventricular preload.

Treatment should be initiated with a bolus injection of 12.5 to 25 μg and should be followed by infusion by pump of 10 to 20 μg/min, with increases of 5 to 10 μg every 5 to 10 min while assessing hemodynamic and clinical responses.[15] Control of symptoms is a major end point; in the case of high left ventricular filling pressure, a decrease of 10 to 30 percent in pulmonary artery wedge pressure is the objective. Limitations of nitroglycerin dosing are a decrease in mean arterial pressure of 10 percent in normotensive patients or a decrease of 30 percent in hypertensive patients, but not below a systolic pressure of 90 mmHg, or an increase in heart rate of 10 beats per minute not to exceed 110 beats per minute.

Doses of nitroglycerin greater than 200 μg/min are associated with an increased risk of hypotension. The development of such high requirements may indicate tolerance, and alternative drugs such as ACE inhibitors or nitroprusside should be considered. If tolerance is the issue, responsiveness should return after a 12- to 18-h period off of nitroglycerin.

Aspirin Recommendations for aspirin therapy[15]:

Class I

1. A dose of 160 to 325 mg should be given on day 1 of AMI and continued indefinitely on a daily basis thereafter.

Class IIb

1. Other antiplatelet agents such as dipyridamol or ticlopidine may be substituted if a true aspirin allergy is present.

Aspirin has become a standard part of the armamentarium for treating not only acute myocardial infarction but also atherosclerotic vascular disease generally. A 23 percent reduction in mortality at 35 days in patients treated with aspirin during the early stages of AMI was observed in the Second International Study of Infarct Survival (ISIS-2).[318] The reduction in mortality due to aspirin in combination with streptokinase was 42 percent. In a summary of a large number of clinical trials, aspirin has been shown to reduce the incidence of vascular events in patients with AMI at 1 month; a prior history of myocardial infarction (2 years); a history of transient cerebral ischemia or stroke; and unstable angina.[319]

Aspirin irreversibly inhibits platelet cyclooxygenase, an enzyme that causes formation of thromboxane A_2, a mediator of platelet aggregation.[320] Its antithrombotic and side effects are discussed in detail in Chap. 52. Aspirin should be avoided in cases of true hypersensitivity. In the case of a history of bleeding from acid peptic disease, aspirin rectal suppositories can be used. Ticlopidine, which is an antiplatelet drug with a mechanism of action different from that of aspirin, can be used (150 mg twice a day) in acute infarction in patients in

whom aspirin is contraindicated. Its actions do not develop immediately. Ticlopidine is also discussed in Chap. 52.

Aspirin is an effective antithrombotic at doses as low as 80 mg, but the rapid, acute effect probably requires 160 mg, which is absorbed and is thus clinically effective more quickly if the tablet is chewed rather than swallowed whole. Thus the patient suspected of having a coronary ischemic syndrome should receive, early in the course, 160 to 325 mg of non-enteric-coated aspirin, which is chewed.

Management after Triage into Electrocardiographic Subgroups

As discussed above, the initial ECG, as a first approximation, permits the assignment of patients with chest pain into subgroups that are distinguishable in terms of therapeutic responsiveness and risk. Thus, those with either ST-segment elevation and presumptively new bundle branch block or those with ST-segment depression and/or T-wave inversion are in high-risk groups, whereas those with either normal ECGs or nonspecific changes are in a lower risk category. Furthermore, the high-risk groups can be subdivided into those (ST-segment elevation or new bundle branch block) who have a favorable therapeutic response to thrombolytics and those who do not (ST-segment depression and/or T-wave inversion). *It must be kept in mind that these initial categorizations do not necessarily define ultimate outcome. Thus, patients with no ST-segment elevation at presentation may, in fact, have unstable angina and ultimately have no infarction or may progress to have either a Q-wave or a non-Q-wave infarction. Similarly, those presenting with ST-segment elevation may have a non-Q-wave infarction, although the majority of these will develop Q waves.* This potential for variable outcomes provides the underlying rationale for close monitoring and continuous reassessment of clinical course, risk, and therapeutic strategies during the period of observation and for monitoring both in the emergency department and subsequently in other hospital units.

APPROACH TO THE PATIENT WITH ST-SEGMENT ELEVATION

The approach to the patient with chest pain and ST-segment elevation is guided heavily by the evidence that this subgroup has a high frequency of epicardial coronary artery occlusion by a thrombus[5,321] and by evidence from animal studies that myocardial necrosis can be halted by prompt reperfusion.[322,323] Furthermore, multiple clinical trials of thrombolytic therapy have shown clinical benefit, as reviewed previously. Among patients with active, unstable coronary syndromes, only those with ST-segment elevation show efficacy in clinical response to thrombolysis (Fig. 47-6[15]). This efficacy, however, has been shown in men, women, and diabetics and is manifest regardless of any history of previous myocardial infarction, existing heart rate, or recorded blood pressure (if less than 175 mmHg).[263] The greatest benefit is seen in patients with anterior myocardial infarction (and inferior infarction with right ventricular involvement), those with signs of a large infarction (systolic blood pressure less 100 mmHg or heart rate greater than 100 beats per minute), and in diabetics. Thus, the evaluation and management of the patient with ischemic chest pain and ST-segment elevation is focused on the rapid assessment of suitability for and delivery of reperfusion therapy.

During the initial evaluation, the patient will have had aspirin given, blood drawn, intravenous access established, a 12-lead ECG showing ST-segment elevation in at least two adjacent leads, nasal oxygen administered, appropriate analgesia, and continuous electrocardiographic monitoring initiated. The appropriate next steps are to administer a beta-adrenergic blocker, if not contraindicated, and to initiate evaluation for reperfusion therapy. Based on the data from nine major clinical trials of thrombolytic therapy summarized by the Fibrinolytic Therapy Trialists Collaborative Group, thrombolytic therapy is efficacious in acute myocardial infarction (although linearly decreasing with the passage of time) for up to 12 h after the onset of symptoms.[263] There was a statisically uncertain benefit from 13 to 18 h. Thus, the 12-h point was chosen as defining the time frame in which the risk/benefit ratio is clearly favorable for administering thrombolytic therapy (Fig. 47-5).

Beta-Adrenergic Receptor Blockers
Recommendations for early therapy[15]:

Class I

1. Patients without a contraindication to beta-adrenergic blocker therapy who can be treated within 12 h of onset of infarction, irrespective of the administration of concomitant thrombolytic therapy
2. Patients with continuing or recurrent ischemic pain
3. Patients with tachyarrhythmias, such as atrial fibrillation with a rapid ventricular response

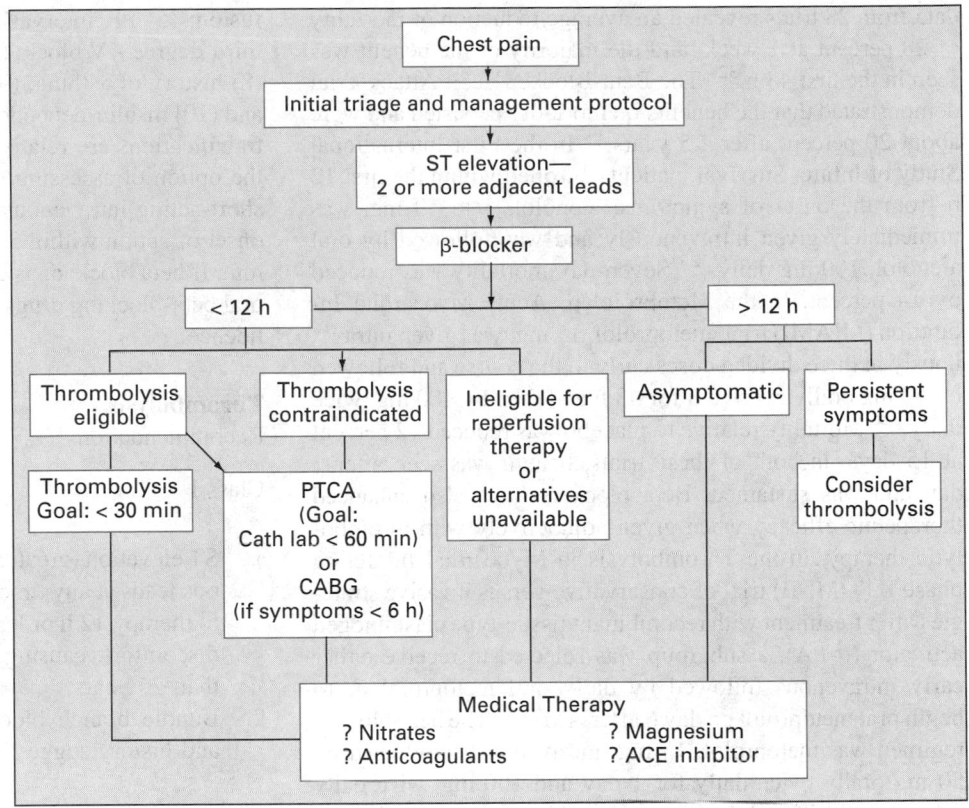

FIGURE 47-6

Evaluation of patients with ST-segment elevation. Algorithm for initial decision making in regard to reperfusion therapy in patients with suspected acute myocardial infarction and ST-segment elevation. Whether or not to administer thrombolytics or to perform primary PTCA is determined by the time from onset of symptoms. For patients in whom more than 12 h have elapsed since the onset of symptoms, reperfusion should be considered only if there are persistent or recurrent symptoms associated with ST-segment elevation. For patients with ST-segment elevation and duration of symptoms between 7 and 12 h, the decision to proceed with a reperfusion strategy requires careful clinical judgment in weighing the risk/benefit issues, as discussed in the text. (From Ryan et al.,[15] with permission.)

Class IIb

1. Non-Q-wave myocardial infarction

Class III

1. Patients with moderate or severe left ventricular failure or other contraindications

Beta-adrenergic receptor blockers interfere with the positive inotropic and chronotropic effects of catecholamines, thus reducing afterload (blood pressure) and therefore myocardial oxygen consumption. In the myocardial ischemia syndromes, these drugs should decrease ischemia and catecholamine-induced arrhythmias and should potentially reduce infarct size, in part by prolonging diastole and by improving subendocardial perfusion. Most of these theoretical advantages have, in fact, been borne out in clinical trials. The pharmacology of beta-adrenergic blockers is discussed in Chap. 54.

Many studies have demonstrated the clinical efficacy of beta blockers in the treatment of AMI. Analysis of pooled data from 28 trials revealed an average reduction of mortality of 28 percent at 1 week, and the majority of the benefit was seen in the first 48 h.[324] The Beta-Blocker Heart Attack Trial demonstrated that the benefits on mortality persisted and were about 20 percent after 2.5 years.[11] In the First International Study of Infarct Survival, patients enrolled within the first 12 h from the onset of symptoms; atenolol, 5 to 10 mg, was immediately given intravenously and was followed by oral atenolol, 100 mg daily.[325] Seven-day mortality was reduced by 14 percent. In the Metoprolol in Acute Myocardial Infarction (MIAMI) trial, metoprolol, 15 mg, was given intravenously in three divided doses early in the course and followed by 50 mg orally every 6 h for 48 h and then by 100 mg twice daily.[326] Mortality relative to placebo was reduced 12 percent at 15 days. In both of these trials, benefit was seen after 1 day and was sustained. Beta blockers have also enhanced therapeutic efficacy when given adjunctively with thrombolytic therapy. In the Thrombolysis in Myocardial Infarction phase II (TIMI-II) trial of conservative versus invasive strategies after treatment with recombinant tissue-type plasminogen activator (rt-PA), a subgroup was selected to receive either early intravenous followed by daily oral metoprolol or to begin oral metoprolol on day 6 after AMI.[327] The beta-blocker regimen was metoprolol, 15 mg, intravenously, followed by 50 mg orally twice daily for 1 day and 100 mg twice daily subsequently. The alternative protocol involved beginning the oral metoprolol regimen on day 6. The immediate intravenous metoprolol regimen was associated with a 45 percent reduction in nonfatal reinfarction and a 27 percent reduction in recurrent ischemic events in comparison with the group beginning beta-blocker therapy on day 6. *Thus, the available data strongly support the use of beta blockers early in the course of acute Q-wave myocardial infarction in the absence of contraindications.* As discussed below, the data supporting the use of beta blockers in non-Q-wave MI are less compelling. The effects of beta blockers in Q-wave MI are summarized in Table 47-9. While metoprolol and atenolol are the only FDA-approved beta blockers for use in the United States in AMI, it is generally thought that *therapeutic efficacy is a class effect of beta blockers lacking intrinsic sympathomimetic activity.*

The relative contraindications to beta-blocker therapy are as follows[15]: (1) heart rate less than 60 beats per minute; (2) systolic blood pressure less than 100 mmHg; (3) moderate or severe left ventricular failure; (4) signs of peripheral hypoper-

fusion; (5) PR interval greater than 240 ms; (6) second- or third-degree AV block; (7) severe chronic pulmonary disease; (8) history of asthma; (9) severe peripheral vascular disease; and (10) insulin-dependent diabetes mellitus. Since these contraindications are relative and not absolute, the clinician has the option of assessing the effects of beta blockade with the short-acting intravenous beta blocker esmolol, which has an onset of action within 5 to 10 min and a half-life of about 30 min. If beta blockade is tolerated by the patient, longer-acting oral beta-blocking drugs can then be used with increased confidence.

Thrombolysis
Recommendations[15]:

Class I

1. ST elevation (greater than 0.1 mV in two or more contiguous leads at any time during the observation period); time to therapy 12 h or less since the onset of continuous chest discomfort, causing hospital presentation; and age less than 75 years
2. Bundle branch block (obscuring ST-segment analysis) and history suggesting acute myocardial infarction

Class IIa

1. ST elevation (as above), age 75 years or older

Persons above age 75 benefit from thrombolytic therapy, but because of the high overall mortality rate, the relative benefit is reduced.[263]

Class IIb

1. ST elevation (as above), time to therapy (as above) greater than 12 to 24 h

Thrombolysis can be considered in the case of ongoing pain and marked ST-segment elevation, although there is only a trend for benefit under these circumstances in clinical trials.

2. Blood pressure on presentation greater than 180 mmHg systolic and/or greater than 110 mmHg diastolic with a high risk of myocardial infarction

The potential for a therapeutic benefit of thrombolysis when the blood pressure is markedly elevated must be carefully considered against the increased risk of intracranial hemorrhage under these circumstances. Lowering the blood pressure pharmacologically before administering thrombolytics has been recommended but is of unproven benefit. If available, coronary artery bypass grafting or primary PTCA should be considered.[15]

TABLE 47-9

EFFECTS OF BETA BLOCKADE IN Q-WAVE AMI

Reduces ventricular ectopy, atrial fibrillation, and nonfatal cardiac arrest

Reduces frequency of progression of threatened infarction to completed infarction

Reduces recurrent ischemia and infarction during first 6 weeks after initial event

Class III

1. ST-segment elevation, time to therapy greater than 24 h, ischemic pain resolved
2. ST-segment depression only

Indications for Thrombolytic Therapy Reperfusion therapy should be given immediate consideration in all patients presenting with acute myocardial infarction. The primary indication for attempts at reperfusion, given an appropriate history, is the findings on the ECG, as discussed above. Patients with ST-segment elevation in two or more contiguous leads or a bundle branch block (BBB) masking ST-segment changes occurring within 12 h of symptoms are candidates for thrombolytic therapy.[263,328] In the ISIS-2 trial,[329] patients with BBB had a mortality of 28 percent when treated with placebo versus 19.8 percent when treated with streptokinase and aspirin. A similar beneficial effect was noted in ISIS-3.[330] Patients of unknown age with BBB and with the clinical features of AMI are candidates for thrombolytic therapy.[328] *Patients with ongoing symptoms suggestive of myocardial ischemia should be repeatedly evaluated by 12-lead ECGs as frequently as every 10 to 15 min in order to identify ST-segment elevation as soon as possible.* Conversely, ST-segment elevation in the absence of suggestive symptoms should raise such possibilities as early repolarization, pericarditis, and previous infarction with aneurysm formation. Elderly patients should not be excluded from thrombolytic therapy primarily because of their age or because of the increased risk of bleeding. In patients over 75 years of age enrolled in the GISSI-2 trial, there were 4.2 fewer deaths per 100 patients in those treated with streptokinase than in controls,[331] while in ISIS-2, there were 3.3 fewer deaths per 100 patients in those patients over 70 years of age who were treated.[318] The results of ISIS-3[330] and GUSTO-I[332] showed benefit regardless of age or site of infarction.

Large, placebo-controlled clinical trials have consistently demonstrated reduced mortality in patients receiving thrombolytic therapy within 6 h of the onset of an AMI.[333] In comparison with conventional medical therapy, thrombolytic therapy reduces the 35-day mortality by 21 percent. It is estimated that 34 lives per 1000 patients treated are saved when thrombolysis is used within the first hour of symptom onset, compared to 16 lives saved per 1000 treated when thrombolytics are given 7 to 12 h after the onset of symptoms.[15] The true benefit of thrombolytic therapy between 6 and 12 h has been somewhat unresolved; however, the ACC/AHA guidelines have indicated acceptance that there may be a definite benefit between 6 and 12 h and have, therefore, recommended that the time limit for therapy be up to 12 h from the onset of symptoms. The EMERAS trial[334] showed an insignificant (14 percent) improvement in survival using streptokinase between 6 and 12 h after an infarction, while the LATE trial[335] observed a significant improvement (22 percent) in patients treated with rt-PA up to 12 h after infarction. Results of pooling the data from the LATE, EMERAS, and ISIS trials indicate a statistically significant improvement in survival with the use of thrombolytics up to 12 h after the onset of symptoms. Thus, the benefit of thrombolytics given between 6 and 12 h postinfarction is greater in patients classified with high-risk infarction, such as those with severe heart failure. In patients with anterior infarction, left BBB, or severe hypotension, thrombolytic therapy should be given even if the precise time of onset of symptoms is unknown. Conversely, the young patient with inferior infarction having ST-T-segment elevation might not benefit greatly from thrombolytic therapy after 6 h from the onset of symptoms.

In contrast, patients with ST-segment depression, T-wave inversion, or no ECG changes have not been shown to benefit from thrombolytic therapy, as noted above.[336] A major problem in patients with nonspecific ST depresson or T-wave inversion is that less than 20 percent will have infarction as opposed to ST-segment elevation, whereas 90 to 95 percent will have infarction. To properly assess thrombolytic therapy in this group of patients, one would need to have some objective marker other than the ECG to triage for infarction upon admission, which, until recently, was not possible (see discussion of MB-CK subforms above). In the TIMI-III trial, the importance of differentiating non-Q-wave infarction from unstable angina was demonstrated, in that patients with unstable angina receiving rt-PA experienced an increased incidence of reinfarction and death compared with conventional therapy, and the trial had to be discontinued.[181] In contrast, rt-PA had no beneficial effect but may even have a deleterious effect on patients with non-Q-wave infarction. However, the mean time of initiating thrombolytic therapy in patients with non-Q-wave infarction was 9 h from the onset of symptoms and was probably too late to have a significant beneficial effect (see "Management of Non-Q-Wave Infarction" below). An appropriate trial in which non-Q-wave infarction is diagnosed upon presentation to the emergency department within 20 to 30 min, as with MB-CK subforms or myoglobin, and is followed by thrombolytic therapy or PTCA is yet to be performed. This would be an important trial, since about 50 percent of infarctions in the United States are now non-Q-wave infarctions.[337]

Contraindications to Thrombolytic Therapy The major contraindication to thrombolytic therapy is a cerebrovascular accident (CVA) within the preceding 3 months. A hemorrhagic CVA in the past is an absolute contraindication, whereas a nonhemorrhagic CVA in the more distant past with complete or nearly complete recovery is only a relative contraindication.[338] Patients who have undergone recent (within 2 weeks) major surgery or vaginal delivery are not candidates for thrombolytic therapy, and neither are those with active internal bleeding or bleeding from a peptic ulcer. Puncture of a noncompressible vessel within the previous 10 days makes thrombolytic therapy inadvisable. Other absolute contraindications to thrombolytic therapy include suspected aortic dissection, recent head trauma or known intracranial neoplasm, and pregnancy. Previous exposure to streptokinase or anistreplase (APSAC) requires the use of rt-PA in subsequent attempts at thrombolysis. Systemic arterial hypertension and cardiopulmonary resuscitation should no longer be regarded as absolute contraindications to thrombolytic therapy. The ISIS-2 trial found that, among patients with a systolic blood pressure greater than 175 mmHg, the mortality rate was lower in those receiving streptokinase than in control subjects (5.7 versus 8.7 percent).[329] Some practitioners consider a recorded blood pressure greater than 200/120 an absolute contraindication. A history of severe chronic hypertension with diastolic blood pressure greater than 100 mmHg, with or without drug therapy, is a relative contraindication. Most clinicians proceed with thrombolytic therapy in a high-risk patient if elevated blood pressure normalizes promptly, with the easing of pain and anxiety through the use of narcotics and more direct therapy, including nitroglycerin and beta blockers. Califf et al. noted that patients who had brief (<10 min), nontraumatic cardiopulmonary resuscitation (CPR) had no evidence of tamponade or hemothorax with thrombolytic therapy.[339] Prior administration of CPR should be considered a relative contraindication, since the risk of further bleeding in the chest may not outweigh the benefit. Other relative contraindications include hemorrhagic retinopathy, trauma or surgery more than 2 weeks previously, active peptic ulcer disease, and bleeding diathesis or current use of anticoagulants. The absolute and relative contraindications for thrombolytic therapy are summarized in Table 47-10.

TABLE 47-10

ABSOLUTE AND RELATIVE CONTRAINDICATIONS
TO THROMBOLYTIC THERAPY

Absolute Contraindications	Relative Contraindications
Active internal bleeding	History of nonhemorrhagic
Intracranial neoplasm or	cerebrovascular accident
recent head trauma	in distant past with
Prolonged, traumatic CPR	complete recovery
Suspected aortic dissection	Recent trauma or surgery
Pregnancy	>2 weeks previously
History of hemorrhagic	Active peptic ulcer disease
cerebrovascular accident	Hemorrhagic retinopathy
or recent nonhemorrhagic	History of severe
cerebrovascular accident	hypertension with
Recorded blood pressure	diastolic blood pressure
>200/120	>100
Trauma or surgery that is a	Bleeding diathesis or
potential bleeding source	concurrent use of
within previous 2 weeks	anticoagulants
Allergy to SK or APSAC	Previous treatment with SK
if being considered	or APSAC if being
	considered (does not
	apply to rt-PA)

Key: CPR = cardiopulmonary resuscitation; SK = streptokinase; APSAC = anistreplase; rt-PA = recombinant tissue plasminogen activator.

Choice of Thrombolytic Agent   Three thrombolytic agents have been approved previously in the United States for routine use: streptokinase (SK), rt-PA, and APSAC. A fourth, reteplase (r-PA), was recently approved. Each has been shown to limit infarct size, preserve ventricular function, and improve survival rates. These drugs and their pharmacologic properties are discussed in detail in Chap. 52.

In angiographic studies,[332,340,341] rt-PA recanalized the coronary artery at 90 min in about 70 to 75 percent of patients, compared with 55 to 60 percent of those receiving SK or APSAC. Patency determined at 24 to 36 h is essentially the same for all four agents. The time course for this "catch-up" phenomenon in vessel patency, as defined by the GUSTO angiographic substudy, occurs within the first 3 h after administration of the lytic agent.[13] Since rapid lysis appears essential for the limitation of infarct size, it was surprising that the initial large trials comparing SK, rt-PA, and APSAC found the reduction in mortality to be identical for each of the three agents. In the GISSI-2 International rt-PA/SK Mortality trial, the mortality rate with SK therapy (8.5 percent) was the same as with rt-PA (8.9 percent).[331] Likewise, the ISIS-3 trial reported a 30-day mortality rate, which was the same for all three agents (10.5 percent for SK, 10.6 percent for APSAC, and 10.3 percent for rt-PA).[330] Conversely, the GUSTO trial found a 30-day mortality rate of 6.3 percent for the accelerated rt-PA regimen, which was significantly less than the 7.2 percent mortality with SK and subcutaneous heparin and less than the 7.4 percent mortality with SK and intravenous heparin (Table 47-11).[342] This absolute reduction of one percent reflects a 14 percent reduction in the risk of death, compared with that of SK or APSAC. The reasons for the discrepancies in these megatrials with regard to survival are probably related both to the more accelerated regimen of rt-PA administration in GUSTO and to the much more aggressive use of intravenous heparin in the rt-PA limb. Initially rt-PA induces patency in a greater percentage of patients than does SK or APSAC, and recent data indicate that the higher patency rate of rt-PA is maintained if the partial thromboplastin time (PTT) is maintained at least 1.5 to 2.0 times that of normal by the use of

TABLE 47-11

30-DAY MORTALITY RATES FROM THE GUSTO TRIAL

Regimen	Mortality, %
SK and subcutaneous heparin	7.2
SK and intravenous heparin	7.4
Accelerated rt-PA and intravenous heparin	6.3[a]
Combination rt-PA and SK with intravenous heparin	7.0

[a] 14% reduction in mortality rate was achieved with the accelerated rt-PA regimen versus the SK strategies ($p = .001$).

Key: SK = streptokinase; APSAC = anistreplase; rt-PA = recombinant tissue plasminogen activator.

heparin. In the GISSI-2 international trial, heparin was not given until 12 h after thrombolytic therapy and was administered in doses of 12,500 U subcutaneously twice a day; in the ISIS-3 trial, it was also given subcutaneously but was initiated 4 h after thrombolytic therapy. It has been shown that heparin given subcutaneously does not reach adequate therapeutic levels for 24 to 36 h and that, at the dose used in these trials, adequate levels even after 24 h occur in only 50 percent of patients.[343] In the rt-PA limb of the GUSTO trial, a bolus of heparin was administered immediately and was followed by intravenous heparin monitored closely by serial determinations of PTT. The 1-year follow-up on the GUSTO-I patients[344,345] showed that the 1 percent lower mortality rate compared with SK was maintained, which provided further evidence that rt-PA is more effective than SK.

Reteplase (r-PA) is a modified recombinant form of rt-PA with a longer half-life (15 min) and can be given as two boluses 30 min apart (see Chap. 52). In the initial open-phase trials (Reteplase Angiographic Phase II International Dose-Finding Trial: RAPID I and RAPID II),[346,347] patency was compared to that of rt-PA. In RAPID I, 60-min patency with r-PA was 78 percent, versus 66 percent for rt-PA, and TIMI-III flow was 51 percent, versus 33 percent for rt-PA. At 90 min after administration, patency was 85 percent for r-PA and 77 percent for rt-PA, with TIMI-III flow being 63 percent for r-PA and 49 percent for rt-PA. These results suggested slightly better patency rates with r-PA than with rt-PA. In the International Joint Efficacy Comparison of Thrombolytics (INJECT) trial of 6000 patients, r-PA was compared with SK.[348] The mortality and the incidence of complications for r-PA was identical to SK. This was followed by the GUSTO-III trial,[349] which compared r-PA with rt-PA, and showed that mortality and bleeding complications were similar. At 30 days, the mortality rate in the r-PA group was 7.43 percent; with rt-PA, it was 7.22 percent. The rate of hemorrhagic strokes was very similar: 0.91 percent for r-PA, versus 0.88 percent for rt-PA. The overall stroke rate was 1.67 for r-PA versus 1.83 for rt-PA. The rate of bleeding events was virtually identical between the two treatments. There remains some lack of clarity, since there were 10,000 patients in the r-PA limb and 5000 in the rt-PA limb, and the confidence limits were somewhat wide, leaving the interpretation open to some extent. Utilizing 95 percent confidence intervals, interpretation may be that rt-PA is 1.1 percent better than r-PA or that r-PA is 0.7 percent better than rt-PA. For this reason, there is still some uncertainty as to whether these drugs are truly equivalent.[349] Nevertheless, the generally accepted conclusion is that the two drugs have similar efficacy and safety. Reteplase has a longer half-life and is given as two boluses, while rt-PA is given as a single bolus followed by a continuous intravenous infusion.

The selection of a thrombolytic agent must be based on its adverse effects as well as upon its efficacy. The major risk with any thrombolytic agent is its propensity for causing bleeding, with the most devastating bleed being a hemorrhagic stroke. In the GUSTO trial, the frequency of hemorrhagic stroke was 0.49 percent for SK and subcutaneous heparin, 0.54 percent for SK and intravenous heparin, 0.72 percent for rt-PA, and 0.94 percent for combined SK and rt-PA. There was a small but significant excess of hemorrhagic strokes for rt-PA and for the combined rt-PA and SK strategy ($p < .001$) compared with the SK arms. The combined end point of death or nonfatal hemorrhagic stroke was, however, significantly reduced in the rt-PA group, compared with the SK groups (6.6 versus 7.5 percent; $p = .004$).[342] One reason to choose rt-PA over SK is the 14 percent decreased risk of mortality. Nevertheless, a 10-fold greater cost of rt-PA must be considered. Choosing between rt-PA and r-PA, since both are equally effective and cost the same, may depend on choosing between monitoring an intravenous infusion of rt-PA versus two bolus injections of r-PA separated by 30 min.

Dose and Administration of Thrombolytic Agents Streptokinase is given in a dose of 1.5 million units intravenously over 30 to 60 min. Since antibodies develop and may persist for several years, a subsequent need for thrombolytic therapy, as for early or late reocclusion, would require the use of rt-PA or r-PA. If the patient has had a streptococcal infection within 3 to 6 months, the use of rt-PA is preferable. Although APSAC is identical to SK as a thrombolytic agent, it can be given as a rapid infusion of 30 U over 5 to 10 min. Its therapeutic half-life is similar to that of SK, which is about 90 min. In contrast, the half-life of rt-PA is about 5 min. The FDA-approved dose of rt-PA is an initial bolus of 15 mg, followed by an infusion of 50 mg or 0.75 mg/kg body weight over the next 30 min, and an infusion of 35 mg or 0.50 mg/kg body weight over the subsequent 60 min, for a total of up to 100 mg given over 90 min. Reteplase is given as an initial bolus of 15 megaunits (MU), followed by a second bolus of 15 MU in 30 min. Thrombolytic therapy is rapidly evolving, and both the specific agent and various combinations as well as the specific doses and regimens of administration are changing rapidly. In addition, urokinase has been used extensively in clinical trials, and although not approved for routine use, is frequently used as an intracoronary as well as an intravenous agent. Urokinase as an agent for thrombolytic therapy appears to be similar in efficacy and safety to SK but is more expensive. Another recombinant product is single-chain prourokinase, which has been studied as a single agent and in combination with either SK or rt-PA but is not approved for routine use. Earlier data suggesting that the combination of SK with rt-PA provided greater benefit than either agent alone was not substantiated by the GUSTO trial.[342]

Overall Strategy for Reperfusion of Patients with Acute Myocardial Infarction

The criteria for initiating thrombolytic therapy are as follows (Table 47-12):

1. Patients presenting with chest pain suggestive of myocardial ischemia, having ST-T-segment elevation greater than 1 mm in two contiguous limb leads or greater than

TABLE 47-12

CRITERIA FOR INITIATING THROMBOLYTIC THERAPY

Chest pain consistent with angina
ECG changes
 ST $\uparrow \geq$ 1 mm, $\geq$2 contiguous limb leads
 ST $\uparrow \geq$ 2 mm, $\geq$2 contiguous precordial leads
 New left bundle branch block
Absence of contraindications

2 mm in two contiguous precordial leads or new left bundle branch block and who are within 6 h of the onset of symptoms should receive thrombolytic therapy if there are no contraindications. In patients presenting between 6 and 12 h of the onset of symptoms, one must weigh more heavily the risk versus the benefit. Patients presenting after 12 h are no longer routinely considered for thrombolytic therapy.

2. Contraindications for thrombolytic therapy are absolute or relative, as discussed earlier (Table 47-10)

3. In patients receiving rt-PA or r-PA, it is recommended that heparin be given as a bolus infusion of 5000 U, followed by a continuous infusion of 1000 U/h, adjusted to keep the PTT at one-half to two times the normal control for 24 to 48 h. Heparin should be given in patients who have received SK or APSAC who are at high risk for systemic embolization. Aspirin (160 to 325 mg) should be administered as soon as possible and continued indefinitely. Beta blockers, nitrates, and occasionally calcium channel blockers may be given as indicated with or without thrombolytic therapy.

4. Patients allergic to SK or APSAC who require thrombolytic therapy should receive rt-PA or r-PA. Patients who received SK or APSAC and who again require thrombolytic therapy should receive rt-PA or r-PA.

5. Patients presenting with ST-T-segment depression and chest pain are not candidates for thrombolytic therapy. These patients need to be triaged, as indicated in Fig. 47-3, as to whether their pain is of cardiac or noncardiac origin, and, if the latter, those with either unstable angina (see Chap. 46) or non-Q-wave infarction should be treated as discussed subsequently.[350] In non-Q-wave infarction, heparin is given together with diltiazem and aspirin, in conjunction with conventional therapy, as needed.

6. As discussed below, PTCA as a primary procedure is an alternative to thrombolytic therapy only if performed in a timely fashion by individuals skilled in the procedure, and supported by experience by personnel in high volume centers (class I). The individual must perform 75 such PTCA procedures per year, and the center a minimum of 200 PTCAs per year. PTCA is indicated in patients with a contraindication to thrombolytic therapy because of a severe bleeding diathesis or in those who are in cardiogenic shock (class IIa).

7. Elective angioplasty should be reserved for patients who develop ischemia or reinfarction or in whom thrombolytic

therapy appears ineffective. In patients in whom angioplasty cannot be performed and who develop recurrent ischemia with possible infarction, the possibility of readministering a thrombolytic agent should be considered; rt-PA may be given in a full dose if the patient has not received it for 24 to 48 h.

Percutaneous Transluminal Coronary Angioplasty as a Primary Therapy for Acute Myocardial Infarction

Recommendations[15]:

Class I

1. As an alternative to thrombolytic therapy only if performed in a timely fashion by individuals skilled in the procedure, and supported by experienced personnel (individuals who perform more than 75 PTCAs per year) in high-volume centers performing more than 200 PTCAs per year

Class IIa

1. As a reperfusion strategy in patients who are candidates for reperfusion, but who have a high risk of a bleeding contraindication to thrombolytic therapy (Table 47-10)
2. Patients in cardiogenic shock

Class IIb

1. As a reperfusion strategy in patients who fail to qualify for thrombolytic therapy for reasons other than a risk of bleeding contraindication

Angioplasty as Primary or Adjunctive Therapy to Thrombolysis Detailed discussions of PTCA and its indications appear in Chap. 48. Direct angioplasty has been compared with thrombolytic therapy in eight randomized trials[351]; in all studies, however, the sample size was inadequate and selection bias may have played a role in the final results. Two large studies of registry data[351,352] raised doubt as to the apparent superiority of angioplasty over thrombolytic therapy, since, in general clinical practice, treatment delays together with technical failures may be more common than in selected centers that have participated in randomized trials. The largest (395 patients) of these studies was the Primary Angioplasty in Myocardial Infarction (PAMI) study,[232] which showed a higher success rate for establishing reperfusion in the angioplasty group. The in-hospital mortality rate was 6.5 percent for the rt-PA group and 2.6 percent for the PTCA group. Higher-risk subgroups had a mortality rate of 10.4 percent with rt-PA versus 2.6 percent with PTCA. Reinfarction or death in the hospital occurred in 12 and 5.1 percent of patients treated with rt-PA and PTCA, respectively. Treatment with PTCA was associated with a lower incidence of intracranial bleeding than was that with rt-PA. There was a higher rein-farction and death rate at 6 months with rt-PA than with PTCA.

In the PAMI trial, the incidence of intracranial hemorrhage in the rt-PA group was 2.5 percent, which is considerably higher than that observed in any other clinical trial and suggests that there may have been a selection bias. Although the PAMI trial was larger than the other primary PTCA trials, the sample size was still relatively small. This limitation, together with the high incidence of hemorrhage in the rt-PA group, made it less than definitive. A more recent study (GUSTO IIB[336]) randomized 1138 patients to PTCA or rt-PA, who presented within 12 h of the onset of symptoms. The primary end point of this study was the composite outcome of death, nonfatal reinfarction, and nonfatal disabling stroke at 30 days. Of the patients assigned to angioplasty, 83 percent had a completely occluded infarct-related artery, and TIMI-III flow was established in 73 percent. This patency is better than the 55 to 60 percent TIMI-III flow expected with rt-PA. In 3.7 percent of the patients who underwent angioplasty, surgery was also performed on the same day. The incidence of the primary end point in the angioplasty group was 9.6 percent and that of rt-PA 13.7 percent, which was highly significant ($p < .032$). However, the individual end points of death, reinfarction, and disabling stroke were not significantly different between the angioplasty and rt-PA groups. In the 6-month follow-up, the favorable effect of angioplasty disappeared, with 14.1 percent in the angioplasty group and 16.1 percent in the rt-PA group reaching the primary end point (insignificant). In summary, this study showed that overall, primary angioplasty had a slight advantage over that of rt-PA at 30 days, with most of the benefit observed between 5 and 10 days after the onset of infarction. This benefit, however, was lost over the next 6 months, such that the overall end points were the same for the two groups. Thus, primary PTCA is an excellent alternative method for myocardial reperfusion in patients with AMI. It is thus recommended as an alternative method only if the medical center performs at least 200 or more cases of primary PTCA per year and if the operator performs at least 75 PTCAs per year. It is concluded that, in most situations, thrombolytic therapy should still be regarded as the preferred strategy and the first choice for reperfusion. However, patients with severe hypertension, advanced age, or symptomatic cerebrovascular disease who are at high risk of intracranial hemorrhage should be treated with angioplasty if a skilled operator is readily available and the patient can be treated rapidly. Angioplasty is also recommended for cardiogenic shock, although definitive evidence for its benefit over conventional therapy is lacking.

Heparin as Conjunctive or Adjunctive Therapy Recommendations for heparin administration postmyocardial infarction[15]:

Class I

1. Patients undergoing percutaneous revascularization.

Class IIa

1. Administer intravenously in patients undergoing reperfusion therapy with rt-PA (alteplase) or r-PA (reteplase).
2. Administer subcutanenously (7500 U twice daily) in all patients not treated with thrombolytic therapy who do not have a contraindication to heparin. Intravenous heparin is acceptable as an alternative and is preferred in patients who have a large or anterior myocardial infarction, atrial fibrillation, a known left ventricular thrombus, or a previous embolus and thus are at high risk for systemic emboli.
3. Administer intravenously in patients treated with nonselective thrombolytic agents (streptokinase, anistreplase, urokinase) who are at high risk for systemic emboli (anterior or large infarction, history of embolus, atrial fibrillation, or demonstrable left ventricular thrombus).

It is recommended that heparin not be started immediately but that an activated partial thromboplastin time (aPTT) be drawn at 4 h and that heparin be started when the aPTT returns to less than twice control (about 70 s).

Lysis of a thrombus by any thrombolytic agent induces a surface that is perhaps the most thrombogenic known.[340,352a] Furthermore, lysis with either rt-PA or SK has been shown to be associated with marked elevation of plasma levels of thrombin, which return to normal after 24 h.[353] Since aspirin has no effect on thrombin-induced platelet aggregation,[354] the use of heparin during the initial 24 to 48 h was assumed to be critical to prevent rethrombosis and reocclusion.

The necessity of heparin for maintaining coronary patency induced by rt-PA was established in the HART trial.[332] In this trial, 208 patients received rt-PA within 4 h of the onset of their infarction. Simultaneously, 50 percent of these patients received heparin administered as a bolus, followed by an intravenous infusion, while the remainder received only oral aspirin in a dose of 81 mg/day. Coronary angiographic studies performed at 18 to 81 h showed a patency of 82 percent in the group receiving heparin and 52 percent in the group receiving aspirin (Fig. 47-7). Stratifying the group on the basis of PTT

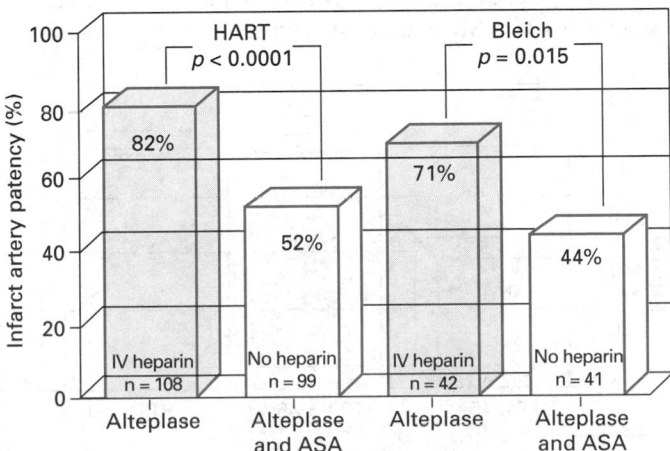

FIGURE 47-7
Influence of effective anticoagulation on early patency rates with rt-PA. Patency assessed angiographically at an average of 18 to 81 h is significantly greater in patients treated with intravenous heparin.

established an excellent correlation between patency and PTT (Fig. 47-8). In patients with a PTT of less than 45 s, the patency was only 45 percent; patency was 83 percent or greater in patients with a PTT over 45 s.[355] The findings of HART were confirmed by Bleich et al.,[356] who showed that rt-PA given with heparin had a patency of greater than 90 percent; without heparin, the patency rate was 44 percent (Fig. 47-7). In the National Heart Foundation of Australia Study,[357] all patients received rt-PA, followed by intravenous heparin for 24 h. They were then randomized to continue heparin for 72 h or were switched to antiplatelet agents. The study found the patency rate at 72 h to be the same for both groups.

Heparin appears to act by preventing early reocclusion, at least after rt-PA.[358,359] The adjunctive heparin therapy in both GISSI-2 and ISIS-3 was administered by the subcutaneous route (12 h after thrombolytic therapy in GISSI-2 and 4 h afterward in ISIS-3). Such a heparin regimen seems to be suboptimal adjunctive therapy for rt-PA and is believed to be the main reason why rt-PA was not shown to be superior over SK in GISSI-2 and ISIS-3. A subcutaneous heparin dose of 12,500 units twice a day used in the megatrials failed to provide therapeutic anticoagulation for at least 24 h in various cohort analytic studies.[343,360] The administration of SK without adjunctive heparin has not been properly tested. However, the ISIS data raise the possibility that it may not be necessary in the early hours, since the marked increase, after SK administration, in plasma levels of fibrinogen breakdown products, which inhibit platelet aggregation, may prevent rethrombosis and reocclusion.[328] In contrast, these platelet-inhibiting breakdown products are not present in high concentrations with the fibrin-selective agents, rt-PA and r-PA. The results of the SCATI trial argue for the existence of a beneficial effect of heparin even in patients treated with SK. In the SCATI trial, patients receiving SK with subcutaneous heparin had a mortality rate of 4.5 percent, while those receiving SK without heparin had a mortality rate of 8.8 percent.[361] The combined data from these studies suggest that heparin is not necessary to achieve reperfusion but is essential in the first 24 h to maintain patency rates with rt-PA. While heparin may be beneficial when SK is used, subcutaneous administration of

heparin appears adequate in this circumstance.[328] At present, heparin is recommended in a bolus of 5000 U intravenously followed by an infusion of 1000 to 1200 U/h to keep the PTT at 1.5 to 2.0 times normal. It is recommended that the PTT not be measured until 4 h after heparin therapy is initiated, because it has not yet reached a steady state. If the PTT has increased more than twofold over normal, the same dose of heparin should be continued; if PTT exhibits less than a twofold increase, the infusion rate of heparin should be increased. Initiation of heparin is recommended either during or following completion of thrombolytic therapy, as discussed above, and should be maintained in uncomplicated cases for 24 to 48 h.

The role of direct-acting antithrombins as a substitute for heparin as conjunctive therapy has been evaluated in several trials. Initial results of the pilot studies with hirudin were promising.[362] In the pilot study of hirudin for improvement of thrombolysis (HIT-I),[363] 40 patients were enrolled and received rt-PA followed by an intravenous infusion of hirudin. Grade 3 TIMI flow was observed in 71 percent at 90 min, but the reocclusion rate was 16 percent. A second open-label dose-finding study was performed (HIT-II),[364] and results were more promising at a lower dose of 0.15 mg/kg/h for 48 h. The pilot study of TIMI-V[365] was performed in 246 patients, with everyone receiving rt-PA followed by heparin or hirudin. Hirudin was associated with greater patency and a lower reocclusion rate than heparin. HIT-III[347] was performed as a randomized double-blind trial to compare heparin with hirudin in 7000 patients with AMI treated with rt-PA, but it was stopped after 302 patients because of a 3.5 percent incidence of intracranial hemorrhage with hirudin versus zero percent with heparin and a death rate of 9.7 percent in the hirudin and 5.2 percent in the heparin arms, respectively. The other two large trials were TIMI-IXA and GUSTO-2A. In TIMI-IXA,[366] patients receiving thrombolysis and aspirin were randomly assigned to receive hirudin (0.6 mg/kg bolus), followed by an infusion (0.2 mg/kg/h) of heparin over 96 h. Enrollment was stopped prematurely after 757 patients because of the high rate of intracranial bleeding in both treatments of 1.7 and 1.9 percent. Similarly, the GUSTO-2A trial,[367] in which the same dose of hirudin was compared with heparin, was discontinued after enrollment of 2584 patients because of an excess of intracerebral bleeding of 1.3 percent with hirudin and 0.9 percent with heparin. TIMI-IXB[368] was started with a lower dose of hirudin—a 0.1-mg/kg bolus—followed by an infusion of 0.1 mg/kg/h as adjunctive therapy to rt-PA or SK, plus aspirin in 3002 patients with AMI. The clinical event rate was 11.9 percent of 1491 patients treated with heparin and 12.9 percent in the 1511 patients treated with hirudin. There was no difference between the death rate or nonfatal reinfarction of the two groups. Similarly, the incidence of major and minor bleeding was the same in both groups. The investigators concluded that hirudin was as effective as heparin but was not superior. The last large trial assessing the role of hirudin as adjunctive or conjunctive therapy was the GUSTO-2B,[369] which was reinitiated with a lower dose of hirudin, similar to that of TIMI-IXB.[368] Over 12,000

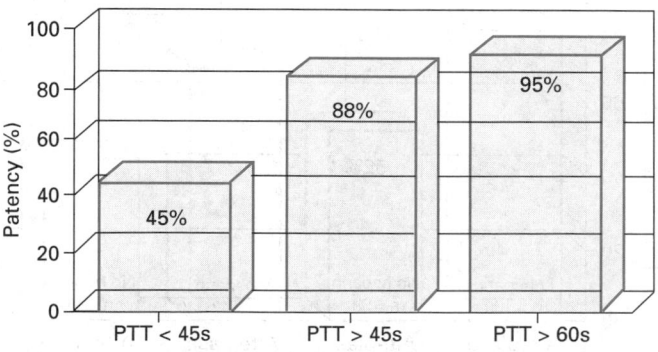

FIGURE 47-8

Retrospective analysis of the HART Trial showing the relationship between increased PTT and coronary artery patency ($n = 94$). This illustrates the importance of heparin.

patients were randomized to at least 72 h of therapy with intravenous hirudin or heparin. The primary end point of death or nonfatal myocardial infarction occurred in 8.9 percent of the hirudin group and 9.8 percent of the heparin group. *The investigators concluded that hirudin offered no benefit over heparin in patients undergoing thrombolytic therapy.* Thus, it is unlikely that hirudin will be used as adjunctive or conjunctive therapy generally in preference to heparin. However, it is clear that at the lower dose, hirudin is as effective as heparin, and in patients that develop thrombocytopenia due to heparin or are known to have had heparin-induced thrombocytopenia, hirudin is the preferred choice over heparin.[370]

The use of heparin has also been recommended conjunctively in patients with AMI who are not being treated with the drug for other reasons, i.e., postthrombolysis or postprimary PTCA. Currently, the American Association of Chest Physicians' guidelines recommend heparin 7500 U twice daily subcutaneously as prophylaxis against deep venous thrombosis.[319] Given the enhanced risk of stroke after AMI in patients with atrial arrhythmias, large and especially anterior and apical infarction, and in those with history of previous stroke,[371] the ACC/AHA guidelines have incorporated this recommendation for broader prophylaxis against systemic embolization.[15] In high-risk patients, the intravenous route is probably preferable. Heparin therapy should be continued for 48 h and judgment should be made at that point about continuation based on individual patient characteristics. Heparin therapy, including precautions concerning the monitoring of platelet counts because of the risk of heparin-induced thrombocytopenia, is discussed in Chap. 52.

EARLY CORONARY ANGIOGRAPHY IN PATIENTS WITH ST-SEGMENT ELEVATION NOT UNDERGOING PRIMARY PERCUTANEOUS TRANSLUMINAL CORONARY ANGIOPLASTY

Recommendations[15]:

Class I
None

Class IIa

1. In the presence of cardiogenic shock or persistent hemodynamic instability

Class IIb

1. In the presence of evolving large or anterior infarction and evidence that thrombolysis has not resulted in arterial patency and if adjuvant PTCA is planned

Class III

1. Routine use of angiography and subsequent PTCA within 24 h of administration of thrombolytic agents

Routine immediate or delayed angioplasty is not recommended as a standard mode of therapy following thrombolysis. The TIMI-IIA AND -IIB trials,[372] the TAMI study,[358] The

European Cooperative Study Group trial,[373] and the Should We Intervene Following Thrombolysis (SWIFT) trial[374] all showed no reduction in the incidence of coronary reocclusion or hospital mortality rates and no evidence of improved ventricular function with routine immediate or delayed angioplasty compared with elective angioplasty in the case of manifest ischemia following thrombolytic therapy. The TIMI-II trial found that angioplasty either performed routinely at 18 to 48 h when anatomically appropriate or in response to induced or spontaneous ischemia did not improve survival or reduce the reinfarction rate at either 6 weeks or 1 year,[375] and neither did it reduce the need for surgery (Fig. 47-9[375]). *At present, the most widely accepted recommendation is to perform cardiac catheterization for possible angioplasty or bypass surgery in patients who develop angina or manifest evidence of myocardial ischemia during submaximal exercise testing or who develop hemodynamic or ischemic instability.* Thus, if intervening with PTCA generally offers no demonstrable benefit after thrombolysis, there is little apparent reason to perform early coronary angiography routinely.

Rescue angioplasty to open occluded arteries after presumptive failed thrombolysis has been advocated and, in fact, recent studies indicate that TIMI grade 3 flow can be achieved in a high percentage of these patients.[376] In the recently reported TIMI-IV trial, however, it was found that although a strategy of rescue angioplasty could restore flow that is superior to that of thrombolysis alone, the incidence of adverse events for the strategy as a whole was the same as for not undertaking PTCA (35 percent adverse event rate whether or not PTCA was performed for an occluded artery). Both rates tended to be higher than the incidence in patients with patent arteries (23 percent, $p = .07$).[377] *Thus, rescue angioplasty as a routine strategy for failed or presumptively failed thrombolysis cannot be recommended.*

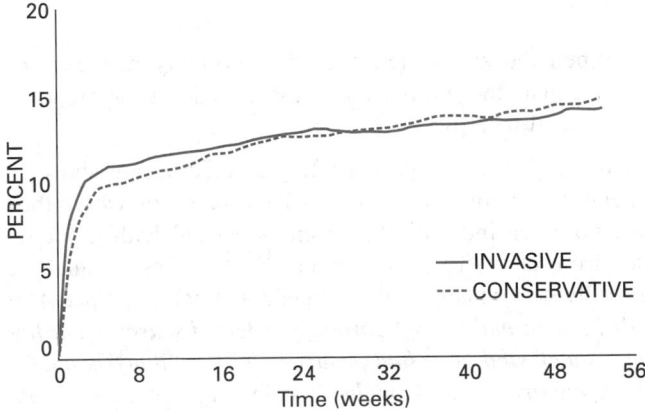

FIGURE 47-9
Kaplan Meier curves for death and infarction in patients assigned to the invasive or conservative strategies in TIMI-2. Routine cardiac catheterization after thrombolytic therapy and revascularization with PTCA or bypass grafting (when anatomically appropriate) was not a superior strategy to catheterization and revascularization when there is development of spontaneous ischemia or ischemia induced by exercise testing. (From Williams et al.,[375] with permission.)

Patients with cardiogenic shock have a very high (>70 percent) mortality with or without thrombolysis, and some rather small series have provided evidence that outcomes are improved with an aggressive reperfusion strategy. Successful PTCA in conventionally treated patients who had cardiogenic shock reduced mortality from greater than 80 to about 30 percent.[378,379] *Thus, based on available data, an aggressive interventional strategy including PTCA seems reasonable in appropriate patients with cardiogenic shock who have failed thrombolytic therapy.*

EMERGENCY OR URGENT CORONARY ARTERY BYPASS SURGERY

Recommendations[15]:

Class I

1. Failed PTCA with hemodynamic instability or persistent pain in patients with coronary anatomy suitable for surgery
2. Acute myocardial infarction with medically refractory recurrent or persistent ischemia in patients who are not candidates for PTCA but who have coronary anatomy suitable for surgery
3. After myocardial infarction, at the time of surgical repair of mitral insufficiency or ventricular septal defect

Class IIa

1. Postinfarction cardiogenic shock with coronary anatomy suitable for surgery

Class IIb

1. Failed PTCA and a relatively small mass of myocardium at risk and if hemodynamically stable

Class III

1. When the anticipated operative mortality rate exceeds or equals the mortality rate associated with appropriate medical therapy

Coronary artery bypass grafting in cardiogenic shock in patients in whom other stategies have failed or where they have not been indicated has been associated with mortality rates from about 10 to 40 percent.[380–382] These results are generally better than those associated with PTCA. *Thus, AMI patients with multivessel coronary artery disease or cardiogenic shock who have had unsuccessful thrombolysis and/or PTCA and are within 4 to 6 h of the onset of symptoms should be considered for emergency coronary artery bypass grafting.*[15]

ARRHYTHMIAS EARLY IN THE COURSE OF ACUTE MYOCARDIAL INFARCTION

Bradycardia

Bradyarrhythmias are relatively common (30 to 40 percent) early in the course of AMI, especially in inferior infarction,

or after reperfusion of the right coronary artery, because of the activation of vagal afferents that ultimately result in enhanced parasympathetic tone.[15] Atropine, because of its anticholinergic effects, can be very useful in this situation, since it enhances the discharge rate of the sinus node and facilitates atrioventricular conduction[383] as well as reversing the peripheral effects of excessive cholinergic activity such as vasodilation with associated hypotension. Parasympathomimetic effects with bradycardia, hypotension, and nausea and vomiting are also produced by morphine and can be reversed by atropine. Atropine should be used sparingly and appropriately in AMI, however, because of the protective effect of vagal stimulation against ventricular fibrillation.[384]

The Use of Atropine Recommendations[15]:

Class I

1. Sinus bradycardia with evidence of low cardiac output and hypoperfusion peripherally or frequent ventricular premature complexes at the onset of symptoms of acute myocardial infarction
2. Acute inferior infarction with type I second- or third-degree atrioventricular (AV) block associated with symptoms of hypotension, ischemic discomfort, or ventricular arrhythmias
3. Sustained bradycardia and hypotension after administration of nitroglycerin
4. Morphine-induced nausea and vomiting
5. Ventricular asystole

Class IIa

1. In patients with inferior infarction and type I second- or third-degree block at the AV-nodal level (narrow QRS complex or known preexisting bundle branch block) who are symptomatic from the low output and/or vagal predominance

Class IIb

1. Vagal symptoms and sinus bradycardia associated with the administration of morphine
2. Patients with inferior infarction who are asymptomatic with type I second-degree heart block or third-degree block at the AV node
3. Second- or third-degree AV block of uncertain mechanism and unavailability of pacing

Class III

1. Asymptomatic sinus bradycardia and a rate of greater than 40 beats per minute with no signs of hypoperfusion or frequent ventricular premature contractions
2. Type II and third-degree AV block and third-degree AV block with new, wide QRS complex (i.e., block below the AV junction)

Sinus Bradycardia, Atrioventricular Block, or Ventricular Asystole Atropine is indicated for the treatment of type I second-degree AV block, especially with complicating inferior myocardial infarction, and is useful at times in third-degree AV block at the AV node in restoring AV conduction or for increasing the junctional response rate.[15] By increasing the sinus node rate or by improving AV conduction, atropine may improve signs or symptoms of congestive heart failure, hypotension, or frequent, complex ventricular arrhythmias associated with AV block or sinus bradycardia; thus, pacemaker insertion may be avoided.[385] Treatment of sinus bradycardia or first- or second-degree AV block is generally not indicated in the absence of hemodynamic compromise,[15] and atropine should seldom be used in the treatment of type II AV block (location of block below the AV node). *Symptomatic bradycardia that is unresponsive to atropine should be treated with pacing.*

Atropine should be administered intravenously at a dosage of 0.5 to 1.0 mg and repeated as necessary to achieve an adequate heart rate every 3 to 5 min, up to a total maximum dose of 2.5 mg, which gives complete vagal blockade.[15] Atropine may also be efficacious in ventricular asystole and should be given intravenously at a dosage of 1.0 mg every 3 to 5 min during cardiopulmonary resuscitation up to a maximum of 2.5 mg if asystole persists.

At doses of 0.5 mg or less, atropine may produce, paradoxically, bradycardia and suppression of AV nodal conduction due to a central or peripheral parasympathomimetic effect.[386] Atropine dosage should be titrated carefully, because tachycardia can be induced and ischemia can be worsened. Thus, atropine should be given in 0.5-mg increments, as noted, to achieve an adequate heart rate of 50 to 60 beats per minute.

Heart Block Heart block develops in about 10 percent of patients with AMI and is associated with an increased mortality during hospitalization, but it does not predict long-term mortality in those who survive to be discharged.[387–389] Intraventricular conduction delay or BBB is also associated with increased in-hospital mortality.[263] The increase in mortality associated with heart block reflects the extent of myocardial damage, not heart block per se. Thus, a heart block in the setting of anterior myocardial infarction reflects extensive infarction and concomitant destruction of the conduction system and is associated with relatively high mortality. In contrast, heart block with inferior myocardial infarction may primarily reflect ischemia of the AV node rather than extensive tissue damage and is associated with a more favorable prognosis. Because of the overwhelming effect of the extent of myocardial damage on prognosis, pacing has not been shown to lessen mortality associated with AV block or BBB.[388,390] It is likely, however, that pacing will benefit subgroups of these patients with severe slowing of ventricular rates but without extensive myocardial damage[390,391] by preventing hypotension, ischemia, and ventricular escape arrhythmias associated with the appearance of a heart block. *In AMI, the risk of developing heart block is augmented by the presence of any evidence of conduction system abnormality including first-degree AV block, Mobitz type I or II AV block, left anterior or posterior hemiblock, or a left or right bundle branch block.*[15]

Temporary Pacing Early in the Course of Acute Myocardial Infarction The most recent "Guidelines for the Management of Patients with Acute Myocardial Infarction"[15] place increased emphasis on transcutaneous pacing in view of the availability of new systems that provide standby status for pacing in AMI patients who do not necessitate immediate pacing and are at intermediate risk for developing heart block. These systems use a single pair of multifunctional electrodes, permitting electrocardiographic monitoring, transcutaneous pacing, and defibrillation.[392] Transcutaneous pacing does not entail the risk and complications of transvenous pacing and, because invasive procedures may thus be avoided or delayed, is well suited for use in the patient who has undergone thrombolysis. Percutaneous pacing is painful; if prolonged pacing is required, the patient should be switched to transvenous systems.

Placement # ***of Transcutaneous Patches and Active (Demand)*** * ***Transcutaneous Pacing*** Recommendations[15,394]:

Class I

1. Sinus bradycardia (rate less than 50 beats per minute) with symptoms of hypotension (systolic blood pressure less than 80 mmHg) unresponsive to drug therapy*
2. Mobitz type II second-degree AV block*
3. Third-degree heart block*
4. Bilateral BBB (alternating left and right BBB or right BBB with alternating left anterior and posterior fascicular block (irrespective of time of onset)#
5. Newly acquired or age-indeterminant left BBB, right BBB, and anterior or posterior fascicular block#
6. Right BBB or left BBB and first-degree AV block#

Class IIa

1. Stable bradycardia (systolic blood pressure greater than 90 mmHg, no hemodynamic compromise, or compromise responsive to initial drug therapy)#
2. Newly acquired or age-indeterminate right BBB#

Class IIb

1. Newly acquired or age-indeterminant first-degree AV block#

Class III

1. Uncomplicated acute myocardial infarction without evidence of conduction system disease

As noted, transcutaneous pacing is intended to be temporary; if prolonged pacing is required, transvenous pacing should be instituted (discussed below). In addition, patients with a high probability of requiring pacing should have it instituted early on.[15] Technical aspects of transcutaneous pacing have been reviewed.[395]

Ventricular Ectopy, Tachycardia, and Fibrillation
Recommendations[15]

Class I

1. Ventricular fibrillation should be treated with an unsynchronized electric shock starting with an energy of 200 J. If the initial shock is unsuccessful, a second shock of 200 to 300 J should be administered, and, if required, a third shock of 360 J should be given.
2. Polymorphic ventricular tachycardia lasting more than 30 s or causing hemodynamic collapse should be treated with an unsynchronized shock, initially of 200 J, and, if necessary, with a second shock of 200 to 300 J, to be followed by a shock of 360 J if the arrhythmia persists.
3. Sustained monomorphic ventricular tachycardia associated with hypotension, with blood pressure of less than 90 mmHg, pulmonary edema, or angina should be treated with a synchronized electric shock of 100 J initially, to be followed by higher-energy shocks if required.
4. Monomorphic ventricular tachycardia that is sustained but not associated with hypotension, angina, or pulmonary edema should be treated with one of the regimens as follows:
   a. Lidocaine bolus of from 1.0 to 1.5 mg/kg intravenously with supplemental boluses of 0.5 to 0.75 mg/kg every 5 to 10 min, up to a maximum loading dose of 3 mg/kg as needed. This loading regimen is followed by an infusion of 2 to 4 mg/min (30 to 50 μg/kg/min).
   b. Procainamide at a loading infusion rate of 20 to 30 mg/min to a maximum of 12 to 17 mg/kg total, which may be followed by infusion of 1 to 4 mg/min.
   c. Amiodarone infused initially at 150 mg over 10 min, followed by a constant infusion of 1.0 mg/min for 6 h, and then at a rate of 0.5 mg/min.
   d. Synchronized electrical cardioversion with an initial starting level of 50 J after anesthesia is induced briefly.

Note that drug metabolism can vary depending upon age, body size, and liver and renal function, and that doses may need to be adjusted accordingly.

Class IIa

1. Antiarrhythmic drug infusions may be utilized after an episode of ventricular tachycardia or fibrillation but should be discontinued after 6 to 24 h, when the need for further management of the arrhythmia is reassessed.
2. Metabolic abnormalities of electrolytes and acid-base balances should be corrected as prophylaxis against recurrence when the initial ventricular arrhythmia has been treated.

Class IIb

1. Polymorphic ventricular tachycardia, which is refractory to drug treatment, should be managed by focusing on relieving the presumptive underlying ischemia with beta blockers, intraaortic balloon pumping, and/or emergency revascularization. Amiodarone infusion, as noted above, may also be useful.

Class III

1. Treatment of isolated ventricular premature beats, couplets, runs of accelerated idioventricular rhythm, and nonsustained ventricular tachycardia.
2. Use of antiarrhythmic drugs prophylactically during administration of thrombolytic agents.

Ventricular rhythm abnormalities are common during the early phases of AMI, with an incidence of ventricular fibrillation (VF) within the first 4 h, so-called *primary VF*, of 3 to 5 percent, which declines rapidly thereafter.[396] Primary VF is thought to be the result of micro reentry mechanisms in the infarct zone.[15] Postulated triggering mechanisms include hypokalemia, hypomagnesemia, enhanced adrenergic tone, acidosis, increased intracellular calcium, increased free fatty acids, and reperfusion-induced production of free radicals.[397–399] Although the relative contribution of each of these factors to early ventricular tachycardia/fibrillation and the effects of their specific treatment are not known,[15] epidemiologic evidence suggests that there has been a decrease in the incidence of primary VF,[400] which may be related generally to more aggressive treatment strategies, including the use of beta blockers. Primary VF is associated with increased in-hospital mortality but not with increased long-term mortality for patients who survive and are discharged.[401]

Post-AMI VT occurs in about 15 percent of patients and is also most commonly manifest during the relatively early period.[396] Ventricular tachycardia is classified according to its electrocardiographic morphology (*monomorphic or polymorphic*) and by its duration and consequences: *sustained (lasting more than 30 s and/or causing hemodynamic compromise earlier, which requires intervention) and nonsustained (not resulting in hemodynamic compromise and lasting less than 30 s).*[15] Short runs (5 beats or less) of nonsustained VT are very common in the early post-MI period and do not require specific treatment.

Because primary VF is one of the major contributors to mortality in the first 24 to 48 h after AMI, a great deal of attention has been paid to attempting to define characteristics of ventricular premature beats that predict VT/VF in order to provide prophylaxis. The hierarchical classification of ventricular arrhythmias according to propensity to cause VT/VF—for example, early coupled R-on-T premature beats as opposed to late-cycle, coupled beats—has fallen out of favor because of the realization that the late-cycle premature beats were equally likely to induce VT/VF.[402]

Accelerated idioventricular rhythm normally occurs frequently during the first hours of AMI,[15] and occurs after thrombolysis as a reperfusion arrhythmia. In neither case is it a premonitory rhythm for VT/VF.[403–405] *Accelerated idioventricular rhythm should ordinarily be observed and not treated specifically.*[15] It has been suggested, however, that if accelerated idioventricular rhythm speeds up to a rate of about 120 beats per minute, it should be considered an automatic rhythm for which suppression with lidocaine should be considered.[402]

Formerly, it was common practice, in order to prevent VT/VF, to treat prophylactically with lidocaine either all patients with AMI or, selectively, those with patterns of premature ventricular contractions thought to predict VT/VF. This approach is no longer common practice, because metaanalysis of trials of lidocaine prophylaxis, although confirming a substantial reduction in primary VF, showed evidence of increased mortality, probably because of episodes of profound bradycardia and asystole.[406] Thus, *routine use of prophylactic lidocaine in AMI in the presence or absence of thrombolysis is not recommended.*

Two prophylactic approaches to the prevention of VT/VF, however, are recommended.[15] Routine administration of beta blockers, as described previously, has been shown to reduce the incidence of VT/VF. Also, since evidence suggests that hypokalemia is a risk factor for VT/VF,[398,399] it is recommended that serum potassium levels be kept above 4.0 meq/L by supplementation as necessary. Although the supporting evidence is less compelling, it is also considered to be good clinical practice to maintain serum magnesium levels above 2.0 meq/L in AMI patients.[15]

Treatment of Ventricular Tachycardia/Fibrillation Electrical cardioversion of VT that is hemodynamically compromising should be performed immediately.[396] Rapid polymorphic VT should be considered the equivalent of VF and cardioverted with an unsynchronized shock of 200 J; monomorphic VT at a rate of greater than 150 beats per minute can be treated initially with a synchronized discharge of 100 J.[15,394] Urgent cardioversion for VT with rates of under 150 beats per minute is usually not needed. Ventricular tachycardia that is tolerated hemodynamically can be approached initially with trials of lidocaine, procainamide, or amiodarone, as outlined above, with attention being paid to need for dose modifications based on age and renal and hepatic function.

Ventricular fibrillation should initially be treated with an unsynchronized shock of 200 J, then incrementally at 200 to 300 J, and finally at 360 J as needed.[394] There are no definitive data concerning appropriate adjunctive therapy for fibrillation that is difficult to cardiovert.[15] The Advanced Cardiac Life Support (ACLS) protocol recommends the following hierar-

chical approach, as needed, to adjunctive therapy of resistant VF[394]: (1) epinephrine (1 mg IV); (2) lidocaine (1.5 mg/kg IV); and (3) bretylium (5 to 10 mg/kg IV). Intravenous amiodarone (150 mg IV bolus) may also be used.[15] In the case of resistant or recurrent ventricular tachycardial/ventricular fibrillation (VT/VF), electrolyte imbalances should be sought and corrected and ongoing ischemia suspected. Beta-adrenergic blockers should be used in recurrent VT or primary VF to decrease both sympathetic input to the heart and ischemia.[15] Intravenous amiodarone should be used in these life-threatening ventricular tachyarrhythmias.[407] *If ongoing ischemia is involved, intraaortic balloon pumping or emergency revascularization should be considered.*

APPROACH TO THE PATIENT WITH ISCHEMIC-TYPE CHEST PAIN AND WITHOUT ST-SEGMENT ELEVATION

As discussed previously, the initial criterion differentiating patients with symptoms compatible with AMI for therapeutic purposes is the presence or absence of ST-segment elevation. This distinction is important, because in the absence of ST-segmentel evation, there is no therapeutic benefit to thrombolysis in the AMI patient (Fig.47-5). Patients without ST-segment elevation are less likely to develop Q waves on the ECG, although about half of those who present with ST-segment elevation as well will not develop Q waves, especially if thrombolysis is utilized.[408,409] Acute myocardial infarction in which Q waves do not develop is categorized as non-Q-wave myocardial infarction (NQWMI), and most patients (90 percent) present with ST-segment depression.[78,147] Non-Q-wave myocardial infarction currently accounts for about 50 percent of all AMIs.[86,337]

Non-Q-wave myocardial infarction, like infarction with Q-waves, is precipitated by plaque disruption.[410,411] Total coronary occlusion demonstrated angiographically is much less common than in Q-wave myocardial infarction.[410] When total occlusion is present, it probably occurs in a well-collateralized vessel.[410,412] These observations—considered together with early data showing that NQWMIs involved loss of a smaller mass of myocardium than in the case of Q-wave myocardial infarctions[413,414]—are consistent with the concept that either NQWMI is associated with less than total compromise of blood flow to a region of myocardium or that early reperfusion occurs. The evidence that early reperfusion is relatively common in NQWMI was reviewed previously. Because of the residual noninfarcted myocardium at risk distal to a disrupted plaque, moreover, patients with NQWMI have a high propensity for recurrent ischemia, infarction, and death[87] and present an opportunity for secondary prevention (Fig.47-10). Nondiagnostic ECGs (ST-segment depression, T-wave inversion) on admission and NQWMI are more common in the elderly and in those with a history of prior AMI.[261,412] Generally, the incidence of NQWMI may be increasing in concert with the aging population and with the increased use of thrombolytic therapy, beta blockers, and aspirin.[15]

No therapeutic benefit of thrombolytic therapy was detected in patients with ST-segment depression in the first

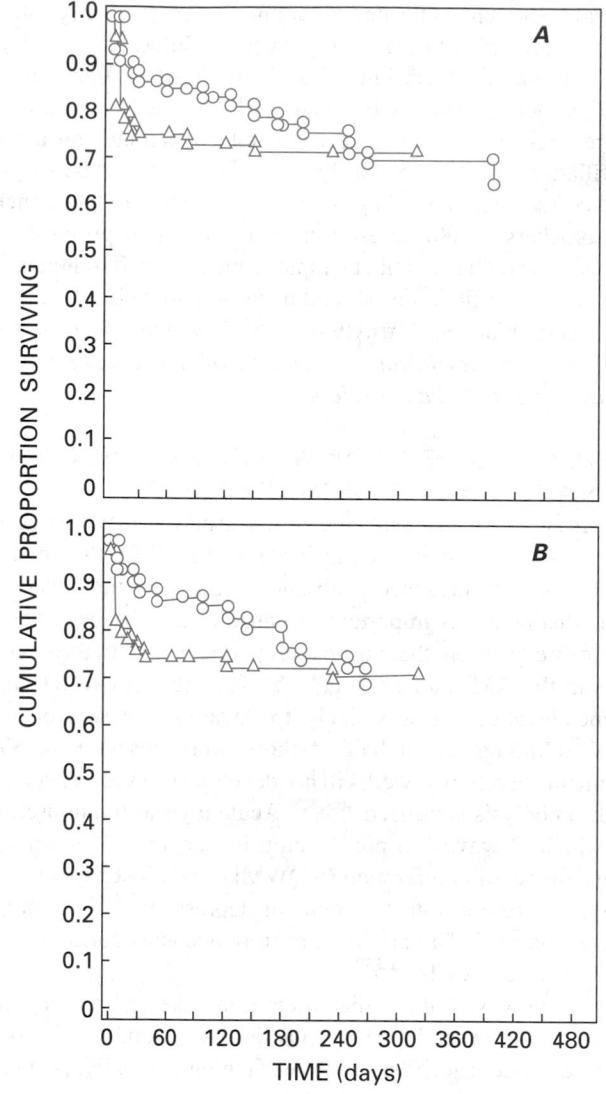

FIGURE 47-10

Comparison of the survival of patients with Q-wave infarction (triangles) to that of patients with non-Q-wave infarction with (circles) and without (squares) early recurrent infarction. Early mortality was higher after Q-wave infarction than after non-Q-wave infarction and no recurrence (*A*), but survival was identical for patients with Q-wave infarction and those with non-Q-wave infarction and an early recurrent infarction (*B*). Longer-term mortality rates are similar in Q-wave infarction and non-Q-wave infarction with or without early recurrence.

GISSI study and, in fact, mortality was slightly higher in the SK-treated group.[12] Patients with less strikingly abnormal ECGs had a lower mortality rate (8 percent) than the control group with ST-segment depression (16.2 percent) but, similarly, there was no benefit to thrombolytic therapy. The ISIS-2 trial illustrated the same principles.[264] ST-segment depression was associated with relatively high mortality and was not decreased by thrombolytic therapy. The mortality rate was relatively low in patients with only T-wave abnormalities and normal ECGs, 5 and 1 to 2 percent, respectively. In the relatively recently reported TIMI-IIIB trial of rt-PA in NQWMI and unstable angina, no benefit was observed with

thrombolysis as compared with aspirin and heparin.[415] Data from this trial do indicate that patients with NWQMI or unstable angina who have elevated troponin I on admission have an increased risk of nonfatal myocardial infarction or death in the ensuing 6 weeks. Two important conclusions can be derived from the available data: *(1) thrombolysis cannot be recommended in AMI patients without ST-segment elevation and (2) in the NQWMI group and based on the admission ECG, there is a graded, decremental spectrum of risk ranging from ST-segment depression to T-wave inversion to normal.*

Management of Non-Q-Wave Myocardial Infarction

Medical Management Beta-Adrenergic Blockers Recommendations[15]:

Class IIb

1. Non-Q-wave myocardial infarction

Calcium Channel Blockers Recommendations[15]:

Class I

1. None

Class IIa

1. Verapamil or diltiazem may be given to patients in whom beta-adrenergic blockers are ineffective or contraindicated (i.e., bronchospastic disease) for relief of ongoing ischemia or control of a rapid ventricular response with atrial fibrillation after acute myocardial infarction in the absence of congestive heart failure, left ventricular dysfunction, or AV block.

Class IIb

1. In infarction without ST-segment elevation, diltiazem may be given to patients without left ventricular dysfunction, pulmonary congestion, or congestive heart failure. It may be added to standard therapy after the first 24 h and continued for 1 year.

Class III

1. Nifedipine (short-acting) is generally contraindicated in the routine treatment of acute myocardial infarction because of its negative inotropic effects and the reflex sympathetic activation, tachycardia, and hypotension associated with its use.

2. Diltiazem and verapamil are contraindicated in acute myocardial infarction with associated left ventricular dysfunction or congestive heart failure.

II.   Invasive and interventional management—early coronary angiography and/or interventional therapy

Class I

1.   Patients with recurrent (stuttering) episodes of spontaneous or induced ischemia or evidence of shock, pulmonary congestion, or left ventricular dysfunction.

Class IIa

1.   Patients with persistent ischemic-type discomfort despite medical therapy and an abnormal ECG or two or more risk factors for coronary artery disease.
2.   Patients with chest discomfort, hemodynamic instability, and an abnormal ECG.

Class III

1.   Patients with chest discomfort and an unchanged ECG.
2.   Patients with ischemic-type chest discomfort and a normal ECG and more than two risk factors for coronary artery disease.

Although the situation may change with the increasing availability of very rapid assays for CK isoforms, it is important to remember that, at present, during the initial evaluation in the emergency department, the NQWMI patient—who by definition does not have diagnostic ST-segment elevation—cannot be distinguished from the patient with unstable angina and no myocardial necrosis. Thus, patients are admitted to the CCU or, if judged to be at relatively low risk, to a unit with continuous electrocardiographic monitoring but of less intensity, and *the initial pharmacologic approach, other than avoiding thrombolytic therapy, is identical* (Fig. 47-3). Serial ECGs and cardiac marker measurements should be performed and, in the case of recurrent pain with the development of ST-segment elevation, thrombolysis or primary PTCA should be performed. If the patient has recurrent, stuttering symptoms, angiography should be performed.

The calcium channel blocker diltiazem (immediate-release form) (see Chap. 54) has been shown to be effective in reducing reinfarction in the Diltiazem Reinfarction Study (DRS) (NQWMI)[78] and in the Multicenter Diltiazem Postinfarction Trial (MDIPIT) (Q-wave myocardial infarction and NQWMI)[416] in patients with preserved left ventricular function and with no evidence of congestive heart failure. The DRS study (Fig. 47-11[745]) was performed during hospitalization only (14 days); diltiazem was given in the initial 24 to 48 h after NQWMI and was shown to reduce the reinfarction rate by 47 percent compared with conventional therapy over a 2-week period. In the long-term prospective, randomized, blinded MDIPIT study, no overall benefit of diltiazem over conventional therapy was observed. In MDIPIT, 20 percent of patients upon entry had pulmonary congestion or clinical cardiac failure, and diltiazem was associated with increased mortality in this subgroup. In the remaining 80 percent of

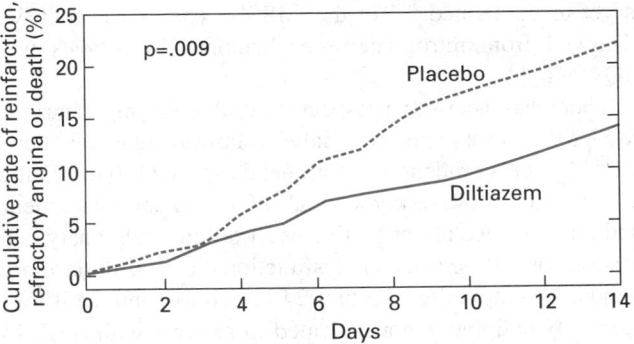

FIGURE 47-11
Life-table cumulative rates of reinfarction, refractory angina, or death according to treatment group in patients receiving diltiazem (*solid line*) or placebo (*dashed line*). This shows a statistical reduction in favor of diltiazem that is maintained throughout the duration of therapy. (From Roberts and Gibson,[745] with permission.)

patients, there was a 27 percent reduction in reinfarction and death in the group receiving diltiazem. Most of this benefit was in the prospective NQWMI substudy of 640 patients in whom diltiazem reduced reinfarction and death by 40 percent at the end of 1 year and 34 percent at the end of 4.5 years in patients without evidence of pulmonary congestion.[417] Analysis in the NQWMI subgroup for either endpoint alone (reinfarction or death) did not show a statistically significant benefit of diltiazem over placebo. A metaanalysis of the heart rate–lowering calcium channel blockers (diltiazem and verapamil) in three randomized, blinded clinical trials involving 5670 patients, with a mean follow-up of 550 days, showed a clinical event rate of 20 percent in the placebo group and 18 percent in the calcium channel blocker group ($p < .01$).[418] A recent observational trial, the VA Non-Q-Wave Infarction Strategies In-Hospital (VANQWISH) trial, comparing PTCA with conventional therapy, also showed that there was a decrease in mortality associated with diltiazem in the arm comparing conventional medical management with or without diltiazem.[349] Parenthetically, there were more deaths in the invasive than in the conservative arm. Verapamil has been studied somewhat less extensively than has diltiazem in the treatment of AMI; but when it is used within 2 weeks, a 16.7 percent reduction in death or myocardial infarction has been observed.[419] Verapamil has adverse effects on patients with heart failure or bradyarrhythmias when used within the first 24 to 48 h after AMI.[420,421] Most of the data on the use of calcium channel blockers in AMI were collected before the widespread use of aspirin, and their precise role in the current management of AMI is somewhat ill defined. The role of sustained-release diltiazem and aspirin is being studied in AMI after thrombolysis in the Incomplete Infarction Trial of European Reasearch Collaborators Evaluating Prognosis Post-Thrombolysis (INTERCEPT).[422]

There has been a lack of new therapies for NQWMI in the past decade despite the increasing proportion of patients with NQWMI (50 percent). Management of NQWMI is still evolving, and the role of antiplatelet or antithrombin agents is yet to be defined.[349] In the GISSI-3 trial, no benefit was observed from nitroglycerin or lisinopril in patients with NQWMI.[314]

There has been no prospective trial assessing aspirin in NQWMI, but retrospective analysis showed significant benefit.[423] It seems prudent to recommend aspirin (160 to 325 mg/day) for non-Q-wave myocardial infarction and—in patients without evidence of congestive heart failure, pulmonary congestion, or left ventricular dysfunction—to add diltiazem to standard therapy after the first 24 h, and to continue it for 1 year.[15] Nifedipine is not indicated in patients with AMI, for cardioprotection, to reduce the reinfarction rate, or to prolong survival.[424] No prospective studies of beta blockers have been performed solely in patients with NQWMI, but retrospective analyses of trials performed prospectively, involving both Q-wave infarction and NQWMI, generally show no effect of beta blockers for the reinfarction rate in patients recovering from NQWMI.[87,425,426] Beta blockers may be given to relieve pain or arrhythmia, as discussed previously for Q-wave myocardial infarction, and have a class IIb recommendation for use in NQWMI, as noted.

PROTOCOLS, CLINICAL PATHWAYS, AND CHEST PAIN EVALUATION UNITS

There are increasing pressures, driven by both economic and clinical imperatives, to improve the management of patients with chest pain. The goal of controlling costs has contributed to the need to triage chest pain patients accurately to levels of care that are appropriate to need and to facilitate evaluation and treatment in the shortest time that is commensurate with good medical care. For example, low-risk patients with normal ECGs frequently do not have to be admitted to the hospital, much less to the intensive care unit (ICU), and can have a total time in the health care facility of hours rather than days. The medical necessity of achieving rapid, accurate diagnoses has been discussed earlier. These two driving forces have led to the development of predictive algorithms to guide triage decisions.[70,278] For example, a recent analysis provided evidence that chest pain patients with ECG changes of ischemia or infarction were, depending on age, the only subgroup with a probability of AMI high enough (21 percent or moderate) to justify admission to the CCU as opposed to an intermediate care unit of reduced intensity.[427] While these algorithms have have been shown to be effective in, for instance, reducing ICU admissions without compromising clinical care,[278,298] they have not been widely adopted for a variety of reasons, including the fact that most experienced clinicians are comfortable with their decision making in triaging chest pain patients.[270]

The continuing need to improve the process of chest pain management has led to the development of clinical pathways, protocols, and practice guidelines that differ from predictive instruments in that they provide structure to the decision-making process rather than influencing decision making.[270,428] A chest pain evaluation unit, which may either be a defined area, frequently near the emergency department, or a virtual entity embracing a team approach to chest pain evaluation and management, is frequently central to the strategy to systematize the approach to the patient with chest pain.

In general, the approach is to triage the patient to evaluation and management pathways according to risk based on electrocardiographic findings, history, and symptoms. For example, and at the opposite end of the clinical spectrum, the patient with ST-segment elevation would receive thrombolytic therapy within 30 min of arrival and be rapidly admitted to the CCU, whereas the low-risk patient with a normal ECG would be evaluated in a unit of lower intensity and acuity and would be discharged within a matter of hours. There is a great deal of interest in the use of imaging modalities such as nuclear scanning with sestamibi or stress echocardiography to guide decision making in cases of intermediate or low probability for AMI during the initial evaluation period.[270] While the results using the systematized approach of a chest pain evaluation unit appear promising, further assessment is needed in large-scale trials to test both clinical value and cost-effectiveness before a specific strategy can be recommended. The general strategy of systematizing the approach to the chest pain patient, however, is strongly encouraged.

MANAGEMENT AFTER HOSPITAL ADMISSION

General Approach

Recommendations[15]:

Class I

1. Selection of electrocardiographic monitoring leads based on infarct location and rhythm to maximize diagnostic utility
2. Bed rest with bedside commode privileges for initial 12 h in hemodynamically stable patients who are free of ischemic-type chest discomfort
3. Avoidance of the Valsalva maneuver and straining
4. Optimization of pain relief

Class IIb

1. Routine use of anxiolytics

Class III

1. Prolonged bed rest (more than 12 to 24 h) in stable patients without complications

The general issues involved in the management of the patient with suspected or manifest AMI in the intensive or moderate care unit are to provide for adequate monitoring for the detection of arrhythmia, ischemia, and hemodynamic instability; to provide the patient with a calm, supportive, and reassuring environment; to control the level of activity; to begin the education process for a lifetime of living with coronary heart disease; to control pain and inappropriate anxiety; and to treat adverse events promptly. It is assumed, as previously discussed, that oxygen therapy, beta-adrenergic blockers, aspirin, thrombolytics, heparin, and nitroglycerin have been begun or given as appropriate in the emergency department.

MONITORING

The patient must have continuous electrocardiographic monitoring and frequent hemodynamic evaluation by the assessment of blood pressure and heart rate. Electrocardiographic monitoring leads should be selected to maximize the ability of the CCU staff to detect and diagnose arrhythmias and recurrent ischemic ST-segment changes. Thus, the lead selected should ideally permit identification of the P wave as well as providing a QRS complex of adequate size. Furthermore, the lead should be selected to interrogate the area of known infarction or ischemia.[15] Blood pressure and pulse rate should be monitored with a frequency to be determined by the perceived level of acuity but generally every half hour until stable and then every 4 h. Pulse oximetry is becoming standard. Precise orders should be given to notify the physician of, for example, systolic pressures of greater than 150 and less than 90 mmHg, heart rates of greater than 110 or less than 60 beats per minute, respiratory rate of greater than 22 or less than 8 per minute, or significant decreases in blood oxygen saturation.[15]

ACTIVITY

Minimizing physical exertion is an important approach, in addition to minimizing sympathetic nervous system drive by administering beta-adrenergic blockers and by controlling pain and excessive anxiety, so as to decrease myocardial oxygen demand and thus decrease myocardial ischemia and necrosis. *Prolonged bed rest and a severe limitation of activities such as self-feeding are no longer recommended except in the case of continuing ischemic pain and/or hemodynamic instability because of evidence that cardiovascular deconditioning and unfavorable shifts in intravascular volume develop very rapidly in immobilized patients in the supine position.*[429] Losses of plasma volume occur that decrease preload and stimulate compensatory reflexes, enhancing sympathetic acitivity. These fluid shifts may be the major cause of cardiovascular dysfunction with prolonged bed rest.[430] It is prudent to prescribe about 12 h of bed rest and a bedside commode for the patient with uncomplicated AMI.[15] Subsequently, low-level activities such as routine self-care, assisted bathing, and brief ambulation should be permitted to prevent deconditioning.

The major coronary precaution that should be strictly adhered to is the avoidance of the Valsalva maneuver, which increases cardiac wall stress becauses of increases in systolic blood pressure and heart rate.[15] These changes in wall stress may cause localized repolarization abnormalities in the infarct zone that may precipitate ventricular arrhythmias.[431,432] Constipation should be avoided and stool softeners routinely pre-

scribed. A bedside commode is preferable to a bedpan in all but the most unstable patients.

ANALGESICS AND ANXIOLYTICS

The importance of controlling chest pain and excessive anxiety and the use of morphine and diazepam were discussed previously (see "Evaluation and Management of the Chest Pain Patient in the Emergency Department"). Morphine is sometimes used in inadequate doses because of fears of side effects, and anxiolytics may be overused. Ischemic chest pain, heart rate, blood pressure, and perceived anxiety level have not been found to be different in patients treated with diazepam or with placebo.[433] Conversely, strong psychological support in hospitals has prolonged effects to prevent anxiety and depression after AMI.[434] Anxiolytics may be useful in treating symptoms of nicotine withdrawal in smokers during hospitalization. Psychosis manifesting as delirium and agitation is not uncommon, particularly in the elderly, with during prolonged stays in ICUs ("ICU psychosis"). Intravenous haloperidol can be useful and safe in this setting. Drug-induced psychosis or delirium caused by lidocaine, for example, should be considered.

EDUCATION

Education of the AMI patient by both the CCU staff and the physician are essential components of the medical management and should be begun early during hospitalization. Presenting the patient with information about the management of symptoms and prevention of a recurrence gives a sense of empowerment associated with changes in behavior[435] and decreased anxiety.[436] Information should be presented in a direct fashion at a relatively simple level and should emphasize issues relevant to patient behavior, such as control of chest pain, diet, smoking, and exercise, rather than the pathophysiology of the disease. Family members, and, in particular, the spouse should participate in the education process. Because of the substantial risk of cardiac arrest in the 18 months after AMI, family members should be taught CPR.[437,438] Ideally, educational materials can be presented in a permanent printed form so that the self-education process can continue after discharge and can supplement that given by health care professionals during cardiac rehabilitation and physician visits.

Adjunctive Therapy during the Early In-Hospital Period

ANGIOTENSIN-CONVERTING ENZYME INHIBITORS
Recommendations[15]:

Class I

1. Patients within the first 24 h of a suspected AMI with ST-segment elevation in two or more anterior precordial leads or with clinical heart failure in the absence of significant hypotension or known contraindications to the use of angiotensin-converting enzyme (ACE) inhibitors

2. Patients with AMI and a left ventricular ejection fraction of less than 40 percent or patients with clinical heart failure on the basis of systolic pump dysfunction during and after convalescence from AMI

Class IIa

1. All other patients within the first 24 h of a suspected or established AMI provided that significant hypotension or other clear-cut contraindications are absent.
2. Asymptomatic patients with mildly impaired left ventricular function (ejection fraction of 40 to 50 percent and a history of old myocardial infarction)

Class IIb

Patients who have recently recovered from myocardial infarction but have normal or mildly abnormal global left ventricular function

A number of clinical trials have shown that ACE inhibitors reduce left ventricular dysfunction and dilatation and slow the progression to congestive heart failure in patients with left ventricular dysfunction after AMI.[439-441]

The ACE inhibitors have also been shown, with few exceptions, to reduce mortality after AMI. Metaanalysis of 4 major and 11 minor trials involving, collectively, more than 100,000 patients showed an odds reduction in the ACE-inhibitor group of 6.5 percent ($2p = 0.006$).[442] Originally, there was some doubt about the timing of initiation of the ACE inhibitor after AMI because of the results of the Cooperative New Scandinavian Enalapril Survival Study (CONSENSUS) II.[443] In this randomized study, patients were assigned to intravenous placebo or enalapril during the first day of AMI and were subsequently given an oral placebo or enalapril. The trial was stopped in its early stages by the Safety Monitoring Committee because it was unlikely to show a positive effect and because of hypotension in elderly patients. The issue of timing of the initiation of ACE inhibitor therapy has been clarified subsequently. In GISSI-3, patients with either ST-segment elevation or depression were given oral lisinopril or were assigned to an open control group starting on the first day of AMI.[314] There was a significant reduction in mortality at 6 weeks (odds ratio 0.88), and the majority (60 percent) of lives saved were in the first 5 days. In ISIS-4, patients were assigned to an oral placebo or to captopril within the first 24 h, and a 7 percent mortality reduction was seen at 5 weeks in the captopril group.[315] The majority of the decrease in deaths was seen in the first 2 days. There was no increase in adverse events in the elderly in ISIS-4 or in GISSI-3. Thus, the hypotension in CONSENSUS II way be attributed to the use of intravenous enalapril.

Initiation of ACE-inhibitor therapy within the first few days after AMI in patients with left ventricular dysfunction and continuation of therapy over the long term was associated with a decrease in mortality and in fatal and severe nonfatal cardiovascular events in three other trials: Survival and Ven-tricular Enlargement (SAVE), captopril[440]; Acute Infarction Ramipril Efficacy (AIRE), ramipril[444]; and Trandolapril Cardiac Evaluation (TRACE), trandolapril.[445]

Thus, trials of ACE inhibitors have shown clear evidence of benefit in AMI from their use early in the course of AMI. Efficacy may be greatest in those at highest risk, i.e., patients with prior myocardial infarction, anterior myocardial infarction, tachycardia, or congestive heart failure. Therapy should begin within the first 24 h after hemodynamic stabilization, whether or not thrombolytic therapy has been administered. Intravenous forms should be avoided, and therapy should be started with low doses. The ACE inhibitors should not be given if systolic blood pressure is below 100 mmHg or if there are contraindications—i.e., bilateral renal artery stenosis, renal failure, history of severe cough, or angioedema with previous treatment.[15] If there is no evidence of left ventricular dysfunction (symptomatic or asymptomatic) at 4 to 6 weeks, therapy can be stopped. In the presence of significant left ventricular dysfunction, therapy should probably be continued indefinitely.

MAGNESIUM
Recommendations[15]:

Class I
None.

Class IIa

1. Correction of documented magnesium (and/or potassium) deficits, especially in patients receiving diuretics before the onset of infarction.
2. Episodes of ventricular tachycardia—torsades de pointes type—associated with a prolonged QT interval should be treated with 1 to 2 g of magnesium administered as a bolus over 5 min.

Class IIb

1. Magnesium bolus and infusion in high-risk patients such as the elderly and/or those for whom reperfusion therapy is not suitable.

The available data are conflicting but suggest that early (<6 h) administration of magnesium in high-risk patients may be associated with mortality reduction.

Magnesium has a number of potential cardioprotective effects, including vasodilatation,[446] inhibition of platelet function,[447] stabilization of cell membranes,[448] and protection against the cardiotoxic effects of catecholamines.[449]

Metaanalysis of seven early randomized trials of the effects of magnesium in AMI was consistent with a significant benefit in mortality (odds ratio 0.44).[450,451] The Second Leicester Intravenous Magnesium Intervention Trial (LIMIT-2) was consistent with this interpretation in that the magnesium-treated patients had a 24 percent reduction in overall mortality ($p < .04$), a 25 percent decrease in the incidence of congestive heart failure in the CCU, and a 21 percent lower rate of coronary artery disease mortality at 4 years.[452,453] The large ISIS-4 trial, however, was negative and even raised the possibility of some harm.[315] Incorporation of the ISIS-4 data with that of the previous randomized trials and performance of metaanalysis resulted in the loss of the benefit that was previously apparent. It has been speculated that the lack of benefit in ISIS-4 was due to the relatively late administration of magnesium,[454] since the time to randomization in ISIS-4 was 8 h, as contrasted with 3 h in LIMIT-2. It may also have been a consequence of the low control-group mortality in ISIS-4 (7.2 percent) and the statistical inability to detect a treatment effect at this level.[455] The fact that only 36 percent of patients in LIMIT-2 received thrombolytic therapy as opposed to 70 percent in ISIS-4 complicates interpretation further. Analysis of subgroups in ISIS-4 in which magnesium was administered within 6 h of the onset of symptoms or within 2 h of thrombolytic therapy also failed to demonstrate a therapeutic effect. A more recent randomized trial of intravenous magnesium in AMI patients who were not candidates for thrombolysis demonstrated a significant reduction of mortality in the treated group (4.2 versus 17.3 percent, $p < .01$), due primarily to a decrease in cardiogenic shock and congestive heart failure.[456]

The conflicting data that are available do not permit a recommendation that magnesium be used as standard general therapy in AMI. Magnesium should be used in situations where it would otherwise be recommended, as in the presence of magnesium deficiency or ventricular tachycardia of the torsades de pointes type ventricular tachycardia with a prolonged QT interval. Intravenous magnesium can be considered in high-risk patients, such as the elderly and in those for whom reperfusion is not suitable.

Management of the Low-Risk Patient

As discussed previously, there are increasing pressures to minimize resource utilization while not compromising safety in the patient with ischemic-type chest discomfort. As a practical matter, this means matching patient acuity and risk appropriately with the hospital facilities required to deal with their situation and to appropriately control time spent in these units. For example, the patient who is at low risk for AMI may be evaluated in the emergency department or in a chest pain evaluation unit, and if AMI or unstable angina are excluded, may be discharged within a matter or hours without having been formally admitted to the hospital. The patient with AMI who has an uncomplicated initial course and is at low risk for development of complications is a candidate for transfer out of the CCU within 24 to 36 h.[457–460] Such low-risk patients do not have a history of prior AMI and have not had recurrent ischemic pain, hypotension, congestive heart failure, persistent sinus tachycardia, heart block, or sustained ventricular tachycardia. These patients may be candidates for early discharge at 3 to 4 days.

Patients who have been treated with thrombolytics are frequently candidates for early discharge from the

CCU.[461–464] In this setting, the *absence* of early sustained ventricular tachycardia or fibrillation, as well as the absence of early sustained hypotension or shock, and the *presence* of a left ventricular ejection fraction of greater than 40 percent and of only one- or two-vessel coronary artery disease are independent predictors of freedom from late complications.[463]

Approaches to risk stratification and noninvasive testing, to guide management decisions in the post-AMI patient, are discussed subsequently (see "Noninvasive Risk Stratification", below). Excessive diagnostic testing in all post-AMI patients, especially those at low risk, should be discouraged. The variability in practice in this regard, without demonstrable correlative changes in outcomes, suggests the need for more rigorous adherence to guidelines and protocols.[15]

As discussed previously, AMI can be diagnosed rapidly using serum cardiac markers. If AMI is effectively ruled out and the patient is at low risk (i.e., normal ECG and absence of the characteristics noted above, especially the absence of prolonged initial pain or the recurrence of pain), then noninvasive testing can establish the safety of early discharge (3 to 12 h) from the emergency department, chest pain evaluation unit, or CCU, for further evaluation as an outpatient.[270] In general, such patients do not necessarily need to be admitted to the CCU unless noninvasive testing is positive for ischemic heart disease. Patients with ischemic-type chest discomfort and intermediate probabilities of AMI—i.e., duration of chest pain greater than 20 to 30 min and nondiagnostic ECG changes (without significant ST-segment elevation or depression, T-wave inversion, or BBB), without known coronary artery disease—should be admitted to an observation unit or to the CCU if an intermediate unit is unavailable. They should be placed on a fast track to rule in AMI or unstable angina, as outlined above. If the clinical course is unrevealing and if early imaging is negative, then stress testing and further evaluation can be planned. Clinical decisions can usually be made within 12 h in this setting.[270]

Management of the High-Risk Patient with Acute Myocardial Infarction

The AMI patient at low risk is defined in the previous section by the absence of certain characteristics. By contrast, the *high-risk AMI patient is defined by the presence of one or more of these clinical features, which include recurrent chest pain; congestive heart failure and low cardiac output; arrhythmias and, in particular, recurrent or sustained VT or VF; mechanical cardiac complications of AMI such as ruptured papillary muscle or intraventricular septum; and/or inducible ischemia and extensive coronary artery disease.*

RECURRENT CHEST PAIN

The most common causes of recurrent chest pain after AMI are coronary ischemia and pericarditis.

Recommendations for diagnosis and treatment of recurrent chest discomfort[15]:

Class I

1. Aspirin for pericarditis
2. Beta-adrenergic blocking drugs (continue or initiate) intravenously, then orally for ischemic-type chest discomfort
3. (Re)administration of thrombolytic therapy (r-PA or rt-PA) for patients with recurrent ST-segment elevation
4. Coronary arteriography for ischemic-type chest discomfort recurring after hours to days after initial therapy and associated with objective evidence of ischemia in patients who are candidates for revascularization

Class IIa

1. Nitroglycerin intravenously for 24 h, then topically or orally for ischemic-type chest discomfort

Class IIb

1. Corticosteroids for pericarditis
2. Indomethacin for pericarditis

Recurrent Ischemia

Recurrence of chest pain in the patient who has had an AMI is a serious development and requires immediate attention to establish the correct diagnosis and initiate treatment, especially if the pain represents recurrent ischemia, which is a more serious development than if the pain is a manifestation of pericarditis. Early postinfarction angina is an important predictor of the severity of coronary artery disease and has an overall incidence of about 18 percent.[465] Postinfarction angina is defined as chest pain that is frequently similar to the original discomfort, occurring at rest or with limited activity during hospitalization 24 h or more after onset of the AMI. The pain may or may not be associated with ST-segment elevation or depression or with pseudonormalization of inverted T waves on the post–myocardial ischemia ECG.[466] The pain is usually a result of ischemia in the territory of the myocardium supplied by the vessel that precipitated the initial myocardial ischemia. At least three categories of patients are at high risk for postinfarction angina: (1) patients with NQWMI; (2) patients who have received thrombolysis; and (3) patients with multiple risk factors.[467–469] The incidence of postinfarction angina is almost twice as high after NQWMI (25 to 35 percent) than after Q-wave myocardial ischemia. Thrombolytic therapy for AMI created a new high-risk group for postinfarction angina (35 to 45 percent incidence), with a 12 to 15 percent incidence of reinfarction during the early experience with lytic therapy for reperfusion.[470] Regardless of whether postinfarction angina occurs after Q-wave myocardial ischemia, NQWMI, or thrombolytic therapy, it is more likely to occur in patients with two- or three-vessel disease than in patients with single-vessel disease.[465] Postinfarction angina is important because it is associated with a twofold increase in the incidence of reinfarction. The 1-year mortality rate and acute risk of reinfarction is two- to fourfold greater in patients with postinfarction angina associated with ECG changes than in patients without chest pain or in patients with chest pain but without associated ST-T changes.[471,472]

The incidence of reinfarction following NQWMI has previously been reported to be as high as 40 percent within the first month following the event,[473] but with treatment with heparin and diltiazem, the incidence is less than 10 percent, as discussed previously. The incidence of reinfarction following thrombolytic therapy has been reduced from 12 to 15 percent to 5 to 7 percent with the use of adjunctive therapy, including heparin, aspirin, nitroglycerin, and beta blockers, as discussed previously. Nevertheless, reinfarction, despite the use of heparin and and aspirin, still accounts for a quarter of all deaths that occur following thrombolytic therapy and thus remains a major concern.[474] Patients with Q-wave myocardial infarction who do not receive thrombolytic therapy were previously likely to have an incidence of postinfarction angina of only about 12 to 15 percent and a reinfarction rate of about 5 to 7 percent, although these absolute rates have probably decreased with the more widespread use of adjunctive therapy with beta blockers, aspirin, and ACE inhibitors. Death, ventricular arrhythmias, and severe congestive heart failure are early sequelae of reinfarction, and there is an increased rate of sudden death and cardiogenic shock.[114,118]

Diagnosis of reinfarction within 18 h after thrombolytic therapy is based upon the recurrence of ischemic-type chest pain, as noted, lasting at least 30 min, which may be associated with ST-T-wave changes. There is a reelevation of CK-MB, and the diagnostic criteria were discussed previously. Adequate beta-adrenergic blockade should be achieved. Sublingual nitroglycerin should be administered, and restarting of intravenous infusion should be considered. Pain should be controlled. Coronary arteriography generally should be performed early after the redevelopment of ischemic chest pain, and it is common that a high-grade stenosis is found. If the lesion is suitable, PTCA should be performed, or additional thrombolysis should be administered if mechanical reperfusion is not feasible or available. With appropriate ECG changes—i.e., ST-segment elevation—thrombolysis should be considered if cardiac catheterization and PTCA are not immediately available. If either APSAC or SK was used originally, it should not be readministered and rt-PA or r-PA should be utilized. These latter agents can be readministered. If multiple high-grade stenoses are found, coronary artery bypass grafting should be considered.

Pericarditis

Pericardial involvement associated with AMI assumes one of two forms. By far the most common type is pericardial inflammation overlying the necrotic segment of a transmural myocardial infarction. This particular pericarditis is usually an incidental finding in the course of a more significant illness. The less frequent form of postinfarction pericarditis is generally a delayed complication, which may represent an immunologic or autoimmune reaction. This pericarditis, a component of Dressler's syndrome, generally represents a major complication that often outlasts the basic illness (see also Chap. 81).

Early Postinfarction Pericarditis The prevalence of early postinfarction pericarditis, as reflected by the presence of typical symptoms and a friction rub, is 6 to 11 percent.[475,476] However, the general consensus among cardiologists is that this entity occurs far more frequently than is clinically recognized. This suspicion is supported by post-mortem studies finding evidence of postinfarction pericarditis when it was not recognized clinically.[477] The pericarditis usually bcomes evident between the second and fourth day following the AMI, but it may occur up to several weeks later. In comparison to post-AMI patients without pericarditis, those who develop the condition have larger infarcts, a lower ejection fraction, and a higher incidence of congestive heart failure.[478,479]

The most common manifestation of pericarditis other than the chest pain is a scratchy two- or three-component friction rub along the left sternal border. The friction rub may have only a single component and may be dismissed erroneously as a systolic murmur. The rub is evanescent, generally lasting 1 to 6 days. The pain of pericarditis is generally perceived by the patient to be different from that of the AMI. The location of the pain may be the same, but any radiation is usually to the neck, shoulder, or scapula rather than to the arms or jaw. Characteristically, the pain is aggravated by inspiration, swallowing, coughing, or recumbency. Fever, usually less than 39°C, frequently accompanies the pericardial inflammation and typically lasts longer than 3 days, unlike the fever in an uncomplicated myocardial infarction.[480] The ECG is frequently not helpful in these patients, partially because it is usually distorted by the infarction and perhaps because of the localized nature of the inflammation. The cardiac rhythm is generally sinus tachycardia, but there is an increased prevalence of atrial fibrillation.[481] Since significant effusion is unusual with this form of pericarditis, the echocardiogram is of limited diagnostic value.

The treatment of choice is aspirin (160 to 325 mg daily), although higher doses (650 mg every 4 to 6 h) may be required.[15,482,483] Indomethacin is effective in relieving symptoms[15] but experimentally causes thinning of scar formation.[484] Corticosteroids and ibuprofen provide pain relief but also have been associated with thinning of scar formation as well as with cardiac rupture.[485,486] The use of anticoagulants is relatively contraindicated in AMI complicated by pericarditis. Situations ordinarily calling for anticoagulation, such as mural thrombosis seen on echocardiography, require excellent clinical judgment in assessing the risk-benefit ratio if pericarditis is also present.

Post–myocardial Infarction Syndrome (Dressler's Syndrome) The clinical features of this syndrome are fever, chest pain, evidence of polyserositis, and a tendency to recur.[482] The reported frequency is 1 to 3 percent of AMIs.[481,482] The incidence, however, has appeared to diminish dramatically in the reperfusion era.[487] While there is usually a latency period of at least 1 week before its appearance, the pleuropericarditis may develop within the first week following the AMI.[488] The syndrome can occur in association with NQWMI, and it is usually associated with fever in the range of 38 to 39°C and occasionally up to 40°C. The chest pain is the most sensitive index of this syndrome and often precedes the fever. Aggravation of the pain by deep inspiration and turning is its most distinctive feature. The pericarditis is manifest by a friction rub, usually occurring between the second and eleventh week after the infarction and lasting from 3 days to 3 weeks. Pericardial effusion is common. While pericarditis is the dominant feature, as many as two-thirds of patients have pleural effusions. These effusions are usually small and are frequently bilateral but may be large and hemorrhagic. About one-quarter of patients have linear or patchy infiltrates in the lung bases.

The clinical features, pathologic findings, and prompt response to steroids all suggest an immunologic or autoimmune reaction. The presence of antimyocardial antibodies has been demonstrated in the majority of patients tested with the syndrome.

Treatment is similar to that of early postinfarction pericarditis but is more likely to require a course of oral corticosteroids. Recurrences are common for several months and require the reinstitution of corticosteroids with a more gradual tapering. Anticoagulants should generally be discontinued in the presence of post–myocardial infarction syndrome.[489]

HEART FAILURE IN ACUTE MYOCARDIAL INFARCTION

Pathophysiology and Hemodynamics

The immediate hemodynamic consequences of myocardial infarction include both systolic and diastolic dysfunction. Systolic dysfunction is secondary to a loss of contractile function of the infarcted and ischemic myocardium.[490] Over a period of 1 to 3 min, the regional disturbance of contraction progresses from dyssynchrony (disturbed temporal sequence of contraction) through hypokinesis (diminished motion) and akinesis (total lack of motion) to dyskinesia (paradoxical systolic expansion).[491] This loss of contractile function results in a decreased systolic ejection, increased end-systolic volume, increased end-diastolic volume, and a secondary increase in diastolic filling pressure caused by the increase in ventricular volume. The diastolic impairment often precedes the systolic dysfunction, which is characterized immediately by a transient increase in left ventricular diastolic distensibility,[492,493] followed by decreased distensibility due in part to ATP depletion and restraint by the pericardium and perhaps ultimately by the infiltration of inflammatory fluid and cells. The hemodynamic consequence of the reduced distensibility is increased diastolic pressure. The systolic stress on the ischemic segment, which contributes to "cell stretch" and "cell slippage," results in expansion of the infarcted segment[494] and provides the stimulus for volume overload hypertrophy, characterized by sarcomere replication, fiber elongation, and chamber enlargement. The chamber enlargement accommodates the increased volume and allows the diastolic pressure to return toward normal.[491]

Cardiac failure develops when left ventricular function is reduced to 30 percent or more of normal and usually occurs within minutes or hours of the onset of a large infarction. Since even with sustained coronary occlusion only 60 to 70 percent of the ischemic region undergoes necrosis, compromise of cardiac function associated with AMI is transient (24 to 72 h) in perhaps more than two-thirds of the cases. *Unlike the situation with chronic heart failure, the circulatory volume is normal or decreased in acute ventricular dysfunction associated with myocardial infarction.* The usual clinical scenario is one of left ventricular dysfunction with pulmonary congestion and without hypoperfusion. There is sometimes biventricular failure, and in about 5 to 10 percent of cases there is predominantly right ventricular failure, as discussed below. The severity of the failure, its duration, and whether or not it is reversible are predominantly dependent on infarct size.[220,221] If more than 40 percent of the myocardium is destroyed, decompensation occurs, resulting in shock.[495–497] In a few patients, failure develops later as a consequence of expansion of the infarcted segment, reinfarction, or ischemia.[492] Less commonly, failure is precipitated by papillary muscle dysfunction or ventricular septal rupture. The compromised heart will also be negatively affected by supraventricular or ventricular arrhythmias, conduction disturbances, drugs with negative inotropic effects, fever, and hypovolemia.

Left ventricular dysfunction with the clinical signs of failure is said to occur in 30 to 40 percent of patients and usually develops when the abnormally contracting segment exceeds 30 percent of the left ventricular circumference.[498] Another factor contributing to cardiac failure is residual scarring from previous episodes of infarction, which limits the extent of compensation. After myocardial infarction, adjacent normal myocardium increases its contractility because of increased stimulation by catecholamines and also utilizes the Starling mechanism in an attempt to maintain cardiac output. The pathophysiology of heart failure is discussed in Chap. 23. The fact that intravascular volume may be normal or decreased in acute heart failure in AMI is important in considering the therapeutic approach to low cardiac output and pulmonary congestion in acute infarction.

Right Ventricular Infarction

Until about 15 to 20 years ago, right ventricular infarction was recognized infrequently and was usually thought not to be of great consequence. Subsequently, it was shown that the majority of patients with acute inferior infarction had abnormal regional function of the right ventricle,[499–501] although typical hemodynamic abnormalities are seen in only 10 to 15 percent of patients.[502,503] Right ventricular function returns to normal in most of these patients, suggesting that substantial stunning, rather than massive infarction, has occurred[15] (see also Chap. 43).

Inferior myocardial infarction associated with right ventricular infarction defines a high-risk subset with a mortality rate of 25 to 30 percent, as opposed to an overall mortality of about 6 percent in inferior myocardial infarction.[502] This group should be approached aggressively with consideration for reperfusion therapy. *Right ventricular involvement should always be considered and should be specifically sought out in inferior myocardial infarction with clinical evidence of low cardiac output because the therapeutic approaches are quite different in the presence of right ventricular involvement from those for predominantly left ventricular failure.*

Pathophysiology of Right Ventricular Infarction Right ventricular infarction is unusual in the absence of inferior infarction because occlusion of the right coronary artery proximal to the right ventricular branches usually also causes infarction in the inferior left ventricle, which is supplied by the distal distribution of the vessel.[504] The infarction usually involves the posterior septum and posterior wall rather than the right ventricular free wall. The relative sparing of the free wall results from the high degree of collateralization of the right ventricular arterial blood supply, from the blood flow derived from Thebesian vessels, and from diffusion of oxygen from the ventricular cavity as well as from the fact that it is thin and has comparatively low oxygen demands because of its mass and low workload.[505–508]

The hemodynamic consequences of right ventricular ischemia or infarction share features previously described for the left ventricle. Thus, there is impairment of contractility and diastolic dysfunction related to dilatation and pericardial restraint. In a low-pressure volume pump, such as the right ventricle, this combination has even more deleterious effects than in the left ventricle and causes substantial increases in diastolic pressure and decreases in systolic pressure. If the right ventricular afterload is also increased because of left ventricular dysfunction, then right-sided output can decrease dramatically and the driving force becomes essentially the right atrial pressure. Under these circumstances, right atrial transport essentially becomes critical, and anything decreasing it, such as diminished volume and filling pressure or loss of AV synchrony, may cause severe decreases of right, and, secondarily, left ventricular output.[469,509,510]

Diagnosis of Right Ventricular Infarction As noted, right ventricular infarction should be considered in all cases of acute inferior myocardial infarction, especially in the setting of low cardiac output. A typical presentation would include inferior myocardial infarction, clear lung fields, and jugular venous distention. Jugular venous distention that is enhanced by inspiration (Kussmaul's sign) in the setting of inferior myocardial infarction is highly suggestive of right ventricular involvement but may not be manifest with volume depletion and might only become apparent with repletion.[511] A right atrial pressure greater than 10 mmHg that is greater than 80 percent of the pulmonary wedge pressure is a sensitive and specific sign of right ventricular infarction.[512]

The differential diagnosis of heart failure or low cardiac output in inferior infarction includes (1) arrhythmia, such as atrial fibrillation, sustained ventricular arrhythmia, or high-degree AV block; (2) ongoing ischemia, such as ischemia at a distance if the occluded artery to the inferior wall was also supplying, through collaterals, the anterior wall; (3) previous infarction at another location; (4) a mechanical complication such as papillary muscle dysfunction or, less commonly, a ventricular septal defect; or (5) right ventricular infarction.[513] This differential diagnosis of causes of congestive heart failure in inferior AMI is summarized in Table 47-13.

ST-segment elevation in lead V_{4R} is the single most powerful predictor of right ventricular involvement in inferior infarction and identifies a patient subset with a markedly increased in-hospital mortality.[502] All patients with inferior infarction should be screened by recording ECG lead V_{4R}. Echocardiography can also be useful as an adjunctive diagnostic approach[203] and can be particularly valuable in detecting right-to-left shunting of blood through the foramen ovale, which can occur because of the high right atrial pressures in right ventricular ischemia. Such shunting can be a cause of hypoxemia unresponsive to oxygen administration in this setting.[514]

Treatment of Right Ventricular Ischemia/Infarction The major objectives in treating right ventricular infarction are to maintain right ventricular preload, provide inotropic support, reduce afterload of the right ventricle, and achieve early reperfusion.[316] The recommendations are summarized in Table 47-14.[15] Venodilators such as nitrates should be avoided, and diuretics should be used with caution. Volume loading with 1 to 2 L of saline will frequently restore cardiac output and correct hypotension; this should be the initial step. Excessive volume loading, however, may dilate the ventricle and decrease output. Inotropic support should be initiated if saline administration does not restore output and correct hypotension.[15] Dobutamine is an ideal initial choice.

The critical role of atrial transport in maintaining output in right ventricular infarction and the need to maintain AV synchrony have been discussed. High-degree AV block occurs in about 50 percent of patients in this setting, and AV sequential pacing can restore cardiac output.[515,516] Atrial fibrillation

TABLE 47-13
DIFFERENTIAL DIAGNOSIS OF CONGESTIVE HEART FAILURE IN INFERIOR AMI

Arrhythmia: high-degree AV block, atrial fibrillation, or sustained ventricular tachycardia
Ischemia at a distance, with the occluded artery to the inferior wall supplying the anterior wall via collaterals
Previous infarction at another location
Mechanical complication, such as papillary muscle dysfunction
Right ventricular infarction

TABLE 47-14
TREATMENT STRATEGY FOR RIGHT VENTRICULAR ISCHEMIA/INFARCTION

Maintain right ventricular preload
  Volume loading (IV normal saline)
  Avoid use of nitrates and diuretics
  Maintain AV synchrony
    AV sequential pacing for symptomatic high-degree heart block unresponsive to atropine
  Prompt cardioversion for hemodynamically significant SVT
Inotropic support
  Dobutamine (if cardiac output fails to increase after volume loading)
Reduce right ventricular afterload with left ventricular dysfunction
  Intra-aortic balloon pump
  Arterial vasodilators (sodium nitroprusside, hydralazine)
  ACE inhibitors
Reperfusion
  Thrombolytic agents
  Primary PTCA
  CABG (in selected patients with multivessel disease)

Key: IV = intravenous; AV = atrioventricular; SVT = supraventricular tachycardia; ACE = angiotensin converting enzyme; PTCA = percutaneous transluminal coronary angioplasty; CABG = coronary artery bypass graft. *Source*: Ryan et al.,[15] with permission.

occurs in up to one-third of these patients, in whom prompt cardioversion should be considered if there is any evidence of hemodynamic compromise.[517] If there is significant left ventricular dysfunction, which may further compromise right ventricular function, as noted, afterload reduction by nitroprusside infusion or intraaortic balloon pumping is indicated.[15]

Reperfusion with thrombolytic therapy or primary PTCA improves right ventricular ejection fraction and hemodynamic status[518] and decreases the incidence of complete heart block.[518-520] Coronary artery bypass grafting should be considered if multivessel disease is found.

Management of Congestive Heart Failure in Acute Myocardial Infarction—General Issues

Hemodynamic Monitoring Recommendations for balloon flotation right—heart catheter monitoring[15]:

Class I

1. Severe or progressive congestive heart failure or pulmonary edema
2. Cardiogenic shock or progressive hypotension
3. Suspected mechanical complications of acute infarction, i.e., ventricular septal defect, papillary muscle rupture, or pericardial tamponade

Class IIa

1. Hypotension that does not respond promptly to fluid administration in a patient without pulmonary congestion

Class III

1. Patients with acute infarction without evidence of cardiac or pulmonary complications

The balloon flotation (Swan-Ganz) catheter fundamentally permits one, in the setting of low cardiac output, to distinguish between inadequate ventricular filling pressures and inadequate systolic function. The former is treated with volume expansion and the latter with inotropic support and frequently afterload reduction. The catheter, even when used correctly, is not totally benign and during manipulation may precipitate ventricular tachycardia and pulmonary hemorrhage or infarction. To minimize the risk of infection, the catheter should not be left in place longer than 5 days.[15]

Recommendations for intraarterial pressure monitoring[15]:

Class I

1. Patients with severe hypotension (systolic arterial pressure less than 80 mmHg) and/or cardiogenic shock
2. Patients receiving vasopressor agents

Class IIa

1. Patients receiving intravenous sodium nitroprusside or other potent vasodilators

Class IIb

1. Hemodynamically stable patients receiving intravenous nitroglycerin for myocardial ischemia
2. Patients receiving intravenous inotropic agents

Class III

1. Patients with acute infarction who are hemodynamically stable

Arterial monitoring in AMI is useful in all hypotensive patients but especially in those who are in shock. The radial artery is the preferred site, although the brachial and femoral arteries can be used. Intraarterial catheters should not be left in place longer than 72 h because of the risk of thrombosis and infection.[15]

Recommendations for intraaortic balloon counterpulsation[15]:

Class I

1. Cardiogenic shock not quickly reversed with pharmacologic therapy as a stabilizing measure for angiography and prompt revascularization

2. Acute mitral regurgitation or ventricular septal defect complicating myocardial infarction as a stabilizing therapy for angiography and repair/revascularization
3. Recurrent intractable ventricular arrhythmias with hemodynamic instability
4. Refractory post–myocardial infarction angina as a bridge to angiography and revascularization

Class IIa

1. Signs of hemodynamic instability, poor left ventricular function, or persistent ischemia in patients with large areas of the myocardium at risk

Class IIb

1. In patients with successful PTCA after failed thrombolysis or those with three-vessel coronary disease, to prevent reocclusion
2. In patients known to have large areas of myocardium at risk, with or without active ischemia

By inflating in the aorta during diastole and by deflating during systole, the intraaortic balloon pump (IABP) reduces afterload during ventricular systole and increases coronary perfusion during diastole. The decrease in afterload and increased coronary perfusion account for its efficacy in cardiogenic shock and ischemia. It is particularly useful as a stabilizing bridge to facilitate diagnostic angiography and revascularization and repair of mechanical complications of AMI. The use of IABP after AMI postthrombolysis or post-PTCA has not been uniformly successful in improving clinical outcome, including reocclusion rate or global or regional left ventricular function.[521] Thus, the routine use of IABP after either drug or mechanical reperfusion cannot be recommended.[15]

Diuretics and Positive Inotropic Agents DIURETICS AND CARDIAC FAILURE IN ACUTE MYOCARDIAL INFARCTION As previously mentioned, patients with failure due to AMI have normal total body water, and the transudation of fluid into the lungs may induce hypovolemia. As ventricular compliance is decreased, an increased left ventricular end-diastolic pressure is necessary to maintain cardiac output, since the heart operates on the steep portion of the ascending limb of Starling's curve.[522,523] The administration of a diuretic in this setting may be associated with a decrease in cardiac output.[524–526] Thus, diuretics should not be the drugs used initially in the treatment of pulmonary congestion in AMI. Their use early in the course should usually be guided by hemodynamic measurements from a Swan-Ganz catheter. Diuretic therapy may become appropriate later if salt and water retention occur and left ventricular filling pressures become excessively high—greater than 18 to 20 mmHg, for example.

INOTROPIC AGENTS IN CONGESTIVE HEART FAILURE ASSOCI-
ATED WITH ACUTE MYOCARDIAL INFARCTION Digoxin is a
relatively weak inotropic agent and is not the drug of choice
in acute heart failure in myocardial infarction. In a direct
comparison, dobutamine was shown to increase cardiac output
by 40 percent and to decrease left ventricular filling pressure,
whereas digoxin increased cardiac output by only 10 percent
and did not decrease filling pressure.[527] Since endogenous
catecholamine levels can be quite elevated, digoxin may contribute little. The primary use of digoxin in AMI is to control
heart rate in atrial fibrillation.

Dobutamine has favorable pharmacologic properties for
use in heart failure in myocardial infarction (see Chap. 23).
It has a rapid onset of action and increases cardiac output
because of its positive inotropic properties. It is a vasodilator
and increases coronary flow. It decreases filling pressure, as
noted. Dopamine has a tendency to increase heart rate more
than dobutamine. With higher doses, it may increase peripheral resistance and filling pressures, offsetting some of the
positive inotropic effects. The phosphodiesterase inhibitor amrinone increases contractility and is a vasodilator that has been
used in patients with heart failure due to AMI. There is concern
that positive inotropic agents may increase infarct size. Evaluation of dobutamine in AMI showed that, as long as heart
rate was not increased more than 10 percent above baseline,
there was no increase in infarct size or in the incidence of
reinfarction or arrhythmia.[528]

***Management of Uncomplicated
Cardiac Failure After Acute
Myocardial Infarction*** The
major determinant of left ventricular dysfunction is the
extent of myocardial in-
jury.[220,221,529] The loss of contractile function in the initial minutes or hours (1 to 4) is
potentially reversible and accounts in part for the transient
nature of cardiac failure in the
setting of uncomplicated AMI, as
noted above. The presence of cardiac failure and its severity depend not only on the extent of
damage but also upon the extent
of injury from previous episodes.

Since the introduction of the
Swan-Ganz catheter, considerable data have accumulated correlating hemodynamics with
clinical features. In 1967, prior to
invasive monitoring, Killip and
Kimball[530] devised a clinical
classification based on physical
findings present on admission
that provided a prognostic guide.

That guide was followed by the classification of Forrester and
colleagues,[531,532] based on extensive data obtained from invasive monitoring of patients with acute AMI (Table 47-15). The
latter classification combined the presence or absence of pulmonary congestion with the presence or absence of systemic
hypoperfusion. Forrester and colleagues added the underlying
hemodynamics to this classification based on the pulmonary
arterial occlusive (wedge) pressure and the cardiac index. These
classifications also provide important diagnostic and therapeutic guidelines, despite the observation that patients frequently cross over from one class to the other and are seldom
restricted to one particular hemodynamic subset. Each classification illustrated that with increasing severity of ventricular
dysfunction, there is an increased risk of mortality. Nevertheless, there is imprecision in predicting mortality rates from hemodynamics. Rackley and coworkers[533] observed that patients
with a ventricular filling pressure above 29 mmHg had a 100
percent mortality rate; those with a filling pressure above 15
mmHg and a cardiac index of less than 2 L/min per square meter
of body surface had a mortality rate of 93 percent; while those
with a ventricular filling pressure less than 15 and a cardiac
index under 2 L/min per square meter of body surface had a
mortality rate of 63 percent.

*In patients with uncomplicated AMI, there is no need to
perform invasive monitoring if careful clinical observations
are made.* There should be repeated assessment of the heart
and lungs; examination of the skin and mucous membranes;

TABLE 47-15

CLINICAL AND HEMODYNAMIC SUBSETS IN AMI

Subset	Clinical Features	Approximate % of Patients with AMI	Hospital Mortality, %
	KILLIP CLASS		
1	No signs of congestive heart failure	40–50	6
2	S$_3$ gallop and bibasilar rales	30–40	17
3	Acute pulmonary edema	10–15	38
4	Cardiogenic shock	5–10	81
	CEDARS-SINAI CLINICAL SUBSETS		
1	No pulmonary congestion or tissue hypoperfusion	25	1
2	Pulmonary congestion only	25	11
3	Tissue hypoperfusion only	15	18
4	Pulmonary congestion and tissue hypoperfusion	35	60
	CEDARS-SINAI HEMODYNAMIC SUBSETS		
	Hemodynamic features		
1	PCW ≤ 18; CI > 2.2	25	3
2	PCW > 18; CI > 2.2	25	9
3	PCW ≤ 18; CI ≤ 2.2	15	23
4	PCW > 18; CI ≤ 2.2	35	51

Key: CI = cardiac index (L/min/m^2); PCW = pulmonary capillary wedge pressure (mmHg).

monitoring of the systemic arterial pressure, cardiac rhythm, and heart rate; and routine laboratory examinations, including chest x-ray and determinations of urine output and arterial blood-gas values. If there are clinical indications of pulmonary congestion and/or decreased peripheral perfusion, invasive monitoring includes the insertion of a Swan-Ganz catheter in order to monitor right ventricular hemodynamics and pulmonary artery occlusive pressure (which will reflect ventricular end-diastolic pressure) and to obtain serial determinations of the cardiac output. Occasionally, it may be necessary to insert an arterial catheter to measure the arterial pressure; however, one can usually follow the pressure adequately with the use of a sphygmomanometer or an automatic blood pressure monitoring device. Frequently, it is also essential to insert a Foley catheter to follow the urine output, particularly in patients with sustained hypotension or cardiogenic shock.

In most patients in whom cardiac failure is not complicated by mechanical factors—such as mitral valve rupture, ventricular septal rupture, pulmonary embolus, or tamponade—the failure is transient and of mild to moderate severity. If the cardiac output is normal, aggressive treatment is often not recommended.[137] In patients with rales at the base of the lungs with only minimal increase in heart rate and no other signs of hypoxemia (Killip class III), conventional therapy with morphine; nasal oxygen; intravenous, oral, or transdermal nitrates; and bed rest is adequate without any specific therapy for failure. In patients with extensive pulmonary edema who are normotensive and exhibit hypoxia and dyspnea (Forrester class II), the treatment of choice is nitroglycerin given intravenously at 0.1 μg/kg per minute and increased in increments of 5 to 10 μg/min, stopping at a dose that does not decrease the systolic blood pressure below 100 mmHg. On the average, nitroglycerin in a dose of 0.5 μg/kg per minute is required in patients with evolving acute infarction and failure. Another vasodilator that has been used extensively in the past in AMI is sodium nitroprusside, which is initiated at 0.5 μg/kg per minute and increased by 10- to 20-μg/min increments every 10 to 15 min until the desired therapeutic point or a maximum of 10 μg/kg per minute is reached. Nevertheless, nitroglycerin is the preferred agent, since it has been shown to offer some cardioprotection when given in the early phase of myocardial infarction and to be both reliable and safe. In contrast, in experimental infarction in the dog, it has been shown that nitroprusside is more likely to redirect coronary flow away from the ischemic area to normal areas and to induce coronary steal.[308] The effect of nitroprusside on cardioprotection has been inconsistent and in one large study was shown to be detrimental.[534] In view of the recent data showing ACE inhibitors to be very effective in cardiac failure, one can anticipate that these agents will be used more generally in this setting. It is preferable that hemodynamics be monitored invasively (by Swan-Ganz catheter) when one gives a vasodilator to reduce the ventricular filling pressure to 15 to 17 mmHg while maintaining adequate cardiac output and coronary perfusion. Whether or not one monitors hemodynamics invasively will depend in part on the confidence that

clinical features reflect the volume status. Mitral valve regurgitation due to papillary muscle dysfunction is commonly an aggravating factor even in mild to moderate cardiac failure and responds well to a vasodilator, as does systemic hypertension. Usually a vasodilator is not adequate, in which case an intravenous inotropic agent should be added. The inotropic agents are generally those of sympathomimetic drugs, including dobutamine, dopamine, and norepinephrine (see Chaps. 23 and 51). Dobutamine, a synthetic direct-acting agent, is preferred, as noted, and has actions that include vasodilatation, increased cardiac output, decreased ventricular filling pressure, and increased coronary flow.[535] The infusion should be initiated at 2 to 5 μg/kg per minute and should be increased such that adequate systemic pressure is maintained and the heart rate does not increase by more than 10 to 15 percent. Dobutamine is preferably titrated to cardiac output and ventricular filling pressure. The ventricular filling pressure should be decreased to a range of 14 to 18 mmHg while maintaining adequate cardiac output and blood pressure. In general, the objective is to maintain adequate cardiac output and blood pressure without inducing tachycardia while maintaining a filling pressure that is normal or minimally increased.

In patients with inferior infarction and low cardiac output, right ventricular infarction should be suspected, as discussed. If it is present, a Swan-Ganz catheter should be inserted to determine the filling pressure. Therapy with a positive inotropic agent, such as dobutamine, should be used after assuring that there is appropriate intravascular volume to facilitate right ventricular filling.[536,536a]

In patients with borderline blood pressure and evidence of peripheral hypoperfusion, therapy should be initiated with an inotropic agent and not a vasodilator. Similarly, in patients with left ventricular failure and frank hypotension (<95 mmHg), a vasodilator must be avoided and initial therapy should be with a positive inotropic agent. Dopamine would frequently be the choice under these circumstances, since it exerts cardiovascular effects similar to those of dobutamine, but it also possesses an alpha$_1$-adrenergic activity and releases endogenous norepinephrine from sympathetic nerve endings. Low doses of dopamine (2 to 7 μg/kg per minute) are associated with an increase in stroke volume, increased cardiac output, increased renal blood flow, and moderate effects to increase peripheral resistance. Higher doses of dopamine induce significant vasoconstriction and may increase the left ventricular filling pressure due to increased afterload, which further exacerbates pulmonary congestion. Dopamine also has a more positive chronotropic effect than does dobutamine, which can be a disadvantage in AMI. Norepinephrine, which produces potent arteriolar and venous constriction, is used for hypotension in other settings but is otherwise relatively contraindicated in AMI. It is seldom used unless patients are hypotensive and do not respond to dopamine, amrinone or milrinone, or dobutamine. It is used in cardiogenic shock after dopamine has failed, since it is the major alternative that can be used for maintaining adequate perfusion pressure.

As indicated above, diuretics should be used with more caution in acute heart failure associated with AMI than in chronic heart failure, since volume expansion is usually not the primary problem. If high filling pressure (>18 to 20 mmHg) persists after adequate output is achieved with positive inotropic agents and/or vasodilators, diuretics may be added. However, this effect can be achieved by vasodilator therapy, which avoids the hypovolemia and hypotension that may occur secondary to the subsequent diuresis (1 to 2 h). The preferred diuretics are intravenous furosemide or ethacrynic acid.[537] These drugs also provide some acute venodilation (see Chap. 24).

Complicated Heart Failure after Myocardial Infarction

Some AMI patients present with acute, fulminating pulmonary edema (with severe respiratory distress; generalized inspiratory crackles and wheezing; expectoration of pink, frothy sputum; cool, clammy, diaphoretic skin; and cyanosis) and require much more aggressive therapy than do patients with uncomplicated AMI. The condition is usually associated with pulmonary artery wedge pressure exceeding 25 mmHg and an in-hospital mortality rate of at least 15 to 20 percent.[538] The systolic blood pressure is usually either low normal or borderline normal (95 to 105 mmHg). The maintenance of adequate oxygenation must be the primary concern. Administration of high concentrations (60 to 100 percent) of oxygen via a face mask is essential. If the patient appears moribund, endotracheal intubation should be performed. While an assessment of arterial blood gases is appropriate, the speed with which clinical events change in these emergent situations may demand that decisions be made without benefit of these values. After the institution of mechanical ventilation, positive end-expiratory pressure (PEEP) may be needed to maintain adequate oxygenation while keeping the inspired oxygen concentration within safe levels ($FI_{O_2} < 60$ percent). Positive end-expiratory pressure should be applied only with an awareness of its risks of pneumothorax and reduction in cardiac output secondary to decreased left ventricular preload.[538] Invasive hemodynamic monitoring is particularly useful in these patients. Therapeutic interventions, however, should not be delayed until the monitoring is established. The therapy for severe pulmonary edema should include intravenous morphine unless the patient is known to have chronic CO_2 retention. From 5 to 10 mg of morphine sulfate should be given slowly with careful observation for evidence of respiratory depression. If the systolic blood pressure is adequate (≥ 100 mmHg), nitroglycerin is administered intravenously. In the patient with severe pulmonary edema, the improvement in left ventricular pump performance afforded by the prompt reduction in systemic vascular resistance by nitroprusside[539] may be essential for the rapid reversal of this life-threatening situation (particularly if systemic hypertension had been present). Either nitroglycerin or nitroprusside will provide a reduction in preload. If the systolic blood pressure is 100 mmHg or less, treatment with a positive inotropic agent should probably be initiated, with the subsequent addition of a vasodilator or an agent to improve cardiac output. The adjunctive use of intravenous diuretics is the same as outlined for milder degrees of heart failure.

Peripheral Hypoperfusion without Pulmonary Congestion

Patients with clinical hypoperfusion without pulmonary congestion (with cool, cyanotic extremities, somnolence or confusion, and decreased urine flow) usually have a cardiac index of less than 2.2 L/min. The mortality rate in these patients is four times greater than that in patients without hypoperfusion.[538] Invasive hemodynamic monitoring of the pulmonary capillary wedge pressure is essential. Volume augmentation is the initial therapeutic step in patients with a pulmonary capillary wedge pressure of less than 15 mmHg. If possible, this pressure should be maintained below the level of pulmonary congestion (>20 mmHg). Vasodilators are usually not indicated at least until adequate filling pressures have been achieved and cardiac output is augmented with positive inotropic agents. This situation is commonly seen with severe biventricular infarction and thus should be suspected with inferior and right ventricular infarction. In this case, bradycardia should be treated with atropine if it is thought to be contributing to the systemic hypoperfusion. Excessive treatment with nitroglycerin and volume contraction from previous diuretic therapy can also contribute to systemic hypotension.

Hypotension and Cardiogenic Shock

Cardiogenic shock may occur when 40 percent or more of the left ventricle is destroyed.[495,496,540] It is the most common cause of in-hospital death with myocardial infarction. The incidence of cardiogenic shock was about 15 percent in the early 1970s, but it has now decreased to approximately 5 to 7 percent.[538] The mortality rate is frequently over 80 percent.[541] The most effective therapy in the treatment of cardiogenic shock is prevention, since its major determinant is infarct size.[220,542] Cardiogenic shock usually occurs within hours of the onset of infarction due to massive ischemia and necrosis.[542] In other cases, a relatively small infarction that is superimposed on extensive previous damage may precipitate cardiogenic shock. Less commonly, cardiogenic shock may develop days after the initial event. This occurrence is almost always due to development of new necrosis (extension or early reinfarction) in the area of the preceding infarction. The decrease in the incidence of cardiogenic shock is believed to be in part due to better treatment of angina and ischemia, together with the widespread use of thrombolytic therapy and other cardioprotective agents. Cardiogenic shock by definition represents a more severe form of cardiac failure, resulting in decreased organ perfusion in addition to the conventional features of pulmonary congestion and left ventricular dysfunction. Cardiac failure with hypoperfusion and that regarded as cardiogenic shock may differ only in the severity of decreased perfusion. Clearly, every effort must be made to treat hypoperfusion whether or not it satisfies the strict criteria of cardiogenic shock. Characteristics of cardiogenic shock are (Table 47-16) (1) evidence of organ hypoperfusion with cold, clammy

TABLE 47-16

CHARACTERISTICS OF CARDIOGENIC SHOCK

Evidence of hypoperfusion: cold clammy skin, especially of feet and hands; impaired mentation; and oliguria
Systolic blood pressure < 80–90 mmHg
LVED pressure (or PCW pressure) ≥ 18 mmHg
Evidence of primary cardiac abnormality
Cardiac index ≤ 1.8 L/m/m^2

skin, especially on the feet and hands, that may be associated with peripheral cyanosis of the nail beds; (2) oliguria, disordered mentation, and systolic blood pressure of less than 80 to 90 mmHg; (3) left ventricular end-diastolic pressure or, more commonly, pulmonary capillary wedge pressure greater than 18 mmHg; (4) evidence of a primary cardiac abnormality; and (5) a cardiac index not greater than 1.8 L/min per square meter of body surface. Hypotension or shock due to a primary abnormality of cardiac rhythm or conduction is not considered cardiogenic shock.

Since the prognosis is extremely poor for patients with cardiogenic shock due primarily to loss of muscle mass, reversible causes associated with a better prognosis must be excluded. Potentially reversible causes include mitral valve rupture, ventricular septal rupture, right ventricular infarction, pulmonary embolus, and cardiac tamponade. While the mortality associated with surgical correction of infarct-associated mitral rupture or ventricular septal defect is still high, it is far less than that associated with cardiogenic shock due solely to myocardial injury. The details of management of these mechanical causes of shock are discussed below. Hypotension may be due to inadequate fluid administration, to vasodilatation induced by such drugs as morphine and vasodilators, and occasionally to depressed contractility due to antiarrhythmic therapy. Inadequate filling pressure is a very important cause of hypotension and should be corrected immediately. It is particularly common in patients with inferior infarction, as noted. A Swan-Ganz catheter should be inserted to determine the circulatory status and assess the response to therapy.

Therapeutic objectives are to establish and maintain a systemic arterial pressure adequate for perfusing the vital organs and for reducing pulmonary congestion. The approaches to pulmonary congestion include the judicious use of morphine, and the maintenance of adequate oxygenation, together with endotracheal intubation and mechanical ventilation if necessary. In addition to instituting hemodynamic monitoring, one should assess urinary output using an indwelling catheter. If the pulmonary artery wedge pressure is less than 15 mmHg, prompt volume expansion to raise the capillary pressure to 18 to 20 mmHg should be initiated. The cornerstones of therapy are inotropic and vasopressor agents. If the systemic arterial vasopressure is below 80 to 90 mmHg, a pressor agent such as dopamine should be infused.[543] At relatively low doses of 2 to 5 μg/kg per minute, increases in stroke volume and cardiac output are mediated by beta-adrenergic stimulation and in-

creases in renal blood flow are mediated by the dopaminergic-specific receptors. The alpha-adrenergic vasoconstrictor effects are manifest progressively at doses above 5 μg/kg per minute. The use of intravenous dopamine requires careful titration, beginning with a low dose and gradually increasing until an adequate (90 to 100 mmHg) systemic pressure is achieved. If high doses of dopamine are necessary to maintain adequate perfusion, a change to norepinephrine infusion should be considered. This drug is a potent arteriolar and venous constrictor that is mediated through alpha-adrenergic stimulation. It demonstrates relatively modest beta-adrenergic stimulation. It is, therefore, a very potent pressor agent with less chronotropic or arrhythmogenic effects than dopamine.[322] The drug should be started at low doses of 1 to 4 μg/min. Extravasation should be avoided, since it will produce tissue sloughing.

When the systemic blood pressure is 90 mmHg or more, dobutamine is frequently the preferred agent. By increasing cardiac output, dobutamine may produce a rise in systemic blood pressure, but this increase would not be expected to be greater than 10 to 15 mmHg.[544,545] Dobutamine will not support arterial pressure except by its effect on cardiac output. As the cardiac output rises, the left ventricular filling pressure should decline. Dobutamine therapy should begin with a dose of 2 to 5 μg/kg per minute with increases every 5 to 10 min. Inappropriate increases in heart rate are unlikely to occur with doses less than 15 to 20 μg/kg per minute.[528]

On occasion, the severity of cardiac pump dysfunction will require the use of two divergent therapeutic modalities in order to facilitate left ventricular emptying.[546] The most commonly utilized of these combined therapies is nitroprusside and dopamine. The principal advantage offered by nitroprusside in this combination is a reduction in left ventricular preload. The cardiac output is not appreciably increased by the addition of nitroprusside to dopamine therapy. The advantage offered by dopamine in this combination is an augmentation of cardiac output and the maintenance of systemic arterial pressure.[547] A less frequently used combination, dobutamine and nitroprusside, has been shown to result in higher cardiac output and lower pulmonary capillary wedge pressures than with either drug alone.[546] Stabilization of the patient with cardiogenic shock may be achieved by mechanical circulatory assist devices, such as the intraaortic balloon. Aortic balloon counterpulsation reduces afterload while simultaneously improving coronary perfusion by increasing diastolic aortic pressure, as discussed. It is the only intervention that will increase diastolic aortic pressure without increasing myocardial oxygen demand. Aortic counterpulsation is usually reserved for patients in cardiogenic shock due to a potentially reversible condition or in whom cardiac transplantation is being considered. Such conditions include an acute but still evolving myocardial infarction or AMI with a severe mechanical complication (e.g., mitral regurgitation or ventricular septal defect). In such cases, aortic counterpulsation should be used to stabilize the patient's condition in preparation for salvage of the jeopardized but still viable myocardium or correction of the mechanical defect.[322] The use of aortic counterpulsation in patients without a reversible defect has been shown not to prolong life significantly or to provide long-term benefit; thus, it should not be instituted unless there is a reasonable expectation of correcting the underlying problem or of transplantation.

Restoration of coronary blood flow will probably be the most effective therapy in salvaging patients with cardiogenic shock who are unresponsive to fluid and pharmacologic management in the early hours after a myocardial infarction. If angioplasty and/or coronary artery bypass grafting are not readily available, thrombolytic therapy should be tried if it has not already been utilized—although it has not been shown to improve survival in this setting.[548,549] These patients should be transferred quickly to a tertiary care center. Blood pressure should be stabilized with an intraaortic balloon pump and cardiac catheterization should be performed as soon as possible. Assessment of correctable mechanical lesions, such as ruptured papillary muscles, can be made together with evaluation of coronary anatomy. Depending upon this anatomy, a judgment can be made as to whether to attempt PTCA or to proceed to coronary artery bypass surgery. Mechanical revascularization appears to improve survival in cardiogenic shock complicating AMI.[550]

Mechanical Dysfunction Contributing to Cardiac Failure—

PAPILLARY MUSCLE RUPTURE   Rupture of the left ventricular papillary muscle occurs in approximately 1 percent of myocardial infarctions and accounts for 0.4 to 5.0 percent of infarct-related deaths.[551] It occurs slightly less frequently than ventricular septal rupture. The posteromedial papillary muscle is involved 6 to 12 times more frequently than is the anterolateral muscle.[552] Thus, papillary muscle rupture with an acute anterior myocardial infarction is uncommon. The rupture may occur distally and may involve one or several of the smaller heads of the muscle or, less commonly, may occur proximally and produce complete dehiscence of the papillary muscle.

Papillary muscle rupture is manifest by the sudden appearance of pulmonary edema, usually 2 to 7 days after the infarction. The abruptness of onset and severity of pulmonary edema are usually greater than seen with ventricular septal rupture. A mid- or holosystolic murmur with wide radiation is usually audible. Although the murmur is generally loud, a thrill is rarely present, and the murmur may seem inconsequential. The diagnosis can be established by Doppler echocardiographic studies (see Chap. 14). The two-dimensional echocardiogram will generally show a flail mitral leaflet and may reveal a portion of the papillary muscle visualized as a mass attached to the chordae. Even when the flail leaflet is not observed, documentation of relatively intact ventricular systolic function in the postinfarction patient with pulmonary edema should suggest the diagnosis. The Doppler study will establish the presence and severity of the mitral regurgitation. Bedside right heart catheterization can be used to exclude an oxygen step-up from the right atrium to the right ventricle, indicative of ventricular septal rupture, and to confirm elevated pulmonary capillary wedge pressures with tall V (regurgitant) waves characteristic of acute mitral regurgitation.

Studies in the presurgical era demonstrated a poor prognosis for these patients, with a 50 percent mortality rate in the first 24 h and a 6 percent survival rate for longer than 2 months.[553] Thus, immediate recognition and treatment are essential. Intraaortic counterpulsation alone or with vasodilator and inotropic therapy may frequently be required for temporary stabilization. During this period, the patient should undergo cardiac catheterization to define coronary anatomy and should be transferred to surgery for mitral valve replacement or repair.

PAPILLARY MUSCLE DYSFUNCTION   The sudden development of an apical systolic murmur after a myocardial infarction is much more often secondary to papillary muscle dysfunction than to rupture. Twenty percent of patients who die from infarction have histologic evidence of papillary muscle necrosis, usually without rupture.[554] Papillary muscle dysfunction is frequently compatible with long-term survival.

The posteromedial papillary muscle is involved with ischemia or infarction more commonly than the anterolateral muscle because the latter receives blood from two arteries (left anterior descending and circumflex), whereas the posteromedial muscle is supplied predominantly from the circumflex.[555] Dysfunction may be transient during ischemia. Papillary muscle ischemia is usually accompanied by ischemia of the contiguous ventricular wall.[556] Involvement of the contiguous ventricular wall is a key factor in the development of significant mitral regurgitation, since isolated papillary muscle ischemia or even infarction is usually not sufficient to cause important mitral regurgitation.[557]

Papillary muscle dysfunction typically presents with an apical systolic murmur. The murmur may be holosystolic, late systolic, or even early systolic. Echocardiographic coupled with Doppler flow studies will confirm the presence of mitral regurgitation, grade its severity, and permit assessment of left ventricular function. There is generally no hemodynamic deterioration associated with the appearance of the murmur. It is the unusual patient who develops pulmonary edema, and these patients usually have concomitant significant left ventricular dysfunction. The ordinary patient with papillary muscle dysfunction will require no specific therapy for the regurgitation, while the unusual patient with severe regurgitation should be treated as in the case of papillary muscle rupture. In intermediate cases with moderate to moderately severe regurgitation where cardiac surgery is not contemplated, afterload reduction with ACE inhibitors should be considered.

VENTRICULAR SEPTAL RUPTURE   Rupture of the interventricular septum is estimated to occur in 1 to 3 percent of AMIs and accounts for approximately 5 percent of all infarct-related deaths.[558] Ventricular septal rupture occurs with an approximately equal frequency between anterior and inferior infarctions. There is a higher prevalence in first infarctions and the majority occur within the first week. Some 20 to 30 percent may develop as early as the first 24 h after the infarction.[559,560]

Septal rupture rarely occurs after 2 weeks. Ventricular septal rupture is usually manifest by the appearance of a new harsh, holosystolic murmur along the left sternal border (often associated with a thrill) and sudden clinical deterioration with hypotension and pulmonary congestion. Right ventricular volume overload secondary to the shunt may produce signs of systemic venous congestion out of proportion to those of pulmonary venous congestion. Often the event is heralded by a recurrence of chest pain.

The diagnosis can be established by two-dimensional and Doppler echocardiographic studies that will demonstrate the site and approximate size of the rupture as well as the left-to-right shunt. Right-sided heart catheterization is useful in confirming the diagnosis (an increase in O_2 saturation of >5 percent from right atrium to right ventricle) and is an aid in managing the patient. The primary diagnostic concern is to exclude rupture of the papillary muscle. The presence of a thrill or an anterior infarction would be unusual with papillary muscle rupture, and results of the Doppler echocardiographic studies and/or the oxygen step-up on right heart catheterization would confirm the presence of septal rupture.

When medical therapy alone is used, most patients with ventricular septal rupture deteriorate rapidly and virtually all patients die, many within 24 h after rupture. Except for the rare case in which there is no clinical or hemodynamic deterioration, medical therapy can be expected to be ineffective. Intravenous sodium nitroprusside may improve forward cardiac output and reduce the shunt, but severe systemic hypotension frequently precludes its use. Inotropic and vasopressor agents may be required to sustain arterial blood pressure but can increase the left-to-right shunt. Prompt but temporary stabilization can be achieved with intraaortic balloon counterpulsation alone or in conjunction with vasodilator and inotropic drug therapy. Cardiac catheterization should be performed in an expeditious manner to define cardiac anatomy, left ventricular function, and mitral valve competence. An aggressive approach of immediate operative repair of these patients results in a short-term survival rate of 42 to 75 percent.[561–563] The 5-year actuarial survival rate for the operative survivors has been reported to be as high as 88 percent.[564] Surgical results are worse when ventricular septal rupture complicates inferior infarction and when there is combined right ventricular and septal dysfunction.[563]

CARDIAC RUPTURE POSTINFARCTION

Cardiorrhexis, or rupture of the heart, occurs in up to 24 percent of fatal AMIs. After cardiogenic shock and arrhythmias, it is the most common cause of death. The free wall of the ventricle is the most common site of rupture.[565]

Rupture of the free wall generally occurs within the first 2 weeks of the infarction and may occur within the first 24 h.[559,560] Rupture occurring after this interval usually represents extension of the infarction or rupture through a false aneurysm.[565a]

The rupture occurs primarily in the left ventricle, with a fairly even distribution between the anterior, inferior, and lateral walls. Given the relatively smaller number of lateral infarctions, the incidence of rupture with lateral wall infarctions would presumably be relatively smaller than at other sites.[566] Free wall rupture is more likely to occur with the initial myocardial infarction, in women, in the sixth decade of life or later, and in patients with systemic arterial hypertension, particularly if there is no associated ventricular hypertrophy.[559] The prolonged use of corticosteroids might predispose a patient to cardiac rupture.

Cardiac rupture generally presents as sudden, unanticipated death. Symptoms such as pain, agitation, sinus tachycardia, or vagally mediated bradycardia seldom precede death by more than minutes. Occasionally, intermittent chest pain and/or transient hypotension may precede and portend the final catastrophic event. Cardiac rupture is diagnosed terminally by the development of electromechanical disassociation in the setting of recurrent chest pain. Few cases, and only those with immediate recognition, can be salvaged. Even these few cases require heroic measures, such as immediate pericardiocentesis, emergency thoracotomy, and surgical repair.

Other Complications of Acute Myocardial Infarction

PULMONARY EMBOLISM The prevalence of deep venous thrombosis (DVT) in AMI is reported to be between 12 and 38 percent. Patients with large infarctions in any location, anterior infarctions, evidence of congestive heart failure, and complicated infarctions have a greater frequency of DVT.[567,568] Reduced cardiac output and immobilization are additional predisposing factors for DVT (see Chap. 100).

Venous thrombosis is usually a minor and frequently unrecognized complication of infarction but is potentially life-threatening. A prevalence of pulmonary embolism of 10 to 15 percent and a prevalence of fatal embolism in 3 to 6 percent of cases has been reported in the past.[569] More recently, pulmonary embolism has been reported to account for less than 1 percent of deaths in myocardial infarction, probably because of earlier ambulation and better therapy of low output.[565a]

Early mobilization combined with therapy directed toward improving cardiac output, when appropriate, is probably the most effective means of preventing pulmonary emboli. Prophylactic anticoagulant therapy is not routinely recommended for all patients after a myocardial infarction but is advisable for patients with increased risk factors for DVT and pulmonary embolism.

SYSTEMIC EMBOLI Emboli to the cerebrovascular, renal, mesenteric, iliofemoral, or other arterial systems may complicate the AMI. The reported prevalence of clinically apparent systemic emboli in patients with myocardial infarction varies from 0.6 to 6.4 percent.[570,571] These emboli result from dislodgement of left ventricular thrombi, which are found in 20 to 40 percent of anterior myocardial infarctions. A ventricular thrombus is unusual in patients with an inferior infarction.[571,572] The predilection of the apical wall for thrombus development appears to be related to a combination of stagnant blood flow and poor wall contractility. Severe depression of left ventricular function is not a prerequisite for thrombus formation. The development of a mural thrombus in a small infarction (CK < 1000 U), however, is unusual.[573,574] Thrombus morphology and mobility would seem to correlate with systemic embolization.[570,575,576] Pedunculated and freely mobile thrombi have been thought to have a greater chance of embolization. At least two studies, however, could not correlate risk of embolization to any particular thrombus morphology.[574,577]

Left ventricular thrombosis usually occurs within the first 3 days after a myocardial infarction[574,578] but may occur at any time during the hospital course. Early mural thrombosis occurs in large infarctions that have an unfavorable prognosis.[574] Systemic embolization occurs an average of 14 days after AMI and is unlikely to occur after more than 4 to 6 weeks.[579] Anticoagulation appears to reduce the incidence of mural thrombus formation[580] and the prevalence of systemic embolization.[570,572,573] All patients with an anterior myocardial infarction should have two-dimensional echocardiography performed within 24 to 72 h following the infarction, with particular emphasis on the two- and four-chamber apical views. Those with a severe apical wall contraction abnormality (akinesis or dyskinesis) should receive heparin for several days, followed by warfarin (INR 2 to 3) for 1 to 3 months. In patients with a left ventricular thrombus demonstrated by echocardiographic studies, chronic warfarin therapy (Chap. 52) is continued for approximately 3 months. Warfarin administration should be maintained indefinitely for atrial fibrillation.

Two-dimensional echocardiography has a sensitivity of 83 to 95 percent and a specificity of 86 to 90 percent in diagnosing a mural thrombus.[571,573,575,581] Angiography has a sensitivity of 20 to 63 percent and a specificity of 67 to 75 percent.[570,582] Occasionally, a technically unsatisfactory echocardiogram may require the use of alternative noninvasive imaging modalities. Both computed tomography (CT) and magnetic resonance imaging (MRI) offer a similar sensitivity and perhaps superior specificity to echocardiography in this setting.[582]

VENTRICULAR ANEURYSM   The true prevalence of ventricular aneurysm after myocardial infarction is not well defined. Probably the best approximation comes from postmortem studies estimating a 3 to 15 percent prevalence.[578,583] The CASS registry documented angiographically defined left ventricular aneurysms in 7.6 percent of patients with coronary artery disease. The location of the aneurysm is usually anterior, anteroapical, or apical. True posterior ventricular aneurysms located in the diaphragmatic wall between the septum and insertion of the posterior papillary muscle have been observed but are quite uncommon.[584]

Pathologically, the aneurysmal area is characterized by a thinned-out transmural scar that has completely lost its trabecular pattern. The scar, which may eventually calcify, is clearly delineated from surrounding ventricular muscle. Aneurysms

characteristically have a wide base (the diameter of the mouth is equal to or larger than its greatest internal diameter), and one-half are lined by a laminated thrombus.[585]

As many as 80 percent of chronic ventricular aneurysms can be diagnosed clinically by the presence of an abnormal precordial impulse; a typical bulge on the left ventricular border on chest x-ray, frequently with calcification around the apex; and ECG evidence of a large anterior infarction with ST-segment elevation persisting beyond 2 weeks following the infarction. Two-dimensional echocardiographic studies can confirm the diagnosis.[577] Left ventricular aneurysms are associated with a reduced survival rate. The prognosis for these patients, however, is primarily related to the left ventricular dysfunction and not to the presence of the aneurysm. True ventricular aneurysms rarely rupture. In fact, the survival rate for patients with an aneurysm is no different than that for patients without an aneurysm but with a similar degree of left ventricular dysfunction. Moreover, the incidence of sudden death is no different. Whether or not clinical recognition of the presence of a ventricular aneurysm is important in the management of the patient after an AMI remains to be answered.[581]

Most patients with ventricular aneurysms should be treated the same as any other postinfarction patient with a similar degree of left ventricular dysfunction. Vasodilators, digoxin, anticoagulants, and antiarrhythmics should be used, based not on the presence of the aneurysm but as dictated by presence of heart failure, mural thrombi, and life-threatening arrhythmias. Occasionally, surgical resection of the aneurysm is justified in order to correct refractory heart failure, recurrent life-threatening arrhythmias, or multiple systemic emboli. The aneurysm resection should usually be combined with coronary bypass grafting and, in cases of ventricular arrhythmias, should be guided by electrophysiologic mapping.

PSEUDOANEURYSM   A pseudoaneurysm is a rare complication of myocardial infarction, the prevalence of which is not known. The probable sequence of events in the development of a pseudoaneurysm is as follows: occurrence of a transmural infarction with localized pericarditis arising at the site of infarction; development of adhesions between the visceral and parietal pericardium; rupture of the infarcted myocardium, with the extravasated blood confined by the adherent pericardium; progressive enlargement of the aneurysmal sac; and development of thrombus within the sac.[565a]

Unlike a true ventricular aneurysm, a pseudoaneurysm has a narrow base (site of rupture). The wall is composed only of a thrombus and pericardium, and the risk of rupture is high.[586] While the neck is small (its diameter is less than 50 percent of the diameter of the fundus), the pseudoaneurysm may progressively enlarge to become larger than the left ventricle. The pseudoaneurysm may be clinically silent or may present as progressively worsening heart failure, an abnormal bulge on the cardiac border, persistent ST-segment elevation in the area overlying the infarction, or systolic murmurs.[587]

The diagnosis can be established by two-dimensional echocardiographic studies, ventriculographic radionuclide studies, MRI, or left ventriculographic contrast studies.[586] Surgical resection is frequently indicated.

Arrhythmias and Conduction Disturbances Complicating Acute Myocardial Infarction ARRHYTHMIAS AND CONDUCTION DISTURBANCES COMPLICATING ACUTE MYOCARDIAL INFARCTION Arrhythmias and conduction disturbances that are likely to be significant problems during the early phases of AMI and their management have been discussed above, under "Evaluation and Management of the Chest Pain Patient in the Emergency Department." The arrhythmias and conduction abnormalties discussed include sinus bradycardia, AV block, idioventricular rhythm, VT, and VF. In general, the acute management of these rhythm disturbances is the same in the early and in the late phases of AMI. Sustained VT and VF are exceptions, however, in that their occurrence after the first 24 h has more ominous implications for long-term electrical instability and sudden cardiac death. Other rhythm and conduction abnormalties that may be manifest throughout the course of AMI and are not characteristically associated with the early phases, are discussed here.

VENTRICULAR ECTOPY, VENTRICULAR TACHYCARDIA, AND VENTRICULAR FIBRILLATION The management of VT and VF after the first 24 h of hospitalization for AMI is similar to that discussed for the early phase. The occurrence of symptomatic, sustained VT or VF in the later phases of the hospital course, however, suggests that a chronic arrhythmogenic focus may be developing in the damaged ventricle. These ventricular arrhythmias are classified as *secondary* and indicate increased risk for subsequent sudden cardiac death. The implications and management of these rhythms are discussed above, under "Risk Stratification and Secondary Prevention in Patients Surviving Acute Myocardial Infarction" (see also Chap. 36).

SINUS TACHYCARDIA OR ATRIAL PREMATURE BEATS Sinus tachycardia following AMI is common and is frequently an unfavorable prognostic sign. The increased heart rate enhances myocardial oxygen demand, while the decreased diastolic time decreases diastolic coronary flow. Patients with a large area of infarcted myocardium may have sinus tachycardia on the basis of left ventricular dysfunction, which causes reflex sympathetic nervous system activation. Other obvious causes of sinus tachycardia—such as fever, anxiety, pain, pulmonary embolism, anemia, hypovolemia, or hypoxemia—must be evaluated and treated. Sinus tachycardia may occur as a result of the effects of drugs, such as dobutamine, dopamine, theophylline, and atropine.[588] In the absence of precipitating causes, a persistent sinus tachycardia most likely reflects progressive left ventricular dysfunction, which should be evaluated and managed accordingly.

Frequent atrial premature complexes are relatively common in AMI and are caused by atrial ischemia or infarction and pericarditis.[588–592] No specific therapy is indicated; rather, attention should be given to the underlying disease process.

PAROXYSMAL SUPRAVENTRICULAR TACHYCARDIA Episodes of paroxysmal supraventricular tachycardia occur rather commonly in AMI and are usually transient.[589] Underlying causes are similar to those of atrial premature complexes. For reasons discussed, the tachycardia may worsen ischemia. Rate control is essential, and the therapeutic approaches—which may include carotid sinus massage, adenosine, digoxin, verapamil, or diltiazem—are discussed in Chaps. 26 and 27.

ATRIAL FLUTTER AND ATRIAL FIBRILLATION Atrial flutter in relatively uncommon in AMI, whereas atrial fibrillation has an incidence of 10 to 15 percent.[589,590] Atrial fibrillation is associated with an increased in-hospital mortality rate, probably because it is associated with large infarcts and is seen relatively more commonly in patients with cardiac failure, complex ventricular arrhythmias, advanced AV block, atrial infarction, and pericarditis.[593] The pathophysiologic implications are similar to those for paroxysmal supraventricular tachycardia in that a rapid ventricular response can worsen ischemia and infarction by increasing oxygen consumption. Furthermore, the loss of atrial transport can worsen cardiac output and lead to hemodynamic instability.

Atrial fibrillation increases in incidence with age; it occurs in less than 5 percent of patients with AMI under the age of 60 and in about 16 percent of those over age 70.[15] The incidence of atrial fibrillation has been reported to be lower in patients receiving thrombolytic therapy than in control patients.[594]

Systemic embolization occurs more commonly in AMI in the presence of atrial fibrillation (1.7 percent) than in its absence (0.6 percent). Fifty percent of these emboli occur during the first hospital day and 90 percent have occurred by the fourth day.[595] Thus, heparin therapy is indicated in patients not already receiving it, in spite of the fact that the rhythm is usually transient.

If the patient experiences new or worsening pain, ischemic ST changes, or hemodynamic instability during atrial fibrillation with a rapid ventricular response rate, immediate electrical cardioversion is indicated. In the conscious patient, brief anesthesia is indicated (see Chap. 27).

If the clinical situation is less urgent, the ventricular rate can be reduced with drugs. Rapid digitalization with intravenous digoxin is effective but will not result in an immediate response, which may take 1 to 2 h. In the absence of contraindications such as congestive heart failure or bronchospastic pulmonary disease, intravenously administered beta-blocking drugs are highly effective in slowing the ventricular rate. Intravenous administration of the calcium channel blockers, verapamil or diltiazem, can also be effective in slowing the ventricular response, but these are not considered to be first-line drugs (except possibly in the setting of NQWMI), because of the general concern about calcium channel blockers in AMI.[15]

Firm recommendations have not been made about the use of class I and III antiarrhythmics to prevent the recurrence of atrial fibrillation in AMI.[15] Since recurrence is associated with a worse prognosis, however, it seems prudent to consider amiodarone or sotalol or, alternatively, quinidine or procainamide. Neither anticoagulation nor antiarrhythmic therapy should be continued for the long term. With stable sinus rhythm, either or both, as the case may be, should be stopped after 6 weeks.

JUNCTIONAL RHYTHM   An escape AV junctional rhythm at a rate of 40 to 60 beats per minute in patients with inferior myocardial infarction and high-degree heart block is not uncommon.[589] Therapy usually is not required. Accelerated junctional rhythms are occasionally seen in AMI, more likely at rates of 70 to 130 beats per minute,[596] but are rarely seen at considerably higher rates. Treatment generally focuses on the underlying conditions, such as ischemia or digitalis toxicity.

HEART BLOCK   First-, second-, and third-degree AV blocks have been discussed briefly. First-degree block is frequently seen in AMI, and especially in inferior myocardial infarction. This is attributable to ischemia or enhanced vagal activity. It can be worsened by drugs such as beta blockers. Treatment is seldom required.

Second-degree AV block is also relatively common, especially Mobitz type I or Wenckebach block. This block, characterized by progressive lengthening of the PR interval before the atrial beat, is not conducted and may occur in as many as 10 percent of AMI patients.[597] It is associated with a narrow QRS and frequently is the result of AV node ischemia in inferior myocardial infarction. It is usually transient, and its presence does not affect the prognosis. Mobitz type II block is uncommon but is associated with more serious complications and a worse prognosis. It usually occurs with anterior myocardial infarction and reflects trifascicular block. It is characterized by a wide QRS and a nonvarying PR interval before a nonconducted atrial beat. Heart block may develop suddenly and is an ominous sign, with a mortality of about 80 percent. It is usually permanent.

Third-degree AV block, or complete heart block, occurs in about 5 percent of patients with AMI and is most commonly seen with inferior infarction, usually with block at the AV node. As indicated, complete heart block in inferior myocardial infarction is usually transient and may occur early or late in the hospital course with the same implications for prognosis. There is some increase in in-hospital mortality rates in this setting, but complete heart block in inferior myocardial infarction is not an independent predictor of poor long-term prognosis.[598] In contrast, patients with anterior infarction who develop third-degree AV block have a mortality rate of 80 percent.[599] Implications for temporary and permanent pacing are discused subsequently.

INTRAVENTRICULAR CONDUCTION DISTURBANCES   The development of BBB during AMI usually signifies an extensive infarct. In one multicenter trial, the presence of BBB was associated with a twofold increase in the in-hospital mortality rate (28 versus 14 percent), compared with the absence of

BBB.[600,601] Data indicate that the presence of BBB identifies patients who (1) are more likely to develop congestive heart failure, (2) are more likely to develop high-degree heart block, (3) are more likely to have an episode of ventricular fibrillation, and (4) have a higher mortality rate[601] (see also Chap. 27).

INDICATIONS FOR TEMPORARY TRANSVENOUS PACING   Recommendations[15]:

Class I

1. Asystole
2. Symptomatic bradycardia (including sinus bradycardia with hypotension and type I second-degree AV block with hypotension not responsive to atropine)
3. Bilateral BBB (alternating or right BBB with alternating left anterior fascicular/posterior fascicular block)(any age)
4. New or indeterminate-age bifascicular block (right BBB with left anterior or posterior fascicular block) with first-degree AV block
5. Mobitz type II second-degree AV block

Class IIa

1. Right BBB and left anterior or left posterior fascicular block (new or indeterminate)
2. Right BBB with first-degree AV block
3. Left BBB, new or indeterminate
4. Incessant VT, for atrial or ventricular overdrive pacing
5. Recurrent sinus pauses (greater than 3 s) not responsive to atropine

Class IIb

1. Bifascicular block of indeterminate age
2. New or age-indeterminant isolated right BBB

Class III

1. First-degree heart block
2. Type I second-degree AV block with normal hemodynamics
3. Accelerated idioventricular rhythm
4. Bundle branch block or fascicular block known to exist before acute myocardial infarction

Cardiac pacing is discussed in Chap. 34. The indications generally agreed on for temporary pacemaker insertion in AMI include asystole, complete heart block in the setting of anterior myocardial infarction, new onset of right or left BBB with persistent Mobitz II second-degree AV block in the setting of anterior myocardial infarction, or other symptomatic bradycardias unresponsive to atropine.[602]

Bundle branch block in the setting of AMI, as noted, identifies a population at risk for both electrical and mechanical complications. Such patients must be monitored for evidence of transient high-degree heart block. Prolonged intermediate care with telemetry monitoring and repeat assessments of heart failure status are important.

PERMANENT PACING   Recommendations[15]:

Class I

1. Persistent second-degree AV block in the His-Purkinje system with bilateral BBB or complete heart block after AMI
2. Transient advanced (second- or third-degree) AV block and associated bundle branch block
3. Symptomatic AV block at any level

Class IIb

1. Persistent advanced (second- or third-degree) block at the level of the AV node

Class III

1. Transient AV conduction disturbances in the absence of intraventricular conduction defects
2. Transient AV block in the presence of isolated left anterior fascicular block
3. Acquired left anterior fascicular block in the absence of AV block
4. Persistent first-degree AV block in the presence of BBB that is old or age-indeterminate

The use of permanent pacemakers is discussed in detail in Chap. 34. The subject is reviewed extensively in the ACC/AHA guidelines for pacemaker implantation.[603] The fact that temporary pacing may have been required in the course of AMI does not necessarily indicate a need for permanent pacing. Patients who have had permanent pacemakers inserted after AMI usually have a relatively unfavorable prognosis primarily related to the extensiveness of the underlying disease and myocardial damage.[15] Thus, these patients are at increased risk for death from progressive congestive heart failure CHF and ventricular tachyarrhythmias. The generally accepted indications for insertion of a permanent pacemaker after AMI are summarized in the recommendations above.

DISCHARGE FROM THE CORONARY CARE UNIT

The length of stay in the CCU should be based on the risk of developing VT and VF. The risk of developing primary VF after AMI decreases exponentially, with the majority of arrhythmic deaths occurring within the first 24 h. After the third day, the episodes of life-threatening arrhythmias are fairly evenly distributed over the remainder of the hospitalization.[604] Thus, a patient with an uncomplicated infarction can

be transferred from the CCU on the third day. Since 31 to 34 percent of in-hospital deaths from AMI occur after discharge from the CCU and half of them are sudden and unexpected, certain patients need more prolonged cardiac monitoring.[605,606] Those patients who are prime candidates for late-hospital sudden deaths manifest, while in the CCU, one or more of the following: (1) the arrhythmias of pump failure (sinus tachycardia, atrial flutter, or atrial fibrillation); (2) the arrhythmias of electrical instability (VT or VF); (3) acute interventricular conduction disturbances; (4) evidence of circulatory failure (CHF, pulmonary edema, or significant hypotension); or (5) large anterior infarction. The effectiveness of prolonged monitoring of this select group of patients in an intermediate care unit following CCU discharge is evident in a doubling of the rate of successful resuscitations.[607,608] Patients who do not fit into these high-risk subgroups can be discharged from the CCU to a medical unit without continuous monitoring. The wide availability of continuous monitoring in many hospitals in non–acute care units, however, permits easy further monitoring even on lower-risk patients and is preferable if available.

The activity permitted the patient with uncomplicated infarction has changed immensely during the last two decades. In an uncomplicated myocardial infarction, the patient does not need to be confined to bed for longer than 24 h. In fact, the patient may use a bedside commode from the time of admission. The safety and benefits of chair rest were initially promoted by Samuel Levine and Bernard Lown in 1951.[609] Upon transfer from a CCU, the patient should be started on a program of progressive ambulation. The speed with which the patient progresses from one stage to the next depends on the severity of the infarction, the presence or absence of complications, the patient's age, and the presence of comorbid conditions. The length of hospitalization following an AMI should likewise depend on these same factors. If the patient has not manifested the arrhythmias of pump failure or electrical instability, evidence of circulatory failure, or advanced AV block during the first 4 days of hospitalization, he or she is very unlikely to do so at any later time.[610] This patient could probably be discharged after 7 or fewer days in the hospital.[611] The last 2 to 3 days of the hospitalization are generally necessary to resolve the questions pertaining to residual ventricular function, the presence or absence of ventricular ectopy, and the adequacy of the remainder of the coronary circulation. In addition, time is needed for instruction in risk-factor modification (see Chap. 55). As discussed previously, time in the hospital is being shortened, especially after successful thrombolysis.

Noninvasive Risk Stratification in Patients Surviving Acute Myocardial Infarction

Survivors of AMI have a substantial risk of facing subsequent cardiovascular events. Noninvasive risk assessment provides useful information to individualize the extent of further workup and therapy: (1) targeting specific long-term therapies, (2) identifying high-risk patients requiring aggressive diagnostic tests, (3) counseling the patient on prognosis, (4) developing an exercise program, and (5) planning modifications of lifestyle.

Three interrelated prognostic factors are the focus of predischarge assessment: (1) assessment of left ventricular function, (2) detection of residual myocardial ischemia (jeopardized myocardium), and (3) assessment of the risk of arrhythmic (sudden cardiac) death. Most proposed algorithms of noninvasive test selection focus on these three important clinical areas.[612–615] High-risk patients can be clinically identified without such noninvasive assessments because of evidence of one or more of the following: decompensated CHF, angina associated with electrocardiographic changes, in-hospital cardiac arrest, spontaneous sustained VT, or the development of a high-degree heart block.[616–620] In contrast to this high-risk group, the majority of patients have a relatively benign hospital course. In these patients, noninvasive testing can accurately identify a group at very low risk whose annual mortality is 1 to 3 percent.[621–625] The practical consequences of identifying a low-risk group is that emphasis is focused on early discharge and lifestyle modification (Chaps. 41 and 53) and targeted prophylactic medical therapy (Chap. 45) rather than expensive, invasive diagnostic testing.

In the recent ACC/AHA guidelines for the management of patients with AMI, there is general agreement that early coronary angiography and aggressive interventional therapy are indicated for patients with recurrent episodes of spontaneous angina or ischemia, as discussed previously.[15] Also, there is general agreement that angiography is indicated and is potentially beneficial in patients with evidence of persistent pulmonary congestion, clinical left ventricular dysfunction, or cardiogenic shock. In addition, many clinicians feel that patients with recurrent ischemic chest discomfort, despite medical therapy or with hemodynamic instability, also merit early coronary angiography. The prevailing opinion is that the weight of evidence is in favor of the usefulness of early angiography in such patients with overt signs and symptoms.[15]

In the following sections, the emphasis is on the noninvasive evaluation of asymptomatic patients. This includes assessments of left ventricular dysfunction, myocardial ischemia and the risk of arrhythmic (sudden cardiac) death. *There is general agreement that in such asymptomatic patients there is not adequate evidence to support routine coronary angiography as the initial assessment; therefore, the guidelines dissuade its use as the primary tool for diagnostic evaluation.*[15]

ASSESSMENT OF LEFT VENTRICULAR FUNCTION AND LEFT VENTRICULAR EJECTION FRACTION

Many clinical features are consistent with an increased risk for the development of clinical CHF. These include patients with anterior and anterolateral infarction, papillary muscle dysfunction, and recurrent myocardial infarction as well as

those who develop transient episodes of high-degree heart block. Congestive heart failure in the setting of inferior AMI associated with right ventricular infarction is a prognostically important category, as discussed previously.

In patients without such obvious left ventricular dysfunction, left ventricular ejection fractions should be assessed by either echocardiographic, radionuclide, or angiographic techniques.[626–629] Ventricular function is an important determinant of long-term survival after AMI regardless of reperfusion status. In-hospital mortality is directly related to the severity of left ventricular dysfunction. Assessment of the left ventricular ejection fraction obtained in the hospital also closely reflects 1- and 2-year survival. In the absence of significant ischemia or ventricular arrhythmias, patients with a left ventricular ejection fraction of ≥ 40 percent have mortality rates in the range of 5 percent over 1 to 2 years, whereas a left ventricular ejection fraction of 30 to 39 percent or <30 percent have mortality rates that increase to 10 to 15 percent and 20 to 25 percent, respectively.[612,626–629] Although measured much less frequently, the end-systolic volume index is also an excellent predictor of survival following AMI.[628–630]

Clinical reflections of the degree of left ventricular systolic dysfunction include the patient's exercise capacity as judged by exercise testing and/or the New York Heart Association's clinical classification, which are independent predictors of outcome. Patients with good exercise capacity, even in the presence of reduced ejection fractions, have a superior long-term outcome in comparison with those who cannot perform mild to moderate exercise.[631,632]

ASSESSMENT OF MYOCARDIAL ISCHEMIA

Exercise Testing in Uncomplicated Patients
Recommendations[15]:

Class I

1. Stress electrocardiography
   a. Before discharge, for prognostic assessment or functional capacity (submaximal at 4 to 6 days or symptom-limited at 10 to 14 days)
   b. Early after discharge for prognostic assessment and functional capacity (14 to 21 days)
   c. Late after discharge (3 to 6 weeks) for functional capacity and prognosis if early stress was submaximal
2. Exercise, vasodilator stress nuclear scintigraphy, or exercise stress echocardiography when baseline abnormalities of the ECG compromise interpretation

Class IIa

1. Dipyridamole or adenosine stress perfusion nuclear scintigraphy or dobutamine echocardiography before discharge, for prognostic assessment in patients judged to be unable to exercise

2. Exercise two-dimensional echocardiography or nuclear scintigraphy (before or early after discharge for prognostic assessment)

Class III

1. Stress testing within 2 to 3 days of AMI.
2. Either exercise or pharmacologic stress testing at any time to evaluate patients with unstable postinfarction angina pectoris.
3. At any time, to evaluate patients with AMI, who have uncompensated CHF, cardiac arrhythmia, or noncardiac conditions that severely limit their ability to exercise.
4. Before discharge, to evaluate patients who have been selected for cardiac catheterization. In this situation, the exercise test may be useful after catheterization to evaluate function or identify ischemia in distribution of lesions of borderline severity.

Timing of Exercise Testing and Protocol Selection During hospitalization, in patients recovering from AMI, a practical and safe approach to exercise testing has been to utilize a submaximal treadmill exercise protocol (modified Naughton or modified Bruce protocol) rather than the standard Bruce protocol. The target for completing the test is often symptom-limited exercise to a specific heart rate goal (e.g., 70 to 75 percent age-predicted) or to a peak work level (e.g., 5 metabolic equivalents, or METs) unless other factors (≥ 2 mm ST depression, ventricular arrhythmia, or hypotension) arise first (see Chap. 15). The exercise ECG most accurately reflects the risk of subsequent ischemic events when baseline ST abnormalities or a BBB is absent. Exercise testing is also useful in planning the exercise prescription for a cardiac rehabilitation program (see Chap. 55). For safety, patients should be angina-free and free of cardiac failure before exercise testing. Patients selected in this fashion under the supervision of a physician are at minimal risk for complications.[621–623,633–636]

Clinical Significance of Predischarge Submaximal Exercise Testing Numerous studies have analyzed the predictive value of predischarge exercise testing during a 6- to 12-month follow-up after AMI.[614,615,621–623] Exercise variables of prognostic significance are exercise-induced ST-segment depression, ST-segment elevation, development of angina during exercise, inadequate blood pressure response to exercise, or exercise of short duration. From the practical standpoint, it is important to consider all of these exercise variables rather than to focus solely on the presence or absence of ST-segment depression. Exercise testing consistently identifies a high-risk group for recurrent cardiac events (myocardial infarction, unstable angina, etc.) or mortality in the first year after the AMI. However, the relative risk for mortality or cardiac events associated with a "positive exercise test" varies greatly between studies (2-fold to more than 15-fold versus a "negative test"). Exercise testing also identifies a very low risk group (1 to 3 percent mortality rate for the first year).[621–623,636] A negative test result is reassuring and should promote early discharge as well as discourage an aggressive diagnostic approach. The ACC/AHA guidelines support the widespread use of submaximal exercise testing in *uncomplicated* patients before discharge.[15]

For patients with a normal exercise test before discharge, symptom-limited maximal exercise testing can be repeated 2 to 6 weeks after AMI. The maximal exercise test can be used to identify additional high-risk patients.[637–639] The magnitude of this additional ischemia detection, however, as compared to a submaximal exercise test prior to hospital discharge, appears to be modest. Since many cardiovascular events can occur in the first 4 to 6 weeks, some type of predischarge assessment of ischemia seems preferred. *The presence of ischemia generally mandates cardiac catheterization to define the coronary anatomy and to consider revascularization (see the ischemia algorithm in Fig. 47-12[15]).*

The majority of data on exercise testing post–myocardial infarction have been acquired in patients who have not received thrombolytic therapy. New therapeutic options have resulted in a lower mortality rate. However, patients who receive thrombolytic therapy presumably have a larger amount of myocardium at risk and have larger amounts of residual myocardial ischemia. The consensus opinion of the ACC/AHA guidelines management group is that exercise testing is still useful in the risk stratification of patients who have received thrombolytic therapy.[15,640,641] There is general agreement that predischarge submaximal testing is beneficial, useful, and effective (class I indication) in uncomplicated patients postinfarction.[15]

Ambulatory Electrocardiographic Detection of Myocardial Ischemia

A number of studies have assessed the presence of silent myocardial ischemia (usually defined as ≥ 1 mm ST-segment depression for ≥ 30 s), using 24-h ambulatory electrocardiographic monitoring in patients who have survived myocardial infarction. Some of the episodes of transient ST-segment depression on ambulatory ECGs are associated with chest pain and typical angina symptoms, but the majority of these ischemic episodes are silent. Many of these episodes of "silent ischemia" occur during levels of low activity and/or mental stress.[642–645] As with other measurements of ischemia, the detection of ambulatory electrocardiographic ischemia has been predictive of a poor outcome in long-term follow-up trials in patients surviving AMI. The correlations between exercise testing, ambulatory ECGs, and ischemia detected by thallium appear to overlap but are not identical.[646,647] While ambulatory electrocardiography appears promising in identifying patients with silent ischemia at higher risk, no studies have been performed to show that the reduction in these episodes of silent ischemia leads to an improved outcome; thus, routine ambulatory electrocardiographic assessment of ischemia is not recommended.[15]

Alternatives for Evaluating Myocardial Ischemia

Thallium-201 Scintigraphy

There are several alternatives to standard exercise testing. One well-studied technique is exercise thallium-201 scintigraphy, as discussed previously (see Chap. 17). Exercise thallium-201 scintigraphy has a number of potential advantages over routine exercise testing: (1) it can be used when the 12-lead ECG is uninterpretable for ischemic ST-segment shifts because of baseline changes such as a left BBB; (2) it allows assessment of reversible and irreversible perfusion defects, both within and outside the vascular region involved in the AMI; (3) the technique of single-photon emission computed tomography (SPECT) thallium scintigraphy provides a semi-quantitative evaluation of ischemia; and (4) exercise thallium-201 scintigraphy it offers superior sensitivity and specificity compared with standard exercise testing.[648–650]

High-risk patients are identified if (1) perfusion defects exist in more than one discrete vascular zone, (2) there is distinct evidence of redistribution, or (3) there was evidence of increased lung uptake. Low-risk patients are defined by thallium scintigraphy showing involvement of a single vascular region without redistribution, with no evidence of increased lung uptake. A high-risk thallium-201 scintigram is correlated with multivessel coronary disease. Thallium scintigraphy has been shown to be excellent at identifying high-grade stenoses of 90 percent or greater, especially high-grade lesions of the left anterior descending coronary artery.[649–651]

As in routine exercise testing, a limited number of studies have evaluated the value of exercise thallium tomography in patients with thrombolytic therapy, with some conflicting results. Provocative pharmacologic studies using thallium-201 tomography also predicted risk of subsequent ischemic events after myocardial infarction.[648,652–654] Adenosine tomography also offers the advantage of allowing the safe assessment of ischemia as early as 3 to 4 days following acute myocardial infarction. In the era of cost containment and pressure for early hospital discharge, this approach, although not proven, may be beneficial in identifying patients who can safely be discharged early.[648]

Other radionuclide techniques are valuable in the evalua-

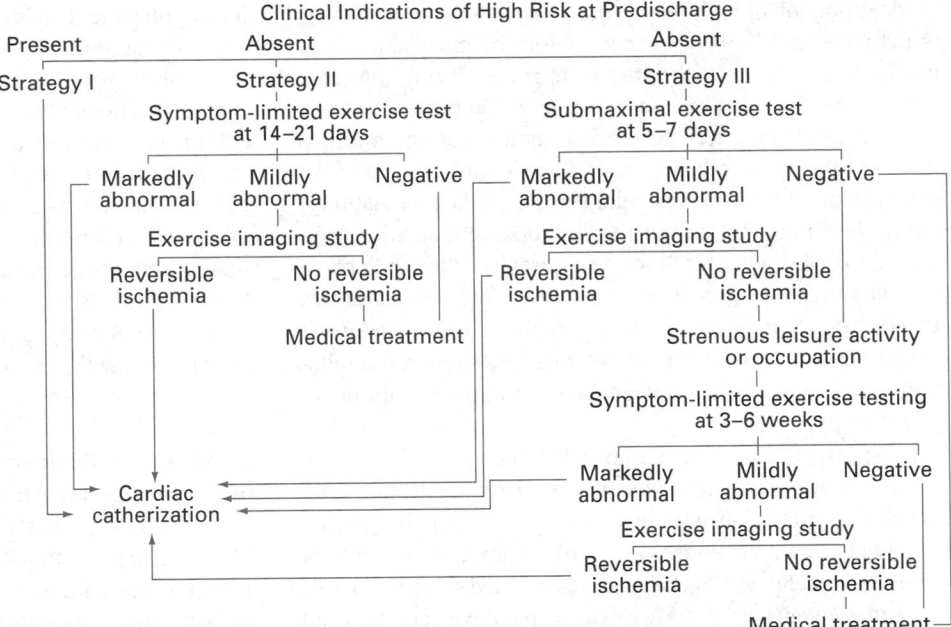

FIGURE 47-12

Strategies for exercise test evaluations soon after myocardial infarction (MI). If patients are at high risk for ischemic events based on clinical criteria, they should undergo invasive evaluation to determine if they are candidates for coronary revascularization procedures (strategy I). For patients initially deemed to be at low risk at time of discharge after myocardial infarction, two strategies for performing exercise testing can be used. One is a symptom-limited test at 14 to 21 days (strategy II). If the patient is on digoxin or if the baseline ECG precludes accurate interpretation of ST-segment changes (e.g., baseline left BBB or left ventricular hypertrophy), then an initial exercise imaging study can be performed. Results of exercise testing should be stratified to determine need for additional invasive or exercise perfusion studies. A third strategy is to perform a submaximal exercise test at 5 to 7 days after myocardial infarction or just before hospital discharge. The exercise test results could be stratified using the guidelines in strategy I. If exercise test studies are negative, a second symptom-limited exercise test could be repeated at 3 to 6 weeks for patients undergoing vigorous activity during leisure or at work. (From Ryan et al.,[15] with permission.)

tion of patients after AMI, but the focus here has been on thallium scintigraphy, which provides the identification of residual myocardial ischemia. Other techniques include the use of radionuclide angiography for the assessment of ventricular function, including the evaluation of right ventricular infarction, and the use of technetium pyrophosphate to estimate myocardial infarct size and hibernating myocardium. These have recently been summarized in the ACC/AHA guidelines for the management of patients with acute myocardial infarction (Table 47-6[15]). Only exercise and pharmacologic thallium studies have a class I indication for the evaluation of ischemia.[15] The choice between this test and standard exercise testing depends on initial ECG interpretability, availability, cost, and clinical experience.

Exercise Echocardiography

Exercise two-dimensional echocardiography is an alternative technique for identifying postinfarction ischemia. A reversible segmental wall motion defect is felt to represent an area of significant ischemia. Studies from specialized centers with expertise in echocardiography have shown that exercise or dobutamine echocardiographic studies have a high sensitivity and specificity in identifying patients with multivessel coronary disease (see Chap. 14).[655–659]

Identification of high risk on dobutamine stress echocardiograms includes (1) the presence of four or more akinetic or diskinetic segments in the infarct territory during low-dose dobutamine (an index of infarct size), (2) the presence of two or more coronary artery territories demonstrating abnormal wall motion at rest or during peak-dose dobutamine, and (3) a lack of improvement in wall thickening (i.e., lack of viability) within the infarct region during low-dose dobutamine infusion.[657,659] As with thallium scintigraphy, the findings of dobutamine stress echocardiograms may provide superior risk stratification than coronary angiography. The procedure is predictive of cardiac events in patients treated with thrombolytic agents as well as in those who did not receive thrombolytic therapy.[659]

Prospective studies to identify the incremental value of exercise echocardiograms over regular exercise testing after myocardial infarction have not been performed. In general, negative tests with exercise echocardiogram, dipyridamole or dobutamine echocardiography are associated with a low rate of cardiac events.[655–659] However, a negative test does not preclude cardiac events in the first 1 to 2 years after myocardial infarction. A great variation among institutions as well as in expertise in study quality are limitations to a widespread recommendation for the preferred use of exercise or pharmacologic echocardiographic studies prior to hospital discharge. In general, these procedures are less costly than radionuclide perfusion scintigraphy.

Suggested Algorithm for the Evaluation of Myocardial Ischemia after Myocardial Infarction

Based on all of the evaluable data, the task force on practice guidelines for the management of acute myocardial infarction created a strategy for the evaluation of myocardial ischemia after myocardial infarction in low-risk patients.[15] Their conclusions are presented in Fig. 47-12. If there are clinical indications of a high-risk patient, as detailed above, such patients are considered for early cardiac catheterization and coronary angiography (strategy I). The evaluation of myocardial ischemia in low-risk patients is alternatively presented for strategies II and III. Strategy III favors using a submaximal exercise test or alternative imaging study prior to hospital discharge. Strategy II alternatively suggests that a symptom-limited exercise test be performed soon after hospital discharge. Regardless of whether exercise testing or a more sophisticated exercise imaging study is ordered in the hospital, a negative test does not preclude the repeat evaluation for myocardial ischemia once the patient is ambulatory, after 3 to 6 weeks.

Assessment of the Risk of Arrhythmic (Sudden Cardiac) Death: Overview

Although the technology to assess the risk of arrhythmic death in patients after AMI has improved in sophistication, antiarrhythmic therapies to reduce risk have thus far proven inadequate. There is general agreement based upon excellent studies that the identification of postinfarction patients with a left ventricular ejection fraction of less than or equal to 40 percent mandates the use of ACE inhibitors.[660–662] Likewise, the identification of asymptomatic post-

infarction patients with ischemia mandates the performance of coronary angiography to assess the potential for PTCA or coronary artery bypass surgery. Unfortunately, the identification of asymptomatic but high-risk patients for arrhythmic death after AMI is not similarly associated with the delineation of a successful treatment strategy. This section addresses those postinfarction patients who are asymptomatic and have not had sustained VT or VF—identifiers that all agree require aggressive management. The presumption is that the majority of postinfarction patients who experience arrhythmic (sudden cardiac) death have developed terminal VT and/or VF.[663] A review of selected clinical trials of antiarrhythmic therapy focusing on patients after myocardial infarction is presented in Table 47-17.[660–662,664–668;669] The percent of the total deaths attributable to arrhythmic or sudden cardiac death varies widely in the placebo groups of these trials. The Cardiac Arrhythmia Suppression (CAST) trials[664,665] and the Canadian Amiodarone Myocardial Infarction Arrhythmia Trial (CAMIAT)[668] identified high-risk patients after myocardial infarction using the criteria of ventricular arrhythmia on ambulatory ECGs. In the placebo groups, the range of death attributable to arrhythmia varied from 48 to 66 percent. The Survival and Ventricular Enlargement (SAVE) trial,[661] the European Myocardial Infarction Amiodarone Trial (EMIAT)[667] and the Survival With Oral D'sotalol (SWORD)[666] trial identified patients after myocardial infarction using only an ejection fraction criterion, yet they found a similar range of deaths attributable to arrhythmia in the placebo group (45 to 67 percent). Patients in trials with a mixture of etiologies of left ventricular dysfunction including old myocardial infarction, such as the Studies of Left Ventricular Dysfunction (SOLVD) prevention and SOLVD treatment trials, have a lower percentage of deaths attributable to arrhythmia.[661,662] The wide discrepancy in arrhythmic death rates and the variety of screening tests used to identify "high-risk" patients highlights a significant problem with arrhythmic death classification.[669]

The changing proportion of deaths attributable to arrhythmia and other causes after myocardial infarction is conceptually depicted in Fig. 47-13. Sustained VT and VF appear to occur most frequently in the first year following myocardial infarction. As ischemic cardiomyopathy develops over many years, deaths attributable to VT/VF decrease and proportionately more "sudden deaths" are attributable to asystole, electromechanical dissociation, or a high-degree heart block.[670] Also, non-cardiac conditions emulate the circumstances of VT or VF (for instance, massive pulmonary embolism, ruptured abdominal or thoracic aortic aneurysm, or massive stroke).[669] Thus, the temporal influence on cause-specific mortality is clinically relevant; it is important to recognize and to consider, especially with the many potential risks for mortality in these patients (Fig. 47-13).

This discussion is limited to tests available for evaluating asymptomatic patients in order to identify individuals at high risk for sudden cardiac death after surviving a recent AMI.

AMBULATORY ELECTROCARDIOGRAPHIC RECORDINGS: VENTRICULAR ARRHYTHMIAS Asymptomatic spontaneous ventricular arrhythmias detected on ambulatory ECGs are predictive of an increased risk of arrhythmic (sudden) death in the first 1 to 2 years following AMI.[612,671,672] The mechanism responsible for the majority of arrhythmic deaths in post–myocardial infarction patients is, as noted, sustained VT or VF.[663] Vulnerability for arrhythmic death appears to be highest in the first year after AMI, probably accounting for one-half of the first-year mortality.[612,671] Thus, it is clinically relevant to attempt to assess potential arrhythmic death risk prior to hospital discharge. The use of ambulatory electrocardiographic recording to identify a "high-risk" group, however, has a very poor positive predictive value.[664,673] As seen in Table 47-18,[11,612,664,671–673] postinfarction patients with no baseline ventricular arrhythmia on ambulatory electrocardiographic recording have a low risk for arrhythmic death.[11,612] Frequent premature ventricular complexes and nonsustained VT are generally associated with a two- and threefold increased risk, respectively.[11,612,671–673] As can be deduced from the data in Table 47-18,[11,612,664,671–673] for every 100 patients identified with "warning arrhythmias," only 4 to 7 are at risk for arrhythmic death in the following 1 to 2 years. Thus, a strategy that would recommend routine prophylactic administration of an antiarrhythmic drug requires a superb safety profile, since approximately ≥95 percent of patients will be exposed to unnecessary, potentially dangerous therapy. Such hazards have been documented in prophylactic antiarrhythmic drug trials.[664–666]

AMBULATORY ELECTROCARDIOGRAM RECORDINGS: HEART RATE VARIABILITY

Heart rate variability, measured by the standard deviation of the RR interval on monitored electrocardiographic leads, is an indirect assessment of proportional autonomic tone. Extensive variability in the heart rate connotes a preponderance of parasympathetic activity, where-

as less variability in the heart rate is consistent with proportionately more sympathetic activity.[674–678] In animal models, enhanced sympathetic activity increases the vulnerability of the ischemic myocardium to the development of ventricular fibrillation (see also Chap. 36).[679,680]

Clinical trials have assessed the relationship of heart rate

TABLE 47-17

REVIEW OF REPRESENTATIVE CLINICAL TRIALS: PLACEBO CAUSE-SPECIFIC MORTALITY

Trial (No. of Placebo Patients), Entrance Criteria	Mean Follow-up (months)	Annualized Mortality, %	Arrhythmia/SCD, %
CAST I[664] (743), VPC≥6/VT/AMI	10	4.2	62
CAST II[665] (574), VPC≥6/VT/ AMI/EF≤40%	18	6.4	66
SAVE[660] (1116), EF≤40%/AMI 3–16 d	42	7.1	45
SOLVD PREV[661] (2117), No CHF/EF≤35%	37	5.3	31
SOVLD Rx[662] (1294), CHF (II/III) + EF≤35%	41	11.7	22
SWORD[666] (1572), MI, EF≤40%	5	1.5	67
EMIAT[667] (743), MI + <40%	21	7.8	49
CAMIAT[668] (596), MI + VPC ≥10 or VT	20	4.7	48

Key: SCD = sudden cardiac death; CAST = Cardiac Arrhythmia Suppression Trial; VPC = ventricular premature complexes; VT = ventricular tachycardia; AMI = acute myocardial infarction; EF = ejection fraction; SAVE = Survival and Ventricular Enlargement; SOLVD = Studies of Left Ventricular Dysfunction; PREV = prevention; CHF = congestive heart failure; Rx = treatment; SWORD = Survival With Oral d-Sotalol; EMIAT = European Myocardial Infarction Amiodarone Trial; CAMIAT = Canadian Amiodarone Myocardial Infarction Arrhythmia Trial.
Source: Adapted from Pratt et al.,[669] with permission.

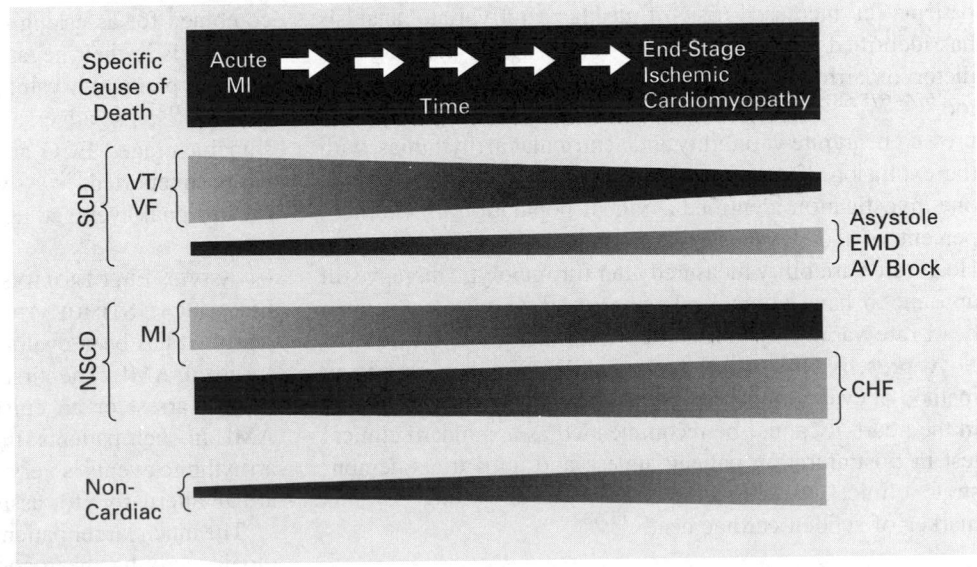

FIGURE 47-13

A theoretical view of approaches to identify a post–myocardial infarction population dying of ventricular tachycardia/fibrillation. This concept is presented in a qualitative fashion and represents estimates based on the literature (see text). (SCD = sudden cardiac death; NSCD = non-sudden cardiac death; VT = ventricular tachycardia; VF = ventricular fibrillation; MI = myocardial infarction; EMD = electromechanical dissociation; CHF = congestive heart failure.)

TABLE 47-18

RISK OF SUDDEN DEATH BASED ON VPCs DETECTED ON AECG IN PATIENTS
SURVIVING ACUTE MYOCARDIAL INFARCTION

Trial	Sample Size	Arrhythmic Death Mortality Rate, %[a]	Total Mortality Rate, %[a]	Actual Follow-up Months
CAST[664] (≥6 VPCs/h)				10
Encainide or flecainide	730	5.4[b]	9.2[b]	
Placebo	725	1.5	3.6	
CAPS[673] (≥10 VPCs/h)				12
All patients	502	4.6	9.0	
Placebo	100	—	7.0	
Bigger et al.[612]				24
All patients	819	3.8	5.9	
0 VPC	112	1.5	3.0	
>3 VPCs/h	2456	6.1	9.8	
>10 VPCs/h	162	6.3	9.4	
>30 VPCs/h	89	7.0	10.5	
BHAT[11] (placebo group)				25
0 VPCs	260	1.2	2.5	
Any VPCs	1380	2.6	5.5	
≤10 VPCs/h	211	4.5	10.0	
≥10 VPCs/h	1429	2.0	4.3	
Moss et al.[671]	759	6.8	11.6	6
Ruberman et al.[672]				24
≤10 VPCs/h	1285	2.3	6.4	
≥10 VPCs/h	454	7.6	13.6	

[a] All corrected to an estimated 1-year mortality rate.
[b] End point of death or cardiac arrest.
Key: VPCs = ventricular premature complexes; AECG = ambulatory ECG.

variability to mortality rate in patients surviving AMI. A depressed heart rate variability identifies postinfarction patients at increased risk of death. Multivariate analysis has identified reduced heart rate variability as a strong predictor of arrhythmic death in the early postinfarction period.[674–678,681] In fact, by selecting patients with both depressed heart rate variability and ventricular arrhythmias, with the exclusion of patients with the lowest ejection fractions, one investigation identified a patient population in whom 75 percent of the deaths were presumed to be arrhythmic.[682] Heart rate variability measured after thrombolytic therapy still appears to have clinical relevance, and an improvement in heart rate variability correlated with TIMI grade 3 flow.[683]

At present, while heart rate variability is a very promising method of evaluating parasympathetic and sympathetic effects in the heart, it cannot be recommended as a standard clinical test in postinfarction patients unless and until trials demonstrate clinical benefits based upon the knowledge of this marker of sudden cardiac death.[15,684]

SIGNAL-AVERAGE ELECTROCARDIOGRAM Time-domain analysis of the signal-averaged ECG can be used to detect low-amplitude, high-frequency potentials at the end of the QRS complex, termed *ventricular late potentials*. The pres-

ence of late potentials identifies patients likely to have inducible sustained monomorphic VT during programmed electrical stimulation and an increased risk of subsequent arrhythmic events.[674,685–691] The predictive value of late potentials is best established in patients with AMI and is of less established value in other patient populations.

In some studies, an abnormal signal-averaged ECG, the presence of frequent ventricular premature complexes on the ambulatory electrocardiographic recording, and the presence of left ventricular aneurysm were independent predictors of ventricular tachycardia, regardless of whether or not a patient had received thrombolytic therapy.[690,691] If results of the signal-averaged ECG are negative—that is, there are no after-depolarizations—the negative predictive value in this population is good and the likelihood of subsequent arrhythmic death is low. As with the evaluation of heart rate variability, the interpretation of the signal-averaged ECG can be improved by combining it with other variables, especially the left ventricular ejection fraction. Even when multiple tests are combined for assessing the risk of sudden cardiac death, the strength is in their negative predictive value rather than their positive predictive value, which usually falls below 50 percent.[685–691] The adverse prognostic consequence of a positive signal-averaged ECG and an occluded infarct-related artery has been reported.[692] As with heart rate variability, the routine use of signal-averaged ECGs is not presently recommended.[15]

INVASIVE ELECTROPHYSIOLOGIC TESTING (PROGRAMMED ELECTRICAL STIMULATION) Invasive electrophysiologic assessment has been evaluated in two distinct populations who survived AMI. The first and relatively small group had a cardiac arrest or an episode of sustained VT following an AMI. In such patients, the risk of recurrent cardiac arrest or arrhythmic events is very high, and electrophysiologic studies are an alternative for assisting in the selection of therapy.[693]

The much larger patient population for whom electrophysiologic study has been considered consists of those identified as having an increased risk of arrhythmic death based upon the results of one or more noninvasive tests, as discussed previously. Performing electrophysiologic studies on all asymptomatic "high-risk" patients is not justified.[15] Reports on the utility of electrophysiologic studies have been inconsistent in predicting total mortality and are only slightly more consistent in identifying patients likely to have subsequent arrhythmic events.[694–699] Recent results from the Multicenter Automatic Defibrillation Implantation Trial (MADIT) are somewhat relevant to this issue.[700] Patients in MADIT had had a prior Q-wave infarction with a left ventricular ejection fraction of <35 percent and were selected if programmed electrical stimulation induced sustained VT that was nonsuppressible with intravenous procainamide. Patients were randomized to an implantable cardioverter-defibrillator group and/or conventional arrhythmic therapy. Although total mortality was less in the cardioverter-defibrillator group, the relevant point is that this invasive screening appeared to identify a high-risk group for subsequent arrhythmic death.[700] This study alone is not sufficient, however, to support the wider use of electrophysiologic testing in asymptomatic postinfarction patients.

ASSESSING ARRHYTHMIC DEATH: CONCLUSIONS In the recent guidelines provided by the ACC/AHA for the assessment of arrhythmic death, none of the noninvasive techniques is generally agreed upon to be beneficial, useful, and effective, either unequivocally (class I) or based upon the weight of evidence or opinion (class IIa). All of these techniques are classified as class IIb indications, meaning that their usefulness and efficacy is less well established by either scientific evidence and/or general opinion.[15] In addition to their poor positive predictive value, no clinical trial has demonstrated that the use of any one or a combination of these modalities of testing identifies a high risk population in whom intervention resulted in clinical benefit. Unless and until such studies are carried out to show that targeting a high-risk population and using the data to direct subsequent prophylactic therapy results in patient benefit, these modalities of risk assessment remain interesting tools for investigational studies and for use on selected individual patients. Other assessments of risk for sudden death, such as QT dispersion and baroreceptor sensitivity, are in an even earlier investigational stage, and at present, there is little supporting evidence that they are useful and effective in improving the management and outcome of post–myocardial infarction patients.[15,701–703]

Coronary Angiography and Percutaneous Transluminal Coronary Angioplasty

Recommendations[15]:

Class I

1. Patients with spontaneous episodes of myocardial ischemia or episodes of myocardial ischemia provoked by minimal exertion during recovery from infarction
2. Before definitive therapy of a mechanical complication of infarction such as acute mitral regurgitation, VSD, pseudoaneurysm, or LV aneurysm
3. Patients with persistent hemodynamic instability

Class IIa

1. When myocardial infarction is suspected to have occurred by a mechanism other than thrombotic occlusion at an atherosclerotic plaque. This would include coronary embolism, certain metabolic or hematologic diseases, or coronary artery spasm.
2. Survivors of AMI with depressed LV systolic function (LV ejection fraction less than or equal to 40 percent), CHF, prior revascularization, or malignant ventricular arrhythmias.
3. Survivors of AMI who had clinical heart failure during the acute episode but subsequently demonstrated well-preserved LV function.

Class IIb

1. Coronary angiography performed in all patients after infarction to find persistently occluded infarct-related arteries in an attempt to revascularize the artery or identify patients with three-vessel disease
2. All patients after a non-Q-wave myocardial infarction
3. Recurrent VT or VF or both, despite antiarrhythmic therapy, in patients without evidence of ongoing myocardial ischemia

Class III

1. Routine use of coronary angiography and subsequent PTCA of the infarct-related artery within days after thrombolytic therapy
2. Survivors of myocardial infarction who are thought not to be candidates for coronary revascularization

The selection of patients for cardiac catheterization and coronary angiographic studies prior to hospital discharge should be based on identifying patients at risk for ischemic events and on whether or not the information provided by cardiac catheterization and coronary angiography will change patient management.

Studies analyzing the prognostic utility of cardiac catheterization prior to hospital discharge are from the prethrombolytic era and demonstrate that the angiographic extent of coronary artery disease was related to survival.[704–706] Other trials have addressed the utility of routine coronary angiographic studies in patients who have received thrombolytic therapy.[707–712] The timing of cardiac catheterization during hospitalization has been addressed in several studies. *In general, studies that have compared acute or early cardiac catheterization to a more conservative approach of performing cardiac catheterization and coronary angiographic studies only for patients with spontaneous recurrent angina or exercise-induced ischemia have demonstrated no benefit to the strategy of routine catheterization.*[15,327]

Figure 47-12 presents a strategy for identifying symptomatic and asymptomatic high-risk patients who should have cardiac catheterization and coronary angiographic studies before discharge. Patients who have a complicated clinical course characterized by refractory cardiac failure, unstable angina, an episode of sustained VT, or cardiac arrest should be studied. An aggressive approach to these patients is justified because of the observed 1-year mortality rate, ranging from 10 to 25 percent.[236,713] In the case of patients with symptomatic cardiac failure, right heart catheterization should be included.

The recommended algorithm for selecting asymptomatic, uncomplicated post-AMI patients for cardiac catheterization is also presented in Fig. 47-12. Decision making focuses on the presence or absence of myocardial ischemia. Because of the high incidence of residual ischemia in patients with a non-Q-wave infarction, the task force for guidelines for coronary angiographic studies after myocardial infarction recommended such studies in all non-Q-wave infarctions.[714] The more conservative recommendation here emphasizes evidence of objective ischemia. Where patients have received thrombolytic therapy, it seems reasonable that those who have evidence of residual ischemia are still at increased risk of future ischemic events and should undergo coronary angiography prior to discharge. Consideration of PTCA following coronary angiographic studies should be based on established clinical and anatomic guidelines[15,715] (see Chap. 48). Coronary artery bypass surgery should be considered in those groups in whom it has been shown to be of proven benefit: patients with triple-vessel disease, patients with ischemia, and those with significant left ventricular dysfunction (see also Chap. 50).[716–718]

SECONDARY PREVENTION AND CARDIAC REHABILITATION

Risk Factor Reduction

The relationship between the level of activity of the inflammatory response in the arterial wall (which is the characteristic feature of atherosclerosis) and the tendency of the structural integrity of the artery to break down, with the resultant exposure of thrombogenic material and clot formation, is discussed in Chap. 44. The inflammatory response is caused and/or exacerbated by the presence of the classic risk factors. It follows that favorably modifying the risk factors would, intuitively, reduce coronary events. There is now abundant evidence that this is the case. Thus, since those who have had AMI are among those at highest risk for recurrence, management strategies to mitigate this risk are very important in patient management.[719]

SMOKING

Smoking has multiple cardiovascular effects that can promote AMI, including enhanced platelet aggregation, coronary vasospasm, and vascular inflammation. Smoking cessation is an essential goal after AMI, since the recurrence rate and death rate after AMI are doubled by the continuation of smoking.[720] After AMI, however, risk associated with smoking declines

rapidly to that of the nonsmoking cohort survivors within 3 years.[721] The psychological and physiologic aspects of smoking should be addressed, and a number of programs have been developed to deal with these needs. Most smokers who have quit, however, have done so without an organized program.[722] The role of the physician in motivating the patient to quit smoking is extremely important and the likelihood of success appears to be directly related to the extent of his or her involvement. Transdermal nicotine patches and oral preparations can be used to aid withdrawal but are not risk-free and should be used temporarily and adjunctively with physician counseling and/or a formal program in behavior modification.[723] The transdermal patches or oral nicotine preparations should not be used during the period just after AMI and should not be used concurrently with smoking. Difficult cases are probably handled best by referral to a formal smoking cessation program. Clonidine hydrochloride has also been used to ameliorate symptoms of smoking withdrawal as well as in conjunction with behavioral intervention.[719]

DYSLIPIDEMIA
Recommendations[15]:

Class I

1. Institute the American Heart Association (AHA) step II diet, which consists of less than 7 percent of total calories as saturated fat and of less than 200 mg/day of cholesterol in all patients after recovery from AMI.
2. Patients with low-density lipoprotein (LDL) cholesterol levels of greater than 125 mg/dL, despite consuming the AHA step II diet, should be placed on drug therapy with the goal of achieving a target LDL cholesterol of less than 100 mg/dL.
3. Patients with normal plasma cholesterol levels who have a high-density lipoprotein (HDL) of less than 35 mg/dL should be placed on a exercise regimen to atttempt to increase it.

Class IIa

1. Drug therapy may be added to diet therapy in patients with LDL cholesterol levels of less than 130 mg/dL but greater than 100 mg/dL after an appropriate trial of the AHA step II diet alone.
2. Patients with normal total cholesterol levels but with HDL cholesterol of less than 35 mg/dL despite dietary and other nonpharmacological therapy, may be started on drugs such as niacin in an attempt to raise HDL levels to more protective levels.

Class IIb

1. Drug therapy using either niacin or gemfibrozil may be added to diet regardless of LDL and HDL levels when triglyceride levels are greater than 400 mg/dL.

The β-hydroxy-β-methylglutaryl-CoA (HMG-CoA) reductase inhibitors are the most effective drugs in lowering LDL cholesterol. Niacin is effective in raising HDL and, in combination with resins, is also effective in lowering LDL. Triple therapy with a reductase inhibitor, niacin, and resin can be useful in resistant cases. Drug therapy of dyslipidemias is discussed in Chap. 53.

As mentioned above, patients who have had an AMI are generally at high risk for recurrence. Furthermore, an abnormally elevated serum cholesterol level is a powerful risk factor for death in this group.[724,725] Early primary prevention studies and relatively small angiographic trials showed decreases in cardiovascular event rates with cholesterol-lowering therapy (see Chaps. 41 and 53). Recent large secondary prevention trials have provided compelling evidence that in patients who have had an AMI, therapy with HMG-CoA reductase inhibitors to lower serum cholesterol levels that were either initially elevated—as in the Scandinavian Simvastatin Survival Study (4S)[726] or within "average" range as in the Cholesterol and Recurrent Events (CARE) trial[727]—was effective in reducing both cardiovascular and total mortality as well as cardiovascular events. In CARE, a treatment effect was not observed in the group with baseline LDL values of less than 125 mg/dL. The guidelines of the expert panel of the National Cholesterol Education Program provide target goals for patients with manifest coronary artery disease. These goals are as follows: LDL cholesterol, 100 mg/dL (2.59 mmol/L; HDL cholesterol, greater than 35 mg/dL (0.91 mmol/L).[728]

Serum lipid levels are decreased within several hours after AMI, presumably by the inflammatory response to tissue necrosis.[729] Evaluation of serum lipid levels should be made within the first 6 to 8 h from onset of symptoms or after recovery at 6 to 8 weeks. *All AMI patients should have serum lipids evaluated and treated intensively in order to achieve target goals.* Treatment should start in the hospital with initiation of the AHA step II diet. With established very high lipid levels (for example, LDL cholesterol > 200 mg/dL), many clinicians would have a low threshold for initiating drug therapy early on, anticipating that diet therapy alone might not be sufficient for achieving target LDL goals. Although low HDL is a powerful risk factor for AMI, the benefit of treating it is unproven. It seems prudent to attempt to raise HDL levels by prescribing an exercise regimen. Niacin is also efficacious in raising HDL levels; it may be used, especially if indicated as adjunctive therapy with HMG-CoA reductase inhibitors or with resins, to lower LDL. There is less certainty about indications for treating elevated triglycerides, but it seems prudent to treat levels of above 400 mg/dL with diet and perhaps with gemfibrozil or niacin (see Chap. 53).

INACTIVITY

There have been numerous studies of post-AMI patients documenting the beneficial effects of aerobic exercise on functional capacity and myocardial oxygen demand at a given submaximal workload.[730,731] Such exercise can decrease angina pecto-

ris and ischemia. Conversely, a sedentary lifestyle is a risk factor for coronary artery disease. Metaanalysis of cardiac rehabilitation studies has shown a reduction in mortality in the exercise group as opposed to a control group.[731] These analyses have not permitted separating the effects of exercise per se from the other beneficial aspects of the programs. *The greatest benefits of exercise are those observed with moderate, regular exercise as contrasted with the nonexercise group.* The benefit can be obtained by exercising about 4200 kJ a week, which can be achieved by walking about 1.5 m (2.4 km) per day. Long-term, regular exercise training can best be sustained by participating in a supervised exercise program beginning several weeks after discharge from the hospital.[719,731] A standard exercise program might involve three 20- to 30-min sessions three to four times per week at 60 to 75 percent of maximal aerobic capacity. This target activity level should be achieved progressively over several weeks, and progress should be monitored by the physician at regular intervals. The exercise regimen should be initiated and guided by monitored exercise testing.

Regular aerobic exercise should be prescribed for post-AMI patients in stable condition at an intensity, duration, and frequency as determined by formal testing and clinical judgment. Optimum benefit is achieved in a supervised program, although asymptomatic, stable patients can exercise without direct supervision but should receive regular monitoring by a physician (see also Chap. 55).

LOW ESTROGEN STATES (FEMALES)
Recommendations[15]:

Class IIa

1. All female post-AMI patients who are postmenopausal should be fully informed about the potential benefits of estrogen replacement therapy (ERT) and be offered the option of receiving ERT.

Estrogen replacement therapy and the primary or secondary prevention of cardiovascular disease continues to be a somewhat contentious and emotional issue that involves weighing the potential efficacy of ERT in reducing cardiovascular risk against the possible increases in breast cancer rates.[732,733] Clinical trials have demonstrated that estrogen with or without progestins lowers both LDL cholesterol and fibrinogen,[734] an effect that would be expected to reduce cardiovascular risk. Analysis of the somewhat limited available data has led to the conclusion that ERT did reduce mortality in women with significant coronary artery disease.[735] Thus, in this high-risk group, the beneficial effects on the cardiovascular system outweighed any adverse effect on the incidence of breast cancer over the time periods studied. A similar conclusion has been reached for the general postmenopausal female population using hypothetical decision analysis modeling.[736] Given the overall uncertainties involved, the decision must be a fully informed one based on patient preference.[15] Hormone replacement therapy should generally be managed in collaboration with a gynecologist or a generalist with special expertise in the area.

Drug Therapy

BETA-ADRENERGIC BLOCKERS

Recommendations for long-term therapy in post-AMI patients[15]:

Class I

1. All post-AMI patients except those at low risk without clear contraindications should receive long-term therapy. Treatment should begin early in the course, preferably acutely, and should be continued indefinitely.

Class IIa

1. Low-risk patients without definite contraindication should be considered for beta-adrenergic blocker therapy.

Class III

1. Patients with a contraindication to beta-blocker therapy.

The benefits of beta-blocker therapy given early in the course of AMI were discussed above. Multiple clinical trials have also demonstrated the benefits of long-term treatment of post-AMI patients with beta blockers.[737] Long-term efficacy has been demonstrated for propranolol,[11] timolol,[738] and metoprolol.[739] Mortality has been shown to be reduced by about 25 to 35 percent. The beneficial effect is highest in high-risk patients with large (usually anterior) myocardial infarction, and compensated left ventricular dysfunction. The beneficial effects in low-risk patients are less clear, but the consensus is that these patients should probably be treated because of the relatively favorable side-effect profile.[15] Beta blockers with intrinsic sympathomimetic activity should not be used in this context (see Chap. 54).

ASPIRIN

The role of aspirin during the early phases of AMI was discussed above. Aspirin use over the long term after AMI is also associated with a reduction in mortality. Metaanalysis of six major trials of aspirin treatment showed an overall reduction in vascular mortality in the treated group of 13 percent, with 31 and 42 percent reductions in nonfatal infarction and nonfatal stroke, respectively.[740] These trials used relatively large aspirin doses (300 to 1500 mg/day), but a relatively recent trial showed efficacy at only 75 mg/day,[741] suggesting that long-term use of more modest doses would be effective. Thus, aspirin at relatively low doses is recommended for all patients with AMI in the absence of contraindications (see also Chap. 52).

ANTICOAGULATION

Anticoagulation can reduce mortality, recurrent myocardial infarction, and stroke after AMI, as indicated by an analysis of multiple trials.[737] Because of relatively high rates of bleeding with warfarin, the need for monitoring, and, in particular, the efficacy and low risk of aspirin, the role of warfarin is rather limited to those at increased risk for developing mural thrombi.[719] In addition, those post-AMI patients with demonstrable left ventricular thrombus and atrial fibrillation should be anticoagulated. The duration of anticoagulation should be limited to 3 months in the case of left ventricular thrombus (see also Chap. 52).

ANGIOTENSIN-CONVERTING ENZYME INHIBITORS

The ACE inhibitors and recommendations for their use early in the course of AMI were discussed above. Recent studies have documented their efficacy in secondary prevention. The reduction in late morbidity and mortality was most obvious in those with large infarctions with reduced ejection fraction and in those with anterior myocardial infarction. In these patients, left ventricular remodeling and progression to heart failure were reduced.[444,660,742] The beneficial effects of ACE inhibitors have been less obvious when low-risk patients were included.[743] The decrease in ischemic events in the SAVE trial[660] and in other ACE-inhibitor trials suggests that the threshold for use of ACE inhibitors for long-term therapy may be lowered by many clinicians to include those with only modest left ventricular dysfunction. Thus, ACE inhibitors are recommended for chronic use after AMI in those patients with significant left ventricular dysfunction, and their use should be considered in those with only mild to moderate left ventricular dysfunction (ejection fraction less than 45 percent).

Modification of Lifestyle and Cardiac Rehabilitation after Acute Myocardial Infarction

Because of the relatively high risk of recurrence and the need for lifelong modification of lifestyles and risk factors, most post-AMI patients should be enrolled in a cardiac rehabilitation program that emphasizes dietary modification, risk factor reduction, and exercise. The low-risk patient does not require prolonged supervised exercise, as previously discussed. All patients, however, can benefit from a structured environment to launch a lifetime of healthy living. Cardiac rehabilitation is discussed in Chap. 55 and risk factors and the prevention of coronary artery disease are discussed in Chap. 41.

REFERENCES

1. Osler W. *The Principles and Practice of Medicine*. New York: Appleton; 1892.
2. Herrick JB. Clinical features of sudden obstruction of the coronary arteries. *JAMA* 1912; 59:2015.
3. Roberts WC, Buja LM. The frequency and significance of coronary arterial thrombi and other observations in fatal acute myocardial infarction. *Am J Med* 1972; 52:425–443.

4. Rentrop KP, Blanke H, Karsch KR, Kreuzer H. Coronary angiographic findings and left ventricular pump function in acute infarction and changes in chronic stage infarction. *Z Kardiol* 1979; 68:335–350.

5. DeWood MA, Spores J, Notske R, Mouser LT, Burroughs R, Golden MS, et al. Prevalence of total coronary occlusion during the early hours of transmural myocardial infarction. *N Engl J Med* 1980; 303:897–902.

6. Bristow JD, Burchell HB, Campbell RW, Ebert PA, Hall RJ, Leonard JJ, et al. Report of the ad hoc committee on the indications for coronary arteriography. *Circulation* 1977; 55:969A–974A.

7. Rentrop KP, Blanke H, Karsch KR, Wiegand V, Kostering H, Oster H. Acute myocardial infarction: intracoronary application of nitroglycerin and streptokinase. *Clin Cardiol* 1979; 2:354–363.

8. European Cooperative Study Group for Streptokinase Treatment in Acute Myocardial Infarction. Streptokinase in acute myocardial infarction. *N Engl J Med* 1979; 301:797–802.

9. Mathey DG, Kuck K-H, Tilsner V, Krebber H-J, Bleifeld W. Nonsurgical coronary artery recanalization in acute transmural myocardial infarction. *Circulation* 1981; 63:489–497.

10. Stampfer MJ, Goldhaber SZ, Yusuf S, Peto R, Hennekens CH. Effect of intravenous streptokinase on acute myocardial infarction: pooled results from randomized trials. *N Engl J Med* 1982; 307:1180–1182.

11. Beta-Blocker Heart Attack Study Group: The beta-blocker heart attack trial. *JAMA* 1981; 246:2073–2084.

12. Gruppo Italiano per lo Studio della Streptochinasi nell'Infarto Miocardico (GISSI). Effectiveness of intravenous thrombolytic treatment in acute myocardial infarction. *Lancet* 1986; 1:397–402.

13. The GUSTO Investigators. An International randomized trial comparing four thrombolytic strategies for acute myocardial infarction. *N Engl J Med* 1993; 329:673–682.

14. Gunnar RM, Passmani ER, Bourdillon PD, Pitt B, Dixon DW, Rapoport E, et al. Guidelines for the early management of patients with acute myocardial infarction. *J Am Coll Cardiol* 1990; 16:249–292.

15. Ryan TJ, Anderson JL, Antman EM, Braniff BA, Brooks NH, Califf RM, et al. ACC/AHA guidelines for the management of patients with acute myocardial infarction: A report of the American College of Cardiology/American Heart Association Task Force on Practice Guidelines (Committee on Management of Acute Myocardial Infarction). *J Am Coll Cardiol* 1996; 28:1328–1428.

16. Herlitz J, Blohm M, Hartford M, Hjalmarsson A, Holmberg S, Karlson BW. Delay time in suspected acute myocardial infarction and the importance of its modification. *Clin Cardiol* 1989; 12:370–374.

17. National Heart, Lung, and Blood Institute. Morbidity and Mortality. Chartbook on Cardiovascular, Lung, and Blood Diseases. Bethesda, MD: U.S. Department of Health and Human Services, Public Health Service, National Institutes of Health; May 1992.

18. Galis ZS, Sukhova GK, Lark MW, Libby P. Increased expression of matrix metalloproteinases and matrix degrading activity in vulnerable regions of human atherosclerotic plaques. *J Clin Invest* 1994; 94:2493–2503.

19. Friesinger GG. The natural history of atherosclerotic coronary heart disease. In: Schlant RC, Alexander RW, eds. *The Heart*, 8th ed. New York: McGraw-Hill; 1994:1185–1204.

20. van der Wal AC, Becker AE, van der Loos CM, Das PK. Site of intimal rupture or erosion of thrombosed coronary atherosclerotic plaques is characterized by an inflammatory process irrespective of the dominant plaque morphology. *Circulation* 1994; 89:36–44.

21. Mounsey P. Prodromal symptoms in myocardial infarction. *Br Heart J* 1951; 215–216.

22. Berk BC, Weintraub WS, Alexander RW. Elevation of C-reactive protein in "active" coronary artery disease. *Am J Cardiol* 1990; 65:168–172.

23. Liuzzo G, Biasucci LM, Gallimore JR, Grillo L, Rebuzzi AG, Pepys MB, et al. The prognostic value of C-reactive protein and serum amyloid a protein in severe unstable angina. *N Engl J Med* 1994; 331:417–424.

24. Ridker PM, Cushman M, Stampfer MJ, Tracy RP, Hennekens CH. Inflammation, aspirin, and the risk of cardiovascular disease in apparently healthy men. *N Engl J Med* 1997; 336:973–979.

25. Spodick DH, Flessas AP, Johnson MM. Association of acute respiratory symptoms with onset of acute myocardial infarction: Prospective investigation of 150 consecutive patients and matched controls. *Am J Cardiol* 1984; 53:481–482.

26. Saikku P. *Chlamydia pneumoniae* infection as a risk factor in acute myocardial infarction. *Eur Heart J* 1993; 14(suppl K):62–65.

27. Miettinen H, Lehto S, Saikku P, Haffner SM, Ronnemaa T, Pyorala K, et al. Association of *Chlamydia pneumoniae* and acute coronary heart disease events in non-insulin-dependent diabetic and non-diabetic subjects in Finland. *Eur Heart J* 1996; 17:682–688.

28. Patel P, Mendall MA, Carrington D, Strachan DP, Leatham E, Molineaux N, et al. Association of *Helicobacter pylori* and *Chlamydia pneumoniae* infections with coronary heart disease and cardiovascular risk factors. *Br Med J* 1995; 311:711–714.

29. Jackson LA, Campbell LA, Schmidt RA, Kuo CC, Cappuccio AL, Lee MJ, et al. Specificity of detection of *Chlamydia pneumoniae* in cardiovascular atheroma: Evaluation of the innocent bystander hypothesis. *Am J Pathol* 1997; 150:1785–1790.

30. Willich SN, Lewis M, Lowel H, Arntz HR, Schubert F, Schroder R. Physical exertion as a trigger of acute myocardial infarction: Triggers and mechanisms of myocardial infarction study group. *N Engl J Med* 1993; 329:1684–1690.

31. Mittleman MA, Maclure M, Tofler GH, Sherwood JB, Goldberg RJ, Muller JE. Triggering of acute myocardial infarction by heavy physical exertion: Protection against triggering by regular exertion. Determinants of Myocardial Infarction Onset Study Investigators. *N Engl J Med* 1993; 329:1677–1683.

32. Mittleman MA, Maclure M, Sherwood JB, Mulry RP, Tofler GH, Jacobs SC, et al. Triggering of acute myocardial infarction onset by episodes of anger. Determinants of Myocardial Infarction Onset Study Investigators. *Circulation* 1995; 92:1720–1725.

33. Rahe RH, Romo M, Siltanen P. Recent life changes, myocardial infarction, and abrupt coronary death. *Arch Intern Med* 1974; 133:221–228.

34. Lundberg U, Theorell T, Linda E. Life Changes and myocardial infarction: Individual differences in life changes scaling. *J Psychosom Res* 1975; 37:27–32.

35. Jenkins CD. Recent evidence supporting psychologic and social risk factors for coronary disease. *N Engl J Med* 1976; 294:1033–1038.

36. Mangano DT. Perioperative cardiac morbidity. *Anesthesiology* 1990; 72:153–184.

37. Leiberman RW, Orkin KF, Jobes DR, Schwartz AJ. Hemodynamic predictors of myocardial ischemia during halothane anesthesia for coronary artery revascularization. *Anesthesiology* 1983; 59:36–41.

38. Nelson AH, Fliesher LA, Rosenbaum SH. The relationship between postoperative anemia and cardiac morbidity in high risk vascular patients in the ICU. *Crit Care Med* 1993; 21:860–866.

39. Frank SM, Beattie C, Christopherson R, Norris EJ, Perler BA, Williams GM, et al. Unintentional hypothermia is associated with post-operative myocardial ischemia. *Anesthesiology* 1993; 78:468–476.

40. Frank SM, Fleisher LA, Breslow MD, Higgins MS, Olson KF, Kelly S, et al. Perioperative maintenance of normothermia reduces the incidence of morbid cardiac events: A randomized clinical trial. *JAMA* 1997; 277:1127–1134.

41. Zainea M, Duvernoy WF, Chauhan A, David S, Soto E, Small D. Acute myocardial infarction in angiographically normal coronary arteries following induction of general anesthesia. *Arch Intern Med* 1994; 154:2495–2498.

42. Moliterno DJ, Willard JE, Lange RA, Negus BH, Boehrer JD, Glamann DB, et al. Coronary-artery vasoconstriction induced by cocaine, cigarette smoking, or both. *N Engl J Med* 1994; 330:454–459.

43. Friedman M, Rosenman RH. Type A behavior pattern: Its association with coronary heart disease. *Ann Clin Res* 1971; 3:300–312.

44. Dimsdale JE. A perspective on type A behavior and coronary disease. *N Engl J Med* 1988; 318:110–112.

45. Muller JE, Stone PH, Turzi ZG, Rutherford JD, Czeisler C, Parker C, et al. Circadian variation in the frequency of onset of acute myocardial infarction. *N Engl J Med* 1985; 313:1315–1322.

46. Mitler MM, Kripke DF. Circadian variation in myocardial infarction. *N Engl J Med* 1986; 314:1187–1188.

47. Petralito A, Mangiafico RA, Giblino S, Cuffari MA, Miano MF, Piore CE. Daily modifications of plasma fibrinogen, platelet aggregation, Howell's time, PTT, PT, and antithrombin III in normal subjects and in patients with vascular disease. *Chronobiologia* 1982; 9:195–201.

48. Rosing DR, Brakma P, Redwood DR, Goldstein RE, Beiser GD, Astrup T, et al. Blood fibrinolytic activity in man: Diurnal variation and the response to varying intensities of exercise. *Circ Res* 1970; 27:171–184.

49. Marshall J. Diurnal variation in occurrence of strokes. *Stroke* 1977; 8:230–231.

50. Sayer JW, Wilkinson P, Ranjadayalan K, Ray S, Marchant B, Timmis AD. Attenuation or absence of circadian and seasonal rhythms of acute myocardial infarction. *Heart* 1997; 77:325–329.

51. Quyyumi AA, Mockus L, Wright, Fox KM. Morphology of ambulatory ST segment changes in patients with varying severity of coronary artery disease: Investigation of the frequency of nocturnal ischemia and coronary spasm. *Br Heart J* 1985; 53:186–193.

52. el-Tamimi H, Mansour M, Pepine CJ, Wargovich TJ, Chen H. Circadian variation in coronary tone in patients with stable angina: Protective role of the endothelium. *Circulation* 1995; 92:3201–3205.

53. Millar-Craig MW, Bishop CN, Raftery EB. Circadian variation of blood pressure. *Lancet* 1978; 1:795–797.

54. Turton MB, Deegan T. Circadian variations of plasma catecholamine, cortisol, and immunoreactive insulin concentrations in supine subjects. *Clin Chim Acta* 1974; 55:389–397.

55. Willich SN, Lowel H, Lewis M, Hormann A, Arntz HR, Keil U. Weekly variation of acute myocardial infarction: Increased Monday risk in the working population. *Circulation* 1994; 90:87–93.

56. Spielberg C, Falkenhahn D, Willich SN, Wegscheider K, Voller H. Circadian, day-of-week, and seasonal variability in myocardial infarction: Comparison between working and retired patients. *Am Heart J* 1996; 132:579–585.

57. Hofgren C, Karlson BW, Herlitz J. Prodromal symptoms in subsets of patients hospitalized for suspected acute myocardial infarction. *Heart Lung* 1995; 24:3–10.

58. Gill JB, Cairns JA, Roberts RS, Costantini L, Sealey BJ, Fallen EF, et al. Prognostic importance of myocardial ischemia detected by ambulatory monitoring early after acute myocardial infarction. *N Engl J Med* 1996; 334:65–70.

59. Maseri A, Crea F, Kaski JC, Davies G. Mechanisms and significance of cardiac ischemic pain. *Prog Cardiovasc Dis* 1992; 35:1–18.

60. Maseri A. The changing face of angina pectoris: Practical implications. *Lancet* 1983; 1:746–749.

61. Everts B, Karlson BW, Wahrborg P, Hedner T, Herlitz J. Localization of pain in suspected acute myocardial infarction in relation to final diagnosis, age and sex, and site and type of infarction in relation to final diagnosis, age and sex, and site and type of infarction. *Heart Lung* 1996; 25:430–437.

62. Herlitz J, Bang A, Isaksson L, Karlsson T. Ambulance dispatchers' estimation of intensity of pain and presence of associated symptoms in relation to outcome in patients who call for an ambulance because of acute chest pain. *Eur Heart J* 1995; 16:1789–1794.

63. Margolis JR, Kannel WB, Feinleich M, Dawber TR, McNamara PM. Clinical features of unrecognized myocardial infarction—silent and symptomatic. *Am J Cardiol* 1973; 32:1–7.

64. Bean, WB. Masquerades of myocardial infarction. *Lancet* 1977; 1:1044–1045.

65. Madias JE, Chintalapaly G, Choudry M, Chalavarya G, Kegan M. Correlates and in-hospital outcome of painless presentation of acute myocardial infarction: A prospective study of a consecutive series of patients admitted to the coronary care unit. *J Invest Med* 1995; 43:567–574.

66. Jaffe AS, Roberts R. Precordial inspection and palpation in patients with acute myocardial infarction. *Pract Cardiol* 1981; 7:46–50.

67. Fowler NO. Physical signs in acute myocardial infarction and its complications. *Prog Cardiovasc Dis* 1968; 10:287–297.

68. Harvey WP. Some pertinent physical findings in the clinical evaluation of acute myocardial infarction. *Circulation* 1969; 40:170.

69. Lee TH, Weisberg MC, Brand DA, Rouan GW, Goldman L. Candidates for thrombolysis among emergency room patients with acute chest pain. *Ann Intern Med* 1989; 110:957–962.

70. Goldman L, Cook EF, Brand DA, Lee TH, Rouan GW, Weisberg MC, et al. A computer protocol to predict myocardial infarction in emergency department patients with chest pain. *N Engl J Med* 1988; 318:797–803.

71. Lee TH, Rouan GW, Weisberg MC, Brand DA, Cook EF, Acampora D, et al. Sensitivity of routine clinical criteria for diagnosing myocardial infarction within 24 hours of hospitalization. *Ann Intern Med* 1987; 106:181–186.

72. Lee TH, Juarez G, Cook EF, Weisberg MC, Rouan GW, Brand DA, et al. Ruling out acute myocardial infarction. *N Engl J Med* 1991; 324:1239–1246.

73. Roberts R. The two out of three criteria for the diagnosis of infarction—Is it passe? *Chest* 1984; 86:511–513.

74. Parker AB III, Waller BF, Gering LE. Usefulness of the 12-lead electrocardiogram in detection of myocardial infarction: Electrocardiographic-anatomic correlations—Part I. *Clin Cardiol* 1996; 19:55–61.

75. Cook RW, Edwards JE, Pruitt RD. Electrocardiographic changes in acute subendocardial infarction: I. Large subendocardial and large transmural infarcts. *Circulation* 1958; 18:603.

76. Gunnar RM, Pietras RJ, Blackaller J, Dadmun SE, Szanto PB, Tobin JR Jr. Correlation of vectocardiographic criteria for myocardial infarction with autopsy findings. *Circulation* 1967; 35:158–171.

77. Ambos HD, Moore P, Roberts R. A database for analysis of patient diagnostic data. In: *Computers in Cardiology*. Long Beach, CA: IEEE Computer Society; 1978.

78. Gibson RS, Boden WE, Therous P, Strauss HD, Pratt CM, Cheorghiade M, et al. Diltiazem and reinfarction in patients with non-Q-wave myocardial infarction: Results of a double-blind, randomized, multicenter trial, *N Engl J Med* 1986; 315:423–429.

79. Pratt CM, Roberts R. Non-Q-wave myocardial infarction: Recognition, pathogenesis, prognosis and management. In: McIntosh HD, ed: *Baylor Cardiology Series*, 8th ed. Houston: Baylor College of Medicine; 1985:5–19.

80. Bodenheimer MM, Banka VS, Trout RG, Hermann GA, Pasdar H, Helfant RH. Relationship between myocardial fibrosis and epicardial and surface electrocardiographic Q-waves in man. *J Electrocardiol* 1979; 12:205–210.

81. Wilson FN, Johnston FD, Hill IGW. The form of the electrocardiogram in experimental myocardial infarction: IV. Additional observations with later effects produced by ligation of the anterior descending branch on the left coronary artery. *Am Heart J* 1935; 10:1025.

82. Spodick DH. Q-wave infarction versus S-T infarction: Nonspecificity of electrocardiographic criteria for differentiating transmural and nontransmural lesions. *Am J Cardiol* 1983; 51:913–915.

83. Roberts R. Nontransmural myocardial infarction. *Newsletter of the Council on Clinical Cardiology, American Heart Association* 1985; 11:1–17.

84. Eaton LW, Bulkley HG. Extension of acute myocardial infarction: Its relationship to infarct morphology in a canine model. *Circ Res* 1981; 49:80–88.

85. Marmor A, Sobel BE, Roberts R. Factors presaging early recurrent myocardial infarction ("extension"). *Am J Cardiol* 1981; 48:603–610.

86. Gibson RS. Non-Q-wave myocardial infarction diagnosis, prognosis and management. *Curr Probl Cardiol* 1988; 13:9–72.

87. Marmor A, Geltman EM, Schechtman K, Soble BE, Roberts R. Recurrent myocardial infarction: Clinical predictors and prognostic implications. *Circulation* 1982; 66:415–421.

88. Schaer DH, Ross AM, Wasserman AG. Reinfarction, recurrent angina and reocclusion after thrombolytic therapy. *Circulation* 1987; 76:II-57.

89. Sgarbossa EB, Pinski SL, Barbagelata A, Underwood DA, Gates KB, Topol EJ, et al. Electrocardiographic diagnosis of evolving acute myocardial infarction in the presence of left bundle branch block. *N Engl J Med* 1996; 334:481–487.

90. Helfant RH, Banka VS, eds. *A Clinical and Angiographic Approach to Coronary Heart Disease*. Philadelphia: Davis; 1978.

91. Fenichel NM, Kugell VH. The large Q wave of the electrocardiogram: A correlation with pathologic observations. *Am Heart J* 1931; 7:235.

92. Rude RE, Poole WK, Muller JE, Turi Z, Rutherford J, Parker C, et al. Electrocardiographic and clinical criteria for recognition of acute myocardial infarction based on analysis of 3697 patients. *Am J Cardiol* 1983; 52:936–942.

93. Bodenheimer MM, Banka VS, Helfant RH. Q-waves and ventricular asynergy: Predictive value and hemodynamic significance of anatomic localization. *Am J Cardiol* 1975; 35:615–618.

94. Schamroth L. Posterior wall myocardial infarction. In: *The 12-Lead Electrocardiogram*. Book 1. Boston: Blackwell; 1989.

95. Geft IL, Shah PK, Rodriguez L, Hulse S, Maddahi J, Berman DS, et al. ST elevations in leads V_1 to V_5 may be caused by right coronary artery occlusion and acute right ventricular infarction. *Am J Cardiol* 1984; 53:991–996.

96. Lopez-Sendon J, Coma-Canella I, Alcasena S, Seoane J, Gamallo C. Electrocardiographic findings in acute right ventricular infarction: Sensitivity and specificity of electrocardiographic alterations in right precordial leads V_{4R}, V_{3R}, V_1, V_2, and V_3. *J Am Coll Cardiol* 1985: 6:1273–1279.

97. Erhardt LR, Sjogren A, Wahlberg I. Single right-sided precordial lead in the diagnosis of right ventricular involvement in inferior myocardial infarction. *Am Heart J* 1976; 91:571–576.

98. Sivertssen E, Hoel B, Bay G, Jorgensen L. Electrocardiographic atrial complex and acute atrial myocardial infarction. *Am J Cardiol* 1973; 31:450–456.

99. Schuster EH, Bulkley BH. Early post-infarction angina: Ischemia at a distance and ischemia in the infarct zone. *N Engl J Med* 1981; 305:1101–1105.

100. Ferguson DW, Pandian N, Kioschos JM, Marcus ML, White CW. Angiographic evidence that reciprocal ST-segment depression during acute myocardial infarction does not indicate remote ischemia: Analysis of 23 patients. *Am J Cardiol* 1984; 53:55–62.

101. Mirvis DM. Physiologic bases for anterior ST segment depression in patients with acute inferior wall myocardial infarction. *Am Heart J* 1988; 116:1308–1322.

102. Muller DWM, Topol EJ, Califf RM, Sigmon KN, Gorman L, George BS, et al. Relationship between antecedent angina pectoris and short-term prognosis after thrombolytic therapy for acute myocardial infarction. *Am Heart J* 1990; 119:224–231.

103. Roberts R, Gowda KS, Ludbrook PA, Sobel BE. Specificity of elevated serum MB CPK activity in the diagnosis of acute myocardial infarction. *Am J Cardiol* 1975; 36:433–437.

104. Lee TH, Goldman L. Serum enzyme assays in the diagnosis of acute myocardial infarction. *Ann Intern Med* 1986; 105:221–233.

105. Grande P, Christiansen C, Pedersen A, Christensen MS. Optimal diagnosis in acute myocardial infarction: A cost effectiveness study. *Circulation* 1980; 61:723–728.

106. Klein MS, Shell WE, Sobel BE. Serum creatine phosphokinase (CPK) isoenzymes after intramuscular injections, surgery, and myocardial infarction: Experimental and clinical studies. *Cardiovasc Res* 1973; 7:412–418.

107. Dawwon DM, Epenberger HM, Kaplan NO. Creatine kinase: Evidence for the dimeric structure. *Biochem Biophys Res Commun* 1965; 21:346.

108. Perryman MB, Kerner SA, Bohlmeyer TJ, Roberts R. Isolation and sequence analysis of a full-length cDNA for human M creatine kinase. *Biochem Biophys Res Commun* 1986; 140:981–989.

109. Villarreal-Levy G, Ma TS, Kerner SA, Roberts R, Perryman MB. Human creatine kinase: Isolation and sequence analysis of cDNA clones for the B subunit, development of subunit specific probes and determination of gene copy number. *Biochem Biophys Res Commun* 1987; 144:1116–1127.

110. Turner DC, Wallimann T, Eppenberger HM. A protein that binds specifically to the M-line of skeletal muscle is identifed as the muscle form of creatine kinase. *Proc Natl Acad Sci USA* 1973; 70:702–705.

111. Wallimann T, Kuhn HJ, Pelloni G, Turner DC, Eppenberger HM. Localization of creatine kinase isoenzymes in myofibrils: II. Chicken heart muscle. *J Cell Biol* 1977; 75:318–325.

112. Tsung JS, Tsung SS. Creatine kinase isoenzymes in extracts of various human skeletal muscles. *Clin Chem* 1986; 32:1568–1570.

113. Wilhelm AH, Albers KM, Toss JK. Creatine phosphokinase isoenzyme distribution in human skeletal and heart muscles. *IRCS Med Sci* 1976; 4:418.

114. Yasmineh WG, Ibrahim GA, Abbasnezhad MA, Awad EA. Isoenzyme distribution of creatine kinase and lactate dehydrogenase in serum and skeletal muscle in Duchenne muscular dystrophy, collagen disease, and other muscular disorders. *Clin Chem* 1978; 24:1985–1989.

115. Roberts R, Henry PD, Witteveen SAGJ, Sobel BE. Quantification of serum creatine phosphokinase (CPK) isoenzyme activity. *Am J Cardiol* 1974; 33:650–654.

116. Apple FS, Rogers MA, Sherman WM, Costill DL, Hagerman FC, Ivy JL. Profile of creatine kinase isoenzymes in skeletal muscles of marathon runners. *Clin Chem* 1984; 30:413–416.

117. Siegel AJ, Silverman LM, Evans WJ. Elevated skeletal muscle creatine kinase MB isoenzyme levels in marathon runners. *JAMA* 1983; 250:2835–2837.

118. Keshgegian AA, Feiberg NW. Serum creatine kinase MB isoenzyme in chronic muscle disease. *Clin Chem* 1984; 30:575–578.

119. Shahangian S, Ash KO, Wahlstrom NO Jr, Warden GD, Saffle JR, Taylor AA, et al. Creatine kinase and lactate dehydrogenase isoenzymes in serum of patients suffering burns, blunt trauma, or myocardial infarction. *Clin Chem* 1984; 30:1332–1338.

120. McBride JW, Labrosse KR, McCoy HG, Ahrenholz DH, Solem LD, Goldenberg IF. Is serum creakine kinase MB in electrically injured patients predictive of myocardial injury? *JAMA* 1986; 255:764–768.

121. Foxall CD, Emery AE. Changes in creatine kinase and its isoenzymes in human fetal muscle during development. *J Neurol Sci* 1975; 24:483–492.

122. Tzvetanova E. Creatine kinase isoenzymes in muscle tissue of patients with neuromuscular diseases and human fetuses. *Enzyme* 1971; 12:279.

123. Sadeh M, Stern LZ, Czyzewski K, Finley PR, Russell DH. Alterations of creatine kinase, ornithine decarboxylase, and transglutaminase during muscle regeneration. *Life Sci* 1984; 34:483–488.

124. Yasmineh WG, Pyle PB, Nicoloff DM. Rate of decay and distribution volume of MB isoenzyme of creatine kinase, intravenously injected into the baboon. *Clin Chem* 1976; 22:1095–1097.

125. Roberts R. Myoglobinemia as an index to myocardial infarction. *Ann Intern Med* 1977; 87:788–789.

126. de Winter RJ, Koster RW, Sturk A, Sanders GT. Value of myoglobin, troponin T, and CK-MB mass in ruling out an acute myocardial infarction in the emergency room. *Circulation* 1995; 92:3401–3407.

127. Adams JE, Bodor GS, Davila-Roman VG, Delmez JA, Apple FS, Ladenson JH, et al. Cardiac troponin I. A marker with high specificity for cardiac injury. *Circulation* 1993; 88:101–106.

128. Bucher EA, Maisonpierre PC, Konieczay SF, Emerson CP Jr. Expression of the troponin complex genes: Transcriptional coactivation during myoblasts differentiation and independent control in heart and skeletal muscles. *Mol Cell Biol* 1988; 8:4134–4142.

129. Wilkinson JM, Grand RJA. Comparison of amino acid sequence of troponin I from different striated muscles. *Nature* 1978; 271:31–35.

130. Bodor GS, Porterfield D, Voss EM, Smith S, Apple FS. Cardiac troponin I is not expressed in fetal and healthy or diseased adult human skeletal muscle tissue. *Clin Chem* 1995; 41:1710–1715.

131. Greaser ML, Gergeley J. Purification and properties of components from troponin. *J Biol Chem* 1973; 248:2125–2133.

132. Staprans I, Takahashi H, Russel MP, Watanabe S. Skeletal and cardiac troponin and their components. *Biochem J* 1972; 72:723–735.

133. Toyota N, Shimada Y. Differentiation of troponin in cardiac and skeletal muscles in chicken embryos as studies by immunofluorescence microscopy. *J Cell Biol* 1981; 91:497–504.

134. Saggin L, Gorza L, Ausoni S, Schiaffino S. Cardiac troponin T in developing, regenerating, and denervated rat skeletal muscle. *Development* 1990; 110:547–554.

135. Kobayashi S, Tanaka M, Tamura N, Hashimoto H, Hirose S. Serum cardiac tropnin T in polymyositis/dermatomyositis. *Lancet* 1992; 340:726.

136. Anderson PAW, Malouf NN, Oakeley AE, Pagani ED, Allen PD. Troponin T isoform expression in humans: A comparison among normal and failing adult heart, fetal heart, and adult and fetal skeletal muscle. *Circulation* 1991; 69:1226–1233.

137. Roberts R. Enzymatic diagnosis of acute myocardial infarction. *Chest* 1988; 93:3S–6S.

138. Bodor GS. Cardiac troponin I: A highly specific biochemical marker for myocardial infarction. *J Immunoassay* 1994; 17:40–44.

139. Selker HP. Coronary care unit triage decision aids: How do we know when they work? *Am J Med* 1989; 87:491–493.

140. Roberts R, From R, Beaudreaux A, Zimmerman J, Meyer D, Wun C, et al. Multicenter blinded trial utilizing multiple diagnostic markers to exclude myocardial infarction in patients presenting consecutively to the ER with chest pain (abstr). *Circulation* 1996; 94:I–322.

141. *Diagnostis Regional Groupings Handbook*. Washington, DC: HCIA; 1993.

142. Guadagnoli E, Hauptman PJ, Ayanian JZ, Pashos CL, McNeil BJ, Cleary PD. Variation in the use of cardiac procedures after acute myocardial infarction. *N Engl J Med* 1995; 333:573–578.

143. Wevers RA, Delsing M, Klein-Gebbink JA, Soons JB. Post-synthetic changes in creatine kinase isoenzymes. *Clin Chim Acta* 1978; 86:323–327.

144. George S, Ishikawa Y, Perryman MB, Roberts R. Purification and characterization of naturally occurring and in vitro induced multiple forms of MM creatine kinase. *J Biol Chem* 1984; 259:2667–2674.

145. Perryman MB, Knell JD, Roberts R. Carboxypeptidase-catalyzed hydrolysis of Cxterminal lysine: Mechanism for in vivo production of multiple forms of creatine kinase in plasma. *Clin Chem* 1984; 30:662–664.

146. Puleo PR, Guadagno PA, Roberts R, Perryman MB. Sensitive, rapid assay of subforms of creatine kinase MB in plasma. *Clin Chem* 1989; 35:1452–1455.

147. Puleo PR, Meyer D, Wathen C, Tawa CB, Wheeler SH, Hamburg RJ, et al. Use of rapid assay of subforms of creatine kinase MB to diagnose

or rule out acute myocardial infarction. *N Engl J Med* 1994; 331:561–566.

148. Puleo PR, Guadagno PA, Roberts R, Scheel MV, Marian AJ, Churchill D, et al. Early diagnosis of acute myocardial infarction based on assay for subforms of creatine kinase-MB. *Circulation* 1990; 82:759–764.

149. Muller JE, Morrison J, Stone PH, Rude RE, Rosner B, Roberts R, et al. Nifedipine therapy for patients with threatened and acute myocardial infarction: A randomized, double-blind, placebo-controlled comparison. *Circulation* 1984; 69:740–747.

150. MILIS Study Group, eds. *National Heart, Lung, and Blood Institute Multicenter Investigation of the Limitation of Infarct Size (MILIS): Design and Methods of the Clinical Trial. An Investigation of Beta-Blockade and Hyaluronidase for Treatment of Acute Myocardial Infarction.* Monograph 100. Dallas: American Heart Association; 1984.

151. Somer H, Dubowitz V, Donner M. Creatine kinase isoenzymes in neuromuscular diseases. *J Neurol Sci* 1976; 29:129–136.

152. Karmen A, Wroblewski F, LaDu. Transaminase activity in human blood. *J Clin Invest* 1954; 34:126.

153. Apple FS, Greenspan NS, Dietzler DN. Elevation of creatine kinase in BB-CK in hospitalized patients. *Ann Clin Lab Sci* 1982; 12:398–402.

154. Kimler SC, Sandhu RS. Circulating CK-MB and CK-BB isoenzymes after prostate resection. *Clin Chem* 1980; 26:55–59.

155. Tsung SH. Several conditions causing elevation of serum CK-MB and CK-BB. *Am J Clin Pathol* 1981; 75:711–715.

156. Laboda HM, Britton VJ. Creatine kinase isoenzyme activity in human placenta and in the serum of women in labor. *Clin Chem* 1977; 23:1329–1332.

157. Somer H, Kaste M, Troupp H, Konttinen A. Brain creatine kinase in blood after acute brain injury. *J Neurol Neurosurg Psychiatry* 1975; 38:572–576.

158. Kaste M, Some K. Brain-type creatine kinase isoenzyme. *Arch Neurol* 1977; 34:142–144.

159. Tsung SH. Creatine kinase activity and isoenzyme pattern in various normal tissues and neoplasms. *Clin Chem* 1983; 29:2040–2043.

160. Goldman J, Matz R, Mortimer R, Freeman R. High elevations of creatine phosphokinase in hypothyroidism: An isoenzyme analysis. *JAMA* 1977; 238:325–326.

161. Urdal P, Landaas S. Macro creatine kinase BB in serum, and some data on its prevalence. *Clin Chem* 1979; 25:461–465.

162. Jaffe AS, Ritter C, Meltzer V, Harter H, Roberts R. Unmasking artifactual increases in creatine kinase isoenzymes in patients with renal failure. *J Lab Clin Med* 1984; 104:193–202.

163. Cummins B, Auckland M, Cummins P. Cardiac-specific troponin I radioimmunoassay in the diagnosis of acute myocardial infarction. *Am Heart J* 1987; 113:1333–1344.

164. Cummings P, Young A, Auckland ML, Michie CA, Stone PCW, Shepstone BJ. Comparison of serum cardiac specific troponin I with creatine kinase, creatine kinase-MB isoenzyme, tropomyosin, myoglobin and C-reactive protein release in marathon runners: Cardiac or skeletal muscle trauma? *Eur J Clin Invest* 1987; 17:317–324.

165. Adams JE, Sicard GA, Allen BT, Bridwell KH, Lenke LG, Davila-Roman VG, et al. Diagnosis of perioperative myocardial infarction with measurement of cardiac troponin I. *N Engl J Med* 1994; 330:670–674.

166. Bhayana V, Gougoulias T, Cohoe S, Henderson AR. Discordance between results for serum troponin T and troponin I in renal disease. *Clin Chem* 1995; 41:312–317.

167. Wu AHB, Valdes R, Apple FS, Gornet T, Stone MA, Mayfield-Stokes S, et al. Cardiac troponin-T immunoassay for diagnosis of acute myocardial infarction. *Clin Chem* 1994; 40:900–907.

168. Katus HA, Looser S, Hallermayer K, Remppis A, Scheffold T, Borgya A, et al. Development and in vitro characterization of a new immunoassay of cardiac troponin T. *Clin Chem* 1992; 38:386–393.

169. Li D, Keffer J, Corry K, Vazquez M, Jialal I. Nonspecific elevation of troponin T levels in patients with chronic renal failure. *Clin Biochem* 1995; 28:474–477.

170. Roberts R. Diagnostic assessment of myocardial infarction based on lactate dehydrogenase and creatine kinase isoenzymes. *Heart Lung* 1981; 10:486–506.

171. Abdelmeguid AE, Topol EJ, Whitlow PL, Sapp SK, Ellis SG. Significance of mild transient release of creatine kinase MB fraction after percutaneous interventions. *Circulation* 1996; 94:1528–1536.

172. Abdelmeguid AE, Ellis SG, Sapp SK, Whitlow PL, Topol EJ. Defining the appropriate threshold of creatine kinase elevation after percutaneous interventions. *Am Heart J* 1996; 131:1097–1105.

173. Abdelmeguid AE, Topol EJ. The myth of the myocardial "infarctlet" during percutaneous coronary revascularization procedures. *Circulation* 1996; 94:3369–3375.

174. Turi ZG, Rutherford JD, Roberts R, Muller JE, Jaffe AS, Rude RE, et al. Electrocardiographic, enzymatic and scintigraphic criteria of acute myocardial infarction as determined from study of 726 patients (a MILIS Study). *Am J Cardiol* 1985; 55:1463–1469.

175. Roberts R. Recognition, diagnosis, and prognosis of early reinfarction: The role of calcium channel blockers. *Circulation* 1987; 75:V-139–V-147.

176. Ohman EM, Armstrong PW, Christenson RH, Granger CB, Katus HA, Hamm CW, et al. Cardiac troponin T levels for risk stratification in acute myocardial ischemia. GUSTO IIA Investigators. *N Engl J Med* 1996; 335:1333–1341.

177. Antman EM, Tanasijevic MJ, Thompson B, Schactman M, McCabe CH, Cannon CP, et al. Cardiac-specific troponin I levels to predict the risk of mortality in patients with acute coronary syndromes. *N Engl J Med* 1996; 335:1342–1349.

178. Lindahl B, Venge P, Wallentin L, FRISC Study Group. Relation between troponin T and the risk of subsequent cardiac events in unstable coronary artery disease. *Circulation* 1996; 93:1651–1657.

179. Ishikawa Y, Saffitz JE, Mealman JE, Grace AM, Roberts R. Reversible myocardial ischemic injury is not associated with increased creatine kinase activites in plasma. *Clin Chem* 1997; 43:467–475.

180. Hamburg RJ, Verani MS, Mahmarian JJ, Puleo PR. Absence of trace MB creatine kinase release following stress-induced myocardial ischemia (abstr). *J Am Coll Cardiol* 1993; 21:161A.

181. TIMI-IIIB Investigators. Effects of tissue plasminogen activator and a comparison of early invasive and conservative strategies in unstable angina and non-Q-wave myocardial infarction: Results of the TIMI-IIIB trial. *Circulation* 1994; 89:1545–1556.

182. Roberts R, Sobel BE. Elevated plasma MB creatine phosphokinase activity: A specific marker for myocardial infarction in perioperative patients. *Arch Intern Med* 1976; 136:421–424.

183. Klein MS, Coleman RE, Weldon CS, Sobel BE, Roberts R. Concordance of electrocardiographic and scintigraphic criteria of myocardial injury after cardiac surgery. *J Thorac Cardiovasc Surg* 1976; 71:934–937.

184. Righetti A, O'Rourke RA, Schelbert H, Henning H, Hardarson T, Daily PO, et al. Usefulness of preoperative and postoperative Tc-99m (Sn)-pyrophosphate scans in patients with ischemic and valvular heart disease. *Am J Cardiol* 1977; 39:43–49.

185. Sullivan W, Vlodaver Z, Tuna N, Long L, Edwards JE. Correlation of electrocardiographic and pathologic findings in healed myocardial infarction. *Am J Cardiol* 1978; 42:724–731.

186. Goldberger AL (ed) *Myocardial Infarction: Electrocardiographic Differential Diagnosis*. St. Louis: Mosby; 1979.

187. Tiefenbrunn AJ, Biello DR, Geltman EM, Sobel BE, Siegel BA, Roberts R. Gated cardiac blood pool imaging and thallium-201 myocardial for detection of remote myocardial infarction. *Am J Cardiol* 1981; 47:1–6.

188. Gore JM, Goldberg RJ, Matsumoto AS, Castelli WP, McNamara PM, Dalen JG. Validity of serum total cholesterol level obtained within 24 hours of acute myocardial infarction. *Am J Cardiol* 1984; 54:722–725.

189. Ryder RE, Hayes TM, Mulligan IP, Kingswood JC, Williams S, Owens DR. How soon after myocardial infarction should plasma lipid values be assessed? *Br Med J* 1984; 289:1651–1653.

190. Ceremuzynski L. Hormonal and metabolic reactions evoked by acute myocardial infarction. *Circ Res* 1981; 48:767–776.

191. Goldberger E, Alesio J, Woll F. The significance of hyperglycemia in myocardial infarction. *NY State Med J* 1945; 45:391.

192. Katz, A S, Harrigan P, Parisi AF. The value and promise of echocardiography in acute myocardial infarction and coronary artery disease. *Clin Cardiol* 1992; 15:401.

193. Nisimura RA. Acute myocardial infarction: The role of echocardiography. In: Fuster V, Ross R, Topol EJ, eds. *Atherosclerosis and Coronary Artery Disease*. Philadelphia: Lippincott-Raven; 1996:855–876.

194. Harrison JK, Bashore TM. Assessment and management of the critically ill patient with valvular heart disease. In: Califf RM, Mark DB, Wagner GS, eds. *Acute Coronary Care*. St. Louis, Mosby–Year Book; 1995:719.

195. Horowitz R, Morganroth J. Immediate detection of early high-risk patients with an acute myocardial infarction using two-dimensional echocardiographic evaluation of left ventricular regional wall abnormalities. *Am Heart J* 1982; 103:814–822.

196. Berning J, Steeensgard-Hanses F. Early estimation of risk by echocardiographic determination of wall motion index in an unselected population with acute myocardial infarction. *Am J Cardiol* 1990; 65:567.

197. Sabia P, Abbott RD, Afrookteh A, Keller MW, Touchstone DA, Kaul S. Importance of two-dimensional echocardiographic assessment of left ventricular function in patients presenting to the emergency room with cardiac-related symptoms. *Circulation* 1991; 84:1615–1624.

198. Hepner AM, Armstrong WF. Echocardiography in acute myocardial infarction. In: Francis GS, Alpert JS, eds. *Coronary Care.* Boston: Little, Brown; 1995:473.

199. Sabia P, Afrookteh A, Touchstone DA, Keller MW, Esquivel L, Kaul S. Value of regional wall motion abnormality in the emergency room diagnosis of acute myocardial infarction: A prospective study using two-dimensional echocardiography. *Circulation.* 1991; 84(suppl I):I-85–I-92.

200. Kuhn MB, Egeblad H, Hojberg S. Prognostic value of echocardiography compared to other clinical findings: Multivariate analysis based on long-term survival in 456 patients. *Cardiology* 1995; 86:157.

201. D'Arcy B, Nanda NC. Two-dimensional echocardiographic features of right ventricular ejection fraction in patients with coronary artery disease. *J Am Coll Cardiol* 1983; 2:911–918.

202. Tice FD, Kisslo J. Echocardiographic assessment and monitoring of the patient with acute myocardial infarction: Prospects for the thrombolytic era. In: Califf RM, Mark DB, Wagner GS, eds. *Acute Coronary Care.* St. Louis: Mosby–Year Book, 1994:49.

203. Cheitlin MD, Alpert JS, Armstrong WF, Aurigemma GP, Beller GA, Bierman FZ, et al. ACC/AHA Guidelines for the Clinical Application of Echocradiography. A report of the American College of Cardiology/ American Heart Association Task Force on Practice Guidelines (Committee on Clinical Application of Echocardiography). Developed in colloboration with the American Society of Echocardiography. *Circulation* 1997; 95:1686–1744.

204. Salustri A, Elhendy A, Garyfallydis P, et al. Prediction of improvement of ventricular function after first acute myocardial infarction using low-dose dobutamine stress echocardiography. *Am J Cardiol* 1994; 74:853.

205. Camarano G, Ragosta M, Gimple LW, et al. Identification of viable myocardium with contrast echocardiography in patients with poor left ventricular cystolic function caused by recent or remote myocardial infarction. *Am J Cardiol* 1995; 75:215.

206. Takeuchi M, Araki M, Nakashima Y, et al. The detection of residual ischemia and stenosis in patients with acute myocardial infarction with dobutamine stress echocardiography. *J Am Soc Echocardiogr* 1994; 7:242.

207. Johnston DL, Gupta VK, Wendt RE, et al. Detection of viable myocardium in segments with fixed defects on thallium-201 scintigraphy: Usefulness of magnetic resonance imaging early after acute myocardial infarction. *Magn Reson Imaging* 1993; 11:949.

208. Holman ER, van Jonbergen HP, van Dijkman PR, et al. Comparison of magnetic resonance imaging studies with enzymatic indexes of myocardial necrosis for quantification of myocardial infract size. *Am J Cardiol* 1993; 71:1036.

209. Kantor HL, Toussaint JF. Acute myocardial infarction: The role of magnetic resonance. In: Fuster V, Ross R, Topol EJ, eds. *Atherosclerosis and Cororonary Artery Disease.* Philadelphia: Lippincott-Raven; 1996; 905–920.

210. Hirose K, Reed JE, Rumberger JA. Serial changes in regional right ventricular free wall and left ventricular septal wall lengths during the first 4 to 5 years after index anterior wall myocardial infarction. *J Am Coll Cardiol* 1995; 26:394.

211. Foster CJ, Sekiya T, Love HG, et al. Identification of intracardiac thrombus: Comparison of computed tomography and cross-sectional echocardiography. *Br J Radiol* 1987; 327.

212. Ritchie JL, Bateman TM, Bonow RO, et al. ACC/AHA guidelines for clinical use of cardiac radionuclide imaging: Report of the American College of Cardiology/American Heart Association Task Force on Assessment of Diagnostic and Therapeutic Cardiovascular Procedures (Committee on Radionuclide Imaging), developed in collaboration with the American Society of Nuclear Cardiology. *J Am Coll Cardiol* 1995; 25:521–547.

213. Coleman RE, Kelin MS, Roberts R, Sobel BE. Improved detection of myocardial infarction with technetium-99m stannous pyrophosphate and serum MB creatine phosphokiase. *Am J Cardiol* 1976; 37:732–735.

214. Corbett JR, Lewis M, Willerson JT, et al. 99mTc-pyrophosphate imaging in patients with acute myocardial infarction: Comparison of planar

215. Johnson LL, Seldin DW, Becker LC, et al. Antimyosin imaging in acute transmural myocardial infarctions: Results of a multicenter clinical trial. *J Am Coll Cardiol* 1989; 13:27–35.

216. Khaw BA, Gold HK, Yasuda T, et al. Scintigraphic quantification of myocardial necrosis in patients after intravenous injection of myosin-specific antibody. *Circulation* 1986: 74:501–508.

217. Reduto LA, Berger HJ, Cohen LS, Gottschalk A, Zaret BL. Sequential radionuclide assessment of left and right ventricular performance after acute transmural myocardial infarction. *Ann Intern Med* 1978; 89:441–447.

218. Kjekshus JK, Sobel BE. Depressed myocardial creatine phosphokinase activity following experimental myocardial infarction in rabbit. *Circ Res* 1970; 27:403–414.

219. Shell WE, Kjekshus JK, Sobel BE. Quantitative assessment of the extent of myocardial infarction in the conscious dog by means of analysis of serial changes in serum creatine phosphokinase (CPK) activity. *J Clin Invest* 1971; 50:2614–2625.

220. Sobel BE, Bresnahan GF, Shell WE, Yoder RD. Estimation of infarct size in man and its relation to prognosis. *Circulation* 1972; 46:640–648.

221. Roberts R, Henry PD, Sobel BE. An improved basis for enzymatic estimation of infarct size. *Circulation* 1975; 52:743–754.

222. Maroko PR, Kjekshus JK, Sobel BE. Factors influencing infarct size following experimental coronary artery occlusion. *Circulation* 1972; 43:67–82.

223. Geltman EM, Roberts R, Sobel BE. Cardiac positron tomography: Current status and future directions. *Herz* 1980; 5:107–119.

224. Sobel BE, Kjckshus KJ, Roberts R. Enzymatic estimation of infarct size. In: Hearst DJ, DeLeiris J, eds. *Enzymes in Cardiology: Diagnosis and Research.* Chichester, England: Wiley; 1979:257–289.

225. Geltman EM, Ehsani AA, Campbell MK, Schechtman K, Roberts R, Sobel BE. The influence of location and extent of myocardial infarction on long-term ventricular dysrhythmia and mortality. *Circulation* 1979; 60:805–814.

226. Roberts R. Creatine kinase isozymes as diagnostic and prognostic indices of myocardial infarction. In: Rattazzi MC, Scandalios JG, Whitt GS, eds. *Isozymes: Current Topics in Biological and Medical Research.* New York: Liss; 1979:115–154.

227. Hackel DB, Reimer KA, Ideker RE, Mikat EM, Hartwell TD, Parker CB, et al. Comparison of enzymatic and antomic estimates of myocardial infarct size in man. *Circulation* 1984; 70:824–835.

228. Roberts R, Ishikawa Y. Enzymatic estimation of infarct size during reperfusion. *Circulation* 1919; 68:I-83–I-89.

229. Maroko PR, Libby P, Covell JW, Sobel BE, Ross J Jr, Braunwald E. Precordial ST-T segment elevation mapping: An atraumatic method for assessing alterations in the extent of myocardial ischemic injury. *Am J Cardiol* 1972; 29:223–230.

230. Lekven J, Chatterje K, Tyberg JV, Parmley WW. Influence of left ventricular dimensions on endocardial and epicardial QRS amplitude and ST segment elevations during acute myocardial ischemia. *Circulation* 1980; 61:679–689.

231. Ideker RE, Wagner GS, Ruth WK, Alonso DR, Bishop SP, Bloor CM, et al. Evaluation of a QRS scoring system for estimating myocardial infarct size: II. Correlation with quantitative anatomic findings for anterior infarcts. *Am J Cardiol* 1982; 49:1604–1614.

232. Roark SF, Ideker RE, Wagner GS, Alonso DR, Bishop SP, Bloor CM, et al. Evaluation of a QRS scoring system for estimating myocardial infarct size: III. Correlation with quantitative anatomic findings for inferior infarcts. *Am J Cardiol* 1983; 51:382–389.

233. Cowan MJ, Bruce RA, Reichenback DD. Validation of computerized QRS criterion for estimating myocardial infarction size and correlation with quantitative morphologic measurements. *Am J Cardiol* 1986; 57:60–65.

234. Bar FW, Vermeer F, deZwaan C. Value of admission electrocardiogram in predicting outcome of thrombolytic therapy in acute myocardial infarction: A randomized trial conducted by The Netherlands Interuniversity Cardiology Institute. *Am J Cardiol* 1987; 59:6–13.

235. Mauri F, Gasparini M, Barbonaglia L, et al. Prognostic significance of the extent of myocardial injury in acute myocardial infarction treated by streptokinase (the GISSI trial). *Am J Cardiol* 1989; 63:1291.

236. The Multicenter Postinfarction Research Group. Risk stratification and survival after myocardial infarction. *N Engl J Med* 1983; 309:331–336.

237. Corbett JR, Dehmer GJ, Lewis SE, et al. The prognostic value of submaximal exercise testing with radionuclide ventriculography before

hospital discharge in patients with recent myocardial infarction. *Circulation* 1981; 64:535–544.

238. Cerqueira MD, Maynard C, Ritchie JL, Davis KB, Kennedy JW. Long-term survival in 618 patients from the Western Washington Streptokinase in Myocardial Infarction Trials. *J Am Coll Cardiol* 1992; 20:1452–1459.

239. Simoons ML, Vos J, Tijssen JG, et al. Long-term benefit of early thrombolytic therapy in patients with acute myocardial infarction: 5-year follow-up of a trial conducted by the Interuniversity Cardiology Institute of The Netherlands. *J Am Coll Cardiol* 1989; 14:1609–1615.

240. Gibson WS, Christian TF, Pellikka PA, Behrenbeck T, Gibbons RJ. Serial tomographic imaging with technetium-99m-sestamibi for the assessment of infract-related arterial patency following reperfusion therapy. *J Nucl Med* 1992; 33:2080–2085.

241. Christian TF, Schwartz RS, Gibbons RJ. Determinants of infarct size in reperfusion therapy for acute myocardial infarction. *Circulation* 1992; 86:81–90.

242. McCallister BD Jr, Christian TF, Gersh BJ, Gibbons RJ. Prognosis of myocardial infarctions involving more than 40% of the left ventricle after acute reperfusion therapy. *Circulation* 1993; 88(4 pt 1):1470–1475.

243. Miller TD, Christian TF, Hopfenspirger MR, Hodge DO, Gersh BJ, Gibbons RJ. Infarct size after acute myocardial infarction measured by quantitative tomographic 99m Tc sestamibi imaging predicts subsequent mortality (see comments). *Circulation* 1995; 92:334–341.

244. Kuller L. Sudden death in arteriosclerotic heart disease: The case for preventive medicine. *Am J Cardiol* 1969; 24:617–628.

245. Fulton M, Julian DG, Oliver MF. Sudden death and myocardial infarction. *Circulation* 1969; 40:182–191.

246. Adgey AAJ, Allen JD, Geddes JS, James RG, Webb SW, Zaidi SA, et al. Acute phase of myocardial infarction. *Lancet* 1971; 2:501–504.

247. Simon AB, Feinleib M, Thompson HK Jr. Components of delay in the prehospital phase of acute myocardial infarction. *Am J Cardiol* 1972; 30:476–482.

248. National Heart, Lung and Blood Institute. 9-1-1: *Rapid Identification and Treatment of Acute Myocardial Infarction*. NIH Publication 94-3302. Bethesda, MD: U.S. Department of Health and Human Services, Public Health Service, National Institutes of Health; 1994.

249. National Heart, Lung and Blood Institute. Patient/bystander recognition and action: Rapid identification and treatment of acute myocardial Infarction. In: *National Heart Attack Alert Program (NHAAP)*. NIH Publication NO. 93-3303. Bethesda, MD: National Institutes of Health; 1993.

250. Pressley JC, Severance HW Jr, Raney MP, McKinnis RA, Smith MW, Hindman MC, et al. A comparison of paramedic versus basic emergency medical care of patients at high and low risk during acute myocardial infarction. *J Am Coll Cardiol* 1988; 12:1555–1561.

251. Kareiakes DJ, Weaver WD, Anderson JL, Feldman T, Gibler B, Aufderheide T, et al. Time delays in the diagnosis and treatment of acute myocardial infarction: A tale of eight cities. Report from the Prehospital Study Group and the Cincinnati Heart Project. *Am Heart J* 1990; 120:773–780.

252. Goldstein S, Moss AJ, Greene W. Sudden death in acute myocardial infarction: Relationship to factors affecting delay in hospitalization. *Arch Intern Med* 1972; 129:720–724.

253. ACC/AHA. ACC/AHA Guidelines for the early management of patients with acute myocardial infarction. *Circulation* 1990; 82:664–707.

254. Lewis RP, Lanese RR, Stang JM, Chirikos TN, Keller MD, Warren JV. Reduction of mortality from prehospital myocardial infarction by prudent patient activation of mobile coronary care system. *Am Heart J* 1982; 103:123–130.

255. Eisenberg MS, Horwood BT, Cummins RO, Reynolds-Haertle R, Hearne TR. Cardiac arrest and resuscitation: A tale of 29 cities. *Ann Emerg Med* 1990; 19:179–186.

256. Cummins RO, Eisenberg MS, Litwin PE, Graves JR, Hearne TR, Hallstrom AP. Automatic external defibrillators used by emergency medical technicians: A controlled clinical trial. *JAMA* 1987; 257:1605–1610.

257. Kerber RE. *Statement on Early Defibrillation: AHA Medical/Scientific Statement*. Emergency Cardiac Care Committee. Chicago: American Heart Association; 1991.

258. Weaver WD, Hill D, Fahrenbruch CE, et al. Use of the automatic external defibrillator in the management of out-of-hospital cardiac arrest. *N Engl J Med* 1988; 319:661–666.

259. Stults KR, Brown DD, Schug VL, Bean JA. Prehospital defibrillation performed by emergency medical technicians in rural communities. *N Engl J Med* 1984; 310:219–223.

260. Weaver WD, Cerqueira M, Hallstrom AP, Litwin PE, Martin JJ, Kudenchuk PJ, et al. Prehospital-initiated vs. hospital-initiated thrombolytic therapy: The Myocardial Infarction Triage and Intervention Trial. *JAMA* 1993; 270:1211–1216.

261. Weaver WD, Litwin PE, Martin JS, Kudenchuk PJ, Maynard C, Eisenberg MS, et al. Effect of age on use of thrombolytic therapy and mortality in acute myocardial infarction: The MITI Project Group. *J Am Coll Cardiol* 1991; 18:657–662.

262. Karagounis L, Ipsen SK, Jessop MR, Gilmore KM, Valenti DA, Clawson JJ, et al. Impact of field-transmitted electrocardiography on time to in-hospital thrombolytic therapy in acute myocardial infarction. *Am J Cardiol* 1990; 66:786–791.

263. Fibrinolytic Therapy Trialists' (FTT) Collaborative Group. Indications for fibrinolytic therapy in suspected acute myocardial infarction: Collaborative overview of early mortality and major morbidity results from all randomized trials of more than one thousand patients. *Lancet* 1994; 343:311–322.

264. ISIS-2 (Second International Study of Infarct Survival) Collaborative Group. Randomized trial of intravenous streptokinase, oral aspirin, both, or neither among 17,187 cases of suspected acute myocardial infarction: ISIS-2. *Lancet* 1988; 2:349–360.

265. Castaigne AD, Herve C, Duval-Moulin AM, Gaillard M, Dubois-Rande JL, Boesch C, et al. Prehospital use of APSAC: Results of a placebo-controlled study. *Am J Cardiol* 1989; 64(suppl 2):30A–33A.

266. Schofer J, Buttner J, Geng G, Gutschmidt K, Herden HN, Mathey DG, et al. Prehospital thrombolysis in acute myocardial infarction. *Am J Cardiol* 1990; 66:1429–1433.

267. GREAT Group. Feasibility, safety, and efficacy of domiciliary thrombolysis by general practitioners: Grapian Region Early Anistreplase Trial. *Br Med J* 1992; 305:548–553.

268. The European Myocardial Infarction Project Group. Prehospital thrombolytic therapy in patients with suspected acute myocardial infarction. *N Engl J Med* 1993; 329:383–389.

269. Gibler WB, Kereiakes DJ, Dean EN, Martin L, Anderson L, Abbottsmith CW, et al. Prehospital diagnosis and treatment of acute myocardial infarction: A North-South perspective. The Cincinnati Heart Project and the Nashville Prehospital TPA Trial. *Am Heart J* 1991; 121:1–11.

270. Jesse RL, Kontos MC. Evaluation of chest pain in the emergency department. *Curr Probl Cardiol* 1997; 22:149–236.

271. Karlson BW, Herlitz J, Wiklund O, Richter A, Hjalmarson A. Early prediction of acute myocardial infarction from clinical history, examination and electrocardiogram in the emergency room. *Am J Cardiol* 1991; 68:171–175.

272. Stark ME, Vacek JL. The initial electrocardiogram during admission for myocardial infarction. *Arch Intern Med* 1987; 147:843–846.

273. Lee TH, Rouan GW, Weisberg MC, Brand DA, Acampora D, Stasiulewicz C, et al. Clinical characteristics natural history of patients with acute myocardial infarction sent home from the emergency room. *Am J Cardiol* 1987; 60:219–224.

274. Tierney WM, Roth BJ, Psaty B, McHenry R, Fitzgerald J, Stump DL, et al. Predictors of myocardial infarction in emergency room patients. *Crit Care Med* 1985; 13:526–531.

275. Rouan GW, Hedges JR, Toltzis R, Goldstein-Wayne B, Brand D, Goldman L. A chest pain clinic to improve the follow-up of patients released from an urban university teaching hospital emergency department. *Ann Emerg Med* 1987; 16:1145–1150.

276. McCarthy BD, Beshansky JR, D'Agostino RB, Selker HP. Missed diagnoses of acute myocardial infarction in the emergency department: Results from a multicenter study. *Ann Emerg Med* 1993; 22:579–582.

277. Rusnak RA, Stair TO, Hansen K, Fastow JS. Litigation against the emergency physician: Common features in cases of missed myocardial infarction. *Ann Emerg Med* 1989; 18:1029–1034.

278. Goldman L, Weinberg M, Weisberg M, Olshen R, Cook EF, Sargent RK, et al. A computer-derived protocol to aid in the diagnosis of emergency room patients with acute chest pain. *N Engl J Med* 1982; 307:588–596.

279. Schroeder JS, Lamb IH, Hu M. Do patients in whom myocardial infarction has been ruled out have a better prognosis after hospitalization than those surviving infarction? *N Engl J Med* 1980; 303:1–5.

280. Kahn JK. Inadvertent thrombolytic therapy for cardiovascular diseases masquerading as acute coronary thrombosis. *Clin Cardiol* 1993; 16:67–71.

281. Butler J, Davies AH, Westaby S. Streptokinase in acute aortic dissection. *Br Med J* 1990; 300:517–519.

282. Eriksen UH, Molgaard H, Ingerslev J, Nielsen TT. Fatal haemostatic complications due to thrombolytic therapy in patients falsely diagnosed as acute myocardial infarction. *Eur Heart J* 1992; 13:840–843.

283. Blankenship JC, Almquist AK. Cardiovascular complications of thrombolytic therapy in patients with a mistaken diagnosis of acute myocardial infarction. *J Am Coll Cardiol* 1989; 14:1579–1582.

284. Katz PO, Dalton CB, Richter JE, Wu WC, Castell DO. Esophageal testing of patients with noncardiac chest pain or dysphagia. *Ann Intern Med* 1987; 106:593–597.

285. Goyal RK. Changing focus on unexplained esophageal chest pain. *Ann Intern Med* 1996; 124:1008–1011.

286. Nevens F, Janssens J, Piessens J, Ghillebert G, DeGeest H, Vantrappen G. Prospective study on prevalence of esophageal chest pain in patients referred on an elective basis to a cardiac unit for suspected myocardial ischemia. *Dig Dis Sci* 1991; 36:229–235.

287. Hewson EG, Sinclair JW, Dalton CB, Richter JE. Twenty-four-hour esophageal pH monitoring: The most useful test for evaluating noncardiac chest pain. *Am J Med* 1991; 90:576–583.

288. Fruergaard P, Launbjerg J, Hesse B, Jorgensen F, Petri A, Eiken P, et al. The diagnoses of patients admitted with acute myocardial infarction: A comparison between patients with and without confirmed myocardial infarction. *Eur Heart J* 1996; 17:1028–1034.

289. Levene DL. Chest pain: Prophet of doom or nagging neurosis? *Acta Med Scand Suppl* 1981; 644:11–13.

290. Ornato JP, Jesse RL, Tatum JL, Nicholson CS, Peberdy MA, Roberts CS. Lack of correlation between relief of chest pain after sublingual nitroglycerin and reversible radionuclide perfusion defects or presence of significant coronary atherosclerosis on coronary angiography (abstr). *J Am Coll Cardiol* 1995; 25A–12A.

291. Cohen M, Hawkins L, Greenberg S, Fuster V. Usefulness of ST-segment changes in greater than or equal to 2 leads on the emergency room electrocardiogram in either unstable angina pectoris or non-Q-wave myocardial infarction in predicting outcome. *Am J Cardiol* 1991; 67:1368–1373.

292. Slater DK, Hlatky MA, Mark DB, Harrell FE Jr, Pryor DB, Califf RM. Outcome in suspected acute myocardial infarction with normal or minimally abnormal admission electrocardiographic findings. *Am J Cardiol* 1987; 60:766–770.

293. Brush JE Jr, Brand DA, Acampora D, Chalmer B, Wackers FJ. Use of the initial electrocardiogram to predict in-hospital complications of acute myocardial infarction. *N Engl J Med* 1985; 312:1137–1141.

294. Goldman L, Cook EF, Johnson PA, Brand DA, Rouan GW, Lee TH. Prediction of the need for intensive care in patients who come to emergency departments with acute chest pain. *N Engl J Med* 1996; 334:1498–1504.

295. Goldberg R, Gore J, Alpert J, Dalen JE. Incidence and case fatality rates of acute myocardial infarction (1975–1984): The Worcester Heart Attack Study. *Am Heart J* 1988; 115:761–767.

296. Gibler W, Lewis L, Erb R, Makens PK, Kaplan BC, Vaughn RH, et al. Early detection of acute myocardial infarction in patients presenting with chest pain and non-diagnostic ECGs: Serial CK-MB sampling in the emergency department. *Ann Emerg Med* 1990; 19:1359–1366.

297. Marin MM, Teichman SL. Use of rapid serial sampling of creatine kinase MB for very early detection of myocardial infarction in patients with acute chest pain. *Am Heart J* 1992; 123:354–361.

298. Pozen MW, D'Agostino RB, Selker HP, Sytkowski PA, Hood WB Jr. A predictive instrument to improve coronary-care-unit admission practices in acute ischemic heart disease. *N Engl J Med* 1984; 310:1273–1278.

299. Selker HP, Griffith JL, D'Agostino RB. A tool for judging coronary care unit admission appropriateness, valid for both real-time and retrospective use. *Med Care* 1991; 29:610–627.

300. Grijseels EWM, Deckers JW, Hoes AW, Hartman JA, Van der Does E, Van Loenen E, et al. Pre-hospital triage of patients with suspected myocardial infarction. *Eur Heart J* 1995; 16:325–332.

301. Antman EM, Tanasijevic MJ, Thompson B, Schactman M, McCabe, CH, Cannon CP, et al. Cardiac-specific troponin I levels to predict the risk of mortality in patients with acute coronary syndromes. *N Engl J Med* 1996; 335:1342–1349.

302. Fillmore SJ, Shapiro M, Killip T. Arterial oxygen tension in acute myocardial infarction: Serial analysis of clinical state and blood gas changes. *Am Heart J* 1970; 79:620–629.

303. Madias JE, Hood WB Jr. Reduction of precordial ST-segment elevation in patients with anterior myocardial infarction by oxygen breathing. *Circulation* 1976; 53(suppl I):I-198–I-200.

304. Lowenstein E. Morphine "anesthesia"—A perspective. *Anesthesiology* 1997; 35:890.

305. Herlitz J. Analgesia in myocardial infarction. *Drugs* 1989; 37:939–944.

306. Antman EM. General hospital management. In: Julian DG, Braunwald E, eds. *Management of Acute Myocardial Infarction*. London: Saunders; 1994:42–44.

307. Mann T, Cohn PF, Holman L, Green LH, Markis JE, Phillips DA. Effect of nitroprusside on regional myocardial blood flow in coronary artery disease: Results in 25 patients in comparison with nitroglycerin. *Circulation* 1978; 57:732–738.

308. Chiariello M, Gold HK, Leinbach RC, Davis MA, Maroko PR. Comparison between the effects of nitroprusside and nitroglycerin on ischemic injury during acute myocardial infarction. *Circulation* 1976; 54:766–773.

309. Flaherty JT, Becker LC, Bulkley BH, Weiss JL, Gerstenblith G, Kallman CH, et al. A randomized prospective trail of intravenous nitroglycerin in patients with acute myocardial infarction. *Circulation* 1983; 68:576–588.

310. Bussmann WD, Passek D, Seidel W, Kaltenbach M. Reduction of CK and CK-MB indexes of infarct size by intravenous nitroglycerin. *Circulation* 1981; 63:615–622.

311. Jugdutt BI, Becker LC, Hutchins GM, Bulkley BH, Reid PR, Kallman CH. Effect of intravenous nitroglycerin on collateral blood flow and infarct size in the conscious dog. *Circulation* 1981; 63:17–28.

312. Jugdutt BI, Khan MI, Jugdutt SJ, Blinston GE. Impact of left ventricular unloading after late reperfusion of canine anterior myocardial infarction on remodeling and function using isosorbide-5-mononitrate. *Circulation* 1995; 92:926–934.

313. Yusuf S, Collins R, MacMahon S, Peto R. Effect of intravenous nitrates on mortality in acute myocardial infarction: An overview of the randomized trials. *Lancet* 1989; 1:1088–1092.

314. GISSI-3. Gruppo Italiano per lo Studio della Streptochinasi nell'Infarto Miocardico. Effects of lisinopril and transdermal glycerol trinitrate singly and together on 6-week mortality and ventricular function after acute myocardial infarction. *Lancet* 1994; 343:1115–1122.

315. ISIS-4. a randomized factorial trial assessing early oral captopril, oral mononitrate, and intravenous magnesium sulphate in 58,050 patients with suspected acute myocardial infarction. *Lancet* 1995; 345:669–685.

316. Kinch JW, Ryan TJ. Right ventricular infarction. *N Engl J Med* 1994; 330:1211–1217.

317. Come PC, Pitt B. Nitroglycerin-induced severe hypotension and bradycardia in patients with acute myocardial infarction. *Circulation* 1976; 54:624–628.

318. ISIS-2 (Second International Study of Infarct Survival) Collaborative Group: Randomised trial of intravenous streptokinase, oral aspirin, both, or neither among 17,187 cases of suspected acute myocardial infarction: ISIS-2. *Lancet* 1988; 2:349–360.

319. Fourth American College of Chest Physicians Consensus Conference on Antithrombotic Therapy. *Chest* 1995; 108(suppl):225S–522S.

320. Monocada S, Vane JR. The role of prostacyclin in vascular tissue. *Fed Proc* 1979; 38:66–71.

321. de Feyter PJ, van Den Brand M, Serruys PW, Wijns W. Early angiography after myocardial infarction: What have we learned? *Am Heart J* 1985; 109:194–199.

322. Reimer KA, Lowe JE, Rasmussen MM, Jennings RB. The wavefront phenomenon of ischemic cell death. I. Myocardial infarct size vs duration of coronary occlusion in dog. *Circulation* 1977; 56:786–794.

323. Reimer KA, Jennings RB. The "wave front phenomenon" of myocardial ischemia cell death: II. Transmural progression of necrosis within the framework of ischemic bed size (myocardium at risk) and collateral flow. *Lab Invest* 1979; 40:633–644.

324. Lau J, Antman EN, Jimenez-Silva J, Kupelnick B, Mosteller F, Chalmers TC. Cumulative meta-analysis of therapeutic trials for myocardial infarction. *N Engl J Med* 1992; 327:248–254.

325. First International Study of Infarct Survival Collaborative Group. Randomised trial of intravenous atenolol among 16,027 cases of suspected acute myocardial infarction: ISIS-1. *Lancet* 1986; 2:57–66.

326. The MIAMI Trial Research Group. Metoprolol in acute myocardial infarction: Patient population. *Am J Cardiol* 1985; 56:1G–57G.

327. The TIMI Study Group. Comparison of invasive and conservative strategies after treatment with intravenous tissue plasminogen activator in acute myocardial infarction: Results of the Thrombolysis in Myocardial Infarction (TIMI) phase II trial. *N Engl J Med* 1989; 320:618–627.

328. Collins R, Peto R, Baigent C, Sleight P. Aspirin, heparin, and fibrinolytic therapy in suspected acute myocardial infarction. *Drug Ther* 1997; 36:847–860.

329. ISIS-2 (Second International Study of Infarct Survival) Collaborative Group. Randomized trial of intravenous streptokinase, oral aspirin, both, or neither among 17,187 cases of suspected acute myocardial infarction: ISIS-2. *J Am Coll Cardiol* 1988; 12:3A–13A.

330. ISIS-3 Collaborative Group: ISIS-3. A randomized comparison of streptokinase vs tissue plasminogen activator vs anistreplase and of aspirin plus heparin vs aspirin alone among 41,299 cases of suspected acute myocardial infarction. *Lancet* 1992; 339:753–770.

331. GISSI-2 Gruppo Italiano per lo Studio della Streptochinasi nell'Infarto Miocardico. A factorial randomised trial of alteplace versus streptokinase and heparin versus no heparin among 12,490 patients with acute myocardial infarction. *Lancet* 1990; 336:65–71.

332. Hsia J, Hamilton WP, Kleiman NS, Roberts R, Chaitman B, Ross AM, et al. A comparison between heparin and low-dose aspirin as adjunctive therapy with tissue plasminogen activator for acute myocardial infarction. *N Engl J Med* 1990; 323:1433–1437.

333. Gurfinkel EP, Manos EJ, Mejail RI, Cerda MA, Duronto EA, Garcia C, et al. Low molecular weight heparin versus regular heparin or aspirin in the treatment of unstable angina and silent ischemia. *J Am Coll Cardiol* 1995; 26:313–318.

334. Piegas LS, Canon SJF, Avezum AJ. Arterial patency and ejection fraction after late thrombolysis with streptokinase. Results from EMERAS (abstr). *Eur Heart J* 1991; 12:97.

335. Wilcox RG. LATE assessment of thrombolytic efficacy: Randomized trial of alteplase or placebo 6–24 hours after symptoms of acute myocardial infarction (abstr). *Eur Heart J* 1992; 13:423.

336. The GUSTO IIb Angioplasty Substudy Investigators. A clinical trial comparing primary coronary angioplasty with tissue plasminogen activator for acute myocardial infarction. *N Engl J Med* 1997; 336:1621–1628.

337. Guadagnoli E, Hauptman PJ, Ayanian JZ, Pashos CL, McNeil BJ, Cleary PD. Variation in the use of cardiac procedures after acute myocardial infarction. *N Engl J Med* 1995; 333:573–578.

338. Grines CL, De Maria AN. Optimal utilization of thrombolytic therapy for acute myocardial infarction: Concepts and controversies. *J Am Coll Cardiol* 1990; 16:223–231.

339. Califf RM, Topol EJ, Kereiakes DJ, Abbottsmith CW, George BS, Candela RJ, et al. Cardiac resuscitation should not be a contraindication to thrombolytic therapy for myocardial infarction. *Circulation* 1988; 78:II-127.

340. Roberts R, Kleiman NS, eds. *The Open Artery: Perspectives on Coronary Reperfusion in Acute Myocardial Infarction*. Hamilton, Ontario, Canada: Decker, 1992.

341. The TIMI Study Group: The Thrombolysis in Myocardial Infarction (TIMI) Trial: Phase I findings. *N Engl J Med* 1985; 312:932–936.

342. Granger CG, Califf RM, Hirsch J, Woodlief LH, Topol EJ, The GUSTO Investigators. APTTs after thrombolysis and standard intravenous heparin are often low and correlate with body weight, age and sex: Experience from the GUSTO trial. *Circulation* 1992; 86:I-258.

343. Hull RD, Raskob GE, Hirsh J, Jay RM, Leclerc JR, Geerts WH, et al. Continuous intravenous heparin compared with intermittent subcutaneous heparin in the initial treatment of proximal vein thrombosis. *N Engl J Med* 1986; 315:1109–1114.

344. Roberts R. La difference: Long-term benefit of one thrombolytic over another. *Circulation* 1996; 94:1203–1205.

345. Califf RM, White H, Van de Werf F, Sadowski Z, Armstrong PW, Vahanian A, et al. One-year results from the global utilization of streptokinase and TPA for occuluded coronary arteries (GUSTO-I) trial. *Circulation* 1996; 94:1233–1238.

346. Smalling RW, Bode C, Kalbfleisch J, Sen S, Limbourg P, Forycki F, et al. More rapid, complete, and stable coronary thrombolysis with bolus administration of reteplase compared with alteplase infusion in acute myocardial infarction. *Circulation* 1995; 91:2725–2732.

347. Bode C, Smalling RW, Berg G, Burnett C, Lorch G, Kalbfleisch JM, et al. Randomized comparison of coronary thrombolysis achieved with double-bolus reteplase (recombinant plasminogen activator) and front-

348. loaded, accelerated alteplase (recombinant tissue plasminogen activator) in patients with acute myocardial infarction. *Circulation* 1996; 94:891–898.

348. Hampton JR, Schroder R, Wilcox RG, Skene AM. Randomised, double-blind comparison of reteplase double-bolus administration with streptokinase in acute myocardial infarction (INJECT): Trial to invesigate equivalence. *Lancet* 1995; 346:329–336.

349. Cody RJ. Results from late breaking clinical trials sessions at ACC '97. *J Am Coll Cardiol* 1997; 30:1–7.

350. Boden WE, Roberts R. Prognosis and management of patients with non-Q-wave myocardial infarction, in Zipes DP, Rowlands DJ, eds: *Progress in Cardiology*. Philadelphia: Lea & Febiger, 1991:143–160.

351. Cropp GJ, Manning GW. Electrocardiographic changes simulating myocardial ischemia and infarction associated with spontaneous intracranial hemorrhage. *Circulation* 1960; 22:25–38.

352. Deantonio HJ, Kaul S, Lerman BB. Reversible myocardial depression in survivors of cardiac arrest. PACE 1990; 13:982–985.

352a. Roberts R. Heparin and aspirin in thrombolysis: Biological and clinical issues. *Clin Chall* 1992; 1:1–7.

353. Francis CW, Markham RE Jr, Barlow GH, Florack TM, Dobrzynski DM, Marder VJ. Thrombin activity of fibrin thrombi and soluble plasmic derivaties. *J Lab Clin Med* 1983; 102:220–230.

354. Funk CD, Funk LB, Kennedy ME, Pong AS, Fitgerald GA. Human platelet/erythroleukemia cell prostaglandin G/H synthase: cDNA cloning, expression, and gene chromosomal assignment. *FASEB J* 1991; 5:2304–2312.

355. Hsia J, Kleiman NS, Aguirre FV, Chaitman BR, Roberts R, Ross AM, et al. Heparin-induced prolongation of partial thromboplastin time after thrombolysis: Relation to coronary artery patency. *J Am Coll Cardiol* 1992; 20:31–35.

356. Bleich SD, Nochols TC, Schumacher RR, Cooke DH, Tate DA, Teichman SL. Effect of heparin on coronary arterial patency after thrombolysis with tissue plasminogen activator in acute myocardial infarction. *Am J Cardiol* 1990; 66:1412–1417.

357. National Heart Foundation of Australia. Coronary thrombolysis and myocardial salvage by tissue plasminogen activator given up to four hours after onset of myocardial infarction. *Lancet* 1988; 1:203–208.

358. Topol EJ, George BS, Kereiakes DJ, Stump DC, Candela RJ, Abbottsmith CW, et al. A randomized controlled trial of intravenous tissue plasminogen activator and early intravenous heparin in acute myocardial infarction. *Circulation* 1989; 79:281–286.

359. Kander NH, Holland KJ, Pitt B, Topol EJ. A randomized pilot trial of brief versus prolonged heparin after successful reperfusion in acute myocardial infarction. *Am J Cardiol* 1990; 65:139–142.

360. Prins MH, Hirsh J. Heparin as an adjunctive treatment after thrombolytic therapy for acute myocardial infarction. *Am J Cardiol* 1991; 67:3A–11A.

361. The SCATI Group. Randomised controlled trial of subcutaneous calcium-heparin in acute myocardial infarction. *Lancet* 1989; 2:182–186.

362. Loscalzo J. Thrombin inhibitors in fibrinolysis. *Circulation* 1996; 94:863–865.

363. Zeymer U, von Essen R, Tebbe U, Michels HR, Jesel A, Vogt A, et al. Recombinant hirudin and front-loaded alteplase in acute myocardial infarction: Final results of a pilot study. HIT-I (hirudin for the improvement of thrombolysis). *Eur Heart J* 1995; 16:22–27.

364. Heuhaus K, Niederer W, Wagner J, Maurer W, von Essen R, Tebbe U, et al. HIT (Hirudin for the Improvement of Thrombolysis): Results of a dose escalation study (abstr). *Circulation* 1993; 88:I-292.

365. Cannon CP, McCabe CH, Henry TD, Schweiger MJ, Gibson RS, Mueller HS, et al. A pilot trial of recombinant desulfatohirudin compared with heparin in conjunction with tissue-type plasminogen activator and aspirin for acute myocardial infarction: Results of the thrombolysis in myocardial infarction (TIMI) 5 trial. *J Am Coll Cardiol* 1994; 23:993–1003.

366. Antman EM. Hirudinn in acute myocardial infarction. Safety report from the Thrombolysis and Thrombin Inhibition in Myocardial Infarction (TIMI) 9A trial. *Circulation* 1994; 90:1624–1630.

367. GUSTO IIa Investigators. Randomized trial of intravenous heparin versus recombinant hirudin for acute coronary syndromes. The Global Use of Strategies to Open occluded Coronary Arteries (GUSTO) IIa investigators. *Circulation* 1994; 90:1631–1637.

368. Ferguson JJ. Meeting Highlights: American Heart Association 68th Scientific Sessions, Anaheim, California, Nov 13–15, 1995. TIMI 9B: Heparin versus hirudin as adjunctive therapy for thrombolysis in acute myocardial infarction. *Circulation* 1996; 93:843–846.

369. GUSTO IIb Investigators: A comparison of recombinant hirudin with heparin for the treatment of acute coronary syndromes. The Global Use of Strategies to Open Occluded Coronary Arteries (GUSTO) IIb investigators. *N Engl J Med* 1996; 335:701–707.

370. Schiele F, Vuillemenot A, Kramarz P, Kieffer Y, Anguenot T, Bernard Y, et al. Use of recombinant hirudin as antithrombotic treatment in patients with heparin-induced thrombocytopenia. Am J Hematol 1995; 50:20–25.

371. Komrad MS, Coffey CE, Coffey KS, McKinnis R, Massey EW, Califf RM. Myocardial infarction and stroke. *Neurology* 1984; 34:1403–1409.

372. Simoons MS, Arnold AER, Betriu A, de Bono DP, Col JJ, Dougherty FC, et al. Thrombolysis with tissue plasminogen activator in acute myocardial infarction: No additional benefit from immediate percutaneous coronary angioplasty. *Lancet* 1988; 1:197–203.

373. Verstraete M, Bory M, Collen D, Erbel R, Lennane RJ, Mathey D, et al. Randomized trial of intravenous recombinant tissue-type plasminogen activity versus intravenous streptokinase in active myocardial infarction: Report from the European Cooperative Study Group for Recombinant Tissue-Type Plasminogen Activator. *Lancet* 1985: I:842–847.

374. SWIFT Trial Study Group. SWIFT trial of delayed elective intervention versus conservative treatment after thrombolysis with anistreplase in acute myocardial infarction. *Br Med J* 1991; 302:555–560.

375. Williams DO, Braunwald E, Knatterud G, Babb J, Bresnahan JF,Greenberg MA, et al. One-year results of the Thrombolysis in Myocardial Infarction (TIMI) phase II trial. *Circulation* 1992; 85:533–542.

376. Juliard JM, Himbert D, Golmard JL, Aubry P, Karrillon GJ, Boccara A, et al. Can we provide reperfusion therapy to all unselected patients admitted with acute myocardial infarction? *J Am Coll Cardiol* 1997; 30:157–164.

377. Gibson CM, Cannon CP, Greene RM, Sequeira RF, Margorien RD, Leya F, et al. Rescue angioplasty in the thrombolysis in myocardial infarction (TIMI) 4 trial. *Am J Cardiol* 1997; 80:21–26.

378. Lee L, Bates ER, Pitt B, Walton JA, Laufer N, O'Neill WW. Percutaneous transluminal coronary angioplasty improves survival in acute myocardial infarction complicated by cardiogenic shock. *Circulation* 1988; 78:1345–1351.

379. Bengtson JR, Kaplan AJ, Pieper KS, Wildermann NM, Mark DB, Pryor DB, et al. Prognosis in cardiogenic shock after acute myocardial infarction in the interventional era. *J Am Coll Cardiol* 1992; 20:1482–1489.

380. Lemmer JH, Ferguson DW, Rakel BA, Rossi NP. Clinical outcome of emergency repeat coronary artery bypass surgery. *J Cardiovasc Surg (Torino)* 1990; 31:492–497.

381. O'Connor GT, Plume SK, Olmstead EM, et al. Multivariate prediction of in-hospital mortality associated with coronary artery bypass graft surgery: Northern New England Cardiovascular Disease Study Group. *Circulation* 1992; 85:2110–2118.

382. Hochman JS, Boland J, Sleeper LA, et al. Current spectrum of cardiogenic shock and effect of early revascularization on mortality: Results of an International Registry. SHOCK Registry Investigators. *Circulation* 1995; 91:873–881.

383. Das G, Talmers FN, Weissler AM. New observations on the effects of atropine on the sinoatrial and atrioventricular nodes in man. *Am J Cardiol* 1975; 36:281–285.

384. Kent KM, Smith ER, Redwood DR, Epstein SE. Electrical stability of acutely ischemic myocardium: Influences of heart rate and vagal stimulation. *Circulation* 1973; 47:291–298.

385. Scheinman MM, Thorburn D, Abbott JA. Use of atropine in patients with acute myocardial infarction and sinus bradycardia. *Circulation* 1975; 52:627–633.

386. Kottmeier CA, Gravenstein JS. The parasympathomimetic activity of atropine and atropine methylbromide. *Anesthesiology* 1968; 29:1125–1133.

387. Berger PB, Ruocco NA Jr, Ryan TJ, Frederick MM, Jacobs AK, Faxon DP. Incidence and prognostic implications of heart block complicating inferior myocardial infarction treated with thrombolytic therapy: Results from TIMI-II. *J Am Coll Cardiol* 1992; 20:533–540.

388. Nicod P, Gilpin E, Dittrich H, Polikar R, Henning H, Ross JJ. Long-term outcome in patients with inferior myocardial infarction and complete atrioventricular block. *J Am Coll Cardiol* 1988; 12:589–594.

389. McDonald K, O'Sullivan JJ, Conroy M, Robinson K, Mulcahy R. Heart block as predictor of in-hospital death in both acute inferior and acute anterior myocardial infarction. *Am J Med* 1990; 74:277–282.

390. Fisch GR, Zipes DP, Fisch C. Bundle branch block in sudden death. *Prog Cardiovasc Dis* 1980; 23:187–224.

391. Hindman MC, Wagner GS, JaRo M, Atkins JM, Scheinman MM, DeSanctis RW, et al. The clinical significance of bundle branch block complicating acute myocardial infarction: I. Clinical characteristics, hospital mortality, and one- year follow-up. *Circulation* 1978; 58:679–688.

392. Zoll PM, Zoll RH, Falk RH, Clinton JE, Eitel DR, Antman EM. External noninvasive temporary cardiac pacing: Clinical trials. *Circulation* 1985; 71:937–944.

393. Harthorne JW, Barold SS. Atherosclerosis, the conduction system, and cardiac pacing. In: Fuster V, Ross R, Topol EF, eds. *Atherosclerosis and Coronary Artery Disease*. Philadelphia: Lippincott-Raven; 1996.

394. Emergency Cardiac Care Committee and Subcomittees, American Heart Association. Guidelines for cardiopulmonary resuscitation and emergency cardiac care: III. Adult advanced cardiac life support. *JAMA* 1992; 268:2199–2241.

395. Wood MA. Temporary transvenous pacing. In: Ellenbogen KA, Kay GN, Wilkoff RL, eds. *Clinical Cardiac Pacing*. Philadelphia: Saunders; 1995:687–700.

396. Campbell RW, Murray A, Julian DG. Ventricular arrhythmias in first 12 hours of acute myocardial infarction: natural history study. *Br Heart J* 1981; 46:351–357.

397. Campbell RWF. Arrhythmias. In: Julian DG, Braunwald E, eds. *Management of Acute Myocardial Infarction*. London: Saunders; 1994:223–240.

398. Nordrehaug JE, von der Lippe G. Hypokalaemia and ventricular fibrillation in acute myocardial infarction. *Br Heart J* 1983; 50:525–529.

399. Higham PD, Adams PC, Murray A, Campbell RW. Plasma potassium, serum magnesium and ventricular fibrillation: A prospective study. *Q J Med* 1993; 86:609–617.

400. Antman EM, Berlin JA. Declining incidence of ventricular fibrillation in myocardial infarction: Implications for the prophylactic use of lidocaine. *Circulation* 1992; 86:764–773.

401. Behar S, Goldbourt U, Reicher-Reiss H, Kaplinsky E. prognosis of acute myocardial infarction complicated by primary ventricular fibrillation: Principal investigators of the SPRINT study. *Am J Cardiol* 1990; 66:1208–1211.

402. Reeder GS, Gersh BJ. Modern management of acute myocardial infarction. *Curr Probl Cardiol* 1996; 21:591–667.

403. Dhurandhar RW, MacMillan RL, Brown KW. Primary ventricular fibrillation complicating acute myocardial infarction. *Am J Cardiol* 1990; 66:1208–1211.

404. Lie KI, Wellens HJ, Durrer D. Characteristics and predictability of primary ventricular fibrillation. *Eur J Cardiol* 1974; 1:379–384.

405. Solomon SD, Ridker PM,Antman EM. Ventricular arrhythmias in trials of thrombolytic therapy for acute myocardial infarction: A meta-analysis. *Circulation* 1993; 88:2575–2581.

406. MacMahon S, Collins R, Peto R, Koster RW, Yusuf S. Effects of prophylactic lidociane in suspected acute myocardial infarction: An overview of results from the randomized controlled trials. *JAMA* 1992; 260:1910–1916.

407. Scheinman MM, Levine JH, Cannom DS, Friehling T, Kopelman HA, Chilson DA, et al. Dose-ranging study of intravenous amiodarone in patients with life-threatening ventricular tachyarrhythmias. *Circulation* 1995; 92:3264–3272.

408. Huey BL, Gheorghiade M, Crampton RS, et al. Acute non-Q wave myocardial infarction associated with early ST segment elevation: Evidence for spontaneous coronary reperfusion and implications for thrombolytic trials. *J Am Coll Cardiol* 1987; 9:18–25.

409. Chouhan L, Hajar HA, George T, et al. Non-Q-wave and Q-wave infarction after thrombolytic therapy with intravenous streptokinase for chest pain and anterior ST-segment elevation. *Am J Cardiol* 1991; 68:446–450.

410. DeWood MA, Stifter WF, Simpson CS, et al. Coronary arteriographic findings soon after non-Q-wave myocardial infarction. *N Engl J Med* 1986; 315:417–423.

411. Fuster V, Badimon L, Badimon JJ, Chesebro JH. The pathogenesis of coronary artery disease and the acute coronary syndromes (2). *N Engl J Med* 1992; 326:242–250, 310–318.

412. Decanay S, Kennedy HL, Uretz E, Parrillo JE, Klein LW. Morphological and quantitative angiographic analyses of progression of coronary stenoses: A comparison of Q-wave and non-Q-wave myocardial infarction. *Circulation* 1994; 90:1739–1746.

413. Kennedy JW. Non-Q-wave myocardial infarction. *N Engl J Med* 1986; 315:451–453.

414. Klein LW, Helfant RH. The Q-wave and non-Q-wave myocardial infarction: Differences and similarities. *Prog Cardiovasc Dis* 1986; 29:205–220.

415. Effects of tissue plasminogen activator and a comparison of early invasive and conservative strategies in unstable angina and non-Q-wave myocardial infarction: Results of the TIMI-IIIB trial. Thrombolysis in Myocardial Ischemia. *Circulation* 1994; 89:1545–1556.

416. Boden WE, Krone RJ, Oakes D, Greenberg H, Dwyer EM Jr, Miller JP, et al. Electrocardiographic subset analysis of diltiazem administration on long-term outcome after acute myocardial infarction. *Am J Cardiol* 1991; 67:335–342.

417. The Multicenter Diltiazem Postinfarction Trial Research Group. The effect of diltiazem on mortality and reinfarction after myocardial infarction. *N Engl J Med* 1988; 319:385–392.

418. Boden WE, Messerli FH, Hansen JF, Schechtman KB. Heart rate-lowering calcium channel blockers (diltiazem, verapamil) do not adversely affect long-term cardiac death or non-fatal infarction in post-infarction patients: Data pooled from 3 randomized, placebo-controlled clinical trials of 5,677 patients (abstr). *J Am Coll Cardiol* 1996; 27:319A.

419. Effect of verapamil on mortality and major events after acute myocardial infarction (the Danish Verapamil Infarction Trial II—DAVIT II). *Am J Cardiol* 1990; 66:779–785.

420. Verapamil in acute myocardial infarction: The Danish Study Group on Verapamil in Myocardial Infarction. *Eur Heart J* 1984; 5:516–528.

421. Gheorghiade M. Calcium channel blockers in the management of myocardial infarction patients. *Henry Ford Hosp Med J* 1991; 39:210–216.

422. Boden WE, Scheldewaert R, Walters EG, et al. Incomplete Infarction Trial of European Research Collaborators Evaluating Prognosis Post-Thrombolysis (diltiazem) (INTERCEPT) Research Group: Design of a placebo-controlled clinical trial of long-acting diltiazem and aspirin versus aspirin alone in patients receiving thrombolysis with a first acute myocardial infarction. *Am J Cardiol* 1995; 75:1120–1123.

423. Klimt CR, Knatterud GL, Stamler J, Meier P. Persantine-aspirin reinfarction study: Part II. Secondary coronary prevention with persantine and aspirin. *J Am Coll Cardiol* 1986; 7:251–269.

424. Roberts R. Preventing recurrent myocardial infarction: Use of calcium-channel blockers. *Postgrad Med* 1988; 83:249–256.

425. Gheorghiade M, Schultz L, Tilley B, Kao W, Goldstein S. Natural history of the first non-Q-wave myocardial infarction in the placebo arm of the Beta-Blocker Heart Attack Trial. *Am Heart J* 1991; 122:1548–1553.

426. Campbell RWF, Murray A, Julian DG. Ventricular arrhythmias and ventricular fibrillation in acute myocardial infarction. *Am J Cardiol* 1979; 45:462.

427. Tosteson ANA, Goldman L, Udvarhelyi, IS, Lee T. Cost-effectiveness of a coronary care unit versus an intermediate care unit for emergency department patients with chest pain. 1996; 94:143–150.

428. Tatum JL, Jesse RL, Kontos MC, et al. Comprehensive strategy for the evaluation and triage of the chest pain patient. *Ann Emerg Med* 1997; 27:1–6.

429. Chobanian AV, Lille RD, Tercyak A, Blevins P. The metabolic and hemodynamic effects of prolonged bed rest in normal subjects. *Circulation* 1974; 49:551–559.

430. Winslow EH. Cardiovascular consequences of bed rest. *Heart Lung* 1985; 14:236–246.

431. Metzger BL, Therrien B. Effect of position on cardiovascular response during the Valsalva maneuver. *Nurs Res* 1990; 39:198–202.

432. Taggart P, Sutton P, John R, Lab M, Swanton H. Monophasic action potential recordings during acute changes in ventricular loading induced by the Valsalva manoeuvre. *Br Heart J* 1992; 67:221–229.

433. Dixon RA, Edwards IR, Pilcher J. Diazepam in immediate post-myocardial infarct period: A double blind trial. *Br Heart J* 1980; 43:535–540.

434. Thompson DR, Meddis R. A prospective evaluation of in-hospital counselling for first time myocardial infarction in men. *J Psychosom Res* 1990; 34:237–248.

435. Duryee R. The efficacy of inpatient education after myocardial infarction. *Heart Lung* 1992; 21:217–225.

436. Fletcher V. An individualized teaching programme following primary uncomplicated myocardial infarction. *J Adv Nurs* 1987; 12:195–200.

437. Dracup K, Moser DK, Guzy PM, Taylor SE, Marsden C. Is cardiopulmonary resuscitation training deleterious for family members of cardiac patients? *Am J Public Health* 1994; 84:116–118.

438. Myerburg RJ, Kessler KM, Castellanos A. Sudden cardiac death: Epidemiology, transient risk, and intervention assessment. *Ann Intern Med* 1993; 119:1187–1197.

439. Pfeffer MA, Lamas GA, Vaughan DE, Parisi AF, Braunwald E. Effect of captopril on progressive ventricular dilatation after anterior myocardial infarction. *N Engl J Med* 1988; 319:80–86.

440. Pfeffer MA, Braunwald E, Moye LA, Basta, Brown EJ Jr, Cuddy TE. Effect of captopril on mortality and morbidity in patients with left ventricular dysfunction after myocardial infarction: Results of the survival and ventricular enlargement trial. The SAVE Investigators. *N Engl J Med* 1992; 327:669–677.

441. The SOLVD Investigators. Effect of enalapril on survival in patients with reduced left ventricular ejection fractions and congestive heart failure. *N Engl J Med* 1991; 325:293–302.

442. Latini R, Maggioni AP, Flather M, Sleight P, Tognoni G. ACE-inhibitor use in patients with myocardial infarction: Summary of evidence from clinical trials. *Circulation* 1995; 92:3132–3137.

443. Sigurdsson A, Swedberg K. Left ventricular remodelling, neurohormonal activation and early treatment with enalapril (CONSENSUS II) following myocardial infarction. *Eur Heart J* 1994; 15(suppl B):14–19.

444. The Acute Infarction Ramipril Efficacy (AIRE) Study Investigators. Effect of ramipril on mortality and morbidity of survivors of acute myocardial infarction with clinical evidence of heart failure. *Lancet* 1993; 342:821–828.

445. Kober L, Torp-Pedersen C, Carlsem JE, et al. A clinical trial of the angiotensin-converting enzyme inhibitor trandolapril in patients with left ventricular dysfunction after myocardial infarction. *N Engl J Med* 1995; 333:1670–1676.

446. Turlapaty P, Altura BM. Magnesium deficiency produces spasms of coronary arteries: Relationship to etiology of sudden death ischemic heart disease. *Science* 1980; 208:198–200.

447. Adams JH, Mitchell JRA. The effect of agents which modify platelet behaviour and of magnesium ions on thrombus formation in vivo. *Thromb Haemost* 1979; 42:603–610.

448. Watanabe Y, Dreifus LS. Electrophysiological effects of magnesium and its interactions with potassium. *Cardiovasc Res* 1972; 6:79–88.

449. Vormann J, Fischer G, Classen HG, Thoni H. Influence of decreased and increased magnesium supply on the cardiotoxic effects of epinephrine in rats. *Arzneimittelforschung* 1983; 33:205–210.

450. Teo KK, Yusuf S, Collins R, Held PH, Peto R. Effects of intravenous magnesium in suspected acute myocardial infarction: overview of randomised trials. *BMJ* 1991; 303:1499–1503.

451. Antman EM, Lau J, Kupelnick B, Mosteller F, Chalmers TC. A comparison of results of meta-analyses of randomized control trials and recommendations of clinical experts: Treatments for myocardial infarction. *JAMA* 1992; 268:240–248.

452. Woods KL, Fletcher S, Roffe C, Haider Y. Intravenous magnesium sulphate in suspected acute myocardial infarction: Results of the second Leicester Intravenous Magnesium Intervention Trial (LIMIT-2). *Lancet* 1992; 339:1553–1558.

453. Woods KL, Fletcher S. Long-term outcome after intravenous magnesium sulphate in suspected acute myocardial infarction: The second Leicester Intravenous Magnesium Intervention Trial (LIMIT-2). *Lancet* 1994; 343:816–819.

454. Antman EM. Magnesium in acute MI: Timing is critical. *Circulation* 1995; 92:2367–2372.

455. Antman EM. Randomized trials of magnesium in acute myocardial infarction: Big numbers do not tell the whole story. *Am J Cardiol* 1995; 75:391–393.

456. Shechter M, Hod H, Chouraqui P, Kaplinsky E, Rabinowitz B. Magnesium therapy in acute myocardial infarction when patients are not candidates for thromblytic therapy. *Am J Cardiol* 1995; 75:321–323.

457. Gheorghiade M, Anderson J, Rosman H, et al. Risk identification at the time of admission to coronary care unit in patients with suspected myocardial infarction. *Am Heart J* 1988; 116:1212–1217.

458. Pozen MW, Stechmiller JK, Voigt GC. Prognosis efficacy of early clinical categorization of myocardial infarction patients. *Circulation* 1977; 56:816–819.

459. Krone RJ. The role of risk stratification in the early management of a myocardial infarction. *Ann Intern Med* 1992; 116:223–237.

460. Kloner RA, Parisi AF. Acute myocardial infarction: Diagnostic and prognostic applications of two-dimensional echocardiography. *Circulation* 1987; 75:521–524.

461. Hopkins LE, Crabbe SJ, Chase SL. Use of a proprietary database to examine lengths of hospital stay of patients who received drug therapy for acute myocardial infarction. *Am J Hosp Pharm* 1989; 46:957–961.

462. Topol EJ, Burek K, O'Neill WW, et al. A randomized controlled trial of hospital discharge three days after myocardial infarction in the era of reperfusion. *N Engl J Med* 1988; 318:1083–1088.

463. Mark DB, Sigmon K, Topol EJ, et al. Identification of acute myocardial infarction patients suitable for early hospital discharge after aggressive interventional therapy: Results from the Thrombolysis and Angioplasty in Acute Myocardial Infarction Registry. *Circulation* 1991; 83:1186–1193.

464. Newby LK, Califf RM, Guerci A, et al. Early discharge in the thrombolytic era: An analysis of criteria for uncomplicated infarction from the Global Utilization of Streptokinase and t-PA for Occluded Coronary Arteries (GUSTO) trial. *J Am Coll Cardiol* 1996; 27:625–632.

465. Bosch X, Theroux P, Waters DD, Pelletier GB, Roy D. Early postinfarction ischemia: Clinical, angiographic, and prognostic significance. *Circulation* 1987; 5:988–995.

466. Oliva PB, Hammill SC. The clinical distinction between regional postinfarction pericarditis and other causes of postinfarction chest pain: Ancillary observations regarding the effect of lytic therapy upon the frequency of postinfarction pericarditis, postinfarction angina, and reinfarction. *Clin Cardiol* 1994; 17:471–478.

467. Kudenchuk PJ, Ho MT, Weaver WD, et al. Accuracy of computer-interpreted electrocardiography in selecting patients for thrombolytic therapy: MITI Project Investigators. *J Am Coll Cardiol* 1991; 17:1486–1491.

468. Rothbaum DA, Linnemeier TJ, Landin RJ, et al. Emergency percutaneous transluminal coronary angioplasty in acute myocardial infarction: A 3 year experience. *J Am Coll Cardiol* 1987; 10:264–272.

469. Ferguson JJ, Diver DJ, Boldt M, Pasternak RC. Significance of nitroglycerin-induced hypotension with inferior wall acute myocardial infarction. *Am J Cardiol* 1989; 64:311–314.

470. Cragg DR, Friedman HZ, Bonema JD, et al. Outcome of patients with acute myocardial infarction who are ineligible for thrombolytic therapy. *Ann Intern Med* 1991; 115:173–177.

471. Gibson RS, Young PM, Boden WE, Schechtman K, Roberts R, and the Diltiazem Reinfarction Study Group. Prognostic significance and beneficial effect of diltiazem on the incidence of early recurrent ischemia after non-Q-wave myocardial infarction: Results of the Diltiazem Reinfarction Study. *Am J Cardiol* 1987; 60:203–209.

472. Schechtman KB, Capone RJ, Kleiger RE, Gibson RS, Schwartz DJ, Roberts R, et al. Differential risk patterns associated with 3 month as compared with 3 to 12 month mortality and reinfarction after non-Q-wave myocardial infarction. The Diltiazem Reinfarction Study Group. *J Am Coll Cardiol* 1990; 15:940–947.

473. Thanavaro S, Krone RJ, Kleiger RE, et al. In-hospital prognosis of patients with first nontransmural and transmural infarctions. *Circulation* 1980; 61:29–33.

474. Loop FD, Lytle BW, Cosgrove DM, et al. Reoperation for coronary atherosclerosis: Changing practice in 2509 consecutive patients. *Ann Surg* 1990; 212:378–385.

475. Krainin FM, Flessas AP, Spodick DH. Infarction-associated pericarditis: Rarity of diagnosis electrocardiogram. *N Engl J Med* 1984; 311:1211–1214.

476. Thadani U, Chopra MP, Aber CP. Pericarditis after acute myocardial infarction. *Br Med J* 1971; 2:135–137.

477. Erhardt LR. Clinical and pathological observation in different types of acute myocardial infarction: A study of 84 patients deceased after treatment in a coronary care unit. *Acta Med Scand* 1974; 560:1–78.

478. Tofler GH, Muller JE, Stone PH, et al. Pericarditis in acute myocardial infarction: Characterization and clinical significance. *Am Heart J* 1989; 117:86–92.

479. Wall TC, Califf RM, Harrelson-Woodlief L, et al. Usefulness of a pericardial friction rub after thrombolytic therapy during acute myocardial infarction in predicting amount of myocardial damage: The TAMI Study Group. *Am J Cardiol* 1990; 66:1418–1421.

480. Barman PC, Krishnaswami V, Geraci AR. Pericarditis in acute myocardial infarction. *NYS J Med* 1973; 73:645–648.

481. Guillevin L, Valere PE. Pericarditis in acute myocardial infarction. *Lancet* 1976; 1:429.

482. Berman J, Haffajee CI, Alpert JS. Therapy of symptomatic pericarditis after myocardial infarction: Retrospective and prospective studies of aspirin, indomethacin, prednisone, and spontaneous resolution. *Am Heart J* 1981; 101:750–753.

483. Lilavie CJ, Gersh PJ. Mechanical and electrical complication of acute myocardial infarction. *Mayo Clin Proc* 1990; 65:709–730.

484. Hammerman H, Schoen FJ, Braunwald E, Kloner RA. Drug-induced expansion of infarct: Morphologic and functional correlations. *Circulation* 1984; 69:611–617.

485. Bulkley BH, Roberts WC. Steroid therapy during acute myocardial infarction: A cause of delayed healing of ventricular aneurysm. *Am J Med* 1974; 56:244–250.

486. Kloner RA, Fishbein MC, Lew H, Maroko PR, Braunwald E. Mummification of the infarcted myocardium by high dose corticosteriods. *Circulation* 1978; 57:56–63.

487. Shahar A, Hod H, Barabash GM, Kaplinsky E, Motro M. Disappearance of a syndrome: Dressler's syndrome in the era of thrombolysis. *Cardiology* 1994, 85:255–258.

488. Dressler W. The post-myocardial-infarction syndrome. *Arch Intern Med* 1959; 103:28–42.

489. Kossowsky WA, Epstein PJ, Levine RS. Post myocardial infarction syndrome: An early complication of acute myocardial infarction. *Chest* 1973; 63:35–39.

490. McKay RG, Pfeffer MA, Pasternak RC, Markis JE, Come PC, Nakao S, et al. Left ventricular remodeling after myocardial infarction: A corollary to infarct expansion. *Circulation* 1986; 74:693–702.

491. Forrester JS, Wyatt HL, da Luz PL, Tyberg JV, Diamond GA, Swan HJC. Functional significance of regional ischemic contraction abnormalities. *Circulation* 1976; 54:64–70.

492. Aroesty JM, McKay RG, Heller GV, Royal HC, Als AV, Grossman W. Simultaneous assessment of left ventricular systolic and diastolic dysfunction during pacing-induced ischemia. *Circulation* 1985; 71:889–900.

493. Tyberg JV, Forrester JS, Wyatt HL, Goldner SJ, Parmley WW, Swan HJC. An analysis of segmental ischemic dysfunction utilizing the pressure-length loop. *Circulation* 1974; 49:748–754.

494. Weisman HF, Healey B. Myocardial infarct expansion, infarct extension, and reinfarction: Pathophysiologic concepts. *Prog Cardiovasc Dis* 1987; 30:73–110.

495. Page DL, Caulfield JB, Kastor JA, DeSanctis RW, Sanders CA. Myocardial changes associated with cardiogenic shock. *N Engl J Med* 1971; 285:133–137.

496. Alonso DR, Scheidt S, Post M, Killip T. Pathophysiology of cardiogenic shock: Quantification of myocardial necrosis, clinical, pathologic and electrocardiographic correlations. *Circulation* 1973; 48:588–596.

497. Harnarayan C, Bennett MA, Pentecost BL, Brewer DB. Quantitative study of infarcted myocardium in cardiogenic shock. *Br Heart J* 1970; 32:728–732.

498. Rigaud M, Rocha P, Boschat J, Farcot JC, Bardet J, Bourdarias JP. Regional left ventricular function assessed by contrast angiography in acute myocardial infarction. *Circulation* 1979; 60:130–139.

499. Marmor A, Geltman EM, Biello DR, Sobel BE, Siegel BA, Roberts R. Functional response of the right ventricle to myocardial infarction: Dependence on the site of left ventricular infarction. *Circulation* 1981; 64:1005–1011.

500. Wackers FJT, Lie KI, Sokole EB, Res J, Van der Schoot B, Durrer D. Prevalence of right ventricular involvement in inferior wall infarction assessed with thallium 201 and technetium 99m pyrophosphate. *Am J Cardiol* 1978; 42:358–362.

501. Rigo P, Murray M, Taylor DR, Weisfeldt ML, Kelly DT, Strauss HW, et al. Right ventricular dysfunction detected by gated scintiphotography in patients with acute inferior myocardial infarction. *Circulation* 1975; 52:268–274.

502. Zehender M, Kasper W, Kauder E, et al. Right ventricular infarction as an independent predictor of prognosis after acute inferior myocardial infarction. *N Engl J Med* 1993; 328:981–988.

503. Berger PB, Ryan TJ. Inferior myocardial infarction: High-risk subgroups. *Circulation* 1990; 81:401–411.

504. Andersen HR, Falk E, Nielsen D. Right ventricular infarction: Frequency, size and topography in coronary heart disease: A prospective study comprising 107 consecutive autopsies from a coronary care unit. *J Am Coll Cardiol* 1987; 10:1223–1232.

505. Lee FA. Hemodynamics of the right ventricle in normal and diseased states. *Cardiol Clin* 1992; 10:59–67.

506. Cross CE. Right ventricular pressure and coronary flow. *Am J Physiol* 1962; 202:12–16.

507. Haupt HM, Hutchins GM, Moore GW. Right ventricular infarction: Role of the moderator band artery in determining infarct size. *Circulation* 1983; 67:1268–1272.

508. Setaro JF, Cabin HS. Right ventricular infarction. *Cardiol Clin* 1992; 10:69–90.

509. Goldstein JA, Barzilai B, Rosamond TL, Eisenberg PR, Jaffe AS. Determinants of hemodynamic compromise with severe right ventricular infarction. *Circulation* 1990; 82:359–368.

510. Goldstein JA, Tweddell JS, Barzilai B, Yagi Y, Jaffe AS, Cox JL. Importance of left ventricular function and systolic ventricular interaction to right ventricular performance during acute right heart ischemia. *J Am Coll Cardiol* 1992; 19:704–711.

511. Dell'Italia LJ, Starling MR, Crawford MH, Boros BL, Chaudhuri TK, O'Rourke RA. Right ventricular infarction: Identification by hemodynamic measurements before and after volume loading and correlation with noninvasive techniques. *J Am Coll Cardiol* 1984; 4:931–939.

512. Cohn JN, Guiha NH, Broder MI, Limas CJ. Right ventricular infarction: Clinical and hemodynamic features. *Am J Cardiol* 1974; 33:209–214.

513. Wellens H. Right ventricular infarction (editorial). *N Engl J Med* 1993; 328:1036–1038.

514. Manno BV, Bemis CE, Carver J, Mintz GS. Right ventricular infarction complicated by right to left shunt. *J Am Coll Cardiol* 1983; 1:554–557.

515. Braat SH, DeZwaan C, Brugada P, Coenegracht JM, Wellens HJ. Right ventricular involvement with acute inferior wall myocardial infarction identifies high risk of developing atrioventricular nodal conduction disturbances. *Am Heart J* 1984; 107:1183–1187.

516. Love JC, Haffajee CI, Gore JM, Alpert JS. Reversibility of hypotension and shock by atrial or atrioventricular sequential pacing in patients with right ventricular infarction. *Am Heart J* 1984; 108:5–13.

517. Sugiura T, Iwasaka T, Takahashi N, et al. Atrial fibrillation in inferior wall Q-wave acute myocardial infarction. *Am J Cardiol* 1991; 67:1135–1136.

518. Braat SH, Ramentol M, Halders S, Wellens HJ. Reperfusion with streptokinase of an occluded right coronary artery: Effects on early and late right and left ventricular ejection fraction. *Am Heart J* 1987; 113:257–260.

519. Schuler G, Hofmann M, Schwarz F, et al. Effect of successful thrombolytic therapy on right ventricular function in acute inferior wall myocardial infarction. *Am J Cardiol* 1984; 54:951–957.

520. Moreyra AE, Suh C, Porway MN, Kostis JB. Rapid hemodynamic improvement in right ventricular infarction after coronary angioplasty. *Chest* 1988; 94:197–199.

521. Griffin J, Grines CL, Marsalese D, et al. A prospective, randomized trial evaluating the prophylactic use of balloon pumping in high risk myocardial infarction patients: PAMI-2 (abstr). *J Am Coll Cardiol* 1995; 25:86A.

522. Parmley WW, Chuck L, Chatterjee K, Swan HJ, Klausner C, Glantz SA. Acute changes in the diastolic pressure-volume relationship of the left ventricle. *Eur J Cardiol* 1976; 4:105–120.

523. Smiseth OA, Rufsum H, Junemann J, Sievers RE, Lipton MJ, Carlsson E, et al. Ventricular diastolic pressure-volume shifts during acute ischemic left ventricular function in dogs. *J Am Coll Cardiol* 1984; 3:966.

524. Dikshit K, Vyden JK, Forrester JS, Chatterjee K, Prakash R, Swan HJC. Renal and extrarenal hemodynamic effects of furosemide in congestion heart failure after acute myocardial infarction. *N Engl J Med* 1973; 288:1087–1090.

525. Biddle TL, Yu PN. Effect of furosemide on hemodynamics and lung water in acute pulmonary edema secondary to myocardial infarction. *Am J Cardiol* 1979; 43:86.

526. Kiel J, Kelly DT, Taylor DR, Pitt B. The role of furosemide in the treatment of left ventricular dysfunction associated with acute myocardial infarction. *Circulation* 1973; 48:581.

527. Goldstein RA, Passamani ER, Roberts R. A comparison of digoxin and dobutamine in patients with acute infarction and failure. *N Engl J Med* 1980; 303:846–850.

528. Gillespie TA, Ambos HD, Sobel BE, Roberts R. Effects of dobutamine in patients with acute myocardial infarction. *Am J Cardiol* 1977; 39:588–594.

529. Kahn JC, Gueret P, Menier R, Giraudet P, Farhat MB, Bourdarias JP. Prognostic value of enzymatic (CPK) estimation of infarct size. *J Mol Med* 1977; 2:223–231.

530. Killip T, Kimball JT. Treatment of myocardial infarction in a coronary care unit: A two year experience with 250 patients. *Am J Cardiol* 1967; 20:457.

531. Forrester JS, Diamond GA, Chatterjee K, Swan HJ. Medical therapy of acute myocardial infarction by application of hempdynamic subsets (first of two parts). *N Engl J Med* 1976; 295:1356–1362.

532. Forrester JS, Diamond GA, Chatterjee K, Swan HJ. Medical therapy of acult myocardial infarction by application of hemodynamic subsets (second to two parts). *N Engl J Med* 1976; 295:1404–1413.

533. Rackley CE, Satler LF, Pearle DL, Del Negro AA, Pallas RS, Kent KM. Use of hemodynamics measurements for management of acute myocardial infarction. *Cardiovasc Clin* 1976; 16:3–15.

534. Cohn JN, Franciosa JA, Francis GS, Archibald D, Tristani F, Fletcher R, et al. Effect of short-term infusion of sodium nitroprusside on mortality rate in acute myocardial infarction complicated by left ventricular failure. *N Engl J Med* 1982; 306:1129–1135.

535. Roberts R, Ambos D. Evaluation of dobutamine in patients with cardiac failure and acute myocardial infarction. In: *International Dobutamine Symposium*. Munich, Urban & Schwarzenberg. 1980:208–216.

536. Clark G, Strauss HD, Roberts R. Dobutamine versus furosemide in the treatment of cardiac failure due to right ventricular function. *Chest* 1980; 77:220–223.

536a. Roberts R. Inotropic therapy for cardiac failure associated with acute myocardial infarction. *Chest* 1988; 93:22S–24S.

537. Young JB, Roberts R. Heart failure. In: Dirks JH, Sutton RAI, eds. *Diuretics: Physiology, Pharmacology and Clinical Use.* Philadelphia: Saunders; 1986:151–167.

538. Schreiber TL, Miller DH, Zola B. Management of myocardial infarction shock: Current status. *Am Heart J* 1989; 117:435–443.

539. Hill NS, Antman EM, Green LH, Alpert JS. Intravenous nitroglycerin: A review of pharmacology, indications, therapeutic effects and complications. *Chest* 1981; 79:69–76.

540. Wackers FJ, Lie KI, Becker AE, Durrer D, Wellens HJ. Coronary artery disease in patients dying from cardiogenic shock or congestive heart failure in the setting of acute myocardial infarction. *Br Heart J* 1976; 38:906–910.

541. Cercek B, Shah PK. Complicated acute myocardial infarction: Heart failure, shock, mechanical complications. *Cardiol Clin* 1991; 9:569–593.

542. Gutovitz AL, Sobel BE, Roberts R. The progressive nature of myocardial injury in selected patients with cardiogenic shock. *Am J Cardiol* 1978; 41:469–475.

543. Goldberg LI. Cardiovascular and renal actions of dopamine: Potential clinical application. *Pharmacol Rev* 1972; 21:1–29.

544. Gunnar R, Mond Loeb HS. Shock in acute myocardial infarction: Evaluation of physiologic therapy. *J Am Coll Cardiol* 1983; 1:154–163.

545. Mikulic E, Cohn JN, Franciosa JA. Comparative hemodynamic effects of inotropic and vasodilator drugs in severe heart failure. *Circulation* 1977; 56:528–533.

546. Miller RR, Awan NA, Joyce JA, Maxwell KS, DeMaria AN, Amsterdam EA, et al. Combined dopamine and nitroprusside therapy in congestive heart failure. *Circulation* 1977; 5:881–884.

547. Richard C, Ricome JL, Rimailho A, Bottineau G, Auzepy P. Combined hemodynamic effects of dopamine and dobutamine in cardiogenic shock. *Circulation* 1983; 67:620–626.

548. Lee L, Erbel R, Brown TM, Laufer N, Meyer J, O'Neill WW. Multicenter registry of angioplasty therapy of cardiogenic shock: Initial and long-term survival. *J Am Coll Cardiol* 1991; 17:599–603.

549. Waller BF, Rothbaum DA, Pinkerton CA, Cowley MJ, Linnemeier TJ, Orr C, et al. States of the myocardium and infarct-related coronary artery in 19 necropsy patients with acute recanalization using pharmacologic (streptokinase, recombinant tissue plasminogen activator), mechanical (percutaneous transluminal coronary angioplasty) or combined types of reperfusion therapy. *J Am Coll Cardiol* 1987; 9:785–801.

550. Brodie BR, Weintraub RA, Stuckey TD, LeBauer EJ, Katz JD, Kelly TA, et al. Outcomes of direct coronary angioplasty for acute myocardial infarction in candidates and noncandidates for thrombolytic therapy. *Am J Cardiol* 1991; 67:7–12.

551. Wei JY, Hutchins GM, Buckley BH. Papillary muscle rupture in fatal acute myocardial infarction: A potentially treatable form of cardiogenic shock. *Ann Intern Med* 1979; 90:149–152.

552. Nishimura RA, Schoff HV, Shub C, Gersh BJ, Edwards WD, Tajik AJ. Papillary muscle rupture complicating acute myocardial infarction: Analysis of 17 patients. *Am J Cardiol* 1983; 51:373–377.

553. Kossowsky WA, Epstein PJ, Levine RS. Post myocardial infarction syndrome: An early complication of acute myocardial infarction. *Chest* 1973; 63:35–39.

554. Lie JT, Wright KE Jr, Titus JL. Sudden appearance of a systolic murmur after acute myocardial infarction. *Am Heart J* 1975; 90:507–512.

555. Shelburne JC, Rubinstein D, Gorlin R. A reappraisal of papillary muscle dysfunction: Correlative clinical and angiographic study. *Am J Med* 1969; 46:862–871.

556. DeBusk RF, Harrison DC. The clinical spectrum of papillary-muscle disease. *N Engl J Med* 1969; 281:1458–1467.

557. Burch GE, DePasquale NP, Phillips JH. The syndrome of papillary muscle dysfunction. *Am Heart J* 1968; 75:399–414.

558. Radford MJ, Johnson RA, Daggett WM, Fallon JT, Buckley MJ, Gold HK, et al. Ventricular septal rupture: A review of clinical and physiologic features and an analysis of survival. *Circulation* 1981; 64:545–553.

559. Rasmussen S, Leth A, Kjoller E, Pedersen A. Cardiac rupture in acute myocardial infarction: A review of 72 consecutive cases. *Acta Med Scand* 1979; 205:11–16.

560. Maker JF, Mallory GK, Laurenz GA. Rupture of the heart after myocardial infarction. *N Engl J Med* 1956; 255:1–10.

561. Held AC, Cole, PL, Lipton B, Gore JM, Antman EM, Hochman JS, et al. Rupture of the interventricular septum complicating acute myocardial infarction: A multicenter analysis of clinical findings and outcome. *Am Heart J* 1988; 116:1330–1336.

562. Gaudiani VA, Miller DG, Stinson EB, Oyer PE, Reitz BA, Moreno-Cabral RJ, et al. Postinfarction ventricular septal defect: An argument for early operation. *Surgery* 1981; 89:48–54.

563. Gray RJ, Sethna D, Matloff JM. The role of cardiac surgery in acute myocardial infarction: I. With mechanical complications. *Am Heart J* 1983; 106:723–728.

564. Moore CA, Nygard TW, Kaiser DS, Cooper AA, Gibson RS. Postinfarction ventricular septal rupture: The importance of location of infarction and right ventricular function in determining survival. *Circulation* 1986; 74:45–55.

565. Bates RJ, Beutler S, Resnekor L, Anagnostopoulos CE. Cardiac rupture —Challenge in diagnosis and management. *Am J Cardiol* 1970; 40:429–437.

565a. Roberts WG, Morrow AG. Pseudoaneurysm of the left ventricle: An unusual sequel of myocardial infarction and rupture of the heart. *Am J Med* 1967; 43:639–644.

566. Cabin HS, Roberts WC. Left ventricular aneurysm, intraaneurysmal thrombus and systemic embolus in coronary heart disease. *Chest* 1980; 77:586–589.

567. Hayes MJ, Morris GK, Hampton JR. Lack of effect of bed rest and cigarette smoking on development of deep venous thrombus after myocardial infarction. *Br Heart J* 1976; 38:981–983.

568. Miller RR, Lies JE, Carretta RF, Wampold DB, DeNardo GL, Kraus JF, et al. Prevention of lower extremity venous thrombus by early mobilization. *Ann Intern Med* 1976; 84:700–703.

569. Emerson PA, Marks P. Preventing thromboembolism after myocardial infarction: Effect of low-dose heparin or smoking. *Br Med J* 1977; 1:18–20.

570. Weinreich DJ, Burke JF, Pauletto FJ. Left ventricular mural thrombi complicating acute myocardial infarction. *Ann Intern Med* 1984; 100:789–794.

571. Visser CA, Kan G, Meltzer RS, Dunning AJ, Roelandt J. Embolic potential of left ventricular thrombus after myocardial infarction: A two-dimensional echocardiographic study of 119 patients. *J Am Coll Cardiol* 1985; 5:1276–1280.

572. Kouvaras G, Chronopoulas G, Soufras G, Sofronas G, Solomos D, Bakirtzis A, et al. The effects of long term antithrombotic treatment of left ventricular thrombi in patients after an acute myocardial infarction. *Am Heart J* 1990; 119:73–78.

573. Keating EC, Gross SA, Schlamowitz RA, Glassman J, Maxur HJ, Pitt WA, et al. Mural thrombi in myocardial infarctions: Prospective evaluation by two dimensional echocardiography. *Am J Med* 1983; 74:989–995.

574. Spirito P, Bellotti P, Chiarella F. Prognostic significance and natural history of left ventricular thrombi in patients with acute anterior myocardial infarction: A two-dimensional echocardiographic study. *Circulation* 1985; 72:774–780.

575. Jugdutt BI, Sivaram CA. Prospective two-dimensional echocardiographic evaluation of left ventricular thrombus and embolism after acute myocardial infarction. *J Am Coll Cardiol* 1989; 13:554–564.

576. Johannssen KA, Nordrehoug JE, Vonder Lippe G, Vollset SE. Risk factors for embolization in patients with left ventricular thrombi and acute myocardial infarction. *Br Heart J* 1988; 60:104–110.

577. Visser CA, Kan G, Meltzer RS, Dunning AJ, Roelandt J. Embolic potential of left ventricular thrombus after myocardial infarction: A two-dimensional echocardiographic study of 119 patients. *J Am Coll Cardiol* 1985; 5:1276–1280.

578. Davis MJE, Ireland MA. Effect of early anticoagulation on the frequency of left ventricular thrombi after anterior wall acute myocardial infarction. *Am J Cardiol* 1986; 57:1244–1247.

579. Lapeyre AC III, Steele PM, Kazmier FJ, Chesebro JH, Vlietstra RE, Fuster V. Systemic embolism in chronic left ventricular aneurysm: Incidence and the role of anticoagulation. *J Am Coll Cardiol* 1985; 6:534–538.

580. Turpie ACG, Robinson JG, Doyle DJ, Mulji AS, Mishkel GJ, Sealey BJ, et al. Comparison of high-dose with low-dose subcutaneous heparin to prevent left ventricular mural thrombosis in patients with acute transmural anterior myocardial infarction. *N Engl J Med* 1989; 320:352–357.

581. Takamoto T, Kim D, Urie PM, Guthaner DF, Gordon HJ, Keren A, et al. Comparative recognition of left ventricular thrombi by echocardiography and cineangiography. *Br Heart J* 1985; 53:36–42.

582. Sechtem U, Theissen P, Heindel W, Hungerberg K, Deutsch HJ, Welslau R, et al. Diagnosis of left ventricular thrombi by magnetic resonance imaging and comparison with angiocardiography, computed tomography and echocardiography. *Am J Cardiol* 1989; 64:1195–1199.

583. Faxon DP, Ryan TJ, Davis KB, McCabe CH, Myers W, Lesperance J, et al. Prognostic significance of angiographically documented left ventricular aneurysm from the coronary artery surgery study (CASS). *Am J Cardiol* 1982; 50:157–164.

584. Loop FD, Effler DB, Webster JS, Groves LK. Posterior ventricular aneurysms: Etiologic factors and surgical treatment. *N Engl J Med* 1973; 288:237–239.

585. Loop FD, Effler DB, Navia JA, Sheldon WC, Groves LK. Aneurysms of the left ventricle: Survival and results of a ten-year surgical experience. *Ann Surg* 1973; 178:399–405.

586. Catherwood E, Mintz GS, Kotler MN, Parry WR, Segal BL. Two-dimensional echocardiographic recognition of left ventricular pseudoaneurysm. *Circulation* 1980; 62:294–303.

587. Martin RH, Almond CH, Saab S, Watson LE. True and false aneurysms of the left ventricle following myocardial infarction. *Am J Med* 1977; 62:418–424.

588. Liberthson RR, Salisbury KW, Hutter AM, DeSanctis RW. Atrial tachyarrhythmias in acute myocardial infarction. *Am J Med* 1976; 60:956–960.

589. Zoni-Berisso M, Carratino L, Ferroni A, Mel GS, Mazzotta G, Vecchio C. Frequency, characteristics and significance of supraventricular tachyarrhythmias detected by 24-hour electrocardiographic recording in the late hospital phase of acute myocardial infarction. *Am J Cardiol* 1990; 65:1064–1070.

590. Gordon S, Finck DR, Perera RD, Levine J, Barne SJ. Atrial infarction complicating an acute inferior myocardial infarction. *Arch Intern Med* 1984; 144:193.

591. Nielsen FE, Andersen HH, Gram-Hansen P, Sorensen JT, Klausen IC. The relationship between ECG signs of atrial infarction and the development of supraventricular arrhythmias in patients with acute myocardial infarction. *Am Heart J* 1992; 123:69–72.

592. James TN. Myocardial infarction and atrial arrhythmias. *Circulation* 1961; 24:761–776.

593. Goldberg RJ, Seeley D, Becker RC, Chen ZY, Osganian V, Gore JM, et al. Impact of atrial fibrillation on the in-hospital and long-term survival of patients with acute myocardial infarction: A community-wide perspective. *Am Heart J* 1990; 119:996–1001.

594. Nielsen FE, Sorensen HT, Christensen JH, Ravn L, Rasmussen SE. Reduced occurrence of atrial fibrillation in acute myocardial infarction treated with streptokinase. *Eur Heart J* 1991; 12:1081–1083.

595. Behar S, Zahavi Z, Goldbourt U, Reicher-Reiss H. Long-term prognosis of patients with paroxysmal atrial fibrillation complicating acute

myocardial infarction: SPRINT Study Group. *Eur Heart J* 1992; 13:45–50.

596. Konecke LL, Knoebel SB. Nonparoxysmal junctional tachycardia complicating acute myocardial infarction. *Circulation* 1972; 45:367–374.

597. Meltzer LE, Cohen HE. The incidence of arrhythmias associated with acute myocardial infarction. In: Meltzer LE, Dunning AJ, eds. *Textbook of Coronary Care*. Philadelphia: Charles Press; 1972.

598. Nicod P, Gilpin E, Dittrich H, Polikar R, Henning H, Ross J Jr. Long-term outcome in patients with inferior myocardial infarction and complete atrioventricular block. *J Am Coll Cardiol* 1988; 12:589–594.

599. Kostuk WJ, Beanlands DS. Complete heart block associated with acute myocardial infarction. *Am J Cardiol* 1970; 26:380–384.

600. Hindman MC, Wagner GS, JaRo M, Atkins JM, Scheinman MM, DeSanctis RW, et al. The clinical significance of bundle branch block complicating acute myocardial infarction: Clinical characteristics, hospital mortality, and one-year follow-up. *Circulation* 1978; 58:679–688.

601. Hindman MC, Wagner GS, JaRo M, Atkins JM, Scheinman MM, DeScantis RW, et al. The clinical significance of bundle branch block complicating acute myocardial infarction: Indications for temporary and permanent pacemaker insertion. *Circulation* 1978; 58:689–699.

602. American College of Cardiology/American Heart Association Task Force: Guidelines for the early management of patients with acute myocardial infarction. *Circulation* 1990; 82:664–707.

603. Dreifus LS, Fisch C, Griffin JC, Gillette PC, Mason JW, Parsonnet V. Guidelines for implantation of cardiac pacemakers and antiarrhythmia devices: A report of the American College of Cardiology/American Heart Association Task Force on Assessment of Diagnostic and Therapeutic Cardiovascular Procedures (Committee on Pacemaker Implantation). *J Am Coll Cardiol* 1991; 18:1–13.

604. Goble AJ, Sloman G, Robinson JS. Mortality reduction in a coronary care unit. *Br Med J* 1966; 1:1005–1009.

605. Graboys TB. In-hospital sudden death after coronary care unit discharge: A high risk profile. *Arch Intern Med* 1975; 135:512–514.

606. Grace WJ, Yarvote PM. Acute myocardial infarction: The course of the illness following discharge from the coronary care unit. A description of the intermediate coronary care unit. *Chest* 1971; 59:15–17.

607. Christensen D, Ford M, Reading J, Castle CH. Sudden death in the late hospital phase of acute myocardial infarction. *Arch Intern Med* 1977; 137:1675–1679.

608. Frieden J, Cooper JA. The role of the intermediate cardiac care unit. *JAMA* 1976; 235:816–819.

609. Levine A, Lown B. The "chair" treatment of coronary thrombosis. *Trans Assoc Am Phys* 1951; 64:316.

610. McNeer JF, Wagner GS, Ginsburg PB, Wallace AG, McCants CB, Conley MJ, et al. Hospital discharge one week after acute myocardial infarction. *N Engl J Med* 1978; 298:229–232.

611. Madsen EB, Hougaard P, Gilpin E, Pedersen A. The length of hospitalization after acute myocardial infarction determined by risk calculation. *Circulation* 1983; 68:9–16.

612. Bigger JT, Fleiss JL, Kleiger R, Miller JP, Rolnitzky LM, the Multicenter Post-Infarction Research Group. The relationships among ventricular arrhythmias, left ventricular dysfunction, and mortality in the 2 years after myocardial infarction. *Circulation* 1984; 69:250–258.

613. Epstein SE, Palmeri ST, Patterson RE. Evaluation of patients after acute myocardial infarction: Indications for cardiac catheterization and surgical intervention. *N Engl J Med* 1982; 307:1487–1492.

614. Iskandrian AS, Hakki AH, Kotler MN, Segal BL, Herling I. Evaluation of patients with acute myocardial infarction: Which test, for whom and why? *Am Heart J* 1985; 109:391–394.

615. Pratt CM, O'Rourke R. Application and interpretation of submaximal exercise testing and ambulatory ECG recordings in patients with acute myocardial infarction. *Chest* 1988; 93:29S–32S.

616. Mavric Z, Zaputovic L, Matana A, Kucic J, Roje J, Marinovic, et al. Prognostic significance of complete atrioventricular block in patients with acute inferior myocardial infarction with and without right ventricular involvement. *Am Heart J* 1990; 119:823.

617. Hillis LD, Forman S, Braunwald E. Risk stratification before thrombolytic therapy in patients with acute myocardial infarction: The Thrombolysis in Myocardial Infarction (TIMI) Phase II co-investigators. *J Am Coll Cardiol* 1990; 16:313–315.

618. Schuster EH, Bulkey BH. Early post-infarction angina: Ischemia at a distance and ischemia in the infarct zone. *N Engl J Med* 1981; 305:1101.

619. Normand SL, Glickman ME, Sharma RG, McNeil BJ. Using admission characteristics to predict short-term mortality from myocardial infarction in elderly patients: Results from the Cooperative Cardiovascular Project. *JAMA* 1996; 275:1322–1328.

620. Lee KL, Woodlief LH, Topol EJ, Weaver WD, Betriu A, Col J, et al. Predictors of 30-day mortality in the era of reperfusion for acute myocardial infarction: Results from an international trial of 41,021 patients. *Circulation* 1995; 91:1659–1668.

621. Krone RJ, Miller JP, Gillespie JA, Weld FM, Multicenter Post-Infarction Research Group. Usefulness of low-level exercise testing early after acute myocardial infarction in patients taking beta-blocking agents. *Am J Cardiol* 1987; 60:23–27.

622. Fioretti P, Brower RW, Simoons ML, Bos RJ, Baardmen T, Beelen A, et al. Prediction of mortality during the first year after acute myocardial infarction from clinical variables and stress test at hospital discharge. *Am J Cardiol* 1985; 55:1313–1318.

623. Krone RJ, Gillespie JA, Weld FM, Miller JP, Moss AJ. Low-level exercise testing after myocardial infarction: Usefulness in enhancing clinical risk stratification. *Circulation* 1984; 71:80–89.

624. Mark DB, Sigmon K, Topol EJ, et al. Identification of acute myocardial infarction patients suitable for early hospital discharge after aggressive interventional therapy: Results from the Thrombolysis and Angioplasty in Acute Myocardial Infarction Registry. *Circulation* 1991; 83:1186–1193.

625. Newby LK, Califf RM, Guerci A, Weaver WD, Col J, Horgan LK, et al. Early discharge in the thrombolytic era: An analysis of criteria for uncomplicated infarction from the Global Utilization of Streptokinase and t-PA for Occluded Coronary Arteries (GUSTO) trial. *J Am Coll Cardiol* 1996; 27:625–632.

626. Van Reet RE, Quiñones MA, Poliner LR, Nelson JG, Waggoner AD, Kanon D, et al. Comparison of two-dimensional echocardiography with gated radionuclide ventriculography in the evaluation of global and regional left ventricular function in acute myocardial infarction. *J Am Coll Cardiol* 1984; 3:243–252.

627. Schiller NB, Shah PM, Crawford M, DeMaria A, Devereux R, Feigenbaum H, et al. Recommendations for quantitation of the left ventricle by two-dimensional echocardiography. *J Am Soc Echocardiogr* 1989; 5:358–367.

628. Becker LC, Silverman KJ, Bulkley BH, Kallman CH, Mellits ED, Weisfeldt M. Comparison of early ^{201}Tl scintigraphy and gated blood pool imaging for predicting mortality in patients with acute myocardial infarction. *Circulation* 1983; 67:1272–1283.

629. White HD, Norris RM, Brown MA, Brandt PWT, Whitlock RML, Wild CJ. Left ventricular end-systolic volume as the major determinant of survival after recovery from myocardial infarction. *Circulation* 1987; 76:44–51.

630. Mahmarian JJ, Moye L, Verani MS, Eaton T, Francis M, Pratt CM. Criteria for the accurate interpretation of changes in left ventricular ejection fraction and cardiac volumes as assessed by rest and exercise gated radionuclide angiography. *J Am Coll Cardiol* 1991; 18:112–119.

631. Pilote L, Silberberg J, Lisbona R, Sniderman A. Prognosis in patients with low left ventricular ejection fraction after myocardial infarction. *Circulation* 1989; 80:1636.

632. Fletcher GF, Balady G, Froelicher VF, Hartley LH, Haskell WL, Pollock ML, et al. Exercise standards: A statement for healthcare professionals from the American Heart Association. *Circulation* 1995; 91:580.

633. DeBusk RF, Haskell W. Symptom-limited vs heart-rate-limited exercise testing soon after myocardial infarction. *Circulation* 1980; 61:738–743.

634. Starling MR, Crawford MH, Kennedy GT, O'Rourke RA. Exercise testing early after myocardial infarction: Predictive value for subsequent unstable angina and death. *Am J Cardiol* 1980; 46:909–914.

635. Sami M, Kraemer H, DeBusk RF. The prognostic significance of serial exercise testing after myocardial infarction. *Circulation* 1979; 60:1238–1246.

636. Weld FM, Chu KL, Bigger JT, Rolnitzky LM. Risk stratification with low-level exercise testing 2 weeks after acute myocardial infarction. *Circulation* 1981; 64:306–314.

637. Senaratne MPJ, Hsu L, Rossall RE, Kappagoda CT. Exercise testing after myocardial infarction: Relative values of the low level predischarge and the postdischarge exercise test. *J Am Coll Cardiol* 1988; 12:1416–1422.

638. Stone PH, Turi ZG, Muller JE, Parker C, Hartwell T, Rutherford JD, et al. Prognostic significance of the treadmill exercise test performance

6 months after myocardial infarction. *J Am Coll Cardiol* 1986; 8:1007–1017.

639. Starling MR, Crawford MH, Kennedy GT, O'Rourke RA. Treadmill exercise tests predischarge and six weeks post-myocardial infarction to detect abnormalities of known prognostic value. *Ann Intern Med* 1981; 94:721–727.

640. Villella A, Maggioni AP, Villella M, Giordano A, Turazza FM, Santoro E, et al. Prognostic significance of maximal exercise testing after myocardial infarction treated with thrombolytic agents: the GISSI-2 data base. Gruppo Italiano per lo Studio della Sopravvivenza Nell'Infarto. *Lancet* 1995; 346:523–529.

641. Chaitman BR, McMahon RP, Terrin M, Younis LT, Shaw LJ, Weiner DA, et al. Impact of treatment strategy on predischarge exercise test in the Thrombolysis in Myocardial Infarction (TIMI) II Trial. *Am J Cardiol* 1993; 71:131–138.

642. Gottlieb SO, Gottlieb SH, Achuff SC, Baumgarden R, Mellits ED, Weisfeldt ML, et al. Silent ischemia on Holter monitoring predicts mortality in high-risk postinfarction patients. *JAMA* 1988; 259:1030–1035.

643. Jerczek M, Andresen D, Schroder J, Voller H, Bruggemann T, Deutschmann C, et al. Prognostic value of ischemia during Holter monitoring and exercise testing after acute myocardial infarction. *Am J Cardiol* 1993; 72:8–13.

644. Currie P, Ashby D, Saltissi S. Prognostic significance of transient myocardial ischemia on ambulatory monitoring after acute myocardial infarction. *Am J Cardiol* 1996; 71:773–777.

645. Langer A, Minkowitz J, Dorian P, Casella L, Harris L, Morgan CD, et al. Pathophysiology and prognostic significance of Holter-detected ST segment depression after myocardial infarction: The Tissue Plasminogen Activator Toronto (TPAT) Study Group. *J Am Coll Cardiol* 1992; 20:1313–1317.

646. Bonaduce D, Petretta M, Lanzillo T, Vitagliano G, Bianchi V, Conforti G, et al. Prevalence and prognostic significance of silent myocardial ischaemia detected by exercise test and continuous ECG monitoring after acute myocardial infarction. *Eur Heart J* 1991; 12:186–193.

647. Mahmarian JJ, Steingart RM, Forman S, Sharaf BL, Coglianese ME, Miller DD, et al. Relationship between ambulatory electrocardiographic monitoring and myocardial perfusion imaging to detect coronary artery disease and myocardial ischemia: An ACIP ancillary study. *J Am Coll Cardiol* 1997; 29:764–769.

648. Mahmarian JJ, Mahmarian AC, Marks GF, Pratt CM, Verani MS. The role of adenosine thallium-201 tomography for precisely defining long-term risk in patients following acute myocardial infarction. *J Am Coll Cardiol* 1995; 25:1333–1340.

649. Mahmarian JJ, Pratt CM, Nishimura S, Abreu A, Verani MS. Quantitative adenosine 201TI single-photon emission computed tomography for the early assessment of patients surviving acute myocardial infarction. *Circulation* 1993; 87:1197–1210.

650. Mahmarian JJ. Prediction of myocardium at risk. Clinical significance during acute infarction and in evaluating subsequent prognosis. *Cardiol Clin* 1995; 13:355–378.

651. Abraham RD, Freedman SB, Dunn RF, et al. Prediction of multivessel coronary artery disease and prognosis early after acute myocardial infarction by exercise electrocardiography and thallium-201 myocardial perfusion scanning. *Am J Cardiol* 1986; 58:423–427.

652. Younis LT, Byers S, Shaw L, Barth G, Goodgold H, Chaitman BR. Prognostic value of intravenous dipyridamole thallium scintigraphy after an acute myocardial ischemia event. *Am J Cardiol* 1989; 64:161–166.

653. Leppo JA, O'Brien J, Rothendler JA, Getchell JD, Lee VW. Dipyridamole-thallium-201 scintigraphy in the prediction of future cardiac events after acute myocardial infarction. *N Engl J Med* 1984; 310:1014–1018.

654. Hendel RC, Gore JM, Alpert JS, Leppo JA. Prognosis following interventional therapy for acute myocardial infarction: Utility of dipyridamole thallium scintigraphy. *Cardiology* 1991; 79:73–80.

655. Ryan T, Armstrong WF, O'Donell JA, Feigenbaum H. Risk stratification after acute myocardial infarction by means of exercise two-dimensional echocardiography. *Am Heart J* 1987; 114:1305–1316.

656. van Daele ME, McNeill AJ, Fioretti PM, Salustri A, Pazzoli MM, el-Said ES, et al. Prognostic value of dipyridamole sestamibi single-photon emission computed tomography and dipyridamole stress echocardiography for new cardiac events after an uncomplicated myocardial infarction. *J Am Soc Echocardiogr* 1994; 7:370–380.

657. Carlos ME, Smart SC, Wynsen JC, Sagor KB. Dobutamine stress echocardiography for risk stratification after myocardial infarction. *Circulation* 1997; 95:1401–1402.

658. Geleijnse ML, Elhendy A, VanDomburg RT, Cornel JH, Rambaldi R, Salustri A, et al. Cardiac imaging for risk stratification with dobutamine-atropine stress testing in patients with chest pain: Echocardiography, perfusion scintigraphy, or both? *Circulation* 1997; 96:137–147.

659. Quiñones MA. Risk stratification after myocardial infarction: Clinical science versus practice behavior. *Circulation* 1997; 95:1352–1354.

660. Pfeffer MA, Braunwald E, Moye LA, Basta L, Brown EJ, Cuddy TE, et al. Effect of captopril on mortality and morbidity in patients with left ventricular dysfunction after myocardial infarction. *N Engl J Med* 1992; 327:669–677.

661. The SOLVD Investigators. Effect of enalapril on mortality and the development of heart failure in asymptomatic patients with reduced left ventricular ejection fraction. *N Engl J Med* 1992; 327:685–691.

662. The SOLVD Investigators. Effect of enalapril on survival in patients with reduced left ventricular ejection fraction and congestive heart failure. *N Engl J Med* 1991; 325:293–302.

663. Pratt CM, Francis MJ, Luck JC, Wyndham CR, Miller RR, Quiñones MA. Analysis of ambulatory electrocardiograms in 15 patients during spontaneous ventricular fibrillation with special reference to preceding arrhythmic events. *J Am Coll Cardiol* 1983; 2:789–797.

664. The Cardiac Arrhythmia Suppression Trial (CAST) Investigators. Preliminary report: Effect of encainide and flecainide on mortality in a randomized trial of arrhythmia suppression after myocardial infarction. *N Engl J Med* 1989; 321:406–412.

665. The Cardiac Arrhythmia Suppression Trial II Investigators. Effect of the antiarrhythmic agent moricizine on survival after myocardial infarction. *N Engl J Med* 1992; 327:227–233.

666. Waldo AL, Camm AJ, deRuyter H, Friedman PL, MacNeil DJ, Pauls JF, et al. Effect of D-sotalol on mortality in patients with left ventricular dysfunction after myocardial infarction. *Lancet* 1996; 348:7–12.

667. Julian DG, Camm AJ, Fragin G, Janse MJ, Munoz A, Schwartz PJ, et al. Randomised trial of effect of amiodarone on mortality in patients with left-ventricular dysfunction after recent myocardial infarction: EMIAT. *Lancet* 1997; 349:667–674.

668. Cairns JA, Connolly SJ, Robert R, Gent M, for the Canadian Amiodarone Myocardial Infarction Arrhythmia Trial Investigators. Randomized trial of outcome after myocardial infarction in patients with frequent or repetitive ventricular premature depolarisations: CAMIAT. *Lancet* 1997; 349:675–682.

669. Pratt CM, Greenway PS, Schoenfeld MH, Hibben ML, Reiffel JA. An exploration of the precision of classifying sudden cardiac death. Implications for the interpretation of clinical trials. *Circulation* 1996; 93:519–524.

670. Luu M, Stevenson WG, Stevenson LW, Baron K, Walden J. Diverse mechanisms of unexpected cardiac arrest in advanced heart failure. *Circulation* 1989; 80:1675–1680.

671. Moss AJ, DeCamilla J, Davis H. Cardiac death in the first 6 months after myocardial infarction: Potential for mortality reduction in the early posthospital period. *Am J Cardiol* 1977; 39:816–820.

672. Ruberman W, Weinblatt E, Goldberg JD, Frank CW, Shapiro S. Ventricular premature beats and mortality after myocardial infarction. *N Engl J Med* 1977; 297:750–757.

673. The Cardiac Arrhythmia Pilot Study (CAPS) Investigators. Effects of encainide, flecainide, imipramine, and moricizine on ventricular arrhythmias during the year after acute myocardial infarction: The CAPS. *Am J Cardiol* 1988; 61:501–509.

674. Farrell TG, Bashir Y, Cripps T, Malik M, Poloniecki J, Bennett ED, et al. Risk stratification for arrhythmic events in postinfarction patients based on heart rate variability, ambulatory electrocardiographic variables and the signal-averaged electrocardiogram. *J Am Coll Cardiol* 1991; 18:687–697.

675. Kleiger RE, Miller JP, Krone RJ, Bigger JT, the Multicenter Postinfarction Research Group. The independence of cycle length variability and exercise testing on predicting mortality of patients surviving acute myocardial infarction. *Am J Cardiol* 1990; 65:408–411.

676. Lombardi F, Sandrone G, Pernpruner S, et al. Heart rate variability as an index of sympathovagal interaction after acute myocardial infarction. *Am J Cardiol* 1987; 60:1239–1245.

677. Bigger JT Jr, LaRovere MT, Steinman RC, Fleiss JL, Rottman JN, Rolnitzky LM, et al. Comparison of baroreflex sensitivity and heart period variability after myocardial infarction. *J Am Coll Cardiol* 1989; 14:1511–1518.

678. Odemuyiwa O, Malik M, Farrell T, Bashir Y, Poloniecki J, Camm J. Comparison of the predictive characteristics of heart rate variability index and left ventricular ejection fraction for all-cause mortality, arrhythmic events and sudden death after acute myocardial infarction. *Am J Cardiol* 1991; 68:434–439.

679. Schwartz PJ, Vanol E, Stramba-Badiale M, De Ferrari GM, Billman GE, Foreman RD. Autonomic mechanisms and sudden death: New insights from analysis of baroreceptor reflexes in conscious dogs with and without a myocardial infarction. *Circulation* 1988; 78:669–679.

680. Lown B, Verrier RL. Neural activity and ventricular fibrillation. *N Engl J Med* 1976; 294:1165–1170.

681. Hartikainen JEK, Malik M, Staunton A, Poloniecki J, Camm AJ. Distinction between arrhythmic and nonarrhythmic death after acute myocardial infarction based on heart rate variability, signal-averaged electrocardiogram, ventricular arrhythmias and left ventricular ejection fraction. *J Am Coll Cardiol* 1996; 28:296–304.

682. Copie X, Hnatkova K, Staunton A, Fei L, Camm AJ, Malik M. Predictive power of increased heart rate versus depressed left ventricular ejection fraction and heart rate variability for risk stratification after myocardial infarction: Results of a two-year follow-up study. *J Am Coll Cardiol* 1996; 27:270–276.

683. Singh N, Mironov D, Armstrong PW, Ross AM, Langer A. Heart rate variability assessment early after acute myocardial infarction: Pathophysiological and prognostic correlates. GUSTO ECG substudy investigators. Global Utilization of streptokinase and TPA for occluded arteries. *Circulation* 1996; 93:1388–1399.

684. American College of Cardiology Cardiovascular Technology Assessment Committee. Heart rate variability for risk stratification of life-threatening arrhythmias. *J Am Coll Cardiol* 1993; 22:948–950.

685. Gomes JA, Winters SL, Martinson M, Machac J, Stewart D, Targonski A. The prognostic significance of quantitative signal-averaged variables relative to clinical variables, site of myocardial infarction, ejection fraction and ventricular premature beats: A prospective study. *J Am Coll Cardiol* 1989; 13:377–384.

686. Turritto G, Fontaine JM, Ursell S, Caref EB, Bekheit S, El-Sherif N. Risk stratification and management of patients with organic heart disease and nonsustained VT: Role of programmed stimulation, LVEF, and the signal-averaged electrocardiogram. *Am J Med* 1990; 88:35N–41N.

687. El-Sherif N, Ursell SN, Bekheit S, Fontaine J, Turrit G, Henkin R, et al. Prognostic significance of the signal-averaged ECG depends on the time of recording in the postinfarction period. *Am Heart J* 1989; 118:256–264.

688. Kuchar DL, Thorburn CW, Sammel NL. Prediction of serious arrhythmic events after myocardial infarction: Signal-averaged electrocardiogram, Holter monitoring and radionuclide ventriculography. *J Am Coll Cardiol* 1987; 9:531–538.

689. Simson MB. Use of signals in the terminal QRS complex to identify patients with ventricular tachycardia after myocardial infarction. *Circulation* 1981; 64:235–242.

690. Hohnloser SH, Franck P, Klingenheben T, Zabel M, Just H. Open infarct artery, late potentials, and other prognostic factors in patients after acute myocardial infarction in the thrombolytic era: A prospective trial. *Circulation* 1994; 90:1747–1756.

691. McClements BM, Adgey AA. Value of signal-averaged electrocardiography, radionuclide ventriculography, Holter monitoring and clinical variables for prediction of arrhythmic events in survivors of acute myocardial infarction in the thrombolytic era. *J Am Coll Cardiol* 1993; 21:1419–1427.

692. Vatterott PJ, Hammill SC, Bailey KR, Wiltgen CM, Gersh BJ. Late potentials on signal-averaged electrocardiograms and patency of the infarct-related in survivors of acute myocardial infarction. *J Am Coll Cardiol* 1991; 17:330–337.

693. Zipes DP, Akhtar M, Denes P, DeSanctis RW, Garson A, Gettes LS, et al. Guidelines for clinical intracardiac electrophysiologic studies: A report of the American College of Cardiology/American Heart Association Task Force on assessment of diagnostic and therapeutic cardiovascular procedures. *J Am Coll Cardiol* 1989; 14:1827–1842.

694. Bourke JP, Richards DAB, Ross DL, Wallace EM, McGuire MA, Uther JB. Routine programmed electrical stimulation in survivors of acute myocardial infarction for prediction of spontaneous ventricular tachyarrhythmias during follow-up: Results, optimal stimulation protocol and cost-effective screening. *J Am Coll Cardiol* 1991; 18:780–788.

695. Kowey PR, Waxman HL, Greenspon A, Greenberg R, Poll D, Kutalek S, et al. Value of electrophysiologic testing in patients with previous myocardial infarction and nonsustained ventricular tachycardia. *Am J Cardiol* 1990; 65:594–598.

696. Bhandari AK, Rose JS, Kotlewski A, Rahimtoola SH, Wu D. Frequency and significance of induced sustained ventricular tachycardia or fibrillation two weeks after acute myocardial infarction. *Am J Cardiol* 1985; 56:737–742.

697. Richards DA, Cody DV, Denniss AR, Russell PA, Young AA, Uther JB. Ventricular electrical instability: A predictor of death after myocardial infarction. *Am J Cardiol* 1983; 51:75–80.

698. Marchlinski FE, Buxton AE, Waxman HL, Josephson ME. Identifying patients at risk of sudden death after myocardial infarction: Value of the response to programmed stimulation, degree of ventricular ectopic activity and severity of left ventricular dysfunction. *Am J Cardiol* 1983; 52:1190–1196.

699. Richards DA, Byth K, Ross DL, Uther JB. What is the best predictor of spontaneous ventricular tachycardia and sudden death after myocardial infarction? *Circulation* 1991; 83:756–763.

700. Moss AJ, Hall J, Cannom DS, Daubert JP, Higgins SL, Klein H, et al. Improved survival with an implanted defibrillator in patients with coronary disease at high risk for ventricular arrhythmia. *N Engl J Med* 1996; 335:1933–1940.

701. Glancy JM, Garratt CJ, Woods KL, deBono DP. QT dispersion and mortality after myocardial infarction. *Lancet* 1995; 345:945–948.

702. Schwartz PJ, LaRovere MT, Vanoli E. Autonomic nervous system and sudden cardiac death: Experimental basis and clinical observations for post-myocardial infarction risk stratification. *Circulation* 1992; 85:I-77–I-91.

703. LaRovere MT, Spoecchia G, Mortara A, Schwartz PJ. Baroreflex sensitivity, clinical correlates, and cardiovascular mortality among patients with a first myocardial infarction: A prospective study. *Circulation* 1988; 78:816–824.

704. Gibson RS, Watson DD, Craddock GB, Crampton RS, Kaiser DL, Denny MJ, et al. Prediction of cardiac events after uncomplicated myocardial infarction: A prospective study comparing predischarge exercise thallium-201 scintigraphy and coronary angiography. *Circulation* 1983; 68:321–336.

705. DeFeyter PJ, Van Eenige MJ, Dighton DH, Visser FC, de Jong J, Roos JP. Prognostic value of exercise testing, coronary angiography and left ventriculography 6–8 weeks after myocardial infarction. *Circulation* 1982; 66:527–536.

706. Taylor GJ, Humphries JO, Mellits ED, Pitt B, Schulze RA, Griffith LS, et al. Predictors of clinical course, coronary anatomy and left ventricular function after recovery from acute myocardial infarction. *Circulation* 1980; 62:960–970.

707. Grines CL, Topol EJ, Bates ER, Juni JE, Walton JA, O'Neill WW. Infarct vessel status after intravenous tissue plasminogen activator and acute coronary angioplasty: Prediction of clinical outcome. *Am Heart J* 1988; 115:1–7.

708. Topol EJ, Califf RM, George BS, Kereiakes DJ, Abbottsmith CW, Candela RJ, et al. A randomized trial of immediate versus delayed elective angioplasty after intravenous tissue plasminogen activator in acute myocardial infarction. *N Engl J Med* 1987; 317:581–588.

709. Muller DW, Topol EJ, Ellis EG, Sigmon KN, Lee K, Califf RM, et al. Multivessel coronary artery disease: A key predictor of short-term prognosis after reperfusion therapy for acute myocardial infarction. *Am Heart J* 1991; 121:1042–1049.

710. Aguirre FV, Kern MJ, Hsia J, Serota H, Janosik D, Greenwalt T, et al. Importance of myocardial infarction artery patency on the prevalence of ventricular arrhythmia and late potentials after thrombolysis in acute myocardial infarction. *Am J Cardiol* 1991; 68:1410–1416.

711. Stack RS, O'Connor CM, Mark DB, Hinohara T, Phillips HR, Lee MM, et al. Coronary perfusion during acute myocardial infarction with a combined therapy of coronary angioplasty and high-dose intravenous streptokinase. *Circulation* 1988; 77:151–161.

712. Stadius ML, Davis K, Maynard C, Ritchie JL, Kennedy JW. Risk stratification for 1 year survival based on characteristics identified in the early hours of acute myocardial infarction: The Western Washington Intracoronary Streptokinase Trial. *Circulation* 1986; 74:703–711.

713. Davis HT, DeCamilla J, Bayer LW, Moss AJ. Survivorship patterns in the posthospital phase of myocardial infarction. *Circulation* 1979; 6:1252–1258.

714. Ross J Jr, Brandenburg RO, Dinsmore RE, Friesinger GC, Hultgren HH, Pepin CJ, et al. Guidelines for coronary angiography: A report of the American College of Cardiology/American Heart Association

Task Force on assessment of diagnostic and therapeutic cardiovascular procedures. *J Am Coll Cardiol* 1987; 10:935–950.

715. Ryan TJ, Faxon DP, Gunnar RM, Kennedy JW, King SB, Loop FD, et al. Guidelines for percutaneous transluminal coronary angioplasty: A report of the American College of Cardiology/American Heart Association Task Force on the assessment of diagnostic and therapeutic cardiovascular procedures. *J Am Coll Cardiol* 1988; 1:889–893.

716. Davis K, Kennedy JW, Kemp HG, Judkins MP, Gosselin AJ, Killip T. Complications of coronary arteriography from the collabroative study of coronary artery surgery (CASS). *Circulation* 1979; 59:1105–1112.

717. European Coronary Surgery Study Group. Coronary artery bypass surgery in stable angina pectoris: Survival at two years. *Lancet* 1979; 1:889–893.

718. European Coronary Surgery Study Group. Prospective randomized study of coronary artery bypass surgery in stable angina pectoris: A progress report on survival. *Circulation* 1982; 65:II-67–II-71.

719. Deedwania PC, Amsterdam EA, Vagelos RH. Evidence-based, cost-effective risk stratification and management after myocardial infarction. *Arch Intern Med* 1997; 157:273–280.

720. Ronnevik PK, Gundersen T, Abrahamsen AM. Effect of smoking habits and timolol treatment on mortality and reinfarction in patients surviving acute myocardial infarction. *Br Heart J* 1985; 54:134–139.

721. Rosenberg L, Kaufman DW, Helmrich SP, et al. The risk of myocardial infarction after quitting smoking in men under 55 years of age. *N Engl J Med* 1985; 313:1511–1514.

722. Ockene JK. Smoking intervention: A behavioral, educational, and pharmacologic perspective. In: Okene IS, Ockene JK, eds. *Prevention of Coronary Heart Disease.* Boston: Little Brown; 1992:201–230.

723. Henningfield JE. Nicotine medications for smoking cessation. *N Engl J Med* 1995; 333:1196–1203.

724. Pekkanen J, Linn S, Heiss G, et al. Ten-year mortality from cardiovascular disease in relation to cholesterol level among men with and without preexisting cardiovascular disease. *N Engl J Med* 1990; 322:1700–1707.

725. Stampfer MJ, Sacks FM, Salvini S, Willett WC, Hennekens CH. A prospective study of cholesterol, apolipoproteins, and the risk of myocardial infarction. *N Engl J Med* 1991; 325:373–381.

726. Scandinavian Simvastatin Survival Study Group. Randomised trial of cholesterol lowering in 4444 patients with coronary heart disease: the Scandinavian Simvastatin Survival Study (4S). *Lancet* 1994; 344:1383–1389.

727. Sacks FM, Pfeffer MA, Moye LA, et al. The effect of pravastatin on coronary events after myocardial infarction in patients with average cholesterol levels. *N Engl J Med* 1996; 335:1001–1009.

728. Expert Panel on Detection, Evaluation, and Treatment of High Blood Cholesterol in Adults. Summary of the second report of the National Cholesterol Education Program (NCEP) Expert Panel on Detection, Evaluation, and Treatment of High Blood Cholesterol in Adults (Adult Treatment Panel II). *JAMA* 1993; 22:933–940.

729. Rosenson RS. Myocardial injury: The acute phase response and lipoprotein metabolism. *J Am Coll Cardiol* 1993; 22:933–940.

730. Laslett L, Paumer L, Amsterdam EA. Exercise training in coronary disease. *Cardiol Clin* 1987; 5:211–225.

731. Haskell WL. Sedentray lifestyle is a risk factor for coronary artery disease. In: Pearson TA, Criqui MH, Leupker RV, et al, eds. *Primer in Preventive Cardiology.* Dallas: American Heart Association; 1994:173–187.

732. Stanford JL, Weiss NS, Voight LF, Daling JR, Havel LA, Rossing MA. Combined estrogen and progestin hormone replacement therapy in relation to risk of breast cancer in middle-aged women. *JAMA* 1995; 274:137–142.

733. Colditz GA, Hankinson SE, Hunter DJ, Willett WC. The use of estrogens and progestins and the risk of breast cancer in postmenopausal women. *N Engl J Med* 1995; 332:1589–1593.

734. Healy B. Effects of estrogen or estrogen/progestin regimes on heart disease risk factors in postmenopausal women: The Postmenopausal Estrogen/Progestin Interventions (PEPI) Trial. *JAMA* 1995; 273:199–208.

735. Lobo RA, Speroff L. International consensus conference of postmenopausal hormone therapy and the cordiovascular system. *Fertil Steril* 1994; 61:592–595.

736. Gorsky RD, Koplan JP, Peterson HB, Thacker SB. Relative risks and benefits of long-term estrogen replacement therapy: A decision analysis. *Obstet Gynecol* 1994; 83:161–166.

737. Yusuf S, Lessem J, Jha P, et al. Primary and secondary prevention of myocardial infarction and strokes: An update of randomly allocated, controlled trials. *J Hypertens* 1993; 11(suppl 4):S61–S73.

738. Anonymous. Timolol-induced reduction in mortality and reinfarction in patients surviving acute myocardial infarction. *N Engl J Med* 1981; 304:801–807.

739. Hjalmarson A, Elmfeldt D, Herlitz J, et al. Effect on mortality of metoprolol in acute myocardial infarction: A double-blind randomised trial. *Lancet* 1981; 2:823–827.

740. Becker RC. Antiplatelet therapy in coronary heart disease: Emerging strategies for the treatment and prevention of acute myocardial infarction. *Arch Pathol Lab Med* 1993; 117:89–96.

741. Juul-Moller S, Edvardsson N, Jahnmatz B, Rosen A, Sorensen S, Omblus R. Double-blind trial of aspirin in primary prevention of myocardial infarction in patients with stable chronic angina pectoris: The Swedish Angina Pectoris Aspirin Trial (SAPAT) Group. *Lancet* 1992; 340:1421–1425.

742. Ambrosioni E, Borghi C, Magnani B. The effect of the angiotensin-converting enzyme inhibitor zofenopril on mortality and morbidity after anterior myocardial infarction. *N Engl J Med* 1995; 332:80–85.

743. Ball SG, Hall AS. What to expect from ACE inhibitors after myocardial infarction. *Br Heart J* 1994; 72(suppl 3):S70–S74.

744. Wagner NB, White RD, Wagner GS. The 12-lead ECG and the extent of myocardium at risk of acute infarction: Cardiac anatomy and lead locations, and the phases of serial changes during acute occlusion. In: Califf RM, Mark DB, Wagner GS, eds. *Acute Coronary Care in the Thrombolytic Era.* Chicago: Year Book, 1988:31–45.

745. Roberts R, Gibson RS. Prevention of reinfarction subsequent to non-Q-wave infarction. *J Cardiovasc Pharmacol* 1989; 13(suppl 1):S36–S46.

48

INTERVENTIONAL CORONARY ARTERY PROCEDURES

John S. Douglas, Jr. / Spencer B. King III

The treatment of patients with coronary heart disease changed dramatically with the advent and refinement of coronary artery surgical techniques in the 1970s and percutaneous coronary intervention in the next decade. This chapter addresses the development and contemporary use of catheter-based coronary artery intervention, including selection of patients and devices, procedural issues, results, complications, and long-term outcome.

Development of Balloon Angioplasty

Percutaneous transluminal coronary angioplasty (PTCA) was conceived and shepherded into worldwide acceptance and application by Andreas R. Gruentzig, but the stage was set by the pioneering effort of others. Gruentzig's ideas were a direct extension of the work of Dotter and Judkins,[1] who, in 1964, mechanically dilated femoral arteries with a coaxial double-catheter system, and of Zeitler,[2] who successfully applied this technique in West Germany and introduced it to Gruentzig. After Gruentzig's introduction of a polyvinyl chloride balloon catheter with fixed maximal inflated diameters in 1974, modern balloon angioplasty evolved rapidly. With further balloon catheter miniaturization and building on the coronary arteriography techniques of Sones and Judkins, Gruentzig succeeded in dilating experimental stenoses in canine coronary arteries,[3–5] and then in dilating human arteries during bypass surgery. In September 1977 the first PTCA was performed in Zurich in a 37-year-old insurance salesman with severe angina pectoris and high-grade stenosis of the proximal left anterior descending (LAD) coronary artery.[6,7] Balloon angioplasty was successful in relieving the stenosis, and on the 10th anniversary of this landmark procedure, coronary arteriography revealed angiographically normal coronary arteries (Fig. 48-1). Over 19 years later, the patient remained asymptomatic.

Following the report of Gruentzig's first five cases in 1978[8] and 50 cases in 1979,[9] worldwide interest in the technique was assured. Under the auspices of the National Heart, Lung, and Blood Institute (NHLBI), multicenter registries were formed to report experiences with the evolving technique of balloon coronary angioplasty.[10,11] Development of an over-the-wire balloon catheter by Simpson et al.[12] combined with advances in guidewire and balloon catheter technology resulted in a steerable balloon catheter system capable of crossing and dilating heretofore unreachable coronary stenoses (Fig. 48-2). The use of percutaneous revascularization increased dramatically, exceeding 130,000 procedures in the United States in 1986 and 400,000 in 1995. At Emory University Hospital, catheter-based revascularization techniques surpassed the frequency of coronary artery bypass surgery for relief from symptoms of ischemic heart disease in 1986 (Fig. 48-3).

Initially, coronary balloon angioplasty was performed for discrete, proximal, noncalcified, subtotal lesions located in one coronary artery. Gruentzig was able to dilate successfully 64 percent of the initial 50 patients and 78 percent of the first 169.[9,13] Most of the patients successfully dilated were symptomatically improved. A 10-year follow-up of Gruentzig's early Zurich series revealed an overall survival rate of 90 percent and of 95 percent for those with single-vessel disease.[13,14] Five-year survival in the NHLBI Registry was 93 percent for single-vessel disease and 87 percent for patients with multivessel disease.[15]

Randomized Trials of Balloon Angioplasty

The favorable results of these observational studies and others reporting mostly multivessel disease patients[16,17] led to a series of randomized trials comparing balloon angioplasty with medical therapy[18] and with coronary artery bypass sur-

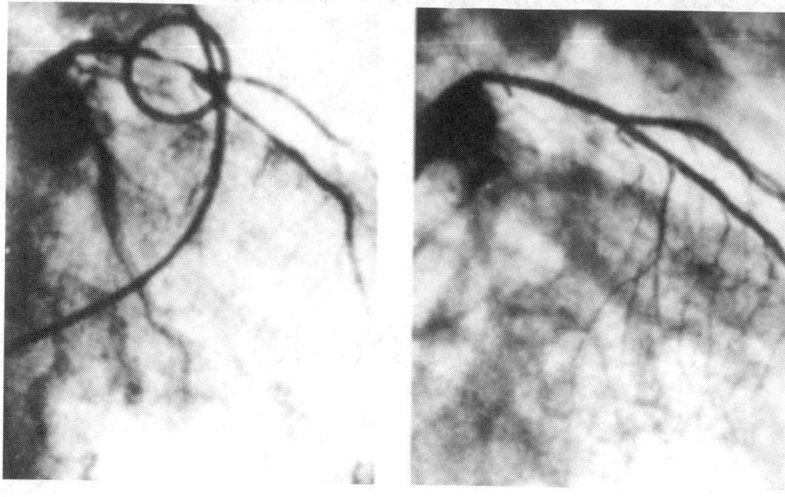

FIGURE 48-1

Right anterior oblique coronary arteriogram of the first patient who underwent transluminal coronary angioplasty on September 16, 1977 (*left*) and on September 16, 1987 (*right*). During this 10-year period, the patient remained completely asymptomatic and the arteriogram at 10 years showed no narrowing in the coronary arteries. Nineteen years later, the patient is free of symptoms.

gery (CABS).[19–24] The Angioplasty Compared to Medical Therapy Evaluation (ACME) involving 212 patients with single-vessel disease and abnormal stress tests revealed greater freedom from angina in the angioplasty group at 6 months (64 versus 46 percent) as well as better treadmill performance (2.1- versus 0.5-min increase). There was no difference in death or myocardial infarction. Over 5000 patients have been randomized in nine trials comparing angioplasty with CABG surgery. Two of these trials were NHLBI-sponsored and performed in the United States. The first, the Emory Angioplasty versus Surgery Trial (EAST), was a single-center study, while the larger Bypass Angioplasty Revascularization Investigation (BARI)[20] involved 18 centers. In-hospital mortality was similar for angioplasty and bypass surgery (approximately 1 percent) in these two studies of patients with multivessel disease, and 5-year survival was also similar (Table 48-1). Repeat revascularization procedures,

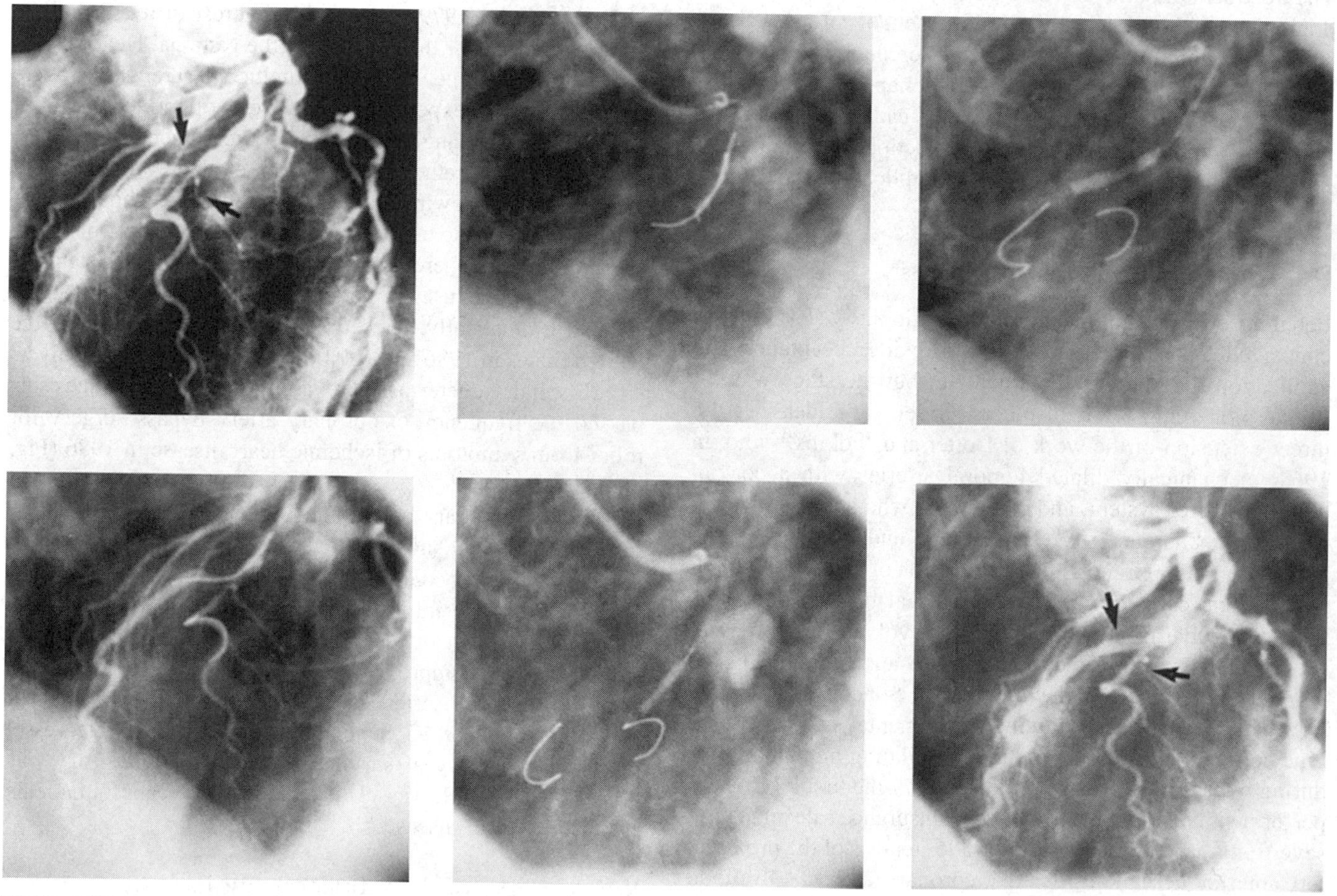

FIGURE 48-2

Angioplasty of high-grade stenoses of the left anterior descending and diagonal bifurcation (*see arrows*) using a single guiding catheter through which two dilatation devices were passed. The left anterior descending artery was dilated with a 2.5-mm balloon (note "waist" of the balloon produced by the lesion), and the diagonal was dilated with a 2-mm balloon. Note the small intimal tear in the left anterior descending artery following the procedure (left anterior oblique views).

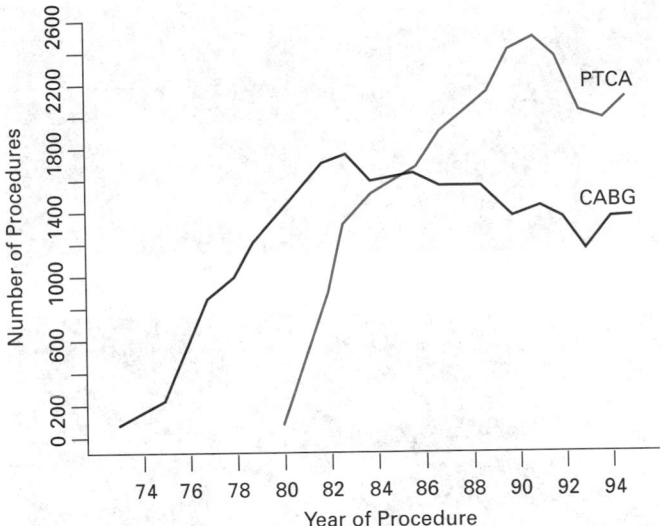

FIGURE 48-3
Coronary revascularization procedures at Emory University Hospitals from 1973 to 1995.

however, were more common in the angioplasty group. A recent metaanalysis of eight randomized published trials (BARI not included) reported no difference in mortality or myocardial at 1 year after angioplasty or CABG, but 18 percent of the angioplasty patients had required bypass surgery and 20 percent had an additional angioplasty, a significantly higher rate of requiring repeat revascularization than in the surgery group.[22] This increased need for additional revascularization procedures in angioplasty patients, largely due to restenosis, eroded the initial cost advantage of angioplasty; by 3 years in the EAST study, angioplasty had been 95 percent as costly as bypass surgery.[24] Although stents were available for failed angioplasty, these studies essentially compared conventional balloon angioplasty with surgery and in ACME with medical therapy.

New Devices and Strategies for Coronary Intervention

The directional atherectomy catheter (Fig. 48-4A) developed by Simpson[29] was, in 1990, the first nonballoon device approved for coronary intervention and the first to undergo randomized comparison with balloon angioplasty. In native coronary artery[26,27] and saphenous vein graft lesions[28] judged suitable for either procedure, however, the more costly directional atherectomy did not show a substantive advantage over balloon angioplasty. Additional trials using techniques to achieve optimal atherectomy (< 20 percent residual stenosis) have been completed and may clarify the role of this technology.[29,30] Excimer laser angioplasty was approved by the Food and Drug Administration (FDA) in 1992 for lesions not favorable for balloon angioplasty, but this technology is infrequently used in most centers. In 1993, the Gianturco-Roubin Flex-Stent (Cook Inc., Bloomington, IN) received approval for acute and threatened vessel closure,[31,32] and this device

continues to be an important adjunct. In 1994, two additional atherectomy devices, the Rotablator (Heart Technologies, Bellevue, WA) (Fig. 48-4B) and the Transluminal Extraction Catheter (TEC, Interventional Technologies, San Diego, CA) (Fig. 48-4C) were approved for marketing by the FDA. The Rotablator's principal advantage is in the treatment of calcified stenoses, while the TEC device is used principally in saphenous vein grafts, where aspiration of thrombus is its unique attribute. None of these devices, however, had the impact on interventional cardiology that was produced by the Palmaz-Schatz stent (Johnson & Johnson Interventional Systems, Warren, NJ) (Fig. 48-5). On the basis of two carefully conducted randomized trials that showed reduced restenosis compared to balloon angioplasty,[33,34] this device was granted FDA approval for marketing in 1994 for the elective treatment of de novo lesions in native coronary arteries. Over 100,000 implantations of this stent were performed in the first year of its availability. The interest in stenting was greatly heightened by a pivotal observation by Colombo that complete stent expansion by high-pressure balloon inflation (Fig. 48-6), confirmed by intravascular ultrasound, yielded a very low thrombosis rate in spite of substitution of aspirin and ticlopidine for warfarin.[35] A recent randomized trial of stent placement without ultrasound guidance comparing aspirin and ticlopidine with phenprocoumon (a warfarin derivative) revealed a low 30-day incidence of cardiac events and bleeding rates

TABLE 48-1
RANDOMIZED COMPARISONS OF PTCA AND CABG

	EAST		BARI	
	PTCA	CABG	PTCA	CABG
Patient characteristics				
Age (years)	62	61	62	61
Ejection fraction, %	61	62	57	58
Heart failure, %	3	4	9	9
Prior MI, %	41	41	54	55
Diseased vessels, %				
Two	60	60	57	58
Three	40	40	41	41
In-hospital outcome, %				
Myocardial infarction	3	10	2.1	4.6
Death	1	1	1.1	1.3
Repeat revascularization				
PTCA	0	0	3.4	0
CABG	10	0	10.2	0.1
Five-year outcome, %				
Death	12.1	8.8	13.7	10.7
Additional PTCA	48.6	15.5	34.0	7.3
Additional CABG	25.1	0.5	31.3	1.1
Any additional revascularization			54.5	8.0

Abbreviations: EAST = Emory Angioplasty Surgery Trial[19,23]; BARI = Bypass Angioplasty Revascularization Investigation[20]; PTCA = percutaneous transluminal coronary angioplasty; CABG = coronary artery bypass graft surgery.

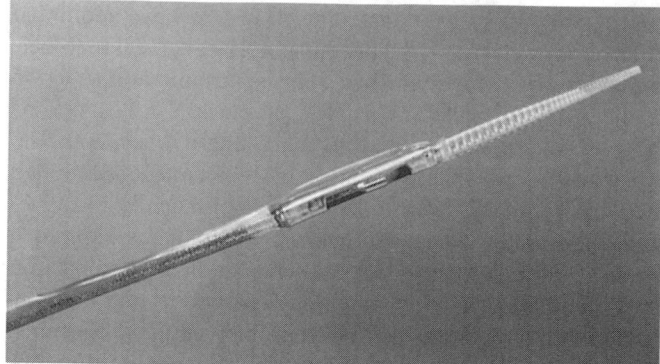

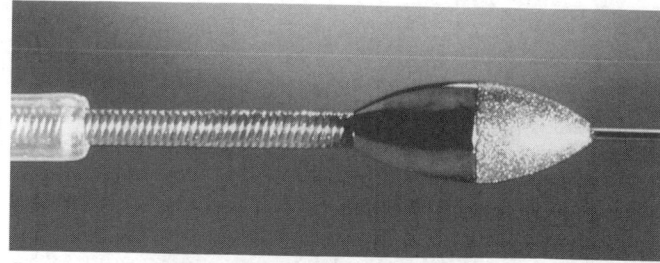

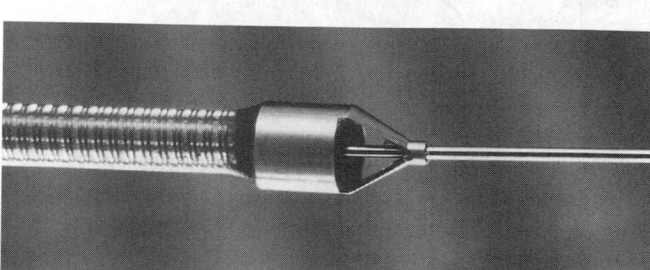

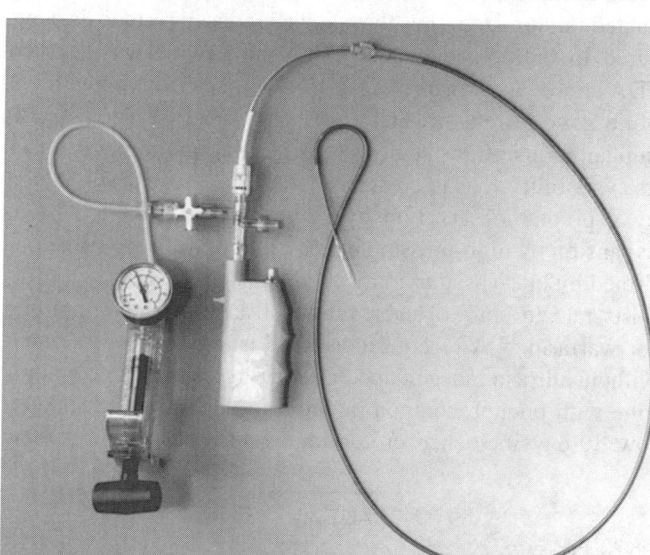

A

B

C

FIGURE 48-4

A. Directional atherectomy device (Simpson Atherocath, Devices for Vascular Intervention, Inc., Redwood City, CA). A battery-powered motor unit drives a cable that spins the cutter at approximately 2500 rpm. *B.* Rotational atherectomy burr (Rotablator, Heart Technologies, Bellevue, WA) and the special 0.009-in stainless steel guidewire over which the diamond-embedded burr spins at 150,000 to 200,000 rpm. *C.* Transluminal extraction catheter (TEC Interventional Technologies, Inc., San Diego, CA). The catheter rotates at 750 rpm over a special 0.014-in TEC guidewire. Vacuum bottles aspirate plaque and thrombus cut by the blades of the conical head.

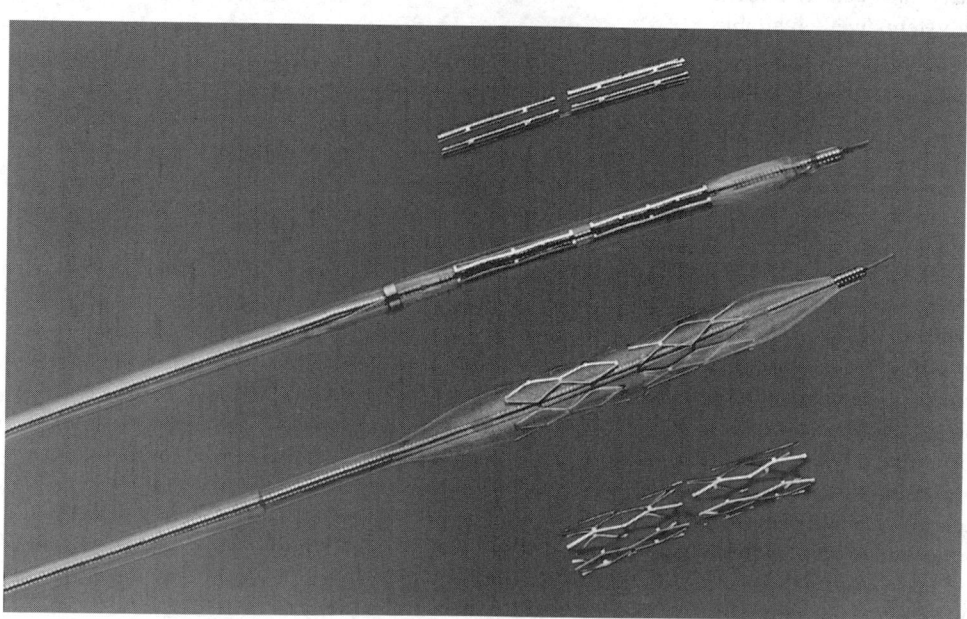

FIGURE 48-5

The Palmaz-Schatz coronary stent (Johnson & Johnson Interventional Systems, Warren, NJ). The free unexpanded stent (*top*) is mounted on a balloon and covered with a sheath. Withdrawal of the sheath and balloon inflation expands the stent (*bottom*).

in the aspirin-ticlopidine patients, supporting this simplified antithrombotic strategy.[36] Several additional randomized trials addressing this issue are in progress.

Intravascular ultrasound has also been used extensively in some centers to evaluate coronary lesions for device therapy and to assess the results of device and balloon treatment, but the increased cost of this approach is a limiting factor. The latest arrow in the quiver of the interventionalist is the availability of new, potent antiplatelet agents. The first approved by the FDA was a monoclonal antibody directed against the platelet glycoprotein IIb/IIIa receptor (see also Chap. 52). This drug has been shown to reduce ischemic complications

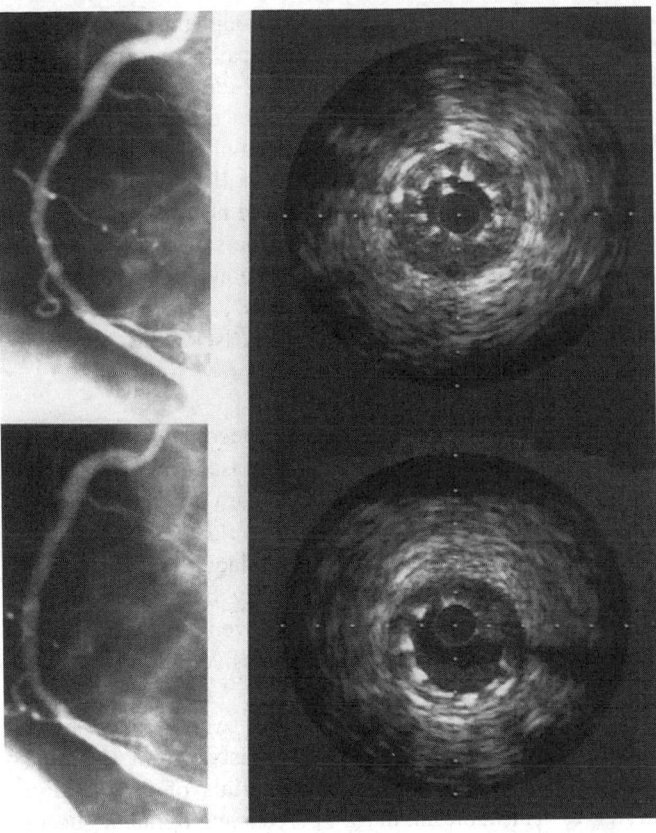

FIGURE 48-6

A 74-year-old woman developed early recurrence of angina after balloon angioplasty of the right coronary artery. Coronary arteriography revealed a severe, long stenosis of the right coronary artery (*top left*). Stenting was advised and a Wallstent was deployed and dilated with a 3.5-mm balloon to 15 atm with an excellent angiographic result (*bottom left*). Intravascular ultrasound, however, showed that the distal end of the stent had been missed with the balloon and was poorly expanded (*top right*). this area was "redilated" to 16 atm with no change in the angiogram but much better stent expansion and wall apposition (*bottom right*). Following repeat dilation, the lumen cross-sectional area increased from 4.2 to 6.4 mm^2.

and late clinical events in high-risk angioplasty.[37] Probably of less importance but also interesting is the availability of new means of sealing femoral artery puncture sites with plugs or sutures. The optimal role of these new and effective but expensive devices and strategies in the day-to-day practice of interventional cardiology is controversial.[38]

INDICATIONS FOR CORONARY INTERVENTION

In general, when one is selecting percutaneous coronary intervention, there should be assurance that the operator can treat, with a high probability of success, the coronary lesion(s) accounting for the symptoms or signs of myocardial ischemia. Further, the associated risk and durability of the revascularization should be acceptable as compared with bypass surgery or medical therapy during both early and long-term follow-up. The latter estimate requires consideration of the likelihood and consequences of abrupt vessel closure, restenosis, and

incomplete revascularization. In addition, one cannot disregard the comparative costs of the initial intervention, its complications, and the need for subsequent revascularization procedures. The American College of Cardiology/American Heart Association Guidelines for Percutaneous Transluminal Coronary Angioplasty provide a detailed analysis of many of these issues.[39,40]

Selection of Patients

SINGLE-VESSEL DISEASE

Percutaneous revascularization is an attractive option for many symptomatic patients who are anatomically suitable, having single-vessel coronary disease. It is important, however, to remember that there are no large studies comparing angioplasty with surgery in this group of patients and none that show a statistically significant survival benefit of angioplasty compared with surgery or medical therapy. Data from Emory University indicate that of 692 single-vessel patients newly diagnosed in 1988, a total of 46 percent underwent angioplasty, 50 percent were treated medically, and 4 percent underwent coronary bypass surgery. Of 7604 patients with single-vessel disease treated at Emory with angioplasty between 1980 and 1991, angiographic success was 90 percent and complications were infrequent [Q-wave myocardial infarction (MI), 0.8 percent; emergency CABG, 1.7 percent; and death, 0.2 percent].[41] In these patients with single-vessel disease, 1-, 5-, and 10-year survival was 0.99, 0.93, and 0.86, respectively, while 0.80, 0.69, and 0.58 were PTCA-free and 0.92, 0.87, and 0.77 were CABG-free at 1, 5, and 10 years. In the Duke data bank experience, 5-year survival with angioplasty in single-vessel disease compared favorably with bypass surgery (95 versus 93 percent with CABG).[42] In a relatively small, randomized trial of angioplasty and internal mammary artery surgery for isolated disease of the LAD coronary artery, there was no difference in mortality or MI, but angioplasty patients had more repeat revascularizations (25 versus 3 percent, $p < .01$).[43]

The ACME study showed that angioplasty in single-vessel disease can lead to improved quality of life compared to medical therapy at 6 months, with reduced angina and improved exercise performance out to 3 years.[18,44,45] Clearly, it is improvement is symptoms rather than prolongation of life that is achieved by angioplasty in this patient subset. The ACME data suggest, however, that using the angioplasty techniques available at that time resulted in a slightly increased risk of acute complications (2 percent emergency CABG, 1 percent Q-wave MI) and repeat revascularization (23 versus 9 percent) at six months, but no difference in late revascularization at 3 years.[45]

Studies from the Cleveland Clinic analyzing the importance of repeat procedures in determining 2-year cardiac cost suggest that coronary intervention is more cost-effective than medical and surgical therapy when the probability of repeat procedures is low.[46] One would infer from this analysis that the presence of multiple or complex lesions, which are likely to recur, may tilt the scale sufficiently to modify adversely the favorable comparative cost-effectiveness of percutaneous intervention in single-vessel disease.

MULTIVESSEL DISEASE

A dramatic increase in utilization of percutaneous intervention in multivessel disease, fueled by improved angioplasty technology and new devices, accounts for the growth in these procedures worldwide. *Rational selection of patients, however, requires a careful analysis of multiple issues, including a risk-benefit assessment of each ischemia-producing lesion, a projection of the possible completeness and durability of the physiologic revascularization, and an estimate of resource consumption compared to surgery and medical therapy.*

In general, as stated in "Guidelines for PTCA,"[40] patients selected for intervention are symptomatic, have evidence of ischemia, need noncardiac surgery, are recovering from cardiac arrest or malignant arrhythmia, or have compelling anatomy. Patient preferences must be considered, since repeat interventions are a common and integral aspect of percutaneous intervention in multivessel disease (see Table 48-1). Complete revascularization, which has been shown in the surgical experience to produce superior long-term results, has been associated with less late intervention after angioplasty,[47] but it is not frequently attained due to the presence of total occlusions, noncritical stenoses, and diffuse disease. In the 1985–1986 NHLBI PTCA Registry, complete revascularization was achieved in 19 percent of patients.[48]

In experience at Emory University with 10,783 patients who underwent coronary intervention, complete revascularization was achieved in 84 percent of patients with single-vessel disease and 25 percent with two-vessel disease but in only 5 percent with triple-vessel disease.[41] In the experience of the Emory Angioplasty Versus Surgery Trial (EAST), 71 percent of index segments were revascularized in PTCA patients.[49] Culprit-lesion angioplasty is clearly an accepted strategy, but care must be taken to avoid significant residual ischemia postintervention. This approach was reflected in EAST, where revascularization was attempted in 96 percent of high-priority lesions in PTCA patients and in 99 percent of surgical patients. (High-priority lesions were defined as 70 to 100 percent stenoses located proximally or in large vessels ≥2.5 mm). This strategy yielded similar 3-year EAST primary clinical end points for CABG and PTCA and an identical frequency of patients with all index segments free of stenosis of 70 to 100 percent (82 versus 82 percent).[49]

The risks of percutaneous coronary intervention are increased in the presence of unstable angina, advanced age, poor left ventricular function, extensive coronary disease, comorbid conditions, and female gender. At Emory, in-hospital mortality for one-, two-, and three-vessel disease was 0.2, 0.4, and 1.2 percent respectively ($p < .0001$) and emergency bypass surgery was needed in 1.7, 3.0, and 3.2 percent respectively.[41] In general, the risk of intervention is directly related to the probability and consequences of abrupt closure; in multivessel disease, both are frequently higher and impaired left ventricu-

lar function is commonly present. Although the major randomized trials of angioplasty versus bypass surgery showed no overall difference in mortality on long-term follow-up, BARI reported that patients being treated for diabetes had significantly worse 5-year mortality with angioplasty compared to surgery (35 versus 19 percent). In a smaller cohort of diabetic patients in EAST, however, there were no differences in outcome. The BARI findings question the safety of angioplasty in the diabetic population who frequently have diffuse multivessel disease and, in many cases, a reduced recognition of recurrent ischemia (increased silent ischemia).

UNSTABLE ANGINA

Patients with unstable angina, who account for a majority of coronary interventions, are at increased risk for ischemia complications, particularly abrupt closure.[39,40,50] These complications, which are presumed to be related to the presence of thrombus and ruptured complex plaque[50,51] (see Chaps. 40 and 44) as demonstrated elegantly by angioscopy,[52,53] have led many operators to defer intervention for a few days while stabilizing the patient on aggressive anti-anginal therapy, including aspirin and heparin[54–56] (particularly in the presence of angiographic thrombus).[57] Alternatively, the favorable results achieved with angioplasty within 18 to 48 h after hospitalization in randomized trials of interventional strategies in unstable angina (96 percent angiographic success, 0.4 percent mortality, 2.9 percent myocardial infarction, 0.7 percent emergency CABG, 2.2 percent abrupt closure)[58] have encouraged some to pursue a more aggressive approach, particularly in patients at highest risk of a coronary event—i.e., those with postinfarction angina[59] and angina refractory to medical therapy.[60] The use of direct antithrombins[61] and platelet glycoprotein IIb/IIIa inhibitors[37] has been shown to be effective in reducing complications of intervention in unstable angina, whereas the routine administration of thrombolytic agents has reduced the thrombus burden but with an unfavorable impact on complications (i.e., in hospital ischemic events, 12.9 versus 6.3 percent without thrombolytics, $p = .02$).[62] At present, the optimal adjunctive therapy in unstable angina is unclear, but recent trials have shown important reduction in complications in high-risk patients with unstable angina or recent infarction undergoing angioplasty who are treated with a IIb/IIIa receptor blocker.[63]

ACUTE MYOCARDIAL INFARCTION

Treatment of patients with MI was revolutionized by the recognition of the primacy of thrombotic occlusion and the potential life-saving benefit of thrombolytic or mechanical reperfusion. Unfortunately, only about half of patients with acute myocardial infarction are candidates for thrombolytic therapy[64] (see Chap. 47). In addition, even using the most aggressive double-bolus strategies (recombinant tissue plasminogen activator (t-PA), patency rates of only 80 percent and thrombolysis in myocardial infarction III (TIMI III) flow rates of 50 to 60 percent are reported at 90 min, and recurrent ischemia or stroke occurs in 10 to 15 percent of patients during the hospitalization. The shortcomings of thrombolytic therapy led to a series of trials of adjunctive angioplasty. These showed that routine angioplasty up to 48 h after t-PA led to higher vessel patency but increased mortality, abrupt closure and reocclusion, and no improvement in ventricular function.[65–67] Identification of thrombolytic failures (those who do not reperfuse) is difficult, since a minority of patients experience complete relief of chest pain and ST-segment resolution. Even when thrombolytic failures are identified, the results of angioplasty are less than optimal (80 percent success rate but high mortality in angioplasty failures of 33 percent).[68–70]

With a direct approach to infarct artery recanalization, primary angioplasty (without thrombolytic agents) performed within 6 h of symptom onset produced angioplasty success rates over 90 percent, less recurrent ischemia than with thrombolytic therapy, and no strokes.[71–74] These favorable outcomes led to a series of randomized trials comparing primary angioplasty with thrombolytic therapy (Table 48-2). Primary angioplasty was more successful in achieving vessel patency and in restoring normal TIMI-III flow (an independent predictor of survival), was associated with less recurrent ischemia, led to improved outlook, and was cost-effective due to reduced hospitalization.[75–80] Myocardial infarction–free survival at 2 years was 86 percent with primary PTCA compared to 79 percent with thrombolytic therapy.[78] Recent reports, however, have indicated that the excellent results reported with primary angioplasty were dependent on short door-to-reperfusion time (optimally <60 min, not immediately attainable in all centers) and were subject to a learning curve even for experienced operators.[81] *Patients most likely to benefit from primary angioplasty include those over age 65 (mortality rate 5.7 versus 15 percent with thrombolytics, p = .06), anterior infarction (mortality 1.4 versus 11.9 percent p = .01), and high-risk patients such as those with inferior MI with anterior ST segment depression and patients in cardiogenic shock, in whom mortality is reduced from the 70 percent reported with thrombolytic therapy to about 50 percent.*[74,75] Improvement in clinical outcome has also been demonstrated with adjunctive intraaortic balloon pumping in high-risk patients undergoing primary PTCA.[82] When primary angioplasty was used in a broader application in the Global Use of Strategies to Open Occluded Arteries (GUSTO) II trial, the advantage of primary PTCA was small. *Best results will be obtained in centers dedicated and committed to primary PTCA, a commitment that is expensive and not always practical.*

Selection of Lesions

The importance of coronary stenosis angiographic morphology in predicting the outcome of coronary angioplasty is reflected in the American College of Cardiology/American Heart Association PTCA Guidelines.[39,40] Lesions were classified as type A for anticipated high success, low risk; type B for anticipated moderate success, moderate risk; and type C for anticipated low success, high risk (Table 48-3). The general validity of this classification in predicting outcome of balloon angioplasty was confirmed in low-risk patients,[83] in patients with multivessel disease,[84] and in directional atherectomy where success and complication rates were 93 and 3 percent for type A lesions, 88 and 6 percent in type B_1, and 75 and 13 percent when more than one B characteristic was present (type B_2).[85] More recent analysis of this lesion scoring system using balloon angioplasty technology of the 1990s suggests rates of 96, 93, and 80 percent can be achieved with A, B, and C lesions, respectively, and that certain morphologic characteristics (long lesions, calcified lesions, stenosis severity 80 to 90 percent, angulated lesions, and presence of thrombus)[86] may have higher predictive value in determining success and complications. The ABC classification, however, continues to be useful in predicting outcome after contemporary angioplasty where early events in a population of unstable angina patients occurred in 4 percent of A, 7.7 percent of B_1 15.3 percent of B_2, and 17.9 percent of C patients treated with heparin.[87] It does appear, however, in many centers that the complexity of lesions being attempted has increased and that new devices (especially stents) and antithrombotic strategies have, to a certain extent, weakened the prognostic value of this scoring system. In one recent report of 1085 lesions treated in the era of new devices (A, 8 percent; B_1, 42 percent; B_2, 35 percent; C, 15 percent), procedural success was 100 percent for A, 97.3 percent for B_1, 97 percent for B_2, 87.4 percent for C. Predictors of procedural failure were lesion length >20 mm, TIMI-I flow, calcification, angle >90 percent, and chronic total occlusion.[88] Similarity, in the Helvetica investigation, the use of hirudin largely neutralized the detri-

---

TABLE 48-2

RANDOMIZED TRIALS OF PRIMARY ANGIOPLASTY VERSUS THROMBOLYSIS IN ACUTE MYOCARDIAL INFARCTION

Trial	PTCA		Thrombolysis	
	Patients	Events, %	Patients	Events, %
IN-HOSPITAL DEATH				
PAMI-1[75]	195	2.5	200	6.5
Mayo[76]	47	4.3	56	3.6
Netherlands[77]	70	0	72	5.6
Total	312	2.2[a]	328	5.8[a]
IN-HOSPITAL REINFARCTION				
PAMI-1	195	2.5	200	6.5
Mayo	47	2.1	56	5.4
Netherlands	70	0	72	12.5
Total	312	1.9[b]	328	7.6[b]

[a] Odds ratio for in-hospital mortality with thrombolysis versus angioplasty = 2.68 (95% confidence limits, 1.16–6.92; p = .023).

[b] Odds ratio for in-hospital reinfarction with thrombolysis versus angioplasty is 4.22 (95% confidence limits, 1.82–11.46; p = .0008).

Source: Reproduced with permission from Simari et al.[79]

TABLE 48-3

AMERICAN COLLEGE OF CARDIOLOGY/AMERICAN HEART ASSOCIATION CLASSIFICATION OF LESIONS

TYPE A LESIONS (HIGH SUCCESS, >85%; LOW RISK)	
Discrete (<10 mm length)	Little or no calcification
Concentric	Less than totally occlusive
Readily accessible	Not ostial in location
Nonangulated segment, <45°	No major branch involvement
Smooth contour	Absence of thrombus

TYPE B LESIONS (MODERATE SUCCESS, 60 TO 85%; MODERATE RISK)	
Tubular (10–20 mm length)	Moderate to heavy calcification
Eccentric	Total occlusions <3 months old
Moderate tortuosity of proximal segment	Ostial in location
Moderately angulated segment, >45°, <90°	Bifurcation lesions requiring double guidewires
Irregular contour	Some thrombus present

TYPE C LESIONS (LOW SUCCESS, <60%; HIGH RISK)	
Diffuse (>2 cm length)	Total occlusion >3 months old
Excessive tortuosity of proximal segment	Inability to protect major side branches
Extremely angulated segments >90°	Degenerated vein grafts with friable lesions

Source: Ryan et al.[40] Reprinted with permission of the authors and the American College of Cardiology.

mental trend in clinical outcome related to lesion severity that was clearly observed in patients treated with heparin.[87]

Lesion characteristics that were associated with increased restenosis rates include length, total occlusion (see Fig. 48-7), thrombus, ostial location, previous angioplasty to the same site, and saphenous vein grafts. The assessment of lesion characteristics by intracoronary ultrasound and angioscopy have also been shown to have prognostic value for determining angioplasty success and long-term outcome[30,35,89–93] and in some centers these strategies are used frequently to guide therapy (see Chap. 49). Selection of lesions for intervention is strongly based on the operator's assessment of his or her ability to treat the ischemic-producing lesion safely, in a cost-conscious manner, and achieve long-term patency and symptomatic benefit.

Selection of Devices

Conventional balloon angioplasty is a simple, relatively low in cost, and effective method of reducing coronary stenosis, but new devices (especially stents) are being used with increasing frequency, particularly in conditions where balloon angioplasty has been proved not to be highly effective (Table

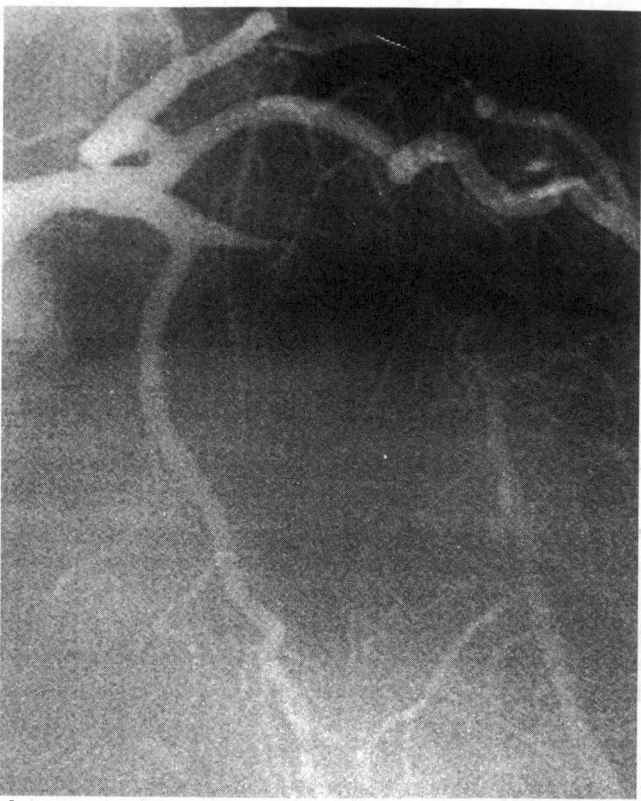

A

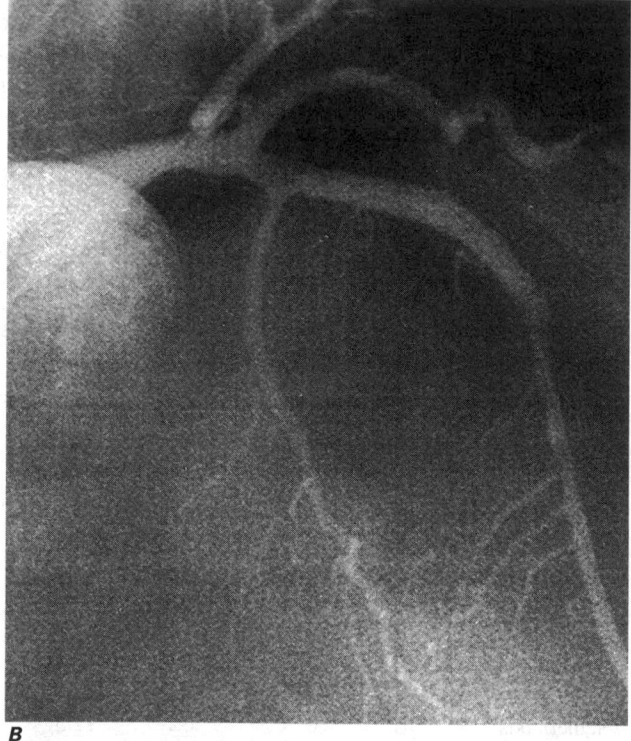

B

FIGURE 48-7

An 82-year-old man with disabling angina and an occluded left anterior descending (LAD) artery of uncertain duration (*A*, right anterior oblique view). It was possible to recanalize the long LAD occlusion (*B*) using a hydrophilic-coated wire (Meditech Terumo Corporation, Piscataway, NJ) and conventional balloon angioplasty followed by placement of two Palmaz-Schatz stents.

48-4). At Emory University Hospital in 1990, balloon angioplasty was the sole technique used in 88 percent of 1863 patients who underwent coronary intervention (directional atherectomy, 3 percent; excimer laser, 3 percent; stents, 2 percent; laser balloon, 1 percent), whereas in 1995 76.5 percent of patients were treated only with balloons, 2.6 percent had extraction atherectomy, 12.2 percent had stents, and none was treated with excimer laser.

The practice of performing balloon angioplasty as an initial strategy in a majority of patients and using stents for suboptimal results is supported by observations from the Benestent trial that stentlike results ($\leq$30 percent residual narrowing) were achievable in 35 percent of patients with balloons and that they had a long-term outcome comparable to that of stented patients.[94] This strategy appears to be cost-effective.[95] Adjunctive stents placed for bailout have been clearly shown to reduce Q-wave infarction and emergency bypass surgery.[31,32] Although subacute thrombosis was substantially higher in patients with stents placed emergently in the early experience, the employment of high-pressure balloon inflations in recent studies has substantially reduced this complication to about 1 percent despite reduced anticoagulation.[96]

In our hospital stents are frequently selected for primary treatment of complex lesions, aortoostial sites, shelflike lesions, early recurrence, total occlusions, and lesions with high restenosis rates (proximal LAD and saphenous vein grafts) (Figs. 48-6, 48-7, and 48-8). It is important to point out that restenosis rates obtained with stents in complex lesions are not as favorable as in simple lesions[97] and that these applications have not been subjected to rigorous comparison with balloon angioplasty. Randomized comparison has been carried out, however, in saphenous vein grafts, where 6-month minimal lumen diameter (MLD) was significantly larger with stents (1.75 versus 1.47 mm, $p = .05$) and a composite end point of death. MI, CABG, or target lesion revascularization was less frequent (26 versus 38 percent, $p = .05$).[98]

Given the superb results recently reported in the Benestent II Pilot Study with heparin-coated stents in relatively ideal lesions (overall clinical success, 99 percent; stent thrombosis, 0; restenosis, 13 percent) and the large number of new stent designs being evaluated, one would anticipate broadened utilization of improved and cheaper stents due to competitive market forces. Decreased cost may permit stenting to rival or prove more cost-effective than simple balloon angioplasty.[99–101]

Directional coronary atherectomy (DCA) is most frequently used as primary therapy but may be applied adjunctively following balloon angioplasty or the use of other devices. Suitable lesions are generally proximal in vessels $\geq$3 mm in diameter and have features that predict poor outcome with balloon angioplasty such as aortoostial location, high-bulk stenoses, and protected left main coronary lesions[102] and include carefully selected bifurcation lesions[103,104] and complex postinfarction lesions, (where histology frequently shows partially organized thrombus (see Fig. 48-8). Pretreatment of calcified lesions with rotational atherectomy may permit successful DCA in selected cases,[105] but in general moderate angiographic calcifi-

TABLE 48-4

NEW CORONARY INTERVENTIONAL STRATEGIES COMPARED TO BALLOON ANGIOPLASTY

Technique	Indications	Contraindications	Advantages and Limitations
Balloon angioplasty	Focal stenosis	Insignificant narrowing, no ischemia, unimportant artery	Broad applicability, lower cost; poor outcome in thrombotic, ostial, and calcified lesions; significant restenosis
Stents	Focal stenosis	Heavy calcification or thrombus, vessel diameter <2.5 mm	Reduced emergency CABG and restenosis; more expensive, rare stent thrombosis, lesion accessibility
Directional atherectomy	Focal noncalcified stenosis, ostial site	Diffuse disease, severe tortuosity or bend	Debulks, ? reduced restenosis; more frequent non-Q-wave MI, more expensive, technically difficult
Rotational atherectomy	Focal calcified stenosis, ostial site	Thrombus, large plaque burden, severe tortuosity or bend	Effective in calcified lesions, reduced elastic recoil; more expensive, similar restenosis, transient left ventricular dysfunction
Laser	Ostial lesion, SVG, ? long lesion	Severe calcification, tortuosity or bend	Debulks effectively; increased cost, similar restenosis
Transluminal extraction atherectomy	Thrombotic lesion, bulky SVG lesion	Severe tortuosity or bend, calcification	Thrombus and plaque removed; high complication rate in native vessels, distal embolization, maximal device diameter 2.5 mm

Abbreviations: CABG = coronary artery bypass graft; MI = myocardial infarction; LV = left ventricular; SVG = saphenous vein graft.

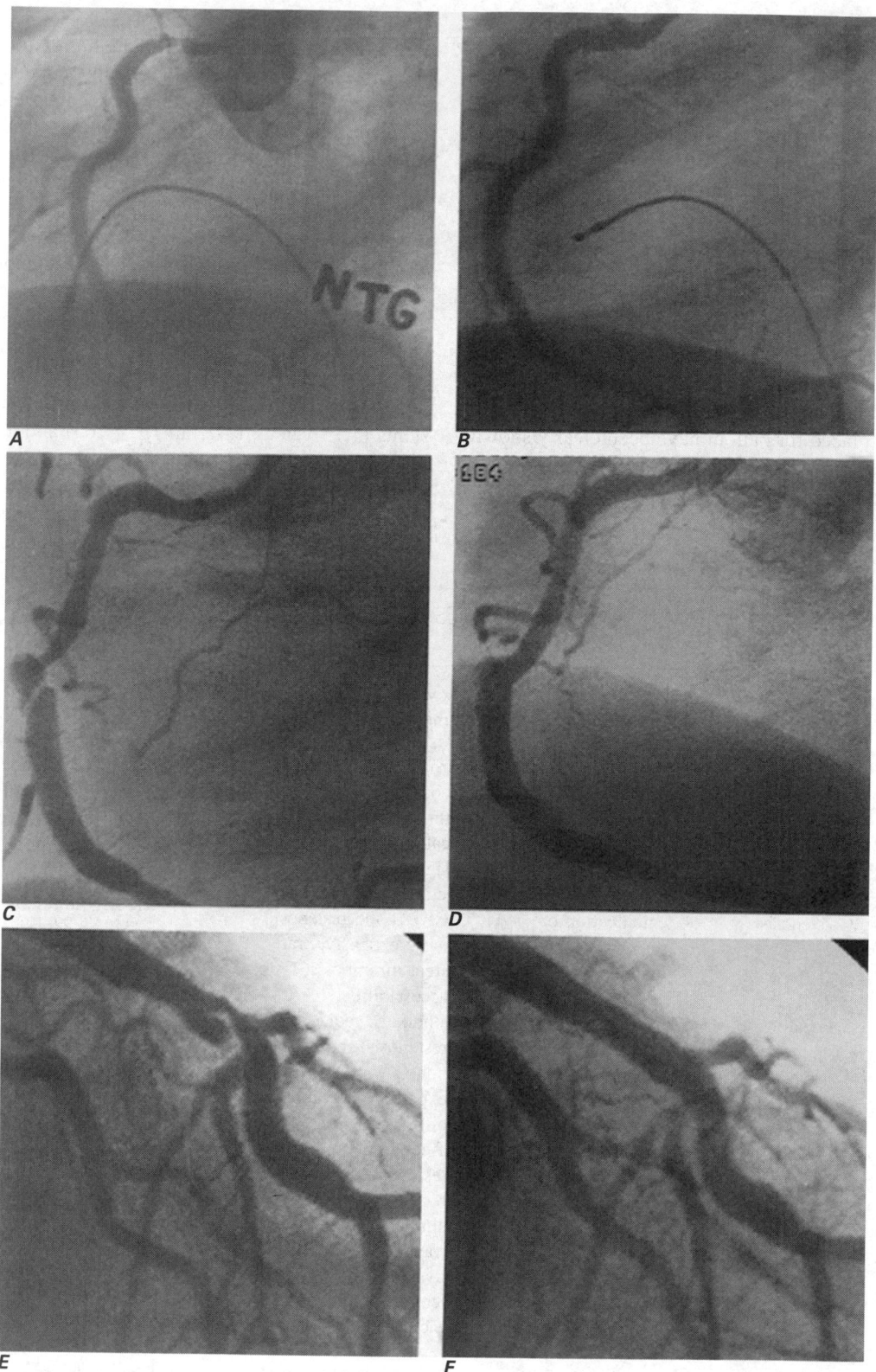

FIGURE 48-8
High-grade de novo stenosis of the ostium of the right coronary in a middle-aged man (*A*) was free of calcification. Directional atherectomy was successful (*B*). This type of lesion is also satisfactory for stenting. A very complex shelflike de novo stenosis of the right coronary artery (*C*) and the site 2 years after successful atherectomy (*D*). Histology showed atheroma and organized thrombus. Flaplike de novo stenosis of the left anterior descending artery (LAD) (*E*). This type of lesion responds well to directional coronary atherectomy or stenting (*F*). Sites *A*, *C*, and *E* are poor lesions for conventional percutaneous transluminal angioplasty.

cation and significant superficial calcification on intracoronary ultrasound are predictors of failure.[90] The Coronary Angioplasty Versus Excisional Atherectomy Trial (CAVEAT) showed improved restenosis rates for directional atherectomy in proximal nonostial lesions of the LAD[106] but not for ostial LAD lesions or saphenous vein intervention (increased acute complications, similar restenosis).[28] In contrast, the Canadian coronary atherectomy study found the restenosis rates of DCA and PTCA were similar even in lesions traditionally selected for DCA (proximal LAD and eccentric, bulky lesions).[107]

Rotational atherectomy has proved useful in the presence of calcium, in treatment of aortoostial and branch ostial lesions, and in nondilatable lesions; in some series, it has been used in long, ulcerated, and complex lesions with excellent acute results.[108,109] Highly angulated or thrombotic lesions or those with impaired distal runoff (recent infarction, fixed thallium defect) and segments with myocardial bridging should be avoided.[108–111] Rotational atherectomy has also been used in total occlusions, but restenosis rates have not been demonstrated to be better than those of balloon angioplasty in any of these groups. Elective intraaortic balloon pump placement has been shown to improve systemic blood pressure and to be associated with a lower non-Q-wave infarction rate in high-risk patients.[112]

The Transluminal Extraction Catheter (TEC), which is unique in its ability to cut and aspirate plaque and thrombus, is used primarily in saphenous vein grafts containing thrombus, where acute success rates are high but embolic myocardial infarction and restenosis are not uncommon.[113–115] In some centers, high-risk patients with MI have been successfully treated with TEC either acutely or following postinfarction angina due to thrombotic coronary occlusion with results comparable with those of balloon angioplasty.[116] When used in the treatment of complex native coronary artery lesions not associated with acute MI, the outcome also appears similar to that of balloon angioplasty,[117] but use of TEC doubles the cost. In carefully selected patients with large intracoronary thrombi and ongoing ischemia, TEC has proved useful, as has the Dispatch catheter (Scimed Life Systems, Maple Grove, MN), a device for localized intracoronary infusion.[118] Thrombectomy devices for intracoronary use are currently under investigation.[119]

Although ablative laser angioplasty (XeCl excimer and holmium Nd:YAG) has been shown to be effective in treatment of aortoostial sites, undilatable lesions, total occlusions, calcification, long lesions, and saphenous vein grafts,[120–123] its superiority to simpler and less costly balloon strategies has not been demonstrated.[124–126] Lesions that should not be selected for ablative laser angioplasty include those on bend points or in tortuous segments, those associated with severe calcification or thrombus, or lesions with a suspected subintimal wire passage. In general, bifurcation lesions should not be selected for ablative laser therapy unless an eccentrically directed device can be used to avoid perforating at the flow divider of the vessel. The use of a laser guidewire to cross total occlusions appears very promising.[127]

PERFORMANCE OF CORONARY INTERVENTION

Operator Proficiency

Current guidelines recommend that cardiologists who wish to become competent in coronary intervention receive special training in diagnostic and therapeutic catheterization during an additional year after the standard fellowship training program and maintain skills by performance of a minimum of 75 procedures per year.[128–132] Adequate case mix is an important aspect of a physician's training in interventional cardiology that has not yet been addressed by practice guidelines.[133,134] Assurance of quality by surveillance of procedural outcomes is made difficult by complex issues including a need to adjust for high-risk patients, low incidence and subjectivity of major adverse events, and low volume of many operators.[135,136]

Interventional Laboratory

Optimal conditions for performance of coronary angioplasty procedures require sophisticated imaging systems; trained personnel; a large inventory of dilation, atherectomy, and stent hardware and software; and a variety of therapeutic safety nets to protect the patient when intervention fails or is complicated. Most studies suggest that laboratory procedural volume is important and inversely related to adverse procedural outcomes.[137–139]

The quality of the video image of the coronary arteries is an important determinant of angioplasty success. A freeze-frame storage and display capability is required for use during the procedure, as is a high-quality video replay with slow-motion and stop-frame capability. The ability to solve specific problems—such as lesion eccentricity or rigidity, vessel tortuosity, and unusual position or orientation of coronary ostia—is often dependent on specific device characteristics. Consequently, it is necessary to have available dilating catheters, atherectomy devices, guidewires, and guiding catheters in a variety of shapes and sizes. Cardiac surgery should be available in the institution if needed for emergency situations.

Interventional Equipment

The over-the-wire steerable catheter system used in most coronary interventions is illustrated in Fig. 48-9. In atherectomy, ablative laser, or stent procedures, the device replaces or is mounted on a balloon catheter. The balloon or device is introduced through a guiding catheter that extends through the arterial puncture site (femoral, brachial, or radial) to the coronary artery or graft ostia, where coaxial alignment of the catheter and vessel is highly desirable. In the past, the Judkins right and left coronary shapes were most frequently used, but many other shapes are currently available to address specific anatomic problems (Figs. 48-10 and 48-11). The size (5 to 11 French) and shape of the guide catheter may be determined by the arterial size at the entry site, the guide catheter lumen

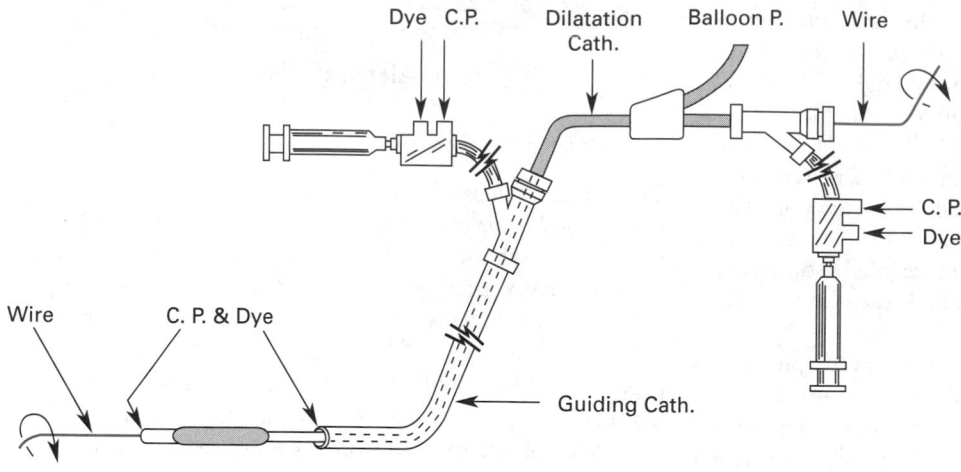

FIGURE 48-9

Diagram of the over-the-wire dilatation catheter with capacity for contract media (dye) injection. The floppy guidewire is steerable. (From Aueron FM, Gruentzig AR. Percutaneous transluminal coronary angioplasty: Indications and current status. *Prim Cardiol* 1984; 10:91. Reproduced with permission of the publisher and authors.)

requirement of the device used, and other factors such as a need for optimal vessel opacification. Directional atherectomy cutters and some stents require a large catheter lumen and a smooth shape.

Balloon catheters for coronary use are available in an array of balloon lengths (9 to 4 mm), diameters (1.5 to 4 mm), shaft sizes, and special features including active and passive perfusion, high-pressure capability, and local intracoronary infusion.

In the United States, the most frequent used stent, the Palmaz-Schatz stent (Fig. 48-5), is provided with a sheath delivery system that necessitates an 8 French guide catheter, whereas in Europe stents are frequently hand-crimped on balloons, which permits 6 French catheters to be used.[140] A large number of new stent designs are undergoing FDA evaluation.

The high-speed rotational atherectomy device (Fig. 48-4*B*), an olive-shaped burr with embedded diamond chips, requires a special 0.009-in. stainless steel guidewire, while the directional atherectomy cutter and laser catheters pass over conventional 0.014-in. steerable guidewires. The transluminal extraction catheter requires a unique 0.014-in. stainless steel guidewire that has a 0.21-in. ball at its tip.

The use of intravascular ultrasound to guide therapy varies widely; it is almost routine practice in some centers and is rarely used in others. Ultrasound assessment of the adequacy of stent deployment (Fig. 48-6), pioneered by Colombo and colleagues,[135] and evaluation of calcified lesions are probably the most frequent applications (see Chap. 49).

The Coronary Interventional Procedure

Prior to coronary intervention, patients receive an explanation of the procedure, including the operator's estimate of success, possible complications, risks, and benefits. A booklet and videotape describing the procedure and an explanation by the nursing staff help to reduce anxiety and ensure that both patient and family are well informed.

Antiplatelet therapy is used routinely. The therapy most widely used is aspirin, 160 to 325 mg daily. Patients in whom stenting is planned receive ticlopidine 250 mg PO bid. In 10 to 15 percent of patients in our hospital, the platelet glycoprotein IIb/IIIa receptor antagonist (c7E3Fab, Eli-Lilly and Co., Indianapolis, IN) is utilized if there is perceived to be an increased risk

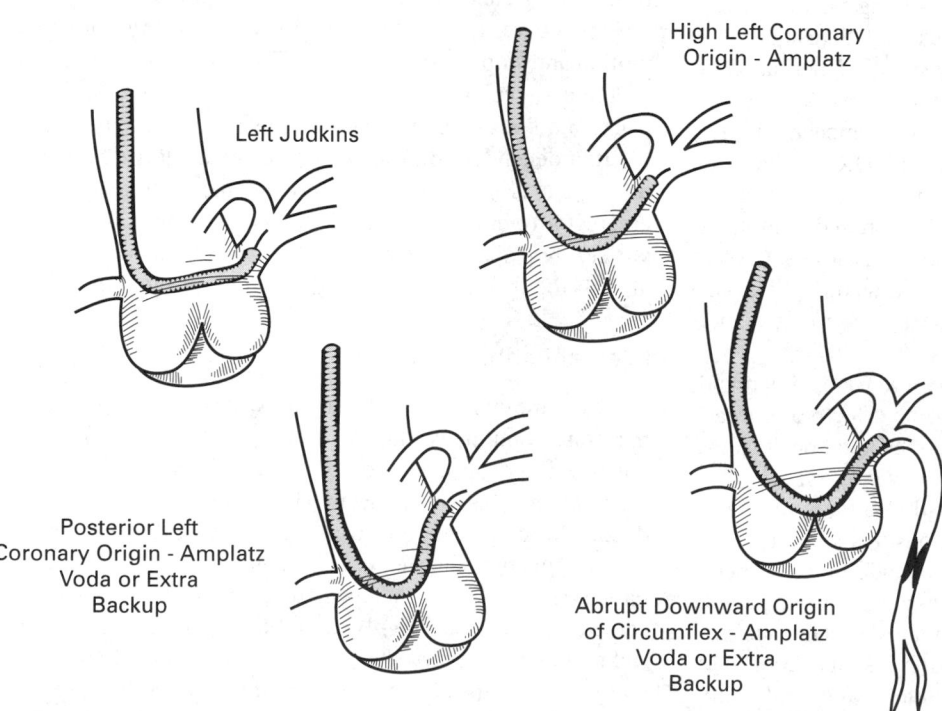

FIGURE 48-10

Guide catheter shapes commonly used for left coronary angioplasty.

of abrupt closure (suspected or definite thrombus, complex lesion).[37] Restenosis trials have failed to show a clear advantage of one antiplatelet regimen over another and have not shown inhibition of restenosis by calcium channel-blocking agents, warfarin anticoagulation, angiotension converting enzyme (ACE) inhibitors, steroids, or many other agents.

A calcium channel blocking agent is commonly given priority to coronary intervention for prophylaxis against coronary artery spasm and to reduce ischemia during the procedure. Once the patient is in the catheterization laboratory, electrocardiographic monitoring leads are applied, a peripheral intravenous line is started, and diazepam 2 to 5 mg or an equivalent drug is given intravenously. In most laboratories a femoral approach is employed. Heparin, either 10,000 U or a weight-based dose, is administered intravenously and either a bolus of 5000 U is repeated hourly during the procedure or a continuous heparin infusion is begun. An activated clotting time (ACT) of greater than 300 s is recommended. Less aggressive heparinization is used in conjunction with c7E3 Fab therapy. Patients with a history of allergy to contrast media are premedicated with prednisone, 60 mg orally, the night before and the day of the procedure and with diphenhydramine (Benadryl), 50 mg

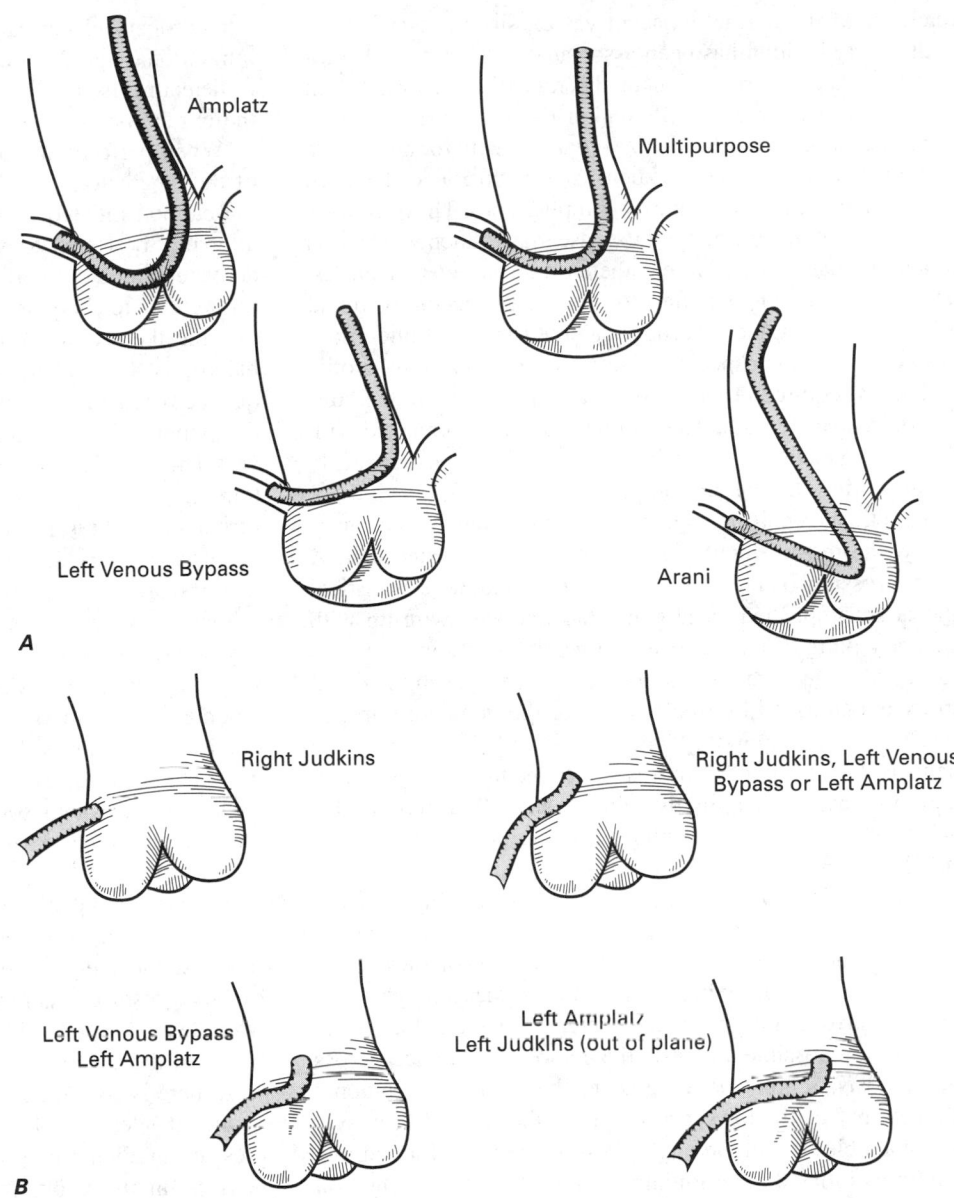

FIGURE 48-11

Guide catheter selection. *A*. Guide catheter shapes that are effective when the right coronary artery has a steep upward initial course. *B*. Guide catheter shapes that are effective when the right coronary artery has an anterior and leftward origin.

intravenously at the time of the procedure. Ionic hyperosmolar contrast medium is used routinely in our hospital for elective coronary angioplasty, due to the extraordinary cost of low-osmolar agents and the lack of proved benefit to warrant their routine use.[141-143] Due to the reported increased thrombotic complications with nonionic agents (attributed to comparatively less thrombin inhibition and enhanced platelet activation), ionic agents are preferred in patients with unstable ischemic syndromes or frank intracoronary thrombus.[142] Contrast-induced bradycardia, more common with ionic agents, is treated with atropine. Patients selected for use of an ionic low-osmolar contrast agent include those with renal insufficiency or severe left ventricular dysfunction. Nonionic agents

are reserved for patients with known allergy to the available ionic agents or with a history of severe bradycardia with ionic agents.

Coronary arteriograms are performed in two approximately orthogonal views selected to demonstrate the lesion(s) to be treated and the course of the parent artery without overlap by other vessels. The angles chosen are recorded, and freeze frames demonstrating the anatomy are stored and displayed during the procedure. A balloon catheter or device is selected based on the diameter of the target coronary artery to be treated, and the length of the stenotic segment is determined by comparison with the guiding catheter of known diameter. The balloon diameter is chosen to approximate closely the diameter of the normal adjacent vessel, since oversizing the angioplasty balloon has been associated with increased complications and no reduction in the rate of restenosis.[144] In general, an over-the-wire dilatation catheter system is preferred because of the ability to exchange easily for alternative balloons or other devices, such as a perfusion catheter or stent, in the event of angioplasty complications. The operator's impression of the difficulty of the case may influence selection of a particularly low-profile catheter to cross severe stenoses, a flexible catheter to negotiate tortuous segments, or rotational atherectomy to treat a fibrotic, calcified lesion. Balloon-on-a-wire devices are especially useful when an ultralow-profile balloon is required or when simultaneous use of two balloons is required (Fig. 48-2). The coronary ostium is engaged with the guiding catheter and the steerable guidewire is cautiously advanced into the target artery.

In patients requiring angioplasty of more than one coronary artery, the most difficult lesion is commonly treated first. A clean crossing of the stenosis with the guidewire is critical and is accomplished by aligning the steerable wire tip with the entry point of the stenosis and gently advancing it across the lesion. The intraluminal position of the wire in the distal artery is confirmed by free rotation of the guidewire tip and by contrast angiography. If there is difficulty in crossing the stenosis with the guidewire, reshaping the tip will commonly lead to success. Changing the wire to one with different characteristics, such as a hydrophilic coating, or to a stiffer wire may be necessary in the case of total occlusions.

With the steerable guidewire securely in the distal coronary artery, injections of contrast medium are made through the guiding catheter to locate and mark the position of the stenosis to be treated. While fixing the position of the guidewire, the operator advances the balloon catheter or device to the lesion. If it is not possible to push the balloon or device across the stenosis, it may be wise to exchange it for rotational atherectomy or the lowest-profile over-the-wire balloon system available. If balloon angioplasty is being performed, the balloon is inflated to an initial pressure of 2 atm. Indentation of the inflated balloon by the lesion confirms proper placement. The balloon is subsequently inflated until the "waist" caused by the lesion is obliterated and the balloon is fully inflated. When using a compliant balloon, the operator may inflate the balloon to higher pressures to produce the balloon diameter desired. During these inflations, an attempt is made not to exceed the burst pressure of the balloon. The balloon is reinflated as needed to achieve an adequate dilation.

There is no clear evidence regarding the optimal number or duration of balloon inflations or the maximal balloon pressure. Occasionally, if two to four inflations of 30 to 60 s do not yield the desired result, prolonged inflations up to 5 to 10 min may be helpful. Tolerance of the longer inflations may be enhanced by distal perfusion of arterial or venous blood through the dilatation catheter or by use of an autoperfusion balloon catheter, a strategy also suitable as a primary approach to many lesions.[145] Balloon inflations are limited by evidence of ischemia, as indicated by symptoms of chest discomfort or by ST-segment elevation. Some investigators have monitored

intracoronary electrocardiograms (ECGs) from the steerable intracoronary guidewire and found these to be more sensitive in detecting ischemia than surface ECGs. One can also use the intracoronary wire for temporary pacing.[146]

When performing directional atherectomy, the "window" of the atherectomy device is oriented toward the lesion and the balloon inflated to 1 atm. The cutter is then withdrawn, allowing the lesion to enter the open window. The motor is activated and a cut performed by slowly advancing the spinning cutter to the distal end of the device housing, thereby packing the shavings into the nose cone of the device. The balloon is then deflated, the window reoriented, and the sequence repeated. To minimize the possibility of perforation, the window is not oriented toward normal portions of the vessel wall. It is important to note that overzealous atherectomy may lead to an increased risk of perforation, aneurysm formation, and restenosis. An ultrasound-guided atherectomy cutter is under development.

Intracoronary stenting may be conducted either as a primary strategy or for suboptimal outcomes after balloon angioplasty or other interventions. Deployment strategies vary depending on stent designs, as some are balloon-mounted and others are self-expanding. Postdeployment dilation with a properly sized balloon is performed (usually to >14 atm) to expand the stent optimally throughout its length. Although some operators advocate intravascular ultrasound guidance, there is no consensus regarding its routine use.[147,148]

With rotational atherectomy and ablative laser procedures, many operators use special infusion or flushing strategies (using saline and/or vasodilators) to optimize laser debulking by blood displacement, reduce acoustic shock and dissection with the laser, and avoid no-reflow phenomena.[108,149] Proper sizing of these debulking devices is under investigation.

If there is concern about the adequacy of the lumen at the treatment site, use of a Doppler flow wire, angioscopy, or pressure gradients may be helpful in addition to ultrasound in assessing the result. Studies suggest that a normal coronary hyperemic flow response and a low transluminal gradient are associated with reduced risk of restenosis. *It is clear that optimizing the lumen size is the goal, since final lumen size is an important determinant of the probability of restenosis.* When the operator is confident that the best possible result has been obtained, the patient is returned to his or her room, where an ECG is obtained and the patient is placed on telemetry. Creatine kinase determinations are performed immediately and every 8 h for three determinations. Because of the dehydrating effect of the osmotic load, most patients receive at least 1 L of intravenous fluids postprocedure. Sheath removal is performed at 2 to 4 h when the activated clotting time is below 150 s. If a large intimal tear, suboptimal result, or intraluminal thrombus is present, heparin is frequently administered overnight or c7E3 Fab may be used. There is evidence that routine heparin administration following uncomplicated angioplasty is not helpful in reducing acute occlusion or restenosis.[150] Postprocedure medications in-hospital include aspirin, a calcium channel-blocking agent, and topical nitrates. Most patients are discharged on the first day following the procedure after receiving instructions on lipid-lowering therapy (see Chap. 53), exercise, and cessation of smoking (see Chap. 41), and are given an outline of follow-up procedures.

RESULTS OF CORONARY INTERVENTION

The results obtained with coronary intervention procedures have been significantly influenced by technologic advances, operator experience, and the difficulty of cases selected. With crude equipment, Gruentzig was able to dilate 64 percent of the initial 50 patients and 78 percent of the first 169 patients.[9,13] Defining primary success as less than 50 percent residual stenosis and freedom from complications, we obtained a success rate of 90 percent in over 20,000 patients treated at Emory University Hospital between 1980 and 1995 (Table 48-5). Note that complication rates generally declined in spite of increasingly difficult cases. Experienced operators should achieve primary success rates in excess of 95 percent in ideal proximal lesions compared to a reduced success rate of approximately 75 percent in recent (<3 months) total occlusions or when attempting to treat fibrotic, calcified, eccentric stenoses located distally in tortuous coronary arteries. In all techniques, including stenting,[97] lesion characteristics are a major determinant of the outcome of the procedure.[39,40,84–88] Long-term outcome has been reported out to 10 years in patients treated in Zurich, Atlanta, and Rotterdam[13–15,41,151] and detailed 5-year follow-up data are available from randomized trials[18–24,49] (see above and Table 48-1).

Complications

Patients undergoing coronary intervention are subject to the same complications encountered with the performance of coronary arteriography. In addition, because instrumentation of the atherosclerotic lesion takes place, coronary artery dissection, thrombus formation, and coronary artery spasm may occur, leading to acute occlusion of the coronary artery or of side branches arising from it. Acute occlusion of the dilated artery is the most common serious complication of coronary angioplasty and accounts for most of the morbidity and mortality related to the procedure.

Of Gruentzig's first 50 patients, 5 experienced an acute deterioration necessitating emergency bypass surgery and 3 showed ECG evidence of MI.[9] The results of 3500 patients undergoing elective balloon angioplasty at Emory were analyzed and reported in detail in 1985.[152] Angioplasty was attempted in 3933 lesions, with a success rate of 91 percent. No complications occurred in 89 percent of cases, minor complications occurred in 6.9 percent, and major complications (emergency surgery, MI, death) in 4.1 percent. Emergency coronary bypass surgery was performed in 2.7 percent of patients, who had an MI rate of 49 percent and a Q-wave infarction rate of 23 percent. In patients sent for emergency surgery, the mortality rate was 2 percent. The overall MI rate was 2.6 percent. There were two nonsurgical deaths, giving a total mortality rate of 0.1 percent (4/3500). *Five preprocedural predictors of a major complication were identified: multivessel coronary disease, lesion eccentricity, presence of calcium in the lesion, female gender, and lesion length. The strongest predictor of a major complication was the appearance of an intimal dissection during the procedure.* Intimal dissection was evident in 29 percent of patients, and its presence resulted in a sixfold increase in the risk of a major complication. Minor complications tabulated in this study included the following: side branch occlusion (1.7 percent), ventricular arrhythmia requiring DC shock (1.5 percent), emergency recatheterization (0.8 percent), femoral artery repair (0.6 percent), transfusion requirement (0.3 percent), coronary embolus (0.1 percent),

TABLE 48-5

RESULTS OF CORONARY ANGIOPLASTY—EMORY UNIVERSITY HOSPITAL

	1980–1983	1984–1987	1988–1991	1992–1995	Total
Patients	2290	4964	6591	6367	20,212
Arterial segments treated	2529	6356	9068	8321	26,274
Initial success, %[a]	87	93	93	94	93
Complication-free success, %[b]	85	89	90	90	90
Single-vessel disease, %	80	61	49	35	51
Multivessel disease, %[c]	20	39	57	65	49
Multivessel PTCA, %[d]	3.1	10	11	9	9
Emergency CABG, %	3.6	3.3	2.1	1.3	2.3
Q-wave MI, %	1.9	1.5	1.0	0.8	1.1
In-hospital death, %	0.1	0.2	0.5	0.6	0.4

[a] Less than 50% residual stenosis.
[b] Less than 50% residual stenosis and freedom from complications.
[c] At least 50% stenosis of LAD + RCA, LAD + CIRC, CIRC + RCA, or LAD + RCA + CIRC.
[d] Dilatation of LAD + RCA, LAD + CIRC, CIRC + RCA, or LAD + RCA + CIRC.

Abbreviations: LAD = left anterior descending; RCA = right coronary artery; CIRC = circumflex coronary artery; PTCA = percutaneous transluminal coronary angioplasty; CABG = coronary artery bypass graft; MI = myocardial infarction.

cardiac tamponade (0.1 percent), and stroke (0.03 percent). This early series of patients was treated with balloon angioplasty alone. In 1995 at Emory University Hospital, over 1600 patients were treated (76 percent with balloon alone), with angiographic success in 94 percent, Q-wave MI in 1.1 percent, non-Q-MI in 2.9 percent, and death in 0.6 percent.

Although angiographic variables are important predictors of abrupt closure, of equal or greater importance is an estimate of the consequences of abrupt closure. This estimate is determined in large part by the amount of myocardium that is supplied by the artery in jeopardy. Occlusion of a small diagonal branch is of little consequence compared, for example, to the occlusion of a large left anterior descending coronary artery that is also supplying collateral vessels to an occluded right coronary artery. In the first case, a small non-Q-wave infarction is likely, whereas in the latter, occlusion would likely result in abrupt anterior and inferior ischemia and be associated with hypotension and possibly cardiogenic shock. Immediate stenting or bypass surgery may be lifesaving, but MI will occur in up to one-half of patients, and there is a significant risk of mortality in this subgroup of patients.

An analysis in 1988 of 294 acute occlusions occurring during 8207 consecutive coronary angioplasty procedures performed in two centers revealed 13 cardiac deaths (4.4 percent of acute occlusions) and an overall cardiac mortality of 0.16 percent.[153] Of 13 patients who died, 12 were women. Multivariate analysis identified three independent predictors of death: collaterals originating from the dilated vessel, female gender, and multivessel disease. In an analysis in 1991 of 32 deaths associated with 8052 PTCA procedures in three centers, left ventricular failure due to vessel occlusion, the most common cause of death, was independently correlated with female sex, "jeopardy score," and PTCA of a proximal right coronary artery (RCA) site but not ejection fraction or presence of multivessel disease.[154] Right ventricular failure due to occlusion of the proximal RCA and left main coronary dissections accounted for the majority of the remaining deaths.

The use of stents in the course of a failing angioplasty and prospectively in patients with unfavorable anatomy has significantly reduced the risk of urgent bypass surgery and Q-wave MI.[31,32,38] The increasing use of stents and adjunctive measures including new, powerful antithrombotic agents may herald a "new era" of coronary intervention.[38]

New complications specifically related to the use of nonballoon devices include coronary perforation, distal atheroembolization, arterial access complications and "domino stenting" (additional stents to treat end-of-stent dissections). The risk of coronary perforation is a limiting factor in achieving optimal atherectomy and significantly restricts use of the TEC device in native vessels. Among 8932 patients treated at Williams Beaumont Hospital, perforation was reported in 0.4 percent (balloon, 0.14 percent; TEC, 1.3 percent; DCA, 0.25 percent; excimer laser 2 percent).[155] This risk of perforation is highest in tortuous and smaller vessels and in laser angioplasty of right coronary lesions. In patients experiencing free perforations, Ellis reported that 75 percent required surgery,

29 percent had a Q-wave MI, and 14 percent died.[156] Perforation has been reported in 10 of 432 stent patients (2.3 percent), resulting in cardiac tamponade (50 percent), MI (40 percent), emergency surgery (50 percent), and death (30 percent).[157] The manifestations of perforation were delayed (5 to 24 h) in 20 percent of patients. *Angiographic features associated with stent-related perforation were complex lesion morphology, small vessel diameter (2.6 ± 0.2 mm), oversized stents (stent/artery ratio 1.4 ± 0.1), tapering vessel (40 percent), and recrossing dissection (20 percent).*[157] *These results should engender a cautious approach to stenting in small vessels and when there is uncertainty regarding wire position.* Prompt application of strategies for the management of vessel perforation can be lifesaving and device angioplasty operators must be facile with them.

Fortunately, the risk of vascular access site complications, a frequent accompaniment of stenting when warfarin (Coumadin) anticoagulation is used adjunctively, has been reduced with less aggressive antithrombotic strategies. In our experience, complications at the femoral artery puncture site were more often related to advanced age, female sex, hypertension, and postprocedure heparin use than to the size of the catheter.[158–160] Prolonged compression of pseudoaneurysms using ultrasound guidance obviates surgery in many patients.[161]

Distal coronary atheroembolization is only occasionally recognized clinically with balloon angioplasty but probably occurs moderately frequently[162] and is a clinically important limitation of debulking strategies such as atherectomy and laser ablation, where its manifestations are slow coronary flow, ischemia, and infarction.[164] Recent reports from CAVEAT also indicate that even mild creatine kinase elevations postprocedure were associated with worse long-term outcomes (death, MI, repeat intervention).[164] Although procedural modifications with rotational atherectomy appear to have reduced the immediate impact of microparticulate embolization,[108] the issue remains a source of concern and needs further study. Patients at increased risk include those with bulky or long native vessel lesions and nonfocal or thrombotic saphenous vein graft lesions, where embolization with TEC was noted in about 20 percent, and about one-third of patients with this complication died.[165,166]

Acute contrast nephropathy requiring dialysis is a costly complication of coronary intervention, which occurred in 15 of 1828 (0.8 percent) patients and was associated with a high (33.8 percent) in-hospital mortality.[167] *Independent predictors of contrast nephropathy included decreased baseline creatinine clearance, diabetes and contrast dose (no dialysis was required in patients receiving <100 mL contrast).*

FUTURE DIRECTIONS

The future of coronary intervention is bright indeed. The problem of subacute stent thrombosis, greatly diminished by current deployment strategies, should be solved by nonthrombogenic stents,[99] thus opening the arena of small-vessel stenting (2- to 2.5-mm vessels) and further expanding intervention for multiple lesions in multiple vessels. The major impediments are cost and restenosis. The former should be ameliorated somewhat by market competition. Restenosis, which has been reduced by stenting of de novo[33,34,99] and restenotic lesions,[168] remains a challenge that is currently being addressed on multiple fronts with good prospects for meaningful solutions.[169-172]

REFERENCES

1. Dotter CT, Judkins MP. Transluminal treatment of arteriosclerotic obstruction: Description of a new technique and a preliminary report of its application. *Circulation* 1964; 30:654–670.

2. Zeitler EJ, Schmidtke J, Schoop W. Die Perkutane Behandlung von Arteriellen Durchbluteungasstorungen der Estremiaten mit Katheter. *Vasa* 1973; 2:401–404.

3. Gruentzig AR, Turina MI, Schneider JA. Experimental percutaneous dilatation of coronary artery stenosis (abstr). *Circulation* 1976; 54(suppl II):II-81.

4. Gruentzig AR, Kumpe DA. Technique of percutaneous transluminal angioplasty with the Gruentzig balloon catheter. *Am J Roentgenol* 1979; 132:547–552.

5. Sheldon WC, Sones FM Jr. Stormy petrel of cardiology. *Clin Cardiol* 1994; 17:405–407.

6. Hurst JW. History of cardiac catheterization. In: King SB III, Douglas JS Jr, eds. *Coronary Arteriography and Angioplasty*. New York: McGraw-Hill; 1985:1–9.

7. King SB III. Angioplasty from bench to bedside to bench. *Circulation* 1996; 93:1621–1629.

8. Gruentzig A. Transluminal dilatation of coronary artery stenosis. *Lancet* 1978; 1:263.

9. Gruentzig AR, Senning A, Siegenthaler WE. Nonoperative dilatation of coronary artery stenosis: Percutaneous transluminal coronary angioplasty. *N Engl J Med* 1979; 301:61–68.

10. Kent KM, Bentivoglio LG, Block PC. Percutaneous transluminal coronary angioplasty: Report from the Registry of the National Heart, Lung, and Blood Institute. *Am J Cardiol* 1982; 49:2011–2020.

11. Detre K, Holubkov R, Kelsey S, Cowley M, Kent K, Williams D, et al. Percutaneous transluminal coronary angioplasty in 1985–1986 and 1977–1981: The National Heart, Lung, and Blood Institute Registry. *N Engl J Med* 1988; 318:265–270.

12. Simpson JB, Baim DS, Robert EW, Harrison DC. A new catheter system for coronary angioplasty. *Am J Cardiol* 1982; 49:1216–1222.

13. Gruentzig AR, King SB III, Schlumpf M, Siegenthaler WE. Long-term follow-up after percutaneous transluminal coronary angioplasty: The early Zurich experience. *N Engl J Med* 1987; 316:1127–1132.

14. King SB, Schlumpf M. Ten year completed follow-up after percutaneous transluminal coronary angioplasty: The early Zurich experience. *J Am Coll Cardiol* 1993; 22:353–360.

15. Detre K, Yeh W, Kelsey S, Williams D, Desvigne-Nickens P, Holmes D, et al. Has improvement in PTCA intervention affected long-term prognosis? The NHLBI PTCA Registry experience. *Circulation* 1995; 91:2868–2875.

16. Cowley MJ, Vetrovec GW, DiSciasio G, Lewis SA, Hirsh PD, Wolfgang TC. Coronary angioplasty of multiple vessels: Short-term outcome and long-term results. *Circulation* 1985; 72:1314–1320.

17. O'Keefe JH Jr, Rutherford BD, McConahay DR, Johnson WL Jr, Giorgi LV, Ligon RW, et al. Multivessel coronary angioplasty from 1980–1989: Procedural results and long-term outcome. *J Am Coll Cardiol* 1990; 16:1097–1102.

18. Parisi AF, Folland ED, Hartigan P. A comparison of angioplasty with medical therapy in the treatment of single-vessel coronary artery disease. *N Engl J Med* 1992; 326:10–16.

19. King SB III, Lembo NJ, Weintraub WS, Kosinski AS, Barnhart HX, Kutner MH, et al. A randomized trial comparing coronary angioplasty with coronary bypass surgery. *N Engl J Med* 1994; 331:1044–1050.

20. The Bypass Angioplasty Revascularization Investigation (BARI) Investigators. Comparison of coronary bypass surgery with angioplasty in patients with multivessel disease. *N Engl J Med* 1996; 335:217–225.

21. Chaitman BR, Schwartz L, Roubin GS, Lytle BW, Hardison RM, Sopko G, et al. Comparative 5 year incidence of ischemic events for PTCA and CABG in the Bypass Angioplasty Revascularization Investigation (BARI), (abstr). *J Am Coll Cardiol* 1996; 27:55A.

22. Pocock SJ, Henderson RA, Rickards AF, Hampton Jr, King SB III, Hamm CW, et al. Metaanalysis of randomized trials comparing coronary angioplasty with bypass surgery. *Lancet* 1995; 346:1184–1189.

23. Kosinski AS, Barnharat HX, Weintraub WS, Guyton RA, King SB III, the EAST Investigators. Five year outcome after coronary surgery or coronary angioplasty: Results from the Emory Angioplasty vs Surgery Trial (EAST), (abstr). *Circulation* 1995; 92:I-543.

24. Weintraub WS, Mauldin PD, Becker E, Kosinski AS, King SB III. A comparison of the costs and quality of life after coronary angioplasty or coronary surgery for multivessel coronary artery disease: Results from the Emory Angioplasty versus Surgery Trial (EAST). *Circulation* 1995; 92:2831–2840.

25. Robertson GC, Simpson JB, Selmon MR, Vetter JW, Bartzokis TC, Rowe MH, et al. Experience of directional coronary atherectomy over four years (abstr). *J Am Coll Cardiol* 1991; 17:384A.

26. Topol EJ, Leya F, Pinkerton CA, Whitlow PL, Hofling B, Simonton CA, et al. A comparison of directional coronary atherectomy with coronary angioplasty in patients with coronary artery disease. *N Engl J Med* 1993; 329:221–227.

27. Adelman AG, Cohen EA, Kimball BP, Bonan R, Ricci DR, Webb JG, et al. A comparison of directional atherectomy with balloon angioplasty for lesions of the left anterior descending coronary artery. *N Engl J Med* 1993; 329:228–233.

28. Holmes DR Jr, Topol EJ, Califf RM, Berdan LG, Leya F, Berger PB, et al. A multicenter, randomized trial of coronary angioplasty versus directional atherectomy for patients with saphenous vein bypass graft lesions. *Circulation* 1995; 91:1966–1974.

29. Baim DS, Kuntz RE, Sharma SK, Fortuna R, Feldman R, Senerchia C, et al. Acute results of the randomized trial of the Balloon versus Optimal Atherectomy Trial (BOAT) (abstr). *Circulation* 1995; 92(suppl I):I-544.

30. Popma JJ, Baim DS, Kuntz RE, Mintz GS, Simonton CS, Hinohara T, et al. Early and late quantitative angiographic outcome from Optimal Atherectomy Restenosis Study (OARS) (abstr). *J Am Coll Cardiol* 1996; 27(suppl A):291A.

31. Roubin GS, King SB III, Douglas JS Jr, Lembo NJ, Robinson KA. Intracoronary stenting during percutaneous transluminal coronary angioplasty. *Circulation* 1990; 81(suppl IV):IV-92–IV-100.

32. Hearn JA, King SB III, Douglas JS Jr, Carlin SF, Lembo NJ, Ghazzal ZMB. Clinical and angiographic outcomes after coronary artery stenting for acute or threatened closure after percutaneous transluminal coronary angioplasty: Initial results with a balloon-expandable, stainless steel design. *Circulation* 1993; 88:2086–2096.

33. Fischman DL, Leon MB, Baim DS, Schatz RA, Savage MP, Penn I, et al. A randomized comparison of coronary-stent placement and balloon angioplasty in treatment of coronary artery disease. *N Engl J Med* 1994; 331:496–501.

34. Serruys PW, de Jaegere P, Kiemeneij F, Macaya C, Rutsch W, Heyndrickx G, et al. A comparison of balloon-expandable-stent implantation with balloon angioplasty in patients with coronary artery disease. *N Engl J Med* 1994; 331:489–495.

35. Colombo A, Hall P, Nakamura S, Almagor Y, Maielli L, Martini G, et al. Intracoronary stenting without anticoagulation accomplished with intravascular ultrasound guidance. *Circulation* 1995; 91:1676–1688.

36. Schoemig A, Newmann FJ, Kastrati A, Schuehlen H, Blasini R, Hadamitzky M, et al. A randomized comparison of antiplatelet and anticoagulant therapy after the placement of coronary artery stents. *N Engl J Med* 1996; 334:1084–1089.

37. The EPIC Investigators. Use of a monoclonal antibody directed against the platelet glycoprotein IIb/IIIa receptor in high-risk coronary angioplasty. *N Engl J Med* 1994; 330:956–961.

38. Ellis SG, Whitlow PL, Guetta V, Sheldon WS, Topol EJ. A highly significant 40% reduction in ischemic complications of percutaneous coronary intervention in 1995: Beginning of a new era (abstr). *J Am Coll Cardiol* 1996; 27(suppl A):253A.

39. Ryan TJ, Faxon DP, Gunnar RM, Kennedy JW, King SB III, Loop ED, et al. Guidelines for percutaneous transluminal coronary angioplasty: A report of the American College of Cardiology/American Heart Association Task Force on Assessment of Diagnostic and Therapeutic Cardiovascular Procedures (Subcommittee of Percutaneous Transluminal Coronary Angioplasty). *J Am Coll Cardiol* 1988; 12:519–540.

40. Ryan TJ, Bauman WB, Kennedy JW, Kereiakes DJ, King SB III, McCallister BD, et al. Guidelines for percutaneous transluminal coro-

nary angioplasty: A report of the American Heart Association/American College of Cardiology Task Force on Assessment of Diagnostic and Therapeutic Cardiovascular Procedures (Committee on Percutaneous Transluminal Coronary Angioplasty). *Circulation* 1993; 88:2987–3007.

41. Weintraub WS, King SB III, Douglas JS Jr, Kosinski AS. Percutaneous transluminal coronary angioplasty as a first revascularization procedure in single, double, and triple-vessel coronary artery disease. *J Am Coll Cardiol* 1995; 26:142–151.

42. Mark DB, Nelson CL, Califf RM, Harrell FE Jr, Lee KL, Jones RH. Continuing evaluation and therapy for coronary artery disease: Initial results from the era of coronary angioplasty. *Circulation* 1994; 89:2015–2025.

43. Goy JJ, Eickhout E, Burnand B. Coronary angioplasty versus left internal mammary artery grafting for isolated proximal left anterior descending artery stenosis. *Lancet* 1994; 343:1449–1454.

44. Strauss WE, Fortin T, Hartigan P, Folland ED, Parisi AF, the Veterans Affairs Study of Angioplasty Compared to Medical Therapy Investigators. A comparison of quality of life scores in patients with angina pectoris after angioplasty compared with after medical therapy. Outcomes of a randomized clinical trial. *Circulation* 1995; 92:1710–1719.

45. Giacomini JC, Parisi AF, Folland ED, Hartigan P. Three year follow-up of patients in the VA ACME Trial (abstr). *Circulation* 1993; 88(suppl I):I-218.

46. Ellis SG, Brown K, Howell G, Kerrick C. Two-year cardiac cost after cardiac catheterization: Profound impact of revascularization after first PTCA compared with initial medical or surgical therapy (abstr). *J Am Coll Cardiol* 1996; 27(suppl A):72A.

47. Cowley MJ, Vandermael M, Topol EJ. Is traditionally defined complete revascularization needed for patients with multivessel disease treated with elective coronary angioplasty. *J Am Coll Cardiol* 1993; 22:1289–1297.

48. Bourassa MG, Holubkov R, Yeh W, Detra KM, Faxon DP, King SBK, et al. Strategy of complete revascularization in patients with multivessel coronary artery disease. (A report from the 1985–86 NHLBI PTCA Registry.) *Am J Cardiol* 1992; 70:174–178.

49. Zhao XQ, Brown BG, Stewart DK, Hillger LA, Barnhart HX, Kosinski AS, et al. Effectiveness of revascularization in the Emory Angioplasty Versus Surgery Trial: A randomized comparison of coronary angioplasty with bypass surgery. *Circulation* 1996; 93:1954–1962.

50. Ellis SG, Roubin GS, King SB III, Douglas JS Jr, Weintraub WS, Thomas RG, et al. Angiographic and clinical predictors of acute closure after native vessel coronary angioplasty. *Circulation* 1988; 77:372–379.

51. Fuster V, Badimon L, Badimon JJ, Chesebro JH. The Pathogenesis of coronary artery disease and acute coronary syndromes. *N Engl J Med* 1991; 326:242–250, 320–328.

52. Mizuno K, Satomura K, Miyamoto A, Arakawa K, Shibuya T, Arai T, et al. Angioscopic evaluation of coronary artery thrombi in acute coronary syndromes. *N Engl J Med* 1992; 326:287–291.

53. Waxman S, Mittleman MA, Manzok, Sassower M, Nesto R. Culprit lesion morphology in subtypes of unstable angina as assessed by angioscopy (abstr). *Circulation* 1995; 92(suppl I):I-79.

54. Laskey MA, Deutsch E, Hirshfield JWJ, Kussmaul WG, Barnathan E, Laskey WK. Influence of herapin therapy on percutaneous transluminal coronary angioplasty outcome in patients with coronary arterial thrombus. *Am J Cardiol* 1990; 65:179–182.

55. Laskey MA, Deutsch E, Barnathan E, Laskey WK. Influence of herapin therapy on percutaneous transluminal coronary angioplasty outcome in unstable angina pectoris. *Am J Cardiol* 1990; 65:1425–1429.

56. Rosenman Y, Gilon D, Zelingher J, Sapoznikov D, Lotan C, Mosseri M, et al. Importance of delaying balloon angioplasty in patients with unstable angina pectoris. *Clin Cardiol* 1996; 19:111–114.

57. Douglas JS Jr, Lutz JF, Clements SD, Robinson PH, Roubin GS, Lembo NJ, et al. Therapy of large intracoronary thrombi in candidates for percutaneous transluminal coronary angioplasty (abstr). *J Am Coll Cardiol* 1988; 11:238.

58. The TIMI-IIIB Investigators: Effects of tissue plasminogen activator and a comparison of early invasive and conservative strategies in unstable angina and non-Q wave myocardial infarction. *Circulation* 1994; 89:1545–1556.

59. Cannon CP, McCabe CH, Stone PH, Thompson B, Rogers W, Gibson RS. Prospective validation of the Braunwald classification of unstable angina: Results from the thrombolysis in myocardial ischemia (TIMI) III Registry (abstr). *Circulation* 1995; 92(suppl I):I-19.

60. Ghigliotti G, Brunelli C, Corsiglia L, Spallorossa P, Iannone A, Caponnetto S. Identification of high-risk patients with unstable angina (abstr). *J Am Coll Cardiol* 1996; 27(suppl A):332A.

61. Serruys PW, Herrman J-PR, Simon R, for the HELVETICA investigators. A comparison of hirudin with herapin in the prevention of restenosis after coronary angioplasty. *N Engl J Med* 1995; 333:757–763.

62. Ambrose JA, Almeida OD, Sharma SK, Torre SR, Marmur JD, Israel DH, et al for the TAUSA investigators. Adjunctive thrombolytic therapy during angioplasty for ischemic rest angina: Results of the TAUSA trial. *Circulation* 1994; 90:69–77.

63. Ferguson JJ. EPILOG and CAPTURE trials halted because of positive interim results. *Circulation* 1996; 93:637.

64. Ellis CJ, French JK, Williams BF, Wyatt S, Poole J, Ingram C. Thrombolytic therapy can be given to half of hospitalized patients with acute myocardial infarction (abstr). *J Am Coll Cardiol* 1996; 27(suppl A):249A.

65. TIMI Research Group. Immediate vs delayed catheterization and angioplasty following thrombolytic therapy for acute myocardial infarction: TIMI IIA results. *JAMA* 1988; 260:2849–2858.

66. Simoons ML, Arnold AER, Betriu A, deBono DP, Col J, Dougherty FC, et al. Thrombolysis with tissue plasminogen activator in acute myocardial infarction: No additional benefit from immediate percutaneous coronary angioplasty. *Lancet* 1988; 1:197–203.

67. Topol EJ, Califf RM, George BS, Kereiakes DJ, Abbotsmith CW, Candela RJ, et al. A randomized trial of immediate versus delayed elective angioplasty after intravenous tissue plasminogen activator in acute myocardial infarction. *N Engl J Med* 1987; 317:581–588.

68. McKendall GR, Forman S, Sopko G, Braunwald E, Williams DO, the Thrombolysis in Myocardial Infarction investigators. Value of rescue percutaneous transluminal coronary angioplasty following unsuccessful thrombolytic therapy in patients with acute myocardial infarction. *Am J Cardiol* 1995; 76:1108–1111.

69. Abbottsmith C, Topol E, George B, Stack R, Kereiakes D, Candela R, et al. Fate of patients with acute myocardial infarction with patency of the infarct-related vessel achieved with successful thrombolysis versus rescue angioplasty. *J Am Coll Cardiol* 1990; 16:770–778.

70. Ellis S, Ribeiro-da Silva E, Heyndrickx G, Talley J, Cernigliaro C, Steg G, et al. Randomized comparison of rescue angioplasty with conservative management of patients with early failure of thrombolysis for acute anterior myocardial infarction. *Circulation* 1994; 90:2280–2284.

71. O'Keefe J Jr, Rutherford BD, McConahay DR, Ligon RW, Johnson WL Jr, Giorgi LV, et al. Early and late results of coronary angioplasty without antecedent thrombolytic therapy for acute myocardial infarction. *Am J Cardiol* 1989; 64:1221–1230.

72. Rothbaum DA, Linnemeier TJ, Landin RJ, Steinmetz EF, Hillis JS, Hallam CC, et al. Emergency percutaneous transluminal coronary angioplasty in acute myocardial infarction: A 3 year experience. *J Am Coll Cardiol* 1987; 10:264–272.

73. O'Neill WW, Brodie B, Knopf W, Ivanhow R, O'Keefe J, Taylor G, et al. Initial report of the Primary Angioplasty Revascularization (PAR) Multicenter Registry (abstr). *Circulation* 1991; 84(suppl 2):II-536.

74. Lieu TA, Gurley RJ, Lundstrom RJ, Parmley WW. Primary angioplasty and thrombolysis for acute myocardial infarction: An evidence summary. *J Am Coll Cardiol* 1996; 27:737–750.

75. Grines CL, Browne KF, Marco J, Rothbaum D, Stone GW, O'Keefe J, et al. A comparison of immediate angioplasty with thrombolytic therapy for acute myocardial infarction. *N Engl J Med* 1993; 328:673–679.

76. Gibbons RJ, Holmes DR, Reeder GS, Bailey KR, Hopfenspirger MR, Gersh BJ. Immediate angioplasty compared with the administration of a thrombolytic agent followed by conservative treatment for myocardial infarction. *N Engl J Med* 1993; 328:685–691.

77. Zijlstra F, De Boer MJ, Hoorntje JCA, Reiffers S, Reiber JHC, Suryapranata H. A comparison of immediate coronary angioplasty with intravenous streptokinase in acute myocardial infarction. *N Engl J Med* 1993; 328:680–684.

78. Nunn C, O'Neill W, Rothbaum D, O'Keefe J Jr, Overlie P, Donohue B. Primary angioplasty for myocardial infarction improves long-term survival: PAMI-1 follow-up (abstr). *J Am Coll Cardiol* 1996; 27(suppl A):153A.

79. Simari RD, Berger PB, Bell MR, Gibbons RJ, Holmes DR Jr. Coronary angioplasty in acute myocardial infarction: Primary, immediate adjunctive, rescue, or deferred adjunctive approach? *Mayo Clin Proc* 1994; 69:346–358.

80. Lundergan CF, Reiner JS, Ross AM. Determinants of 30 day and one year mortality in acute myocardial infarction: Benefit of early angiography (abstr). *J Am Coll Cardiol* 1996; 27(suppl A):153A.

81. Cannon CP, Lambrew CT, Tiefenbrunn AJ, French WJ, Gore JM, Weaver D. Influence of door-to-balloon time on mortality in primary angioplasty results in 3,648 patients in the Second National Registry of Myocardial Infarction (NRMI-1) (abstr). *J Am Coll Cardiol* 1996; 27(suppl A):61A.

82. Stone GW, Marsalese D, Brodie B, Griffin J, Donohue B, Costantini C. The routine use of intra-aortic balloon pumping after primary angioplasty improves clinical outcome in very high risk patients with acute myocardial infarction: Results of the PAMI-2 trial (abstr). *Circulation* 1995; 92(suppl I):I-139.

83. Cragg DR, Friedman HZ, Almany SL, Gangadharan V, Ramos RG, Levine AB, et al. Early hospital discharge after percutaneous transluminal coronary angioplasty. *Am J Cardiol* 1989; 64:1270–1274.

84. Ellis SG, Vandormael MG, Cowley MJ, DiSciascio G, Deligonul U, Topol EJ. Coronary morphologic and clinical determinants of procedural outcome with angioplasty for multivessel coronary disease. *Circulation* 1990; 82:1193–1203.

85. Ellis SG, de Cesare NB, Pinkerton CA, Whitelow P, King SB, Ghazzal ZMB. Relation of stenosis morphology and clinical presentation to the procedural results of directional coronary atherectomy. *Circulation* 1991; 84:644–653.

86. Tan K, Sulke N, Taub N, Sowton E. Clinical and lesion morphologic determinants of coronary angioplasty success and complications: Current experience. *J Am Coll Cardiol* 1995; 25:855–865.

87. Herrman JR, Melkert R, Simon R, Serruys PW, HELVETICA Investigators. ABC-lesion type as a risk factor for the occurrence of early and late clinical events in unstable patients following transluminal coronary angioplasty (PTCA) (abstr). *J Am Coll Cardiol* 1996; 27(suppl A):390A.

88. Fry ET, Hermiller JB, Peters TF, Orr CM, Vantassel J, Berkompas DC. Is ACC/AHA classification predictive of successful coronary intervention in the era of new devices (abstr)? *J Am Coll Cardiol* 1996; 27(suppl A):152A.

89. Topol EJ, Nissen SE. Our preoccupation with coronary luminology: The dissociation between clinical and angiographic findings in ischemic heart disease. *Circulation* 1995; 92:2333–2342.

90. Tuzcu EM, Berkalp B, De Franco AC, Ellis SG, Goormastic M, Whitelow PL, et al. The dilemma of diagnosing coronary calcification: Angiography versus intravascular ultrasound. *J Am Coll Cardiol* 1996; 27:832–838.

91. Mintz GS, Popma JJ, Pichard AD, Kent KM, Satler LF, Chuang YC, et al. Intravascular ultrasound predictors of restenosis after percutaneous transcatheter coronary revascularization. *J Am Coll Cardiol* 1996; 27:1678–1687.

92. Stone GW, Linnemeier T, St Goar FG, Mudra H, Sheehan H, Hodgson JM. Improved outcome of balloon angioplasty with intracoronary ultrasound guidance—Core Lab angiographic and ultrasound results from the Clout study (abstr). *J Am Coll Cardiol* 1996; 27(suppl A):155A.

93. Bauters C, LaBlanche JM, McFadden E, Hamon M, Bertrand ME. Angioscopic thrombus is associated with a high risk of angiographic restenosis (abstr). *Circulation* 1995; 92(suppl I):I-401.

94. Serruys PW, Azar AJ, Sigwart U, Rutsch W, Dejeager P, Kiemenij F. Long term follow-up of "stent-like" (≤30% diameter stent post) angioplasty: A case for provisional stenting (abstr). *J Am Coll Cardiol* 1996; 27(suppl A):15A.

95. Eccleston DS, Eisenberg MJ. Primary, "French" or restenosis stenting or balloon angioplasty? Relative outcome and costs rising a decision analytic model (abstr). *Circulation* 1995; 92(suppl I):I-662.

96. Mak K, Belli G, Ellis SG, Moliterno DJ. Subacute stent thrombosis: Evolving issues and current concepts. *J Am Coll Cardiol* 1996; 27:494–503.

97. Sawada Y, Nosaka H, Kimura T, Nobuyoshi M. Initial and six month outcome of Palmaz-Schatz stent implantation: Stress/Benestent equivalent versus non-equivalent lesions (abstr). *J Am Coll Cardiol* 1996; 27(suppl A):252A.

98. Douglas JS Jr, Savage MP, Bailey SR, Pepine CJ, Werner JA, Overlie PA. Randomized trial of coronary stent and balloon angioplasty in the treatment of saphenous vein graft stenosis (abstr). *J Am Coll Cardiol* 1996; 27(suppl A):178A.

99. Serruys PW, Emanuelsson H, van der Giessen W, Lunn AC, Kiemeney F, Macaya C, et al. Heparin-coated Palmaz-Schatz stents in human coronary arteries: Early outcome of the Benestent-II Pilot Study. *Circulation* 1996; 93:412–422.

100. Cohen DJ, Krumholz HM, Sukin CA, Ho KKL, Siegrist RB, Cleman M, et al. In-hospital and one-year economic outcomes after coronary stenting or balloon angioplasty: Results from a randomized clinical trial. *Circulation* 1995; 92:2480–2487.

101. Eeckout E, Kapenberger L, Goy J. Stents for intracoronary placement: Current status and future directions. *J Am Coll Cardiol* 1996; 27:757–765.

102. Laster SB, Rutherford BD, McConahay DR, et al. Directional atherectomy of the left main coronary artery: Acute and long term results (abstr). *J Am Coll Cardiol* 1994; 23:386A.

103. Lewis BE, Leya FS, Johnson SA, Grassman ED, McKleman TL, Hwang M. Outcomes of angioplasty (PTCA) and atherectomy (DCA) for bifurcation and non-bifurcation lesions in CAVEAT (abstr). *Circulation* 1993; 88(suppl I):I-601.

104. Leya FS, Lewis BE, Sumida CW, McKiernan TL, Grassman ED, Bhatia S, et al. Modified "kissing" atherectomy procedure with dependable protection of side branches by two-wire technique. *Cath Cardiovasc Diagn* 1992; 27:155–161.

105. Mintz GS, Pichard AD, Popma JJ, Kent KM, Satler LF, Leon MB. Preliminary experience with adjunct directional coronary atherectomy after high-speed rotational atherectomy in the treatment of calcific coronary artery disease. *Am J Cardiol* 1993; 71:799–804.

106. Boehrer JD, Ellis SG, Keeler GP, et al. Differential benefit of directional atherectomy over angioplasty for left anterior descending in proximal, non-ostial lesions: Result from CAVEAT (abstr). *J Am Coll Cardiol* 1994; 23:386A.

107. Kimball BP, Cohen EA, Adelman AG, for the Canadian Coronary Atherectomy Trial Investigators. Influence of stenotic lesion morphology on immediate and long-term (6 months) angiographic outcome: Comparative analysis of directional coronary atherectomy versus standard balloon angioplasty. *J Am Coll Cardiol* 1996; 27:543–551.

108. Stertzer SH, Pomerantsev EV, Fitzgerald PJ, Shaw RE, Walton AS, Singer AH, et al. Effects of technique modification on immediate results of high speed rotational atherectomy in 710 procedures on 656 patients. *Cathet Cardiovasc Diagn* 1995; 36:304–310.

109. MacIsaac AI, Bass TA, Buchbinder M, Cowley MJ, Leon MB, Warth DC, et al. High speed rotational atherectomy: Outcome in calcified and non-calcified coronary artery lesions. *J Am Coll Cardiol* 1995; 26:731–736.

110. Ellis SG, Popma JJ, Buchbinder M, Franco I, Leon MB, Kent KM, et al. Relation of clinical presentation, stenosis morphology, and operator technique to the procedural results of rotational atherectomy and rotational atherectomy-facilitated angioplasty. *Circulation* 1994; 89:882–892.

111. Broderick TM, Kereiakes DJ, Whang DD, Toltzis RJ, Abbottsmith CW. Myocardial bridging may predispose to coronary perforation during rotational atherectomy. *J Invas Cardiol* 1996; 8:161–163.

112. O'Murchu B, Foreman RD, Shaw RE, Brown DL, Peterson KL, Buchbinder M. Role of intraaortic balloon pump counterpulsation in high risk coronary rotational atherectomy. *J Am Coll Cardiol* 1995; 26:1270–1275.

113. Moses JW, Tierstein PS, Sketch MH Jr, Siegel RM, Yeh W. Angiographic determinants of risk and outcome of coronary embolus and myocardial infarction (MI) with the transluminal extraction catheter (TEC): A report from the New Approaches to Coronary Intervention (NACI) Registry (abstr). *J Am Coll Cardiol* 1994; 23:220A.

114. Safian RD, Grines CL, May MA, Lichtenberg A, Juran N, Schreiber TL, et al. Clinical and angiographic results of transluminal extraction coronary atherectomy in saphenous vein bypass grafts. *Circulation* 1994; 89:302–312.

115. Baim DS, Kent KM, King SB III, Safian RD, Cowley MJ, Holmes DR, et al. Evaluating new devices: Acute (in-hospital) results from the New Approaches to Coronary Intervention Registry. *Circulation* 1994; 89:471–481.

116. Kaplan BM, O'Neill WW, Safian RD, Schreiber TL, Larkin TJ, Dooris M. Clinical and angiographic follow-up to a prospective study of transluminal extraction atherectomy in high risk patients with myocardial infarction (abstr). *J Am Coll Cardiol* 1995; 25(suppl A):331A.

117. Safian RD, May MA, Lichtenberg A, Schreiber TL, Pavlides G, Meany TB, et al. Detailed clinical and angiographic analysis of transluminal extraction coronary atherectomy for complex lesions in native coronary arteries. *J Am Coll Cardiol* 1995; 25:848–854.

118. Groh WC, Kurnik PB, Matthai WH, Untereker WJ. Initial experience

with an intracoronary flow support device providing localized drug infusion: The Scimed dispatch catheter. *Cathet Cardiovasc Diagn* 1995; 36:67–73.

119. Pajadet J, Bar O, Jordan C. Human percutaneous thrombectomy using the new hydrolyser catheter: Preliminary results in saphenous vein grafts (abstr). *J Am Coll Cardiol* 1994; 23:220A.

120. Douglas JS Jr, Ghazzal ZMG, Ba'albaki HA, Miller SJ, King SB III. Excimer laser coronary angioplasty of ostial lesions: Acute success and complications (abstr). *Cathet Cardiovasc Diagn* 1991; 23:75.

121. Eigler NL, Douglas JS Jr, Margolis JR, Hestrin L, Litvack FL, ELCA Investigators. Excimer laser coronary angioplasty of aorto-ostial stenosis: Results of the ELCA Registry. *Circulation* 1993; 88:2049–2057.

122. de Marchena EJ, Mallon SM, Knopf WD, Parr K, Moses JW, Murphy-Chutorian D, et al. Effectiveness of holmium laser-assisted coronary angioplasty. *Am J Cardiol* 1994; 73:117–121.

123. Litvack F, Eigler N, Margolis J, Rothbaum D, Bresnahan JF, Holmes D, et al. Percutaneous excimer laser coronary angioplasty: Results in the first consecutive 3,000 patients. *J Am Coll Cardiol* 1994; 23:323–329.

124. Appelman YE, Piek JJ, deFeyter PJ, Koolen JJ, Strikwerda S, Margolis JR. Excimer laser coronary angioplasty versus balloon angioplasty used in long-term lesions: The long-term results of the AMRO Trial (abstr). *J Am Coll Cardiol* 1995; 25(suppl A):329A.

125. Appelman JY, Koolen JJ, deFeyter PJ, Strikwerda S, David GK, Redekop K. Long-term outcome of excimer laser angioplasty versus balloon angioplasty in functional and total coronary occlusions (abstr). *J Am Coll Cardiol* 1995; 25(suppl A):330A.

126. Vandormael M, Riefart N, Preusler W. Six month follow-up results following excimer laser angioplasty, rotational atherectomy and balloon angioplasty for complex lesions: ERBAC Study. *Circulation* 1994; 90(suppl I):I-213.

127. Serruys PW, Hamburger J, Fleck E, Koolen JJ, Teunissen Y. Laser guide wire: A powerful tool in recanalization of chronic total coronary occlusion (abstr). *Circulation* 1995; 92(suppl I):I-76.

128. Pepine CJ, Babb JD, Brinker JA, Douglas JS Jr, Jacobs AK, Johnson WL Jr, et al. Task Forec 3: Training in cardiac catheterization and interventional cardiology. *J Am Coll Cardiol* 1995; 25:14–16.

129. Cowley MJ, Faxon DP, Holmes DR Jr. Guidelines for training, credentialing, and maintenance of competence for the performance of coronary angioplasty: A report from the Interventional Cardiology Committee and the Training Program Standards Committee of the Society for Cardiac Angiography and Interventions. *Cathet Cardiovasc Daign* 1993; 30:1–4.

130. Douglas JS Jr, Pepine CJ, Block PC, Brinker JA, Johnson WL, Klinke WP, et al. Recommendations for development and maintenance of competence in coronary interventional procedures. *J Am Coll Cardiol* 1993; 22:629–631.

131. Ryan TJ, Klocke FJ, Reynolds WA, Williams SV, Achord JL, Friesinger GC II, et al. Clinical competence in percutaneous transluminal coronary angioplasty: A statement for physicians from the ACP/ACC/AHA Task Force on Clinical Privileges in Cardiology. *J Am Coll Cardiol* 1990; 15:1469–1474.

132. Conti CR. Credentialing cardiologists who perform therapeutic cardiac interventions. *Clin Cardiol* 1995; 18:689–691.

133. Eisenberg MJ, Rice S, Schiller NB. Guidelines for physician training in advanced cardiac procedures: The importance of case mix. *J Am Coll Cardiol* 1994; 23:1723–1725.

134. Eisenberg MJ, St Claire DA, Mak K, Ellis SG. Importance of case mix during training in interventional cardiology. *Am J Cardiol* 1996; 77:1010–1013.

135. Ellis SG, Nowamagbe O, Bittl JA, Lincoff M, Wolfe MW, Howell G. Analysis and comparison of operator-specific outcomes in interventional cardiology. *Circulation* 1996; 93:431–439.

136. Califf RM, Jollis JG, Peterson ED. Operator-specific outcomes: A call to professional responsibility. *Circulation* 1996; 93:403–406.

137. Ritchie JL, Phillips KA, Luft HS. Coronary angioplasty: Statewide experience in California. *Circulation* 1993; 88:2735–2743.

138. Jollis JG, Peterson ED, DeLong ER, Mark DB, Collins SR, Muhlbaier L, et al. The relation between the volume of coronary angioplasty procedures at hospitals treating Medicare beneficiaries and short-term mortality. *N Engl J Med* 1995; 331:1625–1629.

139. Ryan TJ. The critical question of procedure volume minimums for coronary angioplasty. *JAMA* 1995; 274:1169–1170.

140. Fajadet J, Brunel P, Jordan C, Cassagneau B, Laurent J, Marco J, et al. Transradial approach for interventional coronary procedures:

Analysis of complications (abstr). *J Am Coll Cardiol* 1996; 27(suppl A):392A.

141. Ritchie JL, Nissen SE, Douglas JS Jr, Dreifus LS, Gibbons RJ, Higgins CB, et al. Use of nonionic or low osmolar contrast agents in cardiovascular procedures. *J Am Coll Cardiol* 1993; 21:269–273.

142. Grines CL, Schreiber TL, Savas V, Jones DE, Zidar FJ, Gangadharan V, et al. A randomized trial of low osmolar ionic versus nonionic contrast media in patients with myocardial infarction or unstable angina undergoing percutaneous transluminal coronary angioplasty. *J Am Coll Cardiol* 1996; 27:1381–1386.

143. Lembo NJ, King SB III, Roubin GS, Black AJ, Douglas JS Jr. Effects of nonionic contrast media on complications of percutaneous transluminal coronary angioplasty. *Am J Cardiol* 1991; 67:1046–1050.

144. Roubin GS, Douglas JS Jr, King SB III, Lin S, Hutchinson N, Gruentzig AR. Influence of balloon size in initial success, acute complications and restenosis after percutaneous transluminal coronary angioplasty—A prospective randomized study. *Circulation* 1988; 78:557–565.

145. Waksman R, Ghazzal ZMB, Scott NA, Douglas JS Jr, King SB III. Efficacy and safety of using perfusion dilatation catheter as initial balloon in coronary angioplasty. *Cathet Cardiovasc Diagn* 1994; 32:319–322.

146. Meier B, Rutishauser W. Coronary pacing during percutaneous transluminal coronary angioplasty. *Circulation* 1985; 72:557–561.

147. Tobis JM, Colombo A. Do you need IVUS guidance for coronary stent deployment? *Cathet Cardiovasc Diagn* 1996; 37:360–361.

148. Russo RJ, Teirstein PS, for the AVID Investigators. Angiography versus intravascular ultrasound-directed stent placement (abstr). *J Am Coll Cardiol* 1996; 27(suppl A):306A.

149. Deckelbaum LI, Natarajan K, Bittl JA, Rohlfs K, Scott J, Chisholm R, et al. Effect of intracoronary saline infusion on dissection during excimer laser coronary angioplasty: A randomized trial. *J Am Coll Cardiol* 1995; 26:1264–1269.

150. Ellis SG, Roubin GS, Wilentz J, Lin S, Douglas JS Jr, King SB III, et al. Results of a randomized trial of heparin and aspirin vs aspirin alone for prevention of acute closure and restenosis after angioplasty (abstr). *Circulation* 1987; 76(suppl IV):IV-213.

151. Ruygrok PN, De Jaegere PT, Van Domburg RT, Van Den Brand MJ, Serruys PW, Defeyter PJ. Clinical outcome 10 years after attempted percutaneous transluminal coronary angioplasty in 856 patients. *J Am Coll Cardiol* 1996; 27:1669–1677.

152. Bredlau CE, Roubin GS, Leimbruger PP, Douglas JS Jr, King SB III, Gruentzig AR. In-hospital morbidity and mortality in patients undergoing elective coronary angioplasty. *Circulation* 1985; 72:1044–1052.

153. Ellis SG, Roubin GS, King SB III, Douglas JS Jr, Shaw RE, Stertzer SH, et al. In-hospital cardiac mortality following acute closure after percutaneous transluminal coronary angioplasty—Analysis of risk factors from 8,207 procedures. *J Am Coll Cardiol* 1988; 11:211–216.

154. Ellis SG, Myler RK, King SB III, Douglas JS Jr, Topol EJ, Shaw RE, et al. Causes and correlates of death after unsupported coronary angioplasty: Implications for use of angioplasty and advanced support techniques in high-risk settings. *Am J Cardiol* 1991; 68:1447–1451.

155. Ajluni SC, Glazier S, Blankenship L, O'Neill WW, Safian RD. Perforations after percutaneous coronary interventions: Clinical, angiographic, and therapeutic observations. *Cathet Cardiovasc Diagn* 1994; 32:206–212.

156. Ellis SG, Arnold AZ, Raymond RE, Eigler NL, Sanborn TA, Bittl JA, et al. Increased coronary perforation in the new device era: Incidence, classification, management and outcome (abstr). *Circulation* 1992; 86(suppl I):I-787.

157. Bensuly KH, Glazier S, Grines CL, O'Neill WW, Safian RD. Coronary perforation: An unreported complication after intracoronary stent implantation (abstr). *J Am Coll Cardiol* 1996; 27(suppl A):252A.

158. Waksman R, King SB III, Douglas JS Jr, Shen Y, Ewing H, Mueller L, et al. Predictors of groin complications after balloon and new-device coronary intervention. *Am J Cardiol* 1995; 75:886–889.

159. Moscucci M, Mansour KA, Kent C, Kuntz RE, Senerchia C, Baim DS, et al. Peripheral vascular complications of directional coronary atherectomy and stenting: Predictors, management, and outcome. *Am J Cardiol* 1994; 74:448–453.

160. Popma JJ, Satler LF, Pichard AD, Kent KM, Campbell A, Chuang YC, et al. Vascular complications after balloon and new device angioplasty. *Circulation* 1993; 88:1569–1578.

161. Rocha-Singh KJ, Schwend RB, Otis SM, Schatz RA, Teirstein PS. Frequency and nonsurgical therapy of femoral artery pseudoaneurysm

complicating interventional cardiology procedures. *Am J Cardiol* 1994; 73:1012–1014.

162. Saber RS, Edwards WD, Bailey KR, McGovern TW, Schwartz RS, Holmes DR. Coronary embolization after balloon angioplasty or thrombolytic therapy: An autopsy study of 32 cases. *J Am Coll Cardiol* 1993; 22:1283–1288.

163. Waksman R, Scott NA, Douglas JS Jr, Mays R, Yee-Petersen J, King SB III. Distal embolization is common after directional atherectomy in coronary arteries and vein grafts (abstr). *Circulation* 1993; 88(suppl I):I-299.

164. Harrington RA, Lincoff AM, Califf RM, Holmes DR, Berdan LG, O'Hanesian MA, et al. Characteristics and consequences of myocardial infarction after percutaneous coronary intervention: Insights from the Coronary Angioplasty Versus Excisional Atherectomy Trial (CAVEAT). *J Am Coll Cardiol* 1995; 25:1693–1699.

165. Moses JW, Teirstein PS, Sketch MR Jr, Siegel RM, Yeh W. Angiographic determinants of risk and outcome of coronary embolus and myocardial infarction (MI) with the transluminal extraction catheter (TEC): A report from the New Approaches to Coronary Intervention (NACI) Registry (abstr). *J Am Coll Cardiol* 1994; 23:220A.

166. Safian RD, Grines CL, May MA, Lichtenberg A, Juran N, Schrieber TL, et al. Clinical and angiographic results of transluminal extraction coronary atherectomy in saphenous vein bypass grafts. *Circulation* 1994; 89:302–312.

167. McCullough PA, Wolyn R, Rocher LL, Levine RN, O'Neill WW. Acute contrast nephropathy after coronary intervention: Incidence, risk factors and relationship to mortality (abstr). *J Am Coll Cardiol* 1996; 17(suppl A):304A.

168. Savage M, Fischman D, Teirstein P, Schatz P, Rake R, Gebbhardt S. Utility of coronary stents in the management of incessant restenosis (abstr). *Circulation* 1993; 88(suppl I):I-640.

169. Pratt RE, Dzau VJ. Pharmacological strategies to prevent restenosis. *Circulation* 1996; 93:848–852.

170. Waksman R, Robinson KA, Croker IR, Wang C, Gravanis MB, Cipolla D, et al. Intracoronary low-dose B-irradiation inhibits neointima formation after coronary artery balloon injury in the swine restenosis model. *Circulation* 1995; 92:3025–3031.

171. Waksman R, Robinson KA, Croker IR, Gravanis MB, Palmer SJ, Wang C. Intracoronary radiation before stent implantation inhibits neointima formation in stented porcine coronary arteries. *Circulation* 1995; 92:1383–1386.

172. Hehrlein C, Stintz M, Kinscherf R, Schlosser K, Huttel E, Friedrich L, et al. Pure B-particle-emitting stents inhibit neointima formation in rabbits. *Circulation* 1996; 93:641–645.

49

CORONARY INTRAVASCULAR ULTRASOUND

Steven E. Nissen / E. Murat Tuzcu

For several decades, contrast angiography has served as the principal imaging modality used to assess the anatomic severity of coronary artery disease. Recent technical advances in acoustics and microelectronics have permitted development and refinement of miniaturized ultrasound devices capable of real-time tomographic coronary imaging.[1–5] This approach, intravascular ultrasound, represents an emerging alternative to angiography for direct visualization of coronary anatomy during diagnostic and interventional catheterization. Clinical studies comparing angiography with intravascular ultrasound have demonstrated frequent differences in quantitative or qualitative findings. Accordingly, intraluminal ultrasound imaging is increasingly utilized to confirm, refute, or supplement angiographic data in patients with coronary disease.

The majority of the discrepancies between angiography and intravascular ultrasound can be explained by the inherent characteristics of these two fundamentally different imaging techniques. Unlike angiography, which portrays the vessel as a silhouette of the lumen, ultrasound depicts the coronary artery from a tomographic perspective. This approach provides detailed cross-sectional images that portray not only the lumen, but also the deeper intramural structures within the vessel wall. This ability of ultrasound to penetrate and image soft tissue enables visualization of the extent, distribution, and morphology of coronary atherosclerosis. Images of coronary atheromata provide insights into the pathophysiology of coronary disease not obtainable in vivo by any other technique. Accordingly, intravascular ultrasound is finding diverse applications in both research and clinical practice.

RATIONALE FOR INTRAVASCULAR ULTRASOUND

Limitations of Angiography

Although angiography has endured for several decades as the predominant method for determining the anatomic severity of coronary artery disease (CAD), multiple investigators have questioned the accuracy and reproducibility of coronary arteriography.[6–12] Studies have established that visual interpretation of angiograms exhibited clinically significant intra- and interobserver variability, with differences in the visual estimation of stenosis severity approaching 50 percent.[10,11] Comparisons of angiography to necropsy specimens report major discrepancies between the apparent angiographic severity of lesions and postmortem histologic examination.[6–9] Most studies report that angiography significantly underestimates the extent of atherosclerosis compared with postmortem quantitative measurements. Using functional testing, investigators have demonstrated a prominent discordance between the severity of angiographic lesions and measurements of the physiologic effects of the stenosis.[12]

Several phenomena account for the inaccuracy and high interobserver variability of coronary angiography. Angiography depicts coronary cross-sectional anatomy from a planar two-dimensional silhouette of the contrast-filled vessel lumen. However, both necropsy studies and intravascular ultrasound demonstrate that coronary lesions are often complex, with markedly distorted or eccentric luminal shapes.[13–15] For a com-

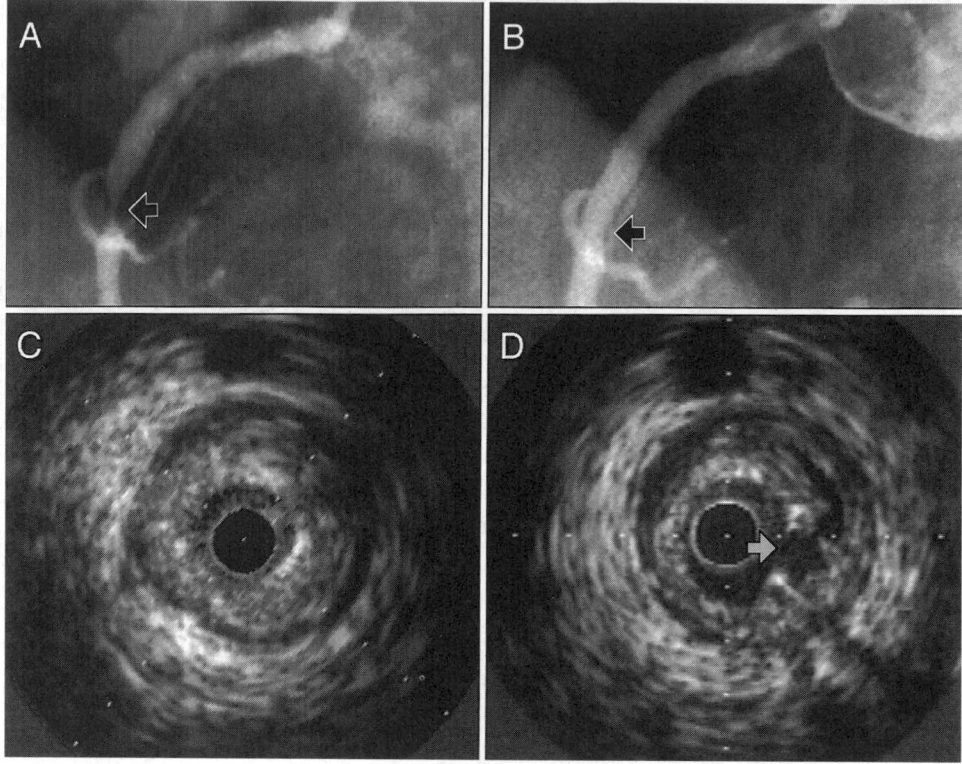

FIGURE 49-1

Angiographic overestimation of the gain in lumen area following balloon angioplasty. *A* and *B*. Improvement in angiographic appearance following PTCA performed at the site indicated by the black arrow. *C* and *D*. Intravascular ultrasound of the same site before and after angioplasty. The gain in lumen area is much less impressive by ultrasound, consisting principally of a plaque fracture indicated by the white arrow in *D*. (From Topol and Nissen,[19] with permission.)

plicated coronary lesion, any arbitrary angle of view may misrepresent the extent of luminal narrowing. Theoretically, two orthogonal angiograms should reflect the severity of many lesions accurately. However, adequate orthogonal views are frequently unobtainable because, at optimal imaging angles, the vessel is obscured by overlapping side branches, disease at bifurcation sites, and/or radiographic foreshortening. Even when unlimited projections are available, the angiographic silhouette cannot accurately depict complex luminal shapes.

In the setting of percutaneous intervention, the complexity of coronary anatomy induced by angioplasty further compromises the assumptions underlying simple projection imaging. Necropsy and ultrasound studies demonstrate that most mechanical interventions exaggerate the extent of luminal eccentricity by fracturing or dissecting the atheroma.[13,16–18] The angiographic appearance of a postintervention vessel often consists of an enlarged although frequently "hazy" lumen. In the setting of extensive plaque fracture, the hazy, broadened angiographic silhouette of the lumen may overestimate the vessel cross section and misrepresent the actual gain in lumen size[19] (Fig. 49-1).

The traditional method for characterizing angiographic lesion severity depends upon visual or computer measurements of the percentage stenosis. This process requires comparison of luminal dimensions within both the lesion and an adjacent,

uninvolved, "normal" reference segment. However, necropsy studies demonstrate that coronary disease is frequently diffuse and contains no truly normal segment from which to calculate the area reduction. In the presence of diffuse disease, calculation of percent stenosis will predictably underestimate disease severity.[7–9,14] In the most dramatic circumstances, diffuse, concentric, and symmetric coronary disease affects the entire vessel, resulting in the angiographic appearance of a small but normal artery[19] (Fig. 49-2).

Angiography is also confounded by the phenomenon of coronary "remodeling," observed histologically as the outward displacement of the external vessel wall in atherosclerotic segments[20] (Fig. 49-3). This adventitial enlargement prevents the disease from encroaching on the lumen, thereby concealing the presence of the atheroma on angiography. Although such lesions do not restrict blood flow, clinical studies have demonstrated that minimal, nonobstructive angiographic lesions represent an important cause of acute coronary syndromes, including myocardial infarction.[21] Angiographically unrecognized disease virtually always underlies an ergonovine-positive response in symptomatic patients with a "normal" coronary angiogram.[22]

Potential Advantages of Ultrasound

Intravascular ultrasound has several unique properties of theoretical value in the detection and quantitation of coronary disease.[19,23–28] The cross-sectional perspective of ultrasound permits visualization of the full 360° circumference of the vessel wall, not just two surfaces. Accordingly, measurement of lumen area is not dependent on the radiographic projection and can be determined by direct planimetry of the image.[25] Because the velocity of sound in soft tissue represents a well-established constant, ultrasound scanners can overlay an electronically generated distance scale within the image. This feature eliminates the troublesome requirement of traditional angiographic methods to correct for radiographic magnification.[19]

The tomographic perspective of ultrasound enables characterization of disease in vessels that are difficult to assess by conventional angiographic techniques, including diffusely diseased segments, bifurcation or ostial lesions, and eccentric

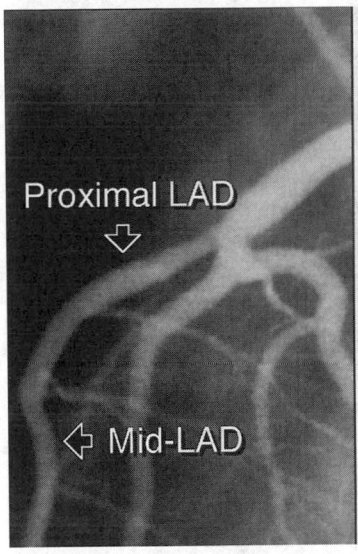
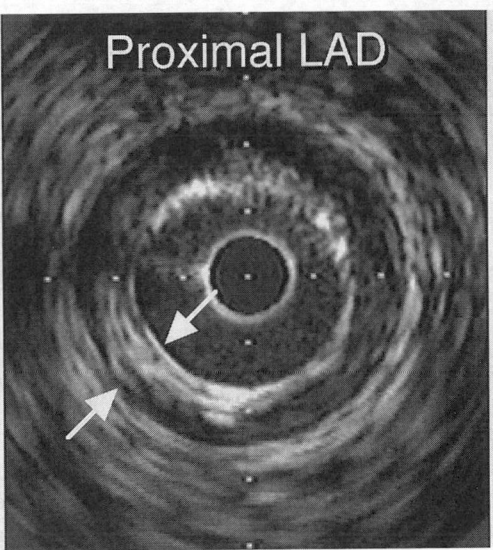
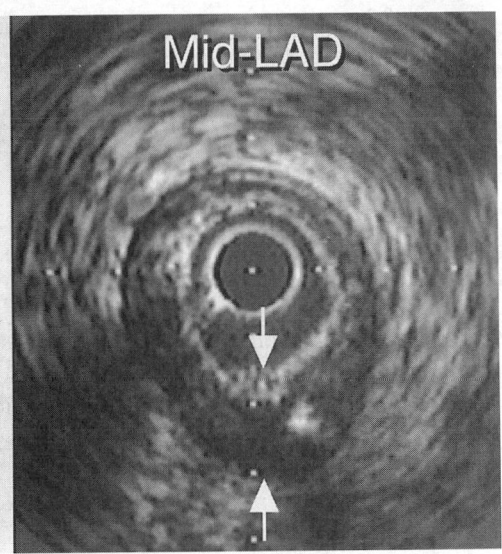

FIGURE 49-2

Angiographic underestimation of diffuse coronary disease. The left panel shows an angiogram with minimal luminal narrowing. In the middle panel, ultrasound from a proximal LAD site is illustrated, showing diffuse concentric atherosclerosis. Atheroma thickness is indicated by the white arrows. In the right panel, a mid-LAD site is illustrated with white arrows also indicating the maximum atheroma thickness. Because the disease is diffuse and concentric, only minimal luminal narrowing is evident by angiography. (From Topol and Nissen,[19] with permission.)

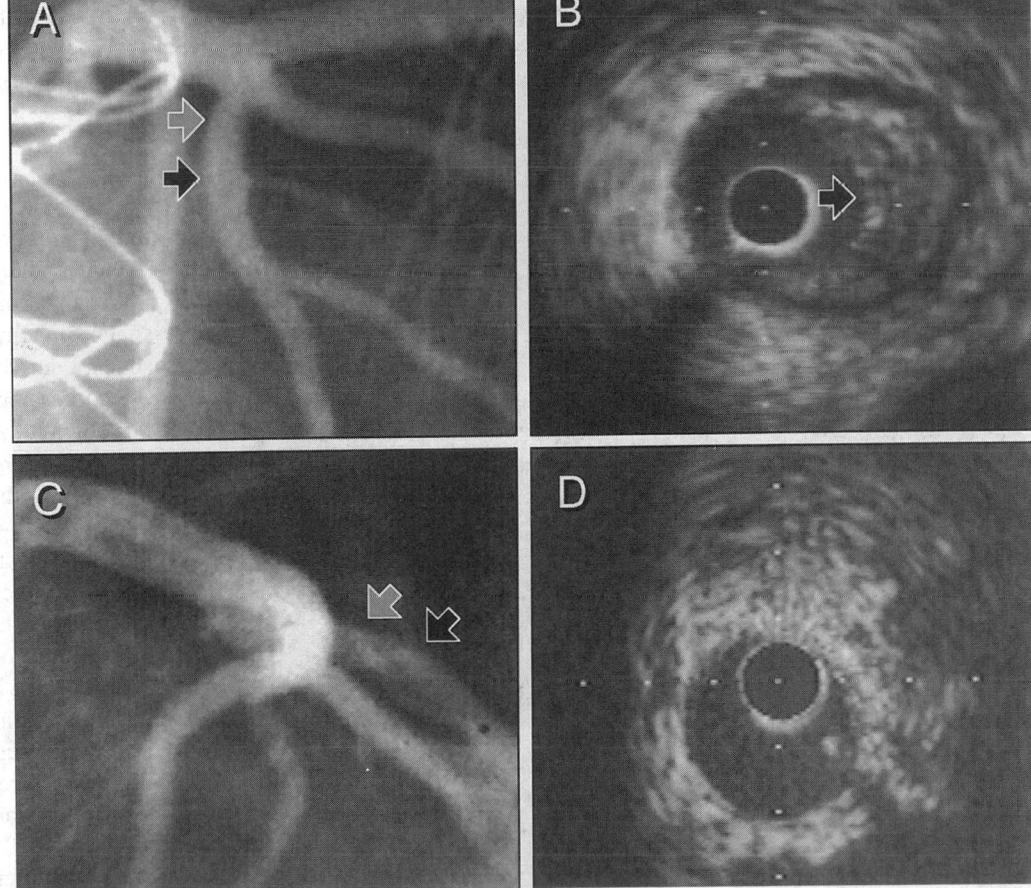

FIGURE 49-3

Coronary remodeling (Glagov phenomenon). The angiograms in panels *A* and *C* illustrate the RAO and LAO views. In each panel, the gray arrow indicates the ultrasound site shown in panel *B* and the black arrow indicates the site shown in panel *D*. Although there is no narrowing on the angiogram, the intravascular ultrasound in panel *B* shows a large crescentic atheroma (*black arrow*). However, the lumen sizes in panels *B* and *D* are similar, resulting in a false-negative angiogram. (From Topol and Nissen,[19] with permission.)

plaques.[19,26] The ability of ultrasound to characterize the intramural anatomy of the vessel wall represents a unique feature, which can yield invaluable insights into the pathophysiology of coronary disease.[27]

INTRAVASCULAR IMAGING TECHNOLOGY

Catheter Design

Intracoronary ultrasound equipment consists of two major components, a catheter incorporating a miniaturized transducer and a console containing the electronics necessary to reconstruct the image. Since the transducer is placed in close proximity to the vessel wall, high frequencies (20 to 50 MHz) can be employed to provide excellent theoretical resolution (axially below 100 μm and laterally less than 250 μm). Initial efforts to develop miniaturized transducers for intraluminal examination began nearly 20 years ago, but practical application required major improvements in the physical properties of imaging catheters.[1] Until recently, devices available for intravascular ultrasound were relatively large, ranging from 4.3 to 5.5 Fr (1.43 to 1.67 mm) and limiting examination to proximal and occasionally midvessel segments imaged after revascularization.

Two dissimilar technical approaches to transducer design have emerged—mechanically rotated devices and multielement electronic arrays.[1–5] Multielement designs generally result in catheters with greater mechanical flexibility, while mechanical probes have, thus far, offered superior image quality. Each design has yielded small intravascular devices suitable for coronary imaging, typically ranging in size from 2.9 to 3.5 Fr (diameter of 0.96 to 1.17 mm). Although the mechanical properties and catheter size have greatly im-

proved, handling characteristics remain distinctly inferior to those of the latest generation of angioplasty equipment. To facilitate subselective coronary cannulation and catheter exchanges, modern ultrasound catheters provide a lumen for a movable guidewire. Most systems employ a monorail design to facilitate rapid catheter exchanges without the necessity for long guidewires or a docking apparatus. Most systems generate images at a temporal frequency of 30 frames per second with archival storage on videotape.

Two different mechanical ultrasound designs have emerged from commercial vendors. In one approach, the distal catheter contains a short monorail segment (5 to 10 mm in length) with the transducer positioned just proximal to the monorail. The operator subselectively cannulates the vessel with a guidewire and advances or retracts the device over the wire to interrogate the vessel. Other catheters employ an alternative approach in which the operator advances a sheath to a distal location in the artery over a guidewire previously placed in the vessel. The guidewire is then removed and the transducer is passed freely within the sheath to image the vessel. Recent sheath-type devices incorporate a distal lumen that is shared by the transducer and guidewire so as to minimize overall device size. Both monorail and sheath-type devices work well, although the monorail design often has difficulty tracking tortuous vessels and the sheath-type device requires leaving a potentially obstructive catheter across the lesion for a longer period of time.

Limitations and Artifacts

All current intravascular ultrasound devices generate artifacts that may adversely affect image quality, alter interpretation, or reduce quantitative accuracy.[29] Visualization of small coronary arteries or stenoses necessitates imaging close to the transducer surface, which requires addressing the troublesome problem of *ring-down artifact,* a defect that appears in virtually all medical ultrasound devices (Fig. 49-4). Ring-down artifacts arise from acoustic oscillations in the piezoelectric transducer material, resulting in high-amplitude ultrasound signals that preclude imaging within a few tenths of a millimeter of the transducer surface. Inability to image structures immediately adjacent to the transducer results in an "acoustic" catheter size slightly larger than its physical size. The most recent designs use carefully chosen transducer and backing materials, specialized coatings, and electronic filtering to suppress ring-down artifacts.

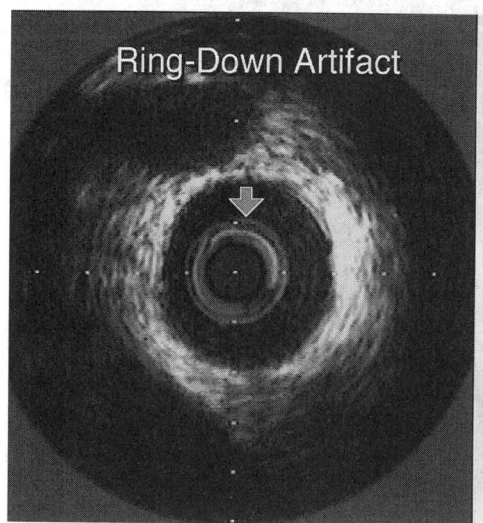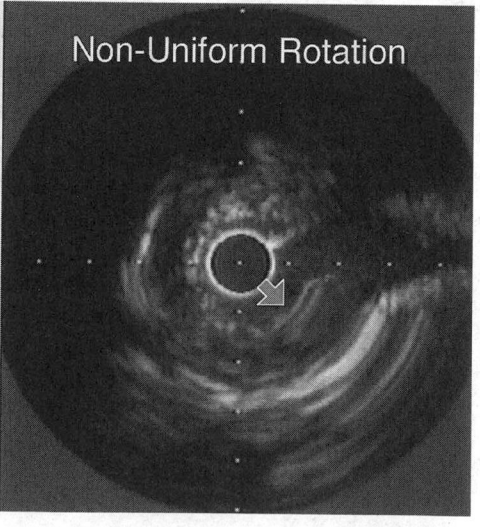

FIGURE 49-4

Two artifacts of intravascular ultrasound imaging. In the left panel, a series of bright concentric rings are evident in close proximity to the ultrasound catheter (*gray arrow*), illustrating a phenomenon known as *ring-down artifact.* In the right panel, the effects of nonuniform rotational distortion are illustrated (*gray arrow*).

In the electronic array design, the transducer is surface mounted and ring-down artifact must be reduced by digital subtraction, which is often incompletely effective.

Normal first-order epicardial coronaries range from 1.0 to 5.0 mm, while atherosclerotic lumina can reach 0.1 mm. Since the minimum size of current devices is approximately 1.0 mm, the operator may be able to deliver the probe to most lesions but cannot fully image severe stenoses prior to intervention. Further reductions in transducer size may be difficult because transducer miniaturization reduces the effective aperture of the device, which limits available acoustic power, reduces lateral resolution, and impairs the signal-to-noise ratio. The resolution limits at small apertures may be overcome using transducers that operate at higher frequencies—an approach under active investigation.

All tomographic imaging techniques, including intravascular ultrasound, are vulnerable to distortion produced by imaging in oblique planes not perpendicular to the long axis of the vessel. This phenomenon increases the maximum but not minimum luminal dimensions and can represent a significant confounding variable in quantitative measurements. Under some circumstances, it is possible to recognize a nonorthogonal catheter position and to manipulate the device to a more coaxial position. Fortunately, the extent of this artifact is self-limiting. The small size of the coronary vasculature geometrically limits the degree of obliquity possible during ultrasound examinations. This artifact can be more troublesome when one is imaging larger vessels such as the aorta or the peripheral vasculature.

Mechanical transducers may exhibit cyclic oscillations in rotational speed, resulting in an artifact known as *nonuniform rotational distortion* (NURD). This artifact arises from differential mechanical drag on the catheter drive shaft during the various portions of its rotational cycle. Nonuniform rotational speed variation produces a readily visible type of distortion recognized as circumferential stretching of a portion of the image with compression of the contralateral vessel wall (Fig. 49-4). NURD is most evident when the drive shaft is bent into a small radius of curvature by a tortuous vessel. Improvements in the mechanical precision of ultrasound devices have reduced the impact of the artifact, but it still remains a troublesome problem during some examinations.

HUMAN CORONARY IMAGING

Laboratory Technique

Standard interventional techniques for catheter delivery are used to enable safe intracoronary ultrasound examination.[30] Intravenous heparin (5000 to 10,000 U) is routinely employed prior to imaging, although there are no controlled studies of the necessity for anticoagulation. The practitioner typically employs a 7- or 8-Fr guiding catheter and a 0.014-in. angioplasty guidewire. Catheter handling procedures include subselective cannulation of the vessel using a steerable guidewire,

followed by careful advancement or retraction of the imaging catheter over the wire. As the transducer is moved to various points along the vessel, the operator examines the vessel in real time, recording images on videotape for subsequent quantitative or qualitative analysis. Monorail designs are commonly employed to facilitate rapid catheter exchanges and allow the guidewire to remain safely in position well beyond any critical coronary stenoses.

Safety of Coronary Ultrasound

Although intravascular ultrasound requires intracoronary instrumentation, studies performed during diagnostic or therapeutic catheterization have demonstrated few serious untoward effects.[13,31] Transient coronary spasm occurs in about 5 percent of patients but usually responds rapidly to administration of intracoronary nitroglycerin. The imaging transducer can reduce coronary blood flow when it is advanced into tight stenoses or small distal vessels, but patients generally do not experience chest pain if the catheter is promptly withdrawn. In interventional practice, operators have safely employed coronary ultrasound following virtually all types of procedures, including balloon angioplasty, directional atherectomy, rotational ablation, and stent deployment. Most protocols avoid instrumentation of patients in whom estimated coronary diameter is too small (2.9 to 3.5 Fr; 0.96 to 1.17 mm) to accommodate the device safely.

Despite the relative safety of coronary ultrasound, any intracoronary instrumentation carries the potential risk of intimal injury or acute vessel dissection. Accordingly, many centers employ intravascular ultrasound during diagnostic catheterization, but most laboratories limit credentialing for intravascular imaging procedures to personnel with interventional training. In the unlikely event of intimal disruption, this safety measure ensures that the necessary personnel and equipment are immediately available to initiate appropriate corrective action.

Normal Coronary Anatomy

A series of investigations have characterized the appearance of normal coronary anatomy by intravascular ultrasound.[13,32–36] At high frequencies (25 MHz and above), the vessel lumen is characterized by faint, finely textured, specular echoes that move in a characteristic swirling pattern during active blood flow. The echogenicity within the lumen arises from the reflection of acoustic energy by circulating blood elements, although the precise origin of this effect remains uncertain. In many situations, blood "speckle" assists image interpretation by providing a means to confirm the communication between dissection planes and the lumen. The pattern of blood speckle is dependent upon the velocity of flow, showing increased intensity and a more coarse appearance when flow is reduced.

Wall morphology in normal arteries consists of two alternative patterns, described as trilaminar when three discrete layers are evident or monolayered if the wall structure does not

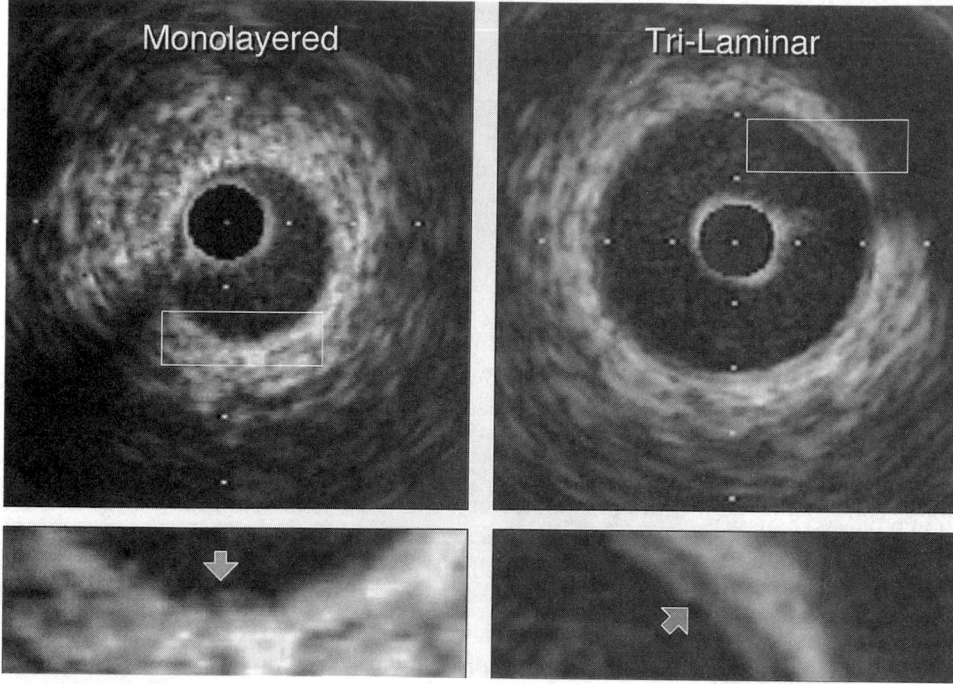

FIGURE 49-5

Two variants of normal morphology by intravascular ultrasound. In the left panel, the arterial wall is principally monolayered; in the right panel, a trilaminar appearance is evident. In both examples, the area within the white box is shown in an enlargement beneath the unmagnified images.

contain distinct laminations (Fig. 49-5). Important determinants of the vessel wall appearance include both the normal arterial structure and the inherent properties of ultrasound. An ultrasound reflection occurs at a tissue boundary whenever there is an abrupt change in acoustic impedance at the interface. Normally, two strong acoustic interfaces are well visualized by ultrasound—the leading edge of the intima (at the interface between the blood-filled lumen and the endothelium) and the outer border of the media (at the junction of media and external elastic membranes). Beneath the trailing edge of the intima a middle sonolucent layer is usually evident, which is composed principally of the media. These three layers (intima, sonolucent medial layer, and external membrane) are the distinct layers seen in trilaminar arteries.

In normal segments without a trilaminar structure, the internal elastic lamina is thin and reflects the ultrasound signal poorly, resulting in a monolayered appearance. The monolayered coronary is particularly common in younger individuals without significant risk factors for coronary atherosclerosis. This finding has led some observers to propose that a trilaminar wall morphology represents evidence of early coronary atherosclerosis.[35] Other investigators have studied normal subjects and report a range of values for the thickness of normal wall components. In normals, the ultrasound-derived intimal thickness typically averages about 0.15 ± 0.07 mm. Accordingly, most investigators use 0.25 to 0.30 mm as an upper limit of normal (2 standard deviations > normal).[13]

Regardless of whether the artery is trilaminar or monolayered, the deepest zones of the arterial wall represent the adventitia and periadventitial tissues, exhibiting a characteristic "onionskin" pattern. The outer border of the vessel is usually indistinct, primarily because there are no clear acoustic differences between the adventitia and other tissues encasing the vessel. Accordingly, total wall thickness cannot be measured using ultrasound except in vessels with a distinct outer border, such as aortocoronary saphenous vein grafts.

Morphology of Coronary Atherosclerosis

Subtle changes that occur early in the development of coronary atherosclerosis, such as fatty streaks, are not visible using current 30-MHz ultrasound devices. Arteries with classical atherosclerosis exhibit a diversity of abnormal features that reflect the distribution, severity, and composition of the atheromata.[13,24,27,32–34] Sites with minimal disease exhibit generalized or focal thickening of the intimal leading edge, while advanced lesions appear as large echogenic masses encroaching upon the lumen (Figs. 49-6 and 49-7). Most classification schemes differentiate coronary atheromata into one of three categories (soft, fibrous, or calcified), according to plaque echogenicity.

The echogenicity of the plaque components is dependent not only on the acoustic properties of tissue but also on the acquisition settings (gain, compression, etc.) of the ultrasound system. Accordingly, most classification schemes compare the echointensity of the plaque to the surrounding adventitia to correct for differences in ultrasound technique. Plaques are usually termed "soft" if they are less echogenic than the adventitia. These soft lesions represent either highly cellular fibromuscular proliferation (e.g., restenosis) or diffuse lipid infiltration, both of which have low echogenicity. Plaques with an echodensity similar to that of the adventitia are described as "fibrous" or "hard." In vitro studies confirm that such lesions have a higher fibrous tissue content, which correlates closely with increasing echogenicity.

"Calcified" lesions are recognized as highly echogenic plaques that attenuate transmission of the ultrasound signal, thereby obscuring deeper layers—a phenomenon known as *acoustic shadowing*.[32,37,38] Obstruction of ultrasound transmission, not merely a high degree of echogenicity, is a requisite for the identification of calcium. Because of the importance of calcium in the selection of interventional devices, most observers further classify the extent of calcification by measuring the circumferential angle subtended by calcified plaque. Commonly, the axial length of the calcified portion of the lesion is also measured and the operator notes whether deposits are single or multiple. The depth of calcification is assessed; it is described as superficial when the calcium remains in contact with the luminal surface and deep if no portion of the calcium deposit is superficial.

Some plaques contain a zone of reduced echogenicity within the main body of the atheroma. In individual cases, one cannot determine whether these represent areas of lipid deposition and necrotic degeneration, both of which can appear as zones of low density. In some cases, the echolucent zone is covered by a distinct "cap" that exhibits greater

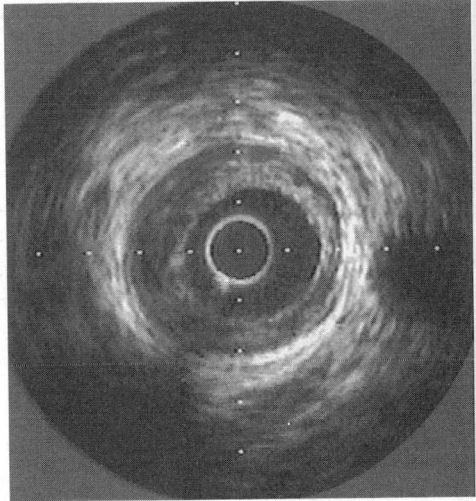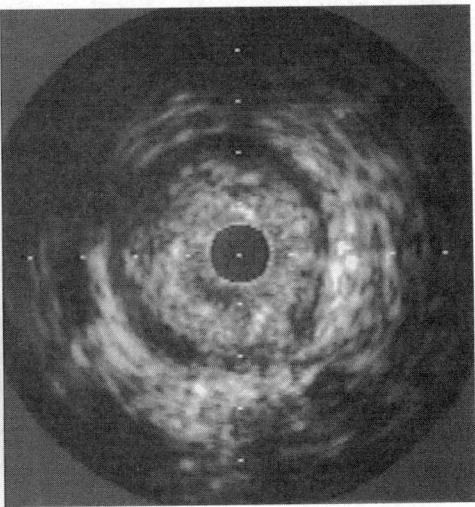

FIGURE 49-6

Soft and fibrous plaque morphology. In the left panel, the atheroma is principally sonolucent, indicating a high lipid content. In the right panel, the atheroma is more echogenic, consistent with a high fibrous tissue content.

echogenicity and presumably represents the classical fibrous cap described by histology. Spontaneous plaque ruptures or fissures associated with unstable coronary ischemic syndromes are sometimes evident in ultrasound examination of the culprit lesions shortly after the event. The detection of multiple channels within the plaque that communicate with the lumen is also highly suggestive of plaque rupture. However, at the typical 30-MHz imaging frequency, organizing thrombus appears visually indistinguishable from other types of plaques. Nevertheless, the presence of mobile intraluminal masses strongly suggest the presence of thrombi.

Some caution is warranted in interpreting intravascular ultrasound images. Although currently available devices produce remarkably detailed views of the vessel wall, interpretation employs visual inspection of acoustic reflections to determine plaque morphology. Methods do not yet exist for objective or automated classification of atheromatous lesions. The echogenicity and texture of different histologic features may exhibit comparable acoustic properties and therefore appear quite similar by intravascular ultrasound. For example, a sonolucent plaque may represent intracoronary thrombus, while a nearly identical appearance may result from an atheroma with a high lipid content. Thus, intravascular ultrasound can delineate

the thickness and echogenicity of vessel wall structures but does not provide actual histology.

Despite these limitations, the general classification of coronary plaques into the categories of soft, fibrous, or calcified has significant clinical implications. Initial experience suggests that these three different categories often respond differently to interventional devices.[39] For example, densely fibrotic or calcified plaques resist removal with the current generation of directional atherectomy devices.[40,41] Armed with this information, the practitioner may choose an alternative revascularization technique, such as rotational atherectomy, for such

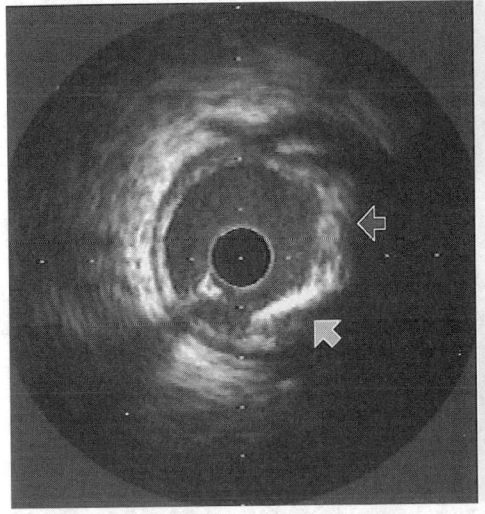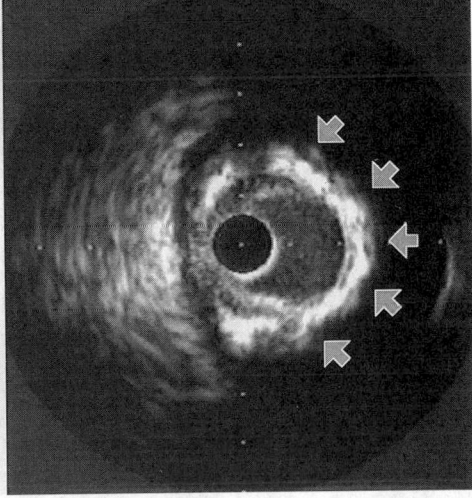

FIGURE 49-7

Appearance of calcified plaque by intravascular ultrasound. In the left panel, an area of highly echogenic material produces acoustic shadowing (*light-gray arrow*), indicating presence of calcium. Similar shadowing is seen at the site marked by a dark gray arrow, but the plaque is less echogenic. In the right panel, five arrows indicate a highly echogenic plaque that shadows all underlying structures and is consistent with extensive calcification.

lesions. Further study will likely refine the application of this approach to permit lesion-specific interventional therapy guided by ultrasound examination.

DIAGNOSTIC CLINICAL APPLICATIONS

Quantitative Luminal Measurements

Many therapeutic decisions hinge upon assessment of coronary luminal dimensions. Practitioners routinely employ luminal measurements to evaluate the severity of stenoses, to determine the size of the "normal" reference segment, and to assess the luminal gain achieved by the revascularization procedure. Thus, in diagnostic and interventional practice, precise quantitation of vascular dimensions from a tomographic perspective represents an important clinical application of intravascular ultrasound. Many studies have validated the accuracy of the luminal measurements of ultrasound by comparing intravascular imaging and quantitative angiography. These studies include both animal investigations and in vivo comparisons performed in normal subjects or patients with coronary disease.[5,13,25]

For vessels without atherosclerosis, studies document a close correlation between angiographic and ultrasonic coronary dimensions. These comparisons typically reveal a linear regression equation with a slope near to the line of identity and an intercept near zero, although a few studies suggest slightly larger measurements by ultrasound. Thus, in disease-free vessels with a circular cross-sectional profile, ultrasound and angiographic measurements of lumen size correlate closely.[13] However, in patients with atherosclerotic arteries, most investigators report only a moderate correlation between ultrasonic and angiographic dimensions, typically a correlation coefficient of approximately $r = 0.7$ to 0.8 and a standard error > 0.5 mm.[13,18] Comparative studies show the greatest disparities between angiography and ultrasound in atherosclerotic vessel segments with a noncircular lumen shape.[19] This reduced correlation is probably explained by the irregular, noncircular cross-sectional profile of atherosclerotic vessels—a configuration that cannot be adequately depicted by angiography. There are also major differences between the ultrasonic and angiographic assessment of stenosis severity. Studies comparing reduction of cross-sectional area as found by both methods revealing only a moderate correlation: $r = 0.5$ to 0.7.[13,18]

Quantitation of Atherosclerosis

Analysis of intravascular ultrasound images permits quantitative measurements of the extent and severity of coronary atherosclerosis.[24,27,32–34] However, the inherent properties of ultrasound require utilization of different anatomic landmarks than those of classical histology. In ultrasound imaging, reflections at the leading edge of any interface are located precisely at the boundary where acoustic impedance changes abruptly. However, location of the trailing edge of any anatomic structure is determined by multiple nonanatomic factors, particularly ultrasound beam properties, such as the imaging frequency. Thus, leading-edge measurements accurately describe the precise location of a boundary, whereas trailing-edge measurements are unreliable.

As previously noted, strong reflections are generally produced at two locations, the interface between the lumen and the leading edge of the intima and the border between the media and the external elastic lamina. In quantitative measurement of atherosclerotic lesions, the boundary at the trailing edge of the intima is not accurately localized in intravascular ultrasound images. Accordingly, quantitative measurements must calculate atheroma cross-sectional area by subtracting the area bounded by the intimal leading edge from the area enclosed by the external elastic lamina (Fig. 49-8). This approach results in a slight overestimation of plaque volume by including the area of the media within the atheroma calculation. Fortunately, in all but the most limited disease, the area of the media is small in comparison to atheroma area, thus limiting the impact of this overestimation.

The tomographic orientation of intravascular ultrasound represents an additional problem in quantifying atherosclerosis. Since each image contains infor-

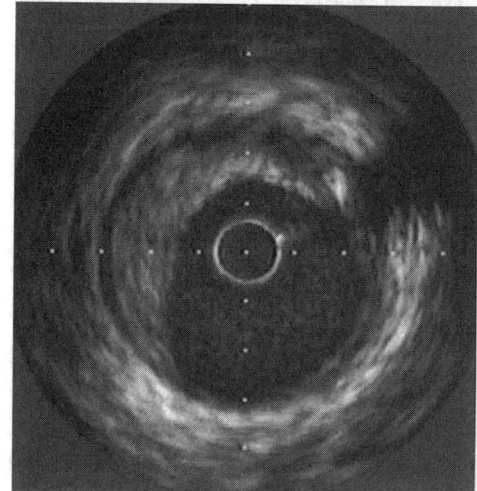
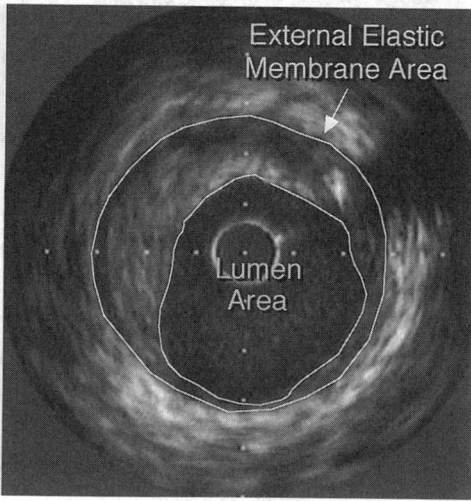

FIGURE 49-8

Intravascular ultrasound measurements. The left panel shows the left main coronary artery with a crescentic atheroma. In the right panel, the tracings indicate the location of the external elastic membrane and the border between the lumen and intima. The area difference between these two measurements represents the plaque volume as measured by intravascular ultrasound.

mation from only a thin "slice" of the vessel, global measures of atheroma burden require integration of multiple cross sections. One successful approach to this conundrum employs a motorized device to steadily and progressively withdraw the ultrasound catheter through the interrogated vessel, typically at 0.5 to 1.0 mm/s. Since motor speed is kept constant, the operator can measure a series of cross sections separated by a constant, recurring time interval. This approach yields a series of tomograms, which are individually measured, and then summated to approximate total atheroma burden. A second approach to atheroma quantitation employs three-dimensional (3D) reconstruction of the vessel from the 2D ultrasound tomograms.[42] Unfortunately, 3D methods are exceedingly complex, have many unresolved confounding variables, and remain largely unvalidated.

Angiographically Unrecognized Disease

In patients with clinical symptoms of coronary disease, intravascular ultrasound commonly detects atherosclerotic abnormalities at angiographically normal sites.[13,43–45] In the presence of any luminal irregularity by angiography, intravascular ultrasound often demonstrates disease at all other examined coronary sites. The extent of disease in angiographically normal vessels confirms the finding, previously reported from necropsy studies, that coronary disease is frequently more diffuse than is apparent by angiography.[7]

There are four principal mechanisms by which angiography may underestimate the presence, extent, or severity of atherosclerotic disease.[19] First, to detect focal narrowing, angiography relies upon comparison of the interrogated site to an adjacent uninvolved segment. However, atherosclerosis is often a diffuse process. The diseased vessel may be reduced in caliber along its entire length, containing no truly normal segment for comparison (Fig. 49-2). In the absence of a focal stenosis, the angiographer could erroneously conclude that the vessel is simply "small in caliber."

Eccentric lesions—plaques that occupy only a portion of the vessel circumference—represent a second important source of false-negative angiography. In many clinical settings, there are limitations that prevent the angiographer from obtaining optimal radiographic projections. For example, at certain angles, overlapping structures such as adjacent vessels can obscure some segments of the coronary, and mechanical limits in positioning of the x-ray gantry may preclude other potentially useful views. Therefore, an eccentric lesion may not be visualized by angiography because the operator cannot obtain an appropriate projection orthogonal to the lesion.

A third important mechanism underlying false-negative angiography results from the phenomenon of coronary remodeling, originally described by Glagov from histology.[20,45,46] At atherosclerotic sites, compensatory enlargement ("remodeling") of the vessel wall overlying the plaque often preserves lumen diameter, resulting in an angiographic lumen size identical to that of adjacent, uninvolved segments (Fig. 49-3). Vessel foreshortening, a fourth mechanism of false-negative

angiography, can conceal short "napkin-ring" lesions (usually less than 1 to 2 mm in length).[19]

For each of these mechanisms of false-negative angiography, ultrasound can confirm the presence and estimate the extent of atherosclerosis.[19] The higher sensitivity of ultrasound in detecting atherosclerosis has important clinical implications. Patients who present with symptoms suggestive of coronary disease but who have "normal" angiograms represent a common and perplexing group. In our experience, ultrasound will demonstrate coronary atherosclerosis in many of these patients—a finding that may affect the choice of therapy. The long-term implications of angiographically occult disease remain uncertain, since no outcomes-based research has demonstrated a worse prognosis for patients with disease detected only by ultrasound. However, Little and others[21] have demonstrated that plaques with minimal to moderate angiographic narrowing are the most likely to lead to myocardial infarction. Accordingly, the presence of angiographically occult coronary disease may have important prognostic significance. Studies are currently under way to determine the predictive value of ultrasound in determining the prognosis in patients with angiographically unrecognized coronary disease.

Lesions of Uncertain Severity

Despite thorough radiographic examination using multiple projections, angiographers commonly encounter lesions that elude accurate characterization.[19] Lesions of uncertain severity often include ostial lesions, bifurcation lesions, and moderate stenoses (angiographic severity ranging from 40 to 75 percent) in patients whose symptomatic status is difficult to evaluate. For these ambiguous lesions, ultrasound provides tomographic measurements, making it possible to assess lesions independent of the radiographic projection. The left main coronary artery represents a particularly difficult site for angiographic quantification.[48] Since the left main coronary artery (LMCA) is short in length, there often exists no normal segment from which to compare a focal narrowing. Furthermore, the ostium may be obscured by radiographic contrast in the aortic cusp, and the distal LMCA is often concealed by the bifurcation or trifurcation into daughter branches. Accordingly, intravascular ultrasound is commonly employed to quantify LMCA when angiographic interpretation is uncertain.[49]

Atheroma Distribution

The circumferential distribution of the atheroma varies from nearly symmetric plaques to very eccentric lesions in which the entire atheroma is located on one side of the artery. Assessed by ultrasound, the majority of plaques are eccentric with a maximum atheroma thickness more than twice the minimum plaque thickness. Studies have demonstrated a poor correlation between the apparent circumferential pattern by angiography and the actual plaque distribution revealed by ultrasound examination.[50] Such studies demonstrate the inaccuracy inherent in determining plaque distribution from a projected 2D silhouette of the lumen (angiography). This observation has important implications for the guidance of coronary interventions, particularly techniques for selective plaque removal such as directional atherectomy.

Atheroma Calcification

Calcification represents an important consequence of coronary disease, generally associated with long-standing atherosclerosis. The presence and extent of calcification represent important determinants of the outcome following percutaneous coronary interventions.[51] Angiographic calcification is associated with increased risk of dissection following balloon angioplasty, typically occurring at the borders of the calcified atheroma. Calcified plaques are more difficult to remove using the currently available directional atherectomy device.[52] The traditional approach to the identification of calcification employs cinefluoroscopy to visualize moving opacities in close proximity to the vessel silhouette. However, this approach is limited by many factors, including the moderate spatial and contrast resolution of radiography and the confounding effects produced by the overlap of other calcium-containing structures, such as ribs or calcified pulmonary lesions.[19]

Intravascular ultrasound has proved highly sensitive in detecting the presence, extent, and location of calcification (Fig. 49-7). Comparative studies have demonstrated poor sensitivity for angiography in detection of coronary calcification, regardless of its severity.[37,38] At lesions targeted for intervention, angiography identifies less than half (45 percent) of the patients with ultrasound-detected calcification. Angiography correctly recognized calcification in only 52 percent of patients with ultrasound-documented involvement subtending more than 90° of the vessel circumference. For patients with extensive calcification (>180° of arc), angiography correctly identified calcium in 63 percent. Although the sensitivity of angiography in detecting calcification is low, its specificity remains high. Studies demonstrate that angiography does not represent an effective method for localizing the depth of calcium deposits. Only one-third of patients with superficial and one-quarter with deep calcium deposits were identified correctly by angiography.

Cardiac Allograft Disease

Transplant coronary artery disease is the leading cause of death beyond the first year after cardiac transplantation, with a reported incidence of 15 to 20 percent per year. Although most transplant centers perform coronary arteriograms annually for screening, these surveillance studies often fail to detect atherosclerosis prior to a clinical event.[53,54] Necropsy studies have demonstrated that angiography systematically underestimates coronary atherosclerosis in transplant recipients.[55,56] These patients may have diffuse vessel involvement that, for reasons already enumerated, conceals the atherosclerosis from the angiographer. Many large centers now routinely perform intravascular ultrasound at the time of annual catheterization in all cardiac transplant recipients. Recent investigations using

ultrasound to detect transplant vasculopathy report a very high incidence of this disease.[57,58] Overall, abnormal intimal thickening is evident in 80 percent of patients at one year and in more than 92 percent of patients studied 4 or more years after transplantation.

Recent studies have revealed two pathways to transplant-associated atherosclerosis. Some patients receive atherosclerotic plaques transmitted via the donor heart, while others develop an immune-mediated vasculopathy.[44,58] Complete interrogation of the coronary arteries using ultrasound reveals a distinctly heterogeneous pattern of longitudinal and circumferential involvement.[58] Available data indicate that the pattern is related to the origins of the disease. Traditional atherosclerosis (usually donor-transmitted) has an eccentric plaque distribution with patchy longitudinal involvement, whereas immune-mediated (acquired) disease is more circumferential and diffuse.

INTERVENTIONAL CLINICAL APPLICATIONS

Luminal Measurements Postintervention

A poor correlation has been reported for comparisons of ultrasound and angiography in assessment of residual stenosis following angioplasty.[13,17,59–61] Measurements of luminal cross-sectional area following angioplasty are generally smaller by ultrasound than by angiography.[61] These differences likely represent enhancement of the apparent angiographic diameter of the vessel produced by extraluminal contrast within cracks or splits in the intima and/or media of the vessel. Because balloon dilatation distorts the vessel lumen and wall, the reported differences between angiographic and ultrasonic measurements probably reflect the differences between silhouette and tomographic imaging of complex, eccentric lumina following angioplasty.

Two factors influence the overly optimistic tendency of angiographic imaging. At the reference site, angiography tends to underestimate the diameter of the normal "reference" vessel because of the frequent presence of unrecognized atherosclerosis. At the target site, angiography tends to overestimate the actual gain in luminal diameter because contrast material penetrates into complex cracks and fissures produced by the intervention, giving the appearance of a more enlarged lumen. To calculate a postprocedure percent diameter stenosis, the diameter at the target site (an overestimate) is divided by the reference diameter (an underestimate), resulting in a more favorable impression of the actual gain in luminal dimensions. Accordingly, when quantitative angiography reports a residual stenosis of 10 to 15 percent, ultrasound not uncommonly reports that 60 to 80 percent of the vessel is still occupied by plaque.

Wall Morphology following Angioplasty

Necropsy studies in patients who have died shortly after balloon angioplasty describe plaque fracturing or disruption as the most common mechanism of successful balloon dilatation.[16] Ultrasound studies have confirmed that plaque fissuring or dissection is the most common mechanism of luminal enlargement, occurring in 40 to 80 percent of patients (Fig. 49-1).[13,17,62,63] The diagnosis of wall dissection or fracture is based on the visualization of blood flow in the newly created lumen, and the injection of saline or iodinated contrast through the guiding catheter opacifies the lumen via microbubbles, which can be helpful in confirming the diagnosis. The severity of wall disruptions can be defined by measuring the circumferential extent and length and the maximal depth of the dissection.

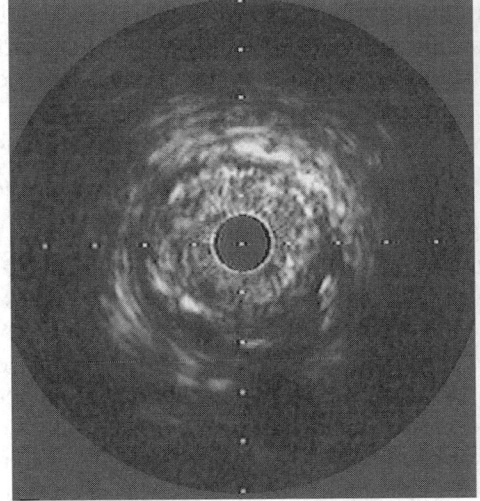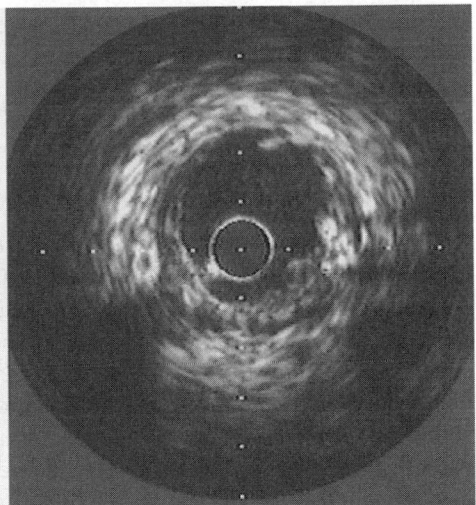

FIGURE 49-9

Intravascular ultrasound before and after directional atherectomy. In the left panel, a dense fibrotic plaque is shown. Following atherectomy, intravascular ultrasound shows extensive plaque removal with some irregularity of the luminal surface (*right panel*).

Ultrasound often shows alternative mechanisms of luminal enlargement after angioplasty that cannot be discerned by angiography.[64,65] Careful pre- and postangioplasty imaging reveals that stretching of the external elastic lamina occurs in at least 25 percent of patients, while apparent reduction of the atheroma area ("compression") at the treated site occurs in another 20 percent. Studies using automatic pullback devices have shown that "compression" actually represents redistribution of plaque along the long axis of the vessel.[65] The prognostic significance of different mechanisms of luminal enlargement is under investigation.

Guidance of Directional Atherectomy

Intravascular ultrasound has been widely employed to guide directional coronary atherectomy. By determining the location and composition of the target atheroma, ultrasound potentially improves preprocedural planning and may aid intraprocedural decision making. As previously described, lesions that appear concentric by angiography are often eccentric by ultrasound and, conversely, angiographically eccentric lesions are often concentric by ultrasound.[50] Thus, ultrasound can confirm or refute angiographic findings with regard to plaque location and circumferential distribution. Such information is used by the interventional operator to direct atherectomy cuts toward the side of the vessel with the greatest plaque thickness. Conversely, areas with a minimal atheroma burden are avoided.

The presence and extent of vessel calcification can also significantly affect the extent of plaque removal using currently available directional atherectomy devices.[41] Studies have demonstrated that extensive superficial calcification prevents effective debulking of atheromata. As previously noted, ultrasound is more sensitive than angiography, frequently demonstrating calcified atheromata despite the absence of any apparent calcification on fluoroscopy.[38] Ultrasound can also determine the depth of calcification in relation to the lumen. Ultrasound studies have demonstrated that target lesions with extensive calcification deep within the atheroma can undergo successful atherectomy if superficial atheroma layers remain uncalcified.

The additional spatial perspective provided by ultrasound can assist in the orientation of atherectomy cuts (Fig. 49-9). However, successful application requires experience, patience, and careful planning, because precise orientation of the intravascular image is difficult. Experienced operators will examine the target vessel prior to atherectomy to locate anatomic features, especially side branches, and use these landmarks to orient the ultrasound image. Subsequently, the operator directs atherectomy cuts toward the appropriate side of the vessel, sometimes repeating ultrasound examinations between passes of the device to determine the extent of plaque removal and the need for additional cuts.

In contrast to balloon angioplasty, ultrasound studies before and after directional atherectomy confirm that plaque removal is the primary mechanism of luminal enlargement.[66] However, ultrasound also reveals that despite a successful angiographic result, 40 to 60 percent or more of the target site is still occupied by atheroma.[67] Some investigators have proposed that a larger lumen after atherectomy would result in a lower restenosis rate (compared to balloon angioplasty). However, it remains untested whether a larger postprocedure lumen can be achieved using ultrasound guidance without a concomitant increase in dissection, perforation, or other complications. Although ultrasound guidance has been reported to favorably affect the extent of plaque removal, the effect on restenosis rates remains uncertain.[68,69] A novel device that combines an ultrasound transducer with an atherectomy device has been developed and is about to enter clinical trials.[70] By enabling the operator to visualize the plaque located directly in the path of the atherectomy cutter, this device should facilitate precise lesional debulking without the necessity for multiple catheter exchanges.

Guidance of Rotational Atherectomy

Rotational ablation (Rotablator, Scimed Life Systems, Maple Grove, MN) employs a high-speed (160,000 to 200,000 rpm) diamond-coated burr to debulk atheromata within coronary stenoses. This approach has proved effective at removing superficial calcium from stenotic vessels.[71–73] However, as noted previously, there is a poor correlation between ultrasound and fluoroscopy in assessment of the presence and extent of calcification. Accordingly, the demonstration of a heavily calcified vessel by ultrasound permits the operator to employ rotational ablation in settings where it is particularly efficacious (Fig. 49-10).

Vessels that are revascularized by rotational ablation are frequently diffusely diseased, and their "normal" dimension can be difficult to determine angiographically. Ultrasound can often be employed to size the vessel and determine the largest burr that can safely be utilized. Observational ultrasound studies to date have confirmed that ablation of plaque constitutes the primary mechanism of rotational atherectomy, particularly the more fibrotic or calcified components of the lesion. The

residual lumen is usually round or ellipsoid and may result in a lumen with a 15 to 20 percent greater area than the largest burr used, presumably due to lateral movement of the burr during the procedure.

Coronary Stent Deployment

Intravascular ultrasound has significantly influenced the application of stenting to the treatment of coronary disease.[74–76] The initial stent studies leading to approval from the Food and Drug Administration (FDA) of the stent employed an articulated slotted-tube design (Palmaz-Schatz, Johnson and Johnson Interventional Systems). In initial trials, these stents were deployed using conventional balloon pressures (6 to 10 atm).[77–78] To prevent subacute stent thrombosis, patients received aggressive anticoagulation during and immediately following the procedure, using both antiplatelet and antithrombotic agents. Long-term management included administration of warfarin for at least 3 to 6 months. These initial studies demonstrated a reduction in the restenosis rate compared to that of balloon angioplasty, but there was a high prevalence of hemorrhagic complications and hospital stays were longer.

A pioneering intravascular ultrasound study detailing the experience of Colombo et al. in Milan, Italy, significantly altered our understanding of the optimal technique for stent deployment and prevention of subacute thrombosis.[76] This large but nonrandomized study employed routine intravascular ultrasound imaging following angiographically guided stent deployment and revealed an average ultrasound-derived residual stenosis of 51 percent comparing minimum stent diameter to reference segment diameter. These authors also frequently observed an absence of complete stent contact with the vessel wall (incomplete apposition) following angiographically guided deployment. Because stents are porous structures, angiographic contrast can flow outside of a partially deployed stent, resulting in the angiographic appearance of full deployment despite the presence of incomplete apposition (Fig. 49-11). In the Milan study, the operators performed additional balloon inflations at higher pressures (typically 18 to 20 atm) or used a larger balloon (or both), resulting in a final ultrasound residual stenosis averaging 34 percent. Importantly, the final angiographic percentage of stenosis

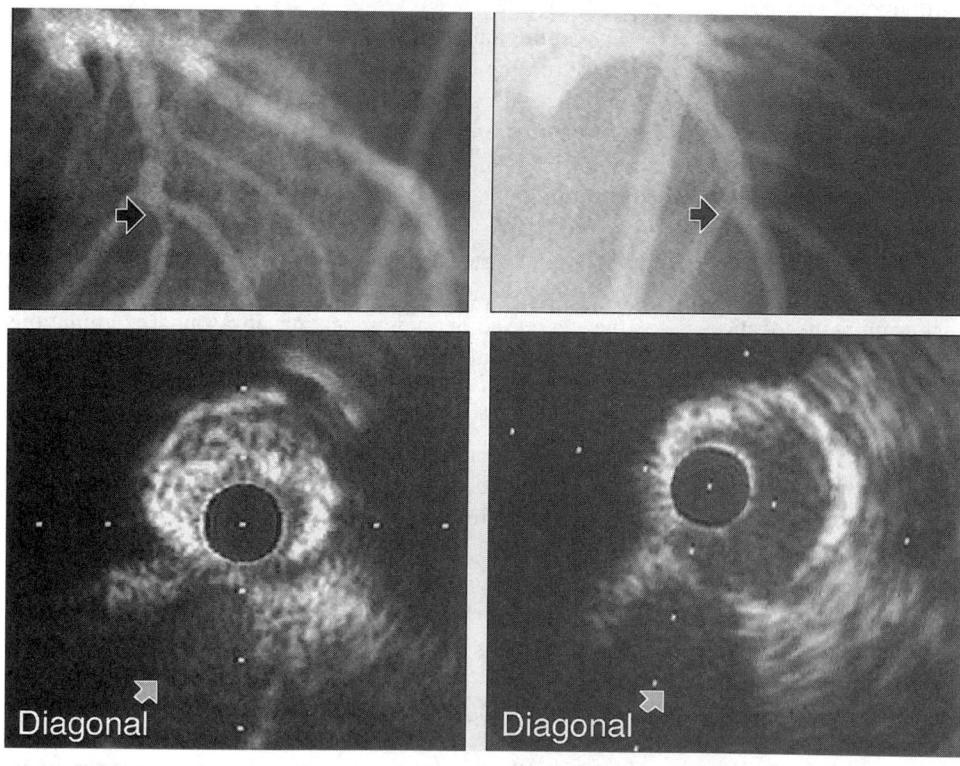

FIGURE 49-10

Angiography and intravascular ultrasound before and after rotational ablation. The top two panels show the angiographic appearance (pre- and post-Rotablator), and the bottom two panels show the same site by intravascular ultrasound. Note that there is dense calcified plaque in the lower left panel. Following rotational ablation, the lower right panel shows an enlarged circular lumen with significant removal of calcium.

was negative (-7.0 percent). Using ultrasound to guide deployment, this study reported a subacute thrombosis rate of only 0.3 percent using no systemic anticoagulation (antiplatelet agents only).

It is now widely accepted that high-pressure deployment of the stents dramatically reduces the incidence of subacute thrombosis and obviates the need for acute and chronic administration of antithrombotic agents.[79] However, it remains uncertain whether intravascular ultrasound imaging is necessary to achieve this benefit.[80] Some observers have advocated routine high-pressure deployment without ultrasound imaging and report low thrombosis rates. However, the effect of the more aggressive dilatation on restenosis rates has not been thoroughly examined by prospective trials. It remains conceivable that increased vessel wall injury from the use of larger high-pressure balloons will yield less favorable long-term results. Optimal procedural goals for ultrasound-guided stent deployment remain to be determined.

In stenting as a bailout for dissection, intravascular ultrasound can prove helpful in determining the true longitudinal extent of a dissection before placement of a stent for vessel salvage. Experienced observers find that intracoronary imaging is more sensitive in detecting the extent of dissection, often revealing a greater true length than is evident from angiography. Although ultrasound appears useful following bailout stenting, there remain questions of safety in passing monorail-type imaging catheters through a fine-wire coil design such as the Gianturco-Roubin (Cook) stent. It is theoretically possible to dislodge the stent by "snagging" a loop of the struts between the monorail catheter and the guidewire.

Intravascular Ultrasound and Restenosis

A more complete understanding of restenosis has evolved from serial ultrasound measurements of plaque and lumen areas at follow-up studies after balloon angioplasty and directional atherectomy.[81] In some studies, serial ultrasound examinations have shown that a late reduction in total vessel area (chronic negative remodeling) is an important mechanism of restenosis after interventional procedures.[81] These observations suggest that mechanical interventions (such as stenting) to prevent chronic recoil may be as important in preventing restenosis as pharmacologic treatment to prevent intimal hyperplasia. If further validated, this concept may explain the lower restenosis rate observed in randomized multicenter studies comparing balloon angioplasty and stent implantation.[77,78]

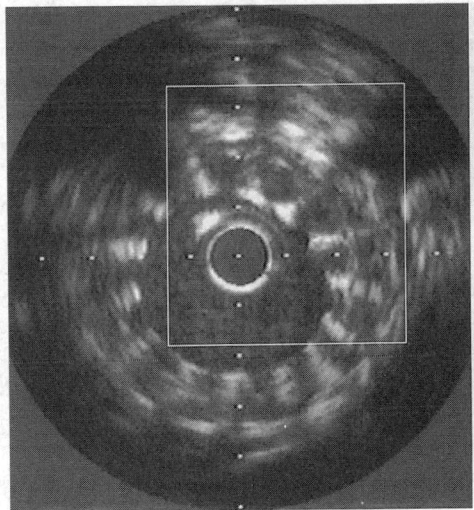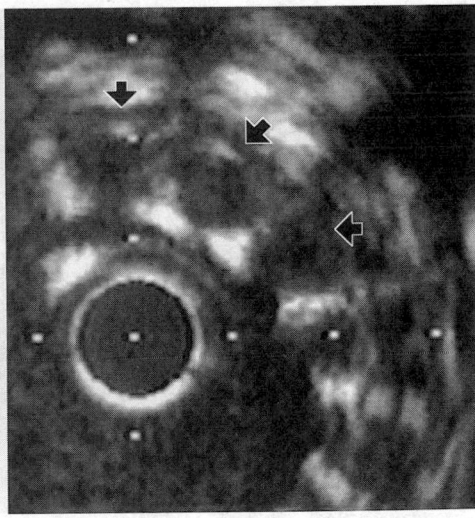

FIGURE 49-11

Intravascular ultrasound showing incomplete apposition of a coronary stent. In the left panel, an unmagnified view shows several stent struts not in full contact with the underlying vessel wall. In the right panel, an enlargement of the area in the white box shows approximately a 1-mm gap between several stent struts and the underlying wall (*black arrows*).

However, other phenomena observed by ultrasound may also play a role in determining the outcome following coronary interventions. The relatively poor correlation between angiographic and ultrasonic dimensions following angioplasty raises a provocative issue. In certain patients, does "restenosis" represent a failure to adequately augment luminal area rather than the subsequent loss of luminal gain? Can ultrasound assessment of the residual lumen predict acute postinterventional complications or identify patients with a high likelihood of poor long-term results? Several multicenter clinical trials, currently under way, are examining whether ultrasound can reliably predict restenosis following various types of intervention.

FUTURE DIRECTIONS

The technology and clinical role of intravascular ultrasound examination of the coronaries are rapidly evolving. During the next several years, technological advances in intravascular imaging are anticipated, including further reductions in the size of imaging catheters to guidewire dimensions (<0.025 in.). This guidewire-sized ultrasound probe will improve the ease and safety of the examination and may also enable simultaneous imaging during the revascularization procedure. Very small devices would also enable imaging of virtually any coronary stenosis prior to treatment. Combination devices are also undergoing refinement, permitting online guidance during revascularization procedures. An angioplasty balloon with an ultrasound transducer (Endosonics—Oracle) is FDA approved, and a transducer combined with an atherectomy device is undergoing initial clinical testing. Imaging catheters that incorporate a tip-mounted Doppler flow probe are also under development; these would allow simultaneous measurements of cross-sectional area and flow velocity.

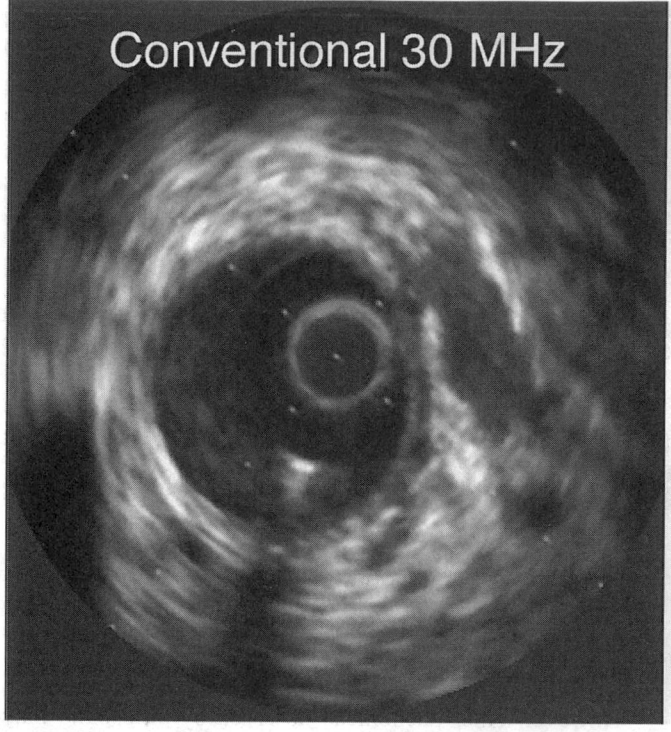

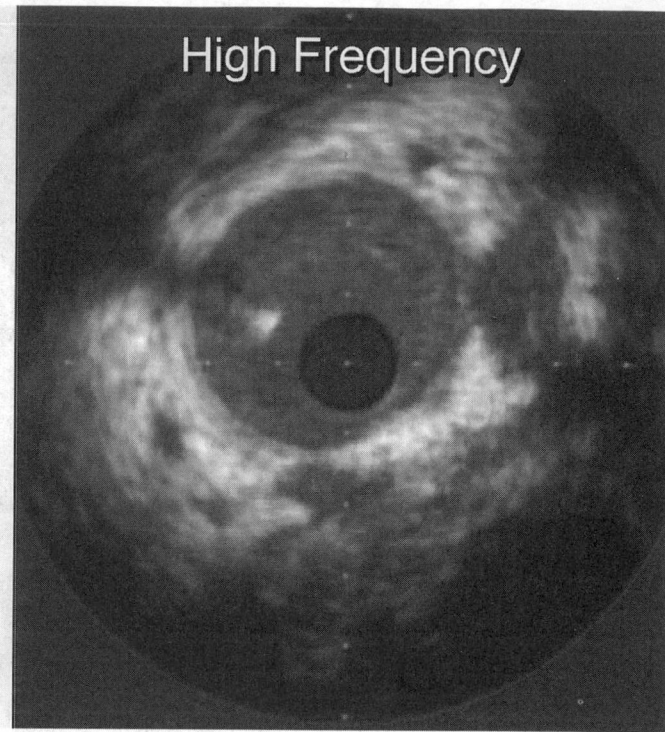

FIGURE 49-12

Improvement in image quality provided by higher-frequency intravascular ultrasound imaging. In the left panel, a porcine coronary is shown imaged using a conventional 30-MHz center frequency. In the right panel, an image obtained at a higher frequency at the same site is illustrated. The right-panel images shows increased structural detail and more intraluminal blood speckle.

Such a device may provide continuous beat-to-beat assessment of coronary blood flow in vivo.

Analysis of backscattered ultrasound signals has been used to perform "tissue characterization" of coronary plaques by several investigators. Preliminary studies have shown that analysis of the unprocessed radiofrequency backscatter from the vessel wall can differentiate the various tissue types within both normal and diseased vessels.[82] Higher-frequency ultrasound catheters are also in an advanced stage of development and will likely yield significantly better spatial resolution, although the incremental clinical benefit remains to be demonstrated (Fig. 49-12).[83] Although high-frequency probes enable better axial and lateral resolution, penetration is likely to be impaired in comparison with that of more conventional 30-MHz devices. It remains apparent that the physical limits of intravascular imaging technology have not been reached. Accordingly, further improvements in the performance of these devices are anticipated.

REFERENCES

1. Bom N, Lancee CT, Van Egmond FC. An ultrasonic intracardiac scanner. *Ultrasonics* 1972; 10:72–76.
2. Yock PG, Johnson EL, Linker DT. Intravascular ultrasound: Development and clinical potential. *Am J Cardiac Imaging* 1988; 2:185–193.
3. Roelandt JR, Bom NY, Serruys PW. Intravascular high-resolution real-time, two-dimensional echocardiography. *Int J Cardiac Imaging* 1989; 4:63–67.
4. Hodgson JM, Graham SP, Savakus AD, Dame SG, Stephens DN, Dhillon PS, et al. Clinical percutaneous imaging of coronary anatomy using an over-the-wire ultrasound catheter system. *Int J Cardiac Imaging* 1989; 4:187–193.
5. Nissen SE, Grines CL, Gurley JC, Sublett K, Haynie D, Diaz C, et al. Application of a new phased-array ultrasound imaging catheter in the assessment of vascular dimensions: In vivo comparison to cineangiography. *Circulation* 1990; 81:660–666.
6. Arnett EN, Isner JM, Redwood CR, Kent KM, Baker WP, Ackerstein H, et al. Coronary artery narrowing in coronary heart disease: Comparison of cineangiographic and necropsy findings. *Ann Intern Med* 1979; 91:350–356.
7. Grodin CM, Dydra I, Pastgernac A, Campeau L, Bourassa MG. Discrepancies between cineangiographic and post-mortem findings in patients with coronary artery disease and recent myocardial revascularization. *Circulation* 1974; 49:703–709.
8. Isner JM, Kishel J, Kent KM. Accuracy of angiographic determination of left main coronary arterial narrowing. *Circulation* 1981; 63:1056–1061.
9. Vlodaver Z, Frech R, van Tassel RA, Edwards JE. Correlation of the antemortem coronary angiogram and the postmortem specimen. *Circulation* 1973; 47:162–168.
10. Zir LM, Miller SW, Dinsmore RE, Gilber JP, Harthorne JW. Interobserver variability in coronary angiography. *Circulation* 1976; 53:627–632.
11. Galbraith JE, Murphy ML, Desoyza N. Coronary angiogram interpretation: Interobserver variability. *JAMA* 1981; 240:2053–2059.
12. White CW, Wright CB, Doty DB, Hirtza LF, Eastham CL, Harrison DG, et al. Does visual interpretation of the coronary arteriogram predict the physiologic importance of a coronary stenosis? *N Engl J Med* 1984; 310:819–824.
13. Nissen SE, Gurley JC, Grines CL, Booth DC, McClure R, Berk M, et al. Intravascular ultrasound assessment of lumen size and wall morphology in normal subjects and patients with coronary artery disease. *Circulation* 1991; 84:1087–1099.

14. Waller BF, Orr CM, Slack JD, Pinkerton CA, Van Tassel JV, Peters T. Anatomy, histology, and pathology of coronary arteries: A review relevant to new interventional and imaging techniques—Part III. *Clin Cardiol* 1992; 15:607–615.

15. Roberts WC, Jones AA. Quantitation of coronary arterial narrowing at necropsy in sudden coronary death. *Am J Cardiol* 1979; 44:39–44.

16. Waller BF. "Crackers, breakers, stretchers, drillers, scrapers, shavers, burners, welders, and melters": The future treatment of atherosclerotic coronary artery disease? A clinical-morphologic assessment. *J Am Coll Cardiol* 1989; 13:969–987.

17. Bessen M, Moriushi M, McLeay L, McRae M, Henry WL. Intravascular ultrasound cross-sectional arterial imaging before and after balloon angioplasty in vitro. *Circulation* 1989; 80:873–882.

18. Tobis JM, Mallery J, Mahon D, Lehmann K, Zalesky P, Griffith J, et al. Intravascular ultrasound imaging of human coronary arteries in vivo. *Circulation* 1991; 83:913–926.

19. Topol EJ, Nissen SE. Our preoccupation with coronary luminology: The dissociation between clinical and angiographic findings in ischemic heart disease. *Circulation* 1995; 92:2333–2342.

20. Glagov S, Weisenberg E, Zarins CK, Stankunavicius R, Koiettis GJ. Compensatory enlargement of human coronary arteries. *N Engl J Med* 1987; 316:1371–1375.

21. Little WC, Constantinescu M, Applegate RJ, Kutcher MA, Burrows MT, Kahl FR, et al. Can arteriography predict the site of a subsequent myocardial infarction in patients with mild-to-moderate coronary artery disease? *Circulation* 1988; 78:1157–1166.

22. Yamagishi M, Miyatake K, Tamai J, Nakatani S, Koyama J, Nissen SE. Detection of atherosclerosis at the site of focal vasospasm in angiographically normal or minimally narrowed coronary segments by intravascular ultrasound. *J Am Coll Cardiol* 1994; 23:352–357.

23. Yock P, Linker D, Angelsen B. Two-dimensional, intravascular ultrasound: Technical development and initial clinical experience. *J Am Soc Echocardiogr* 1989; 4:296–304.

24. Nissen SE, Gurley JC. Application of intravascular ultrasound to detection and quantitation of coronary atherosclerosis. *Int J Cardiac Imaging* 1991; 6:165–177.

25. Nissen SE, Gurley JC. Quantitative assessment of coronary dimensions, lumen shape and wall morphology by intravascular ultrasound. In: Tobis P, Yock P, eds. *Intravascular Ultrasound.* New York: Churchill Livingstone; 1992:71–83.

26. Nissen SE, Gurley JC, DeMaria AN. Assessment of vascular disease by intravascular ultrasound. *Cardiology* 1990; 77:398–410.

27. Nissen SE, DeFranco A, Tuzcu EM. Detection and quantification of atherosclerosis: The emerging role for intravascular ultrasound. In: Fuster, V, ed. *Syndromes of Atherosclerosis: Correlations of Clinical Imaging and Pathology.* Armonk, NY: Futura; 1996:291–312.

28. Nissen SE, Gurley JC, DeMaria AN. Intravascular ultrasound of the coronaries: Current applications and future directions. *Am J Cardiol* 1992; 69:18H–29H.

29. TenHoff H, Korbijn A, Smit TH, Klinkhamer JFF, Bom N. Image artifacts in mechanically driven ultrasound catheters. *Int J Cardiac Imaging* 1989; 4:195–199.

30. Nissen SE, DeFranco AC, Tuzcu EM. Coronary intravascular ultrasound. In: Freed M, Grines C, eds. *Manual of Interventional Cardiology.* Birmingham, MI: Physicians Press; 1996:583–602.

31. Hausmann D, Erbel R, Alibelli-Chemarin MJ, Boksch W, Caraciolo E, Cohn JM, et al. The safety of intracoronary ultrasound: A multicenter survey of 2207 examinations. *Circulation* 1995; 91:623–630.

32. Gussenhoven EJ, Essed CE, Lancee CT, Mastik F, Frietman P, Van Egmond FC, et al. Arterial wall characteristics determined by intravascular ultrasound imaging: An in vitro study. *J Am Coll Cardiol* 1989; 4:947–952.

33. Potkin BN, Bartorelli AL, Gessert JM, Necille RF, Almagor Y, Robert WC, et al. Coronary artery imaging with intravascular high-frequency ultrasound. *Circulation* 1990; 81:1575–1585.

34. Nishimura RA, Edwards WD, Warnes CA, Reeder GS, Holmes DR, Tajik AJ, et al. Intravascular ultrasound imaging: In vitro validation and pathologic correlation. *J Am Coll Cardiol* 1990; 16:145–154.

35. Fitzgerald PJ, St Goar FG, Connolly AJ, Pinto FJ, Billingham ME, Popp RL, et al. Intravascular ultrasound imaging of coronary arteries: Is three layers the norm? *Circulation* 1992; 86:154–158.

36. St Goar FG, Pinto FJ, Alderman EL, Fitzgerald PJ, Stadius ML, Popp RL. Intravascular ultrasound imaging of angiographically normal coronary arteries: An in vivo comparison with quantitative angiography. *J Am Coll Cardiol* 1991; 18:952–958.

37. Mintz GS, Popma JJ, Pichard AD, Kent KM, Satler LF, Chuang YC, et al. Patterns of calcification in coronary artery disease: A statistical analysis of intravascular ultrasound and coronary angiography in 1,155 lesions. *Circulation* 1995; 91:1959–1965.

38. Tuzcu EM, Berkalp B, DeFranco AC, Ellis SG, Whitlow PL, Nissen SE. The dilemma of diagnosing coronary calcification: Angiography versus intravascular ultrasound. *J Am Coll Cardiol* 1996; 27:832–838.

39. Mintz GS, Pichard AD, Kovach JA, Kent KM, Satler LF, Javier SP, et al. Impact of preintervention intravascular ultrasound imaging on transcatheter treatment strategies in coronary artery disease. *Am J Cardiol* 1994; 73:423–430.

40. Popma JJ, Mintz GS, Satler LF, Pichard AD, Kent KM, Chuang YC, et al. Clinical and angiographic outcome after directional coronary atherectomy: A qualitative and quantitative analysis using coronary arteriography and intravascular ultrasound. *Am J Cardiol* 1993; 72:55E–64E.

41. Matar FA, Mintz GS, Pinnow E, Saturnino SP, Popma JJ, Kent JM, et al. Multivariate predictors of intravascular ultrasound end points after directional coronary atherectomy. *J Am Coll Cardiol* 1995; 25:318–324.

42. Gil R, von Birgelen C, Prati F, Di Mario C, Ligthart J, Serruys PW. Usefulness of three-dimensional reconstruction for interpretation and quantitative analysis of intracoronary ultrasound during stent deployment. *Am J Cardiol* 1996; 77:761–764.

43. St Goar FG, Pinto FJ, Alderman EL, Fitzgerald PJ, Billingham ME, Popp RL. Detection of coronary atherosclerosis in young adult hearts using intravascular ultrasound. *Circulation* 1992; 86:756–763.

44. Tuzcu EM, Hobbs H, Rincon G, Bott-Silverman C, De Franco AC, Nissen SE. Occult and frequent transmission of atherosclerosis coronary disease with cardiac transplantation. *Circulation* 1995; 91:1706–1713.

45. Mintz GS, Painter JA, Pichard AD, Kent KM, Satler LF, Popma JJ, et al. Atherosclerosis in angiographically "normal" coronary artery reference segments: An intravascular ultrasound study with clinical correlations. *J Am Coll Cardiol* 1995; 25:1479–1485.

46. Hermiller JB, Tenaglia AN, Kisslo KB, Phillips HR, Bashore TM, Stack RS, et al. In vivo validation of compensatory enlargement of atherosclerotic coronary arteries. *Am J Cardiol* 1993; 71:665–668.

47. Ge J, Erbel R, Zamorano J, Koch L, Kearney P, Gorge G, et al. Coronary artery remodeling in atherosclerotic disease: An intravascular ultrasonic study in vivo. *Coron Artery Dis* 1993; 4:981–986.

48. Isner JM, Kishel J, Kent RM. Accuracy of angiographic determination of left main coronary artery narrowing. *Circulation* 1981; 63:1056–1061.

49. Hermiller JB, Buller CE, Tenaglia AN, Kisslo KB, Phillips HR, Bashore TM, et al. Unrecognized left main coronary artery disease in patients undergoing interventional procedures. *Am J Cardiol* 1993; 71:173–176.

50. Mintz GS, Popma JJ, Pichard AD, Kent KM, Satler LF, Chuang YC, et al. Limitations of angiography in the assessment of plaque distribution in coronary artery disease: A systematic study of target lesion eccentricity in 1446 lesions. *Circulation* 1996; 93:924–931.

51. Fitzgerald PJ, Ports TA, Yock PG. Contribution of localized calcium deposits to dissection after angioplasty in vivo assessed by intravascular imaging. *Circulation* 1992; 86:64–70.

52. Hinohara T, Rowe MH, Robertson GC, Selmon MR, Braden L, Leggett JH, et al. Effect of lesion characteristics on outcome of directional coronary atherectomy. *J Am Coll Cardiol* 1991; 17:1112–1120.

53. Uretsky BF, Kormos RL, Zerbe TR, Lee A, Tokarcyzk TR, Murali S, et al. Cardiac events after heart transplantation: Incidence and predictive value of coronary arteriography. *J Heart Transplant* 1992; 11:S45–S50.

54. O'Neill BJ, Pflugfelder PW, Single NR, Menkis AH, McKenzie FN, Kostuk WJ. Frequency of angiographic detection and quantitative assessment of coronary arterial disease one and three years after cardiac transplantation. *Am J Cardiol* 1989; 63:1221–1226.

55. Dressler FA, Miller LW. Necropsy versus angiography: How accurate is angiography? *J Heart Lung Transplant* 1992; 11(part2):S56–S59.

56. Johnson DE, Alderman EL, Schroeder JS, Gao SZ, Hunt S, DeCampli WM, et al. Transplant coronary artery disease: Histopathological correlations with angiographic morphology. *J Am Coll Cardiol* 1991; 17:449–457.

57. St Goar FG, Pinto FJ, Alderman EL, Valantine HA, Schroeder JS, Gao SZ, et al. Intracoronary ultrasound in cardiac transplant recipients:

In vivo evidence of "angiographically silent" intimal thickening. *Circulation* 1992; 85:979–987.

58. Tuzcu EM, DeFranco AC, Goormastic M, Hobbs RE, Bott-Silverman C, Nissen SE, et al. Dichotomous pattern of coronary atherosclerosis 1 to 9 years after transplantation: Insights from systematic intravascular ultrasound imaging. *J Am Coll Cardiol* 1996; 27:839–846.

59. Nissen SE, Gurley JC. Assessment of coronary angioplasty results by intravascular ultrasound. In: Serruys PW, Strauss BH, King SB, eds. *Restenosis after Intervention with New Mechanical Devices.* Amsterdam: Kluwer; 1992:73–96.

60. Nissen SE, Gurley JC. Assessment of coronary dimensions by intravascular ultrasound: Comparison to quantitative angiography advances. In: Reiber JC, ed. *Quantitative Coronary Angiography.* Hingham, MA: Martinus Nijhoff; 1993:29–51.

61. DeFranco AC, Tuzcu EM, Moliterno DJ, Berkalp B, Whitlow P, Nissen SE, et al. Overestimation of lumen size after coronary interventions: Implications for randomized trials of new devices. (abstr) *Circulation* 1994; 90:I-550.

62. Honye J, Mahon DJ, Jain A, White CJ, Ramee SR, Wallis JB, et al. Morphological effects of coronary balloon angioplasty in vivo assessed by intravascular ultrasound imaging. *Circulation* 1992; 85:1012–1025.

63. Gerber TC, Erbel R, Gorge G, Ge J, Rupprecht HJ, Meyer J. Classification of morphologic effects of percutaneous transluminal coronary angioplasty assessed by intravascular ultrasound. *Am J Cardiol* 1992; 70:1546–1554.

64. Botas J, Clark DA, Pinto F, Chenzbraum A, Fischell TA. Balloon angioplasty results in increased segmental coronary distensibility: A likely mechanism of percutaneous transluminal coronary angioplasty. *J Am Coll Cardiol* 1994; 23:1043–1052.

65. Mintz GS, Pichard AD, Kent KM, Satler LF, Popma JJ, Leon MB. Axial plaque redistribution as a mechanism of percutaneous transluminal coronary angioplasty. *Am J Cardiol* 1996; 77:427–430.

66. Braden GA, Herrington DM, Downes TR, Kutcher MA, Little WC. Qualitative and quantitative contrasts in the mechanisms of lumen enlargement by coronary balloon angioplasty and directional coronary atherectomy. *J Am Coll Cardiol* 1994; 23:40–48.

67. Simonton CA, Leon MB, Kuntz RE, Popma JJ, Hinohara T, Bersin RM, et al. Acute and late clinical and angiographic results of directional atherectomy in the optimal atherectomy restenosis study (OARS). *Circulation* 1995; 92:I-545.

68. Topol EJ, Leya F, Pinkerton CA, Whitlow PL, Hofling B, Simonton CA, et al. A comparison of directional atherectomy with coronary angioplasty in patients with coronary artery disease. *N Engl J Med* 1993; 329:221–227.

69. Adelman AG, Cohen M, Kimball BP, Bonan R, Ricci DR, Webb JG, et al. Canadian Coronary Atherectomy Trial: A randomized comparison of directional coronary atherectomy and percutaneous transluminal coronary angioplasty for lesions of the proximal left anterior descending artery. *N Engl J Med* 1993; 329:228–234.

70. Fitzgerald PJ, Belef M, Connolly AJ, Sudhir K, Yock PG. Design and initial testing of an ultrasound-guided directional atherectomy device. *Am Heart J* 1995; 129:593–598.

71. Mintz GS, Potkin BN, Keren G, Satler LF, Pichard AP, Kent KM, et al. Intravascular ultrasound evaluation of the effect of rotational atherectomy in obstructive atherosclerotic coronary artery disease. *Circulation* 1992; 86:1383–1393.

72. Kovach JA, Mintz GS, Pichard AD, Kent KM, Popma JJ, Satler LF, et al. Sequential intravascular ultrasound characterization of the mechanisms of rotational atherectomy and adjunct balloon angioplasty. *J Am Coll Cardiol* 1993; 22:1024–1032.

73. De Franco AC, Nissen SE, Tuzcu EM, Witlow PL. Incremental value of intravascular ultrasound during rotational coronary atherectomy. *Cathet Cardiovasc Diag* 1996; 3(suppl):23–33.

74. Nakamura S, Colombo A, Galglione S, Almagor Y, Goldberg SL, Maiello K, et al. Intracoronary ultrasound observations during stent implantation. *Circulation* 1994; 89:2026–2034.

75. Goldberg SL, Colombo A, Nakamura S, Almagor Y, Maiello L, Tobis JM. Benefit of intracoronary ultrasound in the deployment of Plamaz-Schatz stents. *J Am Coll Cardiol* 1994; 24:996–1003.

76. Colombo A, Hall P, Nakamura S, Almagor Y, Maiello L, Martini G, et al. Intracoronary stenting without anticoagulation accomplished with intravascular ultrasound guidance. *Circulation* 1995; 91:1676–1688.

77. Serruys PW, de Jaegere P, Kiemeneij, Macaya C, Rutsch W, Heyndrickx G, et al. A comparison of balloon-expandable-stent implantation with balloon angioplasty in patients with coronary artery disease. *N Engl J Med* 1994; 331:489–495.

78. Fischman DL, Leon MB, Baim DS, Schatz RA, Savage MP, Penn IM, et al. A randomized comparison of coronary-stent placement and balloon angioplasty in the treatment of coronary artery disease. *N Engl J Med* 1994; 331:496–501.

79. Morice MC, Breton C, Bunouf P, Cattan S, Eltchaninoff H, Henry M, et al. Coronary stenting without anticoagulation, without intravascular ultrasound: Results of the French registry. *Circulation* 1995; 92(suppl I):I-796.

80. Sandardas MA, McEniery PT, Aroney CN, Bett JNH. Elective implantation of intracoronary stents without intravascular ultrasound guidance or subsequent warfarin. *Cathet Cardiovasc Diagn* 1996; 37:355–359.

81. Mintz GS, Popma JJ, Pichard AD, Kent KM, Satler LF, Wong SC, et al. Arterial remodeling after coronary angioplasty: A serial intravascular ultrasound study. *Circulation* 1996; 94:35–43.

82. Metz JA, Preuss P, Komiyama N, Ramo P, Yock PG, Fitzgerald PJ, et al. Discrimination between soft plaque and thrombus based on radiofrequency analysis of intravascular ultrasound. (abstr) *J Am Coll Cardiol* 1996; 27(suppl A):200A.

83. Lockwood GR, Ryan LK, Gotlieb AI, Lonn E, Haunt JW, Liu P, et al. In vitro high resolution intravascular imaging in muscular and elastic arteries. *J Am Coll Cardiol* 1992; 20:153–160.

50

SURGICAL TREATMENT OF ATHEROSCLEROTIC CORONARY HEART DISEASE

Floyd D. Loop / Derek D. Muehrcke

The development of selective cine coronary arteriography opened a new surgical field. Although there had been previous attempts, in May 1967 Rene G. Favaloro started the first successful series of coronary bypass surgery.[1] Soon afterward, W. Dudley Johnson and colleagues applied the operation to all major vessels.[2] As experience evolved, relative indications and contraindications for coronary artery bypass grafting were developed (Table 50-1), and benefits in certain subsets of patients were documented.[3,4]

The 1980s and 1990s witnessed a virtual explosion in technologic advances, including angioplasty and stenting, to treat coronary artery disease. Bypass surgery is the procedure of choice for diffuse multivessel disease, however, especially for those patients with compromised left ventricular function.

ASSESSMENT OF INDICATIONS

Clinical and Angiographic Indicators

Selection for surgical treatment is based on the arteriographic perception of myocardial jeopardy, vessel characteristics, and left ventricular performance. Narrowing of the left main coronary artery to less than 50 percent of normal diameter is the most powerful arteriographic indicator of adverse prognosis. Apart from such narrowing, a lesion in the proximal anterior descending coronary artery carries the most prognostic weight. Patients with angina/ischemia and two-vessel disease with anterior descending stenosis or proximal three-vessel disease deserve consideration for bypass surgery unless left ventricular regional contraction is irreversibly impaired. The severity of left ventricular dysfunction is the single best indicator of outcome irrespective of the type of treatment. If multivessel disease is identified before left ventricular impairment occurs, longevity, employment, and lifestyle stand to benefit from coronary artery bypass surgery. Increasing left ventricular *dysfunction* may show wider survival differences favorable to surgery, but poor ventricular function reduces overall survival to far less than that with normal left ventricular function.

The benefit of coronary artery bypass surgery depends on (1) severity of angina; (2) severity of ischemia documented by perfusion studies, electrocardiogram, or graded exercise test; (3) number of major coronary vessels with important proximal stenoses, especially with involvement of the left main or proximal anterior descending coronary arteries, or three-vessel disease; (4) extent of left ventricular dysfunction; and (5) existence of coronary atherosclerosis combined with peripheral vascular disease, valve pathology, and complications of myocardial infarction.

Isolated coronary artery surgery is contraindicated when there are no symptoms or signs of ischemia, especially with poor left ventricular function and clinical evidence of heart failure. The very elderly with multiple comorbidities should be evaluated for surgery conservatively. The four "A's"—age, attitude, activity, and associated diseases—may be helpful in discussing risk versus benefit.

Percutaneous Transluminal Coronary Artery Angioplasty as an Alternative to Surgery

Several randomized trials were initiated in the late 1980s to directly compare coronary artery bypass graft surgery with percutaneous transluminal coronary angioplasty. In the only one-vessel trial that considered proximal stenosis of the left

TABLE 50-1

CURRENT INDICATIONS AND CONTRAINDICATIONS
FOR CORONARY ARTERY SURGERY

Indications
  Angina interfering with daily activities
  Evidence of severe ischemia by exercise test or resting electrocardiogram
  Left main coronary artery stenosis of 50% or more
  Proximal left anterior descending artery stenosis of 70% or more in conjunction with
    other major and significant coronary artery stenosis
  Proximal three-vessel disease of 50% or more
  Multivessel stenoses of 50% or more combined with moderate to severe (left ventricular
    ejection fraction ≤0.50) left ventricular impairment
Contraindications
  Advanced age with marked debility and restricted activity
  No angina or ischemia
  Poor left ventricular function (ejection fraction <0.30) and symptoms or signs of heart
    failure only
  Ungraftable coronary arteries
  Noncompliant patient
  Lack of consent

anterior descending coronary artery, Goy and colleagues[5] compared balloon angioplasty to bypass graft surgery using the left internal thoracic artery. At 2-year follow-up, mortality was similar, but the composite primary end points, which included repeat revascularization, death, and myocardial infarction, were higher for the angioplasty group (37 versus 8 percent) ($p < .01$). Patients in the angioplasty group were also receiving substantially more antianginal drugs.

Major prospective randomized trials comparing percutaneous transluminal coronary angioplasty with coronary artery bypass graft surgery in patients with multivessel coronary atherosclerosis have been reported.[6–10] These reports have several similarities in design, patient enrollment characteristics, procedural details, and clinical outcomes. Unfortunately, few of the patients screened for enrollment were actually randomly assigned to the trials (4 to 9 percent), making the results applicable to only a small subset of patients with multivessel coronary artery disease treated clinically. Patients in these randomized trials were relatively young, mostly men, and exhibited modest three-vessel involvement (12 to 45 percent); most had excellent left ventricular function. The eligibility requirements for the studies varied by the extent of revascularization, presence of occluded arteries, and use of adjuvant intervention devices. Outcome at 1 to 5 years revealed comparable survival but better event-free survival (death, myocardial infarction, reintervention) in the surgical group. One important finding of the Bypass Angioplasty Revascularization Investigation (BARI) was an improved survival in diabetic patients with surgery compared to percutaneous transluminal angioplasty.[6] The cumulative health care costs for those assigned to coronary balloon angioplasty appeared to be similar to that of the bypass surgery cohort at 3 to 5 years.[11]

Balloon angioplasty appears to offer equivalent intermediate-term results for one-vessel disease, most two-vessel com-

binations, and selectively for nondiabetic three-vessel disease.[12] Cumulative event rates, including symptom status, are less favorable for angioplasty than for coronary artery bypass surgery, principally as a result of restenosis. Adjuvant therapies, such as stents or platelet IIb–IIIa inhibitors after angioplasty, and the more extensive use of arterial, as opposed to venous, bypass grafts will likely influence future studies.

Asymptomatic Status

Asymptomatic patients and those with no ischemia are rarely candidates for coronary artery surgery. Surgery is indicated in the rare (less than 4 percent of bypass surgeries) circumstance of asymptomatic severe left main disease or severe three-vessel disease with proximal lesions. Bourassa et al.[13] found bypass surgery to be superior to angioplasty in patients suffering from asymptomatic cardiac ischemia. More complete revascularization with surgery is related to better clinical outcomes.

Reversible Impaired Myocardium

"Hibernating" myocardium is a form of painless ischemia caused by chronically reduced myocardial blood flow.[14] The presence of this phenomenon may be confirmed by improved contractility of the left ventricular wall after nitroglycerin administration, by positron emission tomography revealing metabolism in areas of regional ventricular abnormality, and by documented reversible exercise-induced ischemia. Depending on the pathoanatomy, coronary artery surgery may be indicated for its potential to reverse ischemia and thereby improve left ventricular function. Overall, left ventricular segmental wall abnormalities are more often permanent and contractility is improved in only a minority of cases. In contrast, "stunned" myocardium is a condition in which coronary blood flow has been restored after a discrete episode of myocardial ischemia but in which ultrastructural abnormalities persist.[15] Stunned myocardium may occur after myocardial infarction, vasospasm, coronary balloon angioplasty, or coronary bypass surgery performed during acute ischemia. Although surgical revascularization may restore contractility to the stunned myocardium, this objective is rarely the primary indication for surgery.

Unstable Angina

Necropsy studies have shown that unstable angina is often associated with the most severe forms of coronary atherosclerosis. Patients with one-vessel disease are most often treated by coronary angioplasty unless the vessel is not amenable to dilation. Multivessel disease, especially with left ventricular dysfunction or left main disease, is most often treated by coronary artery surgery, preferably when the patient is stable. It is important to recognize that preoperative stability lessens the perioperative infarction rate in coronary bypass surgery and is associated with lower operative risk[16] (see Chap. 46).

Myocardial Infarction

Myocardial infarction patients are candidates for coronary artery surgery mainly when complications ensue. These complications include ventricular aneurysm, left ventricular rupture, ruptured papillary muscle, and postinfarction ventricular septal defect. Formation of a ventricular aneurysm is treated expectantly. If angina, congestive heart failure, ventricular arrhythmia, or, rarely, systemic embolism occurs, aneurysmectomy is considered. These patients frequently have multivessel disease and require combined coronary artery grafting. Repair of left ventricular aneurysms has recently included the use of an endoventricular patch that remodels the left ventricular cavity to a more physiologic geometry. Endoventricular circular patch repair combined with coronary artery bypass grafting improves left ventricular function and clinical status[17] and reduces the incidence of arrhythmia (inducible or sudden death) postoperatively without antiarrhythmic drugs.[18] Left ventricular rupture, ventricular septal defect, and papillary muscle rupture are surgical emergencies. Unless the patient is extremely elderly and in multisystem failure, surgical treatment is better than nonsurgical treatment, which is nearly always fatal.

Since the completion of large, randomized, placebo-controlled trials of thrombolytic therapy, reperfusion therapy for acute myocardial infarction has become a standard of care.[19–26]

Surgery has been advocated and has achieved good results in stable subsets of patients with myocardial infarction. Immediate investigation and surgical treatment of all patients with myocardial infarction, however, is not practical or safe. The role of revascularization and coronary surgery in the myocardial infarction patient is discussed in more detail below and in Chap. 47.

Postinfarction Angina

Postinfarction angina is an indication for coronary arteriography. Many reports attest to the relatively low surgical mortality in this otherwise high-risk group. Poor ventricular function, older age, and cardiogenic shock carry higher risk. Immediate successful revascularization results in an excellent intermediate-term survival rate.

Sudden Cardiac Death

Selection of the therapeutic approach to patients who have been resuscitated from "sudden cardiac death" can be a complicated issue (see Chap. 36). Sudden cardiac death is almost always associated with underlying heart disease, and in this heterogeneous population, a significant portion of which has coronary artery disease, approximately half of the patients have no ischemic symptoms before the event. The prognosis is generally better when cardiac arrest occurs with acute myocardial infarction. Referral to surgery depends on the anatomic diagnosis, left ventricular functional status, and results of electropharmacologic testing. When coronary pathoanatomy is conducive to bypass surgery, surgery appears to reduce the incidence of sudden, unexpected death, but it may not prevent subsequent myocardial infarction.[27]

Peripheral Vascular Disease

Peripheral vascular disease is frequently a marker for coronary atherosclerosis.[28] Although coronary artery bypass graft surgery may improve long-term survival for patients with peripheral vascular disease, the decision to recommend bypass surgery for patients with peripheral vascular disease remains complex and difficult. Abdominal aortic aneurysms are also frequently associated with severe coronary atherosclerosis. If coronary atherosclerosis is suspected on the basis of symptoms or a history of previous myocardial infarction, coronary arteriography should be performed. In most cases, coronary artery surgery is scheduled first and elective peripheral revascularization follows, with the timing dependent on symptoms and pathoanatomy. If a large abdominal aneurysm is detected and the coronary artery is stable, the sequence may be reversed. Rarely, coronary artery bypass surgery and aneurysmectomy are performed simultaneously to treat unstable angina, left main or three-vessel disease, and an enlarging, symptomatic abdominal aneurysm. The risk is less when the procedures are staged.

Internal carotid narrowing is usually detected first by a bruit and confirmed by ultrasound examination, digital subtraction angiography, or conventional brachiocephalic angiography. Recent evidence confirms that patients with severe (70 to 99 percent) carotid artery stenosis face a marked risk of ipsilateral ischemic stroke within a few years[29] (see Chaps. 100 and 101). If the surgical stroke and death rates are within 2 percent, the absolute risk of ipsilateral stroke is greatly reduced in the first 2 years after carotid endarterectomy.[30] If the patient is neurologically asymptomatic and the lesion is unilateral and less than 90 percent narrowed, coronary artery surgery may be staged first and carotid endarterectomy performed electively later (see Chap. 99). For patients with severe unilateral or bilateral disease and a history of transient ischemic attack or stroke, simultaneous carotid endarterectomy and myocardial revascularization may be undertaken. In experienced hands, the stroke and mortality rates for combined treatment are less than 5 percent. In most other instances, myocardial revascularization precedes carotid endarterectomy, which may occur weeks or years later, depending on symptoms. The reverse order may occur when patients are neurologically unstable but have stable angina and coronary pathoanatomy that is not considered dangerous.

Concomitant Valve Disease

Valve disease may accompany severe coronary atherosclerosis. Aortic stenosis is the most frequently associated form of valve dysfunction, probably because it is a form of atherosclerosis. Combining aortic valve replacement with coronary bypass grafting is routine and, for men, the risk is about the same as that for isolated aortic valve replacement. For elderly women, the risk is markedly higher. In cases with coronary atherosclerosis, major coronary vessel bypass should be performed simultaneously with all valve operations. Ischemic mitral regurgitation may result from global left ventricular dysfunction, which may change the spatial relationships of the papillary muscles or compromise papillary muscle blood supply. The majority of these regurgitant valves can be repaired. Preoperative risk factors in combined valve operation and coronary artery bypass grafting include advanced age, female gender, renal failure, New York Heart Association class III or IV functional status, mitral insufficiency, arrhythmia, and impaired left ventricular function.[31]

Coronary atherosclerosis is less frequently associated with other valvular conditions than with aortic stenosis. Coronary arteriography should be included in the preoperative investigation except in young patients, because the absence of angina does not exclude coronary atherosclerosis. Today, valvular aortic regurgitation, mitral stenosis, and mitral regurgitation are frequently corrected by repair rather than by replacement. Mitral valve repair carries a lower operative risk than mitral valve replacement.

Emergency Coronary Artery Surgery

Experience with thrombolytic therapy in acute myocardial infarction indicates that up to 10 percent of patients require immediate surgical treatment because of complications from coronary balloon angioplasty, failure of reperfusion, or discovery of dangerous myocardial jeopardy, especially left main coronary artery disease. Modern methods of myocardial protection allow emergency surgery to be accomplished with an overall hospital mortality rate of approximately 5 percent or less.

Postinfarction angina may be treated surgically when the patient is in relatively stable condition, with risk even lower than 5 percent.[32] Early postinfarction angina emanating from a site distant to the infarct carries a poor prognosis,[33] and these patients should be considered for emergency bypass surgery. Recent studies suggest that surgical mortality is highest immediately after Q-wave infarction. Patients suffering non-Q-wave myocardial infarction may undergo coronary artery bypass graft surgery relatively safely at any time. Acceptable timing for coronary artery bypass graft surgery is 48 h after Q-wave infarction,[34] at which time the operative risk has decreased substantially. Surgery in acute myocardial infarction has decreased considerably since the advent of thrombolytic therapy. Today, patients with postinfarction angina or dangerous coronary pathoanatomy are recommended for early coronary bypass surgery. Balloon dilatation rarely fails, and the risk of emergent surgery is relatively low; however, the mortality related to *reoperation* after balloon angioplasty failure is upward of 20 percent.

THE CHANGING PATIENT POPULATION

In 1995, 30 percent of coronary artery bypass surgery patients at The Cleveland Clinic Foundation were over age 70, 5 percent were over age 80, and 25 percent were women. In comparing patients operated on in the 1970s and 1980s, most investigators have found a significant rise in age, more women surgical candidates, and less severe angina but a greater incidence of recent infarction, more patients with three-vessel disease, more left ventricular dysfunction, a greater incidence of emergency operation, and more comorbidity in the form of diabetes, arrhythmias, heart failure, and peripheral vascular disease.[35,36] Advancing age brings a greater prevalence of previous cerebrovascular events, cardiac enlargement, and more women patients.[37]

Elderly patients tend to have angina preoperatively more often than younger patients. Operative mortality and perioperative stroke rates rise with advancing age. In the absence of major complications, elderly patients react and recover like younger patients. However, the very elderly have less physiologic reserve and seemingly minor events may result in major morbidity. The technology is continuously improving and the safety of surgery in geriatric patients has improved since the 1970s as a result of improved myocardial protection and better overall management.

Because women tend to manifest atherosclerosis after menopause, they, on average, are a few years older than men as surgical candidates. Most studies have shown that the surgical mortality is higher in women. However, in adjusting the population for physical size, weight, or body surface area, gender *per se* is no longer a significant risk factor for operative mortality.[38,39] Smaller patients are at higher risk, probably because of the size of their recipient coronary vessels.

THE OPERATION

The objective of coronary artery surgery is to relieve symptoms, alleviate ischemia, reduce the possibility of subsequent cardiac events, and lengthen life. The first step to achieving these goals is to perform a complication-free operation. The operation begins with preoperative assessment; preoperative stability reduces risk. An experienced anesthesiologist is vital to the team effort.

Intraoperatively, skill and judgment combined with technological support and communication are the fundamental elements that determine risk.[40] Risk may also be predicted and stratified statistically from preoperative characteristics.[41,42] *Emergency status, elevated serum creatinine, advanced age, congestive heart failure, severe peripheral vascular disease, small stature (and low weight), left main coronary artery disease, and severe angina are generally regarded as the main risk factors*. Each advance in myocardial protection has tended to reduce overall risk and change the position or weight of these risk factors. Statistical techniques now in use can stratify risk based on these and other factors, so that high and low probability of mortality and even morbidity may be predicted with enhanced accuracy and conveyed to patients preoperatively.

The conduit of choice is now the internal thoracic artery graft. Use of this conduit may be extended in the form of bilateral thoracic artery grafts, free (aortocoronary) arterial grafts,[43] and sequential usage, which involves one or more side-to-side anastomoses, followed by an end-to-side conduit-to-recipient artery anastomosis. The internal thoracic artery may be applied with no increase in morbidity in either young or older patients. The only caveat is that *bilateral usage in diabetic patients is fraught with a higher rate of wound infection.*

Other arterial conduits that are particularly applicable for patients with diffuse disease and small-sized vessels are the gastroepiploic artery on the greater curvature of the stomach[44] and the inferior epigastric artery,[45,46] which lies behind the rectus muscle. All-arterial-conduit operations are generally reserved for younger patients with premature onset of coronary atherosclerosis. Generally, one or two internal thoracic artery grafts are combined with vein grafts for older patients.

Formerly, the saphenous vein graft was the standard conduit. Atherosclerotic deterioration of this graft and the disproportionately large size of the graft to the coronary artery have relegated the vein graft to secondary roles: revascularization of totally obstructed arteries that have collateral circulation and bypass grafting in very elderly patients or in patients in whom arterial grafts are otherwise unsuitable. Veins may be damaged by rough preparation, which results in separation and desquamation of the vascular endothelium.[47] Endothelial trauma may cause platelet adhesion, fibrin deposition, smooth muscle cell proliferation, vasospasm, and reduced fibrinolytic activity. Endothelial loss may be accompanied by a reduction in prostacyclin and release of endothelium-derived relaxing factor. The delicate vein is best preserved by procurement after heparinization, irrigation with a balanced electrolyte solution and dilute papaverine, low distension pressure, and brief storage.

Endarterectomy is reserved for vessels with compromised runoff that are ungraftable by traditional techniques. A vein graft is used to cover the long arteriotomy. Coronary endarterectomy has undergone a resurgence because of improved myocardial protection and greater technical experience in removing all atheromatous material from the individual side branches. Endarterectomy is not a satisfactory technique for small vessels that have been occluded for many years.

Myocardial Protection

Myocardial protection may be achieved by (1) either crystalloid or blood cardioplegia delivered antegrade into the aortic root below the aortic cross-clamp, alone or combined with retrograde (coronary sinus) delivery; (2) continuous ventricular fibrillation under moderate hypothermia without aortic cross-clamping; (3) hypothermic cardiac arrest using continuous intrapericardial cooling with cold saline solution; (4) intermittent occlusion of the ascending aorta preceded by administration of nifedipine, lidoflazine, or similar drugs; and (5) continuous retrograde warm blood cardioplegia delivered under normothermic core conditions.

Chemical cardioplegia initiates a potassium arrest that allows the oxygen-deprived heart to be protected for increasingly longer periods during complex repairs. Significant reduction of perioperative myocardial infarction, stroke, respiratory distress, and wound complications have been noted with substrate-enhanced blood cardioplegia, including use of a single aortic cross-clamp and warm terminal reperfusate. The reduction in morbid events translates into shorter stays in the intensive care unit and in the hospital, and it decreases length-of-stay outliers and hospital cost.

Recently, warm blood cardioplegia at normothermic core temperature has been delivered continuously through the coronary sinus.[48] Flow rates of warm blood cardioplegia of at least 80 mL/min seem to keep the heart aerobic, reduce lactate production, and improve maintenance of energy stores. If the field is obscured by the installation of blood cardioplegia, the continuous perfusion may be stopped temporarily during anastomotic construction.

Minimally Invasive Surgery

Minimally invasive surgery, the greatest advance of the late 1990s, will set a new standard in the twenty-first century. The evolution of these procedures begins with a minithoracotomy,[49–52] which will evolve into a limited number of ports for telescopic access and instrumentation. Eventually, the instrument access will be barely larger than a needle, and the video cameras will be flexible and provide three-dimensional viewing. Currently, we are in a transitional phase with new and challenging technologies, limited versatility, and a big investment. Nonetheless, valve and coronary artery surgery will be possible through small ports, much smaller than those used in minithoracotomy. To accomplish safe, extensive cardiac surgery by minimal access, optics must advance and the operation must be done through standard cannulation, aortic cross-clamping, and antegrade-retrograde cardioplegia. In other words, the effectiveness of myocardial protection techniques must be equivalent to that obtained today. Fine surgery must be accomplished in a dry, motionless field.

The advantages of minimally invasive surgery compared with traditional approaches are less pain, shorter hospitalization, and an excellent physiologic result with consistent safety. The instrumentation will progressively decrease in size, and new devices for cannulation and cross-clamping will be devised and perfected in the next few years. The goal is to accomplish extended arterial bypass surgery alone or combined with valve repair and placement through minimal access.

COMPLICATIONS

The major complications after coronary artery surgery are bleeding requiring reoperation, myocardial infarction, stroke, respiratory distress, wound infection, and renal failure (see also Chap. 51). Studies have shown that morbidity is not only costly but also life-threatening. Patients who experience one or more complications have an eight- to tenfold greater probability of death than those who sustain no complications.[53] Length of hospital stay and cost are affected by most of these major complications.[54] Important predictors of morbidity include previous cardiac surgery, emergency operation, advanced age, peripheral vascular disease, and preoperative elevated serum creatinine. These indicators affect myocardial and respiratory status but do not predict bleeding or wound infection with the same accuracy.[55]

Bleeding

In our experience, the propensity for bleeding is multifactorial but relates to advanced age, use of antiplatelet drugs preoperatively, prolonged operating time, previous cardiac surgery, and, infrequently, preoperative coagulopathy. Aspirin taken within 7 to 10 days before coronary bypass surgery has been associated with an increased rate of bleeding, increased use of blood and blood products, and longer hospitalization in the intensive care unit.[56] Newer products, such as fibrin glue and aprotinin, are reported to decrease postoperative bleeding. The routine use of preoperative tests in assessing bleeding risk is not justified. The need for transfusions is related to body surface area, preoperative anemia, and advanced age more than any other factors. Erythropoietin has been used to increase red blood cell production after autologous blood donation; however, its role in postoperative anemia is not yet defined.

Myocardial Infarction

In elective coronary bypass surgery, the transmural myocardial infarction rate is approximately 2 percent, and it has declined each decade from the 1970s to the present, presumably because of better myocardial protection. The large Q-wave infarctions seen in the early years of coronary bypass surgery are infrequent today. Transient abnormal Q waves may occur as a result of alterations in ventricular depolarization or may be unmasked by improved function of a contiguous ventricular segment. Patients who experience nonfatal perioperative myocardial damage have essentially the same intermediate-term course as patients without myocardial infarction. The exceptions are those who require intraaortic balloon pumping for ischemia or infarction postoperatively. Although postoperative intraaortic balloon pumping is required in only 1 to 2 percent of elective surgeries today, most studies have shown that its requirement portends a lower survival rate because these patients have experienced myocardial damage and other major complications.

Stroke

The mechanisms of stroke after cardiac surgery include embolization, hypoperfusion, and inflammatory responses stimulated by extracorporeal circulation (see Chap. 96). Ascending aortic atherosclerosis is a major contributor to brain injury and myocardial complications.[57] Aortic disease should be suspected in patients with diffuse brachiocephalic disease, documented peripheral vascular disease, or left main coronary narrowing; it is confirmed by palpable atheroma or plaque discovered during cannulation or construction of aortic anastomoses. Aortic atheroemboli occur more frequently in coronary artery surgery than in other cardiac procedures.[58] An association between increased incidence of atheroembolism, advanced age, and peripheral vascular disease is apparent. The problem may be circumvented by femoral artery, axillary artery, or distal aortic arch cannulation.

If atherosclerosis is discovered during construction of the bypass grafts, most surgeons agree that the ascending aorta should be opened and debrided, possibly under deep hypothermia. Obviously, signs of extensive aortic atherosclerosis contraindicate aortic cross-clamping. In situ internal thoracic arteries should be used if the subclavian vessels are widely patent. Vein grafts or other arterial conduits may be anastomosed directly to the internal thoracic arteries.

Controversy still exists as to whether patients with a previous stroke are at increased risk for neurologic complications after coronary artery bypass graft surgery. The previously injured brain is vulnerable to cardiopulmonary bypass, as evidenced by the reappearance or exacerbation of focal deficits in these patients.[59]

Respiratory Distress

Respiratory distress has been related to lengthy operating time; increased number of blood transfusions; increased amount of crystalloid fluid infused; suboptimal preoperative nutritional status; presence of intrinsic pulmonary disease, neurologic deficit, or phrenic nerve dysfunction; renal failure; and cardiac failure[60] (see Chap. 51). Congestive heart failure in the perioperative period and the amount of blood products used are the most important risk factors for postoperative pulmonary complications. Nosocomial pneumonia may be related to prolonged stay in the intensive care unit, chronic obstructive pulmonary disease, administration of gastric acid–inhibitor drugs, and prolonged mechanical ventilatory support. Pneumonia may be prevented by keeping patients undergoing long stays in the intensive care unit in the head-up position to avoid aspiration, and by maintaining good oral hygiene, frequent sterile suctioning, and use of sucralfate and H_2-antagonists for stress ulcer prophylaxis.[61]

Wound Infection

Sternal wound infection with mediastinitis occurs in approximately 1 percent of elective coronary bypass patients and is usually detected around the seventh to ninth postoperative day. In unusual cases, this complication may arise several weeks postoperatively. The mortality related to mediastinitis is high; in our experience, 14 percent.[62] Wound infections increase hospital cost more than any other nonfatal complication because of the protracted hospitalization related to chest wall reconstruction. Use of the internal thoracic artery is not a risk factor for wound complications except in bilateral usage in diabetic patients, as noted. The sternal blood supply is not reduced in diabetic compared wth nondiabetic patients. Treatment is surgical drainage and either primary closure or treatment with rotational muscle flaps.

Renal Failure

Renal failure may be the result of underlying renal disease, especially when coupled with postoperative cardiac instability. Vasopressor use, intraaortic balloon pumping, excessive bleeding, history of chronic renal disease, and advanced age are predictors of postoperative renal failure. Some studies have supported the use of low-dose dopamine to enhance renal blood flow as a protective measure. Renal failure associated with increasing jaundice and the use of an intraaortic balloon pump carries a particularly poor prognosis.

Abdominal Complications

Although rare, the most common abdominal complication is gastrointestinal hemorrhage caused by esophagitis or gastritis. Pancreatitis is next in frequency and may be associated with low cardiac output and multisystem complications. Patients with a history of pancreatitis and postoperative complications may be more vulnerable to recurring pancreatitis. Transient elevation of bilirubin is noted with vasopressor and intraaortic balloon pump support. The perioperative administration of large doses of calcium chloride is an independent predictor of pancreatic cell injury and may be a cause of it.[63]

Atrial Fibrillation

The incidence of atrial fibrillation after cardiac surgery varies from a low of 4 percent in patients less than 40 years old to more than 50 percent in patients more than 75 years old. Atrial fibrillation may be a source of emboli postoperatively. The risk of incurring new atrial fibrillation appears to be independent of advanced coronary atherosclerosis or even of left ventricular function. A number of factors—including beta-blocker withdrawal, lengthy operation, or postcardiotomy syndrome—have been implicated, but none heralds atrial fibrillation consistently. Electrical reversion to normal sinus rhythm may cause embolization; therefore, prophylactic oral anticoagulation has been advocated (see Chap. 32).

Other Complications

Other infrequent complications include brachial plexus injuries, which may be related to spreading the sternum and compressing the plexus between the clavicle and the first rib (see Chap. 96). There may be associated median nerve trauma,

which usually resolves over several months. Horner's syndrome may result from a fracture of the first rib near the costotransverse articulation, affecting the cervical sympathetic chain. Asymptomatic deep venous thrombosis of the calf is frequent; however, pulmonary embolism is rare. Lower extremity wound complications at the site of saphenous vein procurement are unusual, but cellulitis may occur in diabetic patients with poor circulation.

In the first few months after hospital discharge, the clinician should be vigilant for pericarditis and pleuritis, wound infection, atrial arrhythmias, hepatitis, and recurring angina. Pulmonary embolism is rare but should be suspected in patients who had a protracted hospital course or who have a history of pulmonary embolism or phlebitis.

FACTORS AFFECTING LATE GRAFT PATENCY

The fate of the internal thoracic artery graft and perhaps of some other arterial conduits is different from that of vein grafts. Ten or more years after surgery, the patency rate for the left internal thoracic artery graft to the anterior descending coronary artery is in the 90th percentile, in contrast with the patency of vein grafts, which tend to deteriorate after the fifth to seventh postoperative year.[64] The high patency rate of internal thoracic artery grafts probably relates, at least in part, to the presence of endothelial vasodilatory factors, which may forestall the development of atherosclerosis.[65] Prostacyclin and nitric oxide activities are preserved and the conduit is nourished from the lumen, not the vasa vasorum, as in larger arteries.

Approximately 80 percent of vein grafts are open 5 years after operation. According to studies from the Montreal Heart Institute,[66] The Cleveland Clinic Foundation,[67] and others, this percentage takes into account a 5 to 10 percent graft closure rate in the first month, 10 to 15 percent closure at 1 year, and only slight attrition between postoperative years 1 and 5. After 5 to 7 years, the progression of atheromatous disease in coronary bypass vein grafts appears to increase, so that at 10 to 12 years, only 40 to 60 percent of the grafts are open.[68] Approximately one-half to three-fourths of late patent vein bypass grafts show angiographic evidence of lumen irregularities, presumably atheromatous degeneration. The late occlusion of vein grafts is associated with thrombosis at the site of atherosclerotic lesions. Vein graft atherosclerosis is generally diffuse and has been associated with elevated serum cholesterol, low high-density lipoprotein (HDL) cholesterol, high serum triglycerides, and cigarette smoking.[69]

The classic study from the Mayo Clinic showed that dipyridamole administered preoperatively followed by aspirin and dipyridamole postoperatively significantly improved the patency rate of vein grafts in the first year after surgery.[70,71] Subsequently, it has been shown that one tablet of even low-dose aspirin (81 to 100 mg) may prevent the initiation of platelet thrombi, the release of platelet mediators, and the occurrence of platelet damage in vein grafts. Aspirin started preoperatively offers no additional benefit, and neither does aspirin appear to improve internal thoracic artery graft patency.[72] Long-term antiplatelet therapy is preferable to anticoagulation because it incurs less risk of hemorrhage, does not necessitate laboratory monitoring, and costs less.

Late stenoses in vein grafts appear to be more dangerous prognostically than late stenoses in any of the three major native coronary vessels.[73] Patients recatheterized 5 years or more postoperatively had different survival rates subsequently, depending on whether a lesion was in the vein graft or the native coronary circulation. Late stenoses in saphenous vein grafts to the anterior descending coronary artery predict a high rate of death and cardiac events and are an indication for reoperation. This point is to be emphasized: *vein graft atherosclerosis and native vessel coronary atherosclerosis appear to have different prognoses. For patients who undergo catheterization 5 years or more postoperatively, mortality in the subsequent 2 years is 30 percent for patients with a stenotic vein graft to the anterior descending coronary artery but only 3 percent for those with a stenotic native vessel* (Fig. 50-1).

Progression of Native Vessel Coronary Atherosclerosis

Progression of native vessel coronary atherosclerosis has been studied by serial cardiac catheterization.[74] In the first postoperative year, the rate of progression is higher in grafted arteries, irrespective of whether the grafts are open or closed, and approximately half of the grafted arteries showed progression, compared with only about one-tenth of the ungrafted vessels.

Progression, however, depends on time and is related to the severity of the initial obstruction.[75] The grafted vessels tended to have much more severe obstruction than ungrafted vessels at the time of the initial surgery. At the subsequent 5-year follow-up, progression was found more in previously ungrafted vessels, probably because the proximal lesions in the grafted vessels had become occluded. We have found that proximal native vessel occlusion occurs less frequently after grafting of the internal thoracic artery than after that of the saphenous vein.[76] The most plausible explanation for accelerated proximal closure in bypassed vessels is that graft flow predominates and reduces or eliminates flow across the proximal atherosclerotic narrowing. Surgical error may cause tenting, angulation, or stenosis in the recipient vessel, which may further decrease the flow between the proximal lesion and the distal anastomosis.

OUTCOME

Most of the current information about lifestyle, cardiac events, and survival are confined to the first 10 years after surgery. Some exceptions will be noted. The clinical, angiographic, and surgical variables that predict 10-year survival include age of the patient, left ventricular functional status, type of conduit used, completeness of revascularization, whether cigarette smoking has ceased, and the presence or absence of hypertension, diabetes, and peripheral vascular disease.[77] Other risk factors have been implicated but are less consistently reported. Despite a difference in baseline characteristics, the predictors of long-term mortality in men and women

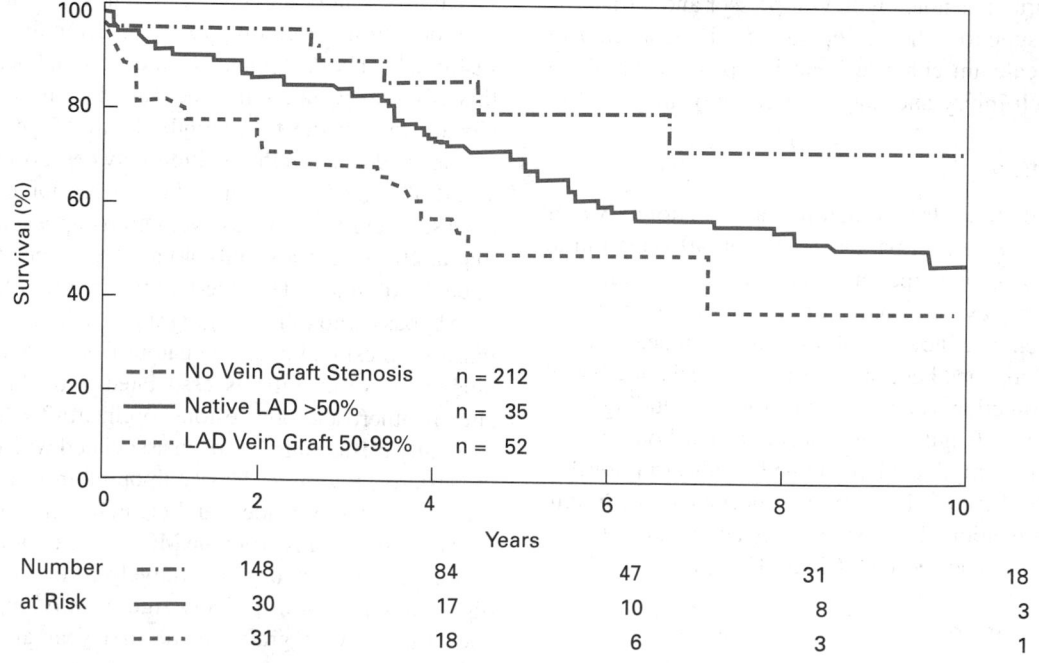

FIGURE 50-1

Patients with 50 to 99 percent stenoses in left anterior descending (LAD) vein grafts had worse survival than either patients with native vessel LAD stenoses (50 to 99 percent) (p = .002) or the control group. Patients with stenotic vein grafts to the LAD had survival rates of 70 and 50 percent at 2 and 5 postoperative years, respectively, compared with 97 and 80 percent for patients with native LAD stenoses. (From Lytle,[73] with permission.)

are nearly identical and depend mainly on preoperative left ventricular function.

Diabetic patients with documented severe coronary atherosclerosis are thought to have a higher frequency of asymptomatic myocardial ischemia than nondiabetic patients. Surgery—as compared with medical therapy—improves survival of diabetic patients with silent ischemia, and the greatest impact is in those with three-vessel disease. Although diabetes tends to increase the complication rate after bypass surgery, it does not affect intermediate-term survival.

Smoking behavior after surgery appears to be an important predictor of clinical events during follow-up.[78] Compared with patients who had stopped smoking after surgery, smokers had more than twice the risk for myocardial infarction and reoperation 1 year after surgery. Patients who were still smoking 5 years after surgery had an even higher risk of myocardial infarction and reoperation and significantly increased risk of angina pectoris. No difference in outcome was found between nonsmokers and smokers who had stopped smoking since surgery.

The preliminary results of the post–coronary artery bypass graft trial[79] revealed a significant reduction in the progression of vein graft atherosclerosis (measured by quantitative angiography), subsequent reoperation, or angioplasty as a consequence of aggressive lowering of cholesterol levels in patients who had undergone coronary bypass graft surgery.

Emergency Operations

Emergency operations may be undertaken in the face of acute myocardial infarction. A report by DeWood and colleagues[80] attests to the good long-term survival (10 years or more) associated with surgical treatment of patients with Q-wave myocardial infarction who were deliberately assigned to surgical or nonsurgical treatment. Medical and surgical groups had similar clinical characteristics. Surgery within 4 h resulted in improved long-term survival and better left ventricular function than traditional medical therapy. This improvement did not extend to those who were operated on later in the course of the infarct. The benefit of surgery applied more to patients with anterior infarction than to those with inferior infarction.[81]

More recently, multicenter trials of thrombolytic therapy have offered another view of emergency myocardial revascularization. As many as one in five patients may undergo emergency or urgent coronary bypass surgery during the initial hospitalization. Despite the fact that many patients were in a high-risk category, the in-hospital and 1-year results—event-free survival, angina status, and general health status—were similar to those in patients who underwent successful thrombolysis and angioplasty.[82] A greater number of grafts per patient and more complete revascularization in the surgical as contrasted with nonsurgical patients portends an excellent long-term prognosis.

Patients who survive an out-of-hospital cardiac arrest generally have a poor outcome. Surgical revascularization may suppress inducible ventricular fibrillation in patients who have reasonably well preserved left ventricular function.[83] Postoperative electrophysiologic evaluation is essential, because bypass surgery suppresses ventricular arrhythmias in only about half the cases—most likely those in whom the rhythm is ischemia-related. Actuarial 5-year survival, cardiac survival, and arrhythmia-free survival have been reported to be 88, 98, and 88 percent respectively. Poor preoperative left ventricular function is predictive of death.

Influence of the Conduit

Influence of the type of conduit on long-term results is evident by contrasting survival after left internal thoracic artery grafting with survival after vein grafting. The arterial conduit grafted to the anterior descending coronary artery, performed either alone or in combination with vein bypass grafts, significantly improves 10-year survival and reduces the incidence of important cardiac events, notably myocardial infarction, rehospitalization for cardiac causes, and reoperation.[84] The 10-year survival of patients who had one internal thoracic artery graft and those who had vein grafts only was 93.4 and 88 percent, respectively, for one-vessel disease; 90.0 and 79.5 percent for two-vessel disease; and 82.6 and 71.0 percent for three-vessel disease. This difference favored the internal thoracic artery graft over the vein graft, irrespective of gender, and held true for good and poor ventricular performance.

Internal Thoracic Artery Grafts

Severe stenosis of the left anterior descending coronary artery is a more important predictor of survival than progression of native coronary atherosclerosis. The relative immunity of the internal thoracic artery graft from atherosclerosis protects the anterior wall longer than its counterpart, the saphenous vein graft. In fact, compared with the use of vein grafts alone, the use of the internal thoracic artery has consistently been associated with better survival rates, regardless of age, gender, degree of stenosis in the left main coronary artery, or preoperative left ventricular functional status. A 15-year study concluded that an internal thoracic artery graft is indicated in most patient groups with few exceptions, because it is the single most important determinant of survival and event-free survival (Fig. 50-2).[85] The exceptions include patients with radiation-induced atherosclerosis of the internal thoracic artery or the brachiocephalic vessels, those with subclavian artery stenosis, and those undergoing reoperation who have a patent large-diameter atherosclerotic vein graft, the replacement of which with a smaller-diameter internal thoracic artery graft might result in hypoperfusion.[86]

More infrequent causes of hypoperfusion include high-dose intravenous vasoconstrictors and the internal thoracic artery malperfusion syndrome. This syndrome is caused by an acute imbalance between myocardial demand and blood flow through the internal thoracic artery.[87] Causes include inadequate flow resulting from spasm; occlusion of the proximal subclavian artery that shunts coronary flow into the distal

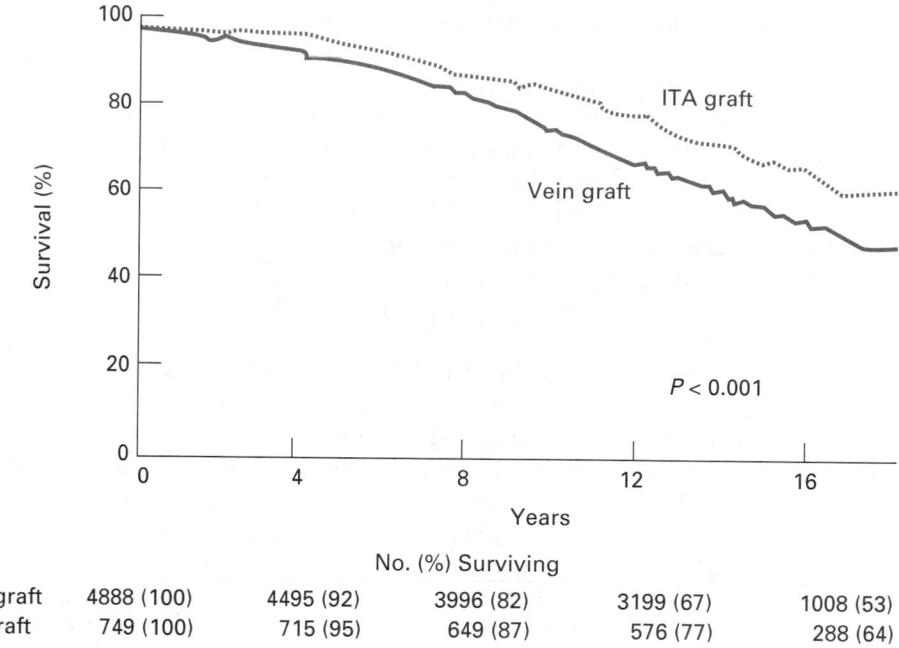

FIGURE 50-2

Actuarial survival for patients with internal thoracic artery bypass grafts and those with vein grafts. After more than 15 years, arterial grafts were associated with a significant survival advantage over vein grafts. Fifteen years is the longest follow-up period in a large literature series. (Adapted from Cameron,[85] with permission.)

	No. (%) Surviving				
Vein graft	4888 (100)	4495 (92)	3996 (82)	3199 (67)	1008 (53)
ITA graft	749 (100)	715 (95)	649 (87)	576 (77)	288 (64)

subclavian distribution (the "subclavian steal" phenomenon); small size of the internal thoracic artery; mismatched diameters between the internal thoracic artery and the recipient coronary vessel in the presence of a technically satisfactory anastomosis; and a large myocardial flow demand in a severely hypertrophied ventricle.[88]

Earlier in the evolution of internal thoracic artery grafting, wound infection was a more frequent complication, and sternal wound infection was especially common in diabetic patients. The sternal blood supply in patients with diabetes is not compromised, as noted, and good surgical technique—namely, minimal use of electrocautery, reasonably short operating time, blood conservation, and meticulous wound closure—have reduced the infection rate substantially to approximately 1 percent. Diabetes is not a contraindication to the use of either or both internal thoracic arteries as bypass grafts.

Patients with single-vessel disease of the left anterior descending coronary artery who underwent coronary artery bypass grafting with either an internal thoracic artery or vein graft have been followed for 18 to 20 years.[89] The patients receiving arterial conduits had better rates of survival, cardiac event-free survival, and intervention-free survival than patients receiving vein grafts. At 18 years, 61 percent of patients with arterial grafts were alive and had had no cardiac events. The presence of noncritical atherosclerosis in other vessels affected the event rates in the patients with vein grafts but not in the patients with arterial grafts to the left anterior descending coronary artery. There appears to be no significant survival advantage of bilateral internal thoracic artery grafting at 5 to 7 years of follow-up.

Predicated on the success of the internal thoracic artery graft, alternative arterial conduits have been pursued. The right gastroepiploic artery graft has been used for over a decade, and 5-year angiographic patency rates of 92 percent have been reported.[90] The gastroepiploic artery is particularly useful for young patients or those with atherosclerotic ascending aortas.

The radial artery graft was introduced into clinical practice in the early 1970s with mixed results. Recently, a 92.5 percent patency rate for 122 radial artery grafts studied at 6 to 13 months postoperatively was reported.[91] Calafiore et al.[92] documented a 94.3 percent conduit patency rate after 12 months of follow-up in 35 patients. Meticulous surgical dissection of the radial artery, which incorporates its surrounding veins, as well as the use of calcium-channel blockers may account for the recently improved patency rates of this conduit. Long-term follow-up studies are needed before this conduit can be employed as widely as the internal thoracic artery or gastroepiploic artery.

The inferior epigastric artery has been proposed as another alternative arterial conduit. The short length of the artery limits its use to the left anterior descending coronary artery or diagonal branches when used as an aortocoronary bypass graft; however, circumflex arteries may be grafted if the inferior epigastric artery is attached proximally to the internal thoracic artery or vein graft.[93]

Long-Term Trials

Few arterial bypass grafts were constructed during the 1970s, when the three most widely reported randomized trials assigned patients to medical or surgical treatment. These important randomized studies were also undertaken in an era when many of the most recent cardiac drugs and lipid-lowering therapies were not available and when myocardial protection was not optimal. In the European Coronary Surgery Study, 10-year survival improved consistently for surgical patients with three-vessel disease or two-vessel disease with involvement of the proximal anterior descending coronary artery.[94] In a 12-year follow-up, the study reported results for patients with respect to treatment received as well as the policy of treatment. Interestingly, the survival was 62 percent at 10 to 12 years for patients adherent to medical treatment and 86 percent for those who had crossed over to surgery. The European Coronary Surgery Study Group concluded that "the time-honored advice of medical care until symptoms deteriorate to an unacceptable level is proved invalid.... surgery was the treatment of choice even when angina pectoris responded adequately to medical management."

The Coronary Artery Surgical Study (CASS) randomized trial of relatively asymptomatic low-risk patients found nearly equal survival after medical or surgical treatment. The exception was the subset of patients with poor ventricular function in whom surgical treatment improved intermediate-term survival. The CASS registry, which followed about 7000 patients operated on at the same time the trial was conducted, found improved 5- to 7-year survival after surgical treatment for three-vessel disease,[95] multivessel disease with poor left ventricular function,[96] three-vessel disease with proximal arterial stenoses, and multivessel disease with severe angina[97] or mild angina[98] in patients 65 years of age or older[99] and in asymptomatic patients with severe ischemia.[100] In all multivessel disease categories, the spread between survival after medical or surgical therapy widens with increasingly worse left ventricular function.[101]

The Veterans Administration Cooperative Study Group has reviewed the management of unstable angina.[102] The 5-year survival for patients with three-vessel disease and all gradations of left ventricular function was better for surgery (89 percent) than for medical treatment (75 percent).[103] Surgery resulted in fewer hospitalizations for cardiac causes, and the difference in favor of surgery widened considerably in categories of reduced ejection fractions.

There are few 15- to 20-year follow-up reports. Given the facts that the distribution of coronary atherosclerosis was more benign and that left ventricular function was generally good in these early series, these reports, based largely on vein graft surgery, provide an important perspective on the evolution of the surgical candidate and the long-term results. Lawrie et al.[104] report actuarial 20-year survival after coronary bypass surgery as follows: for one-vessel disease, 40 percent; two-vessel disease, 26 percent; three-vessel disease, 20 percent; and left main coronary artery disease, 25 percent. Approximately two-thirds of patients were asymptomatic at 20 years, and nearly half of the vein bypass grafts were patent 16 to 20 years postoperatively.

ANGINA RELIEF AND LIFESTYLE

Quality of life refers to symptom relief, well-being, return to full activity, and, where applicable, return to employment. Randomized controlled studies have consistently shown the effectiveness of coronary bypass surgery in alleviating angina.[105] At about the fifth year, however, the slope of the angina-free curve changes, so that the dramatic symptom relief is attenuated in the next 5 years. Only about half of the patients originally angina-free at year 5 remain so by the tenth to twelfth year.[106] The type of conduit is not associated with angina relief. Late return of angina does appear to be associated with factors such as hyperlipidemia and hypertension. Sudden death is related more to preoperative left ventricular function than any other factor and, fortunately, is rare in the first 10 years after surgery.

Angina relief is better in the elderly than among their younger counterparts.[107] In fact, successful bypass surgery in the elderly confers consistent angina relief over the intermediate term and the longevity of these patients exceeds that of the U.S. population matched for age and gender.[108] Most reports indicate that coronary artery surgery does not cause long-term intellectual or neuropsychological dysfunction. The intellectual defects reported immediately after surgery tend to have a short course and generally resolve within 3 months.

According to reports from the CASS registry, myocardial infarction–free survival is significantly improved by coronary artery surgery in both severe and mild angina.[109] Other early reports indicate that freedom from late myocardial infarction is no different than that from medical treatment, but the fatality rate from myocardial infarction is significantly less after surgery than after conservative treatment.[110]

Return to work is a complicated subject. The median age of coronary bypass patients is approaching 65 years and beyond in many communities, so return to full activity may be a more realistic expectation. Nonetheless, factors affecting return to work include preoperative employment status, age, income, gender, self-employment, white collar–blue collar, college education, relief of symptoms, and preoperative left ventricular function. The longer the preoperative unemployment, the less likely the return to full employment. Other factors that adversely affect future employment include comorbidity, physician advice, and disability compensation.

REOPERATION

The incidence of coronary artery *reoperation* tends to increase with time. In our experience, only 3 percent of patients were reoperated on in the first 5 years after their initial bypass surgery; this rate may be even less today with the advent of balloon angioplasty. At 10 to 12 years postoperatively, the rate rises to 12 to 17 percent; at 15 years, it approaches 30 percent among those who survived this interval. The factors that predispose a patient to reoperation include young age, incomplete revascularization at the first operation, use of vein grafts only, one- or two-vessel disease at time of first operation, and good left ventricular function.[111]

The use of more internal thoracic artery grafts at the initial procedure has lengthened the mean interval between the operations, which approaches 10 years today. Vein graft atherosclerosis has become the leading indication for reoperation.[112] Angiography underestimates the severity of vein graft atherosclerosis.[113] Because atherosclerotic disease progresses at a highly unpredictable rate and is associated with a bad prognosis, especially in anterior descending coronary artery grafts, we recommend replacement of vein grafts in most instances when the reoperation occurs more than 5 years postoperatively. In experienced hands, hospital mortality for second operations ranges from 2 to 5 percent. The complication rate is approximately twice that of the first procedure. The Emory University findings[114] coincide with our experience: urgent or emergent surgery, reduced ejection fraction, hypotension, older age, and female gender were multivariate correlates of in-hospital deaths. Multivariate correlates of long-term mortality were older age, reduced ejection fraction, hypertension, diabetes mellitus, congestive heart failure, emergency surgery, and female gender. In the Cleveland Clinic series, 5- and 10-year survival rates after coronary reoperation were 90 and 75 percent, respectively; approximately half of the patients were angina-free postoperatively and about half survived 10 years event-free.

In our experience, patients with a patent internal thoracic artery graft placed during their first operation had a 3 percent incidence of graft damage at reoperation, necessitating regrafting of the internal thoracic artery.[115] All patients with damaged internal thoracic arteries survived. We believe that the use of internal thoracic artery grafting at primary operation did not increase the risk of reoperation and that its use at reoperation did not increase the in-hospital mortality or morbidity.

Coronary artery surgery a third time is still infrequent but rising in some referral centers. The risk is about triple that of the second operation; that is, about 9 percent, according to published reports.

TRANSMYOCARDIAL REVASCULARIZATION

Transmyocardial laser revascularization of the ischemic myocardium is currently being evaluated as an alternative form of revascularization in patients who are otherwise not candidates for surgery or angioplasty. Frazier et al.[116] and Horvath et al.[117] found that transmyocardial laser revascularization improved angina, relative endocardial perfusion, and cardiac function in patients without preoperative congestive heart failure. Transmyocardial laser revascularization is performed through a left thoracotomy and appears to be best suited for patients with ejection fractions above 30 percent who are suffering from angina without congestive heart failure. Septal ischemia cannot be addressed by the laser. Multiple full-thickness laser perforations of the contracting myocardium are confined predominantly to regions determined to exhibit ischemia in viable myocardium. Proof of increased perfusion, improved left ventricular performance, long-term angina relief, and better survival is not yet available.

LONG-TERM MANAGEMENT

Patients who undergo coronary artery bypass surgery tend to have partial or complete alleviation of angina for the first 5 years and improved exercise tolerance. It is generally agreed that platelet-inhibitor drugs should be continued for at least 1 year postoperatively. Recurrent angina requires investigation, and coronary arteriography is the most definitive test. Early recurring angina is unusual, but angiography may reveal anastomotic constriction that may be amenable to coronary balloon angioplasty.

Later on, especially after the fifth postoperative year, progression of coronary and vein graft atherosclerosis becomes increasingly more frequent. Native vessel disease is more likely to progress proximal to the distal anastomosis than to affect the distal arterial runoff. Treatment of late lesions in vein grafts is both risky and fraught with a high rate of restenosis. Atherectomy and stenting are promising treatments but results are preliminary. On an individual basis, progression of disease in the native coronary arteries may be treated by balloon angioplasty, which may spare the patient a reoperation.

Constrictive pericarditis is seen months or years postoperatively and is rare. The causes are obscure. As the condition worsens, pericardiectomy may be required. Even more rarely, chronic pericardial irritation caused by either a reaction to the Teflon felt used in cardiac surgery or by large, loculated, organized intrapericardial hematomas that fail to resolve may require reoperation.

Modification of risk factors applies to all but the very elderly. Advice should be given concerning proper weight, strict abstinence from tobacco, exercise consistent with age and lifestyle, and control of hyperlipidemia. Reduction in serum lipids may reduce progression of disease and improve graft patency. Lipid-lowering drug therapy has been correlated with regression of atherosclerosis and has reduced the progression of coronary lesions in both native vessels and in vein graft atherosclerosis.[79,118] Further, aggressive lipid-lowering in patients who have undergone coronary bypass grafting appears to reduce obstructive changes in vein grafts and the need for reoperation.[119] Blood pressure control and diabetic management affect prognosis and should be attended to regularly. Postoperative management is directed to preventing progressive arterial disease and to prolonging vein graft patency. Abrupt progression of disease in native arteries and grafts emphasizes the need for yearly surveillance after coronary artery bypass surgery.

Too often, especially after the first year, patients return to their bad habits. They should be instructed that the operation is not curative and that risk-factor modification is never-ending. Adherence to a thoughtful program has proved to be beneficial. Failure to observe the guidelines could affect the patient adversely.

REFERENCES

1. Favaloro, RG. Saphenous vein autograft replacement of severe segmental coronary artery occlusion: Operative technique. *Ann Thorac Surg* 1968; 5:334–339.
2. Johnson WD, Flemma RJ, Lepley D Jr, Ellison EH. Extended treatment of severe coronary artery disease: A total surgical approach. *Ann Surg* 1969; 170:460–470.
3. Frye RL, Gibbons RJ, Schaff HV, Vlietstra RE, Gersh BJ, Mock MB. Treatment of coronary artery disease. *J Am Coll Cardiol* 1989; 13:957–968.

4. Kirklin JW, Akins CW, Blackstone EH, Booth RC, Califf RM, Cohen LJ, et al. ACC/AHA Guidelines and Indicators for Coronary Artery Bypass Graft Surgery: A report of the American College of Cardiology/ American Heart Association Task Force on Assessment of Diagnostic and Therapeutic Cardiovascular Procedures (Subcommittee on Coronary Artery Bypass Graft Surgery). *Circulation* 1991; 83:1125–1173.

5. Goy JJ, Eeckhout E, Burnand B, Vogt P, Stauffer JC, Hurni M, et al. Coronary angioplasty versus left internal mammary artery grafting for isolated proximal left anterior descending artery stenosis. *Lancet* 1994; 343:1449–1453.

6. The Bypass Angioplasty Revascularization Investigation (BARI) Investigators. Comparison of coronary bypass surgery with angioplasty in patients with multivessel disease. *N Engl J Med* 1996; 335:217–225.

7. Rodriguez A, Boullon F, Perez-Balino N, Paviotti C, Liprandi MI, Palacios IF. Argentine randomized trial of percutaneous transluminal coronary angioplasty versus coronary artery bypass surgery in multivessel disease (ERACI): In-hospital results and 1-year follow-up. *J Am Coll Cardiol* 1993; 22:1060–1067.

8. King SB III, Lembo NJ, Weintraub WS, Kosinski AS, Barnhart HX, Kutner MH, et al. A randomized trial comparing coronary angioplasty with coronary bypass surgery: Emory Angioplasty vs. Surgery Trial (EAST). *N Engl J Med* 1994; 331:1044–1050.

9. Hamm CW, Reimers J, Ischinger T, Rupprecht HJ, Berger J, Bleifeld W. A randomized study of coronary angioplasty compared with bypass surgery in patients with symptomatic multivessel coronary disease: German Angioplasty Bypass Surgery Investigation (GABI). *N Engl J Med* 1994; 331:1037–1043.

10. RITA Trial Participants. Coronary angioplasty versus coronary artery bypass surgery: The Randomized Intervention Treatment of Angina (RITA) trial. *Lancet* 1993; 341:573–580.

11. Hlatky MA, Rogers WJ, Johnstone I, et al, for the BARI Investigators. Economic and quality of life outcomes after randomization to coronary angioplasty or coronary bypass surgery: A substudy of the Bypass Angioplasty Revascularization Investigation. *N Engl J Med* 1997; 336:92–99.

12. Moliterno DJ, Elliott JM, Topol EJ. Randomized trials of myocardial revascularization. *Curr Probl Cardiol* 1995; 20:121–192.

13. Bourassa MG, Knatterud GL, Pepine CJ, Sopko G, Rogers WJ, Geller NL, et al. Asymptomatic Cardiac Ischemia Pilot (ACIP) study: Improvement of cardiac ischemia at 1 year after PTCA and CABG. *Circulation* 1995; 92(suppl II):11-1–11-7.

14. Rahimtoola SH. The hibernating myocardium. *Am Heart J* 1989; 117:211–221.

15. Braunwald E, Kloner RA. The stunned myocardium: Prolonged, post-ischemic ventricular dysfunction. *Circulation* 1982; 66:1146–1149.

16. Golding LR, Loop FD, Sheldon WC, Taylor PC, Groves LK, Cosgrove DM. Emergency revascularization for unstable angina. *Circulation* 1978; 58:1163–1166.

17. Dor V, Sabatier M, DiDonato M, Maioli M, Toso A, Montiglio F. Late hemodynamic results after left ventricular patch repair associated with coronary grafting in patients with postinfarction akinetic or dyskinetic aneurysm of the left ventricle. *J Thorac Cardiovasc Surg* 1995; 110:1291–1299; discussion, 1300–1301.

18. Grossi EA, Chinitz LA, Galloway AC, Delianides J, Schwartz DS, McLoughlin DE, et al. Endoventricular remodeling of left ventricular aneurysm: Functional, clinical, and electrophysiological results. *Circulation* 1995; 92(suppl II):II-98–II-100.

19. Kennedy JW, Ritchie JL, Davis KB, Fritz JK. Western Washington randomized trial of intracoronary streptokinase in acute myocardial infarction. *N Engl J Med* 1983; 309:1477–1482.

20. Simoons ML, Serruys PW, van den Brand M, Res J, Verheugt FW, Krauss XH, et al. Early thrombolysis in acute myocardial infarction: Limitation of infarct size and improved survival. *J Am Coll Cardiol* 1986; 7:717–728.

21. Schröder R, Neuhaus KL, Leizorovicz A, Linderer T, Tebbe U. A prospective placebo-controlled double-blind multicenter trial of intravenous streptokinase in acute myocardial infarction (ISAM): Long-term mortality and morbidity. *J Am Coll Cardiol* 1987; 9:197–203.

22. Wilcox RG, von der Lippe G, Olsson CG, Jensen G, Skene AM, Hampton JR. Trial of tissue plasminogen activator for mortality reduction in acute myocardial infarction: Anglo-Scandinavian Study of Early Thrombolysis (ASSET). *Lancet* 1988; 2:525–530.

23. Gruppo Italiano per lo Studio della Streptochinasi nell'Infarto Miocardico (GISSI). Effectiveness of intravenous thrombolytic treatment in acute myocardial infarction. *Lancet* 1986; 1:397–402.

24. AIMS Trial Study Group. Effect of intravenous APSAC on mortality after acute myocardial infarction: Preliminary report of a placebo-controlled clinical trial. *Lancet* 1988; 1:545–549.

25. ISIS-2 (Second International Study of Infarct Survival) Collaborative Group: Randomized trial of intravenous streptokinase, oral aspirin, both, or neither among 17,187 cases of suspected acute myocardial infarction: ISIS-2. *Lancet* 1988; 2:349–360.

26. Topol EJ, Califf RM, George BS, Kereiakes DJ, Abbottsmith CW, Candela RJ, et al. A randomized trial of immediate versus delayed elective angioplasty after intravenous tissue plasminogen activator in acute myocardial infarction. *N Engl J Med* 1987; 317:581–588.

27. Brooks R, McGovern BA, Garan H, Ruskin JN. Current treatment of patients surviving out-of-hospital cardiac arrest. *JAMA* 1991; 265:762–768.

28. Hertzer NR, Beven EG, Young JR, O'Hara PJ, Ruschhaupt WF III, Graor RA, et al. Coronary artery disease in peripheral vascular patients: A classification of 1,000 coronary angiograms and results of surgical management. *Ann Surg* 1984; 199:223–233.

29. European Carotid Surgery Trialists' Collaborative Group. MRC European Carotid Surgery Trial: Interim results for symptomatic patients with severe (70–99%) or with mild (0–29%) carotid stenosis. *Lancet* 1991; 337:1235–1243.

30. North American Symptomatic Carotid Endarterectomy Trial Collaborators. Beneficial effect of carotid endarterectomy in symptomatic patients with high-grade carotid stenosis. *N Engl J Med* 1991; 325:445–453.

31. Flameng WJ, Herijgers P, Szecsi J, Sergeant PT, Daenen WJ, Scheys I. Determinants of early and late results of combined valve operations and coronary artery bypass grafting. *Ann Thorac Surg* 1996; 61:621–628.

32. Jones EL, Waites TF, Craver JM, Bradford JM, Douglas JS, King SB, et al. Coronary bypass for relief of persistent pain following acute myocardial infarction. *Ann Thorac Surg* 1981; 32:33–43.

33. Schuster EH, Bulkley BH. Early post-infarction angina: Ischemia at a distance and ischemia in the infarct zone. *N Engl J Med* 1981; 305:1101–1105.

34. Braxton JH, Hammond GL, Letsou GV, Franco KL, Kopf GS, Elefteriades JA, et al. Optimal timing of coronary artery bypass graft surgery after acute myocardial infarction. *Circulation* 1995; 92(suppl II):II-66–II-68.

35. Cosgrove DM, Loop FD, Lytle BW, Baillot R, Gill CC, Golding LA, et al. Primary myocardial revascularization: Trends in surgical mortality. *J Thorac Cardiovasc Surg* 1984; 88:673–684.

36. Miller DC, Stinson EB, Oyer PE, Jamieson SW, Mitchell RS, Reitz BA, et al. Discriminant analysis of the changing risks of coronary artery operations: 1971–1979. *J Thoracic Cardiovasc Surg* 1983; 85:197–213.

37. Jones EL, Weintraub WS, Craver JM, Guyton RA, Cohen CL. Coronary bypass surgery: Is the operation different today? *J Thorac Cardiovasc Surg* 1991; 101:108–115.

38. Fisher LD, Kennedy JW, Davis KB, Maynard C, Fritz JK, Kaiser G, et al. Association of sex, physical size, and operative mortality after coronary artery bypass in the Coronary Artery Surgery Study (CASS). *J Thorac Cardiovasc Surg* 1982; 84:334–341.

39. Loop FD, Golding LR, MacMillan JP, Cosgrove DM, Lytle BW, Sheldon WC. Coronary artery surgery in women compared with men: Analysis of risks and long-term results. *J Am Coll Cardiol* 1983; 1:383–390.

40. Kirklin JW. Technical and scientific advances in cardiac surgery over the past 25 years. *Ann Thorac Surg* 1990; 49:26–31.

41. Parsonnet V, Dean D, Bernstein AD. A method of uniform stratification of risk for evaluating the results of surgery in acquired adult heart disease. *Circulation* 1989; 79(suppl I):I-3–I-12.

42. Higgins TL, Estafanous FG, Loop FD, Beck GJ, Blum J, Paranandi L. Stratification of morbidity and mortality outcome by preoperative risk factors in coronary artery bypass patients: A clinical severity score. *JAMA* 1992; 267:2344–2348. [Published erratum appears in *JAMA* 1992; 268:1860.]

43. Loop FD, Lytle BW, Cosgrove DM, Golding LA, Taylor PC, Stewart RW. Free (aorta-coronary) internal mammary artery graft: Late results. *J Thorac Cardiovasc Surg* 1986; 92:827–831.

44. Pym J, Brown PM, Charrette EJP, Parker JO, West RO. Gastroepiploic-coronary anastomosis: A viable alternative bypass graft. *J Thorac Cardiovasc Surg* 1987; 94:256–259.

45. Puig LB, Ciongoli W, Cividanes GV, Dontos A, Kopel L, Bittencourt D, et al. Inferior epigastric artery as a free graft for myocardial revascularization. *J Thorac Cardiovasc Surg* 1990; 99:251–255.

46. Barner HB, Naunheim KS, Fiore AC, Fischer VW, Harris HH. Use of the inferior epigastric artery as a free graft for myocardial revascularization. *Ann Thorac Surg* 1991; 52:429–436; discussion, 436–437.

47. Baumann FG, Catinella FP, Cunningham JN Jr, Spencer FC. Vein contraction and smooth muscle cell extensions as causes of endothelial damage during graft preparation. *Ann Surg* 1981; 194:199–211.

48. Lichtenstein SV, Abel JG, Salerno TA. Warm heart surgery and results of operation for recent myocardial infarction. *Ann Thorac Surg* 1991; 52:455–458; discussion, 458–460.

49. Calafiore AM, DiGiammarco G, Teodori G, Bosco G, D'Annunzio E, Barsotti A, et al. Left anterior descending coronary artery grafting via left anterior small thoracotomy without cardiopulmonary bypass. *Ann Thorac Surg* 1996; 61:1658–1665.

50. Bennetti FJ, Ballester C, Sani G, Boonstra P, Grandjean J. Video-assisted coronary bypass surgery. *J Cardiol Surg* 1995; 10:620–625.

51. Subramanian VA, Sani G, Bennetti FJ, Calafiore AM. Minimally invasive coronary bypass surgery: A multicenter report of preliminary clinical experience. *Circulation* 1995; 92(suppl I):I-645.

52. Schwartz DS, Ribakove GH, Grossi EA, Stevens JH, Siegel LC, St. Goar FG, et al. Minimally invasive cardiopulmonary bypass with cardioplegic arrest: A closed chest technique with equivalent myocardial protection. *J Thorac Cardiovasc Surg* 1996; 111:556–566.

53. Hammermeister KE, Burchfiel C, Johnson R, Grover FL. Identification of patients at greatest risk for developing major complications at cardiac surgery. *Circulation* 1990; 82(suppl IV):IV-380–IV-389. [Published erratum appears in *Circulation* 1991; 84:446.]

54. Taylor GJ, Mikell FL, Moses HW, Dove JT, Katholi RE, Malik SA, et al. Determinants of hospital charges for coronary artery bypass surgery: The economic consequences of postoperative complications. *Am J Cardiol* 1990; 65:309–313.

55. Higgins TL, ed. Postoperative care of cardiothoracic surgery patients. *Semin Thorac Cardiovasc Surg* 1991; 3(1):1–94.

56. Bashein BG, Nessly ML, Rice AL, Counts RB, Misbach GA. Preoperative aspirin therapy and reoperation for bleeding after coronary artery bypass surgery. *Arch Intern Med* 1991; 151:89–93.

57. Mills NL, Everson CT. Atherosclerosis of the ascending aorta and coronary artery bypass: Pathology, clinical correlates, and operative management. *J Thorac Cardiovasc Surg* 1991; 102:546–553.

58. Blauth CI, Cosgrove DM, Webb BW, Ratliff NB, Boylan M, Piedmonte MR, et al. Atheroembolism from the ascending aorta: An emerging problem in cardiac surgery. *J Thorac Cardiovasc Surg* 1992; 103:1104–1111; discussion, 1111–1112.

59. Redmond JM, Greene PS, Goldsborough MA, Cameron DE, Stuart RS, Sussman MS, et al. Neurologic injury in cardiac surgical patients with a history of stroke. *Ann Thorac Surg* 1996; 61:42–47.

60. Matthay MA, Wiener-Kronish JP. Respiratory management after cardiac surgery. *Chest* 1989; 95:424–434.

61. Gaynes R, Bizek B, Mowry-Hanley J, Dirsh M. Risk factors for nosocomial pneumonia after coronary artery bypass graft operations. *Ann Thorac Surg* 1991; 51:215–218.

62. Loop FD, Lytle BW, Cosgrove DM, Mahfood S, McHenry MC, Goormastic M, et al. Sternal wound complications after isolated coronary artery bypass grafting: Early and late mortality, morbidity, and cost of care. *Ann Thorac Surg* 1990; 49:179–186; discussion, 186–187.

63. Fernandez-del Castillo C, Harringer W, Warshaw AL, Vlahakes GJ, Koski G, Zaslavsky AM, et al. Risk factors for pancreatic cellular injury after cardiopulmonary bypass. *N Engl J Med* 1991; 325:382–387.

64. Grondin CM, Campeau L, Lesperance J, Enjalbert M, Bourassa MG. Comparison of late changes in internal mammary artery and saphenous vein grafts in two consecutive series of patients 10 years after operation. *Circulation* 1984; 70(suppl I):I-208–I-212.

65. Johns RA, Peach MJ, Flanagan T, Kron IL. Probing of the canine mammary artery damages endothelium and impairs vasodilation resulting from prostacyclin and endothelium-derived relaxing factor. *J Thorac Cardiovasc Surg* 1989; 97:252–258.

66. Bourassa MG. Fate of venous grafts: the past, the present and the future. *J Am Coll Cardiol* 1991; 17:1081–1083.

67. Lytle BW, Loop FD, Cosgrove DM, Ratliff NB, Easley K, Taylor PC. Long-term (5 to 12 years) serial studies of internal mammary artery and saphenous vein coronary bypass grafts. *J Thorac Cardiovasc Surg* 1985; 89:248–258.

68. FitzGibbon GM, Kafka HP, Leach AJ, Keon WJ, Hooper GD, Burton JR. Coronary bypass graft fate and patient outcome: Angiographic follow-up of 5,065 grafts related to survival and reoperation in 1,388 patients during 25 years. *J Am Coll Cardiol* 1996; 28:616–626.

69. Campeau L, Enjalbert M, Lesperance J, Bourassa MG, Kwiterovich P Jr, Wacholder S, et al. The relation of risk factors to the development of atherosclerosis in saphenous-vein bypass grafts and the progression of disease in the native circulation: a study 10 years after aortocoronary bypass surgery. *N Engl J Med* 1984; 311:1329–1332.

70. Chesebro JH, Fuster V, Elveback LR, Clements IP, Smith HC, Holmes DR Jr, et al. Effect of dipyridamole and aspirin on late vein-graft patency after coronary bypass operations. *N Engl J Med* 1984; 310:209–214.

71. Chesebro JH, Clements EP, Fuster V, Elveback LR, Smith HC, Bardsley WT, et al. A platelet-inhibitor-drug trial in coronary-artery bypass operations: Benefit of perioperative dipyridamole and aspirin therapy on early postoperative vein-graft patency. *N Engl J Med* 1982; 307:73–78.

72. Goldman S, Copeland J, Moritz T, Henderson W, Zadina K, Ovitt T, et al. Internal mammary artery and saphenous vein graft patency: Effects of aspirin. *Circulation* 1990; 82(suppl IV):IV-237–IV-242.

73. Lytle BW, Loop FD, Taylor PC, Simpfendorfer C, Kramer JR, Ratliff NB, et al. Vein graft disease: The clinical impact of stenoses in saphenouse vein bypass grafts to coronary arteries. *J Thorac Cardiovasc Surg* 1992; 103:831–840.

74. Bourassa MG, Lesperance J, Corbara F, Saltiel J, Campeau L. Progression of obstructive coronary artery disease 5 to 7 years after aortocoronary bypass surgery. *Circulation* 1978; 58(suppl I):I-100–I-106.

75. Bruschke AVG, Kramer JR Jr, Bal ET, Haque IU, Detrano RC, Goormastic M. The dynamics of progression of coronary atherosclerosis studied in 168 medically treated patients who underwent coronary arteriography three times. *Am Heart J* 1989; 117:296–305.

76. Cosgrove DM, Loop FD, Saunders CR, Lytle BW, Kramer JR. Should coronary arteries with less than fifty percent stenosis be bypassed? *J Thorac Cardiovasc Surg* 1981; 82:520–530.

77. Johnson WD, Brenowitz JB, Kayser KL. Factors influencing long-term (10-year to 15-year) survival after a successful coronary artery bypass operation. *Ann Thorac Surg* 1989; 48:19–24; discussion, 24–25.

78. Voors AA, van Brussel BL, Plokker HW, Ernst SM, Ernst NM, Koomen EM, et al. Smoking and cardiac events after venous coronary bypass surgery: A 15-year follow-up study. *Circulation* 1996; 93:42–47.

79. The Post Coronary Artery Bypass Graft Trial Investigators. The effect of aggressive lowering of low-density lipoproteins and cholesterol levels and low-dose anticoagulation on obstructive changes in saphenous-vein coronary-artery bypass grafts. *N Engl J Med* 1997; 336:153–162.

80. DeWood MA, Notske RN, Berg R Jr, Ganji JH, Simpson CS, Hinnen ML, et al. Medical and surgical management of early Q wave myocardial infarction: I. Effects of surgical reperfusion on survival, recurrent myocardial infarction, sudden death and functional class at 10 or more years of follow-up. *J Am Coll Cardiol* 1989; 14:65–77.

81. DeWood MA, Leonard J, Grunwald RP, Hensley GR, Mouser LT, Burroughs RW, et al. Medical and surgical management of early Q wave myocardial infarction: II. Effects on mortality and global and regional left ventricular function at 10 or more years of follow-up. *J Am Coll Cardiol* 1989; 14:78–90.

82. Kereiakes DJ, Topol EJ, George BS, Abbottsmith CW, Stack RS, Candela RJ, et al. Favorable early and long-term prognosis following coronary bypass surgery therapy for myocardial infarction: Results of a multicenter trial. TAMI Study Group. *Am Heart J* 1989; 118:199–207.

83. Kelly P, Ruskin JN, Vlahakes GJ, Buckley MJ Jr, Freeman CS, Garan H. Surgical coronary revascularization in survivors of prehospital cardiac arrest: Its effects on inducible ventricular arrhythmias and long-term survival. *J Am Coll Cardiol* 1990; 15:267–273.

84. Loop FD, Lytle BW, Cosgrove DM, Stewart RW, Goormastic M, Williams GW, et al. Influence of the internal-mammary-artery graft on 10-year survival and other cardiac events. *N Engl J Med* 1986; 314:1–6.

85. Cameron A, Davis KB, Green G, Schaff HV. Coronary bypass surgery with internal-thoracic-artery grafts—effects on survival over a 15-year period. *N Engl J Med* 1996; 334:216–219.

86. Loop FD. Internal-thoracic-artery grafts: Biologically better coronary arteries (editorial). *N Engl J Med* 1996; 334:263–265.

87. Loop FD, Thomas JD. Hypoperfusion after arterial bypass grafting. *Ann Thorac Surg* 1993; 56:812–813.

88. Carrel T, Kujawski T, Zünd G, Schwitter J, Amann FW, Gallino A, et al. The internal mammary artery malperfusion syndrome: Incidence, treatment and angiographic verification. *Eur J Cardiothorac Surg* 1995; 9:190–195; discussion, 196–197.

89. Boylan MJ, Lytle BW, Loop FD, Taylor PC, Borsh JA, Goormastic M, et al. Surgical treatment of isolated left anterior descending coronary stenosis: Comparison of left internal mammary artery and venous autograft at 18 to 20 years of follow-up. *J Thorac Cardiovasc Sug* 1994; 107:657–662.

90. Suma H. Optimal use of the gastroepiploic artery. *Semin Thorac Cardiovasc Surg* 1996; 8:24–28.

91. Acar C, Jebara VA, Portoghese M, Beyssen B, Pagny JY, Grare P, et al. Revival of the radial artery for coronary artery bypass grafting. *Ann Thorac Surg* 1992; 54:652–659; discussion, 659–660.

92. Calafiore AM, DiGiammarco G, Luciani N, Maddestra N, DiNardo E, Angelini R. Composite arterial conduits for a wider arterial myocardial revascularization. *Ann Thorac Surg* 1994; 58:185–190.

93. Buche M, Dion R. Current status of the inferior epigastric artery. *Semin Thorac Cardiovasc Surg* 1996; 8:10–14.

94. European Coronary Surgery Study Group. Long-term results of prospective randomized study of coronary artery bypass surgery in stable angina pectoris. *Lancet* 1982; 2:1173–1180.

95. Kaiser GC, Davis KB, Fisher LD, Myers WO, Foster ED, Passamani ER, et al. Survival following coronary artery bypass grafting in patients with severe angina pectoris (CASS). *J Thorac Cardiovasc Surg* 1985; 89:513–524.

96. Alderman EL, Fisher LD, Litwin P, Kaiser GC, Myers WO, Maynard C, et al. Results of coronary artery surgery in patients with poor left ventricular function (CASS). *Circulation* 1983; 68:785–795.

97. Myers WO, Schaff HV, Gersh BJ, Fisher LD, Kosinski AS, Mock MB, et al. Improved survival of surgically treated patients with triple vessel coronary artery disease and severe angina pectoris: A report from the Coronary Artery Surgery Study (CASS) registry. *J Thorac Cardiovasc Surg* 1989, 97:487–495.

98. Myers WO, Gersh BJ, Fisher LD, Mock MB, Holmes DR, Schaff HV, et al. Medical versus early surgical therapy in patients with triple-vessel disease and mild angina pectoris: A CASS Registry study of survival. *Ann Thorac Surg* 1987; 44:471–486.

99. Gersh BJ, Kronmal RA, Schaff HV, Frye RL, Ryan TJ, Mock MB, et al. Comparison of coronary artery bypass surgery and medical therapy in patients 65 years of age or older: A nonrandomized study from the Coronary Artery Surgery Study (CASS) registry. *N Engl J Med* 1985; 313:217–224.

100. Bourassa MG, Pepine CJ, Forman SA, et al. Asymptomatic Cardiac Ischemia Pilot (ACIP) Study: Effects of coronary angioplasty and coronary artery bypass graft surgery on recurrent angina and ischemia. *J Am Coll Cardiol* 1996; 27:1315–1316.

101. Alderman EL, Bourassa MG, Cohen LS, Davis KB, Kaiser GG, Killip T, et al. Ten-year follow-up of survival and myocardial infarction in the randomized Coronary Artery Surgery Study. *Circulation* 1990; 82:1629–1646.

102. Parisi AF, Khuri S, Deupree RH, Sharma GV, Scott SM, Luchi RJ. Medical compared with surgical management of unstable angina: 5-year mortality and morbidity in the Veterans Administration Study. *Circulation* 1989; 80:1176–1189.

103. Booth DC, Deupree RH, Hultgren HN, DeMaria AN, Scott SM, Luchi RJ. Quality of life after bypass surgery for unstable angina: 5-year follow-up results of a Veterans Affairs Cooperative Study. *Circulation* 1991; 83:87–95.

104. Lawrie GM, Morris GC Jr, Earle N. Long-term results of coronary bypass surgery: analysis of 1,698 patients followed 15 to 20 years. *Ann Surg* 1991; 213:377–385; discussion, 386–387.

105. Rogers WJ, Coggin CJ, Gersh BJ, Fisher LD, Myers WO, Oberman A, et al. Ten-year follow-up of quality of life in patients randomized to receive medical therapy or coronary artery bypass graft surgery: The Coronary Artery Surgery Study (CASS). *Circulation* 1990; 82:1647–1658.

106. Sergeant P, Lesaffre E, Flameng W, Suy R, Blackstone E. The return of clinically evident ischemia after coronary artery bypass grafting. *Eu J Cardiothorac Surg* 1991; 5:447–457.

107. Johnson WD, Brenowitz JB, Kayser KL. Factors influencing long-term (10-year to 15-year) survival after a successful coronary artery bypass operation. *Ann Thorac Surg* 1989; 48:19–24; discussion, 24–25.

108. Loop FD, Lytle BW, Cosgrove DM, Goormastic M, Taylor PC, Golding LA, et al. Coronary artery bypass graft surgery in the elderly: Indications and outcome. *Cleve Clin J Med* 1988; 55:23–34.

109. Myers WO, Schaff HV, Fisher LD, Gersh BJ, Mock MB, Holmes DR, et al. Time to first new myocardial infarction in patients with severe angina and three-vessel disease comparing medical and early surgical therapy: A CASS registry study of survival. *J Thorac Cardiovasc Surg* 1988; 95:382–389.

110. Schaff HV, Gersh BJ, Fisher LD, Frye RL, Mock MB, Ryan TJ, et al. Detrimental effect of perioperative myocardial infarction on late survival after coronary artery bypass. Report from the Coronary Artery Surgery Study—CASS. *J Thorac Cardiovasc Surg* 1984; 88:972–981.

111. Lytle BW, Loop FD, Cosgrove DM, Taylor PC, Goormastic M, Peper W, et al. Fifteen hundred coronary reoperations: Results and determinants of early and late survival. *J Thorac Cardiovasc Surg* 1987; 93:847–859.

112. Loop FD, Lytle BW, Cosgrove DM, Woods EL, Stewart RW, Golding LA, et al. Reoperation for coronary atherosclerosis: Changing practice in 2509 consecutive patients. *Ann Surg* 1990; 212:378–385; discussion, 385–386.

113. Marshall WG Jr, Saffitz J, Kouchoukos NT. Management during reoperation of aortocoronary saphenous vein grafts with minimal atherosclerosis by angiography. *Ann Thorac Surg* 1986; 42:163–167.

114. Weintraub WS, Jones EL, Craver JM, Grosswald R, Guyton RA. In-hospital and long-term outcome after reoperative coronary artery bypass graft surgery. *Circulation* 1995; 92(suppl II):II-50–II-57.

115. Lytle BW, McElroy D, McCarthy P, Loop FD, Taylor PC, Goormastic M, et al. The influence of arterial coronary bypass grafts on the mortality of coronary reoperations. *J Thoracic Cardiovasc Surg* 1994, 107:675–682, discussion, 682–683.

116. Frazier OH, Cooley DA, Kadipasaoglu KA, Pehlivanoglu S, Lindenmeir M, Barasch E, et al. Myocardial revascularization with laser: Preliminary findings. *Circulation* 1995; 22(suppl II):II-58–II-65.

117. Horvath KA, Mannting F, Cummings N. Shernan SK, Cohn LH. Transmyocardial laser revascularization: Operative techniques and clinical results at two years. *J Thorac Cardiovasc Surg* 1996; 111:1047–1053.

118. Brown G, Albers JJ, Fisher LD, Schaefer SM, Lin JT, Kaplan C, et al. Regression of coronary artery disease as a result of intensive lipid-lowering therapy in men with high levels of apolipoprotein B. *N Engl J Med* 1990; 323:1289–1298.

119. Blankenhorn DH, Nessim SA, Johnson RL, Sanmarco ME, Azen SP, Cashin-Hemphill L. Beneficial effects of combined colestipol-niacin therapy on coronary atherosclerosis and coronary venous bypass grafts. *JAMA* 1987; 257:3233–3240. [Published erratum appears in *JAMA* 1988; 259:2698.]

51

MANAGEMENT OF THE PATIENT AFTER CARDIAC SURGERY

Douglas C. Morris / Stephen D. Clements, Jr. / Carl C. Hug, Jr.

The main justification for specialized postoperative care following cardiac surgery is to allow recovery of physiologic systems disrupted by cardiopulmonary bypass (CPB). A number of organ systems are subject to insult during CPB. Much of the insult can be attributed to the generalized inflammatory response caused by blood contact with the synthetic surfaces of bypass equipment.[1] Upon the patient's arrival in the intensive care unit (ICU), these disrupted physiologic systems pose multiple management problems that change over time. The patient's condition on arrival varies, depending on his or her preoperative status, effects of residual anesthetic drugs, length of time on CPB, success of the operative procedure, and intraoperative complications.

THE ROLE OF VASCULAR CANNULAE, LIFE SUPPORT, AND MONITORING IN THE IMMEDIATE POSTOPERATIVE PERIOD

On arrival in the ICU, the patient is still under the effects of anesthesia and hypothermia, often receiving one or more drugs affecting the systemic circulation, and being mechanically ventilated. The patient typically arrives from the operating room with the necessary apparatus for monitoring the following parameters: heart rate and rhythm; arterial, central venous, pulmonary artery, and pulmonary artery occlusion pressures (PAOP); cardiac output; urinary output; mediastinal drainage; body temperature; hemoglobin saturation (pulse oximetry); and end-tidal carbon dioxide tension. While no objective data exist to support the routine use of pulmonary artery catheters, their use to guide therapy in those patients requiring cardiovascular drug therapy postoperatively is the customary standard of care in the majority of centers performing cardiac surgery. Immediately upon arrival in the ICU, reliable monitoring of the above-mentioned variables should be instituted. As appropriate monitoring is being established, the ICU staff's

attention to the patient's condition may be diverted to untangling tubing, connecting bedside monitors, adjusting the ventilator, and verifying drug dosages and infusion rates; it is, therefore, imperative that the operating room staff in attendance remain with the patient until the patient's nurse can attentively receive a report of the patient's intraoperative course and management, after which, the patient's primary ICU nurse can assume responsibility for observing and treating the patient's vital functions. Once the patient is satisfactorily connected to the bedside monitors and ventilator, all the hemodynamic measurements should be recorded, the patient's level of consciousness and comfort should be assessed, a portable supine chest x-ray should be acquired, and a 12-lead electrocardiogram obtained.

Most of the apparatus attached to the patient upon arrival in the ICU serves a dual purpose. The pulmonary artery catheter not only allows monitoring of pulmonary artery pressures but can also be used to estimate the filling pressure of the left ventricle, cardiac output, and body core temperature. The peripheral arterial cannula provides a continuous pulse-wave tracing of systemic blood pressure and ready access to arterial blood sampling for laboratory analysis, especially blood gases and pH, which are essential for adjustments of ventilator settings and calibration of the end-tidal CO_2 monitor. *Regular periodic assessments of arterial blood gases, especially after a major change in ventilator settings, are essential unless continuous end-tidal CO_2 and arterial oxygen saturation (SaO_2) by pulse oximetry are being monitored.* Assessment of volume loss is based on chest and mediastinal tube drainage plus urine output. The endotracheal tube secured in the correct position with an appropriately inflated cuff is essential for positive-pressure ventilation of the lungs. Confirmation of bilateral breath sounds and absence of tracheal air leak versus cuff inflation should be made upon arrival in the ICU after suctioning secretions from the oroparhynx, and the endotracheal tube's position should be ascertained on the initial chest x-ray. The endotracheal tube also allows for suctioning of bronchial secretions and reduces (but does not eliminate) the risk of oropharyngeal and gastric reflux secretions entering the trachea and bronchi. The endotracheal tube can often be removed the evening of surgery if the patient is conscious, is able to protect the airway, has good ventilatory mechanics and muscle strength, and is able to take on the work of breathing. Most patients can have the pulmonary artery catheter removed within 12 to 24 h if cardiovascular drug therapy is at minimum levels. The peripheral arterial cannula can be removed after postextubation blood-gas measurements are satisfactory and the need for blood sampling is at a routine daily level. The urinary catheter is usually removed once the patient is ambulatory unless there is a vigorous diuresis or an increased risk of urinary retention. Chest tubes are generally removed when the total drainage is less than 100 mL per tube over 8 h.

The single factor that differentiates cardiac surgery from other forms of surgery is CPB. With such improvements in extracorporeal technology as membrane oxygenation, arterial blood filtration, and blood sparing techniques, the noncardiac complications have been significantly reduced. Major improvements in myocardial protection technology coupled with changes in anesthetic and CPB techniques now frequently allow extubation within several hours of surgery.[2] Intraoperative management has now evolved to the point of minimizing the need for cardiopulmonary support after surgery, thereby allowing the patient to recover satisfactory vital functions more rapidly than before. As a consequence, mechanical ventilation and other measures can be discontinued much earlier, and the patient can be safely and comfortably transferred from the ICU within the first 6 to 24 h, a process that has been termed *fast-tracking*[3] (see also Chap. 84).

Fast-tracking describes efforts to minimize the duration of the patient's stay in the ICU or postanesthesia care unit and to allow the early, safe transfer of the cardiac surgical patient to a so-called step-down level of monitored care. Early extubation and transfer should require that the patient's status is characterized as follows: awake or easily aroused, neurologically intact, cooperative, and comfortable; stable, satisfactory hemodynamics; normothermia; satisfactory spontaneous ventilation; normal coagulation with minimal chest tube drainage; satisfactory urine output, electrolyte, and acid-base balance.[4]

EARLY POSTOPERATIVE MANAGEMENT

Pathophysiologic Consequences of Cardiopulmonary Bypass

The basic pathophysiology during the early postoperative period revolves around the following variables: transient left ventricular dysfunction, capillary leak, warming from hypothermia, mediastinal bleeding, and emergence from anesthesia.

Clinical evidence of left ventricular dysfunction during the first 24 h postoperatively with a gradual recovery to preoperative levels is substantiated by studies based upon hemodynamic data, nuclear scanning, and metabolic techniques. While improvements in surgical techniques, cardioplegia delivery, and other myocardial protection measures have been achieved, the reported prevalence of early ventricular dysfunction (90 percent) did not change between 1979 and 1990.[5] Myocardial depression in the early postoperative period has been attributed by some authors to inadequate myocardial protection or the effects of cold cardioplegia.[6,7]

CPB induces an inflammatory state that involves platelet–endothelial cell interactions and vasospastic responses that result in low-flow states in the coronary circulation.[8] The inflammatory reaction causes vascular endothelial adhesion molecules to attract inflammatory cells that subsequently adhere to the vascular endothelium. These inflammatory cells mediate much of the subsequent injury by the release of oxygen radicals or proteolytic enzymes.[9] This release of oxygen free radicals in response to reperfusion injury is now generally accepted as the explanation for the transient postoperative ventricular dysfunction.[10–12] Depressed myocardial function seems to be unrelated to CPB time, number of coronary artery grafts, preoperative medications, or postoperative core temperature. Ventricular function is generally depressed by 2 h and is at its worse at 4 to 5 h after CPB. Significant recovery of function usually occurs by 8 to 10 h, and full recovery is reached by 24 to 48 h.[13] Systemic vascular resistance, while not rising immediately after surgery, increases as ventricular function worsens. This rise in systemic vascular resistance is likely secondary to reduced ventricular function and the need to maintain systemic blood pressure and, per se, is not a major causative factor of depressed cardiac contractility. The confounding effect of vasopressor drugs used in an attempt to increase systemic blood pressure must be recognized.

The capillary leak syndrome may last from a few hours up to 1 to 2 days, depending to a large degree on the duration of CPB. Again, the inflammatory response in the vascular endothelium can disturb the "gatekeeper" function of the endothelium and increases capillary permeability, resulting in edema.[9] When the capillary leak ceases, additional fluid does not need to be administered, because fluid tends to remain in the intravascular space and interstitial edema fluid is mobilized from tissues. At this time, diuretics are beneficial to eliminate excessive fluid.

Hypothermia predisposes the patient to cardiac dysrhythmias, increases systemic vascular resistance, precipitates shivering (which increases O_2 consumption and CO_2 production), and impairs coagulation.[13] Hypothermia with the patient's core temperatures below 35°C frequently recurs after rewarming to 37°C at the end of CPB; it reflects the loss of heat from the surgical field after CPB, exposure of the patient to ambient temperature, and incomplete rewarming of peripheral tissues, especially fat and muscle. Nitroprusside or nitroglycerin may have been infused in the operating room to facilitate peripheral perfusion during rewarming on CPB. If the patient is still hypothermic, these agents should be continued at the maximum rate that still allows for an adequate systemic perfusion pressure. Monitoring the temperature of noncore body sites such as a finger or toe can assure complete assessment of rewarming. Hypothermia causes peripheral vasoconstriction and contributes to the hypertension frequently seen after cardiac surgery. Furthermore, hypothermia causes a decrease in cardiac output by producing bradycardia along with the increase in vascular resistance. As the patient is rewarmed, large increases in O_2 consumption, and CO_2 production can occur, with a consequent increase in demand on cardiovascular and pulmonary functions.[14]

Hypercarbia will cause catecholamine release, tachycardia, and pulmonary hypertension. If the patient cannot increase the cardiac output and O_2 delivery, venous hemoglobin desaturation and metabolic acidosis will result. Arterial blood gases should be analyzed as frequently as necessary to guide adjustments in mechanical ventilation to eliminate CO_2 and to determine the need for blood transfusion and inotropic drugs to improve oxygen delivery. Most believe that the patient should be passively rewarmed by warm air (e.g., Bear Hugger) and that shivering should be eliminated by the administration of muscle relaxants.[15] As body temperature increases, the vasoconstriction and hypertension associated with hypothermia are replaced by vasodilatation, tachycardia, and hypotension. Volume loading during the rewarming process helps reduce the rapid swings in blood pressure. Vasopressors (e.g., norepinephrine) may be required to maintain an adequate systemic blood pressure.

The commonly reported frequency of severe postoperative bleeding (more than 10 units of blood transfused) following cardiac surgery is between 3 and 5 percent. In some hospitals, 25 percent of all blood products are dedicated to cardiac surgery.[16] While approximately one-half of the patients who undergo reoperation for excessive bleeding exhibit incomplete surgical hemostasis, the remainder bleed because of various acquired hemostatic defects, most often related to acquired platelet dysfunction.[17] The factors that predispose to bleeding following CPB are residual heparin effect, platelet dysfunction (which may be intensified by preoperative drug therapy, e.g., aspirin), clotting factor depletion, inadequate surgical hemostasis, hypothermia, and postoperative hypertension. CPB decreases both platelet count and function. Hemodilution causes platelet counts to fall rapidly to about 50 percent of preoperative values. Within minutes after instituting CPB, the bleeding time is prolonged and platelet aggregation is impaired. The bleeding time usually normalizes by 2 to 4 h after CPB. The platelet count usually requires several days to return to normal levels. While the exact mechanism responsible for the transient platelet dysfunction remains undefined, it appears to be related to contact of platelets with the synthetic surfaces of the extracorporeal oxygenator and to hypothermia. Reductions in the plasma concentrations of coagulation factors II, V, VII, IX, X, and XIII due to hemodilution occur during CPB, but these coagulation factors remain well above levels considered

adequate for hemostasis and generally normalize within the first 12 h after surgery. Moreover, while bleeding after CPB is often attributed to excessive fibrinolysis, the decrease in both plasminogen and fibrinogen levels during CPB is due to hemodilution and not consumption.[16] Upon returning from the operating room after exploration for bleeding, a common report is that no localized site of bleeding occurred and only diffuse oozing was found. On other occasions, a specific site such as an internal mammary pedicle will be identified.

Management of Common Postoperative Syndromes

VASOCONSTRICTION WITH HYPERTENSION AND BORDERLINE CARDIAC OUTPUT

Vasoconstriction, customarily evident on arrival in the ICU, is usually due to hypothermia. Patients should be rewarmed as noted above, and nitroprusside can be administered to maintain a systolic blood pressure between 100 and 130 mmHg (mean pressure of 80 to 90 mmHg). Nitroprusside is initiated at a dose of 0.1 to 0.25 μg/kg/min and titrated as needed to a maximum dose of 8 μg/kg/min. Intravascular volume should be maintained at a relatively high level (PAOP of 14 to 16 mmHg) in anticipation of vasodilation upon rewarming and to enhance cardiac output and peripheral perfusion. If the cardiac index is marginal ($\leq$2.0 L/min/m^2), an inotropic drug should be administered in addition to the nitroprusside.

VASODILATATION AND HYPOTENSION

This condition, which generally appears during rewarming, is most effectively prevented and best treated by fluid administration. The specific volume expander selected should be based upon a determination of the predominant factor leading to the hypovolemia. If the predominant factor is a capillary leak syndrome with generalized edema, the use of colloids could aggravate the situation as the oncotic elements pass into the interstitium and exacerbate tissue edema. If vasodilatation with increased venous capacitance is the major problem, colloids will provide longer-lasting augmentation of intravascular volume. Hetastarch (administered in 250- to 500-mL increments) provides an equally sustained volume expansion as 5% albumin, at a significant reduction in cost. It does, however, have a tendency to increase bleeding. If fluid administration has increased PAOP appropriately (e.g., 14 to 16 mmHg for a normal ventricle or 18 to 22 mmHg for a noncompliant ventricle) and systemic blood pressure remains marginal, vasopressor or inotropic drugs should be administered. Generally, a PAOP above 15 mmHg in the postoperative period is of little benefit due to a "flattening" of the diastolic function curve, which accompanies the decline in systolic function. An inotropic vasopressor should be infused if more than 1 or 2 L of fluid have been administered and the PAOP is not rising. In some patients after cardiac surgery, fluid administration produces a substantial increase in left ventricular end-diastolic volume without changing PAOP. Whether this is due to an open pericardium with overdistension of the left ventricle or some other factor is unclear.[19] If the blood pressure is marginal and the cardiac index is over 2.0 L/min/m^2, norepinephrine or dopamine is the preferable agent. If the cardiac index is less than 2.0 L/min/m^2, an inotropic agent should be administered initially.

NORMAL VENTRICULAR SYSTOLIC FUNCTION AND LOW CARDIAC OUTPUT

This situation is often noted in small women with systemic hypertension and in patients undergoing aortic valve replacement for aortic stenosis. The cause of the problem in these cases is likely diastolic dysfunction. The problem should be managed by volume expansion with the intent to elevate PAOP to 20 to 25 mmHg. Sinus rhythm and atrioventricular (AV) synchrony are essential and, if not present, should be restored. In the absence of causes of diastolic dysfunction, the possibility of cardiac compression from clots in the mediastinum and pericardial space should be considered as the cause of low cardiac output in the presence of normal systolic function. If volume expansion does not lead to hemodynamic improvement, transesophageal echocardiography (TEE) should be used to establish or exclude the presence of clots or other causes of low output. If the information derived from TEE does not permit explanation and/or resolution of the problem, the patient should return to the operating room for exploration.

A rather characteristic pattern of presentation of cardiac compression is the patient who initially has a large volume of mediastinal bleeding that ceases rather abruptly. The patient then becomes hypotensive, with high PAOP and central venous pressure values and progressively increasing inotropic drug requirements. Cardiac compression from clots in the pericardial space should be suspected and, if time allows, confirmed by TEE. Rapid clinical deterioration demands immediate exploration of the pericardial space, often immediate opening of the sternum in the ICU before transferring the patient to the operating room.

APPROACH TO POSTOPERATIVE CARDIOVASCULAR PROBLEMS

Low Cardiac Output Syndrome

Satisfactory cardiac performance following cardiac surgery is usually indicated by a cardiac index greater than 2.2 L/min/m^2 with a heart rate below 100 beats per minute. Marginal cardiac function is present with a cardiac index between 2.0 and 2.2 L/min/m^2. A cardiac index below 2.0 L/min/m^2 is unacceptably low, and therapeutic intervention is indicated.

ASSESSMENT
The most common causes of low cardiac output postoperatively are related to a decreased left ventricular preload. Hypovolemia (due to bleeding or to vasodilatation as a conse-

quence of warming or drugs), cardiac tamponade, or right ventricular dysfunction are common causes of reduced left ventricular preload. Decreased contractility due to a preexisting low ejection fraction or to intra- or postoperative ischemia or infarction may be the explanation of a low cardiac output. Perioperative myocardial ischemia or infarction is usually due to poor intraoperative myocardial protection, incomplete myocardial revascularization, coronary artery spasm, coronary embolism of atherosclerotic debris or air, prolonged systemic hypotension, or severe acute anemia. Tachy- or bradyarrhythmias decrease cardiac output by reducing ventricular preload (e.g., decreased diastolic filling time, loss of atrial contraction or AV synchrony) or by reducing the number of effective ventricular contractions per minute. Substantial increases in systemic vascular resistance (i.e., vasoconstriction) impede ventricular ejection and lower cardiac output. Vasodilatation from sepsis or anaphylaxis resulting in systemic hypotension could lead to reduced coronary blood flow and myocardial ischemia. Sepsis is also associated with the production of myocardial depressant factors. Anemia may result in reduced blood viscosity (a major determinant of total peripheral resistance), leading to hypotension and decreased oxygen delivery to the heart, which has a high oxygen extraction from oxyhemoglobin. The hypotension in anemia, however, is most often due to changes in effective blood volume rather than to the changes in viscosity.

ETIOLOGY AND MANAGEMENT
The multiple variables being constantly monitored usually provide sufficient clues as to the cause of low cardiac output. If there is no obvious noncardiac cause such as anaphylaxis or anaphylactoid reaction, acidosis, severe anemia, or marked alterations in body temperature, then the first step is to optimize the preload (PAOP of 15 to 18 mmHg.). The next step is to optimize the heart rate by either cardiac pacing or antiarrhythmic drugs. Postoperative myocardial performance is usually best at a rate of 90 to 100 beats per minute. If these measures prove unsuccessful, pharmacologic intervention with inotropic agents, vasodilators, vasopressors, or a combination of these drugs must be considered. The selection of drugs should be based upon the balance of their effects on heart rate, contractility, ventricular preload, and systemic vasculature resistance (Table 51-1). The presence of elevated left- and right-sided filling pressures, a recent cessation of mediastinal drainage, and progressively increasing inotropic drug dosages suggests tamponade, which should be relieved emergently. TEE has been very helpful in clarifying these situations. The final therapeutic step, if the above measures have proven inadequate, is the use of aortic counterpulsation (i.e., intraaortic balloon pump) or another type of cardiac assist device.

Hypertension

MANAGEMENT
A variety of medications are available for control of hypertension, and the drug selected should depend on the hemodynamic

TABLE 51-1

MEDICATIONS USED IN LOW CARDIAC OUTPUT
SYNDROME

Medication	Hemodynamic Properties	Dosage Range
Dopamine	Low dose—dopaminergic effect	2–20 µg/kg/min
	Moderate dose—inotropic effect	
	High dose—vasopressor effect	
Dobutamine	Positive inotropic agent	2–20 µg/kg/min
Epinephrine	Positive inotropic agent	1–4 µg/min
Amrinone	Positive inotropic agent	10–15 µg/kg/min
Isoproterenol	Potent inotropic agent Pronounced chronotropic effect	0.5–10 µg/min
Norepinephrine	Potent vasopressor effect; inotropic effect	1–100 µg/min
Phenylephrine	Potent vasopressor agent	10–500 µg/min

status of the patient, the cardiovascular effects of the drug, and the patient's other medical problems. Systemic hypertension in the presence of a high left ventricular filling pressure and marginal cardiac output is most appropriately treated by an arterial vasodilator. The available choices include sodium nitroprusside, nitroglycerin, nicardipine, and hydralazine. Nitroprusside relaxes vascular smooth muscle in arterial resistance vessels (both systemic and pulmonary) and in venous capacitance vessels. The drug probably should be avoided in the presence of myocardial ischemia or if it is threatened. The concern in this situation is the potential for the drug to dilate the coronary resistance vessels and produce a coronary steal syndrome by shunting blood away from the ischemic areas. The advantages of the drug are its very rapid onset and the rapid dissipation of its effects. The risks with this agent are rapid and excessive hypotension and the potential for either cyanide toxicity acutely or thiocyanate toxicity with prolonged use[19] (see Chap. 23).

Nitroglycerin is primarily a venous dilator, although it produces varying degrees of arterial vasodilatation, especially at high doses. Its major role in treating systemic hypertension is in the patient with high filling pressures and active myocardial ischemia.[20] Nicardipine is a potent systemic and coronary vasodilator without the risk of coronary steal, and it has no significant effect on the venous system. It can, therefore, effectively control postoperative hypertension without reducing the filling pressures or causing a coronary steal. While its onset of action is rapid (1 to 2 min), its elimination half-life is about 40 min. Unlike some calcium channel blockers, this agent lacks a negative inotropic effect and has no effect on AV conduction.[21] Hydralazine is a direct arterial vasodilator, which is usually administered in intermittent intravenous or intramuscular doses. Hydralazine-induced arterial vasodilation may produce a compensatory tachycardia; it is frequently resorted to in patients who are hemodynamically stable but remain hypertensive several days after surgery and cannot yet take or absorb oral medications.

When the hypertension is associated with a normal cardiac output and a relatively rapid sinus heart rate or a propensity toward dysrhythmias, a drug with negative inotropic and chronotropic properties is desirable. Esmolol is a cardioselective, ultrafast short-acting beta blocker, which also produces a rapid and titratable control of the blood pressure accompanied by a decrease in heart rate. The drug is usually tolerated satisfactorily by patients with a history of bronchospasm because of its relatively high selectivity for beta₁-type adrenergic receptors. It is not ideal for patients with impaired cardiac contractility, particularly in the presence of elevated filling pressures.[22] Diltiazem is an arterial vasodilator that has a mild negative inotropic effect and a more potent negative chronotropic effect. Verapamil is a less potent vasodilator but with more potent negative inotropic, chronotropic, and dromotropic effects. It can be administered intravenously be either boluses or continuous infusion (see Chap. 54). Labetalol has both alpha- and beta-blocking properties as well as a direct vasodilatory effect. Its predominant effect is as a beta blocker, especially in the intravenous form. The angiotensin-converting enzyme inhibitor enalaprilat, which is the active form of enalapril, can be administered intermittently by the intravenous route. This agent is usually reserved for the patient who is hemodynamically stable but hypertensive with either a normal or reduced cardiac output (Table 51-2).

Dysrhythmias

GENERAL CONSIDERATIONS AND SINUS TACHYCARDIA

The most common rhythm disturbance after cardiac surgery is sinus tachycardia. This condition is appropriately treated by searching for and treating the underlying cause (pain, anxiety, low cardiac output, anemia, fever, or beta-blocker withdrawal). The second most common arrhythmia is ventricular ectopy. Again, an underlying cause such as myocardial ischemia, hypokalemia, hypomagnesemia, hypoxia, or administration of sympathomimetic drugs must be sought and corrected if possible. It is also important to review the patient's preoperative record to determine if the patient had preexisting ectopy. Patients with chronic ventricular ectopy frequently have their ectopy exaggerated postoperatively.[23] In the presence of active myocardial ischemia, pharmacologic suppression is advisable for complex ventricular ectopy. In the first 12 h after coronary bypass surgery, myocardial ischemia must be suspected and is difficult to exclude; accordingly, the preceding policy for ectopy suppression should be adhered to with the possible exception of those with known chronic ectopy. Lidocaine is the drug of choice in most instances. The loading dose of lidocaine is approximately 3 mg per kilogram of ideal body weight given over 20 min. One approach is to give an initial bolus of 75 mg, following by 50 mg every 5 min to a total dose of 225 mg. An alternative is to give a priming dose of 75 mg, followed by a loading infusion of 150 mg over 20 min. The usual initial maintenance infusion is 1.5 to 2.5 mg/

TABLE 51-2
INTRAVENOUS ANTIHYPERTENSIVE AGENTS

Drug	Peak Effect	Duration	Dosage
Nitroprusside	Immediate	2–5 min	0.3–1.0 μg/kg/min
Nitroglycerine	Immediate	2–5 min	5–100 μg/min infusion
Nicardipine	5–60 min	20–40 min	2.5 mg over 5 min; may repeat times 4 at 10-min intervals; infusion 2–15 mg/h
Esmolol	2–5 min	8–10 min	1-min loading infusion of 0.25–0.5 mg/kg; sustained infusion of 50–200 μg/kg/min
Enalaprilat	15–30 min	6 h or more	0.625–1.25 mg slowly over 5 min every 6 h
Hydralazine	15–20 min	3–4 h	5- to 10-mg bolus may be repeated every 15 min; up to total of 40 mg
Diltiazem	3–30 min	3 h	20- to 25-mg bolus may repeat; infusion of 10–20 mg/h
Verapamil	2–3 min	20–40 min	5- to 10-mg bolus; may repeat in 10 min; infusion of 3–25 mg/h
Labetalol	5–15 min	2–6 h	20-mg bolus over 2 min; then 40- to 80-mg boluses every 15 min until effect achieved (to total dose of 300 mg)

min. If the dysrhythmia is uncontrolled, one can give another bolus of 25 to 50 mg and increase the infusion rate. The chances of toxicity rise significantly at infusion rates above 4 mg/min, especially in older individuals. If the ectopy does not respond to lidocaine, the option is to not use an antiarrhythmic agent unless ventricular tachycardia occurs or to use intravenous amiodarone.

VENTRICULAR DYSRHYTHMIAS

A few patients after cardiac surgery develop sustained ventricular tachycardia (either monomorphic or polymorphic) or ventricular fibrillation. This profound rhythm disturbance may develop in the absence of evidence of acute myocardial ischemia or infarction or electrolyte imbalance. In most cases the patients have had previous myocardial infarction and have undergone "complete" revascularization, including regions likely to be nonviable. Reperfusion of these areas that probably include viable as well as nonviable myofibrils embedded in the healed infarct may lead to altered dispersion of repolarization. These changes support development of reentry arrhythmias.[23] The ventricular tachycardia in these patients uncommonly responds to lidocaine and usually requires amiodarone. In some instances, a combination of amiodarone and a beta blocker is required. In a rare circumstance, aortic counterpulsation has seemed to be of benefit.

Every encounter with a wide complex tachycardia requires careful consideration as to the possibility of supraventricular tachycardia with aberrant conduction. In the presence of atrial fibrillation with a rapid ventricular response, right bundle branch aberrant conduction often mimics ventricular tachycardia. Care must be given to avoid lidocaine in these situations, because it may result in an even more aberrant conduction and a more rapid ventricular rate.

Wide complex tachyarrhythmias in the range of 250 to 300 beats per minute should suggest the presence of an anomalous conduction pathway. The mechanism of this dysrhythmia usually involves atrial flutter, with one-to-one conduction or atrial fibrillation with a very fast ventricular response involving an anomalous pathway. Once this is recognized, procainamide becomes the drug of choice, since it does have favorable therapeutic effects on the bypass track tissue. Lidocaine and verapamil should be avoided if the presence of an anomalous pathway is suspected (see also Chap. 27).

SUPRAVENTRICULAR DYSRHYTHMIAS

The most common supraventricular dysrhythmias, with the exception of sinus tachycardia, are atrial fibrillation and atrial flutter. These rhythm disturbances occur in 10 to 30 percent of patients following cardiac surgery. The most predominant predisposing factor in the development of atrial fibrillation is the patient's age. The prevalence of atrial fibrillation in patients less than 40 years of age is as low as 3.7 percent, while the prevalence is at least 28 percent in patients over age 70. Atrial fibrillation is most likely to appear on the second postoperative day. Eighty percent of these patients will return to sinus rhythm within 1 to 3 days with only digoxin or beta-blocker therapy.[24–26] The prophylactic use of beta blockers has a protective effect against the development of atrial fibrillation or flutter. This beneficial effect has been demonstrated with any one of several beta blockers, administered in low or high doses and starting preoperatively or postoperatively. Neither digoxin nor verapamil has been demonstrated to produce a protective effect against atrial fibrillation or flutter.[27]

Intravenous infusions of either esmolol or diltiazem can be used to control the ventricular rate with atrial fibrillation or flutter, which occasionally will convert to a sinus rhythm. Esmolol is given as a 1-min loading infusion of 0.25 to 0.5 mg/kg, followed by a sustained infusion of 50 to 200 μg/kg/min. Diltiazem is administered as a bolus of 20 to 25 mg (which may be repeated), followed by an infusion of 10 to 15 mg/h.

Atrial epicardial pacing wires provide the means of atrial pacing to convert some cases of atrial flutter to sinus rhythm.[25] Short bursts (15 to 30 s) of atrial pacing at rates of 300 to 600 per minute may be effective in converting atrial flutter. Approximately 10 percent of patients with atrial fibrillation require electrical cardioversion to restore sinus rhythm. If hemodynamic compromise is present and aggravated by a supraventricular tachyarrhythmia, cardioversion should be used earlier rather than later.

CONDUCTION DEFECTS

The prevalence of intraventricular conduction abnormalities after coronary bypass surgery is reported to be from 1 to 45 percent, with approximately 10 percent being the most commonly reported frequency. The most common conduction defect is right bundle branch block, which may be due to selective sensitivity of the right bundle to the effects of hypothermia and the extracorporeal circulation process. Only about 5 percent of the patients are left with a permanent conduction abnormality, and the prognosis for these patients is no worse than for comparable patients with no conduction defect.[28,29] The development of high-degree (second- or third-degree) AV block is an indication for temporary pacing via epicardial pacing wires. AV block is not as common as either bundle branch block or fascicular block, but it does occur, especially after aortic valve surgery where dense calcification is present and the conduction system is encroached upon.

RESPIRATORY MANAGEMENT

Expected Respiratory Changes after Cardiac Surgery

Pulmonary problems are the most significant cause of morbidity following CPB. The pain associated with sternotomy and especially with thoracotomy has a deleterious effect on the patient's willingness to breathe deeply and cough. Pain caused by the presence of chest tubes may also interfere with normal respiratory function. Phrenic nerve damage can result in diaphragmatic dysfunction. More commonly, the diaphragm is passively displaced cephalad by abdominal contents (gastrointestinal intraluminal air and fluid, edematous bowel) in the anesthetized, paralyzed patient supported by mechanical ventilation. Elevated left heart filling pressures may cause alveolar edema, and in some patients increase capillary permeability may exist.

Atelectasis is the most common pulmonary complication, occurring in about 70 percent of patients.[30] During CPB, the lungs are not perfused and are usually allowed to collapse. Once the lungs are reexpanded, a variable amount of atelectasis remains. While the atelectasis might be microscopic, intermediate degrees (subsegmental and segmental) are common. The preponderance of atelectasis occurs in the left lower lobe because of its compression during cardiac surgery, the tendency to suction more thoroughly the right mainstem bronchus during blind naso-orotracheal suctioning, and the frequent surgical practice of opening the left pleural space to facilitate dissection of the left internal mammary artery. Evidence for a depletion of surfactant after cardiopulmonary is lacking.[31]

After thoracotomy, both lung and chest wall compliance decrease significantly. The maximum decrease occurs at approximately 3 days, but the decrease persists to a lesser degree 6 or more days after sternotomy. Alterations in chest wall mechanics lead to a decrease in the forced expiratory volume (FEV_1) and the functional residual capacity (FRC). The changes in the FEV_1 may persist for 6 weeks. In addition to these changes in flows and volumes, reduced inspiratory strength and uncoordinated rib cage expansion occur. These changes result in an increase in respiratory rate and a decrease in tidal volume, decreased respiratory efficiency, and increased oxygen cost of breathing. The atelectasis and decrease in lung volume result in ventilation:perfusion mismatch and shunting. The clinical manifestation is a decrease in arterial P_{O_2} and hemoglobin saturation.[31]

There is little evidence of a significant increase in lung water after routine CPB. When increased capillary permeability exists, it is usually related to elevated cardiac filling pressures.[31]

Basic Concepts of Oxygenation and Alveolar Ventilation

The goals of mechanical ventilation are the maintenance of satisfactory arterial oxygenation and CO_2 removal. Direct measurement of Pa_{O_2} is generally used to assess the overall adequacy of blood oxygenation, while pulse oximetry (Sp_{O_2}) is used to monitor peripheral arterial hemoglobin saturation on a continuous basis. An $Sp_{O_2} \geq 90$ percent is considered to be acceptable, but it may be associated with a marginal Pa_{O_2}. The oxygen-hemoglobin dissociation curve portrays this relationship (Fig. 51-1). The shoulder of this sigmoid curve

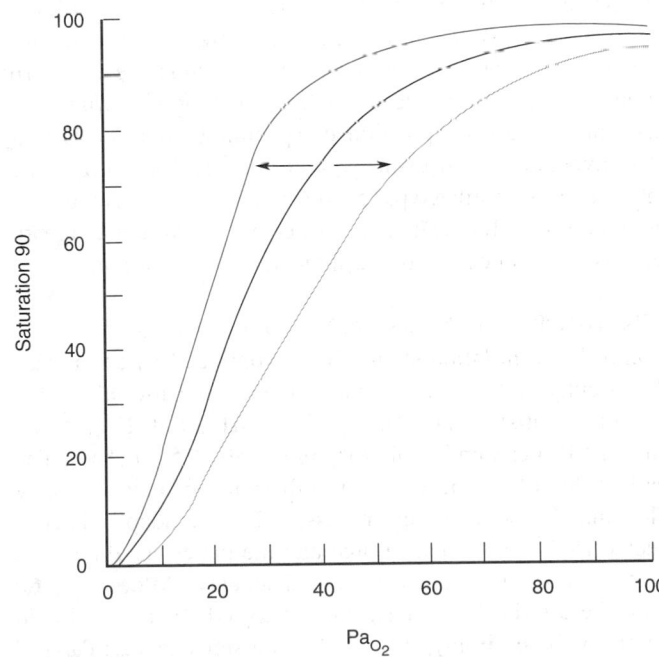

FIGURE 51-1

Oxygen-hemoglobin dissociation curve. The curve depicts the saturation of hemoglobin at increasing levels of Pa_{O_2}. A shift of the curve to the left increases the affinity of hemoglobin for oxygen and a shift to the right decreases the affinity.

lies at a Pa_{O_2} of approximately 65 mmHg. A Pa_{O_2} below this level will result in a precipitous fall in the oxygen saturation of hemoglobin. With hypothermia or with profound respiratory alkalosis, the curve will shift to the left, resulting in more avid binding of oxygen to hemoglobin and less release of oxygen to the tissues. The patient will likely be receiving 100% oxygen during transfer from the operating room to the ICU or postanesthesia care unit. The $F_{I_{O_2}}$ should be gradually decreased to 0.4 as tolerated to minimize adsorption atelectasis and pulmonary O_2 toxicity. Mechanical ventilation is also used to maintain alveolar ventilation, which regulates the arterial blood CO_2 tension (Pa_{CO_2}). Alveolar ventilation is regulated by controlling the tidal volume and the respiratory rate. Generally, the ventilator should maintain an exhaled minute ventilation of 6 to 8 L/min. Decreasing the tidal volume below 8 to 10 mL/kg may result in alveolar hypoventilation and atelectasis. Mild hypocarbia (Pa_{CO_2} of 30 to 35 mmHg) is satisfactory immediately after surgery, but more profound respiratory alkalosis should be avoided because it leads to hypokalemia and a leftward shift of the oxygen-hemoglobin dissociation curve (decreased oxygen release to the tissues). Hypocarbia is best corrected by reducing the ventilator rate.

Hypercarbia in the immediate postoperative period usually indicates that minute ventilation is inadequate. The problem can be rectified primarily by increasing the ventilator rate; in some cases it is appropriate to increase the tidal volume as well. Later, as the patient is being weaned from the ventilator, hypercarbia may reflect opioid analgesia (a necessary side effect of satisfactory analgesia) or compensatory hypoventilation in response to a metabolic alkalosis, most likely due to excessive diuresis. Acetazolamide (Diamox), 250 to 500 mg intravenously every 6 h, is beneficial in correcting a primary metabolic alkalosis. Severe hypercarbia should raise a concern about mechanical problems such as ventilator malfunction, endotracheal tube malposition, or a pneumothorax.[5] Occasionally, hypoxemia and even hypotension may develop in the mechanically ventilated patient due to a tension pneumothorax or hemothorax. If the latter are suspected, assessment of breath sounds and a chest x-ray are indicated for confirmation.

VENTILATORY WEANING AND EXTUBATION

Controlled ventilation should be discontinued when the cardiovascular system has become stable and the arterial oxygen tension is satisfactory [$Pa_{O_2} > 70$ mmHg, with $F_{I_{O_2}} \leq 0.5$ and PEEP (peak end-expiratory pressure) ≤ 5 cmH$_2$O]. The patient should also be alert, normothermic, and have no active bleeding. In the weaning process, a T-piece adapter is connected to the endotracheal tube and the patient is allowed to breathe oxygen-enriched air spontaneously. After 30 to 60 min, the arterial blood gases are analyzed. Weaning should be discontinued if any of the following signs appear: $Pa_{O_2} < 60$ mmHg, $Pa_{CO_2} > 55$ mmHg, pH < 7.30, a 10-mmHg rise in pulmonary artery pressure, respiratory rate > 30, a 20-mmHg rise in systemic blood pressure, or a 20-beat rise in heart rate.[5] An alternative approach to weaning is to reduce the intermittent mandatory ventilation rate by two breaths

every 1 to 2 h as long as the arterial blood gases remain acceptable.

Bronchospasm

Severe bronchospasm during CPB is an unusual event, but it can occur. A few patients cannot have their chest cavity closed at the end of surgery because of hyperinflated lungs. The most likely cause of this fulminant bronchospasm is activation of human C5a anaphylatoxin by the extracorporeal circulation. Other likely causes of bronchospasm in the postoperative period are bronchospasm secondary to cardiogenic pulmonary edema; a simple exacerbation of preexisting bronchospastic disease triggered by instrumentation, secretions, or cold anesthetic gas; beta-adrenergic blockage–induced bronchospasm in susceptible individuals; and allergic reaction to protamine.[30]

The initial therapy of bronchospasm in the postoperative patient, once a diagnosis of heart failure is excluded, should be inhaled beta$_2$-agonists (terbutaline, metaproterenol, albuterol) and/or inhaled cholinergic agents (ipratropium bromide or glycopyrrolate). In the inhaled form these rather potent bronchodilators have minimal cardiovascular effects. In addition to their bronchodilator effect, these agents may augment mucociliary transport and aid in clearing secretions. A combination of beta$_2$-agonists and cholinergic agents should be tried in the patient refractory to a single agent. Even more refractory bronchospasm requires either a short course of systemic steroids or intravenous aminophylline. In addition to being a bronchodilator, aminophylline is a mild diuretic, increases the central nervous system respiratory drive, improves respiratory muscle function, and may decrease the pulmonary artery pressure. It is, however, arrhythmogenic and chronotropic.

POSTOPERATIVE OLIGURIA AND RENAL INSUFFICIENCY

Etiology

The use of radiocontrast agents in the days immediately preceding CPB may embarrass renal function, as manifested by a rise in blood urea nitrogen and serum creatinine values. Following CPB, there is a substantial incidence of postoperative renal dysfunction (up to 30 percent) but a relatively low incidence of severe renal impairment requiring dialysis (1 to 5 percent). Renal blood flow and glomerular filtration rate are reduced by 25 to 75 percent during bypass, with partial but not complete recovery in the first day after CPB. This reduction in renal function is attributed to renal artery vasoconstriction, hypothermia, and the loss of pulsatile perfusion during CPB. Angiotensin II levels are higher with nonpulsatile as opposed to pulsatile flow. While renal dysfunction cannot be consistently related to the systemic blood pressure and pump flow rate during nonpulsatile bypass, there is a definite relationship between the incidence of postbypass renal dysfunction and the duration of CPB. In addition to the duration of CPB, the risk of developing postbypass renal failure seems to be a function of the patient's underlying renal function (also affected by age) and the perioperative circulatory status. The histologic changes that accompany renal impairment after cardiopulmonary bypass are characteristic of tubular necrosis. The tubular cells seem to be the most susceptible to acute reductions in renal perfusion.[31]

Management

There are three agents (so-called renoprotective drugs) that might be used during CPB to prevent an ischemic insult to the kidneys. Mannitol used in the CPB priming fluid may moderate ischemic insult, probably by volume expansion and hemodilution. It also initiates an osmotic diuresis, which prevents tubular obstruction and may serve as a free radical scavenger. Furosemide appears to improve renal blood flow when given during bypass. So-called renal dose dopamine (1 to 2.5 µg/kg/min based on ideal body weight) may maintain renal blood flow and urine output. Once renal failure has developed, none of these drugs is likely to offer any beneficial effect. A megadose of furosemide (200 to 300 mg) may be tried, but if there is no diuretic response, it should not be repeated. Similarly, a single dose of mannitol (12.5 to 25 mg) either with or without furosemide could be tried but not repeated if there is no effect. Whenever possible, it is advisable to avoid potentially nephrotoxic agents in the early postoperative period. Examples of such include radiologic contrast agents, aminoglycoside antibiotics, and angiotensin-converting enzyme inhibitors.

POSTOPERATIVE GASTROINTESTINAL DYSFUNCTION

Gastrointestinal Consequences of Cardiopulmonary Bypass

The gastrointestinal consequences of CPB appear to be minimal. Reviews of the subject report a 1 percent prevalence.[32,33] Most patients are eating within 24 to 48 h after an uncomplicated elective procedure. The limited investigations of the gastrointestinal tract after cardiac surgery have found a slight decrease in hepatic and pancreatic blood flow during cooling and rewarming on bypass and a decrease in gastric pH.[30,34] Transient elevations in liver function tests and hyperamylasemia may occur after cardiac surgery, and the risk factors include long CPB time, multiple transfusions, and multiple valve replacements. Appearance of jaundice portends a poor prognosis.[35] Severe gastrointestinal complications are usually ischemic in nature and are often associated with a low-output syndrome.[30] The use of opioids as part of general anesthesia and postoperative pain management contributes to gastrointestinal dysfunction (cramping, ileus, constipation) and to postoperative nausea and vomiting. The nausea and vomiting can be minimized by use of a naso- or orogastric tube to maintain gastric decompression intraoperatively and early in the post-

operative period, with the additional benefit of improving thoracoabdominal compliance to positive-pressure ventilation.

POSTOPERATIVE METABOLIC DISORDERS

Potassium Imbalance

There are multiple factors that can produce large and rapid shifts in the serum potassium levels during and after CPB. These factors include the following: (1) The patient receives a high-potassium cardioplegia solution during surgery; (2) some degree of renal dysfunction is likely to be present, with associated oliguria and decreased clearance of potassium; (3) low cardiac output states are accompanied by oliguria and acidosis; (4) hemolyzed red cells release potassium; (5) potassium is lost by diuresis; and (6) diabetes mellitus interferes with cellular uptake of potassium unless insulin is infused intra- and postoperatively. The principal detrimental effects of these potassium shifts is on the electrical activity of the heart. The electrocardiographic signs of hyperkalemia and hypokalemia are described in Chap. 12. The electrocardiographic changes of hyperkalemia do not necessarily appear in the classic progressive manner; they are more related to the rate of rise in serum potassium rather than to the absolute serum concentration. The therapy of severe hyperkalemia should include counteracting the toxic cardiac effects of the elevated potassium with intravenous calcium gluconate or calcium chloride and lowering the serum level of potassium with sodium bicarbonate and/or administration of regular insulin and glucose. Hypokalemia does not usually become clinically evident until the serum potassium concentration is less than 2.5 meq/L, and at these levels it can be associated with severe ventricular tachyarrhythmias. Another consequence of potassium depletion is metabolic alkalosis as the hydrogen ions replace potassium ions within the cells. Hypokalemia is treated with the intravenous administration of KCl at a rate of no more than 10 to 15 meq/h. The serum potassium rises approximately 0.1 meq/L for each 2 meq of KCl administered. Large doses of KCl should be administered by a central venous catheter because of the caustic effect of potassium on peripheral veins.

Hypomagnesemia

Hypomagnesemia is common following cardiac surgery using CPB. Magnesium mimics potassium in its effects on the electrical activity of the heart. The cause of the hypomagnesemia is unknown, but it is probably multifactorial. Many patients will be hypomagnesemic preoperatively due to the use of loop diuretics, thiazides, digoxin, or alcohol and to the effects of type I diabetes mellitus. Magnesium is usually lost in the urine during CPB. Patients with postoperative hypomagnesemia develop atrial and ventricular dysrhythmias more frequently and require more prolonged mechanical ventilatory support than do patients with normal magnesium levels.[36] Magnesium administration also seems to improve stroke volume and cardiac index in the early postoperative period.[37] Magnesium can be administered as magnesium sulfate (2 g in 100-mL solution) to raise serum levels to 2 meq/L.

Hyperglycemia

During CPB there is a rise in blood glucose levels. The elevation is modest during hypothermia and becomes more marked during rewarming. This rise in glucose is due in part to increased glucose mobilization related to dramatic increases in cortisol, catecholamine, and growth hormone levels during CPB. Also, there is an apparent failure of insulin secretion, particularly during hypothermia, probably related to inhibition of the insulin secretory response by the elevated catecholamines. This blunting of the insulin response persists for the first 24 h after surgery. These changes are exaggerated in the diabetic patient.[38] Insulin requirements are likely to be seven times greater than the preoperative requirements during the first 4 h postoperatively. Furthermore, such diabetogenic stimuli as catecholamines, diuretics, and blood transfusions are likely to be used in the postoperative period.[39] These multiple factors make the diabetic patient susceptible to hyperosmolar, hyperglycemia, nonketotic diabetic coma.[40]

POSTOPERATIVE FEVER

Fever is a common occurrence in the postoperative patient. It is generally a consequence of pleuropericarditis, atelectasis, or phlebitis. The fact that some 70 percent of patients have atelectasis after cardiac surgery makes it the most likely etiology of postoperative fever.[30] A reasonable assumption in a patient with a core temperature less than 38°C and no evidence of phlebitis or presence of a pericardial or pleural rub is that the source of the fever is atelectasis. The appropriate therapeutic approach is to encourage intensified efforts at incentive spirometry and coughing. Any fever over 38.5°C warrants blood, sputum, and urine cultures. A white blood count (total and differential) and a chest x-ray should also be obtained.

Sternal wound infections occur in 0.4 and 5 percent of patients after sternotomy.[41-43] Multiple factors have been identified as increasing the risk of developing sternal wound infection. These include pneumonia, prolonged mechanical ventilation (especially with tracheostomy), emergency operations, postoperative hemorrhage with mediastinal hematoma, early reexploration, obesity, diabetes mellitus, and use of bilateral internal mammary grafts. While some studies have not found a higher prevalence of sternal wound infections with bilateral mammary grafts, the bulk of the evidence argues to the contrary. Perhaps some of the conflicting results can be explained by the fact that different degrees of devascularization of the sternum occur, depending on the particular internal mammary artery harvesting technique employed. The greatest risk for sternal infection seems to be in diabetic patients who receive bilateral internal mammary grafts.[42] Debate continues as to whether the most appropriate initial treatment is debridement and closure or open packing and subsequent plastic surgical closure with a muscle flap.

Approximately 1 percent of coronary artery bypass surgery patients experience leg wound infections that necessitate extra care. Leg infections seem to occur more frequently in obese women, especially if the thigh veins are harvested.[44]

NEUROLOGIC AND NEUROPHYSIOLOGICAL DYSFUNCTION

Mechanism

The mechanisms thought to account for most cerebral injury during cardiac surgery are macroembolization of air, debris from aortic atheroma, or left ventricular thrombus; microembolization of aggregates of granulocytes, platelets, and fibrin; and cerebral hypoperfusion. Death or disabling stroke occurs in about 2 percent of patients, with another 3 percent experiencing transient or minor functional disability secondary to cerebral infarction. Focal neurologic deficits resulting from intraoperative events are usually noted within the first 24 to 48 h after surgery.

Encephalopathy and Delirium

Alteration of mental status (encephalopathy and delirium) will be seen in approximately 30 percent of patients after cardiopulmonary bypass.[45] While the appearance of these encephalopathic symptoms likely reflects cerebral injury, other causes must be excluded, including drugs, sepsis, fever, hypoxemia, ethanol withdrawal, renal failure, and hyperosmolar state. Postoperative encephalopathic changes, varying from mild confusion and disorientation to protracted somnolence or agitation and hallucinations, may appear at any time during the hospital stay. In fact, some physicians will not accept a diagnosis of postcardiotomy delirium unless the delirium develops following a lucid interval of 2 to 5 days after surgery. Studies of this condition have not identified any consistent risk factors, but advancing age, duration of CPB, and sleep deprivation have been frequently associated. It has been suggested that the insomnia may follow rather than precede the onset of delirium. The prevalence of this condition has remained rather constant since the early days of cardiac surgery involving CPB, but there has been a shift in the clinical presentation. Currently, the condition seems to present with disorientation rather than the hallucinations, paranoid ideation, and agitation noted earlier.[45] Recognition of this entity is important because the family can be assured that the patient's mental status is very likely to be normal by the time of hospital discharge. Agitation and acute psychosis in these patients usually respond to intravenous haloperidol, 2 to 10 mg, repeated as needed to produce adequate sedation.

Some disorientation, especially in elderly patients, is due to their removal from familiar surroundings and the threats implicit in the ICU and hospital settings. Fast-tracking may be beneficial in minimizing situational anxiety and disorientation.

Brachial Plexopathy and Ulnar Nerve Dysfunction

Another serious neurologic complication of cardiac surgery is brachial plexopathy. This neurologic dysfunction, involving C8 and T1, usually results from mechanical trauma secondary to sternal retraction but may be due to penetration by a posterior fractured segment of the first rib or injury during internal jugular cannulation. There is no specific therapy for this condition, and recovery can take as long as 6 months, with a few cases being permanent.[46,47] Ulnar nerve dysfunction may result from malpositioning of the upper extremities during surgery that results in pressure being exerted on the ulnar nerve at the elbow.

REFERENCES

1. Cameron D. Initiation of white cell activation during cardiopulmonary bypass: Cytokines and receptors. *Cardiovasc Pharmacol* 166; 27(suppl 1):S1–S5.
2. Chong JL, Pillai R, Fisher A, Grebenik C, Sinclair M, Westaby S. Cardiac surgery, moving away from intensive care. *Br Heart J* 1992; 68:430–433.
3. Aps C. Fast-tracking in cardiac surgery. *Br J Hosp Med* 1995; 54:139–142.
4. Jindosi A, Aps C, Neville E, Sonmez B, Tun K, Williams BT, et al. Postoperative cardiac surgical care: An alternative approach. *Br Heart J* 1993; 69:59–64.
5. Bojar RM. *Manual of Perioperative Care in Cardiac and Thoracic Surgery*, 2d ed. Boston: Blackwell Scientific; 1994.
6. Levy JH, Salemenpera MT, Bailey JM, Ramsey JG. Postoperative circulatory control. In: Kaplan JA, ed. *Cardiac Anesthesia*, 3d ed. Philadelphia: Saunders; 1993:1168–1193.
7. Swanson DK, Myerowitz PD. Effect of reperfusion temperature and pressure on the functional and metabolic recovery of preserved hearts. *J Thorac Cardiovasc Surg* 1983; 86:242–251.
8. Gold JP, Roberts AJ, Hoover EL, Bland S, Gay WA Jr, Subramanian VA. Effects of prolonged aortic cross clamping with potassium cardioplegia on myocardial contractility in man. *Surg Forum* 1979; 30:252–254.
9. Spiess BD. Ischemia—a coagulation problem? *J Cardiovasc Pharmacol* 1996; 27(suppl 1):538–541.
10. Verrier E. The microvascular cell and ischemia-reperfusion injury. *J Cardiovasc Pharmacol* 1996; 27(suppl 1):S26–S30.
11. Bolli R. Oxygen derived free radical and postischemic myocardial dysfunction. *J Am Coll Cardiol* 1988; 12:239–249.
12. Przyklenk K, Kloner RA. "Reperfusion injury" by oxygen derived free radicals? *Circ Res* 1989; 64:86–96.
13. Breisblatt WM, Stein KI, Wolfe CJ, Follansbee WP, Capozzi J, Armitage JM, et al. Acute myocardial dysfunction and recovery: A common occurrence after coronary bypass surgery. *J Am Coll Cardiol* 1990; 15:1261–1269.
14. Donati F, Maille JG, Blain R, Boulanger M, Sahab P. End-tidal carbon dioxide tension and temperature changes after coronary artery bypass surgery. *Can Anaesth Soc J* 1985; 32:272–277.
15. Ralley FE, Wynando JE, Rams JG, Carli F, MacSullivan R. The effects of shivering on oxygen consumption and carbon dioxide production in patients rewarming from hypothermic cardiopulmonary bypass. *Can J Anaesth* 1988; 35:332–337.
16. Woodman RC, Harker LA. Bleeding complications associated with cardiopulmonary bypass. *Blood* 1990; 76:1680–1697.
17. Harker L. Malpass TW, Branson HE, Hessel EA 2d, Slichter SJ. Mechanism of abnormal bleeding in patients undergoing cardiopulmo-nary bypass: Acquired transient platelet dysfunction associated with selective alpha-granule release. *Blood* 1980; 56:824–834.
18. Ellis RJ, Mangano DT, Van Dyke DC. Relationship of wedge pressure to end diastolic volume in patients undergoing myocardial revascularization. *J Thorac Cardiovasc Surg* 1979; 78:605–613.
19. Palmer RF, Lasseter KC. Drug therapy: Sodium nitroprusside. *N Engl J Med* 1975; 292:294–297.
20. Flaherty JT, Magee PA, Gardner TL, Potter A, MacAllister NP. Comparison of intravenous nitroglycerin and sodium nitroprusside for treatment of acute hypertension developing after coronary bypass surgery. *Circulation* 1982; 65:1072–1077.
21. Lambert CR, Hill JA, Feldman RL, Pepine CJ. Effects of nicardipine on exercise- and pacing-induced myocardial ischemia in angina pectoris. *Am J Cardiol* 1987; 60:471–476.
22. Gray RJ, Bateman TM, Czer LS, Conklin C, Matloff JM. Comparison of esmolol and nitroprusside from acute postcardiac surgical hypertension. *Am J Cardiol* 1987; 59:887–891.
23. Topol EJ, Lerman BB, Baughman KL, Platia EV, Griffith LS. De novo refractory ventricular tachyarrhythmias after coronary revascularization. *Am J Cardiol* 1986; 57:57–59.
24. Leith JW, Thomson D, Baird DK, Harris PJ. The importance of age as a predictor of atrial fibrillation and flutter after coronary artery bypass grafting. *J Thorac Cardiovasc Surg* 1990; 100:338–342.
25. Hashimoto K, Ilstrup DM, Schaff HV. Influence of clinical and hemodynamic variables on risk of supraventricular tachycardia after coronary artery bypass. *J Thorac Cardiovasc Surg* 1991; 101:56–65.
26. Fuller JA, Adams GG, Buxton B. Atrial fibrillation after coronary artery bypass grafting. Is it a disorder of the elderly? *J Thorac Cardiovasc Surg* 1989; 97:821–825.
27. Andrews TC, Reimold SC, Berlin JA, Antman EM. Prevention of supraventricular arrhythmias after coronary artery bypass surgery. A meta-analysis of randomized controlled trials. *Circulation* 1991; 84(suppl III):III-236–III-244.
28. Baerman JM, Kirsch MM, de Buitleir M, Hyatt L, Juni JE, Pitt B, et al. Natural history and determinates of conduction defects following coronary artery bypass surgery. *Ann Thorac Surg* 1987; 44:150–153.
29. Tuzcu EM, Emre A, Goormastic M, Loop FD. Incidence and prognostic significance of intraventricular conduction abnormalities after coronary bypass surgery. *J Am Coll Cardiol* 1990; 16:607–610.
30. Sladden RN, Berkowitz DE. Cardiopulmonary bypass and the lung. In: Gravlee GP, Davis RF, Utley IR, eds. *Cardiopulmonary Bypass*. Baltimore: Williams & Wilkins; 1993:468 487.
31. Ramsey J. The respiratory, renal and hepatic systems: Effects of cardiac surgery and cardiopulmonary bypass. In: Mora CT, ed. *Cardiopulmonary Bypass*. New York: Springer; 1995:147–168.
32. Hanks JB, Curtis SE, Hanks BB, Andersen DK, Cox JL, Jones RS. Gastrointestinal complications after cardiopulmonary bypass. *Surgery* 1982; 92:394–400.
33. Welling RE, Rath R, Albers JE, Glaser RS. Gastrointestinal complications after cardiac surgery. *Arch Surg* 1986; 121:1178–1180.
34. Mori A, Watanabe K, Onoe M, Watarida S, Nakamura Y, Magara Y, et al. Regional blood flow in the liver, pancreas, and kidney during pulsatile and nonpulsatile perfusion under profound hypothermia. *Jpn Circ J* 1988; 52:219–227.
35. Collins JD, Bassendine MF, Ferner R, Blesovsky A, Murray A, Pearson DT, et al. Incidence and prognostic importance of jaundice after cardiopulmonary bypass surgery. *Lancet* 1983; 1:1119–1123.
36. Aglio LS, Stanford GG, Maddi R, Boyd JL 3d, Nussbaum S, Chernow B. Hypomagnesemia is common following cardiac surgery. *J Cardiothorac Anesth* 1991; 5:201–208.
37. England MR, Gordon G, Salem M, Chernow B. Magnesium administration and dysrhythmias after cardiac surgery: A placebo-controlled, double-blind, randomized trial. *JAMA* 1993; 269:2369–2370.
38. Frater RW, Oka Y, Kadish A, Chilukuri S, Becker RM. Diabetes and coronary artery surgery. *Mt Sinai J Med* 1982; 49:237–240.
39. Elliott MJ, Gill GV, Home PD, Noy GA, Holden MP, Alberti KG. A comparison of two regimens for the management of diabetes during open-heart surgery. *Anesthesiology* 1984; 60:364–368.
40. Seki S. Clinical features of hyperglycemia nonketotic diabetic coma associated with cardiac operations. *J Thorac Cardiovasc Surg* 1986; 91:8678–8687.
41. Ulicny KS, Hiradzka SF. The risk factors of median sternotomy infection: A current review. *J Cardiac Surg* 1991; 6:338–351.

42. Hazelrigg SR, Wellons HA, Schneider JA, Kolm P. Wound complications after median sternotomy: Relationship to internal mammary grafting. *J Thorac Cardiovasc Surg* 1989; 98:1096–1099.

43. Grossi EA, Esposito R, Harris LJ, Crooke GA, Galloway AC, Colvin SB, et al. Sternal wound infections and use of internal mammary artery grafts. *J Thorac Cardiovasc Surg* 1991; 102:342–347.

44. De Laria GA, Hunter JA, Goldin MD, Serry C, Javid H, Najafi H. Leg wound complications associated with coronary revascularization. *J Thorac Cardiovasc Surg* 1981; 81:403–407.

45. Smith LW, Dimsdale JE. Postcardiotomy delirium: Conclusions after 25 years? *Am J Psychiatry* 1989; 146:452–458.

46. Breuer AC, Furlan AJ, Hanson MR, Lederman RJ, Loop FD, Cosgrove DM, et al. Central nervous system complications of coronary artery bypass graft surgery: Prospective analysis of 421 patients. *Stroke* 1983; 14:82–87.

47. Shaw PJ, Bates D, Cartlidge NE, Heaviside D, Julian DG, Shaw DA. Early neurological complications of coronary artery bypass surgery. *Br Med J* 1985; 91:1384–1387.

52

THROMBOGENESIS AND ANTITHROMBOTIC THERAPY

Marc Verstraete / Valentin Fuster

HEMOSTASIS, FIBRINOLYSIS, ANTITHROMBOTICS, AND FIBRINOLYTICS

Hemostasis

The arrest of bleeding at the site of blood vessel injury is called *hemostasis;* it is one of the most important host defense mechanisms. Hemostasis serves to preserve the integrity of the closed, high-pressure circulatory system and to limit blood loss. Extensive laboratory research has led to a better understanding of the mechanisms by which both maintenance of blood fluidity and prompt, timely arrest of hemorrhage are achieved. Clinical observations in patients with bleeding or thrombotic disorders have provided important insight into the nature of in vivo hemostasis.

The hemostatic system consists of blood vessels, platelets, procoagulants and anticoagulants, profibrinolytic components, and inhibitors. For clarity, the following sections deal with each component of the hemostatic mechanism individually. It cannot be overemphasized, however, that these processes are intimately related and inseparable.

ROLE OF VESSEL WALL CONTRACTION AND ENDOTHELIUM IN HEMOSTASIS

The immediate control of bleeding from a small severed vessel is vasoconstriction. This primary hemostasis is transient and probably of minor importance in most tissues except in the uterine during menstruation and in arteries, which have a more developed muscular coat than veins. However, the vast majority of vessels are capillaries, which do not have smooth muscle cells and where bleeding immediately stops as the capillaries collapse after transsection. Breaks in arterioles and venules, on the other hand, first but temporarily depend on vascular contraction, soon followed by local perivascular and intravascular activation of platelets and coagulation compo-

nents. What maintains vasoconstriction is only poorly understood. As described in further sections, thromboxane A_2 (TXA_2) produced and released by activated platelets may play a role, as do products released by stimulated endothelium (endothelin) or generated during coagulation (bradykinin generated by activated factor XII and fibrinopeptide B).

One of the unsolved mysteries of hemostasis and thrombosis is why circulating platelets do not or hardly ever adhere to normal (unstimulated) endothelial cells in vivo. One possible answer is that both platelets and endothelium have a negative charge and thus would be mutually repulsive. The negative electrical charge of endothelial cells is due to a pronounced glycocalyx, consisting of proteoglycans, of which heparan sulfate (a heparin-like substance that binds antithrombin III) is the most important. Stimulated or injured endothelial cells lose their negative surface charge or anionic property. The nonthrombogenic nature of endothelium is also partly due to the lack of surface molecules as tissue factor.

The thromboresistance of normal endothelium is also dependent on several substances produced by endothelial cells. They include potent vasodilators and inhibitors of platelet function, such as prostacyclin (PGI_2) and endothelium derived relaxing factor (EDRF), nitrous oxide (NO), which serve to prevent platelet adhesion to endothelium.[1,2] Anticoagulant properties "include" heparin-like glycosaminoglycans (GAG) and a thrombin-binding protein called *thrombomodulin.*

The production of prostacyclin by endothelium is stimulated by contact with activated platelets or leukocytes by stretching of the arterial wall (pulsatile pressure) and by some drugs. PGI_1 has strong antiplatelet and vasodilator properties and thus acts as the biological antagonist of thromboxane A_2. A direct link between impaired biosynthesis of PGI_2 in the vessel wall and thrombosis or atherosclerosis is suggested by the decreased capacity of endothelium to generate prostacyclin with age, atherosclerosis, and risk factors such as high choles-

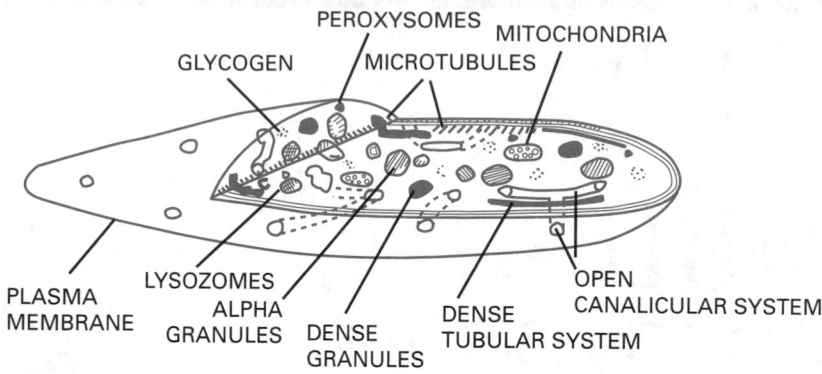

FIGURE 52-1

Platelet structure and main constituents: the dense granules [adenosine diphosphate (ADP), adenosine triphosphate (ATP), calcium, serotonin]; alpha granules [β-thromboglobulin, platelet factor 4, platelet-derived growth factor (PDGF), von Willebrand factor, factor V, fibrinogen, plasminogen activator inhibitor (PAI-1), protease nexin-II, thrombospondin, fibronectin, P-selectin]; lysozomes (acid hydrolases, cathepsin D, E); and peroxysomes (catalase).

terol, heavy smoking, and diabetes. EDRF is formed from L-arginine by an oxidation pathway that requires several cofactors. EDRF relaxes smooth muscle cells through stimulation of guanylate cyclase, which, in turn, generates cyclic guanosine monophosphate (cyclic GMP).[3] By the same mechanism, it is also a potent inhibitor of adhesion and aggregation of platelets. There is a clear synergism between prostacyclin and EDRF in preventing platelet activation. EDRF is effective only in the immediate vicinity of its site of release because hemoglobin almost immediately inactivates any EDRF that enters the

bloodstream. It has been suggested that a deficiency in EDRF production contributes to the pathogenesis of atherosclerosis and to the development of complications of diabetes. Thrombomodulin is a transmembranous protein that serves as an endothelial receptor for free thrombin.[4] In the complex that is formed and which does not require calcium, thrombin loses its procoagulant activity and expresses its anticoagulant role by activating protein C.

Thus, apart from a metabolic function with respect to the synthesis of vasoactive substances, the primary role of endothelium is in maintaining the patency of the blood vessels and the fluidity of blood. However, endothelium also has the potential to enhance and amplify the formation of a hemostatic plug initiated by a local endothelial lesion, as discussed in subsequent sections.

ROLE OF PLATELETS IN HEMOSTASIS

The exterior coat of platelets, the glycocalyx, contains many distinct glycoproteins that are important for platelet function. They include integrins and leucine-rich glycoproteins. These surface glycoproteins mediate platelet adhesion and aggregation as receptors for adhesive proteins and agonists. The platelets contain dense bodies, alpha granules, actin filaments, microtubules, and an open canalicular system, which all have their respective functions in the formation of a hemostatic plug (Fig. 52-1).

In normal conditions, platelets are quiescent and circulate freely in the blood because they do not attach to a normally functioning endothelium. Vessel injury, however, exposes subendothelial connective tissue to various elements to which platelets can adhere.[5,6] This phenomenon, platelet adhesion, is the initial event and one of the most crucial steps in platelet plug formation. The adhesive proteins collagen and fibronectin (and to a lesser extent laminin, microfibrils, and thrombospondin) are present in subendothelium and interact readily with von Willebrand factor, whereby this large protein changes its conformation. This allows platelets to bind to von Willebrand factor via their surface glycoprotein receptors Ia/IIa and Ic/IIa (Figs. 52-2 and 52-3).

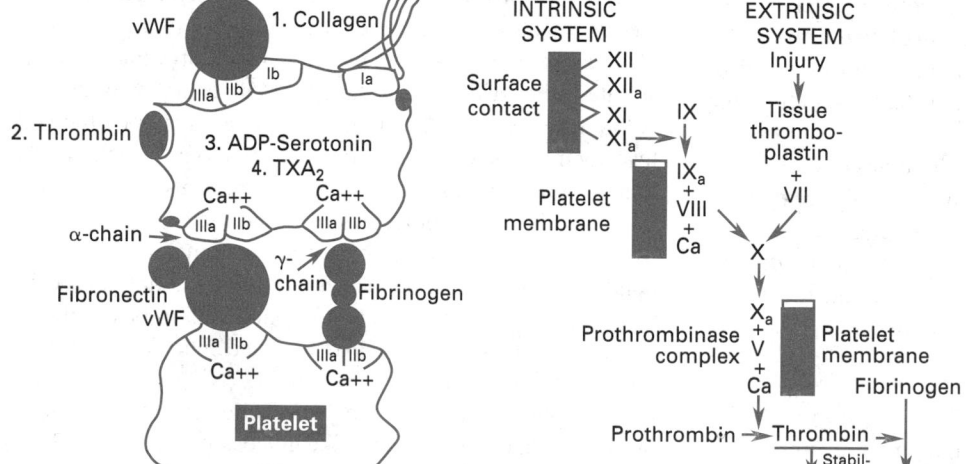

FIGURE 52-2

Interactions among platelet membrane receptors (glycoproteins Ia, Ib, and IIb/IIIa), adhesive macromolecules, and the disrupted vessel wall (*left panel*) and a flowchart of the intrinsic and extrinsic systems of the coagulation cascade (*right panel*). In the left panel, arabic numerals indicate the pathways of platelet activation that are dependent on (1) collagen, (2) thrombin, (3) ADP and serotonin, and (4) thromboxane A₂ (TXA₂); there are also some reports suggesting the binding of von Willebrand factor (vWF) (polymeric protein) to collagen or heparin. Note the interaction of the right panel between clotting factors (XII, XIIa, XI, XIa, IX, IXa, VII, VIII, X, Xa, V, and XIIIa) and the platelet membrane. (From Fuster V, Badimon L, Badimon JH. The pathogenesis of coronary artery disease and the acute coronary syndromes. *N Engl J Med* 1992; 326:315. Copyright Massachusetts Medical Society.)

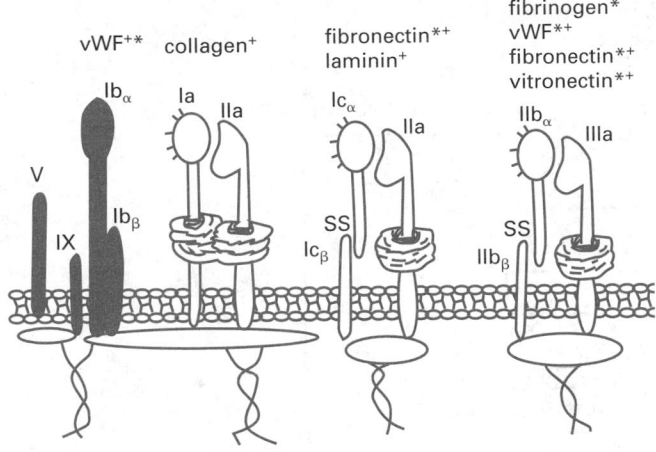

vWF[+*] collagen[+] fibronectin[*+] fibrinogen[*]
laminin[+] vWF[*+]
fibronectin[*+]
vitronectin[*+]

FIGURE 52-3

Interaction among platelet membrane receptors (glycoproteins) and adhesive macromolecules of plasma and/or disrupted vessel wall. * = present in plasma; + = present in vessel wall.

Particularly collagen, a ubiquitous structural component of the vessel wall, is important and may provide a scaffolding on which other adhesive proteins assemble. Von Willebrand factor, which has two collagen binding sites, is an absolute requirement of platelet adhesion, but only at high shear rates; whereas fibronectin plays a significant role in platelet adhesion at lower shear rates. It is interesting to note that platelet adhesion increases progressively as the hemacrit rises in flowing blood. After adhesion, platelets lose their discoid shape, form extended pseudopods, and spread out over the injured surface. Through the action of activators such as collagen and eventually thrombin and norepinephrine, the adhered platelets soon become activated, whereby other platelet receptors are expressed and several mediators stored in platelet granules are released.[7] This release reaction seems to be initiated by contraction of a circumferential band of microtubules. Stored granules are discharged through the open canalicular system after fusion of the granular membrane with the membranes of the open canalicular system. Among the granular agents released are adenosine diphosphate (ADP), serotonin, beta thromboglobulin, platelet factor 4, platelet growth factor, and thromboxane A_2.[8,9]

These released substances, particularly ADP and TXA_2, induce binding of platelets to one another, a phenomenon called *platelet aggregation.* This process increases the size of the hemostatic plug at the site of injury and, by recruiting additional circulating platelets, transforms the initial monolayer of platelets into an aggregate. The platelet surface glycoproteins IIb-IIIa undergo a conformational change in the aggregation process, so that they can interact with plasma fibrinogen and other adhesive proteins as fibronectin and endothelial thrombospondin, which serve to link platelets together into a tighter aggregate.[10,11] In addition, a group of lipids, the prostaglandins, play an important role in mediating the platelet release reaction and aggregation (Fig. 52-3). Collagen and epinephrine appear to trigger the activation of one or more phos-

pholipases in the platelet membrane. Phospholipase A_2 acts on phosphatidylcholine to release arachidonic acid from the platelet membrane. Arachidonic acid is metabolized by cyclooxygenase to unstable proaggregating prostaglandin endoperoxide intermediates (prostaglandins G_2 and H_2). Thromboxane A_2 is formed by the action of thromboxane synthase on prostaglandin H_2; it further promotes platelet activation, thrombus growth, and local vasoconstriction. On the other hand, the vascular endothelial cells synthesize prostacyclin (PGI_2) starting from arachidonic acid or from platelet-derived prostaglandin G_2. Prostacyclin stimulates adenylate cyclase and leads to an increased level of cyclic adenosine monophosphate (cyclic AMP) in the platelet (Fig. 52-4). Cyclic AMP, in turn, inhibits the discharge of calcium from the dense tubular system and thus prevents platelet aggregation and secretion. Phosphodiesterase enhances the breakdown of cyclic AMP.

Arachidonic acid also serves as a substrate for the formation of leukotrienes, a pathway mediated by lipoxygenase in the leukocytes. Thus, eicosanoids derived from arachidonic acid in platelets, endothelial cells, and leukocytes provide short-acting biological mediators that further promote not only platelet activation and local vasoconstriction but also platelet inhibition and vasodilatation. In addition, they intervene in local immune mediated reactions.

ROLE OF BLOOD FLOW IN HEMOSTASIS

The blood flow not only transports platelet and coagulation factors to the site of injury but also removes activated products from the circulation. Blood flow also influences platelet function by shear stress. Exposure of platelets to very high shear stress leads to spontaneous aggregation even in the absence of exogenous agonists. Furthermore, some coagulation reactions are accelerated in the presence of high shear, and the ability of the endothelium to secrete tissue plasminogen activator over the basal level is increased two- to threefold.

ROLE OF BLOOD COAGULATION IN HEMOSTASIS

Activated platelets provide a microenvironment that enhances the acceleration of fibrin formation at the site of injury. They rearrange their surface lipoproteins so that phospholipids, on which coagulation factors can concentrate, are now exposed to the bloodstream. This is accompanied by the exposure of high-affinity binding sites for the activated factors V, VIII, IX, and X. Thus, activated platelets provide a suitable surface on which the activation of prothrombin to thrombin is accelerated dramatically. Thrombin occupies a central position in the coagulation process. It is formed as the end product of a complex chain of reactions that transform, in sequence, a number of coagulation factors present as precursors (*zymogens*) in plasma into activated factors. Table 52-1 lists the well-recognized coagulation factors with their Roman numeral designations and synonyms and some of their properties. The coagulation factors are numbered roughly in the order of their discovery and do not reflect the sequence of reactions. Coagulation factors interact mainly on the membrane of activated platelets and other stimulated cells and tissue factor (a

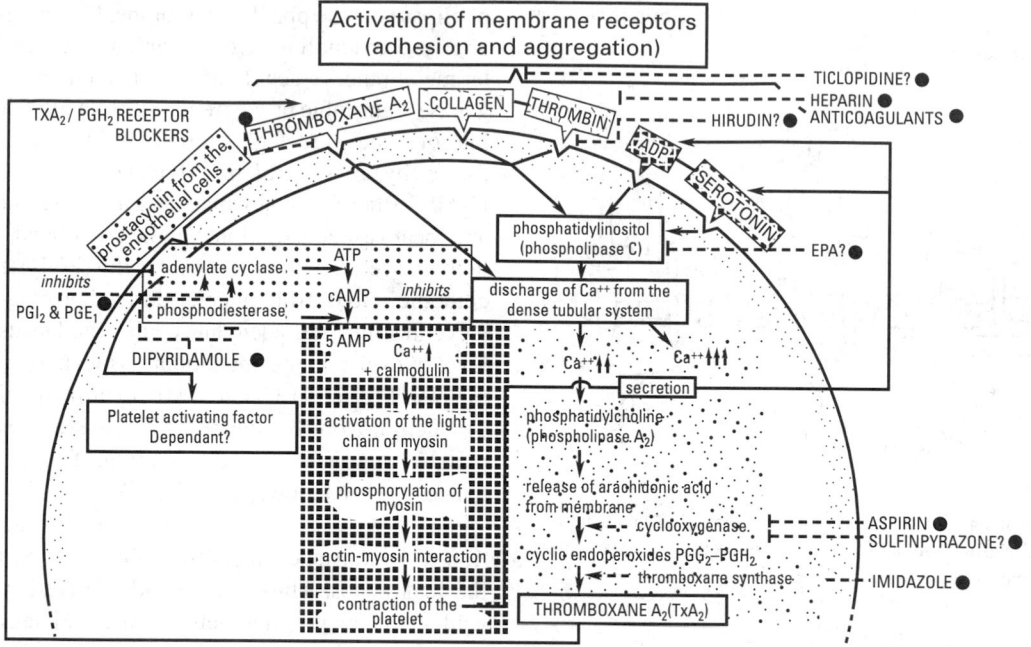

FIGURE 52-4

Mechanism of platelet activation and presumed sites of action of various platelet inhibitor agents. Platelet agonists lead to the mobilization of calcium (Ca^{2+}), which functions as a mediator of platelet activation through metabolic pathways dependent on adenosine diphosphate (ADP), thromboxane A_2 (TXA_2), thrombin, and collagen. Cyclic adenosine monophosphate (cAMP) inhibits calcium mobilization from the dense tubular system. Note that thrombin and collagen may independently activate platelets by means of platelet activating factor. ($\bullet$) = a platelet inhibitor; dashed line = a presumed site of drug action; ATP = adenosine triphosphate; EPA = eicosapentaenoic acid; PGE_1 = prostaglandin E_1; PGH_2 = prostaglandin H_2; PGI_2 = prostaglandin I_2. (From Stein B, Fuster V, Israel DH, Cohen M, Badimon L, Badimon JJ, et al. Platelet inhibitor agents in cardiovascular disease: An update. *J Am Coll Cardiol* 1989; 14:816, with permission.)

TABLE 52-1

GLOSSARY OF THE COAGULATION FACTORS AND SOME OF THEIR PROPERTIES

Factor	Synonyms	Molecular Weight	Plasma Concentration, mg/dL	In Vivo Half-Life, h	Inheritance
I	Fibrinogen	340,000	200–400	100–150	AD
II	Prothrombin	70,000	10	50–80	AD
III	Tissue thromboplastin, tissue factor	44,000	0		
IV	Calcium ion	40	9–10		
V	Proaccelerin, labile factor	330,000	1	24	AR
VII	Serum prothrombin conversion accelerator (SPCA), stable factor	48,000	0.05	6	AR
VIII	Antihemophilic factor (AHF)	330,000	0.01	12	SLR
von Willebrand factor		$(250,000)n^a$	1	24	AD
IX	Christmas factor	55,000	0.3	24	SLR
X	Stuart-Power factor	59,000	1	25–60	AR
XI	Plasma thromboplastin antecedent (PTA)	160,000	0.5	40–80	AR
XII	Hageman factor	80,000	3	50–70	AR
XIII	Fibrin-stabilizing factor (FSF)	320,000	1–2	150	AD
Prekallikrein	Fletcher factor	85,000	5	35	AR
High-molecular-weight kininogen	Fitzgerald, Flaujeac, Williams factor, contact activation cofactor	120,000	6	150	AR

^{a} Multimers of the dimer subunit.

Key: AD = autosomal dominant; AR = autosomal recessive; SLR = sex-linked recessive.

membrane protein exposed to the blood, e.g., after trauma) on which coagulation factors bind. Because of the low concentration of these factors in plasma and the abundant presence of circulating inhibitors, the interaction of procoagulants and their subsequent activation can proceed only slowly in the fluid phase of blood.

Coagulation factors are activated one by one, mainly through limited proteolysis. When the letter "a" accompanies a Roman numeral (e.g., factor VIIa), this indicates that the factor is in its activated form rather than in its naturally occurring precursor form (e.g., factor X). All activated factors are serine proteases: they split arginyl bonds in their specific substrate, and the latter then becomes another activated coagulation factor (waterfall or cascade sequence of events). In contrast, factors V and VIII, tissue factor and high-molecular-weight (HMW) kininogen, are not proenzymes but function rather as cofactors. They can thus be considered as regulatory proteins (cofactors) that influence the reaction rate. These cofactors (except tissue factor) still require activation by minor proteolysis, while tissue factor X, present in extravascular spaces, must make contact with blood to function. The traditional coagulation scheme distinguishes an "intrinsic" from an "extrinsic" activation pathway.

The "Intrinsic" Pathway of the Coagulation System: Activation of Factors XII, XI, X, and IX

All factors participating in the intrinsic pathway are present in circulating blood, and the reaction sequence is initiated by contact of platelets and/or coagulation components with a subendothelial tissue. Antigen-antibody complexes and activated platelets may also serve this purpose, as can fissured atherosclerotic plaques and foreign surfaces, such as those in an extracorporeal circulation or renal dialysis. In vitro, this initial contact phase involves the interaction of factor XII (Hageman factor), factor XI, prekallikrein, and HMW kininogen with a foreign surface (a surface other than normal endothelium or blood cells). However, the precise mechanism of the initial firing spark triggering the contact activation in vivo remains elusive.

When circulating factor XII meets negatively charged surfaces such as glass and kaolin, it binds via its heavy chain to the surface. Upon adsorption, bound factor XII now exerts traces of biological activity. For the mechanisms of this phenomenon, conformation changes of the molecule with exposure of the enzyme site in the light chain have been postulated (Fig. 52-5). Factor XI and prekallikrein exist in plasma as equimolar complexes with HMW kininogen, and these complexes are bound to initiating surfaces via the HMW kininogen moiety. HMW kininogen transports both factor XI and prekallikrein to an appropriate surface. Surface binding is assumed to serve to bring factor XII, prekallikrein, and factor XI to a close spatial orientation. Binding of factor XII to a negatively charged surface also makes the molecule more susceptible to proteolytic cleavage. Initially, traces of factor XIIa presumably generate traces of kallikrein from prekallikrein by splitting of a single peptide bond. Kallikrein will now activate

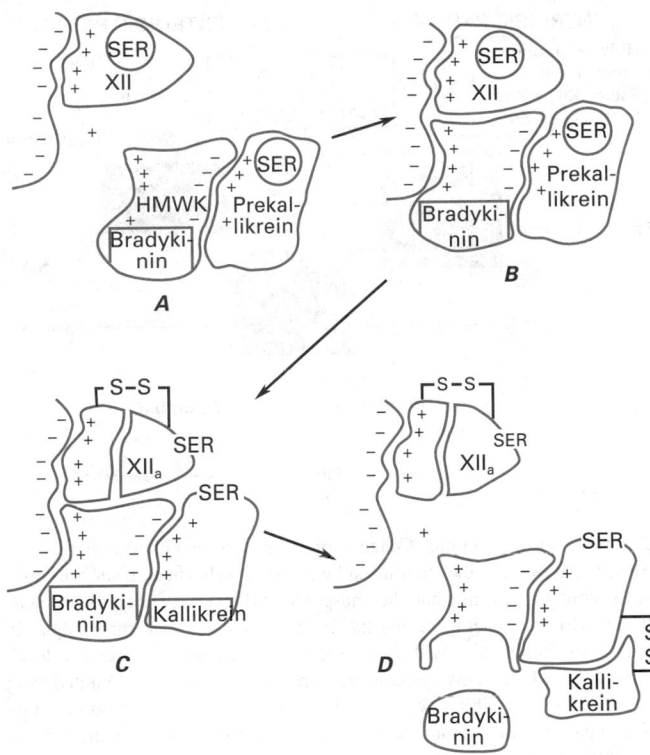

FIGURE 52-5

In the intrinsic pathway of coagulation, *contact activation* refers to a series of reactions following adsorption of factors XII and XI as well as prekallikrein and high-molecular-weight kininogen to highly negatively charged surfaces. The contact activation does not require calcium and results in surface-induced conformational changes of the molecules. *A* to *D:* Sequence of events. SER = serine protease.

more rapidly factor XII in a feedback loop, which, in turn, will generate more kallikrein, and the reciprocal activation of these two surface-bound molecules continues until the substrates are locally exhausted. Of note, a potent vasoactive substance, bradykinin, is released from HMW kininogen upon the activation of factor XII and generation of kallikrein. The latter also activates prourokinase, enhancing fibrinolytic activity.

Factor XIIa converts in vitro the next factor of the coagulation cascade, factor XI, from its zymogen form to its enzymatic constellation. Factor XI also circulates in plasma complexed with HMW kininogen; the latter protein thus serves as helper protein carrying factors XII and XI in the blood (Fig. 52-6). The in vivo activation of factor XI is less clear. It is possible that factor XII–independent activation of factor XI is mediated by thrombin. Both factor XIIa and thrombin cleave the same internal peptide bond (Arg369-Ile) in each of the two chains of the factor XI molecule, leading to the formation of two heavy and two light chains.

Factor XIa bound to the surfaces by HMW kininogen interacts upon activation with factor IX in a calcium-dependent two-step reaction. Each light chain of factor XIa contains a catalytic site, while its heavy chain has the binding site for factor IX and HMW kininogen. Binding of calcium ions to factor IX (a vitamin K–dependent protein) induces a confor-

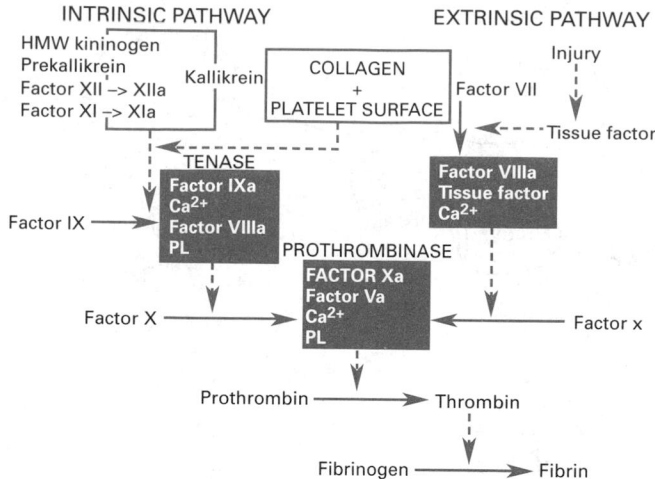

INTRINSIC PATHWAY   EXTRINSIC PATHWAY

FIGURE 52-6

Clotting factor interactions. Coagulation is initiated by either an intrinsic or extrinsic pathway. In the intrinsic pathway, negatively charged surfaces initiate the contact activation and the phospholipid (PL) is furnished by platelets. In the extrinsic system, the phospholipid portion of tissue thromboplastin functions in conjunction with factor VIIa on the activation of factor X. From factor Xa on, both pathways converge upon a common path. Omitted from the diagram are inhibitors of the various steps, the augmentation of action of each pathway by activated factors, and the interaction between the intrinsic and extrinsic systems.

mational change in the molecule which facilitates its binding to the heavy chain of factor XIa, which is essential for the optimal rate of factor IX activation. Platelets can also be reckoned to be important in the intrinsic system as they contain HMW kininogen, which can be expressed when the platelets are activated, as they indeed are on fissured and sclerotic plaques and foreign surfaces.

Activated factor IX, thrombin-modified factor VIII, negatively charged phospholipid (e.g., activated platelets), and calcium ions form a multimolecular complex coined *tenase* because it activates directly factor X; the Gla residues of factors IXa and Xa mediate their binding to phospholipid (Fig. 52-6).

Congenital deficiency of the three contact factors (factor XII, prekallikrein, HMW kininogen) is *not* associated with bleeding, and only half of factor XI–deficient patients have bleeding problems with an intensity not related to the factor XI level. The significance of the contact phase is, therefore, speculative; however, it may become relevant in particular therapeutic settings. Indeed, extracorporeal circuits may be regarded as a giant test-tube condition, and the contact activation becomes important under these circumstances. Beyond the contact phase, the intrinsic activation system is important, already in physiologic conditions, as individuals with a severe deficiency of factor VIII or IX (two forms of hemophilia) have a serious bleeding condition.

The "Extrinsic" (Tissue Factor) Pathway of the Coagulation System: Activation of Factors VII and X

In the "extrinsic" system, membrane-bound tissue factor starts off the chain of events by forming a complex with factor VII in the presence of calcium ions (Fig. 52-6). Tissue factor is

as a dimer composed of two identical subunits with interacting enzyme binding sites.[12,13] It is present on nonvascular cell surfaces and on microvesicles shed from cell surfaces. It was hypothesized that the normal distribution of tissue factor represents a hemostatic envelope ready to activate coagulation when vascular integrity is disrupted. Vascular endothelial cells and monocytes are also able to produce and express tissue factor activity upon stimulation with interleukin 1 or endotoxin, which suggests that cytokines may modulate tissue factor expression and fibrin deposition at the site of inflammation. Tissue factor is an integral membrane protein composed of protein and phospholipid components, both of which are required for its procoagulant activity. Factor VII is a single-chain protein which in this form already has some enzymatic activity and can complex with tissue factor. However, by cleavage of an Arg-Ile bond, the molecule of factor VII splits in a light chain and a heavy chain (containing the active site) linked by two disulfide bonds. This activation increases the coagulant activity of factor VII about 100-fold. However, the activation of factor VII occurs only after it has bound to tissue factor. The tissue factor–factor VIIa complex then combines with the substrate (factor X), producing a further conformational change in factor VIIa, so that it binds still more tightly to tissue factor, precluding dissociation of factor VIIa from tissue factor. The tissue factor–factor VIIa complex activates primarily factor X but also factors IX and XI, which interconnect the intrinsic and extrinsic activation pathways and play a prima ballerina role in the activation of coagulation.[13] Tissue factor accelerates these reactions as a cofactor, apparently by inducing a conformational change in factor VIIa.

It should be noted that phospholipids of the platelet membrane, in conjunction with factor Xa, can also activate factor VII—another bridge between the intrinsic and extrinsic pathways. Thus, the earlier concepts of a clearly separate intrinsic and extrinsic activation system are becoming obsolete. That factor VII is essential to ensure normal hemostasis is underlined by the bleeding condition of patients with severe congenital factor VII deficiency.

The Pathway in Common: The Formation of Prothrombinase, the Enzyme Converting Prothrombin to Thrombin

Factor X stands at the crossroad of the "extrinsic" and "intrinsic" activation pathways.[14] This means that factor X can be activated either by the tenase complex (IXa, phospholipid, VIIIa, and Ca ions) or by the tissue factor–factor VIIa complex (Fig. 52-6). In both instances, activation of factor X results from the cleavage of a single peptide bond between Arg and Ile, releasing an activation peptide and unmasking an active site on the heavy chain.[15] This is brought about by the enzymatic activity residing in factor IXa, which is part of the tenase complex. The presence of proteolytically modified factor VIII—whether by thrombin, factor Xa, or factor IXa—by separation of factor VIII from von Willebrand factor enhances 10,000-fold the rate of activation of factor X by factor IXa. Factor VIIIa has no enzymatic activity and is thus a helper protein (a cofactor) which, to exert its function, binds to phospholipid vesicles, provided phosphatidylserine is available on the platelet membrane.[16] In fact, there are specific binding sites available on activated platelets for factor VIII that are distinct from the binding sites for factor V expressed during stimulation of platelets. As shown below, activated protein C degrades factor VIIIa. Thus, factor VIII must be activated for hemostasis and inactivated for the maintenance of the fluidity of blood.

To be fully active, factor Xa has to form a stoichiometric 1:1 complex with factor Va; the latter molecule enhances the activation of prothrombin by factor Xa 300,000-fold. Normal plasma contains factor V in trace amounts (25 nM, while factor X is about 200 nM) and in an inactive state; its activation requires three specific enzymatic cleavages, which can be brought about by thrombin or less efficiently by factor Xa. The association of factor Va with factor Xa on an anionic phospholipid is termed *prothrombinase*. Factor Va increases the turnover (kcat) 1000-fold, which means that the number of thrombin molecules generated by the enzyme upon saturation by the substrate is multiplied by a factor of approximately 1000. In contrast to the vitamin K–dependent procoagulation factors (prothrombin, factors VII, IX, and X), which bind to phospholipids via calcium bridges with their glutamic acid (Gla) domain, factor Va does not bind to phospholipids via calcium bridges but penetrates into the lipid bilayer.

The Action of Prothrombinase on Prothrombin

The multimolecular complex "prothrombinase" initially cleaves one Arg-Ile bond in the prothrombin molecule, producing meizo-thrombin. This intermediate molecule remains membrane-bound through the retained glutamic acid (Gla)-domain linkage and activates the inhibitor protein C but lacks procoagulant properties either on platelets or on fibrinogen. To obtain the latter property, another arginine bond (Arg-Thr) has to be cleaved, yielding alpha-thrombin, which, lacking a Gla-containing region, is released from the cell surface.

For the different reactions pertaining to the coagulation cascade system, it is being assumed that all coagulation factors immobilize on phospholipids (stimulated platelets, perturbed endothelial or white cells) and that shuttling of reaction products between assembled complexes takes place. An alternative but less efficient possibility is that reaction products dissociate from the phospholipid membranes to become free in solution. Single-membrane channeling protects critical enzymes from inactivation by plasma inhibitors (e.g., antithrombin III) as well as from dilution by blood flow.

The Pivotal Role of Thrombin

Thrombin represents the culmination of the coagulation cascade; its action on fibrinogen is most dramatic, because thrombus formation is a visible process. Thrombin itself is responsible for its own nonlinear generation caused by positive feedback activation, whereby thrombin enhances neoforma-

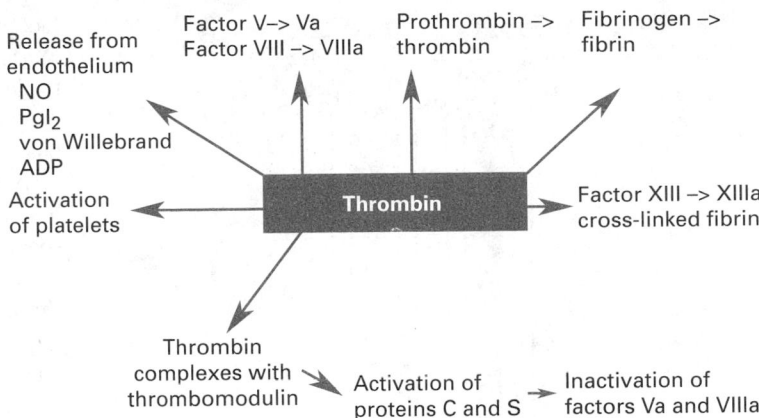

FIGURE 52-7
Thrombin is the pivotal enzyme in coagulation, being responsible for positive feedback activation, rapid activation of platelets and endothelial cells, and indirectly via thrombomodulin for its activation.

tion of thrombin (Fig. 52-7). In addition, thrombin is a pivotal molecule for numerous other functions. The action of thrombin on platelets results in the release of platelet factor V exteriorization and in the transbilayer movement of its inner membrane surface (flip-flop reaction). Thrombin activates three of the four cofactor or helper proteins (factors V and VIII, thrombomodulin, but not tissue factor). Thrombin furthermore activates factor XIII, which increases the strength and renders the fibrin more resistant to thrombolysis. Thrombin can increase the production and release of prostacyclin, nitric oxide (NO, EDRF), ADP, and plasminogen activator inhibitor type 1 (PAI-1) from the normal endothelium, protecting the microcirculation against thrombosis. Thrombin inhibits its own production by a negative feedback mechanism via the thrombomodulin–proteins C and S system. Thrombin is also involved in other biological effects, such as chemotaxis and mitogenesis. It also elicits a potent mitogenic response in fibroblasts and macrophages, thereby modulating inflammatory reactions at the site of vascular injury.

The Conversion of Fibrinogen to Fibrin

Fibrinogen is a large paired molecule held together by disulfide bridges. Each symmetric half-molecule consists of one set of three different polypeptide chains termed Aα, Bβ, and γ. The two half-molecules are joined in the central aminoterminal domain in an antiparallel manner by three interchain disulfide bridges, two of which are between γ chains and the other between α chains. Thrombin splits an arginine-glycine bond, first at the amino end of the two Aα chains and later at the amino end of each of the two Bβ chains so that each molecule releases in sequence two small aminopeptides A (FPA) and two small fibrinopeptides B (FPB) from fibrinogen and thus converts this molecule to fibrin monomers that are still soluble (Fig. 52-8). The FPA release exposes a polymerization site in the central region of the fibrinogen molecule (E domain) that subsequently aligns with a complementary site in the outer region (D domain) of another fibrin monomer to form staggered overlapping two-stranded fibrils. The slower

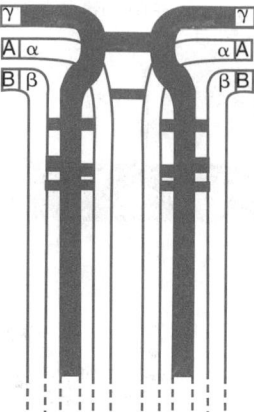

FIGURE 52-8
Structure of fibrinogen. This glycoprotein is a paired molecule, each half consisting of three homologous chains; Aα, Bβ, and γ. The horizontal connecting lines are disulfide bonds. Thrombin cleaves first the A and then the B peptide. The disulfide knot of the dimer fibrinogen is clearly depicted. The entire sequence of 2946 amino acids has been elucidated.

FPB release exposes an independent site for noncovalent intermolecular interaction, resulting in complementary alignment of fibrin monomers. Subsequently, lateral association of fibrin monomers occurs and the network becomes thicker and branched, still through a nonenzymatic process. These coupled monomers of fibrin, called *polymers,* are still soluble unless they become too large and precipitate; the resulting gel of fibrin forms the skeleton of a thrombus and traps red and white cells.

The structural stability of the fibrin network is achieved through covalent cross linking.[17] Thrombin activates factor XIII (*fibrin stabilizing factor*), a transglutaminase which, in the presence of calcium, forms peptide bonds between side chains of suitable lysine (donor) and glutamic acid (acceptor) residues. The result of such a lysine cross link is that the thrombus becomes firmer and more resistant to thrombolysis. It should be noted that fibrin-bound thrombin (approximately 40 percent of the thrombin generated) retains its coagulant and platelet-activating properties and is protected from inactivation by circulating heparin-antithrombin III.[18] During thrombolysis, fibrin-bound thrombin is released and can cause rethrombosis. Hirudin, hirulog, and similar antithrombin III–independent synthetic thrombin inhibitors, which are smaller than heparin, can inhibit fibrin-bound thrombin.

Of note, two other plasma proteins (fibronectin and α_2-plasmin inhibitor) are also covalently cross-linked to fibrin by factor XIIIa and are incorporated in the fibrin mesh.

Connections between the Intrinsic and Extrinsic Pathways of Coagulation

The concept of separating the two pathways of the coagulation system that merge in a common pathway from the activation of factor X on is a didactic schematization that is increasingly blurred as feedback mechanisms and interactions between the two pathways are found.[13] For example, the factor VIIa–tissue

factor complex can activate factors IX and XI directly; factors IXa and Xa can activate factor VII. The extrinsic pathway seems to play a major role in the initiation of in vivo coagulation, while the intrinsic pathway is now thought to be required for continuous growth and maintenance of fibrin formation.

Activation of coagulation factors in successive stages is based on the classical cascade. It will be appreciated that the speed with which these reactions develop increases gradually, as in a system of electronic amplification. Also, here one should realize that nature acts in concert rather than in a sequence of solitary actions. Of course, this is a common feature in biological systems. In the case of the coagulation system, it is the more remarkable because it operates largely outside the cell without the controls imposed by intracellular compartimentation.

Coagulation—A Series of Surface-Catalyzed Events

With the exception of fibrinogen, prothrombin, and plasminogen, the coagulation factors are present in the fluid phase of blood at very low concentrations. Their encounter in solution is possible and their interaction slow, though this can be remarkably accelerated, up to 100,000-fold, after adsorption and concentration on surfaces. Modified endothelium, stimulated platelets, denuded subendothelial structures (e.g., collagen), fissured atherosclerotic plaques, and foreign surfaces (extracorporeal circulation conduits) allow the attachment of passing platelets (adhesion) and the absorption of coagulation proteins. One way for this to occur is by binding mediated through calcium bridges between negatively charged phospholipids (tissue factor, activated platelets, microvesicles) and the γ-carboxyglutamic acid (Gla) residues of the four vitamin K–dependent procoagulants (prothrombin, factors VII, IX, and X), and two endogenous anticoagulants (proteins C and S). Coumarin drugs interfere in the vitamin K cycle, so that less glutamic acid is formed and binding of these proteins to phospholipids is impeded. Assembly on surfaces increases the local concentration of clotting factors considerably and creates an optimal steric relationship (better alignment) for their interaction. This means that a lipid-bound enzyme has a greater affinity for the substrate than the free circulating enzyme. Inhibitors of activated coagulation factors are much less effective in binding to phospholipids surfaces; thus binding of activated coagulation factors to such a surface protects them against endogenous inhibitors.[19] Interaction between coagulation factors is accelerated by the presence of a phospholipid interphase (decrease of Km value) and the efficiency is also improved by the presence of the helper protein factors V and VIII (increase of Kcat).

ROLE OF INHIBITORS OF THE COAGULATION SYSTEM

Several mechanisms help to prevent uncontrolled formation of fibrin in the circulation. First, coagulation remains a strictly localized process because it requires negatively charged surfaces, which are in the first place provided by activated platelets. Platelet activation, in turn, is limited to sites of vessel injury and fissured atherosclerotic plaques. In addition, the flowing blood will rapidly dilute any inadvertently activated clotting factor before it perpetuates the reaction sequence to form fibrin. Finally, a number of proteins circulate in the blood to inhibit the coagulation process at various stages of the cascade. Four of them appear particularly important in preventing thrombosis: antithrombin III, protein C, tissue factor pathway inhibitor, and thrombomodulin.

Antithrombin III inhibits thrombin and the activated forms of several coagulation factors, but inhibition of thrombin and of factor Xa are particularly important and clinically relevant.[20] Thrombin forms a tightly bound, stable complex with antithrombin III; this occurs at a relatively slow rate that is enormously enhanced by heparin (see below) and also appreciably by heparan sulfate, a substance very similar to heparin, which is found on the intraluminal surface of vascular endothelial cells. The inhibition of thrombin is due to ternary complex formation between thrombin, antithrombin III, and heparin. The inhibition of factor Xa is the result of the formation of a binary complex between antithrombin III and factor Xa.

The protein C–thrombomodulin pathway of thrombin inhibition represents the major natural anticoagulant system (Fig. 52-9). Protein C is a proenzyme formed in the liver; vitamin K is required in its synthesis. On the surface of either platelets or endothelium, protein C is activated by thrombin to become a circulating serine protease that inhibits factors Va and VIIIa. Complex formation between thrombin and thrombomodulin, a potent cofactor present on the endothelial surface, catalyzes the activation of protein C. Protein S is another vitamin K–dependent protein that does not possess serine protease properties but appears to function as a cofactor for activated protein C by facilitating its binding to membrane phospholipids.[21] In plasma, protein S circulates free or bound to C4b-binding protein, a component of the complement system. Only free protein S serves as a cofactor of activated protein C. In addition to being a powerful anticoagulant, activated protein C initiates fibrinolysis by releasing tissue plasminogen activator (t-PA) from the endothelium and neutralizing plasminogen activator inhibitor.

Tissue factor–factor VIIa complex is inactivated by the tissue factor pathway inhibitor (TFPI), previously called lipid protein–associated coagulation inhibitor (LACI).[13,14,19] TFPI appears to be the only plasma component inhibiting the catalytic activity of factor VIIa–tissue factor complex. Factor VIIa cannot be neutralized effectively unless it is bound to tissue factor.[13] This is in contrast to other coagulation components, which are neutralized more effectively as free reactants than after they interact in complexes.[22] TFPI first interacts with factor Xa to form Xa-TFPI complexes, which then form a quarternary Xa–TFPI–VIIa–tissue factor complex with resulting loss of the activity of VIIa–tissue factor complex. The plasma concentration of TFPI is low, but a larger pool of

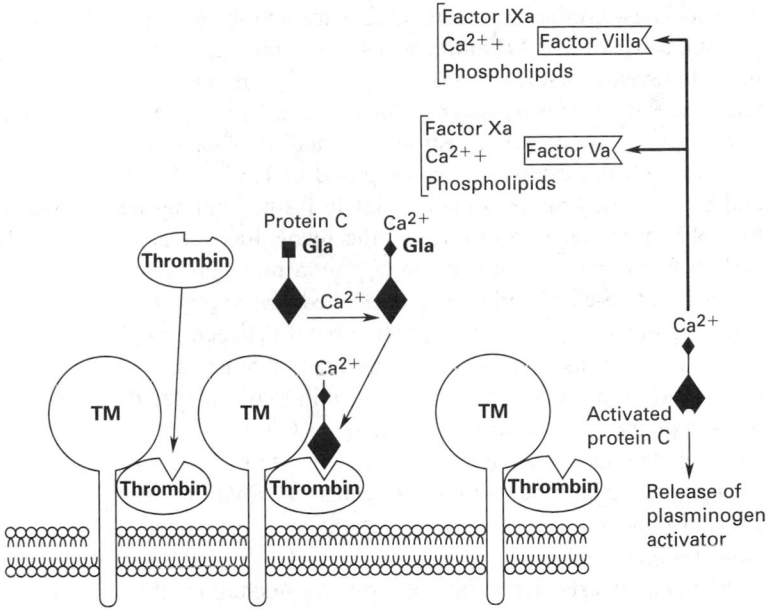

FIGURE 52-9
Thrombin forms a complex with the endothelium-bound protein thrombomodulin (TM). This complex activates circulating protein C, which inhibits factors Va and VIIIa and releases tissue-plasminogen activator from the endothelial cells. Binding of activated protein C to phospholipids is facilitated by protein S. Gla = γ-carboxyglutamic acid.

TFPI bound to vascular endothelium is present from which TFPI can be released into the blood by heparin.

Thrombomodulin is located on the surface of all endothelial cells except those in the microcirculation of the human brain. When thrombin is generated within a vascular space, excess thrombin is bound to thrombomodulin. Thrombomodulin exerts three types of activities: (1) it inhibits thrombin induced activation of platelets, factor V, and fibrinogen; (2) it promotes the activation of protein C after formation of the thrombomodulin-thrombin complex; and (3) it enhances the inhibition of thrombin by antithrombin III. Thus, thrombomodulin modifies the substrate specificity of thrombin; the procoagulant activity is switched off, and at the same time its anticoagulant activity is tremendously increased.

The Fibrinolytic System and Its Control

The fibrinolytic system is essential for removing excess fibrin deposits to preserve vascular patency. The role of fibrinolysis in the maintenance of blood fluidity is well illustrated by an increased incidence of venous thromboembolism in patients with abnormal, nonfunctional plasminogen. Similarly, the overproduction of PAI-1 in transgenic mice leads to an increased risk of venous embolism.

COMPONENTS OF THE FIBRINOLYTIC SYSTEM

Plasminogen

Plasminogen is present in human plasma at a concentration of about 2 μM, which is about twice the concentration of α_2-antiplasmin. The native molecule, denoted Glu-plasminogen, after its NH$_2$-terminal glutamic acid, is a single-chain glycoprotein, consisting of 791 amino acids.[23] Plasminogen is organized in seven structural domains (Fig. 52-10). From the NH$_2$-terminal end, there is a *preactivation peptide,* five sequential, homologous, looped kringle structures, and the T-proteinase domain with the catalytic site composed of His^{603}, Asp^{646}, and Ser^{741}. The kringle domains contain lysine-binding sites that play a crucial role in the specific recognition of fibrin, cell surfaces, and α_2-antiplasmin.[24–26] Plasminogen is converted to a two-chain serine protease called *plasmin* by cleavage of a single Arg^{561}-Val^{562} peptide bond between kringle 5 and the proteinase domain. The serine-containing active site is situated in the B or light chain. Plasmin may catalyze the release of the preactivation peptide from Glu-plasminogen, forming degraded plasminogen with aminoterminal lysine, valine, or methionine commonly called *Lys-plasminogen.* Lys-plasminogen is more easily activated to plasmin than Glu-plasminogen.[26]

Plasmin digests a number of proteins, including fibrin, fibrinogen, and factors V and VIII as well as a number of esters and amides.

Natural Plasminogen Activators

Conversion of plasminogen to plasmin may be achieved by a number of agents called *plasminogen activators.* The principal circulating plasminogen activator in humans is *tissue-type plasminogen activator* (t-PA). This a 70-kDa serine proteinase, which in its native form consists of a single polypeptide chain. t-PA is converted by plasmin to a two-chain form by hydrolysis of the Arg^{275}-Ile^{276} peptide bond. In contrast to most single-chain forms of serine proteinases, single-chain t-PA possesses significant catalytic activity. The amino-terminal region is composed of several domains with homologies to other proteins: a finger domain, a growth factor domain, and two looped kringle structures (Fig. 52-11A). The region constituted by residues 276–527 represents the serine proteinase part with the catalytic site, composed of His^{322}, Asp^{371}, and Ser^{478}.[27] These distinct domains in t-PA are involved in several functions of the enzyme, including its binding to fibrin, fibrin-specific plasminogen activation, rapid clearance in vivo,and binding to endothelial cell receptors. Binding of t-PA to fibrin is mediated via the finger and the second kringle domains. The presence of fibrin markedly enhances the plasminogen-activating property of t-PA, as it not only binds t-PA and plasminogen but also greatly increases the affinity of t-PA for plasminogen. Thus fibrin appears to concentrate both t-PA and plasminogen on its surface and to enhance their interaction (see Refs. 26 and 28). Plasmin so formed on fibrin surfaces has its lysine-binding and active sites occupied and is relatively protected from the inhibitory action of α_2-antiplasmin.

Single-chain urokinase-type plasminogen activator (scu-PA) is a 54-kDa glycoprotein containing 411 amino acids (Fig. 52-11B). The plasma concentration of scu-PA is about 2 ng/mL. Upon proteolytic cleavage of the Lys^{158}-Ile^{159} peptide bond, the molecule is converted to a two-chain derivative (tcu-PA, urokinase). The catalytic triad is located in the carboxy-terminal polypeptide chain and is composed of Asp^{255}, His^{204}, and Ser^{356}. The amino-terminal chain contains an epidermal growth factor domain and one kringle domain. The epidermal

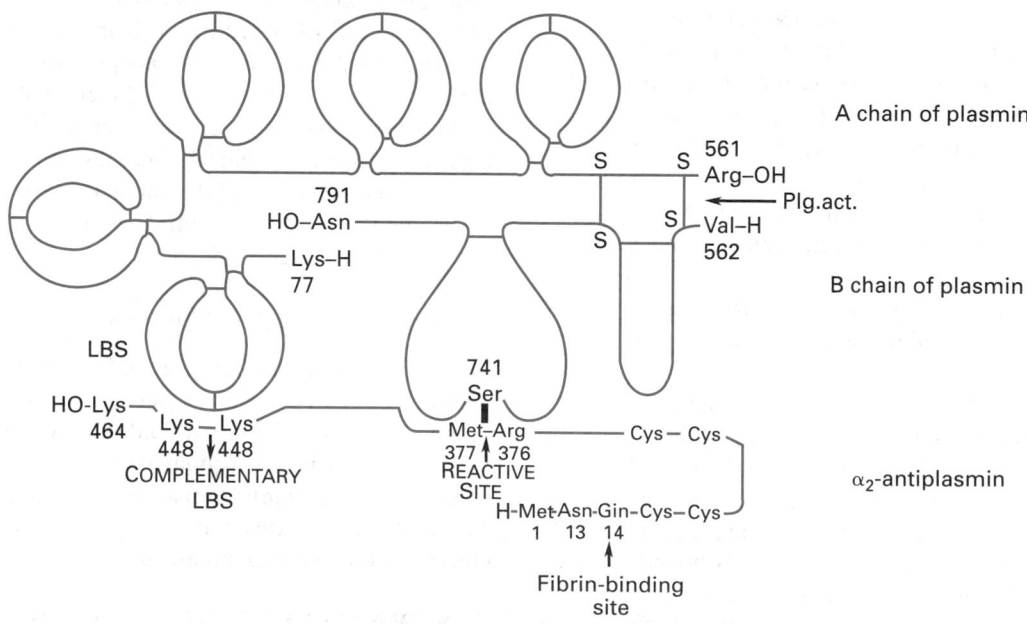

FIGURE 52-10

Schematic visualization of the molecular interactions regulating fibrinolysis. On the fibrin surface, plasminogen is efficiently converted to the proteolytic enzyme plasmin by bound plasminogen activator (Plg. act.). The plasmin generated is partially protected from inactivation by α_2-antiplasmin, while free plasmin in the blood is very rapidly inactivated. The lysine-binding sites (LBS) of plasminogen are important for the interaction between plasmin(o-gen) and fibrin and between plasmin and α_2 antiplasmin. The heavy or A chain of plasminogen originates from the amino-terminal part of the molecule; the light or B chain constitutes the COOH-terminal part; the latter contains the active serine.

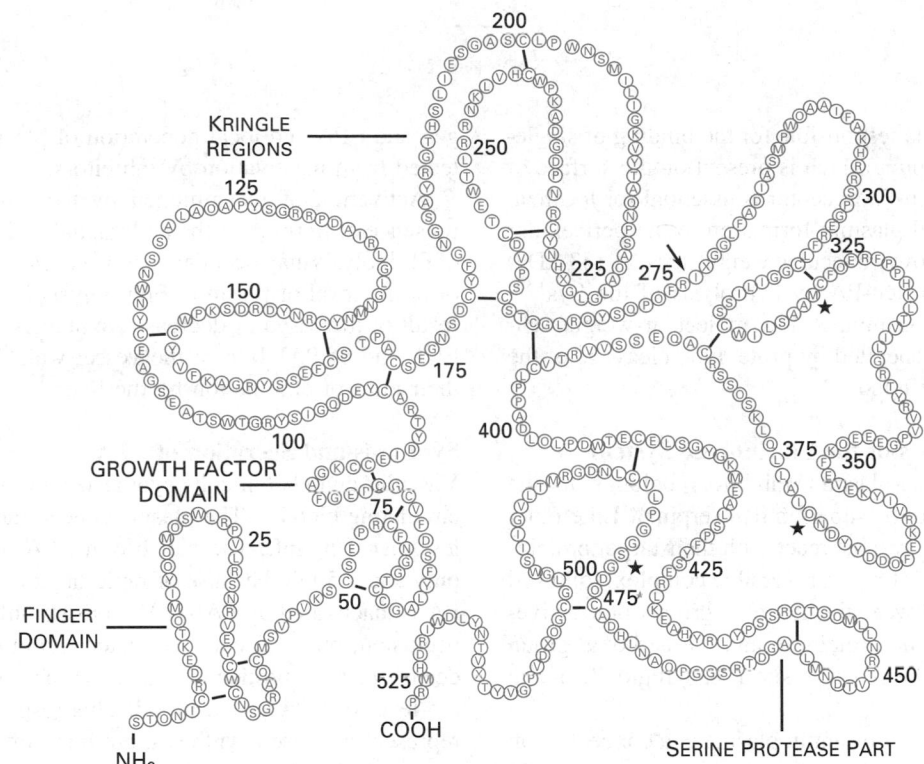

FIGURE 52-11

Primary structure of t-PA (*A*) and prourokinase (*B*). The amino acids are represented by their single-letter symbols, and the black bars indicate disulfide bonds. ★ = active site residues His[322], Asp[371], and Ser[478]; arrow in *A* = plasmin cleavage site for conversion of single-chain t-PA to the two-chain molecule; arrows in *B* = tcu-PA (Lys[158]-Ile[159]), and of 54-kDa tcu-PA (Lys[135]-Lys[136]), the thrombin cleavage site (Arg[156]-Phe[157]) yielding inactive 54-kDa tcu-PA, and the conversion site to 32-kDa scu-PA (Glu[143]-Leu[144]).

growth factor domain is responsible for the binding of single-chain u-PA to its receptor, which is present on the surface of a variety of cells. The u-PA receptor is essential for localization of u-PA–mediated plasmin formation to the pericellular environment.[29,30] A low-molecular-weight tcu-PA (33 kDa) can be generated from tcu-PA by hydrolysis of the Lys^{135}-Lys^{136} peptide with plasmin. A low-molecular-weight scu-PA (32 kDa) can be generated by proteolytic cleavage of the Glu^{143}-Leu^{144} peptide bond.[31]

Endogenous Inhibitors of the Fibrinolytic System

Alpha$_2$-antiplasmin (α_2-plasmin inhibitor) belongs to the serine proteinase inhibitor superfamily (serpins). Like other inhibitors of this class, serpins react with their target proteinases by formation of a 1:1 molar reversible complex, followed by covalent binding between the hydroxyl group of the active-site serine residue of the proteinase and the carboxyl group of the P1 residue at the reactive site ("bait region") of the serpin (Fig. 52-10).

Alpha$_2$-antiplasmin is present in plasma at a concentration of about 1 μM. It is a 67-kDa glycoprotein containing 464 amino acids and about 13 percent carbohydrate.[32] The reactive site of the inhibitor is the Arg^{364}-Met^{365} peptide bond. Alpha$_2$-antiplasmin is unique among serpins by having a carboxy-terminal extension of 51 amino acid residues; this contains a secondary binding site that reacts with the lysine-binding sites of the kringles 1 to 3 of both plasminogen and plasmin. Alpha$_2$-antiplasmin (plasminogen-binding form) becomes partly converted in the circulating blood to a non-plasminogen-binding, less reactive form (about 30 percent of the total), that lacks the 26 carboxy-terminal residues. Two forms of alpha$_2$-antiplasmin are present in about equal amounts in purified preparations of the inhibitor. The aminoterminal Gln^{14} residue of alpha$_2$-antiplasmin can cross-link to Aa chains of fibrin, in a process which requires Ca^{2+} and is catalyzed by activated coagulation factor XIII. This renders the thrombus less sensitive to thrombolysis. Other serpins are alpha$_2$-macroglobulin and alpha$_1$-antitrypsin.

Two principal inhibitors specific for plasminogen activators have been identified in humans, and a number of additional subsidiary inhibitors of this type have been described. They are also members of the serine protease inhibitors (serpin) family.

PAI-1 is a 52-kDa single-chain glycoprotein consisting of 379 amino acids.[33,34] The reactive site of the inhibitor is the Arg^{346}-Met^{347} peptide bond. PAI-1 is stabilized by a tight binding to the cell adhesive protein vitronectin. PAI-2 exists in two different forms with comparable kinetic properties and is detected only in pregnant women.[35]

MECHANISMS INVOLVED IN THE REGULATION OF THE FIBRINOLYTIC SYSTEM

Formed fibrin, whether in normal wound seals or in tissue damaged by any stimulus, is lysed in the body as a result of its unique property of adsorbing small quantities of plasmino-

gen and t-PA and local generation of plasmin, which is protected from inactivation by inhibitors.

Activation of plasminogen by t-PA is enhanced in the presence of fibrin or at the endothelial cell surface. Inhibition of fibrinolysis may occur at the level of plasminogen activation or at the level of plasmin. Fibrinolysis is also regulated as a result of increased or decreased synthesis and/or secretion of t-PA and of PAI-1 from the vessel wall[36] or by changes in their rates of elimination by the liver.[37]

Synthesis and Secretion of t-PA

Vascular endothelial cells synthesize and secrete t-PA to the circulating blood.[36] The plasma concentration of free t-PA is less than 1 ng/mL. The half-life of t-PA in the circulation is only about 5 min because of rapid hepatic clearance; some t-PA is inactivated by PAI-1. Various stimuli—such as venous occlusion, physical exercise, catecholamines, bradykinin, or desmopressin—produce a rapid increase (within minutes) in the level of t-PA in the blood. This response is too rapid to represent increased synthesis, but may reflect release of t-PA from cellular storage pools as well as decrease in hepatic clearance due to a reduced hepatic blood flow.[38] A storage pool of t-PA in endothelial cells has not been conclusively identified.[39]

A variety of agents have been shown to increase the synthesis of t-PA by cultured endothelial cells, including thrombin, histamine, butyrate, phorbol myristate acetate (PMA), basic fibroblast growth factor, activated protein C, butanol and alcohol derivatives, and retinoids. The increase of t-PA induced by histamine, thrombin, and PMA in endothelial cells is paralleled by increased levels of t-PA mRNA as a result of enhanced transcription of the t-PA gene.[39] Overexpression of t-PA in endothelial cells using a retroviral expression vector did not alter the morphology, attachment, proliferation, migration, or invasion in the in vitro systems. Potentially such t-PA transduced cells could increase local fibrinolysis and may thus be useful for in vivo therapeutic interventions.[40]

Synthesis and Secretion of PAI-1

PAI-1 mRNA has been demonstrated in a large variety of tissues, suggesting that common cells in these tissues, such as endothelial or smooth muscle cells, may be the site of production.[41] PAI-1 is found in plasma, platelets, placenta, and extracellular matrix. The concentration in plasma is in the picomolar range but may increase to about 2 nM during pregnancy, most likely as a result of release of the inhibitor from placenta. Both active and latent PAI-1 are cleared rapidly, with half-lives in rabbits of approximately 15 and 5 min.[42,43] For unknown reasons, PAI-1 exhibits a circadian variation; the plasma concentration peaks in the morning and reaches a trough in the late afternoon and evening[44]; t-PA exhibits a diurnal variation, which is opposite to that observed for PAI-1.

PAI-1 mRNA is increased and PAI-1 protein detected in endothelial cells juxtaposed to thrombi, in smooth muscle cells adjacent to the neointima, and in macrophages. The augmented arterial wall expression of PAI-1 induced by thrombosis may shift the local balance between fibrinolysis and thrombosis toward the latter.[45]

Only a few studies have reported a downregulation of PAI-1 synthesis in endothelial cells, either by forskolin or by endothelial cell growth factor combined with heparin.[46] PAI-1 is not stored within cells but is rapidly and constitutively secreted after synthesis. An exception is formed by platelets that store PAI-1 in their alpha granules; activation of platelets thus results in release of PAI-1.

Inhibition of Plasmin by Alpha₂-Antiplasmin

Alpha₂-antiplasmin forms an inactive 1:1 stoichiometric complex with plasmin. The half-life of plasmin molecules on the fibrin surface, which have both their lysine-binding sites and active site occupied, is estimated to be two to three orders of magnitude longer than that of free plasmin (Fig. 52-10).

Inhibition of Plasminogen Activators by Plasminogen Activator Inhibitors

PAI-1 reacts very rapidly with single-chain and two-chain t-PA and with two-chain u-PA (tcu-PA).[47,48] PAI-2 primarily inhibits tcu-PA. The inhibition rate of tcu-PA, single-chain t-PA, and two-chain t-PA by PAI-2 is about 10, 1200, and 150 times slower, respectively, than that by PAI-1. PAI-1 and PAI-2 do not react with scu-PA.[47]

Like other serpins, PAI-1 inhibits its target proteinases by formation of a 1:1 stoichiometric reversible complex, followed by covalent binding between the hydroxyl group of the active-site serine residue of the proteinase and the carboxyl group of the PI residue at the reactive center ("bait region") of the serpin. The rapid inhibition of both t-PA and u-PA by PAI-1 involves a reversible high-affinity second-site interaction that does not depend on a functional active site. In the presence of fibrin, single-chain t-PA is protected from rapid inhibition by PAI-1. It has, however, also been reported that PAI-1 binds to fibrin and that fibrin-bound PAI-1 may inhibit t-PA-mediated fibrin clot lysis.[49]

The active form of PAI-1 converts to a latent form that can be partially reactivated by denaturing agents. In addition, inhibitory PAI-1 may convert not only to latent PAI-1, which can be reactivated, but also to substrate PAI-1, which may be irreversibly degraded by target proteinases, including t-PA, u-PA, and thrombin.[50]

Plasminogen Activation by t-PA at the Fibrin Surface

The main role of t-PA most likely is in the dissolution of fibrin.[51,52] t-PA is a poor enzyme in the absence of fibrin, but the presence of fibrin strikingly enhances the activation rate of plasminogen.[53] Plasmin formed on the fibrin surface has both its lysine-binding sites and active site occupied and is thus only slowly inactivated by alpha₂-antiplasmin (half-life of about 10 to 100 s); in contrast, free plasmin, when formed, is rapidly inhibited by alpha₂-antiplasmin (half-life of about 0.1 s).

During fibrin clot lysis, single-chain t-PA is converted to two-chain t-PA at the fibrin surface. This conversion is probably of little physiologic relevance, since the activity of single-chain t-PA and two-chain t-PA is enhanced to the same extent in the presence of fibrin or fragment-X polymer.[54] Fibrin-bound single-chain t-PA may adopt a conformation similar to that of two-chain t-PA. Whether conversion of Glu-plasminogen to the more easily activatable Lys-plasminogen contributes significantly to the increased plasminogen activation rate during fibrinolysis is still somewhat controversial.

Binding studies[55,56] as well as kinetic studies[57] have revealed that lipoprotein a [Lp(a)] competes with plasminogen for binding to fibrin as a result of binding of Lp(a) to fibrin via its lysine-binding domains. As for plasminogen, binding of Lp(a) to fibrin is enhanced by partial proteolytic degradation of the fibrin surface.[55] As a functional consequence of the competition between Lp(a) and plasminogen for binding to fibrin, the fibrin-dependent enhancement of plasminogen activation by t-PA is inhibited.[56,57]

PATHOPHYSIOLOGY OF FIBRINOLYSIS

Increased levels of PAI-1 activity resulting in a decreased fibrinolytic capacity have been reported in several thrombotic disease states, including venous thromboembolism, obesity, sepsis, coronary artery disease, and acute myocardial infarction.[44,58] Increased levels of PAI-1 have also been found in association with the insulin resistance syndrome in which a significant correlation was found between plasma PAI-1 levels and body mass index, triglyceride levels, insulin levels, and systolic blood pressure. Obese people—particularly those with android obesity—also have high PAI-1 levels.

Increased plasma levels of PAI-1 are one of the major disturbances of the hemostatic system in patients with coronary heart disease, and multiple interrelations with established metabolic risk factors have been observed. Increased PAI-1 levels have also been demonstrated in atherosclerotic lesions within the vessel wall. Therefore, both systemically and locally increased PAI-1 concentrations could have a pathogenic role in the development of atherosclerotic disease (reviewed in Refs. 44 and 63).

Many case-control or cross-sectional studies have demonstrated high plasma PAI-1 levels in patients who have had a myocardial infarction or unstable angina. A relationship between deficient fibrinolysis due to high PAI activity levels and recurrent (within 3 years) myocardial infarction was demonstrated in young men who had survived their first myocardial infarction. On the other hand, PAI-1 activity was not predictive for recurrent infarction (nor was t-PA antigen) in a group of older patients followed over 5 years. In a cohort of patients with angina pectoris, high basal t-PA antigen levels were found to be associated with an increased risk of myocardial infarction, while no correlation was observed with PAI activity.[59,60]

Attempts to demonstrate a relationship between plasma PAI-1 levels and the severity of vessel wall damage have led to conflicting results in cross-sectional studies. Recent analysis of the data of the European Concerted Action on Thrombosis (ECAT) angina pectoris study[61] demonstrated that there was a weak distinction between patients with and patients without significant coronary stenosis; the former had significantly higher plasma levels of PAI-1. No association could be observed with the extent of coronary atherosclerosis.

There are multiple interrelations between plasma PAI-1 levels and other risk factors of atherothrombosis, such as those involved in the metabolic syndrome of insulin resistance. In the ECAT angina pectoris study, in which insulin determination was available for almost 1500 patients, two- to threefold differences in PAI-1 levels were observed in comparing the lowest and the highest quintile of insulin, body mass index, or triglyceride.[62]

In addition, Lp(a) was shown to enhance PAI-1 synthesis by endothelial cells in culture, and it was suggested that Lp(a) binding to endothelium and subsequent increased PAI-1 expression may contribute to the generation of a specific prothrombotic endothelial phenotype.[63]

Antithrombotic Drugs

UNFRACTIONATED HEPARIN, LOW-MOLECULAR-WEIGHT HEPARINS, AND HEPARINOIDS

Unfractionated Heparin

The term *heparin* refers not to a single structure but rather to a family of mucopolysaccharide chains of varying length and composition. Heparin by itself has no anticoagulant property. It accelerates the action of two naturally occurring plasma inhibitors, forming a 1:1 stoichiometric complex with antithrombin III (an inhibitor of thrombin and activated factors X, IX, XI, and XII) and, at very high doses, with heparin cofactor II, which acts only on thrombin decay (Fig. 52-12). Heparin contains a unique pentasaccharide that has a high-affinity binding sequence for antithrombin III. This sequence is present in only one-third of heparin molecules and is not required for binding to heparin cofactor II.

Factor Xa bound to platelets and thrombin bound to the endothelium or to fibrin (thrombus) are protected from inactivation by heparin-antithrombin III complex.[64,65] In plasma, approximately 20 times more heparin is needed to inactivate fibrin-bound thrombin than to inactivate free thrombin.[64] This explains why more heparin is needed to prevent the extension of venous thrombosis than to prevent formation of the initial thrombus.

Heparin is not absorbed by the gastrointestinal mucosa. When in the bloodstream after parenteral administration, heparin binds to endothelial cells, mononuclear macrophages, and numerous plasma proteins. Some of these neutralize anticoagulant activity (e.g., platelet factor 4, vitronectin), while others such as von Willebrand factor lose their function. Elevated levels of these heparin-binding proteins explains the different

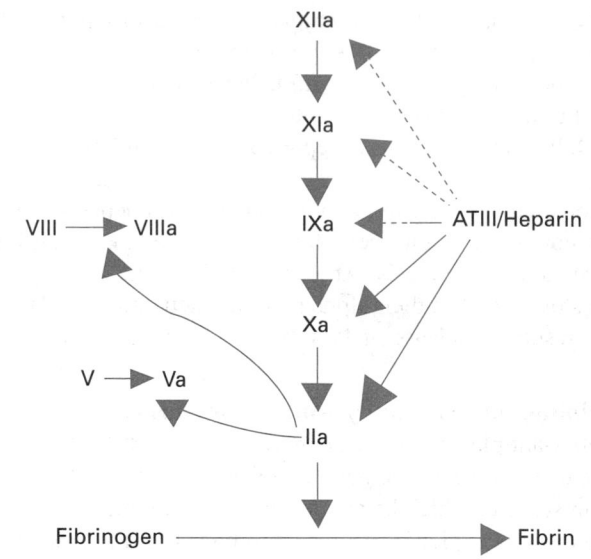

FIGURE 52-12

Heparin/antithrombin III (ATIII) inactivates the following coagulation enzymes: factor XIIa (XIIa), factor XIa (XIa), factor IXa (IXa), factor Xa (Xa), and thrombin (IIa). Thrombin and factor Xa are most sensitive to the effects of heparin/ATIII.

individual heparin dose requirements to obtain the same antithrombotic effect and the so-called heparin resistance in patients with inflammatory and malignant diseases.[65] Binding of heparin to the endothelium and various plasma proteins reduces bioavailability at low concentrations and causes variability of response to fixed doses of anticoagulant[65] (Table 52-2).

The pharmacokinetics of heparin is complicated; suffice it to say that the anticoagulant response increases disproportionately in intensity and duration as the dose increases. This explains why the anticoagulant effect of heparin has to be closely monitored. At present, no completely satisfactory test measuring the generation of thrombin and the levels of antithrombin is available. The most commonly used test is the activated partial thromboplastin time (APTT), which is sensitive to the inhibitory effect of heparin on thrombin, factor X, and factor IX. Unfortunately, the different commercial APTT reagents vary in their response to heparin, and there are technical variables. The therapeutic level of the APTT should therefore be established in each clinical laboratory to correspond to 0.2 to 0.4 U of heparin per milliliter plasma by protamine titration[65] or to 0.2 to 0.7 IU factor Xa per milliliter of plasma by the chromogenic substrate assay for the determination of anti–factor Xa activity. A nomogram may help but should be adapted to the responsiveness of the reagent and APTT test system in use in the local laboratory.[66]

The most common and major side effect of heparin is bleeding. The risk is higher when unfractionated heparin is given by intermittent (14.2 percent) rather than continuous infusion (6.8 percent) or the subcutaneous route (4.1 percent). Also, the dose of heparin, the patient's anticoagulant response, serious concurrent illness, and chronic consumption of alcohol may

TABLE 52-2

ADVANTAGES AND DISADVANTAGES OF UNFRACTIONATED HEPARIN, LOW-MOLECULAR-WEIGHT HEPARIN, AND RECOMBINANT HIRUDIN

Unfractionated Heparin	LMW Heparin	Hirudin
Inhibits to the same extent thrombin and factor VII, much less IXa and XIa	Inhibits mainly factor Xa, thrombin to some extent	Specific and potent inhibitor of thrombin
Antithrombin III–dependent	Antithrombin III–dependent	Antithrombin III–independent
Neutralized by heparinase, several plasma proteins, platelet factor 4, and endothelium	Neutralized by heparinase, weak endothelium binding	Not neutralized by heparinase, endothelium, macrophages, fibrin monomer, and plasma proteins
Does not inactivate clot-bound thrombin and factor VII	Does not inactivate clot-bound thrombin and factor VII	Inactivates clot-bound thrombin
Inhibits platelet function	Inhibits platelet function	Prevents thrombin induced aggregation but not other platelet agonists
Induced thrombocytopenia is not rare	Can induce thrombocytopenia	Does not induce thrombocytopenia
Bioavailability after subcutaneous injection, 30%	Bioavailability after subcutaneous injection, > 90%	Good bioavailability after subcutaneous injection, circa 85%
Poor dose-effect response	Fair dose-effect response	Fair dose-effect response
Not immunogenic	Not immunogenic	Not or barely immunogenic
Transient increase of liver enzymes is common	Transient increase of liver enzymes possible	No liver toxicity
Increases vascular permeability	No increase of vascular permeability	No increase of vascular permeability

predispose to bleeding. Heparin-induced thrombocytopenia (HIT) occurs in 2.4 percent of patients receiving therapeutic heparin and 0.3 percent for prophylactic heparin. In addition, vascular occlusion occurs in 0.4 percent. Rare complications are osteoporosis, alopecia, skin necrosis, urticaria, and transient elevation of hepatic transaminases.

Low-Molecular-Weight-Heparins

Some of the limitations of unfractionated heparin can be overcome with low-molecular-weight (LMW) heparins (mean mol wt 4000 to 5000; range, 1000 to 10,000). These LMW heparins produce their major anticoagulant effect by binding to antithrombin III through the same high-affinity pentasaccharide sequence of unfractionated heparin, which, however, is present in only one-third of the LMW molecules. A minimum additional chain length of 15 saccharides (MW > 5400) is required for the inactivation of thrombin, but the inactivation of factor X requires only the pentasaccharide (Fig. 52-13). Unfractionated heparin has by definition an antifactor Xa to anti-II ratio of 1:1 which is between 4:1 and 2:1 for the various LMW heparins. Drugs with a high anti–factor Xa activity were indeed designed based on the hypothesis that inhibition of earlier steps in the blood coagulation system would be associated

with a more potent antithrombotic effect than inhibition of subsequent steps. This is because of the amplification process inherent in the coagulation cascade; that is, a single factor Xa molecule can lead to the generation of multiple thrombin molecules.

The advantages of LMW heparins over unfractionated heparin are numerous (Table 52-2). Factor Xa bound to the platelet membrane in the prothrombinase complex is resistant to inacti-

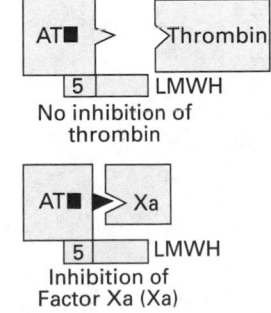
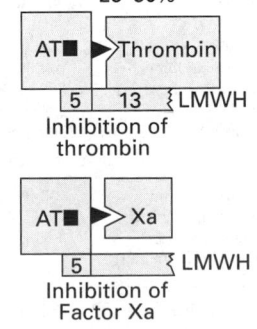

FIGURE 52-13

Low-molecular-weight heparin (LMWH) activity. Approximately 25 to 50 percent of the LMWH molecules of different commercial preparations contain at least 18 saccharide units; these molecules inhibit both thrombin and factor Xa. The remaining 50 to 75 percent of LMWH molecules contain fewer than 18 saccharide units and inhibit only factor Xa.

vation by unfractionated heparin but is not resistant to inactivation by LMW heparins. Also, LMW heparins have lesser binding characteristics to platelet factor 4, other plasma proteins, and endothelial cells, resulting in a higher bioavailability (after subcutaneous injection > 90 versus 30 percent for unfractionated heparin); reduced plasma clearance, which is independent of dose and plasma concentration; a longer half-life (anti–Xa activity between 3 and 4 h for LMW heparins versus 30 to 150 min for unfractionated heparin); and less interindividual variability of the anticoagulant response.[67] LMW heparins have a lower affinity for von Willebrand factor,[68] increase vascular permeability less than unfractionated heparin, and have a weak effect on platelet function. These differences could explain why LMW heparins produce less bleeding than unfractionated heparin with equivalent or higher antithrombotic effect in experimental animals[67] and in some clinical studies.

The long half-life of LMW heparins and their predictable anticoagulant response to weight-adjusted doses allow a once-daily subcutaneous administration without laboratory monitoring.[67] Table 52-3 list the different LMW heparins in clinical use and their recommended dosages in the prevention of deep venous thrombosis.

It has been observed that thrombocytopenia is more common with unfractionated heparin than with LMW heparin.

Heparinoids: Mixture of Low-Molecular-Weight Sulfate Glycosaminoglycans

Danaparoid sodium (Org 10172) is a LMW heparinoid (6 kDa) and consists of a polydisperse mixture comprising sulfated glycosamino-glycuronides derived from animal mucosa; heparan sulfate (83 percent w/w), of which 4 to 5 percent has high affinity for antithrombin III; dermatan sulfate (12 percent w/w); and a minor amount of chondroitin sulfate (5 percent w/w).[69] There is uncertainty whether the low-affinity fraction of danaparoid sodium has an antithrombotic function[70] or not.[71] Danaparoid sodium is more efficacious than heparin and is associated with less and briefer bleeding than heparin in various animal models of thrombosis. The complex mechanism of the antithrombotic activity of danaparoid sodium can so far be only partially explained. Its anticoagulant profile is characterized by a high ratio of anti–factor Xa/antithrombin activity (14 over < 0.5), resulting in an effective inhibition of thrombin generation. The anti-Xa activity is mediated by antithrombin III and is not inactivated by endogenous heparin-

TABLE 52-3

CHARACTERISTICS OF COMMERCIAL LOW-MOLECULAR-WEIGHT HEPARINS AND THEIR THERAPEUTIC DOSAGES IN THE PREVENTION OF DEEP VENOUS THROMBOSIS (DVT)

Generic Name (Brand Name)	MW (Range), daltons	Plasma Half-Life,[a] h	Anti-Xa Activity, U/mg[b]	Anti-IIa Activity, U/mg	Bioavailability,[c] Percent	General Surgery and Other Conditions of Moderate Thrombotic Risk	Orthopedic Surgery and Other Conditions of High Thrombotic Risk	Treatment of DVT, Doses in Anti-Xa, IU or mg
Ardeparin sodium (Normiflo)	6000 (2000–15,000)	IV: 3.3 SC: 2.5–3.3	120	60	88–97	—	50 anti-Xa IU/kg twice daily	
Certoparin (Sandoparin; Monoembolex NM)	6300 (4500–8000)		80	40		3000 anti-Xa IU once daily SC	3000 anti-Xa IU once daily SC	
Dalteparin sodium (Fragmin)	6000 (3000–9000)	IV: 1.8–2.3 SC: 3.8	160	60	87	2500 anti-Xa IU once daily SC	5000 anti-Xa IU once daily SC	100 IU/kg twice daily or 200 IU/kg (max 1800) once daily SC
Enoxaparin sodium (Lovenox; Clexane)	4500 (3000–8000)	IV: 3.8–4.0 SC: 4.6–5.9	90–110	20–40	91	20 mg (2000 anti-Xa IU) once daily SC	40 mg once daily or 30 mg twice daily SC	1 mg (100 IU anti-Xa)/ kg twice daily
Nadroparin calcium (Fraxiparin)	4300 (2000–8000)	IV: 2.2–3.55 SC: 2.3–3.79	95–130[d]	35	98	2850 anti-Xa IU once daily SC	40 anti-Xa IU/kg once daily 3days then 60 anti-Xa IU/ kg once daily SC	85 anti-Xa IU/kg twice daily SC
Parnaparin sodium (Fluxum; Alphaparin)	4500 (2000–8000)	IV: 1.2–1.61 SC: 1.95–5.68	90	40	100	3200 anti-Xa IU once daily SC	6400 anti-Xa IU once daily SC	100 anti-Xa U/kg twice daily
Reviparin sodium (Clivarine)	3900 (3500–4500)	IV: 2.6 SC: 3.3	120	30	90	1750 anti-Xa IU once daily SC	4200 anti-Xa IU once daily SC	2863 IU for patients 35–46 kg; 3436 IU for 46–60 kg; 5153 IU for >60 kg once daily SC
Tinzaparin sodium (Logiparin; Innohep)	4500 (3400–5600)	IV: 1.85 SC: 2.9	90	45	84	3500 anti-Xa IU once daily SC	50 anti-Xa IU/kg once daily SC	175 IU/kg once daily SC
Danaparoid sodium[e] (Lomoparin; Orgaran)	5500	IV: 24 SC: 24	14	<0.5	100	750 anti-Xa IU twice daily SC	750 anti-Xa IU twice daily SC	

[a] Plasma half-life in healthy volunteers measured as anti–factor Xa activity.

[b] Assessed against the First International Standard for Low Molecular Weight Heparins.

[c] Bioavailability based on anti–factor Xa activity.

[d] Anti-Xa international units according to the European Pharmacopoeia Monograph 1997: 1134 for nadroparin calcium.

[e] Danaparoid sodium is a low-molecular-weight heparinoid. It is a polydisperse mixture comprising sulfate glycosaminoglycuronides derived from porcine intestinal mucosa containing heparan sulfate, dermatan sulfate, and a minor amount of chondroitin sulfate.

Abbreviations: IV = intravenous; SC = subcutaneous; MW = molecular weight.

neutralizing factors. The low antithrombin activity is mediated by heparin cofactor II and antithrombin III. The heparan sulfate fraction with low affinity for antithrombin III, despite lacking significant effects on coagulation factors Xa and IIa (thrombin) in vitro, has been shown in animal studies to contribute substantially to the antithrombotic activity. In contrast to heparin, danaparoid sodium shows hardly any or no effect on platelet function in vitro or in vivo. Danaparoid sodium is essentially free of contaminating heparin, has minimal cross reactivity in in vitro assays for heparin-induced thrombocytopenia (HIT), and has been used successfully in patients with this complication.

Pharmacokinetic studies have been primarily based on the kinetics of relevant anticoagulant activities because no specific chemical assay methods are available. In comparison with heparin, danaparoid sodium has a prolonged elimination half-life of anti–factor Xa activity. After intravenous and subcutaneous administration of danaparoid sodium, the antithrombin activity half-life is shorter (1.8 h) than its anti–factor Xa half-life (17.6 h). Danaparoid sodium has an absolute bioavailability of 100 percent after subcutaneous administration. The kidneys play an important role in the elimination of the anti–factor Xa activity of danaparoid sodium, but a cellular metabolism seems unlikely, since the liver does not affect the anti–factor Xa activity and there is only slight and reversible binding to the endothelium.[71]

Danaparoid sodium is effective in the prevention of deep venous thrombosis in patients with thrombotic stroke and after elective hip surgery or hip fracture.[76] The long half-life of danaparoid sodium, which is not effectively neutralized by protamine, has been rather difficult to manage clinically.

COUMARIN-TYPE ANTICOAGULANTS
Warfarin sodium and related coumarin congeners are effective antithrombotic compounds that differ in speed in the inhibition of vitamin K-2,3 epoxide within hepatic chromosomes. These compounds depress the synthesis of four vitamin K–dependent procoagulants (factors II, VII, IX, and X) and of two natural inhibitor proteins C and S (Fig. 52-14). The plasma concentration of these proteins will decrease in accord with their half-lives. The coagulation components with the shortest half-lives

are the procoagulant factor VII and the endogenous anticoagulant protein C. This may cause a frank imbalance between procoagulants and anticoagulants at the start of treatment and lead to thrombosis of skin capillaries and venules with cutaneous necrosis.[73] Coumarin-type anticoagulants are so far the only orally available anticoagulants, but they are not the ideal (Table 52-4).

Monitoring of Coumarin Treatment
The intensity of the effect of warfarin on the synthesis of coagulation factors differs among patients; moreover, in the same individual, it may, over time, vary considerably. This explains the need for close monitoring by having daily blood tests in the first week of treatment with warfarin. The test used is the *prothrombin time*, (PT), a term that leads to confusion because the assay depends in fact on the global activity of five coagulation factors (prothrombin and factors V, VII, IX, and X). Among the six factors whose synthesis is inhibited by coumarin derivatives, three (prothrombin and factors VII and X) are effectively measured by this test, but not factor IX and the anticoagulant proteins C and S. On the other hand, the prothrombin time is also sensitive to factor V, a coagulation protein independent of vitamin K.

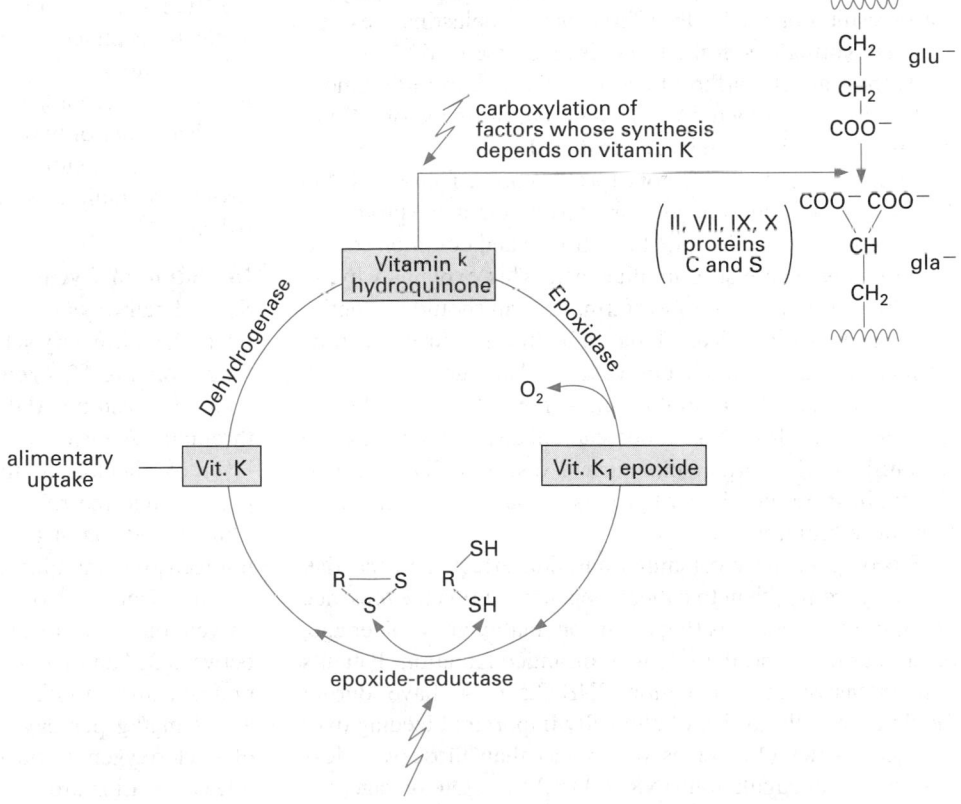

FIGURE 52-14

Vitamin K in its reduced form (vitamin K hydroquinone) is essential for the gamma-carboxylation reaction of glutamic acid (Glu)- to gamma-carboxyglutamic acid (Gla-). In this carboxylation vitamin K hydroquinone is converted to vitamin K_1 epoxide and an epoxide-reductase regenerates active vitamin K hydroquinone. It is this regeneration step which is blocked by all coumarin-type anticoagulant drugs (e.g., warfarin).

TABLE 52-4

DRAWBACKS OF COUMARIN DRUGS AND PROFILE OF
AN IDEAL ANTITHROMBOTIC DRUG

Delayed action
Need for blood monitoring prothrombin time (PT)
PT test does not fully reflect the drug effect
Interaction with many commonly used drugs leading to:
   Potentiation of anticoagulation
   Decreasing anticoagulation level
   Sometimes modifying the activity of the other interacting
    drug
Anticoagulation level influenced by diet
Annual risk of bleeding: Total 6%
                          Major 2%
                          Fatal 0.8%
Narrow benefit-to-risk ratio
Embryotoxicity during first trimester of pregnancy

To perform the prothrombin time, a tissue extract (thromboplastin) and calcium are added to citrated plasma and the time to fibrin formation is measured. Commercial thromboplastin reagents extracted by different methods from various organs and species vary extensively in their sensitivity to reductions in levels of vitamin K–dependent factors. To standardize determinations of prothrombin time and thus allow direct comparison of results obtained with different thromboplastins, the International Normalized Ratio (INR) is recommended.[74]

At the start of warfarin treatment, the prothrombin time is first prolonged by factor VII depletion because factor VII has a half-life much shorter than that of the other vitamin K–dependent coagulation factors (prothrombin, factors IX and X). Thus, in the beginning of warfarin treatment, the prothrombin time is prolonged, while the intrinsic and common coagulation pathways are still uninfluenced. This explains why, in switching from heparin to warfarin, heparin should be continued unabated for at least 1 day after the prothrombin time (INR) has reached therapeutic values. Also, during long-term warfarin therapy, prothrombin times should be checked regularly, as many drugs and foods can enhance or decrease the warfarin effect. Certain intercurrent diseases (liver insufficiency, heart failure, hyperthyroidism) may also modify warfarin dose requirements.

Bleeding is the most important side effect, and the risk may vary from patient to patient, depending upon the presence of comorbid conditions (hypertension, malignancy, older age, recent surgery) and the intensity of anticoagulation. Patients with intensive anticoagulation (INR 2.5 to 4) have, during the first 3 months, a risk of clinically important bleeding over 2 times greater (14 versus 6 percent) than those with less intensive anticoagulation (INR 2.0 to 2.5).[75] On average, the annual overall risk of bleeding is 6 percent, with the incidence of major and fatal bleeding estimated to be 2 and 0.8 percent, respectively (Table 52-4).

A rare, nonhemorrhagic side effect of warfarin is coumarin-induced skin necrosis, an unexplained complication that oc-

curs between the third and eight days of therapy. The rapid decline in protein C level is postulated to play a role in the obscure pathogenesis of thrombosis of skin venules and capillaries within the subcutaneous fat, usually in the lower part of the body. Coumarin drugs readily cross the placenta and may be teratogenic, particularly during the first trimester of pregnancy.

In conclusion, vitamin K antagonists are effective antithrombotic drugs with a narrow risk-benefit ratio that require regular monitoring and a disciplined patient (Table 52-4). Their main virtues are oral administration and low cost.

INHIBITORS OF PLATELET FUNCTION

Several strategies are currently being used to reduce platelet function (Figs. 52-2 and 52-4). These include inhibition of platelet enzyme prostaglandin synthase (aspirin, sulfinpyrazone, flurbiprofen, indobufen), inhibition of thromboxane synthase, blockade of endoperoxide-thromboxane receptors, or inhibition of ADP receptors (ticlopidine, clopidogrel). Inhibition of platelet function was also obtained by modulation of platelet adenylate or guanylate cyclase (stable prostacyclin analogs), interference with the function of the platelet glycoprotein Ib-IX receptor (monoclonal antibodies to GP1b-IX), synthetic peptides to the A1 von Willebrand factor domain, recombinant von Willebrand fragments covering the A1 domain, aurin tricarboxylic acid, specific blockers of the IIb/IIIa receptor (monoclonal antibodies, natural antagonists, synthetic peptides containing the RGD sequence or nonpeptide inhibitors), and peptides that bind to but do not activate the platelet-receptor domain which interacts with thrombin. In this chapter only platelet inhibitors that have been investigated in therapeutic trials are discussed. Several excellent reviews on inhibitors of platelet function were recently published.[75–80]

Inhibition of Cyclooxygenase: Aspirin

Several pathways lead to platelet aggregation (Figs. 52-4 and 52-15). Aspirin very selectively inhibits thromboxane (TXA_2) formation (Fig. 52-4) but only partially impedes platelet aggregation induced by ADP, collagen, and low concentrations of thrombin. Aspirin does not inhibit adherence of the initial layer of platelets to the subendothelium or atherosclerotic plaques, and the release of granule contents is not opposed. Thus the effects of platelet-derived growth factors and other mitogens on smooth muscle cells are not inhibited.[81]

The ideal dose of aspirin for the primary or secondary prevention of cardiovascular disease is not determined. Doses between 324 and 1300 mg/day seem to induce a similar reduction of cardiovascular complications, while doses between 1 and 2 mg/kg per day produce virtually complete inhibition of cyclooxygenase-dependent platelet aggregation.[82] Slow-release aspirins are associated with few gastrointestinal side effects, particularly when an enteric-coated preparation is used. There is increasing evidence that the antithrombotic effect of aspirin is not due only to its inhibition of platelet oxygenase. Aspirin also impairs thrombogenesis by a mechanism that seems to be unrelated to platelet cyclooxygenase,

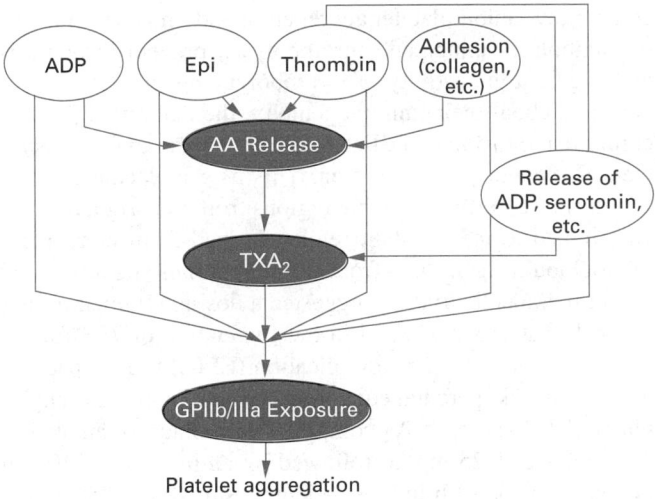

FIGURE 52-15

Exposure of GPIIb/IIIa receptors at the platelet surface is the final common end point of all pathways leading to platelet aggregation.

as, for instance, the acetylation of guanosine triphosphate (GTP) binding proteins, thrombin receptors, and prothrombin.[83] The salicylate moiety of aspirin also antagonizes the lipoxygenase pathway of arachidonate metabolism in platelets, and the demonstration of two cyclooxygenase enzymes (COX-1, COX-2)[84] may further elucidate the antithrombotic mechanism of aspirin.[85]

Inhibition of the ADP Receptor: Ticlopidine, Clopidogrel

These two thienopyridine derivatives can be considered as bioprecursors, since they are inactive in vitro but potent antiaggregating agents in vivo, indicating the importance of at least one active transient metabolite. The metabolic activation takes place in the liver as a portojugular shunt abolishes the antiaggregating effect. Ticlopidine and its chemical analog clopidogrel are noncompetitive but selective antagonists of ADP-induced platelet aggregation and act by specifically blocking GPIIb-IIIa activation (Fig. 52-4) specific for the ADP pathway. Since the two compounds are chemically related, their mechanisms of action are considered similar. Ex vivo studies indicate that the antiaggregating effect is concentration-dependent; the rate of recovery is linked to platelet survival, suggesting a permanent effect on platelets.[86] Both compounds inhibit ADP-induced platelet aggregation by a mechanism that appears to involve effect on 2-methylthio-ADP-binding receptor and the exposure of the fibrinogen binding site of the glycoprotein IIb/IIIa complex. This effect is not due to a direct modification of the glycoprotein complex. Ticlopidine and clopidogrel have no effect on phospholipase A activity or thromboxane A₂ and prostacyclin synthesis. They have no direct effect on either cAMP-phosphodiesterase or adenylate cyclase.

Clopidogrel is approximately 40 to 100 times as active as ticlopidine in inhibiting ADP-induced platelet aggregation in animal models but circa 6 times as potent as ticlopidine in

the inhibition of ADP-induced aggregation of human platelets. Ticlopidine and clopidogrel have been tested in several animal models of platelet-dependent arterial or venous thrombosis and found to be more effective than sulfinpyrazone, dipyridamole, and aspirin (reviewed in Refs. 88 and 89). Other effects are a reduction in fibrinogen levels and blood viscosity and improvement of decreased erythrocyte deformability.

The effectiveness of ticlopidine has been convincingly demonstrated in patients at high risk of arterial thromboembolic events—i.e., those with transient ischemic cerebral attacks and stroke, peripheral arterial, or ischemic heart disease (for review, see Refs. 89 and 90). A trial in more than 3000 patients has shown that ticlopidine has a more pronounced effect on death from all causes or nonfatal stroke than aspirin.[91]

The most common adverse effects associated with ticlopidine are gastrointestinal; diarrhea affects about 20 percent of treated patients. Other effects are skin reactions (urticaria, pruritus, erythema) and hemorrhagic disorders (epistaxis, ecchymoses, menorrhagia). These effects are generally not severe and resolve after discontinuation of ticlopidine. The most potentially serious problem is bone marrow depression (leukopenia, thrombocytopenia, pancytopenia); close monitoring is therefore essential for at least the first 12 weeks of ticlopidine therapy.[89,90] Ticlopidine has also been associated with an increase in total cholesterol levels by 9 percent.[91] Clopidogrel was developed because this compound was not toxic to bone marrow pluripotent stem cells in the mouse (Till and McCullogh test). Also, in the recently finished CAPRIE study, adverse events with clopidogrel were proportionally less frequent than those with ticlopidine.[92] In this trial on 19,185 patients followed up for a mean of 1.91 years, there were 0.10 percent of patients in the clopidogrel group with significant reduction in neutrophil (<1.2 × 10 g/L) and 0.17 percent in the aspirin group. There were 1960 first events included in the outcome cluster on which an intention-to-treat analysis showed that patients treated with clopidogrel had an annual 5.32 percent risk of ischemic stroke, myocardial infarction, or vascular death compared with 5.83 percent with aspirin. These rates reflect a statistically significant ($p = .043$) relative-risk reduction of 8.7 percent in favor of clopidogrel (95 percent CI 0.3–16.5).

Thromboxane Synthase Inhibitors

Thromboxane synthase inhibitors have been developed with the expectation not only of suppressing TXA₂ biosynthesis (Fig. 52-4) but also of sparing or even enhancing the formation of prostacyclin by the vascular endothelium. Thromboxane synthase inhibition offers the advantage over aspirin-type cyclooxygenase inhibitors of reorienting the arachidonic cascade toward an overproduction of inhibitory prostanoids (PGI₂, PGD₂) and a reduction of TXA₂ formation. However, specific inhibition of TXA₂ synthase produces an accumulation of cyclic prostaglandin endoperoxides, which occupy and activate TXA₂ and endoperoxide receptors on platelets and endothelium and thus attenuate the inhibitory effect of PGI₂ and PGD₂.

Most thromboxane synthase inhibitors have moderate potency, short duration of action, and do not result in a sufficiently sustained inhibition of TXA_2 production to be clinically effective. Moreover, some individuals are poor responders to drugs of this type. The increased generation of endoperoxides that share the same receptors as TXA_2 is another problem that will not be solved by more potent and long-acting drugs of this class.[93] Although thromboxane synthase inhibitors have shown some benefit in experimental models, their effects in clinical trials in patients with coronary artery disease have been disappointing.

Thromboxane Receptor Blockers

The more recently developed thromboxane receptor blockers specifically impede the action of both TXA_2 and endoperoxides on their presumed common receptors on platelets (Fig. 52-4) and prevent vasoconstriction induced by TXA_2. These agents leave the normal pattern of thromboxane and prostacyclin formation unaltered. Thromboxane receptor antagonists prolong bleeding time more than thromboxane synthase inhibitors. As expected, TXA_2 synthesis is not inhibited and PGI_2 generation not augmented by specific thromboxane/endoperoxide receptor antagonists. Clinical research with thromboxane receptor antagonists has been slow because the first compounds described had antagonistic effects on platelets but were agonistic on the vessel wall or vice versa. Several of the thromboxane/endoperoxide receptor blockers are also relatively short-acting and the magnitude of their blockade is modest. This is particularly the case for daltroban but not so for vapiprost[94] and fetroban (BMS 180291-1),[95] which are potent TXA_2 receptor blockers with a long duration of action. Unfortunately, the initial clinical studies with vapiprost have been disappointing. The long plasma elimination half-life of BMS 180291-A is most interesting, as are its anti-ischemic effects in canine models of pacing-induced ischemia. However, no therapeutic studies with this compound have been published and it remains to be demonstrated that such agents will offer a relevant advantage over aspirin.

Combined Thromboxane Synthase Inhibitors and Receptor Blockers

Some compounds have a dual activity. Ridogrel is a potent TXA_2 synthase inhibitor with modest additional TXA_2/prostaglandin endoperoxide receptor antagonist properties (at least 100-fold less).[96] Although the animal pharmacology was very promising, the preclinical evaluation is deceptive. Picotamide is a rather weak thromboxane synthase inhibitor and receptor blocker.[97]

BLOCKERS OF THE PLATELET GLYCOPROTEIN IIb/IIIa RECEPTORS

Exposure of GPIIb/IIIa receptors at the platelet surface is the final common end point of all pathways leading to platelet aggregation (Fig. 52-15).

Monoclonal Antibodies against GPIIb/IIIa Receptors

The first platelet GPIIb/IIIa antagonists to be developed were murine monoclonal antibodies.[98] In vitro, these antibodies completely inhibit platelet aggregation and, in animal models of angioplasty injury and thrombolysis, prevent thrombosis and augment the activity of thrombolytic agents. Because of concerns about their immunogenicity, the derivative product chimeric monoclonal 7E3Fab (c7E3Fab, abciximab) was created via genetic recombination. This new molecule consists of the mouse-derived variable regions from the original molecule linked to the constant region derived from human immunoglobulin IgG. Data from a dose-escalation study[99] and a pilot therapeutic trial[100] suggested a dosing regimen for abciximab that was evaluated in the Evaluation of 7E3 for the Prevention of Ischemic Complication (EPIC) trial of patients with high-risk percutaneous transluminal coronary angioplasty (PTCA).[101,102] As compared with placebo, an abciximab bolus of 0.25 mg/kg followed by an infusion of 10 μg/kg per hour for 12 h in 708 patients resulted in a 35 percent reduction in the rate of the primary end points (death, nonfatal myocardial infarction, unplanned surgical revascularization, unplanned repeat PTCA, stent or balloon pump for refractory ischemia). However, bleeding episodes and transfusions were more frequent in abciximab recipients.[101] At 6 months, the absolute difference in patients with a major ischemic event or elective revascularization was 8.1 percent between the placebo group and abciximab bolus-plus-infusion group. The Chimeric 7E3 Anti-Platelet Therapy in Unstable Angina Refractory to Standard Treatment (CAPTURE) study was a randomized, placebo-controlled, multicenter trial to assess whether abciximab can improve outcome in patients with refractory unstable angina who are undergoing PTCA.[103] Predefined stopping rules were met at a planned interim analysis of data for 1050 patients, and recruitment was stopped. After angiography, 1265 patients received a randomly assigned infusion of abciximab or placebo for 18 to 24 h before PTCA, continuing until 1 h afterwards. The primary end point was the occurrence within 30 days of PTCA of death (any cause), myocardial infarction, or urgent intervention for recurrent ischemia. Analyses were by intention to treat. By 30 days, the primary end point had occurred in 71 (11.3 percent) patients who received abciximab compared with 101 (15.9 percent) placebo recipients ($p = .012$). The rate of myocardial infarction was lower in the abciximab than in the placebo group before PTCA [4 (0.6 percent) versus 13 (2.1 percent), $p = .029$] and during PTCA [16 (2.6 percent versus 34 (5.5 percent), $p = .009$]. Major bleeding was infrequent but occurred more often with abciximab than with placebo [24 (3.8 percent) versus 12 (1.9 percent), $p = .043$]. At 6 months follow-up, death, myocardial infarction, or repeat intervention had occurred in 193 patients in each group.

To be effective with abciximab, more than 90 percent of the GPIIb/IIIa receptors have to be blocked. This is associated with a very prolonged bleeding time and risk of bleeding without an antidote being available. Moreover, even chimeric monoclonal antibodies contain some murine proteins and can still be immunogenic. The same drawbacks prevail for cysteine-rich single-chain snake venom peptides binding to GPIIb/IIIa, which, moreover, have a lower potency than chimeric monoclonal abciximab. Their shorter half-life may be an advantage in case of bleeding.

Synthetic Inhibitors of GPIIb/IIIa Receptors

Eptifibatide (Integrelin) is a synthetic cyclic heptapeptide antagonist of GPIIb/IIIa that displays antithrombotic effects in several animal models of thrombosis. Integrin was administered to healthy volunteers as a continuous infusion (0.2 to 1.5 µg/kg per minute) in randomized, double-blind, placebo-controlled studies.[104] Plasma levels of integrin were found to be proportional to its effects on inhibition of ex vivo, ADP-induced platelet aggregation. Complete inhibition of platelet aggregation was observed at infusion rates between 1.0 and 1.5 µg/kg per minute. The half-life of integrin was found to be 50 to 60 min. At the highest infusion rate, bleeding time measurements increased slightly without episodes of clinical bleeding. The bleeding time returned to baseline values within 30 min and platelet aggregation was normal within 2 to 4 h following cessation of drug infusion. The Integrelin to Minimise Platelet Aggregation and Prevent Coronary Thrombosis (IMPACT) study randomized 4010 patients undergoing elective, urgent, or emergency coronary intervention.[105] Patients were assigned to one of three treatments: placebo ($n = 1328$), a bolus of 135 µg/kg eptifibatide followed by an infusion of 0.5 $\mu g\ kg^{-1}\ min^{-1}$ for 20 to 24 h ($n = 1349$), or 135 µg/kg eptifibatide bolus with a 0.75 $\mu g\ kg^{-1}\ min^{-1}$ infusion ($n = 1333$). The coronary procedure was started within 10 to 60 min of the start of study treatment. The primary end point was the 30-day composite occurrence of death, myocardial infarction, unplanned surgical or repeat percutaneous revascularization, or coronary stent implantation for abrupt closure (by intention to treat). The primary safety end point was major bleeding. By 30 days, the composition end point had occurred in 151 (11.4 percent) patients in the placebo group compared with 124 (9.2 percent) in the 135/0.5 eptifibatide group ($p = .063$, and 132 (9.9 percent) in the eptifibatide 135/0.75 group ($p = .22$). Eptifibatide treatment did not increase rates of major bleeding or transfusion.

Fradafiban (BIBU 10 XX) is an orally available synthetic nonpeptide prodrug of the fibrinogen receptor antagonist BIBU 52ZW. Escalating single oral doses of 10, 50, 75, 100, and 150 mg as well as multiple oral doses of 25, 50, 75, and 100 mg fradafibran three times daily for 1 week were administered to healthy volunteers.[106] Fibrinogen receptor occupancy, inhibition of platelet aggregation, and bleeding time increased in a dose-dependent manner. Treatment was well tolerated; only minor events were observed. Clinical trials with fradafibran in patients undergoing coronary angioplasty are under way.

Lamifiban (RO 44-9883), a nonpeptide synthetic compound, binds reversibly to the integrin IIb/IIIa with a K_d 5 nM to approximately 60,000 sites per platelet and is active in several animal models of thrombosis.[107] The inhibition of the ADP-induced aggregation curve parallels the receptor occupancy obtained in in vitro radioligand binding studies (approximately 50 percent inhibition with 50 percent receptor occupancy of

GPIIb/IIIa). The compound is active in several animal models of thrombosis, with a doubling of the bleeding time at 100 percent inhibition of platelet aggregation. The half-life of the free drug is 40 min and of the bound drug 9 h. A dose-finding study was conducted in patients with unstable angina.[108] The dose range resulted in an inhibition of platelet aggregation to ADP up to 100 percent (median, 50 percent) and to thrombin-receptor agonist peptide (TRAP) from up to 76 percent (median, 33 percent). As compared with aspirin/heparin, lamifiban reduced the combined event rate of death, nonfatal myocardial infarction, and recurrent chest pain with ischemic ST changes from 8.2 to 2.5 percent at 1 month. However, bleeding time at effective doses was prolonged to more than 25 min. Phase II (Platelet-IIb/IIIa Aggregation Receptor Antagonist Dose Investigation for Reperfusion Pain in Myocardial Infarction, PARADIGM) and phase III (Platelet IIb/IIIa Antagonism for the Reduction of Acute Coronary Syndromes in a Global Organization network, PARAGON I, II) trials are under way.

Tirofiban (MK383) is another nonpeptide GPIIb/IIIa receptor antagonist. This compound has a short half-life (3 h versus 3 days for abciximab[109] and the potential to be active orally. The plasma concentration yielding 50 percent inhibition of ADP-induced platelet aggregation for tirofiban in healthy volunteers is approximately 13 ng/mL; the plasma concentration doubling the template bleeding time is 30 ng/mL plasma. Intravenous infusion of tirofiban for 1 or 4 h in healthy male volunteers dose-dependently inhibited ADP-, collagen-, arachidonic acid-, U46619- and thrombin-induced platelet aggregation.[109] Bleeding time was significantly increased. In high-risk patients undergoing PTCA, tirofiban dose-dependently inhibited ex vivo ADP-induced platelet aggregation, which was rapidly reversed after 2.8 percent of tirofiban and 5.8 percent of placebo recipients. In this safety and tolerability trial, tirofiban was administered as an intravenous bolus followed by a 16- to 24-h infusion at the following sequential doses: 5 µg/mL + 0.05 µg/mL/min, 10 µg/mL + 0.1 µg/mL min, and 10 µg/mL + 0.15 µg/mL/min.[110]

SC-5468A is a prodrug of a nonpeptide mimetic of the tetrapeptide arginine-glycine-aspartate-serine (RGDS). The active metabolite SC-54701A is a potent inhibitor of GPIIb/IIIa and exhibits specificity for this receptor with respect to other integrins.[111] More than 50 percent of the orally administered prodrug is absorbed in dogs and half that amount is converted to the active agent. Platelet aggregation is completely inhibited for more than 8 h after a single oral dose of 2.5 mg/kg. After intravenous administration, the half-life of the β-phase elimination of the active moiety is 6.5 h (4.7 ± 0.1 h) in dogs, and the total plasma clearance 0.3 L/h per kilogram. The results of a dose-ranging study show that oral administration of the prodrug gives a dose-dependent inhibition of platelet aggregation, which is maintained during a 14-day administration period in dogs without adverse effects.[112] At a dose inhibiting collagen-induced aggregation by 80 percent, bleeding time was increased 2.5-fold. Whether these results will be translated into less bleeding is being investigated in clinical trials.

SPECIFIC THROMBIN INHIBITORS

Hirudin

Natural hirudin is a single-chain, carbohydrate-free polypeptide containing three intramolecular disulfide bridges and a sulfated tyrosine residue. The polypeptide chain contains 65 amino acids with a molecular weight of approximately 7000. Recombinant hirudin has been obtained using *Escherichia coli* bacteria and yeast. With both methods, hirudin is expressed as desulfatohirudin, lacking the sulfate residue on tyrosine 63. The nonsulfated molecules result in about a tenfold reduction in thrombin affinity.[113] Unlike heparin, which requires endogenous cofactors for activity (mainly antithrombin III and heparin cofactor II), hirudin does not need a cofactor for its anticoagulant activity; therefore, it is still active in states of deficiency of these proteins (Table 52-2).

Hirudin is a specific potent inhibitor of thrombin, to which it binds with extraordinary tightness (K_D 2×10^{-14} M) near the active center at the substrate recognition site. In addition, there are multiple other contacts between hirudin and thrombin over an extended area of the molecule, forming a highly stable noncovalent complex. All known functions of thrombin are inhibited. The terminal half-life of r-hirudin in healthy young volunteers is 50 to 65 min,[86,87] with a half-life of its effect on the APTT of about 2 h.[114] In contrast, in older patients with established coronary artery disease with normal renal function (serum creatinine 1.0 ± 0.2 mg/dL), the plasma half-life of hirudin was found to be 2 to 3 h,[115] in agreement with the half-life of the effect of hirudin on the APTT of about 2 to 3 h.

Recombinant hirudin appears to be a weak allergen, and hirudin-specific IgE antibodies were rarely seen in 163 immunocompetent healthy volunteers receiving recombinant hirudin twice at a 1 month interval.[116] No adverse effects occurred. No antibodies to hirudin were detected 2 weeks after the drug administration. The APTT appeared most suited for monitoring r-hirudin administration. In a double-blind pilot trial, 113 low-risk patients with stable angina pectoris undergoing PTCA were randomized to a 24-h infusion of either recombinant hirudin (desirudin) or heparin.[117] All patients received aspirin for at least 4 weeks beginning on the day of PTCA. r-Hirudin was given as a 20-mg bolus followed by an infusion of 0.16 mg/kg per hour and compared with heparin given as a 10,000-IU bolus followed by 12 IU/kg per hour. Dosage of both drugs was adjusted to a target APTT of 85 to 120 s. Acute closure, leading to myocardial infarction and/or coronary bypass surgery, occurred in 10.3 percent of patients randomized to heparin but in only 1.4 percent of patients randomized to r-hirudin. None of the differences in this small pilot trial reached statistical significance.

A randomized, double-blind study of hirudin (40-mg bolus followed by 0.2 mg/kg per hour) and heparin in the prevention of restenosis after coronary angioplasty was conducted in Europe.[118] The primary end point was event-free survival (freedom from cardiac death, myocardial infarction, coronary bypass surgery, bail-out procedure, repeat PTCA, or elective stent placement) within 30 months of PTCA. At 7 months, event-free survival was 67.3 percent in the group receiving heparin, 63.5 percent in the group receiving intravenous hirudin, and 68.0 percent in the group receiving both intravenous and subcutaneous hirudin ($p = .61$). However, the administration of hirudin was associated with a significant reduction in early cardiac events, which occurred in 11.0, 7.9, and 5.6 percent of patients in the respective groups. Although significantly fewer early cardiac events occurred with hirudin than with heparin, hirudin had no apparent benefit with longer-term follow-up.

In a multicenter open-label pilot trial, 166 patients with unstable angina and angiographic thrombus were randomized to a 72- to 120-h infusion of heparin ($n = 50$) or r-hirudin ($n = 116$) at five escalating dosages (0.05 mg/kg to 0.3 mg/kg per hour).[119] A bolus of 0.9 mg/kg preceding the dose of 0.3 mg/kg per hour was abandoned because of minor bleeding, and was replaced by a bolus of 0.6 mg/kg. Heparin was given as a 5000-U bolus, followed by an infusion of 1000 U/h, which was adjusted to an APTT of 65 to 90 s or 90 to 110 s. Hirudin was not adjusted to the ATPP. All patients received aspirin and triple anti-ischemic therapy.

Upon repeat angiography at 72 to 120 h, patients assigned to hirudin (as opposed to heparin) had an improved cross-sectional area of the culprit vessel ($p = .08$), a larger minimum cross-sectional area ($p = .028$), and a smaller diameter stenosis ($p = .071$). The improvement in Thrombolysis in Myocardial Infarction (TIMI) flow grade was not significant ($p = .44$). Importantly, equal angiographic benefit was seen with hirudin at 0.1 to 0.3 mg/kg per hour, suggesting a plateau effect for the benefit of hirudin in this dose range. At similar APTT prolongations, hirudin as compared with high-dose heparin improved the angiographic end points. Clinical outcomes at 30 days did not reach statistical significance, although myocardial infarction developed in 2 percent of hirudin and 8 percent of heparin patients ($p = .11$).

In the open-label TIMI-5 pilot study of acute myocardial infarction in which patients were treated with front-loaded alteplase plus aspirin and randomized to either heparin or hirudin, 162 patients received a 5-day infusion of escalating hirudin dosage (0.05 to 0.2 mg/kg per hour) and 84 patients received heparin adjusted to an APTT of 65 to 90 s.[121] Major spontaneous hemorrhage occurred in 4.7 percent of heparin- versus 1.2 percent of hirudin-treated patients. Intracranial hemorrhage occurred in one heparin patient. Patients in the TIMI-6 pilot trial were treated with streptokinase and aspirin and were randomized to r-hirudin or heparin.[122] A trend toward improved outcome was observed with the higher dose (0.1 and 0.2 mg/kg per hour) of hirudin compared to the lower dose (0.05 mg/kg per hour) of hirudin and heparin.

After these pilot studies, in which the benefit/risk of hirudin appeared to be favorable, the larger trials were launched. The high bleeding risk, particularly of hemorrhagic stroke, of high-dose hirudin and heparin became apparent in the first three large phase III trials: TIMI-9A,[123] Global Use of Strategies to Open Occluded Coronary Arteries (GUSTO)-2A,[120] and Hirudin for the Improvement of Thrombolysis (HIT)-III.[124]

In view of these results, when high doses of hirudin were used and the observation that hirudin at 0.1 mg/kg per hour appeared to be as efficacious as the higher doses of hirudin, both in the unstable angina[119] and the TIMI-5[121] pilot study, GUSTO-IIb[125] and TIMI-9B[126] were restarted at lower hirudin (0.1 mg/kg bolus followed by 0.1 mg/kg per hour) and heparin (1000 IU/h without weight adjustment) dosages. In addition, both the heparin and the hirudin infusions were adjusted to a target APTT range of 55 to 85 s (TIMI-9A) and (GUSTO-IIa) 60 to 85 s to avoid APTTs > 100 s, which are clearly associated with increased risk of intracerebral hemorrhage. In GUSTO-IIb, 12,142 patients with acute coronary syndromes were randomly assigned to 72 h of therapy with either intravenous heparin or hirudin. Patients were stratified according to the presence of ST-segment elevation on the baseline electrocardiogram (4131 patients) or its absence (8011 patients), with the latter characteristic considered to indicate unstable angina or non-Q-wave myocardial infarction. Patients with ST elevation were qualified to receive thrombolytic therapy. At 24 h, the risk of death or myocardial infarction was significantly lower in the group assigned to hirudin therapy than in the group assigned to heparin (1.3 versus 2.1 percent, $p = .001$). The primary end point of death or nonfatal myocardial infarction or reinfarction at 30 days was reached in 9.8 percent of the heparin group as compared with 8.9 percent of the hirudin group (odds ratio for the risk of the end point in the hirudin group, 0.89; 95 percent confidence interval, 0.79 to 1.00, $p = .06$). The predominant effect of hirudin was on myocardial infarction or reinfarction and was not influenced by ST-segment status. There was no significant difference in the incidence of serious or life-threatening bleeding complications, but hirudin therapy was associated with a higher incidence of moderate bleeding (8.8 versus 7.7 percent, $p = .03$). In the TIMI-9 trial, 3002 patients with acute myocardial infarction were treated with aspirin and either accelerated-dose tissue plasminogen activator (t-PA) or streptokinase. They were randomized within 12 h of symptoms to receive either intravenous heparin 5000-U bolus followed by infusion of 1000 U/h) or hirudin (0.1 mg/kg bolus followed by infusion of 0.1 mg/kg per hour). the infusions of both antithrombins were titrated to a target APTT of 55 to 85 s and were administered for 96 h. The primary end point (death, recurrent nonfatal myocardial infarction, or development of severe congestive heart failure or cardiogenic shock by 30 days) occurred in 11.9 percent of the 1491 patients in the heparin group and 12.9 percent of the 151 patients in the hirudin group ($p =$ NS). Subgroup analyses did not reveal any profile of patients who benefited more from one of the antithrombins. The rate of major hemorrhage was similar in the heparin (5.3 percent) and hirudin (4.6 percent) groups; intracranial hemorrhage occurred in 0.9 percent of the heparin and 0.4 percent of the hirudin patients.

Hirulog

Hirulog is a bifunctional 20–amino acid peptide designed on the structure of hirudin. It combines a fragment of the C-terminus of hirudin (interacting with the anion-binding exosite

of thrombin) with an N-terminus fragment [D-Phe-Pro-Arg-Pro-(Gly)], which interacts with the catalytic site of thrombin. Toward thrombin, its K_D is 2.3×10^{-9} M.[127,128] The hirulog-thrombin complex is only transient, as thrombin can slowly cleave the Pro-Arg bond in the N-terminal extension. This metabolic cleavage contributes to its half-life on the APTT of about 40 min. Only 20 percent of hirulog is excreted in the urine, indicating an extensive hepatic catabolism or proteolysis at other sites. Newer hirulogs have been synthesized with noncleavable bonds for hirulog. There is no antidote.

In a dose-escalation pilot study, Lidon et al.[129] evaluated hirulog in 55 patients with unstable angina who also received aspirin and triple anti-ischemic therapy. Hirulog was administered in escalating doses of 0.02 to 0.5 mg/kg per hour increased every 30 min for 72 h. With doses up to 1 mg/kg per hour, only 1 of 20 patients experienced recurrent chest pain. The APTT in angina-free patients averaged 55.6 ± 6 s. Plasma FPA levels were suppressed at doses of 0.25 to 0.5 mg/kg per hour. The APTTs fell to baseline 4 h after discontinuation of hirulog. There was no rebound elevation of FPA at that time. Occult fecal blood was noted in 3 patients.

Pilot trials have evaluated hirulog as an adjunct to thrombolysis. Lidon et al.[130] randomized 45 patients to hirulog (0.5 mg/kg per hour without prior bolus, reduced to 0.1 mg/kg per hour after 12 h) or heparin (1000 U/h) added to streptokinase. At 90 min and 120 min, TIMI grades 2 and 3 flow was observed in 77 and 87 percent of patients treated with hirulog and heparin. TIMI grade 3 flow was present at 120 min in 77 percent of hirulog versus 40 percent of heparin patients. Bleeding complications occurred in 12 percent of hirulog versus 27 percent of heparin patients ($p =$ NS). There was only one intracerebral hemorrhage, which occurred in the heparin group. APTTs peaked at three and four times baseline, respectively, with hirulog and heparin, probably secondary to the fibrinolytic effect of streptokinase, as plasma levels were not higher than predicted from phase I studies.

In a multicenter trial, Topol et al.[131] evaluated hirulog in 291 patients undergoing elective angioplasty and pretreated with aspirin. Following bolus administration, a 4-h infusion of hirulog at 0.6 to 2.2 mg/kg per hour was given. Although there was a trend toward a dose-related increase in APTT prolongation, there was a wide overlap between APTT at different doses. No statistically significant activated clotting time (ACT), level was associated with complete prevention of acute closure. There was no prolongation of the bleeding time and no patient developed life-threatening bleeding. Acute closure within 24 h was inversely related to the hirulog dose and was 3.9 percent for the doses of 1.8 and 2.2 mg/kg per hour combined.[131] Preliminary information on the acute myocardial infarction Canadian Hirulog Early Reperfusion Occlusion (HERO) trial with the use of hirulog combined with thrombolytic therapy is encouraging.

Argatroban

Argatroban (Argipidine), an arginine derivative which binds to thrombin with intermediate affinity (K_D 3.9×10^{-8} M), competitively inhibits fibrinogen cleavage and platelet activation by thrombin. Compared with heparin, argatroban is significantly more effective in the prevention of platelet-rich thrombi after vascular injury and was effective at APTTs of only two to three times baseline control.[132,133]

In a whole-blood thrombolysis study with stenosed femoral arteries in the rabbit, argatroban (100 μg/kg per minute, APTT 2.5- to 3.0-fold baseline) accelerated reperfusion compared to heparin (200 U/kg, APTT > 5-fold baseline), although the incidence of reflow was not increased compared with heparin. Addition of aspirin did not accelerate thrombolysis by either argatroban or heparin.[132]

In a whole-blood clot thrombus model in stenotic canine coronaries, pretreatment with argatroban at 200 μg/kg per minute (yielding APTTs of 6 to 7.6 times control) significantly reduced the time to lysis by alteplase to 23 min, compared with 40 min in the aspirin group. Addition of aspirin to argatroban did not shorten the time to lysis but reduced the incidence of reocclusion by platelet-rich thrombi from 75 to 20 percent, relative to argatroban alone. Argatroban was as effective in this model as abciximab in inhibiting the platelet GPIIb/IIIa receptor.

In a platelet-rich coronary thrombus model after endothelial injury created by electrical current, acceleration of lysis, by alteplase, was observed in dogs pretreated with argatroban at a lower dose (41 μg/kg per minute). However, abolition of cyclic flow reductions, caused by intermittent platelet aggregates, required the addition of a thromboxane A_2/prostaglandin endoperoxide receptor antagonist.[134]

The results with argatroban plus aspirin seems to suggest that additional platelet (thromboxane) inhibition may be necessary when antithrombins of lower affinity are used to prevent early reocclusion after lysis with alteplase. On the other hand, high-affinity antithrombins like hirudin may be as (or more so) effective as antithrombins plus thromboxane blockade without additional antiplatelet agents.[135]

Argatroban combined with aspirin was well tolerated in humans at a dose yielding a mean APTT of 1.6 times baseline and did not prolong the bleeding time. Whether argatroban is effective at this dosage remains to be seen.

Napsagatran

RO46-6240 is a reversible, potent (K_i = 0.3 nM), and selective thrombin inhibitor of low molecular weight (559 Da).[136] Napsagatran was compared with heparin in a canine model of coronary thrombosis and concomitantly in an ex vivo perfusion-chamber model.[137] Occlusive thrombosis of the left circumflex coronary artery was induced by electrical injury. Napsagatran in this model showed arterial antithrombotic effects similar to those of heparin. The chamber experiments suggested that neither compound affects the initiation of platelet thrombus formation. The response to thrombolytic therapy is limited by ongoing platelet activation and thrombin generation. The relative contribution of both was studied in a canine model of coronary thrombolysis induced by t-PA.[138] Coronary thrombosis was induced by electrical injury; 2 h later, t-PA 10 μg/kg per minute was infused. Dose responses were

constructed using the platelet glycoprotein IIb/IIIa antagonist lamifibran (RO44-9883) and napsagatran. Napsagatran dose-dependently shortened the time to reperfusion (70 min at 5 μg/kg per minute versus 17 min at 40 μg/kg per minute), whereas lamifibran had no significant effect. Both drugs dose-dependently inhibited reocclusion. Combination of a subthreshold dose of napsagatran (5 μg/kg per minute) with a low dose of lamifibran (2 μg/kg per minute) reduced the time to reperfusion (40 min) compared with either drug alone. Moreover, the addition of lamifibran to napsagatran 5 μg/kg per minute abolished reocclusion, which persisted on this low dose of thrombin inhibitor alone. Thus, the limited effect of low-dose thrombin inhibitor could be overcome by either addition of a GPIIb/IIIa antagonist or increasing the dose of a thrombin inhibitor. These data suggest that thrombin-dependent activation of platelet GPIIb/IIIa is a major mechanism limiting the response to thrombolytic therapy in vivo. High-dose, specific thrombin inhibition has been associated with an increased risk of cerebral hemorrhage during coronary thrombolysis in humans. Hence, combination of low doses of thrombin inhibition with GPIIb/IIIa antagonism may provide a safer and more optimal approach.

Inogatran

Inogatran is a new, synthetic, active site inhibitor of thrombin with a molecular weight of 439.[139] Inogatran selectively, rapidly, and competitively binds thrombin with a K_i value of 15 nmol/L. In vitro it doubles the plasma thrombin time at a concentration of 23 nmol/L and the APTT at 1.1 μmol/L. Thrombin-induced platelet aggregation is inhibited at an IC_{50} of 17 nmol/L. In healthy volunteers, it was given intravenously as a bolus in doses from 0.002 to 1.1 μmol/kg. The highest peak plasma concentration observed was 7 μmol/L, corresponding to an APTT prolongation of three times. The drug was also given as a constant infusion over 4 h at a dose of 0.73 μmol/kg per hour, which resulted in a mean plasma concentration at steady state of 1.9 μmol/L and an APTT prolongation of 2.3 times. Finally, it was given as a bolus with radiolabeled compound in a total dose of 25 μmol. The drug was well tolerated and without side effects with the exception of slightly increased bleeding tendency at the blood sampling site.

Efegatran

Efegatran sulfate (LY294468) is a tripeptide, direct-acting thrombin inhibitor. The safety and anticoagulant properties of efegatran were studied at three dose levels in 36 patients with unstable angina.[140] Three groups of patients have been treated with a loading dose of 0.1 mg/kg in combination with a 48-h infusion of 0.105, 0.32, and 0.63 mg/kg per hour, respectively. Other patients were randomly allocated to receive standard, APTT-adjusted heparin therapy.

At these dose levels, efegatran has been clinically well tolerated. One of 10 patients at the highest dose received 2 U of packed cells for a hematoma after cardiac catheterization. No clinically significant prolongations of bleeding time have been recorded in any of the patients treated. Results of APTT measurements reveal that efegatran produces a dose-dependent prolongation of APTT (as predicted from both preclinical and human volunteer data). There is no evidence of accumulation of anticoagulant effect over time. In contrast to heparin (5000-IU bolus followed by 1000 IU/h), no APTT overshoot at 0.5 h was apparent. The anticoagulant activity of efegatran is dose-dependent and within the currently accepted clinically effective range at a dose of 0.63 mg/kg per hour. Further studies at these doses are warranted.

DuP714

This boroarginine tripeptide binds to thrombin with moderately high affinity (K_D 4.1×10^{-11} M) and inhibits thrombin-mediated platelet activation and fibrinogen cleavage.[141] DuP 714 reduced the incidence of venous thrombi in rabbits from 100 percent (controls) to 33 percent and arteriovenous shunt thrombosis from 72 to 11 percent. Its anticipated potential for oral administration has not been borne out in experimental or human studies. Because of liver toxicity, presumably related to the boron constituent, human studies were not pursued.

Other Direct Antithrombins

Other antithrombins still in development are peptides against the thrombin receptor of the platelet membrane[142] and hirudisins—hirudin derivatives combining IIb/IIIa receptor and thrombin inhibition. In the hirudisins, residues 32 to 35 of hirudin have been replaced by the integrin motif RGDS and KGDS, obtaining a potent thrombin inhibitor (K_D 0.16–0.26 $\times 10^{-12}$ M, compared with 0.2×10^{-12} M for r-hirudin) with additional dysintegrin activity.[143] In addition to inhibiting GPIIb/IIIa receptor–dependent platelet interactions, the platelet-binding integrin motif is expected to target the antithrombin action of hirudin to platelets, possibly allowing lower and safer doses of hirudin in the treatment of thrombotic disease. Similarly, hirudin targeted to fibrin[144] may allow for highly efficient antithrombotic activity at doses lower than presently required for r-hirudin.

Thrombolytic Drugs

All thrombolytic drugs are plasminogen activators, and, as indicated in Fig. 52-16, some are natural activators endogenous to the human fibrinolytic system and others are not.

STREPTOKINASE

Streptokinase is a nonenzyme protein produced by several strains of hemolytic streptococci; it consists of a single polypeptide chain of 414 amino acids with a molecular weight of about 50,000.[145] Streptokinase cannot directly cleave peptide bonds, but it activates plasminogen to plasmin indirectly, following a three-

step mechanism.[145] In the first step, streptokinase forms an equimolar complex with plasminogen. This complex undergoes a conformational change, resulting in the exposure of an active site in the plasminogen moiety. In the second step, this active site catalyzes the activation of plasminogen to plasmin. In a third step, plasminogen-streptokinase molecules are converted to plasmin-streptokinase complexes.[146] The active-site residues in the plasmin-streptokinase complex are the same as those in the plasmin molecule. However, plasmin is unable to activate plasminogen, whereas the plasmin(ogen)-streptokinase complex is not inhibited by alpha$_2$-antiplasmin.

Most individuals have measurable circulating streptokinase-neutralizing antibodies, which may result from previous infections with β-hemolytic streptococci. Therefore, during thrombolytic therapy, sufficient streptokinase must be infused to neutralize these antibodies. A few days after streptokinase administration, the antistreptokinase titer rises rapidly to 50 to 100 times the preinfusion value and remains high for 4 to 6 months, during which renewed treatment with streptokinase is impracticable.[147]

ANISOYLATED PLASMINOGEN-STREPTOKINASE COMPLEX

Anisoylated plasminogen-streptokinase activator complex (APSAC, anistreplase) was constructed with the aim of controlling the enzymatic activity of the plasmin(ogen)-streptokinase complex by a specific reversible chemical protection of its catalytic center (i.e., by titration with a p-anisoyl group).[148] Anistreplase is an equimolar noncovalent complex between human Lys-plasminogen and streptokinase. It has a catalytic center located in the carboxy-terminal region of the molecule, whereas the lysine-binding sites are found within the amino-terminal region of plasminogen. Reversible acylation of the catalytic center would thus not affect the weak fibrin-binding capacity of Lys-plasminogen in the complex. The plasmin(ogen)-streptokinase complex is an efficient activator of plasminogen. Deacylation of anistreplase uncovers the catalytic

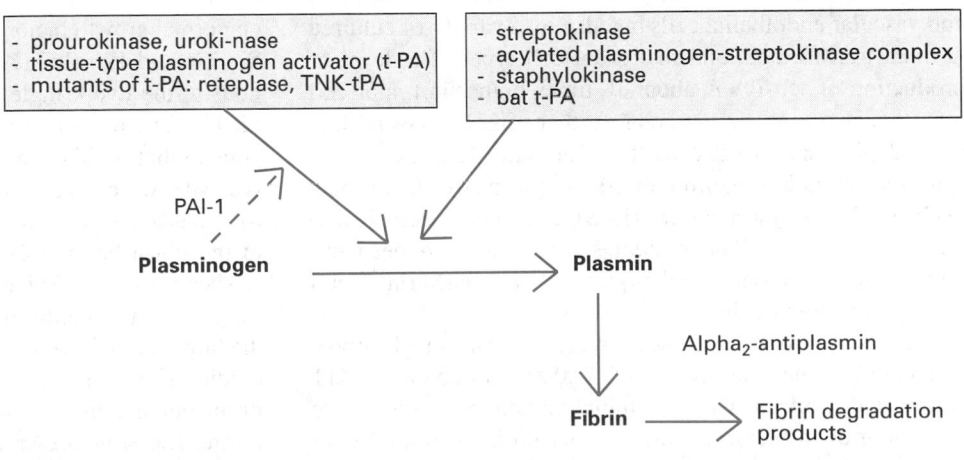

Plasminogen activators

- prourokinase, uroki-nase
- tissue-type plasminogen activator (t-PA)
- mutants of t-PA: reteplase, TNK-tPA

- streptokinase
- acylated plasminogen-streptokinase complex
- staphylokinase
- bat t-PA

PAI-1

Plasminogen → **Plasmin**

Alpha$_2$-antiplasmin

Fibrin → Fibrin degradation products

FIGURE 52-16

Components of the fibrinolytic system. In the left top box, natural plasminogen activators (endogenous to the human fibrinolytic system) and their mutants in clinical use are grouped separately from other plasminogen activators in clinical use (right top box).

center, which converts plasminogen to plasmin. Deacylation of anistreplase does, however, occur both in the circulation and at the fibrin surface, and the fibrin specificity of thrombolysis with anistreplase is only marginal at best. A plasma half-life of 70 min was found for anistreplase, compared with 25 min for the plasminogen-streptokinase complex formed in vivo after administration of streptokinase.[149] Patients with high streptokinase antibodies do not respond to anistreplase, and anistreplase causes a marked increase in the streptokinase antibody titer within 2 to 3 weeks, which persists for months.

UROKINASE

Two-chain urokinase-type plasminogen activator (tcu-PA), a trypsin-like serine proteinase composed of two polypeptide chains (20,000 and 34,000 Da), has been isolated from human urine[150] and from cultured human embryonic kidney cells.[151]

Two-chain urokinase-type plasminogen activator activates plasminogen directly following Michaelis-Menten kinetics but has no specific affinity for fibrin and activates fibrin-bound and circulating plasminogen relatively indiscriminately. Extensive plasminogen activation and depletion of alpha$_2$-antiplasmin may occur following treatment of thromboembolic diseases with tcu-PA, leading to degradation of several plasma proteins, including fibrinogen, factor V, and factor VIII.

PROUROKINASE

Single-chain urokinase-type plasminogen activator (scu-PA, pro-urokinase) is a naturally occurring human protein first isolated from natural sources and then produced through recombinant DNA technology.[152] The human gene responsible for its synthesis is located on chromosome 10 and is about 6.4 kb long, organized in 11 exons; it gives rise to a 2.5-kb-long messenger RNA, which transcribes a single-chain glycosylated polypeptide. Evidence for the signal transduction pathways involved in regulation of the urokinase gene has to date demonstrated three mechanisms, which are dependent respectively on activation of c-AMP protein kinase, protein kinase C, and an as yet uncharacterized protein kinase.[153]

The single-chain protein is synthesized principally by renal and vascular endothelial cells but also by a variety of cultured normal, transformed, and malignant cell types. The level of production of scu-PA is about 10 times higher in tumor cell lines than in normal tissues and is further stimulated by prolactin and pituitary gland extracts, interleukin-1, a number of cytokines including phorbol esters, tumor growth factor beta (TGF-β), lipopolysaccharides (LPS), and tumor necrosis factor-alpha (TNF-α). The protein scu-PA has also been expressed by gene cloning techniques in *E. coli* bacteria[154] and mouse hybridoma cells.

The glycosylated natural scu-PA is a single-chain glycoprotein with a molecular weight of 54,000 Da containing 411 amino acid residues. The N-terminal domain has a homology with the growth factor domain of other proteins, followed by a kringle domain, homologous to plasminogen, t-PA, and other proteins involved in coagulation.[155] However, the single-disulfide-bonded kringle domain of scu-PA does not con-

tain a lysine-binding site, and it does not confer fibrin-binding properties to the enzyme.

The single glycosylation site of the glycoprotein is located at asparagine 302. The molecule expressed by *E. coli* lacks the glycosyl group, which reduces the molecular weight to 47,000 Da.[154]

scu-PA is the native zymogenic precursor of urokinase. Limited hydrolysis by plasmin or kallikrein of the Lys[158]-Ile[159] peptide bond converts the molecule to two-chain urokinase-type plasminogen activator (tcu-PA, urokinase) which is held together by one disulfide bond essential for the thrombolytic activity[156] (Fig. 52-11). A fully active tcu-PA derivative is obtained after additional proteolysis at position Lys[135]-Lys[136]. In purified systems, scu-PA has some intrinsic plasminogen activating potential which is, however, 1 percent of that of tcu-PA. Conversion of scu-PA to tcu-PA in the vicinity of a fibrin clot apparently constitutes a significant positive feedback mechanism for clot lysis in human plasma in vitro.

Specific hydrolysis of the Glu[143]-Leu[144] peptide bond in scu-PA yields an LMW scu-PA of 32,000 (scu-PA-32k). Thrombin, on the other hand, cleaves the Arg[156]-Phe[157] peptide bond in scu-PA, resulting in an inactive double-chain molecule.

TISSUE-TYPE PLASMINOGEN ACTIVATOR

Native tissue–type plasminogen activator (t-PA) is a serine proteinase with a molecular weight of about 70,000, composed of one polypeptide chain containing 527 amino acids with serine as the amino-terminal amino acid.[157] t-PA is converted by plasmin to a two-chain form by hydrolysis of the Arg275-Ile276 peptide bond. The two-chain form is held together by one interchain disulfide bond. t-PA for clinical use is presently produced by recombinant DNA technology (Activase, Genentech Inc.; or Actilyse, Boehringer Ingelheim GmbH, Germany) and consists mainly of the single-chain form.

The NH2-terminal region of t-PA is composed of four domains with homologies to other proteins: residues 4–50 (F domain) are homologous to the "finger domains" in fibronectin, residues 50–87 (E domain) are homologous to human epidermal growth factor, and two regions comprising residues 87–176 and 176–262 (K1 and K2 domains) are both homologous to the five kringle loop structures of plasminogen (Fig. 52-11). The region comprising residues 276–527 is homologous to that of other serine proteinases and contains the catalytic site, which is composed of His322, Asp371, and Ser478. t-PA has a specific affinity for fibrin. The structures involved in the fibrin binding of t-PA are fully contained within the A (heavy) chain. Evidence obtained with deletion mutants suggests that binding of t-PA to fibrin is mediated both via the finger domain and via the second kringle region. A lysine-binding site is involved in the interaction of K2 domain with fibrin but not in the interaction of the finger domain with fibrin. The structures required for the enzymatic activity of t-PA are fully contained within the B chain.

The activation of plasminogen by t-PA, both in the presence and in the absence of fibrin, follows Michaelis-Menten kinetics.[158] There is a consensus that the presence of fibrin enhances the efficiency of plasminogen activation by t-PA by two to three orders of magnitude.[158] The kinetic data support a mechanism in which fibrin provides a surface to which t-PA and plasminogen adsorb in a sequential and ordered way, yielding a cyclic ternary complex. Fibrin essentially increases the local plasminogen concentration by creating an additional interaction between t-PA and its substrate. The high affinity of t-PA for plasminogen in the presence of fibrin thus allows efficient activation on the fibrin clot, while no efficient plasminogen activation by t-PA occurs in plasma. Plasmin formed on the fibrin surface has both its lysine-binding sites and active site occupied and is thus only slowly inactivated by alpha$_2$-antiplasmin (half-life of about 10 to 100 s); in contrast free plasmin, when formed, is rapidly inhibited by alpha$_2$-antiplasmin (half-life of about 0.1 s). The fibrinolytic process thus seems to be triggered by and confined to fibrin.

Mutants and variants of t-PA

Several mutants of recombinant tissue-type plasminogen activator (rt-PA) have been constructed with interesting properties, including slower clearance from the circulation, more selective binding to fibrin, stronger stimulation by fibrin, and resistance to plasma protease inhibitors.

Monteplase (E6010)

This is a modified t-PA constructed by substituting only one amino acid in the epidermal growth factor domain (Cys84 → Ser) has a prolonged half-life of more than 20 min, as compared with 6 min for wild-type t-PA.[159] This molecule has been used successfully for bolus administration in a canine femoral artery thrombosis model and in a multicenter pilot trial in patients with acute myocardial infarction.[160]

Reteplase (Retavase)

This is a single-chain nonglycosylated deletion variant of rt-PA consisting only of the K2 and the protease domains of human t-PA (Fig. 52-17). Production of reteplase in *E. coli* leads to formation of inactive protein aggregates (inclusion bodies). The isolation of the inclusion bodies,

refolding, and chromatographic purification of reteplase have been described.[161,162] The active site of the protease domain of reteplase and of t-PA, and their plasminogenolytic activity in the absence of a stimulator, do not differ, but the plasminogenolytic activity of reteplase in the presence of fragments of fibrinogen as a stimulator was fourfold lower compared to t-PA, whereas the binding of reteplase to fibrin was five times lower. These differences in plasminogenolytic activity and fibrin binding between the two molecules might possibly be due to the missing finger domain in reteplase. It is known that fibrin binding is mediated through both the finger domain and the lysine binding site in the K2 domain of t-PA. Reteplase and t-PA are inhibited by PAI-1 to a similar degree, but the affinity of reteplase for binding to endothelial cells and monocytes is reduced, probably as a consequence of deletion

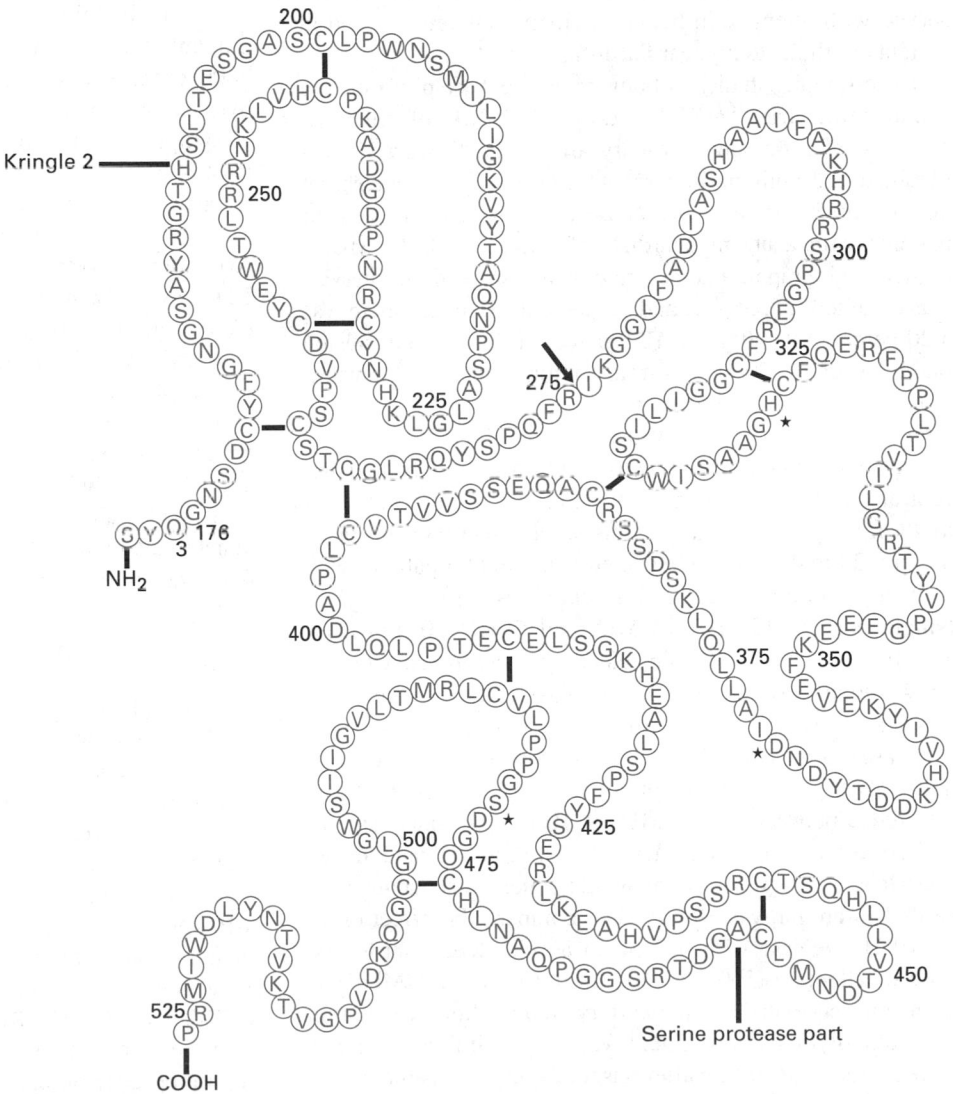

FIGURE 52-17

Schematic representation of the primary structure of reteplase (BM 06.022, retavase) (amino acids Ser^1-Gln^3 and Gly^{176}-Pro^{527} of tissue-type plasminogen activator). The amino acids are represented by their single-letter symbols; black bars indicate disulfide bonds and the asterisks indicate the active-site residues in the protease part. The arrow indicates the plasmin cleavage site.

of the finger and epidermal growth factor domains in reteplase, which seem to be involved in the interaction with endothelial cell receptors. The thrombolytic properties of reteplase and alteplase (recombinant t-PA) were compared in the rabbit jugular vein thrombosis model.[163] The effective dose for 50 percent thrombolysis (ED_{50}) was 163 kU/kg (0.28 mg/kg) for reteplase, and 871 kU/kg (1.09 mg/kg) for alteplase, indicating a 5.3-fold higher potency of reteplase. At equipotent doses (50 percent thrombolysis), the residual concentration of fibrinogen was 74 percent with reteplase and 76 percent with alteplase. Pharmacokinetic analysis of plasma activity at a dose of 400 kU/kg in the rabbit revealed a half-life of 18.9 ± 1.5 min for reteplase and 2.1 ± 0.1 min for alteplase. Plasma clearance for reteplase was 4.3-fold slower than for alteplase (4.7 versus 1.2 mL/min per kilogram).[164] One may therefore conclude that the higher potency of reteplase is due to the slower clearance. An initial half-life of 14 to 18 min was also observed with reteplase in healthy human volunteers[165] and in patients with acute myocardial infarction.[166]

Dose-ranging studies of bolus reteplase were performed in a multicenter trial.[167] With a dose of 10 MU of reteplase, a patent infarct-related coronary artery (TIMI-3 grade) was obtained at 30 min in 46 percent, at 60 min in 48 percent, at 90 min in 52 percent, and at 24 to 48 h in 88 percent of patients with acute myocardial infarction. With 15 MU, a higher angiographic patency rate at the same time intervals was obtained (38, 58, 69, and 85 percent). Because there was a 20 percent (10 MU) and 12.5 percent (15 MU) reocclusion rate between the 30- and 90-min angiograms, the administration of a second smaller bolus of reteplase (5 MU) 30 min after the initial bolus (10 MU) was investigated in an open uncontrolled study.[168] Patency rates (TIMI-3) reached 50 percent at 60 min, 58 percent at 90 min, and 84 percent at 24 to 48 h. Only 1 of the 50 patients studied had reocclusion in the first 24 to 48 h. In a controlled study in 605 patients with acute myocardial infarction, different bolus doses of reteplase (single dose of 15 MU, 10 MU, and 5 MU 30 min later; 10 MU and 10 MU 30 min later) were compared with the conventional dose regimen of alteplase (100 mg over 3 h). TIMI-3 patency rates at 90 min were obtained with the given reteplase regimen in 42.7, 45.4, and 62.9 percent, respectively, and in 47.6 percent of patients treated with alteplase.[169] The difference between the 10 MU + 10 MU reteplase and alteplase arms is significant ($p = .01$). Another randomized open-label angiographic study in 324 patients with acute myocardial infarction was designed to compare the effect of 10 + 10 U reteplase with that of an accelerated, front-loaded dose of alteplase (100 mg over 90 min) on the TIMI grade of the infarct-related coronary artery 90 min after the initiation of thrombolytic therapy. There was no age limit and patients were recruited up to 12 h after onset of symptoms; all received aspirin. The heparin regimen consisted of a 5000-IU intravenous bolus that was administered before thrombolytic therapy, followed by an infusion of 1000 IU/h for at least 24 h. In this study, reteplase achieved earlier and more complete reperfusion than accelerated-dose alteplase. TIMI grades 2 or 3 pat-

ency and TIMI grade 3 flow rates of the infarct-related artery at 90 min were significantly higher for reteplase relative to the alteplase control (83.4 versus 73.3 percent and 59.9 versus 45.2 percent, respectively). At 60 min, both the TIMI grade 2 or 3 patency and the TIMI grade 3 flow rates were significantly higher for reteplase as compared with alteplase. Reteplase-treated patients required significantly fewer additional coronary interventions within the first 6 h of treatment (13.3 versus 26.5 percent). As expected in a trial of this size, there were no significant differences between the reteplase and alteplase groups with respect to 35-day mortality (4.1 versus 8.4 percent) and hemorrhagic stroke (1.2 versus 1.8 percent).

Two mortality trials with reteplase were planned in patients with acute myocardial infarction. The International Joint Efficacy Comparison of Thrombolytics (INJECT) study was designed to determine whether reteplase was at least as effective in mortality reduction as a standard streptokinase regimen.[171] In this double-blind study, 3004 patients were randomized to a double bolus of 10 + 10 U of reteplase 30 min apart and 3006 patients were randomized to 1.5 MU of streptokinase over 60 min. Treatment could be started up to 12 h from onset of symptoms. All patients received intravenous heparin for at least 24 h and aspirin. The 35-day mortality rate was 9.0 percent in the reteplase group and 9.5 percent in the streptokinase group, a nonsignificant difference (95 percent CI, 1.98 to 0.96 percent). At 6 months, mortality rates were 11.0 percent for reteplase and 12.0 percent for streptokinase. Bleeding events were similar in the two groups (0.7 percent for reteplase and 1.0 percent for streptokinase). The in-hospital stroke rates were 1.23 percent for reteplase and 1.0 percent for streptokinase. The incidence of recurrent myocardial infarction was similar in the two groups. In the GUSTO-III mortality trial, reteplase was administered in two bolus injections 30 min apart and compared to front-loaded alteplase (100 mg in 90 min) in up to 12,000 patients treated within 6 h of symptoms of acute myocardial infarction. Although still unpublished, the results were similar in both groups.

TNK-TPA

A mutant of rt-PA in which Thr[103] is substituted by Asn (code rt-PA-T) and the sequence Lys[296]-His-Arg-Arg is mutagenized to Ala-Ala-Ala-Ala (code rt-PA-K) was found to have both a prolonged half-life and resistance to PAI-1. This mutant has an increased potency on platelet-rich arterial thrombi (rich in PAI-1) in a canine model of coronary thrombosis.[172] Additional substitution in this mutant of Asn[117] by Gln (code rt-PA-N) resulted in a t-PA variant with eightfold slower clearance and 200-fold enhanced resistance to PAI-1. These three combinations in a single molecule are referred to as TNK-TPA (Fig. 52-18). In in vivo models of thrombolysis in rabbits, TNK-TPA was shown to have an increased thrombolytic potency on platelet-rich clots, to conserve fibrinogen, and to be effective upon bolus administration at half the dose of rt-PA. Similar results were obtained in a combined arterial and venous thrombosis model in the dog.[173]

A pharmacokinetic study in patients with acute myocardial infarction was conducted with bolus administration of TNK-

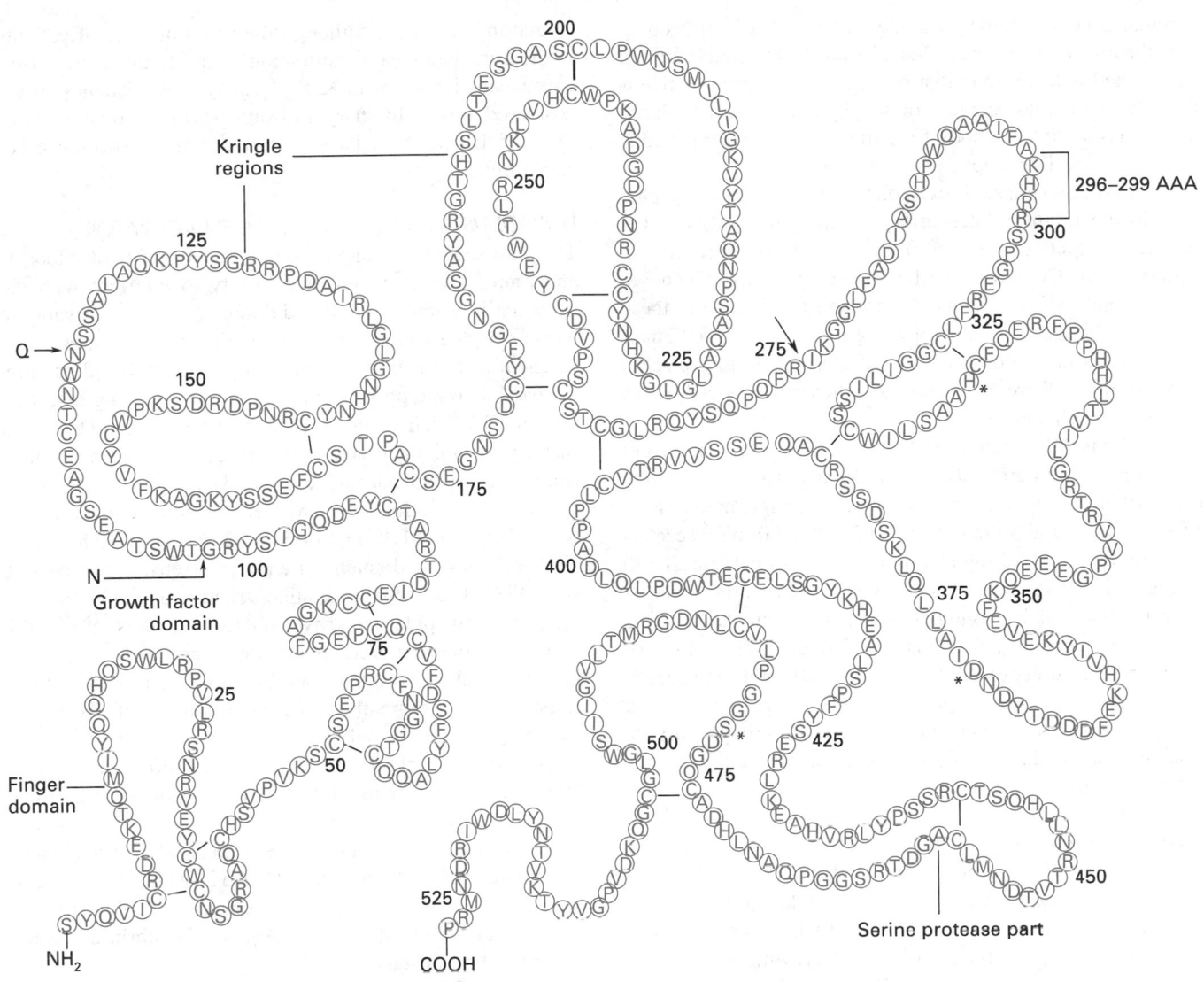

FIGURE 52-18

Schematic representation of the primary structure of recombinant tissue-type plasminogen activator-TNK (TNK-TPA) (substitution on rt-PA of Thr[103] by Asn, Asn[111] by Gln, and Lys[296]-His-Arg-Arg by Ala-Ala-Ala-Ala. The amino acids are represented by their single-letter symbols, black bars indicate disulfide bonds, and the asterisks indicate the active site residues in the protease part. The arrow indicates the plasmin cleavage site.

TPA. Overall the clearance of TNK-t-PA was 151 ± 56 mL/min, which is significantly slower than the clearance of 572 ± 132 mL/min for native t-PA. The clearance ranged from 216 ± 98 to 125 ± 25 over the 5- to 50-mg dose range studied. The initial plasma half-life was from 11 to 20 min as compared with a half-life of 3.5 min for native t-PA. There was a slight decrease in clearance with increasing dose over the 5- to 50-mg dose range studied.[174]

A comparison of the bolus dose of TNK-TPA with the accelerated 90- min infusion of native rt-PA demonstrated a similar plasma concentration profile for the two regimens. Based on pharmacokinetic analysis, it appeared that a 30 mg bolus dose of TNK-TPA could provide a similar plasma exposure to 100 mg of accelerated infusion of t-PA.[174] No decrease was seen in either fibrinogen or plasminogen concentrations as the dose of TNK-TPA was increased from 5 to 50 mg. Similarly, the decreases seen in the alpha₂-antiplasmin levels to approxi-

mately 20 percent below baseline were much less than the 40 to 45 percent decrease seen with recombinant t-PA. Although at even higher doses of TNK-TPA, a further drop in alpha₂-antiplasmin might be expected, it is clear from these data that a generalized fibrinosenolytic effect is not induced.

TNK-TPA also gave encouraging initial indications that it will be angiographically efficacious (TIMI-10A).[174] Beginning with the low doses (7.5 to 15 mg), good 90-min patency rates were seen. The best TIMI-3 flow rates were seen at 30, 40, and 50 mg (57 to 68 percent TIMI-3), which compares favorably with the 54 percent of recombinant t-PA treated patients in GUSTO with TIMI-3 flow.

In the initial phase I study, there were 4 deaths of the 113 patients (mortality = 3.5 percent).[174] No patients experienced a stroke and there were no cases of intracerebral hemorrhages in the study. Six patients (5.3 percent) reported a major hemorrhage and four (3.5 percent) of those occurred at sites of vascular access following catheterization. This is in keeping with the lower rate of surgical-site hemorrhage noted in animal studies and is lower than that of other studies using native t-PA. There were no episodes of anaphylaxis and no evidence of anti-TNK-TPA antibody formation in any of the patients. Overall, TNK-TPA appeared to be well tolerated.

There are two Phase II trials, one for efficacy (angiographic flow in the infarct-related artery as the end point) and the second for safety (safety end points—death and intracerebral hemorrhage). These trials will enroll concurrently. The doses administered will be 30 and 50 mg and the data from these trials will be the basis for selecting a single dose for Phase III. There is an option built into the protocols to replace a dose group if there is a lack of efficacy or safety issues (intracerebral hemorrhage).

The Phase II efficacy trial is a randomized, open-label study and will be performed internationally. This angiography trial will have three treatment groups, two single bolus TNK-TPA arms (30 and 50 mg) compared with a 90-min "accelerated" regimen of 100 mg alteplase. Each arm will enroll 150 patients. The primary end point will be TIMI flow grade at 90 min. There will be a blind evaluation of the cineangiograms by a core laboratory. Secondary end points are patency of infarct-related artery (TIMI flow grade and TIMI frame count), coagulation parameters, pharmacokinetic parameters, and safety parameters. Patients will be followed through hospital discharge and at day 30 (if there are antibodies at day 30, the patient will be reevaluated at 3 months).

The Phase II safety trial is a randomized, open-label trial which will be conducted worldwide. The safety trial will have two dose arms (30 and 50 mg TNK-TPA) and no t-PA arm, since there are well-characterized recent historical data. A total of 3000 patients will be enrolled, 1500 patients per arm. The primary end point for this trial is safety, with intracerebral hemorrhage, death, total stroke, recurrent myocardial infarction, cardiogenic shock, anaphylaxis, pulmonary edema, revascularization, and serious/life-threatening bleeding complications being the prespecified end points.

Based on the patency and safety data from the Phase II trials, Phase III will be designed to compare TNK-TPA to an accelerated (90-min) infusion of Activase. The primary end point of a Phase III trial will likely be "net clinical benefit," defined as mortality plus nonfatal stroke.

RECOMBINANT CHIMERIC PLASMINOGEN ACTIVATORS

Recombinant chimeric plasminogen activators have been constructed primarily using different regions of t-PA and scu-PA, although several alternative combinations have been evaluated to some extent.[175,176] In vivo evaluation of thrombosis in animal models indicated that one of these variants ($K_1K_2P_u$) had a markedly enhanced thrombolytic potency toward venous and arterial thrombi. $K_1K_2P_u$ consists of kringles 1 and 2 of rt-PA (amino acids Ser[1]-Gln[3] and Asp[87]-Phe[274]) and of the serine proteinase part of prourokinase (amino acids Ser[138]-Leu[411]). A small feasibility study of coronary thrombolysis with $K_1K_2P_u$ has been performed in patients with acute myo-

cardial infarction.[177] Although the small number of patients studied precludes valid estimation of the frequency of coronary recanalization with $K_1K_2P_u$ and of the adequacy of the dose used, this preliminary trial suggests that two bolus injections of 10 mg $K_1K_2P_u$ may produce fibrin-specific coronary thrombolysis.

DESMODUS SALIVARY PLASMINOGEN ACTIVATOR

The subsistence of vampire bats on a diet of fresh blood is apparently contingent on their ability to interfere with the hemostatic system of the blood donor. The saliva of vampire bats contains a variety of factors that presumably satisfy two essential requirements: to maintain prolonged bleeding from the wound and to preserve blood fluidity following ingestion of a meal.[178] Different molecular forms of the *Desmodus* salivary plasminogen activator (DSPA) have been purified, characterized, cloned, and expressed. Two high-molecular-weight forms exhibit about 85 percent homology to human t-PA: DSPAα1 (M_r 43) and DSPAα2 (M_r 39) which contain neither a kringle 2 domain nor a plasmin-sensitive processing site. DSPAβ lacks the finger-like structure and DSPAγ lacks the finger and epidermal growth-factor structures.[118–183] The two high-molecular-weight forms exhibit a specific activity in vitro equal to or higher than that of t-PA, a relative PAI-1 resistance, and a greatly enhanced fibrin specificity with a strict requirement for polymeric fibrin as a cofactor.[179,181,182] In animal (rats, rabbits, and dogs) models of thrombolysis, DSPAα1 is superior to t-PA in terms of potency (2.5 times higher), terminal half-life (three times longer), and clearance (four- to eightfold slower).[182] Interestingly, the fibrin cofactor requirement of DSPAα1 and DPSAα2, which both bind to fibrin, may not solely depend on fibrin binding, as the two smaller forms, DPSAβ and DSPAγ, are also fibrin-dependent but lack fibrin affinity.[182]

ZK152387 is recombinant DSPAα1 produced in mammalian cell culture; its amino acid sequence is identical to that of its natural counterpart.[183] DSPAα1 may be suitable for bolus administration; its long half-life and high specific activity may allow a marked reduction of the absolute dose of drug required for effective thrombolysis as compared with t-PA.

STAPHYLOKINASE

Mature staphylokinase consists of 136 amino acids in a single polypeptide chain without disulfide bridges. Staphylokinase, like streptokinase, is not an enzyme but forms a 1:1 stoichiometric complex with plasmin(ogen) that activates other plasminogen molecules. Streptokinase and plasminogen produce a complex that exposes the active site in the plasminogen molecule without proteolytic cleavage, whereas generation of plasmin is required for exposure of the active site in the complex with staphylokinase.[184,185]

Staphylokinase does not bind to fibrin, and fibrin stimulates the initial rate of plasminogen activation by staphylokinase only fourfold as compared with twofold by streptokinase. In purified systems α_2-antiplasmin rapidly inhibits the plasmin-staphylokinase complex (second-order inhibition rate constant of approximately $2 \times 10^6 \text{ M}^{-1}\text{s}^{-1}$), although it does not inhibit the plasmin(ogen)-streptokinase complex. Addition of 6-aminohexanoic acid or of fibrin-like substances (e.g., CNBr-digested fibrinogen) induces a more than 100-fold reduction of the inhibition rate of the plasmin-staphylokinase complex by α_2-antiplasmin. Rapid inhibition by α_2-antiplasmin indeed requires the availability of the lysine-binding sites in the plasminogen moiety of the complex. More detailed studies on the interaction between staphylokinase, plasmin(ogen), and α_2-antiplasmin have shown that neutralization of the plasmin-staphylokinase complex by α_2-antiplasmin results in dissociation of functionally active staphylokinase from the complex, followed by its recycling to other plasminogen molecules.[184]

In plasma, the conversion of plasminogen-staphylokinase to plasmin-staphylokinase complex does not occur at a significant rate because it is prevented by α_2-antiplasmin; without plasmin-staphylokinase complex, no significant plasminogen activation occurs. In the presence of fibrin, generation of the plasmin(ogen)-staphylokinase complex is facilitated and inhibition of plasmin-staphylokinase by α_2-antiplasmin at the clot surface is delayed. Recycling of staphylokinase to fibrin-bound plasminogen, after neutralization of the complex, will result in more efficient generation of the active complex. This mechanism is mediated via the lysine-binding sites of plasminogen and results in a significantly enhanced plasminogen activation at the fibrin surface. These regulatory properties of fibrin and α_2-antiplasmin suggest that the fibrin-specificity of staphylokinase is due to rapid inhibition of generated plasmin-staphylokinase complex by α_2-antiplasmin and by a more than 100-fold reduced inhibition rate at the fibrin surface.[184,186]

Recombinant staphylokinase (STAR)[187] was found to have a potency for venous clot lysis in hamsters and rabbits comparable to that of streptokinase. Additional studies in hamsters and dogs suggested that STAR may be relatively more potent than streptokinase toward platelet-rich clots and potentially less immunogenic. These findings were subsequently confirmed in baboons, where STAR was shown to have a thrombolytic potency toward jugular vein blood clots comparable to that of streptokinase but to be less immunogenic and less allergenic.[188] Indeed, repeated administration of STAR, in contrast to streptokinase, did not induce resistance to clot lysis in this model. In addition, STAR was found to be significantly more efficient than streptokinase for the dissolution of platelet-rich arterial eversion graft thrombi.[187]

These encouraging results have formed the basis for the evaluation, on a pilot scale, of the pharmacokinetic, thrombolytic, and immunogenic properties of STAR in patients with acute myocardial infarction.[189] In 4 of 5 patients with acute myocardial infarction, 10 mg of STAR given intravenously over 30 min was found to induce angiographically documented coronary artery recanalization within 40 min. Plasma fibrinogen and α_2-antiplasmin levels were unaffected and allergic reactions were not observed. In a second series of 5 patients with acute coronary occlusion, intravenous administration of 10 mg of STAR over 30 min induced recanalization

in all patients within 20 min without associated fibrinogen degradation.[190] However, in these patients, neutralizing antibodies were consistently demonstrable in plasma at 14 to 35 days. Thus, with respect to immunogenicity, the initial observations in humans are not as encouraging as the experience in baboons. The experience in patients with myocardial infarction has been expanded to 100 patients with myocardial infarction of < 6 h duration who were allocated to accelerated and weight-adjusted t-PA over 90 min (52 patients) or to recombinant staphylokinase (STAR) (the first 25 patients to 10 mg and the next 23 patients to 20 mg given intravenously over 30 min).[191] All patients received aspirin and intravenous heparin. TIMI 3 flow grade at 90 min was achieved in 62 percent of STAR patients versus 58 percent of t-PA patients (risk ratio, 1.1; 95 percent CI, 0.76 to 1.5). With 10 mg STAR, TIMI-3 patency was 50 percent (risk ratio, 0.86; 95 percent CI, 0.54 to 1.4 versus rt-PA); with 20 mg STAR, it was 74 percent (risk ratio, 1.3; 95 percent CI, 0.90 to 1.2 versus rt-PA). Residual fibrinogen levels at 0 min were 118 ± 47 percent (mean $\pm$ S.D.) of baseline with STAR and 68 ± 42 percent with rt-PA ($p < .0005$). STAR therapy was not associated with an excess mortality or electrical, hemorrhagic, mechanical, or allergic complications. However, patients developed antibody-mediated STAR-neutralizing activity from the second week after STAR treatment.

ANTITHROMBOTIC AND THROMBOLYTIC THERAPY IN CARDIAC DISEASE

A sound understanding of the pathogenesis of the thrombotic processes in cardiovascular disease and the relative risks of thrombosis and thromboembolism is required to develop a rational approach to antithrombotic therapy.[192,193] This review provides guidelines for antithrombotic therapy in the various cardiac syndromes from the perspective of pathogenesis and thrombotic and thromboembolic risk. More specific antithrombotic approaches are described in the chapters devoted to the various disease entities.

Pathogenesis of Thrombosis and Thromboembolism: Predominance of Platelets and/or Fibrin (Table 52-5)

CORONARY ARTERIES

As previously discussed in more detail, vascular injury and thrombus formation are central events in the initiation and progression of the atherosclerotic process leading to the acute coronary syndromes. When there is superficial endothelial injury, the platelets form a monolayer to cover the exposed subendothelium. When injury is more severe, such as plaque rupture during the acute coronary syndromes or immediately after angioplasty, exposure of the vessel wall substrate, such as the lipid pool or smooth muscle cells, appears to lead to fibrin formation and platelet activation and aggregation by exposure of the platelet membrane IIb/IIIa receptors (Fig. 52-2 and Table 52-5). This in turn leads to further activation

TABLE 52-5

RISK STRATIFICATION IN CARDIOVASCULAR DISEASE—ROLE OF ASPIRIN AND ANTICOAGULANTS

Pathogenesis	Thromboembolic Risk		
	High (>6% year)	Medium (2–6% year)	Low (<2% year)
Arterial Platelets and fibrin (PI and/or A/C)	ACS, PTCA ASA + A/C	Stable CAD ASA or A/C	Primary prevent PI?
Chambers	A-fib—emboli A-fib—M. stenosis	A-fib—valv, nonvalv Anterior MI—early Dilated cardiomyopathy	A-fib—lone Chronic LV aneurysm
Fibrin (A/C)	INR 2.5–3.5	INR 2.0–3.0	No therapy
Prostheses Fibrin more than platelets (A/C > PI)	Old mechanical Previous emboli Extensive atherosclerosis INR 3.0–4.5 or INR 2.5–3.5 + ASA	Recent mechanical Bioprosthesis—A-fib Mech—INR 2.5–3.5 Bio—INR 2.0–3.0	Biopr.—NSR No therapy

Key: PI = platelet inhibitor (i.e., aspirin); A/C = anticoagulants; ACS = acute coronary syndrome; ASA = aspirin; PTCA = percutaneous transluminal coronary angioplasty; CAD = coronary artery disease; A-fib = atrial fibrillation; MI = myocardial infarction; LV = left ventricle; INR = International Normalized Ratio.
Source: Modified from Stein et al.,[192] with permission.

of the intrinsic and extrinsic coagulation systems.[194] Specifically, it appears that at the site of plaque damage, the extrinsic pathway is activated through the release of tissue factor from the macrophages present in the arterial wall,[194] and it is the generation of thrombin that leads to fibrin formation and eventually contributes to platelet activation.

Acute Coronary Syndromes

In many patients with unstable angina, plaque rupture leads to thrombus formation and transient occlusion of the coronary artery—with chest pain, usually lasting only 10 to 20 min—followed by reperfusion of the vessel.[194] In non-Q-wave myocardial infarction, there is probably more severe plaque damage and more persistent occlusion of the vessel, often lasting as long as 1 h. In Q-wave infarction, there is persistent occlusion of the coronary artery, which leads to cessation of blood flow for more than 1 h, resulting in transmural cellular necrosis.

The occlusive thrombus may undergo spontaneous lysis. However, the intraarterial surface (i.e., the ruptured plaque and the thrombus) remains very thrombogenic, thus creating a high risk of rethrombosis. Indeed, it appears that the surface of the remaining thrombus exposes tissue factor and thrombin, which activate platelets and the coagulation cascade. Thus, activation of both the coagulation system and platelets plays a pivotal role in thrombus formation and rethrombosis in the acute coronary syndromes.[194]

Coronary Intervention

Percutaneous transluminal coronary angioplasty (PTCA) and other catheter-based interventional techniques are associated with denudation of the endothelium and deep vessel injury. This results in exposure of thrombogenic elements in the atherosclerotic plaque and the vessel wall, which predisposes this area to fibrin formation and platelet deposition, leading to intravascular thrombosis.[195] Therefore, therapy to prevent acute occlusion following coronary intervention should be directed against both platelet activation and the coagulation cascade.

Saphenous Vein Bypass Grafting

Disease of the saphenous vein graft is the most important factor leading to recurrent ischemia following coronary bypass surgery. Occlusion rates are 8 to 18 percent per distal anastomosis 1 month postoperatively and 16 to 26 percent at 12 months.[196] Vein graft disease can be divided into three phases: an early postoperative phase (within 1 month after surgery) related to thrombotic occlusion, in which platelet activation and fibrin formation are implicated; an intermediate phase (within the first postoperative year) characterized by intimal hyperplasia, resulting in a form of accelerated atherosclerosis that may have a superimposed thrombotic tendency; and a late phase (after the first postoperative year) characterized by graft atherosclerosis similar to that of the native coronary arteries.[196] Therefore, the predominant pathogenetic mechanism in saphenous vein bypass grafting is related to both platelet activation and fibrin generation, particularly in the early postoperative phase.

Progression of Chronic Coronary Disease

One might expect atherosclerotic lesions to expand in a linear fashion. However, angiographic studies have shown this not to be the case. Many high-grade lesions often appear in segments of the coronary artery that were previously normal.[197] It is thought that this erratic and unpredictable growth is caused by plaque disruption or fissuring and intracoronary mural thrombosis.[194] Thus, mural thrombus forms by the same mechanism as thrombus in the acute coronary syndromes. However, in the majority of patients, the thrombus is not occlusive. The mural thrombus then undergoes fibrous organization and contributes, often asymptomatically, to the progression of the disease.[194]

CARDIAC CHAMBERS

Below, we relate this brief discussion of intracavitary thrombus formation to that of the left ventricle and left atrium.

Left Ventricle

The development of intracavitary or mural thrombi in patients with acute myocardial infarction, left ventricular aneurysm, and dilated cardiomyopathy is well described. The pathogenesis of intracavitary thrombosis is related to the classical description by Rudolph Vichow, who defined three precipitating factors: endothelial injury, stasis, and hypercoagulability.[198] The last two factors contribute significantly to fibrin deposition and activation of the coagulation system (Fig. 52-2 and Table 52-5). Once a thrombus forms, the clinical significance is mainly related to its potential for embolism.

Endocardial Injury Following an acute myocardial infarction, leukocyte infiltration separates endothelial cells from their basal lamina. This results in exposure of the subendothelial tissue to intracavitary blood, which leads to activation of platelets and the coagulation system and may trigger thrombus formation.

Blood Stasis Blood stasis in areas of akinesis or dyskinesis is an important factor in the predisposition to thrombus formation. Thus, it occurs in a diffuse or segmental dilated ventricle with or without cardiac failure. The three most classic clinical conditions predisposed to blood stasis are dilated cardiomyopathy, anterior myocardial infarction, and left ventricular aneurysm. Stasis triggers activation of the coagulation system, leads to fibrin formation, and accounts for the predominant pathogenetic mechanism in the development of intracavitary thrombus formation.

Hypercoagulable State During an acute myocardial infarction, there is a greater tendency toward systemic coagulation. This is based on observations of increased tendency of deep venous thrombosis and left ventricular thrombus formation and on evidence of systemic elevations of serum fibrinogen levels.

Dynamic Forces of the Circulation Thus, while the combination of the three components of Virchow's triad predisposes to thrombus formation, formation of intracavitary thrombi does not necessarily lead to embolization. Dynamic forces of the chambers determine the propensity toward embolization. For example, in the case of left ventricular aneurysm, the isolation from dynamic circulatory forces may protect from systemic embolization; this in part may explain the relatively low incidence of thromboembolism in segmental ischemic cardiomyopathy. In contrast, in dilated cardiomyopathy, a diffuse process, the mural thrombus is not isolated from the circulation and therefore may be at higher risk of embolization. Therefore, in stratifying risk, one must consider not only the predisposition to thrombus formation but also the risk of subsequent embolization.

Left Atrium

The pathophysiology of thrombus formation in the left atrium is similar to that described above, in which stasis is the pre-

dominant mechanism. In nonvalvular atrial fibrillation, stasis leads to fibrin generation and potentially to thrombus formation (Fig. 52-2 and Table 52-5). Valvular heart disease, particularly mitral stenosis, also predisposes to fibrin generation by increasing stasis in the atria. When atrial fibrillation occurs with mitral stenosis, the risk of thrombus formation in the left atrium becomes high.

Thus, in the cardiac chambers, thrombus formation occurs due to stasis, endocardial injury, and hypercoagulability. The predominant pathophysiologic process is related to generation of fibrin.

PROSTHETIC VALVES

Thrombus formation in mechanical prosthetic heart valves and bioprosthetic valves will be described.

Mechanical Prostheses

Almost immediately after implantation of a mechanical prosthesis, platelet deposition begins, particularly on the endocardium-suture-prosthesis interfaces and on damaged perivascular tissue. Platelet deposition leads to activation of factor XII and initiation of the coagulation cascade.[199] Eventually, stasis and abnormal hemodynamics promote fibrin generation, which predominates over the platelet component of this response (Fig. 52-2 and Table 52-5). This is particularly true when there is left atrial enlargement, which allows for a greater degree of stasis. In recent years, efforts to make lower-profile valves with better flow characteristics have resulted in less fibrin deposition on these valves. Thus, the newer-generation low-profile valves may be less predisposed to thrombus formation.

Bioprostheses

Bioprostheses are considerably less thrombogenic mainly because of the natural properties of the materials used and because of their axial flow properties and leaflet pliability. However, bioprosthetic valves are predisposed to thrombus formation in the immediate postoperative period, with platelet and fibrin deposition, and later, if there is atrial fibrillation and left atrial enlargement, with fibrin generation due to stasis.

In summary, the pathogenesis of arterial thrombosis involves damage to the vessel wall and exposure to a thrombogenic surface leading to both platelet deposition and activation of the coagulation system (Fig. 52-2 and Table 52-5). Intracavitary thrombosis occurs primarily in areas where there is stasis, which predisposes to activation of the coagulation system over platelet deposition. Finally, mechanical prostheses promote activation of the coagulation system and, to a lesser degree, platelet activation. Biological prostheses are significantly less thrombogenic.

Risk Stratification on No Antithrombotics: Implications for Antithrombotic Therapy (Table 52-5)

In the preceding section we described the pathophysiologic basis of thrombus formation in the various clinical syndromes.

It is now imperative to consider the various clinical heart disease syndromes according to absolute and relative risk of developing thromboembolic events. Below, we shall discuss three general risk categories assuming the use of no antithrombotics. The highest-risk category involves more than six episodes per 100 patients per year; the medium-risk range involves two to six episodes per 100 patients annually; and the lower-risk rate involves less than two events per 100 patients per year. In general, for those with high risk, aggressive antithrombotic management is recommended. In contrast, for those with low risk, antithrombotic therapy may not even be recommended. For those in the medium-risk group, an intermediate approach is suggested.[192,193]

CORONARY ARTERIES (Table 52-5)

High Risk (More Than Six Episodes per 100 Patients per Year)

Acute Coronary Syndromes In the absence of thrombolytic therapy, the risk is high for developing an occlusive thrombus in the case of unstable angina or rethrombosis in the case of a lysed thrombus in acute myocardial infarction.[194]

Coronary Intervention As mentioned previously, during the procedure, catheter-based interventions such as PTCA or stenting lead to platelet activation and activation of the coagulation system, with a high risk of thrombotic occlusion. Later on, those who have undergone intervention have a low long-term risk of thrombosis.[192,193]

Saphenous Vein Bypass Grafting As mentioned previously, disease of the saphenous vein graft is the most important factor leading to myocardial ischemia following coronary bypass surgery. Occlusion rates are 8 to 18 percent per distal anastomosis at 1 month postoperatively and 16 to 26 percent at 12 months.[196] Therefore, within the first year (particularly the first few days) after coronary artery bypass surgery, patients are considered to be at high risk for thrombotic complications. Beyond 1 year, patients are considered to be at medium risk for developing thrombotic complications of the saphenous vein graft.[192,193]

Medium Risk (Two to Six Episodes per 100 Patients per Year)

Post–Acute Myocardial Infarction and Chronic Coronary Disease Survivors of acute myocardial infarction are at medium risk of recurrent infarction or cardiac death. Based on data from the Framingham study, those who have survived a myocardial infarction or unstable angina or have chronic coronary disease without infarction are estimated to have a risk of 2.5 to 5 percent of either reinfarction or ischemic death.[192,193]

Low Risk (Less Than Two Episodes per 100 Patients per Year)

Primary Prevention of Coronary Events Individuals who have no risk factors for coronary disease are thought to be at low risk for infarction and ischemic death. However, those populations with a high prevalence of coronary disease—i.e., those with many cardiac risk factors—have a higher inherent risk of an acute coronary syndrome and may therefore be in the intermediate risk category.

CARDIAC CHAMBERS (Table 52-5)

High Risk (More Than Six Episodes per 100 Patients per Year)

Mitral Stenosis with Atrial Fibrillation Atrial fibrillation is a common arrhythmia and is associated with the potentially devastating complication of systemic embolism. The highest risk of systemic thromboembolism in mitral stenosis is in patients with atrial fibrillation. Specifically, the presence of mitral stenosis and atrial fibrillation dramatically increases the risk of thromboembolism, and nearly 75 percent of patients who have emboli are in chronic atrial fibrillation.

Atrial Fibrillation with a History of Previous Thromboembolism In patients with atrial fibrillation, the highest risk is in those patients who have experienced a prior thromboembolism. Those with a prior embolism related to mitral stenosis are at high risk for a recurrent thromboembolism. Specifically, the risk of a recurrent event exceeds 10 percent per year.[193]

Medium Risk (Two to Six Episodes per 100 Patients per Year)

Nonvalvular Atrial Fibrillation The risk of ischemic stroke in nonvalvular atrial fibrillation is about medium, but it is directly related to the presence of coexistent cardiovascular disease. Thus, identification of the subpopulations of patients with higher or lower risk of stroke determines which patients would derive the greatest benefit from anticoagulation.

Two studies, the Stroke Prevention in Atrial Fibrillation study 1 (SPAF)[201] and the Atrial Fibrillation Study Investigators,[245] provide insight into the risk factors for systemic embolism in chronic or intermittent atrial fibrillation. Left ventricular dysfunction, diabetes, hypertension, prior stroke or transient ischemic attack place patients with atrial fibrillation into the highest risk category, particularly those over age 65 years. This translates into a risk of 4 to 5 percent per year.

Mitral Incompetence in Atrial Fibrillation This valvular condition is associated with a lower risk of systemic embolism than mitral stenosis.[202,203] As with mitral stenosis, with mitral regurgitation, risk of systemic thromboembolism increases significantly with atrial fibrillation. In a series by Coulshed and colleagues of over 800 patients with rheumatic mitral disease, the risk of systemic thromboembolism was 7.7 percent in those with predominant mitral incompetence with sinus rhythm, as compared with 22 percent of those with mitral incompetence and atrial fibrillation.[203]

Anterior Myocardial Infarction Left ventricular thrombus develops in approximately 30 percent of patients with anterior myocardial infarction and is associated with a medium risk of subsequent arterial embolization.[204] Other factors that predict left ventricular thrombus formation are ejection fraction, infarct size, and atrial fibrillation. Thrombus formation almost always forms in the anterior, particularly the anteroapical, area of akinesis or dyskinesis.[205,206] Less than 5 percent of patients with infarctions in other areas develop a mural thrombus. The risk of embolization from a detected thrombus may be higher when the thrombus is mobile or protuberant.[204]

Dilated Cardiomyopathy Uncontrolled study patients with dilated cardiomyopathy have an annual incidence of clinically apparent thromboembolism of less than 1 to 12 per 100 patients.[207,208] In a study by Fuster et al., patients not receiving anticoagulation had an overall incidence of thromboembolism of 3.5 percent per year. Over 7 years of follow up, this occurred in 14 percent of patients in sinus rhythm and 33 percent of patients with atrial fibrillation.[207] The risk of thromboembolism is greatest in those with an ejection fraction of less than 35 percent, established or paroxysmal atrial fibrillation, and a history of thromboembolism or echocardiographic evidence of thrombus.[208]

Low Risk (Less Than Two Episodes per 100 Patients per Year)

Lone Atrial Fibrillation The risk of thromboembolism in lone atrial fibrillation, defined as idiopathic atrial fibrillation in the absence of structural heart disease, is low and therefore does not require anticoagulation.

Mitral Valve Disease in Sinus Rhythm As stated previously, mitral incompetence is associated with a somewhat lower risk of thromboembolism than mitral stenosis. Systemic thromboembolism occurs at a rate of one to four events per 100 patient-years, depending on the degree of incompetence and presence or absence of atrial fibrillation.[192,203] Thus, as stated above, in atrial fibrillation the risk is medium while in sinus rhythm the risk is low.

The incidence of thromboembolism complicating mitral stenosis in those in normal sinus rhythm is reported as low to medium, with a rate of 1.5 to 4.7 percent per year. This risk increases with age and correlates inversely with cardiac output. It is unrelated to left atrial size, valve area, or functional class. It is important to monitor patients with mitral stenosis for the onset of atrial fibrillation, since as many as 30 percent of the emboli that occur do so within the first

month and 65 percent within the first year after the onset of atrial fibrillation.[192]

Aortic Valve Disease Few long-term studies are available to confirm what is believed to be a low incidence of thromboembolism in aortic valve disease. Isolated aortic valve disease imparts a low risk of thromboembolism. Aortic valve disease associated with atrial fibrillation or calcification of the aortic valve may be associated with embolic events.

Chronic Left Ventricular Aneurysm Left ventricular aneurysm predisposes to layers of thrombus formation. Intraaneurysmal thrombi are at high risk for thromboembolism during the first 3 weeks following a myocardial infarction and are at low risk beyond 3 months following a myocardial infarction. Specifically, about 5 percent of patients with intraaneurysmal thrombi will embolize within 3 weeks after a myocardial infarction.[202] Beyond 3 months after myocardial infarction, the incidence of thromboembolism is reported to be 0.3 percent per year. This lower risk is presumably due to the presence of an organized thrombus that is somewhat isolated from dynamic forces of the circulation.[209]

PROSTHETIC HEART VALVES (Table 52-5)

High Risk (More Than Six Episodes per 100 Patients per Year)

Old Mechanical Prostheses Without anticoagulation, patients with older mechanical valves are at high risk of thromboembolism. The risk of thromboembolism is cumulative and persistent. Recent observations indicate that even with more modern prosthetic heart valves, there is a medium to high incidence of thromboembolism within the first 30 postoperative days.[204]

Mechanical Valves and Previous Thromboembolism Patients with any type of mechanical prosthesis and a history of thromboembolism appear to be at high risk for recurrent thromboembolic events.[210]

Medium Risk (Two to Six Episodes per 100 Patients per Year)

Newer Mechanical Prostheses Patients with newer prosthetic valves are at medium risk for thromboembolism. Overall, the risk of thromboembolism has been decreasing in recent years, probably as a result of patient factors; earlier operation leading to smaller left atrial size, less atrial fibrillation, and better left ventricular function; as well as the use of mechanical prosthetic valves with less turbulent flow and better hemodynamics.[211]

Bioprosthetic Valves Early Postoperatively or with Atrial Fibrillation Patients with bioprosthetic valves are at medium risk for thromboembolism within the first 30 days following operation. In addition, those with any bioprosthetic valves and atrial fibrillation are at chronic medium risk for thromboembolism.

Low Risk (Less Than Two Episodes per 100 Patients per Year)

Bioprosthetic Valves in Normal Sinus Rhythm Those with bioprosthetic valves and normal sinus rhythm tend to be at low risk for thromboembolic complications beyond the immediate postoperative period.

Antithrombotic Therapy
(Table 52-5)

In coronary artery disease, since thrombotic complications are related to platelet and fibrin deposition, the combination of aspirin and anticoagulants may be considered in the high-risk conditions (i.e., unstable angina), while aspirin or anticoagulants alone may be considered in the medium-risk conditions (i.e., chronic coronary disease). In disease conditions related to the cardiac chambers, since thrombotic complications are primarily related to fibrin deposition, the use of anticoagulants at higher dose may be considered in the high-risk conditions (i.e., mitral stenosis with atrial fibrillation), while a lower dose may be considered in the medium-risk conditions (i.e., valvular atrial fibrillation). In patients with prosthetic heart valves, since thrombotic complications have a predominance of fibrin over platelet deposition, the use of anticoagulants at a higher dose or the combination of lower-dose anticoagulants and aspirin may be considered in the high-risk conditions (i.e., older mechanical prosthetic valves), while a lower dose of anticoagulants alone may be considered in the medium-risk conditions (i.e., recently placed mechanical prostheses). In this last section, we will try to justify such an approach.

CORONARY ARTERIES
(Table 52-5)

High Risk (More Than 6 Episodes per 100 Patients per Year)

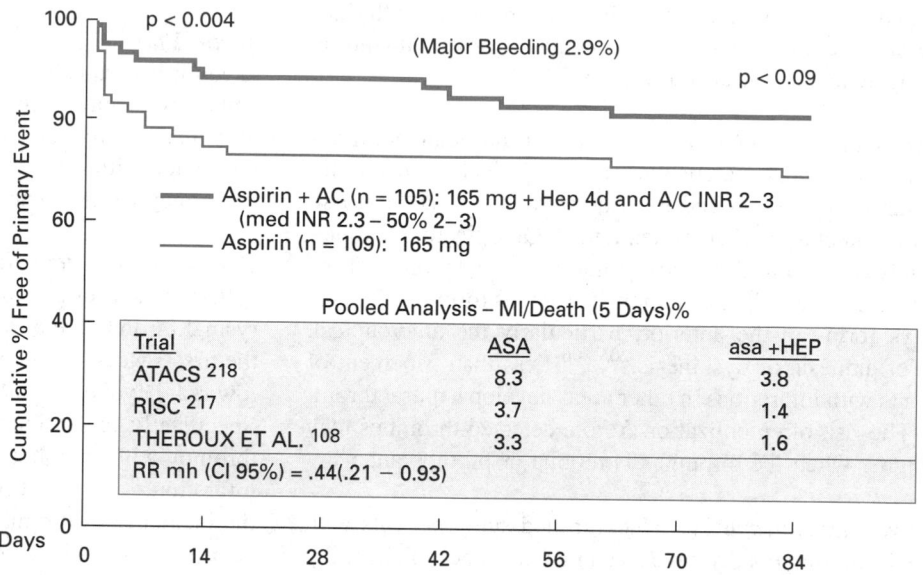

D Holdright, D.Patel, D. Cunningham, et al. JACC 1994; 24:39 — No difference ASA – ASA + Heparin

FIGURE 52-19
Data from the ATACS trial examining the use of aspirin versus aspirin plus anticoagulation in unstable angina and non-Q-wave myocardial infarction demonstrates an improvement in event-free survival in the combination therapy group. Pooled analysis from the ATACS, RISC, and Theroux study groups demonstrates a relative risk reduction (RR) of 0.44 in the combination group.

Unstable Angina As stated previously, unstable angina (Tables 52-6 and 52-7, Fig. 52-19) represents a high thrombotic risk due to fibrin deposition and platelet activation. Therefore, therapy is directed toward both systems. The benefit of aspirin and heparin used independently has been proved and the use of these agents in combination is strongly suggested.

HEPARIN ALONE   The use of heparin (Table 52-6) for the treatment of unstable angina was suggested by Teleford and Wilson.[212] In a 2 × 2 factorial design study, 400 patients

TABLE 52-6
MAJOR ANTICOAGULANT (HEPARIN) TRIALS IN UNSTABLE ANGINA

Trial	No. of Patients	Follow-up	Drug	Reduction in Death or MI, percent	p Value
Teleford and Wilson[212]	214	7 days	Heparin	80	<.05
Theroux et al.[108]	479	6 days	Heparin	89	<.001
			Heparin + aspirin	88	.001
RISC[217]	796	3 months	Heparin	5	NS
			Heparin + aspirin	68	<.0005
ATACS[218]	214	5 days	Aspirin	—	—
			Heparin + aspirin	46	.06
Holdright[219]	285	6 days	Aspirin	—	
			Heparin + aspirin	—	NS

were randomized to atenolol, heparin, both, or neither. The investigators demonstrated an 80 percent reduction in myocardial infarction in patients with unstable angina treated with heparin for 7 days. In the Montreal Heart Institute study,[213] a double-blind placebo-controlled 2 × 2 factorial design study, patients were randomized to heparin alone, aspirin alone, both, or neither. End points of death, myocardial infarction, or severe unstable angina refractory to medical treatment were measured 6 ± 3 days after randomization. Compared with placebo, heparin reduced the total event rate by 57 percent (p = .001). The beneficial effects of aspirin and the results of combining aspirin and heparin are discussed below. There was a trend toward less frequent myocardial infarction in the heparin group as compared with the aspirin group. An extension of this study was subsequently performed that randomized people to either aspirin or heparin. The combined results of these studies demonstrated the superiority of heparin over aspirin in reducing the rate of myocardial infarction.[65] Preliminary results from the ESSENCE trial with the use of subcutaneous LMW heparin enoxporin during hospitalization for unstable angina are very encouraging.[214]

ANTIPLATELET AGENTS ALONE AND WITH HEPARIN Antiplatelet agents (Tables 52-6 and 52-7, Fig. 52-19) have been found to reduce the rate of acute myocardial infarction and short- and long-term death in four large trials of unstable angina. In the Veterans Administration Cooperative Study, 1266 men with unstable angina were randomized to receive 325 mg/day of aspirin or placebo for 12 weeks. During the treatment period, the aspirin group demonstrated a risk reduction of 51 percent, and the overall benefits of aspirin were maintained during the 1-year follow-up period.[215] In the Canadian Multicenter Trial, 55 patients with unstable angina were randomized to receive 1300 mg/day of aspirin, 800 mg/day of sulfinpyrazone, the combination of both, or placebo. After 18 months, the incidence of death and myocardial infarction was reduced in the aspirin groups from 17 to 8.6 percent; sulfinpyrazone demonstrated no benefit.[216]

As previously mentioned, the Montreal Heart Institute study randomized 479 patients with unstable angina to 325 mg twice daily of aspirin, intravenous heparin, the combination of both, or placebo. Compared with placebo, aspirin reduced the rate of myocardial infarction by 72 percent, and the combination of aspirin and heparin was superior to aspirin alone.[207] In the European RISC study group,[217] 794 men with unstable angina or non-Q-wave infarction were randomized to receive 75 mg/day of aspirin for 3 months, intravenous heparin for 5 days, both, or neither. At the end of 3 months, the incidence of death or myocardial infarction was significantly reduced by aspirin and to a greater extent by the combi-

nation of aspirin and heparin. The more recent ATACS[218] trial randomized 214 patients (who were not prior aspirin users) with either unstable angina or non-Q-wave myocardial infarction to receive aspirin alone or aspirin plus anticoagulation. The trial was begun within a mean of 9.5 h after the onset of chest pain and continued for 12 weeks. There was a significant reduction in total ischemic events in the combination group versus aspirin alone (10.5 versus 27 percent, p = .004) at the end of 14 days. At the end of 12 weeks, there was a trend toward reduction in total ischemic events in the combination group (13 versus 25 percent, p = .06).

Ticlopidine was examined in patients with unstable angina.[220] The administration of ticlopidine in a dose of 250 mg twice a day for 6 months was found to reduce the incidence of death and myocardial infarction by 46 percent.

Thus, the efficacy of aspirin and heparin in unstable angina is proved by the above studies. The benefit of combination therapy, although highly suggested by these studies, has not yet been unequivocally demonstrated relative to monotherapy. However, due to the high risk of thrombotic events and the complementary mechanisms of action in preventing platelet and fibrin deposition, the combination of these two agents for initial treatment of unstable angina has been strongly suggested.[221]

DIRECT THROMBIN INHIBITORS AND IIB/IIIA PLATELET BLOCKERS Because patients with unstable angina are at high risk, efforts to develop better antithrombotics have been intensified. Given the central role of thrombin in the coagulation process and the role of IIb/IIIa platelet receptors in the activation of platelets, there is much enthusiasm for the development of direct thrombin inhibitors and IIb/IIIa receptor blockers (Table 52-8) for use in unstable angina. Preliminary results from the OASIS study with the use of the antithrombin hirudin, and, more specifically, from the Platelet Receptor inhibition for Ischemic Syndrome Management Study (PRISM), PRISM PLUS and Platelet IIb/IIIa Underpinning the Receptor for Suppression of Unstable Ischemia Trial (PURSUIT) studies with the use of IIb/IIIa platelet receptor blockers during the hospitalization phase for unstable angina are very encouraging. However, further studies to determine the optimal dosing, route, and length of administration need to be conducted.

TABLE 52-7

MAJOR ASPIRIN TRIALS IN UNSTABLE ANGINA

Study	No. of Patients	Dose, mg/day	Duration of Follow-up	Relative Risk Reduction, percent
Lewis et al.[215]	1338	324	3 months	51
Cairns et al.[216]	555	1300	24 months	51
Theroux et al.[108]	479	650	6 days	72
RISC[217]	796	75	5 days	57
			30 days	46

TABLE 52-8

NEW ANTITHROMBOTICS—ACUTE CORONARY SYNDROME—CLINICAL TRIALS

Agents	Unst Angina	Myoc Infarction	PTCA-Occlusion
Hirudin	GUSTO-IIA[1] GUSTO-IIB[7] OASIS (6 Mo:ASA + A/C)	GUSTO-IIA,[1] TIMI-9A[2] HIT III[3] GUSTO-IIB,[7] TIMI-9B[8] OASIS (non ST↑)	HELVETICA
Hirulog	TIMI-8	HERO (SK)[6]	PTCA
IIb/IIIa Block.	CANADIAN (Pilot)[4] PRISM[9] PRISM PLUS[9] PARAGON PURSUIT	PARADIGM II	IMPACT-II PTCA[6] RESTORE[6] CAPTURE[6] EPIC[5] (& Resten) EPILOG (Resten)[6] ERASER (Stent)

Key : Underline = questionable; Roman = ongoing; Italics = definitive–benefit.
Refs. 1, 2, 3: *Circulation* 1994; 90:1631, 1624, 1638.
Ref. 4: *Circulation* 1996; 94:899; Ref. 5: *NEJM* 1994; 330:956; Ref. 6: *ACC-ESC* 1996; Ref. 7: *NEJM* 1996; 335:775; Ref. 8: *Circulation* 1996; 94:911; Ref 9: *ACC* 1997. *Lancet* 1994; 343:881.
Abbreviations : Unst = unstable; Myoc = myocardial; PTCA = percutaneous transluminal coronary angioplasty; block. = blockers; Resten = Restenosis.

RECOMMENDATIONS   In this high-risk group, with the pathophysiologic processes of both platelet activation and fibrin generation, all patients with unstable angina should receive 325 mg of chewable aspirin and intravenous heparin sufficient to raise the partial thromboplastin time (PTT) to approximately 45 to 70 s. Subcutaneous LMW heparin may be superior to intravenous unfractionated heparin. Ticlopidine can be used as an alternative to aspirin in those who are allergic to or intolerant of aspirin. Evidence of the further beneficial effect of the use of IIb/IIIa platelet receptor blockers or antithrombins instead of heparin is evolving. The use of thrombolytic agents in patients with unstable angina is not recommended.

TABLE 52-9

DATA FROM DIRECT COMPARISON OF ANTITHROMBOTIC REGIMENS: GISSI-2, ISIS-3, AND GUSTO-1

Outcome	GISSI-2 and ISIS-3, Aspirin plus Any Thrombolytic Agent		GUSTO-1, Aspirin plus SK	
	No Heparin (n = 31,050), percent	SC Heparin (n = 31,017), percent	SC Heparin (n = 9971), percent	IV Heparin (n = 10,377), percent
Death	10.2	10.0	7.2	7.4
Reinfarction	3.3	3.0	3.4	4.0
Total stroke	1.2	1.2	1.3	1.4
Hemorrhagic stroke	0.4	0.5	0.5	0.5
Major bleeding	0.7	1.0	0.3	0.5

Source: Hennekens CH et al.[225] with permission.
Abbreviations: SK = streptokinase; SC = subcutaneous; IV = intravenous.

Acute Myocardial Infarction
As stated previously, acute myocardial infarction (Table 52-5) represents a highly thrombotic state for reocclusion and reinfarction due to both platelet activation and fibrin generation. Therefore, therapy is directed toward both the platelet and the coagulation system.

ANTIPLATELET AGENTS AND CLINICAL END POINTS *Aspirin without Thrombolytic Therapy for Patients with Acute Myocardial Infarction (Tables 52-9 and 52-10)* The landmark Second International Study of Infarct Survival (ISIS-2),[222] which included more than 17,000 patients, randomized patients to receive aspirin (160 mg/day for 30 days), intravenous streptokinase, both, or neither. In the group taking aspirin alone, there was a 23 percent reduction in mortality compared with the group taking neither streptokinase nor aspirin; the risk reduction for nonfatal reinfarction was 49 percent and that for nonfatal stroke was 46 percent. Thus, aspirin is critical in the treatment of acute myocardial infarction.

Treatment with Thrombolytic Therapy In International Study of Infarct Survival (ISIS)-2, when aspirin was combined with streptokinase, a 42 percent reduction in vascular mortality was seen. Patients given only aspirin, as previously stated, had a 23 percent reduction in mortality, while those given only streptokinase had a 25 percent reduction. Aspirin with streptokinase compared with streptokinase alone reduced the rate of nonfatal reinfarction (1.8 percent in the combination group compared with 2.8 percent in the streptokinase-alone group). Thus, the effects of aspirin and thrombolytic agents appear to be additive. No significant difference in major bleeding requiring transfusion was seen. However, there was a small but significant increase in minor bleeding in the aspirin group. A recent follow-up study of the ISIS-2 group found that at 4 years there was a persistent mortality benefit.[222]

ANTICOAGULANTS AND CLINICAL END POINTS There have been no clinical trials of aspirin versus heparin during acute myocardial infarction. However, there are studies examining anticoagulants with or without the use of thrombolytic agents, although in the vast majority of these studies patients were on aspirin.

HEPARIN WITH AND WITHOUT THROMBOLYTIC AGENTS The Studio sulla Calciparina nell'Angina e nella Trombosi ventricolare nell'Infarcto (SCATI)[224] group randomized 711 patients to either heparin or no heparin; 433 of these patients also received streptokinase. These patients, unlike those in Gruppo Italiano per lo Studio della Streptochinasi nell'Infarcto miocardico (GISSI)-2, ISIS-3, and GUSTO (described below), did not receive aspirin. This study found a 44 percent reduction in mortality when 12,500 units of subcutaneous heparin was given to patients with acute myocardial infarction. This reduction in mortality was significant both in the group receiving streptokinase and in those who did not receive the thrombolytic agent.

HEPARIN AND ASPIRIN WITH THROMBOLYTIC AGENTS The use of heparin (in those receiving aspirin) as adjunctive therapy with thrombolytic agents (Table 52-9) was examined in many studies, including GISSI-2, ISIS-3, SCATI, and GUSTO. In GISSI-2, patients who received streptokinase and heparin beginning 12 h after the infusion of the thrombolytic agent had a tendency (but there was no statistically significant difference) toward a decrease in mortality as compared with those who received streptokinase alone.[225] Mortality for those receiving t-PA was the same whether or not heparin was added to the regimen.[226] ISIS-3[227] found that heparin (given subcutaneously, 12,500 U every 12 h starting 4 h after the start of thrombolytic therapy) and aspirin, given with t-PA or streptokinase, resulted in a nearly significant decrease in mortality. There was a trend toward a decrease in hospital reinfarction rate in the heparin group. However, this early benefit was lost when the primary end point of 35 days was reached. Also, heparin produced a small excess of extracerebral bleeds (1.0 percent compared with 0.8 percent ($p < .01$) and intracerebral bleeds (0.056 percent compared to 0.40 percent; $p < .05$).

The GUSTO study provided great insight to the issue of anticoagulation as adjunctive therapy to thrombolysis.[228] This study randomized 41,021 patients with myocardial infarctions into four treatment groups: (1) streptokinase and subcutaneous heparin, (2) streptokinase and intravenous heparin, (3) accelerated t-PA and intravenous heparin, or (4) the combination of both agents with intravenous heparin. The results found a significant reduction in mortality in the accelerated t-PA and intravenous heparin group versus the streptokinase groups ($p < .001$). The rates of hemorrhagic stroke were 0.49, 0.54, 0.72, and 0.94 percent, respectively. Since heparin was given in all four groups in conjunction with aspirin, its role alone or in combination with aspirin was not tested. However, it can be stated that there was no advantage to the use of intravenous over subcutaneous heparin with streptokinase.

ASPIRIN AND/OR ANTICOAGULANTS WITH THROMBOLYTIC THERAPY AND ANGIOGRAPHIC END POINTS Angiographic end-point studies are inconclusive in nature, since they do not provide clinical information. Nevertheless, they can provide some insight into the possible role of certain antithrombotics (as adjuncts to thrombolytic therapy) not tested in terms of clinical end points, such as heparin versus aspirin versus the combination of both. Several smaller studies of angiographic patency examined the use of heparin in conjunction with t-PA. The Heparin Aspirin Reperfusion Trial compared heparin with 80 mg of aspirin per day following t-PA administration.[229] Coronary artery patency at 18 h was 82 percent in the heparin group compared with 52 percent in the aspirin-alone group ($p < .002$). Bleich and colleagues found that in patients not receiving aspirin (80 mg/day) during acute myocardial infarction following t-PA administration, patency (as assessed by angiography) of the infarct-related artery at

TABLE 52-10

ASPIRIN IN CARDIOVASCULAR DISEASE

Category of Trial	No. of Trials	MI, Stroke, or Vascular Death		Odds Ratio and Confidence Interval	% Odds Reduction (S.D.)
		Antiplatelet, percent	Controls, percent		
Prior MI	11	13.5	17.1		25% (4)
Acute MI	9	10.6	14.4		29% (4)
Prior stroke/TIA	18	18.4	22.2		22% (4)
Other high risk	104	6.9	9.2		32% (4)
All high risk (4 main categories)	142	11.4	14.7		27% (2)
All low risk (primary prevention)	3	4.46	4.85		10% (6)
All trials (high or low risk)	145	9.5	11.9		25% (2)

0 0·5 1·0 1·5 2·0
Better   Worse
Treatment effect 2p < .00001

Source: Antiplatelet Trialists' Collaboration,[239] with permission.

2 to 3 days was improved by heparin therapy (71 versus 44 percent, $p = .04$).[230] In the European Cooperative Study Group-6, a total of 687 patients received aspirin and t-PA. Half of this group was randomized to heparin, while the other half received no heparin. Patency at 81 h was 80 percent in the heparin group and 75 percent in the no-heparin group ($p < .01$).[231] The Australian National Heart Study[232] determined that after t-PA infusion, there was no difference in patency at 1 week between patients receiving continuous heparin infusion after an initial bolus or a combination of 300 mg of aspirin and 300 mg of dipyridamole after the initial heparin bolus.

In a recent study, the Duke University Clinical Cardiology Studies-1 found no difference in coronary artery patency in those receiving APSAC and heparin versus APSAC alone.[233] All patients were given aspirin.

DIRECT THROMBIN INHIBITORS AND IIb/IIIa PLATELET RECEPTOR BLOCKERS Because patients with acute myocardial infarction are at high risk, efforts to develop better antithrombotics have been intensified (Table 52-8). As already pointed out in unstable angina, thrombin has a central role in the coagulation process and IIb/IIIa platelet receptors in the activation of platelets. Thus, there is much enthusiasm for the development of direct thrombin inhibitors and IIb/IIIa receptor blockers for use in acute myocardial infarction. Preliminary results from the OASIS and GUSTO IIb studies with the use of the antithrombin hirudin and the HERO study with the use of the antithrombin hirulog are very encouraging, particularly when streptokinase is the lytic agent used. However, further studies to determine the optimal dosing, route, and length of administration and the optimal protocol need to be conducted.

RECOMMENDATIONS In summary, the efficacy of aspirin and the efficacy of heparin in acute myocardial infarction is proved. However, the benefit of combining both with thrombolytic therapy versus monotherapy using either aspirin or heparin is suggested if t-PA is used but has not yet been unequivocally demonstrated; at the present time, no study supports the use of either intravenous or subcutaneous heparin as adjunctive therapy to streptokinase when adequate dose (162 to 325 mg/day) of aspirin is used. The same probably applies to the use of heparin in conjunction with APSAC. Based on the data obtained with unstable angina and in myocardial infarction without thrombolytic therapy, the in-hospital use of the combination of aspirin and heparin is justified; however, this approach has not yet been tested. In addition, with the use of thrombolytic therapy, heparin should be used in conjunction with aspirin in patients who would *otherwise* benefit from anticoagulation for preventing systemic embolism (i.e., those with a large anterior myocardial infarction, cardiac failure, or atrial fibrillation). The further beneficial effect of the use of antithrombins, particularly when streptokinase is administered, and of IIb/IIIa platelet receptor blockers has yet to be elucidated.

Coronary Revascularization Procedures Based on several major trials, pretreatment with aspirin combined with adequate heparinization throughout the procedure is strongly recommended.[234] Ticlopidine can be used as an alternative to aspirin in those patients who are allergic to or intolerant of aspirin. Trials of the use of different antiplatelet drugs and anticoagulant agents aimed at reducing the restenosis rate have been disappointing. However, use of the platelet glycoprotein receptor IIb/IIIa antagonist has received much recent attention. The EPIC study showed reduced incidence of acute and delayed complications, including restenosis following PTCA, in the group of patients receiving the 7E3 antibody directed against the glycoprotein IIb/IIIa receptor complex.[101,102] This approach is currently recommended in all patients considered at high risk for ischemic complications following coronary intervention.

In patients undergoing stent implantation, use of aspirin and heparin during the procedure is presently recommended. Subsequent treatment regimens (less aggressive) using aspirin alone or in combination with ticlopidine have been suggested, particularly in conjunction with the use of intravascular ultrasound to guide deployment of the stent.[235]

Saphenous Vein Bypass Grafting Reviews of all reported trials to date have demonstrated the importance of initiating platelet-inhibitor therapy in the perioperative period, preferably before 48 h after surgery. When therapy was not started 48 h after surgery, no reduction in the vein graft occlusion rate was observed.[196,236]

In the Veterans Administration Cooperative Study, patients receiving saphenous vein grafts were randomly assigned into five groups: (1) taking 325 mg aspirin a day, (2) taking 325 mg aspirin three times daily, (3) taking 325 mg aspirin plus 75 mg dipyridamole three times daily, (4) taking 267 mg sulfinpyrazone three times daily, or (5) taking a placebo. Early graft patency at a median of 9 days was significantly higher in the aspirin-treated group (92 percent) than in those receiving placebo (85 percent). At 1 year, benefit was seen in patients at high risk of graft closure (those with grafts placed to vessels <1.5 mm in diameter) taking aspirin. One daily dose of aspirin was as effective as three daily doses. Dipyridamole conferred no benefit over aspirin alone. In another Veterans Administration study, preoperative aspirin use was associated with increased bleeding complications and no additional benefit over aspirin started 6 h after surgery.[237] In a study examining the use of ticlopidine 250 mg twice daily started on the second postoperative day, there was a significant reduction in vein graft occlusion, by approximately 40 percent, as assessed angiographically at 10, 180, and 360 days after surgery.[238] Currently, aspirin should be started immediately after surgery and continued for at least 1 year and probably indefinitely. Ticlopidine can be used as an alternative to aspirin. However, a high rate of occlusion remains; therefore, combination therapy should be tested.

Medium Risk (Two to Six Episodes per 100 Patients per Year)

Post–Myocardial Infarction—Chronic Coronary Artery Disease As stated previously, survivors of acute myocardial infarction are at medium risk of recurrent infarction or cardiac death. Because morbidity and mortality following a myocardial infarction may be related to arrhythmias, left ventricular dysfunction, and recurrent myocardial infarction, it has been difficult to prove that antithrombotic therapy is beneficial in these patients.

ANTIPLATELET AGENTS Multiple trials examining the use of aspirin for the secondary prevention of myocardial infarction have been conducted (Table 52-10). However, no single study has provided definitive results. The results of a metaanalysis that included over 18,000 patients revealed that platelet inhibitor therapy reduced cardiovascular mortality by 13 percent, nonfatal reinfarction by 31 percent, and nonfatal stroke by 42 percent.[82] Aspirin alone was at least as effective as the combination of aspirin and dipyridamole and more effective than sulfinpyrazone. Available data do not justify the additional cost and frequency of administration of drugs other than aspirin in this group of patients.[82] Medium-dose aspirin (75 to 325 mg) was as efficacious as higher-dose aspirin.[239]

In the recent Clopidogrel vs Aspirin in Patients at Risk of Ischemic Events (CAPRIE) study, clopidogrel 75 mg/day was superior to aspirin 325 mg/day in patients who presented with previous myocardial infarction, stroke, or peripheral arterial disease.[92] Despite over 19,185 patients, there was only a reduction from 5.83 to 5.32 percent per year with a modest *p* value of 0.043. As no serious complications were reported, this medication can be considered as an equivalent alternative to aspirin.

ANTICOAGULANTS Numerous studies have assessed the usefulness of anticoagulants (Fig. 52-20) in the secondary prevention of cardiovascular disease after myocardial infarction. The Warfarin and Reinfarction Study (WARIS) is the largest study to date of anticoagulants in the secondary prevention of myocardial infarction.[240] In this placebo-controlled double-blind trial, 1214 patients aged 75 or less were randomized a mean 27 days after initial acute myocardial infarction (AMI) to warfarin (target INR 2.8 to 4.8) or placebo. Only 1 percent of patients received thrombolytic therapy for the initial AMI. Patients were advised not to take aspirin during the trial. At mean follow-up of 37 months, warfarin resulted in significant reduction of mortality, total reinfarctions, nonfatal infarctions, and total strokes. Although four fatal intracranial hemorrhages occurred in the warfarin group compared to none in the placebo group, 10 nonhemorrhagic fatal strokes occurred in the placebo group compared to none in the warfarin group. Efficacy analysis showed even greater benefit to warfarin.

Two clinical trials compared warfarin therapy to antiplatelet therapy in secondary prevention of myocardial infarction.

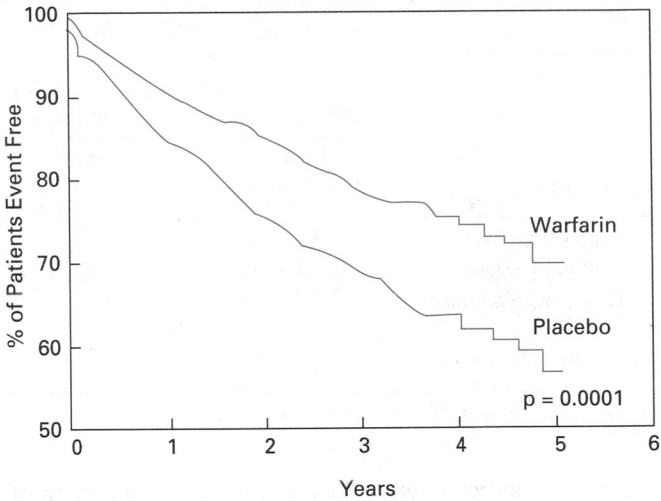

POST MYOCARDIAL INFARCTION: TOTAL MORTALITY, RECURRENT MI, OR CVA

FIGURE 52-20

The WARIS Trial Study of anticoagulants in the secondary prevention of myocardial infarction. Cumulative rates (Kaplan-Meier) of total mortality, recurrent myocardial infarction, and stroke. (From Smith P, Arnesen H, Holme I. *N Engl J Med* 1990; 323:147, with permission.)

In the German Austrian Myocardial Infarction Study (GAMIS), 946 patients 38 to 42 days post-AMI were randomized to open-label phenprocumin (target INR, 2.5 to 5.0), aspirin 1.5 g/day, or placebo.[241] No difference was observed between groups in mortality or reinfarction. The French Enquete de Prevention Secondaire de l'In-farctus de Myocarde (EPSIM) study[243] revealed no difference in death or reinfarction in patients receiving either oral anticoagulants or aspirin. However, there were 54 percent more patients with gastrointestinal events with aspirin and four times more severe hemorrhagic events with warfarin. In the Aspirin versus Coumadin in the Prevention of Reocclusion and Recurrent Ischemia after Successful Thrombolysis (APRICOT) trial, 300 patients were randomized to either 325 mg of aspirin/day or heparin followed by warfarin (target INR, 2.8 to 4.0) after an initial angiogram <48 h after AMI revealed a patent infarct-related artery.[243] At 3 months there was no significant difference in reocclusion rates among the warfarin, aspirin, and placebo arms. Aspirin significantly reduced reinfarction compared with placebo but not with warfarin. Mortality did not differ between the groups.

The combination of fixed low-dose anticoagulants and antiplatelet agents in the secondary prevention of AMI has been the subject of recent examination[244]—the Coronary Artery Reinfarction Study (CARS) planned to study 9000 patients randomized to three treatment regimens: (1) 160 mg/day of aspirin, (2) 80 mg/day of aspirin *plus* 3 mg/day of warfarin, (3) a combination pill of 80 mg of aspirin plus 1 mg of warfarin per day. This trial was stopped, nearing the recruitment of the 9000 patients, following an interim analysis revealing that the combination of fixed low-dose coumadin plus low-dose

TABLE 52-11

ASPIRIN IN PRIMARY PREVENTION (U.S. PHYSICIANS' HEALTH STUDY AND BRITISH DOCTORS' TRIAL RESULTS)

| | Reduction (% ± S.D.) | | | |
| | United States | British | Overview | |
End Point	Physicians' Health Study[243]	Doctors' Trials[244]	Both Trials	p Value
Nonfatal MI	44 ± 9	3 ± 19	32 ± 8	<.0001
Nonfatal stroke	↑19 ± 15	↑13 ± 24	↑18 ± 13	NS
Total cardiovascular deaths	2 ± 15	7 ± 14	5 ± 10	NS
Any vascular event	18 ± 7	4 ± 12	13 ± 6	NS

Sources: V Fuster et al.,[247] with permission.

aspirin is no more effective than aspirin in the prevention of reinfarction, cardiovascular death, and stroke.

The Combination Hemotherapy And Mortality Prevention (CHAMP) study is randomizing patients to receive either 160 mg/day of aspirin or 80 mg of aspirin plus coumadin to achieve an INR of 1.5 to 2.5. Results of this study may definitively settle some of the unanswered questions regarding the use of anticoagulants and antiplatelets for the secondary prevention of AMI.

Low Risk (Less Than Two Episodes per 100 Patients per Year)

Primary Prevention of Acute Myocardial Infarction Two studies examining the use of aspirin in primary prevention of myocardial infarction (Tables 52-10 and 52-11) were con-

ducted. In the United States, in the Physicians' Health Study, more than 22,000 male physicians age 40 to 84 were randomized to receive 325 mg of aspirin every other day or placebo for 5 years. There was a 44 percent relative reduction in acute myocardial infarction in the aspirin-treated group, although the absolute incidence of such event was less than 1 percent in the low-risk population. This effect was limited to those older than 50 years. The incidence of cardiovascular death was not different.[245] In the British primary prevention trial of more than 5000 male physicians aged 50 to 78 years, two-thirds were randomized to receive 500 mg/day of aspirin and one-third were advised to use no aspirin. After 6 years, there was no difference in the rate of myocardial infarction.[246] These two studies evaluated the use of antiplatelet agents in a lower-risk group than the general population, and the use of these agents may, in fact, be beneficial in the high-risk population. Many, therefore, recommend the use of aspirin in the high-risk patient, for the primary prevention of the acute coronary syndromes, and no therapy in the low-risk population.

CARDIAC CHAMBERS—HIGH, MEDIUM, AND LOW RISK

Antithrombotic therapy in the cardiac chambers (Table 52-5) is directed primarily against the deposition of fibrin and consists of antithrombotic therapy. The high-risk situations of atrial fibrillation and a history of thromboembolism or atrial fibrillation and mitral stenosis require a high degree of anticoagulation. Atrial fibrillation and left ventricular dysfunction after an anterior myocardial infarction are medium-risk situations and require a lesser degree of anticoagulation.

Atrial Fibrillation

Given the pathophysiologic basis of thrombosis in the cardiac chambers, predominantly a fibrin-mediated event, the use of anticoagulants has been studied extensively. Five randomized clinical trials using warfarin for the prevention of stroke in atrial fibrillation were recently performed (Tables 52-5 and 52-12, Figs. 52-21 and 52-22).[248] These

TABLE 52-12

RISK STRATIFICATION IN ATRIAL FIBRILLATION[a]: INDEPENDENT PREDICTORS OF THROMBOEMBOLIC RISK

	SPAF I[b] Placebo Patients[201]	AFI[c] Pooled Analysis[248]
Number of patients	568	1236
Number of events	46	81
High-risk variables	History of hypertension Prior stroke/TIA Diabetes Recent heart failure	History of hypertension Prior stroke/TIA Diabetes Age > 65 years
Thromboembolic rate (95% CI)		
Low risk	1.4%/year (0.05–3.7)	1.0%/year (0.3–3.1)
High risk	>7%/year	>5%/year
Percentage of cohort "low-risk"	38%	15%

[a] Large, prospectively acquired data sets analyzed by multivariate techniques. The SPAF-1 placebo data set[201] was included in the pooled analysis of clinical trials by the Atrial Fibrillation Investigators.[248]
[b] SPAF = Stroke Prevention in Atrial Fibrillation study.
[c] AFI = Atrial Fibrillation Investigators.

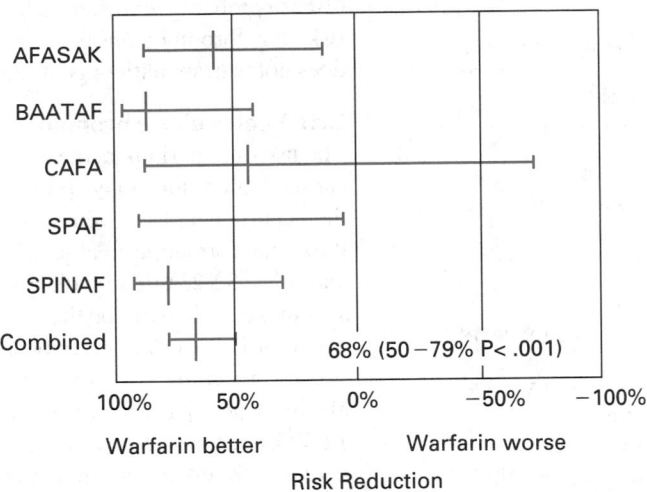

*WARFARIN FOR STROKE PREVENTION IN
ATRIAL FIBRILLATION: RESULTS OF 5 TRIALS*

FIGURE 52-21

Risk-reduction plot of the results of five randomized clinical trials comparing warfarin with control for prevention of ischemic stroke in atrial fibrillation patients: results of 5 trials. Horizontal lines indicate the 95 percent confidence intervals around the point estimates (vertical lines) for each trial. The combined risk reduction was 68 percent (95 percent confidence interval, 50 to 79 percent; $p < .991$). See Atrial Fibrillation Investigators' pooled analysis[114] for specific data. AFASAK = Atrial Fibrillation, Aspirin and Anticoagulant Therapy Study; BAATAF = Boston Area Anticoagulation Trial for Atrial Fibrillation; CAFA = Canadian Atrial Fibrillation Anticoagulation; SPAF = Stroke Prevention in Atrial Fibrillation Study; and SPINAF = Stroke Prevention in Nonrheumatic Atrial Fibrillation Study.

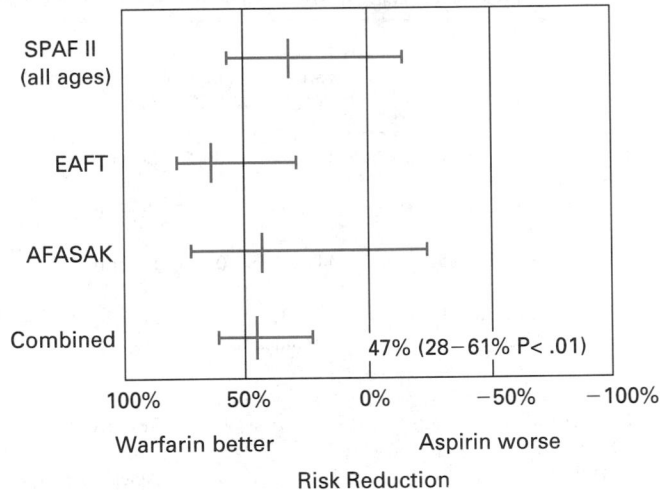

*WARFARIN vs ASPIRIN FOR STROKE IN
ATRIAL FIBRILLATION: RESULTS OF 3 TRIALS*

FIGURE 52-22

Risk-reduction plot of the results of three randomized clinical trials comparing warfarin with aspirin for prevention of ischemic stroke in atrial fibrillation patients: results of 3 trials. Horizontal line indicates the 95 percent confidence intervals around the point estimates (vertical lines) for each trial. The combined estimated risk reduction from published results (intent to treat) was 47 percent (95 percent confidence interval, 28 to 61 percent) by warfarin relative to aspirin. SPAF = Stroke Prevention in Atrial Fibrillation Trial; AFASAK = Atrial Fibrillation, Aspirin and Anticoagulant Therapy Study.

studies demonstrated that an INR of 1.8 to 4.2 translates to a mean reduction in ischemic stroke of nearly 70 percent. This reduction is even more apparent in those patients with a high risk of thromboembolism. The incremental risk of bleeding in those followed closely in these studies was <1 percent per year.[248] Safety in the older age group (>75 years) has not been adequately assessed. One study analyzing safety with patients who had a mean age of 75 demonstrated substantial withdrawal rate: 38.5 percent per year. Recent studies comparing patients over 75 years of age with atrial fibrillation to patients under 75 years of age with atrial fibrillation found that the very elderly had a greater risk of stroke but also had a substantially higher risk of hemorrhage on full-dose anticoagulation (mean INR 2.7).[248,249] It is conceivable that a lower intensity of anticoagulation in this age group may translate into less stroke and lower rates of bleeding complications.[250] This approach is currently being evaluated in several clinical trials. Pooled data examining the efficacy of aspirin in atrial fibrillation patients suggest that it appears to result in risk reduction of approximately 25 percent. However, aspirin was significantly less effective than anticoagulation in these studies.[201] Thus, we currently recommend that low-risk patients, independent of age, should receive 325 mg of aspirin. Those who are at higher risk who can safely receive anticoagulation should receive warfarin with a target INR 2.0 to 3.0; however, those over age 75 should have close

surveillance of the INR levels (and INR closer to 2.0) because of the apparent greater risk of bleeding complications.[251]

As mentioned previously, those who have experienced a thromboembolic event from atrial fibrillation are at a risk exceeding 10 percent per year of developing a recurrent event. A recent large, randomized trial demonstrated anticoagulation (INR 2.5 to 4.0) to be highly effective and relatively safe in the secondary prevention of stroke in atrial fibrillation.[252] Because of the high rate of recurrent stroke, anticoagulation of these patients should begin within 1 to 2 weeks of stroke (depending on the size of the stroke and the risk of hemorrhage) to a target INR 2.5 to 3.5. Those who are unable to receive anticoagulants should receive aspirin, which confers some benefit in secondary prevention.[252]

Valvular Heart Disease (Table 52-5)

Mitral Stenosis No prospective randomized studies have evaluated the effectiveness of anticoagulation in mitral stenosis. However, several descriptive studies report that warfarin is effective in preventing recurrent emboli. Thus, patients with mitral stenosis and atrial fibrillation and those patients with valvular heart disease and a prior thromboembolic event are at higher risk and should receive anticoagulants with an INR of about 2.5 to 3.5.

Mitral Incompetence Patients with mitral incompetence or mixed lesions and atrial fibrillation should receive long-term anticoagulation to maintain the INR at 2 to 3.

TABLE 52-13

THROMBOEMBOLISM IN NONISCHEMIC CARDIOMYOPATHY

Study	Systemic Incidence No A/C[a]	Emboli % A/C	Risk Factors[a]	Relation Thrombo-emboli[a]	Thrombosis Incidence, %, Location
Fuster V et al. (1981) (n = 104)	18	0	Severity ±	—	—
Gottdiener JS et al. (1983) (n = 123)	11		Severity ±	No	36
Kyrle PA et al., (1985) (n = 38)	44	0	Severity ±	—	—
Roberts WC, et al., (1987) (n = 152 autopsy)	39 (clinical)		Severity ±	No	75 LV 40, RV 20 LV 10, RA 5
Ciaccheri M et al. (1989) (n = 126)	8	0	Severity ±	No	
Yokota Y et al. (1989) (n = 40) (n = 17 autopsy)	20	0	Apical akin, dysk Apical flow veloc. Ejection fraction		26 Alive 50 Autopsy
Korin J et al. (1991) (dilated = ischemic)	23	3	—	—	—

[a] Falk RH, et al.[208]

Abbreviations: A/C = anticoagulant; LV = left ventricle; RV = right ventricle; RA = right atrium; akin = akinesis; dysk = dyskinesis; veloc = velocity.

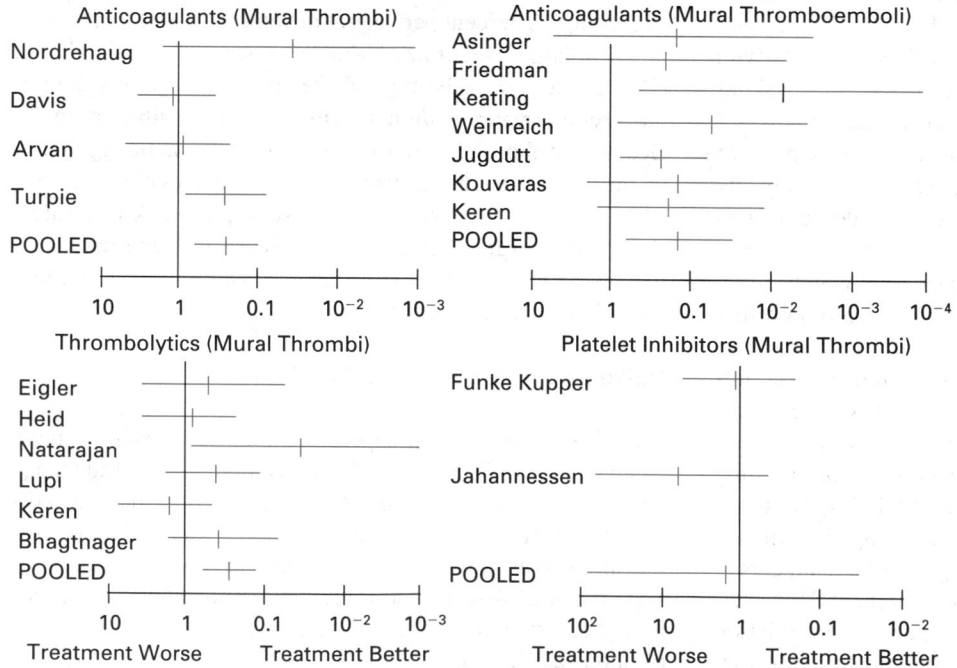

FIGURE 52-23

Metaanalysis of antithrombotic and thrombolytic therapy for the prevention of mural thrombus and systemic emboli after a myocardial infarction. (Modified from Vaitkus PT, Barnathan ES. *J Am Coll Cardiol* 1993; 22:1004, with permission.)

Aortic Valve Disease As mentioned previously, aortic valve disease probably represents a low risk for thromboembolism and does not warrant anticoagulation.

Left Ventricular Thrombus

The use of heparin in acute myocardial infarction may prevent the occurrence of left ventricular thrombus formation (Table 52-5 and Fig. 52-23). The effect of subcutaneous heparin on the incidence of intracardiac thrombosis was evaluated in two clinical trials in which patients receiving 12,500 U every 12 h were compared with either an untreated group or patients taking 5000 U subcutaneously every 12 h. In these two studies the incidence of mural thrombosis detected by two-dimensional echocardiography was 72 and 58 percent lower, respectively, in patients taking a moderate dose (12,500 U) of heparin.[223,253]

During hospitalization, heparin should be used in all anterior myocardial infarctions; at discharge from the hospital, long-term anticoagulation (3 months) should be used in patients with large anterior myocardial infarctions or in those who have visible thrombi at echocardiography. Use of long-term anticoagulation in patients with postinfarction cardiomyopathy and nonischemic cardiomyopathy (Table 52-13) is controversial, but there is full agreement in its use if there is atrial fibrillation. Use of anticoagulation in patients with ventricular aneurysms and mural thrombi is generally not indicated because of the low risk of embolization.

PROSTHETIC HEART VALVES (Tables 52-5 and 52-14, Fig. 52-24)—High, Medium, and Low Risk

Mechanical Valves

As stated previously, thromboembolic complications of pros-

TABLE 52-14

ANTITHROMBOTIC THERAPY FOR PROSTHETIC HEART
VALVES

Mechanical valve	
Routine	MD warfarin
Old prosth, TE,	HD warfarin
Ather	MD warfarin + LD MD ASA or + dip
ACRx problems (bleeding)	LD warfarin
	LD warfarin + dip
Recurrent embolism	Consider other causes
Bioprosthetic valve	
Routine—NSR	LD Warf.—3 months (then ASA?)
AF, LA thrombus, TE	MD Warf.—3 months, then LD Warf.

Warfarin HD = INR 3.0 to 4.5; —MD = INR 2.5 to 3.5; —LD = INR
2.0 to 3.0; ASA MD = 325 mg/day; —LD = 100 mg/day.
D Israel et al.[211]; Freudenberger et al.[193]
Key: MD = medium dose; HD = high dose; LD = low dose; TE =
thromboembolism; prosth = prosthetic valves; Ather = atherosclerosis;
ACRx = atrial fibrillation; LA = left atrium; dip = dipyridamole; ASA
= aspirin; Warf = warfarin.

thetic heart valves are primarily related to fibrin deposition.
The high-risk categories are old prosthetic valves and prosthetic valves with prior thromboembolism. These categories
require a high degree of anticoagulation with an INR of 3
to 4.5.

Recently placed mechanical prostheses and bioprostheses with atrial fibrillation are situations that represent medium risk and require an intermediate degree of anticoagulation.

The optimal anticoagulation regimen has not been fully
defined. Recent retrospective studies have questioned the generally recommended regimen of an INR of 3 to 4.5 for aortic
and mitral valve prostheses.[210,254] Thus, for mechanical prostheses in the aortic and mitral position an INR of 2.5 to
3.5 may be adequate. An INR of 2 to 3 may suffice with
bioprosthetic valves in the presence of atrial fibrillation, and
no anticoagulation at all may be advisable with bioprosthetic
valves and normal sinus rhythm. A large-scale prospective
randomized trial (GELIA) is under way to determine the
optimal level of anticoagulation after valve replacement with
the St. Jude prosthesis.

No randomized placebo-controlled study using platelet inhibitors alone for prevention of thromboembolism with mechanical valve prostheses has been conducted. Other small
studies examining either aspirin alone or in combination with
other antiplatelet agents have failed to demonstrate adequate
protection from thromboembolism.

Although consistent anticoagulation for patients with mechanical heart valves provides a decreased incidence of thromboembolism, there is still a relatively high risk of residual
thromboembolism. Several trials have tried to establish
whether the addition of dipyridamole to warfarin prevents
more episodes of thromboembolism than warfarin alone. In
three trials, the combination of warfarin and dipyridamole
resulted in a 70 to 90 percent reduction in embolic events. In
two other trials, the addition of dipyridamole to warfarin
resulted in a 40 to 50 percent reduction in embolic events.
Because of the low event rates in these trials, these results
were not statistically significant.[211] The addition of aspirin
in doses of 500 to 1000 mg/day to warfarin led to a significant
decrease in embolic events but also to a significant increase
in hemorrhagic events.[211]

In conclusion, in patients with mechanical prosthetic
valves, anticoagulation should be started as soon as possible
after surgery. An INR of 2.5 to 3.5 is currently recommended.
Since the consistency of anticoagulation is critical, we recommend monitoring every 3 to 4 weeks. High-risk patients—
i.e., those with a mechanical valve prosthesis implanted prior
to 1975 and those with prior thromboembolic complications—
should have a target INR of 3 to 4.5 or medium-intensity
anticoagulation (INR 2.5 to 3.5) and the use of a platelet
inhibitor, either aspirin 100 mg/day or dipyridamole 100 mg
four times daily.[202,211] Platelet inhibitor therapy alone is not
advisable in patients with mechanical heart valve prostheses.
In patients who develop an absolute contraindication to anticoagulation after implantation of a mechanical heart valve prosthesis, the combination of dipyridamole 100 mg four times a
day and aspirin 325 mg daily or ticlopidine 250 mg twice
daily may be tried empirically.

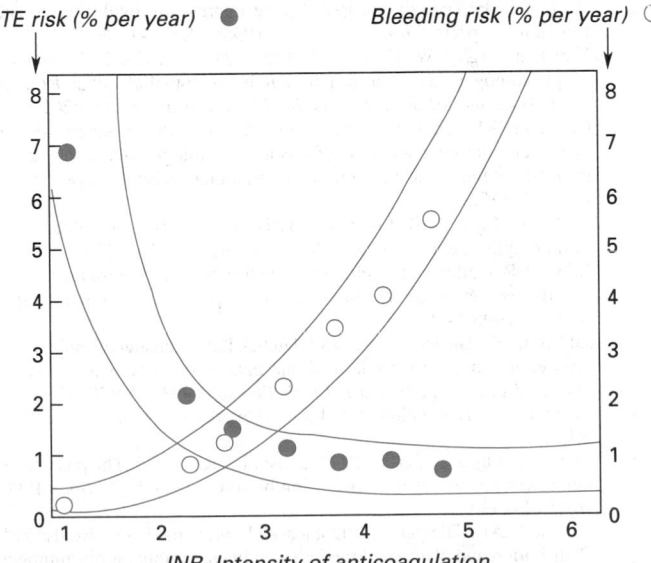

St. Jude Medical Prosthesis (n = 435) (Av 122 months)

TE risk (% per year) ●   Bleeding risk (% per year) ○

INR, Intensity of anticoagulation

FIGURE 52-24

Thromboembolic and bleeding risks with different anticoagulation regimens
in 435 consecutive patients with St. Jude valve replacement. (Modified from
Piper C, et al.[254]

Bioprosthetic Valves

Patients with biological heart valve prostheses should receive
low-intensity oral anticoagulation to an INR of 2.0 to 3.0

beginning as soon as possible after surgery and continuing 3 months postoperatively. Patients with bioprostheses who are at high risk for thromboembolism, including atrial fibrillation and previous thromboembolism, should receive oral anticoagulation indefinitely.[202,211]

Conclusion

Thus, with an understanding of the pathogenesis of and risk of thrombus formation, we can formulate a rational approach to the use of antiplatelet agents, antithrombotic agents, and potentially direct thrombin inhibitors. Those with a high risk for thrombus formation should generally receive a high degree of anticoagulation, and, depending on the pathophysiology of the thrombus, may also benefit from the concomitant use of antiplatelet agents. Those with a medium risk for thrombus formation may benefit from a low degree of anticoagulation or the use of antiplatelet agents alone. Patients at low risk for thrombus formation should not receive anticoagulation.

REFERENCES

1. Vane JR, Anggard EE, Botting RM. Regulatory functions of the vascular endothelium. *N Engl J Med* 1990; 323:27–36.
2. Jaffe EA. Endothelial cell structure and function. In: Hoffmann R, Benz EJ, Shattil SJ, Furie B, Cohen HJ, Silberstein LE, eds. *Hematology: Basic Principles and Practice.* New York: Churchill Livingstone; 1991:1198–1212.
3. Furchgott RF, Vanhoutte PM. Endothelium-deriving relaxing and contracting factors. *FASEB J* 1989; 3:2007–2018.
4. Esmon CT. The roles of protein C and thrombomodulin in the regulation of blood coagulation. *J Biol Chem* 1989; 264:4743–4746.
5. Harker LA. Pathogenesis of thrombosis. In: Williams J, ed. *Hematology,* 4th ed. New York: McGraw-Hill; 1990:1559–1569.
6. Ruoslahti E. Integrins. *J Clin Invest* 1991; 87:1–5.
7. Kieffer N, Philips DR. Platelet membrane glycoproteins: Functions in cellular interactions. *Annu Rev Cell Biol* 1990; 6:329–357.
8. Lapetina EG. The signal transduction induced by thrombin in human platelets. *FEBS Lett* 1990; 268:400–404.
9. Rhee SG. Inositol phospholipids-specific phospholipase C: Interaction of gamma isoform with tyrosine kinase. *Trends Biochem Sci* 1991; 16:297–301.
10. Kieffer N, Phillips DR. Platelet membrane glycoproteins: Functions in cellular interactions. *Annu Rev Cell Biol* 1990; 6:329–357.
11. Turitto VT, Baumgartner HR. Initial deposition of platelets and fibrin on vascular surfaces in flowing blood. In: Colman RW, Hirsh J, Marder VJ, Salzman EW, eds. *Hemostasis and Thrombosis: Basic Principles and Clinical Practice.* Philadelphia: Lippincott; 1994:805–822.
12. Edgington TS, Mackman N, Brand K, Ruf W. The structural biology of expression and function of tissue factor. *Thromb Haemost* 1991; 66:67–79.
13. Rapaport SI, Rao LV. The tissue factor pathway: How it has become a "prima ballerina." *Thromb Haemost* 1995; 74:7–17.
16. Davie EW. Biochemical and molecular aspects of the coagulation cascade. *Thromb Haemost* 1995; 74:1–6.
15. Mann KG, Jenny RJ, Krishnaswamy S. Cofactor proteins in the assembly and expression of blood clotting enzyme complexes. *Annu Rev Biochem* 1988; 57:915–956.
16. Gilbert GE, Furie BC, Furie B. Binding of human factor VIII to phospholipid vesicles. *J Biol Chem* 1990; 265:815–822.
17. Mosesson MW. Fibrin polymerization and its regulatory role in hemostasis. *J Lab Clin Med* 1990; 116:8–17.
18. Hogg PJ, Jackson CM. Fibrin monomer protects thrombin from inactivation by heparin-antithrombin III: Implications for heparin efficacy. *Proc Natl Acad Sci USA* 1989; 86:3619–3623.
19. Harker LA, Mann KG. Thrombosis and fibrinolysis. In: Fuster V, Verstraete M, eds. *Thrombosis in Cardiovascular Disorders.* Philadelphia: Saunders; 1994:837–860.
20. Rosenberg RD, Bauer KA. The heparin-antithrombin system: A natural anticoagulant mechanism. In: Colman RW, Hirsh J, Marder VJ, Salzman EW, eds. *Hemostasis and Thrombosis: Basic Principles and Clinical Practice.* Philadelphia: Lippincott; 1994, 837–860.
21. Dahlbäck B. Protein S and C4b-binding protein: Components involved in the regulation of the protein C anticoagulant system. *Thromb Haemost* 1991; 66:49–61.
22. Rapaport SI. The extrinsic pathway inhibitor: A regulator of tissue factor-dependent blood coagulation. *Thromb Haemost* 1991; 66:6–15.
23. Petersen TE, Martzen MR, Ichinose A, Davie EW. Characterization of the gene for human plasminogen, a key proenzyme in the fibrinolytic serum. *J Biol Chem* 1990; 265:6104–6111.
24. Collen D. On the regulation and control of fibrinolysis. *Thromb Haemost* 1980; 43:77–89.
25. Plow EF, Felez J, Miles LA. Cellular regulation of fibrinolysis. *Thromb Haemost* 1991; 66:32–36.
26. Thorsen S. The mechanism of plasminogen activation and the variability of the fibrin effector during tissue-type plasminogen activator-mediated fibrinolysis. *Ann NY Acad Sci* 1992; 667:52–63.
27. Pennica D, Holmes WE, Kohr WJ, Harkins RN, Vehar GA, Ward CA, et al. Cloning and expression of human tissue-type plasminogen activator cDNA in *E. coli. Nature* 1983; 301:214–221.
28. Lijnen HR, Collen D. Strategies for the improvement of thrombolytic agents. *Thromb Haemost* 1991; 66:88–110.
29. Blasi F. Urokinase and urokinase receptor: A paracrine/autocrine system regulating cell migration and invasiveness. *Bioessays* 1993; 15:105–111.
30. Bachmann F. The plasminogen-plasmin enzyme system. In: Colman RW, Hirsh J, Marder VJ, Salzman EW, eds. *Hemostasis and Thrombosis: Basic Principles and Clinical Practice,* 3d ed. Philadelphia: Lippincott; 1994:1592–1622.
31. Huber R, Carrell RW. Implications of the three-dimensional structure of α_1-antitrypsin for structure and function of serpins. *Biochemistry* 1989; 28:8951–8966.
32. Sumi Y, Ichikawa Y, Nakamura Y, Miura O, Aoki N. Expression and characterization of pro α_2-plasmin inhibitor. *J Biochem (Tokyo)* 1989; 106:703–707.
33. Pannekoek H, Veerman H, Lambers H, Diergaarde P, Verweij CL, van Zonneveld AJ, et al. Endothelial plasminogen activator inhibitor (PAI): A new member of the serpin gene family. *EMBO J* 1986; 5:2539–2544.
34. Kruithof EK, Vassalli JD, Schleuning WD, Mattaliano RJ, Bachmann F. Purification and characterization of plasminogen activator inhibitor from the histiocytic lymphoma cell line U-937. *J Biol Chem* 1986; 261:11207–11213.
35. Bachmann F. The enigma PAI-2 gene expression, evolutionary and functional aspects. *Thromb Haemost* 1995; 74:172–179.
36. Van Hinsbergh VW, Kooistra T, Emeis JJ, Koolwijk P. Regulation of plasminogen activator production by endothelial cells: Role in fibrinolysis and local proteolysis. *Int J Radiat Biol* 1991; 60:261–272.
37. Chandler WL, Levy WC, Veith RC, Stratton JR. A kinetic model of the circulatory regulation of tissue plasminogen activator during exercise, epinephrine infusion, and endurance training. *Blood* 1993; 81:3293–3302.
38. Collen D, Lijnen HR. Molecular basis of fibrinolysis as relevant for thrombolytic therapy. *Thromb Haemost* 1995; 74:167–171.
39. Lijnen HR, Collen D. Regulation of the fibrinolytic system. In: Agnelli G, ed. *Year Book on Thrombolytic Therapy.* Amsterdam: Excerpta Medica; 1995:1–30.
40. Jaklitsch MT, Biro S, Casscells W, Dichek DA. Transduced endothelial cells expressing high levels of tissue plasminogen activator have an unaltered phenotype in vitro. *J Cell Physiol* 1993; 154:207–216.
41. Loskutoff DJ. Regulation of PAI-1 gene expression. *Fibrinolysis* 1991; 5:197–206.
42. Mayer EJ, Fujita T, Gardell SJ, Shebuski RJ, Reilly CF. The pharmacokinetics of plasminogen activator inhibitor-1 in the rabbit. *Blood* 1990; 76:1514–1520.
43. Racanelli AL, Diemer MJ, Dobies AC, Mohamed SN, Reilly TM. Distribution and pharmacokinetics of active recombinant plasminogen activator inhibitor-1 in the rat and rabbit. *Fibrinolysis* 1992; 6:187–191.
44. Wiman B. Plasminogen activator inhibitor 1 (PAI-1) in plasma: Its role in thrombotic disease. *Thromb Haemost* 1995; 74:71–76.
45. Sawa H, Fujii S, Sobel BE. Augmented arterial wall expression of type-1 plasminogen activator inhibitor induced by thrombosis. *Arterioscler Thromb* 1992; 12:1507–1515.

46. Hajjar KA. Cellular receptors in the regulation of plasmin generation. *Thromb Haemost* 1995; 74:294–301.

47. Kruithof EK. Plasminogen activator inhibitors–A review. *Enzyme* 1988; 40:113–121.

48. Thorsen S, Philips M, Selmer J, Lecander I, Astedt B. Kinetics of inhibition of tissue-type and urokinase-type plasminogen activator by plasminogen-activator inhibitor type 1 and type 2. *Eur J Biochem* 1988; 175:33–39.

49. Reilly CF, Hutzelmann JE. Plasminogen activator inhibitor-1 binds to fibrin and inhibits tissue-type plasminogen activator-mediated fibrin dissolution. *J Biol Chem* 1992; 267:17128–17135.

50. Declerck PJ, De Mol M, Vaughan DE, Collen D. Identification of a conformationally distinct form of plasminogen activator inhibitor-1, acting as a non-inhibitory substrate for tissue-type plasminogen activator. *J Biol Chem* 1992; 267:11693–11696.

51. Collen D. On the regulation and control of fibrinolysis. *Thromb Haemost* 1980; 43:77–89.

52. Suenson E, Bjerrum P, Holm A, Lind B, Meldal M, Selmer J, et al. The role of fragment X polymers in the fibrin enhancement of tissue plasminogen activator-catalyzed plasmin formation. *J Biol Chem* 1990; 265:22228–22237.

53. Hoylaerts M, Rijken DC, Lijnen HR, Collen D. Kinetics of the activation of plasminogen by human tissue plasminogen activator: Role of fibrin. *J Biol Chem* 1982; 257:2912–2919.

54. Andreasen PA, Petersen LC, Dan K. Diversity in catalytic properties of single chain and two chain tissue-type plasminogen activator. *Fibrinolysis* 1991; 5:207–215.

55. Harpel PC, Gordon BR, Parker TS. Plasmin catalyzes binding of lipoprotein (a) to immobilized fibrinogen and fibrin. *Proc Natl Acad Sci USA* 1989; 86:3847–3851.

56. Loscalzo J, Weinfeld M, Fless GM, Scanu AM. Lipoprotein (a), fibrin binding, and plasminogen activation. *Arteriosclerosis* 1990; 10:240–245.

57. Edelberg JM, Gonzales-Gronow M, Pizzo SV. Lipoprotein (a) inhibition of plasminogen activation by tissue-type plasminogen activator. *Thromb Res* 1990; 57:155–162.

58. Juhan-Vague I, Alessi MC. Plasminogen activator inhibitor 1 and atherothrombosis. *Thromb Haemost* 1993; 70:138–143.

59. Prins MH, Hirsh J. A critical review of the relationship between impaired fibrinolysis and myocardial infarction. *Am Heart J* 1991; 122:545–551.

60. Jansson JJ, Nilsson TK, Johnson O. Von Willebrand factor in plasma: A novel risk factor for recurrent myocardial infarction and death. *Br Med J* 1991; 66:351–355.

61. Thompson SG, Van de Loo JCW. ECAT angina pectoris study: Baseline associations of haemostatic factors with extent of coronary arteriosclerosis and other coronary risk factors in 3,000 patients with angina pectoris undergoing coronary angiography. *Eur Heart J* 1993; 14:8–17.

62. Juhan-Vague I, Thompson S, Jespersen J. Involvement of the hemostatic system in insulin resistance: A study of 1,500 patients with angina pectoris. *Arterioscler Thromb* 1993; 13:1865–1873.

63. Etingin OR, Hajjar DP, Hajjar KA, et al. Lipoprotein (a) regulates plasminogen activator inhibitor-1 expression in endothelial cells: A potential mechanism in thrombogenesis. *J Biol Chem* 1991; 266:2459–2465.

64. Weitz JL, Hudoba M, Massel D, Maraganore J, Hirsh J. Clot-bound thrombin is protected from inhibition by heparin-antithrombin III but is susceptible to inactivation by antithrombin III-independent inhibitors. *J Clin Invest* 1990; 86:3619–3623.

65. Hirsh J, Fuster V. AHA medical/scientific statement guide to anticoagulant therapy: Part 1: Heparin. *Circulation* 1994; 89:1449–1468.

66. Kandrotas RJ. Heparin pharmacokinetics and pharmacodynamics. *Clin Pharmacokinet* 1992; 22:359–374.

67. Hirsh J, Levine MN. Low molecular weight heparin. *Blood* 1992; 79:1–17.

68. Sobel M, McNeill PM, Carlson PL, Kermode JC, Adelman B, Conroy R, et al. Heparin inhibition of von Willebrand factor–dependent platelet function in vitro and in vivo. *J Clin Invest* 1991; 87:1787–1792.

69. Meuleman DG. Orgaran (Org 10172): Its pharmacological profile in experimental models. *Haemostasis* 1992; 22:58–65.

70. Zammit A, Dawes J. Low-affinity material does not contribute to the antithrombotic activity of Orgaran (Org 10172) in human plasma. *Thromb Haemost* 1994; 71:759–770.

71. Stiekema JC, Wynand HP, Van Danther ThG, Moelker HCT, Dawes J, Vanchenzo A, et al. Safety and pharmacokinetics of the low molecular weight heparinoid ORG 10172 administered to healthy elderly volunteers. *Br J Clin Pharmacol* 1989; 27:39–48.

72. Nurmohamed MT, Fareed J, Hoppensteadt TJM, Walenga JM, ten Cate JW. Pharmacological and clinical studies with Lomoparan, a low molecular weight glycosaminoglycan. *Semin Thromb Haemost* 1991; 17:205–213.

73. Hirsh J, Fuster V. Guide to anticoagulant therapy: Part 2. Oral anticoagulants. *Circulation* 1994; 89:1469–1480.

74. Turpie AGG, Gunstenen J, Hirsh J, Nelson H, Gent M. Randomized comparison of two intensities of oral anticoagulant therapy after tissue heart valve replacement. *Lancet* 1988; 1:1242–1245.

75. Samama MM, Acar J. *Traitements Antithrombolytiques*. Paris: Masson; 1993.

76. Patrono C. Aspirin as an antiplatelet drug. *N Engl J Med* 1994; 3:1287–1294.

77. Lekkovits J, Plow EF, Topol EJ. Platelet glycoprotein IIb/IIIa receptors in cardiovascular medicine. *N Engl J Med* 1995; 332:1553–1559.

78. Verstraete M, Zoldhelyi P. Novel antithrombotic drugs in development. *Drugs* 1995; 49:856–884.

79. Harker LA, Hanson SR, Kelly AB. Antithrombotic benefits and hemorrhagic risks of direct thrombin antagonists. *Thromb Haemost* 1995; 74:464–472.

80. Verstraete M. The long search towards ideal antithrombotic drugs. In: Seghatchian J, Samama MM, Hecker SP, eds. *Hypercoagulable State: Biological Aspects and Clinical Management*. Boca Raton, FL: CRC Press; 1996:433–448.

81. Clowes AW. Prevention and management of recurrent disease after arterial reconstruction: A new prospect for pharmacological control. *Thromb Haemost* 1991; 66:62–66.

82. Antiplatelet Trialists' Collaborative. Secondary prevention of vascular disease by prolonged antiplatelet treatment. *Br Med J* 1988; 296:20–22.

83. Szczeklik A. Thrombin generation in myocardial infarction and hypercholesterolemia: Effects of aspirin. *Thromb Haemost* 1995; 74:77–80.

84. Meade EA, Smith WL, DeWitt DL. Differential inhibition of prostaglandin endoperoxide anti-inflammatory drugs. *J Biol Chem* 1993; 268:610–614.

85. Marcus AJ, Safier LB, Broekman J, Islam N, Fliesbach JH, Hajjar KA, et al. Thrombosis and inflammation as multicellular processes: Significance of cell-cell interactions. *Thromb Haemost* 1995; 74:213–217.

86. Mills DCB, Puri R, Hu CJ, Minniti C, Grana G, Freedman MD, et al. Clopidogrel inhibits the binding of ADP analogues to the receptor mediating inhibition of platelet adenylate cyclase. *Arterioscler Thromb* 1992; 12:430–436.

87. Schrör K. The basic pharmacology of ticlopidine and clopidogrel. *Platelets* 1993; 4:252–261.

88. McTavish D, Faulds D, Goa KL. Ticlopidine: An updated review of its pharmacology and therapeutic use in platelet-dependent disorders. *Drugs* 1990; 40:238–259.

89. Noble S, Goa K. Ticlopidine: A review of its pharmacology, clinical efficacy and tolerability in the prevention of cerebral ischaemia and stroke. *Drugs Aging* 1996; 8:214–232.

90. Verhaeghe R. Prophylactic antiplatelet therapy in peripheral arterial disease. *Drugs* 1991; 42:51–57.

91. Hass WK, Easton JD, Harold P, Adams JR, Pryse-Phillips W, Molonu BA, et al. A randomized trial comparing ticlopidine hydrochloride with aspirin for the prevention of stroke in high-risk patients. *N Engl J Med* 1989; 321:501–507.

92. CAPRIE Steering Committee. A randomized, blinded trial of clopidogrel versus aspirin in patients at risk of ischemic events (CAPRIE). *Lancet* 1996; 348:1329–1339.

93. Verstraete M. Thromboxane synthase inhibition, thromboxane/endoperoxide receptor blockade and molecules with the dual property. *Drugs Today* 1993; 29:221–232.

94. Ritter JM, Doktor HS, Benjamin N, Barrow SE, Stewart-Long P. On the mechanism of the prolonged action in man of GR32191, a thromboxane receptor antagonist. *Adv Prostaglandin Thromboxane Leukot Res* 1991; 21:351–354.

95. Misra RN, Brown BR, Sher PM, Patel MM, Hall SE, Han WC, et al. Thromboxane receptor antagonist BMS-180291: A new pre-clinical lead. *Bioorg Med Chem Lett* 1992; 2:73–76.

96. De Clerck F, Beertens J, De Chaffoy de Courcelles D, Freyne E, Janssen PAJ. R68070: Thromboxane A_2 synthetase inhibition and

thromboxane A$_2$/prostaglandin endoperoxide receptor blockade combined in one molecule: I. Biochemical profile in vitro. *Thromb Haemost* 1989; 61:35–42.

97. Berrettini M, De Cunto M, Parisi F, Grasselli S, Nenci GG. In vitro and ex vivo effects of picotamide, a combined thromboxane A$_2$-synthase inhibitor and -receptor antagonist, on human platelets. *Eur J Clin Pharmacol* 1990; 39:495–500.

98. Coller BS. A new murine monoclonal antibody reports an activation-dependent change in the conformation and/or microenvironment of the platelet glycoprotein IIb/IIIa complex. *J Clin Invest* 1985; 76:101–108.

99. Tcheng JE, Ellis SG, George BS, Kereiakes DJ, Kleiman NS, Talley DJ, et al. Pharmacodynamics of chimeric glycoprotein IIb/IIIa integrin antiplatelet antibody Fab 7E3 in high-risk coronary angioplasty. *Circulation* 1994; 90:1757–1764.

100. Kleiman NS, Ohman E, Califf RM, George BS, Kereiakes D, Aguirre FV, et al. Profound inhibition of platelet aggregation with monoclonal antibody 73E Fab after thrombolytic therapy: Results of the Thrombolysis and Angioplasty in Myocardial Infarction (TAMI) 8 Pilot Study. *J Am Coll Cardiol* 1993; 22:381–389.

101. The EPIC Investigators. Use of a monoclonal antibody directed against the platelet glycoprotein IIb/IIIa receptor in high-risk coronary angioplasty. *N Engl J Med* 1994; 330:956–961.

102. Topol EJ, Califf RM, Weisman HF, Ellis SG, Tcheng JE, Worley S, et al. Randomised trial of coronary intervention with antibody against platelet GPIIb/IIIa integrin for reduction of clinical restenosis: Results at 6 months. *Lancet* 1994; 343:881–886.

103. The CAPTURE Investigators. Randomised placebo-controlled trial of abciximab before and during coronary intervention in refractory unstable angina: The CAPTURE study. *Lancet* 1997; 349:1429–1435.

104. Charo IF, Scarborough RM, Du Mée CP, Wolf D, Phillips DR, Swift RL. Pharmacodynamics of the GPIIb/IIIa antagonist integrelin: Phase I clinical studies in normal healthy volunteers (abstr). *Circulation* 1992; 86:260.

105. The IMPACT-II Investigators. Randomised placebo-controlled trial of effect of eptifibatide on complications of percutaneous coronary intervention: IMPACT-II. *Lancet* 1997; 349:1422–1428.

106. Narjes H, Weisenberger H, Muller TH, Deichsel G, Krause J. Tolerability and platelet fibrinogen receptor occupancy (FRO) after oral treatment with BIBU 104 XX in healthy volunteers (abstr). *Thromb Haemost* 1995; 73:1315.

107. Takiguchi Y, Asai F, Wada K, Nakashima M. Comparison of antithrombotic effects of GPIIb/IIIa receptor antagonist and TXA$_2$ receptor antagonist in the guinea-pig thrombosis model: Possible role of TXA$_2$ in reocclusion after thrombolysis. *Thromb Haemost* 1995; 73:683–688.

108. Théroux P, Kouz S, Knudtson ML, Kel SC, Nasmith J, Roy L, et al. A randomized double-blind controlled trial with the nor peptidic platelet GPI IIb/IIIa antagonist RO 44-9833 in unstable angina (abstr). *Circulation* 1994; 232, part 2.

109. Peerlinck K, De Lepeleire I, Goldberg M, Farrell BA, Barrett J, Hand E, et al. MK-383 (L-700,462), a selective nonpeptide platelet glycoprotein IIb/IIIa antagonist, is active in man. *Circulation* 1993; 88:1512–1517.

110. Kereiakes DJ, Kleiman NS, Ambrose J, Cohen M, Rodriguez S, Palabrica T, et al. Randomized, double-blind, placebo-controlled dose ranging study of tirofiban (MK-383) platelet IIb/IIIa receptor blockade in high risk patients undergoing coronary angioplasty. *J Am Coll Cardiol* 1996; 27:536–542.

111. Nicholson NS, Panzer-Knodle SG, Salyers AK, Taite BB, Szalony JA, Haas NF, et al. SC-54684A: An orally active inhibitor of platelet aggregation. *Circulation* 1995; 91:403–410.

112. Frederick LG, Suleymanov OD, King LW, Salyers AK, Nicholson NS, Feigen LP. The protective dose of the potent GPIIb/IIIa antagonist SC-54701A is reduced when used in combination with aspirin and heparin in a canine model of coronary artery thrombosis. *Circulation* 1996; 93:129–134.

113. Hofsteenge J, Stone SR, Donella-Deane A, Pinna LA. The effect of substituting phosphotyrosine for sulphotyrosine on the activity of hirudin. *Eur J Biochem* 1990; 188:55–59.

114. Marbet GA, Verstraete M, Kienast J, Graf P, Hoet B, Tsakiris DA, et al. Clinical pharmacology of intravenously administered recombinant desulfatohirudin (CGP 39393) in healthy volunteers. *J Cardiovasc Pharmacol* 1993; 22:364–372.

115. Zoldhelyi P, Webster MWI, Fuster V, Grill DE, Gaspar D, Edwards SJ, et al. Recombinant hirudin in patients with chronic, stable coronary artery disease: Safety, half-life and effect on coagulation parameters. *Circulation* 1993; 88:2015–2022.

116. Close P, Bichler J, Kerry R, Ekman S, Bueller HR, Kienast J, et al. Weak allergenicity of recombinant hirudin CGP 39393 (^{TM}Revasc) in immunocompetent volunteers. *Coron Artery Dis* 1994; 5:943–949.

117. van den Bos AA, Deckers JW, Heyndrickx GR, Laarman GJ, Suryapranata H, Zijlstra F, et al. Safety and efficacy of recombinant hirudin (CGP 39393) versus heparin in patients with stable angina undergoing coronary angioplasty. *Circulation* 1993; 88:2058–2066.

118. Serruys PW, Herrman JPR, Simon R, Rutsch W, Bode C, Laarman GJ, et al. A comparison of hirudin with heparin in the prevention of restenosis after coronary angioplasty. *N Engl J Med* 1995; 333:757–763.

119. Topol EJ, Fuster V, Harrington RA, Califf RM, Kleinmann NS, Kereiakes DJ, et al. Recombinant hirudin for unstable angina pectoris. *Circulation* 1994; 89:1557–1566.

120. GUSTO IIa Investigators. Randomized trial of intravenous heparin versus recombinant hirudin for acute coronary syndromes. *Circulation* 1994; 90:1631–1637.

121. Cannon CP, McCabe CH, Henry TD, Schweiger MJ, Gibson RS, Mueller HS, et al. A pilot trial of recombinant desulfatohirudin compared with heparin in conjunction with tissue-type plasminogen activator and aspirin for acute myocardial infarction: Results of the Thrombolysis in Myocardial Infarction (TIMI) 5 trial. *J Am Coll Cardiol* 1994; 23:993–1003.

122. Lee LV, McCabe CH, Animan EM, Koch M, Wilensky R, Stringer K, et al. Initial experience with hirudin and streptokinase in acute myocardial infarction: Results of the TIMI-6 trial. *Am J Cardiol* 1995; 75:7–13.

123. Antman E for the TIMI-9A Investigators. Hirudin in myocardial infarction: Safety report from the thrombolysis and thrombin inhibition in myocardial infarction (TIMI-9A) trial. *Circulation* 1994; 90:1624–1630.

124. Neuhaus KL, von Essen R, Tebbe U, Jessel A, Heinrichs H, Mäurer W, et al. Safety observations from the pilot phase of the randomized r-hirudin for improvement of thrombolysis (HIT-III) study. *Circulation* 1994; 90:1638–1642.

125. The Global Use of Strategies to Open Occluded Coronary Arteries (GUSTO) IIb Investigators. A comparison of recombinant hirudin with heparin for the treatment of acute coronary syndromes. *J Engl J Med* 1996; 335:775–782.

126. Antman EM for the TIMI 9B Investigators. Hirudin in acute myocardial infarction. Thrombolysis and thrombin inhibition in myocardial infarction (TIMI) 9B trial. *Circulation* 1996; 94:911–921.

127. Maraganore JM, Bourdon P, Jablonski J, Ramachandran KL, Fenton JW II. Design and characterization of hirulogs: A novel class of bivalent peptide inhibitors of thrombin. *Biochemistry* 1990; 29:7095–7101.

128. Skrzypczak-Jankun E, Carperos VE, Ravichandran KG, Tulinsky A, Westbrook M, Maraganore JM. Structure of hirugen and hirulog 1 complexes of α-thrombin. *J Mol Biol* 1991; 221:1379–1393.

129. Lidon R-M, Théroux P, Juneau M, Adelman B, Maraganore J. Initial experience with a direct antithrombin, hirulog, in unstable angina. *Circulation* 1993; 1495–1501.

130. Lidon RM, Théroux P, Lesprance J, Adelman B, Bonann R, Duval D, et al. A pilot, early angiographic patency study using a direct thrombin inhibitor as adjunctive therapy to streptokinase in acute myocardial infarction. *Circulation* 1994; 89:1567–1572.

131. Topol EJ, Bonan R, Jewitt D, Sigwart U, Kakkar VV, Rothman M, et al. Use of a direct antithrombin, hirulog, in place of heparin during coronary angioplasty. *Circulation* 1993; 87:1622–1629.

132. Jang I, Gold HK, Ziskind AA, Leinbach RC, Fallon JT, Collen D. Prevention of platelet-rich arterial thrombosis by selective thrombin inhibition. *Circulation* 1990; 81:219–225.

133. Imura Y, Stassen J-M, Collen D. Comparative antithrombotic effects of heparin, recombinant hirudin, and argatroban in a hamster femoral vein platelet-rich mural thrombus model. *J Pharmacol Exp Ther* 1992; 261:895–898.

134. FitzGerald DJ, FitzGerald GA. Role of thrombin and thromboxane A$_2$ in reocclusion following coronary thrombolysis with tissue-type plasminogen activator. *Proc Natl Acad Sci USA* 1989; 86:7585–7589.

135. Zoldhelyi P, Fuster V, Chesebro JH. Antithrombins as conjunctive therapy in arterial thrombolysis. *Coron Artery Dis* 1992; 3:1003–1009.

136. Hilpert K, Ackermann J, Banner DW, Gast A, Gubernator K, Hadvary P, et al. Design and synthesis of potent and highly selective thrombin inhibitors. *J Med Chem* 1994; 37:3889–3901.

137. Roux S, Tschopp T, Baumgartner HR. Effects of napsagatran (Ro 46-6240), a new synthetic thrombin inhibitor and of heparin in a canine model of coronary artery thrombosis: Comparison with an ex vivo annular perfusion chamber model. *J Pharmacol Exp Ther* 1996; 277:71–78.

138. Murphy NP, Pratico D, Jennings L, Doyle C, Fitzgerald DJ. Thrombin-dependent activation of platelet glycoprotein IIb/IIIa during coronary thrombolysis in vivo (abstr). *Circulation* 1995; 92:302.

139. Teger-Nilsson A-C, Eriksson U, Gustafsson D, Byfund R, Fager G, Held P. Phase I studies on inogatran, a new selective thrombin inhibitor (abstr). *J Am Coll Cardiol* 1995; 23:117.

140. Simoons ML, van Mittenburg A, Scheffer MG, Werner H, Leenders CM, Remme WJ, et al. Anticoagulant properties of efegatran, a direct thrombin inhibitor in patients with unstable angina (abstr). *Eur Heart J* 1994; 15:120.

141. Kettner C, Mersinger L, Knabb R. The selective inhibition of thrombin by peptides of boroarginine. *J Biol Chem* 1990; 265:18289–18297.

142. Knapp A, Degenhardt T, Dodt J. Hirudisins: Hirudin-derived thrombin inhibitors with disintegrin activity. *J Biol Chem* 1992; 267:24230–24234.

143. Hung DT, Vu TK, Wheaton VI, Charo IF, Nelken NA, Esmon N, et al. "Mirror image" antagonism of thrombin-induced platelet activation based on thrombin receptor structure. *J Clin Invest* 1992; 89:444–450.

144. Bode C, Hudelmayer M, Mehwald P, Bauer S, Freitag M, von Hodenberg E, et al. Fibrin-targeted recombinant hirudin inhibits fibrin deposition on experimental clots more efficiently than recombinant hirudin. *Circulation* 1994; 90:1956–1963.

145. Jackson KW, Tang J. Complete amino acid sequence of streptokinase and its homology with serine protease. *Biochemistry* 1982; 21:6620–6625.

146. Reddy KNN. Streptokinase—Biochemistry and clinical application. *Enzyme* 1988; 40:78–89.

147. Battershill PE, Benfield P, Goa KL. Streptokinase: A review of its pharmacology and therapeutic efficacy in acute myocardial infarction in older patients. *Drugs Aging* 1994; 4:36–86.

148. Smith RAG, Dupe RJ, English PD, Green J. Fibrinolysis with acyl-enzymes: A new approach to thrombolytic therapy. *Nature* 1981; 290:505–508.

149. Monk JP, Heel RC. Anisoylated plasminogen streptokinase activator complex (APSAC): A review of its mechanism of action, clinical pharmacology and therapeutic use in acute myocardial infarction. *Drugs* 1987; 34:25–49.

150. White WF, Barlow GH, Mozen MM. The isolation and characterization of plasminogen activators (urokinase) from human urine. *Biochemistry* 1966; 5:2160–2169.

151. Barlow GH. Urinary and kidney cell plasminogen activator (urokinase). In: Lorand L, ed. *Methods in Enzymology*: Vol 45. San Diego, CA: Academic Press; 1976:239–247.

152. Nolli ML, Sarubbi E, Corti A, Rabbiati F, Soffientini A, Blasi F, et al. Production and characterization of human recombinant single chain urokinase-type plasminogen activator from mouse cells. *Fibrinolysis* 1989; 3:101–106.

153. Scully MF. Plasminogen activator-dependent pericellular proteolysis. *Br J Haematol* 1991; 79:537–543.

154. Holmes WE, Pennica D, Blaber M, Rey MW, Guenzler WA, Steffens G, et al. Cloning and expression of the gene for pro-urokinase in *Escherichia coli*. *Biotechnology* 1985; 3:923–929.

155. Declerck PJ, Lijnen HR, Verstreken M, Moreau H, Collen D. A monoclonal antibody specific for two-chain urokinase-type plasminogen activator: Application to the study of the mechanism of clot lysis with single-chain urokinase-type plasminogen activator in plasma. *Blood* 1990; 75:1794–1800.

156. Scully MF, Ellis V, Watahiki Y, Kakkar VV. Activation of pro-urokinase by plasmin: Non-Michaelian kinetics indicates a mechanism of negative cooperation. *Arch Biochem Biophys* 1989; 268:438–446.

157. Pennica D, Holmes WE, Kohr WJ, Harkin SRN, Vehar GA, Ward DA, et al. Cloning and expression of human tissue-type plasminogen activator cDNA in *E. coli*. *Nature* 1983; 301:214–221.

158. Hoylaerts M, Rijken DC, Lijnen HR, Collen D. Kinetics of the activation of plasminogen by human tissue plasminogen activator: Role of fibrin. *J Biol Chem* 1982; 257:2912–2919.

159. Suzuki S, Saito M, Suzuki N, Kato H, Nagaoka N, Yoshitake S, et al. Thrombolytic properties of novel modified human tissue-type plasminogen activator (E6010): A bolus injection of E6010 has equiva-

160. Kawai C, Hosoda S, Motomiya T, Kimata S, Yui Y, Kodama K, et al. Multicenter trial of a novel modified t-PA, E6010, by IV bolus injection in patients with acute myocardial infarction (AMI) (abstr). *Circulation* 1992; 86(suppl):I-409.

161. Kohnert U, Rudolph R, Verheijen JH, Weening-Verhoeff EJD, Stern A, Opitz U, et al. Biochemical properties of the kringle 2 and protease domains are maintained in the refolded t-PA deletion variant BM 06.022. *Prot Eng* 1992; 5:93–100.

162. Stern A, Kohnert U, Rudolph R, Fischer S, Martin U. Gewebs-Plasminogenaktivator-Derivat. Eur Patent Appl 38217, 1989.

163. Martin U, Fischer S, Kohnert U, Opitz U, Rudolph R, Sponer G. Thrombolysis with an *Escherichia coli*-produced recombinant plasminogen activator (BM 06.022) in the rabbit model of jugular vein thrombosis. *Thromb Haemost* 1991; 65:560–564.

164. Martin U, Köhler J, Sponer G, Strein K. Pharmacokinetics of the novel recombinant plasminogen activator BM 06.022 in rats, dogs, and non-human primates. *Fibrinolysis* 1992; 6:39–43.

165. Martin U, van Mollendorf E, Akpan W, Kientsch-Engel R, Kaufmann B, Neugebauer G. Dose-ranging study of the novel recombinant plasminogen activator BM 06.022 in healthy volunteers. *Clin Pharmacol Ther* 1991; 50:429–436.

166. Müller M, Haerer W, Ellbrück D, Martin U, Konig R, Seifried E, et al. Pharmacokinetics and effects on the hemostatic system of bolus application of a novel recombinant plasminogen activator in AMI patients (abstr). *Fibrinolysis* 1992; 6(suppl 2):26.

167. Neuhaus K-L, von Essen R, Vogt A, König R, Riess M, Appel KF, et al. Dose finding with a novel recombinant plasminogen activator (BM 06.022) in patients with acute myocardial infarction: Results of the German recombinant plasminogen activator study. *J Am Coll Cardiol* 1994; 24:55–60.

168. Tebbe U, von Essen R, Smolarz A, Limbourg P, Rox J, Rustige J, et al. Open, noncontrolled dose-finding study with a novel recombinant plasminogen activator (BM 06.022) given as a double bolus in patients with acute myocardial infarction. *Am J Cardiol* 1993; 72:518–524.

169. Smalling RW, Bode C, Kalbfleisch J, Sen S, Limbourg P, Forycki F, et al. More rapid, complete, and stable coronary thrombolysis with bolus administration of reteplase compared with alteplase infusion in acute myocardial infarction: A comparison with standard dose alteplase. *Circulation* 1995; 91:2725–2732.

170. Bode C, Smalling RW, Sen S, Kalbfleisch J, Bochm M, Ademheimer DJ, et al. Recombinant plasminogen activator angiographic phase II international dose finding study (RAPID): Patency analysis and mortality endpoints (abstr). *Circulation* 1993; 88:I-292.

171. International Joint Efficacy Comparison of Thrombolytics. Randomised, double-blind comparison of reteplase double-bolus administration with streptokinase in acute myocardial infarction (INJECT): Trial to investigate equivalence. *Lancet* 1995; 346:329–336.

172. Keyt B, Paoni NF, Refino CJ, Berleau L, Nguyen H, Chow A. A faster-acting and more potent form of tissue plasminogen activator. *Proc Natl Acad Sci USA* 1994; 91:3670–3674.

173. Collen D, Stassen JM, Yasuda T, Refino C, Proni N, Keyt B. Comparative thrombolytic properties of tissue-type plasminogen activator and of a plasminogen activator inhibitor-1-resistant glycosylation variant, in a combined arterial and venous thrombosis model in the dog. *Thromb Haemost* 1994; 72:98–104.

174. Cannon CP, McCabe CH, Gibson M, Ghali M, Sequeira RF, McKendall GR, et al. TNK-tissue plasminogen activator in acute myocardial infarction: Results of the thrombolysis in myocardial infarction (TIMI) 10a dose-ranging trial. *Circulation* 1993; 953:351–356.

175. Lijnen HR, Collen D. Development of chimeric tissue-type/urokinase-type plasminogen activators for thrombolytic therapy. *Curr Opin Invest New Drugs* 1993; 2:495–504.

176. Collen D, Stassen JM, Demarsin E, Kieckens L, Lijnen HR, Nelles L. Pharmacokinetics and thrombolytic properties of chimaeric plasminogen activators consisting of the NH2-terminal region of human tissue-type plasminogen activator and the COOH-terminal region of human single chain urokinase-type plasminogen activator. *J Vasc Med Biol* 1989; 1:234–240.

177. Van de Werf F, Lijnen HR, Collen D. Coronary thrombolysis with $K_1K_2P_u$, a chimeric tissue-type and urokinase-type plasminogen activator: A feasibility study in six patients with acute myocardial infarction. *Coron Artery Dis* 1993; 4:929–933.

178. Gardell SJ, Duong LT, Diehl RE, York RE, Habe TR, Register RB, et al. Isolation, characterization, and cDNA cloning of a vampire bat salivary plasminogen activator. *J Biol Chem* 1989; 264:17947–17952.

179. Bergum PW, Gardell SJ. Vampire bat salivary plasminogen activator exhibits a strict and fastidious requirement for polymeric fibrin as its cofactor, unlike human tissue-type plasminogen activator. *J Biol Chem* 1992; 267:17726–17731.

180. Krätzschmar J, Haendler B, Langer G, Boidol W, Bringmann P, Alagon A, et al. The plasminogen activator family from the salivary gland of the vampire bat *Desmodus rotundus:* Cloning and expression. *Gene* 1991; 105:229–237.

181. Gardell SJ, Hare TR, Bergum PW, Cuca GC, O'Neill-Palladino L, Zavodny SM. Vampire bat salivary plasminogen activator is quiescent in human plasma in the absence of fibrin unlike human tissue plasminogen activator. *Blood* 1990; 76:2560–2564.

182. Schleuning WD, Alagon A, Boidol W, Bringmann P, Petri T, KrStzschmar J, et al. Plasminogen activators from the saliva of *Desmodus rotundus* (common vampire bat): Unique fibrin dependence. *Ann NY Acad Sci* 1993; 667:395–403.

183. Witt W, Maass B, Baldus B, Hildebrand M, Donner P, Schleuning WD. Coronary thrombolysis with *Desmodus* salivary plasminogen activator in dogs: Fast and persistent recanalization by intravenous bolus administration. *Circulation* 1994; 90:421–426.

184. Collen D, Lijnen HR. Staphylokinase, a fibrin-specific plasminogen activator with therapeutic potential? *Blood* 1994; 84:680–686.

185. Schlott B, Hartmann M, Guhrs KH, Birch-Hirsch-Feld E, Gase R, Vettermann S, et al. Functional properties of recombinant staphylokinase variants obtained by site specific mutagenesis of methionine-26. *Biochim Biophys Acta* 1994; 1204:235–242.

186. Lijnen HR, Van Hoef B, Vandenbossche L, Collen D. Biochemical properties of natural and recombinant staphylokinase. *Fibrinolysis* 1992; 6:214–225.

187. Schlott B, Hartmann M, Gührs KH, Birch-Hirschfeld E, Pohl HD, Vanderschueren S, et al. High yield production and purification of recombinant staphylokinase for thrombolytic therapy. *Biotechnology* 1994; 12:185–189.

188. Collen D, De Cock F, Stassen JM. Comparative immunogenicity and thrombolytic properties toward arterial and venous thrombi of streptokinase and recombinant staphylokinase in baboons. *Circulation* 1993; 87:996–1006.

189. Collen D, Van de Werf F. Coronary thrombolysis with recombinant staphylokinase in patients with evolving myocardial infarction. *Circulation* 1993; 87:1850–1853.

190. Vanderschueren SMF, Stassen JM, Collen D. On the immunogenicity of recombinant staphylokinase in patients and in animal models. *Thromb Haemost* 1994; 72:297–301.

191. Vanderschueren S, Barrios L, Kerdsinchai P, Van den Heuvel P, Hermans L, Vrolix M, et al. A randomized trial of recombinant staphylokinase versus alteplase for coronary artery patency in acute myocardial infarction. *Circulation* 1995; 92:2044–2049.

192. Stein B, Fuster V, Halperin J, et al. Antithrombotic therapy in cardiac disease—An emerging approach based on pathogenesis and risk. *Circulation* 1989; 80:1501–1513.

193. Freudenberger RS, Fuster V. Fifty years of experience with antithrombotic therapy in cardiac disease: A 1996 approach based on pathogenesis and risk. *Mt Sinai J Med* 1996; 63:342–358.

194. Fuster V, Badimon L, Badimon J, Chesebro J. The pathogenesis of coronary artery disease and the acute coronary syndromes. *N Engl J Med* 1992; 326:242–250, 310–318.

195. Califf R, Willerson J. Percutaneous transluminal angioplasty: Prevention of occlusion and restenosis. In: Fuster V, Vestraete M, eds. *Thrombosis in Cardiovascular Disorders.* Philadelphia: Saunders; 1992:389–408.

196. Fuster V, Chesebro J. Role of platelets and platelet inhibitors in aortocoronary artery vein-graft disease. *Circulation* 1986; 73:227–232.

197. Ambrose J, Tannenbaum M, Alexopoulos D, Hjemdahl-Monsen C, Leavy J, Weiss M, et al. Angiographic progression of coronary artery disease and development of myocardial infarction. *J Am Coll Cardiol* 1988; 12:56–62.

198. Virchow R. Gesammelte Abhandlungen zur wissenschaftlichen Medizin. Frankfurt: Meidinger Sohn; 1856:219–732.

199. Dewanjee M, Fuster V, Rao S, et al. Noninvasive radioisotopic method for detection of platelet deposition in mitral valve prostheses and quantification of visceral microembolism in dogs. *Mayo Clin Proc* 1983; 58:307–314.

200. Stroke Prevention in Atrial Fibrillation Investigators. Predictors of stroke in atrial fibrillation II: Echocardiographic features of patients at risk. *Ann Intern Med* 1992; 116:6–12.

201. Stroke Prevention in Atrial Fibrillation Investigators. The stroke prevention in atrial fibrillation study: Final results. *Circulation* 1991; 84:257.

202. Israel D, Fuster V, Ip J, et al. Intracardiac thrombosis and systemic embolization. In: Colman R, Hirsh J, Marder V, et al, eds. *Hemostasis and Thrombosis: Basic Principles and Clinical Practice*, 3d ed. Philadelphia: Lippincott; 1994:1452–1468.

203. Coulshed N, Epstein E, McKendrick C et al. Systemic embolism in mitral valve disease. *Br Heart J* 1970; 32:26.

204. Kontny F, Dale J, Hegren L, Lem P, Soberg T, Morstol T. Left ventricular thrombosis and arterial embolism after thrombolysis in acute anterior myocardial infarction: Predictors and effects of adjunctive antithrombotic therapy. *Eur Heart J* 1993; 14:1489–1492.

205. Visser C, Kan G, David K, et al. Two-dimensional echocardiography in the diagnosis of left ventricular thrombus. *Chest* 1983; 83:228–232.

206. Penny W, Chesebro J, Heras M, Fuster V. Antithrombotic therapy for patients with cardiovascular disease. *Curr Prob Cardiol* 1988; 13:464–469.

207. Fuster V, Gersh B, Giuliani, et al. The natural history of idiopathic dilated cardiomyopathy. *Am J Cardiol* 1981; 47:525–531.

208. Falk R, Roster R, Coats M. Ventricular thrombi and thromboembolism in dilated cardiomyopathy: A prospective follow up study. *Am Heart J* 1992; 123:136–142.

209. Lapeyere I, Steele P, Kazimer F. Systemic embolism in chronic ventricular aneurysm: Incidence and the role for anticoagulation. *J Am Coll Cardiol* 1985; 6:534.

210. Heras M, Chesebro J, Fuster V, et al. High risk of thromboembolism early after bioprosthetic cardiac valve replacement. *J Am Coll Cardiol* 1995; 25:1111–1119.

211. Israel D, Sharma S, Fuster V. Antithrombotic therapy in prosthetic heart valve replacement. *Am Heart J* 1994; 127:400–411.

212. Teleford A, Wilson C. Trial of heparin versus atenolol in prevention of myocardial infarction in intermediate coronary syndromes. *Lancet* 1981; 1:1225.

213. Théroux P, Ouimet H, McCanu T. Aspirin, heparin or both to treat acute unstable angina. *N Engl J Med* 1988; 319:1105.

214. Cohen M, Demers D, Gurfinkel EP, Turpie GG, Fromell GJ, Goodman S, et al, for the Efficacy and Safety of Subcutaneous Enoxaparin in Non-Q-Wave Coronary Events Study Group. A comparison of low-molecular-weight heparin with unfractionated heparin for unstable coronary artery disease. *N Engl J Med* 1997; 337:447–452.

215. Lewis H, Davis J, Archibald D, Steinke W, et al. Protective effects of aspirin against acute myocardial infarction and death in men with unstable angina: Results of a Veterans Administration Cooperative Study. *N Engl J Med* 1983; 309:396–403.

216. Cairns J, Gent M, Singer J, Finnie K, et al. Aspirin sulfinpyrazone or both in unstable angina. *N Engl J Med* 1985; 313:1369–1375.

217. RISC Investigators. Risk of myocardial infarction and death during treatment with low-dose aspirin and intravenous heparin in men with unstable coronary artery disease. *Lancet* 1990; 336:827–830.

218. Cohen M, Adams P, Parry G, et al. Combination antithrombotic therapy in unstable rest angina and non-Q-wave infarction in nonprior aspirin users. Primary endpoint analysis from the ATACS trial. *Circulation* 1994; 89:81–88.

219. Holdright D, Patel D, Cunningham D, et al. Comparison of the effect of heparin and aspirin versus aspirin alone on transient myocardial ischemia and in-hospital prognosis in patients with unstable angina. *J Am Coll Cardiol* 1994; 24:39–45.

220. Balsano F, Rizzon P, Violoi F, et al. Antiplatelet treatment with ticlopidine in unstable angina: A controlled multicenter clinical trial. The Studio della Ticlopidina nell'Angina Instabile Group. *Circulation* 1990; 82:17–26.

221. Braunwald E, Jones RH, Mark DB, Brown J, Brown L, et al. Diagnosing and managing unstable angina. *Circulation* 1994; 90:613–622.

222. ISIS-2 Collaborative Group. Randomized trial of intravenous streptokinase, oral aspirin, both or neither among 17,187 cases of suspected acute myocardial infarction: ISIS-2. *Lancet* 1988; 2:349–360.

223. Baigent C, Collins R, for the ISIS Collaborative Group. ISIS-2: Four-year mortality follow up of 17,187 patients after fibrinolytic and antiplatelet therapy in suspected acute myocardial infarction. *Circulation* 1993; 88:I-291.

224. The SCATI Group. Randomized controlled trial of subcutaneous calcium heparin in acute myocardial infarction. *Lancet* 1989; 2:182–186.

225. Hennekens CH, Godfried S, Albert C, Gaziano JM, Buring JE: Adjunctive drug therapy of acute myocardial infarction—evidence from clinical trials. *N Engl J Med* 1996; 335:1660–1667.

226. GISSI-2. A factorial randomized trial of alteplase versus streptokinase and heparin versus no heparin among 12,490 patients with acute myocardial infarction. *Lancet* 1990; 336:65–71.

227. ISIS-3 Collaborative Group. ISIS-3: A randomized comparison of streptokinase versus t-PA versus anistreplase and of aspirin plus heparin versus aspirin alone among 41,229 cases of suspected acute myocardial infarction. *Lancet* 1992; 339:753–770.

228. The GUSTO Investigators. An international randomized trial comparing four thrombolytic strategies for acute myocardial infarction. *N Engl J Med* 1993; 329:678–682.

229. Hsia J, Hamilton W, Kleiman N, Roberts R, Chaitman B, Ross A. A comparison between heparin and low dose aspirin as adjunctive therapy with tissue plasminogen activator for acute myocardial infarction: Heparin-Aspirin Reperfusion Trial (HART) Investigators. *N Engl J Med* 1990; 323:1433–1437.

230. Bleich S, Nichols T, Schumacher R, Cooke D, Tate D. The effect of heparin on coronary arterial patency after thrombolysis with tissue plasminogen activator in acute myocardial infarction. *Am J Cardiol* 1990; 66:1412–1417.

231. de Bono D, Simoons M, Tijssen J, Arnold A, European Cooperative Study Group. Effect of early intravenous heparin on coronary patency, infarct size, and bleeding complications after alteplase thrombolysis: Results of double blind European Cooperative Study Group Trial. *Br Heart J* 1992; 67:122–128.

232. Australian Coronary Thrombolysis Group. A randomized comparison of oral aspirin/dipyridamole versus intravenous heparin after rt-PA for acute myocardial infarction. *Circulation* 1989; 80s:114.

233. O'Connor C, Meese R, Camey R. A randomized trial of intravenous heparin in conjunction with APSAC in acute myocardial infarction: The Duke University Clinical Cardiological Study (DUCCS). *J Am Coll Cardiol* 1994; 23:11–18.

234. Popma J, Coller B, Ohman E, et al. Antithrombotic therapy in patients undergoing coronary angioplasty. *Chest* 1995; 108(Suppl Oct): 4865–4925.

235. Colombo A, Hall P, Nakamura S, et al. Intracoronary stenting without anticoagulation accomplished with intravascular ultrasound guidance. *Circulation* 1995; 91:1676–1688.

236. Chesebro J, Goldman S. Coronary artery bypass surgery. In: Fuster V, Verstraete M, eds. *Thrombosis in Cardiovascular Disorders*. Philadelphia: Saunders; 1992:375–388.

237. Goldman S, Copeland J, Moritz T, et al. The Department of Veterans Affairs Cooperative Study Group. Starting aspirin therapy after operation: Effects on early graft patency. *Circulation* 1991; 84:520–526.

238. Limet R, David J, Magotteaux P. Prevention of aortocoronary bypass graft occlusion: Beneficial effect of ticlopidine on early and late patency of venous coronary bypass grafts. A double blind study. *J Thorac Cardiovasc Surg* 1987; 94:773–783.

239. Antiplatelet Trialists' Collaboration. Collaborative overview of randomized trials of antiplatelet therapy. Parts I, II, III. *Br Med J* 1994; 308:159–235.

240. Smith P, Arnesen H, Holme I. The effect of warfarin on mortality and reinfarction after myocardial infarction. *N Engl J Med* 1990; 323:147.

241. Breddin D, Loew D, Lechner K, et al. The German-Austrian Aspirin Trial: A comparison of aspirin, placebo, and phenprocoumon in secondary prevention of myocardial infarction. *Circulation* 1980; 62:63.

242. The EPSIM Research Group. A controlled comparison of aspirin and oral anticoagulants in prevention of death after myocardial infarction. *N Engl J Med* 1982; 307:701.

243. Meijer A, Verheug F, Werter C. Aspirin versus coumadin in the prevention of reocclusion and recurrent ischemia after successful thrombolysis: A prospective placebo-controlled angiographic study: Results of the APRICOT Study. *Circulation* 1993; 87:1524.

244. Coumadin Aspirin Reinfarction Study (CARS) Investigators. Randomised double-blind trial of fixed low-dose warfarin with aspirin after myocardial infarction. *Lancet* 1997; 350:389–396.

245. Steering Committee of the Physician's Health Study Research Group. Final report on the aspirin component of the ongoing Physician's Health Study. *N Engl J Med* 1989; 321:129–135.

246. Peto R, Gary R, Collins R, et al. A randomized trial of the effects of prophylactic daily aspirin among male British doctors. *Br Med J* 1988; 296:313–316.

247. Fuster V, Dyken ML, Vokonas PS, Hennekens C. Aspirin as a therapeutic agent in cardiovascular disease. *Circulation* 1993; 87:659–675.

248. Atrial Fibrillation Investigators. Risk factors for stroke and efficacy of antithrombotic therapy in atrial fibrillation: Analysis of pooled data from five randomized trials. *Ann Intern Med* 1994; 154:1449.

249. Stroke Prevention in Atrial Fibrillation Investigators. Warfarin versus aspirin for prevention of thromboembolism in atrial fibrillation: Stroke prevention in atrial fibrillation II study. *Lancet* 1994; 343:687–691.

250. Veterans' Affairs Stroke Prevention in Nonrheumatic Atrial Fibrillation Investigators. Warfarin in the prevention of stroke associated with nonrheumatic atrial fibrillation. *N Engl J Med* 1992; 327:1406.

251. Prystowsky E, Benson W, Fuster V, et al. Management of patients with atrial fibrillation: A statement for healthcare professionals. *Circulation* 1996; 93:1262–1277.

252. EAFT Study Group. European atrial fibrillation trial: Secondary prevention of vascular events in patients with nonrheumatic atrial fibrillation and recent transient ischemic attack or minor stroke. *Lancet* 1993; 342:1255.

253. Turpie A, Robinson J, Doyle D. A comparison of high dose with low dose subcutaneous heparin to prevent left ventricular mural thrombosis in patients with acute transmural anterior myocardial infarction. *N Engl J Med* 1989; 320:352–357.

254. Piper C, Schulte H, Horstkotte D. Optimization of oral anticoagulation for patients with mechanical heart valve prosthesis. *J Heart Valve Dis* 1995; 4:127–137.

255. Butchart E. Rationalizing antithrombotic management for patients with mechanical heart valves. *J Heart Valve Dis* 1995; 4:106–113.

53

ASSESSMENT AND MANAGEMENT OF LIPID ABNORMALITIES

Peter H. Jones / Scott M. Grundy / Antonio M. Gotto, Jr.

Atherosclerotic coronary heart disease (CHD) is a major health problem in the United States and other industrialized countries. It is the number-one killer of American men and women, taking about 500,000 lives annually.[1] Extensive observational epidemiologic data in single and cross-cultural populations have strongly linked untreated hypertension, cigarette smoking, and elevated total and low-density lipoprotein (LDL) cholesterol concentrations to the development of CHD.[2] Evidence supporting the relation between blood cholesterol concentration and CHD risk has been strengthened by numerous animal studies showing progression and regression of atherosclerotic lesions as cholesterol concentrations rise and fall and by natural history studies of genetic hypercholesterolemias (such as familial hypercholesterolemia), in which marked cholesterol elevations caused premature atherosclerosis even in the absence of other risk factors.[3-6]

Many randomized clinical trials, as discussed later, have shown that diet- and drug-induced reductions in total and LDL cholesterol can significantly reduce CHD morbidity and mortality in both primary and secondary prevention (reviewed in Refs. 6 through 8). Recently, trials with clinical event end points have also demonstrated reductions in all-cause mortality rate in both patients with[9,10] and patients without[11] CHD. In addition, numerous trials monitored by angiography have shown that cholesterol reduction can slow the progression of coronary atherosclerosis and in some cases halt or reverse its course (reviewed in Refs. 7 and 12 through 16). Lowering LDL cholesterol has also been documented, by B-mode ultrasound, to decrease the progression of carotid intimal–medial thickness.[17,18] While the preponderance of the imaging trials were not designed to assess the effects of LDL lowering on clinical events, a number did, nevertheless, demonstrate clinical benefit. Successful cholesterol reductions have been achieved in randomized clinical trials by lifestyle changes with or without single-agent or combination-agent drug therapy,[6-41] including women and the elderly.[9,10,25,30,35,40-42] CHD events and progression were also lowered by partial ileal bypass surgery.[43,44]

There is no longer a question as to whether one should take steps to detect and treat hypercholesterolemia. The second Adult Treatment Panel (ATP II) of the National Cholesterol Education Program (NCEP), a program of the U.S. National Institutes of Health, has provided specific guidelines for the assessment and treatment of hyperlipidemia in adults aged 20 or older.[6] The guidelines include recommendations on how and when to use dietary and drug interventions. A separate NCEP panel developed clinical guidelines for pediatric patients.[45] This chapter reviews the biochemistry and metabolic regulation of lipoproteins as well as the clinical assessment and treatment of lipoprotein abnormalities.

SUMMARY OF LIPID METABOLISM*

Lipoproteins are high-molecular-weight particles that transport water-insoluble nonpolar lipids through the plasma.[46] Ultracentrifugation is one of two classic methods used to separate and identify lipoproteins; the other is electrophoresis. The major plasma lipoproteins (Table 53-1), in order of increasing size and decreasing density, are high-density lipoprotein (HDL), low-density lipoprotein (LDL), intermediate-density lipoprotein (IDL), very low density lipoprotein (VLDL), and the chylomicron. Each is a sphere with a core of various amounts of triglycerides and cholesteryl esters, surrounded by a monolayer of phospholipids, unesterified (or "free") cholesterol, and specialized proteins termed apolipo-

---

* Summary of Lipid Metabolism (except "Mechanisms in Overview") is taken from Gotto AM Jr, Assmann G, Carmena R, Davignon J, Fernández-Cruz A, Paoletti R: *The ILIB Lipid Handbook for Clinical Practice: Blood Lipids and Coronary Heart Disease.* Houston: International Lipid Information Bureau; 1995. Used with permission. The original was prepared with the assistance of Henry J. Pownall, Ph.D., Professor of Medicine and Biochemistry at Baylor College of Medicine.

TABLE 53-1

CLASSIFICATION AND PROPERTIES OF PLASMA LIPOPROTEINS

Lipoprotein Class	Major Lipid Component(s)	Apolipoprotein(s)	Density, g/mL	Diameter, angstroms	Electrophoretic Mobility
Chylomicron	TG	A-I, A-II, A-IV, Cs, B-48, E	<0.95	800–5000	Origin
Chylomicron remnant	Cholesteryl ester, TG	B-48, E	<1.006	>500	Origin
Very low density lipoprotein (VLDL)	TG	B-100, Cs, E	<1.006	300–800	Pre-beta
Intermediate-density lipoprotein (IDL)	Cholesteryl ester	B-100, E	1.006–1.019	250–350	Broad beta
Low-density lipoprotein (LDL)[a]	Cholesteryl ester	B-100	1.019–1.063	180–280	Beta
High-density lipoprotein (HDL)					
HDL$_2$	Cholesteryl ester, phospholipid	A-I > A-II[b]	1.063–1.125	90–120	Alpha
HDL$_3$	Phospholipid	A-I, A-II[b]	1.125–1.210	50–90	Alpha

[a] A usually minor but variable fraction of LDL is complexed to apo[a] and constitutes a lipoprotein subclass termed lipoprotein[a] (Lp[a]).
[b] Minor apolipoproteins of HDL are E, C-I, C-II, C-III, A-IV, and D.
Abbreviation: TG = triglyceride.
Source: From Gotto AM Jr, Assmann G, Carmena R, Davignon J, Fernández-Cruz A, Paoletti R. *The ILIB Lipid Handbook for Clinical Practice: Blood Lipids and Coronary Heart Disease.* Houston: International Lipid Information Bureau; 1995. Used with permission.

proteins. The apolipoproteins mediate lipoprotein catabolism by activating key lipolytic enzymes and associating with cellular receptors that remove lipoproteins from the plasma compartment. The structure and composition of the lipoproteins can be altered by various dyslipidemias (e.g., the small, dense LDL seen in association with hypertriglyceridemia).

The exogenous (chylomicron) and endogenous (VLDL) plasma lipid pathways and HDL maturation are summarized diagrammatically in Fig. 53-1. Chylomicrons are formed in the intestine following the breakdown and absorption of dietary fat; their major protein is apolipoprotein (apo) B-48. VLDL particles are assembled and secreted by the liver; their major protein is apo B-100. At the capillary endothelium, VLDL particles and chylomicrons are converted to IDL particles and chylomicron remnants, respectively, by the enzyme lipoprotein lipase (LPL), which is activated by apo C-II. Concurrently, the apo C proteins are transferred to HDL. LPL occurs at high concentrations in striated muscle and adipose tissue. The fatty acids freed by hydrolysis of chylomicron and VLDL triglycerides are used as energy by muscle tissue or stored in adipose tissue to provide future energy.

In the liver, the IDL particles are further converted to LDL by the action of hepatic lipase (HL), with the simultaneous transfer of apo E to other lipoproteins. LDL, whose sole major apolipoprotein is apo B-100, delivers cholesterol to peripheral cells for use in forming cell membranes and steroid hormones. The chylomicron remnants are removed by specific hepatic receptors ("apo E receptors").[47,48]

The components of HDL are partly derived from the surface monolayer of triglyceride-rich lipoproteins and from peripheral tissue cell membranes. The smallest HDL particles contain free cholesterol, phospholipids, and apolipoproteins. Through the acquisition of additional cholesterol and phospholipids and the action of lecithin:cholesterol acyltransferase (LCAT), a small HDL particle increases in size and forms a core of cholesteryl esters. At least two plasma transfer proteins can exchange lipids between HDL, LDL, and VLDL particles; in the presence of hypertriglyceridemia, efficient transfer of VLDL triglyceride forms triglyceride-rich LDL and HDL particles, which are converted to smaller species (e.g., small, dense LDL) by HL.

Lipoprotein Catabolism

As noted, the liver removes chylomicron remnants through binding of apo E. More than 70 percent of LDL particles in healthy people are removed from plasma by means of the LDL (or B/E) receptor, which recognizes and binds LDL's apo B-100; most of these receptors are active in the liver.[49,50] Hepatic uptake of either LDL particles or chylomicron remnants decreases their respective receptor activities and hepatic cholesterol biosynthesis.

A decrease in the number and/or activity of LDL receptors (e.g., with aging) leads to elevation of serum cholesterol. In the absence of receptor binding, LDL is not efficiently removed from serum; further, without cholesterol uptake, cells continue to produce and secrete more cholesterol, since cholesterol biosynthesis is not downregulated. A diet rich throughout life in cholesterol and saturated fat may lead to chronic suppression of LDL receptor activity. In homozygous familial hypercholesterolemia, functional LDL receptors are absent and total cholesterol concentrations reach 700 to 1200 mg/dL.[51]

LDL particles not removed by the LDL receptor are removed by alternative pathways; removal by cells of the reticuloendothelial system is collectively termed the scavenger cell

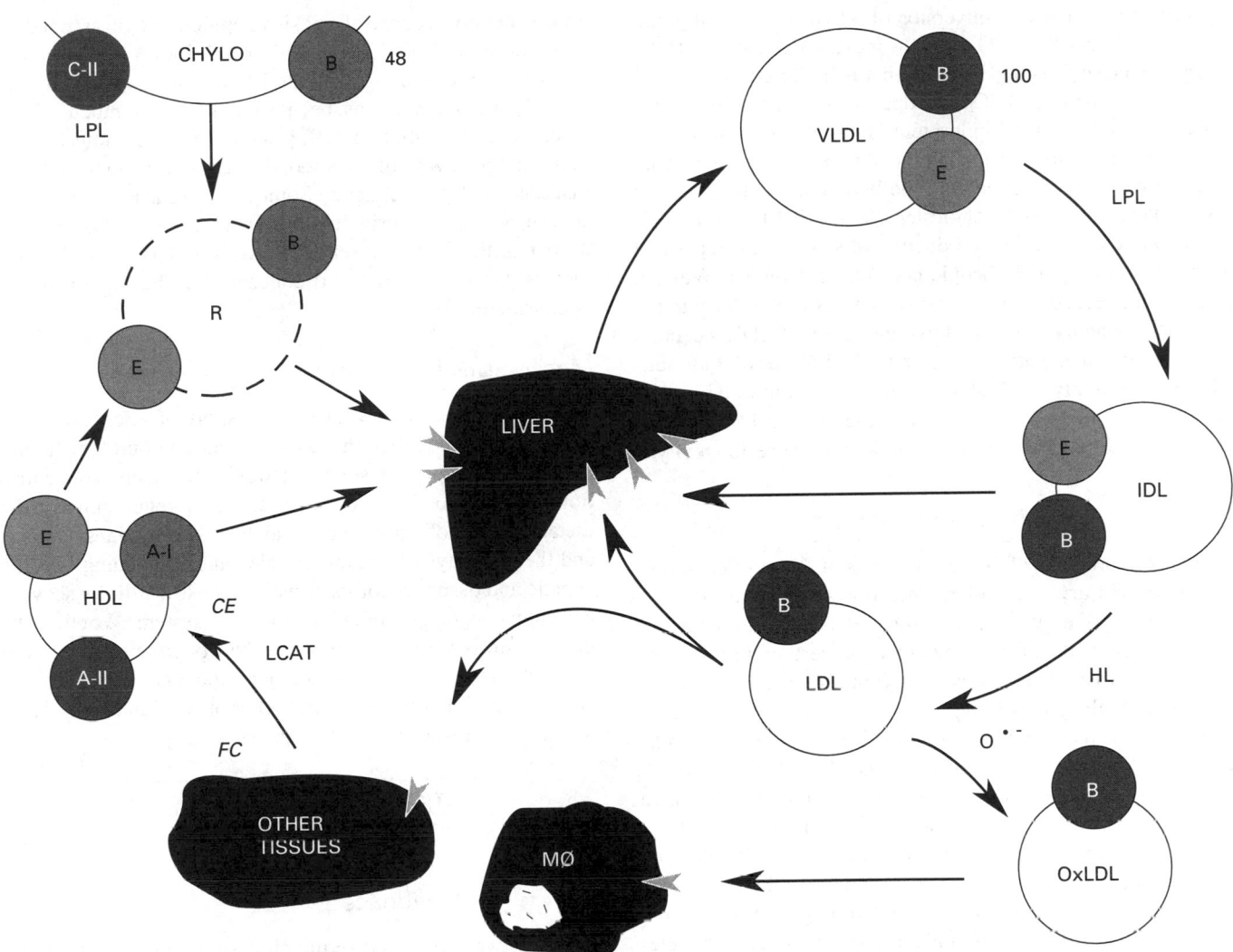

FIGURE 53-1

Diagrammatic summary of the exogenous (chylomicron) and endogenous (VLDL) plasma lipid pathways and HDL maturation, as described in the text. CE = cholesteryl esters; CHYLO = chylomicron; FC = free (unesterified) cholesterol; HDL = high-density lipoprotein; HL = hepatic lipase; IDL = intermediate-density lipoprotein; LCAT = lecithin:cholesterol acyltransferase; LDL = low-density lipoprotein; LPL = lipoprotein lipase; MØ = macrophage; OxLDL = oxidized LDL; R = remnant; VLDL = very low density lipoprotein. The small circles represent apolipoproteins (A-I, A-II, B-48, B-100, C-II, E). (From Gotto AM Jr, Assmann G, Carmena R, Davignon J, Fernández-Cruz A, Paoletti R. *The ILIB Lipid Handbook for Clinical Practice: Blood Lipids and Coronary Heart Disease.* Houston: International Lipid Information Bureau; 1995. Used with permission. Figure designed by Henry J. Pownall, Ph.D., of Baylor College of Medicine, and Jean Davignon, M.D., of the University of Montreal, and prepared by Materia Medica/Creative Annex, New York, under the direction of Barbara Robin Slonevsky.)

pathway.[52,53] The "scavenger receptor" of this alternative route apparently recognizes only lipoproteins that have been chemically modified—for example, oxidized LDL.[54–56] The scavenger receptor, unlike the LDL receptor, is not downregulated by LDL uptake, so that foam cells can form from lipid-laden macrophages. Foam cells are the chief component of the fatty streak, believed to be the precursor lesion of advanced atherosclerosis.

The mechanism of HDL catabolism[57] is not clear. In humans HDL exists in two forms, HDL$_2$ and HDL$_3$, both of which contain apo A-I and apo A-II as their major apolipoproteins. Turnover data on humans are not unequivocal because they are based on exchangeable labels. Data from other species suggest that the larger particle, HDL$_2$, is a precursor of HDL$_3$.

In hypertriglyceridemic subjects, the HDL$_2$, which is triglyceride rich, is a substrate for HL, which converts it to smaller HDL, presumably HDL$_3$. HDL$_3$ is the longest-lived lipoprotein (3 to 5 days), and one could argue that it is removed by nonspecific endocytosis. On the other hand, there is some evidence that HDL associates with cell surface receptors (e.g., liver, adrenals) that affect the translocation of HDL lipids. This can occur through a spontaneous transfer of free cholesterol from HDL to cell membranes, or the selective removal of cholesteryl esters by a mechanism that remains to be defined.

Biosynthesis of Cholesterol

The biosynthesis of cholesterol has been elucidated in considerable detail. The rate-limiting intermediate step in its derivation from acetate is the conversion of 3-hydroxy-3-methylglu-taryl coenzyme A (HMG-CoA) to mevalonic acid by HMG-CoA reductase. It is this key step that is inhibited by the class of drugs termed HMG-CoA reductase inhibitors, or statins (see "Drugs Affecting Lipoprotein Metabolism," below). The liver and intestine are the major sources of endogenously derived cholesterol. Generally, the body can manufacture all the cholesterol it needs; cholesterol is needed for cell membrane biogenesis and the production of steroid hormones and bile salts. However, in people consuming a typical Western diet, the increased intake of dietary cholesterol and saturated fatty acids usually results in downregulation of LDL receptors and subsequent elevation of serum LDL cholesterol. Individuals with extremely low LDL cholesterol (e.g., familial hypobe-talipoproteinemia) exhibit no anomalies in synthesis of bile acids and steroid hormones and may experience longevity.

Lipoproteins and Atherogenesis

Two key hypotheses of the pathogenesis of atherosclerosis are response to injury and lipid modification and infiltration.[58–60] Vascular injury may predispose the endothelium to uptake of lipoproteins, and plasma elevations of certain lipoproteins may lead to vascular injury, so the hypotheses are not mutually exclusive. Pathogenically typical atherosclerosis is generated by diet-induced hypercholesterolemia in experimental models, and lipid-laden foam cells and advanced lesions with lipid-rich cores have been well documented in animals and human subjects in which LDL receptors are decreased or absent.

Derangements in lipid metabolism associated with elevated LDL cholesterol usually lead to premature atherosclerosis. Findings of molecular genetics, cell biology, observational epidemiologic studies, and clinical trials all suggest that elevated LDL cholesterol is involved in atherogenesis. However, the evidence that native LDL itself is an atherogenic lipoprotein is not as compelling, and there has been increased interest in the role of oxidatively modified lipoproteins in the formation of the foam cells that characterize early atherosclerosis.

The inverse correlation between serum HDL cholesterol and premature atherosclerotic disease[61] does not necessarily support HDL as an antiatherogenic lipoprotein, since low HDL cholesterol is frequently associated with hypertriglyceridemia, insulin resistance, low serum LPL, and small, dense LDL, any one of which may be more closely linked to the mechanism for atherosclerosis. "HDL cardioprotection" has been hypothesized to result from reverse cholesterol transport, a model in which cholesterol in peripheral tissues is released into the plasma compartment, where it associates with lipoproteins. It has also been postulated that a protective effect of HDL could be direct—for example, through inhibition of smooth muscle cell proliferation or interference with macrophage uptake of oxidized LDL.

There is also clinical interest in lipoprotein[a] (Lp[a]),[62–65] which is assembled from an LDL particle and a large, hydrophilic glycoprotein termed apo[a], which bears little resemblance to the other apolipoproteins. Research interest has arisen not only because of a positive epidemiologic association between serum Lp[a] concentration and risk for CHD but also because of the striking structural homology between apo[a] and plasminogen. It has been suggested that much of the atherogenic potential of Lp[a] derives from its interference in normal pathways of thrombolysis. Currently, no drugs exist that specifically lower Lp[a]. Some myocardial infarction (MI) survivors exhibit fairly high concentrations of Lp[a] (e.g., >70 mg/dL) in the absence of well-established CHD risk factors. Generally, an Lp[a] concentration below 30 mg/dL is considered desirable.

Mechanisms in Overview

The above brief review of the transport of exogenous and endogenous lipids demonstrates that each lipoprotein family has a specific lipid transport function. The plasma concentrations of lipoproteins are under complex regulation by the dietary intake of cholesterol and fat, lipoprotein synthesis, and the pathways of lipoprotein clearance, including specific hepatic and tissue receptors as well as the low-affinity scavenger pathways of the reticuloendothelial system. Whether the mechanism is an oversynthesis of the lipoprotein, a decrease in catabolism, or a combination of the two, an excess of circulating LDL particles, chylomicron remnants, or VLDL remnants predisposes to atherogenesis.

RATIONALE FOR TREATMENT OF DYSLIPIDEMIA

Clinical Trial Evidence

A link between elevated serum cholesterol concentration and risk for CHD is well established. Numerous observational epidemiologic studies, laboratory investigations, studies in laboratory animals, and genetic forms of hyperlipidemia provide evidence for this connection.[6,66] Observational epidemiologic data come from such studies as the Seven Countries Study,[67] Framingham Heart Study,[68,69] Honolulu Heart Study,[70] Ni-Hon-San Study,[71] and Johns Hopkins Precursors Study[72] as well as screening data of the Multiple Risk Factor Intervention Trial (MRFIT),[73] as reviewed by Gotto and Pownall.[74] However, none of these "prove" that lipid-lowering therapy will prevent CHD. Such evidence can come only from clinical trials. For example, studies in laboratory animals suggest that the effects of cholesterol on atherosclerosis development extend to only the early phases of atherogenesis. If these findings were to be translated to humans, it might be expected that cholesterol lowering in patients with advanced atherosclerosis would be of little benefit. Consequently, clinical trials are needed to determine whether cholesterol lowering in high-risk patients will prove beneficial. Fortunately, many clinical trials have been carried out to address this question, and solid answers have emerged.

Clinical trials of cholesterol lowering generally are divided into three types: primary prevention, secondary prevention, and imaging (imaging trials are sometimes referred to as "regression trials"). Primary prevention trials are designed to determine whether cholesterol lowering will prevent new-onset CHD in patients without clinical evidence of atherosclerotic disease. Secondary prevention trials aim to establish whether cholesterol reduction will prevent recurrent acute coronary events and decrease coronary and total mortality rates in the presence of existing CHD. Finally, angiographic trials employ coronary angiography to ascertain whether cholesterol lowering will retard coronary lesion progression or promote regression; some trials have used B-mode ultrasound to assess effects on carotid or femoral lesions. Some of the imaging trials also have clinical-event end points. A review of the trials is necessary to provide a rationale for treatment of hypercholesterolemia and related disorders. The different classes of lipid-lowering drugs are discussed under "Drugs Affecting Lipoprotein Metabolism" later in this chapter.

NONSTATIN PRIMARY PREVENTION TRIALS

A sizable number of early cholesterol-lowering trials were carried out for the purpose of primary prevention before the introduction of the HMG-CoA reductase inhibitors (statins). These trials employed both diets and drugs for cholesterol reduction. Many of the trials gave suggestive evidence of reduction in coronary events; however, because of their relatively small number of patients, short duration, and only modest cholesterol lowering, their results were not considered definitive (reviewed by Gotto and Pownall[74]). More recently, metaanalysis performed by pooling of data of all trials has provided evidence of CHD risk reduction through cholesterol lowering.[8] In addition, the more recent individual trials in themselves strongly support the benefit of cholesterol-lowering therapy.[6-8,19,20,22,23] The most important of these was the Lipid Research Clinics Coronary Primary Prevention Trial (LRC-CPPT).[19,20] This large trial employed cholestyramine for serum cholesterol reduction; the major effect of cholestyramine is to lower LDL cholesterol concentration. Hypercholesterolemic patients treated with cholestyramine in the LRC-CPPT had significantly lowered rates of MI compared with patients in the placebo group. Another important trial was the Helsinki Heart Study,[22,23] which employed gemfibrozil as the lipid-modifying agent. Again a significant but relatively small reduction in MI rate was achieved with active treatment. Gemfibrozil appears to induce multiple favorable effects on lipoprotein metabolism, as discussed below.

An important result of these primary prevention trials was defining the quantitative relation between cholesterol lowering and CHD risk. The data indicate that every 1 percent lowering of total cholesterol concentration produces a 2 to 3 percent decrease in CHD risk.[2] This finding is consistent with observational epidemiologic data that a 1 percent increase in cholesterol concentration raises CHD risk by about 2 percent.[74,75] In spite of this important finding, these trials left one important question unanswered—namely, whether cholesterol-lowering therapy produces a decrease in total mortality rate. Generally, early trials did not have the statistical power to answer this

question.[76] Consequently, some investigators suggested that these clinical trials did not prove that cholesterol lowering is beneficial overall[77]; indeed, in the absence of documentation of a decrease in total mortality rate, cholesterol-lowering therapy might be detrimental. In sum, prestatin primary prevention trials documented that cholesterol reduction decreases CHD risk, but they did not demonstrate a decrease in total mortality rate.

NONSTATIN SECONDARY PREVENTION TRIALS

During the period when early primary prevention trials were being carried out, there was a parallel series of secondary prevention studies with clinical end points.[6,7,21,24] These trials likewise employed dietary change and/or drug therapy for serum cholesterol reduction. Results of *individual* trials resembled those of primary prevention; in several trials, the findings were suggestive of benefit from cholesterol-lowering therapy, but because of the small size of the trials, results were not definitive. However, when the data from all these trials were pooled and reanalyzed (metaanalysis), a much more definite result emerged.[78] Metaanalysis indicated that cholesterol reduction in patients with established CHD produces a clear-cut benefit. In these studies, a 10 to 15 percent reduction in cholesterol concentration gave an approximately 25 percent reduction in recurrent MI. Metaanalysis further revealed no evidence of an increase in noncardiovascular mortality; overall results support the thesis that cholesterol lowering is safe.[76,79] Metaanalysis further showed a strong trend toward a reduction in total mortality.[78]

ANGIOGRAPHIC TRIALS

The development of angiography made it possible to address the question of whether therapeutic reduction of cholesterol concentration will retard progression of atherosclerotic lesions or promote regression of lesions. A series of cholesterol-lowering trials[26-40,43,44] were carried out in which changes in vessel lumen/atherosclerotic lesions were typically the primary therapeutic end point. These trials generally carried out coronary angiography before and after therapy. Several therapeutic regimens were employed; most combined dietary change and drug therapy to yield a marked reduction in cholesterol concentrations. Drug therapy consisting of or including statin therapy was frequently used. Three major results from these studies have emerged.[6,7,12-16] First, cholesterol-lowering therapy retards progression of coronary atherosclerosis and can even promote regression of some lesions. Second, however, cholesterol reduction does not produce marked regression; most atherosclerotic lesions remained unchanged in size over the course of the trial. Third, cholesterol-lowering therapy produced a marked reduction in rates of new acute thrombotic events—for example, unstable angina and acute MI. Thus, the reduction in clinical events was out of proportion to changes in coronary lesion size.[12,13,15,80,81] This discrepancy strongly suggests that cholesterol-reducing therapy has favorable effects on coronary lesions that are not detected by coronary angiograms.[15,80,81]

The overall results of the angiographic trials have given rise to the concept of the unstable plaque. According to this concept, acute thrombotic events result from rupture of unstable regions of coronary plaques.[15] Pathologic studies suggest that these regions typically are located at the borders of fibrous plaques and are rich in lipid and macrophages. Unstable lesions apparently have a thin, fibrous cap with an underlying inflammatory region.[15] These factors render these areas of the plaque prone to rupture, causing acute coronary events. Seemingly, reducing LDL concentration helps stabilize these regions and reduce the likelihood of plaque rupture.

RECENT STATIN TRIALS

One series of regression trials was carried out with pravastatin,[18,37,38,82] and their data were pooled for metaanalysis.[41] The studies were carried out in Europe and the United States and included 1891 patients treated for an average of 2.3 years. All patients had clinical atherosclerotic disease and moderately elevated cholesterol concentrations. Metaanalysis revealed that pravastatin reduced the rate of fatal or nonfatal MI by 62 percent compared with control. The noncardiovascular mortality rate was not increased. This prospectively planned metaanalysis supports findings of the earlier metaanalysis of secondary prevention trials[78] and suggests benefit from cholesterol lowering over relatively short periods.

The Scandinavian Simvastatin Survival Study (4S), a large, multicenter trial, examined whether simvastatin therapy would decrease rates of mortality, coronary mortality, and recurrent coronary events and revascularization procedures.[9,10] A total of 4444 patients aged 35 to 70 with established CHD (angina pectoris and/or previous MI) were randomized to simvastatin or placebo. Most patients had elevated cholesterol. The cholesterol-lowering goal was total cholesterol below 200 mg/dL. The trial lasted an average of 5.4 years. Simvastatin therapy reduced LDL cholesterol by 35 percent, and the total mortality rate fell by 30 percent. Drug therapy reduced recurrent coronary syndromes by 35 percent, coronary revascularization procedures by 37 percent, and coronary mortality rate by 42 percent. Simvastatin therapy caused no serious side effects, nor was noncardiovascular mortality increased. The women receiving simvastatin showed benefit similar to that achieved in the men. Outcomes in older patients were similar to those of younger patients. Benefit of therapy was not at all reduced in cigarette smokers, in hypertensive patients, or in diabetic patients,[9] and benefit was seen across all quartiles of total, LDL, and HDL cholesterol values.[10]

Another recent secondary prevention trial was the Cholesterol and Recurrent Events (CARE) trial.[25] In this trial, patients were more typical of American CHD patients. Total cholesterol averaged only 209 mg/dL. Many patients had undergone previous revascularization. A total of 4200 patients were randomized to either placebo or pravastatin. Pravastatin therapy produced a 24 percent lower rate of acute MI or coronary death. It decreased the need for coronary artery bypass surgery by 26 percent and the need for coronary angioplasty by 22 percent. The noncardiovascular mortality rate

was not increased with pravastatin therapy. Women had even better outcomes than men.

A recent primary prevention trial employing a statin was the West of Scotland Coronary Prevention Study (WOSCOPS).[11] In WOSCOPS, 6595 hypercholesterolemic men without CHD were randomized to pravastatin or placebo. After 5 years of therapy, pravastatin had lowered serum cholesterol by 20 percent, coronary morbidity and mortality by 32 percent, and total mortality by 22 percent. No significant side effects were observed, nor was noncardiovascular mortality increased.

Thus, statin therapy has proved to be effective and safe in both secondary and primary prevention.[83,84]

TREATMENT CONCEPTS

This section presents an overview of the treatment concepts underlying the NCEP adult guidelines.[6,81,85–87] Detailing of the NCEP algorithmic approach and components of clinical assessment and treatment is provided in later sections.

Very High Risk Prevention (Secondary Prevention)

The presence of clinically manifest atherosclerotic disease confers very high risk for developing recurrent coronary events and dying of CHD. Men with established CHD carry a risk for recurrent MI that is five to seven times higher than that of men without clinical CHD.[78] A similarly high risk of reinfarction occurs in women with existing CHD.[88] A very high risk for developing new CHD extends to patients who have other clinical forms of atherosclerotic disease, whether located in the arteries to the limbs, the carotid arteries, or the aorta. For example, the presence of peripheral vascular disease or symptomatic carotid artery disease confers a four- to sixfold increase in risk of developing new coronary events.[89,90]

The findings of recent clinical trials justify aggressive cholesterol-lowering therapy in patients with established CHD. This evidence includes metaanalyses of secondary prevention trials with clinical end points (including the Program on the Surgical Control of the Hyperlipidemias, or POSCH[43,44]), the data from multiple angiographic trials, and recent large trials with statins (4S and CARE), as described above. Results of recent statin trials indicate that rates of new MI and need for revascularization procedures can be reduced by about one-third in very high risk patients by aggressive cholesterol lowering. This result translates into a decrease in coronary mortality rate without an increase in noncardiovascular mortality rate.

The NCEP identifies LDL cholesterol as the major target of cholesterol-lowering therapy.[6] For patients with established CHD or other atherosclerotic disease, the recommended goal of therapy is LDL cholesterol of 100 mg/dL or less. This target concentration derived in part from the belief that the lower the LDL concentration, the better. The results of several clinical trials suggest benefit from reducing LDL concentrations to this range. In hypercholesterolemic patients of the 4S trial, the target of therapy was an LDL less than approximately 130 mg/dL.[9] This study did not test whether incremental benefit occurs when LDL cholesterol concentrations fall below 100 mg/dL. The results of the CARE study[25] likewise failed to determine whether reducing LDL cholesterol to below 100 mg/dL confers greater benefit than reduction to below about 130 mg/dL. Therefore, the NCEP's recommendation of a target for LDL cholesterol of ≤100 mg/dL is based on theoretical grounds and on data from clinical trials other than 4S and CARE. The latter statin trials nonetheless clearly demonstrate a marked benefit from LDL lowering in CHD patients over a broad range of initial LDL cholesterol concentrations. Thus, clinical trial data taken as a whole justify aggressive LDL-lowering therapy in most patients with CHD or other forms of atherosclerotic disease. It appears that an LDL cholesterol concentration of ≤100 mg/dL is a reasonable target of therapy for secondary prevention.

Recent statin trials, as discussed above, document that cholesterol-lowering therapy reduces the risk for CHD regardless of coexisting risk status. Equal risk reduction from statin therapy occurred in cigarette smokers, hypertensive patients, diabetic patients, women, and older patients. Thus, benefit from cholesterol-lowering therapy extends to all subgroups of patients with atherosclerotic disease. The finding that older patients exhibit significant benefit allows secondary prevention to be used in the elderly population as well.

Although cholesterol lowering drugs produce a striking decrease in recurrent coronary events, the nondrug therapies (Table 53-2) should not be neglected. They potentiate the LDL lowering of drugs and reduce risk by other mechanisms. Cessation of cigarette smoking is of utmost importance. Smoking cessation reduces risk for recurrent thrombotic events by about one-third, similar to that achieved by cholesterol-lowering drugs. Within 2 to 3 years of smoking cessation, risk for MI declines to levels like those in people who have never smoked.[2] Reduced intakes of cholesterol, saturated fat, and total calories combine to lower LDL choles-

terol concentrations. Weight reduction[91–95] and increased physical activity[96–100] produce further benefit: they decrease serum triglyceride, increase HDL cholesterol, reduce insulin resistance, and decrease blood pressure. Regular exercise improves cardiovascular fitness, which may further reduce the danger of cardiovascular complications. Limiting sodium intake often lowers blood pressure.[101–103] Increased intake of vegetables and fruits may convey additional protection against cardiovascular disease.[6,104–106] The last effect may be mediated in part by antioxidant vitamins,[106–112] which reduce the susceptibility of LDL to oxidation. The growing evidence that LDL oxidation promotes atherogenicity[54–56] justifies vitamin C and vitamin E supplementation in patients with established CHD. Recent reports suggest that elevated serum homocysteine predisposes to CHD[113–116]; high concentrations in many patients are reversed by 1 mg/day of folic acid.

Epidemiologic data have shown reduced risk of CHD with moderate alcohol consumption, perhaps mediated through beneficial effects on HDL cholesterol or coagulation factors.[117] However, excessive consumption of alcohol is associated with adverse effects on blood pressure, arrhythmias, and the myocardium and with increased cardiovascular mortality. Maximum benefit for CHD appears to be reached at a limit of one drink daily.[117] Given the inherent problems with alcohol, recommendations to consume alcohol to reduce CHD risk are contraindicated.

Besides maximal nondrug therapy, most CHD patients require cholesterol-lowering drug therapy to achieve target LDL cholesterol, as discussed later in the chapter.

An American Heart Association consensus panel has provided recommendations for comprehensive CHD risk reduction in secondary prevention.[118] Risk reduction measures to be considered include use of antiplatelet agents or anticoagulants, angiotensin-converting enzyme inhibitors, beta blockers, replacement estrogen, and blood pressure control (Table 53-3) in addition to smoking cessation, lipid management, physical activity, and weight management.

High-Risk Primary Prevention

A significant portion of the middle-aged and elderly population even though asymptomatic nonetheless carry a high risk for developing CHD. Many have advanced coronary disease and their chances for developing new coronary events may approach those of patients with known CHD. Unfortunately, effective noninvasive techniques are not available to identify these very high risk patients. Consequently, risk for individuals must be estimated by the number and intensity of risk factors. The NCEP has defined the high-risk status in terms of cholesterol and other risk factors (Table 53-4). Framingham risk scores[119–121] reveal considerable variation in absolute short-term (10-year) risk within this high-risk category. For instance, at any given age below 75 years, men are at higher absolute risk than are women. Absolute risk increases progressively with age. Finally, severe intensity of risk factors (e.g., heavy cigarette smoking or poorly controlled hypertension or

---

TABLE 53-2

NONDRUG THERAPY TO REDUCE RISK FOR CORONARY HEART DISEASE

Smoking cessation
Reduced intake of saturated fatty acids (see Table 53-14)
Reduced intake of cholesterol (see Table 53-14)
Reduced total calories as required to achieve desirable body weight (body mass index <25 kg/m^2)
Increased physical activity (exercise at least 30 min five times per week)
Reduced sodium intake
Increased intake of vegetables and fruits (five servings per day)
Antioxidant vitamins (vitamin C 500 mg/day, vitamin E 1000 mg/day)
Folic acid (1 mg/day)

diabetes mellitus) greatly enhances risk. Of note, high HDL cholesterol reduces absolute risk. These various modifying factors must be kept in mind when estimating absolute risk and crafting a therapeutic regimen.

Support for high-risk primary prevention through cholesterol-lowering therapy comes from the previously mentioned WOSCOPS trial.[11] Patients of this trial generally fell into the high-risk category shown in Table 53-4. Most of the patients in this trial had high-risk LDL cholesterol and multiple CHD risk factors were common. Although absolute short-term risk in WOSCOPS patients was lower than that of hypercholesterolemic patients with CHD in the 4S trial, the marked reduction in new coronary events in WOSCOPS patients undergoing pravastatin therapy justifies drug use in such patients. Therapy appears to be both acceptably safe and cost-effective.

Thus, patients having elevated LDL cholesterol who fall into the high-risk primary prevention category deserve aggressive cholesterol-lowering therapy. In primary prevention, the intensity of drug therapy may be less than in secondary prevention because the target for LDL cholesterol reduction is not as low in primary prevention (see also "Drug Therapy," below).

Moderate-Risk Primary Prevention

A substantial portion of the American public can be considered to be at moderate risk for developing CHD (Table 53-5). In contrast to high-risk patients, individuals at moderate risk are unlikely to develop CHD in the short term (e.g., in the next 10 years). Nonetheless, they are at high relative risk and are more likely to manifest CHD at some time in their lives than low-risk individuals. The list includes young men and premenopausal women with high concentrations of LDL cholesterol. Also included are older individuals (middle-aged and elderly) who have LDL cholesterol in the range of 160 to

TABLE 53-3

AMERICAN HEART ASSOCIATION CONSENSUS PANEL RECOMMENDATIONS FOR SECONDARY PREVENTION: RISK REDUCTION STRATEGIES IN ADDITION TO LIPID MANAGEMENT AND LIFESTYLE CHANGES

Risk Intervention	Recommendations
Antiplatelet agents/anticoagulants	Start aspirin 80–325 mg/day if not contraindicated. Manage warfarin to international normalized ratio = 2–3.5 for post-MI patients not able to take aspirin.
ACE inhibitors post-MI	Start early post-MI in stable high-risk patients (anterior MI, previous MI, Killip class II [S_3 gallop, rales, radiographic congestive heart failure]). Continue indefinitely for all with left ventricular dysfunction (ejection fraction ≤40%) or symptoms of failure. Use as needed to manage blood pressure or symptoms in all other patients.
Beta blockers	Start in high-risk post-MI patients (arrhythmia, left ventricular dysfunction, inducible ischemia) at 5–28 days. Continue 6 months minimum. Observe usual contraindications. Use as needed to manage angina rhythm or blood pressure in all other patients.
Replacement estrogen	Consider estrogen replacement in all postmenopausal women. Individualize recommendation consistent with other health risks.
Blood pressure control Goal: ≤140/90 mmHg	Initiate lifestyle modifications—weight control, physical activity, alcohol moderation, and moderate sodium restriction—in all patients with blood pressure >140 mmHg systolic or >90 mmHg diastolic. Add blood pressure medication, individualized to other patient requirements and characteristics (e.g., age, race, need for drugs with specific benefits) if blood pressure is not <140 mmHg systolic or <90 mmHg diastolic in 3 months or if initial blood pressure is >160 mmHg systolic or >100 mmHg diastolic.

Abbreviations: ACE = angiotensin-converting enzyme; MI = myocardial infarction.
Note: Endorsed by the Board of Trustees of the American College of Cardiology.
Source: From Gotto AM Jr, Assmann G, Carmena R, Davignon J, Fernández-Cruz A, Paoletti R: *The ILIB Lipid Handbook for Clinical Practice: Blood Lipids and Coronary Heart Disease.* Houston: International Lipid Information Bureau; 1995. Format adapted from Smith et al.[118] Used with permission.

TABLE 53-4

HIGH-RISK STATUS IN PRIMARY PREVENTION

LDL cholesterol ≥190 mg/dL (men >45 years old and postmenopausal women)
or
LDL cholesterol 160–189 mg/dL plus two or more other CHD risk factors (see Table 53-6)

Source: Data from National Cholesterol Education Program.[6]

TABLE 53-5

ELEVATED RISK STATUS IN PRIMARY PREVENTION

LDL cholesterol 190–219 mg/dL in young adult men (<35
  years) and premenopausal women
or
LDL cholesterol 160–189 mg/dL plus fewer than two other
  CHD risk factors (see Table 53-6)
or
LDL cholesterol 130–159 mg/dL plus two or more other
  CHD risk factors (see Table 53-6)
(Some patients in this category may be considered to be at
  high risk in the presence of severe risk factors, e.g.,
  diabetes mellitus, heavy cigarette smoking.)

Source: Data from National Cholesterol Education Program.[6]

189 mg/dL combined with fewer than two other CHD risk
factors. Finally, an individual can be said to be at moderate
risk if LDL cholesterol is in the range of 130 to 159 mg/dL
and two or more other risk factors are present; these risk
factors must not be "severe" enough in themselves to place
the patient in the high-risk primary prevention category.

The goal of management in moderate-risk patients is to
retard atherogenesis so as to prevent CHD later in life. An
effort should be made to reduce all risk factors to slow down
atherosclerosis. Part of this effort should extend to LDL lowering, including nondrug therapy and in some cases pharmacotherapy (see "Drug Therapy," below).

CLINICAL ASSESSMENT
OF DYSLIPIDEMIA IN ADULTS

Updated adult clinical guidelines were issued by the NCEP
in 1993—the Adult Treatment Panel II (ATP II).[6] As noted
above, the guidelines algorithmically stratify risk assessment
and treatment by whether CHD or other atherosclerotic disease
is known to be present (i.e., primary versus secondary prevention). Patients considered at highest risk for CHD events are
those with CHD or other atherosclerotic disease. The focus
of the ATP II guidelines is controlling LDL cholesterol concentrations, although HDL cholesterol and triglyceride concentrations also inform risk management decisions.

Evaluation of Patients without Evidence
of Coronary Heart Disease

All adults aged 20 or older should have their total cholesterol
concentration checked at least every 5 years. If accurate methods are available, HDL cholesterol concentration should also
be determined. Both of these measurements may be made in
a nonfasting blood sample. In addition, the examination should
identify major nonlipid risk factors for CHD (Table 53-6);
risk assessment is to determine the patient's overall, or global,
risk for CHD. Fingertip blood and dry chemistry techniques
may be used in lipid screening (total and HDL cholesterol
and triglyceride); however, testing of venous blood is required
for decision making, and the laboratory should participate in

a reliable standardization program. The sample type should
be standardized from one test date to the next; serum lipid
concentrations are about 4 percent higher than plasma concentrations. The patient should have followed his or her current
diet for 3 weeks and have a stable weight, and patient posture
should be standardized (sitting for 5 to 10 min is convenient;
lying down may lower values). Note that cholesterol concentrations fluctuate on a daily basis, by perhaps 3 percent or
more; they also vary seasonally, increasing slightly in spring
and decreasing slightly in autumn. All lipid cutpoints should
be considered flexibly, in the context of total risk for CHD.

In primary prevention, total cholesterol is classified as desirable (<200 mg/dL), borderline high (200 to 239 mg/dL), or
high (≥240 mg/dL), and follow-up is determined by this classification and by HDL cholesterol concentration and the presence
of other risk (Table 53-7). HDL cholesterol <35 mg/dL is considered low for both sexes and is a major risk factor in itself.
HDL cholesterol ≥35 mg/dL is desirable, and HDL cholesterol
≥60 mg/dL is considered a protective factor, or negative risk
factor (e.g., a patient with HDL cholesterol of 60 mg/dL and

TABLE 53-6

OTHER RISK FACTORS[a] FOR CONSIDERATION
IN THE NATIONAL CHOLESTEROL EDUCATION
PROGRAM ADULT TREATMENT PANEL II ALGORITHM

Risk Factor	Notes
Positive	
Age	Male ≥45 years
	Female ≥55 years, or premature menopause without estrogen-replacement therapy
Family history of premature coronary heart disease	Definite myocardial infarction before age 55 in first-degree male relative or before age 65 in first-degree female relative
Current cigarette smoking	
Hypertension	Blood pressure ≥140/90 mmHg confirmed by measurement on several occasions, or taking antihypertensive medication
Low HDL-C	<35 mg/dL confirmed by measurement on several occasions
Diabetes mellitus	
Negative	
High HDL-C	≥60 mg/dL; in primary prevention, subtract one risk factor if HDL-C concentration is high

[a] In addition to presence or absence of atherosclerotic disease and elevation
of low-density lipoprotein cholesterol.

Abbreviation: HDL-C = high-density lipoprotein cholesterol.

Note: Obesity and physical inactivity are not listed but should be targeted
for intervention.

Source: Data from National Cholesterol Education Program.[6]

one other risk factor is considered in the primary prevention treatment algorithm to have no other risk factors). Generally, HDL cholesterol concentrations are higher in women than men; the clinical guidelines of the European Atherosclerosis Society recommend more active risk reduction therapy in women if HDL cholesterol is below 42 mg/dL.[122]

Patients with desirable concentrations of total and HDL cholesterol should be reevaluated in 5 years, although they and all others should be given information on promoting vascular health through a proper diet, exercising, maintaining a proportional body weight, and avoiding tobacco use. Patients with borderline-high total cholesterol, HDL-C ≥35 mg/dL, and fewer than two other risk factors should repeat the examination in 1 to 2 years. Patients with high total cholesterol, low HDL cholesterol, or borderline-high total cholesterol and two or more nonlipid risk factors should undergo fasting lipoprotein analysis (comprising total cholesterol, HDL cholesterol, triglyceride, and LDL cholesterol).

Because a complete lipoprotein analysis requires measurement of triglyceride concentration, the sample must be drawn after a fast of at least 9 to 12 h. Usually, LDL cholesterol is not directly measured but estimated by the Friedewald formula[123]:

$$\text{LDL cholesterol (mg/dL)}$$
$$= \text{total cholesterol} - \text{HDL cholesterol}$$
$$- (\text{triglyceride} \div 5)$$

(The divisor is 2.2 rather than 5 when values are in millimoles per liter.) The formula does not apply if the patient has triglyceride >400 mg/dL, type III hyperlipidemia, or the apo E2/2 phenotype; in each of these circumstances, determination of LDL cholesterol by ultracentrifugation in a specialized laboratory is required for accuracy. Diagnostic lipid evaluation should be deferred for 3 weeks after a minor illness. After an MI (secondary prevention guidelines apply; see below), lipid concentrations should be determined within 12 h of the onset of chest pain, since LDL cholesterol concentrations decrease thereafter for up to 12 weeks. After other major illnesses or surgery, diagnostic lipid evaluation should be deferred for 3 months. With pregnancy, testing is usually deferred until after delivery, since pregnancy is associated with physiologic hyperlipidemia; however, triglyceride should be monitored in a woman with a history of hypertriglyceridemia, since pregnancy can elevate triglyceride to the pancreatitis range.

LDL cholesterol concentration in primary prevention is classified as desirable (<130 mg/dL), borderline high (130 to 159 mg/dL), or high (≥160 mg/dL) (Table 53-7). This risk classification supplants that initially made based on total cholesterol. Individuals who have a desirable LDL cholesterol concentration should be counseled on risk reduction tactics and repeat testing within 5 years.

TABLE 53-7

NATIONAL CHOLESTEROL EDUCATION PROGRAM ADULT TREATMENT PANEL II: RISK ASSESSMENT

Initial Assessment	Results and Action[a]
Macrovascular disease present Fasting lipoprotein analysis[b]	LDL-C ≤100: Individualized instruction on Step II Diet and physical activity; repeat lipoprotein analysis annually LDL-C >100: Clinical evaluation; initiate cholesterol-lowering therapy

Macrovascular disease absent
TC and HDL-C
(nonfasting acceptable)
	TC <200
	  HDL-C ≥35: Repeat TC and HDL-C within 5 years or with physical exam; general educational materials
	  HDL-C <35: Lipoprotein analysis (see below)
	TC 200–239
	  HDL-C ≥35 + <2 other RF: Repeat TC and HDL-C in 1–2 years; instruct in diet, physical activity, RF reduction
	  HDL-C <35 or ≥2 other RF: Lipoprotein analysis (see below)
	TC ≥240: Lipoprotein analysis (see below)

After fasting lipoprotein analysis[c]	LDL-C <130: Repeat TC and HDL-C within 5 years; general educational materials LDL-C 130–159 <2 other RF: Information on Step I Diet and physical activity. Reevaluate annually, including lipoprotein analysis, RF reduction ≥2 other RF: Clinical evaluation; initiate dietary therapy LDL-C ≥160: Clinical evaluation; initiate dietary therapy

[a] All lipid values mg/dL. For list of other risk factors for consideration, see Table 53-6.

[b] Average of two determinations 1–8 weeks apart (three if variation >30 mg/dL); patient should not be in recovery phase from acute coronary or other medical event.

[c] May also be performed at outset. Assignment to last two categories (high risk) should be based on average of at least two determinations, as in previous footnote.

Abbreviations: HDL-C = high-density lipoprotein cholesterol; LDL-C = low-density lipoprotein cholesterol; RF = risk factors; TC = total cholesterol.

Source: Data from National Cholesterol Education Program.[6]

TABLE 53-8

NATIONAL CHOLESTEROL EDUCATION PROGRAM ADULT TREATMENT PANEL II: LDL CHOLESTEROL ACTION LIMITS FOR CONSIDERATION OF DRUG THERAPY

Patient Group	Initiation Concentration, mg/dL	Goal, mg/dL
No CHD, <2 other RF	≥190[a]	<160
No CHD, ≥2 other RF	≥160	<130
With CHD or other atherosclerotic disease	≥130[b]	≤100

[a] Consider delaying drug therapy in both men <35 years old and premenopausal women who have LDL cholesterol 190–220 mg/dL and no other risk.

[b] If LDL cholesterol is 100–129 mg/dL with maximum dietary intervention, use clinical judgment as to whether to use drugs.

Abbreviations: CHD = coronary heart disease; LDL = low-density lipoprotein; RF = risk factors.

Source: Data from National Cholesterol Education Program.[6]

Borderline-high LDL cholesterol is followed up according to the presence of other risk factors. If fewer than two are present, the patient should receive information on the Step I Diet (see below) and risk reduction, and lipoprotein analysis should be repeated in 1 year. If two or more other risk factors are present or if the patient has high LDL cholesterol, lipid-lowering therapy is indicated; a second determination of LDL cholesterol by lipoprotein analysis should be made in 1 to 8 weeks to verify hypercholesterolemia. A variance >30 mg/dL requires that a third determination be made and the average of the three used to define the baseline value. This procedure should compensate enough for the inherent variability in cholesterol values that the baseline achieved can be used with confidence.

If, based on a reliable LDL cholesterol estimate, the patient remains categorized at high or elevated risk (see Tables 53-4 and 53-5), full clinical evaluation (see below) is initiated and a specific lipid intervention program is begun. Lipid-lowering drug therapy may be required if increased risk remains despite lifestyle changes; cutpoints for consideration of drug therapy are shown in Table 53-8, and lipid-lowering therapies are discussed in detail below.

Evaluation of Patients with Coronary Heart Disease

All patients with established CHD or clinical atherosclerotic disease of the aorta, arteries of the limbs, or carotid arteries (Table 53-9) are at high risk for CHD events. A full fasting lipoprotein analysis is required in these patients. As noted above, LDL cholesterol concentrations are lower than normal during the recovery phase after MI and should be interpreted cautiously; diagnostic lipid evaluation is customarily deferred

for 4 to 6 weeks if determinations are not made within 12 h of the onset of chest pain. Optimal LDL cholesterol is defined as ≤100 mg/dL for patients with known atherosclerotic disease, and individuals so classified should receive personalized instruction on diet and physical activity and have a complete lipoprotein analysis annually (Table 53-7). Patients with higher than optimal LDL cholesterol (Table 53-7) should undergo complete clinical evaluation (see below) so that an appropriate regimen may be selected. The NCEP's general LDL cholesterol cutpoint for consideration of drug therapy in secondary prevention is 130 mg/dL, although drug therapy may be selected in some cases of high risk when LDL cholesterol remains >100 mg/dL (Table 53-8), as discussed in more detail below.

Risk from Hypertriglyceridemia

The close metabolic relation between the triglyceride-rich lipoproteins and HDL may account in part for the mixed epidemiologic findings[124–126] regarding elevated serum triglyceride as an independent predictor of CHD. Triglyceride concentration is related to CHD incidence in univariate analyses of data from prospective studies, but the association in

TABLE 53-9

NATIONAL CHOLESTEROL EDUCATION PROGRAM ADULT TREATMENT PANEL II: CLINICAL PRESENCE OF ATHEROSCLEROTIC DISEASE

Vascular Bed	Definitions
Coronary heart disease	Definite clinical and laboratory evidence of myocardial infarction Clinically significant myocardial ischemia History of coronary artery surgery or angioplasty Angiogram demonstrating significant coronary atherosclerosis in the presence of clinical symptoms of coronary heart disease[a]
Peripheral vascular disease	Abdominal aortic aneurysm or clinical signs and symptoms of ischemia of the extremities, either accompanied by significant atherosclerosis on angiography or abnormalities of segment-to-arm pressure ratios or flow velocities
Carotid atherosclerosis	Cerebral symptoms (transient ischemic attacks or stroke) accompanied by ultrasound or angiographic demonstration of significant atherosclerosis

[a] It is not recommended that angiography be performed specifically to classify patients for lipid-lowering therapy.

Source: Data from National Cholesterol Education Program.[6]

some studies weakens or disappears on multivariate analysis, in particular when HDL cholesterol concentration is taken into account.[55,124,125] The difficulty may also lie in the heterogeneity of the triglyceride-rich lipoproteins.[127,128] Chylomicronemia has not been associated with increased rates of atherosclerotic disease, but chylomicron and VLDL remnants appear to be linked to higher risk, and improved risk discrimination may be obtained in the future by lipid assessment in the postprandial state.[57,128,129] Small, dense LDL, related to increased risk for atherosclerosis (see "Clinical Evaluation," below), appears to be caused by impaired triglyceride metabolism.[129] In addition, preliminary evidence suggests that deleterious effects of elevated serum triglyceride on CHD risk may be mediated in part through its effects on clotting and fibrinolytic mechanisms.[125,130–134]

The NCEP defines four categories of fasting triglyceride concentration for adults: normal, <200 mg/dL; borderline high, 200 to 400 mg/dL; high, 400 to 1000 mg/dL; and very high, >1000 mg/dL.[6] Elevated serum triglyceride is most often secondary to an underlying disease or condition, such as diabetes mellitus or the use of certain drugs (see below), and control of the underlying condition may control the hypertriglyceridemia. Borderline-high or high triglyceride may accompany dyslipidemias that increase risk for CHD, such as familial combined hyperlipidemia or type III hyperlipidemia (familial dysbetalipoproteinemia). (As is also the case for HDL cholesterol, clinical trials specifically designed to lower CHD risk through lowering serum triglyceride have not been completed, although indirect data would indicate benefit.) Recent clinical work suggests that fasting hypertriglyceridemia may indicate underlying metabolic abnormalities that increase the potential for atherogenesis, such as prolonged postprandial lipemia, the presence of small, dense LDL, and peripheral insulin resistance with hyperinsulinemia (see below). Also to be considered is the particularly high risk that appears to be conferred, as discussed below, by the conjunction of increased triglyceride, decreased HDL cholesterol, and increased LDL cholesterol. Very high serum triglyceride confers risk for acute pancreatitis, and high triglyceride can be labile and quickly lead to acute pancreatitis. Recognizing chylomicronemia in lipid measurement is discussed below, under "Fredrickson Phenotyping."

Clinical Evaluation

The clinical evaluation includes personal and family histories, a physical examination, and basic laboratory testing to determine whether the condition is more likely to be of primary or secondary origin (see below) and to enable selection of appropriate therapy. The physical examination should include height, weight, calculated body mass index, blood pressure, and examination for manifestations of dyslipidemia (e.g., corneal arcus, xanthomas, hepatosplenomegaly), manifestations of atherosclerosis (e.g., vascular bruits, peripheral pulses), and thyroid abnormalities. Laboratory tests performed in addition to full fasting lipoprotein analysis generally include cre-

atine kinase, fasting blood glucose, alkaline phosphatase, liver function and thyroid tests, urinalysis, and electrocardiography.

A more complete evaluation of risk factor (Table 53-6) and cardiovascular status should be made at this time. High risk is more often due to multiple risk factors than to a single risk factor of severe degree. Risk factor evaluation should include an assessment of diet (including fat, saturated fat, cholesterol, alcohol, simple carbohydrates, and sodium intake) and exercise and smoking habits.

Atherosclerotic disease occurs not only more often in diabetic individuals (causing 75 to 80 percent of deaths in adult diabetics) but also at an earlier age.[135–137] This high risk makes diabetic patients candidates for aggressive CHD risk-reduction intervention. The most common lipid abnormalities in diabetes mellitus are increased serum triglyceride and decreased HDL cholesterol; increased LDL cholesterol may also be present.[138–142] Several lipoprotein compositional abnormalities may contribute to the higher risk for CHD in diabetes, including the tendency to have small, dense LDL and increased susceptibility of LDL in diabetes to oxidation.[139,142] An American Diabetes Association consensus panel has recommended aggressive treatment of dyslipidemia in diabetes, including institution of lipid-lowering measures for serum triglyceride >150 mg/dL in secondary prevention.[138] More aggressive lipid-lowering therapy may also be needed in hypertensive patients.[143,144]

The physician may also wish to consider other risk factors associated with the development of CHD, such as elevations of serum fibrinogen,[145–147] serum homocysteine,[113–116] and Lp[a].[62–65] As noted above, high concentrations of homocysteine can be reversed in many patients by 1 mg/day of folic acid. Epidemiologic evidence suggests that Lp[a] concentrations in the top quartile increase CHD risk anywhere from two- to fivefold.[62–64] Generally, an Lp[a] concentration below 30 mg/dL is considered desirable, as noted earlier. The risk for CHD with increased Lp[a] is enhanced by elevated LDL cholesterol; some recent evidence suggests that Lp[a] may cease to be a risk factor when LDL cholesterol concentrations are low enough.[148] At present, however, Lp[a] measurement is considered to be a research tool, and studies of methods to reduce Lp[a] concentrations are limited. The only treatments that have been associated with reduced Lp[a] are nicotinic acid, oral estrogen, neomycin, certain steroids (e.g., stanozolol), and omega-3 fatty acids.[63,149,150] Further studies on Lp[a]'s origins, metabolism, and physiologic functions and on modulation of its serum concentration are necessary before routine use of this risk factor can be recommended.

A number of clinical studies have focused on the strong correlation of certain apolipoprotein concentrations with the incidence and severity of CHD.[151–154] Apo B, the only protein component of the LDL particle, is the apolipoprotein with the strongest positive correlation with severity of coronary atherosclerosis. In the Familial Atherosclerosis Treatment Study (FATS), the apo B concentration correlated independently on multivariate analysis with regression of coronary lesions, as did systolic blood pressure and HDL cholesterol.[29]

Measurement of apo B may be useful for risk assessment in certain patients, such as those with CHD and LDL cholesterol concentrations <130 mg/dL, and in high-risk primary prevention patients. Apo A-I, the major protein of HDL, has just as strong a negative association with CHD severity. However, most observational epidemiologic studies do not suggest that apo A-I concentration is superior to HDL concentration in predicting CHD risk. Concentrations of these apolipoproteins can be determined on commercially available analyzers; however, there is no standardization of normal ranges and no consensus on predictive or treatment value. Further study is needed to determine the usefulness of such apolipoprotein measurement as an adjunct to risk evaluation by routine lipid measurements.

Central obesity is associated with increased CHD risk and may occur in conjunction with the posited insulin-resistance syndrome (also called metabolic syndrome X), entailing elevated serum triglyceride, reduced HDL cholesterol, increased insulin resistance, hyperinsulinemia, increased glucose concentrations, increased uric acid concentrations, hypertension, microalbuminuria, and increased plasminogen activator inhibitor 1 (PAI-1).[155–157] Another aspect of the syndrome may be the presence of small, dense LDL. A preponderance of small, dense LDL (termed LDL phenotype B or subclass B) as opposed to normal (larger and more buoyant) LDL (LDL phenotype A) in plasma has been associated with increased risk for MI.[158–160] Small, dense LDL also occurs in familial combined hyperlipidemia.[161] Although insulin-resistance syndrome has not yet been directly linked to CHD risk, many of its components are CHD risk factors. The syndrome may help explain the occurrence of CHD in the absence of hypercholesterolemia. Also, findings from the primary prevention

Helsinki Heart Study and the observational Prospective Cardiovascular Muenster (PROCAM) study have linked the conjunction of elevated triglyceride, low HDL cholesterol, and elevated total or LDL cholesterol with very high risk for CHD.[23,162] In the PROCAM study, even though the profile of a high LDL/HDL ratio (>5) plus elevated triglyceride (>200 mg/dL) fit only 4.3 percent of the men studied, it was present in one-fourth of the CHD events during 6-year follow-up.[162]

FREDRICKSON PHENOTYPING

Assigning a Fredrickson phenotype (Table 53-10) according to whether LDL and/or triglyceride-rich lipoproteins are elevated may be useful in characterizing the dyslipidemia, although the Fredrickson classification[163] is not an etiologic classification and does not differentiate primary and secondary hyperlipidemias. In most instances, the standard lipoprotein profile will be sufficient to determine the Fredrickson phenotype. However, elevations of both total cholesterol and triglyceride (the latter exceeding 300 mg/dL) can make the assessment more complicated. Marked hypertriglyceridemia in association with elevated total cholesterol (in an approximately 10:1 triglyceride-to-cholesterol ratio) may be due to VLDL and chylomicron accumulations (type V), which can be detected by one of two methods. Serum stored overnight at 4°C will have a white floating layer (chylomicrons) over a cloudy supernatant (VLDL). Serum lipoprotein electrophoresis will also detect the two lipoproteins. Elevations of cholesterol and triglyceride in fairly equal proportion can be due to increased LDL and VLDL (type IIb) or to the presence of IDL (type III). Again, serum lipoprotein electrophoresis is very helpful in separating these phenotypes; the broad-beta

---

TABLE 53-10

FREDRICKSON CLASSIFICATION OF THE HYPERLIPIDEMIAS

Phenotype	Lipoprotein(s) Elevated	Serum Cholesterol Concentration	Serum Triglyceride Concentration	Atherogenicity	Relative Frequency, %[a]
I	Chylomicrons	Normal to ↑	↑↑↑↑	None seen	<1
IIa	LDL	↑↑	Normal	+ + +	10
IIb	LDL and VLDL	↑↑	↑↑	+ + +	40
III	IDL	↑↑	↑↑↑↑	+ + +	<1
IV	VLDL	Normal to ↑	↑↑	+	45
V	VLDL and chylomicrons	↑ to ↑↑	↑↑↑↑	+	5

[a] Approximate percentages of U.S. patients with hyperlipidemia.

Abbreviations: IDL = intermediate-density lipoprotein; LDL = low-density lipoprotein; VLDL = very low density lipoprotein.

Note: The Fredrickson classification of hyperlipidemias is based on the serum lipoprotein patterns associated with elevated concentrations of cholesterol and/or triglyceride and disregards high-density lipoprotein (HDL) cholesterol concentration. It relies on separation of lipoproteins by electrophoresis and/or ultracentrifugation combined with precipitation. The Fredrickson classification is not an etiologic classification of disease and does not differentiate primary and secondary hyperlipidemias, but it has been useful in characterizing lipoprotein abnormalities. Establishing the lipoprotein phenotype present does not substitute for making a diagnosis of the underlying cause.

Source: From Gotto AM Jr, Assmann G, Carmena R, Davignon J, Fernández-Cruz A, Paoletti R. *The ILIB Lipid Handbook for Clinical Practice: Blood Lipids and Coronary Heart Disease.* Houston: International Lipid Information Bureau; 1995. Used with permission.

band represents IDL (Table 53-1). Specialized laboratories may also use ultracentrifugation for lipoprotein analysis, particularly for the accurate determination of LDL cholesterol, as noted above.

Secondary Dyslipidemia

Beyond lifestyle factors, common causes of secondary dyslipidemia include diabetes mellitus, nephrotic syndrome, chronic renal failure, and hypothyroidism, as well as some pharmacologic therapies. Selected causes of hypercholesterolemia and hypertriglyceridemia are shown in Table 53-11. Decreased HDL cholesterol may be related to obesity, a sedentary lifestyle, hypertriglyceridemia, impaired glucose tolerance, or the use of certain drugs (including isotretinoin, progestins, testosterone, anabolic steroids, and beta blockers without intrinsic sympathomimetic activity). Treatment of the underlying cause of dyslipidemia will often normalize lipid concentrations. When it does not, the dyslipidemia is treated like a primary lipid disorder.

Primary Dyslipidemia

Most cases of dyslipidemia are multifactorial in origin. Various genetic disorders impart a predisposition to dyslipidemia[4–6,51,164–173]; chief examples are shown in Table 53-12. The familial disorders most often encountered in clinical practice are familial combined hyperlipidemia (FCH), polygenic hypercholesterolemia, familial hypercholesterolemia (FH), and type III hyperlipidemia. As noted above, it is important during the physical examination to search for manifestations of dyslipidemia and of atherosclerosis. Family testing is essential to the diagnosis of familial disorders, and evaluation for genetic abnormalities through specialized laboratory methods may be useful in family counseling. Severe or complicated dyslipidemia may require referral to a lipid specialist. As seen in Table 53-12, not all genetic dyslipidemias are associated with increased risk for CHD, although others lead to severe, widespread atherosclerosis at very early ages.

TREATMENT OF
DYSLIPIDEMIA IN ADULTS

Dietary Influences on Lipoprotein Metabolism

The composition of the diet has multiple effects on lipoprotein metabolism. Indeed, according to some authorities, the typical American diet is a major cause of lipoprotein disorders leading to premature CHD. The actions of the diet on lipoprotein metabolism are complex, and they are modified by an individual's overall nutritional status. The nutritional status is most importantly determined by the content of body fat and the state of physical fitness. Thus, a discussion of dietary effects on lipoprotein metabolism is not complete without considering the influence of body weight and exercise. The most important dietary factors affecting the metabolism of lipoproteins are

TABLE 53-11

SELECTED CAUSES OF SECONDARY HYPERLIPIDEMIA

Related to serum cholesterol elevation
  Diet rich in saturated fatty acids
  Hypothyroidism
  Nephrotic syndrome
  Chronic liver disease (mainly primary biliary cirrhosis)
  Cholestasis
  Dysglobulinemia
  Cushing's syndrome
  Oral contraceptives
  Anorexia nervosa
  Acute intermittent porphyria
Related to serum triglyceride elevation
  Diet rich in carbohydrates
  Excessive alcohol consumption[a]
  Obesity
  Pregnancy
  Diabetes mellitus
  Hypothyroidism
  Chronic renal failure
  Pancreatitis
  Bulimia
  Cushing's syndrome
  Hypopituitarism
  Dysglobulinemia
  Glycogen storage disease
  Lipodystrophy
  Acute intermittent porphyria
  Systemic lupus erythematosus
  Diuretic use
  Selected beta-blocker use
  Estrogen use (contraceptive or replacement)
  Glucocorticoid use
  Isotretinoin use

[a] More than 30 g/day ethanol would be considered excessive; 30 g is the amount of alcohol contained in about two drinks, where one drink = 150 mL natural (nonfortified) wine, 360 mL beer, or 45 mL 80-proof liquor, i.e., 5 U.S. fl oz natural wine, 12 U.S. fl oz beer, or 1.5 U.S. fl oz 80-proof liquor.

Source: From Gotto AM Jr, Assmann G, Carmena R, Davignon J, Fernández-Cruz A, Paoletti R. *The ILIB Lipid Handbook for Clinical Practice: Blood Lipids and Coronary Heart Disease.* Houston: International Lipid Information Bureau; 1995. Used with permission.

fat and cholesterol. Other dietary factors, however, such as carbohydrate, also play a role. In the discussion to follow, the effects of each of the major dietary factors are considered. For a more detailed discussion of the dietary factors, see the NCEP adult treatment guidelines.[6] Dietary trials have been well reviewed by Willett.[174]

DIETARY CHOLESTEROL

High intake of dietary cholesterol definitely raises LDL cholesterol concentrations in many humans. Therefore, intake must be kept relatively low. The three major sources of dietary cholesterol are egg yolks, animal fat, and meat. The primary targets for intake reduction should be egg yolk and animal

TABLE 53-12

SELECTED PRIMARY DYSLIPIDEMIAS

Disorder[a]	Fredrickson Phenotype(s)	Transmission and Mechanism	Estimated U.S. Prevalence	Major Clinical Findings	Treatment Principles
Familial chylomicronemia	I	Autosomal recessive; lipoprotein lipase or apo C-II deficiency	Rare	Usually diagnosed in childhood by recurrent abdominal pain and pancreatitis. Lipemia retinalis, eruptive xanthomas, hepatosplenomegaly, and occasionally peripheral neuropathy and reversible mental changes may occur. Heterozygotes: Normal TG or mild HTG in absence of other conditions associated with HTG. Homozygotes: Fasting TG may exceed 1000. Not believed to increase CHD risk.	Diet low in simple carbohydrates and fat (<10% of total energy intake as fat), avoidance of alcohol, weight control; intake of medium-chain TG helpful; drug therapy usually not helpful.
Heterozygous familial hypercholesterolemia (FH)	IIa (IIb rare)	Autosomal dominant; LDL-receptor defect	1/500	TC elevated at birth, eventually reaches 350–500. Tendon xanthomas, corneal arcus, and premature atherosclerosis are typical.	Diet + drug therapy (usually combination resins and statins); LDL apheresis in severe cases.
Homozygous familial hypercholesterolemia (FH)	IIa (IIb rare)	Autosomal dominant; LDL-receptor defect	$1/10^6$	TC elevated at birth; TC reaches 700–1200; cutaneous xanthomas, tendon xanthomas; corneal arcus; severe, widespread early atherosclerosis, including aortic stenosis.	Resistant to diet and most drug therapy (probucol may be used since it can achieve regression of xanthomas); additional therapies such as LDL apheresis, liver transplantation.
Familial defective apo B-100	IIa	Autosomal dominant; apo B mutation	Prevalence varies by ethnicity; rare to 1/600	Lipoprotein values and clinical features can be similar to heterozygous FH; in some cases, may be more moderate; definitive diagnosis by molecular analysis.	Treat as in heterozygous FH; diet + statin and/or resin.
Polygenic hypercholesterolemia	IIa	Mode of transmission unknown; various genetic defects	High, ~1/20	TC elevation generally less than in heterozygous FH, xanthomas are very rare; when elevated HDL-C ruled out, as many as 80% of patients with isolated hypercholesterolemia have polygenic hypercholesterolemia.	Dependent on LDL-C value, gender, age, and CHD status. Severe cases treated as in heterozygous FH (combination-drug therapy may not be necessary).
Familial combined hyperlipidemia (FCH)	IIa, IIb, IV	Unknown if monogenic or polygenic; mechanism unknown; is associated with overproduction of apo B and with serum hyperapo-betalipoproteinemia (hyper–apo B)	~1/100	Elevated TC or TG (or both) in patient and family members. When TC elevated, typically 250–350; when TG elevated, two-thirds of patients have mild to moderate HTG, but elevation may be severe; no unique clinical features; may or may not be expressed in childhood.	Follow standard clinical guidelines for hypercholesterolemia, HTG, or combined hyperlipidemia.

(continued)

TABLE 53-12

SELECTED PRIMARY DYSLIPIDEMIAS (Continued)

Disorder[a]	Fredrickson Phenotype(s)	Transmission and Mechanism	Estimated U.S. Prevalence	Major Clinical Findings	Treatment Principles
Type III hyperlipidemia (familial dysbetalipoproteinemia[b])	III	Usually mimics autosomal recessive mode; an apo E–linked metabolic defect (E2/2 phenotype), usually requiring other metabolic factors for full expression (1% of the general population is homozygous for E2)	1/5000	Typically, TC 300–600, TG 400–800 (TG may be much higher); palmar xanthomas, tuberoeruptive xanthomas may occur; disorder is exacerbated by diabetes mellitus, other disorders; not commonly expressed in childhood; specialized lab can provide definitive diagnosis (apo E isoform); premature CHD, PVD, and stroke.	Diet low in saturated fat, weight control; drug therapy to reduce remnant lipoproteins—fibrates are first-choice drugs; niacin may be considered if diabetes mellitus or prediabetic condition is absent.
Familial endogenous hypertriglyceridemia (FHTG; type IV hyperlipidemia) and familial mixed hypertriglyceridemia (type V hyperlipidemia)	IV, V	Often dominant; mechanism not established	Phenotype IV ~1/300; phenotype V rare	Typically, TG 200–500 in phenotype IV, TG >1000 in phenotype V; uncommonly, "pure" type IV (no chylomicrons) with TG >1000. HDL-C usually decreased; early CHD in some families but not in others. FHTG (type IV hyperlipidemia) is often associated with a modest chylomicronemia, giving a type V pattern in which the VLDL fraction remains predominant; to be distinguished from severe chylomicronemia associated with elevated VLDL (type V hyperlipidemia), a separate entity although probably heterogeneous in origin.	Follow standard clinical guidelines for HTG.
Familial low HDL-C (hypoalphalipoproteinemia)		Usually dominant; molecular basis elucidated for some, but etiology unclear in others	Very rare	*Familial low HDL-C* is an interim term; marked differences in association with premature CHD. Clinical differences include HDL deficiencies with corneal opacities; xanthomatosis; tonsil anomalies, neuropathy, and hepatosplenomegaly; amyloidosis.	Heterogeneous group; refer to lipid specialist.

[a] All hyperlipidemias except familial chylomicronemia are associated with increased risk for CHD (variable in familial HTG). (See also Table 53-10.) Only some of the familial low-HDL-C syndromes described thus far by investigators have been associated with increased risk for atherosclerosis.

[b] Dysbetalipoproteinemia indicates the presence of remnants of chylomicrons and VLDL.

Abbreviations: apo = apolipoprotein; CHD = coronary heart disease; HDL-C = high-density lipoprotein cholesterol; HTG = hypertriglyceridemia; LDL-C = low-density lipoprotein cholesterol; PVD = peripheral vascular disease; TC = total cholesterol; TG = triglyceride; VLDL = very low density lipoprotein.

Note: All lipid values are mg/dL.

Source: From Gotto AM Jr, Assmann G, Carmena R, Davignon J, Fernández-Cruz A, Paoletti R. *The ILIB Lipid Handbook for Clinical Practice: Blood Lipids and Coronary Heart Disease.* Houston: International Lipid Information Bureau; 1995. Used with permission.

fat. If these foods are curtailed, the cholesterol remaining in the flesh of meat usually will not be excessive.

DIETARY FAT

Saturated Fatty Acids

Saturated fatty acids are the major cholesterol-raising fatty acids. Among these, only stearic acid does not raise cholesterol concentrations. The predominant saturated fatty acid is palmitic acid. Most saturated fatty acids come from animal fats (including butterfat). Another source consists of tropical oils (palm oil, coconut oil, and palm kernel oil). Currently, the American diet contains about 12 percent of total calories in the form of saturated fatty acids. This percentage could be reduced one-third to one-half by decreasing intake of animal fats (including butterfat). This can be achieved in large measure by substituting low-fat meat and dairy products for high-fat counterparts currently consumed.

Trans Fatty Acids

Trans fatty acids are produced when vegetable oils are hydrogenated. Currently, about 3 percent of total calories in the American diet come from *trans* fatty acids. Recent studies indicate that they raise LDL cholesterol concentrations to about the same degree as saturated fatty acids. An effort, therefore, should be made to reduce intake of *trans* fatty acids along with saturated fatty acids. The best way to achieve this aim is for the food industry to substitute other types of fats for *trans* fatty acids in food items.

Monounsaturated Fatty Acids

Monounsaturated fatty acids consist mainly of oleic acid, which occurs in both animal fats and plant oils. Animals synthesize oleic acid and incorporate it into triglyceride. Plant oils rich in oleic acid include olive and canola oils. Monounsaturated fatty acids are *neutral* with respect to lipoproteins. They neither raise nor lower concentrations of LDL, HDL, or triglyceride. High intakes of oleic acid appear to be safe. Large amounts are consumed in the traditional Mediterranean diet in the form of olive oil; in the Mediterranean region, rates of both CHD and cancer are relatively low.[175,176]

Polyunsaturated Fatty Acids

Polyunsaturated fatty acids are of two types: omega-6 and omega-3. The former consists largely of linoleic acid, which is present in many vegetable oils. Linoleic acid appears to slightly reduce serum concentrations of LDL, HDL, and triglyceride relative to oleic acid; the degree of reduction, however, is small. Linoleic acid currently contributes about 7 percent of total calories to the American diet. Higher intake is not recommended because of lack of epidemiologic data to support the safety of a higher intake. Moreover, linoleic acid can promote carcinogenesis in some animals and is prone to free radical oxidation in the body.

The omega-3 fatty acids are very long chain polyunsaturates. They are found mostly in fish oils. Relatively large intakes of omega-3 fatty acids reduce triglyceride concentrations and interfere with platelet aggregation. Very small amounts of omega-3 fatty acids may be necessary for normal vision and neurologic function.

DIETARY CARBOHYDRATE

The carbohydrate of the diet consists of sugars and starches. When consumed in large amounts, they, too, can affect lipoprotein metabolism. Like monounsaturates, carbohydrate is *neutral* with respect to LDL cholesterol concentration. However, compared with monounsaturated fatty acids, carbohydrate raises serum triglyceride and reduces HDL cholesterol. The effects of carbohydrate are the same whether in the form of sugars or starches.

EXCESS CALORIES

Consumption of excess calories leading to obesity has several adverse effects on lipoprotein metabolism. Obesity is frequently accompanied by elevations in both serum triglyceride and cholesterol and a reduction in HDL cholesterol. The increasing prevalence of obesity in the United States makes excess caloric intake a major cause of dyslipidemia in this country.

Lifestyle Intervention

The purpose of dietary intervention is to reduce CHD risk by limiting dietary fat, particularly saturated fat, and cholesterol while maintaining a nutritious diet and a suitable calorie level. As noted above, if the patient is obese, weight reduction is an essential element of dietary intervention, and an indispensable part of achieving a proper body weight is exercise. Although LDL cholesterol is the key target of therapy in the ATP II guidelines, weight reduction and exercise also increase HDL cholesterol and reduce serum triglyceride, blood pressure, and risk for diabetes mellitus, thereby improving the patient's total risk status. There are physical activity guidelines that aid the physician in prescribing a safe and appropriate exercise program (Table 53-13).

The NCEP uses a two-step cholesterol-lowering diet (Table 53-14). If at the time of evaluation the patient has been adhering to the Step I Diet (which is the diet recommended for the general population aged 2 years and older) or if the diet proves insufficient to achieve the cholesterol goal, the patient should proceed to the Step II Diet. Also, the Step II Diet is initial dietary therapy in secondary prevention. It more rigorously limits intake of saturated fat and cholesterol but otherwise is identical to Step I. It may require a substantial modification of food choices; the advice of a registered dietitian is valuable in tailoring a diet that avoids less obvious sources of fat and maximizes patient compliance. The goal of lifestyle changes is to bring LDL cholesterol below the NCEP initiation cutpoint—that is, <160 mg/dL for patients without CHD and with fewer than two other risk factors, <130 mg/dL for patients without CHD and with other risk, and ≤100 mg/dL for patients with CHD or other atherosclerotic disease.[6]

TABLE 53-13

AMERICAN HEART ASSOCIATION PHYSICAL ACTIVITY CLASSIFICATIONS[a]

Class A

Definition	Apparently healthy individuals. No evidence of increased CVD risk with exercise.
Individuals included	(1) <40 years with no symptoms or known presence of CHD or major CHD risk factors; (2) any age with no symptoms or known presence of CHD or major CHD risk factors and with normal exercise test.
Activity guidelines	No restrictions other than basic guidelines: (1) Exercise only when feeling well. (2) Do not exercise vigorously soon after eating. (3) Adjust exercise to the weather. (4) Slow down for hills. (5) Wear proper clothing and shoes. (6) Understand personal limitations. (7) Select appropriate exercises. (8) Be alert for symptoms such as discomfort in the upper body, faintness, shortness of breath, and discomfort in bones and joints. (9) Watch for signs of overexercising: inability to finish, inability to converse during the activity, faintness or nausea after exercise, chronic fatigue, sleeplessness, or aches and pains in the joints. (10) Start slowly and progress gradually.
ECG and blood pressure monitoring	Not required.
Supervision required	None.

Class B

Definition	Known, stable CVD with low risk from vigorous exercise but slightly greater risk than in class A. Moderate activity not believed to be associated with increased risk.
Individuals included	(1) CHD (MI, CABG, PTCA, angina pectoris, abnormal exercise test, abnormal coronary angiograms), stable condition, clinical characteristics outlined next; (2) valvular heart disease; (3) congenital heart disease; (4) cardiomyopathy; (5) exercise test abnormalities that do not meet criteria outlined in class C.
Clinical characteristics	(1) New York Heart Association class 1 or 2; (2) exercise capacity >6 METs; (3) no evidence of heart failure; (4) free of ischemia or angina at rest or on the exercise test ≤6 METs; (5) appropriate rise in systolic blood pressure during exercise; (6) no sequential ectopic ventricular contractions; (7) satisfactory ability to self-monitor intensity of activity.
Activity guidelines	Activity individualized with exercise prescription by qualified personnel trained in basic cardiopulmonary resuscitation or with electronic monitoring at home.
ECG and blood pressure monitoring	Only during the early prescription phase of training, usually 6–12 sessions.
Supervision required	Medical supervision during prescription sessions and nonmedical supervision for other exercise sessions until the individual understands how to monitor activity.

Class C

Definition	Moderate to high risk for cardiac complications of exercise and/or unable to self-regulate activity or to understand recommended activity level.
Individuals included	(1) CHD with clinical characteristics outlined next; (2) cardiomyopathy; (3) valvular heart disease; (4) exercise test abnormalities not directly related to ischemia; (5) previous episode of ventricular fibrillation or cardiac arrest that did not occur in the presence of an acute ischemic event or cardiac procedure; (6) complex ventricular arrhythmias that are uncontrolled at mild or moderate work intensities with medication; (7) three-vessel disease or left main disease; (8) low ejection fraction (<30%).
Clinical characteristics	(1) ≥2 MIs; (2) New York Heart Association class 3 or greater; (3) exercise capacity <6 METs; (4) ischemic horizontal or downsloping ST depression ≥4 mm or angina during exercise; (5) fall in systolic blood pressure with exercise; (6) a medical problem that the physician believes may be life-threatening; (7) previous episode of primary cardiac arrest; (8) ventricular tachycardia at workload <6 METs.
Activity guidelines	Activity should be individualized with exercise prescription by qualified personnel.
ECG and blood pressure monitoring	Continuous during exercise until safety is established, usually in 6–12 sessions or more.
Supervision required	Medical supervision during all exercise sessions until safety is established.

(continued)

TABLE 53-13

AMERICAN HEART ASSOCIATION PHYSICAL ACTIVITY CLASSIFICATIONS*a* (Continued)

Class D	
Definition	Unstable disease with activity restriction
Individuals included	(1) Unstable ischemia; (2) heart failure that is not compensated; (3) uncontrolled arrhythmias; (4) severe and symptomatic aortic stenosis; (5) other conditions that could be aggravated by exercise.
Activity guidelines	*No activity is recommended for conditioning purposes.* Attention should be directed to treating the patient and restoring him or her to status of class C or higher. Daily activities must be prescribed on the basis of individual assessment by the patient's personal physician.

a Classifications do not consider accompanying morbidities—such as type 1 diabetes mellitus, morbid obesity, severe pulmonary disease, or debilitating neurologic or orthopedic conditions—that may necessitate closer supervision during training sessions.

Abbreviations: CABG = coronary artery bypass grafting; CHD = coronary heart disease; CVD = cardiovascular disease; ECG = electrocardiography; MET = metabolic equivalent (3.5 mL/kg/min oxygen uptake); MI = myocardial infarction; PTCA = percutaneous transluminal coronary angioplasty.

Note: For minimum conditioning, leisure-time activity should consume a minimum of 700 kcal/week; the activity should be performed on 3 or more nonconsecutive days. Incremental benefits appear to accrue up to 2000 kcal/week (20 miles of walking or jogging). Walking appears to be as beneficial as more vigorous activities. It appears that some benefit is obtained from as little as 20 min of low-intensity exercise performed three times per week. Regular physical activity is beneficial in the presence of CVD if prudent guidelines are followed. More research is needed in women.

Source: From Gotto AM Jr, Assmann G, Carmena R, Davignon J, Fernández-Cruz A, Paoletti R. *The ILIB Lipid Handbook for Clinical Practice: Blood Lipids and Coronary Heart Disease.* Houston: International Lipid Information Bureau; 1995. Based on data from Fletcher et al.[96] Used with permission.

Generally, dietary intervention must be allowed ample time to be effective before any pharmacologic measures are taken. Serum cholesterol should be determined and patient compliance assessed 4 to 6 weeks and 3 months after lifestyle changes are initiated. In most cases, up to 6 months of lifestyle changes is required to evaluate the program's effectiveness; however, patients with severe elevations of LDL cholesterol (≥220 mg/dL) or otherwise at very high risk because of the presence of atherosclerotic disease, diabetes mellitus, or a strong family history of premature CHD may be considered for initial concurrent drug therapy and lifestyle changes. It has recently been recommended that drug therapy not be delayed in patients with CHD, as is discussed below under "Drug Therapy."

Some researchers have argued that dietary intervention can achieve LDL lowering and beneficial arteriographic changes comparable to drug therapy if more intensive lifestyle changes are undertaken than those represented by the Step I or Step II Diet—for example, a very low fat vegetarian diet, a regular exercise program, plus measures designed to promote psychological

health.[28,177] Nevertheless, dietary modification of this degree may pose nutritional hazards for some patients, particularly if professional instruction is insufficient. Also, cholesterol-lowering trials have shown that intensive dietary counseling

TABLE 53-14

DIETARY THERAPY OF ELEVATED BLOOD CHOLESTEROL

Nutrient*a*	Recommended Intake		
	Step I Diet (Primary Prevention*b*)		Step II Diet (Primary or Secondary Prevention*c*)
Total fat		≤30% of total calories	
Saturated fatty acids	8–10% of total calories		<7% of total calories
Polyunsaturated fatty acids		≤10% of total calories	
Monounsaturated fatty acids		≤15% of total calories	
Carbohydrates		≥55% of total calories	
Protein		Approx. 15% of total calories	
Cholesterol	<300 mg/day		<200 mg/day
Total calories		To achieve and maintain desirable weight*d*	

a Calories from alcohol not included.

b The Step I Diet is recommended for the general population (aged 2 years and older).

c The Step II Diet is initial dietary intervention in patients with atherosclerotic disease; it may be initial dietary intervention in primary prevention if the patient has already been adhering to a diet equivalent to the Step I Diet.

d In children and adolescents, sufficient calories to promote normal growth and development and to reach or maintain desirable weight.

Note: The American Heart Association Step I and II Diets are identical to the NCEP Step I and II Diets.

Source: Data from the National Cholesterol Education Program.[6]

consistent with the Step II Diet can halt the progression of CHD and decrease the CHD event rate.[177,178]

Other researchers have suggested that diet is of limited benefit because of the relatively low percentage reductions in cholesterol achieved (about 10 percent in LDL, on average), and that drug therapy should be implemented sooner in patients at high risk. The efficacy of diet varies widely: some patients have dramatic benefit, whereas others do not respond at all.[178]

Drugs Affecting Lipoprotein Metabolism

Four classes of lipid-lowering drugs are currently available in the United States for the treatment of hyperlipidemia[179–185]: HMG-CoA reductase inhibitors (statins), bile-acid sequestrants (resins), nicotinic acid (niacin), and fibric-acid derivatives (fibrates). Each class of drug has unique effects on lipoprotein metabolism. The available lipid-lowering drugs and their usual dosages and side effects are shown in Table 53-15. Their major actions on lipid and lipoprotein metabolism are briefly reviewed next. In addition, oral estrogen-replacement therapy may be considered to improve the lipid profile in postmenopausal women, although it does not yet have a U.S. Food and Drug Administration indication for lipid lowering or CHD risk reduction.

HMG-CoA REDUCTASE INHIBITORS (STATINS)
The statins achieve the greatest LDL lowering of available hypolipidemic drugs.[186–189] Currently available statins are fluvastatin (Lescol),[39,190,191] lovastatin (Mevacor),[17,29,30,33,34,40,192,193] pravastatin (Pravachol),[11,18,25,37,38,41,194] simvastatin (Zocor),[9,10,36,195] and atorvastatin (Lipitor).[196–198] The primary action of these drugs is to inhibit HMG-CoA reductase, the rate-limiting enzyme in the biosynthesis of cholesterol. Because of their high first-pass clearance by the liver, their primary site of action is in the liver. Inhibition of hepatic cholesterol synthesis upregulates the synthesis of LDL receptors. The availability of more LDL receptors on the surface of liver cells reduces circulating concentrations of LDL cholesterol. The decrease in serum LDL cholesterol concentrations results in part from increased hepatic uptake of LDL and in part from removal of VLDL remnants, which are precursors of LDL. VLDL remnants, like LDL, are recognized by LDL receptors.

Reductions of LDL concentrations progressively increase with increasing doses of statins. However, dose–response is curvilinear. The greatest increments in LDL lowering occur at lower doses; increments become smaller with progressively higher doses. The dose–response also varies according to statin. Available data indicate that lovastatin and pravastatin produce similar responses. The same dose of fluvastatin yields about half the response; in contrast, simvastatin evokes about twice the response. However, these relative responses must be considered on the background of the curvilinear response for each statin. Thus, the relative dose–responses, are not simple multiples for all comparisons at all doses. Early published data have shown atorvastatin to lower LDL with greater potency than the other currently available statins.

BILE-ACID SEQUESTRANTS (RESINS)
The bile-acid resins[199] bind bile acids in the intestinal tract. Available drugs are cholestyramine[19,20,26,32] and colestipol.[27,29–31] Removal of bile acids from the intestine stimulates the conversion of cholesterol into bile acids in the liver, decreasing hepatic cholesterol content. Although there is a compensatory increase in cholesterol synthesis, the decrease in hepatic cholesterol is sufficient to evoke an increase in LDL receptor activity. Consequently, LDL cholesterol concentrations decline. Dose–response to sequestrants is curvilinear. This fact makes it possible to achieve significant LDL cholesterol reductions with relatively low dosages of sequestrants. The advantage of low-dose seques-

---

TABLE 53-15

DRUGS AFFECTING LIPOPROTEIN METABOLISM

Category	Drugs	Daily Dose Range	Side Effects
HMG-CoA reductase inhibitors (statins)	Atorvastatin	10–80 mg	Liver function changes, myopathy, skin rash, GI disturbance
	Fluvastatin	20–40 mg	
	Lovastatin	10–80 mg	
	Pravastatin	10–40 mg	
	Simvastatin	10–40 mg	
Bile-acid sequestrants (resins)	Cholestyramine	8–24 g	Constipation, GI distress, drug malabsorption
	Colestipol	10–30 g	
Nicotinic acid (niacin)		1.5–4.5 g	GI distress, liver function abnormalities, glucose intolerance, hyperuricemia, flushing/itching, skin rash
Fibric-acid derivatives (fibrates)	Clofibrate	2.0 g	GI distress, liver function abnormalities (transient), gallstones, myopathy
	Gemfibrozil	1.2 g	
	(Bezafibrate)		
	(Fenofibrate)		

Abbreviation: GI = gastrointestinal.

trants is that they are tolerated by most patients; at moderate to high resin doses, many patients experience gastrointestinal side effects.

NICOTINIC ACID (NIACIN)

The primary mechanism of action for lipid lowering by nicotinic acid[21,24,27,29–31,200–203] is not known. In very small amounts, nicotinic acid serves as a vitamin. At much higher doses, it evokes multiple changes in lipoprotein metabolism, probably from the drug's action in the liver. Lipid effects include a lowering of serum triglyceride, a reduction of LDL cholesterol, and a raising of HDL cholesterol. Nicotinic acid is the best available drug for raising HDL cholesterol. Its action to lower LDL cholesterol is most pronounced in patients with hypercholesterolemia; patients who have lower LDL cholesterol exhibit less lowering. Both lipid responses and side effects are proportional to dosage. Thus, patients who cannot tolerate high dosages of nicotinic acid because of side effects such as flushing and gastrointestinal disturbances may derive some benefit in lipoprotein modification through use of low dosages. Sustained-release preparations of nicotinic acid should be used with caution because of increased risk for hepatotoxicity.[204]

FIBRIC-ACID DERIVATIVES (FIBRATES)

The fibrates[205–208] include clofibrate, gemfibrozil, fenofibrate, and bezafibrate. Only clofibrate[24] and gemfibrozil (Lopid)[22,23] are available in the United States. The primary action of fibrates is to lower triglyceride concentrations, apparently as a result of enhancement of activity of lipoprotein lipase (LPL). Fibrates are largely ineffective in patients who have an absence of LPL. Triglyceride lowering is often accompanied by a modest increase in HDL cholesterol. In patients without hypertriglyceridemia, variable reductions of LDL cholesterol may occur; however, triglyceride lowering in hypertriglyceridemic patients may result in an *increase* in LDL cholesterol. Whether fibrates have other metabolic effects besides enhancing LPL activity is uncertain. The agents often increase secretion of cholesterol into bile, which can induce cholesterol gallstones. Other side effects include gastrointestinal distress and occasional myopathy. One clinical trial suggested that noncardiovascular mortality is increased with clofibrate therapy.[209–212] The nature of side effects responsible for increased deaths has never been defined, nor has this effect been observed in other clinical trials. Nonetheless, since fibrates are relatively poor LDL-lowering drugs, their use is largely limited to treatment of hypertriglyceridemia. They are particularly useful in patients with diabetes (see "Management of Dyslipidemia in Diabetes," below).

ESTROGEN-REPLACEMENT THERAPY

Many large observational epidemiologic studies have shown that postmenopausal oral estrogen-replacement therapy reduces risk for CHD.[213–216] The effect may be at least in part mediated by beneficial effects on the lipid profile, namely, modest reductions in LDL cholesterol and modest increases in HDL cholesterol.[214–217] Oral estrogens may significantly increase serum triglyceride, in particular if triglyceride is already elevated. The clinician may consider use of estrogen replacement for control of dyslipidemia in postmenopausal women; the decision must take into account menopausal symptoms and risks for CHD, osteoporosis, and cancer. Transcutaneously administered estrogens appear to have less effects on lipid concentrations. There is less information about the lipid or CHD effects of combined estrogen–progestin therapy than about estrogen alone, although it appears that the combination blocks some of the harmful lipid effects of progestin while allowing persistence of the beneficial effects of estrogen.[214,218]

Drug Therapy

Table 53-16 outlines a rational approach to drug therapy in patients at very high risk (secondary prevention). As noted above, the most effective agents for lowering LDL cholesterol are the statins. In many patients, LDL cholesterol concentrations fall to below 100 mg/dL with a statin alone. However, if the baseline LDL concentration is substantially elevated, enhanced LDL lowering comes from combining a bile-acid sequestrant with a statin. Even low dosages of bile-acid sequestrants markedly potentiate the action of statins. Pharmacotherapy is often needed in secondary prevention, and the trial of lifestyle interventions may be short.

Given the impressive results of the recent clinical trials of statins, the American Heart Association Task Force on Risk Reduction recently concluded that withholding lipid-lowering drug therapy from patients with CHD in an effort to reach target LDL cholesterol with lifestyle changes is not necessary when LDL exceeds 130 mg/dL, and recommends a 6-week trial of lifestyle therapy when LDL is between 100 and 130 mg/dL.[219] Other clinical experts recommend starting drug therapy as early as the time of hospital discharge after MI when LDL is 130 mg/dL or higher.[220]

A sizable proportion of patients with CHD have low HDL cholesterol. Some of these patients also manifest raised serum triglyceride. For low-HDL patients, the primary aim of therapy remains LDL lowering, and statins are the preferred agents. Treatment of other lipoprotein abnormalities, however, may yield enhanced risk reduction. The most effective drug for raising HDL cholesterol is nicotinic acid. This drug combined with a statin effectively lowers LDL and raises HDL. Since nicotinic acid commonly produces side effects, the lowest effective dosage should be employed, which is usually 1.5 g/day; slow titration of nicotinic acid from 100 mg to 1.5 g/d is recommended, and the response should be monitored at this dosage. If the response is insufficient, the dosage can be slowly titrated up to 3 g/day. If the patient has combined hyperlipidemia (elevated cholesterol and triglyceride), nicotinic acid remains the first choice in combination with a statin. If nicotinic acid is not tolerated, gemfibrozil may be combined

TABLE 53-16

LIPID-LOWERING DRUG THERAPY IN VERY HIGH RISK PREVENTION (SECONDARY PREVENTION)

	LDL Cholesterol Concentration, mg/dL		
	100–129	130–159	≥160
Treatment ⇒	Nondrug therapy ± statin	Nondrug therapy + statin	Nondrug therapy + statin ± sequestrant
	Concomitant Low HDL Cholesterol	Concomitant High Triglyceride	
Optional adjunctive therapy (combined with statin) ⇒	Nicotinic acid	Nicotinic acid or fibric-acid derivative[a]	

[a] There may be an increased risk for myopathy with fibrates combined with statins.
Abbreviations: HDL = high-density lipoprotein; LDL = low-density lipoprotein.

with a statin. Although this combination can be highly effective, there is an increase in risk for myopathy.[221] As a result, these drugs should be employed with the lowest effective dose of statin and should be given only to those individuals at highest risk for recurrent CHD events, such as known CHD patients. Careful monitoring for patient symptoms of myalgias and periodic creatine kinase (CK) measurements are recommended. Discontinuation of these drugs when an elevated CK is found or when myalgias are reported will result in clinical improvement.

In primary prevention in the NCEP guidelines, patients to be considered for drug therapy include those with LDL cholesterol ≥190 mg/dL and fewer than two other risk factors and those who have two other risk factors and LDL cholesterol ≥160 mg/dL (Table 53-8). Patients with less severe LDL cholesterol elevations but with other high risk (e.g., diabetes mellitus or a family history of premature CHD) may also be candidates. Various subgroups differ in the approach to high-risk primary prevention. According to the NCEP,[6] young adults whose LDL cholesterol concentrations range from 190 to 219 mg/dL without other risk factors need not receive drug therapy; long-term toxicity may occur and costs may be high. Some authorities, however, believe that such patients are candidates for bile-acid sequestrants. In young adults, LDL cholesterol concentrations ≥220 mg/dL after maximal nondrug management usually call for cholesterol-lowering drugs. There is growing support for including patients up to age 75 in high-risk primary prevention; in patients >75 years of age, introduction of cholesterol-lowering drugs should be carefully individualized. Finally, drug therapy should be used more readily in high-risk middle-aged men than in women of the same age because of higher absolute risk in men.

The NCEP goals of drug therapy (Table 53-8) are the same as those for dietary intervention, but even lower concentrations of LDL cholesterol are desirable for some patients if feasible.

Clinical judgment is necessary to determine the risk/benefit ratio of treatment options, especially in primary prevention.

Management of Hypertriglyceridemia

Lifestyle interventions are recommended for all individuals with elevated serum triglyceride, particularly weight control by reducing calories and fat in the diet and by exercising. Smoking cessation and restriction of alcohol intake are also urged. Triglyceride elevations are often secondary to a high-carbohydrate diet or a condition such as obesity, excessive alcohol intake, poorly controlled diabetes mellitus, chronic renal failure, nephrotic syndrome, or use of certain drugs such as beta-blocking agents, estrogens, and corticosteroids (Table 53-11). When triglyceride elevation is not severe, modification of underlying conditions should be attempted before any medical therapy is contemplated.

Drug therapy may be indicated for patients with elevated triglyceride (>200 mg/dL) if the patient has increased risk from factors such as established CHD, diabetes mellitus, concomitant high total cholesterol and low HDL cholesterol, or a familial hypertriglyceridemia associated with increased CHD risk, such as FCH or type III hyperlipidemia. As discussed above, reducing LDL cholesterol is again the primary goal of such therapy, although HDL cholesterol concentrations and triglyceride concentrations are secondary targets. Some authorities recommend lower action limits for serum triglyceride in diabetic patients[138]; elevated triglyceride and decreased HDL (with or without elevated LDL) constitute the typical dyslipidemia of diabetes mellitus and, as discussed earlier, are components of the described insulin-resistance syndrome, which combines a variety of CHD risk factors.[155–157]

High triglyceride concentrations (400 to 1000 mg/dL) are often labile, and these patients may quickly develop very high triglyceride, which greatly increases risk for acute pancreatitis, a condition that can cause considerable morbidity and occasional mortality. More aggressive therapy may be necessary in these individuals, particularly if there is a history of acute pancreatitis. Patients who already had very high triglyceride (>1000 mg/dL) should receive immediate triglyceride-lowering therapy to reduce risk for acute pancreatitis, including drug therapy if necessary and if effective drug therapy exists. Effective drug therapy is not available for chylomicronemia, although fish oil supplementation may be helpful. Fish oil supplementation is generally not recommended to lower risk for CHD because neither lowering of risk nor lack of undesirable effects has been clearly established.[6]

Management of Low HDL Cholesterol

While the NCEP adult treatment guidelines[6] incorporate HDL cholesterol as a major aspect of risk determination, they also note that, as for manipulations of triglyceride concentrations, there are not yet direct clinical data on the value of raising HDL cholesterol concentrations to prevent CHD. Isolated low HDL cholesterol concentrations are therefore not a target of drug therapy in primary prevention, although lifestyle changes should be undertaken. However, elevated LDL cholesterol concentrations may be targeted more aggressively if low HDL cholesterol (<35 mg/dL) is present as a risk factor, or a treatment that both lowers LDL cholesterol and raises HDL cholesterol may be selected. Drug therapy may be initiated in cases of isolated low HDL cholesterol if the patient has established CHD. Weight reduction, smoking cessation, and exercise are key to lifestyle management of low HDL cholesterol. Drug therapies that may cause low HDL (e.g., isotretinoin or progestins; see "Secondary Dyslipidemia," above) should be stopped if possible. Observational epidemiologic data show that each 1 mg/dL increase in HDL cholesterol yields a 2 to 3 percent decrease in CHD risk[61]; as noted in Table 53-12, the very rare familial HDL-deficiency disorders show marked differences in association with risk for premature CHD.[222]

Management of Dyslipidemia in Diabetes

Recommendations for the treatment of dyslipidemia in diabetic patients were developed from the 1993 American Diabetes Association (ADA) Consensus Development Conference on the Detection and Management of Lipid Disorders in Diabetes.[138] The physician may wish to consider these recommendations in addition to the NCEP guidelines.

The ADA consensus panel encourages annual performance of a full fasting lipoprotein analysis in all adult diabetics. When cholesterol is elevated, serum thyroid-stimulating hormone should be measured to rule out hypothyroidism. [Children with diabetes should be tested soon after diagnosis; those with any lipid abnormality (see "Management of Dyslipidemia in Children and Adolescents," below) should be reevaluated each year.]

Because the ADA consensus panel concluded that there is considerable evidence that increased triglyceride and reduced HDL cholesterol are intrinsically related to the abnormal physiology produced by insulin resistance or inadequate insulin action and concomitant metabolic disturbances, it defines triglyceride and HDL as independently defining action limits for lipid-lowering therapy. Triglyceride requires attention at 200 mg/dL in primary prevention and at 150 mg/dL in secondary prevention. HDL cholesterol requires attention at <35 mg/dL. If optimized glucose control, diet, exercise, weight control, alcohol control, and smoking cessation do not provide adequate lipid control, drug therapy should be considered if triglyceride remains >150 mg/dL in secondary prevention or ≥400 mg/dL in primary prevention (or ≥200 mg/dL if there is another major risk factor present). The recommendations regarding LDL action limits are in keeping with the NCEP algorithm's lower thresholds as risk rises; the ADA consensus is that lipid-lowering pharmacotherapy should be considered if LDL remains ≥160 mg/dL in primary prevention (or ≥130 mg/dL if there is another major risk factor present) or >100 mg/dL in secondary prevention (compare Table 53-8).

Controlling hyperglycemia may greatly improve abnormal lipid concentrations, particularly in type 1 diabetes mellitus. ADA consensus recommendations regarding total fat, saturated fat, cholesterol, and carbohydrate intake for lipid lowering are those set forth in the NCEP Step I and Step II Diets (Table 53-14), with recognition that choice of carbohydrate sources (i.e., complex carbohydrates) is crucial to glycemic control. Additional dietary modifications are restriction of alcohol and, in hypertensive patients, limitation of sodium to <2400 mg/day. Physical activity recommendations must take into account that many diabetic patients have a low level of fitness. In addition, patients must quit smoking.

The ADA consensus panel considers fibric-acid derivatives to be first-line drug monotherapy in diabetes. It notes that adding a low-dose bile-acid sequestrant may be effective when LDL cholesterol elevation persists. Sequestrants are not considered first-line pharmacotherapy because they can increase triglyceride. Also, they must be used with great care in the diabetic patient with gastrointestinal autonomic neuropathy because they may produce constipation or even fecal impaction. To the ADA recommendations should be added the notation that fibrates are to be used with caution (if at all) in the presence of diabetic nephropathy with renal insufficiency because of the risk of myopathy. Statins may be used to reduce elevated LDL cholesterol in diabetes. Although they have beneficial effects on triglyceride and HDL cholesterol, these effects may be marginal when both concentrations are abnormal. Statins may be used when diabetic nephropathy with renal insufficiency is present. Nicotinic acid is not recommended as first-line pharmacotherapy in diabetic patients because it increases insulin resistance and fasting and postprandial hyperglycemia and hyperinsulinemia. In diabetes, it is reserved for refractory dyslipidemia and used only with close monitoring; inability to maintain glycemic control mandates discontinuation.

MANAGEMENT OF DYSLIPIDEMIA IN CHILDREN AND ADOLESCENTS

Guidelines for the management of dyslipidemia in young people (aged 2 to 19 years) were issued by the NCEP Expert Panel on Blood Cholesterol Levels in Children and Adolescents.[45] Atherosclerosis begins in childhood, and hypercholesterolemic children and adolescents have been shown to be more likely than their peers in the general population to have cholesterol elevation as adults.[223]

The population approach, emphasizing diet and physical

activity, is the major emphasis in cholesterol control for the pediatric population. Screening is selective rather than universal. The panel's screening recommendations are especially directed toward physicians who care for adults, since they are the physicians who know the parents' risk status. It is recommended that total cholesterol be screened if a parent has total cholesterol ≥240 mg/dL. Full fasting lipoprotein analysis is performed if the pediatric patient has total cholesterol >200 mg/dL, total cholesterol averaging >170 mg/dL by two measurements, or a family history of early cardiovascular disease or a familial lipid disorder. The physician may also choose to determine lipid values if a family history is unobtainable, there is other known risk for CHD (e.g., diabetes, obesity, smoking, hypertension, or excess fat consumption), or the patient is taking a drug that can alter lipid concentrations (e.g., isotretinoin, steroids). Blood sampling may be performed any time after age 2 years; before then, more calories as fat are needed for growth. As in adults, lipid testing should be avoided if the patient is actively ill or has an infectious disease, since the values obtained may be misleading.

Total and LDL cholesterol cutpoints for pediatric patients are lower than in adults. Acceptable, borderline-high, and high values are defined at <170, 170 to 199, and ≥200 mg/dL for total cholesterol and <110, 110 to 129, and ≥130 mg/dL for LDL cholesterol. As in adults, HDL cholesterol is considered low if below 35 mg/dL. Triglyceride would be considered quite elevated if above 150 mg/dL or moderately elevated if above 120 mg/dL in a boy or 130 mg/dL in a girl. As in adults, cutpoints are to be interpreted in the context of total risk, and any intervention to lower serum cholesterol requires full clinical evaluation and establishment of LDL cholesterol elevation by at least two fasting determinations. The NCEP values apply expressly to children and adolescents from families with inherited cholesterol problems or premature cardiovascular disease.

Common causes of secondary dyslipidemia in young people are a diet high in saturated fat, overweight, and use of oral contraceptives, isotretinoin (retinoic acid), or anabolic steroids. The two most common genetic dyslipidemias expressed as LDL cholesterol elevation currently recognized in children are familial hypercholesterolemia (FH) and familial combined hyperlipidemia (FCH). Heterozygous FH has been estimated to be present in 1 of 25 children with LDL cholesterol >130 mg/dL[45]; hypercholesterolemia is detectable at birth in heterozygous FH. In the rare homozygous FH (Table 53-12), cutaneous xanthomas may develop within the first few months or years of life. In FCH, hyperlipidemia may or may not be expressed in childhood; FCH has been established to be about three times more common in children and adolescents than heterozygous FH.

Once causes of secondary dyslipidemia have been ruled out or treated, lifestyle therapy—including diet, exercise, and weight control—is the primary intervention (Table 53-17). The diets prescribed are those used in adults (Table 53-14); calorie levels are selected to support growth and development and to reach or maintain desirable body weight. Consultation with a dietitian may

---

TABLE 53-17

NATIONAL CHOLESTEROL EDUCATION PROGRAM: TREATMENT OF HYPERCHOLESTEROLEMIA IN CHILDREN AND ADOLESCENTS AGED 2–19 YEARS

LDL-C Level, mg/dL[a]	Action[b]
<110	*Counsel* on healthy diet and on risk factor reduction; repeat lipoprotein analysis within 5 years.
110–129	*Provide lipid-lowering diet (Step I Diet)* and other risk factor intervention; reevaluate status in 1 year.
≥130	*Perform full clinical evaluation* (family history, physical examination, laboratory tests); assess for causes of secondary dyslipidemia and for familial disorders. Some patients with familial disorders will require referral to a lipid specialist. Screen family members. *Initiate dietary therapy* and other risk reduction.
Refractory >190 *or* >160 + either positive family history of early CVD or ≥2 other persistent risk factors[c,d]	*Consider bile-acid resin to supplement diet in patients ≥10 years of age.* It is usual to provide folic acid supplementation with resins in these patients. Nicotinic acid may be used in a very limited number of pediatric patients, but only by a lipid specialist. Monitor at 6 weeks and then every 3 months by lipoprotein analysis; every 6 months to 1 year after LDL-C goal achieved.
<130, ideally <110	*LDL-C goal* of diet or diet + drug therapy.

[a] For intervention, established by the average of at least two consecutive fasting determinations.

[b] See Table 53-14 for lipid-lowering diet.

[c] Other risk factors for consideration are cigarette smoking, elevated blood pressure, high-density lipoprotein cholesterol <35 mg/dL, severe obesity, diabetes, and physical inactivity.

[d] The NCEP notes that cutpoints that minimize misclassification between pediatric patients with and without familial hypercholesterolemia are about 164 mg/dL for LDL cholesterol and 235 mg/dL for total cholesterol.

Abbreviations: CVD = cardiovascular disease; LDL-C = low-density lipoprotein cholesterol.

Source: From Gotto AM Jr, Assmann G, Carmena R, Davignon J, Fernández-Cruz A, Paoletti R. *The ILIB Lipid Handbook for Clinical Practice: Blood Lipids and Coronary Heart Disease.* Houston: International Lipid Information Bureau; 1995. Used with permission. Data from National Cholesterol Education Program.[45]

be needed to achieve compliance or to ensure adequate nutrition. Drug therapy may be considered in pediatric patients 10 years of age or older when LDL cholesterol concentrations remain very high despite vigorous diet, especially when multiple risk factors are present. Drug therapy may be warranted in younger patients when hyperlipidemia is severe (e.g., in a familial disorder). Familial chylomicronemia may entail risk for pancreatitis.

REFERENCES

1. American Heart Association. *1997 Heart and Stroke Statistical Update.* Dallas: American Heart Association; 1996.
2. Manson JE, Tosteson H, Ridker PM, Satterfield S, Hebert P, O'Connor GT, et al. The primary prevention of myocardial infarction (review). *N Engl J Med* 1992; 326:1406–1416.
3. Marmot M, Elliott P, eds. *Coronary Heart Disease Epidemiology: From Aetiology to Public Health.* Oxford, England: Oxford University Press; 1992.
4. Schaefer EJ, Genest JJ Jr, Ordovas JM, Salem DN, Wilson PWF. Familial lipoprotein disorders and premature coronary artery disease. *Atherosclerosis* 1994; 108:S41–S54.
5. Zannis VI, Kardassis D, Zanni EE. Genetic mutations affecting human lipoproteins, their receptors, and their enzymes. *Adv Hum Genet* 1993; 21:145–319.
6. National Cholesterol Education Program. Second report of the Expert Panel on Detection, Evaluation, and Treatment of High Blood Cholesterol in Adults (Adult Treatment Panel II). *Circulation* 1994; 89:1333–1445.
7. Levine GN, Keaney JF Jr, Vita JA. Cholesterol reduction in cardiovascular disease: Clinical benefits and possible mechanisms (review). *N Engl J Med* 1995; 332:512–521.
8. Law MR, Wald NJ, Thompson SG. By how much and how quickly does reduction in serum cholesterol concentration lower risk of ischaemic heart disease? *Br Med J* 1994; 308:367–373.
9. Scandinavian Simvastatin Survival Study Group. Randomised trial of cholesterol lowering in 4444 patients with coronary heart disease: The Scandinavian Simvastatin Survival Study (4S). *Lancet* 1994; 344:1383–1389.
10. Scandinavian Simvastatin Survival Study Group. Baseline serum cholesterol and treatment effect in the Scandinavian Simvastatin Survival Study (4S). *Lancet* 1995; 345:1274–1275.
11. Shepherd J, Cobbe SM, Ford I, Isles CG, Lorimer AR, MacFarlane PW, et al, for the West of Scotland Coronary Prevention Study Group. Prevention of coronary heart disease with pravastatin in men with hypercholesterolemia. *N Engl J Med* 1995; 333:1301–1307.
12. Gotto AM Jr. Lipid lowering, regression, and coronary events: A review of the Interdisciplinary Council on Lipids and Cardiovascular Risk Intervention, Seventh Council Meeting. *Circulation* 1995; 92:646–656.
13. Superko HR, Krauss RM. Coronary artery disease regression: Convincing evidence for the benefit of aggressive lipoprotein management. *Circulation* 1994; 90:1056–1069.
14. Blankenhorn DH, Hodis HN. Arterial imaging and atherosclerosis reversal: George Lyman Duff Memorial Lecture. *Arterioscler Thromb* 1994; 14:177–192.
15. Brown BG, Zhao X-Q, Sacco DE, Albers JJ. Lipid lowering and plaque regression: New insights into prevention of plaque disruption and clinical events in coronary disease. *Circulation* 1993; 87:1781–1791.
16. Vos J, de Feyter PJ, Simoons ML, Tijssen JGP, Deckers JW. Retardation and arrest of progression or regression of coronary artery disease: A review. *Prog Cardiovasc Dis* 1993; 35:435–454.
17. Furberg CD, Adams HP Jr, Applegate WB, Byington RP, Espeland MA, Hartwell T, et al. Effects of lovastatin on early carotid atherosclerosis and cardiovascular events. *Circulation* 1994; 90:1679–1688.
18. Crouse JR III, Byington RP, Bond MG, Espeland A, Craven TE, Sprinkle JW, et al. Pravastatin, Lipids, and Atherosclerosis in the Carotid Arteries (PLAC-II). *Am J Cardiol* 1995; 75:455–459.
19. Lipid Research Clinics Program. The Lipid Research Clinics Coronary Primary Prevention Trial results: I. Reduction in the incidence of coronary heart disease. *JAMA* 1984; 251:351–364.
20. Lipid Research Clinics Program. The Lipid Research Clinics Coronary Primary Prevention Trial results: II. The relationship of reduction in incidence of coronary heart disease to cholesterol lowering. *JAMA* 1984; 251:365–374.
21. Canner PL, Berge KG, Wenger NK, Stamler J, Friedman L, Prineas RJ, et al. Fifteen-year mortality in Coronary Drug Project patients: Long-term benefit with niacin. *J Am Coll Cardiol* 1986; 8:1245–1255.
22. Frick MH, Elo O, Haapa K, Heinonen OP, Heinsalmi P, Helo P, et al. Helsinki Heart Study: Primary prevention trial with gemfibrozil in middle-aged men with dyslipidemia. *N Engl J Med* 1987; 317:1237–1245.
23. Manninen V, Tenkanen L, Koskinen P, Huttunen JK, Mänttäri M, Heinonen OP, et al. Joint effects of serum triglyceride and LDL cholesterol and HDL cholesterol on coronary heart disease risk in the Helsinki Heart Study: Implications for treatment. *Circulation* 1992; 85:37–45.
24. Carlson LA, Rosenhamer G. Reduction of mortality in the Stockholm Ischaemic Heart Disease Secondary Prevention Study by combined treatment with clofibrate and nicotinic acid. *Acta Med Scand* 1988; 223:405–418.
25. Sacks FM, Pfeffer MA, Moye LA, Rouleau JL, Rutherford JD, Cole TG, et al, for the Cholesterol and Recurrent Events Trial Investigators. The effect of pravastatin on coronary events after myocardial infarction in patients with average cholesterol levels. *N Engl J Med* 1996; 335:1001–1009.
26. Brensike JF, Levy RI, Kelsey SF, Passamani ER, Richardson JM, Loh IK, et al. Effects of therapy with cholestyramine on progression of coronary arteriosclerosis: Results of the NHLBI Type II Coronary Intervention Study. *Circulation* 1984; 69:313–324.
27. Blankenhorn DH, Nessim SA, Johnson RL, Sanmarco ME, Azen SP, Cashin-Hemphill L. Beneficial effects of combined colestipol-niacin therapy on coronary atherosclerosis and coronary venous bypass grafts. *JAMA* 1987; 257:3233–3240. [Published erratum appears in *JAMA* 1988; 259:2698.]
28. Ornish D, Brown SE, Scherwitz LW, Billings JH, Armstrong WT, Ports TA, et al. Can lifestyle changes reverse coronary heart disease? The Lifestyle Heart Trial. *Lancet* 1990; 336:129–133.
29. Brown G, Albers JJ, Fisher LF, Schaefer SM, Lin J-T, Kaplan C, et al. Regression of coronary artery disease as a result of intensive lipid-lowering therapy in men with high levels of apolipoprotein B. *N Engl J Med* 1990; 323:1289–1298.
30. Kane JP, Malloy MJ, Ports TA, Phillips NR, Diehl JC, Havel RJ. Regression of coronary atherosclerosis during treatment of familial hypercholesterolemia with combined drug regimens. *JAMA* 1990; 264:3007–3012.
31. Cashin-Hemphill L, Mack WJ, Pogoda JM, Sanmarco ME, Azen SP, Blankenhorn DH. Beneficial effects of colestipol-niacin on coronary atherosclerosis: A 4-year follow-up. *JAMA* 1990; 264:3013–3016.
32. Watts GF, Lewis B, Brunt JNH, Lewis ES, Coltart DJ, Smith LDR, et al. Effects on coronary artery disease of lipid-lowering diet, or diet plus cholestyramine, in the St Thomas' Atherosclerosis Regression Study (STARS). *Lancet* 1992; 339:563–569.
33. Blankenhorn DH, Azen SP, Kramsch DM, Mack WJ, Cashin-Hemphill L, Hodis HN, et al. Coronary angiographic changes with lovastatin therapy: The Monitored Atherosclerosis Regression Study (MARS). *Ann Intern Med* 1993; 119:969–976.
34. Waters D, Higginson L, Gladstone P, Kimball B, Le May M, Bocuzzi SJ, et al. Effects of monotherapy with an HMG-CoA reductase inhibitor on the progression of coronary atherosclerosis as assessed by serial quantitative arteriography: The Canadian Coronary Atherosclerosis Intervention Trial. *Circulation* 1994; 89:959–968.
35. Haskell WL, Alderman EL, Fair JM, Maron DJ, Mackey SF, Superko HR, et al. Effects of intensive multiple risk factor reduction on coronary atherosclerosis and clinical cardiac events in men and women with coronary artery disease: The Stanford Coronary Risk Intervention Project (SCRIP). *Circulation* 1994; 89:975–990.
36. MAAS Investigators. Effect of simvastatin on coronary atheroma: The Multicentre Anti-Atheroma Study (MAAS). *Lancet* 1994; 344:633–638.
37. Pitt B, Mancini GBJ, Ellis SG, Rosman HS, Park J-S, McGovern ME, for the PLAC I Investigators. Pravastatin Limitation of Atherosclerosis in the Coronary Arteries (PLAC I): Reduction in atherosclerosis progression and clinical events. *J Am Coll Cardiol* 1995; 26:1133–1139.

38. Jukema JW, Bruschke AVG, van Boven AJ, Reiber JHC, Bal ET, Zwinderman AH, et al, on behalf of the REGRESS Study Group. Effects of lipid lowering by pravastatin on progression and regression of coronary artery disease in symptomatic men with normal to moderately elevated serum cholesterol levels: The Regression Growth Evaluation Study (REGRESS). *Circulation* 1995; 91:2528–2540.

39. Herd JA, Ballantyne CM, Farmer JA, Ferguson JJ III, Jones PH, West MS, et al, for the LCAS Investigators. Effects of fluvastatin on coronary atherosclerosis in patients with mild to moderate cholesterol elevations [Lipoprotein and Coronary Atherosclerosis Study (LCAS)]. *Am J Cardiol* 1997; 80:278–286.

40. Waters D, Higginson L, Gladstone P, Boccuzzi SJ, Cook T, Lespérance J, for the CCAIT Study Group. Effects of cholesterol lowering on the progression of coronary atherosclerosis in women: A Canadian Coronary Atherosclerosis Intervention Trial (CCAIT) substudy. *Circulation* 1995; 92:2404–2410.

41. Byington RP, Jukema JW, Salonen JT, Pitt B, Bruschke AV, Hoen H, et al. Reduction in cardiovascular events during pravastatin therapy: Pooled analysis of clinical events of the Pravastatin Atherosclerosis Intervention Program. *Circulation* 1995; 92:2419–2425.

42. LaRosa JC. Dyslipoproteinemia in women and the elderly (review). *Med Clin North Am* 1994; 78:163–180.

43. Buchwald H, Varco RL, Matts JP, Long JM, Fitch LL, Campbell GS, et al. Effect of partial ileal bypass surgery on mortality and morbidity from coronary heart disease in patients with hypercholesterolemia: Report of the Program on the Surgical Control of the Hyperlipidemias (POSCH). *N Engl J Med* 1990; 323:946–955.

44. Buchwald H, Matts JP, Fitch LL, Campos CT, Sanmarco ME, Amplatz K, et al, for the Program on the Surgical Control of the Hyperlipidemias (POSCH) Group. Changes in sequential coronary arteriograms and subsequent coronary events. *JAMA* 1992; 268:1429–1433.

45. American Academy of Pediatrics. National Cholesterol Education Program: Report of the Expert Panel on Blood Cholesterol Levels in Children and Adolescents. *Pediatrics* 1992; 89:525–584.

46. Havel RJ, Kane JP. Structure and metabolism of plasma lipoproteins. In: Scriver CR, Beaudet AL, Sly WS, Valle D, eds. *The Metabolic and Molecular Bases of Inherited Disease II*, 7th ed. New York: McGraw-Hill; 1995:1841–1851.

47. Havel RJ. Chylomicron remnants: Hepatic receptors and metabolism. *Curr Opin Lipidol* 1995; 6:312–316.

48. Lestavel S, Fruchart JC. Lipoprotein receptors (review). *Cell Mol Biol* 1994; 40:461–481.

49. Brown MS, Goldstein JL. A receptor-mediated pathway for cholesterol homeostasis. *Science* 1986; 232:34–47.

50. Javitt NB. Cholesterol homeostasis: Role of the LDL receptor (review). *FASEB J* 1995; 9:1378–1381.

51. Goldstein JL, Hobbs HH, Brown MS. Familial hypercholesterolemia. In: Scriver CR, Beaudet AL, Sly WS, Valle D, eds. *The Metabolic and Molecular Bases of Inherited Disease II*, 7th ed. New York: McGraw-Hill; 1995:1981–2030.

52. Kodama T, Freeman M, Rohrer L, Zabrecky J, Matsudaira P, Krieger M. Type I macrophage scavenger receptor contains alpha-helical and collagen-like coiled coils. *Nature* 1990; 343:531–535.

53. Freeman MW. Macrophage scavenger receptors (review). *Curr Opin Lipidol* 1994; 5:143–148.

54. Berliner JA, Heinecke JW. The role of oxidized lipoproteins in atherogenesis (review). *Free Radic Biol Med* 1996; 20:707–727.

55. Steinberg D. Role of oxidized LDL and antioxidants in atherosclerosis (review). *Adv Exp Med Biol* 1995; 369:39–48.

56. Grundy SM. Role of low-density lipoproteins in atherogenesis and development of coronary heart disease (review). *Clin Chem* 1995; 41:139–146.

57. Patsch W, Gotto AM Jr. High-density lipoprotein cholesterol, plasma triglyceride, and coronary heart disease: Pathophysiology and management. *Adv Pharmacol* 1995; 32:375–426.

58. Fuster V, Gotto AM Jr, Libby P, Loscalzo J, McGill HC Jr. Task Force 1. Pathogenesis of coronary disease: The biologic role of risk factors. *J Am Coll Cardiol* 1996; 27:964–976.

59. Ross R. The pathogenesis of atherosclerosis: A perspective for the 1990s (review). *Nature* 1993; 362:801–809.

60. Fuster V, Badimon L, Badimon JJ, Chesebro JH. The pathogenesis of coronary artery disease and the acute coronary syndromes (parts 1 and 2) (review). *N Engl J Med* 1992; 326:242–250, 310–318.

61. Gordon DJ, Probstfield JL, Garrison RJ, Neaton JD, Castelli WP, Knoke JD, et al. High-density lipoprotein cholesterol and cardiovascular disease: Four prospective American studies. *Circulation* 1989; 79:8–15.

62. Gotto AM Jr, Morrisett JD, eds. Second International Conference on Lipoprotein[a], November 12–14, 1992, New Orleans, Louisiana. *Chem Phys Lipids* 1994; 67/68 (special issue).

63. Utermann G. Lipoprotein(a). In: Scriver CR, Beaudet AL, Sly WS, Valle D, eds. *The Metabolic and Molecular Bases of Inherited Disease II*, 7th ed. New York: McGraw-Hill; 1995:1887–1912.

64. Durrington PN. Lipoprotein(a) (review). *Baillieres Clin Endocrinol Metab* 1995; 9:773–795.

65. Scanu AM, Lawn RM, Berg K. Lipoprotein(a) and atherosclerosis. *Ann Intern Med* 1991; 115:209–218.

66. Jones PH, Gotto AM Jr. Prevention of coronary heart disease in 1994: Evidence for intervention. *Heart Dis Stroke* 1994; 3:290–296.

67. Keys A, ed. Coronary heart disease in seven countries [American Heart Association Monograph 29]. *Circulation* 1970; 41(suppl 1):1–211.

68. Kannel WB, Castelli WP, Gordon T, McNamara PM. Serum cholesterol, lipoproteins, and the risk of coronary heart disease: The Framingham Study. *Ann Intern Med* 1971; 74:1–12.

69. Wilson PWF. Established risk factors and coronary artery disease: The Framingham Study. *Am J Hypertens* 1994; 7:7S–12S.

70. Kagan A, McGee DL, Yano K, Rhoads GG, Nomura A. Serum cholesterol and mortality in a Japanese-American population: The Honolulu Heart Program. *Am J Epidemiol* 1981; 114:11–20.

71. Kagan A, Harris BR, Winkelstein W Jr, Johnson KG, Kato H, Syme SL, et al. Epidemiologic studies of coronary heart disease and stroke in Japanese men living in Japan, Hawaii and California: Demographic, physical, dietary and biochemical characteristics. *J Chronic Dis* 1974; 27:345–364.

72. Klag MJ, Ford DE, Mead LA, He J, Whelton PK, Liang K-Y, et al. Serum cholesterol in young men and subsequent cardiovascular disease. *N Engl J Med* 1993; 328:313–318.

73. Stamler J, Wentworth D, Neaton JD, for the MRFIT Research Group. Is relationship between serum cholesterol and risk of premature death from coronary heart disease continuous and graded? Findings in 356,222 primary screenees of the Multiple Risk Factor Intervention Trial (MRFIT). *JAMA* 1986; 256:2823–2828.

74. Gotto AM Jr, Pownall HJ. *Manual of Lipid Disorders*. Baltimore: Williams & Wilkins; 1992.

75. LaRosa JC, Hunninghake D, Bush D, Criqui MH, Getz GS, Gotto AM Jr, et al. The cholesterol facts: A summary of the evidence relating dietary fats, serum cholesterol, and coronary heart disease. A joint statement by the American Heart Association and the National Heart, Lung, and Blood Institute. *Circulation* 1990; 81:1721–1733.

76. Lewis B, Paoletti R, Tikkanen MJ, eds. *Low Blood Cholesterol: Health Implications*. London: Current Medical Literature; 1993.

77. Hulley SB, Walsh JMB, Newman TB. Health policy on blood cholesterol: Time to change directions. *Circulation* 1992; 86:1026–1028.

78. Rossouw JE, Lewis B, Rifkind BM. The value of lowering cholesterol after myocardial infarction. *N Engl J Med* 1990; 323:1112–1119.

79. Stamler J, Stamler R, Brown WV, Gotto AM, Greenland P, Grundy S, et al. Serum cholesterol: Doing the right thing. *Circulation* 1993; 88:1954–1960.

80. Young AC, Raby KE, Ganz P, Selwyn AP. New insights into the management of myocardial ischemia. *Am J Cardiol* 1992; 70:8G–12G.

81. Gotto AM Jr. Lipid-regulating and antiatherosclerotic therapy: Current options and future approaches (review). *Cleve Clin J Med* 1996; 63:31–41.

82. Salonen R, Nyyssönen K, Porkkala E, Rummukainen J, Belder R, Park J-S, et al. Kuopio Atherosclerosis Prevention Study (KAPS): A population-based primary prevention trial of the effect of LDL lowering on atherosclerotic progression in carotid and femoral arteries. *Circulation* 1995; 92:1758–1764.

83. Oliver MF. Statins prevent coronary heart disease. *Lancet* 1995; 346:1378–1379.

84. Oliver M, Poole-Wilson P, Shepherd J, Tikkanen MJ. Lower patients' cholesterol now: Trial evidence shows clear benefits from secondary prevention. *Br Med J* 1995; 310:1280–1281.

85. Grundy SM. George Lyman Duff Memorial Lecture: Multifactorial etiology of hypercholesterolemia: Implications for prevention of coronary heart disease (review). *Arterioscler Thromb* 1991; 11:1619–1635.

86. Grundy SM, Friedman D. Rationale for cholesterol-lowering strategies (review). *Curr Probl Cardiol* 1995; 20:281–357.

87. Gotto AM Jr. Primary and secondary prevention of coronary artery disease (review). *Curr Opin Cardiol* 1992; 7:553–562.

88. Wenger NK. Gender, coronary artery disease, and coronary bypass surgery. *Ann Intern Med* 1990; 112:557–558.

89. Criqui MH, Langer RD, Fronek A, Feigelson HS, Klauber MR, McCann TJ, et al. Mortality over a period of 10 years in patients with peripheral arterial disease. *N Engl J Med* 1992; 326:381–386.

90. Salonen JT, Salonen R. Ultrasonographically assessed carotid morphology and the risk of coronary heart disease. *Arterioscler Thromb* 1991; 11:1245–1249.

91. Hubert HB, Feinleib M, McNamara PM, Castelli WP. Obesity as an independent risk factor for cardiovascular disease: A 26-year follow-up of participants in the Framingham Heart Study. *Circulation* 1983; 67:968–977.

92. Manson JE, Willett WC, Stampfer MJ, Colditz GA, Hunter DJ, Hankinson SE, et al. Body weight and mortality among women. *N Engl J Med* 1995; 333:677–685.

93. Pi-Sunyer FX. Health implications of obesity. *Am J Clin Nutr* 1991; 53:1595S–1603S.

94. Grundy SM, Barnett JP. Metabolic and health complications of obesity (review). *Dis Mon* 1990; 36:641–731.

95. Council on Scientific Affairs of the American Medical Association. Treatment of obesity in adults. *JAMA* 1988; 260:2547–2551.

96. Fletcher GF, Balady G, Froelicher VF, Hartley LM, Haskell WL, Pollock ML. Exercise standards: A statement for healthcare professionals from the American Heart Association. *Circulation* 1995; 91:580–615.

97. Fletcher GF, Blair SN, Blumenthal J, Caspersen C, Chaitman B, Epstein S, et al. Statement on exercise: Benefits and recommendations for physical activity programs for all Americans. A statement for health professionals by the Committee on Exercise and Cardiac Rehabilitation of the Council on Clinical Cardiology, American Heart Association. *Circulation* 1992; 86:340–344.

98. McHenry PL, Ellestad MH, Fletcher GF, Froelicher V, Hartley H, Mitchell JH, et al. Statement on exercise: A position statement for health professionals by the Committee on Exercise and Cardiac Rehabilitation of the Council on Clinical Cardiology, American Heart Association. *Circulation* 1990; 81:396–398.

99. Pate RR, Pratt M, Blair SN, Haskell WL, Macera CA, Bouchard C, et al. Physical activity and public health: A recommendation from the Centers for Disease Control and Prevention and the American College of Sports Medicine. *JAMA* 1995; 273:402–407.

100. NIH Consensus Development Panel on Physical Activity and Cardiovascular Health. Physical activity and cardiovascular health. *JAMA* 1996; 276:241–246.

101. National High Blood Pressure Education Program. *Working Group Report on Primary Prevention of Hypertension*. NIH publication no. 93-2669. Bethesda, MD: National Institutes of Health; 1993.

102. Haddy FJ, Pamnani MB. Role of dietary salt in hypertension (review). *J Am Coll Nutr* 1995; 14:428–438.

103. Sutton-Tyrrell K, Kuller LH, Wolfson SK Jr. Causes, implications, and treatment of systolic hypertension (review). *Curr Opin Nephrol Hypertens* 1994; 3:264–270.

104. Gillman MW, Cupples LA, Gagnon D, Posner BM, Ellison RC, Castelli WP, et al. Protective effect of fruits and vegetables on development of stroke in men. *JAMA* 1995; 273:1113–1117.

105. Willett WC. Diet and health: What should we eat (review)? *Science* 1994; 264:532–537.

106. Gaziano JM, Manson JE, Branch LG, Colditz GA, Willett WC, Buring JC. A prospective study of consumption of carotenoids in fruits and vegetables and decreased cardiovascular mortality in the elderly. *Ann Epidemiol* 1995; 5:333–335.

107. Jialal I, Grundy SM. Influence of antioxidant vitamins on LDL oxidation (review). *Ann N Y Acad Sci* 1992; 669:237–247.

108. Simon JA. Vitamin C and cardiovascular disease: A review. *J Am Coll Nutr* 1992; 11:107–125.

109. Kushi LH, Lenart EB, Willett WC. Health implications of Mediterranean diets in light of contemporary knowledge: 1. Plant foods and dairy products (review). *Am J Clin Nutr* 1995; 61(suppl):1407S–1415S.

110. Hughes K. Diet and coronary heart disease—A review. *Ann Acad Med Singapore* 1995; 24:224–229.

111. Jha P, Flather M, Lonn E, Farkouh M, Yusuf S. The antioxidant vitamins and cardiovascular disease: A critical review of epidemiologic and clinical trial data (review). *Ann Intern Med* 1995; 123:860–872.

112. Clifton PM. Antioxidant vitamins and coronary heart disease risk (review). *Curr Opin Lipidol* 1995; 6:20–24.

113. Mayer EL, Jacobsen DW, Robinson K. Homocysteine and coronary atherosclerosis (review). *J Am Coll Cardiol* 1996; 27:517–527.

114. Stampfer MJ, Malinow R, Willett WC, Newcomer WC, Upson B, Ullmann D, et al. A prospective study of plasma homocyst(e)ine and risk of myocardial infarction in US physicians. *JAMA* 1992; 268:877–881.

115. Meleady RA, Graham RM. Homocysteine as a risk factor for coronary artery disease (review). *J Cardiovasc Risk* 1995; 2:216–221.

116. Brattstrom L. Vitamins as homocysteine-lowering agents (review). *J Nutr* 1996; 126:1276S–1280S.

117. Criqui MH. Alcohol and coronary heart disease: Consistent relationship and public health implications (review). *Clin Chim Acta* 1996; 246:51–57.

118. Smith SC Jr, Blair SN, Criqui MH, Fletcher GF, Fuster V, Gersh BJ, et al. Preventing heart attack and death in patients with coronary disease: Consensus panel statement. AHA medical/scientific statement. Published simultaneously in *Circulation* 1995; 92:2–4 and *J Am Coll Cardiol* 1995; 26:292–294.

119. Pearson TA, Fuster V. Executive summary [of the 27th Bethesda Conference of the American College of Cardiology, September 14–15, 1995]. *J Am Coll Cardiol* 1996; 27:957–1047.

120. Anderson KM, Wilson PWF, Odell PM, Kannel WB. An updated coronary risk profile: A statement for health professionals. AHA medical/scientific statement. *Circulation* 1991; 83:356–362.

121. Wilson PWF, Evans JC. Coronary artery disease prediction. *Am J Hypertens* 1993; 6:309S–313S.

122. International Task Force. Prevention of coronary heart disease: Scientific background and new clinical guidelines. Recommendations of the European Atherosclerosis Society prepared by the International Task Force for Prevention of Coronary Heart Disease. *Nutr Metab Cardiovasc Dis* 1992; 2:113–156.

123. Friedewald WT, Levy RI, Fredrickson DS. Estimation of the concentration of low-density lipoprotein cholesterol in plasma, without the use of the preparative ultracentrifuge. *Clin Chem* 1972; 18:499–502.

124. Austin MA. Plasma triglyceride and coronary heart disease (review). *Arterioscler Thromb* 1991; 11:2–14.

125. NIH Consensus Development Panel on Triglyceride, High-Density Lipoprotein, and Coronary Heart Disease. Triglyceride, high-density lipoprotein, and coronary heart disease. *JAMA* 1993; 269:505–510.

126. Criqui MH, Heiss G, Cohn R, Cowan LD, Suchindran CM, Bangdiwala S, et al. Plasma triglyceride level and mortality from coronary heart disease. *N Engl J Med* 1993; 328:1220–1225.

127. Castelli WP. Epidemiology of triglycerides: A view from Framingham. *Am J Cardiol* 1992; 70(suppl):3H–9H.

128. Patsch JR, Miesenbock G, Hopferweiser T, Muhlberger V, Knapp E, Dunn JK, et al. Relation of triglyceride metabolism and coronary artery disease: Studies in the postprandial state. *Arterioscler Thromb* 1992; 12:1336–1345.

129. Ebenbichler CF, Kirchmair R, Egger C, Patsch JR. Postprandial state and atherosclerosis (review). *Curr Opin Lipidol* 1995; 6:286–290.

130. Genest J Jr, Cohn JS. Clustering of cardiovascular risk factors: Targeting high-risk individuals (review). *Am J Cardiol* 1995; 76:8A–20A.

131. Miller GJ. Lipoproteins and the haemostatic system in atherothrombotic disorders (review). *Baillieres Clin Haematol* 1994; 7:713–732.

132. Mitropoulos KA. Lipid-thrombosis interface (review). *Br Med Bull* 1994; 50:813–832.

133. Mitropoulos KA. Lipoprotein metabolism and thrombosis (review). *Curr Opin Lipidol* 1994; 5:227–235.

134. Geurian K, Pinson JB, Weart CW. The triglyceride connection in atherosclerosis (review). *Ann Pharmacother* 1992; 26:1109–1117.

135. van Hoeven KH, Factor SM. Diabetic heart disease: The clinical and pathological spectrum—part I. *Clin Cardiol* 1989; 12:600–604.

136. Kannel WB. Lipids, diabetes, and coronary heart disease: Insights from the Framingham Study. *Am Heart J* 1985; 110:1100–1107.

137. Mann JI, Pyörälä K, Teuscher A. *Diabetes in Epidemiological Perspective*. Edinburgh: Churchill Livingstone; 1983.

138. American Diabetes Association. Detection and management of lipid disorders in diabetes. [American Diabetes Association Consensus Development Conference on the Detection and Management of Lipid Disorders in Diabetes, 11–13 January 1993, Dallas, Texas.] *Diabetes Care* 1993; 16(suppl 2):106–112.

139. Stewart MW, Laker MF, Alberti KG. The contributions of lipids to coronary heart disease in diabetes mellitus. *J Intern Med Suppl* 1994; 736:41–46.

140. Laws A, Marcus EB, Grove JS, Curb JD. Lipids and lipoproteins as risk factors for coronary heart disease in men with abnormal glucose tolerance: The Honolulu Heart Program. *J Intern Med* 1993; 234:471–478.

141. Laakso M, Lehto S, Penttila I, Pyorala K. Lipids and lipoproteins predicting coronary heart disease mortality and morbidity in patients with non-insulin-dependent diabetes. *Circulation* 1993; 88:1421–1430.

142. Bierman EL. George Lyman Duff Memorial Lecture: Atherogenesis in diabetes. *Arterioscler Thromb* 1992; 12:647–656.

143. Krone W, Muller-Wieland D. Hyperlipidemia and hypertension (review). *Baillieres Clin Endocrinol Metab* 1990; 4:833–850.

144. Pyörälä K, De Backer G, Graham I, Poole-Wilson P, Wood D, on behalf of the Task Force. Prevention of coronary heart disease in clinical practice: Recommendations of the Task Force of the European Society of Cardiology, European Atherosclerosis Society and European Society of Hypertension. Published simultaneously in *Eur Heart J* 1994; 15:1300–1331 and *Atherosclerosis* 1994; 110:121–161.

145. Ernst E, Resch KL. Fibrinogen as a cardiovascular risk factor: A meta-analysis and review of the literature. *Ann Intern Med* 1993; 118:956–963.

146. Kannel WB, Wolf PA, Castelli WP, D'Agostino RB. Fibrinogen and risk of cardiovascular disease: The Framingham Study. *JAMA* 1987; 258:1183–1186.

147. Heinrich J, Balleisen L, Schulte H, Assmann G, van de Loo. Fibrinogen and factor VII in the prediction of risk: Results from the PROCAM Study in healthy men. *Arterioscler Thromb* 1994; 14:54–59.

148. Maher VMG, Brown BG, Marcovina SM, Hillger LA, Zhao X-Q, Albers JJ. Effects of lowering elevated LDL cholesterol on the cardiovascular risk of lipoprotein(a). *JAMA* 1995; 274:1771–1774.

149. Gotto AM Jr. Postmenopausal hormone-replacement therapy, plasma lipoprotein[a], and risk for coronary heart disease (editorial). *J Lab Clin Med* 1994; 123:800–803.

150. Soma MR, Osnago-Gadda I, Paoletti R, Fumagalli R, Morrisett JD, Meschia M, et al. The lowering of lipoprotein[a] induced by estrogen plus progesterone replacement therapy in postmenopausal women. *Arch Intern Med* 1993; 153:1462–1468.

151. Patsch W, Gotto AM Jr. Apolipoproteins: Pathophysiology and clinical implications. *Methods Enzymol* 1996; 263:3–32.

152. Avogaro P, Bon GB, Cazzolato G, Rorai E. Relationship between apolipoproteins and chemical components of lipoproteins in survivors of myocardial infarction. *Atherosclerosis* 1980; 37:69–76.

153. Maciejko JJ, Holmes DR, Kottke BA, Zinsmeister AR, Dinh DM, Mao SJ. Apolipoprotein A-I as marker of angiographically assessed coronary-artery disease. *N Engl J Med* 1983; 309:385–389.

154. Rader DJ, Hoeg JM, Brewer HB. Quantitation of plasma apolipoproteins in primary and secondary prevention of coronary artery disease. *Ann Intern Med* 1994; 120:1012–1025.

155. DeFronzo RA, Ferrannini E. Insulin resistance: A multifaceted syndrome responsible for NIDDM, obesity, hypertension, dyslipidemia, and atherosclerotic cardiovascular disease. *Diabetes Care* 1991; 14:173–194.

156. Reaven GM. Role of insulin resistance in human disease (syndrome X): An expanded definition. *Annu Rev Med* 1993; 44:121–131.

157. Kaplan NM. The deadly quartet: Upper-body obesity, glucose intolerance, hypertriglyceridemia, and hypertension. *Arch Intern Med* 1989; 149:1514–1520.

158. Krauss RM. Heterogeneity of plasma low-density lipoproteins and atherosclerosis risk (review). *Curr Opin Lipidol* 1994; 5:339–349.

159. Austin MA, Selby JV. LDL subclass phenotypes and the risk factors of the insulin resistance syndrome. *Int J Obes Relat Metab Disord* 1995; 19(suppl 1):S22–S26.

160. Austin MA, Hokanson HE, Brunzell JD. Characteristics of low-density lipoprotein subclasses: Methodologic approaches and clinical relevance (review). *Curr Opin Lipidol* 1994; 5:395–403.

161. Hokanson JE, Krauss RM, Albers JJ, Austin MA, Brunzell JD. LDL physical and chemical properties in familial combined hyperlipidemia. *Arterioscler Thromb Vasc Biol* 1995; 15:452–459.

162. Assmann G, Schulte H. Relation of high density lipoprotein cholesterol and triglycerides to incidence of atherosclerotic coronary artery disease (the PROCAM experience). *Am J Cardiol* 1992; 70:733–737.

163. Fredrickson DS, Levy RI, Lees RS. Fat transport in lipoproteins—An integrated approach to mechanisms and disorders. *N Engl J Med* 1967; 276:34–42, 94–103, 148–156, 215–225, 273–281.

164. Kane JP, Havel RJ. Disorders of the biogenesis and secretion of lipoproteins containing the B apolipoproteins. In: Scriver CR, Beaudet AL, Sly WS, Valle D, eds. *The Metabolic and Molecular Bases of Inherited Disease II*, 7th ed. New York: McGraw-Hill; 1995:1853–1885.

165. Brunzell JD. Familial lipoprotein lipase deficiency and other causes of the chylomicronemia syndrome. In: Scriver CR, Beaudet AL, Sly WS, Valle D, eds. *The Metabolic and Molecular Bases of Inherited Disease II*, 7th ed. New York: McGraw-Hill; 1995:1913–1932.

166. Glomset JA, Assmann G, Gjone E, Norum KR. Lecithin:cholesterol acyltransferase deficiency and fish eye disease. In: Scriver CR, Beaudet AL, Sly WS, Valle D, eds. *The Metabolic and Molecular Bases of Inherited Disease II*, 7th ed. New York: McGraw-Hill; 1995:1933–1951.

167. Mahley RW, Rall SC Jr. Type III hyperlipoproteinemia (dysbetalipoproteinemia): The role of apolipoprotein E in normal and abnormal lipoprotein metabolism. In: Scriver CR, Beaudet AL, Sly WS, Valle D, eds. *The Metabolic and Molecular Bases of Inherited Disease II*, 7th ed. New York: McGraw-Hill, 1995:1953–1980.

168. Breslow JL. Familial disorders of high-density lipoprotein metabolism. In: Scriver CR, Beaudet AL, Sly WS, Valle D, eds. *The Metabolic and Molecular Bases of Inherited Disease II*, 7th ed. New York: McGraw-Hill; 1995:2031–2052.

169. Assmann G, von Eckardstein A, Brewer HB Jr. Familial high density lipoprotein deficiency: Tangier disease. In: Scriver CR, Beaudet AL, Sly WS, Valle D, eds. *The Metabolic and Molecular Bases of Inherited Disease II*, 7th ed. New York: McGraw-Hill; 1995:2053–2072.

170. Goldstein JL, Schrott HG, Hazzard WR, Bierman EL, Motulsky AG. Hyperlipidemia in coronary heart disease: II. Genetic analysis of lipid concentrations in 176 families and delineation of a new inherited disorder, combined hyperlipidemia. *J Clin Invest* 1973; 52:1544–1568.

171. Sniderman AD, Wolfson C, Teng B, Franklin FA, Bachorik PS, Kwiterovich PO Jr. Association of hyperapobetalipoproteinemia with endogenous hypertriglyceridemia and atherosclerosis. *Ann Intern Med* 1982; 97:833–839.

172. Sniderman A, Shapiro S, Marpole D, Skinner B, Teng B, Kwiterovich PO Jr. Association of coronary atherosclerosis with hyperapobetalipoproteinemia. *Proc Natl Acad Sci U S A* 1980; 77:604–608.

173. Soria LF, Ludwig EH, Clarke HR, Vega GL, Grundy SM, McCarthy BJ. Association between a specific apolipoprotein B mutation and familial defective apolipoprotein B-100. *Proc Natl Acad Sci U S A* 1989; 86:587–591.

174. Willett W. *Nutritional Epidemiology*. New York: Oxford University Press; 1990.

175. Sacks FM, Willett W. Chewing the fat: How much and what kind? *N Engl J Med* 1991; 324:121–123.

176. Trichopoulou A, Lagiou P, Trichopoulos D. Traditional Greek diet and coronary heart disease. *J Cardiovasc Risk* 1994; 1:9–15.

177. Ornish D, Denke M. Debate: Dietary treatment of hyperlipidemia. *J Cardiovasc Risk* 1994; 1:283–286.

178. Denke MA. Cholesterol-lowering diets: A review of the evidence (review). *Arch Intern Med* 1995; 155:17–26.

179. Gotto A, Grundy S, section eds. Lipid-lowering drugs. In: Messerli FH, ed. *Cardiovascular Drug Therapy*, 2d ed. Philadelphia: Saunders; 1996:1061–1135.

180. Farmer JA, Gotto AM Jr. Currently available hypolipidaemic drugs and future therapeutic developments. *Baillieres Clin Endocrinol Metab* 1995; 9:825–847.

181. Grundy SM. Cholesterol-lowering drugs as cardioprotective agents (review). *Am J Cardiol* 1992; 70:27I–32I.

182. Denke MA, Grundy SM. Efficacy of low-dose cholesterol-lowering drug therapy in men with moderate hypercholesterolemia. *Arch Intern Med* 1995; 155:393–399.

183. Barth JD, Mancini GB. An update on lipid-lowering therapy (review). *Curr Opin Lipidol* 1995; 6:32–37.

184. Sirtori CR, Manzoni C, Lovati MR. Mechanisms of lipid-lowering agents (review). *Cardiology* 1991; 78:226–235.

185. Farmer JA, Gotto AM Jr. Antihyperlipidaemic agents: Drug interactions of clinical significance. *Drug Safety* 1994; 11:301–309.

186. Davignon J, Montigny M, Dufour R. HMG-CoA reductase inhibitors: A look back and a look ahead (review). *Can J Cardiol* 1992; 8:843–864.

187. Endo A. The discovery and development of HMG-CoA reductase inhibitors (review). *J Lipid Res* 1992; 33:1569–1582.

188. Endo A, Hasumi K. Biochemical aspect of HMG CoA reductase inhibitors (review). *Adv Enzyme Regul* 1989; 28:53–64.

189. Raiteri M, Arnaboldi L, Quarato P, Paoletti R, Fumagalli R, Corsini A. [The pharmacology of the statins: The evidence of a direct anti-atherosclerotic action.] *Ann Ital Med Int* 1995; 10(suppl):35S–42S.

190. Jokubaitis LA. Development and pharmacology of fluvastatin (review). *Br J Clin Pract Symp Suppl* 1996; 77A:11–15.

191. Peters TK. Treatment of dyslipidemias with fluvastatin (review). *Br J Clin Pract Symp Suppl* 1996; 77A:16–19.

192. Frishman WH, Zinetbaum P, Nadelmann J. Lovastatin and other HMG-CoA reductase inhibitors (review). *J Clin Pharmacol* 1989; 29:975–982.

193. Bradford RH, Shear CL, Chremos AN, Dujovne C, Downton M, Franklin FA, et al. Expanded Clinical Evaluation of Lovastatin (EXCEL) Study results: I. Efficacy in modifying plasma lipoproteins and adverse event profile in 8245 patients with moderate hypercholesterolemia. *Arch Intern Med* 1991; 151:43–49.

194. Quion JA, Jones PH. Clinical pharmacokinetics of pravastatin (review). *Clin Pharmacokinet* 1994; 27:94–103.

195. Plosker GL, McTavish D. Simvastatin: A reappraisal of its pharmacology and therapeutic efficacy in hypercholesterolaemia (review). *Drugs* 1995; 50:334–363.

196. Davignon J. Prospects for drug therapy for hyperlipoproteinaemia (review). *Diabete Metab* 1995; 21:139–146.

197. Bakker-Arkema RG, Davidson MH, Goldstein RJ, Davignon J, Isaacsohn JL, Weiss SR, et al. Efficacy and safety of a new HMG-CoA reductase inhibitor, atorvastatin, in patients with hypertriglyceridemia. *JAMA* 1996; 275:128–133.

198. Nawrocki JW, Weiss SR, Davidson MH, Sprecher DL, Schwartz SL, Lupien PJ, et al. Reduction of LDL cholesterol by 25% to 60% in patients with primary hypercholesterolemia by atorvastatin, a new HMG-CoA reductase inhibitor. *Arterioscler Thromb Vasc Biol* 1995; 15:678–682.

199. Ast M, Frishman WH. Bile acid sequestrants (review). *J Clin Pharmacol* 1990; 30:99–106.

200. Brown WV. Niacin for lipid disorders: Indications, effectiveness, and safety (review). *Postgrad Med* 1995; 98:185–189, 192–193.

201. Fattore PC, Sirtori CR. Nicotinic acid and derivatives. *Curr Opin Lipidol* 1991; 2:43–47.

202. Shepherd J. The action of nicotinic acid and its analogues on lipoprotein metabolism. *Atheroscler Rev* 1991; 22:207–212.

203. Drood JM, Zinetbaum PJ, Frishman WH. Nicotinic acid for the treatment of hyperlipoproteinemia (review). *J Clin Pharmacol* 1991; 31:641–650.

204. McKenney JM, Proctor JD, Harris S, Chinchili VM. A comparison of the efficacy and toxic effects of sustained- vs immediate-release niacin in hypercholesterolemic patients. *JAMA* 1994; 271:672–677.

205. Davignon J. Fibrates: A review of important issues and recent findings. *Can J Cardiol* 1994; 10(suppl B):61B–71B.

206. Shepherd J. Mechanism and action of fibrates (review). *Postgrad Med J* 1993; 69(suppl):S34–S41.

207. Sirtori CR, Franceschini G. Effects of fibrates on serum lipids and atherosclerosis (review). *Pharmacol Ther* 1988; 37:167–191.

208. Grundy SM, Vega GL. Fibric acids: Effects on lipids and lipoprotein metabolism (review). *Am J Med* 1987; 83:9–20.

209. A co-operative trial in the primary prevention of ischaemic heart disease. *Br Heart J* 1978; 40:1069–1118.

210. WHO cooperative trial on primary prevention of ischaemic heart disease using clofibrate to lower serum cholesterol: Mortality follow-up. *Lancet* 1980; 2:379–385.

211. WHO cooperative trial on primary prevention of ischaemic heart disease with clofibrate to lower serum cholesterol: Final mortality follow-up. *Lancet* 1984; 2:600–604.

212. Heady JA, Morris JN, Oliver MF. WHO clofibrate/cholesterol trial: Clarifications. *Lancet* 1992; 340:1405–1406.

213. Barrett-Connor E, Laakso M. Ischemic heart disease risk in postmenopausal women. *Arteriosclerosis* 1990; 10:531–534.

214. Knopp RH. Estrogen replacement therapy for reduction of cardiovascular risk in women (review). *Curr Opin Lipidol* 1991; 2:240–247.

215. Martin KA, Freeman MW. Postmenopausal hormone-replacement therapy (editorial). *N Engl J Med* 1993; 328:1115–1117.

216. Kuhn FE, Rackley CE. Coronary artery disease in women: Risk factors, evaluation, treatment, and prevention (review). *Arch Intern Med* 1993; 153:2626–2636.

217. Miller VT. Lipids, lipoproteins, women and cardiovascular disease. *Atherosclerosis* 1994; 108(suppl):S73–S82.

218. The Writing Group for the PEPI Trial: Effects of estrogen or estrogen/progestin regimens on heart disease risk factors in postmenopausal women: The Postmenopausal Estrogen/Progestin Interventions (PEPI) Trial. *JAMA* 1995; 273:199–208.

219. Grundy SM, Balady GJ, Criqui MH, Fletcher G, Greenland P, Hiratzka LF, et al. When to start cholesterol-lowering therapy in patients with coronary heart disease: A statement for healthcare professionals from the American Heart Association Task Force on Risk Reduction. *Circulation* 1997; 95:1683–1685.

220. Ryan TJ, Anderson JL, Antman EM, Braniff BA, Brooks NH, Califf RM, et al. ACC/AHA guidelines for the management of patients with acute myocardial infarction: A report of the American College of Cardiology/American Heart Association Task Force on Practice Guidelines (Committee on Management of Acute Myocardial Infarction). *J Am Coll Cardiol* 1996; 28:1328–1428.

221. Pierce LR, Wysowski DK, Gross TP. Myopathy and rhabdomyolysis associated with lovastatin-gemfibrozil combination therapy. *JAMA* 1990; 264:71–75.

222. Assmann G, Schmitz G, Funke H, von Eckardstein AI. Apolipoprotein A-I and HDL deficiency. *Curr Opin Lipidol* 1990; 1:110–115.

223. Lauer RM, Clarke WR. Use of cholesterol measurements in childhood for the prediction of adult hypercholesterolemia: The Muscatine Study. *JAMA* 1990:3034–3038.

54

BETA-ADRENERGIC BLOCKING DRUGS AND CALCIUM CHANNEL BLOCKERS

William H. Frishman / Edmund H. Sonnenblick

In this chapter, two major classes of cardiovascular drugs are reviewed that have different chemical structures and modes of action but many similar applications in the treatment of cardiovascular disease: the beta-adrenergic blockers and calcium channel blockers. For specific problems, relative efficacy must be judged and contrasted with adverse side effects as well as effects on longer-term morbidity and mortality. This may suggest the advisability of combining more than one agent for optimal benefit.

BETA-ADRENERGIC BLOCKING DRUGS

Beta-adrenergic blocking drugs, which constitute a major pharmacotherapeutic advance, were conceived initially for the treatment of patients with angina pectoris and arrhythmias; however, they also have therapeutic effects in many other clinical disorders including systemic hypertension, hypertrophic cardiomyopathy, supraventricular tachycardias, mitral valve prolapse, silent myocardial ischemia, migraine, glaucoma, essential tremor, and thyrotoxicosis.[1-3] Beta blockers have been effective in treating unstable angina and for reducing the risk of cardiovascular mortality and nonfatal reinfarction in patients who have survived an acute myocardial infarction.[4,5] Beta blockade is also a potential treatment modality, with and without thrombolytic therapy, for reducing the extent of myocardial injury and mortality during the hyperacute phase of myocardial infarction.[6-9] Recently a beta blocker was approved for use in patients with mild to moderate congestive heart failure for reducing the progression of disease and reducing mortality.

The Beta-Adrenergic Receptor

Radioligand labeling techniques have greatly aided the investigation of adrenoreceptors,[10-12] and molecular pharmacologic techniques have positively delineated the beta-adrenoceptor structure as a polypeptide with a molecular weight of 67,000 Å.[11]

In contrast to the older concept of adrenoreceptors as static entities in cells that simply serve to initiate the chain of events, newer theories hold that the adrenoceptors are subject to a wide variety of controlling influences that result in dynamic regulation of adrenoceptor sites and/or their sensitivity to catecholamines. Changes in tissue concentration of receptor sites are probably involved in mediating important fluctuations in tissue sensitivity to drug action.[12] These principles may have significant clinical and therapeutic implications. For example, an apparent increase in the number of beta adrenoceptors, and thus a supersensitivity to agonists, may be induced by chronic exposure to antagonists.[12] With prolonged adrenoceptor-blocker therapy, receptor occupancy by catecholamines can be diminished and the number of available receptors can be increased. When the beta blocker is withdrawn suddenly, an increased pool of sensitive receptors will be open to endogenous catecholamine stimulation. The resultant adrenergic stimulation could precipitate unstable angina pectoris and/or a myocardial infarction.[13]

Using radioligand techniques, investigators have demonstrated a decrease in beta-adrenoceptor sites in the myocardium in patients with chronic congestive heart failure.[14,15] The concentration of beta adrenoceptors in the membrane of mononuclear cells also decreases significantly with age.[10] An apparent reduction in beta adrenoceptors and/or beta-adrenoceptor function has also been associated with the development of refractoriness or desensitization to endogenous and exogenous catecholamines, a phenomenon probably caused by the prolonged exposure of these adrenoceptors to high levels of catecholamines.[16] This desensitization phenomenon or "downregulation" is caused not by a change in receptor formation or degradation but rather by catecholamine-induced changes in the conformation of the receptor sites, thus rendering them ineffective.[17] Beta blocking drugs do not induce desensitization or changes in the conformation of receptors, but they do block the ability of catecholamines to desensitize receptors.[17]

Basic Pharmacologic Differences among Beta-Blocking Drugs

More than 100 beta blockers have been synthesized during the past 35 years and over 30 are available worldwide for clinical use.[18] Selectivity for two subgroups of the beta-adrenergic population has also been taken advantage of: $beta_1$ receptors in the heart and $beta_2$ receptors in the peripheral circulation and bronchi.[1] More controversial has been the introduction of beta-blocking drugs with alpha-adrenergic blocking actions, varying amounts of selective and nonselective intrinsic sympathomimetic activity (partial agonist activity), calcium channel blocker activity, and nonspecific membrane-stabilizing effects.[3] There are also pharmacokinetic differences between beta-blocking drugs that may be of clinical importance.[1]

Fifteen beta blockers are now marketed in the United States for cardiovascular disorders: (1) propranolol for angina pectoris, arrhythmias, systemic hypertension, migraine prophylaxis, essential tremor, and hypertrophic cardiomyopathy and for reducing the risk of cardiovascular mortality in survivors of an acute myocardial infarction; (2) nadolol for hypertension and angina pectoris; (3) timolol for hypertension and for reducing the risk of cardiovascular mortality and nonfatal reinfarction in survivors of myocardial infarction and in topical form for glaucoma; (4) atenolol and (5) metoprolol for hypertension and angina and in intravenous and oral formulations for reducing the risk of cardiovascular mortality in survivors of myocardial infarction; (6) penbutolol; (7) bisoprolol; (8) pindolol for treating hypertension; (9) betaxolol and (10) carteolol for hypertension and in a topical form for glaucoma; (11) acebutolol for hypertension and ventricular arrhythmias; (12) intravenous esmolol for supraventricular arrhythmias; (13) sotalol for ventricular arrhythmias; (14) labetalol for hypertension and in intravenous form for hypertensive emergencies; and (15) carvedilol both for hypertension and for reducing the rate of disease progression and mortality in patients with mild to moderate congestive heart failure.[1,3,19-25] In addition, oxprenolol has been approved for use in hypertension but is not marketed in the United States. Bucindolol is now being evaluated in a clinical trial in patients having moderate to severe congestive heart failure.

Despite the extensive experience with beta blockers in clinical practice, there have been no studies suggesting that any of these agents have major advantages or disadvantages in relation to the others for treatment of many cardiovascular diseases. When any available blocker is titrated properly, it can be effective in patients with arrhythmia, hypertension, or angina pectoris.[1,3,19-25] On the other hand, one agent may be more effective than other agents in reducing adverse reactions in some patients and for managing specific situations.[3]

POTENCY

Beta-adrenoceptor blocking drugs are competitive inhibitors of catecholamine binding at beta-adrenergic receptor sites. The dose-response curve of the catecholamine is shifted to the right; that is, a given tissue response requires a higher concentration of agonist in the presence of beta-blocking drugs.[2] $Beta_1$-blocking potency can be assessed by the inhibition of tachycardia produced by isoproterenol or exercise (the more reliable method in the intact organism); the potency varies from compound to compound (Table 54-1).[2] These differences in potency are of no therapeutic relevance; however, they do explain the different drug doses needed to achieve effective beta-adrenergic blockade in initiating therapy or in switching from one agent to another.[1,3,17]

STRUCTURE-ACTIVITY RELATIONSHIPS

The chemical structures of most beta blockers have several features in common with the agonist isoproterenol (Fig. 54-1), an aromatic ring with a substituted ethanolamine side chain linked to it by an $—OCH_2$ group.[1,3] The beta blocker timolol has a catecholamine-mimicking side chain but a more complex ring. The similarity of the antagonist to the agonist permits it to occupy the receptor site, thus excluding the agonist; however, its altered structure does not permit activation of the receptor, so that it is effectively a blocker of the receptor.

Most beta-blocking drugs exist as pairs of optical isomers and are marketed as racemic mixtures. Almost all the beta-blocking activity is found in the negative $(-)$ levorotatory stereoisomer. The two stereoisomers of beta blockers are useful for differentiating between the pharmacologic effects of beta blockade and membrane-stabilizing activity (possessed by both optical forms). The positive $(+)$ dextrorotatory stereoisomers of beta-blocking agents have no apparent clinical value[1,3] except for d-sotalol, which appears to have type III antiarrhythmic properties.[3] Penbutolol and timolol are marketed only in the levorotatory form. As a result of asymmetric carbon atoms, labetalol has four stereoisomers and carvedilol has two.[26] With carvedilol, beta-blocking effects are seen in the $(-)$ levorotatory stereoisomer and alpha-blocking effects in both the $(-)$ levorotatory and $(+)$ dextrorotatory stereoisomers.

MEMBRANE-STABILIZING ACTIVITY

At concentrations well above therapeutic levels, certain beta blockers have a quinidine-like or local anesthetic membrane-stabilizing effect on the cardiac action potential. This property is exhibited equally by the two stereoisomers of the drug and is unrelated to beta-adrenergic blockade and major therapeutic antiarrhythmic actions. There is no evidence that membrane-stabilizing activity is responsible for any direct negative inotropic effect of the beta blockers, since drugs with and without this property may equally depress left ventricular function. Membrane-stabilizing activity, however, can manifest itself clinically with massive beta-blocker intoxications.[2,27]

TABLE 54-1

PHARMACODYNAMIC PROPERTIES OF BETA–ADRENOCEPTOR BLOCKING DRUGS

Drug	Beta$_1$-Blockade Potency Ratio (Propranolol = 1.0)	Relative Beta$_1$ Selectivity	Intrinsic Sympathomimetic Activity	Membrane–Stabilizing Activity
Acebutolol	0.3	+	+	+
Atenolol	1.0	+ +	0	0
Betaxolol	1.0	+ +	0	+
Bisoprolol	10.0	+ +	0	0
Bucindolol[a]	1.0	0	+	+
Carteolol	10.0	0	+	0
Carvedilol[b]	10.0	0	0	+ +
Esmolol	0.02	+ +	0	0
Labetalol[c]	0.3	0	+	0
Metroprolol	1.0	+ +	0	0
Nadolol	1.0	0	0	0
Oxyprenolol	0.5–1.0	0	+	+
Penbutolol	1.0	0	+	0
Pindolol	6.0	0	+ +	+
Propranolol	1.0	0	0	+ +
Sotalol[d]	0.3	0	0	0
Timolol	6.0	0	0	0
Isomer: D-propranolol	—	—	—	+ +

[a] Bucindolol has additional direct peripheral vasodilatory activity.
[b] Carvedilol has additional alpha$_1$-adrenergic blocking activity without peripheral beta$_2$ agonism.
[c] Labetalol has additional alpha$_1$-adrenergic blocking activity and direct vasodilatory actions (beta$_2$ agonism).
[d] Sotalol has an additional type of antiarrhythmic activity.

Source: From Frishman,[2] with permission.

BETA$_1$ SELECTIVITY

Beta-adrenergic blockers may be classified as selective or nonselective, according to their relative abilities to antagonize the actions of sympathomimetic amines in some tissues at lower doses than those required in other tissues.[1,19] When used in low doses, beta$_1$-selective blocking agents such as acebutolol, betaxolol, bisoprolol, esmolol, atenolol, and metoprolol inhibit cardiac beta$_2$ receptors but have less influence on bronchial and vascular beta adrenoceptors (beta$_2$). In higher doses, however, beta$_1$-selective blocking agents also block beta$_2$ receptors more widely. Accordingly, beta$_1$-selective agents may be safer than nonselective ones in patients with obstructive pulmonary disease, since beta$_2$ receptors remain available to mediate adrenergic bronchodilatation. Even selective beta blockers can aggravate bronchospasm in certain patients; therefore these drugs should generally be used in patients with bronchospastic disease with great caution if at all.

A second theoretical advantage is that unlike nonselective beta$_1$ blockers, beta$_1$-selective blockers in low doses may not block the beta$_2$ receptors that mediate dilatation of arterioles. During infusion of epinephrine, nonselective beta blockers can cause a pressor response by blocking beta$_2$-receptor–mediated vasodilatation, since alpha-adrenergic vasoconstrictor receptors are still operative. Selective beta$_1$ antagonists may not induce this pressor effect in the presence of epinephrine and may lessen the impairment of peripheral blood flow. It is possible that leaving the beta$_2$ receptors unblocked and responsive to epinephrine may be functionally important in some patients with asthma, hypoglycemia, hypertension, or peripheral vascular disease treated with beta-adrenergic blocking drugs.[1,3,19]

INTRINSIC SYMPATHOMIMETIC ACTIVITY (PARTIAL AGONIST ACTIVITY)

Certain beta blockers possess intrinsic sympathomimetic activity (ISA, or partial agonist activity) at beta$_1$-adrenoceptor receptor sites, beta$_2$-adrenoceptor receptor sites, or both. In a beta blocker, this property is identified as a slight cardiac stimulation that can be blocked by propranolol.[1,3,22,23] The beta blockers with this property can partially activate the beta receptor in addition to preventing the access of a natural or synthetic catecholamine agonist to the receptor (Fig. 54-2). Dichloroisoprenaline, the first beta-blocking drug synthesized, exerted such marked partial agonist activity that it was unsuitable for clinical use. Compounds with less partial agonist activity, however, are effective beta-blocking drugs. The partial agonist effects of beta-blocking drugs such as pindolol differ from those of the agonist epinephrine and isoproterenol in that the maximum pharmacologic response that can be obtained is low, although the affinity for the

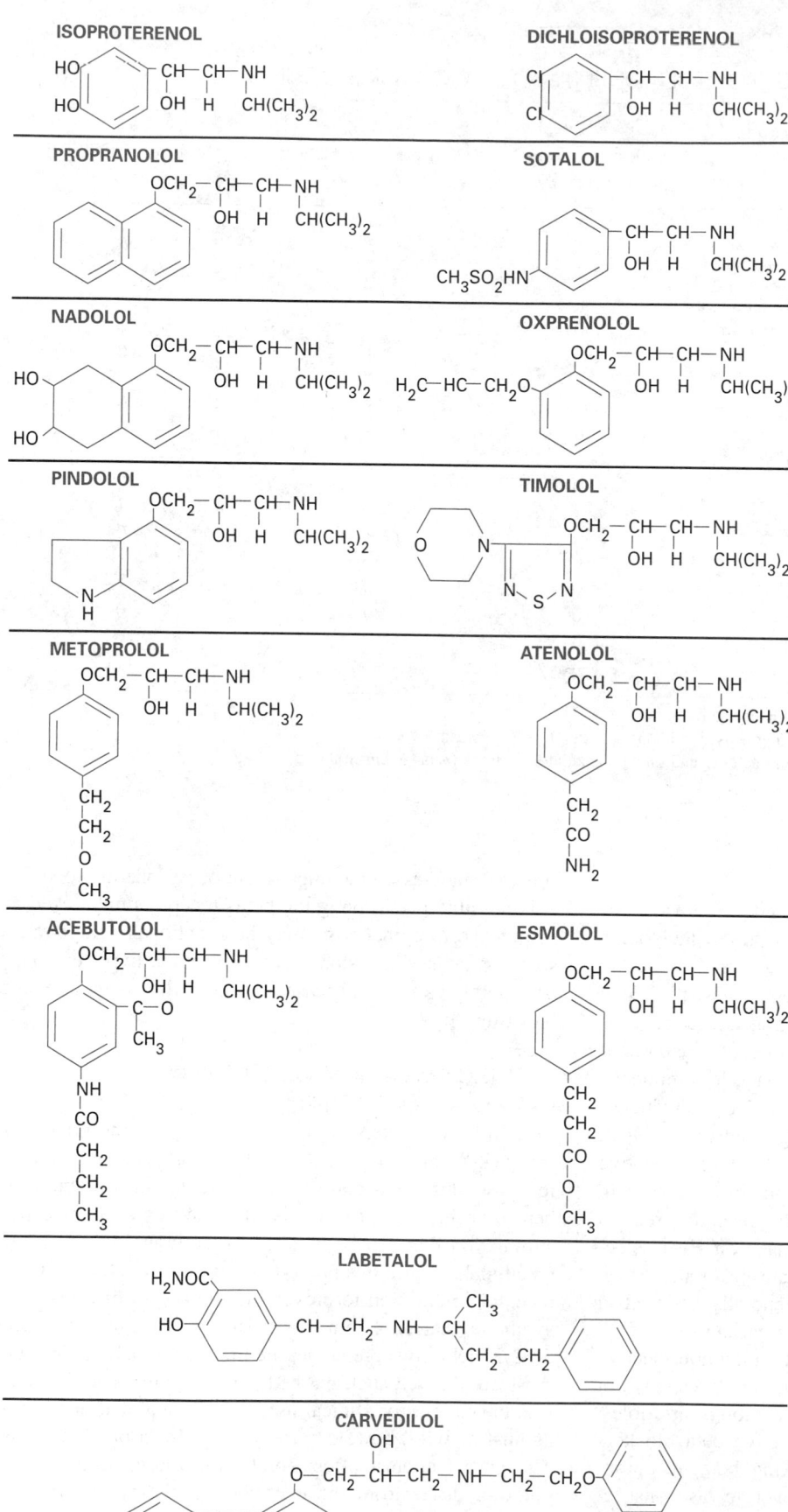

FIGURE 54-1

Molecular structure of the beta-adrenergic agonist isoproterenol and some beta-adrenergic blocking drugs.

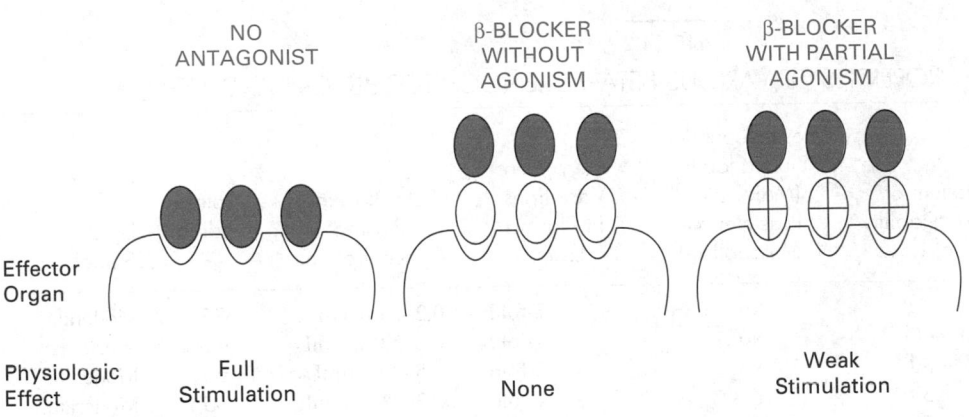

NO ANTAGONIST	β-BLOCKER WITHOUT AGONISM	β-BLOCKER WITH PARTIAL AGONISM

Effector Organ

Physiologic Effect — Full Stimulation — None — Weak Stimulation

FIGURE 54-2

Physiologic effects of beta-blocking drugs with and without partial agonist activity in the presence of circulating catecholamines. When circulating catecholamines (●) combine with beta-adrenergic receptors, they produce a full physiologic response. When these receptors are occupied by a beta blocker lacking partial agonist activity (○), no physiologic effects from catecholamine stimulation can occur. A beta-blocking drug with partial agonist activity (⊕) also blocks the binding of catecholamines to beta-adrenergic receptors, but the drug also causes a relatively weak stimulation of the receptor. (From Frishman,[22] with permission.)

receptor is high. In the treatment of patients with arrhythmias, angina pectoris of effort, and systemic arterial hypertension, drugs with mild-to-moderate partial agonist activity appear to be as efficacious as are beta blockers lacking this property. It is still debated whether the presence of partial agonist activity in a beta blocker constitutes an overall advantage or disadvantage in cardiac therapy.[22] In general, beta blockers can cause a 20 percent reduction in cardiac output both at rest and with maximal exercise. Drugs with partial agonist activity cause less slowing of the heart rate at rest than do propranolol and metoprolol, although the increments in heart rate with exercise are similarly blunted. These beta-blocking agents reduce peripheral vascular resistance and may also cause less depression of atrioventricular conduction compared with drugs lacking these properties.[22,28] Some investigators claim that partial agonist activity in a beta blocker would protect against myocardial depression, adverse lipid changes, bronchial asthma, and peripheral vascular complications, caused by propranolol.[22,28–30] The evidence to support these claims is not conclusive, and more definitive clinical trials will be necessary to resolve these issues.

ALPHA-ADRENERGIC ACTIVITY

Labetalol is a beta blocker with antagonistic properties at both alpha and beta adrenoceptors, and it has direct vasodilator activity.[2,3] Labetalol has been shown to be 6 to 10 times less potent than phentolamine at alpha-adrenergic receptors and 1.5 to 4 times less potent than propranolol at beta-adrenergic receptors; it is itself 4 to 16 times less potent at alpha than at beta adrenoceptors.[2,3] Like other beta blockers, it is useful in the treatment of hypertension and angina pectoris.[2,31] Unlike most beta blockers, however, the additional alpha-adrenergic blocking actions of labetalol lead to an immediate reduction in peripheral vascular resistance that may maintain cardiac output while arterial pressure is reduced.[2] Whether or not concomitant alpha-adrenergic blocking activity

is actually advantageous in a beta blocker remains to be determined.[32,33]

Carvedilol is another beta blocker having additional alpha-blocking activity. Compared to labetalol, carvedilol has a ratio of alpha$_1$ to beta blockade of 1:10. On a milligram-to-milligram basis, carvedilol is about two to four times more potent than propranolol as a beta blocker.[34] In addition, carvedilol has antioxidant and antiproliferative activities.[35] Carvedilol has been used for the treatment of hypertension and angina pectoris, and it was recently approved as a treatment for patients having symptomatic heart failure.[36]

DIRECT VASODILATOR ACTIVITY

Bucindolol is a nonselective beta blocker which, in addition, has direct peripheral vasodilatory activity. It is currently undergoing clinical evaluation as a treatment of symptomatic congestive heart failure.[36]

Pharmacokinetic Properties

Although the beta-blocking drugs as a group have similar therapeutic effects, their pharmacokinetic properties are markedly different (Table 54-2).[3,37] Their varied aromatic ring structures lead to differences in completeness of gastrointestinal absorption, amount of first-pass hepatic metabolism, lipid solubility, protein binding, extent of distribution in the body, penetration into the brain, concentration in the heart, rate of hepatic biotransformation, pharmacologic activity of metabolites, and renal clearance of the drugs and their metabolites, which may influence the clinical usefulness of these drugs in some patients.[1,3,37] The desirable pharmacokinetic characteristics in this group of compounds are a lack of major individual differences in bioavailability and metabolic clearance and a rate of removal of drug from active tissue sites that is slow enough to allow longer dosing intervals.[1,3,38]

The beta blockers can be divided by their pharmacokinetic properties into two broad categories: those eliminated by hepatic metabolism, which tend to have relatively short plasma half-lives, and those eliminated unchanged by the kidney, which tend to have longer half-lives.[1] Propranolol and metoprolol are both lipid-soluble, are almost completely absorbed by the small intestine, and are largely metabolized by the liver. They tend to have highly variable bioavailability and relatively short plasma half-lives.[3,19,37] A lack of correlation between the duration of clinical pharmacologic effect and plasma half-life may allow these drugs to be administered once or twice daily.[1]

TABLE 54-2

PHARMACOKINETIC PROPERTIES OF VARIOUS BETA–ADRENOCEPTOR BLOCKING DRUGS

Drug	Extent of Absorption, % of dose	Extent of Bioavailability, % of dose	Dose-Dependent Bioavailability (Major First-Pass Hepatic Metabolism)	Interpatient Variations in Plasma Levels	Beta-Blocking Plasma Concentrations	Protein Binding, %	Lipid Solubility[a]
Acebutolol	≈70	≈40	No	7-fold	0.2–2.0 μg/mL	25	Moderate
Atenolol	≈50	≈40	No	4-fold	0.2–5.0 μg/mL	<5	Weak
Betaxolol	>90	≈80	No	2-fold	5–20 ng/mL	50	Moderate
Bucindolol	≈90	≈30	Yes	4-fold	0.13–3.0 μg/mL	95	Moderate
Carteolol	≈90	≈90	No	2-fold	40–160 ng/mL	2–30	Weak
Carvedilol	>90	≈30	Yes	5- to 10-fold	10–100 ng/mL	98	Moderate
Esmolol[b]	NA[c]	NA	NA	5-fold	0.15–1.0 μg/mL	55	Weak
Labetalol	>90	≈33	Yes	10-fold	0.7–3.0 μg/mL	≈50	Weak
Metoprolol	>90	≈50	No	7-fold	50–100 ng/mL	12	Moderate
Long-acting metoprolol						92	Moderate
Nadolol	≈30	≈30	No	7-fold	50–100 ng/mL	≈30	Weak
Oxprenolol	≈90	≈40	No	5-fold	80–100 ng/mL	80	Moderate
Penbutolol	>90	≈90	No	4-fold	5–15 ng/mL	98	High
Pindolol	>90	≈90	No	4-fold	50–100 ng/mL	57	Moderate
Propranolol	>90	≈30	Yes	20-fold	50–100 ng/mL	93	High
Long-acting propranolol	>90	≈20	Yes	10- to 20-fold	20–100 ng/mL	93	High
Sotalol	≈70	≈90	No	4-fold	2.4–6.1 μg/mL	0	Weak
Timolol	>90	≈75	No	7-fold	5–10 ng/mL	≈10	

[a] Determined by the distribution ratio between octanol and water.
[b] Ultrashort-acting beta blocker available only in intravenous form.
[c] NA = not applicable.
Source: Adapted from Frishman,[2] with permission.

In contrast, agents such as atenolol and nadolol are more water-soluble, are incompletely absorbed through the gut, and are eliminated unchanged by the kidney.[20,21] They tend to have less variable bioavailability in patients with normal renal function in addition to longer half-lives, allowing one dose a day.[20,21] The longer half-lives may be useful where multidose compliance poses a problem.[20]

Long-acting sustained-release preparations of propranolol and metoprolol are available.[38] Studies have shown that long-acting propranolol and metoprolol can provide a much smoother curve of daily plasma levels than do comparable divided doses of conventional immediate-release formulations.[38,39]

Ultrashort-acting beta blockers may be useful where a short duration of action is desired, as in patients with congestive heart failure. One of these compounds, esmolol, a beta$_1$-selective drug (Tables 54-1 and 54-2) has been useful in the treatment of perioperative hypertension and supraventricular tachycardias.[40] The short half-life of approximately 15 min relates to the rapid metabolism of the drug by esterases in the blood and liver. Metabolism does not seem to be altered by disease states.[40] Currently a propranolol nasal spray that can provide immediate beta blockade is being tested in clinical trials,[41] as well as a new sublingual immediate-release formulation (esprolol).

The specific pharmacokinetic properties of individual beta blockers (first-pass metabolism, active metabolites, lipid solubility, and protein binding) may be clinically important.[3,16,37] When drugs with extensive first-pass metabolism are taken by mouth, they undergo so much hepatic biotransformation that relatively little drug reaches the systemic circulation.[1,3] Depending on the extent of first-pass effect, an oral dose of beta blocker must be larger than an intravenous dose to produce the same clinical effects.[19] Some beta-adrenergic blockers are transformed into pharmacologically active compounds (acebutolol) rather than inactive metabolites.[3] The total pharmacologic effect therefore depends on the amount of the drug administered and its active metabolites.[37] Characteristics of lipid-solubility in a beta blocker have been associated with the ability of the drug to concentrate in the brain,[1,3] and many side effects of these drugs that have not been clearly related to beta blockade may result from their actions on the central nervous system, such as lethargy, mental depression, and hallucinations.[1,21] It is still uncertain, however, whether drugs that are less lipid-soluble cause fewer of these adverse reactions.[16,20,21,42,43]

There are genetic polymorphisms that can influence the metabolism of various beta-blocking drugs, including propranolol, metoprolol, timolol, and carvedilol.[44,45] A single codon difference of CYP2D6 may explain a significant proportion of interindividual variation of propranolol's pharmacokinetics in Chinese subjects.[44] There is no effect of exercise on propranolol's pharmacokinetics.[46]

Relationship among Dose, Plasma Level, and Efficacy

Attempts have been made to establish a relation between the oral dose, the plasma level measured by gas chromatography, and the pharmacologic effect of each beta-blocking drug.[37] After administration of a certain oral dose, beta-blocking drugs that are metabolized mainly in the liver show large interindividual variation in circulating plasma levels.[1,3] Many explanations have been proposed to account for wide individual differences in the relation between plasma concentrations of beta blockers and any associated therapeutic effect. First, patients may have different levels of initial "sympathetic tone" related to circulating catecholamines and active beta-adrenoceptor binding sites and may therefore require different drug concentrations to achieve adequate beta blockade. Second, many beta blockers have flat curves of drug-level response in plasma.[37] Third, active drug isomers and active metabolites are not specifically measured in many plasma assays. Fourth, the clinical effect of a drug may last longer than the period suggested by the drug's half-life in plasma, since recycling of the beta blocker between receptor site and neuronal nerve endings may occur. Fifth, persistent binding to receptors may outlast the plasma level. Despite the lack of correlation between plasma levels and therapeutic effect, there is some evidence that a relation does exist between the logarithm of the plasma level and the beta-blocking effect as demonstrated by blockade of exercise- or isoproterenol-induced tachycardia.[19,37] Plasma levels have little to offer as therapeutic guides except for ensuring compliance and for diagnosis of overdose. Pharmacodynamic characteristics and clinical response should be used as guides in determining efficacy.

Clinical Effects and Therapeutic Applications

The therapeutic efficacy and safety of beta-blocking drugs has been well established in patients with angina pectoris, cardiac arrhythmias, and hypertension and for reducing the risk of mortality and possibly nonfatal reinfarction in survivors of acute myocardial infarction.[1,3,7] These drugs may be useful as a primary protection against cardiovascular morbidity and mortality in hypertensive patients (Chap. 58). The drugs are also used for a multitude of other cardiac (Table 54-3)[2,3,7] and noncardiac[2,3,16] uses.

EFFECTS ON ELEVATED SYSTEMIC BLOOD PRESSURE
Beta blockers are effective in reducing the blood pressure of many patients with systemic arterial hypertension, including elderly patients with isolated systolic hypertension,[47,48] and

TABLE 54-3

REPORTED CARDIOVASCULAR INDICATIONS FOR BETA–ADRENOCEPTOR BLOCKING DRUGS

Hypertension[a] (systolic and diastolic)
Isolated systolic hypertension in the elderly
Angina pectoris[a]
"Silent" myocardial ischemia
Supraventricular arrhythmias[a]
Ventricular arrhythmias[a]
Reducing the risk of mortality and reinfarction in survivors of acute myocardial infarction[a]
Hyperacute phase of myocardial infarction[a]
Dissection of aorta
Hypertrophic cardiomyopathy[a]
Reversing left ventricular hypertrophy
Digitalis intoxication
Mitral valve prolapse
QT interval prolongation syndrome
Tetralogy of Fallot
Mitral stenosis
Congestive cardiomyopathy[a]
Fetal tachycardia
Neurocirculatory asthenia

[a] Indications formally approved by the Food and Drug Administration.

were cited as first-line treatment by the Fifth and Sixth Reports of the Joint National Committee on Detection, Evaluation and Treatment of High Blood Pressure (JNC-V).[49] There is, however, no consensus as to the mechanism or mechanisms by which these drugs lower blood pressure. The immediate effect of beta blockers in hypertensives is a decrease of cardiac output by about 20 percent with no change in arterial pressure and a calculated initial increase in peripheral resistance. When the drug is effective, peripheral resistance falls over the next 12 to 36 h, with a resultant fall in arterial pressure. Labetalol, because of its alpha blockade, may be used to lower blood pressure acutely, which leads to immediate arterial vasodilatation. It is probable that some or all of the proposed mechanisms shown in Table 54-4 play a part. Beta blockers without vasodilatory activity appear to be more efficacious in white patients and younger patients than they are in elderly or black patients.[50]

EFFECTS IN ANGINA PECTORIS
Ahlquist[51] demonstrated that sympathetic innervation of the heart mediates the release of norepinephrine, activating beta adrenoceptors in myocardial cells. This adrenergic stimulation causes an increment in heart rate, isometric contractile force, and maximal velocity of muscle fiber shortening, all of which lead to an increase in cardiac work and myocardial oxygen consumption.[3] The decrease in intraventricular pressure and volume caused by the sympathetic-mediated enhancement of cardiac contractility tends, on the other hand, to reduce myocardial oxygen consumption by reducing myocardial wall tension (LaPlace's law).[52] Although there is a net increase in myocardial oxygen demand, this is normally balanced by an

TABLE 54-4

PROPOSED MECHANISMS TO EXPLAIN THE
ANTIHYPERTENSIVE ACTIONS OF BETA BLOCKERS

Reduction in cardiac output
Inhibition of renin
CNS effects
Effects on prejunctional beta receptors: reductions in
    norepinephrine release
Reduction in peripheral vascular resistance
Improvement in vascular compliance
Reduction in vasomotor tone
Reduction in plasma volume
Resetting of baroreceptor levels
Attenuation of pressor response to catecholamines with
    exercise and stress

Source: From Frishman,[2] with permission.

increase in coronary blood flow. Angina pectoris occurs when oxygen demand exceeds supply, as when coronary blood flow is restricted by coronary atherosclerosis. Since the conditions that precipitate anginal attacks—such as exercise, emotional stress, food, and so on—cause an increase in cardiac sympathetic activity, it might be expected that blockade of cardiac beta-adrenoceptors would relieve the anginal symptoms. It is on this basis that the early clinical studies with beta-blocking drugs in patients with angina pectoris were initiated.[3]

Three main factors—heart rate, ventricular systolic pressure, and the size of the left ventricle—contribute to the myocardial oxygen requirements of the left ventricle. Of these, heart rate and systolic pressure are dominant, so that the product of heart rate and systolic blood pressure is a reliable index to predict the onset of angina in a given patient.[53] Myocardial contractility is also an important contributor to this effect.[54] (See also Chap. 3)

A beta-blockade reduction in heart rate has two favorable consequences: (1) a decease in blood pressure–heart rate product, which reduces myocardial oxygen needs, and (2) a longer diastolic filling time associated with a slower heart rate, which allows for increased coronary perfusion. Beta blockade also reduces exercise-induced blood pressure increments, the velocity of cardiac contraction, and oxygen consumption at any patient workload.[53] Pretreatment heart rate variability or low exercise tolerance may predict which patients will respond best to treatment with beta blockade.[55] Despite the favorable effects on heart rate, the blunting of myocardial contractility with beta blockers may also be an important mechanism for their antianginal benefit.[54,56]

Studies in dogs have shown that propranolol causes a decrease in coronary blood flow.[53] Subsequent experimental animal studies, however, have demonstrated that beta-blocker-induced shunting occurs in the coronary circulation, maintaining blood flow to ischemic areas, especially in the subendocardial region.[53] In human beings, concomitantly with the decrease in myocardial oxygen consumption, beta blockers can reduce coronary blood flow with a rise in coronary vascular resistance.[3] On the basis of coronary autoregulation, the overall reduction in myocardial oxygen utilization caused by beta blockers explains this physiological decrease in coronary blood flow.[53]

Virtually all beta blockers, whether or not they have partial agonist activity, alpha-blocking effects, membrane-stabilizing activity, and general or selective beta-blocking properties, produce some degree of increased work capacity without pain in patients with angina pectoris. Therefore, it must be concluded that this results from their common property: blockade of cardiac beta receptors. Both D- and L-propranolol have membrane-stabilizing activity, but only L-propranolol has significant beta-blocking activity. The racemic mixture (D- and L-propranolol) causes a decrease in both heart rate and force of contraction in dogs, while the D-isomer has hardly any effect.[3] In human beings, D-propranolol, which has "membrane" activity but no beta-blocking properties, has been found to be ineffective in relieving angina pectoris even at very high doses.[3]

Although exercise tolerance improves with beta blockade, the increments in heart rate and blood pressure with exercise are blunted, and the rate-pressure product (systolic blood pressure times heart rate) achieved when pain occurs is lower than that reached during a control run.[57] The depressed pressure-rate product at the onset of pain (about 20 percent reduction from control) is reported to occur with various beta-blocking drugs. Thus, although there is increased exercise tolerance with beta blockade, patients exercise less than might be expected, since cardiac output is reduced about 20 percent at each level of exercise.

COMBINED USE OF BETA BLOCKERS WITH OTHER ANTIANGINAL THERAPIES IN AGINA PECTORIS

Nitrates

Combined therapy with nitrates and beta blockers may be more efficacious for the treatment of angina pectoris than the use of either drug alone.[58] The primary effects of beta blockers are to cause a reduction in both resting heart rate and the response of heart rate to exercise. Since nitrates produce a reflex increase in heart rate and contractility owing to a reduction in arterial pressure, concomitant beta-blocker therapy is extremely effective because it blocks this reflex increment in the heart rate. Similarly, the preservation of diastolic coronary flow with a reduced heart rate is also beneficial.[53] In patients with a propensity for myocardial failure who may have a slight increase in heart size with the beta blockers, the nitrates counteract this tendency by reducing heart size as a result of their peripheral venodilator effects. During the administration of nitrates, the reflex increase in contractility that is mediated through the sympathetic nervous system will be checked by the presence of beta blockers. Similarly, the increase in coronary resistance associated with beta-blocker administration can be ameliorated by the administration of nitrates.[53] Nitrates will also dilate coronary collateral vessels, if present, and this may also help to prevent angina (see also Chap. 45).

Calcium Channel Blockers

Combined therapy with beta-adrenergic and calcium channel blockers (CCBs) can provide clinical benefits for patients with angina pectoris who still remain symptomatic with either agent used alone.[59–61] Because adverse cardiovascular effects can occur, however, patients being considered for such treatment must be carefully selected and observed.[59]

ANGINA AT REST AND VASOSPASTIC ANGINA

Angina pectoris can be caused by multiple mechanisms, including coronary vasospasm, myocardial bridging, and thrombosis, which appear to be responsible for ischemia in a significant proportion of patients with unstable angina and angina at rest.[59,62] Therefore, beta blockers that primarily reduce myocardial oxygen consumption but fail to exert vasodilating effects on coronary vasculature may not be totally effective in patients in whom angina is caused or increased by dynamic alterations in coronary luminal diameter. Despite potential dangers in rest and vasospastic angina, beta blockers have been used successfully as monotherapy and in combination with vasodilating agents in many of these patients[58] (see Chap. 46).

ELECTROPHYSIOLOGIC AND ANTIARRHYTHMIC EFFECTS

Adrenoceptor blocking drugs have two main effects on the electrophysiologic properties of specialized cardiac tissue (Table 54-5).[63] The first effect results from specific blockade of adrenergic stimulation of cardiac pacemaker potentials. In concentrations causing significant inhibition of adrenergic receptors, beta blockers produce little change in the transmembrane potentials of cardiac muscle. By competitively inhibiting adrenergic stimulation, however, beta blockers decrease the slope of phase 4 depolarization and the spontaneous firing rate of sinus or ectopic pacemakers and thus decrease automaticity. Arrhythmias occurring in the setting of enhanced automaticity—as seen in myocardial infarction, digitalis toxicity, hyperthyroidism, and pheochromocytoma—would therefore be expected to respond well to beta blockade.[2,63] Inhomogeneity of catecholamine release in the myocardium, especially

---

TABLE 54-5
ANTIARRHYTHMIC PROPERTIES OF BETA BLOCKERS

Beta blockade
   Electrophysiology: depress excitability and conduction
   Prevention of ischemia: decreased automaticity, inhibit
     reentrant mechanisms
Membrane-stabilizing effects
   Local anesthetic "quinidine-like" properties: depress
     excitability, prolong refractory period, delay conduction
   Clinically: probably not significant
Special pharmacologic properties
   Beta$_1$ selectivity, intrinsic sympathomimetic activity
     (do not appear to contribute to antiarrhythmic
     effectiveness)

Source: From Frishman,[2] with permission.

---

in the ischemic or failing ventricle, may induce or increase ventricular irritability. In this circumstance, beta blockade may reduce ventricular arrhythmias or their evolution.

The second electrophysiologic effect of beta blockers involves membrane-stabilizing action, also known as "quinidine-like" or "local anesthetic" action, which is observed only at very high dose levels. This property is unrelated to inhibition of catecholamine action and is possessed equally by both the D- and L-isomers of the drugs (D-isomers have almost no beta-blocking activity).[63] Characteristic of this effect is a reduction in the rate of rise of the intracardiac action potential without an effect on the spike duration of the resting potential.[63] Associated features include an elevated electric threshold of excitability, a delay in conduction velocity, and a significant increase in the effective refractory period. This effect and its attendant changes have been explained by inhibition of the depolarizing inward sodium current.[63] There is a greater antifibrillatory effect when beta blockers are combined with some other antiarrhythmics[64] (see also Chap 30).

Sotalol is unique among the beta blockers in that it possesses class III antiarrhythmic properties, causing prolongation of the action potential period and thus delaying repolarization.[65] Clinical studies have verified the efficacy of sotalol in control of arrhythmias, but additional investigation will be required to determine whether its class III antiarrhythmic properties contribute significantly to its efficacy as an antiarrhythmic agent. Unfortunately, a recent study has demonstrated an increased mortality risk with *d*-sotalol, the stereoisomer with type III antiarrhythmic activity and no beta-blocking effect.[65]

The most important mechanism underlying the antiarrhythmic effect of beta blockers, with the possible exclusion of sotalol, is believed to be beta blockade with resultant inhibition of pacemaker potentials. The contribution of membrane-stabilizing action does not appear to be clinically significant. In vitro experiments with human ventricular muscle have shown that the concentration of propranolol required for membrane stabilizing is 50 to 100 times the concentration that is usually associated with inhibition of exercise-induced tachycardia and at which only beta-blocking effects occur. Moreover, D-propranolol, which possesses membrane-stabilizing properties but no beta-blocking action, is a weak antiarrhythmic even at high doses, while beta blockers devoid of membrane-stabilizing action (atenolol, esmolol, metoprolol, nadolol, pindolol, etc.) have been shown to be effective antiarrhythmic drugs.[2,3] Differences in overall clinical usefulness of beta blockers for arrhythmia are related to their other associated pharmacologic properties.[2,3]

THERAPEUTIC USES IN CARDIAC ARRHYTHMIAS

Beta-adrenergic blocking drugs have become an important treatment modality for various cardiac arrhythmias (Table 54-6).[2,3,63,66] Although it has long been believed that beta blockers are more effective in treating supraventricular arrhythmias than ventricular arrhythmias, it has only recently been appreciated that this may not be the case.[67,68] These

TABLE 54-6

EFFECTS OF BETA BLOCKERS IN VARIOUS ARRHYTHMIAS

SUPRAVENTRICULAR

Sinus tachycardia: Treat underlying disorder; excellent response to beta blocker if need to control rate (e.g., ischemia).

Atrial fibrillation: Beta blockers reduce rate, rarely restore sinus rhythm, may be useful in combination with digoxin.

Atrial flutter: Beta blockers reduce rate, sometimes restore sinus rhythm.

Atrial tachycardia: Effective in slowing ventricular rate, may restore sinus rhythm; useful in prophylaxis.

VENTRICULAR

Premature ventricular contractions: Good response to beta blockers, especially digitalis-induced, exercise (ischemia-induced, mitral valve prolapse, or hypertrophic cardiomyopathy).

Ventricular tachycardia: Effective as quinidine, most effective in digitalis toxicity or exercise (ischemia)-induced.

Ventricular fibrillation: Electrical defibrillation is treatment of choice. Beta blockers can be used to prevent recurrence in cases of excess digitalis or sympathomimetic amines; they appear to be effective in reducing the incidence of ventricular fibrillation and sudden death after myocardial infarction.

Source: From Frishman,[2] with permission.

agents can be quite useful in the treatment of ventricular tachyarrhythmias in the setting of myocardial ischemia, mitral valve prolapse, and other cardiovascular conditions.[63,69–74] A high prevalence of antibodies against beta$_1$ and beta$_2$ adrenoceptors has been observed in patients with atrial arrhythmias, ventricular arrhythmias, and conduction disturbances[75] (see also Chap. 27).

EFFECTS IN SURVIVORS OF ACUTE MYOCARDIAL INFARCTION

Beta-adrenergic blockers have beneficial effects on many determinants of myocardial ischemia (Table 54-7).[2,3,53,76] The results of placebo-controlled, long-term treatment trials with some beta-blocking drugs in survivors of acute myocardial infarction have demonstrated a favorable effect on total mortality; cardiovascular mortality, including sudden and nonsudden cardiac deaths; and the incidence of nonfatal reinfarction.[7,77,78] These beneficial results with beta-blocker therapy can be explained by both the antiarrhythmic (Table 54-7) and anti-ischemic effects of these drugs.[53,69,79–82] It has also been proposed that beta blockers could reduce the risk of atherosclerotic plaque fissure and subsequent thrombosis.[83] Two nonselective beta blockers, propranolol and timolol, have been approved for reducing the risk of mortality in infarct survivors when started 5 to 28 days after an infarction. Metoprolol and atenolol, two beta$_1$-selective blockers, are approved for the same indication and can both be used intravenously in the hyperacute phase of a myocardial infarction. Beta blockers have also been suggested as a treatment for reducing the extent of myocardial injury[7,84] and mortality during the hyperacute phase of myocardial infarction,[8,85] but their exact role in this situation remains unclear. Intravenous and oral atenolol have been shown to be effective in causing a modest reduction in early mortality when given during the hyperacute phase of acute myocardial infarction.[8] Atenolol and metoprolol reduce early infarct mortality by 15 percent,[8,85] an effect that may be improved upon when beta-adrenergic blockade is combined with acute thrombolytic therapy. Metoprolol combined with acute thrombolysis has been evaluated in the Thrombolysis in Myocardial Infarction (TIMI) trial II.[9] Despite all the evidence showing that beta blockers are beneficial in patients surviving myocardial infarction,[86–89] they are considerably underused in clinical practice. Postinfarction, beta blockade is strongly indicated, especially when the ejection fraction is markedly reduced. With reasonable monitoring, increased heart failure is generally not a problem. Should it occur, it can readily be treated without losing the substantial mortality benefit of beta blockers (see also Chap. 47).

"SILENT" MYOCARDIAL ISCHEMIA

In recent years, investigators have observed that not all myocardial ischemic episodes detected by electrocardiography (ECG) are associated with detectable symptoms.[90] Positron emission imaging techniques have validated the theory that these silent ischemic episodes are indicative of true myocardial ischemia. Compared with symptomatic ischemia, the prognostic importance of silent myocardial ischemia occur-

TABLE 54-7

POSSIBLE MECHANISMS BY WHICH BETA BLOCKERS PROTECT THE ISCHEMIC MYOCARDIUM

Reduction in myocardial consumption, heart rate, blood pressure, and myocardial contractility

Augmentation of coronary blood flow, increase in diastolic perfusion time by reducing heart rate, augmentation of collateral blood flow, and redistribution of blood flow to ischemic areas

Prevention or attenuation of atherosclerotic plaque, rupture, and subsequent coronary thrombosis

Alterations in myocardial substrate utilization

Decrease in microvascular damage

Stabilization of cell and lysosomal membranes

Shift of oxyhemoglobin dissociation curve to the right

Inhibition of platelet aggregation

ring at rest and/or during exercise has not been determined. Beta blockers are as successful in reducing the frequency of silent ischemic episodes detected by ambulatory ECG monitoring as they are in reducing the frequency of painful ischemic events.[90–95]

Other Cardiovascular Applications

Although beta blockers have been studied extensively in patients with angina pectoris, arrhythmias, and hypertension, they have also been shown to be safe and effective in diabetic patients[96] and for other cardiovascular conditions (Table 54-3), some of which are described below.

HYPERTROPHIC CARDIOMYOPATHY

Beta-blocking drugs have been proven effective in therapy for patients with hypertrophic cardiomyopathy and idiopathic hypertrophic subaortic stenosis (IHSS).[97] These drugs are useful in controlling the symptoms: dyspnea, angina, and syncope.[2,3] Beta blockers have also been shown to lower the intraventricular pressure gradient both at rest and with exercise.

The outflow pressure gradient is not the only abnormality in hypertrophic cardiomyopathy; more important is the loss of ventricular compliance, which impedes normal left ventricular function. As shown by invasive and noninvasive methods, propranolol can improve left ventricular function in this condition.[3] The drug also produces favorable changes in ventricular compliance while it relieves symptoms. Moreover, the slowing of the heart rate both at rest and with exercise tends to increase diastolic size of the ventricle, which may decrease filling pressures while also increasing end-systolic volume, so that myocardial obstruction to outflow is reduced. Propranolol has been approved for this condition, and may be combined with the CCB verapamil in patients who do not respond to the beta blocker alone.

The salutary hemodynamic and symptomatic effects produced by propranolol derive from its inhibition of sympathetic stimulation of the heart.[3] There is no evidence that the drug alters the primary cardiomyopathic process; many patients remain in or return to their severely symptomatic state and some die despite its administration[97] (see also Chap. 74).

DILATED CARDIOMYOPATHY

The acute use of intravenous sympathomimetic amines to affect an acute increase in myocardial contractility and ventricular function through stimulation of the beta-adrenergic receptor had prompted the hope that the use of oral catecholamine analogs could provide long-term benefit for patients with severe heart failure.[98] Recent observations concerning the regulation of the myocardial adrenergic receptor and abnormalities of beta-receptor-mediated stimulation of the failing myocardium, however, have caused a critical reappraisal of the scientific validity of sustained stimulation of the beta adrenoceptor.[10,99,100] In contrast, recent evidence suggests that beta-receptor blockade may, when tolerated, have a favorable effect on the underlying cardiomyopathic process.[101]

Enhanced sympathetic activation occurs as congestive heart failure evolves and is associated with decreased exercise tolerance,[102] hemodynamic abnormalities,[103] and increased mortality.[104] Increases in sympathetic tone can potentiate the renin-angiotensin system, leading to increased salt and water retention, arterial and venous constriction, and increments in ventricular preload and afterload.[101] Catecholamines in excess can increase heart rate and cause coronary vasoconstriction.[53] They can adversely influence myocardial contractility on the cellular level[105] while causing myocyte hypertrophy[106] and vascular remodeling. Catecholamines can stimulate growth and provoke oxidative stress in terminally differentiated cardiac cells; these two factors can potentially trigger the process of programmed cell death known as *apoptosis*.[107] Finally, they can increase the risk of sudden death in heart failure by adversely influencing the electrophysiologic properties of the failing heart[108] (see also Chap. 73).

Controlled trials over the last 20 years with several different beta blockers in patients with both ischemic and nonischemic cardiomyopathy have shown that these drugs, as demonstrated primarily with metoprolol and carvedilol, could improve symptoms, ventricular function, and functional capacity while reducing the need for hospitalization.[109–125] A series of placebo-controlled clinical trials with the alpha-beta blocker carvedilol[36,126–129] showed a mortality benefit in patients with New York Heart Association class II–III heart failure when the drug was used in addition to diuretics, angiotensin-converting enzyme inhibitors, and digoxin. Additional placebo-controlled mortality studies are currently in progress in patients with congestive heart failure (CHF), evaluating immediate- and sustained-release metoprolol, bisoprolol, and the vasodilator–beta blockers bucindolol and carvedilol.

The mechanisms of benefit from beta-blocker use are currently not known. Possible mechanisms for beta-blocker benefit in chronic heart failure are listed in Table 54-8 and include the upregulation of impaired beta-receptor expression in the heart[10,130] and an improvement in impaired baroreceptor functioning that can inhibit excess sympathetic outflow.[131]

MITRAL VALVE PROLAPSE

This auscultatory complex, characterized by a nonejection systolic click, a late systolic murmur, or a midsystolic click followed by a late systolic murmur, is associated with various degrees of myxomatous changes primarily in the posterior leaflet of the mitral valve, leading to its systolic motion into the atrium.[132] Atypical chest pain, malignant arrhythmias, and nonspecific ST- and T-wave abnormalities have been observed with this condition. By decreasing sympathetic tone, beta blockers have been shown to be useful for relieving the chest pains and palpitations that many of these patients experience and for reducing the incidence of life-threatening arrhythmias and other ECG abnormalities (see also Chap. 65).

AORTIC DISSECTION

Beta-adrenergic blockade plays a major role in the treatment of acute aortic dissection. During the hyperacute phase, beta-

TABLE 54-8

POSSIBLE MECHANISMS BY WHICH BETA BLOCKERS IMPROVE VENTRICULAR
FUNCTION IN CHRONIC CONGESTIVE HEART FAILURE

Upregulation of beta receptors
Direct myocardial protective action against catecholamine toxicity
Improved ability of noradrenergic sympathetic nerves to synthesize norepinephrine
Decreased release of norepinephrine from sympathetic nerve endings
Decreased stimulation of other vasoconstrictive systems including renin-angiotensin-aldo-
    sterone, vasopressin, and endothelin
Potentiation of kallikrein-kinin system and natural vasodilatation (increase in bradykinin)
Antiarrhythmic effects raising ventricular fibrillation threshold
Protection against catecholamine-induced hypokalemia
Increase in coronary blood flow by reducing heart rate and improving diastolic perfusion
    time; possible coronary dilation with vasodilator–beta blocker
Restoration of abnormal baroreflex function
Prevention of ventricular muscle hypertrophy and vascular remodeling
Antioxidant effects (carvedilol?)
Shift from free fatty acid to carbohydrate metabolism (improved metabolic efficiency)
Vasodilation (e.g., bucindolol, carvedilol)
Antiapoptosis effect
Improved left atrial contribution to ventricular filling

blocking agents reduce the force and velocity of myocardial contraction (*dP/dt*) and hence the progression of the dissecting hematoma.[3] Moreover, such administration must be initiated simultaneously with the institution of other antihypertensive therapy, which may cause reflex tachycardia and increases in cardiac output—factors that can aggravate the dissection process. Initially, propranolol is administered intravenously to reduce the heart rate to below 60 beats per minute. Once a patient is stabilized and long-term medical management is contemplated, the patient should be maintained on oral beta-blocker therapy to prevent recurrence[3] (see also Chap. 98).

Long-term beta-blocker therapy may also reduce the risk of aortic dissection in patients prone to this complication (e.g., Marfan's syndrome)[133] (see also Chap. 85). Systolic time intervals are used to assess the adequacy of beta blockade in children with Marfan's syndrome.[3]

TETRALOGY OF FALLOT

By reducing the effects of increased adrenergic tone on the right ventricular infundibulum in tetralogy of Fallot, beta blockers have been shown to be useful for the treatment of severe hypoxic spells and hypercyanotic attacks.[3] With chronic use, these drugs have also been shown to prevent prolonged hypoxic spells. These drugs should be considered palliative only; definitive surgical repair of this condition is usually required (see also Chap. 70).

QT-INTERVAL PROLONGATION SYNDROME

The syndrome of ECG QT-interval prolongation is usually a congenital condition associated with deafness, syncope, and sudden death.[3] Abnormalities of the sympathetic nervous system in the heart have been proposed as explanations for the electrophysiologic aberrations seen in these patients. Propran-

olol appears to be the most effective drug for treatment of this syndrome. It reduces the frequency of syncopal episodes in most patients and may prevent sudden death. This drug will reduce the QT interval on the ECG (see also Chap. 27).

REGRESSION OF LEFT VENTRICULAR HYPERTROPHY

Left ventricular hypertrophy induced by systemic arterial hypertension is an independent risk factor for cardiovascular mortality and morbidity.[134] Regression of left ventricular hypertrophy with drug therapy is feasible and may improve patient outcome.[134] Beta blockers can cause regression of left ventricular hypertrophy, as determined by echocardiography, with or without an associated reduction in blood pressure.[134]

SYNCOPE

Vasovagal syncope is the most common form of syncope observed. Upright tilt-table testing with isoproterenol can help differentiate vasovagal syncope from other forms.[135] Beta blockers have been shown to be useful for both relieving symptoms and normalizing abnormal tilt-table tests in patients with syncope.[135,136] The mechanism for benefit with beta blockers may be an interruption of the Bezold-Jarisch reflex or an enhancement of peripheral vasoconstriction by blockade of beta$_2$-adrenergic receptors[135] (see also Chap. 35).

Noncardiovascular Applications

Beta-adrenergic receptors are ubiquitous in the human body, and their blockade affects a variety of organ and metabolic systems.[2,3,16] Some noncardiovascular uses of beta blockers—including the treatment of glaucoma, migraine headache, and essential tremor—have been approved by the Food and Drug Administration (FDA).[1,3,137] The combination of nitrates and beta blockers was recently shown to be effective in preventing bleeding from esophageal varices.[138]

Adverse Effects of Beta Blockers

Evaluation of adverse effects is complex because of the use of different definitions of side effects, the kinds of patients studied, study design features, and different methods of ascertaining and reporting adverse side effects from study to study.[139,140] Overall, the types and frequencies of adverse effects attributed to various beta-blocker compounds appear similar.[139,140] The side-effect profiles resemble those seen with concurrent placebo treatments, attesting to the remarkable safety margin of the beta blockers.

Adverse effects fall in two categories: (1) those from known pharmacologic consequences of beta-adrenoceptor blockade and (2) other reactions apart from beta-adrenoceptor blockade. The first type includes asthma, increased heart failure, hypoglycemia, bradycardia and heart block, intermittent claudication, and Raynaud's phenomenon. The incidence of these adverse effects varies with the beta blocker used.[2,139,140] Side effects of the second category are rare. They include an unusual oculomucocutaneous reaction and the possibility of carcinogenesis.[2,139,140]

OVERDOSAGE

Suicide attempts and accidental overdosing with beta blockers are being described with increasing frequency. Since beta blockers are competitive pharmacologic antagonists, their life-threatening effects (bradycardia, myocardial and ventilatory failure) can be overcome with an immediate infusion of beta agonist agents such as isoproterenol and dobutamine.[27] In situations where catecholamines are not effective, intravenous glucagon, amrinone, or milrinone have been used.[27]

Close monitoring of cardiorespiratory function is necessary for at least 24 h after the patient responds to therapy. Patients who recover usually have no long-term sequelae; however, they should be observed for the cardiac signs of sudden beta-blocker withdrawal.[27]

BETA-BLOCKER WITHDRAWAL

After abrupt cessation of chronic beta-blocker therapy, exacerbation of angina pectoris and, in some cases, acute myocardial infarction and death have been reported.[13,141] Observations made in multiple double-blind randomized trials have confirmed the reality of a propranolol withdrawal reaction.[13,142] The mechanism for this reaction is unclear. There is some evidence that the withdrawal phenomenon may be due to the generation of additional beta adrenoceptors during the period of beta-adrenoceptor blockade. When the beta blocker is then withdrawn, the increased beta-receptor population readily results in an excessive beta-receptor stimulation that is clinically important when the delivery and use of oxygen are finely balanced, as occurs in ischemic heart disease. Other suggested mechanisms for the withdrawal reaction include heightened platelet aggregability, an elevation in thyroid hormone activity, and an increase in circulating catecholamines.[13]

Adverse Noncardiac Side Effects Related to Beta-Adrenergic Blockade

EFFECT ON VENTILATORY FUNCTION

The bronchodilatory effects of catecholamines on the bronchial beta$_2$ adrenoceptors are inhibited by nonselective beta blockers, such as propranolol or nadolol.[140] Beta-blocking compounds with partial agonist activity,[22,28] beta$_1$ selectivity,[20] and alpha-adrenergic blocking actions[143] are less likely to increase airways resistance in asthmatics. Beta$_1$ selectivity, however, is not absolute and may be lost with high therapeutic doses, as shown with atenolol and metoprolol. It is possible

in treating asthma to use a beta$_2$-selective agonist (such as albuterol) in certain patients with concomitant low-dose beta$_1$-selective blocker treatment. Alternatively, in some asthmatics, a beta$_2$ inhalant may lead to tachycardia from overflow of the agent into the general circulation. In this circumstance, modest use of an oral beta$_1$ antagonist may allow the more liberal use of a required inhalant. In general, all beta blockers should be avoided in patients with bronchospastic disease.

PERIPHERAL VASCULAR EFFECTS (RAYNAUD'S PHENOMENON)

Cold extremities and absent pulses have been reported more frequently in patients receiving beta blockers for hypertension than in those receiving methyldopa. Among the patients receiving beta blockers, the incidence of these effects was highest with propranolol and lower with drugs having beta$_1$ selectivity or intrinsic sympathomimetic activity. In some instances, vascular compromise has been severe enough to cause cyanosis and impending gangrene.[144] This is probably due to the reduction in cardiac output and blockade of beta$_2$-adrenoceptor-mediated skeletal muscle vasodilatation, resulting in unopposed beta-adrenoceptor vasoconstriction. Beta-blocking drugs with beta$_1$ selectivity or partial agonist activity do not affect peripheral vessels to the same degree as does propranolol.

Raynaud's phenomenon is one of the more common side effects of propranolol treatment. It is more troublesome with propranolol than with metoprolol, atenolol, or pindolol, probably because of the beta$_2$-blocking properties of propranolol.

Patients with peripheral vascular disease who suffer from intermittent claudication occasionally report worsening of their claudication when treated with beta-blocking drugs.[145,146] Whether or not drugs with beta$_1$ selectivity or partial agonist activity can protect against this adverse reaction has not been determined.[147]

HYPOGLYCEMIA AND HYPERGLYCEMIA

Severe hypoglycemic reactions have been described during therapy with beta-blocking drugs.[3] Some of the patients affected were insulin-dependent diabetics, while others were nondiabetic. Studies of resting normal volunteers have demonstrated that propranolol produces no alteration in blood glucose values,[3] although the hyperglycemic response to exercise is blunted.

The enhancement of insulin-induced hypoglycemia and its hemodynamic consequences may be less with beta$_1$-selective agents, where there is no blocking effect on beta$_2$ receptors, or agents with intrinsic sympathomimetic activity that may stimulate beta$_2$ receptors.[3]

There is also marked diminution in the clinical manifestations of the catecholamine discharge induced by hypoglycemia, such as tachycardia.[3] These findings suggest that beta blockers interfere with compensatory responses to hypoglycemia and can mask certain "warning signs" of this condition. Other hypoglycemic reactions, such as diaphoresis, are not affected by beta-adrenergic blockade.

HYPERLIPIDEMIA

The effects of the various beta blockers on plasma lipids and lipoproteins have been well described.[148] Nonselective beta-blocking agents can raise triglycerides and reduce high-density lipoprotein (HDL) cholesterol. This effect may not be seen with agents having partial agonism or alpha-blocking activity.

CENTRAL NERVOUS SYSTEM EFFECTS

Dreams, hallucinations, insomnia, and depression can occur during therapy with beta blockers.[16] These symptoms provide evidence of drug entry into the central nervous system (CNS) and may be more common with the highly lipid-soluble beta blockers (propranolol and metoprolol), which presumably penetrate the CNS better. It has been claimed that beta blockers with less lipid-solubility, such as atenolol and nadolol, cause fewer CNS side effects.[20,21] This claim is intriguing, but its validity has not been corroborated by other extensive clinical experiences.[42] In some patients, beta-adrenergic blockade may have an important beneficial effect in reducing anxiety and promoting a sense of well-being; in others, increased depression may be seen. The former benefits occasionally deserve a trial in selected patients.

MISCELLANEOUS SIDE EFFECTS

Diarrhea, nausea, gastric pain, constipation, and flatulence have occasionally been noted with all beta blockers (2 to 11 percent of patients).[149] Hematologic reactions are rare. Rare cases of purpura and agranulocytosis have been described with propranolol.[3]

A devastating blood pressure rebound effect has been described in patients who discontinued clonidine while being treated with nonselective beta-blocking agents. The mechanism for this may be related to an increase in circulating catecholamines and an increase in peripheral vascular resistance.[3] Whether or not beta$_1$-selective or partial agonist beta blockers have similar effects following clonidine withdrawal has not been determined. This has not been a problem with labetalol or carvedilol.[3]

Drug-Drug Interactions

Beta blockers are commonly employed, and the list of commonly used drugs with which they interact is extensive.[3,150] The majority of the reported interactions have been associated with propranolol, the best-studied beta blocker; the results may not necessarily apply to other drugs in this class.

How to Choose a Beta Blocker

The various beta-blocking compounds given in adequate dosage appear to have comparable antihypertensive, antiarrhythmic, and antianginal effects. Therefore, the beta-blocking drug of choice in an individual patient is determined by the pharmacodynamic and pharmacokinetic differences between the drugs in conjunction with the patient's other medical conditions (Table 54-9).[2,3,22]

CALCIUM CHANNEL BLOCKERS

The calcium channel blockers (CCBs) are a heterogeneous group of drugs with widely variable effects on heart muscle, sinus node function, atrioventricular (AV) conduction, peripheral blood vessels, and the coronary circulation.[151–154] Ten of these drugs—nifedipine, nicardipine, nimodipine, nisoldipine, felodipine, isradipine, amlodipine, verapamil, diltiazem, and bepridil—are approved for clinical use in the United States. An 11th agent, mibefradil, is now being evaluated by the FDA for clinical approval.

Physiologic Background: Basic Principles

Calcium ions play a fundamental role in the activation of cells. An influx of calcium ions into the cell through specific ion channels is required for myocardial contraction, for determining peripheral vascular resistance through calcium-dependent regulated tone of vascular smooth muscle, and for helping to initiate the pacemaker tissues of the heart, which are activated largely by the slow calcium current.[152]

The concept of calcium channel inhibition originated in 1960 when it was noted that prenylamine, a newly developed coronary vasodilator, depressed cardiac performance in canine heart-lung preparations.[155] Initial studies with verapamil showed that it also exerted a negative inotropic effect on the isolated myocardium in addition to having vasodilator properties.[156] These potent negative inotropic effects seemed to differentiate these drugs from the classical coronary vasodilators, such as nitroglycerin and papaverine, which have little if any myocardial depressant activity. Unlike beta-adrenergic antagonists, many of the CCBs depress cardiac contractility without altering the height or contour of the monophasic action potential.[157] Instead, they interfere with excitation-contraction coupling through reversible closure of specific calcium ion channels in the membrane of mammalian myocardial cell.[158] At that time, using effect on atrial and ventricular intracellular potentials,[159] antiarrhythmic compounds were classified as local anesthetics that decreased the maximum rate of depolarization, beta blockers, and a third class that prolonged the duration of the cardiac action potential.[160] None of these electrophysiologic actions, however, could explain the antiarrhythmic effect of verapamil.[160] Thus, a fourth class of antiarrhythmic drug, typified by verapamil, was proposed, with effects separate from those of sodium channel inhibitors and beta blockers.[159] In essence, the antiarrhythmic actions and negative inotropic effects of verapamil are mediated predominantly through interference with calcium conductance.[159]

Chemical Structure and Pharmacodynamics

STRUCTURE OF THE CALCIUM CHANNEL BLOCKERS

The structures of some of the available CCBs are shown in Fig. 54-3. Diltiazem is a benzothiazepine derivative that is

TABLE 54-9

CLINICAL SITUATIONS THAT WOULD INFLUENCE THE CHOICE OF A BETA–BLOCKING DRUG

Condition	Choice of Beta Blocker
Asthma, chronic bronchitis with bronchospasm	Avoid all beta blockers if possible, but small doses of $beta_1$-selective blockers can be used; $beta_1$ selectivity is lost with higher doses; drugs with partial agonist activity and labetalol with alpha-adrenergic blocking properties can also be used.
Congestive heart failure	Drugs with alpha-blocking activity (e.g., carvedilol) may have an advantage, although all beta blockers should be used with caution.
Angina	In patients with angina at low heart rates, drugs with partial agonist activity are probably contraindicated; patients who have angina at high heart rates but who have resting bradycardia may benefit from a drug with partial agonist activity; in vasospastic angina, labetalol may be useful; other beta blockers should be used with caution.
Atrioventricular conduction defects	Beta blockers are generally contraindicated, but drugs with partial agonist activity and labetalol can be tried with caution.
Bradycardia	Beta blockers with partial agonist activity and labetalol have less of a pulse-slowing effect and are preferable.
Raynaud's phenomenon, intermittent claudication, cold extremities	$Beta_1$-selective blocking agents, labetalol, and agents with partial agonist activity may have an advantage.
Depression	Avoid propranolol; substitute a beta blocker with partial agonist activity, or low lipid-solubility.
Diabetes mellitus	$Beta_1$-selective agents and partial agonist drugs are preferable.
Thyrotoxicosis	All agents will control symptoms, but agents without partial agonist activity are preferred.
Pheochromocytoma	Avoid all beta blockers unless an alpha blocker is given; labetalol may be used as a treatment of choice.
Renal failure	Use reduced doses of compounds largely eliminated by renal mechanisms (nadolol, sotalol, and atenolol) and drugs whose bioavailability is increased in uremia (propranolol); also consider possible accumulation of active metabolites (propranolol).
Insulin and sulfonylurea use	There is a danger of hypoglycemia; possibly less using drugs with $beta_1$ selectivity.
Clonidine	Avoid nonselective beta blockers; there is a severe rebound effect with clonidine withdrawal.
Oculomucocutaneous syndrome	Stop drug; substitute with any beta blocker.
Hyperlipidemia	Avoid nonselective beta blockers; use agents with partial agonism or $beta_1$ selectivity, or alpha-blocking activity.

Source: From Frishman,[2] with permission.

structurally unrelated to other vasodilators.[152] Nifedipine is a dihydropyridine derivative that is unrelated to the nitrates; it is lipophilic and is inactivated by light.[152] Nicardipine, amlodipine, felodipine, isradipine, nisoldipine, and nimodipine are also dihydropyridine derivatives similar in structure to nifedipine. Verapamil ([±] verapamil) has some structural similarity to papaverine.[151]

Mibefradil, a drug now approved for use in patients with hypertension and angina pectoris, is from a new structural class of benzomidazolyl-substituted tetraline derivatives (Fig. 54-4). The drug binds competitively at the verapamil binding site and interferes allosterically with the diltiazem site without affecting the dihydropyridine ion-binding site.[161]

Bepridil, which is currently available for treatment of angina pectoris, is not related chemically to other cardioactive drugs.[162]

DIFFERENTIAL EFFECTS ON SLOW CHANNELS

The most important characteristic of all CCBs is their ability to selectively inhibit the inward flow of calcium ions through permeable calcium ion channels on the cell surface membrane. As detailed below under "Electrophysiologic Effects," these agents may differ in their site of action on these channels, resulting in different pharmacologic profiles.[3] Previously, the term *slow channel* was used, but it has recently been recognized that the calcium ion current develops faster than previously thought and that there are at least two types of calcium channels, L and T.[163] The conventional calcium channel, which has been known to exist for a long time, is called the *L channel*. It is blocked by all the CCBs and its permeability is increased by catecholamines. The *T-type channel* appears at more negative potentials than the L-type and probably plays an important role in the initial depolarization of sinus and

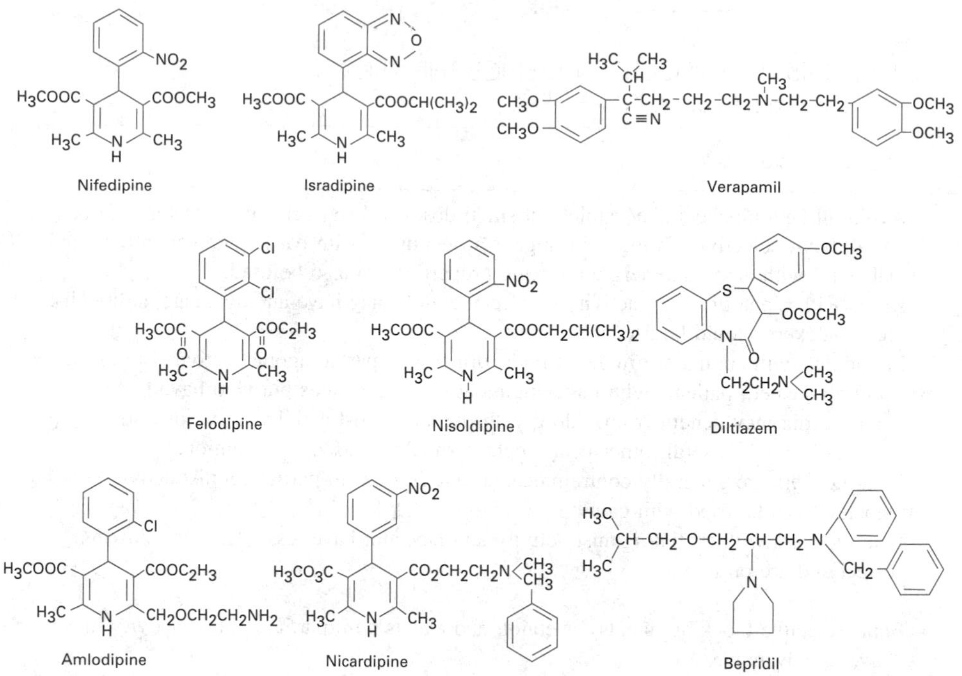

FIGURE 54-3

Chemical structures of diltiazem (a benzothiazepine derivative), nifedipine, felodipine, isradipine, amlodipine, nicardipine, nisoldipine (dihydropyridine derivatives), verapamil (structurally similar to papaverine), and bepridil (structure unlike other cardioactive drugs).

Cardiovascular Effects

EFFECTS ON MUSCULAR CONTRACTION

Calcium is the primary ionic link between neurologic excitation and mechanical contraction of cardiac, smooth, and skeletal muscle.[152] Actin and myosin are the protein filaments that slide past one another in the adenosine triphosphate (ATP)-dependent contractile process of all muscle cells. In myocardial cells, the regulatory proteins *tropomyosin* and *troponin* inhibit this process. When the myocardial cell membrane repolarizes, calcium enters the cell (L channel) and triggers the release of additional calcium from internal stores within the sarcoplasmic reticulum. Calcium released from this large intracellular reservoir then initiates contraction by combining with contraction-inhibiting sites on troponin acting through tropomyosin. With removal of the troponin-tropomyosin inhibition of sites on actin, interaction with myosin ensues, with contraction of the muscle (see also Chap. 3).

AV nodal tissue. The function of the L-type channel is to admit the substantial amount of calcium ions required for initiation of contraction via calcium-induced calcium release from the sarcoplasmic reticulum. Mibefradil is the first CCB that has selective blocking properties on the T-type channel.[164] Specific blockers for the T-type channel are not yet available, but they could be expected to inhibit the sinus and AV nodes profoundly.[163]

Bepridil possesses all the characteristics of the traditional CCBs. In addition, the drug appears to affect the sodium channel ("fast channel") and possibly the potassium channel, producing a quinidine-like effect. Bepridil specifically inhibits maximal upstroke velocity (*dV/dt* max)—that is, the influx of sodium in appropriate load dosages. The effect of bepridil on the maximum rate of depolarization has been examined; the height of the action potential is not changed; however, its duration is extended in a quinidine-like manner.

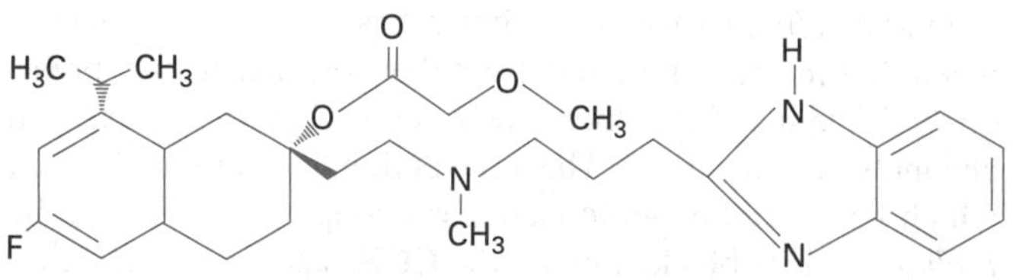

EFFECTS ON CORONARY AND PERIPHERAL ARTERIAL BLOOD VESSELS

The contraction of vascular smooth muscle such as that found in the coronary arteries is slightly different from the contraction of cardiac and skeletal muscles (Table 54-10). Myosin must be phosphorylated, and *calmodulin* is the inhibiting regulatory protein to which calcium binds. In addition, vascular smooth muscle cells have significantly less intracellular calcium stores than do myocardial cells and so rely more heavily on the influx of extracellular calcium for activation.

The observation that CCBs are significantly more effective in inhibiting contraction in coronary and peripheral arterial smooth muscle than in cardiac and skeletal muscle is of great clinical importance. This differential effect is explained by the observation that arterial smooth muscle is more dependent on external calcium entry for contraction, whereas cardiac and skeletal muscle rely on a recirculating internal pool of calcium. Because CCBs are membrane-active drugs, they reduce the entry of calcium into cells and therefore exert a much larger effect on vascular wall contraction. This preferential effect allows CCBs to dilate coronary and peripheral arteries in doses that do not severely affect myocardial contractility or have little if any effect on skeletal muscle.

FIGURE 54-4

Chemical structure of mibefradil (benzimidazolyl-substituted tetraline derivative).

TABLE 54-10

PHARMACOLOGIC EFFECTS OF CALCIUM CHANNEL BLOCKERS

	Heart Rate		Conduction		Myocardial Contractility	Peripheral Resistance	Cardiac Output	Coronary Blood Flow	Myocardial O$_2$ Demand
	Acute	Chronic	SA Node	AV Node					
Diltiazem	↓	↓	↓	↓	↓	↓	V	↑	↓
Bepridil	↓	↓	↓	—	V	—	V	↑	↓
Verapamil	↑	↓	↓	↓	↓↓	↓	V	↑	↓
Mibefradil	↓	↓	↓	↓	—	↓↓	↑ —	↑	↓
Amlodipine	↑	↑ —	—	—	—	↓↓	↑ —	↑	↓
Felodipine	↑	↑ —	—	—	—	↓↓	↑ —	↑	↓
Isradipine	↑	↑ —	—	—	—	↓↓	↑ —	↑	↓
Nicardipine	↑	↑ —	—	—	—	↓↓	↑ —	↑	↓↓
Nifedipine	↑	↑ —	—	—	↓	↓↓	↑ —	↑	↓↓
Nimodipine	↑	↑ —	—	—	—	↓↓	↑ —	↑	↓
Nisoldipine	↑	↑ —	—	—	—	↓↓	↑ —	↑	↓

Key: ↑ = increase; ↓ = decrease; — = no change; V = variable.
Source: From Frishman et al.,[238] with permission.

EFFECTS ON VEINS

The CCBs seem to be less active in veins than in arteries and, in contrast to nitrates, are ineffective at therapeutic doses for increasing venous capacitance.[152]

EFFECTS ON MYOCARDIAL CONTRACTILITY

Force generation during cardiac muscle contraction depends partly on calcium influx during membrane depolarization (Table 54-10).[152] In isolated myocardial preparations, all CCBs have been demonstrated to exert potent negative inotropic effects.[152] In guinea pig atria exposed to a drug concentration of 10^{-6} M, the order of potency for depressing the maximal rate of force development during constant pacing was found to be nifedipine > verapamil > diltiazem.[52] In dog papillary muscle, developed tension was also decreased most markedly by nifedipine; the relative potencies (on a weight basis) of verapamil and diltiazem were 1/15 and 1/40, respectively.[152]

The negative inotropic effect of the CCBs is dose-dependent.[152] The excitation-contraction coupling of vascular smooth muscle is 3 to 10 times more sensitive to the action of CCBs than is that of myocardial fibers.[152] Hence, the relatively low doses of these drugs used in vivo to produce vasodilatation or beneficial antiarrhythmic effects may not produce significant negative inotropic effects.[152] Furthermore, in intact animals and humans, the intrinsic negative inotropic properties of these compounds may be offset by a baroreceptor-mediated reflex augmentation of beta-adrenergic tone consequent to vasodilatation and a decrease in blood pressure.[165] Nifedipine and other dihydropyridines, which exert the greatest vasodilator effects among these agents, produce the strongest reflex beta-adrenergic response, which can counteract the direct negative inotropic effects. This effect, as well as the afterload reduction from arterial dilation, can result in overall enhancement of ventricular performance.[166] While the reflex mechanism plays an important role in patients with normal or nearly normal left ventricular function, it is unlikely to play a similar role in patients with severe CHF, in whom the baroreceptor sensitivity may be markedly attenuated.[167] When the newer CCBs amlodipine and mibefradil were studied in conscious normotensive rats,[161] verapamil and diltiazem were negatively inotropic while amlodipine decreased left ventricular contractility only at the highest dose used and mibefradil was less negatively inotropic than amlodipine.

Electrophysiologic Effects

While verapamil, nifedipine, diltiazem, and bepridil all depress cardiac contractility with only quantitative differences (Table 54-10), their effects on the electrophysiology of the heart are different qualitatively.[168] Local anesthetic actions of bepridil, diltiazem, and particularly of verapamil may account for some of these differences.[169] Nifedipine and other dihydropyridines have a more selective action at the slow channels, while verapamil and diltiazem, at least at higher doses, also inhibit currents in the fast channels in the manner of the local anesthetics.[170] Bepridil has definite class I antiarrhythmic properties.

Verapamil, diltiazem, and mibefradil prolong the conduction and refractoriness in the AV node; the AH interval is lengthened more than is the HV interval.[171] In therapeutic concentrations, there are no demonstrable actions on the rate of depolarization or the repolarization phases of the action potentials in atrial, ventricular, and Purkinje fibers.[168] The rate of discharge of the sinus node, which depends on the calcium ion current, is depressed by all CCBs. In vivo, this effect can be compensated or overcompensated for by activation of baroreceptor reflexes that increase sympathetic nervous activity.[168]

The antiarrhythmic actions of verapamil and diltiazem relate to their effects on nodal cardiac tissues.[168] In sinoatrial (SA) and AV nodal cells, the drugs modify slow-channel electropotentials in three ways: first, there is a decrease in the rate of rise and slope of diastolic slow depolarization and an increase in the membrane threshold potential, which reduces the rate of firing in the cell[172]; second, the action potential upstroke is decreased in amplitude, which slows conduction; and third, the duration of the action potential is increased.[172] These electrophysiologic effects are dose-related, and with doses above the clinical range, electric standstill may occur in SA and AV nodal cells. These observations and others support the concept that slow-channel activity is important in the generation of pacemaker potential in the SA node. Verapamil and diltiazem also exert a depressant effect on the AV node and in low concentrations prolong the effective refractory period.[173] Unlike beta-adrenergic blocking drugs and vagomimetic interventions, which depress AV node transmission by altering autonomic impulse traffic, verapamil and diltiazem prolong AV nodal refractoriness directly.[173] Verapamil may have additional vagomimetic effects.[168]

Bepridil has a modest depressant effect on heart rate and intranodal and infranodal conduction accompanied by a significant increment in the effective and functional refractory periods of the AV node. Unexpected findings that cannot be explained solely on the basis of slow-channel inhibition on the myocardium include lengthening of the QTc interval and significant prolongation of the atrial and ventricular effective refractory periods.

Mibefradil also has a modest depressant effect on heart rate and intranodal and infranodal conduction.[171]

Effects on Nonvascular Tissues

Calcium ions are required for contraction in all smooth muscles, and these drugs can inhibit contractions in the gastrointestinal tract.[174] Calcium is also important in excitation-secretion coupling. There is, however, no evidence that these drugs in clinical doses have significant effects on endocrine organs.[175,176] Although antiadrenergic effects of some CCBs have been suggested, further studies are needed.[142]

Some CCBs may partially inhibit adenosine diphosphate (ADP) and epinephrine-induced platelet aggregation and thromboxane release from platelets.[177–180] Experimental data suggest that verapamil and diltiazem, and to a lesser extent nifedipine, can inhibit platelet aggregation in vitro.[152] The drugs appear to be more efficacious in attenuating aggregation when they are present in the reaction mixture before aggregation begins. This can, however, interrupt or slow the rate of aggregation if added after the beginning of the reaction. In addition, the effect of aspirin in attenuating platelet aggregation appears to be potentiated in vitro in the presence of diltiazem. This has led to considerable speculation as to how much this effect may contribute to the efficacy of CCBs in the treatment of unstable angina. There has been at least one report of a patient with unstable angina being treated with

verapamil who demonstrated decreased platelet aggregability and decreased thromboxane A_2 levels.[152]

Pharmacokinetics

Although classified together, CCBs have differences in their pharmacokinetic properties.[151,181] Differences in completeness of gastrointestinal absorption, amount of first-pass hepatic metabolism, protein binding, extent of distribution in the body, and the pharmacologic actions of different metabolites may influence the clinical usefulness of these drugs in different patients.[151]

Since many of the CCBs are relatively short-acting, they are now available in various sustained-release delivery systems: diffusion type (diltiazem, verapamil), bioerosion (diltiazem, nifedipine, nicardipine), osmosis (verapamil, isradipine, nifedipine), diffusion/erosion (felodipine).[182–184] Nisoldipine was recently approved as a once-daily therapy in a coat-core formulation[185] and verapamil in a delayed-onset sustained-release osmotic drug delivery system.[186]

After administration of a certain oral dose, the CCBs, which are largely metabolized in the liver, show larger interindividual variation in circulating plasma levels.[181,187,188] In angina pectoris and hypertension, wide individual differences also exist in the relation between plasma concentrations of CCBs and their associated therapeutic effect.[187,188]

Various dihydropyridine calcium channel blockers (felodipine, nifedipine, nisoldipine) should not be administered with grapefruit juice, as it has been shown to interfere with the drug's metabolism, resulting in a mean increase in C_{max} of about threefold and mean increase in area under the plasma-concentration–time curve (AUC) of almost twofold.[189]

Cardiovascular Applications

The CCBs are available in the United States for the treatment of patients with angina pectoris (diltiazem, nifedipine, amlodipine, nicardipine, verapamil, bepridil, mibefradil), chronic treatment of systemic hypertension (verapamil, isradipine, diltiazem, amlodipine, nicardipine, nisoldipine, felodipine, mibefradil), the management of hypertensive emergencies and perioperative hypertension (intravenous nicardipine), treatment and prophylaxis of supraventricular arrhythmias (verapamil, diltiazem), and reducing morbidity and mortality in patients with subarachnoid hemorrhage (nimodipine). These drugs have also been evaluated and used for a multitude of other cardiovascular and noncardiovascular conditions.

ANGINA PECTORIS

The antianginal mechanisms of CCBs are complex (Table 54-11).[151,190–193] The drugs exert vasodilator effects on the coronary and peripheral vessels as well as depressant effects on cardiac contractility, heart rate, and conduction; all these actions may be important in mediating their antianginal effects.[190–192] These drugs are only mild dilators of epicardial vessels not in spasm, but they markedly attenuate sympathetically mediated and ergonovine-induced coronary vasocon-

TABLE 54-11

HEMODYNAMIC EFFECTS OF CALCIUM CHANNEL BLOCKERS
ON MYOCARDIAL OXYGEN SUPPLY AND DEMAND

	Verapamil	Nifedipine	Diltiazem	Bepridil	Mibefradil
Demand					
Wall tension	↑↔	↔ reflex	↔	↔	↑↔
Systolic blood pressure	↓	↓	↓	↔	↓
Ventricular volume	↑	↔	↔	↔	↑
Heart rate	↓[a]	↑ reflex	↓	↓	↓
Contractility	↓↓	↓	↓	↓	↔
Supply					
Coronary blood flow	↑	↑↑	↑	↑	↑
Coronary vascular resistance	↓	↓↓	↓	↓	↓
Spasm	↓	↓	↓	↓	↓
Diastolic perfusion time	↑	↓	↑	↑	↑
Collateral blood flow	↔	↑	↑	↔	↑

Key: ↑ = increase; ↓ = decrease; ↔ = no apparent effect
[a] Heart rate may increase sharply but decreases with long-term use.

striction; these actions provide a rational basis for effectiveness of the drugs in vasospastic ischemic syndromes.[192] In patients with exertional angina pectoris, the peripheral vasodilator actions of diltiazem, mibefradil, and verapamil and the inhibitory effects on the sinus node serve to attenuate the increases in double product that normally accompany and serve to limit exercise.[190,191,194]

Stable Angina Pectoris
Multiple double-blind placebo-controlled studies have clearly confirmed the efficacy of diltiazem,[188,193–196] nifedipine,[188,197,198] amlodipine,[199–201] nicardipine,[202] verapamil,[203–205] mibefradil, and bepridil[206] in stable angina pectoris, with patients showing a reduction in attacks of chest pain, decreased nitroglycerin consumption, and improved exercise tolerance.[207] Where reflex tachycardia does not occur, CCBs, for the most part, appear to be as safe and effective as beta blockers and nitrates when used as monotherapies.[207–210] They can also be used as single-dose therapies in hypertensive patients with angina.[207,210,211]

In choosing between a CCB and a beta-blocking drug in the management of patients with effort-related symptoms, it is apparent that some patients do better with one type of drug than with the other. Further, those agents can be used together to great advantage, especially with dihydropyridines. Unfortunately, we know little about how to predict with confidence the superior agent in a specific patient without a therapeutic trial. Verapamil and diltiazem can be used as effective alternatives in patients who remain symptomatic despite therapy with propranolol and other beta blockers and as first-time antianginal drugs in patients with contraindications to beta blockade; the use of nifedipine as a first-line drug in its original formulation was limited by the reflex tachycardia and potential

aggravation of angina that accompanied its use.[188,212] This is probably not a problem with the sustained-delivery nifedipine GITS formulation or with amlodipine.[182,201] Here again, concomitant use of beta blockers to reduce heart rate may add to efficacy and safety. Diltiazem is also approved as a once-daily treatment for angina pectoris in a sustained-delivery formulation.[213] Mibefradil was recently approved in doses of 50 and 100 mg for once-daily treatment of angina pectoris.

Bepridil is available in doses of 200 to 400 mg once daily for use in patients with angina pectoris who are refractory to other antianginal drug therapy.[60] Close monitoring of patients with this drug is necessary at the onset of therapy because a small percentage of patients can have a prolongation of the QT interval on the ECG with a risk of torsades de pointes. Bepridil can be combined with a beta blocker if necessary.[214]

The comparative effects of abrupt withdrawal of verapamil and propranolol in patients with angina pectoris have been studied.[142] Ten percent of patients with stable effort-related symptoms experienced a severe clinical exacerbation of the anginal syndrome upon withdrawal of propranolol; no patient experienced rebound symptoms when verapamil was abruptly discontinued.[42] There also appear to be no major withdrawal reactions with nifedipine, mibefradil, or diltiazem[188] (see also Chap. 45).

Angina at Rest
Patients with angina at rest have a wide spectrum of disorders, ranging from those with variant angina (ST elevation) associated with angiographically normal coronary arteries to those with unstable angina with ST depression or elevation associated with multivessel coronary artery disease.[190,207,211] Coronary vasospasm and/or thrombosis may play a major role in the pathogenesis of ischemia in most patients with angina at rest, regardless of the coronary anatomy.[152] In clinical trials, CCBs have been effective in this syndrome because of their ability to block spontaneous and drug-induced spasm.[215–221]

The comparative efficacy of verapamil and propranolol was assessed in a randomized, blinded crossover trial in rest angina. Only verapamil reduced symptomatic and asymptomatic episodes of ischemia. These findings are consistent with the concept that coronary vasospasm plays a crucial role in patients with angina at rest; in contrast, rather than providing any benefit, propranolol may actually exacerbate vasospastic phenomena.[222] In another study, verapamil and nifedipine

TABLE 54-12

HEMODYNAMIC RATIONALE FOR COMBINING NITRATES AND CALCIUM
CHANNEL BLOCKERS IN ANGINA PECTORIS

	Nitrates	Calcium Blockers	Combination
Heart rate	↑ reflex	↓↔↑	↑ reflex
Blood pressure	↓	↓	↓↓?
Heart size	↓↔	↓↔↑	↔
Contractility	↑ reflex	↓	↔
Venomotor tone	↓	↔	↓
Peripheral resistance	↓	↓	↓↓?
Coronary resistance	↓	↓	↓↓?
Coronary blood flow	↑	↑	↑↑?
Collateral blood flow	↑	↑	↑↑?

Key: ↑ = increase; ↓ = decrease; ↓↓? = questionable additive effects; ↔ = no change.
Source: From Frishman WH. Beta-adrenergic blockade in the treatment of coronary artery disease. In: Hurst JW, ed. *Clinical Essays on the Heart.* New York: McGraw-Hill; 1984:48.

proved equally effective, and neither drug depressed ventricular function at rest or during exercise.[223] Accordingly, in the management of patients with variant angina, the choice of a CCB is likely to be determined not so much by which drug is more effective but by which agent is better tolerated by the individual patient.

The usefulness of CCBs in the long-term management of unstable angina was demonstrated in a double-blind, randomized clinical trial showing that the addition of nifedipine to nitrates and propranolol in patients receiving reduced the number of patients with unstable anginal syndromes requiring surgery for relief of pain; the incidence of sudden death and myocardial infarction was similar in both groups.[224] Clinical benefits, however, were confined largely to patients whose

pain was accompanied by ST-segment elevation (see also Chap. 46).

Combination Therapy with Nitrates in Angina Pectoris
Combination therapy with nitrates may be more efficacious for the treatment of angina pectoris than one drug used alone.[60,190,209] This may relate to the important and unique action of nitrates to dilate coronary collaterals. The hemodynamic effects of combined nitrate/CCB therapy are shown in Table 54-12. Hypotension should be avoided. Different calcium channel blockers may also be combined (nifedipine with verapamil or diltiazem) with added benefit; however, side effects may be prohibitive compared with monotherapy.[188]

Combination therapy with beta blockers was described in the beta-blocker section of this chapter.

ARRHYTHMIAS

Atrial Fibrillation

Except in rare situations, verapamil and diltiazem are ineffective in converting acute and chronic atrial fibrillation to normal sinus rhythm (Table 54-13). Both diltiazem and verapamil (oral and intravenous) are effective for decreasing and controlling ventricular rate during atrial fibrillation by prolonging AV nodal conduction and refractoriness and thereby increasing AV block both at rest and during exercise.[225,226] Clinical trials with verapamil in patients with atrial fibrillation have shown that its ability to decrease ventricular rate appears to be unrelated to the chronicity of the arrhythmia, its etiology, or the patient's age.[227,228] Verapamil appears to be more effective than digoxin in slowing the rapid ventricular rate in response to physical activity.[229] Either diltiazem or verapamil can be used orally in combination with digoxin for control of ventricular rate in treating acute and chronic atrial fibrillation and flutter[168] (see also Chap. 27).

TABLE 54-13

EFFECTS OF DILTIAZEM AND VERAPAMIL IN TREATMENT
OF COMMON ARRHYTHMIAS

Effective	Ineffective
Supraventricular tachycardia	Sinus tachycardia
AV nodal reentrant PSVT[a]	Nonparoxysmal automatic atrial tachycardia
Accessory pathway reentrant PSVT	Atrial fibrillation and flutter in WPW syndrome (ventricular rate may not decrease)
SA nodal reentrant PSVT	Ventricular tachyarrhythmias[b]
Atrial reentrant PSVT	
Atrial flutter (ventricular rate decreases but arrhythmia will only occasionally convert)	
Atrial fibrillation (ventricular rate decreases but arrhythmia will only occasionally convert)	

[a] PSVT = paroxysmal supraventricular tachycardia.
[b] Only limited experience in this area.
Source: From Frishman and LeJemtel,[168] with permission.

Paroxysmal Supraventricular Tachycardia

Virtually all cases of supraventricular tachycardia due to intra-nodal reentry and those related to the circus movement type of tachycardia in preexcitation respond promptly and predict-ably to intravenous verapamil or diltiazem, whereas only about two-thirds of atrial tachycardias from an ectopic focus convert to sinus rhythm after adequate doses of the drug (Table 54-13).[168,230] Intravenous verapamil and diltiazem are highly efficacious in treating reentry paroxysmal supraventricular tachycardia regardless of etiology or age.[168,230] The recom-mended dosage range of verapamil for terminating paroxys-mal supraventricular tachycardia in adults is 0.075 to 1.5 mg/kg infused over 1 to 3 min and repeated at 30 min, as needed.[168] In patients with myocardial dysfunction, the dose should be reduced. Children have safely been treated with a regimen of 0.075 to 0.15 mg/kg.[168] The recommended dose of diltiazem is 0.25 mg/kg infused over 2 min and re-peated at 0.35 mg/kg after 15 min.

There have been few clinical studies comparing intrave-nous verapamil and diltiazem with other standard regimens in the treatment of paroxysmal supraventricular tachycar-dia.[231] In a number of clinical situations, however, verapamil and diltiazem may offer an advantage over either digitalis preparations or beta-adrenergic blockers. For instance, vera-pamil would be preferable in cases where there is an urgent need to terminate paroxysmal supraventricular tachycardia, since it can produce therapeutic responses within 3 min of infusion, whereas the effects of digoxin are not evident for approximately 30 min.[168] Also, if drug therapy fails to achieve normal sinus rhythm, the short duration of action of verapamil and diltiazem permit earlier cardioversion without some of the dangers that accompany electric cardioversion during digoxin therapy. Verapamil and diltiazem also offers distinct advan-tages over beta-adrenergic blocking drugs in patients whose arrhythmias are associated with chronic obstructive lung dis-ease and/or peripheral vascular disease.[168]

Oral verapamil has been approved for prophylaxis against paroxysmal supraventricular tachycardia in doses of 160 to 480 mg/day, and the treatment experiences have yielded favor-able results.[232] Diltiazem is not yet approved in oral form as an antiarrhythmic agent (see also Chap. 27).

Atrial Flutter

The immediate effect of intravenous verapamil and diltiazem in atrial flutter in most patients is an increase in AV block that slows the ventricular response, rarely followed by a return to sinus rhythm (Table 54-13).[168,227] In some, the response occurs through the development of atrial fibrillation with a controlled ventricular response.[168] A single intravenous dose of verapamil or diltiazem has been found to be of diagnostic value in differentiating rapid atrial flutter from paroxysmal supraventricular tachycardia when these two arrhythmias are indistinguishable on the ECG. If the rhythm is atrial flutter, the AV block increases immediately, revealing the true nature of the arrhythmia. Oral verapamil has also been used to convert paroxysmal atrial flutter and to reduce

the rapid ventricular rates associated with this arrhythmia[232] (see also Chap. 27).

Preexcitation

Verapamil and diltiazem have been found to induce reversion of most cases of accessory pathway supraventricular tachycar-dia. From intracardiac recordings of electric activity during programmed electric stimulation of the heart, data have be-come available regarding the actions of verapamil on the electrophysiologic properties of the accessory pathway in overt cases of the Wolff-Parkinson-White (WPW) syn-drome.[233] The drug has a minimal effect on the antegrade and retrograde conduction times and on the refractory pe-riod.[168,172] Verapamil and diltiazem, therefore, terminate ac-cessory pathway paroxysmal supraventricular tachycardia in the same manner as they do an AV nodal reentrant paroxysmal supraventricular tachycardia by slowing AV nodal conduction and increasing refractoriness. The minimal effect of verapamil and diltiazem on the electrophysiologic properties of the by-pass tract is consistent with the observation that these agents are ineffective in atrial fibrillation complicating WPW syn-drome in which fibrillatory impulses conduct predominantly through the anomalous pathway. Under these circumstances, radio-frequency catheter ablation of the accessory pathways appears to be the therapy of choice.[234]

Ventricular Arrhythmias

Intravenous and oral verapamil and diltiazem have no apparent benefit in ventricular arrhythmias.[172] Bepridil, with its class I antiarrhythmic activity, however, has been shown to be effective in the short- and long-term control of ventricular arrhythmias. In humans, mibefradil has been shown to protect against malignant ventricular arrhythmias induced by cocaine in an experimental model.[235] These drugs, however, are not approved in the United States as ventricular antiarrhythmics.

Precautions in Treating Arrhythmias

A diseased SA node is much more sensitive to slow-channel blockers and may be depressed to the point of atrial stand-still.[236] Sinus arrest can also occur without overt evidence of "sick sinus syndrome."[168] Calcium-channel blockade may also suppress potential AV nodal escape rhythms that need to arise if atrial standstill occurs.[168] In patients with the brady-tachy form of sick sinus syndrome, either digoxin or beta-blocking drugs should probably not be combined with either verapamil or diltiazem in the prophylaxis of tachyarrhythmias unless a demand ventricular pacemaker is first inserted (see Chaps. 27 and 34).[168]

SYSTEMIC ARTERIAL HYPERTENSION

CCBs are effective in the treatment of systemic arterial hyper-tension (SAH) and hypertensive emergencies.[237,238] They can be considered potential first-line therapy for initiating treat-ment in many patients with chronic SAH except where discrete inhibition of the renin-angiotensin system is effective.[239]

A vast experience in the United States has been gained in patients with SAH using verapamil,[186,238,239] diltiazem,[240,241] nifedipine,[242] amlodipine,[243] nicardipine,[244] felodipine,[245] and isradipine.[246] Verapamil, nicardipine, nifedipine, felodipine, and diltiazem are available in the United States in both conventional and sustained-release oral formulations, allowing once- and twice-daily dosing. Verapamil is available in a unique delayed-onset sustained-release delivery system[186] to provide a peak blood level at the time of blood pressure elevation during awakening. Whether or not this will influence morbid and mortal events related to SAH has not been determined.[247] Innovative combination antihypertensive formulations have been evaluated in clinical trials and are now available: enalapril/extended-release diltiazem, benazepril/amlodipine,[248] trandolapril/extended-release verapamil,[249] and extended-release felodipine/extended-release metoprolol.[250] By affecting more than one factor that may mediate hypertension in a given individual, such combinations may be very effective.

Studies are now in progress evaluating various CCBs in elderly patients with isolated systolic hypertension. Three such projects include a large outcomes study using (1) a new dihydropyridine, lacidipine, in comparison to chlorthalidone (SHELL—Systolic Hypertension in the Elderly: Lacidipine Long-Term Treatment)[251]; (2) the Study of Mild Isolated Systolic Hypertension (SISH), which is evaluating felodipine and chlorthalidone therapy in elderly patients with systolic blood pressure levels between 140 and 160 mmHg, a clinical situation where, as yet, there are no published treatment outcomes data; and (3) the European Study of Systolic Hypertension (EURO-SYS), which evaluated nitrendipine plus enalapril or hydrochlorothiazide in elderly patients with systolic hypertension. A preliminary report demonstrated the safety and efficacy of nitredipine in this population.

The CCBs reduce both systolic and diastolic pressures with a minimal amount of side effects, including orthostasis.[238] They can cause left ventricular hypertrophy to regress in patients with hypertension.[134,252] These drugs may also exhibit antiadrenergic and natriuretic activities and can normalize the abnormal coronary vasomotion often observed in hypertensive patients.[253–256] They can be combined with other antihypertensive drugs if necessary, such as beta blockers, angiotensin-converting enzyme inhibitors, and diuretics.[238]

CCBs are equally effective in black and white patients[257] and in both the young and the old.[238,257] Women may have greater blood pressure–lowering effects than men with comparable doses of drug.[258] These drugs do not lower the pressures of normotensive patients.[238] The CCBs may be most useful in patients with low-renin, salt-dependent forms of hypertension.[259] In addition, they have been shown to be useful in treating patients with SAH following heart transplantation.[260]

Despite the widespread clinical use of CCBs for the treatment of SAH, there are few long-term studies which evaluate cardiovascular and cerebrovascular morbidity and mortality outcomes with these treatments.[261] In 1995, there were two published reports suggesting an increased risk of myocardial infarction and mortality in hypertensive patients receiving the short-acting CCBs (verapamil, diltiazem, nifedipine) as treatment compared to patients receiving other antihypertensive therapies, which included diuretics and beta blockers.[262,263] These reports were case control studies that have significant methodologic flaws in their experimental designs. Nevertheless, great debate has appeared in the medical literature regarding the safety of CCBs as a class for treating hypertension.[264–271] Based on the available evidence, the FDA has advised physicians not to use the short-acting CCBs for treating hypertension, but it has placed no restrictions on the first-line supplementary use of sustained-release CCB formulations or longer-acting formulations available for this indication, where there appears to be no apparent harm with their use.[272,273] A large number of studies are now in progress comparing CCBs with other antihypertensive treatments to resolve the safety issue with this treatment modality (Table 54-14).[273–277] To enlarge the controversy, in a large cohort study of 11,545 patients with chronic coronary artery disease, it was recently shown that the use of CCBs posed no greater risk of mortality than other drug treatments.[272] This does not detract from the beneficial effects of beta blockers after myocardial infarction (see also Chap. 58).

Hypertensive Emergencies and Perioperative Hypertension

Some CCBs have also been shown to be beneficial in patients with severe hypertension and hypertensive crisis.[238,278,279] Single oral, sublingual, and intravenous doses of these drugs have rapidly and smoothly reduced blood pressure in adults and children with occasional untoward effects, especially with inappropriate use.[242,278–280] The absolute reduction in blood pressure with treatment appears to be inversely correlated with the height of the pretreatment blood pressure level, and few episodes of hypotension have been reported.[278] Continuous hemodynamic monitoring of patients does not seem necessary in most instances.[278] Intravenous nicardipine is approved for clinical use in the treatment of hypertensive emergencies and perioperative hypertension. Its clinical utility compared with other parenteral treatments still needs to be determined.[281–283]

"SILENT" MYOCARDIAL ISCHEMIA

In addition to their favorable effects in relieving painful episodes of myocardial ischemia, the CCBs are also effective in relieving transient myocardial ischemic episodes that are detected by ECG but are unrelated to symptoms ("silent" myocardial ischemia).[284,285] Diltiazem,[188] nifedipine (low-dose), amlodipine,[200] and verapamil alone and in combination with beta blockers and nitrates have all been shown to be effective in reducing the number of ischemic episodes and their duration.[213,286,287] The prognostic importance of relieving silent myocardial ischemia with CCBs and other treatments has been evaluated in a study sponsored by the National Heart, Lung and Blood Institute, the Asymptomatic Coronary Ischemia Pilot (ACIP),[288,289] in which suggestive benefit of drug therapy was observed (see also Chap. 45).

TABLE 54-14

SOME ONGOING CLINICAL TRIALS COMPARING CALCIUM CHANNEL BLOCKERS WITH OTHER ANTIHYPERTENSIVE MEDICATIONS

Trial	Participants	Sample Size	Drugs Compared	Primary Outcome	Length of Study (year completed)
NORDIL	Mild-moderate primary HTN, aged 50–69	12,000	Diltiazem vs. diuretics or beta blockers	Fatal acute MI, fatal stroke, sudden death, other fatal and nonfatal CV disease	5 years (1999)
INSIGHT	HTN higher-risk patients; aged 55–80	6600	Long-acting nifedipine vs. diuretics	Total CV disease	3 years (1999)
HOT	HTN patients; aged 50–80	19,000	Felodipine alone or in combo with other agents	Nonfatal MI, nonfatal stroke, CV death	2.5 years (1996)
CONVINCE	Mild-moderate HTN, higher-risk patients aged >55	15,000	Controlled-onset ER verapamil vs. diuretics or beta blockers	Prevention of fatal and nonfatal MI and stroke, death	4–6 years (2000–2002)
ALLHAT	HTN, higher-risk patients aged >55	40,000	CCB vs. diuretics vs. ACE inhibitors vs. alpha blockers	Mortality and MI	6 years (2002)

Key: NORDIL = Nordic Diltiazem Trial; INSIGHT — International Nifedipine Study Intervention as a Goal in Hypertension Treatment; HOT = Hypertension Optimal Treatment/International Study; CONVINCE = Controlled Onset Verapamil Investigation of Cardiovascular Endpoints; ALLHAT = Antihypertensive and Lipid Lowering to Prevent Heart Attack Trial; HTN = hypertension; MI = myocardial infarction; CV = cardiovascular; CCB = calcium channel blocker; ER = extended release; ACE = angiotensin-converting enzyme.
Source: From Frishman,[152] with permission.

MYOCARDIAL INFARCTION

Although several experimental studies have indicated that nifedipine, verapamil, and diltiazem could reduce the extent of myocardial necrosis in experimental ischemia,[290] these effects have not been obtained clinically. Compared with the established protective actions of some beta-blocking drugs used intravenously or orally in prolonging life and reducing the risk of nonfatal reinfarction in survivors of an acute myocardial infarction,[7] the results with CCBs (diltiazem, lidoflazine, nifedipine, verapamil) have generally not been favorable.[81,290–300] The results of a metaanalysis looking at the effects of immediate-release nifedipine in patients surviving myocardial infarction even suggested the potential for harm,[301] which also prompted a debate in the literature[266,272,273,302] regarding the safety of CCBs as a treatment class for patients surviving myocardial infarction.

The plausibility of these mortality results with CCBs is supported by a failure to show a beneficial effect on infarct size, development of myocardial infarctions, or reinfarctions in most trials of patients with myocardial infarctions or unstable angina.[298] A trial using diltiazem in patients with non–Q-wave infarction reported a reduction in recurrent myocardial infarction in the diltiazem-treated patients but no reduction in mortality.[294] In a larger trial with diltiazem in infarction survivors, no favorable effects on mortality were seen.[297] Indeed, with Q-wave infarctions, diltiazem leads to an increase

in mortality. A subgroup of patients with left ventricular dysfunction did worse with diltiazem therapy than with placebo; on the other hand, chronic diltiazem therapy decreased mortality in patients with relatively normal left ventricular function.[297] Similarly, a more recent study did show a modest benefit of verapamil compared to placebo in infarction survivors, with less benefit observed in patients with left ventricular dysfunction.[298]

A double-blind study is in progress comparing diltiazem and aspirin with aspirin alone [Incomplete Infarction Trial of European Research Collaborators Evaluating Prognosis Post-Thrombolysis (INTERCEPT)] in patients with myocardial infarction who had received thrombolytic therapy. The study is enrolling 920 subjects and will evaluate the effects of treatment on the clinical end points of cardiac death, recurrent nonfatal infarction, and medically refractory ischemia.[303]

Prophylactic use of CCBs to improve patient survival following myocardial infarction cannot be recommended unless there are specific indications for using these drugs.[81,291,299,304,305] Overall, in order to reduce mortality postinfarction, the use of beta blockers rather than CCBs is strongly supported and recommended. In patients with contraindications to beta-adrenergic blockade, however, one can consider using verapamil or diltiazem in survivors of myocardial infarction who have good ventricular function[81] (see also Chap. 47).

HYPERTROPHIC CARDIOMYOPATHY

Propranolol remains the therapeutic agent of choice[306] for symptomatic patients with obstructive hypertrophic cardiomyopathy. The beneficial effects produced by propranolol derive from its blockade of sympathetic stimulation of the heart, resulting in heart rate slowing and a decrease in end-systolic emptying of the ventricle.[307]

Clinical studies have shown that the administration of verapamil can also improve exercise capacity and symptoms in many patients with hypertrophic cardiomyopathy.[308–312] The exact mechanism by which verapamil produces these beneficial effects is not known. Acute and chronic verapamil administration reduces left ventricular outflow obstruction, but examination of indices of left ventricular systolic function during chronic therapy suggests that this effect may not result from a reduction in left ventricular hypercontractility.[308] Since patients with hypertrophic cardiomyopathy also exhibit abnormal diastolic function, it is possible that enhanced diastolic filling may be responsible in part for the benefit conferred by verapamil.[308] Enhanced early diastolic filling and improvement in the diastolic pressure-volume relation might be expected to result in an increase in left ventricular end-diastolic volume, which would decrease the Venturi forces that act to move the anterior mitral valve leaflet across the outflow tract toward the septum.[308] The decrease would cause a diminution of obstruction, reducing left ventricular pressure and myocardial wall stress and thus raising the threshold at which symptoms occur.[308]

In a large study of patients with hypertrophic cardiomyopathy refractory to beta blockers,[308] verapamil proved to be effective on a long-term basis, with almost 50 percent of patients showing either a significant improvement in exercise tolerance, an improvement in symptoms, or a reduction in myocardial ischemia.[309] Approximately 50 percent of patients who were considered to be candidates for surgery because of moderately severe symptoms unresponsive to propranolol showed significant improvement on verapamil, and surgery was no longer considered necessary.[308]

Other studies have reported that not only can chronic administration of verapamil improve symptoms in patients with hypertrophic cardiomyopathy but it can also reduce the left ventricular muscle mass and the ventricular septal thickness measured by echocardiographic and ECG analysis.[310] Verapamil appears to improve the impaired left ventricular filling characteristics,[313,314] whereas propranolol may not.[313]

There may be serious and fatal complications of verapamil treatment in patients with hypertrophic cardiomyopathy,[308] resulting from the accentuated hemodynamic or electrophysiologic effects of the drug. It is unclear whether the fatal complications can occur as a result of verapamil-induced reduction in blood pressure with a resultant increase in left ventricular obstruction or because of the negative inotropic effects of the drug.[308] Verapamil should not be used in patients where ventricular dilatation has ensued with clinical CHF. The loss of sequential atrial ventricular depolarization caused by the electrophysiologic effects of the drug could also compromise cardiac function. The adverse electrophysiologic effects are often transient; however, they could prevent the use of larger drug doses that might provide better relief.[308]

If the CCB effects of verapamil are responsible for its therapeutic actions in hypertrophic cardiomyopathy, other drugs in this class also may be useful. The results of a double-blind trial comparing verapamil with nifedipine, however, indicated that verapamil is more effective than nifedipine in improving exercise tolerance and clinical symptoms.[314] In part, this is probably due to the greater hypotensive effects of nifedipine, which may increase systolic emptying and increase subaortic muscular obstruction. Diltiazem was recently shown to improve active diastolic function in patients with hypertrophic cardiomyopathy; however, certain patients had a marked increase in outflow obstruction[315] (see also Chap. 74).

CONGESTIVE HEART FAILURE

At present, inhibitors of the activated renin-angiotensin system (see Chap. 23) are drugs of choice in reducing peripheral vascular resistance in heart failure, while also reducing morbidity and mortality. The potent systemic vasodilatory actions of nifedipine and other dihydropyridine CCBs should make them potentially useful as afterload-reducing agents in patients with left ventricular failure.[167,316,317] Unlike other vasodilatory drugs, however, nifedipine also exerts a direct negative inotropic effect on the myocardium that is consistent with its ability to block transmembrane calcium transport in cardiac muscle cells.[307] Successful use of nifedipine as a vasodilator in left ventricular failure would be dependent on reduction of ventricular afterload exceeding its direct negative inotropic action, thereby leading to an improvement in hemodynamics and forward flow.[190]

Studies evaluating the effect on hemodynamics of nifedipine used in combination with other vasodilators in patients with heart failure have demonstrated significant reductions in systemic vascular resistance, usually associated with increases in cardiac output[190,318] and an acute increase in resting ejection fraction.[319,320] Reflex increases in heart rate may occur,[319] but most investigators have found heart rate to remain the same[320] and, in isolated cases, to fall.[321] Left ventricular filling pressures usually decrease[320] or do not change significantly,[321] but there are instances where pulmonary capillary wedge pressures rise with the use of nifedipine in heart failure.[322] With nearly normal levels of left ventricular afterload—i.e., disproportionately low wall stress—and with intrinsic fixed mechanical interference to forward flow such as aortic stenosis, nifedipine may be detrimental.[167] Most of the published data have dealt only with the acute hemodynamic effects of the agent after single sublingual dosing, with little information on the use of nifedipine as chronic oral therapy for left ventricular failure. A recent study demonstrated the efficacy and safety of diltiazem in patients with idiopathic dilated cardiomyopathy, but the data are limited.[323]

Since CCBs are potent vasodilators, particularly on the arterial circulation, the combination of an angiotensin-converting enzyme (ACE) inhibitor and a CCB might be useful in further augmenting vasodilation, improving myocardial perfusion and ejection fraction.[167] One limitation to this approach may be insupportable hypotension in some patients. Hence, the third Vasodilator-Heart Failure Trial (V-HeFT III) was conducted to test the efficacy of the combination of felodipine, enalapril, digoxin, and a diuretic in patients with CHF. The end points evaluated were exercise tolerance, quality of life, left ventricular function, plasma norepinephrine and atrial natriuretic factor levels, and reduction in occurrence of arrhythmias and mortality.[324] A similar pilot multicenter, placebo-controlled study was carried out using amlodipine in addition to ACE inhibitors, digoxin, and diuretics. This Prospective Randomized Amlodipine Survival Evaluation (PRAISE) trial found no clear overall mortality effect or harm from the use of the drug in patients with severe congestive heart failure.[325] Contrary to the prior experiences of the investigators, there appeared to be little effect in the large subgroup of patients who had coronary artery disease and a barely significant reduction in morbidity and mortality in the minority of patients who did not have coronary artery disease.[326] Based on the study, the FDA has revised amlodipine's labeling, describing the drug to be safe for use in treating patients with systemic arterial hypertension or angina pectoris who also have CHF. Amlodipine is now being studied in 1800 patients with nonischemic cardiomyopathies who are already receiving digoxin, diuretics, and ACE inhibitors (PRAISE II). Finally, mibefradil, a new nondihydropyridine calcium blocker with little negative inotropic activity, is being evaluated in a similar manner to the PRAISE I trial in patients with class II–III heart failure (NYHA), the Mortality Assessment in Heart Failure (MACH-I) Trial.

In a recent retrospective analysis of the Studies of Left Ventricular Dysfunction, in which enalapril was compared to placebo in patients with class I–III heart failure, it was observed that those patients who were receiving concomitant immediate-release CCB treatment had a higher mortality than those subjects who were receiving concomitant beta-blocker therapy.[327] Thus, long-acting dihydropyridine CCBs as adjunctive vasodilator therapy in patients with left ventricular failure should be used only if additional clinical reasons for their administration exist—i.e., angina pectoris, systemic arterial hypertension, or aortic regurgitation[328]—particularly if these conditions play important contributory roles in the development or exacerbation of left ventricular dysfunction. Some investigators now suggest that CCBs may provide some benefit to patients with predominant diastolic ventricular dysfunction,[329] but more data are needed to substantiate this claim.[330]

PRIMARY PULMONARY HYPERTENSION

Primary pulmonary hypertension is an entity characterized by excessive pulmonary vasoconstriction and increased pulmonary vascular resistance induced by unknown stimuli.[331] Recently, it was suggested that endothelial cell dysfunction and injury may be responsible for the disease process.[332] Typically, the affected patient is a young to middle-aged woman presenting with fatigue, dyspnea, chest discomfort, or syncope. Despite many attempts to develop effective therapy, the results of drug treatment have been generally unsatisfactory. The syndrome is associated with sudden death and continues to bear a very poor prognosis.[331]

Based on the currently available data, some CCBs provide beneficial responses in selected patients with pulmonary hypertension.[331,333] In general, patients with less severe pulmonary hypertension appear to respond better than do those with more advanced disease.[334] Furthermore, early treatment may serve to attenuate progression of the disease (see also Chap. 59).

CEREBRAL ARTERIAL SPASM AND STROKE

A major complication of subarachnoid hemorrhage is cerebral arterial spasm, which may occur several days after the initial event.[335] Such spasm may be focal or diffuse, involving one or more of the larger cerebral vessels, which may cause additional ischemic neurologic deficits. Although the exact etiology of this spasm is unknown, a combination of various blood constituents and neurotransmitters has been postulated to produce a milieu that enhances the reactivity of the cerebral vasculature.[335] The final pathway for the vasoconstriction, however, involves an increase in intracellular calcium concentration in vascular smooth muscle. Accordingly, the CCBs were postulated to have a beneficial effect in reducing cerebral spasm.[336]

Although verapamil and nifedipine have been shown to prevent cerebral arterial spasm in experimental studies, nimodipine and nicardipine, both nifedipine analogs, have an apparent preferential cerebrovascular action in this disorder.[337–339] The lipid-solubility of nimodipine enables it to cross the blood-brain barrier, and this may account for its more potent cerebrovascular effects. In a recent multicenter placebo-controlled study involving 125 patients,[335] nimodipine significantly reduced the occurrence of severe neurologic deficits following angiographically demonstrated cerebral arterial spasm. All patients had a documented subarachnoid hemorrhage and a normal neurologic status within 96 h of entry into the study. While 8 of the 60 placebo-treated patients developed a severe neurologic deficit, only 1 of 55 nimodipine-treated patients suffered such an outcome. Nimodipine is now approved for the improvement of neurologic outcome by reducing the incidence and severity of ischemic deficits in patients with subarachnoid hemorrhage from ruptured congenital aneurysms who are in good neurologic condition postictus. The recommended dose is 60 mg by mouth every 4 h for 21 consecutive days (see also Chap. 99).

Increased cellular calcium concentration may be implicated in neuronal death after ischemia.[340] Nimodipine administered to laboratory animals after global cerebral ischemia had a more favorable effect on neurologic outcome than did placebo.[341] The results of a prospective double-blind, placebo-controlled trial of oral nimodipine administered to 186 patients within 24 h of an acute ischemic stroke showed a reduction in both mortality and neurologic deficit with active treatment. The benefit was confined predominantly to men,[340] and where nimodipine therapy was begun up to 48 h after the onset of symptoms, no benefit of therapy was found.[342,343]

ATHEROSCLEROSIS

Atherosclerosis develops through numerous and interrelated processes involving the accumulation of cholesterol, calcium, and matrix materials in the major arteries and at lesion sites. Many of the intracellular and extracellular processes involved in atherosclerotic plaque formation require calcium, and it has been suggested that large deposits of cholesterol may trigger physiologic changes in membranes that favor uptake of calcium into the vascular smooth muscle.[344] Initial controlled studies employing angiography have suggested that some CCBs may retard the progression of atherosclerosis in humans.[345–347] In the International Nifedipine Trial on Atherosclerosis Coronary Therapy (INTACT) study,[345] while nifedipine reduced the formation of new lesions when compared with placebo, there was no effect on the progression or regression of already existing coronary lesions, and an increased mortality compared to placebo was observed. The administration of nicardipine for 24 months also had no effect on the progression or retardation of advanced stenoses in patients with coronary atherosclerosis, as confirmed by arteriography.[346] The drug, however, did appear to retard the progression of small lesions.

Diltiazem retards the development of coronary artery disease in heart transplant recipients,[348] an action independent of the drug's blood pressure–lowering effect (see also Chap. 25).

In the Multicenter Isradipine Diuretic Atherosclerosis Study (MIDAS),[349] which was a 3-year, double-blind, randomized trial designed to compare the effectiveness of isradipine and hydrochlorothiazide in retarding the progression of atherosclerotic lesions in the carotid arteries, no apparent benefit was seen with either treatment. A similar study to MIDAS is now being carried out with lacidipine, a new dihydropyridine calcium antagonist, in the 4-year European Lacidipine Study on Atherosclerosis (ELSA).[350,351]

CCBs have also been used to treat patients with intermittent claudication and mesenteric insufficiency.[352]

OTHER CARDIOVASCULAR USES

Diltiazem has been used as part of an ice-cold cardioplegia solution in patients undergoing coronary surgical procedures.[353] The addition of diltiazem appeared to preserve high-energy phosphate levels, with an improvement in hemodynamics in the postoperative period.[353] Concomitant use of nifedipine appears to reduce the incidence of myocardial infarction and transient ischemia in patients undergoing bypass surgery.[354]

Intracoronary diltiazem has been used to reduce the severity and delay the onset of ischemic pain in patients undergoing percutaneous transluminal angioplasty.[355] CCBs have also been used as a long-term treatment to prevent restenosis following balloon angioplasty, with questionable benefit.[356]

Microvascular spasm has been shown to be an important pathophysiologic mechanism in experimental cardiomyopathies. Spasm as well as the development of cardiomyopathy

has been prevented by verapamil.[357] The pertinence of these findings to human disease is not established, and effects of verapamil have not been explored in this setting.

CCBs (diltiazem and verapamil) have also been found to preserve the functioning of human renal transplants.[358] The drugs dilate the preglomerular afferent arterioles and appear to possess inherent immunosuppressive properties and the ability to ameliorate the nephrotoxic effects of cyclosporine.[359]

MIGRAINE AND DEMENTIA

Classic migraine is characterized by prodromal symptoms with transient neurologic deficits. Cerebral blood flow is reduced during these prodromes and is then increased during the subsequent vasodilatory phase, causing severe headache. Because the entry of calcium ions into the smooth muscle cells is the final common pathway that controls vasomotor tone, CCBs may prevent or ameliorate the initial focal cerebral vasoconstriction.[360]

Controlled studies have demonstrated that 80 to 90 percent of patients with vascular headaches benefit from nimodipine, confirming the selectivity of this agent for the cerebral blood vessels.[361] Verapamil and nifedipine are also effective in the prophylaxis of migraine, but they are less selective for the cephalic blood vessels and thus cause more systemic side effects.[361,362] Relief from the migraine prodrome usually began 10 to 14 days after initiation of the drugs but could be delayed 2 to 4 weeks.[363] Cerebral vascular resistance was decreased by all three established CCBs, but only nimodipine reduced the cerebral vasoconstriction induced by inhalation of 100 percent oxygen.[361] None of the CCBs are effective against muscle contraction or tension headaches.

Multiple clinical trials are now being carried out to examine the effects of CCBs on the progression of dementing illness, of both the vascular and Alzheimer types. Preliminary results have shown equivocal benefit from treatment.[364]

RAYNAUD'S PHENOMENON

Raynaud's phenomenon is characterized by well-demarcated ischemia of the digits with pallor or cyanosis ending abruptly at one level on the digits.[352] Nifedipine decreases the frequency, duration, and intensity of vasospastic attacks in approximately two-thirds of patients with primary or secondary Raynaud's phenomenon.[352,365] Patients with primary Raynaud's phenomenon usually demonstrate the most improvement; digital ulcers may heal in patients with scleroderma. Doses of 10 to 20 mg of nifedipine thrice daily have been used. Felodipine and isradipine are as effective as nifedipine. Diltiazem, 60 to 360 mg daily, was also useful in patients with primary or secondary Raynaud's phenomenon in multiple placebo-controlled trials (see also Chap. 100).

NONCARDIOVASCULAR USES

Amaurosis Fugax

Hypoperfusion of the retinal circulation may lead to a brief loss of vision in one eye, a syndrome known as *amaurosis fugax.*[366] This brief loss of sight has been attributed to embolism from the heart or great vessels or to carotid occlusive disease. In a small group of patients with amaurosis but no signs of emboli or carotid hypoperfusion, administration of aspirin or warfarin did not relieve symptoms[367]; however, oral doses of either verapamil or nifedipine abolished attacks. In several patients, the attacks returned when the CCB agent was discontinued.

High-Altitude Pulmonary Edema

Hypoxic pulmonary hypertension appears to play a role in the pathogenesis of high-altitude pulmonary edema. Nifedipine has been useful for this condition due to its effectiveness in reducing pulmonary artery pressure[368] (see also Chap. 59).

Adverse Effects

In addition to their widely varying effects on cardiovascular function, these agents also have differing spectra of adverse effects (Table 54-15).[151,190,369] Immediate-release nifedipine has a very high incidence of minor adverse effects (approximately 40 percent), but serious adverse effects are uncommon.[370] The most frequent adverse effects reported with nifedipine and other dihydropyridines include headache, pedal edema, flushing, paresthesias, and dizziness. The most serious adverse effects of this drug include exacerbation of angina, which may occur in up to 10 percent of patients, and occasional hypotension.[188,212] These side effects are reduced in number with the new long-acting formulation of nifedipine[371] and may also be fewer in number with some of the new dihydropyridine CCBs.

Diltiazem, verapamil, and mibefradil can exacerbate sinus node dysfunction and impair AV nodal conduction, particularly in patients with underlying conduction system disease.[151,190,369] The most frequent adverse effect of verapamil is constipation.[151,190,369] The drug may also worsen CHF, particularly when used in combination with beta blockers or disopyramide.[151,190,369] There have been recent reports of verapamil-induced parkinsonism.[372] Most of the adverse effects noted with diltiazem and mibefradil have been cardiovascular, with occasional headache and gastrointestinal complaints.[151,190,369] The side effects of CCBs may increase considerably when these agents are used in combination.[188]

An increased risk of gastrointestinal hemorrhage in older patients has been reported with CCBs, as well as intraoperative bleeding during coronary bypass surgery.[373] An increased risk of developing cancer in older subjects has also been reported.[275]

Bepridil, which has class I antiarrhythmic properties, has the potential to induce malignant ventricular arrhythmias. Because of its ability to prolong the QT interval, torsades de pointes–type ventricular tachycardia can occur. Thus, bepridil should be reserved for patients in whom other antianginal agents do not offer a satisfactory effect.[374] Recently, mibefradil was shown to prolong the QT interval, especially when used with terfanadine, cisapride, and astemizole. This effect is related to inhibition of the hepatic cytochrome P4503A4 by mibefradil.

DRUG WITHDRAWAL

Serious problems have been reported with the abrupt withdrawal of long-term beta-blocker therapy in patients with angina; these may be related to heightened adrenergic activity.[142] Clinical experiences with CCB withdrawal suggest that although patients with angina get worse after treatment when

TABLE 54-15

ADVERSE EFFECTS OF CALCIUM CHANNEL BLOCKERS

	Overall	Headache	Dizziness	GI	Flushing	Paresthesia	Decreased SA and/or AV Conduction	CHF	Hypotension	Pedal Edema	Worsening of Angina
Diltiazem	≈5	+	+	+	+	0	3+	+	+	+	0
Diltiazem SR	≈5	+	+	+	+	0	3+	+	+	+	0
Verapamil	8	+	+	3+	0	0	3+	2+	+	+	0
Verapamil SR	≈8	+	+	3+	0	0	3+	2+	+	+	0
Bepridil	15	0	+	3+	0	0	+	+	0	0	0
Amlodipine	≈15	2+	+	+	+	+	0	0	+	2+	0
Isradipine	≈15	2+	2+	+	+	+	0	0	+	2+	0
Nifedipine	≈20	3+	3+	+	3+	+	0	+	+	2+	+
Nifedipine GITS	≈10	+	+	+	+	+	0	+	+	+	0
Nicardipine	≈20	3+	3+	+	3+	+	0	0	+	2+	+
Nimodipine	15	+	+	+	+	0	0	+	+	+	0
Nisoldipine	≈15	2+	+	+	+	0	0	0	+	2+	0
Felodipine	20	2+	2+	+	2+	+	0	0	+	2+	0
Mibefradil	≈10	+	+	+	+	0	3+	0	+	+	0

Key: GI = gastrointestinal; SA = sinoatrial; AV = atrioventricular; CHF = congestive heart failure; 0 = no report; + = rare; 2+ = occasional; 3+ = frequent; SR = sustained release; GITS = gastrointestinal therapeutic system.

Source: Adapted from Frishman et al.,[238] with permission.

TABLE 54-16

CARDIOVASCULAR TOXICITY WITH CALCIUM CHANNEL BLOCKERS AND
RECOMMENDATIONS FOR TREATMENT

Effects[a]	Suggested Treatment
Profound hypotension	10% calcium gluconate or calcium chloride; norepinephrine or dopamine
Severe LV[b] dysfunction	10% calcium gluconate or calcium chloride; isoproterenol or dobutamine; glucagon; norepinephrine or dopamine
Profound bradycardia	Atropine sulfate (not always effective)
Sinus bradycardia	10% calcium gluconate or calcium chloride
SA node and AV node block	Isoproterenol or dobutamine
Asystole	External cardiac massage and cardiac pacing (if above measures fail)

[a] These effects are seen more frequently in patients who have underlying myocardial dysfunction and/or cardiac conduction abnormalities and who are receiving concomitant treatment with a beta blocker.

[b] LV = left ventricular.

Source: From Frishman WH, Klein NA, Charlap S, Klein P, Cohen MN, Rotmensch HH. Recognition and management of verapamil poisoning. In: Packer M, Frishman WH, eds. *Calcium Channel Antagonists in Cardiovascular Disease.* Norwalk, CT: Appleton-Century-Crofts; 1984:365–370.

a CCB is stopped abruptly, there is no evidence of an "overshoot" in anginal symptoms.[142,188]

DRUG OVERDOSE

CCB overdosage has been described with increasing frequency. The cardiovascular problems associated with this condition are hypotension, left ventricular conduction defects, bradycardia, nodal blocks, and asystole. Treatment approaches are described in Table 54-16.[375]

DRUG-DRUG INTERACTIONS

There are few data on the interactions of diltiazem with other drugs.[151,188] Rifampin severely reduces the bioavailability of oral verapamil by enhancing the first-pass liver metabolism of the drug. Both nifedipine and verapamil increase serum digoxin levels, an observation not made with diltiazem. Verapamil has been reported to increase serum digoxin levels by approximately 70 percent,[376,377] apparently by decreasing renal clearance,[376] nonrenal clearance, and the volume of distribution.[377] Studies of the time course of this effect show that it begins with the first dose and reaches steady state within 1 to 4 weeks. Nifedipine also has been reported to increase serum digoxin concentrations, but to a lesser extent (about 45 percent).[378] The mechanism for this interaction is not clear. Verapamil[377] and diltiazem[379] have additive effects on AV conduction in combination with digitalis. Thus, they can be used to cause further decreases in heart rate compared with digitalis alone in patients who are in atrial fibrillation.

Combinations of drugs are particularly advantageous when they affect different mechanisms to an overall increased benefit. For example, beta blockers may lower heart rate to decrease oxygen needs and increase diastolic time for coronary perfu-sion, while nitrates can dilate collaterals and increase coronary blood flow. Combinations of beta blockers (propranolol, atenolol) with nifedipine or verapamil have shown improved efficacy for the combination compared with any of the drugs used alone.[190,209,380] Hemodynamic studies have shown mild negative inotropic effects of verapamil in patients on a beta blocker.[381] There are also slight decreases in heart rate, cardiac output, and left ventricular ejection fraction.[381] Combinations of nifedipine and propranolol or of metoprolol and verapamil and propranolol are well tolerated by patients with normal left ventricular function, but there may be a greater potential for hemodynamic compromise in patients with impaired left ventricular function with combined verapamil-propranolol treatment.[381] Combinations of diltiazem, nifedipine, or verapamil with nitrates are well tolerated and clinically useful.[190] When diltiazem is combined with nifedipine, blood levels of nifedipine increase significantly, which may contribute to an increased frequency of adverse reactions with this combination.[382] The combination of verapamil with dihydropyridines has not been well studied.

How to Choose a Calcium Channel Blocker

Each CCB exerts its effects through inhibition of slow channel–mediated calcium ion transport. Many of the drugs, however, appear to accomplish this by different mechanisms and with differing effects on various target organs. These differences allow the clinician to select the particular drug most suitable for the patient's specific needs. In addition, the side-effect profiles of these drugs (with little overlap between them) assure that most patients will tolerate at least one of these agents and may benefit from their use along with other therapy.

REFERENCES

1. Frishman WH. β-Adrenoceptor antagonists: New drugs and new indications. *N Engl J Med* 1981; 305:500–506.
2. Frishman WH. *Clinical Pharmacology of the β-Adrenoceptor Blocking Drugs,* 2d ed. Norwalk, CT: Appleton-Century-Crofts; 1984.
3. Frishman WH. Alpha and beta-adrenergic blocking drugs. In: Frishman WH, Sonnenblick EH, eds. *Cardiovascular Pharmacotherapeutics.* New York: McGraw-Hill; 1997:59–94.
4. The Norwegian Multicenter Study Group. Timolol induced reduction in mortality and reinfarction in patients surviving acute myocardial infarction. *N Engl J Med* 1981; 304:801–807.
5. Beta-Blocker Heart Attack Trial Research Group. A randomized trial of propranolol in patients with acute myocardial infarction: I. Mortality results. *JAMA* 1982; 247:1707–1714.
6. Braunwald E. Treatment of the patient after myocardial infarction. *N Engl J Med* 1980; 302:290–293.

7. Frishman WH, Furberg CD, Friedewald WT. β-Adrenergic blockade for survivors of acute myocardial infarction. *N Engl J Med* 1984; 310:830–837.

8. ISIS-I Collaborative Group. Randomized trial of intravenous atenolol among 16,027 cases of suspected acute myocardial infarction: ISIS-I. *Lancet* 1986; 2:57–66.

9. TIMI Study Group. Comparison of invasive and conservative strategies after treatment with intravenous tissue-type plasminogen activator in acute myocardial infarction: Results of the Thrombolysis in Myocardial Infarction (TIMI) trial phase II. *N Engl J Med* 1989; 320:618–627.

10. Insel PA. Adrenergic receptors: Evolving concepts and clinical implications. *N Engl J Med* 1996; 334:580–585.

11. Lefkowitz RJ, Caron MG. Adrenergic receptors: Models for the study of receptors coupled to guanine nucleotide regulatory proteins. *J Biol Chem* 1988; 263:4993–4996.

12. Benovic JL, Bouvier M, Caron MG, Lefkowitz RJ. Regulation of adenyl cyclase-coupled beta-adrenergic receptors. *Annu Rev Cell Biol* 1988; 4:405–428.

13. Frishman WH. Beta-adrenergic blocker withdrawal. *Am J Cardiol* 1987; 59:26F–32F.

14. Colucci WS, Alexander RW, Williams GH, Rude RE, Holman BL, Konstam MA, et al. Decreased lymphocyte beta-adrenergic receptor density in patients with heart failure and tolerance to the beta-adrenergic agonist pirbuterol. *N Engl J Med* 1981; 305:185–190.

15. Gilbert EM, Olsen SL, Renlund DG, Bristow MR. Beta-adrenergic receptor regulation and left ventricular function in idiopathic dilated cardiomyopathy. *Am J Cardiol* 1993; 71:23C–29C.

16. Hausdorff WP, Caron MG, Lefkowitz RJ. Turning off the signal desensitization of beta-adrenergic receptor function. *Fed Am Soc Exp Biol* 1990; 4:2881–2889.

17. Lefkowitz RJ, Caron MG, Stile GL. Mechanisms of membrane-receptor regulation: Biochemical, physiological and clinical insights derived from studies of the adrenergic receptors. *N Engl J Med* 1984; 310:1570–1579.

18. Cruickshank JM, Prichard BNC. *Beta-Blockers in Clinical Practice,* 2d ed. Edinburgh: Churchill Livingstone; 1994:1055.

19. Koch-Weser J. Metoprolol. *N Engl J Med* 1979; 301:698–703.

20. Frishman WH. Atenolol and timolol, two new systemic adrenoceptor antagonists. *N Engl J Med* 1982; 306:1456–1462.

21. Frishman WH. Nadolol: A new β-adrenoceptor antagonist. *N Engl J Med* 1981; 305:678–684.

22. Frishman WH. Pindolol: A new β-adrenoceptor antagonist with partial agonist activity. *N Engl J Med* 1983; 308:940–944.

23. Frishman WH, Covey S. Penbutolol and carteolol: Two new beta-adrenergic blockers with partial agonism. *J Clin Pharmacol* 1990; 30:412–421.

24. Frishman WH, Tepper D, Lazar E, Behrmann D. Betaxolol: A new long-acting β₁-selective adrenergic blocker. *J Clin Pharmacol* 1990; 30:699–703.

25. Frishman WH. Beta-adrenergic blockers. In: Frishman WH, ed. *Current Cardiovascular Drugs,* 2d ed. Philadelphia: Current Medicine; 1995:88–128.

26. Morgan T. Clinical pharmacokinetics and pharmacodynamics of carvedilol. *Clin Pharmacokinet* 1994; 26:335.

27. Frishman W, Jacob H, Eisenberg E, Ribner H. Clinical pharmacology of the new beta-adrenergic blocking drugs: Part VIII. Self-poisoning with beta-adrenoceptor blocking drugs: Recognition and management. *Am Heart J* 1979; 98:798–811.

28. Frishman WH. Clinical perspective on celiprolol. *Am Heart J* 1991; 121:724–729.

29. Johnson BF, Danylchuk MA. The relevance of plasma lipid changes with cardiovascular drug therapy. *Med Clin North Am* 1989; 73:449–473.

30. Taylor SH, Silke B, Lee PS. Intravenous beta-blockade in coronary heart disease: Is cardioselectivity or intrinsic sympathomimetic activity hemodynamically useful? *N Engl J Med* 1982; 306:631–635.

31. Frishman WH, Strom J, Kirschner M, Poland M, Klein N, Halprin S, et al. Labetalol therapy in patients with systemic hypertension and angina pectoris: Effects of combined alpha- and beta-adrenergic blockade. *Am J Cardiol* 1981; 48:917–928.

32. Van Zwieten A. Pharmacology of antihypertensive agents with multiple actions. *Eur J Clin Pharmacol* 1990; 38:577–581.

33. Gilbert EM, Anderson JL, Deitchman D, Yanowitz FG, O'Connell JB, Renlund DG, et al. Long-term β-blocker vasodilator therapy improves cardiac function in idiopathic dilated cardiomyopathy: A double-blind randomized study of bucindolol versus placebo. *Am J Med* 1990; 88:223–229.

34. Frishman WH, Nalamati J. Carvedilol: A new alpha- and beta-adrenergic blocker for heart failure and hypertension. *N Engl J Med* 1997. In press.

35. Yue TL, Lysko PG, Barone FC, Gu JL, Ruffolo RR Jr, Feuerstein GZ. Carvedilol, a new anti-hypertensive with unique antioxidant activity: Potential role in cerebroprotection. *Ann NY Acad Sci* 1994; 738:230–242.

36. Packer M, Bristow MR, Cohn N, Colucci WS, Fowler MB, Gilbert EM. Effect of carvedilol on morbidity and mortality in chronic heart failure. *N Engl J Med* 1996; 334:1349–1355.

37. Frishman WH, Lazar EJ, Gorodokin G. Pharmacokinetic optimization of therapy with beta-adrenergic blocking agents. *Clin Pharmacokinet* 1991; 20:311–318.

38. Frishman WH, Teicher M. Long-acting propranolol. *Cardiovasc Rev Rep* 1983; 4:1100–1102.

39. Abrahamsson B, Lucker P, Olofsson I, Regardh C-G, Sandberg A, Wieselgren I, et al. The relationship between metoprolol plasma concentration and beta₁-blockade in healthy subjects: A study on conventional metoprolol and metoprolol CR/ZOK formulations. *J Clin Pharmacol* 1990; 30:S46–S54.

40. Frishman WH, Murthy VS, Strom JA, Hershman DL. Ultrashort-acting β-adrenoreceptor blocking drug: Esmolol. In: Messerli FH, ed. *Cardiovascular Drug Therapy,* 2d ed. Philadelphia: Saunders; 1996:507–516.

41. Landau A, Frishman WH, Alturk N, Adjei-Poku M, Fornasier-Bongo M, Furia S. Improvement in exercise tolerance and immediate β-adrenergic blockade with intranasal propranolol in patients with angina pectoris. *Am J Cardiol* 1993; 72:995–998.

42. Wurzelmann J, Frishman W, Aronson M, Masur D, Ooi WL. Neuropsychiatric effects of antihypertensive drugs in the old old. *Cardiol Clin* 1987; 5:689–699.

43. Kostis JB, Rosen RC. Central nervous system effects of β-adrenergic blocking drugs: The role of ancillary properties. *Circulation* 1987; 75:204–212.

44. Ward SA, Walle T, Walle UK, Wilkinson GR, Branch RA. Propranolol's metabolism is determined by both mephenytoin and debrisoquin hydroxylase activities. *Clin Pharmacol Ther* 1989; 45:72–79.

45. Fujimaki M. Oxidation of the R(+) and S(−) carvedilol by rat liver microsome: Evidence for stereoselective oxidation and characterization of the cytochrome P450 isozymes involved. *Drug Metab Disp* 1994; 22:700–708.

46. Panton LB, Guillen GJ, Williams L, Graves JE, Vivas C, Cediel M, et al. The lack of effect of aerobic exercise training on propranolol pharmacokinetics in young and elderly adults. *J Clin Pharmacol* 1995; 35:885–894.

47. SHEP Cooperative Research Group. Prevention of stroke by antihypertensive drug treatment in older persons with isolated systolic hypertension: Final results of Systolic Hypertension in the Elderly Program (SHEP). *JAMA* 1991; 265:3255–3264.

48. Kostis JB, Berge KG, Davis BR, Hawkins CM, Probstfield J, for the SHEP Cooperative Research Group. Effect of atenolol and resperine on selected events in the Systolic Hypertension in the Elderly Program (SHEP). *Am J Hypertens* 1995; 8:1147–1153.

49. Joint National Committee on Detection, Evaluation and Treatment of High Blood Pressure. The Fifth Report of the Joint National Committee on Detection, Evaluation and Treatment of High Blood Pressure (JNC V). *Arch Intern Med* 1993; 153:154–183.

50. Saunders E, Weir MR, Kong BW, Hollifield J, Gray J, Vertes V, et al. A comparison of the efficacy and safety of a β-blocker, a calcium channel blocker, and a converting enzyme inhibitor in hypertensive blacks. *Arch Intern Med* 1990; 150:1707–1713.

51. Ahlquist RP. Study of the adrenotropic receptors. *Am J Physiol* 1948; 153:586–600.

52. Sonnenblick EH, Skelton CL. Myocardial energetics: Basic principles and clinical implications. *N Engl J Med* 1971; 285:668–675.

53. Frishman WH. Multifactorial actions of beta-adrenergic blocking drugs in ischemic heart disease: Current concepts. *Circulation* 1983; 67(suppl 1):I11–I18.

54. Frishman WH, Gabor R, Pepine C, Cavusoglu E. Heart rate reduction in the treatment of chronic stable angina pectoris: Experience with a sinus node inhibitor. *Am Heart J* 1996; 131:204–210.

55. Ardissino D, Savonitto S, Egstrup K, Rasmussen K, Bae EA, Omland T, et al. Selection of medical treatment in stable angina pectoris:

PART VI
CORONARY HEART DISEASE

1612

Results of the International Multicenter Angina Exercise (IMAGE) Study. *J Am Coll Cardiol* 1995; 25:1516–1521.

56. Frishman W, Pepine CJ, Weiss R, Baiker WM for the Zatebradine Study Group. Addition of zatebradine, a direct sinus node inhibitor, provides no greater exercise tolerance benefit in patients with angina pectoris taking extended-release nifedipine: Results of a multicenter, randomized, double-blind, placebo-controlled, parallel group study. *J Am Coll Cardiol* 1995; 26:305–312.

57. Frishman WH, Smithen C, Befler B, Kligfield P, Killip T. Noninvasive assessment of clinical response to oral propranolol. *Am J Cardiol* 1975; 35:635–644.

58. Packer M. Combined beta-adrenergic and calcium-entry blockade in angina pectoris. *N Engl J Med* 1989; 320:709.

59. Weiner DA, Klein MD. Calcium antagonists for the treatment of angina pectoris. In: Weiner DA, Frishman WH, eds. *Therapy of Angina Pectoris.* New York: Marcel Dekker; 1986:145–204.

60. Frishman WH, Crawford MH, DiBianco R, Farham J, Katz RJ, Kostis JB, et al. Combination propranolol and bepridil therapy in stable angina pectoris. *Am J Cardiol* 1985; 55:43C–49C.

61. deVries RJM, Dunselman PHJ, van Veldhuisen DJ, van den Heuvel AFM, Wielenga RP, Lie KI. Comparison between felodipine and isosorbide mononitrate as adjunct to beta blockade in patients >65 years of age with angina pectoris. *Am J Cardiol* 1994; 74:1201–1206.

62. Schwarz ER, Klues HG, vom Dahl J, Klein I, Krebs W, Hanrath P. Functional, angiographic and intracoronary Doppler flow characteristics in symptomatic patients with myocardial bridging: Effect of short-term intravenous beta-blocker medication. *J Am Coll Cardiol* 1996; 27:1637–1645.

63. Miura D, Frishman WH, Dangman KH. Class II drugs. In: Dangman KH, Miura D, eds. *Basic and Clinical Electrophysiology and Pharmacology of the Heart.* New York: Marcel Dekker; 1991:665–676.

64. Tisdale JE, Sun H, Zhao H, Fan C-D, Colucci RD, Kluger J, et al. Antifibrillatory effect of esmolol alone and in combination with lidocaine. *J Cardiovasc Pharmacol* 1996; 27:376–382.

65. Cavusoglu E, Frishman WH. Sotalol: A new β-adrenergic blocker for ventricular arrhythmias. *Prog Cardiovasc Dis* 1995; 37:423–440.

66. Wiesfeld ACP, Crijns HJGM, Tuininga YS, Lie KI. Beta-adrenergic blockade in the treatment of sustained ventricular tachycardia or ventricular fibrillation. *PACE* 1996; 19:1026–1035.

67. Antz M, Cappato R, Kuck K-H. Metoprolol versus sotalol in the treatment of sustained ventricular tachycardia. *J Cardiovasc Pharmacol* 1995; 26:627–635.

68. Pitzalia MV, Mastropasqua F, Massari F, Totaro P, DiMaggio M, Rizzon P. Holter-guided identification of premature ventricular contractions susceptible to suppression by β blockers. *Am Heart J* 1996; 131:508.

69. Frishman WH, Cavusoglu E. β-Adrenergic blockers and their role in the therapy of arrhythmias. In: Podrid PJ, Kowey PR, eds. *Cardiac Arrhythmias: Mechanisms, Diagnosis and Management.* Baltimore: Williams & Wilkins; 1995:421–433.

70. Rydén L, Ariniego R, Arnman K, Herlitz J, Hjalmarson A, Holmberg S, et al. A double-blind trial of metoprolol in acute myocardial infarction: Effects on ventricular tachyarrhythmias. *N Engl J Med* 1983; 308:614–618.

71. Szabo BM, Crijns HJGM, Wiesfeld ACP, van Veldhuisen DJ, Hillege HL, Lie KI. Predictors of mortality in patients with sustained ventricular tachycardias or ventricular fibrillation and depressed left ventricular function: Importance of β blockade. *Am Heart J* 1995; 130:281–286.

72. Mason JW, for the Electrophysiologic Study Versus Electrocardiographic Monitoring. A comparison of seven antiarrhythmic drugs in patients with ventricular tachyarrhythmias. *N Engl J Med* 1993; 329:452–458.

73. Kennedy HL, Brooks MM, Barker AH, Bergstrand R, Huther ML, Beanlands DS, et al. Beta blocker therapy in the Cardiac Arrhythmia Suppression Trial. *Am J Cardiol* 1994; 74:674–680.

74. Steinbeck G, Andresen D, Bach P, Haberl R, Oeff M, Hoffmann E, et al. A comparison of electrophysiologically guided antiarrhythmic drug therapy with beta blocker therapy in patients with symptomatic, sustained ventricular tachyarrhythmias. *N Engl J Med* 1992; 327:987–992.

75. Chiale PA, Rosenbaum MB, Elizari MV, Hjalmarson A, Magnusson Y, Wallukat G, et al. High prevalence of antibodies against beta₁- and beta₂-adrenoceptors in patients with primary electrical cardiac abnormalities. *J Am Coll Cardiol* 1995; 26:864–869.

76. Braunwald E, Muller JE, Kloner RA, Maroko P. Role of beta-adrenergic blockade in the therapy of patients with myocardial infarction. *Am J Med* 1983; 74:113–123.

77. Boissel J-P, Leizorovicz A, Picolet H, Peyrieux J-C for the APSI Investigators. Secondary prevention after high risk myocardial infarction with low-dose acebutolol. *Am J Cardiol* 1990; 66:251–260.

78. Park KC, Forman DE, Wei JY. Utility of beta-blockade treatment for older postinfarction patients. *J Am Geriatr Soc* 1995; 43:751–755.

79. Frishman WH. Post infarction survival: Role of β-adrenergic blockade. In: Fuster V, Ross R, Topol EJ, eds. *Atherosclerosis and Coronary Artery Disease.* Philadelphia: Lippincott-Raven; 1996:1205–1214.

80. Frishman WH. Secondary prevention of myocardial infarction: The roles of β-adrenergic blockers, calcium-channel blockers, angiotensin converting enzyme inhibitors, and aspirin. In: Willich SN, Muller JE, eds. *Triggering of Acute Coronary Syndromes.* Dordrecht, The Netherlands: Kluwer; 1996:367–394.

81. Frishman WH, Skolnick AE. Secondary prevention post infarction: The role of beta-adrenergic blockers, calcium-channel blockers, and aspirin. In: Gersh BJ, Rahimtoola SH, eds. *Acute Myocardial Infarction,* 2d ed. New York: Chapman & Hall; 1996:766–796.

82. Kendall MJ, Lynch KP, Hjalmarson A, Kjekshus J. β-Blockers and sudden cardiac death. *Ann Intern Med* 1995; 123:358–367.

83. Frishman WH, Lazar EJ. Reduction of mortality, sudden death and non-fatal reinfarction with beta-adrenergic blockers in survivors of acute myocardial infarction: A new hypothesis regarding the cardioprotective action of beta-adrenergic blockade. *Am J Cardiol* 1990; 66:66G–70G.

84. Hjalmarson A, Elmfeldt D, Herlitz J, Holmberg S, Malik I, Nyberg G, et al. Effect of mortality of metoprolol in acute myocardial infarction: A double-blind randomised trial. *Lancet* 1981; 2:823–827.

85. MIAMI Trial Research Group: Metoprolol in acute myocardial infarction (MIAMI): A randomized placebo-controlled international trial. *Eur Heart J* 1985; 6:199–226.

86. Ayanian JZ, Hauptman PJ, Guadagnoli E, Antman EM, Pashos CL, McNeil BJ. Knowledge and practices of generalist and specialist physicians regarding drug therapy for acute myocardial infarction. *N Engl J Med* 1994; 331:1136–1142.

87. Kennedy HL, Rosenson RS. Physician use of beta-adrenergic blocking therapy: A changing perspective (editorial). *J Am Coll Cardiol* 1995; 26:547–552.

88. ACC/AHA Guidelines for the Management of Patients with Acute Myocardial Infarction. A report of the American College of Cardiology/American Heart Association Task Force on Practice Guidelines. *J Am Coll Cardiol* 1996; 28:1328–1428.

89. Brand DA, Newcomer LN, Freiburger A, Tian H. Cardiologist's practice compared with practice guidelines: Use of beta-blockade after acute myocardial infarction. *J Am Coll Cardiol* 1995; 26:1432–1436.

90. Frishman WH, Teicher M. Antianginal drug therapy for silent myocardial ischemia. *Med Clin North Am* 1988; 72:185–196.

91. Rogers WJ, Bourassa MG, Andrews TC, Bertolet BD, Blumenthal RS, Chaitman BR. Asymptomatic Cardiac Ischemia Pilot (ACIP) Study: Outcome at 1 year for patients with asymptomatic cardiac ischemia randomized to medical therapy or revascularization. *J Am Coll Cardiol* 1995; 26:594–605.

92. Pepine CJ, Cohn PF, Deedwania PC, et al. for the ASIST (Atenolol/ Silent Ischemia Study) Study Group. Effects of treatment on outcome in mildly symptomatic patients with ischemia during daily life. *Circulation* 1994; 90:762–768.

93. Portegies MCM, Sijbring P, Gobel EJA, Viersma JW, Lie KI. Efficacy of metoprolol and diltiazem in treating silent myocardial ischemia. *Am J Cardiol* 1994; 74:1095–1098.

94. von Arnim T for the TIBBS Investigators. Prognostic significance of transient ischemic episodes: Response to treatment shows improved prognosis. Results of the Total Ischemic Burden Bisoprolol Study (TIBBS) follow-up. *J Am Coll Cardiol* 1996; 28:20–24.

95. Madjlessi-Simon T, Mary-Krause M, Fillette F, Lechat P, Jaillon P. Persistent transient myocardial ischemia despite beta-adrenergic blockade predicts a higher risk of adverse cardiac events in patients with coronary artery disease. *J Am Coll Cardiol* 1996; 27:1586–1591.

96. Jonas M, Reicher-Reiss H, Boyko V, Shotan A, Mandelzweig L, Goldbourt U, et al. Usefulness of beta-blocker therapy in patients with non-insulin dependent diabetes mellitus and coronary artery disease. *Am J Cardiol* 1996; 77:1273–1277.

97. Swan DA, Bell B, Oakley CM, Goodwin J. Analysis of symptomatic course and prognosis and treatment of hypertrophic obstructive cardiomyopathy. *Br Heart J* 1971; 33:671–685.

98. Eichhorn EJ, Bristow MR. Medical therapy can improve the biologic properties of the chronically failing heart. *Circulation* 1996; 9:2285–2296.

99. Engelhardt S, Bohm M, Erdmann E, Lohse MJ. Analysis of beta-adrenergic receptor mRNA levels in human ventricular biopsy specimens by quantitative polymerase chain reactions: Progressive reduction of beta$_1$-adrenergic receptor mRNA in heart failure. *J Am Coll Cardiol* 1996; 27:146–154.

100. Wu J-R, Chang H-R, Huang T-Y, Chiang C-H, Chen S-S. Reduction in lymphocyte β-adrenergic density in infants and children with heart failure secondary to congenital heart disease. *Am J Cardiol* 1996; 77:170–174.

101. Sackner-Bernstein JD, Mancini DM. Rationale for treatment of patients with chronic heart failure with adrenergic blockade. *JAMA* 1995; 274:1462–1467.

102. Francis GS, Goldsmith SR, Cohn JN. Relationship of exercise capacity to resting left ventricular performance and basal plasma norepinephrine levels in patients with congestive heart failure. *Am Heart J* 1982; 104:725–731.

103. Viquerat CE, Daly P, Swedberg K, Evers C, Curran D, Parmley WW, et al. Endogenous catecholamine levels in congestive heart failure: Relation to severity of hemodynamic abnormality. *Am J Med* 1985; 78:455–460.

104. Cohn JN, Levin TB, Olivari MT, Garberg V, Lura D, Francis GS, et al. Plasma norepinephrine as a guide to prognosis in patients with chronic heart failure. *N Engl J Med* 1984; 311:819–823.

105. Daley PA, Sole MJ. Myocardial catecholamines and the pathophysiology of heart failure. *Circulation* 1990; 82(suppl I):I-35–I-43.

106. Pauletto P, Vescove G, Scannapieco G, Pessina AC, Dal Palu C. Cardioprotection by beta blockers: Molecular and structural aspects in experimental hypertension. *Drugs Exp Clin Res* 1990; 16:1055.

107. Zimmer HG, Kolbeck-Ruhmkorff C, Zierhut W. Cardiac hypertrophy induced by alpha- and beta-adrenergic receptor stimulation. *Cardioscience* 1995; 6:47.

108. Podrid PJ, Fuchs T, Candinas R. Role of the sympathetic nervous system in the genesis of ventricular arrhythmias. *Circulation* 1990; 82(suppl I):I-103–I-113.

109. Charlap S, Lichstein E, Frishman EH. β-adrenergic blocking drugs in the treatment of congestive heart failure. *Med Clin North Am* 1989; 73:373–385.

110. Waagstein F, Hjalmarson A, Varnauskas E, Wallentin I. Effect of chronic beta-adrenergic receptor blockade in congestive cardiomyopathy. *Br Heart J* 1975; 37:1022–1036.

111. Anderson JL, Lutz JR, Gilbert EM, Sorensen SG, Yanowitz FG, Menlove RL, et al. A randomized trial of low dose beta blockade therapy for idiopathic dilated cardiomyopathy. *Am J Cardiol* 1985; 55:471–475.

112. Engelmeier RS, O'Connell JB, Walsh R, Rad N, Scanlon PJ, Gunnar RM. Improvement in symptoms and exercise tolerance by metoprolol in patients with dilated cardiomyopathy: A double-blind, randomized, placebo-controlled trial. *Circulation* 1985; 72:536–546.

113. Fisher ML, Gottlieb SS, Plotnick GD, Greenberg NL, Patten RD, Bennett SK, et al. Beneficial effects of metoprolol in heart failure associated with coronary artery disease: A randomized trial. *J Am Coll Cardiol* 1994; 23:943–950.

114. Currie PJ, Kelly MJ, McKenzie A, Harper RW, Lim YL, Federman J, et al. Oral beta adrenergic blockade with metoprolol in chronic severe dilated cardiomyopathy. *J Am Coll Cardiol* 1984; 3:203–209.

115. Waagstein F, Bristow MR, Swedberg K, Camerini F, Fowler MB, Silver MA, et al. Beneficial effects of metoprolol in idiopathic dilated cardiomyopathy. *Lancet* 1993; 342:1441–1446.

116. CIBIS Investigators and Committees: A randomized trial of beta blockade in heart failure: The Cardiac Insufficiency Bisoprolol Study. *Circulation* 1994; 90:1765–1773.

117. Ikram H, Fitzpatrick D. Double blind trial of chronic oral beta blockade in congestive cardiomyopathy. *Lancet* 1981; 2:490–493.

118. Pollock SG, Lystash J, Tedesco C, Craddock G, Smucker ML. Usefulness of bucindolol in congestive heart failure. *Am J Cardiol* 1990; 66:603–607.

119. Bristow MR, O'Connell JB, Gilbert EM, French WJ, Leatherman G, Kantrowitz NE, et al. Dose response of chronic β blocker treatment in heart failure from either idiopathic dilated cardiomyopathy or ischemic cardiomyopathy. *Circulation* 1994; 89:1632–1642.

120. Leung WH, Lau CP, Wong CK, Cheng CH, Tai YT, Lim SP. Improvement in exercise performance and hemodynamics by labetalol in patients with idiopathic dilated cardiomyopathy. *Am Heart J* 1990; 119:884–890.

121. Olsen SL, Gilbert EM, Renlund DG, Taylor DO, Yanowitz FD, Bristow MR. Carvedilol improves left ventricular function and symptoms in chronic heart failure: A double-blind randomized study. *J Am Coll Cardiol* 1995; 25:1225–1231.

122. Metra M, Nardi M, Giubbini R, Dei Cas L. Effects of short- and long-term carvedilol administration on rest and exercise hemodynamic variables, exercise capacity, and clinical conditions in patients with idiopathic dilated cardiomyopathy. *J Am Coll Cardiol* 1994; 24:1678–1687.

123. Krum H, Sackner-Bernstein J, Goldsmith RL, Kukin ML, Schwartz B, Penn J, et al. Double-blind, placebo-controlled study of the long-term efficacy of carvedilol in patients with severe chronic heart failure. *Circulation* 1995; 92:1499–1506.

124. Australia/New Zealand Heart Failure Research Collaborative Group: Effects of carvedilol, a vasodilator-β-blocker, in patients with congestive heart failure due to ischemic heart disease. *Circulation* 1995; 92:212–218.

125. Eichhorn EJ, McGhie AA, Bedotto JB, Corbett JR, Malloy CR, Hatfield BA, et al. Effects of bucindolol on neurohormonal activation in congestive heart failure. *Am J Cardiol* 1991; 67:67–73.

126. Australia/New Zealand Heart Failure Research Collaborative Group. Randomised, placebo-controlled trial of carvedilol in patients with congestive heart failure due to ischemic heart disease. *Lancet* 1997; 349:375–380.

127. Colucci WS, Packer M, Bristow MR, Gilbert EM, Cohn JN, Fowler MB, et al. Carvedilol inhibits clinical progression in patients with mild symptoms of heart failure. *Circulation* 1996; 94:2800–2806.

128. Bristow MR, Gilbert EM, Abraham WT, Adams KF, Fowler MB, Hershberger RE, et al. Carvedilol produces dose-related improvements in left ventricular function and survival in subjects with chronic heart failure. *Circulation* 1996; 94:2807–2816.

129. Gilbert EM, Abraham WT, Olsen S, Hattler B, White M, Mealy P. Comparative hemodynamic, left ventricular functional, and anti-adrenergic effects of chronic treatment with metoprolol versus carvedilol in the failing heart *Circulation* 1996; 94:2817–2825.

130. Gilbert EM, Sandoval A, Larrabee P, Renlund DG, O'Connell JB, Bristow MR. Lisinopril flowers cardiac adrenergic drive and increases beta-receptor density in the failing human heart. *Circulation* 1993; 88:472–480.

131. Rahman MA, Hara K, Daly PA, Wigle ED, Floras JS. Reductions in muscle sympathetic nerve activity after long-term metoprolol for dilated cardiomyopathy: Preliminary observation. *Br Heart J* 1995; 74:431–436.

132. Jeresaty RM. Mitral valve prolapse syndrome. *Prog Cardiovasc Dis* 1973; 15:623–652.

133. Silverman DI, Burton KJ, Gray J, Bosner MS, Kouchoukos NT, Roman MJ, et al. Life expectancy in the Marfan syndrome. *Am J Cardiol* 1995; 75:157–160.

134. Hachamovitch R, Strom JA, Sonnenblick EH, Frishman WH. Left ventricular hypertrophy in hypertension and the effects of antihypertensive drug therapy. *Curr Probl Cardiol* 1988; 13:371–421.

135. Mahananda N, Bhuripanyo K, Kangkagate C, Wansanit K, Kulchot B-O, Nademanee K, et al. Randomized, double-blind, placebo-controlled trial of oral atenolol in patients with unexplained syncope and positive upright tilt table test results. *Am Heart J* 1995; 130:1250–1253.

136. Cox MM, Perlman BA, Mayor MR, Silberstein TA, Levin S, Pringle L, et al. Acute and long-term beta-adrenergic blockade for patients with neurocardiogenic syncope. *J Am Coll Cardiol* 1995; 26:1293–1298.

137. Frishman WH, Fuksbrumer M, Tannenbaum M. Topical ophthalmic β-adrenergic blockade for the treatment of glaucoma and ocular hypertension. *J Clin Pharmacol* 1994; 34:795–803.

138. Villaneuva C, Balanzo J, Novella MT, Soriano G, Sainz S, Torras X, et al. Nadolol plus isosorbide mononitrate compared with sclerotherapy for the prevention of variceal bleeding. *N Engl J Med* 1996; 334:1624–1629.

139. Frishman W, Silverman R, Strom J, Elkayam U, Sonnenblick E. Clinical pharmacology of the new beta-adrenoceptor blocking drugs: Part IV. Adverse effects: Choosing a β-adrenoceptor blocker. *Am Heart J* 1979; 98:256–262.

140. Frishman WH. Beta-adrenergic receptor blockers: Adverse effects and drug interactions. *Hypertension* 1988; 11(suppl II):II21–II29.

141. Magjlessi-Simon G, Mary-Krause M, Fillette F, Lechat P, Jaillon P. Persistent transient myocardial ischemia despite beta-adrenergic blockade predicts a higher risk of adverse cardiac events in patients with coronary artery disease. *J Am Coll Cardiol* 1996; 27:1586–1591.

142. Frishman WH, Klein N, Strom J, Cohen MN, Shamoon H, Willens H, et al. Comparative effects of abrupt propranolol and verapamil withdrawal in angina pectoris. *Am J Cardiol* 1982; 50:1191–1195.

143. George RB, Manocha K, Burford JG, Conrad SA, Kinasewitz GT. Effects of labetalol in hypertensive patients with chronic obstructive pulmonary disease. *Chest* 1983; 83:457–460.

144. Frohlich ED, Tarazi RC, Dustan HP. Peripheral arterial insufficiency: A complication of beta-adrenergic blocking therapy. *JAMA* 1969; 208:2471–2472.

145. Radack K, Deck C. β-Adrenergic blocker therapy does not worsen intermittent claudication in subjects with peripheral arterial disease. *Arch Intern Med* 1991; 151:1769–1776.

146. Thadani U, Whitsett TL. β-Adrenergic blockers and intermittent claudication: Time for reappraisal (editorial). *Arch Intern Med* 1991; 151:1705–1707.

147. Hiatt WR, Stoll S, Nies A. Effect of beta-adrenergic blockers on the peripheral circulation in patients with peripheral vascular disease. *Circulation* 1985; 72:1226–1231.

148. Frishman WH, Clark A, Johnson B. The effects of cardiovascular drugs on plasma lipids and lipoproteins. In: Frishman WH, Sonnenblick EH, eds. *Cardiovascular Pharmacotherapeutics.* New York: McGraw-Hill; 1997:1515–1559.

149. Jacob H, Brandt LJ, Farkas P, Frishman WH. Beta-adrenergic blockade and the gastrointestinal system. *Am J Med* 1983; 74:1042–1051.

150. Blaufarb I, Pfeifer TM, Frishman WH. β Blockers: Drug interactions of clinical significance. *Drug Safety* 1995; 13:359–370.

151. Keefe D, Frishman WH. Clinical pharmacology of the calcium-channel blocking drugs. In: Packer M, Frishman WH, eds. *Calcium Channel Antagonists in Cardiovascular Disease.* Norwalk, CT: Appleton-Century-Crofts; 1984:3–19.

152. Frishman WH. Calcium channel blockers. In: Frishman WH, Sonnenblick EH, eds. *Cardiovascular Pharmacotherapeutics.* New York: McGraw-Hill; 1997:101–130.

153. Frishman WH. Current status of calcium channel blockers. *Curr Probl Cardiol* 1994; 19:637–688.

154. Frishman WH, ed. *Current Cardiovascular Drugs,* 2d ed. Philadelphia: Current Medicine, 1995.

155. Lindner E. Phenyl-propyl-diphenyl-prophyl-amin, a new substance with a dilating action in the coronary vessels. *Arzneim Forsch* 1960; 10:569–576.

156. Haas H, Hartfelder G. α-Isopropyl-α(N-methyl-N-homoveratryl)-γ-aminopropyl)-3,4-dimethoxyphenylacetonitrol, a substance with vasodilating properties. *Arzneim Forsch* 1962; 12:549–558.

157. Fleckenstein A, Kammermeier H, Doring H, et al. On the action mechanism of new coronary dilators with oxygen sparing myocardial effects—Prenylamin and Iproveratril. *Z Kreislauf Forsch* 1967; 56:716–744, 839–858.

158. Fleckenstein A. Control of myocardial metabolism by verapamil: Sites of action and therapeutic effects. *Arzneim Forsch* 1970; 20:1317–1322.

159. Singh BN, Vaughan-Williams EM. A fourth class of antidysrhythmic action? Effect of verapamil on ouabain toxicity, on atrial and ventricular intracellular potentials, and on other features of cardiac function. *Cardiovasc Res* 1972; 6:109–119.

160. Vaughan Williams EM. Classification of antiarrhythmic drugs. In: Sande E, Flensted-Jensen E, Olsen KH, eds. *Symposium on Cardiac Arrhythmias.* Elsinor: Astra; 1979:449–501.

161. Veniant M, Clozel JP, Hess P, Wolfgang R. Hemodynamic profile of Ro 40-5967 in conscious rats: Comparison with diltiazem, verapamil and amlodipine. *J Cardiovasc Pharmacol* 1991; 18(suppl 10):S55–S58.

162. Benet LZ. Pharmacokinetics and metabolism of bepridil. *Am J Cardiol* 1985; 55:8C–13C.

163. Opie LH, Frishman WH, Thadani U. Calcium channel antagonists. In: Opie LH, ed. *Drugs for the Heart,* 4th ed. Philadelphia: Saunders; 1995:50–83.

164. Vacher E, Richer C, Fornes P, Clozel J-P, Giudicelli J-F. Mibefradil, a selective calcium T-channel blocker, in stroke-prone spontaneously hypertensive rats. *J Cardiovasc Pharmacol* 1996; 27:686–694.

165. Singh BN, Hecht HS, Nademanee K, Chew CYC. Electrophysiologic and hemodynamic effects of slow channel blocking drugs. *Prog Cardiovasc Dis* 1982; 25:103–132.

166. Ellrodt G, Chew CYC, Singh BN. Therapeutic implications of slow-channel blockade in cardiocirculatory disorders. *Circulation* 1980; 62:669–679.

167. Landau AJ, Gentilucci M, Cavusoglu E, Frishman WH. Calcium antagonists for the treatment of congestive heart failure. *Cor Art Dis* 1994; 5:37–50.

168. Frishman WH, LeJemtel T. Electropharmacology of calcium channel antagonists in cardiac arrhythmias. *PACE* 1982; 5:402–413.

169. Singh BN, Nademanee K, Baky S. Calcium antagonists. *Drugs* 1983; 25:125–153.

170. Nayler WG, Poole-Wilson PH. Calcium antagonists: Definition and mode of action. *Basic Res Cardiol* 1981; 76:1–15.

171. Schmitt R, Kleinbloesem CH, Belz GG, Schroeter V, Feifel U, Pozenel H, et al. Hemodynamic and hormonal effects of the novel calcium antagonist RO 40-5967 in patients with hypertension. *Clin Pharmacol Ther* 1992; 52:314–323.

172. Singh BN, Collet J, Chew CYC. New perspectives in the pharmacologic therapy of cardiac arrhythmias. *Prog Cardiovasc Dis* 1980; 22:243–301.

173. Zipes DP, Fischer JC. Effects of agents which inhibit the slow channel on sinus node automaticity and atrioventricular conduction in the dog. *Circ Res* 1974; 34:184–192.

174. Findling R, Frishman W, Javed MT, Heffer S, Brandt L. Calcium channel blockers and the gastrointestinal tract. *Am J Ther* 1996; 3:383–408.

175. Schoen RE, Frishman WH, Shamoon H. Hormonal and metabolic effects of calcium-channel antagonists in man. *Am J Med* 1988; 84:492–504.

176. Shamoon H, Baylor P, Kamobosos D, Charlap S, Plawes S, Frishman WH. Influence of oral verapamil on glucoregulatory hormones in man. *J Clin Endocrinol Metab* 1985; 60:536–541.

177. Mehta JL. Influence of calcium-channel blockers on platelet function and arachidonic acid metabolism. *Am J Cardiol* 1985; 55:158B–164B.

178. Burns ER, Frishman WH. The anti-platelet effects of calcium channel blockers add to their antianginal properties. *Int J Cardiol* 1983; 4:372–379.

179. Lacoste L, Lam JYT, Hung J, Waters D. Oral verapamil inhibits platelet thrombus formation in humans. *Circulation* 1994; 89:630–634.

180. Frishman WH, Miller KP. Platelets and antiplatelet therapy in ischemic heart disease. *Curr Probl Cardiol* 1986; 11:72–136.

181. Kates R. Calcium antagonists—Pharmacokinetic properties. *Drugs* 1983; 25:113–124.

182. Brogden RN, McTavish D. Nifedipine gastrointestinal therapeutic system (GITS). *Drugs* 1995; 50:495–512.

183. Katz B, Rosenberg A, Frishman WH. Controlled-release drug delivery systems in cardiovascular medicine. *Am Heart J* 1995; 129:359–368.

184. Mitchell J, Frishman W, Heiman M. Nisoldipine: A new dihydropyridine calcium-channel blocker. *J Clin Pharmacol* 1993; 33:46–52.

185. Plosker GL, Faulds D. Nisoldipine coat-core: A review of its pharmacology and therapeutic efficacy in hypertension. *Drugs* 1996; 52:232–253.

186. White WB. A chronotherapeutic approach to the management of hypertension. *Am J Hypertens* 1996; 9:29S–33S.

187. Frishman WH, Kirstein E, Klein M, et al. Clinical relevance of verapamil plasma levels in stable angina pectoris. *Am J Cardiol* 1982; 50:1180–1184.

188. Frishman WH, Charlap S, Kimmel B, Teicher M, Cinnamon J, Allen L, et al. Diltiazem compared to nifedipine and combination treatment in patients with stable angina: Effects on angina, exercise tolerance and the ambulatory ECG. *Circulation* 1988; 77:774–786.

189. Bailey DG, Arnold JMO, Spence JD. Grapefruit juice and drugs. *Clin Pharmacokinet* 1994; 26:91–98.

190. Frishman WH, Sonnenblick EH. Cardiovascular uses of calcium-channel blockers. In: Messerli F, ed. *Current Cardiovascular Drug Therapy,* 2d ed. Philadelphia: Saunders; 1996:891–901.

191. Braun S, van der Wall EE, Emanuelson H, Kobrin I on behalf of the Mibefradil International Study Group. Effects of a new calcium antagonist, mibefradil (RO 40-5967), on silent ischemia in patients with stable chronic angina pectoris: A multicenter placebo-controlled study. *J Am Coll Cardiol* 1996; 27:317–322.

192. Landau AJ, Frishman WH, Alturk A. The pharmacological management of myocardial ischemia. *Curr Opin Cardiol* 1993; 8:629–636.

193. Opie LH. Calcium channel antagonists in the treatment of coronary artery disease: Fundamental pharmacological properties relevant to clinical use. *Prog Cardiovasc Dis* 1996; 38:273–290.

194. Bakx LM, van der Wall EE, Braun S, Emanuelson H, Bruschke AUG, Kobrin I. The effects of the new calcium antagonist mibefradil (RO40-

5967) on exercise duration in patients with chronic stable angina pectoris: A multicenter placebo-controlled study. *Am Heart J* 1995; 130:748–757.

195. Straus WE, McIntyre KM, Parisi AR, Shapiro W. Safety and efficacy of diltiazem hydrochloride for the treatment of stable angina pectoris—Report of a cooperative trial. *Am J Cardiol* 1982; 49:560–566.

196. Weiner DA, Cutler SS, Klein MD. Efficacy and safety of sustained-release diltiazem in stable angina pectoris. *Am J Cardiol* 1986; 57:6–9.

197. Mueller HS, Chahine RA. Interim report of multicenter double-blind placebo-controlled studies of nifedipine in chronic stable angina. *Am J Med* 1981; 71:645–657.

198. Wallace WA, Wellington KL, Chess MA, Liang C-S. Comparison of nifedipine gastrointestinal therapeutic system and atenolol on antianginal efficacies and exercise hemodynamic responses in stable angina pectoris. *Am J Cardiol* 1994; 73:23–28.

199. Cavoretto D, Repossini A, Alamanni F, Fratto PA, Valerio GN, Roberto M, et al. Amlodipine in residual stable exertional angina pectoris after coronary artery bypass surgery: A randomised, placebo-controlled, double-blind, crossover study. *Clin Drug Invest* 1995; 10:22–28.

200. Deanfield JE, Detry J-MRG, Lichtlen PR, et al, for the CAPE Study Group. Amlodipine reduces transient myocardial ischemia in patients with coronary artery disease: Double-bind Circadian Anti-ischemia Program in Europe (CAPE trial). *J Am Coll Cardiol* 1994; 24:1460–1467.

201. Pehrsson SK, Tolagen K, Ulvenstam G. Efficacy and safety of amlodipine compared with diltiazem in patients with stable angina pectoris. *Clin Drug Invest* 1996; 11:313–319.

202. Pepine CJ, Lambert CR. Usefulness of nicardipine for angina pectoris. *Am J Cardiol* 1987; 59:13J–19J.

203. Weiner DA, Klein MD, Cutler SS. Evaluation of sustained-release verapamil in chronic stable angina pectoris. *Am J Cardiol* 1987; 59:215–218.

204. Scheidt S, Frishman WH, Packer M, Mehta J, Parodi O, Bala Subramanian V. Long-term effectiveness of verapamil in stable and unstable angina pectoris: One year follow up of patients treated in placebo-controlled double-blind randomized clinical trials. *Am J Cardiol* 1982; 50:1185–1190.

205. Cutler NR, Anders RJ, Jhee SS, Sramek JJ, Awan NA, Bultas J, et al. Placebo-controlled evaluation of three doses of a controlled-onset, extended-release formulation of verapamil in the treatment of stable angina pectoris. *Am J Cardiol* 1995; 75:1102–1106.

206. Singh BN for the Bepridil Collaborative Study Group. Comparative efficacy and safety of bepridil and diltiazem in chronic stable angina pectoris refractory to diltiazem. *Am J Cardiol* 1991; 68:306–312.

207. Opie LH. Calcium channel antagonists in the management of anginal syndromes: Changing concepts in relation to the role of coronary vasospasm. *Prog Cardiovasc Dis* 1996; 38:291–314.

208. Frishman WH, Klein NA, Strom JA, Willens H, LeJemtel TH, Jentzer J, et al. Superiority of verapamil to propranolol in stable angina pectoris—A double-blind, randomized crossover trial. *Circulation* 1982; 65(suppl I):I51–I59.

209. Frishman WH, Hershman D. Beta-adrenergic blocking drugs in cardiac disorders. In: Messerli F, ed. *Current Cardiovascular Drug Therapy*, 2d ed. Philadelphia: Saunders; 1996:465–474.

210. Frishman WH, Klein N, Klein P, Strom JA, Tawil R, Strair R, et al. Comparison of oral propranolol and verapamil for combined systemic hypertension and angina pectoris: A placebo-controlled double-blind randomized crossover trial. *Am J Cardiol* 1982; 50:1164–1172.

211. Frishman WH, Charlap S. Calcium-channel blockers for combined systemic hypertension and myocardial ischemia. *Circulation* 1988; 75:V154–V162.

212. Boden WE, Korr KS, Bough KW. Nifedipine-induced hypotension and myocardial ischemia in refractory angina pectoris. *JAMA* 1985; 253:1131–1135.

213. Stone PH, Gibson RS, Glasser SP, DeWood MA, Parker JD, Kawanishi DT, et al. Comparison of propranolol, diltiazem, and nifedipine in the treatment of ambulatory ischemia in patients with stable angina: Differential effects on ambulatory ischemia, exercise performance, and anginal symptoms. *Circulation* 1990; 82:1962–1972.

214. Frishman WH. Comparative efficacy and concomitant use of bepridil and beta blockers in the management of angina pectoris. *Am J Cardiol* 1992; 69(suppl):50D–60D.

215. Mehta J, Conti CR. Calcium channel antagonists in the treatment of unstable angina. *Am J Cardiol* 1982; 50:919–922.

216. Theroux P, Waters DD, Affaki GS, Crittin J, Bonan R, Mizgala HF.

Provocative testing with ergonovine to evaluate the efficacy of treatment with calcium antagonists in variant angina. *Circulation* 1979; 60:504–510.

217. Antman E, Muller JE, Goldberg S, MacAlpin R, Rubenfire M, Tabatznik B, et al. Nifedipine therapy for coronary artery spasm experience in 127 patients. *N Engl J Med* 1980; 302:1269–1273.

218. Schroeder JS, Feldman RL, Giles TD, Friedman MJ, DeMaria AN, Kinney EL, et al. Multiclinic controlled trial of diltiazem for Prinzmetal's angina. *Am J Med* 1982; 72:227–232.

219. Feldman RL, Pepine CJ, Whittle J, Conti CR. Short- and long-term responses to diltiazem in patients with variant angina. *Am J Cardiol* 1982; 49:554–559.

220. Prida XE, Gelman JS, Feldman RL, Hill JA, Pepine CJ, Scott E. Comparison of diltiazem alone and in combination in patients with coronary artery spasm. *J Am Coll Cardiol* 1987; 9:412–419.

221. Chahine RA, Feldman RL, Giles TD, Nicod P, Raizner AE, Weiss RJ, et al. Randomized placebo-controlled trial of amlodipine in vasospastic angina. *J Am Coll Cardiol* 1993; 21:1365–1370.

222. Parodi O, Simonetti I, L'Abbate A, Maseri A. Comparative effectiveness of verapamil and propranolol in angina at rest. *Am J Cardiol* 1982; 50:923–928.

223. Johnson SM, Mauritson DR, Willerson JT, Hillis LD. Comparison of verapamil and nifedipine in the treatment of variant angina pectoris—Preliminary observation in 10 patients. *Am J Cardiol* 1981; 47:1295–1300.

224. Gerstenblith G, Ouyang P, Achuff S, Bulkley BH, Becker LC, Mellits ED, et al. Nifedipine in unstable angina: A double-blind randomized trial. *N Engl J Med* 1982; 306:885–889.

225. Pritchett ELC. Management of atrial fibrillation. *N Engl J Med* 1992; 326:1264–1271.

226. Ellenbogen KA, Dias VC, Plumb VJ, Heywood JT, Mirvis DM. A placebo-controlled trial of continuous intravenous diltiazem infusion for 24-hour heart rate control during atrial fibrillation and atrial flutter: A multicenter trial. *J Am Coll Cardiol* 1991; 18:891–897.

227. Klein HO, Pauzner H, DiSegni E, David D. Kaplinsky E. The beneficial effects of verapamil in chronic atrial fibrillation. *Arch Intern Med* 1979; 139:747–749.

228. Weiner I. Verapamil therapy for atrial flutter and fibrillation. In: Packer M, Frishman WH, eds. *Calcium Channel Antagonists in Cardiovascular Disease*. Norwalk, CT: Appleton-Century-Crofts; 1984:257–268.

229. Klein HO, Kaplinsky E. Comparative effectiveness of verapamil and digoxin in atrial fibrillation. *Am J Cardiol* 1982; 50:894–902.

230. Singh BN, Nademanee D, Baky S. Calcium antagonists. Uses in the treatment of cardiac arrhythmias. *Drugs* 1983; 25:125–153.

231. Hartel G, Hartikainen M. Comparison of verapamil and practolol in paroxysmal supraventricular tachycardia. *Eur J Cardiol* 1976; 4:87–90.

232. Mauritson DR, Winniford MD, Walker WS, Rude RE, Cary JR, Hillis LD. Oral verapamil for paroxysmal supraventricular tachycardia: A long-term, double-blind, randomized trial. *Ann Intern Med* 1982; 96:409–412.

233. Matsuyama E, Konishi T, Okazaki H, Matsuda H, Kawai C. Effects of verapamil on accessory pathway properties and induction of circus movement tachycardia in patients with the Wolff-Parkinson-White syndrome. *J Cardiovasc Pharmacol* 1981; 3:11–24.

234. Ruskin J. Catheter ablation for supraventricular tachycardia (editorial). *N Engl J Med* 1991; 324:1660–1662.

235. Billman GE. Effect of calcium channel antagonists on cocaine-induced malignant arrhythmias: Protection against ventricular fibrillation. *J Pharmacol Exp Ther* 1993; 266:407–416.

236. Carrasco HA, Fuenmayor A, Barboza J, Gonzalez G. Effect of verapamil on normal sino-atrial node dysfunction and on sick sinus syndrome. *Am Heart J* 1978; 96:760–771.

237. Cummings DM, Amadio P, Nelson L, Fitzgerald JM. The role of calcium channel blockers in the treatment of systemic hypertension. *Arch Intern Med* 1991; 151:250–259.

238. Frishman WH, Stroh JA, Greenberg SM, Suarez T, Karp A, Peled HB. Calcium-channel blockers in systemic hypertension. *Med Clin North Am* 1988; 72:449–499.

239. Halperin AK, Icenogle MV, Kapsner CO, Chick TW, Roehnert J, Murata GH. A comparison of the effects of nifedipine and verapamil on exercise performance in patients with mild to moderate hypertension. *Am J Hypertens* 1993; 6:1025–1032.

240. Frishman WH, Zawada ET, Smith LK, Sowers J, Swartz SL, Kirkendall W, et al. A comparative study of diltiazem and hydrochlorothiazide as initial medical therapy for mild to moderate hypertension. *Am J Cardiol* 1987; 59:615–623.

241. Materson BJ, Reda DJ, Cushman WC, Massie BM, Freis ED, Kochar MS, et al. Single-drug therapy for hypertension in men: A comparison of six antihypertensive agents with placebo. *N Engl J Med* 1993; 328:914–921.

242. Frishman WH, Garofalo JL, Rothschild A, Rothschild M, Greenberg SM, Soberman J. Multicenter comparison of the nifedipine gastrointestinal system and long-acting propranolol in patients with mild to moderate systemic hypertension receiving diuretics: A preliminary experience. *Am J Med* 1987; 83:15–19.

243. Johnson BF, Frishman WH, Brobyn R, Brown RD, Reeves RL, Wombolt DG. A randomized placebo-controlled, double-blind comparison of amlodipine and atenolol in patients with essential hypertension. *Am J Hypertens* 1992; 5:727–732.

244. Taylor SH, Frais MA, Lee P, Verma SP, Jackson N, Reynolds G, et al. A study of the long-term efficacy and tolerability of oral nicardipine in hypertensive patients. *Br J Clin Pharmacol* 1985; 20(suppl 1):139S–142S.

245. Todd PA, Faulds D. Felodipine: A review of the pharmacology and therapeutic use of the extended-release formulation in cardiovascular disorders. *Drugs* 1992; 44:251–272.

246. Hamilton BP. Treatment of essential hypertension with PN 200-110 (isradipine). *Am J Cardiol* 1987; 59:141–145.

247. Black HR, Smolensky MH, Johnstone MT, White WB. The emerging role of chronotherapeutics in managing hypertension: Panel discussion. *Am J Hypertens* 1996; 9:34S–39S.

248. Frishman WH, Ram CVS, McMahon FG, Chrysant SG, Graff A, Kupiec JW, et al. Comparison of amlodipine and benazepril monotherapy to combination therapy in patients with systemic hypertension: A randomized, double-blind, placebo-controlled, parallel group study. *J Clin Pharmacol* 1995; 35:1060–1066.

249. Messerli F, Frishman WH, Elliott W, and the Trandolapril Study Group. Additive effects of verapamil and trandolapril in the treatment of mild to moderate hypertension. *Am J Hypertens* 1997. In press.

250. Hoffmann J. Comparison of felodipine-metoprolol combination tablet versus each component alone as antihypertensive therapy. *Blood Pressure* 1993; 2(suppl I):30–36.

251. Malacco E. Treatment of isolated systolic hypertension: The SHELL study (abstr). In: Symposium on Diagnostic and Therapeutic Aspects of Hypertension, Nice, June 29–30, 1993.

252. Frishman WH, Skolnick AE. Effects of calcium blockade on hypertension-induced left ventricular hypertrophy. *Circulation* 1989; 80(suppl IV):151–161.

253. Buhler F, DeLeeuw PW, Doyle A, Fleckenstein A, Fleckenstein-Grun G, Frishman WH, et al. Calcium metabolism and calcium-channel blockers for understanding and treating hypertension. *Am J Med* 1984; 77(6B):1–23.

254. Fioretto P, Frigato F, Velussi M, Riva F, Muollo B, Carraro A, et al. Effects of angiotensin converting enzyme inhibitors and calcium antagonists on atrial natriuretic peptide release and action and on albumin excretion rate in hypertensive insulin-dependent diabetic patients. *Am J Hypertens* 1992; 5:837–846.

255. Zanetti-Elshater F, Pingitore R, Beretta-Piccoli C, Riesen W, Heinen G. Calcium antagonists for treatment of diabetes-associated hypertension: Metabolic and renal effects of amlodipine. *Am J Hypertens* 1994; 7:36–45.

256. Frielingsdorf J, Seiler C, Kaufmann P, Vassalli G, Suter T, Hess OM. Normalization of abnormal coronary vasomotion by calcium antagonists in patients with hypertension. *Circulation* 1996; 93:1380–1387.

257. Zing W, Ferguson RK, Vlasses PH. Calcium antagonists in elderly and black hypertensive patients: Therapeutic controversies. *Arch Intern Med* 1991; 151:2154–2162.

258. Kloner RA, Sowers JR, DiBona GF, Gaffney M, Wein M, for the Amlodipine Cardiovascular Community Trial Study Group. Sex- and age-related antihypertensive effects of amlodipine. *Am J Cardiol* 1996; 77:713.

259. Erne P, Bolli P, Bertel O, Hulthen UL, Kiowski W, Muller FB, et al. Antihypertensive monotherapy with calcium antagonists relates to older age, liver pretreatment renin and higher blood pressure: Comparison of nifedipine and verapamil. *Hypertension* 1983; 5(suppl II):II-97–II-102.

260. Brozena SC, Johnson MR, Ventura H, Hobbs R, Miller L, Olivari MT, et al. Effectiveness and safety of diltiazem or lisinopril in treatment of hypertension after heart transplantation. *J Am Coll Cardiol* 1996; 27:1707–1712.

261. Psaty BM, Siscovick DS, Weiss NS, Koepsell TD, Rosendaal FR, Lin

D, et al. Hypertension and outcomes research: From clinical trials to clinical epidemiology. *Am J Hypertens* 1996; 9:178–183.

262. Psaty BM, Heckbert SR, Koepsell TD, Siscovick DS, Raghunathan TE, Weiss NS, et al. The risk of myocardial infarction associated with antihypertensive drug therapies. *JAMA* 1995; 274:620–625.

263. Pahor M, Guralnik JM, Corti M-C, Foley DJ, Carbonin P, Havlik RJ. Long-term survival and use of antihypertensive medications in older persons. *J Am Geriatr Soc* 1995; 43:1191–1197.

264. Furberg CD, Psaty BM. Calcium antagonists: Not appropriate as first line antihypertensive agents. *Am J Hypertens* 1996; 9:122–125.

265. Furberg CD, Psaty BM. Calcium antagonists: Antagonists or protagonists of mortality in elderly hypertensives? (editorial). *J Am Geriatr Soc* 1995; 43:1309–1310.

266. Yusuf S. Calcium antagonists in coronary artery disease and hypertension: Time for reevaluation? *Circulation* 1995; 92:1079–1082.

267. Furberg CD, Psaty BM. Should dihydropyridines be used as first-line drugs in the treatment of hypertension (commentary)? The con side. *Arch Intern Med* 1995; 155:2157–2161.

268. Epstein M. Calcium antagonists should continue to be used for first-line treatment of hypertension (commentary). *Arch Intern Med* 1995; 155:2150–2156.

269. Fagan TC. Calcium antagonists and mortality: Another case of the need for clinical judgement (editorial). *Arch Intern Med* 1995; 155:2145.

270. Epstein M. Calcium antagonists: Still appropriate as first-line antihypertensive agents. *Am J Hypertens* 1996; 9:110–121.

271. Laragh JH, Held C, Messerli F, Pepine C, Sleight P. Calcium antagonists and cardiovascular prognosis: A homogeneous group? *Am J Hypertens* 1996; 9:99–109.

272. Braun S, Boyko V, Behar S, Reicher-Reiss H, Shotan A, Schlesinger Z, et al. Calcium antagonists and mortality in patients with coronary artery disease: A cohort study of 11,575 patients. *J Am Coll Cardiol* 1996; 28:7–11.

273. Messerli F. What happened to the calcium antagonist controversy? *J Am Coll Cardiol* 1996; 28:12–13.

274. Bazunga M, Cho MSS. Reassessing antihypertensive agents in the post-JNC V era. *Formulary* 1996; 31:116.

275. Pahor M, Guralnik JM, Salive ME, Corti M-C, Carbonin P, Havlik RJ. Do calcium channel blockers increase the risk of cancer? *Am J Hypertens* 1996; 9:695–699.

276. Alderman MH. More news about calcium antagonists (editorial). *Am J Hypertens* 1996; 9:710–712.

277. Daling JR. Calcium channel blockers and cancer: Is an association biologically plausible? *Am J Hypertens* 1996; 9:713–714.

278. Frishman WH, Weinberg P, Peled H, Kimmel B, Charlap S, Beer N. Calcium-entry blockers for the treatment of severe hypertension and hypertensive emergencies. *Am J Med* 1984; 77(2B):35–45.

279. Beer N, Gallegos I, Cohen A, Klein N, Sonnenblick E, Frishman W. Efficacy of sublingual nifedipine in the acute treatment of systemic hypertension. *Chest* 1981; 79:571–574.

280. Grossman E, Messerli FH, Grodzicki T, Kowey P. Should a moratorium be placed on sublingual nifedipine capsules given for hypertensive emergencies and pseudoemergencies? *JAMA* 1996; 276:1328–1331.

281. Wallin JD, Fletcher E, Ram CVS, Cook E, Cheung DG, MacCarthy EP, et al. Intravenous nicardipine for the treatment of severe hypertension: A double-blind, placebo-controlled multicenter trial. *Arch Intern Med* 1989; 149:2662–2669.

282. IV Nicardipine Study Group. Efficacy and safety of intravenous nicardipine in the control of postoperative hypertension. *Chest* 1991; 99:393–398.

283. Frishman W. Management of hypertensive urgencies and emergencies. In: Frishman WF, Sonnenblick EH, eds. *Cardiovascular Pharmacotherapeutics*. New York: McGraw-Hill; 1997:1577–1592.

284. Frishman WH, Teicher M. Antianginal drug therapy for silent myocardial ischemia. *Med Clin North Am* 1988; 72:185–196.

285. Deedwania PC, Carbajal EV. Silent myocardial ischemia: A clinical perspective. *Arch Intern Med* 1991; 151:2373–2382.

286. Epstein SE, Quyyumi Aa, Bonow RO. Myocardial ischemia—Silent or symptomatic. *N Engl J Med* 1988; 318:1038–1043.

287. Ardissino D, Savonitto S, Egstrup K, Marraccini P, Slavich G, Rosenfeld M, et al. Transient myocardial ischemia during daily life in rest and exertional angina pectoris and comparison of effectiveness of metoprolol versus nifedipine. *Am J Cardiol* 1991; 67:946–952.

288. Rogers WJ, Bourassa MG, Andrews TC, Bertolet BD, Blumenthal RS, Chaitman BR, et al. Asymptomatic Cardiac Ischemia Pilot (ACIP) Study: Outcome at 1 year for patients with asymptomatic cardiac ischemia randomized to medical therapy or revascularization. *J Am Coll Cardiol* 1995; 26:594–605.

289. Pratt CM, McMahon RP, Goldstein S, Pepine CJ, Andrews TC, Dyrda I, et al. Comparison of subgroups assigned to medical regimens used to suppress cardiac ischemia [The Asymptomatic Cardiac Ischemia Pilot (ACIP) Study]. *Am J Cardiol* 1996; 77:1302–1309.

290. Skolnick AE, Frishman WH. Calcium channel blockers in myocardial infarction. *Arch Intern Med* 1989; 149:1669–1677.

291. Messerli FH. "Cardioprotection"—Not all calcium antagonists are created equal. *Am J Cardiol* 1990; 66:855–856.

292. Wilcox RG, Hampton JR, Banks DC, Birkhead JS, Brooksby IAB, Burns-Cox CJ, et al. Trial of early nifedipine in acute myocardial infarction: The TRENT Study. *Br Med J* 1986; 293:1204–1208.

293. The Danish Study Group on Verapamil in Myocardial Infarction. Verapamil in acute myocardial infarction. *Eur Heart J* 1984; 5:516–528.

294. Gibson RS, Boden WE, Theroux P, Strauss HD, Pratt CM, Gheorghiade M, et al. Diltiazem and reinfarction in patients with non Q-wave-myocardial infarction: Results of a double-blind, randomized, multicenter trial. *N Engl J Med* 1986; 315:423–429.

295. Muller JE, Morrison J, Stone PH, Rude RE, Rosner B, Roberts R, et al. Nifedipine therapy for patients with threatened and acute myocardial infarction: A randomized, double-blind, placebo-controlled comparison. *Circulation* 1984; 69:740–747.

296. Neufeld HN. Calcium antagonists in secondary prevention after acute myocardial infarction: The Secondary Prevention Reinfarction Nifedipine Trial (SPRINT). *Eur Heart J* 1986; 7(suppl B):51–52.

297. The Multicenter Diltiazem Postinfarction Trial Research Group. The effect of diltiazem on mortality and reinfarction after myocardial infarction. *N Engl J Med* 1988; 319:385 392.

298. The Danish Study on Verapamil in Myocardial Infarction. The effect of verapamil on mortality and major events after myocardial infarction: The Danish Verapamil Infarction Trial II (DAVIT II). *Am J Cardiol* 1990; 66:779–785.

299. Yusuf S, Held P, Furberg CD. Update of effects of calcium antagonists in myocardial infarction or angina in light of the second Danish Verapamil Infarction Trial (DAVIT II) and other recent studies. *Am J Cardiol* 1991; 67:1295–1297.

300. Rengo F, Carbonin P, Pahor M, DeCaprio L, Bernabei R, Ferrara N, et al. A controlled trial of verapamil in patients after acute myocardial infarction: Results of the Calcium Antagonist Reinfarction Italian Study (CRIS). *Am J Cardiol* 1996; 77:365–369.

301. Furberg CD, Psaty BM, Meyer JV. Nifedipine: Dose-related increase in mortality in patients with coronary heart disease. *Circulation* 1995; 92:1326–1331.

302. Kostis JB, Wilson AC, Cosgrove NM, Lacy CR. Effects of calcium channel blockers on the incidence of myocardial infarction in patients with left ventricular dysfunction (abstr). *J Am Coll Cardiol* 1996; 27(2, suppl A):36A.

303. Boden WE, Scheldewaert R, Walters EG, Whitehead A, Coltart DJ, Santoni J-P, et al. Design of a placebo-controlled clinical trial of long-acting diltiazem and aspirin versus aspirin alone in patients receiving thrombolysis with a first acute myocardial infarction. *Am J Cardiol* 1995; 75:1120–1123.

304. Yusuf S. Verapamil following uncomplicated myocardial infarction: Promising, but not proven (editorial). *Am J Cardiol* 1996; 77:421–422.

305. Sleight P. Calcium antagonists during and after myocardial infarction. *Drugs* 1996; 51:216–225.

306. Pelliccia F, Cianfrocca C, Romeo F, Reale A. Hypertrophic cardiomyopathy: Long-term effects of propranolol versus verapamil in preventing sudden death in "low-risk patients." *Cardiovasc Drugs Ther* 1990; 4:1515–1518.

307. Seiler C, Hess OM, Schoenbeck M, Turina J, Jenni R, Turina M, et al. Long term follow up of medical versus surgical therapy for hypertrophic cardiomyopathy: A retrospective study. *J Am Coll Cardiol* 1991; 17:634–642.

308. Rosing DR, Bonow RO, Packer M, Epstein SE. Verapamil therapy for the management of hypertrophic cardiomyopathy. In: Packer M, Frishman WH, eds. *Calcium Channel Antagonists in Cardiovascular Disease.* Norwalk, CT: Appleton-Century-Crofts; 1984:313–342.

309. Udelson JE, Bonow RO, O'Gara PT, Maron BJ, VanLingen A, Bacharach SL, et al. Verapamil prevents silent myocardial perfusion abnormalities during exercise in asymptomatic patients with hypertrophic cardiomyopathy. *Circulation* 1989; 79:1052–1060.

310. Kaltenbach M, Hopf R, Kober G, Bussman W-D, Keller M, Petersen Y. Treatment of hypertrophic obstructive cardiomyopathy with verapamil. *Br Heart J* 1979; 42:35–42.

311. Rosing DR, Kent KM, Maron BJ, Epstein SE. Verapamil therapy—A new approach for the pharmacologic treatment of hypertrophic cardiomyopathy: II. Effects on exercise capacity and symptomatic status. *Circulation* 1979; 60:1208–1213.

312. Rosing DR, Kent KM, Borer JS, Seides SF, Maron BJ, Epstein SE. Verapamil therapy—A new approach to the pharmacologic treatment of hypertrophic cardiomyopathy: I. Hemodynamic effects. *Circulation* 1979; 60:1201–1207.

313. Bonow RO, Rosing DR, Bacharach SL, Green MV, Kent KM, Lipson LC, et al. Effects of verapamil on left ventricular systolic function and diastolic filling in patients with hypertrophic cardiomyopathy. *Circulation* 1981; 64:787–796.

314. Rosing DR, Cannon RO, Watson RM, Kent KM, Lakatos E, Epstein SE. Comparison of verapamil and nifedipine effects on symptoms and exercise capacity in patients with hypertrophic cardiomyopathy (abstr). *Circulation* 1982; 66(suppl II):II-24.

315. Betocchi S, Piscione F, Losi MA, Pace L, Boccalatte M, Perrone-Filardi P, et al. Effects of diltiazem on left ventricular systolic and diastolic function in hypertrophic cardiomyopathy. *Am J Cardiol* 1996; 78:451–457.

316. Packer M. Calcium channel blockers in chronic heart failure: The risks of "physiologically rational" therapy (editorial comment). *Circulation* 1990; 82:2254–2257.

317. Charlap S, Frishman WH. Calcium antagonists and heart failure. *Med Clin North Am* 1989; 73:339–360.

318. Elkayam U, Amin J, Mehra A, Vasquez J, Weber L, Rahimtoola SH. A prospective, randomized, double-blind, crossover study to compare the efficacy and safety of chronic nifedipine therapy with that of isosorbide dinitrate and their combination in the treatment of chronic congestive heart failure. *Circulation* 1990; 82:1954–1961.

319. Losardo AA, Klein NA, Beer N, Strom J, Wexler JP, Sonnenblick EH, et al. Beneficial effects of sublingual nifedipine in patients with ischemic heart disease and depressed left ventricular function. *Angiology* 1982; 33:811–817.

320. Klugmann S, Salvi A, Camerini F. Haemodynamic effects of nifedipine in heart failure. *Br Heart J* 1980; 43:440–446.

321. Fifer MA, Colucci WS, Lorell BH, Jaski BE, Barry WH. Comparison of hemodynamic responses to nifedipine in heart failure: Comparison with nitroprusside. *J Am Coll Cardiol* 1985; 5:731–737.

322. Packer M, Lee WH, Medina N, Yushak M, Bernstein JL, Kessler PD. Prognostic importance of the immediate hemodynamic response to nifedipine in patients with severe left ventricular dysfunction. *J Am Coll Cardiol* 1987; 10:1303 1311.

323. Figulla HR, Gietzen F, Zeymer U, Raiber M, Hegelsmann J, Soballa R, et al. Diltiazem improves cardiac function and exercise capacity in patients with idiopathic dilated cardiomyopathy. *Circulation* 1996; 94:346–352.

324. Boden WE, Ziesche S, Carson PE, et al, for the V-HeFT III Investigators. Rationale and design of the third Vasodilator–Heart Failure Trial (V-HeFT III): Felodipine as adjunctive therapy to enalapril and loop diuretics with or without digoxin in chronic congestive heart failure. *Am J Cardiol* 1996; 77:1078–1082.

325. O'Connor CM, Belkin RN, Carson PE, Cropp AB, Frid DJ, Miller AB. Effect of amlodipine on mode of death in severe chronic heart failure: The PRAISE Trial. *Circulation* 1996; 92:676.

326. Packer M, O'Connor CM, Ghali JK, Pressler ML, Carson PE, Belkin RN, et al. Effect of amlodipine on morbidity and mortality in severe chronic heart failure. *N Engl J Med* 1996; 335:1107–1114.

327. Kostis JB, Wilson AC, Cosgrove NM, Lacy CR. Effect of calcium channel blockers on the incidence of myocardial infarction in patients with left ventricular dysfunction (abstr). *J Am Coll Cardiol* 1996; 27(suppl A):36B.

328. Scognamiglio R, Rahimtoola S, Fasoli G, Nistri S, Dalla Volta S. Nifedipine in asymptomatic patients with severe aortic regurgitation and normal left ventricular function. *N Engl J Med* 1994; 331:689–694.

329. Muntinga HJ, van der Vring JAFM, Niemeyer MG, van den Berg F, Knol HR, Bernink PJLM, et al. Effect of mibefradil on left ventricular diastolic function in patients with congestive heart failure. *J Cardiovasc Pharmacol* 1996; 27:652–656.

330. Setaro JF, Zaret BL, Schulman DS, Black HR, Soufer R. Usefulness of verapamil for congestive heart failure associated with abnormal left ventricular diastolic filling and normal left ventricular systolic performance. *Am J Cardiol* 1990; 66:981–986.

331. Dobkin J, Reichel J. Drug treatment of primary pulmonary hypertension. In: Frishman WF, Sonnenblick EH, eds. *Cardiovascular Pharmacotherapeutics.* New York: McGraw-Hill; 1997:1173–1183.

332. Loscalzo J. Endothelial dysfunction in pulmonary hypertension (editorial). *N Engl J Med* 1992; 327:117–119.

333. Rich S, Kaufman E, Levy PS. The effect of high doses of calcium channel blockers on survival in primary pulmonary hypertension. *N Engl J Med* 1992; 327:76–84.

334. Packer M. Vasodilator therapy for primary pulmonary hypertension: Limitations and hazards. *Ann Intern Med* 1985; 103:258–270.

335. Allen GS, Ahn HS, Preziosi TJ, Battye R, Boone SC, Chou SN, et al. Cerebral arterial spasm—A controlled trial of nimodipine in patients with subarachnoid hemorrhage. *N Engl J Med* 1983; 308:619–624.

336. Bussey HI, Talbert RL. Promising uses of calcium-channel blocking agents. *Pharmacotherapy* 1984; 4:137–143.

337. Wadworth AN, McTavish D. Nimodipine: A review of its pharmacological properties, and therapeutic efficacy in cerebral disorders. *Drugs Aging* 1992; 2:262–286.

338. Haley EC, Kassell NF, Torner JC, Kongable G. Nicardipine ameliorates angiographic vasospasm following subarachnoid hemorrhage (abstr). *Neurology* 1991; 41(suppl 1):346.

339. Zornow MH, Prough DS. Neuroprotective properties of calcium-channel blockers. *New Horizons* 1996; 4:107–114.

340. Gelmers HJ, Gorter K. DeWeerdt CJ, Wiezer HJA. A controlled trial of nimodipine in acute ischemic stroke. *N Engl J Med* 1988; 318:203–207.

341. Steen PA, Gisvold SE, Milde JH, Newberg LA, Scheithauer BW, Lanier WL, et al. Nimodipine improves outcome when given after complete cerebral ischemia in primates. *Anesthesiology* 1985; 62:406–414.

342. Trust Study Group. Randomised, double-blind, placebo-controlled trial of nimodipine in acute stroke. *Lancet* 1990; 336:1205–1209.

343. The American Nimodipine Study Group. Clinical trial of nimodipine in acute ischemic stroke. *Stroke* 1992; 23:3–8.

344. Henry PD. Atherogenesis, calcium and calcium antagonists. *Am J Cardiol* 1990; 66:31–61.

345. Lichtlen PR, Hugenholtz PG, Rafflenbeul W, Hecker H, Jost S, Deckers JW on behalf of the INTACT Group Investigators. Retardation of angiographic progression of coronary artery disease by nifedipine. *Lancet* 1990; 335:1109–1113.

346. Waters D, Lesperance J, Francetich M, Causey D. Theroux P, Chiang Y-K, et al. A controlled clinical trial to assess the effect of a calcium channel blocker on the progression of coronary atherosclerosis. *Circulation* 1990; 82:1940–1953.

347. Paoletti R, Bernini F, Corsini A, Soma MR. The antiatherosclerotic effects of calcium antagonists. *J Cardiovasc Pharmacol* 1995; 25(suppl 3):S6–S10.

348. Schroeder JS, Gao S-Z, Alderman EL, Hunt SA, Johnstone I, Boothroyd DB, et al. A preliminary study of diltiazem in the prevention of coronary artery disease in heart transplant recipients. *N Engl J Med* 1993; 328:164–170.

349. Borhani NO, Mercuri M, Borhani PA, Buckalew VM, Canossa-Terris M, Carr AA, et al. Final outcome results of the multicenter isradipine diuretic atherosclerosis study (MIDAS). *JAMA* 1996; 276:785–791.

350. Lee CR, Bryson HM. Lacidipine. *Drugs* 1994; 48:274.

351. Bond MG, Mercuri M for the ELSA Research Group. Potential modification of plaque behavior through the European Lacidipine Study on Atherosclerosis. *J Cardiovasc Pharmacol* 1995; 25(suppl 3):S11–S16.

352. Belch JJF, Ho M. Pharmacology of Raynaud's phenomenon. *Drugs* 1996; 52:682–695.

353. Cristakis GT, Fremes SE, Weisel RD, Tittley JG, Mickle DAG, Ivanov J, et al. Diltiazem cardioplegia: A balance of risk and benefit. *J Thorac Cardiovasc Surg* 1986; 91:647–661.

354. Seitelberger R, Zwolfer W, Huber S, Schwarzacher S, Binder TM, Peschl F, et al. Nifedipine reduces the incidence of myocardial infarction and transient ischemia in patients undergoing coronary bypass grafting. *Circulation* 1991; 83:460–468.

355. Piessens J, Brzostek T, Stammen F, Vanhaecke J, Vrolix M, DeGeest H. Effect of intravenous diltiazem on myocardial ischemia during percutaneous transluminal coronary angioplasty. *Am J Cardiol* 1989; 64:1103–1107.

356. Landzberg BR, Frishman WH, Lerrick K. Pathophysiology and pharmacological approaches for prevention of coronary artery restenosis following coronary artery balloon angioplasty and related procedures. *Prog Cardiovasc Dis* 1997; 34:361–398.

357. Factor SM, Minase T, Cho S, Dominitz R, Sonnenblick EH. Microvascular spasm in the cardiomyopathic Syrian hamster: A preventable cause of focal myocardial necrosis. *Circulation* 1982; 66:342–354.

358. Palmer BF, Dawidson I, Sagalowsky A, Sandor Z, Lu CY. Improved outcome of cadaveric renal transplantation due to calcium channel blockers. *Transplantation* 1991; 52:640–645.

359. Epstein M. Calcium antagonists and renal protection: Current status and future perspectives. *Arch Intern Med* 1992; 152:1573–1584.

360. Meyer JS. Calcium channel blockers in the prophylactic treatment of vascular headache. *Ann Intern Med* 1985; 102:395–397.

361. Meyer JS, Hardenberg J. Clinical effectiveness of calcium entry blockers in prophylactic treatment of migraine and cluster headaches. *Headache* 1983; 23:266–277.

362. Solomon GD, Steele JG, Spaccavento LJ. Verapamil prophylaxis of migraine: A double-blind placebo-controlled study. *JAMA* 1983; 250:2500–2505.

363. Weinberger J. Drug therapy of neurovascular disease. In: Frishman WH, Sonnenblick EH, eds. *Cardiovascular Pharmacotherapeutics*. New York: McGraw-Hill; 1997:1195–1209.

364. Morich FJ, Bieber F, Lewis JM, et al. Nimodipine in the treatment of probable Alzheimer's disease. *Clin Drug Invest* 1996; 11:185.

365. Rodeheffer RJ, Rommer JA, Wigley F, Smith CR. Controlled double-blind trial of nifedipine in the treatment of Raynaud's phenomenon. *N Engl J Med* 1983; 308:880–883.

366. Burger SK, Saul RF, Selhorst JB, Thurston SE. Transient monocular blindness caused by vasospasm. *N Engl J Med* 1991; 325:870–873.

367. Winterkorn JMS, Kupersmith MJ, Wirtschafter JD, Forman S. Brief report: Treatment of vasospastic amaurosis fugax with calcium-channel blockers. *N Engl J Med* 1993; 329:396–398.

368. Bartsch P, Maggiorini M, Ritter M, Noti C, Vock P, Oelz O. Prevention of high-altitude pulmonary edema by nifedipine. *N Engl J Med* 1991; 325:1284–1289.

369. Lewis JG. Adverse reactions to calcium antagonists. *Drugs* 1983; 25:196–222.

370. Terry RW. Nifedipine therapy in angina pectoris: Evaluation of safety and side effects. *Am Heart J* 1982; 104:681–689.

371. Vetrovec GW, Parker VE, Cole S, Procacci PM, Tabatznik B, Terry R. Nifedipine gastrointestinal therapeutic system in stable angina pectoris: Results of a multicenter open-label, crossover comparison with nifedipine. *Am J Med* 1987; 83(6B):24–30.

372. Padrell MD, Navarro M, Faura CC, Horga JF. Verapamil-induced parkinsonism. *Am J Med* 1995; 99:436.

373. Pahor M, Guralnik JM, Furberg CD, Carbonin P, Havlik RJ. Risk of gastrointestinal haemorrhage with calcium antagonists in hypertensive persons over 67 years old. *Lancet* 1996; 347:1061–1065.

374. Funck-Brentano C, Coudray P, Planellas J, Motte G, Jaillon P. Effects of bepridil and diltiazem on ventricular repolarization in angina pectoris. *Am J Cardiol* 1990; 66:812–817.

375. Kenny J. Treating overdose with calcium channel blockers. *Br Med J* 1994; 308:992–993.

376. Klein HO, Lang R, Weiss E, DiSegni E, Libhaber C, Guerrero J, et al. The influence of verapamil on serum digoxin concentrations. *Circulation* 1982; 65:998–1003.

377. Schwartz JB, Keefe D, Kates RE, Kirsten E, Harrison DC. Acute and chronic pharmacodynamic interaction of verapamil and digoxin in atrial fibrillation. *Circulation* 1982; 65:1163–1170.

378. Belz GG, Aust PE, Munkes R. Digoxin plasma concentrations and nifedipine. *Lancet* 1981; 1:844–845.

379. Opie LH. Cardiovascular drug interactions. In: Frishman WH, Sonnenblick EH, eds. *Cardiovascular Pharmacotherapeutics*. New York: McGraw-Hill; 1997:1383–1400.

380. Dargie HJJ for the TIBET Study Group. Medical treatment of angina can favourably affect outcome (abstr). *Eur Heart J* 1993; 14(suppl):304.

381. Packer M, Leon MB, Bonow RO, Kieval J, Rosing DR, Bala Subramanian V. Hemodynamic and clinical effects of combined therapy with verapamil and propranolol in ischemic heart disease. *Am J Cardiol* 1982; 50:903–912.

382. Saseen JJ, Carter BL, Brown TER, Elliott WJ, Black HR. Comparison of nifedipine alone and with diltiazem or verapamil in hypertension. *Hypertension* 1996; 28:109–114.

55

REHABILITATION OF THE PATIENT WITH CORONARY HEART DISEASE

Nanette Kass Wenger

Cardiac rehabilitation is an essential component of the long-term comprehensive management of coronary patients and should include an individualized regimen of physical activity and health education and counseling appropriate for the individual patient's needs and specific cardiac problem.[1] Cardiac rehabilitation is described by the American College of Cardiology as "those exercise and counseling services which reduce symptoms or improve cardiac function"[2] and by the U.S. Public Health Service as "comprehensive, long-term programs involving medical evaluation, prescribed exercise, cardiac risk factor modification, education, and counseling." Previously, these services were recommended for patients following myocardial infarction, coronary artery bypass graft (CABG) surgery, or with chronic stable angina pectoris, but more recently,[3] the Health Care Financing Administration determined that heart transplant patients and patients who had undergone percutaneous transluminal coronary angioplasty (PTCA) could benefit from prescribed cardiac rehabilitation. Provision of these services is physician-directed and is implemented by a variety of health care professionals.

The current short hospital stay for uncomplicated myocardial infarction necessitates early ambulation and an accelerated educational regimen, with deferral of most teaching and counseling to the outpatient setting. Early discharge from the hospital is characteristic for patients after successful myocardial reperfusion by coronary thrombolysis or acute primary angioplasty.[4] Patients recovering from CABG surgery typically undergo rapid ambulation, have a short hospital stay, and constitute an increasing percentage of patients referred for cardiac rehabilitation,[5] particularly patients without prior myocardial infarction who typically have good ventricular function, favorable survival, and are at low risk for proximate coronary events. Others require more protracted guidance for coronary risk reduction,[6,7] and early counseling appears to aid in averting physiologic and psychological disability. Most patients following successful PTCA have brief hospital stays,

good functional status, and early resumption of employment and other activities.[8,9] Patients with stable angina without recent myocardial infarction constitute almost one-fourth of the total coronary population but are underserved in terms of rehabilitative care. They are often not referred for formal rehabilitative services, often due to lack of insurance reimbursement. This population may have a substantial loss of productivity and reduction in the quality of life and requires comprehensive medical management, with needs that can exceed those of patients after uncomplicated infarction. With the aging of the U.S. population, coronary rehabilitative care is now provided to many elderly patients and to many patients with severe and complicated coronary illness.[10,11] There is substantial contemporary emphasis on education and counseling as additional cornerstones of rehabilitative care, using the behavioral approach to assist patients in coronary risk reduction and other cardiovascular health-related goals[6,7,12]; on psychosocial assessment and interventions; and on occupational assessment and vocational counseling.

Each year in the United States, there are almost 1 million survivors of myocardial infarction who are candidates for cardiac rehabilitation services, in addition to more than 7 million patients with stable angina pectoris and patients following revascularization with CABG surgery (309,000 patients in 1993, 45 percent under age 65) or PTCA and other transcatheter interventional procedures (362,000 in 1933, 54 percent younger than age 65). Of these several million patients with coronary heart disease for whom benefits can be anticipated from cardiac rehabilitation, only 11 to 20 percent previously participated in cardiac rehabilitation programs.[13,14] Recently, among patients with acute myocardial infarction enrolled in the Global Utilization of Streptokinase and tPA for Occluded Coronary Arteries (GUSTO) trial, 38 percent of U.S. patients and 32 percent of Canadian patients participated in cardiac rehabilitation programs.[15] In the United States, heart failure is the most common discharge diagnosis for hospitalized Medicare patients and the fourth most common discharge diagnosis for all hospitalized patients. Although coronary heart disease is not the etiology in all these patients, it is a substantial contributor to heart failure. Application of cardiac rehabilitation services to patients with heart failure (as well as after cardiac transplantation) has gained increasing recognition and acceptance as its benefits and safety have been documented. An estimated 4.7 million patients with heart failure are potential candidates for cardiac rehabilitation.[13]

EXERCISE TRAINING

No single randomized trial of exercise training has demonstrated a reduction in mortality and morbidity in patients following myocardial infarction, although favorable trends occurred in several, in part owing to inadequate sample size and/or duration of follow-up, to high dropout rates, etc. Meta-analysis[16,17] of pooled data from large prospective randomized exercise trials suggests that there may be as much as a 25 percent survival advantage for exercising subjects at 3-year follow-up following myocardial infarction. This benefit cannot be attributed solely to exercise training as many studies included coronary risk reduction as well as exercise. The reduction in mortality approaches that resulting from pharmacologic management of patients following myocardial infarction with beta-blocking drugs and of patients with left ventricular systolic dysfunction with angiotensin-converting enzyme (ACE) inhibitor therapy. The reduction in cardiovascular mortality was 26 percent in multifactorial randomized trials of cardiac rehabilitation as compared with 15 percent in trials that involved solely exercise training. There is no evidence that cardiac rehabilitation exercise training changes the rates of nonfatal reinfarction.[7,18–25]

The evidence-based Clinical Practice Guideline *Cardiac Rehabilitation* of the U.S. Department of Health and Human Services[13] highlights the beneficial effect of cardiac rehabilitation exercise training on exercise tolerance as one of the most clearly established favorable outcomes for coronary patients with angina pectoris, myocardial infarction, CABG surgery, and PTCA and for patients with compensated heart failure or a decreased ventricular ejection fraction. This approach particularly benefits patients with decreased exercise tolerance.[26] Improved exercise tolerance was evident for both women and men and occurred in elderly patients as well. The most consistent benefit occurred with exercise training at least three times weekly for 12 or more weeks' duration. The duration of aerobic exercise sessions varied from 20 to 40 min, at an intensity approximating 70 to 85 percent of the baseline exercise test heart rate. Improvement in exercise tolerance, however, was described with lower-intensity exercise as well.[20,27,28] Maintenance of exercise training is required to sustain improvement in exercise tolerance.

No significant increase in cardiovascular complications or other serious adverse outcomes was reported in any random-

ized controlled trial that evaluated exercise training in coronary patients. These randomized controlled trials involved 3932 patients following myocardial infarction, 745 patients with catheterization-documented coronary disease, 215 patients following CABG surgery, and 139 following PTCA. No deterioration in measures of exercise tolerance was reported in any patients undergoing exercise training, nor did any controlled study document significantly greater improvement in exercise tolerance in control patient groups compared with exercising patients.

The improvement in functional capacity with exercise training, averaging 20 percent after recovery from myocardial infarction, is associated with a reduction in activity-related symptoms: angina, dyspnea, fatigue, and at times claudication. Exercise training results in the following: (1) an improvement in oxygen transport, evident as an increase in maximal cardiac output and oxygen consumption; (2) a reduction in heart rate, systolic blood pressure, and thereby myocardial oxygen requirement at rest and at submaximal work levels; and (3) a more rapid return to normal of the exercise heart rate.

Improvement in functional capacity and decrease in activity-related symptoms following usual moderate-intensity exercise training appear to be related primarily to peripheral adaptations. These include an increase in oxygen extraction and utilization by trained skeletal muscle, with a decrease in myocardial oxygen demand and requirement for coronary blood flow at submaximal exercise. The redistribution of cardiac output, decrease in systemic vascular resistance, and autonomic nervous system adaptations (particularly lowering of the heart rate) result in a decreased rate-pressure product at submaximal levels of exertion. High-intensity, long-term endurance exercise may effect cardiac (central) adaptations, possibly including improved ventricular contractility and increased maximal stroke volume in selected coronary patients[29]; such intensive exercise training is feasible for only a small subset of coronary patients. There is no evidence that exercise training as a sole intervention alters the angiographic characteristics of coronary lesions, increases coronary blood flow or myocardial oxygen supply, or stimulates the formation of a coronary collateral circulation in humans. No consistent improvement in cardiac hemodynamic measurements or ventricular systolic function has resulted from exercise training.[30,31] Exercise training, however, may improve skeletal muscle functioning in patients with heart failure.[32] Exercise training can decrease evidence of myocardial ischemia as measured by exercise electrocardiogram (ECG) testing, ambulatory ECG recording, and radionuclide perfusion imaging.[33–35] In several randomized clinical trials, apparently spontaneous improvement in resting ejection fraction after myocardial infarction occurred in both exercising and control populations, rendering suspect the improvements in ejection fraction described in observational studies. There were no consistent changes in ventricular arrhythmia related to exercise rehabilitation.

Exercise training may decrease symptoms of angina pectoris in patients with coronary disease[18,23,34] and symptoms of heart failure in patients with left ventricular systolic dysfunction.[36,37] The improvement in electrocardiographic and nuclear cardiology measures of myocardial ischemia provides objective support for the symptomatic improvement. Exercise training of patients with left ventricular systolic dysfunction provided added symptomatic improvement to that achieved by appropriate medication.[37]

The decrease in symptoms and improvement in functional status that result from exercise training can enable a return to remunerative employment as well as to leisure and recreational activities.[38] For more impaired coronary patients, including many elderly ones, even a modest increase in functional capacity can help maintain independence.[10,11,39–42]

Guidelines for Prescriptive Exercise Training

Individualized medically prescribed physical activity is the hallmark of rehabilitative exercise training. Standards and guidelines have been promulgated by a number of professional organizations.[2,43–49] The prescriptive components of exercise training include its "dosage," determined by the intensity, frequency, and duration of exercise; the types of exercise; and rate of progression of exercise intensity. Coronary patients should not exercise at a level higher than that documented to produce an appropriate cardiovascular response during testing. The prediscovery (or early posthospitalization) exercise test, typically performed for risk stratification, can serve as the basis for initial exercise recommendations. It is inappropriate to use age-predicted target heart rates for coronary patients; disease, therapies, and prior levels of training or fitness may influence the heart rate response to exercise.

Prescription of target heart rate range is based on the results of exercise testing. Although in prior years patients were advised to exercise to a target heart rate range between 70 and 85 percent of the highest level safely achieved at exercise testing,[50] exercise intensities in the 50 to 70 percent heart rate range have produced comparable improvement in functional capacity and endurance and may provide greater safety because of the lower risk of cardiovascular complications with unsupervised exercise.[27,51] These lower rates are less likely to engender discomfort that may deter long-term exercise adherence. This documented efficacy of lower-intensity exercise training to improve aerobic capacity has increased both its applicability and acceptance.[1,27,28] Particularly for unfit patients or those with lower exercise capacities, the increased comfort of lower-intensity exercise may encourage adherence, although increased duration of training may be required. Comparable favorable effects on quality of life occurred with low- and high-intensity exercise.[52] An alternative method for calculating target heart rate involves 70 to 85 percent of the difference between peak exercise test heart rate and resting heart rate, added to resting rate. This method may be advantageous in patients whose heart rate is attenuated by beta-blocking or other drugs.

The basic design of an exercise session involves an initial 5 to 10 min of warm-up exercise: stretching and range-of-motion activities that enable musculoskeletal and circulatory readiness for exercise. This is followed by a 20- to 40-min endurance component that initially involves walk-run sequences or exercise on a stationary bicycle or treadmill; for these activities, skill is a minimal component of the intensity of work demand.

When space for exercise is limited, "station" training may be preferable, with participants serially using bicycle ergometry, arm ergometry, rowing machines, and treadmills. When more space is available, gymnasium-type programs can accommodate larger numbers of patients for walk-jog activities and floor exercises; some facilities have indoor or outdoor tracks. A final 5- to 10-min cool-down period entails a gradual decrease in intensity that allows the heart rate to slow and averts postexercise hypotension. Three exercise sessions weekly appear adequate, and a greater frequency does not significantly improve aerobic capacity. Aerobic games, as a recreational component, add variety to an exercise program and improve adherence; they also provide upper body exercise. Because the oxygen cost of these activities varies with each patient's skills and competitiveness, they should be limited early in exercise training.

As the level of training increases, recreational activities in which skill often influences the intensity of work may add variety to the exercise regimen. Enjoyable, effective endurance activities include rope-skipping, bicycling, skating, swimming, rowing, and aerobic dancing; both rope-skipping and swimming (for unskilled swimmers) impose higher work loads and should be undertaken carefully.

Characteristics of Aerobic (Dynamic) and Strength (Isometric) Exercise Training

Aerobic (dynamic) exercise, rhythmic repetitive movements of large muscle groups, is traditionally prescribed for coronary patients. The physiologic response, an increase in heart rate, parallels the intensity of activity, and an increase in stroke volume occurs in young and middle-aged patients. In most elderly patients, the increase in heart rate predominates, with little increase in stroke volume. Systolic blood pressure increases progressively with exercise intensity, with maintenance of or slight decrease in diastolic blood pressure and widening of the pulse pressure.

By contrast, with strength (isometric) training the increase in heart rate is modest and the increase in cardiac output is slight. There is a substantial increase in systolic blood pressure with high-intensity isometric activity, particularly in unfit individuals; this may provoke angina, ventricular dysfunction, and/or arrhythmias and is the basis for limiting isometric activity in coronary patients with a low exercise capacity. Once a reasonable aerobic capacity is achieved, however, combined aerobic and strength training exercises may produce substantial training effects and improve muscle strength in coronary patients,[53] with resultant improvement in endurance and the ability to return to active occupational and recreational lifestyles.[54] Studies document the effectiveness of mild-to-moderate resistive exercise training in selected patients with coronary heart disease.[55–58] The absence of signs or symptoms of myocardial ischemia, abnormal hemodynamic changes, and cardiovascular complications suggests that resistance exercise training is safe for coronary patients who have previously participated in aerobic exercise training. Most reported studies have involved small numbers of low-risk male patients, 70 years or younger, with minimal functional aerobic impairment and with normal or near-normal left ventricular function. The extent to which the safety and effectiveness of resistance training demonstrated by these studies can be extrapolated to other populations of coronary patients (e.g., women, older patients of both genders with low aerobic fitness, or patients at moderate-to-high cardiovascular risk) is not known.[13]

Arm versus Leg Exercise Training

Because exercise training is predominantly muscle-specific, both arm and leg exercise should be included in exercise rehabilitation.[59] The heart rate and blood pressure responses to leg work decrease following leg training, with only modest improvement in the response to arm work. Following arm training, the predominant decreases in heart rate and blood pressure response occur with arm work. In one study, improvement in exercise response of the untrained limb was only 50 to 75 percent of the trained limb, suggesting that about half of the increase in trained-limb performance is due to a generalized training effect; the remainder reflects predominantly improved oxygen extraction by trained skeletal muscle.

Since walk-run sequences or exercise on a stationary bicycle or treadmill train primarily leg muscles, supplementary arm exercise training is accomplished by selected repetitive calisthenics, shoulder wheels, rowing machines, and arm ergometers. When data from leg exercise testing are used to prescribe arm exercise, a reduction of about 10 beats per minute in target heart rate range is appropriate. The workload for arm training is about half that for leg training.[59] Since most occupational and recreational activities entail both arm and leg work (and often predominantly arm work), arm exercise training should be included in rehabilitative exercise.

The Effect of Cardiovascular Drugs on Exercise Training

Exercise training can occur in patients receiving antianginal drugs, which may lessen symptoms and improve the ability to exercise.[60] Although beta-blocking drugs decrease the heart rate and blood pressure response to exercise, they do not attenuate the improvement in physical work capacity that results from exercise training. Exercise testing undertaken to prescribe exercise should be performed with patients receiving medications that are planned for their training.

The Role of Exercise Testing in Coronary Rehabilitation

Graded exercise testing, using either a treadmill or a bicycle protocol, is safely performed within the initial weeks follow-ing myocardial infarction.[61] Most centers currently test patients to a sign- or symptom-limited endpoint, as heart rate limits are often inaccurate because of antianginal therapy. Treadmill testing typically entails serial 3-min stages of walking, beginning at slow speed, initially on the level, and then at increasing speed and elevations; comparable test protocols are available for a bicycle ergometer (see Chap. 15). Arm testing may be undertaken in patients with claudication or musculoskeletal problems that make leg testing not feasible.[62]

The results of predischarge exercise tests, performed with or without radionuclide studies contribute independent prognostic information for risk stratification.[61] High-risk patients are characterized by having a low exercise capacity [peak workload below 4 to 6 metabolic equivalents (METs)]; the occurrence of angina, ischemic ST-segment abnormalities, and/or exercise-induced hypotension at low levels of exercise; and the development of ventricular arrhythmias at low levels of exercise. Radionuclide evidence of myocardial ischemia or left ventricular dysfunction with exercise also indicates an adverse prognosis. Predischarge exercise testing also identifies low-risk patients with a favorable prognosis who do not require additional diagnostic testing, are well-suited for accelerated rehabilitation, and for whom early discharge home and prompt resumption of preinfarction activities, including return to work, can be recommended.[61,63] The exercise test can help define safe levels of activity and guide the surveillance necessary during exercise rehabilitation. This permits simple, effective, accelerated, and less costly rehabilitation for low-risk coronary patients, reserving financial and personnel resources for high-risk patients who may derive substantial benefit from supervised exercise training. Satisfactory performance of an exercise test, coupled with explanation of its relationship to activities to be undertaken at home, may lessen the common fear of postinfarction patients that physical activity may result in reinfarction or death.[64] Such counseling has also been associated with an earlier return to work.[38]

Safety of Rehabilitative Exercise Training

The Clinical Practice Guideline *Cardiac Rehabilitation*[13] highlights the safety of cardiac rehabilitation exercise training in that randomized controlled trials involving over 4500 coronary patients showed no increase in morbidity or mortality. A questionnaire survey of 142 U.S. cardiac rehabilitation programs, involving patients participating in exercise rehabilitation between 1980 and 1984, reported a low rate of nonfatal myocardial infarction of 1 per 294,000 patient-hours and a cardiac mortality rate of 1 per 784,000 patient-hours.[65] Twenty-one episodes of cardiac arrest occurred, with successful resuscitation of 17 patients. A 1978 report[50] also described a low rate of fatal cardiac events during or immediately following exercise training: 1 per 116,400 patient-hours of participation. Definitive information is not available regarding the effect of levels of supervision and of ECG monitoring of exercise training on safety.

IMPLEMENTATION OF REHABILITATIVE CARE

Inpatient, or Hospital, Phase

The major components of rehabilitative care for patients hospitalized for a coronary event include progressive resumption of physical activity (early ambulation) and education and counseling of both patient and family (see also Chap. 47).

EARLY AMBULATION

Early ambulation is designed to limit the detrimental effects of deconditioning: reduced physical work capacity and maximal oxygen uptake; orthostatic intolerance, characterized by orthostatic hypotension and tachycardia (due both to hypovolemia and to a lessened cardiovascular reflex response); increase in blood viscosity owing to a decrease in plasma volume disproportionate to the decrease in red blood cell mass; and decrease in pulmonary ventilation. The decrease in muscle mass and muscular contractile strength renders muscular contraction inefficient, with more oxygen required for comparable work.

Guidelines[66] for physical activity in the coronary or surgical intensive care unit are for initial low-intensity exercise (1 to 2 METs), with gradual progression in work demand; supervision of progressive ambulation permits detection of inappropriate responses. Patients are encouraged to feed themselves, perform personal care, use a bedside commode, and sit in a bedside chair. Cardiac work is less in the seated than in the supine position. Sitting in a chair two or three times daily limits the hypovolemia of immobilization and resultant orthostatic hypotension. Exposure to gravitational stress, rather than physical activity intensity, appears to be the determinant in limiting hypovolemia, cardiac underfilling, and deterioration of oxygen transport capacity with effort intolerance.[67] Patients perform selected arm and leg exercises designed to maintain muscle tone and increase flexibility and joint mobility. Incentive spirometry is important for postoperative patients.

Disproportionate responses[66] to low-level activity include chest discomfort, dyspnea, or palpitations; a heart rate in excess of 100 beats per minute or lower than 50 beats per minute; ST-segment displacement on the electrocardiographic monitor; appearance of arrhythmias; or a decrease of >10 to 15 mmHg in systolic blood pressure. Although the latter usually indicates ischemic ventricular dysfunction, the vasodilator effect of nitrate or calcium channel blocking drugs must also be considered. A systolic blood pressure response during low-level activity >180 mmHg or a diastolic pressure response >110 mmHg is an indication for antihypertensive therapy. Appropriate responses to ambulation indicate that the patient can progress to higher-intensity activity; disproportionate responses require activity restriction and clinical reassessment for unrecognized cardiac dysfunction.

Most household tasks require a work intensity of 2 to 3 METs. The major prescriptive hospital activity is walking, with stepwise increases in pace and distance. Patients who must climb steps at home should practice this in the hospital. Electrocardiographic telemetry monitoring during ambulation is indicated for selected patients, e.g., those with serious ventricular arrhythmias or asymptomatic myocardial ischemia. A protocol for early ambulation and concomitant educational activities for patients with myocardial infarction is applicable, with minor modifications, to postoperative coronary patients (Table 55-1).

Neither early ambulation nor early hospital discharge adversely affects the short- or long-term morbidity or mortality of appropriately selected coronary patients.[4,68] Benefits include prevention of deconditioning, decrease in pulmonary atelectasis and thromboembolic complications, lessened anxiety and depression, and an enhanced sense of well-being, related to improved functional status. Improved functional status of patients at hospital discharge has been associated with an earlier and more complete return to work.

EDUCATION AND COUNSELING OF HOSPITALIZED PATIENTS AND THEIR FAMILIES[69]

The current abbreviated hospital stay limits the ability of health professionals to address the informational and learning needs of the patient, spouse, and family; to assist them through recovery; and to prepare them adequately for convalescence. Answering the questions or concerns of patients in a coronary or surgical intensive care unit (or during the preprocedure phase for elective coronary angioplasty or bypass surgery) can provide reassurance. Education includes a brief explanation of the medical or surgical problem(s), tests anticipated in subsequent days, and familiarization with procedures and equipment; this information helps patients adjust to a situation perceived as life-threatening. The temporary nature of most restrictions should be emphasized, citing that improved coronary status with recovery lessens the intensity of surveillance and care.

During the remainder of the hospitalization, providing more information and planning for discharge are appropriate. Increased knowledge can lessen anxiety and improve adherence to recommendations. Patients should be instructed about medications—the purpose, dosage, desired effects, and potential adverse responses of each. Many patients have not taken medications prior to a coronary event and may be unfamiliar with the problems of taking medications. Patients and family members should be taught the appropriate response to new or recurrent symptoms and how to gain access to emergency medical care.

Outpatient, or Ambulatory, Phase

About 70 percent of contemporary survivors of myocardial infarction younger than 70 years of age and many patients following successful myocardial revascularization procedures are at low risk for proximate coronary events.[6] Exercise rehabilitation for most low-risk coronary patients, particularly following myocardial revascularization, begins shortly after

TABLE 55-1

IN-PATIENT REHABILITATION: FIVE-STEP MYOCARDIAL INFARCTION PROGRAM (REVISED 1996: GRADY MEMORIAL HOSPITAL/EMORY UNIVERSITY SCHOOL OF MEDICINE)

Step	Date	M.D. Initials	Nurse/ Exer Specialist Notes	Supervised Exercise	CCU/Step Down Unit Activity	Educational Activity
				CCU		
1	———			Active and passive ROM all extremities in bed Teach patient ankle plantar and dorsiflexion—repeat hourly when awake	Partial self-care Feed self Dangle legs on side of bed Use bedside commode Sit in chair 15 min, 1–2 times/day	Orientation to CCU Personal emergencies, social service aid as needed Bedside teaching (CCU staff)
2	———			Active ROM all extremities, sitting on side of bed or bedside chair	Sit in chair 15–30 min, 2–3 times/day Complete self-care	Orientation to rehabilitation team, program Smoking cessation Educational literature if requested Planning transfer from CCU
				STEP DOWN UNIT		

3	———			Warm-up exercises, 2–2.5 METs:
				  Stretching ROM
				  Calisthenics
				
				Walk in hall 50–75 ft and back at slow pace
					Sit in chair ad lib
					Walk in room
					Walk to class with supervision
					Out of bed as tolerated
						Normal cardiac anatomy and function
						Development of atherosclerosis
						What happens when myocardial infarction occurs
						Coronary risk factors and their control
						Diet

4	———			Teach pulse counting, Borg Scale
				ROM and calisthenics, 3 METs
				Practice walking few stairsteps
				Walk 300–500 ft bid
				Instruct on home exercise
					Tepid shower or tub bath, with supervision
					Walk in corridor prn
						Heart attack management:
						  Medications
						  Exercise
						  Surgery
						  Response to symptoms
						  Family, community adjustments on return home
						Work simplification techniques (as needed)

5	———			Continue above activities
				Check pulse counting
				Walk up flight of steps
				Walk 500 ft bid
				Continue home exercise instruction; present information regarding outpatient exercise program
					Continue all previous activities
					Predischarge exercise test (as appropriate)
						Discharge planning
						  Medications, diet, activity
						Return appointments
						  Schedules tests
						  Return to work
						  Community resources
						  Educational literature
						  Medication cards

Source: Reprinted with permission of Grady Memorial Hospital/Emory University School of Medicine.
Note: 1 foot = 0.30 meter.

discharge from the hospital; these patients usually progress rapidly in increasing their intensity and duration of exercise, often without supervision. Coronary patients who are elderly; those with significant comorbidity, myocardial ischemia, heart failure, or serious arrhythmias; those with complications of myocardial infarction or CABG surgery; or those with severe angina may require exercise surveillance of variable duration.[2,43,45,61] Outpatient exercise rehabilitation is best described by the characteristics of the exercise training and the requirements, duration, and complexity of surveillance, based on the patient's clinical and risk factor status, rather than by traditional phases of earlier years that typically had fixed durations and composition. This is concordant with responding to an individual patient's needs for exercise training, rather than requiring a patient to conform to program phases or requirements.

THERAPEUTIC EXERCISE TRAINING

Therapeutic exercise training typically lasts for 8 to 12 weeks. Initial home exercise may involve progressive walking and walk-jog sequences or serial increases in the intensity and duration of use of a stationary bicycle. Videotapes may help guide and pace home exercise and are available for varying intensities of exercise training. Home-based exercise rehabilitation optimally includes planned communication and management by rehabilitation nurses and other specially trained personnel.[6,7]

In the early years of ambulatory exercise rehabilitation, few patients had continuous ECG monitoring because ECG telemetry was not widely available. In subsequent years, complication rates were described as being lower in exercise programs with continuous ECG monitoring.[50] It remains unknown, however, whether ECG monitoring, closer medical supervision, and/or differences in exercise intensity were the safety determinants. More recently, continuous ECG monitoring has not been shown to provide added safety for low-risk patients during supervised exercise[65]; as a result, ECG monitoring is currently recommended only for high-risk patients and other selected patients with problems in exercising,[1,2,45] although others recommend more extensive ECG monitoring. Often, ECG monitoring is undertaken solely owing to its requirement for insurance reimbursement, rather than based on medical need. Many patients in supervised exercise programs without continuous ECG monitoring or patients exercising independently can be taught either to check their heart rate response intermittently to ensure that it remains in the prescribed target heart rate range or to estimate exercise intensity by the rating of perceived exertion as described by Borg.[70] In supervised settings, heart rate response can be documented by intermittent use of defibrillator paddles as ECG leads. A technique of value in maintaining appropriate exercise intensity in unsupervised settings is the "talk test," wherein patients exercise only to the level that permits continued conversation with an exercising companion, a level generally below the anaerobic threshold at which respiratory rate accelerates.

High-risk coronary patients may require supervised and often ECG-monitored exercise. These patients are characterized by having a markedly reduced exercise capacity, severely depressed ventricular function, complex ventricular arrhythmias, exercise-induced angina, ischemia, or hypotension at low exercise intensities and/or the inability to self-monitor exercise heart rate. Because of their increased risk for adverse events, exercise training should occur, at least initially, in a medically supervised and probably ECG-monitored setting.[71] Because exercise-related cardiac complications may be increased not only in proximity to the acute coronary event, the need and duration of ECG surveillance of exercise for these high-risk patients remains uncertain. The uniform success of resuscitation with supervised exercise, despite the rarity of its application, suggests that exercise supervision may be beneficial for selected patients.[65]

Although recent studies document the efficacy of home-based exercise training and risk reduction guided by a specialized cardiac nurse manager, data are not available as to the efficacy of long-term risk reduction or long-term compliance with unsupervised exercise in the absence of management and supervision strategies. Several studies showed that all training regimens appeared to increase functional capacity more rapidly than occurred spontaneously.[7,36,37,53] Supervision of exercise may not entail an "all-or-nothing" approach; intermittent supervision may be feasible in a community facility, there may be periodic telephone transmission of the exercise ECG of patients who exercise at home, patients may use inexpensive heart-rate monitors during home exercise, or a combination of these techniques may be used. It is not known whether or not any of these approaches improves adherence to exercise; several studies of independent exercise showed a lack of coronary risk reduction.

The Clinical Practice Guideline *Cardiac Rehabilitation*[13] highlights alternative approaches to the delivery of cardiac rehabilitation services, other than traditional supervised group interventions, as effective and safe for carefully selected clinically stable patients. Transtelephonic and other means of monitoring and surveillance of patients can extend cardiac rehabilitation beyond the setting of supervised, structured, group-based rehabilitation. The feasibility, safety, and efficacy of these alternative approaches must be assessed in more diverse populations of patients with stable coronary heart disease, particularly elderly patients, those with ventricular dysfunction, and other patients of higher risk status.

MAINTENANCE EXERCISE TRAINING

Once patients attain their initial goals, maintenance exercise training can be undertaken or continued in community recreational facilities or at home. Because lifetime regular physical activity is necessary for the maintenance of physical fitness, patients must achieve reasonable independence in exercising and remain involved in an exercise regimen that is social, enjoyable, convenient, and appropriate. Most coronary patients with prior exercise restrictions who can safely attain a 7- to 8-MET level of performance can progress to unsupervised exercise. Patients leaving supervised exercise programs may require counseling regarding the selection and initiation of long-term exercise in the community or at home.

EDUCATION AND COUNSELING
OF AMBULATORY CORONARY PATIENTS

The behavioral approach to coronary risk reduction encourages and enables coronary patients to manage their illness, adopt and maintain healthy lifestyles, and improve adherence to medications and other recommended regimens.[72,73] Meta-analysis of 28 controlled trials of patient education showed that "education programs have demonstrated a measurable impact on blood pressure, mortality, exercise, diet," and that other parameters are positively affected, although less consistently.[74] A combination of education, counseling, and behavioral intervention strategies seems most effective in promoting health, reducing risk, and favorably altering lifestyle.[6,13,72,75] Whether or not the same interventions are equally effective for men and women and across the life span remains unanswered because few studies have enrolled patients over 70 years of age or included women.

There is no evidence that the performance of CABG surgery per se encourages favorable modification of coronary risk status postoperatively.[76,77] Postoperative recurrence of coronary symptoms or deterioration of function following saphenous vein CABG surgery relates predominantly to progression of the underlying atherosclerosis, both in the graft vessels and in the native circulation. Control of hypertension, diabetes, hyperlipidemia, and obesity and cessation of cigarette smoking,[78] with adoption of a physically active lifestyle, even at advanced age, may slow progression or induce regression of atherosclerosis and decrease the occurrence of subsequent coronary events.

Community resources that may be helpful in rehabilitation should be identified: counseling and guidance services, home-care agencies, vocational rehabilitation facilities and services for job training and placement, services for financial aid, outpatient coronary rehabilitation programs, and postcoronary groups or clubs. Participation in community heart clubs or educational groups may further facilitate rehabilitation; coronary risk reduction and other skills learned and practiced in these settings may encourage health-related behaviors and aid in reinforcing maintenance of these changes. Acquisition of knowledge appears to affect favorably both behaviors involving implementing recommendations for care and coping behaviors.[69]

CORONARY POPULATIONS WITH SPECIAL REHABILITATION NEEDS

Elderly Coronary Patients

Elderly patients constitute a high percentage of those with myocardial infarction, CABG surgery, and PTCA and other transcatheter revascularization procedures. Complications of myocardial infarction and myocardial revascularization are more frequent in the elderly, with prolongation of both immobilization and hospitalization predisposing to deconditioning; early ambulation can limit functional deterioration and decrease depression. In both medical and surgical coronary intensive care settings, the major educational strategy involves concise and repeated explanations, reassurance, and time and place orientation to help avert confusion and delirium. Teaching energy-conserving techniques for self-care and performance of household tasks helps maintain independent living, an outcome valued by elderly patients. Modification of conventional coronary risk factors is feasible and warranted, given the greater prevalence and severity of coronary disease in the elderly.

Elderly patients are also at high risk of disability following a coronary event. Recent trials of exercise rehabilitation have begun to include patients over 65 years of age and to evaluate outcomes in the elderly coronary population specifically. Although few studies and no randomized controlled trials have addressed the efficacy and safety of exercise training and multifactorial rehabilitation in the elderly, the available studies provide important new information for clinical practice.

Elderly coronary patients in posthospital exercise regimens have exercise trainability comparable to that of younger patients participating in similar exercise rehabilitation,[42,79] with elderly women and men showing comparable improvement. One report found that exercise testing before hospital discharge was feasible in about half of patients age 70 years or older with myocardial infarction, enabling accurate risk stratification and exercise prescription.[80] No complications or adverse outcomes of exercise training in the elderly were described in any cardiac rehabilitation study. Nonetheless, rates of entry referral to and participation in exercise rehabilitation were substantially lower among elderly patients than among younger patients,[11,40] and older women were even less likely to be referred than were older men.[41] Elderly patients are less fit after a coronary event, in part because of decreased fitness prior to the events. In the reported studies, adherence to exercise training was high (90 percent),[42] and significant reduction in coronary risk factors occurred in elderly patients who participated in multifactorial cardiac rehabilitation.[11]

For elderly patients who exercise independently, emphasis should be placed on the importance of warm-up and cool-down activities, because of the delayed return of the exercise heart rate to normal in an elderly population. Walking provides an adequate training stimulus for many elderly patients because it constitutes a significant percentage of the decreased aerobic capacity of aging.[81] Running, jumping, and other high-impact activities should be limited to avoid musculoskeletal complications. Walking, bicycle ergometry, and/or walking in a pool in shallow water can favorably modify the decreased joint mobility of aging; enhance neuromuscular coordination, balance, and stability and hence lessen propensity for falls; and improve endurance. Elderly individuals who exercise independently should be cautioned to decrease their exercise intensity in hot and humid environments.

Coronary Patients with Heart Failure

Impairment of exercise capacity with heart failure appears in part due to inadequate nutritive blood flow to skeletal muscle; factors other than lack of increase in cardiac output with exercise seem important, including the ability to decrease peripheral vascular resistance and possibly the adequacy of right ventricular function (see also Chap. 21). The ventricular ejection fraction predicts either exercise capacity or potential for improvement of exercise performance with training poorly; some patients with substantial ventricular dysfunction have a normal exercise capacity.[82]

Most studies of exercise training of patients with heart failure and moderate-to-severe left ventricular dysfunction do not demonstrate deterioration in left ventricular function.[83] Peripheral (skeletal muscle) adaptations appear to mediate the improvement in exercise tolerance, although a combination of left ventricular dysfunction and residual myocardial ischemia may limit trainability. Exercise training may also improve peripheral artery endothelial function in patients with chronic heart failure.[84] Exercise training can augment both the symptomatic and functional benefits of ACE inhibitor therapy.[37] Even small improvements in symptomatic status and functional capacity can exert a substantial favorable impact on quality of life. In both the supervised and at-home setting, low-to-moderate intensity exercise regimens provide benefit, although adverse events may occur in this high-risk patient group.

Although the initial exercise training programs of patients with ventricular dysfunction were predominantly supervised, typically with continuous ECG monitoring, other studies have described moderate intensity, unsupervised exercise as safe and effective.[85,86] The optimal duration of exercise supervision and the duration and need for ECG monitoring of these patients remain uncertain but should be guided by clinical evidence of exercise-related ischemia and/or arrhythmia.[36] In a study of 105 ambulatory cardiac transplant candidates, nonsupervised prescribed walking at a target heart-rate range close to baseline exercise test–determined anaerobic threshold produced significant improvement in peak maximal oxygen consumption and peak exercise tolerance in 38 of 68 clinically stable patients, without adverse effects. After an average of 6 months of such exercise, 31 of these 38 patients improved sufficiently to be removed from the transplant list, with improvement persisting to 2 years.[87]

Additional important components of rehabilitative care for patients with significant activity limitations include teaching work simplification, particularly the pacing of daily living activities; working in a seated rather than standing position; and taking frequent rest periods between activities.

Patients with Implanted Pacemakers and Cardioverter Defibrillators

Exercise prescription is determined by the characteristics of the implanted pacemaker. Because most patients likely to exercise currently receive rate-responsive pacemakers, exercise testing can ascertain the appropriateness of the sensor response to the exercise intensity,[88] and reprogramming can be undertaken as needed.

The exercise target heart-rate range for patients with implanted cardioverter defibrillators should be set at 20 to 30 beats per minute below the threshold rate of the device to fire. This also enables appropriate work-related activities.[89] Coparticipants in the exercise setting must be reassured that they cannot be harmed by physical contact with a patient whose cardioverter defibrillator discharges.

PSYCHOLOGICAL ASPECTS OF CORONARY REHABILITATION

The importance of psychosocial variables in the prognosis of patients with established coronary disease has received increasing attention during the past decade. Although the type A behavior pattern previously received prominent attention, currently the hostility component of type A behavior is regarded as its most adverse feature. High levels of anger and hostility appear associated with increased cardiac morbidity and mortality.[90,91]

Other major psychological problems in coronary patients involve anxiety, depression, denial, and dependence.[92] Denial of presenting symptoms may limit or delay access to care, often with adverse outcomes. "Appropriate" denial, characterized by confidence in a favorable outcome, often an effective coping strategy of patients with a coronary event, is associated with a favorable prognosis. Anxiety, which is often the initial psychological manifestation at hospitalization, is related to a fear of dying and may progress to depression as patients contemplate their potential inability to resume former family, occupational, and community roles. Anxiety and depression, the most common psychological complications of infarction contribute to the failure to make satisfactory life adjustments, to return to work, to return to sexual function, and to engage in social activities subsequent to hospital discharge. Depression is reported to precede myocardial infarction in 30 to 50 percent of patients. Depression is associated with increased morbidity and mortality following myocardial infarction and CABG surgery;[93,94] patients with depression were five times more likely to die during the initial 6 months following myocardial infarction than nondepressed patients.[95] Depression may be associated with social isolation, which may serve as an independent risk factor. The 6-month mortality of patients living alone was double that of patients living with others (16 versus 8 percent); and follow-up study of patients with angiographically documented coronary disease showed a 50 percent 5-year mortality rate among those most socially isolated, compared with 17 percent among those without these characteristics. The impact of social isolation on prognosis appeared independent of ventricular ejection fraction and other physiologic prognostic factors. Interventions against depression and social isolation following myocardial infarction are currently being evaluated.

Many patients with successful physical recovery following myocardial infarction or myocardial revascularization often have residual psychological impairment.[92] Two major strategies that appear to limit this complication are education and counseling and the initiation of a physical activity regimen. Many patients remain psychologically disabled because, inappropriately, they perceive an excessive severity of infarction and vulnerability to sudden death; safe resumption of physical activity provides reassurance and restores self-confidence.[64] In randomized exercise trials, exercising patients returned to sexual activity, to work, and to a near-normal lifestyle more rapidly and had greater improvements in work capacity, income, and job responsibility.[96] Both physical and psychosocial benefits occurred even with low-intensity exercise, particularly among older and sicker coronary patients. Despite the paucity of controlled studies, consistent moderate psychosocial benefit appears to result from combinations of structured exercise, education, and counseling.[69,97] Although the contribution of peer support in a group program has not been ascertained, it may be helpful given the predictive power of social isolation for coronary mortality.[98]

VOCATIONAL ASPECTS OF CORONARY REHABILITATION

A major goal of rehabilitative care for nonelderly patients recovered from myocardial infarction or myocardial revascularization is resumption of gainful employment, a change in occupation if needed, and the resultant economic and psychological benefits. In the 1980s, about 80 percent of patients who recovered from uncomplicated myocardial infarction and who were younger than 65 years of age and employed at the time of infarction returned to work within 2 to 3 months, typically resuming former jobs.[99] Despite this favorable early return to work, subsequent cessation of employment was high, with as much as a 20 percent decrement in continued employment between 6 months and 1 year. Comparable data are not available for patients with complications of infarction or residual functional impairment, although their return to work is estimated as 25 to 33 percent.

These data contrast markedly with work resumption following CABG surgery. Despite a substantial decrease in symptoms, improvement in functional capacity, and reported enhancement of life quality and participation in leisure activities, return to work following coronary bypass surgery has been much less favorable than anticipated.[100,101] No difference in 10-year employment status was described between patients randomized to medical and surgical treatment in the Coronary Artery Surgery Study (CASS).[102] Return to work following PTCA is comparable to that following CABG surgery, although PTCA patients are reported to return to work more promptly.[101] Other reports described lack of confidence in the ability to return to work following PTCA, even when patients were physically able to do so.[103]

Most studies of the return to work have involved predominantly or exclusively men; recent examination of working women with coronary disease showed them to have a longer convalescence and even lesser return to work; whether this is a gender issue or reflects older age or greater occurrence of depression among women warrants study.[104]

For patients younger than 65 years of age following myocardial infarction or myocardial revascularization, the indirect health care costs of disability, including lessened productivity, loss of income, welfare payments, and unemployment insurance costs, must be considered when the cost-effectiveness of rehabilitation is determined.[63,105–107] Coronary heart disease is the leading problem in the United States for which adults receive premature disability benefits under the Social

Security system; almost one-fourth of men and women receiving Social Security disability allowances have permanent disability due to coronary disease. Following both myocardial infarction and myocardial revascularization, symptomatic and functional improvement correlate poorly with the return to work and resumption of preillness lifestyle, with psychosocial status appearing as a more important determinant.[100] Since only about 15 percent of the U.S. labor force currently performs manual labor and this percentage decreases with older age, the severity of angina or heart failure in coronary patients only rarely precludes or delays return to work. Many nonmedical factors negatively influence resumption of employment: older age, adequate nonwork income, anxiety or depression, activity-induced symptoms, lower social class and less education, jobs involving high-level physical activity (more common among blue-collar workers), and perception of the coronary illness as job-related. Patients who fail to resume employment within 6 months after a coronary event are unlikely ever to do so.[108]

Among the medical reasons for failure to return to work are unwarranted medical restrictions or, even more commonly, lack of professional assurance of the safety of so doing.[108] Exercise testing performed for risk stratification can also be used for work evaluation; it permits a relatively precise assessment of function that may help allay the apprehensions of the patient,[64] family,[109] physician, and employer about the capability and safety of return to work.[110] One randomized controlled trial of occupational work assessment in a health maintenance organization population early following myocardial infarction, identifying low-risk patients and counseling them about the appropriateness of prompt return to work, effected a 32-percent reduction in the duration of convalescence.[38] Extrapolation of exercise test data to job requirements should include the analysis of the job to be performed, differences in temperature, environment, intellectual demands, relation to meals, travel requirements, and emotional stress, among others. Nonetheless, patients without evidence of ischemia or arrhythmia during a symptom-limited standard exercise test are typically free of these problems when occupational static and dynamic work are combined.[111] Arm ergometry may be preferable for occupational assessment of patients who perform predominantly arm work.[59]

Further, since most occupational work is intermittent, with brief periods of strenuous activity and longer intervals of low-level activity or rest occupational myocardial work demand is lower than for the same level of steady-state exercise; cardiac output, blood pressure, and oxygen uptake do not approach steady state until about 2 min after the onset of work, explaining the tolerance of patients with modest cardiac impairment and limitation of cardiac output for significant workloads of short duration, when adequate rest periods are interspersed. Recommendations for full-time work should be for work levels approximating 30 percent of measured physical work capacity. Guidelines are available to assist physicians in assessing and establishing the employability of patients with coronary heart disease.[112]

Other nonmedical considerations also influence postinfarction or postrevascularization employment, particularly the financial, social, disability, and compensation benefits of not returning to work. Although appropriate physician and employer attitudes may facilitate reemployment, the viewpoint of the patient appears the major determinant. In a number of studies, the patient's preoperative perception about ability to return to work appeared to be the most important determinant.

Benefits to employers of cardiac rehabilitative care for their employees include earlier return to work, less disability, less absenteeism, reduced financial expenditures for sickness and disability payments, reduced training costs for replacement of personnel, and greater productivity.[1] Employers should thus encourage coronary rehabilitative care as a component of their managed care plans.

REFERENCES

1. Report of a WHO Expert Committee. Wenger NK, Expert Committee Chairman. *Rehabilitation after Cardiovascular Diseases, with Special Emphasis on Developing Countries.* WHO Tech. Rep. Series, No. 831, Geneva: World Health Organization; 1993.

2. American College of Cardiology: Position report on cardiac rehabilitation. Recommendations of the American College of Cardiology on cardiovascular rehabilitation. *J Am Coll Cardiol* 1986; 7:451–453.

3. Agency for Health Care Policy and Research. Cardiac rehabilitation programs. Health technology assessment reports, 1991, no. 3. Rockville, MD: US Department of Health and Human Services, Public Health Service, Agency for Health Care Policy and Research; DHHS publication No. AHCPR 92-0015, December, 1991.

4. Mark DB, Sigmon K, Topol EJ, Kereiakes DJ, Pryor DB, Candela RJ, et al. Identification of acute myocardial infarction patients suitable for early hospital discharge after aggressive interventional therapy. Results from the Thrombolysis and Angioplasty in Acute Myocardial Infarction Registry. *Circulation* 1991; 83:1186–1193.

5. Ben-Ari E, Kellermann JJ, Fishman EZ, Pines A, Peled B, Drory Y. Benefits of long-term physical training in patients after coronary artery bypass grafting—a 58-month follow-up and comparison with a non-trained group. *J Cardiopulm Rehabil* 1986; 6:165–170.

6. DeBusk RF, Houston Miller N, Superko HR, Dennis CA, Thomas RJ, Lew HT, et al. A case-management system for coronary risk factor modification after acute myocardial infarction. *Ann Intern Med* 1994; 120:721–729.

7. Haskell WL, Alderman EL, Fair JM, Maron DJ, Mackey SF, Superko HR, et al. Effects of intensive multiple risk factor reduction on coronary atherosclerosis and clinical cardiac events in men and women with coronary artery disease. The Stanford Coronary Risk Intervention Project (SCRIP). *Circulation* 1994; 89:975–990.

8. Raft D, McKee DC, Popio KA, Haggerty JJ Jr. Life adaptation after percutaneous transluminal coronary angioplasty and coronary artery bypass grafting. *Am J Cardiol* 1985; 56:395–398.

9. Ben-Ari E, Rothbaum DA, Linnemeir TJ, Landin RJ, Steinmetz EF, Hillis SJ, et al: Benefits of a monitored rehabilitation program versus physician care after emergency percutaneous transluminal coronary angioplasty: Follow-up of risk factors and rate of restenosis. *J Cardiopulm Rehabil* 1989; 7:281–285.

10. Ades PA, Waldmann ML, Gillespie C. A controlled trial of exercise training in older coronary patients. *J Gerontol* 1995; 50A:M7-11.

11. Lavie CJ, Milani RV, Littman AB. Benefits of cardiac rehabilitation and exercise training in secondary coronary prevention in the elderly. *J Am Coll Cardiol* 1993; 22:678–683.

12. Schuler G, Hambrecht R, Schlierf G, Niebauer J, Hauer K, Neumann J, et al. Regular physical exercise and low-fat diet. Effects on progression of coronary artery disease. *Circulation* 1992; 86:1–11.

13. Wenger NK, Froelicher ES, Smith LK, Ades PA, Berra K, Blumenthal JA, et al. *Cardiac Rehabilitation.* Clinical Practice Guideline No. 17. Rockville, MD: US Department of Health and Human Services, Public Health Service, Agency for Health Care Policy and Research and the National Heart, Lung, and Blood Institute; AHCPR Publication No. 96–0672, October, 1995.

14. Leon AS, Certo C, Comoss P, Franklin BA, Froelicher V, Haskell WL, et al. Scientific evidence of the value of cardiac rehabilitation services with emphasis on patients following myocardial infarction—Section I: Exercise conditioning component (position paper). *J Cardiopulm Rehabil* 1990; 10:79–87.

15. Mark DB, Naylor CD, Hlatky MA, Califf RM, Topol EJ, Granger CB, et al. Use of medical resources and quality of life after acute myocardial infarction in Canada and the United States. *N Engl J Med* 1994; 331:1130–1135.

16. Oldridge NB, Guyatt GH, Fischer ME, Rimm AA. Cardiac rehabilitation after myocardial infarction. Combined experience of randomized clinical trials. *JAMA* 1988; 260:945–950.

17. O'Connor GT, Buring JE, Yusuf S, Goldhaber SZ, Olmstead EM, Paffenbarger RS Jr, et al. An overview of randomized trials of rehabilitation with exercise after myocardial infarction. *Circulation* 1989; 80:234–244.

18. Carson P, Phillips R, Lloyd M, Tucker H, Neophytou M, Buch NJ, et al. Exercise after myocardial infarction: A controlled trial. *J R Coll Physicians Lond* 1982; 16:147–151.

19. Kallio V, Hamalainen H, Hakkila J, Luurila OJ. Reduction in sudden deaths by a multifactorial intervention programme after acute myocardial infarction. *Lancet* 1979; 2:1091–1094.

20. Rechnitzer PA, Cunningham DA, Andrew GM, Buck CW, Jones NL, Kavanagh T, et al. Relation of exercise to the recurrence rate of myocardial infarction in men. Ontario Exercise-Heart Collaborative Study. *Am J Cardiol* 1983; 51:65–69.

21. Wilhelmsen L, Sanne H, Elmfeldt D, Grimby G, Tibblin G, Wedel H. A controlled trial of physical training after myocardial infarction. Effects on risk factors, nonfatal reinfarction, and death. *Prev Med* 1975; 4:491–508.

22. Hamalainen H, Luurila OJ, Kallio V, Knuts L-R, Arstila M, Hakkila J. Long-term reduction in sudden deaths after a multifactorial intervention programme in patients with myocardial infarction: 10-year results of a controlled investigation. *Eur Heart J* 1989; 10:55–62.

23. Roman O, Gutierrez M, Luksic I, Chavez E, Camuzzi AL, Villalon E, et al. Cardiac rehabilitation after acute myocardial infarction. 9 year controlled follow-up study. *Cardiology* 1983; 70:223–231.

24. P.RE. COR. Group. Comparison of a rehabilitation programme, a counselling programme and usual care after an acute myocardial infarction: Results of a long-term randomized trial. *Eur Heart J* 1991; 12:612–616.

25. Marra S, Paolillo V, Spadaccini F, Angelino PF. Long-term follow-up after a controlled randomized post-myocardial infarction rehabilitation programme: Effects on morbidity and mortality. *Eur Heart J* 1985; 6:656–663.

26. Balady GJ, Jette D, Scheer J, Downing J, and the Massachusetts Association of Cardiovascular and Pulmonary Rehabilitation Database Co-investigators. Changes in exercise capacity following cardiac rehabilitation in patients stratified according to age and gender. Results of the Massachusetts Association of Cardiovascular and Pulmonary Rehabilitation Multicenter Database. *J Cardiopul Rehabil* 1996; 16:38–46.

27. Blumenthal JA, Rejeski WJ, Walsh-Riddle M, Emery CF, Miller H, Roark S, et al. Comparison of high- and low-intensity exercise training early after acute myocardial infarction. *Am J Cardiol* 1988; 61:26–30.

28. Goble AJ, Hare DL, Macdonald PS, Oliver RG, Reid MA, Worcester MC. Effect of early programmes of high and low intensity exercise on physical performance after transmural acute myocardial infarction. *Br Heart J* 1991; 65:126–131.

29. Ehsani AA, Biello DR, Schultz J, Sobel BE, Holloszy JO. Improvement of left ventricular contractile function by exercise training in patients with coronary artery disease. *Circulation* 1986; 74:350–358.

30. Kennedy CC, Spiekerman RE, Lindsay MI Jr, Mankin HT, Frye RL, McCallister BD. One-year graduated exercise program for men with angina pectoris. Evaluation by physiologic studies and coronary arteriography. *Mayo Clin Proc* 1976; 51:231–236.

31. Hung J, Gordon EP, Houston N, Haskell WL, Goris ML, DeBusk RF. Changes in rest and exercise myocardial perfusion and left ventricular function 3 to 26 weeks after clinically uncomplicated acute myocardial infarction: Effects of exercise training. *Am J Cardiol* 1984; 54:943–950.

32. Sullivan MJ, Higginbotham MB, Cobb FR. Exercise training in patients with severe left ventricular dysfunction. Hemodynamic and metabolic effects. *Circulation* 1988; 78:506–515.

33. DeBusk RF, Houston N, Haskell W, Fry F, Parker M. Exercise training soon after myocardial infarction. *Am J Cardiol* 1979; 44:1223–1229.

34. Todd IC, Ballantyne D. Effect of exercise training on the total ischaemic burden: An assessment by 24 hour ambulatory electrocardiographic monitoring. *Br Heart J* 1992; 68:560–566.

35. Sebrechts CP, Klein JL, Ahnve S, Froelicher VF, Ashburn WL. Myocardial perfusion changes following 1 year of exercise training assessed by thallium-201 circumferential count profiles. *Am Heart J* 1986; 112:1217–1226.

36. Coats AJS, Adamopoulos S, Meyer TE, Conway J, Sleight P. Effects of physical training in chronic heart failure. *Lancet* 1990; 335:63–66.

37. Meyer TE, Casadei B, Coats AJS, Davey PP, Adamopoulos S, Radaelli A, et al. Angiotensin-converting enzyme inhibition and physical training in heart failure. *J Intern Med* 1991; 230:407–413.

38. Dennis C, Houston-Miller N, Schwartz RG, Ahn DK, Kraemer HC, Gossard D, et al. Early return to work after uncomplicated myocardial infarction. Results of a randomized trial. *JAMA* 1988; 260:214–220.

39. Ades PA, Grunvald MH. Cardiopulmonary exercise testing before and after conditioning in older coronary patients. *Am Heart J* 1990; 120:585–589.

40. Ades PA, Hanson JS, Gunther PGS, Tonino RP. Exercise conditioning in the elderly coronary patient. *J Am Geriatr Soc* 1987; 35:121–124.

41. Ades PA, Waldmann ML, Polk DM, Coflesky JT. Referral patterns and exercise response in the rehabilitation of female coronary patients aged ≥62 years. *Am J Cardiol* 1992; 69:1422–1425.

42. Williams MA, Maresh CM, Esterbrooks DJ, Harbrecht JJ, Sketch MH. Early exercise training in patients older than age 65 years compared with that in younger patients after acute myocardial infarction or coronary artery bypass grafting. *Am J Cardiol* 1985; 55:263–266.

43. Balady GJ, Fletcher BJ, Froelicher ES, Hartley LH, Krauss RM, Oberman A, et al. Cardiac rehabilitation programs. A statement for healthcare professionals from the American Heart Association. *Circulation* 1994; 90:1602–1610.

44. American College of Sports Medicine Position Stand: Exercise for patients with coronary artery disease. *Med Sci Sports Exerc* 1994; 26:i–v.

45. Health and Public Policy Committee, American College of Physicians. Cardiac rehabilitation services. *Ann Intern Med* 1988; 109:671–673.

46. American Association of Cardiovascular and Pulmonary Rehabilitation. *Guidelines for Cardiac Rehabilitation Programs.* Champaign, IL, Human Kinetics, 1991.

47. Wenger NK, Balady GJ, Cohn LH, Hartley H, King SB III, Miller HS, et al. Ad Hoc Task Force on Cardiac Rehabilitation: Cardiac rehabilitation services following PTCA and valvular surgery. Guidelines for use. *Cardiology* 1990; 19:4–5.

48. Wenger NK, Haskell WL, Kanter K, Squires RW, Yusuf S. Ad Hoc Task Force on Cardiac Rehabilitation: Cardiac rehabilitation services after cardiac transplantation. Guidelines for use. *Cardiology* 1991; 20:4–5.

49. NIH Consensus Development Panel on Physical Activity and Cardiovascular Health. Physical activity and cardiovascular health. *JAMA* 1996; 276:241–246.

50. Haskell WL. Cardiovascular complications during exercise training of cardiac patients. *Circulation* 1978; 57:920–924.

51. DeBusk RF, Haskell WL, Miller NH, Berra K, Taylor CB, Berger WE III, et al. Medically directed at-home rehabilitation soon after uncomplicated acute myocardial infarction: A new model for patient care. *Am J Cardiol* 1985; 55:251–257.

52. Worcester MC, Hare DL, Oliver RG, Reid MA, Goble AJ. Early programmes of high and low intensity exercise and quality of life after acute myocardial infarction. *BMJ* 1993; 307:1244–1247.

53. Kelemen MH, Stewart KJ, Gillilan RE, Ewart CK, Valenti SA, Manley JD, et al. Circuit weight training in cardiac patients. *J Am Coll Cardiol* 1986; 7:38–42.

54. Franklin BA, Bonzheim K, Gordon S, Timmis GC. Resistance training in cardiac rehabilitation. *J Cardiopul Rehabil* 1991; 11:99–107.

55. Kelemen MH. Resistive training safety and assessment guidelines for cardiac and coronary prone patients. *Med Sci Sports Exerc* 1989; 21:675–677.

56. Sparling PB, Cantwell JD, Dolan CM, Niederman RK. Strength training in a cardiac rehabilitation program: A six-month follow-up. *Arch Phys Med Rehabil* 1990; 71:148–152.

57. Stewart KJ, Mason M, Keleman MH. Three-year participation in circuit weight training improves muscular strength and self-efficacy in cardiac patients. *J Cardiopul Rehabil* 1988; 8:292–296.

58. Wilke NA, Sheldahl LM, Levandoski SG, Hoffman MD, Dougherty SM, Tristani FE. Transfer effect of upper extremity training to weight carrying in men with ischemic heart disease. *J Cardiopulm Rehabil* 1991; 11:365–372.

59. Franklin BA. Exercise testing, training and arm ergometry. *Sports Med* 1985; 2:100–119.

60. Wenger NK. Ischemic heart disease: Exercise training, selected aspects of pharmacologic therapy, and drug-exercise interactions. *Emory J Med* 1989; 3:253–259.

61. Ryan TJ, Anderson JL, Antman EM, Braniff BA, Brooks NH, Califf RM, et al. ACC/AHA Task Force Report: Guidelines for the management of patients with acute myocardial infarction: A report of the American College of Cardiology/American Heart Association Task Force on Practice Guidelines (Committee on Management of Acute Myocardial Infarction). *J Am Coll Cardiol* 1996; 28:1328–1428, and (Executive Summary) *Circulation* 1996; 94:2341–2350.

62. Balady GJ, Weiner DA, Rose L, Ryan TJ, Erario M. Physiologic responses to arm ergometry exercise relative to age and gender. *J Am Coll Cardiol* 1990; 16:130–135.

63. Picard MH, Dennis C, Schwartz RG, Ahn DK, Kraemer HC, Berger WE III, et al. Cost-benefit analysis of early return to work after uncomplicated acute myocardial infarction. *Am J Cardiol* 1989; 63:1308–1314.

64. Ewart CK, Taylor CB, Reese LB, DeBusk RF. Effects of early post-myocardial infarction exercise testing on self-perception and subsequent physical activity. *Am J Cardiol* 1983; 51:1076–1080.

65. Van Camp SP, Peterson RA. Cardiovascular complications of outpatient cardiac rehabilitation programs. *JAMA* 1986; 256:1160–1163.

66. Wenger NK. In-hospital exercise rehabilitation after myocardial infarction and myocardial revascularization: Physiologic basis, methodology, and results. In: Wenger NK, Hellerstein HK, eds. *Rehabilitation of the Coronary Patient,* 3d ed. New York: Churchill Livingstone; 1992:351–365.

67. Hung J, Goldwater D, Convertino VA, McKillop JH, Goris ML, DeBusk RF. Mechanisms for decreased exercise capacity after bed rest in normal middle-aged men. *Am J Cardiol* 1983; 51:344–348.

68. Rowe MH, Jelinek MV, Liddell N, Hugens M. Effect of rapid mobilization on ejection fractions and ventricular volumes after acute myocardial infarction. *Am J Cardiol* 1989; 63:1037–1041.

69. Maeland JG, Havik OE. The effects of an in-hospital educational programme for myocardial infarction patients. *Scand J Rehab Med* 1987; 19:57–65.

70. Borg GA. Psychophysical bases of perceived exertion. *Med Sci Sports Exerc* 1982; 14:377–381.

71. Williams RS, Miller H, Koisch FP Jr, Ribisl P, Graden H. Guidelines for unsupervised exercise in patients with ischemic heart disease. *J Cardiac Rehabil* 1981; 1:213–219.

72. Blumenthal JA, Levenson RM. Behavioral approaches to secondary prevention of coronary heart disease. *Circulation* 1987; 76(suppl I):I-130–I-137.

73. Ornish D, Brown SE, Scherwitz LW, Billings LW, Armstrong WT, Ports TA, et al. Can lifestyle changes reverse coronary heart disease? The Lifestyle Heart Trial. *Lancet* 1990; 336:129–133.

74. Mullen PD, Mains DA, Velez R. A meta-analysis of controlled trials of cardiac patient education. *Patient Educ Couns* 1992; 19:143–162.

75. Newton KM, Sivarajan ES, Clarke JL. Patient perceptions of risk factor changes and cardiac rehabilitation outcomes after myocardial infarction. *J Cardiopulm Rehabil* 1985; 5:159–168.

76. CASS Principal Investigators and their Associates. Coronary Artery Surgery Study (CASS): A randomized trial of coronary artery bypass surgery. Quality of life in patients randomly assigned to treatment groups. *Circulation* 1983; 68:951–960.

77. Leaman DM, Brower RW, Meester GT. Coronary artery bypass surgery. A stimulus to modify existing risk factors? *Chest* 1982; 81:16–19.

78. Kottke TE, Battista RN, DeFriese GH, Brekke ML. Attributes of successful smoking cessation interventions in medical practice. A meta-analysis of 39 controlled trials. *JAMA* 1988; 259:2883–2889.

79. Shephard RJ. The scientific basis of exercise prescribing for the very old. *J Am Geriatr Soc* 1990; 38:62–70.

80. Saunamaki KI. Early post-myocardial infarction exercise testing in subjects 70 years or more of age. Functional and prognostic evaluation. *Eur Heart J* 1984; 5(suppl E):93–96.

81. Bruce RA, Larson EB, Stratton J. Physical fitness, functional aerobic capacity, aging, and responses to physical training or bypass surgery in coronary patients. *J Cardiopulm Rehabil* 1989; 9:24–34.

82. Litchfield RL, Kerber RE, Benge JW, Mark AL, Sopko J, Bhatnagar RK, et al. Normal exercise capacity in patients with severe left ventricular dysfunction: Compensatory mechanisms. *Circulation* 1982; 66:129–134.

83. Giannuzzi P, Tavazzi L, Temporelli PL, Corra U, Imparato A, Gattone M, et al. Long-term physical training and left ventricular remodeling after anterior myocardial infarction: Results of the Exercise in Anterior Myocardial Infarction (EAMI) Trial. *J Am Coll Cardiol* 1993; 22:1821–1829.

84. Hornig B, Maier V, Drexler H. Physical training improves endothelial function in patients with chronic heart failure. *Circulation* 1996; 93:210–214.

85. Squires RW, Lavie CJ, Brandt TR, Gau GT, Bailey KR. Cardiac rehabilitation in patients with severe ischemic left ventricular dysfunction. *Mayo Clin Proc* 1987; 62:997–1002.

86. Williams RS. Exercise training of patients with ventricular dysfunction and heart failure. In: Wenger NK, ed. *Exercise and the Heart,* 2d ed. Philadelphia: F.A. Davis; 1985:219–231.

87. Stevenson LW, Steimle AE, Fonarow G, Kermani M, Kermani D, Hamilton MA, et al. Improvement in exercise capacity of candidates awaiting heart transplantation. *J Am Coll Cardiol* 1995; 25:163–170.

88. Tamarisk NK. Enhancing activity levels of patients with permanent cardiac pacemakers. *Heart Lung* 1988; 17:698–707.

89. Kalbfleisch KR, Lehmann MH, Steinman RT, Jackson K, Axtell K, Schuger CD, et al. Reemployment following implantation of the automatic cardioverter defibrillator. *Am J Cardiol* 1989; 64:199–202.

90. Williams RB Jr, Barefoot JC, Haney TL, Harrell FE Jr, Blumenthal JA, Pryor DB, et al. Type A behavior and angiographically documented coronary atherosclerosis in a sample of 2,289 patients. *Psychosom Med* 1988; 50:139–152.

91. Helmers KF, Krantz DS, Howell RH, Klein J, Baircy CN, Rozanski A. Hostility and myocardial ischemia in coronary artery disease patients: Evaluation by gender and ischemic index. *Psychosom Med* 1993; 55:29–36.

92. Razin AM. Psychosocial intervention in coronary artery disease: A review. *Psychosom Med* 1982; 44:363–387.

93. Schleifer SL, Macari Hinson MM, Coyle DA, Slater WR, Kahn M, Gorlin R, et al. The nature and course of depression following myocardial infarction. *Arch Intern Med* 1989; 149:1785–1789.

94. Frasure-Smith N, Lesperance F, Talajic M. Depression and 18-month prognosis after myocardial infarction. *Circulation* 1995; 91:999–1005.

95. Frasure-Smith N, Lesperance F, Talajic M. Depression following myocardial infarction. Impact on 6-month survival. *JAMA* 1993; 270:1819–1825.

96. Stern MJ, Cleary P. National Exercise and Heart Disease Project. Psychosocial changes observed during a low-level exercise program. *Arch Intern Med* 1981; 141:1463–1467.

97. Maeland JG, Havik OE. Psychological predictors for return to work after a myocardial infarction. *J Psychosom Res* 1987; 31:471–481.

98. Orth-Gomer K, Unden A-L, Edwards M-E. Social isolation and mortality in ischemic heart disease. A 10-year follow-up study of 150 middle-aged men. *Acta Med Scand* 1988; 224:205–215.

99. Wenger NK, Hellerstein HK, Blackburn H, Castranova SJ. Physician practice in the management of patients with uncomplicated myocardial infarction: Changes in the past decade. *Circulation* 1982; 65:421–427.

100. Walter PJ (ed): *Return to Work after Coronary Artery Bypass Surgery. Psychosocial and Economic Aspects.* Berlin: Springer-Verlag; 1985.

101. Russell RO Jr, Abi-Mansour P, Wenger NK. Return to work after coronary bypass surgery and percutaneous transluminal angioplasty: Issues and potential solutions. *Cardiology* 1986; 73:306–322.

102. Rogers WJ, Coggin CJ, Gersh BJ, Fisher LD, Myers WO, Oberman A, et al for the CASS Investigators. Ten-year follow-up of quality of life in patients randomized to receive medical therapy or coronary artery bypass graft surgery. The Coronary Artery Surgery Study (CASS). *Circulation* 1990; 82:1647–1658.

103. Fitzgerald ST, Becker DM, Celentano DD, Swank R, Brinker J. Return to work after percutaneous transluminal coronary angioplasty. *Am J Cardiol* 1989; 64:1108–1112.

104. Walling A, Tremblay GJ, Jobin J, Charest J, Delage F, Leblanc M-H, et al. Evaluating the rehabilitation potential of a large population of post-myocardial infarction patients: Adverse prognosis for women. *J Cardiopulm Rehabil* 1988; 8:99–106.

105. Ades PA, Huang D, Weaver SO. Cardiac rehabilitation participation predicts lower rehospitalization costs. *Am Heart J* 1992; 123:916–921.

106. Levin LA, Perk J, Hedback B. Cardiac rehabilitation—a cost analysis. *J Intern Med* 1991; 230:427–434.

107. Oldridge N, Furlong W, Feeny D, Torrance G, Guyatt G, Crowe J, et al. Economic evaluation of cardiac rehabilitation soon after acute myocardial infarction. *Am J Cardiol* 1993; 72:154–161.

108. Almeida D, Bradford JM, Wenger NK, King SB, Hurst JW. Return to work after coronary bypass surgery. *Circulation* 1983; 68(suppl II):II-205–II-213.

109. Taylor CB, Bandura A, Ewart CK, Miller NH, DeBusk RF. Exercise testing to enhance wives' confidence in their husbands' cardiac capability soon after clinically uncomplicated acute myocardial infarction. *Am J Cardiol* 1985; 55:635–638.

110. Hellerstein HK. Vocational aspects of rehabilitation. Work evaluation. In: Wenger NK, Hellerstein HK, eds. *Rehabilitation of the Coronary Patient,* 3d ed. New York: Churchill Livingstone; 1992:523–542.

111. Hung J, McKillip J, Savin W, Magder S, Kraus R, Houston N, et al. Comparison of cardiovascular response to combined static-dynamic effort, postprandial dynamic effort and dynamic effort alone in patients with chronic ischemic heart disease. *Circulation* 1982; 65:1411–1419.

112. 20th Bethesda Conference. Insurability and employability of the patient with ischemic heart disease. October 3–4, 1988. *J Am Coll Cardiol* 1989; 14:1003–1044.

SEVEN

SYSTEMIC ARTERIAL HYPERTENSION

56

PATHOPHYSIOLOGY OF SYSTEMIC ARTERIAL HYPERTENSION

Edward D. Frohlich / Richard N. Re

PRESSOR MECHANISMS IN HYPERTENSION

To understand the pathophysiologic alterations associated with the systemic arterial hypertensive diseases there must first be a clear-cut understanding of the hemodynamic alterations; by definition, hypertension is a hemodynamic derangement.[1–4] The elevated arterial pressure in systemic arterial hypertension (SAH) may be associated with an increased cardiac output or total peripheral resistance. Any changes in blood viscosity would not result in a significant increase in arterial pressure even though they may alter local tissue blood flow in organs. For the most part, however, an increased vascular resistance is the hemodynamic hallmark of the disease; all mechanisms responsible for this increased vascular smooth muscle tone are implicit in the multifactorial nature of SAH disease.[4–6] This chapter considers the factors that may be involved with the pathogenesis, elaboration, and maintenance of hypertensive diseases in essential hypertension as well as in the other forms of hypertension (Table 56-1). The discussion places a major emphasis on essential hypertension, since this is the primary form of hypertension and occurs in approximately 95 percent of all patients with SAH.[3,4] This pathophysiologic discussion, however, is particularly relevant to other (i.e., secondary) clinical forms of hypertension; they will be cited at appropriate points for comparison with those derangements that occur in patients with essential hypertension.

Hemodynamics

SYSTEMIC

As indicated, all patients with hypertension have an increased arterial pressure that is associated with an increased contractile state or increased mass of vascular smooth muscle in both the arterioles and venules. This functional and structural luminal narrowing serves to increase the total peripheral resistance and to reduce total-body venous capacity.[1,3,7] The result of the former is an increase in left ventricular afterload that serves as the major hemodynamic mechanism responsible for the left ventricular hypertrophy (LVH) associated with progression in the severity of hypertensive vascular disease.[8,9] The reduced venous capacity due to active venular constriction has been demonstrated clinically and in experimental forms of hypertension.[10–12] Early in hypertension, this venoconstriction is not associated with contraction in intravascular volume; hence, it serves to redistribute the circulating volume to the cardiopulmonary area from the periphery.[10,13,14] With progression of the vascular disease and more intense vasoconstriction (arteriolar and venular), however, intravascular volume contracts progressively.[15,16] This is reflected in a proportionally diminished right atrial venous return, thereby reducing the cardiac output to a more normal level from, frequently, an elevated level.[13,17] As LVH becomes more manifest, left ventricular function becomes impaired and the resting cardiac output diminishes.[17,18] With these alterations in systemic blood flow there are proportional changes in organ blood flows; these reductions in specific organ flows are in direct relation to the increased organ vascular resistance.[14] Therefore, *the organ or regional vascular resistances seem to be more or less uniformly distributed systemically in proportion to the increased total peripheral resistance.*[1,2,14]

VASCULAR SMOOTH MUSCLE AND WALL

Thus, *the major hemodynamic alteration in hypertensive disease is a progressively increasing vascular resistance, which is achieved through an active increase in the state of tone of vascular smooth muscle in both the arterioles and the venules.* This state of vessel tone can be achieved whether the myocyte

TABLE 56-1

CLASSIFICATION OF THE VARIOUS FORMS OF SYSTEMIC ARTERIAL HYPERTENSION BASED ON CAUSES

PRIMARY (ESSENTIAL) HYPERTENSION (HYPERTENSION OF UNDETERMINED CAUSE)

Borderline (labile) essential hypertension
Essential hypertension (sustained diastolic hypertension)
  Mild severity: diastolic pressures 90 to 104 mmHg
  Moderate severity: diastolic pressures 105 to 114 mmHg
  Severe: persistent diastolic pressures greater than 114 mmHg
Isolated systolic hypertension: systolic pressures greater than
  140 mmHg with diastolic pressures less than 90 mmHg

SECONDARY HYPERTENSION

Coarctation of the aorta
Renal arterial disease (renovascular hypertension)
  Nonatherosclerotic (fibrosing) renal arterial disease
  Atherosclerotic renal arterial disease
  Aneurysm(s) of renal artery
  Embolic renal arterial disease
  Extravascular compression (of renal artery): tumor, fibrosis
  Perinephric hull (Page kidney)
Renal parenchymal diseases
  Chronic pyelonephritis
  Acute glomerulonephritis
  Chronic glomerulonephritis
  Polycystic renal disease
  Diabetic nephropathy
  Others: amyloidosis, ureteral obstruction, etc.
Hormonal diseases
  Thyroid
    Hyperthyroidism
    Hypothyroidism
    Hashimoto's thyroiditis
  Adrenal
    Cushing disease or Cushing syndrome
    Primary hyperaldosteronism
      Adenoma
      Bilateral adrenal hyperplasia
    Adrenal enzyme deficiencies
    Pheochromocytoma
  Ectopic production of hormones
  Growth hormone excess
  Hypercalcemic disease states (including hyperparathyroidism)
Drugs, chemicals, and foods
  Excessive alcohol intake
  Excessive dietary sodium intake
  Exogenously administered adrenal steroids: birth control pills; adrenal steroids for asthma,
    malignancies; anabolic steroids
  Licorice excess (imported)
  Cold preparations: phenylpropanolamine; nasal decongestants
  Milk-alkali syndrome; hypervitaminosis D
  Snuff
Complications from specific therapy
  Antidepressant therapy (tricyclics; monoamine oxidase inhibitors)
  Chronic steroid administration
  Cyclosporine (transplantation and certain diseases requiring immunosuppressive therapy)
  Beta-adrenergic receptor agonists (e.g., for asthma)
  Radiation nephritis, arteritis

is stimulated by enhanced adrenergic input (elevated circulating levels), humoral agents (e.g., catecholamines, angiotensin II, serotonin, vasopressin), local vasoactive peptides (e.g., angiotensin II, vasoactive intestinal polypeptide, endothelin), or ions (e.g., calcium); by a reduced amount of vasoconstrictors (e.g., nitric oxides); or by a decrease in vasodilating agents (e.g., acetylcholine, histamine, nitric oxide, adenosine, prostaglandins), local vasoactive peptides (e.g., insulin, calcitonin gene–related peptide), or ions (e.g., potassium, magnesium, Krebs intermediate metabolites).[1–4] Whatever the myocytic stimulus, there is a consequent rise in cytoplasmic free calcium ions in the resting state and a resulting enhanced phosphorylation of myosin light chains in the contractile state (see Chap. 4). This increased calcium ionic milieu may be achieved either through an inflow of calcium ions through calcium or other (e.g., alpha-adrenergic) receptor-activated membrane channels or by an enhanced release of calcium ions from intracellular organelles (primarily the sarcoplasmic reticulum), although calcium may also be released from the mitochondria or from binding with protein substrates (e.g., calmodulin). The former receptor-operated channels explain the mechanisms of action of the various membrane receptors of naturally occurring humoral substances or of various antihypertensive agents (e.g., calcium antagonists). The intracytoplasmic calcium release seems to be initiated by the formation of inositol triphosphate (IP_3), which serves as the second messenger mediating the calcium ion increase.[19–27] The net effect is the availability of calcium ions for the mechanical coupling that permits the enhanced state of contractility of vascular smooth muscle.

Thus, for examples, serotonin serves to stimulate protein tyrosyl phosphorylation and vascular contraction by means of tyrosine kinase[25]; insulin seems to relax vascular smooth muscle by suppressing secretion of the c-type natriuretic peptide in the endothelium[26]; and angiotensin II increases vascular superoxide production through membrane NADH/NADPH vasomotor tone.[27]

STRUCTURE

As noted, another factor that participates in the increased vascular resistance is an increased wall-to-lumen ratio of the arterial and arteriolar wall. This structural alteration of the vessel wall in hypertension serves to augment vascular responsiveness to constrictor stimuli, thereby serving to perpetuate or maintain the hypertension.[28] The increased arteriolar and arterial wall thickness as well as the increased mass of the left ventricle, which are primarily manifested by myocytic hypertrophy, seem to be initiated (at least in part) by myocytic stretch. Thus, the stretch mechanism stimulates early gene (e.g., c-*myc*) expression, which, in turn, promotes DNA-mediated protein synthesis[29–32] or myocytic protein synthesis through intracellular autocrine/paracrine mechanisms.[33,34] On the other hand, hypertensive arteries undergo structural alteration (remodeling) and, under certain therapeutic circumstances (most particularly with converting enzyme inhibitors), this change can be reversed.[35] This finding is of interest given the fact that angiotensin II, when chronically administered to experimental animals, can produce a long-term effect that is probably the result of structural alterations in the vasculature.[36] Recent investigations have suggested that the hemodynamic stress of vessel stretch may not be the sole responsible mechanism accounting for the vessel wall thickening.[37,38] Thus, recent studies of cultured neonatal cardiac myocytes have revealed that in vitro stretch produces the release of angiotensin II by these cells with secondarily induced hypertrophy of the cells; indeed, after stretch, angiotensinogen gene transcription is augmented in an apparent compensatory manner.[29,30,39] These data taken with other studies suggest that angiotensin II plays an important role in the development of arteriolar smooth muscle and LVH in hypertension. Indeed, numbers of growth factors, such as platelet-derived growth factor, have been shown to participate in this process, some of which are vasoconstrictors (e.g., angiotensin II, endothelin) and are produced within the arteriolar wall.[40–44] Growth factors and vascular smooth muscle cell growth represent common features of hypertension and atherosclerosis.[45,46]

ENDOTHELIUM

Recent years have witnessed a remarkable explosion in our knowledge concerning the role of the endothelium in health and disease. This subject is covered more extensively elsewhere (see Chaps. 4 and 44), but some discussion is also indicated in this chapter. Following the original report by Furchgott and Zawadzki,[47] the endothelium was no longer considered to be merely a lining of cells in the blood vessel but to be an important component of the vasculature that provided an active means for assuring vasodilation and constriction. Thus, intrinsic endothelium-derived relaxing factors promote vasodilation and presently include nitric oxide, prostacyclin and other prostaglandin and related cyclooxygenase substances, bradykinin, and other substances. The endothelial-dependent constricting or contracting factors include endothelin, superoxide anions, endoperoxides, and thromboxane.[48] Nitric oxide, the potent endothelially produced relaxing substance and vasodilator, is synthesized by the metabolism of the amino acid L-arginine through the enzymatic action of nitric oxide synthase.[49] The generated nitric oxide triggers the activation of the intracellular second messenger cyclic GMP and interacts with other intracellular relaxing and constricting substances, including angiotensin II and the kinins, in a complex endothelial modulatory system.[48–50] Several chemicals have been used experimentally to inhibit the enzyme acutely and chemically in order to exacerbate hypertension. Thus, in response to this enzymatic inhibition, less nitric oxide is synthesized in the endothelium and arterial smooth muscle is constricted, resulting in an increased vascular resistance and reduction of blood flow. The net effect systemically is an increased total peripheral resistance and arterial pressure, with a reduction in cardiac output. These changes affect organ and regional circulations, including the kidney,[48,51–53] and mimic the hemodynamic alterations that are associated with aging in experimental animals and in humans.[54–56] Moreover, endothelially derived nitric oxide–mediated function is also impaired in hyperlipidemia,[57,58] in hypertensive coronary arterial disease associated with LVH,[59] and in other systemic arteries in patients with essential hypertension.[60–62] Hence, impaired nitric oxide synthesis and/or its vascular response is impaired with aging, in hypertensive vascular disease, and in hyperlipidemia. Experimental and clinical studies strongly suggest that various types of antihypertensive agents may reverse the pathophysiologic changes associated with endothelial disease. Thus, in the spontaneously hypertensive rat, the renal hemodynamic, glomerular, and pathologic changes of aging and hypertensive nephrosclerosis and proteinuria were reversed within 3 weeks by angiotensin-converting enzyme (ACE) inhibition therapy[53,63] or by L-arginine[64] but were exacerbated by hydrochlorothiazide.[65] These observations have been reported by others[57,66,67] and may be the result of stimulation of local renin-angiotensin systems[53] and/or kinins. At any rate, a new chapter in our understanding of endothelial function in health and disease (and, more specifically, in hypertension) is emerging.

Fluid Volume Partitions

In general, *total-body water is normal in hypertension and seems to be normally distributed between the extracellular and intracellular fluid compartments.*[68] Although there is much epidemiologic evidence for a metabolic derangement in the consumption and handling of sodium in patients with hypertension, there is little evidence to indicate that total-body sodium is increased or that it is associated with abnormal total-body water.[69] Nevertheless, there is good clinical evidence that the extracellular fluid volume is maldistributed.[68] Thus, intravascular (i.e., plasma) volume becomes contracted as arterial pressure and total peripheral resistance increase in patients with essential hypertension[15,16]; it is associated with a greater expansion of the interstitial fluid volume.[70] The pathophysiologic implications of these alterations were extremely important in the earlier days of antihypertensive therapy. Thus, if arterial pressure were reduced by direct-acting smooth muscle vasodilators or antiadrenergic compounds, capillary hydrostatic and renal arterial perfusion pressures would diminish. As a consequence, interstitial fluid would migrate intravascularly to expand (or "reconstitute") the intravascular compartment.[71,72] The net result was an attenuation of the antihypertensive effectiveness and a state of "pseudotolerance." With addition of a diuretic, however, intravascular volume would again become contracted, thereby restoring the antihypertensive drug effectiveness. This, then, provides the physiologic explanation for the phenomenon of pseudotolerance.[71,73] In more recent years, with the introduction of the beta-adrenergic receptor blockers, ACE inhibitors, and calcium antagonist therapies, the induced hypotension is not associated with expanded intravascular volume and pseudotolerance has been of less concern.[74,75] In the intensive care setting, when therapies may still include ganglion-blocking drugs or sodium nitroprusside, however, pseudotolerance may become a very real problem. Thus, with prolonged pressure reduction using these agents, antihypertensive effectiveness may diminish as a result of intravascular volume expansion and not "tachyphylaxis" (or diminished end-organ pharmacologic effectiveness); by adding a diuretic, the desired hypotensive effect may be anticipated.[74–76]

As indicated, most patients with essential hypertension demonstrate an inverse relationship between height of arterial pressure (or total peripheral resistance) and the magnitude of intravascular volume.[15,16,18] Patients with other forms of SAH demonstrate a similar inverse relationship, including those with renal arterial disease and pheochromocytoma.[16] These considerations are of major pathophysiologic significance since inordinate intraoperative hypotension may occur if intravascular volume is not expanded before excision of a pheochromocytoma (e.g., with prior therapy with an alpha-adrenergic receptor inhibitor to lower pressure and expand plasma volume) or with direct intraoperative volume expansion using the patient's own blood (preferably collected prior to surgery). Alternatively, severe hypotension may ensue after removal of the adrenal gland with associated withdrawal of the catecholamine-induced pressure elevation.

In contrast, other patients with hypertension may demonstrate a direct relationship between the height of arterial pressure and intravascular volume.[16] These patients may have steroid-dependent forms of hypertension (e.g., primary aldosteronism, Cushing's disease), renal parenchymal disease, or volume-dependent essential hypertension (which includes a small number of patients having so-called low plasma renin activity that is suppressed by this volume expansion)[16,77–79]

(see Chaps. 57 and 58). In this respect, even in patients with parenchymal renal disease who have normal renal function tests (e.g., serum creatinine and glomerular filtration rate), intravascular volume is expanded.[78] These considerations have important clinical and therapeutic considerations. For example, studies have shown that patients with low plasma renin and essential hypertension, steroid-dependent hypertension, or renal parenchymal disease with hypertension are particularly responsive to diuretic therapy[80] (see Chap. 57).

Sodium Metabolism

Epidemiologic studies have repeatedly demonstrated a high direct correlation between dietary sodium intake of populations and the prevalence of hypertension.[81] Further, other studies have shown that those societies with daily sodium intakes of less than 60 mmol (1.38 g sodium or 3.51 g sodium chloride) also fail to show a rise in arterial pressure with aging. Other studies have demonstrated that there may be genetically determined alterations in sodium transport across cell membranes in different population groups of patients with essential hypertension.[82] Notwithstanding the massive epidemiologic data supporting an important role for the sodium ion in essential hypertension, there is a paucity of pathophysiologic data that have demonstrated this in clinical situations.[74] It remains a major problem to identify which patients with essential hypertension are sodium sensitive and which are not. At this point, therefore, the subject still remains one of great controversy.

Hormonal Alterations

Because of the foregoing issue concerning the role of the sodium ion in essential hypertension, many studies have focused upon the role of adrenal corticosteroids. For the most part, these studies have failed to demonstrate any specific abnormality in the metabolism of the adrenal steroidal hormones. Aldosterone seems to be synthesized, released, and excreted in proportion to the levels of stimulation of the renin-angiotensin system.[83] No clear-cut derangement in adrenal steroid biosynthesis has been demonstrated in patients with essential hypertension. Patients with abnormal levels of steroidal biosynthesis and release have specific adrenal diseases (Cushing's syndrome and disease, primary hyperaldosteronism, hydroxylase deficiencies, etc.)[84] (see Chap. 57).

States of hormonal alteration have been associated with hypertension. There is a high prevalence of hypertension in patients with both hyperthyroidism and hypothyroidism. There also is an increased incidence of hypertension among patients with hypercalcemic diseases (including hyperparathyroidism), although the increased prevalence of hyperparathyroidism observed between 1965 and 1974 seems to be reversing unexpectedly and for unexplained reasons.[85] Furthermore, recent studies have suggested an abnormality in parathyroid hormone in patients with essential hypertension[86]; this observation still requires further confirmation and study. Other hormonal diseases associated with hypertension include acromegaly and gigantism, ectopically produced hormones associated with tumors, and, of course, exogenously administered hormones (e.g., oral contraceptives, androgens).

Neural Mechanisms

The autonomic nervous system participates importantly in the normal control of arterial pressure and may be altered in patients with essential hypertension. One would normally expect that the higher the arterial pressure, the slower the heart rate. On the other hand, most patients with essential hypertension (no matter what the severity) demonstrate a relatively faster heart rate, even if frank tachycardia is not present.[87] This is but one manifestation of the altered baroreceptor sensitivity phenomenon in hypertension.[88] In addition, increased release of, sensitivity to, and excretion of norepinephrine have been demonstrated in many patients with essential hypertension, more frequently in patients with borderline or mild degrees of severity.[89] In addition, other studies have related increased levels of serum catecholamines in proportion to the altered hemodynamics.[90] On the other hand, no abnormalities have been demonstrated in patients with essential hypertension with respect to catecholamine biosynthesis.

A variety of studies have demonstrated increased responsiveness of blood vessels to catecholamine stimulation and stressful stimuli (including cold and physiologic interventions). Thus, several studies, involving patients with essential hypertension, have demonstrated alterations in response to upright tilting, Valsalva maneuver, and tyramine provocation of norepinephrine release from nerve endings.[91,92] Thus, patients with milder forms of hypertension may demonstrate orthostatic hypertension and a greater degree of diastolic pressure overshoot during the Valsalva maneuver, suggesting a greater neural component in this group. By contrast, patients with more severe hypertension (e.g., history of cardiac failure, malignant hypertension) may demonstrate orthostatic hypotension and a lesser degree of pressure/overshoot after the Valsalva maneuver, indicating a less significant neural contribution in the late stages of the disease.[91] Furthermore, patients with essential hypertension who have higher than normal levels of plasma catecholamines will demonstrate an appropriate suppression of these levels with clonidine administration, in contrast to patients with pheochromocytoma.[93] In these latter patients, because the catecholamines are produced by the adrenal tumor, suppression of catecholamine levels does not occur.

Renopressor System

The enzyme renin is released from the juxtaglomerular cells of the kidney for a variety of reasons: stimulation by intravascular volume contraction, decreases in sodium delivery, beta-adrenergically mediated neural input to the juxtaglomerular apparatus, reduced plasma levels of aldosterone, changes in posture, a variety of drugs, hypokalemia, and other causes.[94–96] The released renal enzyme renin acts on a substrate, angiotensinogen, produced principally in the liver. As a result, the decapeptide angiotensin I is released from angiotensinogen. Angiotensin I is rapidly transformed in the pulmonary circulation, and to a lesser extent in the general circulation and the walls of arteries, by ACE, which cleaves a terminal dipeptide to form the powerful pressor octapeptide, angiotensin II. Angiotensin II then acts on its target sites: vascular smooth muscle cells to produce vasoconstriction; adrenal cortex to release aldosterone; adrenal medulla to augment catecholamine release; certain medullary centers of the brain to initiate adrenergic outflow from the brain; and certain thirst centers in the brain. It also produces direct myocardial stimulation and protein synthesis. The amino-terminal amino acid of angiotensin II can be cleaved to generate the heptapeptide angiotensin III.[94,97–102] This compound has many of the same physiologic effects as angiotensin II, though its relative physiologic potency is somewhat different. Recently, it has been discovered that the carboxyl-terminal amino acid can be cleaved from angiotensin II, producing the heptapeptide angiotensin IV.[94,97–101,103] While the precise physiologic role of this peptide remains unclear, it does appear to have effects in the central nervous system and elsewhere.[104–106]

Evidence has accumulated both in experimental models and in humans to suggest that converting enzyme inhibition is beneficial in reducing the rate of glomerular functional decline in diabetic patients.[107–111] Recent evidence suggests that the converting enzyme inhibitors may be similarly beneficial if properly employed in other forms of renal disease.[112] A clinical caveat is that the use of converting enzyme inhibition in patients with renal disease can involve some risk, in that hyperkalemia can occur and persistent diminution of renal function can be seen in patients with significant renal artery stenosis. Nonetheless, these clinical findings support laboratory studies suggesting that inhibition of angiotensin II generation can be beneficial in retarding the progression of diabetic and perhaps other forms of renal disease. In vitro studies suggest a direct effect of angiotensin II on mesangial cell proliferation and physiology, while other studies point to beneficial alterations in glomerular pressure resulting from converting enzyme inhibition as a causative factor.[108,109,111,113–115]

LOCAL GENERATION

Angiotensin II, however, may be produced by means other than this now-classic endocrine mechanism. Recently, alternative means of angiotensin II generation have been demonstrated in the heart.[116] It is now clear that angiotensin II can be generated locally in a number of cellular systems of brain, ovary, salivary gland, uterus, liver, vascular smooth muscle, and cardiac myocytes. The precise roles for these local systems are not yet known fully, but much has been written about the role of the intracellular generation of angiotensin II on muscle protein synthesis and its role in the development and regression of vascular and ventricular hypertrophy[117–122] (see also Chap. 6). This locally generated angiotensin II may be of particular importance: (1) in the function of the cell that produces the peptide (intracrine action); (2) on neighboring cells (paracrine action); or (3) in association (autocrine) with other hormones (e.g., kinins, catecholamines, the atrial natriuretic hormone). In this regard, components of the renin-angiotensin system can be readily identified in multiple tissues.[123] In some instances, these components can be shown to have been taken up from the blood, as, for example, in the case of renin and angiotensin I in selected vascular beds.[123,124] On the other hand, there exists considerable evidence to suggest that local gene expression also plays a role in certain instances.[113,123,125–130] This is most easily seen in the case of ACE gene upregulation during experimental myocardial infarction or left ventricular failure, but it can also be shown for angiotensinogen local gene expression and even in some selected cases for renin gene expression.[36,69,112,115,123,125,127,129–133] Thus, local regulation of components of the renin-angiotensin system and, in particular, of ACE activity seems likely. In this regard it must be pointed out that, although traditional teaching has long held that renin is the rate-regulating enzyme of the renin-angiotensin system, kinetic studies clearly show that angiotensin generation is dependent on angiotensinogen concentration as well.[123] Indeed, it seems likely that ACE concentration similarly can affect angiotensin II production, although the kinetics of converting enzyme are harder to study by virtue of the fact that ACE is in large measure a tissue-bound enzyme. Thus, differential regulation of components of the renin-angiotensin system can be expected to have effects on angiotensin II concentration in tissue. This realization has potentially important clinical implications, as indicated by a variety of experimental models.

The fact that angiotensin II is itself a potent growth regulating hormone suggests that this peptide, whether produced locally or systemically, could have an important role in the abnormal architectural changes seen in the vessels and hearts of patients suffering from hypertension.[35,113,123,134] This possibility is made more vivid by cell culture experiments involving the use of artificially induced stretch to study cultured cardiac myocyte behavior.[29,30,39,112] This work indicates that stretch leads to a release of preformed angiotensin II by cardiac myocytes, with resulting hypertrophy. Angiotensinogen gene upregulation occurs following prolonged stretch. These and other studies suggest that local production of angiotensin II in a paracrine or autocrine fashion could play an important role in vascular and cardiac architecture. This suggestion is further supported by clinical studies involving the use of converting enzyme inhibitors or beta blockers in the treatment of hypertensive patients. Gluteal biopsies performed on patients show a reversal of vascular remodeling in patients treated with converting enzyme inhibitors as opposed to those treated with beta blockers.[35] These studies suggest that the preferential effects of ACE inhibition on lowering angiotensin II levels, be they systemic or local, can have an important effect on vascular architecture.

While the role of local renin-angiotensin systems, as contrasted with the circulating system, is not yet completely worked out, a growing body of experimental and clinical data suggests that these tissue peptide cascades are important mediators of the tissue response to hypertension.

Although controversial, abundant evidence now exists to indicate the presence of components of the renin-angiotensin system in a variety of tissues.[123] While the enzyme renin is not present in every instance, variations in other components of the system have been shown to lead to changes in angiotensin II generation in tissues as well as to architectural changes in tissues secondary to the growth-promoting effects of angiotensin II.[113,123,124,128,131,132,134–140] Moreover, the clinical cardioprotective and renal protective effects of such pharmaceutical agents as converting enzyme inhibitors give additional support to this concept. That is, ACE inhibitors have been shown to improve symptomatology and life expectancy in patients with congestive heart failure, reduce ventricular remodeling following myocardial infarction, reduce the probability of subsequent myocardial infarction, protect against diabetic nephropathy, and rapidly produce regression of hypertension-related LVH.[107–111,141–143] These findings suggest that the vasopressor, angiotensin II, has proliferative effects in the cardiovascular system that can be deleterious and may provide a link between hypertension and pressor agents and structural changes in the vasculature. This latter possibility is also suggested by animal experiments in which, through embryonal stem cell technology, mice were generated possessing different copy numbers of the atrial natriuretic factor genes.[144] In this study, it was found that expression of atrial natriuretic factor provided a resistance to salt-induced hypertension. In additional studies, atrial natriuretic factor has been shown to be antiproliferative; this, taken with the fact that angiotensin is a vasoconstrictor and promotes cell growth, suggests that vasoactivity and effects on vascular structure may be linked.[113,114,123,134,136–140,145] Also of note is the recent evidence indicating that prolonged treatment of hypertensive patients with converting enzyme inhibitors can lead to the reversal of so-called vascular remodeling, a process seen in hypertensive patients and involving the reconfiguration of cells and material in the arteriolar lumen so as to produce a diminished lumen:wall ratio.[35]

RENIN PROFILING

Measurement of plasma renin activity has important clinical implications not only in the classification of patients with essential hypertension[80,83] but also in other hypertensive states. Thus, if an adrenal steroidal form of hypertension is suspected (e.g., primary aldosteronism), plasma renin activity will be suppressed and will be associated with an expanded plasma volume, hypokalemic alkalosis, and increased urinary (or plasma) levels of aldosterone.[84] Moreover, if there are inordinately elevated levels of plasma renin activity and renal arterial disease is suspected, collection of blood from both renal veins with a vena cava sample below the level of the kidneys will be useful in the diagnosis of functionally significant renal arterial disease with hypertension (see also Chap. 57).

Much interest and excitement has been engendered in recent years concerning the role of the renin-angiotensin system in patients with essential hypertension. Sealey and Laragh[83] have suggested that *patients with essential hypertension may be classified (or "profiled") according to the levels of plasma renin activity referenced to daily sodium intake as demonstrated by 24-h urinary sodium excretion.* This categorization has been suggested to be useful not only conceptually with respect to the pathophysiologic alterations producing the disease but also for selecting antihypertensive therapy.[80] In general, the levels of plasma renin activity are directly related to the generated angiotensin II and to the production, release, and excretion of the adrenal cortical hormone aldosterone. As already suggested, *in order to classify these patients reproducibly, however, one must carefully determine their daily sodium intake.* The higher the sodium intake, the lower the plasma renin activity, and vice versa; for a given sodium intake, patients with higher, normal, and lower plasma renin activity may be identified. These investigators have also suggested that those patients with high plasma renin activity seem to be more likely to develop subsequent myocardial infarction.[146] Although no precise physiologic mechanism was offered to explain this association, by employing these physiologic concepts, one mechanism might be suggested. Thus, the higher the arterial pressure or the greater the total peripheral resistance, the more contracted the intravascular volume.[16,42] The more contracted the intravascular volume, the higher the plasma renin activity.[147] It may be argued that patients with high plasma renin activity have a circulation with greater blood and plasma viscosity.[148] These intravascular changes might, in association with potential effects of angiotensin II on atherosclerotic lesions, lead to an increased likelihood of clot formation.

MODULATORY CONSIDERATIONS

It is particularly pertinent to consider that hormones, vasoactive substances, and growth factors not only act at their own "classic" target organs but may also modify the actions of other blood or neurally mediated or local substances in an autocrine/paracrine fashion. Thus, certain agents may exert their physiologic actions very subtly by acting with other substances. As already suggested, angiotensin II is known to amplify adrenergic function by its interaction in certain brain centers as well as at peripheral ganglionic or postganglionic areas.[149,150] Additionally, angiotensin II may interact with kinins and prostaglandins in the kidney, with the atrial peptides at nerve endings or on vascular smooth muscle membrane, and with these or other peptides (e.g., endothelin, neuropeptide Y, or substance P) at the vascular smooth muscle membrane or intracellularly. Another possible example of this modulatory cardiovascular action occurs at the endothelial level to alter local hemodynamic functions (see also Chap. 4). Moreover, as has been previously noted, a variety of ion transport abnormalities have been considered as pathogenetic mechanisms for some form of hypertension, and an intensive investigation is underway utilizing the genes encoding components of these transport processes as candidate genes for hy-

pertension. In this regard, it is interesting to note that the so-called *nonmodulating phenotype of hypertension* is a defined form of sodium-sensitive hypertension that may be related to intrinsic activation of the renin-angiotensin system.[151]

GENETIC CONSIDERATIONS

Essential hypertension has long been clinically appreciated to be genetically predisposed; indeed, it has more recently been estimated that approximately 50 percent of the variance in human blood pressure can be explained by five or so genes (Table 56-2).[94,97–99,103,152] For example, studies have indicated a correlation of blood pressure between monozygotic and dizygotic twins, with the correlation being stronger between monozygotic twins, thereby suggesting a genetic influence on blood pressure. Similarly, studies have indicated a correlation between blood pressure of hypertensive patients with blood pressure seen in their first-degree relatives. Notably, the relatively uncommon hypertensive syndrome of glucocorticoid-remediable hyperaldosteronism has been shown to result from the presence of a genetic chimerism of the genes for 11β-hydroxylase and aldosterone synthase; this chimeric gene is transmitted in a Mendelian-dominant fashion.[100] Genetic testing is now available to detect the presence of this chimeric gene, and, through its use, the spectrum of pathology produced by this syndrome is now being elucidated.

These observations, coupled with a wealth of information regarding heritable hypertension in animals such as rats, has recently led to a major initiative to identify those genetic loci involved in human hypertension. Several approaches have

TABLE 56-2

POTENTIAL GENES RELATED TO HUMAN HYPERTENSION

Causality likely:
11 β-hydroxylase/aldosterone synthase
β subunit epithelial sodium channel
Renal 11 β-hydroxysteroid dehydrogenase
Angiotensinogen
Positive association:
Angiotensin-converting enzyme
Glucocorticoid receptor
Glycogen synthase
Apolipoprotein CIII
Lipoprotein lipase
α-Adducin
MN blood group
Endothelin
Atrial natriuretic peptides
Causality unlikely:
Renin
Angiotensin II AT$_1$ receptor
Endothelial cell nitric oxide synthase
Na-H exchanger
Human SA locus
Insulin receptor

Source: Adapted from Williams and Fisher.[152]

been taken, including the analysis of affected sib pairs and the detailed study of candidate genes. Among the candidate genes for hypertension most intensively studied to date are those encoding components of the renin-angiotensin system.[101,102,153] Although renin is the initiator of the physiologic renin-angiotensin system in humans, studies to date have failed to find an association between renin gene polymorphisms and hypertension in humans, although clinical studies suggest that the high renin phenotype is associated with increased morbidity and mortality.[154] On the other hand, a variety of studies suggest a possible association between the angiotensinogen gene and hypertension as well as preeclampsia, and ACE gene polymorphisms have been associated with the sequelae of hypertension such as myocardial infarction and LVH.[101,102,153–163] Because these associations are not always reproducible in differing populations, it may be that these genotypes are in linkage disequilibrium with disease-causing genes and are not themselves causative.

The possibility, however, that abnormalities in angiotensinogen and ACE concentrations in blood or tissues could contribute to the generation of excessive amounts of angiotensin II and, through the potentially deleterious effects of this vasopressor, produce hypertensive-related morbidity is appealing.

The study of ion transport in the cells of hypertensive patients has also suggested genetically determined mechanisms for the development of high blood pressure. Inhibition of the sodium-potassium pump activity, either by a circulating inhibitor or a genetic defect, has been hypothesized to inhibit sodium-calcium exchange and thereby to raise intracellular calcium, resulting in vasoconstriction and hypertension.[164–169] Other pump abnormalities have been hypothesized to result in hypertension as well. Increased activity of the sodium/lithium countertransporter has been shown in hypertension, but its precise relationship to the pathogenesis of the disease is unknown.[167,168] There appears also to be an association between increased red blood cell sodium/lithium countertransport and a metabolic syndrome of insulin resistance, hypertriglyceridemia, and low high-density lipoprotein cholesterol[170] (see also Chap. 53). These findings, with or without abnormalities of sodium/lithium transport, are associated with hypertension, and it has been argued that the pathogenesis of this form of hypertension is unique. There also exists a more complex subset of patients suffering from both lipid abnormalities and hypertension. So-called familial dyslipidemic hypertension is a syndrome consisting of hypertension at an early age associated with one or more lipid disturbances in at least two siblings of the proband. It has been suggested that this disorder may account for >10 percent of hypertensive patients.[170]

Thus, *while the precise genetic abnormalities that may give rise to high blood pressure are not entirely known, there does appear to be a strong genetic component to the development of the disorder.* A wide variety of candidate genes are being explored, and the prospects for providing a genetic taxonomy of essential hypertension is appealing. If achieved,

this approach, coupled with studies of environmental factors, could shed new light on the mosaic theory of hypertension.

COMPLICATIONS OF HYPERTENSIVE DISEASE

Cardiac Complications

A number of cardiac disorders may complicate SAH. The following discussion concerns primarily those that are directly attributable to the natural history of essential hypertension. Other cardiac abnormalities that complicate hypertension belong to the natural history of other comorbid diseases. For example, myocardial infarction results from occlusion of epicardial coronary arteries as a consequence of atherosclerosis, a disease with its own natural history (see Chap. 38). Nevertheless, SAH not only accelerates but aggravates the progression of atherosclerosis[171,172] (see also Chap. 44) and is a major independent risk factor favoring the development of coronary artery disease[173] (see also Chap. 39). Diabetes mellitus is another disease that is frequently associated with specific cardiac complications, and it also accelerates and aggravates the development of atherosclerotic cardiovascular disease[174,175] (see also Chap. 78). Still other examples are exogenous obesity and hypercholesterolemia—other independent risk factors underlying atherosclerotic coronary arterial disease,[176] which exacerbates hypertensive heart disease.[177]

Left Ventricular Hypertrophy

LVH is the major cardiac alteration associated with SAH, accounting for a risk that is independent of the elevated arterial pressure (whether systolic or diastolic).[178] As already indicated, the left ventricle increases its mass and wall thickness progressively as a direct result of the progressive overload and increased left ventricular wall stress imposed by the increasing arterial pressure and total peripheral resistance.[8,9,17,18] The adaptive structural changes of concentric ventricular hypertrophy that occur in response to this overload[179] serve as a more efficient means for the chamber to provide the forces necessary to maintain stable contractile function and to slow the development of left ventricular failure[6,9,180] (see also Chap. 23). Although Meerson[181] suggested that the functional sequence in this pressure-overload hypertrophy is one of ventricular hyperfunction followed by a stable function and eventually failure, this does not necessarily occur in sequence. More recent studies have supported the concept that simultaneously with the increased functional performance of pressure-overload hypertrophy, there is a concurrent biologic response of the cardiac myocytes to increase protein synthesis and cellular hypertrophy.[182,183] These studies have demonstrated that myocytic stretch stimulus provokes initiation of the growth program, one manifestation of which is the induction of early cellular proto-oncogenes (e.g., c-*myc*) (see also Chap. 6).

This hypertrophic response is also associated with functional changes. One of the earlier changes related to the development of LVH is impaired diastolic filling of the left ventricle. These early changes of LVH are identified clinically and electrocardiographically by the presence of an atrial diastolic gallop rhythm (fourth heart sound) that is highly concordant with left atrial abnormality on the electrocardiogram (ECG), increased prevalence of cardiac dysrhythmias, and a higher arterial pressure.[184,185] Subsequently, echocardiographic studies confirmed actual atrial enlargement in association with diminished distensibility of the hypertrophied left ventricle[18] and impaired left atrial emptying index.[186] Later studies confirmed the earlier reports of impaired left ventricular diastolic filling by nuclear scintigraphy and other means.[187,188] This earlier diastolic functional impairment has been shown to reflect the stiffer and less compliant left ventricle that is associated with hypertrophy. These findings are in contrast with the diastolic dysfunction in hypertension that is seen particularly in elderly patients with hypertension and coexisting ischemic heart disease. Indeed, cardiac failure may be associated with this diastolic dysfunction in the absence of systolic functional impairment; it occurs especially in the elderly but also in other patients with hypertension[189] (see Chaps. 21, 23, and 96). Eventually, left ventricular systolic function becomes impaired following the development of impaired diastolic filling of the ventricle.[17,18] Ultimately, if arterial pressure and ventricular afterload are not reduced, cardiac failure will supervene.[181] Prior to the advent of antihypertensive therapy, hypertension was by far the most common cause of cardiac failure.[190] It still is, but recently, other diseases complicating hypertension (e.g., coronary artery disease) have also become common.

Hemodynamic mechanisms, however, are not the sole cause of the development of LVH, and additional contributing factors have been identified, including the following: the stage of hypertensive heart disease; the age, race, and gender of the patient; the presence of coexisting diseases that frequently complicate hypertensive heart disease (e.g., atherosclerosis, diabetes mellitus, exogenous obesity); vasoactive or humoral substances; growth factors; and whether or not antihypertensive or other therapy has been prescribed.[6,8,9,191–193] While it is generally appreciated that if any type of antihypertensive medication program is utilized for a long enough period of time there will be a reversal of hypertrophy and a decrease in the development of heart failure, certain types of antihypertensive agents have the ability to reverse LVH, at times independently of the hemodynamic effects of the drugs.[9,194–197] This may be demonstrated best following short-term (i.e., 3 to 8 weeks) antihypertensive therapy (clinically or experimentally) with certain centrally acting adrenergic inhibitors, beta-adrenergic blocking agents, calcium antagonists, or the ACE inhibitors.[6,8,9,178,191,193] It must be appreciated that reduced LVH demonstrated by ECG or echocardiographic assessment may not reflect only reduced left ventricular muscle mass; it may also be associated with reduced left ventricular collagen content. Ongoing clinical studies may determine whether or not reversal of ventricular hypertrophy will be associated with reversal of the risk of cardiovascular morbidity and mortality

that is associated with LVH.[194] To date, however, this has not been demonstrated. If this is shown, it will be necessary to know whether or not that reduction in risk is associated with the reduced arterial pressure, improved coronary blood flow, possible antiarrhythmic effects of the drugs employed, or the reversal of LVH itself. For the time being, the best means of decreasing the increased morbidity and mortality is to prevent the development of LVH. This requires early and continuous antihypertensive therapy, even before the hypertrophy becomes clinically manifest[196,198] (see also Chap. 58).

LVH: An Independent Risk Factor

A review of the pathophysiologic mechanisms associated with the risk from LVH is appropriate.[199,200] Although the precise mechanisms imparting that risk are not known, they are suggested, in part, from the clinical diagnoses offered for the deaths that have been associated with LVH. It is reasonable to suggest that the diagnosis of sudden cardiac death, which may have been attributed to coronary heart disease, may actually be related to hypertensive heart disease. Patients with LVH have an increased prevalence of unifocal and multifocal ventricular premature beats as well as ventricular tachycardia.[199–203] Thus, sudden death may be produced by lethal ventricular arrhythmias even if epicardial coronary arterial occlusive disease is not present. There is also abundant evidence that coronary blood flow per gram of tissue is reduced in LVH and that this is associated with an increased minimal coronary vascular resistance and a diminished coronary blood flow reserve.[204–207] This impaired coronary hemodynamics in hypertension is exacerbated further by the endothelial dysfunction of the arterioles and arteries discussed above and confirmed in patients.[59] Each of these factors may be attributable to the coronary arteriolar and small arterial disease that is associated with hypertension per se; each may provide a reasonable pathophysiologic mechanism for acute myocardial ischemia and sudden death. In addition, since LVH provides an adaptive and functional protection against increased myocardial demands (e.g., by physiologic or other interventions), acute left ventricular failure may also provide another pathophysiologic explanation for death.[200] Experimental studies in spontaneously hypertensive rats have shown that more prolonged antihypertensive therapy (involving converting enzyme inhibition and angiotensin II type I receptor antagonism) not only reverses hypertrophy but improves coronary flow and flow reserve.[208] Finally, atherosclerotic coronary artery disease may also be present in patients with LVH and hypertension and may provide a precipitating cause of death.

Myocardial Ischemia and Myocardial Infarction

There are several mechanisms that may explain the presence of angina pectoris or myocardial infarction in the hypertensive patient with LVH. Chest pain may occur in these patients even in the absence of atherosclerotic (epicardial) coronary artery disease. A major determinant of myocardial oxygen demand is systolic wall stress, which is dependent on two factors: left ventricular systolic pressure and the left ventricular chamber diameter[209] (see Chap. 3). Both these functions are increased in the hypertensive patient with LVH; hence, myocardial ischemia often occurs in pure hypertensive heart disease.[17,206,207] Myocardial infarction, especially subendocardial, may also occur. Moreover, since hypertension is an important accelerating factor for the development of atherosclerotic coronary artery disease,[101,102,210,211] this always remains as an important consideration (Fig. 56-1). Finally, since both hypertension and atherosclerosis may be associated with alterations in the endothelium of the coronary arteries, it is possible that local coronary arterial factors may be associated with impaired coronary blood flow (see also Chap. 44). Of course, other factors or a combination of mechanisms may also account for these changes.

In recent years, several explanations have been offered to explain why the incidence of myocardial infarction has not been decreased to the extent that stroke has been diminished in studies of antihypertensive therapy. In part, this discrepancy might be explained on the basis that many of the cardiac deaths in patients with hypertension (in the large number of multicenter clinical studies) may have been due to hypertensive heart disease rather than to what has been typically called "coronary heart disease." Another possible explanation is that most of these studies have been conducted with agents (e.g., diuretics) that may have increased serum lipids, a factor that may have offset the antihypertensive benefits and favored atherogenesis and, hence, occlusive epicardial coronary artery disease.[212] Alternatively, the deaths in these patients could also be attributable to hypokalemia or some other factor discussed above. Supporting this thesis were several recent reports demonstrating that the doses of thiazides employed in the early multicenter antihypertensive trials were sufficient to favor sudden cardiac arrest deaths. Finally, since hypertensive and atherosclerotic heart diseases each have their own natural history, it may require a longer treatment period to reduce the cardiac atherosclerotic complications compared to other complications (e.g., stroke).[213]

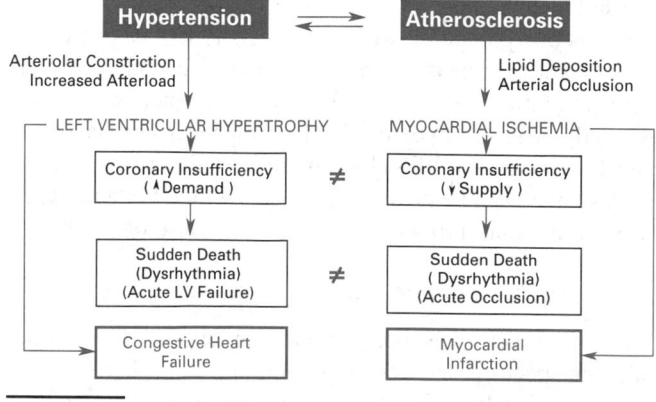

FIGURE 56-1

The natural histories of hypertensive and atherosclerotic disease are independent, but the two diseases also interact with one another to facilitate and exacerbate ischemic heart disease.

J-Shaped Curves Phenomenon

Another controversy is the possibility that mildly hypertensive patients (i.e., those whose pretreatment diastolic pressures ranged from 90 through 94 mmHg) may have the potential of an increased incidence of death coincident with antihypertensive therapy.[214–216] In these patients and in those with more severe hypertension, excessive lowering of blood pressure has been speculated to increase mortality (see also Chap. 58). Although the mechanisms of this so-called J-shaped mortality curve are unknown, several possibilities include the following: impaired autoregulatory flow responses in the hypertensive heart, impaired coronary perfusion during diastole due to excessively vigorous reduction of diastolic pressure, or a combination. This issue will be resolved by prospective studies. Meanwhile, three multicenter studies were conducted in elderly hypertensive and normotensive patients with symptomatic or asymptomatic ischemic heart disease. In those elderly patients having isolated systolic hypertension, deaths from stroke and myocardial infarction were significantly reduced in association with a reduction in diastolic pressure.[217] Moreover, normotensive patients of the SAVE and SOLVD studies having ischemic heart disease were also treated with ACE inhibitors that reduced diastolic pressure.[218,219] These patients also demonstrated a significant reduction in myocardial infarction. At present, however, it is reasonable to suggest that in patients with hypertension and coexisting coronary artery disease particular caution should be exercised in reducing arterial pressure and that diastolic pressure reduction be confined to levels above 75 to 80 mmHg (see also Chap. 58).

Aortic Dissection

Dissecting aneurysms of the thoracic and abdominal aorta were frequent complications of hypertension in the past. In recent years, the prevalence of this complication has diminished with the increased use of antihypertensive therapy. Indeed, such therapy has been advocated for these patients even if they are normotensive. The elevated arterial pressure and the increased force of left ventricular ejection and flow may favor the shearing flow forces that aggravate aortic or other arterial dissection.[220,221] It is for this reason that agents with some negative inotropic action (i.e., beta-adrenergic receptor–blocking drugs) are useful in this condition (see also Chap. 98).

Malignant and Accelerated Hypertension

These forms of hypertension have become less common with the widespread use of antihypertensive therapy. They represent a sudden acceleration in the vascular disease associated with essential hypertension. It is always wise to evaluate the affected patient for a secondary form of hypertension such as occlusive renal arterial disease (fibrosing or atherosclerotic) (see Chap. 57). The clinical course is rapidly progressive, with over 97 percent of the patients dying within 1 year if not treated. Pathologically, there is an onion-skinned appearance of the arterioles throughout the body that is associated with a necrotizing arteriolitis, round cell infiltration in the media of the vessel wall, deposition of protein and complement within the muscle layer, and severe arteriolar spasm. Physiologically, these changes are associated with diminished blood flow, particularly to the kidney, which provokes a state of secondary hyperaldosteronism manifested by hyperreninemia and hyperaldosteronism, hypokalemic alkalosis, and microangiopathic hemolytic anemia. Vigorous antihypertensive therapy will reverse this seemingly positive feedback mechanism that produces a "vicious cycle" toward death.

End-Stage Renal Disease and Nephrosclerosis

More frequently, essential hypertension is associated with renal arteriolar thickening, fibrinoid deposition in the glomeruli, and proteinuria (usually <0.5 g daily).[222] Hyperuricemia that is independent of abnormal purine metabolism or a personal or familial history of gout is frequently associated with untreated hypertension,[223] and the height of serum uric acid levels in these untreated patients is directly related to a decrement in renal blood flow and an increase in renal vascular resistance.[224] These renal changes usually follow the development of echocardiographically demonstrable LVH.[225] Nephrologists have become increasingly concerned with the dramatic increase in end-stage renal failure, particularly in patients with hypertension and even more so in those who are black.[226] For any level of arterial pressure, black patients have lesser renal blood flow and higher renal vascular resistance;[227,228] they are also at greater risk for end-stage renal disease[226] (see also Chap. 94).

There have been few renal hemodynamic studies of patients with nephrosclerosis. Some have demonstrated a reduction in renal blood flow that may not be associated with a reduction in glomerular filtration rate.[222] Most intrarenal hemodynamic studies of experimental hypertension have been concerned with renal micropuncture of an experimental model with a remnant kidney.[229,230] In these studies, reductions in renal blood flow and glomerular filtration rate have been associated with increased renal filtration fraction and proteinuria. These findings suggested that renal functional impairment associated with more advanced nephrosclerosis may be related to glomerular ultrafiltration, proteinuria, and consequent glomerulosclerosis. Renal micropuncture was also accomplished in the spontaneously hypertensive rat (without remnant kidney), and hemodynamics were determined before and after further increase in arterial pressure produced by phenylephrine (an alpha-adrenergic receptor agonist). Pressure elevation was associated with reduction in renal blood flow, efferent arteriolar constriction, increased glomerular hydrostatic pressure, and increased renal filtration fraction.[231,232] Each of these changes was reversed by an alpha-adrenergic receptor inhibitor. Further studies in patients with essential hypertension are necessary to unravel the pathophysiologic alterations involved and to determine whether or not the intrarenal hemodynamic alterations progress to end-stage renal disease.

Finally, the reader is referred to the section above on endothelial dysfunction in hypertension. In that discussion, it was pointed out that naturally occurring hypertension in the spontaneously hypertensive rat is associated with end-stage renal disease from severe nephrosclerosis in the aged rat. The disease is reversed by converting enzyme inhibition therapy and was reproduced in younger rats with chronic nitric oxide synthase inhibition (for 4 weeks). The latter nephrosclerosis mimicked the nephropathy of the old rats and was also reversed and prevented by converting enzyme inhibition therapy.

Parenchymal Renal Disease

Hypertension is a frequent complication of most renal diseases, whether glomerulonephritis, polycystic renal disease, or others. Hypertension associated with parenchymal disease of the kidney should be considered in any hypertensive patient with anemia of undetermined cause, particularly if that patient is black (see also Chap. 57). When such patients are studied hemodynamically, the arterial pressure is found to be related to an increased total peripheral resistance, but not to such an extent as in patients with essential hypertension,[1,2,47] since the cardiac output is increased in proportion to the degree of anemia.[233] In these patients, renal blood flow is diminished and renal vascular resistance is increased (see also Chap. 94).

Strokes

If there is one vascular complication of hypertension that has been dramatically reduced with antihypertensive therapy, it is that due to stroke, whether hemorrhagic, thrombotic, or rupture of small Charcot-Beauchard aneurysms[234] (see also Chap. 99). Since the advent of widespread, effective antihypertensive therapy, there has been at least a 50 percent reduction in fatal strokes, which are also common in the majority of the population who do not have SAH. Other common complications are the so-called small strokes. These may also be the result of embolic disease from the major great vessels or left side of the heart, paradoxic emboli, or rupture of small Charcot-Beauchard cerebral artery aneurysms. They should be considered in any patient with hypertension with unexplained, transient signs and symptoms of sensory, motor, or speech deficits.

REFERENCES

1. Frohlich ED. Hemodynamics of hypertension. In: Genest J, Koiw E, Kuchel O, eds. *Hypertension: Physiopathology and Treatment*. New York: McGraw-Hill; 1977: 15–49.
2. Frohlich ED. Hemodynamic factors in the pathogenesis and maintenance of hypertension. *Fed Proc* 1982; 41:2400–2408.
3. Frohlich ED, Messerli FH, Re RN, Dunn FG. Mechanisms controlling arterial pressure. In: Frohlich ED, ed. *Pathophysiology: Altered Regulatory Mechanisms in Disease*, 3d ed. Philadelphia: Lippincott; 1984: 45–81.
4. Frohlich ED. Mechanisms contributing to high blood pressure. *Ann Intern Med* 1983; 98:709–714.
5. Page IH. The mosaic theory of arterial hypertension—its interpretation. *Perspect Biol Med* 1967; 10:325–333.
6. Frohlich ED: (State of the Art): The first Irvine H. Page lecture. The mosaic of hypertension: Past, present, and future. *J Hypertens* 1988; 6(suppl 4):S2–S11.

7. Freis ED. Hemodynamics of hypertension. *Physiol Rev* 1960; 40:27–54.

8. Frohlich ED. The heart in hypertension: In: Genest J, Kuchel O, Hamet P, Cantin M, eds. *Hypertension: Physiopathology and Treatment*, 2d ed. New York: McGraw-Hill; 1983: 791–810.

9. Frohlich ED. The heart in hypertension: A 1991 overview. *Hypertension* 1991; 18(III):62–68.

10. Ulrych M, Frohlich ED, Dustan HP, Page IH. Cardiac output and distribution of blood volume in central and peripheral circulations in hypertensive and normotensive man. *Br Heart J* 1969; 31:570–574.

11. Trippodo NC, Yamamoto J, Frohlich ED. Whole-body venous capacity and effective total tissue compliance in SHR. *Hypertension* 1981; 3:104–112.

12. Yamamoto J, Trippodo NC, MacPhee AA, Frohlich ED. Decreased total venous capacity in Goldblatt hypertensive rats. *Am J Physiol* 1981; 240:H487–H492.

13. Frohlich ED, Kozul VJ, Tarazi RC, Dustan HP. Physiological comparison of labile and essential hypertension. *Circ Res* 1970; 27:55–69.

14. Messerli FH, de Carvalho JGR, Christie B, Frohlich ED. Systemic and regional hemodynamics in low, normal, and high cardiac output in borderline hypertension. *Circulation* 1978; 58:441–448.

15. Tarazi RC, Frohlich ED, Dustan HP. Plasma volume in men with essential hypertension. *N Engl J Med* 1968; 278:762–765.

16. Tarazi RC, Dustan HP, Frohlich ED, Gifford RW Jr, Hoffman GC. Plasma volume and chronic hypertension. Relationship to arterial pressure levels in different hypertensive diseases. *Arch Intern Med* 1970; 125:835–842.

17. Frohlich ED, Tarazi RC, Dustan HP. Clinical-physiological correlations in the development of hypertensive heart disease. *Circulation* 1971; 44:446–455.

18. Dunn FG, Chandraratna P, de Carvalho JGR, Basta LL, Frohlich ED. Pathophysiologic assessment of hypertensive heart disease with echocardiography. *Am J Cardiol* 1977; 39:789–795.

19. Bond M, Somlyo AP. Calcium regulation of contraction of arterial smooth muscle. In: Aoki K, Frohlich ED, eds. *Calcium in Essential Hypertension*. Tokyo: Academic; 1989: 39–64.

20. Nishimura J, van Breeman C. Regulation of the Ca^{2+} sensitivity of vascular smooth muscle contractile elements. *Adv Exp Med Biol* 1991; 308:9–25.

21. Marche P, Herembert T, Zhu DL. Molecular mechanisms of vascular hypertrophy in the spontaneously hypertensive rat. *Clin Exp Pharmacol Physiol* 1995; 22(suppl 1):114–116.

22. Arendshorst WJ. Role of protein kinase C in angiotensin II-induced renal vasoconstriction in genetically hypertensive rats. *Am J Physiol* 1996; 270:F945–F952.

23. Fardella C, Rodriguesz-Portales JA. Intracellular calcium and blood pressure: Comparison between primary hyperparathyroidism and essential hypertension. *J Endocrinol Invest* 1995; 18:827–832.

24. Lucchesi PA, Bell JM, Willis LS, Byron KL, Corson MA, Berk BC. Ca^{2+}-dependent mitogen-activated protein kinase activation in spontaneously hypertensive rat vascular smooth muscle defines a hypertensive signal transduction phenotype. *Circ Res* 1996; 78:962–970.

25. Watts SW, Yeum CH, Campbell G, Webb RC. Serotonin stimulates protein tyrosyl phosphorylation and vascular contraction via tyrosine kinase. *J Vasc Res* 1996; 33:288–298.

26. Igaki T, Itoh H, Suga S, Komatsu K, Yoshimasa T, Nakao K. Insulin suppresses endothelial secretion of c-type natriuretic peptide, a novel endothelium-derived relaxing peptide. *Diabetes* 1996; 45(suppl 3):62–64.

27. Rajagopalan S, Kurz S, Munzel T, Tarpey M, Freeman BA, Griendling KK, et al. Angiotensin II–mediated hypertension in the rat increases vascular superoxide production via membrane NADH/NADPH oxidase activation. Contribution to alterations of vasomotor tone. *J Clin Invest* 1996; 97:1916–1923.

28. Folkow B. The fourth Volhard lecture. Cardiovascular structural adaptation: Its role in the initiation and maintenance of primary hypertension. *Clin Sci Mol Med* 1978; 55:3–225.

29. Sadoshima J, Xu Y, Slayter HS, Izumo S. Autocrine release of angiotensin II mediates stretch-induced hypertrophy of cardiac myocytes in vitro (abstr). *Circulation* 1993; 88(suppl I):I-190.

30. Sadoshima J, Xu Y, Slayter HS, Izumo S. Autocrine release of angiotensin II mediates stretch-induced hypertrophy of cardiac myocytes in vitro. *Cell* 1993; 75:977–984.

31. Komuro I, Katoh Y, Kaida T, Shibazaki Y, Kurabayashi M, Hoh E, et al. Mechanical loading stimulates cell hypertrophy and specific gene expression in cultured rat cardiac myocytes. *J Biol Chem* 1991; 266:1265–1268.

32. Sadoshima J, Jahn L, Takahashi T, Kulik TJ, Izumo S. Molecular characterization of the stretch-induced adaptation of cultured cardiac cells. *J Biol Chem* 1992; 267:10551–10560.

33. Sadoshima J, Xu Y, Slayter HS, Izumo S. Autocrine release of angiotensin II mediates stretch-induced hypertrophy of cardiac myocytes in vitro. *Cell* 1993; 75:977–984.

34. Sadoshima J, Izumo S. Mechanical stretch rapidly activates multiple signal transduction pathways in cardiac myocytes: Potential involvement of an autocrine/paracrine mechanism. *EMBO J* 1993; 12:1681–1692.

35. Schiffrin EL, Deng LY, Larochell P. Effects of β-Blocker or a converting enzyme inhibitor on resistance arteries in essential hypertension. *Hypertension* 1994; 23:83–91.

36. Lever AF. Slow developing pressor of angiotensin II and vascular structure. *J Hypertens* 1993; 11(suppl):S27–S28.

37. Berk BC, Corson MA. Autocrine/paracrine growth mechanisms in vascular smooth muscle. *Curr Opin Cardiol* 1992; 7:739–744.

38. Owens GK. Influence of blood pressure on the development of medial smooth muscle hypertrophy in spontaneously hypertensive rats. *Hypertension* 1987; 9:178–187.

39. Baker KM, Aceto JF. Angiotensin II stimulation of protein synthesis and cell growth in chick heart cells. *Am J Physiol* 1990; 259:H610–H618.

40. Dzau VJ, Gibbons GH. Endothelium and growth factors in vascular remodeling of hypertension. *Hypertension* 1991; 18(suppl III): III115–III121.

41. Murphy TJ, Alexander RW, Griendling KK, Runge MS, Bernstein KE. Isolation of a cDNA encoding the vascular type-1 angiotensin II receptor. *Nature* 1991; 351:233–235.

42. Hahn AW, Resink TJ, Scott BT, Powell J, Dohi Y, Buhler FR. Stimulation of endothelin mRNA and secretion in rat vascular smooth muscle cells: A novel autocrine function. *Cell Regul* 1990; 1:649–659.

43. Sarzani R, Arnaldi G, Takasaki I, Brecher P, Chobanian AV. Effects of hypertension and aging on platelet-derived growth factor and platelet-derived growth factor receptor expression in rat aorta and heart. *Hypertension* 1991; 18(suppl III):III93–III99.

44. Battegay EJ, Raines EW, Seifert RA, Bowen PDF, Ross R. TGF-beta induces bimodal proliferation of connective tissue cells via complex control of an autocrine PDGF loop. *Cell* 1990; 63:515–524.

45. Ross RC, Bowen-Pope DP, Raines EW. Platelets, macrophages, endothelium, and growth factors. Their effects upon cells and their possible roles in atherogenesis. *Ann NY Acad Sci* 1985; 454:254–260.

46. Libby P, Warner SJC, Salomon RN, Birinyi LK. Production of platelet-derived growth factor–like mitogen by smooth-muscle cells from human atheroma. *N Engl J Med* 1988; 318:1493–1498.

47. Furchgott RF, Zawadzki JV. The obligatory role of the endothelial cells in relaxation of arterial smooth muscle by acetylcholine. *Nature* 1980; 280:373–376.

48. Vanhoutte PM. Endothelial dysfunction in hypertension. *J Hypertens* 1996; 14(suppl 5):83–93.

49. Moncada S, Higgs A. The L-arginine–nitric oxide pathway. *N Engl J Med* 1993; 329:2002–2012.

50. Vanhoutte PM. The endothelium-modulator of vascular smooth muscle tone. *N Engl J Med* 1988; 319:512–513.

51. Ono H, Ono Y, Frohlich ED. Nitric oxide synthase inhibition in spontaneously hypertensive rats. *Hypertension* 1995; 26:249–255.

52. Raij L. Nitric oxide and the kidney. *Circulation* 1993; 87(suppl V):26–29.

53. Frohlich ED. Influence of nitric oxide and angiotensin II on renal involvement in hypertension. *Hypertension* 1997; 29(part 2):188–193.

54. Komatsu K, Frohlich ED, Ono H, Ono Y, Numabe A, Willis GW. Glomerular dynamics and morphology of aged SHR. *Hypertension* 1995; 25:207–213.

55. Tsakada M, Yamazaki Y, Koizami A. Changes in nitric oxide synthase in the cerebellum during development and aging of C57Bl/16 mice. *Tohoku J Exp Med* 1995; 176:69–74.

56. Gerhard M, Roddy MA, Creater SJ, Creager MA. Aging progressively impairs endothelial-dependent vasodilation in forearm resistance vessels of humans. *Hypertension* 1996; 27:849–853.

57. Casino PR, Kilcoyne CM, Quyyumi AA, Hoeg JM, Panza JA. The role of nitric oxide in endothelium-dependent vasodilation of hypercholesterolemic patients. *Circulation* 1993; 88:2541–2547.

58. Gilligan DM, Guetta V, Panza JA, Garcia CE, Quyyumi AA, Cannon RO III. Selective loss of microvascular endothelial function in human hypercholesterolemia. *Circulation* 1994; 90:35–41.

59. Treasure CB, Klein JC, Vita JA, Manoukianu SV, Renwick GH, Selwyn ALP, et al. Hypertension and left ventricular hypertrophy are associated with impaired endothelium-mediated relaxation in human coronary artery resistance vessels. *Circulation* 1993; 87:86–93.

60. Panza JA, Casino PR, Kilcoyne CM, Quyyumi AA. Role of endothelium-derived nitric oxide in the abnormal endothelia-dependent vascular relaxation of patients with essential hypertension. *Circulation* 1993; 87:1468–1474.

61. Panza JA, Casino PR, Badar DM, Quyyumi AA. Effect of increased availability of endothelium-derived nitric oxide precursor on endothelium-dependent vascular relaxation in normal subjects and in patients with essential hypertension. *Circulation* 1993; 87:1475–1481.

62. Panza JA, Garcia CE, Kilcoyne CM, Quyyumi AA, Cannon RO III. Impaired endothelium-dependent vasodilation in patients with essential hypertension. Evidence that nitric oxide abnormality is not localized to a single signal transduction pathway. *Circulation* 1995; 91:1732–1738.

63. Ono H, Ono Y, Frohlich ED. ACE inhibition prevents and reverses L-NAME-exacerbated nephrosclerosis in spontaneously hypertensive rats. *Hypertension* 1996; 27:176–183.

64. Ono Y, Ono H, Frohlich ED. L-arginine reverses severe nephrosclerosis in aged spontaneously hypertensive rats (SHR) (abstr). *Hypertension* 1996; 28:537.

65. Ono Y, Ono H, Frohlich ED. Hydrochlorothiazide exacerbates nitric oxide–blockade nephrosclerosis with glomerular hypertension in spontaneously hypertensive rats. *J Hypertens* 1996; 14:823–828.

66. Vanhoutte PM, Auch-Schwelk W, Biondi ML, Lorenz RR, Schini VB, Vidal MJ. Why are converting enzyme inhibitors vasodilators? *Br J Clin Pharmacol* 1989; 28:955–1045.

67. Mombonli JV, Vanhoutte PM. Kinins and vascular endothelium. *Curr Opin Nephrol Hypertens* 1994; 3:481–484.

68. Tarazi RC. Hemodynamic role of extracellular fluid. *Circ Res* 1976; 38(suppl II):73–83.

69. Frohlich ED, Messerli FH. Sodium and hypertension. In: Papper S, ed. *Cations of Biologic Significance*, vol 2: *Sodium*. Boca Raton, FL: CRC Press; 1982: 144–174.

70. Tarazi RC, Dustan HP, Frohlich ED. Relation of plasma to interstitial fluid volume in essential hypertension. *Circulation* 1969; 40:357–365.

71. Weil JV, Chidsey CA. Plasma volume expansion resulting from interference with adrenergic functions in normal man. *Circulation* 1968; 37:54–61.

72. Dustan HP, Tarazi RC, Bravo EL. Dependence of arterial pressure on intravascular volume in treated hypertensive patients. *N Engl J Med* 1972; 286:861–866.

73. Dustan HP, Tarazi RC, Bravo EL. Diuretic and diet treatment of hypertension. *Arch Intern Med* 1974; 133:1007–1013.

74. The Joint National Committee on the Detection, Evaluation, and Treatment of High Blood Pressure. The 1988 Report of the Joint National Committee on Detection, Evaluation, and Treatment of High Blood Pressure. *Arch Intern Med* 1988; 148:1023–1038.

75. Frohlich ED. Hypertension: Essential. In: Hurst JW, ed. *Current Therapy in Cardiovascular Disease*, 3d ed. Philadelphia: BC Decker; 1991: 297–304.

76. Frohlich ED. Hypertension. In: Rakel RE, ed. *Conn's Current Therapy 1989*. Philadelphia: BC Decker; 1989. 225–241.

77. Bravo EL, Dustan HP, Tarazi RC. Spironolactone as a nonspecific treatment for primary aldosteronism. *Circulation* 1973; 48:491–498.

78. Frohlich ED, Tarazi RC, Dustan HP. Hemodynamic and functional mechanisms in two renal hypertensions: Arterial and pyelonephritis. *Am J Med Sci* 1971; 261:189–195.

79. Dustan HP, Bravo EL, Tarazi RC. Volume-dependent essential and steroid hypertension. *Am J Cardiol* 1973; 31:606–615.

80. Bühler FR, Laragh JH, Baer L, Vaughan ED Jr, Brunner HR. Propranolol inhibition of renin secretion: A specific approach to diagnosis and treatment of renin-dependent hypertensive diseases. *N Engl J Med* 1972; 287:1209–1214.

81. Page LB. Hypertension and atherosclerosis in primitive and accelerating societies. In: Hunt JC, Cooper T, Frohlich ED, Gifford RW Jr, Kaplan NM, Laragh JH, et al, eds. *Hypertension Update: Mechanisms, Epidemiology, Evaluation, Management*. Bloomfield, NJ: Health Learning Systems; 1980: 1–12.

82. Ives H. Ion transport defects and hypertension. Where's the link? *Hypertension* 1989; 14:590–597.

83. Sealey JE, Laragh JH. The renin-angiotensin-aldosterone system for normal regulation of blood pressure and sodium and potassium homeostasis. In: Laragh JH, Brenner BM, eds. *Hypertension: Pathophysiology, Diagnosis and Management*. New York: Raven; 1990: 1287–1317.

84. Bravo EL. Clinical aspects of endocrine hypertension. *Med Clin North Am* 1987; 71:907–920.

85. Nermers RA, Khosla S, Atkinson EJ, Hodgson SF, O'Fallon WM, Melton LJ III. The rise and fall of primary hyperparathyroidism: A population-based study in Rochester, Minnesota, 1965–1992. *Ann Intern Med* 1997; 126:433–440.

86. Resnick LM. Calciotropic hormones in human and experimental hypertension. *Am J Hypertens* 1990; 3:171S–178S.

87. Frohlich ED, Tarazi RC, Dustan HP. Re-examination of the hemodynamics of hypertension. *Am J Med Sci* 1969; 257:9–23.

88. McCubbin JW, Green JH, Page IH. Baroreceptor function in chronic renal hypertension. *Circ Res* 1956; 4:205–210.

89. DeQuattro V, Miura Y. Neurogenic factors in human hypertension: Mechanism or myth? *Am J Med* 1971; 55:362–378.

90. Messerli FH, Frohlich ED, Suarez DH, Reisin E, Dreslinski GR, Dunn FG, et al. Borderline hypertension: Relationship between age, hemodynamics, and circulating catecholamines. *Circulation* 1981; 64:760–764.

91. Frohlich ED, Tarazi RC, Ulrych M, Dustan HP, Page IH. Tilt test for investigation of a neural component in hypertension and its correlation with clinical characteristics. *Circulation* 1967; 36:387–393.

92. Ferrario CM, Averill DB. Do primary dysfunctions in neural control of arterial pressure contribute to hypertension? *Hypertension* 1991; 18(I):38–51.

93. Bravo EL, Tarazi RC, Fouad FM, Vidt DG, Gifford RW Jr. Clonidine-suppression test: A useful aid in the diagnosis of pheochromocytoma. *N Engl J Med* 1981; 305:623–626.

94. Ledingham JM. Genetics of human hypertension. In: Amery A, ed. *Hypertensive Cardiovascular Disease: Pathophysiology and Treatment*. The Hague: Martinus Nijhoff; 1982: 206–216.

95. Tiret L, Rigat B, Visvikis S, Breda C, Corvol P, Cambien F, et al. Evidence, from combined segregation and linkage analysis, that a variant of the angiotensin I-converting enzyme (ACE) gene controls plasma ACE levels. *Am J Hum Genet* 1992; 51:197–205.

96. Re RN. The renin-angiotensin systems. *Med Clin North Am* 1987; 71:5.

97. Pickering GW. The genetic factor in essential hypertension. *Ann Intern Med* 1955; 43:457–464.

98. Mongeau J-G, Brion P, Sing CF. The influence of genetics and household environment upon the variability of normal blood pressure: The Montreal Adoption Survey. *Clin Exp Hypertens* 1986; A8:653–660.

99. Ward R. Familial aggregation and genetic epidemiology of blood pressure. In: Laragh JH, Brenner BM, eds. *Hypertension: Pathophysiology, Diagnosis and Management*. New York: Raven; 1990: 81–100.

100. Lifton RP, Dluhy RG, Powers M, Rich GM, Cook S, Ulrick S, Lalovel JM, et al. Achimaeric 11β-hydroxylase/aldosterone synthase gene causes glucocorticoid-remediable aldosteronism and human hypertension. *Nature* 1992; 355:262–265.

101. White R, Lalouel J-M. Chromosomal mapping with DNA markers. *Sci Am* 1988; 258:40–48.

102. Jeunemaitre X, Soubrier F, Kotelevtsev YV, Lifton RP, Williams CS, Charru A, et al. Molecular basis of human hypertension: Role of angiotensinogen. *Cell* 1992; 71:1–20.

103. Platt R. Heredity in hypertension. *Q J Med* 1947; 16:111–113.

104. Santos RAS, Simoes e Silva AC, Magaldi AJ, Khosla MC, Cesar KR, Passaglio KT, et al. Evidence for a physiological role of angiotensin-(1-7) in the control of hydroelectrolyte balance. *Hypertension* 1996; 27:875–884.

105. Ferrario CM, Barnes KL, Block CH, Brosnihan KB, Diz KI, Khosla MC, et al. Pathways of angiotensin formation and function in the brain. *Hypertension* 1990; 15(suppl I):13–19.

106. Campagnole-Santos MJ, Diz DI, Santos RAS, Khosla MC, Brosnihan KB, Ferrario CM. Cardiovascular effects of angiotensin (1-7) microinjected into the dorsal medulla of rats. *Am J Physiol* 1989; 257:H324–329.

107. Maschio G, Alberti D, Janin G, Locatelli F, Mann JF, Motolese M, et al. Effect of the angiotensin-converting-enzyme inhibitor Benazepril on the progression of chronic renal insufficiency. *N Engl J Med* 1996; 334:939–945.

108. Anderson S, Rennke HG, Brenner BM. Therapeutic advantage of converting enzyme inhibitors in arresting progressive renal disease associated with systemic hypertension in the rat. *J Clin Invest* 1986; 77:1993–2000.

109. Viberti G, Mogensen CE, Groop LC, Paul JF. Effect of captopril on progression to clinical proteinuria in patients with insulin-dependent diabetes mellitus and microalbuminuria. *JAMA* 1994; 271:275–279.

110. Lewis EJ, Hunsicker LG, Bain RP, Rohde RD. The effect of angiotensin-converting-enzyme inhibition on diabetic nephropathy. *N Engl J Med* 1993; 329:1456–1462.

111. Mann FGE, Reisch C, Ritz E. Use of angiotensin-converting enzyme inhibitors for the preservation of kidney function. *Nephron* 1990; 55(suppl 1):38–42.

112. Miyata S, Haneda T, Nakamura Y. The role of cardiac renin-angiotensin system in stretch-induced hypertrophy of cultured neonatal rat heart cells (abstr). *Circulation* 1993; 88(suppl I):614.

113. Cook JL, Chen L, Bhandaru S, Bakris GL, Re RN. The use of antisense oligonucleotides to establish autocrine angiotensin growth effects in human neuroblastoma and mesangial cells. *Antisense Res Dev* 1992; 2:199–210.

114. Bakris GL, Bhandaru S, Akerstrom V, Re RN. ACE inhibitor–mediated attenuation of mesangial cell growth: A role for endothelin. *Hypertension* 1994; 7:538–590.

115. Bakris GL, Re RN. Endothelin modulates angiotensin II-induced mitogenesis of human mesangial cells. *Am J Physiol* 1993; 264(*Renal Fluid Electrolyte Physiol* 33):F937–F942.

116. Santos RAS, Brum JM, Brosnihan KB, Ferrario CM. The renin-angiotensin system during acute myocardial ischemia in dogs. *Hypertension* 1990; 15(I):121–127.

117. Dzau VJ, Re RN. Evidence for the existence of renin in the heart. *Circulation* 1987; 75(suppl I):I134–I136.

118. Dzau VJ, Bart DW, Piatt RE. Molecular biology of the renin-angiotensin system. *Am J Physiol* 1988; 255:F563–573.

119. Re RN, Dzau VJ, Fallon JT, Quay S, Haber E. Renin synthesis by cultured arterial smooth muscle cells. *Life Sci* 1982; 30:99–106.

120. Dzau VJ. Significance of vascular renin-angiotensin pathways. *Hypertension* 1986; 89:544–548.

121. Frohlich ED, Iwata T, Sasaki O. Clinical and physiological significance of local tissue renin-angiotensin systems. *Am J Med* 1989; 87(I):19–23.

122. Unger T, Gohlke P. Tissue renin-angiotensin systems in the heart and vasculature: Possible involvement in the cardiovascular enzyme inhibitions. *Am J Cardiol* 1990; 65(I):3–10.

123. Dzau VJ, Re RN. Tissue angiotensin system in cardiovascular medicine. A paradigm shift? *Circulation* 1994; 89:493–498.

124. Oliver JA, Sciacca RR. Local generation of angiotensin II as a mechanism of regulation of peripheral vascular tone in the rat. *J Clin Invest* 1984; 74:1247–1251.

125. Hirsch AT, Talsness CE, Schunkert H, Paul M, Dzau VJ. Tissue specific activation of cardiac angiotensin converting enzyme in experimental heart failure. *Circ Res* 1991; 69:475–482.

126. Schunkert H, Dzau VJ, Tang SS, Hirsch AT, Apstein CS, Lorell BH, et al. Increased rat cardiac angiotensin converting enzyme activity and mRNA expression in pressure overload left ventricular hypertrophy: Effects on coronary resistance, contractility and relaxation. *J Clin Invest* 1990; 86:1913–1920.

127. Lindpainter K, Lu W, Niedermajer N, Schieffer B, Just H, Ganten D, et al. Selective activation of cardiac angiotensinogen gene expression in postinfarction ventricular remodeling in the rat. *J Mol Cell Cardiol* 1993; 25:133–143.

128. Paul M, Wagner J, Dzau VJ. Gene expression of the renin-angiotensin system in human tissues. Quantitative analysis by the polymerase chain reaction. *J Clin Invest* 1993; 91:2058–2064.

129. Dzau VJ, Ellison KE, Brody T, Ingelfinger J, Pratt RE. A comparative study of the distributions of renin and angiotensin messenger ribonucleic acids in rat and mouse tissues. *Endocrinology* 1987; 120:2334–2338.

130. Mulrow PJ, Franco-Saenz R. The adrenal renin-angiotensin system: A local hormonal regulator of aldosterone production. *J Hypertens* 1996; 14:173–176.

131. Baker KM, Chenin MI, Wixson SK, Aceto JF. Renin-angiotensin system involvement in pressure-overload cardiac hypertrophy in rats. *Am J Physiol* 1990; 259(Pt2):H324–H332.

132. Schunkert H, Dzau VJ, Tang SS, Hirsch AT, Apstein CS, Lorell BH. Increased rat cardiac angiotensin-converting enzyme activity and mRNA expression in pressure overload left ventricular hypertrophy. Effects on coronary resistance, contractility, and relaxation. *J Clin Invest* 1990; 86:1913–1920.

133. Lindpainter K, Ganten D. The cardiac renin-angiotensin system: An appraisal of present experimental and clinical evidence. *Circ Res* 1991; 68:905–921.

134. Dzau VJ. Vascular renin-angiotensin system and vascular protection. *J Cardiovasc Pharmacol* 1993; 22(suppl 5):1–9.

135. Hirsch AT, Talsness CE, Schunkert H, Paul M, Dzau VJ. Tissue-specific activation of cardiac angiotensin-converting enzyme in experimental heart failure. *Circ Res* 1991; 69:475–482.

136. Cook JL, Bhandaru S, Giardina JF, Claycomb WC, Re RN. Identification and antisense inhibition of a renin-angiotensin system in transgenic cardiomyocytes. *Am J Physiol* 1995; 268(*Heart Circ Physiol* 37):H1471–H1482.

137. Geisterfer AA, Peach MJ, Owens GK. Angiotensin II induces hypertrophy, not hyperplasia, of cultured rat aortic smooth muscle cells. *Circ Res* 1988; 62:749–756.

138. Campbell-Boswell M, Robertson AL Jr. Effects of angiotensin II and vasopressin on human smooth muscle cells in vitro. *Exp Mol Pathol* 1981; 35:265–276.

139. Itoh H, Mukoyama M, Pratt RE, Bibbons GH, Dzau VJ. Multiple autocrine growth factors modulate vascular smooth muscle cell growth response to angiotensin II. *J Clin Invest* 1993; 91:2268–2274.

140. Gibbons GH, Pratt RE, Dzau VJ. Vascular smooth muscle cell hypertrophy vs. hyperplasia. Autocrine transforming growth factor-beta 1 expression determines growth response to angiotensin II. *J Clin Invest* 1992; 90:456–461.

141. Pfeffer MA, Braunwald E, Moye LA, Basta L, Brown GJ, Jr, Cuddy TE, et al. Effect of captopril on mortality and morbidity in patients with left ventricular dysfunction after acute myocardial infarction. Result of the survival and ventricular enlargement trial. The SAVE Investigators. *N Engl J Med* 1992; 327:669–677.

142. The Acute Infarction Ramipril Efficacy (AIRE) Study Investigators. Effect of Ramipril on mortality and morbidity of survivors of acute myocardial infarction with clinical evidence of heart failure. *Lancet* 1993; 342:821–828.

143. The SOLVD Investigators. Effect of enalapril on mortality and the development of heart failure in asymptomatic patients with reduced left ventricular ejection fractions. *N Engl J Med* 1992; 327:685–691.

144. John SWM, Krege JH, Oliver PM, Hagaman JR, Hodgin JB, Pang SC, et al. Genetic decreases in atrial natriuretic peptide and salt-sensitive hypertension. *Science* 1995; 267:679–681.

145. Cahall PA, Hassid A. Differential antimitogenic effectiveness of atrial natriuretic peptides in primary versus subcultured rat aortic smooth muscle cells: Relationship to expression of ANF-C receptors. *J Cell Physiol* 1993; 154(1):28–38.

146. Alderman MH, Madhavan S, Ooi WL, Cohan H, Sealey JE, Laragh JH. Association of the renin sodium profile with the risk of myocardial infarction in patients with hypertension. *N Engl J Med* 1991; 324:1098–1104.

147. Dustan HP, Tarazi RC, Frohlich ED. Functional correlates of plasma renin activity in hypertensive patients. *Circulation* 1970; 41:555–567.

148. Chrysant SG, Frohlich ED, Adamopoulos PN, Stein PD, Whitcomb WH, Allen EW, et al. Pathophysiologic significance of "stress" or relative polycythemia in essential hypertension. *Am J Cardiol* 1976; 37:1069–1072.

149. Joy MD, Lowe RD. Site of cardiovascular action of angiotensin II in the brain. *Clin Sci* 1970; 39:327–336.

150. McCubbin JW, Page IH. Neurogenic component of chronic renal hypertension. *Science* 1963; 139:210–215.

151. Williams GH, Dluhy RG, Lifton RP, Moore TJ, Gleason R, Williams RR, et al. Non-modulation as an intermediate phenotype in essential hypertension. *Hypertension* 1992; 20:788–796.

152. Williams GH, Fisher NDL. Genetic approach to diagnostic and therapeutic decisions in human hypertension. *Curr Opin Nephrol Hypertens* 1997; 6:199–204.

153. Ward K, Hata A, Jeunemaitre X, Helin C, Nelson L, Namikawa C, et al. A molecular variant of angiotensinogen associated with pre-eclampsia. *Nature Genet* 1993; 4:59–61.

154. Alderman MH, Madhavan S, Ooi WI, Cohen H, Sealey JE, Laragh JA. Association of renin-sodium profile with the risk of myocardial infarction in patients with hypertension (see comments). *N Engl J Med* 1991; 324:1098–1104.

155. Bohn M, Berge KE, Bakken A, Erikssen J, Berg K. Insertion/deletion (I/D) polymorphism at the locus for angiotensin I-converting enzyme and parenteral history of myocardial infarction. *Clin Genet* 1993; 44:298–301.

156. Badenhop RF, Wang XL, Wilcken DE. Angiotensin-converting enzyme genotype in children and coronary events in their grandparents. *Circulation* 1995; 91:1655–1658.

157. Evans AE, Poirier O, Kee F, Lecerf L, McCrum E, Falconer T, et al. Polymorphisms of the angiotensin converting enzyme gene in subjects who die from coronary heart disease. *Q J Med* 1994; 87:211–214.

158. Schmidt S, van Hooft IM, Grobbee DE, Ritz E. Polymorphism of the angiotensin II converting enzyme gene is apparently not related to high blood pressure: Dutch Hypertension and Offspring Study. *J Hypertens* 1993; 11:345–348.

159. Jeunemaitre X, Lifton RP, Hunt SC, Williams RR, Lalouel JM. Absence of linkage between the angiotensin-converting enzyme loads and human essential hypertension. *Nat Genet* 1992; 1:72–75.

160. Cambien F, Poirier O, Lecerf L, Evans A, Cambou JP, Arveiler D, et al. Deletion polymorphism in the gene for angiotensin-converting enzyme is a potent risk factor for myocardial infarction. *Nature* 1992; 359:641–644.

161. Schunkert H, Hense HW, Holmer SR, Stender M, Perz S, Keil U, et al. Association between a deletion polymorphism of the angiotensin-converting enzyme gene and left ventricular hypertrophy. *N Engl J Med* 1994; 330:1634–1638.

162. Iwai N, Ohmichi N, Nakamura Y, Kinoshita M. DD genotype of the angiotensin-converting enzyme gene is a risk factor for left ventricular hypertrophy. *Circulation* 1994; 90:2622–2628.

163. Berge KE, Gerg K. No effect of inserting/deletion polymorphism at the ACE locus on normal blood pressure level or variability. *Clin Genet* 1994; 45:169–174.

164. Weder AB. Membrane sodium transport. In: Izzo JL, Black HR, eds. *Hypertension Primer. The Essentials of High Blood Pressure.* Dallas: American Heart Association; 1993:36–37.

165. Blaustein M. Sodium ions, calcium ions, blood pressure regulation, and hypertension: A reassessment and a hypothesis. *Am J Physiol* 1977; 232:C165–C173.

166. Haddy FJ. Potassium, $Na^+ - K^+$ pump inhibitor and low-renin hypertension. *Clin Invest Med* 1987; 10:547–554.

167. Canessa ML, Adragna NC, Solomon HS, Connolly TM, Tosteson DC. Increased lithium-sodium countertransport in red cells of patients with essential hypertension. *N Engl J Med* 1980; 302:772–776.

168. Doria A, Fioretto P, Avogaro A, Carraro A, Morocutti A, Trevisan R, et al. Insulin resistance is associated with high sodium-lithium countertransport in essential hypertension. *Am J Physiol* 1991; 261:E684–E691.

169. Lifton RP, Hunt SC, Williams RR, Pouyssegur J, Lalouel JM. Exclusion of the Na^+-H^+ antiporter as a candidate gene in human essential hypertension. *Hypertension* 1991; 17:8–14.

170. William RR, Hunt SC, Hopkins PN, Stults BM, Wu LL, Hasstedt SJ, et al. Familial dyslipidemic hypertension: Evidence for 58 Utah families for syndrome present in approximately 12% of patients with essential hypertension. *JAMA* 1988; 259:3579–3586.

171. Dustan HP. George Lyman Duff Lecture. Atherosclerosis complicating chronic hypertension. *Circulation* 1974; 50:871–879.

172. Wittels EW, Gotto AM Jr. Atherogenic mechanisms. In: Frohlich ED, ed. *Pathophysiology: Altered Regulatory Mechanisms in Disease,* 3d ed. Philadelphia: Lippincott; 1984: 107–118.

173. Kannel WB, Dawber TR, Kagan A, Revotskie N, Stokes J III. Factors of risk in the development of coronary heart disease. Six years' follow-up experience. *Ann Intern Med* 1961; 55:33–50.

174. Ostrander LD Jr, Francis T Jr, Hayer NS, Kjelsberg MD, Epstein FH. The relationship of cardiovascular disease in hyperglycemia. *Ann Intern Med* 1965; 62:1188–1198.

175. Grossman E, Shemesh J, Shemiss A, Thaler M, Carroll J, Rosenthal T. Left ventricular mass in diabetes/hypertension. *Arch Intern Med* 1992; 152(5):1001–1004.

176. Kannel WB, Brand N, Skinner J, Dawber T, McNamara P. Relation of adiposity to blood pressure and development of hypertension: The Framingham Study. *Ann Intern Med* 1967; 67:48–59.

177. Frohlich ED, Reisin E. Hemodynamics in patients with overweight and hypertension. In: Safar ME, Fouad-Tarazi FM, eds. *The Heart in Hypertension.* The Hague: Kluwer Academic; 1989: 105–122.

178. Frohlich ED, Apstein C, Chobanian AV, Devereux RB, Dustan HP,

Dzau V, et al. The heart in hypertension. *N Engl J Med* 1992; 327:998–1008.

179. Linzbach AJ. Heart failure from the point of view of quantitative anatomy. *Am J Cardiol* 1960; 5:370–382.

180. Grossman W. Cardiac hypertrophy: Useful adaptation or pathologic process? *Am J Med* 1980; 69:576–584.

181. Meerson FZ. Compensatory hyperfunction, hyperadaptation, and insufficiency of the heart. In: Katz AM, ed. *The Failing Heart: Adaptation and Deadaptation.* New York: Raven; 1983: 47–66.

182. Komuro I, Kaida T, Shibazaki Y, Kurabayashi M, Katoch Y, Hoh E, et al. Stretching cardiac myocytes stimulates proto-oncogene expression. *J Biol Chem* 1990; 265:3595–3598.

183. Kumuro I, Sibazaki Y, Kurabayashi M, Takaku F, Yazaki Y. Molecular cloning of gene sequences from rat heart rapidly responsive to pressure overload. *Circ Res* 1990; 66:979–985.

184. Tarazi RC, Miller A, Frohlich ED, Dustan HP. Electrocardiographic changes reflecting left atrial abnormality in hypertension. *Circulation* 1966; 34:818–822.

185. Tarazi RC, Frohlich ED, Dustan HP. Left atrial abnormality and ventricular pre-ejection period in hypertension. *Dis Chest* 1969; 55:214–218.

186. Dreslinski GR, Frohlich ED, Dunn FG, Messerli FG, Suarez DH, Reisin E. Echocardiographic diastolic ventricular abnormality in hypertensive heart disease: Atrial emptying index. *Am J Cardiol* 1981; 47:1087–1090.

187. Inouye I, Massie B, Loge D, Topic N, Silverstein D, Simpson P, et al. Abnormal left ventricular filling: An early finding in mild to moderate systemic hypertension. *Am J Cardiol* 1984; 53:120–126.

188. Fouad FM, Slominski JM, Tarazi RC. Left ventricular diastolic function in hypertension: Relation to left ventricular mass and systolic function. *J Am Coll Cardiol* 1984; 3:1500–1506.

189. Topol EJ, Traill TA, Fortulin NJ. Hypertensive hypertrophic cardiomyopathy of the elderly. *N Engl J Med* 1985; 312:377–383.

190. Kannel WB, Castelli WP, McNamara PM, McKee PA, Feinlieb M. Role of blood pressure in the development of congestive heart failure. The Framingham Study. *N Engl J Med* 1972; 287:781–787.

191. Frohlich ED. Hemodynamics and other determinants in development of left ventricular hypertrophy: Conflicting factors in its regression. *Fed Proc* 1983; 42:2709–2715.

192. Frohlich ED, Tarazi RC. Is arterial pressure the sole factor responsible for hypertensive cardiac hypertrophy? *Am J Cardiol* 1979; 44:959–963.

193. Frohlich ED. Overview of hemodynamic and non-hemodynamic factors associated with LVH. *J Mol Cell Cardiol* 1989; 21:3–10.

194. Frohlich ED. Is reversal of left ventricular hypertrophy in hypertension beneficial? *Hypertension* 1991; 18(I):133–138.

195. Pfeffer JM, Pfeffer MA, Weiss AK, Frohlich ED. Development of SHR hypertension and cardiac hypertrophy during prolonged beta blockage. *Am J Physiol* 1977; 232:H639–H644.

196. Frohlich ED. Regression of cardiac hypertrophy and left ventricular pumping ability post-regression. *J Cardiovasc Pharmacol* 1991; 17(suppl 2):81–86.

197. Frohlich ED, Horinaka S. Cardiac and aortic effects of angiotensin converting enzyme inhibitors. *Hypertension* 1991; 18(II):2–7.

198. Frohlich ED, Apstein C, Chobanian AV, Devereux RB, Dustan HP, Dzau V, et al. The heart in hypertension. *N Engl J Med* 1992; 327:998–1008.

199. Kannel WB, Gordon T, Castelli WP, Margolia JR. Electrocardiographic left ventricular hypertrophy and risk of coronary heart disease. The Framingham Study. *Ann Intern Med* 1970; 72:813–822.

200. Frohlich ED. Left ventricular hypertrophy: An independent factor of risk. In: Frohlich ED, ed. *Preventative Aspects of Coronary Heart Disease.* Philadelphia: FA Davis; 1990: 297–304.

201. Messerli FH, Ventura HO, Elizardi DJ, Dunn FG, Frohlich ED. Hypertension and sudden death: Increased ventricular ectopic activity in left ventricular hypertrophy. *Am J Med* 1984; 77:18–22.

202. Levy D, Anderson KM, Savage DD, Balkus SA, Kannel WB, Castelli WP. Risk of ventricular arrhythmias in left ventricular hypertrophy: The Framingham Heart Study. *Am J Cardiol* 1987; 60:560–565.

203. McLenachan JM, Henderson E, Morris KI, Dargie HJ. Ventricular arrhythmias in patients with hypertensive left ventricular hypertrophy. *N Engl J Med* 1987; 317:787–792.

204. Harrison DG, Barnes DH, Diratzka LF, Eastham CL, Kerber RE, Marcus ML. The effect of cardiac hypertrophy on the coronary collateral circulation. *Circulation* 1985; 71:1135–1145.

205. Harrison DG, Florentine MS, Brooks LA, Cooper SM, Marcus ML. The effect of hypertension and left ventricular hypertrophy on the lower range of coronary autoregulation. *Circulation* 1988; 77:1108–1115.

206. Brush JE Jr, Cannon RO, Schenke WH, Bonow RO, Leon MB, Maron BJ, et al. Angina due to coronary microvascular disease in hypertensive patients without left ventricular hypertrophy. *N Engl J Med* 1988; 319:1302–1307.

207. Houghton JL, Frank MJ, Carr AA, vonDohlen TW, Prisant LM. Relations among impaired coronary flow reserve, left ventricular hypertrophy and thallium perfusion defects in hypertensive patients without obstructive coronary artery disease. *J Am Coll Cardiol* 1991; 15:43–51.

208. Nunez E, Hosoya K, Susic D, Frohlich ED. Enalapril and losartan reduces cardiac mass and improves coronary hemodynamics in SHR. *Hypertension* 1997; 29:519–524.

209. Sarnoff SJ, Braunwald E, Welch GH Jr, et al. Hemodynamic determinants of oxygen consumption of the heart with special reference to the tension-time index. *Am J Physiol* 1958; 192:148–156.

210. MacMahon S, Peto R, Cutler J, Collins R, Sorlie P, Neaton J, et al. Blood pressure, stroke, and coronary heart disease. Part I: Prolonged differences in blood pressure: Prospective observational studies corrected for the regression dilution bias. *Lancet* 1990; 335:765–774.

211. Neaton JD, Wentworth D. Serum cholesterol, blood pressure, cigarette smoking, and death from coronary heart disease. Overall findings and differences by age for 316,099 white men. *Arch Int Med* 1992; 152:5664.

212. Weinberger MH. Influence of an angiotensin converting enzyme inhibitor on diuretic-induced metabolic effects in hypertension. *Hypertension* 1983; 5(suppl III):132–138.

213. Frohlich ED. Current issues in hypertension: Old questions with new answers and new questions. *Med Clin North Am* 1992; 76:1043–1056.

214. Cruickshank JM, Thorp JM, Zacharias FJ. Benefits and potential harm of lowering blood pressure. *Lancet* 1987; 1:581–584.

215. Alderman MH, Ooi WL, Madharsn S. Treatment induced blood pressure reduction and the risk of myocardial infarction. *JAMA* 1989; 262:920–924.

216. Farnett L, Mulrow CD, Linn WD, Lucey CR, Tuley MR. The J-curve phenomenon and the treatment of hypertension. *JAMA* 1991; 265:489–495.

217. SHEP Cooperative Research Group. Prevention of stroke by antihypertensive drug treatment in older persons with isolated systolic hypertension. Final results of the Systolic Hypertension in the Elderly Program (SHEP). *JAMA* 1991; 265:3255–3264.

218. Pfeffer MA, Braunwald E, Moye LA, Basta L, Brown EJ Jr, Cuddy TE, et al. Effect of captopril on mortality and morbidity in patients with left ventricular dysfunction after myocardial infarction. Results of the survival and ventricular enlargement trial. *N Engl J Med* 1992; 327:669–677.

219. SOLVD Trial Investigators. Effect of enalapril on survival in patients with reduced left ventricular ejection fractions and CHF. *N Engl J Med* 1991; 325:293–302.

220. Bhatia S, Frohlich ED. Hemodynamic comparison of agents useful in hypertensive emergencies. *Am Heart J* 1973; 85:367–373.

221. Frohlich ED. Hypertensive emergencies. In: Chung EK, ed. *Cardiac Emergency Care*. Philadelphia: Lea & Febiger; 1991: 304–319.

222. Schwartz GL, Strong CG. Renal parenchymal involvement in essential hypertension. *Med Clin North Am* 1987; 71:843–858.

223. Stanton JR, Freis ED. The serum uric acid concentration in essential hypertension. *Proc Soc Exp Biol Med* 1947; 66:193–194.

224. Messerli FH, Frohlich ED, Dreslinski GR, Suarez DH, Aristimuno GG. Serum uric acid in essential hypertension: An indicator of renal vascular involvement. *Ann Intern Med* 1980; 93:817–821.

225. Kobrin I, Frohlich ED, Ventura HO, Messerli FH. Renal involvement follows cardiac enlargement in essential hypertension. *Arch Intern Med* 1986; 146:272–276.

226. Luke RG. Can renal failure due to hypertension be prevented? *Hypertension* 1991; 18(I):139–142.

227. Frohlich ED, Messerli FH, Dunn FG, Oigman W, Ventura HO, Sundgaard-Riise K. Greater renal vascular involvement in the black patient with essential hypertension. A comparison of systemic and renal hemodynamics in black and white patients. *Miner Electrolyte Metab* 1984; 10:173–177.

228. Dustan HP, Curtis JJ, Luke RG, Rostand SG. Systemic hypertension and the kidney in black patients. *Am J Cardiol* 1987; 60(I):73–77.

229. Brenner BM, Meyer TW, Hostetter TH. Dietary protein intake and the progressive nature of kidney disease: The role of hemodynamically mediated glomerular injury in pathogenesis of progressive glomerular sclerosis in aging, renal ablation, and intrinsic renal disease. *N Engl J Med* 1982; 307:652–659.

230. Hostetter TH, Olson JL, Rennke HG, Venkatachalam MA, Brenner BM. Hyperfiltration in remnant nephrons: A potentially adverse response to renal ablation. *Am J Physiol* 1981; 241:F85–F93.

231. Kobrin I, Pegram BL, Frohlich ED. Acute pressure increase and intrarenal hemodynamics in conscious WKY and SHR rats. *Am J Physiol* 1985; 249:H1114–H1118.

232. Uchino K, Frohlich ED, Nishikimi T, Isshiki T, Kardon MB. Spontaneously hypertensive rats demonstrate increased renal vascular alpha$_1$-adrenergic receptor responsiveness. *Am J Physiol* 1991; 260(*Regulatory, Integrative Comp Physiol* 29):R889–R893.

233. Neff MS, Kim KE, Persoff M, Onesti G, Swarz C. Hemodynamics of uremic anemia. *Circulation* 1971; 43:876–883.

234. Roccella EJ, Boroler AE, Horan M. Epidemiologic considerations in defining hypertension. *Med Clin North Am* 1987; 71:785–802.

DIAGNOSTIC EVALUATION OF THE PATIENT WITH SYSTEMIC ARTERIAL HYPERTENSION

W. Dallas Hall

BLOOD PRESSURE MEASUREMENT

The measurement of blood pressure requires precision to avoid erroneous labeling of a normotensive patient as hypertensive.[1,2] False elevations occur often if regular-size blood pressure cuffs are used in adult patients whose midarm circumference exceeds 33 cm.[3,4] Auscultatory measurements can also overestimate intraarterial pressure in some elderly patients, presumably because of "pipe-stem" arteries due to extensive peripheral arteriosclerosis.[5] Cuff measurements of systolic or diastolic blood pressure have been reported to exceed intraarterial levels by more than 20 mmHg in as few as 2 percent to as many as 9 percent of relatively healthy elderly normotensive or hypertensive patients.[6–9]

An "auscultatory gap" is not uncommon in elderly patients with arteriosclerosis; it often causes an underestimation of systolic pressure. It occurs most often in elderly patients with increased arterial stiffness and can be detected by first estimating systolic pressure by palpation and inflating the cuff at least 30 mmHg above that level.[10]

Blood pressure should initially be measured in both arms, and all subsequent determinations should be performed in the arm with the higher pressure. If measurements are made simultaneously with deflation of the cuff at a rate less than 3 mmHg per second, differences greater than 10 mmHg are unusual in the absence of advanced arteriosclerosis of the subclavian artery.[11]

The position of the arm during the blood pressure measurement can be a source of variation in readings. When blood pressure is measured in the sitting or standing position, lowering the arm from a near-horizontal (i.e., "heart level") to a near-vertical position results in an increase in both the systolic and diastolic blood pressure readings.[12] This increase in the measured blood pressure with vertical arm displacement has been attributed to changes in hydrostatic pressure.[13]

Blood pressure should always be measured in the standing as well as the supine or sitting position in patients with hypertension. This is because orthostatic hypotension, especially common in diabetic and elderly patients, can influence the choice of antihypertensive therapy. The normal blood pressure response to standing is a slight decrease in systolic and a slight increase in diastolic pressure, with little change in mean arterial pressure.[14] A standing reduction in systolic pressure of 20 mmHg or more is often used as the criterion for orthostatic hypotension. It occurs in about 17 percent of elderly, untreated hypertensives if the blood pressure is measured after both 1 and 3 min of standing.[15] The finding is not always reproducible, even in symptomatic persons, especially if the measurements are made in the afternoon.[16] Moreover, Masuo and associates[17] reported that normalization of blood pressure in elderly hypertensives, especially with beta blockers, calcium channel blockers, or angiotensin-converting enzyme (ACE) inhibitors, was associated with a lower than pretreatment occurrence of orthostatic hypotension. In general, marked orthostatic decreases in the pretreatment blood pressure indicate a poorer prognosis and are more common in hypertensive patients with target organ complications such as cardiomegaly, congestive heart failure, and associated vascular disease.[18]

Blood Pressure Variability

The variability of blood pressure increases with age and with the level of the blood pressure; it is more striking with systolic than with diastolic pressure.[19,20] Some studies have found that the magnitude of variability in systolic and mean arterial pressure is inversely related to baroreceptor sensitivity,[21] an observation strengthened by the marked variability of blood pressure in some patients following bilateral carotid endarterectomy.

Even for normotensive individuals, however, blood pressure varies considerably throughout a 24-h period; isolated intermittent elevations of systolic pressure to levels above 140 mmHg and diastolic pressure to levels above 90 mmHg are not uncommon.[22] Blood pressure follows a circadian rhythm and is highest in the early morning hours and lowest at night.[23] When two or three consecutive blood pressure readings are taken, the first systolic reading is usually 2 to 4 mmHg higher than the second or third readings.[24] This effect is exaggerated in elderly hypertensives (i.e., those aged 66 to 86 years), in whom Fotherby and Potter[25] reported an average systolic blood pressure decline of 11 mmHg between the first and third readings 4 min later. Daytime ambulatory systolic pressure averaged 17 mmHg below the lowest of the clinic values. Diastolic pressure follows a similar pattern but to a lesser degree.

Souchek et al.[26] found that the mean of two or three consecutive readings at one visit provided a more accurate prediction of blood pressure over an 8-year follow-up period than did a single reading. In the Framingham Study, the mean, maximum, and minimum of three blood pressure measurements obtained during a 1-h examination were equally predictive of subsequent cardiovascular disease.[27] The lowest, or more "basal," of the three blood pressures was no better predictor of cardiovascular disease than the average or the highest of the blood pressure measurements.

Blood pressure is more variable between days than within days.[28] Untreated decreases in systolic pressure of 10 to 30 mmHg and diastolic pressure of 5 to 10 mmHg between the first and subsequent follow-up clinic visits are common.[29] In the Hypertension Detection and Follow-Up Program, over 30 percent of untreated individuals with average diastolic pressures of 95 mmHg or greater on the initial home screening had diastolic pressures below 90 mmHg approximately 1 week later.[30] In the Systolic Hypertension in the Elderly Program (SHEP), 36 percent of elderly individuals with isolated systolic hypertension at the initial visit (i.e., systolic blood pressure of 160 mmHg or more and diastolic blood pressure below 90 mmHg on the average of the last two of three readings) had nonqualifying (lower) blood pressures at the follow-up visit within a few weeks.[31] Of those who did confirm at the second visit, an additional 30 percent did not qualify for randomization at the third visit. Thus, the time of day, the number of measurements during the visit, the variability between visits, and regression toward the mean are all important considerations in making a diagnosis of hypertension.[32] In uncomplicated cases with only modest elevation of blood pressure, a minimum of two measurements on each of three different days is recommended for a diagnosis of hypertension. In patients with only intermittent elevations of blood pressure, additional visits are frequently required to assess blood pressure status accurately.[33]

Home blood pressure measurement and ambulatory monitoring of daytime pressure can assist in evaluation of the patient with borderline levels of blood pressure.[34] Perloff and associates[35] originally demonstrated that patients whose ambulatory blood pressures remained high (as compared with the average of three initial office visit pressures) had more target organ complications and an increased number of cardiovascular events over 5 years than did a group of patients with similar average office pressures but lower ambulatory home pressures. Home or office blood pressure monitoring can also assist in evaluation of the response to antihypertensive therapy and in the detection of "white coat" hypertension, where blood pressure is elevated when measured by the physician in an office setting but is normal during usual daytime activities.[36] Further studies are under way to assess whether white coat "reactors" have normal or increased long-term risks relative to individuals with blood pressures consistently in the normal range.[37,38]

Automated ambulatory blood pressure monitoring with computerized recordings and graphic displays is useful for the diagnosis, prognosis, and treatment of hypertension.[39–42] Current devices use either auscultatory or oscillometric methods and are relatively accurate and reproducible when used properly.[43–47] The most appropriate indication for diagnostic use is the patient with intermittently elevated office readings. Figure 57-1 illustrates hourly average blood pressures in a 69-year-old male with borderline office readings (i.e., 140/88 mmHg). Blood pressure levels rose markedly while driving to work on the expressway; definite hypertension (160 to 170/100 to 114 mmHg) persisted throughout the workday, but blood pressure fell dramatically during a late afternoon nap and subsequently during sleep. The results led to a clinical judgment that a drug with a 12-h duration of action might be appropriate to reduce the persistent daytime hypertension. *Ambulatory blood pressure measurement is more predictive than casual office pressure as an indicator of the presence of target organ damage, including echocardiographically evident left ventricular hypertrophy (LVH),[48–50] impaired diastolic cardiac filling,[51] microalbuminuria,[52] and the presence of lacunae and periventricular hyperintense central nervous system lesions on magnetic resonance imaging (MRI).[53]*

DIAGNOSTIC EVALUATION

The Patient with Stage I, Stage II, or Stage III Hypertension

Table 57-1 provides definitions of stage 1, 2, 3, or 4 hypertension.[54] Important considerations in the patient's history are summarized in Table 57-2. Recommended physical examination and routine laboratory tests are listed in Table 57-3.[55,56] Stage 1 and stage 2 hypertension are widely held to be asymptomatic. On the other hand, Bulpitt et al.[57] compared symptoms in 99 untreated hypertensive subjects with those of 78 normotensive subjects of similar age; unsteadiness, waking headaches, blurred vision, depression, and nocturia were more frequent in untreated hypertensives.

In the initial evaluation, efforts should be made to detect clinical clues to reversible causes of hypertension. For example, coarctation of the aorta is suggested by diminished leg pulses, a delay in the femoral pulse when palpated simultaneously with the radial pulse, a reduced blood pressure in the leg, a coarse systolic murmur at the left sternal border, intercostal pulsations, or rib notching on the chest x-ray. Renovascular hypertension, aldosteronism, renoparenchymal hypertension, Cushing's syndrome, and pheochromocytoma are discussed later in this chapter. Acromegaly, hyperthyroidism, hypothyroidism, sleep apnea,[58,59] and alcoholism should be suspected from the history and general appearance of the patient.

In the baseline evaluation, a search for target organ damage should be made and risk factors for cardiovascular disease assessed (see also Chap. 10). A careful history should be taken for angina, past myocardial infarction, transient ischemic attacks (TIAs), stroke, claudication, cigarette smoking, and a family history of cardiovascular events before age 55. Bruits over the carotid, renal, and femoral arteries should be sought, and the amplitude of arterial pulsations in the limbs graded. An electrocardiogram (ECG) should be obtained for evidence of ischemia or of LVH, and total cholesterol and low-

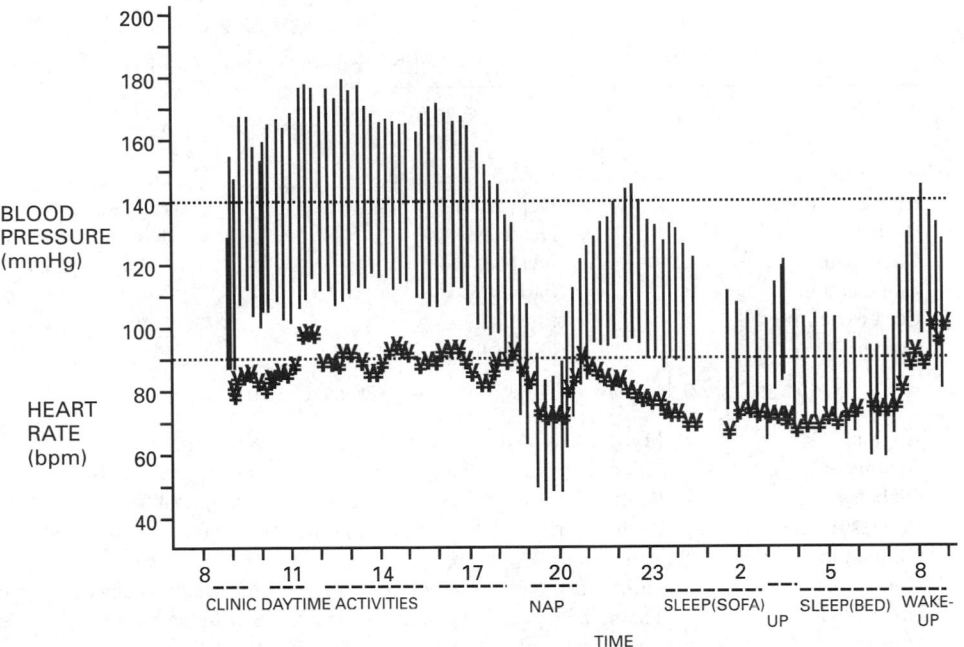

FIGURE 57-1

Twenty-four-hour ambulatory blood pressure monitoring graph of a 69-year-old untreated male with borderline office readings.

and high-density lipoprotein cholesterol levels measured.[60] In addition, the other recommended laboratory tests listed in Table 57-3 should be performed.

Hypertension is a common cause of congestive heart failure, which, in the Framingham Study, was associated with a 5-year mortality of 43 to 62 percent[61] (see Chap. 23). A search should be made for LVH, rales, ventricular gallop, distended neck veins, edema, and other clinical signs of congestive heart failure.

The initial evaluation is also important for the selection of drug therapy, which may be modified if there is a history of diabetes, dyslipidemia, gout, nephrolithiasis, peptic ulcer, severe depression, bronchospasm, edema, angioedema, or a variety of other illnesses. Also, the likelihood must be estimated of proper adherence to medications and compliance in keeping appointments, because long-term control of hypertension depends on good cooperation by the patient. Choice of dosage schedules and cost of medications also influence the choice of therapy.[62–66]

The Patient with Stage 4, Accelerated, or Malignant Hypertension

Diagnostic criteria for "malignant hypertension" include severe hypertension, generally with diastolic pressure of 125 mmHg or more, in conjunction with papilledema. If the fundi show retinal hemorrhages or exudates but no papilledema, the patient has "accelerated" hypertension.[67] If the funduscopic findings are Group II or less (see "Hypertensive Retinopathy," below) but the systolic or diastolic blood pressure exceeds 210 or 120 mmHg, respectively, then the patient has severe, or stage 4, hypertension. Target organ damage

TABLE 57-1

DEFINITIONS OF HYPERTENSION[a]

Category[b]	Systolic Blood Pressure, mmHg		Diastolic Blood Pressure, mmHg
Normal	<130		<85
High normal	130–139		85–89
Hypertension:			
Stage 1	140–159	or	90–99
Stage 2	160–179	or	100–109
Stage 3	180–209	or	110–119
Stage 4	≥210	or	≥120

[a] Based on an average of two or more readings taken at each of two or more visits after an initial screening.

[b] The higher category of systolic or diastolic pressure should be selected to classify the person's blood pressure status.

Source: Adapted from JNC V,[54] with permission.

TABLE 57-2

KEY ITEMS OF THE BASELINE HISTORY IN PATIENTS WITH HYPERTENSION

SYMPTOMS

Angioedema	Daytime sleepiness	Headaches	Sexual dysfunction
Blurred vision	Depression	Hematuria	Skin rash
Bronchospasm	Dizziness	Joint pains	Snoring/gasping
Chest pain	Dyspnea	Muscle cramps	Sweating
Claudication	Fatigue	Nocturia	Unsteadiness
Cold extremities	Flushing	Palpitations	Weakness
Cough	Gingival problems	Polyuria	Weight loss or gain

PAST DISEASE HISTORY | DIET AND DRUG HISTORY | FAMILY HISTORY

Angina	Myocardial	Alcohol	Nasal sprays	Coronary heart	Hypokalemia
Asthma	infarction	Aspirin	Nonsteroidal anti-	disease	Pheochromocytoma
Diabetes	Peptic ulcer	Blood pressure	inflammatory	Diabetes	Polycystic kidney
Congestive heart failure	Pyelonephritis	medications	agents	Hereditary nephritis	disease
Glomerulonephritis	Renal stones/	Cigarettes	Oral contraceptives	Hyperlipidemia	Renovascular
Gout	lithotripsy	Cocaine	Potassium (dietary)	Hyperparathyroidism	hypertension
Heart block	Toxemia	Cold remedies	Salt (dietary)	Hypertension	Thyroid disorders
Hepatitis	Transient	Chewing tobacco	Tricyclic		
Hypertension	ischemic attacks	Cyclosporine	antidepressants		
Lupus erythematosus		Licorice			

often accompanies these conditions and includes heart failure, encephalopathy, and renal insufficiency. Physiologic abnormalities include impaired renal perfusion, elevated plasma renin and aldosterone levels, and increased sympathetic tone. Because of the infrequent occurrence and the morbid prognosis of either accelerated or malignant hypertension,[68] an aggressive diagnostic approach is usually indicated. Diagnostic studies for renal artery stenosis (i.e., angiotensin-converting enzyme renography or renal arteriography) are often indicated if the patient is a candidate for renal artery surgical correction or angioplasty. *Davis et al.[69] identified anatomic renal artery stenosis in 7 percent of African-American and 42 percent of white patients who presented with a diastolic blood pressure of 125 mmHg plus retinal hemorrhages, exudates, or papilledema.* Electrocardiographic estimates of left ventricular anatomy and function and ultrasonic kidney size should also be considered. *Pheochromocytoma can also present with severe or resistant hypertension and can usually be excluded by obtaining plasma or urinary tests for catecholamines or their metabolites.* Appropriate studies to rule out correctable causes of hypertension are discussed in later sections of this chapter.

The Patient with Transient Elevations of Blood Pressure

In these patients, special attention should be given to symptoms suggestive of pheochromocytoma or the abuse of alcohol,[70] diet pills,[71] cocaine,[72–76] chewing tobacco,[77] and nasal decongestants or cold remedies containing stimulants such as phenylpropanolamine.[78] The clinician should inquire about recent stressful events because emotional stress or panic at-

tacks can be associated with intermittent elevations of blood pressure.[79] Rapid heart rate, dilated pupils, and sweating suggest hyperactivity of the sympathetic nervous system. There should be no evidence of target organ damage, and the biochemical profile and urinalysis should be normal in patients with only transient elevations of blood pressure. The presence of any abnormality should be a cause for concern and may indicate that the seemingly intermittent elevations of blood pressure may be more persistent, of longer duration, and/or of greater magnitude than previously appreciated.

The Patient with Isolated Systolic Hypertension

In patients with isolated systolic hypertension, the cardiovascular risks are as great or even greater than in those with elevated diastolic pressure.[80,81] The SHEP trial results documented that pharmacologic treatment of isolated systolic hypertension reduced the 5-year incidence of stroke by 36 percent.[31] Isolated systolic hypertension is associated with an increased prevalence of diabetes mellitus, and particular note should be made of symptoms and laboratory values suggestive of glucose intolerance. Elevation of the systolic blood pressure can also be the first clinical clue to large-vessel atherosclerosis, as well as to more unusual etiologies such as coarctation of the aorta, aortic regurgitation, hyperthyroidism, arteriovenous fistulas, or Paget's disease.

The Athlete with Hypertension

Athletes often present to the clinician for evaluation of an elevated blood pressure detected on a routine screening examination.[82] The usual story is that a physician's clearance is

TABLE 57-3

KEY ITEMS OF THE BASELINE PHYSICAL AND LABORATORY EXAMINATIONS IN PATIENTS WITH HYPERTENSION

PHYSICAL EXAMINATION

General	HEENT[a]	Chest	Abdomen	Extremities	Neurologic
Appearance	Carotid bruit	Aortic regurgitation	Palpable kidneys	Edema	Focal signs
Blood pressure (supine or sitting; standing; both arms)	Fundi	Apex impulse		Peripheral pulses	Proximal muscle strength
	Neck veins	Breast		Peripheral bruits	
Heart rate (supine or sitting; standing)	Temporal arteries	Rales			
	Thyroid gland	S_3			
		S_4			
		Systolic murmur			
		Wheezes			

LABORATORY EXAMINATION

General	Kidney	Metabolic	Miscellaneous
Hemoglobin	Blood urea nitrogen	Calcium	Chest x-ray
Hematocrit	Creatinine	Cholesterol[b]	Electrocardiogram
White blood cell count	Urine dipstick	Glucose (fasting)	Echocardiogram
	Urine sediment	Potassium	
		Uric acid	

[a] HEENT = *Head, Eyes, Ears, Nose,* and *Throat.*
[b] Also obtain fasting triglyceride and low-density and high-density lipoprotein cholesterol levels if the serum cholesterol level is 200 mg/dL or more in patients with other cardiovascular risk factors or 240 mg/dL or more in patients without other cardiovascular risk factors.

needed before the patient can compete in athletic events. The trained athlete's ECG can show evidence of increased vagal tone (sinus bradycardia, first- or second-degree atrioventricular block, junctional rhythm), which sometimes reverts to normal in the standing position. Other changes include high-amplitude R waves, a semivertical QRS axis in asthenic runners, or elevation of the ST segments or inversion of the T waves suggestive of ischemia.[83,84] An S_3 gallop may be heard,[85] and borderline cardiomegaly is often present on the chest x-ray (see also Chap. 95). Isolated systolic hypertension in an unusually tall basketball player can be the first clue to Marfan's syndrome with aortic regurgitation.

Echocardiography frequently reveals increased left ventricular posterior wall and septal wall thickness as well as increased left ventricular mass index (LVMI) in highly trained athletes participating in certain types of isometric exercise such as wrestling, shot-putting, or weight lifting. In contrast, increases in left ventricular end-diastolic internal dimension and volume are characteristic findings in professional athletes participating primarily in isotonic exercises such as competitive running, swimming, or basketball.[86,87]

Almost all of these changes can occur in athletes with normal left-sided heart catheterization and patient coronary arteries.[88] Great caution, however, must be taken in the evaluation of such patients because almost 75 percent of reported sudden deaths in young athletes have occurred during major exertion, especially in athletes with previously undiagnosed hypertrophic cardiomyopathy.[89] Serum antimitochondrial antibodies are found in 30 to 40 percent of patients with hypertrophic cardiomyopathy, but not in athletes with physiologic LVH.[90] Thus, in addition to the usual evaluation, consideration should be given to diagnostic procedures not generally done in the usual asymptomatic patient with hypertension. For example, echocardiography should be considered in athletes who have abnormal ST- and T-wave changes, findings suggestive of LVH on the ECG, and/or clinical findings or a family history suggestive of hypertrophic cardiomyopathy. Echocardiography often reveals physiologic LVH in athletes, although diastolic septal or posterior wall thicknesses of 13 mm or more are uncommon.[91,92] Diastolic left ventricular function is usually normal in athletes with physiologic LVH[93] (see Chap. 95).

Monitoring of blood pressure during a treadmill test usually reveals a marked increase in systolic pressure with little change in diastolic pressure.[94] Occasional patients exhibit an unexpected marked rise in diastolic pressure. These particular patients should be advised not to resume their usual exercise activities until blood pressure is well controlled. Blood pressure monitoring can also be conducted under circumstances that simulate the patient's usual exercise setting (e.g., weight lifting). The blood pressure response to the same exercise can then be reevaluated following institution of selected antihypertensive therapy. In contrast to treadmill-induced rises in diastolic pressure, exercise-induced elevations of peak systolic pressure to ≥190 mmHg in women or 210 mmHg in men, were reported by Lauer et al.[95] to have a benign prognosis with regard to the relative risk of coronary artery disease.

THE DIAGNOSIS OF TARGET ORGAN DAMAGE

Hypertensive Retinopathy

The funduscopic examination helps assess the prognosis and severity of hypertension. Keith and coworkers[96] first noted that patients with groups I (constriction), II (sclerosis, arteriovenous nicking), III (hemorrhages and exudates), and IV (papilledema) retinopathy had untreated 5-year survivals of 85, 50, 13, and 0 percent, respectively. More recent studies suggest that patients with group III and group IV hypertensive retinopathy have an equally poor long-term prognosis.[68] *Advanced hypertensive retinopathy (i.e., groups III and IV) is found in fewer than 10 percent of all hypertensive patients and is an indication for aggressive diagnostic evaluation and treatment.*

Arteriovenous nicking and a copper- or silver-wire appearance of the arterioles often occur in older patients and generally indicate arteriosclerosis.[97] Large inter- and intraobserver variability limits the value of fine distinctions between group I and group II retinopathy, although most agree that both focal and generalized arteriolar narrowing are retinal vascular signs of hypertension (see also Chap. 11).

Hypertensive Cardiovascular Disease

Two major forms of heart disease occur in the patient with hypertension: coronary heart disease and hypertensive heart disease. Criteria for the diagnosis of coronary heart disease are described elsewhere (see Chap. 45). Criteria for the diagnosis of hypertensive heart disease include the presence of hypertension plus LVH when other causes of LVH are reasonably excluded. Hypertension is the most common cause of LVH.[98] Neither a long duration nor any particular level of severity of blood pressure elevation are necessary prerequisites for LVH because factors other than blood pressure elevation are important for its development. *Many hypertensive patients develop a form of heart failure characterized by dyspnea and orthopnea with normal systolic but impaired diastolic function of the left ventricle.*[99–102] (see Chaps. 21 and 23).

Some hypertensive patients also have ischemic chest pain (often with a positive exercise test) but with normal coronary angiography and no evidence of vasospasm.[103] Cannon and Epstein and their associates[104,105] have presented evidence that the myocardial ischemia is related to microvascular angina. A similar syndrome has also been noted in hypertensive patients with LVH (see Chap. 45). Patients with this syndrome typically demonstrate ischemic ST-segment depression with dipyridamole infusion. Picano and associates[106] noted similar ischemic ST-segment changes in 10 of 28 asymptomatic patients with essential hypertension, especially those with higher

LVMIs and longer durations of hypertension. Opherk et al.[107] had earlier shown that in patients with long-standing essential hypertension and LVII, the coronary blood flow response was impaired following coronary vasodilation with dipyridamole. Hence, patients with hypertension and LVH are susceptible to episodes of myocardial ischemia, even in the absence of visible coronary atherosclerosis at catheterization. These observations may help explain the frequently noted ischemic T-wave changes following marked or sudden reductions of blood pressure with minoxidil,[108] nifedipine,[109–111] or sodium nitroprusside.[112]

Noninvasive diagnostic techniques that provide assessment of LVH include the physical examination, chest x-ray, ECG, and echocardiogram. Detection of LVH by physical examination depends on palpation of an enlarged and sustained left ventricular apex impulse.[113] An enlarged apical impulse is defined as one with a diameter greater than that of a quarter (i.e., >2.4 cm); a sustained apical impulse has an outward thrust that lasts one-half to two-thirds or more of the duration of systole. Evaluation is maximized by examining the patient in the left lateral decubitus position where an apical impulse diameter greater than 3 cm is a more sensitive and specific finding of left ventricular enlargement than is the location of the apex impulse 10 cm or more from the midsternal line or lateral to the midclavicular line.[114]

Detection of LVH by chest x-ray is fraught with the problems of defining which portions of the cardiac silhouette belong specifically to the left ventricle. In general, the cardiothoracic ratio should not exceed 0.5 in adults and is usually below 0.45[115] (see Chap. 13).

The criteria of Romhilt and Estes[116] are often used for the electrocardiographic diagnosis of definite or probable LVH. By these ECG criteria, however, left ventricular hypertrophy was detected in only 58 percent of hearts hypertrophied at autopsy, and false-positive results occurred in 3 percent. As defined originally, the "typical" ST-segment shift (i.e., "strain pattern") requires more than a 0.5-mm depression of the ST segment and a 0.5-mm or more inversion of the T wave in the limb or left precordial leads; the resultant ST segments and T-wave vectors are opposite to the direction of the main QRS vector. Refinements in the Romhilt-Estes point-score system have further improved the sensitivity and specificity of the electrocardiographic diagnosis of LVH.[117–119] Electrocardiographic evidence of left atrial abnormality often precedes that of left ventricular abnormality in patients with hypertension[120] (see Chap. 12).

Echocardiography has revolutionized the diagnosis of LVH because echocardiographic evidence of LVH occurs in 30 to 40 percent of hypertensive patients whose ECG and chest x-ray are normal. In fact, Savage et al.,[121,122] in a study of 234 hypertensive patients, found cardiomegaly on chest x-ray or LVH by electrocardiography in fewer than 10 percent of patients who had an abnormal echocardiographic left ventricular mass. Echocardiographic parameters that assess left ventricular muscle anatomy include the interventricular septal thickness (IVST), posterior wall thickness (PWT), and LVMI.

Two-dimensional guided M-mode echocardiography is satisfactory for the assessment of LVH provided that there are no regional wall motion abnormalities[123] (see Chap. 14).

Devereaux and associates[124] correlated LVMI with left ventricular weight at postmortem examination of 55 adult patients. Echocardiographic estimates of left ventricular mass, using both the Penn and American Society of Echocardiography conventions, correlated strongly with anatomic left ventricular mass. Thus, echocardiography is a sensitive and early indicator of anatomic abnormality of the left ventricle in patients with hypertension.[125] Echocardiographic LVH is an important clinical finding because of its association with an excess risk of complex ventricular arrhythmias, coronary heart disease, and sudden death.[126–132] Echocardiography is also used to demonstrate changes in left ventricular anatomy[133–135] and function[136,137] following therapy for hypertension. The current cost of echocardiography, however, is multifold higher than that of electrocardiography and must be considered in the context of diagnostic and therapeutic yields in individual patients with hypertension.[138]

Hypertensive Cerebrovascular Disease

CEREBROVASCULAR ACCIDENTS

Hypertension is the most important risk factor for the development of hemorrhagic or atheroembolic stroke. The incidence of stroke increases with each higher stratum of blood pressure[139] and is florid in young, inner-city African Americans[140] (see Chap. 99).

Microhemorrhage or occlusion of small vessels can result in small areas of infarction, most often in the putamen, thalamus, caudate nucleus, pons, or posterior limb of the internal capsule. These lacunar infarcts are usually associated with neurologic deficits that clear over days to weeks.[141–143] Table 57-4 outlines six distinct neurologic syndromes associated with lacunar infarctions.[144] Pure motor hemiparesis is by far the most common presentation of lacunar infarction. Multiple lacunas can lead to multi-infarct dementia, characterized by lability of affect, dementia, abnormal gait, dysarthria, incontinence, and bilateral long-tract signs.

TABLE 57-4

NEUROLOGIC SYNDROMES ASSOCIATED WITH LACUNAR INFARCTION

1. Pure motor hemiparesis (weakness of the face, arm, and leg)
2. Pure sensory stroke (numbness and sensory loss over the face, arm, trunk, and leg)
3. Ataxic hemiparesis (weakness of the arm or leg with disproportionate ataxia)
4. Dysarthria clumsy hand syndrome (dysarthria, central facial weakness, and mild ipsilateral arm weakness with clumsy hand)
5. Sensorimotor stroke
6. Hemichorea-hemiballismus (arm or leg)

Cerebrovascular accidents of the hemorrhagic and infarctive types are diagnosed on the basis of the neurologic examination, supplemented by the computed tomography (CT) scan. In cerebral infarction, the CT scan may show a sharply marginated, homogeneous, low-density lesion in a specific vascular territory. In intracerebral hemorrhage, the scan usually shows an irregularly shaped, consolidated, high-density mass.[145] The differentiation between a TIA and a small lacunar infarct is often difficult; the CT scan is usually normal in both conditions, but lacunar infarction may be apparent by MRI. Also, TIAs tend to recur in a repetitive pattern, whereas lacunar infarcts, by definition, cannot. Evanescent neurologic symptoms or findings in conjunction with a carotid artery bruit justify carotid duplex Doppler ultrasonography.[146] In a good vascular laboratory, this method should almost always detect >60 percent stenosis of the internal carotid artery.[147]

HYPERTENSIVE ENCEPHALOPATHY

Hypertensive encephalopathy is a syndrome characterized by acute or subacute alterations in neurologic status that occur as the result of elevated arterial pressure and that are reversed by lowering the blood pressure.[148] It usually occurs in the setting of accelerated malignant hypertension, although advanced hypertensive retinopathy can occasionally be absent. This syndrome can occur with almost any variety of hypertension, but it is rare with primary aldosteronism and coarctation of the aorta.

Hypertensive encephalopathy usually presents with severe headache, confusion, and lethargy, frequently accompanied by nausea, vomiting, and visual disturbances. The symptoms generally worsen over 12 to 48 h, and seizures, myoclonus, obtundation, and, in some instances, blindness can develop.

Hypertensive encephalopathy must be differentiated from other disorders that also present with diffuse neurologic findings in patients with hypertension.[149] For example, uremic encephalopathy can also present with hypertension, confusion, lethargy, and seizures. Severe headache and retinal hemorrhages, exudates, or papilledema, however, are more characteristic of hypertensive encephalopathy, whereas uremic encephalopathy is often accompanied by myoclonic jerking. Moreover, the symptoms of hypertensive encephalopathy are usually reversed within 12 to 72 h by effective antihypertensive therapy. In malignant hypertension with renal insufficiency, the encephalopathy may well be due to both. Other causes of encephalopathy (e.g., hyponatremia, meningitis, alcohol or cocaine toxicity, and collagen vascular diseases) should be considered and evaluated as indicated by other signs and symptoms.

Focal seizures and other focal neurologic signs can occur in patients who appear clinically to have hypertensive encephalopathy. In an autopsy study of patients with the clinical diagnosis of hypertensive encephalopathy, however, Chester et al.[149] found that focal neurologic deficits were almost invariably attributable to structural lesions such as cerebral hemorrhage or infarction. Patients who appear to have hypertensive encephalopathy and exhibit focal neurologic signs should undergo further diagnostic evaluation. The CT scan and MRI are the procedures most likely to identify focal areas of intracerebral hemorrhage or infarction.

Severe hypertension can occur in previously normotensive patients who develop intracranial hemorrhage or a wide variety of other primary neurologic disorders. In these settings, considerable caution must be taken to avoid the erroneous diagnosis of hypertensive encephalopathy (see Chap. 99). In general, such patients do not have group III or IV hypertensive retinopathy, LVH, or renal impairment.

Hypertensive Nephrosclerosis

The urinalysis, creatinine clearance, ultrasonic kidney size, pyelogram, and angiogram are relatively normal in patients with essential hypertension. *Special tests are not justified for the prognosis or treatment of hypertension when the usual clinical tests of kidney function are within the normal range.* If the urine sediment, blood urea nitrogen (BUN), and creatinine are normal and proteinuria does not exceed 1 g daily, it can usually be assumed that the hypertension is not secondary to primary renal parenchymal disease.

Both glomerular hyperfiltration[150,151] and microalbuminuria[152,153] are early markers of hypertensive nephropathy. Microalbuminuria is defined as a urinary albumin excretion of >15 μg/min without detectable abnormality on the usual clinical dipstick tests for proteinuria. Its presence in patients with uncomplicated essential hypertension may predict subsequent cardiovascular disease.[154,155]

BENIGN NEPHROSCLEROSIS
Abnormalities of standard kidney function tests in patients with long-standing, poorly controlled hypertension in the absence of intercurrent primary disease of the kidneys are attributable to benign nephrosclerosis. Under these circumstances low-grade proteinuria (<1 g/day) and granular casts may appear, creatinine clearance may fall, and kidneys may shrink. Pyelograms may show poor visualization of the kidneys or delayed excretion of contrast without distortion of the renal contour or collecting system. Advanced nephrosclerosis is characterized by a symmetric reduction in kidney size and increased echogenicity on renal ultrasonography. Kidney biopsy is not indicated unless hematuria, red blood cell casts, heavy proteinuria, or systemic evidence of collagen vascular or neoplastic disease are found. An appreciable number of patients, especially African Americans, develop renal failure as a consequence of long-standing, poorly controlled hypertension causing nephrosclerosis.[156–158]

MALIGNANT NEPHROSCLEROSIS
The renal disease associated with malignant essential hypertension differs in pathology, physiology, and natural history from benign nephrosclerosis. Renal failure from malignant hypertension is usually seen in a clinical context of multiple-target-organ decompensation (i.e., retinopathy, encephalopathy, and congestive heart failure) in association with elevated plasma renin and aldosterone levels and increased sympathetic outflow.

The urinalysis in malignant nephrosclerosis can range from negative, in patients whose lesion is confined to the arterioles, to 4+ proteinuria, hematuria, and red blood cell or pigmented casts, in those with associated glomerulitis or interstitial bleeding. Low-grade proteinuria occurs in about one-third of patients,[159] but nephrotic-range proteinuria occurs in fewer than 5 percent of patients and usually reverses rapidly after lowering of blood pressure.

Elevated levels of plasma renin activity occur in approximately 80 percent of cases and therefore do not provide specific evidence for renal artery stenosis as a cause of the malignant nephrosclerosis. Serum aldosterone levels are elevated in the majority of cases and probably account for the disproportionately low serum potassium concentrations in the setting of mild to moderate renal failure.

THE DIAGNOSIS OF SECONDARY CAUSES OF HYPERTENSION

Estimates of the prevalence of arterial hypertension secondary to an identifiable cause vary considerably. In unselected populations, the best estimate of the prevalence of secondary hypertension would appear to be about 3 percent. Curable etiologies are even less frequent, emphasizing the importance of limiting extensive evaluations to patients in whom the diagnostic yield is likely to be increased.[160]

Renovascular Hypertension

PREVALENCE
Renal artery stenosis is the most common curable cause of hypertension, but it probably occurs in 3 percent or fewer of hypertensive patients. The prevalence depends in part on the demographic characteristics of the hypertensive population. For example, below the age of 40, renovascular hypertension is more frequent in women than men. Renovascular hypertension is less common in African-American patients with hypertension.[161]

CLINICAL FINDINGS
Table 57-5 outlines clinical clues for the diagnosis of renovascular hypertension. It is found more commonly when hypertension begins before age 30 or after age 50. In addition, an abdominal bruit is heard six to nine times more often in patients with renovascular hypertension than in those with essential hypertension. The presence of severe hypertensive retinopathy (hemorrhages, exudates, or papilledema) also increases its likelihood. The sudden onset of severe hypertension or the onset of uncontrolled hypertension in a patient whose blood pressure was previously well controlled is the usual tipoff to renovascular disease. In addition, obesity is less common among patients with renovascular hypertension than in patients with essential hypertension.[162] Little recognized is the association between

TABLE 57-5

CLINICAL CLUES TO THE DIAGNOSIS OF RENOVASCULAR HYPERTENSION

1. Onset <age 30 or >age 50 years
2. Blood pressure resistant to usual drug therapy
3. Abrupt worsening of previously controlled blood pressure
4. Accelerated or malignant hypertension
5. Abdominal bruit with lateral radiation
6. Nonobesity
7. Unexplained episodes of recurrent acute pulmonary edema

TABLE 57-6

SPECIAL TESTS FOR THE DIAGNOSIS OF RENOVASCULAR HYPERTENSION

1. Radioactive renograms
2. Angiotensin-converting enzyme inhibitor renography[a]
3. Digital subtraction angiography or aortography
4. Renal vein renin ratio
5. Post-captopril plasma renin activity
6. Duplex ultrasound scanning
7. Magnetic resonance angiography

[a] Most important special screening test.

renal artery stenosis and the repeated occurrence of unexplained episodes of acute pulmonary edema.[163,164]

Fibrous dysplasia and atherosclerosis of the renal artery account for almost all cases of renovascular hypertension. With fibrous dysplasia, hypertension generally presents before age 35, most often in women. Fibrous dysplasia can involve either or both renal arteries but is usually unilateral when initially diagnosed. An upper abdominal bruit is audible in about 60 percent of patients.[165] Bruits originating from the renal artery are heard best in the midepigastrium; they radiate laterally toward one or both upper quadrants, unlike benign epigastric bruits that radiate vertically. The bruit is high-pitched, often intermittent, and occasionally systolic-diastolic in character. If combined with hypertension of less than 3 years' duration, the presence of a systolic-diastolic bruit is predictive of a favorable response to surgery in patients with fibrous dysplasia.

Atherosclerotic disease accounts for two-thirds or more of patients with renovascular hypertension. Since atherosclerosis is the underlying lesion, the chance of detecting renal artery stenosis rises markedly in smokers[166] and in patients with atherosclerotic heart disease,[167] carotid disease,[168] or lower-extremity claudication.[169] In contrast to fibrous dysplasia, atherosclerotic renovascular disease occurs predominantly in men over age 45. About one-third of patients with atherosclerotic renovascular disease have bilateral lesions at the time of initial diagnosis. Diabetes mellitus is more prevalent in patients with atherosclerotic renal artery disease[170] and should increase the clinician's suspicion of renal artery stenosis. Abdominal bruits are a less specific finding than in fibrous dysplasia because the atherosclerotic process often generates bruits from other abdominal arteries such as the mesenteric or splenic artery. The general approach to the detection, evaluation, and treatment of renovascular hypertension is discussed in an excellent report of the Working Group on Renovascular Hypertension.[171]

SPECIAL DIAGNOSTIC TESTS (TABLE 57-6)

General

When renovascular hypertension is suspected, diagnostic evaluation should generally be conducted in nonobese, young women below age 40, the group with the highest prevalence of fibrous dysplasia of the renal artery. This approach should be automatic for those young women with stage 3 or 4 hypertension of less than 3 years' duration, especially if blood pressure is inadequately controlled on three or more antihypertensive drugs. Evaluation should also be considered in selected older patients who may have atherosclerotic renovascular disease and who are judged to be good candidates for either surgical intervention or angioplasty.[160,172] Diagnostic testing is not usually indicated in patients with advanced renal failure and bilateral small kidneys, although improvement or preservation of renal function following revascularization has been observed in selected patients who generally have only modest impairment of renal function and at least one relatively normal-size kidney.[173-176]

Radioisotopic Renograms

A semiquantitative estimate of kidney size and the symmetry of perfusion can be obtained from the combination of ^{131}I-hippuran (or ^{99}Tc-mercaptoacetyltriglycine, MAG3) and ^{99}Tc-diethylenetriamine pentaacetic acid (DTPA) scintigrams of the kidneys, with measurement of the disappearance rates from the plasma. If plasma flow is symmetric, homogeneous, and markedly reduced in small kidneys, the likelihood of correctable renovascular hypertension is low. Conversely, asymmetry of flow greater than 40 to 60 percent or unilateral delayed isotope appearance but good bilateral renal concentration and excretion is suggestive of large renal artery vascular occlusive disease.

Angiotensin-Converting Enzyme Inhibitor Renography

Isotope renography detects the acute reductions of glomerular filtration rate (GFR) following the administration of oral captopril or intravenous enalapril to patients with functionally significant renal artery stenosis. It is the preferred nuclear medicine screening procedure for renovascular hypertension. The sensitivity of the test, however, is reduced in patients who are unable to withhold diuretics or chronic ACE inhibitor therapy safely for 3 to 5 days prior to the procedure.[177]

Isotope renography, generally using Tc-DTPA (which reflects GFR), is performed immediately before and 60 to 90 min after the administration of a single 25-mg dose of oral captopril or 15 min after a 40-μg/kg (maximum of 2.5 mg) dose of intravenous enalapril. Following ACE inhibition, the uptake of DTPA on the stenotic side is usually decreased from baseline in patients with unilateral renal arterial disease, whereas no consistent decrease is generally observed in the contralateral uninvolved kidney. In contrast, the uptake of hippuran [which reflects renal plasma flow (RPF)] by the stenotic kidney is frequently unchanged (although excretion is delayed). This acute reduction in filtration fraction (i.e., the ratio of GFR/RPF) that occurs in the stenotic kidney following ACE inhibition may be due to interruption of angiotensin II–mediated vasoconstriction of the postglomerular efferent arteriole. Efferent arteriolar vasoconstricton appears to develop initially as a compensatory adaptation to help preserve glomerular capillary filtration pressure in settings, such as renal artery stenosis, that are associated with a reduced renal arterial perfusion pressure.

Digital Subtraction Angiography or Aortography

Vascular anatomic evaluation usually begins with either digital subtraction angiography (DSA) or aortography. The rapid-sequence intravenous program has been abandoned as a screening test because the sensitivity of the test is 80 percent at best.[178,179] Venous DSA combines intravenous urography with angiotomography to create subtraction images of the abdominal arteries following rapid injection of a large bolus of contrast material into the central venous circulation. Lesions of the main renal artery can be detected in up to 90 percent or more of cases if adequate visualization is achieved, although DSA is less reliable for detecting segmental renal artery lesions.[180–182] When the index of clinical suspicion is high or when the risk of complications seems excessive, it is usually more expedient to proceed directly to arterial DSA or renal arteriography. If the serum creatinine is greater than 2 mg/dL, the total amount of contrast material should be limited in combination with adequate hydration and volume expansion.[183] Nonionic, lower osmolality contrast agents may be less toxic in this setting.[184]

Renal Vein Renin Ratio

Once the presence of renal arterial disease has been established, the functional significance of the stenosis can be evaluated to help determine if the renal artery lesion is the likely cause of the hypertension. This assessment is done by measuring the "renal vein renin ratio," i.e., the ratio of plasma renin activity in blood samples obtained from the venous effluent of each kidney. In general, to enhance differential secretion, patients should be free of beta blockers and centrally acting drugs. Administration of a single oral dose of captopril 30 min prior to obtaining renal vein renin studies, however, can enhance lateralization in patients with unilateral renal artery disease, even when other drug therapy is continued.[185–187] ACE inhibitors, however, should be used with caution in this setting because acute renal insufficiency (usually reversible following discontinuation of the drug) can occur during chronic ACE inhibition therapy in patients with severe bilateral renal artery stenosis or renal artery stenosis in a solitary

kidney. A single dose of captopril just prior to the split renin testing is usually tolerated well and can also be useful in improving control of blood pressure during the procedure.

A renal vein renin ratio of 1.5 or greater favoring the stenotic side is abnormal and is generally indicative of a functionally significant renal artery stenosis. Lateralization has additional credence if the peripheral plasma renin activity is also elevated and renin secretion from the unaffected kidney is suppressed; i.e., the renal venous renin activity from the unaffected side is similar to or no more than 30 percent above the renin activity of a sample obtained from the inferior vena cava below the renal veins. In general, when renal vein renins reveal a stenotic-to-nonstenotic ratio of at least 1.5, approximately 90 percent of patients will be improved or relieved of hypertension following technically successful angioplasty, surgical revascularization, or nephrectomy. Up to 50 percent of selected patents with nonlateralizing renal vein renin ratios below 1.5, however, also have a favorable response to surgery. Hence, a lateralizing renal vein renin ratio predicts improvement of hypertension with a high degree of accuracy in patients with unilateral renal arterial disease, whereas a nonlateralizing value is not necessarily a reliable predictor of lack of improvement of hypertension following technically successful surgery or angioplasty.[188] The renal vein renin ratio is frequently not reliable for predicting surgical response in patients with bilateral renovascular disease.

Post-Captopril Plasma Renin Activity

The unstimulated peripheral vein renin activity is not a very useful test for renovascular hypertension because up to 50 percent of patients have values within the normal range. This lack of utility is most likely because renin secretion from the uninvolved kidney is suppressed in patients with unilateral renal artery stenosis or because renin can sometimes be normalized by the sodium retention that occurs with bilateral renovascular disease. In contrast, the peripheral renin response 60 min following a 25- or 50-mg dosage of oral captopril is sometimes a useful and noninvasive screening test for renovascular hypertension.[189] A positive test is defined as a post-captopril renin level that is above 12 ng/mL per hour, increases 10 ng/mL per hour or more and is at least 150 percent above the baseline value (400 percent if the baseline renin is below 3 ng/mL per hour). Optimal interpretation of the test requires that the patient is not receiving antihypertensive medications, especially diuretics. False-positive and negative results are not infrequent in patients with serum creatinine levels of 2.0 mg/dL or more, limiting the overall utility of the test in these patients.[190]

Duplex Ultrasound Scanning

Duplex ultrasound combines B-mode imaging and pulsed Doppler flow analysis. Data are promising with regard to the diagnosis of renal artery stenosis, although the procedure is limited technically by obesity and excess bowel gas and anatomically by the presence of either multiple renal arteries or stenosis of branch vessels.[191–193]

Magnetic Resonance Angiography

The use of magnetic resonance angiography techniques to evaluate renal artery stenosis is an exciting new development (Fig. 57-2).[194,195] Magnetic resonance angiography is noninvasive and uses no radiation but has limitations in detection of stenoses beyond the proximal third of the renal artery. It also has a tendency to overestimate the severity of the stenosis.[196]

Renoparenchymal Hypertension

Two types of renoparenchymal hypertension are the acute form associated with glomerulitis and the chronic form associated with loss of viable nephrons. In neither of these is plasma renin activity usually very elevated. In contrast to essential hypertension associated with nephrosclerosis, the urinalysis is typically abnormal.

HYPERTENSION IN ACUTE RENAL DISEASE

Hematuria with dysmorphic red blood cells, red blood cell casts, proteinuria, and periorbital and/or pedal edema are diagnostic of acute diffuse glomerulitis. If plasma renin is measured, it is often normal or slightly depressed but may be elevated relative to the increased blood volume and pressure. Ultrasonography usually shows the kidneys to be enlarged or at the upper limit of normal size. Other laboratory tests may confirm the etiologic diagnosis: bacteriologic or serologic evidence of streptococcal infection, antinuclear antibodies (ANA), antineutrophilic cytoplasmic antibodies (ANCA), or reduced serum complement. If proteinuria is ≥1+ or is present repeatedly on qualitative testing, 24-h urine protein levels should be measured to determine whether or not a nephrotic type of protein leak is present.

If nephrotic syndrome is diagnosed or if renal function remains severely depressed after initial treatment with appropriate antibiotics and antihypertensive agents, a renal biopsy should be performed if there is no contraindication. Immunologic and ultrastructural classification of the disease will modify diagnosis, prognosis, and therapy.

HYPERTENSION IN CHRONIC RENAL DISEASE

The second major category of renal disease associated with hypertension is that related to loss of nephron population in chronic nephritis. Creatinine clearance is reduced, and urinalysis usually shows moderate proteinuria (0.5 to 2 g/day), moderate numbers of red blood cells, and frequent granular casts with glomerulonephritis. Pyuria, bacteriuria, and white blood cell casts are present with pyelonephritis. Pyuria can also occur with abacterial forms of interstitial nephritis such as analgesic nephropathy.

X-ray and ultrasound studies in chronic nephritis usually show variable degrees of reduction in kidney size (often to 10 cm or less) with increased echogenicity. The kidneys are symmetric and smooth in chronic glomerulonephritis, whereas they are asymmetric and irregular in chronic pyelonephritis and polycystic kidney disease. With uremia, small kidneys indicate irreversibility of the underlying disease. Shrunken kidneys are not usually biopsied because tissue is difficult to obtain and the end-stage histologic pattern is hard to interpret.

When chronic renal failure occurs in conjunction with diabetes mellitus, the pathologic lesion can be intercapillary glomerulosclerosis, large- or medium-vessel atherosclerotic disease, or atrophy with interstitial fibrosis. Ultrasonography usually shows smooth and symmetric kidneys, often of normal or even increased size. Asymmetry of renal size can be a tip-off to coexistent renal artery occlusive disease.

The hypertension of most patients with end-stage renal disease on maintenance hemodialysis is volume-dependent, but about 10 percent of cases are renin-mediated. When hypertension is difficult to control in dialysis patients, plasma renin determinations are of value. The renin level can also be important if kidney transplantation is planned because posttransplant hypertension can be caused by renin secretion from the native kidney as well as acquired stenosis of the implanted renal artery.

Primary Aldosteronism

PREVALENCE

Primary aldosteronism (Conn's syndrome) is an uncommon but

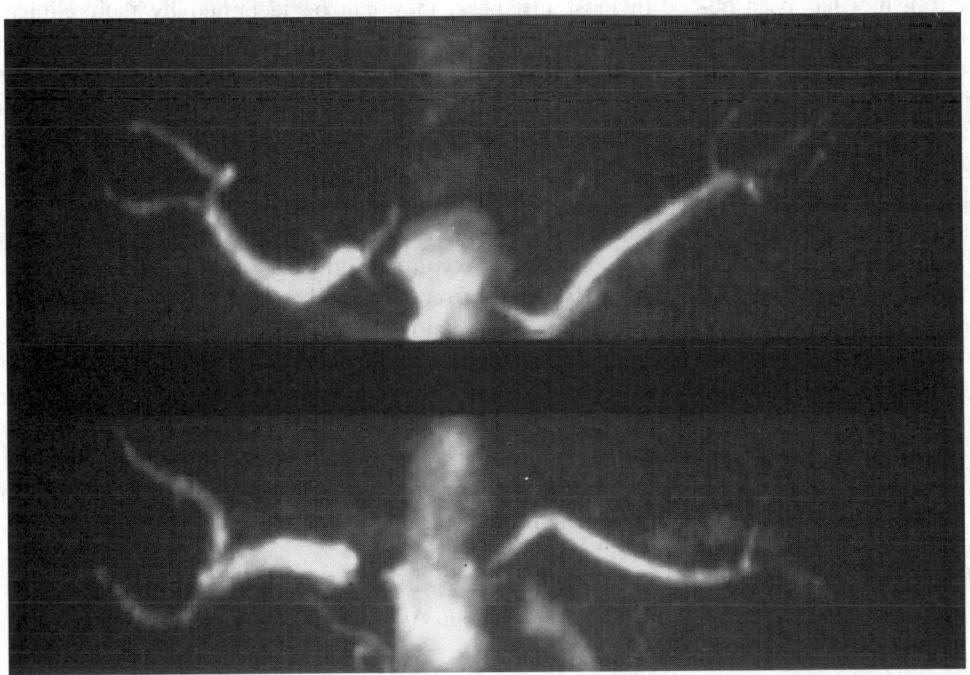

FIGURE 57-2
Magnetic resonance angiography demonstrating bilateral renal artery stenosis.

potentially curable cause of hypertension.[197] In most studies of secondary causes of hypertension, primary aldosteronism is found in 0.5 to 1 percent of patients.

CLINICAL FINDINGS

Table 57-7 outlines clinical clues for the diagnosis of primary aldosteronism. Most cases occur between the ages of 30 and 50 years. The hypertension is usually of mild or moderate severity, although severe hypertension has been observed.[198] Except for hypokalemia, primary aldosteronism does not usually present with clinical manifestations that readily suggest the diagnosis. Occasionally, the presenting feature is nocturia, polyuria, polydipsia, proximal muscle weakness, intermittent paralysis, rhabdomyolysis, paresthesia, or tetany resulting from severe potassium depletion. The manifestations of primary aldosteronism can temporarily ameliorate during pregnancy because of the antimineralocorticoid effect of high levels of progesterone.[199]

Hypokalemia is the most common manifestation of primary aldosteronism and is often associated with metabolic alkalosis and mild hypernatremia. Hypomagnesemia can also occur.[200] Primary aldosteronism can present with either unprovoked or diuretic-induced hypokalemia.[201] Unprovoked hypokalemia occurs in the absence of diuretics, vomiting, diarrhea, alcoholism, or abuse of laxatives or chewing tobacco. It is particularly suggestive of primary aldosteronism because spontaneous hypokalemia is observed in such a small percentage of otherwise healthy, nonalcoholic patients with uncomplicated essential hypertension. Hence, the likelihood of primary aldosteronism is increased markedly in untreated hypertensive patients who present with unexplained hypokalemia.

The presence of a normal serum potassium concentration (i.e., "normokalemic primary aldosteronism") has been observed in as many as 10 to 20 percent of patients who otherwise have the characteristic features of primary aldosteronism. Most patients with normokalemic primary aldosteronism have bilateral hyperplasia rather than adenomas.

There are two major pathologic varieties of primary aldosteronism: adrenocortical adenomas [aldosteronomas, or aldosterone-producing adenomas (APAs)] and bilateral adrenocortical (zona glomerulosa) hyperplasia. APAs account for approximately 60 percent of cases. They are almost invariably benign, and women are affected somewhat more commonly

than men.[202] APAs are usually associated with higher levels of aldosterone and more pronounced hypokalemia and hyporeninemia than bilateral hyperplasia.

Bilateral hyperplasia is sometimes referred to as idiopathic hyperaldosteronism (IHA), or pseudoprimary aldosteronism. Most patients with APAs exhibit a fall in plasma aldosterone levels after 2 to 4 h of upright posture in the morning, whereas those with bilateral hyperplasia usually demonstrate an increase.[203] Cases of unilateral adrenal hyperplasia have also been described.[204] These are referred to as the primary adrenal hyperplasia (PAH) type of primary aldosteronism, and the associated hypertension responds to unilateral adrenalectomy.

A number of young patients have been described with the typical features of primary aldosteronism but whose clinical and laboratory abnormalities were reversed with dexamethasone administration, suggesting supersensitivity to adrenocorticotropic hormone (ACTH).[205,206] The cause has recently been identified as a chimeric duplication of the 11β-hydroxylase/aldosterone synthase gene on chromosome 8, such that aldosterone synthase is activated and facilitates excess aldosterone production.[207] The condition is now referred to as glucocorticoid-remediable aldosteronism (GRA). Bilateral adrenal hyperplasia is the only reported histologic abnormality. More than 150 cases of GRA have now been found. The inheritance is autosomal dominant. GRA is suspected by response to a 2-week course of 1 to 2 mg/day of dexamethasone to patients with the presumptive diagnosis of bilateral adrenal hyperplasia. It can be confirmed by direct genetic testing, which is available free in the United States by calling 1-800-722-5520, extension 8404.

A number of infrequently encountered states are associated with mineralocorticoid hypertension and hypokalemia.[202,208] In most instances, they can be identified by their clinical and laboratory characteristics. Chronic excessive ingestion of licorice-containing candy or chewing tobacco can induce mineralocorticoid hypertension, with elevation of blood pressure caused by glycyrrhizinic acid, a component of licorice extract.[209] Glycyrrhizinic acid directly inhibits 11β-hydroxydehydrogenase (in the kidney and peripheral vasculature), which is necessary for the intrarenal inactivation of steroids with an 11-hydroxy group, primarily cortisol and corticosterone. Hypertensive children and a few adults have now been found with congenital 11β-hydroxydehydrogenase deficiency, and the gene has been localized to chromosome 16q22. These patients present with hypertension, hypokalemia, low plasma renin, low plasma aldosterone, and mildly elevated urinary free cortisol.[210] The abnormality responds to dexamethasone or spironolactone. This condition was previously referred to as the syndrome of apparent mineralocorticoid excess (AME).

SPECIAL DIAGNOSTIC TESTS FOR PRIMARY ALDOSTERONISM (TABLE 57-8)

Plasma Renin Activity

The major criterion for the diagnosis of primary aldosteronism is autonomous overproduction of aldosterone, usually in con-

---

TABLE 57-7

CLINICAL CLUES TO THE DIAGNOSIS OF PRIMARY ALDOSTERONISM

1. Spontaneous hypokalemia (<3.5 meq/L)
2. Exaggerated diuretic-induced hypokalemia (<3.0 meq/L)
3. Hypernatremia (144–148 meq/L)
4. Family history of hypokalemia
5. Inordinate fatigue
6. Unexplained paresthesia
7. Polyuria

TABLE 57-8

SPECIAL TESTS FOR THE DIAGNOSIS
OF PRIMARY ALDOSTERONISM

1. Plasma renin activity
2. Aldosterone suppression tests (saline infusion)[a]
3. Ratio of plasma aldosterone to plasma renin activity
4. Dexamethasone suppression test
5. Postural change in plasma aldosterone
6. Plasma 18-hydroxycorticosterone levels
7. Abdominal CT scan
8. Abdominal MRI scan
9. Adrenal vein aldosterone levels

[a] Most important special screening test.

junction with a low plasma renin activity.[211] Typically, the plasma renin activity is suppressed to low levels and remains subnormal despite volume depletion and upright posture. Under these conditions, a threefold or more increase in baseline plasma renin activity is generally considered normal. The renin levels of patients with primary aldosteronism are usually stimulated minimally or not at all by sodium restriction or diuretic therapy.

Use of the plasma renin activity as a screening test for primary aldosteronism is nonspecific because approximately 30 percent of patients with essential hypertension (i.e., the subgroup with "low renin" essential hypertension) also have subnormal plasma renin activity. Furthermore, a random test of plasma renin activity, obtained without appropriate stimulation, may show that plasma renin activity is not suppressed in 10 percent or more of patients with primary aldosteronism and that it is even increased in patients receiving spironolactone.

Aldosterone Suppression Tests

The diagnosis of primary aldosteronism is confirmed by plasma or 24-h urinary levels of aldosterone that are increased relative to sodium intake and excretion, and that fail to suppress normally with volume expansion. A commonly used method to test aldosterone suppressibility is volume expansion by administration of intravenous saline. The lack of suppression of aldosterone is a critical diagnostic feature because considerable overlap exists in the plasma and urinary aldosterone levels of patients with essential hypertension and primary aldosteronism, particularly when sodium intake has not been controlled. In patients with primary aldosteronism, the plasma aldosterone level usually fails to suppress below 10 ng/dL following the intravenous administration of 2 L of normal saline solution over 4 h.

Ratio of Plasma Aldosterone to Plasma Renin Activity

The ratio of plasma aldosterone to plasma renin activity can also be useful in the diagnosis of primary aldosteronism. Hiramatsu et al.[212] found the ratio of plasma aldosterone concentration (in picograms per deciliter) to plasma renin

activity (in nanograms per milliliter per hour) to be below 200 in patients with essential hypertension and above 400 in patients with APAs. Lyons et al.[213] reported that the ratio of plasma aldosterone concentration to plasma renin activity in blood samples obtained 2 h following the administration of a single 25-mg oral dose of captopril provided better discrimination between essential hypertension and primary aldosteronism than did the baseline values.

LOCALIZATION METHODS

General

Once the diagnosis of primary aldosteronism is established, further tests are indicated in patients judged to be operative candidates. Evaluation must include efforts to distinguish between adenoma and bilateral hyperplasia and to localize the side of any tumor-bearing gland. Adrenal venography is unreliable for identifying bilateral hyperplasia or the 20 percent of adenomas that are smaller than 1 cm in diameter.

Adrenal Vein Aldosterone Levels

A sensitive localization method is that of measuring the aldosterone levels of the venous effluent from each adrenal. Regardless of size, aldosteronomas can be localized with about 90 percent accuracy. The aldosterone levels of venous blood from tumor-bearing glands are often increased 10-fold or more above those from the contralateral uninvolved gland. Bilateral elevation of aldosterone levels suggests bilateral hyperplasia. Adrenal vein epinephrine levels above 1500 pg/mL assure that the sample was indeed from the adrenal vein.[214]

CT and Isotopic Scans

Adenomas larger than 1 cm in diameter can be identified in 60 to 75 percent of cases with the CT scan.[215–217] Adrenal scintillation scanning with ^{131}I-6-iodomethyl-19-norcholesterol (NP-59) is a technique based on the uptake of cholesterol by the adrenal gland. Several reports suggest that adenomas are identified with reasonably good accuracy, but this procedure is not generally available for routine clinical use. Dexamethasone in a dose of 0.5 to 1.0 mg every 6 h suppresses the uptake in glands with bilateral hyperplasia but not in those with adenoma.

Plasma 18-Hydroxycorticosterone Levels

The plasma concentration of 18-hydroxycorticosterone, a precursor of aldosterone, can help distinguish between patients with aldosteronomas and bilateral hyperplasia. Levels are generally higher in patients with APAs than in those with bilateral hyperplasia.[218]

Cushing's Syndrome

PREVALENCE

Cushing's syndrome can be categorized broadly into cases that are ACTH-dependent and those that are not.[219] Examples of the former include pituitary microadenomas (known as

Cushing's disease) and the ectopic ACTH syndrome (such as from small-cell lung carcinomas or bronchial carcinoids). Examples of the latter include primary adrenal abnormalities, such as benign or malignant adrenocortical tumors or, rarely, bilateral micronodular or macronodular hyperplasia. Of all cases of Cushing's syndrome, approximately 70 percent are ACTH-dependent, whereas 30 percent are not.

Previously it was thought that Cushing's syndrome was a cause of hypertension in only about 0.2 percent of cases. This is undoubtedly an underestimate because many cases of pituitary microadenomas are now detected by high-resolution MRI (before and after administration of Gd-DTPA)[220] or by inferior petrosal sinus ACTH sampling.[221] Moreover, many patients may have escaped the diagnosis before it was appreciated that the disease can be cyclical with episodic cortisol secretion.[222,223]

CLINICAL FINDINGS

Table 57-9 outlines clinical clues for the diagnosis of Cushing's syndrome. There are many overweight, hypertensive diabetics who bruise easily but do not have Cushing's syndrome. Their weight gain, however, is usually gradual rather than rapid, and any striae are usually white rather than violaceous. They may have a "buffalo hump" but do not often have prominent supraclavicular fat pads. Acne, if present, rarely extends to areas such as the anterior chest wall. Control of blood glucose is usually not difficult, unlike in the patient with Cushing's syndrome who often requires relatively high doses of insulin because of the insulin resistance associated with hypercortisolism.

SPECIAL DIAGNOSTIC TESTS (TABLE 57-10)

Although the plasma cortisol level is often elevated in Cushing's syndrome, its measurement is not a recommended screening test because secretion may be cyclical or episodic.[222,223] A better screening test, albeit imperfect, is measurement of the excretion of free cortisol and creatinine in two or three consecutive 24-hour urine specimens.[219,224] The urine collection is clearly invalid if the excretion of creatinine

TABLE 57-9

CLINICAL CLUES TO THE DIAGNOSIS OF CUSHING'S SYNDROME

1. Rapid weight gain
2. Truncal obesity
3. Moon facies with plethora
4. Purple striae (>1 cm width)
5. Supraclavicular fat pads
6. Glucose intolerance
7. Hypokalemia
8. Acne, especially nonfacial areas
9. Hirsutism
10. Premenopausal oligomenorrhea or amenorrhea

TABLE 57-10

SPECIAL TESTS FOR THE DIAGNOSIS OF CUSHING'S SYNDROME

1. Plasma cortisol
2. Urinary free cortisol[a]
3. Overnight dexamethasone suppression test (high dose)[a]
4. Plasma ACTH
5. Adrenal CT scan
6. Chest CT scan
7. Pituitary MRI
8. Petrosal vein ACTH levels

[a] Most important special screening tests.

is below 10 mg/kg per day. Another practical and inexpensive screening test is the overnight dexamethasone suppression test.[219,224,225] A baseline serum cortisol measurement is made at 8 A.M., 1 mg dexamethasone is taken by mouth at 11 P.M. that evening, and the plasma cortisol measurement is repeated at 8 A.M. the next morning. If the post-dexamethasone plasma cortisol is suppressed to a level below 5 μg/dL, Cushing's syndrome is unlikely. Although false-positive tests can occur with alcoholism, depression, or acute illness, normal suppressibility of cortisol is unlikely (<5 percent) in patients with Cushing's syndrome.

If the urinary free cortisol is elevated, or plasma cortisol does not suppress adequately with the overnight dexamethasone suppression test, then the patient has a high likelihood of Cushing's syndrome; the next step is to identify whether the cause is ACTH-dependent or not. This involves more sophisticated and expensive testing that is best performed by an endocrinologist. Examples include ACTH radioimmunoassays, the corticotropin-releasing hormone (CRH) stimulation test (with or without dexamethasone), the high-dose dexamethasone suppression test, the metyrapone test, and the plasma ACTH or cortisol responses to hypoglycemic or naloxone stimulation.[226]

LOCALIZATION METHODS

The most common cause of Cushing's syndrome is Cushing's disease due to pituitary microadenomas. The problem is that most lesions are tiny, averaging only 3 to 6 mm in diameter, and hence pituitary CT scans are typically normal. Even Gd-DPTA-enhanced MRI (to detect the focal hypointense abnormality) is negative in up to 30 to 50 percent of patients with surgically proven microadenomas.[220] Venous sampling for CRH-stimulated ACTH levels in the inferior petrosal vein sinuses is helpful in localizing the tumor, but is a complex and invasive test.[221]

In contrast to pituitary microadenomas, the CT scan is excellent for identification of primary adrenal tumors causing Cushing's syndrome, and MRI offers no advantage.[227] Tumors producing the ectopic ACTH or ectopic CRH syndrome can usually be detected by either CT, MRI, or radionuclide imaging with pentreotide labeled with indium-111.[219]

Pheochromocytoma

PREVALENCE

Only about 1 in 1000 hypertensive patients has pheochromocytoma. About 10 percent of pheochromocytomas are inherited. When in the adrenal, familial pheochromocytomas are usually bilateral, but they are also more often extraadrenal or malignant. Multiple endocrine neoplasia (MEN) types IIa and IIb are autosomal dominant disorders, often with mutations in exon 10, 11, or 16 of the *RET* protooncogene located on chromosome 10.[228] MEN IIa includes pheochromocytoma, medullary thyroid carcinoma, and parathyroid hyperplasia. MEN IIb includes pheochromocytoma, medullary thyroid carcinoma, and a phenotype with Marfanoid habitus and mucosal neuromas.

CLINICAL FINDINGS

Table 57-11 outlines clinical clues for the diagnosis of pheochromocytoma. The initial clinical suspicion usually occurs because the patient complains of severe headaches (often of the vascular type), inappropriate sweating, or palpitations.[229] The first hint can occur, however, when the patient has hypertension that is difficult to control; when the patient has neurofibromatosis, café-au-lait spots, von Hipple–Lindau disease, Sturge-Weber disease, or tuberous sclerosis; when the patient exhibits a pressor response to beta blockers; or when the family history reveals hypertension plus either thyroid carcinoma or hyperparathyroidism.

SPECIAL DIAGNOSTIC TESTS (TABLE 57-12)

Urinary Catecholamine Screening Tests

Measurements of the urinary excretion of total catecholamines, metanephrine, and vanillylmandelic acid are the most commonly used screening tests for pheochromocytoma. The 24-h urine measurement of metanephrine and creatinine is the best of these three options.[230]

Gitlow et al.[231] reported that the ratio of urinary metanephrine (expressed in micrograms) to creatinine (expressed in

TABLE 57-11

CLINICAL CLUES TO THE DIAGNOSIS OF PHEOCHROMOCYTOMA

1. Classic symptom triad of headaches, sweating, and palpitations
2. Hypertension difficult to control
3. Inappropriate sinus tachycardia
4. Orthostatic hypotension
5. Recurrent arrhythmias
6. Neurofibromatosis, café-au-lait spots, von Hippel–Lindau disease, Sturge-Weber disease, tuberous sclerosis
7. Previously catastrophic anesthesia or surgery
8. Pressor response to beta blockers
9. Family history of pheochromocytoma, medullary thyroid carcinoma, or hyperparathyroidism

TABLE 57-12

SPECIAL TESTS FOR THE DIAGNOSIS OF PHEOCHROMOCYTOMA

1. Urinary metanephrine to creatinine ratio[a]
2. Plasma catecholamines[a]
3. Plasma normetanephrine
4. Clonidine suppression test
5. Abdominal CT scan
6. Abdominal MRI scan
7. Meta-iodobenzylguanidine scan

[a] Most important special screening tests.

milligrams) was above 2.2 in 90 of 92 patients with pheochromocytoma but in only 2 percent of control subjects without pheochromocytoma. Kaplan et al.[232] documented the usefulness of the metanephrine-to-creatinine ratio from single-voided urine specimens. The highest ratio was 0.56 in 10 untreated adult hypertensive patients without pheochromocytoma, whereas the lowest ratio was 2.8 in multiple urine samples from seven adult patients with pheochromocytoma. A ratio above 1 is strongly suggestive of pheochromocytoma in an untreated patient over 15 years of age with otherwise uncomplicated hypertension.

Elevated urinary metanephrine levels have been noted in patients with coma and increased intracranial pressure as well as in patients with ruptured intracranial aneurysms.[233] False-negative urinary metanephrine levels can occur for 24 to 72 h following the use of methylglucamine contrast media for angiography or intravenous pyelography.[234]

Plasma Catecholamine Levels

Radioenzymatic measurements of plasma catecholamines (usually both norepinephrine and epinephrine) or plasma metanephrines (especially normetanephrine) in the supine and rested state are elevated in 90 to 96 percent of patients with pheochromocytoma.[235–237] Levels may even be abnormal in occasional patients with normal urinary screening tests or when blood pressure is not elevated. In general, there is minimal overlap between catecholamine levels of patients with pheochromocytoma and the highest catecholamine levels of either normotensive subjects or uncomplicated patients with essential hypertension. A common clinical dilemma occurs, however, when samples are drawn from patients with essential hypertension who are undergoing acute stress. For example, marked elevations of plasma catecholamines can accompany acute myocardial infarction,[238,239] subarachnoid hemorrhage,[240] clonidine withdrawal syndrome,[241] volume depletion, and other stressful clinical settings. Less striking but still abnormally elevated plasma catecholamines can also be a consequence of antihypertensive drug therapy including diuretics,[242] hydralazine,[243,244] short-acting calcium channel blockers,[245] labetalol,[246] and alpha blockers.[247,248]

To reduce the effects of stress or ambulation, an indwelling intravenous catheter or heparin lock should be placed, with the patient rested in a quiet area in the supine position for at least 20 min before obtaining the blood sample for plasma catecholamines. Plasma levels of dopamine should be obtained along with the norepinephrine and epinephrine levels, because malignant pheochromocytomas rarely secrete only dopamine.[249] In addition, rare patients with hypertension have episodic surges of dopamine with hypertensive episodes that can mimic pheochromocytoma.[250]

Clonidine Suppression Test

The clonidine suppression test is very useful to differentiate pheochromocytoma from essential hypertension in patients with elevated levels of plasma catecholamines.[251] It is often expedient to proceed directly to this test when plasma catecholamines are first measured. A dose of 0.3 mg of clonidine is given, and plasma catecholamine levels are drawn immediately before and 3 h later. Blood pressure and heart rate are reduced similarly in hypertensive pheochromocytoma and nonpheochromocytoma patients. In patients with pheochromocytoma, elevated levels of plasma norepinephrine (and to a lesser extent epinephrine) are essentially unchanged after clonidine, whereas these are reduced markedly (i.e., by at least 50 percent and to a level below 500 pg/mL) in patients with essential hypertension. This is because the central action of clonidine does not block peripheral production of catecholamines. Elevated plasma catecholamine levels occur in some patients with autonomic epilepsy, but these are also suppressed by clonidine.[252]

Suppression of plasma norepinephrine by clonidine in patients with pheochromocytoma (i.e., a false-negative test) has been noted rarely in metastatic, epinephrine-screening, and otherwise uncomplicated pheochromocytoma.[253,524] Moreover, false-negative clonidine suppression tests are not uncommon in patients with pheochromocytoma whose baseline plasma catecholamine levels are not elevated at the time of testing.[255,256] For optimal interpretation, the clonidine suppression test should be performed under controlled environmental conditions when the patient is not actively receiving concomitant antihypertensive therapy.

LOCALIZATION METHODS

Abdominal CT scans with thin cuts through the adrenals are the primary localization procedure because the average tumor size is large, approximately 4.5 cm.[257] The CT scan is effective in localizing intraabdominal pheochromocytomas in 90 percent or more of cases.[258,259]

MRI is another useful procedure (especially in pregnancy) for the identification of pheochromocytoma, which produces a high signal intensity on T2-weighted images, often described as a "light bulb" appearance (Fig. 57-3).[260,261] False-negative tests occur rarely, however, with either CT or MRI or with scintigraphic imaging with [131]I- or ^{123}I-labeled meta-iodo-benzylguanidine (MIBG), a radiolabeled analogue of guanethidine that is concentrated in adrenergic tissue. MIBG scans have demonstrated pheochromocytoma tumors in occasional patients in whom the CT scan was negative.[262] The MIBG scan, however, should be used as a localizing rather than a screening procedure.[263] It is especially useful in patients suspected of multiple or metastatic pheochromocytomas and in occasional patients with repeatedly abnormal catecholamine levels but a normal abdominal CT scan.

REFERENCES

1. Perloff D, Grim C, Flack J, Frohlich ED, Hill M, McDonald M, et al. Human blood pressure determination by sphygmomanometry. *Circulation* 1993; 88:2460–2470.
2. Kaplan NM. Misdiagnosis of systemic hypertension and recommendations for improvement. *Am J Cardiol* 1987; 60:1383–1386.
3. Nielsen PE, Janniche H. The accuracy of auscultatory measurement of arm blood pressure in very obese subjects. *Acta Med Scand* 1974; 195:403–409.
4. Beevers DG. Sphygmomanometer cuff sizes—new recommendations. *J Hum Hypertens* 1990; 4:587–588.
5. Messerli FH, Ventura HO, Amodeo C. Osler's maneuver and pseudohypertension. *N Engl J Med* 1985; 312:1548–1551.
6. Oster JR, Materson BJ. Pseudohypertension: A diagnostic dilemma. *J Clin Hypertens* 1986; 4:307–313.
7. Vardan S, Mookherjee S, Warner R, Smulyan H. Systolic hypertension: Direct and indirect BP measurements. *Arch Intern Med* 1983; 143:935–938.
8. Kuwajima I, Hoh E, Suzuki Y, Matsushita S, Kuramoto K. Pseudohypertension in the elderly. *J Hypertens* 1990; 8:429–432.

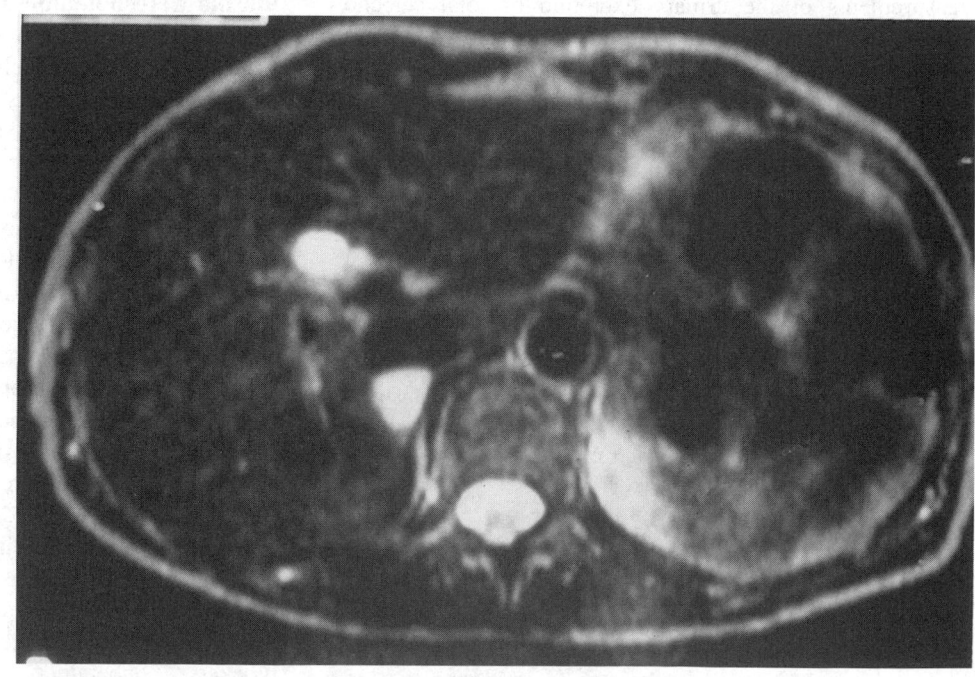

FIGURE 57-3
"Light bulb" appearance of pheochromocytoma on T2-weighted MR image.

9. Belmin J, Visintin J-M, Salvatore R, Sebban C, Moulias R. Osler's maneuver: Absence of usefulness for the detection of pseudohypertension in an elderly population. *Am J Med* 1995; 98:42–49.

10. Cavallini MC, Roman MJ, Blank SG, Pini R, Pickering TG, Devereux RB. Association of the auscultatory gap with vascular disease in hypertensive patients. *Ann Intern Med* 1996; 124:877–883.

11. Goldhill DR. Bilateral simultaneous indirect systolic blood pressure measurements. *Cardiovasc Res* 1986; 20:774–777.

12. Mitchell PL, Parlin RW, Blackburn H. Effect of vertical displacement of the arm on indirect blood-pressure measurement. *N Engl J Med* 1964; 271:72–74.

13. Kahn HS, Bain RP. Vertex-corrected blood pressure in black girls. *Hypertension* 1987; 9:390–397.

14. Currens JH. A comparison of the blood pressure in the lying and standing positions: A study of five hundred men and five hundred women. *Am Heart J* 1948; 35:646–654.

15. Applegate WB, Davis BR, Black HR, Smith WM, Miller ST, Burlando AJ. Prevalence of postural hypotension at baseline in the Systolic Hypertension in the Elderly Program (SHEP) cohorts. *J Am Geriatr Soc* 1991; 39:1057–1064.

16. Ward C, Kenny RA. Reproducibility of orthostatic hypotension in symptomatic elderly. *Am J Med* 1996; 100:418–422.

17. Masuo K, Mikami H, Ogihara T, Tuck ML. Changes in frequency of orthostatic hypotension in elderly hypertensive patients under medications. *Am J Hypertens* 1996; 9:263–268.

18. Davis BR, Langford HG, Blaufox MD, Curb JD, Polk BF, Shulman NB. The association of postural changes in systolic blood pressure and mortality in persons with hypertension: The Hypertension Detection and Follow-up Program experience. *Circulation* 1987; 75:340–346.

19. Gordon T, Sorlie P, Kannel WB. Problems in the assessment of blood pressure: The Framingham Study. *Int J Epidemiol* 1976; 5:327–334.

20. Conway J. Blood pressure and heart rate variability. *J Hypertens* 1986; 4:261–263.

21. Mancia G, Ferrari A, Gregorini L, Parati G, Pomidossi G, Bertinieri G, et al. Blood pressure variability in man: Its relation to high blood pressure, age and baroreflex sensitivity. *Clin Sci* 1980; 59(suppl 6):401–404.

22. Bevan AT, Honour AJ, Scott FH. Direct arterial pressure recording in unrestricted man. *Clin Sci* 1969, 36.329–334.

23. Pickering TG. Ambulatory monitoring and the definition of hypertension. *J Hypertens* 1992; 10:401–409.

24. Armitage P, Fox W, Rose GA, Tinker CM. The variability of measurements of casual blood pressure. II. Survey experience. *Clin Sci* 1966; 30:337–344.

25. Fotherby MD, Potter JF. Variation of within visit blood pressure readings at a single visit in the elderly and their relationship to ambulatory measurements. *J Hum Hypertens* 1994; 8:107–111.

26. Souchek J, Stamler J, Dyer AR, Paul O, Lepper MH. The value of two or three versus a single reading of blood pressure at a first visit. *J Chronic Dis* 1979; 32:197–210.

27. Kannel WB, Sorlie P, Gordon T. Labile hypertension: A faulty concept? The Framingham Study. *Circulation* 1980; 61:1183–1187.

28. Glock CY, Vought RL, Clark EG, Schweitzer MD. Studies in hypertension. II. Variability of daily blood pressure measurements in the same individuals over a three-week period. *J Chronic Dis* 1956; 4:469–476.

29. Watson RDS, Lumb R, Young MA, Stallard TJ, Davies P, Littler WA. Variation in cuff blood pressure in untreated outpatients with mild hypertension—implications for initiating antihypertensive treatment. *J Hypertens* 1987; 5:207–211.

30. Hypertension Detection and Follow-up Program Cooperative Group. Blood pressure studies in 14 communities. A two-stage screen for hypertension. *JAMA* 1977; 237:2385–2391.

31. SHEP Cooperative Research Group. Prevention of stroke by antihypertensive drug treatment in older persons with isolated systolic hypertension. Final results of the Systolic Hypertension in the Elderly Program. *JAMA* 1991; 265:3255–3264.

32. Rosner B, Polk BF. The implications of blood pressure variability for clinical and screening purposes. *J Chronic Dis* 1979; 32:451–461.

33. Rosner B, Polk BF. Predictive values of routine blood pressure measurements in screening for hypertension. *Am J Epidemiol* 1983; 117:429–442.

34. Julius S, Ellis CN, Pascual AV, Matice M, Hansson L, Hunyor SN, et al. Home blood pressure determination. Value in borderline ("labile") hypertension. *JAMA* 1974; 229:663–666.

35. Perloff D, Sokolow M, Cowan R. The prognostic value of ambulatory blood pressures. *JAMA* 1983; 249:2792–2798.

36. White WB. Assessment of patients with office hypertension by 24-hour noninvasive ambulatory blood pressure monitoring. *Arch Intern Med* 1986; 146:2196–2199.

37. Marchesi E, Perani G, Falaschi F, Negro C, Catalano O, Ravetta V, et al. Metabolic risk factors in white coat hypertension. *J Hum Hypertens* 1994; 8:475–479.

38. Cavallini MC, Roman MJ, Pickering TG, Schwartz JE, Pini R, Devereux RB. Is white coat hypertension associated with arterial disease or left ventricular hypertrophy? *Hypertension* 1995; 26:413–419.

39. National High Blood Pressure Education Program Coordinating Committee. National High Blood Pressure Education Program Working Group Report on Ambulatory Blood Pressure Monitoring. *Arch Intern Med* 1990; 150:2270–2280.

40. Grin JM, McCabe EJ, White WB. Management of hypertension after ambulatory blood pressure monitoring. *Ann Intern Med* 1993; 118:833–837.

41. Yarows SA, Khoury S, Sowers JR. Cost effectiveness of 24-hour ambulatory blood pressure monitoring in evaluation and treatment of essential hypertension. *Am J Hypertens* 1994; 7:464–468.

42. Pickering TG, James GD, Boddie JC, Harshfield GA, Blank S, Laragh J. How common is white coat hypertension? *JAMA* 1988; 259:225–228.

43. White WB, Lund-Johansen P, McCabe E, Omvik P. Clinical evaluation of the Accutracker II ambulatory blood pressure monitor: Assessment of performance in two countries and comparison with sphygmomanometry and intra-arterial blood pressure at rest and during exercise. *J Hypertens* 1989; 7:967–975.

44. Santucci S, Cates EM, James GD, Schussel YR, Steiner D, Pickering TG. A comparison of two ambulatory blood pressure monitors, the Del Mar Avionics Pressurometer IV and the Spacelabs 90202. *Am J Hypertens* 1989; 2:797–799.

45. Zachariah PK, Krier JD. Clinical uses of ambulatory blood pressure monitoring. *J Hypertens* 1991; 9(suppl 1):S7–S12.

46. Cox J, O'Malley K, Atkins N, O'Brien E. A comparison of the twenty-four-hour blood pressure profile in normotensive and hypertensive subjects. *J Hypertens* 1991; 9(suppl 1):S3–S6.

47. Staessen JA, Fagard R, Thijs L, Amery A. A consensus view on the technique of ambulatory blood pressure monitoring. *Hypertension* 1995; 26:912–918.

48. Gosse P, Roudaut R, Reynaud P, Jullien E, Dallocchio M. Relationship between left ventricular mass and noninvasive monitoring of blood pressure. *Am J Hypertens* 1989; 2:631–633.

49. Verdecchia P, Schillaci G, Boldrini F, Guerrieri M, Gatteschi C, Benemio G, et al. Risk stratification of left ventricular hypertrophy in systemic hypertension using noninvasive ambulatory blood pressure monitoring. *Am J Cardiol* 1990; 66:583–590.

50. Prisant LM, Carr AA. Ambulatory blood pressure monitoring and echocardiographic left ventricular wall thickness and mass. *Am J Hypertens* 1990; 3:81–89.

51. White WB, Schulman P, Dey HM, Katz AM. Rapid left ventricular filling is more dependent on age and twenty-four-hour blood pressure than on cardiac size. *J Hypertens* 1989; 7(suppl 6):S102–S103.

52. Giaconi S, Levanti C, Fommei E, Innocenti F, Seghieri G, Palla L, et al. Microalbuminuria and casual and ambulatory blood pressure monitoring in normotensives and in patients with borderline and mild essential hypertension. *Am J Hypertens* 1989; 2:259–261.

53. Shimada K, Kawamoto A, Matsubayashi K, Ozawa T. Silent cerebrovascular disease in the elderly. Correlation with ambulatory pressure. *Hypertension* 1990; 16:692–699.

54. Joint National Committee on Detection, Evaluation, and Treatment of High Blood Pressure. The fifth report of the Joint National Committee on detection, evaluation, and treatment of high blood pressure (JNC V). *Arch Intern Med* 1993; 153:154–183.

55. Hall WD. Initial evaluation of the patient with hypertension. In: Wollam GL, Hall WD, eds. *Hypertension Management: Clinical Practice and Therapeutic Dilemmas.* Chicago: Year Book; 1988:145–163.

56. Gifford RW Jr, Kirkendall W, O'Conner DT, Weidman W. Office evaluation of hypertension. A statement for health professionals by a writing group of the Council for High Blood Pressure Research, American Heart Association. *Hypertension* 1989; 13:283–293.

57. Bulpitt CJ, Dollery CT, Carne S. Changes in symptoms of hypertensive patients after referral to hospital clinic. *Br Heart J* 1976; 38:121–128.

58. Fletcher EC. The relationship between systemic hypertension and obstructive sleep apnea: Facts and theory. *Am J Med* 1995; 98:118–128.

59. Strollo PJ Jr, Rogers RM. Obstructive sleep apnea. *N Engl J Med* 1996; 334:99–104.

60. Working Group on Management of Patients with Hypertension and High Blood Cholesterol. National Education Programs Working Group Report on the Management of Patients with Hypertension and High Blood Cholesterol. *Ann Intern Med* 1991; 114:224–237.

61. Kannel WB, Castelli WP, McNamara PM, McKee PA, Feinleib M. Role of blood pressure in the development of congestive heart failure. *N Engl J Med* 1972; 287:781–787.

62. Shulman NB, Martinez B, Brogan D, Carr AA, Miles CG. Financial cost as an obstacle to hypertension therapy. *Am J Public Health* 1986; 76:1105–1108.

63. Roccella EJ. Cost of hypertensive medications: Is it a barrier to hypertension control? *Geriatrics* 1989; 44(suppl B):49–55.

64. Stason WB. Cost and quality trade-offs in the treatment of hypertension. *Hypertension* 1989; 13(suppl I):I145–I148.

65. Shulman NB, Levinson RM, Dever GEA, Porter RS, Owen SL, Hall WD. Impact of cost problems on morbidity in a hypertensive population. *Am J Prev Med* 1991; 7:374–378.

66. Herron RE, Schneider RH, Mandarino JV, Alexander CN, Walton KG. Cost-effective hypertension management: Comparison of drug therapies with an alterative program. *Am J Managed Care* 1996; 2:427–437.

67. Kincaid-Smith P, McMichael J, Murphy EA. The clinical course and pathology of hypertension with papilledema (malignant hypertension). *Q J Med* 1958; 105:117–153.

68. Ahmed MEK, Walker J, Beevers DG, Beevers M. Lack of difference between malignant and accelerated hypertension. *Br Med J* 1986; 292:235–237.

69. Davis BA, Crook JE, Vestal RE, Oates JA. Prevalence of renovascular hypertension in patients with grade III or IV hypertensive retinopathy. *N Engl J Med* 1979; 301:1273–1276.

70. Maheswaran R, Gill JS, Davies P, Beevers DG. High blood pressure due to alcohol. A rapidly reversible effect. *Hypertension* 1991; 17:787–792.

71. Messerli FH, Frohlich ED. High blood pressure. A side effect of drugs, poisons, and food. *Arch Intern Med* 1979; 139:682–687.

72. Virmani R, Robinowitz M, Smialek JE, Smyth DF. Cardiovascular effects of cocaine: An autopsy study of 40 patients. *Am Heart J* 1988; 115:1068–1076.

73. Isner JM, Estes NAM III, Thompson PD, Costanzo-Nordin MR, Subramanian R, Miller G, et al. Acute cardiac events temporally related to cocaine abuse. *N Engl J Med* 1986; 315:1438–1443.

74. Lange RA, Cigarroa RG, Yancy CW Jr, Willard JE, Popma JJ, Sills MN, et al. Cocaine-induced coronary-artery vasoconstriction. *N Engl J Med* 1989; 321:1557–1562.

75. Nademanee K, Gorelick DA, Josephson MA, Ryan MA, Wilkins JN, Robertson HA, et al. Myocardial ischemia during cocaine withdrawal. *Ann Intern Med* 1989; 111:876–880.

76. Brody SL, Slovis CM, Wrenn KD. Cocaine-related medical problems: Consecutive series of 233 patients. *Am J Med* 1990; 88:325–331.

77. Blachley JD, Knochel JP. Tobacco chewer's hypokalemia: Licorice revisited. *N Engl J Med* 1980; 302:784–785.

78. Dietz AJ Jr. Amphetamine-like reactions to phenylpropanolamine. *JAMA* 1981; 245:601–602.

79. White WB, Baker LH. Episodic hypertension secondary to panic disorder. *Arch Intern Med* 1986; 146:1129–1130.

80. Bulpitt CJ. Is systolic pressure more important than diastolic pressure? *J Human Hypertens* 1990; 4:471–474.

81. Hall WD. Management of systolic hypertension in the elderly. *Semin Nephrol* 1996; 16:299–308.

82. Walther RJ, Tifft CP. High blood pressure in the competitive athlete: Guidelines and recommendations. *Phys Sports Med* 1985; 113:93–114.

83. Lichtman J, O'Rourke RA, Klein A, Karliner JS. Electrocardiogram of the athlete. Alterations simulating those of organic heart disease. *Arch Intern Med* 1973; 132:763–770.

84. Huston TP, Puffer JC, Rodney WM. The athletic heart syndrome. *N Engl J Med* 1985; 313:24–32.

85. Roeske WP, O'Rourke RA, Klein A, Leopold G, Karliner JS. Noninvasive evaluation of ventricular hypertrophy in professional athletes. *Circulation* 1976; 52:286–292.

86. Morganroth J, Maron BJ, Henry WL, Epstein SE. Comparative left ventricular dimensions in trained athletes. *Ann Intern Med* 1975; 82:521–524.

87. Morales MC, Gleim GW, Marino ND, Stachenfeld NS, Coplan NL. Left ventricular mass in adolescent basketball players. *Cardiovasc Rev Rep* 1992; 13:60–62.

88. Oakley DG, Oakley CM. Significance of abnormal electrocardiograms in highly trained athletes. *Am J Cardiol* 1982; 50:985–989.

89. Maron BT, Roberts WC, McAllister HA, Rosing DR, Epstein SE. Sudden death in young athletes. *Circulation* 1980; 62:218–229.

90. Autore C, Fiorito S, Pelliccia A, Caselli G, Fragola PV, Picelli A, et al. Antimitochondrial autoantibodies in myocardial hypertrophy: Comparison between hypertrophic cardiomyopathy, hypertensive heart disease, and athlete's heart. *Am Heart J* 1988; 116:496–500.

91. Pelliccia A, Maron BJ, Spataro A, Proschan MA, Spirito P. The upper limit of physiologic cardiac hypertrophy in highly trained elite athletes. *N Engl J Med* 1991; 324:295–301.

92. Spirito P, Pelliccia A, Proschan MA, Granata M, Spataro A, Bellone P, et al. Morphology of the "athlete's heart" assessed by echocardiography in 947 elite athletes representing 27 sports. *Am J Cardiol* 1994; 74:802–806.

93. Colan SD, Sanders SP, MacPherson D, Borow KU. Left ventricular diastolic function in elite athletes with physiologic cardiac hypertrophy. *J Am Coll Cardiol* 1985; 6:545–549.

94. Harshfield GA, James GD, Schlussel Y, Yee LS, Blank SG, Pickering TG. Do laboratory tests of blood pressure reactivity predict blood pressure changes during everyday life? *Am J Hypertens* 1988; 1:168–174.

95. Lauer MS, Pashkow FJ, Harvey SA, Marwick TH, Thomas JD. Angiographic and prognostic implications of an exaggerated exercise systolic blood pressure response and rest systolic blood pressure in adults undergoing evaluation for suspected coronary artery disease. *J Am Coll Cardiol* 1995; 26:1630–1636.

96. Keith NM, Wagener HP, Barker ND. Some different types of essential hypertension: Their course and prognosis. *Am J Med Sci* 1939; 197:332–343.

97. Kagan A, Aurell E, Dobree J, Hara K, McKendrick C, Michaelson I, et al. A note on signs in the fundus oculi and arterial hypertension: Conventional assessment and significance. *Bull WHO* 1966; 34:955–960.

98. Kannel WB, Gordon T, Offutt D. Left ventricular hypertrophy by electrocardiogram. Prevalence, incidence, and mortality in the Framingham Study. *Ann Intern Med* 1969; 71:89–105.

99. Dougherty AH, Naccarelli GV, Gray EL, Hicks CH, Goldstein RA. Congestive heart failure with normal systolic function. *Am J Cardiol* 1984; 54:778–782.

100. Topol EJ, Traill TA, Fortuin NJ. Hypertensive hypertrophic-cardiomyopathy of the elderly. *N Engl J Med* 1985; 312:277–283.

101. Brogan WC III, Hillis LD, Flores ED, Lange RA. The natural history of isolated left ventricular diastolic dysfunction. *Am J Med* 1992; 92:627–630.

102. Goldsmith SR, Dick C. Differentiating systolic from diastolic heart failure: Pathophysiologic and therapeutic considerations. *Am J Med* 1993; 95:645–655.

103. Levy RD, Shapiro LM, Wright C, Mockus L, Fox KM. Syndrome X: The hemodynamic significance of ST segment depression. *Br Heart J* 1986; 56:353–357.

104. Cannon RO III, Epstein SE. "Microvascular angina" as a cause of chest pain with angiographically normal coronary arteries. *Am J Cardiol* 1988; 61:1338–1343.

105. Brush JE Jr, Cannon RO III, Schenke WH, Bonow RO, Leon MB, Maron BJ, et al. Angina due to coronary microvascular disease in hypertensive patients without left ventricular hypertrophy. *N Engl J Med* 1988; 319:1302–1307.

106. Picano E, Lucarini AR, Lattanzi F, Marini C, Distante A, Salvetti A, et al. ST segment depression elicited by dipyrimadole infusion in asymptomatic hypertensive patients. *Hypertension* 1990; 16:19–25.

107. Opherk D, Mall G, Zebe H, Schwarz F, Weihe E, Manthey J, et al. Reduction of coronary reserve: A mechanism for angina pectoris in patients with arterial hypertension and normal coronary arteries. *Circulation* 1984; 69:1–7.

108. Hall D, Charocopos F, Froer K-L, Rudolph W. ECG changes during long-term minoxidil therapy for severe hypertension. *Arch Intern Med* 1979; 139:790–794.

109. O'Mailia JJ, Sander GE, Giles TD. Nifedipine-associated myocardial

ischemia or infarction in the treatment of hypertensive urgencies. *Ann Intern Med* 1987; 107:185–186.

110. Pepi M, Alimento M, Maltagliata A, Guazzi MD. Cardiac hypertrophy in hypertension. Repolarization abnormalities elicited by rapid lowering of pressure. *Hypertension* 1988; 11:84–91.

111. Phillips RA, Goldman ME, Ardeljan M, Eison HB, Shimabukuro S, Krakoff LR. Isolated T-wave abnormalities and evaluation of left ventricular wall motion after nifedipine for severe hypertension. *Am J Hypertens* 1991; 4:432–437.

112. Guazzi MD, Alimento M, Guazzi M, Maltagliati A, Pepi M. Acute blood pressure reduction in the presence of hypertensive cardiac hypertrophy: Any interference with coronary circulation? *Scand J Clin Lab Invest* 1989; 196(suppl):53–61.

113. Davie JC, Langley JO, Dodson WH, Eddleman EE Jr. Clinical and kinetocardiographic studies of paradoxical precordial motion. *Am Heart J* 1962; 63:775–807.

114. Eilen SD, Crawford MH, O'Rourke RA. Accuracy of precordial palpation for detecting increased left ventricular volume. *Ann Intern Med* 1983; 99:628–630.

115. Lusted LB, Keats TE. *Atlas of Roentgenographic Measurement*, 4th ed. Chicago: Year Book; 1978:225.

116. Romhilt DW, Estes EH Jr. A point-score system for the ECG diagnosis of left ventricular hypertrophy. *Am Heart J* 1968; 75:752–758.

117. Murphy ML, Thenabadu PN, Soyza ND, Doherty JE, Meade J, Baker BJ, et al. Reevaluation of electrocardiographic criteria for left, right and combined cardiac ventricular hypertrophy. *Am J Cardiol* 1984; 53:1140–1147.

118. Molloy TJ, Okin PM, Devereux RB, Kligfield P. Electrocardiographic detection of left ventricular hypertrophy by the simple QRS voltage-duration production. *J Am Coll Cardiol* 1992; 20:1180–1186.

119. Norman JE, Levy D, Campbell G, Bailey JJ. Improved detection of echocardiographic left ventricular hypertrophy using a new electrocardiographic algorithm. *J Am Coll Cardiol* 1993; 21:1680–1686.

120. Tarazi RC, Miller A, Frohlich ED, Dustan HP. Electrocardiographic changes reflecting left atrial abnormality in hypertension. *Circulation* 1966; 34:818–822.

121. Savage DD, Drayer JIM, Henry WL, Mathews EC Jr, Ware JH, Gardin JM, et al. Echocardiographic assessment of cardiac anatomy and function in hypertensive subjects. *Circulation* 1979; 59:623–632.

122. Savage DD, Garrison RJ, Kannel WB, Levy D, Anderson SJ, Stokes J III, et al. The spectrum of left ventricular hypertrophy in a general population sample: The Framingham Study. *Circulation* 1987; 75(suppl I):I26–I33.

123. Baker BJ, Bass KM, Scovil JA, Kane JJ, Murphy ML. M-mode echocardiographic correlates of left ventricular mass: An anatomic correlation. *J Cardiovasc Ultrasonogr* 1982; 1:263–266.

124. Devereaux RB, Alonso DR, Lutas EM, Gottlieb GJ, Campo E, Sachs I, et al. Echocardiographic assessment of left ventricular hypertrophy: Comparison to necropsy findings. *Am J Cardiol* 1986; 57:450–458.

125. Levy D, Anderson KM, Savage DD, Kannel WB, Christiansen JC, Castelli WP. Echocardiographically detected left ventricular hypertrophy: Prevalence and risk factors. The Framingham Heart Study. *Ann Intern Med* 1988; 108:7–13.

126. McLenachan JM, Henderson E, Morris KI, Dargie HJ. Ventricular arrhythmias in patients with hypertensive left ventricular hypertrophy. *N Engl J Med* 1987; 317:787–792.

127. Devereux RB. Importance of left ventricular mass as a predictor of cardiovascular morbidity in hypertension. *Am J Hypertens* 1989; 2:650–654.

128. Devereux RB. Echocardiographic insights into the pathophysiology and prognostic significance of hypertensive cardiac hypertrophy. *Am J Hypertens* 1989; 2(6 pt 2):186S–195S.

129. Levy D, Garrison RJ, Savage DD, Kannel WB, Castelli WP. Prognostic implications of echocardiography determined left ventricular mass in the Framingham Heart Study. *N Engl J Med* 1990; 322:1561–1566.

130. Koren MJ, Devereux RB, Casale PN, Savage DD, Laragh JH. Relation of left ventricular mass and geometry to morbidity and mortality in uncomplicated essential hypertension. *Ann Intern Med* 1991; 114:345–352.

131. Ghali JK, Liao Y, Simmons B, Castaner A, Cao G, Cooper RS. The prognostic role of left ventricular hypertrophy in patients with or without coronary artery disease. *Ann Intern Med* 1992; 117:831–836.

132. Zehender M, Faber T, Koscheck U, Meinertz T, Just H. Ventricular tachyarrhythmias, myocardial ischemia, and sudden cardiac death in patients with hypertensive heart disease. *Clin Cardiol* 1995; 18:377–383.

133. Liebson PR. Clinical studies of drug reversal of hypertensive left ventricular hypertrophy. *Am J Hypertens* 1990; 3:512–517.

134. Cruickshank JM, Lewis J, Moore V, Dodd C. Reversibility of left ventricular hypertrophy by differing types of antihypertensive therapy. *J Hum Hypertens* 1992; 6:85–90.

135. Liebson PR, Grandits GA, Dianzumba S, Prineas RJ, Grimm RH Jr, Neaton JD, et al, for the TOMHS Research Group. Comparison of five antihypertensive monotherapies and placebo for change in left ventricular mass in patients receiving nutritional-hygienic therapy in the treatment of mild hypertension study (TOMHS). *Circulation* 1995; 91:698–706.

136. Clement DL, De Buyzere M, Duprez D. Left ventricular function and regression of left ventricular hypertrophy in essential hypertension. *Am J Hypertens* 1993; 6:14S–19S.

137. Kapuku GK, Seto S, Mori H, Mori M, Utsunomia T, Suzuki S, et al. Reversal of diastolic dysfunction in borderline hypertension by long-term medical treatment. Longitudinal evaluation by pulsed doppler echocardiography. *Am J Hypertens* 1993; 6:547–553.

138. Moser M. "Cost containment" in the management of hypertension. *Ann Intern Med* 1987; 107:107–108.

139. Kannel WB, Wolf PA, Verter J, McNamara PM. Epidemiologic assessment of the role of blood pressure in stroke. The Framingham Study. *JAMA* 1970; 214:301–310.

140. Qureshi AI, Safdar K, Patel M, Janssen RS, Frankel MR. Stroke in young black patients. Risk factors, subtypes, and prognosis. *Stroke* 1995; 26:1995–1998.

141. Cuneo RH, Caronna JJ. The neurologic complications of hypertension. *Med Clin North Am* 1977; 61:565–580.

142. Tuszynski MH, Petito CK, Levy DE. Risk factors and clinical manifestations of pathologically verified lacunar infarctions. *Stroke* 1989; 20:990–999.

143. Norrving B, Cronqvist S. Clinical and radiologic features of lacunar versus nonlacunar minor stroke. *Stroke* 1989; 20:59–64.

144. Fisher M, Minematsu K. Lacunar stroke: Diagnosis, evaluation, and management. *Heart Dis Stroke* 1992; 1:353–356.

145. Weisberg LA. Computed tomography in the diagnosis of intracranial disease. *Ann Intern Med* 1979; 91:87–105.

146. Blakeley DD, Oddone EZ, Hasselblad V, Simel DL, Matchar DB. Noninvasive carotid artery testing. A meta-analytic review. *Ann Intern Med* 1995; 122:360–367.

147. Carpenter JP, Lexa FJ, Davis JT. Determination of sixty percent or greater carotid artery stenosis by duplex Doppler ultrasonography. *J Vasc Surg* 1995; 22:697–705.

148. Ram CVS, Khoury AS. Hypertensive emergencies. In: Frohlich ED, Cooke JP, eds. *Current Management of Hypertensive and Vascular Diseases*. Philadelphia: Mosby–Year Book; 1992:35–48.

149. Chester EM, Agamanolis DP, Banker BQ, Victor M. Hypertensive encephalopathy: A clinicopathologic study of 20 cases. *Neurology (NY)* 1978; 28:928–939.

150. Odutola TA, Ositelu SB, D'Almeida EA, Okeiyi JC. Supra-normal creatinine clearance in black mild hypertensive patients in Nigeria. *J Hum Hypertens* 1988; 2:133–134.

151. Schmieder RE, Messerli FH, Garavaglia G, Nunez B. Glomerular hyperfiltration indicates early target organ damage in essential hypertension. *JAMA* 1990; 264:2775–2780.

152. Pedersen EB, Mogensen CE. Effect of antihypertensive treatment on urinary albumin excretion, glomerular filtration rate and renal plasma flow in patients with essential hypertension. *Scand J Clin Lab Invest* 1976; 36:231–237.

153. Palatini P, Graniero GR, Mormino P, Mattarei M, Sanzuol F, Cignacco GB, et al, for the HARVEST Study Group. Prevalence and clinical correlates of microalbuminuria in Stage I hypertension. *Am J Hypertens* 1996; 9:334–341.

154. Cerasola G, Cottone S, D'Ignoto G, Grasso L, Mangano MT, Carapelle E, et al. Micro-albuminuria as a predictor of cardiovascular damage in essential hypertension. *J Hypertens* 1989; 7(suppl 6):S332–S333.

155. Ljungman S. Microalbuminuria in essential hypertension. *Am J Hypertens* 1990; 3:956–960.

156. Whelton PK, Klag MJ. Hypertension as a risk factor for renal disease. Review of clinical and epidemiological evidence. *Hypertension* 1989; 13(suppl I):19–27.

157. Feldman HI, Klag MJ, Chiapella AP, Whelton PK. End-stage renal disease in U.S. minority groups. *Am J Kidney Dis* 1992; 19:397–410.

158. Jones CA, Agodoa L. Kidney disease and hypertension in blacks: Scope of the problem. *Am J Kidney Dis* 1993; 4(suppl 1):6–9.

159. Battey LL, Felner JM, Hall WD. Clinical manifestations of 104 patients with diastolic blood pressure ≥140 mmHg. *Emory Univ J Med* 1988; 2:102–105.

160. Mann SJ, Pickering TG. Detection of renovascular hypertension. State of the art: 1992. *Ann Intern Med* 1992; 117:845–853.

161. Hall WD. Secondary causes of hypertension in blacks. In: Hall WD, Saunders E, Shulman NB, eds. *Hypertension in Blacks: Epidemiology, Pathophysiology and Treatment.* Chicago: Year Book; 1985:144–155.

162. Simon N, Franklin SS, Bleifer KH, Maxwell MH. Clinical characteristics of renovascular hypertension. *JAMA* 1972; 220:1209–1216.

163. Pickering TG, Herman L, Devereux RB, Sotelo JE, James GD, Sos TA, et al. Recurrent pulmonary oedema in hypertension due to bilateral renal artery stenosis: Treatment by angioplasty or surgical revascularisation. *Lancet* 1988; 2:551–552.

164. Missouris CG, Buckenham T, Vallance PJT, MacGregor GA. Renal artery stenosis masquerading as congestive heart failure. *Lancet* 1993; 341:1521–1522.

165. Eipper DF, Gifford RW Jr, Stewart BH, Alfidi RJ, McCormack LJ, Vidt DG. Abdominal bruits in renovascular hypertension. *Am J Cardiol* 1976; 37:48–52.

166. Nicholson JP, Alderman MH, Pickering TG, Teichman SL, Sos TA, Laragh JH. Cigarette smoking and renovascular hypertension. *Lancet* 1983; 2:765–766.

167. Vetrovec EW, Landwehr DM, Edwards VE. Incidence of renal artery stenosis in hypertensive patients undergoing coronary angiography. *J Intervent Cardiol* 1989; 2:64–66.

168. Louie J, Isaacson JA, Zierler E, Bergelin RO, Strandness DE Jr. Prevalence of carotid and lower extremity arterial disease in patients with renal artery stenosis. *Am J Hypertens* 1994; 7:436–439.

169. Missouris CG, Buckenham T, Cappuccio FP, MacGregor GA. Renal artery stenosis: A common and important problem in patients with peripheral vascular disease. *Am J Med* 1994; 96:10–14.

170. Shapiro AP, Perez-Stable E, Moutsos SE. Coexistence of renal arterial hypertension and diabetes mellitus. *JAMA* 1965; 192:813–816.

171. National High Blood Pressure Education Program Working Group. 1995 update of the working group reports on chronic renal failure and renovascular hypertension. *Arch Intern Med* 1996; 156:1938–1947.

172. Olin JW, Vidt DG, Gifford RW Jr, Novick AC. Renovascular disease in the elderly: An analysis of 50 patients. *J Am Coll Cardiol* 1985; 5:1232–1238.

173. Sos TA, Pickering TG, Sniderman K, Saddenki S, Case DB, Silane MF, et al. Percutaneous transluminal renal angioplasty in renovascular hypertension due to atheroma or fibromuscular dysplasia. *N Engl J Med* 1983; 309:274–279.

174. Ying CY, Tifft CP, Gavras H, Chobanian AV. Renal revascularization in the azotemic hypertensive patient resistant to therapy. *N Engl J Med* 1984; 311:1070–1075.

175. Hansen KJ, Starr SM, Sands E, Burkart JM, Plonk GW Jr, Dean RH. Contemporary surgical management of renovascular disease. *J Vasc Surg* 1992; 16:319–331.

176. Novick AC. Renal revascularization for atherosclerotic ischemic renal disease. In: Calligaro KD, Dougherty MJ, Dean RH, eds. *Modern Management of Renovascular Hypertension and Renal Salvage.* Baltimore: Williams & Wilkins; 1996:117–123.

177. Setaro JF, Saddler MC, Chen CC, Hoffer PB, Roer DA, Markowitz DM, et al. Simplified captopril renography in diagnosis and treatment of renal artery stenosis. *Hypertension* 1991; 18:289–298.

178. Pollack HM, Banner MP. Current status of excretory urography. A premature epitaph? *Urol Clin North Am* 1985; 12:585–601.

179. Mushlin AI, Thornbury JR. Intravenous pyelography: The case against its routine use. *Ann Intern Med* 1989; 111:58–70.

180. Buonocore E, Meaney TF, Borkowski GP, Pavlicek W, Gallagher J. Digital subtraction angiography of the abdominal aorta and renal arteries. Comparison with conventional aortography. *Radiology* 1981; 139:281–286.

181. Smith CW, Winfield AC, Price RR, Harding DR, Tucker SW, Witt WS, et al. Evaluation of digital venous angiography for the diagnosis of renovascular hypertension. *Radiology* 1982; 144:51–54.

182. Fiedler V, Peters PE. Digital subtraction angiography of renal arteries—pitfalls and benefits. *Cardiology* 1985; 72(suppl 1):10–12.

183. Cigarroa RG, Lange RA, Williams RH, Hillis LD. Dosing of contrast material to prevent contrast nephropathy in patients with renal disease. *Am J Med* 1989; 86:649–652.

184. Harris KG, Smith TP, Cragg AH, Lemke JH. Nephrotoxicity from contrast material in renal insufficiency: Ionic versus nonionic agents. *Radiology* 1991; 179:849–852.

185. Lyons DF, Streck WF, Kem DC, Brown RD, Galloway DC, Williams GR, et al. Captopril stimulation of differential renins in renovascular hypertension. *Hypertension* 1983; 5:615–622.

186. Thibonnier M, Joseph A, Sassano P, Guyenne TT, Corvol P, Raynaud A, et al. Improved diagnosis of unilateral renal artery lesions after captopril administration. *JAMA* 1984; 251:56–60.

187. Tomoda F, Takata M, Ohashi S, Veno H, Ikeda K, Yasumoto K, et al. Captopril-stimulated renal vein renin in hypertensive patients with or without renal artery stenosis. *Am J Hypertens* 1990; 3:918–926.

188. Marks LS, Maxwell MH, Varady PD, Lupu AN, Kaufman JJ. Renovascular hypertension: Does the renal vein renin ratio predict operative results? *J Urol* 1976; 115:365–368.

189. Muller FB, Sealey JE, Case DB, Atlas SA, Pickering TG, Pecker MS, et al. The captopril test for identifying renovascular disease in hypertensive patients. *Am J Med* 1986; 80:633–644.

190. Hall WD. Diagnosis of renovascular hypertension: The captopril stimulation test. *J Med Assoc Ga* 1990; 79:327–329.

191. Hawkins PG, McKnoulty LM, Gordon RD, Klemm SA, Tunny TJ. Noninvasive renal artery duplex ultrasound and computerized nuclear renography to screen for and follow progress in renal artery stenosis. *J Hypertens* 1989; 7(suppl 6):S184–S185.

192. Taylor DC. Duplex ultrasound in the assessment of vascular disease in clinical hypertension. *Am J Hypertens* 1991; 4:550–556.

193. Olin JW, Piedmonte MR, Young JR, DeAnna S, Grubb M, Childs MB. The utility of duplex ultrasound scanning of the renal arteries for diagnosing significant renal artery stenosis. *Ann Intern Med* 1995; 122:833–838.

194. Belli A-M. New approaches to the diagnosis and management of renal artery stenosis. *J Hum Hypertens* 1994; 8:593–594.

195. Hanna AK, Holland G, Baum RA, Carpenter JP. Diagnosis of renal artery stenosis by magnetic resonance angiography. In: Calligaro KD, Dougherty MJ, Dean RH, eds. *Modern Management of Renovascular Hypertension and Renal Salvage.* Baltimore: Williams & Wilkins; 1996:93–108.

196. Kent CK, Edelman RR, Kim D, Steinman TI, Porter DH, Skillman JJ. Magnetic resonance imaging: A reliable test for the evaluation of proximal atherosclerotic renal artery stenosis. *J Vasc Surg* 1991; 13:311–318.

197. Conn JW, Knopf RF, Nesbit RM. Clinical characteristics of primary aldosteronism from an analysis of 145 cases. *Am J Surg* 1964; 107:159–172.

198. Ferriss JB, Beevers DG, Brown JJ, Davies DL, Fraser R, Lever AF, et al. Clinical, biochemical and pathological features of low-renin ("primary") hyperaldosteronism. *Am Heart J* 1978; 95:375–388.

199. Biglieri EG, Slaton PE Jr. Pregnancy and primary aldosteronism. *J Clin Endocrinol Metab* 1967; 27:1628–1632.

200. Mader IJ, Iseri LT. Spontaneous hypopotassemia, hypomagnesemia, alkalosis and tetany due to hypersecretion of corticosterone-like mineralocorticoid. *Am J Med* 1955; 19:976–988.

201. Kaplan NM. Hypokalemia in the hypertensive patient: With observations on the incidence of primary aldosteronism. *Ann Intern Med* 1967; 66:1079–1090.

202. Biglieri EG. Spectrum of mineralocorticoid hypertension. *Hypertension* 1991; 17:251–261.

203. Bravo EL. The syndrome of primary aldosteronism and pheochromocytoma. In: Schrier RW, Gottschalk CW, eds. *Diseases of the Kidney,* 4th ed. Boston: Little, Brown; 1988:1623–1651.

204. Irony I, Kater CE, Biglieri EG, Shackleton CHL. Correctable subsets of primary aldosteronism. Primary adrenal hyperplasia and renin responsive adenoma. *Am J Hypertens* 1990; 3:576–582.

205. Giebink GS, Gotlin RW, Biglieri EG, Katz FH. A kindred with familial glucocorticoid-suppressible aldosteronism. *J Clin Endocrinol Metab* 1973; 36:715–723.

206. Ganguly A. Glucocorticoid-suppressible hyperaldosteronism: An update. *Am J Med* 1990; 88:321–324.

207. Lifton RP, Dluhy RG, Powers M, Rich GM, Cook S, Ulick S, et al. A chimaeric 11β-hydroxylase/aldosterone synthase gene causes glucocorticoid-remediable aldosteronism and human hypertension. *Nature* 1992; 355:262–265.

208. Dluhy RG, Lifton RP. Glucocorticoid remediable aldosteronism. *Endocrinol Metab Clin North Am* 1994; 23:285–297.

209. Stewart PM, Wallace AM, Valentino R, Burt D, Shackleton CHL, Edwards CRW. Mineralocorticoid activity in licorice: 11-Beta-hydroxysteroid dehydrogenase deficiency comes of age. *Lancet* 1987; 2:821–824.

210. Walker BR, Edwards CRW. Licorice-induced hypertension and syndromes of apparent mineralocorticoid excess. *Endocrinol Metab Clin North Am* 1994; 23:359–377.

211. Weinberger MH, Fineberg NS. The diagnosis of primary aldosteronism and separation of two major subtypes. *Arch Intern Med* 1993; 153:2125–2129.

212. Hiramatsu K, Yamada T, Yukimura Y, Komiya I, Ichikawa K, Ishihara M, et al. A screening test to identify aldosterone-producing adenoma by measuring plasma renin activity. Results in hypertensive patients. *Arch Intern Med* 1981; 141:1589–1593.

213. Lyons DF, Kem DC, Brown RD, Hanson CS, Carollo ML. Single dose captopril as a diagnostic test of primary aldosteronism. *J Clin Endocrinol Metab* 1983; 57:892–896.

214. Levinson PD, Zadik Z, Hamilton BPM, Mersey JH, White RI, Kowarski AA. Adrenal vein epinephrine levels: A useful aid in venous sampling for primary aldosteronism. *Ann Intern Med* 1982; 97:690–693.

215. Gross MD, Shapiro B, Grekin RJ, Freitas JE, Glazer G, Beierwaltes WH, et al. Scintigraphic localization of adrenal lesions in primary aldosteronism. *Am J Med* 1984; 77:839–844.

216. Gross MD, Shapiro B. Scintigraphic studies in adrenal hypertension. *Semin Nucl Med* 1989; 19:122–143.

217. Rossi GP, Chiesura-Corona M, Tregnaghi A, Zanin L, Perale R, Soattin S, et al. Imaging of aldosterone-secreting adenomas: A prospective comparison of computed tomography and magnetic resonance imaging in 27 patients with suspected primary aldosteronism. *J Hum Hypertens* 1993; 7:357–363.

218. Biglieri EG, Schambelan M. The significance of elevated levels of plasma 18-hydroxycorticosterone in patients with primary aldosteronism. *J Clin Endocrinol Metab* 1979; 49:87–91.

219. Orth DN. Cushing's syndrome. *N Engl J Med* 1995; 332:791–803.

220. Hall WA, Luciano MG, Doppman JL, Patronas NJ, Oldfield EH. Pituitary magnetic resonance imaging in normal human volunteers: Occult adenomas in the general population. *Ann Intern Med* 1994; 120:817–820.

221. Oldfield EH, Doppman JL, Nieman LK, Chrousos GP, Miller DL, Katz DA, et al. Petrosal sinus sampling with and without corticotropin-releasing hormone for the differential diagnosis of Cushing's syndrome. *N Engl J Med* 1991; 325:897–905.

222. Van Cauter E, Refetoff S. Evidence for two subtypes of Cushing's disease based on the analysis of episodic cortisol secretion. *N Engl J Med* 1985; 312:1343–1349.

223. Atkinson AB, Kennedy AL, Carson DJ, Hadden DR, Weaver JA, Sheridan B. Five cases of cyclical Cushing's syndrome. *BMJ Clin Res* 1985; 291:1453–1457.

224. Trainer PJ, Grossman A. The diagnosis and differential diagnosis of Cushing's syndrome. *Clin Endocrinol* 1991; 34:317–330.

225. Tyrrell JB, Findling JW, Aron DC, Fitzgerald PA, Forsham PH. An over-night high-dose dexamethasone suppression test for rapid differential diagnosis of Cushing's syndrome. *Ann Intern Med* 186; 104:180–186.

226. Blevins LS Jr, Dobs AS, Wand GS. Naloxone-induced activation of the hypothalamic-pituitary-adrenal axis in suspected central adrenal insufficiency. *Am J Med Sci* 1994; 308:167–170.

227. Kaye TB, Crapo L. The Cushing syndrome: An update on diagnostic tests. *Ann Intern Med* 1990; 112:434–444.

228. Ledger GA, Khosla S, Lindor NM, Thibodeau SN, Gharib H. Genetic testing in the diagnosis and management of multiple endocrine neoplasia type II. *Ann Intern Med* 1995; 122:118–124.

229. Manger WM, Gifford RW Jr. *Clinical and Experimental Pheochromocytoma.* Cambridge, MA: Blackwell; 1996.

230. Bravo EL, Gifford RW Jr. Pheochromocytoma: Diagnosis, localization and management. *N Engl J Med* 1984; 311:1298–1303.

231. Gitlow SE, Mendlowitz M, Bertani LM. The biochemical techniques for detecting and establishing the presence of a pheochromocytoma: A review of ten years' experience. *Am J Cardiol* 1970; 26:270–278.

232. Kaplan NM, Kramer NJ, Holland OB, Sheps SG, Gomez-Sanchez C. Single-voided urine metanephrine assays in screening for pheochromocytoma. *Arch Intern Med* 1977; 137:190–193.

233. Miller R, Stark DCC, Gitlow SE. Paroxysmal hyperadrenergic state. A case during surgery for intracranial aneurysm. *Anaesthesia* 1976; 31:743–749.

234. Gifford RW Jr, Manger WM, Bravo EL. Pheochromocytoma. In: Wollam GL, Hall WD, eds. *Hypertension Management: Clinical Practice and Therapeutic Dilemmas.* Chicago: Year Book; 1988:291–302.

235. Bravo EL, Tarazi RC, Gifford RW, Stewart BH. Circulating and urinary catecholamines in pheochromocytoma. Diagnostic and pathophysiologic implications. *N Engl J Med* 1979; 301:682–686.

236. Bravo EL. Diagnosis of pheochromocytoma. Reflections on a controversy. *Hypertension* 1991; 17:742–744.

237. Lenders JWM, Keiser HR, Goldstein DS, Willemsen JJ, Friberg P, Jacobs M-C, et al. Plasma metanephrines in the diagnosis of pheochromocytoma. *Ann Intern Med* 1995; 123:101–109.

238. Mueller HS, Ayres SM. Propranolol decreases sympathetic nervous activity reflected by plasma catecholamines during evolution of myocardial infarction in man. *J Clin Invest* 1980; 65:338–346.

239. Karlsberg RP, Cryer PE, Roberts R. Serial plasma catecholamine response early in the course of clinical acute myocardial infarction: Relationship to infarct extent and mortality. *Am Heart J* 1981; 102:24–29.

240. Benedict CR, Loach AB. Sympathetic nervous system activity in patients with subarachnoid hemorrhage. *Stroke* 1978; 9:237–244.

241. Hansson L, Hunyor SN, Julius S, Hoobler SW. Blood pressure crisis following withdrawal of clonidine (Catapres, Catapresan), with special reference to arterial and urinary catecholamine levels, and suggestions for acute management. *Am Heart J* 1973; 85:605–610.

242. Weidmann P, Beretta-Piccoli C, Meier A, Kuech G, Gluck Z, Ziegler WH. Antihypertensive mechanism of diuretic treatment with chlorthalidone. Complementary roles of sympathetic axis and sodium. *Kidney Int* 1983; 23:320–326.

243. Murphy MB, Scriven AJ, Brown MJ, Causon R, Dollery CT. The effects of nifedipine and hydralazine induced hypotension on sympathetic activity. *Eur J Clin Pharmacol* 1982; 23:479–482.

244. Lin M-S, McNay JL, Shepherd AMM, Musgrave GE, Keeton TK. Increased plasma norepinephrine accompanies persistent tachycardia after hydralazine. *Hypertension* 1983; 5:257–263.

245. Ruzicka M, Leenan FHH. Relevance of 24-hour blood pressure profile and sympathetic activity for outcome on short- versus long-acting, 1,4-dihydropyridines. *Am J Hypertens* 1996; 9:86–94.

246. Richards DA. Labetalol and urinary catecholamines (letter). *Br Med J* 1979; 1:165.

247. Izzo JL Jr, Horwitz D, Keiser HR. Physiologic mechanisms opposing the hemodynamic effects of prazosin. *Clin Pharmacol Ther* 1981; 29:7–11.

248. Inouye I, Massie B, Benowitz N, Simpson P, Loge D, Topic N. Monotherapy in mild to moderate hypertension: Comparison of hydrochlorothiazide, propranolol and prazosin. *Am J Cardiol* 1984; 53 (Proceedings of a symposium):24A–28A.

249. Proye C, Fossati P, Fontaine P, Lefebvre J, Decoulx M, Wemeau JL, et al. Dopamine-secreting pheochromocytoma: An unrecognized entity? Classification of pheochromocytomas according to their type of secretion. *Surgery* 1986; 100:1154–1162.

250. Kuchel O, Buu NT, Larochelle P, Hamet P, Genest J Jr. Episodic dopamine discharge in paroxysmal hypertension. Page's syndrome revisited. *Arch Intern Med* 1986; 146:1315–1320.

251. Bravo EL, Tarazi RC, Fouad FM, Vidt DG, Gifford RW Jr. Clonidine-suppression test. A useful aid in the diagnosis of pheochromocytoma. *N Engl J Med* 1981; 305:623–626.

252. Metz SA, Halter JB, Porte D Jr, Robertson RP. Autonomic epilepsy: Clonidine blockade of paroxysmal catecholamine release and flushing. *Ann Intern Med* 1978; 88:189–193.

253. Halter JB, Beard JC, Pfeifer MA, Metz SA. Clonidine-suppression test for diagnosis of pheochromocytoma (letter). *N Engl J Med* 1982; 306:49–50.

254. Dupont AG, Velkeniers B, Somers G, Gerlo E, Vanhaelst L. Unusual clonidine-suppression test in an epinephrine-secreting pheochromocytoma (letter). *N Engl J Med* 1984; 310:266.

255. Elliott WJ, Murphy MB. Reduced specificity of the clonidine suppression test in patients with normal plasma catecholamine levels. *Am J Med* 1988; 84:419–424.

256. Grossman E, Goldstein DS, Hoffman A, Keiser GA. Glucagon and clonidine testing in the diagnosis of pheochromocytoma. *Hypertension* 1991; 17:733–741.

257. Stewart BH, Bravo EL, Haaga J, Meaney TF, Tarazi R. Localization of pheochromocytoma by computed tomography. *N Engl J Med* 1978; 299:460–461.

258. Ganguly A, Henry DP, Yune HY, Pratt JH, Grim CE, Donohue JP, et al. Diagnosis and localization of pheochromocytoma. Detection by measurement of urinary norepinephrine excretion during sleep, plasma norepinephrine concentration and computerized axial tomography (CT-scan). *Am J Med* 1979; 67:21–26.

259. Sisson JC, Frager MS, Valk TW, Gross MD, Swanson DP, Wieland DM, et al. Scintigraphic localization of pheochromocytoma. *N Engl J Med* 1981; 305:12–17.

260. Beland SS, Vesely DL, Arnold WC, Beavers HK, Gilbert SR, Henson GN, et al. Localization of adrenal and extra-adrenal pheochromocytomas by magnetic resonance imaging. *South Med J* 1989; 82:1410–1413.

261. Velchik MG, Alavi A, Kressel HY, Engelman K. Localization of pheochromocytoma: MIBG, CT, and MRI correlation. *J Nucl Med* 1989; 30:328–336.

262. Swensen SJ, Brown ML, Sheps SG, Sizemore GW, Gharib H, Grant CS, et al. Use of 131-I-MIBG scintigraphy in the evaluation of suspected pheochromocytoma. *Mayo Clin Proc* 1985; 60:299–304.

263. Clesham GJ, Kennedy A, Lavender JP, Dollery CT, Wilkins MR. Meta-iodobenzylguanidine (MIBG) scanning in the diagnosis of phaeochromocytoma. *J Hum Hypertens* 1993; 7:353–356.

CHAPTER

58

TREATMENT OF PATIENTS WITH SYSTEMIC ARTERIAL HYPERTENSION

Ray W. Gifford, Jr.

Identifying and managing patients with hypertension and other risk factors are important to prevent or postpone morbidity and mortality from cardiovascular disease, including stroke, atherosclerotic heart disease, congestive heart failure, and end-stage renal disease. Many hypertensive patients have additional risk factors such as dyslipidemia, glucose intolerance, cigarette smoking, and obesity that should also be treated. Appropriate management of hypertension requires knowledge of the pharmacology and side effects of the drugs, the severity of hypertension, and the presence or absence of target organ disease. In addition, the physician and the therapeutic team must foster adherence to lifelong regimens by being sympathetic, understanding, patient, and persuasive; office visits must be opportunities not only to measure the blood pressure but also to reinforce the importance of adherence, elicit symptoms of target organ involvement, and inquire about side effects. Although effective treatment of hypertension will reduce cardiovascular morbidity and mortality[1,2] and prevent progression of the disease to more severe stages,[3] only 24 percent of the 43 million hypertensive patients in the United States have their blood pressures controlled to less than 140/90 mmHg.[4]

TREATMENT

Not all hypertensive patients require drug therapy. Recommendations from the report of the fifth and sixth Joint National Committees (JNC) on Detection, Evaluation, and Treatment of High Blood Pressure (JNC-V[5] and JNC-VI[5a]) suggest that a 3- to 12-month trial of lifestyle modifications be prescribed for patients with stage 1 hypertension (Table 58-1) and no evidence of target organ disease or other major risk factors (Table 58-2). If the diastolic blood pressure can be controlled to <90 mmHg and systolic blood pressure to <140 mmHg on a hygienic regimen, drug treatment is unnecessary but close follow-up is required. If blood pressure is unaffected by lifestyle modifications, the addition of an appropriate antihypertensive drug should be considered. In making this decision, the older the patient and the greater the burden of additional risk factors (including male gender, African-American race, and family history of premature cardiovascular disease), the stronger the case for prescribing drugs. Some authorities do not recommend pharmacologic treatment for patients with systolic blood pressure <160 mmHg and/or diastolic blood pressure <95 mmHg in the absence of target organ disease or other risk factors. The Hypertension Detection and Follow-up Program (HDFP) showed a 22 percent reduction in all-cause 5-year mortality comparing the stepped care or intensively treated group to the referred care or control group when pretreatment diastolic blood pressure was 90 to 94 mmHg.[6] Furthermore, it is perilous to wait for evidence of target organ disease before starting drug treatment for patients with stage 1 hypertension because the 5-year mortality rate was more than three times higher for HDFP participants who had evidence of target organ disease before medical treatment was started than it was for those who did not, even in the stepped care or intensively treated group.[6]

It is important to realize that *optimal* blood pressure above which there is increased risk of cardiovascular events is 120/80 mmHg—not 140/90 mmHg, which has been the conventional dividing line between high and "normal" blood pressure.[5,7] More than 30 percent of men who die of coronary disease have systolic blood pressure between 120 and 139 mmHg, and 43 percent have systolic blood pressure between 140 and 159 mmHg.[7] *Systolic blood pressure is a more reliable predictor of cardiovascular events than is diastolic blood*

TABLE 58-1

A NEW CLASSIFICATION SYSTEM
OF BLOOD PRESSURE FOR ADULTS
AGE 18 YEARS AND OLDER[a]

	Systolic, mmHg	Diastolic, mmHg
Optimal[b]	<120	<80
Normal	<130	<85
High-normal	130–139	85–89
Hypertension[c]		
Stage 1	140–159	90–99
Stage 2	160–179	100–109
Stage 3	≥180	≥110

[a] Not taking antihypertensive drugs and not acutely ill. When systolic and diastolic pressures fall into different categories, the higher category should be selected to classify the individual's blood pressure status. For instance, 160/92 mmHg should be classified as stage 2, 180/108 mmHg should be classified as stage 3. Isolated systolic hypertension (ISH) is defined as systolic pressure ≥140 mmHg and diastolic pressure <90 mmHg and staged appropriately (e.g., 170/85 mmHg is defined as stage 2 ISH).

[b] Optimal blood pressure with respect to cardiovascular risk.

[c] Based on the average of two or more readings taken at each of two or more visits following an initial screening.

Note: In addition to classifying stages of hypertension based on average blood pressure levels, the clinician should specify presence or absence of target organ disease and additional risk factors. For example, a patient with diabetes and a blood pressure of 142/94 mmHg plus left ventricular hypertrophy should be classified as "stage 1 hypertension with target organ disease (left ventricular hypertrophy) and with another major risk factor (diabetes)." This specificity is important for risk classification and management.

Source: Adapted from JNC-VI,[5a] with permission.

pressure. At every diastolic blood pressure level, higher systolic blood pressure results in greater cardiovascular risk and curtailment of life expectancy.[7] Contrarily, for any level of systolic blood pressure, the diastolic blood pressure has little effect on survival.

If the decision is made not to prescribe drug treatment for patients with stage 1 hypertension, the physician is obligated to follow them just as closely as if they were on medication because they are at considerable risk of blood pressure rising

TABLE 58-2

INDICATIONS FOR TREATMENT
BY RISK STRATIFICATION

BP Staging	Risk Group		
	A	B	C
High-normal	LM	LM	Drug Rx
1	LM (up to 12 months)	LM (up to 6 months)	Drug Rx
2 and 3	Drug Rx	Drug Rx	Drug Rx

Abbreviations: LM = Lifestyle modification; A = no risk factors, no TOD; B = at least one risk factor other than DM; C = TOD, and/or DM, with or without other risk factors.

Source: Adapted from JNC-VI.[5a]

to higher levels. There is consensus that drug treatment is indicated for most patients with hypertension of stage 2 or greater (Table 58-2), even in the absence of other risk factors or evidence of target organ disease. Persons whose diastolic blood pressure averages 85 to 89 mmHg and/or whose systolic blood pressure averages 130 to 139 mmHg are in a "high-normal" category; they should be under closer surveillance than individuals with lower blood pressure because they are at higher risk for cardiovascular complications and are more likely to develop even higher blood pressures that will require drug treatment. There is some evidence that lifestyle modifications such as dietary sodium restriction, weight reduction when appropriate, reduction of alcohol intake, and aerobic exercise may delay or prevent the onset of hypertension for some people in this group,[5,8,9] but drug treatment is not presently indicated. Elderly patients with isolated systolic hypertension (≥160/<90 mmHg) also benefit from pharmacologic treatment.[10] Lifestyle modifications may be tried initially for those with systolic blood pressure of 160 to 180 mmHg who have no cardiovascular complications and no other risk factors, but if it fails to reduce systolic blood pressure to less than 150 mmHg within 6 months, drugs should be introduced (see section on hypertension in the elderly, below).

Nonpharmacologic Treatment/ Lifestyle Modifications

Although it will have little or no effect on blood pressure, cessation of cigarette smoking will have a proximate and significant impact on risk reduction for cardiovascular disease, especially for the hypertensive patient. Stage 1 hypertension can sometimes be controlled with dietary sodium restriction, weight reduction for the obese, modification of alcohol intake to no more than the equivalent of 1 oz of ethanol daily, and regular exercise.[5,11–15]

In the Treatment of Mild Hypertension Study (TOMHS), lifestyle modifications reduced average blood pressure from 141/91 mmHg to 130/83 mmHg for 234 participants after 4 years.[12] Drug treatment plus the hygienic regimen was more effective in reducing blood pressure and in achieving normotension than was the hygienic regimen plus placebo. The background of nonpharmacologic treatment seemed to make control of hypertension possible with smaller than expected doses of drugs. In the Trial of Antihypertensive Interventions and Management (TAIM) Study, weight loss enhanced the antihypertensive response to both chlorthalidone and atenolol, but dietary sodium restriction did not.[14] Weight reduction in excess of 4.5 kg or sodium restriction to less than 70 meq (1.6 g) daily was equally as effective as drug treatment without dietary modification.[14] Weight reduction, dietary sodium restriction, and increased physical activity have been effective in reducing systolic and diastolic blood pressure for elderly patients with stage 1 hypertension.[15]

Perhaps 50 to 60 percent of hypertensive patients will not respond to dietary sodium control. Nevertheless, a trial of low-sodium diet (<2 g sodium or <5 g sodium chloride) is worthwhile for most patients with hypertension; for responders with stage 1 hypertension, it may obviate the need for drug therapy.[11,16] If diastolic blood pressure is not reduced after 8 to 12 weeks, adherence to the diet should be verified by measuring 24-h urinary sodium excretion. If urinary sodium is below 90 meq per 24 h, it suggests that the patient is indeed adhering to the diet and that the hypertension is not sodium-sensitive. On the other hand, if the patient appears to be noncompliant, this should be discussed and further instructions may be helpful.

Weight reduction for obese patients is often effective in reducing blood pressure, even if dietary sodium is not restricted.[17-20] The beneficial effect on blood pressure is realized before ideal body weight is achieved.[20,21] Behavioral modification is often necessary to motivate patients to reduce their weight, and it is even more important in maintaining weight reduction once achieved.

Increasing the intake of potassium has been shown to have a modest effect on reducing blood pressure in some patients.[22] It seems to enhance the antihypertensive effect of dietary sodium restriction, perhaps by promoting natriuresis.

Although calcium supplementation has been advocated as part of a nonpharmacologic approach to control hypertension, the effectiveness of this cation has not been documented as well as has reduction of dietary sodium.[11] Excessive alcohol intake tends to raise blood pressure and to counteract the antihypertensive effect of drugs, even for patients who are not alcoholics.[23,24] Furthermore, alcoholic patients are often noncompliant with treatment regimens. The effect on blood pressure is reversible, so that excessive alcohol intake is potentially a curable cause of hypertension. Alcohol intake should be restricted to no more than 30 mL (1 oz) of ethanol daily, which is equivalent to 60 mL (2 oz) of 100-proof whiskey, 240 mL (8 oz) of wine, or 720 mL (24 oz) of beer.[5] While some studies have shown that regular aerobic exercise has a modest effect in reducing blood pressure,[25] this is lost if training is not maintained. Exercise is an important adjunct to diet for weight control.

Control of stress by hypnosis, biofeedback, acupuncture, relaxation response, or similar modalities has not been shown to have a lasting or important beneficial effect on blood pressure, but well-controlled studies are lacking.[11,26] In the Trial of Hypertension Prevention, a low-sodium diet and weight reduction were effective in reducing blood pressure, while stress management and supplementation with calcium, potassium, magnesium, and fish oil were not.[9]

A major disadvantage of the nonpharmacologic approaches to management of hypertension is nonadherence to regimens that require lifestyle changes. Most patients would rather take medication than alter their diets. The fact that behavior modification is difficult to achieve and maintain greatly limits the effectiveness of nonpharmacologic/hygienic management.

Pharmacologic Treatment

The concept of stepped care in managing hypertension was introduced in the "Database for Effective Antihypertensive Therapy,"[27] which was the first publication by the National High Blood Pressure Education Program offering guidelines to physicians for treatment of hypertension. It was the forerunner of the JNC reports on detection, evaluation, and treatment. At that time the only available choices among antihypertensive drugs were ganglion-blocking agents, guanethidine, hydralazine, methyldopa, reserpine, and thiazide diuretics. Given the limited choices, it is not difficult to understand that a thiazide diuretic was selected as the step 1 drug of choice. Unfortunately, those not familiar with the genesis of the stepped care approach have come to equate stepped care with "diuretic-based" treatment. Nothing is farther from the truth. The Database Task Force clearly defined stepped care in the original publication as follows: "It calls for beginning therapy with a small dose of an antihypertensive drug, increasing the dose of that drug, and then adding, one after another, additional drugs as needed."[27] This generic definition permits building a regimen, the ingredients of which will change as new agents are introduced and older ones are discarded.

With the advent of additional classes of drugs, such as the beta-adrenergic blockers (Chap. 54), calcium channel blockers (Chap. 54), and angiotensin-converting enzyme (ACE) inhibitors, none of which was available and/or approved for hypertension in 1973, recent JNC reports have broadened the selection for step 1 to include not only the diuretics but also the beta blockers (including the alpha and beta blocker labetalol), the ACE inhibitors, the calcium channel blockers, and the alpha$_1$-adrenergic blockers. Furthermore, subsequent JNC reports have also made stepped care more flexible by offering the option of substituting another step 1 drug if the first choice fails to control hypertension or causes troublesome side effects (sequential monotherapy).[5,28]

Several reports have suggested guidelines for selecting the appropriate initial drug for a given patient,[5,28,29] and these are incorporated in the tables that list the drugs, their doses, and the common side effects for each category of antihypertensive agents. Basically, in making the choice, preference should be given to agents that have been demonstrated to reduce cardiovascular morbidity and mortality in numerous controlled randomized clinical trials. Presently, these include only the diuretics and beta blockers. Consideration should also be given to age and race[30] as well as coexisting symptoms and conditions that might be benefited or aggravated by a given class of drugs (e.g., angina pectoris, myocardial infarction, migraine headache, diabetes mellitus, cardiac arrhythmias, congestive heart failure, constipation).[29] These guidelines are imprecise, are subject to revision as new data become available, and should not contravene the physician's best judgment in selecting the appropriate agent to initiate therapy.

The reliability and cost-effectiveness of measurements of hemodynamic or biochemical parameters such as plasma catecholamines or plasma renin activity have not been great enough to justify their routine use in selecting the appropriate initial drug. While the 1988 JNC report promulgated the concept of "individualized stepped care,"[28] the truth is that our desire to select, prospectively, the appropriate drug for a given patient exceeds our ability to do so.

To enhance adherence, it is preferable to select a long-acting drug that can be given once daily, usually in the morning. The more tablets and the more times a day they are administered, the less likely that a patient will adhere to the regimen.

The TOMHS trial[31] compared in a parallel design as monotherapy a diuretic (chlorthalidone), a beta-adrenergic blocker (acebutolol), a calcium channel blocker (amlodipine), an ACE inhibitor (enalapril), and an alpha-adrenergic blocker (doxazosin). Their effects on blood pressure after 4 years were remarkably similar, the only difference being that the average systolic blood pressure reduction was significantly greater for the diuretic (17.7 mmHg) than it was for doxazosin (14.2 mmHg) ($p = .003$). The systolic reduction fell between these two extremes for the other agents. There was no statistically significant difference in diastolic blood pressure reductions between the five drugs.

DIURETICS

For many years the diuretics were the mainstay of antihypertensive therapy and the only logical choice for step 1 (Tables 58-3 and 24-1). All but one[10a] of the controlled clinical trials

TABLE 58-3

DIURETICS

Agent	Usual Daily Dose, mg[a]	Precautions and Special Considerations	Selected Side Effects[b]
THIAZIDE AND RELATED DIURETICS			
Bendroflumethazide (Naturetin)	2.5–5	May be ineffective in renal failure except for indapamide and metolazone; hypokalemia increases digitalis toxicity; may cause an increase in blood levels of lithium. Decrease urinary calcium excretion. May precipitate acute gout.	Hypokalemia, hypomagnesemia, hyperuricemia, glucose intolerance, insulin resistance, hypercholesterolemia, increased low-density lipoprotein cholesterol, hypertriglyceridemia, hypercalcemia, sexual dysfunction, weakness, photosensitivity (except for ethacrynic acid), leukopenia, allergic skin rash
Chlorothiazide (Diuril)	125–500		
Chlorthalidone (Hygroton, Thalitone)	12.5–50		
Hydrochlorothiazide (Hydro-DIURIL, Esidrix, Oretic)	12.5–50		
Hydroflumethiazide (Diucardin)	25–50		
Indapamide (Lozol)	2.5–5		
Methylclothiazide (Enduron)	2.5–5		
Metolazone (Zaroxolyn)	1.25–10		
(Mykrox)	0.5–1		
Polythiazide (Renese)	1–4		
Trichlormethiazide (Naqua)	1–4		
LOOP DIURETICS[c]			
Bumetanide (Bumex)	0.5–5[d]	Effective in chronic renal failure. Increase urinary calcium excretion	As above, except for hypercalcemia
Ethacrynic acid (Edecrin)	25–100[d]		
Furosemide (Lasix)	20–320[d]		
Torsemide (Demadex)	5–20		
POTASSIUM-SPARING DIURETICS			
Amiloride (Midamor)	5–20	Danger of hyperkalemia in patients receiving a potassium supplement, a potassium-containing salt substitute, an ACE inhibitor, an angiotensin II (type AT_1) receptor blocker and in patients with renal failure; can cause acute renal failure in patients treated with an NSAID (indomethacin and triamterene); may increase blood levels of lithium.	Hyperkalemia for all three agents. For spironolactone only: gynecomastia, mastodynia, gastrointestinal irritation, drowsiness, lethargy, irregular menses or postmenopausal bleeding, hirsutism.
Spironolactone (Aldactone)	25–100	Spironolactone interferes with digoxin immunoassay. Danger of renal calculi (triamterene).	(see above)
Triamterene (Dyrenium)	100–300[d]		

(Continued)

TABLE 58-3

DIURETICS (*Continued*)

Product	Dose, tablets or capsules/day	Product	Dose, tablets or capsules/day
COMBINATIONS OF THIAZIDE AND POTASSIUM-SPARING DIURETICS			
Hydrochlorothiazide 50 mg + triamterene 75 mg (Maxzide)	1/2–1 tablet	Hydrochlorothiazide 25 mg + triamterene 37.5 mg (Maxzide 25)	1/2–2 tablets
Hydrochlorothiazide 25 mg + triamterene 37.5 mg (Dyazide)	1–2 capsules	Hydrochlorothiazide 50 mg + amiloride 5 mg (Moduretic)	1/2–1 tablet
Hydrochlorothiazide 25 mg + spironolactone 25 mg (Aldactazide 25)	1–2 tablets	Hydrochlorothiazide 50 mg + spironolactone 50 mg (Aldactazide 50)	1/2–1 tablet

Special indications: Diuretics or beta blockers should be agents of choice for most patients with uncomplicated hypertension unless contraindicated, ineffective, or unacceptable or unless there are special indications for other agents (see text); especially indicated for African-American, elderly, and obese patients and for patients with congestive heart failure, chronic renal failure (loop diuretics), resistant hypertension, recurrent renal calculi (calcium) (nonloop diuretics).

Contraindications: History of hypersensitivity to diuretics, hypovolemia, hyponatremia, hypochloremia, hypomagnesemia, uncontrolled gout, severe hypertrophic cardiomyopathy, asymmetric septal hypertrophy (idiopathic hypertrophic subaortic stenosis), preeclampsia and eclampsia.

Advantages: Effective in reducing cardiovascular morbidity and mortality, effective in $\geq$50% of mild hypertensives, inexpensive, one dose daily, easy to titrate, well tolerated, enhances potency of all other agents, no pseudotolerance, reduces total peripheral resistance.

Disadvantages: Metabolic side effects: ($K^+\downarrow$, $Mg^{2+}\downarrow$, urate $\uparrow$, $Ca^{2+}\uparrow$, $Na^+\downarrow$, $Cl^-\downarrow$, glucose $\uparrow$, lipids $\uparrow$).

[a] The dosage range may differ slightly from recommended dosage in *Physicians' Desk Reference* or package insert. Drugs are given once daily unless otherwise indicated.

[b] The listing of side effects is not all-inclusive, and health practitioners are urged to refer to the package inserts for a more detailed listing.

[c] Larger doses of loop diuretics may be required in patients with renal failure.

[d] This drug is usually given in divided doses twice daily.

Note: NSAID = nonsteroidal anti-inflammatory drug.

that have shown a reduction in cardiovascular morbidity and mortality have used diuretics or beta-adrenergic blockers as initial therapy.[1,2,10] Nevertheless, it has been postulated that atherogenic and arrythmogenic metabolic side effects of diuretic therapy (dyslipidemia, hyperglycemia, and hypokalemia) may be responsible for the observation that coronary events have not been reduced as much as anticipated or as dramatically as have stroke events.[32] It is interesting that in prospective clinical trials in elderly patients in which a low-dose diuretic was employed, coronary events were reduced to the anticipated level.[1] This is probably because elderly hypertensive patients are at greater risk and will therefore have more events than younger ones will during the course of 3 to 5-year trials, thus making it more likely that a statistically significant conclusion will be reached with regard to coronary end points.[33] The surprising conclusion of the earlier clinical trials was not so much that reduction in coronary events failed to achieve expectations, but that reduction of stroke events did.

The metabolic side effects of diuretics are now well recognized and should be monitored. They are minimized but not eliminated by employing small doses [equivalent to 12.5 to 25 mg of hydrochlorothiazide (HCTZ) or chlorthalidone]. Many patients are not susceptible to the dyslipidemic effects of diuretics, which include an increase in serum cholesterol

concentration of 5 to 10 mg/dL, mostly in the low-density lipoprotein (LDL) fraction, and a rise in triglyceride concentration. This adverse effect can be minimized, if not eliminated, by a low-fat, low-cholesterol diet.[34,35] It has been recommended by the National Education Programs on High Blood Pressure and High Cholesterol that when hypertensive patients receiving diuretics or certain beta blockers present with elevated LDL cholesterol that cannot be controlled with diet, consideration should be given to cautiously discontinuing these antihypertensive medications temporarily, unless otherwise contraindicated, and closely observing the effects of withdrawal on blood cholesterol and blood pressure levels.[36]

Because the rise in serum cholesterol and triglyceride concentrations usually occurs in the first 6 weeks, the patients who are going to respond adversely can often be easily and quickly identified by measuring serum lipids and glucose before and 6 to 8 weeks after initiating diuretic therapy. If no adverse effect has occurred by 6 months, frequent measurement of lipids can be discontinued, although serum potassium and glucose should be monitored at least every 6 months.

At the end of 4 years in the TOMHS trial,[34] in which all participants were asked to follow low-fat, low-cholesterol diets, lose weight if necessary, and increase exercise, total plasma cholesterol had decreased by 5.9 mg/dL compared to pretreatment levels in the group treated with chlorthalidone and by 6.0 mg/dL in the placebo group. For LDL cholesterol, the decline was 4.9 mg/dL in the chlorthalidone group and 5.1 mg/dL in the placebo group. For high-density lipoprotein (HDL) cholesterol, the change was +0.6 mg/dL in the chlorthalidone group compared to a decrease of 0.3 mg/dL in the placebo group. For triglycerides, the change was −7.3 mg/dL in the chlorthalidone group and −2.8 mg/dL in the placebo group.

Several long-term studies have shown that the dyslipidemic effect of diuretics becomes less evident or subsides after the first year of therapy.[34,37–41] Moreover, it is important to recognize that the rise in cholesterol induced by diuretic therapy is inversely proportional to the pretreatment level of serum cholesterol.[37,39] Jeunemaitre et al.[41] have demonstrated a "regression to the mean" phenomenon for both cholesterol and glucose in hypertensive patients treated with diuretics, so that those patients with the highest serum cholesterol and glucose concentrations actually had the largest decreases when diuretics were administered, whereas those with normal pretreatment values had the largest increases. *The clinical implication is that diuretics are not contraindicated de facto for patients with dyslipidemia or diabetes.*

For patients who have left ventricular hypertrophy (LVH) or other resting electrocardiographic abnormalities or who have a history of tachyarrhythmias, it is sometimes preferable to use a combination potassium-sparing/thiazide-type diuretic unless there is a contraindication to the potassium-sparing drug (Tables 58-3 and 24-1) (see also Chap. 24). Diuretics are the least expensive of the recommended drugs for initial therapy, and this is an important consideration because the cost of therapy can detract from compliance to lifelong treatment for many patients.[42] Moreover, the diuretics have an additive, if not synergistic, antihypertensive effect with all of the other classes of drugs for hypertension. Failure to incorporate a diuretic in the regimen is sometimes the cause for suboptimal control of hypertension, and *it is inappropriate to classify hypertension as resistant to treatment unless a diuretic has been included in a multidrug regimen.*[43]

In addition to the JNC-V report,[5] authoritative guidelines from Canada, Great Britain, and New Zealand have recommended that diuretics and beta blockers be given preference in selecting the initial antihypertensive drug.[44] Guidelines from Australia and the World Health Organization/International Society of Hypertension (WHO/ISH), while acknowledging that only diuretics and beta blockers have been shown to reduce cardiovascular morbidity and mortality, were more permissive in their recommendations for initial drug therapy.

BETA-ADRENERGIC BLOCKING AGENTS

Beta-adrenergic blockers were first recommended as an alternative to diuretics for initial therapy of hypertension in the 1984 report of the JNC (Tables 58-4 and 54-2).[45] These agents have been shown to reduce cardiovascular events in randomized, controlled trials.[1,2] Beta blockers have demonstrated a distinct cardioprotective effect compared to placebo following myocardial infarction in randomized studies.[46–48] Compared to placebo, the beta blockers reduced recurrent nonfatal infarctions, sudden death, and total mortality for up to 6 years following myocardial infarction,[46] but without clear benefit following non-Q-wave infarction,[49] (see Chaps. 47 and 54). The beta blockers with intrinsic sympathomimetic activity (ISA) have been less effective than those without ISA.[48] No other classes of antihypertensive drugs have demonstrated this effect so convincingly; consequently, *a non-ISA beta blocker is the drug of first choice for hypertensive patients following a myocardial infarction.*

Although beta blockers can be classified according to the presence or absence of cardioselectivity and the presence or absence of ISA (Table 58-4 and 54-2), they are all equipotent in reducing blood pressure when given in effective doses. Cardioselectivity is lost as dose is increased, and in average antihypertensive doses the cardioselective beta$_1$ blockers may also block beta$_2$ receptors, similar to the nonselective agents (Table 54-xx). Cardioselective agents have marginal advantages over nonselective agents for patients with occlusive arterial disease and intermittent claudication, patients with chronic obstructive pulmonary disease with minimal or no bronchospasm, and diabetic patients who are predisposed to hypoglycemic reactions because they take insulin. The recovery from hypoglycemia is prolonged less by cardioselective beta blockers than by nonselective ones (see also Chap. 54).

Beta-adrenergic blockers of any type are contraindicated for asthmatic patients unless the asthma has been inactive for years, in which case a cardioselective beta-adrenergic blocker may be given cautiously if the indication is strong. One of the disadvantages of beta-adrenergic blockers is the long list of precautions and contraindications noted in (Tables 58-4 and 54-2). The nonselective, non-ISA beta-adrenergic blockers are the only antihypertensive agents that reduce blood pressure primarily by decreasing cardiac output rather than total peripheral resistance. For most patients with primary (essential) systemic arterial hypertension, this is unphysiologic, but nevertheless these drugs have been effective over long periods of time and have reduced cardiovascular mortality. These agents are particularly useful in managing hypertension associated with the hyperdynamic beta-adrenergic circulatory state,[50] which is characterized by an increase in cardiac output and cardiac rate with relatively normal total peripheral resistance, and which is sometimes encountered in adolescents and young adults.

The ISA beta-adrenergic blockers are less likely than non-ISA agents to produce excessive bradycardia and to cause serum lipid abnormalities (hypertriglyceridemia and depressed HDL cholesterol). Nevertheless, ISA beta blockers have not been shown to have as great a cardioprotective effect after a myocardial infarction as non-ISA beta blockers, even though the latter can have an adverse effect on the lipid profile. In TOMHS,[34] the cardioselective, ISA beta-adrenergic blocker acebutolol reduced average total serum cholesterol

TABLE 58-4

BETA-ADRENERGIC BLOCKING AGENTS

Agent	Usual Daily Dose,[a] mg	Precautions and Special Considerations	Selected Side Effects[b]
Cardioselective, with ISA		Should not be used in patients with asthma, chronic obstructive pulmonary disease with bronchospasm, congestive heart failure, heart block (greater than first degree), or sick sinus syndrome; use with caution in insulin-treated diabetics and patients with peripheral vascular disease; should not be discontinued abruptly in patients with ischemic heart disease.	Bronchospasm, peripheral arterial insufficiency, fatigue, insomnia, sexual dysfunction, exacerbation of heart failure, masking of symptoms of hypoglycemia, hypertriglyceridemia, decreased high-density lipoprotein cholesterol (except for drugs with ISA and labetalol)
Acebutolol (Sectral)[c]	200–1200		
Cardioselective, without ISA			
Atenolol (Tenormin)[c]	25–100		
Betaxolol (Kerlone)	10–20		
Bisoprolol (Zebeta)	2.5–20		
Esmolol[e] (Brevibloc)	—		
Metoprolol (Lopressor)	50–200		
Metoprolol XL (Toprol XL)	50–200		
Noncardioselective, with ISA			
Carteolol (Cartrol)[c]	2.5–10		
Penbutolol (Levatol)[c]	20–80		
Pindolol (Visken)[c]	10–60[f]		
Noncardioselective, without ISA			
Labetalol[d] (Normodyne, Trandate)	200–1200[f]		
Nadolol[c] (generic)	40–320[f]		
Propranolol (Inderal)	40–320[f]		
Propranolol, long-acting (Inderal LA)	60–320[f]		
Timolol (Blocadren)	20–60[f]		

Note: ISA = intrinsic sympathomimetic activity; drugs in each category are listed alphabetically, with no preference.

Special indications: Diuretics or beta blockers should be agents of choice for most patients with uncomplicated hypertension unless contraindicated, ineffective, or unacceptable or unless there are special indications for other agents (see text); especially indicated for patients who have had myocardial infarction because of the cardioprotective effect (non-ISA, non-alpha-blocking agents); especially effective for white patients and patients with hyperkinetic circulation, angina pectoris, migraine headache, senile tremor; severe hypertrophic cardiomyopathy of the elderly, severe asymmetric septal hypertrophy with outflow obstruction (idiopathic hypertrophic subaortic stenosis), atrial fibrillation to control ventricular rate, paroxysmal supraventricular tachycardia (non-ISA, non-alpha-blocking agents preferred).

Contraindications: History of hypersensitive reaction to beta-adrenergic blockers, more than first-degree heart block, sick sinus syndrome, left ventricular failure, asthma, chronic obstructive pulmonary disease with bronchospasm. Relative contraindications (see text): insulin-dependent diabetes, remote history of bronchial asthma, intermittent claudication, Raynaud's disease.

Advantages: Effective in reducing cardiovascular morbidity and mortality; cardioprotective after myocardial infarction, antianginal, relatively inexpensive, effective in ~50% of mild hypertensives, reduce CO in hyperkinetic circulation, one dose daily (for most agents), no pseudotolerance, migraine prophylaxis (propranolol), reduces senile tremor (propranolol).

Disadvantages: Many do not reduce total peripheral resistance; central nervous system side effects; metabolic side effects [HDL cholesterol ↓, triglycerides ↑ (except for ISA beta blockers, see text), glucose ↑, insulin resistance ↑]. Multiple contraindications and precautions.

[a] The dosage range may differ slightly from recommended dosage in *Physicians' Desk Reference* or package insert. Drugs are given once daily unless otherwise indicated.

[b] The listing of side effects is not all-inclusive, and health practitioners are urged to refer to the package insert for a more detailed listing.

[c] Drug is excreted by kidney—may require dosage reduction in patients with renal insufficiency.

[d] Combined alpha and beta blocker. Can be given intravenously for hypertensive emergencies—see text.

[e] Esmolol is available only for intravenous infusion. Its duration of action is extremely short, and its dosage is highly variable. Used during operation for pheochromocytoma.

[f] This drug is usually given in divided doses twice daily.

by 11.8 mg/dL at the end of the 4-year trial compared to 6.0 mg/dL for the placebo; LDL cholesterol was reduced by 11.5 mg/dL compared to 5.1 mg/dL for the placebo, and HDL cholesterol was reduced by 0.6 mg/dL compared to 0.3 mg/dL for placebo.

While beta-adrenergic blockers can impair glucose tolerance,[51] they do not often interfere with control of diabetes clinically.[52] Certainly, one would not want to precipitate the need for oral hypoglycemic agents or insulin in a non-insulin-dependent diabetic who is well controlled on diet; if this becomes a problem, a drug from an alternative class of antihypertensive agents should be selected (see also Chap. 54).

CALCIUM CHANNEL BLOCKERS

The last three reports of the JNC have included calcium channel blockers (calcium antagonists) as candidates for initial monotherapy of mild-to-moderate hypertension[28,5,5a] (Table 58-5. See also Chap. 54). The calcium channel blockers differ

TABLE 58-5

CALCIUM CHANNEL BLOCKERS

Agent	Usual Daily Dose,[a] mg	Precautions and Special Considerations	Selected Side Effects[b]
Benzothiazepine derivative			
Diltiazem (sustained release)		Contraindicated in heart failure due	Rash, headache, dizziness,
Cardizem SR	120–360[c]	to systolic dysfunction, sick sinus	asthenia, flushing, ankle edema,
Diltiazem (extended release)		syndrome, or greater than first-	negative inotropic effect
Cardizem CD	120–480	degree heart block; may cause	
Dilacor XR	120–540	liver dysfunction; can increase	
Tiazac	120–540	blood levels of cyclosporine; can	
		aggravate gastroesophageal reflux	
		disease (GERD).	
Diphenylalkylamine derivative			
Verapamil (Calan, Isoptin)	120–360[d]	As above	As above, plus constipation
Verapamil SR (sustained release)			
Calan SR	120–480		
Isoptin SR	120–480		
Verelan	120–480		
Covera HS	120–480[e]		
Dihydropyridines			
Amlodipine (Norvasc)	2.5–10	Nonrandomized studies have shown	Headache, palpitations,
Felodipine (Plendil)	2.5–10	an association between therapy	tachycardia, ankle edema,
Isradipine (DynaCirc)	5–10[c]	with short-acting nifedipine and an	flushing, gastrointestinal
Isradipine (DynaCirc CR)	5–20	increase in myocardial infarction.	symptoms, gingival hyperplasia,
Nicardipine (Cardene)	60–120[d]	Contraindicated in congestive heart	weakness, nausea, heartburn,
Nicardipine XL (Cardene XL)	60–120[e]	failure, with (possible) exception	dizziness
Nifedipine extended release		of amlodipine. Extended release	
Procardia XL	30–90	nifedipine tablets should not be	
Adalat CC	30–90	broken or punctured. May	
Nisoldipine (Sular)	10–60	aggravate angina, myocardial	
		ischemia, and GERD.	

Special indications: Elderly and African-American patients; angina pectoris, hypertension induced by cyclosporine; paroxysmal supraventricular tachycardia (diltiazem or verapamil); migraine, atrial fibrillation to slow atrioventricular conduction (verapamil, diltiazem).

Contraindications: History of hypersensitivity reaction to calcium channel blockers, left ventricular dysfunction with or without congestive heart failure; greater than first-degree heart block, sick sinus syndrome, Wolff-Parkinson-White and Lown-Ganong-Levine syndromes (verapamil, diltiazem).

Advantages: Most preparations are long-acting, reduce total peripheral resistance, effective, no pseudotolerance, antianginal, no metabolic side effects, easy to titrate (sustained-release preparations).

Disadvantages: Expensive, and only one randomized trial has demonstrated long-term efficacy in reducing cardiovascular events.[10a] Short-acting preparations of nifedipine have been associated with increased risk of myocardial infarction and cancer in case control studies (see text).

[a] The dosage range may differ slightly from recommended dosage in *Physicians' Desk Reference* or package insert. Drugs are given once daily unless otherwise indicated.

[b] The listing of side effects is not all-inclusive, and health practitioners are urged to refer to the package insert for a more detailed listing. All calcium channel blockers can cause headache, flushing and edema (see also Chap. 54).

[c] This drug is usually given in divided doses twice daily.

[d] This drug is usually given in divided doses three times daily.

[e] Entire dose should be given at bedtime (see text).

in their action on various vascular beds. Verapamil and, to a lesser extent, diltiazem act on the heart to reduce rate, slow atrioventricular (AV) conduction, and depress contractility. On the other hand, the dihydropyridine calcium channel blockers have very little effect on the myocardium in the intact normal person but are excellent peripheral vasodilators, reducing total peripheral resistance.

The long-acting preparations are preferred, not only to enhance adherence but also because they seem to produce fewer side effects than the shorter-acting formulations. Short-acting preparations of diltiazem and nifedipine have never been approved by the Food and Drug Administration for the treatment of systemic hypertension, and one retrospective, case-control study has suggested an association between the use of short-acting calcium channel blockers, especially nifedipine, and the occurrence of myocardial infarction in hypertensive patients.[53] In one nonrandomized cohort study of elderly hypertensive patients, the use of short-acting nifedipine or diltiazem was associated with an increase in mortality compared with other antihypertensive agents.[54]

Because of their negative inotropic effects, verapamil and diltiazem are contraindicated for patients with left ventricular systolic dysfunction or failure.[55,56] Nifedipine, which may have little or no negative inotropic effect because of reflex sympathetic stimulation, also tends to worsen left ventricular failure,[57] even though it reduces afterload (see also Chap. 54).

Beta blockers should not be prescribed with either verapamil or diltiazem for patients who have left ventricular dysfunction because both classes of drugs have negative inotropic effects. They do have additive effects on blood pressure, however, and can be used together safely when left ventricular function and cardiac conduction are normal. Long-term studies have not demonstrated a convincing cardioprotective effect for the calcium channel blockers after myocardial infarction similar to that shown for beta blockers,[58] and in the case of short-acting nifedipine, there is evidence that they may have a deleterious effect[59] (see also Chap. 54).

Like the diuretics, calcium channel blockers appear to be especially effective in elderly patients and African-American patients,[30] although there are many exceptions to this rule. Like the beta-adrenergic blockers, the calcium channel blockers are effective antianginal drugs and should be considered for initial therapy in hypertensive patients who have angina pectoris, especially when beta blockers are ineffective or contraindicated.

The calcium channel blockers do not have metabolic side effects, but it has been suggested that their use may be associated with an increased incidence of cancer, when compared to other antihypertensive agents in a retrospective study,[60] and of intraoperative and postoperative hemorrhage in a randomized, placebo-controlled trial during cardiac valve replacements.[61] In a prospective cohort study, it was suggested that calcium channel blockers were associated with an increased risk of gastrointestinal hemorrhage in elderly patients when compared to other antihypertensive agents.[62]

An extended-release, controlled-onset formulation of verapamil (Table 58-5) is designed for bedtime administration to be maximally effective in the morning hours, when the diurnal rise in blood pressure and pulse rate may contribute to the excess of cardiovascular and stroke morbidity and mortality from 6:00 A.M. to noon. Timing of medication to coincide with potentially harmful bodily circadian rhythms is known as *chronotherapeutics*.

DRUGS THAT INTERFERE WITH THE RENIN-ANGIOTENSIN SYSTEM

Angiotensin-Converting Enzyme Inhibitors

Although ACE inhibitors (Table 58-6) specifically block the conversion of angiotensin I to angiotensin II, they are effective in reducing blood pressure for a wide spectrum of antihypertensive patients, even when angiotensin II does not seem to be playing a role. Perhaps this is because they also block the degradation of bradykinin, which is a potent vasodilator and also increases the production of prostacyclin and prostaglandin E2.[63]

The ACE inhibitors listed in Table 58-6 are equally effective and have similar side effect profiles. In antihypertensive potency, it does not appear to make a difference whether they are prodrugs or directly active or whether or not they have a sulfhydryl group.[63] Diuretics enhance the hypotensive potency of ACE inhibitors[64] probably more than for any other class of drugs, with the possible exception of the adrenergic neuroeffector blockers (reserpine, guanethidine, and guanadrel). While ACE inhibitors alone seem to be more effective for young and white patients than they are for old and African-American patients,[30] these age and race differences in blood pressure response are obliterated by adding a diuretic to the regimen.

The ACE inhibitors are not direct venodilators, but they do reduce filling pressure of the failing left ventricle and dilate arterioles, thereby reducing preload and afterload. Because of this, they are particularly effective in managing hypertension complicated by left ventricular systolic failure. In fact, the regimen of choice for hypertensive patients with congestive heart failure due to systolic dysfunction includes an ACE inhibitor and a diuretic. Even in the absence of hypertension, ACE inhibitors have been shown to prolong life in patients with moderate-to-severe congestive heart failure when added to conventional regimens[65–67] (see also Chap. 23).

The ACE inhibitors have a unique effect on renal hemodynamics because they selectively dilate the efferent (postglomerular) arteriole, thus reducing pressure within the glomerular capillaries, usually without reducing glomerular filtration rate. Theoretically, this tends to reduce the rate of progression of glomerulosclerosis in various types of glomerulopathies, according to the theory promulgated by Brenner and others.[68] This may not always be beneficial because renal function can deteriorate abruptly when glomerular filtration rate is being maintained by angiotensin II–mediated constriction of the efferent arteriole, as is the case when renal blood flow is jeopardized by renal artery stenosis, congestive heart failure, hypovolemia, and hypotension.[69–72] It is in these situations that ACE inhibitors can cause an abrupt increase in serum creatinine concentration, if not acute renal failure (see also Chap. 23).

After extensive renal ablation in rats, ACE inhibition has been shown to protect animals against hypertension, heavy proteinuria, glomerulosclerosis, and progressive renal failure.[73] This is also true in rats made diabetic by streptozotocin.[74] ACE inhibition with captopril reduced albuminuria in 16 insulin-dependent hypertensive patients with overt diabetic glomerulosclerosis[75] as well as microalbuminuria in insulin-dependent diabetic patients with normal blood pressure.[76] During a 4-year period of observation, 7 of 23 diabetic patients who did not receive ACE inhibitors developed overt diabetic nephropathy with heavy proteinuria, compared to none of 21 patients who were treated with captopril.[76]

In a multicenter, double-blind placebo-controlled trial, Lewis and colleagues demonstrated that captopril reduced

TABLE 58-6

DRUGS THAT INTERFERE WITH THE RENIN-ANGIOTENSIN-ALDOSTERONE SYSTEM

Agent	Usual Daily Dose,[a] mg	Precautions and Special Considerations	Selected Side Effects[b]
ANGIOTENSIN-CONVERTING ENZYME INHIBITORS			
Benazepril (Lotensin)	10–40	*Contraindicated in pregnancy.* Can cause reversible acute renal failure in patients with bilateral renal arterial stenosis or unilateral stenosis in an artery to a solitary kidney. Excreted by the kidney—may require dosage reduction in patients with renal insufficiency. Hypotension has been observed with initiation of treatment, especially in patients with high plasma renin activity or hypovolemia (e.g., in those receiving diuretic therapy).	Cough, rash, angioedema (rare), hyperkalemia (especially when given to patients with renal failure and/or with a potassium-sparing diuretic or an NSAID), dysgeusia, neutropenia (rare), proteinuria (rare at recommended doses)
Captopril (Capoten)	12.5–150[c]		
Enalapril (Vasotec)	2.5–40		
Fosinopril (Monopril)[d]	10–60		
Lisinopril (Zestril, Prinivil)	5–40		
Moexipril (Univasc)	7.5–30		
Quinapril (Accupril)	5–80		
Ramipril (Altace)	1.25–20		
Trandolapril (Mavik)[d]	0.5–4		
ANGIOTENSIN II RECEPTOR (TYPE AT$_1$) ANTAGONISTS			
Losartan (Cozaar)	25–100	*Contraindicated in pregnancy.* With the exception of proteinuria and neutropenia, this class of agents can theoretically produce the same adverse effects on renal function, serum potassium, and blood pressure that are listed above.	Dizziness, angioedema (rare)
Valsartan (Diovan)	80–320		

Special indications: Congestive heart failure (CHF) due to systolic dysfunction, type I diabetes mellitus with nephropathy, young patient, white patient, heavy proteinuria, impotence from other drugs.

Contraindications: Pregnancy, history of hypersensitivity to these agents or history of angioedema; bilateral renal artery stenosis or severe stenosis in an artery to a solitary kidney; hyperkalemia; advanced renal failure (serum creatinine ≥3.0 mg/dL).

Advantages: Beneficial for congestive heart failure with low ejection fraction and diabetic nephropathy (type I), no metabolic side effects (except for hyperkalemia as noted), low side effect profile, effective, long-acting (except captopril), no pseudotolerance, easy to titrate, reduce total peripheral resistance.

Disadvantages: Expensive, risk of acute renal failure and/or hyperkalemia (see text); no long-term trials to demonstrate reduction in cardiovascular morbidity or mortality, except in patients with CHF and type I diabetes with nephropathy.

[a] The dosage range may differ slightly from recommended dosage in *Physicians' Desk Reference* or package insert. Captopril should be given in divided doses twice daily, others can be given once daily but some may require twice daily dosing to control blood pressure for 24 h.

[b] The listing of side effects is not all-inclusive, and health practitioners are urged to refer to the package insert for a more detailed listing.

[c] This drug is usually given in divided doses twice daily.

[d] Fosinopril and trandolapril are excreted by the liver as well as by the kidney; may require dosage reduction in patients with hepatic insufficiency.

proteinuria, slowed progression of renal failure, and postponed the need for dialysis in patients with type I diabetes and nephropathy.[77] Control of hypertension was comparable in both groups. As yet there is no conclusive evidence that ACE inhibitors have similar beneficial effects in patients with type II diabetic nephropathy or that they will prevent diabetic nephropathy.

Ace inhibitors must be prescribed cautiously for patients with chronic renal failure from any cause. They are relatively contraindicated when the serum creatinine level is >3 mg/dL. ACE inhibitors can cause hyperkalemia and abrupt worsening of renal function in some patients with renal insufficiency.[78,79] Consequently, serum creatinine and potassium levels should be measured within 48 h of initiating ACE inhibitor therapy for patients with chronic renal failure and at least once a week for 2 to 3 weeks thereafter. Moreover, it is important to continue to monitor serum creatinine and

potassium at regular intervals for any patient who has chronic renal disease and is receiving an ACE inhibitor. ACE inhibitors do not have adverse effects on lipid or glucose metabolism.

Except for a troublesome, dry, irritative cough that occurs in 5 to 20 percent of patients,[80] ACE inhibitors are relatively free of symptomatic side effects and are least likely of all antihypertensive drugs to cause sexual dysfunction in the male. Unfortunately, they are considerably more expensive than diuretics and many of the beta-adrenergic blockers.

Angiotensin II Receptor (Type AT$_1$) Antagonists

This new class of drugs is listed in Table 58-6 with the ACE inhibitors because these compounds also interfere with the renin-angiotensin system, perhaps more completely than do the ACE inhibitors. Other angiotensin II receptor antagonists are being investigated and will soon become available.

Unlike the ACE inhibitors, the angiotensin II antagonists do not block the degradation of bradykinin and perhaps this may be why they do not cause a dry, irritating cough,[81] which has been a major side effect of ACE inhibition. To the extent that bradykinin may account for some of the hypotensive effect of ACE inhibition, the angiotensin II receptor antagonists may be less effective as antihypertensive agents. To the extent that tissue ACE is not blocked by ACE inhibitors, the angiotensin II receptor blockers may be more effective in reducing blood pressure. In reality, comparative studies have shown that they are equally effective as antihypertensive agents. The angiotensin II receptor antagonists not only avoid the cough but also have not (so far) been implicated in as many cases of angioedema as have the ACE inhibitors, but this is a very rare side effect with either class of drug. Presumably the angiotensin II receptor antagonists will have the same beneficial effects as the ACE inhibitors in patients with left ventricular failure and in patients with type I diabetes with nephropathy, but controlled trials have not been reported. The same precautions as described above for the use of ACE inhibitors in patients with renovascular hypertension, hypovolemia, severe heart failure, and chronic renal failure also apply to the angiotensin II receptor antagonists.[81]

ALPHA-ADRENERGIC BLOCKING DRUGS

The nonselective alpha-adrenergic blockers phentolamine and phenoxybenzamine block both the $alpha_1$ receptor on vascular smooth muscle wall, activation of which causes vasoconstriction, and the $alpha_2$ or presynaptic receptor that mediates a negative feedback to inhibit the release of norepinephrine from the sympathetic nerve terminal (Table 58-7. See also

Chap. 23). These antagonists, therefore, cause release of excessive norepinephrine by blocking the presynaptic $alpha_2$ receptor located on the nerve terminal and thus cause palpitations and tachycardia, among other side effects. They are used primarily in the management of hypertension secondary to pheochromocytoma. Drugs that selectively block the $alpha_1$-adrenergic receptor usually do not produce tachycardia and palpitations because they do not interfere with the negative-feedback mechanism that controls the release of norepinephrine. The 1993 report of the JNC (JNC-V) included the selective $alpha_1$-adrenergic receptor blockers as candidates for initial (step 1) monotherapy.[5] These are the only antihypertensive agents that have a beneficial effect on serum lipids, including reductions in total cholesterol, triglycerides, and LDL cholesterol and an increase in HDL cholesterol.[34,82–84] In the TOMHS trial, doxazosin was the only drug that produced a statistically significant increase in the HDL/total cholesterol ratio compared to placebo.[34] While the magnitude of these beneficial changes in serum lipids is not great, these drugs are particularly useful in patients who have only modest abnormalities in their lipid profiles for whom a drug of this class might control hypertension and dyslipidemia simultaneously.[36] For patients who have major abnormalities in serum lipids, treatment directed at that risk factor will be necessary in addition to whatever antihypertensive drugs are selected.

Selective $alpha_1$-adrenergic blockers also have a favorable effect on glucose metabolism by reducing insulin resistance,[51,82,83,85] which is frequently found in hypertensive patients, especially the obese. There are no contraindications to the use of selective $alpha_1$-adrenergic blocking agents, provided that appropriate caution is exercised in warning

---

TABLE 58-7

ALPHA$_1$-ADRENERGIC BLOCKERS

Agent	Usual Daily Dose,[a] mg	Precautions and Special Considerations	Selected Side Effects[b]
Nonselective		Use cautiously in elderly patients because of orthostatic hypotension. Phentolamine, phenoxybenzamine, and prazosin are more likely to produce orthostatic hypotension than are terazosin and doxazosin.	"First-dose" syncope, orthostatic hypotension, dizziness, headache, weakness, palpitations, nausea
Phentolamine (Regitine)	—[c]		
Phenoxybenzamine (Dibenzyline)	20–80[d]		
Selective			
Prazosin (Minipress)	1–20[d]		
Terazosin (Hytrin)	1–20		
Doxazosin (Cardura)	1–16		

Special indications: Phentolamine and phenoxybenzamine are used almost exclusively for management of patients with pheochromocytoma; the selective alpha$_1$ blockers may also be prescribed as initial therapy for patients with primary hypertension; especially useful for those with diabetes, lipid abnormalities, or symptomatic benign prostatic hyperplasia.

Contraindications: History of hypersensitivity to these agents.

Advantages: No absolute contraindications; beneficial effects on serum lipids and insulin resistance; reduce total peripheral resistance. The selective alpha$_1$ blockers may relieve symptoms of benign prostatic hypertrophy.

Disadvantages: Moderately expensive; unpredictable hypotensive effect after first dose and high side effect profile (especially phenoxybenzamine and prazosin); no trials to demonstrate long-term efficacy in reducing cardiovascular events; can produce pseudoresistance (fluid retention).

[a] The dosage range may differ slightly from recommended dosage in *Physicians' Desk Reference* or package insert. Given once daily unless otherwise indicated.

[b] The listing of side effects is not all-inclusive, and health practitioners are urged to refer to the package insert for a more detailed listing.

[c] Phentolamine is used only parenterally for perioperative management of patients with pheochromocytoma.

[d] This drug is usually given in divided doses two to three times a day.

patients, particularly the elderly, about the possibility of an orthostatic hypotensive response to the first dose ("first-dose effect"). This problem is more likely to occur when an alpha$_1$-blocking agent is added to an existing regimen, especially a diuretic, than when it is given as monotherapy. It is less likely to occur with the long-acting drugs terazosin and doxazosin than with prazosin. Obviously, treatment should be started with the smallest possible "test dose" of whichever drug is selected. Alpha$_1$-adrenergic blockade improves the obstructive symptoms of benign prostatic hyperplasia.[86] A rather high incidence of adverse effects requiring discontinuation of the drug has been found with prazosin in two controlled trials.[30,84] The longer-acting agents seem to be better tolerated.

ALPHA$_2$-ADRENORECEPTOR AGONISTS

The centrally acting sympathetic partial agonists have not been recommended for initial monotherapy because of their high side effect profile and their propensity to cause fluid retention and pseudoresistance (Table 58-8). Usually they are prescribed as step 2 drugs. When they are added to a diuretic, they do not cause fluid retention. Rebound hypertension has been described after sudden withdrawal of these agents, especially oral clonidine.[87] To enhance adherence, the long-acting drug guanfacine is preferred. The transdermal preparation of clonidine has a duration of action of 7 days, but surprisingly it has not been popular with patients, even though it appears to cause fewer side effects than the oral preparation.

Methyldopa, given as monotherapy, is the preferred drug in managing the hypertension associated with preeclampsia.[88]

NEUROEFFECTOR ADRENERGIC BLOCKING DRUGS

Reserpine and guanethidine were among the first antihypertensive drugs introduced more than 35 years ago (Table 58-9). Guanadrel was introduced more recently but shares many of the undesirable side effects of guanethidine, including orthostatic hypotension and sexual dysfunction. At present, none is widely used in the United States because other effective agents with fewer side effects are available.

Reserpine in small doses (0.05 to 0.125 mg daily) combined with a diuretic to prevent pseudotolerance is the least expensive antihypertensive regimen available and was effective and well tolerated in a Veterans Administration (VA) controlled clinical trial.[89] This combination is still widely used in some large inner city clinics where cost is an important consideration.

DIRECT VASODILATORS

Hydralazine and minoxidil are direct vasodilators, the mechanism of action of which is not well understood (Table 58-10). They both cause reflex tachycardia and fluid retention, which can be profound with minoxidil. For this reason, they are usually prescribed with both a sympathetic inhibitor (frequently a beta-adrenergic blocker) to control cardiac rate and a diuretic to control fluid retention. In the case of minoxidil, large doses of a loop diuretic are often required.

Minoxidil is almost exclusively reserved for managing hypertension that is resistant to multidrug regimens and is particularly effective when renal failure is present.[90] Since the advent of ACE inhibitors and calcium channel blockers, minoxidil is less commonly needed.

TABLE 58-8
CENTRALLY ACTING ALPHA$_2$-ADRENORECEPTOR AGONISTS

Agent	Usual Daily Dose,[a] mg	Precautions and Special Considerations	Selected Side Effects[b]
Clonidine (Catapres)	0.1–1.2[c]	Rebound hypertension may occur with abrupt discontinuance (especially oral clonidine), particularly with prior administration of high doses or with continuation of concomitant beta-blocker therapy.	Drowsiness, sedation, lethargy, dry mouth, fatigue, depression, sexual dysfunction, orthostatic hypotension; localized skin reaction to clonidine transdermal therapeutic system (TTS) patch
Clonidine TTS (patch) (Catapres TTS)	0.1–0.3[d]		
Guanabenz (Wytensin)	4–64[c]		
Guanafacine (Tenex)	1–3		
Methyldopa (Aldomet)	250–2000[c]	Methyldopa interferes with fluorometric measurements of urinary catecholamine levels.	Same as above and drug fever, hepatotoxicity, abnormal liver function tests $\pm$ hepatitis, positive Coomb's test with or without hemolytic anemia

Special indications: Elderly patients, usually with a diuretic. Methyldopa: preeclampsia.

Contraindications: History of hypersensitivity reaction to these agents; hepatic dysfunction (methyldopa).

Advantages: Reduce total peripheral resistance, relatively inexpensive, no metabolic side effects.

Disadvantages: High side effect profile, rebound hypertension after sudden withdrawal, especially oral clonidine. Potential to cause fluid retention and pseudotolerance. No trials to demonstrate long-term efficacy in reducing cardiovascular events.

[a] The dosage range may differ slightly from recommended dosage in *Physicians' Desk Reference* or package insert. Drugs are given once daily unless otherwise indicated.

[b] The listing of side effects is not all-inclusive, and health practitioners are urged to refer to the package insert for a more detailed listing.

[c] This drug is usually given in divided doses twice daily.

[d] This drug is administered as a skin patch once weekly.

TABLE 58-9

NEUROEFFECTOR ADRENERGIC INHIBITORS

Agent	Usual Daily Dose,[a] mg	Precautions and Special Considerations	Selected Side Effects[b]
Guanadrel sulfate (Hylorel)	10–75[c]	Use cautiously because of orthostatic hypotension.	Diarrhea (especially guanethidine), sexual dysfunction including retrograde ejaculation, orthostatic hypotension (especially in the morning or after exercise)
Guanethidine (Ismelin)	10–50		
Rauwolfia alkaloids, generic	50–100	Contraindicated in patients with history of mental depression; use with caution in patients with history of peptic ulcer.	Lethargy, lassitude, sedation, nasal congestion, depression, loss of libido, activation of peptic ulcer, Parkinson-like syndrome
Reserpine, generic	0.1 every other day to 0.25 daily		

Special indications: Use with a diuretic to minimize dosage.

Contraindications: Reserpine: history of depression or peptic ulcer; Parkinson's disease. Guanethidine and guanadrel: elderly patients, patients with diabetic autonomic neuropathy, and patients on dialysis (because of the propensity of these drugs to produce orthostatic hypotension).

Advantages: Inexpensive; reduce total peripheral resistance; no metabolic side effects. Reserpine was used with diuretic and hydralazine in first Veterans Administration trial demonstrating reduction of morbidity and mortality.

Disadvantages: High side effect profile. Can cause fluid retention and pseudotolerance. No trials to demonstrate long-term efficacy in reducing cardiovascular events except as noted above. Guanethidine and guanadrel: reduction in blood pressure is primarily orthostatic.

[a] The dosage range may differ slightly from recommended dosage in *Physicians' Desk Reference* or package insert. Drugs are given once daily unless otherwise indicated.

[b] The listing of side effects is not all-inclusive, and health practitioners are urged to refer to the package insert for a more detailed listing.

[c] This drug is usually given in divided doses twice daily.

TABLE 58-10

DIRECT VASODILATORS

Agent	Usual Daily Dose,[a] mg	Precautions and Special Considerations	Side Effects[b]
Hydralazine (Apresoline)	50–300[c]	Minoxidil may cause or aggravate pleural and pericardial effusions. Both may precipitate angina pectoris in patients with coronary disease because of reflex tachycardia. Hydralazine: lupus syndrome. Should be administered with a diuretic to prevent fluid retention and an adrenergic inhibitor (usually a beta-adrenergic blocker) to prevent reflex tachycardia.	Headache, anorexia, nausea and vomiting, diarrhea, palpitations, reflex tachycardia, fluid retention, and aggravation of angina; hydralazine: positive antinuclear antibody test, lupus-like reactions; minoxidil: hirsutism
Minoxidil (Loniten)	2.5–80		

Special indications: Hydralazine: eclampsia or preeclampsia. Minoxidil: severe and resistant hypertension especially with renal failure.

Contraindications: Obstructive coronary artery disease; lupus erythematosus (hydralazine).

Advantages: Minoxidil is one of the most potent antihypertensive agents available. Relatively inexpensive. Reduces total peripheral resistance, no metabolic side effects. Hydralazine was used with a diuretic and reserpine in the first VA Trial to show reduction of cardiovascular events.

Disadvantages: Must be prescribed with a diuretic to prevent fluid retention and a sympathetic inhibiting drug to prevent reflex tachycardia. High side effect profile. No trials with minoxidil to demonstrate long-term efficacy in reducing cardiovascular events.

[a] The dosage range may differ slightly from recommended dosage in *Physicians' Desk Reference* or package insert. Drugs are given once daily unless otherwise indicated.

[b] The listing of side effects is not all-inclusive, and health practitioners are urged to refer to the package insert for a more detailed listing.

[c] This drug is usually given in divided doses two to four times daily.

COMBINATION TABLETS

Some of the tablets containing two antihypertensive agents in combination (usually a beta-blocker or an ACE inhibitor with a diuretic) are listed in Table 58-11. Only two of these (captopril with HCTZ and bisoprolol with HCTZ) are approved by the Food and Drug Administration for initial therapy. Usually it is preferable to initiate antihypertensive therapy for patients with stage 1 or 2 hypertension with a single agent. The combination of bisoprolol and HCTZ, however, contains subtherapeutic doses of each agent, which combined have a definite antihypertensive effect.[91] The combination of captopril and HCTZ contains small doses of each agent, but the presence of HCTZ in the tablet permits once-a-day dosing, whereas captopril by itself is usually given twice daily.

J-Curve

Farnett et al.[92] have summarized 13 publications, nine of which demonstrated that reducing diastolic blood pressure below 85 to 90 mmHg may paradoxically increase the risk of coronary mortality for hypertensive patients and two of which showed a flattening of coronary mortality at the lower end of diastolic blood pressure achieved by treatment, but not actually an upswing. In one of the original reports, Cruickshank et al.[93] stated that the J-curve phenomenon was observed only in those hypertensive patients who had clinical evidence of ischemic heart disease, but others have reported that excess mortality was not limited to patients with ischemic heart disease when the diastolic blood pressure was reduced below 85 to 90 mmHg.[92,94–102] Some authors report that the J-curve is limited to diastolic blood pressure only,[93–95,97,101] while others have also found it for systolic blood pressure (<150 to 155 mmHg).[98,102] Stroke mortality seems to decrease with diastolic blood pressure without a J-curve phenomenon, and there is evidence that maximal protection from end-stage renal failure is achieved when blood pressure is reduced to 130/85 mmHg or below.[103]

The J-curve phenomenon is not confined to hypertensive patients on antihypertensive therapy; it has also been observed in the Framingham observational study,[104,105] in the placebo group in the European Working Party on Hypertension in the Elderly (EWPHE),[102] and in an untreated group of elderly hypertensive patients.[100] In the EWPHE trial, the participants who had the lowest systolic and diastolic blood pressures also had the most pronounced decreases in body weight and hemoglobin concentration, suggesting that they were ill.[102] Noncardiovascular mortality was also highest in patients who were in the lowest third of diastolic pressure.[102] Low blood pressure, with or without therapy, may simply be a marker for chronic illness.

A meta-analysis of observational studies[106] and the large Medical Research Council trial[107] failed to show a J-curve. In the Systolic Hypertension in the Elderly (SHEP) trial, the 5-year average diastolic blood pressure was 68 mmHg for the treated group and 72 mmHg for the placebo group, yet the treated group had significantly fewer coronary and stroke events than did the participants in the placebo group.[10] Fletcher and Bulpitt[108] have concluded a very thoughtful and comprehensive review of this subject with this recommendation: "In conclusion, it appears reasonable to lower diastolic blood pressure to below 85 mmHg. This gives maximal benefit in reducing the risk of stroke, and the risk of myocardial infarction is reduced compared with that at pressures over 100 mmHg. On balance, we consider the J-curve is probably a consequence, not a cause of coronary heart disease. Systolic blood pressure should be lowered to below 125 mmHg, since there is no indication that doing so has any adverse effects." Most patients are not having their blood pressures controlled to this level at the present time.[4,5,5a]

It is equally important to control systolic blood pressure, as noted by Fletcher and Bulpitt.[108] Oxygen consumption of the myocardium is more dependent on systolic blood pressure than it is on diastolic blood pressure, whereas coronary flow (oxygen supply) is dependent on diastolic blood pressure. A disparity, therefore, between oxygen demand and supply might explain the J-curve phenomenon, if indeed there is one.

The J-curve has been a retrospective observation in nonrandomized clinical trials or randomized trials that were not designed to test this hypothesis. A prospective, controlled, randomized trial is needed to settle this issue, and one is in progress.[109]

Treatment of Diabetic and/or Insulin-Resistant Patients

Many hypertensive patients, obese and nonobese, have insulin resistance manifested by higher than normal fasting and post–glucose load plasma insulin levels, even if they are not frankly diabetic.[51,110,111] A direct relationship between diastolic blood pressure and fasting insulin levels has been demon-

TABLE 58-11

TABLETS CONTAINING TWO ANTIHYPERTENSIVE AGENTS

Diuretic with beta blocker
Propranolol hydrochloride and hydrochlorothiazide (HCTZ) (Inderide LA)[a]
Metoprolol tartrate and HCTZ (Lopressor HCT)[a]
Atenolol and chlorthalidone (Tenoretic)[a]
Timolol maleate and HCTZ (Timolide)[a]
Bisoprolol fumarate and HCTZ (Ziac)[b]
Diuretic with ACE inhibitor
Captopril and HCTZ (Capozide)[b]
Benazepril hydrochloride and HCTZ (Lotensin HCT)[a]
Lisinopril and HCTZ (Prinzide, Zestoretic)[a]
Enalapril maleate and HCTZ (Vasoretic)[a]
Calcium antagonists with ACE inhibitor
Amlodipine and benazepril (Lotrel)[a]
Enalapril maleate and felodipine ER (Lexxel)[a]
Trandolapril and verapamil HCl ER (Tarka)[a]

[a] Not approved for initial therapy.
[b] Approved for initial therapy.

strated.[110] Although it has been postulated that insulin may increase blood pressure by promoting sodium retention and increasing sympathetic nervous activity, there is evidence that insulin resistance may be the result rather than the cause of the heightened adrenergic outflow.[51,112] Lipid abnormalities, including high triglyceride and low HDL cholesterol levels in the blood, are often associated with hyperinsulinemia. Indeed, this combination of risk factors has been described as the "deadly quartet"[113]—upper body obesity, hypertension, insulin resistance (glucose intolerance), and hypertriglyceridemia (see also Chap. 78).

Reducing the blood pressure with medication does not necessarily improve insulin resistance, although alpha$_1$-adrenergic blocking agents have been shown to decrease insulin resistance.[51,83,85] The long-term implications of this are not clear. Weight reduction and physical exercise decrease insulin resistance[51,113,114] and should be the cornerstone of therapy for hypertensive patients, whether or not they have diabetes.

In addition to diuretics, beta blockers[51,114] can increase insulin resistance and raise blood glucose in some patients. Diuretic therapy has been associated with increased mortality in diabetic patients with retinopathy in nonrandomized observations in which there was no attempt to allocate treatment regimens prospectively.[115,116]

It should be noted that diuretic-based therapy was used in several of the large prospective randomized trials in which diabetic patients were not excluded (EWPHE,[117] HDFP,[118] SHEP[10]), and no adverse effects were reported. Indeed, in the HDFP trial, diabetic patients had higher mortality rates than nondiabetic patients in both the stepped care and referred care groups, but the benefit of stepped care, although less for diabetic than for nondiabetic patients, was not statistically significantly different between the two groups.[118] Diuretics and beta blockers usually do not adversely affect glucose control and are not contraindicated in patients with diabetes provided that blood glucose and lipids are carefully monitored.[52,119] Long-term beta-blocker therapy was more effective in preventing cardiovascular events and reducing mortality after a myocardial infarction in diabetic than in nondiabetic patients.[120] Randomized trials are needed to determine if drugs that do not have an adverse effect on insulin resistance (calcium channel blockers, ACE inhibitors) or that may actually improve it (alpha$_1$-adrenergic blocking agents) will be more effective than diuretics in reducing cardiovascular morbidity and mortality for diabetic patients. The results of the Antihypertensive Lipid Lowering Heart Attack Trial (ALLHAT)[121] should help answer this question. Unfortunately, the results of that trial will not be available until about 2002. In the meantime physicians should feel comfortable in prescribing diuretics and/or beta blockers for diabetic patients with hypertension, provided they are appropriately monitored.[52,119]

On the other hand, nonselective beta blockers (as well as selective beta blockers in large doses) should be used with caution in patients with type I diabetes mellitus, especially those who are subject to insulin reactions, because they can prolong recovery from insulin-induced hypoglycemia. The benefit of ACE inhibitors in patients with type I diabetic nephropathy was described previously in the section on ACE inhibitors.

MANAGEMENT OF HYPERTENSION IN SPECIAL POPULATIONS

African-American Patients

In the United States, hypertension occurs more frequently, tends to be more severe, and is accompanied by a higher mortality rate in African Americans than in whites, irrespective of age.[5,5a,28,122] For comparable levels of blood pressure, African Americans have LVH (evident on echocardiography) and/or evidence of renal disease more often than do whites.[28,122] The HDFP trial showed that the overall mortality rate was reduced more for African Americans than for whites by stepped care therapy compared to referred care.[118] African-American hypertensive patients seem to respond better to diuretics[14] or calcium channel blockers[30] than they do to beta blockers or ACE inhibitors, although there are many exceptions to this. Because of the obvious racial differences in vulnerability to the complications of hypertension, therapy should be initiated early and should be pursued aggressively for African-American patients, especially young males.

Women

While there is no evidence that women respond any differently than men to the hypotensive effects of antihypertensive drugs, the long-term effect of reducing blood pressure on cardiovascular events for white women has been questioned.[123] It is true that women were not included in the major VA trials showing efficacy of treatment. It is also true that premenopausal hypertensive women have a lower incidence of cardiovascular disease than do hypertensive men of the same age. When hypertensive women are compared to normotensive women of the same age, however, *the relative risk* of cardiovascular morbidity and mortality is about the same for women as it is for men, especially as it relates to systolic blood pressure.[124] In the HDFP trial, the 5-year mortality rate for 908 white women in the stepped care (SC) group with mild hypertension (stratum I; diastolic blood pressure 90 to 104 mmHg) was 27.1 percent lower than for the 917 white women in referred care (RC). This was second only to a 29 percent reduction in mortality enjoyed by African-American women in stepped care. For white men the reduction was 17.6 percent, and for African-American men it was 6.8 percent.[118] In the groups with more severe hypertension (diastolic blood pressure ≥105 mmHg), the white women in stepped care did not fare as well as those in referred care, but this is not necessarily the result of pharmacologic treatment because both groups received antihypertensive agents. The numbers of white women were so small in these groups (SC = 272, RC = 233) that the difference was not statistically significant.

More worrisome is the observation that in the placebo-controlled Medical Research Council trial, all-cause mortality was *increased* by 26 percent for white women on active treatment compared with those on placebo, whereas there was a 15 percent reduction in mortality for men on active treatment.[107] In the HDFP trial, total strokes were reduced by 30.4 percent for white women.[125] In the SHEP trial, white women on active treatment had 27 percent fewer strokes than those on placebo.[10] As yet there is no justification from available evidence that treatment guidelines should be different for the genders, except that ACE inhibitors are contraindicated for pregnant women.[88]

The Elderly

The prevalence of hypertension, both diastolic and isolated systolic, increases with age. If the criteria used for hypertension are ≥ 140 mmHg systolic and/or ≥ 90 mmHg diastolic blood pressures, the prevalence of hypertension was 53 percent for whites and 72 percent for African Americans ages 65 to 74 years in the National Health and Nutrition Examination Survey (NHANES III) of 1988 to 1991.[126] These data were derived either by averaging three blood pressure measurements on a single occasion or by a history of taking antihypertensive medication. Nearly two-thirds (65 percent) of hypertensive individuals ≥ 60 years of age have isolated systolic hypertension (≥ 140 and <90 mmHg), and for hypertensive individuals ≥ 75 years of age, 75 percent have isolated systolic hypertension.[126] Most elderly patients with diastolic hypertension have primary hypertension that started in middle life or earlier.

There is good evidence from randomized controlled trials that treating diastolic hypertension[1,126] as well as isolated systolic hypertension[10] is beneficial in reducing morbidity and mortality for elderly patients. These trials have shown that elderly patients tolerate antihypertensive drugs well and are as adherent to regimens as younger patients. It is advisable to initiate therapy with smaller than average doses and to increase doses or to add new drugs very gradually to avoid reducing blood pressure rapidly and to minimize the risk of orthostatic hypotension.

A trial of lifestyle modifications should be recommended initially for elderly patients with stage 1 hypertension and no evidence of target organ disease or other risk factors and in addition to drug treatment for patients who have more severe hypertension.[15,126]

The drug of choice for most elderly patients is a thiazide-type diuretic in low dose, simply because nearly all the clinical trials that have demonstrated the benefit of treatment have used diuretic-based stepped care.[29,126] Beta-adrenergic blocking agents were also found to be effective in the Swedish Trial in Old Patients with Hypertension[127] and the Hypertension in Elderly Patients trials.[99] Moreover, a VA trial showed that a diuretic as step 1 followed by hydralazine, methyldopa, metoprolol, or reserpine, if needed for step 2, was effective and well tolerated and did not have an adverse effect on cognitive or behavioral function in elderly patients compared

with placebo administered in the pretreatment control period.[128,129] Similarly, in the SHEP Feasibility Trial, participants on diuretic therapy did not have changes in cognitive function or level of depression compared with those on placebo.[130]

Nitrendipine, a dihydropyridine calcium antagonist not available in the United States, has been shown to reduce the incidence of total strokes in elderly patients with isolated systolic hypertension compared to placebo.[10a]

MANAGING PATIENTS WITH COMPLICATIONS OF HYPERTENSION

Cerebrovascular Disease

Controlling diastolic as well as isolated systolic hypertension has had a profound effect on reducing morbidity and mortality from stroke in randomized clinical trials.[1,5,10,10a,125]

Several small trials have shown that control of blood pressure for patients who have already had one stroke will reduce the risk of recurrent stroke, including fatal ones,[131-133] although one large multicenter trial failed to confirm this.[134] Management of hypertension during acute stroke is discussed in the section on hypertensive crises, below. Once a patient has recovered from the acute phase of cerebral infarction or hemorrhage, the neurologic deficit has stabilized, and the patient is ambulatory (usually 3 or 4 weeks after the stroke), hypertension should be treated with the same regimens that would be used for hypertensive patients who have never had a stroke. The goal should be to normalize blood pressure gradually ($<140/90$ mmHg) (see also Chap. 99).

Surprisingly, these patients usually tolerate normotension quite well, including inadvertent orthostatic hypotension, although this is not desirable and should be avoided if at all possible. While none of the antihypertensive agents are absolutely contraindicated, agents that have a proclivity for producing disproportionate orthostatic decreases in blood pressure (e.g., alpha$_1$-adrenergic blockers, guanadrel, guanethidine) should be used with extra caution, and patients should be warned about rising from the seated or recumbent positions rapidly.

If treatment produces symptoms of global cerebral ischemia unrelated to measurable hypotension, the clinician should suspect that the patient has severe occlusive disease in both carotid arteries and/or the vertebral basilar system. Monitoring blood pressure in the standing as well as seated (or supine) position is particularly important for patients with cerebrovascular disease.

In patients with transient ischemic attacks, the treatment of systemic arterial hypertension will not only reduce the frequency of the ischemic episodes but will also lessen the risk of subsequent stroke.[135] Blood pressure should be reduced gradually, with special attention devoted to avoiding orthostatic hypotension. Aspirin should be prescribed in a dose of 325 mg daily. Obviously, a surgically approachable lesion in the extracranial carotid arteries should be sought (see Chap. 99).

Cardiac Complications

ATHEROSCLEROTIC HEART DISEASE

The management of systemic hypertension in patients with unstable angina or acute myocardial infarction is discussed in the section on hypertensive crises, below.

ANGINA PECTORIS

There is a special indication for beta-adrenergic blockers or calcium channel blockers in the management of hypertension in patients with angina pectoris because both classes of drugs are beneficial for relieving angina and controlling hypertension. Their mechanisms for relieving angina pectoris are different, so that there is sometimes an advantage to using these two classes of drugs together when angina is resistant to one. This must be done judiciously because both the beta-adrenergic blockers and the calcium channel blockers verapamil and diltiazem slow conduction and have negative inotropic effects that might lead to heart block or left ventricular failure in patients who already have a conduction defect or left ventricular dysfunction. Drugs that can cause reflexive tachycardia, such as hydralazine and minoxidil, can aggravate angina pectoris and should not be used without an adrenergic inhibitor, usually a beta blocker, in the regimen to prevent tachycardia.

Short-acting calcium channel blockers should be avoided in the management of hypertension (see "Calcium Channel Blockers," above).

POSTMYOCARDIAL INFARCTION

Only the non-ISA beta blockers have been shown conclusively to have a cardioprotective effect following myocardial infarction,[48] and these are the agents of choice for treating hypertension in patients who have had a myocardial infarction, unless there is a bona fide contraindication to their use. The evidence of a cardioprotective effect for verapamil is less impressive than for the beta-adrenergic blockers, and in patients with clinical evidence of left ventricular dysfunction after myocardial infarction, diltiazem had an adverse effect on survival.[56] The dihydropyridine calcium channel blockers have failed to show any cardioprotective effect following myocardial infarction and in some studies have been detrimental[58,59] (see also Chaps. 47 and 54).

LEFT VENTRICULAR HYPERTROPHY

While LVH is an adaptive mechanism to handle the increased workload imposed by high systemic arterial pressure, it nevertheless is an independent risk factor for arrhythmias, myocardial infarction, and sudden death.[136] Because there is as yet no convincing evidence that reversing LVH will eliminate or mitigate this risk, the goal should be to prevent LVH in the first place by treating hypertension before LVH develops. All of the major classes of antihypertensive agents, with the possible exception of the direct vasodilators (hydralazine, minoxidil), will eventually reduce left ventricular mass when it is increased.[137] In a meta-analysis of randomized, double-blind studies, the ACE inhibitors were the most effective in reducing left ventricular mass, followed by the calcium channel blockers, the diuretics, and the beta blockers, in that order.[138] In a meta-analysis of randomized, double-blind studies, the ACE inhibitors were the most effective in reducing left ventricular mass, followed by the calcium channel blockers, the diuretics, and the beta blockers, in that order.[138] In randomized prospective controlled trials comparing the major classes of antihypertensive drugs, the diuretics were more effective than the others in reducing LV mass.[31,138a] Until it has been demonstrated that reversal of LVH will reduce the risk that it imposes, it does not present a special indication or contraindication for any of the antihypertensive drugs recommended for initial therapy. If a diuretic is selected, however, hypokalemia should be avoided since it might enhance the arrhythmogenic potential of LVH. The use of a combination thiazide/potassium-sparing agent is recommended under these circumstances.

CONGESTIVE HEART FAILURE

Agents of choice for hypertensive patients with congestive heart failure due to systolic dysfunction are diuretics and ACE inhibitors, which reduce preload by decreasing venous return and afterload by dilating arterioles. The ACE inhibitors have been shown to improve survival in patients with chronic congestive heart failure and low ejection fraction (<40 percent), with or without hypertension.[65–67] Beta-adrenergic blockers and calcium channel blockers are relatively contraindicated in patients with congestive heart failure due to left ventricular systolic dysfunction and low ejection fraction (see also Chaps. 23 and 54), although some beta blockers have been shown to be beneficial when used judiciously in some cases of left ventricular failure due to systolic dysfunction.[139]

Occasionally, recurrent episodes of left ventricular failure, sometimes with pulmonary edema, are due to diastolic rather than systolic dysfunction, especially in elderly patients. This is characterized by severe concentric LVH that may nearly obliterate the left ventricular cavity, compromising diastolic filling of the ventricle, which relaxes poorly during diastole. The ejection fraction is high, but cardiac index is low in spite of vigorous systolic contractions (see also Chaps. 21 and 23). In this situation, diuretics and vasodilators such as ACE inhibitors, the dihydropyridine calcium antagonists, alpha$_1$-adrenergic blockers, and the direct vasodilators can have an adverse effect by causing hypotension.[140] Drugs of choice are the beta-adrenergic blockers and the calcium channel blockers verapamil or diltiazem because they may improve relaxation of the left ventricle and reduce heart rate, thereby enhancing diastolic filling (see also Chaps. 21, 23, and 54).

CARDIAC ARRHYTHMIAS AND CONDUCTION DISTURBANCES

Certain antihypertensive drugs may be especially indicated or relatively contraindicated when hypertension is complicated by cardiac arrhythmias or conduction disturbances. Non-ISA beta blockers may be helpful in controlling paroxysmal supraventricular tachycardia and premature ventricular contractions due to adrenergic hyperactivity. On the other hand, by slowing the heart rate, they might actually increase premature ventricular contractions in some patients, but there is little evidence that this is clinically important. Verapamil may be more effective than beta blockers in treating and preventing recurrences of paroxysmal supraventricular tachycardia (see Chap. 27). Beta-adrenergic blockers, verapamil, and diltiazem slow AV conduction and therefore are often effective in controlling the ventricular rate in patients with atrial fibrillation or flutter. For the same reason, however, they are contraindicated in the presence of greater than first-degree AV block, although they usually may be used in patients with intraventricular block and bundle branch block. All are contraindicated for patients with "sick sinus syndrome" unless a functioning ventricular pacemaker is in place. Special precautions must be observed in using verapamil, diltiazem, or beta-adrenergic blockers in patients with an accessory bypass tract (Wolff-Parkinson-White or Lown-Genong-Levine syndromes). Verapamil and diltiazem can precipitate reciprocating tachycardias in these patients (see Chap. 27).

VALVULAR HEART DISEASE

Arteriolar vasodilating agents such as the calcium channel blockers and ACE inhibitors are helpful in minimizing the regurgitant flow in hypertensive patients with either mitral or aortic regurgitation[141] (see Chaps. 23, 63, and 64).

Chronic Renal Failure

Treatment of hypertension may prevent or retard progression of renal failure.[103,142] The dramatic increase in the number of patients with diabetes and hypertension coming to end-stage renal failure and requiring dialysis is therefore disturbing. It was the consensus of the National High Blood Pressure Education Program Working Group that efforts to treat hypertension have not been vigorous enough and that reducing blood pressure to 130/85 mmHg or lower may be beneficial to prevent renal failure or to retard its progression[103] (see also Chap. 94). The potential advantages and risks of ACE inhibitors for patients with diabetic nephropathy have already been discussed in the section on ACE inhibitors. Calcium channel blockers, selective alpha$_1$-adrenergic blocking agents, beta-adrenergic blocking agents, alpha$_2$ agonists, and loop diuretics have all been used in managing hypertension in patients with renal failure. Loop diuretics are particularly important when fluid retention seems to be causing or aggravating the hypertension. Minoxidil is especially effective in patients with renal failure and severe hypertension.[143] Appropriate adjustments in dosage of antihypertensive agents that are excreted by the kidney must be made when renal failure is present (see Tables 58-4 and 58-6).

A low-protein diet (40 to 50 g daily) may have a renal protective effect and should be prescribed for most patients with chronic renal failure. Dietary sodium restriction is also important as an adjunct to prevent fluid retention (see also Chap. 94).

Severe and Refractory Hypertension

The more severe the hypertension, the less likely that monotherapy will control it and the greater the urgency for reducing it. Consequently, in the absence of complications that would require immediate reduction of blood pressure (see "Hypertensive Crises," below), it is usually advisable to initiate therapy with two drugs simultaneously for patients with stage 3 hypertension. The selection of drugs should be made on an individualized basis using criteria listed in the tables. Hospitalization is not necessary in the absence of complications, but patients should be seen in the office or clinic at frequent intervals until the blood pressure is controlled. Monitoring blood pressure at home is almost mandatory in this situation. Not all severe hypertension is refractory to treatment, and not all refractory hypertension is severe.[43] *When hypertension does not respond to a rational triple-drug regimen that includes a diuretic, the physician should suspect nonadherence to the regimen as the most likely cause.* This nonadherence may be manifested by failure to take drugs as prescribed or by consuming too much sodium or alcohol or both. Drug-drug interactions should also be suspected. Leading the list of drugs that can interfere with an otherwise effective regimen are nonsteroidal anti-inflammatory drugs and oral contraceptives. Pseudohypertension (related to sclerotic, calcific upper extremity arteries)[144] and "white coat" hypertension[145] should be ruled out. Finally, the physician should reconsider the possibility that a secondary form of hypertension has been overlooked, such as pheochromocytoma, renovascular hypertension, or primary aldosteronism (see Chap. 57). When it is apparent that the hypertension is truly resistant, changes in the regimen can be made empirically.[146] Doses of all the drugs in the regimen should be maximized. Consideration should be given to adding a fourth drug with a different mechanism of action. Minoxidil is one of the most potent agents available.

Sometimes it is necessary to evaluate the mechanism of the hypertension while patients are on their regimen to see which drug or drugs are failing. This strategy could include measurements of plasma renin activity, catecholamines, aldosterone, plasma volume, cardiac output, and total peripheral resistance.

HYPERTENSIVE CRISES

Table 58-12 lists some of the hypertensive emergencies and urgencies that require prompt antihypertensive therapy. True emergencies require immediate reduction of blood pressure to ameliorate target organ damage. Rapid reduction of blood pressure to or toward normal is recommended for patients with acute hypertensive encephalopathy, acute left ventricular failure with pulmonary edema, and acute aortic dissection. It is not desirable to reduce blood pressure rapidly or to normotensive levels for patients with cerebral hemorrhage, subarachnoid hemorrhage, or acute brain infarction[147–149] (see Chap. 99).

The availability of drugs such as short-acting nifedipine, captopril, and clonidine, which can reduce blood pressure within minutes to an hour when given by mouth or sublingually, has blurred the distinction between hypertensive emergencies and urgencies.[150] Sometimes, oral medication will suffice for some emergencies, and parenteral drugs are used for some urgencies, especially when patients are unable to take medication by mouth (e.g., postoperative state). Patients with hypertensive emergencies present with evidence of target organ involvement or are in immediate danger of developing it, whereas patients with hypertensive urgencies have no evidence of target organ involvement, and it is only the height of the blood pressure that is of concern. Usually, reduction of the blood pressure to a safer, though not necessarily normotensive, level over a period of 12 to 24 h is sufficient in managing urgencies. Hospitalization may not even be required, or if it is, monitoring in an intensive care unit is not necessary. Most patients with hypertensive urgencies can be managed on an outpatient basis if they can be seen frequently in the clinic or office for both diagnostic evaluation and therapeutic follow-up. The drugs that can be given parenterally for managing hypertensive emergencies and urgencies are listed in Table 58-13. Sodium nitroprusside is recommended for most of the emergencies listed in Table 58-12 except for eclampsia, acute myocardial ischemia, and post–coronary bypass hypertension.[150] Methyldopa, given intravenously, is the drug of choice for eclampsia,[88] while intravenous nitroglycerin is recommended for patients with acute myocardial ischemia and post–coronary bypass hypertension.[150] A beta-adrenergic blocker must be given orally or parenterally with sodium nitroprusside for managing patients with acute aortic dissection, and the goal of treatment is to maintain systolic blood pressure within the range of 100 to 120 mmHg (see also Chap. 98).

Continuous intravenous infusion of antihypertensive drugs (nitroprusside, nitroglycerin) requires close observation in an intensive care environment, whereas intermittent intravenous administration of drugs (diazoxide, labetalol) can be accomplished on a regular nursing floor or even in the emergency room.

Although it is unusual, administration of antihypertensive agents orally or sublingually can precipitate a rapid and excessive decrease in blood pressure, sometimes to hypotensive levels. This hypotension is particularly deleterious for patients who have severe atherosclerotic disease, especially in the cerebral or coronary circulation. Before administering one of these agents orally, the physician should ensure that effective antidotes are available to raise the blood pressure under these circumstances. The availability of potent antihypertensive drugs that can be given orally to control severe hypertension

---

TABLE 58-12

HYPERTENSIVE EMERGENCIES AND URGENCIES

EMERGENCIES

Require immediate blood pressure reduction, not necessarily to normal:
  Hypertensive encephalopathy
  Acute left ventricular failure with pulmonary edema
  Acute aortic dissection
  Eclampsia
  Post–coronary artery bypass hypertension
  Some cases of hypertension associated with increased circulating catecholamines (pheochromocytoma, clonidine withdrawal hypertension, food or drug interactions with monoamine oxidase inhibitors, ingestion or injection of sympathomimetic agents including cocaine)
Require immediate reduction of blood pressure only when it is excessively high (see text):
  Hypertensive intracerebral bleeding
  Acute subarachnoid hemorrhage
  Some acute brain infarcts
  Unstable angina or acute myocardial infarction

URGENCIES

Require blood pressure reduction within 12–24 h
  Severe systolic hypertension ($\geq$240 mmHg) or severe diastolic hypertension ($\geq$140 mmHg) without complications
  Malignant hypertension without complications
  Perioperative hypertension
  Some cases of hypertension associated with increased circulating catecholamines (pheochromocytoma, clonidine withdrawal hypertension, food or drug interactions with monoamine oxidase inhibitors, ingestion or injection of sympathomimetic agents including cocaine)

Source: Adapted from RW Gifford Jr: Management of hypertensive crises. *JAMA* 1991;266:829–835. Copyright 1991, American Medical Association. With permission from the publisher and author.

---

invites their indiscriminate use for any patient whose blood pressure seems inordinately high, without adequate evaluation of the clinical situation.[151,152] This situation is especially true for short-acting nifedipine, which is extensively employed for hypertensive urgencies but has never been approved by the Food and Drug Administration for treatment of hypertension[153] (see "Calcium Channel Blockers," above).

ACKNOWLEDGMENT

The author gratefully acknowledges the technical assistance of Sandra Stevens in the preparation of this manuscript and Ana Vann, Pharm. D., for reviewing the tables.

TABLE 58-13

PARENTERAL DRUGS FOR TREATMENT OF HYPERTENSIVE EMERGENCIES

Agent	Dose[a]	Onset of Action	Adverse Reactions[b]	Special Indications
		VASODILATORS		
Sodium nitroprusside	0.3–10 μg/kg per min as IV infusion; maximal dose for no more than 10 min	Instantaneous	Nausea, vomiting, muscle twitching, thiocyanate intoxication, methemoglobinemia, cyanide toxicity, hypotension	Hypertensive encephalopathy, acute intracranial hemorrhage, acute cerebral infarction, acute left ventricular failure, acute coronary insufficiency, dissecting aneurysm, catecholamine crisis, head injury, extensive body burns, malignant hypertension, postoperative hypertension
Nitroglycerin	5–100 μg/min as IV infusion	2–5 min	Headache, tachycardia, vomiting, methemoglobinemia	Acute left ventricular failure, acute coronary insufficiency, postoperative hypertension (especially coronary bypass)
Diazoxide	50–150 mg IV bolus, repeated as needed, or 15–30 mg/min by IV infusion	1–2 min	Hypotension, tachycardia, acute MI or stroke, aggravation of angina pectoris, hyperglycemia, fluid retention	Hypertensive encephalopathy, extensive body burns, malignant hypertension, postoperative hypertension
Hydralazine	10–20 mg IV 10–50 mg IM	10 min 20–30 min	Tachycardia, headache, vomiting, aggravation of angina pectoris, fluid retention	Eclampsia, extensive body burns, malignant hypertension, postoperative hypertension
Enalaprilat	0.625–1.25 mg q 6 h IV slowly over 5 min	15–30 min	Hypotension, headache, nausea, fatigue, dizziness, acute MI	Congestive heart failure and whenever oral administration is not feasible
Verapamil	5–10 mg IV repeated, or 0.005 mg/kg per min by infusion	2–3 min	Hypotension, bradycardia, asystole, heart failure, rapid ventricular rate due to antegrade conduction in flutter/fibrillation with Wolff-Parkinson-White and Lown-Ganong-Levine syndromes	Paroxysmal supraventricular tachycardia
		ADRENERGIC INHIBITORS		
Phentolamine	5–15 mg IV	1–2 min	Tachycardia, orthostatic hypotension	Catecholamine crisis
Labetalol hydrochloride	20–80 mg IV bolus every 10 min; 2 mg/min IV infusion	5–10 min	Bronchoconstriction, heart block, orthostatic hypotension, LV dysfunction, sick sinus syndrome	Hypertensive encephalopathy, acute coronary insufficiency, extensive body burns, malignant hypertension, postoperative hypertension
Methyldopa	250–500 mg IV infusion	30–60 min	Drowsiness	Eclampsia, perioperative hypertension

[a] The dosage range may differ slightly from recommended dosage in *Physicians' Desk Reference* or package insert.
[b] The listing of side effects is not all-inclusive, and health practitioners are urged to refer to the package insert for a more detailed listing.
Key: IV = intravenous, MI = myocardial infarction, IM = intramuscular, LV = left ventricular
Source: Reprinted from RW Gifford, Jr.: Management of hypertensive crises. *JAMA* 266:829–835, 1991. Copyright 1991, American Medical Association. With permission from the publisher and author.

REFERENCES

1. Mulrow CD, Cornell JA, Herrera CR, Kadri A, Farnett L, Aguilar CL. Hypertension in the elderly. Implications and generalizability of randomized trials. *JAMA* 1994; 272:1932–1938.

2. Hebert PR, Moser M, Mayer J, Glynn RJ, Hennekens CH. Recent evidence on drug therapy of mild to moderate hypertension and decreased risk of coronary heart disease. *Arch Intern Med* 1993; 153:578–581.

3. Moser M, Hebert PR. Prevention of disease progression, left ventricular hypertrophy and congestive heart failure in hypertension treatment trials. *J Am Coll Cardiol* 1996; 27:1214–1218.

4. Burt VL, Whelton P, Roccella EJ, Brown C, Cutler JA, Higgins M, et al. Prevalence of hypertension in the US adult population. Results from the Third National Health and Nutrition Examination Survey, 1988–1991. *Hypertension* 1995; 25:305–313.

5. Joint National Committee on Detection, Evaluation, and Treatment of High Blood Pressure. The fifth report of the Joint National Committee on Detection, Evaluation, and Treatment of High Blood Pressure (JNC-V). *Arch Intern Med* 1993; 153:154–183.

5a. The sixth report of the Joint National Committee on Detection, Evaluation, and Treatment of High Blood Pressure (JNC-VI). *Arch Int Med* 1997, in press.

6. Hypertension Detection and Follow-up Program Cooperative Group. Results of the Hypertension Detection and Follow-up Program. The effect of treatment on mortality in "mild" hypertension. *N Engl J Med* 1982; 307:976–980.

7. Stamler J, Stamler R, Neaton JD. Blood pressure, systolic and diastolic, and cardiovascular risks. US Population Data. *Arch Intern Med* 1993; 153:598–615.

8. Stamler R, Stamler J, Gosch FC, Civinelli J, Fishman J, McKeever P, et al. Primary prevention of hypertension by nutritional-hygienic means. Final report of a randomized, controlled trial [published erratum appears in *JAMA* 1989 Dec 8;262(22):3132]. *JAMA* 1989; 262:1801–1807.

9. The Trials of Hypertension Prevention Collaborative Research Group. The effects of nonpharmacologic interventions on blood pressure of persons with high normal levels. Results of the Trials of Hypertension Prevention, Phase I. *JAMA* 1992; 267:1213–1220.

10. SHEP Cooperative Research Group. Prevention of stroke by antihypertensive drug treatment in older persons with isolated systolic hypertension. Final results of the Systolic Hypertension in the Elderly Program (SHEP). *JAMA* 1991; 265:3255–3264.

10a. Staessen J, Fagard R, Thijs L, Celis H, Arabidze GG, Birkenhäger WH, et al. Morbidity and mortality in the placebo-controlled European trial on isolated systolic hypertension in the elderly. *Lancet* 1997, in press.

11. Nonpharmacological approaches to the control of high blood pressure. Final report of the Subcommittee on Nonpharmacological Therapy of the 1984 Joint National Committee on Detection, Evaluation, and Treatment of High Blood Pressure. *Hypertension* 1986; 8:444–467.

12. Elmer PJ, Grimm R Jr, Grandits G, Svendsen K, Van Heel N, et al. Lifestyle intervention: Results of the Treatment of Mild Hypertension Study (TOMHS). *Prev Med* 1995; 24:378–388.

13. Stamler R, Stamler J, Grimm R, Gosch FC, Elmer PJ, Dyer A, et al. Nutritional therapy for high blood pressure. Final report of a four-year randomized controlled trial—the Hypertension Control Program. *JAMA* 1987; 257:1484–1491.

14. Wassertheil-Smoller S, Oberman A, Blaufox MD, Davis BR, Langford H. The Trial of Antihypertensive Interventions and Management (TAIM) study. Final results with regard to blood pressure, cardiovascular risk, and quality of life. *Am J Hypertens* 1992; 5:37–44.

15. Applegate WB, Miller ST, Elam JT, Cushman WC, El Derwi D, Brewer A, et al. Nonpharmacologic intervention to reduce blood pressure in older patients with mild hypertension. *Arch Intern Med* 1992; 152:1162–1166.

16. Elmer PJ, Grimm RH Jr, Flack J, Laing B. Dietary sodium reduction for hypertension prevention and treatment. *Hypertension* 1991; 17:I182–I189.

17. Reisin E, Abel R, Modan M, Silverberg DS, Eliahou HE, Modan B. Effect of weight loss without salt restriction on the reduction of blood pressure in overweight hypertensive patients. *N Engl J Med* 1978; 298:1–6.

18. Schotte DE, Stunkard AJ. The effects of weight reduction on blood pressure in 301 obese patients. *Arch Intern Med* 1990; 150:1701–1704.

19. Langford HG, Davis BR, Blaufox D, Oberman A, Wassertheil-Smoller S, Hawkins M, et al, for the TAIM Research Group. Effect of drug and diet treatment of mild hypertension on diastolic blood pressure. *Hypertension* 1991; 17:210–217.

20. Eliahou HE, Iaina A, Gaon T, Shochat J, Modan M. Body weight reduction necessary to obtain normotension in the overweight hypertensive patient. *Int J Obes* 1981; 5(suppl 1):157–163.

21. Cohen N, Flamenbaum W. Obesity and hypertension. Demonstration of a "floor effect." *Am J Med* 1986; 80:177–181.

22. Whelton PK, He J, Cutler JA, Brancati FL, Appel LJ, Follmann D, et al. Effects of oral potassium on blood pressure: Meta-analysis of randomized controlled clinical trials. *JAMA* 1997; 277:1624–32.

23. Grogan JR, Kochar MS. Alcohol and hypertension. *Arch Fam Med* 1994; 3:150–154.

24. World Hypertension League. Alcohol and hypertension—implications for management. A consensus statement by the World Hypertension League. *J Hum Hypertens* 1991; 5:227–232.

25. Kelley G, McClellan P. Antihypertensive effects of aerobic exercise. A brief meta-analytic review of randomized controlled trials. *Am J Hypertens* 1994; 7:115–119.

26. Hunyor SN, Henderson R. The role of stress management in blood pressure control: Why the promissory note has failed to deliver. *J Hypertens* 1996; 14:413–418.

27. National High Blood Pressure Education Program. Report to the Hypertension Information and Education Advisory Committee. Task Force I. Data Base. Recommendations for a national high blood pressure program data base for effective antihypertensive therapy. DHEW Publication No. (NIH) 75-593, September 1, 1973.

28. Joint National Committee on the Detection, Evaluation, and Treatment of High Blood Pressure. Report of the Fourth Joint National Committee (JNC-IV). *Arch Intern Med* 1988; 148:1023–1038.

29. Kaplan NM, Gifford RW Jr. Choice of initial therapy for hypertension. *JAMA* 1996; 275:1577–1580.

30. Materson BJ, Reda DJ, Cushman WC, Massie BM, Freis ED, Kochar MS, et al. Single-drug therapy for hypertension in men. A comparison of six antihypertensive agents with placebo. The Department of Veterans Affairs Cooperative Study Group on Antihypertensive Agents. *N Engl J Med* 1993; 328:914–921 (published correction appears in *N Engl J Med* 1994; 330:1689).

31. Neaton JD, Grimm RH Jr, Prineas RJ, Stamler J, Grandits GA, Elmer PJ, et al. Treatment of Mild Hypertensive Study. Final results. *JAMA* 1993; 270:713–724.

32. Collins R, Peto R, MacMahon S, Hebert P, Fiebuch NH, Eberlein KA, et al. Blood pressure, stroke, and coronary heart disease. Part 2, Short-term reductions in blood pressure: Overview of randomized drug trials in their epidemiological context. *Lancet* 1990; 335:827–838.

33. Gifford RW Jr, Kaplan NM. Thiazides and hypertension in the elderly [commentary]. *Hypertension* 1995; 25:1052.

34. Grimm RH, Flack JM, Grandits GA, Elmer PJ, Neaton JD, Cutler JA, et al. Long-term effects on plasma lipids of diet and drugs to treat hypertension. *JAMA* 1996; 275:1549–1556.

35. Grimm RH Jr, Leon AS, Hunninghake DB, Lenz K, Hannan P, Blackburn H. Effects of thiazide diuretics on plasma lipids and lipoproteins in mildly hypertensive patients: A double-blind controlled trial. *Ann Intern Med* 1981; 94:7–11.

36. National High Blood Pressure Education Program (NHBPEP) and National Cholesterol Education Program (NCEP) Working Group. Report on management of patients with hypertension and high blood cholesterol. *Ann Intern Med* 1991; 114:224–237.

37. Goldman AI, Steele BW, Schnaper HW, Fitz AE, Frohlich ED, Perry HMJ. Serum lipoprotein levels during chlorthalidone therapy. A Veterans Administration–National Heart, Lung, and Blood Institute cooperative study on antihypertensive therapy: Mild hypertension. *JAMA* 1980; 244:1691–1695.

38. Veterans Administration Cooperative Study Group on Antihypertensive Agents. Comparison of propranolol and hydrochlorothiazide for the initial treatment of hypertension. II. Results of long-term therapy. *JAMA* 1982; 248:2004–2011.

39. Williams WR, Schneider KA, Borhani NO, Schnaper HW, Slotkoff LM, Ellefson RD. The relationship between diuretics and serum cholesterol in Hypertension Detection and Follow-up Program participants. *Am J Prev Med* 1986; 2:248–255.

40. Berglund G, Andersson O. Beta-blockers or diuretics in hypertension? A six-year follow-up of blood pressure and metabolic side effects. *Lancet* 1981; 1:744–747.

41. Jeunemaitre X, Charru A, Chatellier G, Degoulet P, Julien J, Plouin PF, et al. Long-term effects of spironolactone and thiazides combined with potassium-sparing agents for treatment of essential hypertension. *Am J Cardiol* 1988; 62:1072–1077.

42. Roccella EJ. Cost of hypertension medications: Is it a barrier to hypertension control? *Geriatrics* 1989; 44(suppl B):49–55.

43. Gifford RW Jr. Resistant hypertension. Introduction and definitions. *Hypertension* 1989; 11(suppl II):II65–II66.

44. Swales JD. Guidelines on guidelines (editorial). *J Hypertens* 1993; 11:899–903.

45. Joint National Committee on Detection, Evaluation, and Treatment of High Blood Pressure. The 1984 Report of the Joint National Committee on Detection, Evaluation, and Treatment of High Blood Pressure. *Arch Intern Med* 1984; 144:1045–1057.

46. Pedersen TR, for the Norwegian Multicenter Study Group. Six-year follow-up of the Norwegian Multicenter Study on Timolol After Acute Myocardial Infarction. *N Engl J Med* 1985; 313:1055–1058.

47. Beta Blocker Heart Attack Trial Research Group. A randomized trial of propranolol in patients with acute myocardial infarction: I. Mortality results. *JAMA* 1982; 247:1707–1714.

48. Yusuf S, Peto R, Lewis J, Collins R, Sleight P. Beta blockade during and after myocardial infarction: An overview of the randomized trials. *Prog Cardiovasc Dis* 1985; 27:335–371.

49. Yusuf S, Wittes J, Probstfield J. Evaluating effects of treatment in subgroups of patients within a clinical trial: The case of non-Q-wave myocardial infarction and beta blockers. *Am J Cardiol* 1990; 66:220–222.

50. Frohlich ED, Tarazi RC, Dustan HP. Hyperdynamic β-adrenergic circulatory state: Increased β-receptor responsiveness. *Arch Intern Med* 1969; 123:1–7.

51. Reaven GM, Lithell H, Landsberg L. Hypertension and associated metabolic abnormalities—the role of insulin resistance and the sympathoadrenal system. *N Engl J Med* 1996; 334:374–381.

52. Moser M, Ross H. The treatment of hypertension in diabetic patients. *Diabetes Care* 1993; 16:542–547.

53. Psaty BM, Heckbert SR, Koepsell TD, Siscovick DS, Raghunathan TE, Weiss NS, et al. The risk of myocardial infarction associated with antihypertensive drug therapies. *JAMA* 1995; 274:620–625.

54. Pahor M, Guralnik JM, Corti MC, Foley DJ, Carbonin P, Havlik RJ. Long-term survival and use of antihypertensive medications in older persons. *J Am Geriatr Soc* 1995; 43:1191–1197.

55. Packer M, Kessler PD, Lee WH. Calcium-channel blockade in the management of severe chronic congestive heart failure: A bridge too far. *Circulation* 1987; 75:V56–V64.

56. Goldstein RE, Boccuzzi SJ, Cruess D, Nattel S. Diltiazem increases late-onset congestive heart failure in postinfarction patients with early reduction in ejection fraction. *Circulation* 1991; 83:52–60.

57. Elkayam U, Amin J, Mehra A, Vasquez J, Weber L, Rahimtoola SH. A prospective, randomized, double-blind crossover study to compare the efficacy and safety of chronic nifedipine therapy with that of isosorbide dinitrate and their combination in the treatment of chronic congestive heart failure. *Circulation* 1990; 82:1954–1961.

58. Yusuf S, Held P, Furberg C. Update of effects of calcium antagonists in myocardial infarction or angina in light of the second Danish Verapamil Infarction Trial (DAVIT-II) and other recent studies. *Am J Cardiol* 1991; 67:1295–1297.

59. Furberg CD, Psaty BM, Meyer JV. Nifedipine. Dose-related increase in mortality in patients with coronary heart disease. *Circulation* 1995; 92:1326–1331.

60. Pahor M, Guralnik JM, Salive ME, Corti M, Carbonin P, Havlik RJ. Do calcium channel blockers increase the risk of cancer? *Am J Hypertens* 1996; 9:695–699.

61. Legault C, Furberg CD, Wagenknecht LE, Rogers AT, Stump DA, Coker L, et al. Nimodipine neuroprotection in cardiac valve replacement: Report of an early terminated trial. *Stroke* 1996; 27:593–598.

62. Pahor M, Guralnik JM, Furberg CD, Carbonin P, Havlik R. Risk of gastrointestinal haemorrhage with calcium antagonists in hypertensive persons over 67 years old. *Lancet* 1996; 347:1061–1065.

63. Williams GH. Converting-enzyme inhibitors in the treatment of hypertension. *N Engl J Med* 1988; 319:1517–1525.

64. Townsend RR, Holland OB. Combination of converting enzyme inhibitor with diuretic for the treatment of hypertension. *Arch Intern Med* 1990; 150:1175–1183.

65. The SOLVD Investigators. Effect of enalapril on survival in patients with reduced left ventricular ejection fractions and congestive heart failure. *N Engl J Med* 1991; 325:293–302.

66. Pfeffer MA, Braunwald E, Moye LA, Basta L, Brown EJ, Cuddy TE, et al. Effect of captopril on mortality and morbidity in patients with left ventricular dysfunction after myocardial infarction. Results of the Survival and Ventricular Enlargement Trial (SAVE). *N Engl J Med* 1992; 327:669–677.

67. Garg R, Yusuf S, for the Collaborative Group on ACE Inhibitor Trials. Overview of randomized trials of angiotensin-converting enzyme inhibitors on mortality and morbidity in patients with heart failure. *JAMA* 1995; 273:1450–1456.

68. Brenner BM, Meyer TW, Hostetter TH. Dietary protein and the progressive nature of kidney disease: The role of hemodynamically mediated glomerular injury in the pathogenesis of progressive glomerular sclerosis in aging, renal ablation, and intrinsic renal disease. *N Engl J Med* 1982; 307:652–659.

69. Hricik DE, Browning PJ, Kopelman R, Goorno WE, Madias NE, Dzau VJ. Captopril-induced functional renal insufficiency in patients with bilateral renal-artery stenoses or renal-artery stenosis in a solitary kidney. *N Engl J Med* 1983; 308:373–376.

70. Coulie P, De Plaen JF, van Ypersele de Strihou C. Captopril-induced acute reversible renal failure. *Nephron* 1983; 35:108–111.

71. Hollenberg NK. Angiotensin-converting enzyme inhibition: Renal aspects. *J Cardiovasc Pharmacol* 1985; 7(suppl 1):S40–S44.

72. Suki WN. Renal hemodynamic consequences of angiotensin-converting enzyme inhibition in congestive heart failure. *Arch Intern Med* 1989; 149:669–673.

73. Meyer TW, Anderson S, Rennke HG, Brenner BM. Converting enzyme inhibitor therapy limits progressive glomerular injury in rats with renal insufficiency. *Am J Med* 1985; 79:31–36.

74. Zatz R, Dunn BR, Meyer TW, Anderson S, Rennke HG, Brenner BM. Prevention of diabetic glomerulopathy by pharmacological amelioration of glomerular capillary hypertension. *J Clin Invest* 1986; 77:1925–1930.

75. Hommel E, Parving HH, Mathiesen E, Edsberg B, Nielsen MD, Giese J. Effect of captopril on kidney function in insulin-dependent diabetic patients with nephropathy. *Br Med J* 1986; 293:467–470.

76. Mathiesen ER, Hommel E, Giese J, Parving HH. Efficacy of captopril in postponing nephropathy in normotensive insulin dependent diabetic patients with microalbuminuria. *Br Med J* 1991; 303:81–87.

77. Lewis EJ, Hunsicker LG, Bain RP, Rohde RD, for the Collaborative Study Group. The effect of angiotensin-converting-enzyme inhibition on diabetic nephropathy. *N Engl J Med* 1993; 329:1456–1462.

78. Toto RD, Mitchell HC, Lee HC, Milam C, Pettinger WA. Reversible renal insufficiency due to angiotensin converting enzyme inhibitors in hypertensive nephrosclerosis. *Ann Intern Med* 1991; 115:513–519.

79. Chapman AB, Gabow PA, Schrier RW. Reversible renal failure associated with angiotensin-converting enzyme inhibitors in polycystic kidney disease. *Ann Intern Med* 1991; 115:769–773.

80. Israili ZH, Hall WD. Cough and angioneurotic edema associated with angiotensin-converting enzyme inhibitor therapy. A review of the literature and pathophysiology. *Ann Intern Med* 1992; 117:234–242.

81. Kang PM, Landau AJ, Eberhardt RT, Frishman WH. Angiotensin II receptor antagonists: A new approach to blockade of the renin-angiotensin system. *Am Heart J* 1994; 127:1388–1401.

82. Khoury AF, Kaplan NM. Alpha-blocker therapy of hypertension. An unfulfilled promise. *JAMA* 1991; 266:394–398.

83. Waite MA. Alpha$_1$ blockers: Antihypertensives whose positive metabolic profile with regard to hyperinsulinaemia and lipid metabolism cannot be ignored. *J Intern Med* 1991; 29(suppl 2):113–117.

84. Stamler R, Stamler J, Gosch FC, Berkson DM, Dyer AR, Hershinow P. Initial antihypertensive drug therapy. Final report of a randomized, controlled trial comparing alpha-blocker and diuretic. *Hypertension* 1988; 12:574–581.

85. Pollare T, Lithell H, Selinus I, Berne C. Application of prazosin is associated with an increase of insulin sensitivity in obese patients with hypertension. *Diabetologia* 1988; 31:415–420.

86. Steers WD, Zorn B. Benign prostatic hyperplasia. *Dis Mon* 1995; 41:437–497.

87. Oster JR, Epstein M. Use of centrally acting sympatholytic agents in the management of hypertension. *Arch Intern Med* 1991; 151:1638–1644.

88. Gifford RW Jr, August P, Chesley LC, Cunningham G, Ferris TF, Lenfant C, et al. National High Blood Pressure Education Program Working Group report on high blood pressure in pregnancy. *Am J Obstet Gynecol* 1990; 163:1689–1712.

89. Participating Veterans Administration Medical Centers. Low doses v standard dose of reserpine. A randomized, double-blind, multiclinic trial in patients taking chlorthalidone. *JAMA* 1982; 248:2471–2477.

90. Pettinger WA. Minoxidil and the treatment of severe hypertension. *N Engl J Med* 1980; 303:922–926.

91. Prisant LM, Weir MR, Papademetriou V, Weber MA, Adegbile IA, Alemayehu D, et al. Low-dose drug combination therapy: An alternative first-line approach to hypertension treatment. *Am Heart J* 1995; 130:359–366.

92. Farnett L, Mulrow CD, Linn WD, Lucey CR, Tuley MR. The J-curve phenomenon and the treatment of hypertension. Is there a point beyond which pressure reduction is dangerous? *JAMA* 1991; 265:489–495.

93. Cruickshank JM, Thorpe JM, Zacharias FJ. Benefits and potential harm of lowering high blood pressure. *Lancet* 1987; 1:581–584.

94. Fletcher AE, Beevers DG, Bulpitt CJ, Butler A, Coles EC, Hunt D, et al. The relationship between a low treated blood pressure and IHD mortality: A report from the DHSS Hypertension Care Computing Project. *J Hum Hypertens* 1988; 2:11–15.

95. Waller PC, Isles CG, Lever AF, Murray GD, McInnes GT. Does therapeutic reduction of diastolic blood pressure cause death from coronary heart disease? *J Hum Hypertens* 1988; 2:7–10.

96. Stewart IM. Relation of reduction in pressure to first myocardial infarction in patients receiving treatment for severe hypertension. *Lancet* 1979; 1:861–865.

97. Alderman MH, Ooi WL, Madharan S, Cohen H. Treatment induced blood pressure reduction and the risk of myocardial infarction. *JAMA* 1989; 262:920–924.

98. Samuelsson O, Wilhelmsen L, Andersson OK, Pennert K, Berglund G. Cardiovascular morbidity in relation to change in blood pressure and serum cholesterol levels in treated hypertension: Results from the Primary Prevention Trial in Goteborg, Sweden. *JAMA* 1987; 258:1768–1776.

99. Coope J, Warrender TS. Randomised trial of treatment of hypertension in elderly patients in primary care. *Br Med J* 1986; 293:1145–1151.

100. Coope J, Warrender TS. Lowering blood pressure (letter). *Lancet* 1987; 1:1380.

101. Cooper SP, Hardy RJ, Labarthe DR, Hawkins CM, Smith EO, Blaufox MD, et al. The relation between degree of blood pressure reduction and mortality among hypertensives in the Hypertension Detection and Follow-up Program. *Am J Epidemiol* 1988; 127:387–403.

102. Staessen J, Bulpitt C, Clement D, De Leeuw P, Fagard R, Fletcher A, et al. Relation between mortality and treated blood pressure in elderly patients with hypertension: Report of the European Working Party on High Blood Pressure in the Elderly. *Br Med J* 1989; 298:1552–1556.

103. National High Blood Pressure Education Program Working Group. 1995 Update of the Working Group Reports on Chronic Renal Failure and Renovascular Hypertension. *Arch Intern Med* 1996; 156:1938–1947.

104. Anderson TW. Re-examination of some of the Framingham blood pressure data. *Lancet* 1978; 2:1139–1141.

105. D'Agostino RB, Belanger AJ, Kannel WB, Cruickshank JM. Relation of low diastolic blood pressure to coronary heart disease death in presence of myocardial infarction: The Framingham Study. *Br Med J* 1991; 303:385–389.

106. MacMahon S, Peto R, Cutler J, Collins R, Sorlie P, Neaton J, et al. Blood pressure, stroke, and coronary heart disease. Part 1, Prolonged difference in blood pressure: Prospective observational studies corrected for the regression dilution bias. *Lancet* 1990; 335:765–774.

107. Medical Research Council Working Party. MRC trial of treatment of mild hypertension: Principal results. *Br Med J* 1985; 291:97–104.

108. Fletcher AE, Bulpitt CJ. How far should blood pressure be lowered? *N Engl J Med* 1992; 326:251–254.

109. Julius S. The Hypertension Optimal Treatment (HOT) Study in the United States. *J Hypertens* 1996; 9:41S–44S.

110. Rocchini AP. Insulin resistance and blood pressure regulation in obese and nonobese subjects. *Hypertension* 1991; 17:837–842.

111. Epstein M, Sowers JR Jr. Diabetes mellitus and hypertension. *Hypertension* 1992; 19:403–418.

112. Julius S, Gudbrandsson T, Jamerson K, Shahab ST, Andersson O. The hemodynamic link between insulin resistance and hypertension. *J Hypertens* 1991; 9:983–986.

113. Kaplan NM. The deadly quartet. Upper-body obesity, glucose intolerance, hypertriglyceridemia, and hypertension. *Arch Intern Med* 1989; 149:1514–1520.

114. Sowers JR Jr, Epstein M. Diabetes mellitus and associated hypertension, vascular disease, and nephropathy. An update. *Hypertension* 1995; 26:869–879.

115. Warram JH, Laffel LMB, Valsania P, Christlieb AR, Krolewski AS. Excess mortality associated with diuretic therapy in diabetes mellitus. *Arch Intern Med* 1991; 151:1350–1356.

116. Klein R, Moss SE, Klein BE, DeMets DL. Relation of ocular and systemic factors to survival in diabetes. *Arch Intern Med* 1989; 149:266–272.

117. Amery A, Birkenhager W, Brixko P, Bulpitt C, Clement D, Deruyttere M, et al. Mortality and morbidity results from the European Working Party on High Blood Pressure in the Elderly Trial. *Lancet* 1985; 1:1349–1354.

118. Langford HG, Stamler J, Wassertheil-Smoller S, Prineas RJ. All-cause mortality in the Hypertension Detection and Follow-up Program: Findings for the whole cohort and for persons with less severe hypertension, with and without other traits related to risk of mortality. *Prog Cardiovasc Dis* 1986; 29(3 Supp 1):29–54.

119. National High Blood Pressure Education Program Working Group. National High Blood Pressure Education Program Working Group report on hypertension in diabetes. *Hypertension* 1994; 23:145–158.

120. Gundersen T, Kjekshus J. Timolol treatment after myocardial infarction in diabetic patients. *Diabetes Care* 1983; 6:285–290.

121. Davis BR, Cutler JA, Gordon DJ, Furberg CD, Wright JT Jr, Cushman WC, et al. Rationale and design for the Antihypertensive and Lipid Lowering Treatment to Prevent Heart Attack Trial (ALLHAT). *Am J Hypertens* 1996; 9:342–360.

122. Saunders E. Hypertension in African Americans. *Circulation* 1991; 83:1465–1467.

123. Anastos K, Charney P, Charon RA, Cohen E, Jones CY, Marte C, et al. Hypertension in women: What is really known? The Women's Caucus, Working Group on Women's Health of the Society of General Internal Medicine. *Ann Intern Med* 1991; 115:287–293.

124. Vokonas PS, Kannel WB, Cupples LA. Epidemiology and risk of hypertension in the elderly: The Framingham Study. *J Hypertens* 1988; 6(suppl):S3–S9.

125. Hypertension Detection and Follow-up Program Cooperative Group. Five-year findings of the Hypertension Detection and Follow-up Program. III. Reduction in stroke incidence among persons with high blood pressure. *JAMA* 1982; 247:633–638.

126. National High Blood Pressure Education Program Working Group, Roccella EJ, Coordinator. National High Blood Pressure Education Program Working Group Report on Hypertension in the Elderly. *Hypertension* 1994; 23:275–285.

127. Dahlof B, Lindholm LH, Hansson L, Schersten B, Ekbom T, Wester PO. Morbidity and mortality in the Swedish Trial in Old Patients with Hypertension (STOP-Hypertension). *Lancet* 1991; 338:1281–1285.

128. Materson BJ, Cushman WC, Goldstein G, Reda DJ, Freis ED, Ramirez EA, et al. Treatment of hypertension in the elderly: I. Blood pressure and clinical changes. Results of a Department of Veterans Affairs cooperative study. *Hypertension* 1990; 15:348–360.

129. Goldstein G, Materson BJ, Cushman WC, Reda DJ, Freis ED, Ramirez EA, et al. Treatment of hypertension in the elderly: II. Cognitive and behavioral function. Results of a Department of Veterans Affairs cooperative study. *Hypertension* 1990; 15:361–369.

130. Gurland BJ, Teresi J, Smith WM, Black D, Hutches G, Edlavitch S. Effects of treatment for isolated systolic hypertension on cognitive status and depression in the elderly. *J Am Geriatr Soc* 1988; 36:1015–1022.

131. Beevers DG, Fairman MJ, Hamilton M, Harpur JE. Antihypertensive treatment and the course of established cerebral vascular disease. *Lancet* 1973; 1:1407–1409.

132. Carter AB. Hypotensive therapy in stroke survivors. *Lancet* 1970; 1:485–489.

133. Marshall J. A trial of long-term hypotensive therapy in cerebrovascular disease. *Lancet* 1964; 1:10–12.

134. Hypertension-Stroke Cooperative Study Group. Effect of antihypertensive treatment on stroke recurrence. *JAMA* 1974; 229:409–418.

135. Whisnant JP, Cartlidge NE, Elveback LR. Carotid and vertebral-basilar transient ischemic attacks: Effect of anticoagulants, hypertension, and cardiac disorders on survival and stroke occurrence—a population study. *Ann Neurol* 1978; 3:107–115.

136. Frohlich ED. The heart in hypertension: A 1991 overview. *Hypertension* 1991; 18(suppl III):III62–III68.

137. Dahlof B, Pennert K, Hansson L. Reversal of left ventricular hypertrophy in hypertensive patients. A metaanalysis of 109 treatment studies. *Am J Hypertens* 1992; 5:95–110.

138. Schmieder RE, Martus P, Klingbeil A. Reversal of left ventricular hypertrophy in essential hypertension. A meta-analysis of randomized double-blind studies. *JAMA* 1996; 275:1507–1513.

138a. Gottdiener JS, Reda DJ, Massie BM, Materson BJ, Williams DW, Anderson RJ, for the VA Collaborative Study Group. Effect of single-drug therapy on reduction of left ventricular mass in mild to moderate hypertension: Comparison of six antihypertensive agents. The Department of Veterans Affairs Cooperative Study Group on Antihypertensive Agents. *Circulation* 1997; 95:2004–2007.

139. Sackner-Bernstein JD, Mancini DM. Rationale for treatment of patients with chronic heart failure with adrenergic blockade. *JAMA* 1995; 274:1462–1467.

140. Topol EJ, Traill TA, Fortuin NJ. Hypertensive hypertrophic cardiomyopathy of the elderly. *N Engl J Med* 1985; 312:277–283.

141. Abrams J. Vasodilator therapy for chronic congestive heart failure. *JAMA* 1985; 254:3070–3074.

142. Pettinger WA, Lee HC, Reisch J, Mitchell HC. Long-term improvement in renal function after short-term strict blood pressure control in hypertensive nephrosclerosis. *Hypertension* 1989; 13:766–772.

143. Mitchell HC, Graham RM, Pettinger WA. Renal function during long-term treatment of hypertension with minoxidil. Comparison of benign and malignant hypertension. *Ann Intern Med* 1980; 93:676–681.

144. Messerli FH, Ventura HO, Amodeo C. Osler's maneuver and pseudohypertension. *N Engl J Med* 1985; 312:1548–1551.

145. Pickering TG, James GD, Boddie C, Harshfield GA, Blank S, Laragh JH. How common is white coat hypertension? *JAMA* 1988; 259:225–228.

146. Gifford RW Jr. An algorithm for the management of resistant hypertension. *Hypertension* 1988; 11(suppl II):II101–II105.

147. Biller J, Godersky JC, Adams HP Jr. Management of aneurysmal subarachnoid hemorrhage. *Stroke* 1988; 19:1300–1305.

148. Brott T, Reed RL. Intensive care for acute stroke in the community hospital setting: The first 24 hours. *Stroke* 1989; 20:694–697.

149. Phillips SJ, Whisnant JP. Hypertension and the brain. The National High Blood Pressure Education Program. *Arch Intern Med* 1992; 152:938–945.

150. Gifford RW Jr. Management of hypertensive crises. *JAMA* 1991; 266:829–835.

151. Fagan TC. Acute reduction of blood pressure in asymptomatic patients with severe hypertension: An idea whose time has come and gone [editorial]. *Arch Intern Med* 1989; 149:2169–2170.

152. Ferguson RK, Vlasses PH. How urgent is "urgent" hypertension? [editorial] *Arch Intern Med* 1989; 149:257–258.

153. Grossman E, Messerli FH, Grodzicki T, Kowey P. Should a moratorium be placed on sublingual nifedipine capsules given for hypertensive emergencies and pseudoemergencies? *JAMA* 1996; 276(16):1328–1331.

PULMONARY HYPERTENSION AND PULMONARY HEART DISEASE

59

PULMONARY HYPERTENSION

Alfred P. Fishman

INTRODUCTION

Unless otherwise specified, the designation *pulmonary hypertension* refers to pulmonary arterial hypertension. This is a hemodynamic abnormality that exerts its predominant clinical effect by increasing inordinately the work of the right ventricle.

The clinical manifestations, natural history, and reversibility of pulmonary hypertension depend heavily on the etiology of the hemodynamic disorder, the nature of the pulmonary arterial lesions, and the level of the pulmonary hypertension. For example, certain etiologies, such as chronic hypoxia, cause increased muscularization of the small muscular pulmonary arteries and arterioles while leaving the intima intact. Relief of the hypoxia reverses the process with little or no pathologic residue.[1,2] In contrast, the lesions of systemic vascular sclerosis (scleroderma), which can be confined to the intima of the small pulmonary arteries and arterioles, are usually poorly reversible and progress to occlusive vascular disease. In contrast to scleroderma and chronic hypoxia, which spare the pulmonary capillary bed, in pulmonary capillary hemangiomatosis, the pulmonary capillary bed is directly involved.[3]

Because of its large capacity, its great distensibility, its low resistance to blood flow, and the modest amounts of smooth muscle in the small arteries and arterioles, the pulmonary circulation is not predisposed to become hypertensive. When total cross-sectional area is decreased, as by amputation of parts of the pulmonary arterial tree, occlusive lesions in the resistance vessels, or both, pulmonary arterial pressures increase, the degree depending on the extent of the perfused pulmonary arterial tree that has been eliminated. Pulmonary hypertension is usually secondary to cardiac or pulmonary disease. Unexplained, or "primary," pulmonary hypertension is rare. Nonetheless, although primary pulmonary hypertension is uncommon, it has attracted considerable attention as a distinctive clinical entity in which intrinsic pulmonary vascular disease is free of the complicating features of secondary pulmonary hypertension contributed by diseases of the heart and/or lungs.

Mild or even moderate pulmonary (arterial) hypertension can exist for a lifetime without becoming evident clinically. For example, native residents at high altitude, in whom mild to moderate pulmonary hypertension is a natural result of unremitting exposure to hypoxia, can transport heavy burdens and play a vigorous game of soccer without undue discomfort. When pulmonary hypertension does become manifest clinically, the symptoms are apt to be nonspecific (Table 59-1).

Definitions

Pulmonary *arterial* hypertension can be either acute or chronic. The acute form is usually a result of either pulmonary embolism (see Chap. 60) of the adult respiratory distress syndrome. This chapter deals with *chronic* pulmonary (arterial) hypertension.

Pulmonary *venous* hypertension is usually encountered clinically as a consequence of left ventricular failure or mitral valvular disease. Occasionally it may occur in the course of fibrosing mediastinitis. Only rarely is the entity known as primary pulmonary veno-occlusive disease encountered. Even though pulmonary hypertension may be confined, at the outset, to the pulmonary veins (e.g., in acute mitral insufficiency), sooner or later pulmonary arterial hypertension supervenes. The hallmarks of pulmonary venous hypertension are pulmonary congestion and edema. For practical purposes, pulmonary

---

TABLE 59-1

SYMPTOMS OF PRIMARY PULMONARY HYPERTENSION

Dyspnea	Palpitations
Fatigue	Orthopnea
Dizziness	Cough
Syncope	Hoarseness
Chest pain	

venous hypertension is said to exist when pulmonary venous (or left atrial) pressure arises above 12 mmHg.

Cor pulmonale merely signifies enlargement of the right ventricle by dilation, hypertrophy, or both.[4] Almost invariably, chronic cor pulmonale is secondary to chronic pulmonary hypertension, i.e. to a sustained increase in right ventricular work due to an increase in its afterload. If the load is inordinate, the right ventricle will fail, i.e., enlargement of the right ventricle (cor pulmonale) will be accompanied by signs of right ventricular failure (e.g., right ventricular gallop rhythm, systemic venous and hepatic congestion, and peripheral edema).

NORMAL PULMONARY CIRCULATION

Structure

Immediately before birth, pulmonary arterial and aortic blood pressures are about equal and of the order of 70/40 mmHg, with a mean of 50 mmHg. Immediately after birth, as the ductus arteriosus closes and the lungs begin breathing air, pulmonary arterial pressure falls rapidly to about one-half of systemic levels. Thereafter, pulmonary arterial pressures gradually decrease over weeks to reach adult levels[5] (see also Chap. 70).

In some neonates, the normal pulmonary hypertension of the fetus fails to recede normally, generally due to either a developmental anomaly or a relentless increase in pulmonary vascular tone. In such infants, the persistent pulmonary hypertension and right ventricular failure may become life threatening. Surgical intervention or a temporizing measure, such as extracorporeal membrane oxygenation (ECMO), may then be required to buy time for regression of the pulmonary vascular abnormalities.[6]

In the normal adult at sea level, the small muscular arteries and arterioles in the lungs are thin walled and sparsely equipped with muscle. In contrast, in the fetus and adult who have lived under hypoxic conditions (e.g., native residents at high altitude), the media of the arterioles are thickened and the muscle extends peripherally into precapillary vessels that are ordinarily devoid of muscle, i.e., the precapillary vessels undergo "remodeling."[7]

Endothelium and Endothelium–Smooth Muscle Interactions

In addition to its role as a semipermeable barrier between blood and interstitium, the endothelium serves a wide array of biologically important functions, the net effect of which is the processing of blood flowing through the lungs. Among these functions are the synthesis, uptake, storage, release, and metabolism of vasoactive substances; transduction of bloodborne signals; modulation of coagulation and thrombolysis; regulation of cell proliferation; engagement in the local inflammatory and proliferative reactions to injury; involvement in immune reactions; and angiogenesis (see also Chap.

4). Some of the enzymes involved in these processes, such as the angiotensin-converting enzyme, are found on the surface of endothelial cells; others, such as 5'-nucleotidase, are found within the cell.[8] Hence it is appropriate to regard endothelium as an organ with diverse metabolic and endocrine functions, one that is unique because of its strategic disposition as a continuous, monolayered lining of blood vessels throughout the body. It is also important to bear in mind that the lungs contain the largest expanse of endothelium in the body.

The cells that comprise the monolayered endothelial lining communicate not only with each other by anatomic junctions and bridges but also with the underlying smooth muscle by way of biologically active substances.[9] This interaction participates in setting normal vasomotor tone as well as in the change in vasomotor tone that follow the administration of vasoactive substances. It is not difficult to imagine that damage to the lining cells, proliferation of the intima, or hypertrophy of the smooth muscle will upset the normal interplay.

Endothelial injury disturbs normal endothelial function. Indeed, a variety of enzyme systems are currently being explored as possible tests for normal and abnormal pulmonary endothelium and, in patients with pulmonary vascular injury and/or occlusion, as a measure of the extent of the total endothelial surface area that is still being perfused (see also Chaps. 4 and 44).

Hemodynamics

For the adult pulmonary circulation, the definition of "normal" depends on the altitude. The normal pulmonary hemodynamics of adults residing at sea level and above sea level are compared in Table 59-2. At *sea level*, a cardiac output of 5 to 6 L/min is associated with a pulmonary arterial pressure of about 20 mmHg systolic and 12 mmHg diastolic, with a mean of about 15 mmHg. At altitude of 15,000 ft, the same level of blood flow is associated with somewhat higher pressures (Table 59-2). Pulmonary arterial pressures tend to increase somewhat with age.

TABLE 59-2

VALUES FOR NORMAL PULMONARY CIRCULATION AT SEA LEVEL AND ALTITUDE

	Sea Level	Altitude (~15,000 ft)
Pulmonary arterial pressure (P_{PA}), mmHg	20/12, 15	38/14, 25
Cardiac output (Q), L/min	6.0	6.0
Left atrial pressure (P_{LA}), mmHg	5.0	5.0
Pulmonary vascular resistance (PVR),[a] (mmHg/L)/min (R units)	1.7	3.3

[a] $PVR = \dfrac{P_{PA} - P_{LA}}{Q} = \dfrac{15 - 5}{6} = 1.67$ R units. To convert R units to CGS units (dynes·s/cm^5), multiply R units by 80.

The large output ejected by the right ventricle is conveyed across the pulmonary circulation with only a modest drop in pressure (e.g., a cardiac output of 5 to 6 L/min is accompanied by a pressure drop of 5 to 10 mmHg between the pulmonary artery and left atrium) (Table 59-2). Determination of pulmonary vascular resistance has proved to be a practical clinical tool for quantifying the hemodynamic state of the pulmonary circulation and for distinguishing between active and passive changes in the pulmonary resistance vessels (e.g., the effect of administering a vasodilator agent to a patient with pulmonary hypertension). It is calculated as the ratio of the difference in mean pressure at the two ends of the pulmonary vascular bed [pulmonary arterial minus left atrial pressures divided by the cardiac output (pulmonary blood flow)] (Table 59-2). In practice, since the left atrium may not be readily accessible, pulmonary wedge pressure is generally substituted for left atrial pressure.

Another approach to defining certain characteristics and the behavior of the pulmonary arterial tree, i.e., elastic properties and geometry, is the calculation of pulmonary arterial input impedance. This approach has more physiologic than clinical value. It takes into account the pulsatile nature of pulmonary arterial pressures and flow. Like vascular resistance, it is defined as a ratio. But instead of a ratio involving *mean* pressures and blood flow, the ratio is of the amplitudes of pulsatile pressure to oscillatory flow near the beginning of the pulmonary artery at a particular frequency. Values for the ratio are obtained by resolving mathematically the pulsatile pressure and flow curves into their sinusoidal components.

Although calculated pulmonary vascular resistance has proved useful in assessing the state of the normal and abnormal pulmonary circulation, and even though a change in calculated resistance can often be helpful in deciding whether pulmonary vasoconstriction or vasodilation has occurred, translation of a calculated ratio into vasomotor activity has to be made with caution.[4] For example, changes in calculated pulmonary vascular resistance are not readily interpretable when a vasodilator agent evokes multiple hemodynamic changes simultaneously (e.g., simultaneous changes in pulmonary vascular pressures and blood flow). Also, a clinical shortcut, such as the substitution in the numerator of the pulmonary arterial pressure for the pressure *drop* between pulmonary artery and left atrium, may be useful empirically but deprives the calculation of any physiologic meaning. Finally, the clinical significance of a value calculated for pulmonary vascular resistance depends heavily on the implications of the hemodynamic changes on the work of the right ventricle. For example, the same decrease in calculated pulmonary vascular resistance brought about by two different pulmonary vasodilators may affect the work of the right ventricle differently: should one agent elicit a *decrease* in pulmonary arterial pressure along with an *increase* in cardiac output (an ideal response), it is more apt to be of long-term benefit than another agent that, while increasing the cardiac output, fails to decrease the pulmonary arterial pressure.

In the normal lung, a considerable increase in cardiac output, i.e., two to three times that at rest, generally increases pulmonary arterial pressure by only a few millimeters of mercury. On the other hand, in pulmonary hypertensive states, in which the distensibility and extent of the pulmonary vascular bed has been restricted by disease, lesser increments in pulmonary blood flow are apt to elicit more striking increases in pulmonary arterial pressure.

Changes in pulmonary blood volume are much more subtle than changes in blood pressure or flow in their hemodynamic effects: they are also much more difficult to quantify. Clinical clues can be helpful in recognizing that the pulmonary blood volume has increased. Often a fullness of the pulmonary vascular pattern on the chest radiograph along with evidences of interstitial edema suggests that pulmonary blood volume has increased acutely. In chronic mitral stenosis or left ventricular failure, the pulmonary blood volume is not only increased but is also redistributed toward the apices of the lungs, i.e., "cephalization."

Autonomic nerves to the pulmonary vascular tree play much less of a role in mediating vasoconstriction or vasodilation than do local stimuli, particularly hypoxia. Indeed, hypoxia can exert its pulmonary pressor effect in the isolated lung, i.e., one that is devoid of external innervation. Acidosis reinforces the hypoxic pressor effect. The mechanism by which hypoxia exerts its local pressor effect is unknown.[2] Hypercapnia also exerts a pulmonary pressor effect, presumably by way of the local acidosis that it generates. Hypercapnia, however, is less powerful than hypoxia as a pulmonary vasoconstrictor agent.

PULMONARY HYPERTENSION: GENERAL FEATURES

Clinical Manifestations

Pulmonary hypertension is a final common hemodynamic consequence of multiple etiologies and diverse mechanisms. As noted above, most cases of pulmonary hypertension are secondary (Table 59-3). Among the underlying causes of pulmonary hypertension are mechanical compression and distortion of the resistance vessels of the lungs (e.g., by widespread pulmonary fibrosis), hypoxic vasoconstriction (e.g., in severe obstructive airways disease), intravascular obstruction (e.g., thromboemboli or tumor emboli), and combinations of mechanical and vasoconstrictive influences. The major importance of pulmonary hypertension, however, is that it leads to cor pulmonale and right ventricular failure. As noted above, not uncommonly, attention is first drawn to the possibility of pulmonary hypertension by the unexpected discovery of right ventricular enlargement, generally a combination of hypertrophy and dilation. When pulmonary arterial pressures climb to systemic levels, right ventricular failure becomes inevitable.

Special Studies

The gold standard for the diagnosis of pulmonary hypertension is right-sided heart catheterization. This technique enables the direct determination of pulmonary arterial pressure, pulmo-

TABLE 59-3

ETIOLOGIES OF CHRONIC PULMONARY (ARTERIAL) HYPERTENSION

I. Secondary
  A. Cardiac diseases
    1. Acquired heart disease associated with pulmonary venous hypertension, e.g., left ventricular failure, mitral valve disease
    2. Congenital heart disease
  B. Pulmonary diseases
    1. Chronic obstructive airways disease (chronic bronchitis and emphysema; chronic obstructive lung disease)
    2. Chronic interstitial lung disease
    3. Pulmonary vascular disease, e.g., thromboembolic disease; collagen vascular disease
  C. Disorders leading to alveolar hypoventilation
    1. Abnormal chest bellows
    2. Disordered respiratory control
    3. Sleep apneas
II. Primary pulmonary hypertension
III. Pulmonary veno-occlusive disease

nary wedge pressure (as an approximation of pulmonary venous pressure), pulmonary blood flow (cardiac output), and the responses of these parameters to interventions (vasodilators, oxygen, exercise). From the measurements and samples obtained during cardiac catheterization, pulmonary vascular resistance can be calculated (Table 59-2). As a rule, noninvasive methods are less reliable and less informative.

CHEST RADIOGRAPHY

The findings on the chest radiograph depend on the duration of the pulmonary hypertension and the etiology. The characteristic findings of pulmonary hypertension are enlargement of the pulmonary trunk and hilar vessels in association with pruning of the peripheral pulmonary arterial tree (Fig. 59-1). Right-sided heart enlargement can be difficult to detect radiographically except when the right ventricle is greatly enlarged. In secondary pulmonary hypertension, changes in the lungs (e.g., hyperinflation) and in the position of the heart and diaphragm often blur the radiologic changes of pulmonary hypertension and cor pulmonale.

Angiography, using contrast dyes, has little role in the workup for pulmonary hypertension unless it is done "selectively" in the search for pulmonary emboli.[10]

THE ELECTROCARDIOGRAM

The electrocardiogram (ECG) can disclose enlargement of the right ventricle with respect to the left ventricle. It is much more reliable in respiratory disorders that do not involve the parenchyma of the lungs (e.g., alveolar hypoventilation and the sleep apneas) than in obstructive airways disease, parenchymal lung disease, or congenital or acquired heart disease.

ECHOCARDIOGRAPHY

The amount of reliable information obtained by Doppler and two-dimensional echocardiography depends greatly on the commitment of individual clinics to standardizing and perfecting these indirect techniques. In general, Doppler techniques have proved useful in providing a measure of right ventricular thickness as an index of cor pulmonale. In some clinics, reliable estimates of the level of pulmonary hypertension have been obtained by determining regurgitant flows across the tricuspid and pulmonic valves using continuous-wave Doppler echocardiography.[11] In patients in whom the pulmonic valve has been visualized, its behavior during the cardiac cycle has also been used to estimate the level of pulmonary arterial pressure. Probably one of the more rewarding applications of echocardiography has been as an alternative to repeated cardiac catheterizations in tracing the course of the disease and in assessing the effects of therapeutic interventions (e.g., pulmonary vasodilators) (see also Chap. 14).

LUNG SCANS

Ventilation-perfusion scans are of most value in the diagnosis and exclusion of pulmonary thromboembolic disease (see below).

RADIONUCLIDE STUDIES

The response of the right ventricular ejection fraction to exercise is assessed in some clinics using radionuclide angiography. Scintigraphy using thallium 201 has also been useful in detecting hypertrophy of the right ventricle, i.e., cor pulmonale due to pulmonary hypertension (see also Chap. 17).

LUNG BIOPSY

The sampling of lung tissue by open thoracotomy is sometimes helpful in identifying the etiology of the pulmonary hypertension and, by excluding known etiologies, establishing the diagnosis of primary pulmonary hypertension. Attempts to predict responsiveness to vasodilators on the basis of lung biopsy have met with limited success.[12]

SECONDARY PULMONARY HYPERTENSION

Cardiac and/or respiratory diseases are the most common causes of secondary pulmonary hypertension. Pulmonary thromboembolic disease ranks third. Cardiac disease leads to pulmonary hypertension by increasing pulmonary blood flow (e.g., large left-to-right shunts) or by increasing pulmonary venous pressure (e.g., left ventricular failure). Almost invariably, secondary influences such as intimal proliferation in the pulmonary resistance vessels add a component of obstructive pulmonary vascular disease.[13] In respiratory disease, the predominant mechanism for the pulmonary hypertension is an increase in resistance to pulmonary blood flow arising from perivascular parenchymal changes coupled with pulmonary vasoconstriction due to hypoxia. In pulmonary thromboembolic disease, clots in various stages of organization and affecting pulmonary vessels of different size increase resistance to blood flow.[13]

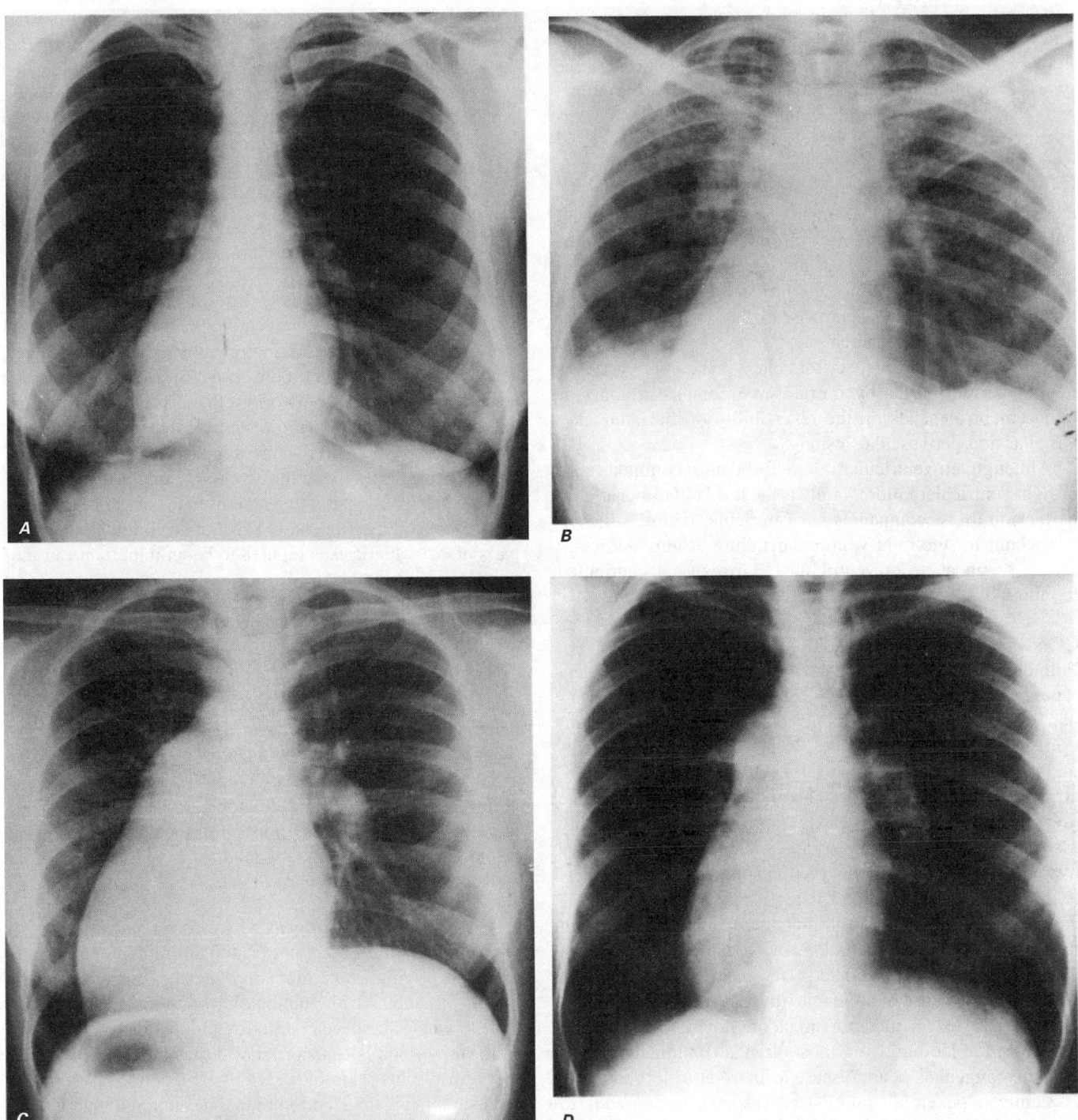

FIGURE 59-1
Cardiac silhouette in four patients with severe pulmonary hypertension on admission to the hospital: *A, B.* Primary pulmonary hypertension showing different stages in the evolution of cor pulmonale. *C.* Widespread pulmonary fibrosis. *D.* Systemic lupus erythematosus proven by lung biopsy. This radiograph is indistinguishable from that of primary pulmonary hypertension.

Cardiac Disease

The mechanisms of pulmonary hypertension are usually quite different in acquired disorders of the left side of the heart from those of congenital heart disease.

ACQUIRED DISORDERS OF LEFT SIDE OF HEART

Left ventricular failure is the most common cause of pulmonary hypertension. Among the various etiologies, myocardial disorders and lesions of the mitral and aortic valves predominate. Both categories of lesions lead to an increase in pulmonary venous pressure that, in turn, evokes an increase in pulmonary arterial pressure. Presumably, the increase in pulmonary arterial pressure is reflex in origin. In time, three types of morphologic changes supervene: (1) occlusive intimal and medial changes, not only in pulmonary venules and veins but also in the precapillary vessels; (2) perivascular interstitial edema and fibrosis that, under the influence of gravity, cause vascular and perivascular changes to be most marked in the dependent portions of the lungs; and (3) occlusion of small pulmonary vessels by emboli or thrombi when the right ventricle fails and cardiac output decreases. The medical management of myocardial failure is considered in Chap. 23. The treatment of congenital heart disease and of mitral valvular disease is usually mechanical (e.g., surgical or balloon mitral valvuloplasty). The prospect for relief of the pulmonary venous hypertension, as by mitral valve commissurotomy or replacement, depends on the reversibility of the pulmonary vascular and perivascular lesions.[14]

Although left ventricular failure is the most common cause of right ventricular failure, rarely is the level of pulmonary hypertension that accompanies left ventricular failure sufficient to account for the right ventricular failure. Right ventricular failure, secondary to left ventricular failure, is usually attributed to failure of the muscle in the shared ventricular septum.

CONGENITAL HEART DISEASE

Pulmonary hypertension is part of the natural history of many types of congenital heart disease and is often a major determinant of the clinical course, the feasibility of surgical intervention, and the outcome (Chaps. 70 and 71). Congenital defects of the heart associated with large left-to-right shunts (e.g., atrial septal defect) or abnormal communications between the great vessels (e.g., patent ductus arteriosus) are commonly associated with pulmonary arterial hypertension. Pulmonary hypertension occurs in both "pretricuspid" congenital defects (e.g., secundum atrial septal defect), and in "posttricuspid" congenital defects (e.g., ventricular septal defect). Important differences exist in the natural history of these two categories. Their differences are considered elsewhere in this book (Chap. 70). The major cause of pulmonary hypertension in congenital heart disease is an increase in blood flow, an increase in resistance to blood flow, or, most often, a combination of the two. In congenital heart disease with right-to-left shunting (systemic hypoxemia), pulmonary vasoconstriction adds to the resistance to blood flow. Erythrocytosis, acting by way of increased viscosity and propensity to thrombosis, also contributes to the increase in resistance. Although the increase in pulmonary vascular tone elicited by hypoxia contributes to the increase in pulmonary vascular resistance, the predominant resistance is offered by anatomic changes in the walls of the small muscular arteries and arterioles. Patients with congenital heart disease and pulmonary hypertension who become pregnant are at increased risk of sudden death both in the course of delivery and immediately post partum.

Depending on the nature of the congenital cardiac defect, vasodilators are sometimes helpful in diminishing heightened pulmonary vasomotor tone. Caution is required in administering such agents to patients with congenital heart disease because of the prospect of inducing imbalances between the systemic and pulmonary pressures and flows. Phlebotomy, with replacement of fluid (e.g., plasma or albumin), is helpful in congenital cyanotic heart disease in which severe hypoxemia has evoked a large increase in red cell mass. Once again, caution is required to avoid depletion of iron stores and to avoid reduction in the circulating blood volume.

THROMBOEMBOLIC DISEASE

Thromboembolic disease is a form of occlusive pulmonary vascular disease. It may be acute or chronic. In the United States and Europe, clots originating in peripheral veins represent a common cause of chronic occlusive pulmonary vascular disease. Elsewhere in the world, other intravascular particulates may cause pulmonary vascular occlusive disease. For example, in Egypt, where schistosomiasis is endemic, pulmonary vascular disease stemming from ova lodged in pulmonary vessels and hypersensitivity reactions to the organism (usually situated outside of the lungs) is not uncommon. In some parts of Asia, filariasis is reputed to be an important cause of pulmonary hypertension. Tumor emboli to the lungs from extrapulmonary sites (e.g., the breast) can cause pulmonary hypertension by invading the adjacent minute vessels of the lungs.

The *syndromes of thromboembolic pulmonary hypertension* can be categorized according to the segments of the pulmonary arterial tree that are primarily affected: (1) small (muscular pulmonary arteries and arterioles), (2) intermediate, and (3) large central arteries. Some overlap among these categories is inevitable because clots lodged in large vessels are fragmented by the churning motion of the heart and both the parent clot and its derivatives tend to move peripherally for final lodging.

1. *Occlusion of small muscular arteries and arterioles by organized thrombi.* At autopsy, small thrombi, predominantly recent in origin, are commonplace in the small pulmonary vessels of patients with pulmonary hypertension and cor pulmonale who have developed heart failure preterminally. As a rule, these spotty occlusions have little clinical significance. In contrast is the syndrome of widespread pulmonary vascular occlusion by organized thrombi in the small pulmonary arteries and arterioles. Once attributed to multiple pulmonary emboli, these lesions are now regarded as organized, in situ thrombi.[15] The syndrome is rare and indistinguishable during life from primary pulmonary hypertension except by lung biopsy. Histologic identification of these lesions serves little purpose in management. After a ventilation-perfusion scan has excluded chronic proximal thromboembolism (see below), treatment consists of long-term anticoagulation to prevent further clotting, using warfarin or related agents, antiplatelet agents, or both.

2. *Occlusion of intermediate pulmonary arteries by emboli.* This syndrome is by far the more common of the three.[15]

It is caused by multiple emboli, almost invariably released from vessels in the upper legs and thighs, that progressively amputate more and more of the pulmonary arterial tree. Ventilation-perfusion scans and selective angiography demonstrate the extent of the pulmonary vascular occlusion (see Chap. 60). Usually, too little of the pulmonary arterial tree is involved to elicit pulmonary hypertension. In some instances, however, repeated emboli may suffice to raise pulmonary arterial pressures to hypertensive levels. The major therapeutic concern in these patients is to exclude chronic proximal pulmonary thromboembolism (see below) and to prevent recurrent thromboemboli. Treatment involves the use of anticoagulants of the warfarin type and antiplatelet agents.

3. *Chronic proximal pulmonary thromboembolism.* In some patients who have survived large to massive pulmonary emboli, resolution fails to occur and the clots become organized and incorporated into the walls of the major pulmonary arteries, leading to pulmonary hypertension (Fig. 59-2). Overwhelming of the local fibrinolytic mechanisms also allows the clot to propagate (antegradely and retrogradely), to obstruct large segments of the pulmonary vascular bed, and to decrease the compliance of the central pulmonary vessels. By the time the diagnosis is made, the obstructing lesions in the central pulmonary arteries have become part of the vessel walls by the processes of organization, fibrosis, endothelialization, and recanalization.[15]

The importance of recognizing *proximal* pulmonary thromboembolism as a cause of pulmonary hypertension is the possibility of relieving the pulmonary hypertension by surgical intervention, i.e., by pulmonary thromboendarterectomy. Ventilation-perfusion lung scanning is the critical diagnostic test. As a rule, patients with proximal pulmonary thromboembolism show two or more segmental perfusion defects. If the perfusion defects are segmental or larger, selective pulmonary angiography is called for to define the location, extent, and number of pulmonary vascular occlusions.[16] Cardiac catheterization for selective pulmonary angiography also enables hemodynamic assessment. Fiberoptic angioscopy and magnetic resonance imaging may be helpful in defining the lesions of proximal thromboembolic pulmonary hypertension[17] (see also Chap. 60).

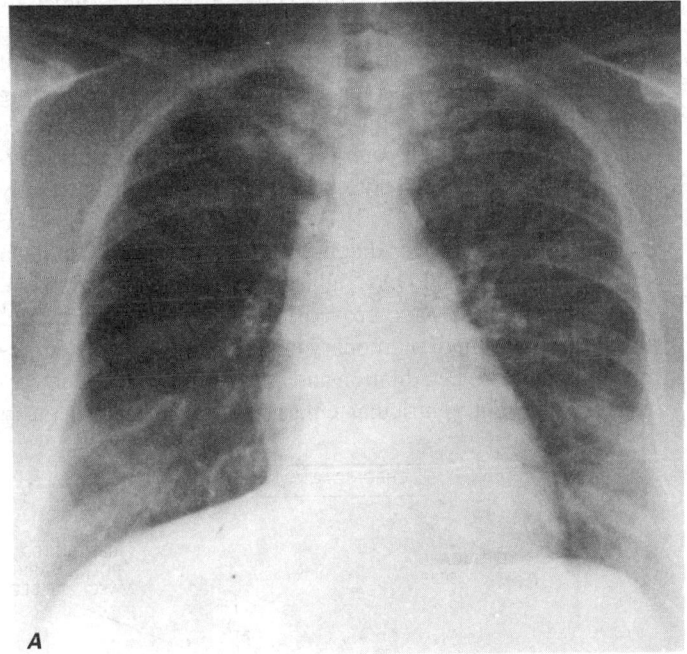

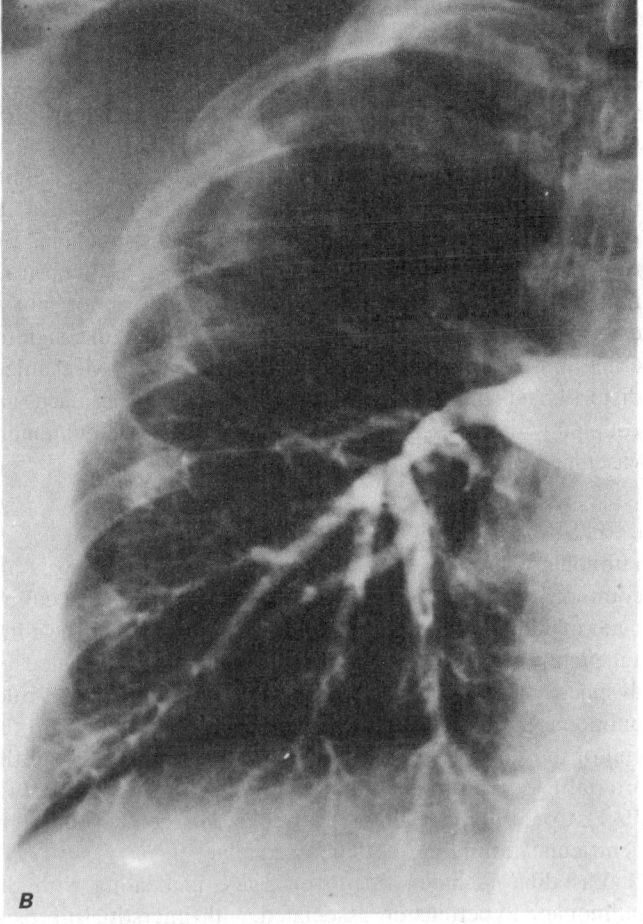

FIGURE 59-2

Pulmonary hypertension due to organized clot in central pulmonary arteries. Dramatic relief after pulmonary thromboendarterectomy. *A.* Chest radiograph. The right upper lobe is strikingly hypoperfused and the vasculature on the left is quite prominent, reflecting redirection of the pulmonary blood flow to open vessels. *B.* Angiogram. The flow to the right upper lung is interrupted by the large central clot.

Surgery is advocated for patients with pulmonary hypertension who have persistent clot in lobar or more proximal pulmonary arteries after at least 6 months of anticoagulation. Thromboendarterectomy is done, generally via a median sternotomy, using deep hypothermic cardiopulmonary bypass with intermittent periods of circulatory arrest. Postoperatively, hemodynamic improvement is usually quite dramatic. Pulmonary edema of the lung that was previously hypoperfused can be a severe complication immediately after the obstruction has been relieved. In experienced hands, mortality is of the order of 6 percent. After the operation, patients are placed on lifelong anticoagulants. A filter is often placed in the inferior vena cava to prevent recurrence.

Respiratory Diseases and Disorders

Not only intrinsic pulmonary diseases but also respiratory disorders, i.e., disturbances in the respiratory muscles or in the control of breathing, can lead to pulmonary hypertension. Among the intrinsic lung diseases are those affecting the airways (e.g., chronic bronchitis) as well as those affecting the parenchyma. Among the respiratory disorders are the syndromes of alveolar hypoventilation and the sleep apneas.

INTRINSIC DISEASES OF LUNGS AND/OR AIRWAYS

Diseases that affect the parenchyma of the lungs or the tracheobronchial tree can elicit pulmonary hypertension in different ways depending on the underlying disease. In widespread interstitial fibrosis and/or inflammation, disease in the vicinity of the minute pulmonary vessels encroaches on vascular lumens, thereby limiting their distensibility and amputating peripheral segments of the pulmonary vascular tree. In obstructive airways disease, ventilation-perfusion abnormalities cause vasoconstriction due to arterial hypoxemia. In conglomerate fibrosis, several mechanisms act in concert: Mechanical distortion, encasement, and obstruction of vascular lumens are coupled with hypoxic vasoconstriction to increase pulmonary vascular resistance.

INTERSTITIAL FIBROSIS

Pulmonary sarcoidosis, asbestosis, and radiation fibrosis are common causes of widespread pulmonary fibrosis that culminates in pulmonary hypertension and cor pulmonale. The clinical picture of interstitial fibrosis is generally dominated by dyspnea and tachypnea; cough is rarely prominent. As a rule, pulmonary hypertension of marked degree occurs toward the end of the illness, when hypoxemia is present at rest and the arterial P_{CO_2} starts its climb toward hypercapnic levels (Fig. 59-1). Cor pulmonale (right ventricular enlargement) and right ventricular failure are common sequelae.

Vasodilators have no proven place in dealing with the pulmonary hypertension associated with interstitial fibrosis. Oxygen therapy, particularly during daily activity or sleep, can be important in avoiding the hypoxic pulmonary pressor response. Glucocorticoids often become the mainstay of therapy and often effect some symptomatic relief. The advent

of lung transplantation has widened greatly the therapeutic horizons for dealing with widespread interstitial fibrosis.

Chronic Obstructive Airways Disease

Chronic bronchitis and emphysema [chronic obstructive pulmonary disease (COPD)] are the most common causes of pulmonary hypertension and cor pulmonale in patients with intrinsic pulmonary disease.[18,19] Even though chronic bronchitis and emphysema generally coexist, the predominant cause of the pulmonary hypertension is alveolar hypoxia resulting from chronic bronchitis; emphysema plays only a minor role, presumably by restricting the extent of the pulmonary vascular bed (Fig. 59-3). Cystic fibrosis illustrates the importance of COPD in evoking pulmonary hypertension since the disease in cystic fibrosis is virtually confined to the airways.

The indiscriminate use of the designation *COPD*, without distinguishing between predominant bronchitis and predominant emphysema, tends to cloud the natural history of this spectrum of obstructive airway diseases. In essence, pulmonary hypertension (generally culminating in cor pulmonale) is encountered in two different settings: *episodically* in the "pink puffer," who only becomes hypoxemic during an acute respiratory infection, and *chronically* in the "blue bloater," within whom unremitting hypoxia is aggravated during an acute respiratory infection. In the blue bloater the course of the pulmonary hypertension is inexorably progressive. During a bout of respiratory failure, clinical distinction between a pink buffer and a blue bloater is often impossible. After recovery from the acute episode, however, distinction is usually quite simple.

The gold standard for diagnosing pulmonary hypertension in patients with COPD is right-sided heart catheterization. Less direct indices have proved useful in some clinics.[20,21] Once cardinal sign of pulmonary hypertension is right ventricular enlargement, i.e., dilation and hypertrophy; however, recognition of right ventricular enlargement can be difficult in

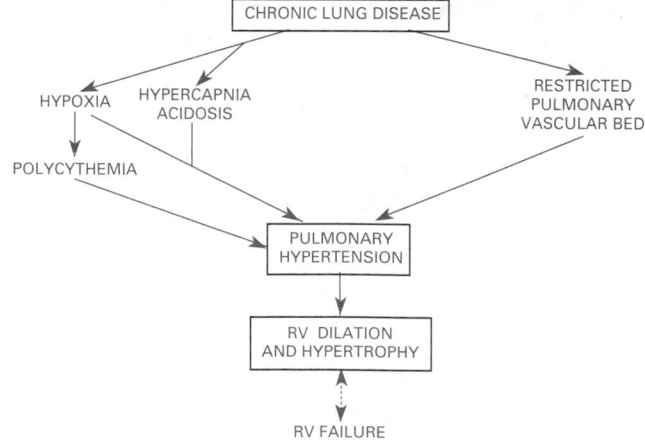

FIGURE 59-3

The evolution of cor pulmonale and right ventricular failure in chronic obstructive airways disease [chronic bronchitis and emphysema; chronic obstructive pulmonary disease (COPD)]. The factors on the left arise primarily from the bronchitis, those on the right from emphysema.

obstructive airways disease because of hyperinflation and cardiac rotation.[22] Once suspicion is raised that the clinical picture of right ventricular failure stems from ventilation-perfusion abnormalities, an arterial blood sample will confirm that the P_{O_2} is low (P_{O_2} < 40 to 50 mmHg), the P_{CO_2} is high (P_{CO_2} > 50 mmHg), and respiratory acidosis is present. Such arterial blood gas tensions are rare in left ventricular failure unless the patient is in frank pulmonary edema.

Electrocardiographic evidence of right ventricular enlargement is also often equivocal in patients with chronic obstructive airways disease (chronic bronchitis and emphysema; COPD) because of rotation and displacement of the heart, widened distances between electrodes and the cardiac surface, and the predominance of dilation over hypertrophy in the cardiac enlargement. Because of these limitations, it is not surprising that standard electrocardiographic criteria for right ventricular enlargement apply in about only one-third of patients with COPD who prove to have cor pulmonale at autopsy. Consecutive changes in the ECG are often more useful than a single ECG in detecting right ventricular overload due to pulmonary hypertension. As the arterial P_{O_2} drops to distinctly subnormal levels (e.g., <60 to 70 mmHg while awake), T waves tend to become inverted, biphasic, or flat in the right, precordial leads (V_1 to V_3); the mean electrical axis of the QRS shifts 30 degrees or more to the right of the patient's usual axis; ST segments become depressed in leads II, III, and aV_F; and right bundle branch block (incomplete or complete) often appears. These changes tend to reverse as arterial oxygenation improves (see also Chap. 12).

In the patient with COPD in whom pulmonary hypertension has been elicited or aggravated by a bout of bronchitis or pneumonia, the goal of therapy is to maintain tolerable levels of arterial oxygenation while waiting for the upper respiratory infection to subside. If the pulmonary hypertension is acute, modest enrichment of inspired air with oxygen, as by 28% oxygen delivered by a Venturi mask, generally suffices to relieve arterial hypoxemia and to restore pulmonary arterial pressures toward normal. Considerable improvement may also be accomplished even in the individual who has chronic pulmonary hypertension by sustained (virtually continuous) breathing of oxygen-enriched air that restores arterial P_{O_2} to nearly normal values.

Once the right ventricle has failed, cardiotonic agents can only be used cautiously because of the threat of arrhythmias posed by arterial hypoxemia and respiratory acidosis. Moreover, after adequate oxygenation has been achieved, the need for digitalis and diuretics often decreases since the hemodynamic burden on the right ventricle, i.e., the pulmonary arterial hypertension, decreases. Even though each episode of acute hypoxia and acidosis seems to elicit about the same increment in pulmonary arterial pressure, each bout of pulmonary hypertension appears to leave behind a slightly higher level of pulmonary hypertension after recovery.[18]

Arterial blood gas composition is the therapeutic compass to the control of pulmonary hypertension in COPD. The degree of hypoxia is usually underestimated by blood sampling since blood is drawn while the patient is awake and at rest, whereas hypoxemia is more marked during sleep and daily activity. In managing ambulatory patients, serial determinations of the hematocrit may serve as a practical clue to the occurrence of covert arterial hypoxemia, i.e., during sleep or activity. Once right ventricular failure has set in, however, there is no substitute for determining arterial P_{O_2} and P_{CO_2} as a guide to therapy. Ensuring the return of arterial oxygenation toward normal is much more vital than is the administration of cardiotonic measures. When respiratory infection has triggered the episode of pulmonary hypertension, a vital strategy for achieving a lasting improvement in arterial oxygenation is the administration of an appropriate antibiotic. While awaiting the salutary effects of antibiotic therapy, attention is paid to hydration, to postural drainage, and to adequate alveolar ventilation. The management of respiratory acidosis is described elsewhere in this text.

Phlebotomy, once popular because of the prospect that increased blood viscosity contributes importantly to the pulmonary hypertension, has fallen into disuse. Polycythemia is rarely severe enough to be a serious problem in cor pulmonale associated with bronchitis and emphysema.

Vasodilators have recently been tried in various types of secondary pulmonary hypertension, including that due to COPD. The agents tried are the same as those outlined for *primary* pulmonary hypertension. They run the risk of aggravating arterial hypoxemia by exaggerating ventilation-perfusion abnormalities. Unfortunately, the efficacy of vasodilator agents in secondary pulmonary hypertension has proved to be far less impressive or predictable than in primary pulmonary hypertension. To date, the safest and most effective approach to pulmonary vasodilation in obstructive arterial hypoxemia is the use of oxygen-enriched inspired air.[22–24]

Conglomerate Fibrosis, Emphysema, and Chronic Bronchitis

Pulmonary hypertension is uncommon in uncomplicated silicosis or tuberculosis. By contrast, in patients in whom smoldering, long-standing tuberculosis or conglomerate massive fibrosis has shrunk and distorted the lungs, pulmonary hypertension is virtually the rule. The likelihood of pulmonary hypertension (and cor pulmonale) is enhanced by chronic pleurisy, fibrothorax, or excisional surgery, which exert their effects by a combination of all of these derangements. Although these combinations are generally complicated, the principles of management are those outlined above for obstructive airways disease. Unfortunately, therapeutic triumphs are uncommon because of the fixed anatomic changes.

CONNECTIVE TISSUE DISEASES

Pulmonary vascular disease is an important component of certain connective tissue diseases. Among these, the more common are systemic lupus erythematosus (SLE), scleroderma (and its variant types), and dermatomyositis.[25] The lesions may take the form of interstitial inflammation and fibrosis, obliterative disease, or vascular disease, either singly or, more often, in combination. Although pulmonary hypertension can complicate many connective tissue diseases, it has been documented most often in SLE and progressive systemic sclerosis (scleroderma) and its variant syndromes. The possibility has been raised that connective tissue diseases may be responsible for some instances of primary pulmonary hypertension. This prospect has gained support from the occasional instances in which the lesions are confined to the pulmonary arterial tree without interstitial involvement and similarities in the histologic appearance of the vascular lesions. The high frequency of both collagen vascular disease and primary pulmonary hypertension in women and the occurrence of Raynaud's phenomenon has been used as additional evidence.[26] Finally, there is a high incidence of positive serologic tests for antibodies in women with primary pulmonary hypertension. With respect to the pathogenesis of the two disorders, the idea has been raised that both the Raynaud's phenomenon and an increase in pulmonary vascular tone represent a widespread, vasoconstrictive pulmonary-systemic disorder. However, this hypothesis has not gained universal support.

The lungs and pleura are frequently involved in SLE, with a reported frequency of up to 70 percent. Patients with pulmonary hypertension and SLE are predominantly women; most of these patients also exhibit Raynaud's phenomenon.[26]

The histopathologic lesions in these patients resemble those of primary pulmonary hypertension. Pulmonary hypertension in these patients may originate in microthrombi secondary to the hypercoagulable state caused by lupus anticoagulant in the blood. Less likely is the hypothesis of generalized vasoconstriction noted above. Unfortunately, treatment of pulmonary hypertension associated with SLE using either anticoagulants or pulmonary vasodilators has had only modest success. This poor outcome contrasts with the results obtained in patients with active pulmonary vasculitis who may either improve or stabilize their vascular disease with immunosuppressive agents.

In progressive systemic sclerosis (scleroderma) and its variants, such as the CREST syndrome (*c*alcinosis, *R*aynaud's syndrome, *e*sophageal involvement, *s*clerodactyly, and *t*elangiectasis) and in overlap syndromes (e.g., mixed connective tissue disease), the incidence of pulmonary vascular disease is high. In these patients, pulmonary hypertension is the cause of considerable morbidity and mortality.[25] In a prospective study involving cardiac catheterization of patients with progressive systemic sclerosis or the CREST syndrome variant, pulmonary hypertension, either as an isolated finding or in association with pulmonary parenchymal or cardiac disease, was found in up to one-third of patients with progressive systemic sclerosis and in up to one-half of patients with the CREST syndrome. The pulmonary vascular disease may be independent of pulmonary or other visceral disease. As in the case of SLE, the pathology of these lesions is often indistinguishable from that of primary pulmonary hypertension. The overlap of findings in patients with pulmonary hypertension and a scleroderma variant, on the one hand, and in those with primary pulmonary hypertension (Raynaud's phenomenon, pulmonary vascular histology, high incidence of positive anti-nuclear antibodies in the blood), on the other, reinforces the idea that a subset of patients with so-called primary pulmonary hypertension actually represents a subset with a scleroderma variant confined to the lungs. Vasodilator therapy has not proved to be highly effective.

ALVEOLAR HYPOVENTILATION IN PATIENTS WITH NORMAL LUNGS

In patients who hypoventilate despite normal lungs ("global" alveolar hypoventilation), the primary pathogenetic mechanism is alveolar hypoxia sometimes reinforced by respiratory acidosis.[19,27] These abnormal alveolar and blood gases play the same role in eliciting pulmonary hypertension in patients with global alveolar hypoventilation as in those in whom the abnormal alveolar and blood gases are the result of ventilation-perfusion abnormalities. In individuals with normal lungs, the global alveolar hypoventilation generally originates from an inadequate ventilatory drive (as after encephalitis), covert obstruction of the upper airways (as in the sleep apnea syndromes), an ineffective chest bellows (as after paralytic poliomyelitis), or lungs entrapped by neoplasm or fibrosis (as in trapped lung caused by asbestosis).

Regardless of etiology, whether pulmonary hypertension will occur in patients with alveolar hypoventilation and normal lungs depends on the whether there is sufficient alveolar and arterial hypoxia to raise pulmonary arterial pressures considerably. In some individuals, such as those with kyphoscoliosis, the stage for arterial hypoxemia and pulmonary hypertension is set by the mechanical limitations imposed by the deformed chest; in these individuals, the activities of daily life aggravate the situation by increasing metabolic demand due to not only the increased activity but also the increase in the oxygen cost of breathing. In the sleep apnea syndromes, severe arterial hypoxemia and pulmonary hypertension that develop initially only during sleep may become self-perpetuating and carry over into wakefulness.[28] As in other types of pulmonary disorders, cor pulmonale is the common sequel to unrelieved pulmonary hypertension. Also, no matter how the alveolar hypoventilation has been initiated, an upper respiratory infection often topples this type of patient into respiratory failure, severe pulmonary hypertension, and right-sided heart failure.

For the patient with global alveolar hypoventilation who is in combined respiratory and cardiac (right ventricular) failure, the highest therapeutic priority is to improve oxygenation. Assisted ventilation, particularly during sleep, may be particularly helpful in improving oxygenation and reducing hypercapnia [e.g., continuous positive airway pressure (CPAP)] breathing. Success in avoiding alveolar and arterial hypoxia decreases pulmonary arterial pressures, thereby relieving the overburdened right ventricle. Recently, potent but short-acting pulmonary vasodilators, such as prostacyclin, have been advocated for urgent relief of right ventricular overload. In patients with global alveolar hypoventilation, however, pharmacologic therapy is rarely needed because of the efficiency of assisted ventilation coupled with oxygen therapy in promoting pulmonary vasodilation.

PRIMARY (UNEXPLAINED) PULMONARY HYPERTENSION

Definition

Primary pulmonary hypertension (PPH) is defined as pulmonary arterial hypertension of unknown cause. It is a diagnosis made by exclusion; all recognizable causes of pulmonary hypertension (Table 59-3) must be ruled out before the diagnosis of PPH can be made. The diagnosis presupposes that the seat of the disorder is intrinsic to the pulmonary arterial tree. Pulmonary veno-occlusive disease (see below) is not included under the rubric of PPH, even though its etiology is also unexplained; although the pulmonary arterial tree does undergo secondary changes that cause pulmonary *arterial* hypertension along with the pulmonary *venous* hypertension, the pathologic features and pathogenetic mechanisms in pulmonary veno-occlusive disease are quite different and distinctive.

PPH is a rare disease. Its prevalence is about 0.1 to 0.2 percent of all patients who come to autopsy. Based on the 194 patients entered into the National Registry for Primary Pulmonary Hypertension, the estimated incidence nationwide in the United States is about 400 new patients per year.[4] A total of about 1000 cases has been reported.

The clinical diagnosis of PPH rests on three different types of evidence: (1) clinical, radiographic, and electrocardiographic manifestations of pulmonary hypertension; (2) hemodynamic features consisting of abnormally high pulmonary arterial pressures and pulmonary vascular resistance in association with a normal pulmonary wedge pressure and a normal or low cardiac output; and (3) exclusion of the causes of secondary pulmonary hypertension.

SPECIAL TYPES

Certain associations of PPH have attracted interest because of their prospects for shedding light on some etiologies. These include so-called dietary pulmonary hypertension; familial pulmonary hypertension; coexistent PPH, human immunodeficiency virus (HIV) infection, and connective tissue disease; and coexistent pulmonary hypertension and hepatic cirrhosis.[29] In each of these, the clinical findings and the histologic appearance of the lungs at autopsy resemble those that characterize the usual types of PPH. This diversity in associations underscores the likelihood that so-called PPH is the final common expression of heterogeneous etiologies.

General Features

After puberty, females predominate, those between 10 and 40 years of age being most often affected. Before puberty, no sex difference is discernible. The textbook picture of a patient with PPH is that of a young woman in the prime of life who develops one or more of the symptoms in Table 59-1 without discernible cause. Sex and age are sometimes useful in distinguishing clinically between the likelihood of PPH and pulmonary thromboembolic disease. The latter generally favors men, particularly in their later years.[30]

As a rule, median survival of patients can be predicted on the basis of the New York Heart Association functional classification: 6 months for class IV; 2 1/2 years for class III; 6 years for classes I and II. Unless interrupted by sudden death, the usual downhill course terminates in intractable right ventricular failure. Although this classification does provide a useful clinical guide, exceptions are not uncommon.[31]

Etiology

The common denominator in the pathogenesis of PPH appears to be injury to the pulmonary endothelium of the small muscular pulmonary arteries and arterioles.[32] In response to injury, the intima of these vessels proliferates so that the endothelium changes from a single flat layer to a piled-up projection that narrows the caliber of the vascular lumen. Along with intimal proliferation, the media of the affected vessels hypertrophy.[33]

This postulated sequence suffers from gaps in understanding. For example, why the localization of intimal proliferation and medial hypertrophy to the small muscular pulmonary arteries and arterioles? Does the piled-up endothelium serve the same functions as single-layered endothelium? Does it have a propensity to form clots? Is communication between endothelium and smooth muscle preserved after occlusive vascular disease sets in? Is the interplay among vasoconstrictor and vasodilator substances, such as endothelin, prostacyclin, and nitric oxide, preserved[34]?

Diverse etiologies seem to be capable of eliciting the syndrome of PPH (Table 59-4).[35] For example, fenfluramine has been implicated in epidemics of so-called PPH, ingestion of toxic oil elicited an outbreak of pulmonary hypertension in Spain,[4] and HIV has also been implicated.[36]

For a long while, virtually all reports of PPH dealt with sporadic cases. An epidemic in Europe between 1967 and 1970 of PPH that was apparently linked to the over-the-counter sale of Aminorex, an anorectic agent, raised the prospect of hereditary predisposition, since only 1 in 1000 who took the drug developed pulmonary hypertension. More recently, fenfluramine and phentermine, taken in combination, have been associated with severe pulmonary hypertension and valvular heart disease.[37,60] The recent toxic oil epidemic in Spain has reinforced the idea of individual susceptibility to toxic agents.[38]

In recent years, an increasing number of patients have been identified in whom PPH is genetically linked.[39] In these individuals, the hereditary pattern is that of autosomal dominance and incomplete penetrance. One major insight provided by the families with PPH is the diversity of pulmonary vascular lesions in members of the same family. The familial incidence has raised questions about whether better family histories would reveal that some cases of PPH currently regarded as sporadic would, on searching inquiry, prove to be familial (see also Chap. 69).

TABLE 59-4

SUGGESTED MECHANISMS FOR PRIMARY PULMONARY HYPERTENSION

Sustained vasoconstriction	Most likely a contributing factor
Autoimmune mechanisms	Based on association with Raynaud's phenomenon and collagen vascular diseases, such as disseminated lupus erythematosus
Persistence of fetal pulmonary vascular bed	Questionably related to the adult syndrome
Dietary pulmonary hypertension	Suggested by outbreaks of pulmonary hypertension after ingestion of anoretic agent, Aminorex, and toxic oil; genetic predisposition seems to be involved
Combined portal and pulmonary hypertension	Pulmonary hypertension occurs in some patients with hepatic cirrhosis; possibly related to dietary pulmonary hypertension
Multiple pulmonary thrombi	Widespread occlusion of small muscular arteries and arterioles in the lungs, possibly due to unidentified endothelial injury
Familial pulmonary hypertension	A well-documented entity; possibility that some sporadic cases are really instances of the familial form of the disease

Pathology

The evolution of PPH depends on progressive attenuation of the pulmonary arterial tree, which gradually increases pulmonary vascular resistance to the point of eliciting right ventricular strain and failure. The seat of the disease is in the small pulmonary arteries (between 40 and 100 μm in diameter) and arterioles. The obliterative lesions can affect one or more layers of these vessels: in some instances, medial hypertrophy predominates; in others, it is the intima that proliferates. In addition, evidence of inflammation is also present (Fig. 59-4).[12,40]

Clinicians have traditionally relied heavily on the pathologist for confirmation of the diagnosis of PPH. The pathologist can be helpful in three ways: (1) identifying a constellation of pulmonary precapillary lesions that are consistent with the clinical diagnosis of PPH, i.e., plexiform lesions, angiomatoid lesions, concentric intimal fibrosis, and necrotizing arteritis; although the full-blown histologic picture is diagnostic, it is also uncommon to see all of these lesions in a single patient; (2) distinguishing between the obliterative vascular disease of PPH and those of pulmonary thromboembolic disease; and (3) excluding etiologies of secondary pulmonary hypertension. Although thromboembolic disease is the cause of the pulmonary hypertension (e.g., as a type of secondary pulmonary hypertension), the pathologist is often hard-pressed to

distinguish between organized clots in small vessels that initiate the pulmonary hypertension and those that result from the obliterative pulmonary vascular disease. Recent clots in small pulmonary arteries and arterioles are not uncommon at autopsy in patients with PPH, particularly when the right ventricle has failed and cardiac output falls. Although similar clots may not have initiated the pulmonary hypertension process in PPH, it seems reasonable that more often they are complicating features that aggravate and exaggerate pulmonary vascular obstruction. The prevalence of clots at autopsy relates clinically to the use of anticoagulants in primary pulmonary hypertension.

Pathophysiology

The hemodynamic hallmarks of PPH in the resting patient have been indicated above: a combination of a high pulmonary arterial pressure, a normal or low cardiac output, and a normal left atrial (pulmonary wedge) pressure. As a result of this hemodynamic pattern, calculated pulmonary vascular resistance is high, generally leading to the logical conclusion that the resistance vessels, i.e., the small muscular arteries and arterioles, are the predominant sites of vascular obstruction. During exercise, as cardiac output increases, pulmonary arterial pressures increase further; the increments in pressure in the pulmonary hypertensive circuit are much more striking than in the normotensive pulmonary circulation.

Pulmonary vasodilators are currently administered acutely for testing the responsiveness of the pulmonary circulation. Among these, prostacyclin has become the gold standard, but other vasodilators are often tried as well. Several clinical and hemodynamic changes are sought as desirable endpoints: (1) improvement in exercise tolerance and in the quality of life; the increase in physical capacity, attributable to an increase in cardiac output, in turn improves oxygen delivery to peripheral organs and tissues; (2) a decrease in the level of pulmonary

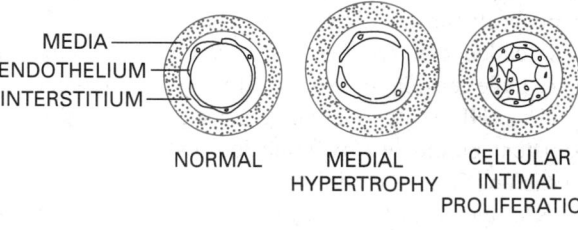

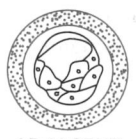 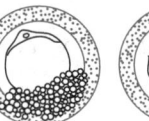 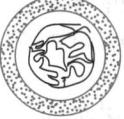 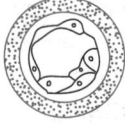

FIGURE 59-4

Vascular lesions in primary pulmonary hypertension. The plexiform lesion, once believed to be the histologic hallmark of primary pulmonary hypertension, has emerged as only one feature of a constellation of lesions.

arterial hypertension, both at rest and during exercise; (3) a decrease in calculated pulmonary vascular resistance; optimally, this decrease should entail an increase in cardiac output (with minimal increase in heart rate) accompanied by a decrease in pulmonary arterial pressure; and (4) since pulmonary vasodilators are also systemic vasodilators, pulmonary vasodilation has to be effected without evoking undue systemic hypotension and tachycardia.

The combination of right-sided heart catheterization and vasodilator testing is particularly useful not only for defining the hemodynamic state of the patient but also in providing a hemodynamic baseline for future noninvasive studies, such as serial echocardiograms.

MD, 56 F

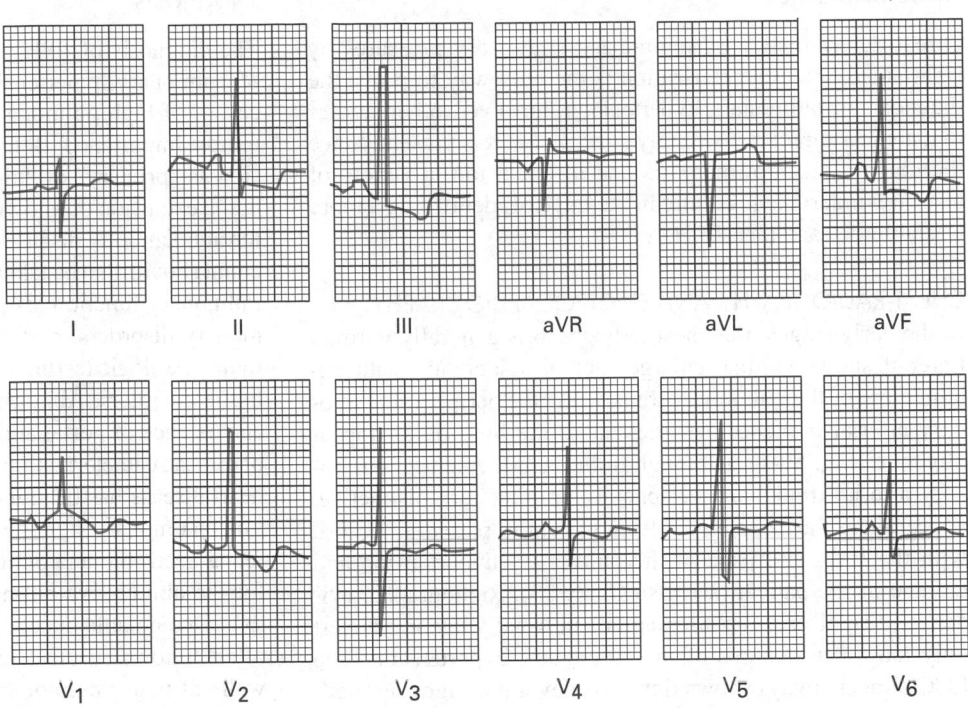

FIGURE 59-5

Electrocardiogram in patients with primary pulmonary hypertension and cor pulmonale.

Clinical Picture

In its early stages, the disease is difficult to recognize. In the sporadic case, the first clue is often an abnormal chest radiograph (Fig. 59-1) or electrocardiograph indicative of right ventricular hypertrophy (Fig. 59-5). Both are late manifestations. The existence of right ventricular enlargement is generally confirmed by echocardiography. By the time these changes appear, however, pulmonary hypertension is moderate to severe and generally long-standing. Initial complaints, particularly easy fatigability and chest discomfort, tend to be discounted, i.e., attributed to being "out of shape" except when the index of suspicion is high, for example, during an "outbreak" of PPH, such as that associated with the ingestion of anorectic agents, or in patients with a history of familial pulmonary hypertension (Table 59-1).

When the disease is advanced, the activities of daily life are progressively circumscribed by increasing nonspecific discomfort. Dyspnea, particularly during exercise, becomes incapacitating. Some patients develop a nondescript type of chest pain along with breathlessness. Other common symptoms are weakness, fatigue, and syncope on effort (Table 59-1). Infrequently, an enlarged pulmonary artery causes hoarseness because of compression of the left recurrent laryngeal nerve. In time, right-sided heart failure develops.

Patients with severe pulmonary hypertension seem prone to sudden death. Death has occurred unexpectedly during normal activities, cardiac catheterization, and surgical procedures and after the administration of barbiturates or anesthetic agents. The mechanisms for sudden death are not clear. In a few instances, severe bradycardia and atrioventricular (AV) dissociation have preceded cardiac arrest.

It was noted above that as far as clinical manifestations and physical examination are concerned, PPH has an advantage over secondary pulmonary hypertension in that its manifestations are not complicated by those of underlying cardiac or respiratory disease. On physical examination, the jugular venous pulse usually shows a prominent *a* wave. Right ventricular hypertrophy causes a heave along the left sternal border, and a distinct systolic impulse is palpable over the region of the main pulmonary artery (Chap. 10). The pulmonic component of the second sound is markedly accentuated, the second heart sound is narrowly split, and an ejection click is heard in the pulmonic area. Often a fourth heart sound emanating from the hypertrophied right ventricle is heard at the lower left sternal border. In some patients, a midsystolic murmur is audible at the pulmonic area; as pulmonary arterial pressures approximate systemic arterial levels, the murmur of pulmonary valvular regurgitation often appears (see also Chap. 10).

The onset of right ventricular failure is accompanied by jugular venous distension and a gallop (S_3); inspiration intensifies the gallop. The liver becomes enlarged and tender, and a hepatojugular reflux can be elicited; in time, dilation of the failing right ventricle leads to tricuspid regurgitation manifested by a holosystolic murmur, best heard in the fourth interspace to the left of the sternum, that increases in intensity during inspiration. Tricuspid regurgitation is a feature of the echocardiographic findings. The liver develops expansile pulsations synchronous with the heart beat. Hydrothorax and ascites are uncommon, even in the face of hepatomegaly and peripheral edema.

Special Studies

Direct determination of pulmonary circulatory pressures by right-sided heart catheterization is the only way to prove the diagnosis of pulmonary hypertension; however, other studies that are less direct can strongly suggest that it is present. Since the diagnosis of "primary" is one of exclusion, a variety of tests are undertaken, usually in the hope of identifying a more treatable disease than PPH.

CHEST RADIOGRAPHY AND ELECTROCARDIOGRAPHY

In the early stages, the chest radiograph is generally normal. Later it shows cardiac enlargement in association with enlargement of the pulmonary trunk while the peripheral pulmonary arterial branches are attenuated; the lung fields appear oligemic (Fig. 59-1). Although fullness of the central pulmonary arterial trunks and peripheral "pruning" are distinctive, appearances vary somewhat from patient to patient in accord with the level and pace of the pulmonary hypertension and the age of the patient (see also Chap. 13). Radiographic evidence of right ventricular enlargement usually becomes overt only late in the course of the pulmonary hypertension. The ECG almost always shows right axis deviation, right ventricular enlargement, and, usually, right atrial enlargement, (Chap. 12).

THE ECHOCARDIOGRAM

Two-dimensional echocardiography confirms the enlargement and hypertrophy of right atrium and ventricle, tricuspid regurgitation, and pulmonic valvular regurgitation. At the same time, left ventricular structure and function are normal. The determination of right ventricular ejection fraction using radionuclide techniques can be helpful in evaluating the extent to which the excessive right ventricular afterload has compromised the right ventricle. This applies not only to PPH but also to other disorders that lead to severe pulmonary hypertension (e.g., COPD and congenital heart disease) (see also Chap. 14).

LUNG SCANS

The lung scan fails to disclose major perfusion defects. Angiography is done in selected cases to exclude pulmonary emboli. Lung scans can be particularly helpful, not only in excluding emboli in distal vessels but also in calling attention to the possibility of large, long-standing organized clots in the major pulmonary arteries; these clots may be amenable to surgical resection.

RIGHT-SIDED HEART CATHETERIZATION

The results of cardiac catheterization are consistent with diffuse obliterative disease of the pulmonary arterial tree (see "Pathophysiology," above). As noted, cardiac catheterization is valuable in quantifying the hemodynamic abnormalities, in excluding cardiac causes of pulmonary arterial hypertension, and in assessing the hemodynamic responses of the heart and of pulmonary circulation to vasodilator agents.[4]

Diagnosis

The diagnosis of PPH rests on two pillars: (1) the detection of pulmonary hypertension, and (2) the exclusion of known causes of high pulmonary arterial pressure. The history is of utmost importance. Before categorizing pulmonary hypertension as "primary" or "unexplained," due regard must be paid to the exclusion of known etiologies (Table 59-3), particularly thromboembolic disease and connective tissue disorders. Account should also be taken of the likelihood of familial disease. Pulmonary function tests are useful in excluding diffuse pulmonary disorders, particularly interstitial fibrosis and granuloma. Serologic testing can point the way to covert connective tissue disorders. Abnormal liver function tests can signal the coexistence of portal and pulmonary hypertension. The value of cardiac catheterization in eliminating acquired or congenital heart disease has been indicated above. Unfortunately, by the time pulmonary hypertension complicating heart disease is recognized, the anatomic lesions are often too far advanced for the obliterative pulmonary vascular disease to be reversible. One notable exception is the dramatic improvement that often follows surgical removal of organized clots from the walls of major pulmonary arteries.

Treatment

For the past few decades, treatment of PPH has repeatedly turned to the use of vasodilators in the hope that an increase in pulmonary vascular tone contributed importantly to the high pulmonary arterial pressures. Although the bulk of the pulmonary vascular obstruction was clearly anatomic, vasodilators offered the prospect not only of decreasing pulmonary arterial pressures somewhat, and therefore the hemodynamic burden on the right ventricle, but also prompting reversibility of the anatomic lesions, such as muscular hypertrophy, that resulted simply from the high pulmonary arterial pressures. Unfortunately, the use of vasodilators, which could affect the systemic as well as the pulmonary circulation and which were often accompanied by undesirable side effects, led to progressive disenchantment with one agent after another.

The situation has changed considerably during the past decade.[41–49] The introduction of acute vasodilator testing for responsiveness helped to confirm the idea that, in about one-third of patients, heightened pulmonary vasomotor tone helped to sustain the pulmonary hypertension. An optimal "responder" to acute testing manifested an increase in cardiac output along with a decrease in pulmonary arterial pressure and in pulmonary vascular resistance without affecting systemic arterial pressure unduly. Improvement in exercise tolerance accompanied the increase in cardiac output. Another landmark was the introduction of calcium channel blocking agents that could be taken orally, and, in general, those who were highly responsive during acute testing could be maintained at lower pulmonary arterial pressures by these agents. A third insight was that even patients who failed to satisfy the criteria for a good hemodynamic response to acute testing might respond to continuous infusion of a pulmonary vasodilator. Indeed, a small number of such patients have been treated in this way for years, and even more have used continuous infusion as a transition to transplantation of the lung or lungs or of heart and lungs. During this evolution, heart-lung and then lung transplantation became increasingly feasible and available, although the donor supply is still a limiting factor.

As a result of these advances, a patient with PPH has several therapeutic options, ranging from oral calcium channel blocking agents to continuous infusion of prostacyclin to lung transplantation. None of these modalities is free of complications. The oral calcium channel blocking agents generally have to be administered in large doses that are often accompanied by undesirable side effects. The continuous infusion of a vasodilator, such as prostacyclin, runs the risks not only of a permanently placed intravenous catheter but also of a refillable pump and tachyphylaxis. Transplantation offers the substitution of immunosuppression and its attendant risk of infection as a better option than chronic cor pulmonale and right ventricular failure. Despite the limitations of each of these therapeutic modalities, together they provide a graduated therapeutic approach that has provided, at each stage, a better quality of life for many individuals with PPH. Moreover, they have prompted the search for agents that can be used instead of prostacyclin, which, until now, has required intravenous infusion; it is currently being tried as an aerosol. Among these new agents is nitric oxide, which can be administered by inhalation.

VASODILATOR AGENTS

Various agents have been tried over the years as pulmonary vasodilators. These include alpha-adrenergic antagonists, beta-adrenergic agonists, diazoxide, hydralazine, nitrates, and angiotensin-converting enzyme inhibitors. In general, these have not withstood the test of time. Experience has taught that untoward reactions can occur with any pulmonary vasodilator, even when low doses are used. Three categories of agents continue to hold promise, however: calcium channel blocking agents, arachidonic acid metabolites, and nitric oxide.

DRUGS THAT BLOCK CALCIUM TRANSPORT

The designation *calcium channel blocker* refers to a heterogeneous group of agents of different structural, pharmacologic, and electrophysiologic properties (see also Chap. 54). The agents in this category currently receiving the most clinical attention as potential pulmonary vasodilators are nifedipine and diltiazem. Of the two, nifedipine is the more popular. Verapamil, once used extensively, has fallen into disuse, largely because of its undesirable negative inotropic effect.

Nifedipine

Nifedipine* is a synthetic agent that is unrelated to other vasoactive or cardiotonic drugs. It is a potent systemic vasodilator that is used for the treatment of coronary vasospasm. Although it has significant direct negative inotropic effects,

---

* This use is not listed in the manufacturer's directive.

these are usually not prominent clinically because of the reflex sympathetic stimulation of the heart; it does not possess antiarrhythmic properties. In an experimental model of pulmonary hypertension in the dog, it was thought to be more effective than either verapamil or diltiazem. It is now the agent of choice for empiric therapy. Both short- and long-acting preparations are available. The dosage is generally titrated to the maximal tolerable level based on avoiding untoward systemic effects, i.e., hypotension, headache, dizziness, and flushing. Considerable caution is necessary in administering the higher dosages, however, because side effects can occur precipitously and be life threatening. In one study, 64 patients with PPH were treated with high doses of calcium channel blockers. Seventeen patients responded to treatment with nifedipine (13 patients) or diltiazem (4 patients) and were alive after 5 years.[44,47]

In some clinics, the trial of nifedipine or diltiazem orally is preceded by use of test doses of prostacyclin (PGI_2; epoprostenol), administered intravenously in increasing doses (starting dose of 1 to 2 ng/kg per minute followed by successive increments every 15 min of 2 ng/kg per minute until a maximal dose of 12 ng/kg per minute is reached). Prostacyclin is generally regarded as the gold standard for acute testing. As an alternative, some clinics substitute adenosine (1 μg/kg per minute administered intravenously, followed by similar increments every 10 min to a maximum of 15 μg/kg per minute). A third alternative is prostaglandin E_1 (PGE_1) which is given in increasing doses intravenously, i.e., 5 to 30 μ/kg per minute. Less commonly used is acetylcholine (1 mg/min intravenously increasing every 15 min to a maximum of 10 to 15 mg/min).

ARACHIDONIC ACID METABOLITES

Epoprostenol (PGI_2), a metabolite of arachidonic acid, continues to be a major focus of experimental attention as a pulmonary vasodilator. The pulmonary endothelium elaborates prostacyclin into the bloodstream, where it has a short biological half-life, i.e., 2 to 3 min. In principle, it is attractive for the treatment of PPH on several accounts: (1) it is a pulmonary vasodilator, (2) it inhibits platelet aggregation, and (3) it inhibits proliferation of vascular smooth muscle. Unfortunately, it suffers the disadvantage of requiring continuous intravenous infusion, which is currently being done using portable pumps.[45,46] Analogues that can be given orally or by other noninvasive routes are being sought. Success in long-term management has recently been reported using aerosolized epoprostenol.[48] Currently, its most effective use, aside from testing for pulmonary vascular responsivity, is either for long-term management in patients who do not respond to calcium channel blockers or as a bridge to transplantation.[43,45,46]

NITRIC OXIDE

Nitric oxide is synthesized in endothelial cells from one of the guanidine nitrogens of L-arginine by the enzyme nitric oxide synthase. It has proved to be the endothelial-derived relaxing factor that contributes to the low initial tone of the pulmonary circulation. It has the advantage of other vasodilators (with the possible exception of acetylcholine) of selectively relaxing pulmonary vessels without affecting systemic arterial pressure. It is currently being tested in a wide variety of pulmonary hypertensive states including PPH.[49,50,51]

ANTICOAGULANT THERAPY

Since 1984, when Fuster et al., in a nonrandomized clinical trial, showed that long-term survival was improved in patients with PPH by anticoagulant therapy (warfarin in low doses), the use of anticoagulants has been incorporated into the therapeutic regimen in patients with PPH.[52] This practice is supported by the high incidence of antemortem clots found at autopsy in the small pulmonary arteries and arterioles of patients with PPH. Moreover, in a recent trial that separated "responders" from "nonresponders" to the acute intravenous injection of prostacyclin, survival was significantly better in those given warfarin than in those who were not anticoagulated.[47] The advent of right ventricular failure increases the propensity for clotting in the pulmonary circulation. The usual regimens of anticoagulation are used (see Chap. 52).

LUNG TRANSPLANTATION

Only one-third of patients with PPH are responsive to short-term pulmonary vasodilator therapy. Some who have failed short-term therapy have done well on long-term continuous therapy using prostacyclin administered intravenously. When pulmonary hypertensive disease has progressed, or threatens to progress, to the stage of right ventricular failure, the physician and patient are left with few therapeutic options other than lung transplantation.[53–56] Lung transplantation is currently being done at specialized centers and is almost invariably handicapped by shortage of donor lungs, which can lead to long delays. Single- or double-lung transplantation has largely replaced heart-lung transplantation. Often, hemodynamic improvement is dramatic, but transplantation for PPH not only poses a considerable surgical risk but also the prospect of opportunistic infections that accompanies life-long immunosuppression. Rejection phenomena, notably bronchiolitis obliterans, occur in up to 50 percent of patients within 2 to 3 years of transplantation.[57]

Two aspects of transplantation merit emphasis: (1) intensive rehabilitation, before and after the surgery, are essential elements in influencing postoperative morbidity and mortality; and (2) serious postoperative complications are common: rejection, infections, and disturbed healing of the airways. Chronic rejection, resulting in bronchiolitis obliterans, is particularly dreaded.[56,57]

Prognosis

The diagnosis of PPH carries with it a poor prognosis for medical management unless pulmonary vasodilators succeed in decreasing pulmonary vascular resistance. Although death usually occurs within a few years after the onset of symptoms, instances of long-term survival do occur. As noted above, exceptions to the rule of a short and fatal course were highlighted by the Aminorex epidemic in patients in whom the drug was stopped. Experience with the toxic oil syndrome in Spain is in keeping with the Aminorex experience. At present, there is no specific medical treatment for PPH. Pulmonary vasodilators have, in about one-third of patients, improved exercise tolerance and the quality of life. The cause of death in patients managed medically is generally right ventricular failure. In some patients, sudden death terminates the illness.

Lung transplantation, single or double, has led to improvement in the quality of life of many patients with PPH. But lung transplantation brings with it the problems associated with immunosuppression and infection; more than 50 percent of transplanted patients experience bronchiolitis obliterans by the third year after surgery. This is an ominous disease, difficult to manage because of its limited response to increasing immunosuppressive therapy.

PULMONARY VENO-OCCLUSIVE DISEASE

This is the least common of all types of unexplained pulmonary hypertension. Not infrequently, the patient is thought to have primary arterial pulmonary hypertension until manifestations inconsistent with pulmonary precapillary disease, such as pulmonary congestion and edema, redirect attention to the pulmonary small veins and venules. Presumably, the disorder begins as an inflammatory-thrombotic process in the small pulmonary veins and venules and ends in fibrous obliteration of the venous and venular lumens. Presumably as a secondary phenomenon, the distal pulmonary arterial tree also develops obstructive lesions that are generally proliferative ("reactive") rather than inflammatory in nature; the intervening capillary bed is remarkably normal. The pulmonary veno-occlusive lesions have been attributed to an inflammatory response to vascular injury, followed by thrombosis and scarring. Among the postulated etiologies (based on exceedingly sparse evidence) are viral illness, chemotherapy, toxins, autoimmune disease, and mediastinal fibrosis.[58–60]

When the pulmonary hypertension is suspected of originating distal to the pulmonary capillary bed, mitral valve disease, myocardial dysfunction, or even left atrial myxoma has a greater likelihood of being the cause than does primary pulmonary veno-occlusive disease. Paracardiac neoplastic neoplasms can produce the same syndrome.[59] More esoteric etiologies for pulmonary venous hypertension to be excluded in arriving at the diagnosis are congenital atresia of pulmonary veins, fibrosing mediastinitis, and coexistent phlebitis of systemic and pulmonary veins.

Clinical Picture

Predominantly children and young adults are affected, but the age has ranged from infancy to 48 years. There seems to be no sex difference. Although hints exist of possibly related familial cardiac disorders, the number of patients is too few to do more than raise suspicion of a familial or common environmental cause.

Clinical suspicion of this disorder generally arises when a patient with congested and edematous lungs proves to have a normal mitral valve and left ventricle. This stereotype is not always encountered, however, and some patients have carried the diagnosis of primary pulmonary arterial hypertension until autopsy disclosed the characteristic pulmonary venous lesions.

The cardinal signs are dyspnea and fatigue on exertion in conjunction with evidence of pulmonary hypertension; the pulmonary venous rather than pulmonary arterial etiology is suggested by radiologic evidence of postcapillary pulmonary hypertension without evidence of involvement of the left side of the heart (Fig. 59-6A). Pleural effusions are common. Cyanosis, syncope, hemoptysis, and finger clubbing have been inconsistent findings. Rarely, systemic embolization may occur.

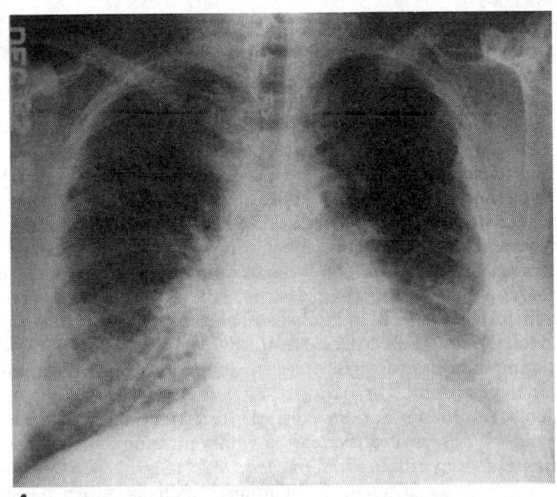

A

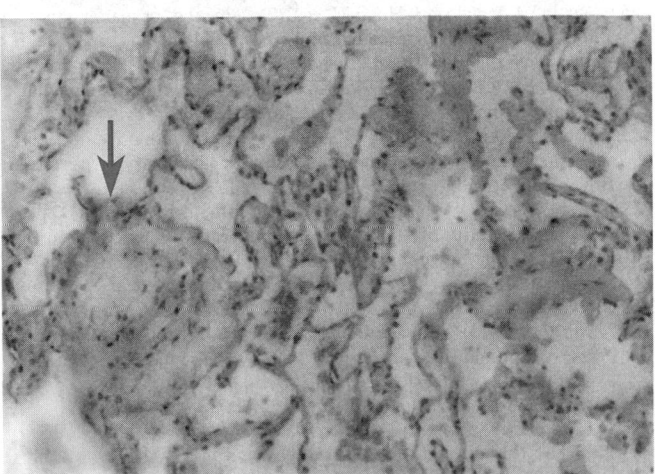

B

FIGURE 59-6

Pulmonary veno-occlusive disease proven by open lung biopsy. *A.* Chest radiography. Pulmonary interstitial edema is marked at both bases. *B.* Lung biopsy. In addition to obliterative pulmonary venular disease, the pulmonary arterioles (*arrow*) showed intimal proliferation and medical hypertrophy. (Courtesy of Dr. G.G. Pietra.)

Hemodynamics

Cardiac catheterization discloses a high pulmonary arterial pressure with a normal pulmonary wedge (and left ventricular end-diastolic) pressure. The low wedge pressure has been attributed to discontinuities and channels of high resistance between the pulmonary capillaries and the pulmonary and bronchial venous channels, so that wedging interrupts all sources of flow distal to the area blocked by the catheter.

Pathology

Few lung biopsies have been done during life. At autopsy, both lungs are involved. The lungs are the seat of congestion, edema, and focal fibrosis, which may become extensive. The venous lesions may be more marked in one region than in another. Although the small pulmonary arteries as well as the small pulmonary veins are affected, the lesions are different Fig. 59-6B). Most striking are the morphologic changes in the pulmonary veins and venules, which are narrowed or occluded by intimal proliferation and fibrosis; up to 95 percent of the veins and venules may be affected in this way, but complete occlusion is uncommon. Bronchial veins and bronchopulmonary anastomoses share in the occlusive process. Hypertrophy in the walls of the pulmonary arteries may be quite striking. In contrast to the pulmonary arterial and venous systems, the pulmonary capillary bed is generally unaffected. Thrombi in the pulmonary arteries are common.[58]

Treatment

Medical management has been disappointing, since the lesions are generally irreversible. An occasional patient has been reported to do well on pulmonary vasodilators. The usual duration after recognition ranges from a few weeks in infants to several years in adults, with 7 years being the maximum. These patients are also candidates for single-lung or heart-lung transplantation.

REFERENCES

1. Fishman AP. Pulmonary circulation. In: Fishman AP, Fisher A, eds. *The Handbook of Physiology;* Section 3; *The Respiratory System;* vol. I: *Circulation and Nonrespiratory Functions.* Bethesda; American Physiological Society; 1985:93–165.
2. Fishman AP. The enigma of hypoxic pulmonary vasoconstriction. In: Fishman AP, ed. *The Pulmonary Circulation: Normal and Abnormal.* Philadelphia: University of Pennsylvania Press; 1990:109–130.
3. Eltorky MA, Headley AS, Winer-Muram H, Garrett HE Jr, Griffin JP. Pulmonary capillary hemangiomatosis: A clinicopathologic review. *Ann Thorac Surg* 1994; 57:772–776.
4. Fishman AP, ed. *The Pulmonary Circulation: Normal and Abnormal.* Philadelphia: University of Pennsylvania Press; 1990:1–551.
5. Harris P, Heath D. The structure of the normal pulmonary blood vessels after infancy. In: Harris P, Heath D, eds. *The Human Circulation, Its Form and Function in Health and Disease.* Edinburgh; Churchill Livingstone; 1986:30–47.
6. Kinsella JP, Abman SH. Recent developments in the pathophysiology and treatment of persistent pulmonary hypertension of the newborn. *J Pediatr* 1995; 126:853–864.
7. Reid LM. Vascular remodeling. In: Fishman AP, ed. *The Pulmonary Circulation: Normal and Abnormal.* Philadelphia: University of Pennsylvania Press; 1990:259–282.

8. Ryan US. Endothelial processing of biologically active materials. In: Fishman AP, ed. *The Pulmonary Circulation: Normal and Abnormal.* Philadelphia: University of Pennsylvania Press; 1990:69–84.

9. Voelkel NF, Tuder RM, Weir EK. Pathophysiology of primary pulmonary hypertension: In Rubin LJ, Rich S, eds. *Primary Pulmonary Hypertension.* New York: Marcel Dekker; 1997:83–133.

10. Nicod P, Peterson K, Levine M, Dittrich H, Buchbinder M, Chappuis F, et al. Pulmonary angiography in severe chronic pulmonary hypertension. *Ann Intern Med* 1987; 107:565–568.

11. Beard JT II, Bryd BF III. Saline contrast enhancement of trivial Doppler tricuspid regurgitation signals for estimating pulmonary arterial pressure. *Am J Cardiol* 1988; 62:486–488.

12. Palevsky HI, Schloo BL, Pietra GG, Weber KT, Janicki JS, Rubin E, et al. Primary pulmonary hypertension. Vascular structure, morphometry, and responsiveness to vasodilator agents. *Circulation* 1989; 80:1207–1221.

13. Edwards WD. The pathology of secondary pulmonary hypertension. In: Fishman AP, ed. *The Pulmonary Circulation: Normal and Abnormal.* Philadelphia: University of Pennsylvania Press; 1990:329–342.

14. Kerstein D, Levy PS, Hsu DT, Hordof AJ, Gersony WM, Barst RJ. Blade balloon atrial septostomy in patients with severe primary pulmonary hypertension. *Circulation* 1995; 91:2028–2035.

15. Fedullo PF, Auger WR, Channick RN, Moser KM, Jamieson SW. Chronic thromboembolic pulmonary hypertension. *Clin Chest Med* 1995; 16:353–374.

16. Ryan KL, Fedullo PF, Davis GB, Vasquez TE, Moser KM. Perfusion scans underestimate the severity of angiographic and hemodynamic compromise in chronic thromboembolic pulmonary hypertension. *Chest* 1988; 93:1180–1185.

17. Ricou F, Nicod PH, Moser KM, Peterson KL. Catheter-based intravascular ultrasound imaging of chronic thromboembolic pulmonary disease. *Am J Cardiol* 1991; 67:749–752.

18. Weitzenblum E, Oswald M, Mirhom R, Kessler R, Apprill M. Evolution of pulmonary haemodynamics in COLD patients under long-term oxygen therapy. *Eur Respir J* 1989; 2(suppl 7):669S–673S.

19. Fishman AP. A century of primary pulmonary hypertension. In: Rubin LJ, Rich S, eds. *Primary Pulmonary Hypertension.* New York: Marcel Dekker; 1997:1–18.

20. Matthay RA, Shub C. Imaging techniques for assessing pulmonary artery hypertension and right ventricular performance with special reference to COPD. *J Thorac Imag* 1990; 5:47–67.

21. Tramarin R, Torbicki A, Marchandise B, Laaban JP, Morpurgo M. Doppler echocardiographic evaluation of pulmonary artery pressure in chronic obstructive pulmonary disease. A European multicentre study. *Eur Heart J* 1991; 12:103–111.

22. Maeda S, Katsura H, Chida K, Imai T, Kuboki K, Watanabe C, et al. Lack of correlation between P pulmonale and right atrial overload in chronic obstructive airways disease. *Br Heart J* 1991; 65:132–136.

23. Weitzenblum E, Sautegeau A, Ehrhart M, Mammoser M, Pelletier A. Long-term oxygen therapy can reverse the progression of pulmonary hypertension in patients with chronic obstructive pulmonary disease. *Am Rev Respir Dis* 1985; 131:493–498.

24. Brown G. Pharmacologic treatment of primary and secondary pulmonary hypertension. *Pharmacotherapy* 1991; 11:137–156.

25. Yousem SA. The pulmonary pathologic manifestations of the CREST syndrome. *Hum Pathol* 1990; 21:467–474.

26. Shuck JW, Oetgen WJ, Tesar JT. Pulmonary vascular response during Raynaud's phenomenon in progressive systemic sclerosis. *Am J Med* 1985; 78:221–227.

27. Fishman AP. Pulmonary hypertension and cor pulmonale. In: Fishman AP, ed. *Pulmonary Diseases and Disorders,* 2d ed. New York: McGraw-Hill; 1988:999–1048.

28. Weitzenblum E, Apprill M, Krieger J, Ehrhart M, Kurtz D. Sleep disordered breathing and pulmonary hypertension. *Eur Respir J Suppl* 1990; 11:523S–526S.

29. Groves BM, Brundage BH, Elliott CG, Koerner SK, Fisher JD, Peter RH, et al. Pulmonary hypertension associated with hepatic cirrhosis. In: Fishman AP, ed. *The Pulmonary Circulation: Normal and Abnormal.* Philadelphia: University of Pennsylvania Press; 1990:359–369.

30. Rich S. NIH Registry on Primary Pulmonary Hypertension: Baseline characteristics of the patients enrolled. In: Fishman AP, ed. *The Pulmonary Circulation: Normal and Abnormal.* Philadelphia: University of Pennsylvania Press; 1990:451–458.

31. D'Alonzo GE, Barst RJ, Ayres SM, Bergofsky EH, Brundage BH, Detre KM, et al. Survival in patients with primary pulmonary hypertension. *Ann Intern Med* 1991; 115:343–349.

32. Albelda SM. Role of growth factors in pulmonary hypertension. In: Fishman AP, ed. *The Pulmonary Circulation: Normal and Abnormal.* Philadelphia: University of Pennsylvania Press; 1990:201–216.

33. Benitz WE. Inhibition of proliferation of vascular smooth muscle cells by heparin. In: Fishman AP, ed. *The Pulmonary Circulation: Normal and Abnormal.* Philadelphia: University of Pennsylvania Press; 1990:187–200.

34. Hajjar KA, Nachman RL. Endothelial cell modulation of coagulation and fibrinolysis. In: Fishman AP, ed. *The Pulmonary Circulation: Normal and Abnormal.* Philadelphia: University of Pennsylvania Press; 1990:231–244.

35. Voelkel NF, Weir EK. Etiologic mechanisms in primary pulmonary hypertension. In: Weir EK, Reeves JT, eds. *Pulmonary Vascular Physiology and Pathophysiology.* New York; Marcel Dekker; 1989:513–539.

36. Weiss JR, Pietra GG, Scharf SM. Primary pulmonary hypertension and the human immunodeficiency virus. Report of two cases and a review of the literature. *Arch Intern Med* 1995.

37. Abenhaim L, Moride Y, Brenot F, et al. Appetite-suppressant drugs and the risk of primary pulmonary hypertension. *N Engl J Med* 1996; 335:609–616.

38. Lopez-Sendon J, Sanchez MAG, De Juan MJM, Coma-Canella I. Pulmonary hypertension in the toxic oil syndrome. In: Fishman AP, ed. *The Pulmonary Circulation: Normal and Abnormal.* Philadelphia: University of Pennsylvania Press; 1990:385–396.

39. Elliott G, Alexander G, Leppert M, Yeates S, Kerber R. Coancestry in apparently sporadic primary pulmonary hypertension. *Chest* 1996; 108:973–977.

40. Pietra GG. The pathology of primary pulmonary hypertension. In: Rubin LJ, Rich S, eds. *Primary Pulmonary Hypertension,* New York: Marcel Dekker; 1996:19–62.

41. Sitbon O, Brenot F, Denjean A, Bergeron A, Parent F, et al. Inhaled nitric oxide as a screening vasodilator agent in primary pulmonary hypertension. A dose-response study and comparison with prostacyclin. *Am J Respir Crit Care Med* 1995; 151:384–389.

42. Fishman AP, Pietra GG. Primary pulmonary hypertension. *Annu Rev Med* 1980; 31:421–431.

43. Barst RJ, Rubin LJ, McGoon MD, Caldwell EJ, et al. Survival in primary pulmonary hypertension with long-term continuous intravenous prostacyclin. *Ann Intern Med* 1994; 121:409–415.

44. Rich S. Medical treatment of primary pulmonary hypertension: A bridge of transplantation? *Am J Cardiol* 1995; 75:63A–66A.

45. Rubin LJ, Mendoza J, Hood M, et al. Treatment of primary pulmonary hypertension with continuous intravenous prostacyclin (epoprostenol). *Ann Intern Med* 1991; 112:485–591.

46. Cremona G, Higenbottam T. Role of prostacyclin in the treatment of primary pulmonary hypertension. *Am J Cardiol* 1995; 75:67A–71A.

47. Rich S, Kaufmann E, Levy PS. The effect of high doses of calcium-channel blockers on survival in primary pulmonary hypertension. *N Engl J Med* 1992; 327:76–81.

48. Olschewski H, Walmrath D, Schermuly R, Ghofrani A, Grimminger F, Seeger W. Aerosolized prostacyclin and iloprost in severe pulmonary hypertension. *Ann Intern Med* 1996; 124:820–824.

49. Lunn RJ. Inhaled nitric oxide therapy. *Mayo Clin Proc* 1995; 70:247–255.

50. Pepke-Zaba J, Higenbottam T, Dinh-Xuan AT, Stone D, Wallwork J. Inhaled nitric oxide as a cause of selective pulmonary vasodilation in pulmonary hypertension. *Lancet* 1991; 338;1173–1174.

51. Weir EK, Archer SL, Reeves JT. *Nitric Oxide and Radicals in the Pulmonary Vasculature.* Armonk, NY: Futura Publishing; 1996.

52. Fuster V, Steele PM, Edwards WD, Gersh BJ, McGoon MD, Frye RL. Primary pulmonary hypertension: Natural history and the importance of thrombosis. *Circulation* 1984; 70:580–585.

53. Medical management. In: Rubin LJ, Rich S, eds. *Primary Pulmonary Hypertension.* New York: Marcel Dekker; 1996:271–286.

54. Badesch DB, Zamora MR, Jones S, Campbell DW, Fullerton DA. Independent ventilation and ECMO for severe unilateral pulmonary edema after SLT for primary pulmonary hypertension. *Chest* 1995; 107:1766–1770.

55. Katayama Y, Cremona G, Wallwork J, Higenbottam T. Transplantation for primary pulmonary hypertension. In: Rubin LJ, Rich S, eds. *Primary Pulmonary Hypertension,* New York: Marcel Dekker; 1996:287–304.

56. Epler GR. Bronchiolitis obliterans organizing pneumonia. *Semin Respir Infect* 1995; 10:65–77.

57. Ren WD, Nicolosi GL, Lestuzzi C, Canterin FA, et al. Role of transesophageal echocardiography in evaluation of pulmonary venous obstruction by paracardiac neoplastic masses. *Am J Cardiol* 1992; 70:1362–1366.

58. Palevsky HI, Pietra GG, Fishman AP. Pulmonary veno-occlusive disease and its response to vasodilator agents. *Am Rev Respir Dis* 1990; 142:426–429.

59. Davis LL, deBoisblanc BP, Glynn CE, Ramirez C, Summer WR. Effect of prostacyclin on microvascular pressures in a patient with pulmonary veno-occlusive disease. *Chest* 1995; 108:1754–1756.

60. Connolly HD, Crary JL, McGoon MD, Hensrud DD, Edwards BS, Edwards WD, Schaff, HV. Valvular heart disease associated with fenfluramine-phentermine. *New Eng J Med* (in press).

60

PULMONARY EMBOLISM

Joseph S. Alpert / James E. Dalen

Each year there are estimated to be approximately 100,000 deaths in the United States due primarily to pulmonary embolism and another 100,000 deaths in patients with other major diseases, in whom pulmonary embolism is a significant contributory cause. The majority of deaths occur in patients who are not treated because the diagnosis is not established.[1–3] *The mortality of untreated pulmonary embolism is 20 to 30 percent.* If the diagnosis is established and appropriate treatment instituted, mortality is less than 10 percent.[3,4]

In nearly all cases, pulmonary embolism originates as deep venous thrombosis (DVT) in the proximal deep venous system in the lower legs.[5–8] Virchow recognized deep venous thrombosis in 1858.[9] Some of the factors that predispose to DVT are shown in Table 60-1. The optimal strategy for preventing fatal pulmonary embolism is to recognize patients who are at increased risk for DVT and to institute appropriate prophylactic treatment. In order to reduce the incidence of pulmonary embolism, DVT must be prevented or, at the very least, recognized and treated.

DEEP VENOUS THROMBOSIS

Pathophysiology and Natural History

Virchow pointed out that three factors underlie the development of venous thrombosis: stasis, injury to the intima of the vein, and a hypercoagulable state. Experimental and clinical observations have subsequently confirmed the role of Virchow's triad in the genesis of DVT.[10–15] All three factors need not be present simultaneously for DVT to occur, although stasis and intimal injury are the most important factors in the usual clinical course that leads to DVT.[14,16] The antiphospholipid syndrome and anticardiolipin antibodies are occasionally associated with venous thrombosis[17,18] (see also Chap. 85).

Venous thrombosis appears to originate as a platelet nidus in the vicinity of the venous valves in the lower extremities. Disordered flow near these valves probably contributes to the formation of the platelet nidi.[14,15,19–21] Abnormal venous endothelial function appears to play an important role in this initial phase of venous thrombosis.[14] Platelet aggregation and activation initiate the clotting cascade, with subsequent formation of a red fibrin thrombus. The thrombus gradually grows

---

TABLE 60-1

RISK FACTORS FOR DEEP VENOUS THROMBOSIS

VENOUS STASIS, VASCULAR INJURY, OR SECONDARY HYPERCOAGULABLE STATES

Surgery (especially involving lower extremities or pelvis)
Trauma (especially fractured hip in the elderly and acute injury of the head and spinal cord)
Bed rest, immobility, stroke, or paralysis
Congestive heart failure, low cardiac output states
Malignancy
Pregnancy
Oral contraceptive agents, estrogen therapy
Obesity
Varicose veins
Inflammatory bowel disease
Advanced age
Prior thromboembolism
Nephrotic syndrome
Sepsis

PRIMARY HYPERCOAGULABLE STATE

Antithrombin III deficiency
Protein C deficiency
Protein S deficiency
Disorders of plasminogen and plasminogen activation
Dysfibrinogenemia
Paroxysmal nocturnal hemoglobinuria
Myeloproliferative disorders
Polycythemia vera
Heparin-induced thrombocytopenia
Lupus anticoagulant/anticardiolipin antibodies
Factor V, Leiden

in size as platelets, fibrin, and red cells are further incorporated. The intrinsic fibrinolytic system is also activated, attacking the fibrin framework of the thrombus. In some instances, the intrinsic fibrinolytic system is successful in dissolving the thrombus; in other situations, pieces of the thrombus break off and embolize to the pulmonary circulation. Residual venous thrombus becomes organized and incorporated into the venous wall[10,11] (see also Chap. 52).

Patients with clinically evident malignancy are often at increased risk for venous thromboembolism, and an unusual form of venous thrombosis, thrombophlebitis migrans, may be a clue to the presence of occult cancer. Thrombophlebitis migrans involves superficial veins, often at atypical sites such as the arms. It may be migratory and resistant to anticoagulant therapy.

More than 90 percent of pulmonary emboli originate in the deep veins of the lower extremities.[5,6] Occasionally, DVT in pelvic veins or thrombi in the right heart give rise to pulmonary emboli. Thrombi localized to the deep venous system of the calf are of limited risk with respect to their tendency to embolize. Once such thrombi propagate into the popliteal vein and/or the veins of the thigh, however, the risk for pulmonary embolism increases markedly.[21–25] The explanation may lie in the fact that calf thrombi are small and offer limited risk, even if they embolize. Thus, symptomatic pulmonary embolism usually stems from recurrent episodes of embolization that arise from thrombi in the proximal veins of the lower extremities.

Most episodes of calf DVT resolve without specific therapy. An occasional symptomatic individual will require anticoagulation. Above the knee, DVT gradually resolves during anticoagulant therapy. Two-thirds of patients will have complete resolution of DVT following 3 months of therapy. Ninety percent of patients will be normal 1 year after an episode of DVT that is treated with 3 months of anticoagulation. *Individuals with DVT who receive no therapy frequently develop pulmonary embolism and/or chronic venous insufficiency of the lower extremities.*[26,27]

Prevention

There are multiple techniques to prevent DVT, as shown in Table 60-2.[26–48] Graduated compression stockings (GCS) are basic prophylaxis against DVT and are useful in most hospitalized patients with a single risk factor, except for those with severe peripheral arterial disease. Prophylactic regimens for specific patient groups are shown in Table 60-3. In medical patients with a factor for increased risk or surgical patients who are over 40 years of age and are undergoing major operations without contraindications, low-dose unfractionated heparin, 5000 units subcutaneously every 8 to 12 h or low-molecular-weight heparin, 50 U/kg twice daily, are very effective in preventing DVT. Elastic stockings and intermittent-pressure calf compression are also effective in preventing DVT in these patients.[27–29,33–35] In patients at higher risk, e.g., in those undergoing hip replacement, in patients with

TABLE 60-2

TECHNIQUES FOR THE PREVENTION OF DEEP VENOUS THROMBOSIS

Graded compression stockings
Intermittent pneumatic compression
Anticoagulation
Intravenous heparin[a]
Adjusted-dose subcutaneous heparin[a]
Low-dose subcutaneous heparin[b]
Low-molecular-weight heparin
Low-dose oral warfarin[c]
Minidose oral warfarin (1 mg/day)
Intravenous dextran
Dihydroergotamine[d]
Hirudin[d]

[a] Activated partial thromboplastin time 1.5–2.5 times control.
[b] 5000 units subcutaneously every 8–12 h.
[c] Prothrombin time of 2.0 to 3.0 INR.
[d] Currently not available in the United States.

hip fracture, and in men undergoing urologic procedures, low-dose subcutaneous heparin does not provide adequate protection. In these circumstances adjusted-dose unfractionated heparin [activated partial thromboplastin time (APTT) 31 to 36 s 6 h after injection], fixed-dose twice daily low-molecular-weight heparin, or low-dose warfarin [International Normalized Ratio (INR) 2.0 to 3.0], combined with elastic stockings or intermittent-pressure calf compression are more appropriate prophylaxis.[27–29,38,48] In patients at increased risk of bleeding, such as those undergoing neurosurgical procedures, intermittent pneumatic compression (IPC) boots have been shown to be effective.[26,27,48] In high-risk neurosurgical patients, low-dose unfractionated heparin given subcutaneously in combination with intermittent pneumatic calf compression may be the most efficacious preventive regimen.[27] In patients undergoing elective surgery, all prophylactic therapies should begin prior to the induction of anesthesia as DVT often begins while patients are anesthetized in the operating room. Aspirin and sulfinpyrazone have not been shown to be effective in preventing DVT. Hirudin appears very promising but is not currently available in the United States.[37]

Diagnosis

If the prophylactic therapies listed above are instituted, the risk of DVT and its potentially lethal complication, pulmonary embolism, is greatly diminished. If prophylactic treatment is not used or if it fails, the clinician must recognize DVT as soon as possible in order to institute treatment to prevent pulmonary embolism. The classic signs of DVT, unilateral leg swelling and tenderness, occur in the minority of cases; most episodes of DVT are clinically silent. Venography or noninvasive tests of venous thrombosis should usually be performed when DVT is suspected.[48–53]

The most sensitive and specific test for the recognition of DVT is venography, but it is invasive and uncomfortable and

TABLE 60-3

PROPHYLAXIS AGAINST DEEP VENOUS THROMBOSIS PULMONARY EMBOLISM FOR SPECIFIC PATIENT GROUPS

Patient Group	Prophylaxis
Medical or surgical patients under 40 years of age with no clinical risk factors	Early ambulation
Medical patients with one or more risk factors (Table 60-1) or surgical patients over 40 years of age undergoing major operations but with no additional risk factors	GCS; LDH every 8–12 h, fixed-dose LMWH, or IPC
Surgical patients over 40 years of age undergoing major operations and with additional risk factors	GCS; adjusted-dose subcutaneous unfractionated heparin or fixed-dose LMWH (IPC is an alternative in patients prone to hematomas or infection)
Very high risk general surgery patients with multiple risk factors	GCS; IPC and adjusted-dose subcutaneous unfractionated heparin or fixed-dose LMWH; in selected patients, perioperative warfarin (INR 2.0–3.0)
Total hip replacement	GCS; adjusted doses of warfarin (INR 2.0–3.0) or unfractionated heparin (APTT 1.5–2.5 times control 6 h after injection); when available, LMWH (without laboratory control)
Hip fractures	GCS; warfarin (INR 2.0–3.0) or LMWH
Knee surgery, neurosurgery	GCS; IPC; LMWH
Acute spinal cord injury with paralysis	GCS; adjusted-dose unfractionated heparin (APTT 31–36 s 6 h after injection); LMWH; low-dose warfarin (INR 2.0–3.0)
Multiple trauma	GCS; IPC; warfarin (INR 2.0–3.0); LMWH
Myocardial infarction	GCS; LDH (IVH if anterior infarct or increased risk factors); IPC if heparin is contraindicated
Ischemic stroke with lower extremity paralysis	GCS; LDH (alternative: LMWH, IPC, warfarin)
Long-term indwelling central vein catheter	GCS; warfarin, 1 mg/day
Hip or knee surgery in high-risk patients with history of serious, previous pulmonary embolism	GCS; warfarin; consider prophylactic inferior vena cava filter

Note: GCS, graded compression stockings; LDH, low-dose subcutaneous heparin; LMWH, low-molecular-weight heparin; IPC, intermittent pneumatic compression; INR, International Normalized Ratio; APTT, activated partial thromboplastin time; IVH, intravenous heparin.
Source: Modified from Dalen and Hirsh.[27]

is therefore seldom performed more than once on a given patient[48–50] (see also Chap. 100).

Impedance plethysmography (IPG) (see Chap. 100) is extremely useful in evaluating patients with suspected DVT and can be performed in 15 to 20 min.[51–53] The correlation between unilaterally positive IPG and venography exceeds 90 percent. A bilaterally normal IPG nearly excludes proximal (above the knee) DVT. The test is less sensitive to DVT confined to the distal leg (below the knee). If the IPG is positive in both legs, venography should be performed (if available) because DVT may or may not be present.[53] The IPG is extremely useful in detecting DVT at the bedside.[51–53]

Scanning the legs after the injection of fibrinogen labeled with ^{125}I is a very sensitive test for the diagnosis of DVT.[50] The disadvantage of this test is that the ^{125}I must be injected prior to the development of DVT. This test can be used preoperatively in patients who are at risk of intra- or postoperative DVT, (see also Chap. 100).

The Doppler technique (Chap. 100) is another noninvasive test for the diagnosis of DVT, but its accuracy is highly dependent on the expertise of the operator. The sensitivity and specificity of this technique in detecting DVT vary widely in different medical centers. The same is true for other tests

that have been suggested for the diagnosis of DVT, including the radionuclide venogram, duplex ultrasonography, and the radionuclide-labeled platelet scan.[26,50]

Treatment

If proximal DVT is detected, treatment usually includes intravenous unfractionated heparin for 7 to 10 days, followed by oral warfarin therapy begun on day 2 to 3.[54,55] Low-molecular-weight heparin can be substituted for unfractionated heparin. Dosing requirements are individualized for the different products.[27,56] Unfractionated heparin is given as an intravenous bolus of 5000 units, followed by an infusion of 1000 units per hour; the dosage is adjusted to produce an APTT between 1.5 and 2.5 times control, which generally corresponds to a plasma heparin level of 0.2 to 0.4 U/mL.[27,57] Warfarin anticoagulation should overlap heparin for 4 to 5 days. Without treatment, pulmonary embolism occurs in 50 percent of patients with proximal DVT. The probability of pulmonary embolism in patients with DVT limited to the distal lower extremity is less than 10 percent, and in this circumstance in an asymptomatic patient, many physicians would not institute heparin treatment. If DVT is limited to the distal lower extremity, it is not treated with heparin; however, repeat IPG is usually indicated to make certain that there has not been extension to the proximal venous circulation. Patients with symptomatic distal lower extremity DVT should be treated with one of the anticoagulation regimens outlined above.[27]

Some authorities advocate thrombolytic treatment with urokinase, streptokinase, or tissue plasminogen activator (TPA) in patients with symptomatic proximal DVT in order to prevent postphlebitic syndrome in the lower extremities. The incidence of postphlebitic syndrome in patients treated with heparin is uncertain, however. *At present, it remains controversial whether or not fibrinolytic therapy prevents the postphlebitic syndrome in patients with DVT.*

PULMONARY EMBOLISM

Pathophysiology and Natural History

Pulmonary embolism produces clinically important hemodynamic and respiratory pathophysiologic alterations. The major hemodynamic consequences of pulmonary embolism result from reduction in the cross-sectional area of the pulmonary vascular bed with associated increases in pulmonary vascular resistance and right ventricular (RV) afterload[58–63] (see also Chap. 61). Because the reserve capacity of the pulmonary vascular bed is substantial, a single large embolic thrombus (or repeated smaller thrombi) must impact the pulmonary vascular bed before pulmonary vascular resistance and RV afterload increase. In general, more than 50 percent of the pulmonary vascular tree must be occluded before pulmonary arterial pressure increases significantly.[58,59] Small increases in pulmonary arterial pressure resulting from hypoxic pulmonary vasoconstriction may be observed with more minor degrees of pulmonary embolism.[63] Patients with advanced cardiopulmonary disease, e.g., marked left ventricular (LV) failure, may develop severe hemodynamic abnormalities following modest episodes of pulmonary embolism.[61]

Increased RV afterload leads to RV dilatation and eventually failure, with decreased cardiac output and systemic arterial hypotension.[60,64,65] Right ventricular wall stress increases as does RV myocardial oxygen consumption. The increased pressure in the right ventricle limits coronary flow to the right ventricle, which is normally perfused throughout both systole and diastole. With cardiac output reduced, arterial pressure falls, further limiting coronary perfusion of the right ventricle and producing ischemia and failure. In patients with preexisting RV hypertrophy, RV subendocardial infarction may develop secondary to the marked increase in RV myocardial oxygen demand accompanied by reduced coronary blood flow.[65] Dilatation of the right ventricle leads to a shift of the intraventricular septum into the LV cavity. The result is a decrease in LV capacitance and a modest reduction in LV compliance.[66] Of course, LV stroke volume decreases pari passu with falling RV stroke volume. Individuals without

prior heart or lung disease who have an episode of acute pulmonary embolism that obstructs more than 50 percent of the pulmonary vascular bed rarely elevate pulmonary arterial or RV systolic pressure above 60 mmHg. Higher values are often observed in patients with chronic, recurrent pulmonary embolism or in individuals with preexisting cardiopulmonary disease and acute pulmonary embolism.

The respiratory consequences of acute pulmonary embolism include the development of increased alveolar dead space, constriction of airway smooth muscle in lung zones with proximal embolism, hypoxemia, and hyperventilation.[67–69] Later in the course of the illness, regional loss of surfactant and pulmonary infarction may occur.[68,69]

As soon as an embolus obstructs a pulmonary artery, blood flow ceases to the alveoli in that lung zone secondary to mechanical obstruction and alveolar hypoxia. Ventilation of these alveoli continues, thereby increasing alveolar dead space. Reduction of carbon dioxide tension in these alveoli results in proximal airway smooth muscle constriction, with a resultant decrease in alveolar ventilation. Teleologically, this is an attempt to correct the initial abnormal increase in alveolar dead space. Unfortunately, this compensatory effect is usually short-lived since carbon dioxide soon arrives in hypoperfused alveoli from adjacent perfused alveoli and/or from bronchial arterial collateral blood flow.[67]

Arterial hypoxemia is quite common in patients with acute pulmonary embolism. Ventilation/perfusion mismatches and reduced cardiac output contribute to shunting of deoxygenated blood across the pulmonary vascular bed. In addition, patients with massive embolism and RV failure may develop an intracardiac right-to-left shunt as right atrial dilatation stretches and opens a previously closed foramen ovale. Because right atrial pressure exceeds left atrial pressure in this setting, a right-to-left shunt of deoxygenated blood results. This opening of the foramen ovale can also allow a subsequent paradoxical embolus to enter the systemic circulation (see Chap. 59).

A minority of patients develop minimal or even no hypoxemia following acute pulmonary embolism, as the result of compensatory hyperventilation. Both the respiratory rate and the depth of respiration increase following acute pulmonary embolism. In general, the larger the embolism, the greater the depth of respiration but the slower the respiratory rate. Hyperventilation usually produces arterial hypocarbia and respiratory alkalosis. An occasional patient with massive embolism may develop hypercarbia despite marked hyperventilation.[67] Hypercarbia in this setting reflects the minimal amount of pulmonary blood flow actually reaching the alveoli. Hyperventilation is probably the result of stimulation of stretch receptors in the pulmonary vascular bed, but this explanation remains controversial.[67] During the first 24 h following an episode of acute pulmonary embolism, alveolar surfactant is depleted, with resultant local atelectasis and edema.[68,69]

Pulmonary infarction or hemorrhage results when distal emboli totally occlude a small pulmonary artery.[70] True infarction following acute pulmonary embolism is often prevented since the pulmonary parenchyma has four sources of oxygen: the airways, the pulmonary arteries, bronchial arterial collateral circulation, and back-diffusion from the pulmonary veins. Some or all of these compensatory mechanisms may be compromised in patients with heart failure or intrinsic lung disease. Consequently, true pulmonary infarction is more common under these circumstances.

Patients who survive an initial episode of pulmonary embolism usually do well if the diagnosis is made and appropriate therapy is instituted. The intrinsic fibrinolytic system of the pulmonary vascular bed initiates dissolution of thrombi. With heparin therapy alone, 36 percent of perfusion lung scan defects resolve within 5 days. At 2 weeks, 52 percent of defects have resolved; at 3 weeks, 73 percent; and at 1 year, 76 percent.[71] Arterial hypoxemia and chest roentgenographic abnormalities improve as the thromboemboli resolve.[72] Persistent pulmonary hypertension and chronic cor pulmonale from unresolved embolism are unusual.[73] In patients with chronic pulmonary thromboembolic disease complicated by pulmonary hypertension, a high incidence of circulating lupus anticoagulant has been observed.[74] Moreover, this chronic syndrome of pulmonary embolism has an association with heparin-related thrombocytopenia.[74]

Diagnosis of Acute Pulmonary Embolus

One reason that *the diagnosis of acute pulmonary embolism is frequently missed is that it may present as one of three different clinical syndromes: pulmonary infarction (or hemorrhage), acute cor pulmonale, or acute "unexplained" dyspnea.*[75] The pathophysiology, signs, and symptoms of these three syndromes are quite different. The differential diagnosis and the appropriate diagnostic workup are also different. *In many patients with acute pulmonary embolism, the presenting clinical picture is so nonspecific that the diagnosis is easily overlooked.*

PULMONARY INFARCTION OR HEMORRHAGE

Pulmonary infarction or hemorrhage is the most common presentation of pulmonary embolism. More than 50 percent of all patients in whom pulmonary embolism is diagnosed have signs or symptoms of pulmonary infarction or hemorrhage. The classic symptom is the abrupt onset of pleuritic chest pain, with or without dyspnea. Hemoptysis occurs in a minority of patients. Pleuritic chest pain in patients with pulmonary infarction or hemorrhage may be caused by intraalveolar hemorrhage due to the influx of blood from the bronchial collateral circulation into obstructed portions of the distal pulmonary circulation.[70] In these patients, pulmonary angiography demonstrates submassive embolism with obstruction of one or more distal pulmonary arterial branches. As noted earlier, true pulmonary infarction is much more likely to occur in patients with preexisting heart or lung disease, particularly if these entities are complicated by heart failure or pulmonary hypertension.

Pulmonary hemorrhage due to bronchial arterial collateral flow or true pulmonary infarction usually causes a pulmonary infiltrate on the chest x-ray. Other chest film abnormalities include an elevated diaphragm due to splinting of respiration or a small pleural effusion that is usually unilateral and may or may not be bloody. One or more of these three chest film abnormalities are present in more than two-thirds of patients with pulmonary infarction or hemorrhage.[76]

On physical examination, tachypnea with a respiratory rate greater than 20 per minute is nearly always present. Signs of RV failure are absent. Examination of the lungs usually reveals rales, wheezes, or evidence of a pleural effusion. A pleural friction rub may be present. Evidence of deep venous thrombosis on physical examination is present in a minority of cases.

The principal differential diagnosis in patients with pulmonary infarction or hemorrhage includes viral or bacterial pneumonitis/pleuritis, which is suggested by a history of a viral prodrome or of a shaking chill with fever or purulent sputum.

The most useful routine laboratory tests in patients with suspected pulmonary infarction or hemorrhage include the chest x-ray, white blood cell count and differential, Gram's stain of sputum if available, and arterial blood gas analysis. The white blood cell count and differential and the sputum examination help to diagnose bacterial pneumonia. Analysis of arterial blood gases in patients with pulmonary infarction or hemorrhage will nearly always demonstrate hypocapnia and respiratory alkalosis secondary to tachypnea. Since pulmonary infarction or hemorrhage usually occurs in patients with submassive pulmonary embolism, however, the arterial P_{O_2} may be in the normal range in patients without prior lung disease. *Therefore, a normal arterial blood gas analysis by itself is not sufficient grounds for dismissing the diagnosis of pulmonary embolism.*[77,78]

The most useful screening test for pulmonary embolism is the ventilation/perfusion ($\dot{V}/\dot{Q}$) lung scan[77,79–82] (see Chap. 17). The most specific finding for acute pulmonary embolism is the presence of large segmental perfusion defects that ventilate normally.[79,80] In the Prospective Investigation of Pulmonary Embolism Diagnosis (PIOPED) study, a normal perfusion scan excluded the diagnosis of pulmonary embolism with an accuracy of 98 percent.[81] A highly probable scan with multiple segmental or lobar perfusion defects that have normal ventilation patterns had a specificity of about 88 percent (Table 60-4). On the other hand, of the 931 patients in PIOPED who

TABLE 60-4

RESULTS OF PULMONARY ANGIOGRAPHY
IN 731 PATIENTS WITH $\dot{V}/\dot{Q}$ SCAN

$\dot{V}/\dot{Q}$ Scan Interpretation	Percent with Angiographic Evidence of Pulmonary Embolism
High probability	88
Intermediate probability	33
Low probability	16
Near normal/normal	9

Source: PIOPED Study.[81]

had a $\dot{V}/\dot{Q}$ scan, only 13 percent were interpreted as high probability and 73 percent were either intermediate probability or low probability (Table 60-5). In addition, of the 251 patients who had pulmonary embolism documented by pulmonary angiography, only 40 percent had a high probability $\dot{V}/\dot{Q}$ scan, 58 percent had scans interpreted as intermediate or low probability, and 2 percent had $\dot{V}/\dot{Q}$ scans interpreted as near normal or normal (Table 60-6). Thus, patients suspected of having a pulmonary embolus who have an intermediate probability $\dot{V}/\dot{Q}$ scan should be considered for either selective pulmonary angiography or additional tests to assess the lower extremities for DVT.[77,81] Pulmonary scintigraphy continues to maintain its diagnostic accuracy, even in patients who are critically ill.[77,83]

As noted earlier, IPG (Chap. 100) is useful in patients with suspected acute pulmonary embolism, in that it is positive in the majority of cases.[23,52,77,84] If the diagnosis remains uncertain after evaluation of the clinical findings, IPG, and $\dot{V}/\dot{Q}$ lung scan, then selective pulmonary angiography is usually indicated for a definitive diagnosis[77,82] (see Table 60-7). Doppler sonography or venography (Chap. 100) are also useful diagnostic modalities for this indication (see below).

ACUTE COR PULMONALE

Acute cor pulmonale, the most dramatic presentation of acute pulmonary embolism, occurs when pulmonary embolism obstructs more than 60 to 75 percent of the pulmonary circulation (see Chap. 61).

The normal response to acute pulmonary embolism is to increase cardiac output and RV systolic pressure in order to overcome the increased resistance in the pulmonary circulation. Acutely, the normal right ventricle can increase its systolic pressure to about 50 to 60 mmHg. Sudden increases in systolic pressure above this level cause acute RV dilatation and increased ventricular filling pressures. As the right ventricle dilates and fails, its stroke volume decreases, leading to decreased cardiac output, hypotension, and possible cardiac arrest. Therefore, in addition to marked, acute dyspnea, patients with acute cor pulmonale may present with signs of decreased cardiac output: hypotension, syncope, or cardiac arrest.[64] On physical examination, there are tachypnea and tachycardia and possibly hypotension. P_2 may be increased in intensity. Signs of acute RV failure—distended neck veins, right-sided S_3 gallop, and a parasternal heave are usually present. The lungs may be clear, but signs of DVT may be present.

TABLE 60-5

INTERPRETATIONS OF $\dot{V}/\dot{Q}$ SCANS IN 931 PATIENTS SUSPECTED OF HAVING PULMONARY EMBOLISM

High probability	13 percent
Intermediate probability	39 percent
Low probability	34 percent
Near normal/normal	14 percent

Source: PIOPED Study.[81]

TABLE 60-6

INTERPRETATIONS OF $\dot{V}/\dot{Q}$ SCANS IN 251 PATIENTS WITH PULMONARY EMBOLISM DOCUMENTED BY PULMONARY ANGIOGRAPHY

High probability	40 percent
Intermediate probability	42 percent
Low probability	16 percent
Near normal/normal	2 percent

Source: PIOPED Study.[81]

The most useful diagnostic tests in patients with suspected acute cor pulmonale are the electrocardiogram (ECG), measurement of central venous pressure, and arterial blood gas analysis. The ECG in patients with acute cor pulmonale will often show a new $S_1Q_3T_3$ pattern, incomplete right bundle branch block, and/or signs of RV ischemia.[85,86] The ECG helps to exclude acute myocardial infarction. Measurement of central venous pressure may be critical in diagnosing acute cor pulmonale in patients who present with systemic hypotension or cardiovascular collapse. If systemic arterial hypotension is due to acute cor pulmonale, right atrial and central venous pressure will be elevated.[87] Arterial blood gas analysis in patients with acute cor pulmonale usually, but not always, demonstrates hypoxemia as well as hypocapnia.[81,88,89] The chest x-ray is not helpful in the diagnosis of acute cor pulmonale and is often unremarkable.

Once the diagnosis of acute cor pulmonale is suspected, it should be confirmed by $\dot{V}/\dot{Q}$ lung scan or pulmonary angiography. In unstable patients in whom surgical or thrombolytic therapy may be indicated, it is usually wise to proceed promptly to pulmonary angiography for definitive diagnosis (see Table 60-7).

ACUTE, UNEXPLAINED DYSPNEA

The diagnosis of pulmonary embolism is most difficult in patients with submassive pulmonary embolism who do not sustain pulmonary infarction. The ECG remains normal, and there are no physical signs of RV failure. If pulmonary infarction or hemorrhage does not occur, pleuritic pain is absent and there is no specific abnormality on chest x-ray. In this circumstance, the primary symptom of acute pulmonary embolism is the sudden onset of dyspnea. The only abnormalities on physical examina-

TABLE 60-7

INDICATIONS FOR PULMONARY ANGIOGRAPHY

When examination of clinical findings, $\dot{V}/\dot{Q}$ scan, and impedance plethysmography are inconclusive
When there are relative contraindications to anticoagulation
When thrombolytic therapy may be indicated
When inferior vena cava interruption or surgical therapy may be indicated
Recurrent pulmonary embolism, despite therapy
Young patient with uncertain predisposition to deep venous thrombosis

tion are tachypnea, possibly tachycardia, and anxiety. The lungs are clear; there are no signs of acute RV failure. Signs of DVT may be present or absent. Thus, many of the commonly obtained clinical variables are not abnormal.

The principal differential diagnoses in patients with acute dyspnea due to pulmonary embolism are LV failure, pneumonia, and the hyperventilation syndrome. Left ventricular failure and pneumonia can usually be excluded by further history, physical examination, and chest x-ray. Patients presenting with dyspnea due to acute pulmonary embolism usually, but not always, have significant hypoxemia.[81,88] Measurement of arterial blood gases while the patient breathes room air may allow one to distinguish between potentially lethal pulmonary embolism and benign hyperventilation. On the other hand, some patients with pulmonary embolism have a normal arterial P_{O_2}.[77,81,89]

As with other syndromes of acute pulmonary embolism, IPG examination is very helpful, and the diagnosis should be confirmed by $\dot{V}/\dot{Q}$ lung scan and/or pulmonary angiography.

Summary of Laboratory Tests in the Diagnosis of Pulmonary Embolism

CHEST X-RAY

The chest x-ray is most useful in evaluating patients with pleuritic chest pain possibly stemming from pulmonary infarction or hemorrhage. Most patients with pulmonary infarction or hemorrhage have an infiltrate, an elevated hemidiaphragm due to splinting, or a pleural effusion that is usually small and unilateral and may or may not be bloody.[70] In patients with acute cor pulmonale or acute unexplained dyspnea and without pulmonary infarction or hemorrhage, the chest x-ray is usually normal or it may show subtle, nonspecific findings. The combination of unexplained dyspnea, arterial hypoxemia, and a normal chest x-ray should suggest the diagnosis of pulmonary embolism.[80]

ELECTROCARDIOGRAM

The ECG is most helpful in evaluating patients who have had massive pulmonary embolism complicated by acute cor pulmonale. In these patients, the ECG helps to exclude myocardial infarction and will usually demonstrate the ECG correlates of acute cor pulmonale, i.e., a new $S_1Q_3T_3$ pattern, a new incomplete right bundle branch block, or signs of RV ischemia. These ECG findings are transient and resolve as RV failure resolves. In patients with submassive pulmonary embolism, the ECG is usually not helpful. It may show nonspecific ST changes or sinus tachycardia. An occasional patient develops atrial fibrillation or flutter following an episode of pulmonary embolism.

ARTERIAL BLOOD GASES

The vast majority of patients with acute pulmonary embolism have tachypnea; therefore, arterial blood gas analysis demonstrates hypocapnia and respiratory alkalosis.[76,81,88] The arterial P_{O_2} (breathing room air) is usually, but not always, decreased in patients with dyspnea due to pulmonary embolism.[76,81,88] In patients with pulmonary infarction or hemorrhage who have submassive pulmonary embolism, the arterial P_{O_2} may be normal or near normal, particularly if there is no prior pulmonary disease. The arterial blood gases should be measured while the patient is breathing room air.[89] In patients receiving supplemental oxygen who do not have overt, significant, coexistent pulmonary disease, it is only necessary to discontinue supplemental oxygen for 5 to 10 min in order to assess baseline values.[89] *It is important to emphasize that arterial blood gas changes are nonspecific and should not be used to make the diagnosis of pulmonary embolism.* Similarly, a normal arterial P_{O_2} does not exclude the diagnosis.[77,81]

VENTILATION/PERFUSION LUNG SCANS ($\dot{V}/\dot{Q}$ SCANS)

Perfusion lung scans are extremely sensitive in detecting pulmonary embolism; a normal multiple-view perfusion scan essentially (96 to 98 percent) excludes acute pulmonary embolism.[75,76,79,81,90–92] Unfortunately, perfusion defects are not specific for pulmonary embolism; they may be the result of a wide variety of other pulmonary abnormalities. The specificity of perfusion lung scanning is increased by the use of a ventilation scan (see Chap. 17).

The scan abnormality most consistent with acute pulmonary embolism is the presence of multiple large segmental perfusion defects that ventilate normally.[75,79–81] The probability of pulmonary embolism with this set of findings exceeds 90 percent.

Unfortunately, as noted above, $\dot{V}/\dot{Q}$ scan findings are very often nonspecific.[76,81,91,92] The perfusion scan may show defects that are nonsegmental, and the ventilation scan may show that these perfusion defects ventilate normally. In this circumstance, the diagnosis of acute pulmonary embolism is neither excluded nor confirmed. When this type of nonspecific lung scan is coupled with a strong clinical picture of pulmonary embolism and there is no other reasonable explanation for the patient's symptoms, it may be appropriate to proceed to selective pulmonary angiography and/or to treat for acute pulmonary embolism. The same nonspecific lung-scan findings coupled with a weak clinical story for pulmonary embolism may be sufficient to make the diagnosis of pulmonary embolism unlikely. The IPG is especially helpful in this setting, i.e., when the lung scan is nonspecific or of intermediate probability. If the IPG is negative, it is appropriate to conclude that the patient does not have pulmonary embolism. If the IPG is unilaterally positive, the diagnosis of pulmonary embolism should be pursued further by performing pulmonary angiography or peripheral venography. *A bilaterally positive IPG is a nonspecific finding, and further diagnostic testing, i.e., pulmonary angiography is usually indicated.*[53]

The diagnosis of acute pulmonary embolism is not made by the results of the lung scan alone. The clinician must evaluate the clinical findings and the IPG (and arterial blood gas analysis, venography, and Doppler sonography, if performed) together with the results of the lung scan.

ECHOCARDIOGRAPHY

Two-dimensional echocardiographic examination of patients with suspected and documented pulmonary embolism often yields clinically useful information[93,94] (see Chap. 14). Echocardiography may reveal thromboemboli trapped in the right heart chambers, RV dilatation and/or dysfunction, shift of the interatrial septum, and shift of the interventricular septum into the LV cavity with resultant diminution of LV volumes. Coexisting valvular and/or myocardial abnormalities are also readily identified. Transesophageal echocardiography may demonstrate the presence of thrombi in the pulmonary arteries. In many patients with suspected pulmonary embolism, an echocardiographic/Doppler examination is of considerable help in establishing the diagnosis.[94]

LABORATORY EXAMINATIONS

Over a period of years, a number of laboratory examinations have been suggested as aids in the diagnosis of pulmonary embolism. At one time, an elevated serum lactate dehydrogenase value, particularly if it occurred together with an elevated serum indirect bilirubin value, was said to be highly suggestive of pulmonary embolism. Subsequent studies demonstrated that these laboratory findings were of minimal or no value in the diagnosis of pulmonary embolism.[76] The determination of D-dimer levels in plasma has also been suggested as a useful diagnostic test in patients with pulmonary embolism.[95] D-Dimer is a degradation product of circulating cross-linked fibrin. Elevated levels suggest that intravascular coagulation and fibrinolysis have occurred. Thus, the finding of elevated plasma D-dimer levels might help the clinician to rule in or out the possible diagnosis of pulmonary thromboembolism. Unfortunately, because of differences in D-dimer assays and lack of standardization, the data obtained up to now fail to support the use of D-dimer levels as an accurate diagnostic test for patients with suspected pulmonary embolism.[95] Future investigation with more standardized assays may yet prove this test useful in the diagnosis of pulmonary embolism.

PULMONARY ANGIOGRAPHY

Pulmonary angiography is the most accurate test for the diagnosis of acute pulmonary embolism.[96] Unfortunately, it is not available in all hospitals and has the disadvantage of being invasive. The mortality from pulmonary angiography is very low when performed by an experienced team[97]; however, the morbidity associated with the test is substantial. Therefore, the authors do not recommend that pulmonary angiography be performed in all patients in whom pulmonary embolism is suspected, but that the test be reserved for those patients with the specific indications noted in Table 60-7.

The primary contraindication to pulmonary angiography is a history of a severe systemic reaction to contrast media. Relative contraindications include the presence of high-grade ventricular ectopy, left bundle branch block, and coexisting life-threatening disease.[97] *Pulmonary angiography should be performed with great caution in patients with suspected primary pulmonary hypertension.* When angiography is per-

formed in such patients, mainstream injections into the central pulmonary artery should be avoided. The use of stiff cardiac catheters is associated with an increased incidence of complications, including perforation of the heart.

Pulmonary angiography should be performed only by properly trained physicians. The complications of pulmonary angiography include those due to right-sided heart catheterization (arrhythmias, cardiac perforation) and reactions to contrast media. The ECG and systemic blood pressure should be monitored continuously. Right-sided heart pressures should be measured and recorded.

In patients with submassive pulmonary embolism, it is not necessary to perform main pulmonary arterial injections to visualize the entire pulmonary circulation. Rather, selective or subselective injections should be made into areas shown to have perfusion defects by lung scan. Injections of contrast medium by hand through a flexible, balloon-tipped catheter are often satisfactory.[98] The artery is occluded with the balloon, and the injection is made distal to the occlusion during cineangiography. The diagnostic finding of acute pulmonary embolism is the visualization of intraluminal clot.[96–98]

In patients with acute cor pulmonale due to massive pulmonary embolism, in whom pulmonary embolectomy or thrombolytic therapy may be indicated, mainstream injection into the main pulmonary artery with the use of cut film or cineangiography is appropriate. In this circumstance, the total pulmonary circulation, including the main and proximal right and left pulmonary arteries, must be visualized.

VENOGRAPHY

Venography, a test more widely available than pulmonary angiography, is useful in several circumstances.[48,49] In patients with nonspecific findings or intermediate probability by $\dot{V}/\dot{Q}$ lung scan but a positive IPG, venography is appropriate. If the venogram demonstrates DVT, the treatment is the same as if acute pulmonary embolism had been documented (see Chap. 100).

Occult Malignancies and Pulmonary Embolism

Deep venous thrombosis and its complication, pulmonary embolism, may be clues to the presence of occult cancer, especially in young patients.[99] Malignancies may be present in a wide variety of locations, including the gastrointestinal tract, lung, breast, uterus, and prostate.

Given this association, the evaluation of the patient with venous thrombosis or pulmonary embolism should obviously include a complete history and physical examination, including breast and pelvic examination in women and examination of the prostate in men. Further diagnostic evaluation will be guided by the results of the history taking and physical examination. In the follow-up of patients with pulmonary embolism, the clinician should be alert to signs or symptoms of early cancer. This is particularly the case if no other factors predisposing to the development of DVT (Table 60-1) are present.

Paradoxical Embolism

Paradoxical embolism of the systemic circulation is a rare complication of DVT that may occur in patients who have an intracardiac defect (atrial septal defect, ventricular septal defect, patent ductus arteriosus, or pulmonary arteriovenous fistula) or a patent foramen ovale.[100–105] Most reported cases of paradoxical embolism have occurred in patients with a patent foramen ovale, which is present in about 27 percent of the adult population.[101] In order for a venous thrombus to cross a patent foramen ovale, the pressure in the right atrium must be greater than in the left atrium. The most common acute cause for right atrial pressure to exceed left atrial pressure is acute cor pulmonale secondary to acute massive pulmonary embolism.[100]

The usual clinical profile in a case of paradoxical embolism is that of massive pulmonary embolism causing acute cor pulmonale in a patient without prior heart disease but with a patent foramen ovale. The increased right atrial pressure causes a right-to-left shunt across the foramen ovale. If another venous thrombus is dislodged from the deep venous system, it may cross the foramen to enter and embolize the systemic circulation. The most common recognized site of systemic embolism is the brain.[102,105] Additional common *recognized* sites include the extremities and the coronary arteries.

Paradoxical embolism should be considered whenever systemic embolism occurs without the usual predisposing causes: atrial fibrillation, mitral valve disease, myocardial infarction, prosthetic heart valves, or cardiomyopathy. In this circumstance, evidence of paradoxical pulmonary embolism should be sought. If there is evidence of acute pulmonary embolism in addition to unexplained systemic embolism, evidence of a right-to-left intracardiac shunt should be sought by means of indicator dilation curves, angiography, transesophageal echocardiography, or contrast echocardiography.[103,104] Paradoxical embolism may occur without clinically important pulmonary embolism in patients with intracardiac defects complicated by right-to-left shunts and in patients with chronic cor pulmonale with RV failure.

Paradoxical embolism tends to recur and is frequently fatal. If the diagnosis is confirmed during life, recurrence can be prevented by means of insertion of a filter in the inferior vena cava, interruption of the inferior vena cava, or closure of the intracardiac defect.

Treatment of Acute Pulmonary Embolism

The therapeutic modalities available for patients with acute pulmonary embolism can be divided into two groups: prophylactic and definitive therapy. *Prophylactic therapy* is based on the concept that the body's intrinsic fibrinolytic system will dissolve thromboembolic material that finds its way into the pulmonary vascular bed. Such dissolution usually leads to resolution of the pathophysiologic changes associated with acute pulmonary embolism over a period of 7 to 14 days.[71–73] Thus, prophylactic therapy aims at preventing further embolic episodes. Examples of prophylactic therapy include anticoag-

ulation with heparin or warfarin and inferior vena cava interruption (see Table 60-3). Prophylactic therapy with anticoagulants is initiated as soon as the clinician has a high index of suspicion for DVT or pulmonary embolism.

Definitive therapy focuses on thromboemboli that have already arrived in the pulmonary vascular bed. Definitive therapy attempts to remove or dissolve such emboli in order to effect a more rapid resolution of the pathophysiologic sequelae of pulmonary embolism. Examples of definitive treatment for pulmonary embolism include use of thrombolytic agents and pulmonary embolectomy. Placement of an inferior vena cava filter is used to prevent further pulmonary emboli. Supportive measures, e.g., fluid and pressor administration, often precede or accompany definitive therapy and are terminated once the patient's hemodynamic status is stable.

ANTICOAGULATION[106–115]

Intravenous unfractionated heparin is the initial treatment of choice for most patients with acute pulmonary embolism.[27,106–109] Heparin in a dosage higher than that required to block thrombin-fibrinogen interaction can relieve bronchoconstriction; heparin may also decrease the high pulmonary vascular resistance associated with acute pulmonary embolism. Several investigators have reported striking success with high-dose intravenous heparin in patients with massive pulmonary embolism in whom the prognosis was guarded. Table 60-8 provides a dosage schedule for heparin tailored to the severity of the thromboembolic process. Low-molecular-weight heparin is also highly effective as a therapeutic agent for patients with pulmonary embolism.[106,107] Indeed, low-molecular-weight heparin in high doses may be safer and more effective than unfractionated heparin for the management of patients with venous thromboembolism.[107]

The incidence of bleeding during heparin therapy is determined not by the dose of heparin but by defects in the walls of blood vessels[112] (see Chap. 52). Therefore, contraindications to anticoagulants include conditions that predispose to bleeding, e.g., active peptic ulcer disease, esophageal varices, hemorrhagic diatheses, severe liver or kidney disease, severe hypertension, intracranial disease, and recent surgery on brain, spinal cord, joints, or genitourinary tract.

As noted in Table 60-8, heparin is continued for 5 to 10 days and should overlap oral warfarin therapy until a prothrombin time of INR = 2.0 to 3.0 (approximately 1.3 to 1.5 times control, using rabbit brain thromboplastin) is achieved. Warfarin is usually started at a dose of 5 mg/day for the first 3 days of therapy. Thereafter, warfarin dosage is adjusted according to the results of the prothrombin time. After the prothrombin time has been in the therapeutic range for 4 to 5 days, heparin is discontinued and fine regulation of the prothrombin time is achieved by altering the dosage of warfarin. Warfarin should be continued for as long as the patient has an underlying predisposition to thromboembolism, e.g., bed rest. In the patient with a fracture, this period of time should be for 2 months after the cast or traction is removed and the individual is ambulatory. If predisposition

TABLE 60-8

HEPARIN REGIMENS FOR THE TREATMENT OF DEEP VENOUS THROMBOSIS AND PULMONARY EMBOLISM

Diagnosis	Heparin Dosage
Deep venous thrombosis without pulmonary embolism or with minor pulmonary embolism	5000 U IV loading dose followed by 1000–1500 U IV per hour; check activated partial thromboplastin time (APTT) 4–6 h after initiating infusion and adjust heparin dose to prolong APTT to 1.5–2.5 times control. Warfarin is started simultaneously with heparin. Heparin is discontinued on day 5 to 10. Heparin and warfarin therapy overlap for 4 to 5 days.
Major pulmonary embolism with or without right ventricular failure and hypotension	10,000 U IV loading dose followed by 1000–2000 U IV per hour; check APTT 4 h after initiating infusion and adjust heparin dose to prolong APTT to 1.5–2.5 times control (employ smaller loading and infusion dosage for smaller individuals or patients with hepatic and/or renal insufficiency). Warfarin is started on day 2 to 3 (if patient is stable) and heparin is discontinued on day 7 to 10.

to thromboembolism is transitory, patients who have suffered an episode of acute pulmonary embolism should receive oral anticoagulation for at least 3 and preferably 6 months.[110] In the individual with permanent predisposition to thromboembolism, anticoagulation should be lifelong.

An alternative to daily oral warfarin is injection of subcutaneous unfractionated or low-molecular-weight heparin every 8 to 12 h for a minimum of 12 weeks.[27] Subcutaneous heparin can be either fixed dose (i.e., 5000 units every 8 to 12 h) or adjusted dose to maintain the predose APTT at one-and-one-half times the control value (see Table 60-2 and Chap. 52). The Fourth ACCP Consensus Conference on Antithrombotic Therapy recommends adjusted-dose heparin as being superior to a fixed-dose regimen.[27]

Some former anticoagulant regimens prolonged the prothrombin time to as much as two-and-one-half times control. Recent experience, however, favors more modest prolongation of the prothrombin time (INR of 2.0 to 3.0) without any resultant loss of therapeutic efficacy and with a decreased risk for hemorrhagic complications.[27] Heparin plasma activity is significantly shortened in some patients with acute pulmonary embolism, presumably as a result of active intravascular coagulation on the surface of pulmonary thromboemboli in the pulmonary vascular bed.[111] Administration of heparin as a continuous infusion results in fewer hemorrhagic complications than administration by the intermittent bolus technique. Hemorrhagic complications of heparin are more common in elderly females than in any other patient group.[112]

Heparin can cause an immunologically mediated thrombocytopenia[113,114] (see Chap. 52). Such decreases in platelet counts are usually asymptomatic but may occur in as many as 5 to 22 percent of patients receiving intravenous heparin. Because the onset of heparin-associated thrombocytopenia usually occurs 6 to 12 days after initiation of therapy, patients begun on heparin should have serial platelet counts. Occasion-

ally, heparin-associated thrombocytopenia develops together with arterial thrombosis, which may be life-threatening.[113,114]

Additional medical therapy is often required in patients with acute pulmonary embolism, regardless of whether prophylactic or definitive treatment is elected. For example, apprehension, pain, and respiratory distress usually respond to intravenous morphine sulfate. Oxygen is administered by nasal cannulae or mask. Hypotension or shock usually requires intravenous infusion of positive inotropic agents such as dobutamine, dopamine, or norepinephrine.

PROPHYLACTIC THERAPY: VENOUS INTERRUPTION

Venous interruption is also a form of prophylactic therapy in that it is performed to prevent additional venous thromboemboli from reaching the pulmonary vascular bed.[115–123] The first form of venous interruption to be performed was bilateral common femoral vein ligation. This type of venous interruption is simple to perform and entails minimal risk for the patient without heart disease as local anesthesia is employed. Further embolism occurs in 5 to 10 percent of cases, however, usually because clot is present above the tie at the time of surgery. Surgical interruption of the vena cava just below the renal veins carries a risk of 2 to 5 percent in patients without heart disease. If the patient has left-sided heart failure, the in-hospital mortality is approximately 20 percent; if left- and right-sided heart failure are present, the risk is 50 percent.[115] Essentially the same risk exists for femoral vein ligation in patients with heart failure because of the high mortality rate from recurrent thromboembolism in patients with prior cardiac decompensation. If a pelvic source of embolism exists, the left ovarian vein must also be ligated. In pregnant patients, this latter procedure does not result in interruption of pregnancy or prevent future pregnancies.

Interruption of the vena cava is highly effective in preventing further episodes of thromboembolism. Interruption of the inferior vena cava is indicated: (1) when embolism occurs in patients receiving appropriate anticoagulant therapy; (2) when anticoagulants are contraindicated; (3) when diseases predisposing to venous thrombosis and pulmonary embolism are prominent and persistent; (4) when septic embolism occurs; (5) when paradoxical embolism occurs; (6) when a large, free-floating vena caval thrombus is present; and (7) in some patients with massive embolism in whom a further episode of embolism would be fatal.

At present, the most common form of venous interruption is not surgery but rather the insertion of a filter or umbrella into the inferior vena cava.[121] In 5000 patients who had undergone insertion of a Mobin-Uddin filter,[117] nonfatal recurrent emboli occurred in 1.8 percent and fatal recurrent embolism developed in 0.5 percent. When the 28-mm filter was employed in 2500 patients, nonfatal embolic recurrences occurred in only 0.5 percent of patients and fatal recurrences were noted in 0.1 percent.[117] Filter migration is also said to be reduced with the 28-mm device.

Another popular inferior vena caval filter is the Kim-Ray–Greenfield stainless-steel wire filter.[118] This device is inserted in a manner similar to that employed for the Mobin-Uddin filter, i.e., via a venous cutdown on the common femoral or internal jugular vein. Both of these approaches utilize local anesthesia, thereby avoiding the risks associated with general anesthesia necessary for inferior vena caval clipping or ligation.

Morbidity following vena caval clipping or filter insertion is largely the result of subsequent total occlusion of the vena cava below the site of the clip or filter. In some series, such occlusion was said to occur in 50 percent or more of patients who underwent these procedures. Occlusion of the inferior vena cava is much less frequent in patients with a Kim-Ray–Greenfield filter than in those who have surgical inferior vena caval clipping or a Mobin-Uddin umbrella.[118,121] Morbid events secondary to total occlusion of the vena cava include postphlebitic limb syndrome, unilateral or bilateral leg swelling, and mild venous claudication.[119,120] Administration of anticoagulants following clip or umbrella insertion may reduce markedly the incidence of vena caval occlusion and the attendant morbid events.[120] Inferior vena caval filters can also be inserted prophylactically in patients undergoing high-risk orthopedic surgical procedures.[122,123]

PROGNOSIS OF PATIENTS TREATED WITH PROPHYLACTIC THERAPY

The excellent prognosis of patients with pulmonary embolism when the diagnosis is suspected and confirmed and prophylactic treatment is initiated has been documented.[4,73,124,125] Indeed, death secondary to pulmonary embolism is almost invariably the result of massive obstruction of the pulmonary vascular bed by thromboembolism.[4] Such patients usually die within minutes or hours following the acute episode, often before diagnosis and therapy are even considered. If the diagnosis is made and appropriate therapy is initiated, however, the outlook is often excellent, even in patients with massive

embolism complicated by RV failure without hypotension.[4] Patients with massive embolism, RV failure, and systemic arterial hypotension are the subgroup who have the highest mortality rate.[4,73,125] As noted below, patients in this subgroup are often given definitive therapy, since the prognosis is excellent for all other patient subgroups treated with less aggressive and invasive therapy, i.e., prophylactic therapy.

The overall hospital mortality rate for all patients treated for acute pulmonary embolism is approximately 8 percent.[4] Individuals with massive pulmonary embolism obstructing 50 percent or more of the pulmonary vascular bed have an in-hospital mortality rate of 16 percent. As noted above, most of the deaths in these latter patients occur in individuals with RV failure and systemic hypotension.[4] Preexisting heart disease also worsens the prognosis in patients with acute pulmonary embolism by predisposing them to the development of RV failure and hypotension following the embolic event.

Resolution of pulmonary embolism occurs by two mechanisms: in vivo fibrinolysis and mechanical changes in the location of clots within the pulmonary vascular bed. The pressurized flow of blood near and around emboli shifts their position in the pulmonary vascular bed to more distal, and hence less obstructive, locations. Embolic obstruction resolves by approximately 10 to 20 percent during the first 24 h after acute pulmonary embolism.[1,79] Complete resolution can occur as soon as 14 days after the acute event, but in most patients it remains incomplete for weeks.[79] The hemodynamic abnormalities associated with pulmonary embolism, i.e., pulmonary hypertension and RV failure in patients with massive embolism, resolve as the pulmonary emboli resolve.[79,126]

Thus, the late prognosis of the patient with acute pulmonary embolism depends on two factors: (1) whether or not the diagnosis of pulmonary embolism is made and appropriate therapy is initiated, and (2) the presence of associated medical illness, e.g., heart disease.

Further modest resolution of pulmonary embolism occurs for 3 to 4 months following discharge from the hospital. Thereafter, little, if any, further resolution occurs. Approximately two-thirds of patients with acute pulmonary embolism have complete resolution of their embolism. The remainder have partial resolution of much of the thromboembolic material. Very few patients with partial resolution of embolism develop chronic cor pulmonale. Only a rare patient with untreated or inadequately treated recurrent pulmonary embolism develops chronic cor pulmonale.[1,73] Recurrences of pulmonary embolism are uncommon in patients who are adequately treated and in whom appropriate prophylactic measures are undertaken.

DEFINITIVE THERAPY

Rationale

As noted earlier, most patients with pulmonary embolism have an excellent prognosis if the diagnosis is suspected and confirmed and prophylactic treatment is initiated. Individuals with massive embolism, RV failure, and hypotension form a subgroup who have a high in-hospital mortality rate (32 percent).[4] One would expect these patients to benefit from a direct, definitive attack on the pulmonary vascular thromboemboli. This small minority of patients appear to benefit from thrombolytic dissolution of thromboemboli or even embolectomy. *To date, however, unequivocal proof is still lacking that definitive therapy, in comparison with prophylactic therapy, leads to decreased mortality.*

Embolectomy[124,127–130]

Pulmonary embolectomy (Trendelenburg's operation) was introduced at the turn of the century but met with only occasional success. The introduction of cardiopulmonary bypass made successful performance of embolectomy more feasible. The surgical mortality rate associated with embolectomy, however, remains high, approximately 30 to 50 percent, because the operation is usually performed on patients who are in profound shock. Most individuals who require embolectomy die before it can be performed. Conversely, many patients who survive embolectomy might have survived with less vigorous therapy.[124]

The primary indications for embolectomy are the presence of RV failure and systemic arterial hypotension requiring vasopressors in a patient with bilateral central pulmonary emboli documented by pulmonary angiography. In this setting, embolectomy can be lifesaving. In the absence of hypotension, pulmonary embolectomy is not indicated even if massive pulmonary embolism is documented by angiography. Such patients survive without embolectomy if further embolism is prevented by the administration of prophylactic therapy.[124]

Contraindications to pulmonary embolectomy include recurrent pulmonary embolism without angiographic evidence of occluded central pulmonary arteries, pulmonary arterial systolic pressure in excess of 70 mmHg, severe underlying heart disease complicated by heart failure, and marked pulmonary insufficiency secondary to severe pulmonary disease, i.e., chronic obstructive lung disease.

An alternative to operative pulmonary embolectomy, which requires a thoracotomy, is percutaneous pulmonary embolectomy employing a special catheter.[129,130] This technique involves percutaneous, transvenous introduction of a steerable suction catheter into the pulmonary artery under fluoroscopic guidance. Emboli are aspirated via the catheter, thereby removing them from the pulmonary vascular bed. Multiple retrievals of embolic material by the catheter are usually required before an improvement occurs in the abnormal pulmonary vascular hemodynamic pattern. A vena caval filter is usually inserted at the end of this procedure.[129] Experience with this technique is modest, and further work is required to define the applicability and success rate of catheter pulmonary embolectomy.

Thrombolytic Therapy[131–148]

The search for an agent to dissolve thromboemboli in humans has been long and complex. The agents that have been studied most extensively are streptokinase, urokinase, and TPA (see Chap. 52).

The efficacy of urokinase in the treatment of acute pulmonary embolism was assessed in a national cooperative trial sponsored by the National Heart, Lung and Blood Institute.[131] In this multicenter trial, half of the patients were treated with a 12-h infusion of urokinase, while the remainder received a 12-h infusion of heparin.[131] After completion of the 12-h infusions, therapy was the same in both groups: intravenous heparin followed by oral warfarin. Repeat pulmonary angiography demonstrated greater, albeit modest, resolution of embolism in the group treated with urokinase. Five days after the initial treatment, however, resolution of embolism as determined by lung scanning was the same in both groups. The in-hospital mortality rate was the same for both groups as well.

Hemorrhagic complications were significant: moderate or severe bleeding occurred in 27 percent of the heparin-treated group and in 45 percent of the urokinase-treated patients.[131]

A second trial sponsored by the National Institutes of Health compared a 24-h infusion of urokinase with an infusion of streptokinase in 167 patients with angiographically documented pulmonary embolism. Urokinase and streptokinase were equally effective.[132] There was no significant benefit derived from 24 h of thrombolytic infusion as compared with 12 h. Significant bleeding occurred in more than one-third of patients treated with urokinase or streptokinase; bleeding was sufficiently severe in 14 percent of patients to require transfusion.[132]

The 1980 National Institutes of Health Consensus Conference on Thrombolytic Therapy and Thrombosis recommended that this form of treatment be widely applied to patients with documented pulmonary embolism with associated hemodynamic abnormalities.[132] Thrombolytic therapy, however, did not alter mortality secondary to pulmonary embolism in either of these two trials. Patients with massive embolism fared just as well with heparin (prophylactic) therapy as with thrombolytic (definitive) therapy. Another study demonstrated reduced morbidity with thrombolytic therapy as compared to routine anticoagulation.[133] In this study, two indices of pulmonary function, pulmonary capillary blood volume and pulmonary diffusing capacity, were significantly better in pulmonary embolism patients treated with thrombolytic therapy than in individuals who received routine anticoagulation.[133]

Major concern persists about the incidence of bleeding complications in patients treated with thrombolytic therapy. Estimates of this incidence in early trials ranged from 5 to 45 percent.[134–137] Because estimates of bleeding complications with thrombolytic therapy varied, contraindications to this therapy were also variable, depending on the investigator's perception of the risk of hemorrhage. On the basis of these early studies, it was difficult to determine firm indications for the use of thrombolytic agents in patients with acute pulmonary embolism. Genton concluded that thrombolytic therapy is potentially most useful in patients with documented massive pulmonary embolism and hemodynamic abnormalities, such as RV failure and/or hypotension.[138] A multicenter randomized trial, however, has documented improved RV function and possibly a reduced number of adverse clinical events in patients with acute pulmonary embolism treated with TPA as compared with intravenous heparin.[139]

The dosage of urokinase for patients with acute pulmonary embolism is an initial intravenous infusion of 4400 IU per kilogram of body weight dissolved in 15 mL of sterile water given over 10 min. Maintenance therapy is then initiated: 4400 IU/kg per hour for a total of 12 h. Streptokinase is given as an initial loading dose of 250,000 IU dissolved in normal saline solution or 5% dextrose in water and administered over 30 min. Maintenance therapy consists of 100,000 IU/h for 24 h. Bell and Meek recommend determination of thrombin time, prothrombin time, partial thromboplastin time, and platelet count before initiating thrombolytic therapy in order to screen for preexisting coagulation disorders. During thrombolytic therapy, these investigators advise that thrombin times be measured every 4 to 8 h.[135] The thrombin time should be prolonged to between two and five times the normal control value in seconds to confirm that adequate fibrinolysis has been achieved.[135]

A number of studies have employed recombinant TPA in the thrombolytic therapy of acute pulmonary embolism.[26,139–148] In general, the studies have demonstrated that in selected patients thrombolytic therapy with recombinant TPA can rapidly lyse pulmonary embolism and that it acts more rapidly and may cause less bleeding than urokinase. The usual dosage is 100 mg given intravenously over 2 h. It has also been administered at a rate of 0.6 mg/kg intravenously over 2 min[148] (see also Chap. 52).

At the present time, thrombolytic therapy is generally reserved for those patients who have hemodynamic embarrassment, RV dysfunction, anatomically large pulmonary embolism, or extensive DVT. Additional data from ongoing clinical trials should document the full effect of thrombolytic therapy on morbidity and mortality. The contraindications to thrombolytic therapy are discussed in Chap. 52.

Pulmonary Embolism in Pregnancy[149–152]

Pulmonary embolism during pregnancy represents a difficult diagnostic and therapeutic problem. Lung scanning and pulmonary angiography involve ionizing radiation exposure for both mother and fetus. Consequently, the diagnosis often remains tentative. Therapy is also problematic since warfarin, which is teratogenic, crosses the placenta and reaches the fetal circulation. It is usually wise to pursue the diagnostic evaluation of pulmonary embolism aggressively, even in pregnancy, because untreated pulmonary embolism carries a 30 percent mortality rate.[4]

The treatment of pulmonary embolism during pregnancy is hazardous.[149] Prophylactic therapy must continue throughout pregnancy and the puerperium. Heparin does not cross the placental barrier, but it is difficult to administer for more than 2 weeks and its use is associated with an increased rate of pregnancy complications, as noted below. Warfarin derivatives cross the placenta and result in significant fetal teratogenesis and mortality. Termination of the pregnancy to avert further embolism is usually not appropriate. Ligation of the femoral veins does not protect against emboli arising from pelvic and gluteal veins. Interruption of the inferior vena cava and left ovarian vein is a highly effective preventive procedure. This operation, however, entails a surgical risk of about 2 percent in experienced hands; there is little risk of miscarriage after the first trimester, and no interference with future pregnancies.[115] When pulmonary embolism occurs in the first trimester, the appropriate treatment is a 10-day course of heparin, followed by adjusted-dose subcutaneous heparin administered by the patient at home.[27] Heparin is used after delivery until the patient is fully ambulatory. In selected cases, inferior vena caval interruption is appropriate.

Hall et al. reviewed the complications associated with anticoagulant therapy during pregnancy.[151] Heparin therapy was associated with hemorrhage (10 percent), spontaneous abortion (2 percent), stillbirths (13 percent), early infant mortality (7 percent), and chronic complications in 1 percent of surviving children. Warfarin therapy was complicated by fetal developmental abnormalities (nasal hypoplasia, mental retardation) in 7 percent of infants, spontaneous abortion (9 percent), and stillbirths (8 percent). Consequently, these authors recommend avoidance or termination of pregnancy in patients who require anticoagulant therapy.[151]

Chronic Pulmonary Embolism and Pulmonary Embolectomy[153–161]

Elective pulmonary embolectomy for chronic, unresolved pulmonary thromboembolism is considerably more successful than is the emergency operation. Daily et al. described four such patients, three of whom survived the operation and were markedly improved.[153] Moser et al. reported good results in 15 and 41 patients.[155–157] Benotti et al. identified 30 patients for whom extensive clinical and hemodynamic data were available.[158] The mean age was 45 years; most complained of dyspnea. Roentgenographic, arterial blood gas, and ECG findings were nonspecific; perfusion lung scans were invariably abnormal. Most patients had mild to moderate pulmonary hypertension at rest. Marked pulmonary hypertension developed during exercise. Operative mortality was 20 percent in the 20 patients who underwent elective pulmonary embolectomy, and operative results ranged from good to excellent.[158]

SPECIAL TYPES OF PULMONARY EMBOLISM

Fat Embolism[162–190]

In 1861, Zenker[188] described the postmortem findings of fat emboli in the lungs, and in 1873, Bergmann[189] described the classic triad for the fat embolism syndrome: dyspnea (respiratory insufficiency), confusion (neurologic dysfunction), and petechiae.

The entrance of free globules of fat into systemic veins most often occurs after fractures of long bones, especially fractures of the tibia and femur in automobile accidents. Fat may also enter the circulation following direct injury to subcutaneous fat tissue by contusion, concussion, burns, childbirth, poisoning, the use of a pump oxygenator, or high-altitude flights. Some less common causes include alcoholism, fatty metamorphosis of the liver, decompression sickness, sickle cell crisis, multiple blood transfusions, sternal-splitting incisions for cardiac surgery, and external cardiac massage.

The exact pathophysiology of fat embolism syndrome is unknown and probably differs between patients.[184] At least some of the fatty emboli causing mechanical obstruction in the pulmonary circulation originate from traumatized bone, as myeloid tissue can occasionally be identified in the pulmonary vessels.[163,170,173] There is also evidence that physiobiochemical alterations in the natural emulsion of circulating fat can result in the production of macroglobules of fat that may act as emboli. Other physiobiochemical mechanisms suggested as contributing to the syndrome include the following: release of thromboplastin from traumatized tissues with resultant platelet aggregation; excess free fatty acidemia from the superimposition of fat on platelet aggregations; liberation of toxic free fatty acids in the lungs by enzymatic hydrolysis of embolic fat with subsequent pulmonary capillary leak and curtailment of lung surfactant activity[172]; release of vasoactive and bronchoactive substances such as bradykinin, histamine, or serotonin from pulmonary microthrombi; traumatic shock; and defects in the coagulation system.[168,169] The commonly observed sudden drop in hematocrit is usually related to blood loss in fractured extremities, extensive pulmonary hemorrhage, or, less frequently, associated disseminated intravascular coagulation (DIC). Thrombocytopenia frequently develops in individuals with fat embolism, probably as a result of platelet adhesion to fat droplets in the lung.[167]

The fat droplets vary in size and may obstruct small pulmonary arterial branches, including arterioles and capillaries. The fat globules may also traverse the pulmonary circulation and block arterioles and capillaries of the brain, skin, kidney, heart, and other organs.

Patients can develop the acute respiratory distress syndrome (ARDS) with extensive intrapulmonary hemorrhage and damage to pulmonary vascular endothelium and parenchyma. Clinically, it is frequently difficult to distinguish fat embolism syndrome from ARDS.

Patients often have a lucid interval of 6 h to several days (typically, 24 to 40 h) following trauma before the first symptoms or signs of fat embolism are recognized. Most features of the syndrome result from fat emboli either to the lungs or to the brain.[177,182] Cardiorespiratory manifestations of pulmonary fat emboli include tachypnea, dyspnea, sinus tachycardia, hypoxemia, and pyrexia to 39.4°C (103°F). Individuals with severe respiratory distress may become cyanotic. Patients with fat embolism syndrome often have copious bronchial secretions, which may be hemorrhagic. The cerebral symptoms, which may occur simultaneously with or after the pulmonary

symptoms, include headache, increasing irritability, disturbances of consciousness, disorientation, delirium, confusion, restlessness, convulsions, apathy, stupor, and coma. Focal cerebral syndromes may also occur.[186] As noted above, patients with fat embolism may present with, or develop, the full clinical picture of ARDS.[180] Oliguria and even anuria may develop.

Signs of systemic fat embolism include petechiae, especially on the anterior chest, axillary folds, neck, fundi, and conjunctivae. Rarely, fat emboli are seen in the retinal vessels. In some patients, the petechiae, whether spontaneous or induced, may be related to the associated thrombocytopenia, although small fat emboli may be found in biopsies of cutaneous capillaries adjacent to the petechiae.[190] The prothrombin time and partial thromboplastin time may be increased, and plasma fibrinogen may be reduced. The serum calcium level is often decreased, presumably because of the interaction between increased serum fatty acids and calcium; serum lipase and tributyrinase concentrations are usually elevated. A frozen section of clotted blood examined for fat may be of some diagnostic value early in the course of the fat embolism syndrome, particularly in patients with an arterial P_{O_2} less than 60 mmHg.[175,179] The findings of fat droplets in sputum or urine are also suggestive, but not diagnostic, of fat embolism.[166] Arterial hypoxemia is one of the earliest and most important laboratory findings. The chest roentgenogram usually shows extensive fluffy infiltrates; occasionally, only hazy, diffuse, fine stippling is seen throughout both lungs. The chest x-ray may also be compatible with pulmonary edema.[181]

There is no specific therapy for fat embolism; the most important principle is maintenance of pulmonary oxygenation and function. It is important to correct the arterial hypoxemia that is usually present and is occasionally quite marked. Supplemental inspiratory oxygen is usually required. Occasionally, assisted ventilation, with or without positive end-expiratory pressure, is needed. Although 100% inspiratory oxygen may be necessary initially, this should later be reduced to 40% to avoid oxygen toxicity. Frequent determinations of arterial blood gas concentration are necessary. Massive doses of glucocorticoids may decrease alveolar damage, although adequate clinical trials are lacking.[164,165,171,174,176–178,183,185] Doses usually employed are: hydrocortisone, 1 to 2 g/day, or methylprednisolone, 13 mg/kg per day, for 3 to 5 days. Schonfeld et al. demonstrated that prophylactic administration of methylprednisolone, 7.5 mg per kilogram of body weight, every 6 h for 12 doses to patients with long bone fractures reduced the development of signs and symptoms of the fat embolism syndrome.[185] Low-dose heparin was formerly recommended in order to decrease platelet adhesiveness. The stimulatory effort of heparin upon lipase activity in the lung is theoretically detrimental, however, since it might increase the amounts of toxic fatty acids in the lungs. Other former therapies that are no longer used include low-molecular-weight dextran,[168] intravenous ethyl alcohol, hypothermia, and various detergents.[167]

Air Embolism[191-200]

Air may enter the circulation during the course of intravenous infusions, pneumoperitoneum, knee-chest position in the puerperium, uterine douches, surgical procedures on the neck or brain, retroperitoneal air injection, irrigation of nasal sinuses, tubal or vaginal insufflation, orogenital sex,[197] rapid pressure decompensation, mechanical ventilation, or heart-lung bypass. The lethal dose varies with the age, condition, and position of the patient and the rapidity of air entry. Fatal air embolism can result from 5 to 15 mL of air per kilogram of body weight. Death results either from an "air lock" in the right ventricle or from air embolism to the lungs with resultant pulmonary vascular obstruction and secondary reflex pulmonary vasoconstriction.[191,192] It is likely that only very minute (if any) volumes of air traverse the pulmonary capillaries. Clinically, air embolism is associated with the sudden onset of dyspnea, shock, and cyanosis. Frequently, there is a loud, continuous churning, or "mill-house," murmur or noise over the precordium produced by the mixing of air and blood in the right ventricle. Venous air embolism can also result in diffuse pulmonary injury with subsequent development of ARDS.[193] Marked ventilation-perfusion abnormalities can result from air in the pulmonary vascular bed.[195] Air bubbles in cardiac chambers can be detected by echocardiography.[198]

Treatment consists of turning the patient onto the left side with the head in a dependent position, in an effort to displace the air bolus from the RV outflow tract to the RV apex or right atrium and to trap the air in the superior portion of the right atrium. The air can then be aspirated through a needle or catheter inserted into the right ventricle. One should also administer 100% inspiratory oxygen.[196] Closed-chest cardiac massage has been used successfully, particularly when air embolism occurs during a neurosurgical or neck operation.[199]

Arterial air embolism can also occur and may produce embolic retinopathy, ventricular fibrillation, myocardial infarction, or cerebral symptoms including coma, confusion, hemiplegia, loss of memory, and seizures.[194,200] Air can enter the arterial system by many routes, including cardiac surgery, pneumothorax, paradoxical air embolism, artificial ventilation with high airway pressures, hemodialysis, and intraaortic balloon counterpulsation. Treatment is supportive, although hyperbaric oxygen has been employed with apparent benefit.

Amniotic Fluid Embolism[201-213]

Amniotic fluid embolism causing maternal mortality was first described in 1926 by Meyer[201] and was more firmly established as a clinical syndrome in 1941 by Steiner and Luschbaugh.[202] The incidence has been variably stated as being from 1 in 8000 to 1 in 80,000 live births. It remains one of the more common causes of maternal death during legal abortion, labor, delivery, and the immediate postpartum period. Predisposing factors are increased age and parity, premature placental separation, intrauterine fetal death, oversized baby, prolonged and vigorous labor with tumultuous uterine contractions, uterine rupture, large doses of oxytocin, meco-

nium contamination of amniotic fluid, and abortion induced by intraamniotic injection of saline or glucose. It may also occur following amniocentesis.[211]

The amniotic fluid contains meconium, epithelial squamae, mucin, amorphous debris, lipids, bile pigments, lanugo, or any combination of these. It enters the maternal circulation either through the venous sinuses of the uroplacental site or through the endocervical veins. The pulmonary embolic manifestations are primarily due to the solid contents of the amniotic fluid, since most experiments have indicated that filtered amniotic fluid produces minimal pulmonary vascular response. Occasionally, amniotic fluid material can be detected in the vessels of the lungs, heart, kidneys, and brain.[203] Recent evidence, however, suggests that cytologic techniques are not helpful in the diagnosis.[212,213]

Clinically, most episodes of amniotic fluid embolism occur near the end of the first stage of labor and are manifested by the abrupt onset of severe dyspnea, hypotension or frank shock, tachypnea, tachycardia, cyanosis, evidence of acute cor pulmonale and pulmonary edema, and apprehension. The latter symptoms may progress rapidly to semicoma or coma. Generalized convulsions, cardiac arrest, and death may occur suddenly. Chest pain is relatively unusual. About 25 to 50 percent of patients die within the first hour, and the survivors are still at great risk of death from either irreversible shock or the subsequent development of profuse vaginal bleeding. There may be bleeding from venipuncture sites and all body orifices or into skin and mucosa. Acute renal failure may develop secondary to hypotension. The mortality in patients with the full-blown amniotic fluid embolism syndrome exceeds 80 percent.[207]

DIC develops in a significant number of patients who survive the initial pulmonary embolic event. It is produced by the entry into the circulation of large amounts of thromboplastic substances contained in the amniotic fluid. The coagulation cascade is initiated, leading to the consumption of factors V and VIII, prothrombin, and fibrinogen. If consumption proceeds more rapidly than repletion, deficiencies of these factors can develop. The fibrinolytic enzyme system is activated as a compensatory mechanism, resulting in the production of large amounts of fibrin degradation products; these act as inhibitors of thrombin, interfere with normal fibrin polymerization, and impair platelet function. This process can result in severe vaginal hemorrhage. Fibrin deposition throughout the microvasculature aggravates the pulmonary embolic manifestations and may produce systemic hypoperfusion with profound alteration in function of almost every organ in the body.

Laboratory findings usually reflect deficiencies of all coagulation factors, especially low fibrinogen levels and a low platelet count.

Treatment[202-208] consists of (1) general supportive measures for thromboembolism with hypotension and/or respiratory distress; (2) immediate evacuation of the uterus to remove the basic cause of the DIC process; (3) administration of fresh frozen plasma, platelets, and packed red blood cells as needed for anemia, hemorrhage, and/or hypotension; and (4) administration of cryoprecipitate (which contains fibrinogen and factor VIII) if bleeding persists and if fibrinogen and factor VIII are low.[207,208] Controversy exists regarding the use of fibrinogen, which promotes clotting and hemostasis, since theoretically it might produce more deposition of fibrin. The management of amniotic fluid embolism is greatly assisted by monitoring intraarterial blood pressure, central venous pressure, pulmonary artery pressure (with a balloon pulmonary artery catheter), and urinary output.[209,210]

Tumor Embolism[214-218]

In addition to pulmonary metastases from malignant tumors, acute and subacute cor pulmonale may result from emboli of malignant tissue cells to the pulmonary arteries and capillaries. These emboli may originate from the primary site of the tumor or from metastatic sites, such as the liver or inferior vena cava. Tumor emboli occur with virtually any type of malignancy but are more common in patients with renal carcinoma, primary hepatic carcinoma, gastric carcinoma, and trophoblastic tumors (chorioepithelioma). Rarely, pulmonary tumor embolism occurs in a patient without apparent malignancy, producing a syndrome of slowly progressive dyspnea and pulmonary hypertension[218] (see also Chap. 86).

Because trophoblastic tumors, even with extensive pulmonary metastases, may respond well to chemotherapy,[215,216] it is imperative to consider this diagnosis whenever a female patient has symptoms of acute dyspnea, pleurisy, cough, and/or hemoptysis or unexplained signs of pulmonary hypertension following a hydatidiform mole, abortion, or normal pregnancy. Occasionally, trophoblastic pulmonary emboli may not occur until several years after the initiating pregnancy, and the patient may have been asymptomatic in the interval. It is most common, however, for patients to describe amenorrhea, excessive menstrual bleeding or discharge, or other disturbance of menses. Since uterine curettage is often negative, the diagnosis is best established by measuring urinary gonadotropin excretion. Radiologic changes in the lungs resulting from metastasis of trophoblastic tumors may take one or more of the following forms: (1) discrete, usually well-defined, rounded opacities; (2) "snowstorm" patterns with multiple, small, less well defined opacities; and (3) changes resulting from embolic occlusion of the pulmonary arteries without invasion of the lung parenchyma. Of interest is one study of 50 asymptomatic puerperal patients, 13 of whom had pulmonary scan defects thought to be due to asymptomatic trophoblastic emboli.[218]

Cor pulmonale, i.e., right-sided heart failure, occasionally results from hematogenous or lymphatic spread of tumor. Cor pulmonale may be subacute, occurring over the course of a week or 10 days, or it may appear more slowly with a clinical picture of chronic right-sided heart failure.[214,218]

Rare Causes of Embolism

Among the many less common forms of pulmonary embolism are those due to cotton fiber, talc, hair, or other particulate matter in contaminated heroin or other illicit drugs; barium sulfate crystals after barium enema; vegetable material; bullets or shotgun shot; cardiac catheters or indwelling venous catheters; bone marrow, brain tissue, parasites, cardiac vegetations; foam cells from rupture of atheromata in an enlarged pulmonary artery; liver cells; and bile thromboembolism.[219,220]

REFERENCES

1. Dalen JE, Alpert JS. Natural history of pulmonary embolism. *Prog Cardiovasc Dis* 1975; 17:259–269.
2. Anderson FA Jr, Wheeler B, Goldberg RJ, Hosmer DW, Patwardhan NA, Jovanovic B, et al. A population-based perspective of the hospital incidence and case-fatality rates of deep vein thrombosis and pulmonary embolism. *Arch Intern Med* 1991; 151:933–938.
3. Alpert JS, Dalen JE. Epidemiology and natural history of venous thromboembolism. *Prog Cardiovasc Dis* 1994; 36:417–422.
4. Alpert JS, Smith R, Carlson J, Ockene IS, Dexter L, Dalen JE. Mortality in patients treated for pulmonary embolism. *JAMA* 1976; 236:1477–1480.
5. Sevitt S, Gallagher NG. Venous thrombosis and pulmonary embolism: A clinicopathologic study in injured and burned patients. *Br J Surg* 1961; 48:475–482.
6. Havig O. Source of pulmonary emboli. *Acta Chir Scand* 1977; 478:42–47.
7. Kakkar V, Howe CT, Flanc C, Clark WD. Natural history of postoperative deep venous thrombosis. *Lancet* 1969; 2:230–232.
8. Carter CJ. The natural history and epidemiology of venous thrombosis. *Prog Cardiovasc Dis* 1994; 36:423–438.
9. Virchow RIK. *Cellular Pathology as Based upon Physiological and Pathohistology*, 7th Am. ed. Chance F, DeWitt RM (trans). New York, 1860, 236.
10. Wessler S, Reiner L, Freiman D, Reimer SM, Lertzman M. Serum-induced thrombosis. *Circulation* 1959; 20:864–876.
11. Freiman D, Wessler S, Lertzman W. Experimental pulmonary embolism with serum-induced thrombi aged in vivo. *Am J Pathol* 1962; 39:95–104.
12. Sevitt S. The structure and growth of valve-pocket thrombi in femoral veins. *J Clin Pathol* 1974; 27:517–521.
13. Wessler S. Studies in intravascular coagulation. III. The pathogenesis of serum-induced venous thrombosis. *J Clin Invest* 1955; 34:647–650.
14. Carter CJ. The pathophysiology of venous thrombosis. *Prog Cardiovasc Dis* 1994; 36:439–446.
15. Shattil SJ, Beunet J. Platelets in hemostasis. *Ann Intern Med* 1981; 94:108–113.
16. Moser KM. Venous thromboembolism. *Am Rev Respir Dis* 1990; 141:235–249.
17. Asherson RA, Khamashta MA, Ordi-Ros J, Derksen RHWM, Machin SJ, Barquinero J, et al. The "primary" antiphospholipid syndrome: Major clinical and serological features. *Medicine (Baltimore)* 1989; 68:366–371.
18. Ginsburg KS, Liang MH, Newcomer L, Goldhaber SZ, Schur PH, Hennekens CH, et al. Anticardiolipin antibodies and the risk for ischemic stroke and venous thrombosis. *Ann Intern Med* 1992; 117:997–1002.
19. Cotton LT, Clark C. Anatomic localization of venous thrombosis. *Ann R Coll Surg Engl* 1969; 36:214–222.
20. Kravis TC, Shibel EM, Brooks JD, Moser KM. Incorporation of radiolabeled fibrinogen into venous thrombi induced in dogs. *Circulation* 1974; 49:158–163.
21. Moser KM, LeMoine JR. Is embolic risk conditioned by location of deep venous thrombosis? *Ann Intern Med* 1981; 94:439–444.
22. Kakkar W, Howe CT, Nicolaides AW, Renney JT, Clarke MB. Deep vein thrombosis: Is there a high risk group? *Am J Surg* 1970; 120:527–530.
23. Huisman MV, Bulla HR, TenCate JW, Vreeden J. Serial impedance plethysmography for suspected deep venous thrombosis in outpatients. *N Engl J Med* 1986; 314:823–828.
24. Philbrick JT, Becker DM. Calf deep venous thrombosis: A wolf in sheep's clothing? *Arch Intern Med* 1988; 148:2131–2138.

25. Lagersted CL, Olsson CG, Fagher BO, Oquist BW, Albrechtsson U. Need for long-term anticoagulation treatment for symptomatic calf vein thrombosis. *Lancet* 1985; 2:515–518.

26. Goldhaber SZ, Morpurgo M. Diagnosis, treatment, and prevention of pulmonary embolism: Report of the WHO/International Society and Federation of Cardiology Task Force. *JAMA* 1991; 268:1727–1733.

27. Dalen JE, Hirsh J (eds): Fourth ACCP consensus conference on antithrombotic therapy. *Chest* 1995; 108(suppl):225S–522S.

28. Kakkar VV. The logistic problems encountered in the multicenter trial of low-dose heparin prophylaxis. *Thromb Haemost* 1979; 41:105–113.

29. Halkin H, Goldberg J, Modan M, Modan B. Reduction of mortality in general medicine in-patients by low-dose heparin prophylaxis. *Ann Intern Med* 1982; 96:561–565.

30. Poller L, McKernon A, Thomson JM, Elstein M, Hirsch PJ, Jones JB. Fixed minidose warfarin: A new approach to prophylaxis against venous thrombosis after major surgery. *Br Med J* 1987; 295:1309–1312.

31. Kakkar VV, Stamatakis JD, Bentley PG, Lawrence D, de-Haas HA, Ward VP. Prophylaxis for postoperative deep-vein thrombosis, synergistic effect of heparin and dihydroergotamine. *JAMA* 1979; 241:39–42.

32. Pedersen B, Christiansen J. Thromboembolic prophylaxis with dihydroergotamine-heparin in abdominal surgery. *Am J Surg* 1983; 145:788–790.

33. Moser G, Krahenbuhl B, Barroussel R, Bene JJ, Donath A, Rohner A. Mechanical versus pharmacologic prevention of deep venous thrombosis. *Surg Gynecol Obstet* 1981; 152:448–450.

34. Coe NP, Collins REC, Klein LA, Bettmann MA, Skillman JJ, Shapiro RM, et al. Prevention of deep vein thrombosis in urological patients: A controlled, randomized trial of low-dose heparin and external pneumatic compression boots. *Surgery* 1978; 83:230–234.

35. Francis CW, Pellegrini VD, Marder VJ, Totterman S, Harris CM, Gabriel KR, et al. Comparison of warfarin and external pneumatic compression in prevention of venous thrombosis after total hip replacement. *JAMA* 1992; 267:2911–2915.

36. Markwardt F. Hirudin and derivatives as anticoagulant agents. *Thromb Haemost* 1991; 66:141–152.

37. Markwardt F (ed): Hirudin. *Semin Thromb Haemost* 1991; 17:79–159.

38. Levine MN, Hirsh J, Gent M, Turpie AG, Leclerc J, Powers PJ, et al. Prevention of deep vein thrombosis after elective hip surgery: A randomized trial comparing low molecular weight heparin with standard unfractionated heparin. *Ann Intern Med* 1991; 114:545–551.

39. Prandoni P, Lensing AWA, Büller HR, Carta M, Cogo A, Vigo M, et al. Comparison of subcutaneous low-molecular-weight heparin with intravenous standard heparin in proximal deep-vein thrombosis. *Lancet* 1992; 339:441–445.

40. Hull RD, Raskob GE, Pineo GF, Green D, Trowbridge AA, Elliott CG, et al. Subcutaneous low-molecular-weight heparin compared with continuous intravenous heparin in the treatment of proximal-vein thrombosis. *N Engl J Med* 1992; 326:975–982.

41. Hirsh J, Levine MN. Low molecular weight heparin. *Blood* 1992; 79:1–17.

42. Nurmohamed MT, Rosendaal FR, Büller HR, Dekker E, Hommes DW, Vandenbroucke JP, et al. Low-molecular-weight heparin versus standard heparin in general and orthopaedic surgery: A meta-analysis. *Lancet* 1992; 340:152–156.

43. Salzman EW. Low-molecular-weight heparin and other new antithrombotic drugs. *N Engl J Med* 1992; 326:1017–1019.

44. Wells PS, Lensing AWA, Hirsh J. Graduated compression stockings in the prevention of postoperative venous thromboembolism: A meta-analysis. *Arch Intern Med* 1994; 154:67–72.

45. Antiplatelet Trialists' Collaboration. Collaborative overview of randomized trials of antiplatelet therapy. III. Reduction in venous thrombosis and pulmonary embolism by antiplatelet prophylaxis among surgical and medical patients. *Br Med J* 1994; 309:235–246.

46. Hull RC, Raskob GE, Pineo GF, Rosenbloom D, Evans W, Mallory T, et al. A comparison of subcutaneous low molecular weight heparin with warfarin sodium for prophylaxis against deep vein thrombosis after hip or knee implantation. *N Engl J Med* 1993; 329:1370–1376.

47. Kearon C, Hirsh J. Starting prophylaxis for venous thromboembolism postoperatively. *Arch Intern Med* 1995; 155:366–372.

48. Rabinov K, Paulin S. Roentgen diagnosis of venous thrombosis in the leg. *Arch Surg* 1972; 104:134–139.

49. Hull R, Hirsh J, Sackett DL, Taylor DW, Carter C, Turpie AGG, et al. Clinical validity of a negative venogram in patients with clinically suspected venous thrombosis. *Circulation* 1981; 64:622–625.

50. Hull R, Hirsch J, Sackett DL, Stoddart G. Cost effectiveness of clinical diagnosis, venography, and noninvasive testing in patients with symptomatic deep-vein thrombosis. *N Engl J Med* 1981; 304:1561–1567.

51. Wheeler HB, O'Donnell JA, Anderson FA Jr, Benedict K Jr. Occlusive impedance phlebography: A diagnostic procedure for venous thrombosis and pulmonary embolism. *Prog Cardiovasc Dis* 1974; 17:199–205.

52. Hull R, Taylor DW, Hirsh J, Sackett DL, Powers P, Turpie AG, et al. Impedance plethysmography: The relationship between venous filling and sensitivity and specificity for proximal vein thrombosis. *Circulation* 1978; 58:898–902.

53. Curley FJ, Pratter MR, Irwin RS. The clinical implications of bilaterally abnormal impedance plethysmography. *Arch Intern Med* 1987; 147:125–129.

54. Hirsh J. Heparin. *N Engl J Med* 1991; 324:1565–1574.

55. Hull RD, Raskob GE, Hirsh J, Jay RM, Leclerc JR, Geerts WH, et al. Continuous intravenous heparin compared with intermittent subcutaneous heparin in the initial treatment of proximal vein thrombosis. *N Engl J Med* 1986; 315:1109–1114.

56. Leizorovicz A, Simonneau G, Decousus H, Boissel, JP. Comparison of efficacy and safety of low molecular weight heparins and unfractionated heparin in initial treatment of deep venous thrombosis: A meta-analysis. *Br Med J* 1994; 309:299–304.

57. Levine MN, Hirsh J, Gent M, Turpie AG, Cruickshank M, Weitz J, et al. A randomized trial comparing activated thromboplastin time with heparin assay in patients with acute venous thromboembolism requiring large daily doses of heparin. *Arch Intern Med* 1994; 154:49–56.

58. Dalen JE, Haynes FW, Hopper FG Jr, Evans GL, Bhardwaj P, Dexter L, et al. Quantitative studies of pulmonary embolism. *Am J Med Sci* 1964; 247:641–650.

59. Dexter L, Smith GT. Quantitative studies of pulmonary embolism. *Am J Med Sci* 1964; 247:641–650.

60. Vlahakes GJ, Turley K, Hoffman JIE. The pathophysiology of failure in acute right ventricular hypertension. Hemodynamic and biochemical correlations. *Circulation* 1981; 63:87–95.

61. McIntyre KM, Sasahara AA. Determinants of right ventricular function and hemodynamics after pulmonary embolism. *Chest* 1974; 65:534–543.

62. Sasahara AA, Cannilla JE, Morse RL, Sidd JJ, Tremblay GM. Clinical and physiologic studies in pulmonary thromboembolism. *Am J Cardiol* 1967; 20:10–20.

63. Alpert JS, Godtfredsen J, Ockene IS, Anas J, Dalen JE. Pulmonary hypertension secondary to minor pulmonary hypertension. *Chest* 1978; 73:795–797.

64. Thames MD, Alpert JS, Dalen JE. Syncope in patients with pulmonary embolism. *JAMA* 1969; 238:2509–2511.

65. Lualdi JC, Goldhaber SZ. Right ventricular dysfunction after acute pulmonary embolism: Pathophysiologic factors, detection, and therapeutic implications. *Am Heart J* 1995; 130:1276–1282.

66. Alpert JS. Effect of right ventricular dysfunction on left ventricular function. In: Kellerman JS, ed. *Advances in Cardiology*. Basel: Karger; 1986:25–34.

67. Widdicombe JG. Reflex mechanisms in pulmonary thromboembolism. In: Moser KM, Stein M, eds. *Pulmonary Thromboembolism*. Chicago: Yearbook; 1973:178–193.

68. Chernick V, Hodson WA, Greenfield LJ. Effect of chronic pulmonary artery ligation on pulmonary mechanisms and surfactant. *J Appl Physiol* 1966; 21:1315–1319.

69. Finley TN, Swensen EW, Clements JA, Gardner RE, Wright RR, Severinghaus JW. Changes in mechanical properties, appearance and surface activity of extracts of one lung following exclusion of its pulmonary artery in the dog. *Physiologist* 1960; 3:56.

70. Dalen JE, Haffajee CI, Alpert JS, Howe JP, Ockene IS, Paraskos JA. Pulmonary embolism, pulmonary hemorrhage and pulmonary infarction. *N Engl J Med* 1977; 296:1431–1435.

71. National Heart, Lung, and Blood Institute. Urokinase pulmonary embolism trial: Phase 1 results. *JAMA* 1970; 214:2163–2172.

72. Prediletto R, Paoletti P, Fornai E, Perissinotto A, Petruzzelli S, Formichi B, et al. Natural course of treated pulmonary embolism. Evaluation of perfusion lung scintigraphy, gas exchange and chest roentgenogram. *Chest* 1990; 97:554–561.

73. Parakos JA, Adelstein SJ, Smith RE, Rickman FD, Grossman W, Dexter L, et al. Late prognosis of acute pulmonary embolism. *N Engl J Med* 1973; 289:55–58.

74. Auger WR, Permpikul P, Moser KM. Lupus anticoagulant, heparin use, and thrombocytopenia in patients with chronic thromboembolic pulmonary hypertension: A preliminary report. *Am J Med* 1995; 99:392–396.

75. Dalen JE, Dexter L. Pulmonary embolism. *JAMA* 1969; 207:1505–1507.

76. Szucs MM Jr, Brooks HL, Grossman W, Banas JS, Meister G, Dexter L, et al. Diagnostic sensitivity of laboratory findings in acute pulmonary embolism. *Ann Intern Med* 1971; 74:161–166.

77. ACCP Consensus Committee on Pulmonary Embolism. Opinions regarding the diagnosis and management of venous thromboembolic disease. *Chest* 1996; 109:233–237.

78. Stein PD, Goldhaber SZ, Henry JW, Miller AC. Arterial blood gas analysis in the assessment of suspected acute pulmonary embolism. *Chest* 1996; 109:78–81.

79. Hull RD, Hirsh J, Carter CJ, Jay RM, Dodd PE, Ockelford PA, et al. Pulmonary angiography, ventilation lung scanning, and venography for clinically suspected pulmonary embolism with abnormal perfusion lung scan. *Ann Intern Med* 1983; 98:891–899.

80. Stein PD, Alavi A, Gottschalk A, Hales CA, Saltzman HA, Vreim CE, et al. Usefulness of noninvasive diagnostic tools for diagnosis of acute pulmonary embolism in patients with a normal chest radiograph. *Am J Cardiol* 1991; 67:1117–1120.

81. PIOPED Investigators. Value of the ventilation/perfusion scan in acute pulmonary embolism: Results of the prospective investigation of pulmonary embolism diagnosis (PIOPED). *JAMA* 1990; 263:2753–2796.

82. Sasahara AA, Sharma GVRK, Parisi AF. New developments in the detection and prevention of venous thromboembolism. *Am J Cardiol* 1979; 43:1214–1224.

83. Henry JW, Stein PD, Gottschalk A, Relyea B, Leeper KV Jr. Scintigraphic lung scans and clinical assessment in critically ill patients with suspected acute pulmonary embolism. *Chest* 1996; 109:462–466.

84. Stein PD, Hull RD, Pineo G. Strategy that includes serial noninvasive leg tests for diagnosis of thromboembolic disease in patients with suspected acute pulmonary embolism based on data from PIOPED. *Arch Intern Med* 1995; 155:2101–2104.

85. McGinn S, White PD. Acute cor pulmonale resulting from pulmonary embolism. *JAMA* 1935; 104:1473–1480.

86. Stein PD, Dalen JE, McIntyre KM, Sasahara AA, Wenger NK, Willis PW. The electrocardiogram in acute pulmonary embolism. *Prog Cardiovasc Dis* 1975; 17:247–257.

87. Dalen JE, Banas J Jr, Brooks H, Evans GL, Paraskos JA, Dexter L. Resolution rate of acute pulmonary embolism in man. *N Engl J Med* 1969; 280:1194–1197.

88. Huet Y, Lemaire F, Brun-Buisson C, Knaus WA, Teisseire B, Payen D, et al. Hypoxemia in acute pulmonary embolism. *Chest* 1985; 88:829–836.

89. Howe JP III, Alpert JS, Rickman FD, Spackman DG, Dexter L, Dalen JE. Return of arterial P$_{O_2}$ values to baseline after supplemental oxygen in patients with cardiac disease. *Chest* 1975; 67:256–258.

90. Kipper MS, Moser KM, Kortman KE, Ashburn WL. Long term follow-up of patients with suspected pulmonary embolism and a normal lung scan. *Chest* 1982; 82:411–415.

91. Kelley MA, Carson JL, Palevsky HI, Schwartz JS. Diagnosing pulmonary embolism: New facts and strategies. *Ann Intern Med* 1991; 114:300–306.

92. Hull RD, Hirsh J, Carter CJ, Raskob GE, Gill GJ, Jay RM, et al. Diagnostic value of ventilation-perfusion lung scanning in patients with suspected pulmonary embolism. *Chest* 1985; 88:819–828.

93. Farfel Z, Shechter M, Vered Z, Rath S, Goor D, Gafni J. Review of echocardiographically diagnosed right heart entrapment of pulmonary emboli-in-transit with emphasis on management. *Am Heart J* 1987; 113:171–178.

94. Nazeyrollas P, Metz D, Jolly D, Maillier B, Jennesseaux C, Maes D, et al. Use of transthoracic Doppler echocardiography combined with clinical and electrocardiographic data to predict acute pulmonary embolism. *Eur Heart J* 1996; 17:779–786.

95. Becker DM, Philbrick JT, Bachhuber TL, Humphries JE. D-Dimer testing and acute venous thromboembolism. A shortcut to accurate diagnosis? *Arch Intern Med* 1996; 156:939–946.

96. Stein PD, O'Connor JF, Dalen JE, Pur-Shahriari AA, Hoppin FG, Hammond DT, et al. The angiographic diagnosis of acute pulmonary embolism: Evaluation of criteria. *Am Heart J* 1967; 73:730–741.

97. Dalen JE, Brooke HL, Johnson LW, Meister SG, Szucs MM, Dexter L. Pulmonary angiography in acute pulmonary embolism: Indications, techniques, and results in 367 patients. *Am Heart J* 1971; 81:175–185.

98. Benotti JR, Alpert JS, Dalen JE. Superiority of balloon-occlusion pulmonary cineangiography in the diagnosis of pulmonary embolism (abstr). *Chest* 1983; 84:341.

99. Gore JM, Appelbaum JS, Green HL, Dexter L, Dalen JE. Occult cancer in patients with acute pulmonary embolism. *Ann Intern Med* 1982; 96:556–560.

100. Meister SG, Grossman W, Dexter L, Dalen JE. Paradoxical embolism. Diagnosis during life. *Am J Med* 1972; 53:292–298.

101. Hagen PT, Scholz DG, Edwards WD. Incidence and size of patent foramen ovale during the first 10 decades of life: An autopsy study of 965 normal hearts. *Mayo Clin Proc* 1984; 59:17–20.

102. Dalen JE. Systemic embolism. In: Rippe JM, Irwin RS, Alpert JS, et al, eds. *Intensive Care Medicine.* Boston: Little, Brown; 1985: 209–217.

103. Banas J Jr, Meister SG, Gazzaniga AB, O'Connor NE, Haynes FW, Dalen JE. A simple technique for detecting small defects of the atrial septum. *Am J Cardiol* 1971; 28:467–471.

104. Higgins JR, Strunk BL, Schiller NB. Diagnosis of paradoxical embolism with contrast echocardiography. *Am Heart J* 1984; 107:375–377.

105. Lechat P, Mas JL, Lascault G, Loron P, Theard M, Klimczac M, et al. Prevalence of patent foramen ovale in patients with stroke. *N Engl J Med* 1988; 318:1148–1152.

106. Thery C, Simonneau G, Meyer G, Helenon O, Bridey F, Armagnac C, et al. Randomized trial of subcutaneous low molecular weight heparin CY 216 (Fraxiparine) compared with intravenous unfractionated heparin in the curative treatment of submassive pulmonary embolism. A dose ranging study. *Circulation* 1992; 85:1380–1389.

107. deValk HW, Banga JD, Wester JWJ, Brouwer CB, van Hessen MWJ, Meuwissen OJATh. Comparing subcutaneous Danaparoid with intravenous unfractionated heparin for the treatment of venous thromboembolism. A randomized controlled trial. *Ann Intern Med* 1995; 123:1–9.

108. Colman RW, Rubin RN. Prophylaxis and treatment of thromboembolism based on pathophysiology of clotting mechanisms. In: Fishman AP, ed. *Pulmonary Diseases and Disorders,* 2d ed. New York: McGraw-Hill; 1988:1049–1057.

109. Hull R, Hirsh J, Jay R, Carter C, England C, Gent M, et al. Different intensities of oral anticoagulant therapy in the treatment of proximal vein thrombosis. *N Engl J Med* 1982; 307:1676–1681.

110. Schulman S, Rhedin AS, Lindmarker P, Carlsson A, Larfars G, Nicol P, et al. A comparison of six weeks with six months of oral anticoagulant therapy after a first episode of venous thromboembolism. *N Engl J Med* 1995; 332:1661–1665.

111. Hirsh J, VanAken WG, Gallus AS, Dollery CT, Cade JF, Yung WL. Heparin kinetics in venous thrombosis and pulmonary embolism. *Circulation* 1976; 53:691–695.

112. Jick H, Sloane D, Borda IT, Shapiro S. Efficacy and toxicity of heparin in relation to age and sex. *N Engl J Med* 1968; 279:284–286.

113. Bell WR, Tomasulo PA, Alving BM, Duffy TP. Thrombocytopenia occurring during the administration of heparin—a prospective study in 52 patients. *Ann Intern Med* 1976; 85:155–160.

114. King DJ, Kelton JG. Heparin-associated thrombocytopenia. *Ann Intern Med* 1984; 100:535–540.

115. Crane C. Venous interruption for pulmonary embolism: Present status. *Prog Cardiovasc Dis* 1975; 17:329–333.

116. Bomalaski JS, Martin GJ, Hughes RL, Yao JS. Inferior vena cava interruption in the management of pulmonary embolism. *Chest* 1982; 82:767–774.

117. Schlosser V. Umbrella filter implantation as prophylaxis against pulmonary embolism. *Eur Soc Cardiovasc Radiol* 1979; 23:329–331.

118. Greenfield LJ. Technical considerations for insertion of vena caval filters. *Surg Gynecol Obstet* 1979; 148:422–426.

119. Askew AR, Gardner AM. Long-term follow-up of partial caval occlusion by clip. *Am J Surg* 1980; 140:441–443.

120. Adelson J, Steer ML, Glotzer DJ, Skillman JJ, Simon M, Salzman EW. Thromboembolism after insertion of the Mobin-Uddin caval filter. *Surgery* 1980; 87:184–189.

121. Becker DM, Philbrick JT, Selby JB. Inferior vena cava filters: Indications, safety, effectiveness. *Arch Intern Med* 1992; 152:1985–1994.

122. Collins DN, Barnes LC, McCowan TC, Nelson CL, Carver DK, McAndrew MP, et al. Vena caval filter use in orthopaedic trauma patients with recognized preoperative venous thromboembolic disease. *J Orthop Trauma* 1992; 6:135–138.

123. Webb LX, Rush PT, Fuller SB, Meredith JW. Greenfield filter prophylaxis of pulmonary embolism in patients undergoing surgery for acetabular fracture. *J Orthop Trauma* 1992; 6:139–145.

124. Alpert JS, Smith RE, Ockene IS, Askenazi J, Dexter L, Dalen JE. Treatment of massive pulmonary embolism: The role of pulmonary embolectomy. *Am Heart J* 1975; 89:413–417.

125. Carson JL, Kelley MA, Duff A, Weg JG, Fulkerson WJ, Palevsky HI, et al. The clinical course of pulmonary embolism. *N Engl J Med* 1992; 326:1240–1245.

126. McIntyre KM, Sasahara AA. Hemodynamic and ventricular responses to pulmonary embolism. *Prog Cardiovasc Dis* 1974; 17:175–190.

127. Sautter RD, Myers WO, Ray JF III, Wenzel FJ. Pulmonary embolectomy: Review and current status. *Prog Cardiovasc Dis* 1975; 17:371–389.

128. Meyer G, Tamisier D, Sors H, Stern M, Vouhé P, Makowski S, et al. Pulmonary embolectomy: A 20-year experience at one center. *Ann Thorac Surg* 1991; S1:232–236.

129. Greenfield LJ, Zocco JJ. Intraluminal management of acute massive pulmonary thromboembolism. *J Thorac Cardiovasc Surg* 1979; 77:402–410.

130. Timsit J-F, Reynaud P, Meyer G, Sors H. Pulmonary embolectomy by catheter device in massive pulmonary embolism. *Chest* 1991; 100:655–658.

131. Urokinase Pulmonary Embolism Study Group. The urokinase pulmonary embolism trial. *Circulation* 1973; 47(suppl 2):1–108.

132. Consensus Development Conference Report. Thrombolytic therapy in thrombosis: A National Institutes of Health consensus development conference. *Ann Intern Med* 1980; 93:141–144.

133. Sharma GVRK, Bueleston VA, Sasahara AA. Effect of thrombolytic therapy on pulmonary-capillary blood volume in patients with pulmonary embolism. *N Engl J Med* 1980; 303:842–845.

134. Marder VJ. Are we using fibrinolytic agents often enough? *Ann Intern Med* 1980; 93:136–137.

135. Bell WR, Meek AG. Guidelines for the use of thrombolytic agents. *N Engl J Med* 1979; 301:1266–1270.

136. Dalen JE. The case against fibrinolytic therapy. *J Cardiovasc Med* 1980; 5:798–804.

137. Sasahara AA. The case for fibrinolytic therapy. *J Cardiovasc Med* 1980; 5:794–797.

138. Genton E. Thrombolytic therapy of pulmonary thromboembolism. *Prog Cardiovasc Dis* 1979; 21:333–341.

139. Goldhaber SZ, Haire WD, Feldstein ML, Miller M, Toltzis R, Smith JL, et al. Alteplase versus heparin in acute pulmonary embolism: Randomized trial assessing right-ventricular function and pulmonary perfusion. *Lancet* 1993; 341:507–511.

140. Goldhaber SZ, Meyerovitz MF, Markis JE, Kim D, Kessler CM, Sharma GVRK, et al. Thrombolytic therapy of acute pulmonary embolism: Current status and future potential. *J Am Coll Cardiol* 1987; 10:96B–104B.

141. Verstraete M, Miller GAH, Bounameaux H, Charbonnier B, Colle JP, Lecorf G, et al. Intravenous and intrapulmonary recombinant tissue-type plasminogen activator in the treatment of acute massive pulmonary embolism. *Circulation* 1988; 77:353–360.

142. Goldhaber SZ, Kessler CM, Heit J, Markis J, Sharma GVRK, Dawley D, et al. Randomized controlled trial of recombinant tissue plasminogen activator versus urokinase in the treatment of acute pulmonary embolism. *Lancet* 1988; 1:293–298.

143. PIOPED Investigators. Tissue plasminogen activator for the treatment of acute pulmonary embolism. *Chest* 1990; 97:528–533.

144. Goldhaber SZ. Thrombolysis for pulmonary embolism. *Prog Cardiovasc Dis* 1991; 34:113–134.

145. Meyer G, Sors H, Charbonnier B, Kasper W, Bassand J-P, Kerr IH, et al. Effects of intravenous urokinase versus alteplase on total pulmonary resistance in acute massive pulmonary embolism: A European multicenter double-blind trial. *J Am Coll Cardiol* 1992; 19:239–245.

146. Dalla-Volta S, Palla A, Santolicandro A, Giuntini C, Pengo V, Visioli O, et al. PAIMS 2: Alteplase combined with heparin versus heparin in the treatment of acute pulmonary embolism. Plasminogen activator Italian Multicenter Study 2. *J Am Coll Cardiol* 1992; 20:520–526.

147. Diehl J-L, Meyer G, Igual J, Collignon MA, Giselbrecht M, Even P, et al. Effectiveness and safety of bolus administration of alteplase in massive pulmonary embolism. *Am J Cardiol* 1992; 70:1477–1480.

148. Levine M, Hirsh J, Weitz J, Cruickshank M, Neemeh J, Turpie AG, et al. A randomized trial of a single bolus dosage regimen of recombinant

149. Evans G, Dalen JE, Dexter L. Pulmonary embolism during pregnancy. *JAMA* 1968; 206:320–326.

150. Hellgren M, Nygards EB. Long-term therapy with subcutaneous heparin during pregnancy. *Gynecol Obstet Invest* 1982; 13:76–89.

151. Hall JG, Pauli RM, Wilson KM. Maternal and fetal sequelae of anticoagulation during pregnancy. *Am J Med* 1980; 68:122–140.

152. Ginsberg JS, Hirsh J. Use of antithrombotic agents during pregnancy. *Chest* 1992; 102(suppl):385S–390S.

153. Daily PO, Johnston GG, Simmons CJ, Moser KM. Surgical management of chronic pulmonary embolism. *J Thorac Cardiovasc Surg* 1980; 79:523–531.

154. DelCampo C. Pulmonary embolectomy: A review. *Can J Surg* 1985; 28:111–113.

155. Moser KM, Spragg RG, Utley J, Dailey PO. Chronic thrombotic obstruction of major pulmonary arteries: Results of thromboendarterectomy in 15 patients. *Ann Intern Med* 1983; 99:299–305.

156. Moser KM, Daily PO, Peterson KL, Dembitsky W, Vapnek JM, Shure D. Thromboendarterectomy for chronic major vessel thromboembolic pulmonary hypertension in 41 patients. Immediate and long-term results. *Ann Intern Med* 1987; 107:560–565.

157. Moser KM, Anger WR, Fedulo PF. Chronic major-vessel thromboembolic pulmonary hypertension. *Circulation* 1990; 81:1735.

158. Benotti JR, Ockene IS, Alpert JS, Dalen JE. The clinical profile of unresolved pulmonary embolism. *Chest* 1983; 84:669–678.

159. Rich S, Levitsky S, Brundage BH. Pulmonary hypertension from chronic pulmonary thromboembolism. *Ann Intern Med* 1988; 108:425–434.

160. Lyerly HK, Sabiston DC. Surgical treatment of chronic pulmonary embolism. *Annu Rev Med* 1991; 42:507–517.

161. Simonneau G, Azarian R, Brenot F, Dartevelle PG, Musset D, Duroux P. Surgical management of unresolved pulmonary embolism. *Chest* 1995; 107:52S 55S.

162. Dudney TM, Elliott CG. Pulmonary embolism from amniotic fluid, fat, and air. 1994; 36:447–474.

163. Gauss H. The pathology of fat embolism. *Arch Surg* 1924; 9:593–604.

164. Ashbaugh DG, Petty TL. The use of corticosteroids in the treatment of respiratory failure associated with massive fat embolism. *Surg Gynecol Obstet* 1966; 123:493–500.

165. Liljedahl S, Westermark L. Aetiology and treatment of fat embolism: Report of five cases. *Acta Anaesthesiol Scand* 1967; 11:177–194.

166. Tedeschi CG, Castelli W, Kropp G, Tedeschi LG. Fat macroglobulinemia and fat embolism. *Surg Gynecol Obstet* 1968; 126:83–90.

167. Warren S. Fat embolism. *Am J Pathol* 1946; 22:69–88.

168. Rokkanen P, Lahdensuu M, Kataja J, Julkunen H. The syndrome of fat embolism: Analysis of thirty consecutive cases compared to trauma patients with similar injuries. *J Trauma* 1970; 10:299–306.

169. Bradford DS, Foster RR, Nossel HL. Coagulation alterations, hypoxemia, and fat embolism in fracture patients. *J Trauma* 1971; 10:307–321.

170. Peltier LF. The diagnosis and treatment of fat embolism. *J Trauma* 1971; 11:661–667.

171. Herndon JH, Riseborough EJ, Fischer JE. Fat embolism: A review of current concepts. *J Trauma* 1971; 11:673–680.

172. Fonte DA, Hausberger FX. Pulmonary free acids in experimental fat embolism. *J Trauma* 1971; 11:668–672.

173. Kerstell J. Pathogenesis of post-traumatic fat embolism. *Am J Surg* 1971; 121:712–715.

174. Fischer JE, Turner RH, Herndon JH, Riseborough EJ. Massive steroid therapy in severe fat embolism. *Surg Gynecol Obstet* 1971; 132:667–672.

175. Dines DE, Linscheid RL, Didier EP. Fat embolism syndrome. *Mayo Clin Proc* 1972; 47:237–240.

176. Rokkanen P, Alho A, Avikainen V, Karaharju E, Kataja J, Lahdensuu M, et al. The efficacy of corticosteroids in severe trauma. *Surg Gynecol Obstet* 1974; 138:69–73.

177. Moylan JA, Evenson MA. Diagnosis and treatment of fat embolism. *Annu Rev Med* 1977; 28:85–90.

178. Alho A, Saikku K, Eerola P, Koskinen M, Hamalainen M. Corticosteroids in patients with a high risk of fat embolism syndrome. *Surg Gynecol Obstet* 1978; 147:358–362.

179. Renne J, Wutheir R, House E, Cancro JC, Hoaglund FT. Fat macroglobulinemia caused by fractures or total hip replacement. *J Bone Joint Surg* 1978; 60A:613–618.

180. Oh WH, Mital MA. Fat embolism: Current concepts of pathogenesis, diagnosis and treatment. *Orthop Clin North Am* 1978; 9:769–779.

181. Curtis AM, Knowles GD, Putnam CE, McLoud TC, Ravin CE, Smith GJ. The three syndromes of fat embolism: Pulmonary manifestations. *Yale J Biol Med* 1979; 52:149–157.

182. Gossling HR, Donohue TA. The fat embolism syndrome. *JAMA* 1979; 241:2740–2742.

183. Guenter CA, Braun TE. Fat embolism syndrome. Changing prognosis. *Chest* 1981; 79:143–145.

184. Gossling HR, Pellegrini VD Jr. Fat embolism syndrome: A review of the pathophysiology and physiological basis of treatment. *Clin Orthop* 1982; 165:68–82.

185. Schonfeld SA, Ploysongsang Y, DiLisio R, Crissman JD, Miller E, Hammerschmidt DE, et al. Fat embolism prophylaxis with corticosteroids. A prospective study in high risk patients. *Ann Intern Med* 1983; 99:438–443.

186. Jacobson DM, Terrence CF, Reinmuth OM. The neurologic manifestations of fat embolism. *Neurology* 1986; 36:847–851.

187. Lindeque BG, Schoeman HS, Dommisse GF, Boeyens MC, Vlok AL. Fat embolism and the fat embolism syndrome. A double-blind therapeutic study. *J Bone Joint Surg Br* 1987; 69:128–131.

188. Zenker FA. *Beitrage zur Anatomie und Physiologie der Lunge.* Dresden: Braunsdorf; 1861.

189. Bergmann EB. Ein Fall tödlicher Fettembolie. *Klin Wochenschr* 1973; 10:385.

190. Whitaker AC. Traumatic fat embolism. Report of two cases with recovery. *Arch Surg* 1939; 38:182–189.

191. Berglund E, Josephson S. Pulmonary air embolization in the dog. I. Hemodynamic changes in repeated embolizations. *Scand J Clin Lab Invest* 1970; 26:97–103.

192. Josephson S. Pulmonary air embolization in the dog. II. Evidence and location of pulmonary vasoconstriction. *Scand J Clin Lab Invest* 1970; 26:113–123.

193. Ence TJ, Gong H Jr. Adult respiratory distress syndrome after venous air embolism. *Annu Rev Respir Dis* 1979; 119:1033–1037.

194. Marini JJ, Culver BH. Systemic gas embolism complicating mechanical ventilation in the adult respiratory distress syndrome. *Ann Intern Med* 1989; 110:699–703.

195. Hlastala MP, Robertson HT, Ross BK. Gas exchange abnormalities produced by venous gas emboli. *Respir Physiol* 1979; 36:1–17.

196. Yee ES, Verrier ED, Thomas AN. Management of air embolism in blunt and penetrating thoracic trauma. *J Thorac Cardiovasc Surg* 1983; 85:661–668.

197. Bray P, Myers RA, Cowley RA. Orogenital sex as a cause of nonfatal air embolism in pregnancy. *Obstet Gynecol* 1983; 61:653–657.

198. Rodigas PC, Meyer FJ, Haasler GB, Dubroff JM, Spotnitz HM. Intraoperative 2-dimensional echocardiography: Ejection of microbubbles from the left ventricle after cardiac surgery. *Am J Cardiol* 1982; 50:1130–1132.

199. Ericsson JA, Gottlieb JD, Sweet RB. Closed-chest cardiac massage in the treatment of venous air embolism. *N Engl J Med* 1964; 270:1353–1354.

200. Dedonis J, Schlant RC, Symbas PN. Arterial air embolism: An update. In: Hurst JW, ed. *Clinical Essays on the Heart*, vol 3. New York: McGraw-Hill; 1984:77–81.

201. Meyer JR. Emboli pulmonar amino-caseosa. *Brasil Med* 1926; 2:301–303.

202. Steiner PE, Luschbaugh CC. Maternal pulmonary embolism by amniotic fluid as a cause of obstetric shock and unexpected death in obstetrics. *JAMA* 1941; 117:1245.

203. Liban E, Raz S. A clinicopathologic study of fourteen cases of amniotic fluid embolism. *Am J Clin Pathol* 1969; 51:477–486.

204. Peterson EP, Taylor HB. Amniotic fluid embolism: An analysis of 40 cases. *Obstet Gynecol* 1970; 35:787–793.

205. Jewett JF. Amniotic-fluid infusion. *N Engl J Med* 1975; 292:973–974.

206. Morgan M. Amniotic fluid embolism. *Anaesthesia* 1979; 34:20–32.

207. Sterner S, Campbell B, Davies S. Amniotic fluid embolism. *Ann Emerg Med* 1984; 13:343–345.

208. Rodgers GP, Heymach GJ III. Cryoprecipitate therapy in amniotic fluid embolization. *Am J Med* 1984; 76:916–920.

209. Hogberg U, Joelsson I. Amniotic fluid embolism in Sweden, 1951–1980. *Gynecol Obstet Invest* 1985; 20:130–137.

210. Clark SL. Amniotic fluid embolism. *Clin Perinatol* 1986; 13:801–811.

211. Paterson WG, Grant KA, Grant JM, McLean N. The pathogenesis of amniotic fluid embolism with particular reference to transabdominal amniocentesis. *Eur J Obstet Gynecol Reprod Biol* 1977; 7:319–324.

212. Clark SL, Pavlova Z, Greenspoon J, Horenstein J, Phelan JP. Squamous cells in the maternal pulmonary circulation. *Am J Obstet Gynecol* 1986; 154:104–106.

213. Giampaola C, Schneider V, Kowalski BH, Bellaver LA. The cytologic diagnosis of amniotic fluid embolism: A critical reappraisal. *Diagn Cytopathol* 1987; 3:126–128.

214. Durhan JR, Ashley PF, Dorenclamp D. Cor pulmonale due to tumor emboli: Review of literature and report of a case. *JAMA* 1961; 175:757–760.

215. Bagshawe KD, Noble MIM. Cardiorespiratory aspects of trophoblastic tumors. *QJ Med* 1966; 35:39–54.

216. Li MC. Trophoblastic disease: Natural history, diagnosis and treatment. *Ann Intern Med* 1971; 74:102–112.

217. Ross M, Nowicki K, Rangarajan NS. Asymptomatic pulmonary embolism during pregnancy. *Obstet Gynecol* 1971; 37:131–133.

218. Margolis ML, Jarrell BE. Pulmonary tumor microembolism. *South Med J* 1985; 78:757–758.

219. Mehta S, Rubenstone AI. Pulmonary bile thromboemboli: A report of two cases. *Am J Clin Pathol* 1967; 47:490–496.

220. Dimmick JE, Bove KE, McAdams AJ, Benzing G. Fiber embolization—hazard of cardiac surgery and catheterization. *N Engl J Med* 1975; 292:685–687.

61

CHRONIC COR PULMONALE

John H. Newman / Joseph C. Ross

DEFINITION

Cor pulmonale is a term that describes the pathologic effects of lung dysfunction on the right side of the heart. Pulmonary hypertension is the link between lung dysfunction and the right side of the heart in cor pulmonale. Because the pulmonary hypertension results from abnormal lung function, cor pulmonale is a form of secondary heart disease. Cor pulmonale occurs as a late manifestation of many diseases of the lung, but the common thread in each case is increased right ventricular afterload. Cor pulmonale can be an elusive clinical diagnosis because pulmonary hypertension can exist without clinical manifestations and because clinical signs may be shared with the underlying disease. Depending on severity and chronicity, the pulmonary hypertension leads to dilatation of the right ventricle with or without hypertrophy. The presence of overt right-sided heart failure is not essential to make the diagnosis of cor pulmonale, but right-sided heart failure is a common consequence. The clinical manifestations of cor pulmonale relate to alterations in cardiac output, salt and water homeostasis, and in most cases, gas exchange in the lung. Right-sided heart dysfunction secondary to left-sided heart failure, valvular dysfunction, or congenital heart disease is excluded in the definition of cor pulmonale.[1] Pulmonary venous obstruction is a cause of cor pulmonale; pulmonary venoocclusive disease is usually considered in the spectrum of primary pulmonary hypertension. As a concept, cor pulmonale was introduced over 200 years ago, but the exact origin of the term is uncertain.[2] Osler[3] commented in the first edition of his textbook that "hypertrophy of the right ventricle . . . results from increased resistance in the pulmonary circulation, as in cirrhosis of the lung and emphysema." McGinn and White[4] apparently were the first to use the term *acute cor pulmonale* in the discussion of a case of acute, massive thromboembolism in 1935. William Harvey's discussion of the relationship of the lung and right side of the heart in *De Motu Cordis*[5] showed remarkable insight into the limitations of that muscular structure.

INCIDENCE, ETIOLOGIES, AND PATHOLOGY

Emphysema and chronic bronchitis cause over 50 percent of cases of cor pulmonale in the United States. The prevalence of cor pulmonale is difficult to determine because cor pulmonale does not occur in all cases of chronic lung disease and because routine physical examination and laboratory tests are relatively insensitive to the presence of pulmonary hypertension. The prevalence of chronic obstructive lung disease in the United States is about 15 million, directly resulting in approximately 70,000 deaths per year and contributing to about 160,000 other deaths.[6] It has been estimated that cor pulmonale accounts for 5 to 10 percent of organic heart disease. Cor pulmonale was present in 20 to 30 percent of admissions for heart failure in one study.[7] It is likely that cor pulmonale is a complication in a high percentage of cases. Gazes[8] found that 9.2 percent of cases of heart disease that came to autopsy had right heart abnormalities.

Chronic cor pulmonale occurs most frequently in adult male smokers, although the incidence in women is increasing as heavy smoking in females becomes more prevalent. A list of all diseases that may lead to cor pulmonale would be extensive and is not included in this chapter, but the major types of disease processes are listed in Table 61-1. Two important causes of cor pulmonale, thromboembolism and primary pulmonary hypertension, are discussed in Chaps. 59 and 60.

Chronic Obstructive Pulmonary Disease

Chronic obstructive lung diseases (COPDs) cause cor pulmonale through several interrelated mechanisms, including hypoventilation, hypoxemia from ventilation/perfusion ($\dot{V}/\dot{Q}$) mismatch, and reduction of perfused surface area.[9,10] Patients with more prominent hypoxemia and alveolar hypoventilation develop erythrocytosis, edema, and early onset of cor pulmo-

TABLE 61-1

ETIOLOGIES OF CHRONIC COR PULMONALE BY
MECHANISM OF PULMONARY HYPERTENSION

I. Hypoxic vasoconstriction
  A. Chronic bronchitis and emphysema, cystic fibrosis
  B. Chronic hypoventilation
    1. Obesity
    2. Sleep apnea
    3. Neuromuscular disease
    4. Chest wall dysfunction
  C. High-altitude dwelling and chronic mountain
    sickness (Monge's disease)
II. Occlusion of the pulmonary vascular bed
  A. Pulmonary thromboembolism, parasitic ova, tumor
    emboli
  B. Primary pulmonary hypertension
  C. Pulmonary venocclusive disease/pulmonary
    capillary hemangioma
  D. Sickle cell disease/sickle crisis/marrow embolism
  E. Fibrosing mediastinitis, mediastinal tumor
  F. Pulmonary angiitis from systemic disease
    1. Collagen vascular diseases
    2. Drug-induced lung disease
    3. Necrotizing and granulomatous arteritis
III. Parenchymal disease with loss of vascular surface area
  A. Bullous emphysema, alpha$_1$ antiproteinase
    deficiency, hyperinflation
  B. Diffuse bronchiectasis, cystic fibrosis
  C. Diffuse interstitial disease
    1. Pneumoconiosis
    2. Sarcoid, idiopathic pulmonary fibrosis,
    histiocytosis X
    3. Tuberculosis, chronic fungal infection
    4. Adult respiratory distress syndrome
    5. Collagen vascular disease (autoimmune lung
    disease)
    6. Hypersensitivity pneumonitis

flattened diaphragms. In some cases, increased bronchovascular markings and air bronchograms suggest the presence of thickened or inflamed airways. On the other hand, the chest roentgenogram may not show characteristic findings or be indicative of the severity of the physiologic impairment. Pulmonary function tests show an increased residual volume (RV) and total lung capacity (TLC), decreased forced vital capacity (FVC), and markedly decreased expiratory flow rates (FEV_1, FEF_{25-75}).[18] Arterial blood studies at rest can be normal when disease is mild but in severe disease show decreased P_{O_2}, increased P_{CO_2}, and decreased pH. With cor pulmonale, P_{O_2} is likely to be below 55 torr. Desaturation increases with exercise and frequently during sleep. The $\dot{V}/\dot{Q}$ inequality and alveolar hypoventilation both contribute to the hypoxemia. A P_{O_2} above 45 torr at rest defines net alveolar hypoventilation. Asthma is a form of COPD that rarely if ever leads to chronic cor pulmonale, probably because asthma is usually a disease of intermittent airway obstruction.

Cor pulmonale in COPD is related to the severity of lung dysfunction, and pulmonary hypertension is a manifestation of advanced disease. Exercise limitation in COPD is usually due to limitation of ventilatory capacity, not cardiac reserve, although sedentary patients develop deconditioning, which reduces exercise performance. No single test of lung function—such as spirometry, lung volumes, carbon monoxide diffusing capacity (DL_{CO}), blood gas tension, or radiography—is highly predictive of cor pulmonale, because abnormalities such as reduced surface area and hypoxic vasoconstriction add independently to pulmonary artery pressure.[10]

Diffuse Interstitial Lung Disease

These patients have dyspnea, tachypnea, exercise intolerance, and occasionally clubbing of the digits. Basilar crackles are frequently heard on auscultation of the chest and may persist throughout inspiration. The *chest roentgenogram* shows diffuse reticular, reticulonodular, or fibrotic lesions, but the appearance does not always correlate well with physiologic impairment. In some disease presentations, such as desquamative interstitial pneumonitis, there may be an alveolar filling pattern with air bronchograms. A lung biopsy is frequently required to identify the basic pathologic process, and even then the exact etiology may not always be determined. Transbronchial biopsy can be diagnostic in some interstitial diseases such as sarcoidosis, and bronchoalveolar lavage may point to a diagnosis in many cases.[13] *Pulmonary function tests* show a restrictive process with reduced lung volumes, decreased compliance, and decreased diffusing capacity without airway obstruction. The vital capacity is reduced, and the forced expiratory volume in 1 s (FEV_1) as a percentage of forced vital capacity (FVC) is usually at least 80 percent. At first, P_{O_2} decreases during exercise but is kept at normal levels at rest by hyperventilation. As the disease becomes more severe, P_{O_2} is low at rest. The course and prognosis of interstitial lung disease depend on the specific etiology, and there is wide variation among and within diseases.[3,14] The presence of cor pulmonale in interstitial lung disease implies extensive lung

nale ("blue bloaters").[11] Patients in whom dyspnea on exertion is the most prominent symptom have less hypoventilation and less hypoxemia at rest and therefore develop cor pulmonale later ("pink puffers"). Some of the differences between blue bloaters and pink puffers may relate to ventilatory drives; patients with low drives may be more likely to fit the blue-bloater category, whereas pink puffers strive to maintain normal arterial pH and gas tensions.[12] Another hypothesis is that blue bloaters have more inflammatory bronchitis and that pink puffers suffer more from pure emphysema.[11] *Physical examination* in all forms of COPD shows an increase in the thoracic diameter, low diaphragms, hyperresonance to percussion, decreased breath sounds with expiratory wheezes, distant heart sounds, distended neck veins during expiration, and a palpable liver. Liver enlargement and leg edema are manifestations of fluid retention and right heart failure and may or may not be present. The *chest roentgenogram* may show characteristic changes of emphysema such as hyperlucent lungs, bullae, increased anteroposterior (AP) diameter, and

dysfunction, perhaps with vascular involvement (as in systemic lupus erythematosus), and cor pulmonale may not occur even in end-stage disease.

Hypoventilation Syndromes

Some disorders (i.e., kyphoscoliosis) may impair or restrict mechanisms of ventilation, causing general alveolar hypoventilation and alveolar hypoxia.[15] Extreme obesity may be associated with hypoventilation, cyanosis, polycythemia, and somnolence (without intrinsic lung disease), often called the *pickwickian syndrome*.[16] Patients with daytime somnolence, morning headaches, and personality disturbances have been found to have periodic apnea during sleep associated with sleep deprivation, loud snoring, hypoxemia, and hypercapnia caused by upper airway obstruction (i.e., by the tongue, enlarged tonsils, or collapse of pharyngeal walls).[17] Brainstem abnormalities such as Arnold-Chiari malformation may also cause respiratory center depression and primary hypoventilation. Neuromuscular diseases such as postpolio syndrome and chronic Guillain-Barre' syndrome may present with cor pulmonale and right heart failure.[18] Diagnosis of hypoventilation is confirmed by blood gas analysis, a depressed ventilatory response to inhaled CO_2, tests of pulmonary hypoventilation, or sleep studies. It has become apparent that disordered ventilation during sleep is a major component of many hypoventilation syndromes.[18] In all cases of hypoventilation, the main stimulus for pulmonary hypertension is hypoxic vasoconstriction, a response of the pulmonary arterioles to alveolar hypoxia. The respiratory acidosis that may accompany hypoventilation augments the vasoconstrictor response to hypoxia.

Pulmonary Vascular Disease

Chronic cor pulmonale is a consequence of several diseases that involve the pulmonary vessels. Primary pulmonary hypertension and recurrent (or unresolved) pulmonary emboli are described in detail in Chaps. 59 and 60. Sickle cell disease, from SS or SC hemoglobinopathy, can cause cor pulmonale after multiple episodes of pulmonary infarction from focal pulmonary sickling, fat embolism, or thromboembolism.[19,20] Venoocclusive disease is a rare disease of the veins that presents with pulmonary hypertension and variable pulmonary infiltrates. There is a least one report of a beneficial response to immunosuppressive therapy in that disease.[21] Cirrhosis of the liver is usually associated with pulmonary vasodilatation, but occasionally a disorder clinically and pathologically identical to primary pulmonary hypertension emerges.[22,23] Human immunodeficiency virus (HIV) infection is a new cause of pulmonary vascular disease resembling primary pulmonary hypertension.[24] Collagen vascular disease can cause cor pulmonale by primary vasculitis as well as by diffuse interstitial fibrosis. Systemic sclerosis, systemic lupus erythematosus (SLE), and rheumatoid arthritis (RA) are the collagen vascular diseases that most commonly cause pulmonary arteritis. Patients with SLE and RA frequently present with primary interstitial lung disease. Occasionally, the presentation is that of cor pulmonale without interstitial disease but with primary

pulmonary arteritis.[25] Cor pulmonale is not reported as a feature of Goodpasture's syndrome or idiopathic pulmonary hemosiderosis. Historically, dietary pulmonary hypertension has occurred as a result of the use of aminorex in Europe, contaminated canola oil in Spain, and in eosinophilia myalgia syndrome in the United States related to contaminated tryptophan.[26] A new anorectic drug, dexfenfluramine, has caused pulmonary hypertension in France and has been approved for use in the United States.[26]

PATHOPHYSIOLOGY

Increased pulmonary vascular resistance (PVR) and pulmonary hypertension are central mechanisms in all cases of cor pulmonale.[10] Physiologic mechanisms of pulmonary arterial pressure are shown in Table 61-2. These variables can partly be described by Poiseuille's law. Fortunately, most pulmonary diseases and disorders do not produce enough pulmonary hypertension to cause cor pulmonale.

Normal Pulmonary Circulation

The primary function of this unique high-flow, low-pressure, low-resistance system is to provide blood for gas exchange, and it is ideally suited to optimize that function. It receives and transmits the entire cardiac output at low hydrostatic pressures primarily because of three characteristics: (1) the pulmonary arteries are thin-walled with little resting muscular tone, (2) there is negligible vasomotor control by the autonomic nervous system at rest in the adult, and (3) many small arterioles and alveolar capillaries are nonperfused at rest and can be recruited when needed to expand the pulmonary vascu-

---

TABLE 61-2

GENESIS OF PULMONARY VASCULAR PRESSURE: POISEUILLE'S LAW

$$Ppa = CO \left(\frac{8}{\pi} \times n \times \frac{1}{N} \times \frac{1}{r^4} \right) + Pla$$

Flow = cardiac output (usually ↑ elevated in COPD; if PRV is fixed, ↑ CO will ↑ PAP).

$\frac{8}{\pi}$ = numerical constant related to tubular structure of vessels.

n = blood viscosity (increased in polycythemia vera, secondary erythrocytosis, and cryoglobulinemia).

N = number of perfused vessels of a particular radius. N is decreased in any occlusive or destructive disease (see Table 61-1). N for pulmonary capillaries is >200 million.

$\frac{1}{r^4}$ = radius of a vessel is a critical determinant of flow (r is decreased by vasoconstriction, luminal obstruction, or hyperinflation. A change in r from 1 to 2 units changes resistance 16-fold).

Pla = left atrial pressure. Passive pulmonary hypertension can result from left atrial pressure elevation due to either LV or valvular disease.

lar bed, resulting in a decreased PVR. Normal mean pulmonary artery pressure (PAP) is about 12 to 17 mmHg; PAP above 20 mmHg at rest suggests pulmonary hypertension. Flow of blood from the main pulmonary artery (PA) through the pulmonary capillaries to the left atrium (LA) is accomplished by a pressure drop of only 5 to 9 mmHg, compared to an arterial to venous gradient of 90 mmHg in the systemic circuit. Thus, normal PVR is 10- to 20-fold less than systemic vascular resistance (SVR).

Pulmonary Hypertension

The effective cross-sectional area of the pulmonary vascular bed must be reduced by 25 to 50 percent before any change in PAP can be detected at rest. Exercise causes increased PAP because of increased pulmonary blood flow in the normal bed, and exercise will dramatically raise PAP if the vascular bed is reduced. Obliterative vascular diseases increase PVR by vascular occlusion, while diffuse interstitial diseases act primarily by compression and obliteration of small vessels. Hyperinflation in COPD increases PVR by compressing intraalveolar vessels, reducing cross-sectional area of the bed. It is now well established, however, that arteriolar constriction resulting from alveolar hypoxia is the predominant cause of pulmonary hypertension in chronic airway diseases.[1,10,27,28]

PULMONARY ARTERIOLAR CONSTRICTION

The most important cause of pulmonary vasoconstriction is alveolar hypoxia. The mechanism of hypoxic pulmonary vasoconstriction is unknown. It is thought to be due either to mediator release from some unknown effector cell or a direct action of hypoxia on pulmonary vascular smooth muscle.[29] The degree of hypoxic vasoconstriction is dependent primarily on the alveolar P_{O_2} and when alveolar P_{O_2} is < 55 torr, PAP rises sharply (Fig. 61-1). When PAP is greater than 40 mmHg due to hypoxia, arterial oxygen saturation is very likely less than 75%.[27] There is large individual variability in the hypoxic pressor response, and hypoxic vasoconstriction is enhanced by acidosis and blunted by alkalosis. Acidosis also has a mild direct pressor effect on the pulmonary circulation.[30] Extensive investigations into the mechanism of hypoxic vasoconstriction have shown that many local and circulating mediators of pulmonary vascular tone are capable of modulating the hypoxic pressor response but that no single mediator yet discovered is solely or predominantly responsible (Table 61-3).[29]

Hypoxic vasoconstriction in a region of lung where ventilation is diminished probably serves to maximize net arterial oxygenation by diverting blood from the hypoxic region to better-ventilated areas. Because the pulmonary vascular bed is capable of large recruitment, localized hypoxic vasoconstriction does not cause pulmonary hypertension. Generalized hypoxia causes generalized hypoxic vasoconstriction and the development of pulmonary hypertension (Fig. 61-2). In COPD, the first episodes of alveolar hypoxia may occur during sleep and gradually become more prevalent thereafter.[31] Any cause of alveolar hypoventilation (Table 61-1) can result in

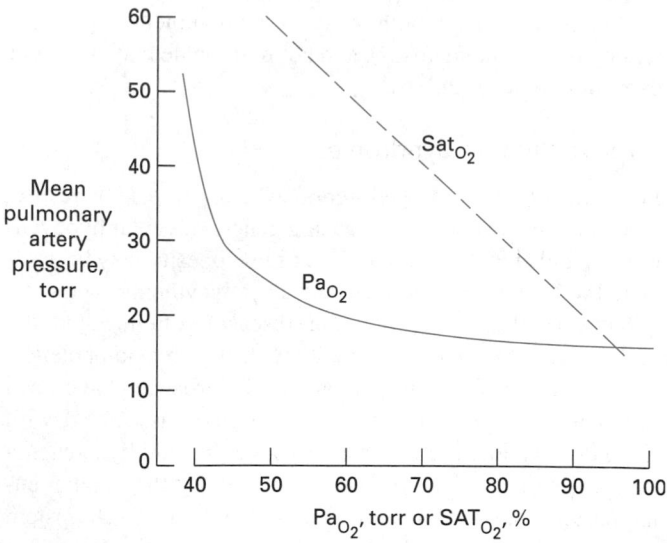

FIGURE 61-1
Pulmonary arterial pressure as a function of Pa_{O_2} or oxyhemoglobin saturation in humans. Pulmonary arterial pressure rises sharply as P decreases below 55 torr. (Redrawn from Reeves JT, Grover RF. High altitude pulmonary hypertension and pulmonary edema. *Prog Cardiol* 1975; 4:105, and from Burrows B. *Am Rev Respir Dis* 1974; 110:64, with permission.)

chronic cor pulmonale through the mechanism of hypoxic pulmonary vasoconstriction from entities as different as diffuse obstructive lung disease and kyphoscoliosis[9,15] (see also Chap. 59).

OTHER FORMS THAT INCREASE PULMONARY HYPERTENSION

Increases in cardiac output and blood volume or direct effects of acidosis and/or hypoxia on the myocardium may contribute to pulmonary hypertension. Increased blood flow such as occurs with exercise engenders an increased PAP, and in such a situation, the effects of hypoxia and acidosis will also be

TABLE 61-3

ENDOGENOUS PULMONARY VASOMOTOR TONE

Dilator	Constrictor
Beta-adrenergic	Alpha-adrenergic agonists
Histamine H_2	Histamine H_1
Prostacyclin (PGI$_2$), PGE$_1$	PGE$_2$, PGF$_{1a}$, Thromboxane A_2PGD$_2$
Acetylcholine[a]	Serotonin
Oxygen	Hypoxia
Bradykinin	Angiotensin II
Vasoactive intestinal polypeptide	Platelet activating factor
Nitric oxide	Endothelin
Atrial natriuretic peptide	Leukotriene C_4/D_4
Adenosine	Vasopressin

[a] The response of the pulmonary vascular bed is tone-dependent. When the pulmonary circulation is preconstricted, acetylcholine is a vasodilator through the release of endothelium-derived NO.

REGIONAL HYPOXIA

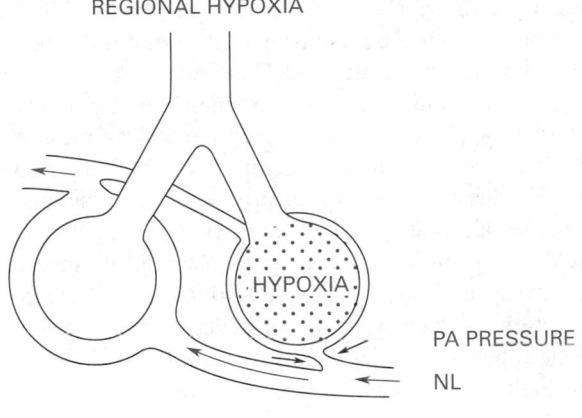

GENERALIZED HYPOXIA

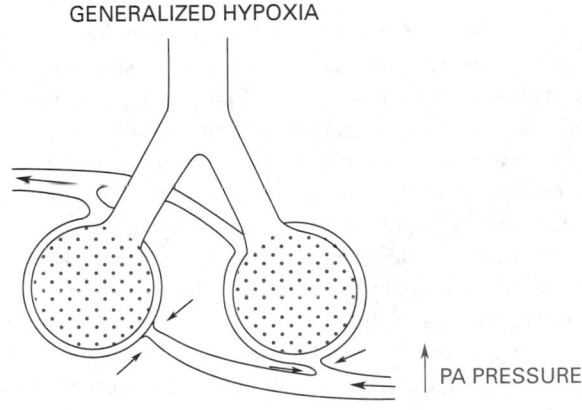

FIGURE 61-2

Hypoxic pulmonary vasoconstriction maximizes arterial oxygenation by diverting blood away from areas of regional hypoxia toward better ventilated zones. Generalized hypoxia causes generalized hypoxic vasoconstriction and results in pulmonary hypertension. (From Newman JH. Pulmonary vascular reactivity in primary pulmonary edema. *Semin Respir Med* 1983; 4:299, reproduced with permission of the publisher. Courtesy of JV Weil.)

exaggerated.[27] Sustained or repetitive severe hypoxemia causes secondary erythrocytosis. Blood viscosity increases rapidly after the hematocrit exceeds about 55 percent, raising PVR and also decreasing cerebral function. If left ventricular failure (LVF) is superimposed on an already reduced pulmonary vascular bed, pulmonary hypertension will be augmented by elevated downstream left atrial pressure. Once established, pulmonary hypertension may be self-perpetuating. A sustained increase in PAP in patients with diffuse lung disease causes muscular hypertrophy in the walls of small arteries, with extension of muscle toward alveolar vessels, further increasing PVR and PAP.[30] Chronic hypoxia alone results in muscularization of pulmonary arterioles and exaggerated increases in PAP with stimuli.[27,32]

Right Ventricular Response to Pulmonary Hypertension

The RV is thin-walled and eccentric and better able to handle an increase in volume load than to meet an increased pressure load.[10] The primary cause of RV strain and failure (RVF), therefore, is a chronic pressure load (afterload). Small increases in PAP may result in large increases in RV work. Pulmonary hypertension at rest indicates a high baseline resistance and small changes in blood flow will cause large increases in PAP.

Response of the right ventricle to pulmonary hypertension depends on the acuteness and severity of the pressure load. Acute cor pulmonale (see Chaps. 59 and 60) occurs after a sudden and severe stimulus (i.e., massive pulmonary emboli) with ventricular dilatation and failure but without hypertrophy. Chronic cor pulmonale, however, is associated with a more slowly evolving and slowly progressive hypertension,[33] and the response may include increased protein synthesis and RV hypertrophy (RVH).[34] The severity of the hypertension, the rapidity with which it becomes severe, and the possible eventual onset of RVF are influenced by factors that intercede intermittently, such as (1) *alterations in ventilatory function*, causing alveolar pressure changes with effects on chamber function.; (2) *alterations in gas exchange* with more or less severe hypoxemia, hypercapnia, and acidosis; and (3) *alterations in volume load* as influenced by exercise, heart rate, polycythemia, or renal retention of salt and water associated with cor pulmonale. At some stage, the myocardium is unable to function at the high pressure load, dilates, and fails. RV failure may occur relatively early in some patients with chronic bronchitis and emphysema because of sustained hypoxemia and hypercarbia, but it occurs later in patients with diffuse interstitial lung disease because the degree of RVH helps to maintain blood flow even when PAP is high.[35] Extreme pulmonary hypertension and RVH can occur in normal persons living at high altitude (>10,000 ft, or 3,033 m) with no evidence for heart failure.[36] Thus the RV can develop into an efficient high-pressure pump over time.

Left Ventricular Function in Cor Pulmonale

Dysfunction of the left ventricle (LV) occurs in some patients with cor pulmonale, but the evidence available indicates that cor pulmonale per se does not cause disease of the left heart. The likelihood in most cases is that left-sided heart dysfunction coexisting with cor pulmonale results from other known causes, such as coronary ischemia or systemic hypertension. LV failure is a serious complication in cor pulmonale because the increase in LA pressure and in lung water further impairs lung function, increases the work of breathing, increases PA pressure, impairs gas exchange, and may induce respiratory failure. When underlying disease of the LV is present, the direct effects of hypoxia, hypercapnia, and acidosis arising from primary lung disease may precipitate LV failure.[10,37,38]

Several lines of evidence point to mechanical effects of lung dysfunction and RV dilatation on performance of the LV.[38,39] Wide swings in transpulmonary pressure in obstructive lung disease can reduce LV filling and increase LV afterload.[40] Hypertrophy and elevated end-diastolic pressure of the RV in cor pulmonale can reduce LV compliance and impair LV filling through effects on the shared ventricular septum.[41,42] Despite these effects, most patients with chronic cor pulmonale demonstrate normal resting cardiac output, normal pulmonary artery wedge pressure, and normal resting LV ejection fraction.[40] The majority of patients with abnormal LV ejection fraction in either compensated or decompensated chronic lung disease probably have demonstrable coronary artery disease.

Edema Formation and Cor Pulmonale

Peripheral edema occurs in some cases of chronic cor pulmonale. The mechanism of edema formation is poorly understood but is probably related to increased systemic venous pressure, hypercarbia, and hypoxemia.[10,43] The presence of pulmonary hypertension per se does not appear to be sufficient to cause fluid retention until RA pressure becomes elevated. Decreased clearance of aldosterone from the passively congested liver contributes to salt retention but is likely not an initiating event. Plasma volume is, however, increased in chronic cor pulmonale.[44]

Hypercarbia stimulates plasma renin activity, and hypercarbic, edematous patients with COPD have increased plasma levels of aldosterone and antidiuretic hormone.[45] This pattern occurs despite oxygen therapy in these patients. Thus, not only increased salt retention but also impaired water excretion contributes to edema in chronic hypercapnia. Atrial natriuretic peptide is elevated in cor pulmonale in response to elevated RA pressure and perhaps acidosis.[10] Severe hypoxemia is associated with reduced renal blood flow and glomerular filtration rate (GFR) and a decrease in urine sodium excretion.[10] Other mechanisms of edema formation are increased systemic capillary hydrostatic pressure, related to increased venous pressure and blood volume; and perhaps inappropriate release of arginine vasopressin.[10] Many mechanisms appear to be operating to produce edema in chronic cor pulmonale, several of which are related to the primary pulmonary dysfunction, especially in COPD. The exact mechanisms and sequence of events leading to edema are difficult to determine in any specific case. Pulmonary edema and pleural effusion are not seen as a consequence of chronic cor pulmonale.

CLINICAL MANIFESTATIONS OF COR PULMONALE

Symptoms

Clinical manifestations of cor pulmonale are often obscured by the signs and symptoms of underlying disease and are, therefore, closely related to the pulmonary disease or disorder. It is necessary first to recognize the type and severity of lung disease and then to look for cor pulmonale.

There is no history that is specific for cor pulmonale. Episodes of leg edema, atypical chest pain, dyspnea on exertion, exercise-induced peripheral cyanosis, prior respiratory failure, and excessive daytime somnolence are all historical

clues suggesting the presence of cor pulmonale. Chest pain may be due to strain or distortion of the chest wall (musculoskeletal) or may be related to RV ischemia. Cough and complaints of easy fatigability are common. Some patients with nocturnal hypoventilation and sleep apnea may present with personality changes, mild systemic hypertension, and headache. Shortness of breath is nearly a universal symptom in cor pulmonale. The degree of activity that leads to dyspnea should be quantified, because patients reduce activities to avoid dyspnea. Thus, the naive question of whether a patient is short of breath may lead to a negative reply because the patient is performing less and less activity. Abdominal pain may result from liver and bowel congestion if RVF is present.

Physical Examination

The earliest signs are those associated with long-standing pulmonary hypertension. The most sensitive sign for pulmonary hypertension is an accentuated pulmonary component of S_2, which may also be palpable in the pulmonic area, and RV lift of the sternum may be seen. With very high PAP, characteristic diastolic and systolic murmurs of pulmonary valvular and tricuspid valvular regurgitation may be heard together with a systolic ejection sound and RV S_3 gallop. In overt RVF, cardiac enlargement, distended neck veins, hepatomegaly, and peripheral edema are present. Symptoms or signs suggestive of heart failure—such as dyspnea, orthopnea, peripheral edema, palpable liver, and distended neck veins—however, can be observed in patients with COPD without RVF. But when neck veins are distended during inspiration as well as expiration, RVF is more likely present. Hyperinflated lungs alter the position of the heart and frequently make the examination difficult. The apical impulse and the RV lift are often not palpable and the RV S_3 gallop may be heard in the epigastrium. The heart sounds may best be heard in the subxiphoid area. Extremities may be warm due to peripheral vasodilatation caused by hypercapnia, or there may be cyanosis due to low flow or hypoxemia.

ELECTROCARDIOGRAM

Electrocardiographic (ECG) patterns are influenced by many factors such as PAP, rotation, and displacement of the heart by hyperinflated lungs, arterial blood gases, myocardial ischemia, and metabolic disturbances. The value of the ECG in diagnosis of cor pulmonale, therefore, is dependent on the underlying disease and complicating conditions. Absence of changes indicating RV disease does not rule out cor pulmonale, since the ECG may be normal in advanced cor pulmonale. The classic RVH pattern is seen more often when there is anatomic restriction of the pulmonary vascular bed. An example of RVH is shown in Fig. 61-3. The standard criteria for RV enlargement were absent in two-thirds of patients with COPD who had RVH on postmortem examination.[1] It has been suggested that when classical RVH changes are absent, diagnosis should be based on the combination of rS in V_5 to V_6, RAD, qR in aVR, and "P pulmonale."[46] Tall peaked P waves in leads II and (AVF) may reflect positional changes rather than right atrial enlargement. Right bundle branch block (RBBB) occurs in about 15 percent of patients.[46] A pattern of S_1, Q_3, and T_3 carries reasonable sensitivity and specificity for cor pulmonale in COPD.[47] Arrhythmias are infrequent in uncomplicated cor pulmonale, but when present, they are mostly supraventricular and may reflect blood gas abnormalities, hypokalemia, or excess of drugs such as digitalis, theophylline, and beta agonists. Multifocal atrial tachycardia is associated with decompensated COPD and is best treated by attention to the underlying disease rather than by antiarrhythmic drugs. Ventricular arrhythmias, when they occur, are associated with a high mortality.

CHEST ROENTGENOGRAM

The radiographic findings of pulmonary hypertension in patients with normal lung parenchyma (such as in primary pulmonary hypertension) are well described (Fig. 61-4).[48,49] Most diseases that cause cor pulmonale have grossly abnormal chest roentgenograms, and the radiologic diagnosis of pulmonary hypertension in these diseases is more difficult. RV enlargement may be difficult to detect in the vertical heart of emphysema, and comparison with previous films may be helpful. In the most obvious cases of cor pulmonale, there is RV and PA enlargement, but pulmonary hypertension precedes RV dilatation. One indicator of pulmonary hypertension is measurement of the dimensions of the right and left PA. Enlargement is considered to exist if the diameter of the right descending PA is greater than 16 mm[47] and the left descending PA is greater than 18 mm.[50] These findings occurred in 43 of 46 patients with known pulmonary hypertension, but the true sensitivity and specificity of these measurements are not known.

ECHOCARDIOGRAM

Advances in echocardiography make this a useful test where cor pulmonale is suspected.[51] The standard M mode reliably detects RV dilatation and is best able to display the anteriormost RV wall near the interventricular septum. Two-dimensional echocardiography allows improved visualization of RV chamber size and wall thickness as well as changes in the interventricular septum resulting from RV hypertrophy.[51,52] Because the RV is asymmetric, measurement of RV

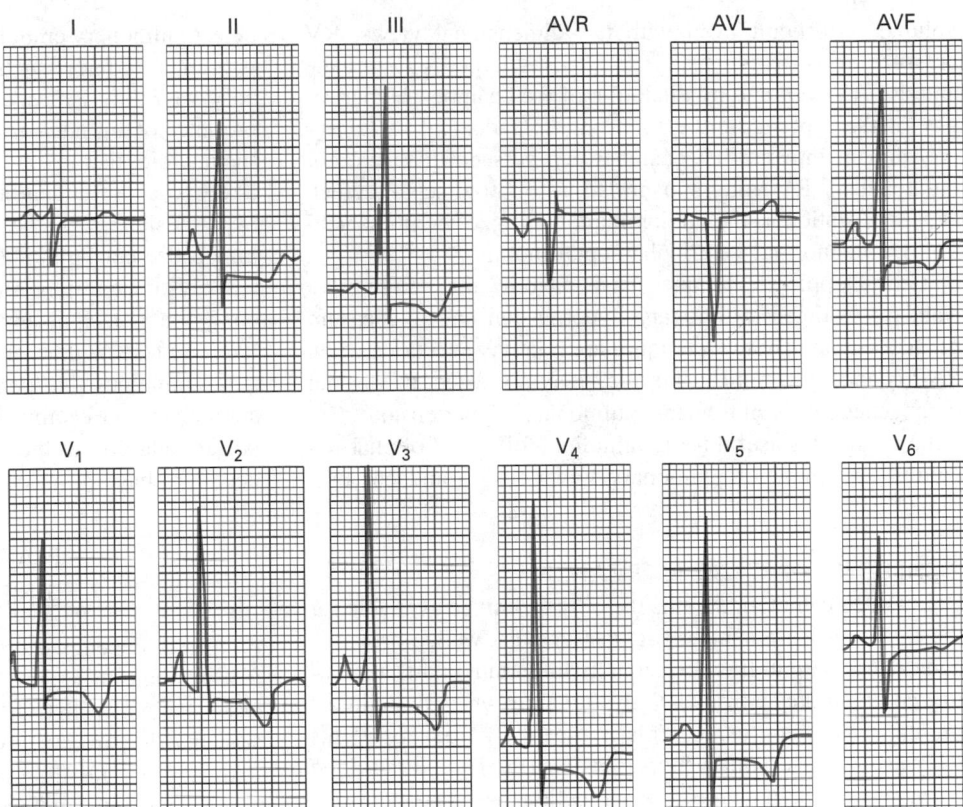

FIGURE 61-3
Electrocardiogram in a patient with cor pulmonale. The mean QRS axis is +120°. The tall, peaked P waves indicate right atrial enlargement. The tall R waves in leads V_1 to V_3 and deep S wave in V_6 and the associated T-wave changes indicate right ventricular hypertrophy. (From Voelkel NF, Reeves JT. Primary pulmonary hypertension. In: Moser KM, ed. *Pulmonary Vascular Diseases.* New York: Marcel Dekker; 1979, reproduced with permission of the publisher and the author. Courtesy of JR Pryor.)

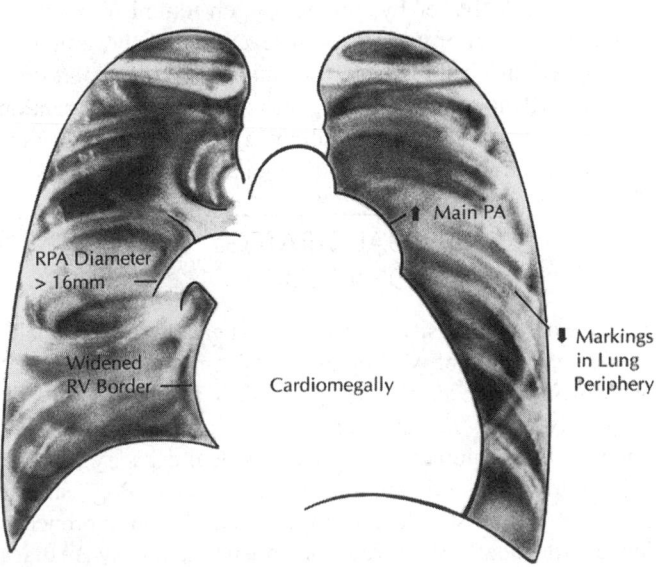

FIGURE 61-4
Classic features of the chest radiograph in severe pulmonary hypertension. The enlarged pulmonary arteries can be mistaken for hilar adenopathy and the large main pulmonary artery obscures the aortic arch. Right descending PA diameter >16 mm suggests severe pulmonary hypertension.

volume is difficult even with two-dimensional views. RV pressure overload is usually detected by hypertrophy of the anterior RV wall and by dilatation of the chamber. Hypertrophy of the septum can be found and paradoxical septal encroachment into the LV chamber can be seen in severe cor pulmonale.[53] RV volume overload, as in atrial septal defect, causes dilatation as the predominant finding, often in association with abnormal ventricular septal motion.[54]

Echo-Doppler techniques have become the noninvasive standard to detect pulmonary hypertension and to measure cardiac output. These techniques are relatively accurate when PAP is above 30 mmHg, but they may not detect milder but pathogenetically significant pulmonary hypertension.[55–57] Echo Doppler is useful for longitudinal follow-up of pharmacologic treatment of pulmonary hypertension and cor pulmonale.

RIGHT-SIDED HEART CATHETERIZATION

Right-sided catheterization is the only technique available for the direct measurement of PA pressure, PA wedge pressure, and cardiac output. It is occasionally important in differentiating cor pulmonale from LV dysfunction when the clinical presentation is confusing. This is especially true in patients with primary pulmonary hypertension (PPH) or unresolved pulmonary emboli, where airway function may appear normal, or with restrictive cardiomyopathy (see Chap. 75). In cor pulmonale, PA diastolic pressure is usually significantly higher than wedge pressure, unlike LVF or mitral stenosis, where the diastolic–wedge pressure gradient is smaller in most patients. Mean PAP can be very high in obliterative vascular diseases but only moderately high in interstitial lung diseases.[38,58] In COPD, PAP is related to the level of hypoxemia; it is not usually as severely increased as in PPH and will generally be decreased by chronic oxygen administration.[28,59] About 50 percent of patients with severe COPD have pulmonary hypertension at rest; in those patients with normal resting values, PAP may rise with exercise.[10,58] Serial catheterization in patients with COPD and pulmonary hypertension has revealed remarkable stability of pulmonary hemodynamics.[60]

USUAL STRATEGY OF WORKUP

Because of the diversity of diseases that cause cor pulmonale, no single strategy of workup exists. When lung parenchymal or airway disease is present, pulmonary function tests will frequently reveal the nature and degree of impairment.[61] Spirometry, lung volumes (functional residual capacity), $D_{L_{CO}}$, and an arterial blood sample for pH, P_{O_2}, and P_{CO_2} should be obtained. Transbronchial biopsy via a fiberoptic bronchoscope, bronchoalveolar lavage, and open lung biopsy are diagnostic options in patients with interstitial lung disease. If the hematocrit is above 50 percent, it gives a clue to the presence of chronic hypoxemia, nocturnal hypoventilation, or polycythemia vera. Patients with cryptogenic pulmonary hypertension should receive a perfusion radionuclide lung scan to detect pulmonary emboli or other causes of obstruction of the pulmonary arteries such as fibrosing mediastinitis. If pulmonary vasculitis is suspected, serum can be screened for the presence of antinuclear antibody, hepatitis B surface antigen, rheumatoid factor, and cryoglobulins. Factor V Leiden is likely to be a frequent abnormality in thrombotic pulmonary hypertension[62] and the antiphospholipid antibody syndrome may cause cor pulmonale.[63]

Polysomnography should be performed in patients with cor pulmonale and any sign or symptoms of sleep apnea. Exercise tests will occasionally reveal desaturation or ventilatory limitations that denote significant lung dysfunction not appreciated on examination at rest. Echo Doppler is an important addition to the noninvasive workup of a patient suspected to have pulmonary hypertension.

NATURAL HISTORY AND PROGNOSIS

Prognosis depends more on control of the underlying lung disease than on control of pulmonary hypertension in most cases. Patients with COPD have hypoxic pulmonary hypertension that is partially reversible, and RVF can be improved with appropriate therapy. Even with repeated episodes of RVF, some patients have long survivals.[1,10] The pink puffers tend to live longer than the blue bloaters.[10] Once RVF occurs, prognosis is poor, but 7- to 8-year survival after the diagnosis of cor pulmonale is reported.[64]

In patients with alveolar hypoventilation but no alteration in lung structure, the natural history is one of progressive worsening of pulmonary hypertension due to sustained hypoxemia, hypercapnia, and eventually, cor pulmonale and RVF. If alveolar ventilation is improved prior to the development of nonreversible changes in vessel walls, the prognosis is good.

MEDICAL TREATMENT

The underlying lung disease is the focus of therapy and is the best way to reduce the RV pressure work associated with the disease. If RVF has not appeared, a major goal is to prevent its onset. When it appears, it should be treated, but the response will be poor unless cardiac work is reduced by control of pulmonary hypertension.

Treatment to Decrease Pulmonary Hypertension

Relief of hypoxia is of prime importance in reducing pulmonary hypertension, both to prevent and to treat cor pulmonale. That may be done in two ways: (1) treatment of the underlying disease and (2) O_2 administration.[1,59] Neither will lower PAP in all patients because hypertension is often intractable in those with an anatomic restriction of the pulmonary vascular bed. Most patients with chronic cor pulmonale have a component of hypoxic pulmonary vasoconstriction, and all patients should be treated with oxygen in amounts adequate to restore arterial O_2 tension to greater than 60 torr. Corticosteroids may be helpful in some patients with interstitial lung disease and in patients with a bronchospastic component of COPD. Measures should be instituted to treat the systemic disease with which obliterative vascular disease is associated or to prevent further pulmonary emboli if that is the problem.

In COPD, the primary focus is relief of hypoxemia by restoration of effective ventilation or by O_2 administration. Net alveolar ventilation may be improved by therapy, including bronchodilators for bronchospasm, antibiotics to prevent or treat acute exacerbations of bronchitis, bronchial toilet for removal of secretions, and avoidance of airway irritants such as tobacco smoke. Nocturnal aspiration of gastric fluid is now known to be a common cause of exacerbation of chronic lung disease. Tranquilizers, sedatives, and narcotics should be avoided in unstable patients and patients with hypoventilation. Correction of hypoxia and acidosis may produce a striking reduction in PAP. In diseases that alter lung function but not structure, effective alveolar ventilation must be restored by treatment of the underlying disease or by use of mechanical ventilation. Short-term ventilatory stimulants may be useful in some cases of decreased ventilatory drives, although nasal continuous positive airway pressure (CPAP) has become the first choice in most cases of sleep apnea.[65]

Adequate oxygenation may prevent the onset of heart failure, both acutely and over a long period of time. Any patient with cor pulmonale and RVF should be given sufficient O_2 to restore P_{O_2} to levels above 60 torr, but it should be given cautiously when P_{CO_2} is high and the threat of respiratory acidosis is present. Oxygen therapy is usually well tolerated in patients with stable lung disease but not in patients with acute acidosis or respiratory muscle fatigue. When low-flow nasal O_2 causes significant increases in P_{CO_2}, mechanical ventilation may be required to relieve hypoxia. Studies have conclusively shown that home oxygen therapy, nocturnal or continuous, is beneficial in keeping patients with severe COPD functioning better for longer periods of time; it may be effective both in treating cor pulmonale and in postponing its onset.[27,28] Continuous 24 h/day oxygen therapy is the desired goal in most patients, because desaturation occurs during both sleep and physical activity.

Treatment of Heart Failure

Cor pulmonale is heart disease, and while treatment of the lung disease and relief of hypoxia are necessary to reduce cardiac work, general principles of management of heart failure apply. Diuretics and phlebotomy can be appropriate measures for treatment of RVF. Pulmonary vasodilators are efficacious in some patients with primary pulmonary hypertension but are of unproven value in cor pulmonale from COPD.[66]

Beneficial effects of digitalis are not as obvious as in LVF, and arrhythmias caused by digitalis may occur at relatively low serum levels in patients with hypoxia and acidosis. Susceptibility to digitalis intoxication is enhanced in pulmonary

disease.[67] Its use in cor pulmonale, therefore, has been controversial. Nevertheless, studies have shown that *digitalis improves RV function in cor pulmonale, and it is an appropriate drug for treatment of RVF when given cautiously and at carefully controlled dosage levels.*[68] It should not be used during the acute phases of respiratory insufficiency when there are large fluctuations in levels of hypoxemia and acidosis but is reserved for the time when the patient is stabilized. Heart rate in this setting cannot be used as a guide for the level of digitalization. It is also reasonable to question whether or not patients with cor pulmonale who continue to have overt RVF after relief of hypoxemia in intensive therapy for the underlying lung disease will benefit from the use of digitalis. Digitalis is appropriate if there is known or suspected concurrent LV systolic dysfunction.

Vasodilator therapy to reduce RV afterload has been recognized as a potential treatment strategy for several years. Vasodilator therapy has the disadvantage of being secondary therapy that is not aimed at the primary lung dysfunction. Vasodilator use has not become widespread because of small observed reductions in pulmonary hypertension and occasional worsening of gas exchange.[66]

Diuretics are effective in the treatment of RVF, and indications for their use are the same as in other forms of heart disease. Pulmonary function is improved by diuretics in patients with COPD who have hypervolemia.[69] The effects of diuretics should be carefully monitored by measurement of arterial P_{O_2}, P_{CO_2}, and pH, since acid-base abnormalities are often present in cor pulmonale. Contraction alkalosis can be a problem in hypercarbic patients with a large buffer base who have had vigorous diuresis.

When the hematocrit is above 55 to 60 percent, phlebotomy may reduce PAP and PVR and possibly improve RV function.[70] The phlebotomy should be in small volumes (200 to 300 mL) and done cautiously.

SURGICAL TREATMENT

There is no surgical treatment for most diseases that cause chronic cor pulmonale. Pulmonary embolectomy is extremely efficacious for unresolved pulmonary emboli causing chronic thrombotic pulmonary hypertension (Chap. 60). Adenoidectomy in children with chronic airway obstruction and uvulopalatopharyngeoplasty in selected patients with sleep apnea can relieve cor pulmonale related to hypoventilation. Single-lung, double-lung, and heart-lung transplantations are all used for salvage in the terminal phase of several diseases complicated by cor pulmonale.[71] *The diseases most commonly treated by lung transplantation are primary pulmonary hypertension, emphysema, idiopathic pulmonary fibrosis, and cystic fibrosis.* Two-year survival for single and double lung transplant has risen to 60 percent, still lower than the approximately 80 percent for heart transplant alone. One interesting finding is that the RV can recover function after lung transplant even after the chronic stress of severe pulmonary hypertension.

Volume-reduction surgery for selected cases of emphysema improves ventilatory function and gas exchange, and the long-term benefit of this approach is under study.[72]

REFERENCES

1. Palevsky HI, Fishman AP. Chronic cor pulmonale. *JAMA* 1990; 263:2347–2354.

2. Richards DW. The right heart and the lung with some observations on teleology: The J. Burns Amberson Lecture. *Am Rev Respir Dis* 1966; 94:691–702.

3. Osler W. *The Principles and Practice of Medicine*. New York: Appleton; 1892:628–640.

4. McGinn S, White PD. Acute cor pulmonale resulting from pulmonary embolism, its clinical recognition. *JAMA* 1935; 104:1473–1480.

5. Harvey W. *Exercitatio de Motu Cordis et Sanguinis in Animalibus*. Francofurti: Guilielem Fitzeri; 1628 (Leake CD, transl). Springfield, IL: Charles C Thomas; 1928.

6. Standards for the Diagnosis and Care of Patients with Chronic Obstructive Pulmonary Disease. ATS Statement. *Am J Respir Crit Care Med* 1995; 152(55):S77–S120.

7. Chronic Obstructive Lung Disease. The health consequences of smoking: A report of the Surgeon General. Rockville, MD: U.S. Department of Health and Human Services; 1984:189.

8. Gazes PC. *Clinical Cardiology: A Bedside Approach*. Philadelphia: Lea & Febiger; 1990:301–320.

9. Thurlbeck WM. Pathophysiology of chronic obstructive pulmonary disease. *Clin Chest Med* 1990; 11:389–403.

10. MacNee W. Pathophysiology of cor pulmonale in chronic obstructive pulmonary disease. State of the art. *Am J Pulm Crit Care Med* 1994; 150(4):833–892, 1158–1163.

11. Filley GF, Beckwitt HJ, Reeves JT, Mitchell RS. Chronic obstructive bronchopulmonary disease. II. Oxygen transport in two clinical types. *Am J Med* 1968; 44:26–38.

12. Mountain R, Zwillich C, Weil J. Hypoventilation in obstructive lung disease. *N Engl J Med* 1978; 298:521–525.

13. Schwarz MI, King TE Jr, eds. *Interstitial Lung Diseases*. St Louis: Mosby-Year Book, 1993.

14. Winterbauer RH, Hammer SP, Hallman KO, Hays JE, Pardee NE, Morgan EH, et al. Diffuse interstitial pneumonitis, clinicopathological correlations in 20 patients treated with prednisone/azathropine. *Am J Med* 1978; 65:661–672.

15. Bergofsky EH. Respiratory failure in disorders of the thoracic cage. *Am Rev Respir Dis* 1979; 119:643–669.

16. Burwell CS, Robin ED, Whaley RD, Bickelmann AG. Extreme obesity associated with alveolar hypoventilation—A Pickwickian syndrome. *Am J Med* 1956; 21:811–818.

17. Sackner MA, Landa J, Forrest T, Greeneltch D. Periodic sleep apnea: Chronic sleep deprivation related to intermittent upper airway obstruction and central nervous system disturbance. *Chest* 1975; 67:164–171.

18. Fanburg BL, Sicilian L, eds. *Respiratory Dysfunction in Neuromuscular Diseases*. Philadelphia: Saunders; 1994.

19. Gerry JL, Buckley BH, Hutchins GM. Clinicopathologic analysis of cardiac dysfunction in 52 patients with sickle cell anemia. *Am J Cardiol* 1978; 42:211–216.

20. Weil JV, Castro O, Malik AB, Rodgers G, Bonds DR, Jacobs TP. Pathogenesis of lung disease in sickle hemoglobinopathies. *Am Rev Respir Dis* 1993; 148:249–256.

21. Wagenvoort CA. Pulmonary venoocclusive disease, entity or syndrome? *Chest* 1976; 69:82–86.

22. Lange PA, Stoller JK. The hepatopulmonary syndrome. *Ann Intern Med* 1995; 122:521–529.

23. Segel N, Kay JM, Bayley TJ, Paton A. Pulmonary hypertension with hepatic cirrhosis. *Br Heart J* 1968; 30:575–578.

24. Coplan N, Shinony R, Ioachim H. Primary pulmonary hypertension associated with human immunodeficiency viral infection. *Am J Med* 1990; 89:96–99.

25. Perez D, Kramer N. Pulmonary hypertension in systemic lupus erythematosus: Report of four cases and review of the literature. *Semin Arthritis Rheum* 1981; 11:177–181.

26. Brenot F, Simonneau G. Risk factors for primary pulmonary hypertension. In: Rubin LJ, Rich S, eds. *Primary Pulmonary Hypertension*: Vol

99. *Lung Biology in Health and Disease*. New York: Marcel Dekker; 1997:131–147.

27. Burrows B. Arterial oxygenation and pulmonary hemodynamics in patients with chronic airways obstruction. *Am Rev Respir Dis* 1974; 110(suppl):64–70.

28. Nocturnal Oxygen Therapy Trial Group. Continuous or nocturnal oxygen therapy in hypoxemic chronic obstructive lung disease: A clinical trial. *Ann Intern Med* 1980; 93:391–398.

29. Voelkel N. Mechanisms of hypoxic pulmonary vasoconstriction. *Am Rev Respir Dis* 1986; 133:1186.

30. Enson Y, Guintini C, Lewis ML, Morris TQ, Ferrer MI, Harvey RM. The influence of hydrogen ion concentration and hypoxia on the pulmonary circulation. *J Clin Invest* 1964; 43:1146–1162.

31. Boysen PG, Block AJ, Wynne JW, Hunt LA, Flick MR. Nocturnal pulmonary hypertension in patients with chronic obstructive pulmonary disease. *Chest* 1979; 76:536–542.

32. Fried R, Meyrick B, Rabinovitch M, Reid L. Polycythemia and the acute hypoxic response in awake rats following chronic hypoxia. *J Appl Physiol* 1983; 55:1167–1172.

33. Enson Y. Pulmonary heart disease: Relation of pulmonary hypertension to abnormal lung structure and function. *Bull NY Acad Med* 1977; 53:551–566.

34. Meerson FX. *The Failing Heart: Adaptation and Maladaptation*. New York: Raven Press; 1983:51.

35. Enson Y, Thomas HM, Bosken CH, Wood JA, Leroy EC, Blanc WA, et al. Pulmonary hypertension in interstitial lung disease: Relation of vascular resistance to abnormal lung structure. *Trans Assoc Am Phys* 1975; 88:248–255.

36. Grover RF. Pulmonary circulation in animals and man in high altitude. *Ann NY Acad Sci* 1965; 127:632–639.

37. Fishman AP. The left ventricle in chronic bronchitis and emphysema. *N Engl J Med* 1971; 285:402–404.

38. Murphy ML, Adamson J, Hutcheson F. Left ventricular hypertrophy in patients with chronic bronchitis and emphysema. *Ann Intern Med* 1974; 81:307–313.

39. Matthay RA, Berger HO. Cardiovascular function in cor pulmonale. *Clin Chest Med* 1983; 4:269–295.

40. Buda AJ, Pinsky MR, Ingels NB, Daughters GT, Stinson EB, Alderman EL. Effect of intrathoracic pressure on left ventricular performance. *N Engl J Med* 1979; 301:453–459.

41. Bermis CE, Sehur JR, Borkenhagen D, Sonnenblick EH, Urschel CW. Influence of right ventricular filling pressure on left ventricular pressure and dimension. *Circ Res* 1974; 34:498–504.

42. Steele PS, Ellis JH, VanDyke D, Sutton F, Creagh E, Davies H. Left ventricular ejection fraction in severe chronic obstructive airways disease. *Am J Med* 1975; 59:21–28.

43. Bichet D, Schrier RS. Cardiac failure, liver disease and nephrotic syndrome. In: Schrier JR, Gottschalk C, eds. *Diseases of the Kidney*. Boston: Little Brown; 1993:2453–2491.

44. Harvey RM, Ferrer MI, Richards DW, Cournand A. Influence of chronic pulmonary disease on the heart and circulation. *Am J Med* 1951; 10:719–738.

45. Farber MO, Roberts LR, Weinberger MH, Robertson GL, Fineberg NS, Manfredi F. Abnormalities of sodium and H_2O handling in chronic obstructive lung disease. *Arch Intern Med* 1982; 142:1326–1330.

46. Padmavati S, Raizada V. Electrocardiogram in chronic cor pulmonale. *Br Heart J* 1972; 34:658–667.

47. Murphy ML, Hutcheson F. The electrocardiographic diagnosis of right ventricular hypertrophy in chronic obstructive pulmonary disease. *Chest* 1974; 65:622–627.

48. Moore CB, Kraus WL, Dork DS. The relationship between pulmonary arterial pressure and roentgenographic appearance in mitral stenosis. *Am Heart J* 1959; 58:576–581.

49. Chang CH. The normal roentgenographic measurement of the right descending pulmonary artery in 1,085 cases. *Am J Roentgenol* 1962; 87:929–935.

50. Matthay RA, Schwarz MI, Ellis JH. Pulmonary artery hypertension in chronic obstructive pulmonary disease: Chest radiographic assessment. *Invest Radiol* 1981; 16:95–100.

51. Cacho A, Prokash R, Sarne R, Kaushik VS. Usefulness of two-dimensional echocardiography in diagnosing right ventricular hypertrophy. *Chest* 1983; 84:154–157.

52. Hagan A, DeMaria A. Diseases of the right heart. In: *Clinical Applications of Two Dimensional Echocardiography*. Boston: Little Brown; 1985:270.

53. Bradley TC. Right and left ventricular functional impairment and sleep apnea. *Clin Chest Med* 1992; 13:459–479.

54. Louie EK, Rich S, Levitshy S, Brundage BH. Doppler echocardiographic demonstration of the differential effects of RV pressure and volume overload on LV geometry and filling. *J Am Coll Cardiol* 1992; 19:84–91.

55. Kitabatake A, Michitoshi I, Asao M, Masuyama T, Tanouchi J, Morita T, et al. Noninvasive evaluation of pulmonary hypertension by a pulsed Doppler technique. *Circulation* 1983; 68:302–309.

56. Schiller N. Pulmonary artery pressure estimation by Doppler and two-dimensional echocardiography. *Cardiol Clin* 1990; 8:277–287.

57. Bishop JM, Cross KW. Use of other physiological variables to predict pulmonary arterial pressure in patients with chronic respiratory disease: Multi-center study. *Eur Heart J* 1981; 2:509–517.

58. Schrijen F, Uffholtz H, Polu JM, Poincelot F. Pulmonary and systemic hemodynamic evolution in chronic bronchitis. *Am Rev Respir Dis* 1978; 117:25–31.

59. Tarpy SP, Edlli BR. Long-term oxygen therapy. *N Engl J Med* 1995; 333:710–715.

60. Weitzenblum E, Loiseau A, Hirth C, Mirhom R, Rasaholinjanahary J. Course of pulmonary hemodynamics in patients with chronic obstructive pulmonary disease. *Chest* 1979; 75:656–662.

61. Crapo RO. Pulmonary function testing. *N Engl J Med* 1994; 331:25–31.

62. Ridker P, Hennekens CH, Lindpaintner K, Stampfer MJ, Eisenberg PR, Miletich JP. Mutation in the gene coding for coagulation factor V and the risk of infarction, stroke, and venous thrombosis in apparently healthy men. *N Engl J Med* 1995; 332:912–917.

63. Asherson RA, Khamashta MA, Ordi-Ros, Derkgen RH, Machin SJ, Barguinero J, et al. The primary antiphospholipid syndrome: Major clinical and serological features. *Medicine* 1989; 68:366–374.

64. Ferrer M. Cor pulmonale (pulmonary heart disease): Present-day status. *Am Heart J* 1975; 89:657–664.

65. Kryger MH. Management of obstructive sleep apnea. *Clin Chest Med* 1992; 13:481–492.

66. Wiedemann H, Matthay R. Cor pulmonale in chronic obstructive pulmonary disease circulatory pathophysiology and management. *Clin Chest Med* 1990; 11:523–545.

67. Green LH, Smith TW. The use of digitalis in patients with pulmonary disease. *Ann Intern Med* 1977; 87:459–465.

68. Smith DE, Bissett JK, Phillips JR, Doherty IE, Murphy ML. Improved right ventricular systolic time intervals after digitalis in patients with cor pulmonale and chronic obstructive pulmonary disease. *Am J Cardiol* 1978; 41:1299–1304.

69. Gertz I, Hedenstierna G, Wester PO. Improvement in pulmonary function with diuretic therapy in the hypervolemic and polycythemic patient with chronic obstructive pulmonary disease. *Chest* 1979; 75:146–151.

70. Weisse AB, Moschos CB, Frank MJ, Levinson GE, Cannilla JE, Regan TJ. Hemodynamic effects of staged hematocrit reduction in patients with stable cor pulmonale and severely elevated hematocrit levels. *Am J Med* 1975; 58:92–98.

71. Patterson GA, Cooper JD. Lung transplantation. *Chest Surg Clin North Am* 3; 1:1995.

72. Cooper JD, Trulock EP, Triantafillon AN, Patterson GA, Pohl MS, Deloney PA, et al. Bilateral pneumectomy (volume reduction) for chronic obstructive pulmonary disease. *J Thorac Cardiovasc Surg* 1995; 109:106–116.

VALVULAR HEART DISEASE

62

ACUTE RHEUMATIC FEVER

Edward L. Kaplan

Acute rheumatic fever, a sequel to group A streptococcal upper respiratory tract infection, ranks among the leading causes of cardiovascular disease in the world today. In the developing countries, which account for approximately two-thirds of the world's population, rheumatic fever is responsible for almost half of cardiovascular disease in all age groups and is the leading cause of cardiovascular death in the first five decades of life.[1-3] The importance of this disease is further emphasized by the mid-1980s resurgence of rheumatic fever in the United States, when increases in the number of cases occurred in many different states.[4-6] The resurgence in middle class families near the close of the 20th century also emphasizes the many remaining unsolved aspects of this unique illnes.[7]

ETIOLOGIC AGENT AND EPIDEMIOLOGY

The epidemiology of acute rheumatic fever (ARF) is that of an infectious disease, group A streptococcal tonsillopharyngitis. Since Lancefield, more than six decades ago, described a method of differentiating the hemolytic streptococci into serologic groups,[8] the association between group A beta-hemolytic streptococci (GAS) and ARF has been recognized. Although a possible role for other etiologic agents, such as viruses, has been considered, the evidence is not supportive.[9]

Rheumatic fever follows only GAS upper respiratory tract infection, not streptococcal pyoderma or impetigo. GAS pharyngitis is primarily, but not exclusively, a disease of children. Just as the highest incidence of group A streptococcal sore throat occurs in children between the ages of 5 and 15, the peak age for attacks of acute rheumatic fever is in this same age range. Although attacks of ARF are concentrated in children, it is not uncommon for outbreaks of streptococcal pharyngitis (and ARF) also to occur in adults, for example, in military recruits.[10]

It has been shown that 3 percent of individuals with true streptococcal infection of the upper respiratory tract develop ARF during epidemics. Other data suggest that, in some in-

stances, the attack rate may be less than 3 percent in children. These latter data probably describe a large percentage of streptococcal carriers, individuals who harbor the organism in their upper respiratory tract but appear to be at minimal danger to themselves of developing ARF and do not appear to readily spread the organism to close family or school contacts.[11]

In the 1940s, 1950s, and early 1960s, ARF was common in the United States. Reliable incidence rates of 20 to 50 per 100,000 population per year were reported from various sources in this country.[12]

Beginning in the mid-1960s, the incidence of ARF in the United States decreased to very low levels, reaching rates of less than 1 per 100,000 population per year by the late 1970s.[13,14] In contrast, the incidence of acute rheumatic fever has remained alarmingly high in many developing countries.[15] It has been suggested that incidence rates in some of these countries have increased with trends toward urbanization; this is not very different from what is thought to have happened at the time of the industrial revolution in Great Britain and the United States. Data collected during the 1970s and 1980s from various areas of the world, particularly developing countries, continue to show incidence rates of over 20 per 100,000 population per year.[15] Furthermore, prevalence rates for rheumatic heart disease among children in many developing countries remain high; figures of over 30 per 1000 schoolchildren have been reported.[16] The economic impact on these countries is significant.

Although the incidence of ARF fell to very low levels in the United States by the late 1970s, beginning in 1984 a resurgence occurred in geographically separated areas of the country.[2,3,6,17-19] The reasons for the resurgence are as yet unexplained. One possible explanation is the appearance of more virulent strains of group A streptococci in the population.[20] In fact, published data suggest that multiple serotypes were involved in the late-1980s resurgence. Of special interest is that ARF has always been considered a disease associated with poverty, but the 1980s resurgence in the United States primarily affected middle-class families with ready access to medical care.[7,17,2]

PATHOGENESIS

Although clearly related to the antecedent group A streptococcal upper respiratory tract infection, the pathogenetic mechanism or mechanisms responsible for the development of ARF after a latent period of several weeks remain unknown. Numerous theories have been proposed. The failure to provide a satisfactory explanation for the pathogenesis of ARF is related to a lack of experimental or clinical evidence of a specific role for any known somatic or extracellular antigen of the group A streptococci. Furthermore, the lack of a suitable experimental animal model for laboratory study has been an important impediment to study of this disease. Because of this, epidemiological approaches can add significant information.[22]

Early hypotheses centered around the organism itself; there was enthusiasm in the late 1930s for implicating direct infection by the group A beta-hemolytic streptococcus of the heart, valves, and tissues. This hypothesis could not be proved, however, and is no longer seriously considered.[23]

A second major group of hypotheses to explain the pathogenesis of ARF involves toxins produced by the group A streptococcus. Among the most frequently considered toxins is the oxygen-labile streptolysin O. This antigen is known to be directly cardiotoxic in experimental animals and in tissue culture.[24] Numerous other toxins and enzymes produced by group A streptococci have been implicated. Injection of many of these antigens into experimental animals has produced tissue damage, but never a clinical syndrome identical to ARF. At the present time, there is no suitable experimental animal model for the laboratory study of ARF.

Perhaps the most widely held group of hypotheses to explain the pathogenesis of ARF is that which includes a qualitatively and/or quantitatively abnormal immunologic response to either extracellular or somatic antigens of the group A streptococcus. For example, it has been shown that the group-specific carbohydrate of the group A streptococcal cell wall is antigenically similar to glycoprotein found in bovine and human heart valves.[25] It has been hypothesized that, with exposure to group A streptococci during infection, "antigenic mimicry" leads to an autoimmune-like reaction by the human host and results in valvulitis, ultimately leading to rheumatic valvular heart disease. In support of the existence of this unusual immune response are studies showing that antibodies to the group A carbohydrate moiety of the streptococcal cell wall appear to persist longer in individuals with rheumatic valvular heart disease than in individuals with only uncomplicated streptococcal pharyngitis or even acute post-streptococcal glomerulonephritis.[26] The finding that group A streptococci carbohydrate antibodies decreased after surgical removal of the rheumatic mitral valve in individuals with chronic rheumatic heart disease provides further support for this concept.[27]

Among the other antigens proposed to play a role in the abnormal immune response in the pathogenesis of ARF are the streptococcal cell membranes, which have been shown to cross-react with myocardial sarcolemma.[28] This cross-reactive or heart-reactive antibody was originally described in the early 1960s as being related to the cell wall, but later studies suggest that the cross-reaction is due to the cell membrane. This hypothesis suggests that an "autoimmune" reaction following a GAS infection results in the carditis seen in patients with ARF. Similarly, a cross-reactive antigen in the brain has been reported, and antibodies to the caudate nucleus have been reported in persons with Sydenham's chorea.

Genetic predisposition to the development of ARF has been very important among the hypotheses proposed to explain this mysterious illness. Numerous investigators have shown that ARF tends to be found in multiple members of some families, but the actual genetics have never been fully explained. Recently, a marker on the surface of non-T lymphocytes has been shown to be present in a majority of patients with ARF or rheumatic heart disease (when compared with control patients).[29,30] Several studies have shown that 75 percent or more of patients with ARF and/or rheumatic heart disease have lymphocytes that test positive for this marker when a monoclonal antibody is used. Furthermore, family studies have indicated a higher prevalence of positivity in families with ARF patients than in control families. It has been suggested that these markers may assist in identifying individuals who process streptococcal antigens in an abnormal, but as yet incompletely defined, fashion. These findings require further confirmation in a variety of populations and ethnic groups.

In summary, although many hypotheses have been suggested to explain how the GAS triggers the pathologic processes of ARF, the pathogenetic mechanisms responsible for the development of this disease remain unexplained.

DIAGNOSIS OF ACUTE RHEUMATIC FEVER

The diagnosis of acute ARF is a clinical one, but requires supporting laboratory confirmation. Although Aschoff bodies have been considered to be pathognomonic of rheumatic heart disease, controversy does exist. They are seldom observed today because deaths during acute ARF are extremely rare. It is important to note again that there is no specific laboratory test that can confirm the diagnosis. This fact is often overlooked.

In 1944, T. Duckett Jones published the Jones Criteria, describing a constellation of clinical and laboratory findings frequently found in association with ARF. Revisions and modifications of the Jones Criteria have been made periodically since the original publication in 1944. The most significant changes were published in 1965 by the American Heart Association, modified slightly in 1984,[31] and most recently updated in 1992.[32] These changes are referred to as the Revised Jones Criteria and are shown in Table 62-1. It should be noted that former guidelines included previous rheumatic fever or rheumatic heart disease as major or minor manifestations. The current (1992) guidelines are intended only for the diagnosis of initial attacks of ARF; therefore, previous ARF and rheumatic heart disease are not included as manifestations.

There are five major criteria and a number of minor criteria. In addition, there is the requirement that supporting evidence of an *antecedent group A beta-hemolytic streptococcal infection must be present*. The presence of one major and two minor criteria *or* two major criteria is necessary for the diagnosis of

TABLE 62-1

GUIDELINES FOR THE DIAGNOSIS OF INITIAL ATTACK
OF RHEUMATIC FEVER (JONES CRITERIA, 1992 UPDATE)[a]

MAJOR MANIFESTATIONS

Carditis
Polyarthritis
Chorea
Erythema marginatum
Subcutaneous nodules

MINOR MANIFESTATIONS

Clinical findings
   Arthralgia
   Fever
Laboratory findings
   Elevated levels of acute-phase reactants
      Erythrocyte sedimentation rate
      C-reactive protein
   Prolonged PR interval

SUPPORTING EVIDENCE OF ANTECEDENT GROUP A
STREPTOCOCCAL INFECTION

Positive throat culture or rapid streptococcal antigen test
  results
Elevated or rising streptococcal antibody titer

[a] If supported by evidence of preceding group A streptococcal infection, the presence of two major manifestations or of one major and two minor manifestations indicates a high probability of acute rheumatic fever. See text for details.

Source: The Special Writing Group of the Committee on Rheumatic Fever, Endocarditis, and Kawasaki Disease of the Council on Cardiovascular Disease in the Young of the American Heart Association.[32] Reproduced with permission from the *Journal of the American Medical Association* and the American Heart Association.

ARF. It must be remembered, however, that there are many diseases that can fulfill the Jones Criteria and yet do not represent ARF. Illnesses such as infective endocarditis, serum sickness, connective tissue diseases, Lyme disease and rheumatoid arthritis are only a few of the many diseases that can mimic ARF and even fulfill the Jones Criteria unless very carefully applied. Of special interest is the fact that ARF may present in unusual ways, and therefore a modification of the Jones Criteria by the World Health Organization may prove clinically helpful.[15] Three categories of patients have been singled out for special consideration: patients in whom chorea is the sole manifestation, those with insidious or late-onset carditis, and those experiencing rheumatic recurrences.

Rheumatic fever produces a *pancarditis*, affecting pericardium, epicardium, myocardium, and endocardium. In very fulminant cases, the cardiac manifestations may mimic viral myocarditis, but often the manifestations may be very subtle. A transient murmur of mitral regurgitation and/or a pericardial friction rub may be all that is evident. Among the more frequent cardiac findings is mitral regurgitation; isolated aortic regurgitation is unusual in first attacks of ARF. Hemodynamically significant stenotic lesions of the aortic or mitral valves also are not seen in first attacks. In contrast, in individuals who have had several previous attacks of ARF and have chronic rheumatic heart disease, both stenosis and regurgitation may be seen. The valves of the right side of the heart are not infrequently involved in patients who have had multiple recurrent attacks. In the patient with previous attacks of ARF the differentiation between acute carditis and congestive cardiac failure may be very difficult. Echocardiography may be helpful for such patients.

The *arthritis* associated with ARF is almost always an exquisitely painful migratory polyarthritis, most often affecting the larger joints such as ankles, knees, elbows, shoulders, and wrists. It is important to recognize the migratory nature. The arthritis may or may not be symmetrical. Involvement of a single joint is rare in ARF. Occasionally, the small joints of the hands or feet may be affected. In the latter instances, other diagnoses should be considered. The arthritis of rheumatic fever does not lead to chronic joint involvement (see "Natural History," below).

Perhaps the most common error made by physicians during the process of establishing a diagnosis of ARF is the administration of salicylates early in the course of the disease, before there is sufficient time for the arthritis to manifest itself completely. Salicylates should be withheld from patients until the diagnosis is clarified. (Some physicians feel that all anti-inflammatory drugs should be withheld.) If the joints are very painful, codeine or a similar drug can relieve the pain without influencing the progression of the disease. The possible beneficial effects of acetaminophen and the nonsteroidal anti-inflammatory agents have not been carefully studied in patients with ARF.

Erythema marginatum, an unusual rash seen primarily on the trunk, is evident in less than 10 percent of cases of ARF. Early in its development, erythema marginatum may look like pink macules, but with time, the rash shows blanching in its center with the outer borders forming an irregular pattern. It may be evanescent and can be accentuated or elicited by application of heat. The lesions are not pruritic, and there is no induration. Although unusual, erythema marginatum may be isolated as a major manifestation of ARF. It is not difficult to confuse erythema marginatum with the skin manifestations of Lyme disease.

Subcutaneous nodules are small, pea-size nodules, appearing over extensor surfaces of joints such as wrists and elbows, and even on the spine (Fig. 62-1). These are painless and nonfixed. These are rare (less than 5 percent of cases) and generally are seen only in persons with significant long-standing rheumatic carditis.

Sydenham's chorea is an unusual manifestation of ARF. There is a long latent period of perhaps several months following the streptococcal infection before this becomes evident. Chorea is often associated with emotional lability, and it may be either bilateral or unilateral. The diagnosis of Sydenham's chorea is one of exclusion. It is imperative that the physician, often in consultation with a neurologist, actively eliminate other causes of chorea. Since there is a prolonged latent period, the evidence of a preceding streptococcal infection is frequently not present, making the diagnosis even more difficult. The *minor manifestations of an initial attack of acute rheu-*

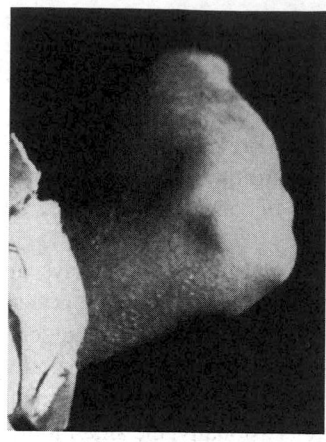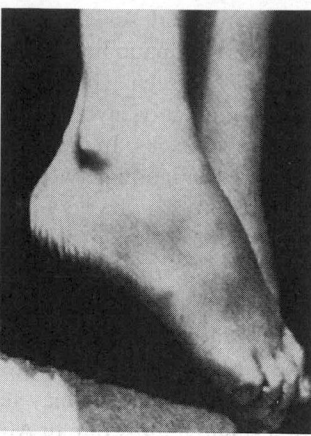

FIGURE 62-1

Photograph showing joints of a child with rheumatic nodules of the elbow, ankle, and foot. Note the nodule on the Achilles tendon. (From White PD. *Heart Disease*. Boston: Macmillan; 1931: facing 336. Reproduced with permission from the publisher and author.)

matic fever include arthralgia, fever, a prolonged PR interval on the electrocardiogram, and elevated levels of acute-phase reactants (such as the erythrocyte sedimentation rate or C-reactive protein). In the 1984 guidelines,[31] which did not differentiate between initial and recurrent attacks of rheumatic fever, a history of rheumatic fever or rheumatic heart disease was also considered a minor criterion. In the 1992 guidelines,[32] which update guidelines only for an initial attack, this is obviously not included.

Minor manifestations are so named because of their lack of specificity. They are included as a part of many clinical syndromes and illnesses. Of particular importance is the differentiation between arthritis and arthralgia. It must be remembered that if arthritis is included as a major criterion, arthralgia cannot be included among the minor criteria in the patient. A prolonged PR interval is very nonspecific and has been associated with many disorders; the same is true for the sedimentation rate and C-reactive protein. In evaluating a patient for rheumatic fever, the minor criteria must be used with caution.

The presence of one major and two minor or two major criteria should make the physician very suspicious of the diagnosis of rheumatic fever. Unless there is *evidence of a preceding group A streptococcal infection*, however, the diagnosis should be entertained with great suspicion.

Evidence of a preceding streptococcal infection may be obtained by means of a positive throat culture for group A streptococci or a history of scarlet fever. Most reliable, however, is elevation of the streptococcal antibody titers such as antistreptolysin O (ASO) titer, antistreptokinase, and antideoxyribonuclease B titer (antiDNase B). Interpretation of streptococcal antibody titers is not always simple. Although a single elevated antibody titer is helpful, a rise between an acute and a convalescent titer is far more reliable. Furthermore, the clinician must remember that "normal" antibody titers vary with the age of the patient, as well as with the population. The latter variations are another reason why both acute and convalescent titers (usually obtained 2 to 4 weeks apart) are

more desirable. Other antibodies may be studied. The antihyaluronidase (AH) antibody test is also commercially available. A rapid agglutination test that tests for antibodies to more than one streptococcal antigen is also used, but results using this test alone must be interpreted with caution because of reported standardization problems with reagents.

No laboratory test is specific for ARF, so the clinician must carefully interpret laboratory studies. For example, presence of a murmur of mitral regurgitation plus an elevated antistreptolysin O test might be compatible with rheumatic fever but also is compatible with presence of mitral valve prolapse in a patient who has had a recent uncomplicated streptococcal infection. In addition to laboratory studies to confirm the presence of a previous streptococcal infection and studies of acute-phase reactants, other blood studies may prove useful in some cases to eliminate other infectious diseases, collagen vascular diseases, and similar disorders.

The echocardiogram is a valuable addition to the workup of a patient suspected of having ARF. For example, it has been reported that patients with isolated manifestations of rheumatic fever such as arthritis or chorea may have "subclinical" carditis.[17] Stretching of the chordae tendineae with "prolapse" of the anterior leaflet of the mitral valve has been reported. This possibility is intriguing, since it may explain those patients without clinical evidence of carditis at the initial attack who later are found to have rheumatic heart disease. Most authorities now feel that patients with acute rheumatic fever in whom there is any question of carditis should undergo echocardiographic examination.

TREATMENT OF ACUTE RHEUMATIC FEVER

The medical therapy for ARF has three objectives: to treat the group A streptococcal infection, to reduce inflammation, and to treat congestive heart failure (when present). Note that therapy is *not* directed toward prevention of development of rheumatic valvular heart disease. Numerous studies have shown that the anti-inflammatory therapy used for an acute attack of ARF does not prevent development of valvular heart disease.

Patients with arthritis as a major component of the clinical syndrome are usually treated and promptly helped with salicylates. Relief is dramatic. Dosage sufficient to give serum salicylate levels of 15 to 20 mg/dL causes the arthritis of rheumatic fever to disappear, usually within 12 to 24 h. This can usually be achieved with total daily doses of aspirin of 100 mg/kg per day, given in four doses daily. In patients with arthritis who do not promptly respond to salicylates, another diagnosis should be seriously considered. As mentioned previously, however, salicylates or corticosteroids should *not* be started until the clinical picture has fully evolved. Withholding anti-inflammatory therapy until the diagnosis is confirmed poses no danger to the patient with ARF. The newer nonsteroidal anti-inflammatory drugs have not been studied in a systematic fashion for use in ARF.

Most physicians do not administer corticosteroids in patients with only arthritis. Corticosteroids are used in patients with carditis, especially when there is evidence of congestive heart failure. It is generally agreed that, although corticosteroids may be clinically helpful during the acute phases of the attack, they have no effect in preventing the development of rheumatic valvular heart disease. The dose of corticosteroids is usually in the range of 2 to 4 mg/kg per day of prednisone and divided into two doses. Short courses of 2 weeks, with a relatively rapid taper of the steroid, are most frequently used. Careful clinical and laboratory monitoring must be performed. If there is clinical relapse, a longer course may be required. Patients who are receiving corticosteroids are frequently given salicylate (aspirin) concomitantly. Maintaining adequate salicylate levels as one is reducing corticosteroid dosage usually prevents rebound.

The treatment of Sydenham's chorea has been helped considerably by the addition of two agents. Diazepam, a benzodiazepine derivative, is now the initial treatment of choice for Sydenham's chorea. Haloperidol, a butyrophenone, has been used with encouraging results but must be monitored very carefully because of potential toxicity.[33]

An essential part of the therapy for ARF is the treatment of the preceding group A streptococcal pharyngitis. Even though GAS can be cultured at the time of the onset of acute rheumatic fever in only about 10 percent of patients, all patients should be treated for streptococcal pharyngitis, and secondary long-term rheumatic fever prophylaxis should be initiated.

Penicillin is the antimicrobial agent of choice for both treatment of the acute streptococcal pharyngitis and long-term secondary prophylaxis.

For the treatment of acute streptococcal pharyngitis, a single dose of penicillin G, 1.2 million units warmed to room temperature, should be injected into a large muscle mass. If the patient will take medication for a full 10-day period, oral penicillin V (phenoxymethyl penicillin), 500 mg every 8 to 12 h, may alternatively be given. For patients allergic to penicillin, oral erythromycin (estolate, 20 to 40 mg/kg per day, divided into two to four doses, or ethyl succinate, 40 mg/kg per day, divided into two to four doses, with a maximum daily dose of either form of 1 g) for 10 days; azithromycin, 500 mg as a single dose on the first day, followed by 250 mg once daily for 4 days; or an oral cephalosporin such as cefadroxil or cephalexin for 10 days may be prescribed. Tetracyclines, sulfadiazine, and chloramphenicol are not recommended for the treatment of active upper respiratory tract streptococcal infections.

For prophylaxis against recurrent ARF, the intramuscular injection of 1.2 million units of benzathine penicillin G every 4 weeks has been recommended by the American Heart Association for many years.[34] Injection every 3 weeks should be considered for high-risk subjects. Because intramuscular injections of penicillin are painful and because of a largely unjustified fear of untoward reactions, however, oral secondary prophalaxis is widely used in the United States. The oral administration of penicillin V, 250 mg twice daily, is the most frequently used method of secondary ARF prophylaxis. For patients allergic to penicillin, oral sulfadiazine, 1 g daily, is an effective substitute. In persons allergic to both penicillin and sulfadiazine, oral

erythromycin, 250 mg twice daily, is recommended. The American Heart Association recommendations provide a more complete discussion of this management.[34]

In patients who develop congestive heart failure, the usual anticongestive measures, including cardiac glycosides and diuretics, have been effective (see also Chap. 23). Of course, in persons with congestive heart failure, bed rest is necessary. In the past, patients with ARF were put to bed for several months, but this is no longer considered necessary unless there is evidence of significant carditis. The purpose of bed rest is to reduce the cardiac work. The arthritis of rheumatic fever does not necessitate bed rest except during the first day or two after the diagnosis is made. Shortly thereafter, aspirin controls the arthritis.

For patients with rheumatic valvular heart disease, bacterial endocarditis prophylaxis is necessary at the time of dental procedures or surgery on infected or contaminated tissues. In contrast, patients who have had rheumatic fever but who do not have rheumatic heart disease do not require endocarditis prophylaxis. A discussion of current recommendations for bacterial endocarditis prophylaxis is provided in Chap. 82.[35]

NATURAL HISTORY

The natural history of individuals who have had documented ARF varies considerably from patient to patient. Continuous antimicrobial secondary prophylaxis generally protects patients from recurrent attacks and therefore from a worsening cardiac status. Thompkins and colleagues demonstrated that if secondary prophylaxis is reliably followed, approximately 70 percent of individuals developing the murmur of mitral regurgitation at the time of the acute attack lose that murmur over the next 5 years.[36]

For this reason, continuous secondary prophylaxis is very important. Patients who have had one episode of rheumatic fever are likely to experience a second attack with a recurrent streptococcal infection. The duration of secondary prophylaxis varies. Some authorities feel that if there is no evidence of rheumatic heart disease, 5 years of secondary prophylaxis may often be sufficient. Most, however, continue secondary prophylaxis until at least the eighteenth birthday. If there is evidence of rheumatic heart disease, prolonged secondary prophylaxis is indicated; some authorities recommend lifelong secondary prophylaxis for these patients. In addition, one must take into consideration the patient's risk of streptococcal infection. Individuals at higher risk of developing streptococcal infection (e.g., schoolteachers, health care workers, and individuals in the military) often are given secondary prophylaxis for longer periods of time.

The prognosis for the arthritis of ARF is excellent. There is no residual arthritis or deformity. Rarely, a patient may have *Jaccoud's arthritis*, with increased ulnar deviation of the fourth and fifth fingers and flexion at the metacarpophalangeal joints. Sydenham's chorea may recur, but this is rare.

Patients with severe valvular heart disease often require cardiovascular surgery, many during the third or fourth decade of life. In some parts of the world, however, an entity known as juvenile or malignant mitral stenosis occurs[37] and results in the need for surgery much earlier, often late in the first or early in the second decade (see Chaps. 63 and 64).

Although methods of prevention are imperfect, the beneficial effects of consistent secondary prophylaxis cannot be too strongly emphasized (see earlier discussion). It is probably the single most effective measure that the physician has to offer patients who have had a previous documented episode of ARF. Because of the complex nature of the GAS, efforts to produce a safe and effective vaccine against GAS infections have been hampered. Advances in molecular biological techniques have provided new knowledge in this regard, and progress is being made in the most important aspect of development in this vaccine, the understanding of the antigenicity and cross-reactivity of the M protein of the group A streptococcus.[38–40] Experimental vaccines have been tried in animals, but they are still in a relatively early stage of development, and sizable human trials have not yet been undertaken.

REFERENCES

1. Markowitz M, Taranta A. *Rheumatic Fever: A Guide to Its Recognition, Prevention and Cure, with Special Reference to Developing Countries*. Boston: MTP Press; 1981:16.
2. Arnigo M-C, Lavin MM, Reyes PA. Acute rheumatic fever. *Rheu Dis Clin N Amer* 1993; 19:333–350.
3. Burge DJ, DeHoratius RJ. Acute rheumatic fever. *Cardiovasc Clin* 1993; 23:3–23.
4. Kavey RW, Kaplan EL. Resurgence of rheumatic fever. *Pediatrics* 1989; 84:585–586.
5. Bisno AL, Shulman ST, Dajani AS. The rise and fall (and rise?) of rheumatic fever. *JAMA* 1988; 259:728–729.
6. Bronze MS, Dale JB. The reemergence of serious group A streptococcal infections and rheumatic fever. *Am J Med Sci* 1996; 311:41–54.
7. Massell BF. *Rheumatic Fever and Streptococcal Infection: Unraveling the Mysteries of a Dread Disease*. Boston, Harvard University Press, 1997.
8. Lancefield RC. A serologic differentiation of human and other groups of hemolytic streptococci. *J Exp Med* 1933; 57:571–595.
9. Limson BM, Chan VR, Guzman SU, Maaba MR, Mendoza MT. Occurrence of infection with group B coxsackie virus in rheumatic and nonrheumatic Filipino children. *J Infect Dis* 1979; 140:415–418.
10. Papadimas T, Escamilla J, Garst P, Oldfield E, Counihan C, Schiffer S, et al. Acute rheumatic fever at a Navy Training Center—San Diego, California. *MMWR* 1988; 37:101–104.
11. Kaplan EL. The group A streptococci upper respiratory tract carrier state: An enigma. *J Pediatr* 1980; 97:337–345.
12. Taranta A, Markowitz M. *Rheumatic Fever*. Dordrecht: Kluwer; 1989.
13. Land MA, Bisno AL. Acute rheumatic fever: A vanishing disease in suburbia. *JAMA* 1983; 249:895–898.
14. Odio A. The incidence of acute rheumatic fever in a suburban area of Los Angeles: A ten-year study. *West J Med* 1986; 144:179–184.
15. World Health Organization. *Rheumatic Fever and Rheumatic Heart Disease*. Geneva, Switzerland, Technical Report Series, No. 764, 1988:1–58.
16. De Oliveira A, de Souza MJ, Benchetrit LC. Rheumatic heart disease and streptococcal carriage in Brazilian children. In: Doyle E, Engle M, Gersony W, Rashkind W, Talner N, eds. *Pediatric Cardiology*. New York: Springer-Verlag; 1986:998.
17. Veasy LG, Wiedmeier SE, Orsmond G, Ruttenberg HD, Boucek MM, Roth SJ, et al. Resurgence of acute rheumatic fever in the intermountain area of the United States. *N Engl J Med* 1987; 316:421–427.
18. Hosier D, Craenen J, Teske DW, Wheller JJ. Resurgence of rheumatic fever. *Am J Dis Child* 1987; 141:730–733.
19. Congeni B, Rizzo C, Congeni J, Sreenivasan VV. Outbreak of acute rheumatic fever in southeast Ohio. *J Pediatr* 1987; 119:176–179.
20. Kaplan EL, Johnson DR, Cleary PP. Group A streptococcal serotypes isolated from patients and sibling contacts during the resurgence of rheumatic fever in the United States in the mid-1980s. *J Infect Dis* 1989; 159:101–103.
21. Markowitz MM, Kaplan EL. Reappearance of rheumatic fever. In: Barness LA, ed. *Advances in Pediatrics*: vol 3. Chicago: Year Book Medical; 1989:339–66.
22. Kaplan EL. Epidemiologic approaches to understanding the pathogenesis of rheumatic fever. *Int J Epidemiol* 1985; 14:499–501.
23. Watson RF, Hirst GK, Lancefield RC. Bacteriological studies of cardiac tissues obtained at autopsy from 11 patients dying with rheumatic fever. *Arthritis Rheum* 1961; 4:74–85.
24. Ginsburg I. Mechanism of cell and tissue injury induced by group A streptococci: Relation to past streptococcal sequelae. *J Infect Dis* 1972; 126:294–340.
25. Goldstein I, Halpern B, Robert L. Immunologic relationship between streptococcus A polysaccharide and the structural glycoproteins of heart valve. *Nature* 1967; 213:44–47.
26. Dudding BA, Ayoub EM. Persistence of streptococcal group A antibody in patients with rheumatic valvular disease. *J Exp Med* 1968; 128:1081–1098
27. Shulman ST, Ayoub EM, Victorica BC, Gessner IH, Tamer DF, Hernandez FA. Differences in antibody response to streptococcal antigens in children with rheumatic and nonrheumatic valve disease. *Circulation* 1974; 50:1244–1251.
28. Zabriskie JB, Freimer EH. The immunological relationship between the group A streptococcus and mammalian muscle. *J Exp Med* 1966; 124:661–678.
29. Patarroyo ME, Winchester RJ, Vejerano A, Gibofsky A, Chalem F, Zabriskie JB, et al. Association of a B-cell antigen with susceptibility to rheumatic fever. *Nature* 1979; 278:173–174.
30. Gray ED, Regelmann WR, Abdin Z, el-Kholy A, Zahers S, Kamel R, et al. Compartmentalization of cells bearing "rheumatic" cell surface antigens in peripheral blood and tonsils in rheumatic heart disease. *J Infect Dis* 1987; 155:242–247.
31. Committee on the Prevention of Rheumatic Fever and Bacterial Endocarditis of the American Heart Association: The Jones Criteria (revised). *Circulation* 1984; 69; 203A–208A.
32. Special Writing Group of the Committee on Rheumatic Fever, Endocarditis, and Kawasaki Disease of the Council on Cardiovascular Disease in the Young of the American Heart Association. Guidelines for the diagnosis of rheumatic fever: Jones Criteria, 1992 update. *JAMA* 1992; 268:2069–2073.
33. Shields WD, Bray PF. A danger of haloperidol therapy in children. *J Pediatr* 1976; 88:301–303.
34. Committee on Rheumatic fever, Endocarditis, and Kawasaki Disease of the Council on Cardiovascular Disease in the Young of the American Heart Association. Treatment of streptococcal pharyngitis and prevention of rheumatic fever: a statement for health professionals. *Pediatrics* 1995; 96:758–764.
35. Dajani AS, Tallbert KA, Wilson W, Bolger AF, Bayer A, Ferrieri P, et al. Prevention of bacterial endocarditis. Recommendations by the American Heart Association. *JAMA* 1997; 277:1794–1801(*Circulation* 1997; 96:358–366).
36. Thompkins DG, Boxerbaum B, Liebman J. Long-term prognosis of rheumatic fever patients receiving regular intramuscular benzathine penicillin. *Circulation* 1972; 45:543–551.
37. Ilyas M, Haidry JG. Juvenile mitral stenosis: A pathogenic puzzle. *J Pak Med Assoc* 1980; 30:254–256.
38. Pruksakorn S, Currie B, Brandt E, Martin D. Galbraith A, Phomphutkul C, et al. Towards a vaccine for rheumatic fever: identification of a conserved target epitope on M protein of group A streptococci. *Lancet* 1994; 344:639–642.
39. Carpetis JR, Carrie BJ, Good MF. Towards understanding the pathogenesis of rheumatic fever (editorial). *Scand J Rheumatol* 1996; 25:127–131.
40. Stollerman GH. Changing streptococci and the prospects for global eradication of rheumatic fever. *Perspec Biol Med* 1997; 40:165–189.

CHAPTER

63

AORTIC VALVE DISEASE

Shahbudin H. Rahimtoola

The assessment and management of patients with valvular heart disease have undergone many changes in the past four decades. The incidence of acute rheumatic fever has declined, and as a result rheumatic heart disease is not the most important cause of valve disease in the developed countries. Prolapse of the mitral valve and congenital aortic valve disease are now the most common valvular lesions. Valve surgery has been the major therapeutic advance in treating patients with severe valve disease; in fact, most patients with severe valve disease are now considered candidates for surgery. Echocardiography/Doppler ultrasound has a very important role in the diagnosis and follow-up of these patients. Cardiac catheterization/angiography remains an extremely important diagnostic procedure that is needed in almost all patients being considered for interventional therapy. Catheter balloon valvuloplasty is a useful technique for the treatment of some stenotic cardiac valves.

AORTIC VALVE STENOSIS

Aortic stenosis (AS) is obstruction to outflow of blood flow from the left ventricle to the aorta. The obstruction may be at the valve, above the valve (supravalvular), or below the valve (subvalvular).[1] Supravalvular AS is a congenital lesion. Subvalvular AS results either from a discrete fibromuscular obstruction, which is a congenital lesion, or from a muscular obstruction (hypertrophic cardiomyopathy).

Etiology

The most common causes of AS are congenital,[2,3] rheumatic, and calcific (degenerative) (Table 63-1). Calcific AS is seen in patients 35 years or older and is the result of calcification of a congenital or rheumatic valve or of a normal valve that has undergone "degenerative" changes.[4] Recent data suggest that degenerative/calcific AS may represent an immune reaction to antigens present in the valve.[5]

Rare causes of AS include obstructive, infective vegetations that are usually large, e.g., those seen in fungal endocarditis. Atherosclerotic AS is seen most frequently in patients with severe hypercholesterolemia and is observed in children and young adults with homozygous type II hyperlipoproteinemia.[6,7] Paget's disease of the bone,[8] end-stage renal disease,[9,10] systemic lupus erythematosus, rheumatoid involvement, ochronosis,[11] and irradiation are other rare causes of AS.

At the present time, calcific AS in the older patient is the most common valve lesion coming to valve replacement.[4,12] Among patients under the age of 70, congenital bicuspid valve accounted for one-half of the surgical cases; degenerative changes were the cause in 18 percent.[4] In contrast, in those aged 70 or older, degenerative changes accounted for almost one-half of the surgical cases, and a congenital bicuspid valve for approximately one-quarter of cases (Fig. 63-1).

Pathology

In congenital AS, the valve may be unicuspid, bicuspid, or tricuspid, depending on the patient's age.[13] In patients under the age of 15 years, over 80 percent of stenotic valves are

TABLE 63-1

ETIOLOGY OF AORTIC VALVE STENOSIS

I. Congenital
II. Acquired
   A. Rheumatic
   B. Calcific (degenerative/autoimmune)
   C. Rare causes
     1. Obstructive infective vegetations
     2. Homozygous type II hyperlipoproteinemia
     3. Paget's disease of bone
     4. Systemic lupus erythematosus
     5. Rheumatoid involvement
     6. Ochronosis (alkaptonuria)
     7. Irradiation

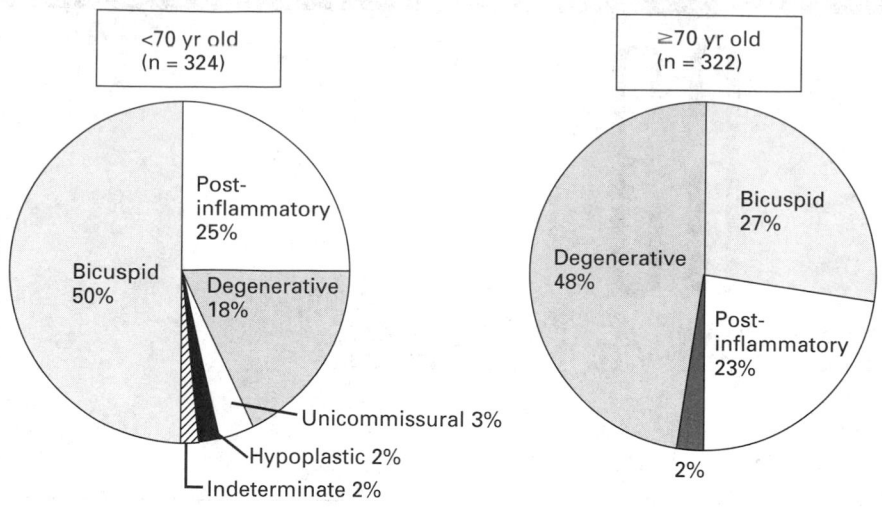

FIGURE 63-1

Etiology of aortic stenosis in patients under the age of 70 years (*left panel*); congenital bicuspid valve accounted for one-half of the surgical cases. In those aged 70 or older (*right panel*), "degenerative" changes accounted for almost one-half of the surgical cases. (From Passik et al.,[4] with permission.)

either unicuspid or bicuspid and 15 to 20 percent are tricuspid. In patients aged 15 to 65 years, 60 percent are bicuspid, 10 percent are unicuspid, and 25 to 30 percent are tricuspid. In patients 65 years of age or over, 90 percent of the valves are tricuspid and 10 percent are bicuspid. Unicuspid valves produce severe obstruction in infancy and are the most frequent malformation found in fatal valvular AS in children under the age of 1 year.[2] Congenital bicuspid valves can produce severe obstruction to left ventricular (LV) outflow after the first few years of life.[3] The valvular abnormality produces turbulent flow, which traumatizes the leaflets and eventually leads to fibrosis, rigidity, and calcification of the valve. In a congenitally abnormal tricuspid aortic valve, the cusps are of unequal size and have some degree of commissural fusion; the third cusp may be diminutive. Eventually, the abnormal structure leads to changes similar to those seen in a bicuspid valve, and significant LV outflow obstruction often results.

Rheumatic AS results from adhesions and fusion of the commissures and cusps. The leaflets and the valve ring become vascularized, which leads to retraction and stiffening of the cusps. Calcification occurs, and the aortic valve orifice is reduced to a small triangular or round opening, which is frequently regurgitant as well as stenotic. Importantly, the heart exhibits other evidence of rheumatic heart disease, namely, involvement of the mitral valve and presence of Aschoff's nodules in the myocardium.

Rheumatoid AS is extremely rare and results from nodular thickening of the valve leaflets and the involvement of the proximal part of the aorta. In severe forms of hypercholesterolemia, lipid deposits occur not only in the aortic wall but also in the aortic valve and occasionally produce AS.

The LV is concentrically hypertrophied.[14] The hypertrophied cardiac muscle cells are increased in size, with their transverse diameters ranging from 15 to 70 μm (normal, 10 to 15 μm). There is an increase of connective tissue,[15–17] and a variable amount of fibrous tissue (collagen fibrils) in the interstitial tissue. Usually, the cardiac muscle cells do not degenerate in patients with AS. Myocardial ultrastructural changes[18] may account for the LV systolic dysfunction that occurs late in the disease; such changes include unusually large nuclei, loss of myofibrils, accumulation of mitochondria, large cytoplasmic areas devoid of contractile material, and proliferation of fibroblasts and collagen fibers in the interstitial space.

Subclinical calcific emboli are commonly found in calcific AS if diligently sought at autopsy.

Pathophysiology

With reduction in the aortic valve area (AVA), energy is dissipated during the transport of blood from the left ventricle to the aorta. The AVA has to be reduced by about 50 percent of normal before a measurable gradient can be demonstrated in humans.[19] When a pressure gradient develops between the left ventricle and the ascending aorta, LV pressure rises; aortic pressure remains within the normal range until end-stage heart failure occurs. The relationship of the AVA to cardiac output and pressure gradient is discussed in Chap. 64. As LV pressure rises, ventricular wall stress increases, which leads to impaired LV function. The heart normalizes wall stress by becoming hypertrophic. Since AS develops slowly, hypertrophy develops in proportion to increased intraventricular pressure, and myocardial stress remains normal.[20] *Thus, the major compensatory mechanism by which the heart copes with LV outflow obstruction is ventricular hypertrophy.* LV mass in patients with severe AS undergoing valve replacement averages 229 g per square meter (normal, 105 g/m²)[20]; at autopsy, left ventricles weighing as much as 1000 g have been reported. LV volume, however, is within the normal range,[20] and so there is a considerable thickening of the LV wall.

The diastolic properties of the LV are affected in AS.[21–25] This diastolic abnormality results from a combination of impaired myocardial relaxation with altered chamber compliance because the hypertrophied LV per se offers increased resistance to filling, and from increased myocardial stiffness because of structural alterations.[25] As a result, LV end-diastolic pressure is elevated, but this is not necessarily a measure of LV failure. Powerful atrial contraction produces the required LV filling and results in an elevated LV end-diastolic pressure (atrial booster pump function).[26,27] The necessary LV filling and fiber length to achieve an adequate stroke volume are achieved by atrial systole, which occupies only a small part of the cardiac cycle. Therefore, there is a transient increase in left atrial pressure due to the large *a* wave, but mean left atrial pressure remains in the normal range or is only minimally increased (Fig. 63-2).

Left atrial contraction is therefore of considerable benefit to these patients. Loss of effective atrial contraction, either because of atrial fibrillation or because of an inappropriately timed atrial contraction [e.g., that associated with first-degree heart block or with atrioventricular (AV) dissociation], results in elevations of mean left atrial pressure, reduction of cardiac output, or both, and may precipitate clinical heart failure with pulmonary congestion.

Patients with severe LV hypertrophy may exhibit LV diastolic dysfunction, which may produce the syndrome of clinical heart failure (paroxysmal nocturnal dyspnea, orthopnea, and even pulmonary edema) even if LV systolic pump function is normal. In patients 60 years of age or older, a higher percentage of women (41 percent) than men (14 percent) have "excessive" hypertrophy, that is, greater amounts of hypertrophy in spite of similar degrees of severity of AS.[28] They have "supernormal" LV systolic pump function (high LV ejection fraction) and a small, thick-walled chamber with lower end-systolic wall stress (Table 63-2).

LV systolic pump function is determined by myocardial (muscle) function and by a combination of LV afterload and preload. Thus, impaired LV systolic pump function (as measured by ejection fraction) may be the result of afterload-preload mismatch,[29] impaired myocardial function, or both. LV systolic pump function is normal in most patients with severe AS. When the LV hypertrophy alone is not adequate to overcome the outflow obstruction, the left ventricle uses the Frank-Starling mechanism (preload reserve) to maintain systolic pump function. When the preload reserve is no longer adequate, a reduction of LV systolic pump function occurs (Fig. 63-2). In AS, major use of the preload reserve is not a good compensatory mechanism. Even small increases in LV volume may result in major increases in LV end-diastolic pressure because the LV is on the very steep portion of its diastolic pressure-volume curve, and the corresponding

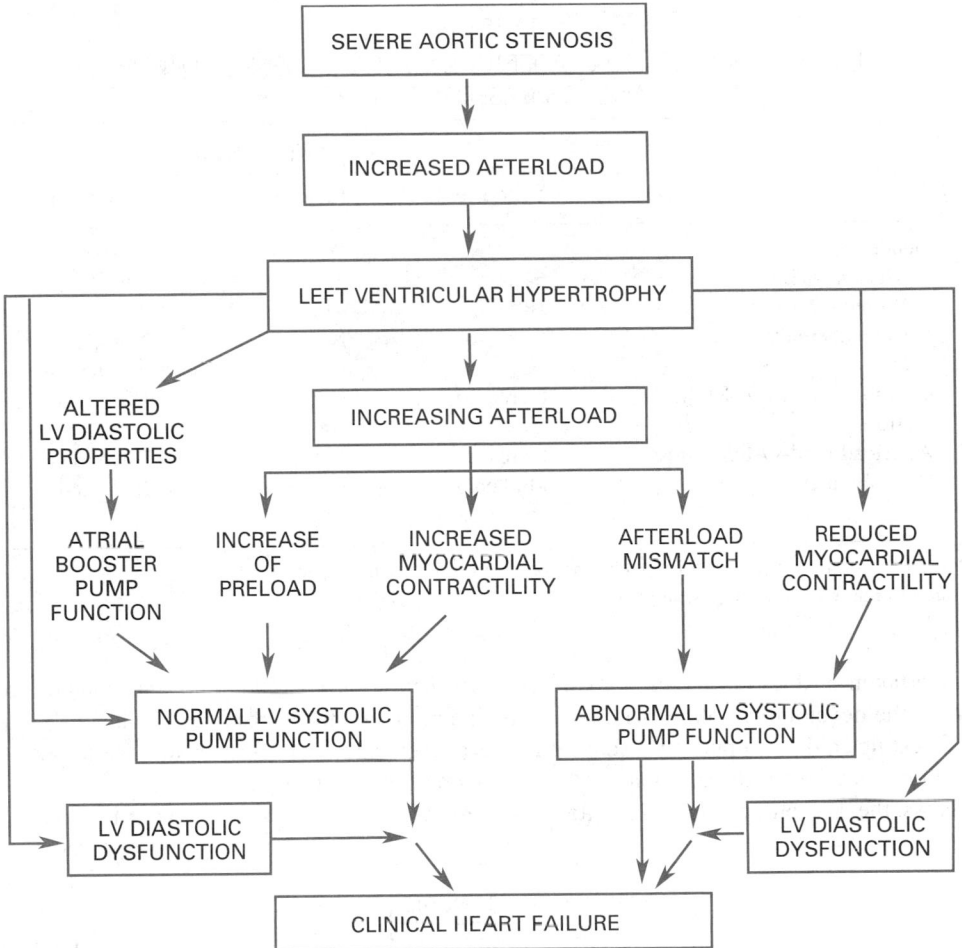

FIGURE 63-2

Illustration of some aspects of the pathophysiology in severe aortic stenosis (see text). The heart responds to AS by hypertrophy, and LV systolic pump function remains normal. LV hypertrophy may alter the LV diastolic properties. As a result, LV end-diastolic pressure is elevated; but powerful atrial contraction produces the required LV filling and fiber length (atrial booster pump function).

As LV afterload continues to increase, the LV uses two additional compensatory mechanisms, namely, increase of preload and increase of myocardial contractility. Both of these help maintain normal LV systolic pump function.

When the limit of the preload reserve has been reached (afterload mismatch) or myocardial contractility is reduced, LV systolic pump function becomes abnormal.

Clinical heart failure is usually a result of abnormal LV systolic pump function; diastolic dysfunction may also be present in some patients. Clinical heart failure in those with normal LV systolic pump function is a result of LV diastolic dysfunction. (Copyright © by S. H. Rahimtoola, M.B., F.R.C.P., M.A.C.P. See Ref. 85.)

increase in mean left atrial pressure produces pulmonary edema. Thus, clinical heart failure may be a result of either LV diastolic dysfunction in the presence of normal LV systolic function or impaired myocardial function producing LV systolic dysfunction, with or without associated LV diastolic dysfunction. Eventually, pulmonary artery, right ventricular, and right atrial pressures are elevated. Peripheral edema results from increases in systemic venous pressure and salt and water retention.

In most patients with AS, cardiac output is in the normal range and initially increases normally with exercise. Later, as the severity of AS increases progressively, the cardiac output remains within the normal range at rest, but, on exercise, it no longer increases in proportion to the amount of exercise

TABLE 63-2

SEVERE AORTIC STENOSIS IN PATIENTS ≥60 YEARS, GENDER DISTRIBUTION
AND CHAMBER PROPERTIES

	LV Systolic Function		
	Subnormal	Normal	Supernormal
Gender			
Men ($n = 29$)	64%	22%	14%
Women ($n = 34$)	18%	41%	41%
LV chamber size	Increased	Normal	Normal to decreased
Chamber geometry (R/Th ratio)	Increased	Normal to decreased	Decreased
Afterload (end-systolic stress)	Increased	Normal	Decreased
Diastolic pressures	Markedly increased	Increased	Increased

Note: LV = left ventricular; R/Th = chamber radius to wall thickness ratio.
Source: From Carroll et al.,[28] with permission.

undertaken or does not increase at all (fixed cardiac output). With the development of heart failure, there is a reduction in the resting cardiac output and a tachycardia. As a result, stroke volume may be so lowered that it results in a small gradient across the LV outflow tract in spite of severe AS. As the patient's age increases, there is a progressive decrease of cardiac output with exercise and a progressive increase of LV end-diastolic pressure at equal levels of AVA. This may be related only to LV diastolic dysfunction and is most marked in the older patient.[30]

In severe AS, myocardial oxygen needs are increased because of an increased muscle mass (hypertrophy), elevations in LV pressures, and prolongation of the systolic ejection time (Fig. 63-3). Total coronary blood flow is increased because of the severe LV hypertrophy; however, coronary blood flow per 100 g of LV mass is reduced.[31] As a result, blood flow to the subendocardium[32] is inadequate at rest; and because coronary vasodilator reserve is reduced,[33] myocardial blood flow is also reduced further, relative to need, on exercise. Coronary blood flow is reduced because of a reduced coronary perfusion pressure (the elevated LV end-diastolic pressure lowers the diastolic aortic–LV pressure gradient) and also because the hypertrophied myocardium compresses the coronary arteries as they traverse the myocardium to supply blood to the subendocardium (systolic "milking" of intramural arteries). As a result, patients may have classic angina pectoris even in the absence of coronary artery disease (CAD). Associated obstructive CAD from atherosclerosis further increases the imbalance between myocardial oxygen needs and supply (Fig. 63-2).

Clinical Findings

HISTORY

Patients with congenital valve stenosis may give a history of a murmur since childhood or infancy; those with rheumatic stenosis may have a history of rheumatic fever. Most patients with valvular AS, including some with severe valve stenosis, are asymptomatic. The symptoms of AS are angina pectoris, syncope, exertional presyncope, dyspnea (on exertion, orthopnea, paroxysmal nocturnal dyspnea, pulmonary edema), and the symptoms of heart failure. Once symptoms occur in a patient with severe AS, the life span of the patient is very short without surgical treatment. Sudden cardiac death is

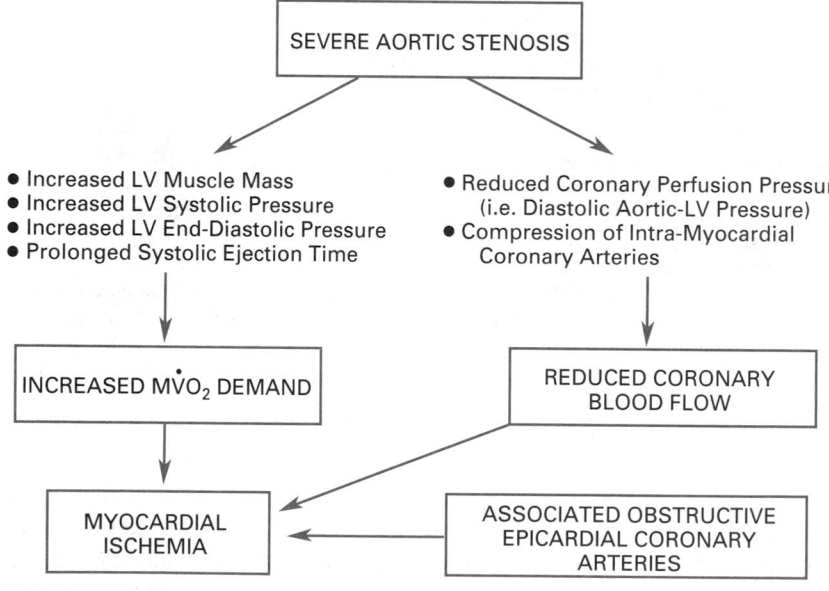

FIGURE 63-3

In severe aortic stenosis, myocardial oxygen needs are increased because of increased muscle mass (hypertrophy), increases in LV pressures, and prolongation of the systolic ejection time. Total coronary blood flow is increased; however, coronary blood flow per 100 g of LV mass is reduced because of a reduction in diastolic aortic–LV pressure gradient and "systolic milking" of the coronary arteries in the hypertrophied LV as they traverse the myocardium from the epicardium to endocardium to supply the subendocardial myocardial region. Thus, these patients may have myocardial ischemia, particularly in the subendocardial region. Coronary vasodilator reserve, i.e., the ability of the coronary blood flow to increase with vasodilatation, is also significantly reduced, and thus the myocardial ischemia can be markedly exacerbated on effort. Associated obstructive coronary artery disease can be expected to further exacerbate the myocardial ischemia. (Copyright © by S. H. Rahimtoola, M.B., F.R.C.P., M.A.C.P. See Ref. 85.)

stated to occur in 5 percent of patients with AS. It occurs only in those with severe valve stenosis, most of whom have had some cardiac symptoms before the fatal episode. Typical angina pectoris occurs with or without associated CAD and results from an imbalance between myocardial oxygen needs and supply (Fig. 63-3).

Syncope is the result of reduced cerebral perfusion. Syncope occurring on effort is caused by either systemic vasodilatation in the presence of a fixed or inadequate cardiac output or an arrhythmia, or by both.[34–36] Syncope at rest is usually due to a transient ventricular tachyarrhythmia, from which the patient recovers spontaneously. Other possible causes of syncope include transient atrial fibrillation or transient AV block, during which the ventricle is deprived of the powerful atrial booster pump function and/or the ventricular rate is slow.

Dyspnea on exertion, orthopnea, paroxysmal nocturnal dyspnea, and pulmonary edema result from varying degrees of pulmonary venous hypertension. Systemic venous congestion with enlargement of the liver and peripheral edema result from increased systemic venous pressure and salt and water retention. There is an increased incidence of gastrointestinal arteriovenous malformations.[37,38] As a result, these patients are susceptible to gastrointestinal hemorrhage and anemia. Calcific systemic embolism may occur.[39,40]

PHYSICAL FINDINGS

There is a spectrum of physical findings in patients with AS, depending on the severity of the stenosis, stroke volume, LV function, and the rigidity and calcification of the valve (Table 63-3). The arterial pulse rises slowly, taking a longer time than normal to reach peak pressure, and the peak is reduced (*parvus et tardus*)[41]; the pulse pressure may be narrowed. The anacrotic notch on the upstroke is best appreciated in the carotid arteries. The more severe the valve stenosis, the lower the anacrotic notch on the arterial pulse. A systolic thrill may be felt in the carotid arteries. The jugular venous pulse is normal unless the patient is in heart failure. In the absence of heart failure, the heart size is normal. The cardiac impulse is heaving and sustained in character, and there may be a palpable fourth heart sound (S_4). An aortic systolic thrill is often present at the base of the heart. In 80 to 90 percent of adult patients with severe AS, there is an S_4 gallop sound, a midsystolic ejection murmur that peaks late in systole, and a single second heart sound (S_2) because A_2 and P_2 are superimposed or A_2 is absent or soft. There is often a faint early diastolic murmur of minimal aortic regurgitation. In the young patient with valvular AS, a systolic ejection sound (systolic ejection click) initiates the systolic murmur but later tends to disappear as AS becomes severe. The S_2 may be paradoxically split due to late A_2, and there may be no early diastolic murmur. In many patients, particularly the elderly, the systolic ejection murmur is atypical, may be soft or cooing, and may be heard only at the apex of the heart. In the presence of heart failure, the jugular venous pressure is often increased, the left ventricle is dilated, a third heart sound is present, and the systolic murmur may be very soft or absent. Thus, the clinical features on physical examination may resemble those of heart failure from a variety of causes, such as dilated cardiomyopathy, rather than AS (see also Chap. 10).

Severe valvular AS is common in patients 60 years of age or older.[12,42] The clinical features in many of these patients tend to be somewhat different from those typical of younger

---

TABLE 63-3

PHYSICAL EXAMINATION OF PATIENTS WITH VARYING SEVERITY OF AORTIC VALVE STENOSIS

	Mild	Moderate	Severe + Normal LV Function	Severe + LV Dysfunction	Severe + Heart Failure[a]
Arterial pulse	Normal	Slowly rising	*Parvus et tardus*	*Parvus et tardus*	Small volume
Jugular venous pulse	Normal	Normal	Normal	Normal	±
Carotid thrill	±	±	±	±	±
Cardiac impulse	Normal	Heaving	Heaving, sustained palpable *a* wave	Heaving	Heaving or reduced
Precordial thrill	±	±	Usually + +	±	−
Auscultation					
S₄	−	±	+ +	+	−
S₃	−	−	−	±	+
ESS	+	±	−	−	−
Peak of ESM	Early systole	Mid-systole	Late systole	Late to mid-systole, soft	Mid-systole, soft or absent
S₂	Normal	Normal or single	Single or paradoxical	Single	Single

[a] There may be signs of mitral and tricuspid regurgitation and of pulmonary hypertension.

Note: S_4 = fourth heart sound (presystolic gallop); S_3 = third heart sound (diastolic gallop); ESS = ejection systolic sound; ESM = ejection systolic murmur; S_2 = second heart sound.

patients.[42] Systemic hypertension is common, being present in about 20 percent of the patients, half of whom have moderate or severe systolic and diastolic hypertension. A fifth of the patients first present in congestive heart failure. The male:female ratio is 2:1. Because of thickening of the arterial wall and its associated lack of distensibility, the arterial pulse rises normally or even rapidly, and the pulse pressure is wide. The S_2 is either absent or single. As noted above, the murmur may be high-pitched and musical and may radiate from the base to the apex or may be heard best at the apex, mimicking mitral regurgitation.

CHEST X-RAY

The characteristic finding is a normal-sized heart with a dilated proximal ascending aorta (poststenotic dilation). Calcium in the aortic valve can be seen on the lateral film but is better appreciated by fluoroscopy with image intensification. In the current era, calcification is most easily recognized on two-dimensional echocardiography. Calcium in the aortic valve is the hallmark of AS in adults 40 to 45 years of age.[43,44] In patients aged 45 years or above, the diagnosis of severe AS is doubtful if there is no calcium in the aortic valve. The presence of calcium, however, does not necessarily mean that the valve is stenotic or that the AS is severe. In patients with heart failure, the cardiac size is increased because of dilatation of the left ventricle and left atrium; the lung fields show pulmonary edema and pulmonary venous congestion with redistribution of blood flow. In the presence of heart failure, the right ventricle and the right atrium may be dilated.

ELECTROCARDIOGRAM

The electrocardiogram (ECG) in severe AS shows LV hypertrophy with or without secondary ST-T-wave changes. It is important to recognize, however, that in about 10 to 15 percent of patients with severe AS, LV hypertrophy cannot be appreciated on the ECG. In fact, the ECG may be entirely normal in some of these patients. The P-wave abnormality (P = 0.12 s) of left atrial enlargement and/or hypertrophy and/or conduction delay is present in over 80 percent.[45] The ECG may show left bundle branch block, right bundle branch block with left or right axis deviation, or, occasionally, isolated right bundle branch block.[46–48] In some patients, the conduction abnormality results from aortic valve calcification extending into the specialized conducting tissue, which may even produce heart block. The patients are usually in sinus rhythm. The presence of atrial fibrillation indicates the presence of either associated mitral valve disease, CAD, or heart failure secondary to aortic valve disease. Atrial fibrillation is relatively common in the elderly with calcific AS, probably because of the increased presence of associated diseases.

Laboratory Investigations

ECHOCARDIOGRAPHY/DOPPLER ULTRASOUND

Echocardiography/Doppler (echo/Doppler) ultrasound (Chap. 14) is an extremely important and useful noninvasive test. On the echocardiogram, the aortic valve leaflets normally are barely visible in systole, and the normal range of aortic valve opening is 1.6 to 2.6 cm. In the presence of a bicuspid aortic valve, eccentric valve leaflets may be seen. The aortic valve leaflets may appear to be thickened as a result of calcification and/or fibrosis; however, the older patient without valve stenosis may also have thickened cusps. The aortic valve may have a reduced opening, but this also occurs in other conditions in which the cardiac output is reduced. The LV hypertrophy often results in thickening of both the interventricular septum and the posterior LV wall. The LV cavity size is normal. All these abnormalities are better appreciated on two-dimensional echocardiography. When LV systolic function is impaired, the left ventricle and left atrium are dilated and the percentage of dimensional shortening is reduced.

In many patients, the severity of AS is incorrectly estimated by M-mode or two-dimensional echocardiography. Neither is a completely reliable technique for assessing the severity of AS. The presence of normal movement of thin aortic leaflets on the echocardiogram, however, is strong evidence against severe AS in adults.

Echo/Doppler, when properly applied, is extremely useful for estimating the valve gradient and AVA noninvasively.[49–54] When compared with results obtained at cardiac catheterization, the standard error of the estimate of mean gradient in the best laboratories is 10 mmHg.[55] Thus, the mean gradient by Doppler can be expected to be within ±20 mmHg (95% confidence level) of that obtained at catheterization.[55] Similarly, the AVA will be within ±0.3 cm² of that obtained at cardiac catheterization.[55] A recent study of 156 patients compared AVA obtained by cardiac catheterization with that obtained by Doppler ultrasound.[56] Of 125 patients with AVA ≤0.8 cm² at cardiac catheterization, in 36 (29 percent) Doppler-estimated AVA was ≥0.9 cm². In all seven patients with AVA >1.0 cm² by cardiac catheterization, Doppler-estimated AVA was ≤1.0 cm²; the findings in these seven patients must be interpreted cautiously because they were likely to be a highly selected subgroup. Guidelines for assessing severity of AS based on Doppler-obtained gradients are shown in Table 63-4.

Transesophageal echo/Doppler ultrasound is very useful

TABLE 63-4

SUGGESTED CONSERVATIVE GUIDELINES FOR RELATING SEVERITY OF AORTIC STENOSIS TO DOPPLER GRADIENTS IN ADULTS WITH NORMAL CARDIAC OUTPUT AND NORMAL AVERAGE HEART RATE

Peak Gradient, mmHg	Mean Gradient, mmHg	Severe AS
≥80	≥70	Highly likely
60–79	50–69	Probable
<60	<50	Uncertain

Source: From Rahimtoola,[55] with permission.

in defining the aortic valve abnormality and in assessing its severity when an adequate examination cannot be obtained with the transthoracic technique.

CARDIAC CATHETERIZATION/ANGIOGRAPHY

Cardiac catheterization remains the standard technique to assess the severity of AS "accurately." This is done by measuring simultaneous LV and ascending aortic pressures and measuring cardiac output by either the Fick principle or the indicator-dilution technique. The AVA can be calculated (see Chap. 16). AS can be considered to be severe when the valve area is 1.0 cm^2 or less or the AVA index is 0.6 cm^2 per square meter or less (Table 63-5).[55] The state of LV systolic pump function can be quantitated by measuring LV end-diastolic and end-systolic volumes and ejection fraction. *It must be recognized that ejection fraction may underestimate myocardial function in the presence of the increased afterload of severe AS.*

The presence of CAD and its site and severity can be estimated only by selective coronary angiography, which should be performed in all patients 35 years of age or older being considered for valve surgery and in those <35 years if they have LV systolic dysfunction, symptoms or signs suggesting CAD, or two or more risk factors for premature CAD (excluding gender) (Table 63-6). The incidence of associated CAD will vary considerably depending on the prevalence of CAD in the population.[55,57] It was reported to be 50 percent in patients with AS and 20 percent in patients with aortic regurgitation.[55] In general, in persons 50 years of age or older, it is about 50 percent (Table 63-7).[42,58-60]

GATED BLOOD POOL RADIONUCLIDE SCANS

Gated blood pool radionuclide scans provide information on ventricular function similar to that provided by two-dimensional echocardiography and LV cineangiography. These studies are of particular value in the occasional patient in whom LV cineangiography is unsuccessful and echocardiographic studies are suboptimal.

EXERCISE TESTS

It is usually recommended that exercise tests of any kind not be undertaken in patients with severe AS unless there is a specific reason for such studies. Exercise tests in these patients

---

TABLE 63-5

A SUGGESTED GRADING OF THE DEGREE OF AORTIC STENOSIS

Aortic Stenosis	AVA, cm^2	AVA Index, cm^2/m^2
Mild	>1.5	>0.9
Moderate	1.1–1.5	>0.6–0.9
Severe[a]	≤0.8–1.0	≤0.4–0.6

[a] Patients with AVAs that are at borderline values between the moderate and severe grades (0.9–1.1 cm^2; 0.55–0.65 cm^2/m^2) should be considered individually.

Note: AVA = aortic valve area.
Source: From Rahimtoola,[55] with permission.

TABLE 63-6

AORTIC VALVE DISEASE: INDICATIONS FOR CORONARY ARTERIOGRAPHY

Patients ≥ 35 years
Patients < 35 years:
    Left ventricular dysfunction
    Symptoms or signs suggesting CAD
    Two or more risk factors for premature CAD (excluding gender)

Note: CAD = coronary artery disease.
Source: From Rahimtoola,[55] with permission.

---

may precipitate ventricular tachyarrhythmias and ventricular fibrillation. If there is doubt about the severity of AS and concern that the patient's symptoms may not be caused by AS, it is usually wise to document the absence of severe AS before performing an exercise test. Occasionally, in a patient with severe AS who denies all symptoms, a closely monitored exercise test may be needed to assess exercise capacity.

AMBULATORY ECG RECORDING

Ambulatory ECG recordings may be needed in an occasional patient suspected of having an arrhythmia[61,62] or painless ischemia. Occasionally, patients with mild or moderate AS who are symptomatic may be suspected of having an arrhythmia or painless ischemia as a cause of the symptoms. At times, in asymptomatic patients with severe AS, one may need to determine if the patient has painless ischemia (see also Chap. 28).

PROVOCATIVE DIAGNOSTIC TEST

In an occasional patient, the severity of the AS may be in doubt because of a small stroke volume and small mean aortic

---

TABLE 63-7

ISOLATED AORTIC VALVE REPLACEMENT: INCIDENCE OF ASSOCIATED CORONARY ARTERY DISEASE

	VA Co-op Study[a]	Mayo Clinic[b]	MGH[c] (80–89 years)
Total number of patients	643	618	64
Patients with coronary artery disease	312	321	37
%	49%	52%	58%
1 VD	17%	22%	27%
2 VD	17%	14%	19%
3 VD	15%	17%	13%
Additional LMCAD	–	5%	3%

[a] Sethi GK et al.[58]
[b] Mullany CJ et al.[59]
[c] Levinson JR et al.[60]

valve gradient. The AS may be severe or mild to moderate, and the calculated AVA may be very small because of severe stenosis or because the small stroke volume only opens the valve to a limited extent; thus, the AVA will be determined to be small even on echo/Doppler ultrasound. Infusion of an inotropic agent such as dobutamine, which results in increases of stroke volume and heart rate, usually helps one to make a correct diagnosis. In these circumstances, it is important to measure cardiac output and LV and aortic pressures simultaneously and meticulously, both before and during dobutamine infusion.

Clinical Decision-Making

There are a number of steps involved in clinical decision-making in patients with valvular heart disease (Table 63-8).[55] The first is a complete clinical evaluation, which includes history, physical examination, ECG, and chest x-ray. Next, disease of all cardiac valves, ventricular function, and hemodynamic effects as well as CAD, other cardiovascular disease, and disease of other organs should be diagnosed and the severity assessed. Before proceeding to additional testing, it is important to list the question(s) to be answered and to be reasonably certain that these questions need to be answered. The test(s) that are most likely to provide these answers *in the clinician's own institution* should then be performed, with the following criteria being kept in mind: reliability, accuracy,

TABLE 63-8

STEPS IN CLINICAL DECISION-MAKING
IN PATIENTS WITH VALVULAR HEART DISEASE

1. Perform a complete clinical evaluation
   History
   Physical examination
   Electrocardiogram
   Chest x-ray film
2. Diagnose and assess severity of disease
   All valves
   Ventricular function
   Hemodynamic effects
   Coronary artery disease
   Other cardiovascular disease
   Effects on other body organs
   Other organ diseases
3. List questions that need answering
4. Be reasonably certain these questions need to be answered
5. Perform test(s) most likely to provide these answers in one's own institution with the following criteria:
   Reliability
   Accuracy
   Lowest risk to patients
   Reasonable (or lowest) cost
6. Review results of test(s)
7. Make an overall assessment of patient
8. Make recommendations regarding management

Source: From Rahimtoola,[55] with permission.

TABLE 63-9

CLINICAL DECISION-MAKING UTILIZING
CLINICAL EVALUATION AND ECHO/DOPPLER
IN PATIENTS WITH AORTIC STENOSIS

	After Clinical Evaluation, %	After Echo/Doppler, %
Diagnosis of AS		
Sensitivity	78	100
Specificity	92	92
Accuracy of diagnosis		
All levels of severity	48	65
Moderate or severe AS	100	100

Source: From Kotlewski et al.,[63] with permission.

lowest risk to patient, and reasonable (lowest) cost. The results of the test(s) should be reviewed as they become available, and an overall evaluation/assessment of the patient and, finally, recommendations regarding management should be made.

In a prospective, blinded study of consecutive patients with valvular heart disease, the sensitivity and specificity of diagnosis of AS and the accuracy of assessment of severity of AS were determined (Table 63-9).[63] This study revealed the following important points: (1) Clinical evaluation was sensitive, highly specific, and reasonably accurate in diagnosing AS and was very accurate in assessing its severity when AS was moderate or severe. This emphasizes the importance of a thorough clinical evaluation of the patient. (2) Echo/Doppler ultrasound improved the accuracy of this assessment to a certain extent. (3) The reason clinical evaluation and echo/Doppler do not have a 100 percent specificity is the inability in an occasional patient to distinguish mild AS from turbulence across a normal or slightly diseased aortic valve. (4) Both clinical evaluation and echo/Doppler ultrasound are excellent in diagnosing the AS as being at least moderate or severe. (5) An important difficulty in diagnosis by clinical evaluation and by echo/Doppler is in not being able to separate accurately all patients with moderate AS from those with severe AS.

Natural History and Prognosis

Valvular AS is frequently a progressive disease, the severity increasing over time.[64–68] The factors that control this progression and the time it takes for severe outflow obstruction to develop are unknown; however, it appears that in the older patient, AS may progress at about twice the rate that it does in the younger patient.[69] In a study of 142 patients with "mild" stenosis (catheterization-proven AVA >1.5 cm²),[70] the rate of progression to severe stenosis was 8 percent in 10 years, 22 percent in 20 years, and 38 percent in 25 years. At 25 years, 38 percent still had mild AS (Table 63-10). The duration of the asymptomatic period after the development of severe

TABLE 63-10

NATURAL HISTORY OF MILD[a] AORTIC STENOSIS ($n = 142$)

	10 Years	20 Years	25 Years
Mild	88%	63%	38%
Moderate	4%	15%	25%
Severe	8%	22%	38%

[a] Mild stenosis is defined here as an aortic valve area >1.5 cm^2.
Source: From Horstkotte and Loogen,[70] with permission.

AS is also unknown; some recent data suggest that it may be less than 2 years. The outcome of the asymptomatic patient with severe AS is not known. The overwhelming majority of adults with severe AS who are seen by cardiologists have symptoms. Severe disease in adults is lethal, particularly if the patient is symptomatic, with a prognosis that is worse than for many forms of neoplastic disease.[55] The 3-year mortality is approximately 36 to 52 percent, the 5-year mortality is about 52 to 80 percent, and the 10-year mortality is 80 to 90 percent.[55] A recent study of elderly patients (average age 77 years) showed 1-year and 3-year mortalities were 44 percent and 75 percent, respectively.[71] With the onset of severe symptoms (angina, syncope, or heart failure) the average life expectancy is 2 to 3 years (Table 63-11).[70,72] Almost all patients with heart failure are dead in 1 to 2 years.[70,72] A combination of symptoms is much more ominous, a sign of a greatly reduced survival. Sudden death, like syncope, occurs in the presence of severe AS. Its exact incidence is difficult to determine but may be about 5 percent.[72] Most, but not all, of these patients have had some cardiac symptoms before the fatal episode; at times, the only symptom has been exertional presyncope.

Management

All patients with AS need antibiotic prophylaxis against infective endocarditis (see Chap. 82). Those in whom the valve lesion is of rheumatic origin need additional prophylaxis

TABLE 63-11

AVERAGE SURVIVAL OF SYMPTOMATIC PATIENTS WITH SEVERE AS

	Autopsy Data,[a] Years	Post Cardiac Catheterization,[b] Months
Overall	3	23
Angina	5	45
Syncope	3	27
Heart failure	<2	11

[a] From Ross and Braunwald.[72]
[b] From Horstkotte and Loogen.[70]

against recurrence of rheumatic fever. Patients with mild or moderate stenosis rarely have symptoms or complications and do not need any specific medical therapy (Table 63-12). In mild stenosis, the patient should be encouraged to lead a normal life. Those with moderate AS should avoid moderate to severe physical exertion and competitive sports. In patients with mild or moderate AS, if atrial fibrillation should occur, it should be reverted rapidly to sinus rhythm. In severe AS, reversion to sinus rhythm often becomes a matter of some urgency.

Operation should be advised for the symptomatic patient who has severe AS. In young patients, if the valve is pliable and mobile, simple commissurotomy or valve repair may be feasible; the operative mortality is <1 percent.[73] It will relieve outflow obstruction to a major degree. In such patients, catheter balloon valvuloplasty is the procedure of choice in experienced and skilled centers. Both of these are palliative procedures that postpone valve replacement for many years. Older patients and even young patients with calcified, rigid valves need valve replacement. The natural history of symptomatic patients with severe AS is dismal, i.e., a 10-year mortality of 80 to 90 percent, but there is good outcome after surgery, particularly in patients without any comorbid cardiac and noncardiac conditions. Given the unknown natural history of the asymptomatic patient with severe AS, which may not be benign,[55] it is reasonable to recommend surgery even to the asymptomatic patient. There is, however, no consensus about valve replacement in the truly asymptomatic patient. Clearly, if the patient has LV dysfunction, then valve replacement should be performed. Some recommend valve replacement in all asymptomatic patients with severe AS, while others would recommend it in those with AVA ≤ 0.75 cm^2 and in selected patients with AVA of 0.76 to 1.0 cm^2 (Table 63-13).

TABLE 63-12

MEDICAL TREATMENT OF PATIENTS WITH AORTIC VALVE STENOSIS

  I. Antibiotic prophylaxis
    A. Infective endocarditis (Chap. 82)
    B. Recurrent rheumatic carditis (Chap. 62)
  II. Restriction of activities
    A. Severe exercise
    B. Competitive sports
  III. Arrhythmias
    A. Prevent and/or control
    B. Restore sinus rhythm, if possible
  IV. Cardiac medications (only if essential)
    A. Avoid negative inotropic and proarrhythmic agents if possible
    B. Diuretics—use cautiously
    C. Arteriolar and venodilators—use cautiously
  V. Follow-up of asymptomatic patients
    A. Mild AS: Every 2–5 years
    B. Moderate AS: Every 6–12 months
    C. Develop symptoms: Immediate

Source: Copyright S. H. Rahimtoola, M.B., F.R.C.P., M.A.C.P. See Ref. 85.

TABLE 63-13

SEVERE AORTIC VALVE STENOSIS:
INDICATIONS FOR SURGERY

I. All symptomatic patients
  A. LV function normal: as soon as possible
  B. LV dysfunction: urgent
  C. Heart failure: emergent
II. Asymptomatic patients
  A. All patients
  B. Alternative strategy
    1. All patients with AVA ≤ 0.75 cm^2
    2. Patients with AVA 0.76–1.0 cm^2
      a. LV dysfunction
      b. Associated significantly obstructive CAD
      c. Patients aged $\geq$ 60–65 years
      d. Severe LV hypertrophy
      e. Painless ischemia
      f. Significant arrhythmias
      g. LV dysfunction on exercise

Note: LV = left ventricular; AVA = aortic valve area; CAD = Coronary artery disease.

Source: Copyright © by S. H. Rahimtoola, M.B., F.R.C.P., M.A.C.P. See Ref. 85.

The operative mortality of valve replacement is about 5 percent or less (see Chap. 68).[55,58,59] In patients without associated CAD, heart failure, or other comorbid factors, it may be ≤ 1 to 2 percent in centers with experienced and skilled staff.[59] Patients with associated CAD should have coronary bypass surgery at the same time as valve surgery because it results in a lower operative and late mortality (Table 63-14). The operative mortality in octogenarians is much higher: up to 8 percent for isolated aortic valve replacement, and up to 13 percent for those undergoing aortic valve replacement and associated coronary bypass surgery.

In severe AS, valve replacement results in an improvement of survival (Fig. 63-4),[70,74] even in those with normal preoperative LV function. LV function remains normal postoperatively if perioperative myocardial damage has not occurred.[20,55,75,76] LV hypertrophy regresses toward normal[20,55,75,76]; after 2 years, the regression continues at a slower rate for up to 8 to 10 years after valve replacement.[76] In those with excessive ventricular hypertrophy preoperatively,[28] the hypertrophy may regress slowly or not at all. These patients may have persistent severe LV diastolic dysfunction, which may be a difficult clinical problem both in the early postoperative period and after hospital discharge. Their clinical picture subsequently resembles that of patients with hypertrophic cardiomyopathy without outflow obstruction, and they may have to be treated as such. Surviving patients are functionally improved. After aortic valve replacement, the 10-year survival is 60 percent or better and the 15-year survival is 45 percent or better.[77] Approximately one-half of the late deaths are not related to the prosthesis but to associated cardiac abnormalities and other comorbid conditions.[77] Thus, the late survival will vary in different subgroups of patients. The older patients ($\geq$65 years) have a relative 10-year survival (actual survival compared to an age- and gender-matched person in the population) after valve replacement that is significantly better than those who are younger (<65 years)—94 percent versus 81 percent (Fig. 63-5).[78]

Patients who present with heart failure should be hospitalized and treated with digitalis, diuretics, and angiotensin-converting enzyme (ACE) inhibitors and should undergo surgery as soon as possible. If heart failure does not respond satisfactorily and rapidly to medical therapy, surgery becomes a matter of considerable urgency.[79] Catheter balloon valvuloplasty can be an important bridge procedure in selected critically ill patients.[79] It usually improves the patient's hemodynamics and makes them better candidates for valve replacement. Valve replacement in patients with AS and heart failure can be performed at an operative mortality of 10 percent or less. Although this is higher than in patients not in heart failure, the risk is justified because late survival in those who survive the operation is excellent and is far superior to that which can be expected with medical therapy; the 7-year survival of patients who survive operation is 84 percent.[80] The impaired LV function improves in all such patients, provided

TABLE 63-14

AORTIC VALVE REPLACEMENT (AVR) OPERATIVE MORTALITY AND LATE SURVIVAL:
EFFECT OF CORONARY BYPASS SURGERY (CBS)

	1982–1983	1967–1976					
	Operative Mortality, %	Operative Mortality, %	All Patients, %	1 VD, %	2 VD, %	3 VD, %	LMCAD, %
AVR + no CAD	1.4	4.5	63	—	—	—	—
AVR + CAD + CBS	4.0	6.3	49	38	28	34	11
AVR + CAD + no CBS	9.4	10.3	36	65	22	13	1

Note: CAD = coronary artery disease, VD = vessel disease, LMCAD = left main coronary artery disease.
Source: From Mullany et al.,[59] with permission.

there has been no perioperative myocardial damage, and becomes normal in two-thirds of the patients. (Fig. 63-6).[81] In addition, the operative survivors are functionally much improved. LV hypertrophy and dilatation (if present preoperatively) regress toward normal. Despite the excellent results of valve replacements in patients with severe AS who are in heart failure, it is important to recognize that surgery should *not* be delayed until heart failure develops.

In the data bases of older patients who underwent catheter balloon valvuloplasty, 6 percent of the patients were in cardiogenic shock.[82,83] The hospital mortality in such patients was very high, almost 50 percent. After hospital discharge, the subsequent mortality is also very high if the patients have not had their stenosis relieved.[83] Thus, these patients need to be treated aggressively with medical therapy with hemodynamic monitoring and need emergent surgery with or without catheter balloon valvuloplasty as a "bridge" procedure[79] (Table 63-15).

The role of catheter balloon valvuloplasty in the older patient has now been clarified.[55,79] In calcific AS after catheter balloon valvuloplasty, the average increase in AVA is 0.3 cm^2 and the final AVA usually averages 0.8 cm^2; thus, many patients continue to have severe AS.[55,79,82] The 30-day, 1-year, and 3-year mortalities average 14, 35, and 71 percent, respectively, in the older patient (average age 78 ± 9 years) with calcific AS,[82] a mortality rate that may be similar to the natural history of this lesion. This technique is indicated[79] as a bridge procedure in those who need emergent noncardiac surgery and in those who are in heart failure (or in cardiogenic shock), who have an expected limited short life span when operative risks are considered to be prohibitively high, and who refuse surgery. When performed as a bridge procedure, valve surgery should not be unduly delayed. On rare occasions, it may be considered as a therapeutic test in patients in whom AS is suspected to be severe but the severity of the AS is in doubt after all standard tests have been performed (Table 63-15), including provocative diagnostic tests to assess mean aortic gradient, stroke volume, and AVA before and after infusion of dobutamine. Catheter balloon valvuloplasty is the procedure of choice in young patients who have pliable, noncalcified valves with commissural fusion (see Chap. 70).

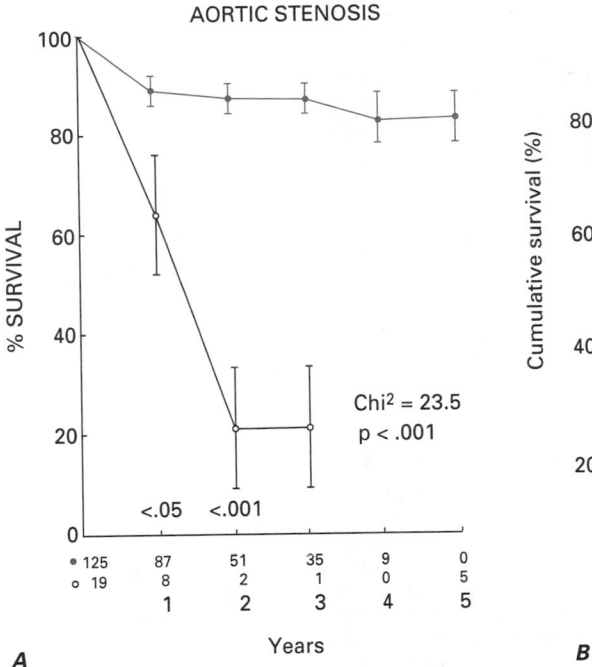

A

B

FIGURE 63-4

There are no prospective randomized trials of aortic valve replacement in severe aortic stenosis, and there are unlikely to be any in the near future. Two studies have compared the results of aortic valve replacement with medical treatment during the same time period in symptomatic patients with normal LV systolic pump function. *Panel A.* Patients who had valve replacement (closed circles) had a much better survival than those treated medically (open circles). (From Schwarz et al.,[74] with permission.) *Panel B.* Patients who were treated with valve replacement (BSA) had a better survival than those treated medically (NH). (From Horstkotte and Loogen,[70] with permission.) These differences in survival between those treated medically and surgically are so large that there is a great deal of confidence that aortic valve replacement significantly improves the survival of those with severe AS.

ACUTE AORTIC REGURGITATION

Etiology

The two most common causes of acute aortic regurgitation (AR) are infective endocarditis and prosthetic valve dysfunction.[84] Other causes include dissection of the aorta, systemic hypertension, and trauma.[85,86] AR associated with dissection of the aorta indicates that the dissection involves the ascending aorta down to the aortic valve annulus/root. AR associated with systemic hypertension is usually mild and transient; it is associated with severe elevation of aortic pressure, and, when the systemic hypertension is controlled, the AR usually disappears unless permanent changes have occurred in the aortic valve annulus/root or valve leaflets.

Pathophysiology

The LV diastolic pressure-volume relationship plays a very important role in the pathophysiology of acute valve regurgitation (Fig. 63-7).[87,88] Two features should be considered:[84] (1) The ability of the left ventricle to dilate acutely is limited; as a result, the volume overload of acute AR produces a rapid

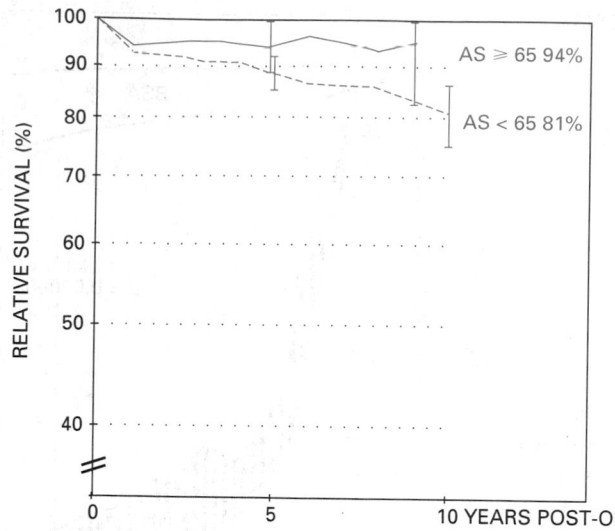

FIGURE 63-5

Data from the Karolinska Institute in Sweden provided an interesting perspective on the long-term survival after valve replacement in patients aged ≥65 years. They examined the relative survival, i.e., compared the survival of the patient who had undergone aortic valve replacement with another age- and sex-matched person in the same population. Patients under the age of 65 had a relative survival of 81 percent, significantly lower than 100 percent. On the other hand, patients aged ≥65 years who underwent valve replacement had a relative survival of 94 percent at the end of 10 years—not significantly different from 100 percent. These data indicate that: (1) survival following valve replacement for AS in patients aged ≥65 years is identical to an age- and sex-matched individual in the population who does not have AS, and (2) the late relative survival of patients aged 65 years or greater is much better than that of patients under the age of 65. (From Lindblom et al.,[78] with permission.)

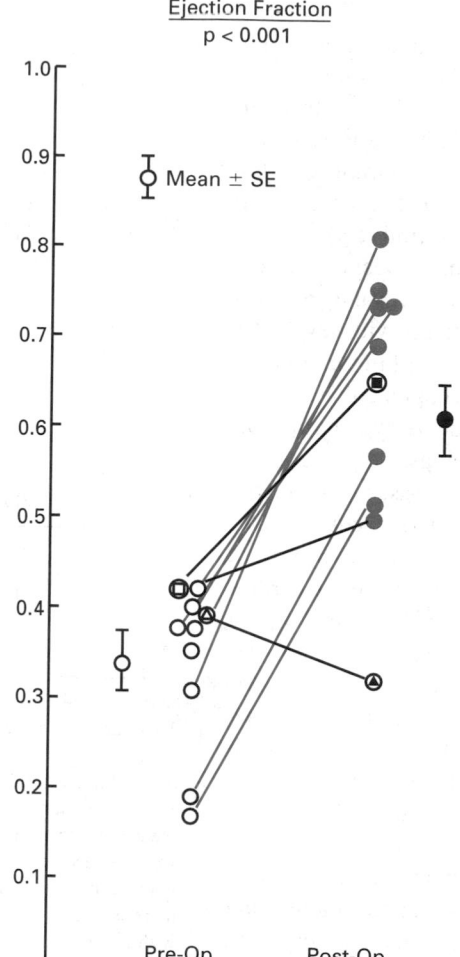

● Peri-Op MI and late CHB
◉ Post-Op Perivalvular Aortic Imcompetence

FIGURE 63-6

Examination of changes in LV ejection fraction in each individual patient in those who had aortic stenosis with LV systolic dysfunction and clinical heart failure showed that after aortic valve replacement the LV ejection fraction improved from 0.34 to 0.63. All but one patient showed an improvement in LV ejection fraction; the only patient who showed a deterioration in ejection fraction suffered a perioperative myocardial infarction and had complete heart block, and the only patient who showed only a small increase in ejection fraction had had a myocardial infarct prior to valve replacement. Note that ejection fraction normalized in two-thirds of the patients, and in the two patients with the lowest ejection fraction (0.18 and 0.19), the ejection fraction normalized in both.

These data indicate that there is probably no lower limit of ejection fraction at which time these patients become inoperable. This also indicates that the lower the ejection fraction, the more urgent the need for valve replacement. (From Smith et al.,[81] with permission.)

TABLE 63-15

SUGGESTED INDICATIONS FOR CATHETER BALLOON VALVULOPLASTY IN PATIENTS WITH SEVERE CALCIFIC AORTIC VALVE STENOSIS[a]

I. "Bridge" procedure to eventual AVR
   A. Cardiogenic shock
   B. Moderate to severe heart failure
   C. Emergent/urgent need for noncardiac therapeutic procedures (e.g., operation)
II. Patient with limited life span
   A. Noncardiac reasons (e.g., carcinoma)
   B. Cardiac reason(s) other than aortic stenosis
III. Others
   A. Patient at extremely high risk for AVR
   B. AVR not desirable for noncardiac reasons or cardiac causes other than aortic stenosis
   C. Patient refuses surgery
IV. Rare
   A. "Therapeutic test": patients with small stroke volume and small valve gradient, with valve stenosis suspected to be severe but severity in doubt even after provocative diagnostic tests

[a] Caution should be exercised in recommending this procedure in asymptomatic patients.

Note: AVR = aortic valve replacement.

Source: Adapted from Rahimtoola,[79] with permission.

increase of LV diastolic pressure (curve B, (Fig. 63-7); and (2) the LV diastolic pressure-volume relationship before the onset of acute AR. If the left ventricle is already stiff or less compliant than normal from an associated lesion (e.g., AS or systemic hypertension), the LV diastolic pressure will rise more precipitously as a result of the volume overload of acute AR (curve A) than if the LV were normal (curve B). On the other hand, if the left ventricle is somewhat dilated from a previous lesion, for example, mild AR (curve C), initially the LV pressure will rise more gradually with acute AR but may subsequently rise to the same high levels as that seen with a normal or stiff LV.

Acute AR that is mild produces little or no hemodynamic abnormality, for example, when associated with systemic hypertension. Increasing severity of regurgitation produces greater degrees of hemodynamic abnormalities, and severe AR often produces the clinical picture of "heart failure."

Acute AR that is severe results in a large volume of regurgitant blood; therefore, the volume of blood in the LV in diastole is increased. In an acute situation, the LV end-diastolic volume can only increase mildly (no more than 20 to 30 percent) and the LV diastolic pressure-volume relationships are particularly important. The LV systolic pump function is initially normal (Fig. 63-8). The increased LV diastolic pressure results

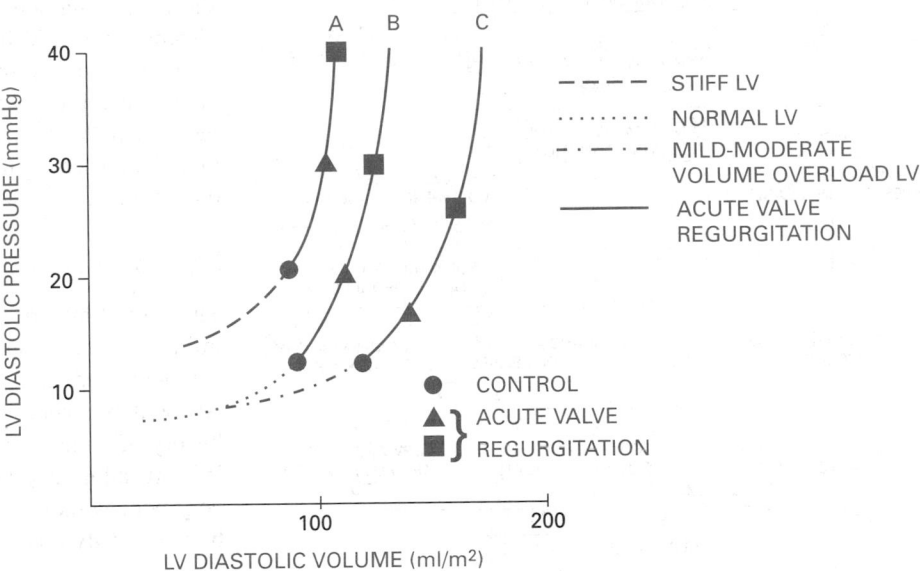

LV DIASTOLIC PRESSURE–VOLUME RELATIONSHIPS

Effects of Acute Valve Regurgitation

FIGURE 63-7
The left ventricular (LV) diastolic pressure-volume (P-V) relationship in acute valve regurgitation. The volume overload of acute AR produces a rapid increase of LV diastolic pressure in a patient with normal LV diastolic P-V prior to the acute AR (curve B). The LV diastolic pressure will rise more or less precipitously as a result of the volume overload of acute AR, depending on whether the LV is already stiff (curve A) or is somewhat dilated from a previous volume overload (curve C). (From Rahimtoola,[90] with permission.)

in increases in mean left atrial and pulmonary venous pressures and produces varying degrees of pulmonary edema.[89] The normal LV systolic pump function in the presence of LV dilatation results in an increase of LV stroke volume. A large percentage of the LV stroke volume is returned to the LV in diastole, however; as a result, the forward stroke volume is reduced. The LV uses two mechanisms: an increase of myocardial contractility and, importantly, a compensatory tachycardia to maintain an adequate forward cardiac output. As a result, the forward cardiac output may be appropriate initially. If the compensatory mechanisms are inadequate, however, forward cardiac output is reduced. Pulmonary edema, with or without an adequate cardiac output, produces the picture of clinical heart failure.[89] Subsequently, LV systolic pump function may become abnormal; when that occurs, the pulmonary edema is further increased and the forward cardiac output is further reduced, leading to more severe manifestations of clinical heart failure.

Clinical Findings

HISTORY, PHYSICAL FINDINGS

The clinical presentations of patients with acute AR are those relating to preexisting disorders that have caused the acute AR. For example, patients may have peripheral signs of infective endocarditis, a history of trauma, or severe chest pain of aortic dissection. The other clinical presentations are those related

to the AR itself. If the AR is mild, the patient is usually asymptomatic. In the symptomatic patient, the symptoms are those of heart failure.

On physical examination, the symptomatic patient with acute severe AR usually has a tachycardia. The arterial pulse shows an increased rate of rise of pressure. Systolic pressure is usually normal unless there is very severe heart failure; however, the diastolic pressure is in the normal range or may be decreased. The pulse pressure is usually normal. Thus, although the classic peripheral signs of chronic, severe AR are often absent, an important diagnostic clue is the rapid rate of rise of arterial pressure. The usual clinical signs of heart failure may be present. On examination of the precordium, the LV impulse is normal or slightly displaced to the left; it is usually hyperkinetic unless LV systolic dysfunction is present. The first heart sound is soft, and the second heart sound is often single and is soft. If pulmonary hypertension is present, P_2 is loud and there is a loud S_3 gallop sound but an S_4 gallop sound is absent. The clinical sine qua non of AR is the AR murmur, an early or immediate, blowing, decrescendo diastolic murmur beginning after A_2 that is best heard with the diaphragm of the stethoscope. Having the patient sit up and lean forward with the breath held in expiration facilitates the audibility of the murmur in difficult cases. The murmur may be short and soft if the ascending aortic pressure equalizes with LV pressure in early or mid-diastole. An Austin Flint murmur, if present, occurs in mid-diastole (see also Chap. 10).

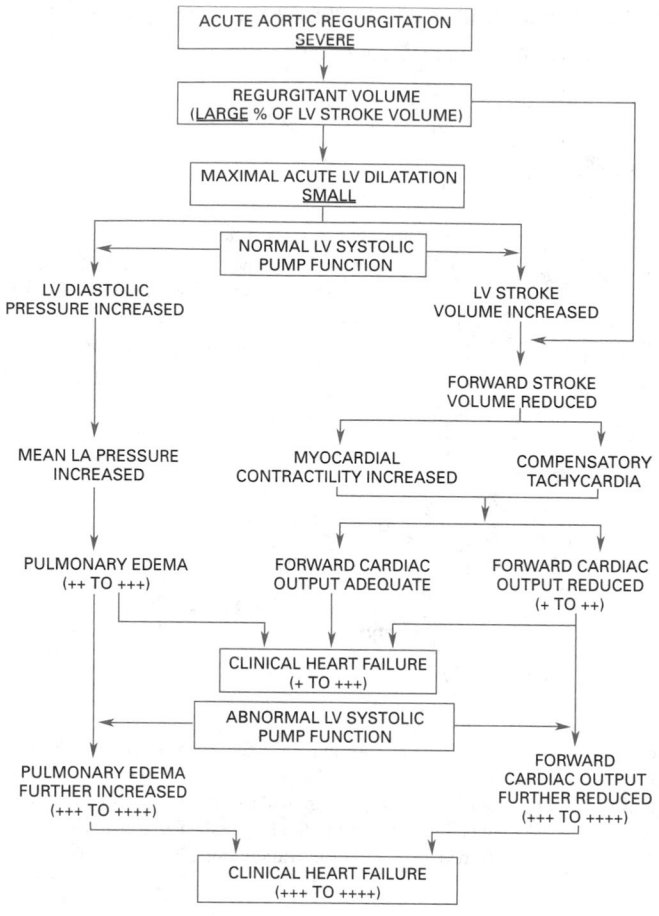

FIGURE 63-8

Pathophysiology of acute severe aortic regurgitation. Acute AR that is severe results in a large volume of regurgitant blood; therefore, the volume of blood in the left ventricle in diastole is increased. In an acute situation, the LV end-diastolic volume can only increase mildly (no more than 20 to 30%) and the LV diastolic pressure-volume relationships are particularly important (see Fig. 64-1). The subsequent findings are dependent on LV systolic pump function, LV diastolic pressure-volume relationship, myocardial contractile state, and compensatory tachycardia (see text for details). (Copyright © by S. H. Rahimtoola, M.B., F.R.C.P., M.A.C.P. See Ref. 85.)

An important clinical picture in intravenous drug abusers[84] includes: (1) a peripheral arterial pulse that has a rapid rate of rise and fall, even though the pulse pressure is small; (2) the telltale signs of intravenous drug abuse; (3) sinus tachycardia; and (4) "normal" heart size with pulmonary edema on chest x-ray.

CHEST X-RAY

The chest x-ray shows a "normal" heart size with pulmonary edema; however, some enlargement of all cardiac chambers and the main pulmonary artery may be present. The aorta is not dilated unless aortic annular/root disease or dissection of the aorta is the cause of the acute AR. The aorta may also be dilated in the older patient and/or in those with an associated disease such as systemic hypertension. The lungs may show the signs of infected pulmonary emboli if there is associated tricuspid valve endocarditis.

ELECTROCARDIOGRAM

The ECG often shows nonspecific ST-T-wave changes and a sinus tachycardia; however, it may be normal. The ECG may show signs that are usually found in the associated causative disorder, e.g., LV hypertrophy with ST-T-wave changes in patients with severe hypertension. The ECG may show a variety of conduction abnormalities (atrioventricular and bundle branch block) including heart block, which, in the presence of infective endocarditis, is a sign of paravalvular/myocardial abscess.

Natural History and Prognosis

The natural history of this condition is variable. If the AR is mild to moderate in severity, these patients are likely to do well with medical therapy. Eventually, the changes of chronic AR will be seen. In patients with severe AR, the natural history depends on whether or not they have heart failure.[90] If heart failure is present, which is common, the prognosis is very poor without valve surgery unless the heart failure can be very easily controlled with medical therapy.

Management

DIAGNOSIS OF AORTIC REGURGITATION

In most instances, the diagnosis can be made by clinical evaluation, which includes the history, physical examination, electrocardiography, and chest x-ray. The diagnosis by physical examination in an acutely ill patient who is *in extremis* may be difficult.

Transthoracic echo/Doppler ultrasound is an important and valuable noninvasive procedure that should be used in every instance. It will demonstrate the AR and its severity and will provide useful information about the size and function of the left ventricle and other valvular and cardiac abnormalities. If the transthoracic method is not adequate, for example, in the very ill patient, then the transesophageal method should be used (see Chap. 14).

Echocardiography shows the diastolic flutter of the anterior leaflet of the mitral valve. In addition, the echocardiogram may show vegetations on the aortic valve, prolapse of an aortic valve leaflet into the left ventricle in diastole, and premature mitral valve closure. The mitral valve may be seen to open for only a short time because the stroke volume is limited. Occasionally, the aortic valve leaflets have been totally destroyed, and none is seen on the echocardiogram. Doppler ultrasound can easily demonstrate the AR and provides an estimate of its severity.

Cardiac catheterization and angiography, including coronary arteriography, show the abnormal physiology described, and aortography shows gross AR. They may be needed to make the diagnosis and are usually indicated before surgical intervention. Coronary arteriography is indicated in the appropriate patient (see above). In the extremely ill patient, there is often a need for clinical judgment with regard to the tests that are essential.

Other tests (cine-computed tomography, including fast cine-computed tomography, radionuclide gated blood scan, or ambulatory ECG) may be needed in very special conditions.

DIAGNOSIS OF THE ETIOLOGY OF ACUTE AORTIC REGURGITATION

The diagnosis of the etiology is usually made during the clinical evaluation by finding the usual clinical characteristics of the underlying lesion. Additional laboratory tests will be needed to confirm the diagnosis, for example, blood cultures in those with suspected infective endocarditis.

Echo/Doppler ultrasound (transthoracic and transesophageal) examination is also extremely valuable in diagnosing the underlying lesion. Its widespread availability and comparative ease of use, especially in the very acutely ill patient, make it the noninvasive procedure of choice. The availability of biplane and omniplane transesophageal probes further enhances its value as a diagnostic tool.

Magnetic resonance imaging (MRI) has a very high specificity for the diagnosis of dissection of the aorta[91,92] and, if available, should be used in all hemodynamically stable patients if the diagnosis has not already been made. The availability of biplane or omniplane transesophageal echocardiography markedly improves the specificity and diagnostic accuracy of transesophageal echocardiography. Angiography is also an effective and time-honored method of diagnosing dissection of the aorta.

In summary, clinical evaluation is available in all institutions; echo/Doppler ultrasound is available in almost all institutions. The use of the other tests depends on the availability of equipment and the skill and experience of personnel using the equipment for this purpose at each institution.

BEDSIDE HEMODYNAMIC MONITORING

In acute disorders affecting the left ventricle, there may be a phase lag between the rise in pulmonary venous pressure and the appearance of pulmonary edema on the chest x-ray film. As a result, the reliability of the chest x-ray in demonstrating the presence and severity of elevated left atrial pressure initially is less than satisfactory in the acutely ill patient.[93] If the assessment of left atrial pressure is made by physical examination and chest x-ray, a significant number of errors may be made in these patients with an acute cardiac problem. Therapeutic decisions based on incorrect assessments may result in significant problems; for example, inappropriate diuresis may result in a fall of cardiac output, or inappropriate volume loading may result in a further increase in left atrial pressure. Furthermore, the optimization of filling pressures and cardiac output may not be made accurately in acute heart failure without measuring their actual values. Thus, use of a balloon flotation catheter for bedside hemodynamic monitoring is required in most if not almost all acutely ill patients with acute AR.

TREATMENT

Treatment of the heart failure is directed toward reducing pulmonary venous pressure and increasing cardiac output. In all patients, treatment is also directed toward correcting or controlling the etiologic disease/disorder and/or the altered pathophysiologic state (Table 63-16).[84,90]

Vasodilators (intravenous nitroprusside for an acute, severe condition) are useful and important in the management of these patients.[94] Vasodilators will produce a reduction of left atrial *v* wave and mean left atrial pressure. They produce a reduction in LV end-diastolic and end-systolic volumes and an increase in LV ejection fraction. The regurgitant fraction and regurgitant volume are reduced; as a result, the forward stroke volume and cardiac output are increased.[94] Digitalis therapy is of significant benefit in the management of heart failure. The combination of various agents (vasodilators, diuretics, and digitalis) tends to produce the maximum benefit in an individual patient; intravenous nitroprusside is often necessary in the acutely ill patient.

Surgical therapy (valve replacement/valve repair or appropriate surgery for dissection of the aorta) is the cornerstone of the most definitive therapy currently available for heart failure in these patients. The management of the patient with heart failure or suspected heart failure is outlined in Fig. 63-9.[90] If the valve regurgitation is due to *dissection of the aorta*, the need for cardiac surgery is an emergency, even if the regurgitation is mild or moderate, because AR indicates involvement of the ascending aorta down to the region of the aortic valve annulus/root (see also Chap. 98). The outcome of the patient with heart failure due to infective endocarditis is very poor with medical therapy but is improved with valve replacement.[95] The indications for surgery in *infective endocarditis* are listed in Table 63-17.[75] Infective endocarditis due to special organisms (e.g., fungi) can only rarely be controlled

---

TABLE 63-16

TREATMENT OF HEART FAILURE IN ACUTE VALVE REGURGITATION

I. Correct or control altered pathophysiologic state
  A. Reduce pulmonary venous pressure
    1. Diuresis
    2. Vasodilation
    3. Control heart rate and maintain sinus rhythm (digitalis, cardioversion, antiarrhythmics)
  B. Increase cardiac output
    1. Reduction of valve regurgitation (vasodilators)
    2. Inotropic stimulation (digitalis, dobutamine)
  C. Improve left ventricular systolic dysfunction
    1. Reduce pulmonary venous pressure
    2. Increase cardiac output
    3. ACE inhibitors
II. Correct or control underlying disease or disorder
  A. Antibiotics for infective endocarditis
  B. Pharmacologic therapy for systemic hypertension
  C. Surgery for valve regurgitation in infective endocarditis, prosthetic valve dysfunction, dissection of the aorta, trauma

Source: From Rahimtoola,[84] with permission.

by pharmacologic therapy alone, and surgery is almost always needed. In these and some other conditions, valve surgery may be needed even if the AR is only mild or moderate. It must be recognized, however, that in 90 to 95 percent of patients needing surgery for endocarditis, the indication for valve surgery is heart failure. When the heart failure is a result of *prosthetic valve dysfunction* or *trauma*, the need for surgery can be an emergency, an urgent situation, or an elective procedure. Prosthetic valves are inherently stenotic. When regurgitation is superimposed, it produces a pressure plus volume overload on the left ventricle that the ventricle may not handle very well acutely. Furthermore, valve regurgitation may be a sign of bioprosthetic valve degeneration or prosthetic endocarditis; in both conditions, prosthetic valve replacement is usually needed even if the valve regurgitation is mild to moderate. Trauma may result in AR from damage to valve leaflets or aortic annulus/root or from dissection of the aorta. If trauma produces dissection of the aorta and AR, the need for surgery may be an emergent one.

In some instances, the heart failure can be controlled completely with pharmacologic therapy, and the left ventricle and left atrium are able to dilate and adapt to the volume overload; in such instances, surgical therapy may be delayed, perhaps for a considerable period of time.

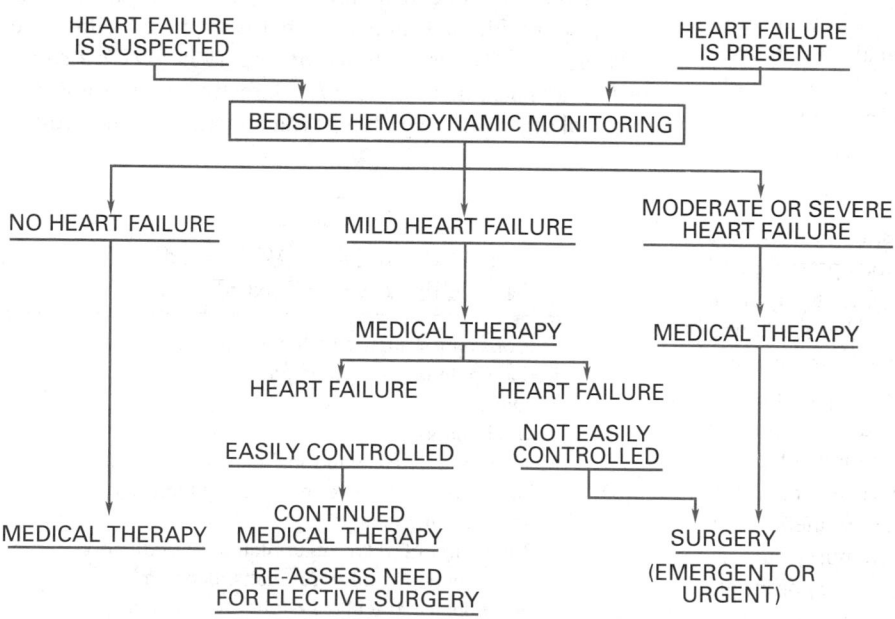

FIGURE 63-9

Role of bedside hemodynamic monitoring in acute aortic regurgitation. All patients with acute AR probably should have this procedure. If the AR is mild and there are no significant hemodynamic abnormalities, then the balloon flotation catheter can be withdrawn. On the other hand, if the AR is moderate to severe and there are significant hemodynamic abnormalities, then the balloon flotation catheter is left in place to guide therapy in the management of these acutely ill patients. If the hemodynamic abnormalities are mild, the patient is treated medically. If these abnormalities are easily controlled, medical therapy is continued and periodic reassessments are made to assess the need for elective surgery. If the hemodynamic abnormalities are not easily corrected, or the hemodynamic abnormalities initially are moderate/severe, then surgery is undertaken either emergently or urgently. (From Rahimtoola,[90] with permission.)

CHRONIC AORTIC REGURGITATION

Etiology

In North America, the most common cause of chronic, isolated severe AR is aortic root/annular dilatation that is presumably the result of medial disease. Other common causes include a congenital (bicuspid) valve, previous infective endocarditis, and rheumatic disease.[85,86] Chronic AR also occurs in association with a variety of other diseases (Table 63-18). Between 40 and 60 percent of the surgically removed valves from patients with isolated severe regurgitation are classified as idiopathic. Half of these (or 20 to 30 percent of all the valves removed) show histologic criteria of myxomatous degeneration.[96]

Pathology

During systole the aortic root/annulus expands by an increase of 14 to 16 percent of the diameter (twice the radius).[97] This causes the commissural attachments to spread apart, initiating the opening of the valves. These movements are continued during LV systole, which produces the forward motion of the blood. The length of the free edge of the cusps equals the diameter of the aortic root/annulus, or roughly one-third of the perimeter. Therefore, dilatation of the aortic root/annulus, if it is not accompanied by an enlargement of the cusps, results in AR.[97]

Depending on the cause, the valve cusps may show thickening, shortening, commissural lesions, or calcification (Fig. 63-10).[98] Regardless of the cause, the LV is dilated and hypertrophied; some of the largest ventricles have been described in association with chronic severe AR. Little pockets may be seen in the LV outflow tract. These are pouches out of the endocardial lining formed by the regurgitant jet(s) striking the left ventricle.

The myocardium is hypertrophied, with replication of sarcomeres in series, elongation of fibers, and wall thickening. The wall is not as thickened as in patients with AS. Ultrastructural changes in the myocardial cells are similar to those seen in AS; an important difference, however, is the frequent presence of degenerated cardiac muscle cells in patients with severe AR. Cardiac muscle cells with mild degeneration show focal myofibrillar lysis, with preferential loss of thick myofilament

TABLE 63-17

INDICATIONS FOR SURGERY IN INFECTIVE ENDOCARDITIS

Congestive heart failure
Infection
  Uncontrolled by antibiotic therapy
  Fungal
    Usually with staphylococcal infection of aortic or mitral valves
  Serratia
    Usually with gram-negative bacillary infection
Recurrent septic systemic emboli despite adequate antibiotic therapy
Perivalvular and myocardial abscesses
Structural damage to valve in association with other catastrophes (e.g., ruptured sinus of Valsalva)
Very large mobile vegetation

Source: From Rahimtoola,[75] with permission.

and focal proliferation of tubules of the sarcoplasmic reticulum. Moderately degenerated muscle cells show a marked decrease in the number of myofibrils and T tubules and proliferation of sarcoplasmic reticulum, mitochondria, or both. Severely degenerated muscle cells usually are present in areas of marked fibrosis; they are often atrophic, have thickened basement membranes, and have lost their intercellular connections. These degenerated cardiac muscle cells may represent the ultrastructural basis for impaired LV function, which is seen more commonly in severe AR than in severe AS.

In patients with rheumatoid arthritis and ankylosing spondylitis, nodules on the outer surface of the anterior leaflet of the mitral valve have been described.

Pathophysiology

In chronic as opposed to acute AR, the AR becomes severe over a period of time; therefore, the LV diastolic pressure-

TABLE 63-18

ETIOLOGY OF CHRONIC AORTIC VALVE REGURGITATION

Aortic root dilatation
Congenital bicuspid valve
Previous infective endocarditis
Rheumatic
In association with other diseases
  Congenital lesions, e.g., supravalvular or discrete subvalvular AS, ventricular septal defect, and aneurysm of the sinus of Valsalva
  Connective tissue disease, e.g., Marfan's syndrome, osteogenesis imperfecta, and Ehlers-Danlos syndrome
  Autoimmune diseases, e.g., ankylosing spondylitis, rheumatoid arthritis, and systemic lupus erythematosus
  Various forms of aortitis and arteritis, e.g., giant-cell arteritis and Takayasu's disease
  Syphilis

volume relationships are different from those seen in acute AR (Fig. 63-7). If the AR is mild to moderate, the LV end-diastolic volume is increased moderately, the LV diastolic pressure-volume curve is moved to the right (curve *B*) of normal (curve *A*), and the LV diastolic pressure is usually normal (Fig. 63-11). In severe AR, the LV diastolic pressure-volume curves are moved further to the right (curves *C* and *D*). If the LV systolic pump function is normal, the LV end-diastolic volume can be quite large without significant elevation of LV end-diastolic pressure (curve *C*). If the LV diastolic volume increases further, however, the LV diastolic pressures will be increased. If LV systolic pump dysfunction supervenes, the LV diastolic pressure-volume curve (curve *D*) relationships are moved even further to the right, with quite marked LV dilatation and increases in LV diastolic pressure.

The increase of LV end-diastolic volume[99] is a result of the regurgitant volume (and is proportional to the amount of regurgitation) and LV systolic dysfunction. As LV systolic dysfunction supervenes and increases in severity, for any severity of regurgitant volume the LV end-diastolic volume increases further in an attempt to maintain LV stroke volume.

Severe chronic AR results in a large regurgitant volume (a large percentage of LV stroke volume). The left ventricle responds by dilating (average LV end-diastolic volume in patients undergoing surgery was 205 mL/m^2)[20]; the dilatation is proportional to the amount of the regurgitant volume. The subsequent large LV stroke volume produces LV systolic hypertension. Both of these increase LV wall stress (afterload), which can result in an impairment of LV function. The heart responds by becoming hypertrophied (average LV mass in patients undergoing valve surgery was 222 g/m^2),[20] and LV systolic pump function remains normal. There is also an alteration of the LV diastolic pressure-volume relationship (Fig. 63-11). As a result, some patients with normal LV systolic pump function become symptomatic[100] because of the abnormal LV diastolic function (Fig. 63-12).

In AR, the left ventricle is ejecting against systemic resistance, and the myocardial tension that is developed to open the aortic valve and eject the huge stroke volume is great. This contrasts with another volume-overload lesion, mitral regurgitation, in which there is a low-resistance chamber into which the LV is also emptying (the left atrium). Thus, for the same degree of regurgitant volume, afterload is higher in AR.

As LV afterload (a combination of LV dilatation, hypertrophy, and systolic hypertension) continues to increase, the LV utilizes two additional compensatory mechanisms, namely, increase of preload and an increase of myocardial contractility. Both of these help maintain normal LV systolic pump function.

When the limit of preload reserve has been reached (afterload mismatch)[29] and/or myocardial contractility is reduced, LV systolic pump function becomes abnormal (see also Chap. 22). At this stage, correction of AR will result in normalization or marked improvement of LV systolic function. The additional LV dilatation also results in further alter-

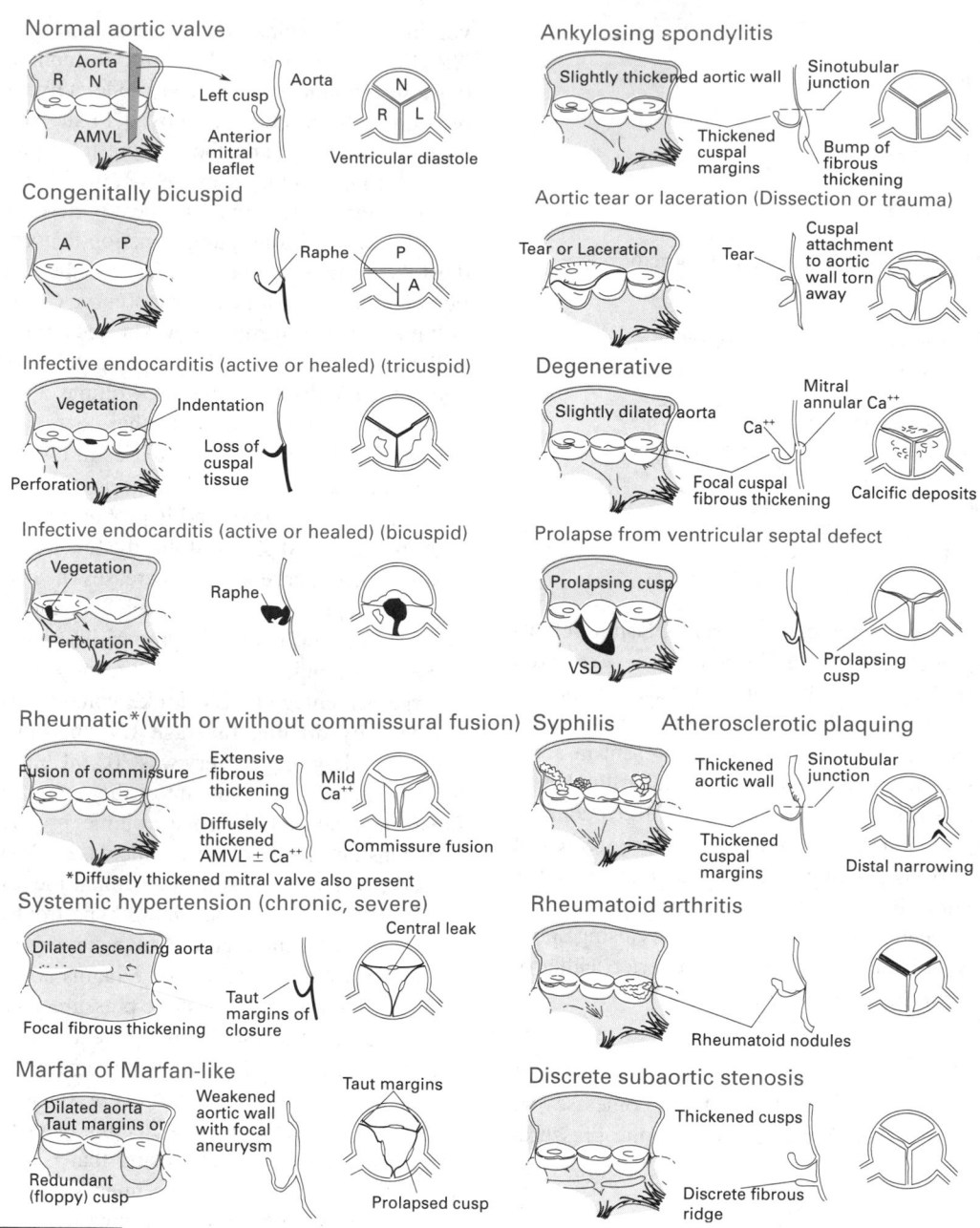

FIGURE 63-10

Pathologic findings in aortic regurgitation depending on the etiology of the AR. (From Waller,[98] with permission.)

ation of the LV diastolic pressure-volume relationship (see Fig. 63-6). Clinical heart failure is usually a result of the abnormal LV systolic pump function. In patients with normal LV systolic pump function, clinical heart failure is a result of LV diastolic dysfunction.

Because of the leak of blood from the ascending aorta to the LV in diastole, the aortic diastolic pressure is reduced. The large LV stroke volume (a combination of forward stroke volume and regurgitant volume) results in elevation of the aortic systolic pressure, and thus the pulse pressure is considerably increased. Reduction or normalization of aortic systolic pressure is suggestive of LV systolic dysfunction in these patients.

LV stroke volume in AR consists of the forward stroke volume (blood delivered to the body tissues and the heart), which, multiplied by heart rate, makes up the forward cardiac output, and the regurgitant volume (the volume of blood that regurgitates back to the left ventricle). In the early stages, even in severe AR, the forward cardiac output and LV ejection fraction are normal at rest. During exercise, as in normal individuals, the systemic vascular resistance is decreased[101] and the heart rate is increased, which reduces the length of diastole. Both these factors reduce the regurgitant volume, and forward stroke volume and cardiac output are increased during exercise.[101] Thus, the ejection fraction on exercise is related to both the myocardial contractile state[102] and the fall

LV DIASTOLIC PRESSURE–VOLUME RELATIONSHIPS
Effects of Chronic Valve Regurgitation

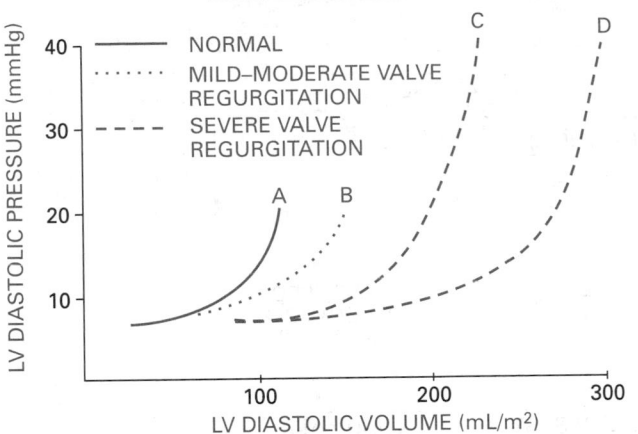

FIGURE 63-11

In chronic aortic regurgitation, as opposed to acute AR, the AR becomes severe over a period of time; therefore, the LV diastolic pressure-volume (P-V) relationships are different from those seen in acute AR (see Fig. 63-7). If the AR is mild to moderate, the LV diastolic P-V curve is moved to the right (curve *B*). In severe AR, the LV diastolic P-V curves are moved further to the right, depending on whether the LV systolic pump function is normal (curve *C*) or abnormal (curve *D*). (From Rahimtoola,[90] with permission.)

in systemic vascular resistance.[101] Accordingly, a decline in ejection fraction on exercise cannot be used as a specific marker of LV function in these patients unless the change in systemic vascular resistance has also been measured. A fall of normal resting ejection fraction to less than 0.50 on exercise, however, has been shown to correlate with reduced total body oxygen consumption[103] and increased left atrial pressure during exercise.[101,103] Further impairment of LV function produces demonstrable abnormalities at rest; there is a further increase in LV end-diastolic volume, which helps to maintain forward stroke volume. The resting LV ejection fraction is reduced, and mean left atrial pressure begins to increase. Even at this stage, the forward cardiac output may be maintained in the normal range. The increases in left atrial pressure may produce various grades of pulmonary edema. Finally, in the state of severe heart failure, the ejection fraction may be low, LV end-diastolic volume is large, and LV end-diastolic pressure is greatly increased and is associated with increases in left atrial, pulmonary, right ventricular, and right atrial pressures. Forward cardiac output is no longer normal. An increase in systemic venous pressure in association with salt and water retention produces engorgement of systemic organs (e.g., the liver) as well as peripheral edema.

In severe AR, myocardial oxygen needs are increased because of increases in LV diastolic and systolic volumes, LV muscle mass (hypertrophy), and LV pressures as well as by prolongation of systolic ejection time. Total coronary blood flow is increased. Coronary reserve, the ability of the coronary blood flow to increase with vasodilatation, however, is significantly reduced,[104–106] probably because of a reduced diastolic aortic-LV pressure gradient and compression of intramyocardial coronary arteries (systolic "milking" of intramural arter-

ies). Therefore, myocardial ischemia is often present on stress in these patients.[104–106] Some patients with severe AR may complain of angina pectoris on effort even in the absence of epicardial CAD. Associated obstructive CAD can be expected to exacerbate further the myocardial ischemia (see Fig. 63-13).

Clinical Features

HISTORY
Patients with mild to moderate AR usually do not have symptoms that can be attributed to the heart. Even patients with severe AR may be asymptomatic. They may complain of pounding of the head or palpitations, which result from their awareness of the beating of a dilated left ventricle that undergoes a large volume change in systole, during either sinus beats or postectopic beats. The main symptoms of severe AR result from elevated pulmonary venous pressures and include dyspnea on exertion, orthopnea, and paroxysmal nocturnal dyspnea. When congestive heart failure occurs, patients complain of fatigue and weakness. Angina pectoris occurs in 20 percent of such patients and may be present even if the coronary arteries are normal. Angina associated with syphilitic AR may be due to associated ostial stenosis of the coronary arteries. In such patients, angina often occurs at rest and is difficult to control.

PHYSICAL EXAMINATION
A variety of interesting but not very useful clinical signs may be present in patients with chronic severe AR. These include *de Musset's sign* (bobbing of the head with each heartbeat), *Traube's sign* (pistol-shot sound heard over the femoral artery), *Duroziez' sign* (systolic murmur over the femoral artery when it is compressed proximally and diastolic murmur when it is compressed distally), and *Quincke's pulse* (capillary pulsations that can be detected by pressing a glass slide on the patient's lip or transmitting a light through the patient's fingertips).

The arterial pulse is very characteristic and consists of an abrupt distension with a rapid rise and a quick collapse (*Corrigan's pulse*). The arterial pulse may be bisferiens, a double impulse during systole. The systolic arterial pressure is increased (in severe AR it averages 145 to 160 mmHg), the diastolic pressure is reduced (in severe AR it averages 45 to 60 mmHg), and the Korotkoff's sounds persist down to 0 mmHg. Even in such instances, however, the recorded intraarterial pressure rarely falls below 30 mmHg. The vasoconstriction that occurs in the presence of heart failure may result in some elevation of the arterial diastolic pressure and should not be interpreted as an improvement in severity of AR. Similarly, LV systolic dysfunction can produce a fall of systolic blood pressure that should not be considered to be an improvement of the AR. The fall of systolic pressure along with elevation of diastolic pressures tends to normalize the pulse pressure. The jugular venous pressure is normal except in heart failure and in those rare instances in which the greatly dilated ascending aorta obstructs the superior vena cava.

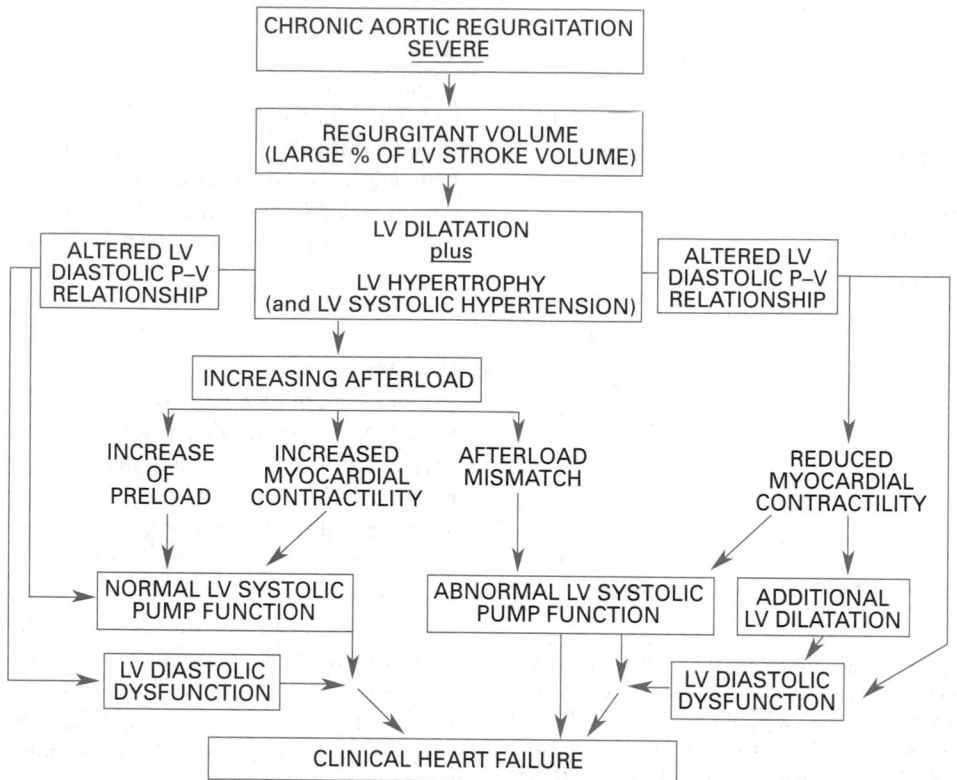

FIGURE 63-12

Severe chronic aortic regurgitation results in a large regurgitant volume (a large percentage of LV stroke volume). The left ventricle responds by dilating; the subsequent large LV stroke volume results in the production of LV systolic hypertension. There is an alteration of the LV diastolic pressure-volume (P-V) relationship. However, some patients with normal LV systolic pump function become symptomatic because of the abnormal LV diastolic function. As LV afterload (a result of LV dilatation, hypertrophy, and systolic hypertension) continues to increase, the LV utilizes two additional compensatory mechanisms, i.e., increase of preload and an increase of myocardial contractility. Both of these help maintain normal LV systolic pump function.

When the limit of preload reserve has been reached (afterload mismatch) and/or myocardial contractility is reduced, LV systolic pump function becomes abnormal. The additional LV dilatation also results in further alteration of the LV diastolic P-V relationship.

Clinical heart failure is usually a result of the abnormal LV systolic pump function; diastolic dysfunction may also be present in some patients. Clinical heart failure in those with normal LV systolic pump function is a result of LV diastolic dysfunction. (Copyright © by S. H. Rahimtoola, M.B., F.R.C.P., M.A.C.P. See Ref. 85.)

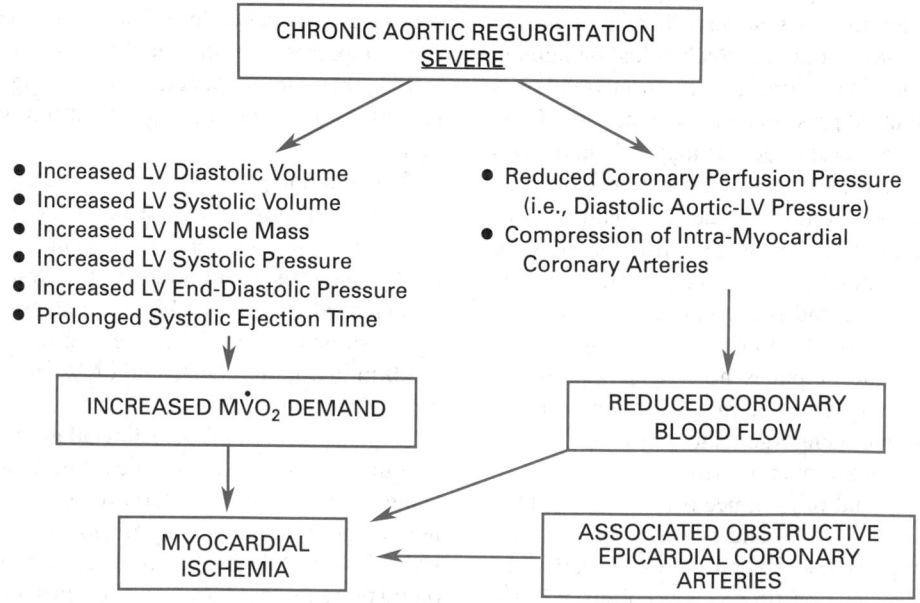

FIGURE 63-13

In severe aortic regurgitation, myocardial oxygen needs are increased. Total coronary blood flow is increased, but coronary reserve, i.e., the ability of the coronary blood flow to increase with vasodilatation, is significantly reduced, probably because of a reduced diastolic aortic–LV pressure gradient and compression (systolic milking) of intramyocardial coronary arteries. There-

fore, myocardial ischemia is often present on stress in these patients. Associated obstructive coronary artery disease can be expected to further exacerbate the myocardial ischemia. (Copyright © by S. H. Rahimtoola, M.B., F.R.C.P., M.A.C.P. See Ref. 85.)

On inspection, the chest may rock and the cardiac impulse may be visible. The cardiac impulse is hyperdynamic (Table 63-19). There may be a systolic thrill at the base of the heart, over the carotids, and in the suprasternal notch. This results from a large LV stroke volume across a diseased aortic valve. A diastolic thrill signifies severe AR. The first heart sound is usually soft because the mitral valve leaflets are close to each other at the onset of systole, or there may be premature valve closure. This is exaggerated if the PR interval is prolonged. The S_2 is usually single because the aortic valve does not close properly[107] or because the LV ejection time is prolonged and the P_2 may not be heard. Often, a systolic ejection murmur, which is sometimes very loud, is present. The clinical sine qua non of AR is an early or immediate, blowing, decrescendo diastolic murmur beginning after A_2. It is best heard with the diaphragm of the stethoscope at the left sternal border or, in difficult instances, by having the patient sit up and lean forward and by auscultating in held respiration at the end of a deep expiration. In severe AR, the murmur may be holodiastolic. When it is soft, its intensity can be increased by having the patient perform isometric exercise, for example, a handgrip, which increases aortic diastolic pressure. At times, this murmur is better heard along the right sternal border, which should draw attention to the possibility that the cause of the AR is aortic root/annular disease (see also Chap. 10). Classically, rupture of the sinus of Valsalva into the right heart chambers produces a continuous murmur.

In many patients with severe AR, an Austin Flint murmur[108] (see Chap. 10) is present in presystole and/or mid-diastole. Two inferences can be drawn from the presence of an Austin Flint murmur: (1) it signifies that the AR is severe, and (2) it requires that associated mitral stenosis be excluded. The most helpful sign at the bedside is the response of the murmur to the inhalation of amyl nitrate. The vasodilatation produced by amyl nitrate increases forward flow, reduces the regurgitant volume, and results in the Austin Flint murmur becoming much softer or disappearing. On the other hand, the increased cardiac output and the tachycardia accentuate or increase the murmur of mitral stenosis. Alternatively, echocardiography can easily demonstrate the presence of organic mitral stenosis.

With severe LV dilatation and/or LV systolic dysfunction, secondary mitral regurgitation may be present with the characteristic holosystolic murmur. Heart failure may be associated with pulmonary congestion/edema, pulmonary hypertension, right ventricular enlargement, tricuspid regurgitation, elevated jugular venous pressure, hepatomegaly, and peripheral edema (see Chap. 23).

TABLE 63-19

PHYSICAL EXAMINATION OF PATIENTS WITH VARYING SEVERITY OF CHRONIC AORTIC VALVE REGURGITATION

	Mild	Moderate	Severe	Severe + LV Systolic Dysfunction	Severe + Heart Failure + LV Systolic Dysfunction
Arterial pulse	Normal	Corrigan's + to + +	Corrigan's + + +	Corrigan's + +	Corrigan's +
Arterial pressure					
Systolic	Normal	Increased + to + +	Increased + + +	Increased + +	Normal/+
Diastolic	Normal	Decreased + to + +	Decreased + + + to + + + +	Decreased + + to + + +	Decreased +
Pulse pressure	Often normal	Increased + to + +	Increased + + + to + + + +	Increased + + to + + +	Increased +
Cardiac impulse	Often normal	Hyperdynamic	Very hyperdynamic visible ± chest may rock	Hyperdynamic	May be hypodynamic
Precordial thrill:					
Systolic	−	±	±	±	−
Diastolic	−	−	±	±	−
Auscultation:					
S_4	−	−	−	−	−
S_1	Normal	Often soft	Soft	Soft	Soft
S_2	Normal	Normal or single	Often single	Often single	Often single
S_3	−	+	+ + to + + +	+ + +	+ + +
ESM	±	+	+ to + +	+ to + +	+
AoDM	+	+ +	+ + + to + + + +	+ + to + + +	+ to + +
Austin Flint murmur	−	−	±	−	−

Note: S_1 and S_2 = first and second heart sounds; S_3 = third heart sound (diastolic gallop); S_4 = fourth heart sound (presystolic gallop); ESM = ejection systolic murmur; AoDM = aortic diastolic murmur; — absent; + + + + most prominent; ± present or absent.

CHEST X-RAY

The LV is increased in size, and this can be appreciated on the chest x-ray by an increase in the cardiothoracic ratio. Since the upper limit of normal of the cardiothoracic ratio is 0.49, many patients with increased LV size have an enlarged ventricular volume and may still have a cardiothoracic ratio within the normal range. A better noninvasive quantification of LV size can be obtained by echocardiography. The ascending aorta is dilated throughout, and there may be calcium in the aortic valve. With increased filling pressures in the later stages, there might be evidence of an enlarged left atrium and an increased left atrial and pulmonary venous pressure, which are manifested in the pulmonary vascular shadows by a redistribution of blood flow, pulmonary congestion, and pulmonary edema. In the presence of heart failure, enlargement of the right atrium and superior vena cava may be appreciated. Calcification that is limited to the ascending aorta is strongly suggestive of luetic aortitis.

ELECTROCARDIOGRAM

The ECG shows LV hypertrophy with or without associated secondary ST-T-wave changes. In a small percentage of patients, ECG evidence of LV hypertrophy is absent in spite of severe AR. Conduction abnormalities, such as atrioventricular block or left or right bundle branch block with or without axis deviation, may be present. The PR interval may be prolonged,[109] particularly in patients with ankylosing spondylitis. The rhythm is usually sinus. The presence of atrial fibrillation should make one suspect the presence of associated mitral valve disease or heart failure.

ECHOCARDIOGRAPHY

The sign of AR on echocardiography is diastolic fluttering of the anterior leaflet of the mitral valve. Echocardiography is of particular value for excluding the presence of associated mitral stenosis in patients with an Austin Flint diastolic murmur. LV dimensions are increased, and if ventricular function is normal, the percentage of dimensional shortening is normal. Because of the increase in LV dimensions caused by volume overload, there is separation between the open anterior leaflet of the mitral valve and the endocardial surface of the interventricular septum (septal–E point separation), but this does not necessarily indicate impaired LV function when AR is present. In AR, as in other volume-overload lesions, the response in mild volume overload is an elongation of the heart. Since M-mode echocardiography takes a pencil look at the short axis of the heart, LV dimensions by M-mode echocardiography may appear to be normal. In such patients, two-dimensional echocardiography is much superior to the M-mode technique for assessing LV volumes and systolic function. A dilated ascending aorta can be detected on echocardiography, as can an enlarged left atrium. Aortic valve vegetations suggest infective endocarditis. Some other conditions can easily be detected by echocardiography, for example, prolapse of the aortic leaflet into the left ventricle in diastole. Doppler ultrasound is useful for diagnosing and assessing the severity of AR.

There is a significant incidence of false-positive mild regurgitation. There is also an overlap between the various grades of severity of assessment of AR by Doppler when compared to angiography. Transesophageal echocardiography is a useful technique when transthoracic echocardiogram is unsatisfactory and in certain instances for identifying the anatomy of the valve leaflets and aortic root/annulus; it is essential to evaluate if the valve is suitable for repair. Echo/Doppler ultrasound is also very useful for assessing disease of other valves.

CARDIAC CATHETERIZATION/ANGIOGRAPHY

Cardiac catheterization allows the measurement of intracardiac and intravascular pressures and cardiac output, both at rest and during exercise, and can demonstrate the changes described under "Pathophysiology." In addition, other valvular disease, for example, mitral stenosis, aortic stenosis, and mitral regurgitation, can be excluded. LV angiography demonstrates enlarged LV volumes and allows the calculation of LV volumes and LV ejection fraction. Angiography performed with injection of contrast medium in the ascending aorta demonstrates AR and allows a semiquantitative assessment of the degree of AR. In addition, the angiogram demonstrates the dimensions of the aortic root and the state of the ascending aorta. The indications for selective coronary angiography are the same as for aortic stenosis (see Table 63-6).

GATED BLOOD POOL RADIONUCLIDE SCANS

Gated blood pool radionuclide scans also allow the measurement of LV volumes and ejection fraction. In addition, with this technique, it is possible to quantify the amount of AR. These scans, however, assess regurgitation present at both the aortic and mitral valves. Thus, if both valves are incompetent, the total amount of regurgitation present at both valves will be measured. This technique also allows measurement of LV ejection fraction on exercise and on serial studies.

TREADMILL EXERCISE TEST

A treadmill exercise test provides an objective assessment of the degree of functional impairment and documentation of arrhythmias related to exertion. In some patients, however, the exercise test may remain normal despite deterioration of LV function.

AMBULATORY ECG RECORDING

Ambulatory ECG recording may be needed in an occasional patient suspected of having an arrhythmia.

MAGNETIC RESONANCE IMAGING

MRI can demonstrate AR but is rarely needed clinically.

Clinical Decision-Making

Please see the equivalent section in "Aortic Valve Stenosis." The sensitivity, specificity, and accuracy of diagnosis of chronic AR are shown in Table 63-20.[63] The following should be noted: (1) The sensitivity, specificity, and accuracy of diagnosing AR after clinical evaluation are good but not quite

CLINICAL DECISION-MAKING UTILIZING CLINICAL EVALUATION VERSUS ECHO/DOPPLER IN PATIENTS WITH AORTIC REGURGITATION

	After Clinical Evaluation, %	After Echo/Doppler, %
Diagnosis of AR		
Sensitivity	66	79
Specificity	76	74
Accuracy of diagnosis		
All levels of severity	43	57
Moderate or severe AR	91	100

Source: From Kotlewski et al.,[63] with permission.

as good as in AS; (2) echo/Doppler ultrasound improves these criteria to a greater extent than in AS; (3) the difficulties lie in accurately distinguishing patients with mild AR from normal individuals and those with moderate AR and in distinguishing between moderate AR and severe AR; and (4) both clinical evaluation and echo/Doppler ultrasound are excellent in diagnosing the AR as being moderate or severe.

Natural History and Prognosis

Patients with mild AR that does not progress should have a normal life expectancy. Their major risk is the development of infective endocarditis and further valve destruction. Patients with moderate AR, if their disease does not progress, would be expected to have a life expectancy that is reasonably close to the normal range. The disease does progress, however, and mortality at the end of 10 years appears to be about 15 percent.

Patients with severe AR are known to have a long asymptomatic period before the condition is discovered. In asymptomatic patients with normal LV function at rest, symptoms and/or LV dysfunction (and/or sudden death) develop at the rate of about 3 to 6 percent per year.[111–113] The predictor of development of symptoms is LV systolic dysfunction at rest. In patients with normal LV systolic function at rest (Table 63-21), the predictors of development of LV systolic dysfunction and/or symptoms are an increased LV size (LV dimension at end-diastole of ≥70 mm and at end-systole of ≥50 mm,[111–113] and LV end-diastolic volume index of ≥150 mL/m²)[114] and abnormal LV ejection fraction on exercise of <0.50.[103] Sudden death in asymptomatic patients appears to occur only in those with a massively dilated left ventricle (LV end-diastolic dimension of ≥80 mm).[111] It is likely that LV dysfunction first appears on exercise and later also at rest; eventually, heart failure ensues. Severe symptoms, however, may occur even when LV systolic pump function is normal at rest (see "Pathophysiology"). The 5-year mortality of symptomatic patients with severe AR is about 25 percent, and the 10-year mortality averages 50 percent.[110] Once symptoms occur in patients with AR, it is likely that the rate of deteriora-

tion will be rapid. Most patients with angina are dead within 4 years.[115] The 2- to 3-year mortality of those with heart failure is 50 to 70 percent.[115]

Management

All patients with AR need antibiotic prophylaxis to prevent infective endocarditis. Patients with AR of a rheumatic origin need antibiotic prophylaxis to prevent recurrences of rheumatic carditis. Patients with syphilitic AR need a course of antibiotics to treat syphilis.

Patients with mild AR need no specific therapy (Table 63-22). They do not need to restrict their activities and can lead a normal life. Patients with moderate AR also usually need no specific therapy. These patients, however, should avoid heavy physical exertion, competitive sports, and isometric exercise.

The value of long-term vasodilators to produce an improvement in LV size and function has been evaluated in two placebo-controlled randomized trials. In the hydralazine trial,[116] 36 percent of the patients were in New York Heart Association (NYHA) functional class II, and patients had moderate to severe AR. Hydralazine produced modest reduction of LV end-diastolic volume and a small increase in ejection fraction at the end of 2 years; however, because of side effects, long-term compliance was poor,[116] which probably accounted for the extremely modest beneficial effects.[117] In asymptomatic patients with severe AR,[118] a calcium channel blocking agent, long-acting nifedipine, produced significant reductions in blood pressure and LV end-diastolic volume and mass and major increases in LV ejection fraction at the end of 1 year. Almost all patients completed the trial. Recently, a prospective randomized trial in *asymptomatic* patients with *normal* LV systolic function[112] showed that at the end of 6 years, 34 ± 6 percent of patients treated with digoxin developed LV systolic dysfunction and/or symptoms and thus needed valve replacement, compared to 15 ± 3 percent of patients treated with long-acting nifedipine ($p < .001$) (Fig. 63-14); 90 percent (23/26) of those who needed valve replacement had developed LV systolic dysfunction with or without symptoms; only three had become symptomatic without

CHRONIC SEVERE AORTIC REGURGITATION: ASYMPTOMATIC + NORMAL LV FUNCTION AT REST

		Likelihood of Symptoms or LV Dysfunction or Death, % per Year
LV end-diastolic dimension	≥70 mm	10
	<70 mm	2
LV end-systolic dimension	≥50 mm	19
	40–49 mm	6
	<40 mm	0

Source: From Bonow et al.,[111] with permission.

TABLE 63-22

MEDICAL TREATMENT OF PATIENTS
WITH AORTIC REGURGITATION

I. Antibiotic prophylaxis
  A. Infective endocarditis
  B. Recurrent rheumatic carditis
II. Restriction of activities (moderate/severe AR)
  A. Severe exercise
  B. Competitive sports
III. Arrhythmias
  A. Prevent and/or control
  B. Restore sinus rhythm, if possible
IV. Cardiac medications
  A. Asymptomatic, normal LV function
    1. Mild AR: None
    2. Moderate AR: ? Nifedipine long-acting
    3. Severe AR: Nifedipine long-acting
  B. Severe AR symptomatic (while waiting for surgery)
    1. Normal LV function: Nifedipine long-acting
    2. LV dysfunction: Digitalis
                    ACE inhibitors
                    Hydralazine ± nitrates, if
                      needed
                    Diuretics, if needed
                    Dobutamine, if needed
  C. Severe AR + heart failure:
    Digitalis, diuretics, ACE inhibitors
    Hydralazine + nitrates
    IV nitroprusside, if IV therapy needed
    Dobutamine, if needed
V. Follow-up of asymptomatic patient
  A. Mild AR: Every 2–5 years
  B. Moderate AR: Every 1–2 years
  C. Severe AR: Every 6–12 months
  D. Develop symptoms: Early or immediate

Source: Copyright © by S. H. Rahimtoola, M.B., F.R.C.P., M.A.C.P. See Ref. 85.

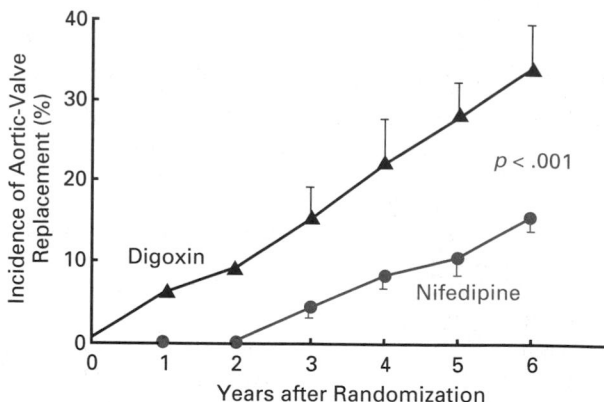

FIGURE 63-14

The role of long-term nifedipine therapy in asymptomatic patients with severe AR and normal LV systolic pump function was evaluated in 143 asymptomatic patients in a prospective randomized trial. By actuarial analysis, at 6 years, 34 ± 6% of patients in the digoxin group underwent valve replacement, versus 15 ± 3% of those in the nifedipine group, *p* <.001.

This randomized trial demonstrates that long-term vasodilator therapy with nifedipine reduces and/or delays the need for aortic valve replacement in asymptomatic patients with severe AR and normal LV systolic pump function. (From Scognamiglio et al.,[112] with permission.)

developing LV systolic dysfunction. Accordingly, all asymptomatic patients with severe AR and normal LV systolic function should be treated with a vasodilator (calcium channel blocking agent, long-acting nifedipine) unless there is a contraindication to its use.

The role of nifedipine in patients with moderate AR has not been studied. In view of its beneficial effects in severe AR, long-acting nifedipine could be used in selected patients with moderate AR if there are no contraindications to its use. An acute study showed that nifedipine was superior to an ACE inhibitor,[119] and a 6-month trial showed that the results with captopril were similar to placebo.[120] One study with quinapril involved 10 patients, many of whom had moderate AR.[121] In another study with enalapril, most patients had mild to moderate AR and many had severe systemic hypertension.[122] Moreover, there are no published data to show that ACE inhibitor therapy reduces the need for valve surgery. In brief, ACE inhibitors are not of proven benefit in asymptomatic patients with AR and with normal LV systolic function.

Symptomatic patients with severe AR need medical and surgical treatment. Medical treatment (Table 63-22) consists of the administration of digitalis, diuretics, and vasodilators. Digitalis acts by increasing myocardial contractility, often reducing LV end-diastolic volume while increasing the LV ejection fraction and also the cardiac output, if it is reduced in the resting state. Digitalis is clearly indicated in patients with symptoms. The need for and benefits of this therapy in asymptomatic patients have not been well documented. Diuretics are of value when the left atrial pressure is elevated and in the presence of heart failure.

Vasodilators are either arterial, venous, or both. Vasodilators act by reducing the peripheral arterial resistance, which favors forward cardiac output and reduces regurgitant volume; initially, the total LV stroke volume remains unchanged. If the left atrial pressure is elevated and LV ejection fraction reduced, vasodilators frequently result in an improvement in both.

Long-term hydralazine therapy in symptomatic patients results in significant benefit in only 20 to 35 percent of patients.[55] Those who are likely to benefit cannot be predicted. Vasodilators are indicated in patients who refuse surgery or are not operative candidates for any reason.

Vasodilators are also indicated for short-term therapy in patients awaiting valve replacement to optimize their hemodynamics (reduce filling pressures and increase cardiac output) and thus reduce their operative risks. If LV systolic function is normal, they can be given long-acting nifedipine. If they have abnormal LV systolic function, they should be treated with digitalis and ACE inhibitors; diuretics and hydralazine, with or without nitrates, can be used if needed. Small doses of hydralazine (≤50 mg) are without therapeutic effect in AR, and larger doses (≥100 mg) need to be given only twice daily[123]; the twice-daily regimen reduces the incidence of side effects. Hydralazine should be started in small doses and gradually increased, depending on patient tolerance of the drug.

Vasodilators are of considerable short-term benefit in patients in functional classes III and IV or heart failure. All such patients need digitalis, diuretics, and ACE inhibitors. In patients in functional class IV with heart failure, vasodilators should ideally be started after the institution of bedside hemodynamic monitoring, that is, measurement of pulmonary artery wedge pressure and cardiac output with the use of balloon flotation catheters. Hemodynamic monitoring accurately identifies patients who need the therapy, since clinical judgments can be wrong. It establishes whether arterial dilators alone will suffice or whether additional venodilators are needed. Finally, it provides information on the optimum dosage of vasodilator therapy. After the initial hemodynamic measurements are made, arterial dilators are given in progressively increasing dosage until an optimum effect on cardiac output has been obtained. If cardiac output does not show any further increase but left atrial pressure is still very high, additional venodilator therapy should be given. If the patient is very ill or the hemodynamic abnormalities are marked, intravenous therapy (e.g., sodium nitroprusside) is the vasodilator of first choice. In this situation, intravenous vasodilator therapy should be used only with bedside hemodynamic monitoring. Inotropic agents, such as dobutamine, may be needed to improve LV function and increase cardiac output. Low-dose dopamine may be of value to increase urinary output.

Patients with severe chronic AR need valve surgery. The correct timing of surgical therapy is now better defined but is not fully clarified. Valve replacement should be performed before irreversible LV dysfunction occurs. The major problem, however, is identifying the precise point at which LV dysfunction will occur. Here, two major difficulties are encountered: (1) patients may already have impaired LV systolic pump function at rest when they first present or at the time of the first symptom, and (2) patients with severe symptoms may have normal LV systolic pump function. Patients may be in NYHA functional class III (symptoms with less than ordinary activity), with a normal LV ejection fraction,[100] or they may be in functional class I (asymptomatic), with a reduced LV ejection fraction.[100] A reduced LV ejection fraction demonstrated by two-dimensional echocardiography and/or radionuclide ventriculography is the best noninvasive indicator of depressed LV systolic function.

Decisions about surgery in AR should be based on the clinical functional class and on the LV ejection fraction at rest (Table 63-23).[124] Patients with chronic severe AR who are symptomatic (NYHA functional class II to IV) need valve replacement. Although there may be some disagreement about recommending valve replacement to patients with normal ejection fraction who are in functional class II, we currently would do so. The benefit from valve replacement has been demonstrated even when the LV ejection fraction is 0.25 or less.[125] As opposed to AS, in which there is no lower level of ejection fraction that indicates inoperability, it is likely that

TABLE 63-23

CHRONIC SEVERE AORTIC REGURGITATION: INDICATIONS FOR SURGERY[a]

I. Symptomatic patients
  A. LV function normal: As soon as possible
  B. LV dysfunction: Urgent
  C. Heart failure: Emergent
  D. Individualize if:
    1. Very severe LV dysfunction (LV EF $\leq$ 0.20)
    2. Severe LV dilatation (LV EDD $\geq$ 80 mm; with severe LV systolic dysfunction: LV EDVI $\geq$ 300 mL/m^2)
    3. Small RgV (RgV/EDV $\leq$ 0.14)
II. Asymptomatic patients
  A. LV dysfunction (LV EF $\leq$ 0.50–0.54)
  B. Normal LV function
    1. Associated severe obstructive CAD
    2. Other valve disease needing cardiac surgery
    3. Any of the following:
      a. LV EDD $\geq$ 70 mm
      b. LV end-systolic dimension $\geq$ 50 mm
      c. LV EDVI $\geq$ 150 mL/m^2 *plus* PAW pressure on exercise $\geq$ 20 mmHg

[a] Valve replacement/valve repair.

Note: CAD = coronary artery disease; EF = ejection fraction; EDD = end-diastolic dimension; EDVI = end-diastolic volume index; RgV = regurgitant volume; EDV = end-diastolic volume; PAW = pulmonary artery wedge.
Source: Copyright © by S. H. Rahimtoola, M.B., F.R.C.P., M.A.C.P. See Ref. 85.

some patients with AR and a very low ejection fraction become inoperable. This level has not been precisely defined but may be about 0.15 or less. There is a need to individualize the need for valve replacement in those with very severe LV systolic dysfunction at rest, in those with very severe LV dilatation (LV end-diastolic volume index $\geq$300 mL/m^2),[126] and in those with a small regurgitant volume, with a ratio of regurgitant volume to end-diastolic volume of $\leq$0.14[127] (Table 63-23). Recent data indicate that patients with severe AR, LV end-diastolic dimension on echocardiography of $\geq$80 mm, and mild to moderate reduction of LV ejection fraction (mean 0.43) can obtain benefit from valve replacement.[128] Postoperatively, they are symptomatically improved, LV ejection fraction increases, and LV size is reduced; the 5- and 10-year survivals are 87 and 71 percent, respectively.

Although the issue is controversial in some countries, we believe that patients who are in NYHA functional class I (asymptomatic) and have a reduced ejection fraction at rest should be offered aortic valve replacement. If the ejection fraction is normal at rest, one should consider valve replacement in NYHA functional class I patients if they have severe obstructive CAD and/or need surgery for other valve disease (Table 63-23). It is suggested that patients undergo an exercise test during right heart catheterization if the left ventricle is large (LV end-diastolic volume $\geq$150 mL/m^2, LV internal dimension on M-mode echocardiography of $\geq$70 mm at end-diastole and ≥50 mm at end-systole) and/or the LV ejection fraction shows a new, persistent reduction to ≤0.54 to 0.60; if the patients have reduced exercise capacity on treadmill testing; or if ambulatory ECG monitoring demonstrates ventricular tachyarrhythmias. Valve replacement is recommended if the pulmonary artery wedge pressure during exercise ≥20 to 24 mmHg. Patients with associated significant CAD should have coronary bypass surgery performed at the time of valvular surgery (see "Aortic Valve Stenosis" and Table 63-14).

Aortic valve replacement, with or without associated coronary bypass surgery for obstructive CAD, can be performed at many surgical centers with an operative mortality of 5 percent or less (see Chap. 68). In those without associated CAD or reduced LV systolic function, the operative mortality may be in the 1 to 2 percent range. If aortic valve replacement is successful and uncomplicated, LV volume and hypertrophy regress but do not return to normal; the beneficial effects on LV size, volume, and mass continue to be seen up to 5 years after surgery.[76,129,130] Impaired LV systolic pump function improves postoperatively in 50 percent or more of patients[125]; this improvement is more likely to occur if LV dysfunction has been present preoperatively for 12 months or less, and in this subgroup LV ejection fraction usually normalizes.[130] Even if LV systolic pump function does not improve, there is a reduction in end-diastolic volume and hypertrophy[125]; from a cardiac point of view, this is advantageous to the patient. The 5-year survival of patients undergoing aortic valve replacement in severe AR is 85 percent (this figure includes operative and late cardiac deaths).[124] The 5-year survival of patients with LV ejection fraction ≥0.45 is 87 percent, versus 54 percent in patients with an ejection fraction <0.45.[124] Late survival after valve replacement for chronic severe AR is best predicted by variables indicative of LV systolic pump function. Both the operative mortality and late survival are dependent on cardiac and LV function and associated noncardiac comorbid factors (see "Aortic Valve Stenosis" and Chap. 68).

New techniques of aortic valve repair are being developed and evaluated, and early results are encouraging in selected subgroups.[97, 131,132] Eventually, it is possible that selected patients may need to have valve repair rather than valve replacement for AR.

REFERENCES

1. Roberts WC. Valvular, subvalvular and supravalvular aortic stenosis. Morphologic features. *Cardiovasc Clin* 1973; 5:97.
2. Moller JH, Nakib A, Elliott RS, Edwards JE. Symptomatic congenital aortic stenosis in the first year of life. *J Pediatr* 1966; 69:728–734.
3. Braunwald E, Goldblatt A, Aygen MM, Rockoff SD, Morrow AG. Congenital aortic stenosis: I. Clinical and hemodynamic findings in 100 patients. II. Surgical treatment and the results of operation. *Circulation* 1963; 27:426–462.
4. Passik CS, Ackerman DM, Pluth JR, Edwards WD. Temporal changes in the causes of aortic stenosis: A surgical pathological study of 646 cases. *Mayo Clin Proc* 1987; 62:119–123.
5. Olsson N, Dalsgaaro C-J, Haegerstrand A, Rosenqvist M, Ryden L, Nilsson J. Accumulation of T lymphocytes and expression of interluken-2 receptors in nonrheumatic stenotic aortic valves. *J Am Coll Cardiol* 1994; 23:1162–1170.
6. Narang NK, Andrew AMR, Chaudhury HR, Gaba BS. Aortic stenosis due to familial hypercholesterolemic xanthomatosis. A case report with brief review of literature. *Indian Heart J* 1978; 30:189–192.
7. Deutscher S, Rockette HE, Krishnaswami V. Diabetes and hypercholesterolemia among patients with calcific aortic stenosis. *J Chron Dis* 1984; 37:407–415.
8. Strickberger SA, Schulman SP, Hutchins GM. Association of Paget's disease of bone with calcific aortic valve disease. *Am J Med* 1987; 82:953–956.
9. Maher ER, Pazianas M, Curtis JR. Calcific aortic stenosis: A complication of chronic uraemia. *Nephron* 1987; 47:119–122.
10. Maher ER, Young G, Smyth-Walsh B, Pugh S, Curtis JR. Aortic and mitral valve calcification in patients with end-stage renal disease. *Lancet* 1987; 2:875–877.
11. Dereymaeker L, Van Parijs G, Bayart M, Daenen W, Lauwerijns J, DeGeest H. Ochronosis and alkaptonuria: Report of a new case with calcified aortic valve stenosis. *Acta Cardiol* 1990; 45:87–92.
12. Selzer A. Changing aspects of the natural history of valvular aortic stenosis. *N Engl J Med* 1987; 31:91–98.
13. Roberts WC. The structural basis of abnormal cardiac function: A look at coronary, hypertensive, valvular, idiopathic myocardial, and pericardial heart disease. In: Levine JJ, ed. *Clinical Cardiovascular Physiology.* New York: Grune & Stratton; 1976.
14. Kennedy JW, Twiss RD, Blackmon JR, Dodge HT. Quantitative angiography. III. Relationships of left ventricular pressure, volume, and mass in aortic valve disease. *Circulation* 1968; 38:838–845.
15. Bertrand ME, LaBlanche JM, Tilmant PY, Thieuleux FP, Delforge MR, Carré AG, et al. Coronary sinus blood flow at rest and during isometric exercise in patients with aortic valve disease. Mechanism of angina pectoris in presence of normal coronary arteries. *Am J Cardiol* 1981; 47:199–205.
16. Bonow RO. Left ventricular structure and function in aortic valve disease. *Circulation* 1989; 79:966–969.
17. Krayenbuehl HP, Hess OM, Monrad ES, Schneider J, Mall G, Turina M. Left ventricular myocardial structure in aortic valve disease before, intermediate, and later after aortic valve replacement. *Circulation* 1989; 79:744–755.
18. Schwarz F, Flameng W, Schaper J, Langebartels F, Sesto M, Hehrlein F, et al. Myocardial structure and function in patients with aortic valve disease and their relation to postoperative results. *Am J Cardiol* 1978; 41:661–669.
19. Tobin JR Jr, Rahimtoola SH, Blundell PE, Swan HJC. Percentage of left ventricular stroke work loss: A simple hemodynamic concept for estimation of severity in valvular aortic stenosis. *Circulation* 1967; 35:868–879.
20. Pantely G, Morton MJ, Rahimtoola SH. Effects of successful, uncomplicated valve replacement on ventricular hypertrophy, volume, and performance in aortic stenosis and aortic incompetence. *J Thorac Cardiovasc Surg* 1978; 75:383–391.
21. Hess OM, Ritter M, Schneider J, Grimm J, Turina M, Krayenbuehl HP. Diastolic stiffness and myocardial structure in aortic valve disease before and after replacement. *Circulation* 1984; 69:855–865.
22. Murakami T, Hess O, Gage JE, Grimm J, Krayenbuehl HP. Diastolic filling dynamics in patients with aortic stenosis. *Circulation* 1986; 73:1162–1174.
23. Dineen E, Brent BN. Aortic valve stenosis: Comparison of patients to those without chronic congestive heart failure. *Am J Cardiol* 1986; 57:419–422.
24. Fifer MA, Borow KM, Colan SD, Lorell BH. Early diastolic left ventricular function in children and adults with aortic stenosis. *J Am Coll Cardiol* 1985; 5:1147–1154.
25. Hess OM, Villari B, Krayenbuehl HP. Diastolic dysfunction in aortic stenosis. *Circulation* 1993; 87(suppl IV):73–76.
26. Braunwald E, Frahm CJ. Studies on Starling's law of the heart. IV. Observations on the hemodynamic functions of the left atrium in man. *Circulation* 1961; 24:633–642.
27. Stott DK, Marpole DGF, Bristow JD, Kloster FE, Griswold HE. The role of left atrial transport in aortic and mitral stenosis. *Circulation* 1970; 41:1031–1041.
28. Carroll JD, Carroll EP, Feldman T, Ward DM, Lang RM, McGaughey D, et al. Sex-associated differences in left ventricular function in aortic stenosis of the elderly. *Circulation* 1992; 86:1099–1107.
29. Ross J Jr. Afterload mismatch and preload reserve: A conceptual framework for the analysis of ventricular function. *Prog Cardiovasc Dis* 1976; 18:255–264.

30. Bache RJ, Wang Y, Jorgensen CR. Hemodynamic effects of exercise in isolated valvular aortic stenosis. *Circulation* 1971; 44:1003.

31. Johnson LL, Sciacca RR, Ellis K, Weiss MB, Cannon PJ. Reduced left ventricular myocardial blood flow per unit mass in aortic stenosis. *Circulation* 1978; 57:582–590.

32. Vinten-Johansen J, Weiss HR. Oxygen consumption in subepicardial and subendocardial regions of the canine left ventric—the effect of experimental acute valvular aortic stenosis. *Circ Res* 1980; 46:139–145.

33. Marcus ML, Doty DB, Horatzka LF, Wright CB, Eastham CL. Decreased coronary reserve: A mechanism for angina pectoris in patients with aortic stenosis and normal coronary arteries. *N Engl J Med* 1982; 307:1362–1366.

34. Grech ED, Ramsdale DR. Exertional syncope in aortic stenosis: Evidence to support inappropriate left ventricular baroreceptor response. *Am Heart J* 1991; 121:603–606.

35. Schwartz LS, Goldfischer J, Sprague GJ, Schwartz SP. Syncope and sudden death in aortic stenosis. *Am J Cardiol* 1969; 23:647–658.

36. Kulbertus HE. Ventricular arrhythmias, syncope and sudden death in aortic stenosis. *Eur Heart J* 1988; 9(suppl E):51–52.

37. Shoenfeld Y, Eldar M, Bedazovsky B, Levy MJ, Pinkhas J. Aortic stenosis associated with gastrointestinal bleeding: A survey of 612 patients. *Am Heart J* 1980; 100:179–182.

38. Love JW. The syndrome of calcific aortic stenosis and gastrointestinal bleeding: Resolution following aortic valve replacement. *J Thorac Cardiovasc Surg* 1982; 83:779–783.

39. Pleet AB, Massey EW, Vengrow ME. TIA, stroke, and the bicuspid aortic valve. *Neurology* 1981; 31:1540–1542.

40. Brockmeier LB, Adolph RJ, Gustin BW, Holmes JC, Sacks JG. Calcium emboli to the retinal artery in calcific aortic stenosis. *Am Heart J* 1981; 101:32–37.

41. Wood P. Aortic stenosis. *Am J Cardiol* 1958; 1:553–571.

42. Murphy ES, Lawson RM, Starr A, Rahimtoola SH. Severe aortic stenosis in the elderly: State of left ventricular function and result of valve replacement on ten-year survival. *Circulation* 1981; 64(suppl II):184–188.

43. Szamosi A, Wassberg B. Radiologic detection of aortic stenosis. *Acta Radiol Diagn* 1983; 24:201.

44. Siegel RJ, Maurer G, Navatpumin T, Shah PK. Accurate noninvasive assessment of critical aortic valve stenosis in the elderly (abstr). *J Am Coll Cardiol* 1983; 1:639.

45. Gooch AS, Calatayud JB, Rogers PA, Garman PA. Analysis of the P wave in severe aortic stenosis. *Dis Chest* 1966; 49:459–463.

46. Thompson R, Mitchell A, Ahmed M, Towers M, Yacoub M. Conduction defects in aortic valve disease. *Am Heart J* 1979; 98:3–10.

47. Nair CK, Aronow WS, Stokke K, Mohiuddin SM, Thomson W, Sketch MH. Cardiac conduction defects in patients older than 60 years with aortic stenosis and without mitral annular calcium. *Am J Cardiol* 1984; 53:169–172.

48. Rosenbaum M, Elizari M, Lazari J. *Los Hemibloques.* Buenos Aires: Paidos; 1968:363.

49. Galan A, Zoghbi WA, Quiñones MA. Determination of severity of valvular aortic stenosis by Doppler echocardiography and relation of findings to clinical outcome and agreement with hemodynamic measurements determined at cardiac catheterization. *Am J Cardiol* 1991; 67:1007–1012.

50. Agatston AS, Chengot M, Rao A, Hildner F, Samet P. Doppler diagnosis of valvular aortic stenosis in patients over 60 years of age. *Am J Cardiol* 1985; 56:106–109.

51. Skjaerpe T, Hegrenaes L, Hatle L. Noninvasive estimation of valve area in patients with aortic stenosis by Doppler ultrasound and two-dimensional echocardiography. *Circulation* 1985; 72:810–815.

52. Yeager M, Yock PG, Popp RL. Comparison of Doppler-derived pressure gradient to that determined at cardiac catheterization in adults with aortic valve stenosis: Implications for management. *Am J Cardiol* 1986; 57:644–648.

53. Currie PJ, Seward JB, Reeder GS, Vlietstra RE, Bresnaham DR, Bresnaham JF, et al. Continuous-wave Doppler echocardiographic assessment of severity of calcific aortic stenosis: A simultaneous Doppler-catheter correlative study in 100 adult patients. *Circulation* 1985; 71:1162–1169.

54. Oh JK, Taliercio CP, Holmes DR Jr, Reeder GS, Bailey KR, Seward JB, et al. Prediction of the severity of aortic stenosis by Doppler aortic valve area determination: Prospective Doppler-catheterization in 100 patients. *J Am Coll Cardiol* 1988; 11:1227–1234.

55. Rahimtoola SH. Perspective on valvular heart disease: Update II. In: Knoebel S, ed. *Era in Cardiovascular Medicine.* New York: Elsevier; 1991:45–70.

56. Roger VL, Tajik AJ, Reeder GS, Hayes SN, Mullany CJ, Bailey KR, et al. Effect of Doppler echocardiography on utilization of hemodynamic cardiac catheterization in the preoperative evaluation of aortic stenosis. *Mayo Clin Proc* 1996; 71:141–149.

57. Enriquez-Sarano M, Klodas E, Garratt KN, Bailey KR, Tajik AJ, Holmes DR Jr. Secular trends in coronary atherosclerosis—analysis in patients with valve regurgitation. *N Engl J Med* 1996; 335:316–322.

58. Sethi GK, Miller DC, Sonchek J, Oprian C, Henderson WG, Hassan Z, et al. Clinical, hemodynamic and angiographic predictors of operative mortality in patients undergoing single valve replacement. *J Thorac Cardiovasc Surg* 1987; 93:884–887.

59. Mullany CJ, Elveback ER, Frye RL, Pluth SR, Edwards WD, Orszulak TA, et al. Coronary artery disease and its management: Influence on survival in patients undergoing aortic valve replacement. *J Am Coll Cardiol* 1987; 10:66–72.

60. Levinson JR, Akins CW, Buckley MJ, Newell JB, Palacios IF, Block PC, et al. Octogenarians with aortic stenosis: Outcome after aortic valve replacement. *Circulation* 1989; 80(suppl I):49–56.

61. Klein RC. Ventricular arrhythmias in aortic valve disease: Analysis of 102 patients. *Am J Cardiol* 1984; 53:1079–1083.

62. von Olshausen K, Schwarz F, Apfelbach J, Röhrig N, Krämer B, Kübler W, et al. Determinants of the incidence and severity of ventricular arrhythmias in aortic valve disease. *Am J Cardiol* 1983; 51:1103–1109.

63. Kotlewski A, Kawanishi DT, McKay CR, Harrison EC, Reid CL, Chandraratna PAN, et al. The relative value of clinical examination, echocardiography with Doppler and cardiac catheterization with angiography in the evaluation of aortic valve disease. In: Bodnar E, ed. *Surgery for Heart Valve Disease.* London: ICR; 1990:66–72.

64. Jonasson R, Jonsson B, Nordlander R, Orinius E, Szamosi A. Rate of progression of severity of valvular aortic stenosis. *Acta Med Scand* 1983; 213:51–54.

65. Nestico PF, DePace NL, Kimbiris D, Hakki A-H, Khanderia B, Iskandrian AS, et al. Progression of isolated aortic stenosis. Analysis of 29 patients having more than one cardiac catheterization. *Am J Cardiol* 1983; 52:1054–1058.

66. Hoagland PM, Cook EF, Wynne J, Goldman L. Value of noninvasive testing in adults with suspected aortic stenosis. *Am J Med* 1986; 80:1041–1050.

67. Cohen LS, Friedman WF, Braunwald E. Natural history of mild congenital aortic stenosis elucidated by serial hemodynamic studies. *Am J Cardiol* 1972; 30:1–5.

68. Cheitlin MD, Gertz EW, Brundage BH, Carlson CJ, Quash JA, Bode RS Jr. Rate of progression of severity of valvular aortic stenosis in the adult. *Am Heart J* 1979; 98:689–700.

69. Wagner S, Selzer A. Patterns of progression of aortic stenosis: A longitudinal hemodynamic study. *Circulation* 1982; 65:709–712.

70. Horstkotte D, Loogen F. The natural history of aortic valve stenosis. *Eur Heart J* 1988; 9(suppl E):57–64.

71. Holmes DR Jr, Nishimura RA, Reeder GS. In-hospital mortality after balloon valvuloplasty: Frequency and associated factors. *J Am Coll Cardiol* 1991; 17:189–192.

72. Ross J Jr, Braunwald E. Aortic stenosis. *Circulation* 1968; 36(suppl IV):61–67.

73. Kirklin JW, Barratt-Boyes BG. Congenital valvular aortic stenosis. In: *Cardiac Surgery.* New York: Wiley; 1986:972–988.

74. Schwarz F, Banmann P, Manthey J, Hoffman M, Schuler G, Mehmel HC, et al. The effect of aortic valve replacement on survival. *Circulation* 1982; 66:1105–1110.

75. Rahimtoola SH. Valvular heart disease: A perspective. *J Am Coll Cardiol* 1983; 1:199–215.

76. Monrad ES, Hess OM, Murakami T, Nonogi H, Corin WJ, Krayenbuehl HP. Time course of regression of left ventricular hypertrophy after aortic valve replacement. *Circulation* 1988; 77:1345–1355.

77. Hammermeister KL, Sethi GK, Henderson WG, Oprian C, Kim T, Rahimtoola S. A comparison of outcomes in men 11 years after heart-valve replacement with a mechanical valve or bioprosthesis. *N Engl J Med* 1993; 328:1289–1296.

78. Lindblom D, Lindblom U, Qvist J, Lundström H. Long-term relative survival rates after heart valve replacement. *J Am Coll Cardiol* 1990; 15:566–573.

79. Rahimtoola SH. Catheter balloon valvuloplasty for severe calcific aortic stenosis: A limited role. *J Am Coll Cardiol* 1994; 23:1076–1078.

80. Rahimtoola SH, Starr A. Valvular surgery. In: Braunwald E, Mock M, Watson J, eds. *Congestive Heart Failure: Current Research and Clinical Applications.* Orlando, FL: Grune & Stratton;1982:89–93.

81. Smith N, McAnulty JH, Rahimtoola SH. Severe aortic stenosis with impaired left ventricular function and clinical heart failure: Results of valve replacement. *Circulation* 1978; 58:255–264.

82. Otto CM, Mickel MC, Kennedy JW, Alderman EL, Bashore TM, Block PC, et al. Three-year outcome after balloon aortic valvuloplasty: Insights into prognosis of valvular aortic stenosis. *Circulation* 1994; 89:642–650.

83. Moreno PR, Jang I-K, Newell JB, Block PC, Palacios IF. The role of percutaneous aortic balloon valvuloplasty in patients with cardiogenic shock and critical aortic stenosis. *J Am Coll Cardiol* 1994; 23:1071–1075.

84. Rahimtoola SH. Recognition and management of acute aortic regurgitation. *Heart Dis Stroke* 1993; 2:217–221.

85. Braunwald E. Valvular heart disease. In: Braunwald E, ed. *Heart Disease,* 4th ed. Philadelphia: Saunders; 1992:1007–1077.

86. Rahimtoola SH. Valvular heart disease. In: Stein J, ed (O'Rourke RA, Cardiology Section ed). *Internal Medicine,* 4th ed. St. Louis: Mosby-Year Book; 1994:202–234.

87. Belenkie I, Rademaker A. Acute and chronic changes after aortic valve damage in the intact dog. *Am J Physiol* 1981; 241:H95–H103.

88. Welch GH Jr, Braunwald E, Sarnoff SJ. Hemodynamic effects of quantitatively varied experimental aortic regurgitation. *Circ Res* 1957; 5:546–551.

89. Rahimtoola SH. Aortic regurgitation. In: Rahimtoola SH, ed. *Atlas of Heart Diseases: Valvular Heart Disease* Vol XI. Philadelphia: Current Medicine; 1997:7.1–7.26.

90. Rahimtoola SH. Management of heart failure in valve regurgitation. *Clin Cardiol* 1992; 15(suppl I):22–27.

91. Nienaber CA, von Kodolitsch Y, Nicholas V, Siglow V, Piepho A, Brockhoff C, et al. The diagnosis of thoracic aortic dissection by noninvasive imaging procedures. *N Engl J Med* 1993; 328:1–9.

92. Cigarroa JE, Isselbacher EM, De Sanctis RW, Eagle KA. Diagnostic imaging in the evaluation of suspected aortic dissection: Old standards and new directions. *N Engl J Med* 1993; 328:35–43.

93. Kostuk W, Barr JW, Simon AL, Ross J Jr. Correlations between the chest film and hemodynamics in acute myocardial infarction. *Circulation* 1973; 48:624–632.

94. Chatterjee K, Parmley WW, Swan HJC, Berman G, Forrester J, Marcus HS. Beneficial effects of vasodilator agents in severe mitral regurgitation due to dysfunction of subvalvular apparatus. *Circulation* 1973; 48:684–690.

95. Richardson JV, Karp RB, Kirklin JW, Dismukes WE. Treatment of infective endocarditis: A 10-year comparative analysis. *Circulation* 1978; 58:589–597.

96. Tonnemacher D, Reid CL, Kawanishi DT, Cummings T, Chandrasoma P, McKay CR, et al. Frequency of myxomatous degeneration of the aortic valve as a cause of isolated aortic regurgitation severe enough to warrant aortic valve replacement. *Am J Cardiol* 1987; 60:1194–1196.

97. Antunes M. Repair for acquired valvular heart disease. In: Rahimtoola SH, ed. *Atlas of Heart Diseases: Valvular Heart Disease* Vol XI. Philadelphia: Current Medicine; 1997:12.1–12.23.

98. Waller BF. Rheumatic and nonrheumatic conditions producing valvular heart disease. In: Frankl WS, Brest AN, eds. *Cardiovascular Clinics. Valvular Heart Disease: Comprehensive Evaluation and Management.* Philadelphia: FA Davis; 1986:30–31.

99. Miller GAH, Kirklin JW, Swan HJC. Myocardial function and left ventricular volumes in acquired valvular insufficiency. *Circulation* 1965; 31:374–384.

100. Karaian CH, Greenberg BH, Rahimtoola SH. The relationship between functional class and cardiac performance in patients with chronic aortic insufficiency. *Chest* 1985; 88:553–557.

101. Kawanishi DT, McKay CR, Chandraratna PAN, Nanna M, Reid CL, Elkayam U, et al. Cardiovascular response to dynamic exercise in patients with chronic symptomatic mild-to-moderate and severe aortic regurgitation. *Circulation* 1986; 73:62–72.

102. Shen WF, Roubin GS, Choong CY-P, Hutton BF, Harris PJ, Fletcher PJ, et al. Evaluation of relationship between myocardial contractile state and left ventricular function in patients with aortic regurgitation. *Circulation* 1985; 71:31–38.

103. Boucher CA, Wilson RA, Kanarek DJ, Hutter AM Jr, Okada RD, Liberthson RR, et al. Exercise testing in asymptomatic or minimally symptomatic aortic regurgitation: Relationship of left ventricular ejection fraction to left ventricular filling pressure during exercise. *Circulation* 1983; 67:1091–1100.

104. Falsetti HL, Carroll RJ, Cramer JA. Total and regional myocardial blood flow in aortic regurgitation. *Am Heart J* 1979; 97:485–493.

105. Uhl GS, Boucher CA, Oliveros RA, Murgo JP. Exercise-induced myocardial oxygen supply-demand imbalance in asymptomatic or mildly symptomatic aortic regurgitation. *Chest* 1981; 80:686–691.

106. Nittenburg A, Foult JM, Antony I, Blanchet F, Rahali M. Coronary flow and resistance reserve in patients with chronic aortic regurgitation, angina pectoris, and normal coronary arteries. *J Am Coll Cardiol* 1988; 11:478–486.

107. Sabbah HN, Khaja F, Anbe DT, Stein PD. The aortic closure sound in pure aortic insufficiency. *Circulation* 1977; 56:859–863.

108. Schaefer RA, McAnulty JH, Starr A, Rahimtoola SH. Diastolic murmurs in the presence of Starr-Edwards mitral prosthesis: With emphasis on the genesis of the Austin Flint murmur. *Circulation* 1975; 51:402–409.

109. Roberts WC, Day PJ. Electrocardiographic observations in clinically isolated, pure, and chronic, severe aortic regurgitation: Analysis of 30 necropsy patients aged 19 to 65 years. *Am J Cardiol* 1985; 55:431–438.

110. Rapaport E. Natural history of aortic and mitral valve disease. *Am J Cardiol* 1975; 35:221–227.

111. Bonow RO, Lakatos E, Maron BJ, Epstein SE. Serial long-term assessment of the natural history of asymptomatic patients with chronic aortic regurgitation and normal left ventricular systolic function. *Circulation* 1991; 84:1625–1635.

112. Scognamiglio R, Rahimtoola SH, Fasoli G, Nistri S, Dalla Volta S. Nifedipine in asymptomatic patients with severe aortic regurgitation and normal left ventricular function. *N Engl J Med* 1994; 331:689–695.

113. Tornos MP, Olona M, Permanyer-Miralda G, Herrejon P, Camprecios M, Evangelista A, et al. Clinical outcome of severe asymptomatic chronic aortic regurgitation. A long-term prospective follow-up study. *Am Heart J* 1995; 130:333–339.

114. Siemienczuk D, Greenberg B, Morris C, Massie B, Wilson RA, Topic N, et al. Chronic aortic insufficiency: Factors associated with progression to aortic valve replacement. *Ann Intern Med* 1989; 110:587–592.

115. McKay CR, Rahimtoola SH. Natural history of aortic regurgitation. In: Gaasch WH, Levine HJ, eds. *Chronic Aortic Regurgitation.* Boston: Kluwer Academic; 1980:1–17.

116. Greenberg B, Massie B, Bristow JD, Cheitlin M, Siemienczuk D, Topic N, et al. Long-term vasodilator therapy of chronic aortic insufficiency: A randomized double-blinded, placebo-controlled clinical trial. *Circulation* 1988; 78:92–103.

117. Rahimtoola SH. Vasodilator therapy in chronic severe aortic regurgitation. *J Am Coll Cardiol* 1990; 16:430–432.

118. Scognamiglio R, Rasoli G, Ponchia A, Dalla-Volta S: Long-term nifedipine unloading therapy in asymptomatic patients with chronic severe aortic regurgitation. *J Am Coll Cardiol* 1990; 16:424–429.

119. Rothlisberger C, Sareli P, Wisenbaugh T. Comparison of single-dose nifedipine and captopril for chronic severe aortic regurgitation. *Am J Cardiol* 1993; 72:799–804.

120. Wisenbaugh T, Sinovich V, Dullabh A, Sareli P. Six month pilot study of captopril for mildly symptomatic, severe isolated mitral and isolated aortic regurgitation. *J Heart Valve Dis* 1994; 3:197–204.

121. Schon HR, Dorn R, Barthel P, Schömig A. Effects of 12 months quinapril therapy in asymptomatic patients with chronic aortic regurgitation. *J Heart Valve Dis* 1994; 3:500–509.

122. Lin M, Chian H-T, Lin S-L, Chang M-S, Chiang BN, Kuo H-W. Vasodilator therapy in chronic asymptomatic aortic regurgitation: Enalapril versus hydralazine. *J Am Coll Cardiol* 1994; 24:1046–1053.

123. McKay CR, Nanna M, Kawanishi DT, Elkayam U, Chandraratna PAN, Weiss JN, et al. Importance of internal controls, statistical methods, and side effects in acute vasodilator trials: A study of hydralazine kinetics in patients with aortic regurgitation. *Circulation* 1985; 72:865–872.

124. Greves J, Rahimtoola SH, McAnulty JH, DeMots H, Clark DG, Greenberg B, et al. Preoperative criteria predictive of late survival following valve replacement for severe aortic regurgitation. *Am Heart J* 1981; 101:300–308.

125. Clark DG, McAnulty JH, Rahimtoola SH. Valve replacement in aortic insufficiency with left ventricular dysfunction. *Circulation* 1980; 61:411–421.

126. Taniguchi K, Nakano S, Hirose H, Matsuda H, Shirakura R, Sakai I, et al. Preoperative left ventricular function: Minimal requirement for successful late results of valve replacement for aortic regurgitation. *J Am Coll Cardiol* 1987; 10:510–518.

127. Levine HJ, Gaasch WH. Ratio of regurgitant volume to end-diastolic volume: A major determinant of ventricular response to surgical correction of chronic volume overload. *Am J Cardiol* 1983; 52:406–410.

128. Klodas E, Enriquez-Sarano M, Tajik AJ, Mullany CJ, Bailey KR, Savard JB. Aortic regurgitation complicated by extreme left ventricular dilation: Long-term outcome after surgical correction. *J Am Coll Cardiol* 1996; 27:670–677.

129. Gaasch WH, Carroll JD, Levine HJ, Criscitiello MG. Chronic aortic regurgitation: Prognostic value of left ventricular end-systolic dimension and end-diastolic radius/thickness ratio. *J Am Coll Cardiol* 1983; 1:775–782.

130. Bonow RO, Dodd JT, Maron BJ, O'Gara PT, White GG, McIntosh CL, et al. Long-term serial changes in left ventricular function and reversal of ventricular dilatation after valve replacement for chronic aortic regurgitation. *Circulation* 1988; 78:1108–1120.

131. Cosgrove DM, Rosenkranz ER, Hendren WG, Bartlett JC, Stewart WJ. Valvuloplasty for aortic insufficiency. *J Thorac Cardiovasc Surg* 1991; 102:571–577.

132. Duran C, Kumar N, Gometza B, Al Halees Z. Indications and limitations of aortic valve reconstruction. *Ann Thorac Surg* 1991; 52:447–454.

64

MITRAL VALVE DISEASE

Shahbudin H. Rahimtoola / Maurice Enriquez-Sarano / Hartzell V. Schaff / Robert L. Frye

MITRAL STENOSIS

Etiology

Mitral stenosis (MS), an obstruction to blood flow between the left atrium (LA) and the left ventricle (LV), is caused by abnormal mitral valve function. In virtually all adult patients, the cause of MS is previous rheumatic carditis.[1] About 60 percent of patients with rheumatic mitral valve disease do not give a history of rheumatic fever or chorea, however, and about 50 percent of patients with acute rheumatic carditis do not eventually have clinical valvular heart disease.[2] Other causes of MS are all uncommon or rare and are listed in Table 64-1.[2-10] Congenital MS is uncommon. It is usually caused by a "parachute" deformity of the valve in which shortened chordae tendineae insert in a large, single papillary muscle. MS, usually rheumatic, in association with atrial septal defect is called *Lutembacher's syndrome*. A rare cause of MS is massive mitral valve annular calcification. This process occurs most frequently in elderly patients and produces MS by limiting leaflet motion. When stenosis is present, it is usually mild in degree. Other causes of obstruction to LA outflow include a LA myxoma, massive LA ball thrombus, and cor triatriatum, in which a congenital membrane is present in the LA.

Pathology

Acute rheumatic carditis is a pancarditis because it involves the pericardium, myocardium, and endocardium. In temperate climates and developed countries, there is usually a long interval (an average of 10 to 20 years) between an episode of rheumatic carditis and the clinical presentation of symptomatic MS. In tropical and subtropical climates and in less developed countries, the latent period is often shorter, and MS may occur during childhood or adolescence (see Chap. 62).

The pathologic hallmark of rheumatic carditis is an Aschoff's nodule. The most common lesion of acute rheumatic endocarditis is mitral valvulitis. The mitral valve has vegetations along the line of closure and the chordae tendineae. Mitral regurgitation may be present during the acute episode of rheumatic carditis.

MS is usually the result of repeated episodes of carditis alternating with healing and is characterized by the deposition of fibrous tissue. MS may result from fusion of the commissures, cusps, or chordae or a combination of these.[9,10] Ultimately, the deformed valve is subject to nonspecific fibrosis and calcification. Lesions along the line of closure result in fusion of the commissures and contracture and thickening of the valve leaflets. The chordal lesions are manifest as shortening and fusion of these structures. The combination of commissural fusion, valve leaflet contracture, and fusion of the chordae tendineae results in a narrow, funnel-shaped orifice, which restricts the flow of blood from the LA to the LV. The rapidity with which patients become symptomatic with this lesion may depend on the number and severity of repeated bouts of rheumatic valvulitis. Frequently, the rheumatic episodes are not clinically apparent.

In pure MS, the LV is usually normal, but there may be evidence of previous carditis with deposition of fibrous tissue. The LA is enlarged and hypertrophied as a consequence of LA hypertension. Mural thrombi are often found in the LA particularly if atrial fibrillation has been present. Calcification of the mitral valve frequently also involves the mitral annulus.

Pathophysiology

The pathophysiologic features of MS all result from obstruction of the flow of blood between the LA and the LV. With reduction in valve area, energy is lost to friction during the transport of blood from the LA to the LV. Accordingly, a pressure gradient is present across the stenotic valve. The relationship between valve area, cardiac output,

TABLE 64 1
CAUSES OF MITRAL STENOSIS

Cause	Leaflet	Chordae	Commissures	Other
Rheumatic fever	+	+	+	
Congenital	+	+		Single papillary muscle
Active infective endocarditis	+			Vegetation
Neoplasm				Mass, pulmonary vein obstruction
Massive annular calcification	+	0	0	Rigid annulus
Systemic lupus erythematosus	+	+	+	Verrucous vegetations may extend into papillary muscles
Carcinoid				Atrial septal defect or lung tumor in order to affect left heart
Methysergide therapy	+	+		Serotonin agonist/antagonist
Hunter-Hurler syndromes				Mucopolysaccharide deposits
Fabry's disease				Aramide trihexoxide deposits
Whipple's disease				PAS-positive macrophage deposits
Rheumatoid arthritis	+	+	+	PAS-positive plasma cell infiltrate

Source: From Kawanishi DT, Rahimtoola SH. Mitral stenosis. In: Rahimtoola SH, ed. *Valvular Heart Disease.* *II.* St. Louis: Mosby; 1996:8.1–8.24.

flow period, and average diastolic gradient between the LA and the LV is defined by the formula of Gorlin and Gorlin (Chap. 16).

It is readily apparent that maintaining cardiac output when the valve area is small requires a large gradient and thus an elevated LA pressure. Similarly, an increased demand for cardiac output, such as occurs during exercise or pregnancy, results in an increase in gradient and high LA pressures. More subtle is the effect of the length of the diastolic flow period on the relationship between output and gradient. The time available for diastole is that part of the cardiac cycle not taken up by isovolumic contraction and relaxation or by ejection. As the heart rate increases, the total amount of time spent during systole increases despite a reduction in the systolic time per beat.[11,12] Thus, time available for diastole decreases as the heart rate increases. Because blood can flow through the mitral valve only during diastole, the flow rate is inversely proportional to the duration of the flow period at a constant stroke volume. Of course, a higher flow rate results in a greater loss of energy to friction and requires a larger gradient and higher LA pressures. It is important to remember that the gradient from LA to LV is a function per beat, not per minute. Thus, the gradient is dependent on the stroke volume and the diastolic filling time as well as the LV diastolic pressure.

The pressure gradient between the LA and the LV, which increases markedly with increased heart rate or cardiac output,

is responsible for LA hypertension. The LA gradually enlarges and hypertrophies. Pulmonary venous pressure rises with LA pressure increase and is passively associated with an increase in pulmonary arterial (PA) pressure (Fig. 64-1). In up to 20 percent of patients, the pulmonary vascular resistance is also elevated,[13] which further increases PA pressure. PA hypertension results in right ventricular (RV) hypertrophy and RV enlargement. The changes in RV function eventually result in right atrial (RA) hypertension and enlargement and systemic venous congestion; frequently, tricuspid regurgitation also occurs. In a small percentage of patients, there may be regional or global LV systolic dysfunction, the cause or causes of which are not fully understood.[14–18]

Pulmonary venous hypertension alters lung function in several ways. Distribution of blood flow in the lung is altered, with a relative increase in flow to the upper lobes and therefore in physiologic dead space. Pulmonary compliance generally decreases with increasing pulmonary capillary pressure, adding to the work of breathing, particularly during exercise. Chronic changes in the pulmonary capillaries and pulmonary arteries include fibrosis and thickening. These changes protect the lungs from the transudation of fluid into the alveoli (alveolar pulmonary edema). Indeed, it is not uncommon to find patients with severe MS whose resting PA wedge pressure (indirect LA pressure) exceeds 25 to 30 mmHg. Capillary and alveolar thickening, which can help protect against pulmonary edema, further add to the abnormalities of ventilation and perfusion. Pulmonary vascular changes result in increasingly elevated pulmonary vascular resistance.

In some patients with high pulmonary vascular resistance and RV dysfunction, cardiac output may be low. The body maintains oxygen consumption by extracting more oxygen from the arterial blood, and the mixed venous oxygen content falls. The hemoglobin-oxygen dissociation curve is shifted to the right, facilitating the unloading of oxygen from hemoglobin to the tissues. The reduced cardiac output may result in a *surprisingly small gradient* across the mitral valve despite severe stenosis. Although pulmonary congestion may be less striking in these patients, the cardiac output does not increase normally with exercise, and, typically, the patients are severely limited by fatigue.

Long-standing MS with severe PA hypertension and resultant RV dysfunction may be accompanied by chronic systemic venous hypertension. Tricuspid regurgitation is frequently present, even in the absence of intrinsic disease of this valve. Functional pulmonic regurgitation may also be present. Dependent edema formation and visceral congestion directly reflect elevated systemic venous pressure and salt and water retention. Chronic passive congestion in the liver leads to central lobular necrosis and eventually to cardiac cirrhosis.

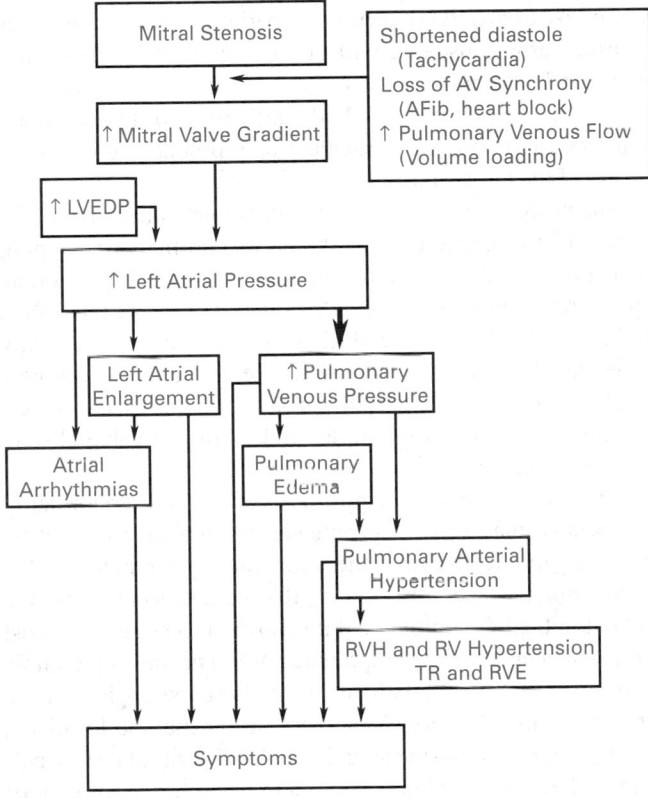

FIGURE 64-1

Pathophysiology of mitral stenosis. Mitral stenosis results in a diastolic pressure gradient from the LA to the LV. The actual gradient is dependent on the mitral valve area and the mitral valve *flow per diastolic second*. As a result, there is an elevation of LA pressure and therefore also of pulmonary venous pressure. Physiologic and pathologic changes—such as tachycardia and atrial fibrillation (which shorten diastole and may also result in loss of effective atrial contraction) or pregnancy, volume loading, and left-to-right shunts (at ventricular and aortopulmonary levels), which increase pulmonary venous flow—will increase the mitral valve gradient as well as LA and pulmonary venous pressures. An increased LV diastolic pressure will also result in further increase of LA pressure. An elevated LA pressure has several important effects; these include enlargement of the left atrium, atrial arrhythmias, and an increase of pulmonary venous pressure. Pulmonary venous hypertension may result in pulmonary edema and pulmonary arterial hypertension. PA hypertension and RV ventricular hypertension results in RV hypertrophy and may result in tricuspid regurgitation and RV enlargement. All of these changes contribute to producing symptoms. In addition, a fixed or even reduced cardiac output will also contribute to the symptomatic state of the patient. [Copyright by S. H. Rahimtoola. M.B., F.R.C.P., M.A.C.P., (Ref. 10).]

Clinical Findings

HISTORY

An asymptomatic interval is usually present between the initiating event of acute rheumatic fever and the presentation of symptomatic MS (an average of 10 to 20 years).[13,19] During this interval, the patient feels well (Table 64-2). Initially, there is little or no gradient at rest, but with increased cardiac output, LA pressure rises and exertional dyspnea develops. As mitral valve obstruction increases, dyspnea occurs at lower work levels. The progression of disability is so subtle and so protracted that patients may adapt by circumscribing their lifestyles. It becomes imperative, then, to document what activities the patient can perform without symptoms and at what activity level symptoms begin; failure to do this often results in an underestimation of disability.

As obstruction progresses, the patients note orthopnea and paroxysmal nocturnal dyspnea that apparently results from redistribution of blood to the thorax on assuming the supine position. With severe MS and elevated pulmonary vascular resistance, fatigue rather than dyspnea may be the predominant symptom. Dependent edema, nausea, anorexia, and right upper quadrant pain reflect systemic venous congestion resulting from elevated systemic venous pressure.

Palpitations are a frequent complaint in patients with MS and may represent frequent premature atrial contractions or paroxysmal atrial fibrillation/flutter. Of patients with severe symptomatic MS, 50 percent or more have chronic atrial fibrillation. Paroxysmal atrial fibrillation may produce pulmonary edema in some patients with MS. The acute increase in LA pressure that produces pulmonary edema results both from a decrease in the diastolic flow period caused by increased heart rate and from a loss of atrial transport function.

Systemic embolism, a frequent complication of MS, may result in stroke, occlusion of extremity arterial supply, occlusion of the aortic bifurcation, and visceral or myocardial infarction. Atrial fibrillation, increasing age of the patient, in-

TABLE 64-2

SYMPTOMS ASSOCIATED WITH MITRAL STENOSIS

On exertion
  Dyspnea, wheezing, cough
  Fatigue
  Diminished activity/or pace of activity
  Palpitations
  Feeling faint, presyncope, syncope
At rest
  Cough, wheezing
  Paroxysmal nocturnal dyspnea
  Orthopnea
  Hemoptysis
  Hoarseness (Ortner's syndrome)
From complications of MS

Source: Copyright S. H. Rahimtoola, M.B., F.R.C.P, M.A.C.P., (Ref. 10).

creasing LA size, and a previous history of embolism are associated with an increased incidence of systemic embolism[13] (Table 64-3).

Hemoptysis may result from a variety of causes. Hemoptysis usually results from increased pulmonary venous pressure. Sputum may be blood-stained with paroxysmal nocturnal dyspnea, pink frothy sputum from rupture of alveolar capillaries can be associated with acute pulmonary edema from pulmonary infarction due to pulmonary embolism, or hemoptysis may be severe and profuse (pulmonary apoplexy). The latter results from rupture of thin-walled, dilated bronchial veins, and although usually not fatal, it may be life-threatening because of aspiration pneumonia or massive hemorrhage. The edematous bronchial mucosa is more likely to be associated with chronic bronchitis, especially in cold and wet climates; it can also result in blood-stained sputum.

Exertional chest pain, typical of angina pectoris, may be present in some patients with severe MS but normal coronary arteries. Severe PA hypertension has been postulated as a cause. Infective endocarditis is an uncommon complication of pure MS.

Progression of symptoms in MS is generally slow but relentless. Thus, a sudden change in symptoms rarely reflects a change in valve obstruction. Rather, there is usually a noncardiac precipitating event or paroxysmal atrial fibrillation. Fever, pregnancy, hyperthyroidism, and noncardiac surgery, all of which increase cardiac output, can precipitate decompensation in patients with moderate to severe MS.

PHYSICAL FINDINGS

During the latent, presymptomatic interval, incidental physical findings may be normal or may provide evidence of mild MS. Frequently, the only characteristic finding noted at rest will be a loud S_1 and a presystolic murmur. A short diastolic decrescendo rumble may be heard only with exercise. In patients with symptomatic stenosis, the findings are more obvious, and careful physical examination usually leads to the correct diagnosis.

TABLE 64-3
COMPLICATIONS OF MITRAL STENOSIS

Arrhythmias
   Atrial flutter/fibrillation
Embolism
   Systemic-cerebral, coronary, abnormal, peripheral,
     pulmonary
Acute pulmonary edema
Pulmonary arterial hypertension
Right ventricular hypertrophy/dilatation
Tricuspid regurgitation
Clinical heart failure
Left ventricular dysfunction
Chest pain/angina
Infective endocarditis

Source: Copyright by S. H. Rahimtoola, M.B., F.R.C.P., M.A.C.P. (Ref. 10).

The general appearance of the patient in MS is usually normal. The MS facies, characterized by malar flush (pinkish-purple patches on the cheeks),[13] is uncommon and is caused by peripheral cyanosis, which is usually associated with a low cardiac output, systemic vasoconstriction, and severe PA hypertension. Tachypnea may be present if LA pressure is high. The arterial pulse is normal except for irregularity in atrial fibrillation and is of low volume when cardiac output is reduced. All peripheral pulses should be carefully examined because of the frequency of systemic embolism. The jugular venous pressure may be normal or may show evidence of elevated RA pressure. A prominent *a* wave is a result of RV hypertension/hypertrophy or of associated tricuspid stenosis. A prominent *v* wave is caused by tricuspid regurgitation. Atrial fibrillation produces an irregular venous pulse with absent *a* waves. The chest findings may be normal or may reveal signs of pulmonary congestion with rales or pleural fluid (dullness and absent breath sounds). Marked LA enlargement may produce egophony at the tip of the left scapula.

The precordium is usually unremarkable on inspection. On palpation, the apical impulse should feel normal or is tapping (palpable mitral valve closure or RV forming the cardiac apex). An abnormal LV impulse suggests disease other than isolated MS. A diastolic thrill is usually appreciated only when the patient is examined in the left lateral decubitus position. When PA hypertension is present, a sustained RV lift along the left sternal border and pulmonic valve closure may be palpable.

On auscultation in the supine position, the only abnormality appreciated may be the accentuated S_1, which is caused by flexible valve leaflets and the wide closing excursion of the valve leaflets[20] (see also Chap. 10). Failure to examine the patient in the left lateral decubitus position accounts for most of the misdiagnoses of symptomatic MS. The diastolic rumble is heard best with the bell of the stethoscope applied at the apical impulse. Nevertheless, the murmur may be localized, and the region around the apical impulse also should be auscultated. The opening snap (OS) occurs when the movement of the domed mitral valve into the LV is suddenly stopped.[20] It is heard best with the diaphragm and is often most easily appreciated midway between the apex and the left sternal border. In this intermediate region, the S_1, the pulmonary component of the second heart sound (P_2), and the OS can be identified. The auscultatory signs of MS in sinus rhythm and in atrial fibrillation are illustrated in Figs. 64-2 and 64-3.

The OS occurs after the LV pressure falls below LA pressure in early diastole. When LA pressure is high, as in severe MS, the snap occurs earlier in diastole (Fig. 64-2). The converse is true with mild MS. The interval between A_2 and the OS varies from 40 to 120 ms. Although the OS is present in most cases of MS, it is absent in patients with stiff, fibrotic or calcified leaflets. Thus, absence of the OS in severe MS suggests that mitral valve replacement rather than commissurotomy may be necessary.

The low-pitched diastolic rumble follows the OS and is best heard with the bell of the stethoscope. In some patients with low cardiac output or mild MS, brief exercise, such as sit-ups or walking, is adequate to increase flow and bring out the murmur. The murmur is low-pitched, rumbling, and decrescendo. In general, the more severe the MS, the longer the murmur (Fig. 64-2). Presystolic accentuation of the murmur occurs in sinus rhythm and has been reported even in atrial fibrillation. In the latter situation, a brief "presystolic" accentuation is due to narrowing of the mitral orifice produced by ventricular systole before the final, complete closure of the mitral valve and the mitral component of S_1. A diastolic rumble is not diagnostic of MS and may be heard with increased flow across a normal mitral valve—for example, in ventricular septal defect with a large left-to-right shunt.

The two most important auscultatory signs of severe MS are a short A_2-OS interval (usually 40 to 60 ms) and a full-length diastolic rumble. The A_2-OS interval may be longer if there is associated moderate/severe aortic regurgitation, and the OS may be absent when the mitral valve is rigid. The diastolic murmur may not be full-length in severe MS if the stroke volume is low and there is no tachycardia.

Systolic murmurs also may be heard in association with the murmur of MS. A blowing, holosystolic murmur at the apex suggests associated mitral regurgitation; whereas a systolic blowing murmur heard best at the lower left sternal border that increases with inspiration usually signifies tricuspid regurgitation. The Graham Steell murmur is a high-pitched diastolic decrescendo murmur of pulmonic regurgitation caused by severe PA hypertension. In most patients with MS, such a murmur usually indicates aortic regurgitation. In general, a left-sided third heart sound (S_3) is not compatible with severe MS with the possible exception of concomitant severe aortic regurgitation and/or significant LV systolic dysfunction. If an S_3 and a rumble are present, mitral regurgitation is usually the predominant lesion (see also Chap. 10).

ROENTGENOGRAM

The posteroanterior and lateral chest films are often so typical that experienced clinicians can make the tentative diagnosis from the film. The thoracic cage is normal. The lung fields show evidence of elevated pulmonary venous pressure. Blood flow is more evenly redistributed to the upper lobes, resulting in apparent prominence of upper lobe vascularity. Increased pulmonary venous pressure results in transudation of fluid into the interstitium. Accumulation of fluid in the interlobular septa produces linear streaks in the bases, which extend to the pleura (Kerley B lines).[21] Interstitial fluid may also be seen as perivascular or peribronchial cuffing (Kerley A lines). With transudation of fluid into the alveolar spaces, alveolar pulmonary edema is seen. These changes are not specific for MS but represent long-standing elevated LA pressure. Chronic hemosiderin deposition can result in an interstitial radiodensity that does not resolve after the relief of stenosis. PA hypertension results in enlargement of the main PA and right and left main pulmonary arteries.

The cardiac silhouette usually does not show generalized cardiomegaly, but the LA is invariably enlarged. This is manifest in the posteroanterior film by a density behind the RA border (double atrial shadow), prominence of the LA appendage on the left heart border between the main PA and LV apex, and elevation of the left main bronchus. The lateral film shows the LA bulging posteriorly. The LV silhouette is normal. The RV may be enlarged if PA hypertension has been

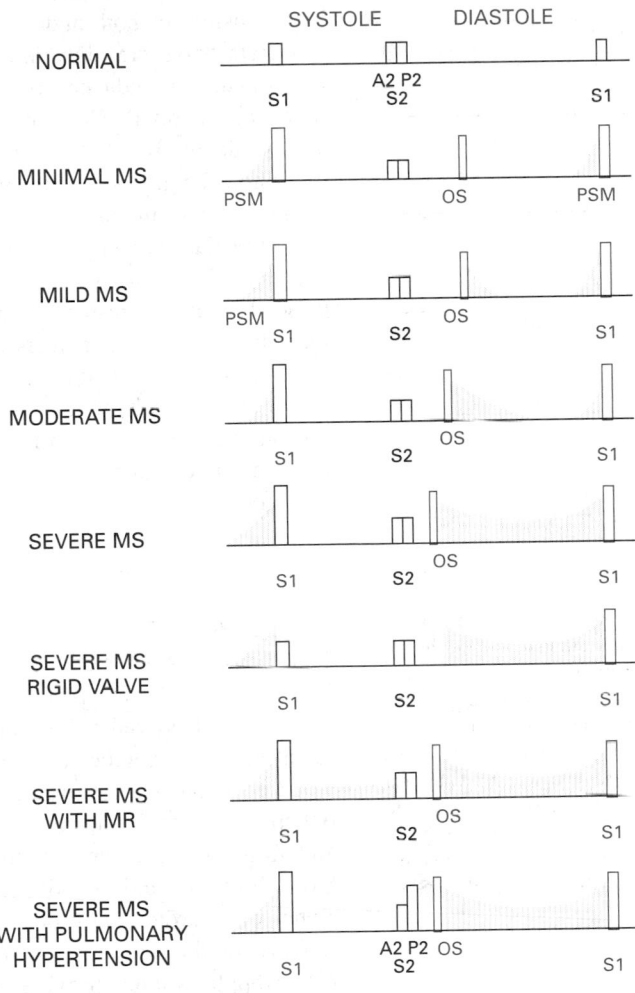

FIGURE 64-2

Auscultatory signs of MS in patients in sinus rhythm are illustrated. These include a presystolic murmur, loud first heart sound (S_1), an opening snap (OS), and a middiastolic murmur (low-pitched, decrescendo diastolic rumble, rumbling murmur). These signs may be accentuated or at times may be heard only by placing the patient in the left lateral decubitus position. Importantly, these signs are helpful in assessing the severity of the MS; as the MS becomes more severe, the S_2-OS interval is shortened and the length of the middiastolic rumble is increased. In mild OS, the S_2-OS interval is long and the diastolic murmur is short. In moderate MS, the S_2-OS interval is shorter, and although the diastolic murmur is longer at rest, there is usually a gap between the end of the murmur and the onset of the presystolic murmur. In severe MS, the S_2-OS interval is short (usually 0.04 to 0.06 s) and the diastolic murmur is a full-length murmur. With PA hypertension, P_2 is increased in intensity. In the presence of a rigid mitral valve (with or without calcification), S_2 is soft and the OS is usually not heard. A holosystolic murmur of mitral regurgitation may be present. (Adapted and modified from Kawanishi DT, Rahimtoola SH. Mitral stenosis. In: Rahimtoola SH, ed. *Valvular Heart Disease II.* St. Louis: Mosby; 1996:8.1–8.24. Copyright by S. H. Rahimtoola, M.B., F.R.C.P., M.A.C.P.)

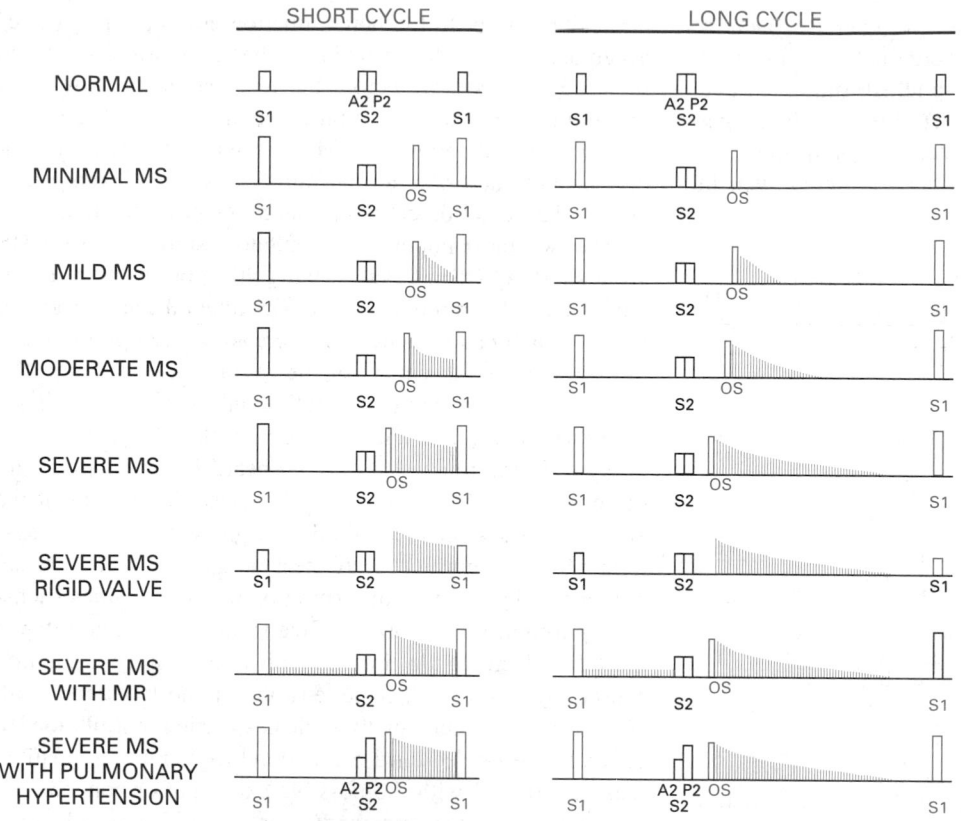

FIGURE 64-3

Auscultatory signs of MS in atrial fibrillation are illustrated. The presystolic murmur is absent. The loud S₁ and the OS are still heard. In the short cycles, the duration of diastole is short and the middiastolic rumble occupies the whole of diastole (*left panel*). In the long cycles (*right panel*), the length of middiastolic murmur is related to the severity of MS. As the MS becomes more severe, the length of this murmur is increased. In atrial fibrillation, with a slow ventricular response and very long R-R intervals, the middiastolic rumble may not occupy the whole diastolic period and the presystolic murmur is usually absent. Thus, one may get the impression that the MS is moderate rather than severe. Increasing the heart rate—for example, with brief physical exertion—may produce more characteristic auscultatory findings. Alternatively, when the ventricular rate in atrial fibrillation is rapid or in short cycles, the auscultatory findings may suggest a more severe degree of MS than is really the case (*left panel*). (Adapted and modified from Kawanishi DT, Rahimtoola SH. Mitral stenosis. In: Rahimtoola SH, ed. *Valvular Heart Disease. II.* St. Louis: Mosby; 1996:8.1–8.24. Copyright 1996 by S. H. Rahimtoola, M.B., F.R.C.P., M.A.C.P.)

present. RV enlargement is usually noted by filling of the retrosternal space, but this is an unreliable sign in adults. The combination of a normal-sized LV, enlarged LA, and pulmonary venous congestion should immediately raise the possibility of MS. Mitral valve calcification is occasionally seen on the plain chest film (see also Chap. 13).

ELECTROCARDIOGRAM

The electrocardiogram (ECG) is not usually as helpful as the chest x-ray. Patients in sinus rhythm may have a widened P wave caused by interatrial conduction delay and/or prolonged LA depolarization. Classically, the P wave is broad and notched in lead II and biphasic in lead V_1; it measures 0.12 s or more. Atrial fibrillation is common. LV hypertrophy is almost never present unless there are associated lesions. RV hypertrophy may be present if PA hypertension is marked (see also Chap. 12).

CLINICAL INDICATIONS OF SEVERE MITRAL STENOSIS

Some clinical features make it virtually certain that MS is severe. These include (1) moderate to severe PA hypertension as indicated by clinical and ECG evidence of RV hypertrophy or PA hypertension, or both and/or (2) moderate to severe elevation of LA pressure as indicated by orthopnea, a short P_2-OS interval, a diastolic rumble that occupies the whole length of a long diastolic interval in patients with atrial fibrillation, and pulmonary edema on the chest x-ray. In both these clinical circumstances, one must be certain that there is no other cause for elevated LA pressure and that LA hypertension is not caused mainly by a correctable transient elevation of LV diastolic pressure.

Laboratory Investigations

ECHOCARDIOGRAPHY/ DOPPLER ULTRASOUND

Echocardiography/Doppler ultrasound has proved to be both sensitive and specific for MS when adequate studies are done (Chap. 14).[22–25] False positives and false negatives are uncommon. M-mode and two-dimensional echocardiography do not reliably predict the severity of MS. Doppler studies provide an estimate of mitral valve area that is within ± 0.4 cm² (prior to interventional therapy) of that obtained by cardiac catheterization.[26] The echographic findings of MS reflect the loss of normal valve function. The fusion of commissures results in movement of the anterior and posterior leaflets anteriorly in parallel during diastole. In patients in sinus rhythm, there is an absence of the further opening of the valve that is normally seen with atrial contraction. Other findings include decreased E-to-F slope, decreased mitral valve leaflet excursion, and multiple echoes, indicating thickening or calcification of the valve. LA enlargement is seen. Abnormal pulmonary valve motion and RV enlargement may signify PA hypertension (see also Chap. 14).

Echocardiography is of great value in patients with equivocal signs, in patients with gross PA hypertension, to differentiate MS from an Austin Flint murmur of aortic regurgitation, and in the rare patient with "silent" MS. It is used to assess

LV, RV, and atrial size and function; to evaluate the aortic and tricuspid valves; and to estimate PA pressure. When transthoracic echocardiography is unsatisfactory, transesophageal echocardiography is a useful technique to assess LA thrombus, the anatomy of the mitral valve and subvalvular apparatus, and to assess the suitability of the patient for catheter balloon commissurotomy or surgical valve repair.

Echocardiography/Doppler ultrasound is a most useful test in MS and should be performed in all patients. It is essential to determine suitability of the valve for commissurotomy and/ or repair and to determine the likely result.

CARDIAC CATHETERIZATION/ANGIOGRAPHY

In the majority of patients with disabling symptoms from presumed MS, right and left heart catheterization should be performed as part of a preoperative assessment. Simultaneous measurement of cardiac output and the gradient between the LA and the LV and calculation of valve area remain the "gold standard" for assessing the severity of MS (Chap. 16). LV angiography assesses the competence of the mitral valve, an important determinant of operability for mitral commissurotomy. Quantification of LV function provides a useful prognostic indicator of operative and late survival and of the expected functional result. Aortic valve function should be evaluated in all patients. Selective supraventricular aortography should be performed in all patients unless there is a contraindication. Tricuspid valve function can be assessed when there is a question of coexisting lesions. In certain circumstances—for example, in a patient with suspected severe MS who has a small gradient and mildly elevated LA pressure—dynamic exercise in the catheterization laboratory with measurement of mitral valve gradient, cardiac output and LA and PA pressures can be extremely useful. Another example is a patient with significant symptoms in whom the findings at rest suggest moderate (or even mild) MS. Selective coronary arteriography establishes the site, severity, and extent of coronary artery disease and should be performed in patients with angina, in those with LV dysfunction, in those with risk factors for coronary artery disease, and in those 35 years of age or older who are being considered for interventional therapy.

OTHER INVESTIGATIONS

In most clinical situations, other investigations are not needed. Occasionally, a treadmill exercise test to evaluate functional capacity may be a very useful test clinically—for example, when a patient denies symptoms in spite of severe hemodynamic abnormalities.

Clinical Decision Making

The reader is referred to the section on aortic stenosis in Chap. 63. In a prospective blinded study of consecutive patients with valvular heart disease, the sensitivity and specificity of diagnosis of MS by clinical evaluation was 86 and 87 percent, respectively. The accuracy of diagnosis of MS for moderate to severe stenosis was 92 percent by clinical evaluation and 97 percent by echocardiography/Doppler ultrasound.[27] This emphasizes the importance of a thorough clinical evaluation. The principal difficulty with both clinical evaluation and echocardiography/Doppler ultrasound is being able to accurately separate in all instances mild from moderate MS and moderate from severe MS.

Natural History and Prognosis

The population presenting with MS is changing because of the sharp decline in the incidence of acute rheumatic fever in the past 40 years (see also Chap. 62). Native-born American citizens with symptomatic MS are presenting at an older age. Young adults in the third and fourth decades with symptomatic MS are more likely to come from low socioeconomic backgrounds and from the inner city or to be immigrants, particularly from Latin America, the Middle East, Southeast Asia, or the Orient. Therefore, the latent period between acute rheumatic fever and symptomatic MS is variable and appears to be related to the presence of repeated streptococcal infection. Women with MS outnumber men by almost two to one. The most important feature of the asymptomatic interval is the susceptibility to repeated bouts of both rheumatic valvulitis and streptococcal infection. The mechanism for the progression from no symptoms to mild to severe symptoms is progressive stenosis of the mitral valve.

With the onset of exertional dyspnea and fatigue, the valve area is usually reduced to one-half to one-third its normal size. Further small reductions in valve area markedly obstruct flow and result in symptoms with minimal exertion. The interval from initial mild symptoms to disabling symptoms may be 10 years. During this time, the patient is at some risk of death (see below). Permanent injury may result from atrial fibrillation with rapid ventricular rate, resulting in pulmonary edema, and from systemic embolus. Unfortunately, it is not possible to predict who is at risk of embolism. When late functional class II or functional class III symptoms are present, the valve area is usually 1.0 cm^2 or less (in an occasional patient the valve area is 1.2 or 1.3 cm^2), and both rest and exercise hemodynamics are deranged.[2] Further small reductions in valve area result in symptoms at rest.

The 10-year survival of patients with MS who are asymptomatic is approximately 84 percent and that of those who are mildly symptomatic is 34 to 42 percent (Fig. 64-4).[28–30] The 10-year survival of patients who are moderately or severely symptomatic and who do not have therapy is 40 percent or less, and the survival at 20 years is less than 10 percent.[28–30] Patients in the New York Heart Association functional class IV have a very poor survival without treatment[28]: 42 percent at 1 year and 10 percent or less at 5 years. All are dead by 10 years (Fig. 64-5).

Management

MS can be prevented through two approaches (Table 64-4). First, all streptococcal infections should be diagnosed rapidly and correctly treated (Chap. 62). This prevents most initial

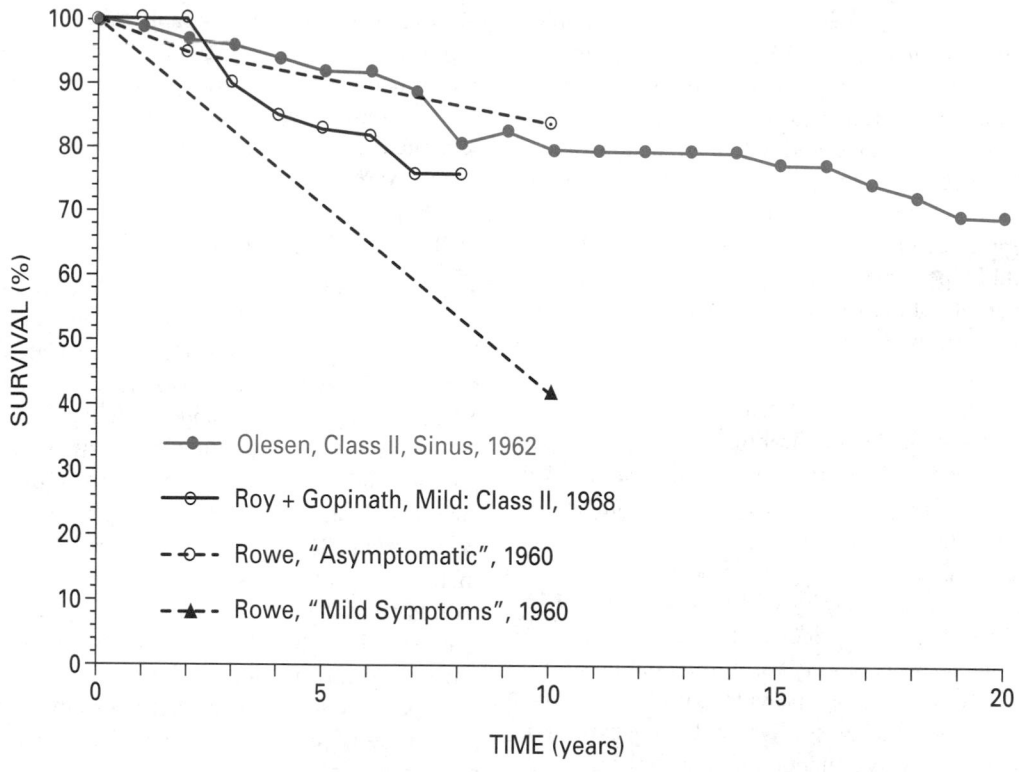

FIGURE 64-4

This figure depicts the survival of patients with MS who initially where asymptomatic or had mild symptoms and were treated medically. In the 1960 study of Rowe and coworkers[30] (*dashed lines*), 52 percent of 250 patients with "auscultatory MS" who presented between 1925 and 1947 were asymptomatic; their 10-year survival was 84 percent. The lower dashed line represents the survival in the 42 percent of patients who had mild symptoms on clinical presentation; their 10-year survival was 42 percent.[30] The data of Olesen, 1962[27] (*upper solid curve connecting solid symbols*), show the survival in the 21 percent of 271 symptomatic MS patients who had class II symptoms. Their 10- and 20-year survival was 34 and 14 percent, respectively. The data of Roy and Gopinath, 1968[29] (*lower solid curve connecting open symbols*), also show the survival in patients with class II symptoms. (From Kawanishi DT, Rahimtoola SH. Mitral stenosis. In: Rahimtoola SH, ed. *Valvular Heart Disease. II*. St. Louis: Mosby; 1996:8.1–8.24).

episodes of acute rheumatic fever. Second, all patients with known previous acute rheumatic fever/rheumatic carditis with or without obvious valve disease should receive appropriate antibiotic prophylaxis against recurrent streptococcal infection (Chap. 62).

Although the incidence of infective endocarditis is low in isolated MS, all patients exposed to bacteremia should receive appropriate prophylaxis against infective endocarditis (Chap. 82). Family and vocational planning should be considered. Women with this disease should consider bearing children before symptoms occur, since pregnancy is usually well tolerated with mild MS. Occupations that require strenuous exertion in middle age and later should probably be avoided if possible. In patients with moderate or severe MS, activities such as strenuous exercise and competitive sports should be restricted.[9]

When patients reach the symptomatic threshold, medical treatment may be of some benefit. Digitalis offers no improvement for the patient with normal sinus rhythm and normal LV function. When atrial fibrillation is present, however, digitalis plays a critical role in controlling ventricular rate. In selected patients, beta-adrenergic blocking agents, diltiazem, or amiodarone may be added if digoxin alone is not satisfactory

in controlling ventricular rate at rest or on exercise. Beta-adrenergic blocking agents should be used with great caution or not at all in patients with impaired LV function, associated significant aortic stenosis, or other associated severe valvular disease. Digoxin and diltiazem or digoxin and low-dose amiodarone are probably the two best combined regimens. Diuretics reduce pulmonary congestion and peripheral edema and allow most patients freedom from severe salt restriction. For the patient with mild symptoms, maintenance of sinus rhythm is desirable. Cardioversion of atrial fibrillation and maintenance of sinus rhythm using antiarrhythmic therapy with either digitalis and quinidine or digitalis and amiodarone should be offered to these patients. In patients who need interventional therapy, cardioversion is usually performed after completion of the procedure. Anticoagulation with warfarin is usually begun about 3 weeks in advance of cardioversion and for 4 weeks after the procedure.[31] Patients with chronic atrial fibrillation and those with a previous history of embolism should receive anticoagulation with warfarin (International Normalized Ratio, or INR, of 2 to 3) unless there is a specific contraindication.

There are no randomized trials of surgery versus medical

TABLE 64-4
MEDICAL TREATMENT OF MITRAL STENOSIS

Prevention
  Primary
    Treatment of streptococcal group A infection
  Secondary (antibiotic prophylaxis)
    Recurrent rheumatic fever
    Infective endocarditis
Restrict activities (moderate/severe MS)
  Severe exercise
  Competitive sports
Arrhythmias
  Prevent and/or control
  Restore sinus rhythm if possible
Cardiac medications
  Use only if essential
  Diuretics—use cautiously
  Anticoagulants for systemic/pulmonary emboli
  Elevated pulmonary venous pressure—diuretics
  Heart failure—digitalis, diuretics, ACE inhibitors
Follow-up of asymptomatic patients

Mild MS	Every 2–5 years
Moderate MS	Every 1–2 years
Severe MS	Every 6–12 months if interventional therapy not performed
Development of symptoms	Early or "immediate"

Source: Copyright by S. H. Rahimtoola, M.B., F.R.C.P., M.A.C.P. (Ref. 10).

therapy. Roy and Gopinath's study[29] showed that in comparable patients, surgical commissurotomy was associated with a better survival than medical therapy in patients with class II symptoms as well as in those with class III and IV symptoms (Fig. 64-6).

Unless there is a contraindication, surgery should be recommended to an MS patient with functional class III or IV

TABLE 64-5
INDICATIONS FOR INTERVENTIONAL THERAPY FOR SEVERE MITRAL STENOSIS

All severely symptomatic patients (functional classes III and IV)
All mildly symptomatic patients (functional class II)[a,b]
Asymptomatic patients[a,b]
  Pulmonary artery hypertension
  Episodic pulmonary edema
  Atrial fibrillation (persistent or repeated episodes)
Thromboembolism (systemic/pulmonary)
Severe mitral stenosis (valve suitable for CBC/surgical valve repair)

[a] Catheter balloon commissurotomy/surgery.
[b] Individualize depending on patient characteristics; suitability of patient for CBC/surgical valve repair versus valve replacement, skill and experience of interventional team.
Source: Copyright by S. H. Rahimtoola, M.B., F.R.C.P., M.A.C.P. (Ref. 10).

symptoms (Table 64-5). For younger patients with a pliable, noncalcified valve and without important mitral regurgitation, this means valve repair. The hemodynamic results of surgical commissurotomy are excellent.[9,32,33] Because of the low morbidity and mortality of mitral commissurotomy/valve repair,[9,32–34] surgery is also offered to those patients when functional class II symptoms are present. The results of successful commissurotomy are excellent; in experienced and skilled centers, surgical mortality is less that 1 percent. Late mortality at 10 years is less than 5 percent, the thromboembolism rate is 2 percent per year or less, and the reoperation rate ranges from 0.5 to 4.5 percent per year. The return of symptoms after commissurotomy/valve repair is usually the result of an incomplete operation, other valvular lesions, refusion of mitral commissures, or deterioration of myocardial function. In less developed countries, excellent results have been reported in a very high percentage of young patients for up to 25 years.[35]

For the older patient with a stiff or calcified valve or when moderate mitral regurgitation is present, mitral valve replacement is usually performed. Valve replacement carries a higher operative mortality than does commissurotomy (up to 5 percent) and the morbidity associated with prostheses (see Chap. 67). Hemodynamic results of mitral valve replacement are often not ideal (Table 64-6).[36,37] Survival at 10 years after mitral valve replacement for functional class III and IV patients is better than 60 percent (see Chap. 67).

TABLE 64-6
MITRAL STENOSIS: RESULTS OF MITRAL VALVE REPLACEMENT IN 33 PATIENTS

	Mitral Stenosis	
	Pre-MVR[a]	Post-MVR
LV end-diastolic pressure, mmHg	11 ± 5	12 ± 6
Mean PA wedge pressure, mmHg	36 ± 15	28 ± 14[b]
Mean systolic PA pressure, mmHg	54 ± 24	42 ± 22[c]
Cardiac index, L/min/m²	2.1 ± 1.5	2.3 ± 0.6
LV EDVI, mL/m²	79 ± 18	72 ± 24
LV ESVI, mL/m²	41 ± 13	39 ± 21
LVEF	0.48 ± 0.10	0.47 ± 0.14
Mitral regurgitant volume, mL	—	—
Regurgitant volume/end-diastolic volume	—	—
Mitral valve gradient, mmHg	15 ± 7	8 ± 3[b]
Mitral valve area, cm²	1.2 ± 0.4	1.8 ± 0.6[b]

[a] MVR = mitral valve replacement.
[b] $p < .001$.
[c] $p < .01$ comparing before and after mitral valve replacement artery.
Source: Crawford MH, et al.[36]

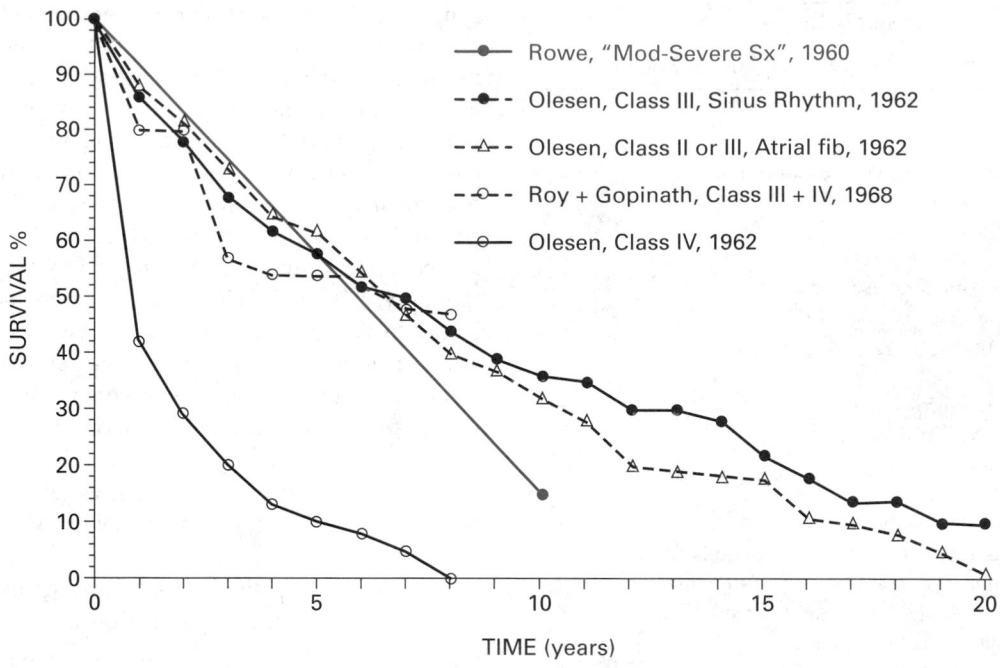

FIGURE 64-5

Survival of patients with MS and moderate or advanced (severe) symptoms is shown. Patients who were in NYHA functional class IV (Olesen, class IV, 1962)[28] had a 42 percent 1-year survival and all patients had died within 8 years. The other four survival curves are of patients who were in functional classes II to IV, and their survival curves are similar, with 5-, 10-, and 15-year approximate survivals of 60, 40, and 20 percent, respectively; at 20 years, less than 10 percent of the patients were still alive.[28–30] Thus, the survival in this group of patients with more advanced symptoms is much worse than that of patients who were initially asymptomatic or minimally symptomatic (see Fig. 64-4). (From Kawanishi DT, Rahimtoola SH. Mitral stenosis. In: Rahimtoola SH, ed. *Valvular Heart Disease. II.* St. Louis: Mosby; 1996:8.1–8.24.)

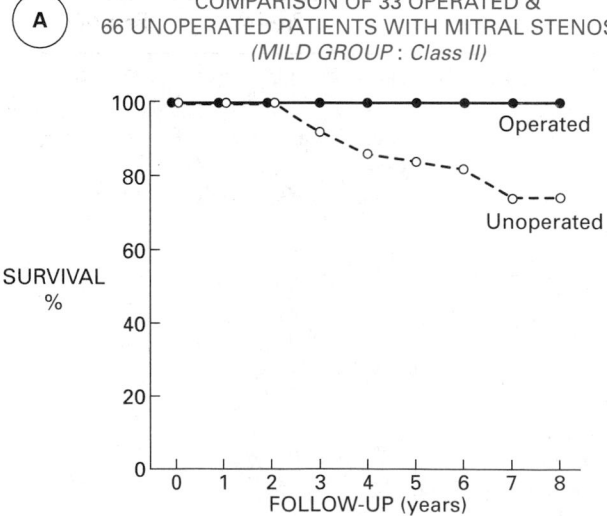

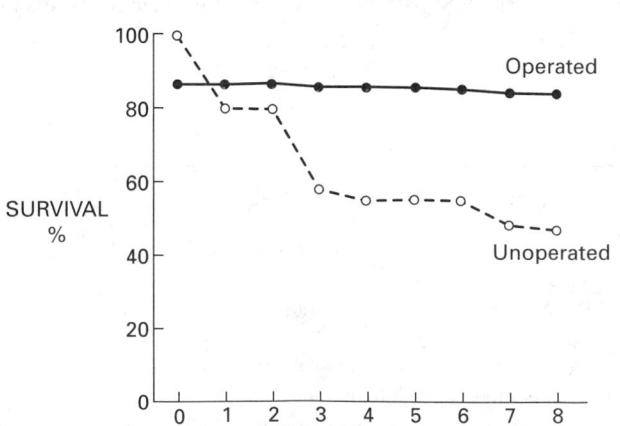

FIGURE 64-6

Compares survival of patients with class II symptoms (*left panel*) and with class III and IV symptoms due to MS (*right panel*).[29] Survival of patients treated medically (unoperated) is indicated by the broken line and with surgical closed mitral commissurotomy (operated) by the solid line. In patients treated by surgical commissurotomy, there were no operative or late deaths in those with mild symptoms and no late deaths in those with class III and IV symptoms. There is a clear improvement in survival in operated patients. The 5-year mortality with medical treatment alone in those with class III and IV symptoms approaches 50 percent (also see Fig. 64-5); with surgery, there is no appreciable mortality following recovery from the procedure. [From Roy SB, Gopinath N. Mitral stenosis. *Circulation* 1968; 38(suppl v):68–76.]

Catheter balloon commissurotomy (CBC) with use of the double balloon technique or the Inoue balloon produces immediate and 3-month hemodynamic and clinical results comparable to those obtained by surgical commissurotomy.[38–41] The mitral valve area increases from a mean of 1.0 to 2.0 cm^2.[26,32,38] There are reductions of LA and PA pressures at rest and on exercise and an increase of exercise capacity.[39] The immediate results of CBC are greatly influenced by the characteristics of the valve and its supporting apparatus, which are best determined by two-dimensional echocardiography (transthoracic and/or transesophageal).[22] Echocardiographic scores of ≤8 or of 0–1 determined by the two different methods provide a clue to the best immediate results. Repeat CBC or mitral valve replacement is needed in 20 percent of patients within 5 to 7 years. Late survival is poorer in those in whom functional class IV, higher echocardiographic score, higher LV end-diastolic pressure, or higher PA systolic pressure is present prior to the CBC.[42–47] In one study, the 7-year survival was 95 ± 1 percent and the event-free survival was 65 ± 6 percent.[47] The 7-year event-free survival ranged from 13 to 90 percent in various subgroups. The 7-year event-free survival was best predicted by the post CBC mitral valve area (≥1.5 cm^2) and PA wedge pressure (≤18 mmHg); the 7-year event-free survival was 90 ± 6 percent.[47] In the appropriate patient and in centers with skilled and experienced staff, CBC is the procedure of first choice for relief of severe MS. Factors to be taken into account choosing between surgery and CBC in an individual patient are shown in Table 64-7.

MITRAL REGURGITATION

Mitral regurgitation (MR) is characterized by an abnormal, reversed blood flow from the LV to the LA. This valvular disease has considerably changed in the last decades in regard to its etiologic profile, which is now dominated by degenerative and ischemic causes in developed countries; to its noninvasive assessment with the recent developments in transesophageal echocardiography, color-flow imaging, and methods of quantitation of regurgitation; and to its management with the improved understanding of the role of LV function in prognosis. Most importantly, advances in conservative surgery have improved its treatment.

Normal Mitral Structure and Function

The mitral valve is a complex structure formed by the following four elements[48–52]:

1. *The annulus* which is asymmetric, with a fixed portion (corresponding to the anterior leaflet) shared with the aortic annulus[50] and a dynamic portion[51] (corresponding to the posterior leaflet) which represents most of the circumference of the annulus.
2. *The anterior and posterior leaflets,* which are asymmetric, the former having the greater length of tissue but occupying a smaller portion of the circumference of the

---

TABLE 64-7

SOME FACTORS TO BE CONSIDERED IN CHOICE OF TYPE OF INTERVENTIONAL THERAPY FOR MITRAL STENOSIS^a

Mitral valve morphology	
Low echo score:	Catheter balloon commissurotomy (CBC)
	Surgical valve repair
High echo score:	Surgery
	CBC in special circumstances
Mitral regurgitation	
≥3+:	Surgery
≤1+:	CBC
2+:	Individualize (CBC versus surgery)
Left atrial thrombus	
Surgery	
CBC in special circumstances	
Need for other cardiac surgery	
Surgery	
CBC in special circumstances	

^{a} In centers with skilled and experienced interventional teams.
Source: Copyright by S. H. Rahimtoola. M.B., F.R.C.P., M.A.C.P. (Ref. 10).

---

annulus than the latter.[48,50] The main mechanism preventing regurgitation is a sufficient area of coaptation of the rough zones of the two leaflets in systole.[50]

3. *The chordae tendineae,* which join each papillary muscle to the corresponding commissure and the adjoining halves of both leaflets[49] and maintain the two leaflets in a position allowing coaptation.
4. *The two papillary muscles and the adjacent wall,* which attach the mitral apparatus to the left ventricle. The fact that the mechanism of MR frequency combines abnormal function of more than one anatomic element underlines the complexity of conservative surgery for restoration of normal mitral function.[52]

During systole, mitral competence is normally ensured by the large area of coaptation between leaflets, allowing high friction resistance to abnormal valve movement, and by the systolic position of the anterior leaflet parallel to the direction of blood flow.

Etiology and Mechanism of Mitral Regurgitation

Although a classification of MR according to the valvular movements has been suggested,[53] the mechanisms of regurgitation are complex and often multiple and therefore should be analyzed with each etiology (Table 64-8).

Pure *rheumatic mitral regurgitation* (Fig. 64-7, Plate 49) represents about 10 percent of rheumatic mitral valve dis-

---

FIGURE 64-7
See color Plate 49.

TABLE 64-8

MITRAL REGURGITATION: MECHANISMS

Etiology	Mechanism	Echocardiographic Appearance

Rheumatic
  Lupus erythematosus
  Anticardiolipin syndrome
  Carcinoid
  Ergot lesions
  Postradiation
	Retraction
	Thickening
		Thickened chordae/leaflets
		Normal or restricted
		  motion

Degenerative
  Marfan
  Ehlers-Danlos
  Traumatic MR
	Prolapsed leaflets
	Ruptured chords
		Prolapsing/flail leaflets
		Redundant tissue
		Ruptured chords

Ischemic (infarction)
  Myocardial disease
  Ischemic (chronic)
  Cardiomyopathies
	Ruptured papillary muscle
	Dilatation of annulus
	Traction anterior leaflet
		Flail leaflet
		Normal leaflets
		Reduced motion of
		  leaflets

Infiltrative disease
  Hypereosinophilic
    syndrome
  Endomyocardial fibrosis
  Hurler's disease
	Thickened leaflet
	Loss of coaptation
		Thickened leaflets
		Reduced motion

Endocarditis	Destructive lesions	Perforations Flail leaflets
Congenital	Cleft leaflet Transposed valve	Cleft leaflet Tricuspid valve

ease.[54] More often, MR is associated with stenosis and fusion of the commissures. Severe rheumatic MR requiring surgical correction is still frequent in developing countries but is now rare in developed ones.[55,56] The underlying lesion is retractile fibrosis of the leaflets and chordae tendineae, causing loss of coaptation.[57] The secondary dilatation of the mitral annulus tends to further decrease the contact between leaflets. Elongated or ruptured chordae are infrequent.

DEGENERATIVE MITRAL REGURGITATIONS

These causes are often associated with valvular prolapse, an abnormal movement of the leaflets into the left atrium during systole due to inadequate chordal support (elongation or rupture), and excessive valvular tissue.[56] In recent years in some Western countries, mitral prolapse represents the most frequent cause leading to surgery for severe MR.[55,56] The degenerative MR can be separated in three categories:

1. The mitral valve prolapse[58] syndrome (Fig. 64-8, Plate 50) which may have an hereditary component.[59] Macroscopically there is a marked increase in valve area and length,[56] with interchordal hooding involving a large area of the leaflets,[60] and secondary ruptured chordae may occur. Microscopically the valves are myxomatous, with deposition of mucopolysaccharides in a thickened spongiosa layer encroaching on the fibrosa layer.[61] Annular myxomatous changes may lead to dilatation and calcification. The myxomatous infiltration may also involve the other cardiac valves and result in regurgitation of these valves (see Chap. 65).

2. The degenerative "primary" ruptured chordae (Fig. 64-9, Plate 51) more often involves the posterior than the anterior leaflet and occur more often in men than in women.[62] There is usually no excessive tissue[56] but enlargement of the annulus may occur, as in any MR. The involved leaflet may present with a myxomatous infiltration,[63] but the other leaflet usually remains normal.[64] Calcification of the mitral annulus[65] or systemic arterial hypertension may precede the occurrence of the ruptured chordae. Isolated ruptured chordae may occasionally be due to blunt thoracic trauma and endocarditis (secondary forms).

3. Degenerative MRs without prolapse are usually mild and are due to sclerosis of the valve or isolated calcification of the mitral annulus,[66] in which the regurgitation is secondary to deformation of the valves or annulus.

INFECTIVE ENDOCARDITIS

Infective endocarditis (Fig. 64-10, Plate 52) accounts for about 5 percent of cases of severe mitral regurgitation. Vegetations can produce some mild regurgitation by interposition between the leaflets. Severe endocarditis regurgitation is usually related to ruptured chords and less frequently to the destruction of mitral tissue involving either the edges of the leaflets or a perforation.[67]

ISCHEMIC AND FUNCTIONAL MITRAL REGURGITATION

Ischemic and functional MR (i.e., due to transient or permanent papillary muscle dysfunction,[68] to left ventricular dilatation[69] isolated or with an aneurysm, to cardiomyopathies, or

FIGURE 64-8
See color Plate 50.

FIGURE 64-9
See color Plate 51.

FIGURE 64-10
See color Plate 52.

to myocarditis) have the same mechanism. The abnormal shape or systolic contraction of the left ventricle produces an abnormal traction on the chordae that is mainly transmitted to the anterior leaflet, resulting in an abnormal anterior position of this leaflet in systole with a resultant reduction of the area of coaptation.[70,71]

Rupture of a papillary muscle (Fig. 64-11, Plate 53) produces regurgitation because of the flail leaflet. It may be traumatic, but usually, in 80 percent of cases, it is due to acute myocardial infarction, involving the posteromedial papillary muscle and is associated with infarction of the adjacent ventricular wall.[72,73] It is the rarest form of cardiac rupture and of ischemic MR. Complete rupture of a papillary muscle is rapidly fatal without surgery; partial or single-head rupture of a papillary muscle more often allows emergency surgery.[73]

OTHER CAUSES OF MITRAL REGURGITATION

MR is observed extremely frequently with color-flow imaging, even in patients without cardiac disease, but clinically significant MR may be found in (1) *connective tissue disorders* (Chap. 85), Marfan syndrome,[74] Ehlers-Danlos syndrome,[75] pseudoxanthum elasticum, osteogenesis imperfecta, Hurler's disease, systemic lupus erythematosus,[76] and anticardiolipin syndrome[77]; (2) penetrating or nonpenetrating *cardiac trauma*[78]; (3) *myocardial disease* such as hypertrophic cardiomyopathy (Chap. 74) or sarcoidosis; (4) *endocardial disease* such as hypereosinophilic syndrome,[79] endocardial fibroelastosis, carcinoid tumors,[80] ergot-related lesions, postradiation lesions; (5) *congenital* lesions such as cleft mitral valve isolated or associated with persistent AV canal (corrected transposition with or without Ebstein's abnormality of the left AV valve may also cause mitral regurgitation); and (6) *cardiac tumors* (Chap 86).

Pathophysiology

The abnormal coaptation of the mitral leaflets creates a *regurgitant orifice* during systole. The systolic pressure gradient between the LV and the LA is the driving force of the regurgitant flow which results in a *regurgitant volume*. This regurgitant volume represents a percentage of the total ejection of the LV and may be expressed as the *regurgitant fraction*. The regurgitant volume creates a volume overload by entering the LA in systole and the LV in diastole and modifies left ventricular loading and function.

CHRONOLOGY OF REGURGITATION

The pressure gradient between the LV and LA normally begins with mitral closure and the mitral component of the first heart sound and persists after the aortic component of the second heart sound until the mitral valve opens.[81] In clinically significant MR, a regurgitant orifice is usually present throughout LV systole, and the regurgitation is holosystolic, beginning

with S_1 and ending after S_2.[81] The statement that most of MR occurs in early systole is not consistent with the small changes in ventricular volumes observed during that period[82] and with the dynamics of the regurgitant orifice.[83] In patients with small regurgitant orifices, however, the progressive decrease in the regurgitant orifice with the decrease of the ventricular volume tends to limit the regurgitation to the early part of systole.[81] Conversely mitral valve prolapse may appear late, when the LV volume is below a specific point during systole. Thus the regurgitant orifice and regurgitant flow are present mainly in mid and late systole.[84]

DEGREE AND CONSEQUENCES OF REGURGITATION

The area of the regurgitant orifice is an essential determinant of the degree of volume overload and the dilatation of left ventricle and left atrium.[85] The resultant volume overload (regurgitant volume) also depends on the magnitude of the regurgitant pressure gradient and its duration. For example, the volume overload observed in patients with MR is usually less severe than in aortic regurgitation,[86,87] although the regurgitant gradient and regurgitant orifice[85] are usually larger than in aortic regurgitation. Some of this difference is related to the shorter duration of mitral regurgitation than of aortic regurgitation.[85]

The degree of MR is not fixed and may vary with interventions.[88] Vasodilators may be beneficial,[89] primarily due to a decrease in regurgitant orifice area rather than a decrease in ventriculoatrial pressure gradient. In both functional[90,91] and organic MR,[92] the regurgitant orifice may be modified by changes in LV afterload, preload, and contractility.[92] The regurgitant orifice increases with increased afterload or ventricular volume; it decreases with decreased afterload or improved contractility but is usually not influenced by short-term moderate changes in heart rate.

With MR, the regurgitant energy produced by the LV translates into two components, the kinetic energy (regurgitant volume) and the potential energy (elevation of atrial pressure). The typical left atrial pressure change is a very prominent V wave with a late systolic peak. The V wave may be extremely high in patients with severe MR and may even transmit through the pulmonary veins and modify the pulmonary artery pressure curves,[93] particularly in acute MR or "small" LA. Nevertheless, the LA V wave is not specific for MR[94] and can be observed solely as a result of changes in the LA pressure-volume relationship. In MR the V wave may increase with tachycardia even with unchanged regurgitation.

The height of the V wave and more generally the LA pressure is mainly determined by the LA compliance.[93] In acute MR, the left atrium is less dilated than in chronic regurgitation and the regurgitant volume produces a marked increase in LA pressure. The rapidly increasing atrial V wave decreases the ventriculoatrial gradient; thus, for any effective regurgitant orifice,[85] it tends to limit the regurgitant volume. In some patients with acute MR, the rapid increase in LA pressure to very high levels causes the MR and its murmur to end prior to the second heart sound (see Chap. 10). When MR becomes

FIGURE 64-11
See color Plate 53.

chronic, the left atrium tends to dilate proportionately to the degree of regurgitation and to become more compliant. Consequently the V wave is less prominent; it does not limit the regurgitant volume, and the left atrial pressure may be normal, or near normal even though the regurgitation is severe.[95] At that stage the cardiac output is usually decreased, but the pulmonary pressures are often normal. Pulmonary hypertension occurs in MR, is related to increases in mean LA pressure and/or in pulmonary vascular resistance, and is usually observed in elderly patients.

LEFT VENTRICULAR FUNCTION

In patients with MR, the LV is dilated, but less so than in aortic regurgitation of comparable degree.[86,96] The LV end-diastolic volume and the end-diastolic wall stress are increased.[96] The end-systolic volume is often increased in chronic MR, but the end-systolic wall stress is nevertheless usually normal.[97,98] The LV is more spherical in diastole and systole than in normal patients,[82] especially with large volumes or reduced function. After correction of the regurgitation, the shape of the ventricle tends to normalize.[99] The myocardial mass is increased in patients with MR usually proportionately to the degree of LV dilatation.[99]

LV function is difficult to characterize because of the changes in preload and afterload. It has been suggested that normalization of the ejection fraction to the preload can provide an appropriate assessment of LV function.[100,101] Afterload is more difficult to assess because the regurgitation into the left atrium may decrease the instantaneous impedance to ejection, but the measure of afterload provided by end-systolic wall stress is within the normal range.[97,98] The usual inverse correlation between end-systolic wall stress and ejection fraction is also observed in MR.[102] Complex indices using the afterload, such as the end-systolic wall stress[103] or maximum elastance[97] normalized to the LV volume, have been proposed and may be sensitive to subtle changes in function (see also Chap. 22).

LV dysfunction is a frequent and dismal complication of MR.[104,105] Although interstitial fibrosis is present in advanced LV failure, the exact mechanism of LV dysfunction remains mysterious. Experimentally, LV dysfunction is not due to changes in coronary blood flow.[106] The changes in myofiber contractility parallel the changes in global LV function[107] and are associated with reduced myofiber content,[108] but the cause of the myofiber dysfunction and the explanation of its high incidence have not been clarified (see Chap. 23).

During diastole, LV relaxation is frequently abnormal but chamber stiffness is usually reduced.[109] Age and decreased systolic function[109] are associated with increased chamber stiffness. The significance of the diastolic abnormalities is unclear.

ISCHEMIC AND FUNCTIONAL MITRAL REGURGITATION

The pathophysiology of ruptured papillary muscles is poorly known. In patients with chronic ischemic or functional MR, the primary disease involves the LV, which is often poorly contracting; but the regurgitation may be determined more by the LV shape than its function. In ischemic or functional as opposed to organic (due to primary valvular disease) MR, the regurgitant volume is usually small[110] and the LV and LA dilatation is not proportional to the degree of regurgitation.[85] Nevertheless, MR may be clinically significant and elevate LA pressure 85; in these patients, the MR *may be a marker* of advanced myocardial disease[111,112] and of sensitivity to vasodilators.[113]

Clinical Presentation

The clinical presentation—including symptoms, physical findings, ECG changes, and radiographic changes—are determined by the degree and rapidity of development and the cause of the regurgitation as well as by the function and compliance of the left atrium and ventricle.

SYMPTOMS

Patients with mild MR usually have no symptoms. Severe MR may be associated with no or minimal symptoms for years.[54] Fatigue due to the low cardiac output and mild dyspnea on exertion are the most usual symptoms and are rapidly improved by rest.[114] More severe symptoms may be reduced by the administration of diuretics and the progressive self-limitation of physical activity. Severe dyspnea on exertion or, more rarely, paroxysmal nocturnal dyspnea, frank pulmonary edema, or even hemoptysis[54,114] may be observed later in the course of the disease. Such severe symptoms may be triggered by the new onset of atrial fibrillation, an increase in degree of regurgitation, endocarditis or ruptured chordae,[115] or a change in LV compliance or function.

In patients with severe regurgitation of acute onset, symptoms are usually more dramatic. They include pulmonary edema or congestive heart failure[115–117] but may progressively subside with administration of diuretic and vasodilator(s) and increased compliance of the left atrium. A syndrome of sudden onset of atypical chest pain and dyspnea may occur with abrupt chordal rupture. Rupture of a papillary muscle usually has a dramatic presentation, with cardiogenic shock or a severe pulmonary edema.[118] Pulmonary edema may be also observed in transient severe papillary muscle dysfunction.[119]

Sudden death as the initial presentation of mitral regurgitation is rare.[120]

The sex distribution has changed in parallel to the changes in etiology of MR.[54] With the decrease in rheumatic heart disease, severe MR is now predominantly seen in males (65 to 75 percent). As degenerative diseases of the mitral valve are more common later in life, the mean age of patients has been steadily increasing (most frequently in the sixth decade of life).

PHYSICAL EXAMINATION

The blood pressure is usually normal. The carotid upstroke is brisk and this impression is further strengthened by a reduced ejection time in patients with severe regurgitation.

The cardiac apex impulse may be laterally displaced, diffuse, and brief in patients with enlarged left ventricle. An apical systolic thrill is characteristic of severe regurgitation. A left sternal border lift is observed in patients with RV dilatation and may be difficult to distinguish from the LA lift due to filling and expansion of the LA, although the latter is more substernal and lower (see Chap. 10).

The first heart sound is difficult to appreciate since it is often obscured by the murmur; usually it is normal, although it may be increased in rheumatic heart disease. The second heart sound is usually normal, but it may be paradoxically split if the LV ejection time is markedly shortened. The presence of a third heart sound is directly related to the volume of the regurgitation in patients with organic MR.[121] It is often associated with an early diastolic rumble due to the increased mitral flow in diastole; at times, the rumble is prolonged even in the absence of MS. The third heart sound and diastolic rumble are low-pitched and may be difficult to detect without careful auscultation performed in the left lateral decubitus position. The S_3 may be increased with expiration. In patients with ischemic and/or functional MR, the third heart sound corresponds more often to restrictive LV filling. An atrial gallop is heard mainly in MR of recent onset,[122] particularly in patients with ischemic/functional MR and maintained sinus rhythm. Midsystolic clicks are markers of mitral valve prolapse, occurring simultaneously to the prolapse,[84] and are due to the sudden tension of the chordae (see Chaps. 10 and 65).

The hallmark of MR is the systolic murmur. In regurgitation of at least moderate degree, the murmur is holosystolic, including the first and second heart sounds. If an opening snap (OS) or a third heart sound are mistakenly interpreted as being the second heart sound, the murmur may appear midsystolic. Only a careful examination, beginning at the base of the heart to identify the second heart sound and progressing toward the apex, will allow clear recognition of the nature of the murmur. The murmur is of the blowing type but may be harsh, especially in mitral valve prolapse. The maximum loudness of the murmur is usually at the apex, and it may radiate to the axilla in patients with rheumatic or anterior leaflet prolapse regurgitation. In patients with prolapse of the posterior leaflet, the jet of regurgitation is usually superiorly and medially directed, and the murmur classically radiates toward the base of the heart.[123] With prolapse or ruptured chordae of the anterior leaflet, the murmur may be heard in the back, in the neck, and sometimes on the skull. In the cases where the murmur radiates to the base, it may difficult to distinguish from the murmurs of aortic stenosis or hypertrophic obstructive cardiomyopathy. With increase of afterload, for example, hand-grip, the murmur is increased. Similarly, within reductions of afterload or LV size, the murmur is reduced. Pharmacologic maneuvers in which the murmur decreases with amyl nitrite and increases with methoxamin strongly suggest MR. The murmur does not increase with postextrasystolic beats, probably because the regurgitant flow is unchanged due to the combination of a decreased regurgitant orifice[92] and increased regurgitant gradient. The murmur in general parallels the degree of regurgitation,[124] but in myocardial infarction, severe MR may be totally silent[125] (see Chap. 10).

Murmurs of shorter duration usually correspond to mild regurgitation; these may be mid- or late systolic in patients with mitral valve prolapse or early systolic in patients with functional MR.

ELECTROCARDIOGRAM

The most frequent feature of MR is atrial fibrillation, which was found in approximately 60 to 75 percent[54] of earlier series and is now present in approximately 50 percent of surgically corrected MR.[126] Patients in sinus rhythm may present with signs of left atrial enlargement (Fig. 64-12). LV hypertrophy is less often seen and may be associated with secondary ST-T abnormalities.[127] RV hypertrophy is uncommon. The ECG especially in acute MR, may be entirely normal. In patients with mitral valve prolapse sydnrome, nonspecific ST-T wave changes may be observed. In patients with ischemic MR, Q waves or a left bundle branch block may often be noted (see also Chap. 12).

CHEST ROENTGENOGRAM

Patients with mitral valve prolapse or Marfan's syndrome may have pectus excavatum or scoliosis. Cardiomegaly (Fig. 64-13) may be present in chronic MR or in patients with ischemic/functional MR. LA and atrial appendage dilatation

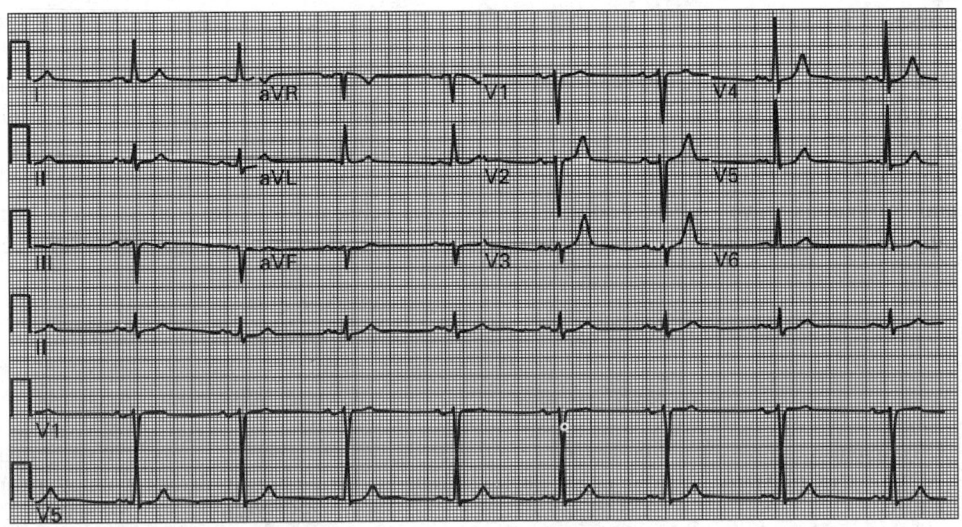

FIGURE 64-12

Electrocardiogram of a patient with severe MR. Note LA enlargement, as indicated by notched p waves.

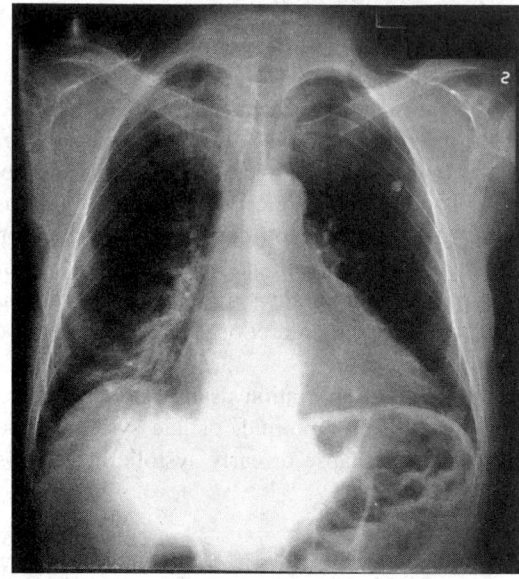

FIGURE 64-13
Chest roentgenogram of a patient with severe mitral regurgitation. Note the cardiomegaly and enlargement of the LA body and appendage.

is frequent in any type of MR. Although valvular calcifications are rare,[65] annular calcifications seen as a C-shaped density below the posterior leaflet are frequent. Giant left atria are usually seen in severe mixed rheumatic mitral valve disease[128] (see also Chap. 13).

Because left atrial pressure is frequently normal even in the presence of severe MR, signs of pulmonary hypertension or pulmonary edema may be absent in patients with isolated chronic MR.

CLINICAL SYNDROMES

The clinical presentation of patients with mitral regurgitation can be schematically separated in four syndromes summarized in Table 64-9.

Laboratory Tests

DOPPLER ECHOCARDIOGRAPHY

Doppler echocardiography has an important role in the assessment of MR using two-dimensional echocardiography with directed M-mode measurements, color-flow imaging, pulsed and continuous-wave Doppler, and transesophageal echocardiography. Quantitative measurements of flow and detailed

hemodynamic assessment should be routinely performed. The goals of Doppler echocardiography are (1) the morphologic assessment of the mitral valve (etiology and mechanism), (2) the assessment of the degree of regurgitation, and (3) the assessment of the ventricular and atrial function (see also Chap. 14).

Morphology

Rheumatic mitral regurgitation is characterized by thickening of the leaflets, mainly at their tips, as well as of the chordae.[129] The posterior leaflet may have reduced mobility, whereas the anterior leaflet may have normal mobility but with doming if there is associated commisural fusion. A valvular prolapse is usually not present unless there is a ruptured chorda or active rheumatic carditis.[130] Similar lesions can be observed in lupus or anticardiolipin syndrome,[76,77] in which transesophageal echocardiography may also show small vegetations on the atrial side of the leaflets.

In *degenerative mitral regurgitations,* prolapse is observed with the passage of valvular tissue beyond the plane of the annulus (Fig. 64-14). Because of the saddle shape of the mitral annulus,[131] the apical four-chamber view may overestimate the presence of valvular prolapse, which should be confirmed on the long-axis view obtained from the apical or parasternal windows. Transesophageal echocardiography can be useful for the diagnosis of prolapse if standard imaging is of mediocre quality.[132] Once the mitral valve prolapse (see Chap. 65) has been clearly diagnosed, the following features should be determined:

- The presence of diffuse myxomatous changes that produce diffusely thickened leaflets[133] with excessive valvular tissue (Fig. 64-15).
- Localization of the prolapse and whether it involves one (usually the posterior) or both leaflets. The initial direction of the jet confirms the predominant lesion,[134] with jets centrally directed in equal bileaflet prolapse, directed inferiorly and externally in predominant anterior leaflet prolapse, or directed superiorly and medially in predominant posterior leaflet prolapse.
- The presence of mitral annular calcification, which may represent a limitation for conservative surgery if the calcification is extensive and severe.
- The presence of flail leaflet is diagnosed by the complete eversion of one leaflet with complete loss of coaptation in the regurgitant area.[134] Flail leaflets can usually be

TABLE 64-9

MITRAL REGURGITATION: CLINICAL PRESENTATIONS

	MVP Syndrome	Chronic MR	Acute MR	Ischemic/Functional MR
Symptoms	Chest pain	Fatigue	Pulmonary edema	CHF
Physical examination	Midsystolic click, murmur	Loud murmur, S_3	Loud murmur, S_4	Soft murmur, S_4, S_3
ECG	ST-T changes	Atrial fibrillation	Normal	Q waves, LBBB
Chest x-ray	Pectus excavatum	Cardiomegaly	Normal heart size, Pulmonary edema	Cardiomegaly, pulmonary edema

diagnosed by transthoracic echocardiography but are more clearly delineated by transesophageal echocardiography. Ruptured chordae may also be better diagnosed by the transesophageal approach[135] (Figs. 64-16 and 64-17).

Endocarditic Mitral Regurgitation The usual mechanism for MR, i.e., flail leaflets, is usually clearly demonstrated by transthoracic echocardiography. Perforations of a leaflet are more difficult to diagnose. Mitral annular abscesses are rare and are best detected by transesophageal echocardiography.[136] Vegetations can be seen on leaflets or on ruptured cords by the transthoracic approach, but transesophageal echocardiography is of superior sensitivity[137] (see also Chap. 14).

Ischemic/Functional Mitral Regurgitation The finding of a dilated annulus[70,71] is nonspecific,[110] but in this type of regurgitation, the amplitude of the annular descent is also reduced.[138] Other features of ischemic heart disease may be observed, such as regional wall motion abnormalities of the free wall or the papillary muscle.[70] The leaflet tissue is usually normal or mildly sclerotic in patients in this age range. The abnormal anterior position of the mitral valve due to the abnormal traction by the principal chordae on the anterior leaflet reduces the area of coaptation of the two leaflets and thereby allows a central jet of mitral regurgitation[70,71] (Fig. 64-18).

In patients with partial or complete rupture of the papillary muscle,[73] the regurgitation is due to the flail leaflet. The diagnosis is based on the visualization of a small mass of muscle attached to a group of chordae and floating freely during the cardiac cycle.[139] If not clearly demonstrated by transthoracic echo, the flail leaflet can be readily demonstrated by transesophageal echocardiography.[140]

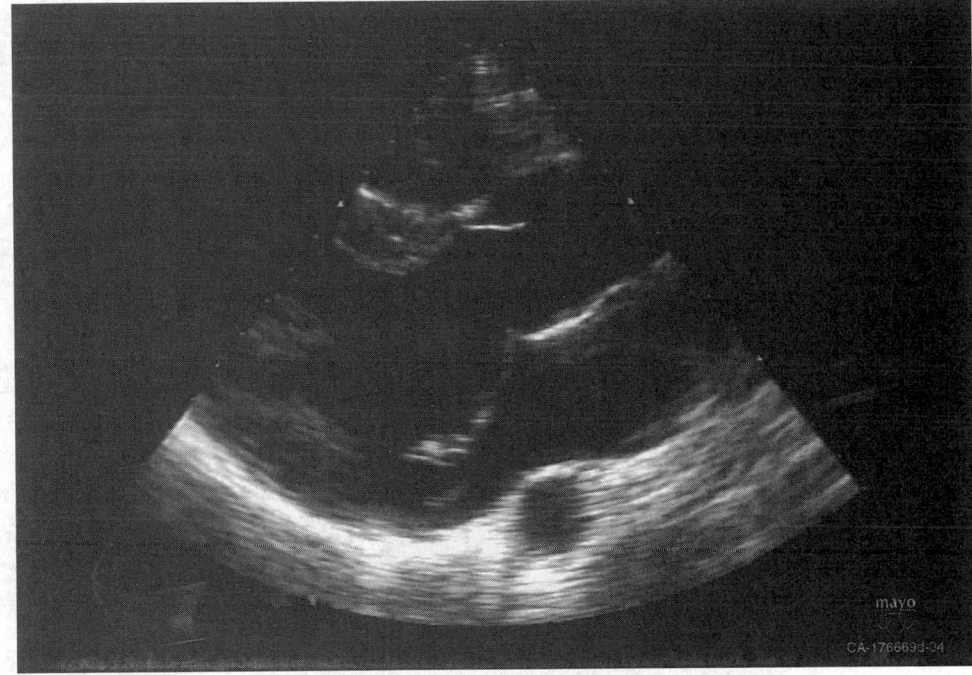

FIGURE 64-14
Echocardiogram of a bileaflet mitral valve prolapse seen from the parasternal long-axis view.

Other Causes of Mitral Regurgitation Some characteristic features may help determine etiology. In hypertrophic obstructive cardiomyopathy, the systolic anterior motion of the mitral valve is associated with a loss of coaptation and the jet of regurgitation is directed inferiorly and laterally. If the jet is directed medially and superiorly, one should strongly suspect ruptured chord of the posterior leaflet.[141] In eosinophilic cardiomyopathies, characteristic infiltration of the region below

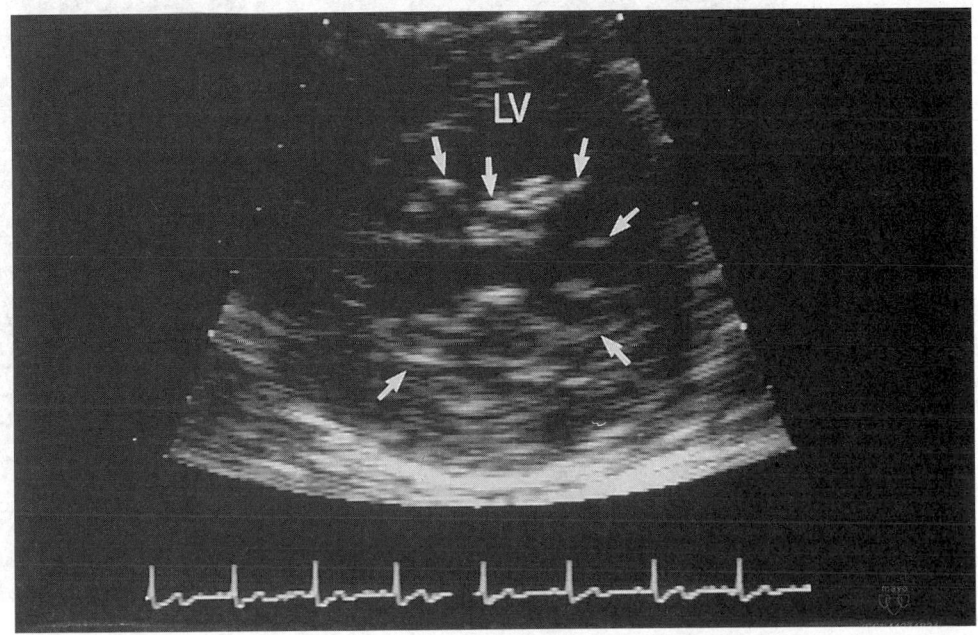

FIGURE 64-15
Echocardiogram of a redundant, myxomatous mitral valve (*arrows*) seen from the parasternal short-axis view.

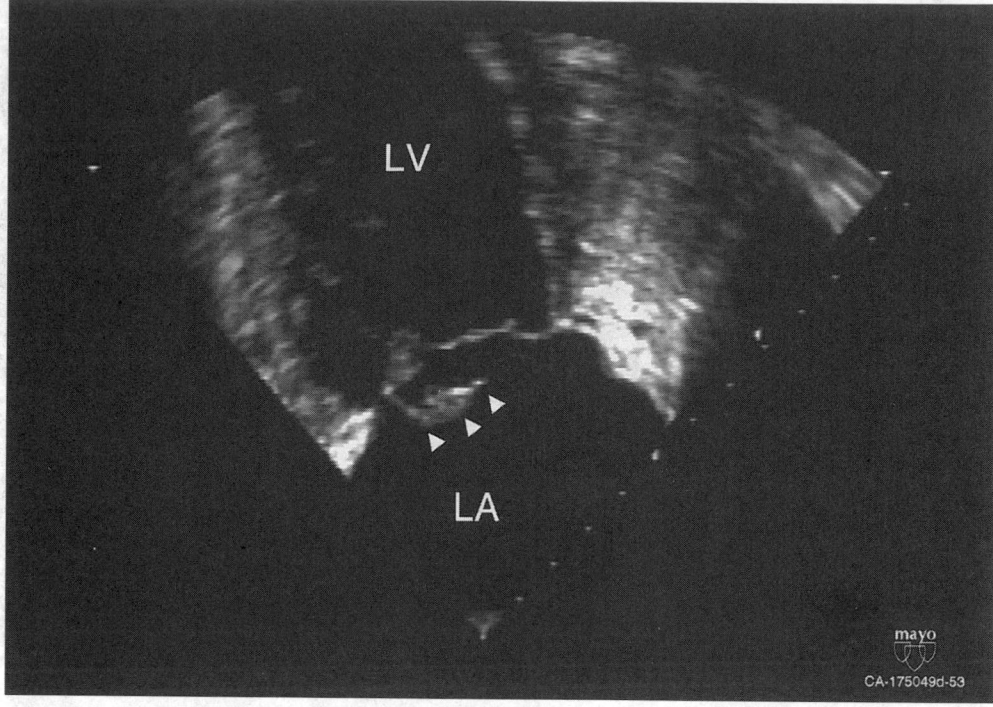

FIGURE 64-16

Transesophageal echocardiography (*sagittal plane*) of a flail posterior leaflet (*arrows*). The ruptured chord is seen at the tip of the posterior leaflet.

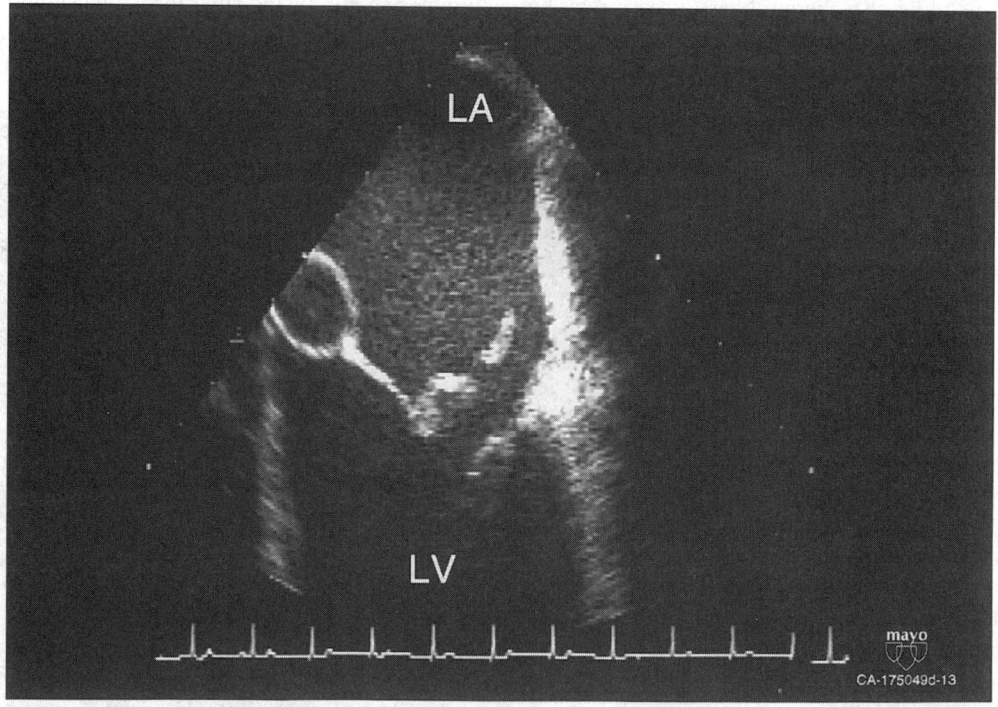

FIGURE 64-17

Transesophageal echocardiography (*horizontal plane*) of a flail anterior leaflet. The ruptured chord is seen at the tip of the anterior leaflet.

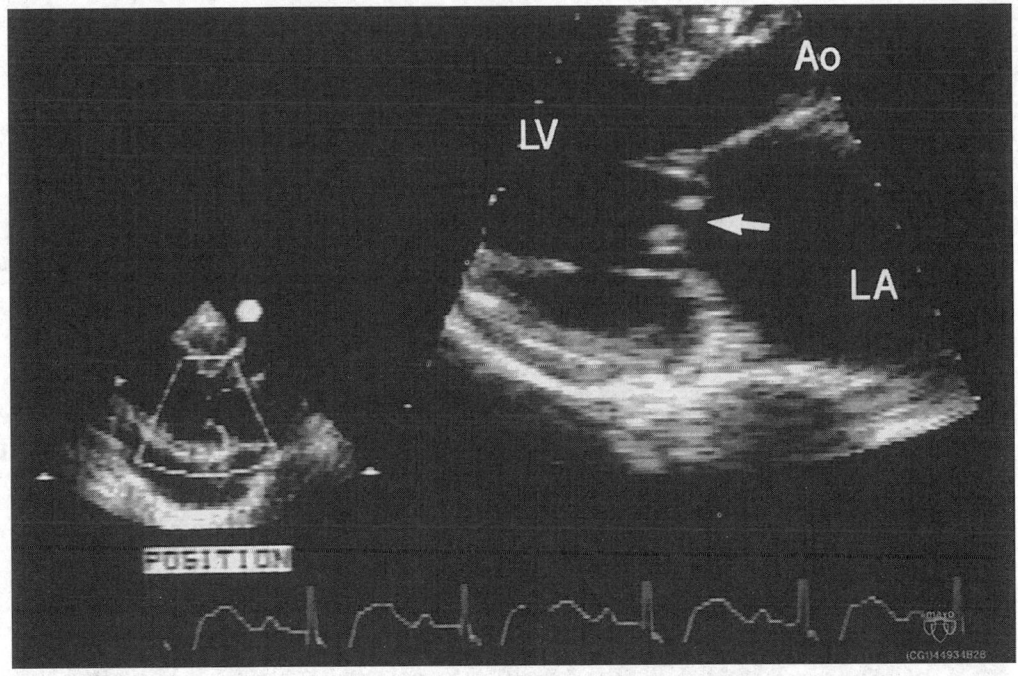

FIGURE 64-18

Echocardiogram of an ischemic MR; note the thinned posterior wall, the tenting of the mitral valve pulled toward the apex by the chordae, and the lack of coaptation (*arrow*). LA = left atrium; LV = left ventricle; Ao = aorta.

the posterior leaflet by thrombus can be demonstrated with immobilization of the posterior leaflet and resultant regurgitation. Other aspects such as calcification of the mitral annulus[142] or sclerosis with nodular calcification of the leaflet, can usually be clearly demonstrated by transthoracic echocardiography.

Assessment of Severity of Regurgitation

Semiquantitative Methods *Color-flow imaging* demonstrates the origin and direction of the jet.[134] The jet length, the ratio of the jet area to the left atrial area,[143] or more simply the jet area[144] have been suggested as good indices of severity of MR. Small jets such as those seen in normal subjects consistently correspond to mild regurgitations.[110] Color-flow imaging has significant technical limitations, in addition to more important limitations that are intrinsically related to the nature of regurgitant jets. The extent of a jet is determined by its momentum, and thus as much by regurgitant velocity as by regurgitant flow. Also, jets are constrained by the LA and expand more in large atria.[110,143] The eccentric jets of valvular prolapse[145] impinge on the left atrial wall[146] and tend to underestimate regurgitation[110,147] (Fig. 64-19, Plate 54). In contrast, the central jets of ischemic and/or functional MR expand markedly in the enlarged left atrium and tend to overestimate regurgitation[110] (Fig. 64-20, Plate 55). Transesophageal echocardiography usually shows larger jets, but it does not eliminate these limitations of color-flow imaging (Fig. 64-19, Plate 54).

Other qualitative indices, such as the width of the jet at the vena contracta or the density of the continuous-wave Doppler signal,[148] have been recommended, but their value needs confirmation.

Pulmonary venous velocity profile is useful to assess the degree of mitral regurgitation.[149,150] Systolic reversal of flow in the pulmonary veins is a strong argument for severe MR. Unfortunately, there is an important interaction between the regurgitation severity, the direction of the jet, and the left atrial pressure, thus, the reversal of flow in the pulmonary veins, which may be absent or asymmetric in severe regurgitation is not specific for severe MR and may be observed in patients with elevated LA pressure or markedly enlarged LA (Fig. 64-21) (see Chap. 14).

Quantitative Methods *The goal* of quantitative methods is to measure parameters that reflect the degree of regurgitation: the volume overload can be expressed as the regurgitant volume (difference between the total and forward stroke volume) per beat or as the regurgitant fraction, which is the proportion of the LV ejection volume regurgitated in the LA. The regurgi-

FIGURE 64-19

See color Plate 54.

FIGURE 64-20

See color Plate 55.

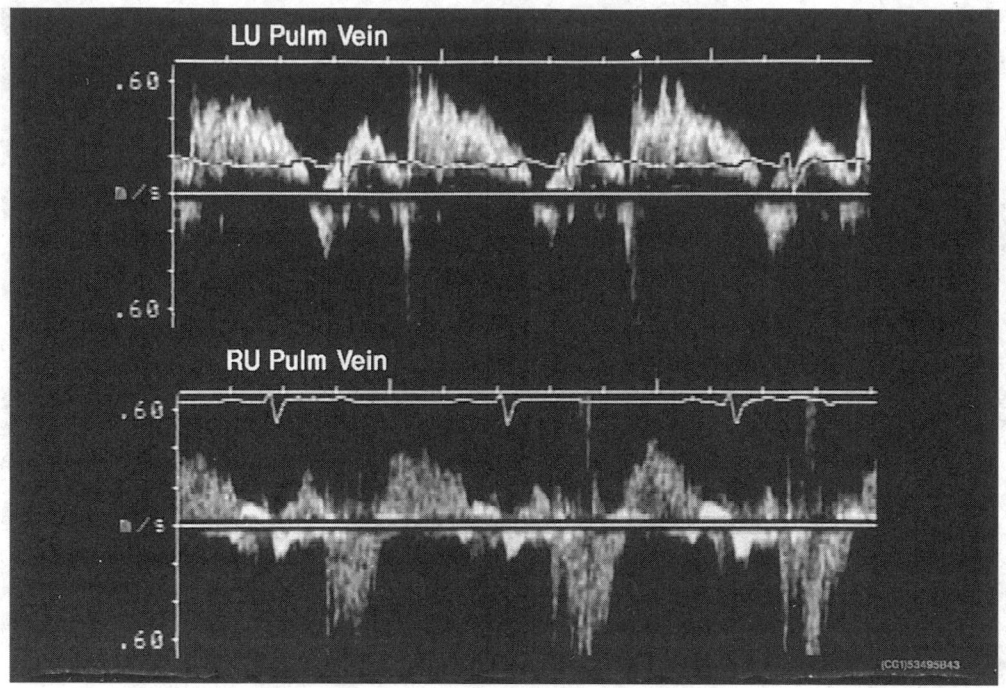

FIGURE 64-21

Pulmonary venous flow of a patient with MR due to a flail posterior leaflet (by transesophageal echocardiography). Note that the flow is asymmetric, with preserved systolic flow in the left upper pulmonary vein and systolic reversal in the right upper pulmonary vein.

tant lesion can be expressed as the effective regurgitant orifice (ERO) area and calculated as follows[85,151]:

$$ERO = \frac{regurgitant\ flow}{regurgitant\ velocity}$$

or

$$ERO = \frac{regurgitant\ volume}{regurgitant\ TV_I}$$

Where the TV_I is the time velocity integral of the regurgitant jet.

The *practical* quantitation of mitral regurgitation can be performed using various methods:

- *Quantitative Doppler* is based on the calculation of the mitral and aortic stroke volumes using pulsed-wave Doppler.[152,153] The principle is simple and applicable in most patients, although the mitral stroke volume calculation is technically demanding, with a significant learning phase.[152]
- *Quantitative two-dimensional echocardiography* is similar but utilizes measurement of LV volumes for total stroke volume.[154]
- The *proximal isovelocity surface area* (PISA) method, conversely directly measures the regurgitant flow by analyzing the flow convergence region proximal to the regurgitant orifice (Fig. 64-22, Plate 56) and is based on the principle of conservation of mass.[155] Color-flow mapping allows precise determination of the velocity in the flow convergence, and the regurgitant flow can be calculated.[156]

Using the regurgitant flow and the regurgitant velocities, the effective regurgitant orifice and the regurgitant volume can be calculated.[151] This method is simple and accurate if the assumptions are respected (see also Chap. 14).

Assessment of Left Ventricular and Atrial Function

Guided M-mode diameters are used for the assessment of the LV size, mass, and wall stress.[126,157–159] LV volumes can now be reliably measured by two-dimensional echocardiography.[160,161] The ejection fraction can be calculated or estimated. The M-mode measurement of the left atrial diameter is limited by the asymmetric shape of that chamber. LA area or volume can be measured simply by two-dimensional echocardiography.

RADIONUCLIDE STUDIES

Radionuclide angiography can be used to estimate the left ventricular end-diastolic and end-systolic volume as well as the right and left ventricular ejection fraction. The detection of exercise-induced LV dysfunction is frequent[162]; however, the significance of such measurements on the long-term prognosis has not been analyzed in large series of patients. The comparison of the counts measured over the RV and LV allows the calculation of the regurgitant fraction.

CARDIAC CATHETERIZATION

Cardiac catheterization is utilized to assess the hemodynamic status, the severity of MR, the left ventricular function, and coronary anatomy (see also Chap. 16).

The major hemodynamic consequences of MR are reduction of cardiac output and elevation of pulmonary artery wedge

FIGURE 64-22
See color Plate 56.

pressure. Marked pulmonary hypertension is rarely present. The large V wave of the pulmonary wedge pressure is more frequent in acute than in chronic MR but can be observed in other conditions such as ventricular septal defect or heart failure with reduced LA compliance without MR[94] (Fig. 64-23).

The assessment of the degree of regurgitation can be obtained by LV selective angiography and can be qualitatively graded in three or four grades on the basis of the degree and persistence of opacification of the LA[163] (Fig. 64-24). Although time-honored, this method has limitations, like all qualitative methods.[164] The quantitation of regurgitation can be obtained by comparing the angiographic stroke volume to the forward stroke volume as calculated by the Fick or thermodilution methods[165] to calculate a regurgitant volume and fraction. The angiographic stroke volume usually overestimates the true stroke volume, and corrections have been used to minimize the overestimation of the regurgitant volume. Of importance, the forward stroke volume must be obtained shortly before the LV angiogram. As with noninvasive meth-

ods, the subtraction of two stroke volumes introduces a potentially greater range of error[166] that cannot be corrected by combined methods or by repeating the measurements. Therefore, this method is not commonly utilized.

The assessment of LV function can be performed using quantitative angiography. LV volumes correlate strongly with the regurgitant volume,[167] duration of regurgitation,[168] etiology of regurgitation, and LV function. The most frequently utilized indices of LV function are the end-systolic volume (in part determined by the degree of regurgitation) and the ejection fraction. Both have been shown to be useful prognostically.[105,169] The addition of high-fidelity pressure recording to LV angiography allows calculation of more complex indices of left ventricular distensibility,[109] wall stress, maximum left ventricular elastance, and LV systolic stiffness. The additional value of these complex measurements has been investigated in small groups of patients and remains to be defined in larger populations, and these measurements are not practical in routine clinical studies.

Regional wall motion abnormalities have been observed in patients with MR even in the absence of coronary lesions. Selective coronary angiography is, at present, the only technique allowing definition of the coronary anatomy. Since coronary stenoses may be present even in the absence of angina, coronary angiography is ordinarily performed in patients older than about 35 years (see also Chap. 63).

STRATEGY OF UTILIZATION OF LABORATORY TESTING

Not all tests should be performed in all patients (see also Chap. 63). The methods used to assess the degree of MR are summarized in Table 64-10 and Fig. 64-25. Because transthoracic Doppler echocardiography allows the confirmation of the diagnosis of MR, analyzes the presence and severity of

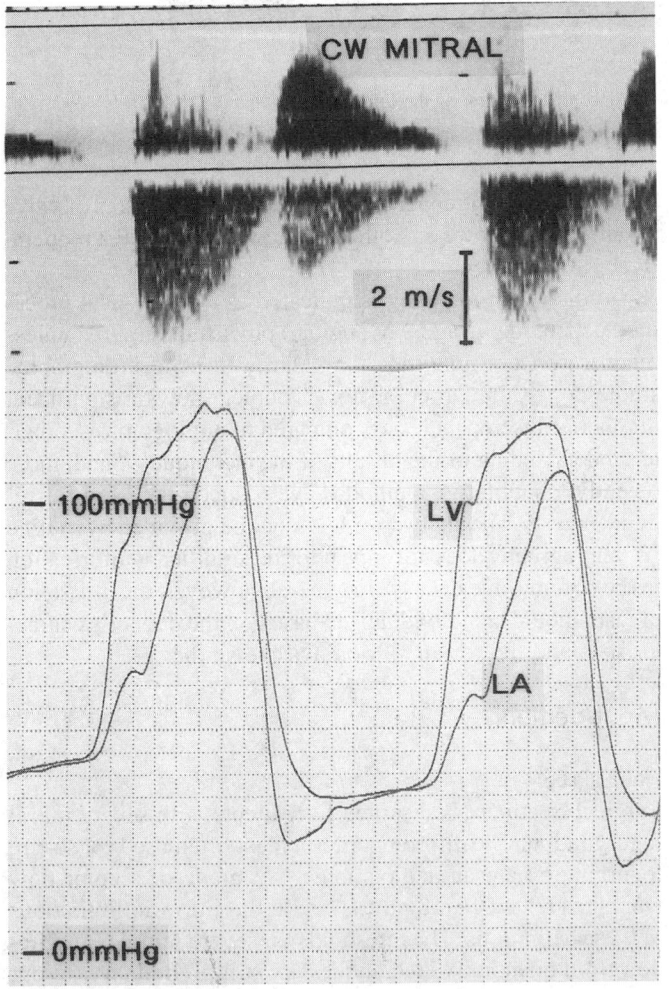

FIGURE 64-23
Simultaneous recording of LV and LA pressures and continuous wave Doppler (CW) in a patient with severe MR. Note the large V wave on the left atrial pressure recording, with a triangular shape of the mitral regurgitant jet obtained by CW. (Courtesy of Dr. Rick Nishimura, Mayo Clinic.)

TABLE 64-10

MITRAL REGURGITATION: ASSESSMENT OF SEVERITY

Clinical
  Systolic thrill
  Murmur intensity
  S_3
  Diastolic rumble
Laboratory
  Qualitative
    Large jet ≥8 cm² (Echo-Doppler)
    Pulmonary vein reversal (Doppler, angiography)
    Dense contrast in LA (angiography)
  Quantitative
    Criteria: Regurgitant volume ≥60 mL
           Regurgitant fraction ≥50%
           Effective regurgitant orifice ≥40 mm²
    Method: Doppler echocardiography
          Quantitative Doppler
          Quantitative 2D echocardiography
          Amplitude-weighted mean velocity
          PISA
      Radionuclide angiography
      Quantitative LV angiography

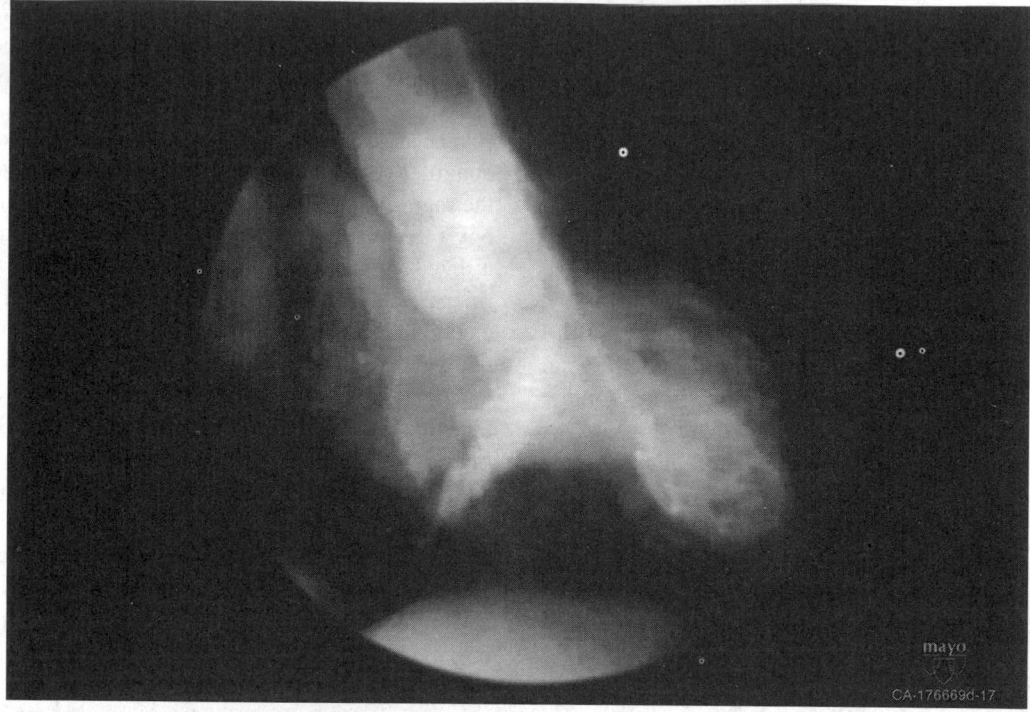

FIGURE 64-24
Left ventricular angiogram in the right anterior oblique view a dense opacification of the left atrium, in this case of severe MR.

associated valvular disease, and provides a unique assessment of the morphologic lesions of the mitral valve, it is performed in all cases for the initial diagnostic assessment, as well as for follow-up and for presurgical assessment. Transesophageal echocardiography provides superior imaging quality, but its incremental value has not been fully documented.[135] We usually reserve TEE preoperatively for patients in whom a doubt persists regarding either the lesions (especially if endocarditis is suspected) or the severity of regurgitation; but we use it

on a large scale intraoperatively to monitor the results of valve repair.[131–134] However, others would obtain TEE preoperatively in all patients.

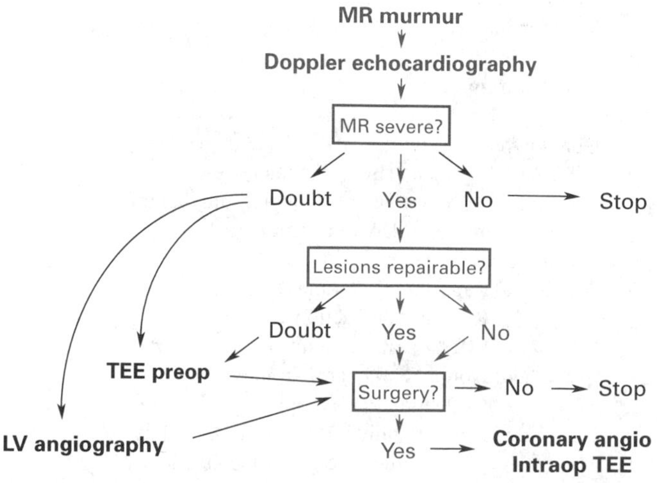

Coronary angiography is indicated as a presurgical procedure depending on age. LV angiography is not required unless there is concern regarding the validity of echocardiographic studies.[170] Although color-flow Doppler shows a significant number of discrepancies as compared to angiography,[171] better understanding of the pitfalls of the technique[110] and, more recently, quantitative methods have reduced the need for redundant tests. The analysis of LV function provided by routine LV angiography does not appear to add significant information to the noninvasive data.[126] In general, however, the utilization of tests should be individualized based on the patient's characteristics and the results of noninvasive studies.

Management

PRINCIPLES

Surgical treatment is reserved for patients with severe mitral regurgitation. The different criteria most often used for severe regurgitation are an angiographic 4+ grade or a color-flow Doppler greater than 8 cm^2,[144] with the intrinsic limitations of these definitions. The thresholds for severe mitral regurgitation from quantitative techniques are still preliminary. In our practice, we use $\geq$60 mL/per beat for regurgitant volumes, 50 percent for regurgitant fraction, and $\geq$40 mm^2 for effective regurgitant orifice[85] if these data are consonant with the clinical assessment of the patient. Patients with severe regurgita-

FIGURE 64-25
Strategy of utilization of tests in patients with mitral regurgitation.

TABLE 64-11

MITRAL REGURGITATION: DETERMINANTS OF OUTCOME

Unoperated Patients	Operated Patients
Symptoms	Age
Pulmonary hypertension	Preoperative symptoms
LV end-diastolic volume	Coronary disease
AV-O$_2$ difference	End-systolic dimensions
Ejection fraction	Ejection fraction
	LA size?
	Valve repair

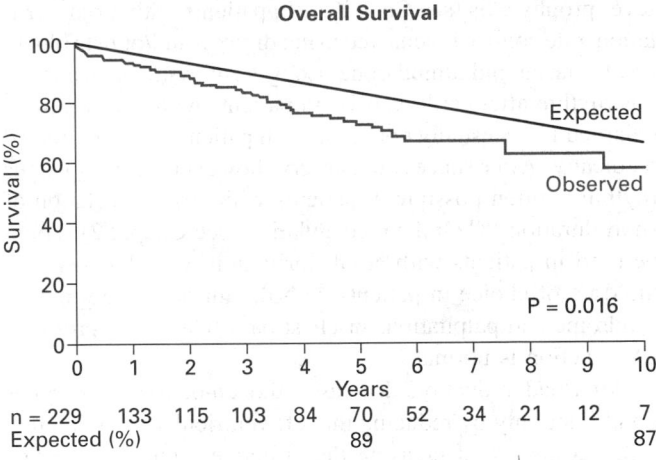

FIGURE 64-26

Survival with medical treatment of patients diagnosed with MR due to flail leaflets. Note the excess mortality in comparison to the expected survival. (Reprinted by permission of the *New England Journal of Medicine* from Ling LH, et al. 1996; 335:1417–1423. Copyright 1996, Massachusetts Medical Society.)

tion will require surgery at some point during their follow-up. In these patients, the most relevant question is the timing of the indication for surgery. This is influenced by the natural history of the disease and by the outcome of any surgical correction of mitral regurgitation. The predictors of outcome are summarized in Table 64-11.

NATURAL HISTORY

Because of the qualitative and imprecise assessment of the degree of regurgitation, the natural history of MR is ill defined. Patients with mild rheumatic MR appear to have a good prognosis.[172] The prognosis of patients with mitral valve prolapse syndrome and no or mild regurgitation is usually excellent.[173] The development of severe mitral regurgitation in patients with mitral valve prolapse occurs usually late (mean = 24 years) after the initial diagnosis of the murmur.[174] Severe regurgitation is rare before the age of 50, but its incidence increases thereafter, especially in men.[62]

It is important to consider the probability of sudden death before delaying surgery. This devastating complication usually occurs in patients with murmurs of regurgitation[175] and more often if the ventricular function is decreased,[120] but it can also occur in patients with normal ejection fraction who are asymptomatic.[176] Of patients who initially are asymptomatic despite severe regurgitation, approximately 10 percent per year develop symptoms,[177] the development of which may be hastened by atrial fibrillation.[54] In patients with unoperated clinically significant MR, the late survival has been found to be as high 60 percent at 10 years[178] or as low as 46 percent[179] or even 27 percent[180] at 5 years. In our experience, patients with flail mitral leaflets have a 10-year survival of 57 percent, which represents an excess mortality as compared to the expected survival (Fig. 64-26). By 10 years heart failure has occurred in 63 percent and atrial fibrillation in 30 percent of patients initially in sinus rhythm.[181] At 10 years 90 percent of the patients had either died or undergone surgery,[181] confirming that in these patients surgery is almost unavoidable (Fig. 64-27).

The predictors of poor outcome in patients medically treated are (1) severe symptoms (NYHA classes III to IV)[179] even if the symptoms are transient,[181] (2) pulmonary hyper-

tension, (3) markedly increased LV end-diastolic volume or arteriovenous differences in O$_2$,[182] and (4) reduced ejection fraction.[181,183] A comparison of the outcome of medically and surgically treated patients shows a trend in favor of the surgical treatment,[176] especially early surgery,[181] with a definite improvement of outcome with surgery in patients who have decreased systolic LV function.[182,184]

The progression, determinants, and most accurate method of monitoring of LV dysfunction in patients medically treated are not well known.

Medical Treatment

Prevention of infective endocarditis using the appropriate prophylaxis is necessary in patients with MR[185] (see Chap. 82). Young patients with rheumatic MR should receive rheumatic

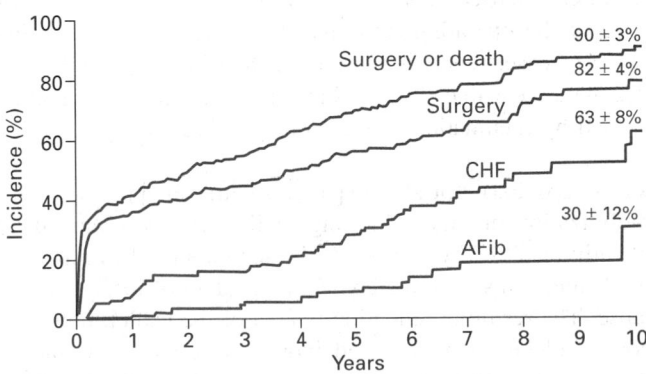

FIGURE 64-27

Cardiac morbidity with medical treatment in patients diagnosed with MR due to flail leaflets. CHF = congestive heart failure, Afib = atrial fibrillation. (Reprinted by permission of the *New England Journal of Medicine* from Ling LH, et al. 1996; 335:1417–1423. Copyright 1996, Massachusetts Medical Society.)

fever prophylaxis (see Chap. 62). In patients with atrial fibrillation, rate control is achieved using digoxin and/or beta blockers, diltiazen and amiodarone. Long-term maintenance of sinus rhythm after cardioversion in patients with severe MR or enlarged LA is usually not possible in patients who are treated medically. After successful surgery, however, return to sinus rhythm is often possible in patients with atrial fibrillation of short duration.[186] Oral anticoagulation (see Chap. 52) should be used in patients with atrial fibrillation. Beta blockers are the drug of choice in patients with the mitral valve prolapse syndrome and palpitations or chest pain (Chap. 65) provided LV function is normal.

Afterload reduction decreases the amount of regurgitation,[89] not only by reducing the left ventricular systolic pressure but also by decreasing the effective regurgitant orifice area.[90,91] The acute utilization of sodium nitroprusside in unstable patients with severe MR, especially in the context of myocardial infarction, may be lifesaving in preparation for surgery.[89] Chronic afterload reduction is more controversial: the hemodynamic effect of either hydralazine or angiotensin converting enzyme (ACE) inhibitors have been analyzed in small series of mostly mild or moderate regurgitations,[187–189] and their long-term efficacy in obtaining large reductions in the regurgitant volume is unclear. In addition, although no change in ejection fraction was observed, a negative inotropic effect is possible.[190] Diuretic treatment is extremely useful for the control of heart failure and for the chronic control of symptoms, especially dyspnea.

Surgical Treatment

There are two main surgical options: mitral valve reconstruction and mitral valve replacement.

Mitral Valve Reconstruction In contrast to management of the incompetent aortic valve, reconstruction of the incompetent mitral valve is almost always possible (approximately 90 percent of patients referred for primary correction of acquired MR at the Mayo Clinic). The frequency with which valve repair can be used in patients with MR varies with the experience of the operating team and the spectrum of underlying valve disease; repair is more often feasible in patients with degenerative valve disease than in those with regurgitation caused by rheumatic valvulitis or endocarditis.

VALVULAR PROCEDURE   In patients with leaflet prolapse, immobilization of this prolapsing section can be obtained by plicating it[191] or by excising[53] the section and then repairing the leaflet. This will overcome the problem of localized prolapse. The resulting reduction in area of the leaflet, however, could reduce coaptation and induce residual regurgitation; therefore, annuloplasty is a routine part of the repair. Resection or plication of prolapsing sections is most successful with posterior leaflet prolapse. In patients with anterior leaflet prolapse, the risk of residual MR is higher if the plication or resection is not combined with subvalvular procedures.[132] Other repairable leaflet abnormalities that can cause valve

regurgitation include congenital clefts and acquired perforation. A perforation in a leaflet as a result of infective endocarditis, especially at the base of the anterior leaflet, may be closed by using a patch of pericardium or synthetic material.

SUBVALVULAR PROCEDURE   In patients with elongated chordae, chordal shortening may be necessary to ensure the appropriate coaptation of the leaflets. A major recent advance has been the introduction of transposition of chordae and of artificial chordae, which have made the anterior leaflet prolapse as repairable as the posterior leaflet prolapse.[192,193]

ANNULAR PROCEDURE   Annular dilatation, almost constantly associated with MR, is treated by reduction in the circumference of the mitral orifice—i.e., annuloplasty. The annuloplasty should be placed in the region of the annulus supporting the posterior leaflet to preserve the area of anterior leaflet. Commissural annuloplasty has been used,[194,195] but this approach tended to distort the valve. The concept of concentrically shortening the posterior mitral annulus by suturing it to a cloth-covered rigid ring was developed by Carpentier.[53] Recently, flexible annuloplasty rings have been developed to preserve the changes in shape of the mitral annulus during systole.[196] In general, results with the Carpentier ring annuloplasty have been favorable, but LV outflow obstruction associated with abnormal systolic anterior motion of the anterior mitral leaflet has been reported in 6 to 10 percent of patients.[197–199] This complication is mainly due to hypovolemia and hypercontractility due to excessive use of inotropes,[132] but the incidence of this complication may be lower with the flexible rings, which may better preserve left ventricular function.[200]

INTRAOPERATIVE ASSESSMENT OF VALVE REPAIR   It is important to assess the adequacy of mitral valve reconstruction before completion of the operation. When satisfactory repair cannot be achieved, it is preferable to replace the valve immediately. To assess if residual MR is present at the end of the operation, two methods are available. Double sampling dye curves use indocyanine green dye injected into the left ventricle while blood is aspirated from the aorta and the left atrium through a densitometer. If less than 20 percent of dye appears in left atrial blood (compared to the aorta), the result can be considered satisfactory. This technique is not commonly used or available. The most recent technique for the intraoperative assessment of the adequacy of mitral repair is transesophageal echocardiography,[131,132] which can be performed without interrupting or interfering with the surgical procedure, and is used routinely.[132]

Valve Replacement When reconstruction of the mitral valve is considered impossible or, if attempted, is unsuccessful, then replacement must be performed. The dilemma is the choice between a mechanical valve of excellent durability but with the hazard of thromboembolism and a biologic valve with undefined long-term durability[201] but less tendency to cause thromboembolism.[202] In patients with atrial fibrillation,[202] chronic anticoagulant therapy is necessary even after replacement with a bioprosthesis, so that avoiding anticoagulation is not relevant in choosing a prosthesis.[203]

Postoperative Outcome

Valve repair, by preserving the normal valvular tissue, is preferable to valve replacement.[53] Compared to prosthetic replacement, mitral valve reconstruction has a lower operative mortality.[204,205] Direct comparison of the results of valve repair and replacement is difficult[205] because the patients undergoing a valve repair are usually at a less advanced stage of the disease than patients undergoing valve replacement.[204] It appears, however, that survival and LV function[206] after mitral valve reconstruction for regurgitation is superior to that observed after insertion of a prosthetic valve[204] even after adjustment for all baseline differences; however, proof that survival is significantly better is more controversial. Better ventricular function with valvuloplasty may be due to preservation of chordae tendineae and papillary muscles.[206,207] Also, valve repair has the same low rate of reoperation as valve replacement.[204] Therefore, valve repair should be the preferred procedure for surgical correction of MR (Fig. 64-28).

In general, patients operated upon for MR have lower survival than do those treated for mitral stenosis. Operative mortality has been reported to be in the range of 5 to 12 percent[201,208] for patients undergoing operation in earlier series, but most patients had prosthetic valve replacement rather than reconstruction. The operative risk is lower in the current era, around 1 to 2 percent in patients younger than 75 years with organic MR operated at the Mayo Clinic, whether they had valve repair or replacement.[126] It should be noted that LV function is not a predictor of operative mortality and that patients with organic MR and with even markedly depressed function have a reasonable chance of surviving surgery.[126] Age, symptoms, and the association of coronary disease are the most important predictors of the operative mortality.[126] Some important points should be noted. First, the risk of surgery has become progressively similar in patients 65 to 75 years old as compared to younger patients. Second, operative mortality has decreased recently in patients aged 75 and older, but it remains relatively high, around 7 percent. Third, in ischemic MR, the operative mortality remains high, around 10 percent.

Reported long-term survivorship ranges from 75 percent[201,208,209] to around 50 percent at 5 years; these numbers are difficult to reconcile because of age differences between the reported series. In our experience, patients undergoing valve replacement between 1963 and 1971 for severely symptomatic, isolated MR had a postoperative probability of survival of about 70 percent at 5 years, 50 percent at 10 years, and 40 percent at 15 years.[210] In our most recent experience, with a population of mean age 62, the 5- and 10-year survivals were 83 and 68 percent after valve repair and 69 and 52 percent after valve replacement. Remarkably, the survival after valve repair is not different from the expected survival, whereas after valve replacement, the survival is only 77 percent of the expected.[204]

A large majority of long-term survivors after mitral valve replacement for MR show symptomatic improvement by at least one functional class and some become asymptomatic.[210] It should be noted, however, that with time, postoperative congestive heart failure with symptomatic deterioration tends to occur at a progressively increasing rate (38 percent at 10 years in operative survivors); it is most often (two-thirds of the cases) due to residual LV dysfunction after surgery.[211] Valvular or prosthetic dysfunction explains the heart failure in approximately one-third of the cases.[211] Postoperative congestive heart failure has a dismal prognosis and should be prevented as much as possible,[211] including by early correction of the regurgitation.

The most frequent cause of mortality after surgical correction of MR is LV dysfunction[126] due to chronic irreversible myocardial damage.[99,104,105,212] LV dysfunction occurs, in our experience, in 40 percent of patients overall and 32 percent of those with organic MR.[104] The majority of patients demonstrate a decrease in total LV ejection fraction after successful valve replacement,[99,100,104,157,208] probably due to the net

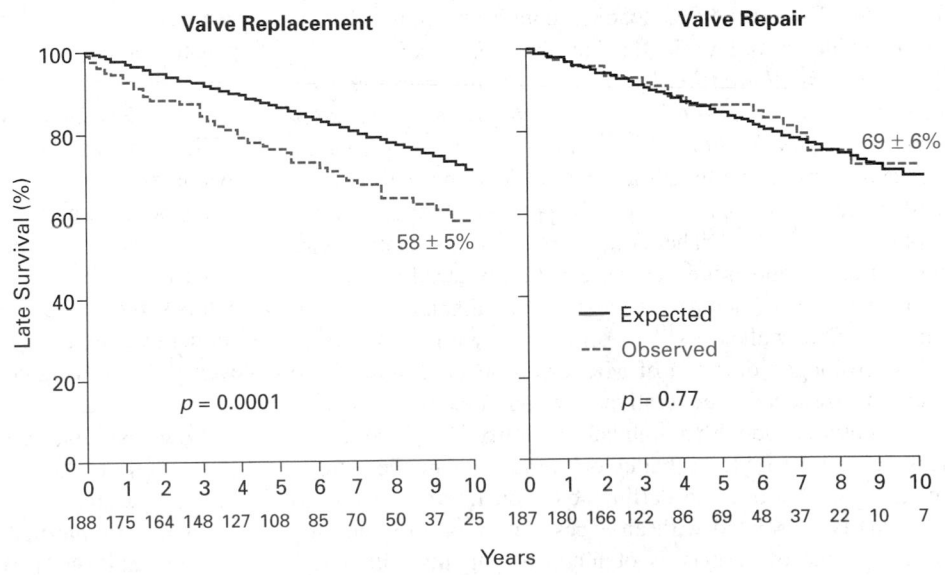

FIGURE 64-28

Late survival after surgical correction of organic MR. Note the excess mortality in comparison to the expected survival after valve replacement (*left*) in contrast to the survival identical to expected after valve repair (*right*). (Reproduced from Enriquez-Sarano et al.,[204] with the authorization of the American Heart Association.)

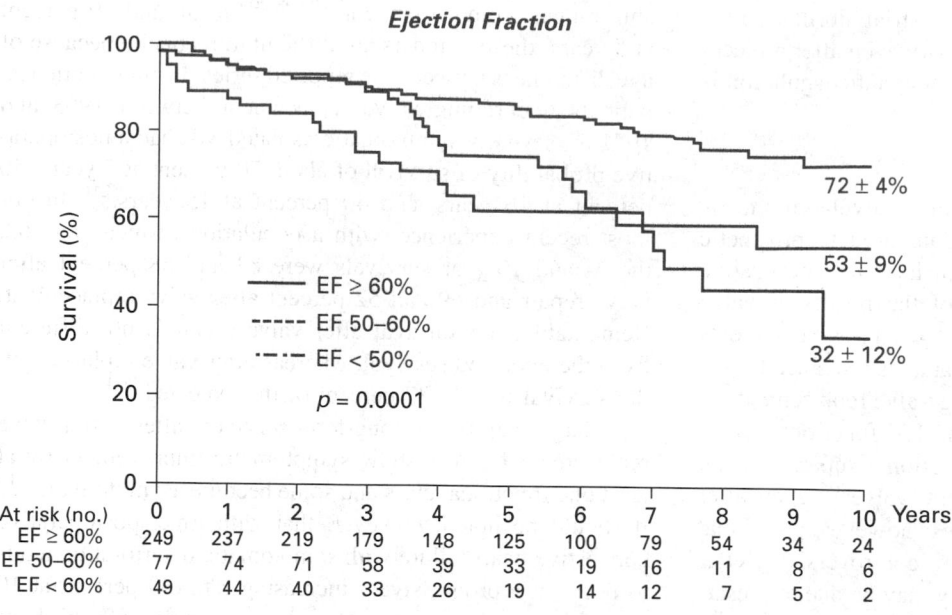

Ejection Fraction

72 ± 4%

53 ± 9%

32 ± 12%

EF ≥ 60%
EF 50–60%
EF < 50%

$p = 0.0001$

At risk (no.)	0	1	2	3	4	5	6	7	8	9	10 Years
EF ≥ 60%	249	237	219	179	148	125	100	79	54	34	24
EF 50–60%	77	74	71	58	39	33	19	16	11	8	6
EF < 60%	49	44	40	33	26	19	14	12	7	5	2

FIGURE 64-29

Survival after surgical correction of organic mitral regurgitation. Note the excess mortality in patients with preoperative ejection fraction above 50 percent but also in patients with preoperative ejection fractions of 50 to 60 percent. (Reproduced from Enriquez-Sarano et al.,[126] with the authorization of the American Heart Association.)

effect of several factors: cumulative permanent myocardial damage, myocardial insult sustained at the time of operation, diminished preload, and probably increase in afterload after surgery, which eliminates the low-impedance pathway. The relationships between pre- and postoperative LV function[97,99,104,105,157,169,213] and between preoperative LV function and postoperative survival[103,126,158,212,214] underline the fact that LV dysfunction is present preoperatively in most patients presenting with this complication postoperatively. Because of the modified loading conditions, multiple and complex indices of LV function have been proposed.[97,100–103] *Despite these altered loading conditions, preoperative ejection fraction is an acceptable independent predictor of postoperative ejection fraction[99,104,105] and survival.[126]* In general, one can estimate that the postoperative ejection fraction likely will decrease by approximately 10 percent early after valve replacement.[99,104,105] There is, however, a significant individual variation, and more decline can be observed in patients with markedly increased end-systolic diameter,[104] volume,[105,169] or wall stress[104,213] or in those with severe symptoms, prolonged duration of MR, or coronary disease.[104] A markedly reduced preoperative ejection fraction (<50 percent) is associated with a high late mortality,[126] but nevertheless surgery provides a better outcome than medical treatment.[182,184] Even a "borderline" ejection fraction (50 to 60 percent) is associated with an excess late mortality, and the best outcome of surgery is obtained in patients with no or minimal symptoms and an ejection fraction ≥60 percent[104,126] (Fig. 64-29).

Atrial fibrillation when present preoperatively usually per-

sists postoperatively unless it is of brief duration,[186] but the excess risk due this arrhythmia appears modest,[126,186] although it requires anticoagulation.

The late risk of thromboembolism after mitral replacement for MR is not different from the risk in other mitral valve diseases.[203] Differences in thromboembolic risk after valve repair and valve replacement have been variably estimated[204,205,209] but appear to favor valve repair. In addition, because following valve repair, anticoagulation is recommended permanently only if atrial fibrillation persists, the occurrence of bleeding is more uncommon in these patients than in those receiving a prosthesis.[204]

Indications for Surgery

Based on the most recent data regarding the natural history of MR treated with and without surgery, the indications for surgery are as outlined below.

Traditional Indications Severe symptoms (patients in NYHA functional class III or IV) even transiently and even if markedly improved by medical treatment.

Advanced Indications No or minimal symptoms (patients in NYHA functional class I or II) but with signs of overt left ventricular dysfunction (left ventricular ejection fraction <60 percent, end-systolic diameter ≥45 mm in our practice).

Early Indications No or minimal symptoms (patients in NYHA functional class I or II) with no sign of left ventricular dysfunction (ejection fraction ≥60 percent). These patients can expect the best results of surgery and, in particular, after the immediate postoperative phase, a survival identical to the expected survival.[126] Therefore, surgery is a reasonable option in this subgroup. Because surgery in these patients is justified neither by symptoms nor by left ventricular dysfunction, however, the following conditions should be fulfilled:

- Low operative risk: Both the operative mortality in the institution where such an indication is contemplated and the operative risk for the individual patients involved should be minimal (1 to 2 percent).
- Repairability: The valvular lesions as determined by echocardiography should in all probability be repairable and the surgeon performing the intervention should have a high degree of experience with all forms of valve repair.

- Intraoperative transesophageal echocardiography should be performed by experienced physicians to monitor the repair procedure and help with decisions warranted by an imperfect result.

- Quantitation of regurgitation should be performed systematically in these patients preoperatively using multiple noninvasive techniques to determine objectively the degree of regurgitation and affirm that surgery is warranted.

Therefore, despite the considerable progress that has recently been made, currently *all patients in all institutions* are not candidates for these early indications for surgical correction of mitral regurgitation, but reparative valve surgery should be considered early in the course of mitral regurgitation when severe regurgitation has been documented.

REFERENCES

1. Waller BE. Rheumatic and nonrheumatic conditions producing valvular heart disease. *Cardiovasc Clin* 1986; 16:3–104.
2. Rahimtoola SH. Valvular heart disease. In: Stein J, ed. *Internal Medicine*, 4th ed. St Louis: Mosby-Year Book; 1994:202–234.
3. Braunwald E. Valvular heart disease. In: Braunwald E, ed. *Heart Disease*, 4th ed. Philadelphia: Saunders; 1992:1007–1018.
4. Davies JJ. Pathology of cardiac valves. London: Butterworth; 1980.
5. Fowler NO. Mitral stenosis and left atrial myxoma. In: *Diagnosis of Heart Disease*. New York: Springer-Verlag; 1991:146–159.
6. Osterberger LE, Goldstein S, Khaja F, Lakier JB. Functional mitral stenosis in patients with massive mitral annular calcification. *Circulation* 1981; 64:472–476.
7. Libman E, Sacks B. A hitherto undescribed form of valvular and mitral endocarditis. *Arch Intern Med* 1924, 33.701–737.
8. Galve E, Candell-Riera J, Pigrau C, Permanyer-Miralda G, Garcia-Del-Castillo H, Soler-Soler J. Prevalence, morphologic types, and evolution of cardiac valvular disease in systemic lupus erythematosus. *N Engl J Med* 1988; 319:817–823.
9. Schoen FJ, St. John Sutton M. Contemporary pathologic considerations in valvular disease. In: Virmani R, Atkinson JB, Fenoglio JJ, eds. *Cardiovascular Pathology*. Philadelphia: Saunders; 1991:334–353.
10. Kawanishi DT, Rahimtoola SH. Mitral stenosis. In: Rahimtoola SH, ed. *Valvular Heart Disease II*. St. Louis: Mosby; 1996:8.1–8.24.
11. Leavitt JL, Coats MH, Falk RH. Effects of exercise on transmitral gradient and pulmonary artery pressure in patients with mitral stenosis or a prosthetic mitral valve: A Doppler echocardiographic study. *J Am Coll Cardiol* 1991; 17:1520–1526.
12. Selzer A. Effects of atrial fibrillation upon the circulation in patients with mitral stenosis. *Am Heart J* 1960; 59:518–526.
13. Wood P. An appreciation of mitral stenosis: Part 1. Clinical features. *Br Med J* 1954; 1:1051–1063. An appreciation of mitral stenosis: Part 2. Investigations and results. *Br Med J* 1954: 1:1113–1124.
14. Gash AK, Carabello BA, Cepin D, Spann JE. Left ventricular ejection performance and systolic muscle function in patients with mitral stenosis. *Circulation* 1983; 67:148–154.
15. Colle JP, Rahal S, Ohayon J, Bonnet J, LeGoff, Besse P. Global left ventricular function and regional wall motion in pure mitral stenosis. *Clin Cardiol* 1984; 7:573–580.
16. Gaasch WH, Folland ED. Left ventricular function in rheumatic mitral stenosis. *Eur Heart J* 1991; 12(suppl B):66–69.
17. Harvey RM, Ferrer MI, Samet P, Bader RA, Bader ME, Cournand A, et al. Mechanical and myocardial factors in rheumatic heart disease in mitral stenosis. *Circulation* 1955; 11:531–551.
18. Mohan JC, Khalilullah M, Arora R. Left ventricular intrinsic contractility in pure rheumatic mitral stenosis. *Am J Cardiol* 1989; 64:240–242.
19. Bowe JC, Bland EF, Sprague HB, White PD. The course of mitral stenosis without surgery: 10 and 20 year perspective. *Ann Intern Med* 1960; 52:741–749.
20. Barrington WW, Bashore T, Wooley CE. Mitral stenosis: Mitral dome excursion at M_1 and the mitral opening snap-the concept of reciprocal heart sounds. *Am Heart J* 1988; 115:1280–1290.
21. Melhem RE, Dunbar JD, Booth RW. The "B" lines of Kerley and left atrial size in mitral valve disease: Their correlation with mean atrial pressure as measured by left atrial puncture. *Radiology* 191; 76:65–69.
22. Reid CL, Chandraratna PAN, Kawanishi DT, Kotlewski A, Rahimtoola SH. Influence of mitral valve morphology on double-balloon catheter balloon valvuloplasty in patients with mitral stenosis: An analysis of factors predicting immediate and 3-month results. *Circulation* 1989; 80:515–524.
23. Gordon PF, Douglas PS, Come PC, Manning WJ. Two-dimensional and Doppler echocardiographic determinants of the natural history of mitral valve narrowing in patients with rheumatic mitral stenosis: Implications for follow-up. *J Am Coll Cardiol* 1992; 19:968–973.
24. Shapiro ML. Echocardiography of the mitral valve. In: Wells PC, Shapiro LN, eds. *Mitral Valve Disease*, 2d ed. London: Butterworths; 1996:47–50.
25. Khandheria BK, Tajik AJ, Reeder GS, Callahan MJ, Nishimura RA, Miller FA. Doppler color flow imaging: A new technique for visualization and characterization of the blood flow jet in mitral stenosis. *Mayo Clin Proc* 1986; 61:623–630.
26. Rahimtoola SH. Perspective on valvular heart disease: An update. *J Am Coll Cardiol* 1989; 14:1–23.
27. Kawanishi DT, Kotlewski A, McKay CR, Harrison EC, Reid CL, Chandraratna PAN. The relative value of clinical examination, echocardiography with Doppler and cardiac catheterization with angiography in the evaluation of mitral valve disease. In: Bodnar E, ed. *Surgery for Heart Valve Disease*. London: ICR Publishers; 1990:73–78.
28. Olesen KH. The natural history of 271 patients with mitral stenosis under medical treatment. *Br Heart J* 1962; 24:349–357.
29. Roy SB, Gopinath N. Mitral stenosis. *Circulation* 1968; 38(suppl V):68–76.
30. Rowe JC, Bland EF, Sprague HB, White P. The course of mitral stenosis without surgery: Ten- and twenty-year perspectives. *Ann Intern Med* 1960; 52:741–749.
31. Prystowsky EN, Benson W Jr, Fuster V, Hart RG, Kay GN, Myerburg RJ, et al. Management of patients with atrial fibrillation: A statement for healthcare professionals from the Subcommittee on Electrocardiography and Electrophysiology, American Heart Association. *Circulation* 1996; 93:1262–1277.
32. Kulick DL, Reid CL, Kawanishi DT, Rahimtoola SH. Catheter balloon commissurotomy in adults: Part II. Mitral and other stenoses. *Curr Probl Cardiol* 1990; 15:403–470.
33. Hickey MSJ, Blackstone EH, Kirklin JW, Dean LW. Outcome probabilities and life history after surgical mitral commissurotomy: Implications for balloon commissurotomy. *J Am Coll Cardiol* 1991; 17:29–42.
34. Scalia D, Rizzoli G, Campanile F, Melacini P, Villanova C, Milano A, et al. Long-term results of mitral commissurotomy. *J Thorac Cardiovasc Surg* 1993; 105:633–642.
35. John S, Bashi VV, Jairaj PS, Muralidharan S, Ravikumar E, Rajarajeswari T, et al. Closed mitral valvotomy: Early results and long-term follow-up of 3724 consecutive patients. *Circulation* 1983; 68:891–896.
36. Crawford MH, Souchek J, Oprian CA, Miller DC, Rahimtoola SH, Giacomini JC, et al. Determinants of survival and left ventricular performance after mitral valve replacement. *Circulation* 1990; 81:1173–1181.
37. Rahimtoola SH. The problem of valve prosthesis—Patient mismatch. *Circulation* 1978; 58:20–24.
38. Turi ZG, Reyes VP, Raju S, Raju AR, Kumar DN, Rajagopal P, et al. Percutaneous balloon versus surgical closed commissurotomy for mitral stenosis: A prospective, randomized trial. *Circulation* 1991; 83:1179–1185.
39. Patel JJ, Shama D, Mitha AS, Blyth D, Hassen F, LeRoux B, et al. Balloon valvuloplasty versus closed commissurotomy for pliable mitral stenosis.
40. Arora R, Nair M, Kalra GS, Nigam M, Khalilullah M. Immediate and long-term results of balloon and surgical closed mitral valvotomy: A randomized comparative study. *Am Heart J* 1993; 125:1091–1094.
41. Reyes VP, Raju BS, Wynne J, Stephenson LW, Raju R, Fromm BS, et al. Percutaneous balloon valvuloplasty compared with open surgical commissurotomy for mitral stenosis. *N Engl J Med* 1994; 331:961–967.

42. NHLBI Valvuloplasty Participants. Multicenter experience with balloon mitral commissurotomy—NHLBI Balloon Valvuloplasty Registry report on immediate and 30-day follow-up results. *Circulation* 1992; 85:448–461.

43. McKay CR, Kawanishi DT, Kotlewski A, Parise K, Odom-Maryon T, Gonzalez A, et al. Improvement in exercise capacity and exercise hemodynamics 3 months after double-balloon catheter balloon valvuloplasty in the treatment of patients with symptomatic mitral stenosis. *Circulation* 1988; 77:1013–1021.

44. Cohen DJ, Kuntz RE, Gordon SPF, Piana RN, Safian RD, McKay RG, et al. Predictors of long-term outcome after percutaneous balloon mitral valvuloplasty. *N Engl J Med* 1992; 327:1329–1335.

45. Palacios I, Tuzcu ME, Weyman AE, Newell JB, Block PC. Clinical follow-up of patients undergoing percutaneous mitral balloon valvotomy. *Circulation* 1995; 91:671–676.

46. Dean LS, Mickel M, Bonan R, Holmes DR, Jr, O'Neill WW, Palacios IF, et al. Four year follow-up of patients undergoing percutaneous balloon mitral commissurotomy: A report from the National Heart, Lung and Blood Institute Balloon Valvuloplasty Registry. *J Am Coll Cardiol* 1996; 28:1452–1457.

47. Orrange SE, Kawanishi DT, Lopez BM, Curry SM, Rahimtoola SH. Actuarial outcome after catheter balloon commissurotomy in patients with mitral stenosis. *Circulation.* 1997; 95:382–389.

48. Rusted I, Scheifley C, Edwards J. Studies of the mitral valve: I. Anatomic features of the normal mitral valve and associated structures. *Circulation* 1952; 6:825–831.

49. Lam J, Ranganathan N, Wigle E, Silver M. Morphology of the human mitral valve: I. Chordae tendineae: A new classification. *Circulation* 1970; 41:449–458.

50. Ranganathan N, Lam J, Wigle E, Silver M. Morphology of the human mitral valve: II. The valve leaflets. *Circulation* 1970; 41:459–467.

51. Ormiston J, Shah P, Tei C, Wong M. Size and motion of the mitral valve annulus in man: II. Abnormalities in mitral valve prolapse. *Circulation* 1982; 65:713–719.

52. Carpentier A. Cardiac valve surgery—The "French Correction." *J Thorac Cardiovasc Surg* 1983; 86:323–337.

53. Carpentier A, Chauvaud S, Fabiani J, Deloche A, Relland J, Lessana A, et al. Reconstructive surgery of mitral valve incompetence: Ten year appraisal. *J Thorac Cardiovasc Surg* 1980; 79:338–348.

54. Selzer A, Katayama F. Mitral regurgitation: Clinical patterns, pathophysiology and natural history. *Medicine* 1972; 51:337–366.

55. Olson L, Subramanian R, Ackermann D, Orszulak T, Edwards W. Surgical pathology of the mitral valve: A study of 712 cases spanning 21 years. *Mayo Clin Proc* 1987; 62:22–34.

56. Waller B, Morrow A, Maron B, Del Negro A, Kent K, McGrath F, et al. Etiology of clinically isolated, severe, chronic, pure mitral regurgitation: Analysis of 97 patients over 30 years of age having mitral valve replacement. *Am Heart J* 1982; 104:276–288.

57. Edwards J, Burchell H. Pathologic anatomy of mitral insufficiency. *Mayo Clin Proc* 1958; 33:497–509.

58. Wooley C, Baker P, Kolibash A, Kilman J, Sparks E, Boudoulas H. The floppy, myxomatous mitral valve, mitral valve prolapse, and mitral regurgitation. *Prog Cardiovasc Dis* 1991; 33:397–433.

59. Pini R, Greppi B, Kramer-Fox R, Roman M, Devereaux R. Mitral valve dimensions and motion and familial transmission of mitral valve prolapse with and without mitral leaflet billowing. *J A Coll Cardiol* 1988; 12:1423–1431.

60. Lucas R, Edwards J. The floppy mitral valve. *Curr Probl Cardiol* 1982; 7:1–48.

61. Guthrie R, Edwards J. Pathology of the myxomatous mitral valve: Nature, secondary changes and complications. *Minn Med* 1976; 59:637–647.

62. Wilcken D, Hickey A: Lifetime risk for patients with mitral valve prolapse of developing severe valve regurgitation requiring surgery. *Circulation* 1988; 78:10–14.

63. Hickey A, Wilcken D, Wright J, Warren B. Primary (spontaneous) chordal rupture: Relation to myxomatous valve disease and mitral valve prolapse. *Am Coll Cardiol* 1985; 5:1341–1346.

64. Van Der Bel-Kahn J, Duren D, Becker A. Isolated mitral valve prolapse: Chordal architecture as an anatomic basis in older patients. *Am Coll Cardiol* 1985; 5:1335–1340.

65. Byram M, Roberts W. Frequency and extent of calcific deposits in purely regurgitant mitral valves: Analysis of 108 operatively excised valves. *Am J Cardiol* 1983; 52:1059–1061.

66. Bloor C. Valvular heart disease in the elderly. *J Am Geriatr Soc* 1982; 30:466–472.

67. Buchbinder N, Roberts W. Left-sided valvular active infective endocarditis: A study of forty-five necropsy patients. *Am J Med* 1972; 53:20–35.

68. Godley R, Wann L, Rogers E, Feigenbaum H, Weyman A. Incomplete mitral leaflet closure in patients with papillary muscle dysfunction. *Circulation* 1981; 63:565–571.

69. Ballester M, Jajoo J, Rees S, Rickards A, McDonald L. The mechanism of mitral regurgitation in dilated left ventricle. *Clin Cardiol* 1983; 6:333–338.

70. Izumi S, Miyatake K, Beppu S, Park Y, Nagata S, Kinoshita N, et al. Mechanism of mitral regurgitation in patients with myocardial infarction: A study using real-time two-dimensional Doppler flow imaging and echocardiography. *Circulation* 1987; 76:777–785.

71. Boltwood C, Tei C, Wong M, Shah P. Quantitative echocardiography of the mitral complex in dilated cardiomyopathy: the mechanism of functional mitral regurgitation. *Circulation* 1983; 68:498–508.

72. Vlodaver Z, Edwards J. Rupture of ventricular septum or papillary muscle complicating myocardial infarction. *Circulation* 1977; 55:815–822.

73. Kishon Y, Oh J, Schaff H, Mullany C, Tajik A, Gersh B. Mitral valve operation in postinfarction rupture of a papillary muscle: Immediate results and long-term follow-up of 22 patients. *Mayo Clin Proc* 1992; 67;1023–1030.

74. Pyeritz R, Wappel M. Mitral valve dysfunction in the marfan syndrome: Clinical and echocardiographic study of prevalence and natural history. *Am J Med* 1983; 74:797–807.

75. Leier C, Call T, Fulkerson P, Wooley C. The spectrum of cardiac defects in the Ehlers-Danlos syndrome, types I and III. *Ann Intern Med* 1980; 92:171–178.

76. Galve E, Candell-Reira J, Pigrau C, Permanyer-Miralda G, Gardia-Del-Castillo H, Soler-Soler J. Prevalence, morphologic types, and evolution of cardiac valvular disease in systemic lupus erythematosus. *N Engl J Med* 1988; 319:817–823.

77. Galve E, Ordi J, Barquinero J, Evangelista A, Vilardell M, Soler-Soler J. Valvular heart disease in the primary antiphospholipid syndrome. *Ann Intern Med* 1992; 116:293–298.

78. Mazzuco A, Rizzoli G, Faggian G, Aru G, Bortolotti U, Sorbara C, et al. Acute mitral regurgitation after blunt chest trauma. *Arch Intern Med* 1983; 143:2326–2329.

79. Gottdiener J, Maron B, Schooley R, Harley J, Roberts W, Fauci A. Two-dimensional echocardiographic assessment of the idiopathic hypereosinophilic syndrome: Anatomic basis of mitral regurgitation and peripheral embolization. *Circulation* 1983; 67:572–578.

80. Pellikka P, Tajik A, Khandheria B, Seward J, Callahan J, Pitot H, et al. Carcinoid heart disease: Clinical and echocardiographic spectrum in 74 patients. *Circulation* 1993; 87:1188–1196.

81. Yellin E, Yoran C, Sonnenblick E, Gabbay S, Frater R. Dynamic changes in the canine mitral regurgitant orifice area during ventricular ejection. *Circ Res* 1979; 45:677–683.

82. Vokonas P, Gorlin R, Cohn P, Herman M, Sonnenblick. E. Dynamic geometry of the left ventricle in mitral regurgitation. *Circulation* 1973; 48:786–796.

83. Schwammenthal E, Chen C, Benning F, Block M, Breithardt G, Levine R. Dynamics of mitral regurgitant flow and orifice area. Physiologic application of the proximal flow convergence method: Clinical data and experimental testing. *Circulation* 1994; 90:307–322.

84. Mathey D, Decoodt P, Allen H, Swan H. The determinants of onset of mitral valve prolapse in the systolic click-late systolic murmur syndrome. *Circulation* 1976; 53:872–878.

85. Enriquez-Sarano M, Seward J, Bailey K, Tajik A. Effective regurgitant orifice area: A noninvasive doppler development of an old hemodynamic concept. *J Am Coll Cardiol* 1994; 23:443–451.

86. Tyrell M, Ellison R, Hugenholtz P, Nadas A. Correlation of degree of left ventricular volume overload with clinical course in aortic and mitral regurgitation. *Br Heart J* 1970; 32:683–690.

87. Dodge H, Baxley W. Left ventricular volume and mass and their significance in heart disease. *Am J Cardiol* 1969; 23:528–537.

88. Borgenhagen D, Serur J, Gorlin R, Adams D, Sonnenblick E. The effect of left ventricular load and contractility on mitral regurgitant orifice size and flow in the dog. *Circulation* 1977; 56:106–113.

89. Chatterjee K, Parmley W, Swan H, Berman G, Forrester J, Marcus H. Beneficial effects of vasodilator agents in severe mitral regurgitation

due to dysfunction of subvalvular apparatus. *Circulation* 1973; 48;684–690.

90. Keren G, Bier A, Strom J, Laniado S, Sonnenblick E, LeJemtel T. Dynamics of mitral regurgitation during nitroglycerin therapy: A Doppler echocardiographic study. *Am Heart J* 1986; 112:517–525.

91. Keren G, Laniado S, Sonnenblick E, LeJemtel T. Dynamics of mitral regurgitation during dobutamine therapy in patients with severe congestive heart failure: A Doppler echocardiographic study. *Am Heart J* 1989; 118:748–754.

92. Yoran C, Yellin E, Becker R, Gabbay S, Frater R, Sonnenblick E. Dynamic aspects of acute mitral regurgitation: Effects of ventricular volume, pressure and contractility on the effective regurgitant orifice area. *Circulation* 1979; 60:170–176.

93. Grose R, Strain J, Cohen M. Pulmonary arterial V waves in mitral regurgitation: Clinical and experimental observations. *Circulation* 1984; 69:214–222.

94. Fuchs R, Heuser R, Yin F, Brinker J. Limitations of pulmonary wedge V waves in diagnosing mitral regurgitation. *Am J Cardiol* 1982; 49:849–854.

95. Braunwald E, Awe W. The syndrome of severe mitral regurgitation with normal left atrial pressure. *Circulation* 1963; 27:29–35.

96. Wisenbaugh T, Spann J, Carabello B. Differences in myocardial performance and load between patients with similar amounts of chronic aortic versus chronic mitral regurgitation. *J Am Coll Cardiol* 1984; 3:916–923.

97. Starling M, Kirsch M, Montgomery D, Gross M. Impaired left ventricular contractile function in patients with long-term mitral regurgitation and normal ejection fraction. *J Am Coll Cardiol* 1993; 22:239–250.

98. Kontos GJ, Schaff H, Gersh B, Bove A. Left ventricular function in subacute and chronic mitral regurgitation: Effect on function early postoperatively. *J Thorac Cardiovasc Surg* 1989; 98:163–169.

99. Enriquez-Sarano M, Hannachi M, Jais J, Acar J: Résultats hémodynamiques et angiographiques après correction chirurgicale de l'insuffisance mitrale: A propos de 51 cathétérismes itératifs. *Arch Mal Coeur* 1983; 76:1194–1203.

100. Wisenbaugh T. Does normal pump function belie muscle dysfunction in patients with chronic severe mitral regurgitation? *Circulation* 1988; 77:515–525.

101. Mirsky I, Corin W, Murakami T, Grimm J, Hess O, Krayenbuehl H. Correction for preload in assessment *Circulation* 1988; 78:68–80.

102. Corin W, Monrad E, Murakami T, Nonogi H, Hess O, Krayenbuehl H. The relationship of afterload to ejection performance in chronic mitral regurgitation. *Circulation* 1987; 76:59–67.

103. Carabello B, Nolan S, McGuire L. Assessment of preoperative left ventricular function in patients with mitral regurgitation: Valve of the end-systolic wall stress-end-systolic volume ratio. *Circulation* 1981; 64:1212–1217.

104. Enriquez-Sarano M, Tajik A, Schaff H, Orszulak T, McGoon M, Bailey K, et al. Echocardiographic prediction of left ventricular function after correction of mitral regurgitation: Results and clinical implications. *J Am Coll Cardiol* 1994; 24:1536–1543.

105. Crawford M, Souchek J, Oprian C, Miller D, Rahimtoola S, Giacomini J, et al. Determinants of survival and left ventricular performance after mitral valve replacement. *Circulation* 1990; 81:1173–1181.

106. Carabello B, Nakano K, Ishihara K, Kanazawa B, Biederman R, Spann JJ. Coronary blood flow in dogs with contractile dysfunction due to experimental volume overload. *Circulation* 1991; 83:1063–1075.

107. Urabe Y, Mann D, Kent R, Nakano K, Tomanek R, Carabello B, et al. Cellular and ventricular contractile dysfunction in experimental canine mitral regurgitation. *Circ Res* 1992; 70:131–147.

108. Spinale F, Ishihra K, Zile M, De Fryte G, Crawford F, Carabello B. Structural basis for changes in left ventricular function and geometry because of chronic mitral regurgitation and after correction of volume overload. *J Thorac Cardiovasc Surg* 1993; 106:1147–1157.

109. Corin W, Murakami T, Monrad E, Hess O, Krayenbuehl H. Left ventricular passive diastolic properties in chronic mitral regurgitation. *Circulation* 1991; 83:797–807.

110. Enriquez-Sarano M, Tajik A, Bailey K, Seward J. Color flow imaging compared with quantitative doppler assessment of severity of mitral regurgitation: Influence of eccentricity of jet and mechanism of regurgitation. *J Am Coll Cardiol* 1993; 21:1211–1219.

111. Hickey M, Smith L, Muhlbaier L, Harrell FJ, Reves J, Hinohara T, et al. Current prognosis of ischemic mitral regurgitation: Implications for future management. *Circulation* 1988; 78:151–159.

112. Lehman K, Francis C, Dodge H. Mitral regurgitation in early myocardial infarction: Incidence, clinical detection, and prognostic implications. *Ann Intern Med* 1992; 117:10–17.

113. Stevenson L, Bellil D, Grover-McKay M, Brunken R, Schwaiger M, Tillisch J, et al. Effects of afterload reduction (diuretics and vasodilators) on left ventricular volume and mitral regurgitation in severe congestive heart failure secondary to ischemic or idiopathic dilated cardiomyopathy. *Am J Cardiol* 1987; 60:654–658.

114. Bentivoglio L, Uricchio J, Goldberg H. Clinical and hemodynamic features of advanced rheumatic mitral regurgitation. *Am J Med* 1961; 30:372–381.

115. Roberts W, Braunwald E, Morrow A. Acute severe mitral regurgitation secondary to ruptured chordae tendineae: Clinical, hemodynamic, and pathologic considerations. *Circulation* 1966; 33:58–70.

116. Ronan JJ, Steelman R, DeLeon AJ, Waters T, Perloff J, Harvey W. The clinical diagnosis of acute severe mitral insufficiency. *Am J Cardiol* 1971; 27:284–290.

117. Selzer A, Kelly JJ, Vannitamby M, Walker P, Gerbode F, Kerth W. The syndrome of mitral insufficiency due to isolated rupture of the chordae tendineae. *Am J Med* 1967; 43:822–836.

118. Austen W, Sokol D, DeSanctis R, Sanders C. Surgical treatment of papillary-muscle rupture complicating myocardial infarction. *N Engl J Med* 1968; 278:1137–1141.

119. Brody W, Criley J. Intermittent severe mitral regurgitation. *N Engl J Med* 1970; 283:673–676.

120. Kligfield P, Hochreiter C, Niles N, Devereux R, Borer J. Relation of sudden death in pure mitral regurgitation, with and without mitral valve prolapse, to repetitive ventricular arrhythmias and right and left ventricular ejection fractions. *Am J Cardiol* 1987; 60:397–399.

121. Folland E, Kriegel B, Henderson W, Hammermeister K, Sethi G. Implications of third heart sounds in patients with valvular heart disease: The Veterans Affairs Cooperative Study on Valvular Heart Disease. *N Engl J Med* 1992; 327:458–462.

122. Cohen L, Mason D, Braunwald E. Significance of an atrial gallop sound in mitral regurgitation: A clue to the diagnosis of ruptured chordae tendineae. *Circulation* 1967; 35:112–118.

123. Antman E, Angoff G, Sloss I. Demonstration of the mechanism by which mitral regurgitation mimics aortic stenosis. *Am J Cardiol* 1978; 42:1044–1048.

124. Desjardins V, Enriquez-Sarano M, Tajik A, Bailey D, Seward J. Intensity of murmurs correlates with severity of valvular regurgitation. *Am J Med* 1996; 100:149–156.

125. Forrester J, Diamond G, Freedman S, Allen H, Parmley W, Matloff J, et al. Silent mitral insufficiency in acute myocardial infarction. *Circulation* 1971; 44:877–883.

126. Enriquez-Sarano M, Tajik A, Schaff H, Orszulak T, Bailey K, Frye R. Echocardiographic prediction of survival after surgical correction of organic mitral regurgitation. *Circulation* 1994; 90:830–837.

127. Glick B, Roberts W. Usefulness of total 12-lead QRS voltage in diagnosing left ventricular hypertrophy in clinically isolated, pure, chronic, severe mitral regurgitation. *Am J Cardiol* 1992; 70:1088–1092.

128. Plaschkes J, Borman J, Merin G, Milwidsky H. Giant left atrium in rheumatic heart disease: A report of 18 cases treated by mitral valve replacement. *Ann Surg* 1971; 174:194–201.

129. Mintz G, Kotler M, Parry W, Segal B. Statistical comparison of M mode and two dimensional echocardiographic diagnosis of flail mitral leaflets. *Am J Cardiol* 1980; 45:253–259.

130. Marcus R, Sareli P, Pocock W, Meyer T, Magalhaes M, Grieve T, et al. Functional anatomy of severe mitral regurgitation in active rheumatic carditis. *Am J Cardiol* 1989; 63:577–584.

131. Dahm M, Iversen S, Schmid F, Drexler R, Erbel R, Oelert H. Intraoperative evaluation of reconstruction of the atrioventricular valves by transesophageal echocardiography. *Thorac Cardiovasc Surg* 1987; 35:140–142.

132. Freeman W, Schaff H, Khanderia B, Oh J, Orszulak T, Abel M, et al. Intraoperative evaluation of mitral valve regurgitation and repair by transesophageal echocardiography: Incidence and significance of systolic anterior motion. *J Am Coll Cardiol* 1992; 20:599–609.

133. Reichert S, Visser C, Moulijn A, Suttorp M, Brink R, Koolen J, et al. Intraoperative transesophageal color-coded Doppler echocardiography for evaluation of residual regurgitation after mitral valve repair. *J Thorac Cardiovasc Surg* 1990; 100:756–761.

134. Sheikh K, Bengtson J, Rankin J, de Bruijn N, Kisslo J. Intraoperative transesophageal Doppler color flow imaging used to guide patient

selection and operative treatment of ischemic mitral regurgitation. *Circulation* 1991; 84:594–604.

135. Hozumi T, Yoshikawa J, Yoshida K, Yamaura Y, Akasaka T, Shakudo M. Direct visualization of ruptured chordae tendineae by transesophageal two-dimensional echocardiography. *J Am Coll Cardiol* 1990; 16:1315–1319.

136. Daniel W, Mugge A, Martin R, Lindert O, Hausmann D, Nonnast-Daniel B, et al. Improvement in the diagnosis of abscesses associated with endocarditis by transesophageal echocardiography. *N Engl J Med* 1991; 324:795–800.

137. Shively B, Gurule F, Roldan C, Leggett J, Schiller N. Diagnostic value of transesophageal compared with transthoracic endocardiography in infective endocarditis. *J Am Coll Cardiol* 1991; 18:391–397.

138. Keren G, Sonnenblick E, LeJemtel T. Mitral annulus motion: Relation to pulmonary venous and transmitral flows in normal subjects and in patients with dilated cardiomyopathy. *Circulation* 1988; 78:621–629.

139. Patel A, Miller FJ, Khandheria B, Mullany C, Seward J, Oh J. Role of transesophageal echocardiography in the diagnosis of papillary muscle rupture secondary to myocardial infarction. *Am Heart J* 1989; 118:1330–1333.

140. Sakai K, Nakamura K, Hosoda S. Transesophageal echocardiographic findings of papillary muscle rupture. *Am J Cardiol* 1991; 68:561–563.

141. Roberts W, Kishel J, McIntosh C, Cannon RI, Maron B. Severe mitral or aortic valve regurgitation, or both, requiring valve replacement for infective endocarditis complicating hypertrophic cardiomyopathy. *J Am Coll Cardiol* 1992; 19:365–371.

142. Schott C, Kotler M, Parry W, Segal B. Mitral annular calcification: Clinical and echocardiographic correlations. *Arch Intern Med* 1977; 137:1143–1150.

143. Helmcke F, Nanda N, Hsiung M, Soto B, Adey C, Goyal R, et al. Color Doppler assessment of mitral regurgitation with orthogonal planes. *Circulation* 1987; 75:175–183.

144. Spain M, Smith M, Grayburn P, Harlamert E, DeMaria A. Quantitative assessment of mitral regurgitation by Doppler color flow imaging: Angiographic and hemodynamic correlations. *J Am Coll Cardiol* 1989; 13:585–590.

145. Pearson A, St. Vrain J, Mrosek D, Labovitz A. Color Doppler echocardiographic evaluation of patients with a flail mitral leaflet. *J Am Coll Cardiol* 1990; 16:232–239.

146. Cape E, Yoganathan A, Weyman A, Levine R. Adjacent solid boundaries alter the size of regurgitant jets on Doppler color flow maps. *J Am Coll Cardiol* 1991; 17:1094–1102.

147. Chen C, Thomas J, Anconina J, Harrigan P, Mueller L, Picard M, et al. Impact of impinging wall jet on color Doppler quantification of mitral regurgitation. *Circulation* 1991; 84:712–720.

148. Utsunomiya T, Patel D, Doshi R, Quan M, Gardin J. Can signal intensity of the continuous wave Doppler regurgitant jet estimate severity of mitral regurgitation? *Am Heart J* 1992; 123:166–171.

149. Castello R, Pearson A, Lenzen P, Labovitz A. Effect of mitral regurgitation on pulmonary venous velocities derived from transesophageal echocardiography color-guided pulsed Doppler imaging. *Am Coll Cardiol* 1991; 17:1499–1506.

150. Klein A, Obarski T, Stewart W, Casale P, Pearce G, Husbands K, et al. Transesophageal Doppler echocardiography of pulmonary venous flow: A new marker of mitral regurgitation severity. *J Am Coll Cardiol* 1991; 18:518–526.

151. Vandervoort P, Rivera J, Mele D, Palacios I, Dinsmore R, Weyman A, et al. Application of color Doppler flow mapping to calculate effective regurgitant orifice area. An in vitro study and initial clinical observations. *Circulation* 1993; 88:1150–1156.

152. Enriquez-Sarano M, Bailey K, Seward J, Tajik A, Krohn M, Mays J. Quantitative Doppler assessment of valvular regurgitation. *Circulation* 1993; 87:841–848.

153. Rokey R, Sterling L, Zoghbi W, Sartori M, Limacher M, Kuo L, et al. Determination of regurgitant fraction in isolated mitral or aortic regurgitation by pulsed Doppler two-dimensional echocardiography. *J Am Coll Cardiol* 1986; 7:1273–1278.

154. Blumlein S, Bouchard A, Schiller N, Dae M, Byrd BI, Ports T, et al. Quantitation of mitral regurgitation by Doppler echocardiography. *Circulation* 1986; 74:306–314.

155. Bargiggia G, Tronconi L, Sahn D, Recusani F, Raisaro A, De Servi S, et al. A new method for quantitation of mitral regurgitation based on color flow Doppler imaging of flow convergence proximal to regurgitant orifice. *Circulation* 1991; 84:1481–1489.

156. Chen C, Koschyk D, Brockhoff C, Heik S, Hamm C, Bleifeld W, et al. Noninvasive estimation of regurgitant flow rate and volume in patients with mitral regurgitation by Doppler color mapping of accelerating flow field. *J Am Coll Cardiol* 1993; 21:374–383.

157. Schuler G, Peterson K, Johnson A, Francis G, Dennish G, Utley J, et al. Temporal response of left ventricular performance to mitral valve surgery. *Circulation* 1979; 59:1218–1231.

158. Wisenbaugh T, Skudicky D, Sarlei P. Prediction of outcome after valve replacement for rheumatic mitral regurgitation in the era of chordal preservation. *Circulation* 1994; 89:191–197.

159. Zile M, Gaasch W, Carroll J, Levine J. Chronic mitral regurgitation: predictive value of preoperative echocardiographic indexes of left ventricular function and wall stress. *J Am Coll Cardiol* 1984; 3:235–242.

160. Schiller N, Shah P, Crawford M, DeMaria A, Devereux R, Feigenbaum H, et al. Recommendations for quantitation of the left ventricle by two-dimensional echocardiography: American Society of Echocardiography Committee on Standards, Subcommittee on Quantitation of Two-Dimensional Echocardiograms. *J Am Soc Echocardiogr* 1989; 2:358–367.

161. Gorge G, Erbel R, Brennecke R, Rupprecht H, Todt M, Meyer J. High resolution two-dimensional echocardiography improves the quantification of left ventricular function. *J Am Soc Echocardiogr* 1992; 5:125–134.

162. Lavie C, Lam J, Gibbons R. Effects of exercise on left ventricular volume and output changes in severe mitral regurgitation: A radionuclide angiographic study. *Chest* 1989; 96:1086–1091.

163. Sellers R: Left retrograde cardioangiography in acquired heart disease: Technic, indications and interpretations in 700 cases. *Am J Cardiol* 1964; 14:437–447.

164. Croft C, Lipscomb K, Mathis K, Firth B, Nicod P, Tilton G, et al. Limitations of qualitative angiographic grading in aortic or mitral regurgitation. *Am J Cardiol* 1984; 53:1593–1598.

165. Sandler H, Dodge H, Hay R, Rackley C. Quantitation of valvular insufficiency in man by angiocardiography. *Am Heart J* 1963; 65:501–513.

166. Lopez J, Hanson S, Orchard R, Tan L. Quantification of mitral valvular incompetence. *Cathet Cardiovasc Diagn* 1985; 11:139–152.

167. Kennedy J, Yarnall S, Murray J, Figley M. Quantitative angiography: IV. Relationships of left atrial and ventricular pressure and volume in mitral valve disease. *Circulation* 1970; 41:817–824.

168. Baxley W, Kennedy J, Feild B, Dodge H. Hemodynamics in ruptured chordae tendinae and chronic rheumatic mitral regurgitation. *Circulation* 1973; 48:1288–1294.

169. Borow K, Green L, Mann T, Sloss L, Braunwald E, Colins J, et al. End systolic volume as a predictor of postoperative left ventricular performance in volume overload from valvular regurgitation. *Am J Med* 1980; 68:655–663.

170. Leitch J, Mitchell A, Harris P, Fletcher P, Bailey B. The effect of cardiac catheterization upon management of advanced aortic and mitral regurgitation. *Eur Heart J* 1991; 12:602–607.

171. Slater J, Gindea A, Freedberg R, Chinitz L, Tunick P, Rosenzweig B, et al. Comparison of cardiac catheterization and Doppler echocardiography in the decision to operate in aortic and mitral valve disease. *J Am Coll Cardiol* 1991; 17:1026–1036.

172. Wilson M, Lim W. The natural history of rheumatic heart disease in the third, fourth, and fifth decades of life: I. Prognosis with special reference to survivorship. *Circulation* 1957; 16:700–712.

173. Nishimura R, McGoon M, Shub C, Miller F, Ilstrup D, Tajik A. Echocardiographically documented mitral-valve prolapse. Long-term follow-up of 237 patients. *N Engl J Med* 1985; 313:1305–1309.

174. Kolibash AJ, Kilman J, Bush C, Ryan J, Fontana M, Wooley C. Evidence for progression from mild to severe mitral regurgitation in mitral valve prolapse. *Am J Cardiol* 1986; 58:762–767.

175. Chesler E, King R, Edwards J. The myxomatous mitral valve and sudden death. *Circulation* 1983; 67:632–639.

176. Delahaye J, Gare J, Viguier E, Delahaye F, De Gevigney G, Milon H. Natural history of severe mitral regurgitation. *Eur Heart J* 1991; 12(suppl B):5–9.

177. Rosen S, Borer J, Hochreiter C, Supino P, Roman M, Devereux R, et al. Natural history of the asymptomatic/minimally symptomatic patient with with severe mitral regurgitation secondary to mitral valve prolapse and normal right and left ventricular performance. *Am J Cardiol* 1994; 74:374–380.

178. Rappaport E. Natural history of aortic and mitral valve disease. *Am J Cardiol* 1975; 35:221–227.

179. Munoz S, Gallardo J, Diaz-Gorrin J, Medina O. Influence of surgery on the natural history of rheumatic mitral and aortic valve disease. *Am J Cardiol* 1975; 35:234–242.

180. Horstkotte D, Loogen F, Kleikamp G, Schulte H, Trampisch H, Bircks W. Effect of prosthetic heart valve replacement on the natural course of isolated mitral and aortic as well as multivalvular diseases: Clinical results in 783 patients up to 8 years following implantation of the Björk-Shiley tilting disc prosthesis. *Z Kardiol* 1983; 72:494–503.

181. Ling H, Enriquez-Sarano M, Seward J, Tajik A, Schaff H, Bailey K, et al. Clinical outcome of mitral regurgitation due to flail leaflets. *N Engl J Med* 1996; 335:1417–1423.

182. Hammermeister K, Fisher L, Kennedy W, Samuels S, Dodge H. Prediction of late survival in patients with mitral valve disease from clinical, hemodynamic, and quantitative angiographic variables. *Circulation* 1978; 57:341–349.

183. Ramanathan K, Knowles J, Connor M, Tribble R, Kroetz F, Sullivan J, et al. Natural history of chronic mitral insufficiency: Relation of peak systolic pressure/end-systolic volume ration to morbidity and mortality. *J Am Coll Cardiol* 1984; 3:1412–1416.

184. Hochreiter C, Niles N, Devereux R, Kligfield P, Borer J. Mitral regurgitation: Relationship of noninvasive descriptors of right and left ventricular performance to clinical and hemodynamic findings and to prognosis in medically and surgically treated patients. *Circulation* 1986; 73:900–912.

185. Shulman S, Amren D, Bisno A, Dajani A, Durack D, Gerber M, et al. Prevention of bacterial endocarditis: A statement for health professionals by the Committee on Rheumatic Fever and Bacterial Endocarditis of the Council on Cardiovascular Diseases in the Young of the American Heart Association. *Am J Dis Child* 1985; 139:232–235.

186. Chua Y, Schaff H, Orszulak T, Morriss J. Outcome of mitral valve repair in patients with preoperative atrial fibrillation: Should the maze procedure be combined with mitral valvuloplasty? *J Thoracic Cardiovasc Surg* 1994; 107:408–415.

187. Greenberg B, Massie B, Brundage B, Botvinick E, Parmley W, Chatterjee K. Beneficial effects of hydralazine in severe mitral regurgitation. *Circulation* 1978; 58:273–279.

188. Schon H, Schroter G, Blomer H, Schomig A. Beneficial effects of a single dose of quinapril on left ventricular performance in chronic mitral regurgitation. *Am J Cardiol* 1994; 73:785–791.

189. Schanzenbacher P, Liebau G. Effect of Captopril on left ventricular dynamics in patients with chronic left ventricular volume overload. *Klin Wochenschr* 1983; 61:343–347.

190. Wisenbaugh T, Essop R, Rothlisberger C, Sareli P. Effects of a single oral dose of captopril on left ventricular performance in severe mitral regurgitation. *Am J Cardiol* 1992; 69:348–353.

191. McGoon D. Repair of mitral insufficiency due to ruptured chordae tendineae. *J Thorac Cardiovasc Surg* 1960; 39:357–362.

192. Frater R, Gabbay S, Shore D, Factor S, Strom J. Reproducible replacement of elongated or ruptured mitral valve chordae. *Ann Thorac Surg* 1983; 35:14–28.

193. Lessana A, Escorsin M, Romano M, Ades F, Vergoni W, Lorenzoni D, et al. Transposition of posterior leaflet for treatment of ruptured main chordae of the anterior mitral leaflet. *J Thorac Cardiovasc Surg* 1985; 89:804–806.

194. Reed G, Fooley R, Moggio R. Durability of measured mitral annuloplasty: Seventeen-year study. *J Thorac Cardiovasc Surg* 1980; 79:321–325.

195. Kay C, Kay J, Zubiate P, Yokoyama T, Mendez M. Mitral valve repair for mitral regurgitation secondary to coronary artery disease. *Circulation* 1986; 74:188–198.

196. Duran C, Revuelta J, Gaite L, Alonso C, Fleitas M. Stability of mitral reconstructive surgery at 10–12 years for predominantly rheumatic valvular disease. *Circulation* 1988; 78:I91–I96.

197. Schiabone W, Cosgrove D, Lever H, Stewart W, Salcedo E. Long-term follow-up of patients with left ventricular outflow tract obstruction after Carpentier ring mitral valvuloplasty. *Circulation* 1988; 78:60–66.

198. Galler M, Kronzon I, Slater J, Lighty GJ, Politzer F, Colvin S, et al. Long-term follow-up after mitral valve reconstruction: Incidence of postoperative left ventricular outflow obstruction. *Circulation* 1986; 74(3 pt 2):I99–I103.

199. Mihaileanu S, Marino J, Chauvaud S, Perier P, Forman J, Vissoat J, et al. Left ventricular outflow obstruction after mitral valve repair (Carpentier's technique): Proposed mechanisms of disease. *Circulation* 1988; 78:178–184.

200. David T, Komeda M, Pollick C, Burns R: Mitral valve annuloplasty: The effects of the type on left ventricular function. *Ann Thorac Surg* 1989; 47:524–528.

201. Cohn L, Allred E, Cohn L, Austin J, Sabik J, DiSesa V, et al. Early and late risk of mitral valve replacement: A 12-year concomitant comparison of the porcine bioprosthetic and prosthetic disc mitral valves. *J Thorac Cardiovasc Surg* 1985; 90:872–880.

202. Pumphrey C, Fuster V, Chesebro J. Systemic thromboembolism in valvular heart disease and prosthetic heart valves. *Mood Concepts Cardiovasc Dis* 1982; 51:131–136.

203. Edmunds LJ. Thromboembolic complications of current cardiac valvular prostheses. *Ann Thorac Surg* 1982; 34:96–106.

204. Enriquez-Sarano M, Schaff H, Orszulak T, Tajik A, Bailey K, Frye R. Valve repair improves the outcome of surgery for mitral regurgitation. *Circulation* 1995; 91:1264–1265.

205. Perier P, Deloche A, Chauvaud S, Fabiani J, Rossant P, Bessou J, et al. Comparative evaluation of mitral valve repair and replacement with Starr, Bjork, and porcine valve prostheses. *Circulation* 1894; 70(3 pt 2):I187–I192.

206. Goldman M, Mora F, Guarino T, Fuster V, Mindich B. Mitral valvuloplasty is superior to mitral valve replacement for preservation of left ventricular function: An intraoperative two-dimensional echocardiographic study. *J Am Coll Cardiol* 1987; 10:568–575.

207. David T, Burns R, Bacchus C, Druck M. Mitral regurgitation with and without preservation of chordae tendineae. *J Thorac Cardiovasc Surg* 1984; 88:718–725.

208. Kay J, Zubiate P, Mendez M, Vanstrom N, Yokoyama T. Mitral valve repair for significant mitral insufficiency. *Am Heart J* 1978; 95:253–262.

209. Orszulak T, Schaff H, Danielson G, Piehler J, Pluth J, Frye R, et al. Mitral regurgitation due to ruptured chordae tendineae: Early and late results of valve repair. *J Thorac Cardiovasc Surg* 1985; 89:491–498.

210. McGoon M, Fuster V, McGoon D, Pumphrey C, Pluth J, Elveback L. Aortic and mitral valve incompetence: Long-term follow-up (10–19 years) of patients treated with the Starr-Edward prosthesis. *J Am Coll Cardiol* 1984; 3:930–938.

211. Enriquez-Sarano M, Schaff H, Orszulak T, Bailey K, Tajik A, Frye R. Congestive heart failure after surgical correction of mitral regurgitation: A long-term study. *Circulation* 1995; 92:2496–2503.

212. Phillips H, Levine F, Carter J, Boucher C, Osbakken M, Okada R, et al. Mitral valve replacement for isolated mitral regurgitation: Analysis of clinical course and late postoperative left ventricular ejection fraction. *Am J Cardiol* 1981; 48:647–654.

213. Zile M, Gaasch W, Levin H. Left ventricular stress-dimension-shortening relations before and after correction of chronic aortic and mitral regurgitation. *Am J Cardiol* 1985; 56:99–105.

214. Reed D, Abbott R, Smucker M, Kaul S. Prediction of outcome after mitral valve replacement in patients with symptomatic chronic mitral regurgitation: The importance of left atrial size. *Circulation* 1991; 84:23–34.

CHAPTER

65

MITRAL VALVE PROLAPSE SYNDROME

Robert A. O'Rourke

Mitral valve prolapse (MVP) syndrome, the most common form of valvular heart disease, occurs in 3 to 8 percent of the population, thus being more common than a bicuspid aortic valve. It is commonly detected by cardiac auscultation, with one or more systolic clicks and/or a mid-to-late systolic murmur detected on a careful physical examination. Often the auscultatory complex is the only clinical manifestation of cardiac disease, and many patients are asymptomatic.

In the late nineteenth century, mid-systolic clicks were first described and were attributed to a pericardial or extracardiac etiology. Subsequently, late systolic murmurs were recognized to be present in apparently healthy individuals and were found to be associated with a benign natural history. Thus, the murmur was also considered to be extracardiac in origin.

In 1961, Reid[1] suggested that the mid-systolic click and the late systolic murmur were due to mitral regurgitation. In 1963, Barlow and associates[2] confirmed this hypothesis by left ventricular cineangiography. Subsequently, intracardiac phonocardiogram studies documented the mitral valve origin of a systolic click and late systolic murmur.

During the past three decades, considerable new data obtained from pathologic studies, echocardiography, and cineventriculography have demonstrated that this common syndrome is associated with prolapse of one or both mitral valve leaflets in the atrium during ventricular systole.

Recognition of the systolic click–late systolic murmur syndrome, which has also been called billowing mitral leaflet syndrome, floppy valve syndrome, and prolapsing mitral valve leaflet syndrome, is often difficult because of the extreme variability in clinical manifestations. It is, however, an important cause of incapacitating chest pain and refractory arrhythmias in certain patients. The abnormal mitral valve apparatus is also a potential site for endocarditis, and some patients, particularly males in their sixties and seventies, can develop severe mitral regurgitation due to ruptured chordae tendineae.

DEFINITION, ETIOLOGY, AND TIMING

Mitral valve prolapse refers to the systolic billowing of one or both mitral leaflets in the left atrium, with or without mitral regurgitation. MVP often occurs as a clinical entity with no or only mild mitral regurgitation, and it is frequently associated with unique clinical characteristics when compared with the other causes of mitral regurgitation.[3–12]

The mitral valve apparatus is a complex structure composed of the mitral annulus, valve leaflets, chordae tendineae, papillary muscles, and the supporting left ventricular, left atrial, and aortic walls.[13] Disease processes involving any one or more of these components may result in dysfunction of the valvular apparatus and prolapse of the mitral leaflets toward the left atrium during systole when left ventricular pressure exceeds left atrial pressure.

The complexity of the mitral valve apparatus provides an explanation for the presence of secondary prolapse in many conditions that affect one or more of the components of the apparatus (e.g., ruptured mitral chordae). There is, however, considerable evidence that a disorder of the mitral valve leaflets exists in which there are specific pathologic changes causing redundancy of the mitral leaflets and their prolapse into the left atrium during systole. This is the primary form of MVP (Table 65-1).

In primary MVP, there is interchordal hooding due to leaflet redundancy that involves both the rough and clear zones of the involved leaflets.[8] The height of the interchordal hooding usually exceeds 4 mm and involves at least one-half of the anterior leaflet or at least two-thirds of the posterior leaflet. The basic microscopic feature of primary MVP is marked proliferation of the *spongiosa*, the delicate myxomatous connective tissue between the *atrialis* (a thick layer of collagen and elastic tissue forming the atrial aspect of the

TABLE 65-1

CLASSIFICATION OF MITRAL VALVE PROLAPSE

Primary mitral valve prolapse
  Familial
  Nonfamilial
  Marfan's syndrome
  Other connective tissue diseases
Secondary mitral valve prolapse
  Coronary artery disease
  Rheumatic heart disease
  Cardiomyopathies
  "Flail" mitral valve leaflet(s)
Normal variant
  Inaccurate auscultation
  "Echocardiographic heart disease"

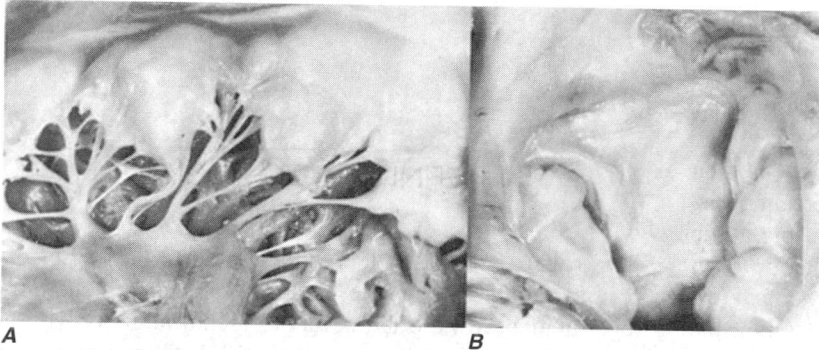

FIGURE 65-1

Myxomatous mitral valve. *A.* The opened mitral valve shows characteristic interchordal hooding and redundancy of the leaflets. *B.* The unopened mitral valve viewed from the left atrial side shows extensive scalloping that is characteristic of a myxomatous mitral valve. From Guthrie and Edwards[14]. Reproduced with permission from the publisher and authors.)

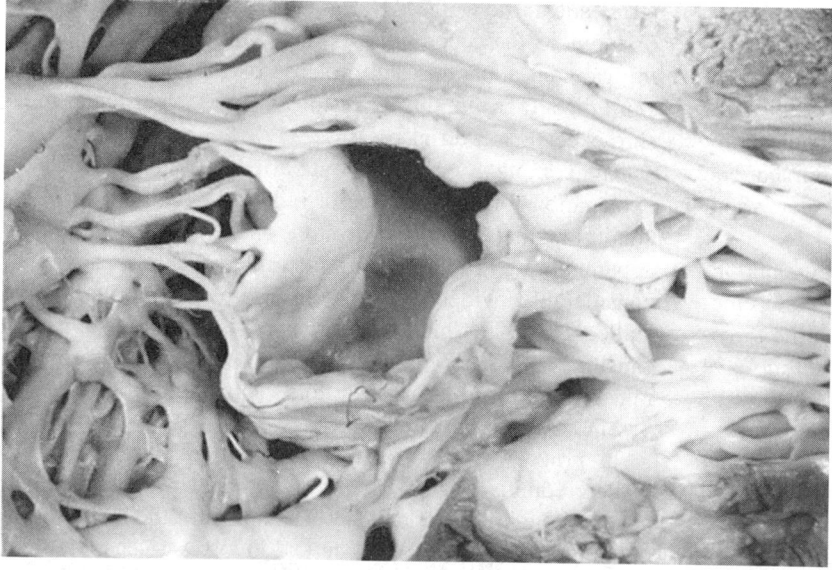

FIGURE 65-2

Myxomatous mitral valve with ruptured posterior leaflet chordae. The central part of the posterior leaflet (lower center) shows fragments of ruptured chordae. The intact chordae are elongated and the leaflets show redundancy and fibrous thickening. (From Edwards F. Pathology of mitral incompetence. In: Silver MD, ed. *Cardiovascular Pathology.* New York: Churchill Livingstone: 1983. Reproduced with permission from the publisher and authors.)

leaflet) and the *fibrosa,* or *ventricularis,* which is composed of dense layers of collagen and forms the basic support of the leaflet.[8,14] In primary MVP, myxomatous proliferation of the acid mucopolysaccharide-containing spongiosa tissue causes focal interruption of the fibrosa.[8,14] Secondary effects of the primary MVP syndrome include fibrosis of the surfaces of the mitral valve leaflets, thinning and/or elongation of chordae tendineae, and ventricular friction lesions.[15,16] Fibrin deposits often form at the mitral valve–left atrial angle (Figs. 65-1 and 65-2).

The primary form of MVP may occur in families, where it appears to be inherited as an autosomal dominant trait with varying penetrance.[17,18] No consistent chromosomal abnormalities have yet been identified in patients with MVP, which also often occurs in isolated cases.[19,20] Primary MVP has been found with increasing frequency in patients with Marfan's syndrome,[8] where it is almost always present, and in other heritable connective tissue diseases such as Ehlers-Danlos syndrome,[21] pseudoxanthoma elasticum,[22] and osteogenesis imperfecta.[23] Marfan's syndrome also has an autosomal dominant mode of inheritance. It is possible that some genetic studies of MVP[17,18] may have been tracking a more general connective tissue disorder such as Marfan's syndrome (see also Chap. 85).

Several clinical observations have led to the speculation that primary MVP syndrome represents a generalized disorder of connective tissue. Thoracic skeletal abnormalities such as straight thoracic spine and pectus excavatum are commonly associated with this syndrome.[24,25] The mitral valve undergoes differentiation between the thirty-fifth and forty-second days of fetal life, when the vertebrae and thoracic cage are beginning chondrification and ossification.[26] Any adverse factors in this period might affect both the mitral valve and the bones of the thoracic cage. Of possible relevance, rats fed a diet containing large amounts of peas of the genus *Lathyrus* develop both bony abnormalities and myxomatous changes in their valve leaflets.[27] Therefore, it has been postulated that the MVP syndrome is a connective tissue disorder resulting from fetal exposure to toxic agents during the early part of pregnancy.[27]

Others have suggested that MVP is a result of defective embryogenesis of cell lines of mesenchymal origin. The association of primary MVP with an increased incidence in patients with von Willebrand disease and other coagulopathies, primary hypomastia, and various connective tissue diseases has been used to support this concept.[28,29]

A secondary form of MVP (Table 65-1) occurs in which myxomatous proliferation of the spongiosa portion of the mitral valve leaflet is absent. Tei and associates [30] were able to produce de novo echocardiographic evidence of MVP, often with mitral regurgitation, in closed chest dogs undergoing transient coronary artery occlusion; MVP was attributed to relative displacement of ischemic papillary muscles. Also, serial studies in patients with known ischemic heart disease have occasionally documented unequivocal MVP following an acute coronary syndrome that was previously absent.[31] In most patients with coronary artery disease (CAD) and MVP, however, the two entities are coincident but unrelated.

Several recent studies[32–34] indicate that valvular regurgitation caused by MVP may result from postinflammatory changes, including those following rheumatic fever. In histologic studies of surgically excised valves, fibrosis with vascularization and scattered infiltration of round cells, including lymphocytes and plasmacytes, were found without myxomatous proliferation of the spongiosa.[32] With rheumatic carditis, the anterior mitral leaflet is more likely to prolapse.[34]

Mitral valve prolapse has been observed in patients with hypertrophic cardiomyopathy in whom posterior MVP may result from a disproportionally small left ventricular cavity, altered papillary muscle alignment, or a combination of factors.[35] The mitral valve leaflet is usually normal. Since left ventricular segmental wall motion abnormalities and sometimes depressed global left ventricular function occur in certain patients with echocardiographic and auscultatory evidence of MVP and regurgitation, nonhypertrophic cardiomyopathy has been listed as a cause of mitral prolapse.[35] This is probably not the case; the ventricular wall motion abnormalities frequently disappear when the mitral valve is repaired or replaced. The MVP in patients with atrial septal defects might be explainable to some extent on the relatively small size of the left ventricle in this disorder, resulting in a mitral apparatus that is relatively large and redundant.

Patients with primary and secondary MVP must be distinguished from those with normal variations on cardiac auscultation or echocardiography; these variations can result in an incorrect diagnosis of mitral prolapse, particularly in patients who are hyperkinetic or dehydrated during the physical examination or two-dimensional echocardiography.[36,37] Other auscultatory findings may be misinterpreted as mid-systolic clicks or late systolic murmurs (see Chap. 10). Patients with mild to moderate billowing of one or more nonthickened leaflets toward the left atrium with the leaflet coaptation point on the ventricular side of the mitral annulus and no or minimal mitral regurgitation by Doppler echocardiography are probably normal. Unfortunately, many such patients with neither a nonejection click nor murmur of mitral regurgitation are frequently overdiagnosed as having the MVP syndrome.[38]

PATHOPHYSIOLOGY

In patients with MVP, there is frequently left atrial enlargement and left ventricular enlargement, depending upon the presence and severity of mitral regurgitation.[39] The supporting apparatus is often involved, and in patients with connective tissue syndromes such as Marfan's syndrome, the mitral annulus is usually dilated, sometimes calcified, and does not decrease its circumference by the usual 30 percent during left ventricular systole. The effects of mild to moderate mitral regurgitation on cardiac function are similar to those from other causes of mitral regurgitation.

Many studies suggest the increased likelihood of autonomic nervous system dysfunction in patients with primary MVP.[40–44] In 1979, Gaffney and associates[40] reported a reduced heart rate slowing with intravenous phenylephrine and an abnormal diving reflex heart rate response in patients with MVP as compared to age-matched controls.[41,42] They also showed that patients with MVP had a less than normal lower extremity pooling of blood in response to lower body negative pressure. There is a higher incidence of increased vagal tone and of prolonged QT interval on the electrocardiogram in patients with MVP. In several studies, measurements of serum and 24-h urine epinephrine and norepinephrine levels were increased in patients with symptomatic MVP as compared to age-matched controls.[41,42] Patients with MVP often have an increased heart rate and contractility response to intravenous isoproterenol.[42,45] An increased incidence of high-affinity beta receptors in the lymphocytes of patients with MVP has been reported, as well as greater than usual increase in cyclic adenosine monophosphate with isoproterenol stimulation as compared to normal individuals.[45] Patients with MVP often have postural phenomena such as orthostatic tachycardia and hypotension. Low intravascular volume and/or an abnormality in the renin-aldosterone axis may contribute to the orthostatic changes.[46,47]

ASSOCIATED CONDITIONS

Tricuspid valve prolapse, with similar interchordal hooding and histologic evidence of mucopolysaccharide proliferation and collagen dissolution, occurs in about 40 percent of patients with MVP.[8] Pulmonic valve prolapse and aortic valve prolapse occur in approximately 10 percent and 2 percent of patients with MVP, respectively.[8] The frequent findings of thoracic skeletal abnormalities in patients with MVP have been noted above. There is an increased incidence of secundum atrial septal defect in patients with MVP, and an increased incidence of MVP in patients with atrial septal defects that cannot be explained by a chance occurrence and does not represent only stretching of a patent fossa ovalis[8,48] (see also Chaps. 70 & 71). An increased incidence of left-sided atrioventricular bypass tracts and supraventricular tachycardias also occurs in patients with MVP.[48]

CLINICAL MANIFESTATIONS

Symptoms

The diagnosis of MVP is most commonly made by cardiac auscultation in asymptomatic patients or by echocardiography being performed for some other purpose. The patient may be evaluated because of a family history of cardiac disease or occasionally may be referred because of an abnormal resting electrocardiogram.

Some patients consult their physicians because of one or more of the common symptoms that occur in patients with this syndrome. The most common presenting complaint is palpitation. The source of palpitation is usually ventricular premature beats, but various supraventricular arrhythmias are also frequent, and the most common sustained tachycardia is paroxysmal reentry supraventricular tachycardia (see Chap. 27). Ventricular tachycardia has been observed in some patients, and others have had symptomatic bradyarrhythmias. Palpitation is often reported by patients at a time when continuous ambulatory electrocardiographic recordings show no arrhythmias.

Chest pain is a frequent complaint in patients with MVP. It is atypical in most patients without coexistent ischemic heart disease and rarely resembles classic angina pectoris. Occasionally, it is recurrent and can be incapacitating. The etiology of the chest pain is unknown; sometimes it may represent true myocardial ischemia produced by abnormal tension on the papillary muscles and supporting ventricular wall by the prolapsing mitral leaflets. In one study, it could be reproduced by elevating the systemic arterial pressure with intravenous phenylephrine.[49] Coronary artery spasm has been reported in patients with MVP, but it is unlikely to be the cause of most episodes of atypical chest pain.[50]

Dyspnea and fatigue are frequent symptoms in patients with MVP, including many without severe mitral regurgitation. Objective exercise testing often fails to show an impairment in exercise tolerance, and some patients exhibit distinct episodes of hyperventilation. Neuropsychiatric complaints are not uncommon in patients with MVP. Some patients have panic attacks (Chap. 90), and others frank manic-depressive syndromes. Transient cerebral ischemic episodes occur with increased incidence in patients with MVP, and some patients develop stroke syndromes.[51–57] Reports of amaurosis fugax, homonymous field loss, and retinal artery occlusion have been described; occasionally the visual loss persists.[58] These signs likely are due to embolization of platelets and fibrin deposits that occur on the atrial side of the mitral valve leaflets.[8,59] *It is important to note that both MVP and panic attacks occur relatively frequently. Accordingly, the occurrence of the two syndromes in the same individual would be expected to occur frequently by chance, rather than panic attacks necessarily being part of the primary MVP syndrome.*

Physical Examination

The presence of thoracic skeletal abnormalities may suggest the diagnosis of MVP, the most common being scoliosis, pectus excavatum, straightened thoracic spine, and narrowed anterior-posterior diameter of the chest.[16] Some patients with MVP may show signs, such as arachnodactyly, more typical of Marfan's syndrome.

The principal cardiac auscultatory feature of this syndrome is the mid-systolic click, a high-pitched sound of short duration (Chap. 16). The click may vary considerably in intensity and location in systole according to left ventricular loading conditions and contractility. It results from the sudden tensing of the mitral valve apparatus as the leaflets prolapse into the left atrium during systole. Multiple systolic clicks may be generated by different portions of the mitral leaflets prolapsing at varying times during systole.[60] The major differentiating feature of the mid-systolic click of mitral prolapse from that due to other causes (e.g., aneurysm of the ventricular septum, atrial myxomas, pericarditis) is that its timing during systole may be altered by maneuvers that change hemodynamic conditions (Table 65-2).

The mid-systolic click is frequently followed by a late systolic murmur, usually medium- to high-pitched and most audible at the apex. Occasionally, the murmur has a musical or honking quality. The character and intensity of the murmur also vary under certain conditions, from brief and almost inaudible to holosystolic and loud (Fig. 65-3).

Dynamic auscultation is often useful for establishing the clinical diagnosis of the MVP syndrome.[7,27] Changes in the left ventricular end-diastolic volume lead to changes in the timing of the mid-systolic click and murmur. When end-diastolic volume is decreased, the critical volume is achieved earlier in systole and the click-murmur complex occurs shortly after the first heart sound (Fig. 65-4).

In general, any maneuver that decreases the end-diastolic left ventricular volume, increases the rate of ventricular contraction, or decreases the resistance to left ventricular ejection of blood causes the MVP to occur early in systole and the systolic click and murmur to move toward the first heart sound (Table 65-2). By contrast, any maneuver that augments the volume of blood in the ventricle, reduces myocardial contractility, or increases left ventricular afterload lengthens the time from the onset of systole to the initiation of MVP, and the systolic click and/or murmur move toward the second heart sound. Maneuvers causing the click and/or murmur to occur earlier in systole include standing from the supine position, submaximal isometric handgrip exercise, the Valsalva maneuver, and amyl nitrite inhalation. Those that cause the click

TABLE 65-2

RESPONSE OF THE MURMUR OF MITRAL VALVE PROLAPSE TO INTERVENTIONS

Intervention	Timing	Intensity
Standing upright	←	↑
Recumbent	→	↓ or 0
Squatting	→	↓ or 0
Handgrip	←	±
Valsalva	←	±
Amyl nitrite	±	↑

Note: ↑ = increase; ↓ = decrease; 0 = no change; ± = variable; ← = earlier; → = later.

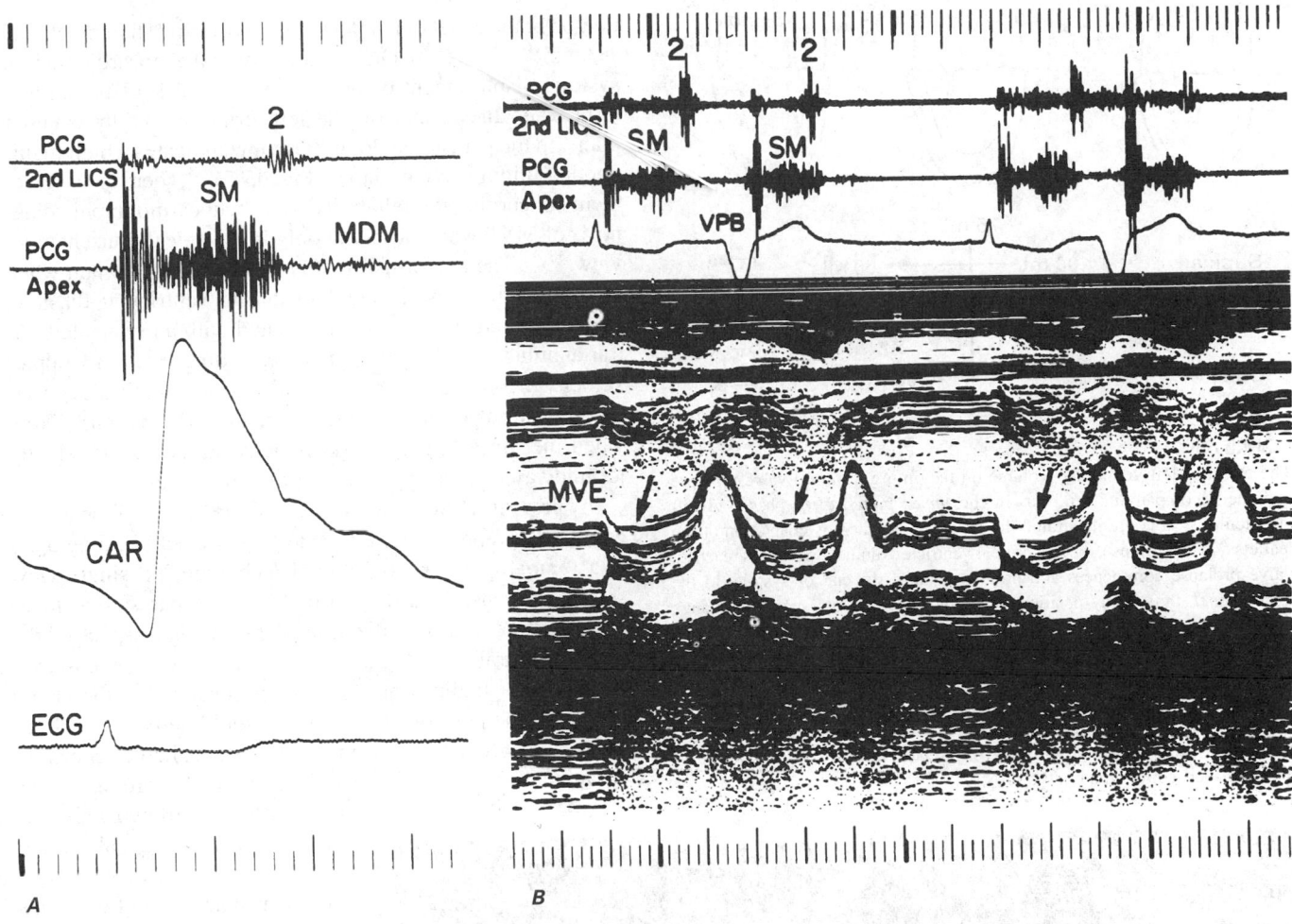

FIGURE 65-3

Phonocardiogram and echocardiogram in mitral valve prolapse. *A.* The phonocardiogram shows a high-frequency holosystolic murmur (SM) with late systolic accentuation. A low-frequency mid-diastolic murmur (MDM) is present at the apex. *B.* The echocardiogram demonstrates a hammock-shaped systolic motion of the valve leaflets. The rhythm is atrial fibrillation with bigeminy. 1 = first heart sound; 2 = second heart sound; MVE = mitral valve echogram. (Courtesy of Dr. Ernest Craige.)

and murmur to move toward the second heart sound include squatting from the upright position and maneuvers that slow the heart rate.

Electrocardiogram

The electrocardiogram is usually normal in patients with MVP. The most common abnormality in the MVP syndrome is the presence of ST-T-wave depression or T-wave inversion in the inferior leads (III, aV$_F$).[61] These changes may reflect ischemia of the inferior wall due to traction on the posteromedial papillary muscle by the prolapsing mitral leaflets. Sometimes ST-T-wave changes are present only during interventions that induce prolapse earlier in systole, as discussed above. More unusual electrocardiographic changes include prominent U waves, peaked T waves in the midprecordial leads, and prolongation of the QT interval.

MVP is associated with an increased incidence of false-positive exercise electrocardiographic results in patients with normal coronary arteries, especially females. Myocardial perfusion imaging with thallium or technetium sestamibi has been useful for differentiating false from true abnormal exercise electrocardiographic findings in patients with MVP (see Chap. 17).

Although arrhythmias may be observed on the resting electrocardiogram or during treadmill or bicycle exercise, they are detected more reliably by continuous ambulatory electrocardiographic recordings (Chap. 28). The reported incidence of documented arrhythmias is higher in patients with MVP, ranging from 40 to 75 percent.[29] Most of the arrhythmias detected, however, are not life-threatening. Patients with ST-T-wave changes in the inferior electrocardiographic leads appear to have a higher incidence of serious ventricular arrhythmias on ambulatory recordings.[27,62]

Echocardiography

Echocardiography (Chap. 14) is the most useful noninvasive test for defining MVP. The M-mode echocardiographic definition of MVP includes ≥2-mm posterior displacement of

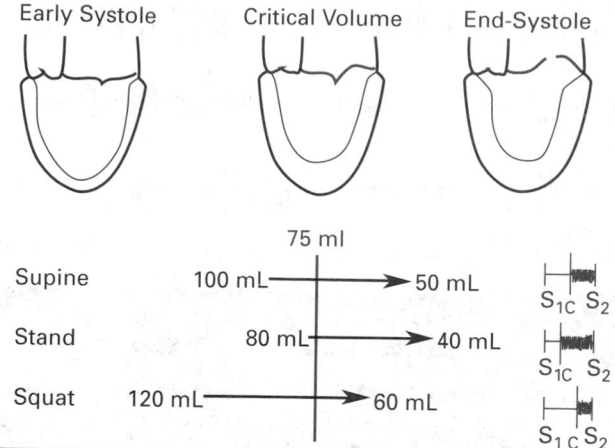

	75 ml		
Supine	100 mL ——→	50 mL	S_{1C} S_2
Stand	80 mL ——→	40 mL	S_{1C} S_2
Squat	120 mL ——→	60 mL	S_{1c} S_2

FIGURE 65-4

The effect of left ventricular volume on the timing of mitral valve prolapse and the accompanying murmur. In the *upper panel*, three phases of left ventricular systole are illustrated. In early systole, there is coaptation of the leaflets and no prolapse; when a critical ventricle volume of 75 mL is reached, valve prolapse commences and progresses until the end of systole. In the *lower panel*, three body positions are indicated; the corresponding change in volume and timing of the click-murmur are shown. The critical volume for prolapse remains constant. When the critical volume occurs earlier, the onset of click-murmur is earlier. When the critical volume occurs later, the onset of the click-murmur is later. (From Crawford MH, O'Rourke RA. In: Isselbacher KJ et al, eds. *Harrison's Principles of Internal Medicine*, 9th ed. New York: McGraw-Hill; 1980: 91–105. Reproduced with permission from the publisher, editors, and authors.)

one or both leaflets or holosystolic posterior "hammocking" >3 mm[10] (Fig. 65-3). On two-dimensional echocardiography, systolic displacement of one or both mitral leaflets, particularly when they coapt on the left atrial side of the annular plane, in the parasternal long-axis view indicates a high likelihood of mitral valve prolapse (Fig. 65-5).[63] There is disagreement concerning the reliability of an echocardiographic diagnosis of MVP when observed only in the apical four-chamber view.[38,63] The diagnosis of MVP is even more certain when the leaflet thickness is >5 mm during ventricular diastole. Leaflet redundancy is often associated with an elongated mitral annulus and elongated chordae tendineae.[10] On Doppler velocity recordings, the presence or absence of mitral regurgitation is an important consideration, and MVP is more likely when the mitral regurgitation is detected as a high-velocity jet midway or more posterior in the left atrium.[38]

At present, there is no consensus on the two-dimensional echocardiographic criteria for MVP. Since echocardiography is a tomographic cross-sectional technique, no single view should be considered diagnostic.[64,65] The parasternal long-axis view permits visualization of the medial aspect of the anterior mitral leaflet and middle scallop of the posterior leaflet. If the findings of prolapse are localized to the lateral scallop in the posterior leaflet, they would be best visualized by the apical four-chamber view.[64,65] All available echocardiographic views should be utilized, with the provision that anterior leaflet billowing alone in the four-chamber apical view is not evidence of prolapse; however, a displacement of the posterior leaflet or the coaptation point in any view including the apical views suggests the diagnosis of prolapse. The echocardiographic criteria for MVP should include structural changes such as leaflet thickening, redundancy, annular dilatation, and chordal elongation.[64,65]

Patients with echocardiographic criteria for MVP but without evidence of thickened/redundant leaflets or definite mitral regurgitation are more difficult to classify. If such patients have auscultatory findings typical of MVP, the echocardiogram confirms the diagnosis. On the other hand, a patient with typical auscultatory findings but a negative echocardiogram likely also has MVP; in the past as many as 10 percent of patients with MVP have had a nondiagnostic echocardiographic study. Currently it is probable that this percentage

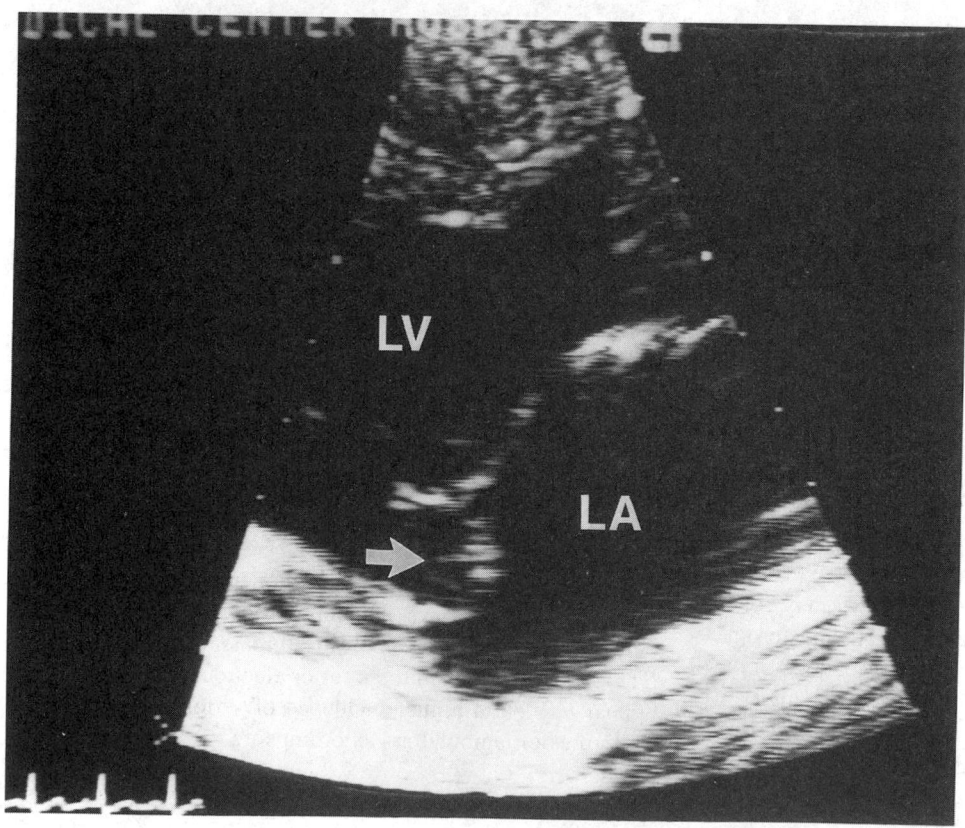

FIGURE 65-5

A parasternal two-dimensional echocardiographic view showing prolapse of a redundant posterior mitral leaflet toward the left atrium during systole. LV = left ventricle; LA = left atrium.

is lower because of more careful and complete echocardiographic studies. In clinical practice, a false diagnosis of MVP occurs too frequently.

The use of echocardiography as a screening test for MVP in patients with and without symptoms who have no systolic click or murmur on serial, carefully performed auscultatory examinations is not recommended.[10] The likelihood of finding a prolapsing mitral valve in such patients is extremely low.[10] Most patients with or without symptoms who have negative dynamic cardiac auscultation and "mild mitral valve prolapse" by echocardiography should not be diagnosed as having MVP.

Echocardiography is also useful for defining left atrial size, left ventricular size and function, and the extent of mitral leaflet redundancy and for detecting associated lesions such as secundum atrial septal defect. Doppler echocardiography is helpful for the detection and semiquantitation of mitral regurgitation as well. Serial echocardiograms are often useful for following patients with murmurs, especially holosystolic murmurs, since quantitation of mitral regurgitation by examination alone is more difficult. In a carefully performed study comparing auscultatory findings with echocardiographic results in patients with clinical evidence of MVP, the amount of billowing of one or both mitral leaflets into the left atrium, the level of the leaflets' coaptation point, and the presence or absence of moderate or severe mitral regurgitation were each important considerations in deciding on the likelihood of MVP.[38]

Chest Roentgenogram

Posterior-anterior and lateral chest x-ray films usually show normal cardiopulmonary findings. The skeletal abnormalities described above can be seen.[26] When severe mitral regurgitation is present, both left atrial and ventricular enlargement often result. Various degrees of pulmonary venous congestion are evident when left heart failure results. Acute chordal rupture with a sudden increase in the amount of mitral regurgitation may present as pulmonary edema without obvious left ventricular or left atrial dilatation. Calcification of the mitral annulus may be seen, particularly in adults with Marfan's syndrome (see Chap. 13).

Myocardial Perfusion Scintigraphy

Exercise myocardial perfusion imaging with thallium or technetium sestamibi has been recommended as an adjunct to exercise electrocardiography for determining the presence or absence of coexistent myocardial ischemia in patients with MVP.[27,65] Most MVP patients with clinical evidence of CAD have an abnormal exercise scintigram. On the other hand, a negative scintigram in these patients does not exclude ischemia as the basis for the chest pain nor does it completely exclude CAD as the etiology (see Chap. 17).

Cardiac Catheterization

Cardiac catheterization is rarely used as a diagnostic technique for MVP. Also, contrast ventriculography is unnecessary for determining left ventricular function since it usually can be quantitated by two-dimensional echocardiography or radionuclide ventriculography. While contrast cineventriculography is often useful for assessing the severity of mitral regurgitation, cardiac catheterization and angiography are most commonly used in patients with MVP to exclude the possibility of CAD.

Intracardiac pressures and cardiac output are usually normal in uncomplicated MVP; however, these measurements become progressively more abnormal as mitral regurgitation becomes more severe.

Left ventricular angiography usually confirms the presence of prolapse of the mitral valve.[7,10] The right anterior oblique projection is best for observing prolapse of the three scallops of the posterior leaflet. The left anterior oblique view is necessary for the adequate evaluation of prolapse of the anterior leaflet.

Left ventricular wall motion is usually normal in patients with primary MVP, but some patients show abnormal contraction patterns in the absence of CAD.[7,35] These contraction abnormalities usually represent indentation of the left ventricle at the point of attachment of the papillary muscles; it is thought to be due to abnormal traction on the papillary muscles and buckling of the ventricular wall. Patients with the most severe prolapse more commonly exhibit misshapen ventricular cavities during systole, and wall motion abnormalities frequently disappear after successful mitral valve replacement or repair.[35]

Coronary arteriography is usually normal in patients with primary MVP, and no congenital anomalies of the coronary vessels have been associated with this syndrome.

Electrophysiologic Testing

The indications for electrophysiologic testing in a patient with MVP are similar to those in general practice (i.e., recurrent unexplained syncope, sudden death survivors, symptomatic complex ventricular ectopy, and the presence of the preexcitation syndromes)[10] (see Chap. 29). Upright tilt studies with monitoring of blood pressure and rhythm may be valuable in patients with light-headedness or syncope and in diagnosing autonomic dysfunction[10] (see Chap. 35).

NATURAL HISTORY, PROGNOSIS, AND COMPLICATIONS

In most patient studies, the MVP syndrome is associated with a benign prognosis (Fig. 65-6).[8,66–70] The age-adjusted survival rate for both males and females with MVP is similar to that in patients without this common clinical entity. The gradual progression of mitral regurgitation in patients with mitral prolapse, however, may result in progressive dilatation of the left atrium and ventricle. Left atrial dilatation often results in atrial fibrillation, and moderate to severe mitral regurgitation eventually results in left ventricular dysfunction and the development of congestive heart failure.[10] Pulmonary

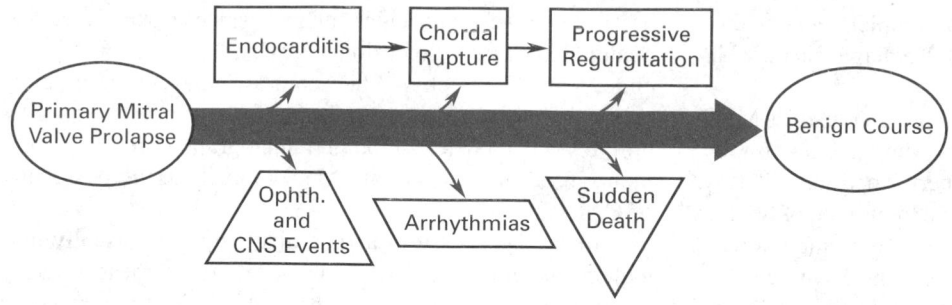

FIGURE 65-6

The course and possible complications of mitral valve prolapse. In most patients the mitral valve prolapse syndrome is associated with a benign prognosis. CNS = central nervous system; Ophth = ophthalmologic. (From Crawford MH, O'Rourke RA. In: Isselbacher KJ et al, eds. *Harrison's Principles of Internal Medicine*, 9th ed. New York: McGraw-Hill; 1980: 91–105. Reproduced with permission from the publisher, editors, and authors.)

hypertension may occur with associated right ventricular dysfunction. In some patients with an initially prolonged asymptomatic interval, the entire process may enter an accelerated phase as a result of left atrial and left ventricular dysfunction, atrial fibrillation, and, in certain instances, ruptured mitral valve chordae.[10] The latter occurs more commonly in males and with increasing age.[8,10]

Several long-term prognostic studies suggest that complications occur most commonly in patients with a mitral systolic murmur, thickened redundant mitral valve leaflets, or increased left ventricular or left atrial size (Fig. 65-7).[39,70,71]

In a prospective follow-up study of 237 asymptomatic or minimally symptomatic patients with MVP documented by echocardiography, sudden death occurred in six patients.[68] In a multivariant analysis of the echocardiographic findings, the presence or absence of redundant mitral valve leaflets by M-mode echocardiography was the only variable associated with sudden death. Ten patients sustained a cerebral embolic event, six of whom were in atrial fibrillation with left atrial enlargement.

Marks et al.[63] confirmed these data in a retrospective two-dimensional echocardiographic study from 456 patients with MVP. Two groups of patients were compared; those with thickening and redundancy of the mitral valve leaflet and those without leaflet thickening. Complications, or a history of complications, were more prevalent in those with leaflet thickening and redundancy compared to those without leaflet thickening. The incidence of stroke, however, was similar in the two groups.

Long-term follow-up studies in patients with MVP associated with a floppy, myxomatous mitral valve permit several conclusions.[10] Serious complications occur in some patients with MVP, predominantly in those with diagnostic auscultatory findings. Also, redundant mitral valve leaflets and increased left ventricular size are associated with a frequency of serious complications. Finally, men and those over 50 years of age are at increased risk of complications, including severe mitral regurgitation requiring surgery.[10]

Sudden death is the least common but obviously the most severe complication of mitral valve prolapse (Table 65-3). While infrequent, the highest incidence of sudden death has been reported in the familial form of MVP. Some of these patients have been noted to have QT prolongation. Also, patients with MVP with severe autonomic dysfunction and excessive vagotonia resulting in bradyarrhythmias and asystole have been reported.[10,72,73] Therefore, arrhythmias are likely to be the usual cause of sudden

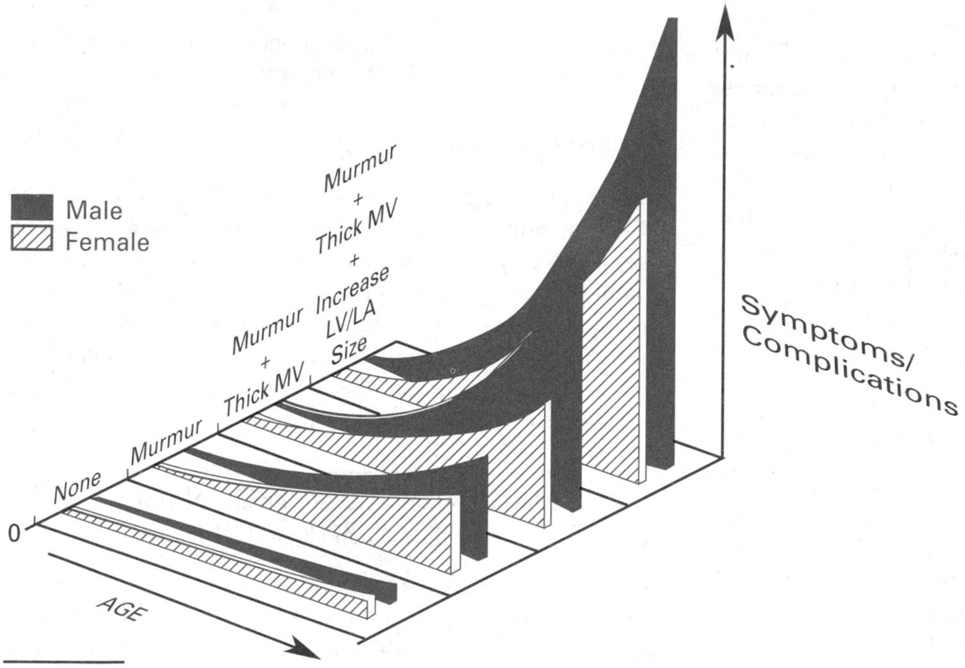

FIGURE 65-7

The relations between cardiac structure, age, and complications in the mitral valve (MV) prolapse syndrome. Patients with mitral valve prolapse, typical auscultatory findings, thickening of the valve leaflets, and left ventricular (LV) or left atrial (LA) enlargement are at risk of developing complications. When two or more of these findings are present, the likelihood of complications is highest. By contrast, the absence of these features can be used to identify patients with mitral valve prolapse who have an exceedingly low risk. In general, complications increase with age and are more common in males than in females. (From Boudoulas H et al.[70] Reproduced with permission from the publisher and authors.)

TABLE 65-3

MITRAL VALVE COMPLICATIONS IN 102 HEARTS
WITH MITRAL VALVE PROLAPSE

	No.	%
Sudden death	0	0
Primary rupture of chordae	7	7
Bacterial endocarditis	7	7
Mitral valve regurgitation	18	18
Primary rupture of chordae	(7)	—
Bacterial endocarditis	(4)	—
Severe prolapse	(4)	—
Entrapped chordae	(3)	—
Fibrin deposits	4	4

Source: Modified from Lucas and Edwards,[8] with permission.

death in patients with MVP, so it seems prudent to limit ambulatory electrocardiographic recordings to those patients at highest risk. Many believe that patients with electrocardiographic ST-T-wave changes are more likely to have complex ventricular arrhythmias.[8,10] Certainly, any patients with symptoms suggestive of arrhythmia or who have arrhythmias noted during physical examination or on the resting electrocardiogram should be evaluated further (see Chap. 27).

Infective endocarditis is a serious complication of MVP,[8,10,74] and MVP is the leading predisposing cardiovascular diagnosis in most series of patients reported with endocarditis. Since the absolute incidence of endocarditis is extremely low for the entire MVP population, there has been much discussion concerning the risk of endocarditis in MVP.[74,75] While there is general agreement that MVP patients with murmurs and/or thickened redundant valves confirmed by echocardiography or cineangiography should receive antibiotic prophylaxis, some authorities state that patients with isolated systolic clicks and no murmurs do not need antibiotic prophylaxis for endocarditis.[76] The dynamic nature of MVP, with variable physical findings on different examinations, makes it difficult to make judgments on the basis of the presence or absence of a systolic murmur. With the increasing use of color-flow echo-Doppler studies, mitral regurgitation has often been observed in patients in whom no murmur is heard.[77,78] Since endocarditis can cause destruction of even a mildly affected valve, prophylaxis would seem warranted in nearly all cases in which the diagnosis of MVP seems certain (see Chap. 82).

As indicated above, progressive mitral regurgitation occurs frequently in patients with long-standing MVP. Fibrin emboli are responsible in some patients for visual problems consistent with involvement of the ophthalmic or posterior cerebral circulation.[58] Several studies have indicated an increased likelihood of cerebral vascular accidents of various types in patients under age 45 who have MVP than would have been expected in a similar population without MVP.[51-57] Therefore, it has been recommended that antiplatelet drugs such as aspirin be administered to patients who have MVP and suspected cerebral nervous system emboli; however, neither antiplatelet drugs nor anticoagulants should be prescribed routinely for patients with MVP because the incidence of embolic phenomena is very low (see also Chap. 99).

It is important to avoid the incorrect diagnosis of MVP syndrome. This mistake is especially likely to occur in patients with neuropsychiatric symptoms in whom an incorrect diagnosis of MVP is made from the echocardiogram. Such an improper diagnosis can form the foundation of a chronic, often disabling cardiac neurosis. Even if the diagnosis of MVP is properly made, it is not necessarily correct to attribute neuropsychiatric symptoms to the MVP (see also Chap. 90).

TREATMENT

The majority of patients with MVP are asymptomatic and lack the high-risk profile described earlier. These patients with mild or no symptoms and findings of milder forms of prolapse should be assured of a benign prognosis. A normal lifestyle and regular exercise are encouraged.[7,10] For most patients in whom the diagnosis of MVP is definite,[7] we recommend antibiotic prophylaxis for the prevention of infective endocarditis while undergoing procedures associated with bacteremia. Patients with MVP and palpitation associated with sinus tachycardia or mild tachyarrhythmias and those with chest pain, anxiety, or fatigue often respond to therapy with beta blockers.[7,10,79] In many cases, however, the cessation of catecholamine stimulants such as caffeine, alcohol, cigarettes, and certain drugs[10] may be sufficient to control symptoms.

Orthostatic symptoms are best treated with volume expansion, preferably by liberalizing fluid and salt intake. Mineralocorticoid therapy may be needed in severe cases, and wearing support stockings may be beneficial.[10] In sudden death survivors and those patients with symptomatic complex arrhythmias, specific antiarrhythmic therapy should be guided by monitoring techniques, including electrophysiologic testing when indicated (Chap. 29).[10]

Daily aspirin therapy (80 to 325 mg/day) is recommended for MVP patients with documented focal neurologic events. Such patients should also avoid cigarettes and oral contraceptives. Some clinicians utilize long-term anticoagulant therapy with warfarin in poststroke patients with prolapse, particularly when symptoms occur on aspirin therapy (see also Chap. 99).

Restriction from competitive sports is recommended when moderate left ventricular enlargement, left ventricular dysfunction, uncontrolled tachyarrhythmias, long QT interval, unexplained syncope, prior sudden death, or aortic root enlargement is present, individually or in combination.[10]

The familial occurrence of MVP should be explained to the patient and is particularly important in those with associated disease who are at greater risk for complications. Screening relatives can uncover high-risk individuals and potentially prevent some complications. There is no contraindication to pregnancy based on the diagnosis of MVP alone.

Patients with severe mitral regurgitation with symptoms and/or impaired left ventricular systolic function require cardiac catheterization studies and evaluation for mitral valve surgery.[80–83] The thickened, redundant mitral valve can often be repaired rather than replaced, with a low operative mortality and excellent long-term results.[84–87] Follow-up studies also suggest lower thromboembolic and endocarditis risk than with prosthetic valves.

Asymptomatic patients with MVP and no significant mitral valve regurgitation can be evaluated clinically every 2 to 3 years. Echocardiography has been suggested every 5 years in such patients to help determine the natural history and the likelihood of complications.[10] Patients with MVP who have high-risk characteristics, including those with moderate to severe regurgitation, should be followed more frequently, even if no symptoms are present.

REFERENCES

1. Reid JV. Mid-systolic clicks. *S Afr Med J* 1961; 35:353–357.
2. Barlow JB, Pocock WA, Marchand P, Denny M. The significance of late systolic murmurs. *Am Heart J* 1963; 66:443–452.
3. Read RC, Thal AP, Wendt VE. Symptomatic valvular myxomatous transformation (the floppy valve syndrome). *Circulation* 1965; 32:897–910.
4. Criley JM, Lewis KB, Humphries JO, Ross RS. Prolapse of the mitral valve: Clinical and cine-angiocardiographic findings. *Br Heart J* 1966; 28:488–496.
5. Barlow JB, Bosman CK, Pocock WA, Marchland P. Late systolic murmurs and non-ejection ("mid-late") systolic clicks: An analysis of 90 patients. *Br Heart J* 1968; 30:203–218.
6. Pomerance A. Ballooning deformity (mucoid degeneration) of atrioventricular valves. *Br Heart J* 1969; 31:343–351.
7. O'Rourke RA, Crawford MH. The systolic click-murmur syndrome: Clinical recognition and management. *Curr Probl Cardiol* 1976; 1(1):1.
8. Lucas RV Jr, Edwards JE. The floppy mitral valve. *Curr Probl Cardiol* 1982; 7:1–48.
9. Cheitlin MD, Byrd RC. Prolapsed mitral valve: The commonest disease? *Curr Probl Cardiol* 1984; 8:1–54.
10. Fontana ME, Sparks EA, Boudoulas H, Wooley CF. Mitral valve prolapse in the mitral valve prolapse syndrome. *Curr Probl Cardiol* 1991; 16:315–375.
11. O'Rourke RA. The mitral valve prolapse syndrome. In: Chizner MA, ed. *Classic Teachings in Clinical Cardiology.* Cedar Grove, NJ: Laennec; 1966; 1049–1070.
12. Devereux RB. Recent developments in the diagnosis and management of mitral valve prolapse. *Curr Opin Cardiol* 1995; 10:107–116.
13. Perloff JK, Roberts WC. The mitral apparatus. Functional anatomy of mitral regurgitation. *Circulation* 1972; 46:227–239.
14. Guthrie RG, Edwards JE. Pathology of the myxomatous mitral valve: Its nature, secondary changes and complications. *Minn Med* 1976; 59:637–647.
15. Salazar AE, Edwards JE. Friction lesions of ventricular endocardium: Relation to chordae tendineae of mitral valve. *Arch Pathol* 1970; 90:364–376.
16. Tamura K, Fukuda Y, Ishizaki M, Masuda Y, Yamanaka N, Ferrans VJ. Abnormalities in elastic fibers and other connective-tissue components of floppy mitral valve. *Am Heart J* 1995; 129:1149–1158.
17. Devereux RB, Brown WT, Kramer-Fox R, Sachs I. Inheritance of mitral valve prolapse: Effect of age and sex on gene expression. *Ann Intern Med* 1982; 97:826–832.
18. Shell WE, Walton JA, Clifford ME, Willis PW III. The familial occurrence of the syndrome of mid-late systolic click and late systolic murmur. *Circulation* 1969; 39:327–338.
19. Savage DD, Garrison RJ, Devereux RB, Castelli WP, Anderson SJ, Levy D, et al. Mitral valve prolapse in the general population. I: Epidemiologic features: The Framingham Study. *Am Heart J* 1983; 106:571–576.
20. Procacci PM, Savran SV, Schrieter SL, Bryson AL. Prevalence of clinical mitral valve prolapse in 1169 young women. *N Engl J Med* 1976; 294:1086–1088.
21. Leier CV, Call TD, Fulkerson PK, Wooley CF. The spectrum of cardiac defects in the Ehlers-Danlos syndrome, types I & III. *Ann Intern Med* 1980; 92:171–178.
22. Lebwohl MG, Distefano D, Prioleau PG, Uram M, Yannuzzi LA, Fleischmajer R. Pseudoxanthoma elasticum and mitral valve prolapse. *N Engl J Med* 1982; 307:228–231.
23. Schwartz T, Gotsman MS: Mitral valve prolapse in osteogenesis imperfecta. *Isr J Med Sci* 1981; 17:1087–1088.
24. Udoshi MB, Shah A, Fisher VJ, Dolgin M. Incidence of mitral valve prolapse in subjects with thoracic skeletal abnormalities—a prospective study. *Am Heart J* 1979; 97:303–311.
25. Salomon J, Shah PM, Heinle RA. Thoracic skeletal abnormalities in idiopathic mitral valve prolapse. *Am J Cardiol* 1975; 36:32–36.
26. Bon Tempo CP, Ronan JA Jr. Radiographic appearance of the thorax in systolic click–late systolic murmur syndrome. *Am J Cardiol* 1975; 36:27–31.
27. Crawford MH, O'Rourke RA. Mitral valve prolapse syndrome. In: Isselbacher KJ, Adams RD, Braunwald E, et al (eds): *Update I. Harrison's Principles of Internal Medicine.* New York: McGraw-Hill; 1981:91–152.
28. Pickering NJ, Brody JI, Barrett MJ. von Willebrand syndromes and mitral valve prolapse. *N Engl J Med* 1981; 305:131–134.
29. Rosenberg CA, Derman GH, Grabb WC, Buda AJ. Hypomastia and mitral valve prolapse. Evidence of a linked embryologic and mesenchymal dysplasia. *N Engl J Med* 1983; 309: 1230–1232.
30. Tei C, Sakamaki T, Shah PM, Meerbaum S, Kondo S, Shimoura K, et al. Mitral valve prolapse in short-term experimental coronary occlusion: A possible mechanism of ischemic mitral regurgitation. *Circulation* 1983; 68:183–189.
31. Crawford MH. Mitral valve prolapse due to coronary artery disease. *Am J Med* 1977; 62:447–451.
32. Tomaru T, Uchida Y, Mohri N. Post-inflammatory mitral and aortic valve prolapse: A clinical and pathological study. *Circulation* 1987; 76:68–76.
33. Lembo NJ, Dell'Italia LJ, Crawford MH, Miller JF, Richards KL, O'Rourke RA. Mitral valve prolapse in patients with prior rheumatic fever. *Circulation* 1988; 77:830–836.
34. Marcus RH, Sareli P, Pocock WA, Meyer TE, Magalhaes MP, Grieve T, et al. Functional anatomy of severe mitral regurgitation in active rheumatic carditis. *Am J Cardiol* 1986; 63:577–584.
35. Crawford MH, O'Rourke RA. Mitral valve prolapse: A cardiomyopathic state? *Prog Cardiovasc Dis* 1984; 27:133–139.
36. Lax D, Eicher M, Goldberg SJ. Mild dehydration induces echocardiographic signs of mitral valve prolapse in healthy females with prior normal cardiac findings. *Am Heart J* 1992; 124:1533–1540.
37. Aufderheide S, Lax D, Goldberg SJ. Gender differences in dehydration-induced mitral valve prolapse. *Am Heart J* 195; 129(1):83–86.
38. Krivokapich J, Child JS, Dadourian BJ, Perloff JK. Reassessment of echocardiographic criteria for the diagnosis of mitral valve prolapse. *Am J Cardiol* 1988; 61:131–135.
39. Fukuda N, Oki T, Iuchi A, Tabata T, Manabe K, Kageji Y, et al. Predisposing factors for severe mitral regurgitation in idiopathic mitral valve prolapse. *Am J Cardiol* 1995; 76(7):503–507.
40. Gaffney FA, Karlsson ES, Campbell W, Schutte JE, Nixon JV, Willerson JT, et al. Autonomic dysfunction in women with mitral valve prolapse. *Circulation* 1979; 59:894–899.
41. Boudoulas H, Reynolds JC, Mazzaferri E, Wooley CF. Metabolic studies in mitral valve prolapse syndrome. *Circulation* 1980; 61:1200–1205.
42. Boudoulas H, Reynolds JC, Mazzaferri E, Wooley CF. Mitral valve prolapse syndrome: The effect of adrenergic stimulation. *J Am Coll Cardiol* 1983; 2:638–644.
43. Davies AO, Mares A, Pool JL, Taylor AA. Mitral valve prolapse with symptoms of beta-adrenergic hypersensitivity. Beta$_2$-adrenergic receptor supercoupling with desensitization of isoproterenol exposure. *Am J Med* 1987; 82:193–201.
44. Gaffney FA, Bastian BC, Lane LB, Taylor WF, Horton J, Schutte JE, et al. Abnormal cardiovascular regulation in the mitral valve prolapse syndrome. *Am J Cardiol* 1983; 52:316–320.
45. Anwar A, Kohn SR, Dunn JF, Hymer TK, Kennedy GT, Crawford MH, et al. Altered beta-adrenergic receptor function in subjects with symptomatic mitral valve prolapse. *Am J Med Sci* 1991; 302:89–97.

46. Santos AD, Puthenpurakal MK, Ahmad H, Wallace WA, Matthew PK, Hilal A. Orthostatic hypotension: A commonly unrecognized cause of symptoms in mitral valve prolapse. *Am J Med* 1981; 71:746–750.

47. Fontana ME, Pence HL, Leighton RF, Wooley CF. The varying clinical spectrum of the systolic click–late systolic murmur syndrome. *Circulation* 1970; 41:807–816.

48. Betriu A, Wigle ED, Felderhof CH, McLoughlin MJ. Prolapse of the posterior leaflet of the mitral valve associated with secundum atrial septal defect. *Am J Cardiol* 1975; 35:363–369.

49. LeWinter MM, Hoffman JR, Shell WE, Kárliner JHS, O'Rourke RA. Phuenylephrine-induced atypical chest pain in patients with prolapsing mitral valve leaflets. *Am J Cardiol* 1974; 34:12–18.

50. Sabom MB, Curry RC Jr, Pepine CJ, Christie LG, Conti CR. Ergonovine testing for coronary artery spasm in patients with angiographic mitral valve prolapse. *Cath Cardiovasc Diagn* 1978; 4:265–274.

51. Barnett HJM, Jones MW, Boughner DR, Kostuck WJ. Cerebral ischemic events associated with prolapsing mitral valve. *Arch Neurol* 1976; 33:777–782.

52. Boughner DR, Barnett HJM. The enigma of the risk of stroke in mitral valve prolapse. *Stroke* 1985; 16:175–177.

53. Barletta GA, Gagliardi R, Benvenuti L, Fantini F. Cerebral ischemic attacks as a complication of aortic and mitral valve prolapse. *Stroke* 1985; 16:219–223.

54. Jones HR Jr, Nagger CZ, Seljan MP, Downing LL. Mitral valve prolapse and cerebral ischemic events. A comparison between a neurology population with stroke and a cardiology population with mitral valve prolapse observed for five years. *Stroke* 1982; 13:451–453.

55. Barnett HJM, Boughner DR, Taylor DW, Cooper PE, Kostuk VJ, Nichol PM. Further evidence relating mitral valve prolapse to cerebral ischemic event. *N Engl J Med* 1980; 302:139–144.

56. Petty GW, Orencia AJ, Khandheria BK, Whisnant JP. A population-based study of stroke in the setting of mitral valve prolapse; risk factors and infarct subtype classification. *Mayo Clin Proc* 1994; 69:632–634.

57. Orencia AJ, Petty GW, Khandheria BK, O'Fallon WM, Whisnant JP. Mitral valve prolapse and the risk of stroke after initial cerebral ischemia. *Neurology* 1995; 45:1083–1086.

58. Wilson LA, Keeling PW, Malcolm AD, Russel RW, Webb-Peploe MM. Visual complications of mitral leaflet prolapse. *Br Med J* 1977; 2:86–88.

59. Chesler E, King RA, Edwards JE. The myxomatous mitral valve and sudden death. *Circulation* 1983; 67:632–639.

60. Weis AJ, Salcedo EE, Stewart WJ, Lever HM, Klein AL, Thomas JD. Anatomic explanation of mobile systolic clicks: Implications for the clinical and echocardiographic diagnosis of mitral valve prolapse. *Am Heart J* 1995; 129:314–320.

61. Bhutto ZR, Barron JT, Liebson PR, Uretz EF, Parrillo JE. Electrocardiographic abnormalities in mitral valve prolapse. *Am J Cardiol* 1992; 70:265–266.

62. Schaal SF. Ventricular arrhythmias in patients with mitral valve prolapse. *Cardiovasc Clin* 1992; 22(1):307–316.

63. Marks AR, Choong CY, Sanfilippo AJ, Ferre M, Weyman AE. Identification of high-risk and low-risk subgroups of patients with mitral valve prolapse. *N Engl J Med* 1989; 320:1031–1036.

64. Shah PM. Echocardiographic diagnosis of mitral valve prolapse. *J Am Soc Echocardiog* 1994; 7(3 pt 1):286–293.

65. Klein GJ, Kostuck WJ, Bougher DR, Chamberlain MJ. Stress myocardial imaging in mitral leaflet prolapse syndrome. *Am J Cardiol* 1978; 42:746–750.

66. Allen H, Harris A, Leatham A. Significance and prognosis of an isolated late systolic murmur: A 9- to 22-year follow-up. *Br Heart J* 1974; 36:525–532.

67. Mills P, Rose J, Hollingsworth J, Amara I, Craige E. Long-term prognosis of mitral valve prolapse. *N Engl J Med* 1977; 297:13–18.

68. Nishimura RA, McGood MD, Shub C, Miller FA Jr, Ilstrup DM, Tajik AJ. Echocardiographically documented mitral-valve prolapse: Long-term follow-up of 237 patients. *N Engl J Med* 1985; 313:1305–1309.

69. Düren DR, Becker AE, Dunning AJ. Long-term follow-up of idiopathic mitral valve prolapse in 300 patients: A prospective study. *J Am Coll Cardiol* 1988; 11:42–47.

70. Boudoulas H, Kolibash BH, Wooley CF. Mitral valve prolapse: A heterogenous disorder. *Prim Cardiol* 1991; 17:29–43.

71. Zuppiroli A, Rinaldi M, Kramer-Fox R, Favilli S, Roman MJ, Devereux RB. Natural history of mitral valve prolapse. *Am J Cardiol* 1995; 75:1028–1032.

72. Stoddard MF, Prince CR, Dillon S, Longaker RA, Morris GT, Liddell NE. Exercise-induced mitral regurgitation is a predictor of morbid events in subjects with mitral valve prolapse. *J Am Coll Cardiol* 1995; 25:693–699.

73. Gooch AS, Vicencio F, Maranbao V, Goldberg H. Arrhythmias and left ventricle asynergy in the prolapsing mitral leaflet. *Am J Cardiol* 1972; 29:611–620.

74. Marshall CE, Shappel SD. Sudden death and the ballooning posterior leaflet syndrome: Detailed anatomic and histochemical investigation. *Arch Pathol* 1974; 98:134–138.

75. Clemens JD, Horwitz RI, Jaffe CC, Feinstein AR, Stanton BF. A controlled evaluation of the risk of bacterial endocarditis in persons with mitral valve prolapse. *N Engl J Med* 1982; 307:776–781.

76. Devereux RB, Frary CJ, Kramer-Fox R, Roberts RB, Ruchlin HS. Cost-effectiveness of infective endocarditis prophylaxis for mitral valve prolapse with or without a mitral regurgitant murmur. *Am J Cardiol* 1994; 74:1024–1029.

77. Dajani AS, Bisno AL, Chung KJ, Durack DT, Freed M, Gerber MA, et al. Prevention of bacterial endocarditis. Recommendations by the American Heart Association. *JAMA* 1990; 264:2919–2922.

78. Bansal RC, Shah PM. Usefulness of echo-Doppler in management of patients with valvular heart disease. *Curr Probl Cardiol* 1989; 14:287–350.

79. Panidis IP, McAllister M, Ross J, Mintz GS. Prevalence and severity of mitral regurgitation in the mitral valve prolapse syndrome; a Doppler echocardiographic study of 80 patients. *J Am Coll Cardiol* 1986; 7:975–981.

80. Winkle RA, Lopes MG, Goodman DJ, Fitzgerald JW, Schroeder JS, Harrison DC. Propranolol for patients with mitral valve prolapse. *Am Heart J* 1977; 93:422–427.

81. Galloway AC, Colvin SB, Baumann FG, Harty S, Spencer FC. Current concepts of mitral valve reconstruction for mitral insufficiency. *Circulation* 1988; 78:1087–1098.

82. Cheitlin MD. The timing of surgery in mitral and aortic valve disease. *Curr Probl Cardiol* 1987; 12:75–149.

83. Cosgrove DM, Stewart WJ. Mitral valvuloplasty. *Curr Probl Cardiol* 1989; 14:359–415.

84. Kirklin JW. Mitral valve repair for mitral incompetence. *Mod Concepts Cardiovasc Dis* 1987; 56:7–11.

85. Cohn LH, Couper GS, Aranki SF, Rizzo RJ, Kinchla NM, Collins JJ Jr. Long-term results of mitral valve reconstruction for regurgitation of the myxomatous mitral valve. *J Thorac Cardiovasc Surg* 1994; 107:143–150.

86. Eishi K, Kawazoe K, Sasako Y, Kosakai Y, Kitoh Y, Kawashima Y. Comparison of repair techniques for mitral valve prolapse. *J Heart Valve Dis* 1994; 3:432–438.

87. Perier P, Clausnizer B, Mistarz K. Carpentier "sliding leaflet" technique for repair of the mitral valve: Early results. *Ann Thorac Surg* 1994; 57:383–386.

66

TRICUSPID VALVE, PULMONIC VALVE, AND MULTIVALVULAR DISEASE

Robert A. O'Rourke / Charles E. Rackley / Jesse E. Edwards / Robert B. Karp / Nevin M. Katz

DEFINITION, ETIOLOGY, AND PATHOLOGY

Tricuspid Valve Disease

Tricuspid regurgitation occurs when the tricuspid valve allows blood to enter the right atrium during a right ventricular (RV) contraction. *Tricuspid stenosis* results from obstruction to diastolic flow across the valve during diastolic filling of the right ventricle.

Diseases causing tricuspid regurgitation are more numerous than those causing tricuspid stenosis. Importantly, the normal tricuspid valve commonly does not completely coapt in systole, as is shown by the frequent occurrence of tricuspid regurgitation jets on Doppler ultrasound. Usually the volume of regurgitant blood is so small that the tricuspid regurgitation is silent; this finding occurs in 24 to 96 percent of normal individuals and thus must be considered a variant of normal by Doppler ultrasound.[1–3]

Pathologic tricuspid valve regurgitation is most commonly due to diseases that cause RV dilatation and failure[4]; left ventricular (LV) failure and/or pulmonary hypertension can result in tricuspid regurgitation (Table 66-1).

Primary diseases of the tricuspid valve apparatus, which includes the tricuspid annulus, the leaflets, the chordae, the papillary muscle, and the RV wall, also cause tricuspid regurgitation (Table 66-1).[5–7] The most common etiology of isolated tricuspid regurgitation is infective endocarditis in drug addicts[8] (see Chap. 82). Less common causes include myocardial infarction, trauma, carcinoid, leaflet prolapse, and congenital abnormalities such as atrial septal defect and Ebstein's

TABLE 66-1

DISEASES CAUSING ACQUIRED TRICUSPID VALVE REGURGITATION

DISEASES CAUSING PULMONARY HYPERTENSION APPARATUS

All left ventricular diseases with left ventricular failure
Mitral stenosis/mitral regurgitation
Pulmonary venous obstruction
Diseases causing an increase in pulmonary vascular resistance
  Primary pulmonary hypertension
  Acquired pulmonary vascular disease (atrial septal defects), ventricular septal defects, patent ductus arteriosus)
  Intrinsic pulmonary disease (chronic obstructive pulmonary disease, pulmonary fibrosis, and pulmonary resection)
  Collagen vascular diseases
Pulmonary emboli, acute and chronic

PRIMARY DISEASES OF THE TRICUSPID VALVE

Rheumatic heart disease
Rheumatoid arthritis
Trauma, penetrating and nonpenetrating
Radiation therapy
Carcinoid heart disease
Right atrial myxoma
Infective endocarditis
Eosinophilic myocarditis
Prosthetic and bioprosthetic valve malfunction, including thrombosis and calcification
Right ventricular myocardial infarction
Myxomatous tricuspid valve (tricuspid valve prolapse)

Source: Modified from Cheitlin and MacGregor.[21]
Reproduced with permission of the publisher and authors.

anomaly[9–13] (see also Chap. 70). Tricuspid valve regurgitation has been reported to occur in patients with rheumatoid arthritis, radiation therapy, and Marfan's syndrome.[5] Primary involvement of the tricuspid valve due to rheumatic fever results in tricuspid stenosis usually associated with tricuspid regurgitation (Fig. 66-1).

The most common cause of tricuspid stenosis is rheumatic fever. This is usually associated with concomitant mitral stenosis. Isolated stenosis of the tricuspid valve can be seen with the carcinoid syndrome, infective endocarditis, endocardial fibroelastosis, endomyocardial fibrosis, and systemic lupus erythematosus among others[5–7] (Table 66-2). It has also been reported to occur in patients with Fabry's disease, Whipple's disease, and in patients receiving methysergide therapy.[5] Mechanical obstruction of the valve can occur with a right atrial myxoma, tumor metastases, and thrombi in the right atrium, each resulting in the hemodynamic abnormalities of tricuspid stenosis.[14,15] Additionally, RV inflow tract obstruction can be due to thrombosis, endocarditis, degeneration, or calcification affecting a prosthetic tricuspid valve.

In rheumatic tricuspid valve disease, alterations in the valve are characterized by fibrosis with contracture of the leaflets and commissural fusion. The former leads to tricuspid regurgitation, and the latter to tricuspid stenosis.[16] The stenotic component of rheumatic tricuspid valve disease is often minor and would go unrecognized clinically if it were not for the high flow across the valve caused by the coexistent regurgitation. Whenever the tricuspid valve is affected by rheumatic disease, there is also involvement of left-sided valves.[17].

Flammang and associates observed that 9.5 percent of cases requiring surgical replacement of both the mitral and aortic valves also had rheumatic involvement of the tricuspid valve.[18] Among cases undergoing mitral commissurotomy,

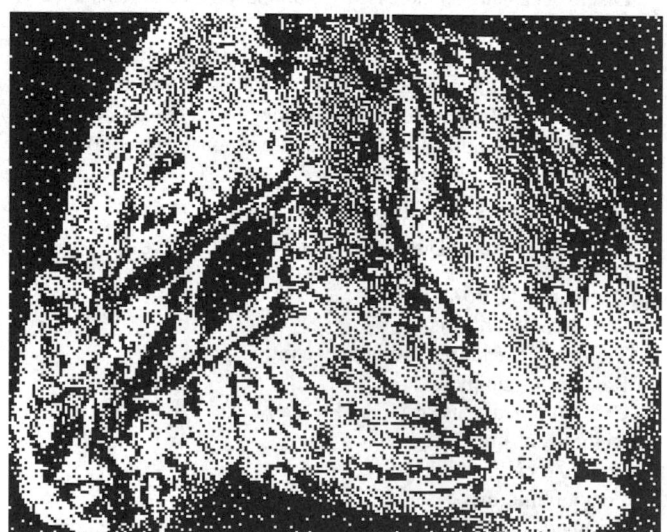

FIGURE 66-1
Tricuspid valves seen from below in chronic rheumatic endocarditis. Although the chordae are relatively uninvolved, there is fusion of the leaflets at the commissures creating a narrow and fixed orifice. The valve is both stenotic and regurgitant.

TABLE 66-2

DISEASES CAUSING ACQUIRED TRICUSPID VALVE STENOSIS

Rheumatic heart disease (usually with mitral stenosis)
Carcinoid heart disease
Fabry's disease
Whipple's disease
Endocardial fibroelastosis
Endomyocardial fibrosis
Methysergide therapy
Systemic lupus endocarditis
Right atrial myxoma or thrombus
Prosthetic valve thrombosis
Prosthetic valve infective endocarditis
Paraprosthetic valve degeneration and calcification

Source: Modified from Cheitlin and MacGregor.[21]
Reproduced with permission of the publisher and authors.

the incidence of clinically evident tricuspid disease was 3 percent. In a series of 217 autopsied cases of rheumatic heart disease, Cooke and White found 47 cases (22 percent) where the tricuspid valve was also involved by rheumatic disease.[19]

Carcinoid heart disease is seen in up to 53 percent of patients with malignant carcinoid tumor (usually originating in the ileum) with extensive metastases[20,21] (see Chap. 86). Carcinoid usually causes tricuspid regurgitation and stenosis and, less often, pulmonic stenosis and regurgitation.[21] Changes include deposits of fibrous tissue on the surfaces of these valves. Fibrous plaques can also develop on the endocardial surfaces of the right atrium and ventricle as well as on the intima of the coronary sinus and the pulmonary artery.[22] The hemodynamic effects result from the ridigity and contracture of the fibrous tissues deposited on the valves. Although tricuspid stenosis may result, the major functional abnormality is usually tricuspid regurgitation.

The most common type of tricuspid regurgitation is the secondary type and results from the enlargement of the orifice and annulus secondary to congestive heart failure with RV dilation due to LV disease (see Table 66-1). Tricuspid regurgitation may diminish when the heart failure is treated successfully but can be permanent with long-standing dilatation of the right ventricle.[23,24]

In infective endocarditis, the tricuspid regurgitation results from improper coaptation of the leaflets because of interposed vegetations (see Table 66-1). Major degrees of regurgitation may be due to rupture of chordae tendineae of the right ventricle or perforation of the valve leaflets.

Until recently, myocardial infarction was not considered a common cause of tricuspid regurgitation except when secondary to chronic congestive heart failure.[25] Rare cases were described from rupture of an RV papillary muscle.[25–28] Currently, RV infarction is being recognized more often and is frequently associated with tricuspid regurgitation, as documented by echocardiography.

Various degrees of prolapse of the tricuspid valve are commonly present in the general population and may occur in 3 to 54 percent in patients with mitral valve prolapse[21] (see also Chap. 65). Reported incidences of *severe* tricuspid regurgitation from prolapse have been relatively uncommon.[29]

External blunt trauma, most commonly occurring in automobile accidents, is a classic cause of tricuspid regurgitation. Isolated instances of rupture of a tricuspid papillary muscle have been described from external cardiopulmonary resuscitation.[30] Traumatic tricuspid regurgitation usually results from rupture of one or more of the components of the tensor apparatus, with disruption of the papillary muscle occurring more often than rupture of the chordae. Less frequently there is a laceration of leaflet tissue, and occasionally more than one of the anatomic elements of the valve are affected.[31,32] Occasionally, traumatic tricuspid regurgitation and ruptured ventricular septum coexist[33] (see also Chap. 87). Tricuspid regurgitation can also occur from iatrogenic trauma produced during an endomyocardial biopsy.[34,35] Mild tricuspid regurgitation often results when a pacemaker is placed across a normally functioning tricuspid valve.

Tolerance of traumatic tricuspid regurgitation varies, with up to 39 years of survival reported.[36–39] Patients with rupture of a papillary muscle tend to tolerate the tricuspid regurgitation less well than those in whom the trauma resulted in rupture of chordae.[37] Among reported cases of tricuspid regurgitation resulting from the rupture of the chordae, a traumatic etiology is more common than infective endocarditis.[40] Primary congenital lesions of the tricuspid valve that cause regurgitation are Ebstein's malformation and valvular dysplasia, as discussed in Chap. 70.

Pulmonic Valve Disease

Acquired lesions of the pulmonic valve generally lead to *pulmonic regurgitation* (Table 66-3). On rare occasions, an

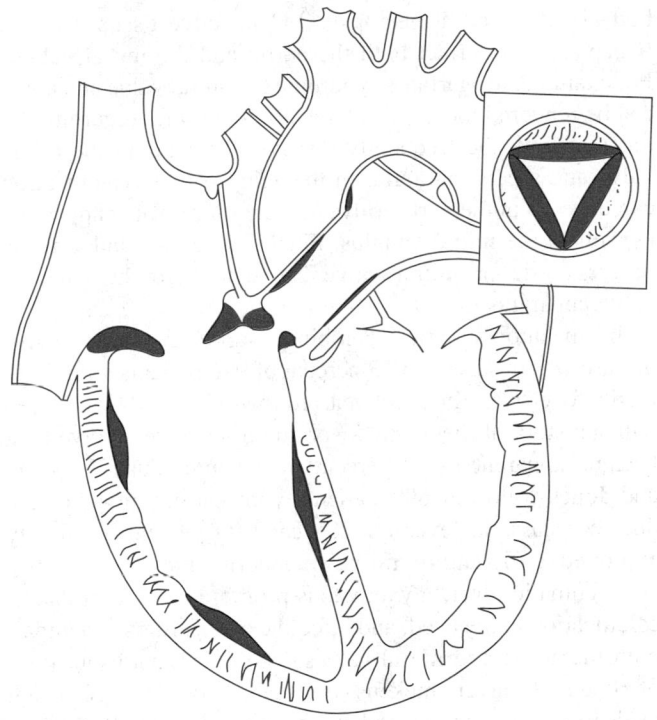

FIGURE 66-2

Carcinoid heart disease. Insert shows pulmonic stenosis. The leaflets of the tricuspid valve are thickened. The valve is predominantly incompetent and causes pulmonary regurgitation. Fibrous plaques are deposited on the lining of the right ventricle and pulmonary trunk. (From Edwards JE. Effects of malignant noncardiac tumors upon the cardiovascular system. *Cardiovasc Clin* 1971; 4:282. Reproduced with permission from the publisher and author.)

inflammatory process can create stenosis and regurgitation of the valve. Pulmonary hypertension from any cause, such as mitral stenosis, chronic lung disease, or pulmonary emboli, can produce pulmonic regurgitation. Inflammatory diseases such as endocarditis, rheumatic fever, and, on rare occasions, tuberculosis can result in pulmonic regurgitation.[41,42]

Pulmonic stenosis is created by obstruction to systolic flow across the valve and is most commonly congenital (see Chaps. 70 and 71). Sarcomas and myxomas can sometimes extend to the pulmonic valve, causing pulmonic stenosis.[43] Previous cardiac surgery on a congenital pulmonic valve lesion can result in pulmonic regurgitation. The carcinoid syndrome with cardiac involvement can create mild pulmonic stenosis and associated regurgitation[44] (Fig. 66-2). Compression of the pulmonary artery can stimulate valvular stenosis and is rarely produced by tumor, aneurysm, or even constrictive pericarditis.

Multivalvular Disease

Rheumatic fever remains an important cause of combined disease of the mitral and aortic valves. Primary involvement of the tricuspid valve in the rheumatic process is unusual, and more commonly tricuspid regurgitation is affected by RV failure secondary to LV decompensation in valvular heart disease. A high incidence of anatomic lesions involving two or more valves is present when the characteristic Aschoff

TABLE 66-3

ACQUIRED LESIONS OF THE PULMONIC VALVE

Pulmonary hypertension with pulmonic regurgitation
   Mitral stenosis
   Chronic lung disease
   Pulmonary emboli
Inflammatory lesions
   Endocarditis
   Rheumatic fever
   Tuberculosis
Tumors
   Sarcoma
   Myxoma
Previous surgery or angioplasty for congenital lesions
Mediastinal lesions
   Tumor
   Aneurysm
   Constrictive pericarditis
Miscellaneous
   Carcinoid syndrome

body is observed at necropsy.[45] Connective tissue diseases (Chap. 85) can affect both the aortic and the mitral valves. For example, in Marfan's syndrome the mitral valve apparatus can be rendered incompetent, resulting in mitral regurgitation together with the frequently observed changes in the aortic valve and ascending aorta. In the aging patient, calcification can develop in the aortic valve and the mitral valve apparatus as well in the mitral annulus. Finally, infective endocarditis of the aortic or mitral valve can extend to the adjacent valve apparatus.

In an autopsy series, combined aortic and mitral valve disease was observed in 33 percent of 996 patients with rheumatic fever.[46,47] In a 30-year follow-up of 1042 children with a history of rheumatic fever, multiple valve involvement became apparent in 50 percent of the individuals.[48] Bland and Jones followed 699 patients with cardiac involvement due to rheumatic fever for 20 years; 99 percent eventually exhibited aortic and mitral valve abnormalities.[49]

Rheumatic fever, myxomatous proliferation and prolapse, calcification in the aged, and infective endocarditis can impair both the aortic and mitral valves. The inflammatory process of rheumatic fever thickens and scars valve leaflets, which leads to fusion, fibrosis, and calcification (Fig. 66-3). Roberts and Virmani reported that histologic evidence of rheumatic fever confirmed by the Aschoff body was frequently associated with anatomic lesions in two or more cardiac valves.[45]

Myxomatous proliferation and valvular prolapse occur in the aortic, tricuspid, and pulmonic valves as well as in the mitral valve (Fig. 66-4). Fusiform aneurysms of the aortic sinus and ascending aorta can develop in Marfan's syndrome, while changes of dilated annulus, prolapse, ruptured chordae, and annular calcification can affect the mitral valve (Fig.

66-5). Annular dilatation, with or without prolapse, is a major cause of mitral regurgitation in Marfan's syndrome,[50] and most of the patients with Marfan's syndrome have mitral valve prolapse (see also Chaps. 65 and 85).

In aging patients, calcification can involve the aortic and mitral valves. Stenosis of the aortic valve is common, whereas mitral annular calcification usually creates regurgitation (Fig. 66-6).

Infective endocarditis can extend from either the aortic or mitral valve to the adjacent valve through the inflammatory process (Fig. 66-7).

PATHOPHYSIOLOGY

Tricuspid Valve Disease

In tricuspid regurgitation, the systolic blood flow into the right atrium elevates the mean right atrial pressure.[51] Regurgitant flow produces a prominent *cv* wave reflected through the venous system. Diastolic volume overload of the right ventricle causes further dilatation of the right ventricle and movement of the intraventricular septum toward the left ventricle during diastole. RV failure further raises the mean right atrial and vena caval pressures and results in systemic venous congestion and signs of RV failure.[21]

Tricuspid stenosis decreases diastolic flow across the valve, elevates the right atrial pressure, and reduces the cardiac output.[52,53] With tricuspid stenosis, there is stiffening of the valve by fibrosis or disease and commissural fusion, both of which narrow the effective valvular orifice.[21] Flow from systemic veins or right atrium into the right ventricle is obstructed, and a pressure gradient develops in diastole between

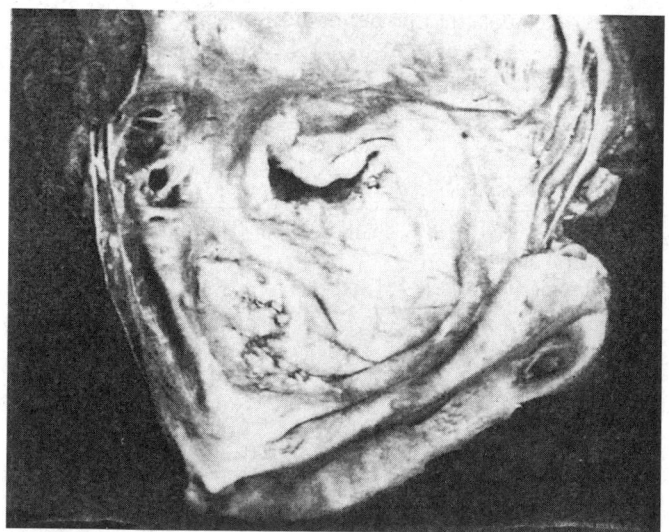

A   *B*

FIGURE 66-3

Rheumatic aortic stenosis and regurgitation and rheumatic mitral stenosis specimens from a 57-year-old woman. *A.* Aortic valve, unopened and viewed from above. Fusion of each of the three aortic valvular commissures, causing reduction in caliber of the orifice of the aortic valve, is apparent. The associated shortening of the cusps results in aortic regurgitation. *B.* Mitral valve, unopened and viewed from above, and opened left atrium. The mitral valve shows fusion at each of the commissures. The orifice is reduced in caliber. The left atrium is large, and calcification of the posterior part of the left atrial wall is present (*lower part of figure*).

the right atrium and right ventricle. The normal area of the tricuspid valve is 7 cm^2, and impairment of RV filling occurs when the valve area is reduced to less than 1.5 cm^2. Elevation of the mean right atrial pressure above 10 mmHg usually results in peripheral edema. Development of atrial fibrillation produces a higher right atrial pressure in tricuspid stenosis than when sinus rhythm and normal right atrial contraction are present. The hemodynamic abnormalities in tricuspid stenosis can be further influenced by the often coexisting mitral stenosis. Reduced RV flow in tricuspid valve obstruction has been proposed as a mechanism for protection against severe pulmonary hypertension.

Pulmonic Valve Disease

Pulmonic regurgitation is the most frequently acquired lesion of the pulmonic valve (see Table 66-3). Regurgitation may be secondary to pulmonary hypertension or may be caused by primary abnormalities in the leaflets. Pulmonic regurgitation imposes a volume overload on the right ventricle, and if pulmonic hypertension preexists, the overload is superimposed on hypertrophied myocardium. Volume overload of the right ventricle may cause an increase in diastolic volume of the chamber, an increase in RV stroke volume, and subsequent RV failure resulting in tricuspid regurgitation.[21] Fortunately, isolated pulmonic valvular regurgitation can usually be tolerated for a long time without cardiac decompensation.[54]

Multivalvular Disease

Multivalvular diseases affecting the mitral and aortic valves can produce a pressure overload, volume overload, or combi-

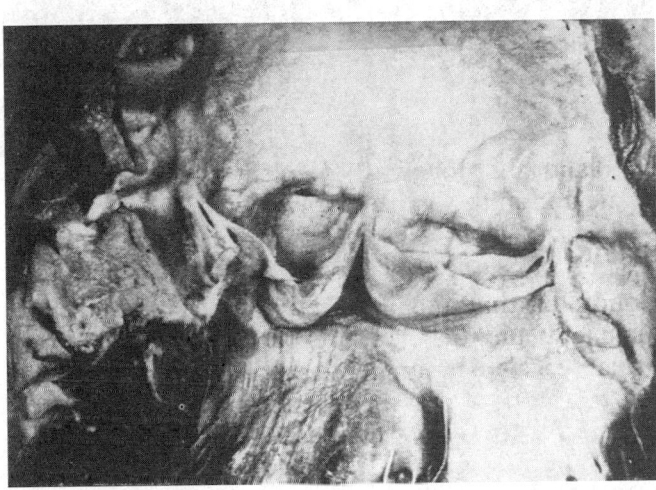

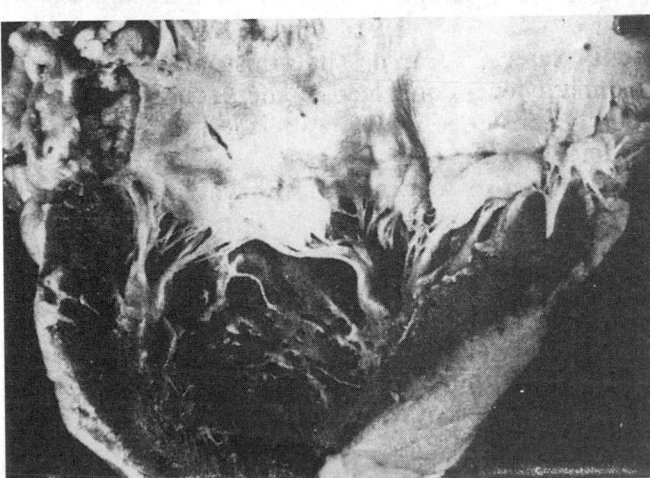

FIGURE 66-4
Prolapsed mitral valve and prolapsed aortic valve. *A.* Specimen of aortic valve from a 61-year-old man. The aortic valve shows redundance or prolapse of its right cusp. *B.* Specimen of mitral valve from a 73-year-old woman. The mitral valve shows prominent evidence of prolapse involving the posterior leaflet (*right*) and the posterior half of the anterior leaflet.

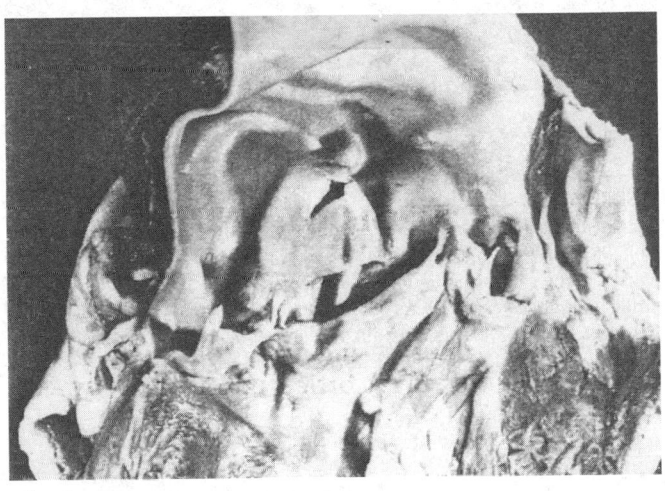

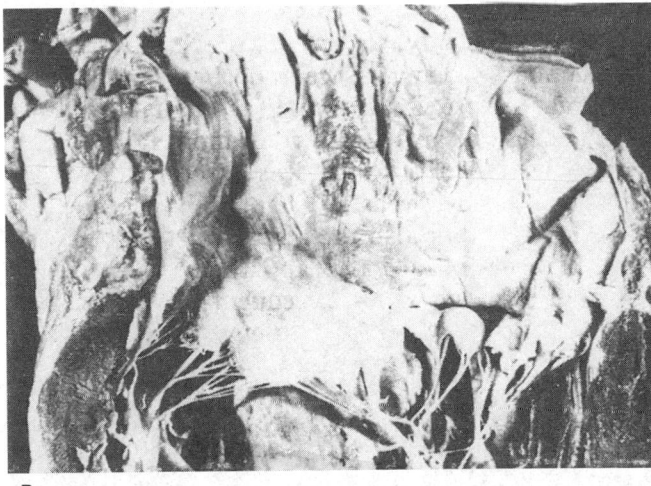

FIGURE 66-5
Floppy mitral valve and limited dissecting aneurysm of ascending aorta leading to aortic regurgitation—specimen from a 60-year-old man. *A.* Ascending aorta and aortic valve. The ascending aorta exhibits a laceration leading to a false channel within the aortic wall in which a hematoma is present (seen on each side of the opened aorta). Secondary distortion of the aortic valvular mechanism caused aortic regurgitation. *B.* Mitral valve, left atrium, and a portion of the left ventricle. The posterior leaflet of the mitral valve (*right*) shows several areas of prolapse.

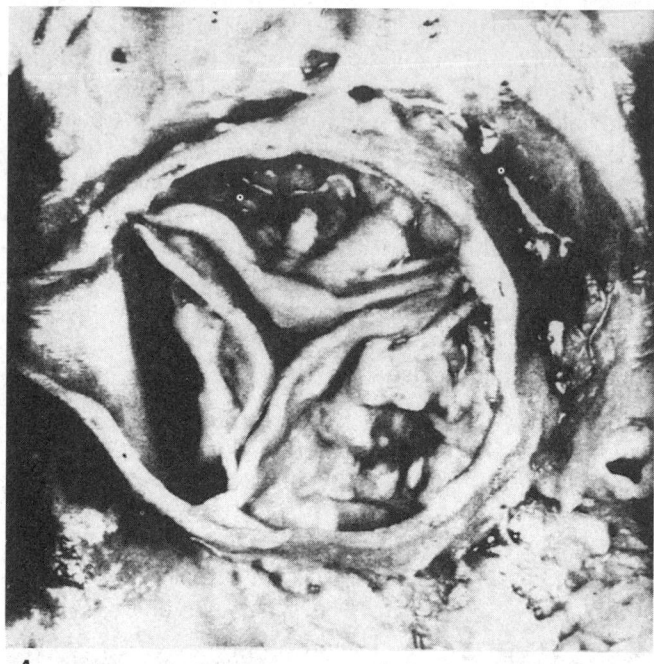

A

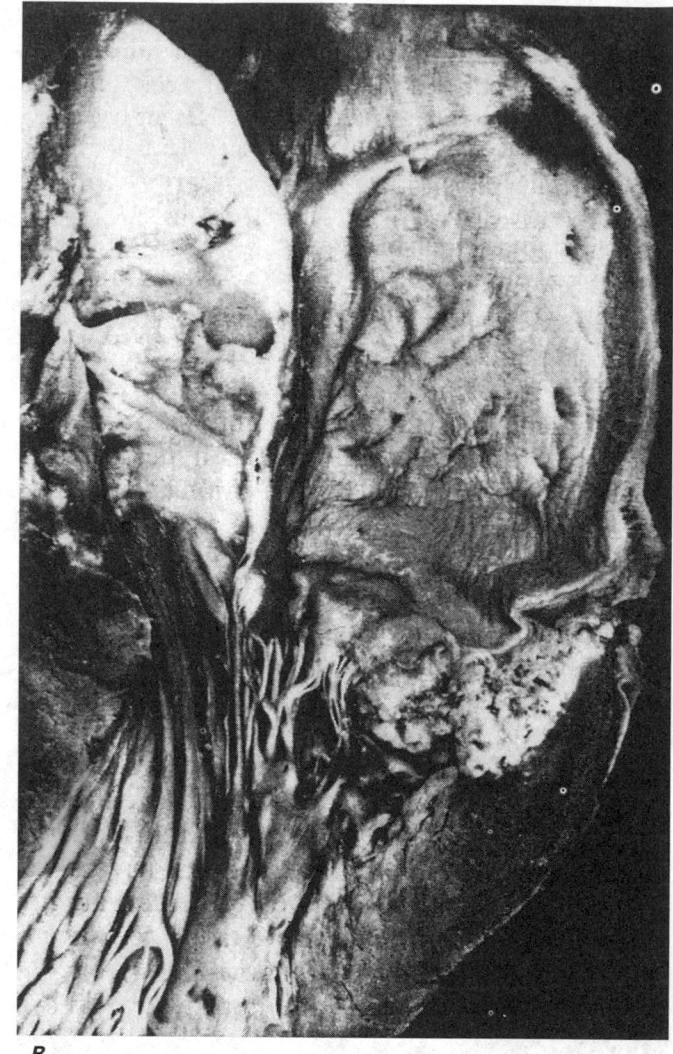

B

FIGURE 66-6
Senile calcific aortic stenosis and calcification of the mitral ring—specimens from two different individuals. *A*. Aortic valve. Classic example of senile calcific aortic stenosis in unopened aortic valve viewed from above. *B*. Left atrium, mitral valve, and lateral wall of left ventricle. Sagittal section through left atrial and left ventricular walls reveals a calcified mass at the junction of the atrium, the left ventricle, and the posterior mitral leaflet.

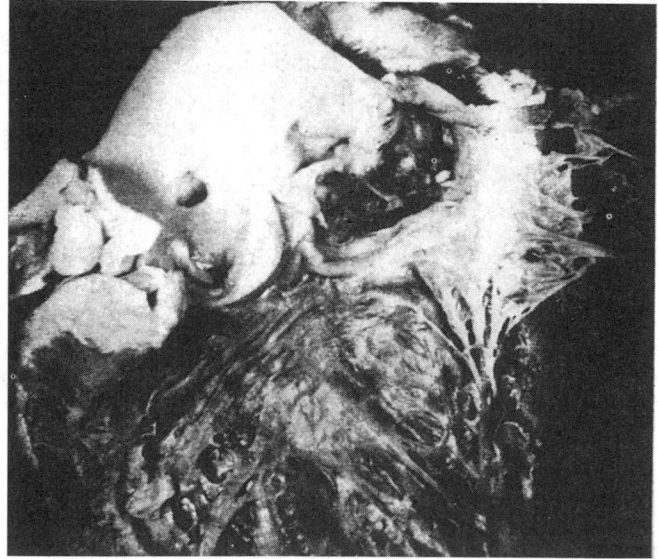

A

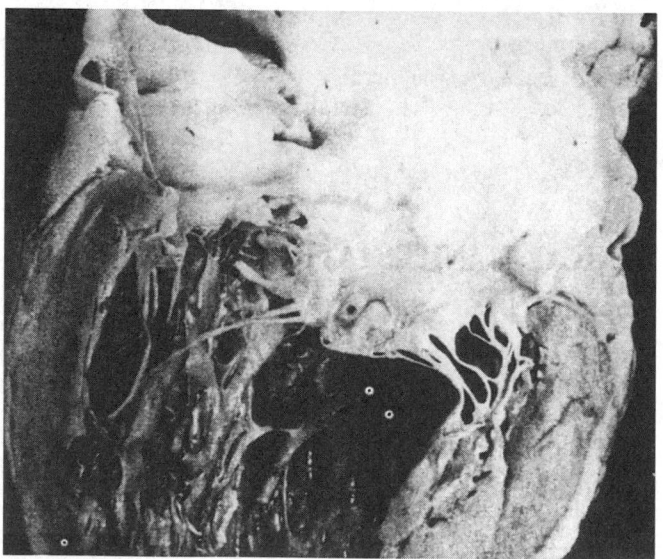

B

FIGURE 66-7
Bacterial endocarditis—specimens from a 36-year-old man. *A*. Aortic valve. The base of the aortic valve shows major destruction of a cusp with extension of inflammation onto the subjacent mitral valve. Near the free edge of the mitral valve, its ventricular aspect shows an ostium of a nonruptured mycotic aneurysm. *B*. Mitral valve, left atrium, and left ventricle. The lobulated mycotic aneurysm of the mitral valve lies near its free edge.

nations of the two.[55] In the presence of combined valvular lesions, the pressure overload will cause concentric LV hypertrophy, even if myocardial failure develops.[56] An LV volume overload will result from aortic and mitral regurgitation, and further dilatation will follow with development of heart failure.[57] The combination of mitral stenosis and aortic regurgitation usually results in a volume overload on the left ventricle associated with LV pressure-volume work and myocardial oxygen consumption.[58,59] Impaired contractility with the development of heart failure decreases the mechanical efficiency of the left ventricle.

Important physiologic considerations in combined valvular disease are the predominance of a single valvular lesion in altering hemodynamics and the potential failure to identify the presence of a second abnormal valve. Mitral stenosis produces left atrial and pulmonary venous hypertension with eventual pulmonary hypertension and RV failure, even though aortic stenosis may also be present. Despite the presence of mitral stenosis, concomitant aortic stenosis can create pressure overload and hypertrophy of the left ventricle. When mitral regurgitation accompanies aortic stenosis, the pressure and volume overloads create both dilatation and hypertrophy of the left ventricle. Left atrial enlargement and elevation of pulmonary artery pressure eventually accompany this condition. In regurgitation of both mitral and aortic valves, severe LV dilatation develops accompanied by compensatory LV hypertrophy.[60] LV compliance increases in mitral and aortic regurgitation, resulting in small elevations of end-diastolic pressure in the left ventricle and left atrium for larger end-diastolic volumes.[61,62] Abnormalities in both early and late diastolic filling can accompany valvular regurgitation.[63] Significant LV hypertrophy can impair filling in both the early and late phases of diastole.

In all combinations of aortic and mitral valve lesions, pulmonary congestion and elevated pulmonary capillary pressure usually follow significant depression of the contractile state of the left ventricle. Left atrial enlargement produced by either stenosis or regurgitation of the mitral valve is often associated with atrial fibrillation. Alterations in pulmonary blood flow and cardiac rhythm commonly accompany the left ventricle pressure-volume overload in combined mitral and aortic valve disease.

Tricuspid regurgitation usually accompanies RV dilatation secondary to pulmonary hypertension from any combination of mitral or aortic valve diseases. Tricuspid stenosis almost invariably is accompanied by disease of the mitral valve and can create significant elevations of the right atrial and central venous pressures.

CLINICAL MANIFESTATIONS

Symptoms

TRICUSPID VALVE DISEASE

Since tricuspid regurgitation generally accompanies LV failure or mitral stenosis, presenting symptoms include dyspnea, orthopnea, and peripheral edema.[64] Even though LV failure is usually present, paroxysmal nocturnal dyspnea is often absent. Tricuspid regurgitation under these conditions may occasionally ameliorate the pulmonary symptoms and provide a physiologic basis for the alleviation of left-sided heart failure by the development of right-sided heart failure. Some patients also have less pulmonary edema due to the development of pulmonary arteriolar disease. If the tricuspid regurgitation is produced by infective endocarditis, symptoms of febrile illness may be accompanied by fatigue and peripheral edema.

The most frequent symptoms in tricuspid stenosis are dyspnea and fatigue. When mitral stenosis coexists, the development of significant tricuspid stenosis can diminish the paroxysmal symptoms of dyspnea, pulmonary congestion, and pulmonary hypertension.[14,15] Occasionally, patients with tricuspid stenosis complain of prominent pulsations in the neck veins, which may precede the development of peripheral edema.

PULMONIC VALVE DISEASE

Clinical manifestations of acquired pulmonic valvular lesions depend on the severity of the hemodynamic impairment as well as on the extent of the underlying disease. Isolated pulmonic regurgitation can be tolerated without symptoms. Severe pulmonary hypertension may cause syncope in addition to shortness of breath and fatigue. With inflammatory lesions of the pulmonic valve, febrile manifestations and pulmonary infection may be present. The carcinoid syndrome is characterized by episodes of facial flushing, increased intestinal activity, diarrhea, and bronchospasm. Tumors involving the pulmonic valve may exert pressure from expansion and metastases that affect the heart and lungs.

MULTIVALVULAR DISEASE

Dyspnea is the most frequent complaint of patients with combined mitral and aortic valve disease.[65] With combined mitral and aortic stenosis, chest discomfort, palpitations, and syncope are frequent clinical manifestations. Symptoms of heart failure result from pulmonary congestion and usually include fluid retention. Although angina pectoris is uncommon in patients with predominant mitral regurgitation, this symptom is more frequent with regurgitation of both the aortic and mitral valves. Also, syncope is rare in predominant mitral regurgitation but may develop when regurgitation involves both aortic and mitral valves. Palpitations are present in the majority of patients.

Angina, dizziness, syncope, and palpitations are common symptoms in aortic stenosis when it is associated with mitral regurgitation. Angina may also be a symptom when aortic regurgitation and mitral stenosis are the predominant lesions; but the more frequent symptoms, dyspnea and fatigue, are attributed to pulmonary congestion and heart failure (see also Chaps. 63 to 65).

Physical Examination

TRICUSPID VALVE DISEASE

In patients with primary tricuspid regurgitation not due to pulmonary hypertension, there are large v waves in the jugular venous pulse. There is a dilated right ventricle with a precordial lift and right-sided third or fourth heart sounds. There is usually a long systolic murmur in the third and fourth intercostal space at the left sternal border that increases with inspiration. The murmur is often confined to early and mid-systole or may not be heard at all when there is small gradient between the right ventricle and right atrium during systole and a large regurgitant orifice (see also Chap. 10). When a large amount of blood returns to the right ventricle in diastole, a short diastolic rumble along the left sternal border may be heard. All of these findings are increased with inspiration (Rivero Carvallo's sign).[66] When RV failure occurs, the mean central venous pressure becomes elevated and the jugular veins are pulsatile and engorged. When tricuspid regurgitation is due to pulmonary hypertension, there is an accentuated pulmonic component of the second heart sound, and a high-pitched decrescendo diastolic murmur of pulmonic valve regurgitation is often heard with a greater intensity during inspiration in the second and third interspace along the left sternal border. In patients with tricuspid regurgitation and atrial fibrillation, there is a prominent *cv* wave in the internal jugular veins produced by the regurgitant flow into the right ventricle. Simultaneous auscultation of the heart remains the best method for timing venous pulsations. The characteristic physical finding of tricuspid regurgitation due to pulmonary hypertension is a holosystolic murmur at the left sternal border that increases during inspiration; there is a right ventricular–right atrial pressure gradient throughout systole. Although the murmur of mitral regurgitation may also be present, respiration exerts a predominant influence on tricuspid regurgitation with little alteration in the intensity of a mitral regurgitation murmur (see also Chap. 10).[66]

Tricuspid stenosis is frequently associated with lesions of the mitral and aortic valves. When sinus rhythm is present, the internal jugular veins will display the prominent *a* wave indicative of impaired RV diastolic filling with atrial systole. The *a* wave in the neck may be of moderate height and sometimes reaches the mandible.[14,15] Auscultation of the heart is required to confirm that the rise of the venous *a* wave is simultaneous with the first heart sound. The *cv* wave is small, and the *y* descent is slow and insignificant (see also Chap. 10).

PULMONIC VALVE DISEASE

If RV failure and tricuspid regurgitation have developed as a result of pulmonic regurgitation, a prominent *cv* wave will be present in the jugular venous pulse. Increased RV activity may be visible and palpable along the left sternal border. If pulmonic hypertension is present, the pulmonic second sound will be accentuated over the left upper sternal border. The murmur of acquired pulmonic regurgitation is a high-pitched diastolic blow along the left sternal border. Thus murmur may be difficult to differentiate from the murmur of aortic regurgitation, but the absence of peripheral findings of aortic regurgitation is useful in identifying regurgitation of the pulmonic valve as the source of the diastolic blow. Congenital

pulmonic regurgitation characteristically is associated with a low-pitched, decrescendo murmur along the left sternal border, the peak of the murmur occurring shortly after the pulmonic component of the second heart sound.

MULTIVALVULAR DISEASE

In combined mitral and aortic stenosis, the LV apical impulse may not be displaced, but a palpable parasternal RV systolic lift is usually present. A mitral diastolic rumble is audible in most patients and can vary from grade III intensity down to a minimum of grade I to II intensity (scale I to VI). The aortic systolic murmur is usually loud, but occasionally may be faint with severe mitral stenosis. A mitral opening snap may not be audible, and in some patients the diastolic rumble of mitral stenosis cannot be heard.

When both aortic and mitral regurgitation exist, the diastolic arterial blood pressure is usually less than 70 mmHg; however, almost half of the patients with combined regurgitant lesions will exhibit diastolic blood pressures above 70 mmHg. Most such patients have a loud holosystolic mitral murmur. If aortic regurgitation is the dominant lesion, the early diastolic murmur is usually prominent, whereas when mitral regurgitation prevails, the aortic murmur becomes less intense. Mitral regurgitation may diminish the aortic regurgitation due to the increased LV diastolic filling from the enlarged left atrium. Depending on the contractile state of the myocardium, loud regurgitant murmurs may be associated with mild regurgitation, whereas faint murmurs may accompany severe valvular regurgitation if myocardial failure has developed. A diastolic "flow murmur" across the mitral valve is heard in the majority of patients with combined mitral and aortic regurgitation. If aortic regurgitation is important, a systyolic murmur produced by the large forward flow across the aortic valve is present (see also Chap. 10).

When aortic regurgitation and mitral stenosis are both present, the apex impulse is also displaced, sustained, and forceful. The early diastolic murmur at the apex may be prominent and may be accentuated by the aortic regurgitant flow striking the anterior leaflet of the stenotic mitral valve. Although the low-pitched diastolic murmur of mitral stenosis and the diastolic flow murmur with aortic regurgitation are usually reliable diagnostic parameters, neither murmur correlates with the hemodynamic measurements when the two lesions coexist.

When aortic regurgitation is combined with mitral stenosis, the systemic pulse pressure may be useful but does not necessarily reflect the severity of aortic regurgitation. A prominent apical impulse in apparently pure mitral stenosis indicates the possibility of associated aortic regurgitation but may not indicate its severity. Finally, the intensity of the aortic diastolic murmur is of little value in predicting the severity of aortic regurgitation in the presence of mitral stenosis (see also Chap. 10).

In the presence of aortic stenosis and possible mitral regurgitation, an apical holosystolic murmur is reasonable evidence for associated mitral regurgitation, but the intensity of the murmur is not a reliable indicator in estimating severity.

While the murmur of tricuspid regurgitation often increases with inspiration (Rivero Carvallo's sign), distinction from a concomitant mitral regurgitant murmur may be difficult. Identification of the rumble of tricuspid stenosis requires careful auscultation during inspiration at the left lower sternal border. Detection by auscultation is more difficult because of the frequent association of mitral and tricuspid stenosis.

Electrocardiogram

TRICUSPID VALVE DISEASE

Atrial fibrillation is frequent in patients with tricuspid regurgitation. When tricuspid regurgitation results from myocardial infarction, acute or chronic electrocardiogram (ECG) changes will be seen in the inferior ECG leads, and ST-segment elevation indicating RV infarction may be present in the right-sided precordial leads. The characteristic ECG finding in tricuspid stenosis is a large P wave of right atrial enlargement in the absence of RV hypertrophy[14,15,67] (see Chap. 12).

PULMONIC VALVE DISEASE

Although there are no characteristic changes with pulmonic valvular lesions, preexisting pulmonary hypertension will produce RV hypertrophy, right-axis deviation, and changes in the P wave, suggesting right atrial enlargement. If pulmonary hypertension is secondary to mitral stenosis, P mitrale with characteristic notches will be presented in lead II (see Chap. 12).

MULTIVALVULAR DISEASE

In combined mitral and aortic valve stenosis, ECG evidence of LV hypertrophy, left atrial enlargement, and atrial fibrillation is often present. Similar findings are observed in mitral and aortic regurgitation, with a high likelihood of left atrial and LV enlargement along with atrial fibrillation. With aortic stenosis and mitral regurgitation, LV hypertrophy is accompanied by a moderate incidence of atrial fibrillation. Mitral stenosis with severe aortic regurgitation also produces LV hypertrophy.

Chest Roentgenogram

TRICUSPID VALVE DISEASE

Tricuspid regurgitation may produce some degree of right atrial enlargement, but there will usually be accompanying RV enlargement.[64] In tricuspid stenosis, the most characteristic radiographic finding is prominence of the right atrium without significant pulmonary arterial enlargement or changes due to pulmonary hypertension[14] (see also Chap. 13).

PULMONIC VALVE DISEASE

Patients with pulmonic valve regurgitation have pulmonary artery prominence along with an increase in RV dimensions. If stenosis of the pulmonary valve is acquired, there may be poststenotic dilatation of prominence of the main pulmonary artery.[54]

MULTIVALVULAR DISEASE

With mitral stenosis and aortic stenosis, the left atrium is always enlarged. LV chamber size may be be significantly elevated; however, prominent RV dimensions are usually present. Valvular calcification at either site is relatively uncommon. In aortic stenosis accompanied by mitral regurgitation, heart size is increased with both LV and left atrial enlargement. In mitral stenosis with aortic regurgitation, marked LV enlargement is often present.

Echocardiogram

TRICUSPID VALVE DISEASE

With tricuspid regurgitation, there may be echocardiographic evidence of systolic prolapse, rupture of the chordae or papillary muscle, or vegetative lesions on the valve.[68] Increased RV dimensions indicate impaired RV function and the likelihood of secondary tricuspid regurgitation. Contrast echocardiography with peripheral venous injection can identify the back-and-forth flow across the valve.[69] The echo Doppler technique can estimate the severity of the regurgitation and the systolic pressure in the right ventricle[70] (Fig. 66-8). Color flow Doppler imaging can delineate the patterns and sites of regurgitation across the valve apparatus[71] (see also Chap. 14).

A characteristic pattern of stenosis of the tricuspid valve can often be recorded with the echocardiogram. Fibrosis and calcification of the valve can be identified. Obstructive lesions such as myxoma, thrombus, or other tumors can be recognized

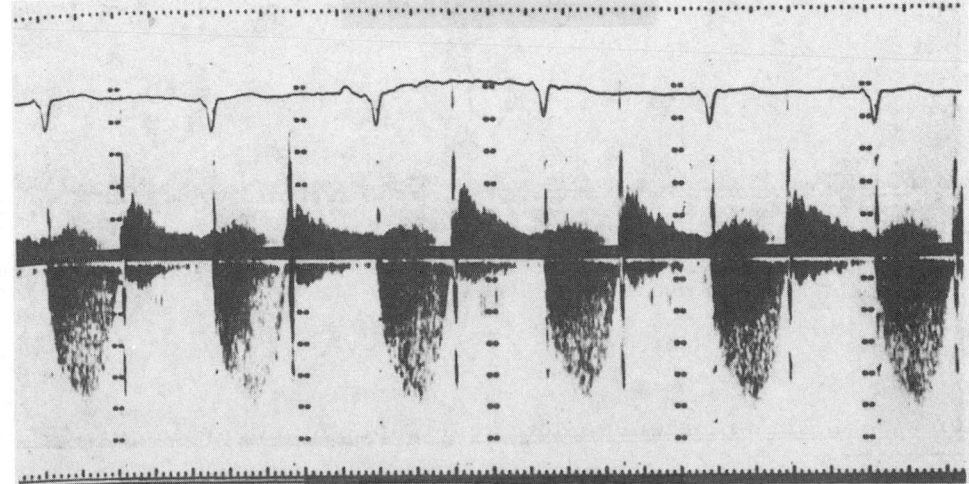

FIGURE 66-8

A continuous echo Doppler recording in a patient with tricuspid valve disease illustrates tricuspid regurgitation in the lower portion and tricuspid stenosis in the upper portion of the tracing. (Reproduced with permission from and courtesy of Dr. Pamela Sears-Rogan.)

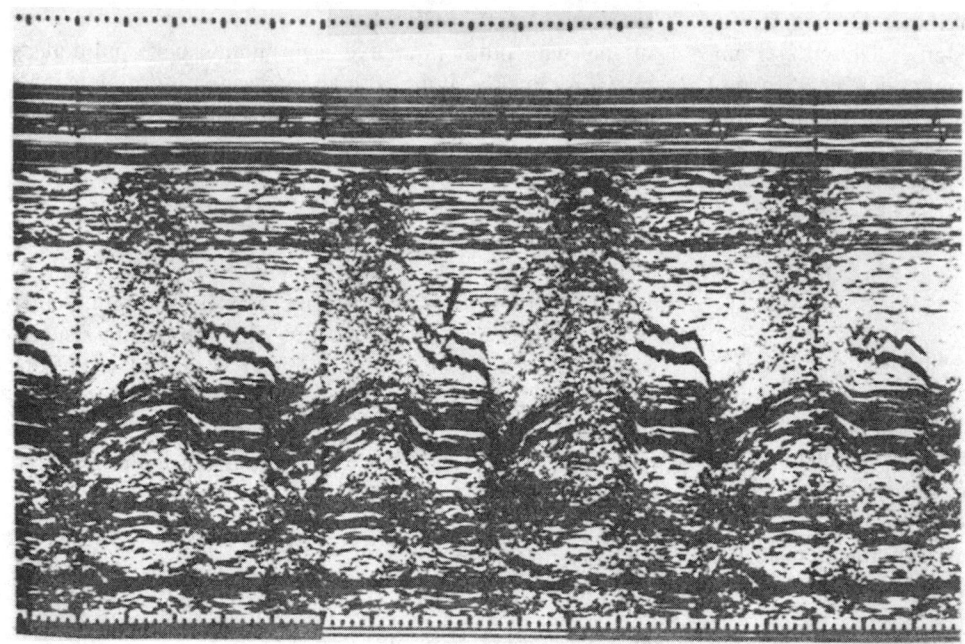

FIGURE 66-9

M-mode echocardiogram in a patient with pulmonary regurgitation illustrates thickening and fluttering of the pulmonic valve, as indicated by the arrow. (Reproduced with permission from Dr. Pamela Sears-Rogan.)

echocardiographically. The echo Doppler technique can be used to estimate the diastolic gradient across the valve with generally good accuracy (see Chap. 14).

PULMONIC VALVE DISEASE

Echocardiography can delineate the anatomy of the pulmonic valve as well as intrinsic or extrinsic lesions impinging on the valve apparatus (Fig. 66-9). Sometimes a vegetative lesion or tumor can be detected in the pulmonary valve area. The echo Doppler technique can estimate both the severity of the regurgitation and the stenosis of the valve,[72] and analysis of echo Doppler recordings can provide estimates of pulmonary artery pressure[73–75] (Fig. 66-10). Color flow imaging can further confirm the patterns of regurgitation in the right ventricular outflow tract (see Chap. 14).

MULTIVALVULAR DISEASE

Echocardiography provides information on valve anatomy, chamber dimensions, pressure gradients, valve size, patterns of regurgitation, and estimates of ventricular function. Stenosis of the mitral and aortic valve produces characteristic echoes (see also Chap. 14). Prolapse of mitral, aortic, and tricuspid valves can be characteristically recognized with echocardiography (Fig. 66-11).[76] The number of aortic cusps can be identified, as can the presence of calcium via the aortic or mitral valve apparatus. Dimensions of the left atrium, left ventricle, and right ventricle together with LV wall thickness measurements and mass are useful in estimating the extent of volume and pressure overload. Two-dimensional and Doppler echocardiographic techniques can assess the orifice size of the aortic and mitral valves and estimate the valve gradients accurately.[77,78] Even in the presence of aortic regurgitation, appropriate modifications in the mathematical analysis of the pressure gradient can yield reasonably accurate estimates of the aortic valve gradients. Color flow Doppler readings can identify patterns and sites of valvular regurgitation across the aortic and mitral valves.[79,80] In addition, thrombus formation in the left atrium and left ventricle can be detected with various echocardiographic methods (see also Chap. 68). Transesophageal echocardiography can accurately assess prosthetic valve function and valvular repair during the operative procedures.

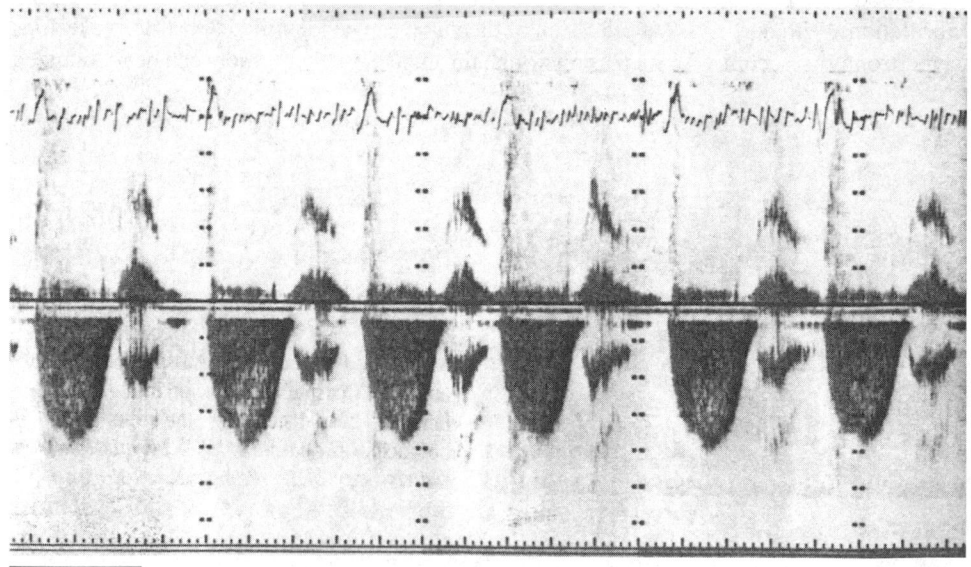

FIGURE 66-10

An echo Doppler continuous tracing in a patient with tricuspid regurgitation. By employing the equation, the systolic gradient across the tricuspid valve can be calculated, and the addition of 10 mmHg yields an estimate of the pulmonary systolic pressure. Thus, in this patient, the level of pulmonary hypertension could be estimated from the echo Doppler tracing of the tricuspid regurgitation. (Reproduced with permission from Dr. Pamela Sears-Rogan.)

Nuclear Techniques

A radionuclide ventriculogram can delineate dimensions of the right atrium and right ventricle, which may help differentiate between stenosis and regurgitation of the tricuspid valve (see Chap. 17). RV size and function can be evaluated in stenotic and regurgitant lesions of the pulmonic valve. Myocardial perfusion imaging techniques are useful in detecting RV infarction as a cause of tricuspid regurgitation as well as providing estimates of RV function. RV size and function can be evaluated in stenotic and regurgitant lesions of the pulmonic valve.

Quantitative information on LV function at rest and during exercise can be provided by radionuclide ventriculography (see also Chap. 17). Segmental wall motion can be assessed at rest and during exercise and may assist in the recognition of underlying coronary artery disease. Since combined lesions of the aortic and mitral valves often create pulmonary hypertension and RV dysfunction, radionuclide ventriculography is useful in estimating the RV ejection franction.[81]

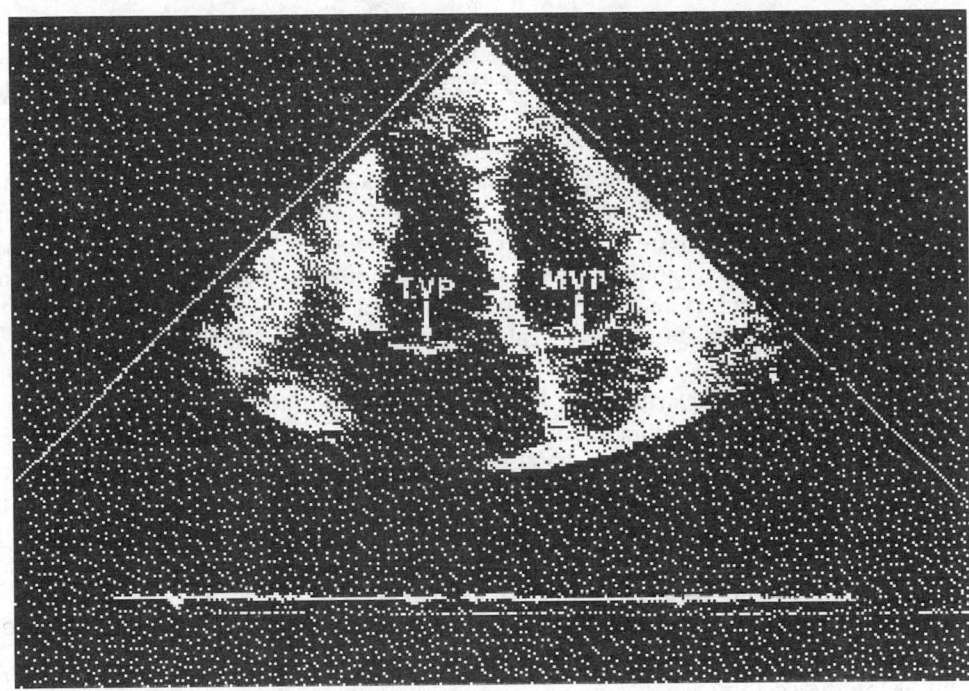

FIGURE 66-11

A four-chamber echocardiograph demonstrates prolapse of both the mitral valve on the right (MVP) and the tricuspid valve on the left (TVP). (Reproduced with permission from Dr. Pamela Sears-Rogan.)

Cardiac Catheterization

TRICUSPID VALVE DISEASE

Accurate angiographic documentation of tricuspid regurgitation is difficult to obtain because the catheter overrides the tricuspid valve, and ventricular irritability with an RV injection can induce tricuspid regurgitation. A prominent *cv* wave in the right atrium suggests tricuspid regurgitation, and an intracardiac phonocardiogram may record a regurgitation murmur in the absence of Rivero Carvallo's sign.[82]

If tricuspid stenosis is clinically suspected, simultaneous pressures should be recorded in the right atrium and in the right ventricle in order to measure the gradient across the valve accurately.[62] Since the normal gradient across the tricuspid valve is less than 1 mmHg, small gradients may not be detected if pullback pressure is recorded from the right ventricle to the right atrium. The area of the tricuspid valve in significant stenosis is usually less than 1.5 cm^2; in severe stenosis it is less than 1 cm^2.

PULMONIC VALVE DISEASE

Pulmonic regurgitation is not readily demonstrated angiographically, but a right-sided injection can outline the pulmonary valve as well as poststenotic dilatation. An aortic root injection can be helpful in the elimination of aortic regurgitation as the etiology of a diastolic murmur along the left sternal border. Nevertheless, this distinction is usually best made by echo Doppler studies. Intracardiac phonocardiography has been employed to detect the diastolic murmur in the RV outflow tract.

MULTIVALVULAR DISEASE

Cardiac catheterization is appropriate for most patients with combined valvular heart disease in order to calculate the stenotic and regurgitant status of each valve as well as to identify the predominant valvular lesion. Delineation of the coronary artery anatomy is also important, because underlying coronary disease must be taken into account in planning the operative approach. Gradients across the valve can be measured with precision, and the valve area calculated. Pulmonary hypertension is commonly present in these patients, and LV end-diastolic pressure is often elevated despite the presence of mitral stenosis (see Chap. 16).

In mitral and aortic regurgitation, the LV end-diastolic pressure is elevated in most patients, and the central aortic pressure will generally be greater than 40 mmHg. As noted, however, in approximately one-third of the patients the central aortic diastolic pressure may be above 70 mmHg. The *v* wave of mitral regurgitation can be recorded in the wedge position, and capillary and pulmonary arterial pressures are abnormally elevated in most of these patients.

In aortic stenosis with mitral regurgitation, LV end-diastolic and pulmonary artery pressures are elevated; however, the extent of pressure elevation does not necessarily reflect the severity of the mitral regurgitation. When it is severe, forward cardiac output may be reduced; thus, a spuriously small pressure gradient may be recorded across a significantly stenotic aortic valve.

In mitral stenosis with aortic regurgitation, the LV end-diastolic pressure is abnormal and the central aortic diastolic pressure is usually less than 70 mmHg.

In combined valvular lesions, the measurement of total angiographic LV stroke volume is useful in calculating the regurgitant volume across each valve.[57] When both valves are regurgitant, it is more difficult to calculate the regurgitant volume across each valve.

Assessment of ventricular function (see Chap. 22) is important in patients with combined valvular lesions; yet the injection fraction may be spuriously elevated in regurgitation across the mitral valve and, to a lesser extent, in aortic regurgitation. Measurements of LV end-systolic pressure, volume, and wall thickness permit calculation of end-systolic wall stress.[83] This parameter has been particularly helpful in pressure and volume overload conditions since the end-systolic pressure-volume wall stress calculation is relatively independent of loading conditions.

Finally, coronary arteriography should be performed at the time of cardiac catheterization in patients above the age of 35, since coronary artery disease may be present without symptoms and may contribute to LV dysfunction.

USUAL STRATEGY OF WORKUP

Tricuspid Valve Disease

The history should identify underlying conditions such as rheumatic fever, systemic disorders, and left-sided heart failure as etiologies for tricuspid valve disease. The physical examination should carefully define the waveforms in the jugular veins. The auscultatory changes of systolic and diastolic murmurs at the left lower sternal border during the respiratory cycle should be carefully observed. In addition, physical findings of left-sided valvular abnormalities, particularly mitral stenosis or evidence of LV failure, should be observed. Peripheral edema as evidence of impaired right-sided filling should be identified.

Although an ECG and chest x-ray should accompany the most recent examination, echocardiography is the most useful noninvasive technique for identifying the presence, severity, and potential etiologies of stenosis and/or regurgitation of the tricuspid valve (see also Chap. 14). If the patient undergoes cardiac catheterization for assessment of left-sided heart disease, right-sided hemodynamics should be recorded and, if clinically indicated, simultaneous pressures recorded in the right atrium and the right ventricle (see Chap. 16).

Pulmonic Valve Disease

The clinical history is important in delineating causes of left-sided heart failure that can lead to pulmonary hypertension and regurgitation of the pulmonic valve. Symptoms of the carcinoid syndrome, tumors, or infectious etiologies involving the pulmonic valve should be determined. The physical examination is important in evaluating the venous pulsations in the neck veins as well as the pulmonic murmurs. RV prominence should be carefully evaluated, as should concomitant left-sided valve lesions and evidence of heart failure. Although an ECG and chest x-ray should be obtained to assess the pulmonic artery, RV outflow tract, and body of the right ventricle, the most useful noninvasive technique is echocardiography. The anatomy, competence of the valve, extent of the regurgitation, and stenosis can be recognized and assessed by an echo Doppler study. In addition, other valve lesions affecting the left side of the heart can be documented. Since pulmonic regurgitation can be relatively well tolerated, this specific lesion does not require such frequent follow-up, but underlying mechanisms for pulmonary hypertension or left-sided heart failure should be monitored closely.

Multivalvular Disease

Symptoms of dyspnea, exercise intolerance, chest discomfort, or syncope should be elicited during a carefully taken clinical history. On physical examination, special attention should be directed to the peripheral and central arterial pulses and the jugular venous pulse waveforms. Heart size, precordial movement, and auscultatory findings should be carefully noted. A 12-lead ECG and posterior-anterior and lateral chest films should be obtained. Echocardiography is indicated to delineate valve anatomy, measure valve gradients, recognize regurgitant patterns, calculate orifice size, and estimate ventricular function and wall motion (see also Chap. 14). A limited exercise test with or without radionuclide studies may help determine the exercise capacity as well as detect functional deterioration, chest pain, arrhythmias, deterioration of ventricular injection fraction, or segmental wall motion abnormalities. If symptoms are atypical and the extent of valvular or LV function cannot be satisfactorily evaluated by noninvasive techniques, cardiac catheterization is indicated. Patients should be seen on a 3- to 6-month basis, depending on their status on initial examination.

NATURAL HISTORY AND PROGNOSIS

Tricuspid Valve Disease

With tricuspid regurgitation due to RV hypertension, the symptoms and clinical course are primarily related to the left-sided heart conditions that produce a pressure-volume overload on the right ventricle. Tricuspid regurgitation virtually always develops with severe RV failure. In infective endocarditis of the tricuspid valve, the type of organism may significantly influence the course and the response to antibiotics (see Chap. 82).

With tricuspid stenosis, the symptoms are usually those of mitral stenosis, and the absence of pulmonary congestion in the presence of peripheral edema should raise the possibility of underlying stenosis of the tricuspid valve. Significant tricuspid stenosis may slow the development of characteristic symptoms of mitral stenosis and result in an underestimation of the severity of mitral valve obstruction.

Multivalvular Heart Disease

When combined aortic and mitral valve disease are due to rheumatic fever, 10 or more years may elapse before the development of significant murmurs and an additional decade (or more) may elapse before symptoms become manifest. If lesions of the aortic and mitral valves are due to degenerative collagen changes, symptoms may develop later in life. When combined lesions are due to calcific changes in the aortic valve and annulus as well as the mitral valve annulus, symptoms develop much later in life. There may, however, be rapid progression of degenerative aortic calcific stenosis over 2- or 3-year periods.

MEDICAL MANAGEMENT

Tricuspid Valve Disease

With tricuspid regurgitation, treatment of RV failure requires digitalis, and diuretics, and vasodilating agents are also required for the management of LV failure (see also Chap. 23). If failure of the right side of the heart is caused by mitral stenosis, early intervention to enlarge or replace the mitral valve is appropriate (see Chap. 64).

In tricuspid stenosis, the usual precautionary measures of antibiotic coverage and prevention of endocarditis apply (see Chap. 81). Peripheral edema may not respond well to administration of digitalis, diuretics, and vasodilator therapy, thus emphasizing the clinical importance of detecting underlying tricuspid stenosis. Tricuspid balloon valvuloplasty has been used successfully in patients with predominant tricuspid stenosis.[84]

Pulmonic Valve Disease

Patients with congenital pulmonic valve stenosis are usually best treated by catheter balloon valvotomy (see Chaps. 70 and 71).

Prophylaxis and Medical Therapy

Antibiotic prophylaxis against endocarditis (Chap. 82) is appropriate for patients with either tricuspid or pulmonic valve lesions. If pulmonary emboli contribute to the pulmonary hypertension, anticoagulation is indicated (Chap. 60). Further treatment of pulmonary hypertension may require management of failure of the left side of the heart, correction of mitral stenosis, or the use of vasodilating agents that can lower pulmonary artery pressure. Vasodilating agents are often ineffective in treating primary pulmonary hypertension (see Chap. 59).

If rheumatic fever is the likely etiology of combined aortic and mitral valve disease, prophylactic penicillin should usually be continued until age 35 years (see Chap. 62). Dental prophylaxis with antibiotic coverage, using either amoxicillin or erythromycin, should be provided in all patient groups prior to dental procedures. For genitourinary or other abdominal procedures, gram-negative antibiotic coverage should be provided (Chap. 82).

Atrial Fibrillation

If atrial fibrillation develops, chronic anticoagulation with low-dose warfarin [International Normalized Ratio (INR) 2.0 to 3.0] is warranted since the accompanying incidence of systemic and cerebral emboli is estimated at 10 to 20 percent (see also Chap. 66).

The early development of atrial fibrillation associated with hemodynamic deterioration warrants an initial attempt at electrical cardioversion. If this is successful, digitalis as well as antiarrhythmic preparations should be administered thereafter for prophylaxis against recurrence (see also Chap. 27). Chronic atrial fibrillation should be controlled with digitalis, beta blockers, and calcium blockers as indicated. The development of symptoms, particularly dyspnea, limitations of exercise activity, chest pain, and syncope, warrants consideration for surgery. It is usually recommended for New York Heart Association (NYHA) class III symptoms despite adequate medical therapy.

SURGICAL MANAGEMENT

Tricuspid Valve Disease

The decision to proceed with valvular heart surgery is usually based on the severity of the aortic and mitral valve disease, rather than on the severity of the disease of the tricuspid valve. The usual decisions to be made regarding the tricuspid valve are: (1) whether or not a procedure should be added to the mitral and/or aortic valve procedures, and if so, (2) which procedure—annuloplasty or valve replacement—should be performed. Patients may present with mild mitral valve disease but severe tricuspid valve dysfunction. Such patients may require an operation on the tricuspid valve only.

INDICATIONS FOR SURGERY

The severity of the symptoms and clinical signs of tricuspid valve disease are used to determine whether or not to perform tricuspid valve surgery. If there are signs of tricuspid stenosis and, particularly, if stenosis is demonstrated by cardiac catheterization and two-dimensional echocardiography, the tricuspid valve is directly visualized at operation with the anticipation of performing commissurotomy or valve replacement.

When there are signs of severe tricuspid regurgitation secondary to mitral stenosis, it is important to document the duration of the regurgitation and the severity and duration of pulmonary artery hypertension. If the tricuspid regurgitation is severe and long-standing and if there is chronic pulmonary artery hypertension, it is unlikely that the tricuspid regurgitation will resolve in the early postoperative period after mitral valve surgery alone. In this circumstance, tricuspid valve surgery is usually indicated. In contrast, if the tricuspid regurgitation and pulmonary artery hypertension are of short duration, mitral valve replacement will usually reduce pulmonary artery pressure in the early postoperative period, and this will result in a decrease in the tricuspid valve regurgitation. In this situation, the surgeon usually waits until discontinuation of bypass after mitral valve surgery to decide whether or not a procedure to reduce tricuspid regurgitation is indicated. Occasionally, severe tricuspid regurgitation will be present with only modest elevation of pulmonary artery pressure. In this circumstance, the tricuspid valve leaflets are usually deformed and valve replacement is necessary.[85]

The appearance of the heart at the time of surgery is helpful in assessing the severity of tricuspid valve disease. A thinned-out right atrial wall together with moderate to marked enlargement of the right atrium and venae cavae are indications of significant disease. The degree of stenosis and regurgitation can be estimated by palpation through the right atrial appendage. If tricuspid valve surgery is not performed as the initial surgical approach, examination through the right atrial appendage can be performed after discontinuation of bypass for mitral valve surgery to evaluate residual tricuspid regurgitation. Intraoperative transesophageal echocardiography (see also Chap. 14) provides more precise information as to the degree of residual valvular regurgitation after repair.

The NYHA class III status is usually an indication for operation in patients with combined aortic and mitral valve disease. Many of these patients, however, are diagnosed at a later stage of this disease.

Surgical intervention is now commonly being performed in patients who have volume overload of the left ventricle even when they remain in functional class II. Thus, in severe aortic regurgitation with moderate mitral valve involvement, or in important mitral regurgitation together with moderate aortic stenosis and regurgitation, surgery may be advised to avert progressive and poorly reversible LV dysfunction associated with dilatation (see also Chaps. 63 and 64).

TRICUSPID VALVE SURGERY

Tricuspid stenosis may be treated successfully by commissurotomy, which is usually performed under direct vision. The procedure may be combined with annuloplasty to correct valve regurgitation. Valve replacement is occasionally necessary if the changes in the leaflets and subvalvular structures are advanced or if severe regurgitation cannot be relieved by annuloplasty. For tricuspid regurgitation, three basic reconstructive techniques have been described. The first procedure is used widely and consists of plication of the posterior leaflet,[86,87] thus converting the tricuspid valve into a functionally bicuspid valve.[84,85] De Vega described a second type of annuloplasty that narrows the annulus along the anterior and posterior leaflets with a purse-string suture.[88,89] The third major technique, described by Carpentier et al., consists of placing a carefully sized semiflexible ring along the anterior and posterior aspects of the annulus.[90] It draws in and supports the tissue evenly. Follow-up studies have shown that annular dilatation occurs in these areas rather than along the leaflets.[91]

When the leaflets and subvalvular apparatus are severely deformed as a result of rheumatic fever, reconstruction may not be feasible. In such cases, replacement is performed with either a mechanical or tissue valve. Anticoagulation with warfarin (see also Chap. 52) is generally advisable in patients with tricuspid valve replacement, and therefore the major advantage of a bioprosthetic valve is negated. Nevertheless, the bioprosthetic valve has been the prosthesis of first choice of many surgeons. If a mechanical valve is preferred and the cavity of the right ventricle is not capacious, a low-profile, tilting disk-type prosthesis seems appropriate. Usually, however, if tricuspid regurgitation is severe, a ball-cage prosthesis functions better.

RESULTS OF TRICUSPID VALVE SURGERY

Mild tricuspid regurgitation does not seem to increase the risk of surgery involving the mitral valve or both aortic and mitral valves. When the tricuspid disease is moderate to severe, however, the risk of operation is significantly increased. Although long-term improvement in tricuspid regurgitation after mitral valve replacement alone has been documented, a tricuspid procedure is generally employed in the setting of moderate to severe tricuspid regurgitation to enhance cardiac function in the critical early days after operation.[92] Mitral valve replacement alone does not invariably decrease tricuspid regurgitation, even several months after operation.[93]

In general, the early and late results of tricuspid annuloplasty have been superior to those of valve replacement, and valve replacement should be avoided when possible. There is a significant incidence of thrombosis with tricuspid prostheses, and the long-term functional results have been less favorable than those of aortic and mitral valve replacements.[94] The less favorable results may be related to more advanced disease but may also be a function of the less favorable position of the prosthesis in relation to the ventricular outflow tract. The risk of annuloplasty in combination with aortic and mitral valve surgery is about 10 percent. Good early results have been obtained with all three methods of annuloplasty.[89,90,95–99] Ring annuloplasty probably gives the best long-term results. When tricuspid valve replacement is necessary, the 30-day operation risk increases to 15 to 20 percent. A study of long-term results after tricuspid valve surgery identified two preoperative factors—severity of edema and mean pulmonary artery pressure—as important predictors of long-term survival.[100] A variety of prostheses have been used for tricuspid valve replacement with variable results.[100–104] The valve of choice remains controversial. Experience with the St. Jude prosthesis in the tricuspid position has generally been favorable[105] (see also Chap. 67).

TRICUSPID VALVE SURGERY FOR INFECTIVE ENDOCARDITIS

Infective endocarditis of the tricuspid valve is relatively common because of incremental drug abuse. In general, the treatment of tricuspid valve endocarditis is medical. When septic pulmonary embolization occurs despite intensive antibiotic treatment, tricuspid valve surgery is indicated. Excision of the valve without replacement has been recommended, and reinfection of the new valve in intravenous drug users is an important risk.[106] Nevertheless, since valvulectomy alone carries an important risk of heart failure, tricuspid valve replacement has been recommended by others.[107] A good result will likely occur if there is no subsequent drug abuse.

POSTOPERATIVE MANAGEMENT

The cardiac output is often marginal after tricuspid valve surgery, a reflection of persistent pulmonary arterial hypertension and long-standing RV dysfunction. Measurements of cardiac output and pulmonary artery pressure are used to guide postoperative care. If annuloplasty is performed, a pulmonary artery catheter can be used for such measurements (see also Chap. 16). Nitroglycerin infused through a central venous catheter is a valuable adjunct in reducing pulmonary artery pressure. Prostaglandin E_1, in combination with pressor agents, may also be employed to treat severe postoperative pulmonary hypertension.[108] Intravenous dopamine and dobutamine may be used to enhance myocardial contractility. If cardiac output remains marginal, an intraaortic balloon pump may be used to reduce left-sided pressures (see also Chap. 23). Pulmonary artery balloon counterpulsation has been employed for acute RV failure.[109] The use of a temporary circulatory assist device, such as a centrifugal pump, to bypass the right ventricle may sustain adequate circulation when RV failure is unresponsive to other measures.

Digitalis and diuretics are usually employed for several months after tricuspid valve surgery. For patients with tricuspid valve replacement, warfarin and dipyridamole are used as anticoagulants.[110] The additional use of antiplatelet agents (such as aspirin, 80 to 160 mg/day) in this setting may improve the long-term results.[111] A serious late complication of tilting disk valves in the tricuspid position is thrombosis. Thrombolytic therapy with streptokinase has been used successfully to restore valve function.[112] Prophylaxis against infective endocarditis is also required (see Chap. 82).

Pulmonic Valve Disease

Pulmonic valve surgery for acquired disease is performed infrequently. Pulmonic valve stenosis on an acquired basis is rare. Although there are a variety of causes of pulmonic valve regurgitation, this hemodynamic condition is relatively well tolerated if pulmonary vascular resistance is normal. Pulmonic valve replacement may be performed for acquired conditions such as carcinoid heart disease and infective endocarditis, but it usually is limited to cases where RV dysfunction has become severe after congenital heart disease surgery[113,114] (see Chaps.

70 and 71). Although pulmonic regurgitation is generally well tolerated for several years after correction of malformations such as tetralogy of Fallot, the regurgitation may become hemodynamically significant, especially if pulmonary artery hypertension is present or develops. In such a case, the placement of a pulmonic valve prosthesis may significantly improve the patient's functional status. In general, bioprosthetic valves have been preferred because of the tendency for mechanical valve thrombosis in this position.[85] Pulmonic valve surgery is currently being performed earlier and more commonly as studies indicate that RV dysfunction may be present in asymptomatic postoperative patients with pulmonic regurgitation.[115]

Infective endocarditis involves the pulmonic valve in about 1 percent cases seen at autopsy.[116] Isolated pulmonic valve infective endocarditis is even more uncommon but may be the cause of metastatic pulmonary infections. In a review of 28 cases of this entity, the overall mortality was 24 percent, with all those treated by operation surviving.[117] Valvulectomy in combination with antibiotic therapy is sometimes the most effective treatment (see also Chap. 82).

Multivalvular Heart Disease

Many patients with clinical evidence of combined disease of the mitral and aortic valves have severe and progressive symptoms. Experience indicates that both valves can be replaced, with a hospital mortality that is now between 5 and 10 percent—considerably less than the 22 percent reported for an earlier period.

Commonly in the presence of aortic and mitral valve disease, repair, rather than replacement, of the stenotic or regurgitant mitral valve can be accomplished (see also Chap. 64). Disease of the aortic valve in adults usually requires valve replacement. The combination of aortic valve replacement with mitral valve repair probably decreases early mortality and improves long-term survival. There has been marked subjective and objective improvements in surviving patients. When tricuspid valve replacement is added, the risk of the operation is higher (up to 20 percent), but even then the long-term results are considerably better than the life history of surgically untreated patients with triple-valve disease. The use, when possible, of tricuspid annuloplasty rather than replacement has greatly improved the early results of operation in this group of patients.

When hemodynamic derangement is significant at both mitral and aortic valves, the decision to repair/replace both is easily made, and the principles of surgical treatment are the same as when one valve alone requires operation.[118,119]

MULTIVALVULAR SURGERY

A median sternotomy is performed. With current techniques of myocardial preservation, using cold potassium cardioplegia, the operation can be done in an unhurried, precise manner with the optimal cardiac performance. On cardiopulmonary bypass, the heart is cooled by the perfusate and by external cardiac cooling. The aorta is cross-clamped. The aorta is opened, and cardioplegic solution is infused into each coronary orifice to attain a myocardial temperature of between 10 and 15°C. Reinfusion of the cardioplegic solution is done every 20 to 30 min or when the myocardial temperature reaches 19 or 20°C. The aortic valve is resected, and attention is then turned to the mitral valve. The left atrium is opened from the right side, and the mitral valve is assessed and resected, if necessary, or repaired. The mitral prosthesis is inserted, and the left atrium is left open while the aortic valve is then sutured into place. If the tricuspid valve is stenotic or regurgitant, the right atrium is opened at this time and either annuloplasty or replacement is done. The aortotomy is then closed, and reperfusion with the perfusate is done while the left atriotomy and right atriotomy are closed. The usual procedures are followed for removing all air from the heart and preventing air embolization as the heart begins to eject.

Often, when the aortic valve is severely diseased and only class II mitral regurgitation (on a scale of I to VI) is evident, it is not necessary to replace the mitral valve. This is true even if left atrial pressure preoperatively was very high, since such pressure can result solely from severe pressure or volume overload of the left ventricle. After repair of the aortic valve disease, the mitral valve regurgitation usually lessens. When there is class II regurgitation of the aortic valve in the presence of severe disease at the mitral valve, however, the aortic valve regurgitation often appears to be of greater magnitude after repair of the mitral valve and may contribute to poor postoperative performance. In these situations, therefore, replacement of both the mitral and aortic valves seem indicated.

RESULTS OF MULTIVALVULAR SURGERY

Long-term survival after replacement of either the aortic or the mitral valve or both is only partially related to factors having to do with the device[120,121] (see also Chap. 67). Other factors, related to the preoperative condition of the patient, intraoperative events, and early postoperative events, also significantly affect late mortality. In particular, patients having had previous valve replacement who need a second replacement, because of xenograft degeneration, paraprosthetic leak, or other complications, do less well than patients with primary valve replacements. Patients who have LV aneurysmectomy along with valve replacement have less satisfactory long-term survival rates. There is, however, no deleterious influence on ischemic heart disease in general, as suggested by the lack of any negative effect on long-term survival associated with coronary artery bypass grafting (see also Chap. 67). Finally, patients in whom treatment of ventricular arrhythmias is necessary in the early postoperative course have less satisfactory survival rates.

Acknowledgment

We are indebted to Dr. Robert B. Wallace for his contribution in the Eighth Edition to areas discussed in this chapter.

REFERENCES

1. Kostucki W, Vandenbossche JL, Friart A, Engbert H. Pulsed Doppler regurgitant flow patterns of normal valves. *Am J Cardiol* 1986; 58:309–313.
2. Sahn DJ, Maciel BC. Physiological valvular regurgitation. Doppler echocardiography and the potential for iatrogenic heart disease. *Circulation* 1988; 78:1075–1077.
3. Yoshida K, Yoshikawa J, Shakudo M. Color Doppler evaluation of valvular regurgitation in normals. *Circulation* 1988; 78:840–847.
4. McMichael J, Shillingford JP. The role of valvular incompetence in heart failure. *Br Med J* 1957; 1:537–542.
5. Waller BF, Howard J, Fess S. Pathology of tricuspid valve stenosis and pure tricuspid regurgitation—Part III. *Clin Cardiol* 1995; 18:225–230.
6. Waller BF, Howard J, Fess S. Pathology of tricuspid valve stenosis and pure tricuspid regurgitation—Part I. *Clin Cardiol* 1995; 18:97–102.
7. Waller BF, Howard J, Fess S. Pathology of tricuspid valve stenosis and pure tricuspid regurgitation—Part II. *Clin Cardiol* 1995; 18:167–174.
8. Glancy DL, Marcus FI, Cuadra M, Ewy GA, Roberts WC. Isolated organic tricuspid valvular regurgitation. *Am J Med* 1969; 46:989–996.
9. Nishimura RA, Smith HC, Gersh BJ. Tricuspid regurgitation after myocardial infarction. *Am J Cardiol* 1994; 74:308.
10. Bonow RO, Carabello B, deLeon AC, Edmunds LH, Fedderly BJ, Freed MD, et al. ACC/AHA Guidelines for Valvular Heart Disease. *Circulation* 1997 (in press).
11. Szyniszewski AM, Carson PE, Sakwa M, Lundstrom T, Boden W. Valve replacement for tricuspid regurgitation appearing late after healing of left ventricular posterior wall and right ventricular acute myocardial infarction. *Am J Cardiol* 1994; 73:616–617.
12. Chiu WC, Shindler DM, Scholz PM, Boyarsky AH. Traumatic tricuspid regurgitation with cyanosis: Diagnosis by transesophageal echocardiography. *Ann Thorac Surg* 1996; 63:992–993.
13. Crumbley AJ 3rd, Van Bakel AB. Tricuspid valve repair for biopsy-induced regurgitation after cardiac transplantation. *Ann Thorac Surg* 1994; 58:1156–1160.
14. Perloff JK, Harvey WP. Clinical recognition of tricuspid stenosis. *Circulation* 1960; 22:346–364.
15. Kitchin A, Turner R. Diagnosis and treatment of tricuspid stenosis. *Br Heart J* 1964; 26:354–379.
16. Edwards JE. The spectrum and clinical significance of tricuspid regurgitation. *Pract Cardiol* 1980; 6:86.
17. Clawson BJ. Rheumatic heart disease: An analysis of 796 cases. *Am Heart J* 1940; 20:454–474.
18. Flammang D, Jaumin P, Kremer R. Organic tricuspid pathology in rheumatic valvulopathics. *Acta Cardiol* 1975; 30:155–170.
19. Cooke WT, White PD. Tricuspid stenosis: With particular reference to diagnosis and prognosis. *Br Heart J* 1941; 3:147–165.
20. Pellikka PA, Tajik AJ, Khandheria BK, Stewart JB, Callahan JA, Pitot HC, et al. Carcinoid heart disease. Clinical and echocardiographic spectrum in 74 patients. *Circulation* 1993; 87:1188–1196.
21. Cheitlin MD, MacGregor J. Acquired tricuspid and pulmonic valve disease. In: Rahimtoola SH, ed. *Atlas of Heart Diseases: Valvular Heart Disease.* St. Louis: Mosby; 1997; 11.2–11.13.
22. Ludwig J. Cardiac vein involvement in carcinoid syndrome: Possible evidence of retrograde blood flow in cardiac veins in tricuspid insufficiency. *Am J Clin Pathol* 1971; 55:617–623.
23. McMichael J, Shillingford JP. The role of valvular incompetence in heart failure. *Br Med J* 1957; 1:537–541.
24. Boucek RJ Jr, Graham TP, Morgan JP, Atwood GF, Boerth RC. Spontaneous resolution of massive congenital tricuspid insufficiency. *Circulation* 1976; 54:795–800.
25. Collins R, Daly JJ. Tricuspid incompetence complicating acute myocardial infarction. *Postgrad Med J* 1977; 53:51–52.
26. Zone DD, Botti RE. Right ventricular infarction with tricuspid insufficiency and chronic right heart failure. *Am J Cardiol* 1976; 37:445–448.
27. McAllister RG Jr, Friesinger GC, Sinclair-Smith BC. Tricuspid regurgitation following inferior myocardial infarction. *Arch Intern Med* 1976; 95:95–99.
28. Eisenberg S, Suyemoto J. Rupture of a papillary muscle of the tricuspid valve following acute myocardial infarction: Report of a case. *Circulation* 1964; 30:588–591.
29. Maranhao V, Gooch AS, Yang SS, Sumathisena DR, Golderg L. Prolapse of the tricuspid leaflets in the systolic murmur-click syndrome. *Cath Cardiovasc Diagn* 1975; 1:81–90.

30. Gerry JL Jr, Bulkley BH, Hutchins GM. Rupture of the papillary muscle of the tricuspid valve: A complication of cardiopulmonary resuscitation and a rare cause of tricuspid insufficiency. *Am J Cardiol* 1977; 40:825–828.

31. Jahnke EJ Jr, Nelson WP, Aaby GV, FitzGibbon GM. Tricuspid insufficiency: The result of nonpenetrating cardiac trauma. *Arch Surg* 1967; 95:880–886.

32. VanGilder JE, Jain AC, Weiss RB, Boyer AF, Tarney TJ. Traumatic right ventricular aneurysm presenting as tricuspid regurgitation. *W V Med J* 1979; 75:93–98.

33. Stephenson LW, MacVaugh H III, Kastor JA. Tricuspid valvular incompetence and rupture of the ventricular septum caused by nonpenetrating trauma. *J Thorac Cardiovasc Surg* 1979; 77:768–772.

34. Williams MJ, Lee MY, DiSalvo TG, Dec GW, Picard MH, Palacios IF, et al. Biopsy-induced flail tricuspid leaflet and tricuspid regurgitation following orthotopic cardiac transplantation. *Am J Cardiol* 1996; 77:1339–1344.

35. Hausen B, Albes JM, Rohde R, Demertzis S, Mugge A. Schafers HJ. Tricuspid valve regurgitation attributable to endomyocardial biopsies and rejection in heart transplantation. *Ann Thorac Surg* 1995; 59:1134–1140.

36. Brandenburg RO, McGoon DC, Campeau L, Giuliani ER. Traumatic rupture of the chordae tendineae of the tricuspid valve: Successful repair twenty-four years later. *Am J Cardiol* 1966; 18:911–915.

37. Morgan JR, Forker AD. Isolated tricuspid insufficiency. *Circulation* 1971; 43:559–564.

38. Marvin RF, Schrank JP, Nolan SP. Traumatic tricuspid insufficiency. *Am J Cardiol* 1973; 32:723–727.

39. Croxson MS, O'Brien KP, Lowe JB. Traumatic tricuspid regurgitation: Long-term survival. *Br Heart J* 1971; 33:750–755.

40. Grubier M, Denis B, Martin-Noel O. Les ruptures de cordages tricuspidiens. *Coeur Med Int* 1976; 15:215–222.

41. Espino Vela J, Contreras R, Rustrian Rosa F. Rheumatic pulmonary valve disease. *Am J Cardiol* 1969; 23:12–18.

42. Roberts WC, Buchbinder NA. Right-sided valvular infective endocarditis. *Am J Med* 1972; 53:7–19.

43. Seymour J, Emanuel R, Patterson N. Acquired pulmonary stenosis. *Br Heart J* 1968; 30:776–785.

44. Rossignol B, Machecourt J, Denis B, Roche J, N'Golet A, Morena H, et al. Cardiopathie carcinoide secondaire a une tumeur du grêle: A propos d'un cas associat insuffisance tricuspidienne et insuffisance pulmonaire. *Arch Mal Coeur Vaiss* 1977; 70:1221–1226.

45. Roberts WC, Virmani R. Aschoff bodies at necropsy in valvular heart disease. *Circulation* 1978; 57:803–815.

46. Clausen BJ. Rheumatic heart disease: An analysis of 796 cases. *Am Heart J* 1940; 20:454–474.

47. Cooke WT, White PD. Tricuspid stenosis: With particular reference to diagnosis and prognosis. *Br Heart J* 1940; 3:147–165.

48. Wilson MG, Lubschez R. Longevity in rheumatic fever. *JAMA* 1948; 138:794–798.

49. Bland EF, Jones TD. Rheumatic fever and rheumatic heart disease: A twenty year report on 1000 patients followed since childhood. *Circulation* 1951; 4:836–843.

50. Roberts WC, Honig HS. The spectrum of cardiovascular disease in the Marfan's syndrome: A clinico-pathologic study of 18 necropsy patients and comparison to 151 previously reported patients. *Am Heart J* 1982; 104:115–135.

51. Hansing CE, Rowe GG. Tricuspid insufficiency: A study of hemodynamics and pathogenesis. *Circulation* 1972; 45:793–799.

52. Killip T, Lukas DS. Tricuspid stenosis: Physiologic criteria for diagnosis and hemodynamic abnormalities. *Circulation* 1957; 16:3–13.

53. El-Sherif N. Rheumatic tricuspid stenosis: A haemodynamic correlation. *Br Heart J* 1971; 33:16–31.

54. Holmes JC, Flowler NO, Kaplan S. Pulmonary valvular insufficiency. *Am J Med* 1968; 44:851–862.

55. Rackley CE, Hood WP Jr, Rolett EL, Young DT. Left ventricular end-diastolic pressure in chronic heart disease. *Am J Med* 1970; 48:310–319.

56. Hood WP Jr, Rackley CE, Rolett EL. Wall stress in the normal and hypertrophied left ventricle. *Am J Cardiol* 1968; 22:550–558.

57. Sandler H, Dodge HT, Hay RE, Rackley CE. Quantitation of valvular insufficiency in man by angiocardiography. *Am Heart J* 1963; 65:501–513.

58. Rackley CE, Bechar VS, Whalen RE, McIntosh HD. Biplane cinean-

giographic determinations of left ventricular function: Pressure-volume relationships. *Am Heart J* 1967; 74:766–779.

59. Baxley WA, Dodge HT, Rackley CE, Sandler H, Pua LD. Left ventricular mechanical efficiency in man with heart disease. *Circulation* 1977; 55:564–568.

60. Jones JW, Rackley CE, Bruce RA, Dodge HT, Cobb LA, Sander H. Left ventricular volumes in valvular heart disease. *Circulation* 1964; 29:887–891.

61. Dodge HT, Hay RE, Sandler H. Pressure-volume characteristics of the diastolic left ventricle in man with heart disease. *Ann Heart J* 1962; 64:503–511.

62. Kern MJ, Aguirre F, Donohue T, Bach R. Interpretation of cardiac pathophysiology from pressure waveform analysis: Multivalvular regurgitant lesions. *Cath Cardiovasc Diagn* 1993; 28:167–172.

63. Rousseau MF, Pouleur H, Charlier AA, Bruseur LA. Assessment of left ventricular relaxation in patients with valvular regurgitation. *Am J Cardiol* 1982; 50:1028–1036.

64. Salazar E, Levine HD. Rheumatic tricuspid regurgitation: The clinical spectrum. *Am J Med* 1962; 33:111–129.

65. Terzaki AK, Cokkinos DV, Leachman RD, Merde JB, Hallman GI, Cooley DA. Combined mitral and aortic valve disease. *Am J Cardiol* 1970; 25:588–601.

66. Rivero Carvallo JM. El diagnostica de la estenosis tricuspides. *Arch Inst Cardiol Mex* 1950; 20:1–11.

67. Killip T, Lukas DS. Tricuspid stenosis: Clinical features in twelve cases. *Am J Med* 1958; 24:836–852.

68. DePace NL, Ross J, Ashandrian AS, Nestico PF, Kottler MN, Mintz GS, et al. Tricuspid regurgitation: Noninvasive techniques for determining causes and severity. *J Am Coll Cardiol* 1984; 3:1540–1550.

69. Meltzer RS, VanHoogenhuyze D, Serruys PW, Haalebos MMP, Hugenholtz PG, Roelandt J. Diagnosis of tricuspid regurgitation by contrast echocardiography. *Circulation* 1981; 63:1093–1099.

70. Yock PG, Popp RL. Noninvasive estimation of right ventricular systolic pressure by Doppler ultrasound in patients with tricuspid regurgitation. *Circulation* 1984; 70:657–662.

71. Suzuki YU, Kambara N, Kadota K, Tamaki S, Yamazato A, Nohara R, et al. Detection and evaluation of tricuspid regurgitation using a real-time two-dimensional color-coded Doppler flow imaging system: Comparison with contrast two-dimensional echocardiography and right ventriculography. *Am J Cardiol* 1986; 57:811–815.

72. Waggoner AD, Quinones MA, Young JB, Brandon TA, Shah AA, Verani MS. Pulsed Doppler echocardiographic detection of right-sided valve regurgitation: Experimental results and clinical significance. *Am J Cardiol* 1981; 47:279–286.

73. Masuyama T, Kodama K, Kitabatake A, Sato H, Nanto S, Inoue M. Continuous-wave Doppler echocardiographic detection of pulmonary regurgitation and its application to noninvasive estimation of pulmonary artery pressure. *Circulation* 1986; 74:484–492.

74. Isobe M, Yazaki Y, Takaku F, Koizumi K, Hara K, Tsuneyoshi H. Prediction of pulmonary arterial pressure in adults by pulsed Doppler echocardiography. *Am J Cardiol* 1986; 57:316–321.

75. Chan KL, Currie PJ, Seward JB, Hagler DJ, Mair DD, Tajik AJ. Comparison of three Doppler ultrasound methods in the prediction of pulmonary artery pressure. *J Am Coll Cardiol* 1987; 9:549–554.

76. Ogawa S, Hayashi J, Sasaki H, Tani M, Akaishi MN, Mitamura H, et al. Evaluation of combined valvular prolapse syndrome by two-dimensional echocardiography. *Circulation* 1982; 65:174–180.

77. Otto CM, Pearlman AS, Comens KA, Reamer RP, Janko CL, Huntzman LL. Determination of the stenotic aortic valve area in adults using Doppler echocardiography. *J Am Coll Cardiol* 1986; 7:509–517.

78. Smith MD, Handshoe R, Handshoe S, Kwan OL, DeMaria AN. Comparative accuracy of two-dimensional echocardiography and Doppler pressure half-time methods in assessing severity of mitral stenosis in patients with and without prior commissurotomy. *Circulation* 1986; 78:100–107.

79. Perry GJ, Helmcke F, Nanda NC, Byard C, Soto B. Evaluation of aortic insufficiency by Doppler color flow mapping. *J Am Coll Cardiol* 1987; 9:952–959.

80. Enriquez-Serano M, Bailey KP, Seward JB, Tajik AJ, Krohn MJ, Mays JM. Quantitative Doppler assessment of valvular regurgitation. *Circulation* 1993; 87:841–848.

81. Winzelberg GG, Boucher CA, Pohost GM, McKusick KA, Bingham JB, Okada RD, et al. Right ventricular function in aortic and mitral valve disease. Relation of gated first-pass radionuclide angiography to clinical and hemodynamic findings. *Chest* 1981; 79:520–528.

82. Cha SD, Gooch AS, Maranhao V. Intracardiac phonocardiography in tricuspid regurgitation: Relation to clinical and angiographic findings. *Am J Cardiol* 1981; 48:573–583.

83. Rackley CE. Quantitative evaluation of left ventricular function by radiographic techniques. *Circulation* 1976; 54:862–879.

84. Patel TM, Sani SI, Shah SC, Patel TK. Tricuspid balloon valvuloplasty: A more simplified approach using Inoue balloon. *Cath Cardiovasc Diagn* 1996; 37:86–88.

85. Scully HE, Armstrong CS. Tricuspid valve replacement. Fifteen years of experience with mechanical prostheses and bioprostheses. *J Thorac Cardiovasc Surg* 1995; 109:1035–1041.

86. Kay JH, Maselli-Campagna G, Tsuji HK. Surgical treatment of tricuspid insufficiency. *Ann Surg* 1965; 162:53–58.

87. Boyd AD, Engelman RM, Isom OW, Reed GE, Spencer FC. Tricuspid annuloplasty: Five and one-half years' experience with 78 patients. *J Thorac Cardiovasc Surg* 1974; 68:344–351.

88. DeVega NF. La annulplastia selectiva: Reguable y permanente. *Rev Esp Cardiol* 1972; 25:555–556.

89. Abe T, Tsukamoto M, Morishita K, Tanaka T, Kuwaki K. 1989: De Vega's annuloplasty for acquired tricuspid disease: Early and late results in 110 patients. Updated in 1996. *Ann Thorac Surg* 1996; 62:1876–1877.

90. Carpentier A, Deloche A, Hanania G, Forman J, Sellier P, Piwnica A. Surgical management of acquired tricuspid valve disease. *J Thorac Cardiovasc Surg* 1974; 67:53–65.

91. Deloche A, Guerino J, Fabiani JN, Morillo F, Caramanian M, Carpentier A, et al. Étude anatomique des valvulopatheis rheumatismales tricuspidiennes. *Ann Chir Thorac Cardiovasc* 1973; 44:343–349.

92. Braunwald NS, Ross J, Morrow AG. Conservative management of tricuspid regurgitation in patients undergoing mitral valve replacement. *Circulation* 1967; 35(suppl 1):163–169.

93. Simon R, Oelert H, Borst HG, Lichtelen PR. Influence of mitral valve surgery on tricuspid incompetence concomitant with mitral valve disease. *Circulation* 1980; 62:1152–1157.

94. Thorburn CW, Morgan JJ, Shanahan MX, Chang VP. Long-term results of tricuspid valve replacement and the problem of prosthetic valve thrombosis. *Am J Cardiol* 1983; 51:1128–1132.

95. Grondin P, Meere C, Limet R, Lopez-Bescos L, Delcan JL, Rivera R. Carpentier's annulus and De Vega's annuloplasty: The end of the tricuspid challenge. *J Thorac Cardiovasc Surg* 1975; 70:852–861.

96. Kay JH, Mendez AM, Zubiate P. A further look at tricuspid annuloplasty. *Ann Thorac Surg* 1976; 22:498–500.

97. Peterffy A. Jonasson R, Szamosi A, Henze A. Comparison of Kay's and De Vega's annuloplasty in surgical treatment of tricuspid incompetence. *Scand J Thorac Cardiovasc Surgery* 1980; 14:249–255.

98. Rabago G, De Vega NG, Castillon L, Moreno T, Fraile J, Azpitarte J, et al. The new De Vega technique in tricuspid annuloplasty: Results in 150 patients. *J Cardiovasc Surg* 1980; 21:231–238.

99. Reed GE, Boyd AD, Spencer FC, Engelman RM, Isom OW, Cunningham JN Jr. Operative management of tricuspid regurgitation. *Circulation* 1976; 54(suppl 3):III96–III98.

100. Baughman K, Kallman C, Yurchak P, Daggett WM, Buckley MJ. Predictors of survival after tricuspid surgery. *Am J Cardiol* 1984; 54:137–141.

101. Breye RH, McClenathan JH, Michaelis LL, McIntosh CL, Morrow AG. Tricuspid regurgitation: A comparison of nonoperative management, tricuspid annuloplasty, and tricuspid valve replacement. *J Thorac Cardiovasc Surgery* 1976; 72:867–874.

102. Jugdutt BI, Fraser RS, Lee SJK, Rossall RE, Callaghan JC. Long-term survival after tricuspid valve replacement: Results with seven different prostheses. *J Thorac Cardiovasc Surg* 1977; 74:20–27.

103. Kouchoukos NT, Stephenson LW. Indications for and results of tricuspid valve replacement. *Adv Cardiol* 1976; 17:199–206.

104. Sanfelippo PM, Giuliani ER, Danielson GK, Wallace RB, Pluth JR, McGoon DC. Tricuspid valve prosthetic replacement: Early and late results with the Starr-Edwards prosthesis. *J Thorac Cardiovasc Surg* 1976; 71:441–445.

105. Singh AK, Christian FD, Williams DO, Georas CS, Riley RR, Nanian KB, et al. Follow-up assessment of St. Jude medical prosthetic valve in the tricuspid position: Clinical and hemodynamic results. *Ann Thorac Surg* 1984; 37:324–327.

106. Arbulu A, Asfaw I. Tricuspid valvulectomy without prosthetic replacement: Ten years of clinical experience. *J Thorac Cardiovasc Surg* 1981; 82:684–691.

107. Stern H, Sisto D, Strom J, Soeiro R, Jones SR, Frater WM. Immediate tricuspid valve replacement for endocarditis. *J Thorac Cardiovasc Surg* 1986; 91:163–167.

108. D'Ambra M, LaRaia P, Philbin D, Watkins WD, Hilgenberg AD, Buckley MJ. Prostaglandin E_1: A new therapy for refractory right heart failure and pulmonary hypertension after mitral valve replacement. *J Thorac Cardiovasc Surg* 1985; 89:567–572.

109. Miller DD, Moreno-Cabral RJ, Stinson EB, Shinn JA, Shumway NE. Pulmonary artery balloon counterpulsation for acute right ventricular failure. *J Thorac Cardiovasc Surg* 1980; 80:760–763.

110. Cannegieter SC, Rosendaal FR, Wintzen AR, van der Meer FJM, Vandenbroucke JP, Briët E. Optimal oral anticoagulant therapy in patients with mechanical heart valves. *N Engl J Med* 1995; 333:11–17.

111. Chesebro JH, Fuster V, Elveback LR, McGoon DC, Pluth JR, Puga FJ, et al. Trial of combined warfarin plus dipyridamole of aspirin therapy in prosthetic heart valve replacement: Danger of aspirin compared with dipyridamole. *Am J Cardiol* 1983; 51:1537–1541.

112. Boskovic D, Elezovic I, Boskovic D, Simin N, Rolovic Z, Josipoulc V. Late thrombosis of the Björk-Shiley tilting disc valve in the tricuspid postion. *J Thorac Cardiovasc Surg* 1986; 91:1–8.

113. DePace NL, Iskandrian AS, Morganroth J, Ross J, Mattleman S, Nestico PF. Infective endocarditis involving a presumably normal pulmonic valve. *Am J Cardiol* 1984; 53:385–387.

114. Misbach GA, Turley K, Ebert PA. Pulmonary valve replacement for regurgitation after repair of tetralogy of Fallot. *Ann Thorac Surg* 1983; 36:684–691.

115. Wessel HU, Cunningham WJ, Paul MH, Bastanier CK, Muster AJ, Idriss FS. Exercise performance in tetralogy of Fallot after intracardiac repair. *J Thorac Cardiovasc Surg* 1980; 80:582–593.

116. Lepeschkin E. On the relation between the site of valvular involvement in endocarditis and the blood pressure resting on the valve. *Am J Med Sci* 1952; 225:318–319.

117. Cassling R, Rogler W, McManus B. Isolated pulmonic valve infective endocarditis: A diagnostically elusive study. *Am Heart J* 1985; 109:558–567.

118. Stephenson LW, Edic RN, Harken AH, Edmunds H Jr. Combined aortic and mitral valve replacement: Changes in practice and prognosis. *Circulation* 1984; 69:640–644.

119. Kumar AS, Chander H, Trehan H. Surgical technique of multiple valve replacement with biological valves: A new option. *J Heart Valve Dis* 1995; 4:45–46.

120. Blackstone EH, Kirklin JW. Death and other time-related events after valve replacement. *Circulation* 1985; 72:753–767.

121. Kirklin JW, Barratt-Boyes BG. Combined aortic and mitral valve disease with and without tricuspid valve disease. In: Kirklin JW, Barratt-Boyes BG, eds. *Cardiac Surgery*, 2d ed. New York: John Wiley; 1993; 573–587.

67

CLINICAL PERFORMANCE OF PROSTHETIC HEART VALVES

Gary L. Grunkemeier / Albert Starr / Shahbudin H. Rahimtoola

A heart valve functions as a check-valve: opening to permit forward blood flow and closing to prevent retrograde flow, about 40 million times per year. Heart valve prostheses consist of an orifice, through which blood flows, and an occluding mechanism that closes and opens the orifice. There are two classes of heart valves: *mechanical prostheses*, with rigid, manufactured occluders, and *biological* or *tissue valves*, with flexible leaflet occluders of animal or human origin. Among the mechanical valves there are three basic types, depending on whether the occluding mechanism is (1) a reciprocating ball, (2) a tilting disk, or (3) two semicircular hinged leaflets. The biological valves include those whose origin is from (1) the patient, (2) another human, or (3) another species. For each type there are several models available from different manufacturers. Selected frequently used valves are described.

PROSTHETIC HEART VALVES

Mechanical Valves

Ball valves appeared in the early 1960s, disk valves in the early 1970s, and bileaflet valves predominantly during the 1980s.

BALL VALVES

The first successful valve replacement devices, which led to long-term survivors and a design that has endured until today, used a ball-in-cage design.[1,2] Several modifications of this design have been used, but only the *Starr-Edwards* valve has endured; it has been used about 200,000 times. The ball is a silicone rubber polymer, impregnated with barium sulphate for radiopacity, which oscillates in a cage of cobalt-chromium alloy (Fig. 67-1, Plate 47). When the valve opens, blood flows

through the circular primary orifice and a secondary orifice (truncated conical frustum) between the ball and the housing. In the aortic position, there is a tertiary orifice between the equator of the ball and the aortic wall.

DISK VALVES

Improvement on the clinical success of the ball valves was sought by developing designs with reduced height. The first successful low-profile design was the *Björk-Shiley* tilting disk valve, introduced in 1969[3] (Fig. 67-2, Plate 48). It evolved through several design refinements,[4] and about 360,000 valves were implanted. These refinements also introduced a structural failure mode caused by strut fracture in the Convexo-Concave model. Some results with the discontinued Björk-Shiley models are included because so many patients are still alive with these valves.

Tilting disk valves employ a circular disk as an occluder. It is retained by wirelike arms or closed loops that project into the orifice. The disks are graphite with a coating of pyrolytic carbon, and the housings are stainless steel or titanium. With the disk open, the primary orifice is separated into two unequal (major and minor) orifices. The *Medtronic Hall* valve has a titanium housing and a carbon-coated disk with a unique central hole. The disk is retained and guided by a guide strut that protrudes through this hole. It has been used clinically since 1977.

BILEAFLET VALVES

Current development in mechanical valves is based on the bileaflet design, introduced by St. Jude Medical in 1977. Unlike the free-floating occluders in ball and disk valves, the two semicircular leaflets of a bileaflet valve are connected to the orifice housing by a hinge mechanism. The leaflets swing

FIGURE 67-1
See color Plate 47.

FIGURE 67-2
See color Plate 48.

apart during opening, creating three flow areas: one central and two peripheral. The *St. Jude* bileaflet valve (Fig. 67-3, Plate 49) has leaflets that open to an angle of 85° from the plane of the orifice and travel from 55 to 60° to the fully closed position, depending on valve size. The original version, whose housing did not rotate within the sewing ring, has been supplemented by a model that does rotate for intraoperative adjustment. It has been used over 600,000 times.

Biological Valves

Biological valves include as wide a variety of models as do mechanical valves:

1. *Autograft* valve refers to a translocation within the same individual, e.g., of the pulmonary valve into the aortic valve position.
2. *Autologous* (or autogenous) tissue valve involves fabricating a valve from the patient's own nonvalvular tissue, e.g., pericardium.
3. *Homograft* (or allograft) valve refers to transplantation from a donor of the same species, e.g., a donor's aortic or pulmonary valve into a recipient's aortic or pulmonary position.
4. *Heterograft* (or xenograft) valve is a transplant from another species, either an intact valve, e.g., a porcine aortic valve, or a valve fashioned from heterologous tissue, e.g., bovine pericardium.

The goal of biological valves is to reduce the complications associated with thromboembolism and the need for anticoagulation. The first successful biological valves were homografts, pioneered by Ross[5] and Barratt-Boyes[6] in 1962.

AUTOGRAFT

The pulmonary autograft procedure consists of an autotransplant of the pulmonary valve to the aortic position; the pulmonary valve is then replaced by an aortic or pulmonary homograft. This operation was first described in 1967[7] and is now called the Ross procedure; it is currently undergoing increased popularity,[8–11] but this operation involves a double valve replacement, with the attendant early and late risks. This procedure uses double valve replacement to solve a single valve problem; however, subsequent problems are possibly likely to be with pulmonary valve replacement, which is easier to remedy.

AUTOLOGOUS PERICARDIAL VALVE

An innovative valve concept has recently been developed.[12] This is a new category of valve developed in an attempt to combine the reproducibility and ease of insertion of a commercial, stented heterograft valve with the benefits of autologous tissue. It is a frame-mounted autologous pericardial valve, which is assembled from a kit in the operating room.

HOMOGRAFT

The homograft valve is considered to be a preferred substitute for aortic valve replacement, especially in younger patients. It achieves excellent hemodynamics; there is no need for anticoagulation and it has low thrombogenicity. The drawbacks are a more technically demanding operation and a low availability; however, the latter drawback has been alleviated by its commercial availability from cryopreservation services.

Several methods of procurement, sterilization, and preservation have been used.[13] Three techniques of aortic valve replacement are used: (1) Replacement of only the valve into the subcoronary position, (2) complete aortic root replacement with reimplantation of the coronary arteries, and (3) miniroot replacement with part of the donor aortic wall inserted within the host aorta.

PORCINE HETEROGRAFT

Glutaraldehyde sterilizes valve tissue, renders it bioacceptable by destroying antigenicity, and stabilizes the collagen cross-links for durability. The use of glutaraldehyde for tissue preservation was pioneered by Carpentier,[14] who introduced the term *bioprosthesis* for nonviable valves of biological origin, such as the *Hancock* and *Carpentier-Edwards* porcine valves (Fig. 67-4, Plate 50).[15]

Most porcine valves are mounted on rigid or flexible stents, to which the leaflets and the sewing ring are attached. Unstented versions have also been devised by several manufacturers, however, and are undergoing clinical evaluation.[16–20] Their goal is to achieve some of the potential benefit of a homograft valve, especially hemodynamics and perhaps durability, with an easily available commercial product. As with homografts, there are potentially three ways of implanting a stentless porcine valve (valve only, aortic root, miniroot). The standard porcine bioprosthesis is inserted into the annulus. The Carpentier-Edwards SupraAnnular valve (Fig. 67-5, Plate 51) is designed to be implanted above rather than within the aortic annulus. It has low pressure fixation and a cone-shaped stent that flares out at the top to improve leaflet durability.

BOVINE PERICARDIAL VALVE

Pericardial valves that are tailored and sewn into a valvular configuration using bovine pericardium as a fabric result in a valve that opens more completely than a porcine valve for better hemodynamics. It might also be expected to have better durability, because there is extra tissue to allow for shrinkage and a higher percentage of collagen to be cross-linked during fixation. Unfortunately, the Ionescu-Shiley, the first commercially available pericardial valve, did not bear out this promise. In fact, it experienced a higher failure rate than porcine valves and was taken off the market after about 10 years. The failures

FIGURE 67-4
See color Plate 50.

FIGURE 67-5
See color Plate 51.

FIGURE 67-3
See color Plate 49.

were partly due to aspects of the design, however, rather than to an intrinsic problem with pericardial tissue itself.

The Carpentier-Edwards pericardial bioprosthesis (Fig. 67-6, Plate 52) has a method of construction that does not require stitches to pass through the leaflets, as did the Ionescu-Shiley pericardial valve. Instead, the leaflets are anchored behind the stent pillars. The Carpentier-Edwards pericardial valve was first used in patients in 1982 and received approval from the U.S. Food and Drug Administration (FDA) for the aortic position in 1991. Other pericardial valves are being tested.

AUTOLOGOUS TISSUE VALVE PROCEDURES

From an immunologic standpoint, autologous tissue might seem to be the best material when a tissue transfer is required.

Valve Repair

When possible, valve repair[21–23] is generally preferable to replacement (see discussion below and Chap. 64).

GUIDELINES FOR REPORTING CLINICAL RESULTS

The analytic aspects of the reporting of clinical results of heart valves has evolved consistently since the first successful implants in 1960. As late (posthospital) experience accumulated near the end of the first decade of implants, the need to analyze time-related events resulted in the introduction of actuarial analysis,[24] which had previously been used to analyze the results of cancer therapy.[25] Later, the use of linearized (constant hazard) rates,[26,27] Cox regression,[28] and multivariable parametric models[29] were advocated. The effectiveness of these refined statistical methods in comparing results from different series, however, was limited by the lack of standardization in definitions and follow-up methods.

AATS/STS Guidelines for Clinical Reporting

In 1988, standards that specified which complications should be collected and how they should be defined were proposed by the Ad Hoc Liaison Committee for Standardizing Definitions of Prosthetic Heart Valve Morbidity, a joint committee of the American Association for Thoracic Surgery (AATS) and the Society of Thoracic Surgeons (STS).[30] These guidelines were revised in 1996.[31,32] The complications that were determined to be of critical importance by these guidelines are as follows:

1. *Structural valvular deterioration* refers to any change in function of an operated valve resulting from an intrinsic abnormality that causes stenosis or regurgitation.
2. *Nonstructural dysfunction* is a composite category that includes any abnormality that results in stenosis or regurgitation of the operated valve that is not intrinsic to the valve itself, exclusive of thrombosis and infection. This

includes inappropriate sizing, also called prosthesis-patient mismatch.[33]

3. *Valve thrombosis* is any thrombus, in the absence of infection, attached to or near an operated valve that occludes part of the blood flow path or that interferes with the function of the valve.
4. *Embolism* is any embolic event that occurs in the absence of infection after the immediate perioperative period (when anesthesia-induced unconsciousness is completely reversed). These include any new, temporary or permanent, focal or global neurologic deficit and peripheral embolic event; emboli proven to consist of nonthrombotic material are excluded.
5. *Bleeding event (formerly anticoagulant hemorrhage)* is any episode of major internal or external bleeding that causes death, hospitalization, or permanent injury (e.g., vision loss) or requires transfusion. The complication "bleeding event" applies to all patients, whether or not they are taking anticoagulants or antiplatelet drugs.
6. *Operated valvular endocarditis* is any infection involving an operated valve. Morbidity associated with active infection, such as valve thrombosis, thrombotic embolus, bleeding event, or paravalvular leak, is included under this category but is not included in other categories or morbidity.

The *consequences* of the above morbid events include reoperation, valve-related mortality, sudden unexpected unexplained death, cardiac death, total deaths, and permanent valve-related impairment.[31,32]

FDA Guidelines for New Valve Approvals

In 1976, medical devices including prosthetic heart valves came under the jurisdiction of the FDA,[34] who subsequently issued various guidelines for submission of Premarket Approval (PMA) applications for heart valves. The FDA issued a Guidance document in December 1993[35] that used the analytical approach to clinical studies adapted from the work of Gersh et al.[36] These authors proposed a method for premarket clinical testing of heart valves that emphasizes confidence interval estimation and comparisons to objective performance criteria (OPC). *OPC are linearized rates for critical complications, representing averages achieved by the best currently used valves.* A *linearized rate* is calculated as the number of events divided by total patient-years and multiplied by 100 to convert it to units of "events per 100 years" or "percent per year."[27]

To determine OPC for contemporary use, the FDA screened the literature, plus data submitted to them from clinical investigations of approved devices, and identified OPC for the major morbidity categories.[35] They determined that these rates were similar for aortic and mitral positions but varied for some complications between mechanical and biological valves. The OPC for complications are given in Table 67-1 for mechanical and biological replacement heart valves. Several observations of these data are significant.

FIGURE 67-6
See color Plate 52.

The category of "Structural Deterioration" was not included in the list of OPC because the clinical PMA investigation is not designed to detect intrinsic valve failure. Structural durability should be evaluated by in vitro testing, and the clinical realization of structural failure should be so small (mechanical valves) that the clinical study is of insufficient size, or so long-term (tissue valves) that the clinical study is of insufficient duration to assess it adequately.

From the "Nonstructural Dysfunction" category, the FDA included only leak, the most common and the most frequently reported subcategory, and derived OPC for major leaks ("as defined by AATS/STS, 1988")[30] and for all leaks.

The FDA separated "Thromboembolism" into the separate categories of valve thrombosis and thromboembolism, as had been strongly advocated,[37,38] and the FDA derived OPC both for major "Anticoagulant-related Hemorrhage" events ("as defined by AATS/STS, 1988")[30] and for all bleeding events.

Based on the OPC values given in Table 67-1, the FDA has set the minimum amount of follow-up required for a PMA study at 800 valve-years.[39] The assumption of constant risk for heart valve complications, as embodied by the OPC formulation, is only an approximation; but if operative events are excluded (the intent of the FDA guidelines) and maximum follow-up is in the 2- to 3-year range, this assumption may be acceptable, at least for the purpose of sample size estimation.

VALVE-RELATED COMPLICATIONS

Actuarial valve failure–free curves[25] are used to describe tissue valve durability, and linearized rates[27] are used for all other complications.

Structural Deterioration

This category, the first one considered in the Guidelines for Reporting, virtually always results in death or valve explant. There is a dual standard with regard to this complication: for biological valves, structural deterioration is probably inevitable if the patient lives long enough; whereas for mechanical valves, the only acceptable rate is zero.

TABLE 67-1

COMPLICATIONS FOR EVALUATING CLINICAL PERFORMANCE OF REPLACEMENT HEART VALVES AND OBJECTIVE PERFORMANCE CRITERIA (OPC)^a VALUES FOR COMPLICATION RATES (PERCENT/YEAR)

Definitions of Morbidity	OPC, %/year	
	Mechanical	Biological
1. *Structural deterioration:* Valve deterioration, wear, stress fracture, poppet escape, calcification, leaflet tear, stent creep; *excludes* infected or thrombosed valves		
2. *Nonstructural dysfunction:* Entrapment by pannus or suture, leak, inappropriate sizing, hemolytic anemia; *excludes* thromboembolism and infection	(leak) 1.2 (major 0.6)	(leak) 1.2 (major 0.6)
3A. *Valve thrombosis:* Thrombosis proved by operation, autopsy, or clinical investigation; *excludes* infection	0.8	0.2
3B. *Thromboembolism:* Neurologic deficit, peripheral arterial emboli, acute myocardial infarction *after* operation in patients with known normal coronary arteries or those <40 years of age; *excludes* septic emboli, hemorrhage, immediate surgical events	3.0	2.5
4. *Anticoagulant-related hemorrhage:* Bleeding that causes death, stroke, operation, hospitalization, or transfusion in patients receiving anticoagulants and/or antiplatelet drugs	3.5 (major 1.5)	1.4 (major 0.9)
5. *Prosthetic valve endocarditis:* Based on blood cultures, clinical signs, and/or histologic evidence at reoperation or autopsy; *includes* valve thrombosis, embolus, or paravalvular leak associated with active infection	1.2	1.2

^{a} Please see text for definition of OPC.

Source: The complications and their definitions are adapted from reference 30; the OPC values are taken from Appendix K of reference 35.

MECHANICAL VALVES

The durability of the currently used mechanical valves is remarkable, given the harsh biological environment in which the valve must perform 40 million cycles per year. For example, the current Starr-Edwards ball valve, now in use for more than 30 years and in almost 200,000 patients, has had fewer than a dozen structural problems reported to the manufacturer, most of which did not cause clinical problems. Even the discontinued Björk-Shiley Convexo-Concave valve, whose strut fracture failures have been highly publicized, had fewer than 1 percent failures reported after 15 years of experience.[40] The Medtronic Hall valve had three leaflet fractures in a version that is not used in the United States. The problem was determined to be related to unequal coatings of pyrolytic carbon on the two faces of the leaflet and to be limited to a very small subset of valves. Since the manufacturing specifications were changed to ensure more equal coatings, the problem has not recurred. The St. Jude valve has had only 24 mechanical failures reported to the FDA, an excellent record considering that over 600,000 have been implanted.

BIOLOGICAL VALVES

Freedom from structural deterioration for several series of aortic and mitral porcine bioprostheses is shown in Fig. 67-7. The mean age of patients in these older series is around 50 years. The current series of porcine valves, together with the tendency to select older patients,[41–44] will no doubt result in improved durability. Design changes in some porcine valves,[45,46] such as stentless configurations,[16–20] may also improve durability.

Although the Carpentier-Edwards pericardial valve has been available for over 15 years, relatively few long-term results of the valve are available. Those that have been reported, however, show improved durability in the aortic position compared to the previously discontinued Ionescu-Shiley pericardial valve (Fig. 67-7). The durability of the Carpentier-Edwards pericardial valve also compares favorably with that of porcine valves (Fig. 67-7; Table 67-2). The patients in the Carpentier-Edwards pericardial valve series were older than patients in previous series of pericardial and porcine valves, however, and it is unknown to what extent this has resulted in apparent improvement in the durability of the Carpentier-Edwards pericardial valve.

Structural durability is considered to be better with *homografts* compared to other bioprostheses. From various published reports[13] for homografts used primarily in the aortic position, it is apparent that the variation among series is wide, the current methods of sterilization/preservation provide better results than those which have been discontinued, and the results do not appear better than those for porcine bioprostheses.

The pulmonary autograft is considered an excellent aortic valve substitute, especially for young patients[10] and in the treatment of patients with endocarditis.[47] Freedom from reoperation has been reported as 100 percent in 33 patients from 8 to 47 years old followed to a maximum of 48 months[11] and 93 percent at 5.5 years in 51 patients from 2 to 21 years old.[10] Data from one center showed 48.5 percent freedom from reoperation at 19 years and, after excluding patients from one clinic, 85 percent freedom from reoperation at 20 years.[48] To evaluate complications of this procedure fully, problems with the valve

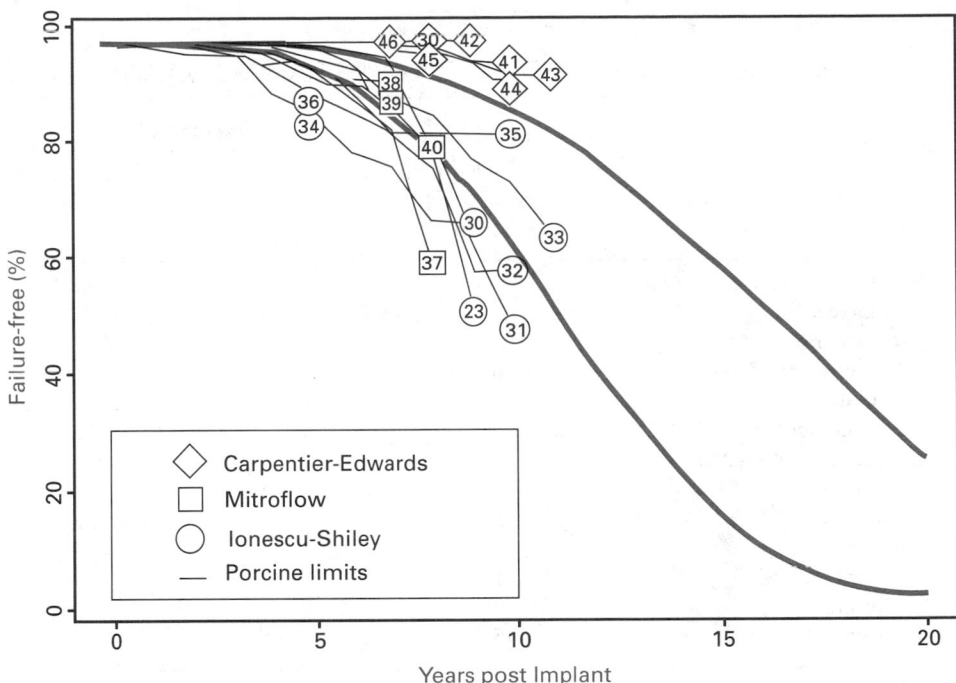

FIGURE 67-7
Reported actuarial curves of freedom from structural aortic valve deterioration. The shape of the symbol at the end of the line indicates the model of the pericardial valve and the numeral inside the symbol corresponds to the reference number in the *original* publication. The Weibull curves indicating the approximate limits of porcine valve failure curves are superimposed for comparison. The Carpentier-Edwards bovine pericardial valve has a much lower failure rate than the Ionescu-Shiley or Mitroflow pericardial valves and also a lower failure rate than the porcine bioprosthesis. (From Grunkemeier and Bodnar.[13] Reproduced by permission of the publisher and authors.)

used to replace the pulmonary valve must be combined with complications of the pulmonary autograft itself.

VALVE REPAIR

Mitral valve repair is considered preferable to replacement, when practicable. It has been shown to improve ejection fraction[49] and to provide good results for treating bacterial endocarditis[50] and in elderly patients.[51,52] It has been suggested strongly that it improves survival; however, there are problems associated with the comparisons.[53]

The weakness of valve repair is durability. The 10-year actuarial reoperation rate has been reported to be 15 percent in non-rheumatic mitral disease.[54] The reoperation rate for patients with rheumatic mitral disease varies from 25 percent reoperation at 5 years[55] to 17 percent at 10 years in a large series in which calcium debridement[56] and anterior leaflet procedures were performed.[57] The reoperation rate at 10 years was 24 percent for patients less than 20 years of age and 9 percent at 10 years for patients over 20 years of age.[58]

The early results of aortic valve repair have been promising,[23,59,60] but further follow-up is needed to assess the long-term results.

Other Valve-Related Complications

Linearized rates are often used to describe the complications required by the AATS/STS guidelines for reporting.[30–32] The

TABLE 67-2

YEAR RESULTS WITH CARPENTIER-EDWARDS PERICARDIAL VALVE

Series	FDA-Mandated Patients,[a] (n = 267) Actuarial %	Cleveland Clinic[b] (n = 310) Actuarial %	Cleveland Clinic[b] (n = 310) Linearized Rate, %/Year
Structural valve deterioration:	—	9	0.3 ± 0.2
<65 years	—	6	—
>65 years	—	3	—
All valve dysfunction	6 ± 3	—	—
Reoperation	8 ± 2	4	—
Thromboembolism	16 ± 3	11 ± 2.1	1.6 ± 0.3
Anticoagulation-related hemorrhage	6 ± 2	9 ± 1.8	1.0 ± 0.2
Endocarditis	5 ± 2	6 ± 1.6	0.8 ± 0.3
Valve related:			
Complications	41 ± 4		
Mortality	10 ± 2		
Total mortality	45 ± 3	45.5	

[a] FDA approval was based on 719 patients at 7 years.[75] Data at 10 years from FDA-mandated longer follow-up of selected patients is shown. (Data from Baxter Laboratories database, reproduced by permission.)

[b] Two-thirds of all deaths were cardiac-related. Multivariate analyses identified age ≥65 years ($p = .0002$) and coronary disease ($p = .0001$) as significant risk factors.

Note: All percentages are ± standard error.

Source: Cosgrove et al.[23]

use of such rates assumes that the risks are constant, which is usually only approximately true. A review of a large number of published reports of the performance of prosthetic heart valves reveals a wide spread of results for every complication for every valve. In 152 series of heart valves covering 194,000 patient-years accumulated by 44,000 patients who had 7 models of valves in 3 positions (aortic, mitral, double), the linearized event rates ranged from 0 to 7.6 percent/year for thromboembolism, 0 to 3.1 percent/year for thrombosis, 0 to 7.2 percent/year for bleeding, 0 to 2.6 percent/year for infection, and 0 to 1.9 percent/year for paravalvular leak.[61] Caution must be exercised in directly comparing event rates among valves for many reasons, including the simplifications involved in the use of linearized rates, varying definitions of complications (many of these reports predate the standardized definitions), and differences in patient characteristics between series.[53,62]

Difficulties in Making Comparisons Between Published Series

As noted above, there is wide variation in the reported complication rates of series using the same valves. Figures 67-8 to 67-11 illustrate the wide range of embolism with use of the same heart valve in different series. This variation must be due to variations between series other than the *valve model.* These include factors associated with the following:

1. *Patients*—age, ventricular function, comorbidities, etc.

2. *Reporting center*—surgical variables, postoperative medical management, method, frequency and thoroughness of follow-up, definitions of complications, etc.

3. Problems with *data analysis*[63,64]—many patient-related factors are known to influence thromboembolism,[53,65] stroke rates in patients with atrial fibrillation and in the elderly are equal to those observed in prosthetic valve series,[66] and standardized definitions[30–32] were not in effect or were not employed when many of the available series were reported, etc.

4. *Published data*—these reports describe only a small fraction of the valves implanted and are probably not a representative subset.

Several types of bias can affect reported results. As examples, selection bias occurs in the collection and analysis of data and the decision to report it[63]; publication bias describes the fact that published series tend to be those with the best (or worst, but not typical) results.[67] If a random allocation of valves had been made among patients within a center, statistical methods could theoretically assess the effect on complication rates due to valve model. For logistic, financial, and ethical reasons, however, the number of randomized studies of valves is small, and the available studies are usually of insufficient size to show differences among valves. Although randomized studies provide the best internal validity or valve-specific comparison within centers, they may lack external validity or generalizability to patients outside of the study.[68]

A theoretically preferable way to answer this bias is to allocate patients randomly to different treatments (valves). Randomized trials, however, also have difficulties,[69] and as noted there are logistic, financial, and ethical arguments against randomization of patients to different heart valves.[70] Consequently, the number of randomized studies of valves is small, and those that exist are usually of insufficient size to add to the knowledge already obtained from careful observational studies.

Major Randomized Trials

The two major randomized clinical trials that have been reported are the Edinburgh Heart Valve Trial[71] and the Veterans

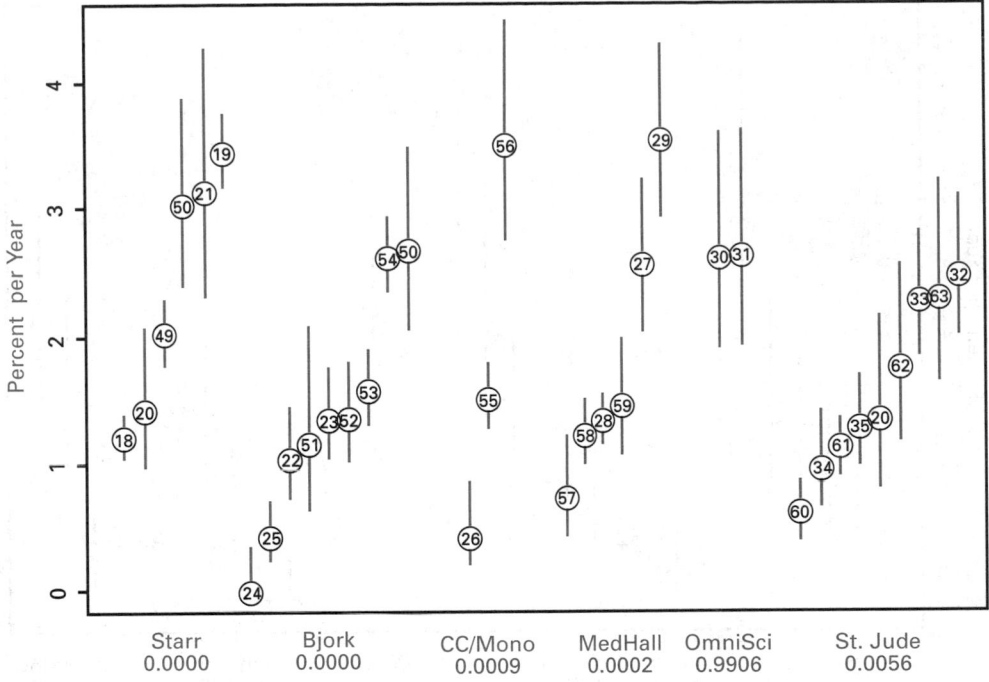

Embolism Rates for Mechanical Aortic Valves
with 70% confidence intervals and comparison *p*-values

FIGURE 67-8

Embolism rates for mechanical aortic valves. Each open symbol represents a different series, and the height of the symbol is the linearized rate for the series. The vertical bar indicates the 70 percent confidence interval. The decimal below each valve model name on the horizontal axis is the *p*-value for the comparison of rates for the series with that model of valve. The numerals inside the open symbols correspond to the cited reference numbers for the series in the *original* publication. Note the large range of embolism in the various studies and the overlap between the different valves. (From Grunkemeier et al.[61] Reproduced by permission of the publisher and authors.)

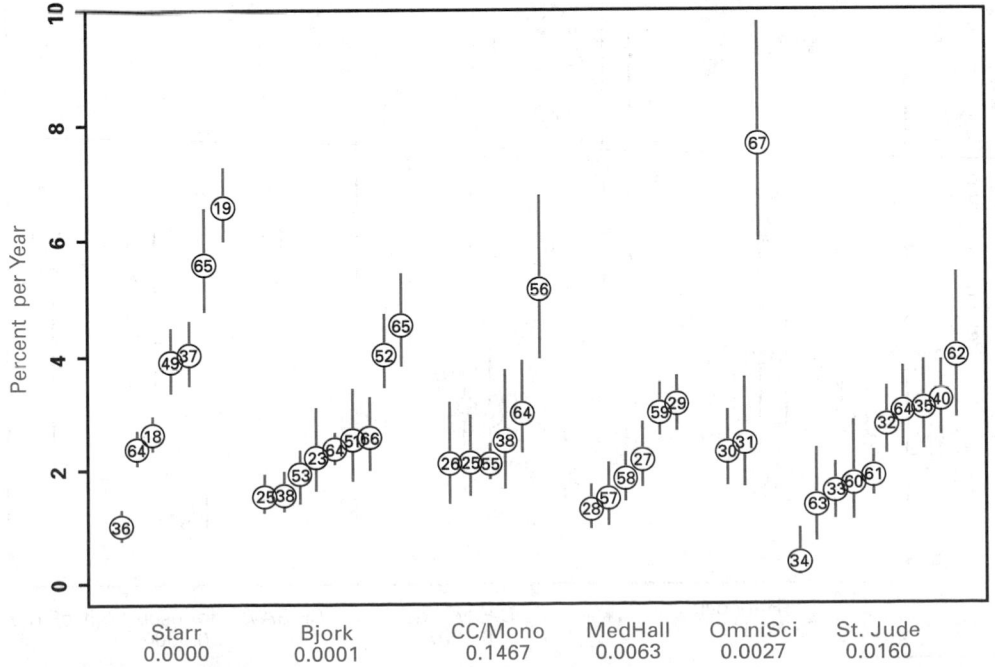

Embolism Rates for Mechanical Mitral Valves
with 70% confidence intervals and comparison *p*-values

FIGURE 67-9

Embolism rates for mechanical mitral valves. For explanation of symbols, see Fig. 67-8. (From Grunkemeier et al.[61] Reproduced by permission of the publisher and authors.)

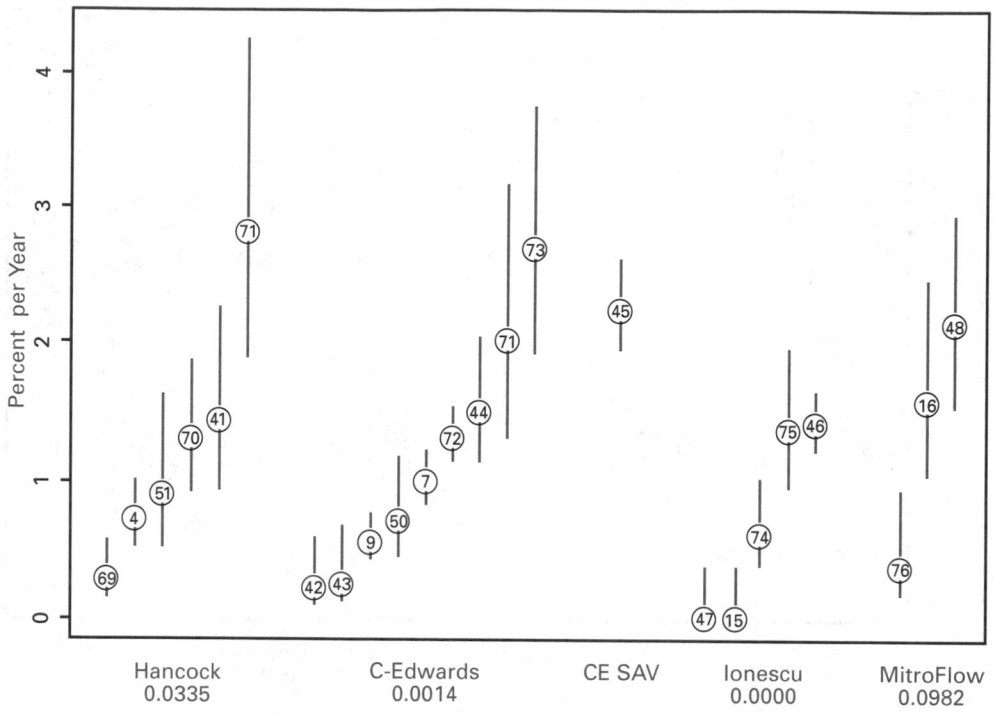

FIGURE 67-10

Embolism rates for biological aortic valves. For explanation of symbols, see Fig. 67-8. (From Grunkemeier et al.[61] Reproduced by permission of the publisher and authors.)

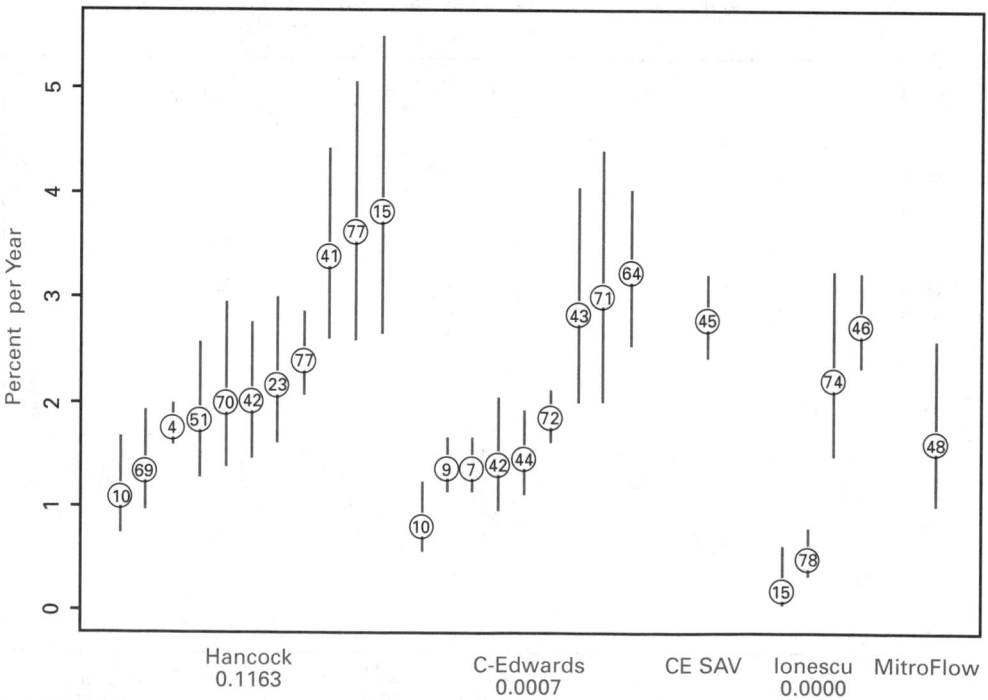

FIGURE 67-11

Embolism rates for biological mitral valves. For explanation of symbols, see Fig. 67-8. (From Grunkemeier et al.[61] Reproduced by permission of the publisher and authors.)

Administration (VA) Cooperative Study on Valvular Heart Disease.[72] Both studies compared mechanical valves to porcine bioprostheses.

The Edinburgh trial compared the Björk-Shiley Standard valve to porcine valves—initially the Hancock and later the Carpentier-Edwards.[71] Table 67-3 contains actuarial comparisons at 5 and 12 years for the 211 aortic and 261 mitral valve patients. The authors concluded that survival with a mechanical valve was better than with the bioprosthetic valve, but that this was somewhat offset by the increased risk of bleeding.

The VA trial compared the standard Björk-Shiley valve to the Hancock Modified Orifice (size 21 to 23 mm aortic) or Hancock Standard (other sizes) porcine valves.[72] Table 67-4 contains actuarial comparisons at 11 years of the endpoint variables. For the event "any valve-related complication," the risk for mechanical valves is higher during the first 5 years, but the cumulative risks converge by about 10 years. The authors concluded that the rates of both survival and all valve-related complications were similar with mechanical and porcine valves, but that the types of complications differed between the two; bleeding rates were higher with mechanical valves, but structural valve deterioration (and reoperation) rates were higher with a bioprosthesis.

Comparison of the 12-year actuarial event rates between these two trials[72] showed that the bleeding and thromboembo-

TABLE 67-3

ACTUARIAL SURVIVAL AND OCCURRENCE OF VALVE-RELATED EVENTS AFTER 5 YEARS AND 12 YEARS IN PATIENTS RECEIVING A BJÖRK-SHILEY OR PORCINE PROSTHESIS[a]

	Mitral Valve Replacement		Aortic Valve Replacement	
	5 Years	12 Years	5 Years	12 Years
SURVIVAL				
All survivors				
Björk-Shiley valve	76.0 ± 4.1	56.1 ± 4.9	67.4 ± 4.1	44.2 ± 4.8
Porcine valve	82.4 ± 3.8	52.3 ± 5.4	69.7 ± 4.0	40.4 ± 4.4
Survivors with original valve				
Björk-Shiley valve	75.1 ± 4.2	55.2 ± 5.0	74.3 ± 4.2	41.6 ± 4.7*
Porcine valve	79.4 ± 4.0	41.1 ± 5.4	77.4 ± 4.1	23.8 ± 3.8
Survivors w/o major events				
Björk-Shiley valve	71.4 ± 4.3	41.1 ± 4.9	63.6 ± 4.2	35.2 ± 4.5*
Porcine valve	77.5 ± 4.1	38.6 ± 5.3	65.9 ± 4.1	21.5 ± 3.7
VALVE-RELATED EVENTS				
Reoperation				
Björk-Shiley valve	4.2 ± 2.1	4.2 ± 2.1**	5.8 ± 2.3	9.9 ± 3.2***
Porcine valve	4.5 ± 2.2	22.6 ± 5.7	4.7 ± 2.1	43.1 ± 6.0
Bleeding				
All episodes				
Björk-Shiley valve	5.5 ± 2.4	32.6 ± 6.1***	4.8 ± 2.1	24.5 ± 5.9
Porcine valve	1.1 ± 1.1	9.7 ± 4.7	2.7 ± 1.6	24.5 ± 7.2
Major episodes				
Björk-Shiley valve	5.5 ± 2.4	22.5 ± 5.0**	4.8 ± 2.1	17.1 ± 4.9
Porcine valve	1.1 ± 1.1	4.2 ± 2.4	2.7 ± 1.6	9.7 ± 4.3
Embolism				
All episodes				
Björk-Shiley valve	6.1 ± 2.4	11.5 ± 4.0	20.2 ± 3.9	31.5 ± 5.1
Porcine valve	8.2 ± 3.0	22.5 ± 4.9	16.0 ± 3.7	32.2 ± 6.0
Major episodes				
Björk-Shiley valve	0.9 ± 0.9	0.9 ± 0.9*	11.5 ± 3.2	16.3 ± 4.1
Porcine valve	4.6 ± 2.2	8.9 ± 3.3	5.7 ± 2.3	10.1 ± 3.4
Endocarditis				
Björk-Shiley valve	2.0 ± 1.4	4.8 ± 2.4	0.8 ± 0.8	2.3 ± 1.7
Porcine valve	1.0 ± 1.0	2.2 ± 1.6	0.9 ± 0.9	7.4 ± 3.4

[a] Values given are actuarial percentages ± standard error.

Note: Symbols for significant differences between mechanical and porcine valves: *, $p < .05$; **, $p < .01$; ***, $p < .001$.

Source: From Bloomfield et al,[71] as summarized in Grunkemeier et al,[73] with permission.

TABLE 67-4

PROBABILITY OF DEATH DUE TO ANY CAUSE, ANY VALVE-RELATED COMPLICATION, AND INDIVIDUAL VALVE-RELATED COMPLICATIONS 11 YEARS AFTER RANDOMIZATION[a]

Event	Mitral Valve			Aortic Valve		
	Mechanical (n = 198)	Porcine (n = 196)	p	Mechanical (n = 88)	Porcine (n = 93)	p
Death from any cause	53 ± 4	59 ± 4	.26	64 ± 5	67 ± 5	.41
Any valve-related complication	62 ± 4	64 ± 4	.64	71 ± 5	79 ± 6	.34
Systemic embolism	16 ± 4	15 ± 3	.49	18 ± 5	15 ± 4	.61
Bleeding	43 ± 4	24 ± 4	***	41 ± 6	28 ± 7	.02
Endocarditis	7 ± 2	8 ± 2	.79	11 ± 4	17 ± 5	.37
Valve thrombosis	2 ± 1	1 ± 1	.33	1 ± 1	1 ± 1	.95
Perivalvular regurgitation	4 ± 2	2 ± 1	.28	17 ± 5	9 ± 6	.05
Reoperation	7 ± 2	16 ± 4	.07	21 ± 5	47 ± 9	.23
Structural valve failure	0 ± 0	15 ± 4	***	0 ± 0	36 ± 8	***

[a] Values given are actuarial percentages ± standard error.

Note: p values are for differences between mechanical and porcine valves; ***, $p < .001$

Source: From Hammermeister et al,[72] as summarized in Grunkemeier et al,[73] with permission.

lism rates were higher in the VA study, but that reoperation rates were higher in the Edinburgh study. These differences could be partially accounted for by the composition of the two patient populations: The Edinburgh patients (1) were younger and less heavily anticoagulated, (2) included women and those with double valve replacements, and (3) had a higher percentage of porcine valves in the mitral position. Late results show a better survival with mechanical valves than with bioprostheses in the mitral position with the original valve (Table 67-3) in the Edinburgh trial (42 percent versus 24 percent, $p < .05$), probably because of the high rate of bioprosthetic degeneration, and in the aortic position in the VA trial (33 percent versus 25 percent, $p = .03$ at 16 years[74]).

VALVE SELECTION CRITERIA

Because of the wide variation in results among and between various valve models, it is impossible to rank valves within valve types on the basis of complication rates. Some general recommendations, however, can be made with regard to valve selection (Table 67-5).[73]

A biological valve should be used when the patient cannot or will not take anticoagulants, desires pregnancy (see Chap. 68), or has a short life expectancy. A mechanical valve should be used if the patient needs anticoagulant therapy (e.g., because of atrial fibrillation), has a mechanical valve in another position, previously had a stroke, requires double valve replacement, or has a long life expectancy. Mechanical valves should be considered for double valve replacement because the risk of structural deterioration for two porcine valves is additive,[76] whereas the thromboembolic risk of two mechanical valves is not additive.[77]

MANAGEMENT OF PATIENTS WITH PROSTHETIC HEART VALVES

Patients who have undergone valve replacement are not cured but still have serious heart disease. They have exchanged native valvular disease for prosthetic valvular disease and must be followed with the same care as patients with native valvular disease. The clinical course of patients with prosthetic heart valves is influenced by several factors.[78]

Ventricular Dysfunction

Despite relief of valvular obstruction or regurgitation, some patients fail to improve after valve replacement, or even deteriorate, because of impaired ventricular function. The cause of dysfunction may be carditis associated with rheumatic disease, myocardial degeneration and fibrosis from long-standing pressure or volume overload, ischemic damage at the time of valve replacement, coronary artery disease, or other associated diseases such as idiopathic dilated cardiomyopathy. Perioperative myocardial damage is an important cause of postoperative ventricular dysfunction. The importance of myocardial protection at the time of valve surgery is now recognized, and current operative techniques reduce myocardial oxygen consumption by hypothermic cardioplegia and use a variety of means for maintaining adequate myocardial perfusion and protection.

Other Cardiac Lesions

Cardiac diseases affecting primarily one valve often affect other valves, the conduction system, the coronary arteries, and the pulmonary vasculature. With the exception of pulmonary

TABLE 67-5

VALVE SELECTION CRITERIA[a,b]

Reasons for preferring mechanical valve
- Quality of life, as perceived by the patient
- Age < 40 years
- Renal failure
- Long expected lifetime
- Composite graft
- Anticoagulated patient
  Coronary bypass using internal mammary artery
  Previous dysfunctional tissue valve
  Double valve replacement
Reasons for preferring bioprosthesis
- Quality of life, as perceived by the patient
- Anticoagulant intolerance
- Unreliable anticoagulant risk
- Age ≥65 years[c]
- Short expected lifetime
  Pregnancy anticipated
  Previous thrombosed mechanical valve

[a] Bulleted items are more compelling.

[b] This table refers only to mechanical and bioprosthetic valves. It does not consider the impact on valve selection of the appropriate use of homograft valves (e.g., endocarditis) or the pulmonary autografts (e.g., children). The indications for these procedures are still evolving, and these procedures are not (currently) universally available options.

[c] If data from newer bioprostheses warrant, or if refinements in selection of patients according to risk factors become more developed, the age may be lowered.

Source: Grunkemeier et al,[73] with permission.

hypertension and functional tricuspid regurgitation, these disorders usually do not improve after isolated valve replacement. Rheumatic disease typically affects both mitral and aortic valves but not necessarily with the same severity at the same time. Therefore, patients who have mitral valve replacement may subsequently require aortic valve replacement years later, or vice versa. Calcification of the aortic and mitral valve annuli may extend to the conduction system. High-degree or complete atrioventricular block may occur at the time of surgery or during the late postoperative period, requiring pacemaker implantation. Coronary artery disease is very common in the age range of patients requiring valve replacement. Preoperative coronary arteriography should be performed in all patients with myocardial ischemic pain, in those with left ventricular dysfunction, in those with risk factors for coronary artery disease, and in those about 35 years of age or older.[78,79] Coronary bypass surgery of technically suitable vessels should be performed at the time of valve surgery.

Prosthesis-Related Problems See Table 67-6

The incidence of problems with each prosthesis was discussed earlier. *Operative mortality* is related to older age of patient, New York Heart Association functional class III or IV, increased left ventricular size, left ventricular dysfunction, heart failure, pulmonary hypertension, low cardiac output, and pres-

ence of associated diseases such as systemic arterial hypertension, diabetes mellitus, peripheral and cerebral vascular disease, prior heart surgery, prior myocardial infarction, chronic obstructive pulmonary disease, and renal and hepatic failure. Coronary bypass surgery performed at the same time as valve replacement increases the operative mortality modestly (from 1.4 to 4.0 percent), but associated coronary artery disease, if not bypassed, significantly increases the operative mortality to 9.4 percent and the 10-year mortality to 64 percent.[80] Other very important factors include the occurrence of perioperative myocardial infarction, the duration of the operation, aortic cross-clamp time, and whether or not the patient needed reoperation within 1 to 2 weeks after the initial operation, and on an elective or emergency basis.

The risk of *prosthetic endocarditis* is about 3 percent in the first year and 0.5 percent in subsequent years. Despite therapy, infections in the early postoperative period (up to 2 to 12 months) are the result of hospital-based organisms. The infections are difficult to cure and have a high mortality rate (about 80 percent)[81,82]; early reoperation is usually recommended. The mortality rate from late (2 to 12 months or later) postoperative infection is approximately 40 percent.[81,82] About half the patients can be treated successfully with medication alone. The infected valve should be replaced in patients who do not respond to medical treatment or who have evidence of heart failure, annular invasion, embolism, prosthetic dysfunction, unstable prosthesis, or gram-negative, staphylococcal, or fungal infection.[64] The importance of adequate antibiotic prophylaxis for the prevention of endocarditis cannot be overemphasized; the prevention and treatment of prosthetic valve endocarditis are discussed in Chap. 82.

Long-term anticoagulant therapy is associated with *bleeding* episodes. The incidence of minor bleeding is about 2 to 4 percent per year or less. The incidence of major bleeding

TABLE 67-6

MAJOR COMPLICATIONS OF VALVE REPLACEMENT

1. Operative mortality
2. Perioperative myocardial infarction
3. Prosthetic endocarditis
4. Prosthetic dehiscence
5. Prosthetic dysfunction
   a. Obstruction: Usually thrombotic, occasionally due to item 3, 4, or 8
   b. Regurgitation
   c. Hemolysis
   d. Structural failure
6. Thromboemboli
7. Hemorrhage with anticoagulant therapy
8. Valve prosthesis-patient mismatch
9. Prosthetic replacement often caused by item 3, 4, or 5; occasionally caused by item 6, 7, or 8
10. Late mortality, including sudden, unexplained death

Source: Rahimtoola.[64] Reproduced with permission of the publisher and author.

is about 1 to 2 percent per year or less, with a mortality rate of about 0.5 percent per year or less. The incidence of these complications is lower in patients who take their medications reliably and in those in whom smooth long-term anticoagulation can be achieved. With oral anticoagulants, low- or mid-dose warfarin therapy is combined with low-dose aspirin. Higher degrees of anticoagulation increase the incidence of bleeding without reducing the incidence of thromboembolism. The management of antithrombotic therapy is discussed in Chap. 68.

Prosthetic dehiscence is the result of sutures pulling out of the cardiac tissues. It may result from infection, inadequate surgical technique, or diseased cardiac tissue (e.g., edema, necrosis, calcification).

Because of the continued proliferation of new types and models of prostheses and their relatively brief history of clinical use, the natural history of *structured valve deterioration* is incompletely determined. Although some mechanical prostheses had initial problems with component failure, the most common cause for dysfunction of mechanical prosthetic valves is thrombotic obstruction. The incidence of thrombotic obstruction with the Björk-Shiley spherical occluder valve is higher than that seen with the Starr-Edwards or St. Jude valves, particularly in the mitral position. Failure of biological valves is more common than failure of mechanical prostheses because of leaflet deterioration or calcification; progressive prosthetic regurgitation and/or stenosis is the rule. Bioprosthesis failure is greater in younger patients, in older patients with chronic renal insufficiency, and in the mitral position. In patients over 50 years old, failure of mitral prostheses usually starts at 5 to 8 years and of aortic prostheses at 8 to 10 years. It is unlikely that the tissue valves currently in use will be able to provide the long-term performance demonstrated by the ball-valve mechanical prosthesis.

Red cells are fractured by turbulence and contact with foreign surfaces. Some degree of *hemolysis* is present with all mechanical prostheses but not with bioprostheses. Important hemolysis, however, may occur with a perivalvular leak or severe prosthetic obstruction regardless of prosthesis type. Serum lactic dehydrogenase (LDH) is usually the simplest and most reliable index of hemolysis to follow in patients with prosthetic valves. A sudden increase in LDH may indicate prosthesis dysfunction, perivalvular leak, or cloth tear. Iron and folate therapy usually correct the anemia. Valve replacement may be required for severe, refractory hemolytic anemia.

Important *systemic embolization* is an unfortunate complication of prosthetic valve replacement. Anticoagulation is recommended for all patients with mechanical prostheses. *Despite long-term anticoagulation, patients with prosthetic valves face an embolic rate from aortic prostheses of 1 to 2 percent or less per year and from mitral prostheses of 3 to 4 percent or less per year.*

No prosthesis currently employed has an effective orifice as large as that of the native valve, and *valve prosthesis-patient mismatch*[33] may occur. *All patients with prosthetic heart valves have mild to moderate stenosis.* Patients with aortic valve prostheses have obstruction to left ventricular outflow (aortic stenosis), and patients with mitral valve prostheses have obstruction to left atrial emptying (mitral stenosis). This is most important in a large patient in whom a small prosthesis must be placed for technical reasons. The resulting patient-prosthesis mismatch[33] contributes to incomplete relief of symptoms. The long-term effect of intrinsic prosthetic stenosis on survival and ventricular dysfunction is unknown but may lead to long-term effects similar to those of aortic or mitral stenosis.[83] The presence of intrinsic prosthetic stenosis must be considered when advising patients with prosthetic heart valves concerning activity.

Reoperation to replace a prosthetic heart valve is a serious complication. It is usually required for moderate to severe prosthetic dysfunction and dehiscence, for prosthetic valve endocarditis, and occasionally for recurrent thromboembolism, severe recurrent bleeding from anticoagulant therapy, or valve prosthesis-patient mismatch.

Late cardiac death may result from ventricular dysfunction, other cardiac lesions, or prosthesis-related causes. Late, sudden death is not uncommon. It may result from a bradyarrhythmia, a tachyarrhythmia that is often associated with ventricular dysfunction, prosthetic dysfunction or mismatch, coronary artery disease, or a combination of these.

Management[78]

All patients with prosthetic valves need appropriate antibiotics for prophylaxis against infective endocarditis (Chap. 82). Patients with rheumatic heart disease continue to need antibiotics as prophylaxis against the recurrence of rheumatic carditis (Chap. 62). Adequate antithrombotic therapy is needed for appropriate patients (Chap. 68).

During the first 4 to 6 weeks after surgery, the physician and surgeon jointly manage the patient, directing their attention toward relieving postoperative discomfort, readjusting cardiac medications, and instituting anticoagulation if not contraindicated. A graduated plan of activity is started that, in most cases, enables the patient to return to full activity in 4 to 6 weeks.

Several syndromes are peculiar to the postoperative period. The *postperfusion syndrome*, which occurs in up to 5 percent of patients, usually appears in the third or fourth postoperative week. It is characterized by fever, splenomegaly, and atypical lymphocytes; it is benign and self-limited. The *postpericardiotomy syndrome* occurs in up to 25 percent of patients and is characterized by fever and pleuropericarditis. It usually develops in the second or third postoperative week but can appear as late as 1 year after surgery and sometimes recurs. Although this syndrome is usually self-limited, most patients benefit from taking anti-inflammatory drugs, such as aspirin or indomethacin, and a short course of glucocorticoids is also required occasionally.

Even though the pericardium is left open at the end of surgery, *cardiac tamponade* has been known to occur during the first 6 weeks. The fact that a critically ill patient may improve promptly with pericardial drainage underscores the need to consider this uncommon postoperative complication. Usually, anticoagulants have been given and the fluid is hemorrhagic.

The *4- to 6-week postoperative visit* is critical, because by this time the patient's physical capabilities and expected improvement in functional capacity can usually be assessed. At this time, the physician should assemble essential records and data for the subsequent office follow-up, including the preoperative history, physical examination, chest roentgenogram, electrocardiogram (ECG) and indication for surgery, preoperative echocardiographic/Doppler ultrasound and cardiac catheterization/angiographic reports, surgeon's operative report, postoperative complications, and hospital discharge summary. The prosthesis model, serial number, and size should be recorded.

The workup on this visit should include an interval or complete initial history and physical examination, ECG, chest x-ray, echocardiography/Doppler ultrasound, complete blood count, and measurement of electrolytes, LDH, and international normalized ratio (INR), if indicated. The examination's main focus is on physical signs that relate to functioning of the prosthesis or suggest the presence of a myocardial, conduction, or valvular disorder. The auscultatory findings to expect with some normally functioning prostheses are listed in Fig. 67-12.[84] Severe perivalvular mitral regurgitation can be inaudible on physical examination, a fact to remember

Type of Valve	Aortic Prosthesis		Mitral Prosthesis	
	Normal Findings	Abnormal Findings	Normal Findings	Abnormal Findings
Caged–Ball (Starr–Edwards)	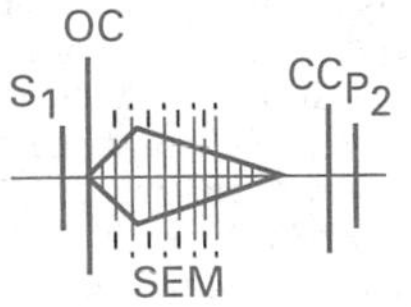	Aortic diastolic murmur Decreased intensity of opening or closing click	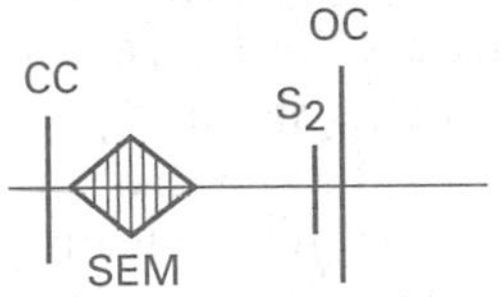	Low-frequency apical diastolic murmur High-frequency holosystolic murmur
Single–Tilting–Disk (Bjork–Shiley or Medtronic–Hall)	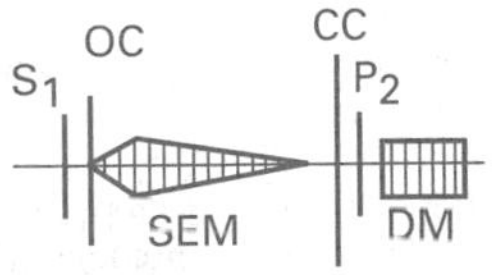	Decreased intensity of closing click	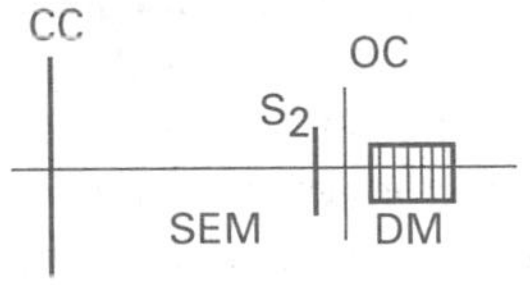	High-frequency holosystolic murmur Decreased intensity of closing click
Bileaflet–Tilting–Disk (St. Jude Medical)	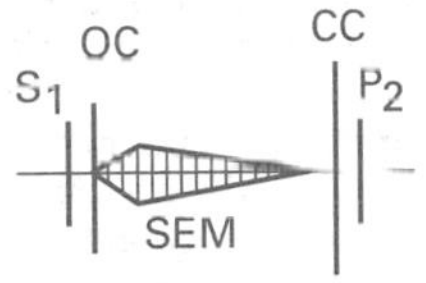	Aortic diastolic murmur Decreased intensity of closing click	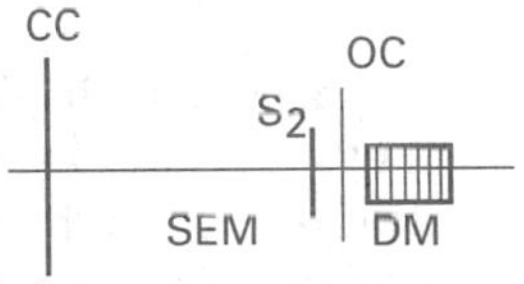	High-frequency holosystolic murmur Decreased intensity of closing click
Heterograft Bioprosthesis (Hancock or Carpentier-Edwards)	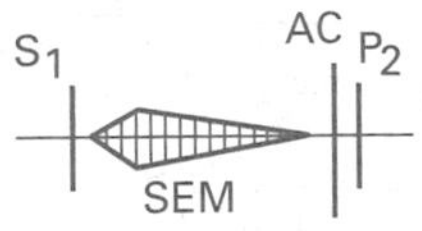	Aortic diastolic murmur	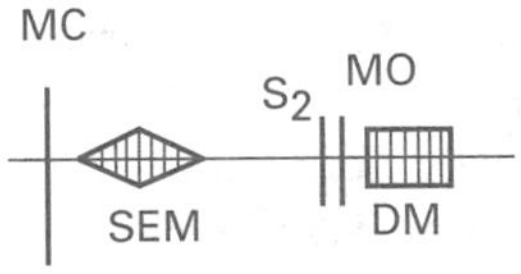	High-frequency holosystolic murmur

FIGURE 67-12

Auscultatory characteristics of various prosthetic valves in the aortic and mitral positions, with schematic diagrams of normal findings and descriptions of abnormal findings. The caged-ball aortic prosthesis produces a loud opening click (OC) after the first heart sound (S_1) and a less prominent closing click (CC); an early-to-mid-peaking systolic ejection murmur (SEM) is audible, along with multiple systolic clicks (broken lines) of the bouncing poppet within the cage. P_2 denotes the pulmonic component of the second heart sound. The caged-ball mitral prosthesis produces a loud opening click after the second heart sound (S_2). An early-to-mid-systolic ejection murmur, usually loudest at the left sternal border, is caused by turbulent flow in the left ventricular outflow tract. The aortic single-tilting-disk valve has a louder closing click than opening click. An early-to-mid-peaking systolic ejection murmur is usually best heard at the base and often radiates to the carotid arteries. A soft diastolic murmur (DM) may be noted in an occasional patient. The mitral single-tilting-disk valve has a louder closing click than opening click. A low-frequency diastolic rumbling murmur, which represents turbulent flow across the open valve, is usually audible. The aortic bileaflet-tilting-disk prosthetic valve produces a loud closing click. An early-to-mid-peaking systolic ejection murmur is best heard at the base and often radiates to the carotid arteries. A diastolic murmur is not audible. The mitral bileaflet-tilting-disk valve has auscultatory characteristics similar to those of the mitral single-tilting-disk valve. The aortic heterograft bioprosthesis has a closing sound (AC) similar to that of a normal valve. An early-to-mid-peaking systolic ejection murmur is audible and often radiates to the carotid arteries. The mitral heterograft bioprosthesis has a closing sound (MC) that may be indistinguishable from a normal first heart sound; an opening sound (MO) is usually audible after the second heart sound, as is an early-to-mid-systolic ejection murmur, representing turbulent flow in the left ventricular outflow tract. A low-frequency diastolic rumbling murmur may also be audible at the apex. (From Vongpatawasin et al.[84] Reproduced by permission of the publisher and authors.)

when considering possible causes of functional deterioration in a patient.

The interval between routine follow-up visits depends on the patient's needs. Anticoagulant regulation usually does not require office physician visits.

Multiple noninvasive tests have emerged for assessing valvular and ventricular function. Fluoroscopy can reveal abnormal rocking of a dehiscing prosthesis or limitation of the occluder if the latter is opaque as well as strut fracture of a Björk-Shiley valve. Phonocardiography can detect variant poppets if "normal" sounds were previously established. Radionuclide angiography, which is useful for determining whether or not functional deterioration is the result of reduced ventricular function, is performed if the same data cannot be obtained by echocardiography.

Echocardiography/Doppler ultrasound is the most useful noninvasive test. It provides information about prosthesis stenosis/regurgitation, valve area, assessment of other valve disease(s), pulmonary hypertension, atrial size, left ventricular hypertrophy, left ventricular size and function, and pericardial effusion/thickening. It is essential at the first postoperative visit because it allows an assessment of the effects and results of surgery and serves as a baseline for comparison should complications and/or deterioration occur later. Subsequently, it is performed as is needed in symptomatic patients and in asymptomatic patients at 1- to 2-year intervals. In patients with a bioprosthesis in the mitral position, echocardiography/Doppler ultrasound should be performed annually after 5 years and in the aortic position annually after 8 years because of the increasing incidence of bioprosthetic structural valve deterioration.

"Heart failure" after valve replacement may be the result of (1) preoperative left ventricular dysfunction that improved partially or not at all, (2) perioperative myocardial damage, (3) progression of other valve disease, (4) complications of prosthetic heart valves, and (5) associated heart disease such as coronary artery disease and systemic arterial hypertension.

Any patient with a prosthetic heart valve who does not improve after the surgery or who later shows deterioration of functional capacity should undergo appropriate testing to determine the cause. Such studies are also usually necessary for patients who require reoperation for endocarditis or repeated embolism to determine the hemodynamics and anatomy.

The indications for reoperating on a patient with prosthetic valve endocarditis have already been discussed. A patient in stable condition, without prosthetic valve endocarditis, can usually undergo reoperation with only slightly greater risk than that of the initial surgery. For the patient with catastrophic dysfunction, surgery is clearly indicated and urgent. The patient without endocarditis or severe dysfunction requires careful hemodynamic evaluation; the decision about reoperation should then be based on the hemodynamic abnormalities, the symptoms, ventricular function, and current knowledge of the natural history of the particular prosthesis.

Acknowledgment

The authors wish to thank Ms. K. Jeanne Zerr, RN, MBA, for valuable assistance in bibliographic management.

REFERENCES

1. Harken D, Soroff HS, Taylor WJ. Partial and complete prosthesis in aortic insufficiency. *J Thorac Cardiovasc Surg* 1960; 40:744–762.
2. Starr A, Edwards M. Mitral replacement: Clinical experience with a ball valve prosthesis. *Ann Surg* 1961; 154:726–740.
3. Björk VO. A new tilting disc valve prosthesis. *Scand J Thorac Cardiovasc Surg* 1969; 3:1–10.
4. Björk VO. The improved Björk-Shiley tilting disc valve prosthesis. *Scand J Thorac Cardiovasc Surg* 1978; 12:81–84.
5. Ross DN. Homograft replacement of the aortic valve. *Lancet* 1962; 2:487.
6. Barratt-Boyes BG. Homograft aortic valve replacement in aortic incompetence and stenosis. *Thorax* 1964; 19:131–135.
7. Ross DN. Replacement of aortic and mitral valves with a pulmonary autograft. *Lancet* 1967; 2:956–958.
8. Elkins RC. Pulmonary autograft—the optimal substitute for the aortic valve? *N Engl J Med* 1994; 330:59–60.
9. Oury JH, Eddy AC, Cleveland JC. The Ross procedure: A progress report. *J Heart Valve Dis* 1994; 3:361–364.
10. Elkins RC, Santangelo K, Randolph JD, Knott-Craig CJ, Stelzer P, Thompson WM Jr, et al. Pulmonary autograft replacement in children. The ideal solution? *Ann Surg* 1992; 216:363–370; discussion, 370–371.
11. Kouchoukos NT, Davila-Román VG, Spray TL, Murphy SF, Perrillo JB. Replacement of the aortic root with a pulmonary autograft in children and young adults with aortic-valve disease. *N Engl J Med* 1994; 330:1–6.
12. Love JW, Schoen FJ, Breznock EM, Shermar SP, Love CS. Experimental evaluation of an autologous tissue heart valve. *J Heart Valve Dis* 1992; 1:232–241.
13. Grunkemeier GL, Bodnar E. Comparison of structural valve failure among different "models" of homograft valves. *J Heart Valve Dis* 1994; 3:556–560.
14. Carpentier A, Lemaigre G, Robert L. Biological factors affecting long-term results of valvular homografts. *J Thorac Cardiovasc Surg* 1969; 58:467–483.
15. Carpentier A, Dubost C. From xenograft to bioprosthesis. In: Ionescu MI, Ross DN, Wooler GH, eds. *Biological Tissue in Heart Valve Replacement.* London: Butterworth; 1971: 515–541.
16. Hazekamp MG, Goffin YA, Huysmans HA. The value of the stentless biovalve prosthesis. An experimental study. *Eur J Thorac Cardiovasc Surg* 1993; 7:514–519.
17. Konertz W, Hamann P, Schwammenthal E, Breithardt G, Scheld HH. Aortic valve replacement with stentless xenografts. *J Heart Valve Dis* 1992; 1:249–252.
18. David TE, Bos J, Rakowski H. Aortic valve replacement with the Toronto SPV bioprosthesis. *J Heart Valve Dis* 1992; 1:244–248.
19. Vrandecic MP, Gontijo BF, Fantini FA, Gutierrez C, Paula E, Silva JA, et al. The new stentless aortic valve: Clinical results of the first 100 patients. *Cardiovasc Surg* 1994; 2:407–414.
20. Hvass U, Chatel D, Ouroudji M, Pansard Y, Laperche T, Depoix JP, et al. The O'Brien-Angell stentless valve. Early results of 100 implants. *Eur J Cardiothorac Surg* 1994; 8:384–387.
21. Carpentier A. Mitral reconstruction in predominant mitral incompetence. In: Duran C, Angell WW, Johnson AD, Oury JH, eds. *Recent Progress in Mitral Valve Disease.* London: Butterworth; 1984:265–276.
22. Duran C. Mitral reconstruction in predominant mitral stenosis. In: Duran C, Angell WW, Johnson AD, Oury JH, eds. *Recent Progress in Mitral Valve Disease.* London: Butterworth; 1984:255–264.
23. Cosgrove DM, Rosenkranz ER, Hendren WG, Bartlett JC, Stewart WJ. Valvuloplasty for aortic insufficiency. *J Thorac Cardiovasc Surg* 1991; 102:571–576; discussion, 576–577.
24. Duvoisin GE, Brandenburg RO, McGoon DC. Factors affecting thromboembolism associated with prosthetic heart valves. *Circulation* 1967; 35,36(suppl I):70–76.
25. Kaplan EL, Meier P. Nonparametric estimation from incomplete observations. *J Am Stat Assn* 1958; 53:457–481.

26. Stinson EB, Griepp RB, Oyer PE, Shumway NE. Long-term experience with porcine xenografts. *J Thorac Cardiovasc Surg* 1977; 73:54–63.

27. Grunkemeier GL, Thomas DR, Starr A. Statistical considerations in the analysis and reporting of time-related events. Application to analysis of prosthetic valve-related thromboembolism and pacemaker failure. *Am J Cardiol* 1977; 39:257–258.

28. Grunkemeier GL, Macmanus Q, Thomas DR, Starr A. Regression analysis of late survival following mitral valve replacement. *J Thorac Cardiovasc Surg* 1978; 75:131–138.

29. Blackstone EH, Naftel DC, Turner ME Jr. The decomposition of time-varying hazard into separate phases, each incorporating a separate stream of concomitant information. *J Am Stat Assn* 1986; 81:615–624.

30. Edmunds LH Jr, Clark RE, Cohn LH, Miller DC, Weisel RD. Guidelines for reporting morbidity and mortality after cardiac valvular operations. *Ann Thorac Surg* 1988; 46:257–259.

31. Edmunds LH Jr, Clark RE, Cohn LH, Grunkemeier GL, Miller DC, Weisel DC. Guidelines for reporting morbidity and mortality after cardiac valvular operations. *Ann Thorac Surg* 1996; 62:932–935.

32. Edmunds LH Jr, Clark RE, Cohn LH, Grunkemeier GL, Miller DC, Weisel DC. Guidelines for reporting morbidity and mortality after cardiac valvular operations. *J Thorac Cardiovasc Surg* 1996; 112:708–711.

33. Rahimtoola SH. The problem of prosthesis-patient mismatch. *Circulation* 1978; 58:20–24.

34. Rahimtoola SH, Rahmoeller GA. The law on cardiovascular devices: The role of the Food and Drug Administration and of physicians in its implementation. *Circulation* 1980; 62:919–924.

35. *Draft Replacement Heart Valve Guidance.* Prosthetic Devices Branch, Division of Cardiovascular, Respiratory and Neurological Devices, Office of Device Evaluation, Center of Devices and Radiological Health, Food and Drug Administration. December 7, 1993.

36. Gersh BJ, Fisher LD, Schaff HV, Rahimtoola SH, Reeder GS, Frater RW, et al. Issues concerning the clinical evaluation of new prosthetic valves. *J Thorac Cardiovasc Surg* 1986; 91:460–466.

37. Nashef SAM. Reporting the results of heart valve operations (letter). *Ann Thorac Surg* 1989; 47:949–950.

38. Bodnar E, Butchart EG, Bamford J, Besselaar AMPH, Grunkemeier GL, Frater RWM. Proposal for reporting thrombosis, embolism and bleeding after heart valve replacement. *J Heart Valve Dis* 1994; 3:120–123.

39. Grunkemeier GL, Johnson D, Naftel DC. Sample size requirements for studying heart valves with constant risk events. *J Heart Valve Dis* 1994; 3:53–58.

40. Grunkemeier GL, Anderson WN. Passive surveillance of heart valve devices: Björk-Shiley outlet strut fracture rates. *J Long-term Effects of Medical Implants* 1995; 5:155–168.

41. Jones LE, Weintraub WS, Craver JM, Guyton RA, Cohen CL, Corrigan VE, et al. Ten-year experience with the porcine bioprosthetic valve: Interrelationship of valve survival and patient survival in 1,050 valve replacements. *Ann Thorac Surg* 1990; 49:370–383; discussion, 383–384.

42. Jamieson WR, Tyers GF, Janusz MT, Miyagishima RT, Munro AI, Ling H, et al. Age as a determinant for selection of porcine bioprostheses for cardiac valve replacement: Experience with Carpentier-Edwards standard bioprosthesis. *Can J Cardiol* 1991; 7:181–188.

43. al-Khaja N, Belboul A, Rashid M, el-Gatit A, Roberts D, Larson S, et al. The influence of age on the durability of Carpentier-Edwards biological valves. Thirteen years' follow-up. *Eur J Cardiothorac Surg* 1991; 5:635–640.

44. Pelletier LC, Carrier M, Leclerc Y, Dyrda I, Gosselin G. Influence of age on late results of valve replacement with porcine bioprostheses. *J Cardiovasc Surg* 1992; 33:526–533.

45. Barratt-Boyes BG, Jaffe WM, Ko PH, Whitlock RM. The zero pressure, fixed Medtronic Intact porcine valve: An 8.5 year review. *J Heart Valve Dis* 1993; 2:604–611.

46. Munro AI, Jamieson WR, Tyers GF, Burr LH. The Medtronic Intact porcine bioprosthesis: Clinical performance to eight years. *J Heart Valve Dis* 1994; 3:634–640.

47. Matsuki O, Okita Y, Almeida RS, McGadrick JP, Hooper TL, Robles A, et al. Two decades' experience with aortic valve replacement with pulmonary autograft. *J Thorac Cardiovasc Surg* 1988; 95:705–711.

48. Ross D, Jackson M, Davies J. Pulmonary autograft aortic valve replacement: Long-term results. *J Cardiac Surg* 1991; 6(suppl 4):529–533.

49. Enriquez-Sarano M, Schaff HV, Orszulak TA, Tajik AJ, Bailey KR, Frye RL. Valve repair improves the outcome of surgery for mitral regurgitation. A multivariate analysis. *Circulation* 1995; 91:1022–1028; comments, 1264–1265.

50. Hendren WG, Morris AS, Rosenkranz ER, Lytle BW, Taylor PC, Stewart WJ, et al. Mitral valve repair for bacterial endocarditis. *J Thorac Cardiovasc Surg* 1992; 103:124–128; discussion, 128–129.

51. Azar H, Szentpetery S. Mitral valve repair in patients over the age of 70 years. *Eur J Cardiothorac Surg* 1994; 8:298–300.

52. Jebara VA, Dervanian P, Acar C, Grare P, Mihaileanu S, Chauvaud S, et al. Mitral valve repair using Carpentier techniques in patients more than 70 years old. Early and late results. *Circulation* 1992; 86(suppl II):53–59.

53. Rahimtoola SH. Lessons learned about the determinants of the results of valve surgery. *Circulation* 1988; 78:1503–1507.

54. Aoyagi S, Tanaka K, Kawara T, Oryoji A, Kosuga K, Oishi K. Long-term results of mitral valve repair for non-rheumatic mitral regurgitation. *Cardiovasc Surg* 1995; 3:387–392.

55. Skoularigis J, Sinovich V, Joubert G, Sareli P. Evaluation of the long-term results of mitral valve repair in 254 young patients with rheumatic mitral regurgitation. *Circulation* 1994; 90(suppl II):167–174.

56. Grossi EA, Galloway AC, Steinberg BM, LeBoutillier M III, Delianides J, Baumann FG, et al. Severe calcification does not affect long-term outcome of mitral valve repair. *Ann Thorac Surg* 1994; 58:685–687.

57. Grossi EA, Galloway AC, LeBoutillier M III, Steinberg B, Baumann FG, Delianides J, et al. Anterior leaflet procedures during mitral valve repair do not adversely influence long-term outcome. *J Am Coll Cardiol* 1995; 25:134–136.

58. Duran CM, Gometza B, Saad E. Valve repair in rheumatic mitral disease: An unsolved problem. *J Cardiac Surg* 1994; 9(suppl 2):282–285.

59. Cosgrove DM, Lytle BW, Taylor PC, Camacho MT, Steward RW, McCarthy PM, et al. The Carpentier-Edwards pericardial aortic valve: Ten year results. *J Thorac Cardiovasc Surg* 1995; 110:651–662.

60. Waller DA, Essop AR, Scott PJ, Nair RU. Repair of asymptomatic aortic valve disease during other cardiac surgery. *Int J Cardiol* 1992; 36:309–314.

61. Grunkemeier GL, Starr A, Rahimtoola SH. Prosthetic heart valve performance: Long-term follow-up. *Curr Probl Cardiol* 1992; 17:329–406.

62. Grunkemeier GL, London MR. Reliability of comparative data from different sources. In: Butchart E, Bodnar E, eds. *Current Issues in Heart Valve Disease: Thrombosis, Embolism and Bleeding.* London: ICR; 1992:464–475.

63. Sackett DL. Bias in analytic research. *J Chron Dis* 1979; 32:51–63.

64. Rahimtoola SH. Valvular heart disease: A perspective. *J Am Coll Cardiol* 1983; 3:199–215.

65. Edmunds LH Jr. Thrombotic and bleeding complications of prosthetic heart valves. *Ann Thorac Surg* 1987; 44:430–445.

66. Bamford J, Warlow C. Stroke and TIA in the general population. In: Butchart EG, Bodnar E, eds. *Thrombosis, Embolism and Bleeding.* London: ICR; 1992:3–15.

67. Berlin JA, Begg CB, Louis TA. An assessment of publication bias using a sample of published clinical trials. *J Am Stat Assn* 1989; 84:381–392.

68. Kramer MS, Shapiro SH. Scientific challenges in the application of randomized trials. *JAMA* 1984; 252:2739–2745.

69. Rahimtoola SH. Some unexpected lessons from large multicenter randomized clinical trials. *Circulation* 1985; 72:449–455.

70. Grunkemeier GL, Starr A. Alternatives to randomization in surgical studies. *J Heart Valve Dis* 1992; 1:142–151.

71. Bloomfield P, Wheatley DJ, Prescott RJ, Miller HC. Twelve-year comparison of a Björk-Shiley mechanical heart valve with porcine bioprostheses. *N Engl J Med* 1991; 324:573–579.

72. Hammermeister KE, Sethi GK, Henderson WG, Oprian C, Kim T, Rahimtoola SH. A comparison of outcomes in men 11 years after heart-valve replacement with a mechanical valve or bioprosthesis. Veterans Affairs Cooperative Study on Valvular Heart Disease. *N Engl J Med* 1993; 328:1289–1296.

73. Grunkemeier GL, Starr A, Rahimtoola SH. Replacement heart valves. In: O'Rourke RA, ed. *The Heart: Update I.* New York: McGraw-Hill; 1996:98–123.

74. Hammermeister K, Sethi GK, Henderson WG, Rahimtoola SH. Comparison of outcomes 16 years after randomization to valve replacement with a bioprosthetic or mechanical prosthetic valve (abstr.) *Circulation* 1996; 94:I-650.

75. Grunkemeier GL, Jamieson WR, Miller DC, Starr A. Actuarial versus actual risk of porcine structural valve deterioration. *J Thorac Cardiovasc Surg* 1994; 108:709–718.

76. Starr A, Grunkemeier GL. Recurrent thromboembolism: Significance and management. In: Butchart EG, Bodnar E, eds. *Current Issues in Heart Valve Disease: Thrombosis, Thromboembolism and Bleeding.* London: ICR; 1992:402–415.

77. Rahimtoola SH. Valvular heart disease. In: Stein J, ed. *Internal Medicine*, 4th ed. *Cardiology*, O'Rourke RA, section ed. St. Louis: Mosby-Year Book; 1994:202–234.

78. Grunkemeier GL, Rahimtoola SH, Starr A. Prosthetic heart valves. In: Rahimtoola SH, ed. *Atlas of Heart Diseases*, 11. Philadelphia: Current Medicine, 1997:13.1–13.27.

79. Rahimtoola SH. Aortic valve stenosis. In: Rahimtoola SH, ed. *Valvular Heart Disease*, II. St. Louis: Mosby; 1997:7.02–7.26.

80. Mullany CJ, Elveback LR, Frye RL, Pluth JR, Edwards WD, Orszulak TA, et al. Coronary artery disease and its management: Influence on survival in patients undergoing aortic valve replacement. *J Am Coll Cardiol* 1987; 10:66–72.

81. Kloster FE. Infective prosthetic valve endocarditis. In: Rahimtoola SH, ed. *Infective Endocarditis.* New York: Grune & Stratton; 1978:291–305.

82. Douglas JL, Cobbs CG. Prosthetic valve endocarditis. In: Kaye D, ed. *Infective Endocarditis*, 2d ed. New York: Raven Press; 1992:375–396.

83. Rahimtoola SH, Murphy E. Valve prosthesis-patient mismatch: A long-term sequela. *Br Heart J* 1981; 45:331–335.

84. Vongpatawasin W, Hillis LD, Lange RA. Prosthetic heart valves. *N Engl J Med* 1996; 335:407–416.

Due to a clerical misunderstanding, the valves illustrated in this chapter (Plates 56-61) do not contain a representative selection of the products of the various manufacturers. All subsequent printings of this chapter will have a different, representative selection.

68

ANTITHROMBOTIC THERAPY AND VALVULAR HEART DISEASE

John H. McAnulty / Shahbudin H. Rahimtoola

The most important reason to address the issue of protection against thromboemboli in every patient with valve disease is the risk of a *stroke,* which is often a devastating complication. In addition, the consequences of valve thrombosis and of emboli to other organs make the risk of antithrombotic therapy reasonable in many patients with valve disease. Treatment has to be individualized, but some issues and principles are widely applicable (Table 68-1). When considering the recommendations given in this chapter, the social context of each patient should also be assessed. While some recommendations are appropriate for affluent American communities, the risk, benefit, and cost ratios may make little sense in poorer areas where the resources and protective measures are simply not available. This does not mean that thromboemboli should be ignored, but alternative therapy—for example, a greater use of antiplatelet agents, in particular aspirin—may, on balance, be more appropriate.

Intracardiac thrombosis most often presents as an embolic event; in over 80 percent of cases this is a cerebrovascular event. Less commonly, thrombosis becomes manifest by interfering with valve function, resulting in valve dysfunction. The physical examination should include careful attention to the peripheral pulses and to the skin, fundi, and soft tissues (mouth, conjunctiva) looking for clues of an embolus. A detailed neurologic assessment for focal deficits is essential. Although thrombosis most often occurs without any change in the cardiac examination, auscultation to assess for a change in a murmur or quality of heart sounds is important. Intracardiac thrombosis is, at times, first diagnosed when cardiac catheterization or echocardiography are performed for other reasons.

It needs to be emphasized that not all emboli are due to an intracardiac thrombus. Infective endocarditis must be considered and excluded as a cause, particularly in individuals with valve disease. Vascular plaque disruption in the ascending aorta, arch, or descending aorta and in the cerebral vessels may be a common cause of peripheral and cerebral emboli in patients with atherosclerotic disease. Intracardiac tumors or calcified emboli from the heart or aorta are other rare causes.

TABLE 68-1

VALVE DISEASE AND ANTITHROMBOTIC THERAPY[a,b]

1. Prevention of thromboemboli should be addressed in all patients with valve disease.
2. Lifelong antithrombotic therapy is required in patients with atrial fibrillation (paroxysmal or persistent) (Table 68-2).
3. Warfarin therapy is required in all patients with a mechanical prosthesis (Table 68-3) and in all patients with prosthetic heart valves who are in atrial fibrillation.
4. Antithrombotic therapy should be started early after valve surgery.
5. Warfarin should be avoided if possible in the first trimester of pregnancy.
6. Antithrombotic therapy should be individualized during noncardiac surgery and cardiovascular procedures (Table 68-4)

[a] See text for discussion.
[b] In general, whenever warfarin/aspirin therapy is recommended, it is assumed there is no specific contraindication to its use.

NATIVE VALVE DISEASE

The risk of thromboembolism in patients with native valve disease is most directly related to certain risk factors, that is, "the company it keeps" (Table 68-2). This "company," or the risk factors, includes atrial fibrillation, a history of thromboembolism, left ventricular (LV) dysfunction, and known hypercoagulability.[1] The risk is increased by the presence of

TABLE 68-2

ANTITHROMBOTIC THERAPY—NATIVE VALVE DISEASE

I. *No therapy* if no thrombosis risk factor
II. *Therapy* if thrombosis risk factor present
   A. *Atrial fibrillation*
     1. Warfarin (INR 2–3) if congestive heart failure, hypertension, or previous thromboembolism
     2. Warfarin (INR 2–3) if valve lesion is mitral stenosis
     3. Aspirin (325 mg/day) or warfarin (INR 2–3) if valve lesion other than mitral stenosis
   B. *Previous thromboembolism*—warfarin (INR 2–3)
   C. *LV dysfunction* (ejection fraction ≤ 0.30)—warfarin (INR 2–3)
   D. *Hypercoagulable state*—warfarin (INR 2–3)

Abbreviation: INR = international normalized ratio.

certain native valve disease, e.g., with mitral stenosis, and with prosthetic heart valves, particularly mechanical prostheses, which put a patient at risk even without other associated risk factors (Fig. 68-1).

Risk of Thromboemboli with Native Valve Disease

ATRIAL FIBRILLATION

Most is known about the stroke risk with atrial fibrillation, which is common even without valve disease. Six recent large, prospective randomized trials have assessed the value of antithrombotic therapy as primary prevention in patients with nonvalvular atrial fibrillation.[1–7] The term *nonvalvular* is not completely accurate, as at least some patients with aortic valve disease and with mitral regurgitation were included in the studies if the valve lesions were considered hemodynamically "insignificant." In essence, "nonvalvular" in these stud-ies implied no mitral stenosis, no prosthetic heart valves, and no other severe valve lesions; some did have some native valve disease.

In these trials, the embolic rate (essentially the rate of a stroke in untreated nonvalvular atrial fibrillation patients) ranged from 3 to 8 percent per year. This was true whether the atrial fibrillation was constant or paroxysmal. Importantly, these trials indicated that warfarin therapy reduced the stroke rate to approximately 0.5 to 2 percent per year. One study, SPAF II,[6] demonstrated equal protection against an adverse neurologic event when aspirin (325 mg daily) was compared to warfarin. In SPAF III,[7] the aspirin was less protective if atrial fibrillation occurred in association with LV dysfunction or uncontrolled hypertension or if the patient was a woman over age 75. Warfarin is indicated in these patients if they are reasonable candidates for the drug, and it is indicated in patients with atrial fibrillation who have had a previous embolic event, i.e., as secondary prevention[5,7]; the international normalized ratio (INR) should be in the 2.0 to 3.0 range (see also Chaps. 52 and 99).

The exclusion of mitral stenosis in these prospective trials implies that the risks of emboli and the benefits of warfarin in these patients with associated atrial fibrillation are well understood; however, these are not thoroughly documented or proven. Retrospective assessment, however, suggests that such patients may have an embolic rate >5 percent per year. Until the role of warfarin is better defined, the authors recommend its use in these patients.

LEFT VENTRICULAR DYSFUNCTION

Systemic or pulmonary thromboemboli occur at a rate of over 5 percent per year in patients with LV dysfunction. The type and degree of dysfunction that put individuals at risk are not well defined, but LV systolic abnormalities have been related to emboli most often. Additionally, antithrombotic therapy is of unproven value in preventing or reducing the embolic rate. Still, the risk is sufficient that, with or without valve disease, consideration should be given to treatment. One approach (including the authors') is to use warfarin if the LV ejection fraction is ≤0.30 and the patient is a reasonable candidate for this treatment.

PREVIOUS THROMBOEMBOLI

In other clinical situations (e.g., in patients with atrial fibrillation[5,7] or with a prosthetic valve[8–10]), a thromboembolic event defines patients at high risk for having an embolic event, i.e., a recurrent event. It is unclear whether or not this is true in patients with native valve disease, but we recommend lifelong warfarin therapy.

Risk of Thromboembolism

High (>2% per year)	Atrial fibrillation LV dysfunction Previous thromboembolism Hypercoagulable condition Mechanical prosthesis	i.e., **"risk factors"** for thromboemboli
Low (<1% per year)	Normal sinus rhythm Normal LV function No previous thromboembolism Tissue prosthesis	

FIGURE 68-1

Risk of thromboembolism. Clinical variables define valve disease patients as being at high or low risk of thromboembolic events.

HYPERCOAGULABLE CONDITIONS

Reasons to consider anticoagulant therapy are the presence of protein C, protein S, or antithrombin III deficiencies; the anticardiolipin antibody syndrome; resistance to activated protein C; or an associated malignancy. This is also true in patients with native valve disease.

Screening for Patients at High Risk for Thromboemboli

The recognition of the risk factors described above defines patients requiring antithrombotic therapy. Transthoracic and transesophageal echocardiography are often performed in patients with valvular heart disease and in those who have had a systemic embolic episode. The use of these procedures in determining which patients are at risk of thromboemboli is not yet well defined; left atrial thrombi, a patent foramen ovale, an atrial septal aneurysm, or spontaneous echo contrast are occasional findings of concern, but the value of treatment is unproven. Until more is known, it does not seem appropriate to screen patients with native valve disease who do not have one of the obvious risk factors listed above.

Antithrombotic Treatment for Native Valve Disease (Table 68-2)

Antithrombotic therapy is not required in patients with native valve disease unless there is an associated risk factor.[11] Theoretically, the risk of thrombosis is greater with mitral valve disease as compared to aortic valve disease: there is more blood stasis, the left atrium may be larger, and the frequency of atrial fibrillation is greater. Still, the presence of mitral valve stenosis or regurgitation by itself is not a reason to initiate antithrombotic therapy. If there is a risk factor, antithrombotic therapy should be considered as defined in Table 68-2. If the patient is a reasonable candidate for warfarin therapy, the use of warfarin (maintaining an INR of 2 to 3) is appropriate if a patient with valve disease has atrial fibrillation (constant or paroxysmal) in combination with reduced LV function (heart failure or a LV ejection fraction ≤0.30) or with associated servere hypertension or if there is a history of thromboemboli. There is a suggestion that women with atrial fibrillation over the age of 75 might be better protected by warfarin than aspirin, but the bleeding rate is significant in this patient population on warfarin; treatment should be individualized and the INR more closely monitored. If a patient with atrial fibrillation has reasonable LV function, has not had a previous thromboembolism, and

does not have other risk factors, aspirin (325 mg/day) is just as likely as warfarin to be protective against thromboemboli, without the associated expense and risk of warfarin therapy.[6] Unrelated to atrial fibrillation, if a patient has had a previous thromboembolism or has LV dysfunction (heart failure and an ejection fraction ≤0.30), warfarin therapy is recommended.

PROSTHETIC HEART VALVES

All patients with mechanical valves require warfarin therapy. Even with the use of warfarin, the risk of thromboemboli in these patients is 1 to 2 percent per year,[12–15] and the risk is considerably higher without treatment with warfarin.[8] Several studies showed that the risk of an embolus in patients with biological valves in sinus rhythm was approximately 0.6 to 0.7 percent per year, and most of these patients were not on warfarin therapy.[12,13,15,16] Almost all studies have shown the risk of embolism is greater with a valve in the mitral position (mechanical or biological) as compared to a valve in the aortic position;[8,12] however, this was not found in one study.[13] With either type of prosthesis or valve location, the risk of emboli is probably higher in the first few days and months after valve insertion,[16] before the valve is fully endothelialized.

Antithrombotic Treatment for Prosthetic Valves (Table 68-3)

MECHANICAL VALVES

All patients with mechanical valves require warfarin, and the INR should be maintained between 2.0 and 3.5.[12,13,17–19] Some valves are thought to be more thrombogenic than others (particularly the tilting disc valves), and a case could be made for increasing the INR to between 3 and 4.5, but this would come at the price of considerable increased risk of bleeding.[17,20] The addition of low-dose aspirin (50 to 100 mg/

TABLE 68-3

ANTITHROMBOTIC THERAPY[a]—PROSTHETIC HEART VALVES

	Mechanical Prosthetic Valves			Biological Prosthetic Valves		
	Warfarin, INR 2–3	Warfarin, INR 2.5–3.5	Aspirin, 50–100 mg	Warfarin, INR 2–3	Warfarin, INR 2.5–3.5	Aspirin, 50–100 mg
First 3 months after valve replacement		+	+		+	+
After first 3 months						
Aortic valve	+		+			+
Aortic valve + risk factor[b]		+	+	+		+
Mitral valve		+	+			+
Mitral valve + risk factor		+	+	+		+

[a] Depending on the clinical status of patient, antithrombotic therapy must be individualized (see special situations in text).

[b] Risk factors (see Fig. 68-1—atrial fibrillation, previous thromboembolus, LV dysfunction, hypercoagulable state).

day) to warfarin therapy may further decrease the risk of thromboembolism.[21,22] The authors recommend the addition of aspirin (50 to 100 mg/day) to warfarin unless there is a contraindication to the use of aspirin (i.e., bleeding or aspirin intolerance). This combination is particularly appropriate in patients who have had an embolus while on warfarin therapy and/or who are known to be particularly hypercoagulable; for example, it is recommended by a committee addressing antithrombotic therapy in women during pregnancy.[23] It is important to note that the thromboembolic risk increases early after the insertion of the prosthetic valve; this is a reason to initiate heparin therapy within the first 24 to 48 h of surgery, with maintenance of the activated partial thromboplastin time (aPPT) between 60 and 80 s until warfarin therapy has achieved an INR of 2.0 to 3.5.

BIOLOGICAL (TISSUE) VALVES

Because of an increased risk of thromboemboli during the first 3 months after implantation of a biological prosthetic valve, anticoagulation with warfarin is indicated.[16] The risk is particularly high in the first few days after surgery, and heparin therapy should be started within 24 to 48 h, with maintenance of the aPTT between 60 and 80 s until an INR of 2.0 to 3.0 is achieved with warfarin. After 3 months, the tissue valve can be treated like native valve disease (see Table 68-2), and warfarin can be discontinued in approximately two-thirds of patients with biological valves.[12,13,16,24] Associated atrial fibrillation or an LV ejection fraction <0.30 are reasons for lifelong warfarin therapy.

SPECIAL CLINICAL SITUATIONS

Altered Native Valves

Valve disease is increasingly being treated by interventional catheter techniques or surgical valve repair. It is difficult to give firm recommendations about antithrombotic therapy in these patients, but the recommendations given for treatment of native valve disease would seem most applicable in patients who have had surgical valve repair or catheter valve procedures (see Table 68-2).

Pregnancy

Pregnancy makes decisions regarding antithrombotic therapy for valve disease more difficult. Warfarin should be avoided if at all possible in the first trimester of pregnancy, particularly in weeks 7 through 12.[23,25,26] It crosses the placental barrier and is associated with, and is the clear cause of, an embryopathy manifest in the live born as mental impairment, ocular atrophy, and facial and digital abnormalities. Therefore, warfarin should be discontinued immediately when pregnancy is recognized, and heparin therapy should be initiated. The value of switching from warfarin to heparin before conception is uncertain. We suggest this when pregnancies are planned,

since little is known about the consequences of warfarin taken in the first 6 weeks of pregnancy; however, this is often not clinically practical or feasible. While a return to warfarin during the second and third trimesters has been recommended, there is concern that this drug may continue to endanger the fetus.

Heparin does not cross the placenta. While not devoid of problems (maternal bleeding, heparin-initiated thrombocytopenia, an increased risk of osteoporosis when used for longer than 1 month), successful pregnancies have occurred when adequate doses of the drug are administered subcutaneously at home throughout gestation.[27] Thromboembolic complications have occurred with heparin use during pregnancy in women with a mechanical prosthesis.[28,29] To minimize this, it is important to maintain an aPPT of at least 60 to 80 s prior to the next dose (this usually requires 15,000 to 30,000 units every 12 h).[23,30]

Low-molecular-weight heparin (LMWH) is currently approved only for treatment of venous thrombosis. Still, there is no reason to suspect that it will not result in effective anticoagulation in patients with valve disease. It has been used safely in pregnancy,[31] does not cross the placenta, can be given once or twice daily, does not require regular blood test monitoring, and is associated with less thrombocytopenia and osteoporosis. Even with the uncertainty associated with incomplete data, the use of LMWH for anticoagulation in preference to standard unfractionated heparin may be reasonable; however, more studies are needed.[31]

Aspirin crosses the placenta and has been implicated as a cause of abortion and fetal growth retardation,[32] but it has been used so frequently without problems and has even been considered for use in all pregnant women as prophylaxis against preclampsia[33] that, when required for valve disease (see Table 68-2), it should be continued.

The concern about the use of antithrombotic therapy during pregnancy makes the decision about management of valve disease more difficult in women of child-bearing age. If a woman of child-bearing age requires valve surgery, commissurotomy or valve repair is preferable because subsequent antithrombotic therapy is not required unless the woman has one of the risk factors for thrombosis (see Fig. 68-1). If a prosthetic valve is required in a woman of child-bearing age, the advantage of a mechanical prosthesis is its durability. On the other hand, it obligates the woman of child-bearing age to anticoagulation with warfarin because aspirin therapy itself does not offer adequate protection again thromboembolism. The theoretical advantage of a biological prosthesis is that, except for the first 3 months after valve replacement, warfarin therapy is not required. Practically, however, there are difficulties. As many as a third of patients with biological valves have associated atrial fibrillation and thus require warfarin antithrombotic therapy. In addition, the rate of degeneration of biological valves accelerates dramatically in young patients and, thus, also in women of child-bearing age.[34] The choice of a prosthesis should be individualized. A young woman capable of safely using warfarin when not pregnant and heparin during pregnancy is best treated with a mechanical valve. If a woman's social situation or attention to her health are questionable in regard to the safe use of anticoagulation therapy, a biological valve is more appropriate.

Surgery and Dental Care (Table 68-4)

The risk of increased bleeding during a procedure performed with a patient on antithrombotic therapy has to be weighed against the increased risk of a thromboembolism caused by stopping the therapy.

The risk of stopping warfarin can be estimated and is relatively slight if the drug is withheld for only a few days. As an example, and using a *worst case* scenario (e.g., a patient with a mechanical prosthesis with previous thromboemboli), the risk of a thromboembolus off warfarin could be as high as 10 to 20 percent per year. Thus, if the therapy were stopped for 3 days, the risk of an embolus would be 3/365 times 0.10 to 0.20, which equals 0.08 to 0.16 percent. There are theoretical concerns that stopping the drug and then reinstituting it might result in hypercoagulability—there might be a thrombotic "rebound." An increase in markers for activation of thrombosis with abrupt discontinuation of warfarin therapy has been observed,[35] but it is not clear that these increase the clinical risk of thromboembolism.[36] In addition, when reinstituting warfarin therapy, there are theoretical concerns

---

TABLE 68-4

ANTITHROMBOTIC THERAPY AT THE TIME OF SURGERY

I. Usual approach
  A. If patient on warfarin
     Stop 72 h before procedure
     Restart on day of procedure or after control of active bleeding
  B. If patient on aspirin
     Stop 1 week before procedure
     Restart the day after procedure or after control of active bleeding
II. Unusual circumstances
  A. Very high risk of thrombosis if off warfarin[a]
     Stop warfarin 72 h before procedure
     Start heparin 48 h before procedure[b]
     Stop heparin 6 h before procedure
     Restart heparin within 24 h of procedure and continue until warfarin can be restarted and the INR is 2–3
  B. Surgery complicated by postoperative bleeding
     Start heparin as soon after surgery as deemed safe and maintain aPTT of 60–80 s until warfarin restarted and the INR is 2–3
  C. Very low risk from bleeding[c]
     Continue antithrombotic therapy

[a] Clinical judgment: consider this approach if recent thromboembolus or if three risk factors are present.
[b] Heparin can be given in outpatient setting before and after surgery.
[c] For example, local skin surgery, dental prophylaxis, and treatment for caries.
Abbreviation: aPTT = activated partial thromboplastin time.

of a hypercoagulable state caused by suppression of proteins C and S before the drug affects the thrombotic factors. While the risks are only hypothetical, in individuals at very high risk, this is a reason to treat with heparin therapy until the INR returns to the desired range.

Management of antithrombotic therapy has to be individualized, but some generalizations apply (see Table 68-4). For procedures where bleeding is unlikely or would be inconsequential if it occurred, antithrombotic therapy should not be stopped. This can apply to surgery on the skin, dental prophylaxis, or simple treatment for dental caries. Eye surgery, in particular surgery for cataracts or glaucoma, is usually associated with very little bleeding; some ophthalmologists perform the procedures without altering antithrombotic treatment. When bleeding is likely or its potential consequences are severe, antithrombotic treatment should be altered. If a patient is on aspirin, it should be discontinued 1 week before the procedure and restarted as soon as it is considered safe by the surgeon or dentist.

For most patients on warfarin, the drug should be stopped 72 h before, and restarted within 24 h after, a procedure; admission to the hospital or a delay in discharge to give heparin is usually unnecessary.[21,36–39] Deciding who is at very high risk of thrombosis and thus should require heparin until warfarin can be reinstated may be difficult; clinical judgment is required. Heparin can usually be reserved for those who have had a recent thrombosis or embolus (arbitrarily within 1 year), those with demonstrated thrombotic problems when previously off therapy, and those with three or more risk factors. When used, unfractionated heparin should be started 24 h after warfarin is stopped (i.e., 48 h before surgery) and stopped 4 to 6 h before the procedure. The heparin should be restarted as early after surgery as bleeding stability allows, and the aPTT maintained at 60 to 80 s until warfarin is restarted and the desired INR can be achieved. Home administration and management of heparin (and warfarin) can be arranged to minimize time in the hospital. LMWH is even more easily utilized outside of the hospital (see also Chap. 83).

Cardiac Catherization and Angiography

Antiplatelet therapy or heparin does not have to be stopped for these procedures. Protamine can be given to the patient on heparin if bleeding occurs. In an emergent or semiemergent situation, cardiac catheterization can be performed with a patient on warfarin, but, preferably, the drug should be stopped 72 h before the procedure and restarted the day of the procedure. This is also true for most patients with prosthetic heart valves (mechanical as well as biological). If a patient is at very high risk of thromboembolism, heparin should be started 48 h before the procedure and continued until warfarin is restarted and the desired INR is achieved. If the catherization procedure is to include a transseptal puncture (especially in a patient who has not had previous opening of the pericardium), patients should be off all antithrombotic therapy and the INR should be ≤1.2—the same is also true if an LV puncture is to be performed.[40]

At the Time of an Active Thromboembolic Event

VALVE THROMBOSIS

Thrombosis of a valve, usually a prosthetic valve, can result in severe hemodynamic compromise. If recognized (transesophageal echocardiography can be diagnostic[41]), this complication may be treated with thrombolytic therapy, although the risk of bleeding and of emboli at the time of treatment is high.[42,43] Furthermore, thrombolytic therapy is likely to be effective for a thrombus, preferably a recent one. Many valves, however, have pannus formation and tissue ingrowth on the valve; therefore, we recommend emergency surgery rather than thrombolytic therapy in the patient with severe hemodynamic compromise. If a patient is a nonsurgical candidate, thrombolysis should be attempted.

THROMBOEMBOLIC EVENT

An embolic event often indicates inadequate therapy for that patient's circumstances. Data and opinions about optimal timing for initiating or continuing anticoagulants in patients in whom an embolus is the presumed cause of a stroke are conflicting.[44–46] Ideally, treatment would be started early to prevent recurrent emboli, but the early use of heparin (within 72 h) is associated with a 15 to 25 percent chance of converting a nonhemorrhagic into a hemorrhagic stroke.[45] While a case can still be made for immediate use of heparin,[44,45] the early recurrence of an embolus in patients with valve disease while off anticoagulants has not been clearly documented. Data are insufficient to provide definitive treatment outlines, but the authors' practice is listed in Table 68-5.

ACUTE MANAGEMENT OF AN EMBOLIC EVENT

Antithrombotic therapy should be withheld or stopped for 72 h. If a computed tomography (CT) scan at that time reveals little or no hemorrhage, heparin should be administered to maintain an aPPT of 45 to 60 s until warfarin, started at the same time, results in the desired INR (see Tables 68-2 and 68-3). If the CT scan demonstrates significant hemorrhage, antithrombotic therapy should be withheld until the bleed is treated or has stabilized (7 to 14 days). Anticoagulation can then be started as just described.

LONG-TERM MANAGEMENT

If the embolic event occurs when a patient is *off* antithrombotic therapy, long-term warfarin therapy is required (see Tables 68-2 and 68-3). An exception may be those with mitral valve prolapse; aspirin (325 mg/day) is recommended for those who are judged to have had a minor event. If the embolic event occurs while the patient is *on* antithrombotic treatment, therapy should be individualized. Those who are on warfarin, but in whom the INR was low at the time of the embolus, should have the dose increased into the high end of the desired range (see Tables 68-2 and 68-3). If the embolus occurs in a patient despite an INR in the desirable range, aspirin (50 to 100 mg/day) should be added to the warfarin. Embolism recurring

TABLE 68-5

ANTITHROMBOTIC THERAPY AT THE TIME OF A THROMBOEMBOLIC EVENT

I. Acute management
  A. *No* antithrombotic treatment for 72 h
  B. CT scan at 72 h
    1. *No (or little) hemorrhage* on CT:
      a. Heparin: aPPT 45–60 s
      b. Warfarin: continue heparin until INR in desired range[a]
    2. *Hemorrhage* on CT:
      a. No treatment until bleed stabilized or treated (7–14 days), then heparin and warfarin as above
II. Chronic management
  A. If embolus occurred *off* antithrombotic therapy:
    1. Treat with warfarin[a]
  B. If embolus occurred *on* antithrombotic therapy:
    1. If patient was on aspirin, switch to warfarin[a]
    2. If patient was on warfarin but INR was low, increase dose until INR in high desired range[a]
    3. If patient was on warfarin and INR was in desired range, add aspirin 80–325 mg/day
    4. If recurrent embolus or bleed on warfarin plus aspirin, assess valve for possible surgery

[a] See Tables 68-2 and 68-3.
Abbreviation: CT = computed tomography.

with this combination should lead to consideration of possible valve surgery if the valve is the likely source of the thrombus.

At the Time of a Bleed

With significant bleeding, antithrombotic therapy should be stopped and, if the patient is at risk, drug effects should be reversed. If possible, the site of bleeding should be corrected, and antithrombotic therapy restarted as soon as possible. If this is not possible, treatment decisions are difficult. In patients with a mechanical prosthesis or multiple risk factors for thromboemboli, acceptance of intermittent bleeding with acute management for the bleeds may be necessary. In valve patients who are at lower risk of emboli or in whom the role of antithrombotic treatment is less clear (e.g., LV dysfunction), it may be optimal to withhold chronic therapy or, if a patient is on warfarin, to switch to aspirin. In some patients with mechanical valves, consideration should be given to replacing the mechanical valve with a biological valve, for example, in those who have had multiple, large life- or organ-threatening bleeds.

Infective Endocarditis

If a patient with valve disease develops endocarditis, antithrombotic therapy should be continued.[21,47] If the patient presents with or develops an embolic event involving the central nervous system, therapy should be as described above for acute embolic events. Additionally, the issue of whether or not the embolus is due to thrombus or infected vegetation should be addressed. If thrombus is likely, the chronic anticoagulation program will also require alteration.

REFERENCES

1. Rahimtoola S. Lessons learned about the determinants of the results of valve surgery. *Circulation* 1988; 78;1503–1506.
2. Petersen P, Boysen G, Godtfredsen J, Andersen ED, Andersen B. Placebo controlled, randomized trial of warfarin and aspirin for prevention of thromboembolic complications in chronic atrial fibrillation. *Lancet* 1989; 1:175–179.
3. The Boston Area Anticoagulation Trial for Atrial Fibrillation Investigators. The effect of low-dose warfarin on the risk of stroke in patients with nonrheumatic atrial fibrillation. *N Engl J Med* 1990; 323:1505–1511.
4. Ezekowitz MD, Bridgers SL, James KE, Carliner NH, Colling CL, Gornick CC, et al. Warfarin in the prevention of stroke associated with nonrheumatic atrial fibrillation. *N Engl J Med* 1992; 327:1406–1412.
5. EAFT (European Atrial Fibrillation Trial) Study Group. Secondary prevention in nonrheumatic atrial fibrillation after transient ischemic attack or minor stroke. *Lancet* 1993; 342:1255–1262.
6. Stroke Prevention in Atrial Fibrillation Investigators. Warfarin versus aspirin for prevention of thromboembolism in atrial fibrillation: Stroke Prevention in Atrial Fibrillation II Study. *Lancet* 1994; 343:687–691.
7. Stroke Prevention in Atrial Fibrillation Investigators. Adjusted-dose warfarin versus low-intensity, fixed dose warfarin plus aspirin for high-risk patients with atrial fibrillation: Stroke Prevention in Atrial Fibrillation III randomized clinical trial. *Lancet* 1996; 348:633–638.
8. Cannegieter SC, Rosendaal FR, Briet E. Thromboembolic and bleeding complications in patients with mechanical heart valve prostheses. *Circulation* 1994; 89:635–641.
9. Starr A, Grunkemeier GL. Recurrent thromboembolism: Significance and management. In: Butchart EG, Bodnar E, eds. *Thrombosis, Embolism and Bleeding*. London: ICR; 1992:402–415.
10. Blackstone EH. Analyses of thrombosis, embolism and bleeding as time-related outcome events. In: Butchart EG, Bodnar E, eds. *Thrombosis, Embolism and Bleeding*. London: ICR; 1992:445–463.
11. Levin HJ, Pauler SG, Eckman MH. Antithrombotic therapy in valve disease. Fourth ACCP conference on antithrombolic therapy; Dalen JE, Hirsh J, eds. *Chest* 1995; 108(suppl):360S–370S.
12. Bloomfield P, Wheatley DJ, Prescott RJ, Miller HC. Twelve-year comparison of a Bjork-Shiley mechanical heart valve with porcine bioprostheses. *N Engl J Med* 1991; 324:573–579.
13. Hammermeister KE, Sethi GK, Henderson WG, Oprian C, Kim T, Rahimtoola S. A comparison of outcomes in men 11 years after heart-valve replacement with a mechanical valve or bioprosthesis. *N Engl J Med* 1993; 328;1289–1296.
14. Cobanoglu A, Fessler CL, Guvendik L, Grunkemeier G, Starr A. Aortic valve replacement with the Starr-Edwards prosthesis: A comparison of the first and second decades of follow-up. *Ann Thorac Surg* 1988; 45:248–252.
15. Vongpatanasin W, Hillis D, Lange RA. Prosthetic heart valves. *N Engl J Med* 1996; 335:407–416.
16. Geras M, Chesebro JH, Fuster V, Penny WJ, Grill DE, Bailey KR, et al. High risk of thromboemboli early after bioprosthetic cardiac valve replacement. *J Am Coll Cardiol* 1995; 25:1111–1119.
17. Cannegieter SC, Rosendaal FR, Wintzen AR, van der Meer FJM, Vandenbroucke JP, Briet E. Optimal oral anticoagulant therapy in patients with mechanical heart valves. *N Engl J Med* 1995; 333:11–17.
18. Jegaden O, Eker A, Delahaye F, Montagna P, Ossette J, Durand de Geuigney G, et al. Thromboembolic risk and late survival after mitral valve replacement with the St. Jude medical valve. *Ann Thorac Surg* 1994; 58:1721–1728.
19. Saour JN, Sieck JO, Mamo LAR, Gallus AS. Trial of different intensities of anticoagulation in patients with prosthetic heart valves. *N Engl J Med* 1990; 322:428–432.
20. Hylek EM, Skates SJ, Sheehan MA, Singer DE. An analysis of the lowest effective intensity of prophylactic anticoagulation for patients with nonrheumatic atrial fibrillation. *N Engl J Med* 1996; 335:540–546.
21. Hyashi J, Nakazawa S, Oguma F, Miyamura H, Equchi S. Combined warfarin and antiplatelet therapy after St. Jude medical valve replacement for mitral valve disease. *J Am Coll Cardiol* 1994; 23:672–677.
22. Turpie AG, Gent M, Laupacis A, Latour Y, Gunstensen J, Basile F, et al. A comparison of aspirin with placebo in patients treated with warfarin after heart-valve replacement. *N Engl J Med* 1993; 329:524–529.
23. Ginsberg JS, Hirsh J. Use of antithrombotic agents during pregnancy. Fourth ACCP conference on antithrombotic therapy; Dalen JE, Hirsh J, eds. *Chest* 1995; 108(suppl):305S–311S.
24. Turpie AGG, Gunstensen J, Hirsh J, Nelson H, Gent M. Randomized comparison of two intensities of oral anticoagulant therapy after tissue heart valve replacement. *Lancet* 1988; 1:1242–1245.
25. Hall JR, Pauli RM, Wilson KM. Maternal and fetal sequelae of anticoagulation during pregnancy. *Am J Med* 1980; 68:122.
26. Iturbe-Alessio I, del Carmen Fonseca M, Mutchinick O, Santos MA, Zajarias A, Salazar E. Risks of anticoagulant therapy in pregnant women with artificial heart valves. *N Engl J Med* 1986; 315:1390–1393.
27. Ginsbert JS, Kowalchuk G, Hirsh J, Brill-Edwards P, Burrows R. Heparin therapy during pregnancy. *Arch Intern Med* 1989; 149:2233–2236.
28. Hanania G, Thomas D, Michel PL, Gabarz E, Age C, Millaire A, et al. Pregnancy and prosthetic heart valves: A French cooperative retrospective study of 155 cases. *Eur Heart J* 1994; 15:1651–1658.
29. Salazar E, Iazguirre R, Verdejo J, Mutchinick O. Failure of adjusted doses of subcutaneous heparin to prevent thromboembolic phenomena in pregnant patients with mechanical cardiac valve prostheses. *J Am Coll Cardiol* 1996; 27:1698–1703.
30. Elkayam U. Anticoagulation in pregnant women with prosthetic heart valves: A double jeopardy (editorial). *J Am Coll Cardiol* 1996; 27:1704–1706.
31. Sturridge F, DeSwiet M, Letsky E. The use of low molecular weight heparin for thromboprophylaxis in pregnancy. *Br J Obstet Gynaecol* 1994; 101:69–71.
32. Corby DG. Aspirin in pregnancy and fetal effects. *Pediatrics* 1978; 62:930–937.
33. DuBard MB, Cutter GR. Low-dose aspirin therapy to prevent preeclampsia. *Am J Obstet Gynecol* 1993; 168:1083–1091.
34. Jamieson WR, Miller DC, Akins CW, Munro AI, Glower DD, Moore KA, et al. Pregnancy and bioprostheses: Influence on structural valve deterioration. *Ann Thorac Surg* 1995; 60:S282–S286.
35. Genewein U, Hasberli A, Werner S, Beer J. Rebound after cessation of oral anticoagulant therapy: The biochemical evidence. *Br J Haematol* 1996; 92:479–485.
36. Eckman MH, Beshansky JR, Durand-Zaleski I, Levine HJ, Pauker SG. Anticoagulation for noncardiac procedures in patients with prosthetic heart valves: Does low risk mean high cost? *JAMA* 1990; 263:1513–1521.
37. Bryan AJ, Butchart EG. Prosthetic heart valves and anticoagulant management during non-cardiac surgery. *Br J Surg* 1995; 82:577–578.
38. Busuttil WJ, Fabr BMI. The management of anticoagulation in patients with prosthetic heart valves undergoing non-cardiac operations. *Postgrad Med J* 1995; 71:390–392.
39. Tinker JH, Tarhan S. Discontinuing anticoagulant therapy in surgical patients with cardiac valve prostheses: Observations in 180 operations. *JAMA* 1978; 239:738–739.
40. Morton MJ, McAnulty JH, Rahimtoola SH, Ahuja N. Risks and benefits of postoperative cardiac catherization in patients with ball-valve prostheses. *Am J Cardiol* 1977; 40:870–875.
41. Gueret P, Vignon P, Fournier P, Chabernaud JM, Gomez M, LaCroix P, et al. Transesophageal echocardiography for the diagnosis and management of nonobstructive thrombosis of mechanical mitral valve prosthesis. *Circulation* 1995; 91:103–110.
42. Silber H, Khan SS, Matloff JM, Chaux A, DeRobertis M, Gray R. The St. Jude valve: Thrombolysis as the first line of therapy of cardiac valve thrombosis. *Circulation* 1993; 887:30–37.
43. Reddy NK, Padmanabhan TNC, Singh S, Raju PR, et al. Thrombolysis in left-sided prosthetic valve occlusion: Immediate and follow-up results. *Ann Thorac Surg* 1994; 58:462–471.

44. Pessin MS, Estol CJ, Lafranchise F, Chaplan LR. Safety of anti-coagulation after hemorrhagic infarction. *Neurology* 1994; 43(7):1289–1303.

45. Chamorro A, Vila N, Saiz A, Alday M, Tolosa E. Early anticoagulation after large cerebral embolic infarction: A safety study. *Neurology* 1995; 45:861–865.

46. Sherman DJ, Dyken ML, Gent M, Harrison MJA, Hart RG, Mohr JP. Antithrombotic therapy for cerebrovascular disorders. Fourth ACCP consensus conference on antithrombolic therapy; Dalen JE, Hirsh J, eds. *Chest* 1995; 108(suppl):444s–456s.

47. Wilson WR, Geraci JE, Danielson GK, Thompson RL, Spittell JA Jr, Washington JR 2d, et al. Anticoagulant therapy and central nervous system complication in patients with prosthetic valve endocarditis. *Circulation* 1978; 57:1004–1007.

CONGENITAL HEART DISEASE

69

CARDIOVASCULAR DISEASES DUE TO GENETIC ABNORMALITIES

Jeffrey A. Towbin / Robert Roberts

Deoxynucleic acid (DNA), the chemical substance that forms the chromosomes and their genes, encodes within the sequence of its bases the hereditary information required as the blueprint for each individual. This information directs the formation of all fetal structures, the potential of each person and his or her unique individuality, as well as the potential of future generations. During the past decade, it has become increasingly clear that genetic factors play a significant role in the pathogenesis of many, if not most, cardiovascular disorders. Many of these disorders have obvious genetic etiologies, such as long QT syndrome (LQTS), familial hypertrophic cardiomyopathy (HCM), or Marfan's syndrome.[1-3] Even diseases such as rheumatic fever and myocarditis will most likely be shown to occur in individuals with certain genetic predispositions. Malformations of the heart and blood vessels account for the largest number of human birth defects, occurring in about 1 percent of all live births; among stillbirths, the prevalence is estimated to be tenfold higher.[4,5]

In conjunction with cytogenetics (the study of chromosomes and their abnormalities), molecular genetics provides an opportunity to decipher the genetic basis of cardiovascular diseases. Isolation of disease-causing genes has led to identification of the specific protein abnormality, which is essential to elucidate the pathogenesis and design specific therapy. Genetic diagnosis and screening for genetic disorders are rapidly being incorporated into standard practice.

The goal of the Human Genome Project[6] is to identify all of the genes by the year 2005; however, the present rate of progress indicates that by the year 2000 the number of genes identified will be so enormous that it will significantly impact on the practice of cardiology. Thus, it will be necessary to understand these disorders to have a better appreciation of the medical, ethical, and moral implications.

BASIS FOR GENETIC TRANSMISSION

All hereditary information is transmitted through DNA, a linear polymer composed of purine (adenine, guanine) and pyrimidine (cytosine, thymine) bases (see Chap. 57). The basic hereditary unit is the *gene,* which consists of a distinct fragment of DNA that encodes for a specific polypeptide. It is estimated that there are only around 67,000 genes, although there is enough DNA to code for several hundred thousand genes. Only about 5 to 10 percent of the DNA, therefore, is used to code for genes. Each individual has two copies of each gene—called *alleles.* The genes are localized in linear sequence along 23 pairs of chromosomes, the rod-shaped bodies derived from the parents of each individual. Each parent contributes one member of each chromosome pair (the pair is referred to as *homologous chromosomes*) and, thus, one copy of each gene. The site at which a gene is located on a particular chromosome is called the *genetic locus.* A given gene always resides at the same specific locus on a particular chromosome, and so the loci on homologous chromosomes are identical but the alleles residing at these loci may be the same or different. When the same loci on two homologous chromosomes have identical alleles, the individual is *homozygous.* When the two genes differ (i.e., two different alleles present at the loci), the individual is *heterozygous* at that locus. Each individual is homozygous at some loci and heterozygous at others, and, based on present knowledge, at least one-third of human genes have polymorphic forms. The gene, transmitted to each offspring during the union of sperm and ova, passes on the genetic information to the offspring (*genotype*), which, through the synthesis of their corresponding proteins, determines the observable characteristics of an individual (*phenotype*). The genetic information carried in the gene's DNA is coded by the sequence of the four bases. Translation of this information into protein is through a translational code passed on through messenger ribonucleic acid (mRNA), whereby each specific amino acid is encoded by three bases referred to as a *codon* (Chap. 7). The mRNA transcribed from the gene serves as the template that determines which amino acids are included and their sequence in the resulting polypeptide.

The 23 pairs of chromosomes include 22 pairs of autosomes (chromosomes 1 to 22) and one pair of sex chromosomes, X and Y. Females have two X chromosomes, while males carry one X and one Y chromosome. Both autosomal alleles are potentially active in specifying RNA copies of their DNA sequences, but the expression of each gene depends on the cell type, developmental stage, and regulatory molecules that interact with *promoter sequences* and *enhancer sequences* that control gene transcription. In cells that carry two X chromosomes, whether these are derived from normal females or XXY individuals with Klinefelter syndrome, only one X is active after early embryogenesis.

ORIGIN
OF GENETIC DISEASE

Hereditary and congenital diseases may be due to chromosomal abnormalities or mutations within a single gene. A *mutation* is a stable, heritable alteration in DNA caused by a number of factors including environmental agents such as radiation, chemicals, and viruses as well as baseline changes in the fidelity of transfer of sequences. Since offspring typically resemble their parents, it is assumed that the DNA nucleotide sequences remain stable. Base sequence changes do occur, however, albeit at a slow rate compared to the overall life span of humans, and these changes occur by a number of different mechanisms. Mutations can involve a visible alteration at the level of the chromosome, such as deletion or translocation of a portion of the chromosome, whereby often several genes are eliminated or altered. Chromosome alterations, especially those involving too many or too few chromosomes (called *aneuploidy*), are quite common in human development. Chromosome aberrations are discussed in "Cardiovascular Disorders Associated with Chromosome Abnormalities," below.

The sequence of each codon determines the amino acid, and the linear sequence of the codons in the mRNA is colinear with the linear sequence of the amino acids in the protein. A change in even one amino acid, if critical to the function of the protein, will result in altered function or lack of function, with a concomitant change in the phenotype. Since proteins are the working molecules derived from genes, mutations in genes exert their deleterious effects via structural alteration of the proteins, whether they be enzymes, regulatory proteins, or structural proteins. On the average, a mutation occurs every 10^6 cell divisions, and, obviously, only mutations occurring in the gametes are transmitted. On the average, a gene undergoes one mutation per 200,000 years.

GENETICS
OF SINGLE-GENE DISORDERS

Types of Mutations and Genetic Heterogeneity

Inherited disorders due to a single abnormal gene are transmitted to offspring in a predictable fashion termed *mendelian transmission*. These inheritance patterns produce phenotypes that are inherited according to Mendel's laws of inheritance. As previously noted, each gene exists in two alternative forms, referred to as alleles, one obtained from the mother and one from the father. Mendel's first law states that each of the two alleles located on separate chromosomes segregates independently and is passed unchanged into different gametes at the formation of the next generation. Thus, the odds of getting the mother's allele versus the father's is by chance alone, namely, 50 percent. Mendel's second law states that genes on the same chromosome also assort themselves independently through the process of crossover between chromosomes (discussed below). The greater the distance between two loci, the more likely they are to be separated during genetic transmission. As a result of gene mutations, abnormal genes located on any of the 22 autosomal pairs or the two sex chromosomes produce phenotypes inherited by simple patterns classified as *autosomal* (dominant or recessive) or *X-linked,* respectively. Single-gene mutations account for most of the disorders in the adult cardiac population; hereditary disorders with a known molecular genetic defect are primarily due to mutations in a single gene. When different genes induce the same phenotype, it is referred to as *genetic heterogeneity,* and most diseases in humans exhibit genetic heterogeneity. The same disease may be due to multiple mutations in the same gene (*allele heterogeneity*) or it may be due to a single or multiple mutations in two or more genes (*gene heterogeneity*). Within any one family, however, the gene and the mutation responsible for the disease are always the same. A good example is familial HCM, in which four different genes have been recognized with multiple mutations in each. Genetic heterogeneity is to be distinguished from *polygenic disorders,* such as atherosclerosis, which are due to the interaction of several genes.

As noted above, mutations can involve a visible alteration, such as *deletion* or *translocation* of a portion of the chromosome, or they can involve a minute change in one purine or pyrimidine base in the DNA sequence of a single codon of a gene. Mutations involving only a single nucleotide are known as *point mutations*. A point mutation may be a substitution of one nucleotide for another, resulting in a different amino acid being encoded (*missense mutation*); or it may change the codon from one encoding for an amino acid to that of a stop codon, which will truncate the protein (*truncated mutant*); or it may eliminate a stop codon so the protein is elongated (*elongated mutant*). Finally, a nucleotide may be deleted or added, which results in a frameshift, and the gene is read entirely differently (*nonsense mutation*), resulting in a nonfunctioning protein. If a purine nucleotide is substituted for a pyrimidine, the mutation is referred to as a *transversion,* while if purine or pyrimidine substitutes for another purine or pyrimidine, respectively, it is called a *transition.* Other mutations may result from deletion or addition of several nucleotides. An example of the latter is the defect responsible for myotonic dystrophy, where a triplet repeat of several thousand nucleotides in length is inserted into the $3'$ end of the gene, which makes the mRNA unstable and presumably leads to the disease. Another type of mutation is known as *gene conversion,* where two genes interact and part of the nucleotide sequence of one gene becomes incorporated into the other. Mutations in genes exert their deleterious effects via structural alteration of enzymes, regulatory proteins, or structural proteins.

The terms *dominant inheritance* and *recessive inheritance* refer to characteristics of the phenotype and are *not* characteristics of the gene per se. Dominant inheritance implies that a person with one copy of a mutant allele and one copy of the normal allele develops a phenotype referred to as heterozygosity. Recessive traits, on the other hand, require a double dose of the mutant allele at the locus to develop a phenotype. Those individuals carrying two identical mutant alleles are called homozygous. This situation usually occurs when the patients are consanguineous, with each carrying mutant alleles, or when the mutant allele is common in the population, such as is seen in sickle cell anemia.

Genetic Penetrance and Expressivity

In some individuals, despite having a disease-related gene, there is no clinical manifestation. The percentage of individuals with a disease-related gene who have one or more features of the disease is referred to as *penetrance.* Penetrance is an all-or-none phenomenon, and any manifestation, however minute, indicates that the gene has full penetrance in that individual. *Nonpenetrance* refers to lack of any observable phenotype. This feature is to be distinguished from *expressivity,* which refers to the variable nature of the clinical features, and thus, by definition, to have expressivity, the trait must be penetrant.

The effect of any gene on any organ such as the heart is highly variable. The manifested phenotype of any given mutant allele can be vastly different, depending on whether an individual is homozygous or heterozygous for the gene. Variability is also due in part to the frequency of a particular pleiotropic manifestation, the severity of clinical expression, and the age of onset of the manifestations. When an individual carries a mutant allele but no phenotypic abnormality, the trait is nonpenetrant. This description, however, relies heavily on the sensitivity of the technique utilized for detection. For instance, the diagnosis of familial HCM by clinical examination will be significantly less sensitive than that from echocardiography. Numerous genetic and environmental factors can affect expression of a gene, making it nearly impossible to determine which factor is most important in a specific individual or specific disease. These factors include: (1) genetic background, (2) age-dependency, (3) sex influence and sex limitation, (4) exogenous factors, (5) maternal factors, (6) modifying loci, and (7) gene alterations.

Patterns of Inheritance

AUTOSOMAL DOMINANT INHERITANCE

Dominant disorders are those that have phenotypic manifestations (disease) in heterozygous individuals—persons carrying only one abnormal allele, with the other allele on the homologous chromosome being normal. In autosomal dominant disorders, both males and females can be affected and since alleles segregate independently at meiosis, there is a 50-50 chance that the offspring of an affected heterozygote will inherit the mutant allele. Not all affected individuals, however, must have an affected parent because, in all autosomal dominant diseases, a certain proportion of cases occur due to a *new mutation* (i.e., they are sporadic). The parent whose germ cells contain the new mutation will be clinically normal, since the mutation affects only a single germ cell, but will, however, transmit the disease-causing allele to half of their offspring. Autosomal dominant inheritance can be misdiagnosed as sporadic if there is low expressivity in the phenotypically normal parent carrying the mutant allele or if extramarital paternity has occurred. The following features are characteristic of autosomal dominant inheritance (Fig. 69-1): (1) each affected individual has an affected parent, unless the disease occurred due to a new mutation or the heterozygous parent has low expressivity; (2) equal proportions (i.e., 50-50) of normal and affected offspring are likely statistically to be born to an affected individual; (3) normal children of an affected individual bear only normal offspring; (4) equal proportions of males and females are affected; (5) both sexes are equally likely to transmit the abnormal allele to male and female offspring, and male-to-male transmission occurs; and (6) vertical transmission through successive generations occurs.

Two other features are characteristically seen in autosomal dominant diseases that help to differentiate this type of inheritance from autosomal recessive disorders: *delayed age of onset and variable clinical expression.* The former is commonly seen in such disorders as familial HCM, while the latter may occur in Holt-Oram syndrome, in which the patient may present with an atrial septal defect (ASD) and skeletal abnormality of the upper extremity in combination or with either of these abnormalities individually. Examples of autosomal dominant primary heart disease include HCM and Romano-Ward LQTS.

AUTOSOMAL RECESSIVE INHERITANCE

Autosomal recessive phenotypes are clinically apparent when the patient carries two mutant alleles (i.e., is homozygous) at the locus responsible for the disease state. The disease-causing gene is found on one of the 22 autosomes, and thus both males and females will be equally affected. Clinical uniformity is typical, and disease onset generally occurs early in life. Recessive disorders are more commonly diagnosed in childhood than are dominant diseases. Only one in four children (25 percent, on average, will be affected. The following are

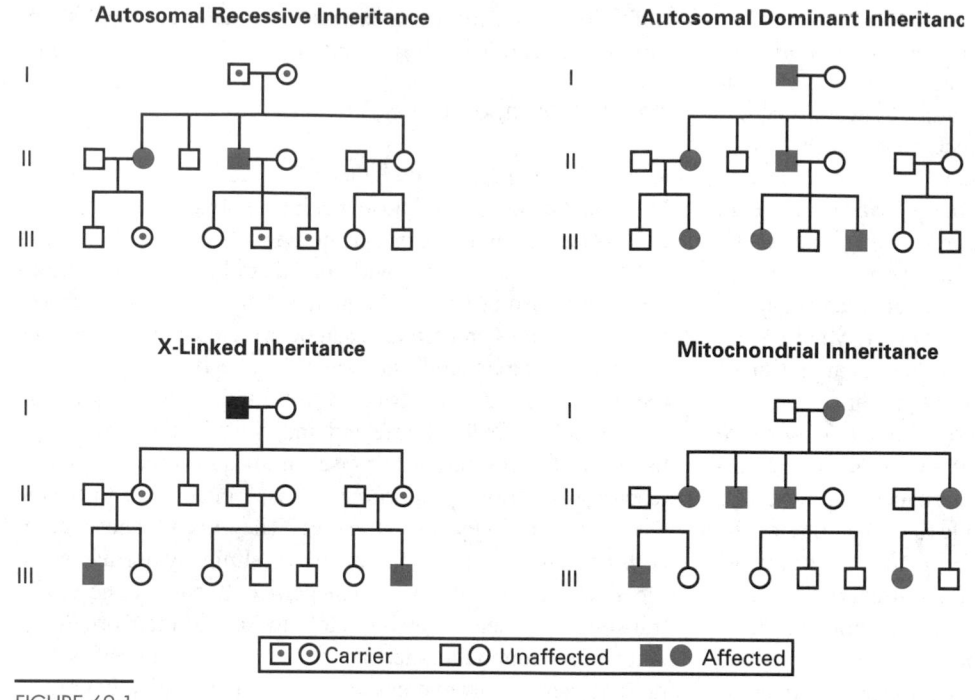

FIGURE 69-1

This typical set of pedigrees outlines the usual inheritance patterns for autosomal dominant and recessive traits, X-linked inheritance, and mitochondrial inheritance. Squares signify males, and females are designated by circles. Filled-in circles and squares are affected females and males, respectively.

characteristics of autosomal recessive disorders (Fig. 69-1): (1) parents are clinically normal heterozygotes; (2) alternate generations are affected, with no vertical transmission; (3) both sexes are affected with equal frequency; and (4) each offspring of heterozygous carriers has a 25 percent chance of being affected, a 50 percent chance of being an unaffected carrier, and a 25 percent chance of inheriting only normal alleles. Examples of autosomal recessive disorders affecting the heart include Jervell and Lange-Nielsen long QT/deafness syndrome and Pompe's (type II glycogen storage) disease.

X-LINKED INHERITANCE

X-linked inherited disorders are caused by genes located on the X chromosome and, therefore, the clinical risk and severity of disease differ between the sexes. Since a female has two X chromosomes, she may carry either one mutant allele (heterozygote) or two mutant alleles (homozygote); the trait may therefore display dominant or recessive expression. Males have a single X chromosome (and one Y chromosome), so they are expected to display the full syndrome whenever they inherit the abnormal gene from their mother. This development of the trait occurs regardless of whether the mother carrying the mutant allele exhibits a recessive (i.e., clinically silent) or dominant (i.e., clinically apparent) trait. Hence, the terms *X-linked dominant* and *X-linked recessive* apply only to the expression of the gene in females. Since males must pass on their Y chromosome to all male offspring, they cannot pass on mutant X alleles to their sons, and, therefore, no male-to-male transmission of X-linked disorders may occur. On

the other hand, males must contribute their one X chromosome to all daughters. All females receiving a mutant X chromosome are known as *carriers,* and those who become affected clinically with the disease are known as *manifesting female carriers.* The characteristic features of X-linked inheritance (Fig. 69-1) include: (1) no male-to-male transmission; (2) all daughters of affected males are carriers; (3) sons of carrier females have a 50 percent risk of being affected, and daughters have a 50 percent chance of being carriers; (4) affected homozygous females occur only when an affected male marries a carrier female; and (5) the pedigree pattern in X-linked recessive traits tends to be oblique because of the occurrence of the trait in the sons of normal carrier sisters of affected males (i.e., uncles and nephews affected). Examples of X-linked disorders of the heart include X-linked cardiomyopathy, X-linked cardioskeletal myopathy (Barth's syndrome) and those X-linked diseases in which the heart is affected, such as muscular dystrophy (MD) (e.g., Duchenne/Becker and Emery-Dreifuss MD).

MITOCHONDRIAL INHERITANCE

Another inheritance pattern recently described in patients with cardiovascular anomalies occurs because of abnormalities of the mitochondrial genome. Energy generation is dependent on the oxidative-phosphorylation process that takes place in mitochondria, which are found in the cytoplasm of most cell types. Within many mitochondria is a single chromosome that encodes for a number of the enzymes of oxidative phosphorylation (i.e., encodes for 13 of the 69 proteins required for oxidative metabolism) and the transfer RNAs (tRNAs and ribosomal RNAs (rRNAs) required for their translation). The remaining enzymes of the oxidative-phosphorylation pathway are encoded by genes on the nuclear chromosomes, and the resultant proteins are transported into the mitochondrion. Genetic defects of oxidative phosphorylation, therefore, can be due either to gene mutations within the X chromosome or autosomes (i.e., nuclear chromosomes), resulting in diseases that behave as mendelian recessive traits, or to mitochondrial genome defects that cause diseases with nonmendelian traits. These differences may be explained by events of conception, since the spermatocyte contributes few or no mitochondria to the zygote (Fig. 69-2). The entire mitochondrial complement present in a fetus must therefore be derived from the mitochondria already pres-

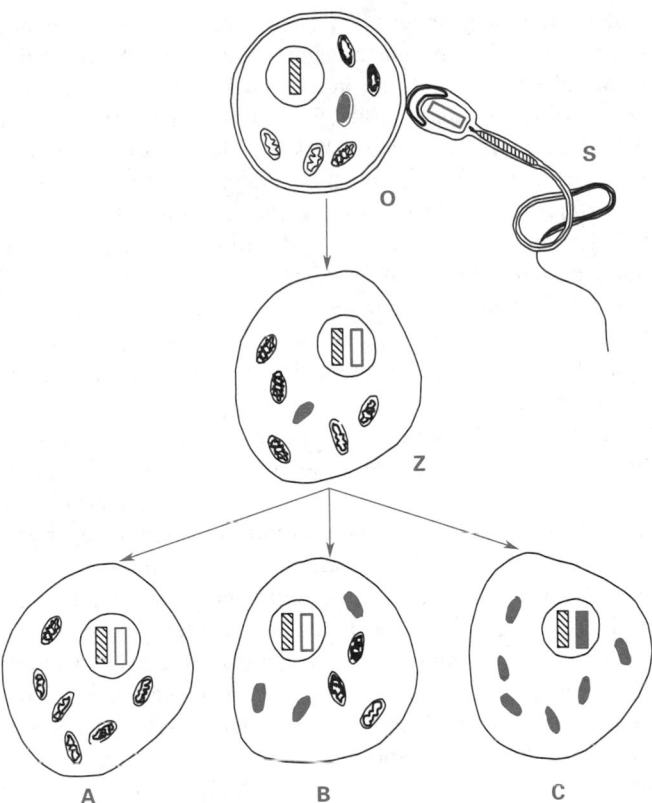

FIGURE 69-2

Cartoon (not to scale) illustrating maternal inheritance of mtDNA, compared with biparental inheritance of nuclear genes, and the random distribution of normal and mutant mitochondrial genomes in daughter cells of the zygote. It is assumed for simplicity that individual mitochondria contain either normal (open mitochondria) or mutant (filled mitochondria) mtDNA, not both. O, oocyte; S, sperm; Z, zygote; A, B, C, daughter cells of zygote, representing stem cells of different tissues. (Reprinted with permission from DiMauro S, et al. *Clin Neurol* 1990;8:494)

ent in the cytoplasm of the oocyte. Thus, phenotypes due to mitochondrial mutations demonstrate maternal inheritance only. The characteristic features of mitochondrial inheritance of disease (Fig. 69-1) include: (1) equal frequency and severity of disease for each sex; (2) transmission through females only, with offspring of affected males being unaffected; (3) all offspring of affected females may be affected; (4) extreme variability of expression of disease within a family (may include apparent nonpenetrance); and (5) phenotypes may be age-dependent. An example of mitochondrial inherited cardiac disease is the cardiomyopathy of Kearns-Sayre syndrome.

Polygenic Inheritance of Cardiac Disease

Disorders such as hypertension or ischemic heart disease are believed to require concomitant mutations in several genes, i.e., they are polygenic hereditary disorders. The genes responsible for polygenic hereditary disorders are difficult to map and identify since computational methods to describe their mode of inheritance are only now being explored.

Over the past two decades, this type of inheritance has been invoked for a large number of disorders, including coro-

nary artery disease and congenital heart disease. In multifactorial, or polygenic, genetic diseases, multiple genes interact in a cumulative fashion to induce the disease or provide an increased risk of developing the disease. This multifaceted process is illustrated by coronary artery disease, in which one common phenotype is myocardial infarction due to thrombosis superimposed on atherosclerosis. There are many single-gene disorders that alter plasma lipoproteins and contribute to atherosclerosis (see Chaps. 39 and 41). In addition, the individual is more likely to develop severe atherosclerosis if he or she inherited the form of the paraoxonase gene that leads to low levels of the enzyme paraoxonase.[7] The phenotype of acute myocardial infarction is more likely if the individual, in addition to atherosclerosis, has a mutant form of fibrinogen[8] or of other clotting factors. When an individual inherits a combination of genes that interacts to create a risk potential above threshold, environmental factors play a major role in determining whether or not he or she is clinically affected and to what extent. Thus, in a family with multifactorial genetic diseases, other family members must inherit the same genetic and environmental combinations to express the same disorder. Since all first-degree relatives of affected individuals (i.e., parents, siblings, and offspring) share one-half of that individual's genes, they are at increased risk of exhibiting the same disorder. Second-degree relatives, such as uncles, aunts, and grandparents, share an average of one-fourth of the affected individual's genes [i.e., $(1/2)^2$], while third-degree relatives (i.e., cousins) share one-eighth [i.e., $(1/2)^3$] of the genes, and so on. Therefore, as the relationship to the affected individual becomes increasingly distant, the likelihood of inheriting the disease decreases significantly, because the chance of any relative inheriting the correct combination of genes decreases as the number of genes required for expression of a given trait increases. Since the precise number of genes responsible for polygenic traits is not known, the precise risk of inheritance cannot be determined. Empiric risk figures—the proportion of affected relatives in previously reported families—must be relied upon in counseling families with polygenic diseases. In contrast to single-gene disorders, which affect 20 to 50 percent of first-degree relatives of an affected proband, multifactorial genetic disorders generally affect no more than 5 to 10 percent of first-degree relatives. In contradistinction to mendelian traits, the recurrent risk varies between families, depending on the number of affected individuals already diagnosed and the severity of the disorder in the index case. The larger the number of affected family members and the more severe the disease, the higher the risk to other relatives. This is distinguished from a single-gene disorder in which the phenotype is influenced by many other genes.

The empiric risk of recurrence of congenital heart disease has increased during the past decade and is consistent with the overall higher incidence of congenital heart disease previously noted. The original study of recurrence risk was performed by Edwards,[9] who developed a method to test the polygenic model. He calculated the incidence of disease to be expected in first-degree relatives of subjects affected with polygenic disease. Nora and coworkers[10] showed that the recurrence risk for first-degree relatives is in the range of 1 to 5 percent and is in agreement with the figures predicted by Edwards' theory. For this reason, the concept of polygenic inheritance of congenital heart disease gained wide acceptance. Additionally, they observed a sex distribution of congenital heart disease that appeared to conform to the distribution predicted by this model. Recent evidence suggests that different anatomic defects may be the result of the same pathogenic mechanisms. Clark[11] suggested that the majority of congenital cardiovascular defects are due to six developmental mechanisms: (1) abnormal ectomesenchymal tissue migration, (2) abnormal intracardiac blood flow, (3) abnormal targeted growth, (4) extracellular matrix abnormalities, (5) endocardial cushion defects, and (6) looping defects.

Overview of Chromosomal Mapping and Identification of a Disease-Related Gene

Identification of a disease-causing gene, in the setting where the protein is unknown, has until recently been nearly impossible. In contrast, in diseases with a known protein abnormality, the possible expressed nucleotide sequences (cDNA sequence) can be deduced from the protein sequences. Probes can then be designed to identify the approximate chromosomal location and ultimately clone and sequence the gene and the specific disease-causing mutation(s). Familial hypercholesterolemia and some of the thalassemias are disorders in which genes were isolated and cloned using this approach. For the majority of diseases, however, neither the defect or protein is known. Technical advances made recently make it possible to map the chromosomal locus of a disease-related gene without knowing the protein.[12] The new techniques aiding chromosomal mapping are: (1) computerized linkage analysis, (2) development of highly informative DNA markers, and (3) detection of markers by polymerase chain reaction (PCR).[12]

The 46 chromosomes of the human genome contain 3 billion base pairs (bp). To locate a particular gene, one must first map the chromosomal location and its relative position. This process requires certain chromosomal landmarks. Identification of a particular locus is made possible by showing that the disease-related gene of interest is on the same chromosome and in close proximity to one of these landmarks, a method referred to as *genetic linkage analysis*. This technique requires a family with a disease that is transmitted over at least two generations (and preferably three) with at least 10 living, affected individuals, although even six or seven affected individuals may be adequate, depending on the structure of the family. A landmark, referred to as a DNA or *chromosomal marker,* is a polymorphic sequence of DNA, the chromosomal position of which is known and can be detected by analyzing an individual's DNA (discussed in detail below). A major limitation until recently was the lack of markers distributed across each of the chromosomes.[13,14] Today there is a marker available at least every 1 million base pairs on all chromosomes.[13,14] This distance is defined as 1 centimorgan (cM),

named after the geneticist T. H. Morgan. Markers, like genes, have two alleles and are transmitted to offspring according to Mendel's law, with the individual being heterozygous or homozygous for that marker. If a marker is homozygous, it is not informative for genetic linkage. Hence, several markers in the same region often must be analyzed to find one that is heterozygous in that individual. Placing all of the markers together on each chromosome and estimating the genetic distance between them is referred to as a *genetic map*. A map of over 5000 highly informative markers has been developed, which has significantly accelerated the mapping of disease-related genes, an achievement that provides the foundation for genetic linkage analysis.[14]

Each gene, allele, or marker is transmitted independently; thus, the odds of any two genes (or a marker and a gene) being coinherited are by chance alone (50 percent), even though they are on the same chromosome. The independent assortment of genes from each other during transmission is nature's means of maintaining biological diversity. The homologous pairs of chromosomes are assorted, and one from each parent transmitted to the offspring by chance. Genetic diversity from homologous chromosomes segregating independently would produce 2^{23} types of gametes; in other words, the probability of an offspring inheriting a set of chromosomes identical to a parent is one in 8,388,608.[15] If this were the only mechanism, however, all of the genes on a particular chromosome would be coinherited in the next progeny. This does not happen. Even genes on the same chromosome are transmitted independently, unless they are on the same chromosome in close physical proximity to each other, in which case they tend to be coinherited. Genes on the same chromosome are transmitted independently by the mechanism of crossover between homologous chromosomes (Fig. 69-3), which provides continual mixing of the genes during every meiosis and is the predominant reason why no two individuals have the same genotype unless they are identical twins. prior to meiosis, the two homologous chromosomes come together and form bridges (chiasmata) such that segments of equal proportion are exchanged between them, giving rise to crossover of various genes. There is no net loss of chromosomal material or genes, but crossover leads to a constant intermixing of the chromosomes such that no two offspring will ever be identical. Crossovers occur only between homologous chromosomes. The loci occupy the same chromosomal position on the homologous chromosome to which they recombined as they had on their original homologous chromosome. On average there are 33 crossovers between homologous chromosome pairs per meiosis.[15] In genetic parlance, crossing-over is referred to as *recombination*.

CONCEPT OF GENETIC LINKAGE ANALYSIS

Despite the independent assortment of chromosomes and even genes, two or more loci are often coinherited because they are so close together that the chance of a bridge forming between them is less likely and, therefore, they tend to be coinherited more often than by chance alone; by definition

Non-Linkage-
Distance Between
Loci Great

Genetic Linkage-
Distance Between
Loci Minimal

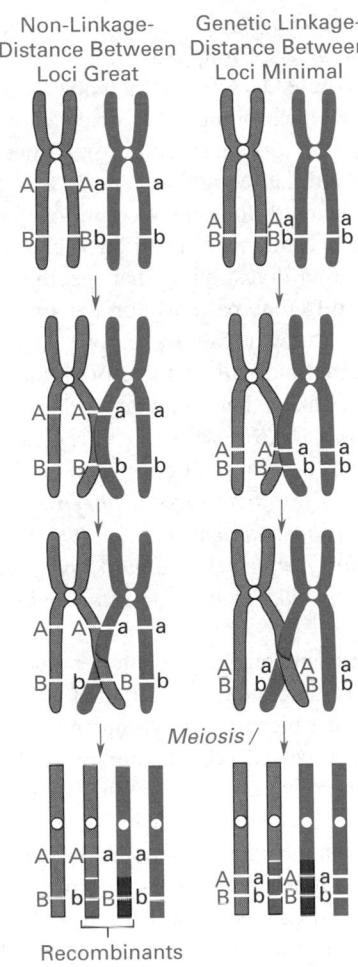

Meiosis /

Recombinants

FIGURE 69-3

Comparison of nonlinked genes (*left*) and linked genes (*right*). In nonlinkage the distance between loci is large, allowing crossing over to occur, resulting in recombinants after meiosis. The distance between linked genes is comparatively small, thereby minimizing the chance for recombinants.

The concept of linkage analysis is illustrated in Fig. 69-3. Shown in the panel at the right is an illustration of genetic linkage between a locus for a DNA marker and that of a disease that is inherited in a mendelian dominant fashion. The locus, designated with an "A," carries the allele responsible for the disease. The corresponding locus "a" on the homologous chromosome has the allele that codes for the same protein but has not undergone a mutation and is thus the normal allele. The loci designated "B" and the other "b" represent alleles of a DNA marker of known location that has nothing to do with the disease. In the panel on the right, the disease and the marker loci are so close that they tend to be coinherited within the family, whereas in the panel on the left, the DNA marker of known location is so far from the locus carrying the disease allele it is not coinherited but separate by chance. The calculation necessary to prove definitively that genetic linkage exists between a marker and a disease-related locus is sophisticated and requires advanced computerized programs. The odds for and against linkage are calculated, and linkage exists if the odds are in favor with a ratio of at least 1000:1. To avoid the cumbersome ratio (1000:1), the logarithm to base 10 is derived, which is 3 (i.e., 10^3), and is referred to as the *LOD score* (log of the odds). If the LOD score is −2 (i.e., 10^{-2} or 100:1 odds against linkage), it excludes linkage.

The likelihood of two genes being separated by recombination increases in proportion to the distance between them. The distance between a marker and a disease-causing gene when genetically linked is quite variable and may be anywhere from 1000 kilobase pairs (kbp) to 50,000 kbp but is usually within 1000 to 10,000 kbp.[16] The inherent resolution of genetic linkage analysis is never better than 1000 kbp. It is possible on the basis of linkage analysis alone to construct a *chromosomal map* of all the markers, with the distance between the various markers estimated in cM. This is a complex calculation derived from the number of recombinations between the markers during meioses. The *recombination frequency* between two markers, two genes, or a gene and a marker is the ratio of the number of crossover events to the total number of meioses. The lower the recombination frequency between the locus of a marker and that of a disease-related gene, the closer those two must be in physical distance on the chromosome. Even though the locus of the marker and that of the disease-related gene are in close enough proximity to be genetically linked, recombination may occur, and the extent to which recombination does occur reflects roughly the physical distance between the two loci. The recombination factor (or Θ) is used to develop a means of estimating the genetic distance (in cM) between genetically linked loci. A recombination frequency or crossover of 1 percent between two loci, whether occupied by two genes or one gene and a marker, reflects a physical distance between them of approximately 1 million bp (1 cM).[16] For a marker and a gene separated by 1 cM, this means the chance of a crossover between them during meiosis is only 1 percent and, thus, the chance of being coinherited is 99 percent. This is a statistically derived genetic map, however, and the distances are only

this means the two loci are in genetic linkage. Linkage analysis takes advantage of the location of a genetic marker on the same chromosome, in close physical proximity to a disease-related gene, which tends to be coinherited in the offspring more often than by chance alone. Any two loci coinherited more than 50 percent of the time are said to be genetically linked. Thus, genetic linkage means that a marker and the gene responsible for the disease are on the same chromosome in reasonably close proximity. To map the chromosomal locus responsible for a disease-related gene, one selects markers that are evenly distributed across the chromosomes. DNA is collected from all the members of a family (normal and affected) and analyzed for these markers. If one or more markers is coinherited in more than 50 percent of the affected individuals, the locus where the marker resides is genetically linked to the locus of the gene that is responsible for the disease. Once a disease is linked to a marker of known chromosomal locus, it follows that the disease locus is on the same chromosome, and its approximate position on the chromosome is also known.

approximate. The correlation between the percent crossover and the physical distance in base pairs varies somewhat from chromosome to chromosome and from region to region, even on the same chromosome. For example, recombination is more frequent in the telomeric than in the centromeric portion of the chromosome. If the marker locus and the disease-related locus are close, such as 5 to 10 cM, then a single crossover may be uncommon and a double crossover rare. Two loci may be 20 to 40 cM apart, however, and a double crossover occurs, which recombines the locus with the original chromosome and leads to coinheritance of the two (linkage of the two loci). When this occurs, the genetic distance is misleading and represents a gross underestimation of the true physical distance between the two loci.

CHROMOSOMAL MARKERS AND THEIR IDENTIFICATION

A chromosomal marker (as defined above) is any DNA sequence of known chromosomal location that is polymorphic for the population (two or more alleles). The greater the number of alleles, the more informative the marker. When compared between individuals in the population, the DNA of the human genome shows a difference in the nucleotide sequence (polymorphism) every 300 to 500 bp. Polymorphisms occur more frequently in the sequence of the unexpressed DNA (intron) than in DNA coding for proteins (exon). Until recently, the most common chromosomal marker was that of restriction fragment length polymorphism (RFLP)[17] identified by Southern blotting. Restriction endonucleases cleave foreign DNA by recognizing specific DNA sequences of three to eight bases. Consequently, digestion of human DNA by a given restriction endonuclease results in a specific pattern of fragments characterized by the number of fragments cleaved and the length of each fragment. These DNA fragments can be separated by size using agarose gel electrophoresis and detected by hybridization using a DNA probe (Southern blotting). If there were a base change that altered the recognition site of a restriction endonuclease or created an additional recognition site in one allele but not in the other, the pattern exhibited by the DNA on gel electrophoresis after digestion by that specific enzyme would give distinctly different patterns for the two alleles[18] (see Chap. 7). If a particular pattern for one of these alleles is detected in affected individuals more often than by chance, it suggests genetic linkage between that marker and the disease-related gene. *The RFLPs as markers represented a major breakthrough for genetic linkage in the 1980s but are seldom used today. These markers have been replaced by what are referred to as short tandem repeat polymorphisms (STRP), which occur more frequently, are more informative, and are more conveniently and rapidly detected than are RFLPs*[19] (Fig. 69-4).

Distributed throughout the human genome are repeats of dinucleotides, trinucleotides, or tetranucleotides that are repeated in tandem (microsatellites) and may vary anywhere from 60 to 300 repeats. The number of tandem repeats of STRPs, which provide for marked polymorphism, occur about every 500 bp throughout the human genome. The dinucleotide repeats of cytosine-adenosine are more common than trinucleotide or tetranucleotide repeats. A major advantage of STRPs is rapid and convenient detection by PCR rather than requiring Southern blotting as is necessary for RFLPs. PCR requires only a nanogram of DNA as opposed to a milligram for RFLPs, and results are available in only 1 to 24 h as opposed to 9 to 10 days for Southern blotting. The resolution of STRPs detected by PCR is much better than by Southern blotting and, since STRPs have multiple alleles (as opposed to RFLPs which have only two alleles), they are much more informative for genetic linkage.

IDENTIFICATION OF THE GENE

Thus, even after mapping the chromosomal locus by genetic linkage analysis, it is a considerable task to identify the gene. Years may pass between the chromosomal localization of a gene and the final identification of the gene and its protein products. Huntington's disease and myotonic dystrophy required

Sequence-based polymorphisms

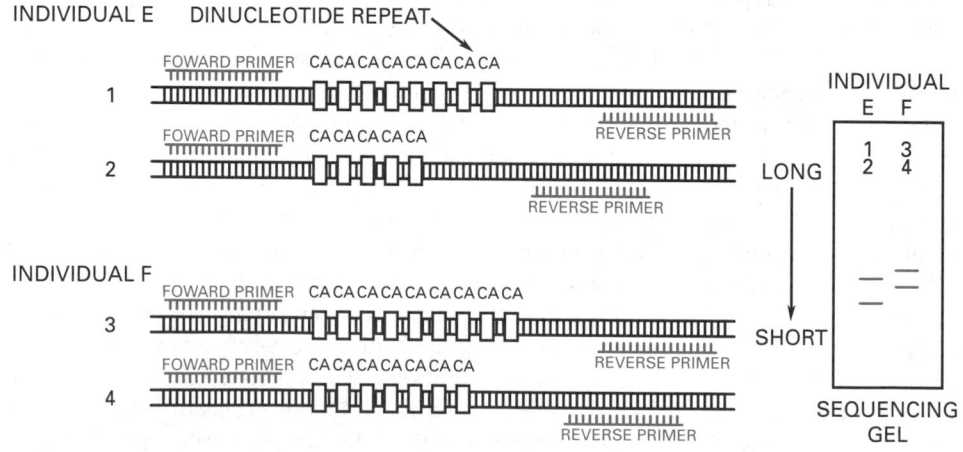

FIGURE 69-4

Sequence-based polymorphisms. This type of polymorphism is based on sequence variations caused by variable numbers of repeat sequence within a population. In this case, variable numbers of CA dinucleotide repeats are shown at one locus. These polymorphisms can be detected by use of specific oligonucleotide primers and polymerase chain reaction (PCR). The resultant PCR products will vary in size and can be detected by polyacrylamide gel electrophoresis. These sequence-based PCR polymorphisms may be highly polymorphic, thus providing increased statistical strength to linkage analysis over 2-allele polymorphisms seen in Southern blot restriction fragment length polymorphisms. (Reprinted with permission from Keating M. *Circulation* 1992; 85:1973–1986.)

about 10 years. It is often necessary to identify other DNA markers that flank the disease locus more closely than the original marker to decrease the distance between the nearest marker locus and that of the disease gene. The first technique in attempting to identify the gene is referred to as the *candidate gene approach*. Over 5000 loci have now been mapped for human genes, and over 1000 genes recorded in a gene bank. These genes and their sequences are entered through a worldwide network with a database in the United States, Europe, and Japan that is updated on a daily basis. Once a locus is identified on a chromosome, genes previously known to be localized to that region become candidate genes for the newly mapped locus. These genes are amplified, usually by PCR, to determine if there is a mutation that segregates with the disease and, if not, as a candidate gene. If none of the candidate genes in the region is shown to have a mutation that cosegregates with the disease, it may be necessary to clone the region. This approach is referred to as *positional cloning,* so named because a region is cloned knowing only its position relative to the genetically linked marker. To prove that the gene causes the disease, the mutation must be identified and shown to cosegregate with the disease and not with the unaffected members in the family. The remaining task would be to determine the gene product (protein) and the pathophysiology of how the mutation induces the disease. In attempting to decipher the pathophysiology, one may transfect cells in culture with normal and mutant forms of the gene and compare the resulting phenotype. The other definitive approaches for determining causality are to overexpress the gene as a transgene in animals such as mice or to do homologous knockout, replacing the normal with the mutant gene to determine whether the disease phenotype is induced.

Chromosomal mapping of hereditary diseases by linkage analysis and subsequent isolation of the gene[20] may be summarized as follows:

1. Identification of a family with a familial disease
2. Collection of clinical data from the family
3. Clinical assessment to provide an accurate diagnosis of the disease using a consistent and objective criterion to separate normal individuals from those affected and from those that are indeterminate or unknown
4. Collection of blood samples for immediate DNA analysis and development of lymphoblastoid cell lines for a renewable source of DNA
5. Development of a family pedigree
6. DNA analysis for markers of known chromosomal loci that span the human genome in an attempt to find a marker locus linked to the disease
7. Identification of the gene
8. Identification of mutation(s) causing the disease
9. Demonstration of a causal relationship between the mutant gene and the disease
10. Development of a convenient test to screen for the mutations

Family History and Evaluation

The most important part of an evaluation for genetic disease is the family history. First, the family history may give clues to the diagnosis of a particular disorder, information about possible inheritance patterns within an individual family, and information about conditions for which family members may be at an increased risk. An individual's ethnic background may, for instance, suggest the need for specific types of genetic screening such as for hemoglobinopathies in individuals of African or Mediterranean ancestry or for Tay-Sachs disease in individuals of eastern European (Ashkenazi) Jewish ancestry.

The individual with the medical problem who brought the family to the attention of the physician is referred to as the proband, or propositus (proposita for females). Information generally should be collected on all individuals who are first-, second-, or third-degree relatives of the proband. First-degree relatives of the proband are the parents and children. Second-degree relatives are aunts and uncles, grandparents, and grandchildren of the proband. Third-degree relatives are first cousins, great aunts and uncles, great-grandparents, and great-grandchildren. A pedigree chart (as shown in Fig. 69-1) is useful in this task. This information should include medical problems and pregnancies. If relatives are deceased, the age at death and the cause of death should be recorded.

With a pedigree chart and specific family information, more general questions are asked including whether other family members have the same or similar problems. Information about various types of birth defects, mental retardation, early infant deaths, miscarriages, stillbirths, or other diseases or handicaps in the family is sought. With some disorders, there may be a variability of a particular condition (i.e., clinical heterogeneity), even within a family. For example, with a possible diagnosis of familial HCM, one should ask about premature death or syncope.

A pregnancy history may provide information to support a possible teratogenic exposure. The date of the last menstrual period, whether the pregnancy was planned, whether contraception was used immediately prior to pregnancy, the time when the pregnancy was recognized, and when the mother sought prenatal care should be noted. Problems during the pregnancy, such as bleeding, spotting, cramping, fevers, rashes, or illnesses; drug exposures (both prescribed and nonprescribed), alcohol intake, or "recreational" drug use; and exposures to potent chemicals in the workplace or while involved in various hobbies should be explored.

Pregnancy and family histories can then be used in conjunction with the findings on physical examination to derive a potential etiologic diagnosis and to plan for further diagnostic studies. The term *etiologic diagnosis* should suggest whether a specific cardiac defect is familial (by family history), genetic but not familial (sporadic), teratogenic (by pregnancy history), or multifactorial. Prognosis and recurrence risk are linked strongly to an accurate diagnosis and its probable etiology.

Genetic Counseling

PRINCIPLES

Genetic counseling should provide information about the diagnosis, its possible etiology, and its prognosis. In addition, psychosocial issues, reproductive options, and the availability of prenatal diagnosis should be discussed. Genetic counseling should be nondirective, providing information in a nonjudgmental, unbiased manner. The family should then be able to make decisions based on medical information in the context of their religious, moral, cultural, and social backgrounds and their financial situation.

Although a genetic counselor may occasionally feel frustrated with a specific couple's decision, an effective counselor does not let personal biases interfere with the counseling role. Conflicts leading to major ethical issues and disputes may arise, however, and may be particularly apparent regarding issues of nonpaternity, sex selection, pregnancy termination, and selective nontreatment of malformed infants. Couples have many reproductive options, but not all may be acceptable religiously or culturally. Nevertheless, potential options should be mentioned in a sensitive manner. A common misunderstanding among families in genetic counseling is the issue of prenatal diagnosis and its relationship to abortion. Prenatal diagnosis does not imply that a parent should or would terminate the pregnancy. In many circumstances, the information from prenatal diagnosis may help to reassure a couple that their risk of having another handicapped child is in fact much lower than expected. Conversely, if defects are found, the subspecialist may use more diagnostic approaches to make rational decisions about medical management of the infant prior to, or immediately after, delivery.

Genetic Diagnosis and Health Insurance

The accelerated pace of gene discovery, molecular medicine, and molecular diagnostics has begun to allow for improved genetic counseling and portends the possibility of future genetic therapy. As knowledge about the genetic basis of disease grows, however, so does the potential for health insurance coverage discrimination to be used to exclude individuals at risk or to change prohibitively high rates on the basis of predetermined illness. For this reason, planners of the Human Genome Project recognized the need to protect individuals who volunteered for genetic study, as well as those diagnosed by molecular methods in the future. For this reason, the National Institutes of Health–Department of Energy (NIH-DOE) Working Group on Ethical, Legal, and Social Implications (ELSI) of the Human Genome Project was developed. The Congress has passed a bill prohibiting companies from using DNA analysis to assess genetic risk as a basis for hiring. Only 11 states, however, prohibit the use of DNA analysis in deciding who should get medical insurance or whether they qualify for high- or low-risk premiums.

CARDIOVASCULAR DISEASE DUE TO SINGLE-GENE MUTATIONS

Compensatory Response of the Heart is Limited to Hypertrophy, Dilatation, or a Combination

The heart responds to stimuli, physiologic or pathologic, which may be inherited or acquired, with hypertrophy, dilation, or a combination of the two.[21] The same mechanisms mediate the growth response to pressure overload, volume overload, or loss of contractile mass (myocardial infarction). In familial HCM, hypertrophy occurs without altered workload. In familial dilated cardiomyopathy (DCM), the heart responds predominantly by dilatation, generally in association with diffuse loss of myocytes and fibrosis. Most inherited defects are associated with hypertrophy. Several mutations in the mitochondrial genome have been associated with cardiac hypertrophy or dilatation.[22,23] In mitochondrial DNA mutations, HCM or DCM is part of a general phenotypic expression of a systemic disease that is characterized by metabolic disorders and usually involves the central nervous and the skeletal muscle systems.

Until the latter half of the 1980s, the accumulated knowledge of cardiomyopathies was mainly clinical and descriptive, since the causes for the vast majority of these primary myocardial diseases were unknown. Despite the fact that myocardial hypertrophy and development of cardiac failure commonly occur, the molecular basis of cardiac growth, hypertrophy, and repair is still incompletely understood. The new technology of recombinant DNA and molecular genetics has provided some new understanding of some of these disorders. *Three clinical categories of primary cardiomyopathies exist: (1) hypertrophic, (2) dilated, and (3) restrictive forms.* Most of the cardiomyopathies other than those caused by infection have a genetic basis, although many of the mutations may occur de novo and are not necessarily familial. Only when a genetic defect is present in the germline and transmitted to one or more generations is it familial. For example, it is estimated that about one-third to one-half of HCM is sporadic, meaning that it occurs because of a de novo mutation that is not transmitted. Until most or all of the genes and their mutations are identified, such estimates await to be verified. Following is a discussion emphasizing the genetics of specific cardiac disorders. For a detailed discussion of the clinical features, diagnosis, and treatment of the cardiomyopathies refer to Chaps. 72, 73, and 74; for congenital diseases such as septal or valvular defects, see Chaps. 70 and 71.

HYPERTROPHY CARDIOMYOPATHY

Familial Hypertrophic Cardiomyopathy

Familial HCM disorder is characterized by myocardial hypertrophy with a wide spectrum of symptoms, including dyspnea, chest pain, and syncope, and an annual mortality rate of 2 to 4 percent due to sudden death, which often occurs in asymptomatic individuals (see Chap. 74). *This disorder is the leading cause of sudden death in the young and in athletes.* The annual incidence of sudden death is higher in younger patients with familial HCM (~6 percent) than in the elderly (1 percent). The diagnosis is based on typical clinical features and the demonstration of unexplained left ventricular, right ventricular, or biventricular hypertrophy on two-dimensional echocardiography. The left ventricular hypertrophy is commonly asymmetric, localized to the septum, but may involve the entire ventricle in a concentric pattern. Isolated right ventricular hypertrophy occurs in fewer than 5 percent of cases. Isolated apical hypertrophy is rare except in Japan where it is claimed to account for 20 to 30 percent of the cases. Dynamic outflow tract obstruction occurs in fewer than 20 percent. Histologically, the myocardial hypertrophy consists of myocyte hypertrophy, cellular and myofibrillar disarray, and myocardial fibrosis. The literature suggests that the hallmark of familial HCM is myocyte and myofibrillar disarray, but this is not unique in that myofibrillar disarray is present in normal hearts during embryogenesis and in congenital heart defects that place a strain on the right-sided circulation, such as pulmonary atresia with intact ventricular septum. The disorder exhibits marked variability of expressivity, even in the same family. The clinical manifestations, including echocardiographically detectable hypertrophy, are seldom observed before puberty. In a small number of cases, mitochondrial inheritance is observed.

Familial HCM was the first primary cardiomyopathy to yield to molecular genetics. Jarcho et al. in 1989 showed genetic linkage of the disease to the chromosomal locus of 14q1 in a large French/Canadian family.[2] The 14q1 locus subsequently was shown to be involved in familial HCM in several other families.[24] The β-myosin heavy chain (βMHC) gene was identified as the responsible gene (Fig. 69-5), and at least 36 missense mutations and 1 deletion[25] in the βMHC gene have been identified.[12,21,26]

Three new chromosomal loci responsible for familial HCM were subsequently mapped to 1q3, 11q11, and 15q2, and the responsible genes were identified to be cardiac troponin T,[27] myosin-binding protein C[28,29] and α-tropomyosin,[27] respectively. A brief description of the loci and the proteins which they encode, together with their function, is summarized in Table 69-1. Mutations in the βMHC, cardiac troponin T, and α-tropomyosin genes have been identified.[27] Mutations in the βMHC gene may account for approximately 20 to 30 percent of the families with familial HCM.[30] While the true incidence of βMHC, cardiac troponin T, and α-tropomyosin mutations remains to be determined, they may account for about 40 to 50 percent of the disease. Two other loci have been identified. The disease in a family with HCM and Wolff-Parkinson-White (WPW) syndrome was mapped to 7q3 (31), and to chromosome 11 in a Japanese family with apical hypertrophy.[32] Furthermore, Poetter et al.[33] recently reported two missense mutations in the essential light chain (3p) and three missense mutations in the regulatory light chain of myosin (12q23-q24.3) of patients with a peculiar form of HCM in which mid–left ventricular chamber thickening occurs due to massive hypertrophy of the papillary muscles and adjacent ventricular tissue, resulting in mid-cavitary obstruction. In addition to the cardiac abnormalities described, the skeletal muscles of these patients were histologically abnormal, and appeared as ragged red fibers. Since all of the genes identified to date involve the sarcomere, it has been proposed that familial HCM is a disease of the sarcomere.[26]

The hypertrophy of familial HCM is markedly variable in its degree, distribution, and age at onset, as well as in the type and severity of its associated clinical manifestations. The natural course of familial HCM in certain families is riddled with sudden cardiac death, whereas in others, sudden cardiac death is almost absent and the life span is essentially normal.[26] Genotype/phenotype correlations[34] have shown that the majority of families with the βMHC mutations Arg^{403}Gln,

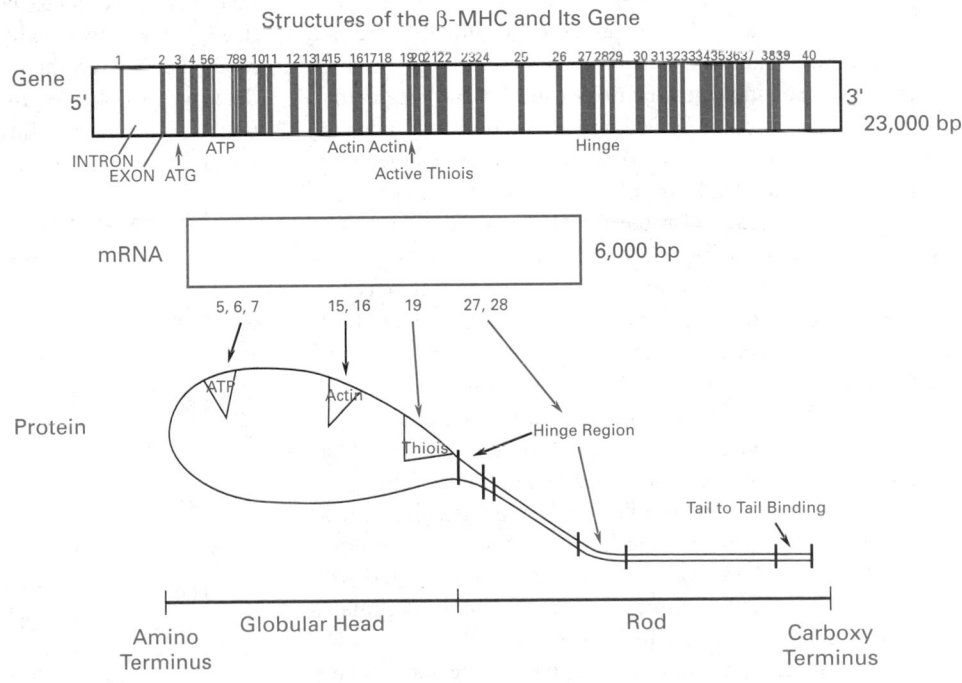

Structures of the β-MHC and Its Gene

FIGURE 69-5
Structure of β-myosin heavy chain (βMHC) and its gene. ATG represents the transcriptional start site. Numbers represent exons and their corresponding translated portion of the protein.

TABLE 69-1

HYPERTROPHIC CARDIOMYOPATHY (HCM) GENES, mRNA, AND PROTEINS

HCM Gene	Chromosomal Location	Length of mRNA, Base Pairs	Protein Size		Function and Location of Protein
			Amino Acids	Molecular Mass, kDa	
βMHC	14q1	6008	1936	223	Contractile molecules that form the thick filaments of the sarcomere
Troponin T	1q3	1200	288	39	Regulation of contraction; part of the sarcomere linking the troponin complex to tropomyosin
α-Tropomyosin	15q2	~1000	284	32	Regulation of contractility; is bound to the actin filaments
Myosin binding protein C	11p11	4575	1318	2137	Binds the tails of myosin heavy chain and titin
Essential myosin light chain	3p	~495	165	~16–25	Unknown
Regulatory myosin light chain	12q23	~495	165	20	Unknown

Note: βMHC, β = myosin heavy chain.

Arg^{453}Cys, and Arg^{719}Trp are associated with a poor prognosis and a high incidence of sudden cardiac death[26,35–37] (Fig 69-6). In contrast, the βMHC mutations Leu^{908}Val, Gly^{256}Glu, and Val^{606}Met are associated with near-normal life expectancy, and mutations Glu^{930}Lys and Arg^{249}Gln are associated with an intermediate risk of sudden cardiac death.[38] The incidence of premature death in affected individuals with Arg^{403}Gln is approximately 50 percent,[26] and the mean age of sudden cardiac death is 33 years. The life expectancy of affected individuals with the βMHC mutation Arg^{719}Gln appears to be about 38 years, and that those with Arg^{453}Cys about 30 years. In contrast, the mutation Leu^{908}Val is associated with low penetrance, a benign course, and a low incidence of sudden cardiac death.[37] The cumulative survival rate at 60 years of age was 92 percent with this mutation. Similarly, the Gly^{256}Glu and Val^{606}Met mutations are associated with a relatively benign course, with most individuals having a near-normal life span. In contrast, the two mutations Glu^{930}Lys and Arg^{249}Gln[36,38] show an intermediary prognosis, with an average age of onset of cardiac failure and severe symptoms around 49 years. These correlations must be interpreted with caution, however, as the number of families studied remains too small for definitive conclusions to be made.

While a single-gene mutation appears to be the primary cause of the disease, there remain significant environmental and other genetic influences that determine whether or not the phenotype develops (penetrance) and its expressivity. A striking example of the influence of environment on familial HCM is the observation that hypertrophy seldom develops in the right ventricle, yet the defective genes and their mutations are present to the same extent in the right as in the left ventricles. Presumably, the increased workload and pressure in the left ventricle stimulate the development of the hypertrophy and phenotypic expression. Moreover, despite identification of abnormal genes, it remains unclear how the genotype explains the phenotype. Similarly, βMHC is the major myosin and contractile unit of many skeletal muscles, yet the latter do not appear to be affected by this disease.[39] Another example of presumably environmental or other genetic influences is the marked variability of the extent and degree of left ventricular hypertrophy that occurs even within the same family with the same mutation. An example of how other genetic factors influence familial HCM is afforded by the angiotensin-converting enzyme (ACE) DD genotype. Patients with familial HCM who happen also to have the ACE DD genotype are found to have a much higher incidence of sudden death[40] and more extensive hypertrophy,[41] which may be mediated through the mitogenic effect of angiotensin II. Cardiac hypertrophy requires the coordination of probably hundreds of genes, and thus it is highly likely that other genes in addition to ACE will influence either the penetrance or

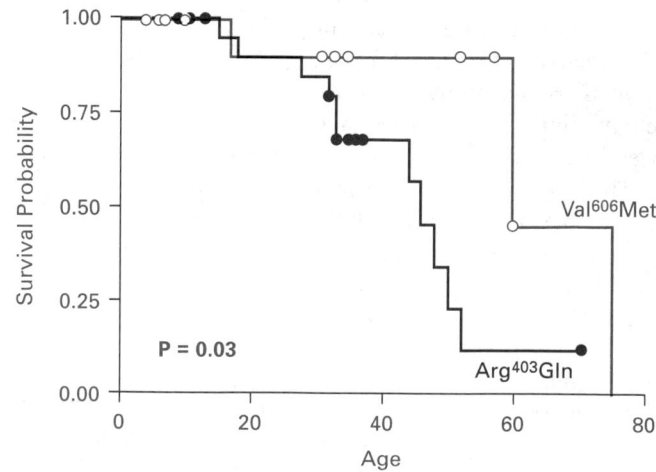

FIGURE 69-6
Kaplan-Meier survival curve in patients with hypertrophic cardiomyopathy depending on myosin heavy chain mutation.

expressivity of the primary genetic defect. The DD genotype is interesting since it has been shown that ACE inhibitors induce some regression of hypertrophy due to pressure overload independently of their afterload effects to reduce afterload. Therefore, it would be intriguing to know whether or not ACE inhibitors could also induce regression of hypertrophy in patients with familial HCM and, perhaps more importantly, prevent hypertrophy in children genetically affected who are identified by genetic testing prior to the development of hypertrophy. The data are insufficient to recommend such therapy for familial HCM at this time.

The mechanism responsible for familial HCM is associated with expression of an abnormal protein that is incorporated into the sarcomere and either prevents sarcomere assembly or induces disassembly. Analysis of a human heart from a patient with the Arg[403]Gln mutation showed the ratio of myosin to actin was normal,[42] indicating there is no deficiency of the βMHC protein, either normal or abnormal. There are data to indicate that expression of a truncated protein, as from nonsense mutations, is not associated with a phenotype, and patients are clinically normal.[43] This observation has therapeutic implications suggesting that if expression of the mutant allele were inhibited, expression of the normal allele would provide a normal phenotype. In vitro motility studies show the mutant βMHC protein to have impaired contractile function and decreased actin-dependent ATPase activity.[44–46] Expression of a full-length human mutant βMHC cDNA in feline (a species known to have βMHC and familial HCM) myocytes is associated with impaired sarcomere assembly and disarray, which is not observed with expression of the normal human βMHC cDNA.[47] Most recently, in a series of experiments in the transgenic mouse, it has been shown that a mutation from the human αMHC inserted into mouse αMHC replaces the normal mouse gene and is associated with a phenotype of hypertrophy and sarcomere disarray.[48] A concern with inducing HCM in the mouse, the usual transgenic animal, is that the mouse heart has αMHC, as opposed to βMHC in humans. The observations in feline myocytes, however, confirm that the mutation of the βMHC present in humans causes familial HCM. *In summary, the impaired contractility resulting from the mutation provides the stimulus for the development of compensatory hypertrophy analogous to hypertrophy secondary to hypertension or myocardial infarction.* The growth stimulus, as in acquired disorders, appears highly localized and mediated by autocrine or intracrine factors, given that the hypertrophy is localized in many patients, primarily to the interventricular septum. The future elucidation of the molecular basis for the pathogenesis of this disease, however, must provide a rationale for three puzzling, consistent features of the pathology of familial HCM: (1) predominance of hypertrophy in the septum, (2) sarcomere and myocyte disarray, and (3) the supernormal systolic function. The diastolic stiffness or decreased compliance is expected with hypertrophy whether it is primary or compensatory, but these other features are not seen in compensatory hypertrophy resulting from myocardial infarction or pressure overload, for example.

Despite the observation that fewer than 50 percent of the genes responsible for familial HCM have been identified, it must be realized that the first gene was not identified until 1990. Screening for mutations in individuals from a family affected with familial HCM is feasible for known mutations but is tedious and expensive. In a family in which the disease is not due to a known mutation, chromosomal mapping and subsequent identification of the gene are required. It is expected, however, that the techniques for mass genetic screening, such as in athletes, to identify known mutations will soon be automated. Within the next few years, physicians should be able to screen and identify genotype-positive individuals routinely. Ultimately, if gene therapy becomes available, genotyping will, of course, be essential. It is conceivable that regression of cardiac hypertrophy can be induced by inhibiting transcription of the mutant allele or translation of the mutant mRNA, thus abolishing synthesis of the mutant peptide. Thus, not only genetic diagnosis but also curative therapy may be possible. Since the heart, even in an adult, is renewed every 2 to 3 weeks, there is a tremendous potential for a cure with subsequent remodeling to normal.

Pompe's Disease (Type II Glycogen Storage Disease)

Genetic deficiency of acid α-1,4 glucosidase production results in a wide clinical spectrum of disease, ranging from the rapidly fatal infantile-onset of type II glycogen storage disease to a slowly progressive adult-onset myopathy. The infantile-onset form (Pompe's disease) typically manifests during the first months of life, and patients usually die before their second year.[49] This rare inborn error of glycogen metabolism occurs in fewer than 1 per 100,000 persons. Massive glycogen accumulation occurs, leading to the clinical findings of enlarged tongue, striking hepatomegaly, hypotonia with decreased deep tendon reflexes, and hypertrophic cardiomyopathy[50] with cardiac failure (Table 69-2). The diagnosis may be predicted from the pathognomonic electrocardiogram (ECG) with massively increased QRS voltage.[49] The disease is inherited as autosomal recessive, and the gene coding for the lysosomal enzyme has been mapped[51,52] to chromosome 17q23-q25. The diagnosis can also be made by analysis of α-glucosidase in blood lymphocytes or skin fibroblasts or by mutation analysis.

Beckwith-Wiedemann Syndrome

The combination of macroglosia, exomphalos, and visceromegaly has been designated the Beckwith-Wiedemann syndrome.[53,54] Multiple other abnormalities have also been described, including fetal adrenocortical cytomegaly, hypoglycemia due to pancreatic islet hyperplasia, transverse linear creases of the ear lobules, hemihypertrophy, and accelerated osseous maturation. Infants with this syndrome are at particularly high risk, cumulatively estimated at between 5 and 20 percent, for development of Wilms' tumor, adrenocortical carcinomas, hepatoblastomas, and rhabdomyosarcomas.[55] The cardiovascular system is also commonly affected with the development of HCM. Beckwith-Wiedemann syndrome occurs with an incidence of 1 per 13,700 live births. Cases

TABLE 69-2

CARDIOVASCULAR ANOMALIES ASSOCIATED WITH SELECTED AUTOSOMAL RECESSIVE SYNDROMES

Syndrome	Cardiovascular Anomaly
Carpenter's syndrome	Patent ductus arteriosus
Cockayne's syndrome	Atherosclerosis
Cutis laxa	Pulmonary hypertension
Cystic fibrosis	Cor pulmonale
Ellis–van Creveld syndrome	Atrial septal defect
Friedreich's ataxia	Hypertrophic cardiomyopathy
Homocystinuria	Thromboses (arterial and venous); occlusive vascular disease
MPS IH (Hurler's syndrome)	Coronary artery disease, aortic and mitral insufficiency, hypertrophic cardiomyopathy
MPS IS (Scheie's syndrome)	Aortic valve disease
MPS IV (Morquio's syndrome)	Aortic valve disease
MPS VI (Maroteaux-Lamy syndrome)	Aortic valve disease
Pompe's disease (GSD II)	Hypertrophic cardiomyopathy
Pseudoxanthoma elasticum	Coronary artery disease, mitral insufficiency
Refsum's disease	Arrhythmias
Smith-Lemli-Opitz syndrome	Ventricular septal defect, patent ductus arteriosus
Thrombocytopenia–absent radii (TAR) syndrome	Atrial septal defect, tetralogy of Fallot

Note: MPS, mucopolysaccharidosis; GSD, glycogen storage disease.

are generally sporadic (~85 percent), but familial disease has been described (15 percent). Most of these familial cases have apparent autosomal dominant inheritance,[56] albeit with reduced, sex-dependent penetrance and variable expressivity. A variety of structural abnormalities of chromosome 11, reminiscent of alterations seen in Wilms' tumor, have been shown, including partial duplication of 11p13, duplication of 11p15 only, deletion of 11p11-13, or deletion of 11p11. Whenever identifiable, the extra chromosomal material was of paternal origin. The breakpoints found in those patients with balanced chromosomal translocation or inversion involving chromosome 11 lie in two regions: (1) close to the insulin/insulin-like growth factor II genes in 11p15.5, or (2) proximal to β-hemoglobin. The recombinant chromosome has been shown to be of maternal origin. Family studies using probes in this region showed that the gene responsible for familial Beckwith-Wiedemann syndrome mapped to 11p15.5. For sporadic Beckwith-Wiedemann syndrome, uniparental paternal disomy for 11p15.5 markers has been found in approximately 20 percent of cases analyzed. Mechanisms of disease include a possible role for genomic imprinting in 11p15, as well as the possibility

that this syndrome is a contiguous gene disorder and not a single-gene disorder.

Leopard Syndrome

This rare autosomal dominant disorder is characterized by the cardinal features leading to the mnemonic LEOPARD (*l*entigenes, *E*CG conduction defects, *o*cular hypertelorism, *p*ulmonic valve stenosis, *a*bnormalities of genitals, *r*etardation of growth, and *d*eafness, sensorineural). Cardiac abnormalities are common and include both anatomic as well as ECG defects. Anatomically, pulmonic stenosis is the most frequent, followed by HCM and endocardial fibroelastosis (Table 69-3). The most common ECG defects include first-degree atrioventricular (AV) block, left anterior hemiblock, and complete heart block. No cytogenetic or molecular genetic abnormalities have been identified.

Friedreich's Ataxia

Friedreich's ataxia is the most common of the hereditary spinal cerebellar degenerations, with an incidence of 1 in 50,000 and carrier frequency of 1 in 110.[57] This autosomal recessive form of spinocerebellar degeneration is characterized by progressive limb ataxia, loss of deep tendon reflexes, sensory abnormalities, and musculoskeletal deformities. The symptoms of Friedreich's ataxia usually appear insidiously

TABLE 69-3

CARDIOVASCULAR ANOMALIES ASSOCIATED WITH SELECTED AUTOSOMAL DOMINANT SYNDROMES

Syndrome	Cardiovascular Anomaly
Albright's hereditary osteodystrophy	Cardiomyopathy
Ehlers-Danlos syndrome	Rupture of large vessels
Holt-Oram syndrome	Atrial and ventricular septal defects
LEOPARD syndrome	Pulmonic stenosis, hypertrophic cardiomyopathy, prolonged PR interval
Marfan's syndrome	Aortic aneurysm, aortic insufficiency, mitral valve prolapse
Myotonic dystrophy	Dilated cardiomyopathy, conduction abnormalities
Neurofibromatosis	Coarctation of the aorta, renal artery stenosis
Treacher Collins syndrome	Atrial and ventricular septal defects, patent ductus arteriosus
Tuberous sclerosis	Myocardial rhabdomyoma, Wolff-Parkinson-White syndrome
Noonan's syndrome	Pulmonic stenosis, hypertrophic cardiomyopathy, atrial septal defect, aortic stenosis

during childhood or early adolescence. Progressive weakness of the upper and lower extremities gradually becomes obvious. Gait difficulties, which progress slowly, are often the first symptom, followed by unsteadiness in the arms and hands. Difficulty in writing and handling eating utensils subsequently becomes apparent.

Cardiac involvement occurs in 50 to 90 percent of patients, and the most common abnormality is HCM (Table 69-2); dilated cardiomyopathy DCM occurs rarely. Thus, the most common cardiac symptoms relate to cardiac failure and arrhythmias. Left ventricular outflow tract obstruction due to asymmetric septal hypertrophy may be evident, and approximately 50 percent of patients die of cardiac disease. Patients are followed for development of arrhythmias and the signs and symptoms of cardiac failure. Treatment consists primarily of conventional drugs to relieve the symptoms and signs of heart failure.

Involvement of the heart is readily detected by electrocardiography and echocardiography. The electrocardiographic abnormalities are found in 90 percent of patients and include repolarization abnormalities manifesting as inverted or biphasic T waves in the inferior limb leads and left precordial leads, a short PR interval, left and right ventricular hypertrophy, as well as left and right axis deviation. Premature atrial contractions, atrial flutter/fibrillation, and premature ventricular contractions are common. Echocardiography detects cardiac involvement in 60 to 100 percent of patients, with the most common finding of concentric hypertrophy, but asymmetric septal hypertrophy accompanied by systolic anterior motion of the mitral valve is also common. Left ventricular chamber diameter may be normal or decreased, and fractional shortening or ejection fraction is usually normal, although DCM (left ventricular dilation and reduced contractility) is seen occasionally (see Chap. 10). There is no specific treatment for the cardiac manifestations except symptomatic treatment if cardiac failure ensues (see Chap. 23).

Friedreich's ataxia is inherited as an autosomal recessive disorder, and parental consanguinity has been noted in some cases. The gene has been mapped to chromosome 9q13-31.1,[58] and recently, Campuzano et al.[59] identified a gene, called *X25,* that mapped within the Friedreich's ataxia critical region on 9q13. This gene is 40 kbp and contains five exons that encode a novel 210-amino acid protein, called *frataxin.* The highest level of expression of X25 was found within the heart, while intermediate levels were seen in liver, skeletal muscle, and pancreas; minimal levels were identified in other tissues, including the brain. The transcript was 1.3 kbp. Although a few affected patients were found to have a point mutation in X25, the majority was homozygous for an unstable GAA trinucleotide expression in the first X25 intron.[59]

DILATED CARDIOMYOPATHY

Idiopathic Dilated Cardiomyopathy

Idiopathic DCM is a disease of unknown cause characterized by increased ventricular size and impaired systolic ventricular function. The prevalence of idiopathic DCM has been estimated to be approximately 40 cases per 100,000 in the population,[60] and many cases are believed to be sporadic. The diagnosis of DCM is typically made by echocardiography (see Chap. 73), and symptoms usually are those of cardiac failure. Familial DCM, while initially considered rare, may represent approximately 20 percent of patients with idiopathic DCM. The differential diagnosis of DCM is relatively large. In a large family with idiopathic DCM, a family history of autosomal dominance was determined and the disease was linked to 1q32.[61] Three other loci have been identified: 9q23,[61,62] 3p22,[63] and 10q21-23.[64] No gene for idiopathic DCM has yet been identified.

X-Linked Dilated Cardiomyopathy

Berko and Swift[65] reported a five-generation kindred with DCM and no clinical evidence of skeletal myopathy. Males presented in their teens or early twenties with clinical evidence of mitral regurgitation and an echocardiographic diagnosis of DCM. Episodes of ventricular tachycardia were noted in several patients. The males progressed rapidly (within 1 or 2 years) to death or cardiac transplantation. Manifesting female carriers developed mild cardiomyopathy in the fourth or fifth decade and progressed slowly. Right ventricular endomyocardial biopsy revealed minimal interstitial fibrosis, while postmortem evaluation showed marked dilatation, widespread patchy fibrosis (worst in the posterior wall), and normal mitochondria on electron microscopy. There were no pathognomonic findings differentiating this cardiomyopathy from other dilated forms, except for the apparent X-linked inheritance.

Towbin and colleagues[66] demonstrated linkage of X-linked DCM to the dystrophin locus at Xp21 (i.e., the gene responsible for Duchenne's and Becker's muscular dystrophy) in the family described above, as well as in a second family. Evaluation of the protein defect in X-linked DCM using antiserum against total cardiac protein showed absence (or low abundance) of the N-terminal and rod portion of the dystrophin protein, while skeletal muscle total protein was normal.[67] The 156-kDa dystrophin-associated glycoprotein (known as α-dystroglycan),[68] a constituent of the dystrophin-associated glycoprotein complex, was decreased in abundance in cardiac tissue as well.[67] Diverse mutations leading to X-linked DCM were shown by Muntoni et al.,[69] Towbin and Ortiz-Lopez,[70] Yoshida et al.,[71] and Milasin et al.[62,72] Treatment is that of congestive failure (See Chap. 23).

X-Linked Cardioskeletal Myopathy (Barth's Syndrome)

Barth and coworkers[73] described an X-linked recessive disease in one large family characterized by DCM and the triad of endocardial fibroelastosis, neutropenia, and skeletal myopathy. All affected males died in infancy or early childhood from cardiac decompensation or septicemia. There were no affected females. Ultrastructural abnormalities were detected in mitochondria from cardiac and skeletal muscle, as well as in neutrophil bone marrow cells. Furthermore, respiratory chain abnormalities were observed, and isolated skeletal muscle mitochondria demonstrated diminished cytochrome concentrations. Lactic acidemia not provoked by prolonged fasting increased plasma and muscle carnitine concentrations, and growth retardation and increased levels of urinary 3-methylglutaconic acid and 2-ethyl-hydracrylic acid have also been seen.

The locus was mapped by linkage to Xq28.[74] The gene[75] codes for a novel protein known as G4.5, the function of which is unclear. The sequence of the novel related protein is unique and was named *tafazzin* after a masochistic comic character on an Italian television sports show. Tafazzin belongs to a family of proteins ranging from 129 to 292 amino acids in length. Direct sequencing of genomic DNA indicated different mutations in G4.5 that interfere with translation of the putative protein. Treatment is that of cardiac failure (see Chap. 23).

Conduction Disturbance with Dilated Cardiomyopathy

A large six-generation family presenting with conduction defects and subsequent development of DCM was mapped to 1p1-1q1.[76] This family demonstrated autosomal dominant transmission and variable expressivity. Transient arrhythmias, which presented in the second or third decade, became sustained and commonplace by the third or fourth decade. The abnormal rhythms included second- or third-degree AV block, atrial fibrillation, or marked bradycardia, commonly requiring a pacemaker. DCM usually developed in the fourth or fifth decade, generally out of proportion to the severity of the rhythm disturbance. Sudden death commonly occurred in the late stages of the disease. On autopsy, marked right and left ventricular dilatation, interstitial fibrosis, myocyte degeneration characterized by cytoplasmic vacuolization, and AV nodal cell replacement by fibrous tissue were noted. The gene and its characteristics have remained elusive. Genetic heterogeneity was recently found by Olson and Keating[63] when they mapped a locus to 3p (3p25-3p22) for a similar family.

Familial Arrhythmogenic Right Ventricular Dysplasia

Familial clusters of arrhythmogenic right ventricular dysplasia have been reported,[77] demonstrating autosomal dominant inheritance, incomplete penetrance, and marked clinical heterogeneity (see Chap. 27). It is characterized by right ventricular dilatation, thinning and fatty infiltration of the right ventricle, ventricular tachycardia with left bundle branch block, ventricular fibrillation, and sudden cardiac death. These patients usually have good exercise tolerance. The electrocardiographic abnormalities include inverted T waves in the right precordial leads, late potentials, and right ventricular arrhythmias. Rampazzo et al.[78] mapped this disease in two families to 1q42-q43, and another locus was identified on chromosome 14q23-q24.[79] A large Greek family with arrhythmogenic right ventricular dysplasia was recently mapped to 17q.[80]

RESTRICTIVE CARDIOMYOPATHY DUE TO AMYLOID

Restrictive cardiomyopathy is the least common in the Western countries of the three major categories of cardiomyopathy (see Chap. 75). The most common cause of secondary restrictive cardiomyopathy in adults is due to myocardial amyloid. Patients manifest exercise intolerance because of their inability to increase cardiac output by tachycardia without further compromising ventricular filling. Weakness and dyspnea are often prominent, and chest pain may also occur. At end-stage, the findings are those of cardiac failure with anasarca. Recently, mutations in the transthyretin (TTR) gene,[81] which codes for the TTR serum protein, were found associated with restrictive cardiomyopathy. This protein contains four subunits, each with 127 amino acids, encoded by four exons within a 7-kbp gene. Many TTR point mutations cause TTR to form amyloid, which occurs primarily in the heart and leads to heart failure. The diagnosis is suspected by echocardiography and confirmed by genetic analysis. Treatment is that of cardiac failure.

Mucopolysaccharidoses

The mucopolysaccharidoses (MPS) are a group of diseases caused by deficiency of lysosomal enzymes involved in the degeneration of glycosaminoglycans.[82] Undegraded glycosaminoglycans accumulate in lysosomes and affect tissue function. MPS have been divided into seven major types. The classification (types I to VII) is based on the deficient enzyme responsible for the disorder. These disorders carry such eponyms as *Hurler, Scheie, Hurler-Scheie, Hunter, Sanfilippo, Morquio, Maroteaux-Lamy,* and *Sly.* They share many clinical features, including multiple system involvement, organomegaly, dysostosis multiplex, facial abnormalities, hearing and vision loss, joint involvement, cardiac involvement, and central nervous system involvement. Cardiac diseases include myocardial hypertrophy, pulmonary and systemic hypertension, valvular disease, coronary occlusion, and myocardial infarction. Congestive heart failure and sudden death are relatively frequent. The most common mucopolysaccharidosis with cardiac involvement is MPS-I (Hurler's syndrome). Valvular disease is prominent in Scheie's syndrome (late-onset form). Less commonly, heart disease has been noted in the Sanfilippo A syndrome with aortic regurgitation as well as in severe Maroteaux-Lamy syndrome with valvular heart disease (see Table 69-2). The diagnosis for either of these disorders is made by assaying the enzyme activity in cultured skin fibroblasts or leukocytes.

HURLER'S SYDNROME

Hurler's syndrome (MPS-I) is an autosomal recessive trait found on chromosome 22 (22q11) and occurs in approximately 1 per 40,000 people. It is caused by a deficiency of α-iduronidase, which is required for the degradation of both heparan sulfate and dermatan sulfate.[83] The result is similar to that of Hunter's syndrome, with both dermatan and heparan sulfate in high concentrations in the urine. Myocardial infarction occurs in childhood (see Table 69-2). *Severe* (Hurler, MPS-IH), *intermediate* (Hurler/Scheie, MPS-IH/S), and *mild* (Scheie) clinical subtypes of MPS-I occur.[82] MPS-IH patients usually present within the first year of life and progress with a combination of hepatosplenomegaly, skeletal deformities, corneal clouding, and severe mental retardation. Obstructive airway disease, respiratory infection, and cardiac complications usually result in death before age 10 years. MPS-IH/S is characterized by little neurologic involvement, but most of the somatic involvement described for MPS-IH develops early in the teenage years, causing considerable loss of mobility. MPS-IS patients, those with the mildest symptoms, have little or no neurologic involvement, normal stature, and normal life span but do develop stiff joints, mild hepatosplenomegaly, aortic valve disease, and corneal clouding.[82] Diagnosis is confirmed in MPS-I by demonstration of mucopolysacchariduria and absence of α-iduronidase activity in leukocytes and fibroblasts. Biochemical differentiation between subtypes is difficult. Isolation of the cDNA by Scott et al.[84] and subsequent gene identification[85] have allowed for mutation analysis. The broad range of clinical phenotypes is related to the types of mutations in the α-iduronidase gene.[86]

HUNTER'S SYNDROME

Hunter's syndrome, an X-linked disorder mapped to the Xq26-Xq28 region, is found in approximately 1 per 30,000 people.[82] It is caused by a deficiency of the enzyme iduronate sulfatase and results in excessive urinary excretion of dermatan and heparan sulfate and accumulation of mucopolysaccharides, which can result in coronary obstruction and subsequent myocardial infarction in childhood. Most patients die before the third decade.

MORQUIO'S DISEASE

Morquio's disease (MPS-IVA),[87] an autosomal recessive disorder caused by a genetic deficiency in N-acetyl-galactosamine-6-sulfatase, is a prototypical chondro-osteodystrophy. The disorder is characterized by specific spondyloepiphyseal dysplasia, short-trunk dwarfism, coxa valga, odontoid hypoplasia, corneal opacities, normal intelligence, and excessive urinary excretion of keratan sulfate and chondroitin 6-sulfate. The deficient N-acetyl-galactosamine-6-sulfatase results in progressive accumulation of mucopolysaccharides in lysosomes of various tissues, leading to vertebral involvement and cardiac disease in the second decade of life (see Table 69-2). Tomatsu et al.[88] isolated and characterized the full-length cDNA of the enzyme gene, and Baker et al.[89] and Masuno et al.[90] localized it to chromosome 16q24. This gene is approximately 50 kbp in size and has 14 exons; mutations have been described.[91]

MAROTEAUX-LAMY DISEASE

The Maroteaux-Lamy syndrome is caused by deficiency of the enzyme arylsulfatase B, which is required for degradation of the glycosaminoglycans, dermatan sulfate, and chondroitin 4-sulfate.[92] It is associated with aortic valve disease. This gene, located on 5q13-q14,[92] has been isolated and characterized.[93] Mutations have been identified, and different mutations cause different clinical phenotypes.[94] The clinical features are quite variable, occurring in infancy and consisting of growth retardation, course facies, corneal clouding, and multiple skeletal changes together with dilated cardiomyopathy and aortic or mitral valve stenosis or insufficiency. Cardiac manifestations usually appear after neurologic manifestations but are usually present by adolescence. Molecular diagnosis is currently available. There is no effective therapy, but bone marrow transplants are being tried. All of these disorders can be diagnosed prenatally by enzyme assay in at-risk pregnancies.

Muscular Dystrophies with Cardiac Involvement

The muscular dystrophies (MD) are a heterogeneous group of diseases, and the primary manifestations include progressive muscle wasting secondary to intrinsic defects of the muscle fiber. These defects have a wide spectrum of clinical expression and include Duchenne's MD, Becker's MD, Emery-Dreifuss' MD, and myotonic dystrophy. Cardiac disease, especially DCM, is central to the morbidity and mortality associated with these disorders (Table 69-4).

DUCHENNE'S MUSCULAR DYSTROPHY

Duchenne's MD is an X-linked disorder characterized by the early onset of progressive, generalized muscle weakness and "pseudohypertrophy" of certain muscle groups.[95,96] The incidence of Duchenne's MD is estimated to be 1 in 3300 live male births, with little ethnic variation, and the calculated mutation rate of 10^4 is an order of magnitude higher than for most other genetic diseases.[95] About one-third of cases arise by spontaneous mutation, with the remaining two-thirds occurring by inheritance of the disease-causing gene from the carrier mother. Female carriers of Duchenne's MD are usually asymptomatic but occasionally have a slowly progressive myopathy of moderate severity. This manifesting female carrier state occurs in approximately 8 percent of carriers and is thought to occur due to random X inactivation. The disease may also be expressed in females with Turner's syndrome having a single X chromosome and in females with X-autosome translocations that disrupt the Duchenne's MD gene. In the latter case, the translocation not only disrupts the gene but also causes the nonrandom inactivation of the normal allele on the other X chromosome, resulting in the expression of the disease phenotype.

Although evidence of skeletal muscle disease in boys with Duchenne's MD is evident in the neonatal period, as seen by high serum levels of muscle enzymes (particularly CK-MM), clinical disease is not. There may be mild developmental delay, particularly walking later than expected, but weakness is usually not appreciated until at least 2 or 3 years of age. Early symptoms reported by parents include difficulty in running or climbing stairs, frequent falling, and enlargement of calf muscles. Pelvic girdle weakness is more obvious than shoulder girdle weakness in the early stages. The gait becomes lordotic and waddling, and the child usually walks with the heels raised slightly off the ground (i.e., toe walking). As pelvic girdle weakness increases, the child has increasing

TABLE 69-4

MANIFESTATIONS OF NEUROLOGIC CARDIAC DISORDERS

Neuromuscu-lar Disorder	Mode of Inheritance	Incidence per 100,000	Age of Onset	Pathology		Clinical	
				Cardiac	Musculoskeletal	Cardiac	Musculoskeletal
Myotonic dystrophy	Autosomal dominant	10	3rd to 4th decade	Atrophy Interstitial fibrosis and fatty infiltration of the conduction system	Atrophy; Interstitial fibrosis and fatty infiltration	AV block Atrial arrhythmias CHF (rare)	Myotonia; Atrophy of strap muscles
Friedreich's ataxia	Autosomal recessive	2.0	Child/ adolescent	Interstitial fibrosis Myocyte hypertrophy	Normal	Abnormal ECG axis and Q waves Atrial arrhythmias Hypertrophic cardiomyopathy Concentric Asymmetric Dilated cardiomyopathy	Ataxia Kyphoscoliosis
Duchenne's muscular dystrophy	X-linked recessive	2.0	2–5 years	Myocardial fibrosis in posterobasal LV free wall Degeneration of conducting fibers Noninflammatory arteriopathy	Myofibril necrosis Interstitial accumulation of fat and fibrous tissue	Dysrhythmias ECG abnormalities Dilated cardiomyopathy	Pseudohypertrophy Proximal limb and neck weakness Contractures Scoliosis and chest cage deformities
Becker's muscular dystrophy	X-linked recessive	0.4	2nd to 3rd decade	Focal areas of fatty infiltration and proliferating connective tissue	Same as Duchenne's	Dilated cardiomyopathy	Pseudohypertrophy Proximal limb girdle weakness and atrophy
Kearns-Sayre syndrome	Maternal, non-Medelian (i.e., mitochondrial)	Rare	Childhood/ adolescence	Ragged red fibers	Ragged red fibers; Glycogen accumulation Proliferation of abnormal mitochondria	Progessive AV block Dilated cardiomyopathy Hypertrophic cardiomyopathy	Ptosis Ataxia
Emery-Dreifuss syndrome	X-linked recessive ?(Autosomal dominant)	Rare	2nd to 3rd decade	Focal myocardial fibrosis	Same as Duchenne's	Atrial standstill Progressive conductive block Malignant ventricular arrhythmias Dilated cardiomyopathy	Contractures of elbow, pericervical muscles, and Achilles tendon Humeroperoneal muscle weakness and atrophy
Fascioscapulo-humeral muscular dystrophy	Autosomal dominant	0.6	2nd to 3rd decade	Unknown	Same as Duchenne's	Atrial abnormalities Conduction delays Atrial fibrillation/ flutter	Proximal shoulder and facial weakness and atrophy Lower extremity weakness
Nemaline myopathy	Autosomal dominant with reduced penetrance	Rare	Birth/ infancy	Nemaline bodies	Nemaline bodies	Dilated cardiomyopathy	Diffuse muscle weakness and hypotonia

Note: CHF, congestive heart failure.

difficulty rising from a seated position. In order to rise from the floor to a standing position, the child must brace the arms against the front of the thighs and climb up the legs, the so-called Gowers' sign. Muscle pseudohypertrophy usually appears by 5 to 6 years of age, with muscle enlargement most commonly occurring in the calf muscles; the quadriceps, infraspinatus, deltoid, and gluteal muscles may also be involved, however. The upper and lower extremities become progressively weaker with age, and joint contractures may appear due to uneven weakness of agonist and antagonist muscles. Contractures of the hip flexors, iliotibial bands, and heel cords develop in 70 percent of patients between 6 and 10 years of age. Most patients are wheelchair-bound by the end of the first decade of life. After ambulation is lost, fixed contractures occur and paraspinal muscle weakness leads to progressive kyphoscoliosis. Significant weakness of the respiratory muscles occurs early in the second decade and is a common cause of demise.

While most cases of Duchenne's MD can be recognized on the basis of the patient's history and clinical signs alone, laboratory evaluation is important to confirm the diagnosis.[95] As previously noted, extremely high levels of CK-MM are found in the early stages of disease, as early as birth, and preceed evidence of clinical involvement. Other muscle enzymes, including aldolase, SGOT, lactic dehydrogenase, and pyruvate kinase are also grossly elevated. In the end stages of the disease, enzyme levels fall but do not reach normal values. Electromyographic examination may also be useful, demonstrating the characteristic features of a myopathy. Insertional activity is normal or increased initially but decreases in the advanced stages of the disease, when fibrosis replaces muscle fibers. Fibrillation potentials and positive sharp waves occur in the early stages of the disease due to the splitting of muscle fibers. The motor unit potentials are small and polyphasic, and an early recruitment pattern with minimal effort is present. Mild intellectual impairment is common in patients with Duchenne's MD. The retardation is present at an early age, is nonprogressive, and does not correlate well with the stage of the disease. Approximately one-third of patients have IQs < 75, characterized primarily by impaired verbal ability.

The heart is commonly involved in Duchenne's MD, with electrocardiographic abnormalities and DCM being most typical. Cardiac symptoms, however, are unusual before the terminal stages of the disease. Congestive heart failure tends to occur. A mid-systolic click and late systolic murmur associated with mitral valve prolapse are also common. In addition, an S_3 or S_4 gallop, sinus tachycardia, and a mitral regurgitation murmur are usually heard, along with cardiomegaly and increased pulmonary vascular markings; at this stage, bilateral diaphragmatic elevations may be seen due to diaphragmatic dystrophy. Unlike the late-onset findings of DCM, the ECG is abnormal early in the course of Duchenne's MD, with a tall R wave and an abnormally increased R/S ratio in the right precordial chest leads and a deep, narrow Q wave in leads I, aV_L, V_5, and V_6. These abnormalities progress over time and are attributed to the finding of the greatest dystrophic

myocardial changes in the posterobasal and contiguous lateral left ventricular myocardium. In addition, P waves with negative terminal deflections in V_1 exceeding 20 ms and 0.1 mV appear in 20 to 45 percent of patients and, in the absence of left atrial enlargement on echocardiogram, are attributed to an intrinsic disorder of left atrial or intraatrial conduction. A short PR interval may be seen in up to 50 percent of patients but is not thought to be due to a bypass tract as seen in WPW syndrome. Infranodal conduction abnormalities, however, may be seen in patients with Duchenne's MD, and these include complete or incomplete bundle branch block and left anterior or posterior fascicular block. Atrial and ventricular premature beats and atrial flutter are seen in some patients.

Echocardiography reveals left ventricular dilatation and dysfunction, with significantly reduced shortening fraction or ejection fraction, and left ventricular hypokinesis of the posterobasal ventricular wall is identified. Doppler and color Doppler commonly demonstrate mitral regurgitation, either secondary to the DCM or to the associated mitral valve prolapse, which occurs secondary to papillary muscle dysfunction. In some patients, systolic function appears normal but diastolic dysfunction is present.

Histopathologic abnormalities of the heart and skeletal muscle are universal in patients with Duchenne's MD, and those of skeletal muscle are widespread even in the early stages of disease.[95] Typical findings are rounding of the muscle fibers, increased variability in fiber size, increased central nucleation, and fiber splitting. Necrotic and regenerating fibers are present along with large, round hyaline fibers. In the late stages, muscle may be virtually replaced by fat and fibrous tissue. In the heart, degenerative changes in muscle fibers and areas of fibrosis in the ventricles, atria, and conduction system occur, with most pronounced changes in the posterobasal region and adjacent lateral wall of the left ventricle. The underlying cause of cardiac disease is not currently known, but it is speculated that the gene defect in Duchenne's MD leads to instability of the translated cytoskeletal protein, leading to weakening of the myocyte membrane and subsequent myocyte death due to mechanical stress.

The dystrophin gene, on the short arm of the X chromosome[97,98] due to mutations, may cause either low-level production of a nonfunctional protein or complete absence of dystrophin in the heart and skeletal muscle of affected patients. It is amongst the largest genes discovered thus far, comprising approximately 2.5 Mbp and transcribing a 14-kbp mRNA molecule. The gene is normally expressed in striated and smooth muscle, as well as in brain. In muscle tissue, the dystrophin protein has been localized to the cytoplasmic surface of the sarcolemma and is believed to be a cytoskeletal protein that is associated with several integral membrane glycoproteins.[99] This glycoprotein/dystrophin complex may be involved in the regulation of intracellular calcium, which in dystrophin-deficient muscle is increased along with increased calcium channel transport.

The dystrophin mRNA transcripts in muscle and brain tissue have sequence differences. The mRNA transcript is alternatively spliced to encode multiple isoforms of the dystrophin protein in a developmental- and tissue-specific manner. Several of these isoforms appear to be unique for the heart; this posttranscriptional modification may result in a functional diversity for the dystrophin protein. Recently; human cardiac Purkinje fibers have been shown to express dystrophin isoforms,[100] and it is speculated that this may be important in the development of cardiac arrhythmias in this disorder. The dystrophin mRNA sequence in skeletal muscle has been sequenced, but the cause of the cardiomyopathy affecting Duchenne's MD patients has not been ascertained.

The diagnostic approaches to Duchenne's MD have changed dramatically over the past 5 years. Previously, serum CK-MM level and muscle biopsy were the standard approaches. Today, Duchenne's MD is diagnosed primarily by Southern blotting and PCR analysis of deletion mutations (which affect approximately one-half of all patients) from blood or by immunoblots of biopsy samples. This allows for very accurate diagnosis and permits speculation as to the severity of the disease. Most commonly, dystrophin mutations that cause a frameshift[101] of the nucleotide sequence result in the severe form of muscular dystrophy, Duchenne's MD.

Management of the congestive heart failure associated with the DCM seen in Duchenne's MD is identical to that used for patients with other causes of heart failure and arrhythmias. Pacing is not usually necessary.

BECKER'S MUSCULAR DYSTROPHY

Becker's MD is an X-linked disorder that differs in both severity and time of onset from Duchenne's MD,[95,102] despite being due to allelic mutations in dystrophin, the gene responsible for Duchenne's MD. Becker's MD appears later and progresses more slowly than Duchenne's, so that survival to middle age is seen. The pattern of muscle weakness, however, is identical to that in Duchenne's MD, with early involvement of the pelvic girdle and proximal lower extremities.[95] The initial signs of weakness usually appear during the second decade but may occur as late as the third decade. The weakness gradually progresses, with the upper extremities becoming involved after 5 to 10 years. Patients generally remain ambulatory until their mid-thirties. Similar to Duchenne's MD, muscle hypertrophy is common; intellectual impairment, however, is less common and less severe. As in Duchenne's, life expectancy is also reduced in Becker's MD, with only 50 percent of patients surviving to 40 years of age.

Cardiac involvement may be seen in adolescence and ultimately affects 80 percent of patients. As in Duchenne's MD, dilated cardiomyopathy and cardiac failure are the usual abnormalities encountered (see Table 69-4) and are often the ultimate cause of death. Conduction abnormalities manifesting as fascicular block or complete heart block are also seen. As in Duchenne's, muscle enzyme activity is markedly elevated in Becker's MD, and preclinical cases may be detected by elevated CK-MM levels. Electromyographic examination shows a "myopathic" pattern with small, polyphasic motor units and early recruitment of motor units.[95] The histology

of Becker's MD is similar to that of other forms of MD. In contrast to Duchenne's MD, hyaline fibers are rarely seen. ECG changes[95] are similar to those seen in Duchenne's MD. Other ECG abnormalities encountered include left axis deviation, right bundle branch block, left bundle branch block, and complete heart block. The echocardiogram may demonstrate the features of DCM.

The gene causing Becker's MD is also located at Xp21 and is also due to different mutations within the dystrophin gene; i.e., it is allelic with Duchenne's MD. As is the case with the latter, more than 30 percent of patients with Becker's MD have no family history of the disease, an indication that their disease results from spontaneous mutations. The phenotypic difference between Duchenne's and Becker's MD patients has been speculated to be due to frameshift mutations leading to more severe disease (Duchenne's), while out-of-frame mutations cause less severe (Becker's) disease.[101] The frameshift hypothesis explains >90 percent of the cases of Duchenne's versus Becker's MD. The cardiac abnormalities in Becker's MD, as with those described for Duchenne's MD, require further study. The treatment of congestive heart failure and arrhythmias is similar to other patients with these signs and symptoms.

EMERY-DREIFUSS MUSCULAR DYSTROPHY

Emery-Dreifuss MD is a relatively rare disorder[103] characterized by weakness in the humeroperoneal distribution, early joint contractures, and dilated cardiomyopathy with X-linked (occasionally, autosomal dominant) inheritance. The onset of disease in these patients occurs between 2 and 10 years of age, with weakness initially noted in the shoulder girdles and upper extremities. Contractures of the elbows and posterior cervical muscles appear early. The disease is slowly progressive, with involvement of the distal leg musculature following that of the upper extremities; contractures of the knees and ankles follow contractures of the elbows. Unlike Duchenne's and Becker's MD, muscle pseudohypertrophy does not occur. The disease evolves slowly and usually stabilizes in the third decade, with most patients remaining ambulatory. DCM is a common occurrence, but the severity of disease varies from family to family. Varying degrees of AV block are common (see Table 69-4), and atrial standstill may occur. These electrical abnormalities may lead to episodes of syncope, transient ischemic attacks, stroke, and sudden death. A pacemaker is commonly required. Atrial fibrillation has also been observed. As in Duchenne's and Becker's MD, muscle enzyme activity is elevated, albeit to a lesser extent. Skeletal muscle biopsy histopathologic findings are similar to those associated with other forms of MD. Type I fiber atrophy has been described in some cases (Fig. 69-7). The gene responsible for Emery-Dreifuss MD was localized to Xq28.[74] Recently the gene, called *emerin* (or STA),[75] was identified and shown to have an open reading frame of 762 nucleotides that encode a serine-rich 254-amino acid protein with uncertain function. Emerin mRNA shows ubiquitous tissue distribution, with the highest expression in skeletal and cardiac muscles. The cDNA se-

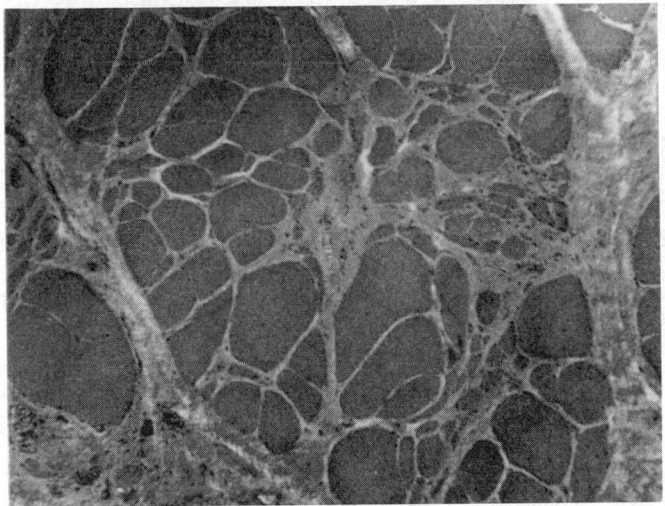

FIGURE 69-7

Skeletal muscle biopsy in Emery-Dreifuss muscular dystrophy. Increased endomysial and perimysial connective tissue, with marked variation in myofiber size, internal nuclei, and myofibers splitting ($\times$153). (Reprinted with permission from *N Engl J Med* 1992; 327:548.)

quence of emerin predicts a new tail-anchored membrane protein with amino acid sequence similar to thymopletins, nuclear lamina-associated proteins.[105] Recently, Nagano et al.[106] and Manilal et al.[107] all showed that emerin is a 34-kDa nuclear membrane protein in skeletal and cardiac muscle. In Emery-Dreifuss MD, this protein is absent.

MYOTONIC DYSTROPHY (STEINERT'S DISEASE)

Myotonic dystrophy is the most common form of inherited MD in adults, with an incidence of 1 in 8000 to 10,000 persons.[108] This autosomal dominant disorder affects multiple organ systems, and its name is derived from the combined myopathy, dystrophy, and myotonia of skeletal muscle. Myotonia, an abnormality in relaxation after muscle contraction, is the primary feature of this disease. Myotonic dystrophy is variably expressed, and individuals may present with signs and symptoms involving many different organ systems. Penetrance varies with age, and the disease may affect different tissues at different periods of life; a severe form of myotonic dystrophy exists with symptoms at birth.

Classically, myotonic dystrophy presents in a young adult with new-onset weakness of the hands or mild foot drop. Asymptomatic myotonia, namely, sustained contraction and depolarization of skeletal muscle in response to a percussive or electrical impulse, may be elicited. Myotonia is usually present in the hands and tongue, while weakness involves the distal extremities predominantly. A typical facies usually accompanies these findings, including loss of temporal muscle and slight weakness of the lips and mouth with a "hatchet-like" shape, frontal balding, and ptosis (Fig. 69-8). The heart and eyes, and central nervous, endocrine, gastrointestinal, and respiratory systems may be involved (Table 69-5). Electromyographic abnormalities are frequent, and subcapsular, punctate iridescent cataracts are common in middle-aged patients.

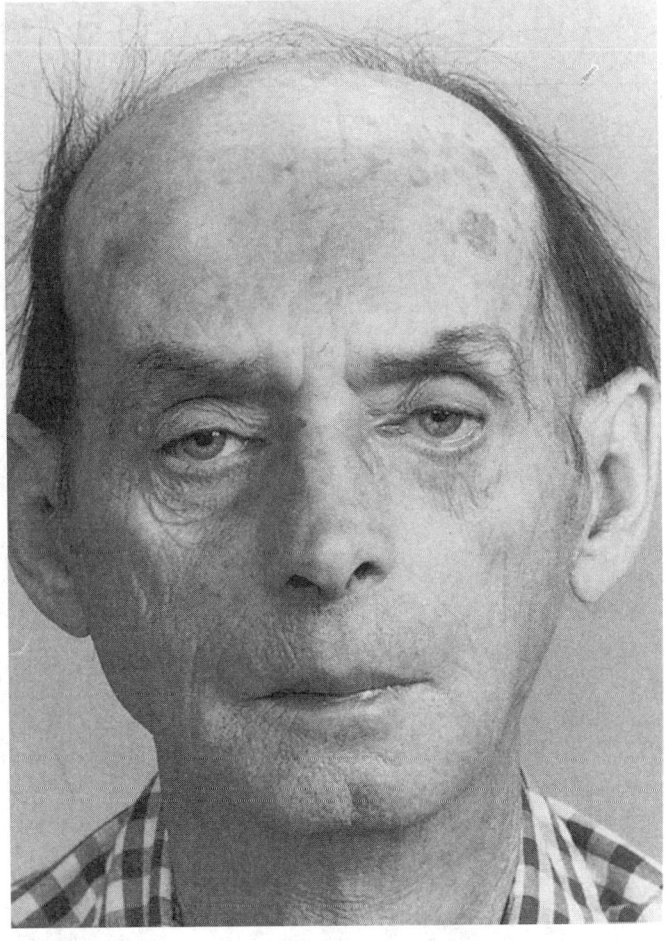

FIGURE 69-8

A 41-year-old man with myotonic dystrophy. Muscle-wasting of temporalis muscles with narrow small chin produces a "hatchet-like" facies. Baldness and ptosis (note droopy eyelids with pupils partially covered and sclerae visible) contribute to characteristic appearance. (Reprinted with permission from Roses AD, Pericak-Vance MA. In: P.M. Conneally, ed. *Molecular Basis of Neurology*. Cambridge, MA: Blackwell Scientific, 1993; 147–159.)

Myotonia is best seen in the small muscles of the hand and in the tongue. Repetitive discharges with gradual and uneven decay of amplitude are seen on electromyography. Myotonic muscles undergo dystrophic changes, which may take years to several decades. In general, the younger the presentation, the more rapid the progression. Only a small percentage of affected individuals, probably <10 percent, progress to requiring a wheelchair for ambulation; many require a brace worn in the shoes to control the presence of foot drop.

Serious complications of myotonic dystrophy involve the heart.[109] Cardiac conduction abnormalities are common (see Tables 69-4 and 69-5) and may be progressive, particularly in younger patients. These are identified by periodic ECG monitoring and usually occur without obvious complaints. Sudden cardiac death in athletically inclined adolescents is relatively frequent. In studies of families with myotonic dystrophy, cardiac findings may be the initial clinical manifestation of the disease, with bradycardia and first-degree heart

TABLE 69 5

SYSTEMIC INVOLVEMENT IN MYOTONIC DYSTROPHY

Organ or System	Clinical	Diagnostic Signs
Muscle	Myotonia, weakness, dystrophy	*EMG:* decreased resting membrane potential; repetitive depolarization ("dive bomber" sound) *Pathology:* sarcoplasmic masses, ringed fibers, internal nuclei, frequent; nuclei often in chains; large variation in fiber size.
Cardiac	Bradycardia common; complete heart block frequent; prolonged PR interval; dilated cardiomyopathy	First-degree heart block, bradycardia on ECG; abnormal vectorcardiogram; SA node, right and left bundle branch dysfunction; increased His-Purkinje conduction (His bundle studies) with progressive conduction system abnormalities; dilated cardiomyopathy
Lens	Posterior subcapsular, iridescent, or scintillating cataracts	Dustlike cataracts may be visible only on slit lamp examination
Eye	Decreased vision (independent of cataracts and diabetic retinopathy); diplopia	Pigmentary disorders of macula keratosis sicca; decreased intraocular pressure; frequent ptosis and extraocular muscle weakness
Central nervous system	Mental retardation (especially congenital myotonic dystrophy); hypersomnia	Possible neuronal heterotopias; suspicious, reticent personality characteristics
Endocrine	Abnormal carbohydrate metabolism; testicular (and ovarian) atrophy	Abnormal glucose tolerance with elevated insulin levels; gonadal fibrosis (pathology); decreased 17-ketosteroids (occasional); decreased metabolic rate, normal thyroid hormone levels
Integument	Frontal balding	Calcifying epitheliomas
Gastrointestinal	Dysphagia, abdominal pain	Disordered esophageal and gastric peristalsis; dilation of bowel
Skeletal	Cranial and facial abnormalities; malocclusion of dentition	Cranial bony abnormalities, hyperostosis of skull (localized or diffuse), small sella turcica, large sinuses, micrognathia
Respiratory	Hypoventilation; postanesthesia respiratory failure	Diaphragmatic and intercostal muscle weakness
Smooth muscle	Dilation of hollow viscous organs and ureters; abnormal bowel motility	Thinned or interrupted smooth muscle

Note: EMG, electromyography.

block being common. Progression to complete heart block may occur over time and is not well tolerated, potentially ending in death and frequently requiring pacing. In some cases, ventricular tachycardia or DCM may also occur (Table 69-5). Typically, however, systolic function is preserved but diastolic dysfunction may occur.

Myotonic dystrophy patients may have a particular psychological profile that includes indifference, reticence, and hostility. Mild mental retardation may be seen, particularly in patients with very early manifestations of myotonic dystrophy. Young and middle-aged patients may be hypersomnolent and indolent, sometimes sleeping up to 20 h daily. Testicular atrophy is common in males, and amenorrhea and ovarian cysts may occur in females (Table 69-5). Increasing debilitation, handicap, and disability may occur in subsequent generations of a family; this increasing disease severity is known as *anticipation.*

The gene for myotonic dystrophy was localized to 19q13.3[110] and encodes for myotonin protein kinase (Mt-PK),

a serine-threonine protein kinase.[111,112] The genetic basis for myotonic dystrophy consists of long stretches of three bases repeated in tandem, referred to as triplet repeats. The triplet repeat present in Mt-PK gene is CTG, which in the mRNA is CUG and is located in the 3′ end of the gene beyond the protein coding region. The severity of disease (neuromuscular, cardiac, and central nervous system) relates to the length of the repeats. A total of fewer than 50 triplet repeats is usually associated with no disease. Usually 100 to 250 are required to cause disease; if more than 250 repeats are present, the disease is usually seen at birth and reflects *genetic anticipation* (increasingly severe expression and earlier onset of disease through generations as a result of the increase in the number of CTG repeats with subsequent generations). Clinical cardiac symptoms (i.e., syncope) and ECG abnormalities (i.e., left bundle branch block) correlate directly with CTG expansion size.[109] In addition, the incidence of malignant ventricular arrhythmias also correlates directly with the size of CTG expansion.

Myotonic dystrophy is one of the many familial neuromuscular diseases due to the genetic defect of multiple triplet repeats.[113] The mechanisms whereby the triplet repeats induce the disease remains an enigma, however. Myotonic dystrophy is somewhat unique since the triplet repeats are in the 3′ end of the gene, beyond the protein coding region. Mt-PK levels are reduced in patients with myotonic dystrophy, but when the gene for Mt-PK is eliminated in knockout mice, muscle weakness results but none of the other organs are involved, such as the eyes or testes, as observed in myotonic dystrophy. This has led to an extensive search for other explanations, including adjacent genes. One by-product of this research was identification of a novel group of proteins that bind specifically to triplet repeats in DNA and RNA[114]; binding is determined by the sequence of the triplet repeat. A specific protein was identified that binds only to the CUG sequence in the mRNA of Mt-PK. The CUG binding protein (CUG-BP) has a molecular weight of 52 kDa and three binding sites for CUG repeats.[114] The protein has several serine and threonine phosphorylation sites, which appear to be regulated by Mt-PK. Further studies indicate that this protein is identical to another protein (NB50) that is known to be responsible for mRNA transport from the nucleus to the cytoplasm.[115] This has given rise to the hypothesis that the CUG-BP is sequestered by the multiple CUG repeats and is not available to other mRNAs for processing or transport from the nucleus. The involvement of several mRNAs would explain the multiple organs involved. This would also explain why in the mouse with the Mt-PK gene knocked out, one observes only muscle weakness—in the absence of the multiple triplet repeats, the other mRNAs are properly transported by the CUG-BP protein and function normally. This hypothesis is now being actively pursued by many investigators. Preliminary findings show an accumulation of the CUG-BP in the nuclei of cells from myotonic dystrophy.[116] Diagnosis of this disorder within families and its prenatal detection can be done by the use of recombinant DNA techniques.[117]

In regard to therapy, conduction disturbances typically require permanent pacemaker implantation, and DCM requires treatment for heart failure.

FASCIOSCAPULOHUMERAL DYSTROPHY

Facsioscapulohumeral,[118] or Landouzy-Dejerine, MD exists as two clinical types. One type has autosomal dominant inheritance, with onset at the end of the first decade of the beginning of the second. The weakness of the facial, shoulder, and upper arm muscles is slowly progressive, but wide variability is seen. The second clinical type of fascioscapulohumeral dystrophy is the infantile form. Onset is within the first 2 years of life, and many patients are wheelchair-bound by 1 year of age. Clinical manifestations of MD generally are absent in the parents.

The cardiac involvement involves progressive atrial dysfunction resulting in permanent paralysis of the atria, beginning with sinus bradycardia, junctional escape rhythm, and AV block (see Table 69-4). Criteria for diagnosis of permanent paralysis of the atria include absence of P waves on surface ECG, esophageal electrogram, and intracardiac ECG; unresponsiveness of the atrium to electrical stimulation; and immobility of the atria on fluoroscopy and echocardiography. Focal abnormalities of the atria precede these events. Nonparalytic regions of the atrium may demonstrate enhanced activity, apparent clinically as atrial tachycardia or flutter. Therapy depends on the clinical features. The chromosomal locus and responsible genes are unknown.

NEMALINE MYOPATHY

Nemaline myopathy is named for the small rodlike particles found in striated muscle. Inheritance is probably autosomal dominant, although autosomal recessive inheritance may occur. Clinical features include hypotonia with truncal and extremity weakness from an early age and a narrow, arched palate. Conduction abnormalities and cardiac dilatation have been described but are unusual (see Table 69-4). Nemaline rods are demonstrable in the myocardium and conduction tissues. The genetic cause of this disease is not known. Therapy is required when the conduction abnormalities or cardiac dilatation cause clinical symptoms.

Endocardial Fibroelastosis

Endocardial fibroelastosis (EFE) is characterized by endocardial thickening, which leads to decreased compliance and impaired diastolic function. Primary forms are typically unassociated with other cardiac anomalies. Most commonly, this disease presents in infancy and early childhood with signs and symptoms of congestive heart failure.[119] The diagnosis is usually made by biopsy. The incidence of primary EFE in the United States in the past was relatively high—approximately one case in 5000 live births.[120] During the past decade, however, this incidence has decreased markedly for unknown reasons. Treatment of children with primary EFE with anticongestive and inotropic measures has been ineffective, and the clinical course usually results in either death or transplantation. Postmortem examination typically demonstrates enlargement of the left ventricle. Histopathologic examination commonly reveals extensive deposition of extracellular matrix, primarily collagen and elastic fibers, in the endocardium. Three inherited forms of EFE have been described: autosomal recessive, autosomal dominant, and an X-linked recessive disorder. The majority of cases, however, occur sporadically. The X-linked form shows mitochondrial abnormalities similar to Barth's syndrome,[73] with the exception that EFE patients have endocardial scarring. It has been hypothesized that EFE is secondary to myocarditis in sporadic cases, in particular, as a result of mumps.[121]

Defects of Metabolism Causing Cardiomyopathy

CARNITINE DEFICIENCY

L-Carnitine is a small, water-soluble molecule containing seven carbon atoms and is important in the shuttling of long-chain fatty acids and activated acetate across the intermitochondrial membrane. A specific translocase facilitates this exchange of long-chain acylcarnitine and acetylcarnitine. Carnitine also serves as the shuttle for the end-products of peroxisomal fatty acid oxidation and for α-ketoacids derived from branch chain amino acids. These metabolites are transferred into the mitochondrial matrix for terminal oxidation.

Primary carnitine deficiency syndrome is characterized by a profound decrease in carnitine in affected tissues. The mechanism underlying the primary disorder is defective transport of carnitine from the serum into the affected cells.[122] End-stage disease of many different organs including the heart may induce depletion of carnitine stores and must be differentiated from the chronic inherited type. Based on carnitine levels, carnitine deficiency is usually divided into two forms: a myopathic form and a systemic form. In the myopathic form, carnitine levels are only decreased in muscle tissue, while in the systemic form multiple tissues are affected, including muscle, liver, and plasma.[122] The systemic form presents in infancy or early childhood with episodes of hypoglycemia, ammonemia, acidemia, hepatomegaly, and EFE. Therapy includes oral carnitine, occasionally reversing the cardiomyopathy. Additional therapy includes bicarbonate to reverse the acidemia, intravenous glucose, and anticongestive measures. Intercurrent illness commonly causes acute decompensation and death.

PHYTANIC ACID STORAGE DISEASE (REFSUM'S DISEASE)

Refsum's disease, characterized by retinitis pigmentosa, cerebellar ataxia, and peripheral neuropathy, is inherited as an autosomal recessive trait. It is due to the absence of an α-hydroxylase that is necessary for metabolizing dietary phytol and phytanic acid. The absence of the enzyme leads to the accumulation of tissue phytanic acid. The disease is occasionally associated with cardiomyopathy, which may be dilated and/or hypertrophic. Conduction disturbances and sudden death may occur. Cardiomyopathy preceding development of the neuropathy has been reported.[123] Plasmapheresis acutely or dietary modification may improve function.

MEDIUM-CHAIN ACYL-CoA DEHYDROGENASE (MCAD) DEFICIENCY

This disorder, first described in 1982, appears to be the most common inborn error of fatty acid oxidation and is estimated to occur in 1 per 6000 to 10,000 live births in Caucasians. It is characterized by recurrent episodes of illness, provoked by fasting >12 h, with the first episode generally occurring between ages 6 and 24 months. The most common symptoms include vomiting and severe lethargy that can progress to coma, as well as the less striking symptoms of muscle weakness and exercise intolerance. Hypoglycemia is often present between episodes, when patients appear normal. Hepatomegaly and DCM (rarely) are also seen. Liver biopsy can show marked fatty infiltrate, ranging from a predominantly microvesicular to a macrovesicular pattern. This autosomal recessive disorder has recently been localized to chromosome 1p31. Human and rat MCAD cDNAs have been cloned and se-

quenced.[124] The coding region is 1263 bp and encodes a precursor protein containing 421 amino acids. An A-to-G (adenosine-to-guanine) nucleotide replacement at position 985 of MCAD cDNA appears to be the most prevalent mutation responsible for MCAD deficiency[125]; a 13-bp tandem repeat insertion at position 999 has also been reported, as have other rare mutations. Recently,[126] investigation of the A-to-G-985 (A985G) mutation in MCAD cDNA was studied in 22 unrelated MCAD-deficient families, 4 of which were compound heterozygotes for the mutation and the other 18 were homozygotes. Utilizing PCR amplification and sequencing of the cDNA product from a compound heterozygote, Ding et al.[126] demonstrated a 4-bp deletion in one MCAD allele and an A985G mutation in the other allele. This resultant 4-bp deletion in MCAD-deficient individuals allowed for a PCR-based screening method to be developed, which allows for improved diagnosis and carrier detection in over 93 percent of all MCAD mutations. This deletion is predicted to result in a truncated protein of 385 amino aids instead of the normal 421-amino acid product. The common A985G mutation appears to be due to a founder effect.

The therapy for these patients incudes treatment of the acidosis and, when present, treatment of heart failure. Glucose therapy is indicated for hypoglycemia, while intravenous fluids are needed during episodes of vomiting.

LONG-CHAIN ACYL-CoA DEHYDROGENASE (LCAD) DEFICIENCY/VERY LONG CHAIN ACYL-CoA DEHYDROGENASE DEFICIENCY

First described in 1985, LCAD manifests as recurrent episodes of coma, vomiting, and hypoglycemia triggered by fasting. Some patients have much more severe illness, with notable involvement of cardiac and skeletal muscle.[23] Both DCM and HCM have been seen. Similar to patients with MCAD, LCAD patients have secondary carnitine deficiency, and their fasting urine organic acid profile is abnormal, with low ketones and increased levels of dicarboxylic acids. The LCAD gene was identified,[127] but unlike the situation in many of the patients with MCAD deficiency, no mutations or abnormal immunoreactive proteins were identified.[128] In addition to the well-known β-oxidation enzymes in the mitochondrial matrix, there are two additional membrane-bound enzymes of β-oxidation.[129,130] One of these has been called very long chain acyl-CoA dehydrogense (VLCAD), while the other is known as a "trifunctional protein." This new understanding of the mitochondrial β-oxidation pathway has led to new insights of the disorder thought to be due to LCAD deficiency but now thought to be VLCAD deficiency.

Therapy for these patients includes aggressive treatment with glucose and hemodynamic support. When cardiac disease persists, chronic therapy for the dilated or hypertrophic heart disease should be instituted.

FABRY'S DISEASE

Fabry's disease is an X-linked recessive disorder with complete penetrance and variable clinical expressivity. This entity is due to a deficiency of the enzyme α-galactosidase A, a lysosomal enzyme that participates in the catabolism of neutral glycosphingolipids, and is found in 1 in 40,000 live births. The disease frequently has its onset in adolescence and typically manifests with sensations of burning pain in the hands and feet. These sensations tend to be associated with fever, heat, cold, and exercise. Multiple angiokeratoma are noticeable with increasing age, with the umbilical area and genitalia the sites most commonly affected (Fig.10-8). Progressive renal failure develops with age, and central nervous system manifestations commonly include seizures, headaches, hemiplegia, and stroke. Corneal opacities are also seen frequently.

The cardiac manifestations of Fabry's disease generally appear in young adulthood. Aortic root dilation, DCM or HCM,[131] valve dysfunction (especially of the mitral valve),[132] and myocardial infarction occur in these patients. Electrocardiographic abnormalities commonly include atrial fibrillation, intraventricular conduction delay, right bundle branch block, ST-T-wave changes, short PR interval, and left ventricular hypertrophy. The short PR interval can shorten progressively over time, probably secondary to lipid deposition in the AV node. Chamber thickness and mitral valve prolapse are evident on echocardiographic examination.[133] Light microscopy shows lipid accumulation in nearly all cardiac tissue. Concentric lamellae are seen within cells and contain the neutral glycophospholipid. Therapy for these cardiac abnormalities does not differ from that typically used for HCM, myocardial ischemia or infarction, or mitral insufficiency found in patients without Fabry's disease.

The disease-causing gene is localized to X121-Xq122. The full-length cDNA has 1393 bp with a 60-nucleotide 5′ untranslated region, encoding for a precursor peptide of 429 amino acids.[134] Three overlapping clones spanning 32-kbp were identified, and contained the 12-kbp chromosomal gene and the 9-kbp and 1-kbp 5′ and 3′ flanking sequences, respectively. The gene was found to contain seven exons. Recently, mutations were described[135,136] and genotype-phenotypic correlation performed.[137] Antenatal and postnatal diagnosis is available. Therapy is symptomatic at present, but enzyme replacement therapy is likely in the future.

HOMOCYSTINURIA

Homocystinuria, inherited as an autosomal recessive defect, occurs with a frequency of 1:75,000. There is a deficiency of cystathionine β-synthase, which leads to elevated levels of methionine in the blood and homocystine and methionine in the urine[138,139] (see Chaps. 39 and 41). In the homozygous individuals, major clinical features include a marfanoid habitus with a thin, tall body build and arachnodactyly, pectus excavatum, kyphoscoliosis, and osteoporosis. Subluxation of the lens, usually in a downward position, is frequently seen by 10 years of age, and myopia is common. Approximately 60 percent of affected individuals are mentally retarded to some degree. Schizophrenic behavior has also been noted in some patients. Cardiovascular abnormalities consist primarily of arterial and venous thrombosis (Table 69-2), with medial degeneration of

the aorta and large arteries, and intimal hyperplasia and fibrosis. It is estimated that about one-third of patients with familial homocystinuria will experience arterial or venous thrombosis. It is interesting that even within the same family with the same mutation there is marked variability among affected siblings, and the reason remains unknown.[140] The thrombotic episodes usually occur before the age of 30 and include deep vein thrombosis, pulmonary embolism, and arterial thrombosis in the cerebral, peripheral, and coronary arteries.[140] When this disease occurs in individuals with other thrombogenic risk factors such as factor V Leiden,[141] however, the incidence of thrombosis, both arterial and venous, is significantly increased. An increased risk of cardiovascular disease has also been observed in carriers of the gene for homocystinuria.

The genetic defect has been assigned to the subtelomeric region of band 21q22.3 by in situ hybridization studies.[142] Three types of cDNAs,[143] differing in both their translated and untranslated regions, have been isolated with the resultant differences due to alternative splicing. The significance of these alternatively spliced forms is presently being investigated.[144] Numerous mutations have now been identified and correlated with the phenotype.[145] The defect can be treated in some cases by pyridoxine supplementation. The percentage of pyridoxine responders ranges between 13 and 47 percent. Betaine, low-methionine diet, and aspirin treatments have also been tried with varying success. Prenatal diagnosis is available by an enzyme assay and gene analysis.

Homocystinuria, while a rare disease, has received increased attention recently because of several studies indicating that homocysteine is an important and independent risk factor for atherosclerosis and thrombosis.[146,147] In one such study performed recently, of 269 patients with the first episode of deep vein thrombosis, 10 percent had elevated plasma homocysteine levels compared to 4 percent in 269 matched controls.[147] Homocystinuria results from impaired enzyme activity in the metabolism of cobalamin but may also occur from a deficiency of vitamin B_6, folate, or vitamin B_{12}.[148,149] A mechanism whereby homocysteine induces atherosclerosis is postulated to be through induction of cyclin A gene, which induces vascular smooth muscle proliferation, a major component of atherosclerosis.[150] The mechanism whereby homocysteine induces thrombosis is probably through its known effect on activation of factor V in endothelial cells, inhibition of protein C, and decreased antithrombin III activity.[151] It remains somewhat controversial as to how common hyperhomocysteinemia is as a risk factor for atherosclerosis and/or thrombosis. It is, however, very important to exclude hyperhomocysteinemia in patients with vascular disease such as myocardial infarction, strokes, or systemic thrombosis, particularly if occurring prematurely or there are no other risk factors; in the acquired form, it is relatively easy to treat by the administration of vitamins.[152]

Mitochondrial Cardiomyopathies

The human mitochondrial genome[153] is a small circular DNA molecule that is maternally inherited. Mitochondrial DNA (mtDNA) encodes 13 of the 69 proteins required for oxidative metabolism, 22 transfer RNAs (tRNAs), and 2 ribosomal RNAs (rRNAs) required for their translation. Since mtDNA has much less redundancy than the nuclear genome (in which essentially identical information is received from both parents), and tRNAs and rRNAs are present in multiple copies, the mitochondrial genome is an excellent target for mutations giving rise to human disease.[154,155] Mitochondria are dependent on nucleocytoplasmic mechanisms for most structural components but do contribute vital peptides that are central to cellular respiration. The 13 mtDNA genes that encode enzymes in the respiratory chain[154,156] include seven complex I subunits (ND1, 2, 3, 4L, 4, 5, and 6), one complex III subunit (cytochrome b), three complex IV subunits (COI, II, III), and two complex V subunits (ATPase 6 and 8). Each cell contains numerous mitochondria, and each mitochondrion contains multiple copies of mtDNA. In most mitochondrial disorders, patients carry a mix of mutant and normal mitochondria—a condition known as *heteroplasmy*—with the proportions varying from tissue to tissue and individual to individual within a pedigree, in a manner correlating with severity of phenotype.[157]

Mitochondrial diseases often produce disturbances of brain and muscle function and are usually evident during infancy or early childhood. Cardiac disease is most commonly seen with respiratory chain defects.[158] Ragged red fibers are present in muscle biopsy specimens almost invariably when the molecular defect involves mtDNA.[159] These defects represent the genetics of ATP production. The diverse clinical syndromes associated with various respiratory chain complexes are thought to result from involvement of tissue-specific isoforms in some cases, involvement of tissue-nonspecific (generalized) subunits in other cases, and the residual enzyme activity in affected tissues. The cardiac diseases seen associated with mitochondrial defects include both HCM and DCM.[22]

Mitochondrial gene mapping, in contrast to the nuclear genome, does not require genetic linkage. One simply has to show that the disease exhibits transmission through all mothers and no fathers in a sufficiently large family. Once this is established, the mitochondrial genome can be sequenced to identify the mutation, which must be shown to segregate with the disease since there are many harmless polymorphisms.

Therapy for these disorders is generally symptom-based. Conduction disturbance generally requires placement of a permanent pacemaker, and heart failure is treated with the usual therapy. In some patients, beta blockers may be useful. Hypertrophic heart disease is usually treated in a fashion similar to that of other forms of HCM. Therapy may include coenzyme Q10, carnitine, or vitamins, but these therapeutic approaches typically do not alter the clinical course.

COMPLEX I DEFICIENCY

Approximately 60 cases of complex I deficiency have been described, about 20 of these representing a myopathic syndrome, and 40 cases representing an encephalomyopathic syndrome. The latter includes: (1) a fatal infantile disorder with involvement of brain, muscle, and heart; (2) a milder version of the above, with clinical manifestations later in childhood or early adulthood; and (3) the MELAS syndrome (*m*itochondrial myopathy, *e*ncephalopathy, *l*actic *a*cidosis, and *S*trokelike episodes) thought to be secondary to NADH CoQ reductase abnormalities.[160] Treatment of these disorders is limited. Riboflavin, succinate supplements (since the metabolite enters the respiratory chain at complex II), ubiquonone, and idebanone have been recommended for therapy in patients with the MELAS syndrome. A mitochondrial mutation was initially described in a patient with MELAS syndrome and fatal infantile cardiomyopathy: this mutation was shown to be due to an A-to-G transition in mitochondrial DNA of the isoleucine tRNA gene.[161] Analysis of enzyme activities and subunits in the heart showed combined defects of complex I and complex IV of the respiratory chain.

COMPLEX III DEFECTS

These defects result in a myopathic or multisystem disorder. Cardiomyopathy has been found both alone or in conjunction with skeletal myopathy.[162] Encephalomyopathy also presents with retinopathy, ataxia, spasticity, dementia, weakness, sensorineural hearing loss, and exercise intolerance.

COMPLEX IV DEFECTS

This abnormality is clinically similar to complex I defects. The mitochondrial genome encodes for three subunits of cytochrome C oxidase, which represents the terminal portion of the respiratory chain and catalyzes conversion of molecular oxygen to water. A benign reversible infantile myopathy,[163] which normalizes by early childhood, may occur, as may a fatal infantile myopathy manifested by profound weakness, hypotonia, respiratory insufficiency, and death. This myopathy may occur alone or in association with severe renal tubular dysfunction or cardiomyopathy with red ragged fibers.

HYPOXEMIA, mtDNA DAMAGE, AND CARDIAC DISEASE

Since cardiac tissue relies on mitochondrial oxidative phosphorylation (ox-phos) for energy production, deficiency of portions of this system or its end-product may cause cardiac abnormalities.[164] Hypoxemia can increase oxygen radical production, which results in elevated mtDNA damage and altered ox-phos gene expression. In addition, these enzymes decline with age while mtDNA deletions increase with age, especially deletion at nucleotide 4977 bp. Ischemic hearts may be more likely to have increased chances of mtDNA deletion due to the effect of hypoxemia.[165] By using PCR amplification across the deletion breakpoint of the common mtDNA4977 deletion, it was shown that mtDNA damage was increased in chronically ischemic hearts as well as in some hearts with other forms of chronic cardiac disease (i.e., DCM, HCM), but this may be an incidental finding and whether or not it affects cardiac function is not known. Similarly, mitochondrial DNA damage increases with age independent of ischemia, but, similarly, it is doubtful whether it alters cardiac function.

KEARNS-SAYRE SYNDROME

This mitochondrial myopathy is characterized by ptosis, chronic progressive external ophthalmoplegia, abnormal retinal pigmentation, and cardiac conduction defects[166,167] as well as DCM.[168] Hearing loss and limb weakness are frequently associated, as are endocrinopathies such as diabetes mellitus, hypoparathyroidism, and growth hormone deficiency. Approximately 20 percent of patients with Kearns-Sayre syndrome have cardiac involvement, and of these, the majority usually have conduction defects causing progressive heart block (see Table 69-4). These patients generally have large heterogeneous deletions in the mitochondrial genome, of which tRNA^leu(UUR)-3243 is most common.

Clinically, conduction abnormalities, bifascicular block, or progressive high-grade block may define the requirement for permanent pacemaker implantation. Symptomatic improvement using mitochondrial-directed therapies may occasionally be seen with coenzyme Q10 therapy. The major function of coenzyme Q10 in mitochondria is to shuttle electrons from complexes I and II to complex III, while stabilizing the respiratory chain complexes. Vitamins such as phylloquinone (vitamin K_1), menadione (vitamin K_3), and ascorbic acid (vitamin C) have been used to donate electrons directly to cytochrome C. In addition, the endocrine abnormalities and heart failure should be treated in the usual way.

MERRF SYNDROME

The characteristics of this syndrome lead to its mnemonic MERRF (*m*yoclonic *e*pilepsy with *r*agged *r*ed muscle *f*ibers). It is caused by a single nucleotide substitution in tRNA^Lys, which apparently interferes with mitochondrial translation.[169] The defining clinical features are myoclonus, generalized seizures, ataxia, and hypertrophic cardiomyopathy. Skeletal muscle biopsy demonstrates ragged red fibers on microscopy. Symptoms usually begin in childhood, but adult onset has been described. Other common manifestations include impaired hearing, demential neuropathy, short stature, optic atrophy, lactic acidosis, and lipomas.

Shoffner et al.[170] showed at A-to-G transition mutation (position 8344) as the cause of the disease, which has been associated with defects in complexes I and IV. This abnormality causes decline in ATP-generating capacity, with a resultant cardiomyopathy. Other reports have outlined various disease-causing mutations. Therapy is similar to other mitochondrial myopathies; anticonvulsant medications may also be indicated.

MELAS SYNDROME

The MELAS syndrome is clinically characterized by stroke before age 40 years; encephalopathy characterized by seizures, dementia, or both; and lactic acidosis, ragged-red fibers, or both.[171] Recurrent headaches and recurrent vomiting are common. Other frequent manifestations include exercise intolerance, limb weakness, short stature, and elevated cerebrospinal fluid protein. HCM or DCM may occur.

Variable respiratory chain defects have been described, but complex I abnormalities are most common. Between 80 and 90 percent of patients have an A-to-G point mutation in tRNA^Leu(UUR) at position 3243. Therapy is similar to that described for MERRF syndrome.

Connective Tissue Disorders

The composition, structure, and function of normal and abnormal connective tissues are gradually being elucidated[172] (see Chap. 85). The annuli fibrosis that separate the atria and ventricles and support the two AV valves are largely type I collagen fiber bundles, while the blood vessel walls are elastin and collagen types I and III (50 percent), with lesser contributions from types IV, V, and VI collagen. Elastin is located at 7q11; Collagen 1A1 at 17q21.13-17q22.05; Collagen 1A2 at 7q21.3-7q22.1; Collagen 2A1 at 12q13.1-12q13.3; Collagen 3A1 at 2q31; and Collagen 5A2 at 2q31.

MARFAN'S SYNDROME

Marfan's syndrome is a heritable disorder of connective tissue that is caused by a defect in fibrillin protein encoded by the fibrillin-1 gene on chromosome 15[173] (see Chap. 85). Marfan's syndrome occurs in approximately 1 in 10,000 individuals and is equally common in males and females. There is marked variation in clinical expression, and the diagnosis can be made at any age from the newborn period through adulthood.[174] Because of the variability in expression, overlap with nonpathologic features (such as tall stature) can be observed in the general population. Since fibrillin[175] is diffuse, Marfan's syndrome affects skeletal, ocular,[176] cardiovascular,[177,178] skin, pulmonary,[179] and central nervous systems (Table 69-6). The skeletal manifestations of Marfan's syndrome include tall stature, thin body build, long arms and legs (dolichostenomelia), long fingers and toes (arachnodactyly), hyperextensibility, pectus deformity, scoliosis, joint contractures, and narrow, high-arched palate. Cardiovascular abnormalities, particularly affecting the mitral apparatus and aorta, are also common (Table 69-6). The requirements for diagnosis are outlined in Table 69-6. There may also be overlap with other disorders that share some of the same phenotype features, such as the condition termed *congenital contractual arachnodactyly*.[180,181] Clinical manifestations of this condition include dolichostenomelia and arachnodactyly, contractures of large joints, and abnormal pinnae formation. Recent data suggest that congenital contractual arachnodactyly is a separate disorder due to a fibrillin-2 gene defect on chromosome 5 (5q23-q31).[182] Marfan's syndrome has been observed in all racial and ethnic groups, and approximately 55 percent of cases are sporadic with no family history. There appears to be an increased effect of paternal age, with the mean age of fathers of patients with sporadic disease being increased.

Some of the skeletal features can be analyzed anthropometrically. For example, the skeletal disproportion is demonstrated by measuring the length of the upper and lower seg-

TABLE 69-6

FEATURES OF MARFAN'S SYNDROME

System Features	System Features
Skeletal	Pulmonary
Tall stature	Pneumothorax
Long arms and legs	Cardiovascular
(dolichostenomelia)	Ascending aorta
Long fingers	dilatation
(arachnodactyly)	Mitral valve prolapse
Narrow, high-arched	Mitral regurgitation
palate	Aortic regurgitation
Joint hyperextensibility	Aortic dissection
Pectus deformity	Dysrhythmia
Scoliosis	Skin
Congenital contractures	Striae distensae
Ocular	Inguinal hernia
Flat cornea	Central nervous system
Myopia	Dural ectasia
Subluxation of lens	Sacral meningocele
(ectopia lentis)	Dilated cisterna magna
Retinal detachment	

Requirements for diagnosis:
1. If family history is positive, features in at least two systems listed above should be present.
2. If family history is negative for affected first-degree relative, skeletal features plus features in at least two other systems should be present.
3. Negative nitroprusside test for hemocystinuria.

Source: Pyeritz RE. The Marfan syndrome. *Am Fam Physician* 1986; 84:83.

ments and by calculating the ratio of the upper segment (US) to the lower segment (LS). The lower segment is measured from the top of the pubic ramus to the floor, and the upper segment is measured from the pubic ramus to the top of the head. US/LS is reduced for classic Marfan's syndrome at all ages. The ratio of arm span to height is usually increased in Marfan's syndrome, although scoliosis may complicate the calculation of both ratios. Arachnodactyly can be assessed by the ratio of the middle finger length to total hand length or by analysis of the metacarpal index on hand radiographs.[183]

Hyperextensibility can be assessed by several simple maneuvers (see Fig. 10-7). The Steinberg (thumb) sign is positive when the thumb projects through the clenched hand on the ulnar side. The Walker-Murdock (wrist) sign is positive when the first and fifth digit of one hand wrap completely around the wrist of the other hand. Pectus excavatum of variable severity is fairly common. Scoliosis can occur at any age and frequently occurs or increases during adolescence. The ocular findings of Marfan's syndrome classically include subluxation of the lenses (ectopia lentis), usually but not always in an upward direction.[176] This occurs in 50 to 60 percent of patients. Myopia is very common, and retinal detachments have also occurred, especially after surgical removal of the lenses. Corneal flattening is also described. Loss of vision occurs in

a significant number of patients. Other manifestations include an increase in the occurrence of inguinal hernias, which may recur, and the development of spontaneous pneumothorax and lung abnormalities in some patients. Sacral meningoceles and dilated cisterna magna have also been reported. A severe neonatal form of Marfan's syndrome has cardiovascular, skeletal, and ocular complications present at birth,[184] and patients typically succumb within the first year of life, often from congestive heart failure.

The majority of cardiac abnormalities associated with Marfan's syndrome affect the ascending aorta, the aortic valve, and the mitral valve[185] (Table 69-3). Physical examination alone is insufficient to detect subtle changes in the heart and in the aorta. The dilatation of the ascending aorta may occur gradually before physical findings occur. Echocardiograms are recommended annually, and beta-blocker therapy should be considered.[186] If the diameter of the aorta corrected for body surface area exceeds the upper limits of normal by 50 percent, the frequency of evaluations should be increased to at least every 6 months. Prophylactic repair with a composite graft including the aortic valve should be performed when ascending aorta dilatation reaches a diameter of 5.5 to 6 cm[187,188] (see Chap. 85). Repair of a severe pectus excavatum may be indicated at an earlier stage, not only of cosmetic reasons but to allow easier and safer aortic surgery, should it be indicated. After surgery, the use of beta blockers and anticoagulants should be maintained, and individuals should avoid contact sports and marked physical exertion. Surveillance of the aorta should continue after surgery. Some evidence suggests that beta blockers may reduce the rate of aortic dilatation and the risk of serious complications.[186] Prophylactic antibiotics should be used on all patients to decrease the risk of bacterial endocarditis. In general, contact sports (e.g., football, basketball) should be avoided, along with isometric exercises, weight lifting, and extreme physical activity, and replaced with noncompetitive sports such as swimming and bicycling. Other abnormalities include mitral valve prolapse, mitral regurgitation, and aortic regurgitation. The cardiovascular abnormalities in neonatal Marfan's syndrome differ somewhat from those seen in older patients, demonstrating significant mitral regurgitation as well as tricuspid and pulmonary valve regurgitation. In addition, these children have significant heart failure, as previously noted.

A special issue involves Marfan's syndrome and pregnancy (see Chaps. 85 and 92). In addition to the 50 percent recurrence risk in offspring, there is also a concern about the stress that pregnancy will put on the aorta. There are at least two dozen case reports of aortic dissection occurring during pregnancy or shortly after delivery,[189] generally occurring with aortic regurgitation or other evidence of aortic dilation. Pregnant women with Marfan's syndrome should have echocardiograms every 6 to 8 weeks during pregnancy and should be followed as high-risk obstetric patients.

The diagnosis of Marfan's syndrome is currently made primarily on clinical grounds, although molecular diagnosis is now feasible.[190] Suspected patients with a positive family history should have positive clinical features in at least two organ systems (see Table 69-6). If the family history is negative for Marfan's syndrome, positive findings should be present in the skeletal system and in at least two other organ systems. Suspected patients should also have a negative urine nitroprusside test to rule out homocystinuria, one of the disorders in the differential diagnosis. Management of patients with a negative family history and only suggestive skeletal features is unclear. It may be unwise to inform such patients with minimal features that they have Marfan's syndrome, in view of its implications. Nonetheless, they should be followed clinically with perhaps periodic echocardiograms and ophthalmologic examinations. In these individuals, strong consideration for molecular genetic evaluation is wise.

In 1990, Marfan's syndrome was mapped to the long arm of chromosome 15(15q15q-q20).[3] Subsequently, a defect in the gene for fibrillin-1 (FBN1)[191-193] was found to be the cause of Marfan's syndrome. This large glycoprotein has a molecular mass of 350 kDa[175] and is a component of microfibrils that are ubiquitous in the connective tissue space. The mRNA transcript of this gene is approximately 10 kbp.[193] Not only do defects in this gene cause Marfan's syndrome, but recently Milewicz[193] also showed that severe neonatal Marfan's syndrome is due to a specific 3-bp insertion in the fibrillin-1 cDNA. Furthermore, fibrillin defects have been found in patients with atypical phenotypes, including autosomal dominant ectopia lentis with skeletal features[194] and milder forms such as the MASS phenotype (*m*itral valve, *a*orta, *s*keleton, and *s*kin)[195] or isolated ascending aortic aneurysm with dissection.[196] Unfortunately, each family appears to have an individual mutation in the gene, making screening difficult and requiring that each new mutation case be studied individually.

In terms of genetic counseling, families should be informed of the autosomal dominant inheritance pattern with 50 percent recurrence in offspring. The rationale for patient follow-up and management should also be explained, along with psychosocial support and medical follow-up. Prenatal diagnosis may be possible.[197]

EHLERS-DANLOS SYNDROMES

There are at least 11 different forms of Ehlers-Danlos syndrome (EDS), which are generally given numerical designations.[198] The most common forms are types I through IV, as discussed here. Type II and type III overlap with the features of type I, but both are progressively less severe; type III is sometimes known as *benign hypermobility syndrome*. The features of EDS type I include hyperextensible and fragile skin, with poor wound healing and "cigarette paper" scarring. Hyperextensibility of the joints (Fig. 10-5) increases susceptibility to dislocation of the hips, shoulders, elbows, knees, and clavicles. The ears tend to be hypermobile and are sometimes described as "lop ears." Scoliosis is a relatively common finding, as are clubfeet in infancy. There is an increased risk of premature birth resulting from premature rupture of membranes.[199] Umbilical and diaphragmatic hernias tend to be relatively common.

The most common cardiac features include mitral valve prolapse, tricuspid valve prolapse, and dilatation of the aortic root and/or sinus of Valsalva. ASDs and abnormalities of the aortic arch and mitral valve have also been seen. Probably the most significant cardiovascular defect is the increased susceptibility to dissecting aortic aneurysm (see Table 69-3), which can lead to death. Poor wound healing and decreased vascular integrity have been noted. Surgical procedures are frequently not tolerated well, and patients should probably avoid unnecessary surgery. In addition, patients should be cautioned to avoid trauma as much as possible. Type I EDS is inherited as an autosomal dominant disorder with variability in expression. The presumed defect in this disorder involves synthesis of normal collagen.

Ehlers-Danlos type IV is sometimes referred to as the "malignant" form of EDS, since there is marked susceptibility to spontaneous rupture of large blood vessels or bowel.[200] The hyperelasticity and hyperextensibility tend to be less obvious than in type I. Easy bruisability and susceptibility to bleeding, however, are very prominent. Spontaneous rupture of any of the major vessels has been reported. Pregnancy-related complications are particularly striking, the overall risk of death with pregnancy being 25 percent. The basic defect in this autosomal dominant disorder is in the type III collagen gene located on chromosome 2 (2q31),[201] and additional defects have been reported.[202,203] Other Ehlers-Danlos defects in collagen genes thus far localized include types VI (1p36.3-1p36.2). VII A1 (17q21.31-q22), and VII A2 (7q22.1).[204]

Patients with types I and IV EDS require yearly cardiac examinations. Initial evaluation with chest radiography and echocardiography will enable the cardiologist to decide the frequency of follow-up and repeat echocardiograms, depending on the level of aortic dilatation and mitral valve prolapse. Annual chest x-rays are cost-effective as a minimal approach, with echocardiograms necessary every 1 to 2 years. Antibiotic prophylaxis for subacute bacterial endocarditis (SBE) is also needed in patients with mitral valve prolapse or aortic abnormalities.

FAMILIAL ANEURYSMS

It has been recognized for some time that certain aneurysms in peripheral and central arteries (see "Marfan's syndrome") have a familial tendency.[205] As data accumulate on genetic defects in fibrillin[206] (Marfan's sydnrome) and in the collagen disorders,[207-209] there appears to be overlap in the genetic defects of fibrillin and procollagen, particularly type III, as causes for aneurysms. Some have a defect in type II procollagen (COL3A1) similar to defects that have been reported in EDS type IV.[210] Familial incidence is said to account for 7 percent of aneurysms.[211] Since EDS is relatively rare, many of the more common familial procollagen abnormalities may represent phenotypic overlap. *These findings have resulted in a reassessment of the traditional teaching that most aortic aneurysms result from atherosclerosis. Family history should be carefully assessed in all patients with aortic or cerebral aneurysms, and, if it is positive, other family members should be assessed. Many should be followed with noninvasive evaluation in a fashion similar to that described for Marfan's syndrome.*

PSEUDOXANTHOMA ELASTICUM

This is a genetic disease of the elastic tissue that involves the skin, eyes, and cardiovascular system. The characteristic lesion is that of the skin consisting of a highly raised, yellowish papule, known as a *pseudoxanthoma,* overlying areas of flexural stress such as the neck, cubital and popliteal fossae, and groin (Fig. 10-6).[212] The eye changes are slate-gray linear bands, representing tears in Bruch's membrane, and subsequent fibrosis leading to loss of central vision in 70 to 80 percent of cases. Calcification of peripheral arteries occurs frequently, most commonly in the femoral artery but also in the coronary arteries. The heart is affected by myocardial ischemia and infarction, secondary to the coronary disease that is the major cause of morbidity and mortality (see Table 69-2). A restrictive cardiomyopathy is common due to endocardial fibrosis.[213] Pseudoxanthoma elasticum is also associated with mitral valve prolapse.[214] Two genetic variants having autosomal dominant inheritance and two others with autosomal recessive inheritance occur. The only difference between the recessive and dominant forms is the presence of affected parents and offspring. Because the basic defect is unknown, no specific treatment is available.

The cardiac features should be followed closely once abnormalities are noted. In stable patients, yearly examinations are required at a minimum. Myocardial dysfunction with or without heart failure requires anticongestive and inotropic support, while SBE prophylaxis is needed for those patients with mitral valve prolapse. Symptoms should be used to direct therapy.

CUTIS LAXA

This designation refers not only to a specific dermatologic sign but to a variety of mendelian and nonmendelian, congenital and acquired syndromes sharing the characteristic feature of lax, nonresilient skin.[212] Two varieties of autosomal recessive cutis laxa exist. Death from pulmonary complicatons may occur in the first months of life, and most patients die by the third year. Signs of right-sided heart failure are often seen in infancy and are generally due to pulmonary disease, although pulmonary artery stenosis also occurs[215] (see Table 69-2). Histopathologically, the pulmonary artery lesions are due to medioelastic fiber paucity. Mitral valve prolapse has also been notable. The gene(s) that cause this spectrum of disease have remained elusive.

Primary Disorders of Rhythm and Conduction

Virtually all rhythm and conduction abnormalities have been reported to be familial. However, many families have been small so that the mode of inheritance (or even whether the inheritance is mendelian) is uncertain. In many cases, these conduction defects have been associated with other cardiac and systemic disorders. For a detailed clinical discussion of arrhythmia and conduction disorders see Chap. 27.

ROMANO-WARD LONG QT SYNDROME

The association of stress-induced syncope, sudden death, and ventricular arrhythmias in families has long been noted, but recently a distinct syndrome was recognized,[216,217] having prolongation of the QT interval and abnormal T waves on ECG. Multiple families with this syndrome have demonstrated autosomal dominant inheritance, with torsades de pointes, polymorphic ventricular tachycardia, bradycardia, and T-wave alternans[218] (see Chap. 36). The diagnosis is made when the QT interval corrected for heart rate (QT$_c$) is greater than 480 ms using Bazzett's formula; T-wave abnormalities are usually seen. In symptomatic patients (i.e., patients with syncope, or "seizures"), the diagnosis may be made with shorter QT$_c$ (i.e., 470 ms). A diagnostic algorithm has been useful.[219]

In 1991, genetic linkage to chromosome 11p (11p15.5) was shown in a large Mormon kindred[1] and subsequently in six other unrelated families.[220] Shortly thereafter, genetic heterogeneity was demonstrated in families with Romano-Ward LQTS.[221] Linkage evidence was found for loci on chromosome 7 (LQTS2)[222] and chromosome 3 (LQTS3), and a gene has been linked to chromosome 4 (LQTS4).[223]

The two most likely hypothetical pathogenetic mechanisms of Romano-Ward LQTS as proposed by Schwartz et al.[218] are (1) sympathetic nervous system abnormalities, and (2) potassium channel (or other ion channel) abnormalities. The HERG gene, an I$_{Kr}$ potassium channel, has been mapped to chromosome 7q35-q36,[224] and mutations in a variety of domains of this channel were shown to be responsible for the disease in LQTS2 families. Another channel gene, the cardiac sodium channel called SCN5A and located at 3p21, has been shown to be responsible for LQTS3.[225] The chromosome 11–linked (LQTS1) gene was recently discovered to be another potassium channel, known as KVLQTS1.[226] Multiple mutations in KVLQTS1 have been identified. The chromosome 4–linked (LQTS4) gene remains undiscovered at this time. Thus, multiple different mutations could result in LQTS (Figs. 69-9 and 69-10). *The long QT syndromes now appear to be due to ion channel abnormalities.*[227] Distinct ECG differences between patients have been demonstrated with the four different genes (LQTS1 to LQTS4).[228] Important prognostic differences are present between various mutations.[229,230] Specific ion channel–based therapy might be possible in LQTS[231]; the sodium channel blocker mexiletine normalized the QT$_c$ in sodium channel–defective patients with LQTS3. Studies using potassium-based therapy are currently ongoing in families with HERG and KVLQTI mutations,[232] while other approaches to sodium channel therapy are also being evaluated[233] (see Chap. 36).

JERVELL AND LANGE-NIELSEN LQTS

This syndrome, described in 1957,[234] is characterized by congenital deafness, syncope, prolonged QT interval, sudden death, and autosomal recessive inheritance[235] (see Chap. 36). Affected individuals are usually diagnosed in childhood with congenital, severe high-tone perceptive bilateral deafness; fainting spells precipitated by exertion, rage, or fright; and ECG evidence of QT-interval prolongation and T-wave abnormalities. As would be expected for rare autosomal recessive traits, the parents of affected individuals are more likely than usual to be consanguineous. At present, neither the cause nor the pathogenesis is known. An interesting possibility that arises is that those families shown to be unlinked to any of the Romano-Ward LQTS genes are actually heterozygotes with Jervell and Lange-Nielsen sydnrome, manifesting long QT interval without deafness.

FAMILIAL ATRIAL FIBRILLATION

Familial atrial fibrillation appears to be rare, but a moderate-sized family was identified and the gene responsible for the disease mapped to 10q22.[236] This family inherited the disease as an autosomal dominant trait, with the average age of onset of atrial fibrillation being 17 years. This family has a highly penetrant form of the disease, with most affected individuals developing atrial fibrillation very early in childhood. The signs and symptoms are those related to atrial fibrillation and include palpitations, syncope, and dyspnea. Several other families with familial atrial fibrillation have since been identified, with the disease mapped to the same locus.

WOLFF-PARKINSON-WHITE SYNDROME

The preexcitation syndromes, including WPW, have been considered to be congenital, but only a small number of patients demonstrate familial occurrence; the majority of cases appear to be sporadic. ECG features of WPW include the presence of a short PR interval and a prolonged QRS with slurred upstroke of the R wave, known as a delta wave[237] (see Chap. 26). Patients with WPW syndrome are prone to episodes of paroxysmal supraventricular tachycardia (see Chap.

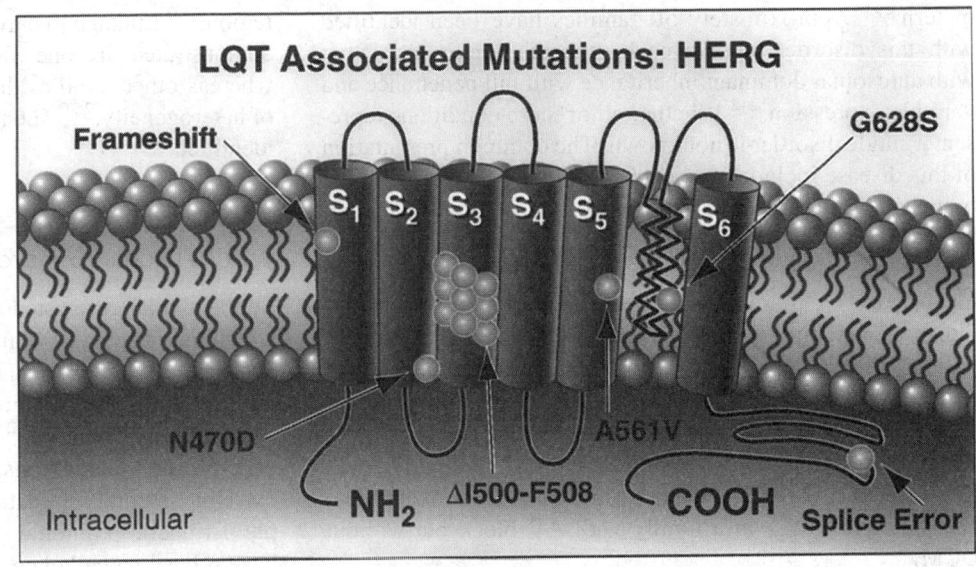

FIGURE 69-9
HERG, a cardiac potassium channel gene that causes LQTS2, contains six α-helical transmembrane segments (S1–S6). Mutations in various segments cause LQTS, as illustrated by the blue circles.

27). An autosomal dominant pattern of inheritance of accessory pathways has been reported[238] based on the first-degree relatives of 383 patients with preexcitation. Autosomal dominant inheritance in children with WPW syndrome and supraventricular tachycardia was previously reported.[239] In a family with familial HCM and WPW syndrome, the locus was mapped to chromosome 7 (7q3).[31]

AUTOSOMAL DOMINANT ATRIOVENTRICULAR BLOCK

This disorder, when familial, presents with adult onset (age 20 to 50 years)[240] and has an autosomal dominant inheritance

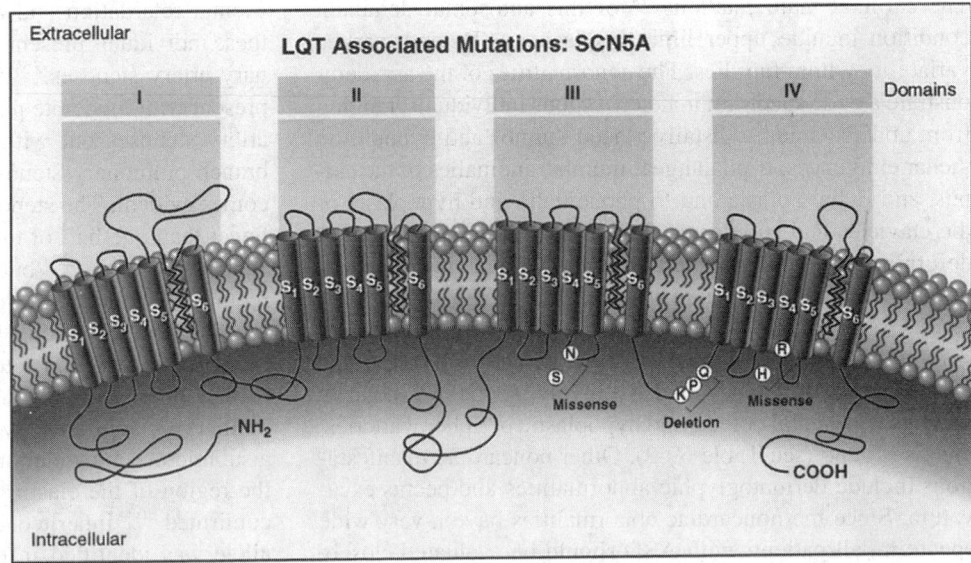

FIGURE 69-10
SCN5A, a cardiac sodium channel gene responsible for LQTS3, contains four domains (I–IV) with six transmembrane segments each (S1–S6); the four domains are connected to form a tetrameric unit. Various mutations result in LQTS.

pattern.[241] Approximately 50 families have been identified with this disorder, and in each, transmission is consistent with autosomal dominant inheritance with full penetrance and variable expression.[242] Whether all of these conditions represent a single disorder is not known. The common presentation of this disease includes one of the following: (1) right bundle branch block alone, (2) left axis deviation alone, (3) right bundle branch block plus left axis deviation, (4) complete heart block. Ten families with pure AV block have been identified,[243] six families with AV block or sinus brachycardia, three with pure sinus brachycardia, and eight with congenital AV block. A six-generation family presenting with a conduction defect and subsequent DCM has been identified,[244] and the gene in this family was mapped to 1p1-1q1.[76] In addition, a family with similar clinical findings[245] was localized to 3p25-p22.[63] Another gene has been mapped to chromosome 19q13 in a family with AV block but without DCM.[246]

Familial Atrial Septal Defect

Two mendelian forms of ASD exist as autosomal dominant traits. One form has no other associated abnormalities and is speculated to be on chromosome 6p, linked to the HLA complex; it is as yet unconfirmed by genetic linkage analysis. The more common form of familial secundum ASD is associated with AV conduction delay,[247] which rarely progresses to heart block. In these patients, attention should be directed to the upper limbs, particularly the thumbs, to rule out the Holt-Oram syndrome, (see below). Another form of familial ASD has also been described, thought to be due to mitochondrial inheritance.[248]

Holt-Oram Syndrome

The cardinal manifestations[249] of this autosomal dominant condition include upper limb dysplasia, ASD, and marked variability within families. The abnormalities of the arm demonstrate a wide spectrum in heterozygous individuals, ranging from undetectable, to distally placed thumbs and hypoplastic thenar eminences, triphalangeal thumbs, anomalies of the carpus, and radial aplasia and to phocomelia and hypoplasia of the clavicles and shoulders (Fig. 10-2). The upper extremity deformity is typically bilateral, but the left side is commonly more severe than the right. In addition to the ASD, other cardiac malformations are occasionally found, the most frequent of which is a ventricular septal defect (VSD). Cardiac conduction disturbances, usually involving the AV node in patients with septal defects and hypoplastic peripheral arteries, are also found (see Table 69-3). Other noncardiac manifestations include dermatoglyphic abnormalities and pectus excavatum. Since the noncardiac abnormalities have a very wide spectrum, all patients with ASD should be evaluated closely for upper limb deformities.

A male with features consistent with Holt-Oram syndrome in addition to mental retardation and other anomalies was found to have a deletion of chromosome 14 in the q23-q24.2

region.[250] Linkage to chromosome 12 (12q213-q22) has been demonstrated in one family with Holt-Oram syndrome, whereas other families did not link to this region, indicative of heterogeneity.[251] The responsible gene at 12q213 has been identified.[252,253]

Supravalvular Aortic Stenosis and Williams' Syndrome

Supravalvular aortic stenosis (SVAS) occurs in three different situations. The most common is associated with Williams' syndrome, which is usually sporadic but may be a highly variable autosomal dominant condition. The full spectrum of Williams' syndrome[254–256] includes dysmorphic facies, often called "elfin" facies (Figs. 10-34 and 69-11), infantile hypercalcemia, mental retardation, short stature, SVAS, and multiple peripheral pulmonic stenoses. Many of these individuals have robust, so-called cocktail party personalities. Late-onset problems may include progressive joint contractures, gastrointestinal dysfunction, and genitourinary dysfunction.

Cardiovascular features of Williams' syndrome are present in about 75 percent of patients,[256,257] the most characteristic of which is SVAS. Other findings include peripheral pulmonic arterial stenosis and pulmonic valvular stenosis. Occasionally, VSD or ASD may be present. Peripheral vascular anomalies, including renal arterial stenosis, diffuse narrowing of the aorta, and coarctation of the aorta, may be present and may be associated with systemic hypertension. Sudden death has occurred in children with Williams' syndrome, especially after cardiac catheterization. Coronary arterial stenosis may occur and lead to myocardial infarction. Histopathology in these patients suggests the possibility of abnormal elastic fibers.[258]

A second setting for SVAS is the autosomal dominant entity, which is distinct from that of Williams' syndrome. Mental retardation and abnormal facies are not found, and these individuals present with SVAS and/or peripheral pulmonary artery stenoses.[259,260] In some cases, family members present with moderate pulmonic valve and branch pulmonary artery stenoses but without SVAS. Later, the valvular and branch pulmonary stenoses may disappear while SVAS becomes evident. The stenotic aortic lesions requires surgery in fewer than one-half of these patients. The diagnosis relies on echocardiography,[261] but cardiac catheterization is sometimes required. Finally, SVAS may present as sporadic cases. Many investigators have long believed that sporadic SVAS, Williams' syndrome, and autosomal dominant SVAS are all interrelated.

In 1993, Williams' syndrome was reported to result from a submicroscopic deletion involving chromosome 7q11.23 in the region of the elastin gene,[262] and this was subsequently confirmed.[263] Inherited or de novo deletion of one elastin allele was identified in each of the patients studied, and it was suggested that hemizygosity at the elastin locus is responsible for the vascular pathology in Williams' syndrome. Concordance in monozygotic twins and occurrence in second cousins has been described, and anecdotal reports of parent and child with Williams' syndrome have been reported. In addition, familial SVAS without Williams' syndrome, which appears to be inherited as an autosomal dominant trait, is well known.[260] This autosomal dominant form of SVAS was found to be linked to the elastin gene at 7q11.23 as well.[264,265] Subsequent studies showed a deletion of the elastin gene in SVAS as well as in patients with Williams' syndrome. Elastin gene deletion is seen in 90 to 95 percent of Williams' syndrome patients, and translocations also occur.[265,266] However, a few patients with classic features of Williams' syndrome, usually without cardiac defects, do not have a deletion involving elastin. This fact suggests that, while deletion of elastin is necessary for the Williams' syndrome phenotype, it may not be necessary for SVAS or other cardiac defects. Furthermore, not all patients with elastin deletions have cardiac defects. It is possible that Williams' syndrome is a contiguous gene syndrome and that the cardiac defects are due to a neighboring gene.

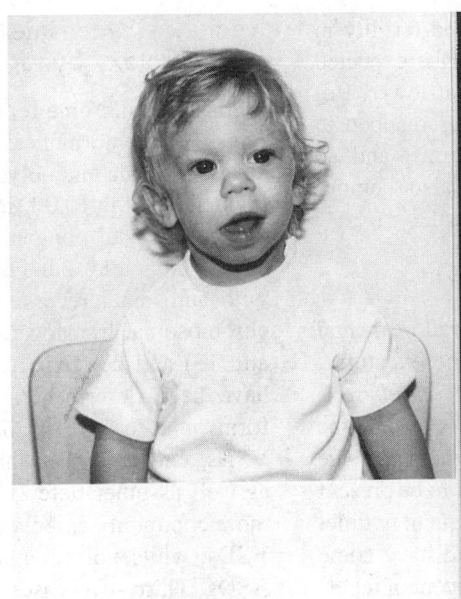
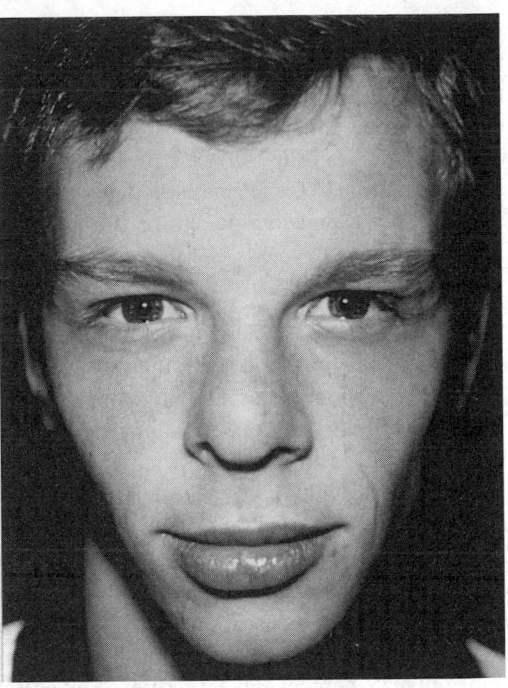

FIGURE 69-11

Williams' syndrome. *Left.* Young child with broad nasal bridge, broad nasal tip with anteverted nares, long philtrum, and prominent lower lip. *Right.* Young adult with Williams' syndrome. (Reprinted with permission from Greenberg F, Rudolph AJ. In: Garson A Jr, Bricker JJ, McNamara DG. (eds.): *The Science and Practice of Pediatric Cardiology.* Philadelphia: Lea & Febiger; Volume 3, 1990; 2397–2413.)

Noonan's Syndrome

In 1963, nine patients with valvular pulmonic stenosis, short stature, mild mental retardation, hypertelorism, and unusual facial features were described.[267] This disorder, sometimes confused with Turner's syndrome, is distinct, and females and males are equally affected (Fig. 10-19). Noonan's syndrome is relatively common, with an incidence of 1 in 1000 to 2500 live births.[268] The diagnosis can sometimes be made prenatally. Postnatal growth, however, is generally delayed and tends to parallel the third percentile with normal growth velocity, although the adolescent growth spurt is usually blunted or absent. Facial features appear to change with age. The main features of the newborn period are hypertelorism with down-slanted palpebral fissures; low-set, posteriorly rotated ears with thickened helices; deeply grooved philtrum; micrognathia; and excess neck skin with low posterior hairline. As the infant ages, the head appears larger, with prominent eyes, thinning of the palpebral fissures, and depression of the nasal root. The face appears more myopathic and becomes more triangular in shape. In some young adults, the eyes become less prominent. The neck length is relatively short, which exaggerates the webbing. Individuals tend to have prominent nasolabial folds, high anterior hairline, and transparent, wrinkled skin. The hair is generally described as being curly or woolly in older children and adolescents. Approximately 60 percent of males have cryptorchidism. Sexual development is variable and may be delayed. Most females appear to be fertile. Pectus carinatum superiorly and pectus excavatum inferiorly appear to be present in about 70 percent of individuals. The chest appears to lengthen with age, giving the appearance of relatively low-set nipples. Other features include cubitus valgus, clinodactyly, vertebral anomalies, dental malocclusion, café-au-lait spots, pigmented nevi, bleeding disorders, lymphatic dysplasia, and pulmonary and intestinal lymphangiectasia. Mental retardation is present in 35 percent of cases.[268,269]

It appears that about two-thirds of patients with Noonan's syndrome have some type of cardiac defect. Approximately half of these patients have valvular pulmonic stenosis.[270] Other relatively common cardiac anomalies include HCM,[270] ASDs, VSDs, and persistent patent ductus arteriosus. Pulmonic arterial branch stenosis, mitral valve prolapse, Ebstein's anomaly, and single ventricle have also been reported (see Table 69-3).

The clinical features of Noonan's syndrome can overlap with a number of other conditions. Chromosome studies should be done in females to rule out Turner's syndrome. Phenotypic overlap with Williams' syndrome, primidone teratogenicity syndrome, fetal alcohol syndrome, Aarskog syndrome, LEOPARD syndrome, neurofibromatosis, and malignant hyperthermia (King's syndrome) have been reported.

Most cases of Noonan's syndrome appear to be sporadic. The majority of inherited cases are apparently inherited from the mother, thought to be the result of decreased fertility in males. Although the recurrence risk for offspring is expected to be 50 percent, it might actually be somewhat lower. Recently, a gene causing Noonan's syndrome was mapped to chromosome 12(12q22-qter)[271] in one large family and 20 smaller families. Genetic heterogeneity was also demonstrated. The responsible gene(s) is not yet known.

Tuberous Sclerosis

Classically, tuberous sclerosis consists of the triad of mental retardation, seizures, and adenoma sebaceum. These features, however, may not be present in all patients. The term *tuberous sclerosis* primarily refers to hamartomatous lesions in the brain as well as intracranial calcifications, primarily in the area of the basal ganglia.[272] These lesions appear to be present in about 90 percent of patients. Seizures are a frequent finding, being seen in about 90 percent of patients, and have some correlation with mental retardation. About 60 percent of tuberous sclerosis patients are mentally retarded, close to 100 percent of whom have seizures; of those without mental retardation, only 75 percent have seizures. Seizures tend to occur earlier in patients with mental retardation than those without mental retardation. Ocular lesions, particularly benign astrocytoma, occur in about 50 percent of patients. Cutaneous lesions are common; 80 percent of patients develop angiofibromas of the face, usually referred to by the misnomer adenoma sebaceum. Depigmented skin patches, which are especially apparent by Wood's light examination, are seen in about 80 percent of patients, frequently from birth. Pulmonary disease may occur primarily in adult females and is likely to be severe and life-threatening. The primary cardiac finding is the presence of rhabdomyomata.[273] WPW syndrome and supraventricular tachycardia have also been reported.[274]

Tuberous sclerosis is an autosomal dominant condition in which about 80 percent of cases are suspected as resulting from new mutations with unaffected parents. A child diagnosed with tuberous sclerosis should be evaluated by computed tomography of the brain and electroencephalography, for the presence of central nervous system lesions, and also have renal ultrasound. Parents should be examined for the presence of depigmented patches (by Wood's light), dental abnormalities, retinal findings, and abdominal ultrasound for renal cysts. It is now apparent that there are at least two genes causing tuberous sclerosis: TSC1 on chromosome 9[275] and TSC2 (Tuberin) on chromosome 16.[276]

Familial Coarctation of the Aorta

Familial coarctation of the aorta (usually with autosomal dominant transmission) has been described, but no locus or gene has been identified. A recessive mutation, called gridlock, in the zebra fish (*Danio rerio*) has been identified in which blood flow to the tail is impeded by a localized vascular defect.[277] There is some question as to whether this mutation is a model for human aortic coarctation,[278] but it may aid in learning about vascular obstruction.

Ivemark's Syndrome (Asplenia/Polysplenia) or Heterotaxy Syndromes

Ivemark's syndrome represents a group of defects that interferes with the normal establishment of laterality.[279] The more severe asplenia and polysplenia syndromes have an estimated incidence of 1 in 10,000 to 20,000 live births, or approximately 1 percent of all congenital heart defects. The occurrence is usually sporadic, but familial cases[280] have been described with autosomal recessive[281] and X-linked transmission[282]; chromosomal translocations (i.e., between chromosomes 12 and 13) and deletions (involving chromosomes 10 and 13) have been described, as has monozygotic twinning. Both forms tend to have similar cardiac defects, including ASDs, VSDs, endocardial cushion defects, and pulmonic stenosis, as well as other defects.[283] Asplenia, however, tends to be more commonly associated with severe AV canal defects and VSDs, while polysplenia tends to be more associated with ASDs. Thirty-two cases of asplenia were identified in 4059 autopsies, and all cases were sporadic, with a male excess.[284]

Several defects relating to situs inversus have been identified in mice but have not yet helped to elucidate defects in humans.[285] In humans, three modes of inheritance have been identified, with most being autosomal recessive. Most cases of human heterotaxy syndrome are sporadic, and mutations in the Connexin 43 gap-junction gene appear responsible for this cardiac abnormality.[286] In four of these children, autosomal recessive inheritance was suggested but not definitively demonstrated. Connexin gene family proteins form membrane-spanning hexameric hemichannels (called *connexons*) when in register in apposed cell membranes, and couple to form a continuous hydrophilic channel through which ions, metabolites, and signal transducing molecules can move between cells. Connexin 43 is a 43-kDa protein that predominates in the heart and acts to unite ventricular myocytes in the electrical syncytium to help regulate synchronized rhythm. Support for this gene as an important determinant of cardiac development has been provided.[287] Neonatal mice lacking Connexin 43 died at birth due to a failure in pulmonary gas exchange caused by a swelling and blockage of the right ventricular outflow tract. Controversy, however, was raised by other authors who analyzed a large number of children with heterotaxy without any Connexin 43 mutations identified.

Other Genetic Syndromes

A variety of other genetic syndromes with associated cardiovascular disease occur primarily in childhood. These include the Ellis–van Creveld syndrome, Treacher Collins' syndrome, Alagille's syndrome, Smith-Lemli-Opitz syndrome, thrombocytopenia–absent radius (TAR) syndrome, Goldenhar's syndrome, Cornelia de Lange's syndrome. Rubinstein-Taybi syndrome, and the VACTERL and CHARGE associations. Since these are primarily pediatric diseases, they are outlined briefly in Table 69-7. For detailed descriptions of these and other pediatric genetic syndromes with cardiovascular abnormalities, see current reviews of this topic.[288]

CARDIOVASCULAR DISORDERS ASSOCIATED WITH CHROMOSOME ABNORMALITIES

Chromosomal Nomenclature

Cytogenetics is the study of chromosomes and chromosomal abnormalities. Chromosomes are classified according to their size and shape. Chromosomes have two arms, one long and one short. The short arm is usually referred to as the "p" arm, and the long arm is usually referred to as the "q" arm. For instance, the long arm of chromosome 22 is designated 22q and the short arm 22p. The arms of the chromosomes meet at the *centromere,* or primary constriction, which is responsible for division of chromosome pairs during meiosis and mitosis. There are three shapes of human chromosomes based on the position of the centromere. *Metacentric chromosomes* have the centromere in a central position, and the long and short arms are approximately equal. *Submetacentric chromosomes* have an eccentric centromere, producing arms of unequal lengths. *Acrocentric chromosomes* have a centromere close to one end of the chromosome. Acrocentric chromosomes have small pieces of chromatin known as satellites attached to their short arms.

Since 1971, banding of chromosomes has become routine, and the banding patterns of each chromosome can be distinguished separately. For this reason, chromosome abnormalities are designated by the actual chromosome number rather than the chromosome group (e.g, trisomy 18 rather than trisomy E).

Classification of Chromosomal Alterations

Chromosome alterations, especially those involving too many or too few chromosomes (aneuploidy), are quite common in human development. Chromosome aberrations most commonly cause structural defects of the cardiovascular system and typically these are evident at birth. Approximately 50 percent of all fetuses conceived are spontaneously aborted (usually in the first trimester), with one-half of these being aneuploid. Among live-born infants, about 1 in 200 (0.5 percent) have a chromosome abnormality. The frequency of chromosome abnormalities among live-born children with congenital heart defects is in the range of 5 to 13 percent.[289–291] Hence, a vast majority of chromosomal aberrations are lost in early fetal life and, in most instances, occur as new mutations. For this reason, with both parents being normal, the risk of recurrence to relatives is usually low.

Aneuploidy, defined as the gain or loss of chromosomes resulting in too many or too few chromosomes, occurs most commonly by nondisjunction (failure of a homologous pair of chromosomes to separate). Nondisjunction occurs during meiosis in one parent (i.e., in spermatogenesis or oogenesis) or in the first mitotic cleavage of the zygote. In meiotic nondisjunction, when a pair of chromosomes does not normally separate, both members of the pair (or neither member of the pair) pass into one gamete. When an additional copy of the chromosome is added during fertilization, three copies of the same chromosome (or only one copy) are found in the new zygote instead of the chromosome pair. Two of the most common chromosomal disorders causing heart disease, Down's syndrome (trisomy 21) and Turner's syndrome (XO), are due to nondisjunction. Absence of one chromosome is called *monosomy;* all autosomal monosomies, as well as those containing only a Y sex chromosome, are lethal for the embryo. The presence of three chromosomes is called *trisomy,* as seen in Down's syndrome, while the presence of an entire extra set of chromosomes is known as *triploidy.*

Chromosomal rearrangements occur when a chromosome breaks and rejoins in a pattern different from normal. This can potentially result in an inversion of genetic material. Typically there is no apparent phenotypic effect in persons carrying an inversion, but their offspring may have severe abnormalities due to the disruption in chromosome pairing during meiosis that can take place.

Chromosome deletion or loss of chromosomal material may be seen by light microscopy, and consists of deletion of $\geq 10^6$ base pairs. If there is a large amount of DNA lost, more than one gene may be affected (disrupted or lost), and a series of abnormalities in a single individual may result due to interruptions in a series of genes within the loci of a single chromosome. These contiguous gene deletion syndromes[292] may be heritable, and the occurrence of the disorder in a family behaves as a dominant disorder (X-linked or autosomal dominant). Most deletions occur de novo. Two breaks in the same chromosome that reunite with the intermediate segment being inverted is referred to as an *inversion.* Isochromes are formed when two short or long arms join with loss of the other arm. *Chromosomal translation* occurs when breaks occur in two chromosomes and they reunite after exchange of segments. These deletions are best appreciated at the DNA level by Southern analysis or PCR analysis.

Chromosome duplications or gain of chromosomal material may also be associated with phenotypic abnormality but most commonly causes no obvious aberration.

Cytogenetics and Techniques

High-resolution cytogenetic techniques allow unambiguous identification of each human chromosome and detection of most structural abnormalities of the chromosomes. These structural abnormalities include translocations, deletions, and duplications. High-resolution chromosome analysis involves synchronization of lymphocyte cultures in order to accumulate all cells at one point in the cell cycle.[293] Other cells that may be used include skin, fibroblasts, and amniotic cells. Enrichment of this cell population in prophase and prometaphase rather than the middle-to-late stages of metaphase, which is characteristic of conventional harvesting techniques, allows improved visualization of the subbanding patterns of chromosomes. Each band seen at metaphase actually represents multiple subbands in earlier stages that have fused

TABLE 69-7

GENETIC SYNDROMES WITH CARDIOVASCULAR ABNORMALITIES PRESENTING PRIMARILY IN CHILDHOOD

Syndrome Eponym	Descriptive Name	Genetic Transmission	Gene or Genetic Locus	Recurrence Risk, %	Cardiac Disease	Patients with Cardiac Disease, %	Life Expectancy
Ellis–van Crevald	Short-limb chondrodysplasia	Autosomal recessive	None	25	Single atrium of first-degree ASD (75%); CoA, hypoplastic left heart or PDA, syndrome, (20%)	>50	Infancy to adulthood
Treacher Collins	Mandibulofacial dysostosis	Autosomal dominant	5q32-5q33.1	50	VSD; ASD; PDA; conotruncal malformations	30	Adulthood
Alagille	Arterial hepatic dysplasia	Autosomal dominant	20p11-20p12	50	Pulmonic stenosis; branch pulmonary artery stenoses	>50	Adolescence to adulthood
Smith-Lemli-Opitz	None	Autosomal recessive	None	25	AV canal; CoA; TOF; VSD; pulmonary atresia/stenosis	>30	Infancy to adolescence
TAR	Thrombocytopenia–absent radii (TAR)	Autosomal recessive	None	25	TOF; ASD	33	Infancy (40%) or young adult
Goldenhar	Facio-auriculo-vertebral spectrum	Sporadic	7p	1	VSD; PDA; TOF; CoA	25	Adulthood
Cornelia de Lange	None	Autosomal dominant or sporadic	3q26.37	1	VSD	30	Late childhood to adulthood
Rubinstein-Taybi	None	Sporadic	16p13.3	1	VSD; PDA; succinylcholine-induced arrhythmias	33	Infancy to adulthood
VACTERL association	None	Sporadic	None	1	VSD		Infancy to adulthood
CHARGE association	None	Autosomal dominant or sporadic	None	1	Conotruncal anomalies	75	Infancy to adulthood
Edwards	Trisomy 18	Sporadic (usually meiotic non-disjunction)	Chromosome 18 trisomy	1–2	ASD; VSD; PDA; PS; TOF; TGA; CoA; Bicuspid aortic valve; pulmonary hypertension	90	Infancy; ≤1% to adulthood (mosaics)
Patau	Trisomy 13	Sporadic; (usually meiotic non-disfunction)	Chromosome 13 trisomy	1–2	VSD; ASD; PS; CoA; PDA; dextrocardia; complex congenital heart disease	80	Infancy

Note: ASD, atrial septal defect; CoA, coarctation of the aorta; PDA, patent ductus arteriosus; PS, pulmonic stenosis; TGA, transposition of great arteries; TOF; tetralogy of Fallot, VSD, ventricular septal defect.

together as the chromosome contracts. Whereas a typical metaphase cell contains 300 to 400 bands per haploid genome, synchronized chromosome preparations make it possible to visualize 500 to 1000 bands per haploid set.[294] With the development of banding methods, the human karyotype could be divided into 300 to 400 discrete bands, or approximately 7×10^6 to 10×10^6 bp per band, and a much greater number of deletions, duplications, and translocations could be detected. High-resolution techniques allow visualization of 500 to 2000 bands per haploid genome and have enabled the delineation of a number of microdeletion or microduplication syndromes (also known as contiguous gene syndromes), including DiGeorge's syndrome and the Beckwith-Wiedemann syndrome.

FLUORESCENCE IN SITU HYBRIDIZATION

A new technique known as fluorescence in situ hybridization (FISH) provides for the detection of submicroscopic chromosomal deletions or duplications. This technique uses DNA probes derived from chromosomal regions that hybridize to the specific chromosomes. The probes are conjugated with a fluorescent dye visible under a fluorescence microscope. This method makes possible direct visualization of single sequences, not only on chromosomes but also within decondensed interphase nuclei, providing a high-resolution (<1 mb) approach to gene mapping and analysis of nuclear organization.

INDICATIONS FOR CHROMOSOMAL ANALYSIS

Chromosomal studies can provide valuable information to the family and the physician and should be considered in any child who has a heart defect with any of the following: (1) minor dysmorphic features, (2) growth retardation that cannot be explained by the heart defect, or (3) developmental delay. In addition, the practitioner might consider chromosome studies more strongly if there is a family history of multiple miscarriages or other infants with birth defects or mental retardation. A genetic consultant can help determine whether or not chromosome studies should be performed and can help to integrate the findings of the chromosome analysis with the clinical picture. The major disadvantage of doing chromosomal studies is the cost (generally between $300 and $500).

Chromosomal Disorders

Many chromosomal disorders have associated cardiovascular disease. The most common of these include Down's syndrome (trisomy 21), Patau's syndrome (trisomy 13), Edwards' syndrome (trisomy 18), and Turner's syndrome. Since trisomy 13 and trisomy 18 usually result in death during infancy, these are outlined briefly in Table 69-7. A significant number of other chromosome abnormalities are also associated with cardiovascular disease (Table 69-7) and are seen primarily as pediatric disorders.[288] These abnormalities include triploidy, aneuploidy (other than trisomy 21, trisomy 18, trisomy 13, and Turner's syndrome), deletions, and duplications. The triploidy syndrome, which include 69,XXX, 69,XXY, or 69,XYY, have

greater than 50 percent incidence of congenital heart disease, the vast majority of which are ASDs and VSDs. The aneuploidy syndromes not discussed thus far are varied and uncommon. These include mosaicism of chromosome 8[295] and chromosome 9,[296] which present clinically with VSDs with or without other associated complex defects. Aortic root dilatation and mitral valve prolapse occur with partial monosomy of chromosome 22.[297] Other cardiovascular abnormalities associated with partial trisomy of chromosome 7q includes VSD, pulmonic stenosis, patent ductus arteriosus, coarctation of the aorta, and L-transposition of the great vessels.[298] Partial trisomy of chromosome 7p also occurs and most commonly is associated with VSD, pulmonic stenosis, or AV canal defects.[299]

Down's Syndrome (Trisomy 21)

Chromosome 21 is the smallest of all human chromosomes, containing less than 2 percent of the genomic DNA. Down's syndrome, however, is the most common phenotype caused by a human chromosome abnormality, occurring approximately once in every 500 to 600 births. This disorder is usually due to the presence of an extra chromosome 21 (Fig. 69-12). In some cases, however, it is caused by the presence of only the distal one-half of chromosome 21, band q22 (i.e., 21q22)— the Down's syndrome critical region—so-called because of the presence of a subset of major phenotypic features of Down's syndrome including mental retardation, congenital heart disease, characteristic facial appearance (Fig. 69-13), and hand and dermatoglyphic changes. In order to produce this syndrome, the region of 21q22 must be triplicated.[300,301] The gene(s) responsible for manifesting Down's syndrome is unknown, but the severity of the disease is believed to depend on the extent of the region q22, and beyond, that is triplicated. Creation of a linkage map of chromosome 21 has allowed for consideration of potential candidate genes.

The typical trisomy 21 occurs in 95 percent of cases of Down's syndrome and results from chromosomal nondisjunction. Two to three percent of Down syndrome cases are mosaics, having one trisomy cell line and one normal cell line, and the remainder (1 to 4 percent) are due to an extra copy of all, or part, of the long arm of chromosome 21 translocated to another chromosome. *The risk of trisomy 21 is exponentially related to maternal age, with the lowest risk for young women, and rises steeply after age 35 years, reaching 4 percent for women older than 45 years.*

The recurrence risk is generally quoted as 1 to 2 percent.[302] When a child with a translocation type of Down's syndrome is discovered, parental chromosomal analysis should always be performed to determine whether the translocation was inherited. If the translocation was not inherited and both parents have normal chromosomes, the recurrent risk is probably low, although prenatal chromosome diagnosis may be considered for future pregnancies. *If the mother carries translocation of chromosome 21, the recurrence risk is approximately 10 percent. If the father is determined to be the carrier of a D;21 translocation, the recurrent risk is about 2 percent.*[203] *If one*

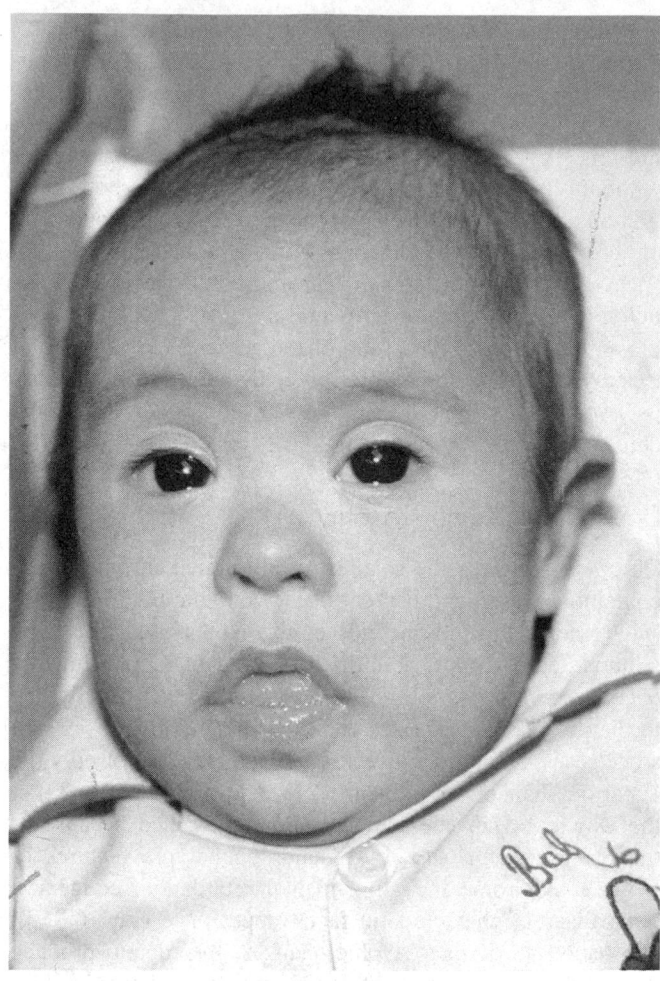

FIGURE 69-12

Three-month-old infant with features of Down's syndrome.

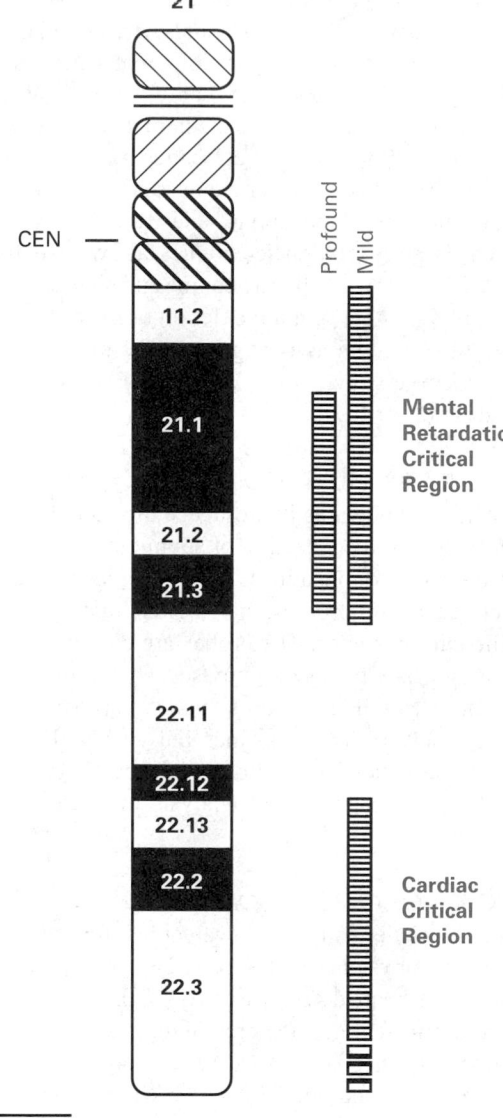

FIGURE 69-13

Ideogram of Down's syndrome phenotypic map. (Modified from Korenberg JR. *Nature Genet* 1995; 11:109–111.)

of the parents is determined to specifically be a 21;21 translocation carrier, the parents have a 100 percent chance of recurrence of Down's syndrome and no possibility of having normal offspring.[303] Luckily, the latter occurs in only about 1 in every 2000 cases of Down's syndrome but clearly has a significant impact on family planning.

Between 40 and 50 percent of patients with Down's syndrome have congenital heart disease and this, hematologic malignant disease, and duodenal atresia are among the most common causes of morbidity and mortality. Patients who escape these problems generally survive into the fifth decade and beyond. *The most characteristic cardiac defect in Down's syndrome is the endocardial cushion defect or AV canal defect* (Table 69-8)[302] (see Chap. 70). In addition to problems of volume overload secondary to left-to-right shunting, these patients are predisposed to early pulmonary hypertension).[304] Elevated pulmonary vascular resistance becomes a significant risk beyond 1 year of age. Once this occurs, these patients become unsuitable for surgical repair. Approximately one-third of patients with Down's syndrome and congenital heart defects have complex heart disease, increasing the morbidity and mortality further. Other clinical features of Down's

TABLE 69-8

CHROMOSOMAL ABNORMALITIES ASSOCIATED WITH SPECIFIC TYPES OF CONGENITAL HEART DEFECTS

Endocardial cushion defect	Trisomy 21
Coarctation of the aorta	Turner's syndrome
Hypoplastic left heart syndrome	Partial trisomy 22q
	49,XXXXX; 49,XXXXX
Total anomalous pulmonary venous return	Partial trisomy 8q
	Monosomy 22q11
Patent ductus arteriosus	Partial trisomy 5q
Tetralogy of Fallot	
Conotruncal abnormalities	
Conduction defect	

syndrome include: hypotonia and decreased Moro reflex with joint hyperextensibility in the newborn period; a flat facial profile with excessive, redundant skin in the posterior neck; anti-Mongoloid slant (upward) of palpebral fissures; and small white Brushfield spots around the circumference of the irides in children with blue irides. The hands and feet may reveal a simian crease (50 percent), clinodyactyly or incurving of the fifth finger, brachydactyly with short metacarpals and phalanges, and a wide gap between the first two toes. Individuals are mentally retarded to varying degrees, with IQs ranging from 25 to 70. Generally, males are infertile.

Turner's Syndrome

This disorder, which is due to a single X chromosome in females (i.e., XO genotype), occurs in approximately 1 female in 2500.[305] The frequency of nonmosaic XO karotypes is significantly higher in spontaneous abortuses than in live-borns, with fewer than 2 percent of such conceptuses reaching term. Clinically, there is a variable and often mild phenotype, and the diagnosis may go unsuspected until a child's short stature is evaluated or a woman complains of amenorrhea. The clinical findings[306] of patients with Turner's syndrome include lymphedema of hands and feet, inguinal hernias, short stature, primary amenorrhea, and facial features including a slightly triangular face with downslated palpebral fissures, epicanthal folds, and ptosis (Fig. 10-10). Ears are frequently low set and posteriorly rotated, and the mandible is commonly micrognathic. The neck is typically short with marked webbing, and the posterior hairline may be low, extending to the upper shoulders. A broad thorax with widely spaced nipples is common, as is cubitus valgus and shortening of the fourth and fifth metacarpals. Abnormalities of sexual development are usually associated, including hypogonadotropic hypogonadism with ovarian dysgenesis. Intelligence is normal. Many cases are mosaic for cell lines with the normal 46XX or 46XY makeup. The frequency of congenital cardiac disease varies from 20 to 50 percent, with at least one-half of these individuals having coarctation of the aorta. A variety of other cardiac defects may also occur either singly or in combination with coarctation of the aorta. The majority of these are other left heart abnormalities, including bicuspid aortic valve, aortic stenosis, dilated ascending aorta,[307] and hypoplastic left heart syndrome. ASD and VSD, as well as partial anomalous pulmonary venous return,[308] have also been reported (Table 69-8).

Coarctation of the aorta can usually be diagnosed clinically due to poor femoral pulses and differential blood pressure; the arm blood pressures are consistently hypertensive, while the leg pressures are typically very low (see Chap. 57). Echocardiography or magnetic resonance imaging will confirm the diagnosis. Therapy may include surgical repair or, in some cases, balloon angioplasty. Infants may require prostaglandin E therapy to keep the ductus arteriosis patent; these young patients may present in heart failure or cardiac collapse if ductal-dependent. Those patients with hypoplastic left heart syndrome are ductal-dependent and will die unless a Norwood operation or cardiac transplant is performed. Bicuspid aortic valves do not usually require therapy unless stenosis occurs. All cardiac defects require prophylaxis for SBE. Chromosomal studies are recommended in all cases of Turner's syndrome since only about 60 percent of cases will have monosomy X.[296] The remaining cases have mosaicism or various abnormalities of the X chromosome. Most cases of Turner's syndrome are sporadic, and the recurrence risk appears to be relatively low. Parents, however, may choose to have prenatal chromosomal diagnosis in subsequent pregnancies.

CATCH-22 Syndromes

DIGEORGE ANOMALY

First described in 1965,[309] the combination of thymic hypoplasia, parathyroid hypoplasia, and cardiac defects has been termed *DiGeorge's syndrome* or the *DiGeorge anomaly*. Because the disorder is of heterogeneous etiology, the term *DiGeorge anomaly* is currently preferred. These thymic, parathyroid, and cardiac defects all result from developmental abnormalities of the third and fourth branchial arches.

Eighty percent of affected infants present with congenital heart defects within the first 48 h of life.[310] According to the classification system of Clark,[11] the two types of defects associated with the DiGeorge anomaly are conotruncal defects and branchial arch mesenchymal tissue defects. Among conotruncal defects, truncus arteriosus is the most common type. Among the branchial arch mesenchymal tissue defects, interrupted aortic arch type b and right aortic arch are the most common. In a series reported by Conley and coworkers, interrupted aortic arch type b occurred in over one-third of the patients, and the DiGeorge anomaly was seen in one-half of autopsy cases with interrupted aortic arch.[310]

The second key feature is persistent hypocalcemia, occurring either as the initial presenting feature or in combination with the cardiac defect. Parathyroid glands may be absent or reduced in size and number, and serum parathyroid hormone levels are decreased. Hypocalcemia may require continuous calcium infusions and/or frequent calcium supplementation. In cases of partial defect, the hypocalcemia may improve over time.

There are multiple etiologies for the DiGeorge anomaly, and they include chromosome abnormalities, single-gene defects, teratogenic exposures, and association with other defects. In 1981, five members of a family with a chromosome 20;22 translocation leading to partial monosomy 22 were reported. Affected infants had evidence of DiGeorge anomaly with conotruncal cardiac defects, thymic aplasia, and parathyroid hypoplasia as well as cleft palate, dysplastic kidneys, and lung malformations. Three additional cases of DiGeorge anomaly have been reported with abnormalities involving chromosome 22.[311] Approximately 5 to 10 percent of infants with features of DiGeorge anomaly will have an obvious abnormality of chromosome 22, with monosomy of the proximal portion of the long arm. Approximately 70 percent of patients, however, will have submicroscopic deletions of

22q11 detectable only by FISH.[312] In addition, many of these patients have features of the Shprintzen velo-cardio-facial (VCF) syndrome and the Takao conotruncal anomaly–face syndrome. These features are currently referred to as a group by the mnemonic of CATCH-22 syndrome for the associated defects (*c*ardiac, *a*bnormal facies, *t*hymic hypoplasia, *c*left palate, *h*ypocalcemia, 22q11 deletions).[225] Approximately 15 percent of infants with the DiGeorge anomaly can be found to have obvious chromosome abnormalities, of which about two-thirds involve a monosomy 22q11.[313] This usually results from an unbalanced translocation involving chromosome 22 and another chromosome. More recent studies using FISH with probes from the critical region have shown that a total of about 85 percent of DiGeorge anomaly patients have deletions, with about 70 percent of patients having submicroscopic, molecular deletions, del22 (q11.21 q11.23). Although patients have different deletion end-points, there is a 1.5-Mbp region deleted in most. Rarely, a syndrome of "partial" DiGeorge syndrome due to balanced translocation has been described. This translocation has been cloned and a disrupted gene identified,[314] with speculation that it is a DNA binding protein. More recently, the minimal DiGeorge critical region of 250 kbp has been defined, and a detailed transcription map of the region constructed.[315]

SHPRINTZEN VELO-CARDIO-FACIAL SYNDROME

This condition was first recognized in 1978, with ascertainment primarily in children with palatal defects[316]; this is the most common syndrome associated with cleft palate and appears to be the same disorder as the Takao conotruncal anomaly–face syndrome.[317] The clinical features include mildly short stature; cleft palate, especially of the secondary palate with submucous clefts; pharyngeal incompetence leading to speech disorders; and speech delay. Most cases are sporadic, but some autosomal cases have been reported.[318]

Cardiac defects are prominent in this disorder, the majority being conotruncal-type defects.[319] VSD occurs in 70 to 75 percent, right-sided aortic arch occurs in about 50 percent, and tetralogy of Fallot is found in 15 to 20 percent of children. Partial DiGeorge anomaly seems to be present in some cases. About 85 percent of VCF syndrome patients have deletions of chromosome 22q11, usually submicroscopic and visible only by FISH techniques.

Takao syndrome (conotruncal face–anomaly syndrome), first described in 1976, has similarities to both the DiGeorge and Shprintzen syndromes clinically[320]; hence, its incorporation in the CATCH-22 association. These Japanese children were noted to have a specific dysmorphic facial appearance in association with conotruncal malformations. Deletions within the 22q11 region in these patients have been found,[317] confirming its similarity to the DiGeorge anomaly and VCF syndrome.

REFERENCES

1. Keating M, Dunn C, Atkinson D, Timothy K, Vincent GM, Leppert M. Linkage of a cardiac arrhythmia, the long QT syndrome, and the Harvey ras-1 gene. *Science* 1991; 252:704–706.

2. Jarcho JA, McKenna W, Pare JAP, Solomon SD, Holcombe RF, Dickie S, et al. Mapping a gene for familial hypertrophic cardiomyopathy to chromosome 14q1. *N Engl J Med* 1989; 321:1372–1378.

3. Kainulainen K, Pulkkinen L, Savolainen A, Kaitila I, Peltonen L. Location on chromosome 15 of the gene defect causing Marfan's syndrome. *N Engl J Med* 1990; 323:935–939.

4. Hoffman JIE. Incidence of congenital heart disease. II. Prenatal incidence. *Pediatr Cardiol* 1995; 16:155–165.

5. Olson EN. Molecular pathways controlling heart development. *Science* 1996; 276:671–676.

6. Dressler D. Studying the Human Genome is one of the great enterprises of 20th Century science. In: Cooper NG, ed. *The Human Genome Project: Deciphering the Blueprint of Heredity.* Mill Valley, CA: University Science Books; 1994:9–10.

7. Serrato M, Marian AJ. A variant of human paraoxonase/arylesterase (HUMPONA) gene is a risk factor for coronary artery disease. *J Clin Invest* 1995; 96:3005–3008.

8. Yu QT, Safavi F, Roberts R, Marian AJ. A variant of β fibrinogen is a genetic risk factor for coronary artery disease and myocardial infarction. *J Invest Med* 1996; 44:154–159.

9. Edwards JG. Familial predisposition in man. *Br Med Bull* 1969; 25:58–64.

10. Nora JJ, McGill CW, McNamara DG. Empiric recurrent risks in common and uncommon congenital heart lesions. *Teratology* 1970; 3:325–330.

11. Clark EB. Mechanisms in the pathogenesis of congenital heart defects. In: Pierpont ME, Moller JM, eds. *The Genetics of Cardiovascular Disease.* Boston: Martinus-Nijhoff; 1985:3–36.

12. Roberts R, Marian AJ, Bachinski LL. Overview: Application of molecular biology to medical genetics. In: Markwald RR, Clark EB, Takao A, eds. *Inborn Heart Disease—Developmental Mechanisms.* Mount Kisco, NY: Futura Press; 1994:87–111.

13. Weissenbach J. A second generational linkage map of the human genome based on highly informative microsatellite loci. *Gene* 1994; 135:275–278.

14. Cooperative Human Linkage Center (CHLC). A comprehensive human linkage map with centimorgan density. *Science* 1994; 265:2049–2054.

15. Cooper NG, ed. *The Human Genome Project: Deciphering the Blueprint of Heredity.* Mill Valley, CA: University Science Books, 1994.

16. Roberts R, Towbin J. Principles and techniques of molecular biology. In: Roberts R, ed. *Molecular Basis of Cardiology.* Cambridge: Blackwell Scientific; 1993:15–112.

17. Botstein D, White RL, Skolnick M, Davis RW. Construction of a genetic linkage map in man using restriction fragment length polymorphisms. *Am J Hum Genet* 1980; 32:314–331.

18. Wells RA. DNA fingerprinting. In: Rickwood D, Hames BD, eds. *Genome Analysis: A Practical Approach.* Oxford: IRL Press; 1988:153–170.

19. Weber JL, May PE. Abundant class of human DNA polymorphisms which can be typed using the polymerase chain reaction. *Am J Hum Genet* 1989; 44:388–396.

20. Hejtmancik JF, Roberts R. Molecular genetics and the application of linkage analysis. In: Roberts R, ed. *Molecular Basis of Cardiology.* Cambridge: Blackwell Scientific; 1993:355–381.

21. Roberts R, Bachinski LL, Yu QT, Kelly DP, Quiñones MA, Young R, et al. Molecular analysis of genotype/phenotype correlations of hypertrophic cardiomyopathy. In: Dhalla NS, Singal PK, Beamish RE, eds. *Heart Hypertrophy and Failure.* Boston: Kluwer Academic; 1995:3–19.

22. Ozawa T, Tanaka M, Sugiyama S, Hattori K, Ito T, Ohno K, et al. Multiple mitochondrial DNA deletions exist in cardiomyocytes of patients with hypertrophic or dilated cardiomyopathy. *Biochem Biophys Res Commun* 1990; 170:830–836.

23. Kelly DP, Strauss AW. Inherited cardiomyopathies. *N Engl J Med* 1994; 330:913–919.

24. Hejtmancik JF, Brink PA, Towbin J, Hill R, Brink L, Tapscott T, et al. Localization of the gene for familial hypertrophic cardiomyopathy to chromosome 14q1 in a diverse U.S. population. *Circulation* 1991; 83:1592–1597.

25. Marian AJ, Yu QT, Mares A Jr, Hill R, Roberts R, Perryman MB. Detection of a new mutation in the β-myosin heavy chain gene in an individual with hypertrophic cardiomyopathy. *J Clin Invest* 1992; 90:2156–2165.

26. Marian AJ, Roberts R. Recent advances in the molecular genetics of hypertrophic cardiomyopathy. *Circulation* 1995; 92:1336–1347.

27. Thierfelder L, Watkins H, MacRae C, Lamas R, McKenna W, Vosberg HP, et al. Alpha-tropomyosin and cardiac troponin T mutations cause familial hypertrophic cardiomyopathy: A disease of the sarcomere. *Cell* 1994; 77:701–712.

28. Bonne G, Carrier L, Bercovici J, Cruaud C, Richard P, Hainque B, et al. Cardiac myosin binding protein-C gene splice acceptor site mutation is associated with familial hypertrophic cardiomyopathy. *Nature Genet* 1995; 11:438–439.

29. Watkins H, Conner D, Thierfelder L, Jarcho JA, MacRae C, McKenna WJ, et al. Mutations in the cardiac myosin binding protein-C gene on chromosome 11 cause familial hypertrophic cardiomyopathy. *Nature Genet* 1995; 11:434–435.

30. Abchee AB, Greve G, Ifegwu J, Joseph A, Bachinski LL, Roberts R. Rapid genetic screen for common β-myosin heavy chain mutations causing familial hypertrophic cardiomyopathy (abstr). *J Am Coll Cardiol* 1995; 25:26A.

31. MacRae C, Ghasia N, Kass S, Donnelly S, Basson CT, Watkins H, et al. Familial hypertrophic cardiomyopathy with Wolff-Parkinson-White syndrome maps to a locus on chromosome 7q3. *J Clin Invest* 1995; 96:1216–1220.

32. Ko Y, Chen J, Tang T, Teng M, Lin S, Kuan P, et al. Mapping the locus for familial hypertrophic cardiomyopathy to chromosome 11 in a family with a case of apical hypertrophic cardiomyopathy of the Japanese type. *Hum Genet* 1996; 97:457–461.

33. Poetter K, Jiang H, Hassenzadeh S, Master SR, Chang A, Dalakas MC, et al. Mutations in either the essential or regulatory light chains of myosin are associated with a rare myopathy in human heart and skeletal muscle. *Nature Genet* 1996; 13:63–69.

34. Roberts R. Molecular genetics: Therapy or terror? *Circulation* 1994; 89:499–502.

35. Anan R, Greve G, Thierfelder L, Watkins HC, McKenna WJ, Solomon S, et al. Prognostic implications of novel β cardiac myosin heavy chain gene mutations that cause familial hypertrophic cardiomyopathy. *J Clin Invest* 1994; 93:280–285.

36. Marian AJ. Sudden cardiac death in patients with hypertrophic cardiomyopathy: From bench to bedside with an emphasis on genetic markers. *Clin Cardiol* 1995; 18:189–198.

37. Epstein ND, Cohn GM, Cyran F, Fananapazir L. Differences in clinical expression of hypertrophic cardiomyopathy associated with two distinct mutations in the β-myosin heavy chain gene: A 908 Leu-Val mutation and a 403 Arg-Gln mutation. *Circulation* 1992; 86:345–352.

38. Watkins H, Rosenzweig A, Hwang D, Levi T, McKenna W, Seidman CE, et al. Characteristics and prognostic implications of myosin missense mutations in familial hypertrophic cardiomyopathy. *N Engl J Med* 1992; 326:1108–1114.

39. Perryman MB, Yu QT, Marian AJ, Mares A Jr, Czernuszewicz G, Ifegwu J, et al. Expression of a missense mutation in the mRNA for β-myosin heavy chain in myocardial tissue in hypertrophic cardiomyopathy. *J Clin Invest* 1992; 90:271–277.

40. Marian AJ, Yu QT, Workman R, Greve G, Roberts R. Angiotensin converting enzyme polymorphism in hypertrophic cardiomyopathy and sudden cardiac death. *Lancet* 1993; 342:1085–1086.

41. Lechin M, Yu QT, Roberts R, Quinones MA, Marian AJ. Angiotensin I converting enzyme geneotypes and left ventricular hypertrophy in patients with hypertrophic cardiomyopathy. *Circulation* 1995; 92:1808–1812.

42. Vybiral T, Roberts R, Deitiker PR, Epstein HF. Accumulation and assembly of myosin in the Arg-Gin β-MHC hypertrophic cardiomyopathy mutant. *Circ Res* 1992; 71:1404–1409.

43. Nishi H, Kimura A, Harada H, Koga Y, Adachi K, Matsyama K, et al. A myosin missense mutation, not a null allele, causes familial hypertrophic cardiomyopathy. *Circulation* 1995; 91:2911–2915.

44. Sweeney HL, Straceski AJ, Leinwand LA, Tikunov BA, Faust L. Heterologous expression of a cardiomyopathic myosin that is defective in its actin interaction. *J Biol Chem* 1994; 269:1603–1605.

45. Cuda G, Fananapazir L, Zhu W, Sellers JR, Epstein ND. Skeletal muscle expression and abnormal function of β myosin in hypertrophic cardiomyopathy. *J Clin Invest* 1993; 91:2861–2865.

46. Lankford EB, Epstein ND, Fananapazir L, Sweeney HL. Abnormal contractile properties of muscle fibers expressing β-myosin heavy chain gene mutations in patients with hypertrophic cardiomyopathy. *J Clin Invest* 1995; 95:1409–1414.

47. Marian AJ, Yu QT, Mann DL, Graham FL, Roberts R. Expression of a mutation causing hypertrophic cardiomyopathy in adult feline cardiocytes disrupts sarcomere assembly in adult feline cardiac myocytes. *Circ Res* 1995; 77:98–106.

48. Geisterfer-Lowrance AA, Christe M, Conner DA, Ingwall JS, Schoen FJ, Seidman CE, et al. A mouse model of familial hypertrophic cardiomyopathy. *Science* 1996; 272:731–734.

49. Towbin JA. Molecular genetic aspects of cardiomyopathy. *Biochem Med Metab Biol* 1993; 49:285–320.

50. Senocak F, Sarclar M, Ozkutlu S. Echocardiographic findings in some metabolic storage diseases. *Jpn Heart J* 1994; 35:635–643.

51. Rauser AJ, Kroos MA, Hermans MM, Bijvoet AG, Verbeet MP, Van Diggelen OP, et al. Glycogenosis Type II (acid maltase deficiency). *Muscle Nerve* 1995; 3:S61–S69.

52. Raben N, Nichols RC, Boerkoel C, Plotz P. Genetic defects in patients with glycogenosis Type II (acid maltase deficiency). *Muscle Nerve* 1995; 3:S70–S74.

53. Wiedemann HR. Complexo malformatif familial avec hernie unbilicate et macroglossie: Un "syndrome nouveau"? *J Genet Hum* 1964; 13:223–232.

54. Beckwith JB. Macroglossia, omphalocele, adrenal cytomegaly, gigantism and hyperplastic visceromegaly. *Birth Defects* 1969; 2:188–196.

55. Sotelo-Avila C, Gonzalez-Crussi F, Fowler JW. Complete and incomplete forms of Beckwith-Wiedemann syndrome: Their oncogenic potential. *J Pediatr* 1980; 96:47–50.

56. Best LG, Hoekstra RE. Wiedemann-Beckwith syndrome: Autosomal dominant inheritance in a family. *Am J Med Genet* 1981; 9:291–299.

57. Barbeau A. Friedreich's ataxia 1978: An overview. *Can J Neurol Sci* 1978; 5:161–165.

58. Chamberlain S, Shaw J, Rowland A, Wallis J, South S, Nakamura Y, et al. Mapping of mutation causing Friedreich's ataxia to human chromosome 9. *Nature* 1988; 334:248–250.

59. Campuzano V, Montermini L, Mooto MD, Pianese L, Cossee M, Cavalcanti F, et al. Friedreich's ataxia: Autosomal recessive disease caused by an intronic GAA triplet repeat expansion. *Science* 1996; 271:1423–1427.

60. Codd MB, Sugrue DD, Gersh BJ, Melton LJ III. Epidemiology of idiopathic dilated and hypertrophic cardiomyopathy: A population-based study in Olmsted County, Minnesota, 1975–1984. *Circulation* 1989; 80:564–572.

61. Durand JB, Bachinski LL, Beiling L, Czernuszewicz GZ, Abchee AB, Yu QT, et al. Localization of a gene responsible for familial idiopathic dilated cardiomyopathy to chromosome 1q32. *Circulation* 1995; 92:3387–3389.

62. Krajinovic M, Pinamonti B, Sinagra G, Vatta M, Severini GM, Milasin J, et al. Linkage of familial dilated cardiomyopathy to chromosome 9. *Am J Hum Genet* 1995; 57:846–852.

63. Olson TM, Keating MT. Mapping a cardiomyopathy locus to chromosome 3p22-25. *J Clin Invest* 1996; 97:528–532.

64. Bowles KR, Gajarski R, Porter P, Goytia V, Bachinski L, Roberts R, et al. Gene mapping of familial autosomal dominant dilated cardiomyopathy to chromosome 10q21-23. *J Clin Invest* 1996; 98:1355–1360.

65. Berko BA, Swift M. X-linked dilated cardiomyopathy. *N Engl J Med* 1987; 316:1186–1191.

66. Towbin JA, Hejtmancik JF, Brink P, Gelb BD, Zhu XM, Chamberlain JS, et al. X-linked dilated cardiomyopathy (XLCM): Molecular genetic evidence of linkage to the Duchenne muscular dystrophy gene at the Xp21 locus. *Circulation* 1993; 87:1854–1865.

67. Towbin JA. Biochemical and molecular characterization of X-linked dilated cardiomyopathy. In: Clark EB, Markwald RR, Takao A, eds. *Developmental Mechanisms of Heart Disease*. New York: Futura Publishing; 1995:121–132.

68. Ohlendieck K, Matsumura K, Ionasescu W, Towbin JA, Bosch EP, Weinstein SL, et al. Duchenne muscular dystrophy: Deficiency of dystrophin-associated proteins in the sarcolemma. *Neurology* 1993; 43:795–800.

69. Muntoni F, Cau M, Ganau A, Congiu R, Mateddu A, Marrosu M, et al. Deletion of the muscle-promoter region associated with X-linked dilated cardiomyopathy. *N Engl J Med* 1993; 329:921–925.

70. Ortiz-Lopez R, Li H, Su J, Goytia V, Towbin JA. Evidence for a dystrophin missense mutation as a cause of X-linked dilated cardiomyopathy (XLCM). *Circulation* 1997; 95:2434–2440.

71. Yoshida K, Ikeda S, Nakamura A, Kagoshima M, Takeda S, Shoji S, et la. Molecular analysis of the Duchenne muscular dystrophy gene in patients with Becker muscular dystrophy presenting with dilated cardiomyopathy. *Muscle Nerve* 1993; 16:1161–1166.

72. Milasin J, Muntoni F, Severini GM, Bartoloni L, Vatta M, Krajinovic M, et al. A point mutation in the 5′ splice site of the dystrophin gene first intron responsible for X-linked dilated cardiomyopathy. *Hum Mol Genet* 1996; 5:73–79.

73. Barth PG, Scholte HR, Berden JA, Van der Klei-Van Moorsel JM, Luyt-Houwen IEM, Van T, et al. An X-linked mitochondrial disease affecting cardiac muscle skeletal muscle and neutrophil leukocytes. *J Neurol Sci* 1983; 62:327–355.

74. Consalez GG, Thomas NST, Stayton CL, Knight SJL, Johnson M, Hopkins LC, et al. Assignment of Emery-Dreifuss muscular dystrophy to the distal region of Xq28: The results of a collaborative study. *Am J Hum Genet* 1991; 48:468–480.

75. Bione S, Maestrini E, Rivella S, Mancini M, Regis S, Romeo G, et al. Identification of a novel X-linked gene responsible for Emery-Dreifuss muscular dystrophy. *Nature Genet* 1994; 8:323–327.

76. Kass S, MacRae C, Graber HL, Sparks EA, McNamara D, Boudoulas H, et al. A gene defect that causes conduction system disease and dilated cardiomyopathy maps to chromosome 1p1-1q1. *Nature Genet* 1994; 7:546–551.

77. Kearney DL, Towbin JA, Bricker JT, Radovancevic B, Frazier OH. Familial ventricular dysplasia (cardiomyopathy). *Pediatr Pathol Lab Med* 1995; 15:181–189.

78. Rampazzo A, Nava A, Erne P, Eberhard M, Vian E, Slomp P, et al. A new locus for arrhythmogenic right ventricular cardiomyopathy (ARVD2) maps to chromosome 1q42-q43. *Hum Mol Genet* 1995; 4:2151–2154.

79. Severini GM, Krajinovic M, Pinamonti B, Sinagra G, Fioretti P, Brunazzi MC, et al. A new locus for arrhythmogenic right ventricular dysplasia on the long arm of chromosome 14. *Genomics* 1996; 31:193–200.

80. Coonar AS, Protonotarios N, Tsatsopoulou A, Needham EWA, Murday VA, Houlston RS, et al. A gene locus for arrhythmogenic right ventricular cardiomyopathy maps to chromosome 17q1-q3 (abstr). *J Am Coll Cardiol* 1997; 29:4A.

81. Nordlile M, Sletten K, Husby G, Ranlov PJ. A new prealbumin variant in familial amyloidotic cardiomyopathy of Danish origin. *Scand J Immunol* 1988; 27:119–122.

82. Neufeld EF, Muenzer J. The mucopolysaccharidoses. In: Scriver CR, Beaudet AL, Sly NS, Valle D, eds. *The Metabolic and Molecular Bases of Inherited Disease*, 7th ed. New York: McGraw-Hill; 1995:2465–2494.

83. Bach G, Freidman R, Weissmann B, Neufeld EF. The defect in Hurler and Scheie syndromes: Deficiency of α-L-iduronidase. *Proc Natl Acad Sci USA* 1972; 69:2048–2051.

84. Scott HS, Anson DA, Osborn AM, Nelson PV, Clements PR, Morris CP, et al. Human α-L-iduronidase: cDNA isolation and expression. *Proc Natl Acad Sci USA* 1991; 88:9695–9699.

85. Scott HS, Guo X, Hopwood JJ, Morris CP. Structural and sequence of the human α-L-iduronidase gene. *Genomics* 1992; 13:1311–1313.

86. Scott HS, Litjens T, Nelson PV, Thompson PR, Brooks DA, Hopwood JJ, et al. Identification of mutations in the α-L-iduronidase gene (IDUA) that cause Hurler and Scheie syndromes. *Am J Hum Genet* 1993; 53:973–986.

87. Morquio L. Sur une forme de dystrophie osseuse familiale. *Bull Soc Pediatr Paris* 1929; 27;145–152.

88. Tomatsu S, Fukuda S, Masue M, Sukegawa K, Fukao T, Yamagishi A, et al. Morquio disease: Isolation, characterization and expression of full-length cDNA for human *N*-acetyl-galactosamine-6-sulfate sulfatase. *Biochem Biophys Res Commun* 1991; 1871:677–683.

89. Baker E, Guo X, Osborn MA, Sutherland GR, Callen DF, Hopwood JJ, et al. The Morquio A syndrome (mucopolysaccharidosis IVA) gene maps to 16q24.4 *Am J Hum Genet* 1993; 52:96–98.

90. Masuno M, Tomatsu S, Nakashima Y, Hori T, Fukuda S, Masue M, et al. Mucopolysacharidosis IVA: Assignment of the human *N*-acetylgalactosamine-6-sulfatase (GALNS) gene to chromosome 16q24. *Genomics* 1993; 16:777–778.

91. Fukuda S, Tomatsu S, Masue M, Sukegawa K, Iwata H, Ogawa T, et al. Mucopolysacchardiosis type IVA *N*-acetyl galactosamine-6-sulfate sulfatase exonic point mutations in classical Morquio and mild cases. *J Clin Invest* 1992; 90:1049–1053.

92. Jackson CE, Yuhki N, Desnick RJ, Haskins ME, O'Brien SJ, Schuchman EH. Feline arylsulfatase B (ARSB):Isolation and expression of the cDNA, comparison with human ARSB, and gene localization to feline chromosome A1. *Genomics* 1992; 14:403–411.

93. Mondaressi S, Rupp K, Von Figura K, Peters C. Structure of the human arylsulfatase B gene. *Biol Chem Hoppe Seyler* 1993; 374:327–355.

94. Voskoboeva E, Isbrandt D, Von Figura K, Krasnopolskaya X, Peters C. Four novel mutant alleles of the arylsulfatase B gene in two patients with intermediate form of mucopolysaccharidosis VI (Maroteaux-Lamy syndrome). *Hum Genet* 1994; 93:259–264.

95. Emery AEH, ed. *Duchenne Muscular Dystrophy: Oxford Monographs on Medical Genetics.* Oxford: Oxford University Press; 1987.

96. Moser H. Duchenne muscular dystrophy: Pathogenetic aspects and genetic prevention. *Hum Genet* 1984; 66:17–40.

97. Davies KE, Pearson PL, Harper PS, Murray JM, O'Brien T, Sarfarazi M, et al. Linkage analysis of two cloned DNA sequences flanking the Duchenne muscular dystrophy locus on the short arm of the human X chromosome. *Nucleic Acids Res* 1983; 11:2303–2312.

98. Verellen-Dumoulin C, Freund M, De Meyer R, Laterre C, Frederic J, Thompson MW, et al. Expression of an X-linked muscular dystrophy in a female due to translocation involving Xp21 and non-random inactivation of the normal X chromosome. *Hum Genet* 1984; 67:115–119.

99. Campbell KP, Kahl SD. Association of dystrophin and an integral membrane glycoprotein. *Nature* 1989; 388:259–262.

100. Bies RD, Friedman DL, Roberts R, Perryman MB, Caskey CT. Expression and localization of dystrophin in human cardiac Purkinje fibers. *Circulation* 1992; 86:147–153.

101. Malhotra SB, Hart KA, Klamut HJ, Thomas NS, Bodrug SE, Burghes AH, et al. Frame-shift deletions in patients with Duchenne and Becker muscular dystrophy. *Science* 1988; 242:755–759.

102. Emery AE, Skinner R. Clinical studies in benign (Becker type) X-linked muscular dystrophy. *Clin Genet* 1976; 10:189–201.

103. Dicky RP, Ziter FA, Smith RA. Emery-Dreifuss muscular dystrophy. *J Pediatr* 1984; 104:555–559.

104. Ridker PM, O'Donnel CJ, Marde VJ, Hennekens CH. A response to "Holding GUSTO up to the light." *Ann Intern Med* 1994; 120:882–885.

105. Harris CA, Andryuk PJ, Cline SW, Matthew S, Siekierka JJ, Goldstein G. Structure and mapping of the human thymopletin (TMPO) gene and relationship of the human TMPO-β to rat lamin-associated polypeptide-2. *Genomics* 1995; 28:198–205.

106. Nagano A, Koga R, Ogawa M, Kurano Y, Kawada J, Okada R, et al. Emerin deficiency at the nuclear membrane in patients with Emery-Dreifuss muscular dystrophy. *Nature Genet* 1996; 12:254–259.

107. Manilal S, thi Man N, Sewry CA, Morris GE. The Emery-Dreifuss muscular dystrophy protein, emerin, is a nuclear membrane protein. *Hum Mol Genet* 1996; 5:801–808.

108. Dodge PR, Gamstorp I, Byers RK, Russell P. Myotonic dystrophy in infancy and childhood. *Pediatrics* 1965; 35:3–19.

109. Tokgozogla LS, Ashizawa T, Pacifico A, Armstrong RM, Epstein HF, Zoghbi WA. Cardiac involvement in a large kindred with myotonic dystrophy: Quantitative assessment and relation to size of CTG repeat expansion. *JAMA* 1995; 274:813–819.

110. Brunner H, Korneluk R, Coerwinkel-Driessen M, Mackenzie A, Smeets H, Lambermon HM, et al. Myotonic dystrophy is closely linked to the gene for muscle-type creatine kinase (CKMM). *Hum Genet* 1989; 81:308–310.

111. Brook JD, McCurrack ME, Harley HG, Buckler AJ, Church D, Aburatani H, et al. Molecular basis of myotonic dystrophy: Expansion of a trinucleotide (CTG) repeat at the 3′ end of a transcript encoding a protein kinase family member. *Cell* 1992; 68:799–808.

112. Fu Y, Pizzuti A, Fenwick RG Jr, King J, Rajnarayan S, Dunne PW, et al. An unstable triplet repeat in a gene related to myotonic muscular dystrophy. *Science* 1992; 255:1256–1258.

113. Timchenko LT, Caskey CT. Trinucleotide repeat disorders in humans: Discussions of mechanisms and medical issues. *FASEB J* 1996; 10:1589–1597.

114. Timchenko LT, Timchenko NA, Caskey CT, Roberts R. Novel proteins with binding specificity for DNA CTG repeats and RNA CUG repeats: Implications for myotonic dystrophy. *Hum Mol Genet* 1996; 5:115–121.

115. Timchenko LT, Miller JW, Timchenko NA, DeVore DR, Datar KV, Lin L, et al. Identification of a (CUG)n triplet repeat RNA-binding protein and its expression in myotonic dystrophy. *Nucleic Acids Res* 1996; 24:4407–4414.

116. Caskey CT, Swanson MS, Timchenko LT. Myotonic dystrophy: Discussion of molecular mechanisms. In: *Function and Dysfunction in the Nervous System.* Cold Spring Harbor, NY: Cold Spring Harbor; 1996: vol 61, 607–614.

117. Maeda M, Taft CS, Bush EW, Holder E, Bailey WM, Neville H, et al. Identification, tissue-specific expression, and subcellular localization of the 80- and 71-kDa forms of myotonic dystrophy kinase protein. *J Biol Chem* 1995; 270:20246–20249.

118. Hanson PA, Rowland LP. Mobius syndrome and facioscapulohumeral muscular dystrophy. *Arch Neurol* 1971; 24:31–39.

119. Sellers FJ, Keith KD, Manning JA. The diagnosis of primary endocardial fibroelastosis. *Circulation* 1994; 29:49–59.

120. Opitz JM. Genetic aspects of endocardial fibroelastosis. *Am J Med Genet* 1982; 11:92–96.

121. Ni J, Bowles NE, Kim Y, Demmler G, Kearney D, Bricker JT, et al. Viral infection of the myocardium in endocardial fibroelastosis: Molecular evidence for the role of mumps virus as an etiological agent. *Circulation* 1997; 95:133–139.

122. Waber LJ, Valle D, Neill C, DiMauro S, Shug A. Carnintine deficiency presenting as familial cardiomyopathy: A treatable defect in carnitine transport. *J Pediatr* 1982; 101:700–705.

123. Leys D, Petit H, Bonte-Adnet C, Millaire A, Fourrier F, Dubois F, et al. Refsum's disease revealed by cardiac disorders (letter). *Lancet* 1989; 1:621.

124. Kelly KP, Kim J, Billadello JJ, Hainline BE, Chu TW, Strauss AW. Nucleotide sequence of medium-chain acyl-CoA dehydrogenase mRNA and its expression in enzyme-deficient human tissue. *Proc Natl Acad Sci USA* 1987; 84:4068–4072.

125. Matsubara Y, Naarisawa K, Miyabyshi S, Tada K, Coates PM, Bachmann C, et al. Identification of common mutation in patients with medium-chain acyl-CoA dehydrogenase deficiency. *Biochem Biophys Res Commun* 1990; 171:498–505.

126. Ding J, Yang B, Bao Y, Roe CR, Chen Y. Identification of a new mutation in medium-chain CoA dehydrogenase (MCAD) deficiency. *Am J Hum Genet* 1992; 50:229–233.

127. Indo Y, Yang-Feng T, Glassberg R, Tanaka K. Molecular cloning and nucleotide sequence of cDNAs encoding human long-chain acyl-CoA dehydrogenase and assignment of the location of its gene (ACADL) to chromosome 2. *Genomics* 1991; 11:609–620.

128. Indo Y, Coates PM, Hale DE, Tanaka K. Immunochemical characterization of variant long-chain acyl-CoA dehydrogenase in cultured fibroblasts from nine patients with long chain acyl-CoA dehydrogenase deficiency. *Pediatr Res* 1991; 30:211–215.

129. Izai K, Uchida Y, Orii T, Yamamoto S, Hashimoto T. Novel fatty acid β-oxidation enzymes in rat liver mitochondria. I. Purification and properties of very long-chain acyl-coenzyme A dehydrogenase. *J Biol Chem* 1992; 267:1027–1033.

130. Uchida Y, Izai K, Orii T, Hashimoto T. Novel fatty acid β-oxidation enzymes in rat liver mitochondria. II. Purification and properties of enoyl-coenzyme A (CoA) hydratase/3-hydroxyacyl-CoA dehydrogenase 3-ketoacyl-CoA thiolase trifunctional protein. *J Biol Chem* 1992; 267:1034–1041.

131. Colucci WS, Lorell BH, Schoen FJ, Warhol MJ, Grossman W. Hypertrophic obstructive cardiomyopathy due to Fabry's disease. *N Engl J Med* 1982; 307:926–928.

132. Becker AE, Schoorl R, Balk AG, van der Heide RM. Cardiac manifestations of Fabry's disease. Report of a case with mitral insufficiency and electrocardiographic evidence of myocardial infarction. *Am J Cardiol* 1975; 36:829–835.

133. Goldman ME, Cantor R, Schwartz MF, Baker M, Desnick RJ. Echocardiographic abnormalities and disease severity in Fabry's disease. *J Am Coll Cardiol* 1986; 7:1157–1161.

134. Bishop DF, Calhoun DH, Bernstein HS, Hantzopoulos P, Quinn M, Desnick RJ. Human alpha-galactosidase A; Nucleotide sequence of a cDNA clone encoding the mature enzyme. *Proc Natl Acad Sci USA* 1986; 83:4859–4863.

135. Eng CM, Desnick RJ. Molecular basis of Fabry disease: Mutations and polymorphisms in the human alpha-galactosidase A gene. *Proc Natl Acad Sci USA* 1994; 3:103–111.

136. Eng CM, Niehaus DJ, Enriquez AL, Burgert TS, Ludman MD, Desnick RJ. Fabry disease: 23 mutations including sense and antisense CpG alterations and identification of a deletion hot-spot in the alpha-galactosidase A gene. *Hum Mol Genet* 1994; 3:1795–1799.

137. Okumiya T, Ishii S, Kase R, Kamei S, Sakuraba H, Suzuki Y. Alpha-galactosidase gene mutation in Fabry disease: Heterogeneous expressions of mutant enzyme proteins. *Hum Genet* 1995; 95:557–561.

138. Kraus JP. Molecular basis of phenotype expression in homocystinuria. *J Inherit Metab Dis* 1994; 17:383–390.

139. Skovby F. Homocystinuria: Clinical, biochemical and genetic aspects of cystathionine beta-synthase and its deficiency in man. *Acta Paediatr Scand* 1985; 321:14–21.

140. Mudd SH, Shovby F, Levy HL, Pettigrew KD, Wilcken B, Pyeritz RE, et al. The natural history of homocystinuria due to cystathionine β-synthase deficiency. *Am J Hum Genet* 1985; 37:1–31.

141. Mandel H, Brenner B, Berant M, Rosenberg N, Lanir N, Jakobs C, et al. Coexistence of hereditary homocystinuria and factor V Leiden: Effect on thrombosis. *N Engl J Med* 1996; 334:763–768.

142. Munke M, Kraus JP, Ohura T, Francke U. The gene for cystathionine beta-synthase (CBS) maps to the subtelomeric region on human chromosome 21q and to proximal mouse chromosome 17. *Am J Hum Genet* 1988; 42:550–559.

143. Kraus JP, Williamson CL, Firgaira FA, Yang Feng TL, Munke M, Francke U, et al. Cloning and screening with nanogram amounts of immunopurified mRNAs: cDNA cloning and chromosomal mapping of cystathionine beta-synthase and the beta subunit of propionyl-CoA carboxylase. *Proc Natl Acad Sci USA* 1986; 83:2047–2051.

144. Kraus JP, Le K, Swaroop M, Ohura T, Tahara T, Rosenberg LE, et al. Human cystathionine beta-synthase cDNA: Sequence, alternative splicing and expression in cultured cells. *Hum Mol Genet* 1993; 2:1633–1638.

145. Shih VE, Fringer JM, Mandell R, Kraus JP, Berry GT, Heidenreich RA, et al. A missense mutation (1278T) in the cystathionine beta-synthase gene prevalent in pyridoxine-responsive homocystinuria and associated with mild clinical phenotype. *Am J Hum Genet* 1995; 57:34–39.

146. Mayer EL, Jacobsen DW, Robinson K. Homocysteine and coronary atherosclerosis. *J Am Coll Cardiol* 1996; 27:517–527.

147. den Heijer M, Koster T, Blom HJ, Bos GMJ, Briet E, Reitsma PH, et al. Hyperhomocysteinemia as a risk factor for deep-vein thrombosis. *N Engl J Med* 1996; 334:759–762.

148. Selhub J, Jacques PF, Wilson PW, Rish D, Rosenberg IH. Vitamin status and intake as primary determinants of homocysteinemia in an elderly population. *JAMA* 1993; 370:2693–2698.

149. Selhub J, Jacques PF, Bostom AG, D'Agostino RB, Wilson PW, Belanger AJ, et al. Association between plasma homocysteine concentrations and extracranial carotid-artery stenosis. *N Engl J Med* 1995; 332:286–291.

150. Tsai J, Wang H, Perrella MA, Yoshizumi M, Sibinga NES, Tan LC, et al. Induction of cyclin a gene expression by homocysteine in vascular smooth muscle cells. *J Clin Invest* 1996; 97:146–153.

151. Lentz SR, Sadler JE. Inhibition of thrombomodulin surface expression and protein C activation by the thrombogenic agent homocysteine. *J Clin Invest* 1991; 88:1906–1914.

152. Landgren F, Israelsson B, Lindgren A, Hultberg B, Andersson A, Brattstrom L. Plasma homocysteine in acute myocardial infarction: Homocysteine-lowering effect of folic acid. *J Intern Med* 1995; 237:381–388.

153. Attardi G. The elucidation of the human mitochondrial genome: A historical perspective. *Bioessays* 1994; 5:34–39.

154. Clarke A. Mitochondrial genome: Defects, disease, and evolution. *J Med Genet* 1990; 27:451–456.

155. Wallace DC. Mitochondrial DNA mutation and neuromuscular disease. *Trends Genet* 1989; 4:9–13.

156. Grivell L. Small, beautiful and essential. *Nature* 1989; 341:569–571.

157. D'Ancona GG, Wurm J, Groce CM. Genetics of type II glycogenosis: Assignment of the human gene for acid a-glucosidase to chromosome 17. *Proc Natl Acad Sci USA* 1979; 76:4526–4529.

158. Mariotti C, Tiranti V, Carrara F, Dallapiccolo B, DiDonato S, Zeviani M. Defective respiratory capacity and mitochondrial protein synthesis of transformant hybrids harboring the tRNA^Leu(UUR) mutation associated with maternally inherited myopathy and cardiomyopathy. *J Clin Invest* 1994; 93:1102–1107.

159. Wallace DC, Zheng X, Lott MT, Shoffner JM, Hodge JA, Kelley RI, et al. Familial mitochondrial encephalomyopathy (MERRF). Genetic, pathophysiological, and biochemical characterization of a mitochondrial DNA disease. *Cell* 1988; 55:601–610.

160. Kobayashi M, Morishita H, Sugiyama N, Yokochi K, Nakano M, Wada Y, et al. Two cases of NADH-coenzyme Q reductase deficiency: Relationship to MELAS syndrome. *J Pediatr* 1987; 110:223–227.

161. Tanaka, Ino H, Ohno K, Hattori K, Sato W, Ozawa T, et al. Mitochondrial mutation in fatal infantile cardiomyopathy. *Lancet* 1990; 1:1452.

162. Papadimitrious A, Neusteon HB, DiMauro S, Stanton R, Bresolin N. Histiocytoid cardiomyopathy of infancy: Deficiency of reducible cytochrome b in heart mitochondria. *Pediatr Res* 1984; 18:1023–1028.

163. DiMauro S, Nicholson JF, Hays AP, Eastwood AB, Papadimitriou A, Koenigsberger R, et al. Benign infantile mitochondrial myopathy due to reversible cytochrome C oxidase deficiency. *Ann Neurol* 1983; 14:226–234.

164. Hatefi Y. The mitochondrial electron transport and oxidative phosphorylation system. *Annu Rev Biochem* 1985; 54:1015–1069.

165. Corral-Debrinski M, Stepien G, Shoffner JM, Lott MT, Kanter K, Wallace DC. Hypoxemia is associated with mitochondrial DNA damage and gene induction: Implications for cardiac disease. *JAMA* 1991; 266:1812–1816.

166. Kearns TP, Sayre GP. Retinitis pigmentosa, external ophthalmoplegia, and complete heart block. *Arch Ophthalmol* 198; 60:280–289.

167. Rowland LP, Blake D, Kirano M, DiMauro S, Schon EA, Hays AP, et al. Clinical syndromes associated with ragged-red fibers. *Rev Neurol* 1991; 147:467–473.

168. Tveskov C, Angelo-Nielsen K. Kearns-Sayre syndrome and dilated cardiomyopathy. *Neurology* 1990; 40:553–554.

169. Fukuhara N, Tokigushi S, Shirakawa K, Tsubaki T. Myoclonus epilepsy associated with ragged-red fibers (mitochondrial abnormalities): Disease entity or syndrome? Light and electron microscopic studies of two cases and review of the literature. *J Neurol Sci* 1980; 47:117–133.

170. Shoffner JM, Lott MI, Lezza AMS, Seibel P, Balliner SW, Wallace DC. Myotonic epilepsy and ragged-red fiber disease (MERRF) is associated with a mitochondrial DNA tRNA^{LYS} mutation. *Cell* 1990; 61:931–937.

171. Pavalakis SG, Phillips PC, DiMauro S, DeVivo DC, Rowland LP. Mitochondrial myopathy, encephalopathy, lactic acidosis, and stroke-like episodes: A distinctive clinical syndrome. *Ann Neurol* 1984; 16:481–487.

172. Byers PH. Disorders of collagen biosynthesis and structure. In: Scriver CR, Beaudett AL, Sly NS, Valle D, eds. *The Metabolic and Molecular Bases of Inherited Disease,* 7th ed. New York: McGraw-Hill; 1995:4039–4078.

173. Tsipouras P, del Mastro R, Sarfarazi M, Lee B, Vitale E, Child AH, et al. Genetic linkage of the Marfan syndrome, ectopiclentis, and congenital contractural arachnodactyly to the fibrillin genes on chromosomes 15 and 5. *N Engl J Med* 1992; 326:905–909.

174. Geva T, Sanders SP, Diogenes MS, Rockenmacher S, Van Praagh R. Two-dimensional and Doppler echocardiographic and pathologic characteristics of the infantile Marfan syndrome. *Am J Cardiol* 1990; 65:1230–1237.

175. Sakai LY, Keene DR, Engvall E. Fibrillin, a new 250-kD glycoprotein, is a component of extracellular microfibrils. *J Cell Biol* 1986; 103:2499–2509.

176. Cross H, Jenson DA. Ocular manifestations of the Marfan syndrome and homocystinuria. *Am J Ophthalmol* 1973; 75:405–420.

177. Shankar KR, Hultgren MK, Lauer RM, Diehl AM. Lethal tricuspid and mitral regurgitation in Marfan's syndrome. *Am J Cardiol* 1967; 20:122–128.

178. Phornphutkul C, Rosenthal A, Nadas AS. Cardiac manifestations of Marfan syndrome in infancy and childhood. *Circulation* 1973; 47:587–596.

179. Day DL, Burke BA. Pulmonary emphysema in a neonate with Marfan syndrome. *Pediatr Radiol* 1986; 16:518–521.

180. Huggon IC, Burke JP, Talbot JF. Contractural arachnodactyly with mitral regurgitation and iridodonesis. *Arch Dis Child* 1990; 65:317–319.

181. Pyeritz RE. Congenital contractual arachnodactyly as a feature of Marfan syndrome (abstr). *Am J Med Genet* 1986; 25:725.

182. Putnam EA, Zhang H, Ramirez F, Milewicz DM. Fibrillin-2 (RBN2) mutations result in the Marfan-like disorder, congenital contractual arachnodactyly. *Nature Genet* 1995; 11:456–458.

183. Eldridge R. The metacarpal index: The useful aid in the diagnosis of Marfan syndrome. *Arch Intern Med* 1964; 113:248–250.

184. Gross DM, Robinson LK, Smith CT, Glass N, Rosenberg H, Duvic M. Severe perinatal Marfan syndrome. *Pediatrics* 1989; 84:83–89.

185. Roberts WC, Honig HS. The spectrum of cardiovascular disease in the Marfan syndrome: A clinico-morphologic study of 18 necropsy patients and comparison to 151 previously reported necropsy patients. *Am Heart J* 1982; 104:115–135.

186. Shores J, Berger KR, Murphy EA, Pyeritz RE. Progression of aortic dilatation and the benefit of long-term beta-adrenergic blockade in Marfan's syndrome. *N Engl J Med* 1994; 330:1335–1341.

187. Gott VL, Pyeritz RE, Magovern GJ, Cameron DE, McKusick VA. Surgical treatment of aneurysms of the ascending aorta in the Marfan syndrome. *N Engl J Med* 198; 314:1070–1074.

188. Gott VL, Gillinov AM, Pyeritz RE, Cameron DE, Reitz BA, Greene PS, et al. Aortic root replacement. Risk factor analysis of a seventeen-year experience with 270 patients. *J Thorac Cardiovasc Surg* 1995; 109:536–544.

189. Pyeritz RE. Maternal and fetal complications in pregnancy in the Marfan syndrome. *Am J Med* 1981; 71:784–790.

190. Tynan K, Comeau K, Pearson M, Wilgengus P, Levitt D, Gasner C, et al. Mutation screening of complete fibrillin-1 coding sequence: Report of five new mutations, including two in 8-cysteine domains. *Hum Mol Genet* 1993; 2:1813–1821.

191. Magenis RE, Maslen CL, Smith L, Allen L, Sakai L. Localization of the fibrillin gene to chromosome 15, band 15q21.1. *Genomics* 1991; 11:346–351.

192. Dietz HC, Cutting GR, Pyeritz RE, Maslen CL, Sakai LY, Corson GM, et al. Marfan syndrome caused by a recurrent de novo missense mutation in the fibrillin gene. *Nature* 1991; 352:337–339.

193. Milewicz DM, Duvic M. Severe neonatal Marfan syndrome resulting from a denovo 3-bp insertion into the fibrillin gene on chromosome 15 *Am J Hum Genet* 1994; 54:447–453.

194. Lonnqvist L, Child A, Kainulainen K, Davidson R, Puhakka L, Peltonen L. A novel mutation of the fibrillin gene causing ectopia lentis. *Genomics* 1994; 19:573–576.

195. Boileau C, Jondeau G, Babron M, Coulon M, Alexandre JA, Sakai L, et al. Autosomal dominant Marfan-like connective tissue disorder with aortic dilation and skeletal anomalies not linked to the fibrillin genes. *Am J Hum Genet* 1993; 53:46–54.

196. Francke U, Berg MA, Tynan K, Brenn T, Liu W, Aoyama T, et al. A Gly1127Ser mutation in an EGF-like domain of the fibrillin-1 gene is a risk factor for ascending aortic aneurysm and dissection. *Am J Hum Genet* 1994; 45:1287–1296.

197. Godfrey M, Vandemark N, Wang M, et al. Prenatal diagnosis and a donor splice site mutation in fibrillin a family with Marfan syndrome. *Am J Hum Genet* 1993; 53:472–480.

198. McKusick VA, ed. *Mendelian Inheritance in man.* Baltimore: Johns Hopkins Press; 1986.

199. Barabas AP. Ehlers-Danlos syndrome: Associated with prematurity and premature rupture of fetal membranes. *Br Med J* 1967; 2:682–684.

200. Byer PH, Holbrook KA, McGillivray B, MacLeod PM, Lowry RB. Clinical and ultrastructural heterogeneity of Type IV Ehlers-Danlos syndrome. *Hum Genet* 1979; 47:141–150.

201. Emanuel BS, Cannizzaro LA, Seyer JM, Myers JC. Human α_1 (III) and α_2 (V) procollagen genes are located on the long arm of chromosome 2. *Proc Natl Acad Sci USA* 1985; 82:3385–3389.

202. Kontusaari S, Tromp G, Kuivaniemi H, Ladda RL, Prockop DJ. Inheritance of an RNA slicing mutation (G^{+1} ^{1V520}) in the type III procollagen gene (COL3A) in a family having aortic aneurysms and Ehlers-Danlos syndrome type IV. *Am J Hum Genet* 1990; 47:112–120.

203. Lee B, D'Alessio M, Vissing H, Ramirez F, Steinmann B, Superti-Furga A. Characterization of a large deletion associated with a polymorphic block of repeated dinucleotides in the Type II procollagen (COL3A1) of a patient with Ehlers-Danlos syndrome Type IV. *Am J Hum Genet* 1990; 47:112–120.

204. Prockop DJ. Mutations in collagen genes as a cause of connective-tissue diseases. *N Engl J Med* 1992; 326:540–546.

205. Kontusaari S, Tromp G, Kuivaniemi H, Romanic AM, Prockop DJ. A mutation in the gene for type II procollagen (COL3A1) in a family with aortic aneurysms. *J Clin Invest* 190; 86:1465–1473.

206. MacSweeney ST, Skidmore C, Turner RJ, Sian M, Brown L, Henney AM, et al. Unravelling the familial tendency to aneurysmal disease; Popliteal aneurysm, hypertension and fibrillin genotype. *Eur J Vasc Endovasc Surg* 1996; 12:162–166.

207. McMillan WD, Patterson BK, Keen RR, Shively VP, Cipollone M, Pearce WH. In situ localization and quantification of mRNA for 92-kD type IV collagenase and its inhibitor in aneurysmal, occlusive, and normal aorta. *Athero Thromb Vasc Biol* 1965; 15:1139–1144.

208. Thromp G, Wu Y, Prockop DJ, Madhatheri SL, Kleinert C, Earley JJ, et al. Sequencing of cDNA from 50 unrelated patients reveals that mutations in the triple-helical domain of type II procollagen are an infrequent cause of aortic aneurysms. *J Clin Invest* 1993; 91:2539–2545.

209. Deak SB, Ricotta JJ, Mariani TJ, Deak ST, Zatina MA, Mackenzie JW, et al. The role of abnormal type II collagen in the development of common aneurysms. *J Vasc Surg* 1992; 15:926–927.

210. Kuivaniemi H, Tromp G, Prockop DJ. Genetic causes of aortic aneurysms: Unlearning at least part of what the textbooks say. *J Clin Invest* 1991; 88:1441–1444.

211. Kuivaniemi H, Kontusaari S, Stolle C, Pope FM, Prockop DJ. Identical G^{+1} to A mutations in three different introns of the type III procollagen gene (COL3A1) produce different patterns of RNA splicing in three variants of Ehlers-Danlos syndrome IV: An explanation for exon skipping with some mutations and not others. *J Biol Chem* 1990; 265:12067–12074.

212. Pyeritz RE, Moller JH. Heritable disorders of connective tissue. In: Pierpont MD, ed. *The Genetics of Cardiovascular Disease.* Boston: Martinus-Nijhoff, 1987:265.

213. Challenor VF, Conway N, Munro JL. The surgical treatment of restrictive cardiomyopathy in pseudoxanthoma elasticum. *Br Heart J* 1988; 59:266–269.

214. Pyeritz RE, Weiss JL, Renie WE, Fine SL. Pseudoxanthoma elasticum and mitral-valve prolapse. *N Engl J Med* 1982; 307:1451–1452.

215. Weir EK, Joffe HS, Blaufuss AH, Beighton P. Cardiovascular abnormalities in cutis laxa. *Eur J Cardiol* 1977; 5:255–261.

216. Romano C. Congenital cardiac arrhythmia. *Lancet* 1965; 1:658–659.

217. Ward OC. A new familial cardiac syndrome in children. *J Indian Med Assoc* 1964; 54:103–106.

218. Schwartz PJ, Bonazzi O, Locati E, Napditano C, Sala S. Pathogenesis and therapy of the idiopathic long QT syndrome. In: Hashiba K, Moss AJ, Schwartz PJ, eds. *QT Prolongation and Ventricular Arrhythmias.* New York: New York Academy of Science; 1992:112–141.

219. Schwartz PJ, Moss AJ, Vincent GM, Crampton RS. Diagnostic criteria for the long QT syndrome: An update. *Circulation* 1993; 88:782–784.

220. Keating M, Dunn C, Atkinson D, Timothy K, Vincent GM, Leppert M. Consistent linkage of the long-QT syndrome to the Harvey ras-1 locus on chromosome 11. *Am J Hum Genet* 1991; 49:1335–139.

221. Towbin JA, Li H, Taggart RT, Lehmann MH, Schwartz PJ, Satler CA, et al. Evidence of genetic heterogeneity in Romano-Ward long QT syndrome. Analysis of 23 families. *Circulation* 1994; 90:2635–2644.

222. Jiang C, Atkinson D, Towbin JA, Splawski I, Lehmann MH, Li H, et al. Two long-QT syndrome loci map to chromosome 3 and 7 with evidence for further heterogeneity. *Nature Genet* 1994; 8:141–147.

223. Schott J, Carpentier F, Peltier S, Foley P, Drouin E, Bouhour JB, et al. Mapping of a gene for long QT syndrome to chromosome 4q25-27. *Am J Hum Genet* 1995; 57:1114–1122.

224. Curran ME, Splawski I, Timothy KW, Vincent GM, Green ED, Keating MT. A molecular basis for cardiac arrhythmia: HERG mutations cause long QT syndrome. *Cell* 1995; 80:795–803.

225. Hall JG: CATCH 22. *J Med Genet* 1993; 3::801–802.

226. Wang Q, Curran ME, Splawski I, Burn TC, Millholland JM, VanRaay TJ, et al. Positional cloning of a novel potassium channel gene: KVLQT1 mutations cause cardiac arrhythmias. *Nature Genet* 1996; 12:17–23.

227. Towbin JA. New revelation about the long-QT syndrome. *N Engl J Med* 1995; 333:384–385.

228. Moss AJ, Zareba W, Benhorin J, Locati EH, Hall WJ, Robinson JL, et al. Electrocardiographic T-wave patterns in genetically distinct forms of the hereditary long-QT syndrome. *Circulation* 1995; 92:2929–2934.

229. Vincent GM, Timothy KW, Leppert M, Keating M. The spectrum of symptoms and QT intervals in carriers of the gene for the long-QT syndrome. *N Engl J Med* 1992; 327:846–852.

230. Roden DM, Lazzara R, Rosen M, Schwartz PJ, Towbin J, Vincent GM. Multiple mechanisms in the long-QT syndrome. Current knowledge, gaps, and future directions. *Circulation* 1996; 94:1996–2012.

231. Schwartz PJ, Priori SG, Loctai EH. Long QT syndrome patients with mutations of the SCN5A and HERG genes have differential responses to Na^+ channel blockade and to increases in heart rate. Implications for gene-specific therapy. *Circulation* 1995; 92:3373–3375.

232. Compton SJ, Lux RL, Ramsey MR, Strelich KR, Sanguinetti MC, Green LS, et al. Genetically defined therapy of inherited long-QT syndrome: Correction of abnormal repolarization by potassium. *Circulation* 1996; 94:1018–1022.

233. An RH, Bangalore R, Rosero SZ, Kass RS. Lidocaine block of LQT-3 mutant human Na^+ channels. *Circ Res* 1996; 79:103–108.

234. Jervell A, Lange-Nielsen F. Congenital deaf-mutism, functional heart disease with prolongation of the Q-T interval and sudden death. *Am Heart J* 1957; 54:59–78.

235. Fraser GR, Froggatt P, Murphy T. Genetical aspects of the cardio-auditory electrocardiographic abnormalities. *Ann Hum Genet* 1964; 28:133–135.

236. Brugada R, Tapscott T, Czernuszewicz GZ, Marian AJ, Iglesias A, Mont L, et al. Identification of a genetic locus for familial atrial fibrillation. *N Engl J Med* 1997; 336:905–911.

237. Wolff L, Parkinson J, White PD. Bundle branch block with short PR interval in healthy young people prone to paroxysmal tachycardia. *Am Heart J* 1930; 5:686–704.

238. Vidaillet HJ Jr, Pressley JC, Henke E, Harrell FE Jr, German LD. Familial occurrence of accessory atrioventricular pathways (preexcitation syndrome). *N Engl J Med* 1987; 317:65–69.

239. Gillette PC, Freed D, McNamara DG. A proposed autosomal dominant method of inheritance of the Wolff-Parkinson-White syndrome and supraventricular tachycardia. *J Pediatr* 1978; 93:257–258.

240. Brink AJ, Torrington M. Progressive familial heart block—two types. *S Afr Med J* 1977; 52:53–59.

241. Waxman MB, Catching JD, Felderhof CH, Downar E, Silver MD, Abbot MM. Familial atrioventricular heart block. An autosomal dominant trait. *Circulation* 1975; 51:226–233.

242. Amat-y-Leon F, Racki AJ, Denes P, Ten Eick RE, Singer DH, Bharati S, et al. Familial atrial dysrhythmia with A-V block: Intracellular microelectrode, clinical electrophysiologic, and morphologic observations. *Circulation* 1974; 50:1097–1104.

243. Sarachek NS, Leonard JJ. Familial heart block and sinus bradycardia: Classification and natural history. *Am J Cardiol* 1972; 29:451–458.

244. Graber HL, Unverferth DV, Baker PB, Ryan JM, Baba N, Wooley CF. Evolution of a hereditary cardiac conduction and muscle disorder: A study involving a family with six generations affected. *Circulation* 1986; 74:21–35.

245. Greenlee PR, Anderson JL, Lutz JR, Lindsay AE, Hagan AD. Familial automaticity-conduction disorder with associated cardiomyopathy. *West J Med* 1996; 144:33–41.

246. Brink PA, Ferreira A, Moolman JC, Weymar HW, van der Merwe PL, Corfield VA. Gene for progressive familial heart block type I maps to chromosome 19q13. *Circulation* 1995; 91:1633–1640.

247. Pease WE, Nordenberg A, Ladda RL. Genetic counseling in familial atrial septal defect with prolonged atrioventricular conduction. *Circulation* 1976; 53:759–762.

248. Sherman J, Angulo M, Boxer RA, Gluck R. Possible mitochondrial inheritance of congenital cardiac septal defects. *N Engl J Med* 1985; 313:186–187.

249. Smith AT, Sack GH, Taylor GJ. Holt-Oram syndrome. *J Pediatr* 1979; 95:538–543.

250. Bonnet D, Pelet A, Legeai-Mallet L, Sidi D, Mathieu M, Parent P, et al. A gene for Holt-Oram syndrome maps to the distal long arm of chromosome 12. *Nature Genet* 1994; 6:405–408.

251. Basson CT, Cowley GS, Solomon SD, Weissman B, Poznanski AK, Traill TA, et al. The clinical and genetic spectrum of the Holt-Oram syndrom (heart-hand syndrome). *N Engl J Med* 1994; 330:885–891.

252. Basson CT, Bachinski DR, Lin RC, Levi T, Elkins JA, Soults J, et al. Mutations in humans cause limb and cardiac malformation in Holt-Oram syndrome. *Nature Genet* 1997; 15:30–35.

253. Li QY, Newbury-Ecog RA, Terrett JA, Wilson DI, Curtis ARJ, Yi CH, et al. Holt-Oram syndrome is caused by mutations in TBX5, a member of the *Brachyury (T)* gene family. *Nature Genet* 1997; 15:21–29.

254. Becroft DMO, Chambers D. Supravalvular aortic stenosis–infantile hypercalcaemia syndrome: In vitro hypersensitivity to vitamin D_2 and calcium. *J Med Genet* 1976; 13:223–228.

255. Preus M. The Williams syndrome. Objective definition and diagnosis. *Clin Genet* 1984; 25:422–428.

256. Hallidie-Smith KA, Karas S. Cardiac anomalies in Williams-Beuren syndrome. *Arch Dis Child* 1988; 63:809–813.

257. Burn J. Williams syndrome. *J Med Genet* 1986; 23:389–395.

258. O'Connor WN, Davis JB, Geissler R, Cottril CM, Noonan JA, Todd EP. Supravalvular aortic stenosis: Clinical and pathological observations in six patients. *Arch Pathol Lab Med* 1985; 109:179–185.

259. Chiarella F, Bricarelli FD, Lupe G. Familial supravalvular aortic stenosis: A genetic study. *J Med Genet* 1989; 26:86–89.

260. Schmidt MA, Ensing GJ, Carter GA, Hagler DJ, Feldt RH. Autosomal dominant supravalvular aortic stenosis: Large three-generation family. *Am J Med Genet* 1989; 32:384–389.

261. Enging GJ, Schmidt MA, Hagler DJ, Michels VV, Carter GA, Feldt RH. Spectrum of findings in a family with nonsyndromic autosomal dominant supravalvular aortic stenosis: A Doppler echocardiographic study. *J Am Coll Cardiol* 1989; 13:413–416.

262. Ewart AK, Morris CA, Atkinson D, Jin W, Sternes K, Spallone P, et al. Hemizygosity at the elastin locus in developmental disorders, Williams syndrome. *Nature Genet* 1993; 5:11–16.

263. Nickerson E, Greenberg F, Keating MT, McCaskill C, Shaffer LG. Deletions of the elastin gene at 7q11.23 occur in about 90% of patients with Williams syndrome. *Am J Hum Genet* 1995; 56:1156–1161.

264. Olson TM, Michels VV, Lindor N, Pastores GM, Weber JL, Schad DJ, et al. Autosomal dominant supravalvular aortic stenosis: Localization to chromosome 7. *Hum Mol Genet* 1993; 2:869–873.

265. Morris CA, Loker J, Ensing G, Stock AD. Supravalvular aortic stenosis cosegregates with a familial 6:7 translocation which disrupts the elastin gene. *Am J Med Genet* 1993; 46:737–744.

266. Curran M, Atkinson D, Ewart A, Morris C, Leppert M, Keating MT. The elastin gene is disrupted by a translocation associated with supravalvular aortic stenosis. *Cell* 1993; 73:159–168.

267. Noonan JA, Ehmke DA. Associated noncardiac malformations in children with congenital heart disease. *J Pediatr* 1963; 63:468–470.

268. Allanson JE. Noonan syndrome. *J Med Genet* 1987; 24:9–13.

269. Sharland M, Burch M, McKenna WM, Paton MA. A clinical study of Noonan syndrome. *Arch Dis Child* 1992; 67:178–183.

270. Van der Hauwaert LG, Fryns JM, Dumoulin M, Logghe N. Cardiovascular malformations in Turner's and Noonan's syndrome. *Br Heart J* 1978; 40:500–509.

271. Jamieson CR, van der Burgt I, Brady AF, van Reen M, Elsawi MM, Hol F, et al. Mapping a gene for Noonan syndrome to the long arm of chromosome 12. *Nature Genet* 1994; 8:357–360.

272. Konishi Y, Ito M, Okuno T, Hojo H, Okuda R, Nakano Y, et al. Tuberous sclerosis: Early neurological manifestations and CT features in 18 patients. *Brain Dev* 1979; 1:31–37.

273. Tsakraklides V, Burke B, Mastri A, Ronge W, Rose E, Anderson R. Rhabdomyomas of heart. A report of four cases. *Am J Dis Child* 1974; 128:639–646.

274. Jayakar PB, Stanwick RS, Seshia SS. Tuberous sclerosis and Wolff-Parkinson-White syndrome. *J Pediatr* 1986; 108:259–260.

275. Murrell J, Troffatter J, Rutter M, Cutone S, Stotler C, Rutter J, et al. A 500-kilobase region containing the tuberous sclerosis locus (TSC1) in a 1.7 megabase YAC and cosmid cloning. *Genomics* 1995 25:59–65.

276. Olsson PG, Sutherland HF, Nowicka U, Korn B, Poustka A, Frischauf AM. The mouse homologue of the tuberin gene (TSC2) maps to a conserved syntheny group between mouse chromosome 17 and human chromosome 16p13.3. *Genomics* 1995; 25:339–340.

277. Weinstein BM, Stemple DL, Driever W, Fishman MC. Gridlock, a localized heritable vascular patterning defect in the zebrafish. *Nature Med* 1995; 1:1143–1147.

278. Towbin JA, McQuinn TC. Gridlock: A model for coarctation of the aorta? *Nature Med* 1995; 1:1141–1142.

279. Zlotogora J, Elian E. Asplenia and polysplenia syndromes with abnormalities of lateralization in a sibship. *J Med Genet* 1981; 18:301–302.

280. Nikawa N, Kohsaka S, Mizumoto M, Hamada I, Kajii T. Familial clustering of situs inversus totalis, and asplenia and polysplenia syndromes. *Am J Med Genet* 1983; 16:43–47.

281. Arnold GL, Bixler D, Girod D. Probable autosomal recessive inheritance of polysplenia, situs inversus and cardiac defects in an Amish family. *Am J Med Genet* 1983; 16:35–42.

282. Mathis RS, Lacro RV, Jones KL. X-linked laterality sequence: Situs inversus, complex cardiac defects, splenic defects. *Am J Med Genet* 1987; 28:111–16.

283. Rose V, Izukawa T, Moes CA. Syndromes of asplenia and polysplenia: A review of cardiac and noncardiac malformations in 60 cases with special reference to diagnosis and prognosis. *Br Heart J* 1987; 37:840–852.

284. Seo J, Brown HA, Ho SY, Anderson RH. Abnormal laterality and congenital cardiac anomalies: Relations of visceral and cardiac morphologies in the iv/iv mouse. *Circulation* 1991; 86:642–650.

285. Yokoyama T, Copeland NG, Jenkins NA, Montgomery CA, Elder FFB, Overbeek PA. Reversal of left-right asymmetry: A situs inversus mutation. *Science* 1993; 260:679–682.

286. Britz-Cunningham SH, Shah MM, Zuppan CW, Fletcher WH. Mutations of the *Connexin43* gap-junction gene in patients with heart malformations and defects of laterality. *N Engl J Med* 1995; 332:1323–1329.

287. Reaume AG, de Sousa P, Kulkarni S, Langille BL, Zhu D, Davies TC, et al. Cardiac malformation in neonatal mice lacking connexin 43. *Science* 1995; 267:1831–1834.

288. Towbin JA, Greenberg F. Genetic syndromes and clinical molecular genetics. In: Bricker JT, Garson A Jr, Fisher DJ, Neish SR, eds. *The Science and Practice of Pediatric Cardiology*. Baltimore: Williams & Wilkins; 1997:In press

289. Nora JJ, Nora AH. Recurrence risks in children having one parent with congenital heart disease. *Circulation* 1976; 53:701–702.

290. Rose VR, Gold RJM, Lindsay G, Allen M. A possible increase in the incidence of congenital heart defects among the offspring of affected parents. *J Am Coll Cardiol* 1985; 6:376–382.

291. Ferencz C, Neill C, Boughman J, Rubin JDA, Brenner JI, Perry LW. Congenital cardiovascular malformations associated with chromosome abnormalities: An epidemiologic study. *J Pediatr* 1989 114:79–86.

292. Emanuel BS. Molecular cytogenetics: Toward dissection of the contiguous gene syndromes. *Am J Hum Genet* 1988; 43:575–578.

293. Yunis JJ. High resolution of human chromosomes. *Science* 1976; 191:1268–1270.

294. Yunis JJ. Mid-prophase human chromosomes. The attainment of 2000 bands. *Hum Genet* 1981; 56:293–298.

295. deGrouchy J, Turleau C, eds. *Clinical Atlas of Human Chromosome*. New York: Wiley; 1984.

296. Schinzel AP, ed. *Catalogue of Unbalanced Chromosome Aberrations in Man*. New York: Walter de Gruyter; 1984.

297. Roche KB, Moore JW, Surana RB, Wilson BE. Aortic root dilatation associated with partial trisomy 7 (q31.2-qter). *Pediatr Cardiol* 1989; 10:53–55.

298. Tiller GE, Watson MS, Duncan LM, Dowton SB. Congenital heart defect in a patient with deletion of chromosome 7q. *Am J Med Genet* 1988; 29:283–287.

299. Talley JD, Dooley KJ, Tuboku-Metzger A, Burgess GH, Wilcox WD, Click LA, et al. The cardiovascular abnormalities associated with duplicated segments of chromosome 7. *Clin Cardiol* 1989; 12:227–232.

300. Korenberg JR, Kawashima H, Pulst S-M, Ikeuchi T, Ogasawara N, Yamamoto K, et al. Molecular definition of a region of chromosome 21 that causes features of the Down syndrome phenotype. *Am J Hum Genet* 1990; 47:236–246.

301. Summit RL. Specific segments that cause the phenotype Down syndrome. In: de la Cruz FF, Gerald PS, eds. *Research Perspectives*. Baltimore: University Park Press; 1981:225.

302. Mikkelsen M, Stene J. Genetic counseling in Down's syndrome. *Hum Hered* 1970; 20:457–464.

303. Nora JJ, Nora AH. Update on counseling the family with a first-degree relative with a congenital heart defect. *Am J Med Genet* 1988; 27:137–140.

304. Clapp S, Perry BL, Farook ZG, Jackson WL, Karpawich PP, Hakimi M, et al. Down's syndrome, complete atrioventricular canal, and pulmonary vascular obstructive disease. *J Thorac Cardiovasc Surg* 1990; 100:115–118.

305. Gerald PS. Sex chromosome disorders. *N Engl J Med* 1976; 294:706–710.

306. Palmer CG, Reichmann A. Chromosomal and clinical findings in 110 females with Turner syndrome. *Hum Genet* 1976; 35:35–49.

307. Allen DB, Hendricks SA, Levy JM. Aortic dilation in Turner syndrome. *J Pediatr* 1986; 109:302–305.

308. Moore JS, Kirby WC, Rogers WM, Poth MA. Partial anomalous pulmonary venous drainage associated with 45,X Turner's syndrome. *Pediatrics* 1990; 86:273–276.

309. DiGeorge AM. Discussions on a new concept of the cellular base of immunology. *J Pediatr* 1965; 67:907–908.

310. Conley ME, Beckwith JB, Mancer JFK, Tenckhoff L. The spectrum of the DiGeorge syndrome. *J Pediatr* 1979; 94:883–890.

311. Kelley RI, Zackai EH, Emanuel BS, Kistenmacher M, Greenberg F, Punnett H. The association of the DiGeorge anomalad with partial monosomy of chromosome 22. *J Pediatr* 1982; 101:197–200.

312. Lindsay EA, Halford S, Wedey R, Scambler PJ, Baldini A. Molecular cytogenetic characterization of the DiGeorge syndrome using fluorescence in situ hybridization. *Genomics* 1993; 17:403–407.

313. Greenberg F, Elder FFB, Haffner P, Northrup H, Ledbetter DH. Cytogenetic findings in a prospective series of patients with DiGeorge anomaly. *Am J Hum Genet* 1988; 43:605–611.

314. Budarf ML, Collins J, Gong W, Roe B, Wang Z, Bailey LC, et al. Cloning a balanced translocation associated with DiGeorge syndrome and identification of a disrupted candidate gene. *Nature Genet* 1994; 10:269–278.

315. Gong W, Emanuel BS, Collins J, Kim DH, Wang Z, Chen R, et al. A transcription map of the DiGeorge and velo-cardio-facial syndrome minimal critical region on 22q11. *Hum Mol Genet* 1996; 5:789–800.

316. Shprintzen RJ, Goldberg RB, Young D, Wolford L. The velo-cardio-facial syndrome: A clinical and genetic analysis. *Pediatrics* 1981; 67:167–172.

317. Burn JA, Takao A, Wilson D, Cross I, Momma K, Wadey R, et al. Conotruncal anomaly face syndrome is associated with a deletion within chromosome 22q11. *J Med Genet* 1993; 30:822–824.

318. Williams MA, Shprintzen RJ, Goldberg RB. Male-to-male transmission of the velo-cardio-facial syndrome: A case report and review of 60 cases. *J Craniofac Genet Dev Biol* 1985; 5:175–180.

319. Young D, Shprintzen RJ, Goldberg RB. Cardiac malformations in the velo-cardiao-facial syndrome. *Am J Cardiol* 1980; 46:643–648.

320. Kiinouchi A, Mori K, Ando M, Takao A. Facial appearance of patients with conotruncal abnormalities. *Pediatr Jpn* 1976:84–86.

70

THE PATHOLOGY, PATHOPHYSIOLOGY, RECOGNITION, AND TREATMENT OF CONGENITAL HEART DISEASE

Michael D. Freed / William H. Plauth, Jr.

INCIDENCE AND ETIOLOGY

The incidence of congenital heart disease in the United States is approximately 8 per 1000 live births.[1,2] Many of the infants born alive with cardiac defects have anomalies that do not represent a threat to life, at least during infancy. Almost one-third, or 2.6 per 1000 live births, however, have critical disease, defined as a malformation severe enough to result in cardiac catheterization, cardiac surgery, or death within the first year of life.[3] Today, with early detection and proper management, the majority of infants with critical disease can be expected to survive the first year of life.[3] Most who now survive infancy will join the increasingly large cohort of adults with congenital heart disease.

Estimates of the incidence of specific lesions vary, depending on whether the data are drawn from infants or older children and whether the diagnosis is based on clinical, catheterization, surgical, or postmortem studies.[1–4] The incidence in other countries is remarkably similar to that reported for the United States.[5,6]

Despite these differences in case material, except for bicuspid aortic valve and mitral valve prolapse, it is apparent that ventricular septal defect (VSD) is the most common malformation, occurring in 28 percent of all patients with congenital heart disease (Table 70-1).

Of 2251 infants with critical congenital heart disease in the New England Regional Infant Cardiac Program,[3] 53.7 percent were male. Certain defects, however, are considerably more common in one sex than in the other.

While previous theories concerning the etiology of congenital heart diseases suggested that most defects were multifactorial, that is, the malformations were caused by a combination of a hereditary predisposition (presumably caused by abnormalities in the genetic code) and an environmental trigger,[7] more recent advances in molecular biology suggest a much higher percentage are caused by point mutations.[8]

Some abnormalities are caused by chromosomal aberrations (see Chap. 69). Trisomy 21 (Down's syndrome) is highly associated with complete atrioventricular (AV) canal, VSDs, and tetralogy of Fallot, and children with Turner's syndrome (XO) frequently have coarctation of the aorta. Other anomalies are caused by teratogens: VSD in fetal alcohol syndrome, Epstein's disease in a fetus with prenatal exposure to lithium, and patent ductus arteriosus (PDA) in mothers who contracted rubella during the first trimester are examples.

Some syndromes are inherited as single-gene defects and have congenital heart disease as one of the manifestations. Holt-Oram syndrome, an association of radial limb abnormalities and atrial septal defects (ASDs), has been mapped to the long arm of chromosome 12, and the DiGeorge syndrome, associated with abnormalities of the conotruncus resulting in truncus arteriosus or interrupted aortic arch, has been found to be due to a deletion on the 22 chromosome[9] (see Chap. 69).

It is clear now that a higher proportion of congenital heart disease than previously thought is due to single-gene defects and that types of congenital heart disease and the same malformation may be caused by mutant genes at different loci.[8] With increasing knowledge of molecular mechanisms, it

TABLE 70-1

INCIDENCE OF SPECIFIC
CONGENITAL HEART DEFECTS

Defect	Percentage of Cases[a] Averaged
Ventricular septal defect	28.3
Pulmonary stenosis	9.5
Patent ductus arteriosus	8.7
Ventricular septal defect with pulmonary stenosis[b]	6.8
Atrial septal defect, secundum	6.7
Aortic stenosis	4.4
Coarctation of aorta	4.2
Atrioventricular canal[c]	3.5
Transposition of great arteries	3.4
Aortic atresia	2.4
Truncus arteriosus	1.6
Tricuspid atresia	1.2
Total anomalous pulmonary venous connection	1.1
Double-outlet right ventricle	0.8
Pulmonary atresia without ventricular septal defect	0.3

[a] Total number of cases = 103,590.
[b] Includes tetralogy of Fallot.
[c] Includes partial and complete.
Source: Refs. 1–3, 5, 6.

seems inevitable that the etiology and pathogenesis of congenital heart disease will be increasingly clarified in the years ahead.

FETAL CIRCULATION AND THE TRANSITION TO NEONATAL AND ADULT CIRCULATION

The fetus obtains all metabolic necessities including oxygen from the placenta. The fetal circulation is an adaptation so that most of the right ventricular output bypasses the lungs and goes instead to the placenta to pick up oxygen. Most of our understanding of this adaptation comes from more than 40 years of research,[10–18] primarily on fetal lambs. The fetal circulation is arranged in parallel rather than in series, with mixing at the atrial (foramen ovale) and great vessel (ductus arteriosus) level (Fig. 70-1). Normally, blood returning from the body goes in the right atrium via the superior vena cava or inferior vena cava. Inferior vena cava blood is diverted by the crista dividens so that approximately 27 percent of combined ventricular output passes through the foramen ovale into the left atrium, with the remainder passing through the tricuspid valve to the right ventricle. Left atrial return is mixed with blood returning from the lungs into the left ventricle and then to the ascending aorta, where it goes to the coronary arteries, head, and upper body vessels, with a small proportion going across the arch into the descending aorta. Right ventricu-

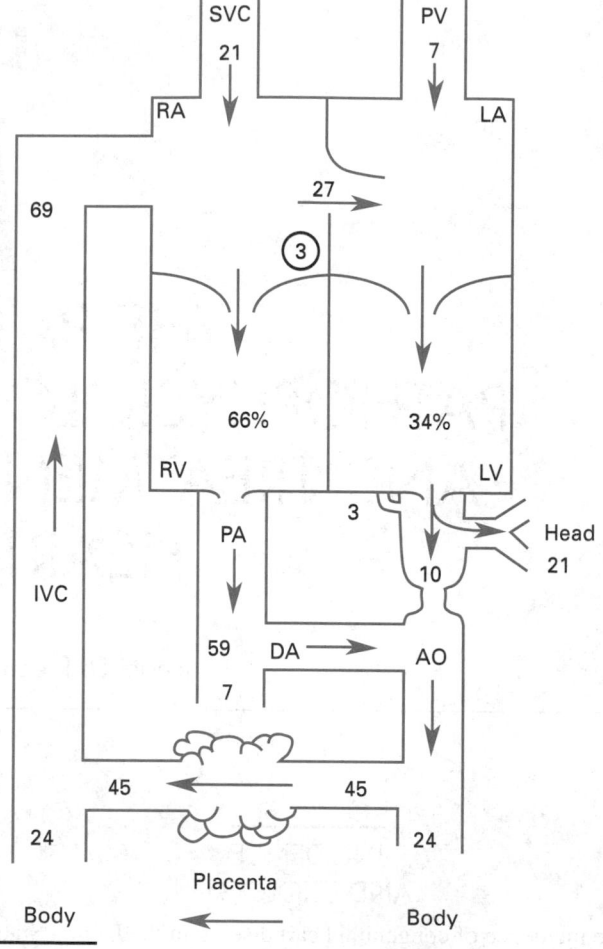

FIGURE 70-1

The course of the circulation in the late-gestation fetal lamb. *The numbers represent the percentage of combined ventricular output.* Some of the return from the inferior vena cava (IVC) is diverted by the crista dividens in the right atrium (RA) through the foramen ovale into the left atrium (LA), where it meets the pulmonary venous return (PV), passes into the left ventricle (LV), and is pumped into the ascending aorta. Most of the ascending aortic flow goes to the coronary, subclavian, and carotid arteries, with only 10 percent of combined ventricular output passing through the aortic arch (indicated by the narrowed point in the aorta) into the descending aorta (AO). The remainder of the inferior vena cava flow mixes with the return from the superior vena cava (SVC) and coronary veins, passes into the right atrium and right ventricle (RV), and is pumped into the pulmonary artery (PA). Because of the high pulmonary resistance, only 7 percent passes through the lungs (PV), with the rest going into the ductus arteriosus (DA) and then to the descending aorta (AO), the placenta, and the lower half of the body. (From Freed MD. Fetal and transitional circulation. In: Fyler DC, ed. *Nadas' Pediatric Cardiology.* Philadelphia: Hanley & Belfus; 1992. Reproduced with permission from the publisher and author.)

lar blood passes out of the pulmonary artery, where approximately 90 percent (59 percent of combined ventricular output) is diverted through the ductus arteriosus into the descending aorta by the elevated pulmonary vascular resistance. Thus, approximately two-thirds of the blood passes through the right side of the heart, and one-third through the left side of the heart.

The oxygen saturation of the fetal blood is considerably lower than that of the newborn or infant because of the lower efficiency of the placenta compared to the lungs as an organ for oxygen exchange (Fig. 70-2). The blood with the highest saturation (approximately 70 percent) is that returning from the placenta. Some of this higher-saturation blood is diverted across the foramen ovale so the saturation on the left side of the heart (65 percent) is somewhat higher than on the right side (55 percent). This allows diversion of the lowest-saturation blood (~55 percent) through the ductus arteriosus to the placenta, increasing the efficiency of oxygen pickup. An additional fetal adaptation to oxygen transport at low oxygen saturation is the presence of high levels of fetal hemoglobin with a higher affinity for oxygen than normal hemoglobin. This leftward shift of the oxygen dissociation curve facilitates oxygen uptake at the relatively low P_{O_2} of the placenta vasculature.

The wide communication at the atrial level (foramen ovale) allows for near equalization of atrial and ventricular end-diastolic pressures. The wide communication at the great vessel

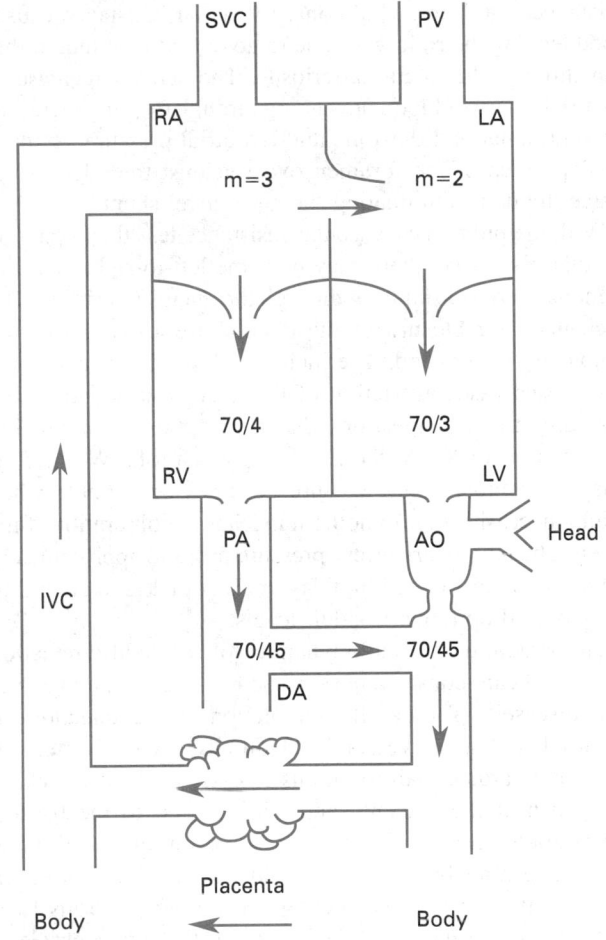

FIGURE 70-3

The numbers indicate the pressures observed in late gestation lambs. Because large communications between the atrium and great vessels are present, the pressures on both sides of the heart are virtually identical. The abbreviations are the same as in Fig. 70-1. (From Freed MD. Fetal and transitional circulation. In: Fyler DC, ed. *Nadas' Pediatric Cardiology*. Philadelphia: Hanley & Belfus; 1992. Reproduced with permission from the publisher and author.)

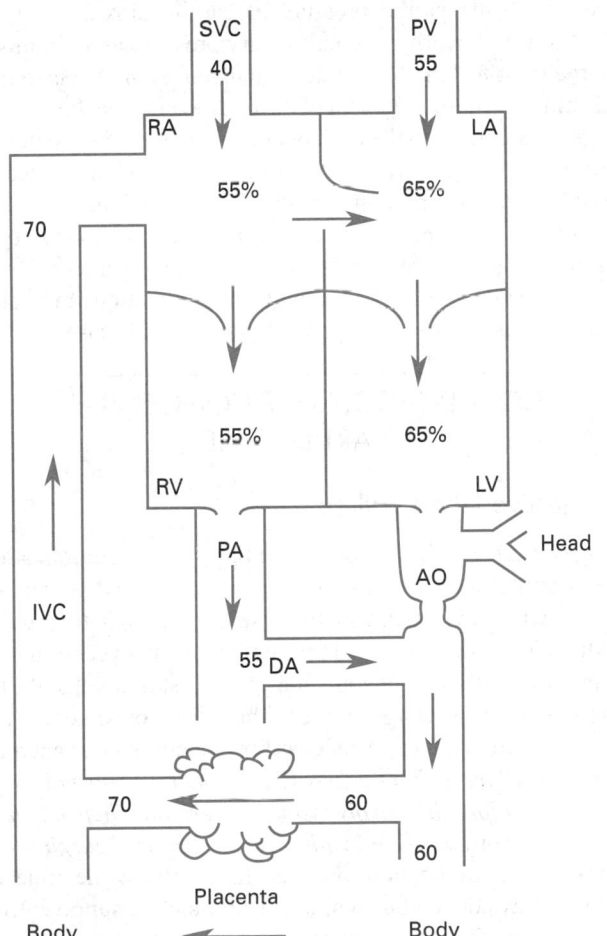

FIGURE 70-2

The numbers indicate the percent of oxygen saturation in the late-gestation lamb. The oxygen saturation is highest in the inferior vena cava, representing that primarily from the placenta. The saturation of blood in the heart is slightly higher on the left side than the right side. The abbreviations in this diagram are the same as in Fig. 70-1. (From Freed MD. Fetal and transitional circulation. In: Fyler DC, ed. *Nadas' Pediatric Cardiology*. Philadelphia: Hanley & Belfus; 1992. Reproduced with permission from the publisher and author.)

level (ductus arteriosus) allows equalization of systolic pressures in the aorta and pulmonary artery and, in the absence of aortic or pulmonic stenosis, at the ventricular level (Fig. 70-3).

Within a few moments of birth, the circulatory physiology must switch rapidly from the placenta to the lung as the organ of oxygen exchange. Failure of any one of a number of a complex series of pulmonary and cardiac events may result in cerebral and then generalized hypoxemia, with lasting damage or death. With the onset of spontaneous respiration, the lungs are expanded and the pulmonary arterioles, which have probably been actively vasoconstricted, dilate. The reduction in pulmonary vascular resistance results from both simple physical expansion of the lung with the onset of respiration and the vasodilation of the pulmonary resistance vessels, probably in part due to the high level of oxygen in alveolar gas. Simultaneously, the placenta is removed from the circulation, either by clamping the umbilical cord or by constriction of the umbilical arteries. This sudden increase in systemic vascular resistance and drop in pulmonary vascular resistance causes blood leaving the right ventricle to go out into the lung rather than through the ductus arteriosus. The sudden increase in left atrial return of blood now going through the lung increases left ventricular end-diastolic and left atrial pressure, shutting the flap valve of the foramen ovale against the edge of the cristae dividens, eliminating the atrial level shunt.

With the pulmonary vascular resistance less than systemic vascular resistance, there may be some left-to-right (aorta to pulmonary artery) shunting through the ductus arteriosus. The mechanism for closure of the ductus arteriosus is still not completely understood. The increased level of oxygen probably causes vasoconstriction of the ductus musculature, but there are strong suggestions that a reduction in circulating prostaglandins (PG) of the E series plays a role. Within 3 or 4 days, the biochemical closure becomes irreversible when cellular necrosis of the endothelium leads to obliteration of the lumen. The pulmonary artery pressure drops to approximately half systemic levels within a day or so but takes another 2 to 6 weeks to drop down to adult levels.

The structure and hemodynamics of the field circulation have significant consequences in the neonate with congenital heart disease.[19] The parallel circulation with connections at the atrial and great vessel level allows a wide variety of congenital cardiac malformations to exist while still picking up oxygen at the placenta and delivering it to the tissues. For example, atresia of the tricuspid or mitral valve, while devastating after birth, does not have a significant effect in utero. Furthermore, since the right ventricle performs two-thirds of the cardiac work before birth, the left ventricle is underloaded, possibly explaining why congestive heart failure is seen not uncommonly with congenital defects. Finally, because the normal flow across the aortic isthmus is relatively small (only about 10 percent of combined ventricular output), this area is especially vulnerable to small changes in flow across the foramen ovale. A somewhat small foramen may result in left-sided hypoplasia, almost always associated with narrowing (coarctation) or atresia (interrupted), at the distal transverse aorta just proximal to ductal insertion.

Since the pulmonary blood flow in utero is less than 10 percent of combined ventricular output and increases four to five times at birth, anomalies obstructing pulmonary venous return may be masked in utero when the pulmonary venous return is low. The low circulating levels of oxygen before birth (P_{O_2} 26 to 38 mmHg) with the saturation at 50 to 60 percent may account for the relative level of comfort in infants with cyanotic heart disease, who may do well, at least in the short run, with a P_{O_2} of 30 mmHg and an aortic saturation of 50 percent, a level that would lead to cerebral and cardiac anoxia, acidosis, and death within a few minutes for the older child and adult.

Persistence of Fetal Circulation

Persistence of fetal circulation[20,21] or persistent pulmonary hypertension in the newborn results in right-to-left shunting through the patent foramen ovale and/or PDA. It most commonly occurs in full-term infants. Severe hypoxia is usually manifested in the first few hours of life with tachypnea and acidosis, and a chest roentgenogram shows diminished vascular flow but no evidence of pulmonary parenchymal disease. Physical examination may reveal a parasternal heave, a loud second heart sound, and a systolic murmur.

Polycythemia, transient myocardial ischemia from hypoglycemia, and cyanotic congenital cardiac defects must be excluded. A greater oxygen level in the right radial artery than in the umbilical artery confirms right-to-left shunting through the ductus arteriosus. Echocardiography and Doppler evaluation are of utmost importance to rule out structural heart disease, especially total anomalous pulmonary venous connection.

Initial treatment[21] includes an increase in the inspired oxygen level and correction of acidosis with sodium bicarbonate. Frequently, artificial ventilation is required. Hyperventilation to diminish the partial pressure of carbon dioxide is often successful in lowering the pulmonary pressure and diminishing the right-to-left shunt. Intravenous infusion of tolazoline, either into the upper segment of the body to enhance flow to the lungs or directly into the pulmonary artery, may be beneficial. Recently, inhaled nitric oxide to reduce pulmonary vascular resistance has been found to be a useful adjunct to other therapies.[22] Treatment of severe disease with an extracorporeal membrane oxygenator is successful in a significant number of patients.[23] Similar hemodynamic alterations may also be seen in newborns with parenchymal lung disease.

COMPLICATIONS OF CONGENITAL HEART DISEASE

Congestive Heart Failure

Congestive heart failure is a potentially lethal complication of congenital heart disease and occurs in over 80 percent of infants who have malformations severe enough to require cardiac catheterization or surgery within the first year of life.[24] Its onset is usually a phenomenon of the first 6 months of life. Onset after 1 year of age is rare without a serious intercurrent problem such as infective endocarditis, pneumonia, or anemia.

Heart failure within the first 12 to 18 h of life is usually due to malformations that involve volume overload independent of pulmonary flow, as occurs with severe valvular regurgitation. Rarely, myocarditis may produce failure from the time of birth, as may congenital complete heart block or supraventricular tachycardia. Other causes in this age group include primary cardiomyopathy, volume overload from a systemic AV fistula, severe polycythemia, or depressed myocardial contractility from neonatal asphyxia, hypocalcemia, hypoglycemia, anemia, or sepsis.

A majority of full-term infants presenting with severe heart failure during the remainder of the first week have critical obstruction to systemic arterial flow, which, in many cases, has been unmasked by narrowing or closure of the ductus arteriosus. Examples are aortic atresia, coarctation of the aorta, interruption of the aortic arch, and critical aortic stenosis. *During the second week of life, aortic atresia and coarctation remain the most common causes of heart failure, but VSD, transposition of the great arteries with a VSD, and truncus arteriosus make their appearance.* These latter malformations require a pulmonary vascular bed with a reduced vascular resistance for full expression of their severity. *Therefore, VSD is the primary cause of congestive failure, followed by transposition, coarctation, complete AV canal, and PDA.*

The most common symptom of congestive heart failure is difficulty in breathing, with rapid, grunting, or gasping breathing or breathlessness with feeding, except in those rare instances of isolated right ventricular failure. Observation of the undisturbed infant reveals dyspnea, the signs of which are nasal flaring and subcostal or intercostal retractions. A respiratory rate consistently above 60 is to be expected, and rates in the range of 90 to 100 are not uncommon. Poor weight gain is the rule. Cool, moist skin; a subdued and rapid arterial pulse; and hepatic enlargement are common accompanying signs. A gallop rhythm, pulmonary rales, and expiratory wheezes may be present. It may be difficult to distinguish the pulmonary findings of heart failure from those of pneumonia or bronchiolitis; indeed, many infants have both heart failure and pulmonary infection. Edema, if present, is usually found in the periorbital area and on the dorsa of the feet and hands. Cardiac enlargement is confirmed by chest roentgenogram. Infants with malformations such as coarctation of the aorta and total anomalous pulmonary venous connection, abnormalities not usually characterized by an impressive murmur, sometimes are referred only after weeks of tachypnea and failure to thrive, when a chest roentgenogram, taken to explore the possibility of lung disease, has revealed cardiac enlargement.

When a sizable systemic-to-pulmonary communication exists in a premature infant, usually due to a patent ductus, signs of heart failure are usually associated with signs of ventilatory failure.

Hospitalization is recommended for all infants with heart failure. Elevation of the head and chest to an angle of approximately 30° and administration of humidified oxygen by techniques that do not disturb the infant help relieve dyspnea and systemic arterial hypoxia as determined by pulse oximetry. Oxygen administration carries the potential dangers of encouraging closure of a PDA, upon which the systemic circulation may be dependent, producing flooding of the pulmonary vascular bed by decreasing pulmonary vascular resistance and, particularly in the premature, increasing the rest of retrolental fibroplasia. Arterial oxygen saturation levels should be monitored in the newborn, particularly the premature, to avoid the risk of retrolental fibroplasia. Rest, aided by sedation, is beneficial. With severe failure, oral feedings should be temporarily suspended and fluid intake restricted to 65 mL/kg per day intravenously for at least the first 24 h. Anemia, acidosis, hypoxia, hypercarbia, hypoglycemia, or hypocalcemia should be corrected; serum sodium, potassium, blood urea nitrogen, and creatinine concentrations should be monitored. A low threshold for the administration of antibiotics is appropriate.

Digoxin is recommended for the management of congestive failure in infants and children because of its excellent absorption when given orally, rapid onset of action, relatively rapid excretion, and convenience of administration. The recommended oral maintenance doses of digoxin for the different age ranges of children, expressed as μg/kg per day, are as follows: for the premature, 5; for the neonate, 10; for the infant between 4 and 24 months of age, 15; for the older child, 10; and for the adolescent, 5. The daily maintenance dose is usually given in two divided doses approximately 12 h apart. The total digitalizing dose is three times the daily maintenance dose. The parenteral doses of digoxin are approximately 75 percent of the oral doses for digitalization and maintenance. Half of the digitalizing dose may be given initially, followed by the remaining two quarter-doses at 4-, 8-, or 12-h intervals, depending upon the desired speed of total digitalization. Maintenance therapy should be started 8 to 12 h after the last digitalizing dose. In the severely ill infant, with decreased perfusion and unpredictable absorption, digitalization by the intravenous route is recommended. Impaired renal function leads to digoxin accumulation and toxicity, so the initial and maintenance doses should be adjusted accordingly. Toxicity, if it is to occur, usually appears within the first week of therapy. If anorexia, nausea or vomiting, or electrocardiographic evidence of either atrial or ventricular ectopy or AV block appears, digoxin should be stopped and the serum digoxin level determined. Toxicity is probable if the level exceeds 3.0 ng/mL in the infant below 6 months of age or 2.0 ng/mL in the older infant or child. If the need for digoxin continues, the dose is adjusted as the patient grows and gains weight.

The diuretic furosemide, used intravenously in doses of 1.0 to 2.0 mg/kg or orally in doses of 1.5 to 2.0 mg/kg, is very effective in the acute management of congestive heart failure. With severe failure, the dose may be increased by increments of 1.0 mg/kg intravenously if no urinary response has been achieved after 45 min. For long-term oral diuretic therapy, 1.5 to 2.0 mg/kg once daily or, if necessary, twice daily is recommended. The diuretic response to furosemide may be very significantly enhanced by the addition of metolazone given orally 30 min prior to furosemide. The dose of metolazone is 0.2 to 0.4 mg/kg every 24 h. Very careful attention to fluid balance and electrolytes is essential with this powerful combination. Chlorothiazide, a slightly less potent diuretic but one with a longer duration of action, may be given orally in a dose of 20 to 50 mg/kg per day. Hypokalemia and hypochloremia can be induced with these potent diuretics, and a daily oral supplement of potassium chloride in the range of 1.0 to 1.5 meq/kg, with adjustment depending on the serum level, is recommended (see Chap. 24). Spironolactone, an aldosterone antagonist, has proved useful in supplementing the diuresis and in preventing the hypokalemia induced by the diuretics described above. It may be given orally in a single daily dose of 2 to 3 mg/kg. A regimen of spironolactone,

2 mg/kg given every day, and chlorothiazide, 20 mg/kg given on alternate days, is usually adequate for long-term diuretic therapy of mild to moderate heart failure and does not require potassium supplementation. With more severe heart failure, chlorothiazide may be given daily, the dose of both diuretics may be increased, or furosemide may be substituted for chlorothiazide. Under these circumstances, potassium supplementation may be necessary (see also Chap. 24).

In emergency situations, it may be necessary to provide an immediate inotropic stimulus in the form of intravenous sympathomimetic amines administered by constant infusion pump. Isoproterenol, in a dose of 0.1 µg/kg per min, exerts a powerful inotropic effect, but its usefulness may be limited by induced tachycardia and peripheral vasodilation, sometimes to the detriment of renal perfusion. Epinephrine, in a dose of 0.1 to 1.0 µg/kg per min, or dobutamine or dopamine, in a dose of 5 to 15 µg/kg per min, generally has been more helpful, with dopamine providing more adequate renal flow. The systemic arterial blood pressure, urinary output, and electrocardiogram (ECG) should be monitored continuously. Vasodilator therapy in the form of intravenous sodium nitroprusside may be of considerable help in patients with severe congestive failure not associated with large left-to-right shunts. The infusion rate at the start should be no greater than 0.5 µg/kg per min, but it may be increased gradually to 4.0 µg/kg per min to achieve the desired effect. Systemic arterial pressure should be monitored continuously to detect serious hypotension. Two oral vasodilators, hydralazine, in a dose of 0.25 to 0.50 mg/kg four times daily for children with normal or only mildly elevated ventricular filling pressure, or prazosin, in a dose of 0.05 to 0.10 mg/kg four times daily if ventricular filling pressures are elevated, have proved beneficial in selected patients. The angiotensin-converting enzyme inhibitors captopril, enalapril, and lisinopril have proven effective in selected patients: captopril starting at doses of 0.1 to 0.4 mg/kg per dose in the neonate and 0.3 to 0.6 mg/kg per dose in the older child given one to four times per day; enalapril, 0.16 to 0.25 mg/kg per day in two divided doses; or lisinopril, 0.16 to 0.25 mg/kg per day in a single daily dose. Hypotension and/or hyperkalemia are the primary adverse effects of these agents.[25]

Infants with potentially exhausting respiratory effort or with hypoxia or hypercapnia secondary to pulmonary edema or respiratory failure benefit from endotracheal intubation and ventilation on a volume-controlled, positive-pressure respirator, usually with the addition of positive end-expiratory pressure. These measures may permit additional therapy, cardiac catheterization, and surgical intervention with a much greater margin of safety.

In newborns who have failure as the result of narrowing or closure of the ductus arteriosus in the presence of critical obstruction to flow from the left side of the heart, dramatic and lifesaving relief can be expected with reopening of the ductus by infusion of PGE$_1$ at a dose of 0.1 µg/kg per min.

Finally, infants or children in whom medical therapy is clearly inadequate or only temporarily successful may require prompt surgical intervention for control of their heart failure. *As a rule, the earlier the onset of congestive failure, the more likely will be the need for surgery.*

Cyanosis

Cyanosis, a bluish tinge to the color of the skin caused by the presence of at least 3 to 5 g/dL of reduced hemoglobin, is one of the more frequent initial signs of congenital heart disease in the infant. It may also be an early sign of pulmonary, central nervous system, or metabolic disease or of methemoglobinemia.[26] Nonsurgical palliation with PGE$_1$ and the rapid development of surgical techniques for infants make prompt distinction between cardiac and noncardiac cyanosis extremely important. *Echocardiography (Chap. 14) is helpful in distinguishing cyanotic heart disease from other causes of cyanosis.*

Cyanosis in congenital heart disease may be due to heart failure with pulmonary edema or to intracardiac right-to-left shunting. Low cardiac output and peripheral vasoconstriction frequently give a grayish discoloration to the skin (or pallor) rather than typical cyanosis. Hypoxia due either to heart failure or to lung disease with intrapulmonary shunting usually responds dramatically to oxygen administration, whereas hypoxia due to cyanotic defects does not. Since many infants are relatively anemic during the first few months of life (hemoglobin concentration 10.4 to 12 g/dL), cyanosis may be subtle.

When cyanosis is present for several months, clubbing occurs. Tachypnea and dyspnea may be due to desaturation and are exaggerated with exercise. Paroxysms of increased cyanosis, occasionally leading to loss of consciousness (cyanotic spells), and squatting may be seen with tetralogy of Fallot. When hypoxemia persists, the children may become polycythemic, which can exaggerate the cyanosis.

The serious complications of hypoxemia frequently result from polycythemia and paradoxical embolism (Table 70-2). The central nervous system may be the target organ, with cerebrovascular accidents and brain abscesses occurring as a result of the effects of polycythemia and paradoxical embolism, especially in the setting of dehydration or febrile states. Paradoxical embolism is a potential complication whenever a right-to-left shunt exists. An infected venous thrombus of unfiltered blood during an episode of bacteremia can cause a cerebral abscess, but this is rare under 2 years of age. The

---

TABLE 70-2

SEQUELAE OF HYPOXEMIA

Cyanosis
Clubbing
Polycythemia
Squatting
Exercise intolerance
Hypoxic spells
Brain abscess
Cerebral vascular accidents

incidence and mortality rates are directly related to the degree of hypoxia.[27] Thrombosis, embolism, and hemorrhage can cause cerebrovascular accidents (see also Chap. 99). A majority of instances occur in infants up to 1 year of age, with relatively few after 4 or 5 years of age. The younger patients very frequently have iron-deficiency anemia relative to the degree of desaturation, whereas the older patients have polycythemia.[28] Acutely increasing hemoglobin concentration in those with relative anemia has significant hemodynamic benefits[29] as well as an effect on tissue oxygen delivery.[30] Prevention of iron deficiency by dietary supplementation in infants and of excessive polycythemia by surgical intervention should decrease the number of cerebrovascular accidents and help prevent the occurrence of brain abscess. In older adolescents or adult patients with prolonged polycythemia, the resultant hyperuricemia can precipitate a secondary form of gout.[31]

Disturbances in hemostasis also occur with polycythemia. Coagulation factors are commonly abnormal in patients with hematocrits in excess of 60 percent.[32] Actual platelet counts may be normal but can be increased initially in some patients, with subsequent decreases related to persistent and worsening desaturation. There is evidence of shortened platelet survival time in patients with cyanotic heart disease.[33] Laboratory evaluation of coagulation status requires that correction be made for the diminished volume of plasma and for the volume of anticoagulant used in the blood samples to avoid false results. Hematologic management of adults with cyanotic congenital heart disease requires special experience and knowledge.[34,35]

The major consequences of cyanosis can be avoided in many instances, although there have been differences in intelligence demonstrated between cyanotic and acyanotic children.[36]

Retardation of Growth and Development

Children having severe cardiac malformations frequently exhibit retardation of growth and development, with height and weight near or below the third percentile or weight 20 percentile points below the mean percentile for height.[37]

Growth retardation is most severe among those children with overt cyanosis and those with large left-to-right shunts causing heart failure. Heart failure tends to cause a greater retardation of weight than of height. Skeletal retardation, reflected by bone age, usually occurs with height and weight retardation and, among children with cyanotic heart disease, correlates with the severity of hypoxemia.

Other factors contribute to growth retardation including insufficient caloric intake, dyspnea, frequent infections, psychological disturbances, malabsorption, or hypermetabolism. Among infants with severe congenital heart disease recognized within the first year of life, there is a significantly increased incidence of subnormal birth weight, intrauterine growth retardation, and major extracardiac anomalies.[38] Finally, a relatively small number of children will have associated syndromes known to be characterized by growth retardation, such as rubella and Noonan's, Turner's, and Down's syndromes.

Growth retardation related primarily to congenital heart disease usually responds to surgical correction or palliation, with an impressive acceleration of growth and a return to or toward normal.

While cardiac surgery is seldom recommended on the basis of growth failure alone, this undesirable trend should be recognized early and, until proved otherwise, considered an index of the severity of the heart disease. In general, the earlier and the more successful the surgery, the less will be the retardation of growth and development, with its sequelae of physical, psychological, and intellectual problems.[39]

Pulmonary Arterial Hypertension and Pulmonary Vascular Obstructive Disease

Pulmonary arterial hypertension (PAH) and pulmonary vascular obstructive disease (PVOH) are serious complications of congenital heart disease. PAH is usually the result of direct transmission of systemic arterial pressure to the right ventricle or pulmonary arteries via a large communication. Less frequently, it is due to severe obstruction to blood flow through the left side of the heart at the pulmonary venous level or beyond. PVOH refers to a process involving structural and developmental changes in the smaller muscular arteries and arterioles of the lung that gradually diminishes and eventually destroys the ability of the pulmonary vascular bed to transport blood from the larger pulmonary arteries to the pulmonary veins without an abnormal elevation of proximal pulmonary arterial pressure.

Pulmonary resistance (R_p) may be as high as 8 to 10 Wood units immediately after birth but falls rapidly throughout the first week. Indexed Wood units, as a measure of resistance to flow across either the pulmonary or systemic vascular beds, are obtained by dividing the mean pressure difference (in millimeters of mercury) across the pulmonary or systemic vascular beds by the blood flow index (expressed in liters per minute per square meter) across those respective beds. By 6 to 8 weeks it has usually reached the normal adult level (1 to 3 Wood units).[40] These changes are accompanied by a gradual dilatation of first the smaller and then the larger muscular pulmonary arteries and then, in the weeks and months that follow, a thinning of their muscular walls, growth of existing arteries, and the development of new arteries and arterioles. The latter process contributes over 90 percent of the smaller or intraacinar pulmonary arterial vessels present in the older child and adult.[41]

Increased pulmonary arterial pressure has an adverse effect on the normal maturation of the pulmonary vascular bed. Such pressure encourages a persistence of the thick muscular medial layer present in the smaller pulmonary arteries of the term newborn, stimulates an extension of smooth muscle into smaller and more peripheral arteries than normal for age, and, lastly, retards the growth of existing acinar arteries and the development of new ones.

In the presence of a large systemic-to-pulmonary communication, pulmonary arterial pressures tend to remain at or near systemic levels, with the result that the diminution in pulmonary muscle mass and pulmonary resistance is less rapid and of less magnitude than it is in the normal infant. Nevertheless, the diminution is usually sufficient to permit a large pulmonary blood flow and, as a result, congestive failure by the end of the first month. Exceptions are found among those infants with a large systemic-to-pulmonary communication but with alveolar hypoxia, a stimulus for pulmonary vasoconstriction, in whom there is less than normal involution of the medial musculature and diminution in pulmonary vascular resistance. Clinically, this is expressed by the lower incidence of congestive failure observed among infants with large VSDs born and living at high altitude. Rarely, an infant will maintain a very high pulmonary vascular resistance in the face of an anatomically large systemic-to-pulmonary communication, without evidence of significant hypoxemia or acidemia, and remain free of the signs and symptoms of congestive failure. In the premature infant, in whom the medial muscle mass is less at birth than it is in the full-term infant, the fall in pulmonary vascular resistance is usually much more rapid than normal.

Chronic PAH or increased flow, or both, produces a characteristic series of histologic changes originally described and graded by Heath and Edwards (grades I through VI below)[42] and, more recently, by Rabinovitch and coworkers[41] (grades A through C below):

- Grade I—medial hypertrophy in the small, normally muscular, pulmonary arteries.
- Grade II—concentric or eccentric cellular intimal proliferation within the smaller pulmonary arteries and arterioles.
- Grade III—relatively acellular intimal fibrosis with accumulation of concentric or eccentric masses of fibrous tissue leading to widespread occlusion of the smaller pulmonary arteries and arterioles.
- Grade IV—progressive, generalized dilatation of the distal muscular arteries and the appearance of plexiform lesions, complex vascular structures composed of a network or plexus of proliferating endothelial tissue, frequently accompanied by thrombus, within a dilated thin-walled sac. Whether these are the result of aneurysms of the media, of vasculitis, or of thrombosis is unclear, but their appearance signifies very severe PVOD.
- Grade V—thinning and fibrosis of the media superimposed upon the formation of numerous complex dilatation lesions.
- Grade VI—necrotizing arteritis within the media with surrounding areas of inflammatory reaction and granulation tissue. This is found most commonly among patients with primary pulmonary hypertension.

- Grade A—extension of muscle into normally nonmuscular peripheral arteries with or without a mild increase in medial wall thickness of normally muscular arteries (less than 1.5 times normal). The former appears related to increased flow rather than pressure and may be noted as early as 4 to 6 weeks of age among infants with a ventricular septal defect.
- Grade B—extension of muscle as above with an even greater increase in medial wall thickness of normally muscular arteries. Grade B is subdivided into: *mild*, in which the medial wall thickness is between 1.5 and 2 times normal, and *severe*, in which medial wall thickness is greater than twice normal.
- Grade C—changes seen in grade B (severe) but with a decreased arterial concentration relative to alveoli. Grade C is also subdivided into: *mild*, in which the arterial number is still half or more than half the normal number, and *severe*, in which less than half the normal number is present.

Grades A and B are partitions of Heath-Edwards grade I. Grade C criteria may be found with grades I and II, are invariable with grade III, and usually preclude a complete return to normal of pulmonary arterial pressures and resistance despite successful surgical correction of the systemic-to-pulmonary communication.

Estimation of pulmonary vascular resistance from data obtained at cardiac catheterization remains the most widely used means of assessing the state of the pulmonary vascular bed. Hypoxemia from oversedation, atelectasis, or pneumonitis at the time of study should be scrupulously avoided. If pulmonary vascular resistance is elevated, its responsiveness to vasodilation induced by the inhalation of 100 percent oxygen, the pulmonary arterial administration of tolazoline, or the inhalation of nitric oxide[43] should be tested.

Values of $R_p \leq 3$ Wood units are considered normal. The status of the pulmonary vasculature can also be expressed as a ratio of pulmonary vascular resistance to systemic vascular resistance (R_p/R_s). *Pulmonary/systemic resistance ratios of less than 0.2:1 are considered normal.*

As pulmonary vascular resistance increases, pulmonary blood flow generally decreases. Eventually, a point is reached where surgical closure of the defect will produce only a small diminution of blood flow, a proportionately small decrease in pulmonary arterial pressure, and no significant change in the factors contributing to the progression of the vascular disease. Patients in this category are considered prohibitive risks for surgery because of the increased mortality associated with the procedure in the early postoperative period. *An R_p/R_s ratio 0.7:1 or an R_p of 11 Wood units with a pulmonary/systemic blood flow ratio 1.5:1 are the criteria generally used to define this situation.* Without surgery, these patients survive as examples of the Eisenmenger syndrome, in which $R_p \geq R_s$ and at least some right-to-left shunting occurs at rest or with exercise. Some of these patients can survive for several decades and lead productive lives, with relatively mild symptoms and few limitations.[44]

The decision regarding surgery for patients with less severe PVOD is a clinical one. The higher the calculated resistance and the greater the structural changes in the pulmonary vasculature, as judged by lung biopsy or quantitative pulmonary arterial wedge angiography, and the older the patient with any given level of elevated resistance or grade of structural change, the less likely it is that the outcome will be satisfactory.[41]

The prevention of PVOD requires the identification of those patients at risk, namely, all patients with a systemic-to-pulmonary communication and a pulmonary arterial systolic pressure greater than half the systemic arterial systolic pressure. Also included would be all patients with transposition, regardless of pressure or flow, with the possible exception of those with severe pulmonary stenosis. Ideally, all patients at risk should undergo correction or pulmonary arterial banding unless there is proof that the pulmonary arterial systolic pressure has fallen to or is less than half the systemic systolic pressure before the end of the first year of life among those with normally related great arteries. Among patients with transposition with a large VSD, action must be taken within the first 3 months of life.

Long-Term Problems with Surgically Corrected Defects

With the advances that have occurred in the surgical treatment of congenital heart defects, more of these patients are becoming adults. This discussion of potential long-term problems is intended for those who follow these children after surgery and through adult life[45] (see also Chap. 71).

First, there are residua, sequelae, and complications that result from most surgical procedures for congenital heart defects. A residual part of the original defects, such as mitral prolapse and repaired ASD, may purposefully not have been approached surgically. Some sequelae are unavoidable consequences of the surgery, such as pulmonary regurgitation after pulmonary valvotomy. There are also complications that occur as unexpected, but related, events after successful surgery, such as late complete heart block. When viewed with these possibilities in mind, only surgical correction of patent ductus is likely to have no long-term problems.

At the simplest level, most patients have residual murmurs after surgery for congenital heart defects. Proper interpretation of the origin of these murmurs and the evaluation of the severity of the hemodynamic abnormalities that they represent are important. Noninvasive diagnostic tools, especially Doppler and two-dimensional echocardiography, are often useful.

In general, the risk of infective endocarditis to patients is not diminished after surgery, with the exception of those who have undergone patent ductus ligation or repair of VSD or secundum ASD in whom there is no residual shunt. Those patients in whom it has been necessary to place an artificial valve are at increased risk.[46,47]

There are specific problems related to some of the more common defects. For those with repaired ASD, VSD, and AV (canal) septal defects, a residual shunt may be present, but ordinarily it is small and not of hemodynamic significance.

Those with repaired AV canal defects may have important AV valvular regurgitation. Repaired coarctation of the aorta can gradually become narrowed again, or patients may develop idiopathic hypertension. Surgery for valvular pulmonary stenosis usually results in mild residual stenosis and regurgitation, which are well tolerated and have little tendency to progress with time. The natural history of valvular aortic stenosis after surgery is not so benign.[48] Because significant regurgitation must be avoided, initial results may not be as good in terms of the severity of residual stenosis. In addition, aortic stenosis tends to worsen with time; thus, proper follow-up is mandatory for these patients.

Few patients enter adulthood with the continued problem of cyanosis. Since those with residual defects amenable to surgical correction should have had surgery well before this time, only patients with complex and uncorrectable defects or those with pulmonary vascular disease should have problems of cyanosis during the adult years. Particularly important among these patients is management of any attendant psychosocial problems (employment, insurability,[49] and learning disabilities) and difficulties related to pregnancy.[50]

Those who have had surgery for cyanotic defects are more likely to have sequelae and complications.[51] Some degree of exercise intolerance is not unusual in this group of patients, and exercise stress testing aids in their management.[52,53]

Dysrhythmias are also particularly frequent among these patients. *In those who have had intraventricular repairs, most commonly for tetralogy of Fallot, late complete heart block and serious ventricular arrhythmias can occur and may result in sudden death.*[54] This risk is highest in those who had transient complete heart block at the time of surgery and who develop right bundle branch block with left anterior hemiblock after surgery.[55] Extensive interatrial surgical procedures for transposition of the great arteries also frequently lead to dysrhythmias, most commonly sick sinus syndrome with bradytachyarrhythmias and atrial flutter, with a high incidence of sudden death.[56] Ambulatory 24-h electrocardiographic monitoring (Chap. 28) and stress testing (Chap. 15) and intracardiac electrophysiologic studies are important in following patients who have had complex repairs.

Serious ventricular dysfunction[57] and venous obstructions may also occur, usually in those who had severe defects. Interatrial repairs for transposition of the great arteries leave the anatomic right ventricle to do the work of the systemic ventricle.[58] In addition, these repairs may lead to pulmonary and/or systemic venous obstruction. Atriopulmonary connections for repair of tricuspid atresia[59] and many types of univentricular hearts frequently leave an anatomically abnormal ventricle as the systemic ventricle. In this group of patients, the right atrium has become the "pulmonary ventricle," with an elevated right atrial pressure that may lead to problems of systemic venous hypertension such as protein-losing enteropathy.[60]

Finally, some children have had repairs utilizing synthetic prostheses. Artificial valves do not grow as the child does, and they must be much more durable in view of the life expectancy. There are also some surgical procedures that require placement of conduits, with or without valves, that can degenerate and become obstructive with time. *Bioprosthetic valves undergo accelerated fibrosis and calcification in patients less than about 30 to 35 years of age.*

It should be kept in mind that in spite of these problems the majority of patients who reach adulthood after surgical repair of congenital defects are relatively asymptomatic; they can and do lead productive lives.

INTRACARDIAC COMMUNICATIONS BETWEEN THE SYSTEMIC AND PULMONARY CIRCULATIONS, USUALLY WITHOUT CYANOSIS

Ventricular Septal Defect

DEFINITION
VSD represents an opening in that part of the ventricular septum that separates the two ventricles.

PATHOLOGY
A defect of the ventricular septum represents the most common alteration among malformed hearts. In some this is the only condition, whereas in others it is part of a complex malformation.

ANATOMIC TYPES
Approximately 80 percent of all defects are paramembranous but may extend into the inlet, trabecular, or outlet sections of the muscular septum. Less common (except among Asians)

are the conal septal or subarterial doubly committed defects (5 to 7 percent), inlet defects lying beneath the septal leaflet of the tricuspid valve in the region of the atrioventricular canal (5 to 8 percent), and finally, defects in the muscular septum whether they lie in the inlet, trabecular, or outlet area[61] (see Fig. 70-4). Multiplicity of muscular defects is characteristic.

The major conduction tissue is most closely related to the paramembranous defects where it lies along the posteroinferior quadrant of the defect and favors the left ventricular side of the septum.

ASSOCIATED CONDITIONS
Cardiac malformations associated with VSD are, in order of decreasing frequency, (1) coarctation of the aorta; (2) additional shunts, most commonly ASD and PDA, and other VSDs; (3) intracardiac obstructions such as subpulmonary or subaortic stenosis, mitral stenosis, and anomalous muscle bundle of the right ventricle; and (4) incompetent atrioventricular valves.

ABNORMAL PHYSIOLOGY
The consequences of a VSD depend upon the size of the defect and the pulmonary vascular resistance. A small defect offers a large resistance to flow. There is no elevation of right ventricular or pulmonary arterial pressures, and the left-to-right shunt may be so small that it can be detected only by selective left ventricular angiography or two-dimensional imaging with Doppler color flow mapping. This type of defect imposes little burden on the heart except for the danger of infective endocarditis.

A defect of moderate size still permits a separation of right and left ventricular systolic pressures with the right ventricular systolic pressure generally being 80 percent or less of the left ventricular systolic pressure, but a large left-to-right shunt may be present with resulting left atrial hypertension and dilatation and left ventricular volume overload. The development of pulmonary vascular disease among these patients is unusual but possible. When the effective area of the defect is large, approximately equal to or greater than the aortic valve orifice, the defect offers virtually no resistance to flow and the systolic pressures in both ventricles, the aorta, and the pulmonary artery are essentially the same. The relative proportion of blood going to the two circulations is directly governed by the relative resistance of the two vascular beds.

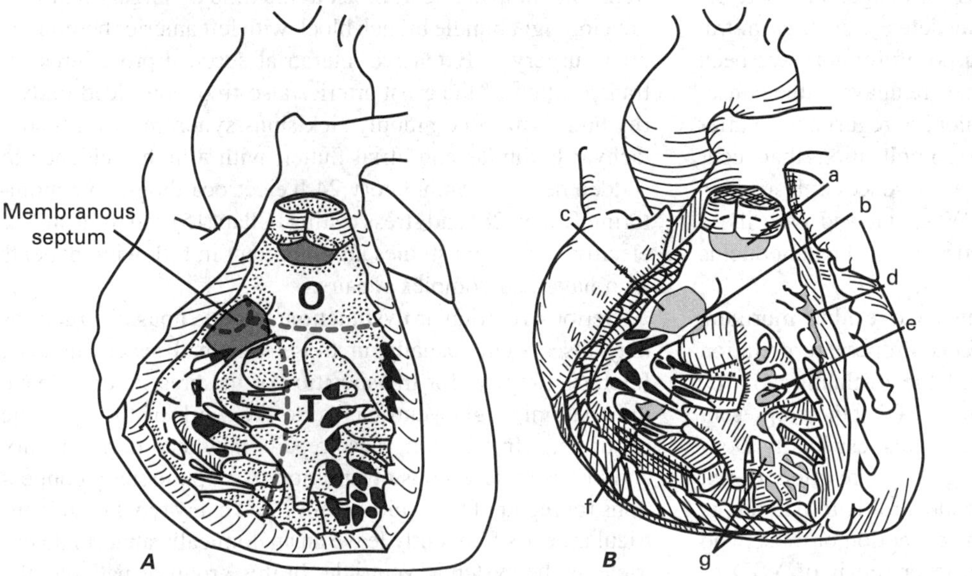

FIGURE 70-4

A. The ventricular septum viewed from the right ventricular side is made up of four components: I, inlet component extends from tricuspid annulus to attachments of tricuspid valve; T, trabecular septum extends from inlet out to the apex and up to smooth-walled outlet; O, outlet septum or infundibular septum, which extends up to the pulmonary valve, and membranous septum. *B.* Anatomic position of defects: a, outlet defect; b, papillary muscle of the conus; c, perimembranous defect; d, marginal muscular defects; e, central muscular defects; f, inlet defect; g, apical muscular defects. (From Graham and Gutgesell.[61] Reproduced with permission from the publisher and authors.)

At birth, pulmonary vascular resistance is high and there is little if any left-to-right shunt despite the presence of a large defect. This resistance to flow gradually falls over the first few weeks of life, permitting a progressively greater amount of blood to flow through the defect, the lungs, and back to the left atrium and left ventricle. The left ventricular volume overload eventually leads, in most infants, to left ventricular "failure" with, in many, markedly elevated left ventricular end-diastolic and left atrial pressures and pulmonary edema.

In term infants born at sea level with a large VSD, clinical deterioration may occur at any time from about 3 to 12 weeks after birth. In premature infants, in whom the less well developed pulmonary vascular hypertrophy regresses more rapidly, failure is frequently noted at 1 to 4 weeks.

CLINICAL MANIFESTATIONS

VSD is a common form of congenital heart disease, second only to a bicuspid aortic valve and mitral valve prolapse (see Chaps. 63 and 65). It occurs as an isolated defect in approximately 23 percent of infants with congenital heart disease and occurs in combination with other malformations in an additional 26 percent.[6] Its incidence is 2 per 1000 live births, its prevalence among school-age children has been estimated as 1 per 1000, and it constitutes about 10 percent of the congenital cardiac malformations found among adults.[62] Males and females are affected equally. It is the most common defect found among infants with chromosomal abnormalities, with the notable exceptions being those with Down's syndrome (trisomy 21) and Turner's syndrome (XO genotype), among whom it ranks second.

History

Infants or children with a small isolated defect are asymptomatic. The murmur of a small defect may be detected within the first 24 to 36 h of life, since the very restrictive opening permits the normal rapid fall in pulmonary arterial resistance and pressures. Infants with larger defects usually present between 3 and 12 weeks of age with congestive failure, frequently with associated lower respiratory tract infections. Parents describe tachypnea, grunting respirations, and fatigue, particularly with feedings. Weight gain is slow, and excessive sweating is common.

Physical Examination

The child with a small defect is comfortable. A systolic thrill at the lower left sternal border is common, although with very small defects this may not be present. The second heart sound is normal. The systolic murmur along the lower left sternal border is characteristically holosystolic but may be decrescendo and limited to early or midsystole. These latter features suggest a defect in the muscular rather than the membranous septum.

Infants with large defects, large flow, and PAH tend to be restless, irritable, and underweight. Moderate respiratory distress may be present. Both the right and left ventricular systolic impulses are impressively hyperdynamic to palpation. A thrill at the lower left sternal border is the rule. The second heart sound is narrowly split, with a loud, frequently palpable pulmonary component. Third heart sound gallops at the apex are common. Characteristically, the systolic murmur is holosystolic at the lower left sternal border and is accompanied by a middiastolic rumble of grade 2 to 3 intensity at the apex, the latter indicating a pulmonary/systemic blood flow ratio (Q_p/Q_s) of 2:1 or greater. Hepatic enlargement can be identified below the right costal margin. Pulmonary rales are common with severe failure.

With the passage of time, one may observe signs of a diminishing left-to-right shunt with an improved rate of weight gain, less dyspnea, a diminution of the precordial hyperactivity, and disappearance of the apical diastolic flow rumble. This clinical improvement may be the result of the defect becoming smaller, the development of subvalvular pulmonary stenosis with little or no appreciable change in the size of the defect, or, most worrisome, the development of PVOD with continued severe PAH. With developing subpulmonary stenosis, the systolic murmur radiates more and more impressively to the upper left sternal border and the second heart sound becomes more widely split, with a progressive diminution in the intensity of the pulmonary component. Decreased flow due to pulmonary vascular disease is characterized by a gradual reduction in the intensity and duration of the systolic murmur, more narrow splitting of the second heart sound, and marked accentuation of the pulmonary component.

The clinical picture of advanced pulmonary vascular disease secondary to a congenital left-to-right shunt, or Eisenmenger syndrome, is that of a relatively comfortable older child, adolescent, or young adult with mild cyanosis and clubbing in whom one finds a prominent *a* wave in the jugular venous pulse, a mild right ventricular lift, and a second heart sound that is narrowly split or virtually single with a very loud, usually palpable pulmonary component. An early pulmonary systolic ejection sound, reflecting dilatation of the main pulmonary artery, may be heard, and there may be no systolic murmur at all. In older adolescents and adults, an early diastolic murmur of pulmonary regurgitation or a holosystolic murmur of tricuspid regurgitation may appear.

Chest Roentgenogram

In the presence of a small defect, the heart size and shape and the pulmonary blood flow are barely altered. With large defects, there will be moderate to marked enlargement of the heart, with prominence of the main pulmonary arterial segment and impressive overcirculation in the peripheral lung fields. The left atrium is dilated in the absence of an associated ASD. With increasing pulmonary vascular disease, there is diminution in heart size toward normal while the central pulmonary arteries remain dilated. The peripheral pulmonary arterial markings become attenuated, and a "pruned" effect is produced in the outer third of the lung fields (see also Chap. 13).

Electrocardiogram

With a small defect, one can expect the normal progression of the mean QRS axis from right to left and the normal gradual diminution of the prominent right ventricular voltages characteristic of the newborn. The left ventricular forces will either remain within normal limits or become slightly augmented as a reflection of the mild left ventricular volume overload. With large defects, the mean QRS axis tends to remain oriented to the right and there is little or no regression in right ventricular voltage. The left ventricular forces gradually increase, resulting in a pattern of biventricular hypertrophy within the first few weeks of life. Left atrial hypertrophy is usually present, and frequently right atrial hypertrophy as well. With the development of pulmonary vascular disease or significant pulmonary stenosis, the mean QRS axis tends to remain oriented to the right, there is no regression in right ventricular voltage, and the evidence of left ventricular and left atrial hypertrophy lessens or disappears.

Echocardiogram

Two-dimensional imaging can distinguish the uncomplicated VSD from more complex malformations and is capable of imaging most defects directly when multiple transducer positions are used. The addition of pulsed-wave Doppler with color flow mapping permits identification of small, multiple, muscular, and other less easily visualized defects.[63] The position and size of the opening can be determined as well as its relationships to the aorta, pulmonary artery, and AV valves. Continuous-wave Doppler echocardiography (Fig. 70-5) can predict right ventricular systolic pressure in the absence of

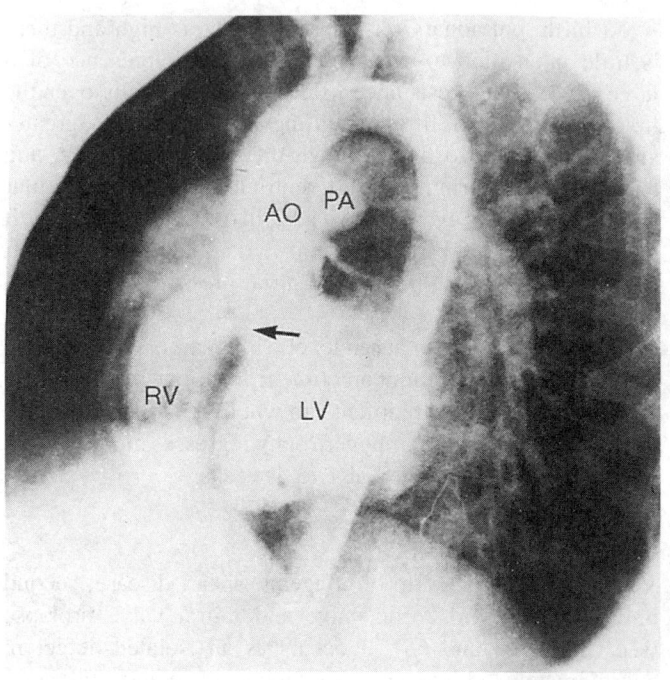

FIGURE 70-6
Left anterior oblique view of the left ventricular angiogram from a 5-year-old child with a small, membranous ventricular septal defect (*arrow*). RV, right ventricle; LV, left ventricle; AO, ascending aorta; PA, pulmonary artery.

aortic stenosis by estimating the interventricular pressure gradient across the defect. An accurate approximation of right ventricular systolic pressure also can be made by estimating the right ventricular to right atrial systolic pressure gradient across the tricuspid valve if tricuspid regurgitation is present.

Cardiac Catheterization

An increase in oxygen saturation at the right ventricular level reflects the left-to-right shunt via the VSD. With small defects, the right ventricular and pulmonary arterial systolic pressures are normal. With large defects, these pressures are at or near systemic levels, and the mean left atrial pressure may be elevated to the 10- to 15-mmHg range.

Selective left ventricular angiography in the anteroposterior, lateral, and oblique views with craniocaudal angulation is recommended to establish the spatial relations of the great arteries to each other and to the ventricles and also to determine the exact site, size, and number of septal defects (Fig. 70-6). Aortography is also recommended to eliminate the possibility of an associated ductus arteriosus or unsuspected coarctation of the aorta.

NATURAL HISTORY AND PROGNOSIS

Fortunately, the majority of VSDs are small and do not present a serious clinical problem. Approximately 24 percent of these small defects close spontaneously by 18 months, 50 percent by 4 years, and 75 percent by 10 years.[64] A spontaneous closure rate approaching 45 percent within the first 12 to 14 months has been observed among infants with an uncomplicated paramembranous or muscular VSD in the neonatal pe-

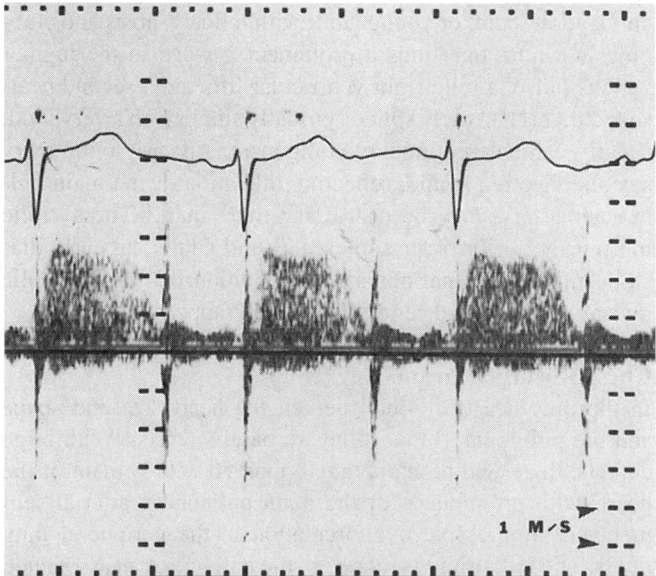

FIGURE 70-5
Continuous-wave Doppler with spectral display from the left lower sternal border of child with a ventricular septal defect that demonstrates holosystolic turbulence with peak velocity = 2.8 m/s across the defect, compatible with an instantaneous systolic pressure difference of 31 mmHg between the ring and left ventricles.

riod.[65,66] Even large defects tend to become smaller, but the likelihood of eventual spontaneous closure is much less (probably in the range of 60 percent if judged large at 3 months of age, and only 50 percent if still large at 6 months).[64]

Congestive failure is a threatening and almost inevitable complication of a large VSD. Almost 80 percent of infants with large defects require hospitalization by the age of 4 months.[3] The risk of death with congestive failure is in the range of 11 percent. Significant subvalvular pulmonary stenosis develops in approximately 3 percent of these individuals and may progress to the point of severe tetralogy of Fallot. PVOD is seldom severe and rarely irreversible in the first 12 months of life, but thereafter it becomes progressively more common and less likely to regress. At risk of this complication are those infants and children with a pulmonary systolic pressure in excess of 50 percent of the systemic arterial systolic pressure beyond the first year of life.[67] A very small number of the infants with large VSDs maintain a high level of pulmonary vascular resistance throughout the first year of life and remain almost entirely free of symptoms and congestive heart failure. In these patients, irreversible pulmonary vascular disease may develop without the usual and expected clinical signs and symptoms described above.

A small number of children, 0.6 percent in a large group of carefully followed patients, will develop aortic regurgitation as a result of prolapse of the right, the posterior, or both aortic valve leaflets into the defect.[68] This complication is more prevalent among males, in a ratio of 2:1, and seems particularly likely to occur with defects of the subarterial type. Shunt size appears unrelated to the development of this complication. The characteristic aortic diastolic murmur may appear at any time between the ages of 6 months and 20 years. Regurgitation is usually progressive, sometimes rapidly so, and predisposes these individuals to infective endocarditis.

The risk of infective endocarditis in patients with an uncomplicated VSD managed medically lies somewhere between 4 and 10 percent for the first 30 years of life.[69] The development of aortic regurgitation more than doubles this risk. Attempts at surgical closure of the defect, with or without aortic regurgitation, reduce the risk to less than half that of unoperated patients.[70]

MEDICAL MANAGEMENT

It is important to identify as early as possible those patients in whom the defect is moderate or large, since these are the patients at special risk of developing congestive failure, pulmonary vascular disease, or serious pulmonary stenosis. Careful and complete two-dimensional Doppler echocardiographic assessment should define the site, size, and number of defects as well as the presence of additional anomalies. The ECG is helpful in identifying those infants in whom the right ventricular systolic pressure is remaining at or near systemic levels, and this can be supported by periodic Doppler reestimation of the interventricular gradient. Heart failure is treated with digoxin and, if necessary, oral diuretics. Anemia

is prevented or corrected, and respiratory infections are treated promptly. Cardiac catheterization is performed on all infants who develop overt congestive heart failure, retain impressive right ventricular or biventricular voltage in the ECG, or fail to thrive despite intensive treatment. If the pulmonary arterial systolic pressure, estimated by two-dimensional Doppler echocardiography in expert hands or measured directly by cardiac catheterization, is greater than half the systemic systolic pressure and congestive failure is difficult to manage medically, the defect should be closed surgically. If congestive failure is not severe, medical management is continued with the hope that spontaneous narrowing of the defect will occur. This trial of medical management is limited to no longer than 6 months, at which point, with or without clinical improvement, the patient undergoes repeat cardiac catheterization. Surgical closure may be postponed in selected patients if clinical improvement during this period has been matched by electrocardiographic evidence of decreasing right ventricular voltages, convincing two-dimensional echocardiographic evidence of a smaller defect, and Doppler estimate of an interventricular pressure gradient of greater than one-half the systemic arterial systolic pressure. If, at restudy, the pulmonary arterial systolic pressure is still greater than half of the systemic systolic pressure, the defect should be closed without delay. If, by the second birthday, the pulmonary arterial pressure has not returned to normal (a mean pulmonary arterial pressure <20 mmHg), as judged by persistent right or biventricular hypertrophy, by two-dimensional Doppler echocardiography, or by direct measurement at catheterization, the defect should be closed. A few children will remain symptomatic or continue to have cardiac enlargement beyond the second year of life due to a large left-to-right shunt (pulmonary/systemic blood flow ratio 1.8:1), despite a normal pulmonary arterial pressure. Surgical closure is recommended in these children as well. Finally, a closure of a defect in an adult is usually recommended if the flow ratio is 1.4:1 and severe pulmonary vascular disease is not present (see Chap. 71).

Unfortunately, not all patients with a large defect are encountered during the first or second year of life, when it would be possible to prevent injury to the pulmonary vascular bed. If significant PAH is allowed to persist, one can expect progression to irreversible pulmonary obstructive disease. For this reason, *prompt surgical closure of defects is recommended in all individuals beyond the age of 2 years if the pulmonary arterial systolic pressure is greater than half the systemic arterial systolic pressure, the mean pulmonary pressure exceeds 25 mmHg, or the R_p/R_s ratio is greater than 0.3:1.* With severe pulmonary vascular disease, a point is eventually reached where the risk of death at operation or in the months or years immediately following operation due to progressive vascular disease more than offsets the possible benefits from surgical closure. At present, surgery is recommended if the calculated R_p is 10 Wood units/m^2 or if the R_p/R_s ratio is 0.7:1, provided the Q_r/Q_s ratio is still 1.5:1. In adults, the upper limit of pulmonary vascular resistance for surgery is approximately 800 dynes, or 10 Wood units.

Those patients in whom the defect is judged clinically to be small at 6 months of age may be reexamined at 1- or 2-year intervals to reassure the patient and family, to reemphasize the importance of antibiotic protection against infective endocarditis, to document the further narrowing or closure of the defect, and (in a very small number of patients) to detect the first signs of aortic valve prolapse.

In patients with Eisenmenger complex,[44] stamina is limited by systemic arterial hypoxemia and, in some, right-sided heart failure. Complications to be anticipated include syncope, hemoptysis, brain abscess, hyperuricemia, and congestive failure. Pregnancy, with a maternal mortality of 30 to 60 percent, and oral contraceptives are contraindicated. Transient symptomatic relief from extreme polycythemia may be achieved by careful erythropheresis. Travel to or living at high altitudes is poorly tolerated, and supplemental oxygen should be provided and used in air travel. The average age of death for individuals with Eisenmenger complex is 33 years, with sudden death the mode of exit in the majority.

Postoperative cardiac catheterization is recommended for individuals with preoperative elevated pulmonary vascular resistance, a persistent loud murmur, unexplained cardiac enlargement, or congestive failure. Following surgical repair, precautions against infective endocarditis are continued indefinitely if there is a residual shunt, and for 6 months in those without a shunt. Symptoms suggesting an arrhythmia should be evaluated at least by 24-h ambulatory monitoring of the ECG (see Chap. 28).

The risk of congenital heart disease for a subsequent sibling of a single affected child is of the order of 1 to 2 percent. The risk to the newborn having one parent with VSD is approximately 3 percent.[71] Pregnancy in the presence of a small defect and normal pulmonary vascular resistance does not appear to carry an increased risk to the patient or infant, although precautions against infective endocarditis should be observed.

SURGICAL MANAGEMENT

Banding of the pulmonary artery to reduce pulmonary blood flow and pressures played an important role in the management of congestive heart failure and the prevention of PVOD before the era of predictably successful closure of VSDs in infants. Complications of pulmonary arterial banding include deformity of the pulmonary arteries and/or pulmonary valve, progressive right ventricular hypertrophy with loss of ventricular compliance, and development of subaortic left ventricular outflow tract obstruction. Banding is now usually reserved for palliation of complex and otherwise uncorrectable defects.[72]

VSDs are closed during total cardiopulmonary bypass with cardioplegic arrest and moderate systemic hypothermia. Total circulatory arrest or minimal perfusion with profound hypothermia (18°C) facilitates closure of defects in infants weighing less than 5 kg.

Paramembranous VSDs may be exposed through the right atrium and tricuspid valve orifice. A transverse or longitudinal right ventriculotomy is preferred for closure of high conal septal defects associated with aortic valve leaflet prolapse.

Care is required to prevent injury to the AV node near the ostium of the coronary sinus and to the bundle of His as it courses inferiorly, passing on the left side of the ventricular septum near the posterocaudal margin of the septal defect. Interoperative transesophageal echocardiography with Doppler color flow assessment is recommended for the detection of significant residual or previously unsuspected problems that may be corrected before leaving the operating room.[73]

Results from primary closure of VSDs are generally excellent, with surgical mortality less than 1 percent in centers with extensive experience, when surgery is performed during the early months of life prior to the evolution of PVOD. Operative risk should be even lower in older children if the pulmonary vascular resistance remains low. The pulmonary vascular bed responds favorably when the systemic-to-pulmonary shunt is eliminated prior to the age of 2 years. Normal life expectancy and functional capabilities should be anticipated postoperatively. Survival 25 years after closure of VSD is approximately 95 percent.[74] The mortality rate is unquestionably higher among patients who are operated upon with $R_p > 7$ Wood units.[72]

Atrial Septal Defect

DEFINITION

An ASD is a through-and-through communication between the atria at the septal level. This is to be distinguished from the valvular-competent foramen ovale, which may persist into adulthood.

PATHOLOGY

ASDs are usually sufficiently large to allow free communication between the atria. They may be subdivided according to anatomic location[75] (Fig. 70-7).

ANATOMIC TYPES

Defect at the Fossa Ovalis (Ostium Secundum)
This defect classically involves the region of the fossa ovalis and is the most common type (70 percent)[75–77] (Fig. 70-7A and C). Atrial septal tissue separates the inferior edge of the defect from the AV valves. Associated partial anomalous pulmonary venous connections are not uncommon, with one or more of the right pulmonary veins draining into the right atrium or one of its tributaries.[78] Mitral valve prolapse is present in some.

Partial Atrioventricular Canal Defects
Defects of the AV septum, which lies inferior to the fossa ovalis, constitute approximately 20 percent of ASDs and are part of a complex malformation known as *common atrioventricular canal defects*, considered later (Fig. 70-7D).

Sinus Venosus Defects
These defects, approximately 6 percent of the total, appear to represent a biatrial connection of the superior vena cava

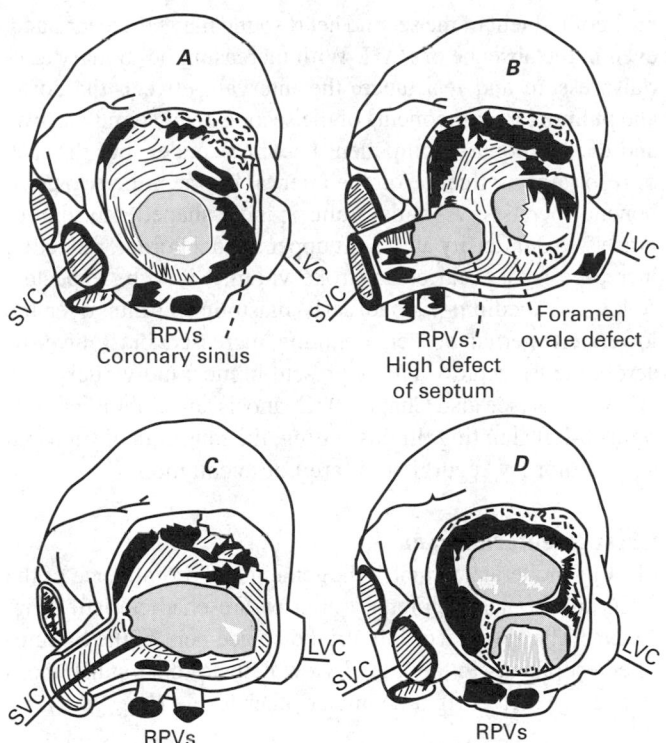

FIGURE 70-7

Types of interatrial communications. *A.* Large ostium secundum type of atrial septal defect. *B.* So-called sinus venosus type of defect—one high in the atrial septum associated with anomalous connection of the right superior pulmonary vein to the junctional area of the superior vena cava and right atrium. *C.* Very large ostium secundum type of atrial septal defect with absence of the posterior rim. *D.* Partial form of common atrioventricular canal with cleft mitral valve. SVC, superior vena cava; RPVs, right pulmonary veins; IVC, inferior vena cava. (From Lewis et al.[75] Copyright 1957, American Medical Association. Reproduced with permission from the publisher and authors.)

(or, in rare instances, the inferior vena cava), which straddles the otherwise normal intact atrial septum. Also involved is an anomalous termination of one or more of the right-sided pulmonary veins, either into the vena cava or into the right atrium near its junction with the vena cava[79] (Fig. 70-7*B*).

Coronary Sinus Defects

A coronary sinus defect is an uncommon type of ASD located in the position normally occupied by the ostium of the coronary sinus. This defect is part of a developmental complex consisting of the absence of the coronary sinus and entry of the left superior vena cava directly into the left atrium.[80]

Conditions Common to All Anatomic Types

The right atrial and ventricular chambers as well as the central pulmonary arteries become enlarged. When pulmonary hypertension intervenes, the right ventricular wall hypertrophies and atherosclerosis may occur in the major pulmonary arteries. Saccular aneurysm and thrombosis with dissecting aneurysm or rupture may occur.

Pulmonary hypertension may develop but usually not be-

fore the third decade. The earliest lesion is cellular fibrous intimal thickening in the proximal segments of arterioles. The pulmonary arterial pressure then rises, followed by the development of medial hypertrophy of muscular arteries and the appearance of plexiform lesions. In the final state, the pulmonary vascular bed may be difficult to distinguish from that in VSD with PVOD.

ABNORMAL PHYSIOLOGY

Usually there is no resistance to blood flow across the defect and no significant pressure difference between the two atria. A left-to-right shunt of blood occurs (Fig. 70-8) because (1) the right atrial system is more distensible than the left, (2) the tricuspid valve is normally more capacious than the mitral valve, and (3) the thinner-walled right ventricular chamber more readily accommodates a larger volume of blood at the same filling pressure than does the left ventricle. A large left-to-right shunt may be found in a neonate or young infant before the right ventricular compliance has had time to change appreciably from that of the left ventricle. Presumably this occurs because a rapid fall in pulmonary vascular resistance encourages a larger right ventricular stroke volume, a smaller end-systolic volume, and hence, an increased ability of the

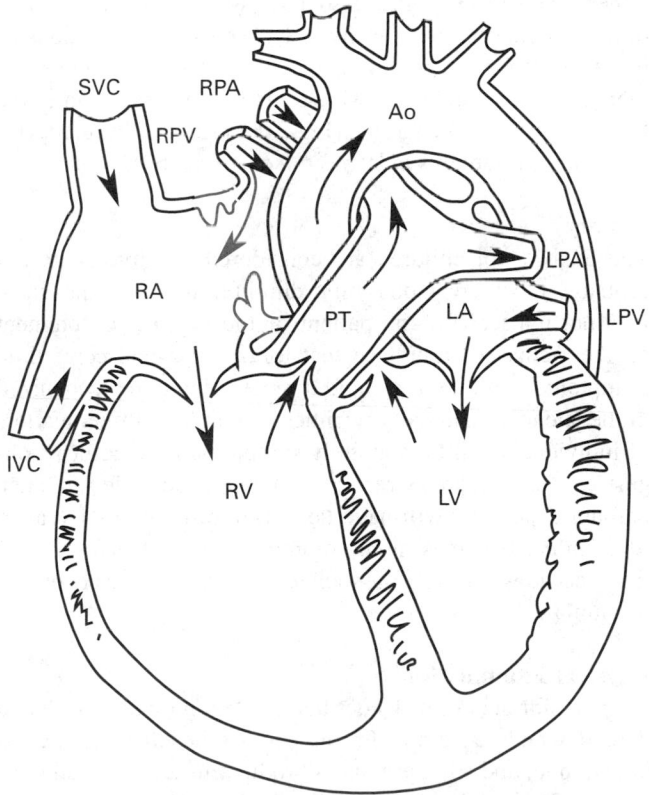

FIGURE 70-8

Atrial septal defect at fossa ovalis, with left-to-right shunt. SVC, superior vena cava; IVC, inferior vena cava; RA, right atrium; RV, right ventricle; PT, main pulmonary arterial trunk; RPA, right pulmonary artery; LPA, left pulmonary artery; RPV, right pulmonary vein; LPV, left pulmonary vein; LA, left atrium; LV, left ventricle; AO, aorta. (From Edwards.[76] Reproduced with permission from the publisher and author.)

right ventricle to accept a larger volume of blood during the diastolic filling phase of the cardiac cycle.[81]

The pulmonary arterial system undergoes normal maturation after birth, with most patients tolerating the large volume load on the right ventricle and pulmonary circuit quite well for many years. With the development of pulmonary vascular disease and PAH, the left-to-right shunt decreases, largely because of the increased thickness and decreased compliance of the right ventricle. In some patients, this process continues until there is eventually shunt reversal, with arterial desaturation and cyanosis.

CLINICAL MANIFESTATIONS

ASD is found in approximately 6 percent of children surviving beyond the first year of life with congenital heart disease.[82] *If one excludes mitral valve prolapse and the congenitally bicuspid aortic valve, it is the most common form of congenital heart disease among adults.*

ASDs are more common among females, with a female/male ratio of approximately 2:1. The mode of transmission is best explained in most instances on a multifactorial basis, where the risk would be approximately 2.5 percent for first-degree relatives of a single affected family member. However, examples of autosomal dominant transmission are recognized, either as an isolated entity, associated with severe AV conduction disturbances, or with upper extremity malformations as in the Holt-Oram syndrome (see Fig. 10-2). Examples of mendelian autosomal recessive transmission are found in the Ellis–van Creveld syndrome (Fig. 10-1) and the thrombocytopenia–absent radius syndrome[83] (see Chap. 69).

History

The majority of children are considered asymptomatic, but probably most have some mild diminution of stamina, since it is not unusual for the patient or the parents to comment on the increased endurance that follows surgical correction. Symptoms of mild fatigue and dyspnea tend to be recognized in the late teens and early twenties, and at least three-quarters of individuals will be definitely symptomatic as adults. Congestive heart failure is rare in childhood, but a few infants, perhaps 5 percent, will have heart failure in the first year of life. Failure becomes more common again in the fourth and fifth decades, usually associated with the onset of arrhythmias.[84]

Physical Examination

Many children have a slender habitus, but normal growth and development are the rule. Prominence of the left anterior chest is common, and a hyperdynamic right ventricular systolic lift can usually be felt. "Left atrialization" of the jugular venous pulse with *v* wave equal to the *a* wave instead of the normal *a* wave predominance is a characteristic feature. The first heart sound may be slightly accentuated at the lower left sternal border. The two components of the second heart sound are characteristically widely split, with the interval of splitting fixed despite expiration or the Valsalva maneuver. The pulmo-

nary component of the second heart sound may be accentuated, even in the absence of PAH. With increasing pulmonary arterial pressure and resistance, the interval between the aortic and pulmonary components of the second heart sound narrows and the pulmonary component becomes louder, but the lack of respiratory influence on the interval between the two components persists. A midsystolic spindle-shaped murmur of grade 2 to 3 intensity at the left upper sternal border, reflecting increased right ventricular stroke volume, is to be expected. A low- to medium-pitched early diastolic murmur over the lower left sternal border, denoting increased diastolic flow across the tricuspid valve, is present in most individuals with large shunts (see also Chap. 10). Cyanosis and clubbing reflect right-to-left shunting. In this setting, the murmurs of tricuspid and pulmonary regurgitation are not uncommon.

Chest Roentgenogram

Mild-to-moderate cardiac enlargement and prominence of the main and branch pulmonary arteries are characteristic (Fig. 13-2*B*). The absence of left atrial displacement of the barium-filled esophagus in the lateral view helps to distinguish ASD from large left-to-right shunts at other levels (Fig. 70-9).

Electrocardiogram

An rsR′ pattern over the right precordium, indicating mild right ventricular conduction delay or mild right ventricular hypertrophy, is characteristic in secundum-type ASD. The mean QRS axis in the frontal plane is 90° or greater in 60 percent of patients. Left-axis deviation is common in primum-type ASD. Abnormal leftward p axis is common in sinus venosus–type ASD. Serious arrhythmias are usually, though not invariably, limited to adults; atrial fibrillation and atrial flutter are the most common.

Echocardiogram

M-mode studies reflect volume overload of the right side of the heart with increased right atrial and right ventricular dimensions and paradoxical ventricular septal motion. Two-dimensional and Doppler echocardiography with color flow mapping (Chap. 14) permit identification and visualization of virtually all secundum and AV canal defects. Visualization of sinus venosus defects is slightly more difficult.[85] The transesophageal approach (Chap. 14) offers excellent images for those patients in whom the transthoracic approach is inadequate.[86]

Cardiac Catheterization

There is a significant increase in oxygen saturation in the blood samples drawn from the right atrium, right ventricle, and pulmonary artery compared to those from the superior or inferior venae cavae. Pulmonary arterial and right ventricular systolic pressures are normal or only slightly elevated. A systolic pressure gradient of up to 20 mmHg across the right ventricular outflow tract is accepted as secondary to flow rather than to organic obstruction. The right and left atrial

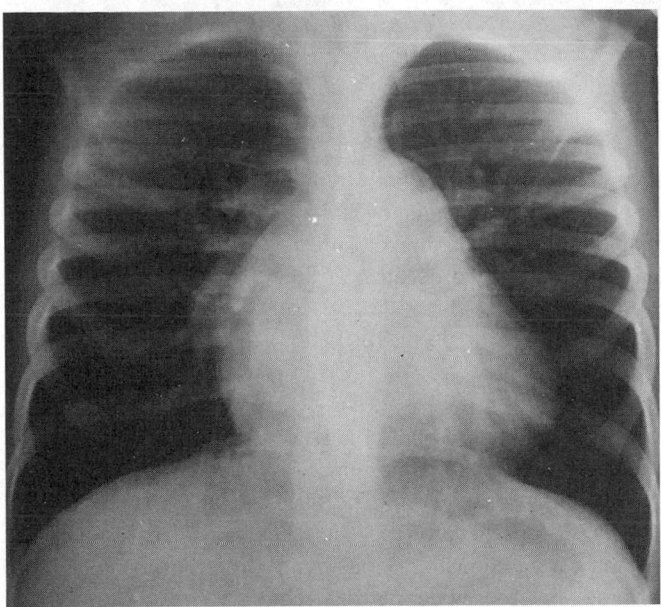

A

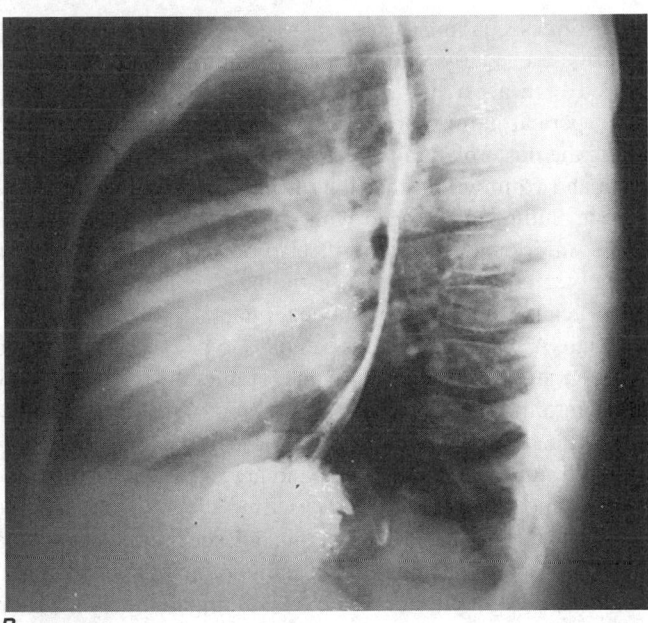

B

FIGURE 70-9

Chest roentgenogram of a 4-year-old child with a secundum atrial septal defect, a large left-to-right shunt, and normal pulmonary arterial pressures. *A.* Frontal. *B.* Lateral. Right ventricular enlargement (seen in the lateral view) accompanies prominence of the main pulmonary arterial segment and increased blood flow. No left atrial dilation is present.

mean and phasic pressures will be virtually identical, with little if any elevation above normal (mean pressure gradient <3 mmHg) unless there are associated abnormalities (see also Chap. 16).

NATURAL HISTORY AND PROGNOSIS

Defects of the secundum type usually go undetected in the first year or two of life because of the lack of symptoms and unimpressive auscultatory findings. A soft systolic murmur is the usual reason for referral. Symptoms become more common in persons in their late teens and twenties, and by age 40 the majority of individuals are symptomatic, some severely so.[87] Pulmonary vascular disease with serious pulmonary hypertension begins to make its appearance in the early twenties. *It affects approximately 15 percent of young adults, particularly women, and may be rapidly progressive, especially with pregnancy.* The incidence of atrial fibrillation or flutter also increases with each decade and is closely linked to the onset of congestive failure. Spontaneous closure of secundum defects is rare beyond the first 2 years of life. The passage of time is associated with a higher mortality and morbidity, with and following corrective surgery.[84] Congestive heart failure is the most common cause of death among unoperated patients. Other causes of death include pulmonary embolism or thrombosis, paradoxical emboli, brain abscess, and infection.

MEDICAL MANAGEMENT

Those few infants presenting with symptoms of congestive failure are treated with digoxin and, if necessary, diuretics and are studied by cardiac catheterization. If the defect is uncomplicated and the symptoms persist despite a trial of therapy, surgical closure is advised without further delay. For asymptomatic infants and children, closure is recommended just prior to their entry into school. Restrictions of activity or exercise are unnecessary. If the physical, laboratory, and echocardiographic findings are completely characteristic, preoperative catheterization is not necessary. Surgery is recommended if the pulmonary/systemic blood flow ratio is >1.5:1, provided no serious malfunction of the left side of the heart is present. Closure is also recommended for those patients with ratios <1.5:1 if PAH is documented by catheterization, provided the systemic arterial saturation is >92 percent and total R_p <15 Wood units.[88] Closure would seem prudent prior to pregnancy or to the use of contraceptives, in view of the tendency to develop rapidly progressive PVOD in this setting. Transcatheter closure of centrally located defects in selected older infants, children, and adults using a double-umbrella ("clamshell") or a buttoned device appears to be an acceptable alternative to surgical closure.[89,90] In the absence of a syndrome transmitted dominantly or recessively in a mendelian pattern and if the patient is the only first-degree relative affected, the risk for the next sibling, or, more importantly, for the patient's parents, is on the order of 2.5 percent.[87] The risk for the child of an affected parent is probably in the 5 percent range, particularly if that parent is the mother.[91] *Infective endocarditis is rare, and antibiotic coverage at times of possible bacteremia is recommended only if associated mitral valve disease is suspected.*

SURGICAL MANAGEMENT

Defects of the interatrial septum are exposed through the lateral wall of the right atrium.

Ostium secundum (fossa ovalis) defects are closed by direct suture; a very large defect or one having tenuous margins is closed with a patch—usually glutaraldehyde-treated autologous pericardium. Anomalous pulmonary veins are sought along the posterolateral aspect of the superior or inferior vena cava and from within the right atrium prior to closure of the defect. Sutures are placed with care along the posterior rim of the inferior vena caval orifice to prevent the creation of a tunnel from the inferior vena cava into the left atrium, which would cause postoperative hypoxemia.

High ASDs of the sinus venosus type, often associated with anomalous drainage of one or more right pulmonary veins into the superior vena cava, are corrected by placement of a pericardial or tubular Dacron patch from above the abnormally draining vein(s) down to and around the ASD (Fig. 70-10). Pulmonary venous blood is thus diverted through the ASD into the left atrium. Pericardial gusset enlargement of the superior vena cava at the cavoatrial junction may be required. Anomalous right pulmonary veins draining to the right atrium are diverted into the left atrium by placement of a patch baffle well anterior and to the right of the pulmonary vein orifices.[78]

Although clinical benefit following closure of ASDs can be anticipated, even in adults having significant physiologic compromise, mortality is higher than in the young and the magnitude of improvement less certain[84,92] (see Chap. 71). Nonetheless, surgical closure of ASDs is advised even when R_p approaches 15 Wood units because of the excessive morbidity and mortality associated with a persistent interatrial communication.[93] *Morbidity in adults and the low risk of surgical closure in young children mandate surgery in the preschool or preadolescent years.*

Although life-threatening complications following closure of ASDs in children are rare, transient postoperative atrial arrhythmias and postpericardiotomy syndrome with pericardial effusions are relatively common. Long-term prognosis for a normal life expectancy and functional capability is excellent for patients having closure of an uncomplicated ASD during the first two decades of life.

Partial Anomalous Pulmonary Venous Connection

PATHOLOGY

In partial anomalous pulmonary venous connection, one or more, but not all, of the pulmonary veins enter the right atrium or its venous tributaries. The atrial septum may be intact, but an ASD is usually present. There are many patterns of anomalous pulmonary venous connection, but the four most common, in order of decreasing frequency, are: (1) pulmonary veins from the right upper and/or middle lobe to the superior vena cava, usually with a sinus venosus ASD; (2) all of the right pulmonary veins to the right atrium, usually in the polysplenia syndrome; (3) all of the right pulmonary veins to the inferior vena cava, entering this systemic vein just above or below the diaphragm; and (4) the left upper or both left pulmonary veins to an anomalous vertical vein draining to the left brachiocephalic vein.

When the right pulmonary veins are connected to the inferior vena cava, the atrial septum may be intact. This venous anomaly may be isolated or may be part of the *scimitar syndrome*. The latter includes hypoplasia of the right lung, bronchial abnormalities, anomalous systemic pulmonary arterial supply to the right lung from branches of the descending thoracic and/or the abdominal aorta, and dextroposition of the heart.

CLINICAL MANIFESTATIONS

In an autopsy series, this malformation occurred in approximately 1 in every 160 individuals, or 0.6 percent of the population.[94] There is no sex predilection. Approximately 15 percent of all ASDs have this coexisting anomaly; however, in the case of the sinus venosus type, the association is in the range of 85 percent.

History

When partial anomalous pulmonary venous connection coexists

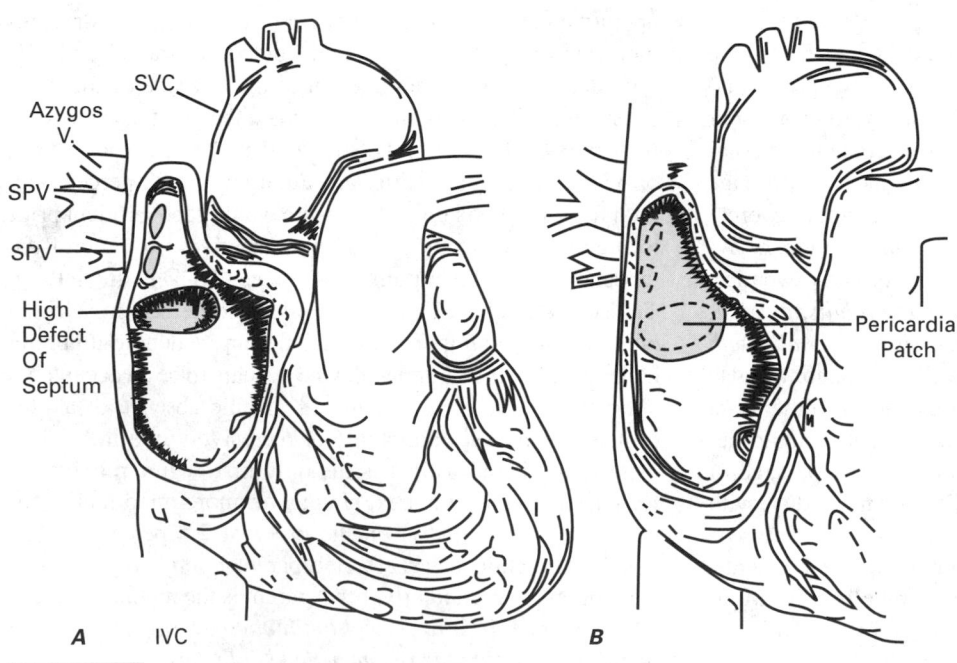

FIGURE 70-10
A. Sinus venosus type of atrial septal defect, with its constantly accompanying anomalous pulmonary venous connection of superior pulmonary vein (SPV) to superior vena cava (SVC) *B.* Repair is effected with a pericardial patch so placed as to divert pulmonary venous blood across the defect into the left atrium and to divert superior vena caval blood to the right atrium. (This illustration appeared originally in the first edition of *The Heart*, in 1966, and in all subsequent editions. It is reproduced here by courtesy of Dr. John W. Kirklin, Birmingham, Alabama.)

with an ASD, the symptoms, as well as the other clinical manifestations, are indistinguishable from those of an isolated ASD. Isolated, uncomplicated anomalous connection of a single pulmonary vein usually goes undetected clinically, since in this circumstance only about 20 percent of the pulmonary venous flow returns to the right atrium or its tributaries. When the entire venous return from one lung or two pulmonary veins is connected anomalously, approximately 65 percent of the pulmonary venous flow returns to the right side of the heart and symptoms are similar to those of an ASD with a comparable increase in pulmonary blood flow.

Physical Examination

The findings are the same as those in patients with an ASD with the exception that *the two components of the second heart sound, though usually widely split, move normally with respiration if the atrial septum is intact.*

Chest Roentgenogram

Right ventricular enlargement, pulmonary arterial dilatation, and increased pulmonary blood flow are characteristic when more than one pulmonary vein connects anomalously. With anomalous connection of the right pulmonary veins to the inferior vena cava, the pulmonary venous pattern may assume a crescent-shaped or scimitar curve in the right lower lung field along the right lower heart border.

Electrocardiogram

The ECG either is normal (in the case of anomalous connection of a single pulmonary vein) or reflects volume overload of the right side of the heart.

Echocardiogram

If more than one pulmonary vein drains anomalously, the volume usually is sufficient to produce the characteristic pattern of right ventricular diastolic overload (Chap. 14). Failure to visualize an atrial septal opening with two-dimensional imaging and color flow mapping from a subcostal coronal or high right-sided parasternal longitudinal view should arouse suspicion of an intact atrial septum. A variety of views supplemented by color flow mapping may be necessary to identify the anomalous connection.[95]

Cardiac Catheterization

Anomalously connected pulmonary veins may be entered directly with the venous catheter. Selective biplane angiograms in these vessels will document their site of connection. Left-to-right shunting with partial anomalous pulmonary venous connection and an intact atrial septum is usually small or moderate and may go undetected by oximetry techniques. Selective indicator dilution curves in the right and left pulmonary arteries with systemic arterial sampling can detect the lung with the anomalous pulmonary venous connection, and selective biplane angiograms in the pulmonary arterial branches will visualize these connections.

NATURAL HISTORY AND PROGNOSIS

Patients with partial anomalous pulmonary venous connection with ASD appear to follow a course similar to, if not identical with, that of patients with an isolated ASD. When the atrial septum is intact, the course depends primarily on the volume of pulmonary venous blood returning to the right side of the heart. Rarely, PVOD may be found, even in the presence of a single anomalously connected pulmonary vein and an intact atrial septum.[96] Finally, increasing left atrial pressure, due either to mitral valve disease or to diminishing left ventricular compliance, will, in the course of time, encourage a greater redistribution of pulmonary arterial blood flow to that portion of the lung drained by the more compliant right atrium. Thus, patients who were initially asymptomatic and had a very modest volume of anomalous pulmonary venous return in youth may become symptomatic and even develop congestive failure in adult life.

MEDICAL MANAGEMENT

Asymptomatic patients with small shunts require no treatment. Those with symptoms, larger pulmonary blood flows, congestive failure, or PAH require surgical correction. With an intact atrial septum, precise preoperative identification of the site of the anomalous venous connection is essential. Long-term follow-up in patients who have not had surgery is indicated to detect increasing flow or the appearance of PAH.

SURGICAL MANAGEMENT

Anomalous connection of right pulmonary vein(s) to the superior vena cava is usually associated with a sinus venosus ASD (Fig. 70-10). (See "Atrial Septal Defect, Surgical Management.") Partial anomalous pulmonary veins draining to the superior vena cava, inferior vena cava, or right atrium are repaired by diverting them through the ASD into the left atrium using an appropriately placed patch baffle. Isolated left-sided anomalous pulmonary veins draining to the left ascending vertical vein or the left superior vena cava are detached and anastomosed directly to the left atrial appendage. Long-term morbidity and mortality are minimal among patients with uncomplicated partial pulmonary venous connections, equivalent to that observed after closure of ASD.[78]

Common Atrioventricular Canal Defects

DEFINITION

The condition called *AV canal* is characterized by an ASD in the lowermost part of the atrial septum, a cleft condition of the mitral valve (either alone or in combination with cleft of the tricuspid valve), and deficiency of ventricular septal tissue. The condition appears to result from incomplete growth of the AV endocardial cushions and atrioventricular septum (see Chap. 8).

PATHOLOGY

The ostium primum type of ASD is characterized by a crescent-shaped upper border and no septal tissue forming the lower border. The lower aspect of the defect is bounded by the atrial surfaces of the AV valves and, in the complete type (see below), in part by the upper edge of the ventricular septum. A small amount of septal tissue separates the defect from the posterior atrial wall.

ANATOMIC TYPES

Variations occur with respect to the nature of the AV valves. The terms *partial* and *complete* were first introduced to describe these types.[97]

Partial Type

The ostium primum ASD is associated with a "cleft" in the anterior mitral leaflet or, probably more accurately, a septal commissure between the superior and the inferior leaflets of the left AV valve (Figs. 70-7*D* and 70-11).[98] The tricuspid valve either is not cleft or shows minor central deficiency. The ventricular aspects of the anterior mitral valve elements are fused to the upper edge of the deficient ventricular septum, precluding an interventricular communication. If there is no atrial septal tissue or if the atrial septum is so rudimentary as

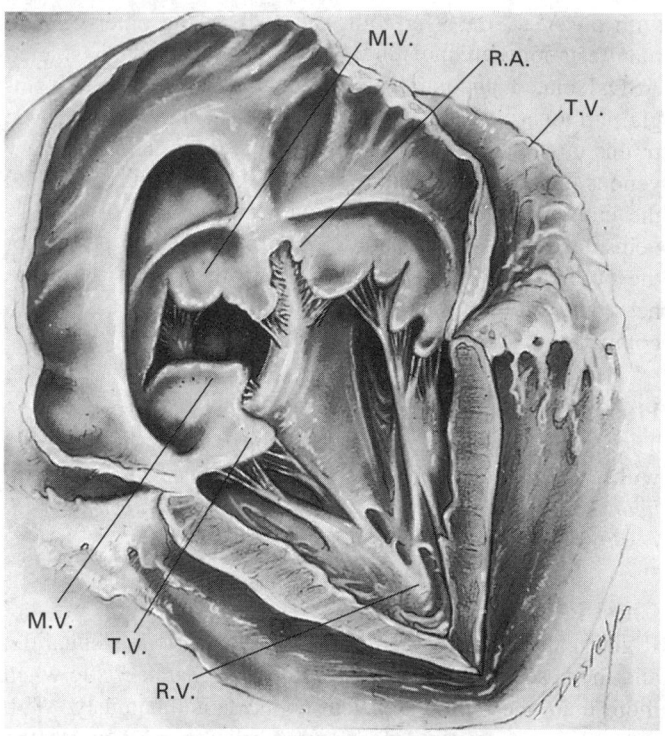

FIGURE 70-12
Complete form of common AV canal type A. The common anterior leaflet has a recognizable mitral component, MV, and tricuspid component, TV. In type B, not illustrated, those components are attached by chordae to a papillary muscle in the right ventricle. In type C, not illustrated, the common anterior leaflet is a single unit without any attachment to the underlying ventricular septum. Type A is most amenable to repair. RV, right ventricle; RA, right atrium. (From Rastelli et al.[99] Reproduced with permission from the publisher and authors.)

to produce a common chamber involving both atria, the term *common atrium* or *single atrium* is applied.

Complete Type

The complete type of common AV canal is characterized by failure of partitioning of the primitive canal into separate AV orifices. The orifice between the atria and the ventricles is guarded by a common valve, of which the anterior leaflet is derived from the ventral AV endocardial cushion and represents the anterior halves of the anterior mitral and septal tricuspid leaflets. The posterior leaflet is derived from the dorsal AV endocardial cushion and represents the posterior halves of the anterior mitral and septal tricuspid leaflets.

Usually, considerable space exists between the anterior and posterior leaflets, above, and the ventricular septum, below, so that in most cases of the complete type there is free communication between the ventricles.

Rastelli and associates subdivided the complete variety into three subgroups—types A, B, and C—on the basis of the structure of the common anterior leaflet and its chordal attachments to the ventricular septum and/or papillary muscles[99] (Fig. 70-12). With regard to the posterior common leaflet, there is variation among the three types as to the

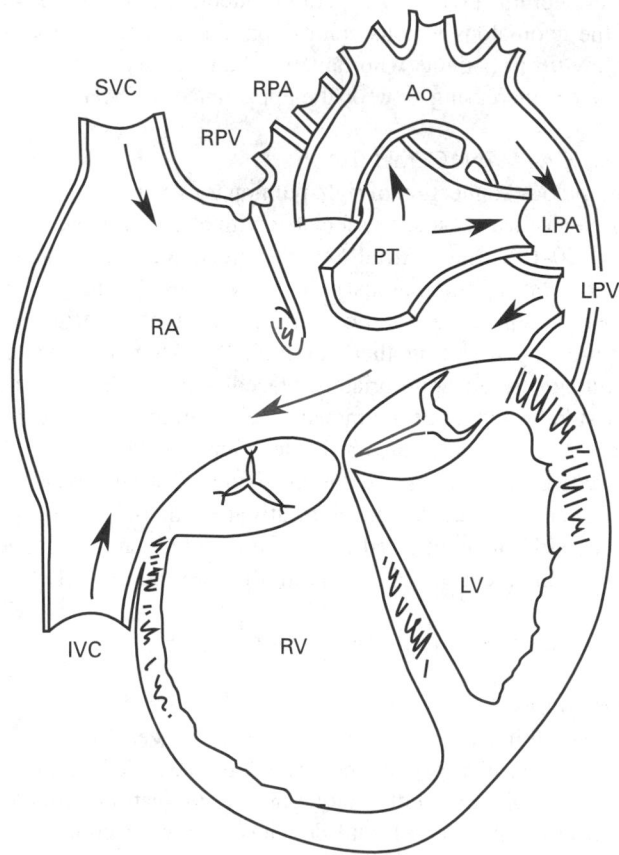

FIGURE 70-11
Common AV canal of the partial type. The mitral valve shows a cleft in its anterior leaflet, while the tricuspid valve is undisturbed. SVC, superior vena cava; IVC, inferior vena cava; RA, right pulmonary artery; LPA, left pulmonary artery; RPV, right pulmonary vein; LPV, left pulmonary vein; LV, left ventricle; Ao, aorta. (From Edwards.[76] Reproduced with permission from the publisher and author.)

presence or absence of subdivision and as to whether the posterior leaflet is attached to the ventricular septum by chordae or by an imperforate membrane.

Variations from the classic types of AV canal defects are recognized, the most frequent being the AV canal type of isolated VSD, isolated ostium primum ASD without malformed AV valves, and isolated cleft of the anterior mitral or septal tricuspid valve leaflets.[100]

ASSOCIATED CONDITIONS

In the asplenia syndrome, the complete variety is almost universal; with polysplenia, it occurs in about one-quarter of cases.[101] An ASD of the secundum type is present in about half of the cases. Double orifice of the mitral valve may be associated with the incomplete type, and tetralogy of Fallot may be associated with the complete type.[100]

ABNORMAL PHYSIOLOGY

If the communication at the ventricular level is large, the right ventricular and pulmonary artery pressures will be elevated. These patients are similar to those with large VSDs. Patients with a communication at the atrial level usually only have normal or slightly elevated systolic pressures in the right side of the heart and a large pulmonary blood flow, as in the secundum type of ASD. Defects in the tricuspid or mitral valve, or both, may result in severe regurgitation or direct shunting of blood from the left ventricle to the right atrium.

CLINICAL MANIFESTATIONS

Approximately 3 percent of infants and children with congenital heart disease have AV canal defects. The majority, some 60 to 70 percent, have the complete form.[102] The female/male ratio is approximately 1.3:1. Well over half of the patients with the complete form have associated Down's syndrome. Among children with Down's syndrome, 45 percent have some form of congenital heart disease. Malformations of the AV canal type, usually of the complete variety, comprise approximately 50 percent of these abnormalities[103] (see also Chap. 69).

History

Only if the mitral valve is incompetent do the symptoms of patients with partial AV canal differ from those associated with a secundum type of ASD. Mitral regurgitation may be associated with poor weight gain, easy fatigue, dyspnea, repeated respiratory infections, and congestive heart failure. Patients with complete AV canal are almost invariably very sick.

Physical Examination

The findings with a partial defect are those of an ASD. If the cleft anterior mitral leaflet is incompetent, the findings of mitral regurgitation will also be present.

The physical findings with the complete canal are those of a very large VSD, usually with full-blown congestive failure, but the second heart sound is split and fixed. The murmur of mitral regurgitation may not be heard or recognized as such.

Chest Roentgenogram

Overall cardiac enlargement, out of proportion to the degree of pulmonary plethora, or a cardiac silhouette suggesting combined ventricular dilatation may serve to distinguish the uncomplicated secundum ASD from the primum defect with significant mitral regurgitation. Marked cardiac enlargement with severe pulmonary overcirculation are features of the complete canal.

Electrocardiogram

One of the most helpful diagnostic features in distinguishing individuals with AV canal defects from those with isolated ASDs or VSDs is the characteristic superior orientation of the mean QRS axis in the frontal plane, with a right bundle branch delay in the precordial leads. Between 92 and 95 percent of both types of canal have a QRS axis lying between 0 and $-150°$.[100] The patterns of atrial and ventricular hypertrophy reflect the underlying hemodynamic abnormalities.

Echocardiogram

Two-dimensional echo is capable of visualizing the extent of septal defects and, with Doppler study and color flow mapping, left-to-right shunting at the atrial and/or ventricular level and associated mitral and/or tricuspid valvular regurgitation (Fig. 70-13). The anatomic features of the anterior AV leaflet and its connections may be visualized with sufficient clarity to permit subdivision of complete AV canal defects into types A, B, and C (see Fig. 70-12).[104] Straddling AV valves, double-orifice mitral valve, single papillary muscles, and hypoplasia or outflow obstruction of the right or left ventricle can also be determined with this technique.[105]

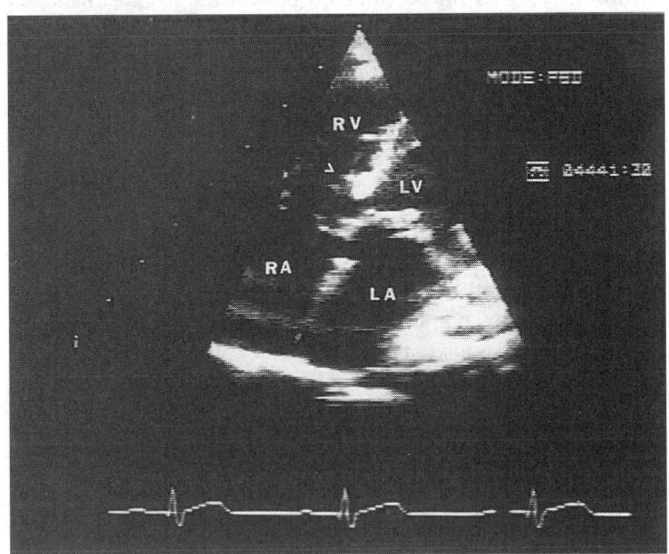

FIGURE 70-13

Two-dimensional echocardiogram in the apical view in a child with atrioventricular canal defect. The defects of the atrial and ventricular septae are clearly outlined. There are attachments from the tricuspid portion of the atrioventricular valve to the interventricular septum (arrowhead). RV, right ventricle; LV, left ventricle; RA, right atrium; LA, left atrium.

Cardiac Catheterization

A significant increase in oxygen saturation between the superior vena cava and the right atrium is present. A right ventricular or pulmonary arterial systolic pressure in excess of 60 percent of the systemic systolic pressure favors the presence of a complete canal. With a large communication between the two ventricles below the AV valves, the right ventricular, pulmonary arterial, and systemic arterial systolic pressures are virtually identical. Left ventricular angiography in the frontal view demonstrates the "gooseneck deformity" of the left ventricular outflow tract characteristic of AV canal malformations and allows a semiquantitative assessment of the degree of mitral regurgitation and shunting from left ventricle to right atrium. The left anterior oblique view with craniocaudal angulation is recommended for visualizing the interventricular defect and judging the extent of ventricular septal deficiency. Aortography is essential to eliminate the possibility of a PDA.

NATURAL HISTORY AND PROGNOSIS

Partial defects without significant mitral regurgitation follow a course similar to that described for the secundum type of septal defects. An exception would be the greater likelihood of infective endocarditis because of the mitral valve deformity. Moderate or severe mitral regurgitation produces heart failure with resulting symptoms and growth retardation. Infants with a complete AV canal without protective pulmonary stenosis quickly develop and continue in congestive failure until the course is altered by death, the development of PVOD, or surgical intervention.

MEDICAL MANAGEMENT

Children with an uncomplicated partial defect are managed in the same manner as children with uncomplicated ASD. Those who are symptomatic should undergo surgical closure of their primum ASD and, if possible, plication of the septal commissure of the left AV ("mitral") valve. Those few patients with significant residual mitral regurgitation following surgery are managed medically until such time as mitral valve replacement is appropriate.

The approach to the infant with complete AV canal is the same as for infants with a large VSD but is tempered by the knowledge that spontaneous improvement is very unlikely except at the expense of the pulmonary vascular bed. Repair is recommended between 4 and 10 months of age if the pulmonary arterial systolic pressure is greater than half the systemic arterial systolic pressure. Elevation of the pulmonary vascular resistance in the first year of life warrants surgical intervention without delay.

Antibiotic coverage at times of special risk of bacteremia is indicated indefinitely for all forms of AV canal, with or without surgery.

With regard to genetic counseling, the risk of a subsequent sibling having heart disease in the presence of a single affected family member is in the range of 2 percent; it is probably higher, perhaps as high as 10 percent, for the offspring of an affected parent, particularly if the affected parent is the mother.[106] Concordance for AV canal defects among affected siblings or offspring is much higher than with other forms of congenital heart disease and approaches 90 percent.

SURGICAL MANAGEMENT

The remarkable clinical improvement following anatomic repair of complete common AV septal defects in infancy encourages early correction within the first year of life. Banding of the pulmonary artery in the critically ill infant having a large interventricular defect was used in the past but has been replaced by a more reparative operation in most centers. Specifics of repair are dictated by anatomic detail: individual variation is considerable (Fig. 70-14), but creation of a competent, nonstenotic left-sided AV ("mitral") valve is essential for acceptable early and long-term prognosis.

A patch is usually sutured to the right side of the ventricular septum to obliterate the interventricular communication. The anterior and posterior components of the mitral valve are sutured to the patch at an appropriate level. The "cleft" be-

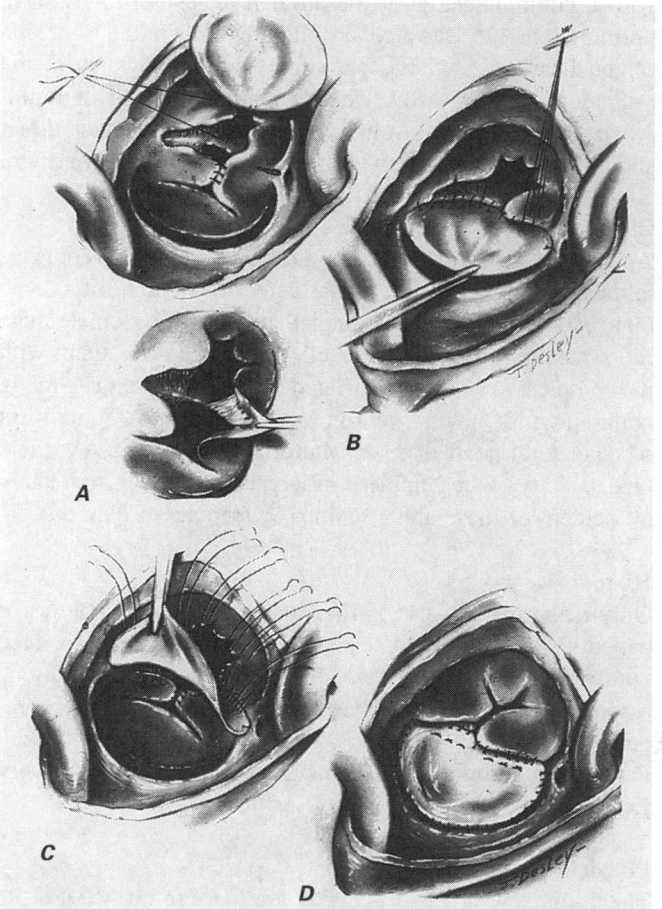

FIGURE 70-14

Steps in the repair of the complete form of common AV canal, type A. *A, B.* A pericardial patch is sutured to the ventricular septum. *C, D.* The anterior leaflet of the mitral valve is reconstructed and attached to the patch. A portion of the tricuspid leaflet is attached to the patch. (From Rastelli et al.[99] Reproduced with permission from the publisher and authors.)

tween the left anterior and left posterior leaflets should be closed by suture if approximation of these edges appears to increase competence without creation of stenosis. Prosthetic valve implantation is rarely required during primary anatomic repair.[107] The right-sided AV ("tricuspid") apparatus, although less critical to survival, is repaired using the same principles. The interatrial communication is usually closed with a separate piece of pericardium to minimize hemolysis in the presence of residual mitral regurgitation.[107] Mitral valve competence is assessed by gentle distention of the left ventricle with cold saline.

Partial AV canal is repaired through a right atriotomy. The cleft may be closed with a few simple interrupted sutures to encourage inversion and coaptation of the leaflet margins. The ASD is usually closed with a pericardial patch.

Permanent complete heart block contributed substantially to early mortality and morbidity but is now rare. Patients undergoing repair of partial AV canal should be observed for the possible development of subaortic left ventricular outflow tract obstruction caused by redundant or residual endocardial cushion tissue.

In-hospital mortality following correction of complete AV canal in infancy ranges from 3 to 10 percent[108,109]; the highest mortality is encountered during the first few months of life and in those infants having severe AV valve regurgitation, elevated pulmonary vascular resistance, hypoplasia of the left or right ventricle, or other cardiac malformations.[107] A 10-year survival of 91 percent, including operative mortality, for patients undergoing total correction has been reported.[110] Successful correction of complete AV canal can be accomplished despite associated common ventricle, tetralogy of Fallot, double-outlet ventricle, and other complex anomalies.[107]

EXTRACARDIAC COMMUNICATIONS BETWEEN THE SYSTEMIC AND PULMONARY CIRCULATIONS, USUALLY WITHOUT CYANOSIS

Patent Ductus Arteriosus

DEFINITION
Patent ductus arteriosus, the most common type of extracardiac shunt, represents persistent patency of the vessel that normally connects the pulmonary arterial system and the aorta in the fetus (Fig. 70-15).

PATHOLOGY
The ductus arteriosus usually closes within 2 or 3 days after birth and becomes the *ligamentum arteriosum*, but it may remain patent as long as 8 weeks postnatally.[111] It runs from the origin of the left pulmonary artery, below, to the lower aspect of the aortic arch just beyond the level of origin of the left subclavian artery, above. The recurrent branch of the left vagus nerve hooks around its lateral and inferior aspects. Closure postnatally is a complex interaction of increased oxygen tension in the blood and circulating prostaglandins. Exog-

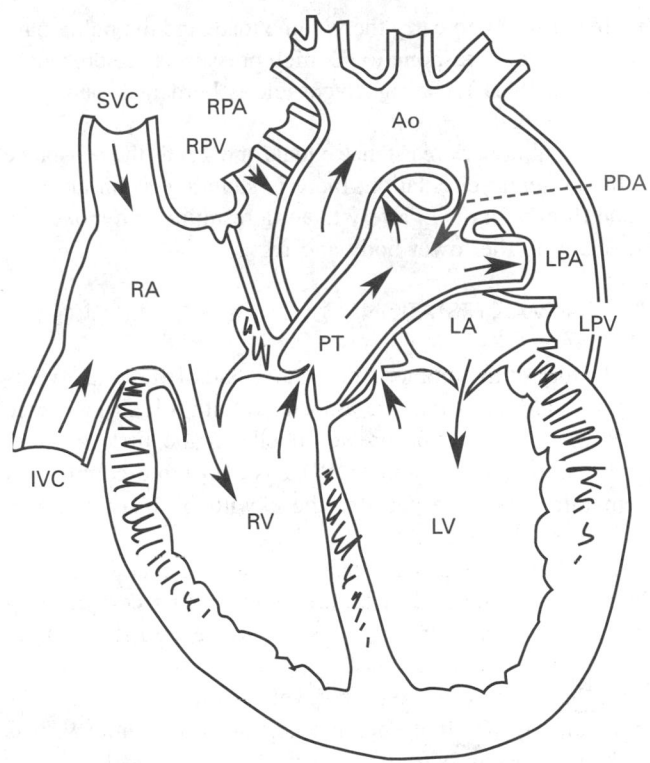

FIGURE 70-15

Patent ductus arteriosus (PDA). SVC, superior vena cava; IVC, inferior vena cava; RA, right atrium; RV, right ventricle; PT, main pulmonary arterial trunk; RPA, right pulmonary artery; LPA, left pulmonary artery; RPV, right pulmonary vein; LPV, left pulmonary vein; LA, left atrium; LV, left ventricle; Ao, aorta. (From Edwards.[76] Reproduced with permission from the publisher and author.)

enous PGE_1 has been used extensively to keep the ductus open postnatally,[112] and indomethacin, a prostaglandin inhibitor, can close the ductus in many premature infants in whom persistent patency is disadvantageous.[113]

ABNORMAL PHYSIOLOGY
Patients with PDA may be divided into groups according to whether the vascular resistance through the ductus itself is low, moderate, or high. The resistance of the ductus is related not only to its cross-sectional area but also to its length. In patients with a very small ductus that offers high resistance, the flow across the ductus is relatively small. The extra volume of work on the left ventricle is small, and the pulmonary pressure and resistance are not elevated. Patients with only moderate resistance in the ductus have some increase in pulmonary artery pressure, with a moderately greater volume of shunting across the ductus.

In patients with a large patent ductus, the aorta and pulmonary artery are essentially in free communication; the systolic pressure in the pulmonary artery will be equal to that in the aorta. The volume load of blood recirculating through the lungs is on the left ventricle, with pulmonary congestion resulting from increased pulmonary flow and/or left ventricular failure. With time, the left ventricle compensates with dilation and hypertrophy to carry the volume load, and the pulmonary vasculature may respond to the high pressure. (See preceding section on PAH.) The right ventricle is burdened mainly by a pressure load.

If the pulmonary resistance equals or exceeds the resistance of the systemic circulation, there is shunting of unsaturated blood from pulmonary artery to aorta resulting in hypoxemia, especially in the lower body and legs.

CLINICAL MANIFESTATIONS

History
The history of the mother's pregnancy and of perinatal events may provide clues that are associated with a high incidence of PDA, such as exposure to rubella in the first trimester by a nonimmunized mother. PDA is also more common in premature infants, especially those with birth asphyxia or respiratory distress.[114–117]

Symptoms are usually restricted to patients with large shunts that produce heart failure or with other complicating problems, such as respiratory distress in the premature infant. The symptoms related to heart failure were discussed earlier. Heart failure is most likely to develop in the first few weeks or months of life. If it does not appear during infancy, it is unlikely to occur before the third decade. Growth may be affected in those with large shunts and failure. The clinical presentation in the premature infant is usually very different from that in the full-term infant. This is particularly true in those with a birth weight under 1.5 kg, who are more likely to have moderate to severe respiratory distress. In these infants, the clinical features of respiratory distress often blend over the course of several days into those of heart failure. Increasing ventilatory or oxygen requirements with carbon dioxide retention or episodic apnea and bradycardia are often the first signs that a PDA may be complicating the picture.

Physical Examination
In the full-term infant or child with PDA, there is frequently a systolic thrill over the pulmonary artery and in the suprasternal notch. The peripheral pulses are generally brisk and bounding, especially with the larger shunts secondary to runoff from the aorta to the pulmonary artery in diastole. The patient with elevated pulmonary vascular resistance and shunt reversal will have "differential cyanosis," with cyanosis and clubbing of the toes and occasionally clubbing of the fingers on the left due to right-to-left shunting from the pulmonary artery into the descending aorta. The apex impulse may be increased or displaced in those with large shunts. The right ventricular impulse is increased in the premature infant with respiratory distress and in infants and children with significant pulmonary hypertension. The typical murmur is a continuous, or "machinery," murmur that is best heard at the left upper sternal border and below the left clavicle. It is usually a rough murmur with eddy sounds, which are helpful in making the diagnosis, and it peaks at or near the second heart sound. In patients with at least a moderate shunt, there is a middiastolic rumble at the apex due to increased flow across the mitral valve. The second heart sound may be difficult to hear due to the continuous murmur, but it is usually normal. The pulmonary component will be accentuated in those with pulmonary hypertension.

Chest Roentgenogram
Findings on chest roentgenogram are also dependent on the magnitude of the shunt. In patients with a small shunt, the chest roentgenogram is normal. With larger shunts, the left atrium and left ventricle are enlarged. Increases in pulmonary arterial flow on x-ray parallel the magnitude of the shunt. In the presence of heart failure, there are signs of pulmonary edema. In older patients who have developed Eisenmenger physiology, the only abnormality may be marked prominence of the central pulmonary arteries, with rapid tapering to the periphery of the lung fields.

Electrocardiogram
With a small shunt, the ECG is normal. Left atrial hypertrophy is probably the most common abnormality found, but left ventricular hypertrophy of the volume overload type, with deep Q waves and increased R-wave voltage in the left precordial leads, is also common. Right ventricular hypertrophy is seen with pulmonary hypertension.

Echocardiogram
There is left atrial enlargement, and the left ventricular end-diastolic dimension and mean velocity of circumferential fiber shortening are significantly increased.[118] Small shunts can be detected with color Doppler imaging with a typical spectral flow pattern, while a larger ductus can be visualized with two-dimensional echocardiography (Fig. 70-16).

Cardiac Catheterization
In those with typical, uncomplicated PDA, cardiac catheterization is not necessary. When catheterization is performed, the catheter usually passes quite easily from the pulmonary artery, compared to the right atrium and ventricle, to the descending aorta, except when the ductus is too small. The saturation will be increased in the pulmonary artery to a degree relative to the size of the shunt. The pulmonary arterial and right ventricular pressures are elevated in those with a large ductus. The pulmonary vascular resistance will be elevated in older patients who have developed changes in the pulmonary vascular bed. These patients will also have diminished saturation in the descending aorta once the pulmonary resistance reaches a level that will reverse the shunt. Aortography will opacify the ductus and pulmonary arteries.

NATURAL HISTORY AND PROGNOSIS
The complications related to PDA include infective endarteritis, heart failure, and pulmonary hypertension with vascular damage. Infection of the ductus is a risk regardless of its size. The risk increases with length of survival. This can lead to development of a mycotic aneurysm with the potential of

compressing the recurrent laryngeal nerve, embolizing septic material to the lungs, or rupturing. Calcification of the ductal wall is common in adults.

In patients with large shunts, heart failure can cause significant morbidity and mortality, particularly in the premature and young infant, and sudden death can occur. Progressive damage to the pulmonary vascular bed can occur in some, but it rarely occurs to an irreversible degree in the first year or two of life. Once irreversible damage occurs, premature death in late adolescence or early adulthood can be anticipated.

MEDICAL MANAGEMENT

Interruption of flow through the PDA is the ultimate goal of management. For those in congestive heart failure, usually premature infants, medical management with digoxin and diuretics with fluid restriction may have a minor role,[119] but the ultimate aim is closure to prevent heart failure and promote growth in the infant and prevent infective endarteritis and pulmonary vascular disease in the older child.

For premature infants, treatment with indomethacin is usually the first line of therapy.[113] Successful closure depends on both dosage and timing of treatment, although the major determinants seem to be gestational and postnatal age rather than the concentration of the drug. Because of ductal reopening, serial treatment regimens may be necessary, especially in those weighing less then 1000 g at birth. There is increasing evidence that administration of "prophylactic" indomethacin in those infants weighing less than 1000 g may be associated with a higher closure rate and a better outcome.[120] Indomethacin therapy has been associated with increased bleeding tendency due to platelet dysfunction, decreased urine output secondary to renal dysfunction, and necrotizing enterocolitis.[113] For the very premature with a PDA, however, a trial of indomethacin is preferable to the other options.

For premature infants who failed to close their PDA with a course of indomethacin or for term infants with a persistent PDA, closure has been recommended. If the PDA is large, there is usually a large left-to-right shunt with congestive heart failure. In these infants, the indication for closure is heart failure and usually failure to thrive. Even in the absence of these indications, when a large PDA is associated with PAH, closure is recommended to prevent PVOD. In children with a smaller PDA, with an audible murmur but no evidence of significant hemodynamic embarrassment, closure is usually recommended because of the incidence of bacterial endarteritis, which over a lifetime is in the range of 30 percent. For children with a PDA without a heart murmur, usually discovered incidentally when an echocardiogram is performed for other reasons, the authors do not currently recommend closure.

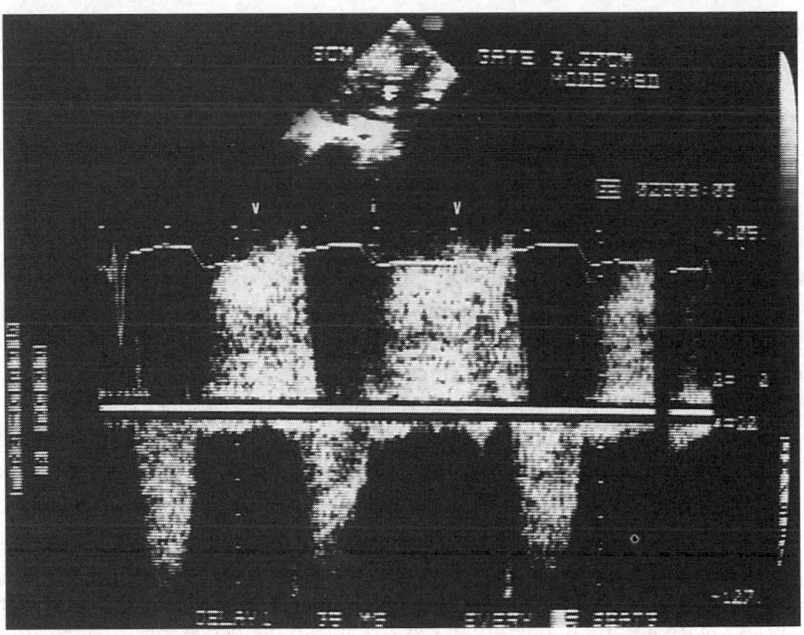

FIGURE 70-16

Pulsed-wave Doppler with spectral display and sampling volume in the pulmonary artery in a patient with a patent ductus arteriosus outlines pandiastolic reversal (*arrowheads*) of flow with spectral broadening.

SURGICAL AND INTERVENTIONAL CATHETER CLOSURE

Surgery for a persistent PDA was first reported more than 55 years ago and is now done routinely in most centers. The safety and efficacy of this procedure even in very young children is well established, with risks that are very low (well under 1 percent) and success at interrupting flow almost universal.

Recently two methods have been popularized that substitute for this method—closure by interventional cardiac catheterization and video-assisted thorascopic surgical repair. In 1971, Portsmann and Wierny introduced a rather complex methodology to plug a PDA by a transarterial and transvenous approach using very large catheters.[121] More recently, Rashkind and Cuaso introduced, and others have popularized, the use of a double-umbrella device to plug a PDA.[122] While the delivery sheath of the Rashkind device is smaller than those initially utilized, it is still large, requiring either a no. 8 or no. 11 French sheath, depending upon the size of the device, making it inapplicable to young and very small children. In spite of a fair amount of experience among interventional cardiologists, there continues to be some problem with residual shunts, hemolysis, and occasional protrusion of the device into the left pulmonary artery or aorta.

Gianturco coils, thin metallic wires glossed with Dacron that assume a coil configuration when released from a catheter, become an attractive alternative, since they can be delivered via relatively small catheters and have been found to be quite effective, although their utility is limited to PDAs that are less than 3.5 or 4.0 mm at their narrowest point.[123,124] In groups using these coils, the results have been very promising, with a 95 percent success rate.

The conventional historical approach has been surgical. The PDA is exposed and mobilized through a small left thoracotomy in the fourth intercostal space.[125] Ductus obliteration is accomplished by division or ligation. A short, broad, or thin-walled ductus is divided between vascular clamps. The ends are closed with continuous suture. A long, narrow, thick-walled ductus can be divided or ligated with two or three sutures spaced a few millimeters apart. The suture ligatures at each end are anchored superficially in the ductus wall to prevent migration and to assure thrombosis and obliteration.

The fragile and thin-walled PDA of the premature infant is obliterated by gentle ligation with a thick suture to minimize disruption or, if small, by occlusion using metallic surgical clips.[126] Extrapleural exposure is preferred by some surgeons. Ligation in the neonatal intensive care unit, avoiding transport to the operating room, is common. Transport from a remote intensive care unit to a cardiac surgical unit for ductus ligation on a "day-stay" basis is also efficacious.[127] Ductus obliteration offers clinical improvement in infants weighing as little as 500 g, with minimal operative risk, reduced incidence of necrotizing enterocolitis, reduced duration of intubation, and improvement in late survival.[128]

Closure of a PDA in an adult requires particular caution; calcification and rigidity of the ductus wall complicate clamping. Placement of a Dacron patch over the aortic orifice of the ductus from within the aorta may be advisable.[129]

Recently, advances in less invasive surgery have been applied to closure of a PDA via several small incisions using video-assisted thorascopic surgery. A miniaturized camera is inserted into the thorax, and through a separate tiny incision, a surgical stapler is inserted and a clip placed across the PDA, interrupting flow. Among 230 patients, there was only one with minimal residual flow; one with persistent recurrent laryngeal nerve dysfunction; and no deaths, transfusions, or chylothoraces. The mean operating time was 20 min, and the hospital stay was only a couple of days.[130] At Children's Hospital, Boston, this has been applied to premature infants as small as 575 g, with discharge from the hospital the day following the procedure in full-term infants or children.[131] With several highly successful, low-risk, inexpensive, and minimally traumatic procedures available to close a persistent PDA in the neonate child, adolescent, or adult without pulmonary vascular disease, local experience is likely to be the best guide as to which option is preferable in an individual child.

Sinus of Valsalva Fistula

PATHOLOGY

Sinus of Valsalva fistula is uncommon; it is also referred to as *aortic sinus aneurysm*. Because of an assumed intrinsic weakness at the union of the aorta with the heart, the aortic media may separate from the aortic annulus and retract upward. The structure that lies between becomes aneurysmal and may rupture to form a fistula. The usual sites of the defects are the posterior (noncoronary) sinus aneurysms that rupture through the atrial septal wall into the right atrium (Fig. 70-17A) and those of the right sinus that rupture into the right ventricular infundibulum (Fig. 70-17B).[132,133] The aneurysm is represented by a gray pouch with multiple perforations in the wall. The principal associated condition is a supracristal VSD in cases with aneurysms of the right sinus (about 50 percent).

CLINICAL MANIFESTATIONS

Sinus of Valsalva fistulas are most common in adults.[134] When the rupture is secondary to bacterial endocarditis,[135] evidence of preceding infection is found. If the rupture occurs slowly, a small fistulous tract into the right atrium or ventricle develops and presents recent-onset findings of a small left-to-right shunt. With sudden rupture, there is usually a tearing pain in the midchest associated with dramatically rapid development of pulmonary congestion due to the sudden onset of a large shunt. Characteristically, the murmur is loud and continuous but heard lower on the chest than the murmur of PDA. A to-and-fro murmur rather than a continuous one may be heard at times. The apex impulse is hyperdynamic, and the pulse pressure is widened. VSD may complicate the clinical picture. Cardiac catheterization will confirm the level of the shunt. A pressure difference across the right ventricular outflow tract may be present if the right sinus is involved. Aortography or Doppler echocardiography[136] will confirm the diagnosis.

NATURAL HISTORY AND PROGNOSIS

With slow rupture and a small shunt, the major risk is infective endocarditis or extension of the rupture with an increasing shunt. With a large shunt, the heart failure is usually rapidly progressive and may result in death very quickly. A few patients seem to stabilize in this situation.[137]

MEDICAL MANAGEMENT

Appropriate cultures should be drawn and antibiotics begun if endocarditis is suspected. Treatment of heart failure should be instituted rapidly. *Because of the natural history, all patients should have this condition corrected surgically.*[138]

SURGICAL MANAGEMENT

Aneurysms or fistulae from the noncoronary or right coronary sinuses are repaired through the aortic root while the patient is supported on total cardiopulmonary bypass with moderate hypothermia, using techniques similar to those employed for aortic valve replacement. The aortic valve leaflets, the margins of the aneurysm, and the coronary arterial orifices must be precisely visualized. Aneurysms of the noncoronary sinus can be repaired through the right atrium; those arising from the right coronary sinus are accessible through the right ventricle. In most cases, the orifice of the aneurysmal fistula is surgically obliterated using a Dacron patch.[139]

A conal, or supracristal (type I), VSD must be sought and closed through either the aortic valve or the right ventricular outflow tract when an aneurysm of the right coronary sinus extends into the right ventricle. Aortic valve replacement was

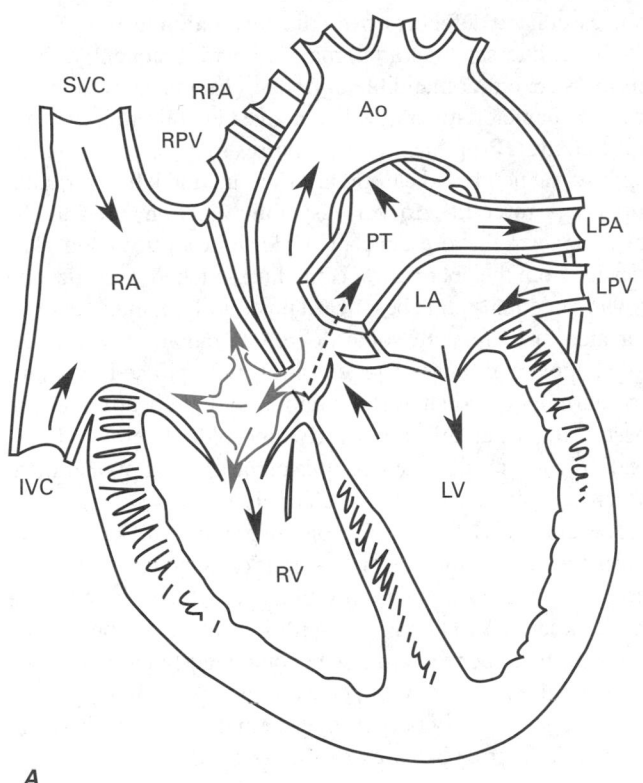

A

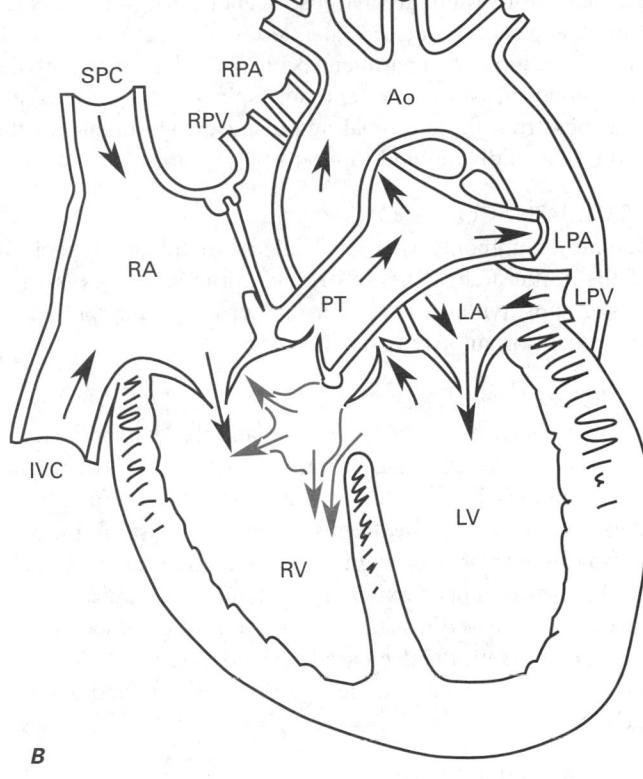

B

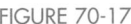

FIGURE 70-17

Sinus of Valsalva fistula. *A*. Aneurysm involves the posterior sinus and ruptures into the right atrium. *B*. Aneurysm involves the right aortic sinus and ruptures into the right ventricle. A ventricular septal defect is commonly associated, as illustrated. SVC, superior vena cava; IVC, inferior vena cava; RA, right atrium; RV, right ventricle; PT, main pulmonary arterial trunk;

RPA, right pulmonary artery; LPA, left pulmonary artery; RPV, right pulmonary vein; LPV, left pulmonary vein; LA, left atrium; LV, left ventricle; Ao, aorta. (From Edwards.[76] Reproduced with permission from the publisher and author.)

required to correct associated aortic regurgitation in 24 of 45 patients.[138]

In a review of 176 cases of aortic fistula to the heart, 126 were repaired, with success in 108 (86 percent).[140] In another series, correction of ruptured aneurysm of the aortic sinuses was accomplished in 51 patients by exposure through the cardiac chamber into which rupture occurred; survival rate was 88 percent.[141] Improved survival can probably be anticipated on the basis of the 21 patients operated upon at the Mayo Clinic and reviewed in 1971,[142] all of whom survived even though 3 patients required secondary operations to repair dehiscence of the repair.

VALVULAR AND VASCULAR MALFORMATIONS OF THE LEFT SIDE OF THE HEART WITH RIGHT-TO-LEFT, BIDIRECTIONAL, OR NO SHUNT

Coarctation of the Aorta

PATHOLOGY

Coarctation of the aorta is a discrete narrowing of the distal segment of the aortic arch. The characteristic lesion is a deformity of the media of the aorta, involving the anterior, superior,

and posterior walls, and is represented by a curtain-like infolding of the wall that causes the lumen to be narrowed and eccentric.[143]

In infants, the lesion lies either opposite the ductus or in a preductal location. In adolescents and adults, it is usually distal to the ligamentum arteriosum. An aberrant right subclavian artery may be associated. In about one-half of such cases, the vessel arises proximal to the coarctation and is distal to the coarctation in the other half. In rare cases, the lesion lies proximal to the origin of the left common carotid artery or involves a segment of the abdominal aorta.[144]

The principal cardiac abnormality is left ventricular hypertrophy. In some infants, left ventricular endocardial fibroelastosis may be associated. Tubular hypoplasia of the distal aortic arch and isthmus is very common and appears directly related to the presence and severity of associated cardiac anomalies.[145] The proximal aorta may show moderate degrees of cystic medial necrosis (see also Chap. 98). Beyond the coarctation, the lining may show a localized jet lesion.

Prominent collaterals are characteristic in the older infant, child, and adolescent. These may be divided into anterior and posterior systems, with the anterior system originating with the internal mammary arteries and making use of the epigastric arteries in the abdominal wall to supply the lower extremities.

The posterior system involves parascapular arteries connected with the posterior intercostal arteries and carries blood to the distal aortic compartment principally for supply of the abdominal viscera. The anterior spinal artery, receiving branches from the proximal and distal compartments of the aorta, is also dilated and tortuous.

ASSOCIATED CONDITIONS

The most commonly associated defects are tubular hypoplasia of the aortic arch, PDA, VSD, and aortic stenosis (valvular and/or subvalvular).[146] A bicuspid aortic valve is present in 46 percent of autopsy cases.[143]

ABNORMAL PHYSIOLOGY

In most instances, both the systolic and the diastolic arterial pressures above the coarctation are elevated above normal levels. Below the coarctation, the systolic pressure is lower than that in the upper extremities, and the diastolic pressure is usually near or only slightly below the normal range. The mechanism of upper extremity hypertension appears to involve the increased resistance to aortic flow produced by the coarctation itself, the decreased capacity and distensibility of the vessels into which the left ventricle ejects, and humoral factors.[147]

CLINICAL MANIFESTATIONS

Coarctation of the aorta occurs in approximately 8 to 9 percent of all infants and children with congenital heart disease and is the predominant lesion in approximately 8 percent of infants presenting with critical heart disease in the first year of life. It ranks behind only VSD, dextrotransposition of the great arteries, and tetralogy of Fallot.[148] Of all individuals born with coarctation, approximately half present within the first month or two of life with heart failure. About 50 percent of infants so admitted have uncomplicated coarctation; the remaining half can be expected to have at least one complicating cardiac abnormality. VSD is the most common (64 percent), followed by left ventricular outflow tract obstruction (31 percent).[146] The timing of ductal tissue constriction, both in terms of ductal closure and, perhaps, aortic constriction, appears to play a decisive role in the onset or worsening of symptoms in most of these patients. The male/female ratio is approximately 3:1 for isolated coarctation but is only 1.1:1 for complicated coarctation. Approximately 45 percent of children with Turner's syndrome (Fig. 10-19) have coarctation. Familial occurrence has been described.[149]

History

The clinical picture in the symptomatic infant is one of dyspnea, difficulty in feeding, and poor weight gain. Older children are for the most part asymptomatic, although a few will complain of mild fatigue, dyspnea, or symptoms of claudication in their legs when running.

Physical Examination

In the symptomatic infant, signs of congestive heart failure are characteristic. A gallop rhythm is common, and a murmur

from associated defects or from the coarctation itself (posteriorly in the interscapular area) may be heard. Frequently, these murmurs are either inaudible or nondescript on admission and become characteristic only when congestive failure is brought under control. Prominent arterial pulses may be visible in the suprasternal notch and carotid arteries, and the left ventricular impulse is forceful. An early systolic ejection click at the apex suggests the presence of a bicuspid aortic valve. The murmur from the coarctation is medium-pitched, systolic, and blowing in quality. It is best heard posteriorly in the interscapular area, usually with some degree of radiation to the left axilla, apex, and anterior precordium. Low-pitched, continuous murmurs of collateral circulation may be heard over the chest wall, particularly posteriorly, but seldom before adolescence. A short middiastolic rumble at the apex without clinical evidence of mitral disease is relatively common.

The characteristic systolic blood pressure difference between the upper and lower extremities may be difficult to appreciate or measure in infants with severe congestive failure or with a large VSD or PDA. With improved compensation, pulses in the upper extremities become readily palpable. The femoral pulses remain weak, delayed, or absent. In these very young infants, it is important that the pulses in both brachial and carotid arteries be assessed. Weak or absent pulses in all sites are characteristic of critical aortic stenosis or aortic atresia.

In older children and adults, the radial arterial pulses typically are strong; those in the femoral arteries are either diminished, delayed, or absent. A measured systolic or mean pressure difference between the upper and lower extremities of greater than 10 mmHg is diagnostic. The pulse pressure in the leg is reduced, and in some patients no pressure can be measured by auscultation. Approximately one-third will have mild to severe hypertension, with the latter defined as a systolic pressure above 150 mmHg, a diastolic pressure above 100 mmHg, or both. Some patients have only a mild pressure difference between the arms and legs at rest but a much larger difference during treadmill exercise. A systolic pressure difference between the two arms suggests that the origin of one subclavian artery is at or below the obstruction.

Given the simplicity of measuring the blood pressure in the upper and lower extremities of children and the importance of early detection, it is surprising and disappointing that approximately 95 percent of children and adolescents with coarctation are referred by pediatricians and other health-care providers to a pediatric cardiologist for evaluation of a heart murmur and/or hypertension without this serious underlying malformation being recognized.[150]

Chest Roentgenogram

For the symptomatic infant, the pattern is one of impressive cardiac enlargement and venous congestion. In the older and asymptomatic child, the heart size is generally at the upper limits of normal with a left ventricular prominence. A figure-three configuration of the left margin of the aorta at the level of the coarctation may be seen in overpenetrated films, with the upper curve formed by the slightly dilated aorta just above the coarctation, the central indentation by the coarctation itself, and the lower curve by the poststenotic dilatation below the coarctation (Fig. 13-1C). Notching of the inferior margin of the ribs by tortuous intercostal arteries acting as collaterals is seldom present before 7 or 8 years of age.

Electrocardiogram

The ECG of the symptomatic infant reflects right or biventricular hypertrophy during the first 3 months of life. T-wave inversion in the left precordial leads is common. In older children, the ECG is usually normal or may indicate mild left ventricular and left atrial hypertrophy.

Echocardiogram

Echocardiography is useful in assessing left ventricular function. Two-dimensional echocardiographic imaging of the aortic arch from the suprasternal notch permits visualization of the coarctation and detection of anatomic variations, such as isthmic or transverse arch hypoplasia. The precordial and subxiphoid views are of great value in assessing the presence and severity of associated defects. Doppler flow studies are helpful for diagnostic confirmation.[151]

Cardiac Catheterization

Study of symptomatic infants characteristically reveals left atrial and left ventricular hypertension and a significant systolic pressure difference between the left ventricle and the femoral artery, particularly if the coarctation is isolated. In the presence of a large VSD or PDA, the left ventricular hypertension and the systolic pressure difference between the left ventricle and femoral artery are less impressive and may not exist at all. Every attempt should be made to define the nature and severity of associated defects. Imaging is recommended in older children to demonstrate the exact site and length of the coarctation as well as to show unusual features of the collateral circulation that may be of importance to the surgeon. Magnetic resonance imaging (Chap. 19) is an excellent and, in most instances, preferable alternative to angiography today for demonstrating the site and length of the coarctation (Fig. 70-18).

NATURAL HISTORY AND PROGNOSIS

Approximately one-half of infants admitted with heart failure within the first weeks of life will have coarctation without significant associated defects.[146] The majority of these infants will respond well to medical management and, usually, reach a stage at 2 or 3 years of age where they are indistinguishable from those asymptomatic children of the same age whose coarctation is first detected on a routine physical examination. Upper extremity hypertension usually increases during the first several months of life and then tends to diminish again as collateral circulation improves, while signs of failure diminish at the same time. For infants with severe failure and any serious associated defects, surgery provides virtually the only chance of survival.

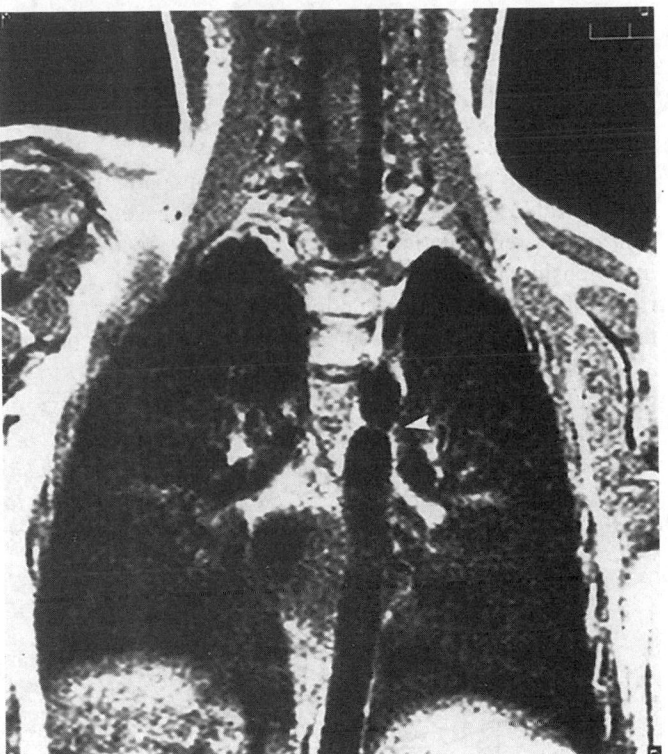

FIGURE 70-18
Selected frame from magnetic resonance imaging study in coronal plane in child with coarctation of the aorta. The proximal aorta is not in the imaging plane, but the isthmus and descending thoracic aorta are clearly imaged with a discrete coarctation (*arrow*) in the common position.

The consequences of persistent hypertension in the individual who has not undergone surgery appear in the second and third decades in the form of hypertension, aortic rupture, or intracranial hemorrhage from an aneurysm of the circle of Willis. Congestive heart failure, often complicated by mitral or aortic valve disease, dissecting aneurysm of the aorta, or atherosclerosis, is seen in the fourth decade. The risk of endocarditis on the aortic or mitral valves or endarteritis at the site of coarctation appears spread relatively evenly over the years. The average age of death of patients surviving childhood with coarctation without surgery is 34 years[152] (see Chap. 71).

MEDICAL MANAGEMENT

Vigorous medical treatment is indicated for infants with severe heart failure. The newborn with severe failure may experience dramatic relief with the intravenous infusion of PGE_1 to reopen the closing ductus. Prompt surgical correction of the coarctation is recommended for all infants in whom there is one or more associated defects and for all infants with isolated coarctation unless the response to medical management has been dramatic and sustained. Balloon dilation angioplasty of unoperated coarctation is still a debated issue and is not currently recommended. The incidence of recoarctation at follow-up in infants undergoing end-to-end anastomosis or subclavian flap angioplasty of the aorta in the first year of life is of the order of 20 percent.[153] Infants not requiring immediate surgery generally improve steadily but develop impressive hypertension in the first months of life. *For this reason the authors recommend surgical repair of the coarctation in all symptomatic infants upon discovery.*

Residual or recurrent hypertension among patients without demonstrable recurrent coarctation, renal disease, or significant aortic regurgitation appears related to the duration of hypertension prior to surgery. This complication is in the range of 6 percent among individuals operated upon before the age of 6 years but becomes progressively more common as surgery is delayed; it may be present in from 45 to 50 percent of individuals operated upon at 20 years of age or beyond.

Elective correction of coarctation has been recommended for children between the ages of 1 and 4 years in order to avoid (1) the relatively high rate of recoarctation found among *patients with coarctation corrected before 1 year of age, and (2) the complication of persistent or recurrent hypertension, without demonstrable recoarctation, among those individuals having surgery after 6 years of age.* With advances in surgical techniques, many centers are now performing elective surgery in children under 1 year of age. Restriction from strenuous sports or exercise is recommended prior to correction. Older children and adults should undergo correction without delay.

Patients who have had coarctation should be followed indefinitely. For those with significant recoarctation, expressed as a systolic pressure gradient between the upper and lower extremities of 20 mmHg or more at rest, balloon angioplasty or reoperation is recommended.[146] Those who have insignificant or small resting gradients but who manifest abnormal upper extremity hypertension and significant gradients with exercise probably should undergo balloon angioplasty or reoperation as well. Patients with persistent hypertension without gradients either at rest or with exercise and those patients described above in whom reoperation seems unjustified or unduly hazardous will probably benefit from restricted activity and antihypertensive medication.

Pregnancy carries a mortality rate of approximately 10 percent and a complication rate of 90 percent among women with uncorrected coarctation. After correction, the mortality rate does not differ significantly from the normal, while complications are of the order of 15 percent.[154] The risk of congenital heart disease in the offspring of one affected parent or in a sibling of a single affected family member is estimated at 2 percent, with about a 50 percent chance of the defect being coarctation.[155]

SURGICAL MANAGEMENT

The coarctation is exposed and mobilized through a left posterolateral thoracotomy. It is usually possible to resect the narrow segment and restore continuity by direct end-to-end anastomosis (Fig. 70-19). Repair by subclavian flap aortoplasty in the first few years of life probably offers the greatest likelihood of long-term cure, although the choice of specific operation in infancy remains controversial.[153]

Occasionally a tubular vascular prosthesis is required to bridge the gap between the two ends of the aorta when the coarctation is unusually long, the aortic isthmus is hypoplastic, or there is an associated aneurysm. In adults with a relatively nonelastic or calcified aorta and in secondary repairs, a tubular vascular prosthesis can be used to bypass the unresected coarctation or the previous repair. Dacron patch repair of coarctation in older children has an unacceptably high incidence of late aneurysm formation and is no longer advised.[156] Tension-free suture lines are

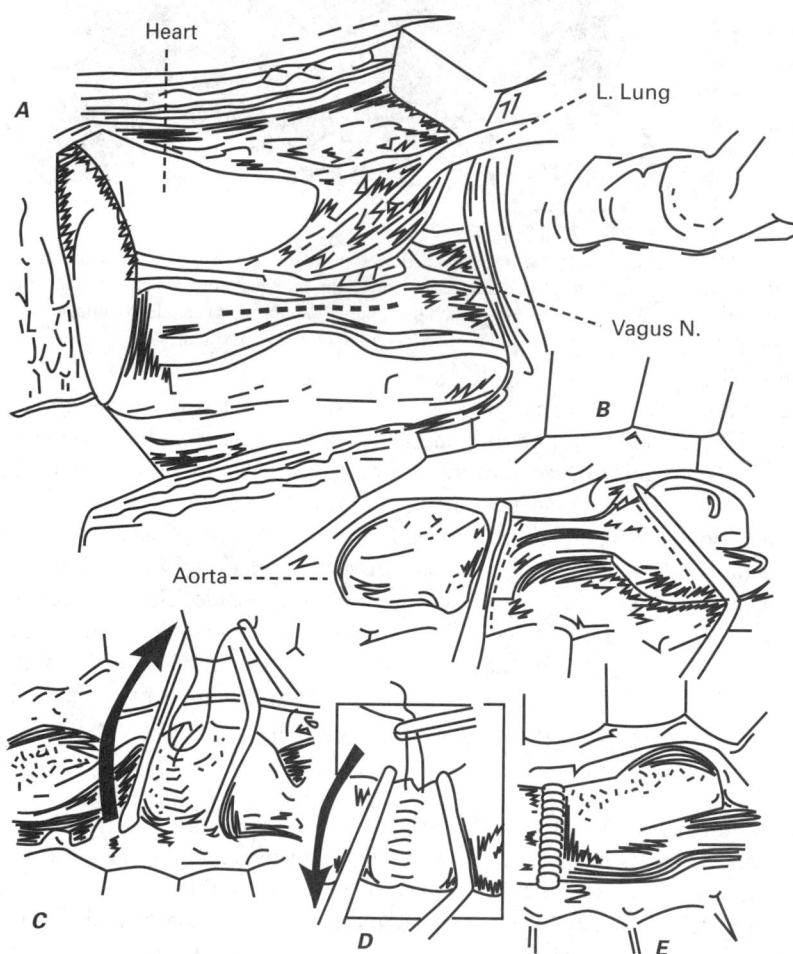

FIGURE 70-19

Steps in operative repair of coarctation of the aorta. *A.* Mediastinal pleura is opened over the upper part of the descending thoracic aorta. *B.* After appropriate mobilization of the coarctation area and division of ligamentum arteriosum, appropriate clamps are placed above and below the structure. At times the distal clamp must be placed farther downstream than is shown here, and then the intercostal arteries are temporarily controlled with bulldog clamps. *C, D,* and *E.* End-to-end anastomosis is made with interrupted simple suture of no. 5-0 silk. (This illustration appeared originally in the first edition of *The Heart,* in 1966, and in all subsequent editions. It is reproduced here by courtesy of Dr. John W. Kirklin, Birmingham, Alabama.)

essential. Postoperative bleeding, chylothorax, paraplegia, and injury to the phrenic and recurrent laryngeal nerves remain potential complications.[157]

If a significant VSD is also present, a pulmonary arterial band is placed at the time of coarctation repair during infancy. The VSD may then be repaired electively during the following several months when the child's congestive heart failure is well controlled. VSD closure following shortly after or simultaneously with coarctation repair is a viable alternative.[158]

Adequacy of collateral circulation is crucial for safe repair of coarctation. A rise in proximal systemic arterial pressure of more than 20 mmHg when the aorta is clamped above the coarctation suggests a marginal collateral circulation. Pressure in the descending aorta can be measured, and, if necessary, a cardiopulmonary bypass or shunt can be used to provide adequate distal perfusion.[159] Mild systemic hypothermia is a simple and useful adjunct for spinal cord protection. Aortic occlusion time should obviously be kept to a minimum, but neurologic sequelae have occurred regardless of the methods used to maintain distal perfusion. Monitoring of somatosensory cortical evoked potentials may warn of impending ischemic insult to the spinal cord.[160]

Postoperative paradoxical hypertension is common between the 2d and 10th postoperative days and may contribute to the *postcoarctation syndrome* in which ileus, abdominal pain, mesenteric vasculitis, and even visceral infarction can occur. This syndrome is not encountered if the postoperative diastolic blood pressure is maintained within normal range for age with sodium nitroprusside, propranolol, or captopril and if nasogastric tube decompression of the gastrointestinal tract is maintained postoperatively for 48 h. Preoperative treatment with propranolol appears to minimize paradoxical hypertension following repair of coarctation.[161]

Operative mortality for infants with isolated coarctation is in the 0 to 3 percent range[153,157,158] and is 20 percent or higher when other cardiovascular defects are present. Subsequent deaths are uncommon for surviving infants with isolated coarctation but are more problematic for those with complicated associated defects.

Valvular Aortic Stenosis

DEFINITION
Aortic stenosis is defined as subtotal obstruction of varying severity in the channel of left ventricular outflow. In order of decreasing frequency, the sites of obstruction by congenital lesions are (1) valvular, (2) subvalvular, and (3) supravalvular (see also Chap. 63).

PATHOLOGY
Most commonly, the aortic valve is bicuspid with two commissures, one or both of which are fused to varying degrees. A third rudimentary commissure, or raphe, is frequently present in the larger of the leaflets. The valve opening is eccentric. Less frequently encountered is the unicuspid, unicommissural, or noncommissural valve in which the orifice is often slitlike,

at first glance suggesting a bicuspid valve. Uncommonly, a true dome is present, resembling the valve of congenital isolated pulmonary stenosis. Rarely, the valve is tricuspid with fusion of one or more of the three commissures. When survival to adult life occurs, calcification may appear in the valvular tissue, leading to rigidity of the valve. Poststenotic dilation of the ascending aorta occurs in all cases to some degree. Coarctation of the aorta is the most common associated anomaly.

ABNORMAL PHYSIOLOGY
The hemodynamics of congenital valvular aortic stenosis are similar to those of acquired aortic stenosis (Chap. 63), except that a persistent PDA or stretched foramen ovale in the immediate postnatal period may lessen the severity of pulmonary edema by diverting blood away from the left ventricle.

Severity is usually judged by the peak systolic pressure gradient (PSPG) across the aortic valve, determined at cardiac catheterization, and the calculated aortic valve area. In the presence of a normal cardiac output, a PSPG ≥ 75 mmHg or an aortic valve area <0.5 cm^2/m^2 is considered severe; PSPG between 50 and 75 mmHg or a valve area between 0.5 and 0.8 cm^2/m^2 is considered moderate; a PSPG <50 mmHg or a valve area >0.9 cm^2/m^2 is considered mild[162] (see also Chaps. 63 and 71).

CLINICAL MANIFESTATIONS
About 7 percent of infants and children with congenital heart disease have aortic stenosis in one of its several forms, and approximately 80 percent of these patients have valvular aortic stenosis. Valvular stenosis is much more common among males than females, in a ratio of 4:1.

History

The detection of a systolic murmur leads to the discovery of this malformation in most patients, the vast majority of whom are asymptomatic. Easy fatigue, dyspnea, syncope, or angina suggest severe obstruction, but severe obstruction may exist in the absence of any symptoms. Sudden death may occur from this malformation, but in most such cases death is preceded by either symptoms or electrocardiographic changes. Infants with critical stenosis from birth present with congestive failure within the first week or two of life and represent true emergencies. A similar small number of patients with less critical but still very severe obstruction are detected over the course of the next 4 to 6 months.

Physical Examination

The arterial blood pressure and the quality of the peripheral arterial pulses of the older infant and child are usually normal. A measured pulse pressure <20 mmHg suggests severe stenosis. The cardiac apex impulse may be forceful and sustained, and a systolic thrill along the right upper sternal border and over the carotid arteries is present in most patients. The absence of such a thrill at the right upper sternal border suggests a PSPG ≤ 30 mmHg. Paradoxical splitting of the second heart sound is rare and is associated with either very severe obstruction or coexisting myocardial disease. An early systolic ejection click at the apex is characteristic and serves to distinguish valvular aortic stenosis from other forms of left ventricular outflow tract obstruction. The classic auscultatory finding is a harsh systolic spindle-shaped murmur, loudest at the right upper sternal border with radiation into the carotid arteries and down the left sternal border to the apex (see also Chap. 10). Among infants with critical obstruction, there may be no palpable peripheral pulses and no distinctive murmur, with a return of weak pulses and typical murmur only after decongestive therapy.

Chest Roentgenogram
The overall heart size is normal, but infants with failure will have generalized cardiac enlargement and varying degrees of pulmonary edema. Poststenotic dilatation of the ascending aorta is characteristic.

Electrocardiogram
Left ventricular hypertrophy, as indicated by voltage criteria in the left precordial leads, is seldom helpful in distinguishing those patients with severe obstruction from those with mild to moderate obstruction. On the other hand, diminished anterior forces in the right precordial leads and a deep $SV_1 \geq 30$ mm suggests severe stenosis, as does absence of the Q wave in V_6. Fifty percent of patients with severe obstruction have a flat, biphasic, or inverted T wave in V_6 (Fig. 70-20). Severe

and even critical obstruction may be present with none of the electrocardiographic abnormalities mentioned above. Monitoring of the ST segment in leads V_5 through V_7 during cautious exercise testing appears to be a reliable method of detecting those children in whom a significant PSPG (>50 mmHg) has developed and in whom that gradient might represent a threat of sudden death.[163] Symptomatic infants may show right, left, or biventricular hypertrophy, frequently with T-wave inversion over the left precordium.

Echocardiogram
Continuous-wave Doppler echocardiography guided by two-dimensional echocardiographic imaging predicts very accurately the peak and mean instantaneous systolic pressure gradient across discrete forms of left ventricular outflow tract obstruction (see Chap. 41). Two-dimensional echocardiography can distinguish valvular from supravalvular or subvalvular obstruction and identify those critically ill infants in whom the size of the left ventricle, mitral valve annulus, or aortic root is hypoplastic to a degree that would preclude survival.[164,165]

Cardiac Catheterization
Infants symptomatic with severe aortic obstruction often have a left-to-right shunt through a stretched foramen ovale, PAH, and a right-to-left shunt through a PDA. A marked increase in left ventricular end-diastolic pressure is usually present. The PSPG between the left ventricle and the central aorta should be documented whenever possible. If left ventricular output is markedly diminished, this gradient may be relatively small, even in the presence of severe obstruction. Left ventricular angiography will confirm the site of obstruction and outline the size of the left ventricular cavity.

In older infants and children, pressures on the right side of the heart are usually normal. Simultaneous recording of central aortic and left ventricular pressures or a pressure tracing upon catheter withdrawal from the left ventricle to the aorta, coupled with an accurate estimate of cardiac output, are necessary for reliable assessment of severity. Left ventricular angiography will document the site of obstruction. The aortic leaflets typically will be thickened and domed, with a central or eccentric jet of contrast material entering the ascending aorta. Poststenotic dilatation is characteristic. Supravalvular aortography is recommended to assess the presence and severity of aortic regurgitation.

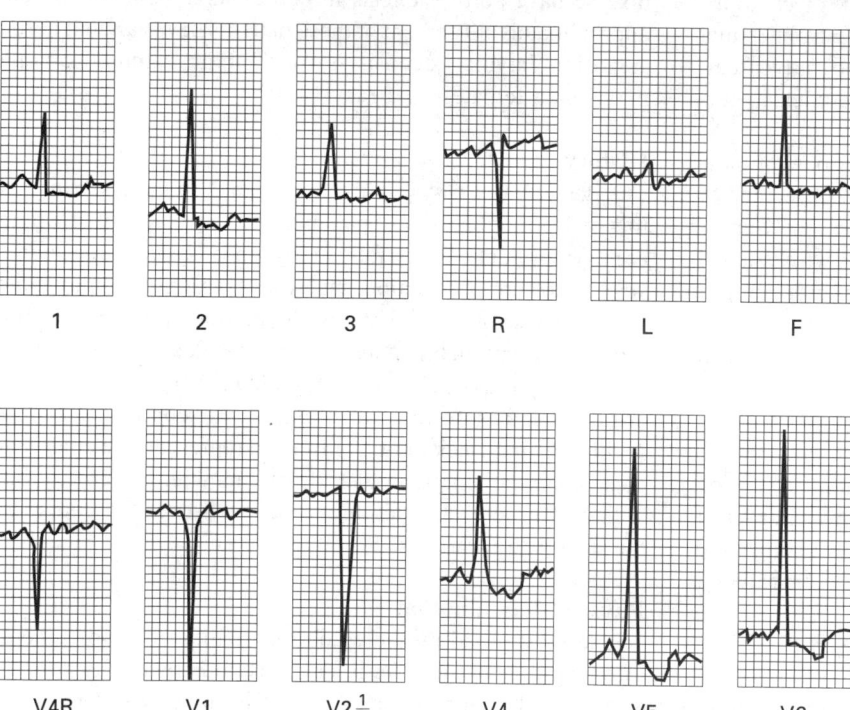

FIGURE 70-20
Electrocardiogram from an 8-year-old boy with valvular aortic stenosis and a 94-mmHg peak systolic pressure gradient. The small anterior QRS forces, abnormally large posterior forces, absent Q waves in leads V_5 and V_6, and abnormal T waves and ST segments reflect severe left ventricular systolic pressure overload with ischemia.

NATURAL HISTORY AND PROGNOSIS
About half the infants born with severe valvular aortic stenosis are symptomatic enough to require hospitalization within

the first week of life. The remainder develop congestive failure over the course of the next 6 months. Not uncommonly, the murmur is mistaken for that of a VSD. Failure beyond infancy and before adolescence is not usually seen without the presence of complicating factors. Symptomatic infants require prompt relief of obstruction, by either balloon or surgical valvotomy, but the mortality rate remains significant. Endocardial fibroelastosis, papillary muscle necrosis, associated intra- and extracardiac deformities, and a small left ventricular cavity contribute to this mortality rate. Survivors may have significant aortic regurgitation, but the majority can be managed medically until such time as valve replacement is feasible.

Most infants beyond the newborn period or children with mild aortic valvular stenosis (PSPG at catheterization <25 mmHg or a Doppler mean pressure gradient <25 mmHg) will remain stable, with only a 21 percent likelihood of progression in severity and the need for intervention within the subsequent 25 years. For those patients with a PSPG between 25 and 49 mmHg, this likelihood rises to 41 percent, and with a PSPG >50 mmHg, it rises to 71 percent.[166] Patients with a PSPG >50 mmHg are judged to be at risk of serious ventricular arrhythmias and sudden death. Infective endocarditis on the aortic valve (Chap. 82) poses an extremely serious complication in the form of systemic arterial emboli and the production of serious, sometimes catastrophic, aortic regurgitation with congestive failure, shock, and death.[70]

MEDICAL MANAGEMENT

Infants with the characteristic murmur detected in the first weeks of life should be evaluated very carefully to be certain the obstruction is not severe, nor becomes severe within the next few weeks or months.[167] Those who develop heart failure should be operated upon or undergo balloon valvuloplasty without delay. In the critically ill neonate, intravenous PGE_1 infusion to open the ductus may provide temporary relief of pulmonary edema en route to the operating room or the catheterization laboratory. Beyond infancy, a plan of reexamination with careful questioning regarding symptoms and an ECG each year, an echocardiogram with Doppler assessment of the mean and maximum pressure gradient every 2 years, exercise testing, and 24-h ECG monitoring about every 3 years should suffice to prevent progression from going unrecognized. Indications for cardiac catheterization include the appearance of symptoms or syncope, an arterial pulse pressure <20 mmHg on physical examination, cardiac enlargement demonstrated by chest roentgenogram, small anterior forces with an $SV_1 \geq 30$ mm or flattening or inversion of the T wave in V_6 in the resting ECG, abnormal ST-T segments on exercise testing, or an estimated PSPG of 50 mmHg or a mean pressure gradient ≥ 27 mmHg by echocardiographic Doppler techniques.[168] Transluminal catheter balloon valvuloplasty has become an alternative to surgery. In skilled hands, it can provide effective reduction of the transvalvular gradient while producing only a mild increment in aortic regurgitation in most instances.[169,170] Elective balloon dilation is recommended

if the PSPG >50 mmHg at catheterization and aortic regurgitation is mild or nonexistent. For the neonate with critical valvular obstruction, some centers continue to rely on surgical intervention, but catheter balloon valvuloplasty has become a very competitive alternative[171] and, in the authors' institution, is the procedure of choice for these very sick infants.

Relief of aortic valve obstruction, whether it be by balloon valvuloplasty or surgical valvotomy, is palliative rather than curative. Gradual restenosis is the rule, with almost one-third of those infants undergoing valvotomy requiring a second operation, usually valve replacement, within the next two decades. Aortic regurgitation, a well-recognized complication of valvuloplasty, valvulotomy, and/or infective endocarditis, may require surgical intervention as well. Endocarditis is a serious and lifelong hazard, with an incidence among patients followed for 20 years of approximately 5 percent, a mortality rate of just over 25 percent, and a predilection for those patients in their second, rather than first, decade of life and with PSPGs >50 mmHg.[70,166]

Children with more than mild aortic stenosis are restricted from strenuous organized athletics, isometric exercises, and activities that require a good deal of stamina and produce shortness of breath. For genetic counseling, the risk of congenital heart disease is estimated at 3 percent for a subsequent sibling and offspring of an affected father, but it may be as high as 13 to 18 percent for the offspring of an affected mother.[172]

SURGICAL MANAGEMENT

When surgical intervention is required for critical aortic stenosis during infancy, the heart is exposed through a median sternotomy and the aortic valve is visualized through the ascending aorta during a brief period of low-flow perfusion with mild hypothermia. Standard cardiopulmonary bypass, mild hypothermia, and cardioplegia are used in older children.[173] The surgeon must discriminate between true commissures and abnormal raphes, incision of the latter producing intolerable aortic valvular regurgitation. Relief of valvular stenosis is accomplished by a carefully placed incision in the middle of each fused but well-supported true commissure[174] (Fig. 70-21).

A conservative attitude is essential during operation for aortic stenosis in the infant or small child. Mild valvular regurgitation almost always occurs consequent to commissurotomy but is usually well tolerated. Moderate residual stenosis is preferred to intolerable aortic valvular regurgitation, especially in infants in whom valve implantation is technically difficult. If valve replacement is necessary in the infant or small child, reconstruction using a cryopreserved, valve-containing aortic homograft has been the procedure of choice.[173] Recent experience with the use of the autograft pulmonary valve in the aortic position, however, offers the attractive possibility of continuing growth of this neoaortic valve that may parallel that of the patient.[175]

The risk of operation is high in critically ill infants, in the range of 13 to 18 percent, particularly those having a low

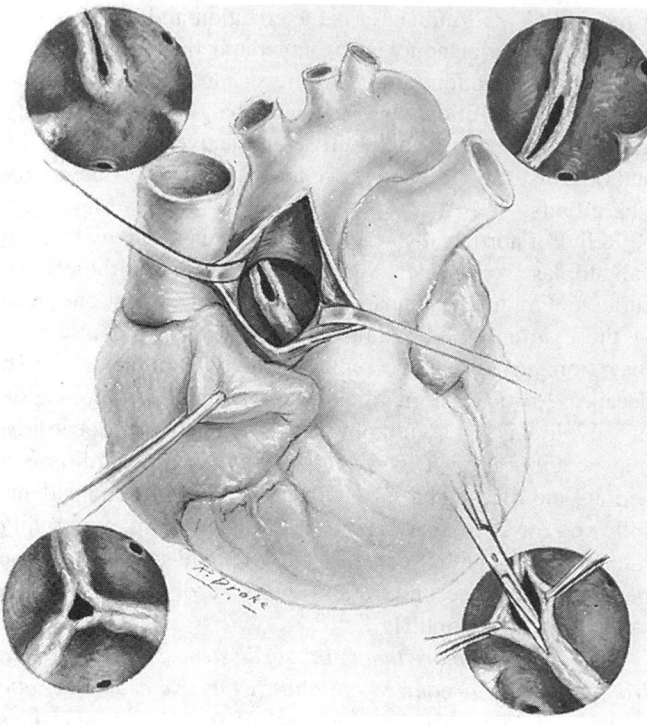

ejection fraction, high left ventricular end-diastolic pressure, endocardial fibroelastosis, marked congestive failure, or features of left ventricular hypoplasia.[176,177] Morbidity following aortic valvotomy in the older child is rare, and the likelihood of relief of left ventricular outflow tract obstruction and survival is good. If the aortic valve has tricuspid configuration, a good result can be anticipated. Satisfactory results with some reduction in left ventricular pressure are usually obtained even when the valve is bicuspid, but moderate aortic regurgitation is usually present postoperatively. The Natural History Study of Congenital Heart Defects, reporting on 133 children undergoing aortic commissurotomy after the age of 2 years, found only 27 percent required a second operation during the course of the subsequent 20 years, with 78 percent of these operations consisting of valve replacement. Aortic regurgitation was the indication for operation in 14 percent of the valve replacements.[166]

Secondary valvulotomy for recurrent or residual stenosis can be attempted, but calcification and restenosis eventually force aortic valve replacement in almost all those requiring surgery on the aortic valve in infancy or childhood. A small aortic annulus severely limits the relief of left ventricular hypertension without resorting to Konno's operation, in which the annulus is divided, a VSD is created and patched with prosthetic material, and a prosthetic valve, a homograft aortic valve or a pulmonary autograft valve, is implanted. The ascending aorta and anterior right ventricular wall are reconstructed using a prosthetic graft and, in the case of the auto-graft, the main pulmonary artery and pulmonary valve are replaced with a cryopreserved pulmonary homograft.[178]

Supravalvular Aortic Stenosis

PATHOLOGY
The obstruction in the ascending aorta includes the following three types: (1) hourglass, (2) hypoplastic, and (3) membranous. Associated obstructions in the pulmonary trunk, peripheral pulmonary arteries, and branches of the aortic arch are common.[179] Hypertrophy of the coronary arterial walls and premature coronary atherosclerosis have been described.[180]

CLINICAL MANIFESTATIONS
Supravalvular stenosis may be familial, associated with characteristic facies and mental retardation, sporadic, or (rarely) the result of congenital rubella. All forms may be, and usually are, associated with varying degrees of peripheral or branch pulmonary arterial stenosis. The familial form is transmitted as an autosomal dominant trait with variable expression (see Chap. 69). Mental retardation is not present, and there are no characteristic facial features.[181] Supravalvular aortic stenosis associated with mental retardation, frequently called *Williams' syndrome*, is associated with a high and prominent forehead, epicanthal folds, underdevelopment of the bridge of the nose and mandible, and a broad, overhanging upper lip (Fig. 10-34). It has been linked with idiopathic hypercalcemia of infancy, but in the majority of patients recognized beyond infancy, hypercalcemia is not present.[182]

The symptoms of supravalvular aortic stenosis are similar to those of subvalvular aortic stenosis (see below). Patients with the familial form usually have a distinctive family history, but one which seldom emerges in its entirety on initial questioning. The physical findings are also similar to subvalvular aortic stenosis, although a systolic blood pressure difference may be recorded between the two arms on occasion, with the right arm pressure being greater than the left. Chest roentgenogram and ECG are not distinctive unless associated pulmonary arterial stenosis leads to right ventricular hypertrophy. Echocardiography can identify the narrowed aortic lumen just above the aortic valve and provide an estimate of the severity of the obstruction in terms of the Doppler-derived instantaneous pressure gradient.[183]

At cardiac catheterization, a systolic pressure gradient can be demonstrated just above the aortic valve by careful pull-back. Supravalvular aortography or left ventricular angiography will visualize the supravalvular narrowing. Pressure recordings in the branch pulmonary arteries should be obtained, and pulmonary arterial angiography performed in the presence of any significant stenoses.

NATURAL HISTORY AND PROGNOSIS
The sequence of progressive obstruction, the appearance of symptoms and electrocardiographic changes, and the possibility of sudden death appear to apply for supravalvular aortic stenosis as well as for valvular aortic stenosis.[184] Infective

endocarditis represents a threat to these patients throughout life.

MEDICAL MANAGEMENT

The indications for cardiac catheterization surgery and follow-up are the same as for valvular aortic stenosis.

SURGICAL MANAGEMENT

Discrete supravalvular aortic stenosis is relieved by one or more incisions through the narrow segment of the ascending aorta, usually at the level of the sinotubular ridge at the top of the commissures. Incisions are extended well down into the aortic sinuses[185] (Fig. 70-22). Ridges of obstructing fibrous tissue are excised. The aorta is enlarged by the insertion of a gusset of prosthetic vascular graft material or pericardium to increase the circumference.[173] Rigidity and fibrous thickening of the aortic wall may prevent the aorta from opening up adequately even after insertion of the usual oval gusset in the noncoronary sinus of Valsalva. In this situation, an extended aortoplasty in which the fibrous ring is incised at two points and the aorta augmented with a pants-shaped tailored Dacron prosthesis is used.[186] A favorable outcome can be anticipated postoperatively in most patients having supravalvular aortic stenosis if the arterial wall abnormality is localized. Intimal obstruction of the coronary arterial ostia may require debridement, dilation, or even saphenous vein bypass grafting.

Diffuse tubular hypoplasia of the ascending aorta is a technically challenging problem associated with a high mortality rate and, usually, poor postoperative hemodynamic results. Use of a conduit from the apex of the left ventricle to the descending or abdominal aorta is appealing, although most attempts at repair have used an extensive prosthetic or homograft enlargement of the ascending aorta.[187]

Subvalvular Aortic Stenosis

PATHOLOGY

Three classic varieties of subvalvular aortic stenosis involve the left ventricular outflow tract. These are the discrete, the tunnel, and the muscular types. The discrete type is characterized by a localized fibrous encirclement of the left ventricular outflow tract a short distance below the aortic valve. The fibromuscular tissue usually extends onto the mitral leaflet and may also attach to the aortic cusps.[188] The tunnel type involves hypoplasia of the aortic annulus and a channel with a fibrous lining in the subjacent left ventricular outflow tract.[189] The muscular type is also known as *hypertrophic cardiomyopathy* (or idiopathic hypertrophic subaortic stenosis) and is discussed in Chap. 74.

More than half the patients have associated malformations, of which PDA, VSD, or coarctation are most common.[190]

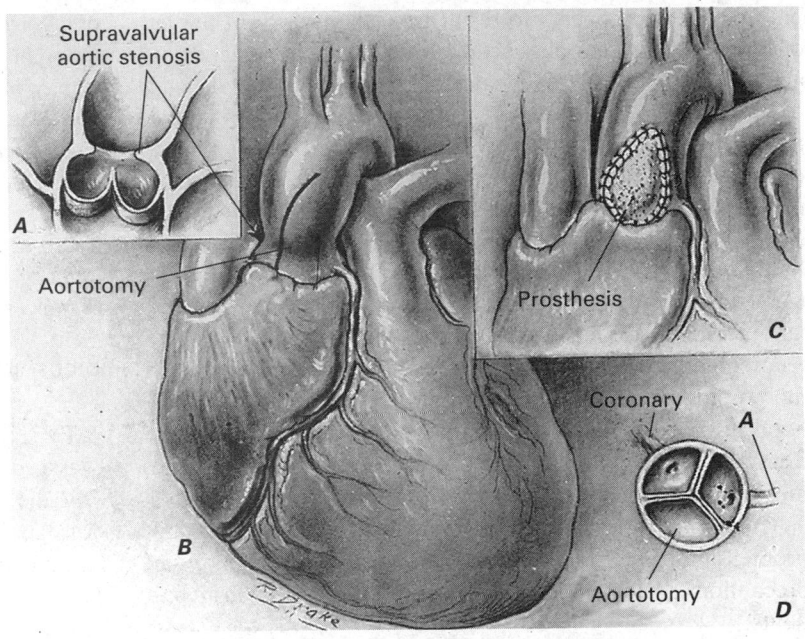

FIGURE 70-22

A to *D.* Supravalvular aortic stenosis and its repair. Obstruction is almost diaphragmatic in nature (*A*) and is not easily recognized externally (*B*). The complete repair is shown (*C*). (From McGoon et al.[185] Reproduced with permission from the publisher and authors.)

CLINICAL MANIFESTATIONS

Discrete stenosis is more frequent among males, with a male/female ratio of approximately 2.5:1. In the isolated forms, the majority of patients are referred because of the detection of a murmur that, not uncommonly, is mistaken initially for that of a VSD. Symptoms have the same implications as they do for valvular aortic stenosis.

The physical examination is similar to that of valvular aortic stenosis with two exceptions: an early systolic ejection click is not heard and an early diastolic murmur of aortic regurgitation is present in approximately one-half of these patients.

The roentgenographic features and ECG are also similar to those of valvular aortic stenosis except for absence of poststenotic dilatation of the ascending aorta. Two-dimensional echocardiography permits excellent visualization of the anatomy of the obstruction.[191] Estimation of the systolic pressure gradient can be obtained from Doppler echocardiographic studies.

At catheterization, a careful pullback pressure tracing across the left ventricular outflow tract will document the severity of the gradient and establish the site of the obstruction. Left ventricular biplane angiography will outline the nature of the obstruction.[192] Aortography is recommended to evaluate the degree of aortic regurgitation.

NATURAL HISTORY AND PROGNOSIS

Severe congestive failure in infancy is unusual and, if present, is almost invariably associated with complicating defects.[189] The obstruction is progressive in most instances, sometimes rapidly so. Associated aortic regurgitation also tends to be progressive and appears to result from damage from the jet of blood through the obstruction, with secondary thickening and deformity of the valve leaflets. Results of surgery depend on the extent of involvement of the left ventricular outflow tract, with the best results being obtained in patients with a thin, discrete subvalvular membrane. The least satisfactory results occur in patients with tunnel obstruction.

MEDICAL MANAGEMENT

Medical management is similar to that of patients with valvular aortic stenosis, but surgery for the discrete type is usually recommended for pressure gradients ≥30 mmHg because of the possibility of rapid progression of obstruction, the likelihood of progressive aortic valvular deformity and regurgitation, and the likelihood of complete and lasting relief if the membrane can be removed in its entirety.[193]

Continued follow-up for assessment of reobstruction and progression of aortic regurgitation and for reemphasis of the precautions against infective endocarditis is essential in all patients.[194]

SURGICAL MANAGEMENT

Subvalvular fibromuscular (membranous) left ventricular outflow tract obstruction is exposed through the aortic root as described for aortic valvular stenosis[195] (Fig. 70-23). A nasal speculum, a transparent glass ear speculum, and small flat retractors protect the aortic valve leaflets. Small half-circle needles and sutures or hooks are placed into the abnormal fibromuscular tissue, pulling it into view for precise excision from the underlying ventricular septum and the anterior mitral valve leaflet. The area of the bundle of His, usually just beneath the anterior commissure between the right and noncoronary leaflets, is avoided. An additional septal myectomy

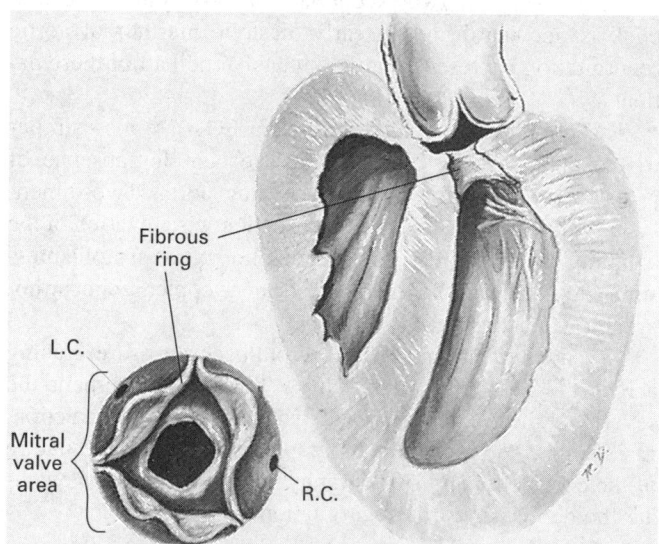

Fibrous ring

L.C.

Mitral valve area

R.C.

FIGURE 70-23

Localized subvalvular aortic stenosis. Obstruction is immediately upstream from the aortic valve. LC and RC, left and right coronary arteries. (From Kirklin and Ellis Jr.[195] Reproduced with permission from the publisher and authors.)

or myotomy beneath and to the left of the commissure between the right and left leaflets may be required if secondary hypertrophy is significant.[173] Immediate and early operative outcome is generally good, but *residual, recurrent, and progressive subaortic obstruction occurs in up to 25 percent of patients, demanding long-term follow-up.*[196]

Diffuse tunnel obstruction in the left ventricular outflow tract poses a difficult technical problem requiring aortoseptoplasty, reconstruction of the left ventricular outflow (Konno's operation or a modification thereof).[193]

Bicuspid Aortic Valve

PATHOLOGY

Classically, the two cusps are oriented anteriorly and posteriorly, the anterior or conjoined cusp being the larger. A raphe, or ridge, is present along the aortic aspect of the larger cusp, running from the aortic wall to the free edge of the cusp. The most common associated condition of significance is coarctation of the aorta. The most common complication is calcification of the valve. *In about 85 percent of cases of calcific aortic stenosis in patients below the age of 70, the fundamental valve is congenitally bicuspid.* Aortic regurgitation from prolapse of the larger cusp is a less common complication and is usually not evident until adolescence or adult life.

CLINICAL MANIFESTATIONS

The incidence in the general population approaches 2 percent; therefore it is the most common congenital abnormality of the heart or great vessels except for mitral valve prolapse (Chap. 65). Its importance lies in its frequent association with other forms of congenital heart disease, the predisposition of the valve to become stenotic as a result of fibrosis and deposition of calcium over the course of years, the tendency of the valve to become regurgitant, its association with aortic root dilatation and dissection,[197] and, finally, the susceptibility of the valve to infective endocarditis. It is found in 60 percent of patients with valvular aortic stenosis between the ages of 15 and 65 years.[198] It is also common among patients with isolated or dominant aortic regurgitation, among patients with infective endocarditis with or without a history of predisposing heart disease, and, probably most frequently, among otherwise normal individuals who come to the physician's attention because of unrelated illnesses. Patients with uncomplicated bicuspid aortic valve are asymptomatic. The incidence among males is approximately 2.5 times that among females (see also Chap. 63).

The characteristic feature is auscultatory and consists of an early systolic ejection click, which is best heard at the apex and which does not vary with respiration. A soft, early, or midsystolic murmur is frequently present at the right upper sternal border. Less commonly, a soft murmur of aortic regurgitation may be heard.[199] Two-dimensional echocardiography, with adequate images, can identify the bicuspid valve with a sensitivity of 78 percent and a diagnostic accuracy of 96 percent[200,201] (Fig. 14-41).

NATURAL HISTORY AND PROGNOSIS

The majority of congenitally bicuspid aortic valves are nonobstructive at birth, but with the passage of time a few of these valves will become fibrotic, stiffer, and more obstructive and will eventually be the site of calcium deposition, primarily among individuals between the ages of 15 and 65. Important calcium deposition is unusual before the age of 30, whereas grossly visible deposits of calcium are present in the valves of virtually all patients with severe stenosis beyond that age. A much smaller number of individuals born with a bicuspid aortic valve develop isolated aortic regurgitation. In approximately one-third, this is the result of fibrosis, prolapse, or retraction of one or both of the leaflets; in the remainder, regurgitation results from infective endocarditis on an apparently functionally normal bicuspid valve (see also Chaps. 63 and 82).

Right Aortic Arch

Right aortic arch is characterized by the arch passing over the right, rather than the left, bronchus. Mirror-image branching is the most common arrangement. Less commonly, the left subclavian artery arises anomalously as the fourth branch from the aortic arch. In combination with a ductus or its ligament, tracheal and esophageal compression can occur (Figs. 13-21C and D). Barium swallow will demonstrate the typical filling defects, which are confirmed by bronchoscopy. This condition is relieved by division of the ductus or its ligament surgically.

Aberrant Right Subclavian Artery

The right subclavian artery may arise anomalously as the fourth branch of a normal left aortic arch. It runs posterior to the esophagus to assume its normal course thereafter. Posterior indentation on a barium-filled esophagus is diagnostic.

Congenital Mitral Regurgitation

PATHOLOGY

Mitral regurgitation may be due to a primary valve abnormality or secondary to a more complex defect (see "Common Atrioventricular Canal Defects," above). There are a variety of rare primary malformations including isolated cleft, fenestration, and double orifice. Mitral regurgitation also occurs frequently with conditions that cause left ventricular dilatation and failure.

CLINICAL MANIFESTATIONS

Poor growth, frequent respiratory infections, and failure occur with significant mitral regurgitation. Physical findings are generally similar to those with mitral regurgitation of other causes (see Chap. 64). There may be a prominent left precordial bulge if cardiomegaly has been present from infancy. The systolic murmur may radiate to the base of the heart. Left atrial and left ventricular enlargement correlate with the degree of volume overload. Echocardiography with Doppler color flow mapping will demonstrate these as well as left ventricular function and the severity of regurgitation. The specific defect may be outlined, such as an isolated cleft or double orifice valve. Findings at cardiac catheterization substantiate the hemodynamic alterations (see also Chap. 16).

NATURAL HISTORY AND PROGNOSIS

Mild and even moderate mitral regurgitation may be well tolerated, but severe regurgitation leads to progressive deterioration. Endocarditis is a risk.

MANAGEMENT

Vigorous medical treatment of heart failure and infections is warranted. Every attempt should be made to control symptoms to a degree that will allow growth in infants. In infants and young children, only those with very severe and uncontrollable failure are subjected to surgery. In the adolescent, continued symptoms justify surgery.

At surgery, the valve and its apparatus are carefully inspected. Numerous individualized plastic procedures have been described. Reconstruction is not possible in many, and replacement (Chap. 67) is necessary. Currently, the St. Jude medical prosthesis is often utilized. Lifelong anticoagulation with warfarin (Chap. 68) is required. With body growth, replacement with a larger prosthesis may be difficult, and no good annular enlarging operation exists.

VALVULAR AND VASCULAR MALFORMATIONS OF THE RIGHT SIDE OF THE HEART WITH RIGHT-TO-LEFT, BIDIRECTIONAL, OR NO SHUNT

Pulmonary Stenosis with Intact Ventricular Septum

PATHOLOGY

Valvular pulmonary stenosis with intact ventricular septum is usually characterized by the so-called dome-shaped stenosis of the pulmonary valve and less commonly by dysplasia of the valve. The valve may be unicuspid, bicuspid, or tricuspid. The annulus may also be narrow. The pulmonary trunk exhibits poststenotic dilatation. In adult patients, calcification of the valve may appear.[202]

In pulmonary valvular dysplasia, the annulus of the valve may be abnormally narrow, but the most dramatic changes are related to the cusps, of which three are identifiable. The cusps are exceedingly thickened by mucoid and dense connective tissue.[203]

Concentric hypertrophy of the right ventricle is present, its degree reflecting the degree of obstruction at valve level. *The hypertrophy of the infundibular musculature may cause secondary infundibular stenosis.*

Less commonly, there may be isolated subvalvular pulmonary stenosis due to infundibular narrowing or an anomalous muscle bundle across the middle of the right ventricle.[204] Both types are usually associated with a VSD.

Isolated supravalvular pulmonary stenosis, or pulmonary arterial coarctations, may also occur. From angiographic studies, these are classified into four types: (1) *localized stenosis with poststenotic dilatation*, (2) *segmental stenosis*, (3) *diffuse hypoplasia,* and (4) *multiple peripheral stenoses*. The stenosis may be localized to any segment of the pulmonary arterial system. The process is unilateral in about one-third of cases and bilateral in two-thirds. Pulmonary arterial stenosis is commonly (about 75 percent), though not universally, associated with other cardiovascular abnormalities such as tetralogy of Fallot. It may also be seen as a sequela of congenital rubella[205] or Williams',[206] Noonan's,[207] or Alagille[208] syndromes.

ABNORMAL PHYSIOLOGY

There is a pressure difference during systole between the main right ventricular cavity and the pulmonary artery. The area of the pulmonary valve orifice is normally 2 cm^2/m^2; it is about 0.5 cm^2 at birth and increases in size with body growth. In general, the effective valve area must be decreased by about 60 percent before there is hemodynamically significant obstruction to flow. The PSPG may reach 150 to 240 mmHg in severe cases. The degree of obstruction is assessed by the peak and mean systolic pressure gradients and the amount of flow across the valve. In neonates, severe stenosis can be associated with a relatively small pressure difference if the flow is very low as a result of right ventricular failure. If pulmonary flow is normal, most patients with PSPG at rest of less than 40 mmHg have mild stenosis, and patients with PSPG >75 mmHg have severe stenosis.

When the pulmonary stenosis is severe, the right ventricle may fail and the cardiac output may be decreased, even at rest; this is associated with elevation of both the right ventricular end-diastolic pressure and the right atrial mean pressure. This may cause the foramen ovale to open and allow shunting of blood from the right to the left atrium, resulting in arterial oxygen desaturation and cyanosis. In most adolescent or adult patients with significant pulmonary stenosis, the resting cardiac output is within normal limits but usually does not increase normally during exercise. In contrast, younger children may be able to increase cardiac output during exercise, even with significant obstruction.[163,209]

CLINICAL MANIFESTATIONS

Pulmonary stenosis is one of the most common congenital heart defects and accounts for about 10 percent of patients in most large study populations. The stenosis is at the level of the pulmonary valve in most instances, but it can occur within the right ventricle, in the pulmonary arteries, or in combination. Approximately one-quarter of patients with stenosis of the pulmonary valve also have an atrial shunt,[210] but this frequency is dependent on the age group studied.

History

Most infants and children are asymptomatic, but a small percentage with very severe obstruction will manifest symptoms, usually mild fatigue or shortness of breath with exertion.

Young infants with critical obstruction present with symptoms related to heart failure and may have cyanosis if there is a patent foramen ovale or ASD. Squatting and syncope are rare in childhood.

Physical Examination

Patients with a dysplastic valve and occasional supravalvular stenosis have consistent noncardiac abnormalities in a familial syndrome described by Noonan. They frequently have short stature, hypertelorism, ptosis, low-set ears, and mental retardation[207] (see Chap. 69). Patients with rubella syndrome[205] have supravalvular stenoses and PDA, along with cataracts, sensorineural deafness, and microcephaly. Supravalvular stenoses can occur in Williams' syndrome[206] or in idiopathic hypercalcemia of infancy. These patients have characteristic facies, dental anomalies, mental retardation, and supravalvular aortic stenosis (see Chap. 69). There is also a familial occurrence of supravalvular pulmonary and aortic stenosis without these other features.

In patients with valvular pulmonary stenosis, cyanosis is uncommon, except with severe obstruction and an atrial communication. Hepatomegaly and the murmur of tricuspid regurgitation may be present in infants with severe obstruction. In older children with at least moderate obstruction, a prominent *a* wave is seen on examination of the jugular venous pulse. A systolic thrill in the suprasternal notch and at the left upper sternal border is present with significant obstruction unless there is isolated subvalvular stenosis. The right ventricular parasternal impulse becomes increasingly forceful with more severe obstruction. *An early systolic click, accentuated with expiration, at the left upper sternal border is the hallmark of valvular stenosis unless the obstruction is severe or the valve is dysplastic.* A click is not present with isolated stenosis at other levels. As the obstruction increases in severity, the pulmonary component of the second heart sound becomes progressively softer and more delayed. When the right ventricular pressure reaches systemic levels or greater, it becomes inaudible. The second heart sound is normal with supravalvular stenosis. A fourth heart sound is heard if obstruction is severe. The characteristic systolic murmur is harsh, crescendo-decrescendo in shape, and best heard at the left upper sternal border with radiation toward the left clavicle. The murmur radiates more to the axillae and back with supravalvular stenosis. The duration of the murmur and the timing of peak intensity correlate well with the severity of obstruction. With mild to moderate stenosis, the murmur peaks in midsystole and ends at or before the aortic component of the second heart sound. In patients with severe stenosis, the murmur peaks late in systole and extends beyond the aortic component of the second heart sound (see also Chaps. 10 and 63).

Chest Roentgenogram

Most patients have a normal or only slightly increased heart size, primarily of the right ventricle. Significant enlargement is seen with critical obstruction and is an ominous sign. Characteristically, the main and proximal left pulmonary arteries are prominent as a result of poststenotic dilatation when the stenosis is valvular. This finding may be absent with very severe obstructions, with a dysplastic valve, in very young infants, or with stenosis above or below the valve. The pulmonary vascular pattern is normal in most, but the vascularity is diminished in those with right-to-left shunt at atrial level.

Electrocardiogram

Right ventricular forces in the anterior precordial leads correlate reasonably well with the degree of obstruction.[211] They are normal or demonstrate mild hypertrophy with an rsR' pattern if there is mild obstruction. With severe stenosis, there are right axis deviation, right atrial hypertrophy, and very tall pure R waves in the anterior precordial leads. The presence of a qR pattern in these leads is almost always a sign of very severe obstruction. Those with a dysplastic valve frequently have a superior QRS axis.

Echocardiogram

Two-dimensional imaging allows identification of the level of obstruction, and Doppler studies provide an excellent measure of severity.[212] Shunting at the atrial level can also be evaluated.

Cardiac Catheterization

There is an elevated right ventricular systolic pressure with a distinct systolic pressure difference across the narrowed segment, which can be shown by slow withdrawal of the catheter from the distal pulmonary arterial branches to the proximal right ventricle. If critical obstruction is suspected, it may be wise not to attempt to advance the catheter into the pulmonary artery because of the risk of compromising an already marginal opening. Simultaneous measurement of systemic arterial and right ventricular pressures with measurement of flow is necessary to assess severity accurately. The right ventricular end-diastolic pressure and right atrial *a* wave may be elevated. Systemic oxygen saturation is diminished only in those with more severe obstruction and a patent foramen ovale or, less commonly, a true ASD. A left-to-right shunt at atrial level is detected in some patients with mild to moderate obstruction. With valvular stenosis, right ventricular angiography demonstrates thickened and doming valve leaflets and a jet of contrast material entering the dilated pulmonary artery (Fig. 70-24). Doming is not characteristic of the dysplastic valve. Infundibular subvalvular narrowing due to muscular hypertrophy may occur secondary to the valvular stenosis or rarely as an isolated anomaly. Isolated anomalous muscle bundles in the right ventricle may also be seen. Pulmonary arterial angiography best demonstrates the sites of obstruction with supravalvular stenoses. Ventricular volume studies have demonstrated depressed ventricular function in patients with right-to-left shunts. Balloon dilation is discussed below under "Medical Management."

NATURAL HISTORY AND PROGNOSIS

The clinical course of valvular stenosis is favorable in most patients with mild to moderate obstruction. In a national coop-

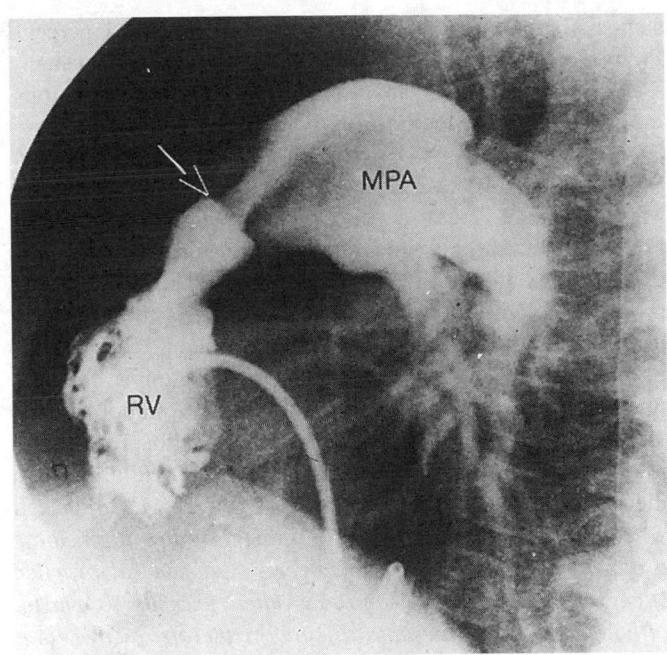

FIGURE 70-24
Lateral view of a right ventricular (RV) angiogram demonstrating the typical features of valvular pulmonary stenosis with doming of the pulmonary valve (*arrow*) and a narrow jet of contrast entering the dilated main pulmonary artery (MPA).

erative study,[213] 86 percent of patients had no significant increase in their pressure gradients over a 4- to 8-year interval. Those with a significant increase were less than 4 years of age and had at least moderate stenosis initially. Progression during the period of growth seems the likely explanation for most of the increases, but a few patients developed subvalvular muscular hypertrophy, which increased the obstruction. Even mild obstruction may progress significantly in some infants during the first year of life. The prognosis of those with severe obstruction without intervention is poor, especially for infants with critical obstruction. With severe obstruction, right ventricular damage and dysfunction can ensue over the years, and heart failure or arrhythmias can cause premature death in adults.[214] Tricuspid regurgitation may also result. Obstruction of the subvalvular type frequently increases with time, while supravalvular stenosis does not usually progress. Brain abscess can occur if a right-to-left shunt is present. Infective endocarditis with vegetations on the valve, pulmonary arterial wall, or infundibular region is also a risk. The children originally followed as part of the national cooperative study above[213] were reevaluated 15 to 25 years later.[215] Of the 580 patients alive at the completion of the previous study, new data were available on 464 (78.4 percent). Probability of 25-year survival was 95.7 percent compared to an expected age- and sex-matched control group survival of 96.6 percent. Ninety-seven percent were asymptomatic. Although cardiac catheterization studies were not repeated, clinical examination and echocardiography at follow-up suggested no pulmonary stenosis in 2 percent, mild stenosis in 93 percent, moderate stenosis in 3 percent, and severe stenosis in only 1 percent. Pulmonary regurgitation was present in 40 percent, usually secondary to surgical valvotomy. Endocarditis was uncommon, as were ventricular arrhythmias.

MEDICAL MANAGEMENT

Management obviously depends on the severity of obstruction. For those with mild to moderate valvular pulmonary stenosis, periodic reexamination is indicated to detect any evidence of progression, with more frequent evaluation for those under 1 year of age. Measures to treat heart failure should be instituted in the infant with critical stenosis, but prompt intervention is mandatory. Cyanosis or a right ventricular systolic pressure well above systemic levels also is an indication for prompt intervention. Intervention is warranted in older children when the gradient exceeds 75 mmHg and is clearly not indicated when the gradient is less than 25 mmHg. *In the intermediate group there is still some controversy, but general practice suggests valvuloplasty when the gradient exceeds 40 mmHg, although the objective data to support therapy at this level are lacking.*

Balloon valvuloplasty has replaced surgical therapy as a first approach. Via the femoral vein, a balloon catheter is advanced across the valve and inflated to about 120 percent the size of the pulmonary annulus, ripping the domed valve and thereby relieving the obstruction.

Recently the Valvuloplasty and Angioplasty of Congenial Anomalies Registry has published the combined results on 822 children.[216] Valvuloplasty resulted in improvement in most children with valvular obstruction, reducing the gradient from 71 ± 33 mmHg to 28 ± 24 mmHg. Valvuloplasty is, not surprisingly, less effective in those children with a dysplastic pulmonary valve.[216,217] Complications were uncommon (5/822, or 0.6 percent) including two deaths. Valvuloplasty has also been performed in critical neonatal pulmonary stenosis with cyanosis due to right-to-left shunting at the atrial level with a high success rate.[218,219] Subvalvular obstruction is less amenable to dilatation.

Peripheral pulmonic stenosis associated with rubella or Noonan's, Williams', or Alagille syndromes has also been occasionally amenable to dilatation, although the results are frequently less dramatic because of the multiple areas of stenosis and the complications, including pulmonary artery rupture, being higher.[220,221] Recently, coronary artery stents have been used, with promising results,[222] in those with peripheral pulmonary artery stenosis in an attempt to keep open vessels that recoil back to normal size after the balloon is deflated. For those in whom there is isolated subvalvular stenosis or associated defects or in whom balloon dilatation has failed, surgical intervention is recommended.

Exercise studies during the catheterization in children have demonstrated that the altered cardiac function observed in some children is reversible by surgery. This does not appear to be true for adults, so *intervention should be carried out relatively early in childhood.* Prophylaxis against infective endocarditis is recommended for all patients, whether or not

surgery is performed, although the risks seem lower than with many other congenital anomalies.

SURGICAL MANAGEMENT

Operation is rarely indicated for isolated pulmonary valvular stenosis; balloon valvuloplasty is virtually always successful in eliminating clinically significant obstruction. A thickened, immobile, dysplastic pulmonary valve, however, is best treated by complete surgical excision (valvectomy). A small annulus is augmented with a pericardial or Dacron gusset.[223]

Subvalvular pulmonary stenosis is relieved through a right ventriculotomy, a main pulmonary arteriotomy, or a right atriotomy. Hypertrophic parietal and septal muscle bands constituting the fibrous orifice of the os infundibulum and obstructing moderator bands or muscle bundles within the body of the right ventricle are excised. Care is exercised to avoid injury to major coronary arterial branches. The right ventriculotomy can usually be closed by direct suture, but a small oval patch of pericardium or Dacron can be used to prevent constriction of the outflow tract. Right ventricular function is minimally compromised by a small patch that does not extend across the annulus; larger patches to the pulmonary arterial bifurcation probably impair ventricular performance but may be necessary when there is associated annular or main pulmonary arterial hypoplasia. When possible, excision from the pulmonary artery or the right atrium is preferred to avoid ventricular injury.

Excellent relief of right ventricular outflow tract obstruction can be expected following resection. Mortality and significant morbidity are rare. Repair during childhood reduces the likelihood of complications related to severe right ventricular hypertrophy, diminished ventricular compliance and function, subendocardial ischemia, tricuspid regurgitation, and supraventricular dysrhythmias associated with right atrial hypertrophy.

Stenoses of main or extraparenchymal branch pulmonary arteries can be relieved by pericardial, synthetic, or homograft aortic or pulmonary arterial patches if poststenotic dilatation is present. Proximal coarctations in the larger portion of the arterial tree are more readily corrected than those located in small distal branches beyond the bifurcation of either the right or left pulmonary artery, where results are poor.[224] Tubular conduits can be placed to bypass obstructions, but these are generally not needed unless there is absence of confluence of the arteries centrally.[225] An artery treated by excision of a discrete stenosis with repair by primary anastomosis is subject to restenosis as the child grows and may result in moving the gradient distally as stenoses remote from the mediastinum are revealed.

Catheter balloon angioplasty, although certainly not without risk, offers nonsurgical relief of obstruction even in the small pulmonary arterial branches and should be considered the procedure of choice for distal pulmonary arterial stenoses, unless other major cardiac reconstruction is also required.[220,221]

Tetralogy of Fallot

PATHOLOGY

Tetralogy of Fallot is characterized by biventricular origin of the aorta above a large VSD (Fig. 70-25), obstruction to pulmonary blood flow, and right ventricular hypertrophy. Fibrous continuity of the aortic origin and the anterior mitral valve is maintained.[226]

The right ventricular infundibulum lies anterior to the position of the VSD and is bounded by the anterior and septal walls anteriorly and medially; the posterior wall is said to be a vertical crista supraventricularis or displaced conus septum.[227] The right ventricular infundibulum is a distinctive channel, but the caliber varies widely from only mild obstruction to atresia. Usually, it exhibits a significant degree of stenosis and is the dominant site of the obstruction to pulmonary flow characteristic of tetralogy.

The pulmonary valve is often malformed, usually being either bicuspid or unicuspid. The valve may contribute to pulmonary stenosis, but only uncommonly will it be the only site of significant obstruction to pulmonary flow. Characteristically, the pulmonary trunk is thin-walled and its lumen is more narrow than normal, but usually it is wider than either the right ventricular infundibulum or the orifice of the pulmonary valve. The aorta is wider than normal, its change in caliber roughly opposite to that of the pulmonary trunk. The foramen ovale is frequently patent in patients of all ages. In all cases of tetralogy with significant pulmonary obstruction, collateral branches to the lungs arise from the aorta.

There is invariably a large malalignment VSD. Anterior, mid, or apical muscular defects are also present in up to 5 percent of children seen as infants. Many close spontaneously, but if corrective surgery is to be successfully performed, they must be evaluated.

Coronary artery abnormalities are not uncommon. The anterior descending coronary artery in the interventricular septum may arise from the right instead of the left coronary artery.[228] While physiologically unimportant preoperatively, the course across the right ventricular outflow tract makes the usual site of right ventriculotomy and outflow patch unavailable during reparative surgery, frequently necessitating a conduit to "jump over" the vessel. The anatomy of the coronary circulation used to require angiography to establish, but more recently echocardiography with Doppler color flow has been sufficient to detail the distribution of the proximal coronary circulation in most cases.

ASSOCIATED CONDITIONS

The condition most commonly associated with tetralogy of Fallot is right aortic arch (about 30 percent).[229] A persistent left superior vena cava has been described in 10.6 percent of cases. When an associated ASD exists, this anomaly is referred to as *pentalogy of Fallot.* The ductus arteriosus may be absent, present unilaterally on either right or left side, or bilateral.

ABNORMAL PHYSIOLOGY

Since the VSD is usually large, with an area about as large as that of the aortic valve, both ventricles and the aorta have essentially the same systolic pressures. The most important hemodynamic factor is the ratio between the resistance to flow into the aorta and the resistance to flow across the stenotic right ventricular infundibulum. If the resistance to right ventricular outflow is not large, the pulmonary flow may be twice the systemic flow and the arterial oxygen saturation may be normal (this is so-called acyanotic tetralogy of Fallot). On the other hand, the resistance to the pulmonary flow may be markedly increased, causing right-to-left shunting, arterial unsaturation, and subsequent polycythemia. When the pulmonary stenosis is very severe, much or most of the pulmonary blood flow may be by way of collateral blood flow. The infundibular obstruction, which may be very dynamic, is increased by drugs, heart rate maneuvers, or activities that increase myocardial contractility or that decrease right ventricular volume. In addition, the infundibular hypertrophy may gradually increase.[230] Since the systolic pressure in the right ventricle cannot exceed that in the left ventricle because of the large VSD, the right ventricle is "protected" from excessive pressure-work, so congestive heart failure is uncommon.

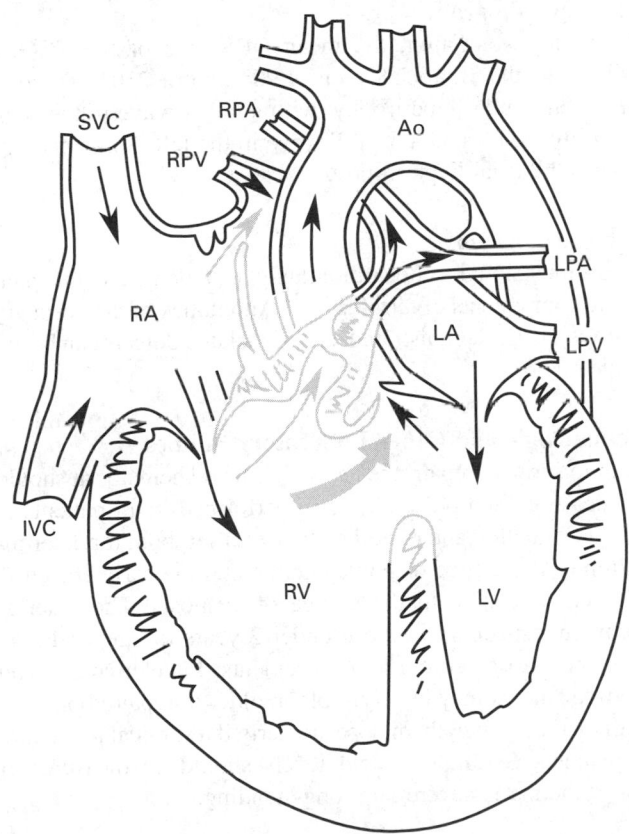

FIGURE 70-25

Classic tetralogy of Fallot. There are infundibular and pulmonary valvular stenoses. There is also right-to-left shunting at the atrial level. SVC, superior vena cava; IVC, inferior vena cava; RA, right atrium; RV, right ventricle; RPA, right pulmonary artery; LPA, left pulmonary artery; RPV, right pulmonary vein; LPV, left pulmonary vein; LA, left atrium; LV, left ventricle; Ao, aorta. (From Edwards.[76] Reproduced with permission from the publisher and author.)

The precise mechanism by which squatting relieves breathlessness and faintness after exercise in patients with tetralogy of Fallot is complex. It is known that the arterial saturation returns to its resting value more rapidly if the patient squats after exercise. In normal individuals, squatting produces increases in systemic arterial blood pressure, venous return to the heart, and systemic cardiac output. In patients with tetralogy, these same changes occur plus a possible increase in peripheral resistance by compression and kinking of the femoral arteries. Squatting also usually increases venous return from the abdomen to the heart, with increases in right ventricular stroke volume, pressure, and pulmonary blood flow.

Hypercyanotic episodes (spells) in patients with tetralogy are of uncertain origin. It is likely that some episodes are caused by unusual hyperactivity of muscular fibers in the right ventricular outflow tract producing, or exaggerating, the infundibular stenosis. Some spells may be caused by a decrease in peripheral resistance and in systemic arterial pressure, which causes the right-to-left shunt to increase and pulmonary blood flow to decrease.

CLINICAL MANIFESTATIONS

Tetralogy of Fallot is one of the most common congenital cardiac defects causing cyanosis. Tetralogy with an associated ASD, or pentalogy of Fallot, is not distinguishable clinically. For a discussion on the hypoxemia and the consequences in tetralogy, see the section on cyanosis and its complications earlier in this chapter.

History

Most patients are now diagnosed prenatally by ultrasound or present in the first days or weeks of life with a heart murmur. If the right ventricular obstruction is severe, cyanosis is present at birth and is exacerbated when the ductus closes. If the obstruction is milder, the infant may be acyanotic with left-to-right flow through the VSD and may occasionally develop congestive heart failure. In this group, gradually increasing right ventricular obstruction reduces the left-to-right shunt, and eventually, when infundibular and pulmonary resistance exceed systemic resistance, right-to-left shunting develops, resulting in cyanosis.

Dyspnea with exertion occurs commonly in toddlers and older children with unrepaired defects. Attacks of suddenly increasing cyanosis associated with hyperpnea, or hypoxic spells,[231,232] are common between the ages of 2 months and 2 years. There are many precipitating events, including infection, exertion, and summer heat. They occur most often in the morning, with increasing irritability. Frequency and duration vary widely, but prolonged episodes can lead to syncope, seizures, and death. Squatting with exercise is common from 1½ to 10 years of age in those not previously repaired.

Physical Examination

Growth is usually normal unless cyanosis is extreme.[233] Clubbing occurs after 3 months of age and is proportional to the level of cyanosis. Signs of congestive heart failure do not appear in tetralogy of Fallot during childhood unless there is a superimposed illness such as anemia or infective endocarditis.

Increased right ventricular activity is observed. A systolic thrill may be palpable at the left midsternal border, with a harsh midsystolic murmur in this location. Softer murmurs signal more severe obstruction and are common when presentation is in the newborn period or during hypoxic spells. The murmur ends before the second heart sound, which is characteristically single. A continuous murmur is heard if a PDA or large bronchial collateral vessels are present. An early systolic ejection sound at the left sternal border and apex is common; its presence suggests valvular pulmonic stenosis.

Chest Roentgenogram

The total heart size is usually normal on chest roentgenogram, but right ventricular enlargement is present in the lateral view. The aorta arches to the right in many cases. Pulmonary flow is diminished. The pulmonary segment is concave and the apex elevated, giving the *coeur en sabot* (boot-shaped) contour. The very young infant may have only diminished pulmonary flow.

Electrocardiogram

In tetralogy of Fallot, the mean QRS axis of the ECG is usually to the right, between $+90°$ and $+210°$. There is right ventricular hypertrophy, with a tall R wave in the right precordial leads and a deep S wave in the left. Some patients have right atrial hypertrophy.

Echocardiogram

Two-dimensional echocardiography can delineate the anatomic components of tetralogy.[234] Anomalies of the coronary arteries can be demonstrated, and associated defects can be excluded.

Hematologic and Other Laboratory Studies

Prior to surgical repair, the hemoglobin and hematocrit should be measured and pulse oximetry performed in all patients at initial evaluation and periodically thereafter, both for determination of the degree of polycythemia and the early detection of anemia relative to the degree of cyanosis. The latter is common, especially in those under 2 years of age, and may predispose to cerebrovascular accidents. Platelet counts and clotting studies may be advisable in older unrepaired patients with marked polycythemia, particularly if a surgical procedure is planned. Serum uric acid levels should be measured if polycythemia is severe and long-standing.

Cardiac Catheterization

In an increasing number of centers, the quality of echocardiography (especially when done in neonates or infants) is sufficiently diagnostic to outline the right ventricular and proximal pulmonary artery anatomy, rule out additional muscular VSDs, and establish the proximal coronary circulation. As a consequence, cardiac catheterization and angiography are less commonly performed preoperatively in children with tetralogy of Fallot.

In those in whom the study is performed, the right ventricular systolic pressure is equal to that in the left ventricle and aorta. If the pulmonary artery can be entered, the pressure will be normal or low. The level(s) of obstruction can be evaluated by careful pullback to the right ventricle. Caution should be observed if the pulmonary artery is entered, as the catheter may critically reduce the pulmonary flow and cause a hypoxic episode. It is unnecessary to attempt to enter the pulmonary artery in patients with severe cyanosis or with a history of severe hypoxic spells. Systemic arterial oxygen saturation is low because of right-to-left shunting from the right ventricle. If a patent foramen ovale or ASD is present, there will be an additional right-to-left or bidirectional shunt at the atrial level. Selective biplane right ventricular angiography is extremely valuable to demonstrate levels of obstruction, continuity and size of the pulmonary arteries, and size and position of the ventricular defect. If not demonstrated by echocardiography or aortography, selective coronary arteriography should be performed on all patients preoperatively to demonstrate the coronary arterial pattern.[235,236]

MEDICAL MANAGEMENT

Although the definitive treatment of tetralogy of Fallot is surgical, medical management plays a role prior to surgery and in the postoperative period. For the severely cyanotic newborn, prostaglandin administration is of benefit[112] to open the ductus until surgery can be done. Prior to surgery, the hematocrit and hemoglobin should be monitored and iron-deficiency anemia should be promptly treated to prevent strokes. Fever or other illness that would lead to dehydration and possible thrombotic complications should be treated promptly.

Hypoxic spells in infants should be treated initially by placing the infant in the knee-chest position and administering a high concentration of oxygen and morphine sulfate. If acidosis is present and does not correct spontaneously and promptly, intravenous sodium bicarbonate should be given. Propranolol is useful in the acute treatment and possibly in the prevention of hypoxic spells.[237]

Bacterial endocarditis is a serious complication, especially in those who have had a systemic-to-pulmonary artery shunt.[238] Meticulous care should be taken to maintain good dental hygiene, and prophylactic antibiotics at times of predictable risk[239] are mandatory (see Chap. 82).

SURGICAL MANAGEMENT

Historically, the approach to tetralogy of Fallot has been either palliation or corrective surgery. The introduction of an aorta-to-pulmonary artery shunt for the treatment of tetralogy of Fallot[240] could truly be called the beginning of effective treatment for pediatric cardiovascular disease. When the cardiopulmonary bypass was initiated in the 1950s, tetralogy of Fallot was among the first lesions corrected.[241] Over the years, the age at which corrective surgery can be performed has dropped, so that in many centers primary repair is the procedure of choice at any age.[242] Palliation, when it is now performed, almost inevitably involves a modified Blalock-Taussig shunt interposing a graft between the subclavian artery and the ipsolateral pulmonary artery, usually on the side opposite the aortic arch.[243] Even in the perinatal period, the placement of a 4-mm tube will result in satisfactory palliation for a year in more than 90 percent of the infants.[244]

Surgical correction involves closing the VSD, usually through a right ventriculotomy, resecting infundibular muscle, and, if the infundibulum, pulmonary valve, and main pulmonary artery are hypoplastic, using a pericardial patch to open the narrowed area. Care must be taken to avoid heart block while closing the VSD and to avoid cutting a major branch of the coronary artery. If a patent foramen ovale is present, it is usually left open to allow decompression in the perioperative period. If a true ASD is present (pentology of Fallot), this should be closed to avoid left-to-right shunting once the right ventricle has recovered from the perioperative period.[245]

Children with tetralogy of Fallot and pulmonary atresia with good-sized pulmonary arteries are usually repaired by closing the VSD and interposing a conduit, frequently an aortic homograft, between the right ventricle and pulmonary artery.[246] If this is done in children under 7 or 8 years of age, replacement of the conduit is to be expected secondary to somatic growth. Children with tetralogy of Fallot and hypoplastic and/or discontinuous pulmonary arteries need an individualized approach, frequently involving balloon dilation of hypoplastic vessels, unifocalization of discontinuous vessels, and, it is to be hoped, eventual repair with a conduit closing the VSD.[247] Operative and early mortality rates for repair of tetralogy of Fallot are now quite low in most centers. Kirklin and coworkers[243] have reported mortality rates of 1.6 percent with operations at 5 years of age to 4.1 percent at 1 year of age. At Children's Hospital, Boston, there was a 4.2 percent mortality rate among 330 children under 1 year of age operated upon between 1973 and 1990, with a mortality rate of only 2.5 percent in the past 6 years.[245] Late complications have included residual, peripheral pulmonary stenosis, a small incidence of residual VSDs, and, rarely, aortic regurgitation. The long-term survivors have had atrial or, more commonly, ventricular arrhythmias and continue to be at risk for infective endocarditis.

Physicians at the Mayo Clinic, the first center to use cardiopulmonary bypass to repair tetralogy of Fallot in the 1950s, reported a 30-year follow-up of the 30-day survivors of surgery.[248] The 32-year actuarial survival rate was 86 percent, with subgroup survival rates of those less then 5 years old, 5 to 7 years old, and 8 to 11 years old at the time of surgical repair being 90, 93, and 91 percent, respectively. Late sudden death from cardiac causes occurred in 10 patients during the 32-year period. The performance of some previous palliative operation (Waterston or Pott's shunts), but not a palliative Blalock-Taussig shunt, was associated with higher mortality. With earlier surgery and less utilization of palliative procedures, it is hoped that the surgical results will be even better for children born in the 1980s and 1990s and beyond.

Ebstein's Anomaly

PATHOLOGY

In Ebstein's anomaly, the anterior leaflet of the tricuspid valve is attached normally to the annulus, while varying portions of the posterior and septal leaflets are displaced downward, being attached to the ventricular wall below the annulus. The proximal part of the right ventricle is thin-walled and continuous with the right atrium. The functional right ventricle is small and made up of the apical and infundibular portions of the right ventricle.[249] An additional common finding is that the papillary muscles and chordae are highly malformed, with great variation in the manner of attachment of the two involved leaflets to the right ventricular wall. Commonly, multiple direct attachments of valvular tissue to the right ventricular mural endocardium occur.[250]

An interatrial communication is present in most cases, usually taking the form of a patent foramen ovale. Continuity of right atrial and right ventricular myocardial tissues, in addition to the usual connections by way of the main conduction pathways, has been observed. *The presence of Ebstein's anomaly has been associated with maternal lithium use during pregnancy, although the risk ratio remains unclear.*[251]

ABNORMAL PHYSIOLOGY

Ebstein's anomaly results in obstruction to the right ventricular filling because of a decrease in size of the right ventricle, part of which is incorporated into the huge right atrium. The deformed tricuspid valve also frequently allows tricuspid regurgitation with a right-to-left shunt through the foramen ovale. In the perinatal period when the pulmonary vascular resistance is high, the tricuspid regurgitation may be severe. This results in an increased right atrial pressure and, when the patent foramen ovale is open, severe cyanosis. As the pulmonary vascular resistance falls, the right-to-left shunting is decreased and hypoxemia improves. In older children, right-sided congestive heart failure with edema and/or ascites may develop.

CLINICAL MANIFESTATIONS

History

Approximately one-half of reported cases develop symptoms of cyanosis and right-sided heart failure in early infancy.[252] The remainder present because of a murmur or abnormal chest roentgenogram, but with no symptoms, in early childhood or because of gradual progression of symptoms through late childhood or adult life.[253] The most common symptom is dyspnea on exertion. The spectrum of exercise intolerance has been described.[254] Palpitations due to supraventricular tachyarrhythmias occur in 20 to 30 percent of children. Occasionally, syncope occurs due to arrhythmia or low cardiac output if the atrial septum is intact.

Physical Examination

The newborn with elevated pulmonary vascular resistance has severe cyanosis. In older infants and children, cyanosis and clubbing are mild. Only a small percentage do not have an ASD or patent foramen ovale and thus are not cyanotic. The precordium is generally quiet, even in those with striking cardiomegaly. The liver is enlarged, and the jugular venous pulse may be elevated. The holosystolic murmur of tricuspid regurgitation is heard at the lower left sternal border and may be accompanied by a "scratchy" diastolic murmur of tricuspid stenosis. The first heart sound is split and loud, and the second heart sound is widely and persistently split. Loud third and fourth heart sounds are usual, especially in older patients.

Chest Roentgenogram

Heart size, as shown by chest roentgenogram, varies but is ordinarily very large, due to the very dilated right atrium. In those with cyanosis, pulmonary blood flow is diminished correspondingly.

Electrocardiogram

Giant, peaked P waves are common, along with a prolonged PQ interval and right ventricular conduction delay or complete right bundle branch block. Electrophysiologic correlates of these abnormalities have been reported.[255] In approximately 10 percent, the pattern of Wolff-Parkinson-White syndrome (with a short PQ interval and slurring of the initial QRS forces, or a delta wave) is seen.[253]

Echocardiogram

Two-dimensional echocardiography is very helpful in diagnosis (Fig. 70-26). Studies in the fetus and neonate have identified features associated with high risk.[256]

Cardiac Catheterization

There is a higher risk than usual associated with cardiac catheterization because of the frequency of rhythm distur-

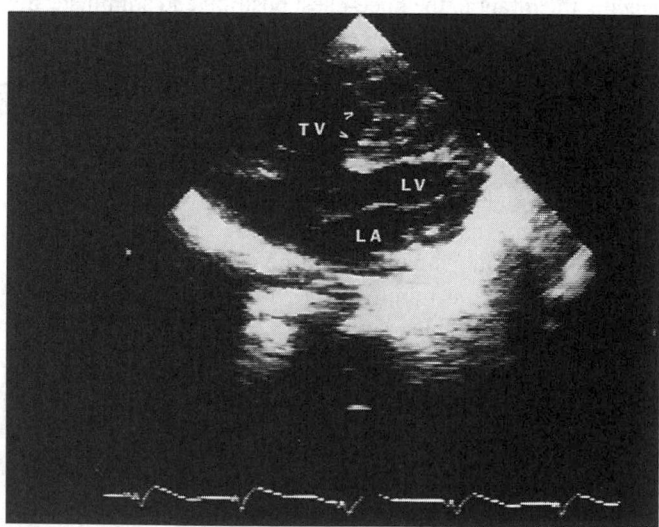

FIGURE 70-26

Two-dimensional echocardiogram in parasternal view in a patient with Ebstein's anomaly of the tricuspid valve (TV). Numerous attachments of the tricuspid valve (*arrowheads*) to the interventricular septum and right ventricular apex are seen. LV, left ventricle; LA, left atrium.

bances. Proper precautions and prompt use of cardioversion when necessary minimize this risk. In most cases, echocardiography and color Doppler evaluation are sufficient, and catheterization is now less commonly performed than previously.

There is usually right-to-left shunting at atrial level. Right atrial hypertension is present. The characteristic right ventricular pressure recording is not obtained until the catheter is advanced to the apex or outflow tract. An intracardiac ECG[257] demonstrates, on pullback from the right ventricle, an area where the ECG is ventricular but the pressure is atrial in contour. This method is not infallible, but it is good evidence of tricuspid displacement with an "atrialized" portion of the right ventricle.

NATURAL HISTORY AND PROGNOSIS

The natural history varies greatly with the severity of the abnormality. In one study of 50 patients who presented in the neonatal period, 9 (18 percent) died in the perinatal period, with late deaths in another 15 (9 due to hemodynamic deterioration, 5 sudden, and 1 noncardiac)—a 10-year actuarial survival of 61 percent.[258] In a study that included more children who presented after the perinatal period, the probability of survival was 50 percent at 47 years of age.[259] Predictors of poor outcome were New York Heart Association class II or IV, cardiothoracic ratio >65 percent, and atrial fibrillation.[259]

For women who survive into adulthood without significant arrhythmias or cyanosis, successful pregnancy with good fetal outcome is possible.[260]

MEDICAL MANAGEMENT

Medical therapy varies depending upon the severity of disease and age at presentation. For those presenting with cyanosis in the perinatal period, procrastination until the pulmonary vascular resistance has decreased may be the best strategy. For those severely hypoxemic, maintaining patency of the ductus with PGE_1[112] may be lifesaving. Reducing the pulmonary vascular resistance with nitric oxide may reduce right-to-left shunting and improve oxygenation.[261] Persistence of severe cyanosis beyond 1 week of age suggests pulmonic stenosis or pulmonic atresia in addition to the Ebstein's deformity of the tricuspid valve.

For children with arrhythmias, electrophysiologic study may be indicated. Pharmacologic treatment is occasionally appropriate, but more recently radiofrequency catheter ablation of the bypass tract usually responsible has been used[262] (see Chap. 31).

In older children who develop right-sided congestive heart failure, anticongestive measures with digoxin and diuretics may be tried, although this level of deterioration is usually an indication for surgical intervention.

SURGICAL MANAGEMENT

The surgical management of Ebstein's disease remains problematic. In the perinatal period, when the pulmonary vascular resistance is high, watchful waiting is probably the best approach. If after the pulmonary vascular resistance falls the child remains severely hypoxemic (saturations <75 percent), palliation with a Blalock-Taussig shunt to improve pulmonary blood flow may be sufficient to relieve hypoxemia, which should allow growth to an age where other procedures can be considered.[263] For children in whom hypoxemia remains a significant problem, three approaches have been used. The first is a Glenn anastomosis connecting the superior vena cava to the right pulmonary artery, allowing inferior vena cava blood to go through the right atrium and ventricle to the pulmonary artery.[264] This improves hypoxemia but does not eliminate the right-to-left shunting at the atrial level. A more definitive procedure that eliminates hypoxemia, used primarily for children with single ventricle but now applied in this situation, is the modified Fontan. In this approach, the tricuspid valve is oversewn and the patent foramen ovale closed. The superior vena cava is divided, with the cephalad portion connected to the top of the right pulmonary artery. An intraatrial tunnel is constructed so that inferior vena caval blood is diverted to the superior vena cava. The caudad portion of the superior vena cava is then connected to the bottom of the right pulmonary artery. This diverts all systemic venous blood away from the right ventricle directly into the pulmonary artery. In a small group of patients, this has been done with success.

The more common approach has been tricuspid valve reconstruction or replacement, usually with a bioprosthesis. Among 189 patients operated on at the Mayo Clinic over an almost 20-year period, there were 12 hospital deaths (6.3 percent) and an additional 10 late deaths. Of those followed more than 1 year after operation, more than 90 percent were in the New York Heart Association class I or II.[265] More recently, other approaches have been suggested, including reconstruction of the normally shaped right ventricle with repositioning of the displaced leaflet of the tricuspid valve at the normal level[266] or reimplantation of the tricuspid valve leaflets with a vertical plication of the atrialized portion of the right ventricle to reduce its size (Fig. 70-27).[267] *Although the newer approaches seem promising in small numbers of patients over the short run, many patients with the milder form of the disease can live well into adulthood,[268] so that indications for the newer operation in patients who are asymptomatic or only mildly limited remain problematic.*

ABNORMALITIES OF THE PULMONARY VENOUS CONNECTIONS

Total Anomalous Pulmonary Venous Connection

PATHOLOGY

When all pulmonary veins terminate in a systemic vein or the right atrium, the term *total anomalous pulmonary venous connection* or *return* is applied (Fig. 70-28). The usual veins leave the lung and then join a chamber-like confluence posterior to the left atrium. From the confluence of veins, one vessel leads to the anomalous termination. Less commonly, two or more vessels lead to multiple sites of termination.

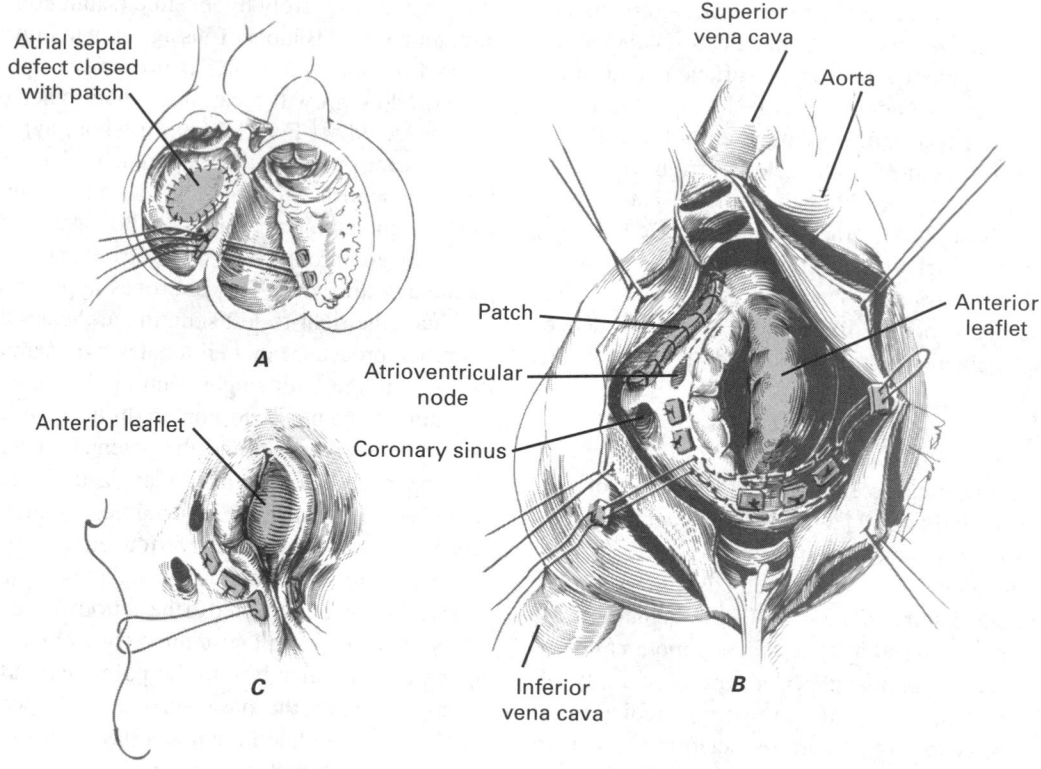

FIGURE 70-27

Danielson repair of Epstein's malformation. *A.* Anterior cutaway drawing. The atrial septal defect is closed securely with a patch. Pledgeted sutures are placed so as to position the posterior leaflet at the annulus and imbricate the "atrialized" right ventricular chamber. *B* and *C.* Drawing of the right atrium showing the annuloplasty suture passed through two pledgets. Tying of this suture reduces dilation of the tricuspid valve so that the large anterior leaflet can meet the two smaller cusps and constitute a functional, essentially monocusp valve.

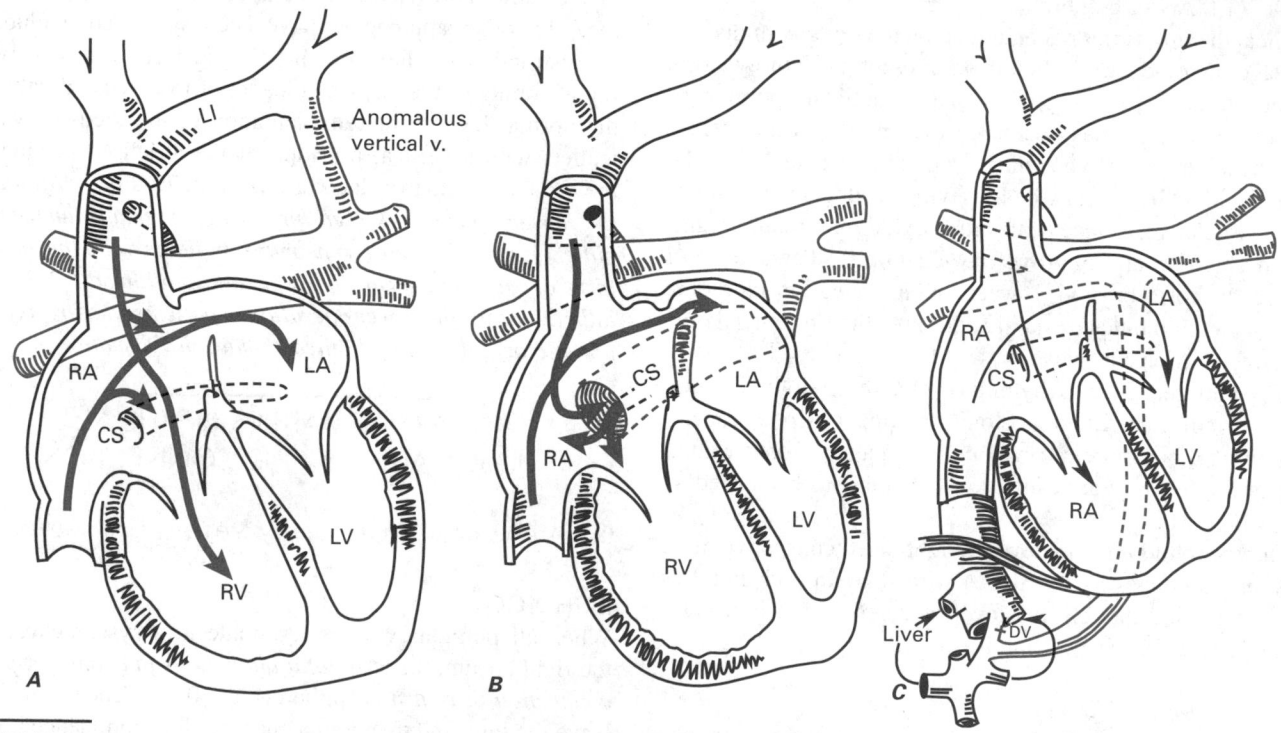

FIGURE 70-28

Three common types of total anomalous pulmonary venous connection. *A.* Total anomalous pulmonary venous connection to the left brachiocephalic (innominate) vein (LI) *B.* Total anomalous pulmonary venous connection to the coronary sinus (CS). *C.* Total anomalous pulmonary venous connection of the infradiaphragmatic type to the ductus venosus (DV). RA, right atrium; RV, right ventricle; LA, left atrium; LV, left ventricle.

Sites of supradiaphragmatic termination, in order of decreasing frequency, are the left brachiocephalic vein, the coronary sinus, the right atrium, the superior vena cava, and the azygous vein.[269] Supradiaphragmatic termination is not usually associated with pulmonary venous obstruction.[270]

The site of termination may also be infradiaphragmatic, with connection to the portal venous system or the inferior vena cava. The anomalous vein leaves the confluence of pulmonary veins and descends into the abdomen along the esophagus to join the ductus venosus, the portal vein, or the left gastric vein. *Pulmonary venous obstruction is present in virtually all cases of infradiaphragmatic connection.*[270,271]

In all cases of total anomalous pulmonary venous connection, there is a patent foramen ovale. The atrium and ventricle of the left side are small in comparison with the right-sided chambers but are within normal limits as to absolute size.

In the absence of asplenia or polysplenia syndromes, associated anomalies are not common.

ABNORMAL PHYSIOLOGY

In this anomaly, all the blood from both pulmonary and systemic circulations returns to the right atrium. It is compatible with life only if there is a communication between the right and left sides of the heart. In neonates with the connection below the diaphragm, the increase in pulmonary flow after birth cannot be accommodated and the obstruction to flow causes a marked increase in pulmonary venous pressure, resulting in a very high pulmonary vascular resistance. If the ductus arteriosus is still open, the pulmonary vascular resistance exceeds systemic vascular resistance with a right-to-left shunt at the ductal level. When the ductus closes, the increased pulmonary resistance results in an increased right ventricular pressure. If the right ventricle fails, the right atrial pressure will increase, and right-to-left shunting at the atrial level may be present, often with profound hypoxemia.

In older children with unobstructed damage above the diaphragm (supracardiac), the pulmonary resistance is usually low. The low resistance facilitates a high pulmonary flow. With mixing of all pulmonary and systemic flow in the right atrium, the oxygen saturation is usually relatively high, resulting in physiology similar to an ASD and mild cyanosis.[272]

CLINICAL MANIFESTATIONS

Total Anomalous Pulmonary Venous Connection with Pulmonary Venous Obstruction

Neonates with total anomalous pulmonary venous connection below the diaphragm who have pulmonary venous obstruction present with cyanosis, which may be severe, and dyspnea. Symptoms frequently develop beyond 12 h of age, allowing differentiation from respiratory distress syndrome. In addition to dyspnea, feeding difficulties and cardiac failure are seen.

Physical findings are usually unimpressive. The heart is not hyperactive and thrills are absent. The second heart sound may be split, with an increased pulmonic component. Significant murmurs are uncommon.

Total Anomalous Pulmonary Venous Connection without Pulmonary Venous Obstruction

These patients are usually asymptomatic at birth, although some may develop transient tachypnea. Presentation is typically during the first year of life. Some children have tachypnea and feeding difficulties, with frequent respiratory infections. Cyanosis is frequently mild and may be clinically inapparent. Other children may be asymptomatic and present with a heart murmur.

On physical examination, the right ventricular impulse is usually hyperactive. The jugular venous pulse is elevated, and hepatomegaly appears early. There is a diffuse and hyperdynamic right ventricular impulse. The second heart sound is split and relatively fixed; the loudness of the pulmonary component is usually increased. There is usually a grade 2 or 3 midsystolic murmur at the left sternal border. At the lower sternal border, there are a middiastolic rumble and prominent third and fourth heart sounds. Rales may be heard over the lung fields, and periorbital edema is frequent. A continuous murmur may be heard over the common venous channel.

Chest Roentgenogram

With the unobstructed types, the heart is enlarged with the pulmonary flow. Pulmonary edema is uncommon. In those patients with return to the left innominate vein, there may be a characteristic bulging of the superior mediastinum bilaterally, producing a "snowman," or figure-of-eight, contour. With obstructed types, the heart size is near normal; there is very marked pulmonary edema, which may give a granular appearance to the lungs, making differentiation from respiratory distress syndrome difficult in the newborn.

Electrocardiogram

There is right axis deviation and right atrial and right ventricular hypertrophy. Commonly, there is a qR pattern in the right precordial leads.

Echocardiogram

Echocardiography with color Doppler is specific in defining the anomaly and the site of drainage.[273]

Cardiac Catheterization

If echocardiography is inconclusive at delineating the site of the pulmonary venous connection, catheterization may be necessary. There is an increase in oxygen saturation at the level of the abnormal connection, with similar saturations in the remainder of the chambers on both sides of the heart. Pulmonary arterial pressure is elevated to a variable degree, but it may be above systemic pressure if there is marked pulmonary venous or pulmonary vascular obstruction. Pulmonary capillary wedge pressures are elevated in proportion to the degree of venous obstruction. The atrial communication may rarely be obstructive,[272] and balloon atrial septostomy may occasionally be helpful.[274] Pulmonary arteriography will usually show the anomalous venous connection. Angiography directly in the common venous channel, if it is entered, will outline its course and any sites of obstruction optimally.

NATURAL HISTORY AND PROGNOSIS

The clinical course is commonly that of progressive congestive heart failure, with death in the first year of life.[272] There are significant differences among patients with varying degrees of pulmonary hypertension. The majority of those with severe pulmonary hypertension and pulmonary venous obstruction die by the age of 3 months, whereas those with significant pulmonary hypertension alone may survive to 1 year of age or more. The best clinical course is seen in those with pulmonary pressures lower than one-half of systemic pressure. The majority of patients survive to 1 year, and some do not develop congestive heart failure. Severe growth failure occurs in all but a few of this latter group. At postmortem examination, structural changes in the pulmonary vascular bed are present to some degree at all ages, but changes are more severe in those with venous obstruction.[275]

MEDICAL MANAGEMENT

Medical management involves vigorous treatment of congestive heart failure and intercurrent respiratory infections and prevention of endocarditis.

Because of the poor outlook with medical management alone, surgery is being recommended soon after diagnosis. Any newborn or young infant with severe obstruction or pulmonary edema should have prompt surgical correction. Failure to grow is also an indication for surgery. For infants with less than one-half systemic pressure in the pulmonary artery who grow, surgery may be deferred for a few months.

SURGICAL MANAGEMENT

Correction of total anomalous pulmonary venous connection requires: (1) creation of a large communication between the left atrium and the pulmonary venous system, (2) obliteration of the anomalous pulmonary venous connection to the systemic circulation, and (3) closure of the associated interatrial communications.[276,277]

Supracardiac anomalous connection to the left brachiocephalic (vertical) vein and infracardiac connections to the portal venous system or the inferior vena cava are corrected by the creation of a wide anastomosis between the posterior aspect of the left atrium and the common transverse pulmonary vein.[277] The stretched foramen ovale is closed. The ascending or descending anomalous pulmonary venous connection to the systemic circulation is ligated, as is the PDA.

Anomalous pulmonary venous connection to the coronary sinus is repaired by creation of a large fenestration in the common wall between the coronary sinus and the left atrium. The coronary sinus is diverted into the left atrium by placement of an intracardiac patch, which also closes the interatrial communication.

Total anomalous pulmonary venous connection to the right atrium is repaired by excision of the atrial septum and placement of a patch diverting the opening of the anomalous pulmonary venous connection into the left atrium.

Mixed forms of total anomalous pulmonary venous connection pose particular technical difficulties, requiring individualized operations. Mortality rates are slightly higher after early repair of symptomatic neonates having mixed types of total anomalous pulmonary venous connections.

While the results of repair of total anomalous pulmonary venous connection without obstruction in the older child have always been quite good, until recently those neonates with obstructed total venous return have been problematic. In the 1960s and early 1970s, the surgical mortality rate exceeded 50 percent.[278] Between 1970 and 1980, surgical techniques improved and the mortality rate was reduced to between 10 and 20 percent.[279] More recently, surgical results have continued to improve, with no mortality among 27 infants who underwent reparative surgery at Children's Hospital, Boston, in the late 1980s.[280]

After a satisfactory operative course, the prognosis has been excellent in those in whom a large common pulmonary vein can be attached to the back wall of the left atrium with a relatively large anastomosis. For those initially with obstructed total anomalous pulmonary venous return, the left atrium may be small and the anastomosis may be more difficult. Late obstruction of one or more pulmonary veins has been seen. When present, the obstruction can be approached by balloon dilation, stent placement, or repeat surgery.[280,281]

MALPOSITION OF THE CARDIAC STRUCTURES

Definition and Terminology

The *segmental approach* to the diagnosis of complex congenital heart disease[282] provides an orderly, effective method for determining the anatomic and hemodynamic interrelationships of the cardiac chambers, valves, and great vessels. In order for this approach to be better understood, certain definitions will be helpful. Positioning of viscera is described as situs solitus, inversus, or ambiguous. In *situs solitus* (S), distribution of all the organs is recognized as normal, as, for example, a left-sided stomach and spleen, a predominantly right-sided liver, a trilobed right lung, and a bilobed left lung. In *situs inversus (totalis)* (I), the organs show a perfect mirror image, as regarding left and right, to that of situs solitus. Anteroposterior relations are not disturbed. When neither situs solitus nor situs inversus can be identified, *situs ambiguous* (A) is said to be present. This usually applies in cases of asplenia or polysplenia.

With the rarest of exceptions, the *atria follow the body situs* and are so designated (morphologic right atrium to the right of the left atrium in atrial situs solitus and to the left of the left atrium in atrial situs inversus). The AV canal consists of the tricuspid valve, the mitral valve, and the septum of the AV canal and connects the atrial with the ventricular portion of the heart. As a rule *each AV valve is part of the specific ventricle into which it leads*. The valve situs may be solitus, inversus, or ambiguous.

The alignment or type of atrioventricular (AV) or ventriculoarterial (VA) connection addresses the issue of what flows into what. The connection may be described at the AV or VA level as concordant (e.g., right atrium to right ventricle, left ventricle to aorta), discordant (e.g., right atrium to left ventricle, left ventricle to pulmonary artery), or an arrangement that requires a special description. In the case of AV alignment where the atria are not lateralized, the alignment would be ambiguous. In the univentricular heart, the designation would be double-inlet, absent right or absent left AV connection. Special descriptions in the case of VA alignment or type of VA connection include double-outlet or single-outlet VA connection. The mode of connections, either AV or VA, on the other hand, addresses the structural makeup of the connecting segments, namely, the AV canal and the infundibulum or conus. The mode of AV connection may be normal, common, stenotic, imperforate, atretic, double-orifice, overriding, straddling, or unguarded. The mode of VA connection may be expressed in terms of the position and development of the conus or infundibulum, which, although normally incorporated into the right ventricle, is not an intrinsic part of the true right ventricle. It may be described as subpulmonary, subaortic, very deficient, or bilaterally present or absent.[283]

The position of the ventricles may be described by the terms *d loop* and *l loop*. When the morphologic right ventricle lies to the right of the morphologic left ventricle, the ventricular portion of the heart is said to exhibit a d loop (D). The ventricles are said to be noninverted or in the solitus position. When the ventricular relations are reversed, l loop (L) is said to be present. The ventricles are inverted or in the inversus position. *These relationships are independent of the visceral or atrial situs as well as the position of the heart or its chambers within the chest.*

The great arteries may deviate from the usual with respect to both their anteroposterior and their lateral (left to right) relationships. In solitus (S) or *normally related great arteries* (NRGA), the aortic origin lies to the right of and posterior to the position of the pulmonary valve. In the inversus (I) relationship, the anteroposterior relationships are not disturbed but the aortic origin lies to the left of the pulmonary arterial origin. In *transposition of the great arteries* (TGA), the aorta arises from the anatomic right ventricle, the pulmonary artery from the anatomic left ventricle, and, usually, the aortic origin is more anterior than that of the pulmonary artery.

When the aortic origin lies to the right of the pulmonary origin, the transposition is called *dextro* or *d transposition* (D-TGA) (see discussion of complete transposition of great arteries, below). When the aortic origin lies to the left of the pulmonary origin, *levo transposition* (L-TGA) is said to be present (see the section on congenitally corrected transposition, below).

When the abnormal relationship of the great arteries is neither complete nor corrected transposition, the term *malposition of the great arteries* (MGA) may be used. Malpositions are designated as D-MGA or L-MGA, depending on the laterality in the relation between the origins of the two great arteries.[283] Within this group will be found examples of the abnormal VA alignment, where one great artery arises from

the appropriate ventricle and the other great artery also arises from the same (or inappropriate) ventricle. These will be examples of *double-outlet right ventricle* (DORV) or *double-outlet left ventricle* (DOLV). Also included will be the arterial malposition termed *anatomically corrected malposition* (ACM). This is characterized by the great arteries having a normal VA alignment (concordant), but with the aorta anterior to the pulmonary artery by virtue of an abnormal mode of VA connection, namely, the presence of a well-developed conus lying beneath both the aorta and the pulmonary artery or only beneath the aorta. The route for the flow of blood in ACMs may be normal or abnormal, depending on the atrioventricular alignment.[283]

The Segmental Approach to Diagnosis

The segmental, or step-by-step, approach is a valuable tool for arriving at the correct diagnosis in patients with complex congenital heart disease and is independent of cardiac position. In order, one determines: (1) the locations of the right and left atria and their venous connections, (2) the location of the right and left ventricles and their alignment with the atria, (3) the mode of connection of the AV valves to the ventricles, (4) the position of the great arteries and their alignment with the ventricles, and (5) the location and status of the infundibulum. In addition, one must search for associated malformations between and within each of these segments.

Determining atrial situs can be accomplished in most instances by taking advantage of the high degree of abdominal visceroatrial concordance. With abdominal situs solitus (S), the liver is on the right and the right atrium will almost invariably be on the right as well; with abdominal situs inversus (I), the liver is on the left and the right atrium will almost invariably be on the left. With abdominal situs ambiguous (A), the liver may be almost symmetrically placed across the midline and the atria may be normally located or inverted or both atria may have morphologic characteristics of either the right or the left atrium (Fig. 13-4). A symmetric liver is found in approximately 60 percent of patients with situs ambiguous. Lateralization of the liver, evident in the remainder, may simulate either situs solitus or situs inversus.

When both atria have characteristics of a right atrium,[284] *dextroisomerism*, or "bilateral right-sidedness," is said to be present. This situation is usually, though not invariably, accompanied by asplenia. When both atria have characteristics of a left atrium,[284] *levoisomerism*, or "bilateral left-sidedness," is said to exist. This usually, but again not invariably, is accompanied by polysplenia.

Bronchial situs, determined by overpenetrated chest roentgenogram or bronchial tomography, is an excellent predictor of atrial situs, but the most accurate technique appears to be two-dimensional echocardiography with Doppler color flow mapping. The hepatic portion of the inferior vena cava, which almost always enters the morphologic right atrium, usually can be easily identified, as can the connections and structural details of the superior vena cava, coronary sinus, pulmonary veins, atrial septum, and atrial appendages.[285]

Additional clinical clues to atrial situs may be obtained from the ECG, where a superior and leftward orientation of the P-wave vector suggests levoisomerism and polysplenia. Howell-Heinz and Howell-Jolly bodies in the peripheral blood smear are characteristic of dextroisomerism or asplenia.

For determination of the AV, ventricular, and VA relationships, high-quality, selective biplane angiography supplemented by equally high quality two-dimensional echocardiography with Doppler color flow mapping are essential.[284] Symbols used to designate the combination or sequence of segments are arranged in order as follows: (1) the visceroatrial or bronchoatrial situs, (2) the ventricular loop, and (3) the relations of the great arteries. These may be included within parentheses and preceded by abbreviations that indicate the VA alignment, for example, TGA, DORV, or single ventricle (SV). Associated malformations such as VSD, pulmonary stenosis, and straddling tricuspid valve may be listed after the parentheses. Thus, the typical or usual transposition of the great arteries with situs solitus, d-ventricular loop, and aorta arising from the right ventricle and to the right of the pulmonary artery, with an intact ventricular septum (IVS), would be designated TGA (SDD) IVS. The designation for typical corrected transposition (TGA) with situs solitus (S), l-ventricular loop (L), aorta arising from the morphologic right ventricle and lying to the left of the pulmonary artery (L), with ventricular septal defect (VSD) and pulmonary stenosis (PS), would be TGA (SLL), VSD, PS. This designation would apply to transposition with situs solitus, whether the heart lay in the right or left chest (dextrocardia or levocardia, respectively). It should be noted that the description of the position of the heart within the chest would offer no additional information referable to the intracardiac anatomy or great-vessel alignment.[282]

Levocardia, Dextrocardia, and Mesocardia

The position of the cardiac apex indicates a condition of levocardia, dextrocardia, or mesocardia.

The trend today is to discard the terms *dextroposition, dextroversion, mirror-image dextrocardia,* and *isolated dextrocardia* because they do not provide any significant information beyond what is already known, namely, that the cardiac apex is in the right chest, and to use the broad term *dextrocardia* for all right-sided hearts, followed by a description of the visceroatrial situs. In the case of those patients in whom the heart appears to have been pulled or pushed into the right chest by massive atelectasis or hypoplasia of the right lung, diaphragmatic hernia, eventration of the diaphragm, pleural effusion, obstructive emphysema, or pneumothorax, an appropriate descriptive phrase should be added. The term *isolated levocardia* is applied to all left-sided hearts with situs inversus or situs ambiguous, and a description of the visceroatrial situs should follow.

Dextrocardia with complete situs inversus occurs in approximately 2 per 10,000 live births. *The incidence of congenital heart disease is relatively low among these individuals and is estimated to be about 3 percent.* Dextrocardia with

situs solitus or situs ambiguous is considerably less common and occurs in perhaps 1 per 20,000 live births. The incidence of congenital heart disease is extremely high in this situation, however, and is probably in the range of 90 percent or greater. From these figures, one could project that approximately 12 percent of individuals found to have dextrocardia and congenital heart disease would have complete situs inversus. This estimate compares favorably with the figure of 18 percent observed in large autopsy series. About 50 percent of patients with dextrocardia and heart disease have situs solitus, and the remainder, perhaps 30 percent, have situs ambiguous.[282] An l-ventricular loop is found in the majority of patients with dextrocardia regardless of situs but is most common, as one might expect, among those patients with situs inversus, where it approaches 80 percent. Cardiac malformations usually, although not invariably, are severe and complex. The most common lesions and their approximate frequency are as follows: transposition of the great arteries, 50 to 75 percent; double-outlet right ventricle, 10 to 18 percent; VSD, 60 to 80 percent; single ventricle, 15 to 40 percent; and pulmonary stenosis or atresia, 70 to 80 percent.[282] Approximately three-quarters of the transposed great arteries will have the segmental arrangement of corrected transposition. Tetralogy of Fallot is distinctly uncommon. Polysplenia or asplenia is found in about one-third of patients with dextrocardia and almost invariably with situs ambiguous. Kartagener's syndrome, the triad of situs inversus, sinusitis, and bronchiectasis, results from impaired ciliary movement. It is present in approximately 20 percent of patients with dextrocardia and situs inversus totalis.[285] The incidence of isolated levocardia is estimated at approximately 0.6 per 10,000 live births. It is estimated that over 90 percent of affected individuals will have associated heart disease. Situs inversus is present in approximately 15 percent, while the remainder have situs ambiguous, with the ratio of asplenia to polysplenia or accessory spleens being from 2.5:1 to 1.5:1. The associated defects are comparable in complexity and severity to those associated with dextrocardia. *Mesocardia* may exist either as a variant position of the normal heart or as a variant position of dextrocardia or isolated levocardia.

MEDICAL AND SURGICAL MANAGEMENT

Medical management of patients with cardiac malposition is similar to that of patients with normally located hearts, with the exceptions of continuous daily antibiotic coverage and pneumococcal vaccine for patients with asplenia and the particular attention to detail that is necessary to establish the correct diagnosis in those individuals with unusual and complex malformations. Surgical management differs in the technical considerations imposed by the malposition of the heart itself, the frequency of occurrence of the l-ventricular loop, and the variability of the intracardiac conduction system.

Dextro Transposition of the Great Arteries

DEFINITION

In this condition, the aorta and the pulmonary artery are misplaced in relation to the ventricular septum, with the aorta arising from the right ventricle and the pulmonary artery arising from the left ventricle (discordant VA connection).

PATHOLOGY

In the majority of cases there are situs solitus of the atria and viscera (S) and concordance of the AV connection, and the right ventricle lies to the right of the left ventricle (d loop, D) (Fig. 70-29). The aorta lies to the right of the pulmonary arterial origin (d transposition, D) and is anterior. Of the communications between the two sides of the circulation, a narrow patent foramen and PDA are common in very young infants. The ventricular septum is intact in approximately half the patients, and another 10 percent will have only a very small VSD. The remainder will have a large or multiple VSDs.[286]

Pulmonary stenosis of significance is very uncommon among neonates with intact ventricular septum but develops with the passage of time in approximately one-third of those patients in whom the right ventricle continues as the systemic ventricle. In most cases it is mild and usually, though not invariably, is the result of a bulging of the ventricular septum into the left ventricular outflow area. Approximately one-third of patients with a large VSD will have significant left ventricular outflow tract obstruction. Causes of this obstruction include leftward malalignment of the infundibular septum, presence of a membranous collar or ridge encircling the left ventricular outflow tract, anomalous adhesion of the anterior mitral leaflet to the ventricular septum, stenotic defor-

mity of the pulmonary valve, and, rarely, an aneurysm of endocardial tissue related to the VSD.[287]

The coronary arteries usually arise from the two aortic sinuses adjacent to the pulmonary trunk, the "facing sinuses," with the most common arrangement being the right coronary artery arising from the rightward sinus and the left coronary artery, with its anterior descending and circumflex branches, arising from the leftward sinus.

Hypertensive pulmonary vascular disease may occur at an inordinately early age and may occur even in patients with an intact ventricular septum and initially low left ventricular pressures. Three-quarters of more of patients with d transposition, situs solitus, and d loop [TGA (SDD)] either have no significant associated cardiac defects or have relatively simple malformations in the form of VSD, ASD, PDA, or pulmonary stenosis. The remainder have more complicated lesions and will not be discussed in this section.

ABNORMAL PHYSIOLOGY

The systemic and pulmonary circulations are arranged so that the systemic venous return is conducted back to the systemic arterial system and the pulmonary venous return back to the pulmonary arterial system, with no obligatory mixing or interchange. For survival, there must be communication between the two circulations in the form of a patent foramen ovale, a PDA, or a VSD. The hemodynamics are dependent on the combination of defects present and particularly on the amount

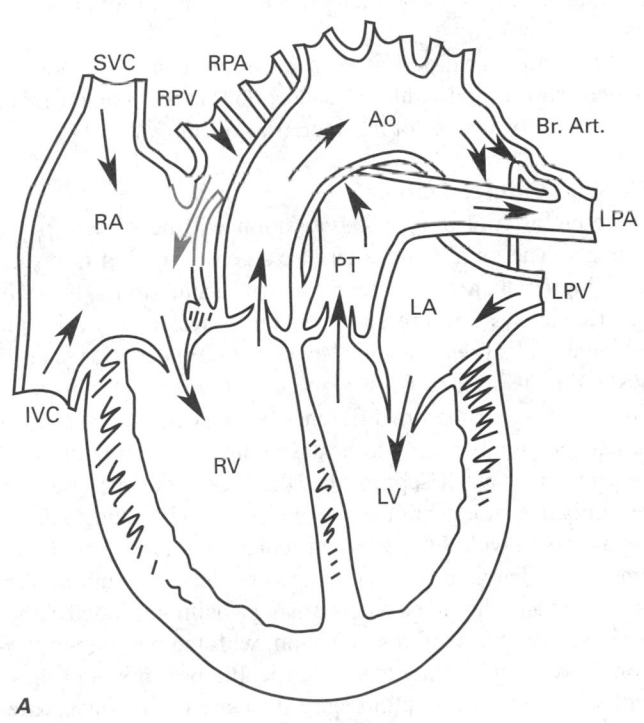

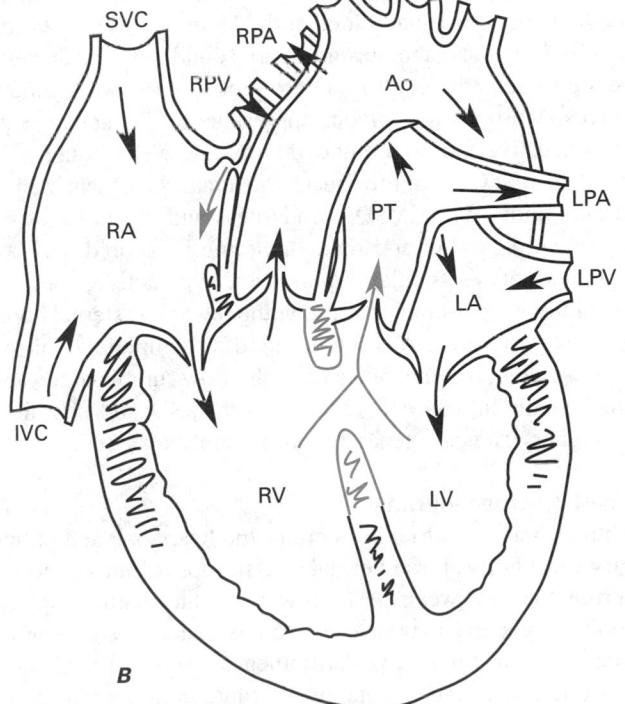

FIGURE 70-29

Complete D-transposition of the great arteries. *A.* With intact ventricular septum. A patent foramen ovale and enlarged bronchial arteries (Br. Art.) are present. *B.* With ventricular septal defect and without pulmonary stenosis.

SVC, superior vena cava; IVC, inferior vena cava; RA, right atrium; RV, right ventricle; Ao, aorta; LA, left atrium; LV, left ventricle.

of mixing between the systemic and pulmonary circulations. The right ventricle is the systemic ventricle, and its systolic pressure will be the same as systemic arterial pressure.

CLINICAL MANIFESTATIONS

Approximately 5 to 7 percent of children with recognized congenital heart disease have transposition of the great arteries.[287] Males are more commonly afflicted than females in a ratio between 2:1 and 3:1.

History

Among infants with intact ventricular septum, very early, severe, and progressive cyanosis is the presenting sign, making its clinical appearance within the first hour in over half and by the end of the first 24 h in over 90 percent of neonates so afflicted.[287] In a very few, a persistent PDA in combination with an incompetent foramen ovale or a small VSD permits survival for several weeks, but narrowing or closure of any of the three communications produces critical hypoxemia. Infants with a sizable VSD present with severe congestive failure and only mild or barely detectable cyanosis toward the middle or latter part of the first month of life. Infants with a large VSD and significant pulmonary stenosis may present within the first days of life with cyanosis if stenosis is severe; with more moderate stenosis, they may present with cyanosis and little if any congestive failure somewhat later within the first year.

Physical Examination

Among infants with an intact ventricular septum, the most prominent feature is intense cyanosis. Tachypnea and mild dyspnea are present. The right ventricular lift is forceful, and the first sound is usually loud at the lower left sternal border. In most patients, the second heart sound may be heard to be split narrowly, confirming the presence of two semilunar valves. Murmurs are seldom impressive or distinctive. Signs of congestive failure are uncommon unless the infant is beyond the first week of life and a large ductus is present. Among infants with a large VSD, slenderness and mild cyanosis or a grayish pallor are apparent. Breathing is labored, and both right and left ventricular impulses are hyperactive. A thrill is uncommon. A systolic murmur at the lower left sternal border is usually present but is seldom loud or completely holosystolic. A gallop rhythm and a diastolic flow rumble at the apex are typical. Infants and children with VSD and significant pulmonary stenosis generally are severely cyanotic.

Chest Roentgenogram

With an intact ventricular septum, the heart size and pulmonary vascularity appear normal or at the upper limits of normal during the first week. A narrow base due to the displaced pulmonary artery may give rise to the characteristic "egg-on-side" contour. Impressive cardiomegaly, pulmonary plethora, and this characteristic contour are more common during the second week and beyond. With a large VSD, marked cardiac enlargement involving all chambers, impressive pulmonary plethora, and the egg-on-side contour are present. With sig-

nificant pulmonary stenosis, the heart resembles that of a patient with tetralogy of Fallot, but it is usually slightly larger and the pulmonary vascularity less diminished than one would expect for a comparable degree of clinical cyanosis. A right aortic arch is present in 4 to 16 percent of patients.

Electrocardiogram

If the ventricular septum is intact, the ECG may reveal tall or peaked P waves by the second or third day of life; however, clearly abnormal right ventricular forces are not usually apparent until the latter part of the first week. The persistence of an upright T wave in leads V_1 and V_{3R} beyond 4 days of age would provide an early clue that the right ventricular systolic pressure is at systemic levels. The older infant will have abnormal right axis deviation and marked right ventricular hypertrophy. A large VSD with a large pulmonary blood flow will usually produce biatrial and biventricular hypertrophy. If pulmonary blood flow is reduced toward normal, whether by significant pulmonary stenosis, pulmonary arterial banding, or severe PVOD, the pattern becomes one of right ventricular and right atrial hypertrophy.

Echocardiogram

Two-dimensional study with Doppler color flow mapping is the diagnostic procedure of choice. The pulmonary artery can be seen arising from the left ventricle, and the aorta from the right ventricle. The presence or absence of VSDs, anomalies of the AV connections, status of the left ventricular outflow tract, and, in very skilled hands, the coronary arterial pattern can be identified.[288]

In addition, balloon atrial septostomy can be performed under echocardiographic guidance, and an assessment made of the size of the resulting interatrial opening.

Cardiac Catheterization

Systemic arterial oxygen desaturation will be present in all patients. The pulmonary arterial oxygen saturation is invariably higher than the systemic arterial saturation. The right ventricular systolic pressure will be at systemic levels; the left ventricular pressure will also be at systemic levels if a large VSD, ductus arteriosus, or significant pulmonary stenosis is present. A wide pressure difference between the two ventricles or between the two atria indicates an intact or virtually intact ventricular or atrial septum, but the lack of such a gradient certainly does not guarantee the presence of an adequate opening at either level. Selective ventricular angiography will document the diagnosis and associated defects. The pulmonary artery can and should be entered using a balloon-guided catheter in all patients with transposition, with the possible exception of very small infants with critical hypoxemia and those with extremely severe pulmonary stenosis. The coronary arterial pattern should be established.[289] *All newborns with transposition will benefit from balloon atrial septostomy at initial catheterization by virtue of the increased mixing of the pulmonary and systemic venous circulations and the decompression of the left atrium.*

NATURAL HISTORY AND PROGNOSIS

Without balloon septostomy or surgical intervention, 50 percent of infants with transposition will die within the first month and 90 percent within the first year of life.[287] Those with an intact ventricular septum die very early from hypoxemia. Those with a large VSD usually live somewhat longer, but the majority die in the first months of congestive failure; the few survivors will have severe PVOD. Those with a large VSD and pulmonary stenosis have the best outlook, but the average life expectancy is barely 5 years even with this combination of defects. With an adequate interatrial opening, whether it be natural, balloon-induced, or surgically created, infants with an intact ventricular septum do relatively well during the first year. Increasing cyanosis during the first year in these patients may be due to a gradual diminution of the size of the atrial septal opening, narrowing or closure of a persistent PDA or small VSD, the gradual development of subvalvular pulmonary stenosis, or the development of PVOD. Below the age of 2 years, cerebrovascular accidents are a hazard to these hypoxemic infants and occur, almost invariably, in a setting of relative anemia rather than extreme polycythemia. The appearance of PVOD is unusual but can occur within the first 12 months of life. It becomes more frequent, approaching 40 percent, in the second year of life and thereafter.[287] Infants with a large VSD and no significant pulmonary stenosis will develop PVOD and become prohibitive risks for corrective surgery by the end of the first year of life. Those with a VSD and severe pulmonary stenosis usually become progressively more cyanotic.

Palliative and subsequent corrective operations have enabled a relatively large group of patients to survive beyond infancy and early childhood. Among the survivors of the atrial switch operations, such as the Mustard and Senning procedures, will be found such residual abnormalities as pulmonary stenosis or PVOD, as well as complications that are the result of surgery. These include residual intraatrial baffle leaks, systemic and/or pulmonary venous obstruction, and arrhythmias. Late sudden death has been described in about 3 percent of survivors and is very possibly the result of arrhythmias. Finally, right ventricular dysfunction, with or without progressive tricuspid regurgitation, has been documented in many of the somewhat older survivors of the atrial inversion operations and raises the question of whether or not the right ventricle can function adequately as the systemic arterial ventricle beyond adolescence and early adult life. Survivors of the arterial switch operation may develop supravalvular pulmonary or aortic stenosis at the site of the anastomoses, but these are usually mild and amenable to balloon dilatation.[290]

MEDICAL MANAGEMENT

The first step in treatment of infants with intact ventricular septum is to provide without delay an adequate systemic arterial oxygen saturation. This can be achieved in almost all instances by establishing an adequate interatrial opening with balloon atrial septostomy and providing adequate systemic arterial-to-pulmonary arterial shunting via the ductus with the use of intravenous PGE_1 infusion; the latter is frequently supplemented by endotracheal intubation to compensate for prostaglandin-related apnea. The adequacy of the atrial septostomy opening can be determined by a sustained increase in the systemic arterial oxygen saturation to above 60 percent and verified by direct visualization with two-dimensional echocardiography. If the relief of hypoxemia is unsatisfactory, if the interatrial opening is judged by echocardiography to be small, or if an unacceptable systemic arterial oxygen saturation returns upon withdrawal of the PGE_1 infusion, the alternatives are to perform a surgical atrial septectomy without delay in those infants in whom an atrial inversion repair is planned at 4 to 8 months of age, or to proceed directly with corrective surgery in the form of the arterial switch operation. Today, if the infant were less than 3 weeks of age or the left ventricular systolic pressure was known to be 60 percent or more of the systemic arterial or right ventricular systolic pressure, the authors would recommend the arterial switch operation.

Once an adequate ASD has been created, infants with transposition, an intact septum, or a very small VSD in whom an atrial inversion repair is anticipated should be followed carefully over the intervening 4 to 8 months. Care is taken to prevent anemia or infective endocarditis. Increasing hypoxemia or a suspicion of increasing pulmonary arterial pressure is an indication for prompt recatheterization. Even if the course is uncomplicated, these infants are recatheterized electively at 3 to 7 months of age and the defect repaired shortly thereafter, using either the Senning or Mustard operation or the two-stage arterial switch operation.

Arterial switch repair is now the preferred surgical alternative to the atrial inversion procedures for the neonate with an intact ventricular septum and for the slightly older infant with a large VSD and without significant structural pulmonary stenosis. Arterial switching should be performed within the first 2 to 3 weeks of life, before left ventricular systolic pressure falls significantly below that of the right ventricle. For infants beyond 3 weeks of age, if the ratio of left ventricular to right ventricular pressure has fallen below 0.60, a pulmonary arterial band may be applied with or without a systemic-to-pulmonary arterial shunt and the arterial switch operation performed approximately 1 week later.[287] Most patterns of coronary arterial origin and course appear to be amenable to the operation, and infants as small as 2.5 kg may be successfully repaired. Repair is usually preceded by cardiac catheterization, balloon atrial septostomy, and infusion of PGE_1 to keep the ductus open and the left ventricular systolic pressure at or near systemic levels until the switch can be accomplished. Expert echocardiography and immediate surgery may make catheterization and septostomy unnecessary.[287]

In some centers the surgical risks have been reduced to about 5 to 10 percent,[291] although in other centers the surgical mortality continues to be higher.[292] Short- and midterm prognosis is good,[293] but longer-term studies are awaited.

For infants with transposition, a large VSD, and pulmonary hypertension, the arterial switch technique with VSD closure or banding of the pulmonary artery must be carried out within the first 2 months of life if severe PVOD is to be prevented. The authors' current preference is for repair. Infants with a large VSD and severe pulmonary stenosis usually may be palliated with a systemic-to-pulmonary arterial shunt and repaired in later infancy or as young children,[246] although some centers are doing reparative surgery in infancy.[291] Finally, the severe hypoxemia present in those children with a large VSD and severe PVOD may be reduced, in selected patients, by an intraatrial repair performed as a palliative procedure, with no attempt at closure of the VSD.[294]

Double-Outlet Right Ventricle

PATHOLOGY

In this malformation, more than 50 percent of the semilunar valve orifices of both great arteries arise from the morphologic right ventricle. In most cases, the ventricles display a d loop, and the pulmonary arterial origin is normally positioned, arising from a conus above the right ventricle. The aorta also arises from the right ventricle above conal tissue. The two semilunar valves are at about the same level, and there is no fibrous continuity between the semilunar and mitral valves (Fig. 70-30).

In most cases, the aortic origin is to the right (d malposition) of the pulmonary arterial origin, the two vessels usually displaying a side-by-side relationship. Uncommonly, the aortic origin is distinctly anterior to the pulmonary origin or the aorta arises to the left (l malposition) of the pulmonary artery.[295]

With rare exceptions, there is a VSD. The condition may be further subdivided on the basis of the relation of the VSD to the origin of the great arteries. The VSD will be subaortic in approximately two-thirds of patients, subpulmonary (*Taussig-Bing heart*) in 18 percent, related to both great arteries (*doubly committed*) in 3 percent, and remote or unrelated to either great artery in about 7 percent.[295]

ASSOCIATED CONDITIONS

Pulmonary stenosis occurs in over half of cases, the condition usually resulting from a narrow subpulmonary conus. ASD, subaortic stenosis, and coarctation of the aorta are also relatively common, with the latter particularly associated with the subpulmonary defect. Obstruction at the mitral valve may be observed in about one-fifth of cases of double-outlet right ventricle. Mitral valve straddling of the VSD and varying degrees of left ventricular hypoplasia are also encountered.

CLINICAL MANIFESTATIONS

Double-outlet right ventricle, or origin of both great arteries from the right ventricle, is a relatively rare malformation found in only 0.5 percent of patients with congenital heart disease.[296] It is of considerable importance, however, because its clinical and laboratory features frequently resemble those of more common and more easily correctable malformations.

History and Physical Examination

Patients with a subaortic VSD without pulmonary stenosis (Fig. 70-30A) have the same findings on examination as do patients with a large isolated VSD. Congestive failure appears within a few weeks of birth, and cyanosis is seldom described. Those with a subaortic VSD and pulmonary stenosis (Fig. 70-30B) usually present after the newborn period and follow a course similar to patients with tetralogy of Fallot. Patients with a subpulmonary defect without pulmonary stenosis (Fig. 70-30C), the Taussig-Bing malformation, resemble patients with transposition of the great arteries and a large VSD without pulmonary stenosis. The finding are those of severe congestive failure and impressive cyanosis.

Chest Roentgenogram

Cardiomegaly with pulmonary overperfusion is characteristic of all types of this anomaly without pulmonary stenosis. Dou-

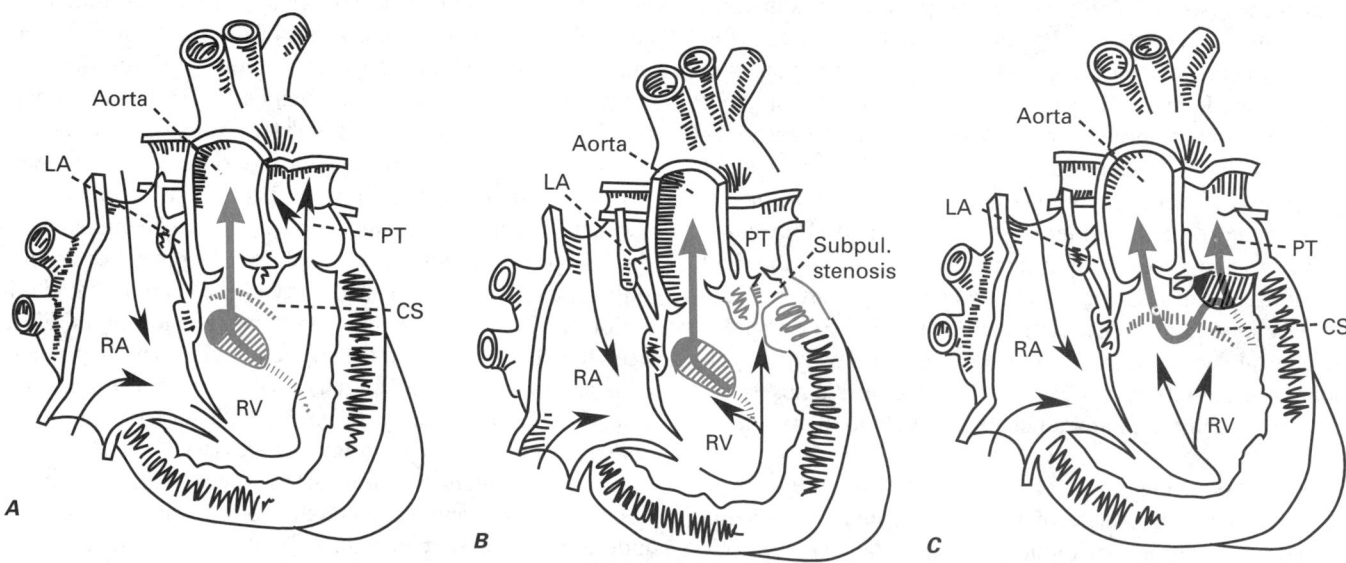

FIGURE 70-30
Double-outlet right ventricle. *A*. With subaortic ventricular septal defect without pulmonary stenosis. *B*. With subaortic ventricular septal defect and subpulmonary stenosis (Subpul. stenosis). *C*. With subpulmonary, supracristal ventricular septal defect. The so-called Taussig-Bing complex. RA, right atrium; RV, right ventricle; CS, crista supraventricularis; LA, left atrium; PT, main pulmonary arterial trunk.

ble-outlet right ventricle with subaortic VSD and pulmonary stenosis resembles tetralogy of Fallot. In the case of subpulmonary VSD without pulmonary stenosis, the pulmonary artery usually lies beside rather than posterior to the aorta; this clearly visible, dilated main pulmonary artery may permit distinction of this malformation from transposition, which it mimics so closely.

Electrocardiogram

Right axis deviation and right atrial and right ventricular hypertrophy are characteristic of double-outlet right ventricle.

Echocardiogram

Two-dimensional echocardiography is capable of demonstrating the anatomic components and associated defects.[295,297]

Cardiac Catheterization

There is an increase in oxygen saturation at the right ventricular level. The pulmonary arterial saturation is lower than that of the aorta in patients with a subaortic VSD and is invariably higher than that of the aorta in those with a subpulmonary septal defect. Left ventricular systolic pressure may be higher than the right if the VSD is small and restrictive. Selective right and left ventricular biplane angiography as well as an aortogram are recommended.

NATURAL HISTORY AND PROGNOSIS

The clinical course of each variety of double-outlet right ventricle is determined by the associated defects. Without surgical intervention, those with an unguarded pulmonary artery either die in infancy with congestive failure or develop PVOD. Spontaneous narrowing or closure of the VSD may occur and is life-threatening. Increasing dyspnea, increasing intensity of the systolic murmur, and progressive left ventricular hypertrophy suggest this complication. Patients with pulmonary stenosis tend to have progressive obstruction and cyanosis.

MEDICAL MANAGEMENT

Vigorous treatment of heart failure is required for those without pulmonary stenosis. Essentially all cases are best treated with surgical palliation or correction in infancy. If there is pulmonary hypertension, banding or correction should be done by 3 to 4 months of age. Patients having ventricular hypoplasia, mitral stenoses, straddling AV valves, or a remote VSD are usually not candidates for biventricular repair, and initial palliation should prepare the child for a modification of Fontan's operation.[295,298] Whether or not corrective surgery has been performed, all patients in whom the left ventricular output must pass through the VSD should be observed continuously for the possibility of spontaneous narrowing and obstruction at that site.

SURGICAL MANAGEMENT

Great variability exists in the morphologic spectrum of double-outlet right ventricle. Although primary total repair of most forms of double-outlet right ventricle is now performed and preferred in infancy, palliation (pulmonary arterial banding, repair of aortic coarctation, atrial septal excision, or the creation of systemic arterial-to-pulmonary arterial or systemic venous-to-pulmonary arterial shunts) to adjust pulmonary blood flow and thus preserve the pulmonary vascular bed, ventricular function, and AV valve competence may be considered in complex variants.

In all forms of double-outlet ventricle, the relation of the VSD to the great arteries and the magnitude of ventricular outflow tract obstruction dictate management.[299] Surgical correction requires (1) obliteration of the interventricular communication, (2) relief of pulmonary stenosis when present, (3) diversion of oxygenated pulmonary venous blood to the aorta, and (4) diversion of hypoxemic systemic venous blood to the pulmonary artery.[299] When the VSD is committed to the aorta, a Dacron semiconduit or tunnel-shaped patch is placed to obliterate the interventricular communication while diverting the left ventricular blood through the VSD to the aorta. Pulmonary stenosis is corrected by a valvotomy, with excision of obstructive muscle bundles and placement of a transannular patch when necessary. Otherwise, an extracardiac conduit is placed between the right ventricle and the pulmonary artery.[300,301]

When the great arteries are transposed or the VSD is not committed to the aorta, the arterial switch operation, using the concepts of Jatene and Le Compte, permits patch closure of the VSD, directing left ventricular blood into the neoaorta.[302] Further consideration of repair of double-outlet right ventricle associated with more complex defects is beyond the scope of this discussion. For patients who are not candidates for biventricular repair, initial palliation should prepare the child for a modification of Fontan's operation.

In a 10-year review of repair of double-outlet right ventricle in 73 patients,[300] early mortality was 11 percent, with an overall actuarial survival estimate at 8 years of 81 percent. Twenty-six percent required reoperation, and there was one death; 79 percent of operative survivors required no restriction of physical activity, and 83 percent required no cardiac medications.[300]

Corrected Transposition of the Great Arteries

DEFINITION

AV discordance and VA discordance form the characteristics of corrected transposition.

PATHOLOGY

Usually situs solitus is present, but the ventricles are inverted (an l loop). The great arteries are transposed and in the l position, so that the pulmonary artery arises posteriorly from the right-sided morphologic left ventricle and the l-transposed aorta arises anteriorly from the left-sided right ventricle (SLL) (Fig. 70-31). If situs inversus is present, the segmental pattern is IDD. Along with the ventricular inversion there is AV valvular inversion. The two coronary arteries arise from the right and left (posteriorly facing) sinuses, with the right-sided

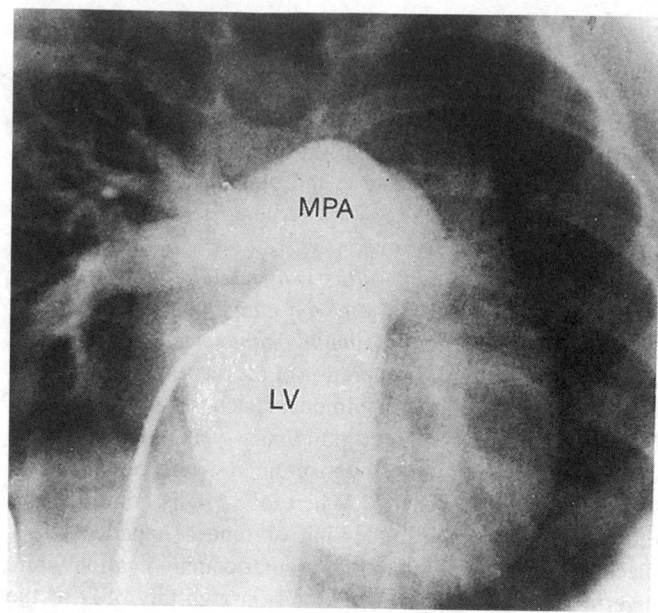

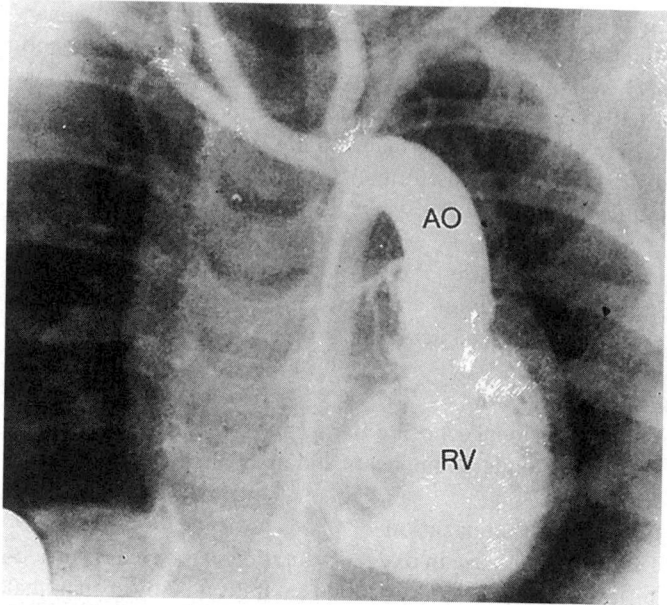

FIGURE 70-31

A. Posteroanterior view of the left ventricular (LV) angiogram in a child with corrected transposition of the great arteries. The main pulmonary artery (MPA) arises from the smooth-walled left ventricle, which receives the systemic venous blood. *B.* Posteroanterior view of the right ventricular angiogram (RV). The ascending aorta (AO) arises to the left of the pulmonary artery from the more heavily trabeculated right ventricle, which receives the pulmonary venous blood. The ventricular septum, seen here perpendicular to the frontal plane, is intact.

coronary artery giving off the anterior descending and the circumflex branches.[303]

ASSOCIATED CONDITIONS

Rarely, no associated conditions are present and the circulation is normal. In the majority of cases (about 75 percent), a VSD is present. It may be in any location, but a perimembranous subpulmonary defect is most common.

The inverted left-sided systemic tricuspid valve frequently shows some degree of abnormality, usually leading to incompetence. The most common abnormality is an Ebstein-like displacement of the septal and posterior leaflets, but dysplasia, clefts, and straddling of the ventricular septum are also described.

Pulmonary atresia or stenosis is present in about 40 percent of cases, usually associated with a VSD.[303] This obstruction is usually subvalvular, rarely only valvular, and may characteristically result from attachments of accessory mitral valve tissue.[303]

CLINICAL MANIFESTATIONS

Corrected transposition is an uncommon malformation, occurring in slightly fewer than 1 percent of children with congenital heart disease. The importance of this anomaly lies in its frequent association with serious AV conduction disturbances, the intracardiac malformations, and the medical and surgical implications of the ventricular inversion. The clinical picture is determined primarily by the associated anomalies. Approximately half of patients can be expected to develop complete AV block if followed for a 20-year period.[304]

History

A slow, irregular heart rate is often detected in utero, and 10 percent of patients with congenital complete block prove to have corrected transposition. Those patients with a large VSD without pulmonary stenosis usually present within the first month or so of life with symptoms indistinguishable from those of infants with a large VSD alone. Patients with VSD and pulmonary stenosis may present with symptoms of cyanosis and resemble patients with tetralogy of Fallot.

Physical Examination

The murmur of left AV valve regurgitation may be best heard either at the apex or at the lower left sternal border. Most cases have a murmur of VSD or pulmonary stenosis. Occasionally, an inordinately accentuated second heart sound at the upper left sternal border suggests the presence of PAH, although in reality it represents the sound of aortic valve closure augmented to auscultation by the anterior and superior displacement of the aorta.

Chest Roentgenogram

A straight or gently curved convex upper left heart border, representing the contour of the transposed ascending aorta, is characteristic and is most easily recognized in those patients with a VSD and pulmonary stenosis, in whom there is a mild dilatation of the ascending aorta.

Electrocardiogram

Varying degrees of AV conduction delay are present in almost a third of patients. The initial forces of ventricular depolarization are characteristically oriented anteriorly and to the left, with Q waves in the right precordial leads and not in leads I, V_5, and V_6. With normal or near-normal pressure in the systemic venous or morphologic left ventricle, a QS pattern in the right and an RS pattern in the left precordial leads are usual.

Echocardiogram

Two-dimensional echocardiography permits identification of the anatomic components and associated defects.[303,305]

Cardiac Catheterization

From the right atrium, the morphologic left ventricle is entered, and, in the presence of a VSD, the catheter may cross the defect, traverse the morphologic right ventricle, and enter the ascending aorta in the position normally occupied by the pulmonary artery. Entry into the medially placed pulmonary artery may be much more difficult, but the use of flow-guided catheters will permit successful entry for measurement of pressure in most instances. Selective angiography in both ventricles will outline the defects. The ventricular septum usually lies in the anteroposterior plane, and frequently a VSD may be imaged best angiographically in the frontal view (Fig. 70-31). Gentle manipulation of the catheter within the heart is indicated, since the production of varying degrees of transient AV block is not uncommon, and, in a rare instance, the block may prove permanent.

NATURAL HISTORY AND PROGNOSIS

The clinical course is determined primarily by the severity of the associated defects. It is estimated that only about 1 percent of individuals with corrected transposition have an otherwise normal heart. Even with complicating anomalies, survival to adulthood is possible.[306] Congestive heart failure associated with a large VSD has been the most common cause of death, with most fatalities occurring within the first year of life. AV conduction abnormalities tend to be progressive, and complete AV block may appear at any age. Similarly, left AV valve regurgitation may present at any age and significantly alters long-term outcome.[307] Finally, the morphologic right ventricle may not be capable of sustaining adequate cardiac output over a normal life span.[304]

MEDICAL MANAGEMENT

Management of corrected transposition includes the treatment of congestive failure, cyanosis, and AV block and the prevention of infective endocarditis. Patients with severe pulmonary hypertension or congestive heart failure should undergo early banding of the pulmonary artery or repair of the defect. Similarly, those patients with a VSD, severe pulmonary stenosis, and cyanosis benefit from systemic-to-pulmonary artery shunting procedures or total correction. The vulnerability of the ventricular conduction system and the difficulty in visualization of the septal defect in the subpulmonary region of the morphologic left ventricle have influenced the authors to recommend the palliative approach in both groups of patients,

especially during infancy. Those with congenital block require prompt pacemaker therapy. Patients with significant left AV valve regurgitation require valve replacement. Regularly scheduled follow-up examinations are recommended for all patients to detect progressive AV conduction disorders and the progression or late appearance of left AV valve incompetence. Antibiotic coverage as protection against infective endocarditis is recommended, as is the introduction of an afterload reducer at the first appearance of AV valve regurgitation.[308]

SURGICAL MANAGEMENT

VSD closure, relief of pulmonary stenosis, and correction of systemic AV valve regurgitation are sometimes required in patients having corrected transposition of the great arteries.[309] The specialized electrical conduction system is particularly at risk in these patients because of its location on the right (left ventricular) side of the VSD and its abnormal anatomic course arching over the subpulmonary outflow tract and lying anterior to the defect. An approach to the VSD through the right atrium and right (mitral) AV valve or through the aorta, or a combined right atrial–mitral valve and aortic approach, placement of sutures through the VSD on the left side of the septum, and the use of intracardiac mapping appear to reduce the incidence of complete heart block.

Relief of valvular pulmonary stenosis may be technically complicated by the fact that additional subvalvular obstruction may exist in the form of obstructing tags, membranous redundant right AV, valve tissue, or simply a narrow subpulmonary left ventricular outflow tract. Again, the conduction system is vulnerable. Left ventricular-to-pulmonary arterial conduits are advised when subvalvular pulmonary stenosis is severe.[309]

Despite recent advances, operative mortality rates for VSD or VSD and pulmonary stenosis or atresia remain in the 4 to 15 percent range, with postoperative heart block in the 14 to 33 percent range.[310,311] The 10-year actuarial survival was 83 percent in one study[310] and 55 percent in the other.[311]

Replacement of a regurgitant left AV valve at the earliest sign of progressive ventricular dysfunction is recommended to preserve systemic ventricular function.[312]

Other possible surgical options for selected patients include the combined atrial and arterial switch procedure, which leaves the left ventricle as the systemic ventricle,[313] and the Fontan approach for those patients in whom biventricular repair is either not possible or the risk is considered prohibitive.[310]

Univentricular Heart

DEFINITION

The univentricular heart, or single ventricle, is characterized by the entire flow from the two atria being carried directly through the left and right AV valves into the single ventricular chamber (Fig. 70-32). This double-inlet type of AV connection may take the form of either one common or two separate AV valves; straddling of one AV valve is sometimes included. The VA connections may be concordant (pulmonary artery

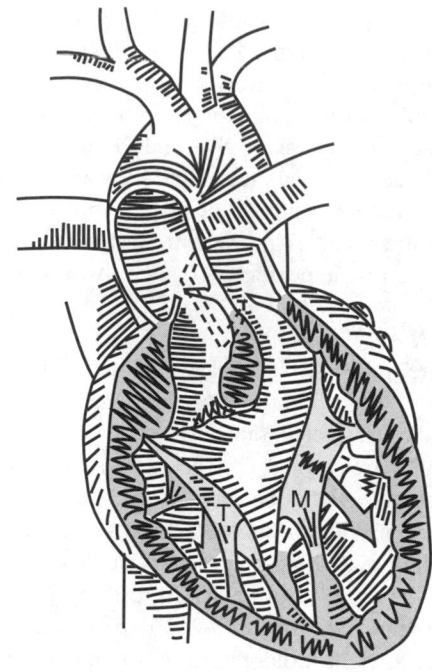

FIGURE 70-32
Common ventricle with dextro malposition and without pulmonary stenosis. T, tricuspid valve; M, mitral valve.

from the right ventricle and aorta from the left ventricle), discordant (pulmonary artery from the left ventricle and aorta from the right ventricle), double-outlet (both great arteries from either the left or right ventricle), or single-outlet (atresia of one great artery). By this definition, cases of mitral or tricuspid atresia are excluded, as are those of pulmonary or aortic atresia with an intact ventricular septum.

PATHOLOGY

The most common type of univentricular heart (65 to 70 percent of cases),[314] is that in which the dominant ventricular chamber has the trabecular pattern of a left ventricle and communicates through an opening, the bulboventricular foramen, with a rudimentary right ventricle.[315] The VA connection is discordant (transposition of the great arteries) in about 90 percent of patients. In about 20 percent of cases, the dominant ventricle shows the trabecular features of a right ventricle and the rudimentary chamber those of a left ventricle. The majority of these patients have a double-outlet VA connection from the main chamber, and a smaller number have a single-outlet connection, with pulmonary atresia.[316] In 10 to 14 percent, neither ventricular sinus can be identified; this is the so-called primitive ventricle.

The term *Holmes' heart*, of historical interest, refers to double-inlet left ventricle with situs solitus, normally related great arteries (SDS), absent right ventricular sinus, and a subpulmonary infundibular outlet chamber communicating with the left ventricle via a restrictive bulboventricular foramen.[317]

ASSOCIATED CONDITIONS

Pulmonary stenosis or atresia is common. Subaortic stenosis may result from a narrow bulboventricular foramen.

CLINICAL MANIFESTATIONS

This complex and challenging malformation is relatively rare. The clinical picture is determined largely by the associated defects, of which pulmonary stenosis or atresia, present in a little over half of the patients, and obstruction to aortic flow are the most important.

History

All patients will have some degree of systemic arterial oxygen desaturation, although cyanosis, appreciated clinically, may range from barely detectable to severe. Congestive failure is common. The majority will require hospitalization in the first month of life.

Physical Examination

The findings on palpation and auscultation are quite variable and not distinctive.

Chest Roentgenogram

Almost all patients have at least some degree of cardiac enlargement. Those with little or no pulmonary stenosis generally have very large hearts with marked pulmonary plethora. Only those patients with very severe pulmonary stenosis or atresia show a near-normal heart size and diminished pulmonary arterial blood flow.

Electrocardiogram

Evidence of right or left ventricular hypertrophy is common.

Echocardiography

Two-dimensional echocardiography with Doppler color flow studies can identify virtually all of the morphologic and functional features of this malformation necessary to establish the diagnosis and make a plan for clinical management.[318]

Cardiac Catheterization

A degree of systemic arterial oxygen desaturation is present in all patients, although the severity appears to be related mainly to the volume of pulmonary blood flow. Careful recording of intracardiac and arterial pressures is essential in order to detect significant or potentially significant obstruction to blood flow across either AV valve, across the atrial septum, or between the ventricle and the aorta or pulmonary artery. The morphologic features of the ventricle, relation of the aorta and pulmonary artery, and other features can be established by high-quality selective ventricular angiography using specially angled views to supplement conventional views.[319]

NATURAL HISTORY AND PROGNOSIS

Patients usually present as newborns with cyanosis, congestive failure, or a combination of both. Those in whom the pulmonary arterial pressure and blood flow are increased require surgery to prevent death from congestive heart failure or progressive PVOD. Patients with severe pulmonary stenosis or atresia require systemic-to-pulmonary arterial shunting procedures. Among patients with univentricular heart, there is a propensity for the development of subaortic obstruction[320] and AV valve regurgitation.[321] Both threaten ventricular compliance and diminish the likelihood of successful long-term palliation.[322] Survivors are subject to the threats of infective endocarditis, brain abscess, and progressive PVOD.

MEDICAL MANAGEMENT

Early recognition and identification of patients with these complex defects are important if successful palliative surgical procedures are to be carried out for the relief of congestive failure or cyanosis. PGE$_1$ is useful in neonates with ductal-dependent defects.[112] An adequate interatrial communication is essential. Ventricular function and AV valvular competence are preserved by early creation of a bidirectional modified Glenn anastomosis (superior vena cava–to–undivided pulmonary artery); subaortic stenosis or obstruction at the bulboventricular foramen can be bypassed by anastomosis of the proximal pulmonary artery to the lateral aspect of the ascending aorta while pulmonary blood flow is delivered to the distal pulmonary arterial tree through a systemic arterial or systemic venous shunt.[323,324] Digitalis and diuretics may be necessary for those patients with continuing heart failure. Care should be taken that anemia or severe polycythemia does not develop and that these patients are adequately protected against infective endocarditis. The pulmonary vascular bed must be protected and ventricular function and compliance must be carefully preserved if more definitive procedures are to be considered. The long-term outlook for the survivors has yet to be determined.

SURGICAL MANAGEMENT

Palliation for patients with univentricular AV connections requires adjustment of pulmonary blood flow with (1) a pulmonary arterial band when it is excessive, or (2) creation of a shunt when it is diminished. The modified Blalock-Taussig shunt is preferred in the neonate. An adequate interatrial communication is essential. Prognosis is adversely affected by a single ventricle of the right ventricular type[325] and the evolution of AV valvular regurgitation[326] or subaortic obstruction.[327] Ventricular function and AV valvular competence are preserved by early creation of a bidirectional modified Glenn anastomosis, in which the superior vena cava is divided with the caudad portion patched closed; the cephalad portion is sutured to the top of the right pulmonary artery. If pulmonary atresia is not present, the main pulmonary artery is closed.[328] Subaortic stenosis or obstruction at the bulboventricular foramen can be palliated by anastomosis of the proximal pulmonary artery to the lateral aspect of the ascending aorta, while pulmonary blood flow is delivered to the distal pulmonary arterial tree through a systemic arterial or systemic venous shunt (the Damus-Kaye-Stansel operation). Other surgical options for relief of subaortic obstruction are direct enlargement of the bulboventricular foramen (VSD), the modified Norwood operation, or the arterial switch operation.[329,330]

In the past, correction was accomplished in a small number of patients by septation of the single ventricle using a woven Dacron patch.[329] Today, long-term palliation is accomplished by exclusion of the pulmonary circulation from the systemic

ventricular outflow using modifications of Fontan's operation to direct systemic venous blood directly to the pulmonary arteries. First, a bidirectional Glenn anastomosis is constructed (see above), then an intraatrial tunnel is constructed to divert the inferior vena caval blood to the caudad portion of the superior vena cava, which is then connected to the underside of the right pulmonary artery (Fig. 70-33). The single ventricle is thus relieved of the burden of the volume overload and ventricular hypertrophy required to maintain the pulmonary circulation and is asked only to deliver systemic cardiac output.[328] Repair by Fontan's concepts early in life, usually between the ages of 1 and 3 years, minimizes the development of PVOD, AV valvular regurgitation, and congestive heart failure and relieves the child of the burden of hypoxemia. Experience with atresia of the aortic tract (the hypoplastic

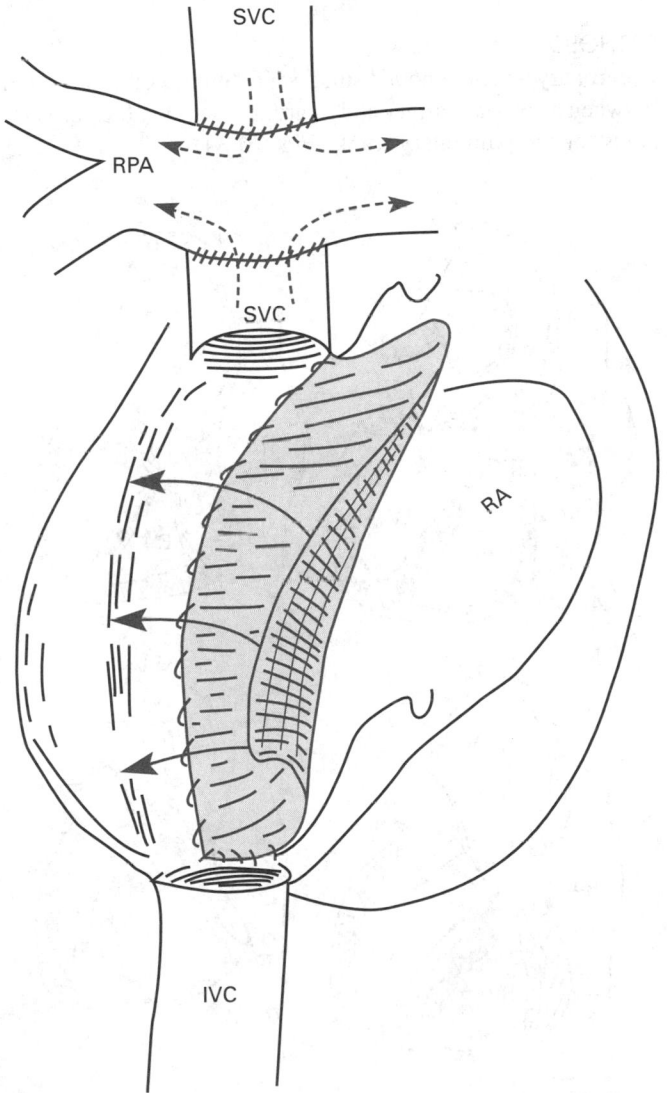

FIGURE 70-33

The modified Fontan operation. The superior vena cava (SVC) is divided. The cephalad portion is anastomosed to the superior aspect of the right pulmonary artery (RPA), and an intraatrial baffle is constructed from the inferior vena cava (IVC) to the superior vena cava along the lateral wall of the right atrium (RA). The caudad portion of the SVC is then connected to the inferior aspect of the right pulmonary artery.

left heart syndrome) has encouraged early cavopulmonary connection, usually between 4 and 8 months, followed by modifications of Fontan's operations between 15 and 24 months of age.[331]

Quality and length of life are clearly improved, but persistent problems include AV valvular regurgitation, systemic embolization, limitation of exercise tolerance, protein-losing enteropathy, atrial arrhythmias, and deterioration of ventricular function.[332] For those patients with progressive deterioration, cardiac transplantation is recommended.

CONGENITAL ABNORMALITIES OF THE CORONARY ARTERIAL CIRCULATION

Coronary Arteriovenous Fistula

PATHOLOGY

A coronary arteriovenous fistula is a fistulous communication between a coronary artery and a cardiac chamber, the coronary sinus, or the pulmonary trunk (Fig. 70-34).

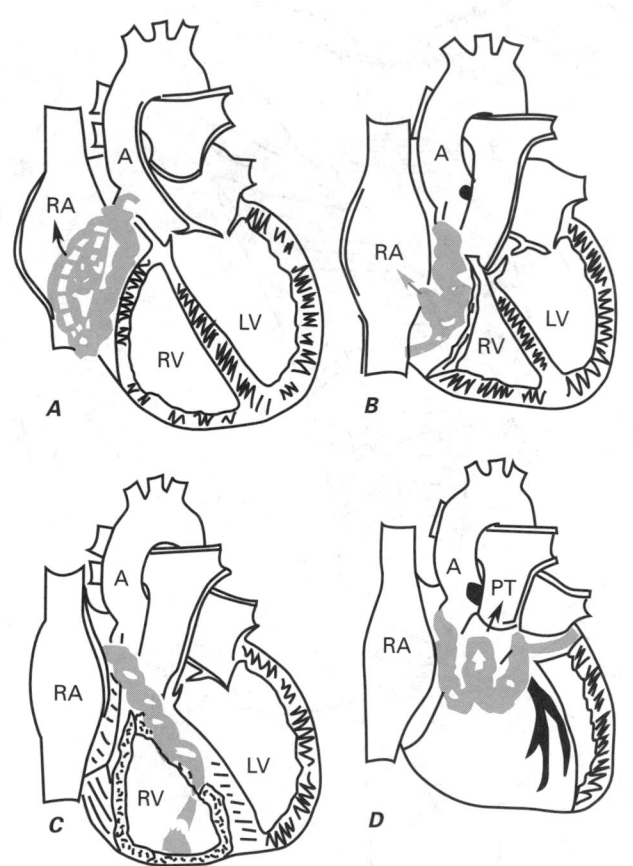

Anomalous communications of coronary arteries. *A*. Right coronary artery communicates with coronary sinus. *B*. Right coronary artery communicates with right atrium (RA). *C*. Anomalous communication of right coronary artery with right ventricle (RV). *D*. Two coronary arteries arise from the aorta (A) and make collateral communication with accessory coronary artery arising from pulmonary trunk (PT). LV, left ventricle.

The site of origin may involve any of the epicardial coronary arteries. *The right coronary artery is the site of origin in somewhat over half the cases, and the two most common sites into which the fistula feeds are a cardiac vein (usually the coronary sinus) and the right ventricle.* Although solitary communication is the rule, there may be multiple sites of termination.[333] A fistula into the pulmonary trunk is usually characterized by one or more vessels opening into the pulmonary trunk and connecting with branches of each of the two main coronary arteries. The artery or arteries feeding the fistula are grossly enlarged and tortuous. Saccular aneurysms may develop in segments of dilated vessels; such aneurysms are usually observed in the adult and frequently show calcification of the wall.

CLINICAL MANIFESTATIONS

Many patients with a coronary arteriovenous fistula are asymptomatic.[334–336] In some, the magnitude of the shunt into the right side of the heart is great enough to cause congestive heart failure, with a tendency for this to occur in early infancy or after 40 years of age. The classic finding is that of continuous murmur with an unusual location, since it is loudest over the fistula. It may have a louder diastolic component, especially if communication is with the right ventricle. In those with large shunts, there may be cardiomegaly and increased pulmonary flow shown by chest roentgenogram and right ventricular hypertrophy shown by ECG. Transthoracic echocardiography is usually diagnostic in children[337]; transesophageal studies may be necessary in adults.[335] At cardiac catheterization, an increase in oxygen saturation may be encountered, usually in the right atrium or right ventricle, if the shunt is large enough. Selective coronary arteriography will demonstrate the involved coronary artery and site of entry of the fistula. The most common complication is infective endocarditis, but thrombosis, myocardial ischemia, and rupture may occur.

SURGICAL MANAGEMENT

Except for very small fistulas, closure is recommended, since the flow tends to increase with age and the patients are at risk for infective endocarditis, congestive heart failure, or myocardial ischemia. Until relatively recently, closure was invariably surgical. Occasionally, closure was done without coronary bypass by placing obliterating mattress sutures across the fistula beneath the coronary artery as it passes over the surface of the heart.[338] More commonly, cardiopulmonary bypass is preferred for safe exposure of large or multiple fistula, such as those entering the right atrium near the junction of the superior vena cava and right atrium, those arising from the artery to the sinoatrial node, and those between the left coronary artery and the left ventricle.[339] The orifice of the fistula is obliterated by direct suture or placement of a Dacron or pericardial patch. Fistulas have been closed from within the open coronary artery; the artery is then repaired by direct suture.

Only 4 deaths occurred in 116 reported cases of coronary fistulas that were closed surgically[340]; the long-term results have been favorable.[341]

Recently fistulas have been closed by interventional catheterization techniques. Perry and associates[342] have attempted to close fistulas in nine patients, four from the left circumflex artery, three from the left anterior descending artery, and two from the right coronary artery. Gianturco coils were used in six patients, and a double-umbrella in two, with coils and an umbrella in one. All were completely occluded. In three patients with multiple fistulas, no attempt was made in the catheterization laboratory and the patients were referred for surgery. This "noninvasive" technique seems to be applicable to some children and adults with coronary AV fistulas, although long-term follow-up is necessary to be certain the fistulas do not recur.

Origin of the Left Coronary Artery from the Pulmonary Artery

In this anomaly, the right coronary artery arises from the aorta, while the left coronary artery arises from the pulmonary artery (Fig. 70-35). This is also known as the *Bland-White-Garland syndrome*. The course and branching of the vessel are normal. In the young, the coronary arteries are of normal size, but if the patient survives beyond infancy, there is noticeable dilatation of these vessels. In cases of infant death from this condition, the left ventricle is dilated and may show sites of infarction with calcification of affected myocardium. In

patients surviving infancy, there is often scarring of the left ventricular papillary muscles and of the left ventricular wall, particularly in the distribution of the left coronary artery. The left ventricular cavity is dilated, and the chamber shows endocardial fibroelastosis. The mitral valve may become incompetent.[343] Associated conditions are uncommon (see also Chaps. 16 and 42).

The clinical spectrum and mode of presentation in patients with this abnormality vary.[344,345] The majority of patients present at a few months of age. Acute episodes of irritability, profuse cold sweating, pallor, and respiratory distress occur, with evidence of heart failure. Less often, the patients present at any age with mitral regurgitation and heart failure. A few reach adolescence or adulthood with relatively few symptoms other than occasional exertional angina or palpitations. Sudden death may be the first and only sign of this condition.

On physical examination, the heart is enlarged, with an abnormal left ventricular apex impulse. Other signs of failure are usually present. Pallor and clammy skin are common. In some, a soft continuous murmur is heard at the upper left sternal border. This murmur is more prominent in older patients, presumably due to development of a more extensive collateral circulation. The murmur of mitral regurgitation may be heard at the apex, radiating to the axilla; however, in young infants with heart failure, there can be a surprising degree of regurgitation without a distinctive murmur.

The chest roentgenogram typically shows marked enlargement of the heart with posterior displacement of the esophagus by a large left atrium. There is pulmonary edema, and there may be atelectasis of the left lower lobe due to bronchial compression.

The ECG demonstrates the pattern of anterolateral infarction, with deep Q wave in leads I and aV_L and abnormal R-wave progression across the precordium. Arrhythmias are frequent. The horizontal loop of the vectorcardiogram is clockwise and posteriorly oriented. The echocardiogram shows marked enlargement of the left atrium and ventricle with little or no left ventricular wall motion. The origin of the coronary artery can be imaged, and flow can be seen towards the great artery instead of towards the heart.[346,347] Myocardial perfusion imaging with thallium 201 can help distinguish an anomalous coronary artery from congestive cardiomyopathy.[348]

At cardiac catheterization, there may be an increase in saturation in the pulmonary artery if there is enough retrograde flow. There is usually some pulmonary hypertension, with very elevated pulmonary wedge pressure. Aortography or selective right coronary arteriography demonstrates the collateral circulation filling the left coronary artery retrogradely, with at least faint opacification of the main pulmonary artery.

The natural history and prognosis are related by the modes of presentation. Those that present in infancy die without surgical intervention. Medical management is aimed at control of congestive heart failure and arrhythmias prior to surgical procedure.

Four approaches have been used for surgical repair. The first, of historical interest only, is ligation of the left coronary

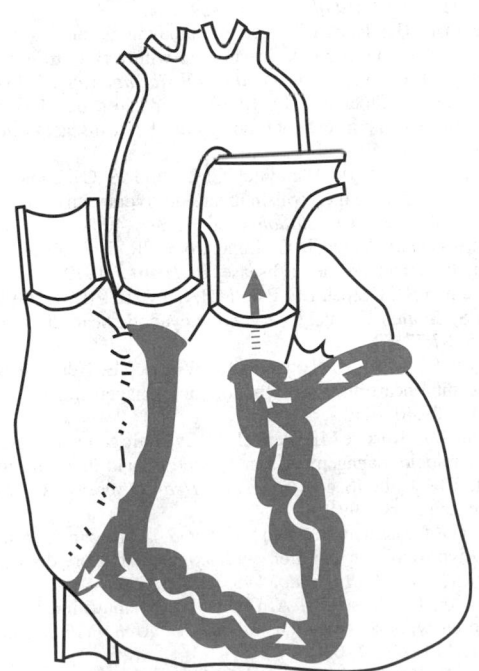

FIGURE 70-35

Anomalous origin of the left coronary artery from the pulmonary trunk. With time, wide collaterals develop between the two coronary systems, so that right coronary arterial blood is shunted into the left coronary system and thence into the pulmonary trunk.

artery to eliminate the coronary artery–to–pulmonary artery shunt that acts as a coronary artery steal.[349] Many children benefited from this procedure, but there continued to be myocardial ischemia, and late sudden death was not eliminated.[350] The second approach was to tunnel the coronary artery inside the pulmonary artery to the wall of the aorta and to create an aortopulmonary window.[351] This usually required an external roofing of the pulmonary artery to allow egress of flow from the right ventricle. While this surgical approach has the advantage of making a two-coronary system, a high proportion of children developed supravalvular pulmonary stenosis at the site of the intrapulmonary artery tunnel. More recently, as coronary artery reimplantation has become more common in the arterial switch operation for transposition of the great arteries, surgeons have removed the anomalous coronary artery with a button of pulmonary artery and reimplanted it on to the aorta.[352] Finally, in a few older patients, saphenous vein grafting or internal mammary artery implantation has been used.[353]

The late results after surgery have been quite good.[354] The congestive heart failure frequently improves, the heart becomes smaller, left ventricular shortening fraction improves, and mitral regurgitation tends to regress. Interestingly, the infarction pattern on ECG with deep anterolateral Q waves frequently disappears, suggesting that the poor function is due to extreme ischemia rather than infarction.

REFERENCES

1. Mitchell SC, Korones SB, Berendes HW. Congenital heart disease in 56,109 births. Incidence and natural history. *Circulation* 1971; 43:323–332.
2. Hoffman JIE, Christianson R. Congenital heart disease in a cohort of 19,502 births with long-term follow-up. *Am J Cardiol* 1978; 42:641–647.
3. Fyler DC. Report of the New England Regional Infant Cardiac Program. *Pediatrics* 1980; 65:II375–II461.
4. Perry LW, Neill CA, Ferencz C, Rubin JD, Loffredo CA. Infants with congenital heart disease: The cases. In: Ferencz C, Rubin JD, Loffredo CA, Magee CA, eds. *Epidemiology of Congenital Heart Disease: The Baltimore-Washington Infant Heart Study 1981–1989*. Mount Kisco, NY: Futura; 1993:33–61.
5. Fyler DC, ed. *Nadas' Pediatric Cardiology*. Philadelphia: Hanley & Belfus; 1992:273.
6. Keith JD. Prevalence, incidence and epidemiology. In: Keith JD, Rowe RD, Vlad P, eds. *Heart Disease in Infancy and Childhood*, 3d ed. New York: Macmillan; 1978:3–13.
7. Nora JJ. Causes of CHD—old and new modes, mechanisms and models. *Am Heart J* 1993; 125:1409–1418.
8. Payne RM, Johnson MC, Grant JW, Strauss AW. Toward a molecular understanding of congenital heart disease. *Circulation* 1995; 91:494–504.
9. Hall JG. Catch 22. *J Med Genet* 1993; 30:801–802.
10. Dawes GS. *Foetal and Neonatal Physiology: A Comparative Study of the Changes at Birth*. Chicago: Year Book; 1968:90–101, 160–187.
11. Lind J, Wegelius C. Human fetal circulation: Changes in the cardiovascular system at birth and disturbances in the postnatal closure of the foramen ovale and ductus arteriosus. Cold Spring Harbor Symposium. *Quant Biol* 1954; 19:109–125.
12. Rudolph AM, Heymann MA. The circulation of the fetus in utero. *Circ Res* 1967; 21:163–184.
13. Rudolph AM, Heymann MA. Circulatory changes with growth in the fetal lamb. *Circ Res* 1970; 26:289–299.
14. Rudolph AM, Heymann MA. Cardiac output in the fetal lamb: The

effects of spontaneous and induced changes of heart rate on right and left ventricular output. *J Obstet Gynecol* 1976; 124:183–192.
15. Teitel DF, Iwamoto HS, Rudolph AM. Effects of birth-related events on central flow patterns. *Pediatr Res* 1987; 22:557–566.
16. Clyman RI, Mauray F, Roman C, Heymann MA, Payne B, et al. Factors determining the loss of ductus arteriosus responsiveness to prostaglandin E. *Circulation* 1983; 68:433–436.
17. Coceani F, Olley PM. Role of prostaglandins, prostacyclin, and thromboxanes in the control of prenatal patency and postnatal closure of the ductus arteriosus. In: Heymmann MA, ed. *Prostaglandins in the Perinatal Period*. New York: Grune & Stratton; 1980:109.
18. Rudolph AM. Fetal and neonatal pulmonary circulation. *Annu Rev Physiol* 1979; 41:383–395.
19. Heymann MA, Rudolph AM. Effects of congenital heart disease on fetal and neonatal circulations. *Prog Cardiovasc Dis* 1972; 15:115–143.
20. Levin DL, Heymann MA, Kitterman JA, Gregory GA, Phibbs RH, Rudolph AM. Persistent pulmonary hypertension in the newborn infant. *J Pediatr* 1976; 89:626–630.
21. Fox WW, Duara S. Persistent pulmonary hypertension in the neonate: Diagnosis and management. *J Pediatr* 1983; 103:505–514.
22. Kinsella JP, Abman SH. Clinical pathophysiology of persistent pulmonary hypertension of the newborn and the role of inhaled nitric oxide therapy. *J Perinatol* 1996; 16:S24–S27.
23. Kirkpatrick BV, Krummel TM, Mueller DG, Ormazabal MA, Greenfield LJ, Salzberg AM. Use of extracorporeal membrane oxygenation for respiratory failure in term infants. *Pediatrics* 1983; 72:872–876.
24. Talner NS. Heart failure. In: Emmanouilides GC, Riemenschneider TA, Gutgesell HP, eds. *Moss and Adams Heart Disease in Infants, Children, and Adolescents Including the Fetus and Young Adult*, 5th ed. Baltimore: Williams & Wilkins; 1995:1746–1772.
25. Seguchi M, Nakazawa M, Momma K. Effect of enalapril on infants and children with congestive heart failure. *Cardiol Young* 1992; 2:14–19.
26. Avery GB. *Neonatology: Pathophysiology and Management of the Newborn*. Philadelphia: Lippincott; 1975.
27. Fischbein CA, Rosenthal A, Fischer EG, Nadas AS, Welch K. Risk factors of brain abscess in patients with congenital heart disease. *Am J Cardiol* 1974; 34:97–102.
28. Phornphutkul C, Rosenthal A, Nadas AS, Berenberg W. Cerebrovascular accidents in infants and children with cyanotic congenital heart disease. *Am J Cardiol* 1973; 32:329–334.
29. Beekman RH, Tuuri DT. Acute hemodynamic effects of increasing hemoglobin concentration in children with a right to left ventricular shunt and relative anemia. *J Am Coll Cardiol* 1985; 5:357–362.
30. Gidding SS, Stockman JA III. Effect of iron deficiency on tissue oxygen delivery in cyanotic congenital heart disease. *Am J Cardiol* 1988; 61:605–607.
31. Ross EA, Perloff JK, Danovitch GM, Child JS, Canobbio MM. Renal function and urate metabolism in late survivors with cyanotic congenital heart disease. *Circulation* 1986; 73:396–400.
32. Henriksson P, Varendh G, Lundstrom NR. Haemostatic defects in cyanotic congenital heart disease. *Br Heart J* 1979; 41:23–27.
33. Waldman JD, Czapek EE, Paul MH, Schwartz AD, Levin DL, Schindler S. Shortened platelet survival in cyanotic heart disease. *J Pediatr* 1975; 87:77–79.
34. Perloff JK, Rosove MH, Child JS, Wright GB. Adults with cyanotic congenital heart disease: Hematologic management. *Ann Intern Med* 1988; 109:406–413.
35. Territo MC, Rosove MH, Perloff JK. Cyanotic congenital heart disease: Hematologic management, renal function, and urate metabolism. In: Perloff JK, Child JS, eds. *Congenital Heart Disease in Adults*. Philadelphia: Saunders; 1991:93.
36. Aram DM, Ekelman BL, Ben Shachar G, Levinsohn MW. Intelligence and hypoxemia in children with congenital heart disease: Fact or artifact? *Am J Coll Cardiol* 1985; 6:889–893.
37. Cameron JW, Rosenthal A, Olson AD. Malnutrition in hospitalized children with congenital heart disease. *Arch Pediatr Adolesc Med* 1995; 149:1098–1102.
38. Levy RJ, Rosenthal A, Fyler DC, Nadas AS. Birthweight of infants with congenital heart disease. *Am J Dis Child* 1978; 132:249–254.
39. Rosenthal A, Castaneda A. Growth and development after cardiovascular surgery in infants and children. *Prog Cardiovasc Dis* 1975; 18:27–37.
40. Kulik TJ. Pulmonary hypertension. In: Fyler DC, ed. *Nadas' Pediatric Cardiology*. Philadelphia: Hanley & Belfus; 1992:83–100.

41. Rabinovitch M. Pathophysiology of pulmonary hypertension. In: Emmanouilides GC, Riemenschneider TA, Allen HD, Gutgesell HP, eds. *Moss and Adams Heart Disease in Infants, Children, and Adolescents,* 5th ed. Baltimore: Williams & Wilkins; 1995:1659–1695.

42. Heath D, Edwards JE. The pathology of hypertensive pulmonary vascular disease: A description of six grades of structural changes in the pulmonary arteries with special reference to congenital cardiac septal defects. *Circulation* 1958; 18:533.

43. Berner M, Beghetti M, Sparhr-Schopfer I, Oberhansli I, Friedli B. Inhaled nitric oxide to test the vasodilator capacity of the pulmonary vascular bed in children with long-standing pulmonary hypertension and congenital heart disease. *Am J Cardiol* 1996; 77:532–535.

44. Nihill MR. Clinical management of patients with pulmonary hypertension. In: Emmanouilides GC, Riemenschneider TA, Allen HD, Gutgesell HP, eds. *Moss and Adams Heart Disease in Infants, Children, and Adolescents,* 5th ed. Baltimore: Williams & Wilkins; 1995:1695–1711.

45. Gersony WM. Long-term follow-up of operated congenital heart disease. *Cardiol Clin* 1989; 7:915–923.

46. Freed MD. Infective endocarditis in the adult with congenital heart disease. *Cardiol Clin* 1993; 11:589–602.

47. Dajani AS, Taubert KA, Wilson W, Bolger AF, Bayer A, Ferrieri P, et al. Prevention of bacterial endocarditis: Recommendations by The American Heart Association. *JAMA* 1997; 277:1794–1801.

48. Keane JF, Driscoll DJ, Gersony WM. Second Natural History Study of Congenital Heart Defects. Results of treatment of patients with aortic valvar stenosis. *Circulation* 1993: 87(suppl):I16–I27.

49. Hart EM, Garson A Jr. Psychosocial concerns of adults with congenital heart disease: Employability and insurability. *Cardiac Clin* 1993: 11:711–715.

50. Sciscione AC, Callan NA. Pregnancy and contraception. *Cardiac Clin* 1993; 11:701–709.

51. Leung MP, Benson LN, Smallhorn JF, Williams WG, Trusler GA, Freedom RM. Abnormal cardiac signs after Fontan type of operation: Indicators of residua and sequelae. *Br Heart J* 1989; 61:52–58.

52. Rowe SA, Zahka KG, Manolio TA, Horneffer PJ, Kidd L. Lung function and pulmonary regurgitation limit exercise capacity in postoperative tetralogy of Fallot. *J Am Coll Cardiol* 1991; 17:461–466.

53. Zellers TM, Driscoll DJ, Mottram CD, Puga FJ, Schaff HV, Danielson GK. Exercise tolerance and cardiorespiratory response to exercise before and after the Fontan operation. *Mayo Clin Proc* 1989; 64:1489–1497.

54. Chandar JS, Wolff GS, Garson A Jr, Bell TJ, Beder SD, Bink Boelkens M, et al. Ventricular arrhythmias in postoperative tetralogy of Fallot. *Am J Cardiol* 1990; 65:655–661.

55. Krongrad E. Prognosis for patients with congenital heart disease and postoperative intraventricular conduction defects. *Circulation* 1978; 57:867–870.

56. Gelatt M, Hamilton RM, McCrindle BW, Connelly M, Davis A, Harris L, et al. Arrhythmia and mortality after the Mustard procedure: A 30-year single-center experience. *J Am Coll Cardiol* 1997; 29:194–201.

57. Moreau GA, Graham TP Jr. Clinical assessment of ventricular function after surgical treatment of congenital heart defects. *Cardiol Clin* 1989; 7:439–452.

58. Turina MI, Siebenmann R, von Segesser L, Schonbeck M, Senning A. Late functional deterioration after atrial correction for transposition of the great arteries. *Circulation* 1989; 80:I162–I167.

59. Girod DA, Fontan F, Deville C, Ottenkamp J, Choussat A. Long-term results after the Fontan operation for tricuspid atresia. *Circulation* 1987; 75:605–610.

60. Driscoll DJ, Offord KP, Feldt RH. Five to fifteen year follow-up after Fontan operation. *Circulation* 1992; 85:469–496.

61. Graham TP, Gutgesell HP. Ventricular septal defects. In: Emmanouilides GC, Riemenschneider TA, Allen HD, Gutgesell HP, eds. *Moss and Adams Heart Disease in Infants, Children, and Adolescents,* 5th ed. Baltimore: Williams & Wilkins; 1995:724–746.

62. Engle MA, Kline SA, Borer JS. Ventricular septal defect. In: Roberts WC, ed. *Adult Congenital Heart Disease.* Philadelphia: Davis; 1987:409–441.

63. Silverman NH. *Pediatric Echocardiography.* New York: Williams & Wilkins; 1993.

64. Alpert BS, Cook DH, Varghese PJ, Rowe RD. Spontaneous closure of small ventricular septal defects: Ten-year follow-up. *Pediatrics* 1979; 63:204–206.

65. Moe DG, Guntheroth WG. Spontaneous closure of uncomplicated ventricular septal defect. *Am J Cardiol* 1987; 60:674–678.

66. Trowitzsch E, Braun W, Stute M, Pielmeier W. Diagnosis, therapy, and outcome of ventricular septal defects in the 1st year of life: A two-dimensional colour-Doppler echocardiography study. *Eur J Pediatr* 1990; 149:758–761.

67. Weidman WH, Blount SG Jr, DuShane JW, Gersony WM, Hayes CJ, Nadas AS. Clinical course in ventricular septal defect. *Circulation* 1977; 56:I156–I169.

68. Rhodes L, Keane JF, Keane JP, Fellows KE, Jones RA, Castaneda AR, et al. Long follow-up (to 43 years) of ventricular septal defect with audible aortic regurgitation. *Am J Cardiol* 1990; 66:340–345.

69. Gersony WM, Hayes CJ. Bacterial endocarditis in patients with pulmonary stenosis, aortic stenosis or ventricular septal defect. *Circulation* 1977; 56:I84–I87.

70. Gersony WM, Hayes CJ, Driscoll DJ, Keane JF, Kidd L, O'Fallon WM, et al. Bacterial endocarditis in patients with aortic stenosis, pulmonary stenosis or ventricular septal defect. *Circulation* 1993; 8F(suppl I):I121–I126.

71. Driscoll DJ, Michels VV, Gersony WM, Hayes CJ, Keane JF, Kidd L, et al. Occurrence risk for congenital heart defects in relatives of patients with aortic stenosis, pulmonary stenosis, or ventricular septal defect. *Circulation* 1993; 8F(suppl I):I114–I120.

72. Kirklin JW, Barratt-Boyes BG. Ventricular septal defect. In: Kirklin JW, Barratt-Boyes BG, eds. *Cardiac Surgery,* 2d ed. New York: Churchill Livingstone; 1993:749–824.

73. Stevenson JG. Role of intraoperative transesophageal echocardiography during repair of congenital cardiac defects. *Acta Pediatr Suppl* 1995; 410:23–33.

74. Moller JH, Patton C, Varco RL, Lillehei CW. Late results (30–35 years) after operative closure of isolated ventricular septal defect from 1954–1960. *Am J Cardiol* 1991; 68:1491–1497.

75. Lewis FJ, Winchell P, Bashour FA. Open repair of atrial septal defects: Results in sixty-three patients. *JAMA* 1957; 165:922.

76. Edwards JE. Classification of congenital heart disease in the adult. In: Roberts WC, ed. *Congenital Heart Disease in Adults.* Cardiovasc Clin Series 10/1. Philadelphia: Davis; 1979:1–26.

77. Bedford DE. The anatomical types of atrial septal defect: Their incidence and clinical diagnosis. *Am J Cardiol* 1960; 6:568.

78. Kirklin JW, Barrett-Boyes BG. Atrial septal defect and partial anomalous pulmonary venous connection. In: Kirklin JW, Barrett-Boyes BG, eds. *Cardiac Surgery,* 2d ed. New York: Churchill Livingstone; 1993:609–644.

79. Van Praagh S, Carrera ME, Sanders SP, Mayer JE, Van Praagh R. Sinus venosus defects: Unroofing of the right pulmonary veins, anatomic and echocardiographic findings, and surgical treatment. *Am Heart J* 1994; 128:365–379.

80. Kirklin JW, Barrett-Boyes BG: Unrooted coronary sinus syndrome. In: Kirklin JW, Barrett-Boyes BG, eds. *Cardiac Surgery,* 2d ed. New York: Churchill Livingstone; 1993:683–692.

81. Mahoney LT, Truesdell SC, Krzmarzick TR, Lauer RM. Atrial septal defects that present in infancy. *Am J Dis Child* 1986; 140:1115–1118.

82. Fyler DC. Atrial septal defect secundum. In: Fyler DC, ed. *Nadas' Pediatric Cardiology.* Philadelphia: Hanley & Belfus; 1992; 513–524.

83. Noonan JA. Syndromes associated with cardiac defects. In: Engle MA, Brest AN, eds. *Pediatric Cardiovascular Disease.* Philadelphia: Davis; 1981:97–116.

84. Murphy JG, Gersh BJ, McGoon MD, Mair DD, Porter CJ, Ilstrup DM, et al. Long-term outcome after surgical repair of isolated atrial septal defect. Follow-up at 27–32 years. *N Engl J Med* 1990; 323:1645–1650.

85. Porter CJ, Feldt RH, Edwards WD, Seward JB, Schaff HV. Atrial septal defects. In: Emmanouilides GC, Riemenschneider TA, Allen HD, Gutgesell HP, eds. *Moss and Adams Heart Disease in Infants, Children and Adolescents,* 5th ed. Baltimore: Williams & Wilkins; 1995; 687–703.

86. Seward JB, Tajik AJ. Transesophageal echocardiography in congenital heart disease. *Am J Card Imaging* 1990; 4:215–222.

87. Hamilton WT, Hattajee CE, Dalen JE, Dexter L, Nadas AS. Atrial septal defect secundum: Clinical profile with physiologic correlates. In: Roberts WC, ed. *Adult Congenital Heart Disease.* Philadelphia: Davis; 1987:395–407.

88. Steele PM, Fuster V, Cohen M, Ritter DG, McGoon DC. Isolated atrial septal defect with pulmonary vascular obstructive disease, long-term follow-up and prediction of outcome after surgical correction. *Circulation* 1987; 76:1037–1042.

89. Rome JJ, Keane JF, Perry SB, Spevak PJ, Lock JE. Double umbrella closure of atrial defects. Initial clinical applications. *Circulation* 1990; 82:751–758.

90. Rao PS, Sideris EB, Hausdorf G, Rey C, Lloyd TR, Beekman RH, et al. International experience with secundum atrial septal defect occlusion by the buttoned device. *Am Heart J* 1994; 128:1022–1035.

91. Nora JJ, Nora AH. Update on counseling the family with a first-degree relative with a congenital heart defect. *Am J Med Genet* 1988; 29:137–142.

92. Konstantinides S, Geibel A, Olschewski M, Gornandt L, Roskamm H, Spiller G, et al. A comparison of surgical and medical therapy for atrial septal defect in adults. *N Engl J Med* 1995; 333:469–473.

93. St. John-Sutton MG, Tajik AJ, McGoon DC. Atrial septal defect in patients ages 60 years or older: Operative results and long-term postoperative follow-up. *Circulation* 1981; 64:402–409.

94. Krabill KA, Lucas RV Jr. Abnormal pulmonary venous connections. In: Emmanouilides GC, Riemenschneider TA, Allen HD, Gutgesell HP, eds. *Moss and Adams Heart Disease in Infants, Children, and Adolescents*, 5th ed. Baltimore: Williams & Wilkins; 1995:839–874.

95. Silverman NH: Anomalous pulmonary venous connections. In: Silverman NH, ed. *Pediatric Echocardiography*. New York: Williams & Wilkins; 1993:179–193.

96. Saalouke MG, Shapiro SR, Perry LW, Scott LP III. Isolated partial anomalous pulmonary venous drainage associated with pulmonary vascular obstructive disease. *Am J Cardiol* 1977; 39:439–444.

97. Rogers HM, Edwards JE. Incomplete division of the atrioventricular canal with patent interatrial foramen primum (persistent common cardioventricular ostium): Report of five cases and review of the literature. *Am Heart J* 1948; 36:28.

98. Edwards JE. Classification of congenital heart disease in the adult. In: Roberts WC, ed. *Congenital Heart Disease in Adults*, Cardiovasc Clin Series 10/1. Philadelphia: Davis; 1979:1–26.

99. Rastelli GC, Ongley PA, Kirklin JW, McGoon DC. Surgical repair of the complete form of persistent common atrioventricular canal. *J Thorac Cardiovasc Surg* 1968; 55:299–308.

100. Feldt RH, Porter CJ, Edwards WD, Puga FJ, Seward JB. Atrioventricular septal defects. In: Emmanouilides GC, Riemenschneider TA, Allen HD, Gutgesell HD, eds. *Moss and Adams Heart Disease in Infants, Children, and Adolescents*, 5th ed. Baltimore: Williams & Wilkins; 1995:704–724.

101. Rose V, Izukawa T, Moes CA. Syndromes of asplenia and polysplenia: A review of cardiac and non-cardiac malformations in 60 cases with special reference to diagnosis and prognosis. *Br Heart J* 1975; 37:840–852.

102. Fyler DC. Endocardial cushion defects. In: Fyler DC, ed. *Nadas' Pediatric Cardiology*. Philadelphia: Hanley & Belfus; 1992:577–587.

103. Lacro RV. Dysmorphology. In: Fyler DC, ed. *Nadas' Pediatric Cardiology*. Philadelphia: Hanley & Belfus; 1992:37–55.

104. Sewart JB, Tajik AJ, Edwards WD, Hagler DJ. *Two-Dimensional Echocardiographic Atlas*, vol 1, *Congenital Heart Disease*. New York: Springer; 1987:270–292.

105. Silverman NH. *Pediatric Echocardiography*. New York: Williams & Wilkins; 1993:143–166.

106. Nora JJ, Nora AH. Maternal transmission of congenital heart diseases: New recurrence risk figures and the questions of cytoplasmic inheritance and vulnerability to teratogens. *Am J Cardiol* 1987; 59:459–463.

107. Kirklin JW, Barratt-Boyes BG. Atrioventricular canal defect. In: Kirklin JW, Barratt-Boyes BG, eds. *Cardiac Surgery*, 2d ed. New York: Churchill Livingstone; 1993:693–747.

108. Hanley FL, Fenton KN, Jonas RA, Mayer JE, Cook NR, Wernowsky G, et al. Surgical repair of complete atrioventricular canal defects in infancy: Twenty-year trends. *J Thorac Cardiovasc Surg* 1993; 106:387–397.

109. Alexi-Meskishvili V, Ishino K, Dahnert I, Uhlemann F, Weng Y, Lange PE, et al. Correction of complete atrioventricular septal defects with the double-patch technique and cleft closure. *Ann Thorac Surg* 1996; 62:519–525.

110. Bando K, Turrentine MW, Sun K, Sharp TG, Ensing GJ, Miller AP, et al. Surgical management of complete atrioventricular septal defects: A twenty year experience. *J Thorac Cardiovasc Surg* 1995; 110:1543–1554.

111. Christie A. Normal closing time of the foramen ovale and the ductus arteriosus. *Am J Dis Child* 1930; 40:323.

112. Freed MD, Heymann MA, Lewis AB, Roehl SL, Kensey RC. Prosta-glandin E-1 in infants with ductus arteriosus-dependant congenital heart disease. *Circulation* 1981; 64:899–905.

113. Gersony WM, Peckham GJ, Ellison RC, Miettinen OS, Nadas AS. Effects of indomethacin in premature infants with patent ductus arteriosus: Results of a national collaborative study. *J Pediatr* 1983; 102:895–906.

114. Danilowicz D, Rudolph AM, Hoffman JI. Delayed closure of the ductus arteriosus in premature infants. *Pediatrics* 1966; 37:74–78.

115. Kitterman JA, Edmunds LH Jr, Gregory GA, Heymann MA, Tooley WH, Rudolph AM. Patent ductus arteriosus in premature infants: Incidence, relation to pulmonary disease and management. *N Engl J Med* 1972; 287:473–477.

116. Thibeault DW, Emmanouilides GC, Nelson RJ, Lachman RS, Rosengart RM, Oh W. Patent ductus arteriosus complicating the respiratory distress syndrome in preterm infants. *J Pediatr* 1975; 86:120–126.

117. Siassi B, Blanco C, Cabal LA, Coran AG. Incidence and clinical features of patent ductus arteriosus in low-birthweight infants: A prospective analysis of 150 consecutively born infants. *Pediatrics* 1976; 57:347–351.

118. Liao P, Su W, Hung J. Doppler echocardiographic flow characteristics of isolated patent ductus arteriosus: Better delineation by Doppler color flow mapping. *J Am Coll Cardiol* 1988; 12:1285–1291.

119. Stevenson JD. Fluid administration in the association of patent ductus arteriosus complicating respiratory distress syndrome. *J Pediatr* 1977; 90:257–261.

120. Varvarigou A, Bardin CL, Beharry K, Chemtob S, Papageorgiou A, Aranda JV. Early Ibuprofen administration to prevent patent ductus arteriosus in premature newborn infants. *JAMA* 1996; 275:539–544.

121. Portsmann W, Wierny L. Percutaneous transfemoral closure of the patent ductus arteriosus: An alternative to surgery. *Semin Roentgenol* 1981; 16:95–102.

122. Rashkind WJ, Cuaso CC. Transcatheter closure of patent ductus arteriosus. *Pediatr Cardiol* 1979; 1:3–7.

123. Lloyd TR, Fedderly R, Mendelsohn AM, Sandhu SK, Beekman RH. Transcatheter occlusion of patent ductus arteriosus with Gianturco coils. *Circulation* 1993; 88(part 1):1412–1420.

124. Rothman A, Lucas VW, Skalnsky MS, Cocalis MW, Kashani IA. Percutaneous coil occlusion of patent ductus arteriosus. *J Pediatr* 1992; 130:447–454.

125. Hallman GL, Cooley DA, Gutgesell HP. *Surgical Treatment of Congenital Heart Disease*. Philadelphia: Lea & Febiger; 1987.

126. Adzick NS, Harrison MR, deLorimier AA. Surgical clip ligation of patent ductus arteriosus in premature infants. *J Pediatr Surg* 1986; 21:158.

127. Satur CR, Walker DR, Dickinson DF. Day case ligation of patent ductus arteriosus in preterm infants: A 10-year review. *Arch Dis Child* 1991; 66:477–480.

128. Hubbard C, Rucker RW, Realyvasquez F, Sperling DR, Hicks DA, Worcester CC, et al. Ligation of the patent ductus arteriosus in newborn respiratory failure. *J Pediatr Surg* 1986; 21:3–5.

129. Bell Thomson J, Jewell E, Ellis FH Jr, Schwaber JR. Surgical technique in the management of patent ductus arteriosus in the elderly patient. *Ann Thorac Surg* 1990; 30:80–83.

130. Laborde F, Folligvet T, Batisse A, Dibie A, Da-Cruz E, Carbognani D. Video-assisted thorascopic surgical interruption: The technique of choice for patent ductus arteriosus. *J Thorac Cardiovasc Surg* 1995; 110:1681–1685.

131. Burke RP, Wernovsky G, van der Velde M, Hansen D, Castaneda AR. Video-assisted thorascopic surgery for congenital heart disease. *J Thorac Cardiovasc Surg* 1995; 109:499–507.

132. Edwards JE, Burchell HB. Pathologic anatomy of deficiencies between the aortic root and the heart including aortic sinus aneurysms. *Thorax* 1957; 12:125–139.

133. Sakakibara S, Konno S. Congenital aneurysm of the sinus of Valsalva: Anatomy and classification. *Am Heart J* 1962; 63:405–424.

134. Burakovsky VI, Podsolkov VP, Sabirow BN, Nasedkina MA, Alekian BG, Dvinyaninova NB. Ruptured congenital aneurysm of the sinus of Valsalva: Clinical manifestations, diagnosis, and results of surgical corrections. *J Thorac Cardiovasc Surg* 1988; 95:836–841.

135. Shumaker HB Jr. Aneurysms of the aortic sinuses of Valsalva due to bacterial endocarditis with special reference to their operative management. *J Thorac Surg* 1972; 63:896–902.

136. Shaffer EM, Snider AR, Beekman RH, Behrendt DM, Peschiera AW. Sinus of Valsalva aneurysm complicating bacterial endocarditis in an

infant: Diagnosis with two-dimensional and Doppler echocardiography. *J Am Coll Cardiol* 1987; 9:588–591.

137. Kakos GS, Kilman JW, Williams TE, Hosier DM. Diagnosis and management of sinus of Valsalva aneurysms in children. *Ann Thorac Surg* 1974; 17:474–478.

138. Meyer J, Wukasch DC, Hallman GL, Cooley DA. Aneurysm and fistula of the sinus of Valsalva: Clinical considerations and surgical treatment in 45 patients. *Ann Thorac Surg* 1975; 19:170–179.

139. Doty DB. *Cardiac Surgery: A Looseleaf Notebook and Update Service.* Chicago: Year Book; 1985: Sinus V 1–4.

140. Norwicki ER, Aberdeen E, Friedman S, Rashkind WJ. Congenital left aortic sinus-left ventricle fistula and review of aortocardiac fistulas. *Ann Thorac Surg* 1977; 23:378–388.

141. Pan-Chih O, Ching-Heng T, Chen-Chun O, Chieh-Fu L. Surgical treatment of ruptured aneurysm of the aortic sinuses. *Ann Thorac Surg* 1981; 32:162–166.

142. Bonfils-Roberts EA, DuShane JW, McGoon DC, Danielson GK. Aortic sinus fistula—surgical considerations and results of operation. *Ann Thorac Surg* 1971; 12:492–502.

143. Clagett OT, Kirklin JW, Edwards JE. Anatomic variations and pathologic changes in 124 cases of coarctation of the aorta. *Surg Gynecol Obstet* 1954; 98:103.

144. Rees AH, Elbl F, Villafane J, Solinger R, Mavroudis C, Harrison H. Surgical repair of atypical coarctation of the abdominal aorta in an infant. *Kentucky Med Assoc J* 1990; 88:62–65.

145. Bharati S, Lev M. The surgical anatomy of the heart in tubular hypoplasia of the transverse aorta (preductal coarctation). *J Thorac Cardiovasc Surg* 1986; 91:79–85.

146. Beekman RH. Coarctation of the aorta. In: Emmanouilides GC, Riemenschneider TA, Allen HD, Gutgesell HP, eds. *Moss and Adams Heart Disease in Infants, Children, and Adolescents,* 5th ed. Baltimore: Williams & Wilkins; 1995:1111–1133.

147. Gardiner HM, Celermajer DS, Sorensen KE, Georgakopoulos D, Robinson J, Thomas O, et al. Arterial reactivity is significantly impaired in normotensive young adults after successful repair of aortic coarctation in childhood. *Circulation* 1994; 89:1745–1750.

148. Fyler DC. Coarctation of the aorta. In: Fyler DC, ed. *Nadas' Pediatric Cardiology.* Philadelphia: Hanley & Belfus; 1992:535–556.

149. Beekman RH, Robinow M. Coarctation of the aorta inherited as an autosomal dominant trait. *Am J Cardiol* 1985; 56:818–819.

150. Ing FF, Starc TJ, Griffiths SP, Gersony WM. Early diagnosis of coarctation of the aorta in children: A continuing dilemma. *Pediatrics* 1996; 98:378–382.

151. Silverman NH. *Pediatric Echocardiography.* New York: Williams & Wilkins; 1993:409 414.

152. Campbell M. Natural history of coarctation of the aorta. *Br Heart J* 1970; 32:633–640.

153. Zehr KJ, Gillinov AM, Redmond JM, Greene PS, Kan JS, Gardner TJ, et al. Repair of coarctation of the aorta in neonates and infants: A thirty-year experience. *Ann Thorac Surg* 1995; 59:33–41.

154. Barash PG, Hobbins JC, Hook R, Stansel HC Jr, Whittemore R, Hehre FW. Management of coarctation of the aorta during pregnancy. *J Thorac Cardiovasc Surg* 1975; 69:781–784.

155. Nora JJ, Nora AH. *Genetics and Counseling in Cardiovascular Diseases.* Springfield, IL: Charles C Thomas; 1978.

156. Parks WJ, Ngo TD, Plauth WH, Bank ER, Sheppard SK, Pettigrew RI, et al. Incidence of aneurysm formation after Dacron patch aortoplasty repair for coarctation of the aorta: Long-term results and assessment utilizing magnetic resonance angiography with three-dimensional surface rendering. *J Am Coll Cardiol* 1995; 26:266–271.

157. Kirklin JW, Barratt-Boyes BG. Coarctation of the aorta and interrupted aortic arch. In: Kirklin JW, Barratt Boyes BJ, eds. *Cardiac Surgery,* 2d ed. New York: Churchill Livingstone; 1993:1263–1325.

158. Quaegebeur JM, Jonas RA, Weinberg AD, Blackstone EH, Kirklin JW. Outcomes in seriously ill neonates with coarctation of the aorta: A multi-institutional study. *J Thorac Cardiovasc Surg* 1994; 108:841–854.

159. Moreno NN, deCampo T, Kaiser GA, Pallares VS. Technical and pharmacologic management of distal hypotension during repair of coarctation of the aorta. *J Thorac Cardiovasc Surg* 1980, 80:182–186.

160. Pollock JC, Jamieson MP, McWilliam R. Somatosensory evoked potentials in the detection of spinal cord ischemia in aortic coarctation repair. *Ann Thorac Surg* 1986; 41:251–254.

161. Gidding SS, Rocchini AP, Beekman R, Szpunar CA, Moorehead C,

Behrendt D, et al. Therapeutic effect of propranolol on paradoxical hypertension after repair of coarctation of the aorta. *N Engl J Med* 1985; 312:1224–1228.

162. Friedman WF. Aortic stenosis. In: Emmanouilides GC, Riemenschneider TA, Allen HD, Gutgesell HP, eds. *Moss and Adams Heart Disease in Infants, Children, and Adolescents,* 5th ed. Baltimore: Williams & Wilkins; 1995:1087–1111.

163. Driscoll DJ, Wolfe RR, Gersony WM, Hayes CJ, Keane JF, Kidd L, et al. Cardiorespiratory responses to exercise of patients with aortic stenosis, pulmonary stenosis, and ventricular septal defect. *Circulation* 1993; 87(suppl I):I102–I113.

164. Silverman NH: *Pediatric Echocardiography.* New York: Williams & Wilkins; 1993:386–394.

165. Rhodes LA, Colan SD, Perry SB, Jonas RA, Sanders SP. Predictors of survival in neonates with critical aortic stenosis. *Circulation* 1991; 84:2325–2335.

166. Keane JF, Driscoll DJ, Gersony WM, Hayes CJ, Kidd L, O'Fallon WM, et al. Second Natural History Study of Congenital Heart Defects: Results of treatment of patients, with aortic valvular stenosis. *Circulation* 1993; 87(suppl I):I16–I27.

167. Yetman AT, Rosenberg HC, Joubert GI. Progression of asymptomatic aortic stenosis identified in the neonatal period. *Am J Cardiol* 1995; 75:636–637.

168. Bengur AR, Snider AR, Serwer GA, Peters J, Rosenthal A. Usefulness of the Doppler mean gradient in evaluation of children with aortic valve stenosis and comparison to gradient at catheterization. *Am J Cardiol* 1989; 64:756–761.

169. McCrindle BW, for the Valvuloplasty and Angioplasty of Congenital Anomalies (VACA) Registry Investigators. Independent predictors of immediate results of percutaneous balloon aortic valvotomy in childhood. *Am J Cardiol* 1996; 77:286–293.

170. Moore P, Egito E, Mowrey H, Perry SB, Lock JE, Keane JF. Midterm results of balloon dilatation of congenital aortic stenosis: Predictors of success. *J Am Coll Cardiol* 1996; 27:1257–1263.

171. Gatzoulis MA, Rigby ML, Shinebourne EA, Redington AN. Contemporary results of balloon valvuloplasty and surgical valvotomy for congenital aortic stenosis. *Arch Dis Child* 1995; 73:66–69.

172. Nora JJ, Nora AH. Maternal transmission of congenital heart disease: New recurrence risk figures and the questions of cytoplasmic inheritance and vulnerability to teratogens. *Am J Cardiol* 1987; 59:459–463.

173. Kirklin JW, Barratt-Boyes BG. Congenital aortic stenosis. In: Kirklin JW, Barratt-Boyes BH, eds. *Cardiac Surgery,* 2d ed. New York: Churchill Livingstone; 1993:1195–1237.

174. Ellis FHJ, Kirklin JW. Congenital valvular aortic stenosis: Anatomic findings and surgical technique. *J Thorac Surg* 1962; 43:199.

175. Elkins RC, Knott-Craig CJ, Ward KE, McCue C, Lane MM. Pulmonary autograft in children: Realized growth potential. *Ann Thorac Surg* 1994; 57:1387–1394.

176. Turley K, Bove EL, Iannettoni M, Yeh J, Cotroneo JV, Galdieri RJ. Neonatal aortic stenosis. *J Thorac Cardiovasc Surg* 1990; 99:679–684.

177. Gildein HP, Kleinert S, Weintraub RG, Wilkinson JL, Karl TR, Mee RB. Surgical commissurotomy of the aortic valve: Outcome of open valvulotomy in neonates with critical aortic stenosis. *Am Heart J* 1996; 131:754–759.

178. Frommelt PC, Lupinetti FM, Bove EL. Aortoventriculoplasty in infants and children. *Circulation* 1992; 86(suppl II):II176–II180.

179. Fyler DC. Aortic outflow abnormalities. In: Fyler DC, ed. *Nadas' Pediatric Cardiology.* Philadelphia: Hanley & Belfus; 1992:506–507.

180. Van Son JA, Edwards WD, Danielson GK. Pathology of coronary arteries, myocardium, and great arteries in supravalvular aortic stenosis. *J Thorac Cardiovasc Surg* 1994; 108:21–28.

181. Ensing GJ, Schmidt MA, Hagler DF, Michels VVR, Carter GA, Feldt RH. Spectrum of findings in a family with nonsyndromic autosomal dominant supravalvular aortic stenosis. A Doppler echocardiographic study. *J Am Coll Cardiol* 1989; 13:413–419.

182. Zalzstein E, Moes CA, Musewe NN, Freedom RM. Spectrum of cardiovascular anomalies in Williams-Beuren syndrome. *Pediatr Cardiol* 1991; 12:219–223.

183. Silverman NH. *Pediatric Echocardiography.* New York: Williams & Wilkins; 1993:405–407.

184. Friedman WF. Aortic stenosis. In: Emmanouilides GC, Riemenschneider TA, Allen HD, Gutgesell HP, eds. *Moss and Adams Heart Disease in Infants, Children, and Adolescents,* 5th ed. Baltimore: Williams & Wilkins; 1995:1087–1111.

185. McGoon DC, Mankin HT, Vlad P, Kirklin JW. The surgical treatment of supravalvular aortic stenosis. *J Thorac Cardiovasc Surg* 1961; 41:125–133.

186. Permut LC, Laks H. Surgery for valvular and supravalvular aortic stenosis. *Prog Pediatr Cardiol* 1994; 3:177–187.

187. Folliguet TA, Mace L, Dervanian P, Casasoprana A, Magnier S, Neveux JY. Surgical treatment of diffuse supravalvar aortic stenosis. *Ann Thorac Surg* 1996; 61:1251–1253.

188. Feigl A, Feigl D, Lucas RV Jr, Edwards JE. Involvement of the aortic valve cusps in discrete subaortic stenosis. *Pediatr Cardiol* 1984; 5:185–189.

189. Wright GB, Keane JF, Nadas AS, Bernhard WF, Castaneda AR. Fixed subaortic stenosis in the young: Medical and surgical course in 83 patients. *Am J Cardiol* 1983; 52:830–835.

190. Choi JY, Sullivan ID. Fixed subaortic stenosis: Anatomic spectrum and nature of progression. *Br Heart J* 1991; 65:280–286.

191. Snider AR, Serwer GA. *Echocardiography in Pediatric Heart Disease*. Chicago: Year Book; 1990:250–254.

192. Freedom RM, Culham JAG, Moes CAF. *Angiocardiography of Congenital Heart Disease*. New York: Macmillan; 1989.

193. Drinkwater DC, Laks H. Surgery for subvalvular aortic stenosis. *Progr Pediatr Cardiol* 1994; 3:189–201.

194. Maginot KR, Williams RG. Fixed subaortic stenosis. *Prog Pediatr Cardiol* 1994; 3:141–149.

195. Kirklin JW, Ellis FH Jr. Surgical relief of diffuse subvalvular aortic stenosis. *Circulation* 1961; 24:739.

196. DeVries AG, Hess J, Witsenburg M, Frohn-Mulder IM, Bogers JJS, Bos E. Management of fixed subaortic stenosis: A retrospective study of 57 cases. *J Am Coll Cardiol* 1992; 19:1013–1017.

197. Braverman AC. Bicuspid aortic valve and associated aortic wall abnormalities. *Curr Opin Cardiol* 1996; 11:501–503.

198. Roberts WC. Anomalies usually silent until adulthood. In: Roberts WC, ed. *Adult Congenital Heart Disease*. Philadelphia: Davis; 1987:646–656.

199. Leech G, Mills P, Leatham A. The diagnosis of a nonstenotic bicuspid aortic valve. *Br Heart J* 1978; 40:941–950.

200. Brandenburg RO Jr, Tajik AJ, Edwards WD, Reeder GS, Shub C, Seward JB. Accuracy of a 2-dimensional echocardiographic diagnosis of congenitally bicuspid aortic valve: Echocardiographic anatomic correlation in 115 patients. *Am J Cardiol* 1983; 51:1469–1473.

201. Snider RA, Serwer GA. *Echocardiography in Pediatric Heart Disease*. Chicago: Year Book; 1990:242–245.

202. Hardy WE, Gnoj J, Ayres SM, Giannelli S Jr, Christianson LC. Pulmonic stenosis and associated atrial septal defect in older patients: Report of three cases including one with calcific pulmonic stenosis. *Am J Cardiol* 1969; 24:130–134.

203. Koretzky ED, Moller JH, Korns ME, Schwartz CJ, Edwards JE. Congenital pulmonary stenosis resulting from dysplasia of valve. *Circulation* 1969; 40:43–53.

204. Li MD, Coles JC, McDonald AC. Anomalous muscle bundle of the right ventricle: Its recognition and surgical treatment. *Br Heart J* 1978; 40:1040–1045.

205. Emmanouilides GC, Linde LM, Critenden IH. Pulmonary artery stenosis associated with ductus arteriosus following maternal rubella. *Circulation* 1964; 29:51.

206. Vernant P, Corone P, Rossignol AM, Bielman C. Etude de 120 observations de syndrome de Williams et Beuren. *Arch Mal Coeur* 1980; 73:661–666.

207. Noonan JA. Hypertelorism with Turner phenotype, a new syndrome associated with congenital heart disease. *Am J Dis Child* 1968; 116:373–380.

208. Alagille D, Odievre M, Gautier M, Dommergues JP. Hepatic ductular hypoplasia associatd with characteristic facies, vertebral malformations, retarded physical, mental, and sexual development and cardiac murmur. *J Pediatr* 1975; 86:63–71.

209. Stone FM, Bessinger FB Jr, Lucas RV Jr, Moller JH. Pre- and postoperative rest and exercise hemodynamics in children with pulmonary stenosis. *Circulation* 1974; 49:1102–1106.

210. Roberts WC, Shemin RJ, Kent KM. Frequency and direction of interatrial shunting in valvular pulmonic stenosis with intact ventricular septum and without left ventricular inflow or outflow obstruction: An analysis of 127 patients treated by valvulotomy. *Am Heart J* 1980; 99:142–148.

211. Cayler CG, Ongley P, Nadas AS. Relation of systolic pressure in the right ventricle to the electrocardiogram. *N Engl J Med* 1958; 258:979.

212. Lima CO, Sahn DJ, Valdez-Cruz LM, Goldberg SJ, Barron JV, Allen HD, et al. Noninvasive prediction of transvalvular pressure gradient in patients with pulmonary stenosis by quantitative two-dimensional echocardiographic Doppler studies. *Circulation* 1983; 67:866–871.

213. Nadas AS, ed. Pulmonary stenosis, aortic stenosis, ventricular septal defect: Clinical course and indirect assessment (report from the Joint Study on the Natural History of Congenital Heart Defects). *Circulation* 1977; 56:I1–I87.

214. Mody MR. The natural history of uncomplicated valvular pulmonic stenosis. *Am Heart J* 1975; 90:317–321.

215. Hayes CJ, Gersony WM, Driscoll DJ, Keane JF, Kidd L, O'Fallon M, et al. Second natural history of congenital heart defects: Results of treatment of patients with pulmonary valvular stenosis. *Circulation* 1993; 87(suppl I):I28–I37.

216. Stanger P, Cassidy SC, Girod DA, Kan JS, Lababidi Z, Shapiro SR. Balloon pulmonary valvuloplasty: Results of the Valvuloplasty and Angioplasty of Congenital Anomalies Registry. *Am J Cardiol* 1990; 65:775–783.

217. Marantz PM, Huhta JC, Mullins CE, Murphy DJ Jr, Nihill MR, Ludomirsky A, et al. Results of balloon valvuloplasty in typical and dysplastic pulmonary valve stenosis: Doppler echocardiographic follow-up. *J Am Coll Cardiol* 1988; 12:476–479.

218. Ali Khan MA, al-Yousef S, Huhta JC, Bricker JT, Mullins CE, Sawyer W. Critical pulmonary valve stenosis in patients less than 1 year of age: Treatment with percutaneous gradational balloon pulmonary valvuloplasty. *Am Heart J* 1989; 117:1008–1014.

219. Ladysans EJ, Qureshi SA, Parsons JM, Arab S, Baker EJ, Tynan M. Balloon dilation of critical stenosis of the pulmonary valve in neonates. *Br Heart J* 1990; 63:362–367.

220. Ring JC, Bass JL, Marvin W, Fuhrman BP, Kulik TJ, Lock JE, et al. Management of congenital stenosis of a branch pulmonary artery with balloon dilation angioplasty. Report of 52 procedures. *J Thorac Cardiovasc Surg* 1985; 90:35–44.

221. Kan JS, Marvin WJ Jr, Bass JL, Muster AJ, Murphy J. Balloon angioplasty—branch pulmonary artery stenosis: Results from the Valvuloplasty and Angioplasty of Congenital Anomalies Registry. *Am J Cardiol* 1990; 65:798–801.

222. O'Laughlin MP, Perry SB, Lock JE, Mullins CE. Use of endovascular stents in congenital heart disease. *Circulation* 1991; 83:1923–1939.

223. Vancini M, Roberts KD, Silove ED, Singh SP. Surgical treatment of congenital pulmonary stenosis due to dysplastic leaflets and small valve annulus. *J Thorac Cardiovasc Surg* 1980; 79:464–468.

224. McGoon MD, Fulton RE, Davis GD, Ritter DG, Neill CA, White RI Jr. Systemic collateral and pulmonary artery stenosis in patients with congenital pulmonary valve atresia and ventricular septal defect. *Circulation* 1977; 56:473–479.

225. Barbero-Marcial M, Atik E, Baucia JA, Pradel HO, Macruz R, Jatene AD. Reconstruction of stenotic or nonconfluent pulmonary arteries simultaneously with a Blalock-Taussig shunt. *J Thorac Cardiovasc Surg* 1988; 95:82–89.

226. Edwards JE. Classification of congenital heart disease in the adult. In: Roberts WC, ed. *Congenital Heart Disease in Adults*, Cardiovasc Clin Series 10/1. Philadelphia: Davis; 1979:1–26.

227. Becker AE, Connor M, Anderson RH. Tetralogy of Fallot: A morphometric and geometric study. *Am J Cardiol* 1975; 35:402–412.

228. McManus BM, Waller BF, Jones M, Epstein SE, Roberts WC. The case for preoperative coronary arteriography in patients with tetralogy of Fallot and other complex heart diseases. *Am Heart J* 1982, 103:451–456.

229. Rao BN, Anderson RC, Edwards JE. Anatomic variations in the tetralogy of Fallot. *Am Heart J* 1971; 81:361–371.

230. Roberts WC, Friesinger GC, Cohen LS, Mason DT, Ross RS. Acquired pulmonic atresia: Total obstruction to right ventricular outflow after systemic to pulmonary arterial anastomoses for cyanotic congenital cardiac disease. *Am J Cardiol* 1969; 24:335–345.

231. Morgan BC, Guntheroth WG, Bloom RS, Fyler DC. A clinical profile of paroxysmal hyperpnea in cyanotic congenital heart disease. *Circulation* 1965; 31:66–69.

232. Guntheroth WG, Morgan BC, Mullins GL. Physiologic studies of paroxysmal hyperpnea in cyanotic congenital heart disease. *Circulation* 1965; 31:70–76.

233. Danilowicz DA. Delay in bone age in children with cyanotic congenital heart disease. *Radiology* 1973; 108:655–658.

234. Hagler DJ, Tajik AJ, Seward JB, Mair DD, Ritter DG. Wide-angle two-

dimensional echocardiographic profiles of conotruncal abnormalities. *Mayo Clin Proc* 1980; 55:73–82.

235. Formanek A, Nath PH, Zollikofer C, Moller JH. Selective coronary arteriography in children. *Circulation* 1980; 61:84–95.

236. Dabizzi RP, Caprioli G, Aiazzi L, Castelli C, Baldrighi G, Parenzan L, et al. Distribution and anomalies of coronary arteries in tetralogy of Fallot. *Circulation* 1980; 61:95–102.

237. Ponce FE, Williams LC, Webb HM, Riopel DA, Hohn AR. Propanolol palliation of tetralogy of Fallot: Experience with long-term drug treatment in pediatric patient. *Pediatrics* 1973; 52:100–108.

238. Taussig HB, Crocetti A, Eshaghpour E, Keinomen R, Yap KN, Bachman D, et al. Long time observations on the Blalock-Taussig operation III: Common complications. *John Hopkins Med J* 1971; 129:274–289.

239. Dijani AS, Taubert KA, Wilson W, et al. Prevention of bacterial endocarditis: Recommendations by the American Heart Association. *JAMA* (in press).

240. Blalock A, Taussig HB. The surgical treatment of malformations of the heart in which there is pulmonary stenosis or pulmonary atresia. *JAMA* 128:129:1945.

241. Lillehei CW, Cohen M, Warden HE, Read RC, Aust JB, Dewall RA, et al. Direct vision intracardiac surgical correction of the tetralogy of Fallot, pentalogy of Fallot, and pulmonary atresia defects: Report of the first 10 cases. *Ann Surg* 1955; 142:418–442.

242. Castaneda AR, Freed MD, Williams RG, et al. Repair of tetralogy of Fallot in infancy. *J Thorac Cardovasc Surgery* 1977; 74:372–381.

243. Kirklin JW, Blackstone EH, Kirklin JK, Pacifico AD, Aramendi J, Bargeron LM Jr. Surgical results and protocols in the spectrum of tetralogy of Fallot. *Ann Surg* 1983; 198:251–265.

244. Castaneda AR, Jonas RA, Mayer JE. Surgery for infants with congenital heart disease. In: Fyler DC, ed. *Nadas' Pediatric Cardiology.* Philadelphia: Hanley and Belfus; 1992:731.

245. Castaneda AR, Jonas RA, Mayer JE, Hanley FL. Tetralogy of Fallot. In: *Cardiac Surgery of the Neonate and Infant.* Philadelphia: Saunders; 1994: Chapter 13.

246. Rastelli GC, Wallace RB, Ongley PA. Complete repair of transposition of the great arteries with pulmonary stenosis: A review and report of a case corrected by using a new surgical technique. *Circulation* 1969; 39:83–95.

247. Kreutzer J, Perry SB, Jonas RA, Mayer JE, Cataneda AR, Lock JE. Tetralogy of Fallot with diminutive pulmonary arteries: Preoperative pulmonary valve dilation and transcatheter rehabilitation of pulmonary arteries. *J Am Coll Cardiol* 1996; 27:1741–1747.

248. Murphy JG, Gersh BJ, Mair DD, Fuster V, McGoon MD, Ilstrup DM, et al. Long-term outcome in patients undergoing surgical repair of tetralogy of Fallot. *N Engl J Med* 1993; 329:593–599.

249. Lev M, Liberthson RR, Joseph RH, Seten CE, Eckner FA, Kunske RD, et al. The pathologic anatomy of Ebstein's disease. *Arch Pathol* 1970; 90:334–343.

250. Becker AE, Becker MJ, Edwards JE. Pathologic spectrum of dysplasia of the tricuspid valve. Features in common with Ebstein's malformation. *Arch Pathol* 1971; 91:167–178.

251. Cohen LS, Friedman JM, Jefferson JW, Johnson EM, Wiener ML. A reevaluation of risk of in utero exposure to lithium. *JAMA* 1994; 271:146–150.

252. Kumar AE, Fyler DC, Miettinen OS, Nadas AS. Ebstein's anomaly: Clinical profile and natural history. *Am J Cardiol* 1971; 28:84–95.

253. Watson H. Natural history of Ebstein's anomaly of tricuspid valve in childhood and adolescence: An international co-operative study of 505 cases. *Br Heart J* 1974; 36:417–427.

254. Driscoll DJ, Mottram CD, Danielson GK. Spectrum of exercise intolerance in 45 patients with Ebstein's anomaly and observations on exercise tolerance in 11 patients after surgical repair. *J Am Coll Cardiol* 1988; 11:831–836.

255. Kastor JA, Goldreyer BN, Josephson ME, Perloff JK, Scharf DL, Manchester JH, et al. Electrophysiologic characteristics of Ebstein's anomaly of the tricuspid valve. *Circulation* 1975; 52:987–995.

256. Roberson DA, Silverman NH. Ebstein's anomaly: Echocardiographic and clinical features in the fetus and neonate. *J Am Coll Cardiol* 1989; 14:1300–1307.

257. Hernandez FA, Richkind R, Cooper HR. The intracavitary electrocardiogram in the diagnosis of Ebstein's anomaly. *Am J Cardiol* 1958; 1:181–190.

258. Celermajer DS, Cullen S, Sullivan ID, Spiegelhalter DJ, Wyse RK, Deanfield JE. Outcome in neonates with Ebstein's anomaly. *J Am Coll Cardiol* 1992; 19:1041–1046.

259. Gentles TL, Calder AL, Clarkson PM, Neutze JM. Predictors of long-term survival with Ebstein's anomaly of the tricuspid valve. *Am J Cardiol* 1992; 69:377–381.

260. Donnelly JE, Brown JM, Radford DJ. Pregnancy outcome and Ebstein's anomaly. *Br Heart J* 1991; 66:368–371.

261. Kulik TJ. Inhaled nitric oxide in the management of congenital heart disease. *Curr Opin Cardiol* 1996; 11:75–80.

262. Van Hare GF, Lesh MD, Stanger P. Radiofrequency catheter ablation of supraventricular arrhythmias in patients with congenital heart disease: Results and technical considerations. *J Am Coll Cardiol* 1993; 22:883–890.

263. Starnes VA, Pitlick PT, Bernstein D, Griffin ML, Choy M, Shumway NE. Ebstein's anomaly appearing in the neonate. A new surgical approach. *J Thorac Cardiovasc Surg* 1991; 101:1082–1087.

264. Scott LP, Dempsey JJ, Timmis HH, McClenathan JE. A surgical approach to Ebstein's disease. *Circulation* 1963; 27:574–577.

265. Danielson GK, Driscoll DJ, Mair DD, Warnes CA, Oliver WC Jr. Operative treatment of Ebstein's anomaly. *J Thorac Cardiovasc Surg* 1992; 104:1195–1202.

266. Carpentier A, Chauvaud S, Mace L, Relland J, Mihaileanu S, Marino JP, et al. A new reconstructive operation for Ebstein's anomaly of the tricuspid valve. *J Thorac Cardioasc Surg* 1988; 96:92–101.

267. Quaegebeur JM, Sreeram H, Fraser AG, Bogers AJ, Stumper OF, Hess J. Surgery for Ebstein's anomaly: The clinical and echocardiographic evaluation of a new technique. *J Am Coll Cardiol* 1991; 17:722–728.

268. Radford DJ, Graff RF, Neilson GH. Diagnosis and natural history of Ebstein's anomaly. *Br Heart J* 1985; 54:517–522.

269. Blake HA, Hall RJ, Manion WC. Anomalous pulmonary venous return. *Circulation* 1965; 32:406–414.

270. Lucas RV Jr, Lock JE, Tandon R, Edwards JE. Gross and histologic anatomy of total anomalous pulmonary venous connections. *Am J Cardiol* 1988; 62:292–300.

271. Lucas RV Jr, Adams P Jr, Anderson RC, Varco RL, Edwards JE, Lester RG. Total anomalous pulmonary venous connection to the portal venous system: A cause of pulmonary venous obstruction. *Am J Roentgenol* 1961; 86:561.

272. Gathman GE, Nadas AS. Total anomalous pulmonary venous connection: Clinical and physiologic observations of 75 pediatric patients. *Circulation* 1970; 42:143–154.

273. Chin AJ, Sanders S, Sherman F, Lang P, Norwood WI, Casteneda AR. Accuracy of subcostal two-dimensional echocardiography in prospective diagnosis of total anomalous pulmonary venous connection. *Am Heart J* 1987; 113:1153–1159.

274. Galioto FJ Jr, Fyler DC, Chameides L. Total anomalous pulmonary venous drainage (TAPVD): A 5 year review in New England (abstr). *Am J Cardiol* 1975; 35:138.

275. Newfeld EA, Wilson A, Paul MH, Reisch JS. Pulmonary vascular disease in total anomalous pulmonary venous drainage. *Circulation* 1980; 61:103–109.

276. Harlan BJ, Starr A, Harwin FM. Total anomalous pulmonary venous connection. In: Harlan BJ, Harwin FM, eds. *Manual of Cardiac Surgery*, vol 2. New York: Springer; 1981:333.

277. Kirklin JW. Surgical treatment for total anomalous pulmonary venous connection in infancy. In: Barratt-Boyes BG, ed. *Heart Disease in Infancy: Diagnosis and Surgical Treatment*. Edinburgh: Churchill Livingstone; 1973:89–100.

278. Behrendt DM, Aberdeen E, Waterson DJ, Bonham-Carter RE. Total anomalous pulmonary venous drainage in infants. I. Clinical and hemodynamic findings, methods, and results of operation in 37 cases. *Circulation* 1972; 46:347–356.

279. Norwood WI, Hougen TJ, Castaneda AR. Total anomalous pulmonary venous connection: Surgical considerations. *Cardiovasc Clin* 1981; 11:353–364.

280. VanderVelde M, Parness IA, Colan SD, Spevak PJ, Lock JE, Mayer JE, et al. Two-dimensional echocardiography in the pre- and postoperative management of total anomalous pulmonary venous connection. *J Am Coll Cardiol* 1991; 18:1746.

281. Lupinetti FM, Kulik TJ, Beekman RH III, Crowley DC, Bove EL. Correction of total anomalous pulmonary venous connection in infancy. *J Thorac Cardiovasc Surg* 1993; 106:880–885.

282. Van Praagh R, Weinberg PM, Smith SD, Foran RB, Van Praagh S. Malpositions of the heart. In: Adams FH, Emmanouilides GC, Riemenschneider TA, eds. *Moss' Heart Disease in Infants, Children, and Adolescents*, 4th ed. Baltimore: Williams & Wilkins; 1989:530–580.

283. Van Praagh R. Segmental approach to diagnosis. In: Fyler DC, ed. *Nadas' Pediatric Cardiology*. Philadelphia: Hanley & Belfus; 1992; 27–35.

284. Van Praagh S, Santini F, Sanders SP. Cardiac malpositions with special emphasis on visceral heterotaxy (asplenia and polysplenia syndromes). In: Fyler DC, ed. *Nadas' Pediatric Cardiology*. Philadelphia: Hanley & Belfus; 1992:589–608.

285. Rooklin AR, McGeady SJ, Mikaelian DO, Soriano RZ, Mansmann HC Jr. The immotile cilia syndrome: A cause of recurrent pulmonary disease in children. *Pediatrics* 1980; 66:526–531.

286. Fyler DC. D-transposition of the great arteries. In: Fyler DC, ed. *Nadas' Pediatric Cardiology*. Philadelphia: Hanley & Belfus; 1992:557–575.

287. Paul MH, Wernovsky G. Transposition of the great arteries. In: Emmanouilides GC, Riemenschneider TA, Allen HD, Gutgesell HD, eds. *Moss and Adams Heart Disease in Infants, Children, and Adolescents*, 5th ed. Baltimore: Williams and Wilkins; 1995:1154–1224.

288. Silverman NH. *Pediatric Echocardiography*. New York: Williams & Wilkins; 1993:245–366.

289. Yoo S, Burrows PE, Moes CAF, MacDonald C, Williams WG, Houde C, et al. Evaluation of coronary arterial patterns in complete transposition by laidback aortography. *Cardiol Young* 1996; 6:149–155.

290. Hurwitz RA, Caldwell RL, Girod DA, Brown J. Right ventricular systolic function in adolescents and young adults after Mustard operation for transposition of the great arteries. *Am J Cardiol* 1996; 77:294–297.

291. Norwood WI, Dobell AR, Freed MD, Kirklin JW, Blackstone EH. The Congenital Heart Surgeons Society: Intermediate results of the arterial switch repair: A 20 institution study. *J Thorac Cardiovasc Surg* 1988; 96:854–863.

292. Gutgesell HP, Massaro TA, Kron IL. The arterial switch operation for transposition of the great arteries in a consortium of University Hospitals. *Am J Cardiol* 1994; 74:959–960.

293. Wernovsky G, Freed MD. Transposition of the great arteries: Results and outcome of the arterial switch operation. In: Freedom RM, ed. *Atlas of Heart Diseases*, vol XII, *Congenital Heart Disease*. Philadelphia: Current Medicine; 1997.

294. Sagin-Saylam G, Somerville J. Palliative Mustard operation for transposition of the great arteries: Late results after 15–20 years. *Heart* 1996; 75:72–77.

295. Hagler DJ. Double-outlet right ventricle. In: Emmanouilides TA, Riemenschneider TA, Allen HD, Gutgesell HP, eds. *Moss and Adams Heart Disease in Infants, Children, and Adolescents*, 5th ed. Baltimore: Williams & Wilkins; 1995:1246–1270.

296. Fyler DC. Trends. In: Fyler DC, ed. *Nadas' Pediatric Cardiology*. Philadelphia: Hanley & Belfus; 1992:273–280.

297. Snider AR, Serwer GA. *Echocardiography in Pediatric Heart Disease*. Chicago: Year Book; 1990:190–195.

298. Fyler DC. Double-outlet right ventricle. In: Fyler DC, ed. *Nadas' Pediatric Cardiology*. Philadelphia: Hanley & Belfus; 1992:643–648.

299. Kirklin JW, Barratt-Boyes BG. Double outlet right ventricle. In: Kirklin JW, Barratt-Boyes BG, eds. *Cardiac Surgery*, 2d ed. New York: Churchill Livingstone; 1993:1469–1500.

300. Aoki M, Forbess JM, Jonas RA, Mayer JE Jr, Castaneda AR. Result of biventricular repair for double-outlet right ventricle. *J Thorac Cardiovasc Surg* 1994; 107:338–349.

301. Belli E, Serraf A, Lacour-Gayet F, Inamo J, Houyel L, Bruniaux J, et al. Surgical treatment of subaortic stenosis after biventricular repair of double-outlet right ventricle. *J Thorac Cardiovasc Surg* 1996; 112:1570–1580.

302. Mavroudis C, Backer CL, Muster AJ, Rocchini AP, Rees AH, Gevitz ML. Taussig-Bing anomaly: Arterial switch versus Kawashima intraventricular repair. *Ann Thorac Surg* 1996; 61:1330–1338.

303. Freedom RM, Dyck JD. Congenitally corrected transposition of the great arteries. In: Emmanouilides GC, Riemenschneider TA, Allen HD, Gutgesell HD, eds. *Moss and Adams Heart Disease in Infants, Children, and Adolescents*, 5th ed. Baltimore: Williams & Wilkins; 1995:1225–1245.

304. Fyler DC. "Corrected" transposition of the great arteries. In: Fyler DC, ed. *Nadas' Pediatric Cardiology*. Philadelphia: Hanley & Belfus; 1992:701–706.

305. Sneider AR, Serwer GA. *Echocardiography in Pediatric Heart Disease*. Chicago: Year Book; 1990:186–190.

306. Connelly MS, Liu PP, Williams WG, Webb GD, Robertson P, McLaughlin PR. Congenitally corrected transposition of the great arteries in the adult: Functional status and complications. *J Am Coll Cardiol* 1996; 27:1238–1243.

307. Lundstrom U, Bull C, Wyse RK, Somerville J. The natural and "unnatural" history of congenitally corrected transposition. *Am J Cardiol* 1990; 65:1222–1229.

308. Warnes CA: Congenitally corrected transposition: The uncorrected misnomer (editorial comment). *J Am Coll Cardiol* 1996; 27:1244.

309. Kirklin JW, Barratt-Boyes BG. Congenitally corrected transposition of the great arteries. In: Kirklin JW, Barratt-Boyes BG, eds. *Cardiac Surgery*, 2d ed. New York: Churchill Livingstone; 1993:1511–1533.

310. Sano T, Riesenfeld T, Karl TR, Wilkinson JL. Intermediate term outcome after intracardiac repair of associated cardiac defects in patients with atrioventricular and ventriculoarterial discordance. *Circulation* 1995; 92(suppl II):II272–II278.

311. Termignon JL, Leca F, Vouhe PR, Vernant F, Bical OM, LeCompte Y, et al: "Classic" repair of congenitally corrected transposition and ventricular septal defect. *Ann Thorac Surg* 1996; 62:199–206.

312. Van Son JA, Danielson GK, Huhta JC, Warnes CA, Edwards WD, Schaff HV, et al. Late results of systemic atrioventricular valve replacement in corrected transposition. *J Thorac Cardiovasc Surg* 1995; 109:642–653.

313. Imai Y, Sawatari K, Hoshino S, Ishihara K, Nakazawa M, Momma K. Ventricular function after anatomic repair in patients with atrioventricular discordance. *J Thorac Cardiovasc Surg* 1994; 107:1272–1283.

314. Hagler DJ, Edwards WD. Univentricular atrioventricular connection. In: Emmanouilides GC, Riemenschneider TA, Allen HD, Gutgesell HD, eds. *Moss and Adams Heart Disease in Infants, Children, and Adolescents*, 5th ed. Baltimore: Williams & Wilkins; 1995:1278–1306.

315. Fyler DC. Single ventricle. In: Fyler DC, ed. *Nadas' Pediatric Cardiology*. Philadelphia: Hanley & Belfus; 1992:649–657.

316. Shinebourne EA, Lau KC, Calcaterra G, Anderson RH. Univentricular heart of right ventricular type: Clinical, angiographic and electrocardiographic features. *Am J Cardiol* 1980; 46:439–445.

317. Dobell ARC, Van Praagh R. The Holmes heart: Historic associations and pathologic anatomy. *Am Heart J* 1996; 132:437–445.

318. Silverman NH. *Pediatric Echocardiography*. New York: Williams & Wilkins; 1993:279–302.

319. Freedom RM, Culham JAG, Moes CAF. *Angiocardiography of Congenital Heart Disease*. New York: Macmillan; 1989.

320. George BL, Kaplan S. Single ventricle and subaortic obstruction. *Prog Pediatr Cardiol* 1994; 3:167–176.

321. Moak JP, Gersony WM. Progressive atrioventricular valvular regurgitation in single ventricle. *Am J Cardiol* 1987; 59:656–658.

322. Donofrio MT, Jacobs ML, Norwood WI, Rychik J. Early changes in ventricular septal defect size and ventricular geometry in the single left ventricle after volume-unloading surgery. *J Am Coll Cardiol* 1995; 26:1008–1015.

323. Mainwaring RD, Lamberti JJ, Moore JW. The bidirectional Glenn and Fontan procedures—integrated management of the patient with a functionally single ventricle. *Cardiol Young* 1996; 6:198–207.

324. Van Son JA, Reddy VM, Haas GS, Hanley FL. Modified surgical techniques for relief of aortic obstruction in (SLL) hearts with rudimentary right ventricle and restrictive bulboventricular foramen. *J Thorac Cardiovasc Surg* 1995; 110:909–915.

325. Mayer JE, Bridges ND, Lock JE, Hanley FL, Jonas RA, Castaneda AR. Factors associated with marked reduction in mortality for Fontan operation in patients with single ventricle. *J Thorac Cardiovasc Surg* 1992; 103:444–452.

326. Moak JP, Gersony WM. Progressive atrioventricular valvular regurgitation in single ventricle. *Am J Cardiol* 1987; 59:656–658.

327. Matitiau A, Geva T, Colan SD, Sluysmans T, Parness IA, Spevak PJ, et al. Bulboventricular foramen size in infants with double-inlet left ventricle or tricuspid atresia with transposed great arteries: Influence on initial palliative operation and rate of growth. *J Am Coll Cardiol* 1992; 19:142–148.

328. Jacobs ML, Rychik J, Rome JJ, Apostolopoulou S, Pizzaro C, Murphy JD, et al. Early reduction of the volume work of the single ventricle: The hemi-Fontan operation. *Ann Thorac Surg* 1996; 62:456–462.

329. Kirklin JW, Barratt-Boyes BG. Double inlet ventricle and atretic atrioventricular valve. In: Kirklin JW, Barratt-Boyes BG, eds. *Cardiac Surgery*, 2d ed. New York: Churchill Livingstone; 1993:1549–1580.

330. Van Son JA, Reddy VM, Haas GS, Hanley FL. Modified surgical techniques for relief of aortic obstruction in (SLL) hearts with rudimentary right ventricle and restrictive bulboventricular foramen. *J Thorac Cardiovasc Surg* 1995; 110:909–915.

331. Mainwaring RD, Lamberti JJ, Moore JW. The bidirectional Glenn and Fontan procedures—integrated management of the patient with a functional single ventricle. *Cardiol Young* 1996; 6:198–207.

332. Cetta F, Feldt RH, O'Leary PW, Mair DD, Warnes CA, Driscoll DJ, et al. Improved early morbidity and mortality after Fontan operation the Mayo Clinic experience, 1987 to 1992. *J Am Coll Cardiol* 1996; 28:480–486.

333. McNamara JJ, Gross RE. Congenital coronary artery fistula. *Surgery* 1969; 65:59–69.

334. Liberthson RR, Sagar K, Berkoben JP, Weintraub RM, Levine FH. Congenital coronary arteriovenous fistula: Report of 13 patients, review of the literature and delineation of management. *Circulation* 1979; 59:849–854.

335. Tkebuchava T, Von Segesser LK, Vogt PR, Jenni R, Arbenz U, Turina M. Congenital coronary fistulas in children and adults: Diagnosis, surgical technique and results. *J Cardiovasc Surg* 1996; 37:29–34.

336. Vavuranakis M, Bush CA, Boudoulas H. Coronary artery fistulas in adults: Incidence, angiographic characteristics, natural history. *Cathet Cardiovasc Diagn* 1995; 35:116–120.

337. Velvis H, Schmidt KG, Silverman NH, Turley K. Diagnosis of coronary artery fistula by two-dimensional echocardiography, pulsed Doppler ultrasound and color flow imaging. *J Am Coll Cardiol* 1989; 14:968–976.

338. Urruita SCO, Falashci G, Ott DA, Cooley DA. Surgical management of 56 patients with congenital coronary artery fistulas: Report of three cases. *Ann Thorac Surg* 1983; 35:300–307.

339. Pezzella AT, Falaschi G, Ott DA, Cooley DA. Congenital coronary artery–left heart fistulas: Report of three cases. *Cardiovasc Dis Bull Texas Heart Inst* 1981; 8:355–363.

340. Oldham HN Jr, Ebert PA, Young WG, Sabiston DC Jr. Surgical management of congenital coronary artery fistula. *Ann Thorac Surg* 1971; 12:503–513.

341. Blanche C, Chaux A. Long-term results of surgery for coronary artery fistulas. *Int Surg* 1990; 75:238–239.

342. Perry SB, Rome J, Keane JF, Baim DS, Locke JE. Transcatheter closure of coronary artery fistulas. *J Am Coll Cardiol* 1992; 20:205–209.

343. Noren GR, Raghib G, Moller JH, Amplatz K, Adams P Jr, Edwards JE. Anomalous origin of the left coronary artery from the pulmonary trunk with special reference to the occurrence of mitral insufficiency. *Circulation* 1964; 30:171–179.

344. Hurwitz RA, Caldwell RL, Girod DA, Brown J, King H. Clinical and hemodynamic course of infants and children with anomalous left coronary artery. *Am Heart J* 1989; 118:1176–1181.

345. Wesselhoeft H, Fawcett JS, Johnson AL. Anomalous origin of the left coronary artery from the pulmonary trunk: Its clinical spectrum, pathology, and pathophysiology, based on a review of 140 cases with seven further cases. *Circulation* 1968; 38:403–425.

346. Caldwell RL, Hurwitz RA, Girod DA, Weyman AE, Feigenbaum H. Two-dimensional echocardiographic differentiation of anomalous left coronary artery from congestive cardiomyopathy. *Am Heart J* 1983; 106:710–716.

347. Schmidt KG, Cooper MJ, Silverman NH, Stanger P. Pulmonary artery origin of the left coronary artery: Diagnosis by two-dimensional echocardiography, pulsed Doppler ultrasound and color flow mapping. *J Am Coll Cardiol* 1988; 11:396–402.

348. Gutgesell HP, Pinsky WW, DePuey EG. Thallium-201 myocardial perfusion imaging in infants and children: Value in distinguishing anomalous left coronary artery from congestive cardiomyopathy. *Circulation* 1980; 61:596–599.

349. Sabiston DC Jr, Neill CA, Taussig HB. The direction of blood flow in anomalous left coronary artery arising from the pulmonary artery. *Circulation* 1960; 22:591–597.

350. Shrivastava S, Castaneda AR, Moller JH. Anomalous left coronary artery from pulmonary trunk: Long-term follow-up after ligation. *J Thorac Cardiovasc Surg* 1978; 76:130–134.

351. Takeuchi S, Imamura H, Katsumoto K, Hayashi I, Katoghi T, Yozu R, et al: New surgical method for repair of anomalous left coronary artery from pulmonary artery. *J Thorac Cardiovasc Surg* 1979; 78:7–11.

352. Vouhe PR, Baillot-Vernant F, Trinquet F, Sidi D, de Geeter B, Khoury W, et al. Anomalous left coronary artery from the pulmonary artery in infants. Which operation? When? *J Thorac Cardiovasc Surg* 1987; 94:192–199.

353. el-Said GM, Ruzyllo W, Williams RL, Mullins CE, Hallman GL, Cooley DA, et al. Early and late results of saphenous vein graft for anomalous origin of left coronary artery from pulmonary artery. *Circulation* 1973; 48(suppl III):2–6.

354. Rein AJ, Colan SD, Parness IA, Sanders SP. Regional and global left ventricular function in infants with anomalous origin of the left coronary artery from the pulmonary trunk: Preoperative and postoperative assessment. *Circulation* 1987; 75:115–123.

71

CONGENITAL HEART DISEASE IN ADULTS

John E. Deanfield / Bernard J. Gersh / Carole A. Warnes / Douglas D. Mair

Congenital heart disease occurs in 5 to 10 per 1000 live births.[1] Without early treatment, the majority of patients would die in infancy or childhood, with only 5 to 15 percent surviving until puberty.[2] The advent of surgical procedures, from ligation of a patent arterial duct[3] in 1939 to the innovations of the 1990s, as well as advances in medical treatment, has transformed the outlook for children with even complex defects. The majority now survive into adolescence and adult life (Chap. 70). This success story has radically altered both the size and complexity of the population of young adults with congenital heart disease. In the United States alone, well over a half million patients with functionally important congenital cardiac malformations have reached adulthood in the past three decades.[4] Despite the fact that most patients now surviving to adult life will have undergone surgery during childhood, "total correction" is not the rule.[5] The majority if not all require long-term surveillance, and many need reoperation. Other adults may require their first operation for congenital heart lesions that were well tolerated during childhood.

Both the "natural" survivors and the postoperative patients require specialized medical care. Arrhythmia is common, as are residual or deteriorating hemodynamic problems and endocarditis. Although cardiologists specializing in the care of adults may be expert in one or more of these areas, the critical relationship between rhythm and hemodynamic status in hearts with complex circulations (as after a Fontan operation or after intraatrial repair for transposition) may lead to treatment errors by those inexperienced in the treatment of congenital heart defects. Patients with cyanosis require special care because of erythrocytosis, bleeding, renal problems, and arthropathy; moreover, they require specific counseling and management regarding pregnancy. In addition to the medical problems, psychosocial problems such as the search for employment, life and health insurance, participation in sports, sexual activity, and contraception are of great importance to adolescents and young adults with congenital heart disease. Many of the "normal" ordeals of growing up are more difficult for this group, in whom chronic illness, embarrassing scars, and/or exercise limitation may inhibit normal social intercourse and maturation.

Over the last few years, the specialist needs of this growing population have begun to be appreciated. In addition to the challenge of continuing the expert care of their complex cardiac problems, from the pediatric environment into the much wider adult medical community, knowledge of the long-term fate of patients with congenital heart disease is essential for pediatric cardiologists in order to refine initial management strategy. A rather short-term view of "success" or "failure" has been encouraged by rapid changes in medical and surgical policies over the last three decades. Nevertheless, there are clear examples, such as the management of transposition of the great arteries, where awareness of long-term problems has altered the primary surgical approach. The Mustard or Senning procedures (see below) provide a physiologic repair at acceptably low risk but may result in long-term systemic ventricular dysfunction, arrhythmias, and sudden death. This has enabled the introduction of anatomic repair by the arterial-switch procedure, despite high surgical mortality in the early series, with the expectation of a more satisfactory long-term outcome. Other debates, over such issues as the place of Fontan operations, cavopulmonary anastomosis, and systemic-to-pulmonary shunts, are not yet resolved and will be strongly influenced by the accumulation of rigorously collected outcome data, not merely for survival but also for morbidity and quality of life.

The optimal solutions for delivery of care to the adult with congenital heart disease will depend on the different medical systems in operation around the world. The common requirements include collaboration between pediatric and adult cardiologists, the establishment of a few specialist centers with appropriate medical, surgical, anesthetic, and nonmedical staff together with investigational facilities, the establishment of treatment guidelines, and centralization of accumulating knowledge. The report of a consensus conference on adult congenital heart disease, commissioned by the Canadian Cardiovascular Society, represents an important step forward.[6] This includes recommendations for training and a hierarchy of care from the community to the specialist center. Similar training guidelines have been published in the United States.[7]

MEDICAL CONSIDERATIONS

Many young adults with congenital heart disease have mild lesions that have not required and may not ever require surgery. The commonest defects in this category are small ventricular septal defect, mild pulmonary valve stenosis, mild aortic valve stenosis, and mitral valve prolapse (Table 71-1). Such patients need infrequent follow-up (e.g., biannual) to assess any progression in severity of the lesion, to reinforce the need for antibiotic prophylaxis against infective endocarditis (Chap. 82), and to obtain psychosocial advice. Other patients reach adult life with more complex defects that are still uncorrected. Some may still be candidates for palliative or definitive surgery, whereas in others surgery may no longer be possible, often because of the presence of irreversible pulmonary vascular disease. More and more survivors of surgery in childhood are now reaching adult life; they now form the largest group of patients (Table 71-2). The majority need continuing medical surveillance, as late cardiovascular problems may result from hemodynamic disturbances, arrhythmia, and endocarditis.

TABLE 71-1

COMMON CONGENITAL HEART DEFECTS COMPATIBLE WITH SURVIVAL TO ADULT LIFE WITHOUT SURGERY OR INTERVENTIONAL CATHETERIZATION

Mild pulmonary valve stenosis
Peripheral pulmonary stenosis
Bicuspid aortic valve
Mild subaortic stenosis
Mild supravalvar aortic stenosis
Small atrial septal defect
Small ventricular septal defect
Small patent ductus arteriosus
Mitral valve prolapse
Ostium primum atrial septal defect (atrioventricular septal defect)
Marfan's syndrome
Ebstein's anomaly
Corrected transposition (atrioventricular-ventriculoatrial discordance)
Balanced complex lesions (e.g, double-inlet ventricle with pulmonary stenosis)
Defects with pulmonary vascular obstructive disease (Eisenmenger's syndrome)

TABLE 71-2

COMMON CONGENITAL HEART DEFECTS SURVIVING TO ADULT LIFE AFTER SURGERY/INTERVENTIONAL CATHETERIZATION

Aortic valve disease, valvotomy or replacement
Pulmonary stenosis, valvotomy
Tetralogy of Fallot
Atrial septal defect
Ventricular septal defect
Atrioventricular septal defect
Transposition of the great arteries, atrial redirection
Complex transposition of the great arteries
Total anomalous pulmonary venous connection
Pulmonary atresia/ventricular septal defect
Fontan operation for complex congenital heart disease
Ebstein's anomaly
Coarctation of the aorta
Mitral valve disease

Such patients can also develop noncardiac problems as a consequence of their heart disease (e.g., secondary to cyanosis) and are, of course, susceptible to all the potential acquired "medical problems" of adulthood.

Hemodynamics

Study of the hemodynamic consequences of repaired and unrepaired congenital heart disease is a crucial aspect of long-term follow-up. Progressive congestive cardiac failure secondary to myocardial deterioration is the most common cause of disability and death in patients whose ventricles may have been subjected to many years of volume and pressure loading, often with chronic hypoxia. A significant number of the adult postoperative patients with congenital heart disease have been repaired at older ages than is the current practice. This may result in greater preoperative damage and pulmonary vascular disease, which may persist postoperatively. In the early era of open-heart surgery, myocardial protection was sometimes less than optimal, resulting in myocardial damage.

It should also be appreciated that postoperative circulations created by the repair of many congenital heart defects result in an adequate physiologic repair (e.g., deoxygenated blood to lungs and oxygenated blood to the body) but often have very far from normal anatomy. For example, after the Mustard and Senning operation for transposition of the great arteries, the right ventricle remains on the systemic side of the circulation. Some of these patients have evidence of deteriorating right ventricular function, and there is increasing concern that this will become a major life-threatening problem with longer follow-up.[8] Similar concerns have been expressed for systemic ventricular function after the Fontan operation.[9] The different morphology and loading conditions for these ventricles suggest that standard indices of ventricular function, derived from studies of structurally normal hearts, may be inappropriate for such patients[10] (see also Chap. 22). Prospective serial studies are beginning to define "normal ranges" for congenital heart defects and to examine their "natural" and "unnatural" history.[11,12]

Residual hemodynamic defects are often present in repaired patients and may cause problems even many years after surgery. These may be amenable to further surgery (see below) or require long-term medical treatment. Medical management of cardiac failure in patients with congenital heart disease is adopting newer therapies shown to be of benefit in recent large-scale clinical trials of patients with heart failure from predominantly cardiomyopathy or ischemic heart disease.[13–15] Appreciation of ventricular "remodeling" and the effect of neurohumeral responses on symptoms and disease progression has led to increasing and earlier use of angiotensin-converting enzyme inhibitors and, in some cases, beta blockers and long-acting calcium antagonists in addition to standard therapy with digoxin and diuretics (see Chap. 23). These may also slow the rate of progressive deterioration in ventricular function reported in certain congenital heart diseases even when they have been adequately "corrected."

Cyanosis

Adults with congenital heart disease may have central cyanosis from right-to-left shunting secondary to their uncorrected cardiac defect or to pulmonary vascular disease (Eisenmenger's syndrome) (see Chap. 70). The latter complication should be seen less frequently in years ahead as a result of the trend to early recognition and repair of congenital heart disease in infancy. Currently, however, a significant number of patients reach adult life with pulmonary vascular disease as a result of lesions such as large ventricular septal defect, atrioventricular septal defect, truncus arteriosus, and double-outlet right ventricle. Their pulmonary vascular resistance may already have been too high for surgical repair at the time of diagnosis; in others, pulmonary vascular disease may have progressed despite repair of the congenital heart defect.

Chronic cyanosis may lead to erythrocytosis and hyperviscosity.[16] Many patients with cyanotic congenital heart disease establish a stable high hematocrit but few symptoms of hyperviscosity.[17] They have a low risk of stroke and do not require venesection.[18] In others, the hemoglobin concentration may rise progressively. Once it exceeds 20 g/dL, they are at risk from thromboembolic complications and may suffer from headache, dizziness, and fatigue.[19] Symptoms may be improved by judicious venesection to hemoglobin levels of 17 to 18 g/dL. This can be performed by the removal of 500 mL of blood and volume replacement with normal saline.[18,20] Overzealous venesection, however, may result in both acute and chronic problems, including cardiovascular collapse in patients with Eisenmenger's syndrome, iron depletion, microcytosis, and hyperviscosity in its own right.[21] The paradoxical anemia of erythrocytotic patients with iron deficiency due to repeated phlebotomy may be missed and indeed has been shown to increase the risk of stroke.[22] This study demonstrated

that phlebotomies and microcytosis were strongly associated with stroke, perhaps due to the fact that iron-deficient red blood cells are less deformable than normal red blood cells and do not pass through the microcirculation as readily as iron-replete cells.[23]

Patients with chronic cyanosis also develop defective hemostasis from abnormalities in platelet function and in the coagulation and fibrinolytic systems,[24] especially in patients with marked erythrocytosis. The risk of hemorrhage, especially at surgery, is well recognized and may be fatal. Hyperuricemia is common because of increased red cell turnover and renal dysfunction.[25] Arthralgia is well recognized, but gouty arthritis is rare and may be misdiagnosed. Other important problems include acne and renal impairment, which can deteriorate to renal failure as a result of relatively minor interventions, such as injection of contrast medium at angiography.[26] Patients with right-to-left shunts are at risk of paradoxic embolus, which may cause a cerebrovascular accident or renal infarction. A cerebral abscess is a well-known complication of a septic embolus and must always be considered in the cyanotic patient with sudden onset of headache, somnolence, other neurologic symptoms, or low-grade fever. A specific concern has been the safety of air travel in adults with cyanotic congenital heart disease, as in-flight atmospheric conditions on commercial jets approach altitude equivalents of 6000 to 8000 ft (1829 to 2438 m). In a recent report, however, only modest (approximately 6 percent) decreases in systemic arterial oxygen saturation were found, with no adverse effects.[27]

The prognosis for patients with Eisenmenger's syndrome depends to a great extent on their management. A number of vasodilator drugs—including calcium channel blockers, angiotensin converting enzyme inhibitors, hydralazine, and nitrates—have been used, but no treatment has been shown to produce regression or to alter the progress of pulmonary vascular disease.[28–30] Death may result from right-sided heart failure,[31] pulmonary hemorrhage, or arrhythmia.[31,32] It can also occur prematurely due to potentially avoidable complications such as inappropriate drug therapy or injudicious general anesthesia.

Progressive kyphoscoliosis has been recognized for many years as a complication of congenital heart disease.[33] This is common in cyanotic patients and in those with previous thoracotomy. The degree of deformity, if left untreated, may become profound and compromise pulmonary function. Treatment with bracing or insertion of a Harrington rod may be indicated even if the patient has an uncorrectable cardiac lesion, since the kyphoscoliosis may significantly reduce both the quality and quantity of life.

Infective Endocarditis

Patients with both unoperated and operated congenital heart disease are at risk from infective endocarditis. Lifelong antibiotic prophylaxis is recommended, but the specific indications and optimal regimens are still debated.[34,35] The American

Heart Association Special Report on Prevention of Infective Endocarditis has stratified risk groups for the various lesions.[35] Prophylaxis is advocated for all lesions except secundum atrial septal defect closed by direct suture or a divided patent ductus arteriosus (see Chap. 82). The wide variety of portals of entry include dental work, skin sepsis, obstetric and gynecologic procedures, genitourinary and gastrointestinal interventions, cardiac catheterization, transesophageal echocardiography, and surgery.[36–40] There is also a risk of bacteremia and infective endocarditis in young adults who have their ears pierced or acquire a tattoo. Patients must be educated and preferably should carry an information card with them. The symptoms of endocarditis may be subtle, and the diagnosis must be considered in any patient who experiences unexplained malaise or fever. Injudicious prescription of antibiotics without previous blood culture may mask the problem and make bacteriologic diagnosis and appropriate treatment difficult. Both general measures—such as oral hygiene as well as skin and nail care—and appropriate antibiotic treatment are important. Among 102 patients with congenital heart disease who filled in a questionnaire, there was a disturbing lack of knowledge about endocarditis prevention measures and indeed about their cardiac lesion in general.[41]

Electrophysiologic Problems

Arrhythmias and conduction defects have a major impact on the prognosis and management of both unoperated and operated patients and have been linked to sudden death in a number of conditions.[42–44] The principles of diagnosis and treatment are similar to those employed in patients with arrhythmia due to other causes (see Chap. 27). In unoperated patients, chamber dilatation, myocardial hypertrophy, and fibrosis may all contribute to the genesis of arrhythmia. In operated patients, additional sinus or atrioventricular node damage and atrial and/or ventricular scarring may cause electrophysiologic problems. The etiology is multifactorial and the clinical significance of arrhythmia depends very much on the hemodynamic context in which it occurs. Rhythm disturbances that might be benign in a structurally normal heart may be life-threatening in congenital heart disease.

Supraventricular arrhythmia and sinus node injury, not surprisingly, occur most often in conditions with "atrial defects" or those requiring atrial surgery.[43,45,46] Abnormalities of sinus node function are common in patients with atrial septal defect, particularly the sinus venosus type,[47] and are often seen after Mustard or Senning operation for transposition of the great arteries.[48] Sinus node dysfunction has also been reported after surgery for tetralogy of Fallot, the Fontan procedure, and many other operations for congenital heart lesions.[49,50] Clinical manifestations include sinus bradycardia, sinoatrial block, sinus arrest, and occasionally the tachybradycardia syndrome with paroxysmal atrial flutter and fibrillation. Although bradycardia has been postulated as the cause of sudden death in some conditions, current evidence indicates that tachyarrhythmia is usually a more likely explanation[48] (see below).

In sinus node disease, insertion of a pacemaker is indicated for patients with symptoms resulting from a slow heart rate such as tiredness, dizziness, and syncope or for an extremely low heart rate (see Chap. 34). Indications in asymptomatic individuals are still controversial, since the arrhythmia is benign in many cases. It should be noted that pacing may be difficult because of the complex underlying anatomy and lack of a suitable site for endocardial lead fixation. The choice of pacemaker will depend on the precise indication. The simplest VVI pacemaker may be adequate prophylaxis against bradycardia-related sudden death. In general, however, rate-responsive pacemakers are preferable and dual-chamber pacing may provide the best hemodynamics[51,52] (see also Chap. 34).

Injury to the atrioventricular (AV) node and proximal conduction tissue may result from surgery for lesions such as ventricular septal defect, AV septal defect, or tetralogy of Fallot. High-grade AV block was seen more commonly in the early era of surgery.[53] Transient complete AV block in the postoperative period has been shown to have prognostic significance in some reports, particularly if the site of damage is below the bundle of His. In a recent 30-year follow-up of ventricular septal defect repair at the Mayo Clinic, the development of transient complete heart block for over 72 h followed by resumption of sinus rhythm was a strong independent predictor of late mortality.[54] Whether or not transient perioperative AV block warrants permanent pacing and whether or not an invasive electrophysiologic study can help stratify risk are unresolved.[45] Postoperative right bundle branch block is frequent after ventriculotomy and may be due to injury related to closure of a ventricular septal defect or to interruption of distal Purkinje fibers by ventriculotomy or muscle resection.[43–45] Occasionally, the electrocardiographic pattern of right bundle branch block with left axis deviation occurs (bifascicular block), and there may also be PR interval prolongation (trifascicular block).[55,56] Early reports suggested that these findings were harbingers of sudden cardiac death due to complete heart block.[57] More recent studies, however, have not substantiated this adverse prognosis.[58]

Tachyarrhythmias can be life-threatening. Late sudden death has been reported in several lesions, both before and after repair. In general, the worse the disease (i.e., more complex anatomy and/or more extensive surgery), the greater the incidence of sudden death.[45] The identification of patients at risk and their management are important but controversial issues. After the Mustard and Senning operation, atrial flutter with a rapid ventricular response is dangerous, especially when it occurs in association with right ventricular dysfunction or venous pathway obstruction.[59] Medical or electrical cardioversion should be promptly used to restore sinus rhythm, and drug therapy may need to be accompanied by pacemaker insertion. Recently, ablation (surgical or catheter) has been advocated for certain cases of atrial flutter (see Chap. 31). Atrial tachyarrhythmias are also common after the Fontan operation; sinus node injury, atrial suturing, and a dilated hypertensive right atrium probably contribute.[45,50] Modification of the operation to exclude the right atrium from the

Fontan circuit, the total cavopulmonary connection, may reduce the incidence of potentially serious early and late rhythm disturbances.[60,61]

Ventricular arrhythmias are known to occur after open-heart surgery, particularly repair of tetralogy of Fallot.[56,62–64] Studies using ambulatory electrocardiographic (ECG) monitoring in postoperative patients have documented asymptomatic complex ectopy and nonsustained ventricular tachycardia in up to 50 percent of patients,[63–65] and up to 30 percent have inducible ventricular tachycardia at electrophysiologic study.[66] Experimental and clinical studies have shown that the electrical substrate for reentry arrhythmia is present in the right ventricle.[67] In several reports, older age at surgery is a predisposing factor,[65,68] an observation that suggests factors present at the time of repair may be involved in the genesis of postoperative arrhythmia in addition to the myocardial damage occurring at the time of surgery or during postoperative follow-up.[69] This is consistent with morphologic studies that have documented increasing fibrosis of the right ventricle as part of the natural history of defects such as tetralogy of Fallot.[70,71] The current practice of early surgical repair for tetralogy of Fallot may reduce the incidence of such postoperative ventricular arrhythmia, and encouraging preliminary data support this view.[69,72] Other postulated risk factors include elevated right ventricular systolic pressure, reduced right ventricular ejection fraction, pulmonary regurgitation, and a ventriculotomy scar.[66,73,74] The clinical significance of nonsustained ventricular tachycardia and especially the indications for prophylactic antiarrhythmic therapy remain unclear.[59] There is a disparity between the high frequency of ventricular arrhythmia and the much lower incidence of sudden death.[62,75,76] In the 30-year follow-up series from the Mayo Clinic, the risk of sudden death was highest in the first few years after repair without any evidence of an increasing hazard with time. The predictive value of an abnormal ambulatory ECG or of electrophysiologic study has not been established. Furthermore, prophylactic antiarrhythmic therapy has not been shown to be of value in asymptomatic patients with congenital heart defects. Such therapy may have proarrhythmic potential, be negatively inotropic, or have serious extracardiac side effects. As a result, there is insufficient evidence to advocate prophylactic treatment for asymptomatic individuals with nonsustained arrhythmia. On the other hand, there are a few cases of sudden death, out of hospital ventricular fibrillation, and/or sustained ventricular tachycardia in almost all large series of patients after repair of tetralogy of Fallot. Identification of "at risk" individuals and appropriate treatment remains a challenge. Recent reports have indicated a link between the electrical and mechanical properties of the right ventricle, which may have clinical relevance.[77] Restrictive right ventricular physiology can be detected in a proportion of patients late after repair and this is associated with reduced pulmonary regurgitation, smaller right ventricular dimensions, and improved exercise tolerance. The QRS duration on the surface ECG correlates well with cardiothoracic ratio and, in a retrospective review, a QRS of >180 ms was a sensitive and specific marker for sudden death or out-of-hospital cardiac arrest.[78] This simple measurement may be useful for risk stratification and is being tested in prospective multicenter clinical studies. Further refinements in risk stratification in adults with tetralogy of Fallot or other congenital heart lesions will involve hemodynamic and electrophysiologic testing both at rest and after exercise, evaluation of ventricular late potentials (Chap. 29), and heart rate variability. It should be remembered, however, that despite the attention given to ventricular arrhythmia after repair of tetralogy of Fallot, a major source of morbidity in such patients is from atrial arrhythmia.[79] Radiofrequency ablation, so successfully used to treat arrhythmia in patients with structurally normal hearts (Chap. 31), is being applied to patients with congenital heart disease. These represent some of the most challenging electrophysiologic procedures because of the complex cardiac anatomy, enlarged chamber size, and abnormal localization of the underlying conduction system. Nevertheless, ablation may have a role, not merely in subjects with accessory pathways or atrioventricular reentry tachycardia but also in intra-atrial reentry arrhythmias that may be present after operations such as Fontan and Mustard or Senning procedures.[80–82]

Pregnancy

An increasing number of women with complex and postoperative congenital heart defects are reaching childbearing age. Advice is sought on both maternal and fetal risk as well as on the incidence of congenital heart disease in the offspring. Firm recommendations for many conditions are difficult, as most experience has been gathered for patients with relatively simple defects such as secundum atrial septal defect and patent ductus arteriosus.[83] It has been estimated that congenital heart disease accounts for approximately 10 percent of heart disease cases in pregnancy and up to 1 percent of maternal deaths.[84]

There are profound changes in the maternal cardiovascular system during pregnancy, including a large (30 to 40 percent) increase in blood volume, a fall in peripheral vascular resistance, and an increase in cardiac output (approximately 40 percent)[85] (see also Chap. 92). In general, women with left-to-right shunts or valvular regurgitation tolerate pregnancy well, whereas those with right-to-left shunts or valvular stenosis do less well. Asymptomatic young women with small or moderate left-to-right shunts and normal pulmonary artery pressures can expect an uncomplicated pregnancy and labor. In the presence of a large left-to-right shunt, however, heart failure may be provoked or aggravated by pregnancy. Patients with cyanosis have the most problems in carrying a fetus to term and have a high incidence of early spontaneous abortion. Early studies showed that with higher degrees of cyanosis (as reflected by the maternal hemoglobin), the incidence of spontaneous abortion increased and the handicap to fetal growth became more pronounced. Infants are unlikely to survive if the maternal hemoglobin is >18 g/dL.[86] A recent study from Presbitero et al. demonstrated a clear relationship between the degree of hypoxia and fetal loss.[87] (Table 71-3).

TABLE 71-3

FETAL OUTCOME IN CYANOTIC
CONGENITAL HEART DISEASE
AND ITS RELATION WITH MATERNAL CYANOSIS

Hemoglobin, g/dL[a]	Pregnancy, no.	Live Births, no.	Live Born, %
≤16	28	20	71
17–19	40	18	45
≥20	26	2	8

Arterial Oxygen Saturation, %[b]	Pregnancy, no.	Live Births, no.	Live Born, %
≤85	17	2	12
85–89	22	10	45
≥90	13	12	92

[a] Hemoglobin level unknown in two pregnancies.
[b] Arterial oxygen saturation unknown in 44 pregnancies.
Source: From Presbitero P, Somerville J, Stone S, et al. Pregnancy in cyanotic congenital heart disease: Outcome of mother and fetus. *Circulation* 1994; 89:2673–2676. Reproduced with permission from the publisher and authors.

When the maternal oxygen saturation was ≤85 percent, only 2 out of 17 pregnancies (12 percent) resulted in live-born infants. Only 41 of 96 pregnancies (43 percent) produced a live birth in 45 cyanosed mothers. There were 49 spontaneous abortions and 6 stillbirths in this series, again reflecting the high risk that maternal cyanotic congenital heart disease poses for the fetus. Meticulous care during pregnancy and delivery lessened the maternal complication rate, but this was still considerable. Such patients require rest and a short labor as well as avoidance of dehydration and sepsis. In such situations, the decision as to whether or not to continue with the pregnancy depends on an assessment of the risk to the mother and fetus as compared with the patient's desire to have children. An elevated pulmonary vascular resistance, from either Eisenmenger's syndrome or primary pulmonary hypertension, is a clear contraindication to pregnancy.[86] Pregnancy for women with Eisenmenger's syndrome carries approximately a 50 percent mortality.[88] Termination of pregnancy is always preferable; ideally, this should be done with cardiac anesthesia. If such patients are seen late in pregnancy and termination is not feasible, management should concentrate on maintenance of adequate preload and avoidance of vasodilation. The ideal management around the time of delivery is controversial because individual experience is small. Vaginal delivery is usually associated with less blood loss than cesarean section. The latter, however, can be done quickly with all medical personnel in attendance. One report has suggested an approach of elective delivery by cesarean section under general anesthesia.[89] The use of prophylactic heparin before and after delivery is also controversial, and there is no established consensus.[89,90] Even after successful delivery, however, death frequently occurs within the few days following from deteriorating hemodynamics or pulmonary infarction.[88,91] Patients with Marfan's syndrome and aortic root dilation and those with severe aortic stenosis are also at increased risk. While early reports suggested a high risk of aortic rupture and cerebral hemorrhage in patients with aortic coarctation,[92] more recent data have been more encouraging.[93] Fetal risk is increased, however, presumably as a result of compromised placental blood supply.

The management of pregnant women with prosthetic cardiac valves is a special problem because of the risk to the mother of thromboembolism and the risk to the fetus of anticoagulants (warfarin crosses the placenta and is teratogenic).[94–97] Depending on the condition involved and the mother's motivation and compliance, the use of subcutaneous heparin in the first and third trimesters and warfarin in midtrimester is one treatment option. Heparin, however, is a poor anticoagulant during pregnancy; even with meticulous control of anticoagulation, there is still an increased risk of valve thrombosis.[98] In addition, there is also an increased risk of fetal loss with this approach. Because of the poor results with heparin, some authors have advocated the use of warfarin throughout pregnancy despite the risk of fetal teratogenicity.[99] This risk may be less if the dose of warfarin is <5 mg/day.[100] Nonetheless, this approach is still very controversial despite the fact that fetal teratogenicity with warfarin may have been overemphasized[101] (see Chap. 52). Before prescribing any cardiovascular drug during pregnancy, the effects on both mother and fetus must be considered. Management of labor should be specifically directed toward avoidance of rapid changes in circulatory volume, blood pressure, or cardiac output. In most cases vaginal delivery is recommended, with careful attention to maternal position and analgesic agents. The American Heart Association no longer recommends endocarditis prophylaxis for vaginal delivery.[35] This, however, is not based on controlled data, and most cardiologists recommend antibiotics under these circumstances for almost all congenital heart defects.

Genetic Counseling

The risk of recurrence is an increasingly important issue as more males and females with congenital heart disease reach reproductive age, and genetic counseling should be provided for all potential parents. Recent genetic advances are clarifying the etiology of a number of congenital heart diseases. It has been estimated that the cause of congenital heart disease is genetic in approximately 8 percent of cases (e.g. velocardiofacial syndrome and Holt-Oram syndrome with autosomal dominant transmission) and environmental in 2 percent (e.g., congenital rubella syndrome).[102] In the remainder, genetic and environmental factors are thought to interact.[103] The greater the number of affected first-degree relatives within the family, the greater the recurrence risk. Recurrence risks in siblings of patients with congenital heart disease are well documented and range between 1 and 8 percent.[104] For the affected potential parents, however, the risk of recurrence in offspring is the key information, and fewer data exist. Early reports suggested that recurrence risks were considerably higher in offspring compared to siblings. In a series of 233 women with congenital heart disease followed through 482 pregnancies, the overall incidence of heart disease in offspring was 16.1 percent.[105] More recent studies, such as the Second Natural History of Congenital Heart Defects (NHS-2), have suggested a much lower risk (1.2 percent for aortic stenosis, 2.8 percent for pulmonary stenosis and 2.9 percent for ventricular septal defects).[106] A number of factors inherent in the study design and nature of follow-up may account for the differences in recurrence risks reported. In addition, certain forms of congenital heart disease recur more frequently than others (e.g., left ventricular outflow tract obstruction) and the recurrence risk appears to be higher in pregnancies with affected mothers rather than fathers. Accumulation of further information will be invaluable for patient counseling.

Investigation and Imaging

Transthoracic echocardiography and cardiac catheterization with

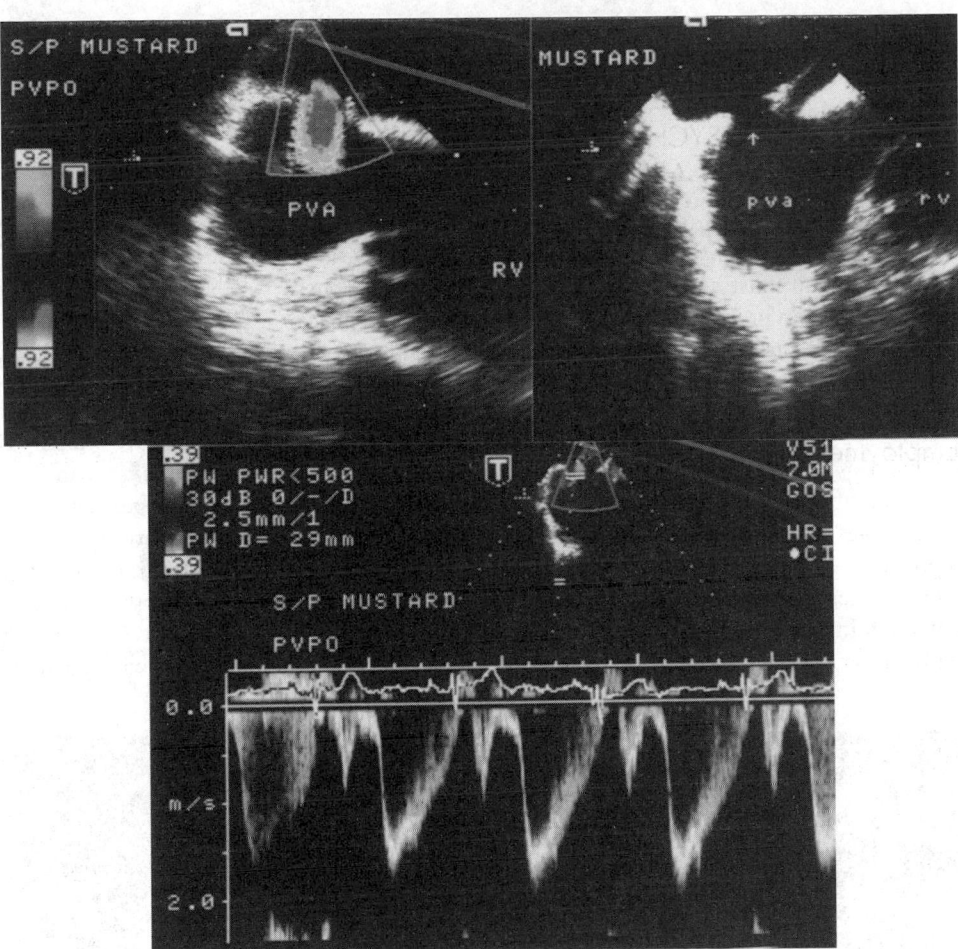

FIGURE 71-1
Transoesophageal echocardiogram and Doppler evaluation after Mustard operation for transposition of the great arteries. There is moderate pulmonary venous obstruction indicated by the accelerated flow through the narrowing indicated by the arrow. pva = pulmonary venous atrium; RV = right ventricle. (Courtesy of Dr ID Sullivan, Great Ormond Street Hospital for Children, London.)

angiocardiography are the principal investigations in pediatric cardiology. In adults, transoesophageal echocardiography is becoming increasingly important for the definition of cardiac structure and function. Precordial imaging becomes more difficult in the older patient with the natural reduction in the size of the ultrasound window further compromised by chest wall abnormalities as a result of surgery and cardiac malposition. Multiplane probes with color-flow Doppler allow simultaneous assessment of anatomy and physiology. Specific areas of the heart that are well imaged in this way include systemic and pulmonary venous drainage, atrial lesions (including baffle function), AV valve morphology and function, left ventricular outflow tract lesions (including the ascending aorta in Marfan's syndrome), as well as intracavity thrombus or vegetations (Fig. 71-1).

Magnetic resonance imaging can also provide valuable anatomic information, which in some cases is superior to that from ultrasound even via a transesophageal approach. Rapid technologic advances—including three-dimensional image reconstruction, software to study hemodynamics such

as velocity mapping, and cine magnetic resonance imaging—may reduce the need for invasive investigation (Fig. 71-2). The expertise required both to acquire and interpret MRI information is likely to be confined to specialized regional centers, but access to the MRI facility should be available to all units managing adult patients with congenital heart disease.

In parallel with the decreasing need for diagnostic cardiac catheterization, there has been a dramatic rise in the indications for and scope of interventional procedures in adult patients with congenital heart disease. Residual defects after repair that are amenable to treatment in the catheterization laboratory include coronary fistulas, paravalvular leaks, and pulmonary artery stenoses. Optimum management of patients with complex congenital heart disease can often be achieved by planned collaboration between surgeon and interventional cardiologist. In other patients with a range of relatively simple lesions—including patent ductus arteriosus, aortic valve stenosis, pulmonary valve stenosis, atrial septal defect/patent foramen ovale, and certain forms of ventricular septal defect—

definitive treatment avoiding surgery may be achieved by interventional catheterization.

PSYCHOSOCIAL ASPECTS

During adolescence, a crucial transition occurs for the patient with congenital heart disease. By the end of the teenage years, the young adult must understand the nature and implications of his or her heart problem. Sensible advice and guidance must be available regarding employment, insurance, socialization, contraception, exercise, and sports.

Employment

Most patients can work and should have access to employment appropriate to their physical and intellectual capabilities. The report of the Natural History Study of Congenital Heart Defects suggested that among patients with ventricular septal defect, pulmonary stenosis, and aortic stenosis, in comparison with national normal standards, a greater percentage achieved higher levels of education (college and beyond).[107] No similar data are yet available for large groups of patients with more complex defects, although their situation will undoubtedly prove worse.

Despite the excellent potential of many adults with congenital heart disease, job discrimination is frequently encountered, even when a patient has been cleared by a cardiologist. In the United States, the National Rehabilitation Act of 1973 seeks to prevent job discrimination by employers with ≥10 employees by obliging them to consider only the present capacity of applicants to perform a given job and not projections of future deterioration. In other countries, employers frequently take into account future prospects for absenteeism or premature career curtailment. In these circumstances, young adults with congenital heart defects are often at a disadvantage, particularly if they apply for jobs with long training periods.

Restrictions for employment exist for jobs in which the safety of others is the direct responsibility of an individual, such as driving a bus or truck. Most armed services exclude applicants with a cardiac history. The regulations for commercial airline pilots are clearer and subject to regular review. In Europe, a risk of sudden cardiac death or acute disability below 1 percent per annum is the maximum considered acceptable for multicrew flights and 0.1 percent for solo flights.[108] The number of congenital heart defects in which such low risk rates are clearly defined remains small.[109]

Insurance

Possession of adequate life insurance is often a prerequisite for a home mortgage. Insurance companies are of necessity fiscally conservative. As a result, life insurance is difficult to obtain for many young adults in the absence of adequate long-term survival data for their congenital heart lesions. Most of the data used to assess risk are either incorrect or out of date and do not apply to currently performed medical or surgical procedures. In 1986, a survey in the United States recorded that only patients with very simple lesions were insured at regular rates.[110] These included mild pulmonary valve stenosis, uncomplicated corrected atrial septal defect, ventricular septal defect, and patent ductus

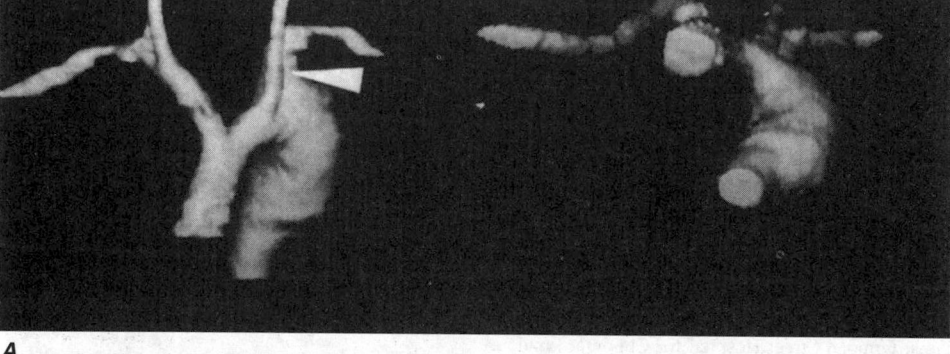

A

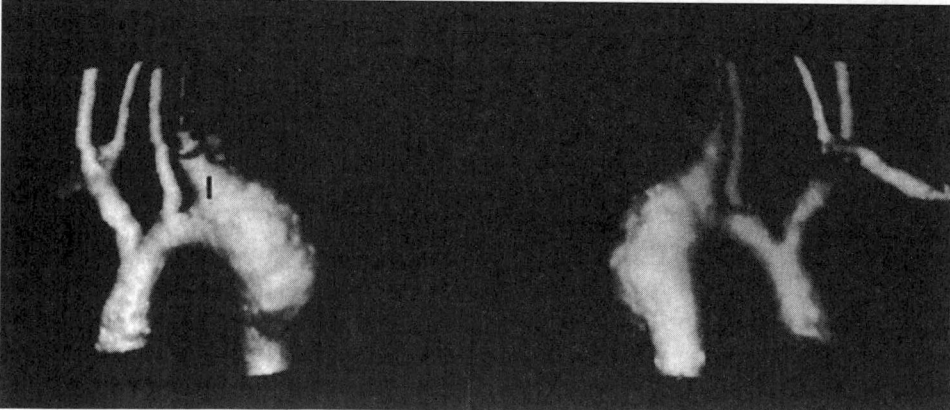

B

FIGURE 71-2

Three-dimensional surface MR image of the aorta in a 21-year-old man 15 years after repair of coarctation involving insertion of a Dacron patch. A large aneurysm is shown in multiple views involving the base of the left subclavian artery. (From Parks WJ, Ngo TD, Plauth WH, Bank ER, Sheppard SK, Pettigrew RI, et al. Incidence of aneurysm formation after Dacron patch aortoplasty repair for coarctation of the aorta: Long-term results and assessment utilizing magnetic resonance angiography with three-dimensional surface rendering. *J Am Coll Cardiol* 1995; 26:266–271. Reproduced with permission from the publisher and authors.)

arteriosus. A similar survey in the United Kingdom in 1993 evaluated both employment status and insurability of young adults with congenital heart disease.[111] In general, policies were as restrictive as those in the earlier survey, with mitral valve prolapse (without regurgitation), postoperative patent ductus arteriosus, and coarctation insurable at standard rates and all other lesions being either insurable at higher rates or not insurable at all. Marked inconsistencies were found, making "shopping around" mandatory. This situation is likely to improve when health care professionals are able to provide high-quality follow-up data on morbidity and mortality relevant to current treatment protocols (see Chap. 104).

Despite surgical repair, long-term cardiac care into adult life is usually required for patients with congenital heart disease. In many countries, health care provision and financing are changing rapidly, with costs spiraling dramatically.[112] There are particular problems in systems that rely on private health insurance. Medical expenses incurred during childhood are usually reimbursed as part of the parents' policy. This coverage often ceases to be available once the patient reaches the age of majority. A new policy sought at this stage at best excludes benefits for medical or surgical treatment of the cardiac condition itself. As a result, the level of medical surveillance of the adult patient with congenital heart disease drops dramatically after age 21 years. This is a major problem as, with adequate regular follow-up, costs for adults with congenital heart disease are considerably lower than those for other chronic diseases.

Psychosocial Development

Large controlled longitudinal studies of the psychosocial consequences of congenital heart disease are rare and difficult to interpret.[113] Most patients with congenital heart disease appear well adjusted but have subtle feelings of "difference" from their peers. Lack of self-esteem and fear of isolation are common.[114] These feelings are often compounded by frequent reminders that they are different through limitation of their activities compared with those of their peers, the presence of scars, cardiac symptoms, hospital visits, and family anxiety. As a result, adolescents and adults with congenital heart disease should be encouraged to lead as normal a life as possible and to discuss their heart disease openly. Anxieties about sexual activity, marriage, and childbirth are common, but patients often find these aspects difficult to discuss, particularly with the doctor in a regular clinic.[115] Often, such issues are best handled by the team caring for the patient, which may include a nurse, social worker, and psychologist. As the child with congenital heart disease matures, one of the most potent effects on his or her life is parental overprotection. In adolescents and young adults, this may result in enormous resentment and rebellion against all adult authority figures, including the doctor. Compliance with medical treatment and advice can be affected.

The impact of congenital heart disease on intellectual development is controversial. Interpretation of testing must take into account the very abnormal childhood experienced by many patients, with absences from school for medical reasons as well as decreased social interaction. In addition, patients have often had an overprotected childhood, and their attitude to testing procedures may be different. All studies of intellect exclude patients with genetic syndromes and other dysmorphic, somatic, or neurologic defects, but subtle abnormalities are easily missed.[116] Certain aspects of development appear to be more specifically affected by congenital heart disease. For example, walking is delayed in cyanotic children, but speech is not. This will affect the relevance of early IQ testing on later performance. Currently, data suggest that cyanosis is associated with mild intellectual impairment.[117–119] This is reduced by early corrective surgery even involving cardiopulmonary bypass.

Contraception

Sexually active adolescents and young adults should be given appropriate advice about contraception.[120] In general, the low-dose estrogen oral contraceptive pill is safe for young women with congenital heart disease.[121] Exceptions include women with hypertension (e.g., associated with coarctation of the aorta) and those with pulmonary vascular disease or cyanosis with associated erythrocytosis. Progesterone preparations are alternatives, although they have a lower contraceptive efficacy.[122] They are, however, inappropriate for patients with cardiac failure because of the tendency for fluid retention; moreover, progesterone-only pills can cause depression in adolescents. Barrier methods, either using condom or diaphragm, are safe and effective, but intrauterine devices should probably not be used because of the risk of endocarditis and of increased bleeding, particularly in cyanotic women.[123] In women with severe pulmonary vascular disease or with lesions in which pregnancy would result in high maternal risk, laparoscopic sterilization should be considered.

Exercise/Sports

Exercise is of both physical and psychological benefit. It leads to improved cardiovascular fitness and decreased likelihood of obesity, hypertension, and ischemic heart disease.[124–126] Furthermore, participation in exercise and sports is part of normal socialization in adolescent and adult life. In many adults with congenital heart disease, exercise capacity is diminished, even after surgery. Reduced performance may also reflect lack of regular exercise in protected individuals with congenital heart defects. This is often reinforced by doctors who, if in doubt, tend to limit exercise.

The Sixteenth Bethesda Conference provided recommendations for competition in athletics by patients with cardiovascular abnormalities,[127] but it remains difficult to make dogmatic recommendations.[128] In some cases, exercise capacity is clearly normal and the risk is minimal, as after closure of a small patent ductus arteriosus. In others, exercise capacity is limited and the risk is high, as in severe left ventricular hypertrophy. Between these extremes is a gray area in which recommendations must take into account the individual, the underlying cardiac defect, hemodynamic status, and the type of sport and form of exercise contemplated (e.g., isotonic or isometric, social or competitive, contact or noncontact). Formal testing should be performed (preferably including measurement of oxygen uptake), both as a measure of the effects of submaximal and maximal exercise and also as a reassurance to the patient. A 12-min walking test gives a good guide to functional capacity, whereas a treadmill protocol with more strenuous effort is employed to assess risk by revealing occult arrhythmia, ischemia, or fall in blood pressure (Chap. 15). Subjective estimates of exercise capacity are often inaccurate.

In general, volume overload, valve regurgitation, and left-to-right shunts are associated with good exercise tolerance, whereas pressure overload, valve stenosis, and right-to-left shunt are not. Recommendations for individual lesions are given in Tables 71-4 to 71-6. These should be considered as guidelines only, as adequate information to assess capacity and associated risk is not yet available for many conditions. Patients with fixed, elevated pulmonary vascular resistance have limited exercise capacity, and for them exercise has considerable risk. As a result, most forms of active exercise should be avoided. The most controversial recommendations are those for aortic stenosis and Marfan's syndrome. It could be argued that exercise has an adverse effect on sudden death or the progression of left ventricular hypertrophy in the former (see Chap. 63) and may increase the risk of progressive aortic dilatation in the latter (see Chap. 85). In the absence of formal data, however, we currently allow such patients to take part in a noncompetitive sport. In patients with Marfan's syndrome, we measure the aortic root dimensions at frequent intervals. Patients with Marfan's syndrome and normal dimensions of the aortic root for age and size appear to have normal exercise capacity and no additional cardiovascular risk. Supervised training programs for adults with congenital heart disease can improve aerobic fitness and increase the safe level at which they can participate in sports. Such programs also improve psychological adjustment and self-esteem.

TABLE 71-4

CONGENITAL CONDITIONS IN WHICH EXERCISE ORDINARILY SHOULD NOT BE LIMITED OTHER THAN BY THE PATIENT'S OWN DESIRE

Left-to-right shunts without ventricular dysfunction or pulmonary vascular disease

Mild-to-moderate valvular regurgitation

Mild valvular stenosis

Marfan's syndrome with normal aorta

Most arrhythmias in the structurally normal heart, including Wolff-Parkinson-White syndrome

Postoperative patients with excellent hemodynamic repairs, such as closure of atrial septal defect or some cases of tetralogy of Fallot

TABLE 71-5

CONGENITAL CONDITIONS IN WHICH STRENUOUS SPORTS SHOULD BE RESTRICTED BUT IN WHICH LESSER LEVELS OF EXERCISE MAY USUALLY BE ALLOWED

Mild hypertrophic cardiomyopathy

Mild left ventricular outflow tract obstruction

Marfan's syndrome with aortic root dilatation less than 5 cm

Ventricular dysfunction with ejection fraction less than 40%

Postoperative atrial redirection for transposition of the great arteries

Hearts with univentricular atrioventricular connection (preoperative and postoperative)

Some arrhythmias

Some treated hypertensive patients after coarctation repair

SURGICAL CONSIDERATIONS

Reoperations

Reoperations in adults with congenital heart disease provide a particular challenge.[129] The risks are often higher than for primary procedures. Careful preoperative planning should include complete understanding of the cardiac anatomy and its relations and study of previous operative reports. In a multicenter study using a questionnaire, catastrophic hemorrhage occurred in 144 patients during sternal reentry, with a 37 percent mortality. Eighty-eight percent occurred in situations where the pericardium was not closed at the time of the first operation.[130] Sternal reentry is particularly risky when the ventricle immediately beneath the sternum is a high-pressure chamber or when an extracardiac conduit lies in this position. Reentry via a different surgical approach (e.g., thoracotomy after sternotomy) can avoid adhesions and thus minimize bleeding. The current use of Gore-Tex membranes under the sternum may reduce the difficulties of future repeat proce-

TABLE 71-6

CONGENITAL CONDITIONS IN WHICH ALL MODERATE AND STRENUOUS EXERCISE SHOULD BE RESTRICTED

Moderate and severe hypertrophic cardiomyopathy

Moderate and severe pulmonary vascular disease

Severe valvular stenosis

Marfan's syndrome with aortic root more than 5 cm in diameter

Long-QT syndrome with exercise-induced ventricular tachycardia

Postoperative patients with exercise-induced ventricular tachycardia

dures. Postoperative hemodynamic and respiratory problems are particularly common after reoperation because of the increased duration of surgery, previously scarred myocardium and/or lung disease, and greater use of blood products. The need for reoperation may come as a shock to patients and relatives who may have believed that childhood surgery was curative. As a result, resentment is frequent and tact is required. Indications for reoperation are shown in Table 71-7.

Inevitable Reoperation

Early repair of congenital heart defects that have involved insertion of a prosthetic valve or extracardiac conduit commonly results in a need for reoperation to replace prostheses that are either too small or have undergone degeneration. Extracardiac conduits are commonly used for repair of pulmonary atresia with ventricular septal defect, truncus arteriosus, transposition with left ventricular outflow tract obstruction and/or ventricular septal defect, congenitally corrected transposition with left ventricular outflow tract obstruction, and/or ventricular septal defect and were used in early Fontan operations. Development of obstruction is influenced by the type of conduit, technique of insertion, and timing of the original operation. Heterografts have shown a high incidence of early obstruction. In one series, replacement of 55 of 86 (64 percent) of heterograft conduits used for repair of truncus arteriosus was necessary after a mean interval of 4 years.[131] In another series of 143 survivors of conduit insertion, all had to be replaced by 10 years.[132] A homograft aorta or pulmonary artery and valve have also been used for the repair of pulmonary atresia with ventricular septal defect.[133] Homografts, fresh or frozen, in childhood, have not performed as well as initially hoped.[134,135] Calcification and obstruction remain significant complications. However, because of their favorable

handling characteristics, homografts remain the conduits of choice for most reconstructions.[136,137] Besides the conduit itself, improved operative technique and the use of a large conduit have clear beneficial influence on the need for early replacement. Patients with right-sided conduits need careful follow-up, particularly toward the end of the expected life of the conduit. Although conduit obstruction may be suspected from clinical examination, the signs of severe obstruction may be subtle and may be missed. As a result, replacement may be performed too late. The consequent major deleterious effects on right ventricular function increase the risk of surgery and may not be fully reversible. Regular, noninvasive evaluation by transthoracic or transesophageal echocardiography or magnetic resonance imaging is indicated in selected patients and may provide the information usually obtained by cardiac catheterization/angiography. Reoperation is usually indicated if the right ventricular pressure is near systemic or if there is evidence of deteriorating ventricular function.[138]

Residual/Recurrent Defects

Residual or recurrent defects may be difficult to distinguish unless careful assessment after the original repair has been performed. They may have a major impact on morbidity and mortality, as when major left AV valve regurgitation persists after repair of AV septal defect.[139] Much more long-term follow-up data are needed before guidelines for reoperation for relatively minor residual abnormalities, such as mild left AV valve regurgitation, in this situation can be established.

The reported need for reoperation after the commonly performed "corrective" operation for tetralogy of Fallot varies between 1.8 and 13 percent over a follow-up of up to 31 years.[140,141] Ventricular septal defect and right ventricular outflow tract obstruction are the commonest residual abnormalities. Pulmonary regurgitation is extremely common and inevitable after transannular patching as part of the original repair. The hemodynamic consequences of pulmonary regurgitation for the right ventricle are greater in the presence of other defects such as residual obstruction and/or ventricular septal defect. Pulmonary valve replacement has not been frequently required in the first two decades after repair but may become increasingly performed because of the late deleterious effects of pulmonary regurgitation on the right ventricle.[142] Current indications include progressive right ventricular dilatation and a decrease in exercise tolerance.[143] When surgery is performed before the development of right ventricular failure (often with tricuspid regurgitation and atrial flutter/fibrillation), both clinical status and right ventricular function improve.[144] The optimal method for assessing pulmonary regurgitation in serial follow-up has not been determined; therefore appropriate guidelines for intervention are still not established.

Several studies have emphasized the palliative nature of aortic valvotomy in childhood.[145–147] Isolated aortic stenosis most frequently results from a bicuspid aortic valve, although in neonates and infants the structural abnormality of the aortic valve is more severe and the results of surgery even worse

---

TABLE 71-7

INDICATIONS FOR REOPERATION IN ADULTS WITH CONGENITAL HEART DISEASE

1. Inevitable reoperation after definitive repair: prosthetic valves, extracardiac conduits placed at an early age, and body size that becomes of inadequate size because of body growth
2. Residual defects after definitive repair: ventricular septal defect after tetralogy of Fallot and left AV valve regurgitation after AV septal defect repair
3. New/recurrent defects after definitive repair: subaortic stenosis, restenosis of aortic valve, pulmonary regurgitation in tetralogy of Fallot
4. Staged repair of complex defects: pulmonary atresia with ventricular septal defect
5. Unexpected complications: infective endocarditis
6. Heart/heart-lung transplantation for uncorrectable congenital heart disease
7. Patient operated on for congenital heart disease with new acquired heart disease: coronary disease

(see Chap. 70). In a series of 59 patients who underwent open aortic valvotomy at over 1 year of age, actuarial survival was 94 percent at 5 years but only 77 percent at 22 years. Reoperation was carried out in 36 percent, and the actuarial probability of reoperation was 44 percent at 22 years.[148] When serious events comprising death, reoperation, and endocarditis were grouped together, 92 percent were free of events at 5 years but only 39 percent at 22 years. Others have reported a similar long-term outcome.[145] The causes of restenosis have not been studied in detail but appear to be related to the degree of residual obstruction. The management of patients with aortic stenosis is likely to be influenced by balloon valvotomy in the young adult, in contrast to the disappointing impact of this technique in elderly patients[148] (see also Chap. 63).

Staged Repair

For complex congenital heart disease, definitive repair may not be possible until the anatomy and physiology of the circulation have been improved by one or more palliative procedures as part of a staged approach to "correction." This course is often necessary for patients with pulmonary atresia and ventricular septal defect, hypoplastic pulmonary arteries, and multifocal pulmonary blood supply. Palliative procedures to increase flow to the central pulmonary arteries and unifocalization of pulmonary flow by anastomosis (direct or indirect) of collateral vessels to the pulmonary arteries may eventually result in the ability to perform a repair (conduit insertion between the right ventricle and pulmonary artery and ventricular septal defect closure) with an acceptable postoperative right ventricular/left ventricular pressure ratio.[149,150] Excellent surgical results have been reported from such an approach, but the long-term outcome is not yet available.[151]

Other situations in which definitive repair may be indicated in the young adult include complex congenital heart defects with one functioning ventricle palliated by a systemic-pulmonary shunt or pulmonary artery banding in childhood. In selected patients who fulfill the stringent criteria for a Fontan operation, it is likely that long-term results will be better after a Fontan operation than when the ventricle is left with a chronically increased load secondary to a systemic pulmonary shunt.[12] The Fontan operation, however, should be considered palliative rather than curative: long-term problems are frequent and increase with duration of follow-up[152,153] (Table 71-8). Arrhythmia is a particularly common problem and occurs in approximately 20 percent of patients at 10-year follow-up[152] (Table 71-9). Protein-losing enteropathy (PLE) is another important complication and probably results from elevated systemic venous pressure, which subsequently causes lymphangiectasia. PLE is associated with fluid accumulation, such as pleural effusion, ascites, and peripheral edema. The cumulative risk for the development of PLE by 10 years in one reported large series was approximately 13 percent[154]; once this complication had developed, the 5-year survival was

TABLE 71-8

INDICATIONS FOR HOSPITALIZATIONS AFTER FONTAN PROCEDURE FOR 215 SURVIVING PATIENTS WHO RETURNED A QUESTIONNAIRE

Indication	Patients Hospitalized (No.)[a]
Cardiac operation	62
Other	57
Arrhythmia	52
Pacemaker insertion or replacement	22
Heart failure	14
Abdominal swelling	10
Leg edema	9
Endocarditis	7
Protein-losing enteropathy	6
Hypoproteinemia	4
Stroke	4
Liver problems	1
Brain abscess	1

[a] *A patient may have provided multiple indications for one hospitalization.*
Source: Driscoll DJ, Offord KP, Feldt RH, et al. Five- to fifteen-year follow-up after Fontan operation. *Circulation* 1992; 85:469–496. Reproduced with permission from the publisher and authors.

approximately 50 percent. Therapy includes sodium restriction, dietary modification, and anticongestive measures such as diuretics and afterload-reducing agents. Many patients require periodic albumin infusion, but medical management of PLE is usually only partially successful. Obstruction in the Fontan circuit should always be ruled out as a potential cause, since reoperation may result in resolution of the PLE. Isolated reports have suggested that percutaneous atrial fenestration may also resolve the PLE.[155,156] Despite these complications, more and more modifications of the Fontan operation are being performed, and more long-term data are necessary to see whether or not important complications can be reduced in this way.

Unexpected Reoperations

Indications for unexpected reoperation include thrombosis in a low-flow circulation such as the Fontan, prosthetic valve failure or thrombosis, and infective endocarditis. The latter may be particularly difficult to diagnose in complex congenital heart disease where the site of vegetations may not be easy to image (e.g., in a Blalock-Taussig shunt). Reoperation in the patient with uncontrolled endocarditis carries a particularly high risk.

Heart/Heart-Lung Transplantation

Despite the major successes of the last three decades, an increasing number of patients survive to adult life with deteriorating clinical status. Their only remaining prospect may be a heart or heart-and-lung transplant (see Chap. 25). These patients often present specific surgical problems of multiple previous chest incisions, complex venous anatomy, and borderline pulmonary vascular resistance. In addition, the young adult with end-stage heart disease may not have the ideal social milieu to cope with the demands of transplantation and may require considerable psychological support. The shortage of donors and the ability to monitor rejection in a single organ have stimulated great interest in single-lung transplantation for patients with primary pulmonary hypertension and Eisenmenger's syndrome (in conjunction with closure of the shunt). Such patients accounted for 23 percent of the single-lung transplants performed in 1990, and the use of this approach is increasing.[157]

TABLE 71-9

ARRHYTHMIAS IN 215 SURVIVORS OF THE FONTAN OPERATION

Results from Follow-up Questionnaire	5 years Postop Patients		Current Patients	
	No.	%	No.	%
Syncope	18	8	17	8
Rapid heart rate (tachycardia)	44	20	45	21
Slow heart rate (bradycardia)	17	8	15	7
Palpitations	51	24	60	28
Atrial flutter or fibrillation	26	12	41	19
Premature ventricular contractions	13	6	15	7
Ventricular tachycardia	9	4	13	6
Pacemaker	[b]	[b]	22	10
Number of antiarrhythmic medications[a]				
0	179	83	167	78
1	31	13	40	19
2	5	2	8	4

[a] Excluding digitalis.
[b] "Presence of a pacemaker" asked only for patient's current status.
Source: From Driscoll DJ, Offord KP, Feldt RH, et al. Five-to-fifteen-year follow-up after Fontan operation. *Circulation* 1992; 85:469–496. Reproduced with permission from the publisher and authors.

First Operations for Congenital Heart Disease in Adults

The first surgical repair of a congenital heart defect may be required in the teenager or adult. This may be because the lesion has been mild and of little hemodynamic significance in childhood but has progressed in severity with time. Examples include a bicuspid aortic valve with progressive stenosis (see Chap. 63), Marfan's syndrome with aortic root dilatation (see Chap. 85), and Ebstein's anomaly with worsening symptoms. Alternatively, lesions such as small-to-moderate atrial septal defects may have been missed or misdiagnosed until adult life. In certain complex congenital heart defects, the combination of lesions produces a balanced hemodynamic state compatible with prolonged survival without intervention. Patients with double-inlet ventricle and pulmonary stenosis, complex pulmonary atresia, and tetralogy of Fallot may remain well until the second and even third decades of life before deteriorating.[158] The contemplation of heart surgery in an adolescent or young adult is often terrifying, implying the acceptance of the presence of a serious heart problem by the patient and his or her immediate friends and family. The scar on the chest may cause embarrassment, and the patient may be discriminated against both socially and at work. All these issues need to be dealt with sympathetically by the physician.

Noncardiac Surgery

When performed without adequate preparation, noncardiac surgery in adults with congenital heart disease is a major cause of avoidable morbidity and mortality. All the anesthetic risks encountered for cardiac reoperation apply equally to noncardiac surgery, but in the latter the patient may be managed by medical staff who may be unfamiliar with the significance of the congenital heart disease. Many patients with congenital heart defects are at increased risk for arrhythmia and from agents that depress ventricular function. The surgeon must be aware of the presence of a pacemaker or pacing leads that may affect the safe use of diathermy. Prophylaxis against infective endocarditis is usually indicated, and the choice of antibiotic regimen is dictated by the surgical procedure/intervention being undertaken (see Chap. 82). In patients with pulmonary vascular disease, general anesthesia may have disastrous consequences, with a sudden fall in systemic vascular resistance. Similar hemodynamic changes may induce a severe hypercyanotic spell in a patient with uncorrected tetralogy of Fallot, and meticulous pre-, intra-, and postoperative hemodynamic monitoring is mandatory together with the avoidance of vasodilating anesthetic agents, hypoxia, hypoventilation, and blood or volume loss. Cyanotic patients also have impaired hemostasis, and some patients may be taking anticoagulants. Intravenous lines, drugs, and infusions must be managed carefully in patients with intracardiac shunts, as air or emboli may reach the systemic circulation. The safety of noncardiac surgery in adults with congenital heart disease is greatly increased when physicians, anesthesiologists, and surgeons familiarize themselves with these issues, seek specialized advice, and, if necessary, refer the patient to a team with more experience.

SPECIFIC LESIONS

General Considerations

Some lesions that are commonly seen in adult congenital heart disease, both as a result of natural and unnatural survival, are listed in Tables 71-1 and 71-2.

Interpretation of the literature on long-term outcome of congenital heart defects is hampered by a number of difficulties. First, follow-up is still short and numbers of survivors are small for many defects. The era of open-heart surgery for congenital heart defects only began in the 1950s, and "correction" has only been attempted much more recently for many categories of patients now beginning to reach adult life (e.g., the Fontan operation). Second, surgical practice has undergone a process of evolution during this time, with new operations for some lesions (e.g., transposition of the great arteries) or major change in operative technique for others (e.g., the Fontan operation). Third, major advances in cardiopulmonary bypass and myocardial protection have accompanied improved preoperative diagnosis and recognition of intracardiac anatomy, particularly of the disposition of the conduction tissues. Finally, for almost all lesions, the management philosophy has changed, with a trend to early primary correction as opposed to initial palliation. For many defects, therefore, long-term outcome data relevant to current practice are not available.

Correct application of survival analysis is essential for interpretation of follow-up data.[159] In particular, the use of hazard functions providing an estimate of *instantaneous risk* is particularly valuable. The following section deals with some specific defects seen in adults with congenital heart disease.

Atrial Septal Defect

Atrial septal defects are among the most common congenital anomalies in adolescents and adults, accounting for up to 30 percent of congenital heart disease in this age group.[160,161] Approximately 75 percent of defects are ostium secundum defects, 20 percent are ostium primum defects (discussed below), and 5 percent sinus venosus defects; defects at other sites are rare[162,163] (see Chap. 70). Associated lesions include pulmonary stenosis, mitral valve prolapse, and mitral regurgitation. Atrial septal defects may be associated with other syndromes, including the Holt-Oram syndrome[164] (Fig. 10-2), and may be familial.[165] In the latter, conduction disease manifesting as prolongation of the PR interval and rarely heart block have been described.[165] Lutembacher syndrome (atrial septal defect coexisting with mitral stenosis) is now very uncommon.

NATURAL HISTORY

Survival into adulthood is the rule, and patients living into their eighties and nineties have been reported.[160] Life expectancy, however, is not normal. Death during the first 20 years of life is infrequent, but after the age of 40 years, the mortality

increases to about 6 percent per year.[166-168] Defects may go unrecognized for many years because symptoms are rare until later life and physical signs may be subtle. Later, the natural history is characterized by progressive symptoms and cardiomegaly, the development of atrial arrhythmias, right ventricular hypertrophy, and pulmonary hypertension. The mechanisms for the development of symptoms are multifactorial[160] and include the following:

1. Change in left ventricular compliance from superimposed hypertension or coronary artery disease that increases the shunt with age. Long-standing right ventricular volume overload, although relatively well tolerated, ultimately leads to right ventricular failure, and a marked increase in right ventricular volume can further compromise the left ventricle.
2. Supraventricular arrhythmias, particularly atrial fibrillation and flutter, increase with time and may cause symptoms and cardiac failure (Fig. 71-3).
3. Progressive pulmonary vascular disease after the third decade of life.
4. Rarer complications, including systemic and pulmonary emboli, recurrent chest infections, and infective endocarditis (in patients with coexisting mitral valve disease).

MANAGEMENT

Surgical closure either by direct suture or use of a patch has been performed for almost 40 years (Chap. 70). Surgery carries a low risk (<1 percent operative mortality) provided that the pulmonary vascular resistance is not significantly elevated.[163] In older patients, the indication for closure is a little more controversial. Shah et al. compared the outcome of patients treated medically and surgically when diagnosed after the age of 25 years.[169] This unrandomized study followed

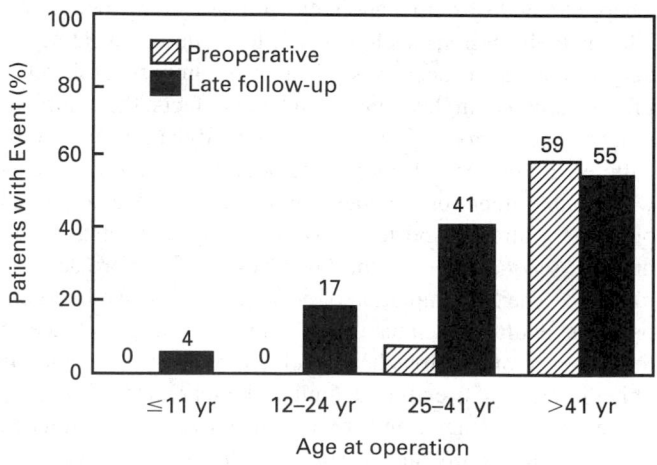

FIGURE 71-3

Incidence of atrial flutter or atrial fibrillation preoperatively and at late follow-up according to the age at operation after repair of atrial septal defect. (From Murphy JG, Gersh BJ, McGoon MD, et al. Long-term outcome after surgical repair of isolated atrial septal defects: Follow-up at 27–32 years. *N Engl J Med* 1990; 323:1645. Reproduced with permission from the publisher and authors.)

patients for more than 20 years and concluded that there was no difference in survival or symptoms between the two groups and no difference in the incidence of new arrhythmia, stroke, or other embolic phenomena in the follow-up period. Notably, however, more than 70 percent of patients in both the medical and surgical groups were asymptomatic at presentation, which may partly explain the favorable outcome of the medically treated group, who had a 91 percent survival. Konstantinides et al. evaluated 179 patients with secundum atrial septal defect ≥40 years of age and compared the outcome of medically and surgically treated groups.[170] They demonstrated a reduced mortality after surgical closure with a 95 percent surgical survival versus an 84 percent medical survival at 10 years. Nonfatal cardiovascular complications, however, were similar with atrial fibrillation and flutter occurring with a similar incidence in both groups. The functional status of the medically treated group deteriorated in 34 percent of patients and improved in many of the surgical patients, particularly those in class III or IV. It thus seems reasonable to conclude that symptomatic adult patients will improve after surgical repair, and the only real contraindication is severe pulmonary vascular disease. When surgery is delayed, symptoms are likely to be progressive and surgical repair is less likely to prevent problems with atrial fibrillation and thromboembolic events. The management of the asymptomatic adult patient is less clear, but certainly closure of the defect halts progression of right ventricular volume overload, tricuspid regurgitation, and progression of pulmonary vascular disease, and it can be accomplished with low surgical risk. The standard surgical approach remains a midline sternotomy, but patients should be made aware of the alternatives of thoracotomy or inframammary incision. Although morbidity may be higher, the resulting scar may be less offensive, especially to young women.

Closure of atrial septal defect has been achieved in selected patients by use of a variety of occlusion devices inserted at cardiac catheterization.[171,172] Despite the encouraging early results, the first generation "clamshell" occluders required modification because of a high incidence of strut fracture and a low but significant incidence of embolization. Several alternatives have been evaluated, but no large series with adequate follow-up are yet available for comparison with surgery. The attractions of closing defects without open-heart surgery are obvious. Eventually, the transcatheter technique may supplant surgery as the method of closure for atrial septal defects of appropriate size, morphology, and location. In addition, the presence of a patent foramen ovale has been suggested as a risk factor for cerebral embolus. Determining the risk of clinical events in asymptomatic subjects with patent foramen ovale and indications for treatment are highly controversial areas. Catheter treatment is likely to be the method of choice for patients who have a clear indication for intervention.

LATE RESULTS

In a recent study of patients undergoing surgical repair of an atrial septal defect between 1956 and 1960, late survival of patients undergoing operation at below 24 years of age was not significantly different from an age- and sex-matched control population. Late survival in patients aged 25 to 41 years was good but less than that of the control population, whereas repair after age 41 years was associated with significantly poorer late survival (Fig. 71-3). The combination of older age at operation and pulmonary hypertension had an additive effect on late mortality.[173] In this and other series, the propensity for atrial fibrillation and flutter increased as a function of age both before and after operation (Fig. 71-4).[173,174] Twenty-two percent of late deaths were due to stroke, and all occurred in patients with postoperative atrial fibrillation or flutter. These data support the current policy of repair at a preschool age (Chap. 70). A separate study of 66 patients who underwent closure of atrial septal defect between 60 and 78 years of age implied a benefit in survival in patients discharged from the hospital compared with unoperated historical age- and sex-matched controls.[175]

The near-normal survival and low morbidity in patients undergoing repair within the first two decades of life have important implications for employment and insurance recommendations. Such patients should be encouraged to lead a normal life, and competitive sports should not be restricted in the absence of hemodynamic or electrophysiologic sequelae. The risk of endocarditis in the absence of mitral valve disease is minimal. Patients who have undergone repair in the third decade of life or later require careful regular surveillance. Although late survival is good, the development of supraventricular arrhythmia and risk of cerebrovascular accident are of concern. Anticoagulation is indicated in patients with atrial fibrillation and should be considered in those with supraventricular tachycardia or atrial flutter in the absence of other contraindications (see also Chaps. 27 and 52). Long-term follow-up is recommended for patients repaired in adult life who have increased pulmonary artery pressure at the end of operation, pre- and postoperative arrhythmia, ventricular dysfunction, or coexisting heart disease.

Ventricular Septal Defect

Isolated ventricular septal defect, although one of the commonest congenital abnormalities in infants and children, is far less frequent in the adolescent and adult for several reasons.[160] First, most patients with a hemodynamically significant defect will have undergone repair in childhood; second, spontaneous decrease in size and closure are common for small or moderate perimembranous or muscular defects (this decreases in frequency with increasing age); finally, patients with large, unoperated defects may die earlier in life.[176] The spectrum of isolated ventricular septal defects in the adult is thus limited to the following four groups of patients: (1) those with small, restrictive defects that were either small to begin with or have partially closed; (2) those with Eisenmenger syndrome and a predominant right-to-left shunt with cyanosis[177] who need to be distinguished from those who develop secondary infundibular pulmonary stenosis, which can also decrease the left-to-right shunt and may result in cyanosis with shunt reversal[178] (see Chap. 70); (3) the occasional patient with a moderately restrictive defect in whom the diagnosis has been overlooked or who has not had closure in childhood; and (4) those who have had their defects closed in childhood.

NATURAL HISTORY

The natural history of small, restrictive ventricular septal defects is very favorable.[161] Nevertheless, the risk of infective endocarditis persists (developing in almost 4 percent of patients with ventricular septal defect), and lifelong prophylaxis is required. Spontaneous closure may occasionally still occur in adult life. A subset of patients with perimembranous defects or defects in the outlet septum may develop aortic cusp prolapse and aortic regurgitation. This may be progressive and is often severe by the end of the second decade of life. As incompetence increases, the ventricular septal defect may become "closed" by the prolapsing cusp; if it is left to develop, however, aortic valve replacement may be necessary.[179] Such defects are associated with a high risk of infective endocarditis. Severe and progressive pulmonary vascular disease is a feature of older patients with nonrestrictive large defects. Eisenmenger's syndrome is compatible with survival into young adult life, but the complications of right-sided heart failure, paradoxical emboli, and erythrocytosis usually result in death by the third decade (see Chap. 70). Occasionally, patients with moderate-sized ventricular septal defects and left-to-right shunts who did not develop pulmonary vascular disease present in adolescence and young adult life with symptoms of fatigue, effort intolerance, and respiratory infections.

MANAGEMENT

Patients with small ventricular septal defects are asymptomatic and should be managed conservatively. Continued medical follow-up is, however, helpful to remind patients about the need for prophylaxis against infective endocarditis and to minimize inappropriate discrimination during the search for employment and insurance. Ventricular septal defects associated with aortic cusp prolapse and aortic regurgitation should be repaired even when the shunt is small in an effort to prevent progressive deterioration of the aortic valve. Surgical repair is indicated in the rare adult with a significant left-to-right shunt (pulmonary to systemic flow ratio exceeding 2:1) and a low pulmonary vascular resistance. The management of patients with large defects and infundibular narrowing causing right-to-left shunting and cyanosis is similar to that for tetralogy of Fallot (see below). A rather unique approach using a unidirectional valve patch to allow right-to-left but not left-to-right shunting has been described.[180]

Unfortunately, adults are still seen with a large ventricular septal defect and pulmonary vascular disease. In those with borderline pulmonary vascular resistance (7 to 10 U/m^2), surgery may be attempted, but the benefits are unpredictable as the pulmonary vascular disease may progress despite closure of the defect[181] (see Chap. 70). Medical management and consideration for heart-lung or single-lung transplantation are the only realistic options for patients with established severe pulmonary vascular disease.

LATE RESULTS

Late results of surgery are good, but the life expectancy for the whole group is not normal. In a study of 179 operative survivors between 1956 and 1959, 30-year survival was 82 percent, compared with 97 percent in age- and sex-matched controls.[178] Only 25 percent of patients in the series were over 10 years of age at surgery, and their 30-year survival of 70 percent was substantially lower than the 88 percent in patients under 2 years of age at operation. Thirty-year survival was 83 percent for patients aged 3 to 10 years at surgery. Older age at repair and preoperative pulmonary vascular disease are important predictors of late outcome. Postoperative conduction defects, especially right bundle branch block, are common, but complete heart block, which was seen in the early surgical experience, is now rare. Late ventricular arrhythmia has been reported, as after repair of tetralogy of Fallot.[182] The incidence of late sudden death, however, is extremely low, and prophylactic antiarrhythmic therapy in asymptomatic patients is not indicated.

Certain selected ventricular septal defects may be closed with transcatheter devices. A recent report described closure of 21 muscular ventricular septal defects in 12 patients, half of whom had complex heart defects.[183] All the defects were closed successfully, and subsequent cardiac surgery for associated lesions was performed in 11 of 12 patients.

In postoperative patients, the risk of late infective endocarditis is very small provided that the defect is isolated and is completely closed. Antibiotic prophylaxis, however, is often advised, particularly for 6 months postoperatively. Recommendations regarding physical activity and competitive sports require detailed evaluation, which may include exercise testing, cross-sectional echocardiography, and ambulatory electrocardiographic monitoring. The presence of abnormal left ventricular function, a more than trivial residual shunt, arrhythmia, or any degree of pulmonary hypertension mandates some restriction of physical activity.

Atrioventricular Septal Defect

The term *atrioventricular septal defect* describes the spectrum of lesions that involve a defect at the site of the normal AV septum, resulting in an abnormality involving the AV valves, ventricular architecture, and left ventricular outflow tract. A variety of different classifications have been used (Chap. 70), but the defects are usefully divided into "partial" and "complete" forms. In the former, there is a large defect in the primum or inferior part of the atrial septum but no direct intraventricular communication (ostium primum defect). In the latter, there is a large ventricular component beneath either or both the superior or inferior bridging leaflets of the AV valve. The deficiency of ventricular septum together with the abnormal AV valve(s) produces an elongated left ventricular outflow tract characteristically described as having a "goose neck" appearance at angiography (Fig. 16-7). The morphologic and functional features, together with the associated cardiac and noncardiac abnormalities, determine the natural history.

NATURAL HISTORY

In the New England Regional Cardiac Registry, 5 percent of newborns with cardiac disease had AV septal defects, with two-thirds being the "complete" form.[184] Down's syndrome is very frequently associated, especially with complete defects. The noncardiac features, especially mental retardation, have a major influence on management in adolescence and adult life.

The natural history of partial AV septal defects with little left AV valve regurgitation is similar to that of large secundum atrial septal defects (see above). A small number develop pulmonary vascular disease, and symptomatic deterioration in unoperated adults is often due to the onset of supraventricular arrhythmia. If the left AV valve is more than mildly regurgitant, the natural history is much worse, with a large left-to-right shunt, often with at least moderate pulmonary hypertension and early symptoms of cardiac failure. Patients with complete defects do even worse. Their course is characterized by the early development of pulmonary vascular disease (especially in patients with Down's syndrome who may have irreversible damage before their first birthday) with consequent right-to-left shunting and all the problems of patients with Eisenmenger's syndrome. As a result, surgery needs to be undertaken early if it is to be successful, and most uncorrected patients seen by the adolescent or adult cardiologist will have a pulmonary vascular resistance that is too high for repair (greater than 8 to 10 U/m^2) (see Chaps. 70 and 16). Their outcome is poor, but survival into their thirties is possible. Uncorrected patients with partial AV septal defects may present to the adult cardiologist for consideration of surgery, which should be recommended for those with a significant left-right shunt in the absence of other contraindications.

MANAGEMENT

Surgical repair involves closure of the atrial and ventricular septal defects and restoration of a competent left AV valve as far as is possible.[185] (Chap. 70). Surgical mortality in experienced centers is approximately 10 percent for complete defects and less than 5 percent for partial defects.[163]

LATE RESULTS

Patients with repair of both partial and complete forms of AV septal defect have now been followed for more than 20 years. Late results are good in the absence of pulmonary vascular disease and significant residual left AV valve regurgitation. Some patients with complete defects who were corrected later in childhood, before the need for correction in early infancy was appreciated, have developed progressive pulmonary vascular disease. This late complication should be greatly reduced in patients undergoing repair in the first 6 months of life, as is now technically feasible (see Chap. 70). Even patients who are repaired late in adult life ($\geq$40 years of age) can have excellent results with an early mortality of only 6 percent and a good chance of left AV valve repair in experienced hands.[186]

During long-term follow-up, careful attention must be paid to the status of the left AV valve. If the regurgitation increases in severity, reoperation and mitral valve replacement may be necessary.[139] Monitoring for arrhythmia at intervals is also currently recommended; in general, little intervention is usually required apart from lifelong infective endocarditis prophylaxis. Surgically repaired non-Down's patients without pulmonary vascular disease can often enjoy life without cardiovascular disability and should not be discouraged from competitive sports, pregnancy, or employment. Restrictions are clearly required for those with pulmonary vascular disease, left AV valve regurgitation, or mitral valve replacement on anticoagulants. Patients with Down's syndrome, both operated and unoperated, are demanding, and their families require considerable support from the physician as well as from the educational and social services. The recurrence risk of congenital heart disease in offspring of mothers with AV septal defect is higher than average, and potential parents should be counseled.

Tetralogy of Fallot

Tetralogy of Fallot is the most common form of cyanotic congenital heart disease seen in the adult. Nonetheless, in the developed world the unoperated patient with tetralogy of Fallot has fortunately become a rarity since the overwhelming majority of patients will have undergone palliation or more usually repair in childhood. From an anatomic and pathophysiologic standpoint, the manifestations of tetralogy of Fallot are similar in all age groups, although hypercyanotic spells, which are often seen in infants and young children, are rare in adults. The development of systemic hypertension with age is a problem as this increases the afterload to both ventricles.[160,187] Although pulmonary blood flow may improve, this occurs at the expense of right ventricular failure. Acquired calcific aortic stenosis has similar effects. Aortic regurgitation may occur as a result of cusp prolapse in patients with aortic defect. If exacerbated by infective endocarditis, the volume overload is transmitted to both ventricles. The development of chronic obstructive lung disease is another manifestation of an acquired cardiopulmonary disease that may place the adult patient with tetralogy of Fallot at particular risk.

NATURAL HISTORY

Survival into the seventh decade is described,[188] but the natural history in the unoperated patient, which is determined by the severity of obstruction of the right ventricular outflow tract and pulmonary vasculature, is poor. Only 25 percent of patients reach the age of 10 years, 11 percent are alive at 20 years, 6 percent at age 30 years, but only 3 percent at age 40 years.[160,163,189] Complications of right-to-left shunting and erythrocytosis, which include stroke and cerebral abscess, are common and in many instances fatal. Patients are at continuing risk of infective endocarditis; the development of congestive heart failure in adolescence or early adult life is a major cause of death, as is arrhythmia. Myocardial fibrosis resulting from long-standing right ventricular pressure overload and hypoxemia are postulated mechanisms.[190] Prior palliative surgery with a Cooley or Waterston shunt (between the ascending aorta and right pulmonary artery) or a Potts shunt (between the descending aorta and the left pulmonary artery) can lead to the late development of pulmonary vascular disease.[191]

MANAGEMENT

The focus of medical treatment in unoperated patients is on the elevated hematocrit, bleeding disorders, and abnormal uric acid metabolism and the complications of pregnancy. Repair is indicated in all suitable patients, and the principles and techniques are not significantly different in adults from those in children[162] (see Chap. 70). Most adults are suitable for repair, but the occasional patient with an underdeveloped pulmonary vascular bed may require a palliative shunt procedure. Intracardiac repair consists of closure of the ventricular septal defect and relief of right ventricular outflow tract obstruction. In some patients, this may require excision of the pulmonary valve and patch reconstruction of the annulus and outflow tract. In the occasional patient with an anomalous origin of the left coronary artery from the right coronary artery, a conduit between the right ventricle and pulmonary artery may be required.[163]

LATE RESULTS

Late survival is excellent, even in patients who underwent repair during the very early years of open heart surgery.[163] At the Mayo Clinic, the cumulative 30-year survival for patients undergoing successful surgery between 1956 and 1960 was 86 percent compared to 95 percent in age- and sex-matched controls (Fig. 71-4).[192] In a previous series of 396 hospital survivors of repair between 1955 and 1962 at the same institu-

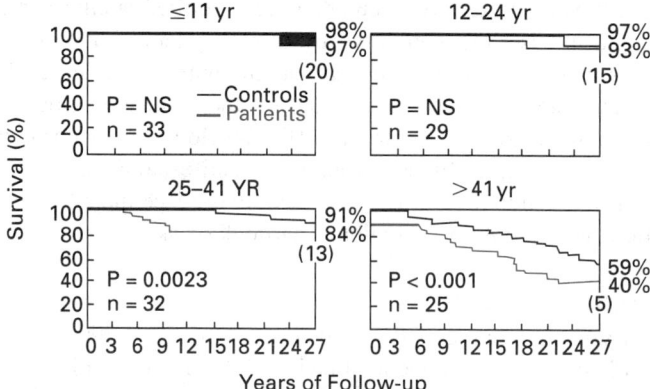

FIGURE 71-4

Long-term survival of perioperative survivors of atrial septal defect repair by age at time of operation. Controls are survival in an age- and sex-matched population. (From Murphy JG, Gersh BJ, McGoon MD, et al. Long-term outcome after surgical repair of isolated atrial septal defects: Follow-up at 27–32 years. *N Engl J Med* 1990; 323:1645. Reproduced with permission from the publisher and authors.)

tion 91 percent were alive at 20 years. At 30 years, 77 percent of the initial cohort of 106 patients undergoing surgery between 1954 and 1960 by Lillehei and associates were alive, including one patient who was 45 years of age at the time of operation.[193] Surgery cannot be considered "curative" as survival even in excellent series is slightly but significantly worse than for a matched control population. The risk factors for an adverse late outcome include older age at surgery, preoperative congestive heart failure, a previous Potts shunt, persistent right ventricular systolic hypertension, and a residual ventricular septal defect.[191,192] Late death may be sudden, due to tachyarrhythmia or, very rarely in the current era, due to conduction disease[194] (see above). Left and right ventricular failure due to right ventricular pressure overload or left ventricular volume overload is another important cause of late mortality in older patients.[160] In some patients, isolated right ventricular restrictive physiology may paradoxically improve exercise performance and reduce cardiac enlargement due possibly to shortening of the duration of pulmonary regurgitation.[77]

The late functional outcome is excellent for the majority of patients. Most lead normal lives, but the results appear to be better in those undergoing surgery at a younger age.[195] Persistent or recurrent symptoms are usually the result of incomplete relief of right ventricular systolic hypertension or recurrent/residual ventricular septal defects. These problems are often manifest within the first few years after surgery and may require reoperation. Although pulmonary regurgitation does not appear to increase mortality, it may be associated with late impairment of exercise capacity and persistent cardiomegaly.[196] It may well become an increasing problem with very long follow-up, but the precise indications for pulmonary valve insertion are not yet clear.

Recent information links pulmonary regurgitation, cardiomegaly, QRS duration and potentially life-threatening ventricular arrhythmia.[77,78] This may be important for identification of risk of late sudden death, which has been a rare event in most long-term follow-up series. Asymptomatic ventricular arrhythmia is very common during long-term follow-up. It is again related to older age at repair, but the link between nonsustained ventricular arrhythmia and adverse clinical outcome is uncertain (see above).[68,69] Objective testing has emphasized the effects of older age at operation on subsequent exercise performance. This is essentially normal for children repaired at below 5 years of age but is usually impaired when surgery is undertaken in adolescence or adulthood.[197]

Before unrestricted physical activity after repair of tetralogy of Fallot can be recommended, careful evaluation—including cross-sectional echocardiography, ECG monitoring, and exercise testing should be undertaken. Normal activity including competitive sports seems reasonable if surgery has been performed at a young age, right and left ventricular function and size are normal, and there is no residual ventricular septal defect or significant right ventricular outflow tract obstruction and no worrisome arrhythmia. In those who do not fulfill these stringent criteria, the degree to which physical activity should be restricted must be individualized. Currently, long-term follow-up of all patients with tetralogy of Fallot is recommended.

Pulmonary Stenosis

Isolated pulmonary valve stenosis is a common form of adult congenital heart disease and is characterized typically by a trileaflet valve with fused commissures. A dysplastic valve without commissural fusion occurs infrequently in otherwise normal children, but more commonly in patients with Noonan's syndrome[160] (Fig. 10-13). Subvalvar stenosis due to infundibular hypertrophy is usually a secondary phenomenon in response to obstruction to right ventricular outflow but may occur as a rare isolated entity. Supravalvular or peripheral pulmonary artery stenosis is also extremely uncommon as an isolated entity but is associated with tetralogy of Fallot and supravalvar aortic stenosis in Williams' syndrome (Fig. 10-25).

NATURAL HISTORY

Prolonged survival into adult life is common and depends upon the severity of obstruction. In patients with severe pulmonary stenosis, symptoms of right-sided failure increase with time because of progressive obstruction and alterations in right ventricular compliance.[198,199] In the Joint Study of the Natural History of Congenital Heart Disease, 19 percent of patients with severe stenosis aged 2 to 11 years and 37 percent aged 12 to 21 years were symptomatic. The natural history of moderate pulmonary stenosis in older patients is more favorable, with less tendency to progression. Patients with mild pulmonary stenosis (in contrast to those with mild aortic stenosis) at ages exceeding 2 years rarely have symptoms and rarely develop progressive obstruction.[199] Associated right ventricular cavity hypoplasia, which is an important prognostic factor in neonates and infants, is much less relevant in those surviving to adulthood.

MANAGEMENT

Patients with mild stenosis are asymptomatic and require no intervention other than antibiotic prophylaxis against infective endocarditis. In patients with more severe stenosis (>40 mm gradient between the right ventricle and pulmonary artery), intervention to reduce severity should be considered even if there are no symptoms.

Surgical valvotomy for isolated pulmonary stenosis has been successfully performed for more than 40 years. Perioperative morbidity and mortality are minimal beyond the neonatal period in patients without severe congestive cardiac failure or right ventricular dysplasia.[163] Late results are also excellent. In a study from the Mayo Clinic of patients undergoing surgery between 1956 and 1957, late survival for those undergoing valvotomy who are over 21 years of age was similar but not identical to that of an age- and sex-matched control population (Fig. 71-5). Among patients undergoing surgery

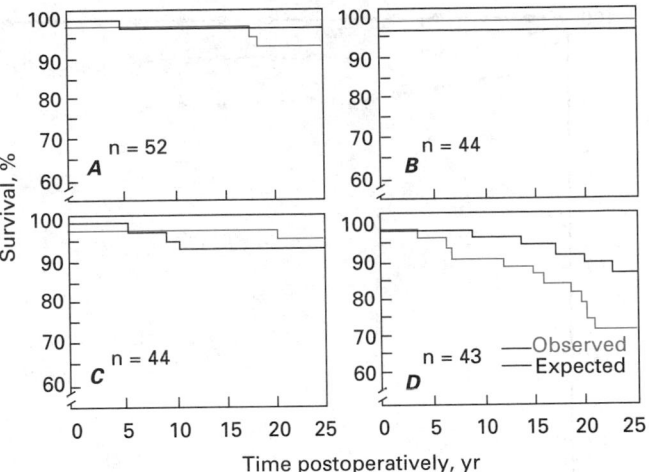

FIGURE 71-5

Long-term survival of perioperative survivors of surgical repair of pulmonary valve stenosis by age at time of operation. *A*. Ages 0 to 4 years. *B*. Ages 5 to 10 years. *C*. Ages 11 to 20 years. *D*. Ages 21 to 68 years. Expected is survival in an age- and sex-matched population. Values of *p* for comparison between the expected and observed survivals: .07, .34, .16, and <.002 for panels *A*, *B*, *C*, and *D*, respectively. (From Kopecky SL, Gersh BJ, McGoon MD, et al. Long-term outcome of patients undergoing surgical repair of isolated pulmonary valve stenosis: Follow-up at 20–30 years. *Circulation* 1988; 78:1150. Reproduced with permission from the publisher and authors.)

at an older age, late survival, although still good, was less than that of the control population (Fig. 71-6).[200] This effect of age on late outcome, which was independent of the use of ventriculotomy and outflow patches and pulmonary regurgitation, is likely the result of long-standing pressure overload on the right ventricle. Late functional results are excellent, and pulmonary regurgitation is well tolerated in the short and medium term. More severe pulmonary regurgitation may result when a pulmonary valvectomy or transannular patch is required, as may be the case for a small or dysplastic valve; the long-term consequences on the right ventricle and functional capacity are not yet well documented (see "Tetralogy of Fallot," above).

Surgical valvotomy is now rarely required after infancy because of the advent of catheter balloon pulmonary valvotomy.[201] In many institutions, balloon valvotomy is the initial procedure of choice at all ages even though most accumulated data apply to younger patients. In the series of 822 patients in the Valvuloplasty and Angioplasty of Congenital Heart Abnormalities (VACA) registry, gradient reduction was substantially worse in patients with dysplastic valves.[202] Interventional catheter procedures should be confined to centers with experienced operators.

Long-term follow-up data are not yet available. It appears that the excellent early results are maintained for at least 5 years, especially in older patients.[203] The late effects of pulmonary regurgitation resulting from the use of large balloons need to be determined. The risk of infective endocarditis in patients with mild pulmonary stenosis or in those with mild gradients after surgical or balloon valvotomy is low. Long-

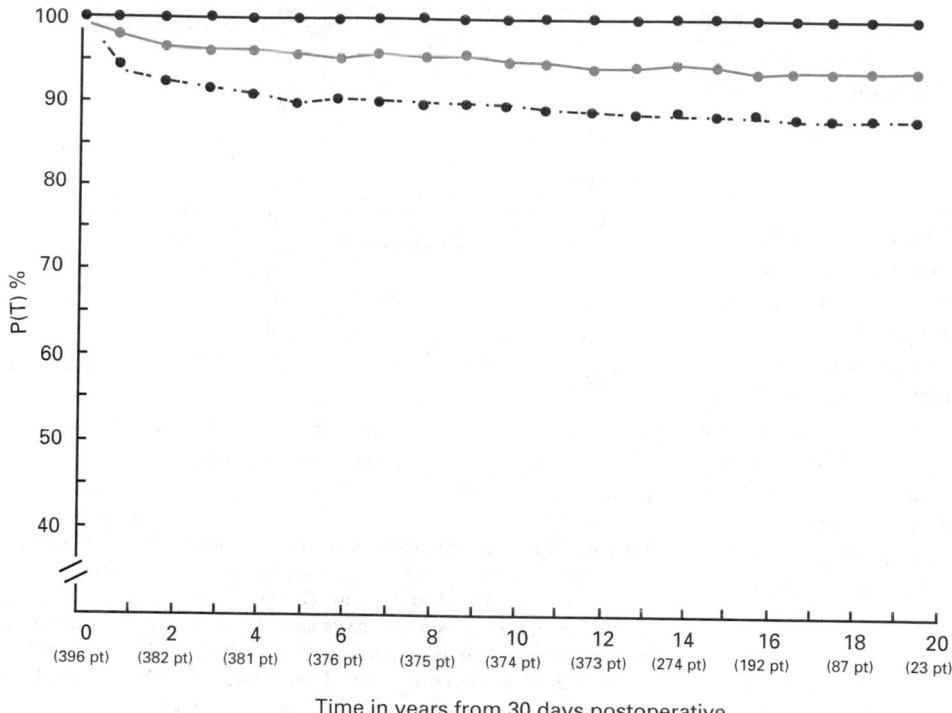

FIGURE 71-6

Probability of deterioration in operative survivors after repair of tetralogy of Fallot plotted against time in years. Time of deterioration is defined as the postoperative year in which late death (*middle curve*) or in which death, reoperation, or symptoms occurred (*bottom curve*). The top curve represents the controlled expected survival on the basis of an age- and sex-matched distribution. The number of patients at each follow-up interval is denoted in parentheses. (From Fuster V, McGoon DC, Kennedy M, et al. Long-term evaulation (12–22 years) of open heart surgery for tetralogy of Fallot. *Am J Cardiol* 1980; 46:635. Reproduced with permission from the publisher and authors.)

term follow-up is recommended to evaluate not only the right ventricular outflow tract gradient but also pulmonary regurgitation, right ventricular function, and exercise performance. In patients with good relief of pulmonary stenosis, no restriction of physical activities, including competitive sports, is required. In those with moderate residual obstruction or right ventricular dysfunction, exercise intensity should be reduced (see also Chap. 86).

Left Ventricular Outflow Tract Obstruction

Congenital left ventricular outflow tract obstruction may occur at valvular, subvalvular, and supravalvular levels (see Chap. 95). Aortic valve stenosis is a common abnormality in adults with congenital heart disease. It may either be an isolated defect or be associated with other lesions such as coarctation or ventricular septal defect. It is usually due to a bicuspid aortic valve, which may be present in 1 to 2 percent of the total adult population and is three to four times more common in males than in females.[204] Unicuspid and tricuspid stenotic valves are less common.[163] Subvalvar stenosis is due either to a discrete "membrane" below the aortic valve or less commonly to a fibromuscular tunnel.[205] Supravalvar stenosis is the least common variety of left ventricular outflow tract obstruction in adolescents and adults except in the context of Williams' syndrome.[206]

NATURAL HISTORY

The natural history of congenital valvar aortic stenosis in adults is variable but is characterized by progressive stenosis with time (Fig. 71-7)[160] (see Chap. 63). By the age of 45 years, approximately half of all bicuspid aortic valves have some degree of narrowing. The severity of obstruction at the time of diagnosis correlates with the pattern of progression (Fig. 71-8).[207] Bacterial endocarditis is relatively uncommon (1.8 to 2.7 cases per 100 patient-years).[208] Slowly progressive aortic regurgitation is well recognized in young adulthood, but sudden deterioration is rare except as a sequel to infection.[209,210]

Discrete subaortic stenosis may cause rapidly progressive obstruction in childhood and young adulthood. Progressive aortic regurgitation is common, and infective endocarditis is considered to be a particular hazard[209,210] (see Chap. 70). The natural history of supravalvular aortic stenosis is poor and survival to adulthood is exceptional.[160] The presence of associated congenital abnormalities and possibly premature coronary artery disease with systolic hypertension is likely a contributory factor to this adverse outcome.

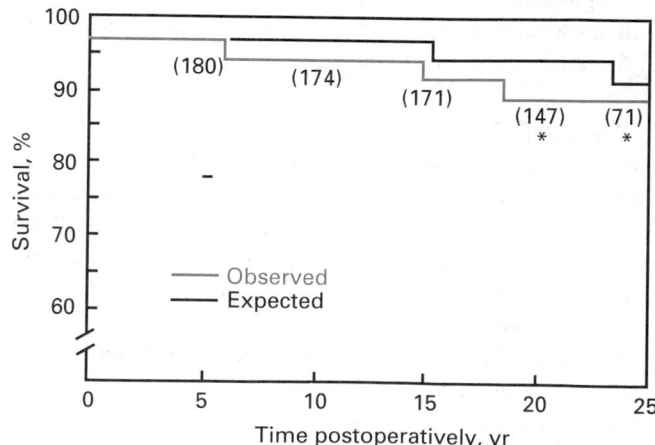

FIGURE 71-7

Long-term survival of perioperative survivors following surgical repair of isolated pulmonary stenosis and expected survival of age- and sex-matched control populations. Difference between expected and observed p < .002. (From Kopecky SL, Gersh BJ, McGoon MD, et al. Long-term outcome of patients undergoing surgical repair of isolated pulmonary valve stenosis: Follow-up at 20–30 years. *Circulation* 1988; 78:1150. Reproduced with permission from the American Heart Association and authors.)

MANAGEMENT

The development of symptoms (e.g., angina, exertional dyspnea, and syncope) mandates prompt intervention in aortic valve stenosis (see Chap. 63). In asymptomatic younger individuals, however, the documentation of severe aortic stenosis is in itself an indication for intervention.[211,212] Mild aortic stenosis in asymptomatic patients with gradients below 50 mm warrants careful surveillance. The management of patients in the intermediate group (gradients 50 to 75 mmHg) is more controversial, but evidence argues in favor of elective intervention. Calculation of aortic valve area is important as left ventricular–aortic gradients may be misleading if there is reduced cardiac output.

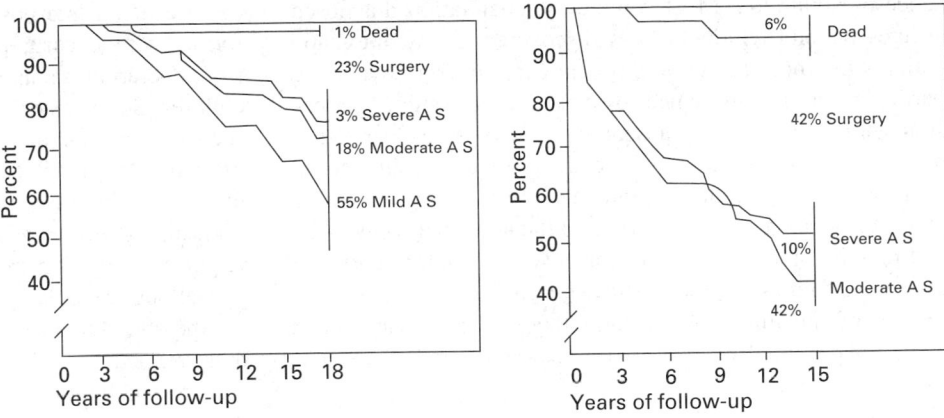

FIGURE 71-8

Left: Cumulative actuarial curves of 153 patients presenting with *mild* aortic stenosis. Bars show ±1 standard error in age at presentation 6.5 years (range 1 to 25 years); mean follow-up 8.8 years (range, 1 to 26 years). *Right:* Cumulative actuarial curves of 54 patients presenting with *moderate* aortic stenosis. Conventions as in left-hand figure. Mean age at presentation 11.8 years (range, 1 to 25 years). Mean follow-up 8.5 years (range, 1 to 24 years). (From Hossack KF, Neutze JM, Lowe JB, Barratt-Boyes BG. Congenital valvar aortic stenosis: Natural history and assessment for operation. *Br Heart J* 1980; 43:561. Reproduced with permission from the publisher and authors.)

Surgery in the young adult with congenital aortic stenosis must be considered as palliative.[147,213] In the absence of calcification, aortic valvotomy is the procedure of choice (see also Chaps. 63 and 70). Perioperative mortality in adolescents and adults is extremely low and late survival is excellent. A large proportion (35 to 45 percent), however, will require reoperation, including aortic valve replacement, over a follow-up period of 20 to 25 years.[145,147] As surgical valvotomy is palliative, catheter balloon valvotomy (Chap.70) has obvious attractions as the initial procedure or as treatment for restenosis.[214] The feasibility of this technique has been well documented in several series, with restenosis less of a problem than in patients with degenerative aortic stenosis. It is encouraging that any resulting aortic regurgitation has rarely required intervention in the short term. Balloon valvotomy, however, is unlikely to be applicable to all patients because of the variable changes in the aortic valve. It is difficult to compare the results of surgical and balloon valvotomy, as long-term follow-up data for the catheter balloon technique are not available and there are no controlled trials of the two approaches.

Valve replacement is the only option for valves unsuitable for valvotomy, including those with significant calcification and regurgitation. The pulmonary autograft ("Ross") operation represents an attractive surgical alternative to prosthetic or homograft aortic valve replacement. The choice of operation is discussed elsewhere (Chap. 63), but the age and size of the patient are major considerations, as well as individual characteristics that determine the safety of anticoagulation, such as the desire for future pregnancies.

Subaortic stenosis is usually amenable to more definitive surgical repair. This fact, in conjunction with the potential for progressive aortic regurgitation, justifies a more aggressive approach even in asymptomatic patients with lesser gradi-ents.[215] Excision of the obstructive membrane together with a myectomy or myotomy is usually required. Subaortic stenosis occasionally recurs, and persistent or progressive aortic regurgitation may develop. Operative mortality is low, but the risks are greater in patients with "tunnel" forms of obstruction and in patients with obstruction at several levels. Some centers have reported promising results for catheter balloon dilatation of subaortic stenosis over short-term follow-up, but further evaluation of this technique is required.[216]

Hospital mortality for repair of supravalvular aortic stenosis is low, and late morbidity and mortality rates are also excellent. Nevertheless, residual abnormality such as aortic regurgitation or stenosis may persist after aortoplasty.

Medical follow-up of patients who have undergone surgical or balloon valvotomy should focus on the development of restenosis, the severity and progression of aortic regurgitation, and the constant hazard of infective endocarditis. Echocardiography has facilitated serial evaluation of gradients, valve areas, ventricular dimensions, function, and mass. The acceptable level of physical activity in patients with left ventricular outflow tract obstruction remains very controversial. It is debatable whether or not any patient who has had significant obstruction should be allowed to participate in competitive sports. We consider a residual gradient greater than 20 mmHg or persistent left ventricular hypertrophy to be contraindications to vigorous physical activity.[128] Before one approves strenuous activity in others, evaluation should include ECG monitoring and maximal exercise testing (Chap. 15).

Coarctation of the Aorta

Although coarctation of the aorta is a congenital malformation, nearly 20 percent of the cases presenting at the Mayo Clinic over a 20-year period were diagnosed initially in adolescence or adulthood. Most commonly, coarctation diagnosed at ages beyond childhood was discovered in asymptomatic patients in whom a routine physical examination for athletic participation or employment disclosed upper limb hypertension with diminished or absent femoral pulses. Coarctation of the aorta may occur anywhere along the descending aorta, even below the diaphragm, but in more than 95 percent of cases it is located below the origin of the left subclavian artery and may involve the origin of this vessel. Usually, there is a discrete infolding of the aortic wall causing eccentric narrowing of the lumen. Frequently there is secondary aortic dilatation proximal and distal to the coarcted area (Fig. 13-1C).

NATURAL HISTORY

Isolated, severe aortic coarctation may cause congestive heart failure as early as the neonatal period. More frequently, however, coarctation producing symptoms during early infancy is associated with other congenital cardiovascular abnormalities such as ventricular septal defect, left ventricular outflow tract obstruction, or mitral valve abnormality. Many patients with undetected coarctation will remain symptom-free until adolescence or early adulthood, when symptoms such as headaches related to hypertension, leg fatigue, or leg cramps may develop. Occasionally, a major catastrophic event such as a cerebrovascular accident, infective endocarditis, or even rupture of the aorta is the first recognized symptom. A bicuspid aortic valve is found in approximately 25 to 50 percent of patients with coarctation, and these abnormal valves have a tendency to calcify in early or middle adult life, producing aortic stenosis. Calcific aortic stenosis may be the presenting condition, and subsequent investigation may disclose an additional coarctation of the aorta. In the era before surgical intervention, approximately 50 percent of patients with coarctation died within the first three decades, and 75 percent were dead by age 50.[217] Death was most frequently caused by a complication of hypertension such as stroke or aortic dissection, but other causes included endocarditis, endarteritis, and congestive heart failure.

MANAGEMENT

Infrequently, a mild degree of coarctation may be present which would not justify intervention. In the great majority of cases, however, symptoms or the presence of significant upper-body hypertension mandate surgical repair. On occasion, an asymptomatic adolescent or adult patient with a severe coarctation will be normotensive at rest because of well-developed collaterals around the coarctation site. Such patients have inappropriate hypertension with exercise, however, and should be repaired. There is evidence that residual hypertension and late complications are directly related to age at the time of repair.[218]

Surgery for coarctation has been available since 1945.[219] Various techniques have been used, including end-to-end anastomosis, patch grafting, and the use of the subclavian flap technique.[220] Aneurysmal or atherosclerotic changes in the aorta found in adolescents or adults may occasionally mandate the use of an interposition prosthetic graft. Surgery is performed without cardiopulmonary bypass, and the risk of death from operation is small, although it is higher in adults than in children. Serious morbidity is rare, but occasionally paraplegia secondary to spinal cord ischemia and bowel ischemia or infarction occur.[221] Some patients require antihypertensive medication because of transient postoperative hypertension for a short period, whereas in others hypertension may persist, requiring long-term treatment.

Balloon angioplasty of native coarctation has been utilized, but the role of this technique remains controversial.[222] Immediate reduction of the degree of obstruction and gradient is usually possible but is achieved at the price of tearing both the aortic intima and media. Late aneurysm formation, presumably secondary to the disruption of the media, has been observed.[223] Currently, most centers do not perform catheter balloon angioplasty as the primary procedure for coarctation, reserving it for recoarctation, where it appears to have a much greater role.

LATE RESULTS

The Mayo Clinic has published late results in 646 patients with coarctation operated upon between 1946 and 1981.[218] The median age at operation was 16 years (range, 1 week to 72 years) with 72 patients (11 percent) over age 35 years of age. Although survival was good (91 percent at 10 years, 72 percent at 30 years), the mean age of death was 38 years, confirming the previous finding that life expectancy is reduced, even after repair. In this and other series reporting long-term follow-up, the most common cause of death was premature coronary artery disease with secondary myocardial infarction.[224,225] Other causes included congestive heart failure, stroke, and ruptured aortic aneurysm. Age at operation was a powerful prognostic factor. The older the patient, the greater the probability of premature death, making it highly likely that the duration of preoperative obstruction and hypertension is important in the etiology of arterial disease and subsequent cardiovascular events.

The incidence of recoarctation with all surgical techniques is low for repairs performed after infancy, but surgery in later years for associated abnormalities such as aortic and mitral valve disease may be required. The majority of survivors are asymptomatic, but there is a high incidence of late hypertension, despite satisfactory early fall in blood pressure after surgery and good relief of obstruction. In one series, only 32 percent of patients were normotensive 30 years after repair and 25 percent were significantly hypertensive.[225] Long-term blood pressure surveillance including blood pressures with exercise is therefore mandatory as hypertension is directly related to many of the late vascular complications.[218,224,225] This incidence may decline significantly as more patients are diagnosed and repaired during infancy or early childhood. Long-term regular follow-up should also include surveillance of the repaired aorta (magnetic resonance imaging is very suitable), assessment of the aortic valve, and endocarditis prophylaxis.

Transposition of the Great Arteries

In complete transposition of the great arteries, the aorta arises from the right ventricle and the pulmonary artery from the left ventricle (discordant ventriculoarterial connection). As a result, the systemic and arterial circulations run "in parallel" rather than "in series" and predominantly desaturated blood enters the aorta. Oxygenation and survival depend on mixing between the systemic and pulmonary circulations at the atrial level in simple transposition (via a patent foramen ovale or atrial septal defect) (see Chap. 70). In approximately half the cases, there are associated anomalies: ventricular septal defect (30 percent), left ventricular outflow tract obstruction (5 to 10 percent), ventricular septal defect with left ventricular outflow tract obstruction (10 percent), patent ductus arteriosus, and, more rarely, coarctation of the aorta or AV valve anomalies.[226] These associated conditions affect both the natural history and surgical management.

NATURAL HISTORY

Transposition of the great arteries is relatively common, but the natural history is so poor that very few patients survive past childhood without intervention. For all varieties, actuarial survival at 1 month is 55 percent and at 1 year 10 percent.[227,228] The outlook is even worse for simple transposition, with only 4 percent natural survival at 1 year.[229] Death is usually due to profound hypoxia and its hematologic consequences. In transposition of the great arteries with large ventricular septal defect, severe hypoxia is rare, but patients do badly as a result of heart failure from excessive pulmonary flow and early pulmonary vascular disease.[121] Transposition with ventricular septal defect and left ventricular outflow tract obstruction presents with early hypoxia. Occasionally, prolonged survival into adult life may occur with a large atrial septal defect, ventricular septal defect, and/or patent ductus arteriosus with the development of pulmonary vascular disease (Eisenmenger's syndrome) or with associated ventricular septal defect and left ventricular outflow tract obstruction.

MANAGEMENT

The outlook has been transformed by the use of catheter balloon atrial septostomy.[230] In the late 1950s and early 1960s, the Senning[231] and Mustard[232] operations involving atrial redirection of the systemic and pulmonary venous returns were introduced. These operations are usually performed between 3 and 12 months of age, with a trend over the years to earlier surgery. Both procedures have been undertaken with excellent early mortality (approximately 2 percent operative mortality and less than 10 percent for the whole early management protocols). Long-term follow-up for both procedures is now available, with comparable late results apart from a lower incidence of baffle obstruction after the Senning operation.[233] Survival into adult life is common; therefore cardiologists are likely to see patients who have undergone these types of atrial redirection. Late problems, however, are now recognized, with sudden death, arrhythmia, tricuspid regurgitation, and right

(systemic) ventricular dysfunction being the major concerns. These late complications have led to the increasing acceptance of the arterial switch operation as the operation of choice.[234] This procedure involves transection and reanastomosis of the great arteries (aorta to left ventricle, pulmonary artery to right ventricle) with coronary artery transfer. The mortality for this procedure has decreased, but the long-term results into adult life are not yet available. For transposition with ventricular septal defect, the mortality for atrial repair with ventricular septal defect closure has always been higher than for simple transposition, and arterial switch is the operation of choice. Transposition with ventricular septal defect and left ventricular outflow tract obstruction is usually palliated in infancy with a systemic-to-pulmonary shunt followed by repair by the Rastelli procedure in later childhood.[235] This involves closure of the ventricular septal defect to connect the left ventricle to the aorta and insertion of a valved conduit from the right ventricle to the pulmonary artery. Long-term results are good, but further surgery to replace the extracardiac conduit in adolescent and adult life is inevitable (see "Surgical Considerations," above).

LATE RESULTS

Two specific problems after atrial redirection have caused concern during long-term follow-up: arrhythmia and systemic ventricular dysfunction. Loss of sinus rhythm is progressive and has not been prevented by modification of surgical technique for either the Mustard or Senning operation.[48,236] In most cases, it is asymptomatic, but occasionally profound bradycardia may necessitate pacemaker insertion. There appears, however, to be no relation between loss of sinus rhythm and risk of sudden death. More worrisome is the development of atrial tachyarrhythmias, including atrial flutter. This arrhythmia has profound hemodynamic consequences after intraatrial repair and is a risk factor for sudden death, especially in the presence of right ventricular dysfunction. Deteriorating performance of the right ventricle supporting the systemic circulation has been reported in some patients, but the precise basis for this problem remains unclear.[237,238] Although a major concern, it is not yet known whether or not ventricular performance will inevitably deteriorate in the majority of patients, and if so, over what period.[239]

As most patients who have undergone intraatrial repair are well, clinical follow-up is directed largely at attempts to stratify risk for sudden death, which is currently difficult. Late death cannot be predicted merely from serial ECGs or ambulatory monitoring.[48] This difficulty underscores the need for a more sophisticated approach involving both electrophysiologic and hemodynamic measurements. Assessment should include evaluation of cardiac performance at rest and exercise and evaluation of systemic and venous pathways. Transesophageal echocardiography appears useful in this situation. Heart transplantation should be considered in the patient who has severe right ventricular failure or disabling arrhythmias. An alternative approach is to perform pulmonary artery banding as preparation for conversion of the atrial repair to an arterial switch. Published results have indicated a significant surgical mortality for this approach. As a result, case selection and timing, as well as optimal surgical strategy, remain unclear.[240] The rather limited information after arterial switch operation suggests that electrophysiologic problems are much less prevalent.[241] More recent studies confirm the theoretical advantages of anatomic repair over atrial repair with respect to preservation of sinus node function and lower prevalence of clinically relevant tachyarrhythmias.[242] The systemic left ventricle after the switch is at risk from the surgical procedure itself, potential myocardial ischemia from coronary distortion, as well as aortic regurgitation. Early results, however, are encouraging, but few patients have yet reached adult life.[243] Because of the high incidence of observed and potential medical problems, all patients who have had both atrial or arterial repair of transposition of the great arteries should have lifelong follow-up by a cardiologist at a center specializing in adult congenital heart disease.

Congenitally Corrected Transposition (Atrioventricular and Ventriculoarterial Discordance)

In congenitally corrected transposition of the great arteries, there is a discordant AV connection (right atrium to left ventricle and left ventricle to right atrium) and a discordant ventriculoarterial connection (left ventricle to pulmonary artery and right ventricle to aorta). As a result of this "double discordance," the systemic and pulmonary venous returns flow to the appropriate great arteries, hence the potentially confusing term *corrected transposition*.

NATURAL HISTORY

In a small proportion of cases (approximately 10 percent in reported series, but this is probably an underestimate) there are no associated cardiac defects.[244,245] Such individuals are pink and asymptomatic and may survive undiagnosed until adult life. The only specific difference from normal hearts is the tendency to develop AV conduction problems and complete heart block. Complete heart block may be present from birth ($\approx$10 percent)[246] and is said to develop in about 2 percent of patients per year.[247] It is not clear whether or not the systemic right ventricle in patients with corrected transposition can maintain function over extended periods and whether or not this has an impact on outcome, since few studies have examined enough patients without associated defects over a long enough period. The majority of cases have a ventricular septal defect (90 percent) and/or pulmonary stenosis (80 percent).[244] Abnormalities of the tricuspid valve (systemic AV valve) are common and may be due to an intrinsic tricuspid valve abnormality such as Ebstein's malformation. These defects influence the natural history and surgical strategy required.

MANAGEMENT

Strategies and indications for surgery differ from those in patients with normal connections because of the potential for the operation to aggravate systemic ventricular dysfunction, systemic AV valve incompetence, or conduction problems. Palliative surgery in childhood is sometimes performed, as definitive repair may involve insertion of an extracardiac conduit. In a large retrospective study of 111 patients managed over a 20-year period, it was concluded that patients with symptomatic heart failure should be repaired before the systemic ventricle dilates and the tricuspid regurgitation becomes severe.[245] Patients with more than mild tricuspid regurgitation whose valves were not replaced did very poorly. In contrast, the patients with cyanosis did much better and the timing of intracardiac surgery can be delayed and be determined by the patient's symptoms. Left AV valve regurgitation is common in adults with congenitally corrected transposition and may be related to Ebstein's malformation of the left AV valve. These valves, however, in contrast to Ebstein's anomaly of the right AV valve, cannot be repaired adequately and always need to be replaced. Left AV valve replacement should always be performed before there is compromise of systemic (morphologic right) ventricle function. In one series of 40 patients, left AV valve replacement was accomplished without surgically induced complete heart block, an early mortality of 10 percent ($N=4$), and 8 late deaths.[248] The principal cause of death in all 12 patients was systemic ventricular failure. Survival correlated with preoperative systemic ventricular ejection fraction of $\geq$44 percent. It thus seems appropriate to refer these patients for valve replacement at the earliest signs of ventricular dysfunction.

Recently, alternative surgical strategies involving a "double switch" have been adopted by some units. These involve an atrial repair by Mustard or Senning operation, together with connection of the left ventricle to the aorta (via a patch through the ventricular septal defect) or an arterial switch.[249,250] The advantage of these approaches is that the morphologic left ventricle (with mitral valve) supports the systemic circulation. While this is an attractive option, it should be stressed that few patients who have received double-switch procedures have reached adolescence, and long-term follow-up data are not yet available for comparison with the conventional surgical approach.

LATE RESULTS

The long-term outcome for well-corrected patients is good, whereas those with severe symptomatic heart failure preoperatively do badly. Atrial arrhythmias are common in long-term follow-up and in one recent series occurred in 36 percent of survivors.[251] Since repairs may involve insertion of an extracardiac conduit, prosthetic AV valve, and pacemaker, careful long-term follow-up is mandatory.

Complex Lesions

A number of complex congenital heart defects involve structural abnormalities that preclude the creation of a biventricular circulation. The changing nomenclature and classification that has been applied to these defects over the years is a major source of confusion (see Chap. 70). This group of patients includes those with double-inlet ventricle (single ventricle), absent right or left AV connection (tricuspid or mitral atresia), some cases of pulmonary atresia/intact ventricular septum and Ebstein's anomaly, and cases with straddling of an AV valve and hypoplastic left or right ventricles. The natural history of these defects is highly variable and depends to a large extent on the impact of the associated defects. In a recent report of 191 patients with double-inlet ventricle presenting in the first year of life, actuarial survival before definitive repair for the whole group was 57 percent at 1 year and 42 percent at 10 years.[158] On multivariate analysis, pulmonary stenosis, balanced pulmonary flow, and older age at presentation were factors favoring survival, whereas right atrial isomerism, common AV orifice, pulmonary atresia, obstruction to systemic output, and anomalous pulmonary venous return were detrimental. Despite the complex morphologic defects, prolonged natural survival is possible, particularly if the physiology is well balanced.[252] The patients with double-inlet left ventricle with discordant ventriculoarterial connection and pulmonary stenosis with balanced pulmonary flow do best, with predicted actuarial survivals of 96 percent at 1 year and 91 percent at 10 years. Such patients may remain well past the third decade of life without intervention.[158]

MANAGEMENT

For most patients with complex congenital heart disease prolonged survival into adult life is possible only with one or more palliative operations (such as systemic to pulmonary shunt, Glenn shunt, pulmonary artery banding, and relief of systemic outflow obstruction) or after a Fontan-type procedure. With palliative surgery alone, clinical deterioration usually begins in the second decade of life and is often due to progressive ventricular dysfunction and/or AV valve regurgitation.[253–255]

The goals of management during childhood have been to maintain suitable anatomy and physiology for the Fontan circulation. A number of modifications of Fontan's original operation have been introduced.[156,256–258] (Fig. 71-9). The basic principle is to separate the systemic and pulmonary circuits by returning systemic venous blood to the pulmonary artery without incorporating a subpulmonary ventricle. This circulation is less "flexible" than one with two functioning ventricles; the operative risk and postoperative status are largely dependent on the patient's suitability. Most important are a low pulmonary vascular resistance and adequate ventricular function (both systolic and diastolic), allowing the circulation to operate with an acceptably low systemic venous pressure.[259] Careful preoperative hemodynamic assessment is vital to optimize patient selection. The operative risk varies considerably between institutions.

LONG-TERM RESULTS

The early and medium-term results of the successful Fontan operation are excellent when compared to the preoperative status of the patients. Improvement in arterial saturation and exercise tolerance have been confirmed by objective testing.[258] The patients with the best hemodynamics can perform well at submaximal levels of exercise equivalent to most normal daily activities[259]; however, less encouraging long-term data are beginning to appear. Fontan's own analysis of 334 patients revealed a premature decline in survival and functional status and a late rise in hazard for which no risk factors could be identified other than the Fontan state per se.[153] Late problems include supraventricular arrhythmia, thrombus in the atria, and declining ventricular function.[152,153,260] Other concerns are the effects of nonpulsatile pulmonary flow favoring the development of pulmonary arteriovenous malformations as seen after the Glenn anastomosis.[261] Extrapolation of these data to current practice is difficult, but the Fontan procedure should be considered to be palliative, not curative.

Certain interesting surgical modifications have been introduced that may improve early and late hemodynamics and the functional results. Perforation of the patch at surgery (fenestrated Fontan) allows a hypertensive right atrium to decompress via a right-to-left shunt at the atrial level.[262] These holes may be closed later with an occlusion device at catheterization. Recent "Fontan" operations have excluded the right atrium from the circulation, creating a total cavopulmonary connection (superior vena cava to right pulmonary artery via a bidirectional Glenn anastomosis and inferior vena cava blood channeled to the pulmonary artery).[263] Data suggest improved flow and energy characteristics compared to the standard atriopulmonary connection and fewer early supraventricular arrhythmias.[54] Anticoagulation policy differs widely even between specialist centers. The increasing concerns regarding stasis of blood in the right atrium and thrombus formation has led to wider routine use of long-term anticoagulants, but this is not standard practice. Patients with a history of documented atrial arrhythmias, a fenestration in the Fontan connection, and "smoke" in the right atrium on echocardiography have the strongest indications for anticoagulation.

All patients who have complex congenital heart defects palliated by systemic to pulmonary shunt, cavopulmonary anastomosis (bidirectional Glenn), or Fontan should have lifelong regular cardiac follow-up at a specialist center. Particular attention should be paid to ventricular function, detection of thrombus in the right atrium, residual shunts, systemic AV valve regurgitation, AV malformations in the lung, obstruction at the Fontan anastomosis (especially in early operations involving a right atrium to pulmonary artery conduit), and protein-losing enteropathy (see above).

Ebstein's Anomaly of the Tricuspid Valve

Ebstein's anomaly is characterized by displacement of the proximal attachments of the tricuspid valve from the AV ring into the right ventricle (see Chap. 70). This structural abnormality divides the right ventricle into an "atrialized" portion and distal "ventricularized" portion. The severity is

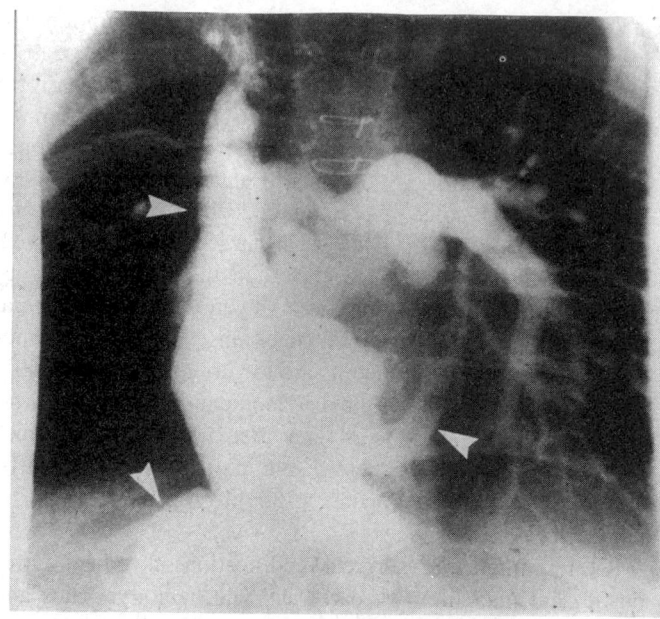

A

FIGURE 71-9

Angiograms showing (*A*) fontan conduit from right atrium to pulmonary artery. There is dilatation of the right atrium with filling of the inferior vena cava, superior vena cava, and coronary sinus. (*B*) Total cavopulmonary connection. The superior vena cava is connected to the right pulmonary artery ("bidirectional Glenn"), and the inferior vena cava is baffled to the pulmonary artery. (Courtesy of Dr ID Sullivan, Great Ormond Street Hospital for Children, London.)

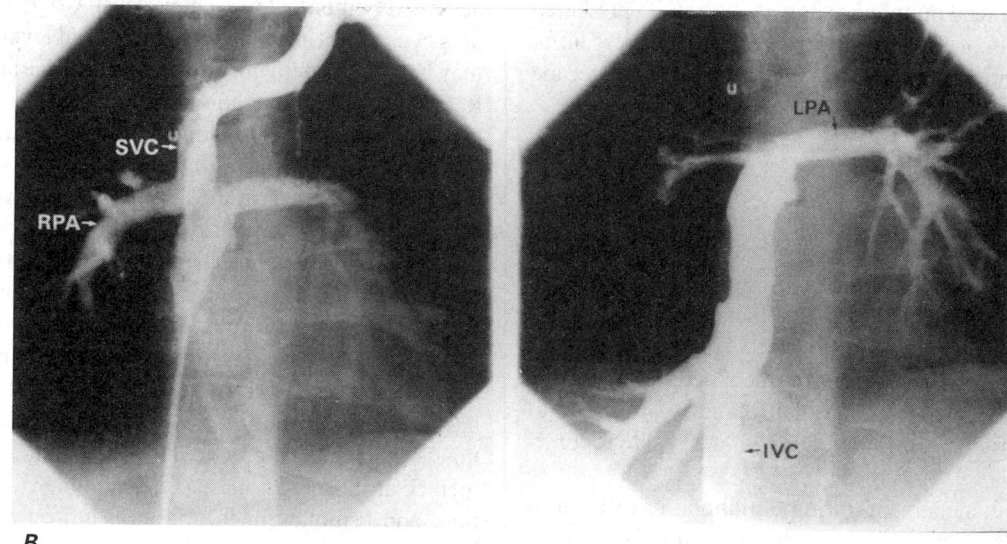

B

variable and accounts for the broad clinical spectrum, from severe disease causing fetal or neonatal death to mild disease compatible with natural survival as late as the eighth decade of life.[264] Ebstein's anomaly is an uncommon defect occurring in less than 1 percent of patients with congenital heart disease, but it is disproportionately represented in the adult congenital heart disease population because of its favorable natural history.

NATURAL HISTORY

The diagnosis of Ebstein's anomaly is now much easier with echocardiography, which has altered our understanding of the natural history. In a large collaborative study of Ebstein's anomaly reported in 1974, only 7 percent of patients were under 1 year of age.[264] Neonates presenting with Ebstein's anomaly represent, not surprisingly, the worst end of the spectrum, with a severe anatomic defect and a high incidence of associated abnormalities, particularly right ventricular outflow tract obstruction. Their poor outcome is predictable from their anatomy.[265] Those who survive this period with or without surgery may live into adult life, although there is continued morbidity and mortality throughout childhood. Many patients are minimally symptomatic in childhood and do not present until adolescence or adult life. Symptoms and signs, when they develop, include cyanosis due to right-to-left shunting at the atrial level, dyspnea secondary to hypoxia, and palpitation due to supraventricular arrhythmia. Ebstein's anomaly is often associated with ventricular preexcitation, which may involve one or more, usually right-sided, accessory pathways.[266] Approximately 25 to 30 percent of adults will have symptomatic arrhythmias that may be difficult to treat and can result in sudden death.[267] Progressive heart failure may develop with time and may be related not only to right-sided problems but also to left-sided abnormalities. Excessive fibrosis has been reported in the left ventricle, and left venticular dysfunction may be induced on exercise.[265,268] Only 50 percent of adults with Ebstein's anomaly that were over 50 years old were cyanotic in one report,[269] and early cyanosis is an adverse risk factor for survival, as is congestive cardiac failure.[270]

MANAGEMENT

Surgery may consist of repair or replacement of the tricuspid valve together with closure of the atrial septal defect to prevent cyanosis.[271] (Fig. 71-10). In 189 patients aged 11 months to 64 years (mean 19.1 years), a tricuspid valve reconstruction was possible in 58.2 percent, and in 36.5 percent a prosthetic valve, usually a bioprosthesis, was inserted. In the occasional patient, the atrial septal defect may be responsible for a left-to-right shunt and can be closed as the sole procedure. In others, the functioning right ventricle is too small for a biventricular circulation, and a Fontan procedure may be the only option. Cross-sectional echocardiography is very useful in determining whether the tricuspid valve is amenable to repair, delineating the mobility or tethering of the enlarged anterior leaflet and the presence or absence of fenestration. The results of surgery are affected by the presence of arrhythmia. Uncontrolled preoperative supraventricular arrhythmia is a risk factor for early postoperative rhythm problems that may have serious hemodynamic consequences.[267] It is usually recommended that division of an accessory pathway be performed at the time of tricuspid valve surgery. The pathways are usually in the posteroseptal or right free wall position and may be multiple. A prolonged electrophysiologic procedure on top of difficult tricuspid valve surgery may result in a very long operation. An alternative approach is to perform catheter radiofrequency ablation of the accessory pathway (Chap. 31) before surgery. Thus far, few such procedures have been done in patients with Ebstein's anomaly. In hearts with marked enlargement of the right atrium, catheter ablation is challenging and, in the setting of an atrial communication, poses the additional risk of a paradoxical embolus and stroke. If there are no accessory pathways, a right-sided maze procedure at the time of tricuspid valve surgery may successfully control supraventricular arrhythmia.[272]

Marfan's Syndrome

Although this autosomal dominant syndrome is congenital in the sense that the patient is born with an abnormal gene (genes), the heart defect is usually ac-

quired. The typical phenotypic features—tall, thin stature, pectus deformities, arachnodactyly, and high-arched palate—by which the condition is currently diagnosed, may be obvious, subtle, or absent (Fig. 10-7). Cardiovascular complications occur in 30 to 60 percent of patients and are the cause of a decreased life expectancy.[273] Mitral valve prolapse is the commonest finding in the pediatric population,[274] but aortic root dilation with a potential for aortic dissection or severe aortic valve regurgitation is the most serious later complication.[275] In a review of 257 patients seen between 1939 and 1972, the average age of death of the 72 patients who died was 32 years, with aortic root problems accounting for three-fourths of the deaths (see also Chap. 85).[273]

MANAGEMENT

The risk of dissection is broadly related to the degree of dilation of the aortic root. Dilation can be followed serially by regular cross-sectional echocardiography, which should be performed at least annually. Particularly close monitoring is necessary during puberty and the rapid-growth phase of adolescence. Treatment with beta blockade has been advocated for patients with evidence of aortic root enlargement, and elective aortic root surgery is recommended when the aorta exceeds 5 to 6 cm in diameter. The aortic valve may also need to be replaced. As regular long-term follow-up visits are required, patients with the Marfan's syndrome are not uncommon in adult "congenital" heart clinics. In addition to their cardiac care, patients need expert help with skeletal and ocular problems, genetic counseling, advice on physical activity (see above), and general psychosocial support.

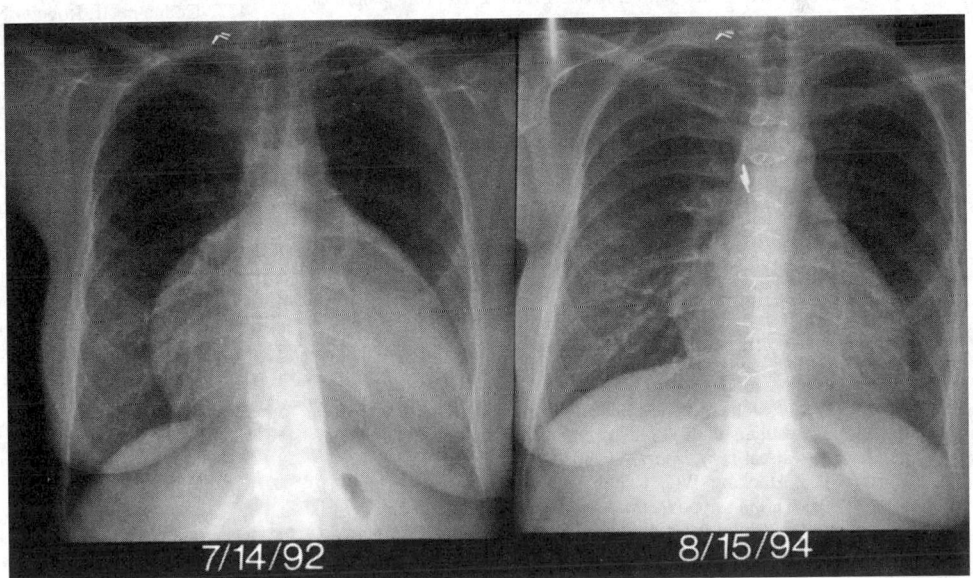

7/14/92   8/15/94

FIGURE 71-10

The chest radiograph on the left shows severe cardiac enlargement associated with Ebstein's anomaly in a 32-year-old woman. She had had a right Blalock-Taussig shunt at age 12. Following tricuspid valve repair and closure of a secundum atrial septal defect, there has been dramatic reduction in the size of the heart, shown on the right.

REFERENCES

1. Ferencz C, Rubin JD, McCarter RJ, Neill CA, Perry LW, Harper SI, et al. Congenital heart disease: Prevalence at live birth. *Am J Epidemiol* 1985; 121:31–36.

2. MacMahon B, McKeown T, Record RG. The incidence and life expectation of children with congenital heart disease. *Br Heart J* 1953; 15:121–129.

3. Gross RE, Hubbard JP. Surgical ligation of a persistent ductus arteriosus. *JAMA* 1939; 112:729–731.

4. Perloff JK. Congenital heart disease in adults. In: Kelly WN (ed). *Textbook of Internal Medicine*. Philadelphia: Lippincott; 1989:223–235.

5. Stark J. Do we really correct congenital heart defects? *J Thorac Cardiovasc Surg* 1989; 97:109.

6. *1996 Consensus Conference on Adult Congenital Heart Disease*. Montreal: Canadian Cardiovascular Society, 1996.

7. Skorton DJ, Cheitlin MD, Freed MD, Garson A, Pinsky WW, Sahn DJ, et al. Task Force 9: Training in the care of adult patients with congenital heart disease. *J Am Coll Cardiol* 1995; 25:1–34.

8. Graham TP, Atwood GF, Boucek RJ, Boerth RC, Bender HW. Abnormalities of right ventricular function following Mustard's operation for transposition of the great arteries. *Circulation* 1975; 52:678–684.

9. Penny DJ, Redington AN. Angiographic demonstration of incoordinate motion of the ventricular wall after the Fontan operation. *Br Heart J* 1991; 66:456–459.

10. Redington AN. Functional assessment of the heart after corrective surgery for complete transposition. *Cardio Young* 1991; 1:84–90.

11. Graham TP, Franklin RCG, Wyse RKH, Gooch V, Deanfield JE. Left ventricular wall stress and contractile function in transposition of the great arteries after the Rastelli operation. *J Thorac Cardiovasc Surg* 1987; 93:775–784.

12. Gewillig MH, Lundstrom UR, Deanfield JE, Gooch VM, Franklin RCG, Graham TP, et al. Impact of the Fontan operation on left ventricular size and contractility. *Circulation* 1990; 81:118–127.

13. Packer M, O'Connor CM, Ghali JK, Pressler ML, Carson PE, Belkin RN et al. Effect of amlodipine on morbidity and mortality in severe chronic heart failure. *N Engl J Med* 1996; 335:1107–1114.

14. CIBIS Investigators and Committees. A randomized trial of β-blockade in heart failure: The Cardiac Insufficiency Bisprolol Study (CIBIS). *Circulation* 1994; 90:1765–1773.

15. Pfeffer MA, Braunwald E, Moyé LA, Basta L, Brown EJ Jr., Cuddy TE, et al. on behalf of the SAVE Investigators. Effect of captopril on mortality and morbidity in patients with left ventricular dysfunction after myocardial infarction. Results of the Survival and Ventricular Enlargement Trial. *N Engl J Med* 1992; 327:669–677.

16. Rudolph AM, Nadas AS, Borges WH. Hematologic adjustment to cyanotic congenital heart disease. *Pediatrics* 1953; 11:454–464.

17. Territo MC, Rosove M, Perloff JK. Cyanotic congenital heart disease: Haematologic management, renal function, and urate metabolism. In: Perloff JK, Child JS (eds). *Congenital Heart Disease in Adults*. Philadelphia: Saunders; 1991:94–95.

18. Perloff JK, Rosove MH, Child JS, Wright GB Adults with cyanotic congenital heart disease: Haematological management. *Ann Intern Med* 1988; 109:406–413.

19. Linderkamp O, Klose HJ, Betke K, Brodherr-Heberlein S, Buhlmeyer K, Kelson S, et al. Increased blood viscosity in patients with cyanotic congenital heart disease and iron deficiency. *J Pediatr* 1979; 59:567–569.

20. Oldershaw PJ, St John Sutton MS. Haemodynamic effects of haemocrit reduction in patients with polycythaemia secondary to cyanotic congenital heart disease. *Br Heart J* 1980; 44:584–588.

21. Rosove MH, Hocking WG, Canobbio MM, Perloff JK, Child JS, Skorton DJ. Chronic hypoxaemia and decompensated erythrocytosis in cyanotic congenital heart disease. *Lancet* 1986; 2:313–315.

22. Ammash NM, Warnes CA. Cerebrovascular events in adult patients with cyanotic congenital heart disease. *J Am Coll Cardiol* 1996; 28:768–772.

23. Cottrill CM, Kaplan S. Cerebral vascular events in cyanotic heart disease. *Am J Dis Child* 1973; 125:484–487.

24. Lusher JM. Diseases of coagulation: The fluid phase. In: Nathan DG, Oski FA (eds). *Haematology in Infancy and Childhood*, 3d ed. Philadelphia: Saunders; 1987:1328–1329.

25. Young D. Hyperuricemia in cyanotic congenital heart disease. *Am J Dis Child* 1980; 134:902–903.

26. Ross EA, Perloff JK, Danovitch GM, Child JS, Canobbio MM. Renal function and urate metabolism in late survivors with cyanotic congenital heart disease. *Circulation* 1986; 73:396–400.

27. Harinck E, Hutter PA, Hoorntje TM, Simons M, Benatar AA, Fischer JC, et al. Air travel and adults with cyanotic heart disease. *Circulation* 1996; 93:272–276.

28. Packer M. Therapeutic application of calcium channel antagonists for pulmonary hypertension. *Am J Cardiol* 1985; 55:196–198.

29. Packer M. Vasodilation therapy for primary pulmonary hypertension: Limitations and hazards. *Ann Intern Med* 1985; 103:258–270.

30. Rich S, Kaufmann E, Levy PS. The effect of high doses of calcium-channel blockers in survival in primary pulmonary hypertension. *N Engl J Med* 1992; 327:76–81.

31. Morrison D, Sorenson S, Caldwell J, Ritchie J, Goldman S, Wright AL, et al. The effect of pulmonary hypertension on systolic function of the right ventricle. *Chest* 1983; 84:250–257.

32. Rounds S, Hill NS. Pulmonary hypertensive disease. *Chest* 1984; 85:397–405.

33. Jordan CE, White RC Jr, Fischer KC, Neill C, Dorst JP. The scoliosis of congenital heart disease. *Am Heart J* 1972; 84:463–469.

34. Working Party of the British Society for Antimicrobial Chemotherapy. The antibiotic prophylaxis of infective endocarditis. *Lancet* 1982; 2:1323–1326.

35. Dajani AS, Talbert KA, Wilson W, Bolger AF, Bayer A, Ferrieri P, et al. Prevention of bacterial endocarditis: Recommendations by the American Heart Association. *JAMA* 1997; 277:1794–1801.

36. Sullivan NM, Sutter VL, Mims MM, Marsh VH, Finegold SM. Clinical aspects of bacteremia after manipulation of the genitourinary tract. *J Infect Dis* 1973; 127:49–55.

37. DeSwiet M, Ramsey ID, Rees GM. Bacterial endocarditis after insertion of intrauterine contraceptive device. *Br Med J* 1975; 2:76–77.

38. Shull HJ Jr, Greene BM, Allen SD, Dunn GD, Schenker S. Bacteremia with upper gastrointestinal endoscopy. *Ann Intern Med* 1975; 83:212–214.

39. Görge G, Erbel R, Henrichs J, Wensschel H, Werner J, Meyer J. Positive blood cultures during transesophageal echocardiography (abstr). *J Am Coll Cardiol* 1990; 15:62A.

40. Sande MA, Levison ME, Lukas DA, Kaye D. Bacteremia associated with cardiac catheterization. *N Engl J Med* 1969; 281:1104–1106.

41. Cetta F, Warnes CA. Adults with congenital heart disease: Patient knowledge of endocarditis prophylaxis. *Mayo Clin Proc* 1995; 70:50–54.

42. Godman MJ, Roberts NK, Izukawa T. Late postoperative conduction disturbances after repair of ventricular septal defect and tetralogy of Fallot. *Circulation* 1974; 49:214–221.

43. Stevenson WG, Klitzner T, Perloff JK. Electrophysiologic abnormalities: Natural occurrence and postoperative residua and sequelae. In: Child JS, Perloff JK (eds). *Congenital Heart Disease in Adults*. Philadelphia: Saunders; 1991:259–295.

44. Vetter VL, Horowitz LN. Electrophysiologic residua and sequelae of surgery for congenital heart defects. *Am J Cardiol* 1982; 50:588–604.

45. Garson A Jr. Chronic postoperative arrhythmia. In: Gillette PC, Garson A Jr (eds) *Pediatric Arrhythmia: Electrophysiology and Pacing*. Philadelphia: Saunders; 1990:667–678.

46. Dodo H, Gow RM, Hamilton RM, Freedom RM. Chaotic atrial rhythm in children. *Am Heart J* 1995; 129:990–995.

47. Boelens M, Friedli B. Sinus node function and conduction system before and after surgery for secundum atrial septal defect: An electrophysiologic study. *Am J Cardiol* 1984; 53:1415–1420.

48. Deanfield J, Camm J, Macartney F, Cartwight T, Douglas J, Drew J, et al. Arrhythmia and late mortality after Mustard and Senning operation for transposition of the great arteries: An eight year prospective study. *J Thorac Cardiovasc Surg* 1988; 96:569–576.

49. Weber HS, Hellenbrand WE, Kleinmann CS, Perlmutter RA, Rosenfeld LE. Predictors of rhythm disturbances and subsequent morbidity after the Fontan operation. *Am J Cardiol* 1989; 64:762–767.

50. Gewillig M, Wyse RK, de Leval MR, Deanfield JE. Early and late arrhythmia after the Fontan operation: Predisposing factors and clinical consequences. *Br Heart J* 1992; 67:72–79.

51. Ward DE, Clarke B, Schofield PM, Jones S, Dawkins K, Bennett D. Long term transvenous ventricular pacing in adults with congenital abnormalities of the heart and great arteries. *Br Heart J* 1983; 50:325–329.

52. Stewart WJ, DiCola VL, Hawthorne JW. Doppler ultrasound measurement of cardiac output in patients with physiologic pacemakers: Effects of left ventricular function and retrograde ventriculoatrial conduction. *Am J Cardiol* 1984; 54:308–312.

53. Fryda RJ, Kaplan S, Helmsworth JA. Postoperative complete heart block in children. *Br Heart J* 1971; 33:456–462.

54. Murphy JG, Gersh BJ, Warnes CA, McGoo MD, Mair DD, Porter CJ et al. The late survival after surgical repair of isolated ventricular septal defect (VSD). *Circulation* 1989; 80(suppl II):490.

55. Kulbertus HE, Coyne JJ, Hallidie-Smith KA. Conduction disturbances before and after surgical closure of ventricular septal defect. *Am Heart J* 1969; 77:123–131.

56. Deanfield JE, McKenna WJ, Hallidie-Smith KA. Detection of late arrhythmia and conduction disturbance after correction of tetralogy of Fallot. *Br Heart J* 1980; 44:577–583.

57. Wolff GS, Rowland TW, Ellison RC. Surgically induced right bundle branch block with left anterior hemiblock. *Circulation* 1972; 46:587–594.

58. Deanfield JE. Late ventricular arrhythmias occurring after tetralogy of Fallot: Do they matter? *Int J Cardiol* 1991; 30:143–150.

59. Gewillig M, Cullen S, Mertens B, Lesaffre E, Deanfield J. Risk factors for arrhythmia and death after Mustard operation for simple transposition of the great arteries. *Circulation* 1991; 84(suppl IV):187–192.

60. Balaji S, Gewillig M, Bull C, de Leval MR, Deanfield JE. Arrhythmias after the Fontan procedure: Comparison of total cavopulmonary connection and atriopulmonary connection. *Circulation* 1991; 84(suppl IV):162–167.

61. Gardiner HM, Dhillon R, Bull C, de Leval MR, Deanfield JE. Prospective study of the incidence and determinants of arrhythmia after total cavopulmonary connection. *Circulation* 1996; 94(suppl II):II-17–II-21.

62. Quattlebaum TG, Varghese J, Neill CA, Donahoo JS. Sudden death among postoperative patients with tetralogy of Fallot: A follow-up study of 243 patients for an average of twelve years. *Circulation* 1976; 54:289–293.

63. Garson A, Nihill MR, McNamara DG, Cooley DA Status of the adult and adolescent after repair of tetralogy of Fallot. *Circulation* 1979; 59:1232–1240.

64. Kavey RE, Blackman MS, Sondheimer HM. Incidence and severity of chronic ventricular dysrhythmia after repair of tetralogy of Fallot. *Am Heart J* 1982; 103:342–350.

65. Vaksmann G, Fournier A, Davignon A, Ducharme G, Houyel L, Fouron J-C. Frequency and prognosis of arrhythmias after operation "correction" or tetralogy of Fallot. *Am J Cardiol* 1990; 66:346–349.

66. Garson A Jr, Porter CB, Gillette PC, McNamara DG. Induction of ventricular tachycardia during electrophysiologic study after repair of tetralogy of Fallot. *J Am Coll Cardiol* 1983; 1:1493–1502.

67. Deanfield JE, McKenna W, Rowland E. Local abnormalities of right ventricular depolarization after repair of tetralogy of Fallot: A basis for ventricular arrhythmia. *Am J Cardiol* 1985; 55:522–526.

68. Deanfield JE, McKenna WJ, Presbitero P, England D, Graham GR, Hallidie-Smith K. Ventricular arrhythmia in unrepaired and repaired tetralogy of Fallot: Relation to age, timing of repair and haemodynamic status. *Br Heart J* 1984; 52:77–86.

69. Sullivan ID, Presbitero P, Gooch VM, Aruta E, Deanfield JE. Is ventricular arrhythmia in repaired tetralogy of Fallot an effect of operation or a consequence of the course of the disease? A prospective study. *Br Heart J* 1987; 58:40–44.

70. Jones M, Ferrans VJ. Myocardial degeneration in congenital heart disease: Comparison of morphologic findings in young and old patients with congenital heart disease associated with muscular obstruction to right ventricular outflow. *Am J Cardiol* 1977; 39:1051–1063.

71. Hegerty A, Anderson RH, Deanfield JE. Myocardial fibrosis in tetralogy of Fallot: Effect of surgery or part of the natural history? (abstr). *Br Heart J* 1988; 59:123.

72. Walsh ED, Rockenmacher S, Keane JF, Hougen TJ, Lock JE, Castaneda AR. Late results in patients with tetralogy of Fallot repaired during infancy. *Circulation* 1988; 77:1062–1067.

73. Kobayashi J, Hirose H, Nakano S, Matsuda H, Shirakura R, Kawashima Y. Ambulatory electrocardiographic study of the frequency and cause of ventricular arrhythmia after correction of tetralogy of Fallot. *Am J Cardiol* 1984; 54:1310–1313.

74. Horowitz LN, Vetter VL, Harken AH, Josephson ME. Electrophysiologic characteristics of sustained ventricular tachycardia after repair of tetralogy of Fallot. *Am J Cardiol* 1980; 46:446–452.

75. Dunnigam A, Pritzker MR, Benditt DG, Benson DW Jr. Life threatening ventricular tachycardias in later survivors of surgically corrected tetralogy of Fallot. *Br Heart J* 1984; 52:198–206.

76. Deal BJ, Scagliotti D, Miller SM, Gallastegni JL, Harriman RJ, Levitsky S. Electrophysiologic drug testing in symptomatic ventricular arrhythmias after repair of tetralogy of Fallot. *Am J Cardiol* 1987; 59:1380–1385.

77. Gatzoulis MA, Clark AL, Newman CG, Redington AN. Right ventricular diastolic function 15–35 years after repair of tetralogy of Fallot: Restrictive physiology predicts superior exercise performance. *Circulation* 1995; 91:1775–1781.

78. Gatzoulis MA, Till JA, Sommerville J, Redington AN. Mechanoelectrical interaction in tetralogy of Fallot: QRS prolongation relates to right ventricular size and predicts malignant ventricular arrhythmias and sudden death. *Circulation* 1995; 92:231–237.

79. Roos-Hesselink J, Perlroth MG, McGhie J, Spitaels S. Atrial arrhythmias in adults after repair of tetralogy of Fallot: Correlations with clinical, exercise, and echocardiographic findings. *Circulation* 1995; 91:2214–2219.

80. Rodefeld MD, Gandhi SK, Huddleston CB, Turken BJ, Shuessler RB, Boineau JP, Cox JL, Bromberg BI. Anatomically based ablation of atrial flutter in an acute canine model of the modified Fontan operation. *J Thorac Cardiovasc Surg* 1996; 112:898–907.

81. Kalman JM, VanHare GF, Olgin JE, Saxon LA, Stark SI, Lesh MD. Ablation of "incisional" reentrant atrial tachycardia complicating surgery for congenital heart disease: Use of entrainment to define a critical isthmus of conduction. *Circulation* 1996; 93:502–512.

82. Triedman JK, Saul JP, Weindling SN, Walsh EP. Radiofrequency ablation of intraatrial reentrant tachycardia after surgical palliation of congenital heart disease. *Circulation* 1995; 91:707–14.

83. de Swiet M. Management of congenital heart disease in pregnancy. In: Anderson RH, Macartney FJ, Shinebourne EA, Tynan M (eds), *Paediatric Cardiology.* Edinburgh: Churchill Livingstone; 1987:1353–1361.

84. Naeye RL, Hagstrom JW, Talmadge BA. Postpartum death with maternal congenital heart disease. *Circulation* 1967; 36:304–312.

85. Perloff JK. Pregnancy in congenital heart disease. In: Perloff JK, Child JS (eds), *Congenital Heart Disease in Adults.* Philadelphia: Saunders; 1991:124–140.

86. Neill CA, Swanson S. Outcome of pregnancy in congenital heart disease (abstr). *Circulation* 1961; 24:1003.

87. Presbitero P, Somerville J, Stone S, Aruta E, Spiegelhalter D. Pregnancy in cyanotic congenital heart disease: Maternal complications and factors influencing successful fetal outcome. *J Am Coll Cardiol* 1992; 19(suppl A):288A.

88. Gleicher N, Midwall J, Hochberger D, Jaffin H. Eisenmenger's syndrome and pregnancy. *Obst Gynecol* 1975; 34:721–741.

89. Avila WS, Grinberg M, Snitcowsky R, Faccioli R, Dahuz PL, Bellotti G, et al. Maternal and fetal outcome in pregnant women with Eisenmenger's syndrome. *Eur Heart J* 1995; 16:460–464.

90. Pitts JA, Crosby WM, Basta LL. Eisenmenger's syndrome in pregnancy: Does heparin prophylaxis improve the maternal mortality rate? *Am Heart J* 1977; 93:321–326.

91. Lieber S, Dewilde PH, Huygens L, Tray E, Gepts E. Eisenmenger's syndrome in pregnancy. *Acta Cardiol* 1985; 40:421–424.

92. Mendelson CL. Pregnancy and coarctation of the aorta. *Am J Obstet Gynecol* 1940; 39:1014–1021.

93. Deal K, Colley CF. Coarctation of the aorta and pregnancy. *Ann Intern Med* 1973; 78:706–710.

94. Limet R, Grondin CM. Cardiac valve prosthesis, anticoagulation, and pregnancy. *Ann Thorac Surg* 1977; 23:337–341.

95. Lutz DJ, Noller KL, Spittell JA, Danielson GK, Fish CR. Pregnancy and its complications following cardiac valve prothesis. *Am J Obstet Gynecol* 1978; 131:460–468.

96. Hall JG, Pauli RM, Wilson KM. Maternal and fetal sequelae of anticoagulation during pregnancy. *Am J Med* 1980; 68:122–140.

97. Iturbe-Alessio I, Del Carmen Fonseca M, Mutchinik O, Santos MA, Zajarias A, Salazar E. Risks of anticoagulant therapy in pregnant women with artificial heart valves. *N Engl J Med* 1986; 315:1390–1393.

98. Salazar E, Izaguirre R, Verdejo J, Mutchinick O. Failure of adjusted doses of subcutaneous heparin to prevent thromboembolic phenomena

in pregnant patients with mechanical cardiac valve prostheses. *J Am Coll Cardiol* 1996; 27:1698–1703.

99. Sbarouni E, Oakley CM. Pregnancy and prosthetic heart valves. *Br Heart J* 1994; 71:196–201.

100. Cotrufo M, deLuca TSL, Calabro R, Mastrogiovanni G, Lama D. Coumarin anticoagulation during pregnancy in patients with mechanical valve prostheses. *Eur J Cardiothorac Surg* 1991; 5:300–305.

101. Elkayam U. Anticoagulation in pregnant women with prosthetic heart valves: A double jeopardy. *J Am Coll Cardiol* 1996; 27:1704–1706.

102. Nora JJ, Nora AH. The evolution of specific genetic and environmental counseling in congenital heart disease. *Circulation* 1978; 57:205–213.

103. Burn J. The aetiology of congenital heart disease. In: Anderson RH, Macartney FJ, Shinebourne EA, Tynan M (eds). *Paediatric Cardiology*. Edinburgh: Churchill Livingstone, 1987:15–63.

104. Allan LD, Crawford DC, Chita SK, Anderson RH, Tynan MJ. Familial recurrence of congenital heart disease in a prospective series of mothers referred for fetal echocardiography. *Am J Cardiol* 1986; 58:334–337.

105. Whittlemore R, Hobbins JC, Engle MA. Pregnancy and its outcome in women with and without surgical treatment of congenital heart disease. *Am J Cardiol* 1982; 50:641–651.

106. Driscoll DJ, Michels VV, Gersony WM, Hayes CJ, Keane JF, Kidd L, et al. Occurrence risk for congenital heart defects in relatives of patients with arotic stenosis, pulmonary stenosis, or ventricular septal defect. *Circulation* 1993; 87(suppl I):I-114–I-120.

107. Weidman WH, Lenfant C, Hayes CJ, Kidd L, Keane JF, Gersony WM, et al. Symposium: The Report of the Natural History Study of Congenital Heart Defects: A 20-year follow-up. Presented at 61st Scientific Session of the American Heart Association, Washington DC: 1988.

108. Tunstall-Pedoe H. Acceptable risk in aircrew. *Eur Heart J* 1988; 9(suppl G):9–11.

109. Deanfield JE. Adult congenital heart disease with special reference to the data on long term follow-up of patients surviving to adulthood with or without surgical correction. *Eur Heart J* 1992; 13(suppl H):111–116.

110. Truesdell SC, Skorton DJ, Lauer RM. Life insurance for children with cardiovascular disease. *Pediatrics* 1986; 77:687.

111. Celermajer DS, Deanfield JE. Employment and insurance for young adults with congenital heart disease. *Br Heart J* 1993; 69:539–543.

112. Garson AJ, Allen HD, Gersony WM, Gillette PC, Hohn AR, Pinsky WW, et al. Cost of congenital heart disease in children and adults: Sources of variation assessed by multicenter study (abstr). *Circulation* 1991; 84(suppl II):II-385.

113. Mahoney LT, Truesdell SC, Hamburgen M, Skorton DJ. Insurability, employability, and psychosocial considerations. In: Perloff JK, Child JS (eds). *Congenital Heart Disease in Adults*. Philadelphia: Saunders; 1991:178–189.

114. Kellerman J, Zeltzer L, Ellenberg L, Dash J, Rigler D. Psychological effects of illness in adolescence: I. Anxiety, self-esteem, and perception of control. *J Pediatr* 1980; 97:126–131.

115. Zeltzer L, Kellerman J, Ellenberg L, Dash J, Rigler D. Psychologic effects of illness in adolescence: II. Impact of illness in adolescents—crucial issues and coping styles. *J Pediatr* 1980; 97:132–138.

116. Myers-Vando R, Steward MS, Folkins CH, Hines P. The effects of congenital heart disease on cognitive development, illness causality concepts, and vulnerability. *Am J Orthopsychiatr* 1979; 49:617–625.

117. Silbert A, Wolff P, Mayer B, Rosenthal A, Nadas A. Cyanotic heart disease and psychological development. *Pediatrics* 1969; 43:192–200.

118. Aram DM, Ekelman BL, Ben-Shachae G, levinsohn MW. Intelligence and hypoxemia in children with congenital heart disease; Fact or artifact? *J Am Coll Cardiol* 1985; 6:889–893.

119. Newburger JW, Silbert AR, Buckley LP, Fyler DC. Cognitive function and age at repair of transposition of the great arteries in children. *N Engl J Med* 1984; 310:1495–1499.

120. Huffman JW. Sex and the teenager. In: Huffman JW, Dewhurst JC, Capuaro VJ (eds). *The Gynecology of Childhood and Adolescence*, 2d ed. Philadelphia: Saunders; 1981:527–542.

121. Bonnar J. Coagulation effects of oral contraception. *Am J Obstet Gynecol* 1987; 157:1042–1048.

122. Fraser IS. Progestogens for contraception. *Austr Fam Phys* 1988; 17:882–885.

123. Whittemore R. Pregnancy and congenital heart disease. In: Adams FH, Emmanoulides GC, Riemenschneider TA (eds). *Heart Disease in Infants, Children and Adults*, 4th ed. Baltimore: Williams & Wilkins; 1989: 684–690.

124. Mayer JA, Bullen BA. Nutrition, weight control and exercise. In: Johnson WR, Buskurk ER (eds), *Science and Medicine of Exercise and Sport*. New York: Harper & Row; 1974:259–275.

125. Rocchini AP, Katch V, Anderson J, Hinderliter J, Becque D, Martin M, et al. Blood pressure in obese adolescents: Effects of weight loss. *Pediatrics* 1988; 82:16–23.

126. Powell KE, Thompson PD, Casperen CJ, Kendrick KS. Physical activity and the incidence of coronary heart disease. *Annu Rev Public Health* 1987; 8:281–287.

127. Maron BJ, Epstein SE, Mitchell JH. Sixteenth Bethesda Conference. Cardiovascular abnormalities in the athlete: Recommendations regarding eligibility for competition. *J Am Coll Cardiol* 1985; 6:1185–1232.

128. Cullen S, Celermajer DS, Deanfield JE. Exercise in congenital heart disease. *Cardiol Young* 1991; 1:129–135.

129. Stark J, Pacifico AD (eds) *Reoperations in Cardiac Surgery*. Berlin: Springer-Verlag; 1989.

130. Dobell ARC, Jain AK. Catastrophic hemorrhage during redo sternotomy. *Ann Thorac Surg* 1984; 37:273–278.

131. Ebert PA, Turley K, Stanger P, Hoffman JIE, Hyemann MA, Rudolph AM. Surgical treatment of truncus arteriosus in the first 6 months of life. *Ann Surg* 1984; 200:451–456.

132. Jonas RA, Freed MD, Mayer JE Jr, Castaneda AR. Long-term follow-up of patients with synthetic right heart conduits. *Circulation* 1985; 72(suppl II):77–83.

133. Ross DN, Somerville J. Correction of pulmonary atresia with a homograft aortic valve. *Lancet* 1966; 2:1446–1447.

134. Merin G, McGoon DC. Reoperation after insertion of aortic homograft as a right ventricular outflow tract. *Ann Thorac Surg* 1973; 16:122–126.

135. Park SC, Neches WH, Lenox CC, Zuberbuhler JR, Bahnson HT. Massive calcification and obstruction in a homograft after the Rastelli procedure for transposition of the great arteries. *Am J Cardiol* 1973; 32:860–864.

136. Shabbo FP, Wain WH, Ross DN. Right ventricular outflow reconstruction with aortic homograft conduit: Analysis of the long-term results. *Thorac Cardiovasc Surg* 1980; 28:21–25.

137. Di Carlo D, de Leval MR, Stark J. "Fresh" antibiotic sterilized aortic homografts in extracardiac valved conduits: Long-term results. *Thorac Cardiovasc Surg* 1984; 32:10–14.

138. Stark J. Reoperations in patients with extracardiac valved conduits. In: Stark J, Pacifico AD (eds). *Reoperations in Cardiac Surgery*. Berlin: Springer-Verlag; 1989:271–290.

139. Studer M, Blackstone EH, Kirklin JW, Pacifico AD, Soto B, Chung GKT, et al. Determinants of early and late results of repair of atrioventricular septal (canal) defects. *J Thorac Cardiovasc Surg* 1982; 84:523–542.

140. Poirier RA, McGoon DC, Danielson GK, Wallace RB, Ritter DG, Moodie DS, et al. Late results after repair of tetralogy of Fallot. *J Thorac Cardiovasc Surg* 1977; 73:900–908.

141. Zhao H, Miller DC, Reitz BA, Shumway NE. Surgical repair of tetralogy of Fallot: Long-term follow-up with particular emphasis on late death and reoperation. *J Thorac Cardiovasc Surg* 1985; 89:204–220.

142. Ebert PA. Second operation for pulmonary stenosis or insufficiency after repair of tetralogy of Fallot. *Am J Cardiol* 1982; 50:637–640.

143. Wessel HU, Cunningham WJ, Paul MH, Nastanier CK, Muster AJ, Idriss FS. Exercise performance in tetralogy of Fallot after intracardiac repair. *J Thorac Cardiovasc Surg* 1980; 80:582–593.

144. Ilbawi MN, Idriss FS, Muster AJ, Wessel HU, Paul MH, De Leon SY. Tetralogy of Fallot with absent pulmonary valve: Should valve insertion be part of the intracardiac repair? *J Thorac Cardiovasc Surg* 1981; 81:906–915.

145. Presbitero P, Somerville J, Revel-Chion R, Ross D. Open aortic valvotomy for congenital aortic stenosis: Late results. *Br Heart J* 1982; 47:26–34.

146. Stewart JR, Paton BC, Blunt SG Jr, Swan H. Congenital aortic stenosis: Ten to twenty years after valvulotomy. *Arch Surg* 1978; 113:1248–1252.

147. Hsieh K, Keane JF, Nadas AS, Bernhard WF, Castaneda AR. Long term follow-up of valvulotomy before 1968 for congenital aortic stenosis. *Am J Cardiol* 1986; 58:338–341.

148. Rao PS, Thapar MK, Wilson AD, Levy JM, Chopra PS. Intermediate-term follow-up results of balloon aortic valvuloplasty in infants and children with special reference to causes of restenosis. *Am J Cardiol* 1989; 64:1356–1360.

149. Puga FJ, Leoni FR, Julsrud PR, Mair DD. Complete repair of pulmonary atresis, ventricular septal defect and severe peripheral arborization abnormalities of the central pulmonary arteries: Experience with preliminary unifocalization procedures in 38 patients. *J Thorac Cardiovasc Surg* 1989; 6:1018–1029.

150. Sullivan ID, Wren C, Stark J, de Leval M, Macartney FJ, Deanfield JE. Surgical unifocalisation in pulmonary atresia and ventricular septal defect: A realistic goal? *Circulation* 1988; 78(suppl III):5–13.

151. Watterson KG, Wilkinson JL, Karl TR, Mee RBB. Very small pulmonary arteries: The central end-to-side shunt. *Ann Thorac Surg* 1991; 52:1132–1137.

152. Driscoll DJ, Offord KP, Felot RH, Schaff HV, Puga FJ, Danielson GK. Five to fifteen year follow-up after Fontan operation. *Circulation* 1992; 85:469–496.

153. Fontan F, Kirklin JW, Fernandez G, Costa F, Naftel DC, Tritto F, et al. Outcome after a "perfect" Fontan operation. *Circulation* 1990; 81:1520–1536.

154. Feldt RH, Driscoll DJ, Offord KP, Cha RH, Perraoult J, Schaff HV, et al. Protein-losing enteropathy after the Fontan operation. *J Thorac Cardiovasc Surg* 1991; 112:672–680.

155. Mertens L, Dumoulin M, Gewillig M. Effective percutaneous fenestration of the atrial septum on protein-losing enteropathy after the Fontan operation. *Br Heart J* 1994; 72:591–592.

156. Warnes CA, Feldt RH, Hagler DJ. Protein-losing enteropathy after the Fontan operation: Successful treatment by percutaneous fenestration of the atrial septum. *Mayo Clin Proc* 1996; 71:378–379.

157. Kaiett JM, Kaye MP. The Registry of the International Society for Heart and Lung Transplantation: Eighth official report. *J Heart Transplant* 1991; 10:491–498.

158. Franklin RCG, Spiegelhalter DJ, Anderson RH, Maccartney FJ, Filho RIR, Douglas JM, et al. Double inlet ventricle presenting in infancy: I. Survival without definitive repair. *J Thorac Cardiovasc Surg* 1991; 101:767–776.

159. Kaplan EL, Meier P. Nonparametric estimation from incomplete observations. *J Am Stat Assoc* 1958; 53:457–481.

160. Child JS, Perloff JK. Natural survival patterns: A narrowing base. In: Child JS, Perloff JK (eds), *Congenital Heart Disease in Adults*. Philadelphia: Saunders; 1991:21–59.

161. Borow KM, Braunwald E. Congenital heart disease in the adult. In: Braunwald E (ed), *Heart Disease*, 3d ed. Philadelphia. Saunders; 1988:976–1002.

162. Warnes CA, Fuster V, Driscoll DJ. McGoon DC, Atrial septal defect. In: Giuliani ER, Fuster V, Gersh BJ, McGoon MD, McGoon DC (eds), *Cardiology Fundamentals and Practice*, 2d ed. St Louis: Mosby–Year Book; 1991:1622–1638.

163. Kirklin JW, Barratt-Boyes BG (eds). *Cardiac Surgery*, New York: Wiley; 1986:463–497.

164. Massumi RA, Nutter DO. The syndrome of familial defects of the heart and upper extremities (Holt-Oram syndrome). *Circulation* 1966; 34:65–76.

165. Nora JJ, McNamara, Fraser FC. Hereditary factors in atrial septal defect. *Circulation* 1967; 35:448–456.

166. Perloff JD. Ostium secundum atrial septal defect—Survival for 87–94 years. *Am J Cardiol* 1984; 53:388–389.

167. Craig RJ, Selzer A. Natural history and prognosis of atrial septal defects. *Circulation* 1968; 37:805–815.

168. Campbell M. Natural history of atrial septal defect. *Br Heart J* 1970; 32:820–826.

169. Shah D, Azhar M, Oakley CN, Cleland JGF, Nihoyannopoulos P. Natural history of secundum atrial septal defect in adults after medical or surgical treatment: A historical prospective study. *Br Heart J* 1994; 71:224–228.

170. Konstantinides S, Geibel A, Olschewski M, Grnandt L, Roskamm H, Spillner G, et al. A comparison of surgical and medical therapy for atrial septal defects in adults. *N Engl J Med* 1995; 333:469–473.

171. Lock JE. The adult with congenital heart disease: Cardiac catheterization as a therapeutic intervention. *J Am Coll Cardiol* 1991; 18:330–331.

172. Hellenbrand WE, Fahey JT, McGowan FX, Welton GG, Kleinman CS. Transesophageal echocardiographic guidance of transcatheter closure of atrial septal defect. *Am J Cardiol* 1990; 66:207–213.

173. Murphy JG, Gersh BJ, McGoon MD, Mair DD, Porter CJ, Ilstrup DM, et al. Long term outcome after surgical repair of isolated atrial septal defect. Follow up at 27 to 32 years. *N Engl J Med* 1990; 323:1645–1697.

174. Brandenburg RO Jr, Holmes DR Jr, Brandenburg RO, McGoon DC. Clinical follow-up study of paroxysmal supraventricular arrhythmias after operative repair of a secundum type atrial septal defect in adults. *Am J Cardiol* 1983; 51:273–276.

175. St John Sutton MG, Tajik AJ, McGoon DC. Atrial septal defect in patients aged 60 years or older: Operative results and long-term postoperative follow-up. *Circulation* 1981; 64:402–409.

176. Engle MA, Kline SA, Borer JS. Ventricular septal defect. In: Roberts WC (ed). *Adult Congenital Heart Disease*. Philadelphia: Davis; 1987:409–441.

177. Wood P. The Eisenmenger syndrome or pulmonary hypertension with reversed central shunt. *Br Med J* 1958; 2:701–709.

178. Warnes CA, Fuster V, Driscoll DJ, McGoon DC. Ventricular septal defect. In: Giuliani ER, Fuster V, Gersh BJ, McGoon MD, McGoon DC (eds). *Cardiology: Fundamentals and Practice*, 2d ed. Vol 2. St Louis: Mosby–Year Book, 1991:1639–1652.

179. Tatsuno K, Konno S, Sakakibara S. Ventricular septal defect with aortic insufficiency: Angiocardiographic aspects and a new classification. *Am Heart J* 1973; 85:13–21.

180. Zhou Q, Lai Y, Wei H, Sorg R, Wu Y, Zhang H. Unidirectional valve patch for repair of cardiac defects with pulmonary hypertension. *Ann Thorac Surg* 1995; 60:1245–1249.

181. Cartmill TB, DuShane JW, McGoon DC, Kirklin JW. Results of repair of ventricular septal defect. *J Thorac Cardiovasc Surg* 1966; 52:486–499.

182. Blake RS, Chung EE, Wesley H, Hallidie-Smith KA. Conduction defects, ventricular arrhythmias and late death after surgical closure of ventricular septal defect. *Br Heart J* 1982; 47:305–315.

183. Bridges ND, Perry SB, Keane JF, Goldstein SAN, Mandell V, Mayer JE Jr, et al. Preoperative transcatheter closure of congenital muscular ventricular septal defects. *N Engl J Med* 1991; 324:1312–1317.

184. Report of the New England Regional Infant Cardiac Program. *Pediatrics* 1980; 65(suppl):441–444.

185. Rastelli GC, Ongley PA, Kirklin JW, McGoon DC. Surgical repair of the complete form of persistent common atrioventricular canal. *J Thorac Cardiovasc Surg* 1968; 55:299–308.

186. Bergin ML, Warnes CA, Tajik AJ, Danielson GK. Partial atrioventricular canal defect: Long-term follow-up after initial repair in patients ≥40 years old. *J Am Coll Cardiol* 1995; 25:1189–1194.

187. Abraham KA, Cherian G, Rao VD, Sukumar IP, Krishnaswami S, John S. Tetralogy of Fallot in adults: A report on 147 patients. *Am J Med* 1979; 66:811–816.

188. Phadke AR, Phadke SA, Handy M, Junnarkar RV. Acyanotic Fallot's tetralogy with survival to the age of 70 years: Case report. *Indian Heart J* 1977; 29:46–49.

189. Bertranou EG, Blackstone EH, Hazelrig JB, Turner ME, Kirklin JW. Life expectancy without surgery in tetralogy of Fallot. *Am J Cardiol* 1978; 42:458–466.

190. Deanfield JE, Ho S-Y, Anderson RH, McKenna WJ, Allwork SP, Hallidie-Smith KA. Late sudden death after repair of tetralogy of Fallot: A clinico-pathological study. *Circulation* 1983; 67:636–641.

191. Katz NM, Blackstone EH, Kirklin JW, Pacifico AD, Bargeron LM Jr. Late survival and symptoms after repair of tetralogy of Fallot. *Circulation* 1982; 65:403–410.

192. Murphy JG, Gersh BJ, McGoon MD, Mair DD, Ilstrup D, Porter CJ, et al. Long term (30 year) survival of patients undergoing complete repair of tetralogy of Fallot (abstr). *J Am Coll Cardiol* 1990; 15:205A.

193. Lillehei CW, Varco RL, Cohen M, Warden HE, Gott VL, DeWall RA, et al. The first open heart corrections of tetralogy of Fallot: A 26–31 year follow-up of 106 patients. *Ann Surg* 1986; 204:490–501.

194. Deanfield JE. Late ventricular arrhythmias occurring after repair of tetralogy of Fallot: do they matter? *Int J Cardiol* 1991; 30:143–150.

195. Wennevold A, Rygg I, Lauridsen P, Efsen F, Jacobsen JR. Fourteen-to nineteen-year follow-up after corrective repair for tetralogy of Fallot. *Scand J Thorac Cardiovasc Surg* 1982; 16:41–45.

196. Piccoli GP, Dickinson DF, Musumeci F, Hamilton DI. A changing policy for the surgical treatment of Fallot: Early and late results in 235 consecutive patients. *Ann Thorac Surg* 1982; 33:365–373.

197. Bjarke B. Oxygen uptake and cardiac output during submaximal and maximal exercise in adult subjects with totally corrected tetralogy of Fallot. *Acta Med Scand* 1975; 197:177–186.

198. Nugent EW, Freedom RM, Nora JJ, Ellison RC, Rowe RD, Nadas AS. Clinical course in pulmonary stenosis. *Circulation* 1977; 56(suppl I):I-38–I-47.

199. Mody MR. The natural history of uncomplicated valvular pulmonic stenosis. *Am Heart J* 1975; 90:317–321.

200. Kopecky SL, Gersh BJ, McGoon MD, Mair DD, Porter CH, Ilstrup DM, et al. Long-term outcome of patients undergoing surgical repair of isolated pulmonary valve stenosis: Follow-up at 20 to 30 years. *Circulation* 1988; 78:1150–1156.

201. Kan JS, White RI Jr, Mitchell SE, Gardner TJ. Percutaneous balloon valvuloplasty: A new method for treating congenital pulmonary valve stenosis. *N Engl J Med* 1982; 307:540–542.

202. Mullins CE, Latson LA, Neches WH, Colvin EV, Kan J. Balloon dilatation of miscellaneous lesions: Results of Valvuloplasty and Angioplasty of Congenital Anomalies Registry. *Am J Cardiol* 1990; 65:802–803.

203. Sullivan ID, Robinson PJ, Macartney FJ, Taylor JFN, Rees PG, Bull C, et al. Percutaneous balloon valvuloplasty for pulmonary valve stenosis in infants and children. *Br Heart J* 1985; 54:435–441.

204. Friedman WF, Johnson AD. Congenital aortic stenosis. In: Roberts WC (ed). *Adult Congenital Heart Disease*. Philadelphia: Davis; 1987:357–374.

205. Kelly DT, Wulfsberg BA, Rowe RD. Discrete subaortic stenosis. *Circulation* 1972; 46:309–322.

206. Williams JCP, Barratt-Boyes BG, Lowe JB. Supravalvular aortic stenosis. *Circulation* 1961; 24:1311–1318.

207. Mills P, Leech G, Davies M, Leatham A. The natural history of a non-stenotic bicuspid aortic valve. *Br Heart J* 1978; 40:951–957.

208. Gersony WM, Hayes CJ. Bacterial endocarditis in patients with pulmonary stenosis, aortic stenosis or ventricular septal defect. *Circulation* 1977; 56(suppl I):I-84–I-87.

209. Fontana RS, Edwards JE *Congenital Cardiac Disease: A Review of 357 Cases Studied Pathologically*. Philadelphia: Saunders; 1962.

210. Muna WFT, Ferrans VJ, Pierce JE, Roberts WC. Discrete subaortic stenosis in Newfoundland dogs: Association of infective endocarditis. *Am J Cardiol* 1978; 41:746–754.

211. Cohen LS, Friedman WF, Braunwald E Natural history of mild congenital aortic stenosis elucidated by serial hemodynamic studies. *Am J Cardiol* 1972; 30:1–5.

212. Wagner HR, Ellison RC, Keane JF, Nadas AS, Bernhard WF, Castaneda AR. Long-term follow-up of valvotomy before 1968 for congenital aortic stenosis. *Am J Cardiol* 1986; 58:338–341.

213. Kugelmeier J, Egloff L, Real F, Rothlin M, Turina M, Senning A. Congenital aortic stenosis: Early and late results of arotic valvotomy. *Thorac Cardiovasc Surg* 1982; 30:91–95.

214. Bull C. Interventional catheterisation in infants and children (editorial). *Br Heart J* 1986; 56:197–200.

215. Somerville J, Stone S, Ross D. Fate of patients with fixed subaortic stenosis after surgical removal. *Br Heart J* 1980; 43:629–647.

216. Suarez de Lezo J, Pan M, Sancho M, Herrera N, Arizon J, Franco M, et al. Percutaneous transluminal balloon dilatation for discrete subaortic stenosis. *Am J Cardiol* 1986; 58:619–621.

217. Campbell M. Natural history of coarctation of the aorta. *Br Heart J* 1970; 32:633–640.

218. Cohen M, Fuster V, Steele PM, et al. Coarctation of the aorta: Long term follow-up and prediction of outcome after surgical correction. *Circulation* 1989; 80:840–845.

219. Gross RE, Hufnagel CA. Coarctation of the aorta: Experimental studies regarding its surgical correction. *N Engl J Med* 1945; 233:287–293.

220. Waldhausen JA, Whitman V, Werner JC, et al. Surgical intervention in infants with coarctation of the aorta. *J Thorac Cardiovasc Surg* 1981; 81:323–325.

221. Keen G: Spinal cord damage and operations for coarctation of the aorta: Aetiology, practice and prospects. *Thorax* 1987; 42:11–18.

222. Sperling DR, Dorsey TJ, Rowen M, Gazzaniga AB. Percutaneous transluminal angioplasty of congenital coarctation of the aorta. *Am J Cardiol* 1983; 51:562–564.

223. Ritter SB. Coarctation and balloons: Inflated or realistic? *J Am Coll Cardiol* 1989; 13:696–699.

224. Maron BJ, Humphries J, Rowe RD, et al. Prognosis of surgically corrected coarctation of the aorta: A 20 year postoperative appraisal. *Circulation* 1973; 47:119–126.

225. Presbitero P, Demarie D, Villani M, et al. Long-term results (15-30 years) of surgical repair of aortic coarctation. *Br Heart J* 1987; 57:462–467.

226. Fyler DC. Report of the New England regional cardiac infant program. *Pediatrics* 1980; 65:375–460.

227. Miller RA. Complete transposition of the great arteries. In: Morse DP (ed). *Congenital Heart Disease: Pathogenic Factors, Natural History, Diagnosis and Surgical Treatment*. Philadelphia: Davis; 1962:74–75.

228. Keith JD, Neill CA, Vlad P, Rowe RD, Chute AL. Transposition of the great vessels. *Circulation* 1953; 7:830–838.

229. Leibman J, Cullum L, Belloc NB. Natural history of transposition of the great arteries: Anatomy and birth and death characfteristics. *Circulation* 1969; 40:237–262.

230. Rashkind WJ, Miller WW. Creation of an atrial septal defect without thoracotomy: A palliative approach to complete transposition of the great arteries. *JAMA* 1966; 196:991–992.

231. Senning A. Surgical correction of transposition of the great vessels. *Surgery* 1959; 45:966–980.

232. Mustard WT. Successful two-stage correction of transposition of the great vessels. *Surgery* 1964; 55:469–472.

233. Turina MI, Seibenmann R, Segesser L, Schonbeck M, Senning A. Late functional deterioration after atrial correction for transposition of the great arteries. *Circulation* 1989; 80(suppl I):162–167.

234. Jatene AD, Fontes VF, Paulista PP, Souza LCB, Neger F, Galantier M, et al. Successful anatomic correction of transposition of the great vessels: A preliminary report. *Arg Braz Cardiol* 1975; 28:461–464.

235. Rastelli GG, Wallace RB, Ongley PA. Complete repair of transposition of the great arteries with pulmonary stenosis: A review and report of a case corrected by using a new surgical technique. *Circulation* 1969; 39:83–95.

236. Flinn CJ, Wolff GS, Dick M, Campbell RM, Borkal G, Casta A, et al. Cardiac rhythm after the Mustard operation for complete transposition of the great arteries. *N Engl J Med* 1984; 310:1635–1638.

237. Graham TP, Arwood GF, Boucek RJ, Boerth RF, Bender HW. Abnormalities of right ventricular function following Mustard's operation for transposition of the great arteries. *Circulation* 1975; 52:678–684.

238. Hagler DJ, Ritter DG, Mair DD, Tajik AJ, Seward JB, Fulton RE, et al. Right and left ventricular function after the Mustard procedure for transposition of the great arteries. *Am J Cardiol* 1979; 44:276–283.

239. Graham TP, Burger J, Bender HW, Hammon JW, Boucek RJ, Appleton S. Improved right ventricular function after intraatrial repair of transposition of the great arteries. *Circulation* 1985; 72:1145–1151.

240. Mee RBB. Severe right ventricular failure after Mustard or Senning operation: Two-stage repair: Pulmonary artery banding and switch. *J Thorac Cardiovasc Surg* 1986; 92:385–390.

241. Wernovsky G, Hougen TJ, Walsh EP, Scholler GF, Colan SD, Sanders SP, et al. Mid-term results after the arterial switch operation for transposition of the great arteries with intact ventricular septum: Clinical, hemodynamic, echocardiographic and electrophysiologic data. *Circulation* 1988; 77:1333–1344.

242. Rhodes LA, Wernovsky CT, Keane JF, Mayer JE Jr, Shuren A, Dindy C, et al. Arrhythmias and intracardiac conduction after the arterial switch operation. *J Thorac Cardiovasc Surg* 1995; 19:303–310.

243. Colan Sd, Trowitzsch E, Wernovsky G, Sholler GF, Sanders SP, Castaneda A. Myocardial performance after arterial switch operation for transposition of the great arteries with intact ventricular septum. *Circulation* 1988; 78:132–141.

244. Allwork SP, Bentall HH, Becker AD, Cameron H, Gerlis LM, Wilkinson JL, et al. Congenitally corrected transposition of the great arteries: Morphologic study of 32 cases. *Am J Cardiol* 1976; 38:910–923.

245. Lundstrom U, Bull C, Wyse RKH, Somerville J. The natural and "unnatural" history of congenitally corrected transposition. *Am J Cardiol* 1990; 65:1222–1229.

246. Friedberg DZ, Nadas AS. Clinical profile of patients with congenitally corrected transposition of the great arteries: A study of 60 cases. *N Engl J Med* 1970; 282:1053–1059.

247. Huhta JC, Maloney JE, Ritter DG, Ilstrup DM, Feldt RH. Complete atrioventricular block in patients with atrioventricular discordance. *Circulation* 1983; 67:1374–1377.

248. van Son JAM, Danielson GK, Huhta JC, Warnes CA, Edwards WD, Schaff HV, et al. Late results of systemic atrioventricular valve replacement in corrected transposition. *J Thorac Cardiovasc Surg* 1995; 109:642–653.

249. Yagihari T, Kishimoto H, Isobe F et al. Double switch operation in cardiac anomalies with atrioventricular and ventriculoarterial discordance. *J Thorac Cardiovasc Surg* 1994; 107:351–358.

250. Ilbawi MN, DeLeon SY, Backer CL, et al. An alternative approach to the surgical management of physiologically corrected transposition with ventricular septal defect and pulmonary stenosis or atresia. *J Thorac Cardiovasc Surg* 1990; 100:410–415.

251. Connelly MS, Piu PP, Williams WG, Webb GD, Robertson P, McLaughlin PR. Congenitally corrected transposition in the adult: Functional status and complications. *J Am Coll Cardiol* 1996; 27:1238–1243.

252. Ammash NS, Warnes CA. Survival into adulthood of patients with unoperated single ventricle. *Am J Cardiol* 1996; 77:542–544.

253. LaCorte MA, Dick M, Scheer G, LaFarge CG, Flyer DC. Left ventricular function in tricuspid atresia: Angiographic analysis in 28 patients. *Circulation* 1975; 52:996–1000.

254. Moodie DS, Ritter DG, Tajik AH, McGoon DC, Danielson GK, O'Fallon WM. Long-term follow-up after palliative operation for univentricular heart. *Am J Cardiol* 1984; 53:1648–1651.

255. Moodie DS, Ritter DG, Tajik AH, O'Fallon WM. Long-term follow-up in the unoperated univentricular heart. *Am J Cardiol* 1984; 53:1124–1128.

256. Fontan F, Baudet E. Surgical repair of tricuspid atresia. *Thorax* 1971; 26:240–248.

257. Choussat A, Fontan I, Besse P, Vallot F, Cahuve A, Bricand H. Selection criteria for Fontan's procedure. In Anderson RH, Shineborune EA (eds): *Paediatric Cardiology*. Edinburgh: Churchill Livingstone; 1978: chap 64.

258. Fontan F, Deville C, Quagebeur J, Ottenkamp J, Sourdille N, Choussat A, et al. Repair of tricuspid atresia in 100 patients. *J Thorac Cardiovasc Surg* 1983; 85:647–660.

259. Gewillig MH, Lundstrom UR, Bull C, Wyse RKH, Deanfield JE. Exercise responses in patients after Fontan repair: Patterns and determinants of performance. *J Am Coll Cardiol* 1990; 15:1424–1432.

260. Matsuda H, Kawashima Y, Kishimoto H, Hirose H, Nakano S, Kato H, et al. Problems with the modified Fontan operation for univentricular heart of the right ventricular type. *Circulation* 1987; 76(suppl II):II-45–II-52.

261. Mathur M, Glenn WWL. Long term evaluation of cavopulmonary artery anastomosis. *Surgery* 1973; 74:889–916.

262. Bridges ND, Lock JE, Castaneda AR. Baffle fenestration with subsequent transcatheter closure: Modifications of the Fontan operation for patients at higher risk. *Circulation* 1990; 82:1681–1689.

263. de Leval MR, Kilner P, Gewillig M, Bull C. Total cavopulmonary connection: A logical alternative to atriopulmonary connection for complex Fontan operations. *J Thorac Cardiovasc Surg* 1988; 96:682–695.

264. Watson H. Natural history of Ebstein's anomaly of the tricuspid valve in childhood and adolescence: An internation cooperative study of 505 cases. *Br Heart J* 1974; 36:417–427.

265. Celermajer DS, Dodd SM, Greenwald SE, Wyse RK, Deanfield JE. Morbid anatomy in neonates with Ebstein's anomaly of the tricuspid valve: Pathophysiologic and clinical implications. *J Am Coll Cardiol* 1992; 19:1049–1053.

266. Lev M, Gibson S, Millar RA. Ebstein's disease with Wolff-Parkinson-White syndrome: Report of a case with histopathologic study of possible conduction pathways. *Am Heart J* 1955; 49:724–741.

267. Till J, Celermajer D, Deanfield J. The natural history of arrhythmias in Ebstein's anomaly. *J Am Coll Cardiol* 1992; 19(suppl A):273A.

268. Saxena A, Fong LV, Tristram M, Ackery DM, Keeton BR. Late noninvasive evaluation of cardiac performance in mildly symptomatic older patients with Ebstein's anomaly of the tricuspid valve: Role of radionuclide imaging. *J Am Coll Cardiol* 1991; 17:182–186.

269. Genton E, Blount G. The spectrum of Ebstein's anomaly. *Am Heart J* 1967; 73:395–425.

270. Kumar AJ, Fyler DC, Miettinen OS, Nadas AS. Ebstein's anomaly: Clinical profile and natural history. *Am J Cardiol* 1981; 28:84–95.

271. Danielson GK, Driscoll DJ, Mair DD, Warnes CA, Oliver WC. Operative treatment of Ebstein's anomaly. *J Thorac Cardiovasc Surg* 1992; 104:1195–1202.

272. Theodoro DA, Danielson GK, Porter CJ, Warnes CA. Right-sided maze procedure: A surgical treatment for atrial fibrillation and atrial flutter in right-sided congenital heart disease. *Annals Thorac Surg.* In press.

273. Murdoch JL, Walker BA, Halpern BI, Kuzma JW, McKusick VA. Life expectancy and causes of death in the Marfan syndrome. *N Engl J Med* 1972; 286:804–808.

274. Pyerlitz RE, Wappel MA. Mitral valve dysfunction in the Marfan syndrome. *Am J Med* 1983; 74:797–807.

275. Gott VL, Pyerlitz RE, Magovern GJ Jr, Cameron DE, McKusick VA. Surgical treatment of aneurysms of the ascending aorta in the Marfan syndrome: Results of composite graft repair in 50 patients. *N Engl J Med* 1986; 314:1070–1074.

CARDIOMYOPATHY AND SPECIFIC HEART MUSCLE DISEASES

72

CLASSIFICATION OF CARDIOMYOPATHIES

Jay W. Mason

Despite controversy in classifying the cardiomyopathies, there is general agreement on the definition. Cardiomyopathy is a primary disorder of the heart muscle that causes abnormal myocardial performance and is not the result of disease or dysfunction of other cardiac structures. Thus, the term *cardiomyopathy* excludes cases of myocardial failure due to myocardial infarction (so-called ischemic cardiomyopathy, a misnomer), systemic arterial hypertension, and valvular stenosis or regurgitation. Although cardiomyopathy is easily defined, classification of its various forms is difficult. This difficulty results because the great majority of cases of cardiomyopathy are associated with generalized cardiac dilatation and ventricular systolic dysfunction, in which the etiology is unknown.

CLASSIFICATION SCIENCE

Physicians and biomedical scientists use classification schemes to draw relationships and distinctions between diseases. This process promotes understanding and aids recollection. Even disorders we know little about can be understood if appropriately placed in a class with other disorders we do know about.

The science of classification requires that all items within the domain being classified be included and that each item appear in only one class. Inability to make clear distinctions between biologic systems makes this latter requirement the most demanding. Classification must be based on those features of the individual units within the domain that are understood or recognizable and that permit a useful distinction between groups.

Thus, the classification of cardiomyopathies should be based on an extensive, current category of knowledge about heart diseases and should be as useful as possible to physicians and scientists.

CATEGORIES OF KNOWLEDGE ABOUT CARDIOMYOPATHIES

Our knowledge about cardiomyopathies falls into several categories: Etiology, gross anatomy, histology, genetics, biochemistry, immunology, hemodynamic function, prognosis, treatment, and others. No single classification scheme can utilize all of these areas of knowledge because there is so much overlap between them.[1]

The best classifications use a single category of knowledge with which to separate items in the domain. On the other hand, the most useful knowledge category differs among users of the classification. A histologic classification will be useful to the pathologist, while a functional categorization is more valuable to the treating physician. If only one classification is to be used by both clinicians and scientists, etiologic categorization seems to be most successful. It must be recognized, however, that no single classification can serve all users and all purposes.

Several commonly employed classifications of cardiomyopathy are discussed below. For clarity, the primary categories of each classification are displayed in the accompanying tables (72-1 to 72-6), but only a few representative diseases are mentioned within each category. The exceptions are the etiologic classification (Table 72-3) and the International Classification of Disease, Ninth Revision (ICD-9) classification (Table 72-5), in which more nearly complete listings are provided.

THE WORLD HEALTH ORGANIZATION CLASSIFICATION

The only currently used clinical classification of cardiomyopathy that was developed by consensus is that of the World Health Organization (WHO) and the International Society and

TABLE 72-1

WORLD HEALTH ORGANIZATION CLASSIFICATIONS
OF CARDIOMYOPATHIES

I. Former WHO classification[a]
  A. Heart muscle diseases of unknown cause
    1. Dilated cardiomyopathy
    2. Hypertrophic cardiomyopathy
    3. Restrictive cardiomyopathy
    4. Unclassified cardiomyopathy
  B. Specific heart muscle disease
    1. Infective
    2. Metabolic
      a. Endocrine
      b. Familial storage disease and infiltrations
      c. Deficiency
      d. Amyloid
    3. General system disease
      a. Connective tissue disorders
      b. Infiltrations and granulomas
    4. Heredofamilial
      a. Muscular dystrophies
      b. Neuromuscular disorders
    5. Sensitivity and toxic reactions
II. New WHO classification[b]
  A. Functional classification of cardiomyopathy
    1. Dilated cardiomyopathy
    2. Hypertrophic cardiomyopathy
    3. Restrictive cardiomyopathy
    4. Arrhythmogenic right ventricular
       cardiomyopathy
    5. Unclassified cardiomyopathies
  B. Specific cardiomyopathies
    1. Ischemic cardiomyopathy
    2. Valvular cardiomyopathy
    3. Hypertensive cardiomyopathy
    4. Inflammatory cardiomyopathy
      a. Idiopathic
      b. Autoimmune
      c. Infectious
    5. Metabolic cardiomyopathy
      a. Endocrine
      b. Familial storage disease and infiltrations
      c. Deficiency
      d. Amyloid
    6. General system disease
      a. Connective tissue disorders
      b. Infiltrations and granulomas
    7. Muscular dystrophies
    8. Neuromuscular disorders
    9. Sensitivity and toxic reactions
   10. Peripartal cardiomyopathy

[a] This dates from 1980; see reference 2.
[b] This dates from 1995; see reference 3.

Note: These are listings of major categories only; specific disorders are not listed.

Federation of Cardiology.[2,3] This scheme is outlined in Table 72-1. Because it was developed by a panel of experts and has the implied backing of the WHO, it is widely recognized and frequently used. Although it has been in existence since 1980, it has not gained general acceptance.

The 1980 WHO committee[2] reserved the term *cardiomyopathy* for myocardial disease of unknown cause. This somewhat restricted usage has not been adopted widely and is not fully adhered to in this text. The more common usage includes all forms of heart disease in which the myocardium is primarily involved, as defined at the start of this chapter, but excluding valvular heart disease, systemic arterial hypertension, and coronary atherosclerosis. In its new 1995 classification, however, the WHO committee, entirely new except for one member, moved toward this more common usage, stating "With increasing understanding of etiology and pathogenesis, the difference between cardiomyopathy and specific heart muscle disease has become indistinct."[3]

Examination of the 1980 and 1995 WHO classifications reveals that they are, in fact, somewhat awkward schemes that employ two separate categorizations in series, one based primarily on left ventricular morphology and function and the other based on etiology. A resultant disadvantage is that diseases are placed in two schema that overlap.

FUNCTIONAL CLASSIFICATION OF CARDIOMYOPATHIES

The most widely used functional classification of cardiomyopathy recognizes three disturbances of function: dilatation, hypertrophy, and restriction (Table 72-2). *Dilatation* is dominated by left ventricular cavity enlargement and systolic failure. *Hy-*

TABLE 72-2

FUNCTIONAL CLASSIFICATION
OF CARDIOMYOPATHIES

I. Cardiac dilatation
  A. With systolic failure
    1. Idiopathic dilated cardiomyopathy
    2. Late cardiac amyloidosis
    3. Tachycardia-induced congestive failure
  B. Without systolic failure
    1. High cardiac output state
    2. Bradycardia-induced congestive failure
II. Cardiac hypertrophy
  A. With obstruction
    1. Hypertrophic obstructive cardiomyopathy
  B. Without obstruction
    1. Hypertrophic cardiomyopathy
    2. Left ventricular hypertrophy due to systemic
       hypertension
III. Cardiac restriction
  A. Early cardiac amyloidosis
  B. Endomyocardial fibrosis

Note: This is a complete listing of primary categories, but only a few specific examples are provided for illustration.

pertrophy includes both obstructive and nonobstructive forms. *Restriction* is characterized by inadequate compliance causing restriction of diastolic filling. The value of this scheme is that virtually all cardiomyopathies are readily placed in one of the three categories and the therapeutic approaches to each category are distinctly different. For example, left ventricular afterload reduction is a cornerstone of therapy for dilated cardiomyopathies with systolic failure but is of little benefit in the restrictive forms. There are, however, some shortcomings of the functional classification. Many diseases are physiologically heterogeneous. Almost all hypertrophic conditions have an element of diastolic restriction. Most dilated ventricles display myocyte hypertrophy. Some diseases change from one category to another during their course; the best example is cardiac amyloidosis, which initially exhibits diastolic stiffness, with complete preservation of systolic performance, followed years later by dilatation and systolic failure.

The functional scheme also associates diseases that have vastly different causes, some of which require special therapeutic interventions. For example, the primary therapy for cardiac hemochromatosis, often an initially restrictive disease, is removal of excessive iron stores; this would not, of course, be effective treatment for other diseases similarly classified. Despite its shortcomings, the functional classification of cardiomyopathy remains the most popular among clinicians because it is based on easily understood physiology and is relevant to therapy.

ETIOLOGIC CLASSIFICATION

This scheme utilizes our knowledge about cardiomyopathies more extensively than all the others. It has the most primary categories as a result of the fact that there are numerous known causes that are not interrelated. The table included here (Table 72-3) categorizes the diseases covered in Chaps. 69, 73 to 80, 85, 86, and 91 to 94. The general outline established by the WHO in 1980 is followed roughly. In many cases the etiologic agent is poorly understood (e.g., uremic "cardiomyopathy"), or the cardiomyopathy is associated with another disease but the mechanism responsible for heart failure is not known (e.g., cardiomyopathy of systemic neoplasia).

While this classification has the advantage of being inclusive, it has the disadvantage of being awkwardly long. It has 7 primary and 40 secondary categories. In addition, most similarly classified disorders are anatomically, physiologically, and therapeutically unrelated. Thus, this classification is not used routinely by clinicians. It has been used most frequently as an organizational scheme in textbooks and reviews concerning heart muscle disease and cardiomyopathy.

ENDOMYOCARDIAL BIOPSY CLASSIFICATION

Because the heart can be safely biopsied, antemortem histologic diagnosis can be used to classify cardiomyopathies.

TABLE 72-3

ETIOLOGIC CLASSIFICATION OF CARDIOMYOPATHIES

I. Infective/inflammatory
    Idiopathic lymphocytic myocarditis
    Peripartum myocarditis
    Eosinophilic myocarditis
    Giant-cell myocarditis
    Viral myocarditis
    Rickettsial myocarditis
    Bacterial myocarditis
    Mycobacterial heart disease
    Spirochetal heart disease
    Fungal myocarditis
    Protozoal myocarditis
    Metazoal myocarditis
II. Metabolic
    A. Endocrine
      1. Thyroid disease
        Thyrotoxicosis
        Hypothyroidism
      2. Pheochromocytoma
      3. Acromegaly
      4. Diabetes mellitus
      5. Carcinoid heart disease
    B. Uremia
    C. Hyperoxaluria
    D. Gout
    E. Storage diseases and infiltrative processes
      1. Lysosomal storage diseases
        GM1 gangliosidosis
        Tay-Sachs disease and variants
        Sandhoff's disease
        Niemann-Pick disease
        Gaucher's disease
        Fabry's disease
        Farber's disease
        Fucosidosis
        Hurler's syndrome
        Scheie's syndrome
        Hunter's syndrome
        Sanfilippo
        Morquio
        Moroteaux-Lamy
      2. Glycogen storage diseases
        Pompe's disease
        Cori's disease
        Andersen's disease
        Dominantly inherited cardioskeletal myopathy with lysosomal glycogen storage and normal acid maltase levels
      3. Refsum's syndrome
      4. Hand-Schuller-Christian
      5. Adipositos cordis
      6. Hemochromatosis
    F. Deficiencies
      1. Electrolyte
        Hypocalcemia
        Hypophosphatemia

(continued)

TABLE 72-3

ETIOLOGIC CLASSIFICATION OF CARDIOMYOPATHIES (Continued)

2. Nutritional
    Kwashiorkor
    Beriberi
    Pellagra
    Scurvy
    Selenium
    Carnitine
III. Amyloid
    AL (primary amyloid, myeloma-associated amyloid)
    AA (secondary amyloid, familial Mediterranean fever-associated amyloid)
    AF (familial amyloid)
    SSA (senile cardiac amyloid, senile systemic amyloid)
    IAA (atrial amyloid)
IV. General system disorders
    A. Collagen vascular (connective tissue)
        Systemic lupus erythematosus
        Polyarteritis nodosa
        Rheumatoid arthritis
        Scleroderma
        Dermatomyositis
        Whipple's disease
        Kawasaki's disease
    B. Sarcoidosis
    C. Neoplastic
V. Muscular dystrophies, myopathies, and neuromuscular disorders
    A. Muscular dystrophies
        Duchenne's muscular dystrophy
        Becker's muscular dystrophy
        Myotonic dystrophy
        Facioscapulohumeral muscular dystrophy
        Limb girdle dystrophy
        Scapuloperoneal dystrophy, including Emery-Driefuss
        Congenital muscular dystrophy
        Distal muscular dystrophy
    B. Congenital myopathies
        Central-core disease
        Nemaline myopathy
        Myotubular myopathy (centronuclear)
        Congenital fiber-type disproportion
    C. Mitochondrial myopathies, including Kearns-Sayre syndrome
    D. Neuromuscular disorders, Friedreich's ataxia
VI. Toxicity, hypersensitivity, and physical agent effects
    A. Toxic effects
        1. Caused by drugs, heavy metals, and chemical agents
            Alcohol (ethyl)
            Amphetamine/methamphetamine
            Anthracyclines
            Antidepressants
            Antimony
            Arsenic
            Arsine gas
            Carbon monoxide

            Catecholamines
            Chloroquine
            Cobalt
            Cocaine
            Cyclophosphamide
            Emetine
            5-Fluorouracil
            Hydrocarbons
            Interferon
            Lead
            Lithium
            Mercury
            Methysergide
            Paracetamol
            Phenothiazines
            Phosphorus
            Reserpine
        2. Caused by scorpions, spiders, arthropods, and snakes
            Scorpions
            Arthropods
            Black widow spider
            Snakes
    B. Hypersensitivity reactions
        Acetazolamide
        Amitriptyline
        Amphotericin B
        Ampicillin
        Carbamazepine
        Chlorthalidone
        Hydrochlorothiazide
        Indomethacin
        Isoniazid
        Methyldopa
        Oxyphenbutazone
        Para-Aminosalicylic acid
        Penicillin
        Phenindione
        Phenylbutazone
        Phenytoin
        Streptomycin
        Sulfadiazine
        Sulfisoxazole
        Sulfonylureas
        Tetracycline
    C. Physical agents
        Heat
        Hypothermia
        Radiation
VII. Miscellaneous
    Peripartum heart disease
    Tachycardia-induced cardiomyopathy
    Ectodermal dysplasia-associated cardiomyopathy
    Idiopathic endocardial fibrosis
    Endocardial fibroelastosis
    Infantile cardiomyopathy

Note: This is an essentially complete listing of cardiomyopathies of known cause.

Dozens of specific myocardial diseases can be detected by biopsy (Table 72-4). The great strength of histologic diagnosis is that it is definitive and unequivocal when a specific disease is observed. On the other hand, numerous deficiencies make this method of classification relatively restricted in use. The foremost problem is that although the number of specific histologic diagnoses is large, they represent a small proportion of all cases—certainly fewer than 15 percent. The histology in most patients with cardiomyopathy is nonspecific and nondiagnostic. Hypertrophy, or fiber attenuation, and fibrosis may be seen in varying degrees in almost any disorder and are the only findings in most cases of idiopathic dilated cardiomyopathy and hypertrophic cardiomyopathy (as well as in many instances of heart failure due to myocardial infarction and valvular dysfunction). Furthermore, completely normal histology may occasionally be seen on biopsy in cases of severe dilatation and systolic failure.

Myocardial biopsy samples can be subjected to several additional analytic techniques that expand the potential for classification using endomyocardial biopsy. While at present these analyses are only investigational and none can be generally applied, it is likely that one or more of them will become clinically useful in the future and could form the basis of a classification with wide appeal.

ICD-9 CLASSIFICATION

ICD-9-CM stands for International Classification of Disease, Ninth Revision, Clinical Modification. This system was developed by the WHO in 1948 for registering disease incidences. In 1977, the U.S. National Center for Health Statistics modified the ICD-9 code to allow coding of medical records. That modification is the current ICD-9-CM. In 1989 it became mandatory for physicians in the United States to include an ICD-9-CM code on their Medicare claims. A majority of the codes applicable to heart diseases are listed in Table 72-5 in numerical order. It is fascinating to see how utterly different a classification system intended for governmental statistics and claims payment is in comparison to those intended for scientific or clinical purposes! The code is a remarkable hodgepodge, combining multiple categories of knowledge into one classification system. Diseases are variously defined according to one or more features such as etiology, anatomy, physiology, comorbidity, symptoms, and even method and extent of diagnosis. It is no wonder that this code is impossible to remember and notoriously ambiguous and difficult to use. In Table 72-5, the codes describing cardiomyopathies are listed in boldface; they appear in several groups scattered throughout the listing. Some of the groups contain entirely unrelated disorders. Relatively few—21—cardiomyopathy diagnoses are coded, and these represent only 9 specific entities. Some well-recognized diseases are completely ignored, such as arrhythmogenic right ventricular dysplasia and long QT syndrome. This classification system and the method of classification it represents are certainly not recommended to physicians and scientists. ICD-9-CM should remain in the bailiwick of bureaucrats and serve as a paragon of classification chaos.

TABLE 72-4

ENDOMYOCARDIAL BIOPSY HISTOLOGY CLASSIFICATION OF CARDIOMYOPATHIES

I. Inflammatory/immune cardiomyopathy
   Lymphocytic myocarditis
   Rheumatic carditis
   Sarcoidosis
   Giant cell myocarditis
   Cardiac allograft rejection
   Chagas' cardiomyopathy
   Hypersensitivity myocarditis
II. Infectious cardiomyopathy
   Toxoplasmosis
   Lyme carditis
   Cytomegalovirus
III. Infiltrative cardiomyopathy
   Glycogen storage
   Hemochromatosis
   Right ventricular lipomatosis
   Amyloidosis
IV. Cardiac tumors
   Cardiac origin
   Noncardiac origin
V. Miscellaneous specific cardiomyopathies
   Anthracycline cardiotoxicity
   Endocardial fibrosis
   Endocardial fibroelastosis
   Fabry's disease
   Carcinoid disease
   Irradiation injury
   Kearns-Sayre syndrome
   Henoch-Schönlein purpura
   Chloroquine cardiomyopathy
   Carnitine deficiency
   Hypereosinophilic syndrome
VI. Nonspecific abnormalities
   Idiopathic dilated cardiomyopathy
   Other cardiomyopathies of unknown cause
VII. No histologic abnormality

Note: This represents a relatively complete listing of diagnoses that have been made by endomyocardial biopsy and reported in the literature.

THERAPEUTIC CLASSIFICATION

A classification based on specific therapies borrows heavily from the functional and the etiologic classifications of cardiomyopathy. This classification adds information regarding treatment that is not available in other schemes and therefore may be useful to clinicians.

Nevertheless, this classification has several shortcomings. First, often more than one class of therapy is appropriate for a disease. Therefore, the classification must categorize

TABLE 72-5

ICD-9 CLASSIFICATION OF HEART DISEASE

ICD-9 Code	Description	ICD-9 Code	Description
306.2	Neurocirculatory asthenia	424.0	Mitral valve disorders, nonrheumatic
394.0	Rheumatic mitral stenosis	424.1	Aortic valve disorders, nonrheumatic
394.1	Rheumatic mitral insufficiency	424.2	Tricuspid valve disorders, nonrheumatic
394.2	Rheumatic mitral stenosis and insufficiency	424.3	Pulmonary valve disorders, nonrheumatic
395.0	Rheumatic aortic stenosis	424.9	Endocarditis, valve unspecified, unspecified cause
395.1	Rheumatic aortic insufficiency	**425.0**	**Endomyocardial fibrosis**
395.2	Rheumatic aortic stenosis and insufficiency	**425.1**	**Hypertrophic obstructive cardiomyopathy**
396.0	Rheumatic tricuspid disease	**425.2**	**African endomyocardial disease**
401.0	Malignant hypertension	**425.3**	**Endomyocardial fibroelastosis**
402.00	**Hypertensive heart disease, malignant, w/o CHF**	**425.4**	**Idiopathic cardiomyopathy**
402.01	**Hypertensive heart disease, malignant, w CHF**	**425.5**	**Alcoholic cardiomyopathy**
402.10	**Hypertensive heart disease, benign, w/o CHF**	426.0	Complete AV block
402.11	**Hypertensive heart disease, benign, w CHF**	426.10	AV block, unspecified
402.90	**Hypertensive heart disease, unspecified, w/o CHF**	426.11	First degree AV block
402.91	**Hypertensive heart disease, unspecified, w CHF**	426.12	Mobitz II AV block
410.0	Acute anterolateral MI	426.13	Other second-degree AV block
410.1	Acute anterior MI	426.2	Left hemiblock
410.2	Acute inferolateral MI	426.3	LBBB
410.3	Acute inferoposterior MI	426.4	RBBB
410.4	Acute inferior MI	426.51	RBBB + LPFB
410.6	Acute true posterior MI	426.52	RBBB + LAFB
410.7	Acute subendocardial MI	426.53	Other bilateral bundle branch block
410.8	Acute other site MI	426.6	Other heart block
410.9	Acute unspecified site MI	426.7	Ventricular preexcitation
411.0	Dressler's syndrome	426.81	Lown-Ganong-Levine syndrome
411.1	Unstable angina	426.89	AV dissociation or nonparoxysmal AV nodal tach
412	Old MI	426.9	Conduction disorder, unspecified (e.g., Stokes-A)
413.0	Angina decubitus	427.0	Paroxysmal SVT
413.1	Prinzmetal angina	427.1	Paroxysmal VT
413.9	Unspecified angina	427.31	Atrial fibrillation
414.00	Coronary atherosclerosis, unspecified vessel	427.32	Atrial flutter
414.01	Coronary atherosclerosis, native vessel	427.41	Ventricular fibrillation
414.02	Coronary atherosclerosis, vein graft	427.42	Ventricular flutter
414.1	Aneurysm of heart wall	427.5	Cardiac arrest
414.11	Aneurysm of coronary artery	427.60	Premature beats, unspecified
414.9	Chronic ischemic heart disease, unspecified	427.61	Supraventricular premature beats
415.0	Acute cor pulmonale	427.62	Ventricular premature beats
415.11	Pulmonary embolism and infarction	427.81	Sinoatrial node dysfunction
416.0	Primary pulmonary hypertension	427.9	Cardiac arrhythmia, unspecified
416.8	Secondary pulmonary hypertension	**428.0**	**CHF**
416.9	Chronic cor pulmonale	**428.1**	**Left heart failure**
420.90	Acute pericarditis, unspecified	**428.9**	**Heart failure, unspecified**
420.91	Acute idiopathic pericarditis	**429.0**	**Myocarditis, unspecified**
421.0	Acute and subacute bacterial endocarditis	**429.1**	**Myocardial disease related to CAD**
421.9	Acute endocarditis, unspecified	**429.3**	**Cardiomegaly**
422.90	**Acute myocarditis, unspecified**	429.5	Rupture of chordae tendineae
422.91	**Idiopathic myocarditis**	429.6	Papillary muscle rupture
422.92	Septic myocarditis	429.82	Hyperkinetic heart syndrome
423.0	Hemopericardium	**674.84**	**Postpartum cardiomyopathy**
423.2	Constrictive pericarditis	745.10	Complete transposition of the great vessels *(cont.)*
423.9	Pericardial disease, unspecified		

TABLE 72-5
ICD-9 CLASSIFICATION OF HEART DISEASE *(Continued)*

ICD-9 Code	Description
745.12	Corrected transposition of the great vessels
745.2	Tetralogy of Fallot
745.4	Ventricular septal defect
745.5	ASD, ostium secundum
745.61	ASD, ostium primum
746.02	Congential pulmonic stenosis
746.2	Ebstein's anomaly
746.3	Congenital AS
746.4	Congenital AI
746.5	Congenital MS
746.85	Coronary anomaly
746.86	Congenital heart block
747.0	PDA
747.10	Coarctation of the aorta
759.82	Marfan's syndrome
785.0	Tachycardia, unspecified
785.1	Palpitations
785.2	Undiagnosed cardiac murmur
785.3	Other abnormal heart sounds
785.50	Shock, unspecified
785.51	Shock, cardiogenic
786.50	Chest pain, unspecified
786.51	Precordial pain
786.59	Chest discomfort, or pressure or tightness
996.01	Complication of pacemaker lead
996.04	Complication of ICD
996.62	Infection due to pacemaker or ICD
996.83	Heart transplant rejection

Note: Codes describing cardiomyopathies are in bold.

TABLE 72-6
THERAPEUTIC CLASSIFICATION OF CARDIOMYOPATHIES

I. Reduce ventricular afterload
   Idiopathic dilated cardiomyopathy
   Late cardiac amyloidosis
II. Reduce ventricular preload
   Endocardial fibrosis
   Early cardiac amyloidosis
III. Increase ventricular compliance
   Hypertrophic cardiomyopathy
IV. Relieve ventricular obstruction
   Hypertrophic obstructive cardiomyopathy
V. Improve cardiac rhythm
   Cardiomyopathy of persistent tachycardia
VI. Specific therapy
   A. Replace deficiency
      Carnitine deficiency cardiomyopathy
   B. Remove toxic agent
      Hemochromatosis
      Hypersensitivity
   C. Immunosuppression
      Giant cell myocarditis
      Lymphocyte myocarditis(?)
   D. Correct systemic disease
      Uremic cardiomyopathy
      Cardiomyopathy of cancer
      Systemic lupus erythematosus

Note: This is a complete listing of primary categories with a few specific examples for illustration.

diseases on the basis of their *primary* therapy. This introduces some instability to the classification, since therapeutic preferences are subject to variance in opinion and to change with new research. The greatest fault of therapeutic categorization is that when new therapies are introduced, the existing classification becomes obsolete. The therapeutic classification shown in Table 72-6 illustrates the sensitivity of this approach to opinion. Some might argue, for example, that diuretic therapy remains the primary treatment for dilated cardiomyopathy.

Note that some commonly employed therapies, such as inotropic agents and cardiac transplantation, do not appear in Table 72-6 because they are often not the initial or primary therapies.

GENE-BASED CLASSIFICATION

Aside from traumatic, iatrogenic, infectious, and certain other secondary cardiac disorders, most heart diseases result from an abnormality of gene function. Most of us think of inherited diseases as the entirety of the genetics of heart disease. Indeed, many diseases caused by adverse gene behavior are due to inherited or acquired genetic mutations. Several diseases are now defined genetically, including hypertrophic cardiomyopathy, long QT syndrome, forms of dilated cardiomyopathy, muscular dystrophies involving the heart, arrhythmogenic right ventricular dysplasia, and others. But in the future, most cardiac diseases will be shown to be due to genes functioning at the extremes of normal behavior. A classification system based upon adverse gene behavior is diagnostically and therapeutically useless unless the biochemical and resultant physiologic aberrations are understood. When they are understood, gene-based classification will become the best classification system for cardiomyopathies, because it will at once precisely and uniquely define the disease and make evident the necessary diagnostic and therapeutic actions.

SUMMARY

No single classification of cardiomyopathy is generally accepted within the biomedical community. An attempt to gain a consensus for one of the many classifications in current use is not likely to succeed because we are unable to subdivide meaningfully cases of idiopathic dilated cardiomyopathy, which constitute the large majority of all cases. At present, it seems best for the individual health practitioner or scientist to use the classification scheme that best serves his or her purpose. For clinicians, this will often be the functional classification.

In the future, a widely acceptable classification may develop that is based on the molecular genetics of myocardial disease. Although this field is only beginning to develop, it is the discipline most likely to contribute to our understanding of causes and our development of new treatments for myocardial disease.

REFERENCES

1. Abelmann WH. Classification and natural history of primary myocardial disease. *Prog Cardiovasc Dis* 1984; 27:73–94.
2. Report of the WHO/ISFC task force on the definition and classification of cardiomyopathies. *Br Heart J* 1980; 44:672–673.
3. Richardson P, McKenna W, Bristow M, Maisch B, Mautner B, O'Connell J, et al. Report of the 1995 World Health Organization/International Society and Federation of Cardiology task force on the definition and classification of cardiomyopathies. *Circulation* 1996; 93:841–842.

73

DILATED CARDIOMYOPATHY

Michael R. Bristow / Teresa J. Bohlmeyer / Edward M. Gilbert

Heart failure is an enormously important clinical problem that, if not contained or solved, may ultimately overwhelm health care resources.[1] As discussed in Chap. 21, the clinical syndrome of heart failure is a complex process where the primary pathophysiology is quickly obscured by a variety of superimposed secondary adaptive, maladaptive, and counter-regulatory processes. Heart failure is best understood and approached from the vantage point of *myocardial failure,* because the secondary and primary cardiomyopathies[2] cause the majority of cases of clinical heart failure.[3] As an indication of the importance of the problems of cardiomyopathy and heart failure, the cardiomyopathies have been recently reclassified by a World Health Organization (WHO) subcommittee,[2] as described in Chap. 72 and elaborated on further below.

IMPORTANCE OF HEART FAILURE

Because of its high prevalence (1 to 1.5 percent of the adult population) and high morbidity, including frequent hospitalizations, the clinical syndrome of heart failure is among the most costly medical problems in the United States.[1] Despite improvements in the treatment of heart failure introduced in the past 10 years, including the general availability of cardiac transplantation and better medical treatment, clinical outcome following the onset of symptoms has not changed substantially.[3] That is, mortality remains high (median survival of 1.7 years for men and 3.2 years for women),[3] the natural history remains progressive,[3] the cost is excessive,[1] and disability[4] and morbidity[3,4] are among the highest of any disease or disease syndrome.

RELATIONSHIP OF MYOCARDIAL FAILURE TO THE CLINICAL SYNDROME OF HEART FAILURE

The vast majority of the cases of heart failure are caused by heart muscle disease (cardiomyopathy). Within the WHO categorization[2] (Table 73-1) of cardiomyopathy, the most common cause of the clinical syndrome of heart failure is a secondary (ischemic, valvular, hypertensive, etc.) or a primary (e.g., idiopathic, familial) dilated cardiomyopathy, defined as a left ventricular (LV) chamber exhibiting increased diastolic and systolic volumes and a low (<0.40) ejection fraction. The natural history of the clinical syndrome of heart failure is dependent on the course of myocardial failure because of the following factors: (1) the most powerful single predictor of outcome is the degree of LV dysfunction as assessed by the LV ejection fraction[5]; (2) treatment that improves intrinsic ventricular function improves the natural history of heart failure[6]; and (3) treatment that ultimately worsens intrinsic function, such as many types of positive inotropic agents, is associated with an adverse effect on outcome.[6]

THE WHO CLASSIFICATION OF CARDIOMYOPATHIES

The WHO classification of cardiomyopathies was recently revised[2] to accommodate several rapidly emerging realities. The first was that the molecular genetic basis of previously unknown types of heart muscle disease is rapidly being elucidated, and so it really makes no sense to reserve the classification for "unknown etiologies" of cardiomyopathy.[7] The second consideration was that many of the mechanisms responsible for the natural history of myocardial dysfunction are qualitatively similar in primary versus secondary dilated cardiomyopathies,[8] which accurately predicted a qualitatively similar response to treatment targeted at these mechanisms.[9–11] This made the exclusion of secondary, or "known cause,"[7] cardiomyopathies inappropriate, and their inclusion in the new classification allows all cardiomyopathies to be classified under one scheme.

As shown in Table 73-1, the WHO cardiomyopathy classification utilizes two separate methods to define the individual categories. The first is based on the global anatomic description of chamber dimensions in systole and diastole. Thus the

TABLE 73-1

THE WORLD HEALTH ORGANIZATION CLASSIFICATION OF THE CARDIOMYOPATHIES

Category	Definition

I. Dilated (DCM)
  1. Primary
  2. Secondary
	↑ EDV, ↑ ESV; low EF

II. Restrictive (RCM)
  1. Primary
  2. Secondary
	↓ EDV, ↔ ESV; ↑ FP, ↔ EF

III. Hypertrophic (HCM)	↑↑ Septal and ↑ posterior wall thickness, myofibrillar disarray Mutation in sarcomeric protein, autosomal dominant inheritance
IV. Arrhythmogenic RV (ARVC)	Fibrofatty replacement of RV myocardium Autosomal dominant (most) and recessive inheritance

V. Unclassified
  1. Primary
  2. Secondary
	Not meeting criteria for other categories
	Features of > one category

Note: EDV, (end-diastolic volume; ESV, end-systolic volume; EF, LV ejection fraction; FP, LV filling pressure.

Source: From Richardson et al.,[2] with permission of the publisher and authors.

dilated and restrictive categories have definitions based on LV dimensions or volume, which also define function using the calculated ejection fraction (Table 73-1). The justification for this is that these two groups have distinct natural histories and respond distinctly differently to medical treatment. The second method of creating individual categories within the WHO classification is for cardiomyopathies that are genetically based, have unique myocardial phenotypic features, and do not exhibit extracardiac phenotypes. Thus, hypertrophic cardiomyopathy (HCM), caused by mutations in contractile proteins manifesting as a unique phenotype, merits a separate category (Chaps. 69 and 74). The same is true for arrhythmogenic right ventricular dysplasia, which also has a unique phenotype and will likely turn out to be completely genetic in basis, as has HCM (Chap. 27). On the other hand, genetic cardiomyopathies without unique phenotypes, such as the dilated cardiomyopathy of Becker-Duchenne, are included as one form of the anatomic/chamber dimension category (category I).

The WHO classification includes another assignment of nomenclature in "secondary" cardiomyopathies, i.e., those associated with known cardiac or systemic processes. These are referred to as *specific cardiomyopathies,* named for the disease process with which they are associated. Thus an *ischemic cardiomyopathy* would be a specific cardiomyopathy related to previous myocardial infarctions (MI) and the subsequent remodeling process, which would usually be categorized within the dilated class. On the other hand, a *hypertensive*

cardiomyopathy might be classified as either dilated or restrictive depending on the chamber dimensions. Therefore, the correct term for these cardiomyopathies would be *ischemic dilated cardiomyopathy* and *hypertensive dilated (or restrictive) cardiomyopathy,* respectively.

GENERAL PATHOPHYSIOLOGY

Molecular Mechanisms in Cardiomyopathies and Myocardial Failure

OVERVIEW

As shown in Table 73-2, there are three general categories of mechanisms whereby altered gene expression can lead to a phenotypic change in cardiac myocytes. These are as follows: (1) a single gene defect, for example as present in β-myosin heavy chain codon 403 in familial HCM[12] and in an analogous region of α-myosin heavy chain in HCM transgenic mouse models[13,14]; (2) polymorphic variation in modifier genes, such as is present in many components of the renin-angiotensin system (RAS)[15–19]; and (3) maladaptive regulated expression of completely normal genes, such as for the mechanisms responsible for progressive myocardial dysfunction and remodeling in secondary dilated cardiomyopathies[6] (see also Chap. 69).

SINGLE GENE DEFECTS AS THE CAUSE OF CARDIOMYOPATHIES IN HUMANS AND ANIMAL MODELS

The ability to manipulate the cardiovascular system genetically has made it possible to investigate the role of a number of genes in the developing and adult mouse heart (for a review, see Robbins[20]). The discovery that mutations in sarcomeric proteins lead to HCM has made it possible to generate animal

TABLE 73-2

GENERAL CATEGORIZATION OF MYOCARDIAL FUNCTION

Intrinsic[a]	Modulated[b]
Contractile proteins	R-G-adenylyl cyclase pathways
E-C coupling mechanisms	
R-G-adenylyl cyclase pathways	R-G-phospholipase C pathways
Bioenergetics	
Cytoskeleton	
Sarcomere and cell remodeling	

[a] Function in the absence of neural or hormonal influence.

[b] Function that may be stimulated or inhibited by extrinsic factors, including neurotransmitters, cytokines, or hormones.

Note: E-C, excitation-contraction; R-G, receptor–G protein.

models for this disease.[13,14] In the case of myosin mutations, a single genetic defect initiates a pathway that ultimately leads to hypertrophy and then in males results in late decompensation and ventricular dilatation.[14]

A serendipitous genetic model of dilated cardiomyopathy and heart failure ("*myf* 5 mice") has been generated by activation of a skeletal muscle genetic program in the heart.[21] These mice have a dilated cardiomyopathy phenotype characterized by progressive myocardial dysfunction and dilatation. They develop the clinical syndrome of heart failure and have an extraordinarily high (>90 percent at 260 days) heart failure–related mortality.[21] These characteristics make this model very useful in assessing the mechanisms that lead to the development and progression of myocardial failure. There are several additional genetic models of cardiomyopathy that may be more relevant to the production of a dilated phenotype in humans. Two of them involve overexpression of components of the beta₁-adrenergic receptor pathway: a $G_{\alpha s}$ overexpressor transgenic animal[22,23] and a beta₁-receptor overexpressor mouse.[24] The $G_{\alpha s}$ and beta₁-receptor transgenic mouse models exhibit similar histopathology, consisting of myocyte hypertrophy and increased fibrosis.[22,24] The $G_{\alpha s}$ animal ultimately develops dilatation,[23] while the beta₁ receptor overexpressor has not been followed for a long enough period to determine if it undergoes remodeling. This transgenic mouse develops both systolic and diastolic dysfunction,[23] however, and exhibits an increased mortality that appears to be due to sudden death (Port JD and Bristow MR, unpublished observations). The $G_{\alpha s}$ mouse also exhibits evidence of myocardial cell apoptosis.[25] Another recently produced transgenic model of dilated cardiomyopathy is the MLP-deficient mouse model.[26] MLP is *muscle LIM protein*, a regulator of myogenic differentiation that is involved in maintaining the integrity of the actin cytoskeleton.[26] Targeted ablation of the MLP gene produces hypertrophy and a cardiomyopathy,[25] illustrating the importance of the cytoskeleton in maintaining both structure and function of the heart.

Several transgenic models of concentric or symmetric LV hypertrophy have now been reported, including overexpression of *ras,*[27] *myc,*[28] and alpha₁-adrenergic receptors.[29] The mechanisms for the induction of increased ventricular size are diverse, inasmuch as the *ras* and alpha₁-receptor overexpressors exhibit true cellular hypertrophy with an increase in cell size,[27,29] while the *myc* animal exhibits cardiac myocyte hyperplasia.[28] As for the HCM phenotypes discussed above, this illustrates that apparently diverse signals can culminate in the same phenotype, presumably by converging on final common pathways.

POLYMORPHIC VARIATION IN MODIFIER GENES
Genes exhibit polymorphic variation; that is, normal variants of genes exist in the population that are of slightly different size or sequence.[30] Some of these variations are associated with differences in function of the expressed protein gene product, and some of these differences in function likely account for some of the "biologic variation" routinely encoun-

tered in population studies of disease susceptibility or clinical response to treatment.

Examples of "modifier" genes that may impact on the natural history of a cardiomyopathy include the angiotensin-converting enzyme (ACE) *DD* genotype, where individuals are homozygous for the "deletion" variant, which is associated with increased circulating[15] and cardiac tissue[31] ACE activity. The *DD* genotype appears to increase the extent of hypertrophy in HCM[32] and may be a risk factor for early remodeling post-MI[33] and for the development of end-stage ischemic or idiopathic dilated cardiomyopathy (IDC).[16,34] Other potentially important polymorphic variants that may influence the natural history of a cardiomyopathy involve the angiotensin AT_1 receptor[18,35] and beta₂-adrenergic receptors.[36]

ALTERED, MALADAPTIVE EXPRESSION
OF A COMPLETELY NORMAL GENE
The third way in which altered gene expression can contribute to the development of a cardiomyopathy is altered, maladaptive expression of a completely normal gene. This most commonly occurs in the context of progression of heart muscle disease and myocardial failure, which is the natural history of virtually all cardiomyopathies once they are established.

General Mechanisms of Myocardial Dysfunction and its Progression

Tissue preparations and myocytes isolated from failing human hearts exhibit evidence of decreased contractile function.[37] Assuming that loading conditions and ischemia are not adversely affecting cardiac myocyte function, in the setting of chronic systolic dysfunction from a dilated cardiomyopathy progressive myocardial failure is caused by myocardial cell loss or changes in myocyte gene expression. Figure 73-1 summarizes these general points and emphasizes the central

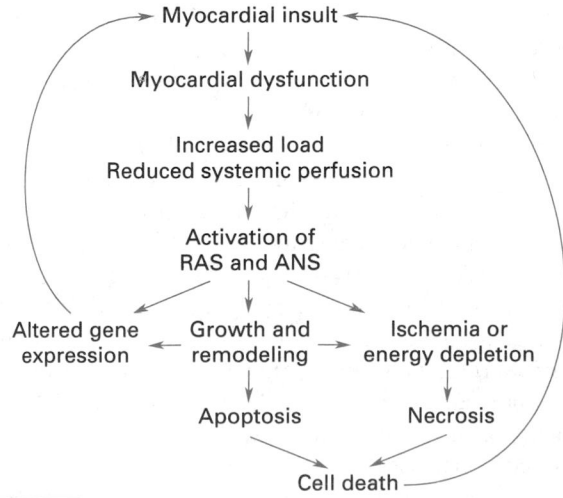

FIGURE 73-1
Relationship of neurohormonal activation and production of cardiac myocyte loss due to apoptosis and necrosis and altered gene expression. Cell loss and altered gene expression result in more myocardial dysfunction, and a vicious cycle is established. RAS, renin-angiotensin system; ANS, adrenergic nervous system.

roles of the RAS and adrenergic nervous system (ANS) in promoting cell loss, growth and remodeling, and altered gene expression.[6]

Altered Cardiac Myocyte Gene Expression in Human Cardiomyopathies and Myocardial Failure

If one defines gene expression in its broadest sense as the expression of either a fully or normally functional protein gene product or the steady-state abundance of a gene's mRNA transcript, numerous abnormalities of gene expression have been demonstrated in the failing human heart. In order to characterize the abnormalities that may account for progressive myocardial dysfunction and remodeling, it is useful to subdivide them into two general categories,[38] as shown in Table 73-2. The first category encompasses mechanisms that subserve *intrinsic* function, or the mechanisms responsible for contraction and relaxation of the heart in the basal or resting state. *Intrinsic function* is defined as myocardial contraction and relaxation in the absence of extrinsic influences, such as neurotransmitters or hormones. The second general category is *modulated* function, which comprises the mechanisms responsible for the remarkable ability of the heart to increase or decrease its performance dramatically (by two- to tenfold) and rapidly in response to various physiologic or physical stimuli. Other critical organs such as the brain, kidney, and liver do not exhibit this quality. *Modulated function* is defined as stimulation or inhibition of myocardial contraction or relaxation by endogenous bioactive compounds, including neurotransmitters, cytokines, autocrine/paracrine substances, and hormones.

In the failing human heart, changes are present in the expression of genes potentially responsible for both general types of myocardial function depicted in Table 73-2.[6,38] Abnormalities of intrinsic function include the factors responsible for an altered length-tension relation,[39–41] a blunted force-frequency response,[42,43] and/or the signals responsible for abnormal cellular and chamber remodeling.[44,45] In the case of the abnormal force-frequency and length-tension responses, the evidence favors abnormal contractile function of individual cardiac myocytes.[37] As shown in Table 73-2, these abnormalities likely reside in the contractile proteins or their regulatory elements,[46–49] various mechanisms involved in excitation-contraction coupling, or perhaps the cytoskeleton.[26,50–52] Within these possibilities for altered intrinsic function, however, there is not currently a consensus as to which specific abnormalities are present in IDC, the most common form of heart failure studied in humans. For cellular remodeling, in both human ventricles[53,54] and animal models[45,55] the assembly of sarcomeres in series leads to a myocyte that is markedly increased in length but not in diameter, which contributes to remodeling at the chamber level. Such remodeling places the chamber and the myocyte at an energetic disadvantage because of the attendant increase in wall stress,[56] which is one of the major determinants of myocardial oxygen consumption. Inadequate myocyte energy production, particularly associated with key subcellular ion flux mechanisms or the myosin ATPase cycle,[57] in turn would contribute to myo-

cyte contractile dysfunction. On the other hand, cardiac myocyte contractile dysfunction likely plays a role in the remodeling process, inasmuch as medical treatment that improves intrinsic myocardial function can reverse remodeling.[6] Thus contractile dysfunction and remodeling at the cellular level are intimately related to the progressive contractile dysfunction and chamber enlargement that define the natural history of myocardial failure[58] (see also Chap. 21).

In contrast to abnormalities of intrinsic function, a consensus has been reached on several specific abnormalities in the stimulation component of modulated function. Most of these changes concern beta-adrenergic signal transduction.[38] The ability of beta-adrenergic stimulation to increase heart rate and contractility is markedly attenuated in the failing heart due to multiple changes at the level of receptors, G proteins, and adenylyl cyclase. This produces a major abnormality in the stimulation component of modulated function. In addition, the inhibition component of modulated function is also abnormal in the failing heart, due to a reduction in parasympathetic drive.[59]

There is obviously overlap between the two major subdivisions of myocardial function. Recent data indicate that even in the absence of adrenergic stimulation, beta-adrenergic receptors have intrinsic activity.[60–63] That is, a small percentage of receptors are in an activated state without agonist occupancy, and as such can support intrinsic myocardial function.[61,62] Thus overexpression of human beta$_2$-adrenergic receptors is able to increase intrinsic myocardial function markedly,[62] as is enhancement of sarcoplasmic reticulum (SR) calcium uptake and release by genetic ablation of the phospholamban gene.[64] The recent realization that active state, agonist unoccupied beta-adrenergic receptors can modulate intrinsic myocardial function is the reason why the "R-G-adenylyl cyclase" mechanism appears in both categories in Table 73-2.

The third general mechanism for producing myocardial dysfunction discussed above, loss of cardiac myocytes, may also play a role in the progression of ventricular dysfunction in dilated cardiomyopathies. That is, apoptosis (programmed cell death) has been described in end-stage IDC[65] as well as in the G$_{\alpha s}$ overexpressor mouse[25] and in models of hypertrophy.[66] The human hearts with IDC or ischemic cardiomyopathy were taken from very late stage, literally dying patients maintained on multiple powerful intravenous inotropic medications,[65] however, and it is not clear if apoptosis plays a significant role in remodeling and/or chamber systolic dysfunction until this point in the natural history of the dilated cardiomyopathies.

Importance of "Compensatory" Mechanisms in the Progression of Myocardial Failure

As depicted in Figs. 73-1 and 73-2, there is now a large body of information supporting the idea that activation of the adrenergic and renin-angiotensin compensatory mechanisms contributes to, or is responsible for, the progressive nature of both myocardial failure and the natural history of the heart

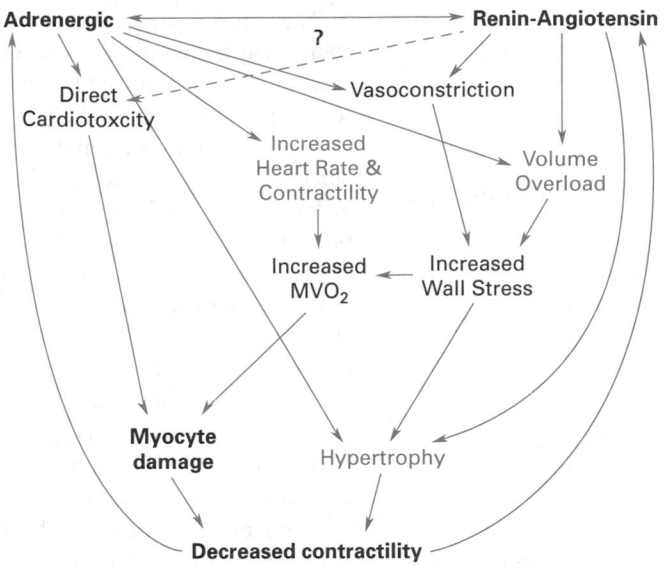

FIGURE 73-2

Heart failure compensatory mechanisms that are activated to support the failing heart. Color blue indicates physiologic mechanisms that stabilize pump function.

failure clinical syndrome.[6] This evidence includes the observations that activation of both these systems is associated with progression of myocardial dysfunction and the heart failure syndrome, and clinical trial data that consistently demonstrate that inhibition of these systems can prevent deterioration in or improve myocardial function as well as reduce mortality.[6] Despite the fact that in human heart failure we now know that chronic activation of the ANS and RAS contributes to the progressive nature of myocardial dysfunction, we know virtually nothing about how these systems adversely affect the biology of the cardiac myocyte. What we do know is that mechanisms within both general categories outlined in Table 73-2 must be involved in the adverse myocardial effects mediated by the ANS and RAS. This is because of the following: (1) modulated function may be improved by treatment with ACE inhibitors or beta-blocking agents; (2) progressive myocardial dysfunction and remodeling are attenuated by both beta-blocking agents and ACE inhibitors; and (3) in cardiomyopathies, intrinsic myocardial function is improved and remodeling is reversed by chronic treatment with beta-blocking agents.[6] Additionally, mortality in chronic heart failure is directly related to activation of the ANS[67,68] and RAS[69] and, as discussed in Chap. 21, may be related to the activation of other neurohormonal or autocrine/paracrine systems as well.

DEFINITIONS, SPECIFIC PATHOPHYSIOLOGY, CLINICAL PROFILES, AND MANAGEMENT OF DILATED CARDIOMYOPATHIES

Definition and Pathophysiology

The dilated phenotype is by far the most common form of cardiomyopathy, comprising over 90 percent of cases referred to specialized centers.[70] It is defined by an increase in ventric-

ular diastolic diameter [on echocardiography or magnetic resonance imaging (MRI)] or volume (on MRI or radionuclide or contrast angiography) combined with a decreased LV ejection fraction. In the United States, the most common dilated cardiomyopathy is ischemic cardiomyopathy,[3] or the cardiomyopathy that follows MI. Other common secondary dilated cardiomyopathies are hypertensive and valvular cardiomyopathies, both produced in part by chronically increased wall stress. The primary cardiomyopathy, IDC, is another relatively common dilated phenotype,[71,72] as discussed below.

Regardless of the type or cause of dilated cardiomyopathy, an initial myocardial result resulting in this phenotype exhibits common pathophysiologic features that are summarized in Fig. 73-1. That is, a myocardial insult that produces systolic dysfunction will be followed by the initiation of processes designed to temporarily stabilize pump function. The possible mechanisms available for such stabilization are in fact limited. As shown in Fig. 73-2 they are, in chronologic order of their action, an increase in heart rate and contractility mediated by an increase in cardiac beta-adrenergic signaling (produced within seconds of the onset of pump dysfunction), volume expansion in order to utilize the Frank-Starling mechanism to increase stroke volume (evident within hours of the onset of pump dysfunction), and cardiac myocyte hypertrophy to increase the number of contractile elements (evident within days to weeks of the onset of pump dysfunction). As shown in Fig. 73-2, these compensatory adjustments are largely accomplished by activation of the RAS and ANS. Despite the short-term (days-months) stability achieved through these mechanisms, however, they ultimately prove harmful.[6] The best evidence that chronic, continued activation of the RAS and ANS contributes to progressive myocardial dysfunction and remodeling comes from clinical trials where both inhibitors of the RAS (ACE inhibitors) and ANS (beta-adrenergic receptor blocking agents) prevent these two phenomena, and beta-blocking agents actually may reverse remodeling and progressive systolic dysfunction.[6]

Much current work is focused on the precise pathophysiologic mechanisms by which activation of the RAS and ANS produces remodeling and adverse effects on myocardial function. Some of the possibilities are given in Fig. 73-1, and they include an exacerbation of ischemia and/or energy depletion leading to cell loss through necrosis, cell loss by programmed cell death, direct promotion of hypertrophy and remodeling through stimulation of cell growth, and alterations in cardiac myocyte gene expression.[6] A key feature of the schema shown in Fig. 73-1, the process of *remodeling*, is discussed in more detail in Chap. 21. Virtually all dilated cardiomyopathies undergo this process, which is characterized by progressive dilatation, progressive myocardial systolic dysfunction in viable segments, and a chamber shape change whereby the ventricle becomes less elliptical and more round.[6,44] As shown in Fig. 73-3, this places the ventricle at an energetic disadvantage,[6,44,56] which likely contributes to further myocardial dysfunction and then contributes to progressive remodeling. The latter observation is based on data with beta-adrenergic blocking agents, which produce an improvement in systolic

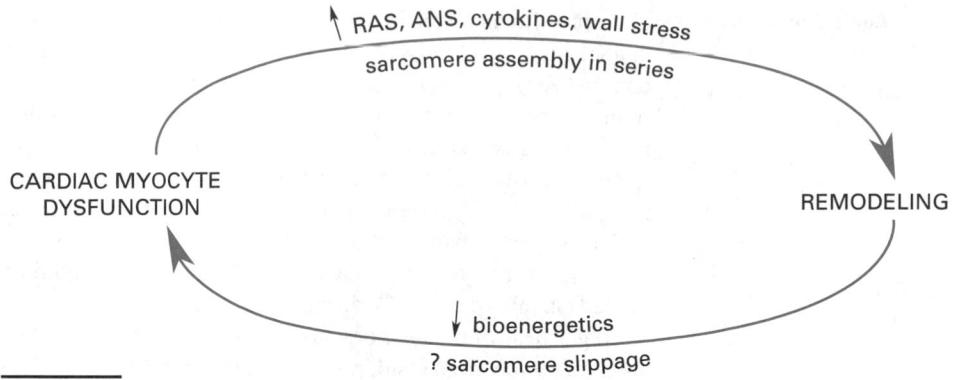

FIGURE 73-3
Relationship between progressive myocardial dysfunction and remodeling. RAS, renin-angiotensin system; ANS, adrenergic nervous system.

dysfunction that can be detected prior to a reversal in remodeling.[6] As emphasized by Fig. 73-3, each myocardial degenerative process likely begets the other, leading to an inexorably progressive deterioration in myocardial performance and clinical condition.

Specific Types of Dilated Cardiomyopathy

The number of cardiac or systemic processes that can produce or are associated with a dilated cardiomyopathy are plentiful and remarkably varied, as shown in Table 73-3.

Selected, Common Types of Dilated Cardiomyopathy

ISCHEMIC CARDIOMYOPATHY

Definition/Diagnosis
Ischemic cardiomyopathy is defined as a dilated cardiomyopathy in a patient with a history of MI or evidence of clinically significant (i.e., ≥ 70 percent narrowing of a major epicardial artery) coronary artery disease, in whom the degree of myocardial dysfunction and ventricular dilatation is not explained solely by the extent of previous infarction or the degree of ongoing ischemia.[2] In other words, an ischemic cardiomyopathy is present when a post-MI left ventricle experiences remodeling and a significant drop in ejection fraction. Dilatation of the left ventricle and a decrease in ejection fraction occur in 15 to 40 percent of patients within 12 to 24 months following an anterior MI[73,74] and in a smaller percentage of patients following an inferior infarction.[74] Based on limited data,[33] it is tempting to speculate that the patients who undergo the remodeling process and develop an ischemic cardiomyopathy are individuals with particularly heightened compensatory mechanisms (Fig. 73-1 and 73-2), perhaps as a result of polymorphic variation in these systems.[16] As discussed above, the remodeling process is an attempt of the compromised ventricle to increase its performance by increasing stroke volume. Although this adjustment undoubtedly is effective in the short term, in the long term it correlates with an adverse outcome.[6,44]

The gross pathology of ischemic cardiomyopathy includes transmural or subendocardial scarring representing old MI(s), which may comprise up to 50 percent of the LV chamber. The histopathology of the noninfarcted regions is similar to changes that occur in IDC,[59] as discussed below.

Prognosis
Several studies have concluded that ischemic cardiomyopathy patients have a worse prognosis than those with a "nonischemic" dilated cardiomyopathy,[11,75,76] probably because the risk of ischemic events is added to the risk of having a dilated cardiomyopathy.

Treatment
The treatment of ischemic cardiomyopathy and chronic heart failure is covered in detail in Chaps. 23 to 25. In general, treatment consists of the use of ACE inhibitors in asymptomatic or symptomatic patients, the use of diuretics in volume-overloaded patients, and the use of digoxin in those who remain symptomatic on the former medications. An emerging treatment strategy is the use of beta-adrenergic blocking agents in symptomatic individuals,[6,9,10,11,77–79] where in both ischemic and nonischemic cardiomyopathies at least the "third-generation" compounds involve LV function,[6,9–11] reduce hospitalizations,[10,11] and may lower mortality.[10,11] Additional, adjunctive therapy includes anticoagulation in subjects with lower left ventricular ejection fractions (LVEFs) to prevent thromboembolic complications, amiodarone to treat symptomatic arrhythmias, maintenance of potassium levels in the high normal (4.3 to 5.0 meq/L) range to prevent sudden death, frequent clinic visits to adjust medications, and an aggressive approach to treating ischemia including revascularization (see also Chaps. 23 and 45).

HYPERTENSIVE CARDIOMYOPATHY

Definition/Diagnosis
A hypertensive dilated cardiomyopathy is diagnosed when myocardial systolic function is depressed out of proportion to the increase in wall stress. In other words, a person presenting in heart failure with a hypertensive crisis would not carry this diagnosis unless ventricular dilatation and depressed systolic function remained after correction of the hypertension. In addition to its "pure" form of hypertensive cardiomyopathy, hypertension is a major risk factor for heart failure from any cause.[80] Within the WHO classification, hypertensive heart disease may present in the dilated, restrictive, or unclassified categories.

Prognosis

The prognosis depends on the presence of other comorbid conditions, such as diabetes mellitus and coronary artery disease, as well as on the extent of control of afterload. Compared to other forms of cardiomyopathy, in the absence of comorbid conditions the prognosis of hypertensive cardiomyopathy in individuals whose afterload is controlled is probably better than for most other types of dilated cardiomyopathy.[81]

Treatment

The treatment is as for ischemic cardiomyopathy (see above), except that afterload must be vigorously controlled. This consists of the addition of pure vasodilators, such as amlodipine or alpha-blocking agents, to standard heart failure therapy (see also Chaps. 23 and 58).

VALVULAR CARDIOMYOPATHY

Definition/Diagnosis

A valvular cardiomyopathy occurs when a valvular abnormality is present and myocardial systolic function is depressed out of proportion to the increase in wall stress. This occurs most commonly with left-sided regurgitant lesions (mitral regurgitation and aortic regurgitation), less commonly with aortic stenosis, and never with pure mitral stenosis.

Prognosis

The prognosis is variable and depends on the number of associated conditions, the nature and extent of the valvular abnormality, and most importantly the severity of the cardiomyopathy at the time of surgical correction (see below). In general, severely depressed myocardial function will not improve much with surgical repair of aortic regurgitation or mitral regurgitation, but the prognosis is often improved

TABLE 73-3

KNOWN CAUSES OF DILATED CARDIOMYOPATHY

Ischemic insult (ischemic cardiomyopathy)
Valvular disease (mitral regurgitation, aortic regurgitation, aortic stenosis); (valvular cardiomyopathy)
Chronic hypertension (hypertensive cardiomyopathy)
Tachyarrhythmias (supraventricular, ventricular, atrial flutter)
Familial (autosomal dominant, X-linked)
Idiopathic
Toxins
  Ethanol
  Chemotherapeutic agents (anthracyclines such as doxorubicin and daunorubicin)
  Cobalt
  Antiretroviral agents (zidovudine, didanosine, zalcitabine)
  Phenothiazines
  Carbon monoxide
  Lithium
  Lead
  Cocaine
  Mercury
Metabolic abnormalities
  Nutritional deficiencies (thiamine, selenium, carnitine, protein)
  Endocrinologic disorders (hypothyroidism, acromegaly, thyrotoxicosis, Cushing's disease, pheochromocytoma, catecholamines, diabetes mellitus)
  Electrolyte disturbances (hypocalcemia, hypophosphatemia)
Infectious
  Viral (coxsackie virus, cytomegalovirus, human immunodeficiency virus)
  Rickettsial
  Bacterial
  Mycobacterial
  Spirochetal
  Fungal
  Parasitic (toxoplasmosis, trichinosis, Chagas' disease)
Systemic disorders
  Systemic lupus erythematosus
  Juvenile rheumatoid arthritis
  Polyarteritis nodosa
  Kawasaki's disease
  Collagen vascular disorders (scleroderma, lupus erythematosus, dermatomyositis)
  Hemochromatosis
  Amyloidosis
  Sarcoidosis
  Pseudoxanthoma elasticum
  Hypereosinophilic syndrome
Hypersensitivity myocarditis
Peri/postpartum dysfunction
Arrhythmogenic right ventricular dysplasia or cardiomyopathy
Infantile histiocytoid
Neuromuscular dystrophies
  Beckel's or Duchenne's muscular dystrophy, X-linked cardioskeletal myopathy
Facioscapulohumoral muscular dystrophy
Erb's limb-girdle dystrophy
Myotonic dystrophy
Friedreich's ataxia
Emery-Dreifuss muscular dystrophy
Inborn errors of metabolism
Mitochondrial cardiomyopathies
Keshan's cardiomyopathy

because of elimination of the some of the hemodynamic insult. Replacement of the mitral valve in patients with severe mitral regurgitation and LEVFs < 25 percent is associated with high operative perioperative mortality rates (see Chap. 64). On the other hand, there is seldom an impairment of LV systolic function severe enough to preclude valve replacement of severe aortic stenosis, because function will usually improve on relief of the hemodynamic insult and the prognosis is relatively good (see Chap. 63).

Treatment

The treatment of a valvular cardiomyopathy is surgical valve replacement when significant cardiomyopathy is detected. Catheter valvuloplasty may be an option for a few patients with severe aortic stenosis who are not good surgical candidates for reasons other than heart failure.[82] In those with aortic or mitral regurgitation whose LV function is severely impaired, medical treatment may be the only option. The medical treatment of either disorder should be as above for ischemic cardiomyopathy plus aggressive afterload reduction, usually hydralazine/nitrates in addition to ACE inhibitors. The calcium channel blocker amlodipine is another option for afterload reduction,[83] particularly for aortic regurgitation where calcium blocker therapy has been shown to prolong the time to surgery in patients with normal left ventricular function[84] (see also Chaps. 23, 63, and 64).

IDIOPATHIC DILATED CARDIOMYOPATHY, INCLUDING FAMILIAL DILATED FORMS

Definition/Diagnosis

IDC is diagnosed by excluding significant coronary artery disease and valvular and other causes. IDC is a relatively common cause of heart failure, with a prevalence rate of 0.04 percent[71] and incidence rates varying from 0.005 to 0.006 percent.[71,72] The true incidence of IDC is undoubtedly higher, and many individuals may remain asymptomatic until marked ventricular dysfunction has occurred. The incidence of IDC increases with age, and males are afflicted at a higher rate.[71] As discussed below, histologic features are nonspecific and consist of myocardial cell hypertrophy and varying amounts of increased interstitial fibrosis. Although the diagnosis is not difficult, problems arise when a person with an apparent IDC presents with a history of hypertension or excessive alcohol intake. In such cases, it is best to reassign the etiology to alcohol only when the intake has exceeded 100 g/day for a substantial (years) period of time, and to hypertensive heart disease when blood pressure has been uncontrolled and high (>160/100 mmHg) as well as sustained (for years). All patients with an unexplained dilated cardiomyopathy need a thyroid stimulating hormone measurement to exclude hypo- or hyperthyroidism, and those with diastolic dysfunction need to have an infiltrative process excluded. As discussed below, this is frequently best done by performing an endomyocardial biopsy.

IDC may be familial in as many as 50 percent of the cases

when first-degree relatives are carefully screened.[85,86] Several chromosomal assignments for gene location have been made for autosomal dominant patterns of inheritance, including one on chromosome 9[87] and one on chromosome 1.[88] No candidate genes have been proposed as yet. In cases of familial dilated cardiomyopathy, it is important to exclude X-linked inheritance,[89] which will likely turn out to be Becker's (subclinical or mild skeletal muscle involvement) or Duchenne's (clinically apparent skeletal myopathy) muscular dystrophy presenting predominantly in the heart.[90–92] Abnormalities of myocardial dystrophin gene expression are best detected by immunohistochemical or immunochemical quantification of dystrophin protein gene expression on endomyocardial biopsy,[93] and candidates for such a diagnostic test can be identified by screening for an elevated serum total creatine kinase level[91] (see also Chap. 69).

The major morphologic feature of IDC on postmortem examination is dilatation of the cardiac chambers.[94,95] One ventricle (usually the left) may be more dilated than the other ventricle. The weight of the heart is increased in IDC, with a mean cardiac weight of 551 g for women and 632 g for men.[95] Although there is an increase in muscle mass and myocyte cell volume in IDC, LV wall thickness is usually not increased because of the marked dilatation of the ventricular cavities. Grossly visible scars may be present in either ventricle. While most scars are small, some may be large and transmural. Scarring occurs in the absence of significant narrowing of the epicardial coronary arteries. In most cases, the degree of fibrosis does not appear to be extensive enough to cause changes in systolic or diastolic function. Intracardiac thrombi and mural endocardial plaques (from the organization of thrombi) are present at necropsy in more than 50 percent of patients with IDC.[94,95] The effect of anticoagulation on the incidence of thrombi has not been carefully studied, but systemic and pulmonary emboli are more frequently in patients with ventricular thrombi or plaques.[95]

The characteristic findings of IDC on microscopy are marked myocyte hypertrophy and very large, bizarre-shaped nuclei[95–98] (Fig. 73-4). Myocyte atrophy and myofilament loss are also seen.[95,99] In isolated cardiac myocytes, the major cellular phenotypic change is marked increase in cell length without a concomitant increase in diameter. As described earlier, this cellular lengthening or remodeling contributes to the chamber remodeling/dilatation that characterizes IDC and other cardiomyopathies. These morphologic changes in IDC are not specific and are generally found in secondary cardiomyopathies such as in the noninfarcted regions of ischemic dilated cardiomyopathy or in valvular cardiomyopathy. Also, the morphometric changes in IDC do not correlate with the severity of illness.[98,99] Ultrastructural abnormalities such as mitochondrial changes, T-tubular dilatation, and intracellular lipid droplets may be observed in IDC but can also be observed in other forms of heart disease.[98] There may be interstitial parenchymal and perivascular focal infiltrates of small lymphocytes.[97–101] The lymphocytic infiltrates present on histologic examination in IDC are not associated with adjacent myocyte damage, in contrast to myocarditis, where adjacent myocyte necrosis may be observed. Fibrosis is nearly always present in IDC,[95–101] and its pattern is quite variable—from a fine perimyocytic distribution to coarse scars indistinguishable from those present in chronic ischemia. Small intramural arteries and capillaries, however, are normal in IDC.[98]

A number of immune regulatory abnormalities have been identified in IDC, including humoral and cellular autoimmune reactivity against myocytes,[102] decreased natural killer cell activity,[103] and abnormal suppressor cell activity.[104,105] These abnormalities suggest that immune defects may be important etiologic factors in the development of IDC. These findings, however, are not universally present in patients with IDC, and some abnormalities are also present in other types of heart muscle disease. For example, an increase in the cardioselective M7 antimitochondrial antibodies is found in both IDC and HCM but not in heart failure from coronary artery disease.[106] The incidence of some autoreactive antibodies, such as antinuclear and antifibrillary antibodies, increases with the severity of heart failure.[107] It is likely that many of the antibodies detected in IDC and other myocardial diseases do not have pathogenic relevance but rather are secondary to the primary degenerative process. It is possible, however, that certain antibodies present in IDC may have important functional implications. For example, anti-beta$_1$-adrenergic receptor antibodies[108,109] could modify beta-adrenergic receptor activity[110] and produce chronic increases in signal transduction that are harmful to the failing heart. Another potential pathogenetic autoimmune mechanism is disturbed energy metabolism from antibodies to the ADP/ATP carrier of the inner mitochondrial membrane.[111] These antibodies are present in some individuals with IDC,[112] and they have been shown to impair metabolism and myocardial function.[111]

There has been great interest in histocompatibility locus antigens (HLAs) in IDC since these antigens are known to be associated with immune regulatory functions and many autoimmune diseases are found to have positive HLA antigenic associations. HAL associations have also been identified in IDC; the frequency of HLA-B27, HLA-A2, HLA-DR4, and HLA-DQ4 is increased compared to controls, and the frequency of HLA-DRw6 is decreased compared to controls.[113] Genetic abnormalities in the HLA region could potentially alter immune response and thereby increase disease

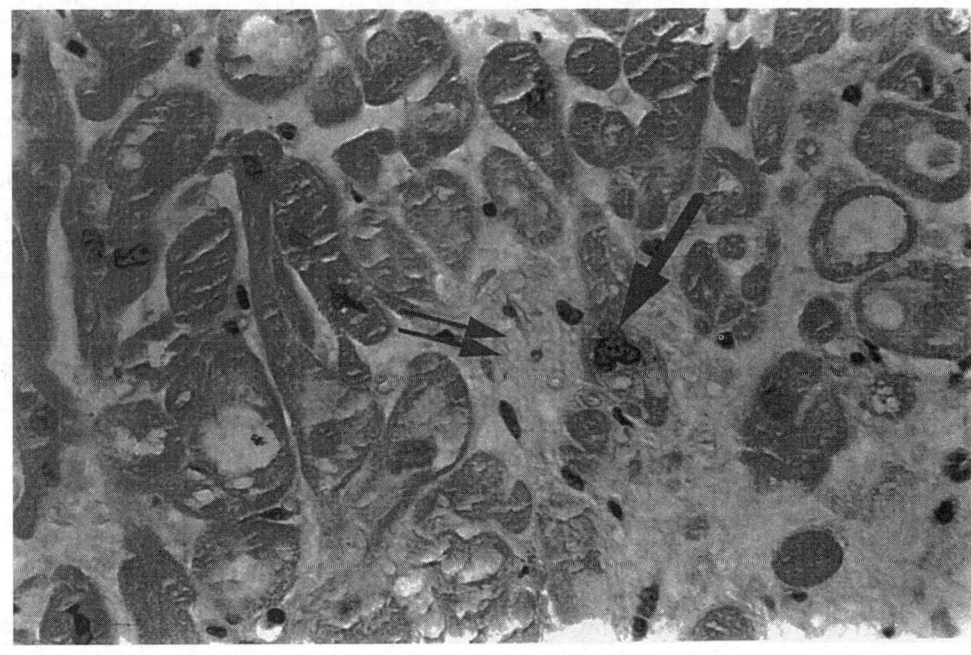

FIGURE 73-4

Right ventricular endomyocardial biopsy from a 42-year-old male patient with idiopathic dilated cardiomyopathy, with left and right ventricular ejection fractions of 0.31 and 0.36, respectively. Note the myocyte hypertrophy with marked nuclear pleomorphism (*thick arrow*), and interstitial fibrosis (*double arrows*).

susceptibility to infectious agents such as enteroviruses. Thus, the association in IDC with specific HLAs suggests a possible immunologic etiology for this disease. These specific HLAs, however, are present in fewer than 50 percent of patients with IDC, and the heterogeneity of these antigens does not point to a unique site for a putative disease-associated gene. Further investigation will be necessary to understand the significance of these findings.

A clinical and pathologic syndrome that is similar to IDC may develop after resolution of viral myocarditis in animal models and biopsy-proven myocarditis in humans.[114] This has led to speculation that IDC may develop in some individuals as a result of subclinical viral myocarditis. Theoretically, an episode of myocarditis could initiate a variety of autoimmune reactions that injure the myocardium and ultimately result in the development of IDC. The abnormalities in immune regulation and the variety of antimyocardial antibodies present in IDC are consistent with this hypothesis. On the other hand, it is generally not possible to isolate an infectious virus or to demonstrate the presence of viral antigens in the myocardium of patients with IDC.[114,115] Enteroviral RNA sequences are found in heart biopsy samples in IDC, but only in approximately zero to one-third of patients.[115–117] Furthermore, active myocardial inflammation is usually not detected in IDC.[100,101] Finally, glucocorticoid therapy of patients with IDC does not result in significant clinical improvements.[118] Thus, while the viral infection–autoimmune hypothesis is an attractive candidate for the etiology of some cases of IDC, it remains unproved.

As noted in Chaps. 25 and 72, endomyocardial biopsy of the right or left ventricle may be a valuable diagnostic adjunct for diagnosing specific myocardial processes that can produce a dilated phenotype, such as myocarditis and infiltrative cardiomyopathies. Because several of these other dilated cardiomyopathies may have specific treatments and/or a different prognosis than IDC, endomyocardial biopsy may be warranted in many individuals presenting with a dilated cardiomyopathy. In the future, biopsy may be used more frequently to identify genetic disorders resulting in abnormal gene expression,[119] such as can now be done to diagnose Becker-Duchenne cardiomyopathy.[93] Since special staining, electron microscopy, or molecular analysis of the biopsy material may be necessary, endomyocardial biopsy is best performed in specialized cardiomyopathy/heart failure centers.

Prognosis

Several studies of the natural history of IDC have been conducted.[118,119] The prognosis is generally considered to be better than for ischemic cardiomyopathy,[75,76] and prior to the routine use of ACE inhibitors the survival was approximately 50 percent at 5 years.[120] The prognosis has been substantially improved since then,[121] as ACE inhibition,[122] cardiac transplantation,[123] and beta-adrenergic blockade[10,11,77,124] are all effective treatments in this cardiomyopathy.

Treatment

The treatment of IDC is similar to that discussed above for ischemic cardiomyopathy, except there is no issue of revascularization. The risk of thromboembolic complications may be higher than in ischemic cardiomyopathy, resulting in a lower threshhold for anticoagulation. Beta-adrenergic blockade produces a quantitatively greater degree of improvement in LV function compared to that in ischemic cardiomyopathy,[125,126] because either there is a greater degree of adrenergic activation[8] or there is more viable myocardium to work with in IDC. Approximately 10 percent of IDC patients treated with beta-adrenergic blockade will normalize their myocardial function, and this form of treatment should be offered to all IDC patients who do not have a contraindication before considering cardiac transplantation[77] (see Chap. 23).

SELECTED SPECIFIC DILATED CARDIOMYOPATHIES WITH UNIQUE MANAGEMENT ISSUES

Anthracycline Cardiomyopathy

Definition/Diagnosis

The commonly used and highly efficacious anthracycline antibiotic anticancer agents doxorubicin and daunorubicin produces a dose-related cardiomyopathy[127–132] that may limit their clinical application (see also Chaps. 80 and 86). Within the WHO classification, an anthracycline cardiomyopathy would most likely be in the dilated category, but because the extent of dilatation may initially be minimal (see below), it could also be in the unclassified category. The cardiomyopathy

produced by these agents depends on the total cumulative dose, and for the more widely used compound doxorubicin (Adriamycin), the incidence of heart failure due to cardiomyopathy increases dramatically above total cumulative doses of 450 mg per square meter of body surface area in patients without underlying cardiac problems or other risk factors.[128] Prior mediastinal radiation involving the heart is a powerful risk factor for anthracycline cardiomyopathy,[129] and the risk is also evident if radiation treatment follows chemotherapy.[132,133] In patients with risk factors, anthracycline cardiomyopathy can present at cumulative doses lower than 450 mg/m^2 (see also Chap. 80).[128]

Although the diagnosis of anthracycline cardiomyopathy can be made clinically, the definitive diagnosis depends on the demonstration of a substantial number of cardiac myocytes exhibiting the characteristic anthracycline effect.[129–132] Tissue sampling is best done by endomyocardial biopsy, which allows for "thin section" electron-microscopic processing of the sample and more definitive resolution of the anthracycline effect with light microscopy.[129,130] As shown in Fig. 73-5, the anthracycline cardiac myocytic lesion consists of cell vacuolization progressing to cell dropout, and when 15 to 25 percent of the total number of sampled cells exhibit this morphology, myocardial dysfunction results.[129] It is not clear whether this abnormality represents a toxic effect of anthracyclines, disordered cell cycle regulation and apoptosis, or both.

In the absence of a tissue diagnosis, anthracycline cardiomyopathy may be diagnosed clinically by exclusion of other causes of cardiomyopathy in a patient who has had at least 350 mg/m^2 of doxorubicin or the equivalent amount with another anthracycline. Additionally, there are some distinguishing clinical features of anthracycline cardiomyopathy that may aid in making the diagnosis. These include a relative absence of hypertrophy and dilatation and a higher heart rate (110 to 130 beats per minute) than is usually encountered in ambulatory heart failure. The reasons for these features are that the onset of symptoms may be relatively acute (remodeling takes time to develop) and the anthracycline inhibits contractile protein synthesis,[133] reducing the amount of compensatory dilatation and remodeling. In this situation the only option available for stabilizing cardiac output is increasing heart rate, because increasing stroke volume via a larger end-diastolic volume has been precluded. The increased heart rate is produced by a greater than expected hyperadrenergic state, and so these patients may be exceptionally dependent on adrenergic support.

Prognosis

The prognosis of anthracycline cardiomyopathy is variable and depends on numerous factors, including the age and underlying prechemotherapy cardiac status of the patient and the time of presentation relative to the last dose of drug. Those who present late (several months) or very late (years) after the last dose have a better prognosis, because the anthracycline myocardial effect takes at least 60 days to become fully manifest.[134] That is, patients who develop heart failure within a few days of the last dose of drug have an additional cardiomyopathic burden to face because the last one to two doses produce their full morphologic effect over the next 1 to 2 months.

Treatment/Prevention

Patients who develop anthracycline cardiomyopathy should be treated aggressively with conventional heart failure treatment, as some degree of reversibility is likely. Conventional treatment consists of ACE inhibitors, digoxin, and diuretics. Beta-adrenergic blockade has been used successfully in some individuals,[135,136] but because of the high adrenergic drive it may be difficult to achieve. On the other hand, the heightened adrenergic mechanism may be producing a commensurate amount of adverse effect on the myocardium, and so the potential for a favorable response to beta blockers may be even greater than in other kinds of cardiomyopathy. In severe, refractory cases cardiac transplantation may be performed, provided that the patient's cancer is in complete remission and is not likely to recur (≥70 percent chance of cure).

Several strategies have been shown to lower the risk of developing anthracycline cardiomyopathy without compromising the chemotherapy response rate. These include using endomyocardial biopsy and right heart catheterization with exercise to assess risk, which can virtually eliminate clinical cardiomyopathy and allow more anthracycline to be administered to less susceptible subjects.[137] An alternative approach uses serial radionuclide angiography with[138] or without[139] exercise as a monitoring strategy, which may be useful, but because of a low specificity, it reduces the total amount of chemotherapy that can safely be administered to some patients.[137] Other strategies include giving the agents as low-dose weekly[140] or 48- to 72-h infusions[141] rather than as boluses every 3 to 4 weeks, using a liposomal formulation,[142] or concomitantly administering a second agent that reduces toxicity.[143] Unfortunately, none of these strategies completely eliminates the risk of developing a clinical cardiomyopathy (see also Chap. 80).

Postpartum Cardiomyopathy

Definition/Diagnosis

Post- or peripartum cardiomyopathy is defined as the presentation of systolic dysfunction and clinical heart failure during the last trimester of pregnancy or within 6 months of delivery.[144]

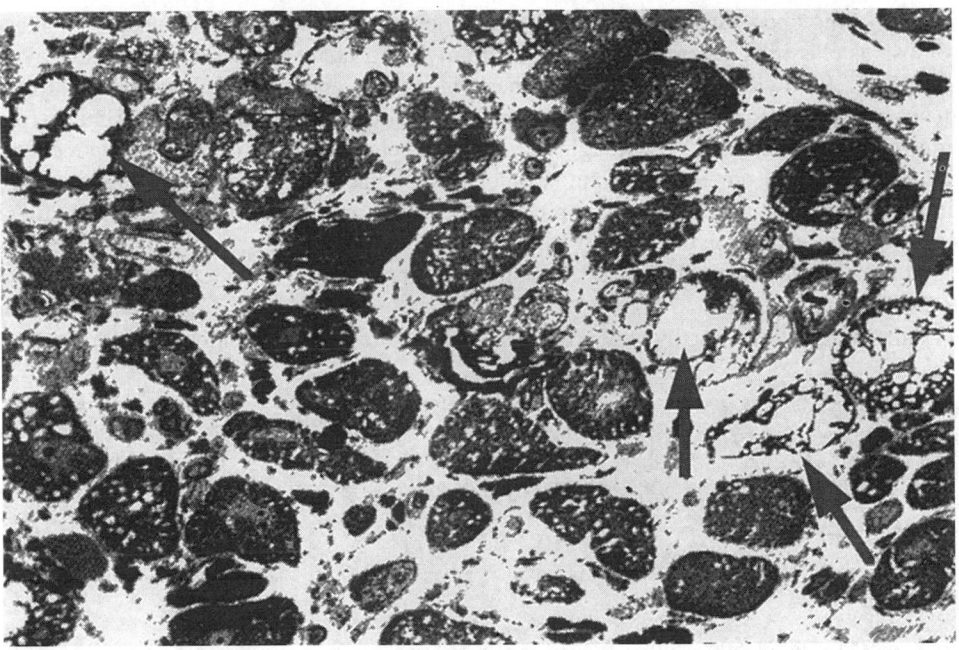

FIGURE 73-5
Cardiac myocyte vacuolization in cases of doxorubicin cardiomyopathy classified on endomyocardial biopsy as grade 3 by the Billingham classification.[126,133,134]

Given the extreme hemodynamic load produced by pregnancy, it is perhaps surprising that postpartum cardiomyopathy is not more common. Postpartum cardiomyopathy will most likely be in the dilated category of the WHO classification but occasionally will be listed as unclassified because dilatation and remodeling have not had time to occur. Postpartum cardiomyopathy is likely a heterogeneous group of disorders, consisting of the addition of the hemodynamic load of pregnancy to a variety of underlying myocardial processes, including hypertensive heart disease, familial or idiopathic dilated cardiomyopathy, and myocarditis[145] (see also Chap. 92).

Prognosis

Approximately half of the patients who develop postpartum cardiomyopathy will recover completely,[146] and most of the rest will improve. Those who have developed postpartum cardiomyopathy should never become pregnant again, even if myocardial function has fully recovered.

Treatment

Treatment should be aggressive and as for IDC. In severely compromised patients who do not improve, cardiac transplantation may be required (see also Chap. 92).

Amyloid Cardiomyopathy

Definition/Diagnosis

As discussed in Chaps. 75 and 76, amyloidosis is a group of diseases characterized by extracellular deposition of proteins characterized by their unique β-pleated sheet conformation and recognized on electron microscopy as randomly arranged nonbranching fibers ranging from 8 to 14 nm in length. Amyloidosis is classified according to the type of amyloid protein involved.[147] Amyloidosis involving the heart is not rare and in autopsy studies accounts for up to 10 percent of all nonischemic cardiomyopathies.[148] Although the source and chemical nature of amyloid protein differ among the various types of amyloidosis, the tissue/organ pathophysiology is the same, i.e., the slow destruction of the heart by the inexorable deposition of a β-pleated sheet fibril that is insoluble and impervious to proteolytic digestion.[149]

Amyloid cardiomyopathy may present in the WHO restrictive, dilated, or unclassified categories. Most commonly it presents as a restrictive cardiomyopathy with conduction system abnormalities. In the setting of systemic amyloidosis (secondary or primary forms), the presence of increased wall thickness on echocardiogram plus electrocardiogram (ECG) voltage is highly suggestive of cardiac involvement.[150] In primary systemic amyloidosis, a monoclonal immunoglobulin spike is detectable in urine or serum in approximately 80 percent of patients.[151] The definitive diagnosis of amyloid cardiomyopathy is made by tissue examination, ideally premortem by endomyocardial biopsy.[152] In systemic forms, the tissue diagnosis may be made by rectal, skin, or tongue biopsy of any abnormal tissue in these locations coupled with an unexplained myocardial process. As shown in Fig. 73-6, the characteristic histologic signature of amyloid is extracellular deposition of a fibrillar protein with a characteristic periodicity on electron microscopy.[152] although a Congo red stain can identify most cases, electron microscopy is more sensitive and specific and should be used routinely when amyloid is suspected.

Prognosis

The prognosis is uniformly bad regardless of the type of amyloidosis, and the majority of patients with amyloid cardiomyopathy are dead within 2 years of diagnosis.

Treatment

There is no definitive treatment of amyloid cardiomyopathy. Treatment of amyloid cardiomyopathy is completely empiric and consists of diuretics when needed, pacemaker treatment of bradyarrhythmias, and the avoidance of digoxin, which may be arrhythmogenic in any infiltrative cardiomyopathy. Cardiac transplantation should be avoided even in primary localized amyloid cardiomyopathy, because the amyloidosis will invariably recur in the heart or in other organs. The exception may be familial forms of amyloidosis where the abnormal protein is a transthyretin, or prealbumin,

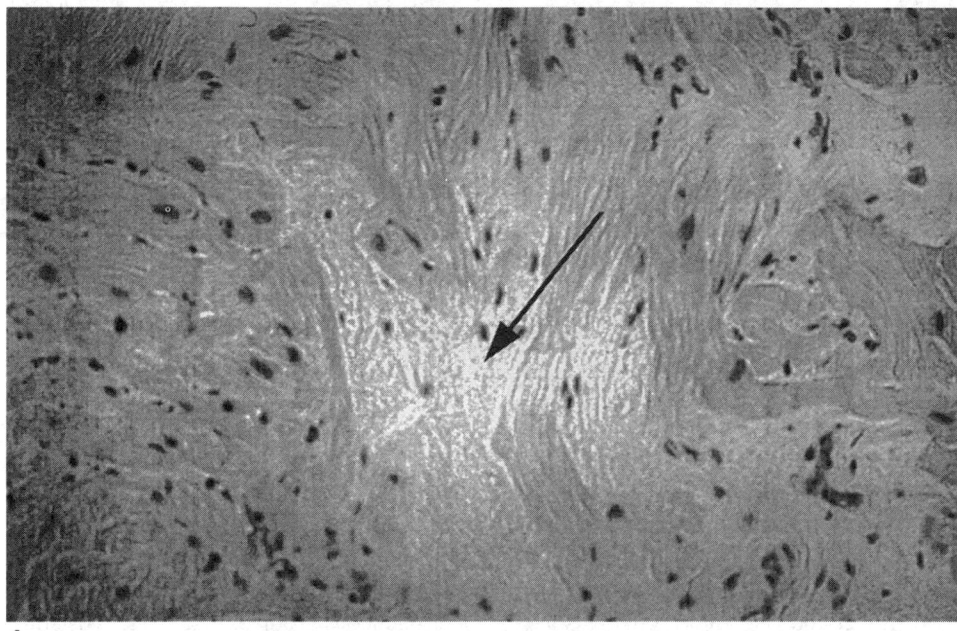

A

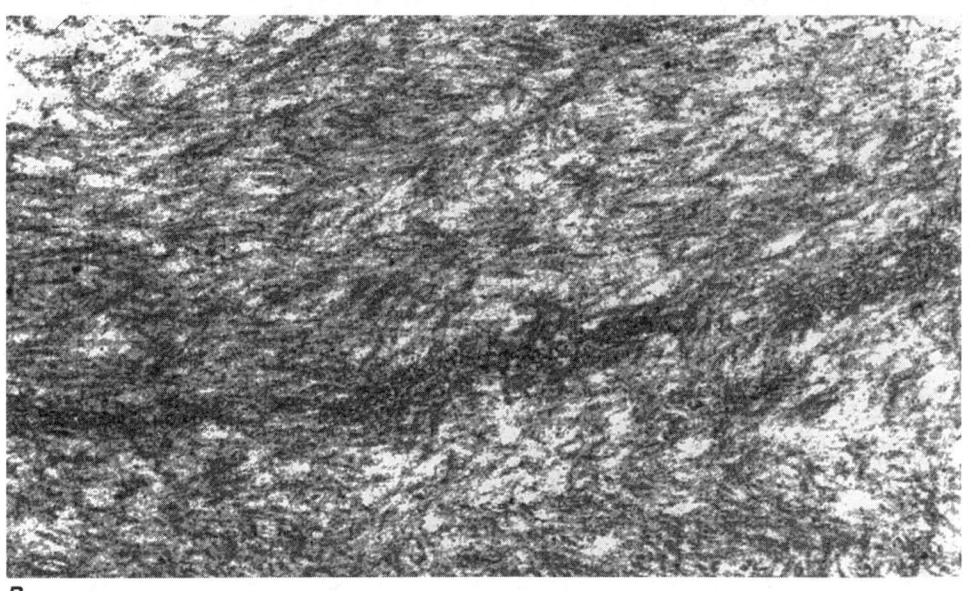

B

FIGURE 73-6

A. Right ventricular endomyocardial biopsy demonstrating interstitial amyloid deposition (H&E, 100×). *B.* Electron micrograph of the same biopsy specimen illustrating the characteristic 8- to 14-nm, nonbranching, randomly oriented amyloid fibrils.

variant synthesized in the liver. In this situation combined liver and heart transplantation can be curative[153] (see also Chap. 75).

Alcohol Cardiomyopathy

Definition/Diagnosis

An alcohol cardiomyopathy is said to be present when other causes of a dilated cardiomyopathy have been excluded and there is a history of heavy, sustained alcohol intake. The usual requirement in terms of alcohol amount is 100 g of alcohol per day, typically over several years. In susceptible individuals, however, it is likely that lower amounts of intake can produce a cardiomyopathy. The histologic features of alcohol cardiomyopathy are nonspecific and do not differ from those of IDC. Other than history, the only potentially distinguishing feature between IDC and alcohol cardiomyopathy is that the latter may present with a relatively high cardiac output.

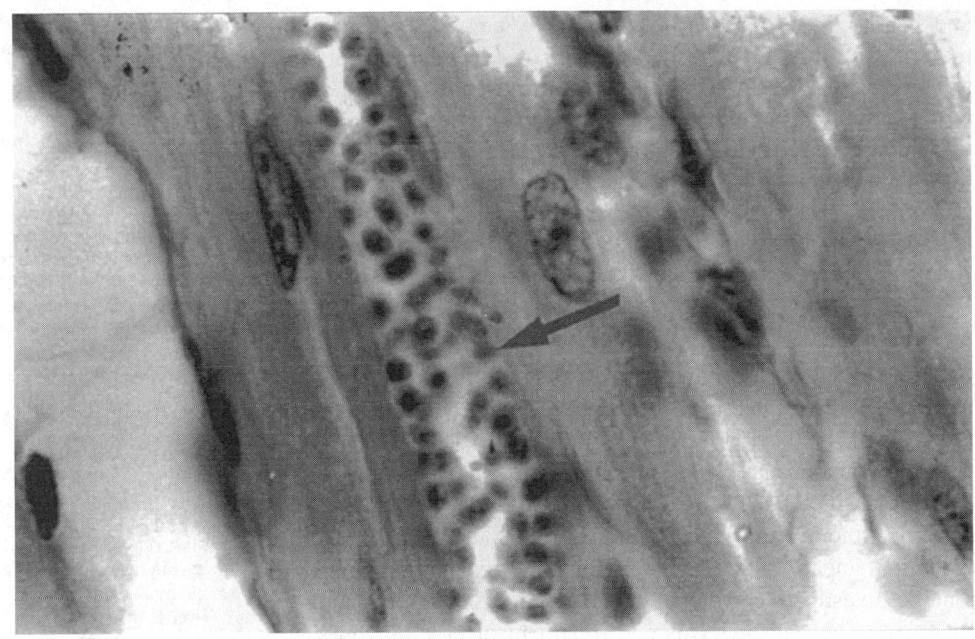

FIGURE 73-7

Leishmanial forms of *Trypanosoma cruzi* within the swollen cytoplasm of a cardiac myocyte (Chagas' cardiomyopathy) (H&E, 250×). (Courtesy of Dr. Elmer Koneman.)

Prognosis

The prognosis depends on the degree of impairment of myocardial function and the extent of abstinence from alcohol. There is evidence that the prognosis is somewhat better than for IDC.[154]

Treatment

The treatment of alcohol cardiomyopathy does not differ from that of IDC, except for the inclusion of total abstinence from alcohol. Obviously, these patients are not good candidates for cardiac transplantation because of the high relapse rate to alcoholism (see also Chap. 77).

Chagas' Cardiomyopathy

Definition/Diagnosis

Chagas' disease is discussed in Chap. 76 as a cause of myocarditis. In addition, Chagas' disease is the most common cause of nonischemic cardiomyopathy in South and Central America, with over 10 million people afflicted.[155] It is caused by a parasite, the leishmanial or tissue form of the protozoan *Trypanosoma cruzi*. Although in the United States the vector (*Triatoma*, or kissing bug) is found only in the southwest, Chagas' disease may be transmitted by blood transfusions; as a result, it could become relatively more important in this country. The natural history consists of an initial myocarditis, most commonly presenting in childhood, associated with acute myocardial infection, followed by recovery; in some individuals, the development of a dilated cardiomyopathy follows 10

to 30 years later. The basis for the chronic cardiomyopathy is unknown but may be immunologic, whereby antibodies generated against *T. cruzi* cross-react with cardiac myocyte antigens including myosin.[156]

The diagnosis of Chagas' cardiomyopathy is based on clinical (history, LV function, and ECG) criteria and a positive serologic test for *T. cruzi*.[157] ECG abnormalities consist of bundle branch or hemiblocks (indeed, hemiblocks were first described by Rosenbaum and colleagues[158] in Chagas' afflicted hearts with discrete foci of involvement), LV hypertrophy, and first- or second-degree atrioventricular block.[159] The histologic lesion of chronic Chagas' cardiomyopathy consists of mononuclear infiltrates, fibrosis, and, as shown in Fig. 73-7, foci of the leishmanial form of *T. cruzi* in myocardial fibers.[159] The LV functional abnormalities may be initially segmental and may include an apical aneurysm; later, however, they become more global.[157,159]

Prognosis

The prognosis is relatively good for a dilated cardiomyopathy and similar to IDC; the 5-year survival in Chagas' cardiomyopathy with heart failure is around 50 percent.[157] Compared to IDC, death probably occurs more commonly due to an arrhythmic mechanism.[157] As for IDC and most other dilated cardiomyopathies, however, mortality risk is directly dependent on the degrees of ventricular dysfunction and exercise intolerance.[157]

Treatment

There is no definitive treatment for Chagas' cardiomyopathy, and treatment includes pacemaker implantation for heart block and heart failure treatment as for IDC. The one exception may be the more frequent use of amiodarone, which appears to be particularly effective in treating arrhythmias associated with Chagas' cardiomyopathy and in one study reduced mortality compared to standard treatment.[160] The role of cardiac transplantation is still somewhat uncertain but can be done at acceptable risk,[161] especially when coupled with trypanocidal agents.[162]

SUMMARY

Cardiomyopathies are important because they are currently the most common cause of heart failure, which is the single most costly medical problem in the adult U.S. population. Cardiomyopathies are a heterogeneous group of diseases and can be classified under a newly modified WHO classification system; although imperfect, this system should be of great value in standardizing the terminology and encouraging systematic investigative and clinical approaches to diagnosis and treatment. Current diagnosis and treatment of cardiomyopathies vary considerably among the various types, and in many cases are best left to specialized centers that routinely deal with these disorders.

Genetic causes and influences over the natural history of the cardiomyopathies are the new frontier in this field, and their elucidation is almost certain to lead to new therapeutic and diagnostic approaches to the treatment of cardiomyopathies. In the near future, molecular genetic testing will be performed routinely for many cardiomyopathies that may be due to a single gene defect and for many other cardiomyopathies, as we learn more about the influence of polymorphic genetic variation on the natural history and selection of specific medical therapy.

REFERENCES

1. O'Connell JB, Bristow MR. Economic impact of heart failure in the United States: Time for a different approach. *J Heart Lung Transplant* 1994; 13:S107–S112.
2. Richardson P, McKenna W, Bristow MR, Maisch B, Mautner B, O'Connell J, et al. Report of the 1995 World Health Organization/ International Society and Federation of Cardiology Task Force on the definition and classification of cardiomyopathies. *Circulation* 1996; 93:841–842.
3. Ho KKL, Anderson KM, Kannel WB, Grossman W, Levy D. Survival after the onset of congestive heart failure in Framingham Heart Study subjects. *Circulation* 1993; 88:107–115.
4. Guccione AA, Felson DT, Anderson JJ, Anthony JM, Zhang Y, Wilson PW, et al. The effects of specific medical conditions on the functional limitations of elders in the Framingham Study. *Am J Public Health* 1994; 84:351–358.
5. Cohn JN, Johnson GR, Shabetai R, Loeb H, Tristani F, Rector T, et al. for the V-HeFT VA Cooperative Studies Group. Ejection fraction, peak exercise oxygen consumption, cardiothoracic ratio, ventricular arrhythmias, and plasma norepinephrine as determinants of prognosis in heart failure. *Circulation* 1993; 87(suppl VI):VI5–VI16.
6. Eichhorn EJ, Bristow MR. Medical therapy can improve the biologic properties of the chronically failing heart: A new era in the treatment of heart failure. *Circulation* 1996; 94:2285–2296.
7. WHO/ISFC Task Force on Cardiomyopathies. Report of the WHO/ ISFC Task Force on the definition and classification of cardiomyopathies. *Br Heart J* 1980; 44:672–673.
8. Bristow MR, Anderson FL, Port JD, Skerl L, Hershberger RE, Larrabee P, et al. Differences in β-adrenergic neuroeffector mechanisms in ischemic vs idiopathic dilated cardiomyopathy. *Circulation* 1991; 84:1024–1039.
9. Bristow MR, O'Connell JB, Gilbert EM, French WJ, Leatherman G, Kantrowitz NE, et al. for the Bucindolol Investigators. Dose-response of chronic β blocker treatment in heart failure from either idiopathic dilated or ischemic cardiomyopathy. *Circulation* 1994; 89:1632–1642.
10. Packer M, Bristow MR, Cohn JN, Colucci WS, Fowler MB, Gilbert EM, et al. Effect of carvedilol on morbidity and mortality in patients with chronic heart failure. *N Engl J Med* 1996; 334:1349–1355.
11. Bristow MR, Gilbert EM, Abraham WT, Adams KF, Fowler MB, Hershberger RE, et al. Carvedilol produces dose-related improvements in left ventricular function and survival in subjects with chronic heart failure. *Circulation* 1996; 94:2807–2816.
12. Geisterfer-Lawrence AA, Kass S, Tanigawa G, Vosberg HP, McKenna W, Seidman CE, et al. A molecular basis for familial hypertrophic cardiomyopathy: A beta-cardiac myosin heavy chain missense mutation. *Cell* 1990; 62:999–1006.
13. Geisterfer-Lawrence AA, Christe M, Conner DA, Ingwall JS, Seidman CE, Seidman JG. A mouse model of familial hypertrophic cardiomyopathy. *Science* 1996; 272:731–735.
14. Vikstrom KL, Factor SM, Leinwand LA. Mice expressing mutant myosin heavy chains are a model for familial hypertrophic cardiomyopathy. *Mol Med* 1996; 2:556–567.
15. Tiret L, Rigat B, Visvikis S, Breda C, Corvol P, Cambien C, et al. Evidence, from combined segregation and linkage analysis, that a variant of the angiotensin I-converting enzyme (ACE) gene controls plasma ACE levels. *Am J Hum Genet* 1992; 51(1):197–205.
16. Raynolds MV, Bristow MR, Bush E, Abraham WT, Lowes BD, Zisman LS, et al. Angiotensin-converting enzyme *DD* genotype in patients with ischaemic or idiopathic dilated cardiomyopathy. *Lancet* 1993; 342:1073–1075.
17. Jeunemaitre X, Charru A, Rigat B, Hout A-M, Soubrier F, Corvol P. Sib-pair linkage analysis of renin gene haplotypes in human essential hypertension. *Hum Genet* 1992; 88:301–306.
18. Bonnardeaux A, Davies E, Jeunemaitre X, Fery I, Charru A, Clauser E, et al. Angiotensin II type 1 receptor gene polymorphisms in human essential hypertension. *Hypertension* 1994; 24:63–69.
19. Jeunemaitre X, Soubrier F, Kotelevtsev Y, Lifton RP, Williams CS, Charru A, et al. Molecular basis of human hypertension: Role of angiotensinogen. *Cell* 1992; 71:169–180.
20. Robbins J. Gene targeting and animal models of cardiovascular disease. *Circ Res* 1993; 73:3–9.
21. Edwards JG, Lyons GE, Micales BK, Malhorta A, Factor S, Leinwand LA. Cardiomyopathy in transgenic *myf5* mice. *Circ Res* 1996; 78:379–387.
22. Iwase M, Bishop SP, Uechi M, Vatner DE, Shannon RP, Kudej RK, et al. Adverse effects of chronic endogenous sympathetic drive induced by cardiac $G_{\alpha S}$ overexpression. *Circ Res* 1996; 78:517–524.
23. Iwase M, Uechi M, Vatner DE, Asai K, Shannon RP, Kudej RK. Dilated cardiomyopathy induced by cardiac $G_{\alpha S}$ overexpression (abstr). *Circulation* 1996; 94:I16.
24. Bisognano JD, Pende A, Tremmel KD, Dutcher DL, Knudson OA, Bohlmeyer TJ, et al. Preliminary characterization of a transgenic mouse over-expressing the human β_1 adrenergic receptor. *J Invest Med* 1997; 45:210A.
25. Geng Y-J, Ishikawa Y, Vatner DE, Wagner TE, Bishop SP, Vatner SF, et al. Overexpression of $G_{\alpha S}$ accelerates programmed death (apoptosis) of myocardiocytes in transgenic mice (abstr). *Circulation* 1996; 94:I282.
26. Arber S, Hunter JJ, Ross J, Hongo M, Sansig G, Borg J, et al. MLP-deficient mice exhibit a disruption of cardiac cytoarchitectural organization, dilated cardiomyopathy, and heart failure. *Cell* 1997; 88:393–403.
27. Hunter JJ, Tanaka N, Rockman HA, Ross J, Chien KR. Ventricular expression of a MLC-2v-*ras* fusion gene induces cardiac hypertrophy and selective diastolic dysfunction in transgenic mice. *J Biol Chem* 1995; 270:23173–23178.
28. Robbins RJ, Swain JL. C-*myc* protooncogene modulates cardiac hypertrophic growth in transgenic mice. *Am J Physiol* 1992; 62:H590–H597.
29. Milano CA, Dolber PC, Rockman HA, Bond RA, Venable ME, Allen LF. Myocardial expression of a constitutively active α_{1B}-adrenergic receptor in transgenic mice induces cardiac hypertrophy. *Proc Natl Acad Sci USA* 1994; 91:10109–10113.

30. Lander ES, Schork NJ. Genetic dissection of complex traits. *Science* 1994; 265:2037–2048.

31. Jan Danser AH, Maarten ADH, Schalekamp MD, Bax WA, Maasen van den Brink A, Saxena PR, et al. Angiotensin-converting enzyme in the human heart: Effect of the deletion/insertion polymorphism. *Circulation* 1995; 92:1387–1388.

32. Lechin M, Quinones MA, Omran A, Hill R, Yu Q-T, Rakowski H, et al. Angiotensin-I converting enzyme genotypes and left ventricular hypertrophy in patients with hypertrophic cardiomyopathy. *Circulation* 1995; 92:1808–1812.

33. Pinto YM, van Gilst WH, Kingma JH, Schunkert H, for the Captopril and Thrombolysis Study Investigators. Deletion-type allele of the angiotensin-converting enzyme gene is associated with progressive ventricular dilatation after anterior myocardial infarction. *J Am Coll Cardiol* 1995; 25:1622–1626.

34. Andersson B, Sylven C. The DD genotype of the angiotensin-converting enzyme gene is associated with increased mortality in idiopathic dilated cardiomyopathy. *J Am Coll Cardiol* 1996; 28:162–167.

35. Raynolds MV, Roden RL, Blain-Nelson P, Bristow MR, Perryman MB. Association of genetic variants in the angiotensin II type 1 receptor and angiotensinogen with end-stage heart muscle disease. *J Am Coll Cardiol* February 1996:27A.

36. Green SA, Cole G, Jacinto M, Innis M, Liggett SB. A polymorphism of the human β_2-adrenergic receptor within the fourth transmembrane domain alters ligand binding and functional properties of the receptor. *J Biol Chem* 1993; 268(31):23116–23121.

37. Davies CH, Davia K, Bennett JG, Pepper JR, Poole-Wilson PA, Harding SE. Reduced contraction and altered frequency response of isolated ventricular myocytes from patients with heart failure. *Circulation* 1995; 92:2540–2549.

38. Bristow MR, Gilbert EM. Improvement in cardiac myocyte function by biologic effects of medical therapy: A new concept in the treatment of heart failure. *Eur Heart J* 1995; 16(suppl F):20–31.

39. Ross J, Braunwald E. Studies on Starling law of the heart. IX. The effects of impeding venous return on performance of the normal and failing ventricle. *Circulation* 1964; 30:719–727.

40. Schwinger RHG, Bohm M, Koch A, Schmidt U, Morano I, Eissner H-J, et al. The failing human heart is unable to use the Frank-Starling mechanism. *Circ Res* 1994; 74:959–969.

41. Holubarsch C, Thorsten R, Goldstein DJ, Ashton RC, Nickl G, Pieske B, et al. Existence of the Frank-Starling mechanism in the failing human heart: Investigations on the organ, tissue, and sarcomere levels. *Circulation* 1996; 94:683–689.

42. Feldman MD, Gwathmey JK, Phillips P, Schoen F, Morgan JP. Reversal of the force-frequency relationship in working myocardium from patients with end-stage heart failure. *J Appl Cardiol* 1988; 3:273–283.

43. Muleiri LA, Hasenfuss G, Leavitt B, Allen PD, Alpert NR. Altered myocardial force-frequency relationship in the human heart failure. *Circulation* 1992; 85:1743–1750.

44. Cohn JN. Structural basis for heart failure: Ventricular remodeling and its pharmacological inhibition. *Circulation* 1995; 91:2504–2507.

45. Gerdes AM, Capasso JM. Structural remodeling and mechanical dysfunction of cardiac myocytes in heart failure. *J Mol Cell Cardiol* 1995; 27:849–856.

46. Nadal-Ginard B, Mahdavi V. Molecular basis of cardiac performance. *J Clin Invest* 1989; 84:1693–1700.

47. Hirzel HO, Tuchschmid CR, Schneider J, Krayenbuhl HP, Schaub MC. Relationship between myosin isoenzyme composition, hemodynamics, and myocardial structure in various forms of human cardiac hypertrophy. *Circ Res* 1985; 57:729–740.

48. Anderson PAW, Malouf NN, Oakley A, Pagani ED, Allen PD. Troponin T isoform expression in humans: A comparison among normal and failing adult heart, fetal heart, and adult and fetal skeletal muscle. *Circ Res* 1991; 69:1226–1233.

49. Lowes BD, Minobe WA, Abraham WT, Roden RL, Port JD, Gilbert EM, et al. Downregulation of α- and upregulation of β-myosin heavy chain in intact, failing human left ventricles. *J Am Coll Cardiol* 1997; 29(suppl A):422A.

50. Tsutsui H, Ishihara K, Cooper GIV. Cytoskeletal role in the contractile dysfunction of hypertrophied myocardium. *Science* 1993; 260:682–687.

51. Yoshida K, Ikeda S, Nakamura A, Kagoshima M, Takeda S, Shoji S, et al. Molecular analysis of the Duchenne muscular dystrophy gene in patients with Becker muscular dystrophy presenting with dilated cardiomyopathy. *Muscle Nerve* 1993; 16:1161–1166.

52. Maeda M, Holder E, Lowes B, Valent S, Bies RD. Dilated cardiomyopathy associated with deficiency of the cytoskeletal protein metavinculin. *Circulation* 1997; 95:17–20.

53. Gerdes AM, Kellerman SE, Moore JA, Muffly KE, Clark LC, Reaves PY. Structural remodeling of cardiac myocytes from patients with chronic ischemic heart disease. *Circulation* 1992; 86:426–430.

54. Gerdes AM, Kellerman SE, Schocken DD. Implications of cardiomyocyte remodeling in heart dysfunction. In: Dhalla NS, Beamish RE, Takeda N, Nagano N, eds. *The Failing Heart.* New York: Raven Press; 1995:197–205.

55. Gerdes AM, Odera T, Wang X, McCune SA. Myocyte remodeling during progression to failure in rats with hypertension. *Hypertension* 1996; 28:609–614.

56. Zhang J, McDonald KM. Bioenergetic consequences of left ventricular remodeling. *Circulation* 1995; 92:1011–1019.

57. Sata M, Sugiura S, Yamashita H, Momomura S, Serizawa T. Coupling between myosin ATPase cycle and creatine kinase cycle facilitates cardiac actomyosin sliding in vitro: A clue to mechanical dysfunction during myocardial ischemia. *Circulation* 1996; 93:310–317.

58. Cintron C, Johnson G, Francis G, Cobb F, Cohn JN. Prognostic significance of serial changes in left ventricular ejection fraction in patients with congestive heart failure. *Circulation* 1993; 87(suppl VI):V117–VI23.

59. Binkley PF, Nunziata E, Haas GH, Nelson SD, Cody RJ. Parasympathetic withdrawal is an integral component of autonomic imbalance in congestive heart failure: Demonstration in human subjects and verification in a paced canine model of ventricular failure. *J Am Coll Cardiol* 1991; 18:464–472.

60. Chidiac P, Hebert TE, Valiquette M, Dennis M, Bouvier M. Inverse agonist activity of β-adrenergic antagonists. *Mol Pharmacol* 1994; 45:490–499.

61. Mewes T, Dutz S, Ravens U, Jakobs KH. Activation of calcium currents in cardiac myocytes by empty β-adrenoceptors. *Circulation* 1993; 88:2916–2922.

62. Milano CA, Allen LF, Rockman HA, Dolber PC, McMinn TR, Chien KR, et al. Enhanced myocardial function in transgenic mice overexpressing the β_2-adrenergic receptor. *Science* 1994; 264:562–566.

63. Bond RA, Leff P, Johnson TD, Milano C, Rockman H, McMinn TR, et al. Physiological effects of inverse agonists in transgenic mice with myocardial overexpression of the β_2-adrenoceptor. *Nature* 1995; 374:272–276.

64. Luo W, Grupp IL, Harrer J, Ponniah S, Grupp G, Duffy JJ, et al. Targeted ablation of the phospholamban gene is associated with markedly enhanced myocardial contractility and loss of β-agonist stimulation. *Circ Res* 1994; 75:401–409.

65. Narula J, Haider N, Virmani R, DiSalvo TG, Kolodgie FD, Hajjar RJ, et al. Apoptosis in myocytes in end-stage heart failure. *N Engl J Med* 1996; 335:1182–1189.

66. Teiger E, Dam T-V, Richard L, Wisnewsky C, Tea B-S, Sgaboury L, et al. Apoptosis in pressure overload–induced heart hypertrophy in the rat. *J Clin Invest* 1996; 97:2891–2897.

67. Cohn JN, Levine TB, Olivari MT, Garberg V, Lura D, Francis GS, et al. Plasma norepinephrine as a guide to prognosis in patients with chronic congestive heart failure. *N Engl J Med* 1984; 311:819–823.

68. Kaye DM, Lefkovits J, Jennings GL, Bergin P, Broughton A, Esler D. Adverse consequences of high sympathetic nervous activity in the failing human heart. *J Am Coll Cardiol* 1995; 26:1257–1263.

69. Swedburg K, Eneroth P, Kjekshus J, Wilhelmsen L. Hormones regulating cardiovascular function in patients with severe congestive heart failure and their relation to mortality. *Circulation* 1990; 82:1730–1736.

70. Bristow MR, O'Connell JB. Myocardial diseases. In: Kelly WN, ed. *Textbook of Internal Medicine,* 3d ed. Philadelphia: Lippincott; 1977:398–405.

71. Codd MB, Sugrue DD, Gersh BJ, Melton LJ. Epidemiology of idiopathic dilated and hypertrophic cardiomyopathy: A population based study in Olmstead County, MN 1975–1984. *Circulation* 1989; 80:564–572.

72. Torp A. Incidence of congestive cardiomyopathy. *Postgrad Med J* 1978; 54:435–439.

73. McKay RG, Pfeffer MA, Pasternak RC, Markis JE, Come PC, Nakao S, et al. Left ventricular remodeling after myocardial infarction: A corollary to infarct expansion. *Circulation* 1986; 74:693–702.

74. Mitchell GF, Lamas GA, Vaughan DE, Pfeffer MA. Left ventricular remodeling in the year after myocardial infarction: A quantitative analysis of contractile segment lengths and ventricular shape. *J Am Coll Cardiol* 1992; 19:1136–1144.

75. Franciosa JA, Willen M, Ziesche S, Cohn JN. Survival in men with severe chronic left ventricular failure due to either coronary heart disease or idiopathic dilated cardiomyopathy. *Am J Cardiol* 1983; 51:831–836.

76. Likoff MJ, Chandler SL, Kay HR. Clinical determinants of mortality in chronic congestive heart failure secondary to idiopathic dilated or to ischemic cardiomyopathy. *Am J Cardiol* 1987; 59(6):634–638.

77. Waagstein F, Bristow MR, Swedberg K, Camerini F, Fowler MB, Johnson M, et al. Beneficial effects of metoprolol in idiopathic dilated cardiomyopathy. *Lancet* 1993; 342:1441–1446.

78. Fowler MB, Bristow MR. Rationale for beta-adrenergic blocking drugs in cardiomyopathy. *Am J Cardiol* 1985; 55(10):D120–D124.

79. Bristow MR. Pathophysiologic and pharmacologic rationales for clinical management of chronic heart failure with beta-blocking agents. *Am J Cardiol* 1993; 71:12C–22C.

80. Levy D, Larson MG, Vasan RS, Kannel WB, Ho KK. The progression from hypertension to congestive heart failure. *JAMA* 1996; 275:1557–1562.

81. Nielsen I. The natural history of hypertensive heart disease as suggested by echocardiography. *Acta Med Scand Suppl* 1986; 714:165–169.

82. Moreno PR, Jang IK, Block PC, Palacios IF. The role of percutaneous balloon valvuloplasty in patients with cardiogenic shock. *J Am Coll Cardiol* 1994; 23:1071–1075.

83. Packer M, O'Conner CM, Ghali JK, Pressler ML, Carson PE, Belkin RN, et al. Effect of amlodipine on morbidity and mortality in severe chronic heart failure. *N Engl J Med* 1996; 335:1107–1114.

84. Scognamiglio R, Rahimtoola SH, Fasoli G, Nistri S, Dalla Volta S. Nifedipine in asymptomatic patients with severe aortic regurgitation and normal left ventricular function. *N Engl J Med* 1994; 331:689–694.

85. Michels VV, Moll PP, Miller FA, Tajik AJ, Chu JS, Driscoll DJ, et al. The frequency of familial dilated cardiomyopathy in a series of patients with idiopathic dilated cardiomyopathy. *N Engl J Med* 1992; 326:77–82.

86. Gregori D, Rocco C, DiLenarda A, Sinagra G, Miocic S, Camerini F, et al. Estimating the frequency of familial dilated cardiomyopathy and the risk of misclassification errors (abstr). *Circulation* 1996; 94:I270.

87. Krajinovic M, Pinamonti B, Sinagra GF, Vatta M, Severini GM, Milasin J, et al. Linkage of familial idiopathic dilated cardiomyopathy to chromosome 9. *Am J Hum Genet* 1995; 57:846–852.

88. Durand J-B, Bachinski LL, Bieling LC, Czernuszewicz GJ, Abchee AB, Yu QT, et al. Localization of a gene responsible for familial dilated cardiomyopathy to chromosome 1q32. *Circulation* 1995; 92:3387–3389.

89. Towbin JA, Hejtmancik JF, Brink P, Gelb BD, Zhu XM, Chamberlain JS, et al. X-linked cardiomyopathy. Molecular genetic evidence of linkage to the Duchenne muscular dystrophy (dystrophin) gene at the Xp21 locus. *Circulation* 1993; 87:1854–1865.

90. Muntoni F, Wilson L, Marrosu G, Marrosu MG, Cianchetti C, Mestrone L, et al. A mutation in the dystrophin gene selectively affecting dystrophin expression in the heart. *J Clin Invest* 1995; 96:693–698.

91. Melacini P, Fanin M, Danieli GA, Villanova C, Martinello F, Miorin M, et al. Myocardial involvement is very frequent among patients affected with subclinical Becker's muscular dystrophy. *Circulation* 1996; 94:3168–3175.

92. Bies RD, Holder E, Maeda M. X-linked cardiomyopathy: Selective deficiency of dystrophin MRNA and protein in the heart. *J Am Coll Cardiol* 1995; 25:277A.

93. Maeda M, Nakao S, Miyazato H, Setoguchi M, Arima S, Higuchi I, et al. Cardiac dystrophin abnormalities in Becker muscular dystrophy assessed by endomyocardial biopsy. *Am Heart J* 1995; 129:702–707.

94. Silver MA. Anatomy of the failing heart in dilated cardiomyopathy. In: Engelmeier RS, O'Connell JB, eds. *Drug Therapy in Dilated Cardiomyopathy and Myocarditis.* New York: Marcel Dekker; 1988:1–12.

95. Roberts WC, Siegel RJ, McManus BM. Idiopathic dilated cardiomyopathy: Analysis of 152 necropsy patients. *Am J Cardiol* 1987; 60:1340–1355.

96. Rowan R, Maesk MA, Billingham ME. Ultrasound morphometric analysis of endomyocardial biopsies. *Am J Cardiovasc Pathol* 1988; 2:137–144.

97. Baandrup U, Olsen EG. Critical analysis of endomyocardial biopsies from patients suspected of having cardiomyopathy. *Br Heart J* 1981; 45:475–486.

98. Arbustini E, Pucci R, Pozzi R, Grasso M, Graziano G, Campani C. Ultrastructural changes in myocarditis and dilated cardiomyopathy. In: Baroldi G, Camerini F, Goodwin JF, eds. *Advances in Cardiomyopathies.* Berlin: Springer-Verlag; 1990:274–289.

99. Schwarz F, Mall G, Zebe H, Schmitzer E, Manthey J, Scheurlen H, et al. Determinants of survival in patients with congestive cardiomyopathy: Quantitative morphologic findings and left ventricular hemodynamics. *Circulation* 1984; 70:923–928.

100. Tazelaar HD, Billingham ME. Leukocytic infiltrates in idiopathic dilated cardiomyopathy. *Am J Surg Pathol* 1986; 10:405–412.

101. Hammond EH, Anderson JL, Menlove RL. Diagnostic and prognostic value of immunofluorescence and electron-microscopic findings in idiopathic dilated cardiomyopathy. In: Bavoldi G, Camerini F, Goodwin JF, eds. *Advances in Cardiomyopathies.* Berlin: Springer-Verlag; 1990:290–301.

102. Kawai C, Takatsu T. Clinical and experimental studies on cardiomyopathy. *N Engl J Med* 1975; 293:592–597.

103. Anderson JL, Carlquist JF, Hammond EH. Deficient natural killer cell activity in patients with idiopathic dilated cardiomyopathy. *Lancet* 1982; 2:1124–1127.

104. Fowles RE, Bieker CP, Stinson EB. Defective in vitro suppressor cell function in idiopathic congestive cardiomyopathy. *Circulation* 1979; 59:483–491.

105. Gerli R, Rambotti P, Spinozzi F, Bertotto A, Chiodini V, Solinas P, et al. Immunologic studies of peripheral blood from patients with idiopathic dilated cardiomyopathy. *Am Heart J* 1986; 112:350–355.

106. Klein R, Maisch B, Kochsiek K, Berg PA. Demonstration of organ specific antibodies against heart mitochondria (anti-M) in sera from patients with some forms of heart disease. *Clin Exp Immunol* 1984; 58:283–292.

107. Maisch B, Deeg P, Liebau G, Kichsiek K. Diagnostic relevance of humoral and cytotoxic immune reactions in primary and secondary dilated cardiomyopathy. *Am J Cardiol* 1983; 52:1071–1078.

108. Limas CJ, Goldenberg IF, Limas C. Autoantibodies against β-adreno-receptors in human idiopathic dilated cardiomyopathy. *Circ Res* 1989; 64:97–103.

109. Magnusson Y, Marullo S, Hoyer S, Waagstein F, Andersson B, Vahlne A, et al. Mapping of a functional autoimmune epitope on the β_1-adrenergic receptor in patients with idiopathic dilated cardiomyopathy. *J Clin Invest* 1990; 86:1658–1663.

110. Magnusson Y, Wallukat G, Waagstein F, Hjalmarson A, Hoebeke J. Autoimmunity in idiopathic dilatated cardiomyopathy. Characterization of antibodies against the β_1-adrenoceptor with a positive chronotropic effect. *Circulation* 1994; 89:2760–2767.

111. Schultheiss H-P. Disturbance of the myocardial energy metabolism in dilated cardiomyopathy due to autoimmunological mechanisms. *Circulation* 1993; 87(suppl IV):IV43–IV48.

112. Schultheiss H-P, Bolte HD. Immunological analysis of autoantibodies against the adenine nucleotide translocator in dilated cardiomyopathy. *J Mol Cell Cardiol* 1985; 17:603–617.

113. Anderson JL, Carlquist JF, Lutz JR, DeWitt CW, Hammond EH. HLA A, B, and DR typing in idiopathic dilated cardiomyopathy: A search for immune response function. *Am J Cardiol* 1984; 33:1326–1330.

114. Gilbert EM, Mason JW. Immunosuppressive therapy of myocarditis. In: Engelmeier RS, O'Connell JB, eds. *Drug Therapy in Dilated Cardiomyopathy and Myocarditis.* New York: Marcel Dekker; 1987:233–263.

115. Archard LC, Freeke CA, Richardson PJ, Olsen EGJ. Persistence of enterovirus RNA in dilated cardiomyopathy: A progression from myocarditis. In: Shultheiss H-P, ed. *New Concepts in Viral Heart Disease.* Berlin: Springer-Verlag; 1989:347–359.

116. Giacca M, Severini GM, Mestroni L, Salvi A, Lardieri G, Falaschi A, et al. Low frequency of detection by nested polymerase chain reaction of enterovirus ribonucleic acid in endomyocardial tissue of patients with idiopathic dilated cardiomyopathy. *J Am Coll Cardiol* 1994; 24:1033–1040.

117. Bowles NE, Richardson PJ, Olsen ECJ, Archard LC. Detection of coxsackie-B virus specific RNA sequences in myocardial biopsy samples from patients with myocarditis and dilated cardiomyopathy. *Lancet* 1986; 1:1120–1128.

118. Parrillo JE, Cunnion RE, Epstein SE, Parker MF, Suffredini AF, Brenner M, et al. A prospective, randomized, controlled trial of prednisone for dilated cardiomyopathy. *N Engl J Med* 1989; 321:1061–1067.

119. Feldman AM, Ray PE, Silan CM, Mercer JA, Minobe WA, Bristow MR. Selective gene expression in failing human heart. Quantification of steady-state levels of messenger RNA in endomyocardial biopsies using the polymerase chain reaction. *Circulation* 1991; 83:1866–1872.

120. Fuster V, Gersh BJ, Giuliani ER, Tajik AJ, Brandenburg RO, Frye RL. The natural history of idiopathic dilated cardiomyopathy. *Am J Cardiol* 1981; 47:525–531.

121. Redfield MM, Gersh BJ, Bailey KR, Ballard DJ, Rodeheffer RJ. Natural history of idiopathic dilated cardiomyopathy: Effect of referral bias and secular trend. *J Am Coll Cardiol* 1993; 22:1921–1926.

122. The SOLVD Investigators. Effect of angiotensin converting enzyme inhibition with enalapril on survival in patients with reduced left ventricular ejection fraction and congestive heart failure: Results of the Treatment Trial of the Studies of Left Ventricular Dysfunction (SOLVD): A randomized double-blind trial. *N Engl J Med* 1991; 325:293–302.

123. Hosenpud JD, Novick RJ, Bennett LE, Keck BM, Fiol B, Daily OP. The registry of the international society for heart and lung transplantation: Thirteenth official report—1996. *J Heart Lung Transplant* 1996; 15:655–674.

124. CIBIS Investigators. A randomized trial of beta-blockade in heart failure: The cardiac insufficiency bisoprolol study (CIBIS). *Circulation* 1994; 90:1765–1773.

125. Woodley SL, Gilbert EM, Anderson JL, O'Connell JB, Deitchman D, Yanowitz FG, et al. β-Blockade with bucindolol in heart failure due to ischemic vs idiopathic dilated cardiomyopathy. *Circulation* 1991; 84:2426–2441.

126. Bristow MR, Colucci WS, Fowler MB, Gilbert EM, Lukas MA, Young ST, et al. Effect of carvedilol on survival and hospitalization in patients with ischemic or nonischemic cardiomyopathy (abstr). *Circulation* 1996; 94:I338.

127. Bristow MR, Mason JW, Billingham ME, Daniels JR. Doxorubicin cardiomyopathy: Evaluation by phonocardiography, endomyocardial biopsy, and cardiac catheterization. *Ann Intern Med* 1978; 88:168–175.

128. Von Hoff DD, Layard MW, Basa P, Davis HL, Von Hoff AL, Rozencweig M, et al. Risk factors for doxorubicin-induced congestive heart failure. *Ann Intern Med* 1979; 91:710–717.

129. Bristow MR, Mason JW, Billingham ME, Daniels JR. Dose-effect and structure function relationships in doxorubicin cardiomyopathy. *Am Heart J* 1981; 102:709–718.

130. Bristow MR, Billingham ME, Mason JW, Daniels JR. The clinical spectrum of anthracycline antibiotic cardiotoxicity. *Cancer Treat Rep* 1978; 62:873–879.

131. Billingham ME, Bristow MR, Glatstein J, Mason JW, Masek MA, Daniels JR. Adriamycin cardiotoxicity: Endomyocardial biopsy evidence of enhancement by irradiation. *Am J Surg Pathol* 1977; 1:17–23.

132. Kantrowitz NE, Bristow MR. Cardiotoxicity of antitumor agents. *Prog Cardiovasc Dis* 1984; 27:195–200.

133. Lewis W, Kleinerman J, Puszkin S. Interaction of Adriamycin in vitro with myofibrillar proteins. *Circ Res* 1982; 50:547–553.

134. Jaenke RS. Delayed and progressive myocardial lesions after Adriamycin administration in rabbits. *Cancer Res* 1976 36:2958–2966.

135. Eiswirth CC, Bowden RE, Kazamias T, Fowler M, Bristow MR. Treatment of Adriamycin cardiomyopathy with metoprolol. *Circulation* 1986; 74(suppl II):1236.

136. Shaddy RE, Olsen SL, Bristow MR, Taylor DO, Bullock EA, Tani LY, et al. Efficacy and safety of metoprolol in the treatment of doxorubicin-induced cardiomyopathy in pediatric patients. *Am Heart J* 1995; 129:197–199.

137. Bristow MR, Lopez MB, Mason JW, Billingham ME, Winchester MA. Efficacy and cost of cardiac monitoring in patients receiving doxorubicin. *Cancer* 1982; 50(1):32–41.

138. McKillop JH, Bristow MR, Goris ML, Billingham ME, Bockemuehl K. Sensitivity and specificity of radionuclide ejection fractions in doxorubicin cardiotoxicity. *Am Heart J* 1983; 105:1048–1056.

139. Alexander J, Dainiak N, Berger HJ, Goldman L, Johnstone D, Reduto L, et al. Serial assessment of doxorubicin cardiotoxicity with quantitative radionuclide angiocardiography. *N Engl J Med* 1979; 300:278–283.

140. Torti FM, Bristow MR, Howes AE, Ashton D, Stockdale FE, Kohler M, et al. Endomyocardial biopsy evidence of reduced cardiotoxicity of doxorubicin delivered on a weekly schedule. *Ann Intern Med* 1983; 99:745–749.

141. Legha SS, Benjamin RS, Mackay B, Ewer M, Wallace S, Valdivieso M, et al. Reduction of doxorubicin cardiotoxicity by prolonged continuous intravenous infusion. *Ann Intern Med* 1982; 96:133–139.

142. Rahman A, More N, Schein PS. Doxorubicin-induced chronic cardiotoxicity and its prevention by liposomal administration. *Cancer Res* 1982; 42:1817–1825.

143. Speyer JL, Green MD, Kramer E, Rey M, Sanger J, Ward C, et al. Protective effect of the bispiperazinedione ICRF-187 against doxorubicin-induced cardiac toxicity in women with advanced breast cancer. *N Engl J Med* 1988; 319(12):745–752.

144. Julian DG, Szekely P. Peripartum cardiomyopathy. *Prog Cardiovasc Dis* 1985; 27:223–240.

145. Midei MG, DeMent SH, Feldman AM, Hutchins GM, Baughman KL. Peripartum myocarditis and cardiomyopathy. *Circulation* 1990; 81:922–928.

146. O'Connell JB, Costanzo-Nordin MR, Subramanian R, Robinson JA, Wallis DE, Scanlon PJ, et al. Peripartum cardiomyopathy: Clinical, hemodynamic, histologic and prognostic characteristics. *J Am Coll Cardiol* 1986; 8:52–56.

147. Jacobson DR, Busbaum JN. Genetic aspects of amyloidosis. *Adv Hum Genet* 1991; 20:69–75.

148. Kyle RA, Griepp PR. Amyloidosis (AL): Clinical and laboratory features in 229 cases. *Mayo Clin Proc* 1983; 58:665–672.

149. Glenner GG. Amyloid deposits and amyloidosis. *N Engl J Med* 1980; 302:1283–1292.

150. Hamer JP, Janssen S, van Rijswik MH, Lie KI. Amyloid cardiomyopathy in systemic nonhereditary amyloidosis. Clinical, echocardiographic and electrocardiographic findings in 30 patients with AA and 24 patients with AL amyloidosis. *Eur Heart J* 1992; 13:623–627.

151. Stone MJ. Amyloidosis: A final common pathway for protein deposition in tissues. *Blood* 1990; 75:531–545.

152. Schroeder JS, Billingham ME, Rider AK. Cardiac amyloidosis: Diagnosis by transvenous endomyocardial biopsy. *Am J Med* 1975; 59:269–273.

153. Holmgren G, Ericzon B-G, Groth C-G. Clinical improvement and amyloid regression after liver transplantation in hereditary transthyretin amyloidosis. *Lancet* 1993; 341:1113–1116.

154. Prazak P, Pfisterer M, Osswald S, Buser P, Burkart F. Differences of disease progression in congestive heart failure due to alcoholic as compared to idiopathic dilated cardiomyopathy. *Eur Heart J* 1996; 17(2):251–257.

155. World Health Organization Expert Committee. Chagas' disease. *World Health Organ Tech Rep Ser* 1984; 697:50–55.

156. Tibbetts RS, McCormick TS, Rowland EC, Miller SD, Engman DM. Cardiac antigen-specific autoantibody production is associated with cardiomyopathy in *Trypanosoma cruzi*–infected mice. *J Immunol* 1994; 152(3):1493–1499.

157. Mady C, Cardoso RHA, Barretto ACP, da Luz PL, Bellotti G, Pileggi F. Survival and predictors of survival in patients with congestive heart failure due to Chagas' cardiomyopathy. *Circulation* 1994; 90:3098–3102.

158. Rosenbaum MB. The hemiblocks: Diagnostic criteria and clinical significance. *Mod Concepts Cardiovasc Dis* 1970; 39:141–146.

159. Laranja FS, Dias E, Nobrega G, Miranda A. Chagas' disease: A clinical, epidemiological, and pathological study. *Circulation* 1956; 14:1035–1060.

160. Nul DR, Grancelli HO, Perrone SV, Bortman GR, Curiel R. Randomised trial of low-dose amiodarone in severe congestive heart failure. *Lancet* 1994; 344:493–498.

161. Bocchi EA, Bellotti G, Mocelin AO, Uip D, Bacal F, Higuchi ML, et al. Heart transplantation for chronic chagas' heart disease. *Ann Thorac Surg* 1996; 61:1727–1733.

162. Blanche C, Aleksic I, Takkenberg JJM, Czer C, Fishbein MC, Trento A. Heart transplantation for Chagas' cardiomyopathy. *Ann Thorac Surg* 1995; 60:1406–1409.

74

HYPERTROPHIC CARDIOMYOPATHY

Barry J. Maron

Hypertrophic cardiomyopathy (HCM) is a genetically transmitted primary cardiac disease that has been of great interest to clinicians and laboratory scientists because of its particularly diverse clinical, morphologic, pathophysiologic, and molecular genetic manifestations.[1–21] Because of the broad and complex spectrum of HCM disease, as well as its relatively low prevalence in cardiologic practice, a measure of confusion and uncertainty has persisted regarding this condition.

HISTORICAL CONSIDERATIONS

There is some uncertainty regarding the first gross anatomic description of HCM. About 1900, French and German authors reported four patients at autopsy in whom striking hypertrophy involving the ventricular septum appeared to be responsible for obstruction to left ventricular ejection.[22,23] The first unequivocal description of HCM was the detailed pathologic report of Teare,[24] which stimulated widespread interest in this disease among cardiologists, pathologists, and surgeons. Teare described a condition in eight patients (seven of whom died suddenly) characterized by an asymmetric pattern of left ventricular wall thickening and nondilated ventricular cavities. The striking ventricular septal hypertrophy and bizarre arrangement of muscle bundles observed in these patients was thought to represent a benign tumor.

NOMENCLATURE AND PREVALENCE

Over the past 40 years, numerous studies have led to a dramatic evolution of our concepts concerning the clinical and pathologic spectrum of HCM; in the process, the disease has acquired a myriad of names[6] (Fig. 74-1). This multiplicity of descriptive terms largely reflects the enormous clinical, functional, and morphologic diversity of this disease. However, many of the terms that have been used to describe HCM are somewhat misleading in emphasizing the presence of left ventricular outflow obstruction, a clinical feature that occurs in only a minority of patients with HCM.[2]

The prevalence of HCM appears to be about 0.2 percent in the general population[25] and 0.5 percent in primary medical practice[26] based on identification of the disease phenotype with two-dimensional (2D) echocardiography. It is possible, however, that many individuals with HCM go undetected in the community because they manifest no or only mild symptoms and are not referred for echocardiographic studies.[27,28] Reports from a large number of diverse geographic areas suggest that HCM has extensive if not worldwide occurrence; there is also some evidence that the morphologic expression of the disease may differ in certain ethnic or racial groups (such as the Japanese).[29–31]

DEFINITION AND CRITERIA FOR DIAGNOSIS

The clinical diagnosis of HCM is based on definition of the most characteristic morphologic feature of the disease—i.e., thickening of the left ventricular wall associated with a nondilated cavity in the absence of another cardiac or systemic disease capable of producing the magnitude of hypertrophy present (e.g., hypertension or aortic stenosis)[6] (Fig. 74-2). Because the nonobstructive form of HCM is predominant, the well-described clinical features of dynamic obstruction to left ventricular outflow—such as systolic anterior motion of the mitral valve, partial premature closure of the aortic valve, and a loud systolic ejection murmur—are not required for diagnosis. Also, not all individuals harboring a genetic abnormality capable of producing the clinical and morphologic abnormalities of HCM show left ventricular hypertrophy at all phases of life.[9,32] Some children with HCM will not have left ventricular wall thickening identifiable by 2D echocardiogram prior to about age 16,[33] and a few adults with incomplete penetrance may also show little or no hypertrophy.[9,34]

Asymmetrical hypertrophic cardiomyopathy
Asymmetrical hypertrophy of the heart
Asymmetrical septal hypertrophy
Brock's disease
Diffuse muscular subaortic stenosis
Diffuse subvalvular aortic stenosis
Dynamic hypertrophic subaortic stenosis
Dynamic muscular subaortic stenosis
Familial hypertrophic cardiomyopathy
Familial hypertrophic subaortic stenosis
Familial muscular subaortic stenosis
Familial myocardial disease
Functional aortic stenosis
Functional hypertrophic subaortic stenosis
Functional obstructive cardiomyopathy
Functional obstruction of the left ventricle
Functional obstructive subvalvular aortic stenosis
Functional subaortic stenosis
Hereditary cardiovascular dysplasia
HYPERTROPHIC CARDIOMYOPATHY
Hypertrophic constrictive cardiomyopathy
Hypertrophic hyperkinetic cardiomyopathy
Hypertrophic infundibular aortic stenosis
Hypertrophic nonobstructive cardiomyopathy
Hypertrophic obstructive cardiomyopathy
Hypertrophic stenosing cardiomyopathy
Hypertrophic subaortic stenosis
Idiopathic hypertrophic cardiomyopathy
Idiopathic hypertrophic obstructive cardiomyopathy
Idiopathic hypertrophic subaortic stenosis

Idiopathic hypertrophic subvalvular stenosis
Idiopathic muscular hypertrophic subaortic stenosis
Idiopathic muscular stenosis of the left ventricle
Idiopathic myocardial hypertrophy
Idiopathic stenosis of the flushing chamber of the left ventricle
Idiopathic ventricular septal hypertrophy
Irregular hypertrophic cardiomyopathy
Left ventrical muscular stenosis
Low subvalvular aortic stenosis
Muscular aortic stenosis
Muscular hypertrophic stenosis of the left ventricle
Muscular stenosis of the left ventricle
Muscular subaortic stenosis
Muscular subvalvular aortic stenosis
Non-dilated cardiomyopathy
Nonobstructive hypertrophic cardiomyopathy
Obstructive cardiomyopathy
Obstructive hypertrophic aortic stenosis
Obstructive hypertrophic cardiomyopathy
Obstructive hypertrophic myocardiopathy
Obstructive myocardiopathy
Pseudoaortic stenosis
Stenosing hypertrophy of the left ventricle
Stenosis of the ejection chamber of the left ventricle
Subaortic hypertrophic stenosis
Subaortic idiopathic stenosis
Subaortic muscular stenosis
Subvalvular aortic stenosis of the muscular type
Teare's disease

FIGURE 74-1
Terms used to describe HCM.

MORPHOLOGIC CHARACTERISTICS

Gross Features

Left ventricular hypertrophy is the gross anatomic marker and likely determinant of many of the clinical features of HCM in most patients with this disease[2-4,6] (Figs. 74-3 and 74-4). Since the left ventricular cavity is usually small or normal in size, the increased left ventricular mass is due almost entirely to an increase in wall thickness. Although a symmetric (concentric) pattern of left ventricular hypertrophy can be observed,[11,17,35] the distribution of hypertrophy is almost always asymmetric; i.e., all segments of the left ventricular wall are not thickened to a similar degree, with the ventricular septum showing the greatest magnitude of hypertrophy.[11,17,36] Gross examination of the heart at necropsy in patients with HCM also typically shows enlargement of the atria, enlargement and elongation of the mitral valve leaflets, and areas of fibrosis in the left ventricular wall.[16,20] In addition, most hearts show a characteristic fibrous plaque on the mural endocardium of the left ventricle in apposition to the thickened anterior mitral leaflet, presumably resulting from contact between mitral valve and septum[16] (Fig. 74-3).

Based on both echocardiographic and necropsy analyses in large numbers of patients, it is apparent that the HCM disease spectrum is characterized by vast structural diversity with regard to the patterns and extent of left ventricular hypertrophy[11,17,35] (Figs. 74-5 and 74-6). Indeed, no single phenotypic expression can be considered "classic" or typical of this disease. Thickness of the left ventricular wall varies greatly, although the average reported value is usually 21 to 22 mm. Wall thickness is markedly increased in many patients, with some showing the most severe hypertrophy observed in any cardiac disease[36,37]; 60 mm is the most extreme dimension reported to date.[37] On the other hand, the HCM phenotype is not invariably expressed as a particularly thickened left ventricle; some show only a mild increase of ≤15 mm, including a very few genotypically affected individuals with normal thicknesses (≤12 mm).[9,34] Often the pattern of wall thickening is strikingly heterogeneous, involving noncontiguous segments of left ventricle (i.e., with areas of normal thickness evident in between), or showing marked differences in wall thickness in adjacent

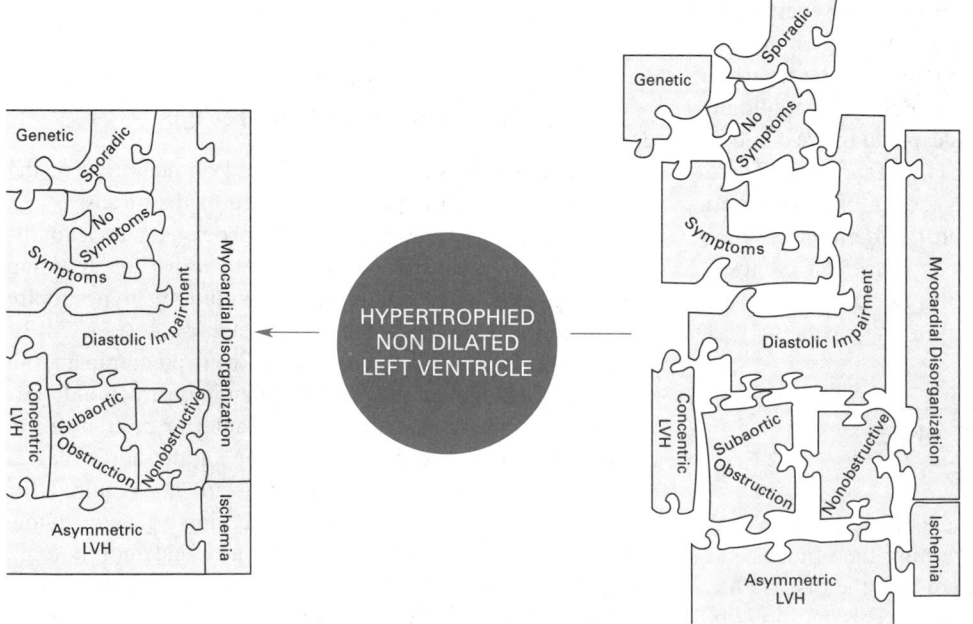

FIGURE 74-2
Diagrammatic representation of the basic morphologic definition of HCM (*dark circle*), as it unifies the clinical and morphologic diversity characteristic of the disease spectrum.

segments. Transitions between thickened areas and regions of normal thickness are often sharp and abrupt, not infrequently creating right-angled contours of the wall. The variable morphologic expression of HCM is underlined by the fact that even first-degree relatives with the disease usually show great dissimilarity in the pattern of left ventricular wall thickening.[10]

In most patients the pattern of hypertrophy is diffuse, involving both septum and substantial portions of the lateral free wall, while the posterior segment of free wall is usually least affected by the hypertrophic process.[11,17] In others, hypertrophy involves only the ventricular septum while sparing the free wall. In an important proportion of patients (about one-third), wall thickening may be relatively mild and localized to a single segment of left ventricle. Such segmental hypertrophy is usually confined to the anterior septum but may also involve only posterior septum, anterolateral free wall, posterior free wall, or even the most apical portion of the left ventricle. Therefore, the ventricular septum is usually but not always prominently involved in the hypertrophic process. Hypertrophy confined to the left ventricular apex ("apical HCM") has been reported most commonly by Japanese investigators,[29,30] who have described the condition of this subgroup of HCM patients to be clinically benign and with a "spade" deformity of the left ventricular cavity on angiography and a distinctive ECG pattern of deep ("giant") T-wave inversion.

In some young athletes, segmental hypertrophy of the anterior ventricular septum (wall thicknesses of 13 to 15 mm), consistent with a relatively mild morphologic expression of HCM, may often be difficult to distinguish from the physiologic left ventricular hypertrophy that may be an adaptation to intense forms of athletic training.[38] In asymptomatic individuals within this morphologic "gray zone," the differential diagnosis between athlete's heart and HCM can often be resolved by clinical assessment and noninvasive testing (Fig. 74-7).

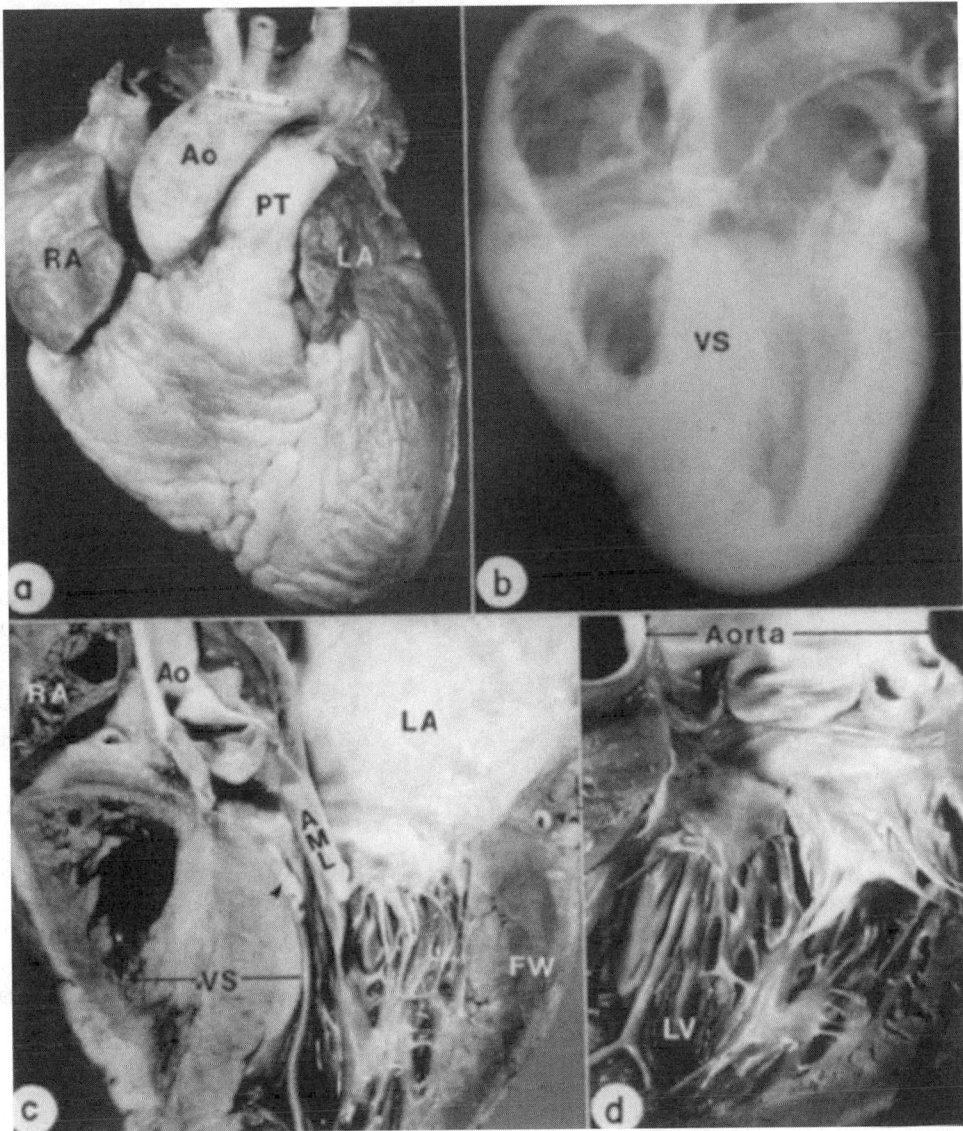

FIGURE 74-3

Anatomic features of HCM are demonstrated on the heart of a 26-year-old man. *A*. Exterior view; both right atrium (RA) and left atrium (LA) are dilated. Ao = aorta; PT = pulmonary trunk. *B*. Radiography of specimen showing asymmetric thickening of ventricular septum (VS). *C*. Coronal section; the septum is clearly thicker than left ventricular free wall (F); an endocardial mural contact plaque (*arrowhead*) is present in the left ventricular outflow tract in apposition to the anterior mitral leaflet (AML). *D*. Closer view of plaque and thickened anterior leaflet. (From Roberts WC, Ferrans VJ. Pathologic anatomy of the cardiomyopathies. Idiopathic dilated and hypertrophic types, infiltrative types, and endomyocardial disease with and without eosinophilia. *Hum Pathol* 1975; 6:287–342. Reproduced with permission from the authors and the publisher.)

HCM can represent a congenital heart malformation in which phenotypic expression in the form of left ventricular wall thickening begins during fetal development and is evident at or shortly after birth. Indeed, HCM has been reported in a small number of very young children, including a few infants under 6 months of age.[2,39,40] When HCM presents in infancy, the disease is usually associated with marked septal hypertrophy as well as severe progressive congestive heart failure and biventricular outflow obstruction.

Later in childhood, serial echocardiographic investigations have shown left ventricular hypertrophy in HCM to have a

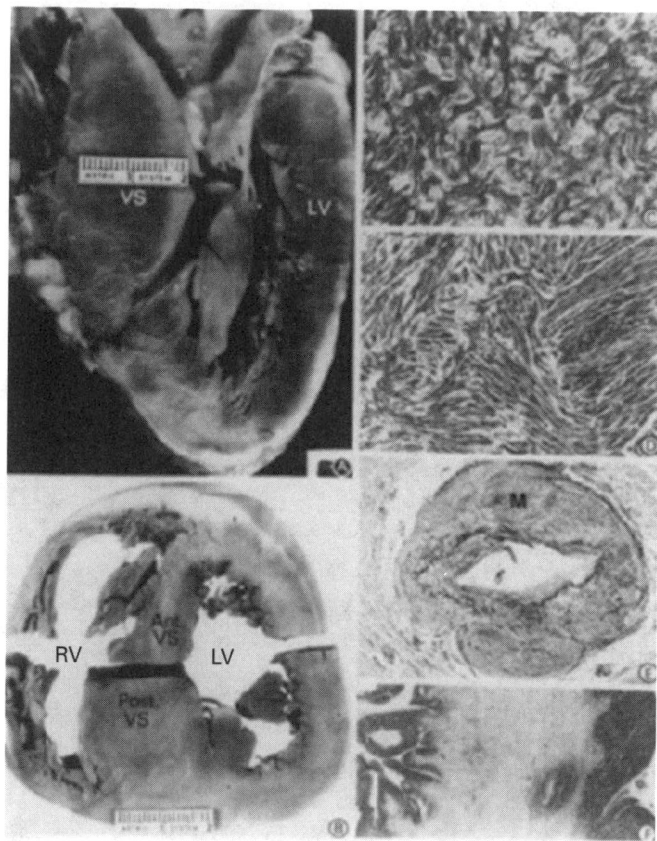

FIGURE 74-4

Morphologic components of the underlying disease process in HCM. *A.* Gross heart specimen sectioned in a cross-sectional plane similar to that of the echocardiographic (parasternal) long axis. The pattern of left ventricular hypertrophy is asymmetric, with wall thickening confined primarily to the anterior ventricular septum (VS), which bulges into the left ventricular outflow tract. *B.* Heart specimen illustrating a different pattern of hypertrophy, in which marked left ventricular wall thickening is localized to the posterior portion of the ventricular septum (Post. VS), while the anterior septum (Ant. VS) is only mildly thickened. *C.* and *D.* Histology characteristic of the left ventricle in HCM. In *C,* septal myocardium shows markedly disordered architecture, with adjacent hypertrophied cardiac muscle cells arranged at perpendicular and oblique angles to each other. In *D,* bundles of hypertrophied cells show a disorganized, "interwoven" arrangement. *E.* Intramural coronary artery with apparently narrowed lumen and thickened wall due primarily to medial (M) hypertrophy. *F.* Extensive scarring of ventricular septum, which is transmural in distribution. LV = left ventricular free wall. (From Maron et al.,[2] with permission from the authors and publisher.)

dynamic nature. Morphologic expression of HCM is not usually complete until adulthood,[33] and children often show striking spontaneous increases in wall thicknesses (i.e., of about 100 percent) and more extensive distribution of hypertrophy with increasing age, including de novo development of wall thickening during adolescence, when body growth and maturation are accelerated (Fig. 74-8). In some young children, abnormalities on the 12-lead ECG may be the initial clinical manifestation of HCM, preceding the appearance of hypertrophy on the echocardiogram.[32,40] Such remodeling of left ventricular structure is not consistently associated with develop-

ment or progression of symptoms or sudden death and appears to be an expression of the predetermined morphologic evolution of the disease; once full growth and maturation are achieved (at about age 18), further progression of left ventricular hypertrophy does not usually occur.[41] Progression of basal septal hypertrophy associated with a developmentally small left ventricular outflow tract appear to be the major determinants for development of mitral valve systolic anterior motion and outflow obstruction during childhood.[42]

In adult symptomatic patients with HCM, the magnitude of left ventricular hypertrophy appears to *decrease* with aging[43]; very marked degrees of hypertrophy (e.g., wall thickness >30 mm) appear to be largely limited to patients under age 40, while older patients over age 60 generally have more modest degrees of hypertrophy and rarely show wall thickness >25 mm. The explanation for this inverse relation between age and magnitude of hypertrophy could be a higher rate of premature death in younger patients with more severe morphologic forms or, alternatively, to a gradual process of wall thinning and remodeling occurring in many patients.[44]

Histologic Features

Several histologic features of the left ventricular myocardium represent components of the primary cardiomyopathic disease process in HCM[45–55]: (1) disarray of cardiac muscle cells, (2) replacement fibrosis, and (3) abnormal small intramural coronary arteries (Fig. 74-4). Marked distortion of cellular architecture, described prominently by Teare in his initial report of HCM,[24] is a characteristic feature of the left ventricle.[46–50] Many cardiac muscle cells in both the ventricular septum and left ventricular free wall show increased transverse

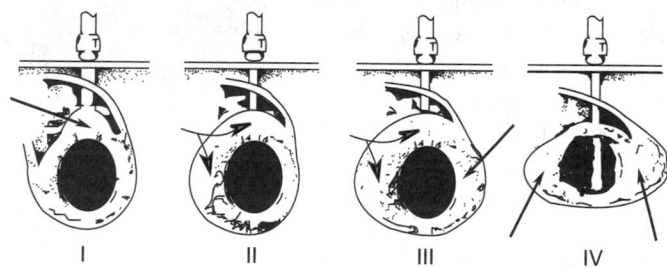

FIGURE 74-5

Morphologic variability in HCM, based on observations made from two-dimensional echocardiography; areas of hypertrophy are indicated by arrows. All images are drawn in the standard short-axis cross-sectional plane at mitral valve level with anterior chest wall and transducer to the top, posterior free wall to the bottom, posterior septum to the left, and anterolateral free wall to the right. *I.* Relatively mild left ventricular hypertrophy confined to anterior portion of ventricular septum. *II.* Hypertrophy of anterior and posterior septum in the absence of free-wall thickening. *III.* Diffuse hypertrophy of substantial portions of both ventricular septum and anterolateral free wall. *IV.* Includes more unusual patterns of hypertrophy in which M-mode echo beam does *not* traverse the thickened portions of left ventricle present in posterior septum or anterolateral free wall (as shown here) or at the left ventricular apex. (From Maron BJ. Asymmetry in hypertrophic cardiomyopathy: The septal free wall ratio revisited. *Am J Cardiol* 1985; 55:835–838, with permission from the author and the American Journal of Cardiology).

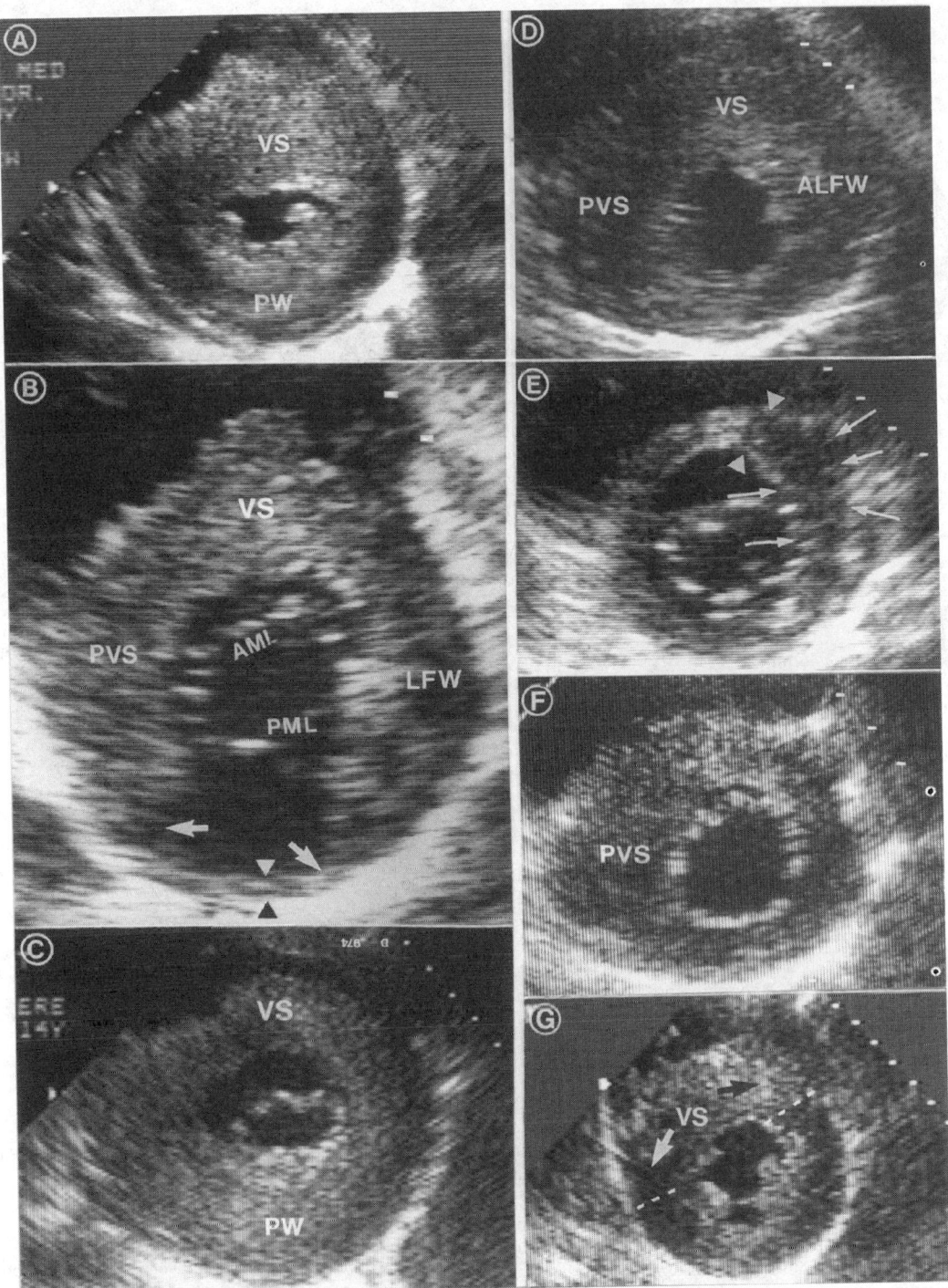

FIGURE 74-6

Variability of patterns of left ventricular hypertrophy in patients with hypertrophic cardiomyopathy, shown in a composite of diastolic stop-frame images in the parasternal short-axis plane. *A, B, D*. Wall thickening is diffuse, involving substantial portions of ventricular septum and free wall. At the papillary muscle level (*A*), all segments of the left ventricular wall are hypertrophied, including the posterior free wall (PW), but the pattern of thickening is asymmetric, with the anterior portion of ventricular septum (VS) massive (i.e., 50 mm). *B*. Hypertrophy is diffuse, involving three segments of the left ventricle but with the posterior wall spared and thin (< 10 mm) (*arrowheads*) and with particularly abrupt changes in wall thickness evident (*arrows*). *C*. Marked hypertrophy in a pattern distinctly different from that in *A, B,* and

D in which the thickening of the posterior wall is predominant, and the ventricular septum is of nearly normal thickness. *D*. Diffuse distribution of hypertrophy involving three segments of the left ventricle similar to that in *B* but without sharp changes in the contour of the wall. *E*. Hypertrophy predominantly of lateral free wall (*arrows*) and only a small portion of contiguous anterior septum (*arrowheads*). *F*. Hypertrophy predominantly of posterior ventricular septum (PVS) and, to a lesser extent, the contiguous portion of the anterior septum. *G*. Thickening of anterior and posterior septum to a similar degree but with sparing of the free wall. Calibration dots are 1 cm apart. AML = anterior mitral leaflet; LVW = lateral free wall; PML = posterior mitral leaflet.

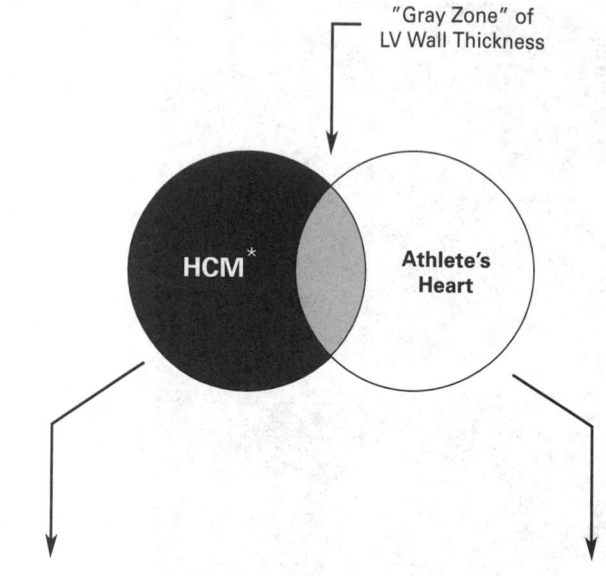

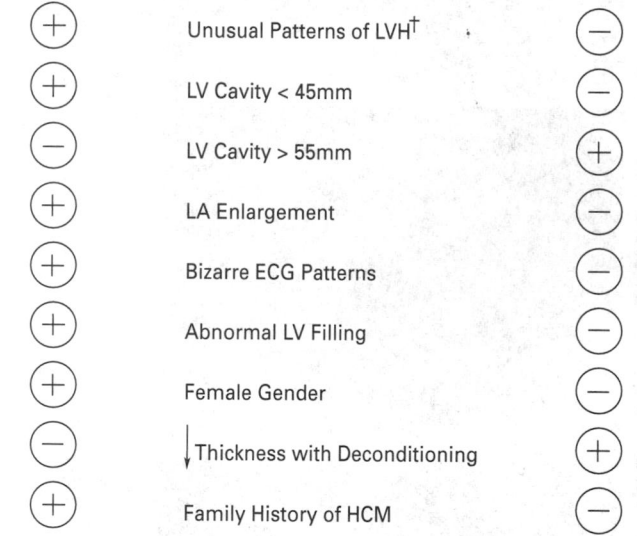

FIGURE 74-7

Criteria used to distinguish HCM from athlete's heart when left ventricular (LV) wall thickness is within the shaded gray zone of overlap, consistent with both diagnoses. *Assumed to be the nonobstructive form, since substantial mitral valve systolic anterior motion would confirm, per se, the diagnosis of HCM in an athlete. †May involve a variety of abnormalities, including heterogeneous distribution of LV hypertrophy in which adjacent regions may be of greatly different thicknesses, with sharp transitions evident between segments; also, asymmetric patterns in which anterior ventricular septum is spared from the hypertrophic process and the region of predominant thickening may be in the posterior septum or anterolateral or posterior free wall. ↓ = decreased; LA = left atrial. (From Maron et al.[38] with permission from the authors and the American Heart Association.)

diameter, have bizarre shapes, maintain intercellular connections with several adjacent cells, and are arranged in a disorganized pattern at oblique and perpendicular angles to each other. This cellular disarray is present in about 95 percent of patients dying of HCM and usually occupies substantial portions of myocardium (about 33 percent of septum and 25 percent of free wall) (see Fig. 74-4C and D). However, there

is virtually no correlation between absolute wall thickness and the amount of disorganized myocardium in HCM.[53]

The clinical relevance of disordered myocardial architecture in HCM remains largely unresolved. Possibly, the disorganized cells dispersed throughout the left ventricular myocardium impair transmission of normal electrophysiologic impulses, predispose toward disordered patterns of electrical depolarization and repolarization, and thereby serve as an arrhythmogenic substrate. Alternatively, it is also possible

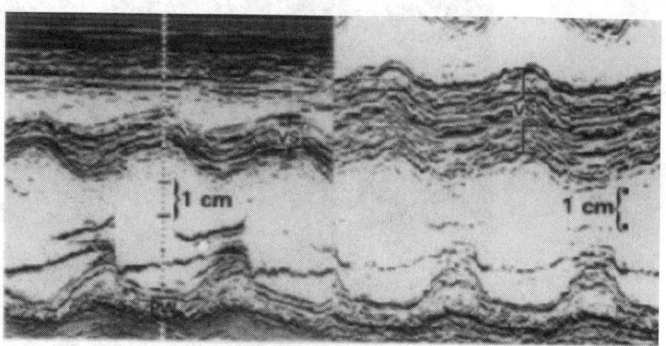

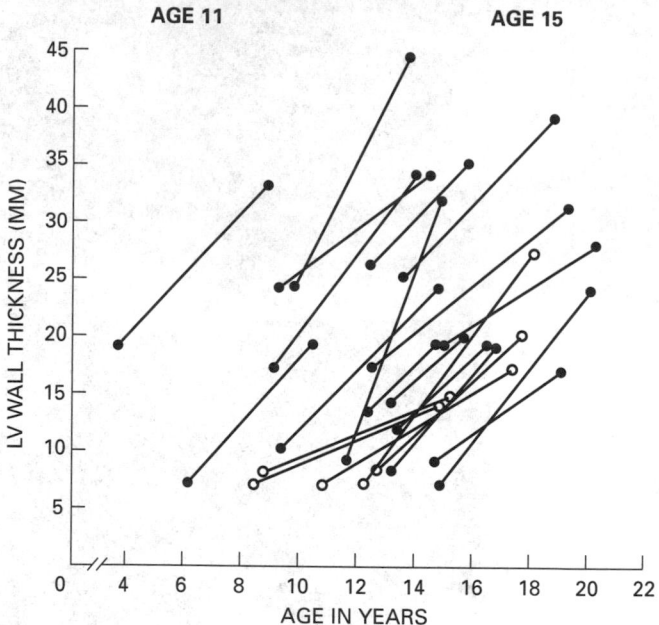

FIGURE 74-8

Development and progression of left ventricular hypertrophy in children with HCM. *Upper panel*: Development of marked hypertrophy of the anterior basal ventricular septum (VS). M-mode echocardiograms shown here were obtained at the same cross-sectional level in a girl with a family history of HCM. At age 11, ventricular septal thickness was at upper limit of normal (10 mm); at age 15, septal thickness had increased markedly (to 33 mm), and appearance of the echocardiogram is typical of HCM. The patient remained asymptomatic throughout this period of time but died suddenly and unexpectedly at age 17. PW = posterior left ventricular free wall. *Lower panel*: Dynamic, striking changes in left ventricular wall thickness with age in 22 children; each patient is represented by the left ventricular segment that showed the greatest change in wall thickness. Open symbols denote 5 patients who had no evidence of hypertrophy in any segment of the left ventricle at the initial evaluation but subsequently developed de novo hypertrophy typical of HCM. (From Maron et al.,[33] with permission from the authors and publisher.)

that this distorted cellular architecture could contribute to diastolic or systolic dysfunction.[2,47,48]

Patients with HCM (but without atherosclerotic coronary artery disease) often exhibit fibrous tissue formation in the left ventricle at necropsy.[45,49,51,54,55] A spectrum of severity and distribution is observed ranging from mild to moderate degrees of interstitial (matrix) and perivascular connective tissue to grossly visible replacement scarring that may be extensive[55] or even transmural[54] (Fig. 74-4F). These areas of fibrosis, which likely result from prior episodes of myocardial ischemia[56,57] or are related in some other way to the underlying cardiomyopathic disease process, are identifiable during life as irreversible thallium-201 myocardial perfusion abnormalities[58] and may well be responsible for the increased ventricular chamber stiffness and impaired relaxation identifiable in most patients with HCM.[2,3,59,60]

Abnormal intramural coronary arteries are present in about 80 percent of patients with HCM studied at necropsy; such abnormalities are most commonly evident in the ventricular sep-

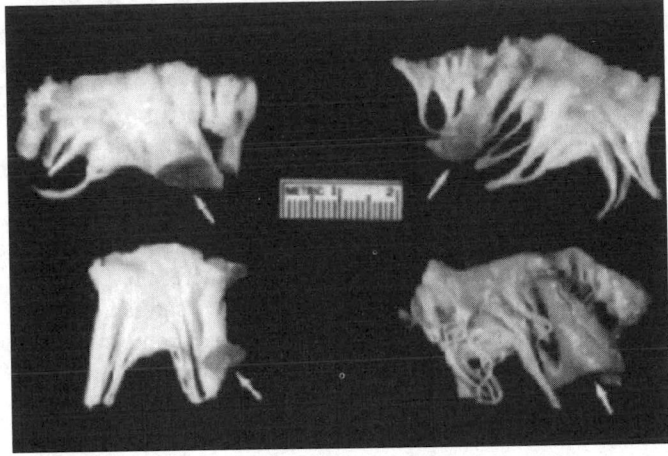

FIGURE 74-10

Mitral valve specimens (with ventricular aspect exposed) excised at operation from four patients with obstructive HCM showing anomalous papillary muscle insertion directly into anterior mitral leaflet (*arrows*). Papillary muscles are of various sizes and insert into the region of either the posteromedial (valve at upper right) or anterolateral commissure (the other three valves). (From Klues et al.,[18] with permission of the authors and the American Heart Association.)

tum.[51,52] The walls of these intramural vessels are thickened (because of increased smooth muscle cells, collagen, elastic fibers, and mucoid deposits in the intima and/or media), and frequently the lumen appears narrowed and compromised (Fig. 74-4E). Increased numbers or clusters of abnormal intramural arteries are often observed within or at the margins of sizable areas of fibrosis.[51,54] This association between abnormal intramural coronary arteries and myocardial scarring suggests that a form of "small-vessel disease" present in patients with HCM may be responsible for myocardial ischemia and necrosis.[51]

Mitral Valve Abnormalities

Morphometric analysis of mitral valves removed at operation or necropsy from patients with outflow obstruction supports the concept that primary structural abnormalities of the mitral valve are also characteristic of many patients with HCM[18,19] (Fig. 74-9). About two-thirds of patients show alterations in mitral valve size and shape, with an increased mitral valve area (up to twice normal) due primarily to leaflet elongation (but without evidence of "floppy" mitral leaflets). These enlarged valves demonstrate considerable structural variability, with both the anterior and posterior leaflets increased in size or asymmetric and segmental enlargement of only one leaflet.

In addition, other HCM patients show a congenital malformation of the mitral apparatus due to an arrest in embryonic development, with anomalous insertion of papillary muscle directly into the anterior mitral leaflet (without the interposition of chordae tendineae)[18] (Fig. 74-10). Greatly enlarged mitral valves and anomalous papillary muscle insertion represent a constellation of structural malformations of the mitral apparatus (in >50 percent of patients studied at necropsy) that expands the morphologic definition of HCM.

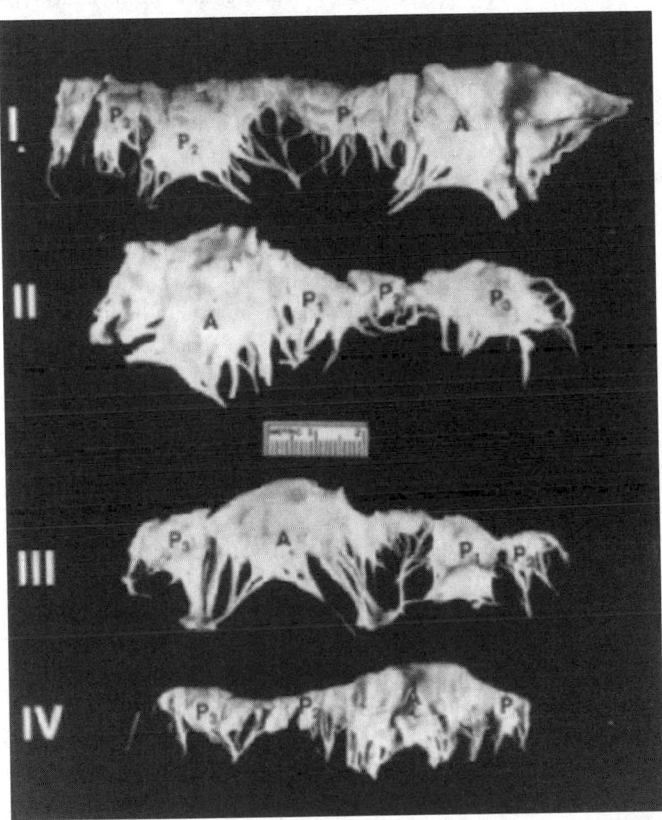

FIGURE 74-9

Mitral valves from three patients with obstructive HCM, aged 31, 29, and 60 years (I, II, and III), and from a normal control patient without cardiovascular disease (IV), showing variation in valvular size and structure present in HCM. Valves are opened with the circumference displayed in a horizontal orientation, exposing the atrial surface, with annular margin to top and chordal attachments to bottom. *I.* Large valve (area 22 cm²) in which both the anterior (A) and posterior (P) leaflets are greatly elongated and increased in area. *II.* Large valve in which increased valve size (area 18 cm²) is due primarily to elongation and enlargement of the anterior leaflet (A). *III.* Segmental elongation and increased area confined to a scallop of posterior leaflet. (From Klues et al.,[19] with permission of the authors and the American Heart Association.)

ETIOLOGY
AND GENETICS

HCM commonly demonstrates genetic transmission with an autosomal pattern of inheritance.[1–4,7–10,34,61] Molecular studies that have defined the genetic alterations responsible for this disease also provide insights into its clinical heterogeneity. HCM can be caused by a mutation in one of four genes that encode proteins of the cardiac sarcomere: the β-myosin heavy-chain gene on chromosome 14,[7,8,62] cardiac troponin T on chromosome 1,[9] α-tropomyosin on chromosome 15,[9] and myosin binding protein C on chromosome 11.[63] This complexity is further compounded by intragenic heterogeneity; more than 75 HCM-causing mutations have now been identified in these genes of the sarcomere.[7,8]

Available data suggest that β-myosin heavy-chain mutations may account for about 30 percent of familial HCM.[7,8] All the known mutations in this gene have proved to be missense mutations that alter a single amino acid residue in the head or head-rod junction of the protein.[7,8,62] Most adult patients with these mutations have overt cardiac hypertrophy and typical clinical features. However, survival in patients with different myosin mutations may vary; some are benign (Val606Met), while others are associated with premature death due to either heart failure or sudden catastrophic events (Arg403Gln).[7,8,62]

Cardiac troponin-T mutations account for an estimated 10 to 20 percent of familial HCM.[9] Several different gene defects have been identified, including missense mutations and small deletions. Despite this diversity, the clinical manifestations of HCM associated with the eight reported cardiac troponin-T mutations are similar. Cardiac hypertrophy is relatively mild (and can be subclinical in some adults), and life expectancy appears to be reduced.

The increasing availability of gene-based diagnosis will lead to the identification of a greater number of children and adults with a preclinical diagnosis of HCM (i.e., who have a gene defect but not phenotypic manifestations of HCM).[9,32,63–65] At present, the clinical implications of such gene abnormalities and appropriate management for these individuals are largely unresolved.

Occurrence of premature sudden cardiac death in a family with HCM should dictate an echocardiographic and clinical genetic evaluation in surviving relatives, since sudden death can be repetitive and clinical expression may be particularly virulent in certain families (e.g., "malignant" HCM).[66,67] Also, because HCM is the leading cause of sudden unexpected death in young competitive athletes,[68] young family members should be screened for HCM prior to participating in competitive athletic training. Because phenotypic expression may not be complete until adulthood,[33] a single screening echocardiogram may not definitively exclude HCM. Therefore, those children with the potential to harbor a genetic defect for HCM (but without left ventricular hypertrophy on echocardiogram) should have periodic echocardiographic examinations until full growth and maturation are achieved.

Although the aforementioned mutations are regarded as disease-causing for HCM, many of the abnormal and primary structural characteristics of this disease do not appear to greatly involve sarcomeric proteins; these features include mitral valve enlargement and elongation, abnormal intramural coronary arteries, and increased matrix collagen. This fact, together with the observation that much of the left ventricular wall is free of hypertrophy or only mildly thickened in many patients with HCM, suggests that phenotypic expression is importantly influenced by other genetic factors (such as modifying genes)[7] or by undefined environmental variables in addition to the causal mutation.

PATHOPHYSIOLOGY

The symptoms of HCM are varied and include those of pulmonary congestion—such as exertional dyspnea, orthopnea, and paroxysmal nocturnal dyspnea—as well as fatigue, chest pain (which may be typical of angina pectoris), palpitations, and impairment of consciousness including dizziness, near-syncope, and syncope.

A number of pathophysiologic components of the HCM disease process dictate the clinical course and outcome that patients experience[2–5,56,57,59,60,69–71]: (1) left ventricular outflow obstruction, (2) diastolic dysfunction, (3) myocardial ischemia, and (4) a variety of arrhythmias. Other such mechanisms may well exist but have not yet been identified. However, consistent with the heterogeneity of HCM, cardiac symptoms do not always show a direct (one-to-one) correlation with a particular pathophysiologic mechanism in the individual patient, and the relative contributions of each component to symptoms appear to vary considerably among patients.

Outflow Obstruction

The dynamic form of obstruction to left ventricular outflow exhibited by patients with HCM (due to systolic anterior motion of the mitral valve and midsystolic contact with the ventricular septum)[2,3,69–73] characteristically shows spontaneous variability.[1] Interventions or circumstances that decrease myocardial contractility (administration of beta-blocking drugs) or increase ventricular volume or arterial pressure (squatting or vasoconstrictor agents) have the effect of reducing or abolishing subaortic obstruction. Interventions or circumstances that increase contractility (exercise or infusion of isoproterenol) or decrease arterial pressure or ventricular volume (Valsalva maneuver or administration of a hypotension-producing agent) will increase or provoke obstruction. Not uncommonly, patients with little or no obstruction to left ventricular outflow under basal conditions are capable of generating substantial "labile" gradients with physiologic or pharmacologic provocations[1–3]; also, such gradients may be evident only after the cessation of exercise.[74]

The increase in systolic intraventricular pressure caused by outflow obstruction may augment myocardial oxygen demand. It is generally conceded that dynamic outflow obstruction in HCM can, in some patients, have long-term detrimental consequences for left ventricular function and be responsible for the genesis of symptoms.[2,3,5,69] The magnitude of the systolic pressure gradient can be estimated noninvasively by the degree of mitral valve systolic anterior motion on M-mode echocardiogram or, more quantitatively, by continuous-wave Doppler interrogation[75] (Chap. 14).

The mechanism by which the subaortic gradient is produced in patients with HCM involves several morphologic and hemodynamic factors[2,3,5,69,71–73,75]: (1) reduced diastolic outflow tract dimension; (2) substantial hypertrophy involving the anterior basal ventricular septum; (3) anterior displacement of mitral valve and papillary muscles within the ventricular cavity; (4) increased size and length of the mitral leaflets; (5) hyperdynamic left ventricular ejection, creating a high-velocity jet that streams through a narrowed outflow, pulling the mitral leaflets toward the septum (i.e., Venturi effect) or creating substantial flow-drag; and (6) primary geometric abnormalities of the papillary muscle–mitral valve apparatus, producing altered distribution of tension to the mitral leaflets. Malposition of the mitral valve and systolic anterior motion almost invariably interfere with normal valve closure, resulting in mitral regurgitation[35]; while mitral incompetence is usually mild in HCM, it may be much more marked when it is associated with primary intrinsic abnormalities of the valve (e.g., floppy mitral valve with prolapse).[76]

Although outflow obstruction is due to mitral systolic anterior motion in most patients with HCM (>95 percent), occasional patients demonstrate a peak systolic outflow gradient that is due to muscular midcavity obstruction (in the absence of systolic anterior motion)[18,77]; such gradients may result from anomalous papillary muscle insertion directly into the anterior mitral leaflet[18] (Fig. 74-10) or from other forms of muscular apposition, which in some instances are associated with segmental apical or generalized ventricular hypokinesia.[78]

In infants and young children with HCM, obstruction to right ventricular outflow is common and usually occurs in association with subaortic obstruction.[39,69,79] Right ventricular outflow obstruction in HCM is probably produced by greatly hypertrophied right ventricular musculature (crista supraventricularis, moderator band, or trabeculae) projecting into the relatively small outflow tract as part of an excessive hypertrophic process.[80]

Diastolic Dysfunction

Echocardiographic, Doppler, contrast, or radionuclide angiographic and hemodynamic studies of left ventricular diastolic function have identified characteristic abnormalities in relaxation and filling that are present in about 80 percent of patients with HCM[2,3,59,60] and are presumed to be responsible for symptoms of fatigue, exertional dyspnea, and angina pectoris.[81] These investigations have shown that the rapid filling phase of diastole is significantly prolonged and associated with a decreased rate and volume of rapid filling. Associated with this abnormality is a compensatory increase in the contribution of atrial systole to overall left ventricular filling. Diastolic dysfunction may occur in the absence or presence of symptoms or outflow obstruction and appears unrelated to the severity or distribution of ventricular hypertrophy.[59]

Myocardial Ischemia

There is abundant evidence that myocardial ischemia occurs in HCM as part of the underlying cardiomyopathic process and unrelated to extramural coronary artery disease.[45,49,51,52,54–58] Patients with HCM may have angina and ECG abnormalities consistent with ischemia and infarction. When patients with HCM and anginal chest pain undergo right atrial pacing, the characteristic chest pain usually develops, the induced increase in coronary flow is less than normal, and lactate is often produced.[56] Also, such patients may have exercise-induced reversible thallium-201 defects indistinguishable from those in patients with myocardial ischemia secondary to coronary artery disease.[58]

Myocardial ischemia and impaired vasodilator reserve in HCM may be due to several potential mechanisms: (1) compromised coronary blood flow to the left ventricular myocardium due to abnormal intramural coronary arteries, (2) excessive myocardial oxygen demand that exceeds the capacity of the coronary system to deliver oxygen, or (3) prolonged diastolic relaxation, resulting in elevated myocardial wall tension.

ELECTROCARDIOGRAPHIC FEATURES

The 12-lead ECG is abnormal in about 90 percent of patients with HCM and shows a wide variety of patterns, often bizarre in appearance.[3,14,15,82] However, no particular ECG alteration is characteristic of most patients with HCM; common abnormalities are left ventricular hypertrophy, ST-segment changes and T-wave inversion, left atrial enlargement, abnormal Q waves, and diminished or absent R waves in the right precordial leads. Infants and young children often have the paradoxic finding of right ventricular hypertrophy on ECG, which may reflect obstruction to right ventricular outflow.

NATURAL HISTORY AND SUDDEN CARDIAC DEATH

Predicting the clinical course and outcome for *individual* patients with HCM has proved to be difficult due to the substantial variability in natural history and the complexity of disease expression.[70,83–88] Also, because most of the considerable published literature on HCM is based on studies performed at tertiary referral centers,[27] the clinical picture of HCM that has emerged is profoundly influenced by biases in highly selective patient referral patterns,[28,89–92] which may have overestimated the overall risk for premature death. This concept is substantiated by the fact that annual mortality figures from such referral centers are considerably higher (3 to 4 percent and up to 6 percent in children)[2,86–89,93,94] than those more recently reported in unselected populations (≤1 percent).[27,89–92,95,96] Therefore, while HCM is a complex disease capable of having important clinical consequences and causing premature death in some patients, the disease has a more favorable overall clinical course than previously believed, with many patients living their natural lives (and even achieving statistical life expectancy) with little or no disability and often without the aid of therapeutic intervention.

Sudden death is most common in children and young adults 12 to 35 years of age, based on referral center data[2–5,66–68,70,79,86–88,93,94]; it may also occur in older patients, but reports in very young children and infants are exceedingly rare (Fig. 74-11). Sudden death in HCM usually occurs in patients who have been previously asymptomatic (or only mildly symptomatic); therefore such catastrophes are often the first clinical manifestation of the disease, even in those remaining free of symptoms through midlife.[85] Although most patients die while sedentary or during mild exertion, a substantial proportion collapse during or just after vigorous physical activity.[66] The latter observation—as well as the evidence that HCM is the most common cause of sudden death in young competitive athletes (Fig. 74-12) and that athletes with HCM usually collapse during training or competition[68]—supports the view that intense physical activity represents a trigger for sudden death and that it is prudent to recommend the disqualification of athletes with HCM from intense competitive sports.[97] Standard preparticipation athletic screening with history and physical examination (but without noninvasive testing) is not likely to systematically identify athletes with unsuspected HCM, since most such individuals do not have evidence of outflow obstruction producing a loud heart murmur, symptoms, or obvious family history of the disease.[98]

The mechanisms responsible for sudden death in HCM are probably multiple and complex.[2,99–102] No particular symptom complex has been shown to be reliably associated with subsequent sudden death in HCM with the possible exception of recurrent syncope in selected patients.[70,87] Furthermore, the magnitude of the outflow gradient has not been associated with increased risk for sudden death; patients with or without subaortic obstruction may die suddenly, and some patients appear to tolerate marked outflow obstruction for virtually their entire lives without incurring adverse consequences. However, other disease variables have been associated with an increased likelihood of sudden death. The most important of these proposed "risk factors"[9,62,67,70,87,103–111] include prior cardiac arrest, sustained ventricular tachycardia, massive left ventricular hypertrophy, "malignant" genotype or family history of multiple premature deaths, multiple-repetitive bursts of nonsustained ventricular tachycardia on ambulatory ECG, and early onset of symptoms in childhood.

The data available at this time do not provide convincing evidence that programmed electrical stimulation has a major role in risk stratification in HCM. Particularly aggressive programmed stimulation protocols with triple ventricular premature depolarizations seldom induce monomorphic ventricular

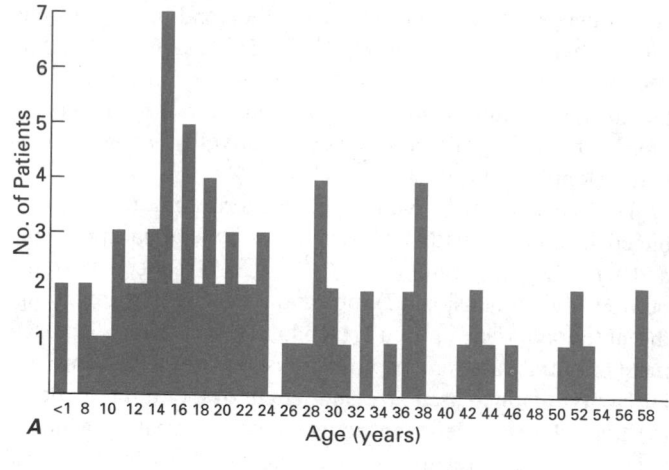

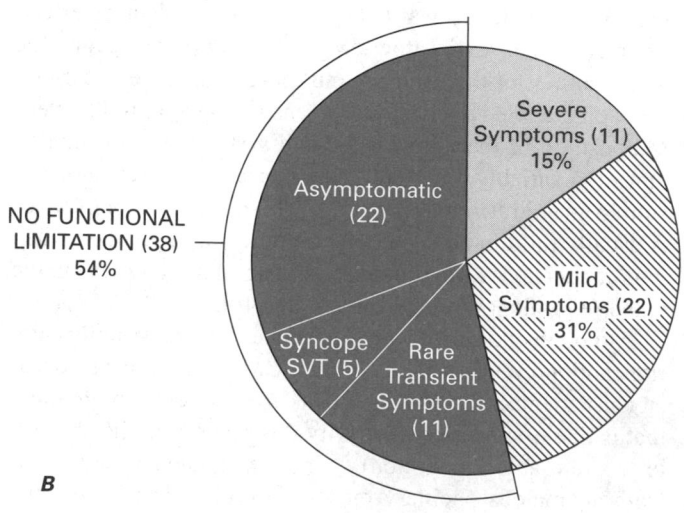

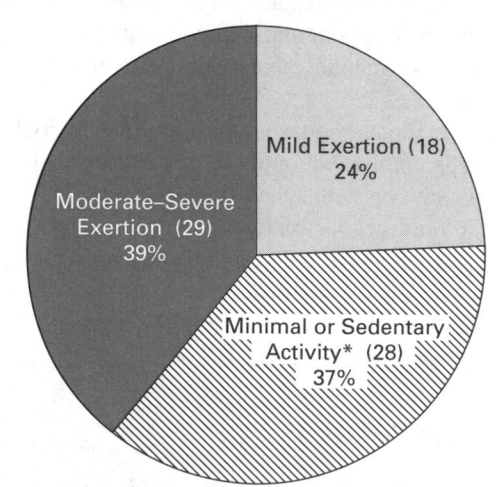

FIGURE 74-11

Clinical profile of patients with HCM and sudden death from a referral center population. *A.* Age distribution for 78 patients who died suddenly or experienced cardiac arrest; of note, the true incidence of sudden death by age is not defined because the frequency with which HCM occurs in each age group is not known. *B.* Functional state before sudden death or cardiac arrest; SVT = supraventricular tachycardia. *C.* Activity at time of sudden death or arrest: * includes four patients who died during sleep. (From Maron et al.,[66] with permission of the authors and the American Heart Association.)

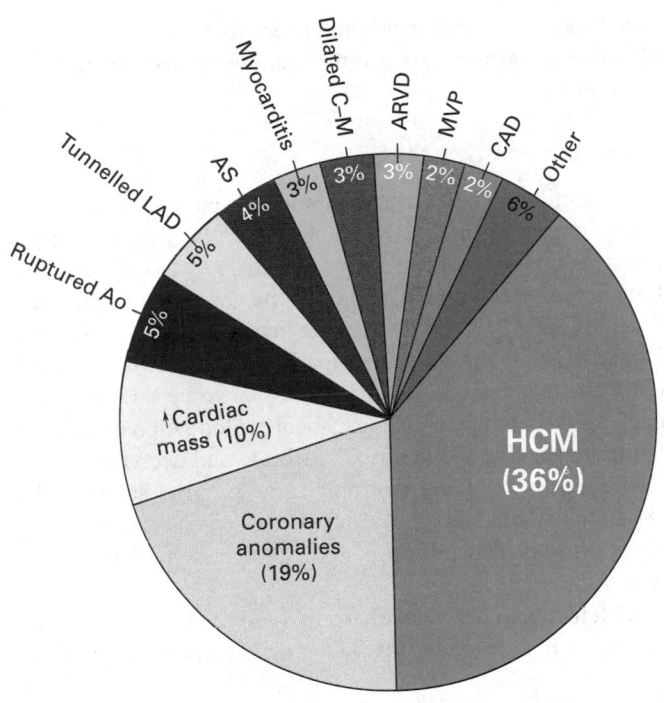

FIGURE 74-12

Causes of sudden cardiac death in young competitive athletes (median age, 17), based on systematic tracking of 158 athletes in the United States, 1985 to 1995. In an additional 2 percent, no evidence of cardiovascular disease sufficient to explain death was found at necropsy; ↑ (increased) cardiac mass = hearts with increased weight and some morphologic features consistent with (but not diagnostic of) HCM. Ao = aorta; LAD = left anterior descending coronary artery; AS = aortic stenosis; C-M = cardiomyopathy; ARVD = arrhythmogenic right ventricular dysplasia; MVP = mitral valve prolapse; CAD = coronary artery disease; HCM = hypertrophic cardiomyopathy. (Adapted from Maron et al.,[98] with permission of the American Heart Association.)

tachycardia but frequently trigger polymorphic ventricular tachycardia or ventricular fibrillation in patients with HCM[112]; these latter arrhythmias are generally regarded as nonspecific responses on the basis of experience in HCM as well as in coronary artery disease and dilated cardiomyopathy.[113]

END-STAGE PHASE

A distinctive final phase of disease evolution occurring in about 10 to 15 percent of symptomatic patients with HCM in a referral-based population has been variously referred to as the "end-stage," "burned-out," or "dilated" phase of HCM[2,5,44,54,70,78,114] (Fig. 74-13). This clinical course is characterized by progressive congestive symptoms with exercise limitation and atrial arrhythmias, associated with substantial left ventricular remodeling—i.e., enlarging left ventricular cavity size (occasionally with marked absolute dilatation), thinning of portions of the wall, systolic dysfunction, and—in a few selected patients—spontaneous reduction of the subaortic gradient. Therefore, the disease in such end-stage patients is transformed from the typical morphologic and functional

appearance of HCM (hyperdynamic, hypertrophied, and non-dilated left ventricle) to a clinical state that is more suggestive of a dilated form of cardiomyopathy (Chap. 73) in which the thickness of the left ventricular wall may be virtually normal. Many such patients exhibit irreversible thallium-201 myocardial perfusion abnormalities, which undoubtedly represent areas of extensive myocardial scarring.[45,49,51,54,58] It is possible that the morphologic and functional changes that result in end-stage depression of left ventricular contractile function are due to impaired coronary blood flow and myocardial ischemia resulting from small-vessel coronary artery disease. Patients evolving into the end-stage phase of HCM or experiencing sudden cardiac death may coexist in the same family (and share the identical disease-causing mutation).[114] Also, a few patients with aborted episodes of cardiac arrest have themselves died many years later in the end-stage phase.[115]

HYPERTROPHIC CARDIOMYOPATHY IN THE ELDERLY

Older patients (over age 60) with morphologic and clinical features consistent with HCM have been re-

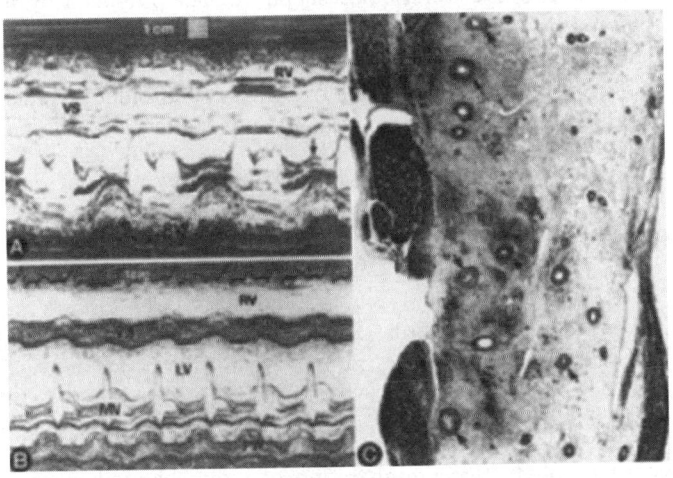

FIGURE 74-13

Studies in patients with HCM and normal extramural coronary arteries showing changes occurring concomitantly with progressive congestive cardiac failure and transmural myocardial infarction (end-stage phase). *A.* Echocardiographic study from a 26-year-old patient with exertional chest pain and dyspnea. Ventricular septum (VS) is markedly thickened (23 mm) and pattern of hypertrophy is asymmetric. Left ventricular end-diastolic dimension is reduced (38 mm), and there is a trivial degree of mitral systolic anterior motion (*arrow*). PW = posterior wall; RV = right ventricle. *B.* From same patient at 30 years of age (9 months before death) after clinical deterioration with progressive cardiac failure, pulmonary edema associated with chronic atrial fibrillation, and cardiopulmonary collapse. Appearance of left ventricle has changed dramatically. Septum has thinned considerably (to 13 mm) and is about as thick as the posterior wall; left ventricular (LV) and right ventricular cavities have enlarged substantially. MV = mitral valve. *C.* Low-power photomicrograph of a specimen from a patient with a clinical course similar to that of the patient in *A* and *B* showing transmural scarring of the septum and numerous abnormal intramural coronary arteries, some with thickened walls and narrowed lumen (*arrows*). (Magnification ×6) (From Maron et al.,[2] with permission from the authors and the publisher.)

ported.[2,21,70,116–118] In some of these patients, HCM may be well tolerated to particularly advanced ages (80 to 90 years and above) and therefore must be regarded as a condition compatible with normal longevity. In other elderly patients, symptoms are not present early in life, but severe functional limitation and heart failure may intervene abruptly for the first time after age 60 to 65. This prolonged period of symptomatic latency is perhaps unusual for a disease expressed morphologically by age 20 and in which symptoms are usually evident by age 40 to 50.

Elderly patients with the morphologic features of HCM differ in many respects from many younger patients having more "typical" expressions of the disease.[3,5,11,17,35–37] Older patients characteristically have relatively small hearts with only modestly increased left ventricular wall thickness (usually ≤20 mm)[21,118]; outflow tract morphology is severely distorted, with greatly reduced dimension and exaggerated anterior displacement of a normal-sized mitral valve. Substantial deposits of calcium in the mitral annular region are frequently present and may contribute to anterior displacement of the valve. Outflow obstruction often occurs in the presence of restricted systolic anterior motion of the anterior leaflet, with mitral valve–ventricular septal contact produced by a combination of anterior mitral valve excursion toward the septum and posterior excursion of septum toward the mitral valve.[21] It is uncertain whether HCM in such older patients has the same genetic etiology as in other patients within the clinical spectrum.

MEDICAL TREATMENT

Asymptomatic Patients and Prevention of Sudden Death

Therapeutic strategy for asymptomatic patients with HCM remains largely unresolved.[70] Some investigators have favored prophylactic administration of either beta-adrenergic blocking drugs or calcium channel blockers (such as verapamil) in an effort to prevent or delay progression of the disease process or the occurrence of sudden death. However, evidence is lacking that these drugs influence left ventricular hypertrophy or clinical course, and other therapeutic modalities have been introduced for prevention of sudden death in those selected patients who can be judged to be at high risk for life-threatening tachyarrhythmias—i.e., amiodarone or the implantable cardioverter-defibrillator (ICD). For example, in one nonrandomized study in which amiodarone was administered in relatively low doses (100 to 300 mg/day) to largely asymptomatic or mildly symptomatic patients with nonsustained ventricular tachycardia, it was suggested that this drug diminished the risk of sudden death compared to standard antiarrhythmic therapy.[119]

The ICD has been used selectively, but with increasing frequency, in high-risk HCM patients. Although systematic data are not presently available on the efficacy of the ICD in this disease, it is reasonable to expect that the device will be effective in terminating life-threatening ventricular tachyarrhythmias.

Alleviation of Symptoms

Therapeutic strategies for symptomatic patients with HCM are summarized in Fig. 74-14. Historically, beta-adrenergic blocking drugs have been utilized extensively to relieve symptoms in patients with either the obstructive or nonobstructive form of HCM.[2–5,70,120,121] The beneficial effects of beta blockers on symptoms (principally exertional dyspnea and chest pain) and exercise capacity appear to be due largely to decreased heart rate, with consequent prolongation of diastole, increased passive left ventricular filling, and decreased filling pressures. By reducing inotropic state, propranolol may also lessen myocardial oxygen demand and decrease left ventricular outflow gradient during exercise when sympathetic tone is increased.

Calcium channel blockers (principally verapamil) are also important therapeutic agents in the management of symptom-

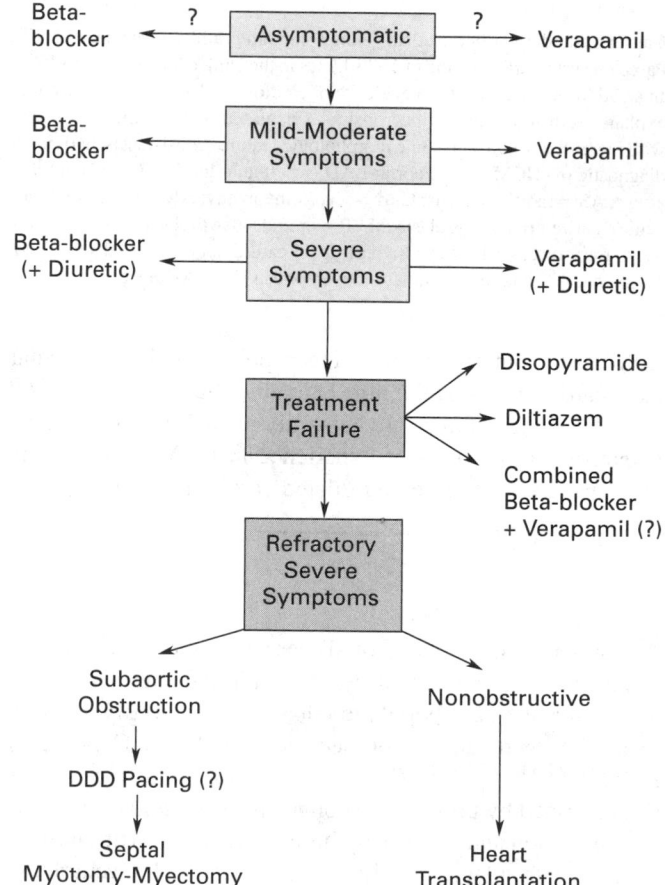

FIGURE 74-14

Therapeutic strategies for patients with HCM. Question marks indicate treatment recommendations that are largely unresolved. (Adapted from Maron BJ, Epstein SE. Heart disease: Update. In: Braunwald E, ed. *Textbook of Cardiovascular Medicine, 3d ed.* London: Saunders; 1990:157–168, with permission from the authors and the publisher.)

atic patients with HCM.[2–5,70,122,123] Orally administered verapamil provides improvement in cardiac symptoms and exercise tolerance for many patients with HCM, including those who have failed to benefit from beta blockers. This symptomatic improvement with verapamil appears to be due largely to normalization of left ventricular filling parameters.[60] There is no evidence that the use of beta blockers and verapamil together is superior to that of either drug alone.

Some patients with particularly severe symptoms of heart failure despite treatment with beta blockers or verapamil may show symptomatic improvement with the judicious addition of diuretic agents.[2,70] At selected centers, disopyramide has been an alternative treatment for patients with obstructive HCM and severe symptoms otherwise unresponsive to standard therapy.[124,125] This drug has the potential to reduce outflow gradient and improve symptoms by virtue of its negative inotropic properties.

The aforementioned therapeutic considerations apply to those patients with HCM in whom symptoms typically occur in the presence of normal or hyperdynamic systolic performance. Conversely, in the subgroup of patients experiencing congestive symptoms secondary to systolic dysfunction (i.e., end stage of HCM),[2,5,44,54,70,78,114] therapeutic strategy is similar to that for heart failure in other diseases with impaired systolic function, using diuretics, angiotensin-converting enzyme inhibitors, and digitalis; ultimately, cardiac transplantation may be considered[126] (see Chap. 25).

Prevention of Bacterial Endocarditis

Infective endocarditis is a recognized complication of HCM, with vegetations most commonly located on the anterior mitral leaflet.[127] Predisposing valvular damage is a likely consequence of the high-velocity outflow jet. Consequently, antimicrobial prophylaxis for endocarditis is indicated primarily for patients with the obstructive form of HCM.

Atrial Fibrillation

Atrial fibrillation is a particularly important arrhythmia in HCM,[128] reportedly occurring in up to 25 percent of patients followed longitudinally with this disease.[95] Atrial fibrillation is associated with an increased risk of systemic thromboembolism, heart failure, and death.[2–5,70] Of note, HCM patients with atrial fibrillation usually show substantial left atrial enlargement but, paradoxically, only relatively mild left ventricular hypertrophy.[129] Onset of atrial fibrillation may importantly impair the clinical course in HCM, since absence of the atrial systolic contribution to ventricular filling is critical to cardiac function in patients with such poorly compliant ventricles. In many patients, however, chronic atrial fibrillation appears to be reasonably well tolerated as long as ventricular rate is controlled (and anticoagulation is instituted).[128] A beta-adrenergic blocking agent or verapamil is usually efficacious in controlling heart rate in patients with chronic atrial fibrillation; however, ablation of the atrioventricular node and implantation of a pacemaker may be necessary in selected

patients. Recurrent atrial fibrillation is managed either by restoring sinus rhythm with cardioversion if possible or, alternatively, by adequate ventricular rate control. Amiodarone is probably the most effective antiarrhythmic agent for prevention of paroxysmal atrial fibrillation. Because of the risk of peripheral embolism and stroke, anticoagulant therapy should be administered (and continued indefinitely) in most patients once atrial fibrillation has been documented.

SURGICAL TREATMENT

Operation for HCM is performed to relieve incapacitating symptoms and subaortic obstruction and normalize markedly increased systolic intraventricular pressures.[70,121,130–142] Surgical intervention is reserved for those patients with severe symptoms refractory to standard medical therapy in whom marked obstruction to left ventricular outflow is present (gradient $\geq$ 50 mmHg under basal conditions or with provocative maneuvers). General agreement is lacking, however, as to whether symptomatic patients with marked gradients present only under provocable conditions require operation.[3,5,70]

Ventricular septal myotomy-myectomy (Morrow operation)[130] (Fig. 74-15) is the surgical procedure of choice. However, mitral valve replacement has been employed[133,136] in selected patients when the operative site for muscular resection in the basal/anterior portion of the ventricular septum is relatively thin ($\leq$ 18 mm), the distribution of septal hypertrophy is atypical, or when the outflow gradient is due to anomalous papillary muscle insertion.[18] Suture plication of the anterior mitral leaflet (in combination with myotomy-myectomy) has also been introduced in patients judged to have a greatly enlarged mitral valve to reduce the likelihood that mitral valve systolic anterior motion will persist postoperatively.[143]

Intraoperative echocardiography, using a sterile transducer placed directly on the right ventricle, is an important guide to mapping the distribution and magnitude of septal hypertrophy[136,144] and determining how the muscle resection should be tailored to the distribution of septal hypertrophy present in the individual patient in order to achieve the desired hemodynamic result and avoid iatrogenic ventricular septal defect. Transesophageal echocardiography (Chap. 14) may also be useful in assessing morphologic and functional abnormalities during surgery in patients with obstructive HCM.

Results from several centers employing primarily septal myotomy-myectomy over the past 35 years have demonstrated salutary hemodynamic as well as symptomatic effects.[121,130–142] Operative mortality at selected centers has improved over the past several years and is presently as low as $\leq$ 1–2 percent,[70,132,141] exclusive of patients >age 65 with associated cardiac lesions such as coronary artery disease requiring bypass grafting.[145]

Several important effects of operation have been defined in patients with HCM.[121,130–142] First, in more than 90 percent of patients, myotomy-myectomy (or mitral valve replacement) abolishes or substantially reduces the basal subaortic gradient

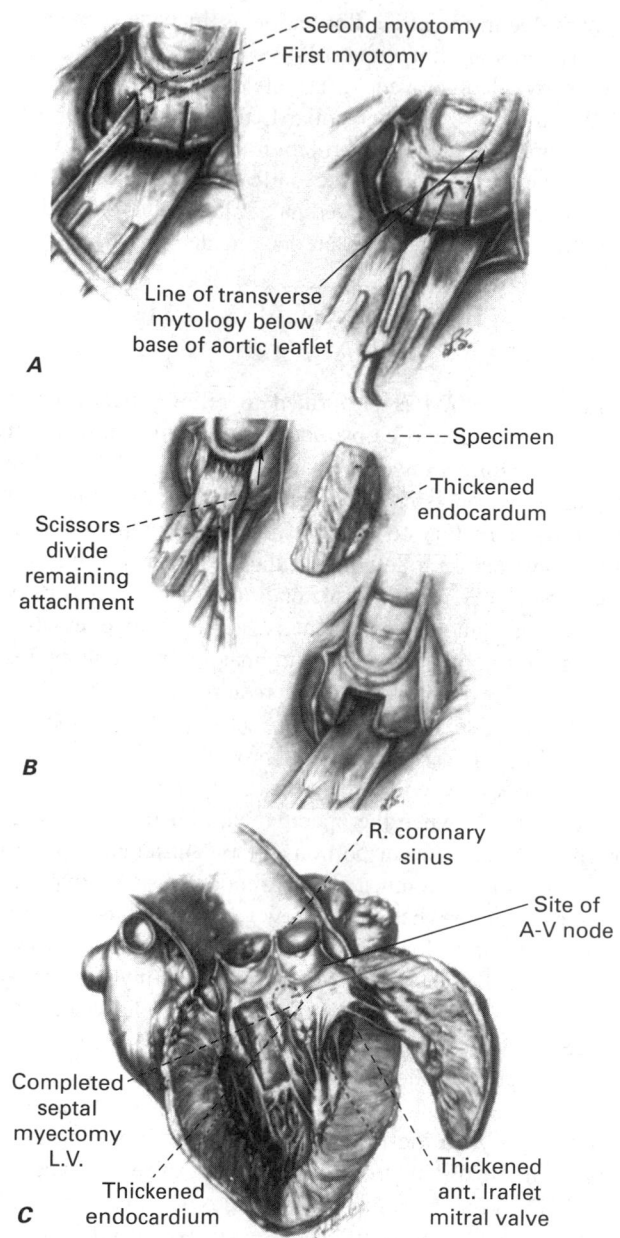

FIGURE 74-15

Illustration of ventricular septal myotomy-myectomy operation (Morrow procedure). *A*. Two vertical parallel myotomies are made in the cephalad portion of the septum about 1 cm apart. A transverse incision is then made, connecting the two parallel myotomies. *B*. Attachments of the muscle bar to the septum are divided; this segment of muscle is isolated and then excised. *C*. After completion of the myotomy-myectomy, a rectangular channel about 4 cm long and 2 cm wide is evident extending from the aortic annulus to a point just distal to the caudal margins of the mitral leaflets. (From Maron et al.,[131] with permission from the authors and the publisher.)

and mitral valve systolic anterior motion without importantly compromising left ventricular function; this consequence of surgery appears to be permanent with no evidence that the gradient recurs postoperatively or that spontaneous growth of septal musculature occurs in the area of the resection. Second, the reduction in left ventricular systolic pressure is associated with a significant and persistent improvement in symptoms

and exercise capacity in 70 percent of patients ≥ 5 years after operation, as well as a demonstrable decrease in myocardial oxygen consumption and improvement in lactate metabolism.[146] Even after surgical relief of outflow obstruction, symptoms may nevertheless recur (e.g., due to persistently impaired left ventricular filling or ischemia, atrial fibrillation, or conduction abnormalities), and premature cardiac death can still ensue many years postoperatively.[131] Traditionally, surgery has not been recommended for asymptomatic (or mildly symptomatic) patients with outflow obstruction because, in addition to the operative risk, definitive evidence is lacking that prophylactic relief of outflow obstruction prolongs survival, diminishes risk for sudden death, or mediates the onset of symptoms.

ALTERNATIVES TO SURGERY

Over the past several years there has been interest in the application of permanent dual-chamber pacing, as an alternative to operative intervention, for severely symptomatic patients with obstructive HCM who become refractory to drug therapy.[147–150] Some uncontrolled study designs have shown pacing to be associated with impressive reductions in outflow gradient and amelioration of symptoms in many patients.[148,149] However, this reported symptomatic benefit has occurred over a relatively short period of time (generally ≤ 2 years), and not consistently accompanied by objective measures documenting improved exercise tolerance (e.g., treadmill exercise duration and measured oxygen consumption). In one randomized study, pacing was associated with a more modest decrease in gradient and no objective evidence of improved exercise capacity, suggesting that the subjectively perceived symptomatic improvement reported by patients is largely due to a placebo effect.[151] Other catheterization laboratory studies show dual-chamber pacing to have deleterious effects on left ventricular function.[152,153] Because the basic HCM disease process and risk for sudden death is unlikely to be affected by permanent dual-chamber pacing, this potential treatment modality cannot be regarded as a panacea for the diverse clinical and functional abnormalities of HCM,[154] although it is possible that a therapeutic role may be defined for relief of symptoms in some patients with this disease.

A potential new method of treating severely symptomatic patients with hypertrophic obstructive cardiomyopathy using selective intracoronary alcohol injection to induce localized septal infarction has recently been reported.[155] Whether this technique will provide an alternative to surgical myotomy-myectomy in selected patients remains to be proven and this procedure must be considered experimental at the present time.

REFERENCES

1. Braunwald E, Lambrew CT, Rockoff D, Ross J Jr, Morrow AG. Idiopathic hypertrophic subaortic stenosis: I. A description of the disease based upon an analysis of 64 patients. *Circulation* 1964; 30(suppl IV):3–217.

2. Maron BJ, Bonow RO, Cannon RO, Leon MB, Epstein SE. Hypertrophic cardiomyopathy: Interrelation of clinical manifestations, pathophysiology, and therapy. *N Engl J Med* 1987; 316:780–789, 844–852.

3. Wigle ED, Sasson Z, Henderson MA, Ruddy TD, Fulop J, Rakowski H, et al. Hypertrophic cardiomyopathy: The importance of the site and extent of hypertrophy. A review. *Prog Cardiovasc Dis* 1985; 28:1–83.

4. Louie EK, Edwards LC. Hypertrophic cardiomyopathy. *Prog Cardiovasc Dis* 1994; 36:275–308.

5. Wigle ED, Rakowski H, Kimball BP, Williams WG. Hypertrophic cardiomyopathy: Clinical spectrum and treatment. *Circulation* 1995; 92:1680–1692.

6. Maron BJ, Epstein SE. Hypertrophic cardiomyopathy: A discussion of nomenclature. *Am J Cardiol* 1979; 43:1242–1244.

7. Marian AJ, Roberts R. Recent advances in the molecular genetics of hypertrophic cardiomyopathy. *Circulation* 1995; 92:1336–1347.

8. Schwartz K, Carrier L, Guicheney P, Komajda M. Molecular basis of familial cardiomyopathies. *Circulation* 1995; 91:532–540.

9. Watkins H, McKenna WJ, Thierfelder L, Suk HJ, Anan R, O'Donoghue A, et al. The role of cardiac troponin T and α tropomyosin mutations in hypertrophic cardiomyopathy. *N Engl J Med* 1995; 332:1058–1064.

10. Ciró E, Nichols PF, Maron BJ. Heterogeneous morphologic expression of genetically transmitted hypertrophic cardiomyopathy: Two-dimensional echocardiographic analysis. *Circulation* 1983; 67:1227–1233.

11. Maron BJ, Gottdiener JS, Epstein SE. Patterns and significance of distribution of left ventricular hypertrophy in hypertrophic cardiomyopathy: A wide-angle, two-dimensional echocardiographic study of 125 patients. *Am J Cardiol* 1981; 48:418–428.

12. Spirito P, Maron BJ, Bonow RO, Epstein SE. Severe functional limitation in patients with hypertrophic cardiomyopathy and only mild localized left ventricular hypertrophy. *J Am Coll Cardiol* 1979; 44:401–412.

13. Webb JG, Sasson Z, Rakowski H, Liu P, Wigle ED. Apical hypertrophic cardiomyopathy: Clinical follow-up and diagnostic correlates. *J Am Coll Cardiol* 1990; 15:83–90.

14. Alfonso F, Nihoyannopoulos P, Steward J, Dickie S, Lemery R, McKenna WJ. Clinical significance of giant negative T waves in hypertrophic cardiomyopathy. *J Am Coll Cardiol* 1990; 15:965–971.

15. Louie EK, Maron BJ. Apical hypertrophic cardiomyopathy: Clinical and two-dimensional echocardiographic assessment. *Ann Intern Med* 1987; 106:663–670.

16. Roberts CS, Roberts WC. Morphologic features. In: Zipes DP, Rowlands DJ, eds. *Progress in Cardiology 2/2*. Philadelphia: Lea & Febiger, 1989:3–22.

17. Klues HG, Schiffers A, Maron BJ. Phenotypic spectrum and patterns of left ventricular hypertrophy in hypertrophic cardiomyopathy: Morphologic observations and significance as assessed by two-dimensional echocardiography in 600 patients. *J Am Coll Cardiol* 1995; 26:1699–1708.

18. Klues HG, Roberts WC, Maron BJ. Anomalous insertion of papillary muscle directly into anterior mitral leaflet in hypertrophic cardiomyopathy: Significance in producing left ventricular outflow obstruction. *Circulation* 1991; 84:1188–1197.

19. Klues HG, Maron BJ, Dollar AL, Roberts WC. Diversity of structural mitral valve alterations in hypertrophic cardiomyopathy. *Circulation* 1992; 85:1651–1660.

20. Olsen EG: Anatomic and light microscopic characterization of hypertrophic obstructive and non-obstructive cardiomyopathy. *Eur Heart J* 1983; 4(suppl F):1–8.

21. Lewis JF, Maron BJ. Elderly patients with hypertrophic cardiomyopathy: A subset with distinctive left ventricular morphology and progressive clinical course late in life. *J Am Coll Cardiol* 1989; 13:36–45.

22. Liouville, H. Rètrècissement ventriculo-aortique. *Gazette Med Paris* 1869; 24:161–163.

23. Schmincke A. Über linseitige muskulöse Conusstenosen. *Dtsch Med Wochenschr* 1907; 33:2082.

24. Teare D. Asymmetrical hypertrophy of the heart in young adults. *Br Heart J* 1958; 20:1–18.

25. Maron BJ, Gardin JM, Flack JM, Gidding SS, Kurosaki TT, Bild E. Prevalence of hypertrophic cardiomyopathy in a general population of young adults: Echocardiographic analysis of 4111 subjects in the CARDIA study. *Circulation* 1995; 92:785–789.

26. Maron BJ, Peterson EE, Maron MS, Peterson JE. Prevalence of hypertrophic cardiomyopathy in an outpatient population referred for echocardiographic study. *Am J Cardiol* 1994; 73:577–580.

27. Spirito P, Chiarella F, Carratino L, Zoni-Berisso M, Bellotti P, Vecchio C. Clinical course and prognosis of hypertrophic cardiomyopathy in an outpatient population. *N Engl J Med* 1989; 320:749–755.

28. Shapiro LM, Zezulka A. Hypertrophic cardiomyopathy: A common disease with a good prognosis: Five year experience of a district general hospital. *Br Heart J* 1983; 50:530–533.

29. Yamaguchi H, Ishimura T, Nishiyama S, Nagasaki F, Nakanishi S, Takatsu F, et al. Hypertrophic nonobstructive cardiomyopathy with giant negative T waves (apical hypertrophy): Ventriculographic and echocardiographic features in 30 patients. *Am J Cardiol* 1979; 44:401–412.

30. Sakamoto T, Tei C, Murayama J, Ichiyasu H, Hada Y, Hayashi T, et al. Giant T wave inversion as a manifestation of asymmetrical apical hypertrophy (AAH) of the left ventricle: Echocardiographic and ultrasono-cardiotomographic study. *Jpn Heart J* 1976; 17:611–629.

31. Ando H, Imaizumi T, Urabe Y, Takeshita A, Nakamura M. Apical segmental dysfunction in hypertrophic cardiomyopathy: Subgroup with unique clinical features. *J Am Coll Cardiol* 1990; 16:1579–1588.

32. Rosenzweig A, Watkins H, Hwang D-S, Miri M, McKenna W, Traill TA, et al. Preclinical diagnosis of familial hypertrophic cardiomyopathy by genetic analysis of blood lymphocytes. *N Engl J Med* 1991; 325:1753–1760.

33. Maron BJ, Spirito P, Wesley Y, Arce J. Development and progression of left ventricular hypertrophy in children with hypertrophic cardiomyopathy. *N Engl J Med* 1986; 315:610–614.

34. Solomon SD, Wolff S, Watkins H, Ridker PM, Come PC, Seidman CE, et al. Left ventricular hypertrophy and morphology in familial hypertrophic cardiomyopathy associated with mutations of the β-myosin heavy chain gene. *J Am Coll Cardiol* 1993; 22:498–505.

35. Shapiro LM, McKenna WJ. Distribution of left ventricular hypertrophy in hypertrophic cardiomyopathy: A two-dimensional echocardiographic study. *J Am Coll Cardiol* 1983; 2:437–444.

36. Louie EK, Maron BJ. Hypertrophic cardiomyopathy with extreme increase in left ventricular wall thickness: Functional and morphologic features and clinical significance. *J Am Coll Cardiol* 1986; 8:57–65.

37. Maron BJ, Gross BJ, Stark SI. Extreme left ventricular hypertrophy. *Circulation* 1995; 92:2748.

38. Maron BJ, Pelliccia A, Spirito P. Cardiac disease in young trained athletes: Insights into methods for distinguishing athlete's heart from structural heart disease with particular emphasis on hypertrophic cardiomyopathy. *Circulation* 1995; 91:1596–1601.

39. Maron BJ, Tajik AJ, Ruttenberg HD, Graham TP, Atwood GF, Victorica BE, et al. Hypertrophic cardiomyopathy in infants: Clinical features and natural history. *Circulation* 1982; 65:7–17.

40. Panza JA, Maron BJ. Relation of electrocardiographic abnormalities to evolving left ventricular hypertrophy in hypertrophic cardiomyopathy. *Am J Cardiol* 1989; 63:1258–1265.

41. Spirito P, Maron BJ. Absence of progression of left ventricular hypertrophy in adult patients with hypertrophic cardiomyopathy. *J Am Coll Cardiol* 1987; 9:1013–1017.

42. Panza JA, Maris TJ, Maron BJ. Development and determinants of dynamic obstruction to left ventricular outflow in young patients with hypertrophic cardiomyopathy. *Circulation* 1992; 85:1398–1405.

43. Spirito P, Maron BJ. Relation between extent of left ventricular hypertrophy and age in patients with hypertrophic cardiomyopathy. *J Am Coll Cardiol* 1989; 13:820–823.

44. Spirito P, Maron BJ, Bonow RO, Epstein SE. Occurrence and significance of progressive left ventricular wall thinning and relative cavity dilatation in patients with hypertrophic cardiomyopathy. *Am J Cardiol* 1987; 60:123–129.

45. Tanaka M, Fujiwara H, Onodera T, Wu D-J, Hamashima Y, Kawai C. Quantitative analysis of myocardial fibrosis in normals, hypertensive hearts, and hypertrophic cardiomyopathy. *Br Heart J* 1986; 55:575–581.

46. Ferrans VJ, Morrow AG, Roberts WC. Myocardial ultrastructure in idiopathic hypertrophic subaortic stenosis: A study of operatively excised left ventricular outflow tract muscle in 14 patients. *Circulation* 1972; 45:769–792.

47. Maron BJ, Roberts WC. Quantitative analysis of cardiac muscle cell disorganization in the ventricular septum of patients with hypertrophic cardiomyopathy. *Circulation* 1979; 59:689–706.

48. Maron BJ, Anan TJ, Roberts WC. Quantitative analysis of the distribution of cardiac muscle cell disorganization in the left ventricular wall of patients with hypertrophic cardiomyopathy. *Circulation* 1981; 63:882–894.

49. St. John Sutton MG, Lie JT, Anderson KR, O'Brien PC, Frye RL. Histopathological specificity of hypertrophic obstructive cardiomyopathy. *Br Heart J* 1980; 44:433–443.

50. Fujiwara H, Kawai C, Hamashima Y: Myocardial fascicle and fiber disarray in 25 μ-thick sections. *Circulation* 1979; 59:1293–1298.

51. Maron BJ, Wolfson JK, Epstein SE, Roberts WC. Intramural ("small vessel") coronary artery disease in hypertrophic cardiomyopathy. *J Am Coll Cardiol* 1986; 8:545–557.

52. Tanaka M, Fujiwara H, Onodera T, Wu D-J, Matsuda M, Hamashima Y, et al. Quantitative analysis of narrowings of intramyocardial small arteries in normal hearts, hypertensive hearts, and hearts with hypertrophic cardiomyopathy. *Circulation* 1987; 75:1130–1139.

53. Maron BJ, Wolfson JK, Roberts WC. Relation between extent of cardiac muscle cell disorganization and left ventricular wall thickness in hypertrophic cardiomyopathy. *Am J Cardiol* 1992; 70:785–790.

54. Maron BJ, Epstein SE, Roberts WC. Hypertrophic cardiomyopathy and transmural myocardial infarction without significant atherosclerosis of the extramural coronary arteries. *Am J Cardiol* 1979; 43:1086–1102.

55. Factor SM, Butany J, Sole MJ, Wigle ED, Williams WC, Rojkind M. Pathologic fibrosis and matrix connective tissue in the subaortic myocardium of patients with hypertrophic cardiomyopathy. *J Am Coll Cardiol* 1991; 17:1343–1351.

56. Cannon RO, Rosing DR, Maron BJ, Leon MB, Bonow RO, Watson RM, et al. Myocardial ischemia in hypertrophic cardiomyopathy: Contribution of inadequate vasodilator reserve and elevated left ventricular filling pressures. *Circulation* 1985; 71:234–243.

57. Pasternac A, Noble J, Streulens Y, Elie R, Henschke C, Bourassa MG. Pathophysiology of chest pain in patients with cardiomyopathies and normal coronary arteries. *Circulation* 1982; 65:778–789.

58. O'Gara PT, Bonow RO, Maron BJ, Damske BA, Van Lingen A, Bacharach SL, et al. Myocardial perfusion abnormalities in patients with hypertrophic cardiomyopathy: Assessment with thallium-201 emission computed tomography. *Circulation* 1987; 76:1214–1223.

59. Maron BJ, Spirito P, Green KJ, Wesley YE, Bonow RO, Arce J. Noninvasive assessment of left ventricular diastolic function by pulsed Doppler echocardiography in patients with hypertrophic cardiomyopathy. *J Am Coll Cardiol* 1987; 10:733–742.

60. Bonow RO, Fredrick TM, Bacharach SL, Green MV, Goose PW, Maron BJ, et al. Atrial systole and left ventricular filling in patients with hypertrophic cardiomyopathy: Effect of verapamil. *Am J Cardiol* 1983; 51:1386–1391.

61. Maron BJ, Nichols PF, Pickle LW, Wesley YE, Mulvihill JJ. Patterns of inheritance in hypertrophic cardiomyopathy: Assessment of M-mode and two-dimensional echocardiography. *Am J Cardiol* 1984; 53:1087–1094.

62. Watkins H, Rosenzweig A, Hwang D-S, Levi T, McKenna WJ, Seidman CE, et al. Characteristics and prognostic implications of myosin missense mutations in familial hypertrophic cardiomyopathy. *N Engl J Med* 1992; 326:1108–1114.

63. Watkins H, Conner D, Thierfelder L, Jarcho JA, Suk HJ, MacRae C, et al. Mutations in the cardiac myosin binding protein-C gene on chromosome 11 cause familial hypertrophic cardiomyopathy. *Nature Genet* 1995; 11:434–437.

64. McKenna WJ, Stewart JT, Nihoyannopoulos P, McGinty F, Davies MJ. Hypertrophic cardiomyopathy without hypertrophy: Two families with myocardial disarray in the absence of increased myocardial mass. *Br Heart J* 1990; 63:287–290.

65. Maron BJ, Kragel AH, Roberts WC. Sudden death due to hypertrophic cardiomyopathy in the absence of increased left ventricular mass. *Br Heart J* 1990; 63:308–310.

66. Maron BJ, Roberts WC, Epstein SE. Sudden death in hypertrophic cardiomyopathy: A profile of 78 patients. *Circulation* 1982; 67:1388–1394.

67. Maron BJ, Lipson LC, Roberts WC, Savage DD, Epstein SE. "Malignant" hypertrophic cardiomyopathy: Identification of a subgroup of families with unusually frequent premature death. *Am J Cardiol* 1978; 41:1133–1140.

68. Maron BJ, Shirani J, Poliac LC, Mathenge R, Roberts WC, Mueller FO. Sudden death in young competitive athletes: Clinical, demographic and pathological profiles. *JAMA* 1996; 276:199–204.

69. Maron BJ, Epstein SE. Clinical significance and therapeutic implications of the left ventricular outflow tract pressure gradient in hypertrophic cardiomyopathy. *Am J Cardiol* 1986; 11:752–756.

70. Spirito P, Seidman CE, McKenna WJ, Maron BJ. Management of hypertrophic cardiomyopathy. *N Engl J Med* 1997; 30:775–785.

71. Pollick C, Rakowski H, Wigle ED. Muscular subaortic stenosis: The quantitative relationship between systolic anterior motion and pressure gradient. *Circulation* 1984; 69:43–49.

72. Cape EG, Simons D, Jimoh A, Weyman AE, Yoganathan AP, Levine RA. Chordal geometry determines the shape and extent of systolic anterior motion. *J Am Coll Cardiol* 1989; 13:1438–1448.

73. Klues HG, Roberts WC, Maron BJ. Morphologic determinants of echocardiographic patterns of mitral valve systolic anterior motion in obstructive hypertrophic cardiomyopathy. *Circulation* 1993; 87:1570–1579.

74. Klues HG, Leuner C, Kuhn H. Hypertrophic obstructive cardiomyopathy: No increase of the gradient during exercise. *J Am Coll Cardiol* 1991; 19:527–533.

75. Panza JA, Petrone RK, Fananapazir L, Maron BJ. Utility of continuous wave Doppler in noninvasive assessment of the left ventricular outflow tract pressure gradient in patients with hypertrophic cardiomyopathy. *J Am Coll Cardiol* 1992; 19:91–99.

76. Petrone RK, Klues HG, Panza JA, Peterson EE, Maron BJ. Significance of the occurrence of mitral valve prolapse in patients with hypertrophic cardiomyopathy. *J Am Coll Cardiol* 1992; 20:55–61.

77. Falicov R, Resnekov L, Bharati S, Lev M. Mid-zone ventricular obstruction: A variant of obstructive cardiomyopathy. *Am J Cardiol* 1976; 37:432–437.

78. Fighali S, Krajcer Z, Edelman S, Leachman RD. Progression of hypertrophic cardiomyopathy into a hypokinetic left ventricle: Higher incidence in patients with midventricular obstruction. *J Am Coll Cardiol* 1987; 9:288–294.

79. Fiddler GI, Tajik AJ, Weidman WH, McGoon DC, Ritter DG, Giuliani ER. Idiopathic hypertrophic subaortic stenosis in the young. *Am J Cardiol* 1978; 42:793–799.

80. Maron BJ, McIntosh CL, Klues HG, Cannon RO, Roberts WC. Morphologic basis for obstruction to right ventricular outflow in hypertrophic cardiomyopathy. *Am J Cardiol* 1993; 71:1089–1094.

81. Nihoyannopoulos P, Karatasakis G, Frenneaux M, Mckenna WJ, Oakley CM. Diastolic function in hypertrophic cardiomyopathy: Relation to exercise capacity. *J Am Coll Cardiol* 1992; 19:536–540.

82. Maron BJ, Wolfson JK, Ciró E, Spirito P. Relation of electrocardiographic abnormalities and patterns of left ventricular hypertrophy identified by two-dimensional echocardiography in patients with hypertrophic cardiomyopathy. *Am J Cardiol* 1983; 51:189–194.

83. Newman H, Sugrue DD, Oakley CM, Goodwin JF, McKenna WJ. Relation of left ventricular function and prognosis in hypertrophic cardiomyopathy: An angiographic study. *J Am Coll Cardiol* 1985; 5:1064–1074.

84. Frenneaux MP, Counihan PJ, Caforio ALP, Chikamori T, McKenna WJ. Abnormal blood pressure response during exercise in hypertrophic cardiomyopathy. *Circulation* 1991; 82:1995–2002.

85. Hecht GM, Panza JA, Maron BJ. Clinical course of middle-aged asymptomatic patients with hypertrophic cardiomyopathy. *Am J Cardiol* 1992; 69:935–940.

86. Adelman AG, Wigle ED, Ranganathan N, Webb GD, Kidd BSL, Bigelow WG, et al. The clinical course in muscular subaortic stenosis: A retrospective and prospective study of 60 hemodynamically proved cases. *Ann Intern Med* 1972; 77:515–525.

87. McKenna WJ, Deanfield JE, Faroqui A, England D, Oakley C, Goodwin JF. Prognosis in hypertrophic cardiomyopathy: Role of age and clinical electrocardiographic and hemodynamic features. *Am J Cardiol* 1981; 47:532–538.

88. Shah PM, Adelman AG, Wigle ED, Gobel FL, Burchell HB, Hardarson T, et al. The natural (and unnatural) history of hypertrophic obstructive cardiomyopathy. *Circ Res* 1973; 34,35(suppl II):II-179–II-195.

89. Maron BJ, Spirito P. Impact of patient selection biases on the perception of hypertrophic cardiomyopathy and its natural history. *Am J Cardiol* 1993; 72:970–972.

90. Kofflard MJ, Waldstein DJ, Vos J, ten Cate FJ. Prognosis in hypertrophic cardiomyopathy: A retrospective study. *Am J Cardiol* 1993; 72:939–943.

91. Spirito P, Rapezzi C, Autore C, Bruzzi P, Bellone P, Ortolani P, et al. Prognosis in asymptomatic patients with hypertrophic cardiomyopathy and nonsustained ventricular tachycardia. *Circulation* 1994; 90:2743–2747.

92. Cannan CR, Reeder GS, Bailey KR, Melton LJ III, Gersh BJ. Natural history of hypertrophic cardiomyopathy: A population-based study, 1976 through 1990. *Circulation* 1995; 92:2488–2499.

93. Frank S, Braunwald E. Idiopathic hypertrophic subaortic stenosis: Clinical analysis of 126 patients with emphasis on the natural history. *Circulation* 1968; 37:759–788.

94. McKenna WJ, Deanfield JE. Hypertrophic cardiomyopathy: An important cause of sudden death. *Arch Dis Child* 1984; 59:971–975.

95. Cecchi F, Olivotto I, Montereggi A, Santoro G, Dolara A, Maron BJ. Hypertrophic cardiomyopathy in Tuscany: Clinical course and outcome in an unselected regional population. *J Am Coll Cardiol* 1995; 26:1529–1536.

96. Maron BJ, Poliac LC, Casey SA, Lange SK, Aeppli D. Clinical significance and consequences of hypertrophic cardiomyopathy assessed in an unselected patient population: Evidence for the relatively benign nature of the true disease state in adulthood (abstr). *Circulation* 1996; 94:I-84.

97. Maron BJ, Isner JM, McKenna WJ. Hypertrophic cardiomyopathy, myocarditis and other myopericardial disease, and mitral valve prolapse. Task Force 3. In: 26th Bethesda Conference. Recommendations for determining eligibility for competition in athletes with cardiovascular abnormalities. *J Am Coll Cardiol* 1994; 24:880–885.

98. Maron BJ, Thompson PD, Puffer JC, McGrew CA, Strong WB, Douglas PS, et al. American Heart Association Medical Scientific Statement: Cardiovascular preparticipation screening of competitive athletes. *Circulation* 1996; 94:850–856.

99. Nicod P, Polikar R, Peterson KL. Hypertrophic cardiomyopathy and sudden death. *N Engl J Med* 1988; 318:1255–1257.

100. Stafford WJ, Trohman RG, Bilsker M, Zaman L, Catellanos A, Myerburg RJ. Cardiac arrest in an adolescent with atrial fibrillation and hypertrophic cardiomyopathy. *J Am Coll Cardiol* 1985; 7:701–704.

101. Krikler DM, Davies MJ, Rowland E, Goodwin JF, Evans RC, Shaw DB. Sudden death in hypertrophic cardiomyopathy: Associated accessory atrioventricular pathways. *Br Heart J* 1980; 43:245–251.

102. DeRose JJ, Banas JS, Winters SL. Current perspectives on sudden cardiac death in hypertrophic cardiomyopathy. *Prog Cardiovasc Dis* 1994; 36:475–484.

103. Gilligan DM, Nihoyannopoulos P, Chan WL, Oakley CM. Investigation of a hemodynamic basis for syncope in hypertrophic cardiomyopathy: Use of a head-up tilt test. *Circulation* 1992; 85:2140–2148.

104. Maron BJ, Cecchi F, McKenna WJ. Risk factors and stratification for sudden cardiac death in patients with hypertrophic cardiomyopathy. *Br Heart J* 1994; 72(suppl):S-13–S-18.

105. Spirito P, Maron BJ. Relation between extent of left ventricular hypertrophy and occurrence of sudden cardiac death in hypertrophic cardiomyopathy. *J Am Coll Cardiol* 1990; 15:1521–1526.

106. Maron BJ, Savage DD, Wolfson JK, Epstein SE. Prognostic significance of 24-hour ambulatory monitoring in patients with hypertrophic cardiomyopathy: A prospective study. *Am J Cardiol* 1981; 48:252–257.

107. McKenna WJ, England D, Doi JL, Deanfield JE, Oakley OM, Goodwin JF. Arrhythmia in hypertrophic cardiomyopathy: I. Influence on prognosis. *Br Heart J* 1981; 46:168–172.

108. Mckenna WJ, Camm AJ. Sudden death in hypertrophic cardiomyopathy: Assessment of patients at high risk. *Circulation* 1989; 80:1489–1492.

109. Anan R, Greve G, Thierfelder L, Watkins H, McKenna WJ, Solomon S, et al. Prognostic implications of novel β cardiac myosin heavy chain gene mutations that cause familial hypertrophic cardiomyopathy. *J Clin Invest* 1994; 93:280–285.

110. Maron BJ, Kogan J, Proschan MA, Hecht GM, Roberts WC. Circadian variability in the occurrence of sudden cardiac death in patients with hypertrophic cardiomyopathy. *J Am Coll Cardiol* 1994; 23:1405–1409.

111. Cecchi F, Maron BJ, Epstein SE. Long-term outcome of patients with hypertrophic cardiomyopathy successfully resuscitated after cardiac arrest. *J Am Coll Cardiol* 1989; 13:1283–1288.

112. Fananapazir L, Chang AC, Epstein SE, McAreavey D. Prognostic determinants in hypertrophic cardiomyopathy: Prospective evaluation of therapeutic strategy based on clinical, Holter, hemodynamic and electrophysiologic findings. *Circulation* 1992; 86:730–740.

113. Kuck K-H, Kunze KP, Schlueter M, Nienaber CA, Costard A. Programmed electrical stimulation in hypertrophic cardiomyopathy: Results in patients with and without cardiac arrest or syncope. *Eur Heart J* 1988; 9:177–185.

114. Hecht GM, Klues HG, Roberts WC, Maron BJ. Coexistence of sudden cardiac death and end-stage heart failure in familial hypertrophic cardiomyopathy. *J Am Coll Cardiol* 1993; 22:489–497.

115. Maron BJ, Hecht G, Klues HG, Kunkes SH, Rosenfeld LE, Cecchi F. Both aborted sudden cardiac death and end-stage phase in hypertrophic cardiomyopathy. *Am J Cardiol* 1993; 72:363–365.

116. Fay WP, Taliercio CP, Ilstrup DM, Tajik AJ, Gersch BJ. Natural history of hypertrophic cardiomyopathy in the elderly. *J Am Coll Cardiol* 1990; 16:821–826.

117. Lever HM, Kuram RF, Currie PH, Healy BP. Hypertrophic cardiomyopathy in the elderly: Distinctions from the young based on cardiac shape. *Circulation* 1989; 79:580–589.

118. Chikamori T, Doi YL, Yonezawa Y, Dickie S, Ozawa T, McKenna WJ. Comparison of clinical features in patients ≥ 60 years of age to those ≤ 40 years of age with hypertrophic cardiomyopathy. *Am J Cardiol* 1990; 66:875–877.

119. McKenna WJ, Oakley CM, Krikler DM, Goodwin JF. Improved survival with amiodarone in patients with hypertrophic cardiomyopathy and ventricular tachycardia. *Br Heart J* 1985; 53:412–416.

120. Adelman AG, Shah PM, Gramiak R, Wigle ED. Long-term propranolol therapy in muscular subaortic stenosis. *Br Heart J* 1970; 32:804–811.

121. Seiler C, Hess OM, Schoenbeck M, Turina J, Nenni R, Turina M, et al. Long-term follow-up of medical versus surgical therapy for hypertrophic cardiomyopathy: A retrospective study. *J Am Coll Cardiol* 1991; 17:634–642.

122. Kaltenbach M, Hopf R, Kober G, Bussman W-D, Keller M, Petersen Y. Treatment of hypertrophic obstructive cardiomyopathy with verapamil. *Br Heart J* 1979; 42:35–42.

123. Rosing DR, Condit JR, Maron BJ, Kent KM, Leon BM, Bonow RO, et al. Verapamil therapy: A new approach to the pharmacologic treatment of hypertrophic cardiomyopathy. III. Effects of long-term administration. *Am J Cardiol* 1981; 48:545–553.

124. Sherrid M, Delia E, Dwyer E. Oral disopyramide therapy for obstructive hypertrophic cardiomyopathy. *Am J Cardiol* 1988; 62:1085–1088.

125. Pollick C. Muscular subaortic stenosis: Hemodynamic and clinical improvement after disopyramide. *N Engl J Med* 1982; 307:997–999.

126. Shirani J, Maron BJ, Cannon RO, Shahin S, Roberts WC. Clinicopathologic features of hypertrophic cardiomyopathy managed by cardiac transplantation. *Am J Cardiol* 1993; 72:434–440.

127. Roberts WC, Kishel JC, McIntosh CL, Cannon RO, Maron BJ. Severe mitral or aortic valve regurgitation, or both, requiring valve replacement for infective endocarditis complicating hypertrophic cardiomyopathy. *J Am Coll Cardiol* 1992; 19:365–377.

128. Robinson KC, Frenneaux MP, Stockins B, Karatasakis G, Poloniecki JD, McKenna WJ. Atrial fibrillation in hypertrophic cardiomyopathy: A longitudinal study. *J Am Coll Cardiol* 1990; 15:1279–1285.

129. Spirito P, Lakatos E, Maron BJ. Degree of left ventricular hypertrophy in chronic atrial fibrillation in hypertrophic cardiomyopathy. *Am J Cardiol* 1992; 69:1217–1222.

130. Morrow AG, Reitz BA, Epstein SE, Henry WL, Conkle DM, Itscoitz SB, et al. Operative treatment in hypertrophic subaortic stenosis: Techniques and the results of pre- and postoperative assessments in 83 patients. *Circulation* 1975; 52:88–102.

131. Maron BJ, Epstein SE, Morrow AG. Symptomatic status and prognosis of patients after operation for hypertrophic obstructive cardiomyopathy: Efficacy of ventricular septal myotomy and myectomy. *Eur Heart J* 1983; 4(suppl F):175–185.

132. Williams WG, Wigle ED, Rakowski H, Smallhorn J, LeBlanc J, Trusler GA. Results of surgery for hypertrophic obstructive cardiomyopathy. *Circulation* 1987; 76(suppl V):104–108.

133. Krajcer Z, Leachman RD, Cooley DA, Coronado R. Septal myotomy-myectomy versus mitral valve replacement in hypertrophic cardiomyopathy: Ten-year follow-up in 185 patients. *Circulation* 1989; 80(suppl I):I-57–I-64.

134. Bircks W, Schulte HD. Surgical treatment of hypertrophic obstructive cardiomyopathy with special reference to complications and to atypical hypertrophic obstructive cardiomyopathy. *Eur Heart J* 1983; 4(suppl F):187–190.

135. Mohr R, Schaff HV, Danielson GK, Puga FJ, Pluth JR, Tajik AJ. The outcome of surgical treatment of hypertrophic obstructive cardiomyopathy: Experience over 15 years. *J Thorac Cardiovasc Surg* 1989; 97:666–674.

136. McIntosh CL, Maron BJ. Current operative treatment of obstructive hypertrophic cardiomyopathy. *Circulation* 1988; 78:487–495.

137. Cohn LH, Trehan H, Collin JJ. Long-term follow-up of patients undergoing myotomy-myectomy for obstructive hypertrophic cardiomyopathy. *Am J Cardiol* 1992; 70:657–660.

138. Schulte HD, Bircks WH, Loesse B, Godehardt SE, Schwartzkopff B. Prognosis of patients with hypertrophic cardiomyopathy after transaortic myectomy: Late results up to twenty-five years. *J Thorac Cardiovasc Surg* 1993; 106:709–717.

139. ten Berg JM, Maarten JS, Knaepen PJ, Ernst SM, Vermeulen FE, Jaarsma W. Hypertrophic obstructive cardiomyopathy: Initial results and long-term follow-up after Morrow septal myectomy. *Circulation* 1994; 90:1781–1785.

140. Heric B, Lytle BW, Miller DP, Rosenkranz ER, Lever HM, Cosgrove DM. Surgical management of hypertrophic obstructive cardiomyopathy: Early and late results. *J Thorac Cardiovasc Surg* 1995; 110:195–208.

141. Robbins RC, Stinson EB. Long-term results of left ventricular myotomy and myectomy for obstructive hypertrophic cardiomyopathy. *J Thorac Cardiovasc Surg* 1996; 111:586–594.

142. Schoendube FA, Klues HG, Reigh S, Flachskampf FA, Hanrath P, Messmer B. Long-term clinical and echocardiographic follow-up after surgical correction of hypertrophic obstructive cardiomyopathy with extended myectomy and reconstruction of the subvalvular mitral apparatus. *Circulation* 1995; 92(suppl II):II-122–II-127.

143. McIntosh CL, Maron BJ, Cannon RO, Klues HG. Initial results of combined anterior mitral leaflet plication and ventricular septal myotomy-myectomy for relief of left ventricular outflow tract obstruction in patients with hypertrophic cardiomyopathy. *Circulation* 1992; 86:II-60–II-67.

144. Marwick TH, Stewart WJ, Lever HM, Lytle BW, Rosenkranz ER, Duffy CI, et al. Benefits of intraoperative echocardiography in the surgical management of hypertrophic cardiomyopathy. *J Am Coll Cardiol* 1992; 20:1066–1072.

145. Siegman IL, Maron BJ, Permut LC, McIntosh CL, Clark RE. Results of operation for coexistent obstructive hypertrophic cardiomyopathy and coronary artery disease. *J Am Coll Cardiol* 1989; 13:1527–1533.

146. Cannon RO, McIntosh CL, Schenke WH, Maron BJ, Bonow RO, Epstein SE. Effect of surgical reduction of left ventricular outflow obstruction on hemodynamics, coronary flow, and myocardial metabolism in hypertrophic cardiomyopathy. *Circulation* 1989; 79:766–775.

147. McDonald KM, Maurer B. Permanent pacing as treatment for hypertrophic cardiomyopathy. *Am J Cardiol* 1991; 68:108–110.

148. Jeanrenaud X, Goy J-J, Kappenberger L. Effects of dual-chamber pacing in hypertrophic obstructive cardiomyopathy. *Lancet* 1992; 339:1318–1323.

149. Fananapazir L, Epstein ND, Curiel RV, Panza JA, Tripodi D, McAreavey D. Long-term results of dual-chamber (DDD) pacing in obstructive hypertrophic cardiomyopathy: Evidence for progressive, symptomatic and hemodynamic improvement and reduction of left ventricular hypertrophy. *Circulation* 1994; 90:2731–2742.

150. Slade AKB, Sadoul N, Shapiro L, Chojnowska L, Simon JP, Saumarez RC, et al. DDD pacing in hypertrophic cardiomyopathy: A multicentre clinical experience. *Heart* 1996; 75:44–49.

151. Nishimura RA, Trusty JM, Hayes DL, Ilstrup DM, Larson DR, Hayes SN, et al. Dual-chamber pacing for hypertrophic cardiomyopathy: A randomized, double-blind, crossover trial. *J Am Coll Cardiol* 1997; 29:435–441.

152. Nishimura RA, Hayes DL, Holmes DR, Tajik AJ. Effects of dual-chamber pacing on systolic and diastolic function in patients with hypertrophic cardiomyopathy: Acute Doppler echocardiographic and catheterization hemodynamic study. *J Am Coll Cardiol* 1996; 27:427–430.

153. Betocchi S, Losi M-A, Piscione F, Boccalatte M, Pace L, Golino P, et al. Effects of dual-chamber pacing in hypertrophic cardiomyopathy on left ventricular outflow tract obstruction and on diastolic function. *Am J Cardiol* 1996; 77:498–502.

154. Maron BJ. Appraisal of dual-chamber pacing therapy in hypertrophic cardiomyopathy: Too soon for a rush to judgment (editorial)? *J Am Coll Cardiol* 1996; 27:431–432.

155. Knight C, Kurbaan AS, Seggwiss H, Henein M, Gunning M, Harrington D, et al. Nonsurgical septal reduction for hypertrophic obstructive cardiomyopathy. Outcome in the first series of patients. *Circulation* 1997; 95:2075–2081.

75

RESTRICTIVE, OBLITERATIVE, AND INFILTRATIVE CARDIOMYOPATHIES

Ralph Shabetai

RESTRICTIVE CARDIOMYOPATHY

Definition

Restrictive cardiomyopathy is considerably less common than classical congestive heart failure. Its importance therefore lies primarily in properly distinguishing it from constrictive pericarditis, because of the dire consequences of mistakenly treating a case of constrictive pericarditis as though it were inoperable.

Restrictive cardiomyopathy must be considered within the broader spectrum of diastolic dysfunction (see Chaps. 3, 21, and 23). Diastolic dysfunction of some degree and of one or other type is common to many disorders of the heart.[1] Congestive heart failure may be produced by systolic dysfunction, diastolic dysfunction, or combined systolic and diastolic ventricular dysfunction that may affect one or both ventricles, in the latter instance either symmetrically or asymmetrically. The principal hemodynamic manifestations of ventricular systolic dysfunction are reduction of cardiac output and failure of cardiac output to respond normally to the increased demand of exercise (see Chap. 21).

The major clinical and hemodynamic manifestations of diastolic dysfunction are congestion and increased diastolic pressure. In some cases of heart failure, ventricular systolic function is normal or nearly so, whereas diastolic dysfunction is prominent, a syndrome that has been called diastolic heart failure.[2] Diastolic dysfunction may also occur because the loading conditions of the heart are abnormal. The ventricles are unloaded when there is severe mitral or tricuspid stenosis. Perhaps the most dramatic clinical picture of unloading the heart is that of constrictive pericarditis or cardiac tamponade, in which the basic pathophysiology is an impediment to diastolic filling. Severe diastolic dysfunction can also occur when the ventricles hypertrophy in the face of severe increase in their afterload, as in outflow obstruction or hypertension of

the systemic or pulmonary circulation. Diastolic dysfunction is also an important component of hypertrophic cardiomyopathy. Details concerning the pathophysiology, quantification, classification, and clinical manifestations of diastolic dysfunction are to be found in Chaps. 21 to 23.

In the past, erroneous concepts regarding restrictive cardiomyopathy have arisen and spurious claims have been made that restrictive cardiomyopathy can easily be distinguished from constrictive pericarditis. Thus, it is necessary to define restrictive cardiomyopathy quite specifically, albeit somewhat arbitrarily.[3]

A workable definition of *restrictive cardiomyopathy is a systemic or idiopathic disorder of the myocardium manifest by a clinical and hemodynamic picture that simulates constrictive pericarditis.* To meet the criteria, there should be increased jugular venous pressure with prominent *x* and *y* descents, a small or normal-sized heart, pulmonary congestion, and the absence of ventricular hypertrophy or dilatation. Ventricular systolic function should be normal, and there cannot be a stenotic valvular lesion or outflow tract obstruction. Although it is generally unwise to define clinical entities by rigid numbers, patients with a left ventricular end-diastolic dimension of 7 cm or more, myocardial wall thickness of 1.7 cm or more, left ventricular end-diastolic volume of 150 mL/m^2 or more, or an ejection fraction below 20 percent cannot be considered to have restrictive cardiomyopathy. The closer these values are to normal, the more likely is the diagnosis of restrictive cardiomyopathy to be correct. As a rough guideline, left ventricular end-diastolic volume should not be more than 110 mL/m^2 per minute and left ventricular end-diastolic dimension certainly should not exceed 6 cm.

Etiology

Restrictive cardiomyopathy may be either idiopathic, and thus be a true cardiomyopathy in the strict sense of the term,[4] or secondary to an infiltrative disease of the myocardium, in which case it actually is a systemic myocardial disorder or heart muscle disease rather than a primary cardiomyopathy. Unfortunately, these cases are usually referred to as restrictive cardiomyopathy, the advice of the World Health Organization report notwithstanding.[4] Idiopathic cases may be manifest by extensive fibrosis, but in some cases no pathologic substrate for the abnormal diastolic behavior of the heart is apparent.[5] Cardiac amyloidosis is the most common systemic cause, but not all cases of cardiac amyloidosis present as restrictive cardiomyopathy; some have a diastolic abnormality that differs from that of classical restrictive cardiomyopathy, and they also have major impairment of systolic function. Hemochromatosis can also produce restrictive cardiomyopathy,[6] although more commonly the cardiac manifestation of hemochromatosis is dilated cardiomyopathy,[7] which is often reversible when the iron load has been removed or decreased. Typical pathophysiology of restrictive cardiomyopathy is usual in the transplanted heart soon after operation and in 15 percent persists for at least a year.[8] Late occurrence or recurrence is thought to be evidence of late rejection. It may be confused or even associated with constrictive pericarditis[9] (see Chap. 25). Restrictive physiology characterizes a minority of cases of acute myocarditis. Other less common causes of restrictive cardiomyopathy have been reviewed recently.[10] They include *scleroderma,* in which the cardiopulmonary-pericardial hemodynamic abnormalities are complex (see Chap. 85); *carcinoid,* in which the restrictive pattern may be due to subacute tricuspid regurgitation, causing the heart to engage the pericardium (see Chaps. 76 and 86); and *sarcoidosis,* which usually presents with arrhythmia or conduction disturbances (see also Chap. 76). The infiltrative cardiomyopathies and endomyocardial disorders are discussed later in this chapter.

History

Unfortunately, many patients present when the disease process is far advanced and they already have pronounced symptoms of pulmonary and systemic congestion. The leading complaints usually include dyspnea, orthopnea, nocturnal dyspnea, or pulmonary edema, together with ankle swelling, abdominal discomfort, and increase in abdominal girth. In patients in whom the restrictive cardiomyopathy is secondary to a systemic disease, symptoms of other organ involvement may be elicited, but the heart may be the only organ involved even in what is more commonly a systemic disorder.

Clinical Examination

On examination, the patients have the classical findings of raised filling pressure on the two sides of the heart. Right-sided heart filling pressure judged from the jugular venous pulse is strikingly elevated. Commonly, neither the *a* nor the *v* wave is particularly prominent, but the *x* and *y* descents are often dramatic. Which of these two inward motions of the jugular pulse predominates varies among patients, but more

commonly it is the *y* descent. The central venous pressure can be assessed at the bedside by skilled analysis of the jugular venous pulse (see Chap. 10). The patient's thorax must be placed at an angle from the horizontal that optimizes the jugular pulsation. The *x* and *y* descents appear as sharp inward movements, the *x* synchronous and the *y* out of phase with the carotid pulse. In severe cases the peripheral arterial pulses reflect the tachycardia and the low stroke volume with diminished pulse pressure and, occasionally, a prominent dicrotic wave. The apex impulse is usually in a normal location and is of normal character, without left or right ventricular heave. In most cases there is no systolic murmur, but sometimes there is a systolic murmur of mitral or tricuspid regurgitation. A third heart sound marking the abrupt cessation of early rapid filling may be present.

When restrictive cardiomyopathy is secondary to a systemic disorder such as amyloidosis, extracardiac manifestations may be detected upon careful general physical examination, although one frequently has to rely upon abnormal laboratory findings.

Electrocardiogram

The electrocardiogram is almost always abnormal. Left bundle branch block is common, but some patients may have right bundle branch block. When restrictive cardiomyopathy is secondary to amyloidosis, generalized low voltage characteristically is present in the electrocardiogram, a finding that is in contrast to the apparent increase of wall thickness of the left ventricle demonstrated by the echocardiogram[11] (Fig. 75-1). In this instance, much of the increased wall thickness of the left ventricle represents infiltration with amyloid rather than hypertrophy. In idiopathic restrictive cardiomyopathy, sinus rhythm is often maintained until the end stages of the disorder, whereas a variety of major arrhythmias commonly occur in patients with cardiac amyloidosis.[12]

Chest Radiogram

The three major features that characterize the chest radiogram are absence of ventricular enlargement, left or biatrial enlargement, and the presence of the various manifestations of pulmonary venous hypertension and pulmonary congestion (see Chap. 13).

Echo-Doppler Cardiography

Echo-Doppler cardiography can provide crucial information pertinent to both the anatomic and physiologic abnormalities of restrictive cardiomyopathy. The study should show that neither the left nor the right ventricle is severely dilated and there should be no apparent thickening of the pericardium. Pericardial effusion may be detected, however, either as a manifestation of severe systemic congestion or because of pericardial involvement in some cases of cardiac amyloidosis. There should be no severe valvular abnormality, although some thickening of the mitral or aortic valve or minor calcification, presumably unrelated to the restrictive cardiomyopathy, may be found in older patients. When restrictive cardiomyopathy is secondary to an infiltrative disorder, the walls of the heart may appear grossly thickened; but in the idiopathic cases, ventricular wall thickness is well within normal limits. Frequently, both atria are moderately enlarged, and this enlargement usually exceeds that observed in constrictive pericarditis.[13] Careful observation of the image throughout diastole or, better yet, computer-assisted analysis shows a restrictive pattern of filling, in which early rapid filling is even more rapid than normal, but little or no further increase in ventricular size occurs throughout the latter two-thirds of diastole. This filling pattern is also characteristic of constrictive pericarditis. It has been proposed that restrictive cardiomyopathy can be distinguished from constrictive pericarditis because in restrictive cardiomyopathy early rapid filling is slower than normal, whereas in constrictive pericarditis it is more rapid.[14–16] While this observation is true of some cases, especially those least typical of restrictive cardiomyopathy, it is not true in the many cases of restrictive cardiomyopathy where the filling pattern is indistinguishable from that of constrictive pericarditis.[17]

Typically, the Doppler echo signal at the tips of the mitral or tricuspid valve shows a very prominent E wave, reflecting the abnormally rapid filling in early diastole (Fig. 75-2). The E wave also has a severely reduced deceleration time, indicating elevated left atrial pressure. Details of Doppler ventricular inflow and outflow signals have also been used to help differentiate constrictive pericarditis from restrictive cardiomyopathy (see Chap. 14). This subject is discussed later in this chapter and also in Chap. 81.

Other Imaging Modalities

Computed tomography[18] and nuclear magnetic resonance imag-

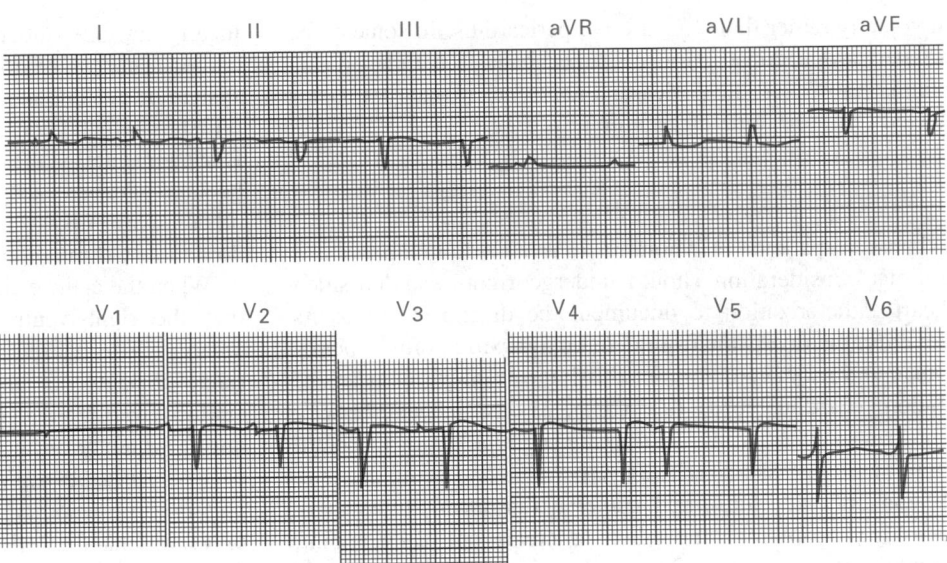

FIGURE 75-1

Electrocardiogram of a 62-year-old woman with cardiac amyloidosis. Portions of the echo Doppler study of the same patient are shown in Fig. 75-7. Note the low voltage, which is in striking contrast to the increased left ventricular wall thickness shown echocardiographically. There is also a ventricular conduction disturbance.

ing[19] are frequently used in these patients to help differentiate their condition from constrictive pericarditis. Obvious thickening of the pericardium greatly favors constrictive pericarditis or at least a major contribution by the pericardium. Conversely, the demonstration that the pericardial image by these techniques appears normal strongly favors restrictive cardio-

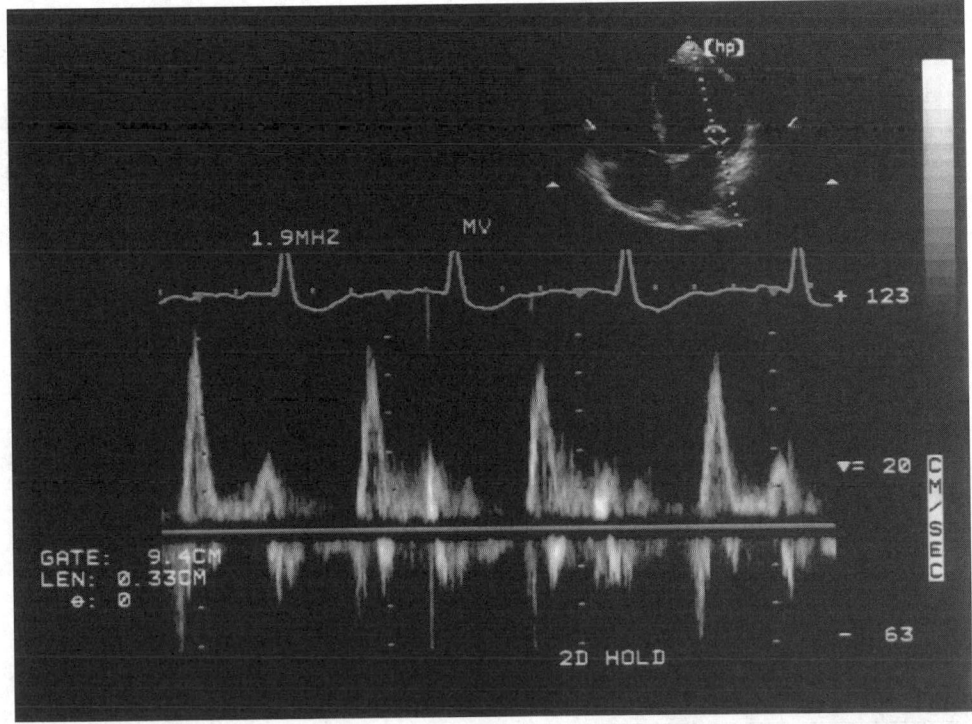

FIGURE 75-2

Doppler record of mitral inflow velocity from a patient with idiopathic restrictive cardiomyopathy. Note marked E dominance.

myopathy rather than constrictive pericarditis. In some cases of pericardial constriction produced by a thin tight epicardium,[20] however, the pericardial abnormality may not be detected by these imaging techniques.

Cardiac Catheterization

Almost all patients in whom restrictive cardiomyopathy is a serious consideration should undergo right- and left-sided heart catheterization to document the diagnosis, assess its severity, distinguish it from constrictive pericarditis if possible, and, in some patients, establish the etiology by means of endomyocardial biopsy (see Chap. 25). As in patients with constrictive pericarditis, extra care must be taken to obtain high-quality pressure recordings, particularly during diastole. If conventional fluid-filled catheter-transducer systems are employed, care must be taken to create optimal damping conditions—i.e., as close as possible to critical. The catheters should be short, the stopcocks and other interconnections as few as possible, and the connecting tubing rigid, short, and of relatively large bore insofar as possible. Transducer height and system calibration should be carefully double checked to ensure that simultaneously recorded pressures are strictly comparable.

When the catheter is introduced into the right atrium, the abnormalities of venous pressure detectable at the bedside are confirmed and can be more precisely quantified. Typically, the venous pressure is elevated, frequently to the high teens or even low twenties. The deep and steep nature of the y descent in the right atrium is the most striking feature of the tracing (Fig. 75-3). Since tachycardia is frequent, the record may need to be obtained at higher than normal chart speed.

Ideally, an independent marker of respiration should be recorded. This can be done either through a separate transducer system or by simultaneously recording the pulmonary wedge pressure, which should track the respiratory cycle faithfully. During inspiration the descent of the y wave in the right atrium becomes deeper, steeper, and more pointed,[21] whereas the other waves of the venous pulse and the mean atrial pressure do not vary throughout the respiratory cycle.[22]

When the catheter is advanced through the tricuspid valve into the right ventricle, a highly characteristic pressure emerges. The right ventricular systolic pressure is within the range of 35 to 45 mmHg. The early portion of diastole is characterized by a deep, sharp dip followed by a plateau, during which no further increase in right ventricular pressure occurs[23] (Fig. 75-4). When right ventricular and right atrial pressures are recorded simultaneously, the early diastolic dip of ventricular diastolic pressure is seen to correspond with the y descent of right atrial pressure, marking early rapid filling. Also, the plateau of right ventricular diastolic pressure is equal to the right atrial pressure throughout the remainder of diastole. Characteristically, these pressures are elevated considerably above the upper limits of normal for right atrial pressure. These features are identical to those of constrictive pericarditis (Chap. 81). Most authors concur, although one report has stated that the dip and plateau do not occur in restrictive cardiomyopathy.[24]

There is usually modest pulmonary hypertension with no pressure difference in systole across the pulmonary valve. Pulmonary arterial diastolic pressure is a few millimeters higher than the pulmonary wedge pressure, indicating a normal transpulmonary pressure gradient. The pulmonary wedge pressure is elevated, often to extreme levels. Contrary to earlier publications,[25] it is not uncommon for the pulmonary wedge and the right atrial pressures to be identical. The finding of equal filling pressures in the left and right ventricles, therefore, does not necessarily indicate that a patient has constrictive pericarditis (Fig. 75-5). On the other hand, a left ventricular filling pressure appreciably above right-sided heart filling pressure strongly favors the diagnosis of restrictive cardiomyopathy rather than constrictive pericarditis.[26] Left ventricular systolic pressure is normal, while the left ventricular diastolic pressure tracing shows the same abnormalities as those of the right ventricle. Severe pulmonary hypertension, in contrast to some earlier reports, does not occur in restrictive cardiomyopathy.[17,26] Because of

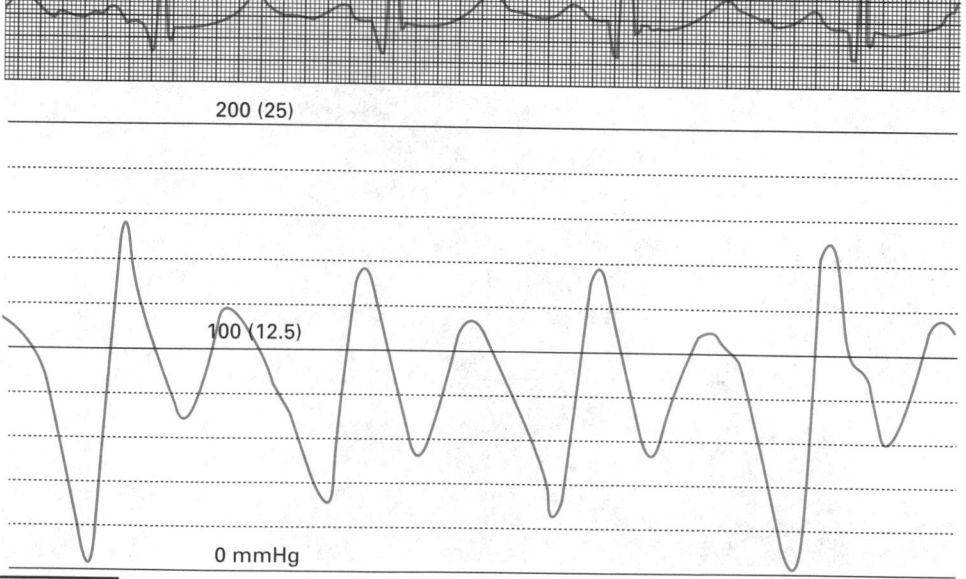

200 (25)

100 (12.5)

0 mmHg

FIGURE 75-3

Right atrial pressure tracing in restrictive cardiomyopathy. Respiratory variation is absent and the y descent is prominent.

suboptimal damping characteristics of the pressure recording systems, catheter motion, and different levels of intracardiac catheters, the *y* descent of atrial pressure and the early diastolic dip of the corresponding ventricular diastolic pressures are frequently not exactly equal. On the other hand, right atrial and right ventricular pressures equilibrate in mid- and late diastole, as do the pulmonary wedge and left ventricular diastolic pressures. In those cases that most closely simulate constrictive pericarditis, all four pressures equilibrate during this phase of the cardiac cycle.

Left ventriculography usually shows a normal ejection fraction[17,18] and the absence of major regional wall motion abnormalities. In the most characteristic cases, frame-by-frame analysis of the left ventriculogram shows unduly rapid filling in early diastole followed by little if any additional filling after middiastole. In some atypical cases, the early rapid filling is slow,[15] and many of these patients do not have the typical clinical picture of restrictive cardiomyopathy. Endomyocardial biopsy is an integral part of the workup of many patients with restrictive cardiomyopathy.[26] In cases where distinction from constrictive pericarditis is particularly difficult, the biopsy may furnish proof of myocardial disease or, by absence of such proof, lend support to the diagnosis of constrictive pericarditis. The biopsy may establish the cause of restrictive cardiomyopathy—for instance, cardiac amyloidosis (see also Chaps. 25 and 76).

Differentiation from Constrictive Pericarditis
(see also Chap. 81)

HISTORY

The history can provide important clues to this often difficult differential diagnosis (Table 75-1). A history of tuberculosis, trauma, or previous episodes of pericarditis or systemic diseases that frequently involve the pericardium, particularly collagen vascular disorders, favors constrictive pericarditis. A history of prior radiation lends more weight to constrictive pericarditis, but in many cases there is considerable myocardial radiation damage as well. Indeed, after extensive mediastinal radiation, as for treatment of lymphoma or in preparation for bone marrow transplantation, some patients subsequently

TABLE 75-1

DISTINGUISHING BETWEEN CONSTRICTIVE PERICARDITIS AND RESTRICTIVE CARDIOMYOPATHY: HISTORY

Constrictive Pericarditis	Restrictive Cardiomyopathy	Both
Tuberculosis	Amyloidosis	Radiation
Prior acute pericarditis	Transplant	
Trauma	Pseudoxanthoma	
Collagen vascular disease		
Prior cardiac surgery		
Neoplasm		

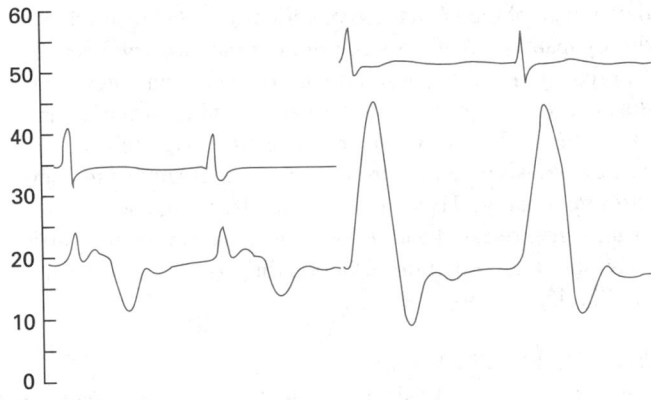

FIGURE 75-4
High-fidelity pressure tracing from the right ventricle and right atrium in a case of restrictive cardiac amyloidosis. Note the "dip and plateau" of right ventricular pressure and the deep *y* descent of right atrial pressure. The *y* descent was easily observed in the jugular venous pulse.

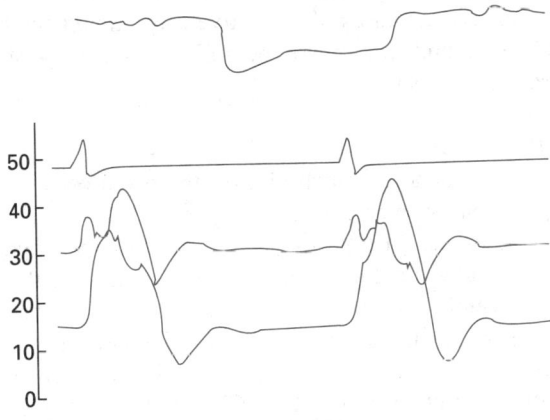

LV and RV

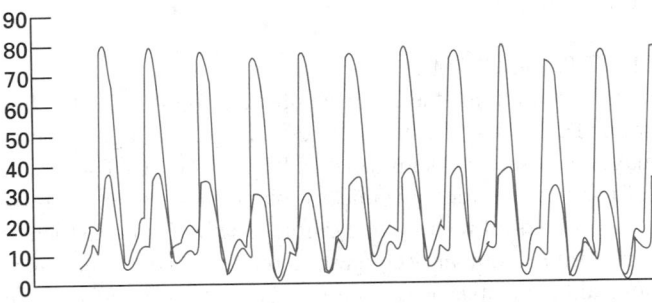

FIGURE 75-5
Top: Right-sided heart hemodynamic data from a patient with typical restrictive amyloid cardiomyopathy recorded with a high-fidelity catheter. Tracings from above down, the phase of respiration, the electrocardiogram, and right ventricular pressure with superimposed first derivative of right ventricular pressure. Note the characteristic dip and plateau configuration. The patient displayed a prominent *y* descent of venous pressure corresponding with the early diastolic dip of right ventricular pressure. *Bottom:* Simultaneous right and left ventricular pressure tracings from another patient with cardiac amyloidosis. In this patient, the typical restrictive dip and plateau pattern was not present, but diastolic pressure rose steeply throughout diastole and culminated in a prominent *a* wave reflecting atrial systole. Note also that during inspiration left and right ventricular diastolic pressures are equal, making differentiation from constrictive pericarditis more difficult.

develop combined constrictive pericarditis and restrictive cardiomyopathy.[27] A history of prior cardiac surgery favors constrictive pericarditis, but impaired myocardial preservation during cardiopulmonary bypass can result in restrictive cardiomyopathy. A history of disorders that involve the heart, such as amyloidosis or hemochromatosis, strongly favors restrictive cardiomyopathy. Hypertension and ischemic heart disease usually give rise to diastolic heart failure that does not particularly simulate constrictive pericarditis (see also Chaps. 21, 22, 23, 45, and 56).

PHYSICAL EXAMINATION

The results of the physical examination described above are the same as those found in patients with constrictive pericarditis and are therefore not helpful in differentiating these two conditions (Table 75-2). Some authorities claim that the third heart sound is usually not present in restrictive cardiomyopathy[28] but that a fourth heart sound is fairly frequent. Nevertheless, some typical cases of restrictive cardiomyopathy have a third heart sound, which may be difficult to distinguish from a pericardial knock.

ELECTROCARDIOGRAPY

Left or right bundle branch blocks strongly favor restrictive cardiomyopathy over constrictive pericarditis (Table 75-3). The same is true for left or right ventricular hypertrophy and atrioventricular conduction disturbances, although the latter are rare even in restrictive cardiomyopathy. Atrial fibrillation may supervene in either condition. Complex arrhythmias, however, are more common in restrictive cardiomyopathy than in constrictive pericarditis. Chronic, especially calcific, constrictive pericarditis can involve the epicardial coronary arteries and produce electrocardiographic changes that are otherwise more frequently found in patients with restrictive cardiomyopathy.[29]

CHEST RADIOGRAM

In both conditions, the cardiac silhouette on the chest radiogram (Table 75-4) is usually of normal size, although the heart may sometimes be somewhat enlarged. Atrial enlargement sufficient to be recognizable by plain chest radiography is more in favor of restrictive cardiomyopathy than constrictive pericarditis. Pulmonary congestion is a feature of either condition, although it is less pronounced in constrictive than in restrictive disease or classical congestive heart failure. A heavy, large ring of calcification is much more likely to be present in patients with constrictive pericarditis. Care should be taken not to mistake a calcified ventricular aneurysm (Fig.

TABLE 75-2

DISTINGUISHING BETWEEN CONSTRICTIVE
PERICARDITIS AND RESTRICTIVE CARDIOMYOPATHY:
PHYSICAL EXAMINATION

By definition is not helpful

TABLE 75-3

DISTINGUISHING BETWEEN CONSTRICTIVE
PERICARDITIS AND RESTRICTIVE CARDIOMYOPATHY:
ELECTROCARDIOGRAM

Constrictive Pericarditis	Restrictive Cardiomyopathy	Either
Repolarization changes	LBBB, RBBB, Q waves Atrioventricular block	Atrial fibrillation P mitrale

---

75-6) for pericardial calcification. Intracardiac calcification should be absent in both conditions unless the patient is old, in which case incidental calcification of the aortic valve or the mitral valve ring may be present. Calcification is best assessed by cardiac fluoroscopy. Striking radiographic left or right ventricular enlargement is not a feature of either condition (see also Chap. 13).

OTHER IMAGING MODALITIES

The contributions made by computed tomography and nuclear magnetic resonance[30] (Table 75-5 and Fig. 75-7) have already been mentioned. Echocardiography is a relatively insensitive means of detecting constrictive pericarditis except when pericardial thickness is greatly increased and especially when it is heavily calcified. Restricted motion of the coronary arteries is a feature of constrictive pericarditis but not of restrictive cardiomyopathy.[31] Furthermore, when the pericardium is greatly thickened, the epicardial coronary arteries are never located at a border of the cardiac shadow.[32]

ECHO DOPPLER CARDIOGRAPHY

The preceding sections emphasize similarities in the hemodynamic features of constrictive pericarditis and restrictive cardiomyopathy. It is therefore not unexpected that the two conditions share a number of Doppler characteristics, notably a restrictive ventricular filling pattern denoted by striking E dominance and an abbreviated deceleration time. On the other hand, in constrictive pericarditis, the ventricular septum is spared, and the constricting pericardium strongly enhances ventricular interaction,[33] thereby accounting for differences in the Doppler findings in the two disorders. In constrictive pericarditis, inspiration causes a more profound drop in pulmonary wedge pressure than in left ventricular diastolic pressure because the pericardial scar limits or, in severe cases, prevents transmission of variations in intrathoracic pressure to the ventricles. The pressure gradient that determines ventricular filling, therefore, is less during inspiration than during expiration. This abnormal hemodynamic effect of inspiration explains why left ventricular filling velocity drops substantially during inspiration. Pericardial space is invariate in constrictive pericarditis and therefore reciprocal changes are manifest in right ventricular filling—i.e., respiratory variation is

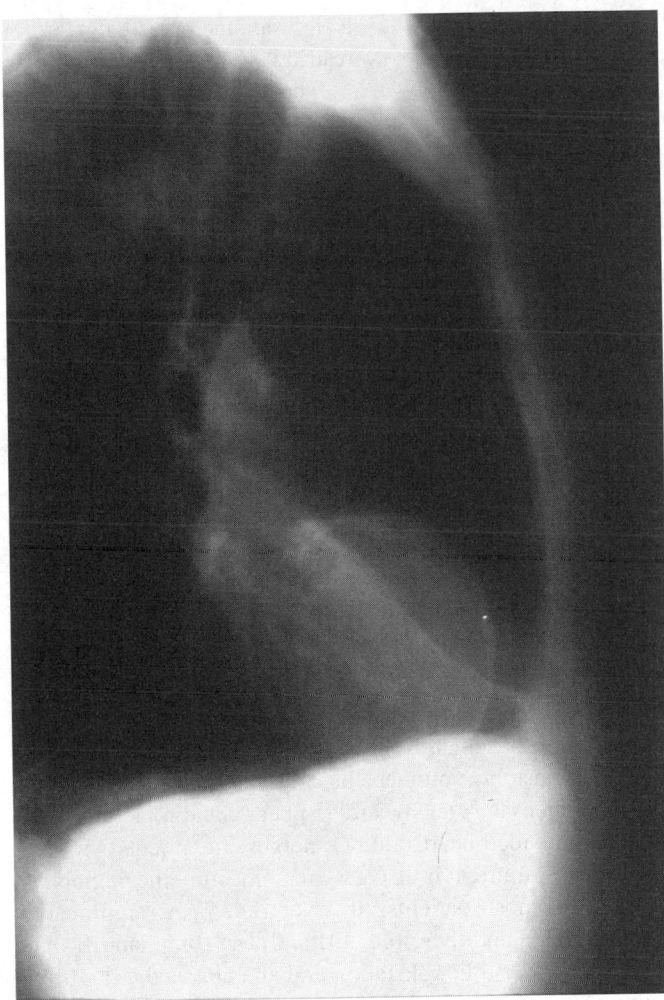

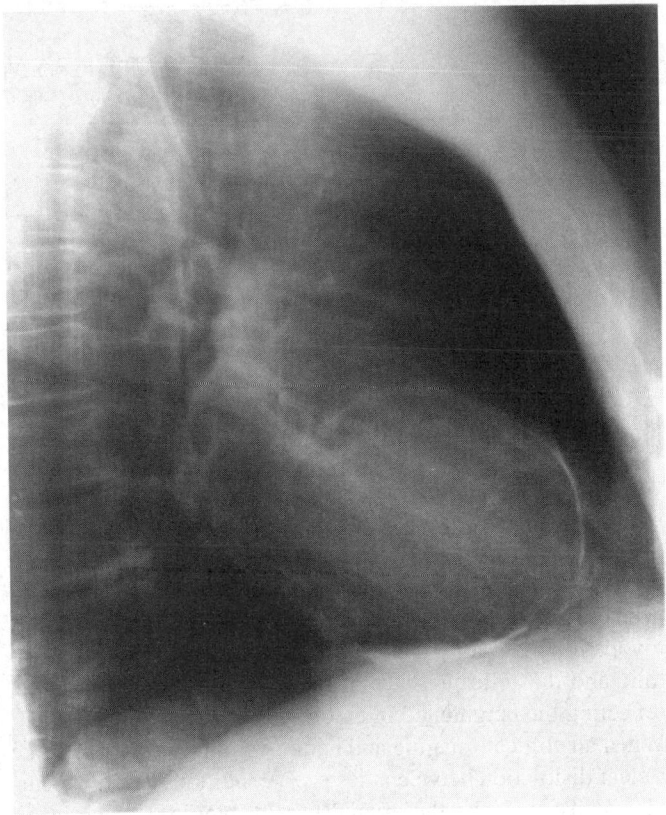

FIGURE 75-6
Lateral chest radiograms. *Left:* Calcified left ventricular aneurysm. *Right:* Calcified pericardium.

greatly exaggerated, showing a pronounced increase with the first cardiac cycle after inspiration begins. In normal subjects, respiratory variation in left ventricular filling velocity is less than 10 percent. In constrictive pericarditis, it may be as much as 30 percent and is uniformly at least 15 percent in patients with significant pericardial constriction.[34,35] Another consequence of the inspiratory decrease in the pressure gradient responsible for left ventricular filling is delayed mitral valve opening, which lengthens isovolumic relaxation during inspiration. In restrictive cardiomyopathy, isovolumic relaxation is also prolonged but is constant through the respiratory cycle.

In constrictive pericarditis, the rigid pericardium determines left and right ventricular diastolic compliance. Furthermore, no change in total cardiac volume is possible, but there is no impediment to transfer of volume from the atria to the ventricles. In restrictive cardiomyopathy, the stiff ventricles are responsible for massive dilation and ultimate failure of the atria. Consequently, the atrial contribution filling is impaired and diastolic flow reversal is a prominent feature. In constrictive pericarditis, flow reversals either are limited to systole or are both systolic and diastolic.[33,34]

In patients with restrictive cardiomyopathy, motion of the ventricular septum is restricted and ventricular interdependence is not increased. The pressure gradient for ventricular filling is therefore much less influenced by respiration and consequently respiratory variation in left ventricular filling velocity is normal or only slightly increased.

CARDIAC CATHETERIZATION

The important features detectable by hemodynamic and angiographic studies (Table 75-6) and their relative frequency in constrictive pericarditis and restrictive cardiomyopathy are described in Chap. 81. It should be reemphasized that *the demon-*

TABLE 75-4

DISTINGUISHING BETWEEN CONSTRICTIVE PERICARDITIS AND RESTRICTIVE CARDIOMYOPATHY: CHEST RADIOGRAM

Constrictive Pericarditis	Restrictive Cardiomyopathy	Either
Calcification	Absence of calcification	Absence of calcification
Moderate atrial enlargement	Massive atrial enlargement	

TABLE 75-5

DISTINGUISHING BETWEEN CONSTRICTIVE PERICARDITIS AND RESTRICTIVE CARDIOMYOPATHY: IMAGING

Constrictive Pericarditis	Restrictive Cardiomyopathy	Either
Increased pericardial thickness ⇑ Early rapid filling rate	Normal appearance of the pericardium ⇑ Early rapid filling rate	Absence of increased pericardial thickness ⇑ Early rapid filling rate

stration that left and right ventricular diastolic pressures are equal does not rule out restrictive cardiomyopathy, nor does it prove that a patient has constrictive pericarditis.[26] Contrary to a commonly held belief, the severity of pulmonary arterial systolic hypertension is not greater in restrictive cardiomyopathy than in constrictive pericarditis. For both conditions, a pulmonary systolic pressure approximating 40 mmHg is typical.[26] In constrictive pericarditis but not in restrictive cardiomyopathy, respiration has an opposite effect on both the systolic and diastolic pressure of the left versus right ventricle, reflecting the heightened interaction between the chambers.[36] When all clinical imaging and hemodynamic data fail to make a clear distinction between these two conditions, endomyocardial biopsy may be the crucial test (Table 75-7). The result may be obvious myocardial disease or an entirely normal biopsy. In the latter circumstance, surgical exploration should be carried out even if imaging techniques fail to show a thickened pericardium. As in the interpretation of most laboratory tests, however, clinical judgment is still of prime importance; nowhere is this more true than when the studies yield data compatible with mixed constrictive pericarditis and restrictive cardiomyopathy. In these patients, the clinician must make a decision whether to explore or to treat conservatively on the basis of the hemodynamic findings and the morphologic abnormalities found on biopsy. It is important to appreciate that in many cases, except for cardiac transplantation, there

is no satisfactory treatment for restrictive cardiomyopathy.

The literature documents at least one autopsy-proven case in which amyloidosis actually was the cause of constrictive pericarditis. Myocardial involvement in that case was minimal. At pericardiectomy, constrictive pericarditis was confirmed, but the patient died during the operation.[37]

Treatment

The clinician diagnoses restrictive cardiomyopathy with reluctance, since there is no satisfactory medical treatment. It is difficult to understand the pathophysiologic basis of the diastolic disorder characterizing restrictive cardiomyopathy. Not surprisingly, therefore, it is difficult to devise logical therapy. By comparison, the pathophysiology of constrictive pericarditis is simple (Chap. 81). The scarred, noncompliant, shrunken pericardium limits cardiac size from the end of early rapid filling until the end of diastole, thereby producing a marked increase in ventricular diastolic pressures and limiting ventricular end-diastolic volumes. In consequence, stroke volume falls, compensatory tachycardia appears, and a picture simulating right-sided heart failure emerges. In patients with diastolic heart failure, it is also easy to conjecture the pathophysiology. In most patients, the ventricles are significantly hypertrophied and therefore stiff and less compliant. If there is also slow diastolic relaxation and an enhanced atrial filling velocity, one has the rudiments of diastolic heart failure (see also Chap. 21). Since the hemodynamics and ventricular filling characteristics in restrictive cardiomyopathy are the same as those found in constrictive pericarditis, it is necessary to postulate that the myocardial disorder allows normal or even increased ventricular diastolic compliance in early diastole but that there is an almost infinitely stiff ventricle in mid- and late diastole. Since the structural basis for this behavior of the myocardium, be it in the myocytes or the collagen, is often not known, treatment is empirical.

When the filling pressures are extremely high with systemic and pulmonary congestion, significant benefit can be obtained from the use of diuretics. More caution in the diuretic dosage is advised in the treatment of restrictive cardiomyopathy than in that of conventional heart failure, because a relatively high level of ventricular filling pressure must be maintained in restrictive cardiomyopathy if ventricular filling is to be

TABLE 75-6

DISTINGUISHING BETWEEN CONSTRICTIVE PERICARDITIS AND RESTRICTIVE CARDIOMYOPATHY: HEMODYNAMICS

Constrictive Pericarditis	Restrictive Cardiomyopathy	Either
Equal diastolic pressures	Unequal diastolic pressures	Pulmonary arterial systolic pressure 40 mmHg Dip and plateau configuration of ventricular diastolic pressure Diastolic pressure equilibration
Discordant effect of respiration on ventricular pressures	Concordant effect of respiration on ventricular pressures	

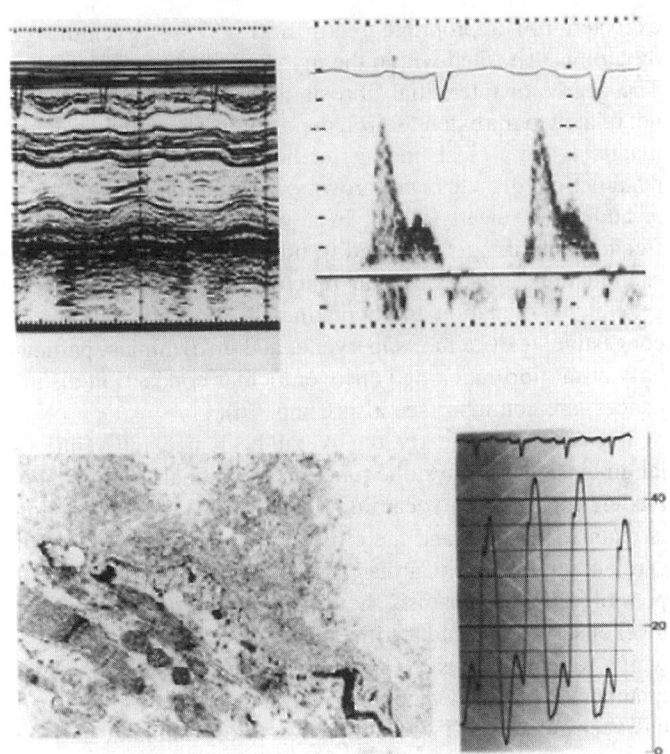

FIGURE 75-7

Data from the patient whose electrocardiogram is illustrated in Fig. 75-1. *Top left:* M-mode echocardiogram showing increased thickness of the left ventricular myocardium, which ordinarily would have suggested left ventricular hypertrophy. Calibration marks 1 cm. *Top right:* Doppler tracing of mitral inflow velocity. Note that velocity is maximum at middiastole. The atrial contribution to mitral blood flow velocity is considerably reduced. Calibration: single mark, 0.2 m; double mark, 1 m/s. *Bottom left:* Electromicrograph showing extensive replacement of myocardium by amyloid. *Bottom right:* Right ventricular pressure tracing. Note that the early diastolic dip and plateau of amyloid restrictive cardiomyopathy is not present because of tachycardia.

sustained. Digitalis and other agents with positive inotropic activity are not indicated if systolic pump function and contractility are not impaired. Vasodilatation should also be applied very cautiously, lest it further decrease ventricular filling and cause deterioration of the clinical condition. There is some evidence that in patients with hypertrophic cardiomyopathy, diastolic compliance may be increased by administration of calcium channel blocking agents[38] (see Chaps. 54 and 74). Extrapolation of these data from hypertrophic cardiomyopathy to restrictive cardiomyopathy is fraught with hazard. Nevertheless, attempts to treat the restrictive cardiomyopathy with these agents in the hope of improving diastolic compliance

TABLE 75-7

DISTINGUISHING BETWEEN CONSTRICTIVE
PERICARDITIS AND RESTRICTIVE CARDIOMYOPATHY:
ENDOMYOCARDIAL BIOPSY

Performed when diagnosis remains uncertain after following the paradigm

can be justified. On the whole, however, the results have been disappointing, and it remains extremely difficult to obtain a therapeutic benefit with the combined use of low-dose diuretics and agents such as verapamil.

THE INFILTRATIVE CARDIOMYOPATHIES

Amyloid Heart Disease

The most commonly encountered infiltrative cardiomyopathy is amyloid, the biochemical features of which have recently been reviewed.[39] Electron microscopy identifies amyloid as rigid, nonbranching fibrils. Endomyocardial biopsy, in addition to providing the diagnosis, establishes the histochemistry and quantifies myocardial damage and atrophy.[40] In primary amyloidosis, there is no coexisting disease except, in some cases, multiple myeloma; on the other hand, in secondary amyloidosis, a chronic disease such as tuberculosis or rheumatoid arthritis may be present. Rarely, multiple myeloma may be the cause of diastolic heart failure even when amyloidosis is not present.[41] The pathologic counterpart of reduced compliance is a stiff, rubbery heart that does not collapse when placed on the autopsy table. Although the coronary vessels and cardiac valves may be involved, this involvement seldom produces clinical manifestations. Amyloid deposits in the atria may allow atrial thrombus formation even in patients whose cardiac rhythm is still sinus. This unusual phenomenon is attributed to electromechanical dissociation.[42] So-called senile cardiac amyloidosis is common in the very elderly[43] but is often not detected until a postmortem examination is performed. When the amyloid is deposited between myocytes, classic restrictive cardiomyopathy results, but systolic failure may supervene if there is extensive myocardial replacement[44] (see Chap. 23). Calcium channel blockers should be used cautiously or not at all, to stave off systolic failure, because verapamil has been reported to precipitate this development in patients who have cardiac amyloidosis.[45] The severity of the combined systolic and diastolic abnormalities can be assessed by echo Doppler cardiography because both isovolumic contraction and relaxation are slow, whereas ejection time is short. Hence, the ratio of the sum of the two isovolumic periods divided by ejection time is greatly increased.[46]

The clinical and hemodynamic findings have been described above. The echocardiogram shows thickening of both left and right ventricular myocardium. In the earlier literature, the "sparkling" appearance of the myocardium was said to be diagnostic of amyloidosis,[47] but this finding has very poor specificity and should not be relied upon for diagnosis[48] (see also Chap. 14). In general, the prognosis is poor and treatment, for the most part, is ineffective.[49] Cardiac transplantation has been successful in a small number of cases, but in some, amyloidosis reappears in the transplanted heart.[50] Many cardiologists believe that the amyloid heart is highly sensitive to digitalis, which should therefore be employed with caution when systolic failure or atrial fibrillation supervenes. Chemotherapy with melphalan[51] has been tried, but its place in therapy has not yet been established.

Carcinoid Heart Disease

The picture of restrictive cardiomyopathy may develop in carcinoid heart disease due to infiltration of the myocardium by carcinoid. In some cases the restrictive pattern is produced by subacute tricuspid regurgitation with consequent dilatation of the right ventricle and engagement of the enlarged heart against the normal pericardium (see also Chaps. 76 and 86).

Hemochromatosis

Primary hemochromatosis is an inborn error of metabolism associated with HLA-A3 and HLA-B14 (see also Chap. 69). Large amounts of iron are deposited in the reticuloendothelial system, where they are harmless, as well as in the liver, heart, and pancreas, where they cause bronzed diabetes and heart disease. In addition to iron deposition in the heart, secondary myocardial fibrosis may also develop. Dilated heart failure is far more common than restrictive cardiomyopathy,[7] although the latter has been reported on several occasions[52] and may precede the advent of frank systolic heart failure. Unlike the situation in amyloid cardiomyopathy, excellent results can be expected from appropriate treatment (Fig. 75-8), even though the iron is deposited within the myocardial fibers themselves. The degree of interstitial fibrosis is variable and apparently not related to the extent of iron deposition. The patient usually manifests the typical findings of hemochromatosis—hepatic dysfunction, diabetes, and brown pigmentation of the skin—in addition to heart failure. In advanced cases, the heart is frequently strikingly enlarged to both clinical and radiologic examination. Left ventricular function tests show significant generalized dilatation and hypokinesis. Typical symptoms of congestive heart failure supervene, and arrhythmias, particularly atrial fibrillation and atrioventricular conduction disturbances, are common (see also Chap. 76).

In cases detected early, the overall heart size, left ventricular dimensions, and systolic function are normal. At this stage, the left ventricular myocardium is thickened, the dysfunction is mainly diastolic, and the clinical picture simulates that of cardiac amyloidosis. Cardiac dysfunction in the presence of possible hemochromatosis should lead to determination of the level of serum iron and ferritin and to endomyocardial biopsy, which reliably shows the typical findings. The fundamental treatment is repeated venesection until the excessive iron load has been removed. Two or more years of treatment may be required. Chelation therapy has been advocated, but its role remains dubious. Effective treatment is repeated phlebotomy,[51] during which iron metabolism and cardiac function are monitored long term. Secondary hemochromatosis may result from disorders such as a blood dyscrasia, which require enormous numbers of blood transfusions. The cardiac manifestations are identical to those found in primary hemochromatosis. Patients with sickle cell anemia may have preexisting cardiac dilation and hypertrophy prior to the development of hemochromatosis. In such patients, treatment consists of chelation therapy rather than phlebotomy.

Pseudoxanthoma Elasticum

Endocardial fibroelastosis is one of the many lesions that may be found in this rare but striking inherited disorder of elastic tissue metabolism. The endocardium is thick and may even calcify (Fig. 75-9) and be visible under fluoroscopy, resulting in severe restrictive cardiomyopathy.[53] Surgical resection of calcified bands of endomyocardium combined with mitral valve replacement resulted in medium-term improvement in a reported case[54] (see also Chap. 85).

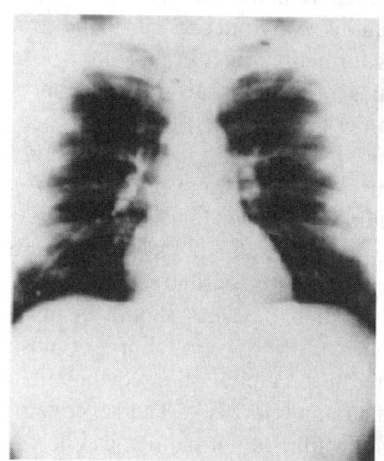
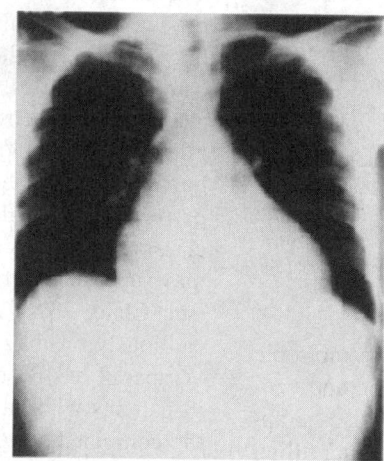
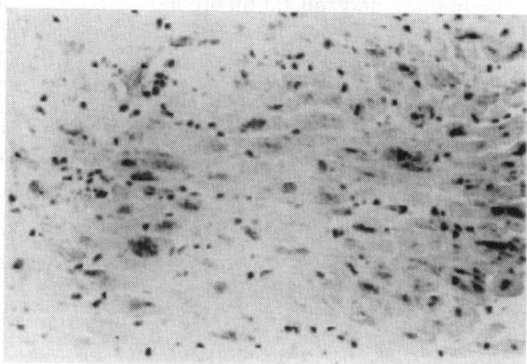

FIGURE 75-8

Chest radiograph of a patient with cardiac hemochromatosis. *Top right:* Before treatment. *Top left:* After several months of regular venesection. *Bottom:* Endomyocardial biopsy that established the diagnosis of cardiac hemochromatosis.

Sarcoidosis

Sarcoidosis is a noncaseating granulomatous infiltration primarily affecting the lungs, skin, and reticuloendothelial system but involving the heart in perhaps 25 to 50 percent of cases at autopsy, although much less commonly clinically. Roughly half the fatalities are caused by cardiac involvement.[55] Rarely, sarcoidosis is confined to the heart, but sometimes the combination of extracardiac sarcoidosis and cardiac abnormalities permits a presumptive diagnosis without biopsy.[55] The principal manifestations are arrhythmia and atrioventricular conduction disturbances, but restrictive cardiomyopathy has been reported,[56] presumably secondary to the granulomatous infiltration of myocardium. In one series of 88 patients with systemic sarcoidosis, 9 had heart muscle disease resembling idiopathic dilated cardiomyopathy, but one had restrictive cardiomyopathy.[57] In addition to granulomata, fibrosis may be present. Sarcoid granulomata appear to have a predilection for the basal myocardium,[58] with the twin results that a strategically placed lesion may produce atrioventricular block and that endomyocardial biopsies taken near the right ventricular apex may fail to reveal the lesion. Magnetic resonance imaging may detect scar or mass lesions due to sarcoid within the myocardium.[59] Radiolabeled technetium may be taken up by the hila when the hilar structures are infiltrated. When this finding is observed in patients who also have a myocardial filling defect, the diagnosis of cardiac sarcoidosis becomes a strong possibility.[60]

The prognosis is poor. Sudden death from ventricular tachycardia or fibrillation or the sudden onset of complete heart block is common. Cardiac sarcoidosis should be distinguished from giant cell myocarditis, which frequently pursues a more rapidly fatal course.[61] Prednisone has been advocated for treatment, as the granulomata in the heart are said to be sensitive. At present, the reported cases are too few to permit an authoritative statement on the value of this treatment, but they are frequent enough to justify a trial of corticosteroids in all proven or highly suspicious cases. Cardiac transplantation is an appropriate consideration in some cases.[62] Sarcoid may recur in the allograft but may be controlled by intensified corticosteroid treatment[63] (see also Chap. 76).

Glycogen Storage Disease of the Heart

A number of metabolic inherited disorders cause massive infiltration of the myocardium in infants and children. The best known is Pompe's disease, otherwise known as type II glycogenesis, which is an autosomal recessive disorder caused by a deficiency of acid maltase. In this disorder, absence of the enzyme alpha-glucosidase causes glycogen to be deposited in massive amounts in the cardiac and skeletal musculature. Manifestations appear in the first few months of life and almost invariably before the age of 11 years. Failure to thrive, weakness, and hyperreflexia are observed early in infancy.[64] The myocardium may become so infiltrated that the pathophysiology may resemble that of hypertrophic cardiomyopathy. Usually, however, the heart is massively dilated.[65] In either case, in spite of the heavy infiltration, the picture of restrictive cardiomyopathy does not appear. The diagnosis can be made from a skeletal muscle biopsy, which confirms the absence of alpha-glucosidase activity. The electrocardiogram shows left ventricular hypertrophy, at times with extremely high voltage, and the massively thickened ventricular myocardium is obvious on echocardiography. Regrettably, no satisfactory treatment has been developed and most patients die in the first year of life (see also Chap. 76).

A number of other rare abnormalities of glycogen metabolism may affect the heart. Nodular glycogenic infiltration occurs in the pediatric age group and is associated with tuberous sclerosis in half of the cases (see Chaps. 69 and 76).

Endomyocardial Fibrosis: Hypereosinophilic Syndrome

Two forms of the eosinophilic syndrome are recognized: *tropical eosinophilic endomyocardial* fibrosis and *nontropical eosinophilic endomyocardial disease,* sometimes referred to as *Löffler's disease.*[66] The major characteristics of the syndrome

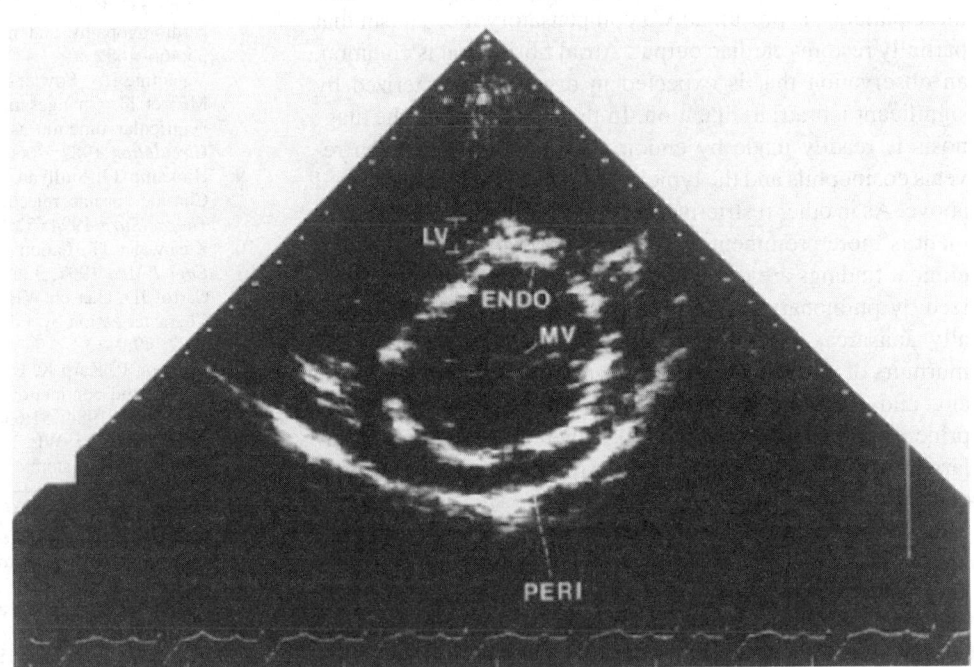

FIGURE 75-9
Short-axis view of the left ventricle (LV) of a young man with pseudoxanthoma elasticum. This echocardiogram was made at the level of the mitral valve (MV) and shows the calcified endomyocardium (ENDO) and an echodense pericardium (PERI). The endocardial calcification was clearly visible by fluoroscopy. (Courtesy Brian Hoit, M.D.)

are eosinophilia in the peripheral blood and an endocardial disease consisting of eosinophilic infiltration, fibrosis, and eventually virtual occlusion of the ventricular cavity by scar and thrombus formation. This results in a very severe form of restrictive myocardial disease, sometimes referred to as *obliterative myocardial disease*.[67]

It should be noted that the eosinophil responsible for endomyocardial disease is itself an abnormal cell. When compared with normal eosinophils, the cells appear to have fewer granules and to contain vacuoles. Adjacent to the abnormal eosinophil, myocardial necrosis is intense, indicating that the cells are toxic to the myocardium. Thus, Löffler's endomyocardial disease is considered to be an immunologic disorder caused by clones of abnormal eosinophils.[68] Endomyocardial fibrosis may affect either one or both ventricles. There does not appear to be a clear distinction between Löffler's syndrome and endomyocardial involvement in eosinophilic leukemia. In the acute stage, the endomyocardium is infiltrated with eosinophils and shows severe adjacent necrosis. This stage is followed by a thrombotic stage and, finally, the fibrosis stage, with virtual elimination of the ventricular cavity. As in many other restrictive diseases of the ventricle, the atria become greatly enlarged and the mitral and tricuspid valves are frequently incompetent.

Hemodynamic studies reveal the typical findings of restrictive cardiomyopathy, with pressures in the left and right ventricles characterized by an early diastolic dip followed by a plateau occupying the last two-thirds of diastole. The reduction in ventricular end-diastolic volume is responsible for a reduction in cardiac stroke volume, even when systolic function remains normal. Sinus tachycardia, a frequent finding in these patients, is presumably a compensatory mechanism that partially restores cardiac output. Atrial fibrillation is common, an observation that is expected in disease characterized by significant left atrial dilatation. In the earlier stages, the diagnosis is readily made by endomyocardial biopsy, which reveals eosinophils and the typical pathologic changes described above. As in other restrictive cardiomyopathies, atrial enlargement is more prominent than in constrictive pericarditis. The clinical findings are those of diastolic heart failure, characterized by pulmonary congestion, dyspnea, edema, and eventually anasarca, often with a large pericardial effusion. The murmurs of mitral and tricuspid regurgitation are usually present, and enlargement of the heart on chest radiography is principally produced by biatrial rather than ventricular enlargement. Pleural effusions are frequently visible on the chest radiogram.

Two-dimensional echocardiography shows the diminished volume of the ventricles, frequently associated with complete obliteration of the apices of both ventricles.[67] The ventricular diastolic filling pattern is that of restrictive cardiomyopathy, with early rapid filling predominating. In some cases, the endocardium, as in pseudoxanthoma elasticum, may show a speckled appearance on echocardiography. Nontropical eosinophilic endomyocardial fibrosis is not a common disease. Even though the author has a special interest in cardiomyopathy, and particularly restrictive cardiomyopathy, he has personally encountered only two or three well-documented cases in the United States. Most of the information concerning the syndrome therefore derives from major referral centers at which the staff has a particular interest in this syndrome. The work of Olsen[69] has been particularly useful to cardiologists encountering sporadic cases. The prognosis is poor, perhaps justifying resection of the endocardium, which has been performed in a few cases with some degree of success.[70]

Restrictive cardiomyopathy characterized by infiltration of the endocardium with toxic eosinophils has been described in the eosinophilia-myalgia syndrome (toxic oil syndrome).[71,72] This syndrome can be expected to disappear, because oils containing L-tryptophan were withdrawn from the market after they were discovered to be a cause of the syndrome.

REFERENCES

1. Grossman W. Diastolic dysfunction in congestive heart failure. *N Engl J Med* 1991; 325:1557–1564.
2. Soufer R, Wohlgelernter D, Vita NA, Amuchestegui M, Sostman HD, Berger HJ, et al. Intact systolic left ventricular function in clinical congestive heart failure. *Am J Cardiol* 1985; 55:1032–1036.
3. Goodwin JF, Oakley CM. The cardiomyopathies. *Br Heart J* 1972; 34:545–552.
4. WHO/ISFC Task Force. Report of the WHO/ISFC Task Force on the definition and classification of cardiomyopathies. *Br Heart J* 1980; 44:672–673.
5. McManus BM, Bren GB, Robertson EA. Hemodynamic cardiac constriction without anatomic myocardial restriction or pericardial constriction. *Am Heart J* 1981; 102:134–136.
6. Cutler DJ, Isner JM, Bracey AW, Hufnagel CA, Conrad PW, Roberts WC, et al. Hemochromatosis heart disease: An unemphasized cause of potentially reversible restrictive cardiomyopathy. *Am J Med* 1980; 69:923–928.
7. Skinner C, Kenmure CF. Hemochromatosis presenting as congestive cardiomyopathy and responding to venesection. *Br Heart J* 1973; 35:466–468.
8. Valantine HA, Fowler MB, Hunt SA, Naasz C, Hatle LK, Billingham ME, et al. Changes in Doppler echocardiographic indexes of left ventricular function as potential markers of acute cardiac rejection. *Circulation* 1987; 76(suppl V):V86–V92.
9. Hinkamp TJ, Sullivan HJ, Montoya A, Park S, Bartlett L, Pifarre R. Chronic cardiac rejection masking as constrictive pericarditis. *Ann Thorac Surg* 1994; 57:1579–1583.
10. Kushwaha JT, Fallon JT, Fuster V. Restrictive cardiomyopathy. *N Engl J Med* 1997; 336:267–276.
11. Carrol JD, Gaasch WH, McAdam KPWJ. Amyloid cardiomyopathy: Characterization by a distinctive volume/mass relation. *Am J Cardiol* 1982; 49:9–13.
12. Eriksson P, Karp K, Bjerle P, Olofsson BO. Disturbances of cardiac rhythm and conduction in familial amyloidosis and polyneuropathy. *Br Heart J* 1984; 51:658–662.
13. Borer JS, Henry WL, Epstein SE. Echocardiographic observations in patients with systemic infiltrative disease involving the heart. *Am J Cardiol* 1977; 39:184–188.
14. Tyberg TI, Goodyer AV, Hurst VW III, Alexander J, Langou RA. Left ventricular filling in differentiating restrictive amyloid cardiomyopathy and constrictive pericarditis. *Am J Cardiol* 1981; 47:791–796.
15. Janos GG, Arjunan K, Meyer RA, Engel P, Kaplan S. Differentiation of constrictive pericarditis and restrictive cardiomyopathy using digitized echocardiography. *Am J Coll Cardiol* 1983; 1:541–549.
16. Gerson MC, Colthar MS, Fowler NO. Differentiation of constrictive pericarditis and restrictive cardiomyopathy by radionuclide ventriculography. *Am Heart J* 1989; 118:114–120.
17. Meaney E, Shabetai R, Bhargava V, Shearer M, Weidner C, Mangiardi LM. Cardiac amyloidosis, constrictive pericarditis and restrictive cardiomyopathy. *Am J Cardiol* 1976; 38:547–556.
18. Isner JM, Carter BL, Bankoff MS, Pastore JO, Ramaswamy K, McAdam KP, et al. Differentiation of constrictive pericarditis from restric-

tive cardiomyopathy by computed tomographic imaging. *Am Heart J* 1983; 105:1019–1025.

19. Sechtem U, Higgins CB, Sommerhoff BA, Lipton MJ, Huycke EC. Magnetic resonance imaging of restrictive cardiomyopathy. *Am J Cardiol* 1987; 59:480–482.

20. Tuna IC, Danielson GK. Surgical management of pericardial diseases. *Cardiol Clin* 1990; 8:683–696.

21. Reddy PS, Curtiss EI, O'Toole JD, Shaver JA. Cardiac tamponade: Hemodynamic observations in man. *Circulation* 78; 58:265–272.

22. Shabetai R, Fowler NO, Gunheroth WG. The hemodynamics of cardiac tamponade and constrictive pericarditis. *Am J Cardiol* 1970; 26:480–489.

23. Hansen AT, Eskildsen P, Gotzsche H. Pressure curves from the right auricle and right ventricle in chronic constrictive pericarditis. *Circulation* 1951; 3:881–885.

24. Hirota Y, Kohriyama T, Hayashi T, Kaku K, Nishimura H, Saito T, et al. Idiopathic restrictive cardiomyopathy: Differences of left ventricular relaxation and diastolic wave forms from constrictive pericarditis. *Am J Cardiol* 1983; 52:421–423.

25. Wood P. Chronic constrictive pericarditis. *Am J Cardiol* 1961; 7:48–61.

26. Schoenfeld MH, Supple EW, Dec EW, Fallon JT, Palacios IF. Restrictive cardiomyopathy versus constrictive pericarditis: Role of endomyocardial biopsy in avoiding unnecessary thoracotomy. *Circulation* 1987; 75:1012–1017.

27. Applefield M, Wiernik PH. Cardiac disease after radiation therapy for Hodgkin's disease: Analysis of 48 patients. *Am J Cardiol* 1983; 51:1679–1681.

28. Chew C, Ziadi GM, Raphael MJ, Oakley CM. The functional defect in amyloid heart disease: The "stiff heart syndrome." *Am J Cardiol* 1975; 36:438–444.

29. Levine HO. Myocardial fibrosis in constrictive pericarditis: Electrocardiographic and pathologic observations. *Circulation* 1973; 48:1268–1281.

30. Rienmuller R, Gurgan M, Erdmann E, Kemkes BM, Kreutzer E, Weinhold C. CT and MR evaluation of pericardial constriction: A new diagnostic and therapeutic concept. *J Thorac Imaging* 1993; 8:108–121.

31. Alexander J, Kelley MHJ, Cohen LS, Cohen LS, Langou RA. The angiographic appearance of coronary arteries in constrictive pericarditis. *Radiology* 1979; 131:609–617.

32. Ramsay HW, Sbar S, Elliott LP, Eliot RS. The differential diagnosis of restrictive myocardiopathy and chronic constrictive pericarditis without calcification: Value of coronary arteriography. *Am J Cardiol* 1970; 25:635–638.

33. Santamore WP, Bartlett R, VanBuren SJ, Dowd MK, Kutcher MA. Ventricular coupling in constrictive pericarditis. *Circulation* 1986; 74:597–602.

34. Hatle LK, Appleton CP, Popp RL. Differentiation of constrictive pericarditis and restrictive cardiomyopathy by Doppler echocardiography. *Circulation* 1989; 79:357–370.

35. Oh JK, Hatle LK, Seward JB, Danielson GK, Schaff HV, Reeder GS, et al. Diagnostic role of Doppler echocardiography in constrictive pericarditis. *J Am Coll Cardiol* 1994; 23:154–162.

36. Hurrell DG, Nishimura RA, Higano ST, Appleton CP, Danielson GK, Holmes DR, et al. Value of dynamic respiratory changes in left and right ventricular pressures for the diagnosis of constrictive pericarditis. *Circulation* 1996; 93:2007–2013.

37. Daubert JP, Gaede J, Cohen HJ. A fatal case of constrictive pericarditis due to a marked, selective pericardial accumulation of amyoid. *Am J Med* 1993; 9:335–340.

38. Bonow RO, Ostrow HG, Rosing DR, Cannon RO III, Lipson LC, Maron BJ, et al. Effects of verapamil on left ventricular systolic and diastolic function in patients with hypertrophic cardiomyopathy: Pressure-volume analysis with a non-imaging scintillation probe. *Circulation* 1983; 68;1062–1073.

39. Hawkins PM, Lavender JP, Pepys MB. Evaluation of systemic amyloidosis by scintigraphy with labelled serum amyloid P component. *N Engl J Med* 1990; 323:508–513.

40. Arbustini E, Merlini G, Gavazzi A, Grasso M, Diegoli M, Fasani R, et al. Cardiac immunocyte-derived (AL) amyloidosis: An endomyocardial biopsy study in 11 patients. *Am Heart J* 1995; 130:528–536.

41. Schattner A, Epstein M, Berrebi A, Caspi A. Case report: Multiple myeloma presenting as a diastolic heart failure with no evidence of amyloidosis. *Am J Med Sci* 1995; 310:256–257.

42. Dubrey S, Pollak A, Skinner M, Falk RH. Atrial thrombi occurring during sinus rhythm in cardiac amyloidosis: Evidence for atrial electro-mechanical dissociation. *Br Heart J* 1995; 74:541–544.

43. Hodkinson HM, Pomerance A. The clinical significance of senile cardiac amyloidosis: A prospective clinico-pathological study. *Q J Med* 1977; 46:381–387.

44. Swanton RH, Brooksby IAB, Davies MJ, Coltarte JD, Jenkins SB, Webb-Peploe MM. Systolic and diastolic ventricular function in cardiac amyloidosis: Studies in six cases diagnosed with endomyocardial biopsies. *Am J Cardiol* 1977; 39:658–664.

45. Pollak A, Falk RH. Left ventricular systolic dysfunction precipitated by verapamil in cardiac amyloidosis. *Chest* 1993; 104:618–620.

46. Tei C, Dujardin KS, Hodge DO, Kyle RA, Tajik AJ, Seward JB. Doppler index combining systolic and diastolic myocardial performance: Clinical value in cardiac amyloidosis. *J Am Coll Cardiol* 1996; 28:658–664.

47. Bhandari AK, Nanda NC: Myocardial texture characterization by two dimensional echocardiography. *Am J Cardiog* 1982; 51:817–825.

48. Falk RH, Plehn JF, Deering T, Shick EC, Boinay P, Rubinow A, et al. Sensitivity and specificity of the echocardiographic features of cardiac amyloidosis. *Am J Cardiol* 1987; 59:418–422.

49. Kyle RA, Bayrd ED. Amyloidosis: Review of 236 cases. *Medicine* 1975; 54:271–299.

50. Hosenpud JD, DeMarco T, Frazier OH, Griffith BP, Uretsky BF, Menkis AH, et al. Progression of systemic disease and reduced long-term survival in patients with cardiac amyloidosis undergoing heart transplantation. Follow-up results of a multicenter survey. *Circulation* 1991; 84(suppl III):III-338–III-343.

51. Skinner M, Anderson J, Simms R, Falk R, Wang M, Libbey C, et al. Treatment of 100 patients with primary amyloidosis: A randomized trial of melphalan, prednisone, and colchicine versus colchicine only. *Am J Med* 1996; 100:290–298.

52. Short EM, Winkle RA, Billingham ME. Myocardial involvement in idiopathic hemochromatosis, morphological and clinical improvement following venesection. *Am J Med* 1981; 70:1275.

53. Rosenzweig BP, Guarneri E, Kronzon I. Echocardiographic manifestations in a patient with pseudoxanthoma elasticum. *Ann Intern Med* 1993; 119:487–491.

54. Challenor VF, Conway N, Monro JL. The surgical treatment of restrictive cardiomyopathy in pseudoxanthoma elasticum. *Br Heart J* 1988; 59:266–269.

55. Perry A, Vuitch F. Causes of death in patients with sarcoidosis: A morphologic study of 38 autopsies with clinicopathologic correlations. *Arch Pathol Lab Med* 1995; 119:167–172.

56. Tan LB, Dickie S, McKenna WJ. Left ventricular diastolic characteristics of cardiac sarcoidosis. *Am J Cardiol* 1986; 58:1126–1127.

57. Wenger NK, Abelmann WH, Roberts WC. Cardiomyopathy and specific heart muscle disease. In: Hurst JW, Schlant RC, Rackley CE, Sonnenblick EH, Wenger NK, eds. *The Heart,* 7th ed. New York: McGraw-Hill; 1990:1278–1347.

58. Fawcett FJ, Goldberg MJ. Heart block resulting from myocardial sarcoidosis. *Br Heart J* 1974; 36:220–223.

59. Chandra M, Silverman ME, Oshinski J, Pettigrew R. Diagnosis of cardiac sarcoidosis aided by MRI. *Chest* 1996; 110:562–565.

60. Nakamura T, Sugihara K, Narihara R, Adachi N Nakagawa M. Antemortem diagnosis of cardiac sarcoidosis by abnormal uptake of 201Tl in bilateral hilar lymph nodes. *Ann Nuc Med* 1994; 8:295–298.

61. Cooper LT Jr., Berry GJ, Rizeq M, Schroeder JS. Giant cell myocarditis. *J Heart Lung Transplant* 1995; 14:394–401.

62. Valantine HA, Tazelaar H, Macoviak J, Mullin AV, Hunt SA, Fowler MB, et al. Cardiac sarcoidosis: Response to steroids and transplantation. *J Heart Transplant* 1987; 5:244–250.

63. Oni AA, Hershberger RE, Norman DJ, Ray J, Hovaguimian H, Cobanoglu AM, et al. Recurrence of sarcoidosis in a cardiac allograft: Control with augmented corticosteroids. *J Heart Lung Transplant* 1992; 11:367–369.

64. Bordiuk JM, Legato MJ, Lovelace RE, Blumenthal S. Pompe's disease: Electromyographic, electron microscopic, and cardiovascular aspects. *Arch Neurol* 1970; 23:113–119.

65. Hwang B, Meng CC, Lin CY, Hsu HC. Clinical analysis of five infants with glycogen storage disease of the heart—Pompe's disease. *Jpn Heart J* 1986; 27:25–34.

66. Davies J, Spry CJ, Sapsford R, Olsen EG, de Perez G, Oakley CM, et al. Cardiovascular features of 11 patients with eosinophilic endomyocardial disease. *Q J Med* 1983; 52(new series LII):23–39.

67. Acquatella H, Schiller NB, Puigbo JJ, Gomez-Mancebo JR, Suarez C, et al. Value of two dimensional echocardiography in endomyocardial disease with and without eosinophilia: A clinical and pathologic study. *Circulation* 1983; 67:1219–1226.

68. Spry CJ, Tai PC. Studies on blood eosinophilia: 11 patients with Löffler's cardiomyopathy. *Clin Exp Immunol* 1976; 24:423–434.

69. Olsen EGJ. Morphologic overview and pathogenetic mechanism in endomyocardial fibrosis associated with eosinophilia in restrictive cardiomyopathy and arrhythmias. In: Olsen EGJ, Sekiguchi M, eds. *Restrictive Cardiomyopathy and Arrhythmias.* Tokyo: University of Tokyo Press; 1990:1–8.

70. Davies J, Sapsford R, Brooksby I, Olsen EGJ, Spry CJF, Oakley CM, et al. Successful surgical treatment of two patients with eosinophilic endomyocardial disease. *Br Heart J* 1981; 46:438–445.

71. Bolster MB, Silver RM. Eosinophilia-myalgia syndrome, toxic-oil syndrome, and diffuse fasciitis with eosinophilia. *Curr Opin Rheumatol* 1994; 6:642–649.

72. Berger PB, Duffy J, Reeder GS, Karon BL, Edwards WD. Restrictive cardiomyopathy associated with eosinophilia-myalgia syndrome. *Mayo Clin Proc* 1994; 69:162–165.

76

MYOCARDITIS AND SPECIFIC CARDIOMYOPATHIES

John B. O'Connell / Dale G. Renlund

Specific cardiomyopathies (also known as secondary cardio-myopathies; see Chap. 72 and Table 72-3), previously defined as specific heart muscle diseases, are cardiac muscle abnormalities associated with specific cardiac or systemic disorders.[1] Excluded from consideration are cardiac disorders caused by systemic or pulmonary hypertension and congenital cardiac anomalies. The specific cardiomyopathies represent a fascinating array of diseases with widely divergent pathogenic mechanisms. Cardiomyopathies associated with general systemic disease, neuromuscular disorders, sensitivity and toxic reactions, and the peripartum state are included in the category of specific cardiomyopathies. While more than 70 specific cardiomyopathies have been described, they are infrequent when considered as a group; when considered individually, they are rare. This chapter includes the inflammatory cardiomyopathies and cardiomyopathies associated with hyperoxaluria, gout, hemochromatosis, amyloidosis, Whipple's disease, and sarcoidosis.

MYOCARDITIS

Since myocarditis was initially defined by autopsy as any inflammation or degeneration of the heart,[2] unexplained heart diseases were commonly mistaken as myocarditis in the nineteenth and early twentieth centuries. While a relationship between infection and chronic heart disease (diphtheria) was postulated as early as 1806, the diagnosis of myocarditis could not be established during life because of lack of precise diagnostic tools until the 1970s. Even though the use of endomyocardial biopsy in patients with symptomatic heart disease of unknown etiology has provided greater insights into the pathogenesis, etiology, and treatment of myocarditis (Chaps. 25 and 72), the majority of patients with active myocarditis will likely remain unsuspected because the cardiac dysfunction is subclinical, asymptomatic, and self-limited.

Etiology

Multiple infectious agents have been associated with myocarditis[3–36] (see Table 76-1). The most commonly identified cause of myocarditis is coxsackie B virus infection. Neutralizing antibodies against two serotypes of coxsackie B virus were detected in 86 percent of sera from normal adults,[37] indicating that most adults have been infected by cardiotropic viruses. Sera from patients with idiopathic dilated cardiomyopathy have a six- to sevenfold greater likelihood of containing coxsackie B virus IgM than controls.[38] Electrocardiographic abnormalities were identified in 9 to 13 percent of those with symptoms due to influenza infection of sufficient severity to require attention by a physician during two separate epidemics.[39,40] Histologic evidence of myocarditis following traumatic death was identified in 1 to 3 percent of autopsies,[41,42] suggesting that the frequency of myocarditis is underestimated by analyzing data only from symptomatic patients.

Pathogenesis

The association of cardiac disease with infection by cardiotropic viruses prompted the hypothesis that the viral infection was responsible for the myocardial injury. Corvisart, as early as 1806, noted that a smoldering inflammatory process could result in progressive abnormalities in cardiac function after all evidence of the infective agent had disappeared.[43] Woodruff noted that histologic evidence of cardiac injury in coxsackie B virus–induced murine myocarditis only developed after virus was no longer detected in the myocardium.[44] Furthermore, elimination of T cell–mediated immune responses by antithymocyte serum or bone marrow irradiation with reconstitution following viral clearance attenuated inflammation with improved survival, less cellular infiltrate, and less necrosis. These observations led to the proposal that infective agents

TABLE 76-1

IMPORTANT CAUSES OF MYOCARDITIS

I. Infection
  A. Viral
    Coxsackie (A,B)
    ECHO
    Influenza (A,B)
    Polio
    Herpes simplex
    Varicella zoster virus
    Epstein-Barr virus
    Cytomegalovirus
    Mumps
    Rubella
    Rubeola
    Vaccinia
    Coronavirus
    Rabies
    Hepatitis B
    Hepatitis C
    Arbovirus
    Junin virus
    Human immunodeficiency virus
  B. Bacterial, rickettsial, spirochetal
    Corynebacterium diphtheriae
    Salmonella typhi
    Beta-hemolytic streptococci
    Neisseria meningitidis
    Legionella pneumophila
    Listeria monocytogenes
    Campylobacter jejuni
    Coxiella burnetii (Q fever)
    Chlamydia trachomatis
    Mycoplasma pneumoniae
    Chlamydia psittaci (psittacosis)
    Rickettsia rickettsii (Rocky Mountain spotted fever)
    Borrelia burgdorferi (Lyme disease)
    Mycobacterium tuberculosis
  C. Protozoal
    Trypanosoma cruzi (Chagas' disease)
    Toxoplasma gondii
  D. Metazoal
    Trichinosis
    Echinococcosis
  E. Fungal
    Aspergillosis
    Blastomycosis
    Candidiasis
    Coccidioidomycosis
    Cryptococcosis
    Histoplasmosis
    Mucormycosis
II. Toxic
  Anthracyclines
  Catecholamines
  Interleukin 2
  Alpha$_2$ interferon
III. Hypersensitivity

induce adverse immunologic responses that persist despite the eradication of the infective agent.

The specific immune responses that lead to the myocardial injury are incompletely defined. When serial sections of murine myocardium following infection with coxsackie B3 virus were analyzed, macrophages were present in the infiltrate until day 8.[45] After macrophage activity decreased, both effector (CD8) and helper (CD4) T cells were identified within myocardial lesions. At peak infiltration, some murine strains showed a predominance of CD8-positive cells while in others CD4 cells predominated, suggesting participation of both humoral- and cell-mediated immune responses.[46] In human subjects, T-lymphocyte and macrophage infiltration characterizes the immunohistochemical picture, whereas B lymphocytes and natural killer cells are absent.[47] T-lymphocyte subset analysis of human serum does not demonstrate consistency in dominance of CD4 or CD8 cells.

The mechanisms of injury when lymphocytes infiltrate the myocardium are unknown. Cardiac function improves in most patients as myocarditis resolves histologically. Cytotoxic injury alone cannot explain these reversible abnormalities. In the murine model, messenger ribonucleic acid (m-RNA) of perforin, the pore-forming protein mediating cytotoxicity, was identified in cytoplasmic granules of infiltrating cells by in situ hybridization.[48] Biopsy samples from patients with active myocarditis contain perforin granules in infiltrating cells.[49] Interleukin 1, interleukin 6, interleukin 8, tumor necrosis factor alpha, and other cytokines may cause reversible depression of myocardial contractility without resulting in cell death.[50] Whole-mount preparations and beating heart cell cultures of cardiac myocytes verify reversible depression of cardiac function when these mediators are infused in physiologic concentrations.[51] The effect of T cell–mediated immune injury, therefore, may be either irreversible as a result of cell death through cytotoxicity (perforin) or reversible as a result of injury mediated by cytokines.

Observations before safe endomyocardial biopsy techniques were developed suggested that antiheart antibodies in serum are common but reflect myocardial damage nonspecifically.[52] The addition of vital adult cardiocytes as a target in vitro has improved the specificity by identification of antimyolemmal antibodies in heart muscle disease.[53] When serum from patients with myocarditis was screened for autoantibodies, high-titer immunoglobulin G (IgG) with cardiac specificity was detected in 59 percent of patients with myocarditis and in none of the normal samples.[54] Antibodies with specificity for contractile and energy-transport proteins have recently been identified. Cardiac myosin antibodies develop in select murine strains following coxsackie B virus infection.[55] Injection of cardiac α-myosin, specifically, in these strains without infection results in myocarditis that is histologically similar to that seen following coxsackie B3 virus infection.[56,57] In sera from patients with active myocarditis, Western immunoblotting demonstrated reactivity of the 190- to 199-kDa fraction, which includes antibody to the heavy chain of cardiac myosin.[54] Autoantibodies against the beta receptor with a strong association to human leukocyte antigen (HLA) DR4 and DR1 phenotype have been detected in patients with dilated cardiomyopathy.[58] Antibodies to the adenine nucleotide translocator and branch-chain alpha ketoacid dehydrogenase have been identified.[59,60] Additionally, the antiadenine nucleotide translocator protein antibody cross-reacts with calcium channel proteins in the plasma membrane of normal cardiac myocytes. By blocking the calcium channel and interrupting high-energy phosphate transport, these autoantibodies may impair cardiac function, providing an attractive hypothesis to explain the reversibility of functional abnormalities following resolution of myocarditis.[61]

The precise role of the virus is unclear. Attempts to culture virus from human myocardial tissue have been frustrating. Coxsackievirus has been identified in a myocardial biopsy specimen obtained during life in a single adult case report.[62] While the role of the virus had been deemphasized following the popularization of the immune injury hypothesis, the identification of viral genomic fragments in myocardial samples from patients with myocarditis and dilated cardiomyopathy by in situ hybridization and polymerase chain reaction has caused reassessment of the role of the virus (Table 76-2).[63-80] Additionally, the prognostic significance of enteroviral positivity has not been resolved.[81,82] The variability in the clinical reports emphasizes the controversial nature of the methodology. Even if present, these genomic fragments may not necessarily be capable of replicating as intact cardiotropic virus but may serve as a persistent source of antigen to drive the deleterious immune responses.[83]

While infection of the heart with cardiotropic virus is probably common, progressive cardiac disease is unusual. In addition to the tropism of the virus, host immune responses play an important role in determining the severity of the clinical disease. When quantitative peripheral T- and B-lymphocyte populations were analyzed in patients with dilated cardiomyopathy and myocarditis, no consistent changes were detected.[84,85] However, immunologic assays demonstrate a reduction in the function of natural killer cells, antibody-dependent cellular cytotoxic cells, and suppressor cells and an increase in circulating levels of interleukin 1 and tumor necrosis factor alpha.[86-88] These immunoregulatory defects may predispose the host with a high antigenic load to develop immune responses that are not modulated by the natural inhibitory immunoregulatory mechanisms.

Clinical Manifestations

The clinical manifestations of myocarditis are variable and reflect abnormalities in left ventricular function, systolic or diastolic, and/or electrical activation with arrhythmias and heart block. In most instances, however, active myocarditis is clinically silent, with neither symptoms nor physical findings to suggest the diagnosis.

The most obvious symptom suggesting myocarditis is an antecedent viral syndrome. Flulike symptoms occur in approximately 60 percent of patients with active myocarditis.[89] Chest pain may occur and be typically ischemic, somewhat atypical, or pericardial in character. Approximately 35 percent of patients with myocarditis and congestive heart failure will have chest discomfort.[89] Occasionally patients will present with a clinical syndrome identical to an acute myocardial infarction, with left ventricular asynergy, electrocardiographic evidence of injury or Q waves, and ischemic cardiac pain.[90] In this syndrome at autopsy, the coronary arteries are widely patent, although viral coronary arteritis has been reported.[91,92] Coronary vasospasm has also been associated with acute myocarditis.[93] The clinical presentation in a large series of subjects with active myocarditis is summarized in Table 76-3.[93]

Left ventricular dysfunction and a syndrome compatible with idiopathic dilated cardiomyopathy identify a significant proportion of patients with active myocarditis.[94] These patients, who may or may not have an antecedent viral syndrome, typically have no clinical signs or symptoms specific for active myocarditis.

TABLE 76-2

MOLECULAR IDENTIFICATION OF ENTEROVIRAL RNA IN IDIOPATHIC DILATED CARDIOMYOPATHY AND MYOCARDITIS IN ADULTS

Investigator/Year	Method	IDC[a]	Myocarditis	Controls
Easton and Eglin,[63] 1988	ISH	6/13 (46%)	—	—
Kandolf and Hofschneider,[64] 1989	ISH	8/27 (30%)	19/81 (23%)	0/31 (%)
Bowles et al.,[65] 1990	S-B	6/21 (29%)	—	1/19 (5%)
Tracy et al.,[66] 1990	ISH	1/8 (12%)	2/9 (22%)	—
Jin et al.,[67] 1990	PCR	4/23 (17%)	1/25 (4%)	0/9 (0%)
Weiss et al.,[68] 1991	PCR	0/11 (0%)	1/5 (20%)	0/21 (0%)
Grasso et al.,[69] 1992	PCR	0/21 (0%)	—	0/20 (0%)
Keeling et al.,[70] 1992	PCR	6/50 (12%)	—	13/75 (17%)
Petitjean et al.,[71] 1992	PCR	22/45 (49%)	3/10 (30%)	9/23 (39%)
Schwaiger et al.,[72] 1993	PCR	6/19 (32%)	—	0/21 (0%)
Severini et al.,[73] 1993	PCR	1/10 (10%)	1/1 (100%)	—
Katsuragi et al.,[74] 1993	PCR	3/11 (27%)	0/1 (0%)	1/10 (10%)
Liljeqvist et al.,[75] 1993	PCR	0/35 (0%)	—	0/8 (0%)
Satoh et al.,[76] 1994	PCR	—	12/36 (33%)	0/10 (0%)
Nicholson et al.,[78] 1994	PCR	—	5/6 (83%)	0/8 (0%)
Ueno et al.,[79] 1995	PCR	7/42 (17%)	4/5 (80%)	—
Fujioka et al.,[80] 1996	PCR	6/31 (19%)	5/28 (18%)	5/23 (22%)
Andreoletti et al.,[81] 1996	PCR	11/19 (58%)	8/14 (57%)	—

[a] Positivities/total.

Key: IDC = idiopathic dilated cardiomyopathy; ISH = in situ hybridization; S-B = slot-blot hybridization; PCR = polymerase chain reaction.

TABLE 76-3

CLINICAL CHARACTERISTICS OF PATIENTS WITH ACTIVE MYOCARDITIS[a]

Age	42 ± 14 years
Sex	62% male
Ejection fraction	0.24 ± 0.10
Chest pain	35%
Increased MB fraction of creatine kinase (MB-CK)	12%
Flulike symptoms	59%
Increased erythrocyte sedimentation rate (ESR)	61%
Elevated white blood cell count	24%
Fever	18%

[a] Data are expressed as mean ±S.D.
Source: The Myocarditis Treatment Trial.[89,165] Reproduced with permission.

Patients may present with syncope or palpitations with atrioventricular (AV) block or ventricular arrhythmia. Myocarditis is a known cause of sudden death. In a 20-year review of sudden death among Air Force recruits, 20 percent had myocarditis documented at autopsy.[95]

Systemic or pulmonary thromboembolic disease is associated with myocarditis.[96,97] Myocarditis may be identified in multiple family members; in one report, a suppressor cell defect was detected predisposing to development of active myocarditis.[98] Patients with peripartum cardiomyopathy have a high frequency of myocarditis on endomyocardial biopsy.[99] The immunoregulatory changes during and following pregnancy may heighten susceptibility to viral myocarditis, and exposure to trophoblastic antigens may predispose to immune-mediated myocardial injury.

Laboratory Evaluation

BLOOD STUDIES

An elevated erythrocyte sedimentation rate occurs in 60 percent of patients with active myocarditis, and an elevated white blood cell count in 25 percent.[89] While elevated titers to enteroviruses or other cardiotropic viruses may be present, a fourfold rise in IgG titer over a 4- to 6-week period is required to document acute infection. Elevated IgM antibody titer to enterovirus may denote an acute infection more specifically than a rise in IgG antibody titer. Unfortunately, a rise in antibody titer documents only the response to a recent viral infection and does not indicate active myocarditis.

Abnormalities in peripheral T- and B-lymphocyte counts have been reported. The T helper-suppressor ratio (CD4/CD8) may be abnormal in some patients with active myocarditis. Peripheral lymphocyte subpopulations vary and the abnormalities lack specificity. While functional abnormalities in antibody-dependent cytotoxicity, natural killer cells, and T-suppressor cells have been noted, these findings have not been consistent and cannot be used as diagnostic adjuncts. Heart-specific antibody may occur in peripheral blood with myocarditis but also in many patients with dilated cardiomyopathy in the absence of myocarditis.

Creatine kinase MB release occurs in approximately 12 percent of patients.[89] Abnormalities in other cardiac enzymes, such as serum aspartate transaminase and lactic dehydrogenase (LDH), may also be present, but superimposed mild viral hepatitis or myositis may cloud the interpretation of these abnormalities.[100] In patients with acute pericarditis, elevation of creatine kinase MB fraction may be helpful in suggesting myocardial involvement.

Cardiac Studies

ELECTROCARDIOGRAM

The most common electrocardiographic abnormality is sinus tachycardia. The 12-lead electrocardiogram (ECG) may suggest myocarditis when diffuse ST-T-wave changes occur in the setting of a viral syndrome.[101] The possibility of a superimposed pericarditis complicates the interpretation of ECG abnormalities. Prolongation of the QTc interval and/or low voltage has been noted in patients with myocarditis compared to controls. A myocardial infarction pattern may occur in some patients (Fig. 76-1). Conduction delay is common,[102] and left bundle branch block is identified in at least 20 percent of patients. Complete AV block is also common, particularly in Japan, where acute myocarditis often presents with Stokes-

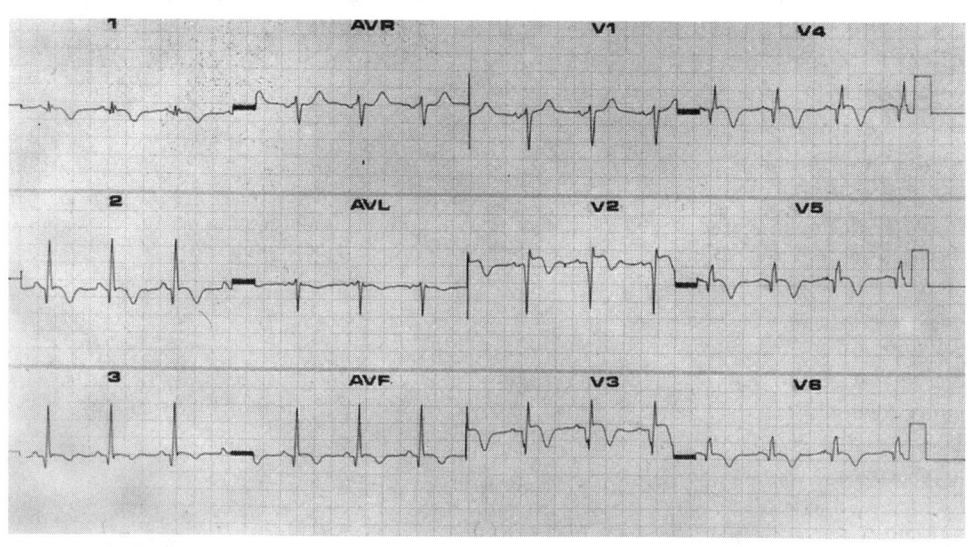

FIGURE 76-1

Twelve-lead ECG suggesting acute anterior myocardial infarction in a patient with active myocarditis. (From Costanzo-Nordin et al.[90] Reproduced with permission.)

Adams attacks from complete heart block. The complete heart block is generally transient and rarely requires a permanent pacemaker.[103]

Supraventricular arrhythmias are common, particularly when myocarditis presents with congestive heart failure or when pericardial inflammation is present. Ventricular arrhythmias may occur in patients with active myocarditis.[104] While the frequency is unknown, sudden cardiac death occurs in myocarditis. The cause of death in most cases is unclear, but both complete heart block and ventricular tachycardia have been postulated. Patients with recurrent uncontrolled ventricular tachycardia in whom no other etiology has been identified may have myocarditis when careful diagnostic analysis is completed.

ECHOCARDIOGRAPHY

Echocardiography is a useful tool in managing patients with active myocarditis. Left ventricular systolic dysfunction is common in patients with congestive heart failure. Segmental wall motion abnormalities occur, and left ventricular asynergy simulating a myocardial infarction may be identified.[105] The size of the left ventricular cavity is typically normal to only mildly dilated. Wall thickness may be increased, particularly if the diagnosis is established early in the course of the disease and inflammation is fulminant.[106] Ventricular thrombi are detected in 15 percent of those studied.[107] Digital image analysis may help differentiate the image texture alterations in active myocarditis from pure fibrosis.[108] These textural changes, however, are distinctly uncommon. The echocardiographic findings in active myocarditis may, therefore, mimic restrictive, hypertrophic, or dilated cardiomyopathy. Following resolution of inflammation, these functional abnormalities may persist.

CARDIAC CATHETERIZATION
AND HEMODYNAMIC ANALYSIS

The left ventricular end-diastolic pressure may be elevated in association with depression of cardiac output. In some patients, a restrictive hemodynamic pattern may occur early in the disease. Left ventriculographic studies confirm the segmental wall motion abnormalities detected on noninvasive analysis. Left ventricular angioscopy demonstrates white, light yellow, and reddish patches of the endocardium.[109] The angioscopy-guided biopsy is most apt to demonstrate the characteristic histologic change of active myocarditis in portions of the myocardium that appear red on visual analysis.

ENDOMYOCARDIAL BIOPSY

The development and refinement of percutaneous, intravascular endomyocardial biopsy techniques enable the repetitive sampling of the human myocardium during life with minimal discomfort and minor morbidity.[94,110,111] Essentially two techniques are available to sample right ventricular myocardium involving access through the right internal jugular or femoral vein. Intravascular biopsy of the left ventricle may also be employed, but potential morbidity limits its use. The right ventricular bioptome is positioned under fluoroscopy or echocardiography so that the interventricular septum is sampled.[112] A minimum of four to six fragments are obtained. Using the Stanford bioptome, typical samples are 2 to 3 mm in maximal diameter and 5 mg in wet weight. Samples are processed, paraffin imbedded, sectioned, and stained with hematoxylin-eosin and trichrome (Fig. 76-2). Special stains are employed if other diagnoses are considered, such as amyloidosis. The cardiac pathologist is careful to examine several levels of all fragments removed.

A number of investigators have applied endomyocardial biopsy to patients with unexplained congestive heart failure and/or ventricular arrhythmia.[94,113–143] As demonstrated in Table 76-4, the percentage of biopsies interpreted as myocarditis varies widely. A major reason for this variability is the different diagnostic criteria for active myocarditis. The number of lymphocytes necessary and the intensity of the infiltrate before the diagnosis is established are also a source of confusion. Leukocytic infiltrates are common in explanted hearts with dilated cardiomyopathy; i.e., more than 50 percent of these hearts have small foci not characteristic of myocarditis.[144] The variability of endomyocardial biopsy interpretation prompted a consensus panel of cardiac pathologists to propose a working standard, the Dallas criteria, to define active myocarditis as "an inflammatory infiltrate of the myocardium with necrosis and/or degeneration of adjacent myocytes not typical of the ischemic damage associated with coronary artery disease."[145] A sample is technically adequate only when four to six fragments are available for interpretation. "Borderline" myocarditis is applied when the inflammatory infiltrate is too sparse or myocyte injury is not demonstrated. Repeat biopsy is suggested. Dec et al. demonstrated a high frequency (four of six fragments) of active myocarditis confirmed by repeat biopsy in patients whose initial histologic samples demonstrated borderline myocarditis.[146] Critics of this definition

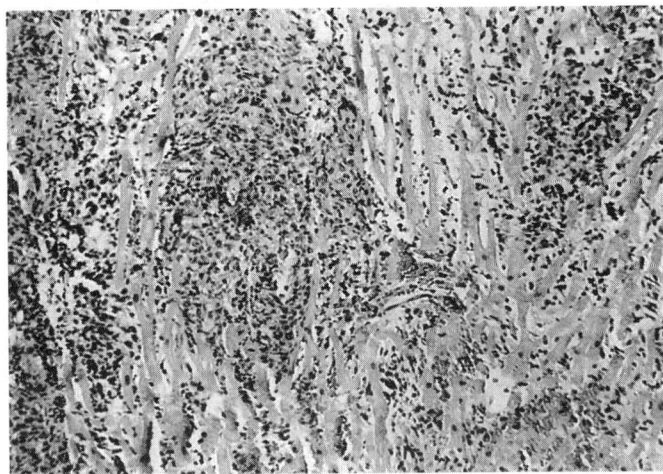

FIGURE 76-2

Photomicrograph showing the extensive lymphocytic infiltrates and myocyte necrosis of active myocarditis (H&E, ×20). (From O'Connell JB, Mason JW. Immunosuppressive therapy in experimental and clinical myocarditis. *Pathol Immunopathol Res* 1988; 7:292–304. Reproduced with permission.)

TABLE 76-4

UNCONTROLLED REPORTS OF IMMUNOSUPPRESSION
IN BIOPSY-PROVEN MYOCARDITIS

Investigators	Year	Total n	Improved n	Therapy
Mason et al.[94]	1980	10	5	CS, AZA
Sekiguchi et al.[158]	1980	3	2	CS
Edwards et al.[159]	1982	4	2	CS
Fenoglio et al.[117]	1983	19	8	CS, AZA
Zee-Cheng et al.[120]	1984	11	5	CS, AZA, ATG
Daly et al.[122]	1984	9	7	CS, AZA
Vignola et al.[141]	1984	6	5	CS, AZA
Fenely et al.[160]	1984	2	2	CS, AZA
Dec et al.[125]	1985	9	4	CS, AZA
Mortensen et al.[127]	1985	12	8	CS, AZA, CYA
Hosenpud et al.[128]	1985	14	8	CS, AZA
Salvi et al.[161]	1989	14	8	CS, AZA
Hobbs et al.[135]	1989	34	25	CS, AZA
Chan et al.[162]	1990	13	6	CS, AZA
Jones et al.[163]	1991	9	4	CS, AZA
Total		161	91 (56%)	

Key: CS = corticosteroids; AZA = azathioprine; ATG = antithymocyte globulin; CYA = cyclosporine.

have expressed concern that the criteria are too stringent and that myocyte necrosis is not necessary to establish the diagnosis.

Endomyocardial biopsy samples primarily the right side of the ventricular septum. Myocarditis may be focal or patchy. In cardiac allograft rejection, sampling error is less than 5 percent when four to six samples are analyzed.[147] Reports defining the sampling error of myocarditis have used autopsy hearts that are not comparable to the state of the myocardium at the time of endomyocardial biopsy during life.[148,149] When right ventricular endomyocardial biopsy has failed to establish the diagnosis, sampling the left ventricle may improve diagnostic yield. Myocarditis cannot be ruled out with complete certainty by biopsy but can be ruled in by morphologic features (see Chap. 25).

Endomyocardial biopsy must be applied as quickly as possible to maximize the diagnostic yield. Patients with peripartum cardiomyopathy have the highest yield when biopsy is performed early after onset of symptoms.[99] Resolution of active myocarditis has been documented within 4 days of initial biopsy, with progressive clearing over several weeks on serial biopsy.[150] Progression of active myocarditis to dilated cardiomyopathy has been documented when serial biopsies are performed.[151]

NONINVASIVE STUDIES

While technetium-99m-pyrophosphate scintigraphy, thallium-201 myocardial imaging, and gated blood pool scanning have not shown diagnostic potential in myocarditis, imaging with gallium 67, an inflammation-avid radioisotope, has shown promise as a screening method for active myocarditis.[121]

Technical variations in imaging have precluded its application to a large population. Indium 111–antimyosin monoclonal antibody is an isotope that is avid for the injured myocardium. Application of this technique to patients with suspected myocarditis has demonstrated a sensitivity of 83 percent, a specificity of 53 percent, and a positive predictive value of a normal scan of 92 percent.[152] In those patients who were antimyosin antibody–positive and biopsy-negative, the possibility of inflammation undetected by biopsy has been considered. Antimyosin imaging, however, detects myocyte injury independent of etiology, and noninflammatory causes of heart muscle injury in young patients may cause false-positive scans (see also Chap. 17).

Tissue alterations associated with myocarditis may be identifiable using magnetic resonance imaging.[153] Preliminary results suggest that myocardial inflammation may induce abnormal signal intensity of the myocardial walls. Analysis in a large patient population has not been reported, and consequently the reliability cannot be judged. Despite the promise of noninvasive techniques, endomyocardial biopsy remains the diagnostic standard.

Natural History

In all likelihood the majority of patients have a self-limited disease that is asymptomatic at onset and produces no residual evidence of cardiac functional impairment. Some patients, however, will die suddenly and unpredictably. Before the widespread application of endomyocardial biopsy, it was recognized that approximately one-third of patients who recover from active myocarditis will have residual functional abnormalities ranging from minor ECG changes to congestive heart failure. Histologic and clinical findings of progression from active myocarditis to dilated cardiomyopathy have been documented in patients who undergo endomyocardial biopsy to document myocarditis, presumably those with a more severe form of the disease.[154] Because endomyocardial biopsy has been applied to only a small percentage of the patients with this disease, however, the frequency of progression cannot be ascertained and is probably overestimated.

Treatment

If the patient presents with left ventricular dysfunction, the management is similar to that of other forms of congestive heart failure (Chap. 23). Sodium restriction, digitalis glycosides, diuretics, and vasodilators should be administered. In profound hemodynamic compromise, an aggressive approach to the management of shock should be employed, including intravenous inotropic and vasodilator agents, intraaortic balloon pump, and mechanical left ventricular assistance. Spontaneous improvement may occur despite rather profound abnormalities of hemodynamic function; therefore, cardiac transplantation should be considered only when aggressive left ventricular support has been attempted and an adequate time for recovery allowed. Cardiac transplantation in patients with active immune-mediated myocardial injury is associated with a high early postoperative mortality due to rejection (Fig. 76-3).[155] The immunologic milieu of activated T lymphocytes and humoral antibodies committed to myocyte antigens offers a donor heart an aggressive immune system from the very onset.

Laboratory animals forced to perform regular physical exercise following infection with cardiotropic viruses experienced an increased intensity of the inflammatory response, with increased necrosis and higher mortality.[156] In vitro study of the infected hearts demonstrated cardiac dilatation, deposition of antiheart antibody, and lymphocyte activation to heart-specific antigen.[157] Either augmented immune responses or intensification of virus-mediated injury is thought to account for this phenomenon. It is prudent, therefore, to suggest that patients with active myocarditis restrict their physical activity until resolution of inflammatory infiltrate is documented.

A higher risk of mural thrombosis with subsequent thromboemboli has been observed in the animal model and isolated human reports.[96,97] It has been suggested that patients with active myocarditis receive anticoagulant therapy even when left ventricular dysfunction is only mild and that patients with histologically proved active myocarditis should receive oral anticoagulation (warfarin) until resolution of myocarditis.

Twenty-four-hour ambulatory monitoring demonstrates runs of nonsustained ventricular tachycardia in 25 percent of patients with even mild myocarditis.[104] Myocarditis may present with recurrent episodes of ventricular tachycardia and syncope or even sudden death. Although antiarrhythmic therapy has not been studied carefully in this population, controlling ventricular arrhythmia temporarily until the myocardial inflammation subsides may be warranted. Antiarrhythmic agents that adversely affect left ventricular function should be avoided, and long-term treatment of the ventricular arrhythmia by amiodarone or an implantable cardioverter/defibrillator (ICD) should be applied only after all other attempts at controlling arrhythmia have failed and adequate time for improvement in the histology has passed. A temporary pacemaker should be considered for complete AV block (see Chaps. 33 and 34).

Following the initial demonstration that 5 of 10 patients with biopsy-proved myocarditis responded when treated with prednisone and azathioprine,[94] a number of uncontrolled and nonrandomized investigations suggested a possible role for immunosuppression.[94,117,120,122,125,127,128,135,141,158-163] Unfortunately, most of these reports antedated the Dallas criteria—i.e., the histologic standards for entry were inconsistent, and immunosuppressive therapy was not standardized within or among the trials. A prospective randomized trial of prednisone in patients with dilated cardiomyopathy who did not meet Dallas criteria for active myocarditis identified early improvement in a "reactive" group that was not sustained by 6 months.[164] The natural history of active myocarditis is unknown, and the reported improvement rates could conceivably reflect only the natural history of the disease. Unfortunately, the significant morbidity associated with immunosuppression was not emphasized in these reports.

To determine prospectively whether or not immunosuppression is beneficial in myocarditis, the multicenter Myocarditis Treatment Trial was organized.[165] Eligible subjects with a histopathologic diagnosis of myocarditis and a left ventricular ejection fraction below 0.45 were randomized to receive conventional therapy of heart failure alone or conventional therapy combined with a 24-week regimen of immunosuppression. Immunosuppressive therapy consisted of either prednisone and azathioprine or prednisone and cyclosporine. The change in left ventricular ejection fraction 28 weeks after randomization was the primary end point. The results indicated that patients with active myocarditis who did not receive immunosuppression were as likely to show an improvement in ejection fraction as those who received immunosuppression (Fig. 76-4).[166] Ejection fraction improved from 0.25 to 0.34. There was also no significant difference in mortality between the two groups (Fig. 76-5). The variables that predicted an improvement in left ventricular ejection fraction included a higher baseline ejection fraction, less intensive conventional drug therapy requirement, and a shorter duration of the disease. However, the treatment assignment was not predictive of improvement.

These data do not support the routine administration of immunosuppression in patients with active myocarditis. However, no patient in the group treated with immunosuppression deteriorated. Consequently, these results do not preclude the use of immunosuppression in patients with a deteriorating clini-

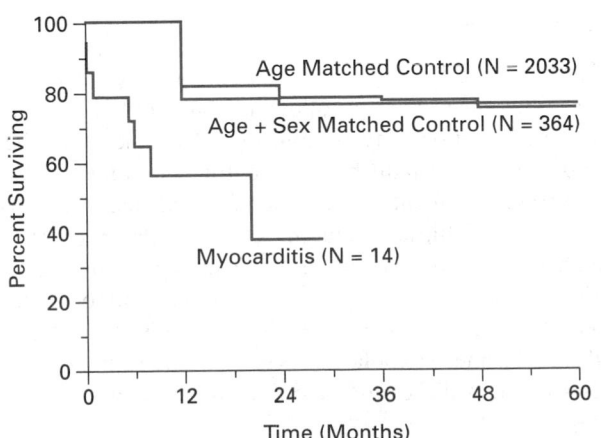

FIGURE 76-3

Actuarial survival of 14 patients with active myocarditis following cardiac transplantation. (From O'Connell et al.[155] Reproduced with permission.)

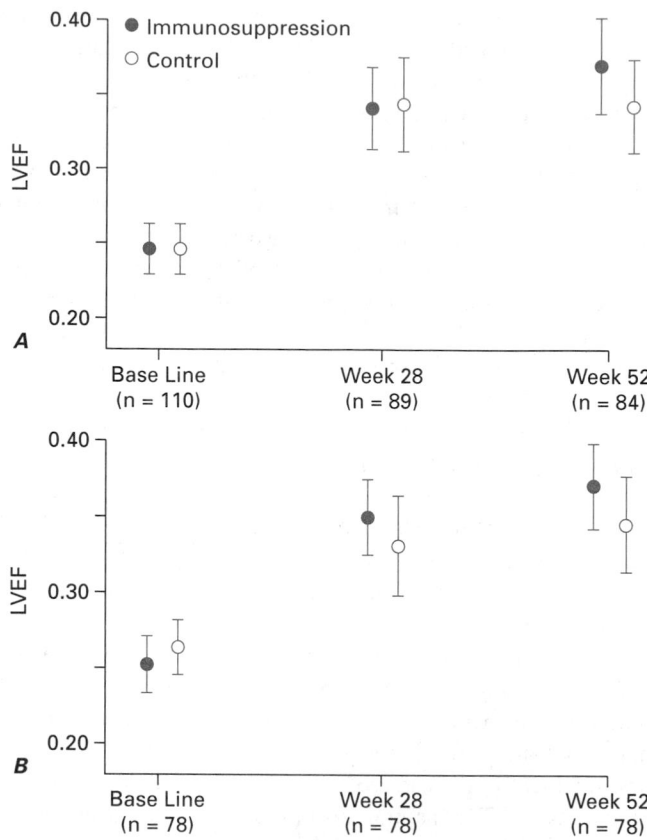

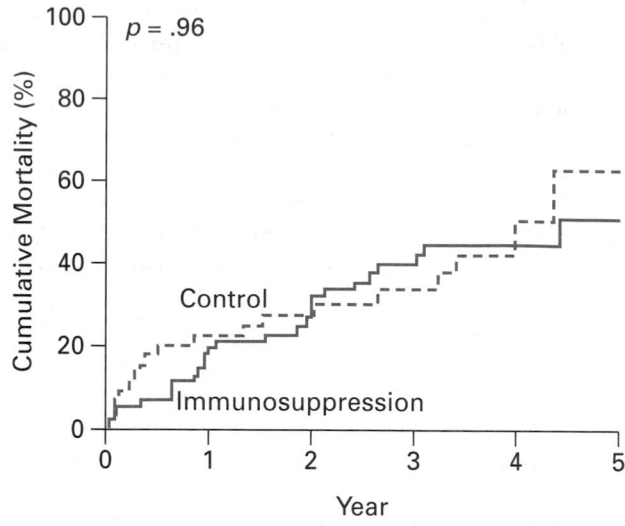

FIGURE 76-5
Actuarial mortality from the Myocarditis Treatment Trial indicating no difference between treatment groups. (From Mason et al.[166] Reproduced with permission.)

FIGURE 76-4
Sequential changes in left ventricular ejection fraction (LVEF) from all subjects (*A*) and only those in whom three serial studies were available (*B*), indicating equal improvement in both treatment groups of the Myocarditis Treatment Trial. (From Mason et al.[166] Reproduced with permission.)

cal state. The role of antiviral therapy or other immunologic modalities such as interferon or tacrolimus has not been studied in sufficient numbers of patients to be considered at this time.

SPECIFIC CAUSES OF MYOCARDITIS

Chagas' Disease

American trypanosomiasis, or Chagas' disease, is the most common cause of congestive heart failure in the world.[31] This condition results from infection with *Trypanosoma cruzi* and is endemic to rural South and Central America. In the chronic form of the illness, the autonomic ganglia of the gastrointestinal tract are affected, leading to megacolon and megaesophagus. The characteristics of the cardiac disease include congestive heart failure, heart block, and arrhythmia.

Although the presence of the trypanosomes can be documented, cellular and humoral immune responses may be responsible for the myocardial injury.[167] Various antiheart antibodies have also been detected in high frequency in patients with Chagas' disease. Endomyocardial biopsy may show active myocarditis using the Dallas criteria.[168] Noninvasive as-

sessment commonly shows segmental wall motion abnormalities, specifically apical aneurysms. The ECG may show complete heart block, AV block, or right bundle branch block with or without fascicular block in 11 percent of infected individuals.[169] Elevated antibody titers to *T. cruzi* may lead to suspicion of the diagnosis. Ventricular arrhythmias may require antiarrhythmic drugs, including amiodarone.[170]

The treatment of Chagas' disease includes a pacemaker if warranted for complete heart block and standard therapy for congestive heart failure as outlined for other forms of myocarditis. Nifurtimox should be administered if the disease has not previously been treated and may be used as prophylaxis if there is a high likelihood of recurrence, such as following immunosuppressive therapy. The role of immunosuppression therapy for Chagasic myocarditis is controversial.

Toxoplasmosis

Acute infection by *Toxoplasma gondii* may result in active myocarditis, particularly following cardiac transplantation when the infection may be transmitted by the donor heart. The diagnosis is established by identification of *Toxoplasma* cysts in areas of focal myocyte necrosis, edema, and a mixed inflammatory infiltrate including plasma cells, macrophages, lymphocytes, and eosinophils.[171] The organisms are ordinarily seen within the myocytes. A rise in antibody titer to *T. gondii* is commonly detected. Treatment is pyrimethamine and sulfadiazine. Toxoplasmosis is a curable form of myocarditis when it is discovered and treated early.

Cytomegalovirus

Cytomegalovirus may lead to myocarditis in the general population, but ordinarily the myocarditis is self-limited and asymptomatic. In the cardiac transplant recipient, however, cytomegalovirus myocarditis may become a more serious disease resulting in cardiac dysfunction.[172] The treatment of cytomegalovirus myocarditis is intravenous ganciclovir, which effectively eradicates the virus. Early cytomegalovirus infection correlates with the development of allograft coronary artery disease, the major cause of death beyond the first year after cardiac transplantation. It is proposed that infection of either subintimal fibroblasts or endothelial cells results in immunologic injury that predisposes to this potentially fatal condition.

Lyme Carditis

Infection with the spirochete *Borrelia burgdorferi* introduced by a tick bite may result in Lyme disease, which is characterized by erythema chronica migrans, myalgias, arthralgias, headache, fever, lymphadenopathy, and fatigue. The treatment of choice is tetracycline during the early phase. Occasionally the disease may progress to Lyme carditis, which presents with complete heart block.[29,173] Left ventricular dysfunction is unusual. Endomyocardial biopsy may reveal active myocarditis, and in one report spirochetes were identified in the myocardium. Administration of corticosteroids has been successful in treating Lyme carditis following therapy with tetracycline.[174]

Acquired Immunodeficiency Syndrome

See Chap. 79.

Eosinophilic Myocarditis

The diagnosis of eosinophilic myocarditis is established when the dominant cells infiltrating the myocardial interstitium are eosinophils. The major basic protein of the eosinophil granule may be detected in the presence of acute necrotizing myocarditis, suggesting toxicity of the contents of these granules.[172] Although endocardial thickening and restrictive myocardial disease are associated with peripheral eosinophilia, eosinophilic myocarditis may occur in the absence of elevations in the total eosinophil count. The cardiac dysfunction in this condition is similar to that of active myocarditis, with a predominance of lymphocytes infiltrating the biopsy. Prompt improvement in cardiac function and resolution of histologic abnormalities have been reported following administration of corticosteroids in uncontrolled trials.[173]

Giant Cell Myocarditis

Giant cells in endomyocardial biopsies identify a particularly aggressive form of myocarditis (Fig. 76-6). This histologic abnormality may be associated with autoimmune disease such as myasthenia gravis, autoimmune hemolytic anemia, or polymyositis. Brady- and tachyarrhythmias are common manifestations and may precede left ventricular dysfunction in giant cell myocarditis.[174] Although isolated reports have been optimistic with regard to response to immunosuppression, the

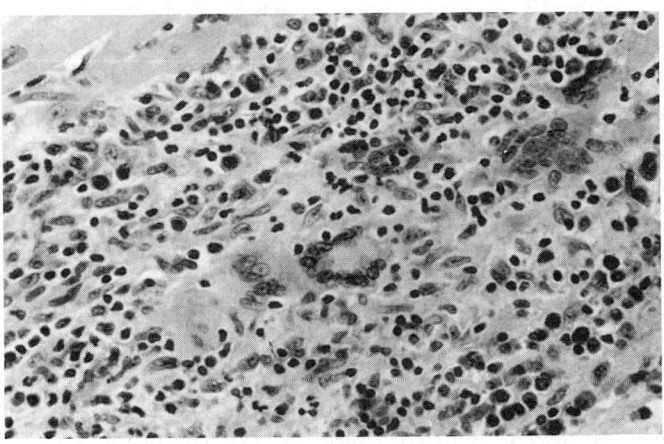

FIGURE 76-6

Photomicrograph showing mixed cellular infiltrate and giant cells characteristic of giant cell myocarditis. H&E, ×50. (From Gries W et al. Giant cell myocarditis: First report of recurrence in the transplanted heart. *J Heart Lung Transplant* 1992; 11:370–374. Reproduced with permission.)

overall experience is that of progressive disease unabated by medical therapy. Giant cell myocarditis has recurred in the allograft following cardiac transplantation.

THE HEART AND ENDOCRINE DISEASE

See Chap. 78.

PHEOCHROMOCYTOMA AND THE HEART

Pheochromocytomas, usually found in the adrenal medulla or in association with sympathetic ganglia, produce, store, and secrete catecholamines,[178–180] which cause a variety of clinical presentations including signs and symptoms of ventricular dysfunction (see Chaps. 57 and 78). Hypertension, while common, may be sustained or intermittent, and orthostatic hypotension can be present due to abnormal neural control of vascular tone. Sinus tachycardia, sinus bradycardia, supraventricular arrhythmias, and premature ventricular depolarizations are seen. Ischemic manifestations may occur even in the absence of coronary artery disease. When congestive heart failure occurs, ventricular dilatation and systolic dysfunction are present, usually associated with spotty myocardial fibrosis. Occasionally concentric or asymmetric hypertrophy is seen. The catecholamine-induced myocardial damage is multifactorial, but medical therapy to decrease circulating catecholamine levels and tumor removal are associated with hemodynamic, ECG, and clinical improvement in the cardiomyopathy.[176,177]

CARCINOID HEART DISEASE

Carcinoid tumors usually arise from argentaffin cells in the gastrointestinal tract and may secrete large amounts of serotonin (5-hydroxytryptamine), which is subsequently metabolized to 5-hydroxyindoleacetic acid (5-HIAA) by monoamine oxidase in the vascular endothelium of the lungs and the liver. The carcinoid syndrome—which is characterized by flushing, telangiectasias, diarrhea, and bronchoconstriction—occurs with less than 10 percent of carcinoid tumors. The primary tumors are generally located in the ileum but may infrequently be found in a bronchus and rarely in the jejunum, rectum, a Meckel's diverticulum, or ovary.[178]

Carcinoid heart disease occurs in approximately half of the patients with a classic carcinoid syndrome. The myofibromatous cardiac lesions usually involve the right side of the heart, causing dysfunction of the tricuspid and pulmonary valves. Severe tricuspid regurgitation (Chap. 66) with right-sided volume overload can dominate the presentation. The tricuspid valve may be thickened, with the valve leaflets fixed in a partially open position. Extensive involvement of the mural endocardium may cause restrictive physiology in some affected individuals. The superficial and right-sided cardiac location of the valvular and endocardial lesions leads to the suggestion that a blood-borne product of the tumor is responsible for the cardiac disease.

Although the severity of right-sided involvement correlates with plasma levels of serotonin and the tachykinins, neuropeptide K, and substance P as well as higher urinary excretion of the serotonin metabolite 5-HIAA, it does not correlate with disease duration. The major causes of death include hepatic failure, right ventricular failure, bowel obstruction, and bowel perforation; 5-year survival rates of 70 to 80 percent have been achieved using interferon and somatostatin analogs. Surgical management of the abnormal right-sided heart valves is encouraging.

THE HEART
AND KIDNEY DISEASE

See Chap. 94.

INFLAMMATORY
CARDIAC DISEASE

Hyperoxaluria

Both primary oxalosis, a rare autosomal recessive disorder, and secondary hyperoxaluria are characterized by calcium oxalate deposition in body tissues, including the myocardium.[179–181] Primary oxalosis is caused by an abnormality in alanine glyoxylate aminotransferase activity, the enzyme that converts glyoxylate to glycine in the liver. In the setting of normal renal function, primary oxalosis manifests itself as relatively benign hyperoxaluria. Unfortunately, nephrolithiasis and nephrocalcinosis may occur, producing renal insufficiency. As renal function deteriorates, urinary excretion of oxalate decreases, causing further renal deposition of calcium oxalate and destroying the remaining renal function. The progressive disease that subsequently develops is associated with painful arthropathy, pe-

ripheral neuropathy, retinopathy, osteodystrophy, and ischemic vasculopathy, with digital and limb necrosis, frequently requiring amputation. The causes of secondary oxalosis include chronic renal failure, ingestion of oxalates or of substances metabolized to oxalates (including ethylene glycol, intravenous feeding with xylitol, anesthesia with methoxyflurane), and enteric hyperoxaluria occurring in patients with extensive disease of the small bowel and pyridoxine deficiency.

In all types of oxalosis, oxalate crystals frequently deposit in the conducting system of the heart, causing heart block, and occasionally in the myocardium and the coronary arteries. Calcium oxalate crystals appear in hematoxylin and eosin (H&E) staining as a light brown, strongly birefringent crystal and cause variable degrees of cellular reaction, including necrosis, fibrosis, and mononuclear cell infiltration. Foreign-body giant cells and myocardial granulomas can be seen. Congestive heart failure and cardiac arrhythmias may occur. Interestingly, the cardiac dysfunction seen in primary oxalosis has been reported to reverse after combined kidney/liver transplantation.[181–183]

Gout

While atherosclerosis and coronary artery disease are the most common cardiovascular manifestations associated with gout, cardiovascular lesions can be found in gout and include uric acid crystals in the walls of blood vessels, myocardial interstitium, pericardium, conducting system, mitral annulus and in mitral, aortic, and tricuspid valve leaflets. Such deposits can calcify and cause a foreign-body type of granulomatous response, including the formation of multinucleated giant cells.[183,184] Heart muscle disease associated with hyperuricemia is rare.[186]

LYSOSOMAL
STORAGE DISEASES

See Chap. 69.

GLYCOGEN
STORAGE DISEASES

See Chap. 69.

REFSUM'S
SYNDROME

See Chap. 69.

CARNITINE
DEFICIENCY

See Chap. 69.

Hemochromatosis

Hemochromatosis is the progressive overload of iron in tissues leading to cirrhosis, diabetes, hyperpigmentation, and cardiac dysfunction (see Fig. 76-7).[184,187–193] Hemochromatosis may be inherited (genetic) or may be acquired, secondary to another process associated with iron loading. In genetic hemochromatosis, the metabolic defect is associated with an abnormal gene tightly linked to the A locus of the HLA complex on chromosome 6 and may affect the relationship between ferritin mRNA and transferrin receptor mRNA expression in the intestinal mucosa cell.[192,193] When the condition is inherited as an autosomal recessive disease, homozygotes usually develop severe iron overload, whereas heterozygotes show either no abnormalities or develop only minor abnormalities in iron metabolism. Determination of both transferrin saturation (22 to 40% in normals; 80 to 100% in hemochromatosis patients) and serum ferritin concentration (3 to 180 μ/dL in normals; 900 to 6000 μg/dL in hemochromatosis) detects genetic hemochromatosis with 95 percent specificity and sensitivity.[194]

Congestive heart failure is the leading cause of death in genetic hemochromatosis. About 15 percent of hemochrotic

matosis patients have cardiac symptoms as the presenting complaints and about one-third subsequently develop symptoms referable to the heart.[193]

Acquired hemochromatosis occurs primarily in chronic disorders of erythropoiesis, such as in sideroblastic anemia and thalassemia. In these disorders, not only is the absorption of iron increased but iron and transfusions are commonly administered. Acquired hemochromatosis may also result from excessive iron ingestion over many years.

The ECG in hemochromatosis may show low voltage and nonspecific ST-T changes. The most common disturbances in rhythm are supraventricular arrhythmias, although premature ventricular depolarizations and ventricular tachycardia can be seen. The cardiomyopathy associated with hemochromatosis is usually a mixed dilated/restrictive type with both systolic and diastolic dysfunction. Early on, increased left ventricular mass with normal function may be present, but progressive dilatation and dysfunction ensue. A transition from a restrictive cardiomyopathy to dilated cardiomyopathy may occur.

Although the iron deposition causes fibrosis in a majority of patients, the fibrosis tends to be mild. Iron deposits are most prominent in the ventricles and more epicardial than endocardial in location. The atria tend to be less involved and the conducting system least involved with iron deposition. Even in the conducting system, differences exist, since the sinus node is usually less involved than the AV node and His bundle. Since cardiac iron deposition tends to be greater in the subepicardial than in the subendocardial regions, endomyocardial biopsy may underestimate myocardial iron overload. While endomyocardial biopsy has been shown to be an insensitive method for the determination of early myocardial iron deposition in transfusion-related hemochromatosis associated with thalassemia major, histologically demonstrable myocardial iron is a consistent finding in endomyocardial biopsy tissue from patients with iron overload and associated cardiac dysfunction.[190] Hemochromatosis does not appear to affect the coronary vasculature.[195]

Treatment of genetic hemochromatosis involves removal of the excess body iron and supportive treatment for the damaged organs. While removal of iron is cheaply done by phlebotomy, chelation therapy with deferoxamine can be used. After iron removal by either phlebotomy or chelation, cardiac dysfunction can normalize, left ventricular dimensions may decrease and resting and exercise left ventricular function may improve.

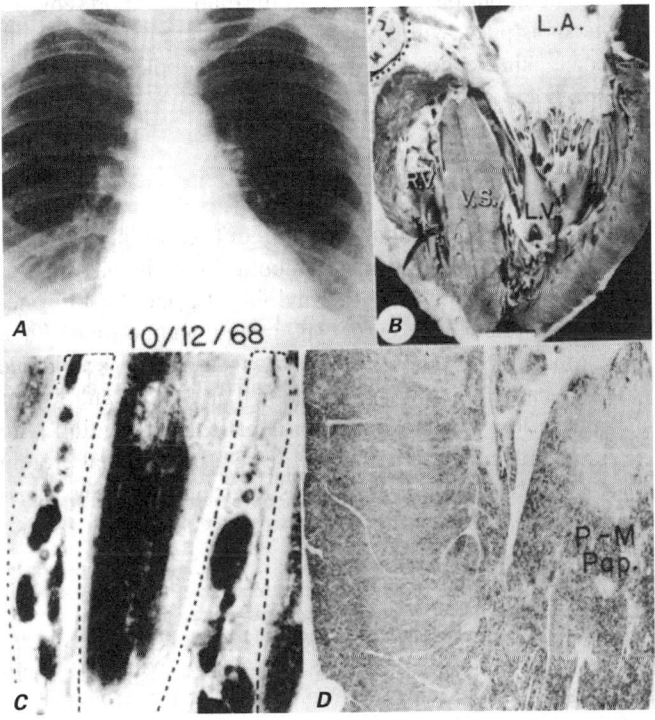

FIGURE 76-7

Cardiac hemosiderosis in a 42-year-old woman with sickle cell anemia. She had received 260 units of blood when congestive heart failure developed 6 years before her death. *A.* Chest roentgenogram showed cardiomegaly. By the time of death, she had received 359 units of blood (90 g iron). *B.* At necropsy, the walls of the right and left ventricles and left atrium were rusty brown due to extensive iron deposits. In contrast, the right atrial wall was tan and only minute particles of iron were detected in it by histologic examination. *C.* Photomicrograph of several myocardial cells showing huge deposits of iron in them. Despite large deposits of iron in the working myocardium, no iron deposits were observed in conducting myocardium. *D.* Longitudinal section of left ventricular wall including posteromedial (P-M) papillary muscle. Foci of necrosis and fibrosis are present. The necrotic and fibrotic areas are probably anatomic indicators of chronic myocardial hypoxia, a result of the chronic anemia. Prussian blue iron stains; $\times 628$ (*C*), $\times 3$ (*D*). (From Wenger et al.[184] Reproduced with permission.)

NUTRITIONAL DISEASE AND THE HEART

See Chap. 77.

SELENIUM DEFICIENCY AND KESHAN'S DISEASE

See Chap. 77.

AMYLOID HEART DISEASE

Amyloid cardiomyopathy is caused by the deposition of abnormal protein in the interstitium of the myocardium, resulting in increased ventricular wall thickness and the eventual development of congestive signs and symptoms (see Figure 76-8).[184] Systolic left ventricular function is usually preserved until late in the disease; once cardiomegaly, pulmonary edema, or systolic dysfunction has occurred, marked amyloid deposition in the myocardium is usually present.[196–203] The clinical presentation is that of congestive heart failure, with a more frequent occurrence of right-sided symptoms. Sudden death and myocardial infarction may result from vascular involvement.

While the ECG may show low voltage and a pseudoinfarct or postinfarct pattern,[204] echocardiography is the most effective noninvasive screening tool for amyloid heart disease. Echocardiography can demonstrate symmetric thickening of the left ventricular wall and qualitative (diffuse hyperrefractile, granular sparkling appearance of the myocardium) and even quantitative texture analysis may identify amyloid

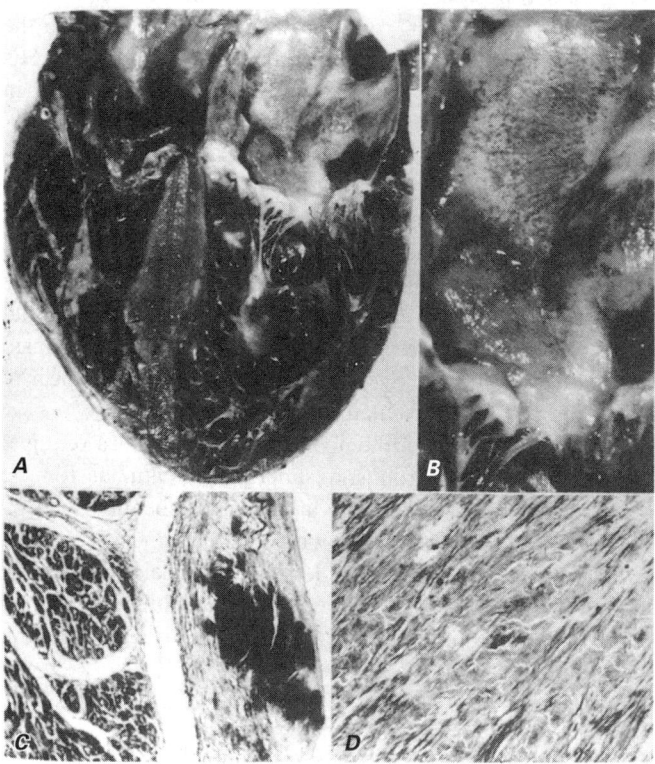

FIGURE 76-8

Cardiac amyloidosis. *A.* Posterior half of the heart in an 86-year-old man who had angina pectoris and healed myocardial infarction as well as large amyloid deposits. *B.* Close-up of left atrial endocardium. The waxy lesions on this endocardium represent amyloid deposits and are indicative of extensive ventricular amyloid deposit. *C.* Photomicrograph of left atrial endocardial amyloid deposit, ×107. *D.* Amyloid has infiltrated extensively a left ventricular papillary muscle, ×32. C.D. Crystal violet stain. (From Wenger et al.[184] Reproduced with permission.)

and distinguish it from hypertrophic cardiomyopathy. Abnormal left ventricular diastolic filling manifested by reduction in the rate, in the volume of rapid diastolic filling with enhanced atrial contraction can be seen very early in cardiac amyloidosis.[205]

While technetium-99m-pyrophosphate scintigraphy may identify early amyloid heart disease, reported most often in patients with familial amyloid polyneuropathy, amyloid is detected easily in endomyocardial biopsy specimens. Amyloid may be deposited in the interstitium in a pericellular or nodular pattern, in the endocardium, or in myocardial blood vessels. Since Congo red staining may not be satisfactory in endomyocardial biopsy specimens, sulfated alcian blue, methyl violet, and thioflavine T stains may be required. Immunoperoxidase stains for kappa and lambda light chains and for prealbumin may categorize the type of cardiac amyloid. Electronmicroscopic examination of biopsy specimens is likely the most sensitive method of recognizing amyloidosis.

Prognosis clearly depends on the extent of myocardial involvement, but once failure and fibrillation are present, the prognosis is poor, with a 5-year survival less than 5 percent. It appears that echocardiography with Doppler assessment can provide prognostic information.[206–208]

Amyloid AL (Myeloma-Associated and Primary Systemic Amyloid)

The amyloid protein subunit of amyloid AL is the ammonia terminal portion of an immunoglobulin light chain (kappa or lambda).[196] Of patients with amyloid AL, one-third to one-half have cardiac involvement and more than one-fourth have symptomatic heart failure. The median survival in individuals with any cardiac involvement is less than 1 year, and 5-year survival is less than 10 percent. In patients presenting with cardiac involvement, the majority have a monoclonal protein spike in the serum or urine.[196] Results following heart transplantation have proved disappointing.

Amyloid AA (Secondary Amyloidosis and Familial Mediterranean Fever)

Amyloid AA results from the deposition of amyloid A protein and is seen in chronic inflammatory disorders (rheumatoid arthritis, juvenile rheumatoid arthritis, ankylosing spondylitis, Crohn's disease, paraplegia associated with decubitus ulcers, cystic fibrosis, and heroin use with chronically infected cutaneous injection sites) and in familial Mediterranean fever, an autosomal recessive inherited disease of Sephardic Jews, Armenians, and other Mediterranean peoples. In general, aside from amyloid A protein deposition in the intima and media of arterioles, the heart is not involved.

Amyloid AF (Familial Amyloidosis)

Familial amyloidosis can manifest initially with progressive neuropathy, cardiomyopathy, or renal involvement. The abnormal protein deposited is designated amyloid AF and is a variant of prealbumin known as transthyretin. The familial amyloidoses are inherited as autosomal dominant disorders, unlike familial Mediterranean fever, which is inherited in an autosomal recessive fashion. All known variant forms of transthyretin can be produced by the alteration of a single nucleotide in the DNA sequence that codes for the protein. The heart disease in amyloid AF is variable. In some of families, cardiac amyloidosis is not even symptomatic, while in others cardiac symptoms predominate. Although ventricular function can appear normal in most members of some families with familial amyloid polyneuropathy, many affected individuals have detectable reductions in peak filling rates and in time to peak filling by radionuclide scanning, suggesting myocardial amyloid deposition.

Amyloid SSA (Senile Cardiac Amyloid and Senile Systemic Amyloid)

Amyloid SSA, like amyloid AF, is also related to the deposition of an abnormal transthyretin, albeit in older individuals. One form of amyloid SSA appears to affect only the atria and another form only the aorta; a third form is commonly known as senile systemic amyloidosis. This latter form of amyloid SSA may involve the lungs, liver, and kidneys as well as the myocardium. It should be noted that amyloid deposition is seen in one-fourth of individuals older than 70 years of age. While amyloid SSA has not been felt to be a frequent cause of cardiac symptoms, senile cardiac amyloid has been retrospectively associated with antemortem congestive heart failure and cardiac arrhythmias. While it appears that those with senile amyloidosis have a much better prognosis than those with immunoglobulin-derived amyloidosis, cardiac involvement by senile systemic amyloidosis may be an important although uncommon cause of cardiovascular morbidity.

Amyloid IAA (Isolated Atrial Amyloid)

Amyloid IAA has been found to be derived from atrial natriuretic polypeptide, the clinical consequences of which are unknown.

Amyloid CAA (Cerebral Amyloid Angiopathy)

Amyloid CAA is seen in the cerebral vessels and neurofibrillatory tangles of patients with senile dementia and Down's syndrome. The subunit protein has been called A4 or beta.

COLLAGEN VASCULAR AND CONNECTIVE TISSUE DISORDERS

See Chap. 85.

WHIPPLE'S DISEASE

Whipple's disease is a rare disorder associated with diarrhea/malabsorption, weight loss, polyarthritis, fever, and central nervous system involvement. Caused by *Tropheryma whippelii*,[209] a rod-shaped bacterium, the microscopic lesions in Whipple's disease have large macrophages with PAS-positive granules present. *Tropheryma whippelii* may be found either free in the affected tissues or phagocytosed in macrophages.[210–212] The course is characterized by progression and leads to death unless the patient receives antimicrobial therapy.[213]

Cardiac involvement is common, resulting from a pancarditis that causes fibrous thickening of cardiac valves with thickening and fusion of the chordae tendineae. The mitral valve is more commonly affected than the tricuspid valve and aortic valve involvement is sometimes seen. In the past, diagnosis has been made by histologic examination, but identification of the gene that encodes the 16s RNA of *T. whippelii* by a polymerase chain reaction may enable the diagnosis to be established more easily, sensitively, and accurately.[209,214] Various antibiotic regimens have been used, including tetracycline or ampicillin. Trimethoprim-sulfamethoxazole has been recommended and may be associated with fewer relapses than tetracycline.[213] Valve replacement may be required to improve hemodynamics and protect ventricular function.

SARCOIDOSIS

Sarcoidosis is a systemic granulomatous disease of unknown etiology characterized by enhanced cellular immune responses at sites of involvement. The initial lesion is an inflammatory infiltrate consisting of activated helper-inducer T lymphocytes and abundant macrophages that secrete cytokines. The resultant noncaseating granuloma consists of pale pink epithelioid cells, occasional multinucleate giant cells, and a scanty rim of lymphocytes. Virtually any organ except the adrenal gland may be involved. Lymphoid, pulmonary, cardiovascular, hepatobiliary, and hematologic systems are the most commonly involved, with the lungs being affected in over 90 percent of patients.[215–217] Cor pulmonale may occur due to extensive pulmonary sarcoidosis with interstitial fibrosis.

Cardiac sarcoid is more common than previously recognized, found in one-third of autopsy cases of patients with sarcoidosis.[218] Cardiac sarcoid is more likely fatal and less likely to be diagnosed antemortem than pulmonary sarcoid. In myocardial sarcoid, portions of the myocardial wall are replaced by sarcoid granulomas, which preferentially involve the cephalad portion of the ventricular septum or the left ventricular papillary muscles (see Fig. 76-9).[184] Granulomas can also affect the right or left ventricular free walls. The granulomas may be confluent and extensive or microscopic and diffuse. Fibrous scar tissue may form, occasionally resulting in wall thinning and infrequently in aneurysm formation. Myocardial involvement is much more common than pericardial involvement.[215,219–222]

Less than 10 percent of patients with sarcoid have symptoms referable to the cardiovascular system; however, because of the varied extent and location of the myocardial granulomas, presenting signs and symptoms are varied, ranging

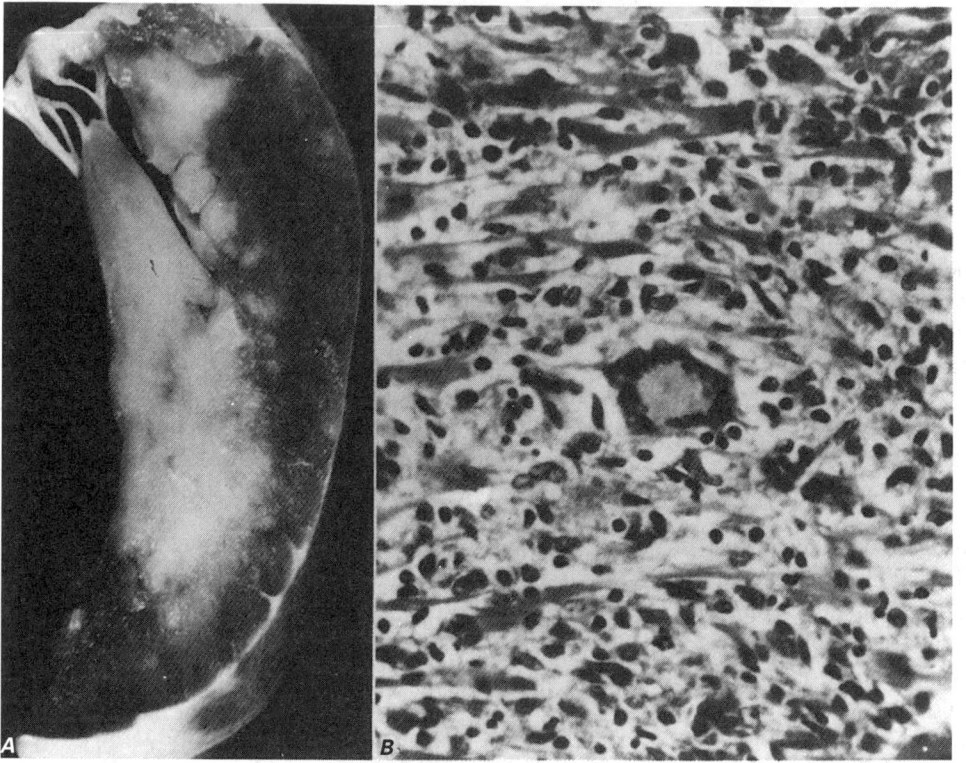

FIGURE 76-9

Cardiac sarcoidosis. *A.* Longitudinal section through anterolateral papillary muscle in a 26-year-old woman who had been asymptomatic until 10 days before her death, when dyspnea appeared. The dyspnea rapidly worsened, and when hospitalized on the day of death, she was in acute pulmonary edema. The blood pressure was 80/80 mmHg, heart rate 160 beats per minute, and a grade 3 to 4/6 holosystolic blowing murmur, which radiated to the axilla, was audible. Chest roentgenogram showed congested lungs, cardiomegaly, and prominent hilar adenopathy. The ECG showed nonspecific ST-T-wave changes and atrial hypertrophy. She developed complete heart block and died shortly thereafter. *A.* At necropsy, large, firm, white deposits were present in the walls of all four cardiac chambers and completely replaced both left ventricular papillary muscles. *B.* On histologic section, the firm white areas represented hard granulomas typical of sarcoidosis. H&E, ×400. Similar hard granulomas were present in lymph nodes, liver, spleen, and lung. Stains for acid-fast organisms, other bacteria, and fungi did not show evidence of infection. (From Wenger et al.[184] Reproduced with permission.)

from first-degree heart block to fulminant heart failure.[223] Myocardial involvement peaks between the third and sixth decades of life. As presenting features of cardiac sarcoid, first-degree AV block, bundle branch block, complete heart block, ventricular arrhythmias, sudden death, and heart failure all occur with a frequency of 10 to 20 percent.[223] Heart failure can present as a cardiomyopathy with restrictive hemodynamics. In patients dying due to cardiac sarcoid, heart failure accounts for one-quarter of the deaths, while sudden death accounts for one-third to one-half of the deaths.

In diagnosing cardiac sarcoid, evidence of other organ system involvement—including lymphadenopathy, hepatomegaly, splenomegaly, or pulmonary findings—should be sought. In cases where the heart is involved to a much greater degree than are other organs, little or no evidence of extracardiac sarcoidosis may be found. Chest x-ray, ECG, and echocardiography findings will depend on the extent and location of involvement. Myocardial imaging with thallium 201 and technetium-99m-sesta-methoxy-isobutyl-isonotrile (sest-

amibi) have been used in patients with suspected cardiac sarcoidosis. Segmental areas of decreased radionuclide uptake in the ventricular myocardium correspond to areas of fibrogranulomatous replacement. In the presence of normal coronary arteries, the perfusion defects on thallium-201 or sestamibi imaging in a patient with known systemic sarcoid strongly suggests cardiac involvement.[224] During exercise or after an infusion of dipyridamole, the perfusion defects seen on thallium or sestamibi scanning may decrease in size—a finding that differentiates the defects from those due to ischemia. The decrease in defect size with exercise or dipyridamole may portend improvement with corticosteroid therapy. Similarly, active uptake of gallium 67 at sites corresponding to thallium defects may also predict improvement with therapy. Due to the scattered nature of the granulomas, endomyocardial biopsy lacks sensitivity and seldom makes the diagnosis despite high specificity.

While no controlled trials have been performed, high-dose corticosteroids are usually given in the hope that the course of disease may be altered, even though concern has been raised that corticosteroids may predispose to aneurysm formation. Administration of corticosteroids improves cardiac symptoms, reverses ECG disturbances, and normalizes thallium scan defects in over half of patients treated with corticosteroids.[225] Antiarrhythmic drugs should be used as necessary, although drug therapy of ventricular tachycardia in patients with sarcoidosis, even when guided with programmed ventricular stimulation, is associated with a high rate of arrhythmia recurrence or sudden death.[226] Automatic internal cardioverter defibrillators have been advocated. Prognosis after the diagnosis of cardiac sarcoid is variable but can be poor.[216] In one series of 247 patients, survival was 41 percent at 5 years and 15 percent at 10 years.[215,227]

MUSCULAR DYSTROPHIES, MYOPATHIES, AND NEUROMUSCULAR DISORDERS

See Chap. 69.

TOXICITY, HYPERSENSITIVITY, AND PHYSICAL AGENT EFFECTS

See Chaps. 77, 80, and 88.

ALCOHOL

See Chap. 77.

PERIPARTUM HEART DISEASE

See Chap. 92.

REFERENCES

1. Richardson P, McKenna W, Bristow M, Maisch B, Mautner B, O'Connell J, et al. Report of the 1995 World Health Organization/International Society and Federation of Cardiology Task Force on the Definition and Classification of Cardiomyopathies. *Circulation* 1996; 93:841–842.

2. Olsen EGJ. Myocarditis—A case of mistaken identity? *Br Heart J* 1983; 50:303–311.

3. O'Connell JB, Robinson JA. Coxsackie viral myocarditis. *Postgrad Med J* 1985; 61:1127–1131.

4. Sainani GS, Krompotic E, Slodki SJ. Adult heart disease due to the Coxsackie virus B infection. *Medicine* 1968; 47:133–147.

5. Proby CM, Hackett S, Gupta S, Cox TM. Acute myopericarditis in influenza A infection. *J Med* 1986; 60:887–892.

6. Bell RW, Murphy WM. Myocarditis in young military personnel. *Am Heart J* 1967; 74:309–323.

7. Lorber A, Zonis A, Maisuls E, Dembo L, Palant A, Iancu TC. The scale of myocardial involvement in varicella myocarditis. *Int J Cardiol* 1988; 20:257–262.

8. Millett R, Tomita T, Marshall HE, Cohen L, Hannah H III. Cytomegalovirus endomyocarditis in a transplanted heart. *Arch Pathol Lab Med* 1991; 115:511–515.

9. Frishman W, Kraus ME, Zahkar J, Brooks V, Alonso D, Dixon LM. Infectious mononucleosis and fatal myocarditis. *Chest* 1977; 72:535–538.

10. Chaudary S, Jaski BE. Fulminant mumps myocarditis. *Ann Intern Med* 1989; 110:569–570.

11. Ainger LE, Lawyer NG, Fitch CW. Neonatal rubella myocarditis. *Br Heart J* 1966; 28:691–697.

12. Datta D, Zaidi A, Brendan DH. Carditis associated with coronavirus infection (letter). *Lancet* 1980; 2:100–101.

13. Raman GV, Prosser A, Spreadbury PL, Cockcroft PM, Okubadejo OA. Rabies presenting with myocarditis and encephalitis. *J Infect* 1988; 17:155–158.

14. Ursell PC, Habib A, Sharma P, Mesa-Tejada R, Lefkowitch JH, Fenoglio JJ Jr. Hepatitis B virus and myocarditis. *Hum Pathol* 1984; 15:481–484.

15. Matsumori A, Mtoba Y, Sasayama S. Dilated cardiomyopathy associated with hepatitis C virus infection. *Circulation* 1995; 92:2519–2525.

16. Obeyesekere I, Hermon Y. Arbovirus heart disease: Myocarditis and cardiomyopathy following dengue and chikungunya fever—A follow-up study. *Am Heart J* 1973; 85:186–194.

17. Milei J, Bolomo NJ. Myocardial damage in viral hemorrhagic fevers. *Am Heart J* 1982; 104:1385–1391.

18. Burch GE, Sun S-C, Sohal RS, Chu K-C, Colcolough HL. Diphtheritic myocarditis. *Am J Cardiol* 1968; 21:261–268.

19. Shalit M, Braverman AJ, Eliakim M. Congestive heart failure in the course of typhoid fever. *J Infect* 1982; 4:81–84.

20. Karjalainen J. Streptococcal tonsillitis and acute nonrheumatic myopericarditis. *Chest* 1989; 95:359–363.

21. Brasier AR, Macklis JD, Vaughan D, Warner L, Kirshenbaum JM. Myopericarditis as an initial presentation of meningococcemia. *Am J Med* 1987; 82:641–644.

22. Gross D, Willens H, Zeldis SM. Myocarditis in legionnaires' disease. *Chest* 1981; 79:232–234.

23. McCue MJ, Moore EE. Myocarditis with microabscess formation caused by *Listeria monocytogenes* associated with myocardial infarct. *Hum Pathol* 1979; 10:469–472.

24. Florkowski CM, Ikram RB, Crozier IM, Ikram H, Berry ME. *Campylobacter jejuni* myocarditis. *Clin Cardiol* 1984; 7:558–559.

25. Willey RF, Matthews MB, Peutherer JF, Marmion BP. Chronic cryptic Q-fever infection of the heart. *Lancet* 1979; 2:270–272.

26. Ringel RE, Brenner JI, Rennels MB, Huang S-W, Wang S, Grayston T, et al. Serologic evidence for *Chlamydia trachomatis* myocarditis. *Pediatrics* 1982; 70:54–56.

27. Lewes D, Rainford DJ, Lane WF. Symptomless myocarditis and myalgia in viral and *Mycoplasma pneumoniae* infections. *Br Heart J* 1974; 36:924–932.

28. Marin-Garcia J, Barrett FF. Myocardial function in Rocky Mountain spotted fever: Echocardiographic assessment. *Am J Cardiol* 1983; 51:341–343.

29. McAlister HF, Klementowicz PT, Andrews C, Fisher JD, Feld M, Furman S. Lyme carditis: An important cause of reversible heart block. *Ann Intern Med* 1989; 110:339–345.

30. Horn H, Saphir O. The involvement of the myocardium in tuberculosis. *Am Rev Tuberc* 1935; 32:492–506.

31. Marsden PD. South American trypanosomiasis (Chagas' disease). *Int Rev Trop Med* 1971; 4:97–121.

32. Leak D, Meghji M. Toxoplasmic infection in cardiac disease. *Am J Cardiol* 1979; 43:841–849.

33. Bessoudo R, Marrie TJ, Smith ER. Cardiac involvement in trichinosis. *Chest* 1981; 79:698–699.

34. Perez-Gomez F, Duran H, Tamames S, Perrote JL, Blanes A. Cardiac echinococcosis: Clinical picture and complications. *Br Heart J* 1973; 35:1326–1331.

35. Samlowski WE, Ward JH, Craven CM, Freedman RA. Severe myocarditis following high-dose interleukin-2 administration. *Arch Pathol Lab Med* 1989; 113:838–841.

36. Cohen MC, Huberman MS, Nesto RW. Recombinant alpha interferon–related cardiomyopathy. *Am J Med* 1988; 85:549–551.

37. Eggers HJ, Mertens Th. Viruses and myocardium: Notes of a virologist. *Eur Heart J* 1987; 8(suppl J):129–133.

38. Keeling PJ, Lukaszyk A, Poloniecki J, Caforio AL, Davies MJ, Booth JC, et al. A prospective case-control study of antibodies to coxsackie B virus in idiopathic dilated cardiomyopathy. *J Am Coll Cardiol* 1994; 23.593–598.

39. Gibson TC, Arnold J, Craige E, Curnen E. Electrocardiographic studies in Asian influenza. *Am Heart J* 1959; 57:661–668.

40. Karjalainen J, Nieminen MS, Heikkila J. Influenza A1 myocarditis in conscripts. *Acta Med Scand* 1980; 207:27–30.

41. Stevens PJ, Underwood Ground KE. Occurrence and significance of myocarditis in trauma. *Aerospace Med* 1970; 41:776–780.

42. Gravanis MB, Sternby NH. Incidence of myocarditis. *Arch Pathol Lab Med* 1991; 115:390–392.

43. Wenger NK, Abelmann WH, Roberts WC. Myocardial disease. In: Hurst JW, Logue RB, Rackley CE, Schlant RC, Sonnenblick EH, Wallace AG, et al (eds). *Diseases of the Heart and Blood Vessels,* 5th ed. New York: McGraw Hill; 1982:1278–1299.

44. Woodruff JF. Viral myocarditis: A review. *Am J Pathol* 1980; 101:427–479.

45. Godeny EK, Gauntt CJ. In situ immune autoradiographic identification of cells in heart tissues of mice with coxsackie virus B3-induced myocarditis. *Am J Pathol* 1987; 129:267–276.

46. Lodge PA, Herzum M, Olszewski J, Huber SA. Coxsackievirus B3 myocarditis. *Am J Pathol* 1987; 128:455–463.

47. Chow LH, Ye Y, Linder J, McManus BM. Phenotypic analysis of infiltrating cells in human myocarditis. *Arch Pathol Lab Med* 1989; 113:1357–1362.

48. Seko Y, Shinkai Y, Kawasaki A, Yagita H, Okumura K, Takaku F, et al. Expression of perforin in infiltrating cells in murine hearts with acute myocarditis caused by coxsackievirus B3. *Circulation* 1991; 84:788–795.

49. Young LHY, Joag SV, Zheng L-M, Lee C-P, Lee Y-S, Young JD. Perforin-mediated myocardial damage in acute myocarditis. *Lancet* 1990; 336:1019–1021.

50. Satoh M, Tamura G, Segawa I, Tashiro A, Hiramori K, Satodate R. Expression of cytokine genes and presence of enteroviral genomic

RNA in endomyocardial biopsy tissues of myocarditis and dilated cardiomyopathy. *Virchows Arch* 1996; 427:503–509.

51. Woodley SL, McMillan M, Shelby J, Lynch DH, Roberts LK, Ensley RD, et al. Myocyte injury and contraction abnormalities produced by cytotoxic T lymphocytes. *Circulation* 1991; 83:1410–1418.

52. Camp TF, Hess EV, Conway G, Fowler NO. Immunologic findings in idiopathic cardiomyopathy. *Am Heart J* 1969; 77:610–618.

53. Maisch B, Trostel-Soeder R, Stechemesser E, Berg PA, Kochstek K. Diagnostic relevance of humoral and cell-mediated immune reactions in patients with acute viral myocarditis. *Clin Exp Immunol* 1982; 48:533–545.

54. Neumann DA, Burek CL, Baughman KL, Rose NR, Herskowitz A. Circulating heart-reactive antibodies in patients with myocarditis or cardiomyopathy. *J Am Coll Cardiol* 1990; 16:839–846.

55. Neu N, Craig SW, Rose NR, Alvarez F, Beisel KW. Coxsackievirus induced myocarditis in mice: Cardiac myosin autoantibodies do not cross-react with the virus. *Clin Exp Immunol* 1987; 69:566–574.

56. Neu N, Rose NR, Beisel KW, Herskowitz A, Gurri-Glass G, Craig SW. Cardiac myosin induces myocarditis in genetically predisposed mice. *J Immunol* 1987; 139:3630–3636.

57. Pummerer CL, Luze K, Grässl G, Bachmaier K, Offner F, Lenz DM, et al. Identification of cardiac myosin peptides capable of inducing autoimmune myocarditis in BALB/c mice. *J Clin Invest* 1996; 97:2057–2062.

58. Limas CJ, Goldenberg IF, Limas C. Influence of anti-beta-receptor antibodies on cardiac adenylate cyclase in patients with idiopathic dilated cardiomyopathy. *Am Heart J* 1990; 119:1322–1328.

59. Schulze K, Becker BF, Schauer R, Schultheiss HP. Antibodies to ADP-ATP carrier—an autoantigen in myocarditis and dilated cardiomyopathy—impair cardiac function. *Circulation* 1990; 81:959–968.

60. Ansari AA, Wang Y-C, Danner EJ, Gravanis MB, Mayne A, Neckelmann N, et al. Abnormal expression of histocompatibility and mitochondrial antigens by cardiac tissue from patients with myocarditis and dilated cardiomyopathy. *Am J Pathol* 1991; 139:337–354.

61. Schulze K, Becker BF, Schultheiss HP. Antibodies to the ADP-ATP carrier, an autoantigen in myocarditis and dilated cardiomyopathy, penetrate into myocardial cells and disturb energy metabolism in vivo. *Circ Res* 1989; 64:179–191.

62. Sutton GC, Harding HB, Trueheart LRP, Clark HP. Coxsackie B4 myocarditis in an adult: Successful isolation of virus from ventricular myocardium. *Aerospace Med* 1967; 38:66–69.

63. Easton AJ, Eglin RP. The detection of coxsackievirus RNA in cardiac tissue by in situ hybridization. *J Gen Virol* 1988; 69:285–291.

64. Kandolf R, Hofschneider PH. Viral heart disease. *Springer Semin Immunopathol* 1989; 11:1–13.

65. Bowles NE, Rose ML, Taylor P, Banner NR, Morgan-Capner P, Cunningham L, et al. End-stage dilated cardiomyopathy. *Circulation* 1989; 80:1128–1136.

66. Tracy S, Chapman NM, McManus BM, Pallansch MA, Beck MA, Carstens J. A molecular and serologic evaluation of enteroviral involvement in human myocarditis. *J Biol Cell Cardiol* 1990; 22:403–414.

67. Jin O, Sole MJ, Butany JW, Chia W-K, McLaughlin PR, Liu P, Liew C-C. Detection of enterovirus RNA in myocardial biopsies from patients with myocarditis and cardiomyopathy using gene amplification by polymerase chain reaction. *Circulation* 1990; 82:8–16.

68. Weiss LM, Movahed LA, Billingham ME, Cleary ML. Detection of coxsackievirus B3 RNA in myocardial tissues by the polymerase chain reaction. *Am J Pathol* 1991; 138:497–503.

69. Grasso M, Arbustini E, Silini E, Diegoli M, Percivalle E, Ratti G, et al. Search for coxsackievirus B3 RNA in idiopathic dilated cardiomyopathy using gene amplification by polymerase chain reaction. *Am J Cardiol* 1992; 69:658–664.

70. Keeling PJ, Jeffery S, Caforio ALP, Taylor R, Bottazzo GF, Davies MJ, McKenna WJ. Similar prevalence of enteroviral genome within the myocardium from patients with idiopathic dilated cardiomyopathy and controls by the polymerase chain reaction. *Br Heart J* 1992; 68:554–559.

71. Petitjean J, Kopecka H, Freymuth F, Langlard JM, Scanu P, Galateau F, et al. Detection of enteroviruses in endomyocardial biopsy by molecular approach. *J Med Virol* 1992; 37:76–82.

72. Schwaiger A, Umlauft F, Weyrer K, Larcher C, Lyons J, Mühlberger V, et al. Detection of enteroviral ribonucleic acid in myocardial biopsies from patients with idiopathic dilated cardiomyopathy by polymerase chain reaction. *Am J Heart* 1993; 126:406–410.

73. Severini GM, Mestroni L, Falaschi A, Camerini F, Giacca M. Nested polymerase chain reaction for high-sensitivity detection of enteroviral RNA in biological samples. *J Clin Microbiol* 1993; 31:1345–1349.

74. Katsuragi M, Yutani C, Mukai T, Arai Y, Imakita M, Ishibashi-Ueda H, et al. Detection of enteroviral genome and its significance in cardiomyopathy. *Cardiology* 1993; 83:4–13.

75. Liljeqvist J-Å, Bergström T, Holmström S, Samuelson A, Yousef GE, Waagstein F, et al. Failure to demonstrate enterovirus aetiology in Swedish patients with dilated cardiomyopathy. *J Med Virol* 1993; 39:6–10.

76. Satoh M, Tamura G, Segawa I. Enteroviral RNA in endomyocardial biopsy tissues of myocarditis and dilated cardiomyopathy. *Pathol Int* 1994; 44:345–351.

77. Nicholson F, Ajetunmobi JF, Li M, Shackleton EA, Starkey WG, Illavia SJ, et al. Molecular detection and serotypic analysis of enterovirus RNA in archival specimens from patients with acute myocarditis. *Br Heart J* 1995; 74:522–527.

78. Ueno H, Yokota Y, Shiotani H, Yokoyama M, Itoh H, Ishido S. Significance of detection of enterovirus RNA in myocardial tissues by reverse transcription-polymerase chain reaction. *Int J Cardiol* 1995; 51:157–164.

79. Fujioka S, Koide H, Kitaura Y, Deguchi H, Kawamura K, Hirai K. Molecular detection and differentiation of enteroviruses in endomyocardial biopsies and pericardial effusions from dilated cardiomyopathy and myocarditis. *Am Heart J* 1996; 131:760–765.

80. Andreoletti L, Hober D, Decoene C, Copin M-C, Lobert P-E, Dewilde A, et al. Detection of enteroviral RNA by polymerase chain reaction in endomyocardial tissue of patients with chronic cardiac diseases. *J Med Virol* 1996; 48:53–59.

81. Why HJF, Meany BR, Richardson PJ, Olsen EGJ, Bowles NE, Cunningham L, et al. Clinical and prognostic significance of detection of enteroviral RNA in the myocardium of patients with myocarditis or dilated cardiomyopathy. *Circulation* 1994; 89:2582–2589.

82. Figulla HR, Stille-Siegener M, Mall G, Heim A, Kreuzer H. Myocardial enterovirus infection with left ventricular dysfunction: A benign disease compared with idiopathic dilated cardiomyopathy. *J Am Coll Cardiol* 1995; 25:1170–1175.

83. Gauntt CJ, Pallansch MA. Coxsackievirus B3 clinical isolates and murine myocarditis. *Vir Res* 1996; 41:89–99.

84. Gerli R, Rambotti P, Spinozzi F, Bertotto A, Chiodini V, Solinas P, et al. Immunologic studies of peripheral blood from patients with idiopathic dilated cardiomyopathy. *Am Heart J* 1986; 112:350–355.

85. Huber KC, Gersh BJ, Sugrue DD, Frye RL, Bailey KR, Ritts RE Jr. T-lymphocyte subsets in patients with idiopathic dilated cardiomyopathy. *Int J Cardiol* 1989; 22:59–66.

86. Fowles RE, Bieber CP, Stinson EB. Defective in vitro suppressor cell function in idiopathic congestive cardiomyopathy. *Circulation* 1979; 59:483–491.

87. Anderson JL, Fowles RE, Bieber CP, Stinson EB. Idiopathic cardiomyopathy, age, and suppressor-cell dysfunction as risk determinants of lymphoma after cardiac transplantation. *Lancet* 1978; 2:1174–1177.

88. Matumori A, Yamada T, Suzuki H, Matoba Y, Sasayama S. Increased circulating cytokines in patients with myocarditis and cardiomyopathy. *Br Heart J* 1994; 72:561–566.

89. Myocarditis Treatment Trial Investigators: Incidence and clinical characteristics of myocarditis (abstr). *Circulation* 1991; 84(suppl II):II–2.

90. Costanzo-Nordin MR, O'Connell JB, Subramanian R, Robinson JA, Scanlon PJ. Myocarditis confirmed by biopsy presenting as acute myocardial infarction. *Br Heart J* 1985; 53:25–29.

91. Saffitz JE, Schwartz DJ, Southworth W, Murphree S, Rodriguez ER, Ferrans VJ, et al. Coxsackie viral myocarditis causing transmural right and left ventricular infarction without coronary narrowing. *Am J Cardiol* 1983; 52:644–647.

92. Burch GE, Shewey LL. Viral coronary arteritis and myocardial infarction. *Am Heart J* 1976; 92:11–14.

93. Ferguson DW, Farwell AP, Bradley WA, Rollings RC. Coronary artery vasospasm complicating acute myocarditis. *West J Med* 1988; 148:664–669.

94. Mason JW, Billingham ME, Ricci DR. Treatment of acute inflammatory myocarditis assisted by endomyocardial biopsy. *Am J Cardiol* 1980; 45:1037–1044.

95. Phillips M, Robinowitz M, Higgins JR, Boran KJ, Reed T, Virmani R. Sudden cardiac death in Air Force recruits: A 20-year review. *JAMA* 1986; 256:2696–2699.

96. Tomioka N, Kishimoto C, Matsumori A, Kawai C. Mural thrombus in experimental viral myocarditis in mice: Relation between thrombosis and congestive heart failure. *Cardiovasc Res* 1986; 20:665–671.

97. Kojima J, Miyazaki S, Fujiwara H, Kumada T, Kawai C. Recurrent left ventricular mural thrombi in a patient with acute myocarditis. *Heart Vessels* 1988; 4:120–122.

98. O'Connell JB, Fowles RE, Robinson JA, Subramanian R, Henkin RE, Gunnar RM. Clinical and pathologic findings of myocarditis in two families with dilated cardiomyopathy. *Am Heart J* 1984; 107:127–135.

99. O'Connell JB, Costanzo-Nordin MR, Subramanian R, Robinson JA, Wallis DE, Scanlon PJ, et al. Peripartum cardiomyopathy: Clinical, hemodynamic, histologic and prognostic characteristics. *J Am Coll Cardiol* 1986; 8:52–56.

100. Karjalainen J, Heikkila J. Acute pericarditis: Myocardial enzyme release as evidence for myocarditis. *Am Heart J* 1986; 111:546–552.

101. Karjalainen J. Functional and myocarditis-induced T-wave abnormalities. *Chest* 1983; 83:868–864.

102. Toshima H, Ohkita Y, Shingu M. Clinical features of acute coxsackie B viral myocarditis. *Jpn Circ J* 1979; 43:441–444.

103. Kimby AG, Sodermark T, Volpe U, Zetterquist S. Stokes-Adams attacks requiring pacemaker treatment in three patients with acute nonspecific myocarditis. *Acta Med Scand* 1980; 207:177–181.

104. Karjalainen J, Viitasalo M, Kala R, Heikkila J. 24-Hour electrocardiographic recordings in mild acute infectious myocarditis. *Ann Clin Res* 1984; 16:34–39.

105. Chandraratna PAN, Nimalasuriya A, Reid CL, Cohn S, Rahimtoola SH. Left ventricular asynergy in acute myocarditis. *JAMA* 1983; 250:1428–1430.

106. Arvan S, Manalo E. Sudden increase in left ventricular mass secondary to acute myocarditis. *Am Heart J* 1988; 116:200–202.

107. Pinamonti B, Alberti E, Cigalotto A, Dreas L, Salvi A, Silvestri F, et al. Echocardiographic findings in myocarditis. *Am J Cardiol* 1988; 62:285–291.

108. Ferdeghini EM, Pinamonti B, Picano E, Lattanzi F, Bussani R, Slavich G, et al. Quantitative texture analysis in echocardiography: Application to the diagnosis of myocarditis. *J Clin Ultrasound* 1991; 19:263–270.

109. Uchida Y, Nakamura F, Oshima T, Fujimori Y, Hirose J. Percutaneous fiberoptic angioscopy of the left ventricle in patients with dilated cardiomyopathy and acute myocarditis. *Am Heart J* 1990; 120:677–687.

110. Konno S, Sakakibara S. Endomyocardial biopsy. *Chest* 1963; 44:345–350.

111. Caves PK, Schultz WP, Dong E Jr, Stinson EB, Shumway NE. New instrument for transvenous cardiac biopsy. *Am J Cardiol* 1974; 33:264–267.

112. Miller LW, Labovitz AJ, McBride LA, Pennington DG, Kanter K. Echocardiography-guided endomyocardial biopsy. *Circulation* 1988; 78(suppl III):III-99–III-102.

113. Noda S. Histopathology of endomyocardial biopsies from patients with idiopathic cardiomyopathy: Quantitative evaluation based on multivariate statistical analysis. *Jpn Circ J* 1980; 44:95–116.

114. Baandrup V, Olsen EGJ. Critical analysis of endomyocardial biopsies from patients suspected of having cardiomyopathy: I. Morphological and morphometric aspects. *Br Heart J* 1981; 45:475–486.

115. Das JP, Rath B, Das S, Sarangi A. Study of endomyocardial biopsies in cardiomyopathy. *Indian Heart J* 1981; 33:18–26.

116. Nippoldt TB, Edwards WD, Holmes DR Jr, Reeder GS, Hartzler GO, Smith HC. Right ventricular endomyocardial biopsy. *Mayo Clin Proc* 1982; 57:407–418.

117. Fenoglio JJ Jr, Ursell PC, Kellogg CF, Drusin RE, Weiss MB. Diagnosis and classification of myocarditis by endomyocardial biopsy. *N Engl J Med* 1983; 308:12–18.

118. Unverferth DV, Fetters JK, Unverferth BJ, Leier CV, Magorien RD, Arn AR, et al. Human myocardial histologic characteristics in congestive heart failure. *Circulation* 1983; 68:1194–1200.

119. Parrillo JE, Aretz HT, Palacios I, Fallon JT, Block PC. The results of transvenous endomyocardial biopsy can frequently be used to diagnose myocardial diseases in patients with idiopathic heart failure. *Circulation* 1984; 69:93–101.

120. Zee-Cheng C-S, Tsai CC, Palmer DC, Codd JE, Pennington DG, Williams GA. High incidence of myocarditis by endomyocardial biopsy in patients with idiopathic congestive cardiomyopathy. *J Am Coll Cardiol* 1984; 3:63–70.

121. O'Connell JB, Henkin RE, Robinson JA, Subramanian R, Scanlon PJ, Gunnar RM. Gallium-67 imaging in patients with dilated cardiomyopathy and biopsy-proven myocarditis. *Circulation* 1984; 70:58–62.

122. Daly K, Richardson PJ, Olsen EGJ, Morgan-Capner P, McSorley C, Jackson G, et al. Acute myocarditis: Role of histological and virological examination in the diagnosis and assessment of immunosuppressive treatment. *Br Heart J* 1984; 51:30–35.

123. Rose AG, Fraser RC, Beck W. Absence of evidence of myocarditis in endomyocardial biopsy specimens from patients with dilated (congestive) cardiomyopathy. *S Afr Med J* 1984; 66:871–874.

124. Regitz V, Olsen EGJ, Rudolph W. Histologisch nachweisbare Myokarditis bei Patienten mit eingeschrankter linksventrikularer Funktion. *Herz* 1985; 10:27–35.

125. Dec GW Jr, Palacios IF, Fallon JT, Aretz HT, Mills J, Lee DC-S, et al. Active myocarditis in the spectrum of acute dilated cardiomyopathies. *N Engl J Med* 1985; 312:885–890.

126. Salvi A, Silvestri F, Gori D, Klugmann S, Tanganelli P, Camerini F. La biopsia endomiocardica: Un'esperienza relativa a 156 pazienti. *G Ital Cardiol* 1985; 15:251–259.

127. Mortensen SA, Baandrup U, Buch J, Bendtzen K, Hvid-Jacobsen K. Immunosuppressive therapy of biopsy proven myocarditis: Experiences with corticosteroids and cyclosporin. *Int J Immunother* 1985; 1:35–45.

128. Hosenpud JD, McAnulty JH, Niles NR. Lack of objective improvement in ventricular systolic function in patients with myocarditis treated with azathioprine and prednisone. *J Am Coll Cardiol* 1985; 6:797–801.

129. Cassling RS, Linder J, Sears TD, Waller BF, Rogler WC, Wilson JE, et al. Quantitative evaluation of inflammation in biopsy specimens from idiopathically failing or irritable hearts: Experience in 80 pediatric and adult patients. *Am Heart J* 1985; 110:713–720.

130. French WJ, Siegel RJ, Cohen AH, Laks MM. Yield of endomyocardial biopsy in patients with biventricular failure. *Chest* 1986; 90:181–184.

131. Hammond EH, Menlove RL, Anderson JL. Predictive value of immunofluorescence and electron microscopic evaluation of endomyocardial biopsies in the diagnosis and prognosis of myocarditis and idiopathic dilated cardiomyopathy. *Am Heart J* 1987; 114:1055–1065.

132. Maisch B, Bauer E, Hufnagel G, Pfeifer U, Rohkamm R. The use of endomyocardial biopsy in heart failure. *Eur Heart J* 1988; 9(suppl H):59–71.

133. Chow LC, Dittrich HC, Shabetai R. Endomyocardial biopsy in patients with unexplained congestive heart failure. *Ann Intern Med* 1988; 109:535–539.

134. Leatherbury L, Chandra RS, Shapiro SR, Perry LW. Value of endomyocardial biopsy in infants, children and adolescents with dilated or hypertrophic cardiomyopathy and myocarditis. *J Am Coll Cardiol* 1988; 12:1547–1554.

135. Hobbs RE, Pelegrin D, Ratliff NB, Bott-Silverman C, Rincon G, Sterba R, et al. Lymphocytic myocarditis and dilated cardiomyopathy: Treatment with immunosuppressive agents. *Cleve Clin J Med* 1989; 56:628–635.

136. Latham RD, Mulrow JP, Virmani R, Robinowitz M, Moody JM. Recently diagnosed idiopathic dilated cardiomyopathy: Incidence of myocarditis and efficacy of prednisone therapy. *Am Heart J* 1989; 117:876–882.

137. Popma JJ, Cigarroa RG, Buja LM, Hillis LD. Diagnostic and prognostic utility of right-sided catheterization and endomyocardial biopsy in idiopathic dilated cardiomyopathy. *Am J Cardiol* 1989; 63:955–958.

138. Vasiljevic JD, Kanjuh V, Seferovic P, Sesto M, Stojsic D, Olsen EGJ. The incidence of myocarditis in endomyocardial biopsy samples from patients with congestive heart failure. *Am Heart J* 1990; 120:1370–1381.

139. Lieberman EB, Hutchins GM, Herskowitz A, Rose NR, Baughman KL. Clinicopathologic description of myocarditis. *J Am Coll Cardiol* 1991; 18:1617–1626.

140. Strain JE, Grose RM, Factor SM, Fisher JD. Results of endomyocardial biopsy in patients with spontaneous ventricular tachycardia but without apparent structural heart disease. *Circulation* 1983; 68:1171–1181.

141. Vignola PA, Aonuma K, Swaye PS, Rozanski JJ, Blankstein RL, Benson J, et al. Lymphocytic myocarditis presenting as unexplained ventricular arrhythmias: Diagnosis with endomyocardial biopsy and response to immunosuppression. *J Am Coll Cardiol* 1984; 4:812–819.

142. Sugrue DD, Holmes DR Jr, Gersh BJ, Edwards WD, McLaran CJ, Wood DL, et al. Cardiac histologic findings in patients with life-threatening ventricular arrhythmias of unknown origin. *J Am Coll Cardiol* 1984; 4:952–957.

143. Hosenpud JD, McAnulty JH, Niles NR. Unexpected myocardial disease in patients with life threatening arrhythmias. *Br Heart J* 1986; 56:55–61.

144. Tazelaar HD, Billingham ME. Leukocytic infiltrates in idiopathic dilated cardiomyopathy. *Am J Surg Pathol* 1986; 10:405–412.

145. Aretz HT, Billingham ME, Edwards WD, Factor SM, Fallon JT, Fenoglio JJ Jr, et al. Myocarditis: A histopathological definition. *Am J Cardiovasc Pathol* 1986; 1:3–14.

146. Dec GW, Fallon JT, Southern JF, Palacios I. "Borderline" myocarditis: An indication for repeat endomyocardial biopsy. *J Am Coll Cardiol* 1990; 15:283–289.

147. Spiegelhelter DJ, Stovin TGI. An analysis of repeated biopsies following cardiac transplantation. *Stat Med* 1983; 2:33–40.

148. Chow LH, Radio SJ, Sears TD, McManus BM. Insensitivity of right ventricular endomyocardial biopsy in the diagnosis of myocarditis. *J Am Coll Cardiol* 1989; 14:915–920.

149. Hauck AJ, Kearney DL, Edwards WD. Evaluation of postmortem endomyocardial biopsy specimens from 38 patients with lymphocytic myocarditis: Implications for role sampling error. *Mayo Clin Proc* 1989; 64:1235–1245.

150. Keogh AM, Billingham ME, Schroeder JS. Rapid histological changes in endomyocardial biopsy specimens after myocarditis. *Br Heart J* 1990; 64:406–408.

151. Billingham ME, Tazelaar HD. The morphological progression of viral myocarditis. *Postgrad Med J* 1986; 62:581–584.

152. Dec GW, Palacios I, Yasuda T, Fallon JT, Khaw BA, Strauss HW, et al. Antimyosin antibody cardiac imaging: Its role in the diagnosis of myocarditis. *J Am Coll Cardiol* 1990; 16:97–104.

153. Gagliardi MG, Bevilacqua M, Di Renzi P, Picardo S, Passariello R, Marcelletti C. Usefulness of magnetic resonance imaging for diagnosis of acute myocarditis in infants and children, and comparison with endomyocardial biopsy. *Am J Cardiol* 1991; 68:1089–1094.

154. Quigley PJ, Richardson PJ, Meany BT, Olsen EGJ, Monaghan MJ, Jackson G, et al. Long-term follow-up of acute myocarditis: Correlation of ventricular function and outcome. *Eur Heart J* 1987; 8(suppl J):39–42.

155. O'Connell JB, Dec GW, Goldenberg IF, Starling RC, Mudge GH, Augustine SM, et al. Results of heart transplantation for active lymphocytic myocarditis. *J Heart Transplant* 1990; 9:351–356.

156. Ilback N-G, Fohlman J, Friman G. Exercise in coxsackie B3 myocarditis: Effects on heart lymphocyte subpopulations and the inflammatory reaction. *Am Heart J* 1989; 117:1298–1302.

157. Hosenpud JD, Campbell SM, Niles NR, Lee J, Mendelson D, Hart MV. Exercise induced augmentation of cellular and humoral autoimmunity associated with increased cardiac dilatation in experimental autoimmune myocarditis. *Cardiovasc Res* 1987; 21:217–222.

158. Sekiguchi M, Hiroe M, Take M, Hirosawa K. Clinical and histopathological profile of sarcoidosis of the heart and acute idiopathic myocarditis: Concepts through a study employing endomyocardial biopsy. II. Myocarditis. *Jpn Circ J* 1980; 44:264–273.

159. Edwards WD, Holmes DR Jr, Reeder GS. Diagnosis of active lymphocytic myocarditis by endomyocardial biopsy: Quantitative criteria for light microscopy. *Mayo Clin Proc* 1982; 57:419–425.

160. Feneley MP, Gavaghan TP, Ralston M, Hickie JB, Baron DW. Diagnosis and management of acute myocarditis aided by serial myocardial biopsy. *Aust NZ J Med* 1984; 14:826–830.

161. Salvi A, Di Lenarda A, Dreas L, Silvestri F, Camerini F. Immunosuppressive treatment in myocarditis. *Int J Cardiol* 1989; 22:329–338.

162. Chan KY, Iwahara M, Benson LN, Wilson GJ, Freedom RM. Immunosuppressive therapy in the management of acute myocarditis in children: A clinical trial. *J Am Coll Cardiol* 1991; 17:458–460.

163. Jones SR, Herskowitz A, Hutchins GM, Baughman KL. Effects of immunosuppressive therapy in biopsy-proved myocarditis and borderline myocarditis on left ventricular function. *Am J Cardiol* 1991; 68:370–376.

164. Parrillo JE, Cunnion RE, Epstein SE, Parker MM, Suffredini AF, Brenner M, et al. A prospective, randomized, controlled trial of prednisone for dilated cardiomyopathy. *N Engl J Med* 1989; 321:1061–1068.

165. Hahn EA, Hartz VL, Moon RE, O'Connell JB, Herskowitz A, McManus BM, et al. The Myocarditis Treatment Trial: Design, methods and patient enrollment. *Eur Heart J* 1995; 16:162–167.

166. Mason JW, O'Connell JB, Herskowitz A, Rose NR, McManus BM, Billingham ME, et al. A clinical trial of immunosuppressive therapy for myocarditis. *N Engl J Med* 1995; 333:269–275.

167. Sadigursky M, von Kreuter BF, Ling P-Y, Santos-Buch CA. Association of elevated anti-sarcolemma, anti-idiotype antibody levels with the clinical and pathologic expression of chronic Chagas myocarditis. *Circulation* 1989; 80:1269–1276.

168. Higuchi MDL, De Morais CF, Barreto ACP, Lopes EA, Stolf N, Bellotti G, et al. The role of active myocarditis in the development of heart failure in chronic Chagas' disease: A study based on endomyocardial biopsies. *Clin Cardiol* 1987; 10:665–670.

169. Maguire JH, Mott KE, Lehman JS, Hoff R, Muniz TM, Guimaraes AC, et al. Relationship of electrocardiographic abnormalities and seropositivity to *Trypanosoma cruzi* within a rural community in northeast Brazil. *Am Heart J* 1983; 105:287–294.

170. Chiale PA, Halpern MS, Nau GJ, Tambussi AM, Przybylski J, Lazzari JO, et al. Efficacy of amiodarone during long-term treatment of malignant ventricular arrhythmias in patients with chronic Chagasic myocarditis. *Am Heart J* 1984; 107:656–665.

171. Luft BJ, Billingham M, Remington JS. Endomyocardial biopsy in the diagnosis of toxoplasmic myocarditis. *Transplant Proc* 1986; 18:1871–1873.

172. Gonwa TA, Capehart JE, Pilcher JW, Alivizatos PA. Cytomegalovirus myocarditis as a cause of cardiac dysfunction in a heart transplant recipient. *Transplantation* 1989; 47:197–199.

173. Steere AC, Batsford WP, Weinberg M, Alexander J, Berger HJ, Wolfson S, et al. Lyme carditis: Cardiac abnormalities of Lyme disease. *Ann Intern Med* 1980; 93:8–16.

174. Olson LJ, Okafor EC, Clements IP. Cardiac involvement in Lyme disease: Manifestations and management. *Mayo Clin Proc* 1986; 61:745–749.

175. Spry CJF, Tai P-C. The eosinophil in myocardial disease. *Eur Heart J* 1987; 8(suppl J):81–84.

176. Kim CH, Vlietstra RE, Edwards WD, Reeder GS, Gleich GJ. Steroid-responsive eosinophilic myocarditis: Diagnosis by endomyocardial biopsy. *Am J Cardiol* 1984; 53:1472–1473.

177. Davidoff R, Palacios I, Southern J, Fallon JT, Newell J, Dec GW. Giant cell versus lymphocytic myocarditis: A comparison of their clinical features and long-term outcomes. *Circulation* 1991; 83:953–961.

178. Scully RE, Mark EJ, McNeely WF, McNeely BU, Samuel MA. Case records of the Massachusetts General Hospital. *N Engl J Med* 1988; 319:970–981.

179. Danpure CJ. Recent advances in the understanding, diagnosis, and treatment of primary hyperoxaluria type 1. *J Inher Metab Dis* 1989; 12:210–224.

180. Boquist L, Lindqvist B, Ostberg Y, Steen L. Primary oxalosis. *Am J Med* 1973; 54:673–681.

181. Rodby RA, Tyszka TS, Williams JW. Reversal of cardiac dysfunction secondary to type 1 primary hyperoxaluria after combined liver-kidney transplantation. *Am J Med* 1991; 90:498–504.

182. Solmos GR, Ali A, Rodby RA, Fordham EW. Rapid reversal of bone scan abnormalities in a patient with type 1 primary hyperoxaluria and oxalosis. *Clin Nucl Med* 1994; 19:769–772.

183. Fyfe BS, Israel DH, Quish A, Squire A, Burrows L, Miller C, et al. Reversal of primary hyperoxaluria cardiomyopathy after combined liver and renal transplantation. *Am J Cardiol* 1995; 75:210–212.

184. Wenger NK, Abelmann WH, Roberts WC. Cardiomyopathy and specific heart muscle disease. In: Hurst JW, Schlant RC, Rackley CE, Sonnenblick EH, Wenger NK (eds). *The Heart*, 7th ed. New York: McGraw-Hill; 1990:1278–1347.

185. Mavrikakis ME, Sfikakis PP, Kontoyannis DA, Antoniades LG, Tsankanikas C. Gout and neurological abnormalities associated with cardiomyopathy in a young man. *Ann Rheum Dis* 1990; 49:942–943.

186. Rosenberg AL, Bergstrom LV, Troost BT, Bartholomew BA. Hyperuricaemia and neurologic deficits: A family study. *N Engl J Med* 1970; 282:992–997.

187. Dabestani A, Child JS, Perloff JK, Figueroa WG, Schelbert HR, Engel TR. Cardiac abnormalities in primary hemochromatosis. *Ann NY Acad Sci* 1988; 526:234–243.

188. Strohmeyer G, Niederau C, Stremmel W. Survival and causes of death in hemochromatosis. *Ann NY Acad Sci* 1988; 526:245–257.

189. Barosi G, Arbustini E, Gavazzi A, Grasso M, Pucci A. Myocardial iron grading by endomyocardial biopsy. A clinicopathologic study on iron overloaded patients. *Eur J Haematol* 1989; 42:382–388.

190. Olson LJ, Edwards WD, Holmes DR, Miller FA, Nordstrom LA, Baldus WP. Endomyocardial biopsy in hemochromatosis: Clinicopathologic correlates in six cases. *J Am Coll Cardiol* 1989; 13:116–120.

191. Weintraub LR, Edwards CQ, Krikker M (eds). *Hemochromatosis: Proceedings of the First International Conference.* New York: New York Academy of Sciences, 1988, vol 526.

192. Edwards CQ, Griffen LM, Goldgar D, Drummond C, Skolnick MH, Kushner JP. Prevalence of hemochromatosis among 11,065 presumably healthy blood donors. *N Engl J Med* 1988; 318:1355–1362.

193. Powell LW, Isselbacher KJ. Hemochromatosis. In: Wilson JD, Braunwald E, Isselbacher KJ, Petersdorf RG, Martin JB, Fauci AS, et al (eds). *Harrison's Principles of Internal Medicine*, 12th ed. New York: McGraw-Hill; 1991:1825–1829.

194. Bonkovsky HL, Slaker DP, Bills EB, Wolf DC. Usefulness and limitation of laboratory and hepatic imaging studies in iron-storage disease. *Gastroenterology* 1990; 99:1079–1091.

195. Miller M, Hutchins GM. Hemochromatosis, multiorgan hemosiderosis, and coronary artery disease. *JAMA* 1994; 272:231–233.

196. Cohen AS. Amyloidosis. In: Wilson JD, Braunwald E, Isselbacher KJ, Petersdorf RG, Martin JB, Fauci AS, et al (eds). *Harrison's Principles of Internal Medicine*, 12th ed. New York: McGraw-Hill; 1991:1417–1421.

197. Cohen AS. Amyloidosis. *N Engl J Med* 1967; 277:522–530.

198. Kyle RA, Greipp PR. Amyloidosis (AL): Clinical and laboratory features in 229 cases. *Mayo Clin Proc* 1983; 58:665–683.

199. Roberts WC, Waller BF. Cardiac amyloidosis causing cardiac dysfunction: Analysis of 54 necropsy patients. *Am J Cardiol* 1983; 52:137–146.

200. Olson LJ, Gertz MA, Edwards WD, et al. Senile cardiac amyloidosis with myocardial dysfunction: Diagnosis by endomyocardial biopsy and immunohistochemistry. *N Engl J Med* 1987; 317:738–742.

201. Nichols WC, Liepnieks JJ, Snyder EL, Benson MD. Senile cardiac amyloidosis associated with homozygosity for a transthyretin variant (ILE-122). *J Lab Clin Med* 1990; 117:175–180.

202. Nordlie M, Sletten K, Husby G, Ranlov PJ. A new prealbumin variant in familial amyloid cardiomyopathy of Danish origin. *Scand J Immunol* 1988; 27:119–122.

203. Gertz MA, Kyle RA, Greipp PR. Response rates and survival in primary systemic amyloidosis. *Blood* 1991; 77:257–262.

204. Gertz MA, Kyle RA. Primary systemic amyloidosis: A diagnostic primer. *Mayo Clin Proc* 1989; 64:1505–1519.

205. Click RL, Olson LJ, Edwards WD, Miller FA, Khandheria BK, Seward JB, et al. Echocardiography and systemic diseases. *J Am Soc Echocardiogr* 1994; 7:201–216.

206. Klein AL, Hatle LK, Taliercio CP, Oh JK, Kyle RA, Gertz MA, et al. Prognostic significance of Doppler measures of diastolic function in cardiac amyloidosis: A Doppler echocardiography study. *Circulation* 1991; 83:808–816.

207. Klein AL, Hatle LK, Taliercio CP, Taylor CL, Kyle RA, Bailey KR, et al. Serial Doppler echocardiographic follow-up of left ventricular diastolic function in cardiac amyloidosis. *J Am Coll Cardiol* 1990; 16:1135–1141.

208. Klein AL, Hatle LK, Burstow DJ, Taliercio CP, Seward JB, Kyle RA, et al. Comprehensive Doppler assessment of right ventricular diastolic function in cardiac amyloidosis. *J Am Coll Cardiol* 1990; 15:99–108.

209. Relman DA, Schmidt TM, MacDermott RP, Falkow S. Identification of the uncultured bacillus of Whipple's disease. *N Engl J Med* 1992; 327:293–301.

210. Pelech T, Fric P, Huslarova A, Jirasek A. Interstitial lymphocytic myocarditis in Whipple's disease. *Lancet* 1991; 337:553–554.

211. McAllister HA Jr, Fenoglio JJ Jr. Cardiac involvement in Whipple's disease. *Circulation* 1975; 52:152–156.

212. Southern JF, Moscicki RA, Margo C, Dickersin GR, Fallot JT, Bloch KJ. Lymphedema, lymphocytic myocarditis, and sarcoid-like granulomatosis: Manifestation of Whipple's disease. *JAMA* 1989; 261:1467–1470.

213. Feurle GE, Marth T. An evaluation of antimicrobial treatment for Whipple's disease: Tetracycline versus trimethoprim-sulfamethoxazole. *Dig Dis Sci* 1994; 39:1662–1648.

214. Wendler D, Mendoza E, Schleiffer T, Zander M, Maier M. *Tropheryma whippelii* endocarditis confirmed by polymerase chain reaction. *Eur Heart J* 1995; 16:424–425.

215. Bascom R, Johns CJ. The natural history and management of sarcoidosis. *Adv Intern Med* 1986; 31:213—241.

216. Roberts WC, McAllister HA, Ferrans VJ. Sarcoidosis of the heart: A clinicopathologic study of 35 necropsy patients and review of 78 previously described necropsy patients. *Am J Med* 1977; 63:86–106.

217. Silverman KJ, Hutchins GM, Bulkley BH. Cardiac sarcoid: A clinicopathologic study of 84 unselected patients with systemic sarcoidosis. *Circulation* 1978; 58:1204–1211.

218. Valantine H, McKenna WJ, Nihoyannopoulos P, Mitchell A, Foale RA, Davies MJ, et al. Sarcoidosis: A pattern of clinical and morphological presentation. *Br Heart J* 1987; 57:256–263.

219. Stein E, Stimmel B, Siltzbach LE. Clinical course of cardiac sarcoidosis. *Ann NY Acad Sci* 1976; 278:470–474.

220. Matsui Y, Iwai K, Tackibana T, Frrie T, Shigematsu N, Izumi T, et al. Clinicopathologic study of fatal cardiac sarcoidosis. *Ann NY Acad Sci* 1976; 278:455–469.

221. Burstow DJ, Tajik J, Bailey KR, DeRemee RA, Taliercio CP. Two-dimensional echocardiographic findings in systemic sarcoidosis. *Am J Cardiol* 1989; 63:478–482.

222. Johns CJ (ed). *Tenth International Conference on Sarcoidosis and Other Granulomatous Disorders.* New York: New York Academy of Sciences, 1986, vol 465.

223. Fleming HA. Cardiac sarcoidosis. *Semin Respir Med* 1986; 8:65–71.

224. Le Guludec D, Menad F, Faraggi M, Weinmann P, Battesti J-P, Valeyre D. Myocardial sarcoidosis: Clinical value of technetium-99m sestamibi tomoscintigraphy. *Chest* 1994; 106:1675–1682.

225. Schaedel H, Kirsten D, Schmidt A, Schmidt H, Strauss H-J. Sarcoid heart disease: Results of follow-up investigations. *Eur Heart J* 1991; 12(suppl D):26 27.

226. Winters SL, Cohen M, Greenberg S, Stein B, Curwin J, Pe E, et al. Sustained ventricular tachycardia associated with sarcoidosis: Assessment of the underlying cardiac anatomy and the prospective utility of programmed ventricular stimulation, drug therapy and an implantable antitachycardia device. *J Am Coll Cardiol* 1991; 18:937–943.

227. Fleming HA. Sarcoidosis heart disease. *Br Med J* 1986; 292:1095–1096.

77

ALCOHOL AND NUTRITION

Timothy J. Regan

HEART DISEASE IN ALCOHOLISM

Alcoholism is one of the more common etiologic factors identified with cardiomyopathy. In a series from an urban setting, a postmortem investigation revealed an association with chronic alcohol abuse in 40 percent.[1] Although many addicted to ethanol exhibit no heart disease, a prospective study of middle-aged Swedish males registered for the addiction revealed a frequency of clinical presentation twofold greater for cardiac events than for liver cirrhosis.[2]

Evidence for heart disease related to abuse of ethyl alcohol has been derived from a variety of disciplines including epidemiology, cardiac physiology, and pathology. As with other causes of primary myocardial disease, a diffuse abnormality of the myocardium is present that is unrelated to coronary atherosclerosis, systemic arterial hypertension, valvular or congenital heart disease. Although symptoms of congestive heart failure may be the most common presentation in primary myocardial disease of multiple etiologies, congestive heart failure may appear in fewer than half of the patients when they are first seen.[3] Arrhythmias without congestive heart failure may be the first abnormality to arise in a significant proportion. Chest pain is not uncommon, and classic angina pectoris may be the only symptom despite normal coronary arteriograms (see also Chap. 45).

Since the cardiovascular system may be affected by chronic alcohol abuse in a variety of ways, careful history taking is essential for patients with unexplained abnormalities related to any degree of cardiac decompensation, transient hypertension, arrhythmias, or chest pain. Clinical reports of cardiomyopathy have emphasized the problem of denial in eliciting a history of alcoholism. There is male predominance, and suggestive diagnostic aspects include a family history of chronic alcoholism, social disruption, or accident-proneness. The major positive diagnostic feature is the history of ethanol ingestion in intoxicating amounts for many years, frequently marked by periods of "spree drinking." Often this information can be obtained only through persistent questioning of the patient, communication with relatives, and evaluation of circulating hepatic enzymes. That subclinical cardiac abnormalities can be present in the absence of other causes of heart disease has been suggested in multiple clinical studies.

Subclinical Dysfunction

Noninvasive evaluation of heart function has enabled evaluation of cardiac involvement in subjects who abuse alcohol but have not yet developed clinical abnormalities. Regional wall motion abnormalities[4] and impaired diastolic relaxation of the left ventricle appear to be early manifestations of the subclinical abnormality.[5] Diminished diastolic compliance has also been described. A further stage of progression includes left ventricular hypertrophy with increased wall thickness and normal internal diameter, which may progress to a modest degree of dilatation.[6] In the asymptomatic patient, contractility may be diminished,[7] and there may be low-grade conduction abnormalities.[8] The type of beverage used does not appear to be a determinant, since these abnormalities have been observed in individuals using predominantly wine, beer, or spirits.

Heart Failure

As cardiac dysfunction in an alcoholic progresses to low-output failure, pulmonary congestion may lead to dyspnea on exertion or during sleep. Cardiomegaly may be moderate during an initial episode of decompensation in the absence of the mitral regurgitation related to papillary muscle dysfunction. After correction of heart failure, heart size may return to near normal. Occasionally a peripheral arterial or pulmonary embolism is the initial manifestation. No consistent pattern of alcohol abuse is associated with the onset of heart failure. A period of intensified drinking may be reported, but in some patients recurrent illness can apparently occur after a period of abstinence. Since the addicted person may commonly delay seeking medical assistance for weeks or months, evidence of right-sided heart failure is not uncommon. Clinical evidence of peripheral neuropathy or hepatic cirrhosis is not usually associated with alcoholic cardiomyopathy. The electrocardiogram (ECG) at this stage may be normal or may show nonspecific changes. Poor progression of the R wave across the pericardium is fairly common, presumably a result of progression of ventricular disease and intramural conduction delay. Evidence of left ventricular and atrial enlargement is common, but left anterior fascicular block or left or right bundle branch block appear in a minority of patients.

Systemic Arterial Hypertension

The diagnosis of alcoholic heart muscle disease is often obscured when the patient presents with elevated arterial blood pressure. When seen in association with other causes of heart failure, hypertension is usually considered to be secondary to compensatory peripheral vasoconstriction during cardiac decompression. In the alcoholic, hypertensive episodes may be frequent, particularly if measurements are performed close to a period of ethanol intake. This response has also been reported during the late intoxication–early withdrawal period in up to one-half of noncardiac alcoholics observed in an outpatient setting, usually without the development of a classical withdrawal illness.[9] Other evidence of hypertension, such as retinopathy, are usually absent.

Arterial pressure may be moderately elevated for several days, with spontaneous decline thereafter to a normal level (Table 77-1). Substantial elevations may require up to a week for spontaneous normalization and are usually associated with moderate sinus tachycardia. After a sustained period of abstinence, arterial pressure is normalized in all but 10 percent of noncardiac alcoholics, no greater than the incidence of the general population. In a 1-year follow-up, the normotensive state was found to persist in patients who remained abstinent. In general, alcoholism is also considered a risk factor for the development of systemic arterial hypertension (see also Chap. 56).

TABLE 77-1

ARTERIAL BLOOD PRESSURES IN CHRONIC ALCOHOLICS[a]

	Group A		Group B	
Day 1	186	115	148	97
	±4	±6	±3	±5
Day 3	158	96	132	80
	±7	±5	±4	±4
Day 7	126	77	128	75
	±3	±4	±2	±3

[a] Systolic and diastolic pressures (mmHg) in chronic alcoholics on day 1, the first day after interruption of alcohol intake and on day 7 without antihypertensive medication. Transient hypertensive responses were marked (group A, n = 8) or moderate (group B, n = 6). (From Regan TJ, et al,[9] with permission of the publisher and authors.)

TABLE 77-2

LEFT VENTRICULAR FUNCTION IN CHRONIC ALCOHOLISM WITH HEART FAILURE[a]

	Control	1 h	2 h	3 h
End-diastolic pressure, mmHg	15	17	27	22
End-diastolic volume, mL/m^2	124	144	200	174
Stroke/volume, mL/m^2	34	38	44	40

[a] Patient with compensated heart failure was fed 6 oz of Scotch whisky over a 2-h period. By 2 h, end-diastolic parameters were abnormal. [From Regan T, Haider B. Ethanol abuse and heart disease. *Circulation* 1981 (supp 3), III:14–19. With permission of the publisher and authors.]

Pathogenic Cofactors

Clinically evident malnutrition is not usually present in the cardiac patient, although it is commonly associated with liver disease. In females, alcoholism-related heart failure is rare before menopause. Cigarette smoking is very common among persons addicted to alcohol. Since myopathic responses to chronic cigarette smoking have been seen experimentally,[10] this factor may be more important than is generally recognized. Additionally, small, isolated outbreaks appear to occur from time to time in association with a combination of ethanol abuse and trace metal excess (lead, cobalt, or arsenic).

The course of alcoholic cardiomyopathy is variable, depending to a large degree on the extent of cardiac involvement. The outlook is relatively poor for patients who continue to ingest ethanol in substantial amounts. As illustrated in Table 77-2, a dose of alcohol that has no significant effect in the noncardiac alcoholic elicits a substantial increase of left ventricular filling pressure and volume in the decompensated patient. In one study, 64 alcoholic patients were followed over a 4-year period.[11] Of those who remained actively alcoholic, more than one-half succumbed. Fully one-third remained abstinent, and the mortality rate in this group was 9 percent, although only a minority exhibited clinical improvement, paralleling the response to abstinence in persons with hepatic cirrhosis.

Presumably, at certain stages of the disease, the pathogenic mechanisms may continue unabated despite traditional pharmacologic management and abstinence from alcohol. The encouraging results of abstinence may well have been exaggerated, since this group of individuals seemed to have relatively mild cardiac disease on entrance into the study. Nevertheless the response to abstinence supports the view that the major etiologic element in this disease process is ethyl alcohol.

The choice of pharmacologic therapy for cardiac decompensation depends on the state of cardiac disease when the patient is first encountered. During the initial episode of heart failure, if the patient has only modest cardiomegaly and pulmonary congestion, he or she may be managed initially by diuretics to diminish volume overload. As the disease progresses, there is a role for preload- and afterload-reducing agents and for digitalis, which is particularly useful in the control of atrial fibrillation (see also Chap. 27).

The role of cardiac transplantation in the treatment of alcoholic cardiomyopathy must be judged case by case. Obviously the patient should have discontinued the use of alcohol, and there should be no organic disease except the heart disease (see also Chap. 25).

Arrhythmias

Individuals addicted to alcohol may experience dizziness or syncope, which can be confused with the inebriated state; but a rhythm disorder can be revealed on the ECG. A series of such patients with a long background of alcoholism have been reported, who presented during or after acute intoxication.[8] Atrial fibrillation was the most common arrhythmia in a report of 32 separate dysrhythmias in 24 patients. Blood chemistries and cardiac anatomy were generally in the normal range. Restoration of sinus rhythm occurred spontaneously in some; cardioversion or pharmacologic intervention was required for others. With sustained drinking the patient may develop chronic fibrillation. Often related to drinking over a long weekend, this phenomenon has been characterized as "holiday heart syndrome," an acute cardiac rhythm disturbance associated with heavy alcohol consumption.[8]

To assess occult electrophysiologic abnormalities analogous to the subclinical mechanical dysfunction, high-fidelity electrocardiograms were performed. Conduction abnormalities of moderate extent were found when the patient has returned to normal sinus rhythm, with prolongation of PRc, QRS, and QTc (Table 77-3). There was an increased notching and slurring of the QRS complex consistent with primary myocardial disease. These conduction changes appeared to be independent of increased ventricular mass.

A unique opportunity to analyze the effects of chronic alcohol intake on cardiac rhythm in a more general population has been provided by a health maintenance organization.[12] The prevalence of acute arrhythmias in 1322 persons reporting six or more drinks per day was compared with the prevalence in 2644 subjects who reported drinking monthly, on average less than 1 drink daily. The relative risk for atrial fibrillation, atrial flutter, supraventricular tachycardia, and atrial premature beats was increased in the former group at least twofold.

In patients who abuse alcohol, ventricular arrhythmias appear to contribute to the incidence of sudden death even without a clinically recognized form of heart disease. Heterogeneous conduction and refractory periods are probable pathogenic factors. Potential contributing variables seen in alcoholics include cigarette smoking, electrolyte deficiencies, sleep apnea, and oxygen desaturation. Chronic ethanol use alone has been shown to be sufficient to reduce the ventricular fibrillation threshold in an animal model of chronic alcoholism.[13] Enhanced sympathetic activity is considered to be a major factor in pathogenesis.

A unique investigation of sudden death at the Pathology Institute in Moscow revealed that 17 percent of all witnessed

TABLE 77-3
CONDUCTION TIMES IN SUBCLINICAL DISEASE

	Normals (n = 10)	"Holiday Heart" (n = 17)	p Value
Heart rate (beats per minute)	63 ± 3	82 ± 3	<0.001
PRc (ms)	153 ± 6	179 ± 7	<0.01
QRS (ms)	80 ± 2	98 ± 3	<0.001
QTc (ms)	377 ± 6	430 ± 9	<0.001

(From Ettinger PO, et al,[8] with permission of the publisher and authors.)

cases of cardiac arrest were related to alcohol abuse.[14] Most patients were under 50 years of age and had significant concentrations of ethanol in blood or urine. Significant coronary artery disease was generally absent, but evidence of subclinical cardiomyopathy by light microscopy and electron microscopy was present in specimens taken within hours of death.

Prospective studies of large populations have buttressed the view that alcohol abuse can lead to sudden cardiac death. A system of registration with social authorities for alcoholism has been used in Sweden to evaluate the role of alcohol in both general and cause-specific mortality.[15] The incidence of sudden death over 11 years was almost doubled in the group registered for alcoholism compared to the unregistered. This association between alcohol and sudden coronary death was detected in men in the presence or absence of coronary heart disease.

To explore the pathogenesis of sudden death related to intoxication, dogs in a canine model were fed 36 percent of total calories as ethanol for 1 year.[13] Myocyte action potentials were assessed in vitro in a superfusion bath. Resting membrane potential, maximal amplitude, and repolarization were normal. These variables were unaffected by ethanol in the perfusate at 100 to 300 mg/dL. In contrast, normal controls exhibited a shortened repolarization time after ethanol.

In vivo chronic exposure to ethanol elicited a reduced threshold for ventricular fibrillation in the basal state as well as during acute ethanol administration,[13] consistent with the view that the myocardium may be susceptible to spontaneous ventricular arrhythmias. A major role for the sympathetic system in pathogenesis may be assumed in view of the substantial increase in the concentration of norepinephrine in the coronary venous effluent as a reflection of neurohormone concentrations in the myocardial synaptic gap (Table 77-4). Paradoxically, there was a reduced sensitivity to administered catecholamines in the chronic animal in terms of in vivo and in vitro electrophysiologic effects.[13] The high basal levels of plasma norepinephrine suggest that there may be a substantial occupation of beta-adrenergic receptors, so that the dose-response curve reflects a reduced activation in vivo as well as in the superfused tissue. The basis for the substantial norepinephrine levels may relate to enhanced sympathetic stimulation with neuronal release of norepinephrine. Reduced reuptake of the neurohormone could contribute to enhanced levels available to the beta receptor.

TABLE 77-4

BASAL PLASMA NOREPINEPHRINE (pg/mL)
AFTER 1 YEAR OF ETHANOL[a]

Group	Arterial			Coronary Sinus–Arterial		
Control, mean	392 ±46	405 ±38	384 ±42	76 ±22	112 ±22	108 ±35
Alcohol, mean	3,150 ±914	3,008[b] ±846	3,217[b] ±973	1410[b] ±388	1794[b] ±258	1483[b] ±394

[a] Three steady state samples were taken at 5-min intervals in fasting anesthetized animals.
[b] Nonpaired test of paired samples versus control group: $p < 0.01$.
(From Patel R, et al,[13] with permission of the publisher and authors.)

Presumably arrhythmogenesis is related to the association of acute neurohormonal and cation alterations in myocardium with structural alterations. The latter include the dilated intercalated disk at the myocyte[16] and collagen accumulation in extracellular matrix.[10]

Determinants of Alcoholic Heart Disease

The evidence that ethanol and/or its metabolites are the etiologic basis for alcoholic cardiomyopathy is circumstantial. The major positive feature supporting this idea is the history of ethanol ingestion in intoxicating amounts over many years, frequently marked by periods of spree drinking.

Animal models have been shown to develop functional, biochemical, and morphologic abnormalities, but congestive heart failure has not been reported. This may be related to an insufficient duration of ethanol exposure. Clinically, the reduced mortality rate in patients who become abstinent supports the view that ethanol is the major factor in development of the disease.[11]

It is noteworthy that development of the subclinical state is consistent with living in a family setting and stable employment.[7] In this study, 60 percent of subjects were skilled laborers or office workers. The others were unskilled, but none were considered indigent. The duration of excessive intake averaged 16 years, while the quantity of alcohol consumed appeared to approximate the more than six drinks per day reported for occurrence of atrial arrhythmias.[12]

In addition to ethanol abuse, several other factors have been considered to be potentially important. Cigarette use is common in persons addicted to alcohol and may be contributory.[10,15] Clinically evident malnutrition, though often seen in association with alcoholic cirrhosis, particularly at the subclinical stage of the disease,[7] is not usually present in the cardiac patient.[8] In females, alcoholic heart disease is rare prior to menopause.

Pathophysiology

With regard to mechanism, there appears to be a direct effect of ethanol or its metabolites on cardiac function as well as a long-term neurohumoral influence on the heart; this may inter-

act with adaptive processes that tend to mitigate pathologic effects. The early decrease of diastolic compliance of the left ventricle seen experimentally is most likely related to alteration of interstitium.[10,17] Collagen accumulates in a largely insoluble state due to the process of advanced glycosylation, resulting in greater cross links. After several years, left ventricular contractility may be impaired.[17,18] There is an associated accumulation of water and Na^+ in cardiac cells without a reduction of K^+, perhaps related to the altered membrane phospholipid composition. In view of the dilatation of sarcoplasmic reticulum observed by electron microscopy,[17] it has been postulated that dysfunction of the tubular membranes may limit the rate of Ca^{2+} availability to contractile protein, and thus diminish contractile performance, without a change in total Ca^{2+}.[18] Although high-energy phosphate levels are not altered, an inhibitory effect of long-term ethanol use on myosin adenosinetriphosphatase (ATPase) and Ca^{2+}-activated myofibrillar ATPase has been demonstrated.

One might expect protein synthesis in the cardiac cell to be adversely affected by chronic ethanol exposure. In experiments to determine the ability of chronic ethanol feeding to affect the process of myocardial hypertrophy during chronic aortic pressure overload,[19] the hypertrophic response was unimpaired. Moreover, ribonucleic acid, a determinant of protein synthesis, was not found to be diminished in alcoholic animals over a period of 14 weeks.[19]

When the disease is clinically evident, there appears to be some degree of impaired synthesis, or accelerated degradation, of contractile protein, since lysis of myofibrils is frequently observed on morphologic study of advanced alcoholic cardiomyopathy. This may precede the appearance of rapid clinical deterioration. In examination of biopsy specimens from patients and of autopsied tissue, no distinctive features have been revealed in patients with alcoholic heart disease as compared with dilated cardiomyopathy from other causes.[20]

Moderate Ethanol Intake and Prevention of Coronary Disease

A series of epidemiologic studies have suggested that one to two drinks a day of any alcoholic beverage provides a protective function in terms of coronary artery disease. Three or more drinks per day can raise blood pressure.[21] The apparent protective effect is of relatively low strength and raises concern about the influence of confounding variables compared to controls. The latter include physical activity as well as educational and economic status. Observations that protective effects are observed in people who have only one drink a month support this view.

Further analysis of the population subsets among females has revealed that only those with coronary risk factors experience a benefit from low-dose ethanol.[22] Whether or not this benefit is additive to the influence of standard cardiac care is not clear. Similar data on males are not available. A down side to the "moderate intake" prescription is the association with an increased risk of cancer[23] and premature mortality.[24]

Studies of peripheral arteries have revealed discordant results.[25,26] Thus, the relative disease risk requires assessment in each subject. Moreover, the use of alcohol for cardioprotective purposes has been discouraged as a general public health measure, since alcohol abuse appears to correlate with average alcohol consumption in populations[27] (see Chap. 41).

VITAMIN DEFICIENCIES[28]

Thiamine

The key features of beriberi, or thiamine deficiency, though not readily reproducible in animals, include a high cardiac output associated with arteriolar vasodilatation. Although it has been the classic view that right ventricular failure is dominant when symptoms develop, several studies have documented a significant elevation of left ventricular end-diastolic and pulmonary capillary wedge pressures. The hemodynamic abnormalities are reversible with thiamine therapy.

Other Vitamins

Unequivocal direct effects of vitamin A and niacin deficiencies on heart muscle in humans have not been established. Scurvy, however, can be associated with sudden death. Human volunteers on a vitamin C-deficient diet have reported dyspnea and chest pain associated with PR interval prolongation and ST-segment abnormalities. ECG alterations can be reversed rapidly with parenteral vitamin C. In experimental vitamin B_6 deficiency in rats, cardiomyopathic changes were found postmortem, but the human counterpart has yet to be described. Excess doses of vitamin D in humans have been associated with deposits of calcium as well as with the shortened QT interval of hypercalcemia. Mild excesses of vitamin D_3 have been shown to intensify atherosclerosis in nonhuman primates.

Vitamin E and Selenium

In recent years a cardiomyopathy (Keshan's disease) affecting infants and children has been described in China. The disease is characterized by local myocardial necrosis, fibrosis, and hypercontraction bands. The disease has a regional distribution in agricultural areas where the selenium content of the staple grains and soil is reduced. Supplementation of the diet with selenium has been found effective as a preventive. In view of a seasonal variation, other factors may also be important. Although isolated selenium deficiency that produces cardiomyopathy has not been described in experimental animal models, a combined deprivation of selenium and vitamin E has been shown to produce diffuse patchy necrosis of the myocardium in young swine. An abnormality of cell lipid peroxidation has been thought to affect membrane lipids, with resultant disturbance of intracellular electrolyte and water composition as well as energy production.

CACHEXIA

Severe weight loss in individuals of relatively normal initial body weight may have important cardiovascular consequences, particularly in infants and children. In an analysis of 93 malnourished children studied at autopsy in Costa Rica, 14 were considered to have primary congestive heart failure resulting from either marasmus or kwashiorkor.[29] On histologic examination, interstitial edema was frequently observed. Substantial degrees of vacuolization within myocardial fibers with apparent disorganization of myofibrillar structure were observed.

The nutritional deficiency that characterizes protein-calorie undernutrition in more mature individuals has been studied by a number of investigators.[30] In human adult volunteers on a semistarvation regimen, significant reductions of heart rate, stroke volume, cardiac output, and heart size were observed during the development of cachexia. Cardiac output, however, did not appear to fall out of proportion to the diminished metabolic requirements. In addition, an echocardiographic study of patients with undernutrition secondary to a variety of chronic disease states found that the reduced cardiac output was associated with a diminished left ventricular end-diastolic diameter and mass. When the cardiac index was adjusted for body weight, however, it was higher than that of normal control subjects.

Anorexia nervosa influences the cardiovascular system in several respects. Observations of a group of individuals with anorexia nervosa showed that the systolic ejection-phase indices of left ventricular function were normal and responded normally to exercise. The patients in this study were considered to have an adult marasmus-type syndrome that did not significantly affect cardiac function; however, on two-dimensional echocardiography, the left ventricular mass was found to be reduced to between one-half and two-thirds that of age- and sex-matched control subjects. This reduction was even greater when left ventricular mass was considered in relation to total body weight. Left ventricular afterload was reduced, while resting left ventricular function was normal. With the change in skeletal muscle mass the response to exercise was limited, with a lower peak oxygen consumption. In addition, there were reduced increments in heart rate and systolic blood pressure.

Analysis of substrates in systemic blood showed normal glucose responses to exercise; however, free fatty acid concentrations, which doubled in control patients during exercise, showed no change in the anorexic group. The ECG in anorexia nervosa is generally unremarkable, but some patients exhibit nonspecific ST- and T-wave changes. Although the QT interval is usually normal, prolongation has been described in association with sudden death, despite normal plasma electrolyte levels, as an apparently unusual event.

In primary protein-calorie undernutrition, the weight of the evidence indicates that the adult heart, though atrophied, will usually function normally prior to refeeding. Patients who recover from anorexia show improvement in heart rate, posterior wall dimension, systolic wall stress, and left ventricular internal dimension.[5] Studies of young children, supported by some experimental data, suggest that substantial histologic abnormalities of the myocardium may occur. In some of the children studied, heart failure may be attributable to the undernutrition. A potential for arrhythmias and sudden death resulting from undernutrition has been postulated, but this has not been well established.

HYPERALIMENTATION

Therapeutic feeding by the enteric or parenteral route has assumed increasing importance in the treatment of a variety of acute illnesses. Although the initial hemodynamic changes during such therapy have not been delineated, the acute responses to oral feeding in normally nourished persons—particularly the cardiovascular changes—are of interest.

During oral feeding in human beings, a diet of mixed caloric composition induces an increase of cardiac output associated with a decline in systemic vascular resistance within 20 min after completion of a meal.[31] The rise in cardiac output is essentially due to an increase in stroke volume without a change in left ventricular filling pressure, implying an increase in contractility. In patients who have postprandial angina pectoris at rest, stroke volume is diminished while pulmonary wedge pressure is elevated.[31]

Patients with chronic cardiac disease may suffer forms of malnutrition similar to those described for the general hospital population.[32] An extreme form, the syndrome of *cardiac cachexia*, is attributable to anorexia, decreased intestinal absorption of food, and perhaps a change in the distribution of substrates absorbed into the circulatory system. Patients with cardiac cachexia appear to have increased morbidity and mortality rates in comparison to noncachectic patients similar in age, sex, and severity of heart disease. In a prospective study of cardiac patients undergoing surgery, the effects of short-term forced feeding of up to 1500 calories were evaluated.[33] The lack of effect on morbidity and mortality rates was perhaps related to the fact that feeding was begun just prior to operation and continued for approximately 5 days. The effects of longer-term preparation of patients before surgery require investigation.

Adults with chronic undernutrition without underlying heart disease may develop heart failure during hyperalimentation.[30] Under the conditions of rapid repletion, a state resembling congestive heart failure may develop that is characterized by hypermetabolism and ventricular gallop but with augmented cardiac output and normal left ventricular ejection fraction. Rapid resolution follows administration of diuretic therapy, slowing of the rate of hyperalimentation, and reduction of the daily intake of sodium.

During hyperalimentation, some patients may develop hypophosphatemia. As in other circumstances producing this anion deficit, significant cardiac effects may ensue. In a study of patients with hypophosphatemia whose echocardiograms showed no mechanical defects, a significant increase in the incidence of arrhythmias was observed, without reduction in the plasma concentrations of other electrolytes.[34] Patients who exhibited nonsustained ventricular tachycardia were improved by normalization of plasma phosphate levels by oral supplements.

REFERENCES

1. Roberts WC, Siegel RJ, McManus BM. Idiopathic dilated cardiomyopathy: Analysis of 152 necropsy patients. *Am J Cardiol* 1987; 60:1340–1355.
2. Rosengren A, Wilhelmsen L, Pennert K, Berglund G, Elmfeldt D. Alcoholic intemperance, coronary heart disease and mortality in middle aged Swedish men. *Acta Med Scand* 1987; 222:201–213.
3. Shirey EK, Proudfit WL, Hawk WA. Primary myocardial disease: Correlation with clinical findings, angiographic and biopsy diagnosis. *Am Heart J* 1980; 99:198–207.
4. Bertolet BD, Freund G, Martin CA, Perchalski DL, Williams CM, Pepine CJ. Unrecognized left ventricular dysfunction in an apparently healthy alcohol abuse population. *Drug Alcohol Depend* 1991; 28:113–119.
5. Kupari M, Koskinen P, Suokas A, Ventila M. Left ventricular filling impairment in asymptomatic chronic alcoholics. *Am J Cardiol* 1990; 66:1473–1477.
6. Mathews EC Jr, Gardin JM, Henry WL, Del Negro A, Fletcher R, Snow J. Echocardiographic abnormalities in chronic alcoholics with and without overt congestive heart failure. *Am J Cardiol* 1981; 47:570–578.
7. Urbano-Marquez A, Estruch R, Navarro-Lopez F, Grau JM, Mont L, Rubin E. The effects of alcoholism on skeletal and cardiac muscle. *N Engl J Med* 1989; 320:409–415.
8. Ettinger PO, Wu CF, DeLa Cruz CL Jr, Weiss AB, Ahmed SS, Regan TJ. Arrhythmias and the "holiday heart": Alcohol-associated cardiac rhythm disorders. *Am Heart J* 1978; 95:555–562.
9. Regan TJ, Pathan A, Weiss AB, Eaddy C, Torres R. The contribution of arterial pressure to the cardiac dysfunction of chronic alcoholism. *Acta Med Scand* 1986; 703(suppl):273–280.
10. Rajiyah G, Agarwal R, Avendano G, Lyons M, Soni B, Regan TJ. Influence of nicotine on myocardial stiffness and fibrosis during chronic ethanol use. *Alcohol: Clin Exp Res* 1996; 20:985–989.
11. Demakis JG, Proskey A, Rahimtoola SH, Jamil M, Sutton GC, Rosen KM et al. The natural course of alcoholic cardiomyopathy. *Ann Intern Med* 1974; 80:293–297.
12. Cohen EJ, Klatsky AL, Armstrong MA. Alcohol use and supra-ventricular arrhythmia. *Am J Cardiol* 1988; 62:971–973.
13. Patel R, McArdle JJ, Regan TJ. Increased ventricular vulnerability in a chronic ethanol model despite reduced electrophysiologic responses to catecholamines. *Alcohol: Clin Exp Res* 1991; 15:785–789.
14. Vikhert AM, Tsiplenkova VG, Cherpachenka NM. Alcoholic cardiomyopathy and sudden cardiac death. *J Am Coll Cardiol* 1986; 8:3A–11A.
15. Rosengren A, Wilhelmsen L, Wedel H. Separate and combined effects of smoking and alcohol abuse in middle aged men. *Acta Med Scand* 1988; 223:111–118.
16. Ettinger PO, Lyons M, Oldewurtel HA, Regan TJ. Cardiac conduction abnormalities produced by chronic alcoholism. *Am Heart J* 1976; 91:66–78.
17. Thomas G, Haider B, Oldewurtel HA, Lyons MM, Yeh CK, Regan TJ. Progression of myocardial abnormalities in experimental alcoholism. *Am J Cardiol* 1980; 46:233–241.
18. Sarma JSM, Shigeaki I, Fischer R, Maruyama Y, Weishaar R, Bing BJ. Biochemical and contractile properties of heart muscle after prolonged alcohol administration. *J Mol Cell Cardiol* 1976; 8:951–972.
19. Whitman V, Schuler HG, Musselman J. Effects of chronic ethanol consumption on the myocardial hypertrophic response to a pressure overload in the rat. *J Mol Cell Cardiol* 1980; 12:519–572.
20. Olsen EGJ. The pathology of cardiomyopathies: A critical analysis. *Am Heart J* 1979; 98:385–392.
21. Friedman GD, Klatsky AL. Is alcohol good for your health? *N Engl J Med* 1993; 329:1882–1883.
22. Fuchs CS, Stampfer MJ, Colditz GA, et al. Alcohol consumption and mortality among women. *N Engl J Med* 1995; 332:1245–1250.

23. Boffetta P, Garfinkel L. Alcohol drinking and mortality among men enrolled in American Cancer Society prospective study. *Epidemiology* 1990; 1:342–348.

24. Zureik M, Ducimentiere P. High alcohol related premature mortality in France; Concordant estimates from a prospective cohort study and national mortality statistics. *Alcohol Clin Exp Res* 1996; 20:428–433.

25. Demirovic J, Nabulsi A, Folsom AR, et al. Alcohol consumption and ultrasonographically assessed carotid artery valve thickness and distensibility. The Atherosclerosis Risk in Communities. (ARIC) Study Investigators. *Circulation* 1993; 88:2787–2793.

26. Camargo CA, Stamfer MJ, Glynn RJ, et al. Prospective study of moderate alcohol consumption and risk of peripheral arterial disease in US male physicians. *Circulation* 1997; 95:577–580.

27. Criqui MH, Ringel BL. Does diet or alcohol explain the French paradox? *Lancet* 1994; 344:1719–1723.

28. Watson R, ed. *Nutrition and Heart Disease II*. Boca Raton, FL: CRC Press; 1987:19–71.

29. Piza J, Troper L, Cespedes R, Miller JH, Berenson GS. Myocardial lesions and heart failure in infantile malnutrition. *Am J Trop Med Hyg* 1971; 20:343–355.

30. Moodie DS. Anorexia and the heart: Results of studies to assess effects. *Postgrad Med* 1987; 81:46–55.

31. Figueras J, Singh GN, Ganz W, Swan HJC. Hemodynamic and electro-cardiographic accompaniments of resting postprandial angina. *Br Heart J* 1979; 42:402–409.

32. Bistrian BR, Blackburn GL, Vitale J, Cochran D, Naylor J. Prevalence of malnutrition in general medical patients. *JAMA* 1976; 235:1567–1570.

33. Abel RM, Fischer JE, Buckley MJ, Barnett GO, Austen WG. Malnutrition in cardiac surgical patients: Results of a prospective randomized evaluation of early post-operative parenteral nutrition. *Arch Surg* 1976; 111:45–50.

34. Venditti F, Panezai F, Marotta C, Oldewurtel H, Regan TJ. Hypophosphatemia and cardiac arrhythmias. *Min Electrolyte Metab* 1987; 13:19–25.

78

ENDOCRINE DISEASES AND THE CARDIOVASCULAR SYSTEM

Joel Zonszein / Edmund H. Sonnenblick

DIABETES MELLITUS, INSULIN RESISTANCE, AND ATHEROSCLEROTIC HEART DISEASE

Metabolic abnormalities found in the insulin resistance syndrome (IRS) and diabetes mellitus (DM) constitute a distinctive milieu for the development of atherosclerotic cardiovascular disease. With concurrent small- and large-vessel disease, the "diabetic heart" becomes a common focus of ischemic states resulting in myocardial infarction and congestive heart failure, with a slower and limited potential for recovery. Therefore, prevention or delay in the onset of heart disease remains the most important, but as yet an elusive, goal in the diabetic patient.

Prevalence

Close to 8 million people in the United States have been diagnosed as having DM. Of these, about 90 to 95 percent appear to have type 2 diabetes (type 2 DM), or non-insulin-dependent diabetes mellitus (NIDDM), a disease characterized by insulin resistance with inadequate compensatory insulin secretion. The reminder have mainly an autoimmune-mediated form of primary pancreatic islet beta-cell defect or failure, known as insulin-dependent diabetes mellitus (IDDM), or type 1 (type 1 DM). The prevalence of type 2 DM increases with age, with rates as high as 10 to 11 percent in the general population at the age of 65. Based on oral glucose tolerance tests, the total prevalence is estimated to be 16 million people. Further, about 20 million people have impaired glucose tolerance (IGT), a condition in which blood glucose levels are not normal but are not in the diabetic range. When IGT is also included, rates of total glucose intolerance in the United States core population approach 50 percent at age 65 years[1] (Fig. 78-1). Atherosclerotic heart disease in DM appears earlier in life, affects women almost as often as men, and is more often fatal. The risk ratio incidence of coronary heart disease (CHD) in the diabetic population is 1.7 to 2.3 higher in men and 2.9 to 3.2 higher in women, with a higher mortality risk of 1.5 to 3.8 for men and 2.6 to 4.7 in women. Also, patients with DM have a poorer prognosis after a myocardial infarction, with 1.4 to 3.1 higher risk for reinfarction and 1.5 to 3.0 higher risk for death.[1]

Endogenous Hyperinsulinemia as a Cardiovascular Risk Factor

Glucose metabolism and insulin have multiple effects on the cardiovascular system and the development of cardiovascular disease. Resistance to insulin-mediated disposal of glucose, and compensatory hyperinsulinemia, is present in most patients with either IGT or type 2 DM.[2] The high prevalence of CHD in newly discovered diabetics[3] and in individuals with IGT without significant hyperglycemia[4,5] favors the hypothesis that hyperinsulinemia and not hyperglycemia per se may play a central role in the pathogenesis of CHD.[3–5] Hyperinsulinemia can be found in nondiabetic first-degree relatives of type 2 DM patients, and hyperinsulinemic individuals often develop type 2 DM. This observation and the high incidence of premature CHD have led to the speculation that this is a singular entity, caused by common genetic and environmental factors.[6] Syndrome X, or IRS, describes individuals with IGT with additional resistance to insulin-stimulated glucose uptake and hyperinsulinemia, along with dyslipidemia (increased triglycerides, decreased high-density lipoprotein cholesterol) and hypertension.[2] Abdominal, or central, obesity has been added to this syndrome.[7] The direct atherogenic properties of insulin have been demonstrated in experimental[8] and observational clinical studies.[9–14] The association between hyperinsulinemia and CHD is less strong when other factors such as age and ethnicity are taken into account.[15–22] For instance, hyperinsulinemia is associated with athero-

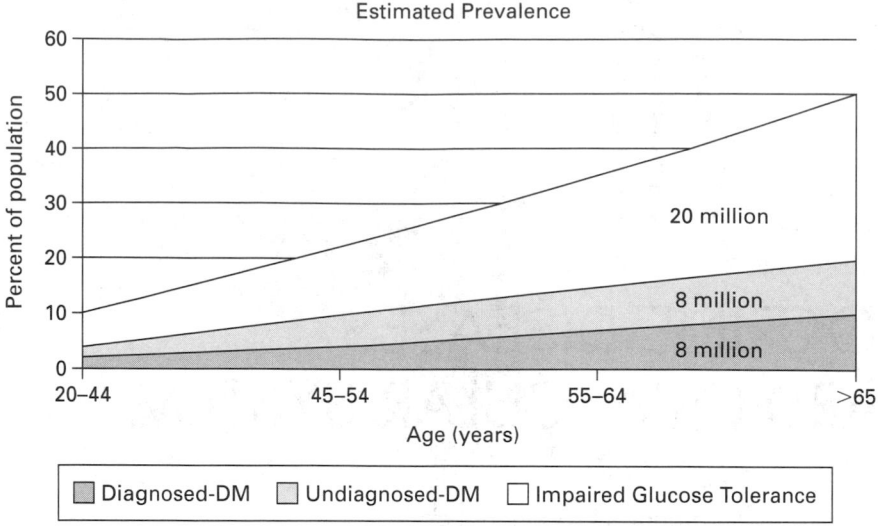

Estimated Prevalence

FIGURE 78-1

Estimated prevalence of diagnosed non-insulin-dependent diabetes mellitus (type 2 DM) and impaired glucose tolerance (IGT) in the U.S. population in 1996. (Adapted from Harris et al.[1])

sclerotic heart disease in the Caucasian population, which has a characteristic apolipoprotein phenotype,[21] and constitutes a greater risk factor in men with apo E 3/2 phenotype, rather than the more common apo E 3/3 phenotype.[22]

While the role that hyperinsulinemia plays in the pathogenesis of atherosclerosis remains unclear,[8] it is an independent predictive risk factor for CHD.[14] Acute administration of insulin produces vasodilatation with a hyperdynamic circulatory state due to reflex sympathetic nervous system activation. It has been postulated that the increased heart rate, a widened pulse pressure, and increased cardiac output can lead to cardiovascular disease in IRS or type 2 DM.[23]

Since standard insulin assays may overestimate "true insulin levels" due to cross-reactivity with intact proinsulin and split insulin products, it has been suggested that proinsulin and/or split proinsulin products, rather than insulin itself, may lead to vascular disease.[24] It is the markedly elevated true insulin levels that appear to be associated with acute myocardial infarction (AMI), however, while increased insulin production also results in increased levels of partially processed proinsulin.[25] Clearly, increased basal C-peptide concentration (an indicator of insulin secretion), proinsulin, and hyperinsulinemia are important markers of vascular disease, but their possible role in the pathogenesis of vascular disease is intriguing and warrants further definition.[26]

Other Risk Factors Associated with Cardiovascular Disease

Hyperinsulinemia appears to be only one of several and more complex factors affecting the cardiovascular system in syndrome X and type 2 DM. Hyperinsulinemia and the other risk factors described initially as the "metabolic syndrome X"[27] for the development of accelerated cardiovascular disease appear to represent only the central core of a larger, more

complex multifactorial syndrome. The IRS and type 2 DM form a continuum of a disease entity affected by an expanding list of genetic and environmental factors[26–29] (Table 78-1).

The great variability in the prevalence of cardiovascular disease in different ethnic populations supports the concept of a *genetic predisposition*. For instance, the Pima Indians, a population with the highest incidence of type 2 DM and adverse lipid profile, are less susceptible to cardiovascular events.[30] The prevalence of IRS and type 2 DM has become apparent in young individuals of certain susceptible populations, such as Native Americans and Mexican Americans, due to a rapid exposure to adverse environmental factors.

Hyperinsulinemia is closely associated with visceral obesity, elevated triglyceride levels, and lowered high-density lipoprotein cholesterol levels. Increases in low-density lipoprotein (LDL) cholesterol are less common, although LDL cholesterol in this syndrome is formed by small dense LDL particles, which are more atherogenic.[31] The *dyslipidemia* of diabetes is highly atherogenic, particularly when associated with other risk factors such as hypertension (see also Chaps. 41 and 53).

Hypertension is another major risk factor for CHD in IGT and type 2 DM,[2,32] independent of the degree of obesity, hyperinsulinemia, and/or antihypertensive therapy. The interrelationship between hyperinsulinemia and hypertension appears unique in this syndrome since other models of hypertension, such as renal artery stenosis, or primary hyperaldosteronism, are not accompanied by hyperinsulinemia.[33,34]

Obesity, IRS, and type 2 DM seem to share common genetic factors and can be adversely affected by lifestyle habits.[6] In nondiabetic individuals or different ethnic backgrounds (European and Native Americans), only less than 50 percent of the total variance of insulin-mediated glucose utilization can be attributed to obesity.[35] Central obesity, also known as "android" or "apple" obesity, is associated with IRS and type 2 DM and a high prevalence of CHD. Measuring the waist-hip ratio, i.e., the circumference at the umbilicus divided by the circumference at the public symphysis, is easy and practical. Values greater than 0.85 are considered to represent android obesity in white populations.

Severity and duration of *hyperglycemia* are involved in the pathogenesis of microvasculopathy.[36–38] Hyperglycemia is also an excellent predictor of CHD morbidity and mortality, particularly in women and in the elderly.[37] While hyperglycemia is an important marker of disease progression, the benefits of normalization of glycemic levels in advanced large-vessel disease is less clear than in microvasculopathy.[36–38]

A state of *increased coagulation* occurs in type 2 DM through several mechanisms.[39] Fibrinogen levels are in-

TABLE 78-1

CARDIOVASCULAR RISK FACTORS AND MARKERS IMPLICATED IN HYPERINSULINEMIA AND TYPE 2 DIABETES MELLITUS

Genetic
Adverse environmental factors
Increased age
Sex
Metabolic syndrome "X"
   Hyperinsulinemia
   Resistance to insulin-stimulated glucose uptake
   Impaired glucose tolerance
   Dyslipidemia
      High triglycerides
      Low HDL-cholesterol
      Elevated dense LDL-cholesterol subparticles
      Increased lipoprotein(a)
      Increased apolipoprotein B
   Central obesity
   Hypertension
Hyperglycemia
Hypercoagulability state
   Platelet hyperaggregability
      Decreased platelet cAMP, cGMP
      Increased platelet-dependent thrombin generation
   Increased von Willebrand factor procoagulant activity
   Elevated fibrinogen
   Impaired fibrinolysis
      Increased plasminogen activator inhibitor type-1 activity
      Decreased plasminogen activator activity
Hyperhomocysteinemia
Endothelial dysfunction
Sex steroids
   Increased androgens
   Low estrogens
   Low dehydroepiandosterone
Others
   Elevated proinsulin and insulin propeptides
   Low sex hormone–binding protein
   Low insulin-like growth factor binding protein-1
   Hyperuricemia
   Albuminuria
   Cardiac syndrome "X"
   Medications

creased, a major risk factor for thrombotic complications, in part due to excessive release of fibrinogen by the liver, responding to cytokine signals such as tumor necrosis factor and interleukin 1. Hyperglycemia is also associated with increased platelet-dependent thrombin generation, an important index of coagulopathy that can be readily reversed with improved glycemic control.[40] Tissue plasminogen activator (tPA) activates the fibrinolytic system by converting plasminogen to plasmin and by the degradation of the fibrin polymer located on the surface clots. This effect is blocked by plasminogen activator inhibitor 1 (PAI-1), and impaired endogenous

fibrinolytic activity can accelerate atherosclerosis. This process may take place by exposing the vascular luminal wall surfaces to persistent and recurrent thrombi and clot-associated mitogens. In type 2 DM individuals, there is a threefold elevation of plasma concentration of PAI-1 with decreased fibrinolytic activity. Increased PAI-1 activity is directly correlated with hyperinsulinemia, and elevated levels are found in type 2 DM,[41] hypertension,[42] hypertriglyceredemia, and obesity. The inverse relationship between tPA activity and insulin concentrations[43] and the high PAI-1/tPA ratios suggest hypercoagulability and may contribute to accelerated CHD in these populations.

Hyperhomocysteinemia is another metabolic risk factor for atherosclerosis that has been associated with type 2 DM.[44] Homocysteine appears to have toxic effects on the vascular endothelium, with adverse effects on the clotting cascade. Elevated homocysteine levels are associated with deficiencies in folic acid, vitamin B_6, and vitamin B_{12}. Vitamin supplementation lowers homocysteine concentrations in almost all patients.[44]

Endothelial dysfunction occurs with atherosclerosis in DM and is associated with decreased availability of endothelium-derived nitric oxide. Nitric oxide also inhibits platelet aggregation and proliferation of vascular smooth muscle. Postulated mechanisms include decreased synthesis or increased inactivation of nitric oxide, decreased responsiveness of the nitric oxide–guanylate cyclase pathway in smooth muscle, and increased release of vasoconstrictor prostanoids preventing the vasodilator effect of nitric oxide. Nitric oxide–mediated vasodilatation is impaired in type 2 DM, related either to decreased nitric oxide release or to decreased reactivity of the vascular smooth muscle.[45]

The role of *sex hormones* in the development of atherogenic changes is suggested by their protective effect in premenopausal women and the high incidence of atherogenic disorders in men. Hyperandrogenism is associated with obesity and insulin resistance[46] and occurs with the syndrome of polycystic ovaries.[47] The causal relation between hyperinsulinemia and androgen excess is difficult to elucidate; while there is improvement in insulin resistance with antiandrogen treatment,[48] decreasing serum insulin concentrations can also ameliorate hyperandrogenism.[47]

Dehydroepiandrosterone (DHEA) *sulfate* is the most abundantly produced adrenal steroid, but a biological role has not yet been clearly established. Low serum DHEA sulfate concentration reflects an insulin-resistant state, however, and is associated with an increased incidence of atherosclerosis.[49] DHEA sulfate and its parent steroid, DHEA, appear to exert antiatherogenic and cardioprotective actions in men but not in women.[50] Further, weight loss is associated with a marked rise in serum DHEA sulfate levels in men, whereas in women, serum DHEA sulfate levels are not changed.[49] Although the concept is speculative, it appears that insulin acts in a sex-specific fashion, reducing circulating DHEA sulfate in men only.

Insulin also regulates hepatocyte production of *sex hormone–binding globulin* (SHBG), and *insulin-like growth fac-*

tor–binding protein 1 (IGFBP-1). Decreased SHBG is an indirect measurement of androgenicity, is closely associated with hyperinsulinemia, and is an important independent risk factor and predictor for the development of type 2 DM in women; SHBG is lower in conditions such as obesity and polycystic ovarian syndrome. Thus SHBG and IGFBP-1 can also serve as markers for insulin sensitivity.[51]

Angiotensin I-converting enzymes (ACE) activate angiotensin I to the vasoactive angiotensin II and degrade bradykinin. The ACE gene may be involved in vascular tone regulation, with the ACE *D/D* genotype being associated with CHD, and ACE *I/D* gene polymorphism being associated with CHD in the NIDDM population. While deletion polymorphism of the ACE gene is associated with increased plasma-converting enzyme activity, however, it has not been found to be an independent predictor of CHD.[52] Further, contrary to the hypothesis that angiotensin II may cause insulin resistance, as is the case with other vasoconstrictive hormones such as catecholamines, infusion of angiotensin II increases insulin-mediated glucose disposal in healthy and in type II DM individuals. Increased skeletal muscle blood flow has been postulated as a possible explanation, although a direct metabolic effect of angiotensin II remains an intriguing possibility.[53] Paradoxically, ACE inhibitors such as captopril as well as other long-acting non-sulfhydryl-containing ACE inhibitors can also enhance insulin-stimulated glucose transport activity. The insulin-sensitive skeletal muscle glucose transport system, GLUT4, is enhanced through bradykinin or one of its metabolites. Inhibition of angiotensin II action results in decreased GLUT4 protein expression induced by diabetes, an effect that may be important in the ischemic diabetic heart, where glucose replaces free fatty acids as a favored energy substrate[54] but where less glucose is available because of the depletion of the GLUT4 glucose transporter.

Elevated uric acid levels, even in the absence of gout, can also be used as a simple marker of insulin resistance and may be an added risk factor for accelerated CHD.[55] Furthermore, caution is needed for diuretic use in these individuals, as diuretics cannot only worsen carbohydrate and lipid metabolism but also further increase uric acid levels.

Albuminuria is also an important marker of CHD.[56] Slight elevation of the urinary albumin excretion rate (AER), termed *microalbuminuria* (AER between 30 and 300 mg/24 h), is an independent predictor of cardiovascular mortality.[57] The combination of poor glycemic control and the degree of albuminuria is linearly related to cardiovascular morbidity and mortality.[57] Microalbuminuria in patients with type 2 DM is closely related to abnormalities of hemostasis, coagulation, and glucose and lipid metabolism. Microalbuminuria may precede and even predict the onset of type 2 DM. The urinary AER should therefore be monitored frequently in all patients with DM.

The metabolic syndrome X of IRS should not be confused with the *cardiology syndrome X*, used to describe patients with angina-like chest pain syndromes but without significant coronary obstruction demonstrated by angiography.[58] Abnormal electrocardiograms (ECG) and a positive exercise stress test may be present in the latter. The etiology of this syndrome is unclear, but it appears to be linked to insulin resistance and hyperinsulinemia.[59] Thus, the metabolic syndrome X and the cardiology syndrome X may be closely interrelated (see also Chap. 45).

Medications such as diuretics, β-adrenergic blocking agents, and glucocorticoids can adversely affect the hyperinsulinemic state, while agents such as ACE inhibitors have been found to have favorable metabolic results.

Diabetic Heart Disease

A variety of adverse genetic and environmental factors exert a direct effect on the cardiovascular system in individuals with DM. These elements, previously discussed and illustrated in Table 78-1, constitute an adverse milieu that results in a process of accelerated obstructive small- and large-vessel disease as well as nonischemic cardiomyopathy; autonomic dysregulation can also contribute to cardiovascular disease. With concomitant hypertension, the development and acceleration of atherosclerosis can be even more pronounced,[7,27,34] with an even higher incidence and severity of coronary artery disease.[60] While many factors contribute to ischemic heart disease, poor glycemic control in the hypertensive patient is associated with increased episodes of ST-segment depression as well as an increased left ventricular (LV) mass index.[61]

The existence of a distinct diabetic cardiomyopathy independent of coronary atherosclerosis has been documented clinically, experimentally, and by pathologic reports.[62,63] In diabetes, there is an increased incidence of congestive heart failure even without overt coronary artery or valvular heart disease, particularly in women.[64] Most of the pathologic studies have also noted the associated effects of hypertension in the diabetic heart. While the significance of small-vessel disease involving intramural coronary arteries, arterioles, and capillaries is still controversial,[62–64] microvascular abnormalities with capillary microaneurysms have been demonstrated in histologic studies.[65] Pathologically, diabetic cardiomyopathy is characterized by cellular hypertrophy and myocytolytic necrosis with replacement fibrosis.[66,67] The diabetic heart commonly has a great amount of microscopic fibrosis, with distribution of interstitial connective tissue throughout the myocardium.[9]

Experimentally, diabetes induced in dogs is associated with reduced LV compliance and increased interstitial connective tissue.[68] Similarly, in diabetic rats LV papillary muscles studied in vitro show marked slowing and prolongation of contraction with delayed relaxation.[69] This is associated with a decrease in myosin ATPase, with a shift in the isoenzyme form of myosin from the faster V*1* form to the slower V*3* form[70]; this accounts for the decreased speed of muscle shortening. The delayed and slowed myocardial relaxation also correlates with a reduction in the rate of Ca^{2+} binding of isolated sarcoplasmic reticulum.[71] All of these changes are reversed by the administration of insulin with a normalization of ventricular contraction.[69]

When hypertension is superimposed on diabetes, irreversible myocardial damage ensues.[72] This is characterized by microvascular stenoses, with resultant focal areas of myocyte necrosis and replacement fibrosis.[73] With progressive myocardial loss, ventricular dilation ensues, with a clinical presentation as a dilated cardiomyopathy. Clinically, in early stages of diabetes, particularly in type 1 DM, ventricular relaxation may be delayed but with a preserved ejection fraction. This is characterized by a decreased E/A wave ratio on echocardiogram (see also Chap. 14). Hemodynamic studies in diabetic patients with overt congestive heart failure have shown either a restrictive (diastolic dysfunction) or congestive (systolic dysfunction) cardiomyopathy.[63] Early in the disease process, systolic time intervals, especially preejection period/LV ejection time, are frequently abnormal, reflecting decreased contractility and/or a reduction in diastolic volume, possibly due to diminished LV compliance.[74] Patients with microangiopathy are also more likely to have abnormal systolic time intervals.[74]

M-mode echocardiography has also shown prolongation of isovolumic relaxation and slowing of ventricular filling in diabetes.[75] Systolic function is frequently abnormal with concomitant hypertension but is less commonly affected in the normotensive patient.[75] Radionuclide studies have generally shown normal resting ejection fractions but a less-than-expected increase in ejection fraction in response to dynamic exercise.[76] These abnormalities have been correlated with the presence of microangiopathy or autonomic neuropathy. Moreover, patients with diabetic autonomic neuropathy are more likely to have abnormal filling dynamics.[77] Young patients with type 1 DM and chronic complications demonstrate an increased frequency of diastolic dysfunction as shown with pulsed Doppler echocardiography, where the ratio of early (E wave) to late (A wave) ventricular filling is reduced, indicating a decrease in ventricular compliance.[78] With later ventricular dilation, the echocardiographic studies are those of a dilated cardiomyopathy (see Chap. 14).[76,78] Even in the absence of congestive failure, echocardiographic studies have also shown increased LV mass in patients with hypertension and diabetes,[79] with a prevalence of LV hypertrophy of 72 percent in diabetic hypertensive patients compared to 32 percent in nondiabetic hypertensive patients.[79] Patients with diabetes and hypertension have a thicker interventricular septum[80] when compared with nondiabetic hypertensive patients.

In summary, diabetic cardiomyopathy represents the end result of a pathologic process that may involve large-vessel artherosclerosis with occlusions producing relatively large areas of myocardial loss as well as small-vessel vasospastic disease producing focal tissue loss. Both processes result in fibrous scarring, reactive hypertrophy of remaining myocytes, and ultimate ventricular dilation. In general, hypertension accelerates these processes. Early on, diastolic dysfunction with a normal ejection fraction is common, while late stages with a reduced ejection fraction provide the usual picture of systolic dysfunction added to the features of diastolic dysfunction.

Cardiac Autonomic Neuropathy

The neuropathy associated with diabetes mellitus is a generalized disorder. Initially, it involves vagal nerves; later, sympathetic pathways are affected. The evolving autonomic neuropathy alters the phasic changes that normally occur in the heart rate, termed *heart rate variability* (HRV). These heart rate fluctuations can be evaluated quantitatively with high-frequency (HF) 24-h multichannel digital ECG reorders and provide an evaluation of autonomic dysfunction.[81] Oscillations or changes in heart rate are regulated by autonomic control. Using spectral analysis, three main frequency bands can be discerned: very low frequency (VLF; 0.033 to 0.04 Hz), low frequency (LF; 0.04 to 0.15 Hz), and high frequency (0.15 to 0.4 Hz). The HF range reflects parasympathetic or vagal stimulation, whereas the VLF range is thought to reflect sympathetic stimulation. A change in HRV characterized by a decrease in the HF rate and an increase in the VLF rate is an early manifestation of diabetic autonomic dysfunction. Early in the disease process, no significant changes in the VLF/HF ratio is found, probably because there is minimal involvement in both sympathetic and parasympathetic limbs. In the course of diabetes, however, a low VLF/HF ratio represents clear development of an autonomic neuropathy and constitutes a poor prognostic sign.[82,83]

HRV with respiration and standing is decreased in diabetic patients, especially in those with evidence of peripheral or autonomic neuropathy.[82,84] Defects in parasympathetic innervation, expressed as an increased resting heart rate and a decreased respiratory variation in heart rate, are more frequent and occur relatively early in DM.[85] Defects in sympathetic innervation, expressed as a decrease in rise of the heart rate during standing, are less frequent and tend to occur later in the disease.[85] A prospective study of patients with DM and without autonomic neuropathy has revealed a markedly diminished rate of survival in those with neuropathy, with a substantial incidence of sudden death.[83] This may relate to an increased tendency to develop ventricular arrhythmias in diabetic patients. Further, in diabetic patients with autonomic neuropathy, there is a high incidence of QT prolongation at rest and especially after exercise, possibly reflecting autonomic imbalance,[86] which is ultimately associated. The relationship of autonomic neuropathy to silent ischemia also remains uncertain. With autonomic neuropathy, postural hypotension is often symptomatic and sometimes disabling in individuals, especially after bed rest or when diuretics and/or other antihypertensive medications are used.

While measurement of HRV is becoming more available and represents a promising market of autonomic dysfunction, its direct clinical application remains to be evaluated. In the meantime, more practical and simple bedside tests are helpful in detecting autonomic neuropathy. A patient can be considered to have cardiac autonomic neuropathy if two or more of the following findings are present:

1. An increased resting heart rate. This is determined after the patient is supine for 15 min, and a rate in excess of 100 beats per minute is considered abnormal.

2. Decreased beat-to-beat HRV. This is determined by the difference between the minimum and maximum heart rate, as taken from ECG tracings obtained during periods of inspiration and expiration with the patient breathing six times per minute. A variability of less than 10 beats per minute is considered abnormal.

3. An abnormal Valsalva maneuver is determined by having the patients blow into a manometer and maintaining 40 mmHg for 15 s. Using ECG tracings, one calculates the ratio of the longest R-R interval after the maneuver to the shortest R-R interval during the maneuver. The ratio is abnormal if it is ≤1.10.

4. An abnormal heart rate response to standing. During ECG monitoring, the ratio of the R-R interval at the thirtieth beat after standing to the R-R interval at the fifteenth beat is determined abnormal if the ratio is ≤1.00.

5. An excessive fall in blood pressure with standing. The fall in systolic blood pressure after 1 min of standing is determined by cuff sphyngomanometry and is abnormal if it is ≥30 mmHg.[87]

As noted above, the diagnosis of an autonomic neuropathy in diabetic patients carries an adverse prognosis.[87] Moreover, such changes in autonomic activity, especially characterized by decreased parasympathetic activity but with increased sympathetic tone, occur with heart failure associated with a diabetic cardiomyopathy. Decreased sensitivity to ischemic pain in these patients may also produce unrecognized ischemia with myocardial damage.

Treatment of Diabetes Mellitus

HISTORICAL BACKGROUND AND ANTIDIABETIC AGENTS

Insulin provided the first form of hormone replacement therapy, and remains essential for survival of the type 1 DM patient, and has been extended to the more common type 2 DM patient population. In the majority of individuals with type II DM, insulin is given not as a replacement hormone but as a supplementation to overcome the insulin-resistant state. More recently, it has also been used intermittently to treat "glucose toxicity," a concept in which hyperglycemia is thought to worsen metabolic control by impairing insulin secretion and action.[88,89] As soon as insulin therapy became available, controversy developed about how best to utilize it. Some felt that insulin treatment in conjunction with exercise and a proper dietary regimen was important for prevention of complications; others thought that insulin was needed merely to ameliorate symptoms of poor metabolic control, as there was no proof that "tight" glycemic control was beneficial. This argument led to the development of a prospective clinical trial, called the University Group Diabetes Study

(UGDP).[90] This well-intended, but poorly planned, study not only failed to give a clear answer but further fueled this controversy. The results suggested a high rate of cardiovascular-related deaths associated with tolbutamide and claimed a high mortality rate due to lactic acidosis in patients treated with phenformin, a biguanide. These findings, however, were largely ignored by the majority, who thought that the benefit of sulfonylureas was more important than their potential side effects. In the early 1980s, the second generation of sulfonylureas became available and continue to be widely used. Metformin was approved in 1995 for use in the United States. While good glycemic control continued to be recommended by the majority of diabetologists, the controvesy of the beneficial effects remained. The Diabetes Control and Complication Trial (DCCT) demonstrated that tight metabolic control in patients with type I DM can significantly decrease the onset and progression of diabetic retinopathy, nephropathy, and neuropathy.[38] A clear beneficial effect on large-vessel disease, however, was not shown. The results of the DCCT were immediately extrapolated to the most common population with type 2 DM, but how best to achieve tight metabolic control in this insulin-resistant population remains controversial. Several prospective studies are currently under way to try to answer this question,[91,92] and a new multicenter trial, the Diabetes Prevention Program (DPP), has been started to address the possibility of primary prevention of type 2 DM and treatment of IRS.

Lifestyle changes remain pivotal for prevention and treatment of IRS. In type 2 DM, however, if diet and exercise alone fail to normalize hyperglycemia, pharmacotherapy is needed. Management has shifted from just treating hyperglycemia to attempts to ameliorate insulin resistance, along with more aggressive and earlier treatment of other risk factors such as hypertension and dyslipidemia. Even mild elevation of blood sugars should not be tolerated since hyperglycemia begets hyperglycemia[88,89] and causes chronic diabetic complications (see Fig. 78-2). With the diversity of antidiabetic agents now available, a more aggressive glycemic control is now attainable. When the set goal for glycemic control is not achieved, intervention with a new antidiabetic agent or combination with other agents is recommended in order to avoid glucose toxicity and chronic diabetic complications (see Table 78-2).

Sulfonylurea agents are commonly used for treatment of type 2 DM. They improve glycemic control by enhancing pancreatic insulin secretion. Failure to respond occurs because of protracted hyperglycemia (glucose toxicity)[88,89] or β-cell failure. Often, pancreatic β-cell function can be improved after glycemic control is achieved by other means such as temporary insulin therapy. When lack of response is caused by β-cell "demise" rather than glucose toxicity, higher doses or switching to other sulfonylureas is rarely beneficial, and continued insulin treatment is required. Treatment with sulfonylureas may be associated with weight gain, with little or no beneficial effect on dyslipidemia and/or hypertension. Hypoglycemia remains the most common side effect of therapy, particularly in the elderly and in those with organ failure.

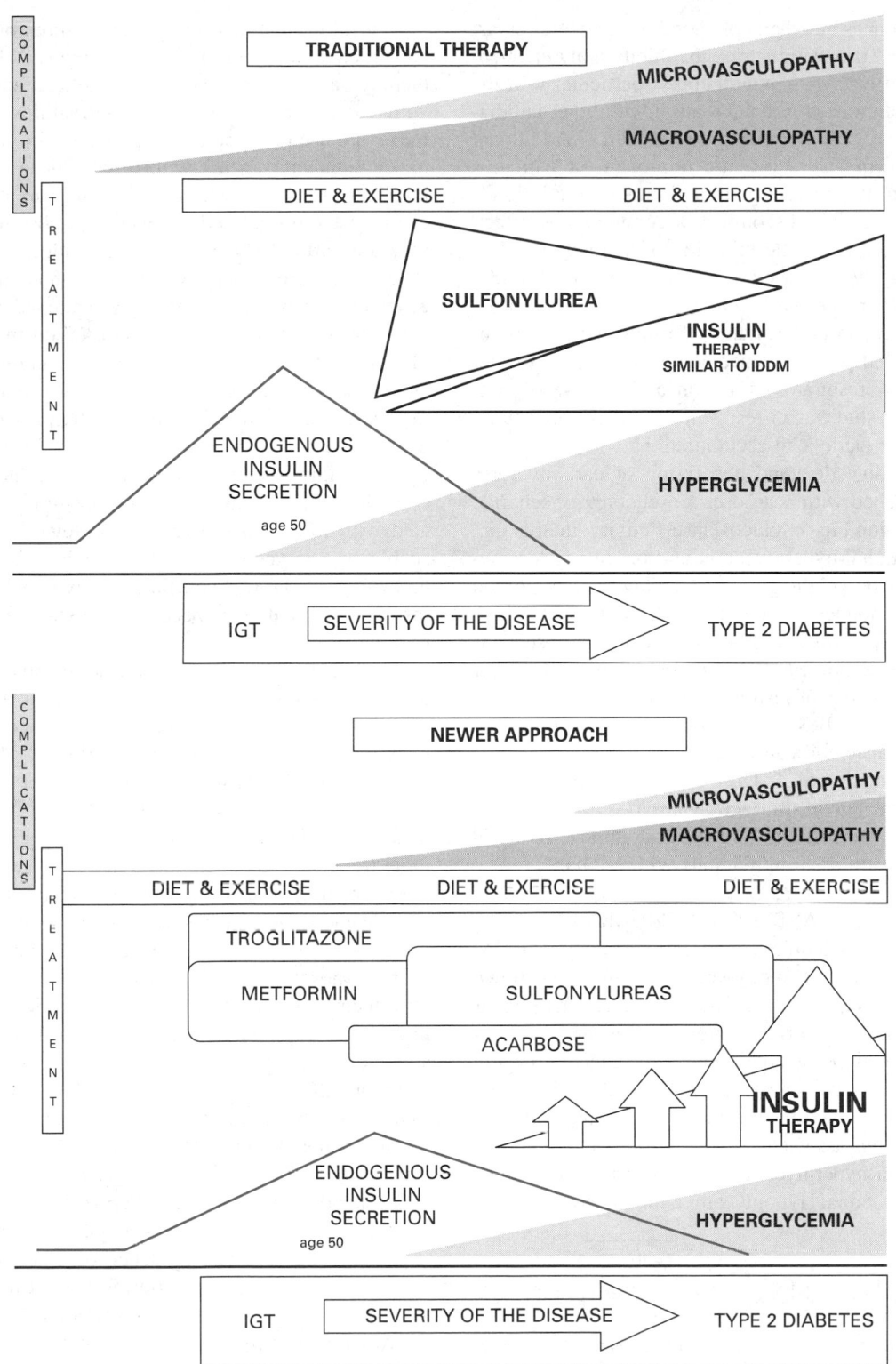

FIGURE 78-2

Theoretical simplified illustration of the development and progression of impaired glucose tolerance (IGT) and type 2 diabetes (non-insulin-dependent diabetes mellitus—NIDDM) as the disease progresses with age. Please note the difference in treatment between the *upper panel* with only two antidiabetic agents and the *lower panel* with a more aggressive and early treatment with several and newer medications. The physiopathology of the disease is illustrated by hyperinsulinemia and IGT. A decrease in islet β-cell function is illustrated by a progressive fall in insulin secretion; the inability to compensate results in hyperglycemia. Note that macrovasculopathy can be found before hyperglycemia, while microvasculopathy is associated with hyperglycemia. An adequate diet and exercise are necessary in order to prevent the disease, and not only when complications ensue. Early intervention with medications may further delay the progression of hyperinsulinemia, the onset of diabetes mellitus, and hopefully the incidence of macrovasculopathy. Also, a more aggressive glycemic control will decrease the onset and progression of microvascular complications.

Metformin reduces blood glucose levels chiefly by decreasing hepatic glucose production through inhibition of gluconeogenesis[93]; it is effective as monotherapy, particularly in the obese, but it is often used in combination with other antidiabetic agents such as sulfonylurea and/or insulin.[94] Additional benefits of metformin are glycemic improvement with less hyperinsulinemia, less weight gain, and a favorable lipid effect.[91,94] Gastrointestinal discomfort, a common side effect, may be ameliorated by gentle initiation of therapy. The risk of lactic acidosis, which occurs in ~3 cases per 100,000 patient/years, is found primarily with impaired renal function, where the drug is contraindicated. Metformin should be withheld in hospitalized patients, since acute illness may further compromise cardiorespiratory function and the use of contrast-radiographic studies can result in decreased renal function and therefore lactic acid accumulation.

Reduction in digestion and absorption of carbohydrates can be accomplished with acarbose, a pseudotetrasaccharide that specifically inhibits α-glucosidase activity in the gut, reducing postprandial hyperglycemia and producing less hyperinsulinemia and weight gain.[95] The lowering of blood sugar is more pronounced when used in combination.

Insulinomimetic drugs, or "insulin sensitizers," such as troglitazone, a thiazolidinedione agent, can reverse the major metabolic abnormalities of insulin resistance. Troglitazone is ideal for treatment of IRS as it improves glucose tolerance and insulin resistance and causes a decrease in both systolic and diastolic blood pressure.[96] The exact mechanism of action remains unknown, but insulin action has been found to be enhanced in the liver, skeletal muscle, and adipose tissue in nondiabetic[96] as well as in individuals with NIDDM.[97]

INSULIN REPLACEMENT AND SUPPLEMENTATION

Insulin replacement is required for treatment of type 1 DM as well as for the insulinopenic type 2 DM patient. As shown by the DCCT,[38] adequate physiologic replacement is labor intensive and far from perfect. Intensive insulin regimens with multiple injections or continuous subcutaneous insulin infusion are necessary since adequate control is rarely achieved with one or two insulin injections a day.[38] Insulin replacement is often associated with periods of hypoinsulinemia resulting in hyperglycemia, and hyperinsulinemia resulting in hypoglycemia. Hypoglycemia, the tradeoff of intensive insulin treatment, is at least threefold higher when compared to conventional insulin therapy.[38] Intensive insulin therapy has so far proven to be beneficial and not associated with adverse cardiovascular abnormalities. Insulin supplements are used in type 2 DM patients who fail to respond to oral antidiabetic agents, with higher doses required due to insulin resistance.[98] Short-term insulin treatment regiments can be used to treat and/or reverse glucose toxicity,[88,89] and they are particularly helpful in individuals with a catabolic state and severe hyperglycemia and when sudden elevations of blood glucose are caused by acute adverse conditions. When insulin supplementation is used during longer periods of time, either as sole therapy or in combination with oral agents, suppression of hepatic glucose production with normalization of fasting glycemias is the primary goal. This is often achieved with a single dose of intermediate insulin given at night (bedtime), with results similar to that of more complicated regimens or multiple insulin doses. It is associated with lower insulin levels and fewer adverse reactions such as hypoglycemia and weight gain.[70] In the natural history of type 2 DM, β-cell failure may eventually ensue, and insulin treatment may become necessary as a replacement hormone.

The fear that exogenous insulin administration may contribute to acceleration of atherosclerosis, hypertension,[99] and weight gain[100] derives from the adverse effects of endogenous hyperinsulinemia in IRS and type 2 DM.[2–16] This same concept has been reinforced by epidemiologic observations in patients from different ethnic backgrounds.[16,18,20–22] Inference from noncontrolled studies is difficult, however, since insulin is used more frequently in patients with more severe disease and with a longer duration of illness. Thus, a clear atherogenic effect of exogenous insulin has yet to be established in properly done prospective, randomized clinical trials.[101] Neither the DCCT[38] nor the UGDP[90] trials showed adverse cardiovascular affects of insulin therapy; however, the DCCT was done in a young population with short-term duration of diabetes, and the UGDP was a flawed study.[102] After 9 years, the ongoing U.K. Prospective Diabetes Study Group (UKPDSG) trial has not been able to find any adverse cardiac effects in insulin-treated individuals.[91] On the other hand, reports from the Feasibility Trial of the VA Cooperative Study on Glycemic Control and Complications in Type II Diabetes are disturbing as they have found a higher incidence of cardiovascular disease during a short-term intensive insulin treatment.[92,103] In view of the benefits of good glycemic control (see Table 78-2), insulin should continue to be used when other therapeutic options fail in type 2 DM. On the other hand, the benefits of chronic use of large insulin doses in patients with poor response and persistent hyperglycemia need to be carefully assessed.

TABLE 78-2

INDICES OF GLYCEMIC CONTROL[a]

Biochemical Index	Nondiabetic	Goal	Action Suggested[b]
Preprandial glucose (mg/dL)	<115	80–120	<80 or >140
Bedtime glucose (mg/dL)	<120	100–140	<100 or >160
HbA$_{1C}$ (%)[c]	<6	<7	>8

[a] These values are for nonpregnant individuals.
[b] Action suggested depends on individual patient.
[c] Hemoglobin A$_{1C}$ (HbA$_{1C}$) is referenced to a nondiabetic range of 4 to 6%.
Source: From The pharmacological treatment of hyperglycemia in NIDDM. Modified from the American Diabetes Association Clinical Practice Guidelines. *Diabetes Care* 1995; 18:1510–1518.

MANAGEMENT OF MYOCARDIAL INFARCTION IN PATIENTS WITH DIABETES MELLITUS

AMI remains the most important cause of death in patients with DM,[104] particularly in women.[105] This is independent of other traditional risk factors[106] and may be related to the higher frequency of a more diffuse, extensive, and distal obstructive coronary disease process.[107] Some may also have associated "diabetic cardiomyopathy" and/or autonomic dysregulation that will contribute to the high morbidity and mortality.[108] Further, poor glycemic control is associated with increased mortality,[109] and tight metabolic control appears to be beneficial[110] (see also Chap. 47).

Insulin administration during AMI as well as glucose and potassium have been proposed to limit the extent of myocardial damage in the nondiabetic population,[111] with claims of improved LV function.[112] This therapeutic modality has now been replaced by myocardial reperfusion.[113] During AMI, patients with DM become more insulin-resistant and have more electrolyte abnormalities. Lack of adequate insulin administration can further aggravate these changes and contribute to an increased morbidity and mortality,[114] in spite of the use of beta-blocker agents[115] and thrombolytic therapy.[113,116] The acute administration of insulin in these patients reduces myocardial protein degradation[117] and may help preserve global LV function.[112] In addition, insulin administration can also improve the hypercoagulable state by improving platelet function[118] and decreasing PAI-1 activity.[119] During AMI, higher insulin doses are required; nevertheless, insulin is commonly withheld or given inappropriately as "sliding-scale coverage." Properly done prospective studies with intensive insulin are difficult. Recently a large study with insulin-glucose infusion in the diabetic patient with AMI (DIGAMI) demonstrated a 30 percent mortality rate reduction after 1 year with intensive insulin therapy during the acute event and thereafter. The patients with a low profile of cardiovascular disease and milder hyperglycemia benefitted the most.[110]

In addition to adequate glycemic control, beta blockers are also beneficial during AMI, as they control heart rate, limit oxygen needs, and reduce the extent of ischemia.[115,120] ACE inhibitors during AMI may be helpful in those with compromised LV function,[121] but their specific role in the diabetic population is still to be determined. Timely introduction of thrombolytic therapy has been shown to reduce in-hospital mortality by 42 percent in patients with DM,[113] an observation confirmed by larger studies.[122] Coronary artery bypass graft surgery (CABG) in the diabetic population is associated with increased short-term morbidity and a higher rate of sternotomy infections and renal failure, in addition to an increased incidence of congestive heart failure, cardiogenic shock, arrhythmias, and myocardial rupture.[123,124] This population has at least a twofold increase in mortality rate during the 2-year period following CABG.[125] Because of this high incidence of complications, percutaneous transluminal coronary angioplasty (PTCA) became an attractive alternative. While the acute closure after single-vessel angioplasty does not represent a problem in patients with diabetes,[126] those with multivessel coronary disease, which is more common, often experience procedural failure with ischemic complications and restenosis.[127] In the Bypass Angioplasty Revascularization Investigation (BARI)[128] study, it was observed that patients with diabetes with multivessel disease have a better outcome with surgery than with angioplasty, and that the latter should be considered only as a second alternative. The survival rate in the diabetic population was as much as 50 percent higher with CABG as compared to PTCA.[128] Nevertheless, because of small numbers and patient selection this conclusion remains tentative. Advances in interventional cardiology, such as the use of blockers of platelet glycoprotein IIb/IIIa receptors,[129] the use of minimally invasive surgical techniques, and the increased use of internal thoracic-artery grafts, may further improve long-term surgical outcome in patients with DM.[130] Finally, the use of low-dose aspirin has so far not been found useful for primary or secondary prevention in the type 2 DM population. Since these patients require higher doses to inhibit platelet aggregation,[131] studies using higher doses are necessary to establish their potential use.

ANTIHYPERTENSIVE THERAPY IN DIABETES MELLITUS

Systemic arterial hypertension is more common in NIDDM and constitutes a major risk factor for cardiovascular disease including CHD, heart failure, and stroke.[132] The association between systemic arterial hypertension and renal disease is particularly significant in type 1 DM patients, where one-third develop nephropathy that eventually evolves into end-stage renal disease. Renal failure in the type 2 DM population is lower, with only approximately 8 percent advancing to end-stage renal disease.[133] Albuminuria in the latter group not only serves as a marker for renal disease but can also be used as a predictor of cardiovascular morbidity and mortality.[56,57] Weight reduction, adequate diet, and increased physical activity may decrease insulin resistance, but when these modalities fail, pharmacotherapy is needed. Antihypertensive medications in the diabetic population not only need to be effective in lowering blood pressure but should also have favorable metabolic, cardioprotective, and nephroprotective effects. Thus the antihypertensive agents used as first-line therapy in the nondiabetic population are not necessarily the drugs of choice in DM. For instance the commonly used β-adrenergic antagonists and diuretics have been found to be associated with an increased incidence of type 2 DM,[134] reflecting their known adverse metabolic effects.[135] On the other hand, ACE inhibitors[136] and calcium channel blocker agents[137] have favorable metabolic effects and may also be organ-protective. In spite of these observations, no reliable data are available for the assessment of the impact that each of these agents or their combinations may have on the prevention or progression of macrovascular complications in the diabetic population. While no antihypertensive agent is specifically contraindicated in the diabetic population, ACE inhibitors are favored as first-line agents (see also Chap. 58).

The antihypertensive effect of ACE inhibitors is variable, but due to their favorable metabolic effects and preservation of renal function, they are preferred as first-line agents in both type 1 and type 2 DM patients, particularly in those with albuminuria. Captopril therapy can result in a 50 percent reduction of combined end points of mortality and renal replacement (dialysis or transplantation) in the type 1 DM patient population with proteinuria.[136] The sparing effects on proteinuria appear to be independent of the antihypertensive properties of ACE inhibitors, as similar declines in blood pressure obtained with metoprolol or hydrochlorothiazide have not been found to be accompanied with protein preservation,[138] and small doses of ACE inhibitors without hypotensive effect can also reduce microalbuminuria.[139] ACE inhibitors have a favorable effect on carbohydrate metabolism,[140] at times permitting lower insulin doses and decrease or discontinuation of oral hypoglycemic agents.[141] Both decreased hepatic glucose production and increased insulin-mediated glucose utilization may account for these changes.[142] Other possible mechanisms by which insulin sensitivity may take place include increased skeletal muscle blood flow caused by reduced angiotensin II or increased levels of bradykinin and/or prostaglandins. The angiotension II receptor antagonist, losartan, is not associated with increased bradykinin levels and therefore does not produce cough, the most common limiting side effect of ACE inhibitors. In small studies, losartan has also been found to improve insulin resistance, prevent cardiac hypertrophy, and decrease proteinuria.[143] Unfortunately no large clinical studies are yet available to demonstrate these effects or to show an improvement in morbidity or mortality. ACE inhibitors should be used cautiously, if at all, in patients with renal artery stenosis, hyperkalemia, severe azotemia, and angioedema, and they are contraindicated in pregnant women or those planning a pregnancy.

Calcium channel blocking agents are also effective and can be used as first-line antihypertensive medications in type 2 DM, since they have no adverse metabolic consequences[144] and may have possible nephroprotective effects.[145] They are particularly useful in patients with coronary artery disease, renal stenosis, or advanced renal failure and in patients during pregnancy. The long-acting preparations are preferable, since the short-acting agents are claimed to be associated with an increased incidence of myocardial infarction.[146]

Thiazide diuretics remain effective and inexpensive but are associated with unfavorable metabolic abnormalities such as dyslipidemia, hyperglycemia, and hyperuricemia.[147] Both thiazide and loop diuretics can produce hyperglycemia by causing insulin resistance and decreasing insulin secretion.[148] Diuretic-induced hypokalemia can often be reversed after proper potassium restoration.[148] In spite of their common use, the beneficial effects of diuretics in type 2 DM are yet to be shown; instead, increased cardiac-related mortality has been observed.[147–149] Since 12.5 mg of hydrochlorothiazide can substantially increase the efficacy of ACE inhibitors and beta blockers, low-dose thiazide treatment is under current evaluation. In the meantime, thiazides are best used in conjunction with other antihypertensive agents, particularly for the treatment of fluid retention.

Treatment with β-adrenergic antagonists in the general population may cause a threefold increase in the incidence of diabetes mellitus; when diuretics are added, the risk rate may increase to fivefold.[150] The unfavorable metabolic consequences, as well as other side effects, makes these agents unpopular among patients with DM. Further, hypoglycemic symptoms may be masked, particularly when tight metabolic control is stressed. The cardioselectivity of β-adrenergic antagonists is limited clinically, particularly when high doses are used. The nonselective β-adrenergic antagonists such as propranolol, without intrinsic sympathetic activity, are associated with more insulin resistance, hyperglycemia, and hypertriglyceridemia than pindolol or dilevalol, which have intrinsic sympathetic activity.[151] An undisputable indication for β-adrenergic antagonists in patients with diabetes, however, is following myocardial infarction, when they favorably affect survival rates.[115,120]

The α_1-adrenergic antagonist agents have favorable metabolic and cardiovascular effects. Both prazosin and doxazosin increase insulin sensitivity and have a beneficial effect on lipids.[152] Orthostatic hypotension, which is often found during the initial treatment, may persist, particularly in the elderly and in those with autonomic neuropathy, limiting this form of therapy. Central adrenergic inhibitors produce little metabolic alterations but are also accompanied by orthostatic hypotension, erectile dysfunction, and fluid retention. Vasodilators decrease peripheral vascular resistance directly and result in increased cardiac output, which can precipitate or aggravate coronary ischemia. In patients with autonomic neuropathy, the increased cardiac workload may not be sustained because of a denervated heart and can result in fluid retention. The use of combination regimens with very low dose diuretic and beta blockers,[153] or diuretics and α-adrenergic blockers—a modality that causes little or no carbohydrate abnormalities since each drug has opposite metabolic effects[135]—may be good alternative regimens for some.

TREATMENT OF OTHER RISK FACTORS

Cardiovascular mortality can be reduced in the diabetic population by aggressive correction of hypertension, hyperglycemia, dyslipidemia, and amelioration of other traditional risk factors.[106] Unfortunately, the exclusion of subjects with diabetes from most major intervention trials has resulted in a lack of trial-based evidence of the particular benefits of each of these interventions. The Multiple Risk Factor Intervention Trial study has provided insight into relations between hypercholesterolemia, blood pressure, smoking, and cardiovascular disease in diabetes and has further confirmed the increased mortality rate risk that diabetes itself represents.[154] Lowering cholesterol levels with simvastatin, a powerful HMG CoA reductase inhibitor, in patients with type 2 DM and known coronary artery disease has resulted in significant reduction in AMI, with a 54 percent decrease in heart-related deaths.[155] The high risk of hypertension and hypercholesterolemia argues for a greater focus on these treatable risk factors.[156] With this in mind, it has been recommended that target values for blood pressure and cholesterol be lower in the diabetic population, perhaps with a diastolic pressure <85 mmHg and an LDL-cholesterol level <100 mg/dL.

THYROID DISEASE

The cardiovascular system is highly susceptible to thyroid hormone, which directly alters heart rate and velocity of myocardial contraction. Indirectly, thyroid hormone regulates tissue metabolism and extracellular fluid volume and distribution.[157] Both deficiency and excess of thyroid hormone can cause striking cardiovascular derangements, particularly in the elderly and in those with underlying intrinsic heart disease. Thyroxine (T_4), the primary secretory product of the thyroid, is converted to the active hormone, triiodothyronine (T_3), by thyroxine 5'-deiodinase enzymes. The direct myocardial actions result primarily from the interaction of T_3 with its nuclear receptor proteins, which can modify gene expression. These receptors are members of a family of hormone-responsive nuclear transcription factors, with similar structure and mechanism of action.[158] Two T_3-receptor genes, α and β, are located on chromosomes 17 and 3 respectively, with at least two alternative messenger RNA (mRNA) splice products for each gene. The T_3-receptor α gene includes α_1 and α_2 receptors, but the latter does not bind T_3. Products of the T_3-receptor β gene are β_1 and β_2 receptors.[158] The clinical manifestations of thyroid dysfunction are T_3-regulated. Excessive thyroid hormone increases myocardial transcription of the myosin heavy chain (MHC) α gene while decreasing transcription of the MHC-β gene. This leads to increased myosin adenosinetriphosphatase (ATPase) activity and increased velocity of contraction.[159] The T_3-responsive (mRNAs) increase sarcolemmal sodium pump sites by stimulating Na^+- and K^+-ATPase[160] and are responsible for the increased number of calcium channels.[161]

In addition to the direct myocardial effect, thyroid hormone can also interact with the sympathetic nervous system by altering responsiveness to sympathetic stimulation. Thus, many of the manifestations of the hyperthyroid state, such as tachycardia, palpitations, tremor, sweating, and central nervous system hyperactivity, mimic adrenergic hyperfunction. Conversely, many of the symptoms of hypothyroidism resemble those of depressed sympathetic tone.[157] This correlation led to the assumption that in thyrotoxicosis there may be excessive catecholamine secretion and resulted in the clinical use of β-adrenergic receptor blocking agents for the symptomatic management of hyperthyroidism. There is no evidence that thyroid hormone alters catecholamine plasma levels, however, nor is there increased content of catecholamines in myocardium. Thyroid hormone increases the cardiac sensitivity to a β-adrenergic agonist by an increased number of, as well as affinity to, β-adrenergic receptors; high doses of thyroid hormone, however, do not increase metabolic and hemody-namic response to epinephrine in spite of increased β-adrenergic receptors. Thus, increased catecholamine sensitivity cannot be the sole explanation for the clinical and metabolic features of hyperthyroidism.[157]

Although the long-term cardiac effect of thyroid hormone can cause changes in myocardial gene expression, attention has been shifted recently to the nonnuclear-mediated actions of T_3. Intravenous administration of T_3 has been postulated as treatment for severe hypothyroidism and for euthyroid patients undergoing cardiac surgery. This treatment may improve cardiac output and reduce systemic and pulmonary vascular resistance, perhaps as a direct effect of T_3 on blood vessels to reduce peripheral vascular resistance, perhaps as a direct effect of T_3 on blood vessels to reduce peripheral vascular resistance.[162] Nevertheless, the clinical value of this form of therapy remains to be determined.

Hyperthyroidism

Hyperthyroidism, or thyrotoxicosis, is the clinical state resulting from chronic elevation of thyroid hormone levels. Common types include autoimmune hyperthyroidism (Graves' disease), toxic multinodular goiter (Plummer's disease), single hyperfunctioning adenoma, and excessive exogenous thyroid hormone treatment. The clinical manifestations of hyperthyroidism are quite protean and include weight loss with appetite preservation, diaphoresis, exertional dyspnea, heat intolerance, palpitations, easy fatigability, emotional lability, and weakness. These symptoms may be so mild or subtle that the patient is unaware of them. The most striking symptoms of hyperthyroidism are reflected by the cardiovascular system and are often the only manifestation, particularly in the elderly. Physical examination frequently reveals a nervous and hyperkinetic individual with a hyperdynamic cardiovascular state. Fine tremor of the hands is common, the skin is warm and moist, and palmar erythema may be present. The hair is fine and silky, and onycholysis (separation of distal nail from its bed), acropachy ("drumstick" appearance of the fingers), and proximal muscle weakness are signs of severe disease and chronic duration. Lid retraction ("stare") and lid-lag are ophthalmic manifestations of thyroid hormone excess. A soft and symmetric goiter is characteristic of autoimmune disease (Graves' disease), often present in the young. In some a bruit may be audible due to increased vascularity. The autoimmune disorder is responsible for ophthalmopathy characterized by protruding eyes, pretibial myxedema, vitiligo, hepatosplenomegaly, and peripheral adenopathy. A nodular goiter with increased consistency is indicative of Plummer's disease, while a single palpable nodule suggests a "toxic adenoma" ("hot" nodule by nuclear scintiscan).

The signs and symptoms of hyperthyroidism are variable and do not always correlate with thyroid hormone serum levels. In older individuals, the manifestations can be subtle, e.g., tachycardia, anxiety, and weight loss. *Apathetic hyperthyroidism* is the term used to describe the condition in the elderly who do not manifest the obvious signs and symptoms. These patients rarely have a goiter and may present with apathetic, placid facies; such patients can be diagnosed erroneously as having a malignancy or heart disease. Mild, or "subclinical," hyperthyroidism may manifest mainly by cardiac abnormalities such as atrial fibrillation (AF).[163] These patients also have increased LV mass index and rates of ventricular contraction[164] and have mild clinical signs, but the diagnosis is often established by the laboratory finding of a low serum level of thyrotropin, a thyroid-stimulating hormone (TSH), often with normal serum levels of T_4 and T_3. Cardiovascular abnormalities can also be found in those receiving excessive amounts of exogenous thyroid hormone for treatment of thyroid cancer or nontoxic nodular goiter.[165] While the beneficial effects of thyroid suppression in thyroid cancer are clear, this has not been the case in nontoxic nodular goiter, and therefore this therapeutic modality needs to be evaluated properly. The cardiovascular changes observed in mild hyperthyroidism are not necessarily associated with increased morbidity or mortality and can be treated with β-adrenergic blockers with normalization of LV mass, restoration of normal resting heart rate, and symptomatic improvement.[165]

CARDIOVASCULAR MANIFESTATIONS OF THYROTOXICOSIS

The most common cardiovascular complications are tachyarrhythmias, thromboembolic accidents, and heart failure. As a general rule, AF occurs in 15 percent of thyrotoxic patients,[166–168] hyperthyroidism accounts for 15 percent of all newly diagnosed AF,[169] and 15 percent of patients with thyrotoxic AF can develop thromboembolism.[170] Clinical manifestations vary, but palpitations and exertional dyspnea are common. The circulation is hyperdynamic, with a full bounding and rapid pulse even at rest. Peripheral vasodilatation is accompanied by systolic hypertension and a low diastolic pressure. The precordial impulse is forceful and often visible. A short, high-pitched systolic murmur may be heard to the left of the sternal border, especially in the pulmonic valve area, and functional mitral valve regurgitation is more frequent in hyperthyroid patients.[171] Dependent edema may be present in severe and chronic cases and should be properly differentiated from that arising from congestive heart failure or from pretibial myxedema.

Congestive heart failure is uncommon but may develop or worsen with underlying intrinsic heart disease. The severity of cardiovascular complications is related to the underlying heart disease as well as patient age.[172] Heart failure occurs more often in hyperthyroid patients with AF in whom the rapid ventricular response and loss of the atrial kick may impair diastolic filling. Most importantly, hyperthyroidism may greatly increase myocardial oxygen consumption, which, in the presence of obstructive coronary artery disease, may result in ischemia or ventricular failure. In some, congestive heart failure is associated with LV dilatation and functional mitral regurgitation. In the absence of overt congestive heart failure, the cardiac index is increased at rest and can be further elevated during exercise. In contrast, thyrotoxic patients with congestive heart failure have a high normal cardiac index that decreases after exercise. While most hyperthyroid patients with heart failure have intrinsic heart disease, a few thyrotoxic young adults may demonstrate reversible ventricular disfunction once the hyperthyroid state is corrected, supporting the concept of a specific thyrotoxic cardiomyopathy. Premature atrial contractions and AF are common in hyperthyroidism, but paroxysmal atrial tachycardia and atrial flutter are less common. When ventricular arrhythmias are found, they often indicate underlying heart disease.[173] Left atrial enlargement often implicates previous impairment of diastolic ventricular filling and is more prevalent in patients with AF than in those with sinus tachycardia.[174] In hyperthyroidism, AF is more frequent in men, increases with age, and is often the major or only manifestation.[175] Thyroid function remains well preserved until the eighth decade of life in healthy individuals. TSH levels remain normal or slightly elevated, whereas reduction of serum levels of free T_3 may be observed in extreme aging. The elderly with low TSH levels may have a transient, innocent abnormality that may or may not progress to overt hyperthyroidism. Individuals 60 years or older with low serum TSH concentrations have a threefold higher risk of AF during the subsequent decade.[176]

Thromboembolic disease is common in these patients, especially with concomitant AF.[177] The incidence increases with age, and thromboembolic disease is more likely in those with congestive heart failure, a dilated left atrium, and mitral valve disease as well as in those with spontaneous or induced cardioversion. Mitral valve prolapse syndrome is often found in women with autoimmune thyroid disease and may persist after correction of the hyperthyroid state. Significant mitral regurgitation, arrhythmias, or thromboembolism, however, are rare.

DIAGNOSIS

The diagnosis is suspected clinically and confirmed by elevated serum levels of T_4 and T_3 and suppressed TSH levels. Virtually all patients with primary hyperthyroidism have suppressed TSH levels, whereas TSH serum concentration is normal in euthyroid patients. Measuring TSH serum concentration is a cost-effective method for confirming or excluding hyperthyroidism. A single TSH determination is not reliable in the management of patients with hypothalamic-pituitary disorders or of hospitalized patients with nonthyroidal illnesses, particularly when receiving medications such as dopamine, which can affect serum TSH levels. In all these situations, determination of other thyroid hormone levels is necessary. In some complex cases, measurement of free thyroid hormone by dialysis methods may also be required.

TREATMENT OF HYPERTHYROIDISM

The main therapeutic goal is the rapid achievement of the euthyroid state while avoiding therapeutic complications. Therapy remains empiric, and whereas hyperthyroidism can be controlled, treatment often results in changing one disease state, hyperthyroidism, for another, hypothyroidism. There is a diversity of opinion regarding the optimal management of thyrotoxic Graves' disease,[178] but treatment should be tailored individually. The current armamentarium consists of drugs affecting production or release of thyroid hormone, such as thionamides and iodide; medications that may improve symptomatology and decrease cardiovascular manifestations, such as β-adrenergic blockers; and thyroid ablation, either surgical subtotal thyroidectomy or radioiodine (^{131}I) therapy. Thionamides such as methimazole and propylthiouracil (PTU) inhibit thyroid hormone synthesis, with the latter having the additional advantage of inhibiting the conversion of T_4 to T_3. High doses of PTU totally block new hormone synthesis, but the stored thyroid hormone continues to be released so that metabolic improvement and euthyroidism may take up to 6 weeks. Iodide blocks the secretion of thyroid hormone, as well as conversion of T_4 to T_3, and acts faster than thionamides. Sodium iodate, an organic iodide agent used as a radio contrast material, is the most effective preparation. Since hyperthyroid glands avidly incorporate more iodine for new synthesis of thyroid hormone, thionamide therapy should be started several hours earlier to prevent iodide incorporation into thyroid hormones. The combination of inhibitors of synthesis, secretion, and conversion of T_4 and T_3 results in progressive clinical improvement with remission within 3 to 4 weeks.

The use of β-adrenergic antagonists is critical for the rapid improvement of the cardiovascular manifestations. Since these agents are rapidly metabolized during hyperthyroidism, frequent and higher doses are required. The longer acting preparations are also effective and can be given with less frequency. β-Adrenergic blockers, including those that are more cardioselective, should be used with great care in patients with asthma, obstructive pulmonary disease, heart block, or overt congestive heart failure. In severe hyperthyroidism or thyroid storm, the use of β-adrenergic blockers in addition to thionamides and iodide results in better outcomes. While beta blockers may control clinical symptoms and tachycardia, they do not reverse the hypermetabolic state. Treatment of other underlying medical conditions, normalization of fluid and electrolyte imbalance, and proper correction of other cardiopulmonary abnormalities are also crucial.

Thyroid ablation with radioactive iodine is effective in the great majority, with surgery being favored in toxic nodular goiters, particularly in those with large thyroid glands, and in patients with solitary toxic nodules. Preoperative therapy with β-adrenergic antagonists alone is effective both for radioiodine therapy and for preoperative preparation.[179]

Control of hyperthyroidism reduces ischemia and may improve congestive heart failure. Management of AF includes slowing of the ventricular rate, anticoagulation, and cardioversion. The high ventricular rate can be controlled with β-adrenergic antagonists; treatment with calcium channel blockers and/or digitalis may be used when β-adrenergic antagonists are contraindicated. Myocardial sensitivity to digitalis glycosides is reduced in thyrotoxicosis, and large doses may be required. As hyperthyroidism lessens, digoxin clearance

decreases, increasing the chance of toxicity. Unless contraindicated, β-adrenergic antagonists are more effective and a better choice than calcium channel blockers (see also Chap. 27).

Achievement of a euthyroid state often results in spontaneous reversion to sinus rhythm, within 3 months. When AF persists for longer than 3 to 4 months after attaining a euthyroid state, medical or electrical cardioversion may be necessary. Early cardioversion is not recommended because of a high rate of recurrence.[180] Anticoagulation is necessary for prevention of ischemic stroke in patients with AF; although prospective, randomized, control studies are not available in hyperthyroidism, the beneficial effects of oral anticoagulation in the general population with AF have been extrapolated.[181] Warfarin-treated patients have a decreased rate of embolic phenomena, while low-dose aspirin appears to be less effective.[182] On the other hand, younger patients with no risk factors have a low rate of stroke and can therefore be treated with aspirin. Thus, the patient's age and inherent risk of thromboembolism should be carefully considered when choosing antithrombotic therapy[183] (see also Chap. 52).

Hypothyroidism

Hypothyroidism, or myxedema, is the clinical syndrome that results from decreased production of T_4 and T_3. Most patients have primary hypothyroidism, but it may also be caused by pituitary (secondary) or hypothalamic (tertiary) disease. The etiology of adult primary hypothyroidism includes autoimmune hypothyroidism (Hashimoto's thyroiditis), ablation of the thyroid gland after radioactive iodine, thyroid surgery, and drugs such as amiodarone and lithium. Manifestations are variable and proportionate to the degree and duration of thyroid hormone deficiency as well as the age of onset. They include weight gain, dry skin, weakness, cold intolerance, memory impairment, deepening of the voice, constipation, lethargy, and menstrual abnormalities. Physical examination reveals a dull expression, slow pulse, mild hypertension, dry yellowed skin, dry hair, periorbital puffiness, hair loss at the lateral aspects of the eyebrows, and delayed relaxation of the deep tendon reflexes. The presence of a goiter is common in younger patients (Hashimoto's) but often absent in the elderly. Clinical features of hypothyroidism are insidious and often missed, particularly in the elderly.

CARDIOVASCULAR MANIFESTATIONS OF HYPOTHYROIDISM

Cardiac manifestations of hypothyroidism are the reverse of those seen in hyperthyroidism. Diastolic relaxation of the heart is prolonged due to decreased rates of cytosolic calcium removal, which is mediated by fast and slow forms of calcium ATPase in the sarcoplasmic reticulum. In patients with hypothyroidism and heart failure, the cardiac content of MHC-α mRNA is low, but the levels increase soon after therapy, with improved cardiac function. This illustrates the role that thyroid hormone plays in regulating MHC genes, although the relative influence of direct and indirect effects is not known.

In hypothyroidism, there is decreased total body oxygen consumption, sinus bradycardia, reduced cardiac output, and elevated total peripheral vascular resistance. The pulse pressure tends to be narrow, with mild hypertension especially in older individuals. Plasma renin activity and plasma aldosterone levels are decreased in the hypertensive hypothyroid patient.[184] In severe chronic myxedema, distinct cardiac anatomic abnormalities include a dilated, pale, and flabby ventricle with myofibrillar swelling and fibrosis. There is a hypodynamic state characterized by reduced cardiac output, stroke volume, heart rate, and plasma volumes[185]; myocardial contraction and relaxation are slowed, and systolic time intervals and LV contraction times are prolonged. The reduced cardiac output coupled with an enlarged cardiac silhouette on chest x-ray, with pleural and peritoneal effusions, often lead to confusion of hypothyroidism with congestive heart failure. In contrast to patients with reduced cardiac output from primary myocardial disease, in hypothyroidism, cardiac output increases in response to exercise.[186] Although circulation times are prolonged, left- and right-sided intracardiac pressures are normal. Thus, in uncomplicated hypothyroidism, congestive heart failure is rare. During aggressive thyroid replacement, congestive heart failure can be precipitated, particularly when underlying myocardial disease or obstructive coronary disease limits the ability to increment cardiac output. The typical ECG changes are sinus bradycardia, low-amplitude P waves and QRS complexes, and atrioventricular or intraventricular conduction disturbances, with occasional nonspecific ST- and T-wave abnormalities and QT prolongation.[187]

Hypercholesterolemia and hypertriglyceridemia are found in the majority, with all cholesterol subfractions being increased, including LDL, very low density lipoprotein, and the protective high-density lipoprotein (HDL) cholesterol. The elevation of LDL-cholesterol results from decreased concentrations of LDL receptors, and the accumulation of very low density lipoprotein is caused by decreased lipoprotein lipase activity, which is not sufficiently reduced to cause fasting chylomicronemia. Reduced hepatic triglyceride lipase is probably responsible for the high HDL-cholesterol. The disproportion elevation of LDL-cholesterol results in an unfavorable LDL/HDL ratio. All these lipid anomalies can be readily reversed with thyroid replacement. A direct association between hypothyroidism and CHD is controversial since no direct correlation between cholesterol levels, coronary artery disease, and mild hypothyroidism has been found.[188] The concomitant elevation of LDL cholesterol levels and hypertension has been associated with diffuse atherosclerosis and coronary obstructions, a condition that becomes evident when therapy is undertaken. Aggressive thyroid replacement increases oxygen requirements, at times leading to ischemia, myocardial infarction, and even death. Although coronary artery disease is common pathologically, angina pectoris is present in only 7 percent,[189] and the incidence of autopsy-proven myocardial infarction is not higher in the hypothyroid population.[190] The low prevalence of angina pectoris can be explained by the protective effect of lower oxygen consumption.[191] In some individuals with severe myxedema, serious coronary atherosclerosis can be found even in the absence of other risk factors. Therefore, it is recommended that thyroid hormone replacement should be given very cautiously, as it may cause myocardial ischemia if the increased heart rate is not matched by a corresponding increase in coronary blood flow. Evaluation of the hypothyroid patient with chest pain is complicated by elevated creatine kinase levels, which may implicate a cardiac origin.[192] Isoenzyme analysis, however, shows skeletal muscle to be the main source, and total creatine kinase levels are disproportionately elevated and do not fluctuate rapidly, as is the case after myocardial damage. In the past, pericardial effusion was a leading manifestation of hypothyroidism and was often confused with congestive heart failure. The prevalence of pericardial effusion is now lower, most likely because of earlier diagnosis and treatment, and serious hemodynamic consequences such as cardiac tamponade are uncommon, since demands for cardiac output are low.

DIAGNOSIS

It is important to entertain the possibility of hypothyroidism since its presentation is often insidious, with noncharacteristic symptoms that may be overlooked. In most cases, the diagnosis is confirmed by a low T_4 level coupled with an elevated plasma TSH level. The T_3 levels are not very helpful and may be depressed in ill patients without thyroidal disease.[193] The degree of hypothyroidism often correlates with the depression in serum T_4 concentration and elevation in plasma TSH. Hence, minimal elevation in TSH levels alone will not explain major clinical findings. While routine testing for hypothyroidism has a low yield in community screening programs, evaluation for thyroid dysfunction is useful and recommended particularly in the elderly.[194] Only a minority of patients have secondary hypothyroidism (hypopituitarism), in which T_4 is depressed and TSH levels range from low to minimally elevated. In these patients and in other difficult clinical settings, TSH determinations alone are not sufficient and measurement of other thyroid function studies may be needed.[193]

EUTHYROID SICK SYNDROME

Seriously ill patients, such as those in critical care units, may have low total T_4, but normal free T_4; hence they are euthyroid. The TSH can also be slightly above or below the normal range in critically sick individuals. With recovery from the critical illness, T_4 and TSH levels normalize; therefore repeat determinations of hormone levels are very useful. In view of the rarity of secondary hypothyroidism and the high frequency of low T_4 levels in euthyroid critically ill patients, the finding of a normal TSH level is often sufficient to exclude the diagnosis of hypothyroidism.[195]

TREATMENT OF HYPOTHYROIDISM

Therapy of hypothyroidism involves replacement with thyroid hormone. Since T_3 is primarily derived from the extrathyroidal production from T_4, L-thyroxine is the preparation of choice. The full daily replacement dose of L-thyroxine will range from 1.5 to 2.0 μg/kg per day, with elderly patients often needing less. During L-thyroxine replacement, TSH determinations alone can provide a satisfactory and cost-effective assessment of dose adequacy in nearly all cases.[196] Reversal of the clinical manifestations of hypothyroidism may take months. Therapy requires considerable prudence, particularly in the elderly or in those with underlying cardiovascular disease. Since coronary blood flow may be limited during the period of increased cardiac demand, ischemia may develop in those being treated aggressively. Also, with valvular heart disease, valvular gradients will increase along with cardiac output. The development of angina, arrhythmias, and AMI are complications that can occur during vigorous thyroid hormone replacement therapy. The most prudent approach in patients with ischemic heart disease is to give low doses (12.5 to 25 μg daily) with very small increments. Myxedema coma is a rare medical emergency that has a high mortality rate when untreated.[192] It represents an extreme stage of decompensated hypothyroidism and is often precipitated by coexisting medical conditions. Clinical hallmarks of myxedema coma include hypothermia, lethargy, respiratory acidosis, cardiovascular shock, and coma. Controversial aspects of its management include the choice of thyroid hormone (T_4 or T_3), dosage, and route of administration. Because of its rarity, no controlled clinical trials have been done comparing these various regimens. Patients have been successfully treated with T_3 alone, the combination of T_3 and T_4, as well as with T_4 alone.[197,198] Despite the theoretical benefit of T_3 therapy, higher serum T_3 levels have been associated with fatal outcome in the elderly.[199] Since the benefits of T_3 therapy have not been clearly documented, it is therefore not routinely recommended. Reversal of heart failure after intravenous T_3 administration has been reported in hypothyroidism[200] and in euthyroid patients undergoing cardiac surgery. Administration of T_3 results in improved cardiac output and reduced systemic and pulmonary vascular resistance, perhaps by a direct, prompt effect of T_3 on blood vessels.[162] The immediate administration of an intravenous bolus dose of levothyroxine is designed to raise the serum T_4 level to 77 to 90 nmol/L (6 to 7 μg/dL). Usually about 500 μg is needed, followed by a daily administration of 75 to 100 μg until the patient's vital signs become stable and gastrointestinal function returns to normal, permitting one to switch to oral administration. Glucocorticoids should also be administered until coexistent adrenal insufficiency can be ruled out. In addition, cardiorespiratory, neurologic, and renal function must be appropriately monitored and treated. Concomitant use of antianginal drugs, such as nitrates, calcium channel blockers, and β-adrenergic blockers, may be helpful but should be used with caution since symptomatic bradycardia and worsening of congestive heart failure may develop. Bypass surgery or angioplasty are preferable in patients with unstable coronary disease. Revascularization can be done successfully before thyroid replacement is given.[172] With good anesthesia technique and careful monitoring, surgery can be done without increased morbidity, mortality, and/or prolonged hospital stay. Revascularization with PTCA has also been performed in hypothyroid patients, without increased mortality or major morbidity.[201]

Amiodarone-Induced Thyroid Dysfunction

Amiodarone is an effective class II antiarrhythmic agent whose use often results in abnormal thyroid function.[202] It has a high fat solubility, with a long half-life that ranges from 25 to 100 days. It is an important source of exogenous iodine, with each 200-mg tablet releasing approximately 6 mg/day of iodine, altering thyroid hormone production in some.[202] It can inhibit the various 5′-deiodinase isoenzymes, including hepatic type I iodothyronine 5′-deiodinase that converts T_4 to T_3, resulting in decreased serum levels of T_3 and increased serum T_4 levels. Amiodarone also reduces iodothyronine uptake by the liver, contributing to T_4 elevation and decreased clearance of reverse T_3 (rT_3), a biologically inactive hormone. Levels of rT_3 are closely correlated with both the cumulative dose of amiodarone and drug-induced side effects. In addition, amiodarone can directly affect the regulation of TSH secretion by inhibiting T_3 binding to its thyrotrope nuclear receptor and by inhibiting the type II 5′-deiodinase enzyme that converts pituitary T_4 to T_3, resulting in increased TSH levels. Elevated TSH concentration stimulates T_4 production, reaching a new equilibrium with elevated T_4, normal or slightly decreased T_3, and a euthyroid patient. The ability of amiodarone to block nuclear T_3 receptors has also been observed in the heart and may contribute to its antiarrhythmic effect.

Amiodarone may induce hypothyroidism in as many as 20 percent[203] and thyrotoxicosis in approximately 10 percent of patients.[202] The incidence of amiodarone-induced hypothyroidism is higher in iodine-sufficient areas such as North America, and the condition more often affects patients with underlying thyroid disease, many with positive antithyroid antibodies. While the role of autoimmunity has been implicated, the likely pathogenesis appears to be related to the inhibitory effects of excessive iodine. The large quantities of iodine inhibit intrathyroidal hormonal synthesis, a phenomenon known as *acute Wolff-Chaikoff effect*. While escape from this effect usually occurs within 72 h under normal circumstances, this escape does not take place in patients with autoimmune thyroid disease, who can therefore develop iodine-induced hypothyroidism. The diagnosis may be difficult to establish since sinus bradycardia, which is suggestive of hypothyroidism, almost invariably occurs with high doses of amiodarone. Unfortunately, measurements of TSH, the most helpful test for primary hypothyroidism, may also give misleading results. In this particular situation, identification of high serum levels of rT_3 concentration may be helpful, with normal or low serum levels indicating hypothyroidism. Amiodarone withdrawal results in spontaneous remission of thyroid dysfunction in approximately half of the patients, but it may persist for several months in the remainder.

Hyperthyroidism occurs more often in iodine-deficient areas. The pathogenesis may also be related to iodine overload, particularly in patients with preexisting thyroid abnormalities.

Amiodarone and its major metabolite, desethylamiodarone, can also exert a direct cytotoxic effect, causing a thyroiditis-like syndrome with leakage of thyroid.[204] Since follicular injury can cause increased serum interleukin 6 levels, its determination may be useful in the differential diagnosis of amiodarone-induced hyperthyroidism.[205] Treatment may require the prolonged use of thionamides; some patients are refractory, and potassium perchlorate, a drug that competitively inhibits iodide uptake by the thyroid gland, may need to be added.[206] Potassium perchlorate should be given cautiously due to the toxic effects, particularly when used in large doses and for long periods of time. Glucocorticoids can also be helpful because of their inhibitory effect on the peripheral generation of T_3 as well as their possible anti-inflammatory effect. When all medical trials have failed and amiodorone treatment needs to be continued, surgical treatment with a near-total thyroidectomy is a rapid and effective modality that may need to be considered[207] (see also Chaps. 27 and 30).

PARATHYROID DISEASE AND DISORDERS OF CALCIUM AND MAGNESIUM METABOLISM

Parathyroid Hormone Effects on the Cardiovascular System

Although calcium has a positive inotropic myocardial effect, most patients with chronic hypercalcemia or hypocalcemia have little or no clinical evidence of altered myocardial contractility. Parathyroid hormone can act directly on cultured heart cells, and prolonged exposure has been associated with increased myocardial calcium content, decreased energy production, and transient decline in cardiac performance.[208] Chronic hypercalcemia can also result in calcium deposition in the coronary arteries, valves, and myocardial fibers.[209] Chronic hypocalcemia, on the other hand, has been associated with low cardiac contractility and congestive heart failure, which can be refractory to diuretic and digitalis therapy but rapidly responsive to calcium restoration.[210] Calcium infusion increases both cardiac output and blood pressure in hypoparathyroid patients, suggesting a subclinical direct cardiac dysfunction. In hypercalcemia, the plateau of the cardiac fiber action potential is abbreviated, resulting in electrocardiographic shortening of the ST segment and the QT interval; in hypocalcemia, a prolongation of the ST segment and QT interval is often found (see also Chap. 12).

The incidence of hypertension is increased in hyperparathyroid patients,[211] but it remains uncertain whether or not there is a true association. Surgical correction of hyperparathyroidism does not seem to reverse hypertension in the majority of patients,[212] but it may facilitate their management. Thiazide diuretics can cause transient hypercalcemia; however, when it persists, it often unmasks hyperparathyroidism.[213] Thiazide diuretics should be avoided in hyperparathyroidism, and loop diuretics should be used instead when necessary (see Chap. 24).

Magnesium Deficiency

Magnesium (Mg) deficiency is the most unrecognized, undiagnosed, and undertreated electrolyte disorder[214]; the relevance it has in the cardiovascular system is well established.[215] Magnesium is critical for oxidative phosphorylation and enzymatic reactions involving adenosine triphosphate (ATP), and it is required for action of membrane Na^+, K^+-ATPase, allowing intracellular potassium flux across cell membranes.[216] Magnesium can act as a calcium antagonist either on intracellular sites or in membrane channels, in both vascular and cardiac smooth muscle. Magnesium deficiency can alter myocardial membrane potential and result in cardiac arrhythmias.[217] Magnesium losses are particularly common in DM,[218] congestive heart failure,[219] and diuretic use.[220] While recognition of potassium deficiency and the need for replacement is common, this is not the case with magnesium. Further, adequate potassium repletion can be impaired in some, unless magnesium deficits are also corrected.[221]

In DM, excessive glycosuria is the main cause of magnesium loss, and its severity is inversely correlated to glycemic control. Magnesium deficiency has also been found during acute metabolic decompensation, due in part to increased fat and protein mobilization. The prevalence and severity of magnesium deficiency can be further aggravated by other concomitant conditions such as congestive failure, diuretic use, and chronic alcoholism. While hypomagnesemia is associated with arrhythmias and refractory treatment for hypokalemia,[219] magnesium deficiency does not constitute an independent risk factor for increased mortality.[222]

The myocardial irritability related to magnesium losses can be effectively reversed by intravenous administration of either $MgSO_4$[223] or $MgCl$.[224] Oral magnesium replacement can also reduce ventricular irritability in individuals treated for congestive heart failure.[225] Hypomagnesemia-induced cardiac arrhythmias are particularly important during digitalis treatment because of a synergistic adverse effect on the Na^+,K^+-ATPase pump.[226] Electrolyte disturbances have been implicated in the increased mortality rate observed in patients being treated with diuretics and in the higher prevalence of ventricular arrhythmias in those without apparent heart disease, after examining for other risk factors.[227] Magnesium deficiency is quite common in hospitalized patients, particularly in those with associated conditions that may aggravate magnesium losses or in those receiving medications such as diuretics and/or aminoglycoside antibiotics, which may cause more magnesium losses.

Establishing the diagnosis of magnesium deficiency may be difficult because of the minimal or often absent clinical manifestations and lack of reliable laboratory tests. The clinical manifestations are nonspecific and mostly confined to mental changes or neuromuscular irritability. Tetany, a striking and better known presentation, is only rarely found. Instead, less specific signs such as tremor, muscle twitching, bizarre movements, focal seizures, generalized convulsions, delirium, or coma are found. Magnesium deficiency should be suspected when other electrolyte abnormalities coexist and when changes in the ECG (prolongation of the Q-T and P-R intervals, widening of the QRS complex, ST-segment depression, and low T waves) are also present. Supraventricular or ventricular tachyarrhythmias may further lead to diagnosis and treatment.[228] Once deficiency is suspected, measurement of serum magnesium concentration continues to be the "routine screening test" but has poor reliability, since it does not reflect intracellular magnesium. A more effective clinical probe is the "magnesium loading test," which is both therapeutic and diagnostic.[214] It consists of the parenteral administration of $MgSO_4$ and assessment of urinary magnesium retention. Individuals with normal magnesium balance should eliminate at least 75 percent. This approach is recommended in all patients for whom one has a high index of suspicion, particularly those with ischemic heart disease or cardiac arrhythmias. Magnesium administration is contraindicated in anuric individuals and in those with significant renal impairment. Restoration of normal magnesium concentration is often achieved after eliminating the causative factors and restarting a normal diet. Parenteral administration, however, is more effective and the best route when replacement is necessary during medical emergencies. The recommended regimen is 2 g of $MgSO_4$ (16.3 meq) given intravenously over 30 min, followed by a constant infusion rate of 1 meq of magnesium per kilogram of body weight for the first day and 0.5 meq/kg per day for 3 to 5 more days. The intramuscular route is painful and should be avoided when an intravenous infusion is possible.

Magnesium Therapy During Acute Myocardial Infarction

The pharmacologic effect of magnesium administration in the non-Mg-deficient patient with ischemic heart disease and cardiac arrhythmias remains controversial. While low serum and myocardial magnesium levels have been found in AMI,[229] magnesium is given in these patients not as replacement but for its pharmacologic qualities, i.e., coronary vasodilation, platelet inhibition, antiarrhythmic characteristics, and possible role in preservation of damaged ischemic myocardium. Intravenous $MgSO_4$ given immediately to patients with suspected AMI in a large prospective double-blind trial (LIMIT-2) was associated with a lower mortality of 7.8 percent, versus 10.3 percent in the placebo-treated group.[230] The routine administration of magnesium during AMI was widely discontinued, however, after an even larger study, the ISIS-4 study, found no beneficial effects.[231] Early treatment is essential since serum magnesium concentrations must be raised by the time of reperfusion.[232] The timing of magnesium administration in relation to thrombolytic therapy or spontaneous reperfusion has been offered as an explanation for this discrepancy. The beneficial effect of magnesium treatment appears to be greater in patients undergoing AMI who are unable to receive thrombolytic therapy, a patient population with a high in-hospital mortality rate. Magnesium can reduce both the incidence of

arrhythmias and, presumably by preserving LV ejection fraction, the incidence of congestive heart failure.[233] Similarly, a beneficial effect has been reported in patients with unstable angina undergoing bypass grafting,[234] but other studies have not confirmed these cardioprotective effects.[235] The disparate results between the two large clinical trials (LIMIT-2 and ISIS-4) remain unexplained. The ISIS-4 trial was not specifically designed to test the hypothesis that magnesium may limit reperfusion injury, and the time at which magnesium was given is a factor that needs to be clarified further. It is important to determine if patients with magnesium deficiency benefit from its administration or whether or not magnesium should be used as a true cardioprotective agent in all non-Mg-deficient individuals. At this time, with the evidence we have, magnesium therapy cannot be recommended routinely in the management of AMI (see Chap. 47).

PITUITARY DISEASE

Pituitary Insufficiency

Pituitary tumors are the most common cause of hypopituitarism, and they can manifest by deficiency of the individual hormones or by symptoms of a space-occupying lesion. Pituitary ischemia and necrosis, which in Sheehan's syndrome occur during acute illness, are a common cause of hypopituitarism. Pituitary necrosis can also occur after major cardiac surgery,[236] and pituitary infarcts can be found in 18 to 33 percent of patients maintained on mechanical respirators, particularly in those with compromised circulatory function.[237] While mild and transient hypopituitarism is not uncommon, a more severe form of pituitary insufficiency may have grievous consequences, requiring prompt recognition and treatment.

Acromegaly

The most common cause of acromegaly is a pituitary adenoma that produces human growth hormone (hGH). The clinical consequences of advanced acromegaly are not limited to the cosmetic disfigurement and incapacitating arthropathy, as previously thought. A shortened life expectancy with doubled mortality rate occurs as a result of respiratory, cardiovascular, and malignant complications.[238] The diagnosis can be established by clinical manifestations and the findings of elevated plasma hGH levels, which fail to suppress after a glucose load. High plasma levels of insulin-like growth factor I (IGF-I) are also diagnostic.

The finding of cardiovascular abnormalities without concomitant hypertension or coronary heart disease has led to the concept of a distinct "acromegalic cardiomyopathy,"[239] an entity that was previously questioned due to lack of distinct pathologic findings[240] or a cause-effect relationship between hGH hypersecretion and cardiovascular complications.[241] The extent of cardiomegaly is disproportional to the degree of hypertension, however, and LV hypertrophy is often associated with congestive heart failure.[242] Ventricular hypertrophy, either concentric or asymmetric septal hypertrophy, initially has a preserved systolic function that can be readily demonstrated by echocardiography.[243] Hypertension, which is three times more common than in the general population,[241] tends to be mild and responsive to conventional therapy; it is associated with sodium retention and low plasma renin.[244] The possibility of hyperaldosteronism or pheochromocytoma must be kept in mind, as they may represent a variant of the multiple endocrine neoplasia syndromes. Thyrotoxicosis should also be suspected when tachyarrhythmias are present.[241]

Role of Human Growth Hormone and Insulin-Like Growth Factor I in Atherogenesis

Both hGH and IGF-I have been implicated in the development of accelerated atherogenesis. Most of the hGH effects appear to be mediated through IGF-I, which may be a promoter of cardiac enlargement.[245] IGF-I is structurally homologous to proinsulin and can exert insulin-like metabolic effects. It can also induce proliferation and differentiation of numerous cell types and, since it is a potent mutagen for arterial and capillary cells, may therefore contribute to the coronary artery disease of acromegaly. This is further supported by the observation that hGH-deficient dwarfs with DM are free of atherosclerotic disease.[246]

Acromegalic tumors are generally removed surgically through a transphenoidal approach. Anesthesia and perioperative care can be difficult due to increases in lung volume, tracheal thickness, and tongue size—changes that may be responsible for obstructive sleep apnea. Since patients with acromegaly frequently have large pituitary tumors, surgical intervention often results in anterior pituitary insufficiency. The surgical cure rate remains low, and the remnant tumor often continues to produce excessive hGH secretion. When the surgical approach is not possible or successful, medical or radiation therapy is necessary, since persistent elevated hGH levels (>5 mU/L) are associated with increased mortality.[247]

Medical treatment with somatostatin analogues with longer half-lives, such as ocetreotide, is effective in reducing hGH levels as well as reducing tumor size in some. Octreotide treatment is also beneficial in the cardiac failure of acromegaly, increasing cardiac output and decreasing systemic vascular resistance.[248] Paradoxically, in patients with idiopathic dilated cardiomyopathy and congestive heart failure,[249] short-term treatment with hGH was found to increase LV ejection fraction, improve isovolumic relaxation, and increase LV muscle mass while improving functional capacity. The potential clinical use of this form of therapy for congestive heart failure, however, remains to be evaluated properly with larger and longer studies (see also Chap. 23).

ADRENAL DISEASE

Adrenal Insufficiency

Cortisol deficiency occurs from impaired adrenocorticotropic hormone (ACTH) secretion, as in hypopituitarism, or following withdrawal of long-term treatment with pharmacologic doses of glucocorticoids. The most common form of isolated aldosterone deficiency is hyporeninemic hypoaldosteronism, or type IV renal tubular acidosis, found in certain patients with mild renal disease, especially in the presence of DM. Another cause of aldosterone deficiency is primary destructive adrenal disease (Addison's disease), where both cortisol and aldosterone production are impaired.

Treatment with glucocorticoid replacement potentiates the vasoconstrictor response to catecholamines[250] and results in a rapid reversal of hypotension. The rapidity of this effect precludes changes in plasma volume and is not related to any increase in myocardial catecholamine receptor number.[251] Aldosterone deficiency causes impaired sodium reabsorption and potassium secretion in the renal distal tubule. This leads to the inability to conserve sodium and the propensity for volume depletion, especially when sodium intake is low and during acute or stressful events. Low blood pressure and low cardiac output are found with both glucocorticoid and aldosterone deficiency, and vascular collapse may result when these patients are stressed.[250,251] The small cardiac size, as judged by chest x-ray, and the hyperkalemia-associated electrocardiographic changes are characteristics of cortisol deficiency and may be of help in establishing the diagnosis (see Chap. 37).

Cushing's Syndrome

Cushing's syndrome results from chronic exposure to elevated plasma levels of cortisol (hypercortisolism), most commonly caused by therapy with glucocorticoids for nonendocrine disorders. The most frequent cause of endogenous hypercortisolism is Cushing's disease caused by a pituitary tumor and bilateral, diffuse adrenal hyperplasis. Tumor hypercortisolism, from adrenal adenoma, adrenal carcinoma, or ectopic production of ACTH or corticotropin-releasing hormone, is another, less common cause. Clinical features include central obesity in 90 percent, hypertension in 85 percent, and glucose intolerance in 80 percent. The extremities are thin, with muscle wasting and proximal muscle weakness. Other catabolic effects include atrophy of the skin and underlying tissues, manifest by violaceous and wide striae, easy bruising, and a decreased skin barrier with propensity to infections. Osteopenia and osteoporosis may result in pathologic fractures. Excessive androgen production, more characteristic of adrenal carcinoma, can account for menstrual irregularities, hirsutism, and acne. Clitoromegaly is the most reliable clinical manifestation of excessive androgens. Hypokalemic alkalosis is often indicative of ectopic ACTH–induced hypercortisolism, where the very high cortisol production manifests with a mineralocorticoid-like effect. Patients with hypercortisolism often have impaired glucose tolerance, overt diabetes, hyperinsulinemia, hypertension, obesity, and dyslipidemia and are therefore at a higher risk to develop accelerated atherosclerosis. When untreated, it can be associated with ischemic-related cardiovascular events with a high mortality rate.[252] A rare form of Cushing's syndrome is "Carney's complex," consisting of primary pigmented nodular adrenocortical disease with hypercortisolism, cardiac myxomatous lesions, and cutaneous pigmentous lentigines. It is found in families with an inherited autosomal X-linked dominant gene.[253]

DIAGNOSIS AND TREATMENT

Simple tests are now available for screening and diagnosis.[254] When Cushing's syndrome is suspected, an overnight dexamethasone suppression screening test can be obtained by giving 1 mg of dexamethasone orally at midnight; normal individuals will have a plasma cortisol level of less than 5 µg/dL the morning after. In those failing to suppress, a more extensive evaluation is needed. Increased cortisol production can best be demonstrated by determination of urinary free cortisol. After a positive screening test and documentation of hypercortisolism, the different causes of increased cortisol production can be determined. This is done by manipulations of the hypothalamic-pituitary-adrenal axis, either by suppression studies with dexamethasone or by stimulation studies with corticotropin-releasing hormone.[255] After the biochemical workup, localization of the source of hypercortisolism can also be established with contrast computerized tomography and magnetic resonance imaging.[255] In some, measurement of plasma ACTH levels from the inferior petrosal sinuses can distinguish corticotropin-secreting pituitary adenomas from other causes of Cushing's syndrome. Transphenoidal pituitary adenomectomy has emerged as the treatment of choice for Cushing's disease.[256] When a pituitary lesion is not localized by imaging studies, petrosal sinus sampling may be helpful for lateralization of the source of excessive ACTH production, in order to enable the neurosurgeon to perform a partial hypophysectomy.[256]

HYPERALDOSTERONISM AND PHEOCHROMOCYTOMA

(See Chap. 57)

Sex Steroids

Sex steroids affect the vascular system, primarily through changes in lipid metabolism, but since estrogen receptors are present in the vasculature, a direct effect may also be likely.[257] Estrogen decreases LDL-cholesterol and raises HDL-cholesterol, particularly the HDL_2 subfraction. In contrast, exogenous androgens, especially those that cannot be metabolized to estrogen (i.e., nonaromatizable androgens), cause unfavorable lipid effects by decreasing plasma HDL-cholesterol and HDL_2.[258]

Androgens in Men

The most common indication for androgen therapy is hypogonadism in men; however, many other potential uses are being constantly explored, and androgen abuse is common among athletes and bodybuilders. Supraphysiologic doses of testosterone, especially when combined with exercise training, result in a favorable anabolic effect with increased fat-free mass and muscle size.[259] Because short-term administration of high doses has not been found to be associated with adverse effects, the potential use in patients with debilitating disorders such as human immunodeficiency virus or cachexia or in patients with cancer is currently being evaluated. Androgen replacement in aging men when physiologic decline in testosterone occurs is associated with increased energy, restoration of body weight and lean body mass, and beneficial bone effects.[260] The extended use of androgens in the elderly, as well as in other non-androgen-deficient populations, should not be routine because of their potential serious side effects on the cardiovascular system, prostate gland, and lipid metabolism. Nevertheless, physiologic doses of androgen replacement should be given to documented hypogonadal individuals, as androgen deficiency may also have serious consequences in men. When administered properly, they are safe and permit normal sexual function, growth and development, and the maintenance of secondary sexual characteristics in men.

Effects of Oral Contraceptives

Complications associated with oral contraceptives, such as venous thromboembolism, myocardial infarction, ischemic and hemorrhagic stroke, and worsening of hypertension and DM, have been significantly lessened by decreasing the dosage of estrogen. Most preparations now contain 35 µg or less of estrogen; the reduction in the dose of estrogen has been directly associated with a reduction in side effects.[261] In order to minimize the associated androgenic side effects, the type of synthetic progestogen has also been changed. The so-called third-generation progestogens (i.e., desogestrel, gestodene, and norgestimate) are extremely potent and have weak estrogen antagonist or androgenic effects; they also result in fewer adverse changes in carbohydrate and lipoprotein metabolism.[261] The risk of adverse cardiovascular events in premenopausal women results not from atherogenesis but from thrombogenesis, which is caused by factors such as altered serum lipoproteins, changes in procoagulants, and platelet aggregation.[262] Combined oral contraceptives can cause a state of increased coagulability that is most significant in women who smoke, since smoking also increases the risk of thrombogenesis. Oral contraceptive administration in young women who smoke has been associated with an increased risk of myocardial infarction.[263] In women over the age of 35, smoking is also associated with high risk for developing coronary artery disease, especially when combined with other factors such as hypertension, DM, and hyperlipidemia. Nonsmokers under the age of 45 or smokers under the age of 35 who use oral contraceptives show no increased likelihood of dying from myocardial infarction. Thus, women under the age of 35 may continue to use oral contraceptives but should be strongly advised to discontinue smoking. Those between the ages of 35 and 45 should use oral contraceptives only if they do not smoke or do not have other underlying risk factors for vascular disease.

The older combinations of oral contraceptives can cause hypertension in about 4 to 5 percent of normotensive women and increased blood pressure in 9 to 16 percent of those with preexisting hypertension.[264] This is probably the effect of both hormones in a susceptible population; however, the third-generation progestogens may have an antimineralocorticoid effect and they are not associated with a high risk for hypertension. The newest third-generation progestines, particularly desogestrel or gestodene, were found to have a higher risk for venous thrombosis and pulmonary embolism.[265] However, fatal pulmonary embolism is still a rare event occurring in less than 1 in a million women using these preparations, and no association has been found between low estrogen oral contraceptives and strokes.[266] On the other hand, the use of lower estrogen oral contraceptives has an added benefit of a reduction in the risk of myocardial infarction, due in part to a decrease in LDL-cholesterol and an increase in the levels of HDL (see also Chap. 41).

Postmenopausal Estrogen Replacement

The average woman in North America will be postmenopausal during one-third of her life. Each year, approximately 2.5 million U.S. women are hospitalized for cardiovascular problems, with 50,000 deaths annually, of which half are caused by coronary artery disease. The benefits of estrogen in postmenopausal women include relief of menopausal symptoms and reduction of bone loss, with a 60 percent decline of hip fracture. Another major benefit is a 50 percent reduction in the risk of heart disease, with a decrease in both nonfatal and fatal myocardial infarctions.[267–270] The mortality can be reduced by 20 percent, mainly by lowering the rate of myocardial infarction among elderly women by using estrogen replacement.[269] Large cross-sectional angiographic studies have also demonstrated a strong association of estrogen use with reduction of atherosclerosis.[270]

Whereas estrogen therapy has favorable lipid effects, the addition of progestin was thought to antagonize these effects, particularly when using progestins derived from testosterone, such as levonorgestrel. Medroxyprogesterone acetate, the most commonly used progestin in the United States, has no adverse effects, however, and when used in combination with estrogen has been found to be associated with an even better profile than estrogen alone.[271] The concern that progestin might weaken the protective effect of estrogen was alleviated by a recent trial that showed that estrogen replacement therapy or combined hormone-replacement therapy improves the lipoprotein profile and lowers fibrinogen levels, without appreciable effects on blood pressure or post–glucose challenge insulin levels.[272] Estrogen shows a more favorable effect on HDL-cholesterol than any form of combined therapy.[272] The favorable estrogen-like effects on bone and lipids and the protective

effect for breast cancer caused by the synthetic antiestrogen tamoxifen have raised the possibility of its clinical use. In normal postmenopausal women, tamoxifen produced greater reductions than estrogens in the levels of atherogenic lipids and fibrinogen, thus offering a superior cardioprotective effect.[273] The increased risk of endometrial carcinoma caused by tamoxifen has made this agent unsuitable for present use, however, but the benefits of tamoxifen raise the possibility of developing other analogues in the future.

Women and their physicians must balance the benefit of hormone-replacement therapy against the possible side effects, which include a somewhat higher incidence of breast and uterus carcinoma.[274] The PEPI trial also found that women treated with estrogens alone had a 34 percent increased risk of these carcinomas, while it was only 1 percent in those treated with an estrogen-progestin combination.[272] It has also been estimated that the risk for breast cancer after 10 years of estrogen therapy is increased by 15 to 30 percent.[275] While the combination of estrogen plus progestin can decrease endometrial carcinoma, it may increase the risk of breast cancer even more than estrogen alone. Similarly, in the Nurses' Health Study cohort, the relative risk of breast cancer was 1.32 for women receiving estrogen alone, with most women taking conjugated equine estrogens, versus 1.41 for women receiving estrogens plus progestin.[276] Mammography before therapy and studies at intervals recommended by the American Cancer Society remain imperative for the early detection of breast carcinoma (see also Chap. 53).

While we await further information from prospective clinical trials such as the Women's Health Initiative study of the National Institutes of Health, it is recommended that all postmenopausal women be considered candidates for hormone-replacement therapy and that all be educated about its risk and benefits, following the guidelines given by the America College of Physicians.[277] Women who have had hysterectomies should receive estrogen alone. Those with a uterus should take conjugated estrogen in conjunction with progestins.

REFERENCES

1. Harris MI, Cowie CC, Reiber G, Boyko E, Stern M, Bennett P, eds. *Diabetes in America*, 2d ed. NIH Publication No. 95-1468. Washington, DC: U.S. Government Printing Office; 1995.
2. Reaven GM. Role of insulin resistance in human disease. *Diabetes* 1988; 37:1595–1607.
3. Fontbonne A, Charles MA, Thibult N, Richard JL, Claude JR, Warnet JM, et al. Hyperinsulinemia as a predictor of coronary heart disease mortality in a healthy population: The Paris Prospective Study, 15-year follow up. *Diabetologia* 1991; 34:356–361.
4. Jarrett RJ, Shipley MJ. Type 2 (non-insulin dependent) diabetes mellitus and cardiovascular disease: Putative association via common antecedents; further evidence from the Whitehall Study. *Diabetologia* 1988; 31:720–737.
5. Ferranini E, Haffner SM, Mitchell BD, Stern MP. Hyperinsulinemia: The key of a cardiovascular and metabolic syndrome. *Diabetologia* 1991; 34:416–422.
6. Stern MP. Diabetes and cardiovascular disease. The "common soil" hypothesis. *Diabetes* 1995; 44:369–374.
7. Kaplan NM. The deadly quartet: Upper-body obesity, glucose intolerance, hypertriglyceridemia, and hypertension. *Arch Intern Med* 1989; 149:1514–1520.

8. Stout RW. Insulin and atheroma: 20 years perspective. *Diabetes Care* 1990; 13:631–654.

9. Laws A, Reaven GM. Evidence for an independent relationship between insulin resistance and fasting plasma HDL-cholesterol, triglyceride and insulin concentrations. *J Intern Med* 1992; 231:25–30.

10. Pyörälä K. Relationship of glucose tolerance and plasma insulin to the incidence of coronary heart disease: Results from two population studies in Finland. *Diabetes Care* 1979; 2:131–141.

11. Welborn TA, Wearne K. Coronary heart disease incidence and cardiovascular mortality in Busselton with reference to glucose and insulin concentrations. *Diabetes Care* 1979; 2:154–160.

12. Eschwège E, Richard JL, Thibult N, Cudimetiere P, Warnet JM, Claude JR, et al. Coronary heart disease mortality in relation with diabetes, blood glucose and plasma insulin level: The Paris Prospective Study, ten years later. *Horm Metab Res Suppl* 1985; 15:41–46.

13. Yarnell JWG, Sweetnam PM, Marks V, Teale JD, Bolton CH. Insulin in ischemic heart disease: Are associations explained by triglyceride concentrations? The Caerphilly prospective study. *Br Heart J* 1994; 171:293–296.

14. Després J-P, Lamarche B, Mauriège P, Cantin B, Deganais GR, Moorjani S, et al. Hyperinsulinemia as an independent risk factor for ischemic heart disease. *N Engl J Med* 1996; 334:952–957.

15. Wingard DL, Barrett-Connor EL, Ferrara A. Is insulin really a heart disease risk factor? *Diabetes Care* 1995; 18:1299–1304.

16. Welin L, Eriksson H, Larsson B. Ohison LO, Svärdsudd K, Tibblin G. Hyperinsulinemia is not a major coronary risk factor in elderly men: The study of men born in 1913. *Diabetologia* 1992; 35:766–770.

17. Liu QZ, Knowler WC, Nelson RG, Saad MF, Charles MA, Liebow IM, et al. Insulin treatment, endogenous insulin concentration, and ECG abnormalities in diabetic Pima Indians. *Diabetes* 1992; 41:1141–1150.

18. Rewers M, Shetterly SM, Baxter J, Mamman RF. Insulin and cardiovascular disease in Hispanics and non-Hispanic whites (NHW): The San Luis Valley Diabetes Study (abstr). *Circulation* 1992; 85:865A.

19. Ferrara A, Barrett-Conner E, Edelstein SL. Hyperinsulinemia does not increase the risk of fatal cardiovascular disease in elderly men or women without diabetes: The Rancho Bernardo Study, 1984 to 1991. *Am J Epidemiol* 1994; 140:857–869.

20. Orchard TJ, Eichner J, Kuller LH, Becker DJ, McCallum LM, Grandits GA. Insulin as a predictor of coronary heart disease: Interaction with apolipoprotein E phenotype; a report from Multiple Risk Factor Intervention Trial. *Ann Epidemiol* 1994; 4:40–45.

21. Pyorala K, Savolainen E, Kaukola S, Happakoski J. Plasma insulin as coronary heart disease risk factor: Relationship to other risk factors and predictive value during 9½-year follow-up of the Helsinki Policemen study population. *Acta Med Scand* 1985; 701 (suppl):38–52.

22. Orchard TJ, Eichner J, Kuller LH, Becker DJ, McCallum LM, Grandits GA. Insulin as a predictor of coronary heart disease: Interaction with apo E phenotype; a report from MRFIT. *Ann Epidemiol* 1994; 4:40–45.

23. Tack CJJ, Smith P, Willemsen JJ, Lenders JWM, Thien T, Lutterman JA. Effects of insulin on vascular tone and sympathetic nervous system in NIDDM. *Diabetes* 1996; 45:15–22.

24. Temple RC, Clark PM, Nagi DK, Schneider AE, Yudkin JS, Hales CN. Radioimmunoassay may overestimate insulin in the non-insulin dependent diabetics. *Clin Endocrinol (Oxf)* 1990; 32:689–693.

25. Bvenholm P, Proudler A, Tornvall P, Godsland I, Landou C, De Faire U, et al. Insulin, intact and split proinsulin, and coronary artery disease in young men. *Circulation* 1995; 92:1422–1429.

26. Stern MP. Do non-insulin-dependent diabetes mellitus and cardiovascular disease share common antecedents? *Ann Intern Med* 1996; 124:110–116.

27. Reaven GM. Syndrome X. *Clin Diabetes* 1994; 12:32–36.

28. Davidson MB. Clinical implications of insulin resistance syndromes. *Am J Med* 1995; 99:420–426.

29. Reaven GM. Role of insulin resistance in human disease (Syndrome X): An expanded definition. *Annu Rev Med* 1993; 44:121–131.

30. Nelson RG, Sievers ML, Knowler WC, Swinburn BA. Low incidence of fatal coronary heart disease in Pima Indians despite high prevalence of non-insulin dependent diabetes mellitus. *Circulation* 1990; 81:987–995.

31. Tchernof A, Lamarche B, Prud'Homme D, Nadeau A, Moorjani S, Labrie F. The dense LDL phenotype: Association with plasma lipoprotein levels, visceral obesity, and hyperinsulinemia in men. *Diabetes Care* 1996; 19:629–637.

32. Ferrannini E, Buzzigoli G, Bonadonna R, Giorico MA, Oleggini M, Graziadei L. Insulin resistance in essential hypertension. *N Engl J Med* 1987; 317:350–357.

33. Reaven GM, Ho H. Renal vascular hypertension does not lead to hyperinsulinemia in Sprague-Dawley rats. *Am J Hypertens* 1992; 5:314–317.

34. Shamiss A, Carroll J, Rosenthal T. Insulin resistance in secondary hypertension. *Am J. Hypertens* 1992; 5:26–28.

35. Bogardus C, Lilloja S, Mott DM, Hollenbeck C, Reaven GM. Relationship between degree of obesity and in vivo insulin action in man. *Am J Physiol* 1985; 248:E286–E291.

36. Nathan DM. The pathophysiology of diabetes complications: How much does the glucose hypothesis explain? *Ann Intern Med* 1996; 124:86–89.

37. Laakso M. Glycemic control and the risk for coronary heart disease in patients with non-insulin dependent diabetes mellitus. *Ann Intern Med* 1996; 124:127–130.

38. The Diabetes Control and Complications Trial Research Group. The effect of intensive treatment of diabetes on the development and progression of long-term complications in insulin-dependent diabetes mellitus. *N Engl J Med* 1993; 329:977–986.

39. Van Wersch JWJ, Westerhuis LWJJM, Venekamp WJRR. Coagulation activation in diabetes mellitus. *Haemostasis* 1990; 20:263–269.

40. Aoki I, Shimoyama K, Aoki N, Homori M, Yanagisawa A, Nakhara K. Platelet-dependent thrombin generation in patients with diabetes mellitus: Effects of glycemic control on coagulability in diabetes. *J Am Coll Cardiol* 1996; 27:560–566.

41. Eliasson M, Asplund K, Evrin PE, Lindhal B, Lundblad D. Hyperinsulinemia predicts low tissue plasminogen activator activity in a healthy population: The Northern Sweden MONICA study. *Metab Clin Exp* 1994; 43:1579–1586.

42. Landin K, Tengborn I, Smith U. Elevated fibrinogen and plasminogen activator (PAI 1) in hypertension are related to metabolic risk factors for cardiovascular disease. *J Intern Med* 1990; 227:273–278.

43. Juhan-Vague I, Alessi MC, Vague P. Increased plasminogen activator inhibitorI levels. A possible link between insulin resistance and atherothrombosis. *Diabetologia* 1991; 34:457–462.

44. Ueland PM, Refsum H, Brattstrom L. Plasma homocysteine and cardiovascular disease. In: Frances RB Jr, ed. *Atherosclerotic Cardiovascular Disease, Hemostasis, and Endothelial Functions*. New York: Marcel Dekker; 1993:183–236.

45. Williams SB, Cusco JA, Roddy M-A, Johnstone MT, Creager MA. Impaired nitric oxide–mediated vasodilation in patients with non-insulin dependent diabetes mellitus. *J Am Coll Cardiol* 1996; 27:567–574.

46. Poretsky L. On the paradox of insulin-induced hyperandrogenism in insulin-resistant states. *Endocr Rev* 1991; 12:3–13.

47. Nestler JE, Jakubowicz DJ. Decreases in ovarian cytochrome P450c17α activity and serum free testosterone after reduction of insulin secretion in polycystic ovary syndrome. *N Engl J Med* 1996; 335:617–623.

48. Moghetti P, Tosi F, Castello R, Magnani CM, Negri C, Brun E, et al. The insulin resistance in women with hyperandrogenism is partially reversed by antiandrogen treatment: Evidence that androgens impair insulin action in women. *J Clin Endocrinol Metab* 1996; 81:952–960.

49. Jakubowicz DJ, Beer NA, Beer RM, Nestler JE. Disparate effects of weight reduction by diet on serum dehydroepiandrosterone-sulfate levels in obese men and women. *J Clin Endocrinol Metab* 1995; 80:3373–3376.

50. Nafziger AN, Herrington DM, Bush TL. Dehydroepiandrosterone and dehydroepiandrosterone sulfate: Their relation to cardiovascular disease. *Epidemiol Rev* 1991; 13:267–293.

51. Nestler JE. Editorial: Sex-hormone binding globulin: a marker for hyperinsulinemia and/or insulin resistance? *J Clin Endocrinol Metab* 1993; 76:273–274.

52. Winkelmann BR, Nauck M, Klein B, Russ AP, Böhm BO, Siekmeier R, et al. Deletion polymorphism of the angiotensin I-converting enzyme gene is associated with increased plasma angiotensin-converting enzyme activity but not with increased risk for myocardial infarction and coronary artery disease. *Ann Intern Med* 1996; 125:19–25.

53. Morris AD, Donnelly T. Angiotensin II: An insulin-sensitizing vasoactive hormone? *J Clin Endocrinol Metab* 1996; 81:1303–1306.

54. Taegtmeyer H, Passmore JM. Defective energy metabolism of the heart in diabetes. *Lancet* 1985; 1:139–141.

55. Vuorinenen-Markkola H, Yki-Jarvinen H. Hyperuricemia and insulin resistance. *J Clin Endocrinol Metab* 1994; 78:25–29.

56. Morgensen CE. Microalbuminuria predicts clinical proteinuria and early mortality in maturity-onset diabetes. *N Engl J Med* 1984; 310:356–360.

57. Gall MA, Borch-Johnsen K, Hougaard P, Nielsen FS, Parving HH. Albuminuria and poor glycemic control predict mortality in NIDDM. *Diabetes* 1995; 44:1303–1309.

58. Kemp HG. Left ventricular function in patients with the anginal syndrome and normal coronary arteriograms. *Am J Cardiol* 1973; 32:375–376.

59. Botker HR, Moller N, Ovesen P, Mengel A, Schmitz O, Orskov H, et al. Insulin resistance in microvascular angina (Syndrome X). *Lancet* 1993; 342:136–140.

60. Assman G, Schulte H. The Prospective Cardiovascular Munster (PRO-CAM) study: Prevalence of hyperlipidemia in persons with hypertension and/or diabetes mellitus and the relationship to coronary heart disease. *Am Heart J* 1988; 116:1713–1724.

61. Melina D, Colivicchi F, Melina G, Pristipino C. Prevalence of silent ST-segment depression during long-term ambulatory electrocardiographic monitoring in asymptomatic diabetic patients with essential hypertension. *Minerva Med* 1993; 84:301–305.

62. Rubler S, Dlugash J, Yuceoglu YZ, Kumral T, Branwood AW, Grishman A. New type of cardiomyopathy associated with diabetic glomerulosclerosis. *Am J Cardiol* 1972; 30:595–602.

63. Regan TJ, Lyons MM, Ahmed SS, Levinson GE, Oldewurtel HA, Ahmad MR, et al. Evidence for cardiomyopathy in familial diabetes mellitus. *J Clin Invest* 1977; 60:885–899.

64. Kannel WB, Hjortland M, Castelli WP. Role of diabetes in congestive heart failure: The Framingham study. *Am J Cardiol* 1974; 34:29–34.

65. Factor SM, Okun EM, Minase T. Capillary microaneurysms in the human diabetic heart. *N Engl J Med* 1980; 302:384–388.

66. Yoarom R, Zirkin H, Stammler G, Rose AG. Human coronary microvessels in diabetes and ischemia. Morphometric study of autopsy material. *J Pathol* 1992; 166:265–270.

67. van Hoeven KH, Factor SM. A comparison of the pathological spectrum of hypertensive diabetic, and hypertensive diabetic heart disease. *Circulation* 1990; 82:848–855.

68. Regan TJ, Ettinger PO, Kahn MI, Jesrani MV, Lyons MM, Oldewurtel HA, et al. Altered myocardial function and metabolism in chronic diabetes mellitus without ischemia in dogs. *Circ Res* 1974; 35:222–237.

69. Fein F, Strobeck JE, Malhotra A, Scheuer J, Sonnenblick EH. Reversibility of diabetic cardiomyopathy with insulin in rats. *Circ Res* 1981; 49:1251–1261.

70. Malhotra A, Penpargkul S, Fein FS, Sonnenblick EH, Scheuer J. The effect of streptozotocin-induced diabetes in rats on cardiac contractile proteins. *Circ Res* 1981; 49:1242–1250.

71. Penpargkul S, Fein F, Sonnenblick EH, Scheuer J. Depressed cardiac sarcoplasmic reticular function from diabetic rats. *J Mol Cell Cardiol* 1981; 13:303–309.

72. Frohlich ED, Apstein C, Chobanian AV, Devereux RB, Dustan HP, Dzau V, et al. The heart in hypertension. *N Engl J Med* 1992; 327:998–1008.

73. Gibbons GH, Dzau VJ. The emerging concept of vascular remodeling. *N Engl J Med* 1994; 330:1431–1438.

74. Seneviratne BI. Diabetic cardiomyopathy: The preclinical phase. *Br Med J* 1977; 1:1444–1446.

75. Shapiro LM, Howat AP, Calter MM. Left ventricular function in diabetes mellitus: I. Methodology and prevalence and spectrum of abnormalities. *Br Heart J* 1981; 45:122–128.

76. Vered A, Battler A, Segal P, Liberman D, Yerushalmi Y, Berezin M, et al. Exercise-induced left ventricular dysfunction in young men with asymptomatic diabetes mellitus (diabetic cardiomyopathy). *Am J Cardiol* 1984; 54:633–637.

77. Kahn JK, Zola B, Juni JE, Vinik AI. Radionuclide assessment of left ventricular diastolic filling in diabetes mellitus with and without cardiac autonomic neuropathy. *J Am Coll Cardiol* 1986; 7:1303–1309.

78. Zarich SW, Arbuckle BE, Cohen LR, Roberts M, Nesto RW. Diastolic abnormalities in young asymptomatic diabetic patients assessed by pulsed Doppler echocardiography. *J Am Coll Cardiol* 1988; 12:114–120.

79. Grossman E, Shemesh J, Shamiss A, Thaler M, Carroll J, Rosenthal T. Left ventricular mass in diabetes-hypertension. *Arch Intern Med* 1992; 122:164–170.

80. Venco A, Grandi A, Barzizza F, Finardi G. Echocardiographic features of hypertensive diabetic heart muscle disease. *Cardiology* 1987; 74:28–34.

81. Task Force of the European Society of Cardiology and the North American Society of Pacing and Electrophysiology. Heart rate variability. Standards of measurement, physiological interpretation, and clinical use. *Circulation* 1996; 93:1043–1065.

82. Lloyd-Mostyn RH, Watkins, PJ. Defective innervation of heart in diabetic autonomic neuropathy. *Br Med J* 1975; 3:15–17.

83. Ewing DJ, Campbell IW, Clarke BF. The natural history of diabetic autonomic neuropathy. *Q J Med* 1980; 193:95–108.

84. Wheeler T, Watkins PJ. Cardiac denervation in diabetes. *Br Med J* 1973; 4:584–586.

85. Oikawa N, Umetsu M, Toyota, T, Goto Y. Quantitative evaluation of diabetic autonomic neuropathy by using heart rate variations: Relationship between cardiac parasympathetic or sympathetic damage and clinical conditions. *Tohuku J Exp Med* 1986; 148:125–133.

86. Kahn JK, Sisson JC, Vinik AI. QT interval prolongation and sudden cardiac death in diabetic autonomic neuropathy. *J Clin Endocrinol Metab* 1987; 64:751–754.

87. Ewing DJ, Marty CN, Young RJ, Clarke BF. The value of cardiovascular autonomic function tests: 10 years experience in diabetes. *Diabetes Care* 1985; 8:491–498.

88. Rossetti L, Giaccari A, DeFronzo RA. Glucose toxicity. *Diabetes Care* 1990; 13:610–630.

89. Yki-Järvinen H. Glucose toxicity. *Endocr Rev* 1992; 13:415–431.

90. Prout TE. A prospective view of the treatment of adult onset diabetes: With special reference to the University Group diabetes program and oral hypoglycemic agents. *Med Clin North Am* 1971; 554(4):1065–1075.

91. Turner R, Cull C, Holman R. United Kingdom Prospective Diabetes Study 17: A 9-year update of a randomized, controlled trial on the effect of improved metabolic control on complications in non-insulin-dependent diabetes mellitus. *Ann Intern Med* 1996; 124:136–145.

92. Abraira C, Johnson N, Colwell J, the Veterans Administration of CSDM Group. VA Cooperation Study on Glycemic Control and Complications in Type II Diabetes (VA CSDM): Results of the completed feasibility trial (abstr). *Diabetes* 1994; 43(suppl 1):59A.

93. Stumvoli M, Nurjhan N, Perriello G, Dailey G, Gerich J. Metabolic effects of metformin in non-insulin-dependent diabetes mellitus. *N Engl J Med* 1995; 333:550–554.

94. DeFronzo RA, Goodman AM, the Multicenter Metformin Study Group. Efficacy of metformin in patients with non-insulin-dependent diabetes mellitus. *N Engl J Med* 1995; 333:541–549.

95. Chiasson JA, Josse RG, Hunt JA, Palmason C, Wilson Roger N, Ross SA, et al. The efficacy of Acarbose in the treatment of patients with non-insulin-dependent diabetes mellitus. *Ann Intern Med* 1995; 121:928–935.

96. Nolan JJ, Ludvik B, Beerdsen P, Joyce M, Olefsky J. Improvement in glucose tolerance and insulin resistance in obese subjects treated with troglitazone. *N Engl J Med* 1994; 33:1188–1193.

97. Iwamoto Y, Kosaka K, Kuzuya T, Akanuma Y, Shigeta Y, Kaneko T. Effects of troglitazone. A new hypoglycemic agent in patients with NIDDM poorly controlled by diet therapy. *Diabetes Care* 1996; 19:151–156.

98. Yki-Järvinen H, Kauppila M, Kujansuu E, Lahti J, Marjanen T, Niskanen L, et al. Comparison of insulin regimens of patients with non-insulin dependent diabetes mellitus. *N Engl J Med* 1992; 327:1426–1433.

99. Modon M, Halkin H, Almg S, Lusky A, Eshkol A, Shefi M, et al. Hyperinsulinemia: A link between hypertension, obesity and glucose intolerance. *J Clin Invest* 1985; 75:809–817.

100. Carlson MG, Cambell PH. Intensive insulin therapy and weight gain in ISSM. *Diabetes* 1993; 42:1700–1707.

101. Genuth S. Exogenous insulin administration and cardiovascular risk in noninsulin-dependent and insulin-dependent diabetes mellitus. *Ann Intern Med* 1996; 124:104–109.

102. Knatterud GL, Klimt CR, Levine ME, Jacobson ME, Goldner MG. Effects of hypoglycemic agents on vascular complications in patients with adult-onset diabetes. *JAMA* 1978; 240:37–42.

103. Colwell John A. The feasibility of intensive insulin management in non-insulin-dependent diabetes mellitus. Implications of the Veterans Affairs Cooperative Study on glycemic control and complications in NIDDM. *Ann Intern Med* 1996; 124:131–135.

104. Pyorala K, Laakso M, Uusitupa M. Diabetes and atherosclerosis: An epidemiological view. *Diabetes Metab Rev* 1987; 3:463–524.

105. Abbott RD, Donahue RP, Kannel WB, Wilson PWF. The impact of diabetes on survival following myocardial infarction in men vs women. The Framingham Study. *JAMA* 1988; 260:3456–3460.

106. Kannel WB. Lipids, diabetes, and coronary heart disease: Insights from the Framingham Study. *Am Heart J* 1985; 110:1100–1107.

107. Abadie E, Masquet C, Guiomard A, Passa P. Coronary angiography in diabetic and non-diabetic patients with severe ischemic heart disease. *Diabete Metab* 1983; 9:53–57.

108. Shapiro L. Specific heart disease in diabetes mellitus. *Br Med J* 1982; 284:140–141.

109. Oswald GA, Corcoran S, Yudkin JS. Prevalence and risks of hyperglycemia and undiagnosed diabetes in patients with acute myocardial infarction. *Lancet* 1984; 1:1264–1267.

110. Malmberg K, Rydén L, Efendic S, Herlitz J, Nicol P, Waldenström A, et al, on behalf of the DIGAMI Study Group. Randomized trial of insulin-glucose infusion followed by subcutaneous insulin treatment in diabetic patients with acute myocardial infarction (DIGAMI Study): Effects on mortality at 1 year. *J Am Coll Cardiol* 1995; 26:57–65.

111. Sodi-Pallares D, Testelli M, Fishleder F. Effects of an intravenous infusion of a potassium-insulin-glucose solution on the electrocardiographic signs of myocardial infarction. *Am J Cardiol* 1962; 9:166–181.

112. Rogers W, Segal P, McDaniel H, Mantel J, Russel R, Rackley C. Prospective randomized trial of glucose-insulin-potassium in acute myocardial infarction. *Am J Cardiol* 1979; 43:801–808.

113. Lynch M, Gammage M, Lamb P, Nattrass M, Penecost B. Acute myocardial infarction in diabetic patients in the thrombolytic era. *Diabet Med* 1994; 71:162–165.

114. Karlson BW, herlitz J, Hjalmarson A. Prognosis of acute myocardial infarction in diabetic and non-diabetic patients. *Diabet Med* 1993; 10:449–454.

115. Beta-blocker Heart Attack Trial Research Group. A randomized trial of propranolol in patients with acute myocardial infarction. I. Mortality results. *JAMA* 1982; 287:1707–1714.

116. ISIS-2 Collaborative Group. Randomized trial of intravenous streptokinase, oral aspirin, both, or neither among 17,187 cases of suspected acute myocardial infarctions: ISIS-2. *Lancet* 1988; 2:349–360.

117. McNulty PH, Louard RJ, Deckelbaum LI, Zaret B, Young LH. Hyperinsulinemia inhibits myocardial protein degradation in patients with cardiovascular disease and insulin resistance. *Circulation* 1995; 92:2151–2156.

118. Davi G, Catalan I, Averna M, Notarbartolo A, Strano A, Ciabattoni G, et al. Thromboxane biosynthesis and platelet function in type II diabetes mellitus. *N Engl J Med* 1990; 322:1769–1774.

119. Gray RP, Patterson DL, Yudkin JS. Plasminogen activator inhibitor activity in diabetic and nondiabetic survivors of myocardial infarction. *Arterioscler Thromb* 1993; 13:415–420.

120. Kjekshus J, Gilpin E, Cali G, Blackely A, Hennin H, Ross J Jr. Diabetic patients and beta-blockers after acute myocardial infarction. *Eur Heart J* 1990; 11:43–50.

121. The Acute Infarction Ramipril Efficacy (AIRE) Study Investigators. Effect of ramipril on mortality and morbidity of survivors of acute myocardial infarction with clinical evidence of heart failure. *Lancet* 1993; 342:821–827.

122. Indications for fibrinolytic therapy in suspected acute myocardial infarction: collaborative overview of early mortality and major morbidity results from all randomized trials of more than 1000 patients. Fibrinolytic Therapy Trialists' (FTT) Collaborative Group. *Lancet* 1994; 343:311–322.

123. Partamian JO, Bradley RF. Acute myocardial infarction in 258 cases of diabetes. Immediate mortality and five-year survival. *N Engl J Med* 1965; 273:455–461.

124. Margolis JR, Kannel WS, Feinleib M, Dawber TR, McNamara PM. Clinical features of unrecognized myocardial infarction—silent and symptomatic. Eighteen year follow-up: The Framingham Study. *Am J Cardiol* 1973; 32:1–7.

125. Herlitz J, Brandrup Wognsen G, Emanuelsson H, Haglid M, Karlson BW, Karlsson T, et al. Mortality and morbidity in diabetic and non-diabetic patients during a 2-year period after coronary artery bypass grafting. *Diabetes Care* 1996; 19:698–703.

126. Ellis SG, Roubin GS, King SB, Douglas JS, Weintraub WS, Thomas RG, et al. Angiographic and clinical predictors of acute closure after native vessel coronary angioplasty. *Circulation* 1988; 77:372–379.

127. Ellis SG, Vandormael MG, Cowley MJ, DiSciascio G, Deligonul V,

128. The Bypass Angioplasty Revascularization Investigation (BARI) Investigators. Comparison of coronary bypass surgery with angioplasty in patients with multivessel disease. *N Engl J Med* 1996; 335:217–225.

129. The EPIC Investigators. Use of a monoclonal antibody directed against the platelet antiprotein IIb/IIIa receptor in high-risk coronary angioplasty. *N Engl J Med* 1994; 330:956–961.

130. Borst C, Jansen EWL, Tulleken CAF, Grundeman PF, Mansvelt Beck HJ, van Dongen JW, et al. Coronary artery bypass grafting without cardiopulmonary bypass and without interruption of native coronary flow using a novel anastomosis site restraining device ("Octopus"). *J Am Coll Cardiol* 1996; 27:1356–1364.

131. Barbash GI, White HD, Modan M, Van de Werf F. Significance of diabetes mellitus in patients with acute myocardial infarction: Data from the GISSI-s study. *J Am Coll Cardiol* 1993; 22:707–713.

132. Kannel WB, McGee DL. Diabetes and cardiovascular disease: The Framingham Study. *JAMA* 1979; 241:2035–2038.

133. Tung P, Levin SR. Nephropathy in non-insulin-dependent diabetes mellitus. *Am J Med* 1988; 85(suppl 5A):131–136.

134. Samuelsson O, Hedner T, Persson B, Andersson O, Berglund G, Wilhelmsen L. The role of diabetes mellitus and hypertriglyccridaemia as coronary risk factors in treated hypertension: 15 years of follow-up of antihypertensive treatment in middle-aged men in the Primary Prevention Trial in Goteborg, Sweden. *J Intern Med* 1994; 235:217–227.

135. Frishman WH, Johnson BF, Pulos G, Danylchuk MA, Brown M, Lazar EJ. The effects of cardiovascular drugs on plasma lipids and lipoproteins. In, Frishman WH, ed. *Medical Management of Lipid Disorders.* New York: Futura Publishing; 1992:253–299.

136. Williams GH. Converting-enzyme inhibitors in the treatment of hypertension. *N Engl J Med* 1988; 319:1517–1525.

137. ter Wee PM, De Micheli AG, Epstein M. Effects of calcium antagonists on renal hemodynamics and progression of nondiabetic chronic renal disease. *Arch Intern Med* 1994; 154:1185–1202.

138. Jauch KW, Hartl W, Guenther B, Wicklmaym M, Rett K, Dietze G. Captopril enhances insulin responsiveness of forearm muscle tissue in non-insulin diabetes mellitus. *Eur J Clin Invest* 1987; 17:448–454.

139. Marre M, Hallab M, Billard A, LeJeane JJ, Bled F, Girault A, et al. Small doses of ramipril to reduce microalbuminuria in diabetic patients with incipient nephropathy independently of blood pressure changes. *J Cardiovasc Pharmacol* 1989; 13(suppl 1):S165–S168.

140. Alkharouf J, Nalininikumari K, Corry D, Tuck M. Long-term effect of the angiotensin converting enzyme inhibitor captopril on metabolic control in non-insulin-dependent diabetes mellitus. *Am J Hyperteus* 1993; 6:337–343.

141. Rett K, Wicklmayr M, Dietze GJ. Hypoglycemia in hypertensive diabetic patients treated with sulfonylureas, biguanides, and captopril. *N Engl J Med* 1988; 319:1609.

142. Pollare T, Lithell H, Berne C. A comparison of the effects of hydrochlorothiazide and captopril on glucose and lipid metabolism in patients with hypertension. *N Engl J Med* 1989; 321:868–873.

143. Iyer SN, Katovich MJ. Effect of acute and chronic losartan treatment on glucose tolerance and insulin sensitivity in fructose-fed rats. *Am J Hypertens* 1996; 9:662–668.

144. Schoen RE, Frishman WH, Shamoon H. Hormonal and metabolic effects of calcium-channel antagonists in man. *Am J Med* 1988; 84:492–504.

145. Velussi M, Brocco E, Frigato F, Zolli M, Muollo B, Maioli M, et al. Effects of cilazapril and amlodipine on kidney function in hypertensive NIDDM patients. *Diabetes* 1996; 45:216–222.

146. Lenfant C. The calcium channel blocker scare: Lessons for the future. *Circulation* 1995; 91:2855–2856.

147. Psaty BM, Heckert SR, Koepsell TD, Siscovik DS, Raghunathan TE, Weiss NS, et al. The risk of myocardial infarction associated with antihypertensive drug therapies. *JAMA* 1995; 274:620–625.

148. Amery A, Birkenhager W, Brixko P, Bulpitt C, Clement D, Deruyttere M, et al. Glucose intolerance during diuretic therapy in elderly hypertensive patients: A second report from the European Working Party on High Blood Pressure in the Elderly (EWPHE). *Postgrad Med J* 1986; 62:919–924.

149. Siscovick DS, Raghunathan TE, Psaty BM, Koepsell TD, Wicklund KG, Lin X, et al. Diuretic therapy for hypertension and the risk of primary cardiac arrest. *N Engl J Med* 1994; 330:1852–1857.

150. Pollare T, Lithell H, Selinus I, Berne C. Sensitivity to insulin during treatment with atenolol and metoprolol: A randomized, double-blind study of effects of carbohydrate and lipoprotein metabolism in hypertensive patients. *Br Med J* 1989; 298:1147–1152.

151. Lithell H, Pollare T, Vessby B. Metabolic effects of pindolol and propranolol in a double-blind cross-over study in hypertensive patients. *Blood Press* 1992; 1:92–101.

152. Pollare T, Lithell H, Selinus I, Berne C. Application of prazosin is associated with an increase of insulin sensitivity in obese patients with hypertension. *Diabetologia* 1988; 31:415–420.

153. Frishman WH, Burris JF, Mroczek WJ, Weir MR, Alemayehu D, Simon JS, et al. First line therapy option with low-dose bisoprolol fumarate and low-dose hydrochlorothiazide in patients with Stage I and Stage II hypertension. *J Clin Pharmacol* 1995; 35:182–188.

154. Multiple Risk Factor Intervention Trial Research Group. Baseline rest electrocardiographic abnormalities, antihypertensive treatment, and mortality in the Multiple Risk Factor Intervention Trial. *Am J Cardiol* 1985; 55:1–15.

155. Pyorala K, Pedersen TR, Kjekshus J, Faergeman O, Olsson AG, Thorgeirsson G, et al. Cholesterol lowering with simvastatin improves prognosis of diabetic patients with coronary heart disease. A subgroup analysis of the Scandinavian Simvastatin Survival Study (4S). *Diabetes Care* 1997; 20:614–620.

156. Andersson DKG, Svardsudd K. Long-term glucemic control related to mortality in type II diabetes. *Diabetes Care* 1995; 18:1534–1543.

157. Levey GS, Klein I. Catecholamine-thyroid hormone interactions and the cardiovascular manifestations of hyperthyroidism. *Am J Med* 1990; 88:642–646.

158. Lazar MA. Thyroid hormone receptors: Multiple forms, multiple possibilities. *Endocr Rev* 1993; 14:184–193.

159. Morkin E, Flink IL, Goldman S. Biochemical and physiological effects of thyroid hormone on cardiac performance. *Prog Cardiovasc Dis* 1983; 25:435–464.

160. Gick GG, Ismail-Beigi F, Edelman IS. Thyroidal regulation of rat renal and hepatic Na,K-ATPase gene expression. *J Biol Chem* 1988; 263:16610–16618.

161. Kim D, Smith TW, Marsh JD. Effect of thyroid hormone on slow calcium channel function in cultured chick ventricular cells. *J Clin Invest* 1987; 80:88–94.

162. Klemperer JD, Ojamaa K, Klein I. Thyroid hormone therapy in cardiovascular disease. *Prog Cardiovasc Dis* 1996; 38(4):329–336.

163. Sawin CT, Geller A, Wolf PA, Belanger AJ, Baker E, Bacharach P, et al. Low serum thyrotropin concentrations as a risk factor for atrial fibrillation in older persons. *N Engl J Med* 1994; 331:1249–1252.

164. Polikar R, Burger AG, Scherrer U, Nicod P. The thyroid and the heart. *Circulation* 1993; 87:1435–1441.

165. Biondi B, Fazio S, Carella C, Amato G, Cittadini A, Lupoli G, et al. Cardiac effects of long-term thyrotropin-suppressive therapy with levothyroxine. *J Clin Endocrinol Metab* 1993; 77:334–338.

166. Kannel WB, Abbott RD, Savage DD, McNamara PM. Epidemiologic features of chronic atrial fibrillation: The Framingham Study. *N Engl J Med* 1982; 306:1018–1022.

167. Petersen P, Godtfredsen J. Atrial fibrillation—a review of course and prognosis. *Acta Med Scand* 1984; 216:5–9.

168. Wolf PA, Abbott RD, Kannel WB. Atrial fibrillation: A major contributor to stroke in the elderly: The Framingham Study. *Arch Intern Med* 1987; 147:1561–1564.

169. Furszyfer J, Kurland LT, McConahey WM, Elveback LR. Graves' disease in Olmstead County, Minnesota, 1935 through 1967. *Mayo Clin Proc* 1970; 45:636–644.

170. Presti CF, Hart RG. Thyrotoxicosis, atrial fibrillation, and embolism, revisited. *Am Heart J* 1989; 117:976–977.

171. Bruaman A, Algom M, Gilboa Y, Ramot Y, Golik A, Stryjer D. Mitral valve prolapse in hyperthyroidism of two different origins. *Br Heart J* 1985; 53:374–377.

172. Ladenson PW. Recognition and management of cardiovascular disease related to thyroid dysfunction. *Am J Med* 1990; 88:638–641.

173. Ladenson PW. Thyrotoxicosis and the heart: Something old and something new. *J Clin Endocrinol Metab* 1993; 77:332–333. Editorial.

174. Iwasaki T, Naka M, Hiramatsu K, Yamada T, Niwa A, Aizawa T, et al. Eechocardiographic studies on the relationship between atrial fibrillation and atrial enlargement in patients with hyperthyroidism of Graves' disease. *Cardiology* 1989; 76:10–17.

175. Ciaccheri M, Cecchi F, Arcangeli C, Dolara A, Zuppiroli A, Pieroni

176. C. Occult thyrotoxicosis in patients with chronic and paroxysmal isolated atrial fibrillation. *Clin Cardiol* 1984; 7:413–426.

176. Sawin CT, Geller A, Wolf PA, Belanger AJ, Baker E, Bacharach P, et al. Low serum thyrotropin concentrations as a risk factor for atrial fibrillation in older persons. *N Engl J Med* 1994; 331:1249–1252.

177. Bar-sela S, Ehrenfeld M, Eliakim M. Arterial embolism in thyrotoxicosis with atrial fibrillation. *Arch Intern Med* 1981; 141:1191–1192.

178. Wartofsky L, Glinoer D, Solomon B. Differences and similarities in the diagnosis and treatment of Graves' disease in Europe, Japan and the United States. *Thyroid* 1991; 1:129–135.

179. Zonszein J, Santangelo RP, Mackin JF, Lee TC, Coffey RJ, Canary JJ. Propranolol therapy in thyrotoxicosis. A review of 84 patients undergoing surgery. *Am J Med* 1979; 66:411–416.

180. Nakazawa HK, Sakurai K, Hamada N, Momotani N, Ito K. Management of atrial fibrillation in the post-thyrotoxic state. *Am J Med* 1982; 72:903–906.

181. Golzari H, Cebul RD, Bahler RC. Atrial fibrillation: Restoration and maintenance of sinus rhythm and indications for anticoagulation therapy. *Ann Intern Med* 1996; 125:311–323.

182. Stroke prevention in Atrial Fibrillation Study Group Investigators. Preliminary report of the Stroke Prevention in Atrial Fibrillation Study. *N Engl J Med* 1990; 322:863–868.

183. Petersen P, Boyesen G, Godtfredsen J, Andersen ED, Andersen B. Placebo controlled, randomized trial of warfarin and aspirin for prevention of thromboembolic complications in chronic atrial fibrillation: The Copenhagen AFASAK study. *Lancet* 1989; 1:175–179.

184. Laragh JH, Sealey JE, Brunner HR. The control of aldosterone secretion in normal and hypertensive man. Abnormal renin-aldosterone patterns in low-renin hypertension. In: Laragh JH, ed. *Hypertension Manual*. New York: Yorke Medical; 1975:197–225.

185. Graettinger JS, Muenster JJ, Checchia CS, Grisson RL, Campbell JA. A correlation of clinical and hemodynamic studies in patients with hypothyroidism. *J Clin Invest* 1958; 37:502–510.

186. Forfar JC, Muir AL, Toft AD. Left ventricular function in hypothyroidism. Responses to exercise and beta adrenoreceptor blockade. *Br Heart J* 1982; 48:278–284.

187. Tajiri J, Morita M, Higashi K, Fuji H, Nakamura N, Sato T. The cause of low voltage QRS complex in primary hypothyroidism. Pericardial effusion or thyroid hormone deficiency? *Jpn Heart J* 1985; 26:539–547.

188. Tunbridge WMG, Evered DC, Hall R, Appleton D, Bresis M, Clark F, et al. Lipid profiles and cardiovascular disease in the Whickham area with particular reference to thyroid failure. *Clin Endocrinol* 1977; 7:495–508.

189. Keating FR, Parkin TW, Selby JB, Dickinson LS. Treatment of heart disease associated with myxedema. *Prog Cardiovasc Dis* 1960; 3:364–381.

190. Steinberg AD. Myxedema and coronary artery disease. A comparative autopsy study. *Ann Intern Med* 1968; 68:338–344.

191. Becker C. Hypothyroid and atherosclerotic heart disease: Pathogenesis, medical management and the role of coronary artery bypass surgery. *Endocr Rev* 1985; 6:432–440.

192. Goldman J, Matz R, Mortimer R. High elevations of creatinine phosphokinase in hypothyroidism. *JAMA* 1977; 238:325–326.

193. Gavin LA. The diagnostic dilemmas of hyperthyroxinemia and hypothyroxinemia. *Adv Intern Med* 1988; 33:185–203.

194. Helfand M, Lawrence MC. Screening for thyroid disease. *Ann Intern Med* 1990; 112:840–849.

195. Wartofsky L, Burman KD. Alterations in thyroid function in patients with systemic illnesses: The "euthyroid sick syndrome." *Endocr Rev* 1982; 3:164–217.

196. Mandel SJ, Brent GA, Larsen PR. Levothyroxine therapy in patients with thyroid disease. *Ann Intern Med* 1993; 119:492–502.

197. Holvey DN, Goodner CJ, Nicoloff JT, Dowling JT. Treatment of myxedema coma with intravenous thyroxine. *Arch Intern Med* 1964; 113:139–146.

198. Jordan RM. Myxedema coma. *Med Clin North Am* 1995; 79:185–194.

199. Hylander B, Rosenquist U. Treatment of myxoedema coma—factors associated with fatal outcome. *Acta Endocrinol (Copenh)* 1985; 108:65–71.

200. Becker C. Hypothyroid and atherosclerotic heart disease: Pathogenesis, medical management and the role of coronary artery bypass surgery. *Endocr Rev* 1985; 6:432–440.

201. Sherman SI, Ladenson PW. Percutaneous transluminal coronary angioplasty in hypothyroidism. *Am J Med* 1991; 90:367–370.

202. Martino E, Safran M, Aghini-Lomardi F, Rajatanavin R, Lenziardi M, Fay M, et al. Environmental iodine intake and thyroid dysfunction during chronic amiodorone therapy. *Ann Intern Med* 1984; 101:28–34.

203. Martino E, Aghini-Lombardi F, Mariotti S, Bartalena L, Lenziardi M, Ceccarelli C, et al. Amiodorone iodine-induced hypothyroidism: Risk factors and follow-up in 28 cases. *Clin Endocrinol* 1987; 26:227–237.

204. Lambert M, Unger J, De Nayer P, Brohet C, Gangji D. Evidence of thyroid damage in amiodarone-induced thyrotoxicosis suggestive of thyroid damage. *J Endocrinol Invest* 1990; 13:527–530.

205. Bartalena L, Grasso L, Brogioni S, Aghini-Lomardi F, Braverman LE, Martino E. Serum interleukin-6 in amiodarone-induced thyrotoxicosis. *J Clin Endocrinol Metab* 1994; 78:423–427.

206. Martino E, Aghini-Lombardi F, Mariotti S, Lenziardi M, Morabito S, Baschieri L, et al. Treatment of amiodarone-associated thyrotoxicosis by simultaneous administration of potassium perchlorate and methimazole. *J Endocrinol Invest* 1986; 9:201–207.

207. Farwell AP, Abend SL, Huang SK, Patwardhan NA, Braverman LE. Thyroidectomy for amiodarone-induced thyrotoxicosis. *JAMA* 1990; 263:1526–1528.

208. Morgan JP. Abnormal intracellular modulation of calcium as a major cause of cardiac contractile dysfunction. *N Engl J Med* 1991; 325:625–632.

209. Roberts WC, Waller BF. Effect of chronic hypercalcemia on the heart: An analysis of 18 necropsy patients. *Am J Med* 1981; 71:371–384.

210. Levine SN, Rheams CN. Hypocalcemic heart failure. *Am J Med* 1985; 78:1033–1035.

211. Health H III, Hodgson SF, Kennedy MA. Primary hyperparathyroidism. *N Engl J Med* 1980; 302:189–193.

212. Lueg MC. Hypertension and primary hyperparathyroidism: A five-year case review. *South Med J* 1982; 75:1371–1374.

213. Christensson T, Hellstrom K, Wengle B. Hypercalcemia and primary hyperparathyroidism: Prevalence in patients receiving thiazides as detected in a health screen. *Arch Intern Med* 1977; 137:1138–1142.

214. McLean RM. Magnesium and its therapeutic uses: A review. *Am J Med* 1994; 96(1):63–76.

215. Burch GE, Giles TD. The importance of magnesium deficiency in cardiovascular disease. *Am Heart J* 1977; 94:649–656.

216. Wacker WEC, Parisi AF. Magnesium metabolism. *N Engl J Med* 1968; 278:658–663.

217. Reinhart RA. Clinical correlates of the molecular and cellular actions of magnesium on the cardiovascular system. *Am Heart J* 1991; 121:1513–1521.

218. Jackson ECH, Meier DW. Routine serum magnesium analysis. Correlation with clinical state of 5100 patients. *Ann Intern Med* 1968; 69:743–748.

219. Leier CV, Dei Cas L, Metra M. Clinical relevance and management of the major electrolyte abnormalities in congestive heart failure: Hyponatremia, hypokalemia, and hypomagnesemia. *Am Heart J* 1994; 128(3):564–574.

220. Whang R, Oei TO, Aikawa JK, Watanabe A, Vannatta J, Fryer A, et al. Predictors of clinical hypomagnesemia, hypokalemia, hypophosphatemia, hyponatremia and hypocalcemia. *Arch Intern Med* 1984; 144:1794–1796.

221. Wester PO, Dyckner T. Diuretic treatment and magnesium losses. *Acta Med Scand* 1981; 647(suppl):145–152.

222. Eichhorn EJ, Tandon PK, DiBianco R, Timmis GC, Fenster PE, Shannon J, et al. Clinical and prognostic significance of serum magnesium concentration in patients with severe chronic congestive heart failure: The PROMISE Study. *J Amer Coll Cardiol* 1993; 213:634–640.

223. Gottlieb SS, Fisher ML, Pressel MD, Patten RD, Weinberg M, Greenberg N. Effects of intravenous magnesium sulfate on arrhythmias in patients with congestive heart failure. *Am Heart J* 1993; 125(6):1645–1650.

224. Sueta CA, Clarke SW, Dunlap SH, Jensen L, Blauwet MB, Koch G, et al. Effect of acute magnesium administration on the frequency of ventricular arrhythmia in patients with heart failure. *Circulation* 1994; 89(2):660–666.

225. Bashir Y, Sneddon JF, Staunton HA, Haywood GA, Simpson IA, McKenna WJ, et al. Effects of long-term oral magnesium chloride replacement in congestive heart failure secondary to coronary artery disease. *Am J Cardiol* 1993; 72(15):1156–1162.

226. Cohen L, Kitzes R. Magnesium sulfate and digitalis-toxic arrhythmias. *JAMA* 1983; 249:2803–2810.

227. Tsuji H, Venditti FJ Jr, Evans JC, Larson MG, Levy D. The associations of levels of serum potassium and magnesium with ventricular premature complexes (the Framingham Heart Study). *Am J Cardiol* 1994; 74(3):232–235.

228. Bailie DS, Inone H, Kaseda S, Ben-David J, Zipes DP. Magnesium suppression of early after-depolarizations and ventricular tachyarrhythmias induced by cesium in dogs. *Circulation* 1988; 77(6):1395–1402.

229. Johnson CJ, Peterson DR, Smith EK. Myocardial tissue concentrations of magnesium and potassium in mey dying suddenly from ischemic heart disease. *Am J Clin Nutr* 1979; 32:967–970.

230. Woods KL, Fletcher S, Roffe C, Haider Y. Intravenous magnesium sulphate in suspected acute myocardial infarction: Results of the second Leicester Intravenous Magnesium Intervention Trial (LIMIT-2). *Lancet* 1992; 339:1553–1558.

231. ISIS-4 (Fourth International Study of Infarct Survival) Collaborative Group. ISIS-4: A randomized factorial trial assessing early oral captopril, oral mononitrate, and intravenous magnesium sulphate in 58,050 patients with suspected acute myocardial infarction. *Lancet* 1995; 345:669–685.

232. Woods KL, Fletcher S. Long-term outcome after intravenous magnesium sulphate in suspected acute myocardial infarction: The second Leicester Intravenous Magnesium Intervention Trial (LIMIT-2). *Lancet* 1994; 343:816–819.

233. Shechter M, Hod H, Chouraqui P, Kaplinsky E, Rabinowitz B. Magnesium therapy in acute myocardial infarction when patients are not candidates for thrombolytic therapy. *Am J Cardiol* 1995; 75(5):321–323.

234. Caspi J, Rudis E, Bar I, Safadi T, Saute M. Effects of magnesium on myocardial function after coronary artery bypass grafting. *Ann Thorac Surg* 1995; 59(4)942–947.

235. Demmy TL, Haggerty SP, Boley TM, Curtis JJ. Lack of cardioplegia uniformity in clinical myocardial preservation. *Ann Thorac Surg* 1994; 57(3):648–651.

236. Kovacs K, Yao J. Pituitary necrosis following major heart surgery. *Z Cardiol* 1975; 64:52–57.

237. Daniel PM, Spicer EJF, Treip CS. Pituitary necrosis in patients maintained on mechanical respirators. *J Pathol* 1973; 111:135–138.

238. Bates AS, Hoff WV, Jones JM, Clayton RN. Does treatment of acromegaly affect life expectancy? *Metabolism* 1995; 44:1–5.

239. Jonas EA, Aloia JF, Lane FJ. Evidence of subclinical heart muscle dysfunction in acromegaly. *Chest* 1975; 67:190–194.

240. Lie JT, Grossman SJ. Pathology of the heart in acromegaly: Anatomic findings in 27 autopsied patients. *Am Heart J* 1980; 100:41–52.

241. McGuffin WL Jr, Sherman BM, Roth J, Gorden P, Kahn CR, Roberts WC, et al. Acromeagaly and cardiovascular disorders: A prospective study. *Ann Intern Med* 1974; 81:11–18.

242. Rodrigues EA, Caruana MP, Lahiri A, Nabarro JDN, Jacobs HSS, Raftery EB. Subclinical cardiac dysfunction in acromegaly: Evidence for a specific disease of heart muscle. *Br Heart J* 1989; 62:185–192.

243. Savage DD, Henry WL, Eastman RC, Borer JS, Gordon P. Echocardiographic assessment of cardiac anatomy and function in acromegalic patients. *Am J Med* 1979; 67:823–829.

244. Cain JP, Williams GH, Dluhy RG. Plasma renin activity and aldosterone secretion in patients with acromegaly. *J Clin Endocrinol* 1972; 34:73–81.

245. Friberg P, Adams MA, Isgaard J, Wickmann A, Wahlander H. Right but not left ventricular insulin-like growth factor 1 (IGF-1) and growth hormone (GH)-receptor levels increase after induction of volume overload (abstr). *Hypertension* 1993; 22:418 (A65).

246. Merimee TJ. Metabolic and clinical studies in growth hormone deficient dwarfs: A ten year follow-up. *N Engl J Med* 1978; 298:1217–1222.

247. Melmed S, Ho K, Klibanski A, Reichlin S, Throner M. Clinical review 75: Recent advances in pathogenesis, diagnosis, and management of acromegaly. *J Clin Endocrinol Metab* 1995; 80:3395–3402.

248. Lim MJ, Barkan AL, Buda AJ. Rapid reduction of left ventricular hypertrophy in acromegaly after suppression of growth hormone hypersecretion. *Ann Intern Med* 1992; 117:719–726.

249. Fazio S, Sabatini D, Capaldo B, Vigoritto C, Giordano A, Guida R. A preliminary study of growth hormone in the treatment of dilated cardiomyopathy. *N Engl J Med* 1996; 334:809–814.

250. Yard AC, Kadowitz PJ. Studies on the mechanism of hydrocortisone potentiation of vasoconstrictor responses to epinephrine in the anesthetized animal. *Eur J Pharmacol* 1972; 20:1–9.

251. Abrass IB, Scarpace PJ. Glucocorticoid regulation of myocardial beta-receptors. *Endocrinology* 1981; 108:977–980.

252. Plotz CM, Knowlton AI, Ragan C. The natural history of Cushing's syndrome. *Am J Med* 1952; 13:597–614.

253. Danoff A, Jormark S, Lorber D, Fleischer N. Adrenocortical micronodular dysplasia, cardiac myxomas, lentigines, and spindle cell tumors. *Arch Intern Med* 1987; 147:443–448.

254. Crapo L. Cushing's syndrome: A review of diagnostic tests. *Metabolism* 1979; 28:955–977.

255. Kaye TB, Crapo L. The Cushing's syndrome: An update on diagnostic tests. *Ann Intern Med* 1990; 112:434–444.

256. Mampalalm TJ, Tyrell BJ, Wilson CB. Transsphenoidal microsurgery for Cushing disease. *Ann Intern Med* 1988; 109:487–493.

257. Lin AL, McGill HC Jr, Shain SA. Hormone receptors of the baboon cardiovascular system: Biochemical characterization of aortic and myocardial cytoplasmic progesterone receptors. *Circ Res* 1982; 50:610–616.

258. Bagatell CJ, Heiman JR, Matsumoto AM, Rivier JE, Bremnaer WJ. Metabolic and behavioral effects of high dose, exogenous testosterone in healthy men. *J Clin Endocrinol Metab* 1994; 79:561–567.

259. Bhasin S, Storer TW, Berman N, Callegari C, Clevenger B, Phillips J, et al. The effects of supraphysiologic doses of testosterone on muscle size and strength in normal men. *N Engl J Med* 1996; 335:1–7.

260. Tenover JS. Effects of testosterone supplementation in the aging male. *J Clin Endocrinol Metab* 1992; 75:1092–1098.

261. Godsland IF, Crook D, Simpson R, Proudler T, Felton C, Lees B, et al. The effects of different formulations of oral contraceptive agents on lipid and carbohydrate metabolism. *N Engl J Med* 1990; 323:1375–1381.

262. Foster DC. Low-dose monophasic and multiphasic oral contraceptives: A review of potency, efficacy, and side effects. *Semin Reprod Endocrinol* 1989; 7:205–212.

263. Mann JI, Vessey MP, Thorogood M, Doll SR. Myocardial infarction in young women with special reference to oral contraceptive practice. *Br Med J* 1975; 2:241–245.

264. Russell RP, Sullivan MA. The pill and hypertension. *Johns Hopkins Med J* 1970; 127:287–293.

265. World Health Organization Collaborative Study of Cardiovascular Disease and Steroid Hormone Contraception. Venous thromboembolic disease and combined oral contraceptives: Results of international multicentre case-control study. *Lancet* 1995; 246:157–182.

266. Petitti DB, Sidney S, Bernstein A, Wolf S, Quesenberry C, Ziel HK. Stroke in users of low-dose oral contraceptives. *N Engl J Med* 1996; 335:8–15.

267. Barrett-Connor E, Bush TL. Estrogen and coronary heart disease in women. *JAMA* 1991; 265:1861–1867.

268. Stampfer MJ, Colditz GA, Willett WC, Manson JE, Rosner B, Speizer FE, et al. Postmenopausal estrogen therapy and cardiovascular disease. Ten-year follow-up from the Nurses' Health Study. *N Engl J Med* 1991; 325:756–762.

269. Henderson BE, Ross RK, Paganini-Hill A, Mack TM. Estrogen use and cardiovascular disease. *Am J Obstet Gynecol* 1986; 154:1181–1186.

270. McFarland KF, Boniface ME, Hornung CA, Earnhardt W, Humphries JO. Risk factors and noncontraceptive estrogen use in women with and without coronary artery disease. *Am Heart J* 1989; 117:1209–1214.

271. Nabulsi AA, Folsom AR, White A, Patsch W, Heiss G, Wu KK. Association of hormone-replacement therapy with various cardiovascular risk factors in postmenopausal women. *N Eng J Med* 1993; 328:1069–1075.

272. The Writing Group for the PEPI trial. Effects of estrogen or estrogen/progestin regimens on heart disease risk factors in postmenopausal women: The Postmenopausal Estrogen/Progestin Interventions (PEPI) Trial. *JAMA* 1995; 273:199–208.

273. Grey AB, Stapleton JA, Evans MC, Rein IR. The effect of the anti-estrogen tamoxifen on cardiovascular risk factors in normal postmenopausal women. *J Clin Endocrinol Metab* 1995; 80:3191–3195.

274. Belchetz PE. Hormonal treatment of postmenopausal women. *N Engl J Med* 1994; 330:1062–1071.

275. Steinberg KK, Smith SJ, Tacker SB, Stroup DF. Breast cancer risk and duration of estrogen use: The role of study design in meta-analysis. *Epidemiology* 1994; 5:415–421.

276. Colditz GA, Hankinson SE, Hunter DJ, Willett WC, Manson JE, Stampfer MJ, et al. The use of estrogens and progestins and the risk of breast cancer in postmenopausal women. *N Engl J Med* 1995; 332:1589–1593.

277. American College of Physicians. Guidelines for counseling postmenopausal women about preventive hormone therapy. *Ann Intern Med* 1992; 117:1038–1041.

79

AIDS AND THE CARDIOVASCULAR SYSTEM

Melvin D. Cheitlin

The pandemic of acquired immunodeficiency syndrome (AIDS), after some 15 years, is now well into its adolescence. It has taken a tragic toll in lives in the United States and threatens a catastrophe in Africa and Southeast Asia. An estimated 10 million people worldwide are infected with the human immunodeficiency virus (HIV), and at least another 12 million have full-blown AIDS.[1] In the United States, over a million people are HIV-positive and about 2 million have been diagnosed with AIDS.[2,3]

AIDS is caused by infection with a virus of the family Retroviridae. This group of retroviruses comprises enveloped ribonucleic acid (RNA) viruses possessing an RNA-dependent deoxyribonucleic acid (DNA) polymerase (reverse transcriptase). There are two classes of AIDS viruses, known as HIV-1 and HIV-2.

The most specific definition of infection by HIV is by identification of the HIV organism in the host's tissues. Since isolation of the virus is not easily done and therefore lacks sensitivity, a patient with repeated positive screening tests for antibodies to HIV, as with an enzyme-labeled immunoabsorbent assay (ELISA), confirmed by a supplemental test such as the Western blot immunofluorescence assay, should be considered to be infected by HIV.

The following classification system for the different stages of HIV infection as proposed by the Centers for Disease Control (CDC) is helpful[4]:

Group I: Acute infection
Group II: Asymptomatic infection
Group III: Persistent generalized lymphadenopathy (PGL)
Group IV: Chronic disease—AIDS with constitutional disease (such as unexplained diarrhea, weight loss, or fever over 1 month), neurologic disease, secondary infectious diseases, secondary cancers (Kaposi's sarcoma, non-Hodgkin's lymphoma, primary lymphoma of the brain).

In January 1993, the CDC, together with other state and territorial health departments, broadened the surveillance definition for AIDS in adolescents and adults to add a measure of immunosuppression (a CD4+ T-lymphocyte count <200/μL or a CD4+ percentage <14) as well as three additional clinical conditions: pulmonary tuberculosis, recurrent pneumonia (two or more episodes within a year), or invasive cervical cancer.[5]

The recognition of human infection by HIV in 1981 represented the startling development of a modern epidemic with many of the aspects of epidemics of the past, such as those of poliomyelitis and the black plague. This infection is due to a retrovirus that invades the nucleus of certain cells containing a specific receptor on their cell membranes and incorporates the DNA copy of HIV in the host's genetic material or genome. After an apparent incubation (dormant) period of a mean of 8 to 10 years, the virus can eventually express itself by releasing into the cytoplasm double-stranded DNA copies of the virus, thus killing the cell and invading other immune cells, usually T-helper lymphocytes, to the point that the host's immune defense mechanisms are compromised.[6] Recent studies have demonstrated a high rate of viral replication in the lymph nodes during this quiescent period, indicating active progression of the disease, despite the low levels of infectious HIV in the plasma of some patients.[7]

A long-term prospective study showed the actuarial rate of progression from the time of infection to the appearance of AIDS to be 54 percent at 10 years after infection, with an increasing progression after 5 years of infection.[8] About 30 percent of patients with PGL will progress to AIDS in 5 years.[9] A minority of patients have an accelerated course and develop full-blown AIDS in 1 or 2 years.[10] Small groups of patients have also been described who have had HIV infection for over 10 years without any symptoms.[11] At some point, there is a breakdown of the body's defense against certain neoplastic changes, resulting in the development of non-Hodgkin's lymphoma and Kaposi's sarcoma. These complications lead inevitably, at least in a very high percentage of cases, to death.

At the beginning of the epidemic in the United States, the HIV organism struck mainly at the male homosexual population. Later it was found to be transmitted not only through sexual intercourse but also through blood-borne contamination, soon affecting the population using intravenous drugs and other populations receiving blood products and blood transfusions, such as hemophiliacs. The disease is also transmitted perinatally, so that an increasing number of pediatric patients with AIDS are being seen.

From work with HIV-1, it has been found that the usual way in which the virus attacks cells is through interaction with a receptor on the surface membrane of the cell, the so-called CD4 receptor. This is present in T-helper lymphocytes. Macrophages, microglia, and Langerhan's cells may have specific receptors for HIV other than CD4. Other cells seem to lack an HIV receptor and therefore are much less often found to be sites of infection; the myocardial cell is one such cell.

From the beginning of the epidemic it was recognized that the heart could be involved but that significant clinical involvement of the heart was unusual. Originally it was believed, through autopsy studies, that the heart was involved mainly because of pericarditis or metastatic Kaposi's sarcoma.[12,13] A few patients with nonbacterial thrombotic endocarditis (NBTE) were reported, but this could be nonspecific, since many of these patients have a wasting disease in which NBTE is not unusual.[14] On further review of autopsy series and clinical series and especially with the study of patients with AIDS who had echocardiography, it was apparent that abnormalities of the heart were seen frequently, even though clinical manifestations of heart disease still remained unusual.

AUTOPSY FINDINGS

The incidence of cardiac involvement at autopsy varies, depending on the definition of cardiac disease. In 15 autopsy series, the incidence of cardiac involvement varies from none to 70 percent of the hearts, depending on whether or not lymphocytic infiltration with or without myocardial necrosis is included.[12–20] The presence of autopsy-proven cardiac involvement in patients who, during life, had clinically significant cardiac involvement is less impressive, especially if one includes the patients with localized, isolated collections of myocardial lymphocytes.

In evaluating autopsy reports, it is often difficult to discern how many patients had clinically significant abnormalities during life. In the large series of consecutive autopsies of AIDS patients, between 5 and 20 percent appear to have had cardiac lesions of potential clinical importance. These include patients with myocarditis with clinical manifestations, mainly with known pathogens—such as toxoplasmosis, clinically evident pericarditis, or nonbacterial endocarditis—which can cause systemic emboli.[21]

More important are the relatively few patients in whom cardiac abnormality was listed as the cause of death. The most common cause of death is respiratory failure and infection.[18,20,22] Neoplasm, lymphoma, and encephalopathy are also frequent causes of death.[23] Of 858 autopsied patients with AIDS from 15 series in the literature, only 9 (1 percent) had the cause of death listed as cardiac. If the cases with a recognized etiology for heart disease are removed, only 0.5 percent of deaths were possibly due to HIV "myocarditis."

Right ventricular hypertrophy and/or dilatation was reported in 12 of 71 patients (16.9 percent)[19] and in 18 of 115 patients (15.7 percent).[18] Pericarditis varied in frequency from 3 of 41 (7.3 percent)[14] to 3 of 101 (3 percent).[16]

ECHOCARDIOGRAPHIC FINDINGS

Echocardiography in patients with either AIDS or PGL has been reported in a number of studies.[24–40] The prevalence of echocardiographic abnormalities varies from 15 to 60 percent and would be higher if the finding of mitral valve prolapse, an echocardiographic abnormality that may be related to cachexia, is included. The prevalence of left ventricular hypokinesis also varies from 12.5 to 41 percent in three large series.[26,27,29] In one series,[26] 4 of the 8 patients had congestive heart failure; 1 died and at autopsy had a dilated cardiomyopathy without evidence of inflammatory myocarditis or cardiac opportunistic infections. Only in this study[26] was clinical congestive heart failure mentioned. Dilated cardiomyopathy was seen only in the hospitalized patients. In a large prospective echocardiographic study in 296 HIV-infected adults conducted over 4 years, Currie and colleagues found 13 (4 percent) with dilated cardiomyopathy.[41]

The finding of pericardial effusion was common, varying from 20 to 40 percent.[27,29,30] The incidence of tamponade varies: In one series[27] of 18 patients with pericardial effusion, 5 (28 percent) had tamponade. In this report of 300 patients with AIDS, 16 (5 percent) had clinically apparent heart disease, due in most cases to opportunistic infection or tumor.[27] Over a period of 3 years at the San Francisco General Hospital, Rapaport found that of 1171 patients hospitalized with AIDS, an echocardiogram was ordered for 88 (7.5 percent) because of suspicion of cardiac disease (personal communication). Of these echocardiograms, 52 (59 percent) showed at least one abnormality. Of the 88 echocardiograms, 16 (18 percent) showed either left ventricular dilatation and/or left ventricular hypokinesis, and 26 (30 percent) showed pericardial effusion. There were no control subjects.

A recent study[31] reported the results of echocardiography in 151 HIV-seropositive patients collected prospectively, 92 percent of whom were men with a median age of 37 years. Seventy-three percent were homosexual men. Of these, 13 percent were intravenous drug users, of whom 74 percent were in Walter Reed stages IV to VI, a classification using counts of T4 helper cells and clinical data.[12,32] One hundred seven patients (71 percent) had normal echocardiograms.

Echocardiographic abnormalities attributed to HIV infection were present in 31 patients (20 percent). There was an association of abnormal echocardiographic findings with advanced clinical stages of the disease. The mortality during follow-up was the same for those with normal echocardiograms (35 of 102) as for those with abnormal echocardiograms (12 of 29) ($p = 48$). Even in those with the most advanced clinical disease, there was no independent prognostic significance of the echocardiographic cardiac involvement, with 44 percent of both echo-normal and echo-abnormal patients dying. This study shows a remarkably low incidence of HIV-associated echocardiographic abnormalities, most often asymptomatic pericardial effusion.

These studies suggest that the prevalence of echocardiographic abnormalities in HIV-positive patients depends on the stage of their clinical illness, with the sickest patients having the most abnormalities.

PERICARDIAL INVOLVEMENT

In general, pericardial effusion and pericarditis constitute the most commonly recognized cardiac involvement in AIDS. At autopsy, Kaposi's sarcoma involvement and lymphoma may be clinically silent, accompanied by asymptomatic pericardial effusion, or they may be clinically important because of pericardial tamponade.[33] Pericarditis due to specific organisms has frequently been reported. These organisms are most commonly *Mycobacterium tuberculosis*[27,34,42] or *Mycobacterium avium–intracellulare*.[28,43] One study[27] reported pericardial tamponade in five patients and large pericardial effusions in six. Of the patients with clinical heart disease in this study, 22 percent had echocardiographic evidence of tamponade, and another 33 percent had large pericardial effusions.

At San Francisco General Hospital, experience has been similar. In a consecutive series of 88 in-hospital AIDS patients who had echocardiograms, 36 (41 percent) had normal echocardiograms, whereas the most common abnormality, seen in 26 (30 percent), was pericardial effusion. We have recognized a total of 25 patients with AIDS or PGL who have pericardial disease. Ten of these patients had pericardiocentesis, of whom 8 (32 percent) presented with tamponade, 2 had pericardial windows, and 1 died and was autopsied. Another 2 patients, who had neither pericardiocentesis nor pericardial windows, died and were autopsied. No etiology was found on examination of either fluid or tissue in any of the 12 patients.

In a prospective echocardiographic study among patients recruited over a 4-year period, the prevalence of pericardial effusion for AIDS patients entering into the study was 5 percent. Over the follow-up time the incidence of pericardial effusion was 11 percent per year. Eighty percent of these were small and asymptomatic. The survival of the AIDS patients who developed pericardial effusion was significantly shorter than those who did not, 36 percent versus 93 percent at 6 months. This shortened survival period remained significant

even after adjustment for lead time bias and was independent of CD4+ T-cell count.[44] Since death was not due directly to the pericardial effusion, the development of pericardial effusion in the setting of HIV infection probably suggests end-stage HIV disease.

Recently Flum and colleagues also reported that AIDS-associated pericardial effusion was a grave prognostic sign. They reported 29 patients who had surgical windows for large effusions; only in 2 patients did this result in a change in clinical management. The mortality was 69 percent at 8 weeks post–pericardial window.[45] They concluded that pericardial biopsy for diagnosis provided little practical therapeutic information and that "surgical windows" were justified only to relieve tamponade.

The etiology of pericardial effusion or pericarditis is not obvious; it may be HIV infection or other opportunistic viral infections with Coxsackie virus or cytomegalovirus. In one recent report of 14 AIDS patients with pericardial effusion, 10 (71 percent) had tamponade.[36] Of the 14 patients, 8 (57 percent) had suggestive evidence of mycobacterial disease. Occasionally pericarditis has been reported to be caused by common organisms such as *Staphylococcus*,[37] *Cryptococcus neoformans*,[38] or herpes simplex virus.[39]

MYOCARDIAL INVOLVEMENT

For a number of years, involvement of the pericardium and myocardium with both common and unusual opportunistic infections and neoplasms, such as Kaposi's sarcoma and lymphoma, has been recognized. At times this involvement appears to be incidental and associated with the presence of organisms in many tissues, including the heart. Often this involvement is not accompanied by signs of cell necrosis or even inflammation. At other times the infection is accompanied by an intense myocarditis. Opportunistic infection has included viruses (herpes simplex, cytomegalovirus, and Coxsackie virus), bacteria, protozoa (*Toxoplasma gondii*), and fungi (*Candida albicans, C. neoformans,* and *Aspergillus fumigatus*).[40,46,47] Diagnosis of these specific infections have been made at autopsy but have also been made during life with myocardial biopsy. The importance of identifying a specific organism as the cause of the myocarditis rests in the potential for treatment[48]; for instance, amphotericin B and flucytosine may be used to treat cryptococcosis. Grange and colleagues[49] reported a case of *T. gondii* myocarditis in a 58-year-old man with AIDS who was treated successfully with pyrimethamine and clindamycin. A similar case was reported by Albrecht and colleagues.[50]

The most common neoplasms are Kaposi's sarcoma and lymphoma of the non-Hodgkin's type.[12,13,18] With Kaposi's sarcoma, the tumor involvement of the myocardium or pericardium is most frequently an incidental finding. On occasion, a diagnosis of myocardial involvement by lymphoma is made on needle biopsy of the myocardium.

One study reported a collection of 21 cases of lymphoma in AIDS patients, 3 Hodgkin's and 18 non-Hodgkin's lymphoma of various histologic types, almost all of which were in the high-grade categories.[51] Unfortunately, these tend to be histologically aggressive tumors involving many organs, and they respond poorly to treatment. At times the patient presents with pericardial tamponade or even superior vena cava syndrome.[52-54] Echocardiography revealing infiltration into the myocardium and/or myocardial or pericardial masses is most helpful in establishing a diagnosis.

CARDIOMYOPATHY

In 1986 Cohen and colleagues[55] reported three patients with AIDS who had clinical, echocardiographic, and morphologic findings of dilated cardiomyopathy. All had a decreased ejection fraction, and two had congestive heart failure. All three died, and two had findings at autopsy compatible with myocarditis resulting in cardiomyopathy. Microscopic examination in both showed focal collections of inflammatory cells together with myofibrillar atrophy and myocardial necrosis. A subsequent report described 58 consecutively autopsied patients.[56] Seven (12 percent) had major clinical cardiovascular abnormalities, including four with congestive heart failure and others with ventricular tachycardia. All were late in the course of their disease. All patients with these major clinical cardiac abnormalities had focal myocarditis at autopsy. The etiology in these cases was not obvious but was believed to be viral myocarditis.

In another study of 71 patients with AIDS, 8 had left ventricular dilatation and decreased contractility and 4 had congestive heart failure.[26] In a similar echocardiographic study, none of 102 AIDS patients had congestive heart failure, although 41 percent had left ventricular hypokinesia.[29]

In autopsy studies reported in the literature, cardiac causes of death have been rare; clinically, the incidence of congestive heart failure has been extremely small, although microscopic focal myocarditis is frequently described. In 14 studies reported in the literature, 1009 patients with AIDS were reported. A total of 8 died of cardiac involvement. One had cryptococcal myocarditis and one had toxoplasmic myocarditis; five came from one institution.[19]

Symptomatic cardiomyopathy in association with HIV-1 infection is apparently unusual; however, echocardiographic evidence of left ventricular dysfunction is more common, especially in patients who are the furthest along in the course of the HIV disease. Individual reports of one to five cases of patients with either dilated left ventricle, hypokinetic left ventricle, or both have been frequent enough to require explanation.[55,57,58] Furthermore, the occurrence of cardiomyopathy in children, in whom a disease unrelated to HIV infection would be rare, further suggests a relationship between HIV disease and cardiomyopathy.[59] Furthermore, children with AIDS who have abnormal left ventricular function have improvement of function when treated with 30 days of intravenously administered immunoglobulin.[60]

Prospective echocardiographic studies have recently been reported that show a high prevalence of myocardial dysfunction. DeCastro and colleagues did serial echocardiograms prospectively on 136 HIV-positive patients over a mean follow-up time of 415 ± 220 days. Seven AIDS patients developed clinical and echocardiographic findings of global left ventricular dysfunction. Of the six who died, five were autopsied; three had acute lymphocytic myocarditis, one had cryptococcal myocarditis, and one had myocardial fibrosis.[61]

Blanchard and colleagues did serial echocardiograms on 70 HIV-positive outpatients. Of the 50 patients with AIDS, 7 (14 percent) had echocardiographic evidence of left ventricular dysfunction. On repeat echocardiogram, 3 of the 7 had improved left ventricular function, implying a transient problem that caused a transient decrease in left ventricular function.[62]

At San Francisco General Hospital, 74 AIDS outpatients were prospectively followed using serial quantitative Doppler echocardiography every 4 months. Control populations included HIV-positive patients without disease, HIV-positive patients with AIDS-related complex, and HIV-negative gay men. Over the follow-up period of 16.5 ± 12 months, no differences in left ventricular systolic or diastolic function were detected between the groups and no differences in mean values from the first to the last echocardiogram.[63]

Possible Reasons for Cardiomyopathy

There are many theories on the etiology of congestive heart failure with a dilated, poorly contracting left ventricle found in the occasional patient. These explanations may well be related also to the more frequently observed echocardiographic reduction in left ventricular function with or without left ventricular dilatation. The most frequently mentioned etiology is that of myocarditis or postmyocarditis cardiomyopathy. There are occasional reports of virus being grown from cardiac muscle. In 1987 Calabrese and colleagues[64] were the first to report the culturing of HIV from a right ventricular myocardial biopsy from a patient with a hypokinetic right ventricle and a normal left ventricle.

There is little evidence that HIV itself invades the myocardial cell. The myocyte has no CD4+ receptors, which are the major way by which the virus enters the cell. Although there are other ways and possibly other receptors by which the virus could invade the cell, no one has convincingly shown the virus or a portion of the viral DNA or RNA within the genome of the myocardial cell.[65] One recent study reported detecting HIV nucleic acid sequences by in situ hybridization in cardiac tissue sections from 6 of 22 patients examined who died of AIDS.[57] The hybridization target was thought to be myocytes, but this could not be proved by this technique. Furthermore, the myocardial cells showing the positive hybridization signal were sparse, comprising only one or a few cells per section; the myocardium was normal by light microscopy; and none of the patients had clinical evidence of cardiac disease.

Other Theories for the Development of Cardiomyopathy

OPPORTUNISTIC INFECTIONS

Patients with AIDS are exposed to and susceptible to multiple bacterial, viral, mycotic, and protozoal infections. Epstein-Barr virus and cytomegalovirus are both known to cause myocarditis in AIDS patients.[66,67] *Cryptococcus neoformans* and *T. Gondii* myocarditis have been well described.[48,49,68] Myocarditis due to *M. avium–intracellulare* has been reported.[14] *Aspergillus* endocarditis and myocarditis have been reported.[69]

DILATED CARDIOMYOPATHY AS A POSTVIRAL DISORDER

The study of patients with myocarditis without AIDS has shown that the myocarditis can be precipitated by viral infection and that the inflammatory reaction can progress when the virus is no longer recoverable from either the heart or even the patient. The viral infection precipitates an immune reaction either to viral antigen that cross reacts with a myocardial protein or to altered myocardial protein, which acts as a foreign antigen, thus precipitating the immune reactions that continue the myocardial necrosis and inflammatory cell infiltration.[70] (See also Chaps. 73 and 76).

The evidence that congestive cardiomyopathy is precipitated by a previous viral myocarditis includes the biopsy finding of inflammatory infiltrate in some patients with dilated cardiomyopathy[71,72] and detection of increased elevated viral antibody titers and viral-specific RNA sequences in myocardial biopsies.[73] Thus, the cardiomyopathy can result from a previous infection with a number of organisms that are no longer recoverable from the myocardium.

Herskowitz and colleagues reported the histologic and immunopathologic results of 37 endomyocardial biopsy samples from patients infected with HIV-1 who developed unexplained global left ventricular dysfunction. Twenty-eight patients had New York Heart Association (NYHA) class III and IV congestive heart failure. Four patients had myocarditis secondary to known etiologies. Of the remaining 33 patients, 17 (51 percent) had histologic evidence of idiopathic active or borderline myocarditis. Specific hybridization within myocytes was abnormal in 5 patients with HIV-1 antisense riboprobe and in 16 of the 33 with cytomegalovirus immediate early (IE-2) antisense riboprobe. This study is compatible with the possibility that cardiotropic virus infection and myocarditis may be important in the pathogenesis of HIV-associated cardiomyopathy.[74]

IMPAIRMENT OF THE IMMUNE MECHANISM LEADING TO CARDIOMYOPATHY

Humorally mediated autoimmune reactions involving antimyosin antibodies may also be implicated in the development of cardiomyopathy.[75] Circulating cardiac autoantibodies have been identified in four of six AIDS patients with cardiomyopa-

thy and in none of the HIV-positive patients without cardiomyopathy. In situ hybridization with genomic probes failed to show evidence of HIV or any other viruses within the heart muscle. Results of ELISA showed a high titer of immunoglobulin G antibody to myosin and to cardiac mitochondrial adenine nucleotide. In this study it was concluded that the cardiomyopathy may be related not to HIV infection of the heart but rather to autoimmunity. Apparent improvement of left ventricular function in children with AIDS using intravenously administered immunoglobulin is also suggestive of an immunologic etiology for the left ventricular dysfunction.[60]

ROLE OF CYTOKINES IN MYOCARDITIS

Ho and colleagues[76] proposed a primary role for neuroglial cell damage from the cytolytic effect of release of substances termed cytokines from HIV-infected monocytes, the "innocent bystander" destruction mechanism. Cytokines are biologically active mediators and are soluble proteins released by immune cells. Reversible myocardial depression is well documented in human and canine septic shock.[77,78] This was subsequently demonstrated to be due to a "myocardial depressant factor."[79] The exact nature of this myocardial depressant factor is not agreed upon, but it could be related to a variety of mediators of sepsis: endotoxin, cytokines, tumor necrosis factor (TNF), and interleukin-2.[80]

Other studies showed that the administration of endotoxin-released TNF caused depression of left ventricular function independent of left ventricular volume or loading conditions,[81] and elevated circulating levels of TNF have been noted in patients with severe chronic heart failure.[82] Increased circulating levels of TNF have been noted in patients with advanced HIV-1 infection.[83] This finding is consistent with a finding of increased production of the cytokine TNF by peripheral myocytes of patients with AIDS.[84] The increased levels of cytokines—including tumor necrosis factor, interleukins-1 and 2, and alpha-interferon—may lead to myocardial dysfunction either acting locally in a paracrine fashion on adjacent myocardium or systemically causing a decrease in myocardial function.[85,86]

CACHEXIA

Many patients with AIDS have marked weight loss and cachexia. In patients with anorexia nervosa, wall motion as assessed by two-dimensional echo Doppler was found to be abnormal in 8 of 14 patients but not in control subjects; also, lower stroke volume was found in patients compared to controls, possibly because of decreased heart size.[87] Starvation and refeeding studies in animals have demonstrated myofibrillar atrophy and cardiac interstitial edema that is accompanied by a decrease in left ventricular compliance and decreased peak systolic force.[88] These changes are thought to be due to protein-calorie malnutrition. Congestive heart failure may occur, especially during refeeding and recovery.[89,90]

VITAMIN AND SELENIUM DEFICIENCY STATES

Cachectic people can have vitamin deficiency states; it is doubtful if many patients with cardiomyopathy have this as a prime etiology. Selenium deficiency has been described, together with reduced cardiac selenium levels in AIDS, similar to the Keshan's disease seen in Chinese with selenium deficiency. In one study, 10 patients with AIDS who had decreased left ventricular fractional shortening on echocardiography received sodium selenite for 23 days.[91,92] Six of eight showed a return toward normal of left ventricular fractional shortening within 21 days. Selenium deficiency has been reported to be common in malnourished pediatric patients with AIDS.[93]

DRUG-INDUCED CARDIOMYOPATHY

The effect of drugs, both recreational and therapeutic, on myocardial function is not well delineated in patients with AIDS. In most patients with AIDS and cardiomyopathy, however, drugs do not seem to be the cause[57,94]; nevertheless, in patients with AIDS, drugs such as doxorubicin, alpha$_2$-interferon, and interleukin-2 have been shown to produce cardiomyopathy that is sometimes reversible. Recombinant alpha$_2$-interferon–related cardiomyopathy in patients treated for primary renal cancer has been reported.[95] One report described three cases of reversible cardiac dysfunction associated with alpha-interferon therapy in AIDS patients with Kaposi's sarcoma.[96]

Cocaine use has been associated with myocarditis and dilated cardiomyopathy, which occasionally has been reported to be reversible.[97,98] Pentamidine has been reported to cause ventricular tachycardia.[99] The most common currently used drug in AIDS, zidovudine (AZT), a nucleoside analog, is a drug that inhibits replication of HIV in vitro, probably by inhibiting the reverse transcriptase enzyme, which is essential to the replication of the retrovirus. No adverse cardiac effects have been reported in phase 1 clinical trials, and one study failed to show cardiotoxicity;[100] however, a toxic mitochondrial myopathy caused by long-term AZT after 12.8 months of therapy has been reported.[101] This myopathy is characterized by abnormal mitochondria with paracrystalloid inclusions. Whether or not this can occur in cardiac muscle in some patients is not clear. Foscarnet therapy for the treatment of cytomegalovirus infection has also been reported to produce a reversible cardiomyopathy.[102]

Conclusions

Clinical heart muscle disease and heart failure in AIDS are unusual. When this condition occurs, there may be explanations other than direct infection with HIV. The exact incidence of heart muscle disease in AIDS is as yet unknown but must be small, and the mechanisms that can cause failure are probably multiple.

CLINICAL WORKUP AND THERAPY

The workup of the patient with AIDS and suspected cardiac involvement begins with the history and physical examination for symptoms and signs of cardiac disease. Since there is no therapeutic advantage to finding subclinical cardiovascular involvement, there is no justification for screening electrocardiograms or echocardiograms. If there are signs or symptoms suggesting cardiovascular disease—such as a friction rub, an S$_3$ gallop, or other evidence of congestive heart failure—an echocardiogram is useful in identifying pericardial effusion and in evaluating right and left ventricular function. Invasive diagnostic studies are rarely necessary.

If left ventricular dilatation and hypokinesis are found with or without clinical evidence of heart failure, consideration should be given to stopping all drugs that are not absolutely essential.[103] If, in a 2-week follow-up, echocardiography reveals improvement, the suspected drug should be eliminated.

The question of whether or not a myocardial biopsy is helpful is controversial. The finding of a treatable cause of biopsy-proved myocarditis is rare. Furthermore, there is no evidence that treating biopsy-proved focal myocarditis with steroids or antimetabolites is effective.[104] Therefore, by available evidence, myocardial biopsy is of little value.

The potential cardiotoxic roles of opportunistic infection drugs as well as other known etiologies—such as hypertension, hypertrophic cardiomyopathy and coronary artery disease—should be considered. The treatment of congestive heart failure is similar to that of the treatment of heart failure from other etiologies, e.g., diuretics, digoxin, and angiotensin converting enzyme inhibitors (see Chap. 23).

CARDIOVASCULAR SURGERY IN AIDS PATIENTS

There has been an increased interest in the danger to the AIDS health care worker of becoming infected or of infecting patients and in the possibility of accelerating the disease through surgery. The problem is illustrated by the following questions:

1. Are we doing an expensive procedure that will cause prolonged hospitalization and probably not affect the outcome in AIDS patients?
2. What is the risk of accelerating the disease by surgery?
3. What is the risk of HIV infection to health care workers?
4. What is the risk of getting HIV infection during open-heart surgery?

In general it is not wise to do expensive procedures with some degree of morbidity and mortality that result in prolonged hospitalization of patients with a limited life span due to their underlying disease. For this reason, patients with AIDS should not be subjected to surgery that will most probably not significantly affect their survival. It is probable that 70 percent of patients found to have AIDS will die within 3 to 4 years of the diagnosis.[105] On the other hand, if patients with AIDS have medically uncontrollable symptoms, invasive procedures that can ameliorate these symptoms may be indicated.

The most frequent problem in which the question of cardiovascular surgery arises in a relatively young subgroup involves the intravenous drug user with infective endocarditis and congestive heart failure. The presence of HIV disease in these patients, who overall have poor results from surgery, would suggest that the patient be treated medically for as long as possible.

HIV-positive patients and patients with PGL who have not had an opportunistic infection or cancer can have a prolonged course over many years and, in general, should be treated like patients without HIV disease. In fact, it is possible that life span will be prolonged after HIV infection by combinations of drugs, including reverse transcriptase inhibitors and the new protease inhibitors. In this subgroup, cardiovascular surgery should be considered for the usual indications.

The possibility that progression of the HIV disease is accelerated by the immunologic challenge that occurs from cardiopulmonary bypass is largely unanswered. Instances of HIV-positive patients who developed AIDS shortly after open-heart surgery have been reported. It is known that cardiopulmonary bypass produces temporary depression of phagocytic function and immune globulin production.[106] Cardiopulmonary bypass per se in HIV-negative patients causes prolonged abnormalities in the CD4+/CD8+ T-cell ratio up to 6 days postoperatively.[107] There is, therefore, a basis for concern that cardiopulmonary bypass surgery could accelerate the progression of HIV disease, and this must be taken into consideration.

Whether or not all patients undergoing cardiovascular surgery or other invasive procedures should have HIV testing is a matter of heated debate. Although the risk to health care personnel is small, HIV infection is usually tantamount to fatal infection; fear is great among both health care workers and the public. On the other hand, AIDS is an emotional subject, and patients who are known to be HIV-positive may be subjected to prejudice and discrimination. At present, HIV testing of both health care workers and patients is voluntary; however, there are proposed recommendations requiring disclosure to patients that a health care worker is HIV-positive and informed consent from the patient before any invasive procedure is done. At present, there is only one instance of transmission of disease by a health care worker, that of an HIV-positive dentist who is believed to have infected five patients, probably from reuse of inadequately sterilized instruments. This matter is still under considerable debate.

Because of this risk, some cardiovascular surgeons and cardiologists are refusing to operate on or catheterize an HIV-positive person or a patient who will not allow an HIV test to be done. A survey was done of the attitudes of cardiac surgeons in the United States concerning operating on HIV-positive patients.[108] More than half responded, and two-thirds of these were reportedly willing to perform open heart surgery on HIV-positive patients no matter how they had acquired their HIV infection. One-quarter of the surgeons would not operate no matter how the HIV infection was acquired, and the rest were uncertain. Once the patient has gone from the HIV carrier state to AIDS, two-thirds of the cardiac surgeons would not operate. Ninety percent of those responding want to be able to test all their patients for HIV status.

The physician's fear of becoming infected with HIV is understandable, but as in the case of other professions that involve personal dangers, the profession of the physician requires performance. Both the American College of Physicians and the American Medical Association currently have standards stating that a physician may not ethically refuse to treat a patient solely because he or she is HIV-positive.

As of 1990, the literature has reported 18 health care workers who had no other risk factors and were known to be HIV-negative at exposure who have seroconverted after exposure. The danger to health care personnel is greatest when there is exposure to blood and the chance of accidental needle or knife perforation or blood splash into the eyes or mouth. In one prospective study of 1307 consecutive procedures, accumulated exposure, parenteral or cutaneous, occurred in only 84 procedures (6.4 percent).[109] Parenteral exposure occurred in 1.7 percent. Knowledge of the patient's HIV status or awareness of the patient's high-risk status for such infection did not appear to influence the rate of exposure, suggesting that preoperative testing for HIV infection would not decrease the frequency of accidental exposure to blood.

In combined data from 14 prospective studies of the risk of HIV-1 transmission to health care workers, there were 2042 parenteral exposures in 1948 subjects. The chance of seroconversion was 0.29 percent per exposure (95 percent confidence interval, 0.13 to 0.7 percent); in 668 people with 1051 total mucous membrane exposures, there were no seroconversions (95 percent confidence limits, upper bound is 0.28 percent per exposure). The risk of a health care worker developing HIV seroconversion from work-related activities was very low, approximately one infection in 300 documented exposures to HIV-positive blood.[110]

REFERENCES

1. Chu SY, Berkelman RL, Curran JW. Epidemiology of HIV in the United States. In: De Vita VT, Hellman S, Rosenberg SA, eds. *AIDS: Etiology, Diagnosis, Treatment and Prevention*, 3d ed. Philadelphia: Lippincott; 1992:99–109.
2. Centers for Disease Control and Prevention. HIV/AIDS surveillance report. Atlanta: CDC 1994; 6(2):7.
3. Steele FR. A moving target: CDC still trying to evaluate HIV-1 prevalence. *J NIH Res* 1994; 6:25–26.
4. Centers for Disease Control. Classification system for human T-lymphotropic virus type III/lymphadenopathy-associated virus infections. *MMWR* 1986; 35:334–339.
5. Centers for Disease Control. 1993 Revised classification system for HIV infection and expanded surveillance case definition for AIDS among adolescents and adults. *MMWR* 1992; 41(RR-17):1–19.

6. Bacchetti P, Moss AR. Incubation period of AIDS in San Francisco (letter). *Nature* 1989; 338:251–253.

7. Feinberg MB, Greene WC. Molecular insights into human immunodeficiency virus type 1 pathogenesis. *Curr Opin Immunol* 1992; 4:466–474.

8. Lifson A, Hessol N, Rutherford GW, Buchbinder S, O'Malley P, Cannon L, et al. The natural history of HIV infection in a cohort of homosexual and bisexual men: Clinical manifestations, 1978–1989 (abstr). International Conference on AIDS, Montreal 1989; 5:60(T.A.O. 32).

9. Osmond D. Progression to AIDS in persons testing seropositive for antibody to HIV. In: Cohen PT, Sande MA Volberding PA, eds. *The AIDS Knowledge Base*. Waltham, MA: Medical Publishing Group; 1990:1.1.6.

10. Piatak M Jr, Saag MS, Yang LC, Clark SJ, Kappes JC, Luk KC, et al. High levels of HIV-1 in plasma during all stages of infection determined by competitive PCR. *Science* 1993; 259:1749–1754.

11. Lifson AR, Buchbinder SP, Sheppard HW, Mawle AC, Wilber JC, Stanley M, et al. Long-term human immunodeficiency virus infection in asymptomatic homosexual and bisexual men with normal CD4 + lymphocyte counts: immunologic and virologic characteristics. *J Infect Dis* 1991; 163:959–965.

12. Silver MA, Macher AM, Reichert CM, Levens DL, Parrillo JE, Longo DL, et al. Cardiac involvement by Kaposi's sarcoma in acquired immune deficiency syndrome (AIDS). *Am J Cardiol* 1984; 53:983–985.

13. Welch K, Finkbeiner W, Alpers CE, Blumenfeld W, Davis RL, Smuckler EA, et al. Autopsy findings in the acquired immune deficiency syndrome. *JAMA* 1984; 252:1152–1159.

14. Cammarosano C, Lewis W. Cardiac lesions in acquired immune deficiency syndrome (AIDS). *J Am Coll Cardiol* 1985; 5:703–706.

15. Roldan EO, Moskowitz L, Hensly GT. Pathology of the heart in acquired immunodeficiency syndrome. *Arch Pathol Lab Med* 1987; 111:943–946.

16. Wilkes MS, Fortin AH, Felix JC, Godwin TA, Thompson WG. Value of necropsy in acquired immunodeficiency syndrome. *Lancet* 1988; 2:85–88.

17. Baroldi G, Corallo S, Moroni M, Repossini A, Mutinelli MR, Lazzarin A, et al. Focal lymphocytic myocarditis in acquired immunodeficiency syndrome (AIDS): A correlative morphologic and clinical study in 26 consecutive fatal cases. *J Am Coll Cardiol* 1988; 12:463–469.

18. Lewis W. AIDS: Cardiac findings from 115 autopsies. *Prog Cardiovasc Dis* 1989; 32:207–215.

19. Anderson DW, Virmani R, Reilly JM, O'Leary T, Cunnion RE, Robinowitz M, et al. Prevalent myocarditis at necropsy in the acquired immunodeficiency syndrome. *J Am Coll Cardiol* 1988; 11:792–799.

20. Magno J, Margaretten W, Cheitlin M: Myocardial involvement in acquired immunodeficiency syndrome: Incidence in a large autopsy study (abstr). *Circulation* 1988; 78(suppl II):II-459.

21. Garcia I, Fainstein V, Rios A, Luna M, Mansell P, Reuben J, et al. Nonbacterial thrombotic endocarditis in a male homosexual with Kaposi's sarcoma. *Arch Inter Med* 1983; 143:1243–1244.

22. Moskowitz L, Hensley GT, Chan JC, Adams K. Immediate causes of death in acquired immunodeficiency syndrome. *Arch Pathol Lab Med* 1985; 109:735–738.

23. Murray JF, Garay SM, Hopewell PC, Mills J, Snider GL, Stover DE. Pulmonary complications of the acquired immunodeficiency syndrome: An update: Report of the second National Heart, Lung and Blood Institute workshop. *Am Rev Respir Dis* 1987; 135:504–509.

24. Fink L, Reichek N, St. John Sutton MG. Cardiac abnormalities in acquired immune deficiency syndrome. *Am J Cardiol* 1984; 54:1161–1163.

25. Kinney EL, Brafman D, Wright RJ II. Echocardiographic findings in patients with acquired immunodeficiency syndrome (AIDS) and AIDS-related complex (ARC). *Cathet Cardiovasc Diag* 1989; 16:182–185.

26. Himelman RB, Chung WS, Chernoff DN, Schiller NB, Hollander H. Cardiac manifestations of human immunodeficiency virus infection: A two-dimensional echocardiographic study. *J Am Coll Cardiol* 1989; 13:1030–1036.

27. Monsuez JJ, Kinney EL, Vittecoq D, Kitzis M, Rozenbaum W, d'Agay MF, et al. Comparison among acquired immune deficiency syndrome patients with and without clinical evidence of cardiac disease. *Am J Cardiol* 1988; 62:1311–1313.

28. Levy WS, Simon GL, Rios JC, Ross AM. Prevalence of cardiac abnormalities in human immunodeficiency virus infection. *Am J Cardiol* 1989; 63:86–89.

29. Corallo S, Mutinelli MR, Moroni M, Lazzarin A, Celano V, Repossini A, et al. Echocardiography detects myocardial damage in AIDS: Prospective study in 102 patients. *Eur Heart J* 1988; 9:887–892.

30. Hecht SR, Berger M, Van Tosh A, Croxson S. Unsuspected cardiac abnormalities in the acquired immune deficiency syndrome: An echocardiographic study. *Chest* 1989; 96:805–808.

31. Steffen HM, Müller R, Schrappe-Bächer M, Salzberger B, Fätkenheuer G, Wagner-Klein S, et al. Prevalence of echocardiographic abnormalities in human immunodeficiency virus 1 infection. *Am J Noninvas Cardiol* 1991; 5:280–284.

32. Redfield RR, Wright DC, Tramont EC. The Walter Reed staging classification for HTLV-III/LAV infection: Special report. *N Engl J Med* 1986; 314:131–132.

33. Steigman CK, Anderson DW, Macher AM, Sennesh JD, Virmani R. Fatal cardiac tamponade in acquired immunodeficiency syndrome with epicardial Kaposi's sarcoma. *Am Heart J* 1988; 116:1105–1107.

34. D'Cruz IA, Sengupta EE, Abrahams C, Reddy HK, Turlapati RV. Cardiac involvement, including tuberculous pericardial effusion, complicating acquired immune deficiency syndrome. *Am Heart J* 1986; 112:1100–1102.

35. Woods GL, Goldsmith JC. Fatal pericarditis due to *Mycobacterium avium-intracellulare* in acquired immunodeficiency syndrome. *Chest* 1989; 95:1355–1357.

36. Reynolds M, Berger M, Hecht S, Kolokathis A, Horowitz SF. Large pericardial effusions associated with the acquired immune deficiency syndrome (AIDS) (abstr.) *J Am Coll Cardiol* 1991; 17:221A.

37. Decker CF, Tuazon CU. Staphylococcus aureus pericarditis in HIV-infected patients. *Chest* 1994; 105:615–616.

38. Zuger A, Louie E, Holzman RS, Simberkoff MS, Rahal JJ. Cryptococcal disease in patients with acquired immunodeficiency syndrome: Diagnostic features and outcome of treatment. *Ann Intern Med* 1986; 104:234–240.

39. Freedberg RS, Gindea AJ, Dieterich DT, Greene JB. Herpes simplex pericarditis in AIDS. *NY State J Med* 1987; 87:304–306.

40. Francis CK. Cardiac involvement in AIDS. *Curr Probl Cardiol* 1990; 15:571–639.

41. Currie PF, Jacob AJ, Foreman AR, Elton RA, Brettle RP, Boon NA. Heart muscle disease related to HIV infection: Prognostic implications. *Br Med J* 1994; 309:1605–1607.

42. Serrano-Heranz R, Camino A, Vilacosta I, Lopez-Castellanos A, Roca V. Tuberculous cardiac tamponade and AIDS. *Eur Heart J* 1995; 16:430–432.

43. Choo PS, McCormack JG. Mycobacterium avium: A potentially treatable cause of pericardial effusions. *J Infect* 1995; 30:55–58.

44. Heidenreich PA, Eisenberg MJ, Kee LL, Somelofski CA, Hollander H, Schiller NB, et al. Pericardial effusion in AIDS: Incidence and survival. *Circulation* 1995; 92:3229–3234.

45. Flum DR, McGinn JT Jr, Tyras DH. The role of the "pericardial window" in AIDS. *Chest* 1995; 107:1522–1525.

46. Zuger A, Louie E, Holzman RS, Simberkoff MS, Rahal JJ. Cryptococcal disease in patients with the acquired immunodeficiency syndrome: Diagnostic features and outcome of treatment: Clinical review. *Ann Intern Med* 1986; 104:234–240.

47. Hofman P, Drici MD, Gibelin P, Michiels J-F, Thyss A. Prevalence of toxoplasma myocarditis in patients with the acquired immunodeficiency syndrome. *Br Heart J* 1993; 70:376–381.

48. Kinney EL, Monsuez JJ, Kitzis M, Vittecoq D. Treatment of AIDS-associated heart disease. *Angiology* 1989; 40:970–976.

49. Grange F, Kinney EL, Monsuez JJ, Rybojad M, Derouin F, Khuong MA, et al. Successful therapy for *Toxoplasma gondii* myocarditis in acquired immunodeficiency syndrome. *Am Heart J* 1990; 120:443–444.

50. Albrecht H, Stellbrink HJ, Fenske S, Schäfer H, Greten H. Successful treatment of *Toxoplasma gondii* myocarditis in an AIDS patient. *Eur J Clin Microbiol Infect Dis* 1994; 13:500–504.

51. Ioachim HL, Cooper MC, Hellman GC. Lymphomas in men at high risk for acquired immune deficiency syndrome (AIDS): A study of 21 cases. *Cancer* 1985; 56:2831–2842.

52. Lloyd EA, Curcio CA. Lymphoma of the heart as an unusual cause of pericardial effusion: A case report. *S Afr Med J* 1980; 58:937–939.

53. Levitt LJ, Ault KA, Pinkus GS, Sloss LJ, McManus BM. Pericarditis and early cardiac tamponade as a primary manifestation of lymphosarcoma cell leukemia. *Am J Med* 1979; 67:719–723.

54. Goldfarb A, King CL, Rosenzweig BP, Feit F, Kamat BR, Rumancik

WM, et al. Cardiac lymphoma in the acquired immunodeficiency syndrome. *Am Heart J* 1989; 118:1340–1344.

55. Cohen IS, Anderson DW, Virmani R, Reen BM, Macher AM, Sennesh J, et al. Congestive cardiomyopathy in association with the acquired immunodeficiency syndrome. *N Engl J Med* 1986; 315:628–630.

56. Reilly JM, Cunnion RE, Anderson DW, O'Leary TJ, Simmons JT, Lane HC, et al. Frequency of myocarditis, left ventricular dysfunction and ventricular tachycardia in the acquired immune deficiency syndrome. *Am J Cardiol* 1988; 62:789–793.

57. Kaminski HJ, Katzman M, Wiest PM, Enler JJ, Gifford DR, Rackley R, et al. Cardiomyopathy associated with the acquired immune deficiency syndrome. *J AIDS* 1988; 1:105–110.

58. Corboy JR, Fink L, Miller WT. Congestive cardiomyopathy in association with AIDS. *Radiology* 1987; 165:139–141.

59. Lipshultz SE, Orav EJ, Sanders SP, Hale AR, McIntosh K, Colan SD. Cardiac structure and function in children with human immunodeficiency virus infection treated with zidovudine. *N Engl J Med* 1992; 327:1260–1265.

60. Lipshultz SE, Orav J, Sanders SP, Colan SD. Immunoglobulins and left ventricular structure and function in pediatric HIV infection. *Circulation* 1995; 92:2220–2225.

61. DeCastro S, d'Amati G, Gallo P, Cartoni D, Santopadre P, Vullo V, et al. Frequency of development of acute global left ventricular dysfunction in human immunodeficiency virus infection. *J Am Coll Cardiol* 1994; 24:1018–1024.

62. Blanchard DG, Hagenhoff C, Chow LC, McCann HA, Dittrich HC. Reversibility of cardiac abnormalities in human immunodeficiency virus (HIV)-infected individuals: A serial echocardiographic study. *J Am Coll Cardiol* 1991; 17:1270–1276.

63. Cheitlin MD. Cardiovascular complications of HIV infection. In: Sande MA, Volberding PA, eds. *The Medical Management of AIDS*, 4th ed. Philadelphia: Saunders; 1995:332–344.

64. Calabrese LH, Proffitt MR, Yen-Lieberman B, Hobbs RE, Ratliff NB. Congestive cardiomyopathy and illness related to the acquired immunodeficiency syndrome (AIDS) associated with isolation of retrovirus from myocardium. *Ann Intern Med* 1987; 107:691–692.

65. Grody WW, Cheng L, Lewis W. Infection of the heart by the human immunodeficiency virus. *Am J Cardiol* 1990; 66:203–206.

66. Lafont A, Marche C, Wolff M, Perronne C, Witchitz S, Régnier B, et al. Myocarditis in acquired immunodeficiency syndrome (AIDS): Etiology and progress (abstr). *J Am Coll Cardiol* 1988; 11:196A.

67. Stewart JM, Kaul A, Gromisch DS, Reyes E, Woolf PK, Gowitz MH. Symptomatic cardiac dysfunction in children with human immunodeficiency virus infection. *Am Heart J* 1989; 117:140–144.

68. Acierno LJ. Cardiac complications in acquired immunodeficiency syndrome (AIDS): A review. *J Am Coll Cardiol* 1989; 13:1144–1154.

69. Cox JN, di Dió F, Pizzolato GP, Lerch R, Pochon N. Aspergillus endocarditis and myocarditis in a patient with the acquired immunodeficiency syndrome (AIDS): A review of the literature: Case report. *Virchows Archiv A (Pathol Anat Histopathol)* 1990; 417:255–259.

70. Lowry PJ, Thompson RA, Littler WA. Cellular immunity in congestive cardiomyopathy: The normal cellular immune response. *Br Heart J* 1985; 53:394–399.

71. Zee-Cheng CS, Tsai CC, Palmer DC, Codd JE, Pennington DG, Williams GA. High incidence of myocarditis by endomyocardial biopsy in patients with idiopathic congestive cardiomyopathy. *J Am Coll Cardiol* 1984; 3:63–70.

72. Parrillo JE, Aretz HT, Palacios I, Fallon JT, Block PC. The results of transvenous endomyocardial biopsy can frequently be used to diagnose myocardial diseases in patients with idiopathic heart failure: Endomyocardial biopsy in 100 consecutive patients revealed a substantial incidence of myocarditis. *Circulation* 1984; 69:93–101.

73. Bowles NE, Richardson PJ, Olsen EGJ, Archard LC. Detection of Coxsackie-B-virus–specific RNA sequences in myocardial biopsy samples from patients with myocarditis and dilated cardiomyopathy. *Lancet* 1984; 1:1120–1123.

74. Herskowitz A, Wu T-C, Willoughby SB, Vlahov D, Ansari AA, Beschorner WE, et al. Myocarditis and cardiotropic viral infection associated with severe left ventricular dysfunction in late-stage infection with human immunodeficiency virus. *J Am Coll Cardiol* 1994; 24:1025–1032.

75. Herskowitz A, Ansari AA, Neumann DA, Beschorner WE, Oliveira M, Chaisson RE, et al. Cardiomyopathy in acquired immunodeficiency syndrome: Evidence for autoimmunity (abstr). *Circulation* 1989; 80(suppl II):II-322.

76. Ho DD, Pomerantz RJ, Kaplan JC. Pathogenesis of infection with human immunodeficiency virus. *N Engl J Med* 1987; 317:278–286.

77. Parker MM, Shelhamer JH, Bacharach SL, Green MV, Natanson C, Frederick TM, et al. Profound but reversible myocardial depression in patients with septic shock. *Ann Intern Med* 1984; 100:483–490.

78. Natanson C, Fink MP, Ballantyne HK, MacVittie TJ, Conklin JJ, Parrillo JE. Gram-negative bacteremia produces both severe systolic and diastolic cardiac dysfunction in a canine model that simulates human septic shock. *J Clin Invest* 1986; 78:259–270.

79. Parrillo JE, Burch C, Shelhamer JH, Parker MM, Natanson C, Schuette W. A circulating myocardial depressant substance in humans with septic shock: Septic shock patients with a reduced ejection fraction have a circulating factor that depresses in vitro myocardial cell performance. *J Clin Invest* 1985; 76:1539–1553.

80. Cunnion RE, Parrillo JE. Myocardial dysfunction in sepsis: Recent insights (editorial). *Chest* 1989;95:941–945.

81. Suffredini AF, Fromm RE, Parker MM, Brenner M, Kovacs JA, Wesley RA, et al. The cardiovascular response of normal humans to the administration of endotoxin. *N Engl J Med* 1989; 321:280–287.

82. Levine B, Kalman J, Mayer L, Fillit HM, Packer M. Elevated circulating levels of tumor necrosis factor in severe chronic heart failure. *N Engl J Med* 1990; 323:236–241.

83. Lähdevirta J, Maury CPJ, Teppo AM, Repo H. Elevated levels of circulating cachectin/tumor necrosis factor in patients with acquired immunodeficiency syndrome. *Am J Med* 1988; 85:289–291.

84. Wright SC, Jewett A, Mitsuyasu R, Bonavida B. Spontaneous cytotoxicity and tumor necrosis factor production by peripheral blood monocytes from AIDS patients. *J Immunol* 1988; 141:99–104.

85. Odeh M. The role of tumour necrosis factor-alpha in acquired immunodeficiency syndrome. *J Intern Med* 1990; 228:549–556.

86. Yamamoto N. The role of cytokines in the acquired immunodeficiency syndrome. *Int J Clin Lab Res* 1995; 25:29–34.

87. Goldberg SJ, Comerci GD, Feldman L. Cardiac output and regional myocardial contraction in anorexia nervosa. *J Adolesc Health Care* 1988; 9:15–21.

88. Abel RM, Grimes JB, Alonso D, Alonso M, Gay WA Jr. Adverse hemodynamic and ultrastructural changes in dog hearts subjected to protein-calorie malnutrition. *Am Heart J* 1979; 97:733–744.

89. Heymsfield SB, Bethel RA, Ansley JD, Gibbs DM, Felner JM, Nutter DO. Cardiac abnormalities in cachectic patients before and during nutritional repletion. *Am Heart J* 1978; 95:584–594.

90. Schocken DD, Holloway JD, Powers PS. Weight loss and the heart: Effects of anorexia nervosa and starvation. *Arch Intern Med* 1989; 149:877–881.

91. Dworkin BM, Antonecchia PP, Smith F, Weiss L, Davidian M, Rubin D, et al. Reduced cardiac selenium content in the acquired immunodeficiency syndrome. *J Parenter Enter Nutr* 1989; 13:644–647.

92. Zazzo JF, Chalas J, Lafont A, Camus F, Chappuis P. Is nonobstructive cardiomyopathy in AIDS a selenium deficiency-related disease (letter)? *J Parenter Enter Nutr* 1988; 12:537–538.

93. Kavanaugh-McHugh AL, Ruff A, Perlman E, Hutton N, Modlin J, Rowe S. Selenium deficiency and cardiomyopathy in acquired immunodeficiency syndrome. *J Parenter Enter Nutr* 1991; 15:347–349.

94. Kaul S, Fishbein MC, Siegel RJ. Cardiac manifestations of acquired immune deficiency syndrome: A 1991 update. *Am Heart J* 1991; 122:535–544.

95. Cohen MC, Huberman MS, Nesto RW. Recombinant alpha$_2$ interferon-related cardiomyopathy. *Am J Med* 1988; 85:549–551.

96. Deyton LR, Walker RE, Kovacs JA, Herpin B, Parker M, Masur H, et al. Reversible cardiac dysfunction associated with interferon alfa therapy in AIDS patients with Kaposi's sarcoma. *N Engl J Med* 1989; 321:1246–1249.

97. Chokshi SK, Moore R, Pandian NG, Isner JM. Reversible cardiomyopathy associated with cocaine intoxication. *Ann Intern Med* 1989; 111:1039–1040.

98. Brown J, Kind A, Francis CK. Cardiovascular effects of alcohol, cocaine, and acquired immune deficiency. *Cardiovasc Clin* 1991; 21:341–376.

99. Wharton JM, Demopulos PA, Goldschlager N. Torsade de pointes during administration of pentamidine isethionate. *Am J Med* 1987; 83:571–576.

100. Richman DD, Fischl MA, Grieco MH, Gottlieb MS, Volberding PA, Laskin OL, et al. The toxicity of azidothymidine (AZT) in the treatment of patients with AIDS and AIDS-related complex: A double-blind,

placebo-controlled trial. *N Engl J Med* 1987; 317:192–197.

101. Dalakas MC, Illa I, Pezeshkpour GH, Laukaitis JP, Cohen B, Griffin JL. Mitochondrial myopathy caused by long-term zidovudine therapy. *N Engl J Med* 1990; 322:1098–1105.

102. Brown DL, Sather S, Cheitlin MD. Reversible cardiac dysfunction associated with foscarnet therapy for cytomegalovirus esophagitis in an AIDS patient. *Am Heart J* 1993; 125:1439–1441.

103. Herskowitz A, Willoughby SB, Baughman KL, Schulman SP, Bartlett JD. Cardiomyopathy associated with antiretroviral therapy in patients with HIV infection: A report of six cases. *Ann Intern Med* 1992; 116:311–313.

104. Mason JW, O'Connell JB, Herskowitz A, Rose NR, McManus BM, Billingham ME, et al. A clinical trial of immunosuppressive therapy for myocarditis: The Myocarditis Treatment Trial Investigators. *N Engl J Med* 1995; 333:269–275.

105. Centers for Disease Control. Acquired immunodeficiency syndrome—United States: Update. *MMWR* 1986; 35:17–21.

106. Utley JR. The immune response. In: *Pathophysiology and Techniques of Cardiopulmonary Bypass I.* Baltimore: Williams & Wilkins; 1982:132–144.

107. Pollock R, Ames F, Rubio P, Jones J, Reuben J, Wong W, et al. Protracted severe immune dysregulation induced by cardiopulmonary bypass: A predisposing etiologic factor in blood transfusion-related AIDS? *J Clin Lab Immunol* 1987; 22:1–5.

108. Condit D, Frater RWM. Human immunodeficiency virus and the cardiac surgeon: A survey of attitudes. *Ann Thorac Surg* 1989; 47:182–186.

109. Gerberding JL, Littell C, Tarkington A, Brown A, Schecter WP. Risk of exposure of surgical personnel to patients' blood during surgery at San Francisco General Hospital. *N Engl J Med* 1990; 322:1788–1793.

110. Henderson DK, Fahey BJ, Willy M, Schmitt JM, Carey K, Koziol DE, et al. Risk for occupational transmission of human immunodeficiency virus type 1 (HIV-1) associated with clinical exposures: A prospective evaluation. *Ann Intern Med* 1990; 113:740–746.

80

EFFECT OF NONCARDIAC DRUGS, ELECTRICITY, POISONS, AND RADIATION ON THE HEART

Andrew L. Smith / Robert C. Schlant

This chapter deals with a number of deleterious side effects of treatments and environmental agents on the heart. Toxic effects may occur acutely and require emergent intervention or may be chronic and not be manifest until days or years after exposure.

NONCARDIAC DRUGS

Chemotherapeutic Agents

Chemotherapeutic agents may result in acute or chronic cardiovascular toxicity. The heart, composed of nonproliferating myocytes, was traditionally thought to be protected from the effects of drugs on rapidly dividing cells. A variety of agents are now recognized to cause cardiovascular complications including cardiomyopathy, myocarditis, pericarditis, myocardial ischemia, arrhythmias, and peripheral hypotension or vasospasm (see Table 80-1).[1]

Cardiovascular alterations in the patient receiving chemotherapy may be the result of a specific drug or combination of drugs or be related to tumor-associated factors such as hypercoagulability or release of myocardial depressant factors. Correlating a specific therapy with a particular adverse event may be difficult[2]; however, knowledge of side effects of each agent should be considered when prescribing therapy.

ANTHRACYCLINES

The anthracycline antineoplastics, doxorubicin and daunorubicin, are the leading cause of chemotherapy-related heart disease. These agents may cause cardiac problems during therapy, weeks after completion of therapy, or, unexpectedly, years later.[3] During acute therapy, electrocardiographic

changes occur in approximately 30 percent of patients and usually regress within weeks.[4] *Findings include ST-T changes, decreased QRS voltage, prolongation of the QT interval, and atrial and ventricular ectopy.* Sustained atrial or ventricular arrhythmias are rare. The occurrence of early electrocardiogram (ECG) abnormalities does not predict cardiomyopathy and is not an indication to discontinue therapy.[1] The development of persistent sinus tachycardia in an otherwise stable oncology patient, however, (although nonspecific), may raise

TABLE 80-1

CHEMOTHERAPEUTIC AGENTS COMMONLY ASSOCIATED WITH CARDIOVASCULAR TOXICITY

Drug	Associated Toxicity
Anthracyclines	
Doxorubicin	Cardiomyopathy
Daunorubicin	
Epirubicin	
Idarubicin	
Mitoxantrone	
Alkylating agents	
Cyclophosphamide	Reversible systolic dysfunction, hemorrhagic myocarditis
Cisplatin	Raynaud's phenomenon
Antimetabolites	
5-Fluorouracil	Coronary vasospasm
Other	
Amsacrine	Dysrhythmias
Paclitaxel	Dysrhythmias
Interleukin 2	Hypotension, myocarditis
Interferon alpha	Hypotension, cardiomyopathy

the suspicion of ventricular dysfunction and impending congestive heart failure.[2]

Congestive heart failure is related to the cumulative dose of the anthracycline administered. The incidences at specific doses of doxorubicin include: 0.4 percent at 400 mg/m^2 of body surface area, 7 percent at 550 mg/m^2, and 18 percent at 700 mg/m^2 (see Fig. 80-1). Traditionally, the cardiac limiting dose has been described as 550 mg/m^2 because of the acute rise in heart failure seen above this dose. There is great individual variability, however, with reports of heart failure occurring with doses less than 100 mg/m^2 and, conversely, with some patients tolerating greater than 1000 mg/m^2 without cardiac compromise.[5,6] Risk factors for anthracycline-induced cardiomyopathy are debated but include prior chest radiation,[6–8] age greater than 70,[3,6] and preexisting heart disease.[6] Young females may be at particularly increased risk for late cardiac dysfunction.[9] Rapid infusion schedules associated with higher peak drug concentration appear to result in greater cardiotoxicity.[10]

The pathogenesis of anthracycline-induced cardiotoxicity is not known. Theories generally implicate free radical damage. One proposal is that enzymatic reduction of the anthracycline-quinone ring results in lipid peroxidation and cell membrane damage. Another theory involves the formation of an anthracycline-iron complex, which undergoes "redoxcycling" that results in oxygen radicals and degradation of microsomal, mitochondrial, and membrane lipids. Disturbances of calcium exchange have also been noted.[11–13]

The average time to clinical development of heart failure symptoms is 1 month from the end of therapy but may occur anytime within 1 year. Patient presentation is similar to that for other dilated cardiomyopathies (see Chap. 73). Biventricular systolic dysfuncton occurs, and restrictive hemodynamics have been described.[14,15] The clinical course varies from fulminant heart failure to gradually progressive deterioration. Some patients have reversibility of systolic dysfunction.[16]

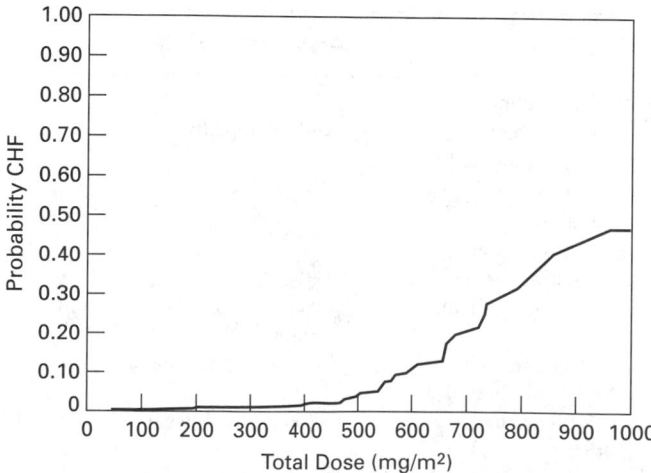

FIGURE 80-1
The development of doxorubicin-induced heart failure is related to cumulative dose. Toxicity may occur at any dose, but at 550 mg/m^2 the probability increases significantly. (From Von Hoff et al.,[5] with permission.)

Therapy, in addition to withholding further anthracycline dosing or other myocardial toxins, is generally considered the same as recommended for patients with heart failure from dilated cardiomyopathy (Chap. 23).

Noninvasive assessment of left ventricular function has been utilized to guide anthracycline dosing and prevent cardiac toxicity. Serial echocardiography in children[17] and radionuclide angiography in adults[3,18] (see Chap. 17) are most commonly used. Improved echocardiographic technologies are likely to increase the use of echocardiography in the adult population. The most commonly used parameter is resting left ventricular ejection fraction. Recognition that resting left ventricular ejection fraction is relatively insensitive for detecting early cardiotoxicity[3] has resulted in investigation of other variables (exercise or dobutamine echocardiography,[19] Doppler velocities,[20] and systolic time intervals) in assessing this problem. These methods have generally been evaluated in small-sized studies and have not gained widespread acceptance in current therapy guidelines.[3] Adult guidelines for serial assessment have been developed.[21] A drop in left ventricular ejection fraction greater than 10 percent (EF units) and to below a normal value of 50 percent is an indication to discontinue therapy. A baseline left ventricular ejection fraction less than 30 percent has generally been considered a contraindication to initiating anthracycline therapy.[21]

Endoyocardial biopsy is considered more specific and provides earlier sensitivity compared to the noninvasive methods in detection of anthracycline cardiotoxicity.[22,23] The Billingham score assessing cytoplasmic changes and the percent of myocytes damaged has been utilized to assess the risk of congestive heart failure.[23] Clinical utility has been limited because of the invasive nature of this procedure and the special expertise required in obtaining and reading the specimens. Additionally, variability of histologic changes and the potential for sampling error have been noted.[14,24]

There is growing recognition of the occurrence of cardiac dysfunction years after completion of anthracycline therapy. This is particularly of concern in children. One study reported a 23 percent incidence of late cardiac abnormalities (decreased systolic function by noninvasive testing) in survivors of pediatric malignancies treated with anthracycline therapy.[25] The incidence of abnormalities was higher in the patients with the longer elapsed times since therapy, with a 38 percent incidence in patients with a follow-up period greater than 10 years. This study, as well as others,[26,27] suggests that subclinical myocardial damage may not become clinically evident until years after therapy. Although fewer than 5 percent of these patients had developed clinical heart failure, the potentially progressive nature of systolic dysfunction raises the issue of need for long-term clinical follow-up. There are presently no accepted guidelines, however, in either the pediatric or adult population for chronic monitoring. Early treatment of systolic dysfunction with angiotensin-converting enzyme inhibitors may be warranted in asymptomatic patients.[3] Additionally, patients presenting late after anthracycline therapy with exertional fatigue and normal resting ejection fractions have been noted to have abnormalities on dobutamine echocardiography. This observation suggests abnormalities in cardiac reserve that may lead to symptoms.

Clinical strategies for preventing anthracycline cardiotoxicity have had to balance the need for antineoplastic efficacy. Lower clinical toxicity has been noted with prolonged infusions of doxorubicin over 48 to 96 h in order to avoid high peak concentrations.[28] Several antioxidants have been evaluated but with inconclusive results.[29,30] *Dexrazoxane*[31], an iron-chelating agent, reduces free-radical generation by anthracyclines and was approved for use in women with breast cancer after a cumulative dose of doxorubicin of 300 mg/m[2]. Studies demonstrate a decrease in cardiotoxicity and most, but not all, trials have suggested preserved efficacy of antitumor activity.[3] New anthracyclines, including epirubicin and idarubicin, appear to have diminished cardiotoxic effects, although long-term results cannot presently be assessed.[3]

OTHER CHEMOTHERAPEUTIC AGENTS

Mitoxantrone, an anthracendione lacking the amino sugar of anthracyclines, causes cardiotoxicity with features similar to anthracycline-induced cardiomyopathy.[1] This drug appears to have less cardiotoxicity than doxorubicin at equal myelotoxic doses. Cumulative doses above 160 mg/m[2] are associated with an increasing incidence of congestive heart failure.[32]

High-dose *cyclophosphamide* (120 to 240 mg/kg over several days) used in bone marrow transplantation may cause acute cardiac toxicity.[1,33,34] Asymptomatic systolic dysfunction, usually reversible with drug discontinuation, is associated with decreased QRS voltage on the ECG. Pericardial effusions have been noted, and a hemorrhagic myocarditis may result in death. Necropsy data demonstrate endothelial injury with resultant interstitial fibrin deposition and capillary microthrombosis.[33] Cyclophosphamide may also potentiate the cardiotoxic effects of the anthracyclines.[1]

5-Fluorouracil may occasionally cause angina, electrocardiographic changes, and rarely myocardial infarction.[1,35] The majority of episodes occur during the first cycle of therapy and resolve spontaneously after discontinuation. Dysrhythmias and systolic dysfunction have been observed. The understanding of 5-fluorouracil toxicity is complicated because combination chemotherapy is generally utilized, patients may be systemically ill, and many receiving this medication have preexisting coronary artery disease.[35] The incidence of cardiac toxicity is uncertain but ranges from 1 to 8 percent.[36] Patients with known coronary artery disease are at higher risk for serious cardiotoxicity.[35] The mechanism of toxicity remains unclear, although coronary vasospasm has been suspected. Coronary catheterization has generally failed to demonstrate vasomotor hyperreactivity with 5-fluorouracil or ergonovine challenge.

Amsacrine (AMSA) has been associated with prolongation of the QT interval. Malignant ventricular arrhythmias may occur in 1 percent of patients and are exacerbated by hypokalemia.[37,38]

Paclitaxel (taxol) has been associated with arrhythmias, most notably bradycardias. Atrioventricular block and bundle branch block have also been reported.[39]

The biologic response modifiers, *interleukin (IL) 2* and *interferon alpha* have been associated with cardiovascular toxicity predominantly secondary to peripheral vasodilatation.[1] IL-2 causes tachycardia, hypotension, as well as a capillary leak syndrome. Myocarditis has been reported in patients who died soon after initiation of therapy. IL-2 therapy requires pretreatment assessment of cardiovascular risks and close monitoring during drug administration.[1,40,41] Interferon alpha may cause supraventricular tachyarrhythmias. A reversible cardiomyopathy has been described.[42]

Psychotropic Agents

Psychiatric illness, particularly depression, is common in patients with cardiovascular disease[43] (see Chap. 89). Morbidity and mortality following cardiac events are increased in patients with depression, particularly if untreated.[44,45] A variety of psychotropic agents have conduction or vascular effects. A thorough understanding of these therapeutic, but potentially toxic, agents is necessary in the treatment of patients with preexisting cardiac disease.[46] Intentional overdose with these drugs may result in serious cardiac manifestations.

TRICYCLIC ANTIDEPRESSANTS

The tricyclic antidepressants, including the tertiary (amitryptyline, clomipramine, doxepin, imipramine, trimipramine) and secondary (desipramine, nortriptyline, protriptyline) amines, have potentially serious cardiovascular effects. These effects include increased heart rate, orthostatic hypotension, ECG changes, and possible depression of ventricular function. These drugs have electrophysiologic properties similar to the type IA antiarrhythmics. Recent concerns have surfaced about the potential for late proarrhythmia in patients with structural heart disease who are taking these agents.[46]

The tricyclic antidepressants have several properties that account for the majority of cardiovascular effects. These drugs inhibit uptake of both norepinephrine and serotonin, resulting in greater toxicity compared to the selective serotonin reuptake inhibitors (SSRIs).[47] A hyperadrenergic state may result in tachycardia.[48] Alpha blockade occurs at higher drug levels and may cause marked hypotension in the setting of overdose.[49] The anticholinergic effects result in tachycardia, dry mouth, and constipation, and in overdose they may delay gastrointestinal absorption of the drug. Sodium channel blockade, typical of the type IA antiarrhythmic compounds, results in conduction abnormalities[50] and the potential to suppress ventricular function.

The most frequent side effect of tricyclic antidepressant treatment, orthostatic hypotension, is common in older patients and does not generally improve with reducing doses to lower levels that will still maintain antidepressant effects.[50] Orthostasis, mediated predominantly by alpha$_1$ blockade, may occur with all of these drugs but is less likely with nortriptyline.[51]

The most common electrocardiographic changes include nonspecific ST-T changes and prolongation of the QT interval,

PR interval, and QRS duration.[52] PR prolongation is due to prolonged infranodal conduction.[52,53] Patients with preexisting conduction disease, particularly bundle branch block, are at increased risk of toxicity.[54] The tricyclic antidepressants have type IA antiarrhythmic properties, and may potentially suppress ventricular ectopy. The results of recent antiarrhythmic studies, however, including those with type I agents, suggest the potential for a proarrhythmic effect for these drugs at therapeutic doses in patients with serious structural heart disease.[46,55,56] *Tricyclic antidepressants are generally contraindicated in the recovery phase following myocardial infarction. Although tricyclic antidepressant therapy may be indicated in the treatment of severely depressed patients, the threshold for use should rise as the severity of heart disease increases[46] or when there is QT prolongation.*

Tricyclic antidepressants may impair left ventricular function in patients with severe systolic dysfunction; however, decreases in left ventricular ejection fraction have generally not been noted in patients with moderately impaired function.[8] Severe orthostatic hypotension, especially with imipramine, may be more common in patients with myocardial dysfunction.[51]

Tricyclic antidepressant overdose carries a mortality of 2 to 3 percent, which is generally related to cardiac complications.[49] Clinical status at initial presentation and serum drug levels are not predictive of prognosis.[49] QRS prolongation is a sign of toxicity but may be absent in the patient with serious cardiac complications. Rightward deviation of the terminal 40 ms of the frontal plane QRS axis is a more sensitive marker. This finding, manifested by a terminal R wave in lead aV_R, has an 83 percent sensitivity and 63 percent specificity for toxicity.[57]

Aggressive support measures in tricyclic antidepressant overdose should be initiated immediately and include airway maintenance, gastric lavage, and repeated dosing of activated charcoal. Alkalinization with intravenous sodium bicarbonate decreases unbound drug and reverses cardiac and central nervous system conduction defects. Alkalinization is indicated in cardiac arrest, hypotension, arrhythmias, acidosis, and QRS duration ≥ 0.16 s.[49] Hypotension refractory to volume loading and bicarbonate therapy should be treated with vasopressors, including norepinephrine and phenylephrine, and with vasopressor doses of dopamine. *Type I antiarrhythmics (quinidine, procainamide, disopyramide) should not be used. Sodium bicarbonate is the initial therapy for ventricular dysrhythmias.*[49]

The duration of monitoring after tricyclic overdose is controversial. Signs of major toxicity generally occur within 6 h of presentation in the emergency department. If clinical or ECG evidence of toxicity is absent and two doses of activated charcoal have been given, patients may not require admission for medical monitoring.[58] Fluoxetine increases tricyclic antidepressant serum levels, and additional monitoring is recommended in patients receiving this medication.[59] Patients with cardiac disease or other serious medical problems may require a longer period of observation.

OTHER ANTIDEPRESSANTS

SSRIs have not been extensively studied in patients with cardiac disease. Case reports of cardiac toxicity are rare, despite the increasing popularity of these agents in the treatment of depression. These agents have rarely been associated with orthostatic hypotension and with bradycardia.[60] *The SSRIs may affect the cytochrome P450 system and may therefore alter the metabolism of a variety of drugs, including agents used in cardiovascular disease such as antiarrhythmic medications, beta blockers, calcium channel blockers, and warfarin.*

The monoamine oxidase (MAO) inhibitors have little effect on cardiac conduction or myocardial contractility. Orthostatic hypotension is common, particularly in elderly patients. The major concern with these agents is interaction with other drugs or tyramine-containing substances, resulting in hypertensive crisis.[61,62]

Lithium, used commonly in the treatment of bipolar disorder, is generally well tolerated in patients with cardiac disease. Suppression of sinus node automaticity, resulting in bradycardias, is the most common complication.[63,64] In patients free of known heart disease, clinically significant sinus node dysfunction occurs in fewer than 1 percent.[64] Preexisting sinus node disease or concomitant therapy with drugs altering sinus node function, however, may result in sinus bradycardia. Pacemaker therapy may be required to allow continuation of lithium therapy.

Lithium therapy has been associated with electrocardiographic changes simulating hypokalemia. T-wave inversion, prominent U waves, and QT prolongation may occur. PR prolongation, bundle branch block, and complete heart block are rare.[63,64] Overdose with lithium may result in severe bradycardias requiring temporary pacemaker therapy. *A low anion gap may suggest the presence of lithium toxicity*[65].

ANTIPSYCHOTIC AGENTS

The phenothiazine antipsychotic agents have potential cardiac toxicity similar to that of the tricyclic antidepressants.[66] These drugs may cause sinus tachycardia, PR and QT prolongation, and disturbances of intraventricular conduction. Chlorpromazine and thioridazine[67] are the most commonly implicated phenopthiazines as causes of torsades de pointes. The butyrophenone, haloperidol, is also associated with torsades de pointes at high doses given intravenously.[68]

Noncardiac Drugs and Toxic Antidepressants Causing Torsades de Pointes

As discussed above, the tricyclic, phenothiazine, and other psychotropic agents may prolong the QT interval and induce torsades de pointes. A variety of antiarrhythmic agents, particularly the type I agents, are most strongly associated with this potentially fatal arrhythmia. Other toxic causes of torsades de pointes[69–72] are listed in Table 80-2.

The antibiotics erythromycin and trimethoprim-sulfamethoxazole[70,71] have only rarely been associated with torsades

TABLE 80-2

NONCARDIAC DRUGS AND TOXINS KNOWN TO CAUSE TORSADES DE POINTES

Psychotropic Agents
   Tricyclic antidepressants
   Tetracyclic antidepressants
   Phenothiazines
   Haloperidol
   Chloral hydrate
Antibiotics
   Erythromycin
   Trimethoprim-sulfamethoxazole
Antihistamines
   Terfenadine
   Astemizole
Other
   Cisapride
   Pentamidine
   Probucol
   Arsenic
   Organophosphates
   Liquid protein diets

de pointes, the exception being the effect of erythromycin on the metabolism of terfenadine, astemizole, and cisapride. Liquid protein diets and starvation[73,74] may cause marked electrolyte and chemical disturbances, triggering QT prolongation. Probucol,[75] particularly in females, may prolong the QT interval, resulting in torsades de pointes.

The QT prolongation and torsades de pointes reported with the antihistamines terfenadine and astemizole[76] and with cisapride.[77] have been associated with high drug levels from excessive dosing or altered metabolism. These drugs are metabolized by the cytochrome P450 3A.[78,79] A variety of agents inhibit this isoenzyme including antifungals (ketoconazole, fluconazole, itraconazole), erythromycin or clarithromycin (not azithromycin), SSRIs (fluvoxamine, nefazodone, fluoxetine, sertaline), quinine, and grapefruit juice.[79] Serious cardiac arrhythmias have been reported in patients taking terfenadine, astemizole, or cisapride with drugs that inhibit cytochrome P450 3A isoenzyme. Patients with a history of prolonged QT interval or those with serious underlying cardiac disease are at higher risk for this problem.[76,77,80]

Methylxanthines and Beta-Adrenergic Agonists

The methylxanthines, caffeine and theophylline, have pharmacologic actions of central nervous system stimulation, bronchial smooth muscle relaxation, and cardiac muscle stimulation and have diuretic effects on the kidneys. At therapeutic doses, or those consumed in xanthine-containing beverages, these agents competitively inhibit adenosine receptors. At higher doses, they exhibit phosphodiesterase inhibition.[81] The effect of caffeine consumption on the cardiovascular system is variable and depends on chronicity of use, dose exposure, and individual responsiveness. Although elevations of catecholamines may occur with acute administration, this effect resolves with chronic usage.[81] At higher concentrations, caffeine may cause tachycardia and dysrhythmias. Despite the concern that caffeine may be detrimental in patients predisposed to cardiac rhythm disturbances,[82] it appears that moderate amounts of caffeine consumption may be well tolerated in patients with ventricular arrhythmias.[83] The role of coffee, with or without caffeine, as a risk factor for coronary artery disease has been debated. While heavy coffee drinking (>4 cups a day) has been suggested as a potential risk factor for cardiovascular mortality, the data are inconclusive.[81]

Theophylline has the potential to cause a slight increase in heart rate with minimal effects on blood pressure. Patients with obstructive lung disease commonly have atrial and ventricular arrhythmias, which can be exacerbated by theophylline therapy.[84] Theophylline toxicity is associated with sinus tachycardia, atrial and ventricular arrhythmias, and hypotension.[85] Hypokalemia, hypercalcemia, hyperglycemia, hypophosphatemia, and metabolic acidosis may occur.[85–87] Esmolol may be useful in the management of refractory arrhythmias.[86] Dialysis may be helpful in patients with refractory arrhythmias or hypotension.[87]

The beta-adrenergic agonists, terbutaline and albuterol, are commonly used to treat asthma and premature labor. Although adverse reactions are uncommon with aerosol therapy, they can cause tachycardia and atrial and ventricular arrhythmias and, rarely, may worsen angina pectoris.[88,89] Intravenous therapy may cause hypokalemia and acidosis.[90] Controversy exists over the safety of long-term aerosol therapy with beta-adrenergic agonists in asthma. These concerns, however, relate predominantly to airway hyperresponsiveness and not to direct cardiac toxicity.[91,92]

Ergotamine

The ergot alkaloids are commonly used in the treatment of migraine headaches. Ergotamine causes constriction of smooth muscle, and its effect on vascular smooth muscle may result in hypertension and increased peripheral vascular resistance.[93] Ergonovine maleate may be used in the catheterization laboratory to diagnose coronary artery spasm. Chronic use of ergotamine may result in variant angina[94] or myocardial infarction.[95] Severe circulatory disturbances of the upper and lower extremities and abdominal arteries have been described.[95] Ergotamine and methysergide have similar chemical structures. Valvular heart disease has been reported with both agents. Either may cause pericardial, pleural, or peritoneal fibrosis or multivalvular heart disease. The occurrence of these side effects is less frequent with ergotamine.[96,97]

Methysergide

Methysergide, used in treating vascular headaches, can cause retroperitoneal, pulmonary, and cardiac fibrosis. Cardiac involvement most commonly affects the valves but may affect the endocardium, myocardium, and rarely the aorta.[98–100] Regurgitant valvular lesions are most common,[99] affecting the mitral and aortic valves more commonly than the tricuspid and pulmonary valves.[98,99] Patients receiving methysergide therapy should be monitored for the development of murmurs. Therapy should be discontinued if a new murmur is detected. Regression of valvular lesions may occur, although valve replacement is occasionally required.[99] Patients with known valvular disease should not be given methysergide.[98]

Histamine H₂-Receptor Antagonists

The histamine H_2-receptor antagonists have rarely been associated with cardiac effects. Episodes of severe bradycardia have been reported as well as hypotension, asystole, and ventricular arrhythmias. These complications have generally occurred with large doses given intravenously.[101–103] Electrophysiologic studies have not demonstrated any direct effect on sinus node function.[104] It has been hypothesized that effects on cardiac H_2-receptors are the source of these infrequent problems.[105]

Chloroquine

The antimalarial agent, chloroquine, is commonly used to treat collagen vascular and dermatologic disorders. Irreversible retinal damage is the primary concern with long-term or high-dose therapy. Skeletal myopathy and less commonly cardiomyopathy may occur.[106,107] With cardiac involvement, features of restrictive cardiomyopathy are most common.[106] Myocardial biopsy with electron microscopy showing curvilinear and myeloid bodies is diagnostic. These findings may be seen on skeletal muscle biopsy.[106,107] The ECG may demonstrate T-wave changes and conduction abnormalities.[107] Acute chloroquine poisoning results in hypotension, tachycardia, and prolongation of the QRS and is often fatal.[108]

Oral Contraceptive Agents

Epidemiologic studies prior to the 1980s demonstrated that women using oral contraceptives had an increased risk of cardiovascular disease including venous thromboembolism, myocardial infarction, hypertension, and stroke.[109] Oral contraceptive formulations used in the 1960s and 1970s consisted of relatively high-dose estrogen. Although rare, the risk of myocardial infarction was increased approximately fourfold.[110] Women smokers, particularly those older than age 35, had a dramatically increased risk of infarction.[109] Coronary angiography done postinfarction not uncommonly demonstrated a discrete lesion in a single vessel or no obstructive lesions, suggesting acute thrombosis as a possible mechanism.[111,112] The risk of venous thromboembolism was 4 to 10 times that of nonusers during this era.[113]

Recent formulations of oral contraceptives consist of less than 50 μg of ethinyl estradiol in combination with a low-dose progestin. Recent studies suggest that these second- and third-generation combined oral contraceptives are much safer in terms of cardiovascular complications.[114] The risks of venous thromboembolism and myocardial infarction are significantly reduced compared to the first-generation agents.[115]

Hypertension is rare, and the risk of stroke in otherwise healthy women is only minimally increased.[116]

Third-generation oral contraceptives that contain desogestrol or gestodene reportedly have a 1.5 to 2.5 increased risk of venous thromboembolism compared with the second-generation agents. The significance of this finding has generated controversy, but generally, the cardiovascular risk profile of these agents is considered favorable.[114,115,117]

Anabolic Steroids

Illicit use of androgens has been identified as a problem in competitive athletes and body builders. It is estimated that 300,000 persons in the United States have had recent steroid use and over 1 million have had prior use.[118,119] Anabolic steroids, including testosterone, stanozolol, and nandrolone, are frequently used in combination and at high doses for intermittent periods of several weeks to months. Doses commonly exceed 100 times the doses used for medical purposes.[118,120] Animal data indicate that these agents can cause abnormal lipids, left ventricular hypertrophy, increased blood volume, and hypertension.[121] Data on human toxicity are limited. Stanozolol and nandrolone reduce total high-density lipoprotein levels by over 50 percent and increase low-density lipoprotein levels by over 30 percent.[122] Isolated reports of young men (<age 35) developing severe coronary atherosclerosis, myocardial infarctions, or stroke exist in the literature.[118,121,123] Because of the secrecy surrounding the use of these agents, the full clinical significance of abuse is not known.

Cocaine

Cocaine is a common drug of abuse and has potentially lethal cardiac toxicity. It is estimated that over 30 million Americans have used cocaine at least once and that 5 million use it regularly.[124] Cocaine may be swallowed, inhaled nasally, smoked, or injected intravenously. Cardiovascular toxicity is broad, ranging from sudden death to chronic cardiomyopathy.[125] A summary of the cardiovascular syndrome associated with illicit cocaine use is shown in Table 80-3. Use of cocaine with other drugs such as ethanol[126] or tobacco[127] may have combined detrimental effects.

Cocaine has a generalized sympathomimetic effect and has local anesthetic properties.[125] Cocaine blocks the reuptake of norepinephrine and dopamine on preganglionic sympathetic nerve terminals. This produces sympathetic stimulation both centrally and peripherally. These catecholamine effects acutely result in tachycardia, hypertension, increased myocardial contractility, and vascular constriction. The local anesthetic effect, occurring through blockade of the fast sodium channel, results in slowed conduction in myocardial tissues. This may result in electrocardiographic abnormalities including prolongation of the PR, QRS, and QT intervals similar to that seen with toxicity from type I antiarrhythmic agents. These effects increase the vulnerability to reentrant ventricular arrhythmias.[124,125,128]

Cocaine may result in increased thrombogenicity.[125,127]

TABLE 80-3

CARDIOVASCULAR COMPLICATIONS OF COCAINE

Sudden death
Acute myocardial infarction
Chest pain without myocardial infarction
Accelerated coronary atherosclerosis
Intimal hyperplasia of coronary vessels
Electrocardiographic abnormalities
   Sinus tachycardia
   Premature ventricular complexes
   Ventricular tachycardia
   Torsades de pointes
   Ventricular fibrillation
   Prolongation of QT interval
   Early repolarization (ST-segment changes)
Acute reversible myocarditis
Dilated cardiomyopathy
Acute severe hypertension
Acute aortic dissection, rupture
Pneumopericardium
Stroke
Subarachnoid hemorrhage
Endocarditis (intravenous use)

Platelet aggregation is enhanced and endothelial function is altered, resulting in the potential for development of coronary thrombosis in the absence of coronary atherosclerosis. Chronic use of cocaine is associated with premature coronary atherosclerosis.[125,129] Cocaine indirectly causes constriction of both diseased and nondiseased coronary artery segments, but its effect is more marked in diseased vessels.[130] Ethanol use and tobacco smoking may worsen the potential for vasospasm.[126,127] Up to one-third of reported cases of patients with cocaine-induced myocardial infarctions have normal coronary arteries.[125] The combined cardiac effects, including early coronary atherosclerosis, coronary vasospasm, increased thrombogenicity, increased myocardial oxygen demands, and proarrhythmic effects, make this drug a lethal threat to users of all ages.

Cocaine may have direct or indirect myocardial toxicity. Animal studies suggest a direct negative inotropic effect on the heart, possibly related to its local anesthetic properties.[125] Chronic dosing has demonstrated myocardial contraction bands, myofibrillar disorganization, interstitial edema, and mitochondrial swelling. Mononuclear infiltrates have been noted.[125,131] Myocardial changes may mimic those seen with catecholamine excess as in pheochromocytoma. Clinical case reports have described transient toxic cardiomyopathy, acute myocarditis, and permanently dilated cardiomyopathy.[125]

Chest pain is the most common reason for cocaine users to seek medical attention. Over 64,000 patients are evaluated annually for cocaine-related chest pain, of whom over half are admitted to the hospital.[132] The evaluation of cocaine-related chest pain is difficult. Prospective studies demonstrate that approximately 6 percent of patients presenting to the emergency room with cocaine-related chest pain have myocar-

dial infarction.[124] These patients are often young men without other risk factors for coronary artery disease except for tobacco smoking. The duration and quality of discomfort does not readily distinguish those eventually noted to have enzyme documentation of infarction. Many young patients have early repolarization patterns, with ST elevation in leads V_1 to V_3, a normal variant that may be confused with acute infarction. Infarction has been noted in patients with normal or nonspecific ECGs. Because of the difficulty in excluding myocardial infarctions, patients are often monitored for a period of at least 12 h until enzymes have excluded infarction.[124]

Treatment strategies for cocaine-induced myocardial ischemia have been developed based on the known cardiac and nervous system toxicity of the drug.[124,128] Randomized prospective trials of therapy do not exist. Patients presenting with anxiety, tachycardia, or hypertension may respond well to benzodiazepines. Nitroglycerin may reverse coronary vasoconstriction induced by cocaine. Aspirin may prevent thrombus formation. Patients not responding to these measures may benefit from the alpha-adrenergic antagonist phentolamine or from calcium channel blocker therapy with verapamil.[124] Beta-adrenergic antagonists should be avoided because of enhanced coronary vasoconstriction and the potential for unopposed alpha-mediated hypertensive crisis.[124,133] Combined alpha and beta blockade with labetalol has been utilized to treat tachyarrhythmias, but is not an accepted therapy for myocardial ischemia.[124]

In documented myocardial infarction, thrombolytic therapy is highly effective; however, over 40 percent of patients without infarction will meet accepted electrocardiographic criteria for use of lytic therapy.[134] The early repolarization pattern common in young men makes diagnosis difficult, particularly when a prior ECG is not available. Thrombolytic therapy carries increased risk of hemorrhagic stroke in patients with recently uncontrolled hypertension. Therefore, emergent coronary angiography may be necessary to document coronary occlusion and direct strategies such as primary angioplasty or thrombolysis[124] (see Chap. 47).

Management of supraventricular or ventricular tachyarrhythmias may be facilitated by administration of benzodiazepines. Beta blockade with propranolol or esmolol should be avoided. Rhythm disturbances may be exacerbated by acidosis or electrolyte disorders. Intravenous sodium bicarbonate and magnesium may be beneficial. Lidocaine should be used cautiously because of concerns of lowered seizure threshold and potential proarrhythmic effects following recent cocaine use.[128]

Patients with cocaine-associated chest pain not related to myocardial infarction have a favorable 1-year prognosis, particularly if cocaine use is discontinued. Urgent diagnostic cardiac evaluation is not generally recommended. Unfortunately, recurrent cocaine use after cocaine-associated chest pain occurs in over 60 percent of cases.[124]

Metamphetamines

The biologic effects of metamphetamines are similar to cocaine, but vasoconstriction is less.[135] Cardiovascular toxicity is common and includes tachycardia, hypertension, and arrhythmias. Chest pain and myocardial infarction are less common than with cocaine.[136] Chronic use may result in a catecholamine-mediated dilated cardiomyopathy.[137]

Ethanol

(See Chap. 77)

ELECTRICITY INJURY

Environmental Accidents

Accidental contact with electricity may occur in the home, where young children are particularly vulnerable.[138] Job-related electrical injuries are most common in construction and electrical workers but also on any job in which electrical equipment is used, including the healthcare setting. Approximately 1200 deaths related to domestic electrical injury occur each year in the United States.[139] There are two to three times as many serious injuries, including burns and neurologic complications.[139,140] Lightning kills at least 100 people per year in the United States, representing a 30 percent mortality rate in reported cases. Lightning injuries generally occur between May and September in the late afternoon hours and affect predominantly young people involved in outdoor recreational activities.[141] Death following electrical shock is usually secondary to immediate cardiac rhythm disturbances, although later cardiac complications secondary to internal injury may occur.

PATHOPHYSIOLOGY

The degree of total body injury from electricity is determined by the amount of current delivered, tissue resistance, and duration of contact.[140] Specific organs or tissues injured are in part determined by the path of the current. Electrical injuries are classified as high voltage ($>$1000 V) or low voltage ($<$1000 V). High-voltage electrical wires and household current (120 or 220 V) are alternating currents (AC) that may result in prolonged exposure due to tetatanic muscle contractions and inability to the victim to "let go." The frequencies of domestically generated AC (50 to 60 cycles per second) result in an increased risk for ventricular fibrillation even at household voltages.[139] Sources of domestic direct current (DC) are usually low voltage (3 to 24 V), including batteries, appliance transformers, and portable emergency generators, and are less likely to cause injury. Lightning is extremely high-voltage, direct current of brief duration.

Heat injury tissue necrosis is more severe with high-voltage AC. These burns are often internal and may mimic crush injuries.[142] Tissue resistance to current flow is least in nervous and vascular tissues, and therefore the heart and neurovascular bundles may serve as conduits for electrical current through the thorax.[143] Arm-to-arm pathway of current is associated with greater risk for cardiac injury, followed by arm-to-leg pathways determined by entry and exit sites. A stride potential, leg-to-leg, is infrequently associated with cardiac effects.[139]

CARDIOVASCULAR EFFECTS

Lightning injuries result from brief, high-voltage direct current. Immediate death may be secondary to asystole or ventricular fibrillation or result from apnea secondary to injury of the central respiratory centers. Lightning strikes may occur by a direct hit, side splash, or ground strike. Direct hits cause mechanical trauma to organs secondary to dissipated energy.[140] Strikes to the chest can result in severe, often reversible global myocardial dysfunction or localized myocardial contusion. Electrocardiographic abnormalities, including QT_c prolongation and ST-T abnormalities, may be the result of cardiac or neurologic injury. ST elevation has been noted with direct strikes. Other conduction abnormalities, including right bundle branch block and complete heart block, have been noted.[141] Pericardial effusions may develop following direct strikes. Elevated levels of CK-MB are generally noted.[140,141] Splash strikes in which a tree or other object is hit prior to the victim being hit are associated with CK-MB release in two-thirds of patients and nonspecific ST-T changes. Severe myocardial injury is unlikely unless there is a short distance between the directly hit object and the victim. Ground strikes generally do not cause a significant cardiac injury but may be associated with nonspecific ST-T abnormalities.[141]

Domestic alternating current accidents may cause myocardial necrosis and conduction abnormalities. An injury pattern mimicking infarction may be seen on the ECG but is generally related to direct myocardial injury and not coronary thrombosis.[139] Household voltages (120 to 220 V) may cause sudden death, particularly when they involve arm-to-arm pathways or low skin resistance in a wet victim. Serious myocardial damage is rare.[138]

Treatment for cardiac arrest should be initiated immediately after the patient is disconnected from the current source, and resuscitation efforts should be continued for a prolonged period. In lightning strikes involving multiple victims, attention should be directed first to those who are "apparently dead."[143,144] This is because there is a higher resuscitation rate for these individuals compared to those with medical cardiac arrest, and lightning victims with vital signs generally survive without immediate medical attention.

Patients surviving high-voltage injuries generally require admission, usually for attention to neurologic complications and internal or external burn injuries or for cardiac monitoring. *An initially normal ECG carries a favorable cardiac prognosis* leading some authors to question the need for 24-h electrocardiographic monitoring. Patients with arm-to-arm or arm-to-leg passage of current may be at risk for postadmission rhythm disturbances, and a higher index of suspicion is required in such patients.[145]

Adults and children presenting to the emergency department following low-voltage shocks of less than 240 V have a low incidence of myocardial injury, and most do not require further monitoring.[138]

Electroconvulsive Therapy

Electroconvulsive therapy (ECT) is accepted therapy for a variety of psychiatric illnesses including depression resistant to pharmacologic therapy, severe suicidal ideation with vegetative signs, acute mania, and depression with intolerance to medication side effects secondary to cardiac problems.[146] ECT is performed with a brief unilateral or bilateral electrical stimulus to the brain while the patient is under short-acting anesthesia with a hypnotic drug and a muscle depolarizing agent.[147] ECT produces brief, intense stimulation of the central nervous system. Cardiovascular complications may result from this stimulation or from the drugs used to modify the response.[148–150]

Initially, the ECT stimulus activates the vagus nerve and may produce bradycardia, hypotension, and rarely asystole.[151,152] Sympathetic discharge occurs, which is amplified by a 15-fold rise in epinephrine and 3-fold rise in norepinephrine levels, resulting in tachycardia and hypertension.[151] Transient atrial and ventricular tachyarrhythmias may occur in approximately 10 percent of patients with known or suspected cardiovascular disease.[152] Transient electrocardiographic alterations, including ST-T-wave changes, QRS changes, QT prolongation, and peaked T waves, may occur.[151–155]

The mortality rate of ECT is less than 3 in 10,000, and the complication rate is approximately 0.3 percent.[150] Patients with severe heart disease may successfully undergo ECT with acceptable risk.[151] Prior to ECT, electrolyte abnormalities should be corrected and systemic hypertension should be controlled. Patients with pulmonary disease require special evaluation because hypoxia and respiratory acidosis may precipitate cardiovascular events.[146]

Following ECT, hypertension and tachycardia may be controlled with adrenergic blockade with intravenous labetolol[156] or esmolol.[150] Other antihypertensive agents such as clonidine or calcium channel blockers may be utilized. Sustained ventricular arrhythmias are treated with lidocaine, but pretreatment with lidocaine is not indicated.[146] Patients with cardiac pacemakers can safely undergo ECT.[157,158] Currently used pacemakers are not likely to be affected by ECT current.[157] Although these newer devices have not been systematically studied, the 50 to 100 W delivered to the scalp during ECT are probably inadequate to reprogram current pacemakers.

Lithotripsy

Extracorporeal shock wave lithotripsy used to treat renal stones and gallstones has the potential to cause cardiac arrhythmias. Rhythm disturbances may be related to electrical stimulus from the shock wave or from enhanced vagal tone associated with the procedure.[159–163] Electrocardiographic monitoring is recommended for patients with cardiac disease. Gating of the shock waves to the QRS cycle may be necessary in high-risk patients, although ungated lithotripsy with newer devices is reportedly safe in most patients.[161]

POISONS

Plants

A variety of plants contain active cardiac glycosides. Ingestion of these plants may result in a clinical presentation similar to digoxin toxicity, including gastrointestinal and visual disturbances as well as dysrhythmias. Plants with cardiac glycoside–like effects[163,164] are listed (Table 80-4).

Aconite is a herb that activates sodium channels in excitable tissues. Ingestion of Chinese herbs containing aconite alkaloids may cause bradyarrhythmias, ventricular arrhythmias, and sudden death.[165] The larkspur (*Delphinium*) contains delphinine and may cause myocardial depression and arrhythmias.[164]

Snakes and Scorpions

Snake bites cause fewer than 15 deaths per year in the United States but over 40,000 deaths per year worldwide. The majority of lethal snake bites occur in Asia, South America, and Africa.[166] Snake venoms contain a variety of enzymes and toxins that may affect the nervous system, blood vessels, coagulation systems, or the heart.[166,167] The majority of deaths are from the elapids (cobra, mamba, coral snake, taipan), which cause severe neuromuscular toxicity. Cardiotoxins are present in variable amounts in snake venom. Cobra venoms may cause augmentation of myocardial contraction at low concentration and asystole at high concentration.[166] Rattlesnake venom may affect myocardial sodium channels and depress myocardial contractility.[166,168] These venoms may cause pulmonary hypertension.[168]

Scorpion stings are a common medical problem in areas including India, Southeast Asia, the southwestern United States, Mexico, and Israel.[169] Venoms from different families have different toxicities. The *Buthidae* venoms, primarily neurotoxic, result in spontaneous sympathetic and parasympathetic depolarization. Massive catecholamine release may cause cardiac toxicity including tachycardia, hypertension, arrhythmias, and myocardial impairment.[166,169,170]

Arthropods

Direct cardiac effects related to bee, hornet, and wasp stings are difficult to establish.[171] Cardiac complications, including arrhythmias, are generally related to anaphylaxis or epineph-

---

TABLE 80-4

PLANTS WITH CARDIAC GLYCOSIDE EFFECTS

Foxglove (*Digitalis purpurea, D. Lanata*)
Oleander (*Nerium oleander*)
Lily-of-the-valley (*Convallaria majolis*)
Christmas rose (*Helleborus niger*)
Wallflower (*Cheirina cheiri*)
Milkweed (*Asclepias* sp.)

rine administration.[171] Animal studies of bee venom toxicity suggest direct cardiac effects.[172]

Marine Toxins

Marine toxin exposure may have serious cardiovascular effects.[173] Scorpion fish cause envenomation that may result in sympathetic and parasympathetic discharges. Rhythm disturbances and heart failure may result. Stingray venom contains phosphodiesterases and has rarely been associated with cardiac rhythm disturbances. Ingestion of sea cucumber, which contains holothurin, may result in cardiac glycoside toxicity. Ingestion of pufferfish, which contains tetrodotoxin, may result in vascular collapse and severe bradycardia.[173]

Halogenated Hydrocarbons

Halogenated hydrocarbons are used in fire extinguishers, solvents, and refrigerants and in the manufacture of pesticides and plastics. Heavy acute exposure to these compounds may result in cardiac arrhythmias and sudden death.[174] Direct cardiac effects include depression of myocardial contractility[175] and sensitization to the arrhythmogenic effects of catecholamines. Indirect cardiotoxicity may result from hypoxia or central nervous system toxicity.

Organophosphates

Organophosphates, used commercially in pesticides, are powerful inhibitors of acetylcholinesterase, and this inhibition can result in parasympathetic overstimulation. Deaths are generally related to respiratory failure. Cardiac arrhythmias have been noted up to 15 days after exposure. Cardiac toxicity is generally associated with QT prolongation. Torsades de pointes, atrioventricular conduction disturbances, and ST-T abnormalities have been noted. Direct myocardial toxicity has been postulated, in addition to cholinergic hyperactivity.[176]

Carbon Monoxide

Toxicity from carbon monoxide is related to tissue hypoxia. Carbon monoxide has a much higher affinity for hemoglobin than does oxygen, preventing adequate oxygen exchange. Carbon monoxide exposure worsens angina pectoris and increases the risk of myocardial infarction.[177] Carbon monoxide poisoning results in electrocardiographic abnormalities, including sinus tachycardia, atrial fibrillation, atrioventricular block, and ST-T abnormalities. Cardiac enzyme elevation may occur. Severe exposure can result in myocardial necrosis and cardiomyopathy.[178] Transient evidence of cardiac toxicity, however, is not necessarily associated with long-term sequelae.[179]

RADIATION

Mediastinal radiation, commonly used to treat Hodgkin's disease, lung cancer, breast cancer, and seminoma, may result in acute or late cardiac sequelae. Prior to the 1960s, the heart was thought to be resistant to the effects of clinical radiation.[180] It is now recognized that a variety of cardiac problems may result from radiation, including acute or chronic pericardial disease, coronary atherosclerosis, myocardial dysfunction, conduction defects, and, occasionally, valvular dysfunction[181–185] (Table 80-5).

The incidence of radiation-induced heart disease is influenced by several factors, including total radiation dose, fraction size, volume of heart irradiated, concomitant anthracycline use, and presence of mediastinal tumor.[181] Improved radiation techniques have diminished the occurrence of acute or chronic cardiac toxicity.[184] Cardiac injury has generally been associated with doses above 40 Gy.[181] Increased toxicity is associated with radiation for Hodgkin's disease, where larger volumes of the heart are irradiated, compared to the small cardiac exposure given as adjuvant treatment for breast carcinoma. Large doses per fraction and anterior-weighted fields result in greater toxicity.[184]

Pericardial disease is the most common manifestation of radiation toxicity to the heart. With the current techniques of subcarinal shielding, equal weighting of anterior and posterior ports, and limiting the dose to less than 30 Gy, the incidence of clinical pericarditis is approximately 2.5 percent.[184] Anatomic changes of the pericardium occur in the majority of patients but are clinically silent. Clinically apparent pericarditis is most frequent 4 to 6 months after therapy. Acute pericarditis, asymptomatic pericardial effusion, or pericardial tamponade may occur. Other etiologies of pericarditis should be considered, particularly malignant involvement of the pericardium. Pericarditis occurring during treatment of a mediastinal mass contiguous to the heart is generally secondary to tumor effects and does not correlate with late pericardial complications.[186,187]

Radiation may cause an exudative pericarditis. Cellular infiltrate is uncommon. Pericardial fibrosis may follow secondary to fibroblast proliferation and collagen deposition. The majority of patients with pericardial effusion clear spontaneously.[181] Constrictive pericarditis may occur months to years after pericardial effusion or may develop in patients without previously recognized pericardial disease.

The majority of patients with pericardial disease have a relatively benign course. Treatment is based on symptoms, including pericardiocentesis for tamponade and antipyretics for fever. Animal data suggest possible benefit from steroids.[181]

TABLE 80-5

RADIATION-INDUCED CARDIAC DISEASE

Pericardial
  Acute pericarditis
  Chronic pericarditis
  Pericardial constriction
Coronary atherosclerosis
Restrictive cardiomyopathy
Dilated cardiomyopathy (concomitant anthracyclines)
Conduction disease
Valvular abnormalities

The surgical management of postirradiation constrictive pericarditis is difficult. Extensive mediastinal and pericardial fibrosis make pericardiectomy technically challenging. Surgical morbidity and mortality are significant.[188] Radiation-induced constriction is often associated with coronary atherosclerosis, myocardial dysfunction, or conduction and valvular abnormalities. Comorbid cardiac or general medical conditions should be considered when selecting patients for pericardiectomy.

Clinically important myocardial dysfunction related to radiation generally occurs in combination with pericardial disease.[181] Asymptomatic patients may have varying degrees of myocardial fibrosis. The anterior right ventricle is most susceptible. Areas of fibrosis may be patchy or diffuse. Noninvasive techniques such as echocardiography may show mild impairment of systolic function; however, this is usually not clinically significant.[189] Diastolic abnormalities may occur due to fibrosis. Restrictive cardiomyopathy has been reported but is rare.[181] Premature coronary artery disease may result from radiation therapy, particularly in patients who were irradiated in an era when cardioprotective techniques were not used. Several series have reported a significant increased risk of coronary artery disease years following therapeutic radiation involving cardiac exposure.[190–193] The Stockholm Trial demonstrated increased mortality secondary to coronary artery disease in women receiving high-dose radiation to the heart as adjuvant therapy for carcinoma of the left breast.[192] A review of 635 patients at Stanford treated for Hodgkin's Disease before age 21 between the years 1961 and 1991 showed a significantly increased risk for myocardial infarction.[193] It is not clear, however, whether present techniques of mediastinal radiation will result in a clinically significant increase in coronary events.[181] Percutaneous angioplasty and coronary bypass surgery have been successful in selected patients. The commonly associated mediastinal and pericardial fibrosis, however, make surgical revascularization more difficult.

Clinically significant valvular heart disease secondary to radiation is rare but, when present, usually involves the aortic or mitral valves.[181,182] Fibrous thickening of the cardiac valves has been noted at autopsy. This fibrous thickening often causes asymptomatic aortic or mitral regurgitation.[184] Coexisting pericardial disease is the rule. Symptoms related to valvular dysfunction have been noted to occur 15 to 40 years after radiation treatment. Surgical reports are rare and most commonly are for replacement of the aortic valve due to aortic stenosis.[182]

Radiation may result in fibrosis of the nodal and infranodal pathways. Complete atrioventricular block, right bundle branch block, and, less commonly, left bundle branch block may occur. Progression to complete heart block is rare.[184,190]

REFERENCES

1. Frishman WH, Sung HM, Yee HCM, Liu LL, Keefe DL, Einzig AI, et al. Cardiovascular toxicity with cancer chemotherapy. *Curr Probl Cardiol* 1996; 21:225–288.

2. Speyer JL, Freedberg R. Toxicities of therapy: Cardiac complications. In: Abeloff MD, Armitage JO, Lichter AS, Niederhuber JE, eds. *Clinical Oncology*. New York: Churchill Livingstone; 1995; 809–819.

3. Shan K, Lincoff AM, Young JB. Anthracycline-induced cardiomyopathy. *Ann Intern Med* 1996; 125:47–58.

4. Antibiotics: Doxorubicin HCl In: Cada DJK, eds. *Drug Facts and Comparisons*, 48th ed. St. Louis: Facts and Comparisons; 1994:2705.

5. Von Hoff DD, Layard MW, Basa P, Davis HL Jr, Von Hoff AL, Rozencweig M, et al. Risk factors for doxorubicin-induced congestive heart failure. *Ann Intern Med* 1979; 91:710–717.

6. Bristow MR, Mason JW, Billingham ME, Daniels JR. Doxorubicin cardiomyopathy: Evaluation of phonocardiography, endomyocardial biopsy, and cardiac catheterization. *Ann Intern Med* 1978; 88:168–175.

7. Minow RA, Benjamin RS, Lee ET, Gottlieb JA. Adriamycin cardiomyopathy—risk factors. *Cancer* 1977; 39:1397–1402.

8. Fisher B, Redmond C, Wickerham DL, Bowman D, Schipper H, Wolmark N, et al. Doxorubicin-containing regimens for the treatment of stage II breast cancer: The National Surgical Adjuvant Breast and Bowel Project experience. *J Clin Oncol* 1989; 7:572–582.

9. Lipschultz SE, Lipsitz SR, Mone SM, et al. Female sex and higher drug dose as risk factors for late cardiotoxic effects of doxorubicin therapy for childhood cancer. *N Engl J Med* 1995; 332:1738–1743.

10. Torti FM, Bristow MR, Howes AE, Aston D, Stockdale FE, Carter SK, et al. Reduced cardiotoxicity of doxorubicin delivered on a weekly schedule. Assessment by endomyocardial biopsy. *Ann Intern Med* 1983; 99:745–749.

11. Olson RD, Mushlin PS. Doxorubicin cardiotoxicity: Analysis of prevailing hypotheses. *FASEB J* 1990; 4:3076–3086.

12. Mimnaugh EG, Trush MA, Bhatnagar, Gram TE. Enhancement of reactive oxygen-dependent mitochondrial membrane lipid peroxidation by the anticancer drug adriamycin. *Biochem Pharmacol* 1985; 34:847–856.

13. Muindi JR, Sinha BK, Gianni L, Myers CE. Hydroxyl radical production and DNA damage induced by anthracycline-iron complex. *FEBS Lett* 1984; 172:226–230.

14. Mortensen SA, Olsen HA, Baandrup U. Chronic anthracycline cardiotoxicity: Hemodynamic and histopathological manifestations suggesting a restrictive endomyocardial disease. *Br Heart J* 1986; 55:274–282.

15. Moreg JS, Oglon DJ. Outcomes of clinical congestive heart failure induced by anthracycline chemotherapy. *Cancer* 1992; 70:2637–2641.

16. Cohen M, Kronzon I, Lebowitz A. Reversible doxorubicin-induced congestive heart failure. *Arch Intern Med* 1982; 142:1570–1571.

17. Steinherz J, Graham T, Hurwitz R, Sondheimer HM, Schwartz RG, Shaffer EM, et al. Guidelines for cardiac monitoring of children during and after anthracycline therapy: Report of the Cardiology Committee of the Children's Cancer Study Group. *Pediatrics* 1992; 89:942–949.

18. Alexander J, Dainiak N, Berger HJ, Goldman L, Johnstone D, Reduto L, et al. Serial assessment of doxorubicin cardiotoxicity with quantitative radionuclide angiocardiography. *N Engl J Med* 1979; 300:278–283.

19. Weegner KM, Bledsoe M, Chauvenet A, Wofford M. Exercise echocardiography in the detection of anthracycline cardiotoxicity. *Cancer* 1991; 68:435–438.

20. Stoddard MF, Seeger J, Liddell NE, Hadley TJ, Sullivan DM, Kupersmith J. Prolongation of isovolumetric relaxation time as assessed by doppler echocardiography predicts doxorubicin-induced systolic dysfunction in humans. *J Am Coll Cardiol* 1992; 20:62–69.

21. Schwartz RG, McKenzie WB, Alexander J, Sager P, D'souza A, Mantunga A, et al. Congestive heart failure and left ventricular dysfunction complicating doxorubicin therapy: Seven-year experience using radionuclide angiocardiography. *Am J Med* 1987; 82:1109–1118.

22. McKillop JH, Bristow MR, Goris ML, Billingham ME, Bockemuehl K. Sensitivity and specificity of radionuclide ejection fraction in doxorubicin cardiotoxicity. *Am Heart J* 1983; 106:1048–1056.

23. Mason JW, Bristow MR, Billingham ME, Daniels JR. Invasive and noninvasive methods of assessing adriamycin cardiotoxic effects in man: Superiority of histopathologic assessment using endomyocardial biopsy. *Cancer Treat Rep* 1978; 62:857–864.

24. Isner JM, Ferrans VJ, Cohen SR, Witkind BG, Virmani R, Gott-Diener JS, et al. Clinical and morphologic cardiac findings after anthracycline chemotherapy: Analysis of 64 patients studied at necropsy. *Am J Cardiol* 1983;51:1167–1174.

25. Steinherz LJ, Steinherz PG, Tan CTC, Heller G, Murphy ML. Cardiac toxicity 4 to 20 years after completing anthracycline therapy. *JAMA* 1991; 266:1672–1677.

26. Leandro J, Dyck J, Poppe D, Shore R, Airhart C, Greenberg M, et al. Cardiac dysfunction late after cardiotoxic therapy for childhood cancer. *Am J Cardiol* 1994; 74:1152–1156.

27. Klewer SE, Goldberg SJ, Donnerstein RL, Berg RA, Hutter JJ Jr. Dobutamine stress echocardiography, a sensitive indicator of diminished myocardial function in asymptomatic doxorubicin-treated long term survivors of childhood cancer. *J Am Coll Cardiol* 1992; 19:394–401.

28. Legha SS, Benjamin RS, MacKay B, Ewer M, Wallace S, Valdivieso M, et al. Reduction of doxorubicin cardiotoxicity by prolonged continuous intravenous infusion. *Ann Intern Med* 1982; 89:133–139.

29. Myers C, Bonow R, Palmeri S, Jenkins J, Corden B, Locker G, et al. A randomized control trial assessing the prevention of doxorubicin cardiomyopathy by *N*-acetylcysteine. *Semin Oncol* 1983; 10:53–55.

30. Siveski-Iliskovic N, Hill M, Chow DA, Signal PK. Probucol protects against adriamycin cardiomyopathy without interfering with its antitumor effect. *Circulation* 1995; 91:10–155.

31. Seifert CF, Nesser ME, Thompson DF. Dexrazoxane in the prevention of doxorubicin-induced cardiotoxicity. *Ann Pharmacother* 1994; 28:1063–1072.

32. Benjamin RS. Rationale for the use of mitoxantrone in the older patient: Cardiac toxicity. *Semin Oncol* 1995; 22:11–13.

33. Ayash LJ, Wright JE, Tretyakov O, Gonin R, Elias A. Cyclophosphamide pharmacokinetics: Correlation with cardiac toxicity and tumor response. *Clin Oncol* 1992; 10:995–1000.

34. Gottdiener JS, Appelbaum FA, Ferrans VJ, Deisseroth A, Ziegler J. Cardiotoxicity associated with high-dose cyclophosphamide therapy. *Arch Intern Med* 1981; 141:758–763.

35. Robben NC, Pippas AW, Moore JO. The syndrome of 5-fluorouracil cardiotoxicity: An exclusive cardiopathy. *Cancer* 1993; 71:493–509.

36. Akhtar SS, Salim KP, Bano ZA. Symptomatic cardiotoxicity with high dose 5-fluorouracil infusion: A prospective study. *Oncology* 1993; 50:441–445.

37. McLaughlin P, Salvador PG, Cabanillas F, Legha SS. Ventricular fibrillation following AMSA. *Cancer* 1983; 52:557–558.

38. Weiss RB, Grillo-Lopez AJ, Marsoni S, Posada JG Jr, Hess F, Ross BJ. Amsacrine-associated cardiotoxicity: An analysis of 82 cases. *J Clin Oncol* 1986; 4:918–928.

39. Biadi O, Mengozzi G, Gherarducci G, Strata G, Mariani M, Baldini F, et al. Evaluation of taxol cardiotoxicity in metastatic breast cancer. *Ann NY Acad Sci* 1993; 698:403–405.

40. Kruit WH, Punt KJ, Goey H, de Mulder PH, Hoogenhuyze DC, Henzen-Logmans SC, et al. Cardiotoxicity as a dose-limiting factor in a schedule of high dose bolus therapy with interleukin-2 and alpha-interferon. *Cancer* 1994; 74:2850–2856.

41. DuBois JS, Udelson JE, Atkins B. Severe reversible, global and regional ventricular dysfunction associated with high-dose interleukin-2 immunotherapy. *J Immunother* 1995; 18:119–123.

42. Vial T, Descotes J. Clinical toxicity of the interferons. *Drug Safety* 1994; 10:115–150.

43. Roose SP, Dalak GW. Treating the depressed patient with cardiovascular problems. *J Clin Psychiatry* 1992; 53(9, suppl):25–31.

44. Fraser-Smith N, Lesperance F, Talajic M. Depression following myocardial infarction: Impact on 6-month survival. *JAMA* 1993; 270:1819–1825.

45. Carney RM, Rich MW, Freedland KE, Saini J, Te Velde A, Simeone C, Clark K. Major depressive disorder predicts cardiac events in patients with coronary artery disease. *Psychosom Med* 1988; 50:627–633.

46. Glassman AH, Roose SP, Bigger JT. The safety of tricyclic antidepressants in cardiac patients—risk benefit reconsidered. *JAMA* 1993; 269:2673–2675.

47. Franco-Bronson K. The management of treatment-resistant depression in the medically ill. *Psychiatr Clin North Am* 1996; 19:329–348.

48. Cole JO, Bodkin JA. Antidepressant drug side effects. *J Clin Psychiatry* 1990; 51(1, suppl):21–26.

49. Pimentel L, Trummer L. Cyclic antidepressant overdoses: a review. *Emerg Med Clin North Am* 1994; 12:533–547.

50. Glassman AH, Preud'home XA. Review of the cardiovascular effects of heterocyclic antidepressants. *J Clin Psychiatry* 1983; 54(2, suppl):16–22.

51. Roose SP, Glassman AH, Siris SG, Walsh BT, Bruno BT, Wright LB. Comparison of imipramine- and nortriptyline-induced orthostatic hypotension: A meaningful difference. *J Clin Psychopharmacol* 1981; 1:316–319.

52. Jefferson JW. Cardiovascular effects and toxicity of anxiolytics and antidepressants. *J Clin Psychiatry* 1989; 50:368–378.

53. Rawling DA, Fozzard HA. Electrophysiological effects of imipramine on cellular electrophysiological properties of cardiac Purkinje fibers. *J Pharmacol Exp Ther* 1979; 209:371–375.

54. Roose SP, Glassman AH, Gardina EGV, Walsh BT, Woodring S, Bisser JT. Tricyclic antidepressants in depressed patients with cardiac conduction disease. *Arch Gen Psychiatry* 1987; 44:273–275.

55. The Cardiac Arrhythmia Suppression Trial II Investigators. Effect of the antiarrhythmic agent moricizine on survival after myocardial infarction. *N Engl J Med* 1992; 327:227–233.

56. Morganroth J, Goin JE. Quinidine-related mortality in the short-to-medium term treatment of ventricular arrhythmias: A meta analysis. *Circulation* 1991; 84: 1977–1983.

57. Wolfe TR, Caravati EM, Rollin DE. Terminal 40-ms frontal plane QRS axis as a marker for tricyclic antidepressant overdose. *Ann Emerg Med* 1989; 18:348–351.

58. Tokarski G, Young MJ. Criteria for admitting patients with tricyclic antidepressant overdose. *J Emerg Med* 1988; 6:121.

59. Ciraulo DA, Shader RI. Fluoxetine drug-drug interactions: I. Antidepressants and antipsychotics. *J Clin Psychopharmacol* 1990; 48:1990.

60. Sheline YI, Freedland KE, Carney RM. How safe are serotonin reuptake inhibitors for depression in patients with coronary heart disease? *Am J Med* 1997; 102:54–59.

61. Goldman LS, Alexander RC, Luchins DJ. Monoamine oxidase inhibitors and tricyclic antidepressants: Comparison of their cardiovascular effects. *J Clin Psychiatry* 1991; 148:512–516.

62. Rudorfer MV, Manji HK, Potter WZ. Comparative tolerability profiles of the newer versus older antidepressants. *Drug Safety* 1994; 10:18–46.

63. Guttmacher LB, Goldstein MG. Treatment of the cardiac-impaired depressed patient. Part II: Lithium, carbamazine, and electroconvulsive therapy. *Psychiatr Med* 1988; 6:34–51.

64. Rosenqvist M, Bergfeldt L, Aili H, Mathe AA. Sinus node dysfunction during long-term lithium treatment. *Br Heart J* 1993; 70:371–375.

65. Simard M, Gumbiner B, Lee A, Lewis H, Norman D. Lithium carbonate intoxication: A case report and review of the literature. *Arch Intern Med* 1989; 149:36–46.

66. Risch SL, Groom GP, Janowsky DS. Interfaces of psychopharmacology and cardiology, part 2. *J Clin Psychiatry* 1981; 42:47–59.

67. Kemper AJ, Dunlap R, Pietro DA. Thioridazine-induced torsade de pointes. Successful therapy with isoproterenol. *JAMA* 1983; 249:2931–2934.

68. Di Salvo TG, O'Gara PT. Torsades de pointes caused by high-dose intravenous haloperidol in cardiac patients. *Clin Cardiol* 1995; 18:285–290.

69. Haverkamp W, Shenasa M, Borggrefe M, Breithardt G. Torsades de pointes. In: Zipes DP, Jalife J, eds. *Cardiac Electrophysiology: From Cell to Bedside* 2nd ed. Philadelphia: Saunders; 1995:885–899.

70. Orban Z, MacDonald LL, Peters MA, Guslits B. Erythromycin-induced cardiac toxicity. *Am J Cardiol* 1995; 75:859–861.

71. Lopez JA, Harold JG, Rosenthal ML, Oseran DS, Schapira JN, Peter T. QT prolongation and torsades de pointes after administration of trimethoprim-sulfamethoxazole. *Am J Cardiol* 1987; 59:376–377.

72. Mitchell P, Dodek P, Lawson L, Russell J. Torsades de pointes during intravenous pentamidine isethionate therapy. *Can Med Assoc J* 1989; 140:173–174.

73. Atkinson RL. Low and very low calorie diets. *Med Clin North Am* 1989; 73:203–215.

74. Pringle TH, Scorbie IN, Murray RG, Kesson CM, Maccuish AC. Prolongation of the QT interval during therapeutic starvation: A substrate for malignant arrhythmias. *Int J Obes* 1983; 7:253–261.

75. Reinoehl J, Frankovich D, Machado C, Kawasaki R, Baga JJ, Pires LA. Probucol-associated tachyarrhythmic events and QT prolongation: Importance of gender. *Am Heart J* 1996; 131:1184–1191.

76. Smith SJ. Cardiovascular toxicity of the antihistamines. *Otolaryngol Head Neck Surg* 1994; 111:348–354.

77. Bran S, Murray WA, Hirsch IB, Palmer SP. Long QT syndrome during high-dose cisapride. *Arch Intern Med* 1995; 155:765–768.

78. Nemeroff CB, DeVane CL, Pollack BG. Newer antidepressants and the cytochrome P450 system. *Am J Psychiatry* 1996; 153:311–320.

79. Cupp MJ, Tracy TS. Role of cytochrome P450 3A subfamily in drug interactions. *US Pharmacist* 1997; 22:HS9–HS21.

80. Pratt CM, Hertz RP, Ellis BE, Crowell SP, Louv W, Moye L. Risk of developing life-threatening ventricular arrhythmia associated with terfenadine in comparison with over-the-counter antihistamines, ibuprofen and clemastine. *Am J Cardiol* 1994; 73:346–352.

81. Chen TM, Benowitz NL. Caffeine and coffee: Effects on health and cardiovascular disease. *Comp Biochem Physiol* 1994; 109C:173–189.

82. Dobmeyer DJ, Stine RA, Leir CV, Greenberg R, Schaal SF. The arrhythmogenic effects of caffeine in human beings. *N Engl J Med* 1983; 308:814–816.

83. Graboys, Blatt CM, Lown B. The effect of caffeine on ventricular ectopic activity in patients with malignant ventricular arrhythmia. *Arch Intern Med* 1989; 149:637–639.

84. Van Dellen, RG. Theophylline: Practical applications of new knowledge. *Mayo Clin Proc* 1979; 54:733–745.

85. Sessler CN, Cohen MD. Cardiac arrhythmias during theophylline toxicity: A prospective continuous electrocardiogrqphic study. *Chest* 1990; 98:672–678.

86. Seneff M, Scott J, Friedman B, Smith M. Acute theophylline toxicity and the use of esmolol to reverse cardiovascular instability. *Ann Emerg Med* 1990; 19:671–673.

87. Greenberg A, Piraino BH, Kroboth PD, Weiss J. Severe theophylline toxicity: Role of conservative measures, antiarrhythmic agents and charcoal hemoperfusion. *Am J Med* 1984; 76:854–860.

88. Whitsett TL, Manion CV, Wilson MF. Cardiac, pulmonary and neuromuscular effects of clenbuterol and terbutaline compared with placebo. *Br J Clin Pharmacol* 1981; 12:195–200.

89. Lee H, Izquierdo R, Evans HE. Cardiac response to oral and aerosol administration of beta agonists. *J Pediatr* 1983; 103:655–658.

90. Gross TL, Sokol RJ. Severe hypokalemia and acidosis: A potential complication of beta-adrenergic treatment. *Am J Obstet Gynecol* 1980; 138:1225–1226.

91. Spitzer WD, Suissa S, Ernest P, Horwitz RI, Habbick B, Cockcroft D, et al. The use of β-agonists and the risk of death and near death from asthma. *N Engl J Med* 1992; 326:501–506.

92. Taylor DR, Sears MR, Cockcroft DW. The beta-agonist controversy. *Med Clin North Am* 1996; 80:719–748.

93. Tfelt-Hansen P, Kanstrup I-L, Christensen NJ, Winkler K. General and regional hemodynamic effects of intravenous ergotamine in man. *Clin Sci* 1983; 65:599–604.

94. Koh KK, Roe IH, Lee M, Cho SK, Kim SS. Variant angina complicating ergot therapy of migraine. *Chest* 1994; 105:1259–1260.

95. Roithinger FX, Punzengruber C, Gremmel F, Hinterreiter M, Holzner F, Pachinger O. Myocardial infarction after chronic ergotamine abuse. *Eur Heart J* 1993; 14:1579–1581.

96. Redfield MM, Nicholson WJ, Edwards WD, Tajik AJ. Valve disease associated with ergot alkaloid: Echocardiographic and pathologic correlations. *Ann Intern Med* 1992; 117:50–52.

97. Allen MB, Tosh G, Walters G, Muers MF. Pleural and pericardial fibrosis after ergotamine therapy. *Respir Med* 1994; 88:67–69.

98. Mason JW, Billingham ME, Friedman JP. Methysergide-induced heart disease: a case of multivalvular and myocardial fibrosis. *Circulation* 1977; 56:889–890.

99. Bana DS, MacNeal PS, Le Compte PM, Shah Y, Graham JR. Cardiac murmurs and endocardial fibrosis associated with methysergide therapy. *Am Heart J* 1974; 88:640–655.

100. Salner AL, Mullany LD, Cole SR. Methysergide-induced mitral valvular insufficiency. *Conn Med* 1980; 44:6–8.

101. MacMahon B, Bakshi M, Walsh MJ. Cardiac arrhythmias after intravenous cimetidine. *N Engl J Med* 1981; 305:832–833.

102. Hulisz DT, Welco JR, Heiselman DE. Sinus arrest associated with continuous-infusion cimetidine. *Pharmacotherapy* 1993; 13:64–67.

103. Koch-Weser J. Ranitidine: A new H₂-receptor antagonist. *N Engl J Med* 1983; 309:1368–1373.

104. Gould L, Reddy CVR, Singh BK, Zen B. Electrophysiologic properties of cimetidine in man. *Pacing Clin Electrophysiol* 1981; 4:3–7.

105. Cardiovascular histamine H₂ receptors (editorial). *Lancet* 1982; 2:421–432.

106. Cubero GI, Reguero JJ, Ortega JM. Restrictive cardiomyopathy caused by chloroquine. *Br Heart J* 1993; 69:451–452.

107. Ratliff NB, Estes ML, Myles JL, Shirey EK, McMahon JT. Diagnosis of chloroquine cardiomyopathy by endomyocardial biopsy. *N Engl J Med* 1987; 316:191–193.

108. Riou KB, Barriot P, Rimailho A, Baud FJ. Treatment of severe chloroquine poisoning. *N Engl J Med* 1988; 318:1–6.

109. Stadel BV. Oral contraceptives and cardiovascular disease. *N Engl J Med* 1981; 305:672–677.

110. Slone D, Shapiro S, Kaufman DW, Rosenberg L, Miettinen OS, Stolley PD. Risk of MI in relation to current and discontinued use of oral contraceptives. *N Engl J Med* 1981; 305:420–424.

111. Engle HJ, Lichtlen PR. Coronary atherosclerosis and myocardial infarction in young women—role of oral contraceptives. *Eur Heart J* 1983; 4:1–8.

112. Jugdutt BI, Stevens GF, Zacks DJ, Lee SJ, Taylor RF. Myocardial infarction, oral contraception, cigarette smoking, and coronary artery spasm in young women. *Am Heart J* 1983; 106:757–761.

113. Dalen JE, Hickler RB. Oral contraceptives and cardiovascular disease. *Am Heart J* 1981; 101:626–639.

114. Rosenberg L, Begaud B, Bergan U, Brown B, Buist AS, et al. What are the risks of third generation oral contraceptives? *Hum Reprod* 1996; 11:687–693.

115. Jick H, Jick SS, Gurewich V, Myers MW, Vasilatis C. Risk of idiopathic cardiovascular death and nonfatal venous thromboembolism in women using oral contraceptives with differing progestagen compounds. *Lancet* 1995; 346:1589–1593.

116. World Health Organization Collaborative Study of Cardiovascular Disease and Steroid Hormone Contraception. Haemorrhagic stroke, overall stroke risk, and combined oral contraceptives: Results of an international, multicentre, case-control study. *Lancet* 1996; 348:505–510.

117. Weiss N. Third-generation oral contraceptives: How risky? *Lancet* 1995; 346:1570.

118. Bagatell CJ, Brewner WJ. Androgens in men—uses and abuses: *New Engl J Med* 1996; 334:707–714.

119. Yesalis CE, Kennedy NK, Kopstein AN, Bahrke MS. Anabolic-adrogenic steroid use in the United States. *JAMA* 1993; 270:1217–1221.

120. Wilson JD. Androgen abuse by athletes. *Endocr Rev* 1988; 9:181–199.

121. Rockhold RW. Cardiocascular toxicity of anabolic steroids. *Annu Rev Pharmacol Toxicol* 1993; 33:497–520.

122. Glazer G. Atherogenic effects of anabolic steroids on serum lipid levels: A literature review. *Arch Intern Med* 1991; 151:1925–1933.

123. Mewis C, Spyridopulous I, Kuhlkamp V, Seipel L. Manifestation of severe coronary heart disease after anabolic drug abuse. *Clin Cardiol* 1996; 19:153–155.

124. Hollander JE. The management of cocaine-associated myocardial ischemia. *New Engl J Med* 1995; 333:1267–1272.

125. Kloner RA, Hale S, Alker Rezkalla S. The effects of acute and chronic cocaine use on the heart. *Circulation* 1992; 85:407–419.

126. Pirwitz MJ, Willard JE, Landau C, Lange RA, Glamann B, Kessler DJ, et al. Influence of cocaine, ethanol, or their combination epicardial coronary arterial dimensions in humans. *Arch Intern Med* 1995; 155:1186–1191.

127. Moliterno DJ, Willard JE, Lange RA, Wegus BII, Bochrer JD, Glamann BD, et al. Coronary-artery vasoconstriction induced by cocaine, cigarette smoking, or both. *N Engl J Med* 1994; 330:454–459.

128. Om A, Ellahham S, Disciascio G. Management of cocaine-induced cardiovascular complications. *Am Heart J* 1993; 125:469–475.

129. Hollander JE, Hoffman RS, Burstein JL, Shih RD, Thode HC. Cocaine-associated myocardial infarction: Mortality and complications. *Arch Intern Med* 1995; 155:1081–1086.

130. Flores ED, Lange RA, Cigarroa RG, Hillis LD. Effect of cocaine on coronary artery dimensions in atherosclerotic coronary artery disease: Enhances vasoconstriction at sites of significant stenosis. *J Am Coll Cardiol* 1990; 16:74–79.

131. Virami R, Robinowitz M, Smialek JE, Smyth DF. Cardiovascular effects of cocaine: An autopsy analysis of 40 patients. *Am Heart J* 1988; 115:1062–1075.

132. Hollander JE, Hoffman RS, Gennis P, Fairweather P, DiSano MJ, Jehumb DA, et al. Prospective multicenter evaluation of cocaine associated chest pain. *Ann Emerg Med* 1994; 1:330–339.

133. Lange RA, Cigarroa RG, Flores ED, McBride W, Kim AS, Wells PJ, et al. Potentiation of cocaine-induced coronary vasoconstriction by beta-adrenergic blockade. *Ann Intern Med* 1990; 112:897–903.

134. Gitter MJ, Goldsmith SR, Dunbar DN, Sharkey SW. Cocaine and chest pain: Clinical features and outcome of patients hospitalized to rule out myocardial infarction. *Ann Intern Med* 1991; 115:277–282.

135. Pitts DK, Marwah J. Cocaine and central monoaminergic neurotransmission: A review of electrophysiologic studies and comparison to amphetamine and antidepressants. *Life Sci* 1988; 42:949–968.

136. Derlet RW, Rice P, Horowitz BZ, Lord RV. Amphetamine toxicity: Experiences with 127 cases. *J Emerg Med* 1989; 7:157–161.

137. Hong R, Matsuyama E, Nur K. Cardiomyopathy associated with the smoking of crystal amphetamine. *JAMA* 1991; 265:1152–1154.

138. Bailey B, Gaudreauh HP, Thivierge RL, Turgeon JP. Cardiac monitoring of children with household electrical injuries. *Ann Emerg Med* 1995; 25:612–617.

139. Carleton SC. Cardiac problems associated with electrical injury. *Cardiol Clin* 1995; 13:263–277.

140. Browne BJ, Gaasch WR: Electrical injuries and lightning. *Emerg Med Clin North Am* 1992; 10:211–229.

141. Lichtenberg R, Dries D, Ward K, Marshall W, Scanlon P. Cardiovascular effects of lightning strikes. *J Am Coll Cardiol* 1993; 21:531–536.

142. Artz CP. Electrical injury simulates crush injury. *Surg Gynecol Obstet* 1967; 125:1316.

143. Robinson NMK, Chamberlain DA. Electrical injury to the heart may cause long-term damage to conducting tissue: A hypothesis and review of the literature. *Int J Cardiol* 1966; 53:273–277.

144. Cooper MA. Lightning injuries: Prognostic signs for death. *Ann Emerg Med* 1980; 9:134–138.

145. Jenson PJ, Thomsen PEB, Bagger JP, Worgaard A, Baandrup U. Electrical injury causing ventricular arrhythmias. *Br Heart J* 1987; 57:279–283.

146. Banazak DA. Electeroconvulsive therapy: A guide for family physicians. *Amr Fam Physician* 1996; 53:273–278.

147. Sackeim HA, Devanand DP, Prudic J. Stimulus intensity, seizure threshold, and seizure duration: Impact on the efficacy and safety of electroconvulsive therapy. *Psychiatr Clin North Am* 1991; 14:803–843.

148. Weiner RD. The psychiatric use of electrically induced seizures. *Am J Psychiatry* 1979; 136:1507–1517.

149. Rice EH, Sombrotto LB, Markowitz JC, Leon AC. Cardiovascular morbidity in high-risk patients during ECT. *Am J Psychiatry* 1994; 151:1637–1641.

150. O'Connor CJ, Rothenberg DM, Soble JS, Maclioch JE, McCarthy R, Newmann A, et al. The effect of esmolol pretreatment on the incidence of regional wall motion abnormalities during electroconvulsive therapy. *Anesth Analg* 1996; 82:143–147.

151. Welch C, Drop L. Cardiovascular effects of ECT. *Convuls Ther* 1989; 5:35–53.

152. Hay DP. Electroconvulsive therapy in the medically ill elderly. *Convuls Ther* 1989; 5:8–16.

153. Gerring JP, Shields HM. The identification and management of patients with a high risk for cardiac arrhythmias during modified ECT. *J Clin Psychiatry* 1982; 43:140–143.

154. Gould L, Copalaswamy C, Chandy F, Kim B. Electroconvulsive therapy induced ECG changes simulating a myocardial infarction. *Arch Intern Med* 1983; 143:1786–1787.

155. Graybar G, Goethe J, Levy T, Phillips J, Youngberg J, Smith G. Transient large upright T-wave on the electrocardiogram during multiple monitored electroconvulsive therapy. *Anesthesiology* 1983; 59:467–469.

156. Leslie JB, Kalayjiam RW, Sirgo MA, Plachetks JR, Watkins WD. Intravenous labetolol for the treatment of postoperative hypertension. *Anesthesiology* 1987; 67:413–421.

157. Abiusa P, Dunkelman R, Proper M. Electroconvulsive therapy in patients with pacemakers. *JAMA* 1978; 240:2459–2462.

158. Blitt CD. Electroconvulsive therapy with a cardiac pacemaker. *Anesthesiology* 1976; 45:580.

159. Jensen PJ, Thomsen PEB, Bagger JP, Norgaard A, Baandrup U. Electrical injury causing ventricular arrhythmias. *Br Heart J* 1987; 57:279–283.

160. Ector H, Jansens L, Baert L, DeGeest H. Extracorporeal shock wave lithotripsy and cardiac arrhythmias. *Pacing Clin Electrophysiol* 1989; 12:1910–1917.

161. Greenstein A, Kaver I, Lechtman V, Braf V. Cardiac arrhythmias during nonsynchronized extracorporeal shock wave lithotripsy. *J Urology* 1995; 154:1321–1322.

162. Zeng ZR, Lindstedt E, Roijer A, Olsson SB. Arrhythmia during extracorporeal shock wave lithotripsy. *Br J Urology* 1993; 71:10–16.

163. Ellis MD. Poisonous plants. In: Ellis MD, ed. *Dangerous Plants, Snakes, Arthropods, and Marine Life.* Hamilton, IL: Hamilton Press; 1975:3–81.

164. Akera T, Brown BS. Cardiovascular toxicology of cardiotonic drugs and chemicals. In: Van Stee EW, ed. *Cardiovascular Toxicology* New York: Raven; 1982; 109–134.

165. Tai Y-T, But PP-H Young K, Lau C-P. Cardiotoxicity after accidental herb-induced aconite poisoning. Lancet 1992; 340:1254–1256.

166. Karalliedde L. Animal toxins. *Br J Anaesth* 1995; 75:319–327.

167. Charak BS, Charak KS, Ram PV, Parikh PM, Gupta VK. Coagulopathies in viper bites. *J Postgrad Med* 1988; 34:80–83.

168. Christopher DG, Rodning CB. Crotalidae envenomation. *South Med J* 1986; 79:159–162.

169. Gueron M, Ilia R, Sofer S. The cardiovascular system after scorpion envenomation: A review. *Clin Toxicol* 1992; 30:245–258.

170. Blum A, Lubezki A, Sclarovsky S. Black scorpion envenomation: Two cases and review of the literature. *Clin Cardiol* 1992; 15:377–378.

171. Horen WP. Insect and scorpion sting. *JAMA* 1972; 221:894–898.

172. Lefer AM, Curtis MT. Cardiotoxicity of naturally occurring animal peptides. In: Van Stee EW, ed. *Cardiovascular Toxicology*. New York: Raven; 1982; 221–258.

173. Brown CK, Shepherd SM. Marine trauma, envenomations and intoxications. *Emerg Med Clin North Am* 1992; 10:385–408.

174. Weill H. Cardiorespiratory effects of inhalant occupational exposures. *Circulation* 1981; 63:250A–252A.

175. Zakhari S, Aviado DM. Cardiovascular toxicology of aerosol propellants, refrigerants, and related solvents. In: Van Stee EW, ed. *Cardiovascular Toxicology*. New York: Raven; 1982:281–314.

176. Roth A, Zellinger I, Arad M, Atsmon J. Organophosphates and the heart. *Chest* 1993; 103:576–578.

177. Anderson RF, Allensworth DC, DeGroot WJ. Myocardial toxicity from carbon monoxide poisoning. *Ann Intern Med* 1967; 1172–1182.

178. Marius-Nunez AL. Myocardial infarction with normal coronary arteries after acute exposure to carbon monoxide. *Chest* 1990; 97:491–494.

179. Roberts JR, Bain M, Klachko MN, Seigel EG, Wason S. Successful heart transplantation from a victim of carbon monoxide poisoning. *Ann Emerg Med* 1995; 26:652–655.

180. Leach JE. Effect of roentgen therapy on the heart: A clinical study. *Arch Intern Med* 1943; 72:715–745.

181. Stewart JR, Fajardo LF, Gillette SM, Constine LS. Radiation injury to the heart. *Int J Radiation Oncol Biol Phys* 1995; 31:1205–1211.

182. Mittal S, Berko B, Bavaria J, Herrmann HC. Radiation-induced cardiovascular dysfunction. *Am J Cardiol* 1996; 78:114–115.

183. Om A, Ellahham S, Vetrovek GW. Radiation-induced coronary artery disease. *Am Heart J* 1992; 124:1598–1602.

184. Arsenian MA. Cardiovascular sequelae of therapeutic thoracic radiation. *Prog Cardiovasc Dis* 1991; 33:299–311.

185. Carlson RG, Mayfield WR, Norman S, Alexander JA. Radiation-associated valvular disease. *Chest* 1991; 99:538–545.

186. Stewart JR, Fajardo LF. Radiation-induced heart disease: An update. *Prog Cardiovasc Dis* 1984; 27:173–194.

187. Fajardo FL, Stewart JR, Cohn KE. Morphology of radiation-induced heart disease. *Arch Pathol* 1968; 86:512–519.

188. Ni Y, von Segesser LK, Turina M. Futility of pericardiectomy for postirradiation constrictive pericarditis. *Ann Thorac Surg* 1990; 49:4452–448.

189. Applefeld MN, Wiernik PH. Cardiac disease after radiation therapy for Hodgkin's disease: Analysis of 48 patients. *Am J Cardiol* 1983; 51:1679–1681.

190. Hancock SL, Donaldson SS. Radiation-related heart disease: risks after treatment of Hodgkin's disease during childhood and adolescence. In: Bricker JT, Green DM, D'Angio GJ (eds): *Cardiac Toxicity After Treatment for Childhood Cancer*. New York: Wiley–Liss; 1993:35–43.

191. McEniery PT, Dorosti K, Schiavone WA, Pedrick TJ, Sheldon WC. Clinical and angiographic features of coronary artery disease after chest irradiation. *Am J Cardiol* 1987; 60:1020–1024.

192. Rutqvist LE, Lax I, Fornancler T, Johansson H. Cardiovascular mortality in a randomized trial of adjuvant radiation therapy vs surgery alone in primary breast cancer. *Int J Radiat Oncol Biol Phys* 1992; 22:887–896.

193. Hancock SL, Donaldson SS, Hoppe RT. Heart disease after Hodgkin's treatment in children and adolescents. *J Clin Oncol* 1993; 11:1208–1215.

TWELVE

PERICARDIAL DISEASES AND ENDOCARDITIS

81

DISEASES OF THE PERICARDIUM

Ralph Shabetai

ANATOMY OF THE PERICARDIUM

The pericardium consists of a tough, fibrous outer coat with discrete attachments to the sternum, great vessels, and diaphragm and an inner membranous coat. The fibrous coat is lined by a serosal layer of cuboidal cells one layer thick. Together, the fibrous pericardium and its serosal membrane make up the *parietal pericardium*. The serosal membrane is reflected over the epicardial surface of the heart, together with which it forms the *visceral pericardium*. The pericardial cavity is enclosed between these two serosal layers and normally contains from 15 to 50 mL of clear fluid,[1] which is an ultrafiltrate of blood plasma.[2] The parietal pericardium contacts the flat ventricular surfaces so as to leave only a potential space. Where the cardiac surfaces are more curved—especially in the grooves—a true fluid-filled pericardial space exists.[3] The pericardium has a number of recesses, the most important of which is the oblique sinus. The left atrium lies anterior to the oblique sinus and is, strictly speaking, largely an extrapericardial chamber. This relationship explains why pericardial effusion behind the posterior wall of the left ventricle is usually not seen behind the left atrium.

The phrenic nerves are embedded in the parietal pericardium; this relationship is the reason why diaphragmatic paralysis may complicate pericardial resection.

The superior and inferior pericardiosternal ligaments attach the pericardium to the sternum. Ligaments also attach the pericardium firmly to the diaphragm. The connective tissue of the pericardium becomes contiguous with the adventitia of the great vessels to provide the superior tether. These attachments maintain the heart in its normal position and are so arranged that external forces exerted on the pericardium by respiration or changes in body posture tend to cancel each other and maintain a constant heart position.[3]

Histology

The major constituent of the parietal pericardium is the fibrosa, the chief component of which is compactly arranged collagen fibers disposed in three layers oriented approximately at equal angles to each other.[4] The collagen bundles have an accordion-like appearance. The elastin fibers are much less numerous, do not occur in dense bundles, and tend to be oriented at right angles to adjacent collagen fibers. The predominance of collagen and its anatomic configuration are important to the viscoelastic properties of pericardium.

Ultrastructure

Scanning electron micrographs disclose that the pericardium is far from being an inert mass of connective tissue but rather is highly organized, with microvilli and cilia for production and absorption of fluid and facilitation of movement of the serosal surfaces over each other.[5]

MECHANICAL (VISCOELASTIC) PROPERTIES

The pressure-volume curve of the pericardium is characterized by an initial flat portion during which volume is increased with little or no change in pressure, followed by a "knee" leading to the final portion, during which pressure rapidly increases with little or no increase in volume[6] (Fig. 81-1). Normally, conventionally measured pericardial pressure is subatmospheric and thus several millimeters of mercury lower than the pressure in the atria and the ventricular diastolic pressures. This suggests that although the pericardium appears to fit the heart quite snugly, the heart is not normally engaged by the pericardium. Experimental studies, however, are not all congruent with this interpretation (see subsequent section Functions of the Pericardium). There is appreciable day-to-

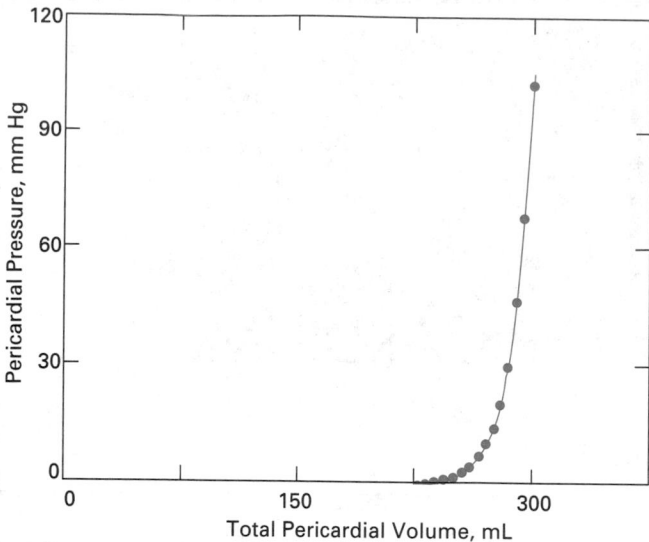

FIGURE 81-1

Pericardial pressure-volume curve (canine). (From Holt JP. The normal pericardium. *Am J Cardiol* 1970; 26:455. Reproduced with permission from the publisher and author.)

day and moment-to-moment variation in cardiac volume, but the pericardial volume exceeds cardiac volume by perhaps 10 to 20 percent, the difference constituting the *pericardial reserve volume*, which allow physiologic changes in cardiac volume to occur without restriction by the pericardium.

The pericardium limits or prevents acute pathologic distension of the heart once the pericardial reserve volume has been exceeded and the pericardium is stretched. The pericardium has then reached the steep portion of its pressure-volume relation and the wavy bundles of pericardium have straightened out and become inextensible. The stress-strain curve of excised pericardium is similar to the pressure-volume curve of the whole pericardium.[7] Most investigators consider the pericardium anisotropic, a finding that can be explained by the directionality of the collagen bundles. The pericardium stretches more in the short than in the long axis of the heart, and this anisotropy persists after the pericardial attachments are cut.

When the pericardium is subjected to constant stretching over a period of time, the tension in it drops slightly. This stress relaxation allows for slight relief of pericardial pressure in acute cardiac tamponade. It has been suggested that with growth of the heart, the collagen fibers are rearranged within the intracellular substance, allowing the pericardium to creep (increase its volume while stretch remains constant) and so adapt to the increased cardiac size,[8] but the magnitude of creep is unlikely to be sufficient to account for this adaptation. More important is that in response to chronic cardiac enlargement, the pericardium undergoes hypertrophy and becomes more compliant.[9]

Pericardial Pressure

Pericardial pressure measured by a catheter in the pericardial cavity is subatmospheric and essentially equal to pleural pressure throughout the respiratory cycle.[10] Superimposed on the large respiratory fluctuations of pericardial pressure are smaller fluctuations related to the events of the cardiac cycle, pericardial pressure being lowest during ventricular ejection. Liquid pressure within the pericardial cavity is lower than pericardial surface pressure measured by an intrapericardial balloon, which some investigators believe provides a more accurate estimate of pericardial restraint on the heart.[11] Under which circumstances liquid versus contact pressure is more relevant is controversial among physiologists, but this is less relevant to pericardial disease, because clinicians measure pericardial pressure only when there is a pericardial effusion.

Normal Pericardial Fluid: Amount and Turnover

As little as 15 mL of pericardial fluid can be detected by echocardiography.[12] On the other hand, the average amount of pericardial fluid found routinely at autopsy in patients free from pericardial and cardiac disease has been reported to be as much as 50 mL.[13]

There are no published data on the turnover of normal human pericardial fluid, but in patients with pericardial effusion, it was noted that losses of albumin from pericardial cavity averaged 1.86 g/day. The albumin disappeared from the pericardial cavity exponentially and accumulated in corresponding concentration in the blood.[14] The membrane characteristics of the pericardium favor removal rather than accumulation, of fluid.[15] Erythrocytes labeled with a radiopharmaceutical can be detected in the peripheral blood within a few hours, but it may take several days for all the cells to be absorbed.

FUNCTIONS OF THE PERICARDIUM

Cardiac Restraint

Numerous experiments have demonstrated that the pericardium restrains cardiac volume; yet no adverse consequences follow congenital absence or surgical removal of the pericardium. The thin-walled right ventricle and atrium are more subject to the influence of the pericardium than the more resistant, thick-walled, left ventricle.[16] Interactions among the cardiac chambers, especially in diastole but also in systole, are more pronounced with the pericardium intact.[17] The pericardium exerts a powerful restraining effect on the size of the heart in situations of acute volume overload, particularly those that involve all four cardiac chambers; but the role of the pericardium in normal physiology and in chronic cardiac enlargement remains controversial. Conventional liquid pressure within the pericardium suggests that pericardial influence on the heart in these circumstances is small,[18] but pericardial surface pressure, measured by an intrapericardial balloon, suggests that pericardial restraint may be important in chronic heart failure, in which right atrial pressure may closely approximate intrapericardial pressure.[11] The controversy regarding how pericardial pressure should be measured has made it difficult to assess the magnitude of external constraint by the pericardium. A recent study[19] that avoids this problem by using a method to estimate external restraint without the need to measure intrapericardial pressure is therefore particularly welcome. The investigators measured left ventricular diastolic pressure in 29 patients, some with normal left ventricle, some with hypertrophy, and some with a dilated left ventricle. Employing transient inferior venal caval balloon occlusion, they measured left ventricular diastolic pressure and volume at closely matched volumes, reasoning that the pressure drop associated with venous occlusion represented the magnitude of external restraint, not the intrinsic stiffness of the left ventricle. The external force would include but not be limited to that exerted by the pericardium. Not surprisingly however, the few attempts to treat congestive heart failure by pericardiectomy have not met with resounding success. Certainly, pericardiectomy is not an acceptable treatment for heart failure. Pericardial pressure is strongly influenced by the intrathoracic pressure, which must be kept normal or itself be measured when measuring ventricular diastolic compliance.

Other Functions

The pericardium maintains the heart in a relatively fixed position and functionally optimal shape within the mediastinum. The thin layer of pericardial fluid reduces friction on the epicardium and is thought to equalize gravitational forces over the surface of the heart; transmural cardiac pressures, therefore, do not change during acceleration or differ regionally within cardiac chambers.[20] Negative pressure in the pericardium augments atrial filling during ventricular systole. These concepts were developed using conventionally measured liquid pressure in the pericardium and do not hold for surface contact pressure, which may vary in different locations on the heart's surface.[11] The pericardium acts as a barrier to inflammation from contiguous structures and may buttress the thinner portions of the myocardium. The pericardium synthesizes and metabolizes prostaglandins.

ACUTE VIRAL AND IDIOPATHIC PERICARDITIS

Like the squeak of leather on a new saddle under a rider, or grating in the knee joint on moving the patella over the femoral condyles

V. Collin, 1955[21]

Acute fibrinous or dry pericarditis is a syndrome associated with characteristic chest pain, pericardial friction rub, and specific electrocardiographic changes. A great variety of conditions are associated with acute pericarditis (Table 81-1). The following description refers to viral and idiopathic pericarditis without significant effusion. Viral infection is often presumed rather than proved, many cases being classified as idiopathic. Epicardial biopsy via a pericardioscope is a promising new investigative technique for establishing the etiology of acute pericarditis.[22] Common viral infections causing acute pericarditis are those due to echovirus and Coxsackievirus.

Pathology

The acute fibrinous deposits give rise to the characteristic bread-and-butter appearance of the pericardium described by Laennec: "The knobbed appearance of this exudation is very like what would result from the sudden separation of two pieces of slab joined by a pretty thick layer of butter." In addition to fibrin deposition, the usual changes of acute inflammation are found.[23]

History

There may be a prodromal phase characterized by fever and myalgia. The characteristic symptom is chest pain, the nature of which varies appreciably among patients and perhaps with etiology as well. In some cases the pain is indistinguishable from that of myocardial infarction; in others it strongly simulates pleurisy. Often the pain of acute pericarditis lies between these extremes, being retrosternal without radiation to the arms but exacerbated by respiration. Characteristically, pericardial pain is relived by sitting up, and a typical, although not common, radiation is to the trapezius ridge.

Physical Examination

The characteristic physical finding of acute pericarditis is the pericardial friction rub, which is superficial, scratchy, or creaky and is often heard anywhere or everywhere over the precordium but most commonly between the lower left sternal edge and the cardiac apex. Pericardial friction rubs are usually best appreciated with the diaphragm of the stethoscope applied firmly and with respiration suspended. Sometimes they are best heard with the patient in the sitting position. Most pericardial friction rubs are independent of the respiratory cycle, but on occasion they are louder during inspiration. The classic pericardial friction rub is triphasic, with components in atrial systole, ventricular systole, and ventricular diastole,[24] but frequently the rub is biphasic, and occasionally there is only a single component. Pericardial friction, especially when of uremic origin, may be palpable. The triphasic pericardial friction rub is virtually unmistakable, but biphasic rubs must be distinguished from the to-and-fro murmur of aortic valve disease, and monophasic rubs are often mistaken for systolic murmurs. In the differential diagnosis, one must consider, in addition to cardiac murmurs, mediastinal crunch and artifacts produced by rubbing of the skin against the stethoscope (see also Chap. 10).

Pericardial friction rubs vary in intensity from hour to hour and from day to day, sometimes transiently disappearing altogether. Pericardial fluid does not prevent the rub. Depending on etiology, there may be fever and other signs of inflammation or systemic illness. Atrial arrhythmias, perhaps owing to the subepicardial location of the sinus node,[25] may

TABLE 81-1

ETIOLOGY OF PERICARDITIS[a]

I. Trauma
  A. Pericardiotomy
  B. Direct or indirect trauma to chest
  C. Transseptal catheterization
  D. Pressure injection of contrast medium
  E. Perforation of right ventricle by indwelling catheter
  F. Implantation of epicardial pacemaker
  G. Blow to chest
  H. Perforation of right ventricle with catheter for parenteral nutrition
II. Viral infections
  A. Coxsackie virus B5, B6
  B. Echovirus
  C. Adenovirus
  D. Infectious mononucleosis
  E. Influenza
  F. Lymphogranuloma venereum
  G. Chickenpox
  H. *Mycoplasma pneumoniae*
  I. Acquired immunodeficiency syndrome
III. Bacterial infections
  A. *Staphylococcus*
  B. *Pneumococcus*
  C. *Meningococcus*
  D. *Streptococcus*
  E. *Haemophilus influenzae*
  F. *Chlamydia psitacci*
  G. *Salmonella*
  H. *Mycobacterium tuberculosis*
IV. Amebiasis
V. *Echinococcus* cysts
VI. Fungal infections—histoplasmosis, aspergillosis, blastomycosis, coccidioidomycosis
VII. Rickettsia
VIII. Radiation
IX. Amyloidosis

X. Tumors
  A. Primary
    1. Mesothelioma
      a. Rhabdomyosarcoma
      b. Teratoma
      c. Fibroma
      d. Leiomyofibroma
      e. Lipoma
      f. Angioma
    2. Metastatic
      a. Bronchogenic carcinoma
      b. Carcinoma of breast
      c. Lymphoma
      d. Leukemia
      e. Melanoma
  B. Sarcoid
    1. Collagen disease
      a. Rheumatic fever
      b. Lupus erythematosus
      c. Rheumatoid arthritis
      d. Vasculitis
      e. Polyarteritis nodosa
      f. Scleroderma
      g. Dermatomyositis
XI. Anticoagulants
  A. Heparin
  B. Warfarin
XII. Myocardial infarction—post–post–myocardial infarction pericarditis (Dressler's syndrome)
XIII. Idiopathic thrombocytopenic purpura
XIV. Drugs
  A. Procainamide
  B. Cromolyn sodium
  C. Hydralazine
  D. Dantrolene
  E. Methysergide
XV. Dissecting aneurysm
XVI. Infective endocarditis with valve-ring abscess
XVII. Thymic cyst

[a] Principal causes of pericardial disease and pericardial heart disease. Most can cause pericardial effusion, cardiac tamponade, and/or constrictive pericarditis. The more common causes of these syndromes are mentioned under the syndromes and under specific disorders.

be observed, but they are rare in the absence of concomitant heart disease.[26]

Electrocardiogram

Electrocardiographic (ECG) changes of acute pericarditis evolve through four stages.[27] In the first, which occurs within hours or days of the onset of pericarditis, there is widespread ST-segment elevation, commonly involving all three standard limb leads and most of the precordial leads. Reciprocal depression is usually found in leads aVR and VI. ST-segment elevation seldom reaches 5 mm, and monophasic patterns are seldom if ever seen. In some cases the PR segment is depressed[28] except in lead aVR (Fig. 81-2); this is a useful sign in differentiating acute pericarditis from early repolarization variants.[29] During the succeeding several days, the ST and PR segments return toward isoelectric status and the ECG becomes normal (stage 2). There may be no further progression, but the T waves may become inverted (stage 3). Abnormal T waves may be permanent or the ECG may revert to normal for a second time (stage 4).

The ST-segment elevation seen in acute pericarditis can usually be distinguished from that of acute myocardial infarction by the absence of Q waves, the upwardly concave

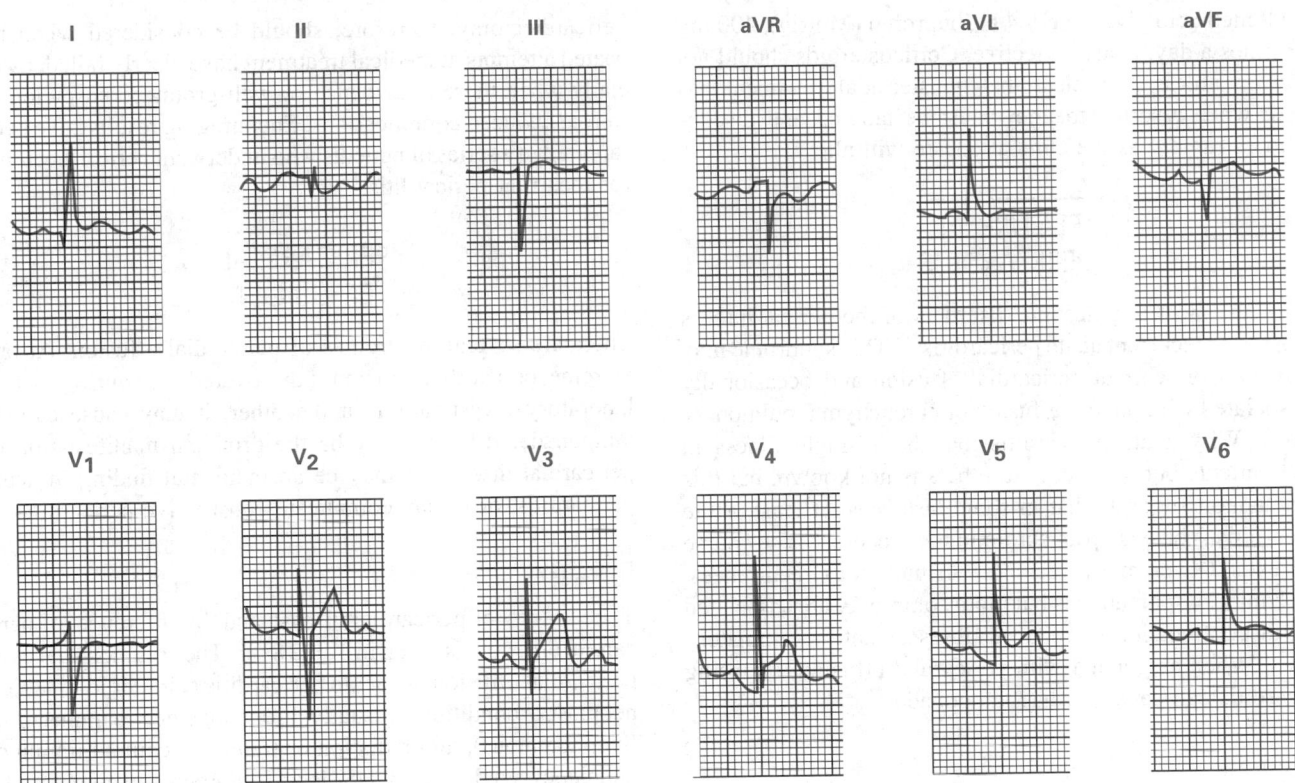

FIGURE 81-2

Electrocardiogram in acute pericarditis showing PR-segment depression and ST-segment elevation. (From Shabetai R. *The Pericardium.* New York: Grune & Stratton; 1981:359. Reproduced with permission from the publisher.)

ST segments, and the absence of associated T-wave inversion. During evolution, the ECG of acute myocardial infarction does not pass through a normal pattern before T-wave inversion occurs. The acute ST-segment elevation of Prinzmetal's variant of angina is more transitory and is associated with transient ischemic pain. The early repolarization variant common in young individuals, especially blacks and athletes and among patients in psychiatric institutions, may simulate the ECG of acute pericarditis. In these cases PR-segment depression is not seen and the ECG pattern does not evolve in a manner consistent with pericarditis (see also Chap. 12).

Other Laboratory Findings

The erythrocyte sedimentation rate is almost always elevated. Leukocytosis is present early but, depending on etiology, may give way to lymphocytosis. Cardiac enzyme levels are usually normal but may be elevated when there is extensive epicarditis. The results of pyrophosphate and gallium scintigraphy may be positive when there is associated myocarditis.[30]

ECG changes in acute pericarditis imply inflammation of the epicardium. The epicardium is frequently spared in uremic pericarditis, in which fibrin deposition may be extensive while inflammatory changes are minimal. In these cases ECG signs of pericarditis do not appear. The occurrence of first-degree heart block or bundle branch block suggests more widespread myocarditis (myopericarditis).

In the absence of pericardial effusion or severe myocarditis, the QRS complex and the chest radiogram remain normal. Computed tomography is seldom resorted to, but in difficult cases it can be relied on to demonstrate the inflamed pericardium,[31] which appears thicker than normal because of edema and fibrin deposition.

Differential Diagnosis

The early stages of acute pericarditis may be confused with acute myocardial infarction. In cases of doubt, the issue is clarified over the subsequent 24 to 36 h by the clinical course and by serial changes in the ECG and the plasma level of cardiac enzymes and troponin I (see Chap. 47). Aortic dissection may be misdiagnosed as pericarditis or, alternatively, may be the cause of pericarditis (see Chap. 98).

Treatment

When acute pericarditis is of known etiology, it may respond to treatment of the underlying cause. For viral and idiopathic pericarditis, the patients should be given an analgesic and, if the pain is severe, should be confined to bed. The patient should be observed for pericardial effusion and cardiac tamponade. Usually aspirin suffices for the control of pain, but it may have to be given every 3 or 4 h for the first 48 h. The pain of acute pericarditis usually responds to 25 to 100 mg of indomethacin given every 4 h. Ibuprofen (Motrin), 400 mg four times a day, is also effective. Corticosteroids should not be given unless it is clear that nonsteroidal treatment has failed; when resorted to, they must be tapered and discontinued as rapidly as the clinical course will allow.

RECURRENT PERICARDITIS

One of the most troublesome disorders of the pericardium is relapsing or recurrent acute pericarditis.[32] This syndrome may occur with or without pericardial effusion and occasionally is associated with pleural effusion or parenchymal pulmonary lesions. Why acute pericarditis may be a single illness in some patients but may recur in others is not known, but this phenomenon suggests that in some instances, at least, acute pericarditis is or sets up an autoimmune process.[33] The course may extend over many years[34] with numerous recurrences, which may be spontaneous but more commonly are associated with discontinuation or reduced doses of anti-inflammatory agents. When associated with pericardial effusion, relapsing pericarditis can cause cardiac tamponade.

Treatment

Recurrences are usually so severe that treatment must be given. Quite commonly, chest discomfort, fever, or dyspnea are not controlled by large doses of nonsteroidal anti-inflammatory drugs but yield only to steroid therapy, usually with prednisone. Once steroids are administered, there is real danger of dependency and the development of steroid-induced abnormalities.[35] When the physician is forced to use steroids, every effort must be made to establish the minimal dose that will control pericarditis. In very ill patients, prednisone is begun at a high dose such as 60 to 80 mg/day, but rapid tapering must be begun within a few days of clinical resolution. Tapering may be easier when prednisone is combined with a nonsteroidal agent. It has been suggested that administering prednisone on alternate days is helpful, but more likely this modification fails to reduce the total dose. In the most difficult cases, relapse occurs every time the dose of prednisone is reduced below 5 to 20 mg/day. When this occurs, the patient should be maintained for several weeks on the lowest suppressive dose before the next taper commences. Some steroid-resistant cases respond to the addition of 50 to 100 mg/day of azathioprine. Colchicine, 1 to 2 mg/dL, has been advocated,[36,37] but its effectiveness remains to be proved. There are no reports to cyclosporine treatment for recurrent pericarditis, and this strategy cannot be recommended except possibly as a last resort. When serious side effects such as osteoporosis with spinal compression or fractures develop, or when severe mental changes appear, pericardiectomy may be considered. It must, however, be recognized that pericardiectomy may abbreviate rather than end the course of relapsing pericarditis and may be followed by troublesome pleural and pulmonary manifestations that require vigorous treatment.

Pericardiectomy, therefore, should be considered when repeated attempts at medical treatment have clearly failed, especially when there is evidence or well-grounded suspicion of steroid-induced complications. Encouraging results have been reported in a series of patients who underwent pericardiectomy for recurrent pericarditis.[38]

PERICARDIAL EFFUSION

There are several syndromes of pericardial effusion. At one extreme, pericardial effusion is discovered only during routine laboratory investigation; at the other, it may cause cardiac tamponade. Effusion may be the principal manifestation of pericardial disease, it may be an incidental finding in acute pericarditis, or it may complicate constrictive pericarditis.

Etiology

The etiology of pericardial disease and, by inference, of pericardial effusion, is given in Table 81-1. The common causes of pericardial effusion are acute pericarditis (viral or idiopathic), neoplastic conditions (usually bronchogenic, mammary, or lymphomatous), and radiation or trauma. Acquired immunodeficiency syndrome (AIDS) is an important newcomer in the causation of pericarditis with effusion and is rapidly becoming a common cause of this condition. Somewhat less common are pericardial effusions induced by drugs and occurring with collagen vascular diseases, particularly rheumatoid arthritis and lupus erythematosus. Pericardial effusion is an important component of the postpericardiotomy syndrome and of many cases of Dressler's syndrome.

Diagnosis

There are no specific symptoms. Likewise, clinical signs such as a quiet precordium, an increased area of cardiac dullness, and cardiac dullness percussible beyond the apex beat are so nonspecific and so rarely employed that the diagnosis of pericardial effusion has become a matter of knowing when to suspect it and to confirm its presence by echocardiography (Chap. 14). On occasion, pericardial effusion is found by chance on the chest radiograph, a radionuclide ventriculogram, an echocardiogram, or an abdominal ultrasound examination or during cardiac catheterization.

Pericardial effusion must be kept in mind whenever a patient with a disorder that may affect the pericardium is encountered, and it should be strongly suspected in such patients when they manifest evidence of pericardial involvement. Particularly suspect are patients with cancer of the lung or breast, those undergoing hemodialysis, those with unexplained enlargement of the cardiopericardial silhouette, those with unexplained increased venous pressure, and those with AIDS.

The most specific and sensitive test is echocardiography,[39] which should be performed whenever there is reasonable suspicion of a pericardial effusion (see Chap. 14). Pericardial liquid appears on the M-mode echocardiogram as an echo-

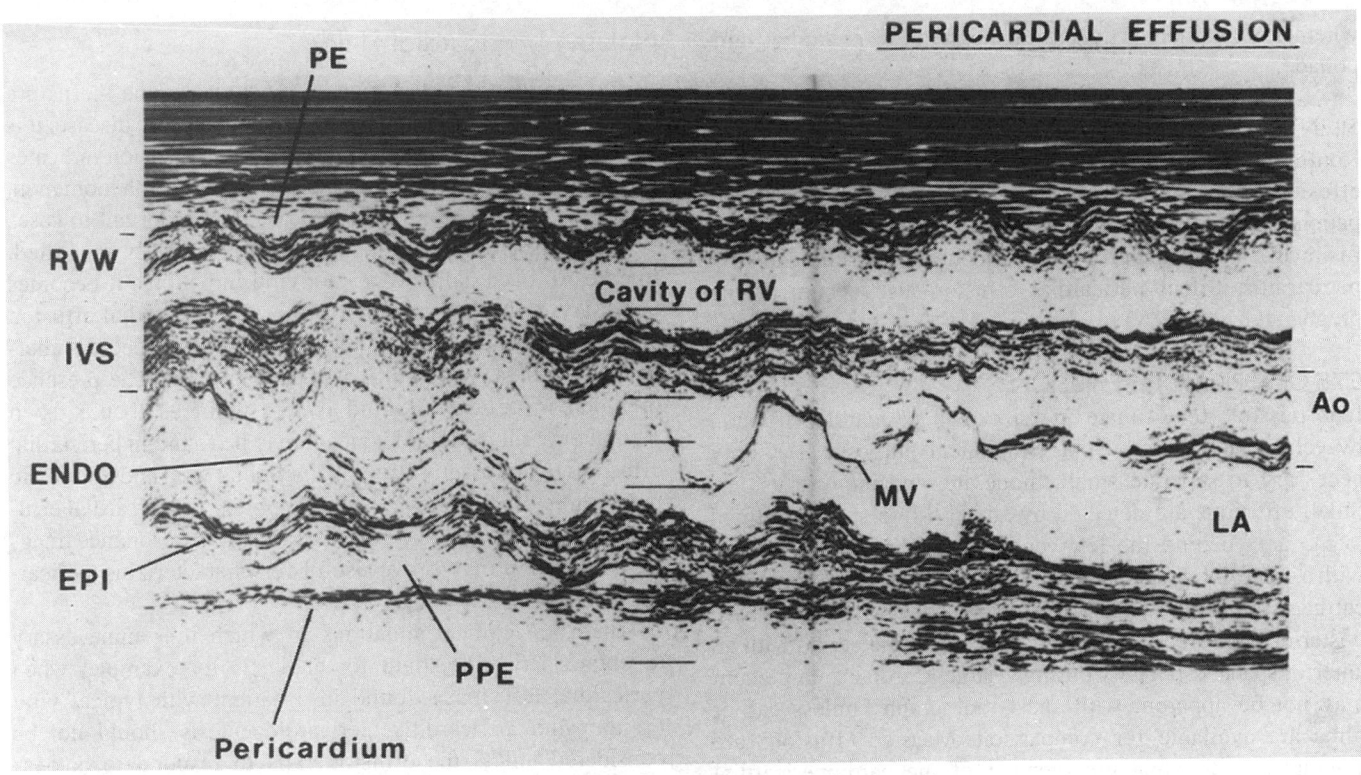

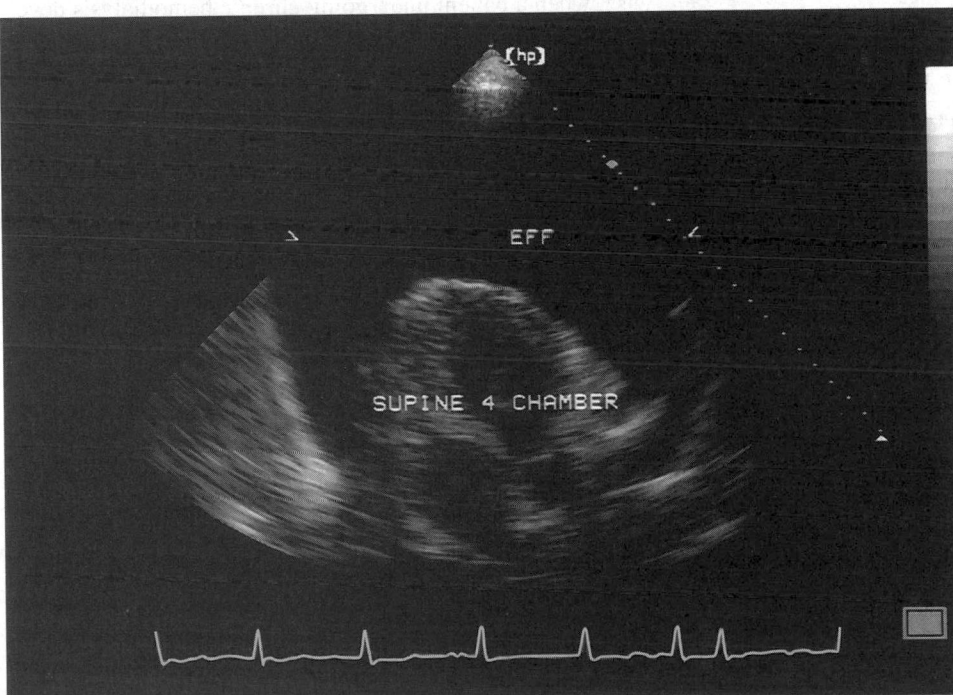

FIGURE 81-3

Echocardiographic features of cardiac tamponade. *A.* M-mode echocardiogram showing moderate pericardial effusion. Pericardial fluid is present anteriorly (PE) and posteriorly (PPE). RVW = right ventricular wall; IVS = interventricular septum; endo = endocardium; epi = epicardium; MV = mitral valve; LA = left atrium. (From Shabetai R. *The Pericardium.* New York: Grune & Stratton; 1981. Reproduced with permission from the publisher.) *B.* Two-dimensional image of a huge pericardial effusion that developed 3 months after mitral valve repair.

free space. In smaller effusions the echo-free space is behind the left ventricle, but larger effusions are associated with an additional space in front of the right ventricle (Fig. 81-3*A*). Two-dimensional echocardiography (Fig. 81-3*B*) has for some time been the method of choice and serves to quantify further the amount and distribution of pericardial effusion[40] and also may demonstrate fibrinous adhesions.[41] Echocardiography

may also indicate whether or not the pericardium is thickened. In analyzing the echocardiogram of a patient with pericardial effusion, one can estimate, by determining the dimensions of the cardiac chambers, whether apparent enlargement of the heart can be entirely accounted for by pericardial effusion or whether there is underlying enlargement of the heart itself. By assessing wall motion, one can determine whether or not there is underlying heart failure or cardiac tamponade.

SILENT PERICARDIAL EFFUSION

Routine echocardiography has shown that silent pericardial effusions are quite common,[42,43] especially in hemodialysis patients. Similarly, echocardiography reveals pericardial effusion in a significant proportion of patients with clinically dry pericarditis. Silent pericardial effusion also occurs during pregnancy.

SIZE OF PERICARDIAL EFFUSION

It is possible to estimate the size of a pericardial effusion by echocardiography,[44] but for clinical purposes it is only necessary to separate small, moderate, and large effusions. Small effusions are detected by an echo-free space confined to the area behind the left ventricle and are not associated with an anterior clear space or enlargement of the radiographic cardiac silhouette. Moderate effusions are characterized by a posterior echo-free space larger than a centimeter and with an anterior space, especially during systole. Cardiac enlargement may not be apparent with chest radiography unless earlier films are available for comparison. Massive effusions are associated with great enlargement of the cardiopericardial silhouette by x-ray and a large echo-free area around the heart visible throughout the cardiac cycle and in all projections. Radiographs show lung fields as disproportionately clear in relation to apparent cardiomegaly (see Chap. 13).

TECHNIQUE

To identify pericardial effusion by M-mode echocardiography (Fig. 81-3A), the controls are adjusted to damp out all cardiac structures except the pericardium and are then adjusted to display, in addition, the epicardium, myocardium, and endocardium.[45] Normal structures and spaces may mimic pericardial effusion[46,47]; these include the space between vertebrae and myocardium, the gap between papillary muscle and free wall, pleural effusion,[48] cyst, hematoma (especially postoperative), giant left atrium,[48] calcified mitral valve annulus,[49] and tumors.[50] Two-dimensional echocardiography (Fig. 81-3B) allows much better identification of normal and abnormal structures with corresponding reduction of false-positive diagnosis[51] (Chap. 14). Two dimensional imaging, which provides much more information than M-mode echocardiography on the distribution of fluid and concerning the underlying cardiac morphology and function, is the preferred technique.

Chest radiography is not specific. There is overall enlargement of the cardiac silhouette, and the lung fields are less congested than in cardiac failure. This combination is difficult to distinguish from four-chamber cardiac enlargement with tricuspid regurgitation, a common manifestation of severe biventricular heart failure. Rarely, the pericardium and cardiac edge can be distinguished as separate shadows along the left border of the heart[52] (see also Chap. 13).

Nature of Pericardial Fluid

In certain situations it is mandatory to determine the nature of the pericardial fluid. In patients with neoplastic disease, it is necessary to determine whether pericardial effusion indicates invasion of the pericardium or a postradiation phenomenon. Cytologic examination of the fluid is also important in cases in which the primary tumor has not been clearly identified. In cases of bacterial or other nonviral infections, it becomes necessary to discover whether or not the pericardial effusion is an exudate and to culture pericardial fluid; suspected tuberculous or fungal pericarditis is a case in point. The presence of blood in pericardial fluid is less ominous than it is in pleural or peritoneal fluid, since it may be found in pericardial effusions of almost any etiology, including viral and idiopathic pericarditis. Hemorrhagic fluid is common in pericardial effusion association with renal disease. Magnetic resonance imaging (Chap. 19) may prove useful for characterizing pericardial fluid.[53]

There are clinical situations in which it is unnecessary to obtain pericardial fluid for analysis; for example, when pericardial effusion is found in a patient with typical viral or idiopathic pericarditis, pericardiocentesis should not be considered unless the effusion fails to respond to anti-inflammatory treatment or cardiac tamponade develops. Likewise, when a patient undergoing chronic hemodialysis develops pericardial effusion, pericardial fluid need be obtained only when the clinical course suggests a different etiology or when there is suspicion of hemodynamic embarrassment.

Readers who wish to employ a paradigm regarding whether or not to recommend pericardiocentesis or pericardial biopsy are referred to the numerous publications of Soler et al.; these options are well summarized in their review of 231 consecutive patients.[54] Here it is emphasized that the yield from so-called diagnostic pericardiocentesis is disappointingly low, whereas a correct diagnosis of the etiology is a common outcome of pericardiocentesis performed for tamponade or to evacuate an effusion though to be purulent (so-called therapeutic pericardiocentesis).

ACQUIRED IMMUNODEFICIENCY SYNDROME

Acquired immunodeficiency syndrome (AIDS) has become an important cause of pericardial disease, sometimes associated with myocardial involvement.[55] In urban hospitals, AIDS has now surpassed malignancy as the commonest cause of pericardial effusion.[56] Pericarditis may be associated with late manifestations of AIDS, including tuberculosis and other mycobacterial infections, lymphoma, and Kaposi's sarcoma,[57] but often the inflammation is nonspecific.[58] Large effusions are less common, but tamponade,[59] sometimes fatal,[60] has been reported. In a 5-year prospective study of 231 subjects with AIDS, the incidence of pericardial effusion was high and effusion was associated with shortened survival even when small and apparently clinically innocuous. Pericardial effusion was more sensitive than the count of CD4 + T cells as a marker of end-stage disease[61] (see also Chap. 79).

THE PERICARDIAL COMPRESSIVE SYNDROMES

Richard Lower (1631–1691), a colleague of William Harvey in his later years at Oxford University and a pulmonary physiologist and practicing physician, possessed an astonishing comprehension of the physiology of cardiac tamponade and constrictive pericarditis. In 1669, he wrote:

It sometimes happens that a profuse effusion oppresses and inundates the heart. The envelope becomes filled in hydrops of the heart; the walls of the heart are compressed by the fluid circling everywhere, so that the heart cannot dilate sufficiently to receive the blood; then the pulse becomes exceedingly small, until finally it becomes utterly suppressed by the great inundation of fluid, thence succeed syncope and death itself.[62]

Norman Chevers, in 1842, described constrictive pericarditis:

The principal cause of dangerous symptoms appears to arise from the occurrence of gradual contraction in the layers of adhesive matter which have been deposited around the heart, compressing its muscular tissue and embarrassing its systolic and diastolic movements, but *more particularly the latter*. The patient becomes incapable of continued muscular exertion and always liable to suffer from dropsy and other serous effusions.[63]

Pathophysiology

Constrictive pericarditis, cardiac tamponade, and restrictive cardiomyopathy are three conditions that restrict diastolic filling. Impaired cardiac filling is manifest by reduced ventricular volumes, elevated ventricular diastolic pressure, and reduced diastolic chamber compliance. Secondarily, cardiac output is reduced.[64]

In cardiac tamponade and constrictive pericarditis, the heart is surrounded either by pericardial fluid under increased pressure or by a noncompliant scar that prevents the heart from attaining its normal diastolic dimensions. The generalized nature of compression by constrictive pericarditis or cardiac tamponade equilibrates the filling pressures of the two sides of the heart. In both conditions, left ventricular and right ventricular diastolic pressures are equal to each other and to the pressure in both atria. Cardiac compression rarely induces reactive pulmonary hypertension; therefore the pulmonary arterial diastolic pressure is virtually the same as the common ventricular filling pressure.

CENTRAL VENOUS PRESSURE
When the filling pressure of the right ventricle is increased by the pericardial fluid or constrictive pericarditis, the central venous pressure must increase if circulation is to be maintained. *The diagnosis of significant constriction or tamponade is hardly tenable when the central venous pressure is normal.*

CARDIAC OUTPUT
In both constrictive pericarditis and cardiac tamponade, cardiac output is reduced—if not at rest, then in response to exercise, and in both conditions left ventricular end-diastolic volume may be diminished,[65] sometimes to as little as 25 to 30 mL/m^2, which is less than the normal stroke volume. Compensatory tachycardia ensues but is often insufficient to maintain cardiac output at rest, and almost invariably cardiac output cannot be adequately increased during exercise. Tachycardia and elevated vascular resistance[66] are mediated by increased sympathetic tone.[67]

The syndrome of raised ventricular diastolic pressure, low cardiac output, and increased systemic vascular resistance mimics cardiac failure. In cardiac failure, however, raised ventricular diastolic pressure is a manifestation of myocardial insufficiency, whereas in constrictive pericarditis and cardiac tamponade it is an expression of increased external restraint.[64] Likewise, decreased cardiac output in the pericardial compressive disorders reflects not systolic pump failure but reduced preload.[64] Cardiac tamponade and constrictive pericarditis thus greatly impair the diastolic function of the heart; when impairment of systolic performance occurs, it is a late manifestation.

DIFFERENCES IN PATHOPHYSIOLOGY BETWEEN TAMPONADE AND CONSTRICTION
Knowledge of the similarities between constrictive pericarditis and cardiac tamponade (Table 81-2) is fundamental to understanding compressive disorders of the heart, and distinction between their pathophysiologies is crucial to understanding their respective clinical and laboratory findings (Table 81-3).

In cardiac tamponade, intrapericardial pressure is elevated and can be reliably measured. The elevated intrapericardial pressure is exerted on the heart throughout the cardiac cycle with slight momentary relief during ventricular ejection, when

---

TABLE 81-2

HEMODYNAMIC SIMILARITIES: CARDIAC TAMPONADE AND PERICARDIAL CONSTRICTION

Ventricular diastolic dysfunction
Preserved ventricular systolic function
Diastolic pressure equilibration
Raised central venous pressure
Diminished cardiac output
Increased respiratory variation of ventricular filling velocity

TABLE 81-3

HEMODYNAMIC DIFFERENCES: CARDIAC TAMPONADE VERSUS PERICARDIAL CONSTRICTION

	Tamponade	Constriction
Central venous pressure (CVP)	Absent *y* descent	Prominent *x* and *y* descents
Inspiration	CVP declines	Kussmaul's sign
Dip and plateau	Absent	Present
Pulsus paradoxus	Common	Rare
Pericardial pressure	Can be measured	Cannot be measured
Respiratory variation in thoracic pressure	Mostly transmitted into cardiac chambers	Not transmitted into cardiac chambers

lar ejection marked by the χ descent of venous pressure and a drop in intrapericardial pressure; a second surge occurs in diastole when the tricuspid valve opens and the γ descent is inscribed.[68] The venous return in cardiac tamponade is unimodal and confined to ventricular systole and corresponds with the χ descent of venous pressure.[69] The γ descent is therefore absent, being replaced by an abnormal upsloping phase of the venous pressure pulse in early diastole. Pericardial pressure and right atrial pressure are elevated above normal and are equal to each other (Fig. 81-5).

intrapericardial pressure falls slightly as cardiac volume diminishes. In severe cardiac tamponade, venous return is halted in diastole, when cardiac volume and intrapericardial pressure are maximal (Fig. 81-4).

It is helpful to recall the normal bimodal pattern of venous return. A surge of venous return occurs at the onset of ventricu-

The waveform of venous pressure in constrictive pericarditis differs from that of cardiac tamponade. In constrictive pericarditis, cardiac volume is set by the scarred pericardium and under no circumstances can the heart exceed this set volume, which is attained near the end of the first third of

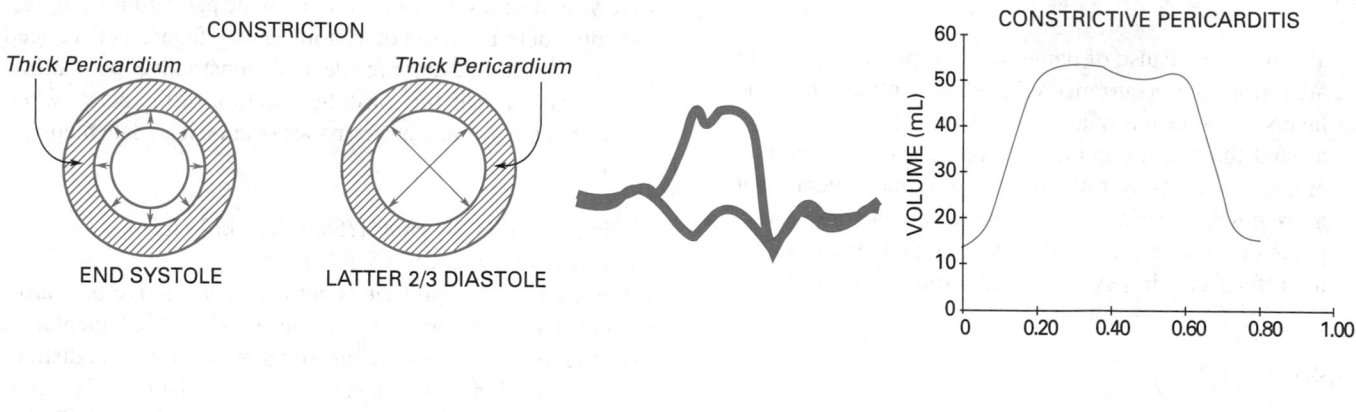

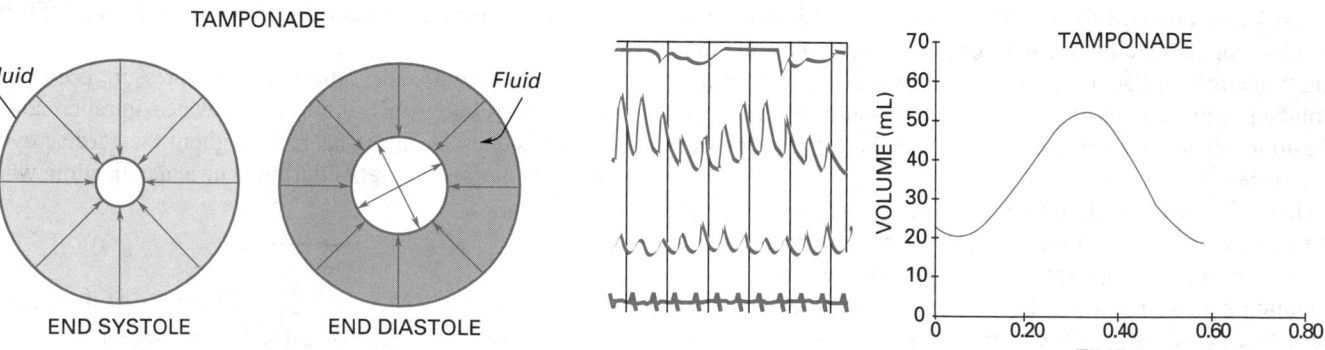

FIGURE 81-4

Diagram illustrating differences between constrictive pericarditis and cardiac tamponade. In constrictive pericarditis, the heart is not restricted at end systole, so the heart fills rapidly during early diastole, creating the dip of ventricular pressure and the γ descent of atrial pressure. When cardiac volume reaches the limit set by the diseased pericardium, further filling cannot take place; thus is created the late plateau of ventricular diastolic pressure. Atrial filling is bimodal, so atrial pressure displays sharp χ and γ descents. In cardiac tamponade, the heart is compressed throughout the cardiac cycle by the pressure of pericardial fluid. Pulsus paradoxus occurs, and the early diastolic dip of ventricular pressure and the γ descent of atrial pressure are absent. In constrictive pericarditis, early diastolic filling is abnormally rapid, but no filling occurs in mid- and late diastole. (Modified from Shabetai R. *The Pericardium.* New York: Grune & Stratton; 1981. Reproduced with permission from the publisher.)

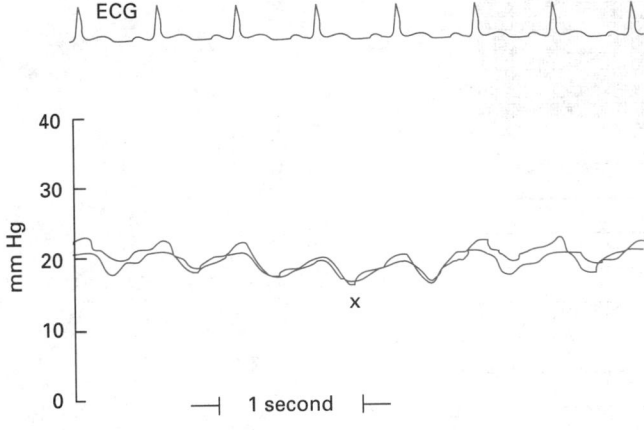

Pressures recorded simultaneously from the right atrium and the pericardial cavity in a patient with severe cardiac tamponade. The two pressures are greatly elevated and are equal to one another, a key hemodynamic observation that should be made during pericardiocentesis. Note also that the χ descent is the single negative deflection; the γ descent is absent. The pressures falls normally during inspiration. (Modified from Shabetai R. *The Pericardium*. New York: Grune & Stratton; 1981:266. Reproduced with permission from the publisher.)

diastole (Fig. 81-4). During ejection, venous return is not significantly impeded; therefore the normal systolic surge of venous return and the χ descent of venous pressure are preserved. Cardiac compression is still insignificant at end systole, so that when the tricuspid valve opens, blood rushes into the ventricles at a supranormal rate, registering a precipitous γ descent of venous pressure. Thus, in constrictive pericarditis the venous return is bimodal, as in normal physiology, but the diastolic surge and γ descent are equal to or greater than the χ descent and the systolic surge[69] (Fig. 81-6A).

Respiratory Variation and Central Venous Pressure

In cardiac tamponade, the inspiratory fall in intrathoracic pressure is transmitted to the pericardial space. Thus, although intrapericardial pressure is elevated, it falls during inspiration almost as much as the pleural pressure, increasing transmural pericardial pressure (pericardial minus pleural pressure) by only 1 or 2 mmHg.[70] The inspiratory drop in pericardial pressure is transmitted into the right-sided heart chambers, so that, despite the elevated intrapericardial pressure, the normal inspiratory increase in systemic venous return is preserved.[70] In constrictive pericarditis, however, the intrapericardial space is obliterated. Thus, during inspiration, the decreased intrathoracic pressure is not transmitted to the heart; therefore, venous pressure does not fall, and systemic venous return fails to rise.

In constrictive pericarditis, early diastolic filling is faster than normal; consequently the ventricular diastolic pressure is characterized by a dip in early diastole[71] (Fig. 81-6B). In normal physiology, the early diastolic filling period is followed by diastasis and a second period of rapid filling associated with atrial systole. In constrictive pericarditis, however, the ventricles are completely filled by the end of the rapid filling phase. Diastasis therefore persists throughout the remainder of diastole and, except in the mildest cases, rapid filling during atrial systole cannot occur. Corresponding to the prolonged diastasis, the ventricular diastolic pressure remains unchanged but is elevated for the latter two-thirds of diastole. The pattern of ventricular diastolic pressure in constrictive pericarditis is frequently referred to as the "dip-and-plateau pattern" or the "square-root sign" (Fig. 81-6C).

Small ventricles and impeded venous return favor filling by suction.[72] In constrictive pericarditis, the end-systolic volumes of the ventricles are reduced[69] and their recoil is rapid. The prominent early diastolic pressure dip indicates increased suction during early diastole.

In cardiac tamponade, ventricular diastolic filling is reduced throughout diastole; an early diastolic dip in ventricular pressure, the γ descent of venous pressure,[73] and abnormally rapid early diastolic filling[69] are absent (Fig. 81-4), denoting a major pathophysiologic difference from constrictive pericarditis.

MECHANISM OF REDUCED LEFT VENTRICULAR VOLUME IN CARDIAC TAMPONADE

The thick-walled left ventricle resists reduction of its volume by direct compression.[74] Several experimental observations support this idea. In dogs, when systemic venous return is diverted and returned by a pump at a slow rate to the right atrium, pericardial pressure can be raised to 20 mmHg without inducing pulmonary congestion or arterial hypotension.[70] This suggests that a major cause of reduced left ventricular volume in cardiac tamponade is decreased pulmonary venous return secondary to compression of the thinner-walled right ventricle. In fresh postmortem canine hearts, fluid injected into the pericardial sac displaces a greater volume from the right ventricle than from the left. Finally, when cardiac tamponade is abruptly induced in dogs, pulmonary arterial flow declines immediately, but aortic flow remains normal for several cardiac cycles.[74] In spite of these results in experimental cardiac tamponade, clinicians must recognize that pericardial effusion located behind the heart can cause echocardiographic left ventricular, not right ventricular, diastolic collapse, particularly in postoperative patients.[75]

PULSUS PARADOXUS

Pulsus paradoxus is an abnormally large inspiratory decline in systemic arterial systolic pressure and pulse pressure (Fig. 81-4). In healthy individuals, systolic blood pressure may decline by as much as 10 mmHg during quiet inspiration. A number of normal and abnormal mechanisms combine to create pulsus paradoxus in cardiac tamponade.

In cardiac tamponade, systemic arterial pressure and left ventricular stroke volume fall during inspiration, while pulmonary arterial pressure and right ventricular stroke volume increase.[76] Minimal aortic pressure and flow, however, do not correspond exactly with maximal pulmonary arterial pressure

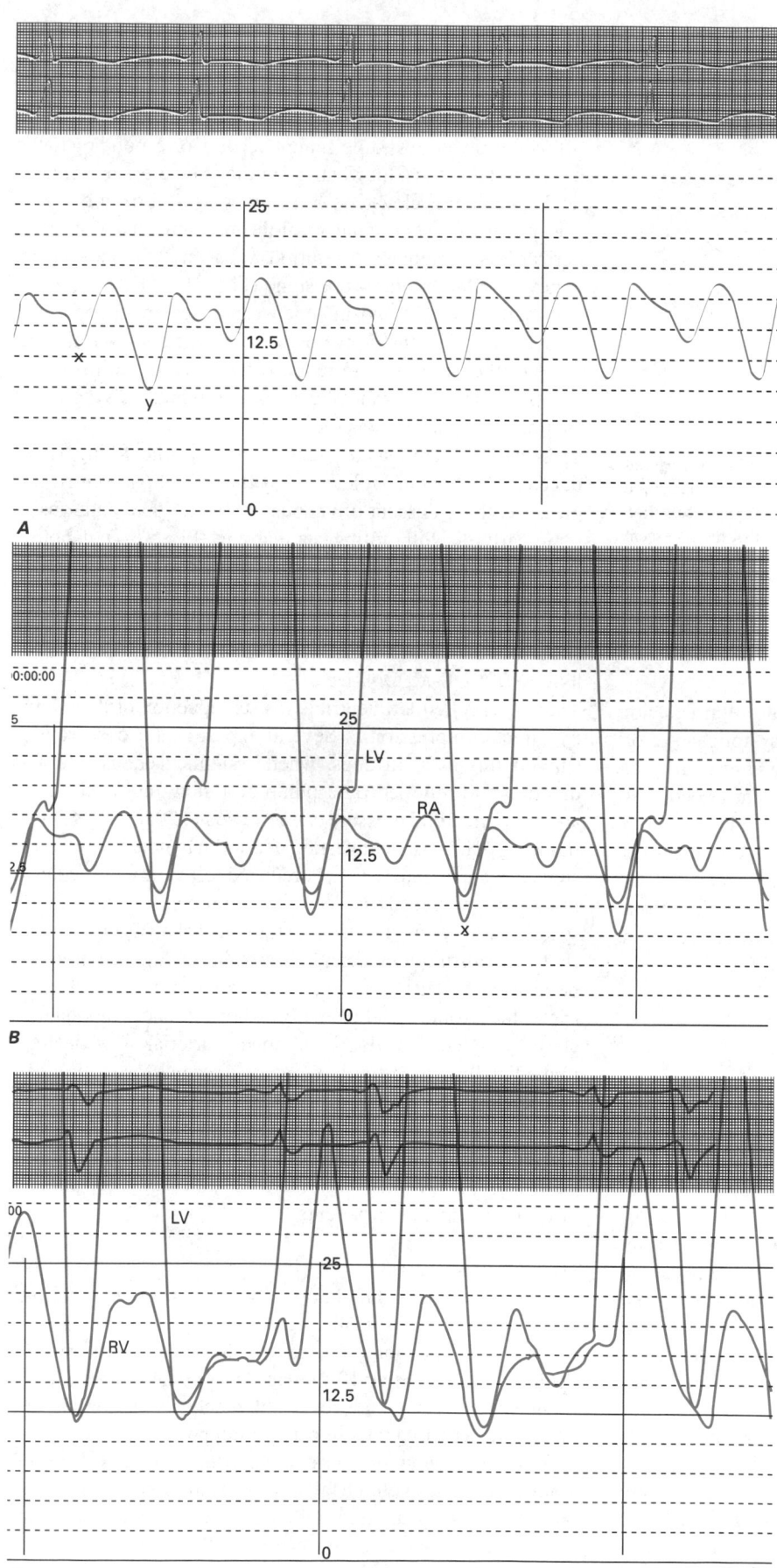

FIGURE 81-6

Intracardiac pressures recorded from a young man with tuberculous pericarditis. *A.* Right atrium. Note the extreme prominence of the γ descent. The χ descent is well preserved and respiratory variation is limited to the γ descent. *B.* Right atrial and left ventricular pressures recorded simultaneously and equisensitively. The γ descent of atrial pressure is synchronous with the early diastolic dip of ventricular pressure. The difference between left ventricular diastolic pressure and right atrial pressure is small. *C.* During recording of the previous panels, the rhythm was sinus tachycardia, which did not allow time for the plateau of late ventricular diastolic pressure. A ventricular extrasystole induced by the catheter while recording the two ventricular diastolic pressures is followed by a postextrasystolic pause that clearly demonstrates the dip and plateau and that the pressures equilibrate during the plateau.

and flow. Rather, maximal pulmonary arterial pressure and flow precede maximal aortic pressure and flow by one to three beats.[77] This observation is not compatible with the hypothesis that competition between the two sides of the heart for fixed pericardial space is the sole cause of pulsus paradoxus in cardiac tamponade.[70] In normal dogs, intrapleural and intrapericardial pressures fall equally during inspiration. In tamponade, however, transmural pericardial pressure rises slightly with inspiration[70] (Fig. 81-7). Inspiratory augmentation of systemic venous return in cardiac tamponade increases the volume of the right side of the heart at the expense of the left side. The volume of the left side of the heart may be decreased in part by bulging of the intraventricular septum from right to left[78] and in part by increased transmural pericardial pressure.

The hemodynamic effect of inspiration has been simulated by rapidly adding a small volume of blood to the venous return of dogs studied during apnea while the right side of the heart was supported by a constant-flow pump.[70] As long as intrapericardial pressure was normal, the addition of blood to the venous return caused an immediate increase in pulmonary arterial pressure but no corresponding fall in aortic pressure. Two or three cycles later, aortic pressure increased, but pericardial pressure did not increase. When the experiment was repeated in the presence of cardiac tamponade, the sudden increase in systemic venous return was again followed by an early increase in pulmonary arterial pressure, but now there was a simultaneous increase in intrapericardial pressure and a drop in aortic pressure. Aortic pressure rose two or three beats later. This experiment confirms the importance of inspiratory expansion of the volume of the right side of the heart and the transit time of the resulting augmented right heart stroke volume in the genesis of pulsus paradoxus when pericardial pressure is elevated.

In cardiac tamponade, pulsus paradoxus appears when both ventricles fill against a common resistance. Therefore, when left ventricular diastolic pressure is elevated by coexisting left ventricular disease, pulsus paradoxus does not develop in cardiac tamponade.[79] Atrial septal defect prevents reciprocal inspiratory changes in the filling of the two sides of the heart; therefore, in this condition too, cardiac tamponade can occur without pulsus paradoxus.[80] In patients with aortic regurgitation, cardiac tamponade may also occur without pulsus paradoxus.

The increased volume of the right side of the heart with inspiration, occurring when the pericardium is overstretched, causes the ventricular septum to bulge to the left. The changed size and shape of the left ventricle decreases its compliance at the same time that transmural pericardial pressure is increased. Pulmonary venous return is diminished and negative thoracic pressure is transmitted to the aorta, increasing left ventricular afterload. Two or three cardiac cycles after the inspiratory augmentation of right ventricular stroke volume, the augmented volume appears in the aorta, but by this time the respiratory phase has shifted to expiration. Finally, left ventricular stroke volume falls more sharply than normal in response to decreased ventricular filling in cardiac tamponade because the small ventricle is operating on the steep ascending limb of the Starling curve.[81] The already complex effect of inspiration on aortic pressure in cardiac tamponade is modified by additional factors, including inspiratory traction by the diaphragm on the already taut pericardium,[82] reflex changes in vascular resistances and cardiac contractility,[83] and increased respiratory effort owing to pulmonary congestion.

Pulsus paradoxus is much less common in constrictive pericarditis than in cardiac tamponade, perhaps because in constrictive pericarditis inspiratory increases in venous return[70] and in the volume of the right side of the heart seldom occur. When pulsus paradoxus does occur in constrictive pericarditis, it may be because there is pericardial effusion in addition[84] or its mechanism differs, inasmuch as the intrapericardial space is obliterated and the position of the ventricular

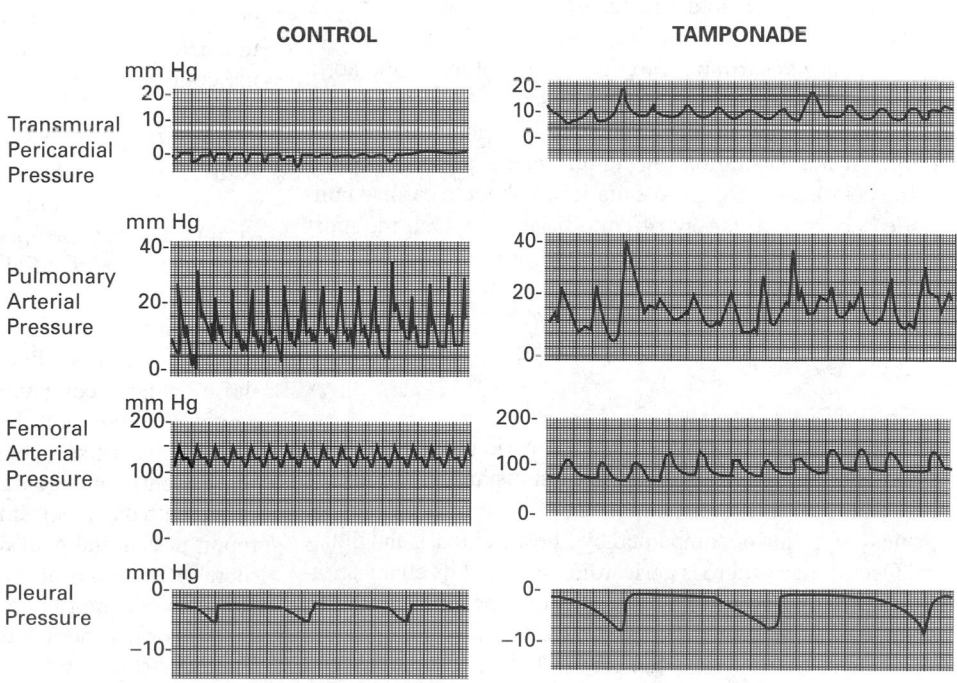

FIGURE 81-7

Tracings made during a study of experimental cardiac tamponade. The top panel shows that during inspiration, transmural pericardial pressure increases when tamponade exists but not otherwise. The third column shows the appearance of pulsus paradoxus with tamponade. Note also that during tamponade, pulmonary arterial pressure is neither exactly in phase nor 180° out of phase with aortic pressure. (From Shabetai R, et al. Pulsus paradoxus. *J Clin Invest* 1965; 11:1898. Reproduced with permission from the publisher.)

septum relative to the two ventricles is not altered by respiration[85] in the same manner as in tamponade. The "septal bounce" is caused by decreased left ventricular filling during inspiration.[85a]

VENTRICULAR FUNCTION AND CORONARY BLOOD FLOW

Systolic left ventricular function is usually unimpaired in both constrictive pericarditis and cardiac tamponade.[64] Longstanding calcific constrictive pericarditis may invade the myocardium and coronary vessels, leading to conduction disturbances[86] and impaired ventricular function.

In cardiac tamponade systolic ventricular function remains normal and is often supranormal. Unrelieved extreme tamponade is fatal because circulation ceases when venous pressure cannot increase to equal the pericardial pressure. In these cases, diminution of myocardial perfusion is aggravated by direct compression of the major coronary arteries[87] and abnormal transmyocardial distribution.[88]

CLINICAL FEATURES
OF CARDIAC TAMPONADE

Etiology

Virtually any disease that can affect the pericardium may cause pericardial effusion, and tamponade may complicate virtually any pericardial effusion; however, the common causes are few.

Acute tamponade is usually caused by trauma, which may be iatrogenic, or by rupture of the heart or aorta. The trauma may be penetrating or blunt. Rupture of the heart may occur during acute myocardial infarction, and rupture of the aorta may complicate aneurysm or aortic dissection. Iatrogenic injuries include perforation during cardiac catheterization or pacing, cardiac laceration during attempted pericardiocentesis, and contusion during resuscitation. Subacute cardiac tamponade occurs in a variety of conditions, of which the most common are idiopathic or viral pericarditis and neoplastic and dialysis-related pericardial disease.

Syndromes of Cardiac Tamponade

ACUTE CARDIAC TAMPONADE

Tamponade may be so sudden that the patient does not complain of symptoms. In less drastic circumstances, victims of chest trauma with cardiac tamponade may complain of severe shortness of breath accompanied by chest tightness and dizziness. Occasionally there is pericardial pain, but its characteristics are usually obscured by the pain of other injuries.

The venous pressure is greatly elevated, and the systemic arterial pressure severely depressed. Pulsus paradoxus can usually be appreciated except when hypotension is extreme. When pulsus paradoxus is not obvious in the radial pulse, it may be detected in larger vessels. In striking contrast to these abnormalities of both venous and arterial pressure, the precordium is quiet, cardiac activity often being impalpable (Beck's triad). In the most severe cases, consciousness may be impaired; but for the raised venous pressure, such patients appear to be in shock.

When cardiac tamponade complicates a diagnostic procedure, the patient complains of discomfort, generalized uneasiness, and precordial pain. Systemic arterial pressure falls, pulsus paradoxus appears, venous pressure rises, and severe tissue hypoperfusion appears. Fluoroscopy shows that the cardiac silhouette has increased and that its pulsations have diminished or disappeared.

Cardiac tamponade should be suspected in any likely victim of recent chest trauma who appears to be in shock. The suspicion is increased when venous pressure is high and pulsus paradoxus is present. When circumstances are at their most pressing, an immediate therapeutic trial of rapid infusion of fluid and diagnostic pericardiocentesis should be carried out. If the threat of death is more remote, pericardiocentesis should be delayed until the presence of pericardial fluid can be demonstrated by prompt echocardiography. On the other hand, when tamponade occurs in the diagnostic laboratory, where pressures are being monitored and fluoroscopy is on hand, one can safely establish the diagnosis without waiting for echocardiography.

Another cause of acute tamponade is cardiac rupture complicating acute myocardial infarction (Chap. 47). This catastrophe must be differentiated from cardiogenic shock (see "Specific Pericardial Disease," below). Acute cardiac tamponade is a life threatening complication of rupture of a dissecting hematoma of the proximal aorta (Chap. 98). A unique feature of this complication is that successful pericardiocentesis may, by permitting increased hemorrhage, lead to the patient's death.[89] If tamponade is severe enough to be considered a threat to survival, a limited pericardiocentesis is the rational compromise.

SUBACUTE CARDIAC TAMPONADE

A disconcertingly large number of diseases can cause cardiac tamponade. The common ones, however, are idiopathic or viral pericarditis, neoplastic invasion of the pericardium, and nephrogenic pericardial disease.

Symptoms

Symptoms may be divided into those of the underlying illness, those of the accompanying pericardial disease, and those of cardiac compression. Many patients with inflammatory pericarditis give a history of prodromal fever, myalgia, and arthralgia. Patients with neoplastic disease may have symptoms associated with the neoplasm itself and its treatment. Some patients report pericardial pain similar to that of acute pericarditis, but more often pain is absent. The symptoms of cardiac compression include rapidly progressive dyspnea accompanied by fullness or tightness in the chest, occasionally with dysphagia. The course may be less rapid, allowing time for increase in weight and abdominal girth and the rapid onset and progression of edema.

Physical Examination

The examination shows raised venous pressure and lowered systemic arterial pressure with pulsus paradoxus.[90] When there is underlying cardiac disease, the precordium is not necessarily unusually quiet, the apex beat may be palpated, and even cardiac enlargement may be present[91] (see Chap. 10).

The abnormalities of venous pressure described under "Pathophysiology," above, can often be recognized at the bedside. The mean pressure is elevated. When the patient's thorax and neck are placed at the elevation that maximizes the jugular venous pulsations, inspiratory decline in the height of pulsations can be appreciated. The χ descent is recognized as an inward pulsation of the internal jugular pulse coincident with the carotid pulse. These abnormalities, together with equal diastolic pressure on the two sides of the heart and reduced ventricular volumes, can also be demonstrated by cardiac catheterization. Catheterization, at least of the right side of the heart (Fig. 81-8), with comparisons of right atrial and pulmonary wedge

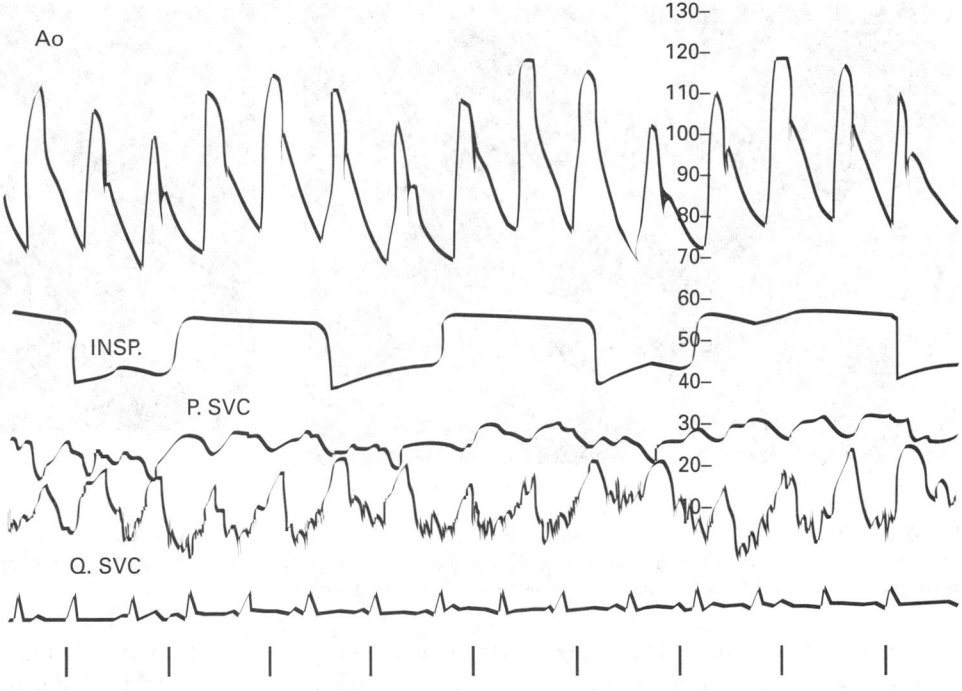

FIGURE 81-8

Cardiac catheterization of a patient with tamponade. From above, aortic pressure showing pulsus paradoxus, respiration, superior vena cava pressure (P SVC), and blood flow velocity (Q SVC). During inspiration (insp.), pressure declines and flow increases in the SVC. The SVC pressure shows a sharp χ but no γ descent. The SVC flow is monophasic, peaking at the χ descent. SVC pressure (and pericardial pressure, not shown) were 27 mmHg.

pressures, should be carried out if there is doubt about the diagnosis or if underlying heart disease is suspected. In the latter instance a full cardiac catheterization and angiographic procedure are required.[91]

Severe pulsus pradoxus is recognized as disappearance of the arterial pulse at the height of inspiration. Less severe pulsus pradoxus is felt as a decrease in pulse amplitude during inspiration. Pulsus paradoxus is difficult to evaluate or may be absent when the patient is in shock,[92] and its identification is also confounded by labored rapid breathing, atrial fibrillation, and frequent extrasystoles. The severity of pulsus paradoxus can be best estimated with the sphygmomanometer. The cuff must be deflated evenly and slowly while the patient's respirations are observed. In pulsus paradoxus, the first Korotkov sound is initially heard only during expiration. As the cuff pressure falls, this sound becomes audible throughout the respiratory cycle. The difference in systolic pressure between these events is an estimate o pulsus paradoxus. The "paradox" of pulsus paradoxus is that the arterial pulse weakens or may disappear while the loudness and regularity of the heart sounds do not vary.

In some cases it is necessary to document venous and arterial pressure by intravascular recordings. In all cases or whenever possible, direct measurement of central venous pressure and systemic arterial pressure should precede and accompany pericardiocentesis. The inspiratory drop in systemic arterial systolic and pulse pressure can then be accurately

quantified, and the initial portion of the χ descent of venous pressure can be identified as coinciding with the QT interval. The tracing verifies the inspiratory decline in venous or right atrial pressure and the absence or severe attenuation of the γ descent.

Echocardiogram

The diagnosis of cardiac tamponade is seldom secure without echocardiographic demonstration of pericardial effusion. Only under exceptional circumstances should pericardial drainage be undertaken without prior echocardiography to document the effusion and perhaps corroborate tamponade. Two-dimensional echocardiography has proved the value of compression of the right atrium[93] and diastolic collapse of the right ventricle[94] as highly reliable evidence of cardiac tamponade (Fig. 81-9) (see also Chap. 14). These two echocardiographic signs appear when cardiac tamponade is hemodynamically significant but before the advent of pulsus paradoxus or profound hypotension, which mark decompensated cardiac tamponade.[95] Less specific signs include exaggerated respiratory variation in ventricular dimensions[78] and the E-F slope of mitral valve closure[96] and pseudoprolapse of the mitral valve. More specific but less common is pendular swinging of the heart within the pericardial fluid.[97] This phenomenon can be recognized by M-mode studies but is dramatically demonstrated by two-dimensional echocardiography and is frequently associated with electrical alternans.[98]

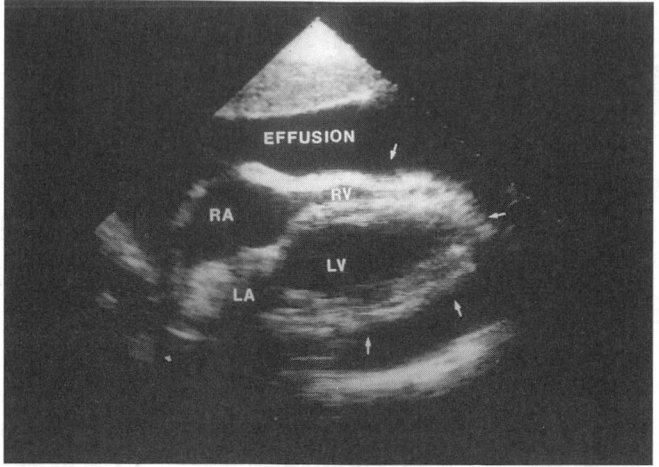

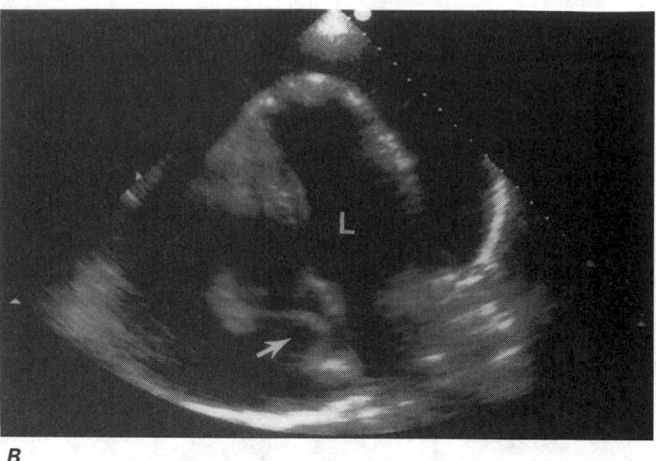

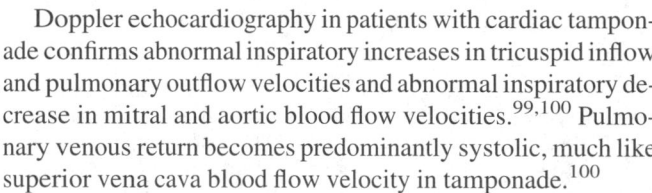

FIGURE 81-9

Echocardiographic features of cardiac tamponade. *A*. Subcostal view demonstrating a large effusion (*arrows*) and severe right ventricular compression.

B. Four-chamber view showing right atrial compression (*arrow*). L = left ventricle.

Doppler echocardiography in patients with cardiac tamponade confirms abnormal inspiratory increases in tricuspid inflow and pulmonary outflow velocities and abnormal inspiratory decrease in mitral and aortic blood flow velocities.[99,100] Pulmonary venous return becomes predominantly systolic, much like superior vena cava blood flow velocity in tamponade.[100]

Electrocardiogram

Frequently, there are no diagnostic ECG findings. Electrical alternans of the P wave, QRS complex, and T wave are highly suggestive of cardiac tamponade but are uncommon. Alternation of the QRS complex alone (Fig. 81-10) is more common but less specific.[101] Pericardial fluid tends to lower QRS voltage, and there may be associated abnormalities of the T waves.[102]

Less Common Syndromes of Cardiac Tamponade

LOW-PRESSURE CARDIAC TAMPONADE

Cardiac tamponade may develop when pericardial pressure is only modestly increased.[103] The clinical picture is subtle. The

venous pressure is increased only a few centimeters of water above normal, although inspection reveals absence or diminution of the γ descent. The blood pressure is normal and pulsus paradoxus is not striking and may be absent. There may be no symptoms. Causes include severe dehydration, overly vigorous diuresis, and massive extrapericardial blood loss.

One makes the diagnosis by keeping in mind the possibility of pericardial effusion in diseases that may reasonably involve the pericardium. Echocardiography can then confirm the effusion and sometimes tamponade and leads to examination of the neck veins. The diagnosis is established when catheterization of the right atrium and pericardial sac shows equal pressures, and hemodynamic improvement follows removal of pericardial fluid (Fig. 81-11).

EFFUSIVE-CONSTRICTIVE PERICARDITIS

When the pericardium is scarred but also contains fluid under pressure, cardiac tamponade results, but pulsus paradoxus may be absent. On the other hand, the venous pressure tends not to show striking γ dominance or Kussmaul's sign, and a pericardial knock is not present. When the pericardial fluid is aspirated, the hemodynamic features of constrictive pericarditis are unmasked.[84] This syndrome may occur in tuberculous pericarditis and in patients undergoing hemodialysis (see subsequent section "Constrictive Pericarditis"). If right atrial pressure fails to return to normal and shows abnormal cardiac and respiratory generated contours, the differential diagnosis is between effusive-constrictive pericarditis, right-sided heart failure, and tricuspid valve disease.

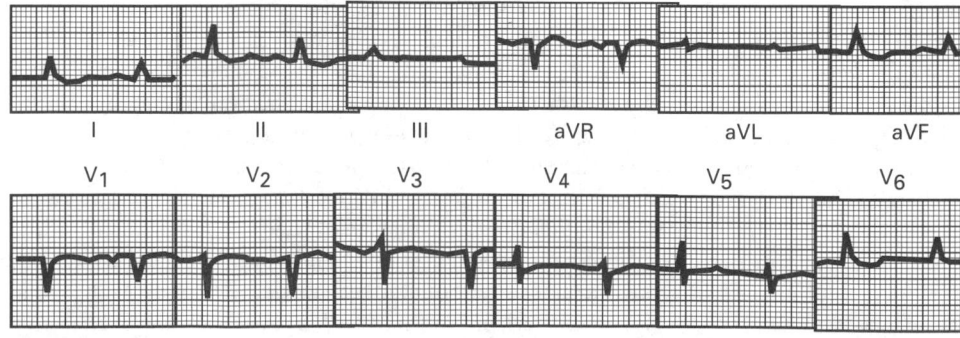

FIGURE 81-10

Alternans of QRS in cardiac tamponade. (From Shabetai R. *The Pericardium*. New York: Grune & Stratton; 1981. Reproduced with permission from the publisher.)

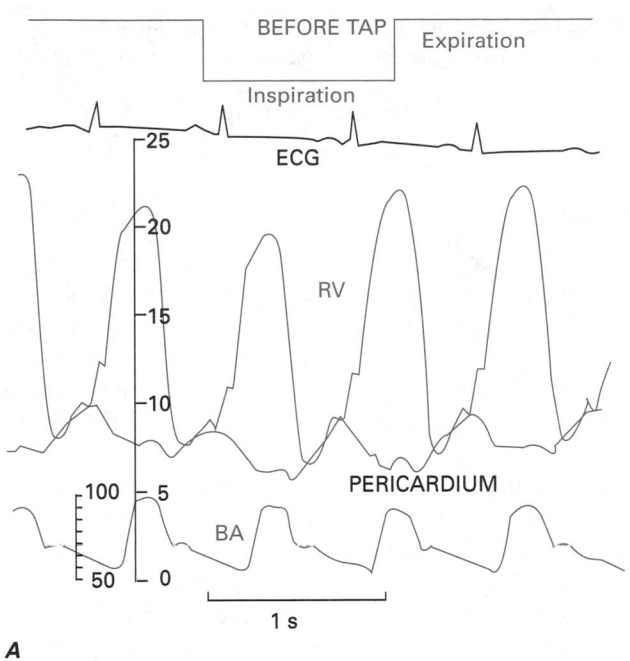

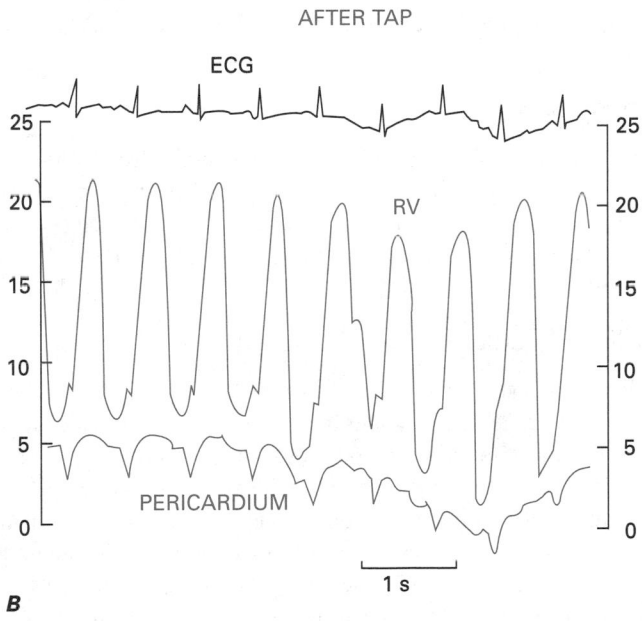

FIGURE 81-11

A. Low-pressure cardiac tamponade; tracing obtained during cardiac catheterization. Right ventricular diastolic pressure is only slightly elevated but is equal to pericardial pressure. Hypotension and pulsus paradoxus are absent. *B.* After pericardiocentesis, pericardial pressure is consistently lower than ventricular diastolic pressure. RV = right ventricle.

TAMPONADE COMPLICATING PREEXISTING HEART DISEASE

A commonly encountered example of cardiac tamponade modified by preexisting cardiac abnormalities is furnished by the population undergoing hemodialysis, in whom hypertrophy, fibrosis, and decreased compliance of the left ventricle are common.[104] The venous pressure may be affected by abnormalities unrelated to the pericardium; in these patients,

hypertension is common and cardiac output may be elevated by anemia and the access shunt. A third or fourth heart sound, cardiac murmurs, cardiac enlargement, and a left ventricular heave may be present in spite of cardiac tamponade. The ECG frequently suggests ischemic, hypertensive, or myocardial disease, which can obscure the findings of pericardial disease. The echocardiogram discloses enlargement and impaired function of the cardiac chambers in addition to the pericardial effusion. Furthermore, pulsus paradoxus is absent.[79] In patients undergoing dialysis, one must not require the classical presentation of cardiac tamponade before making the diagnosis. Rather, any rise in venous pressure that is not explained by fluid overload or a fall in blood pressure that is not explained by overdialysis should lead to the suspicion of cardiac tamponade, especially when there is unexplained enlargement of the heart by chest radiography (see Chap. 13 and subsequent section on "Specific Pericardial Disorders").

Cardiac tamponade is difficult to recognize in patients with severe right ventricular hypertrophy or right-sided failure because the cardiac abnormality and the raised pericardial pressure both contribute to the increase in jugular venous pressure and both can modify its waveform. Increased right ventricular diastolic pressure prevents diastolic collapse of the free wall of the right ventricle and compression of the right atrium.[94] Specific criteria for the diagnosis have not been established.

ATYPICAL CARDIAC TAMPONADE

Fluid in the pericardial space or mediastinum may be localized, compressing one side of the heart or one cardiac chamber.[105] Selective compression of the right side is the more common; but localized left-sided compression has also been reported[106] and can be associated with left atrial compression or left ventricular diastolic collapse. Localized cardiac tamponade from blood clots occurs after surgical operations on the heart.[107] Recognition may be difficult, and echocardiography may be inconclusive. In cases of clinical doubt, surgical exploration may be justified; when it confirms the diagnosis, it produces dramatic relief.

Differential Diagnosis

The differential diagnosis depends to a great extent on associated abnormalities. Many cases are confused with cardiac failure, since the two conditions both produce raised venous pressure, low cardiac output, and apparent cardiac enlargement. Abnormalities of jugular venous pressure in such cases may be wrongly attributed to cardiac failure and tricuspid regurgitation. The correct diagnosis can be arrived at by echocardiography and careful analysis of the jugular pulsations. Many cases are confused with shock, particularly after acute myocardial infarction; indeed, both can be present. The superior vena cava syndrome may be mistaken for cardiac tamponade, especially when the obstructing mass is mistaken for pericardial effusion, but in this case, although venous pressure is increased, pulsations are absent.

Treatment

He had ... in a case which was believed to be one of pericardial effusion, once inserted a trochar and cannula somewhat boldly, and the withdrawal of the trochar had been followed by a jet of blood which gave him great anxiety, but happily relieved the patient

S. West, 1883[108]

PERICARDIOCENTESIS VERSUS OPEN DRAINAGE

Most often, the only effective treatment is to drain the fluid, although early cardiac tamponade complicating idiopathic or viral pericarditis may remit with anti-inflammatory treatment. The pericardium may be drained via pericardiocentesis or by limited pericardiectomy.[109] The choice depends on the cause of effusion, the patient's general health, the physician's experience and preference, and the facilities available. Pericardiocentesis permits exact hemodynamic diagnosis and evaluation of the effects of pericardial drainage.[110] Simultaneous pressure recordings from the pericardial space, the right atrium, and a systemic artery, before and after removal of pericardial fluid, are often the most efficient way of diagnosing effusive-constrictive pericarditis. Pericardiocentesis is less expensive and consumes fewer resources than surgical drainage procedures. On the other hand, even in good hands, pericardiocentesis is associated with morbidity and occasional mortality.[111] The risk is reduced by echocardiographic localization of the fluid or echocardiographic guidance.[112]

Surgical drainage is performed under direct vision in a more controlled environment and permits pericardial biopsy. If it is done from the subxiphoid route, local anesthesia may suffice, but general anesthesia is usually preferred. If a more extensive procedure is needed, the incision can be extended cephalad for pericardiectomy. Intraoperative hemodynamic measurements are seldom satisfactory, although when fluid spurts from a pericardiotomy, cardiac tamponade is a reasonable supposition. Recently pericardiotomy has been performed percutaneously using a balloon.[113-115] it is too early to know how applicable this technique will prove to be.

The need for repeated pericardiocentesis is an indication for open drainage. In effusive-constrictive pericarditis, fluid drainage alone does not suffice but must be followed by pericardiectomy, almost always involving wide resection of the visceral pericardium. In patients with neoplastic pericardial disease, however, the benefits of pericardiectomy must be considered in the light of the total clinical picture (see also Chap. 86).

PHARMACOLOGIC INTERVENTION

Experimental studies[66] to the contrary notwithstanding, pharmacologic treatment of cardiac tamponade should not be thought of as anything but a temporizing measure. Often, the most important step is to expand the intravascular volume with blood, plasma, dextran, or even saline solution. Agents such as isoproterenol may be given to sustain venous and arterial pressures, and a vasodilator such as nitroprusside can be given to overcome the intense arterial vasoconstriction.[66]

CONSTRICTIVE PERICARDITIS

Etiology

Constrictive pericarditis may follow almost any pericardial reaction and should be suspected in any patient who has had pericardial disease and who develops increased central venous pressure. Again, a few causes account for the vast majority of cases. Many are idiopathic and some are posttraumatic. There is a small but definite incidence of constrictive pericarditis complicating operations on the heart and pericardium.[116] Neoplasia may invade the pericardium and is an important cause of constrictive pericarditis, effusive-constrictive pericarditis, and cardiac tamponade. Constrictive pericarditis may appear months or years after mediastinal radiation (see subsequent section on "Radiation-Induced Pericardial Disease"). In the United States, tuberculosis was previously a common etiology[117]; currently it is progressively less important as a cause of constrictive pericarditis,[118] but cases following tuberculosis and other infections of the pericardium are still encountered.

Symptoms

The usual symptoms are indistinguishable from those of congestive heart failure, but there may have been prior pericarditis. Dyspnea and fatigue[117,119] are common; in long-standing cases, weight gain, edema, and ascites make their appearance.[119]

Clinical Features

Signs suggesting congestive heart failure in patients who lack an appropriate etiology and in whom there is no evidence of cardiac abnormalities should arouse suspicion of constrictive pericarditis. This suspicion is heightened by evidence of pre-existing pericardial disease or disorders that affect the pericardium. The venous pressure is almost invariably elevated and is characterized by the preservation of both χ and γ descents. Frequently the γ descent, an inward jugular pulsation asynchronous with the carotid pulse, is dominant. Peripheral edema is common, the liver is enlarged, and ascites may be disproportionate.

In some cases the apex beat is impalpable; in others systolic retraction of the apex impulse may be present. Since there may be preexisting cardiac enlargement, displacement of the apex beat must not be taken as evidence against the presence of constrictive pericarditis. Likewise, systolic murmurs are common, and the pericardial knock may be difficult to distinguish from a third heart sound of heart failure.

In chronic cases the pericardium may be calcified[117] (Fig. 81-12), but it may not be in subacute pericarditis, which in the United States is increasingly replacing chronic pericarditis in the spectrum of pericardial disease.[118] A wide bifid P wave,

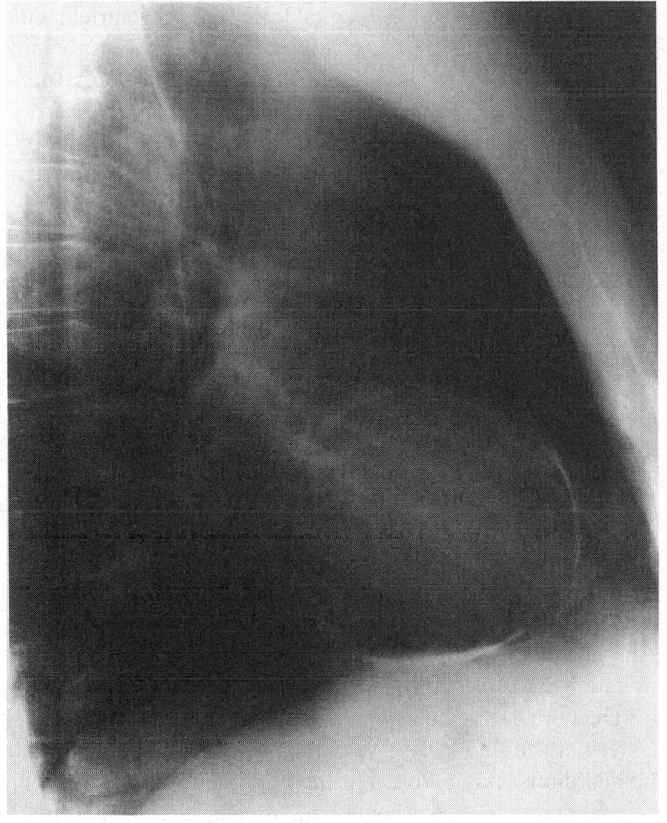

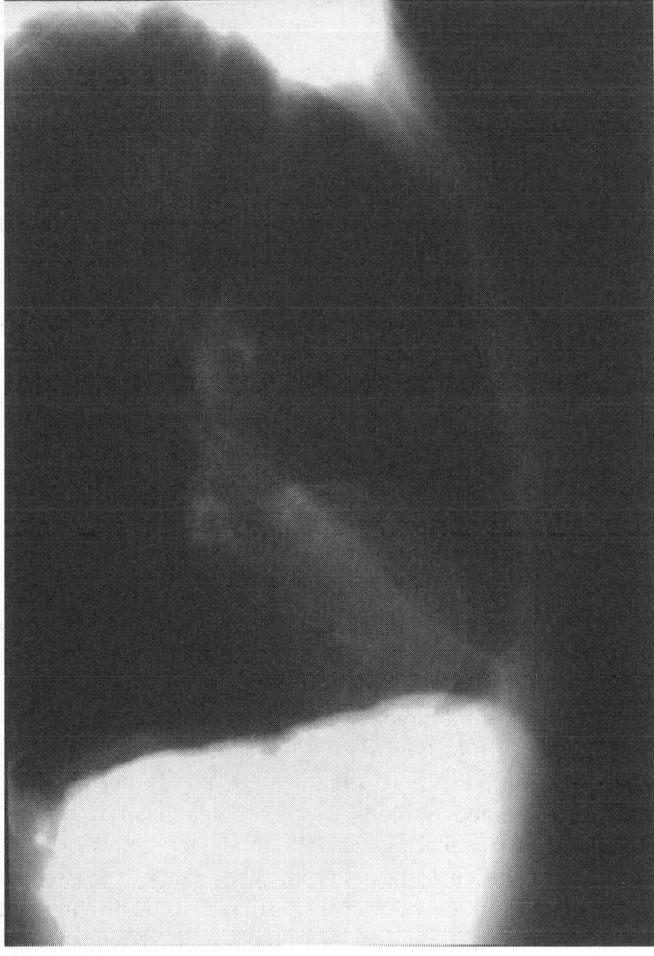

FIGURE 81-12
Calcification around the cardiac silhouette. *A.* Calcific constrictive pericarditis. *B.* Calcified left ventricular aneurysm. This finding can be mistaken for pericardial calcification.

like that of mitral stenosis, is common as long as sinus rhythm is maintained, but in chronic cases atrial fibrillation is the rule.[120] Nonspecific repolarization changes consist for the most part of widespread T-wave inversion[27] (Fig. 81-13). When the scar involves the myocardium or coronary arteries, depolarization changes, such as bundle branch block, and conduction delay between atrium and ventricle may be found[86] (see also Chap. 12). Liver function tests are often abnormal, sometimes grossly so.

Cardiac Catheterization

Catheterization and angiography are done to help assess the severity of constriction, determine cardiac function, discover underlying heart disease and, most importantly, exclude restrictive cardiomyopathy. The findings are those discussed under "Pathophysiology," above, and illustrated in Figs. 81-6 and 81-14.

Differential Diagnosis

The most commonly encountered erroneous diagnosis is cirrhosis of the liver. In cirrhosis, however, the central venous pressure is not much increased. Differentiation from right-sided heart failure with tricuspid regurgitation can be difficult:

There is systemic congestion in both disorders, and both are characterized by a prominent γ descent of venous pressure. Furthermore, severe tricuspid regurgitation can be present without a loud murmur, and the ν wave may not be impressive when the atrium is greatly enlarged and highly compliant. Tricuspid regurgitation can mitigate pulmonary congestion, leading to further confusion with constrictive pericarditis. In right-sided heart failure, the etiology is usually apparent and there is right ventricular hypertrophy and enlargement. The ECG may show tall, narrow P waves in the right precordial leads and limb lead 2, right axis deviation, and right ventricular hypertrophy. Echocardiography or other imaging techniques show enlargement and dysfunction of the right side of the heart.

Right ventricular infarction can produce a hemodynamic picture indistinguishable from that of constrictive pericarditis, with a prominent γ descent, absent respiratory variation in central venous pressure, early diastolic dip of ventricular pressure, and equal diastolic pressures on the two sides of the heart.[121,122] This differential diagnosis is particularly difficult when this condition arises in patients who have undergone saphenous vein bypass grafting operations, because they are at risk for both postoperative constrictive pericarditis and right ventricular infarction. Severe lesions of arteries supplying the

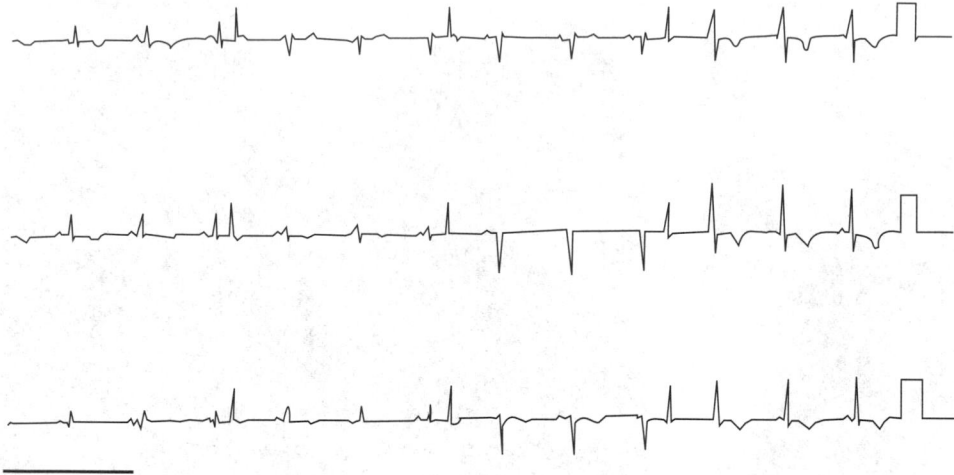

FIGURE 81-13

Electrocardiogram of a patient with tuberculous constrictive pericarditis showing widespread inversed polarity of the T waves. The leads are mounted in the conventional sequence.

right ventricle and evidence of right ventricular dysfunction found by imaging techniques are good clues to right ventricular infarction.

Restrictive cardiomyopathy may also reproduce the hemodynamic picture of constrictive pericarditis (see Table 81-4 and Chap. 75). Restrictive cardiomyopathy is not common but may characterize some cases of amyloid heart disease,[123] idiopathic myocardial disease, and other storage diseases.[124] When left ventricular diastolic pressure greatly exceeds right ventricular diastolic pressure, the diagnosis is usually not in doubt,[120] but exceptional cases of localized constrictive pericarditis can occur.[125] It is restrictive cardiomyopathy with

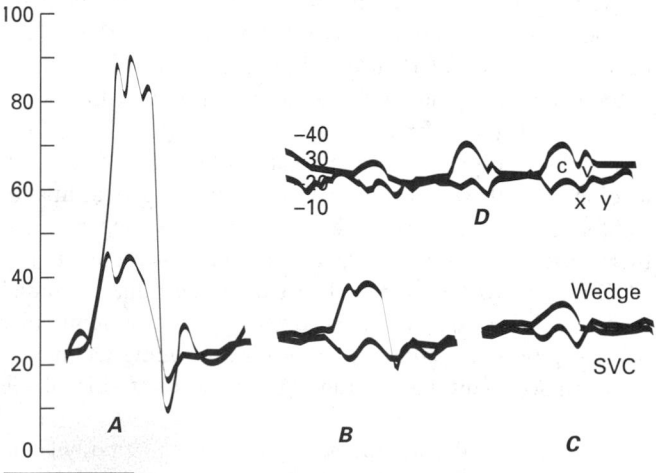

FIGURE 81-14

Cardiac catheterization tracings from a patient with constrictive pericarditis. *A.* Pressures recorded simultaneously from both ventricles. *B.* Simultaneous right atrial and ventricular pressures showing early diastolic dip and χ and γ descents. *C.* Simultaneous pulmonary wedge and superior vena cava (SVC) pressures. *D.* Simultaneous pulmonary arterial and SVC pressures. (From Shabetai R, Grossman W. Profiles in constrictive pericarditis, restrictive cardiomyopathy and cardiac tamponade. In: Grossman W, ed. *Cardiac Catheterization and Angiography*, 2d ed. Philadelphia: Lea & Febiger; 1980:360. Reproduced with permission from the publisher and editor.)

equal left and right ventricular diastolic pressure that must be distinguished from constrictive pericarditis without pericardial calcification. This situation is considerably more common than was previously thought. Exercise,[126] pharmacologic interventions,[127] and fluid challenge may be used to try to induce separation between left and right ventricular diastolic pressures, but experience is so limited that neither the specificity nor the sensitivity of these tests is well established. The same reservation applies to the observation that the rate of early diastolic filling is abnormally rapid in constrictive pericarditis but abnormally slow in restrictive pericarditis.[128] Another major difficulty is that entities such as mediastinal radiation can affect both the pericardium and the myocardium.

The correct diagnosis can sometimes be arrived at by discovery of a systemic disease with a predilection for either the myocardium (amyloidosis) or the pericardium (tuberculosis). Major conduction disturbances and depolarization abnormalities, while possible in constrictive pericarditis,[86] favor the diagnosis of cardiomyopathy.

The thickened adherent parietal pericardium may be visualized by echocardiography[129] (Fig. 81-15), magnetic resonance imaging, or by computed tomography[130] (Fig. 81-16), but current imaging techniques may not be helpful when constriction is produced by a thin, tight visceral pericardium. The analog of the hemodynamic early diastolic dip followed by plateau of pericardial pressure may be recognized echocardiographically by a rapid expansion of ventricular dimensions in early diastole followed by a long period during which there is little or no change. This abnormality is present in both restrictive cardiomyopathy and constrictive pericarditis, but the diagnosis of constrictive pericarditis is favored by preservation of motion of the interventricular septum, notching of the motion of the septum[85] in patients with P mitrale, and motion of the pericardium synchronous with the myocardium.

Attention to the preceding points usually serves to distinguish constrictive pericarditis from restrictive cardiomyopathy. In summary, the history often points to the pericardium or myocardium, the examination by definition is not helpful, and calcification of the pericardium and ECG depolarization abnormalities favor myocardial disease, but their absence is nondiagnostic. Grossly different filling pressures on the left and right sides of the heart favor myocardial disease, but equal filling pressures are nondiagnostic. This problem is addressed in more detail in Chap. 75. When doubt remains, endomyocardial biopsy may disclose myocardial disease.[131] When an experienced cardiologist remains in doubt after full investigation, exploratory thoracotomy with a view to possible pericardiectomy is fully justified, though fortunately this is seldom required.

Syndromes of Constrictive Pericarditis

CHRONIC CALCIFIC CONSTRICTIVE PERICARDITIS

Classic constrictive pericarditis is now encountered less frequently. The clinical picture is striking, with severe cachexia, anasarca, massively increased venous pressure, and atrial fibrillation. Calcium frequently surrounds the whole pericardium and is best seen in lateral or oblique projections of the chest radiograph (Fig. 81-8). Liver dysfunction is severe, amounting to failure, with spider angiomata, bilirubin retention, and even altered states of consciousness.

SUBACUTE CONSTRICTIVE PERICARDITIS

This form of constrictive pericarditis is becoming more common at the expense of chronic constrictive pericarditis. Frequently, the pericardium is not calcified and the course may be a matter of weeks or months to 2 or 3 years. Subacute constrictive pericarditis may occur in rheumatoid arthritis[132] and following *Haemophilus influenzae* infections, the latter especially in children. The diagnosis depends on careful evaluation of venous pressure in patients with systemic diseases that may involve the pericardium.

POSTOPERATIVE CONSTRICTIVE PERICARDITIS

In view of the nature of intrapericardial surgical operations, it is surprising that the incidence of postoperative constrictive pericarditis does not exceed the 0.2 percent reported in a careful retrospective study.[133] In these operations the pericardium is subject to cellular injury and is exposed

TABLE 81-4

FEATURES DISTINGUISHING RESTRICTIVE CARDIOMYOPATHY FROM CONSTRICTIVE PERICARDITIS

Observation	Restrictive Cardiomyopathy	Constrictive Pericarditis
History	Systemic disease that may affect the myocardium	Prior acute pericarditis Prior cardiac surgery Prior radiation therapy Prior chest trauma Systemic disease that may involve the pericardium
Chest radiogram	Not discriminating when pericardial calcification is absent	Discriminates only when pericardial calcification is present
Electrocardiogram	LBBB, RBBB, AV block Q waves Ventricular arrhythmia	Abnormal repolarization, normal depolarization
CT or MRI	Normal appearance of pericardium	Pericardium thick
Hemodynamics	Unequal left and right heart filling pressures	May fail to distinguish
Endomyocardial biopsy	Fibrosis Hypertrophy Infiltrative disease Abnormal nuclei	Normal

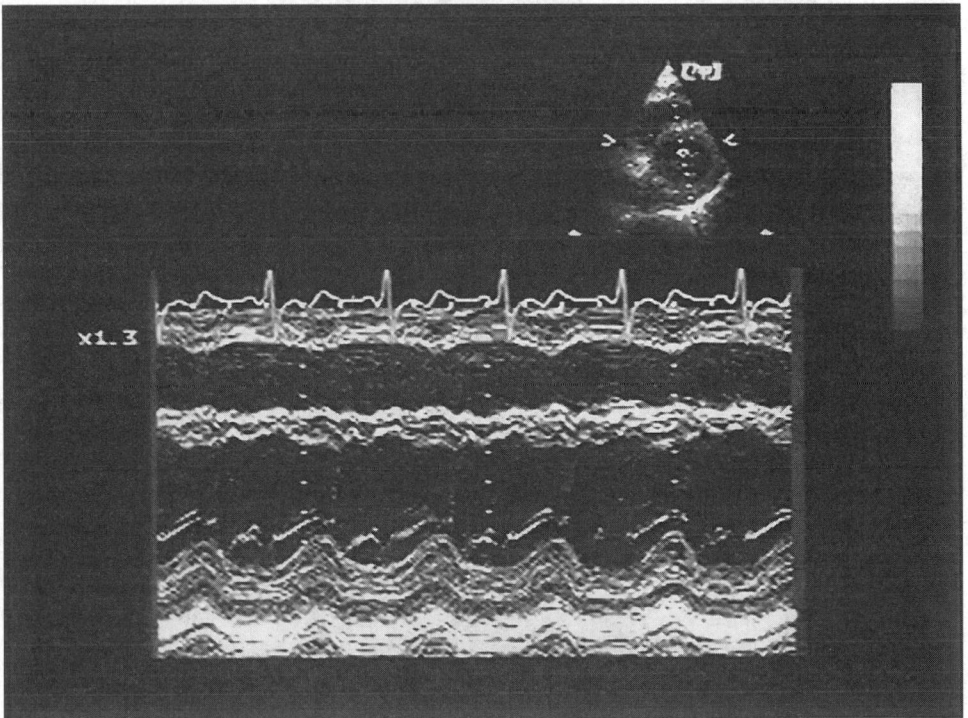

FIGURE 81-15

M-mode echocardiogram from the patient with tuberculous constrictive pericarditis illustrated in Fig. 81-6. Note the thick, echodense pericardium (thick wavy lines along bottom edge of figure). The pericardium moves with the heart, indicating its abnormal adherence to the myocardium.

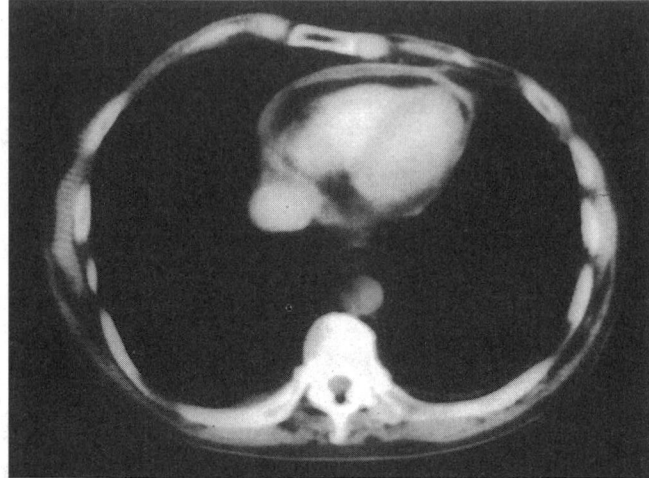

A

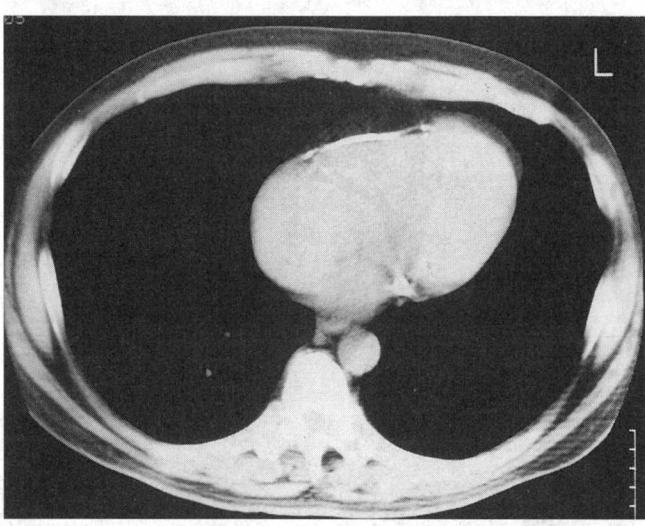

B

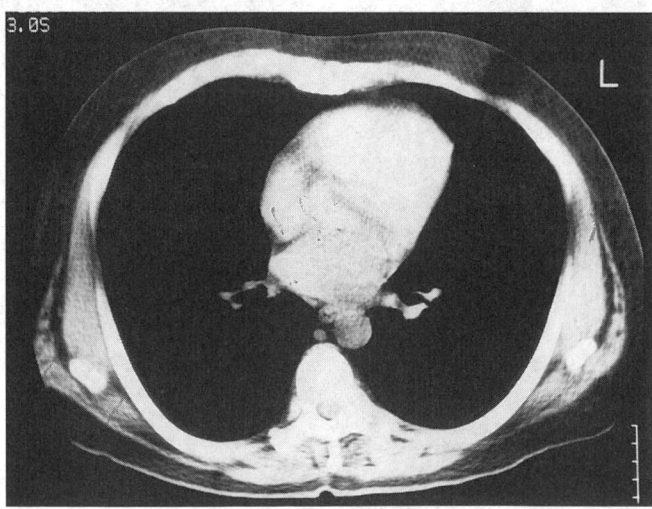

C

FIGURE 81-16

Computed tomography images of the heart taken to image the pericardium. *A.* Greatly thickened pericardium with small effusion. *B.* A less severe case of constrictive pericarditis. *C.* A case of radiation-induced restrictive cardiomyopathy in which the pericardium was not visualized.

to blood, foreign materials, and local hypothermia, all of which may induce inflammation. There is considerable variation in whether or not and how the pericardium is closed after cardiac operations and in the techniques employed for myocardial preservation; yet no specific factors, save possibly the now discontinued use of iodine solutions,[134] have been implicated as etiologic.

OCCULT CONSTRICTIVE PERICARDITIS

This is defined as constrictive pericarditis so mild that it is not detectable without fluid challenge.[135] In the first series reported, the patients complained of nondescript chest pain, for which they underwent cardiac catheterization and coronary arteriography. Many reported previous acute pericarditis. hemodynamic studies revealed normal atrial and ventricular pressures, but following the infusion of approximately 1 L of saline solution in roughly 10 min, the right atrial pressure waveform assumed the characteristics of constrictive pericarditis and the diastolic pressures in the two ventricles became equal. At subsequent operation, the pericardium was thickened and fibrosed—findings that were confirmed by histologic examination.

This form of constrictive pericarditis must be rare, and its existence, though frequently sought, is seldom confirmed. Caution is advised in applying rapid, large fluid challenges to patients undergoing cardiac catheterization; furthermore, the induction of hemodynamic changes suggesting constrictive pericarditis by this technique should seldom if ever be taken alone as indication for pericardiectomy.[136]

EFFUSIVE-CONSTRICTIVE PERICARDITIS

This condition results from combined cardiac tamponade and constrictive pericarditis[84] and may occur in tuberculous pericarditis and in neoplastic or postradiation pericardiopathy. The clinical and hemodynamic presentation is that of cardiac tamponade. Studies of the venous pulse before and after pericardiocentesis, however, reveal persistence of raised venous pressure and absent respiratory variation of the venous pulse but a prominent γ descent that was less apparent before pericardiocentesis (Fig. 81-17).

LOCALIZED CONSTRICTION

Localized constrictive pericarditis is rare, but occasionally a localized band constricts the inflow or outflow region of one or more of the cardiac chambers. The clinical picture then simulates valve disease or venous obstruction[137] (Fig. 81-18).

TRANSIENT CONSTRICTIVE PERICARDITIS

In a series of 117 patients with acute effusive pericarditis, evidence of constriction developed in 16 but disappeared spontaneously.[138] The possibility that pericardial constriction may be transient should be considered before pericardiectomy is embarked upon.

Treatment

The treatment of constrictive pericarditis is usually surgical pericardiectomy. The mildest cases can be followed without

CHAPTER 81
DISEASES OF THE PERICARDIUM

2191

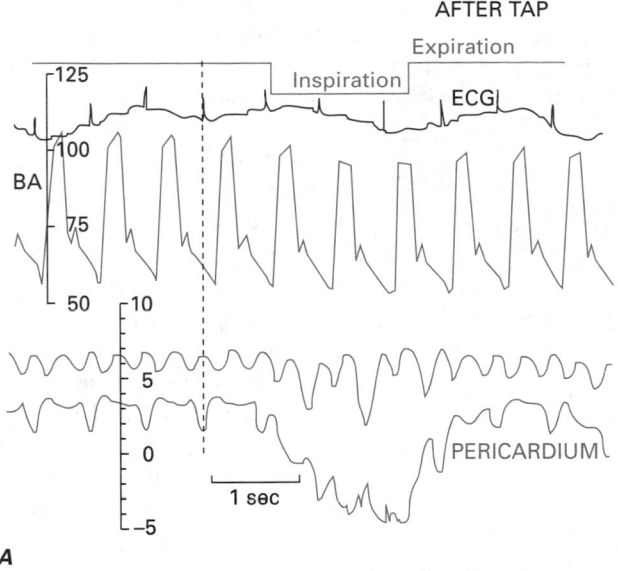

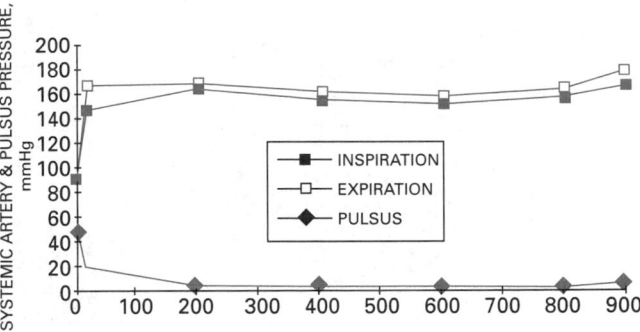

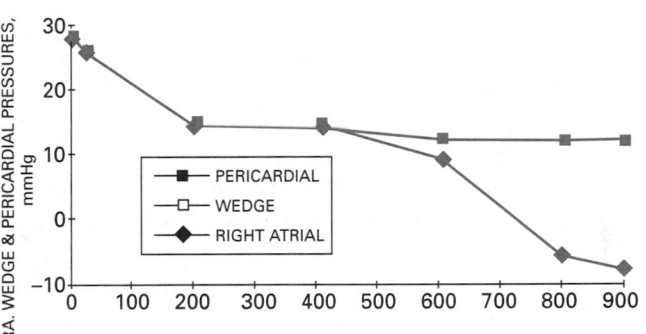

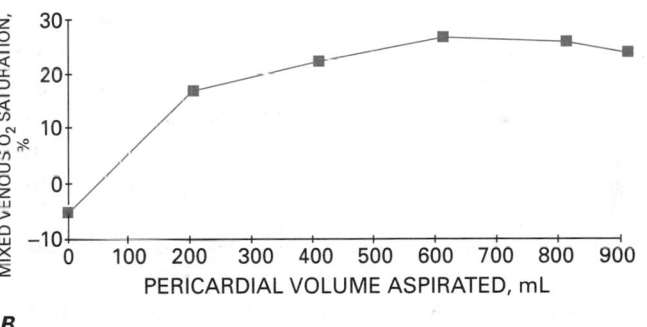

FIGURE 81-17

A. Recording made during cardiac catheterization of a patient with effusive-constrictive pericarditis due to bronchogenic carcinoma. The tracings were obtained during the pericardiocentesis, which has lowered pericardial pressure; however, right atrial pressure elevation persists and the tracing shows prominent χ and γ descents and absent respiratory variation. (From Shabetai R. *The Pericardium.* New York: Grune & Stratton; 1981:273. Reproduced with permission from the publisher.) *B.* Hemodynamic variables recorded from a 62-year-old man with metastatic, far advanced bronchogenic carcinoma who presented with ankle swelling, abdominal distension, and shortness of breath. Pericardiocentesis yielded bloody effusion and abundant malignant cells. When the needle was introduced, pulsus paradoxus (*upper panel, closed circles*) was 50 mmHg and the pericardial, right atrial, and pulmonary wedge pressures were 29 mmHg. During aspiration of the first 400 mL via catheter, the three pressures fell equally, and the mixed venous oxygen saturation rose from 35 to 60 vol %. During aspiration of the next 500 mL, pericardial pressure fell to subambient, but right atrial and pulmonary wedge pressures continued to be equal and elevated to 14 mmHg. Mixed venous oxygen saturation failed to reach normal. These findings indicated effusive-constrictive pericarditis, which was confirmed at necropsy.

surgical treatment, but when jugular venous pressure is consistently raised beyond 7 or 8 mmHg or edema requires medical treatment for its control, pericardiectomy should be carried out. In the most extreme cases of severe long-standing constrictive pericarditis with profound cachexia and liver dysfunction, it has been argued that treatment with a diuretic and digitalis is preferred,[136] because operative mortality can be as high as 30 to 40 percent and many patients fail to improve significantly.

Pericardiectomy is commonly carried out via a median sternotomy, although some surgeons prefer thoracotomy. The risk of mortality has declined but is still in the range of 5 to 15 percent.[139,140] The risk is increased by heavy calcification, especially involving the epicardium, and by the need to remove the visceral pericardium. Recovery of normal venous pressure and cardiac performance may be delayed for weeks or months; it occurs sooner when the operation is carried out before the disease is too chronic and when the pericardiectomy

is almost complete and all constricting bands have been resected.[141] Left ventricular systolic dysfunction may occur after decortication of a severely constricted heart. This condition may require treatment for several months, but then it usually resolves completely.

SPECIFIC PERICARDIAL DISEASE

Congenital Malformation

ABSENCE AND PARTIAL ABSENCE OF THE PERICARDIUM
The most important congenital malformation of the pericardium is partial absence of the left pericardium; complete absence is less common. This anomaly may be associated with congenital malformations of the heart,[142] including patent ductus arteriosus, atrial septal defect, mitral stenosis,

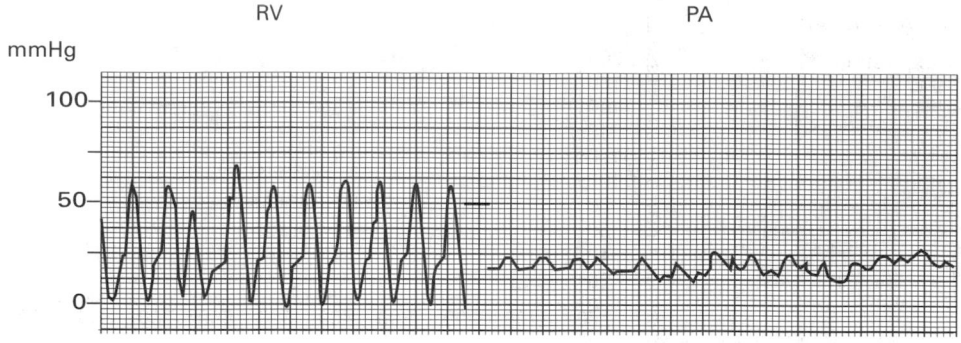

FIGURE 81-18

Pressure tracing from the pulmonary artery (PA) and right ventricle (RV) of a patient with extrinsic pulmonary stenosis caused by a localized band of pericardial constriction that developed after rupture of the esophagus. (From Shabetai R. *The Pericardium*. New York: Grune & Stratton; 1981:208. Reproduced with permission from the publisher.)

tetralogy of Fallot, tricuspid regurgitation, and Eisenmenger physiology. An association with mitral valve prolapse has also been reported.

Diagnosis

Most cases are suspected first because of an abnormality on the chest roentgenogram.[143] The heart tends to be shifted to the left, and its left border is elongated, showing prominent separation between the aorta and the pulmonary artery. Lucencies caused by interposition of lung may be seen between the pulmonary artery segment and the aortic knob and between the left hemidiaphragm and the base of the heart (see Chap. 13). Magnetic resonance imaging detects lesions missed by chest radiography and echocardiography and reliably establishes the anatomy of the defect.[144]

Most patients are symptomless, but chest pain is reported by a significant proportion, perhaps in part because of torsion of the great vessels. Recurrent pulmonary infections may be a significant feature. Physical findings are not often helpful, but a conspicuous left ventricular heave in the anterior or midaxillary line may be found when the deficiency is substantial. A systolic murmur may be present; on occasion, diastolic murmurs have been described.

Laboratory Findings

The ECG in patients with complete absence of the left side of the pericardium usually shows incomplete right bundle branch block. In the presence of induced or spontaneous pneumothorax, air can enter the pericardial space and outline the pericardium.

Clinical Course and Treatment

Total and very small deficiencies are not associated with pathophysiologic changes. medium-size defects may allow herniation of the left atrium, and the rare apical defect may allow herniation of the cardiac apex. Strangulation may then ensue, requiring surgical closure or enlargement of the defect

to reduce the herniation and prevent recurrence. The procedure can sometimes be accomplished via a thoracoscope.[145]

Pericardial Cysts

Pericardial cysts vary greatly in size, are smooth and rounded, and most commonly are found in the right cardiophrenic angle. They are benign and produce no local or general symptoms. Their importance lies in differentiation from neoplasm. The roentgenographic appearance of pericardial cysts is highly characteristic, and the nature of the lesion can be confirmed by computed tomography (see Chap. 13).

Dialysis-Related and Uremic Pericardial Disease

ETIOLOGY

The association of pericardial disease with renal failure has been widely recognized since its description by Richard Bright in 1836.[146] Bright's report referred to end-stage renal disease in which pericarditis still occurs, but today pericarditis complicating chronic dialysis is of greater importance. The mechanism, in spite of considerable investigation and speculation, remains unknown. The theory that uremic pericarditis is a chemical reaction to retained products of metabolism fails to account for the lack of relationship between the level of blood urea nitrogen or other nitrogenous metabolites and the frequency of pericarditis. Pericarditis is less common in patients undergoing peritoneal dialysis than in those undergoing hemodialysis. This suggests a possible role for "middle molecules." The hemorrhagic diathesis, an important component of the uremic syndrome, may predispose to pericarditis, a predisposition that may be aggravated by even regional heparinization. Nephrogenic pericarditis is highly vascular; consequently, uremia or dialysis-related pericardial effusion is usually bloody. The clinical manifestation may be acute fibrinous pericarditis, pericardial effusion, or cardiac tamponade. Classic constrictive pericarditis is a rare sequel (see also Chap. 94).

The etiology in dialyzed patients may be different from that in end-stage renal failure. It is possible that some cases are caused by living agents introduced into the bloodstream during hemodialysis or that pericarditis is an immune response to a component of the hemodialysis equipment of fluid.[147] In recent years pericarditis, pericardial effusion, and cardiac tamponade are encountered much less often in dialysis units, perhaps owing to changes in the material of which the dialysis membranes are made. Renal insufficiency is associated with increased susceptibility to infection; therefore the possibility of viral, tuberculous, or even bacterial pericarditis must not be neglected. Since neoplasia, ischemic heart disease, and thyroid disease occur in this population, it is wise to consider these in the differential diagnosis before making a presumptive diagnosis of dialysis-related pericarditis.

DIAGNOSIS

Fibrinous pericarditis is manifested by a pericardial friction rub, which may be coarse and sometimes is palpable. Chest pain occurs in about two-thirds of patients and fever in the vast majority.[147] The ECG is of little value, since the classic ST-segment elevation may not be present, reflecting sparing of the epicardium.[148]

Pericardial effusion should be suspected whenever there is a sudden unexplained increase in the apparent size of the heart in a dialysis patient, but differentiation from fluid overload or congestive heart failure is important. Unexplained cardiac enlargement or hemodynamic deterioration suggests either cardiac tamponade, fluid imbalance, or heart failure. Physicians caring for patients undergoing hemodialysis must constantly be on the alert for cardiac tamponade, especially since the clinical manifestations may be atypical and difficult to distinguish from cardiac and cardiovascular deterioration. Recognition and good treatment are essential, as cardiac tamponade remains one of the principal causes of hemodialysis-associated morbidity and in 20 percent of cases terminates fatally.[149]

TREATMENT

Acute pericarditis without hemodynamic manifestations is treated by intensified dialysis.[104] Nonsteroidal anti-inflammatory agents may accelerate resolution but can aggravate bleeding. Pericardial effusion without associated changes in venous or arterial pressure is usually treated in the same way; a salutary response may be anticipated.

Considerable controversy exists regarding the optimal management of large, persistent, or recurrent pericardial effusion and especially of cardiac tamponade. A conservative approach to early cardiac tamponade is intensification of hemodialysis combined with either nonsteroidal agents or prednisone. More severe tamponade is an indication for pericardial drainage. The instillation of nonabsorbable steroids directly into the pericardial space has been advocated[150] but is now seldom employed.

The Pericardium and Myocardial Infarction

PERICARDIAL FRICTION RUB IN ACUTE MYOCARDIAL INFARCTION

A pericardial friction rub occurs in approximately 10 percent of patients with acute myocardial infarction[151] and perhaps more commonly, since it is often transitory. Shaggy fibrinous pericarditis may be found overlying transmural or Q-wave infarction. Pericarditis, however, can occur in non-Q-wave infarction, and sometimes a pericardial friction rub is audible in patients with inferior wall myocardial infarction, suggesting that pericarditis may sometimes be an immune reaction to myocardial damage.

The pain may be difficult or impossible to distinguish from angina, extension of infarction, or pulmonary embolism. Similarly, it is often impossible to recognize pericarditis on the ECG during evolution of an acute myocardial infarction. Pericarditis, however, may further increase ST elevation in acute myocardial infarction and can cause ST elevation where reciprocal depression is anticipated. Evolution of T-wave changes is also modified, the T wave remaining or becoming positive when T-wave inversion would have been expected[152] (see Chap. 12). Echocardiography has demonstrated that silent pericardial effusion may accompany myocardial infarction.

The most important practical aspect of acute pericarditis in myocardial infarction is the extent to which it contraindicates or modifies treatment with anticoagulants. A pericardial friction rub occurring in the first 2 or 3 days and not accompanied by pericardial effusion or evidence suggesting cardiac tamponade need not modify standard practice, which in any case is variable. Pericarditis occurring later in the course or accompanied by pericardial effusion or tamponade is a contraindication to anticoagulant therapy. Thrombolytic therapy is almost always begun before pericarditis develops, thereby lessening the need for clinical decision making. The GISSI-2 investigators found that thrombolysis, rather than being a cause of pericardial bleeding, halved the incidence of pericardial involvement in acute myocardial infarction.[153] On the other hand and not surprisingly, thrombolytic therapy given when acute pericarditis is mistaken for acute myocardial infarction can result in serious tamponade.[154] Acute pericarditis does not of itself alter the prognosis but tends to be associated with larger infarctions and hence with a higher incidence of arrhythmia and a higher mortality.[155] In an important study,[156] echocardiography disclosed pericardial effusion in 28 percent of 138 patients with acute myocardial infarction. An association between pericardial effusion and early pericarditis was not demonstrated. Resorption was surprisingly slow, persistence of effusion up to 6 months being found by serial study in 8 of 98 patients (see Chap. 47).

DRESSLER'S SYNDROME

Dressler described a syndrome following myocardial infarction, comprising chest pain, pleurisy, pericardial friction rub, fever, and leukocytosis, sometimes associated with pulmonary infiltrate.[157] This complication, described almost in its entirety in the title of the original description,[157] usually occurs weeks or months after the causative infarction but may occur while the patient is still in the hospital. Most authorities consider it a separate entity from acute pericarditis occurring within the first 48 h,[158] but pericarditis associated with myocardial infarction may be an immune reaction to myocardial damage.[159] The post–myocardial infarction syndrome may be caused by a combination of viral activation and myocardial antibodies,[160] bringing it into line with the clinically similar postpericardiotomy syndrome, for which there is strong evidence supporting this dual etiology.[161]

Diagnosis is scarcely tenable without a pericardial friction rub, and it is strengthened by the presence of pericardial effusion. When Dressler's syndrome occurs soon after infarction, the differential diagnosis must include extension of the infarction, or pulmonary embolism. Later cases must be distinguished from a second infarction and unstable angina. Symptoms and signs usually subside rapidly with treatment with nonsteroidal anti-inflammatory drugs, but more resistant cases need prednisone or a comparable corticosteroid. Over the succeeding months or years, there may be several recurrences that require treatment (see also Chap. 47). The post–myocardial infarction syndrome appears to be decreasing in prevalence,[160] possibly reflecting the decreased use of warfarin in acute myocardial infarction.

POSTPERICARDIOTOMY SYNDROME

This syndrome, with features indistinguishable from those of acute idiopathic pericarditis or Dressler's syndrome, occurs after operations in which the pericardium is opened. The syndrome occurs in children and adults and is not, as previously thought, more common in those undergoing operation for rheumatic heart disease. Epidemiologic studies have shown high levels of both antiheart antibody and viral titers.[161] The differential diagnosis includes overt postoperative complications associated with pleurisy, pleural effusion, pericardial effusion, chest pain, and fever.

TREATMENT

Treatment is with nonsteroidal anti-inflammatory agents. Prednisone should be withheld unless simpler treatment fails. Recurrences are possible and require reinitiation of treatment.

Posttraumatic Pericardial Syndrome

A virtually indistinguishable syndrome may follow blunt or sharp chest trauma. Common to all these conditions are injury to the pericardial mesothelium, myocardial injury, and blood in the pericardial space.[162] Treatment is with anti-inflammatory drugs.

Neoplastic Pericardial Disease

A number of primary and secondary neoplasms may involve the myocardium and pericardium. Secondary neoplasia of the pericardium is much more common than primary, the leading offenders being carcinoma of the breast and lung, lymphoma, and leukemia. Mesothelioma is the most common primary pericardial neoplasm and may respond to treatment with doxorubicin and cyclophosphamide.[163] Melanoma may involve the myocardium extensively yet seldom produces clinical findings except when the pericardium is involved. Echocardiography may demonstrate the pericardial mass and help to differentiate it from a nonneoplastic mass (Fig. 81-19) (see also Chap. 86).

UNCOMMON NEOPLASMS

Rare metastatic neoplasms of the pericardium include carcinomas of the colon, esophagus, kidney, ovary, prostate, and stomach as well as sarcoma.[164] Rare primary neoplasms include lymphangioma, hemangioma,[165] and teratoma.[166]

CLINICAL FEATURES

The most common manifestation is pericardial effusion; indeed, the most common cause of cardiac tamponade observed on medical wards today is neoplasm. Occasionally tamponade is the initial finding, but sometimes the differential diagnosis in patients with raised jugular pressure and an intrathoracic mass lies between cardiac tamponade and the superior vena cava syndrome. In the former, the characteristic pulsations of the jugular veins can be observed, whereas in the latter, the distended neck veins do not pulsate. Respiratory distress, pulsus alternans, and tachycardia may obscure pulsus paradoxus, which otherwise occurs in cardiac tamponade but not in the superior vena cava syndrome. A pericardial friction rub may be present, but electrocardiographic signs of pericarditis are usually lacking. The pericardial fluid is almost always bloody.

The pericardium itself is frequently normal in gross appearance but may be thickened, sometimes sufficiently to encase the heart, causing constrictive pericarditis. Less commonly, effusive-constrictive pericarditis is found. Neoplastic cells can be recovered from the pericardial fluid in many of the cases, especially when the services of a skilled exfoliative cytologist are available.[167] Cytology is more sensitive than pericardial biopsy.[168] Rarely, sympathetic pericardial effusion occurs in thoracic neoplasms that do not involve the pericardium. Quite commonly, even after screening for infection, radiation, and pericarditis, no cause for the development of pericardial effusion is discovered in patients with underlying malignancy.[168]

TREATMENT

Metastatic pericardial effusion almost invariably indicates an inoperable lesion. Treatment is therefore palliative, with the goals being to ameliorate symptoms and prevent death from cardiac tamponade except in otherwise terminal individuals. Procedures should be as limited as possible and yet meet these goals. There is considerable controversy over the relative merits of pericardiocentesis and open drainage with biopsy. In the latter, the less extensive subxiphoid incision should be used whenever possible. The need for frequently repeated pericardiocenteses can be reduced by draining the fluid via an intrapericardial catheter for several hours. Malignant pericardial effusion may often be palliated satisfactorily by balloon pericardiotomy.[113–115,169] Although the procedure saves the patient from having to undergo surgery, it is painful. Contrast medium, needed to establish the anatomy, should be diluted to half strength. In the hands of an experienced interventional cardiologist, balloon pericardiotomy is an acceptable alternative treatment for malignant pericardial effusion.

The ultimate choice depends upon the extent of neoplasia, the patient's general condition, and local preferences. The decision is best made jointly by the patient's physician, an oncologist, and a cardiologist or cardiac surgeon. Pericardiotomy, or the creation of a fistula between the pericardial and peritoneal cavities,[170] is commonly employed to relieve tamponade. Tetracycline or other sclerosing agents can be instilled via an intrapericardial catheter and may succeed in preventing recurrences of pericardial effusion or cardiac tamponade.[171] This form of treatment is usually followed by transient pain and fever, but, surprisingly, not by constrictive pericarditis. Few controlled trials involving the instillation of chemotherapeutic agents are available because this strategy is not commonly used, clinical presentations vary, and there is often a need for emergency treatment. As mentioned above, pericardiotomy can be accomplished by inserting a balloon-bearing catheter into the pericardial space, inflating the balloon when its distal portion is intrapericardial, and pulling it back so as to rent the pericardium[114] (see also Chap. 86).

Radiation-Induced Pericardial Disease

Exposure of the mediastinum to radiation involves the risk of pericardial and myocardial damage. By far the greatest experience has been in patients treated for Hodgkin's disease.[172] The acute reaction of the pericardium to radiation is fibrinous inflammation,[173] often accompanied by

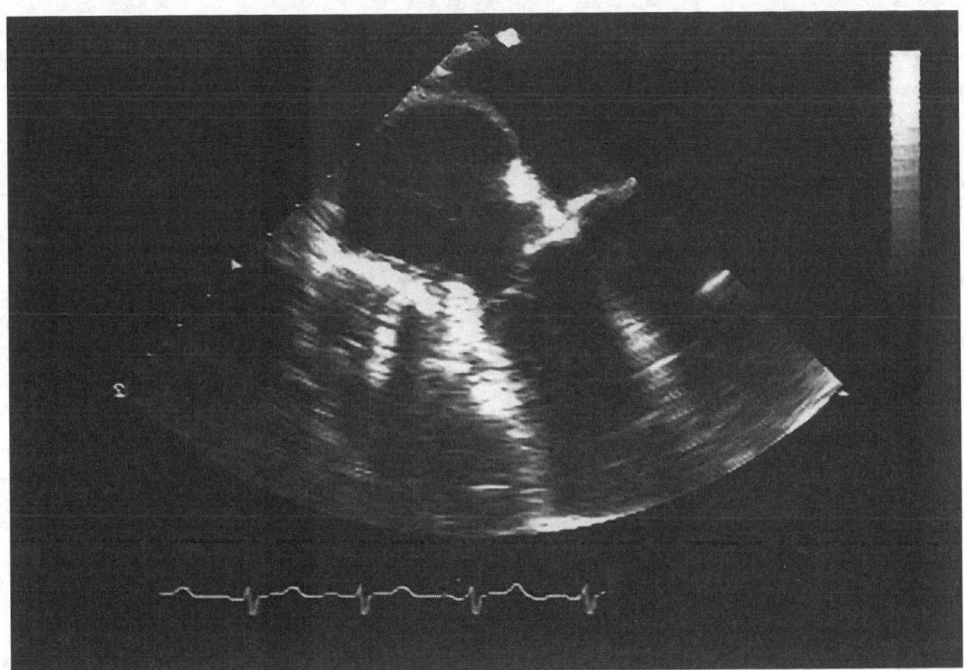

A

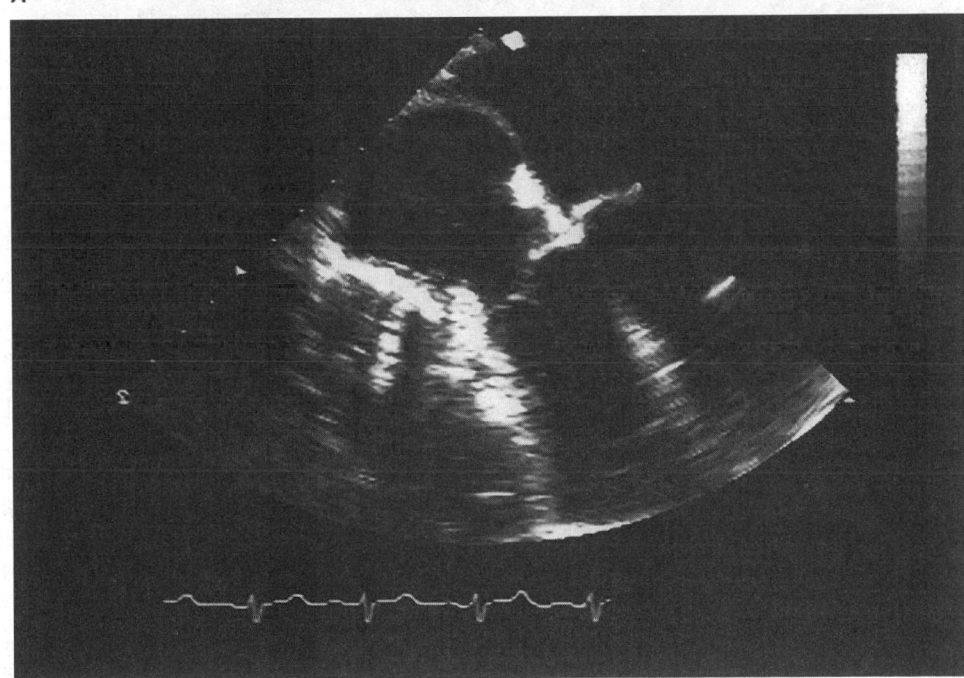

B

FIGURE 81-19
Calcified hematoma presenting as a pericardial mass as seen by transesophageal echocardiography. *A*. Gastric view. *B*. Midesophageal view. (Figure courtesy of Bruce Kimura, MD.)

effusion. The less common chronic response usually takes the form of constrictive pericarditis, sometimes effusive-constrictive pericarditis. The latency between exposure and constriction is often remarkably long. In one series of seven patients, the lesion developed between 51 and 268 months after radiotherapy.[174]

The pathophysiology is unknown. The acute lesion has been studied mainly in experimental animals[175] and only occasionally in humans.[176] The myocardial and, by inference, the pericardial microcirculation is extensively damaged, resulting in ischemic injury to the tissue. The common opinion that the chronic lesion occurs only after 4000 rads has been delivered is not backed by good statistical evidence. The incidence increases when anteriorly weighted thoracic-mantle-field techniques are employed. It has been suggested that reactivation of a latent virus in the pericardium may occur and that radiation may damage the pericardial lymphatics.[175] The lesion appears to be more common in patients who have also received adjunctive chemotherapy[175] (see also Chap. 80).

The acute lesion usually subsides within 2 years without sequel. The chronic lesion produces the typical picture of constrictive pericarditis or effusive-constrictive pericarditis. In the effusive stage, the differential diagnosis includes recurrence of the neoplasm. Examination of pericardial fluid is then helpful, as the fluid is positive in about 30 percent of cases.[177] Cytologic examination of pericardial fluid is reliable in breast and lung cancer but less so in lymphoma and leukemia, where pericardial biopsy may be needed.[178] Acute radiation-induced pericarditis can be managed symptomatically along the same lines as acute idiopathic pericarditis; the response is usually gratifying. Pericardial effusion, when not causing tamponade, can also be managed conservatively. Constrictive pericarditis requires pericardiectomy unless biopsy discloses prohibitive associated endomyocardial fibrosis. Significant impairment of left ventricular systolic function indicates severe myocardial damage, but frequently systolic function is preserved in spite of extensive myocardial fibrosis. In case of doubt, endomyocardial biopsy may be helpful, but good results can accrue from pericardiectomy even when the biopsy shows mild endomyocardial fibrosis[178] (see also Chap. 75).

Hypersensitivity and Collagen-Vascular Pericardial Disease

RHEUMATOID ARTHRITIS

Necropsy studies yield an overall incidence of pericardial disease associated with rheumatoid disease of about 30 percent,[179] a prevalence that was known to Charcot.[180] The clinical incidence is appreciably lower except when ECGs are performed on patients with rheumatoid arthritis who have no symptoms of pericardial disease.[181] Rheumatoid pericardial disease is usually self-limiting but may lead to acute or chronic pericardial effusion, subacute or chronic constrictive pericarditis, or cardiac tamponade (see also Chap. 85).

Rheumatoid pericardial disease appears to be more common in middle-aged males in whom the arthritis was of acute onset. Serologic tests for rheumatoid disease are usually positive, and typical rheumatoid nodules are common. The pericardium was infiltrated with CD8+ lymphocytes in two patients studied after pericardiectomy.[182] Associated cardiac abnormalities, including mitral valve involvement[181] and heart block,[183] are important but less common.

Constrictive pericarditis is usually subacute and seldom calcified. Pericardiectomy may be required within months of the first diagnosis of acute pericarditis[184] and is almost always required within 5 years.

SYSTEMIC LUPUS ERYTHEMATOSUS

Pericardial disease develops in nearly all patients when life is prolonged by steroid treatment. The usual lesion is fibrinous pericarditis, but large pericardial effusions may develop.[185]

Both cardiac tamponade[186] and constrictive pericarditis[187] have been described. Rarely, pericarditis is the initial manifestation.[188] The pericardial fluid usually has a high protein content and a normal or slightly reduced glucose content. As in rheumatoid arthritis, the complement level is low; also, lupus erythematosus cells may be found (see also Chap. 85).

OTHER CONNECTIVE TISSUE DISEASES

Pericardial involvement may be found in systemic sclerosis (scleroderma); often there is an association with cardiomyopathy. The pericardial fluid does not contain antibodies, immune complexes, or low levels of complement. There may be associated cardiac disease, and in some of the cases pericardial involvement is secondary to uremia.[189] In one series of 95 patients with constrictive pericarditis, connective tissue disease accounted for 4 percent of the cases[190] (see also Chap. 85).

Drug-Induced Pericardial Disease

Pericardial abnormalities may develop in response to a number of drugs, of which the more important are hydralazine, procainamide, and daunorubicin.[191] Pericardial abnormalities have also been reported with psicofuranine, isonicotinic acid, and isoniazid. Pericarditis induced by penicillin is presumably a hypersensitivity reaction. Cardiac tamponade has been reported after administration of cromolyn sodium[192] and methysergide.[193] In patients with lupus nephritis treated with hydralazine, it may be difficult to know whether pericarditis is drug-induced or is a manifestation of the disease. Minoxidil may cause pericardial effusion.[194]

Infectious (Nonviral) Pericarditis

TUBERCULOUS PERICARDITIS

The pericardium is infected via lymphatic, hematogenous, or direct spread. Other lesions, including pulmonary, are not always present. Tuberculosis of the pericardium is now rare in the western hemisphere. In a series of 72 pericardiectomies performed between 1974 and 1980, none was performed for tuberculous constrictive pericarditis.[195] Likewise, in two reviews of pericardiocentesis, tuberculosis was proved in only 3 of 173[110] and 4 of 52 cases.[111] Unfortunately, the prevalence of tuberculous pericarditis is again increasing because of its association with AIDS[196] and immigration of individuals with tuberculosis that is often resistant to antibiotics.

Most of the detailed descriptions antedate chemotherapy. Furthermore, the features emphasized in those years of plentiful clinical material—such as insidious onset, lack of constitutional symptoms, thick pericardium found by air contrast, and bloody pericardial effusion—are not sufficiently specific to be of use to the modern clinician.[197] On the other hand, when untreated, tamponade, effusive-constrictive pericarditis, and chronic calcific constriction may result.[198] Cardiac tamponade complicating tuberculous pericardial effusion is frequently followed by effusive-constrictive pericarditis and then the development, usually within a few months, of constrictive pericarditis, which, if not treated surgically, is progressively severe.[199] Consequently, the possibility of tuberculosis must be considered in virtually every case of acute pericarditis, pericardial effusion, cardiac tamponade, or constrictive pericarditis, especially in patients with AIDS (see Chap. 79).

A definitive diagnosis is difficult because of the fastidious nature of the tubercle bacillus and the inherent difficulties in the interpretation of tuberculin skin tests.[200] The dire consequences of missing the diagnosis have led to the common practice of making a presumptive diagnosis based on such indirect evidence as contact with individuals known to be infectious, skin tests, chronicity, and therapeutic trial. It is often difficult to know how many patients treated for tuberculous pericarditis really had the disease. Tubercle bacilli may fail to grow from the pericardial fluid of patients who subsequently proved to have had tuberculous pericarditis,[201] and even pericardial biopsy can be negative in such patients.[202] Growth on conventional culture media is notoriously slow, but newer media require less time.[203] Adenosine deaminase activity in pericardial fluid is elevated,[204] but information on the utility of this enzyme determination is limited. Polymerase chain reaction technology is sometimes successful in proving infection of the pericardium by *Mycobacterium tuberculosis*.[205]

ATYPICAL MYCOBACTERIAL INFECTION

Purulent pericarditis may result from infection with avian mycobacterial complex. This opportunistic infection, from organisms ordinarily confined to the gastrointestinal tract, is particularly apt to occur in patients with AIDS and a low count of CD8+ T cells.[206]

CLINICAL COURSE

A minority of patients present with a large pericardial effusion that is not sanguinous and without thickening of the pericardium. These patients can be considered to have a primary tuberculous pericardial effusion and they respond well to antituberculous chemotherapy with the addition of prednisone to prevent constriction.[207] More often, the constricting process has already begun when the patient comes to medical attention and the fluid is bloody. In the past, the prognosis was poor, but in recent series managed with initial antituberculous chemotherapy and timely pericardiectomy, survival without recurrence has been the rule.[200,208]

TREATMENT

A potent triple-drug regimen—such as rifampin, 600 mg; isoniazid, 300 mg; and ethambutol, 15 mg/kg—should be prescribed. After several months, isoniazid should be discontinued, but the two other drugs are given for 18 months after activity has subsided. Concurrent treatment with corticosteroids has been proposed,[209] but their role remains unsettled. In southern Africa, tuberculosis remains a common cause of pericarditis. In a series of 240 patients with tuberculous pericardial effusion studied in Transkei, quadruple antituber-

culous chemotherapy was given for only 6 months. The patients were randomized to receive prednisolone or placebo for the first 11 weeks. The investigators concluded that the shorter regimen was effective and that prednisolone improved survival and lessened the need for pericardiectomy.[207] Adjunctive steroid therapy can therefore be recommended for tuberculous effusive-constrictive pericarditis and for primary pericardial effusion, but it is unlikely to be helpful in established chronic constrictive pericarditis.

Histoplasmosis

Most cases of histoplasmosis of the pericardium occur in the Ohio and Mississippi Valleys and western Appalachia.[210] Rarely, *Histoplasma* can be recovered from pericardial fluid,[211] but more commonly the diagnosis depends on serology, which must be tested before it is modified by intradermal injections of histoplasmin. A titer exceeding 1:32 suggests recent or active infection. Distinction from tuberculosis can be difficult using clinical criteria. Furthermore, neither *Histoplasma* nor *M. tuberculosis* is easy to culture, but adenopathy favors histoplasmosis. Calcific constrictive pericarditis is a documented outcome.[212]

TREATMENT

Proven active disease, especially with tamponade, should be treated with a total course of 35 to 40 mg/kg of amphotericin B.[213]

Other Organisms and Combined Infections

Tuberculosis may occur in association with histoplasmosis.[214] When disseminated, these diseases may cause adrenal insufficiency.[215] The pericardium may also be infected by *Blastomyces* and by *Candida albicans*, the latter usually after immunosuppressive or broad-spectrum antibiotic treatment. *Actinomyces israelii* and *Nocardia asteroides* may also affect the pericardium and can cause constriction.[216] Purulent pericarditis may complicate pulmonary asperigillosis. Sporotrichosis and mucormycosis were not included in a review[217] to which the reader is referred for references regarding specific pericardial infections.

TREATMENT

Unlike histoplasmosis, these infections do not remit spontaneously; therefore, pericardiectomy should be carried out whenever possible.

Bacterial and Other Pyogenic Infections of the Pericardium

Purulent pericarditis has decreased in frequency because of effective antibiotics, but when it occurs, it is serious, carrying a high risk of mortality in spite of the availability of modern antibiotics[218] Symptoms and signs of pericardial involvement in the clinical picture of a critically ill infected patient are often lacking or subtle[219]; therefore any suspicion of pericarditis in a patient with septicemia demands a relentless search for the causative organism and the presence of pus in the pericardial space. It is most important to obtain at least four blood cultures, which should be tested on a wide range of media so that fastidious organisms as well as the more common pyrogens will grow, and to follow the course with serial echocardiography to detect pericardial fluid or increasing echodensity and thickness of the pericardium. Immunologic studies for *M. tuberculosis*, *H. influenzae*, *Streptococcus*, *Toxoplasma*, and *Entamoeba histolytica* should also be done.

The antibiotic control of common infections has led to a change in the spectrum of bacterial pericarditis. The previously common pneumococcal pericarditis, a direct consequence of pneumococcal pneumonia and streptococcal pericarditis, has given way to infections caused by resistant *Staphylococcus*, anaerobes, fungi, and commensal organisms. Consequently, the population at risk has shifted to the extremes of age, the debilitated, and the immunosuppressed.[220]

TREATMENT

Infections due to penicillin-sensitive organisms can be brought under control by large doses of penicillin, because they achieve therapeutic concentration in the pericardial fluid.[221] The definitive treatment of purulent pericarditis includes surgical drainage, although an occasional success has been reported for prolonged catheter drainage.[222] Meningococcal pericarditis is a metastatic infection, usually from the nasopharynx. Meningococcal pericarditis may occur in the absence of meningitis,[223] and frequently the purulent serosanguineous pericardial exudate is sterile because of previous antibiotic treatment; but in some cases sterile pericardial effusion is thought to be an immune reaction.[224] The disease should yield to penicillin, but surgical drainage is often required, and constrictive pericarditis needing pericardiectomy may occur acutely.[225]

Staphylococcal pericarditis is an extremely serious and frequently fatal illness, especially when it is a complication of cardiac surgery or staphylococcal endocarditis. Systemic illness is profound and the pericardial exudate tenacious and loculated. Vigorous and aggressive treatment must be directed at every aspect of the disease, including control of the primary infection, removal of infected venous and arterial catheters, administration of appropriate antibiotics, and surgical drainage. Pericardiocentesis seldom suffices; surgical decompression must be carried out.[226]

Gram-negative organisms such as *Pseudomonas aeruginosa*, *Klebsiella pneumoniae*, and *Escherichia coli* produce pericarditis by hematogenous spread in the gravely debilitated.[227] Antibiotic treatment is beset with difficulties in selection and toxicity, and surgical drainage may be required. Pericarditis may result from hematogenous spread or by direct extension of anaerobic infections.[228] Treatment must include drainage of both the primary focus and the pericardium.

Purulent pericarditis in children carries a high mortality and may lead rapidly to constrictive pericarditis.[228] *H. influenzae* and meningococci are the most common offenders, but pneumococcal pericarditis still occurs in infants and children. Prognosis remains poor despite modern treatment.

Miscellaneous Diseases of the Pericardium

MYXEDEMATOUS PERICARDIAL DISEASE

Pericardial effusion occurs in about one-third of patients with myxedema. There is no correlation between pericardial effusion and the level of thyroid activity. Cardiomegaly is often the first clue, but it may be due to coexisting heart disease. The pericardial effusion rarely causes symptoms, although tamponade has been reported.[229] The pericardial fluid is usually clear, but it may be myxomatous and is high in cholesterol until restoration of the euthyroid state.

CHOLESTEROL PERICARDITIS

Cholesterol pericarditis may be idiopathic, but more commonly it is found in myxedema, tuberculosis, or rheumatoid disease. The effusions are often large, but because they develop slowly, tamponade is uncommon. The associated inflammation can provoke constrictive pericarditis.[230] The cholesterol may be liberated from injured pericardial cells or lysed from red corpuscles, or it may develop as a consequence of lymphatic obstruction.[231]

CHYLOPERCARDIUM

Chylopericardium is usually idiopathic but may be associated with surgical or traumatic injury of the thoracic duct or neoplastic obstruction of the lymphatic drainage. The diagnosis is established by examination of the pericardial fluid, which is milky-white when allowed to stand and contains fat globules and increased levels of cholesterol and triglycerides. The milky appearance clears promptly after the addition of ether. Treatment is by drainage, and if the thoracic duct is injured, it must be ligated. Intractable cases can be treated with a valved shunt connecting the pericardial to the peritoneal cavity. Lymphopericardium is less common than chylopericardium and is usually secondary to lymphangioma. Pericardial involvement has also been reported in echinococcosis,[232] Degos' disease,[233] and pseudomyxoma peritonei.[234]

OTHER UNCOMMON CAUSES OF PERICARDIAL DISEASE

There are a number of syndromes associated with pericardial effusion, although the mechanism is unclear. These include Reiter's syndrome,[235] ulcerative colitis,[236] Whipple's disease,[237] thalassemia,[238] atrial septal defect,[239] and Sipple's syndrome.[240] Pericardiopathy may also occur as part of mechanical disorders such as the chylous reflux syndrome,[241] inversion of the diaphragm, and pancreatic fistula[242,243] as well as diabetic ketoacidosis.[244]

Constrictive pericarditis is a component of mulibrey nanism. *Mulibrey* is an acronym for *muscle-liver-brain-eye*, the organs principally affected by this autosomal recessive disorder, which is found mainly in Finland.[245] Other features include yellow dots on the ocular fundi, fibrous dysplasia of the long bones, and an abnormally shaped skull and sella turcica.

A patient with Behçet's syndrome with pericardial effusion and mixed cryoglobulinemia who responded to treatment with indomethacin has been reported.[246] There is also a report of pericardial perforation of a gastric ulcer into the pericardium secondary to a phytobezoar in an oligophrenic man.[247] Increasingly, pericardial involvement in AIDS is being recognized[61] (see Chap. 79). Myopericarditis has been reported in Lyme disease.[248]

REFERENCES

1. Roberts WC, Spray TL. Pericardial heart disease: A study of its causes, consequences, and morphologic features. In: Spodick DH, ed. *Pericardial Diseases*. Philadelphia: Davis; 1976:11–65.

2. Gibson AT, Segal MB. A study of the composition of pericardial fluid with special reference to the probable mechanism of fluid formation. *J Physiol (Lond)* 1978; 277:367–377.

3. Santamore WP, Constantinescu MS, Bogen D, Johnston WE. Nonuniform distribution of normal pericardial fluid. *Basic Res Cardiol* 1990; 85:541–549.

4. Elias H, Boyd LJ. Notes on the anatomy, embryology and histology of the pericardium. *J. NY Med Coll* 1960; 2:50–75.

5. Ishihara T, Ferrans VJ, Jones M, Boyce SW, Kawanami O, Roberts WC. Histologic and ultrastructural features of the normal human parietal pericardium. *Am J Cardiol* 1980; 46:744–753.

6. Holt JP. The normal pericardium. *Am J Cardiol* 1970; 26:455–465.

7. Rabkin SW, Hsu PH. Mathematical and mechanical modeling of stress-strain relationship of pericardium. *Am J Physiol* 1975; 229:896–900.

8. Lee JM, Boughner DR. Tissue mechanics of canine pericardium in different test environments. *Circ Res* 1981; 49:533–544.

9. Freeman GL, LeWinter MM. Pericardial adaptations during cardiac dilatation in dogs. *Circ Res* 1984; 54:294–300.

10. Morgan BC, Guntheroth WG, Dillard DH. The relationship of pericardial to pleural pressure during quiet respiration and quiet respiration and cardiac tamponade. *Circ Res* 1965; 16:493–498.

11. Shabetai R. Pericardial and cardiac pressure. *Circulation* 1988; 77:1–5.

12. Horowitz MS, Schultz CS, Stinson EB, Harrison DC, Popp RL. Sensitivity and specificity of echocardiographic diagnosis of pericardial effusion. *Circulation* 1974; 50:239–247.

13. Holt JP, Rhode EA, Kines H. Pericardial and ventricular pressure. *Circ Res* 1960; 8:1171–1181.

14. Hollenberg M, Dougherty J. Lymph flow and ^{131}I-albumin resorption from pericardial effusions in man. *Am J Cardiol* 1969; 24:514–522.

15. Pegram BL, Bishop VS. An evaluation of the pericardial sac as a safety factor during tamponade. *Cardiovasc Res* 1975; 9:715–721.

16. Ditchey R, Engler RL, LeWinter MM, Pavelec R, Bhargava V, Courell J, et al. The role of the right heart in acute cardiac tamponade in dogs. *Circ Res* 1981; 48:701–710.

17. Janicki JS, Weber KT. The pericardium and ventricular interaction distensibility and function. *Am J Physiol* 1980; 238:H494–H503.

18. Tyson GS, Maier GW, Olsen CO, Davis JW, Rankin JS. Pericardial influences on ventricular filling in the conscious dog: An alalysis based on pericardial pressure. *Circ Res* 1984; 54:173–184.

19. Dauterman K, Pak PH, Maughan WL, Nussbacher A, Arie S, Liu C-P, Kass DA. Contribution of external forces to left ventricular diastolic pressure: Implications for the clinical use of the Starling law. *Ann Intern Med* 1995; 122:737–742.

20. Banchero N, Rutishauser WJ, Tsakiris AG, Wood EH. Pericardial pressure duing transverse acceleration in dogs without thoracotomy. *Circ Res* 1967; 20:65–77.

21. Collin V, quoted in Boyd LJ, Elias H. Contributions to diseases of the heart and pericardium: I. Historical introduction. *Bull NY Med Coll* 1955; 18:1–37.

22. Maisch B, Bethge C, Drude L, Hufnagel G, Herzum M, Schönian U. Pericardioscopy and epicardial biopsy—new diagnostic tools in pericardial and perimyocardial disease. *Eur Heart J* 1994; 15(suppl C):68–73.

23. Laennec RTH. A *Treatise on Diseases of the Chest* (J Forbes, trans). London: Underwood; 1821:264.

24. Spodick DH. Acoustic phenomena in pericardial disease. *Am Heart J* 1971; 81:114–124.

25. James TN. Pericarditis and the sinus node. *Arch Intern Med* 1962; 110:305–311.

26. Spodick DH. Frequency of arrhythmias in acute pericarditis determined by Holter monitoring *Am J Cardiol* 1984; 53:842–845.

27. Surawicz Ba, Lasseter KC. Electrocardiogram in pericarditis. *Am J Cardiol* 1970; 26:471–474.

28. Spodick DH. Diagnostic electrocardiographic sequences in acute pericarditis: Significance of PR segment and PR vector changes. *Circulation* 1973; 48:575–580.

29. Wanner WR, Schaal SF, Bashore TM, Norton VJ, Lewis RP, Fulkerson PK. Repolarization variant versus acute pericarditis: A prospective electrocardiographic and echocardiographic evaluation. *Chest* 1983; 83:180–184.

30. O'Connell JB, Robinson JA, Henkin RE, Gunnar RM. Gallium-67 citrate scanning for noninvasive detection of inflammation in pericardial diseases. *Am J Cardiol* 1980; 46:879–884.

31. Hackney D, Slutsky R, Mattrey R, Peck WW, Abraham JL, Shabetai R, et al. Experimental pericardial effusion evaluated by computed tomography. *Radiology* 1984; 151: 145–148.

32. Fowler NO. Recurrent pericarditis. *Cardiol Clin* 1990; 8:621–626.

33. Fowler NO, Harbin AD III. Recurrent acute pericarditis: Follow-up study of 31 patients. *J Am Coll Cardiol* 1986; 7:300–305.

34. Burchell HB. Problems in the recognition and treatment of pericarditis. *Lancet* 1954; 74:465–470.

35. Connolly DC, Burchell HB. Pericarditis: A ten year survey. *Am J Cardiol* 1961; 7:7–14.

36. Marcolongo R, Russo R, Laveder F, Noventa F, Agostini C. Immunosuppressive therapy prevents recurrent pericarditis. *J Am Coll Cardiol* 1995; 26:1276–1279.

37. Guindo J, de la Serna AR, Ramio J, de Miguel Diaz MA, Subirana MT, Perez Ayuso MJ, et al. Recurrent pericarditis: Relief with colchicine. *Circulation* 1990; 82:1117–1120.

38. Tuna IC, Danielson GK. Surgical management of pericardial diseases. *Cardiol Clin* 1990; 8:683–696.

39. Teicholz LE. Echocardiographic evaluation of pericardial diseases. *Prog Cardiovasc Dis* 1978; 21:133–140.

40. Haaz WS, Mintz GS, Kotler MN, Parry W, Segal BL. Two dimensional echocardiographic recognition of the descending thoracic aorta: Value in differentiating pericardial from pleural effusions. *Am J Cardiol* 1980; 46:739–743.

41. Martin RP, Bowden R, Fily K, Popp RL. Intrapericardial abnormalities in patients with pericardial effusion: Findings by two-dimensional echocardiography. *Circulation* 1980; 61:568–572.

42. Riba AL, Morganroth J. Unsuspected substantial pericardial effusions detected by echocardiography. *JAMA* 1976; 236:2623–2625.

43. Goldstein DH, Nagar C, Srivastava N, Schacht RA, Ferris FZ, Flowers NC. Clinically silent pericardial effusions in patients on long term hemodialysis. *Chest* 1977; 72:744–747.

44. Horowitz MS, Schultz CS, Stinson EB, Harrison DC, Popp RL. Sensitivity and specificity of echocardiographic diagnosis of pericardial effusion. *Circulation* 1974; 50:239–247.

45. Feigenbaum H. Echocardiographic diagnosis of pericardial effusion. *Am J Cardiol* 1970; 26:475–479.

46. Hagan AD. Evaluation of pericardial diseases by M mode and two dimensional echocardiography. In: Mason DT, ed. *Advances in Heart Disease* III. New York: Grune & Stratton; 1980:699–702.

47. Come PC, Riley MF, Fortuin NJ. Echocardiographic mimicry of pericardial effusion. *Am J Cardiol* 1981; 47:365–370.

48. Shah PM. Echocardiography in pericardial diseases. In: Reddy PS, Leon DF, Shaver JA, eds. *Pericardial Disease*. New York: Raven Press; 1982:127–136.

49. Hirschfield DS, Emilson BB. Echocardiogram in calcified mitral anulus. *Am J Cardiol* 1975; 36:354–356.

50. Foote WC, Jefferson CM, Price HL. False positive echocardiographic diagnosis of pericardial effusion: Result of tumor encasement of the heart simulating constrictive pericarditis. *Chest* 1977; 71:546–549.

51. Martin RP, Rakowski H, French J, Popp RL. Localization of pericardial effusion with wide angle phased array echocardiography. *Am J Cardiol* 1978; 42:904–912.

52. Tehranzadeh J, Kelley MJ. The differential density sign of pericardial effusion. *Radiology* 1979; 133:23–30.

53. White CS. MR evaluation of the pericardium. *Top Magn Reson Imaging* 1995; 7:258–266.

54. Permanyer-Miralda G, Sagrista-Sauleda J, Soler-Soler J. Primary acute

pericardial disease: A prospective series of 231 consecutive patients. *Am J Cardiol* 1985; 56:623–630.

55. Lewis W. AIDS: Cardiac findings from 115 autopsies. *Prog Cardiovasc Dis* 1989; 32:207–215.

56. Mirri A, Rapezzi C, Iocopi F, Ortolani P, Binetti G, Fabbri M, et al. Cardiac involvement in HIV infection: A prospective, multicenter clinical and echocardiographic study. *Cardiologia* 1990; 35:203–209.

57. Reynolds MM, Hecht SR, Berger M, Kolokathis A, Horowitz SF. Large pericardial effusions in the acquired immunodeficiency syndrome. *Chest* 1992; 102:1746–1747.

58. Zakowski MF, Ianuale-Shanerman A. Cytology of pericardial effusions in AIDS patients. *Diagn Cytopathol* 1993; 9:266–269.

59. Turco M, Seneff M, McGrath BJ, Hsia J. Cardiac tamponade in the acquired immunodeficiency syndrome. *Am Heart J* 1990; 120:1467–1468.

60. Steigman CK, Anderson DW, Macher AM, Sennesh JD, Virmani R. Fatal cardiac tamponade in acquired immunodeficiency syndrome with epicardial Kaposi's sarcoma. *Am Heart J* 1988; 116:1105–1107.

61. Heidenreich PA, Eisenberg MJ, Kee LL, Somelofski CA, Hollander H, Schiller NB, et al. Pericardial effusion in AIDS: Incidence and survival. *Circulation* 1995; 92:3229–3234.

62. Lower R. *Tractatus de Corde, Item de Motu et Colare Sanguinis et Chyli in Sum Transitu.* London: J Allestry, 1669.

63. Chevers N. Observations of diseases of the orifice and valves of the aorta. *Guy's Hosp Rep* 1842; 7:387–439.

64. Gaasch WH, Peterson KL, Shabetai R. Left ventricular function in chronic constrictive pericarditis. *Am J Cardiol* 1974; 34:107–110.

65. Craig RJ, Whalen RE, Behar VS, McIntosh HD. Pressure and volume changes of the left ventricle in acute pericardial tamponade. *Am J Cardiol* 1968; 22:65–74.

66. Fowler NO, Gabel M, Holmes JC. Hemodynamic effects of nitroprusside and hydralazine in experimental cardiac tamponade. *Circulation* 1978; 57:563–567.

67. Pegram BL, Kardon MB, Bishop VS. Changes in left ventricular internal diameter with increasing pericardial pressure. *Cardiovasc Res* 1975; 9:707–714.

68. Brecher GA. *Venous Return.* New York: Grune & Stratton; 1956:111.

69. Shabetai R, Fowler NO, Guntheroth WG. The hemodynamics of cardiac tamponade and constrictive pericarditis. *Am J Cardiol* 1970; 26:480–489.

70. Shabetai R, Fowler NO, Fenton JC, Masangkay M. Pulsus paradoxus. *J Clin Invest* 1965; 44:1882–1889.

71. Hansen AT, Eskildsen P, Gotzsche H. Pressure curves from the right auricle and the right ventricle in chronic constrictive pericarditis. *Circulation* 1951; 3:881–888.

72. Brecher GA. Critical review of recent work on ventricular diastolic suction. *Circ Res* 1958; 6:554–566.

73. DeCristofaro D, Liu CK. The hemodynamics of cardiac tamponade and blood volume overload in dogs. *Cardiovasc Res* 1969; 3:292–298.

74. Ditchey R, Engler RL, LeWinter MM, Pavelec R, Bhargava V, Couell J, et al. The role of the right heart in acute cardiac tamponade in dogs. *Circ Res* 1981; 48:701–710.

75. D'Cruz IA, Kensey K, Campbell C, Replogle R, Jain M. Two-dimensional echocardiography in cardiac tamponade occurring after cardiac surgery. *J Am Coll Cardiol* 1985; 5:1250–1252.

76. Shabetai R, Fowler NO, Gueron M. The effects of respiration on aortic pressure and flow. *Am Heart J* 1963; 65:525–533.

77. Shabetai R, Fowler NO, Braunstein JR, Gueron M. Transmural ventricular pressures and pulsus paradoxus in experimental cardiac tamponade. *Dis Chest* 1961; 39:557–568.

78. Settle HP, Adolph RJ, Fowler NO, Engel P, Agruss NS, Levenson NI. Echocardiographic study of cardiac tamponade. *Circulation* 1977; 56:951–959.

79. Reddy PS, Curtis EI, O'Toole JD, Shaver JA. Cardiac tamponade: Hemodynamic observations in man. *Circulation* 1978; 58:265–272.

80. Kronzon I, Winer HE. Absence of paradoxical pulse in patients with atrial septal defect and cardiac tamponade (abstr). *Am J Cardiol* 1978; 41:446.

81. Friedman HS, Sakurai H, Choe S-S, Lajam F, Celis A. Pulsus paradoxus: A manifestation of marked reduction of left ventricular end-diastolic volume in cardiac tamponade. *J Thorac Cardiovasc Surg* 1980; 79:74–82.

82. Dock W. Inspiratory traction on the pericardium. *Arch Intern Med* 1961; 108:837–840.

83. Friedman HS, Lajam F, Zaman Q, Gomes JA, Calderon J, Marino ND, et al. Effect of autonomic blockade on the hemodynamic findings in acute cardiac tamponade. *Am J Physiol* 1977; 232:H5–H11.

84. Hancock EW. Subacute effusive-constrictive pericarditis. *Circulation* 1971; 43:183–192.

85. Tei C, Child JS, Tanaka H, Shah PM. Atrial systolic notch on the interventricular septal echogram: An echocardiographic sign of constrictive pericarditis. *J Am Coll Cardiol* 1983; 1:907–912.

85a. Holt BD. Pericardial heart disease. *Curr Probl Cardiol* 1997; 22:353–404.

86. Levine HD. Myocardial fibrosis in constrictive pericarditis: Electrocardiographic and pathologic observations. *Circulation* 1973; 48:1268–1281.

87. Jarmakani JMM, McHale PA, Greenfield JC. The effect of cardiac tamponade on coronary hemodynamics in the awake dog. *Cardiovasc Res* 1975; 9:112–117.

88. Wechsler AS, Auerbach BJ, Graham TC, Sabiston DC. Distribution of intramyocardial blood flow during pericardial tamponade: Correlation with microscopic anatomy and intrinsic myocardial contractility. *J Thorac Cardiovasc Surg* 1974; 68:847–856.

89. Isselbacher EM, Cigarroa JE, Eagle KA. Cardiac tamponade complicating proximal aortic dissection: Is pericardiocentesis harmful? *Circulation* 1994; 90:2375–2378.

90. Katz LN, Gauchat HW. Observations on pulsus paradoxus (with special reference to pericardial effusions). *Arch Intern Med* 1924; 33:371–393.

91. Guberman BA, Fowler NO, Engel PJ, Gueron M, Allen JM. Cardiac tamponade in medical patients. *Circulation* 1981; 64:633–640.

92. Cohn JN, Pinkerson AL, Tristani FE. Mechanism of pulsus paradoxus in clinical shock. *J Clin Invest* 1967; 46:1744–1755.

93. Gillam LD, Guyer DE, Gibson TC, King ME, Marshall JE, Weyman AE. Hydrodynamic compression of the right atrium: A new echocardiographic sign of cardiac tamponade. *Circulation* 1983; 68:294–301.

94. Leimgruber PP, Klopfenstein HS, Wann LS, Brooks HL. The hemodynamic derangement associated with right ventricular diastolic collapse in cardiac tamponade: An experimental echocardiographic study. *Circulation* 1983; 68:612–620.

95. Klopfenstein HS, Schuchard GH, Wann LS, Palmer TE, Hartz AJ, Gross CM, et al. The relative merits of pulsus paradoxus and right ventricular diastolic collapse in the early detection of cardiac tamponade: An experimental echocardiographic study. *Circulation* 1985; 71:829–833.

96. D'Cruz IA, Cohen HC, Prabhu R, Glick G. Diagnosis of cardiac tamponade by echocardiography. Changes in mitral valve motion and ventricular dimensions, with special reference to paradoxical pulse. *Circulation* 1975; 52:460–465.

97. Feigenbaum H, Zaky A, Grabhorn LL. Cardiac motion in patients with pericardial effusion: A study using reflected ultrasound. *Circulation* 1966; 34:611–619.

98. Price EC, Dennis EW. Electrical alternans, its mechanism demonstrated (abstr). *Circulation* 1969; 39/40(suppl 3):165.

99. Appleton CK, Hatle LA, Popp RL: Cardiac tamponade and pericardial effusion: Respiratory variation in transvalvular flow velocities studied by Doppler echocardiography. *J Am Coll Cardiol* 1988; 11:1020–1030.

100. Hoit B. Imaging the pericardium. *Cardiol Clin* 1990; 8:587–600.

101. Littman D, Spodick DH. Total electrical alternation in pericardial disease. *Circulation* 1958; 17:912–917.

102. Toney JC, Kolmen SN. Cardiac tamponade: Fluid and pressure effects on electrocardiographic changes. *Proc Soc Exp Biol Med* 1966; 121:642–648.

103. Antman EM, Gargill V, Grossman W. Low pressure cardiac tamponade. *Ann Intern Med* 1979; 91:403–406.

104. Shabetai R, Rostand SG. Nephrogenic pericardial disease: Contemporary issues in nephrology, 13. In: O'Rourke RA, Brenner BM, Stein JH, eds. *The Heart and Renal Disease.* New York: Churchill Livingstone; 1984:89–125.

105. hardesty RL. Delayed postoperative cardiac tamponade: Diagnosis and management. In: Reddy PS, Leon DF, Shaver JS, eds. *Pericardial Disease.* New York: Raven Press; 1981:341.

106. Yacoub MH, Cleland WP, Deal CW. Left atrial tamponade. *Thorax* 1966; 21:305–309.

107. Engleman RM, Spencer FC, Reed GE, Tice DA. Cardiac tamponade following open heart surgery. *Circulation* 1970; 41(suppl 2):II-165–II-171.

108. West S. Purulent pericarditis treated by paracentesis and free incision with recovery. *Br Med J* 1883; 1:814.

109. Naunheim KS, Flore AC, Turrentine M, Hammell LM, Brown JW, Kesler KA, et al. Pericardial drainage subxiphoid vs. transthoracic approach. *Eur J Cardiol Thorac Surg* 1991; 5:99–104.

110. Krikorian JG, Hancock EW. Pericardiocentesis. *Am J Med* 1978; 65:808–814.

111. Wong B, Murphy J, Chang CJ, Hassenein K, Dunn M. The risk of pericardiocentesis. *Am J Cardiol* 1979; 44:1110–1114.

112. Clarke DP, Cosgrove DO. Real-time ultrasound scanning in the planning and guidance of pericardiocentesis. *Clin Radiol* 1987; 38:119–122.

113. Palacios IF, Tuzcu EM, Ziskind AA, Younger J, Block PC. Percutaneous balloon pericardial window for patients with malignant pericardial effusion and tamponade. *Cathet Cardiovasc Diag* 1991; 22:244–249.

114. Ziskind AA, Pearce AC, Lemmon CC, Burstein S, Gimple LW, Herrmann HC, et al. Percutaneous balloon pericardiotomy for the treatment of cardiac tamponade and large pericardial effusions: Description of technique and report of the first 50 cases. *J Am Coll Cardiol* 1993; 21:1–5.

115. Galli M, Politi A, Pedretti F, Castiglioni B, Zerboni S. Percutaneous balloon pericardiotomy for malignant pericardial tamponade. *Chest* 1995; 108:1499–1501.

116. Ng AS, Dorosti K, Sheldon WC. Constrictive pericarditis following cardiac surgery—Cleveland Clinic experience: Report of 12 cases and review. *Cleve Clin Q* 1984; 50:39–45.

117. Andrews GWS, Pickering GW, Sellors TH. The aetiology of constrictive pericarditis with special reference to tuberculous pericarditis, together with a note on polyserositis. *Q J Med* 1948; 17:291–321.

118. Shabetai R. The pericardium: An essay on some recent developments. *Am J Cardiol* 1978; 42:1036–1043.

119. Fowler NO. Constrictive pericarditis: Its history and current status. *Clin Cardiol* 1995; 18:341–350.

120. Wood P. Chronic constrictive pericarditis. *Am J Cardiol* 1961; 7:48–61.

121. Goldstein JA, Barzilai B, Rosamond TL, Eisenberg PR, Jaffe AS. Determinants of hemodynamic compromise with severe right ventricular infarction. *Circulation* 1990; 82:359–368.

122. Lorel B, Leinbach RC, Pohost GM, Gold HR, Dinsmore RE, Hutter AM. Right ventricular infarction: Clinical diagnosis and differentiation from cardiac tamponade and pericardial constriction. *Am J Cardiol* 1979; 43:465–471.

123. Meany E, Shabetai R, Bhargava V, Shearer M, Weidner C, Mangiardi LM, et al. Cardiac amyloidosis, constrictive pericarditis and restrictive cardiomyopathy. *Am J Cardiol* 1976; 38:547–556.

124. Goodwin JP, Oakley CM. The cardiomyopathies. *Br Heart J* 1972; 34:545–552.

125. Schrire V, Gotsman MS, Beck W. Unusual diastolic murmurs in constrictive pericarditis and constrictive endocarditis. *Am Heart J* 1968; 76:4–12.

126. Mchenry MM, Ord JW, Johnson RR, Shoener JA. Exercise performance and stroke volume changes in two patients with constrictive pericarditis. *Am Heart J* 1965; 70:180–185.

127. Nakhjavan FK, Goldberg H. Hemodynamic effects of catecholamine stimulation in constrictive pericarditis. *Circulation* 1970; 42:487–490.

128. Tyberg TI, Goodyer AVN, Hurst VW, Alexander J, Langou RA. Left ventricular filling in differentiating restrictive amyloid cardiomyopathy and constrictive pericarditis. *Am J Cardiol* 1981; 47:791–796.

129. Ling LH, Oh JK, Teic, Click RL, Breen JF, Seward JB, Tajik AJ. Pericardial thickness measured with transeophageal echocardiography: Feasibility and potential clinical usefulness. *J Am Coll Cardiol* 1997; 29:1317–1323.

130. Doppman JL, Rienmuller R, Lissner J, Cyran J, Boh HD, Strauer BE, et al. Computed tomography in constrictive pericardial disease. *J Comput Assist Tomogr* 1981; 5:1–11.

131. Schoenfeld MH, Supple EW, Dec GW, Fallon JT, Palacios IF. Restrictive cardiomyopathy versus constrictive pericarditis: Role of endomyocardial biopsy in avoiding unnecessary thoracotomy. *Circulation* 1987; 75:1012–1017.

132. Keith TA. Chronic constrictive pericarditis in association with rheumatoid disease. *Circulation* 1962; 25:477–483.

133. Kutcher MA, King SB III, Alimurung BN, Craver JM, Logue RB. Constrictive pericarditis as a complication of cardiac surgery: Recognition of an entity. *Am J Cardiol* 1982; 50:742–748.

134. Marsa R, Mehta S, Willis W, Bailey L. Constrictive pericarditis after myocardial revascularization. *Am J Cardiol* 1979; 44:177–183.

135. Bush CA, Stang JM, Wooley CF, Kilman JW. Occult constrictive pericardial disease: Diagnosis by rapid volume expansion and correction by pericardiectomy. *Circulation* 1977; 56:924–930.

136. Fowler NO. Constrictive pericarditis: New aspects. *Am J Cardiol* 1982; 50:1014–1017.

137. Shabetai R. *The Pericardium*. New York: Grune & Stratton; 1981:206–208.

138. Sagrista-Sauleda J, Permanyer-Miralda G, Candell RJ, Angel J, Soler-Soler J. Transient cardiac constriction: An unrecognized pattern of evolution in effusive acute idiopathic pericarditis. *Am J Cardiol* 1987; 59:961–966.

139. Culliford AT, Lipton M, Spencer FC. Operation for chronic constrictive pericarditis: Do the surgical approach and degree of pericardial resection influence the outcome significantly? *Ann Thorac Surg* 1980; 29:146–152.

140. DeValeria PA, Baumgartner WA, Casale AS, Greene PS, Cameron DE, Gardner TJ, et al. Current indications, risks and outcome after pericardiectomy. *Ann Thorac Surg* 1991; 52:219–224.

141. Somerville W. Constrictive pericarditis with special reference to the change in natural history brought about by surgical intervention. *Circulation* 1968; 37/38(suppl 5):V-102–V-111.

142. Nasser WK. Congenital absence of the left pericardium. *Am J Cardiol* 1970; 26:466–470.

143. Nasser WK, Helmen C, Tavel ME, Feigenbaum H, Fisch C. Congenital absence of the left pericardium: Clinical, electrocardiographic, radiographic, hemodynamic, and angiographic findings in six cases. *Circulation* 1970; 41:469–478.

144. Gassner I, Judmaier W, Fink C, Lener M, Waldenberger F, Scharfetter H, et al. Diagnosis of congenital pericardial defects, including a pathognomic sign for dangerous apical ventricular herniation, on magnetic resonance imaging. *Br Heart J* 1995; 74:60–66.

145. Risher WH, Rees AP, Ochsner JL, McFadden PM. Thoracoscopic resection of pericardium for symptomatic congenital pericardial defect. *Ann Thorac Surg* 1993; 56:1390–1391.

146. Bright R. Tabular view of the morbid appearances in a hundred cases connected with albuminous urine. *Guy's Hosp Rep* 1836; 1:380–400.

147. Comty CM, Cohen SL, Shapiro FL. Pericarditis in chronic uremia and its sequels. *Ann Intern Med* 1971; 75:173–183.

148. Beaudry C, Nakamoto S, Kolff WJ. Uremic pericarditis and cardiac tamponade in chronic renal failure. *Ann Intern Med* 1966; 64:990–995.

149. Comty CM, Wathen RL, Shapiro FL. Uremic pericarditis. In: Spodick DH, ed. *Pericardial Diseases*. Philadelphia: Davis; 1976:219–235.

150. Buselmeier TJ, Simmons RL, Najarian JS, Mauer SM, Matas AJ, Kjellstrand CM. Uremic pericardial effusion. *Nephron* 1976; 16:371–380.

151. Parkinson J, Bedford DE. Cardiac infarction and coronary thrombosis. *Lancet* 1928; 1:4–11.

152. Oliva PB, Hammill SC, Talano JV. T wave changes consistent with epicardial involvement in acute myocardial infarction: Observations in patients with a postinfarction pericardial effusion without clinically recognized postinfarction pericarditis. *J Am Coll Cardiol* 1994; 24:1073–1077.

153. Correale E, Maggioni AP, Romano S, Ricciardiello V, Battista R, Salvarola G, et al. Comparison of frequency, diagnostic and prognostic significance of pericardial involvement in acute myocardial infarction treated with and without thrombolytics. *Am J Cardiol* 1993; 71:1377–1381.

154. Heymann TD, Culling W. Cardiac tamponade after thrombolysis. *Postgrad Med J* 1994; 70:455–456.

155. Khan AH. Pericarditis of myocardial infarction: Review of the literature with case presentation. *Am Heart J* 1975; 90:788–794.

156. Galve E, Garcia-del-Castillo H, Evangelista A, Battle J, Permanyer-Miralda G, Soler-Soler J. Pericardial effusion in the course of myocardial infarction: Incidence, natural history, and clinical relevance. *Circulation* 1986; 73:294–299.

157. Dressler W. A post-myocardial-infarction syndrome: Preliminary report of a complication resembling idiopathic recurrent, benign pericarditis. *JAMA* 1956; 160:1379–1383.

158. Lichstein E, Arsura E, Hollander G, Greengart A, Sanders M. Current incidence of postmyocardial infarction (Dressler's) syndrome. *Am J Cardiol* 1982; 50:1269–1271.

159. Kossowsky WA, Lyon AF, Spain DM. Reappraisal of the post-myocardial infarction Dressler's syndrome. *Am Heart J* 1981; 102:954–956.

160. Burch GE, Colcolough HL. Postcardiotomy and postinfarction syndromes—A theory. *Am Heart J* 1970; 80:290–291.

161. Engle MA, Zabriskie JB, Senterfit LB, Gay WA, O'Loughlin JE, 85.Ehlers KH. Viral illness and the postpericardiotomy syndrome: A prospective study in children. *Circulation* 1980; 62:1151–1158.

162. Khan AH. The postcardiac injury syndromes. *Clin Cardiol* 1972; 15:67–72.

163. Antman KH. Current concepts: Malignant mesothelioma. *N Engl J Med* 1980; 303:200–202.

164. Applefeld MM, Pollock SH. Cardiac disease in patients who have malignancies. *Curr Probl Cardiol* 1980; 4:5–37.

165. Syed S, Jung RT. Cardiac tamponade caused by metastasising haemangioendothelial sarcoma of the liver. *Br Heart J* 1978; 40:697–699.

166. Arciniegas E, Hakimi M, Farooki ZQ, Green EW. Intrapericardial teratoma in infancy. *J Thorac Cardiovasc Surg* 1980; 79:306–311.

167. Wiener HG, Kristensen IB, Haubek A, Kristensen B, Baandrup U. The diagnostic value of pericardial cytology: An analysis of 95 cases. *Acta Cytol* 1991; 35:149–153.

168. Wilkes JD, Fidias P, Valckus L, Perez RP. Malignancy-related pericardial effusion: 127 cases from the Roswell Park Cancer Institute. *Cancer* 1995; 76:1377–1387.

169. Kouvaras G, Polydorou A, Hatziantoniou G. Percutaneous balloon pericardiotomy for management of cardiac tamponade in patient with lung cancer and large pericardial effusion. *Acta Cardiol* 1994; 49:549–553.

170. Olson JE, Ryan MB, Blumenstock DA. Eleven years' experience with pericardial-peritoneal window in the management of malignant and benign pericardial effusions. *Ann Surg Oncol* 1995; 2:165–169.

171. Davis S, Sharma SM, Blumberg ED, Kim CS. Intrapericardial tetracycline for the management of cardiac tamponade secondary to malignant pericardial effusion. *N Engl J Med* 1978; 299:1113–1114.

172. Hancock SL, Donaldson SS, Hopps RT. Cardiac disease following treatment of Hodgkin's disease in children and adolescents. *J Clin Oncol* 1993; 11:1199–1203.

173. Benoff LJ, Schweitzer P. Radiation therapy-induced cardiac injury. *Am Heart J* 1995; 129:1193–1196.

174. Applefeld MM, Slawson RG, Hall-Craigs M, Green DC, Singleton RT, Wiernik PH. Delayed pericardial disease after radiotherapy. *Am J Cardiol* 1981; 47:210–213.

175. Ruckdeschel JC, Chang P, Martin RG, Byhardt RW, O'Connell MJ, Sutherland JC, et al. Radiation-related pericardial effusions in patients with Hodgkin's disease. *Medicine* 1975; 54:245–259.

176. Schneider JS, Edwards JE. Irradiation induced pericarditis. *Chest* 1979; 75:560–564.

177. King DT, Nieberg RK. The use of cytology to evaluate pericardial effusions. *Ann Clin Lab Sci* 1979; 9:18–23.

178. Hancock EW. Pericardial disease in patients with neoplasm. In: Reddy PS, Leon DF, Shaver JA, eds. *Pericardial Disease*. New York: Raven Press; 1982:325.

179. Bywaters EGL. The relation between heart and joint disease including "rheumatoid heart disease" and chronic post-rheumatic arthritis (type Jaccoud). *Br Heart J* 1950; 12:101–131.

180. Charcot JM. *Clinical Lectures on Senile and Chronic Diseases* (NS Tuke, trans). London: New Sydenham Society; 1881:172–175.

181. Prakash R, Atassi A, Poske R, Rosen KM. Prevalence of pericardial effusion and mitral valve involvement in patients with rheumatoid arthritis without cardiac symptoms: An echocardiographic evaluation. *N Engl J Med* 1973; 289:597–600.

182. Travaglio-Encinoza A, Anaya J-M, Dupuy D'Angeac A, Rème T, Sany J. Rheumatoid pericarditis: New immunopathological aspects. *Clin Exp Rheumatol* 1994; 12:313–316.

183. Gelson A, Sanderson JM, Carson P. Rheumatoid pericardial effusion with heart block treated by pericardiectomy and implantation of permanent pacemaker. *Br Heart J* 1977; 39:113–115.

184. Burney DP, Martin CE, Thomas CS, Fisher RD, Bender HW. Rheumatoid pericarditis. *J Thorac Cardiovasc Surg* 1979; 77:511–515.

185. Brigden W, Bywaters EGL, Lessof MH, Ross IP. The heart in systemic lupus erythematosus. *Br Heart J* 1960; 22:1–16.

186. Bergen SS Jr. Pericardial effusion: A manifestation of systemic lupus erythematosus. *Circulation* 1960; 22:144–150.

187. Bulkley BH, Roberts WC. The heart in systemic lupus erythematosus and the changes induced in it by corticosteroid therapy: A study of 36 necropsy patients. *Am J Med* 1975; 58:243–264.

188. Kahl LE. The spectrum of pericardial tamponade in systemic lupus erythematosus: Report of ten patients. *Arthritis Rheum* 1992; 35:1343–1349.

189. Sackner MA, Heinz ER, Steinberg AJ. The heart in scleroderma. *Am J Cardiol* 1966; 17:542–559.

190. Cameron J, Oesterle SN, Baldwin JC, Hancock EW. The etiologic spectrum of constrictive pericarditis. *Am Heart J* 1987; 113:354–360.

191. Fowler NO. *Cardiac Diagnosis and Treatment*, 3d ed. New York: Harper & Row; 1980:978.

192. Slater EE. Cardiac tamponade and peripheral eosinophilia in a patient receiving cromolyn sodium. *Chest* 1978; 73:878–879.

193. Orlando RC, Moyer P, Barnett TB. Methysergide therapy and constrictive pericarditis. *Ann Intern Med* 1978; 88:213–214.

194. Houston MC, McChesney JA, Chatergee K. Pericardial effusion associated with minoxidil therapy. *Arch Intern Med* 1981; 141:69–71.

195. Logue RB. Etiology, recognition and management of pericardial disease. In: Hurst JW, ed. *The Heart*, 5th ed. New York: McGraw-Hill; 1982:1371–1393.

196. Cegielski JP, Lwakatare J, Dukes CS, Lema LE, Lattinger GJ. Kitinya J, et al. Tuberculous pericarditis in Tanzanian patients with and without HIV infection. *Tuber Lung Dis* 1994; 75:429–434.

197. Gleckman RA. Nonviral infectious pericarditis. In: Spodick DH, ed. *Pericardial Diseases*. Philadelphia: Davis; 1976:159–175.

198. Sagrista-Sauleda J, Permanyer-Miralda G, Soler-Soler J. Tuberculous pericarditis: Ten year experience with a prospective protocol for diagnosis and treatment. *J Am Coll Cardiol* 1988; 11:724–728.

199. Suwan PK, Potjalongsilp S. Predictors of constrictive pericarditis after tuberculous pericarditis. *Br Heart J* 1995; 73:187–189.

200. Fowler NO. Tuberculous pericarditis. *JAMA* 1991; 266:99–103.

201. Suzman S. Tuberculous pericardial effusion. *Br Heart J* 1943; 5:19–23.

202. Cheitlin MD, Serfas LJ, Sbar SS, Glasser SP. Tuberculous pericarditis: Is limited pericardial biopsy sufficient for diagnosis? *Am Rev Respir Dis* 1968; 98:287–291.

203. Roberts GD, Goodman NL, Heifets L, Larsh HW, Lindner TH, McClatchy JK, et al. Evaluation of the BACTEC radiometric method for recovery of mycobacteria and drug susceptibility testing of *Mycobacterium tuberculosis* from acid-fast smear-positive specimens. *J Clin Microbiol* 1983; 18:689–696.

204. Koh KK, Kim EJ, Cho CH, Choi MJ, Cho SK, Kim SS, et al. Adenosine deaminase and carcinoembryonic antigen in pericardial effusion diagnosis, especially in suspected tuberculous pericarditis. *Circulation* 1994; 89:2728–2735.

205. Seino Y, Ikeda U, Kawaguchi K, Yamamoto K, Sekiguchi H, Nakayama T, et al. Tuberculous pericarditis presumably diagnosed by polymerase chain reaction analysis. *Am Heart J* 1993; 126:249–251.

206. Choo PS, McCormack JG. *Mycobacterium avium*: A potentially treatable cause of pericardial effusions. *J Infect* 1995; 30:55–58.

207. Strang JIG, Gibson DG, Mitchison DA, Girling DJ, Kakaza HHS, Allen BW, et al. Controlled clinical trial of complete open surgical drainage and of prednisone in treatment of tuberculous pericardial effusion in Transkei. *Lancet* 1988; 2:759–764.

208. Desai HN. Tuberculous pericarditis: A review of 100 cases. *S Afr Med J* 1979; 55:877–880.

209. Lyons HA, Rooney JJ, Crocco JA. Tuberculous pericarditis. *Ann Intern Med* 1968; 68:1175.

210. Kirchner SG, heller RM, Sell SH, Altemeier WA. The radiological features of *Histoplasma* pericarditis. *Pediatr Radiol* 1978; 7:7–9.

211. Young EJ, Vainrub B, Musher DM. Pericarditis due to histoplasmosis. *JAMA* 1978; 240:1750–1751.

212. Wooley CF, Hosier DM. Constrictive pericarditis due to *Histoplasma capsulatum*. *N Engl J Med* 1961; 264:1230–1232.

213. Bennett JE. Chemotherapy of systemic mycoses. *N Engl J Med* 1974; 290:30–32.

214. Goodwin RA Jr, Snell JD Jr, Hubbard WW, Terry RT. Relationships in combined pulmonary infections with *Histoplasma capsulatum* and *Mycobacterium tuberculosis*. *Am Rev Respir Dis*. 1967; 96:990–997.

215. Sarosi GA, Voth DW, Dahl BA, Doto IL, Tosh FE. Disseminated histoplasmosis: Results of long-term follow-up. *Ann Intern Med* 1971; 75:511–516.

216. Chavez CM, Causey WA, Conn JH. Constrictive pericarditis due to infection with *Nocardia asteroides*. *Chest* 1972; 61:79–81.

217. Fowler NO, Manitsas GT. Infectious pericarditis. *Prog Cardiovasc Dis* 1973; 16:323–336.

218. Lema LEK. Surgical management of pyopericardium. *East Afr Med J* 1993; 70:140–142.

219. Rubin RH, Moellering RC. Clinical, microbiologic and therapeutic aspects of purulent pericarditis. *Am J Med* 1975; 59:68–78.

220. Klacsmann PG, Bulkley BH, Hutchins GM. The changed spectrum of purulent pericarditis: An 86 year autopsy experience in 200 patients. *Am J Med* 1977; 63:666–673.

221. Tan JS, Holmes JC, Fowler NO, Manitas GT, Phair JP. Antibiotic levels in pericardial fluid. *J Clin Invest* 1974; 53:7–12.

222. Friedland JS, Smith S, Ledingham JGG. Continuous catheter drainage of *Streptococcus pneumoniae* pericardial effusion. *J R Soc Med* 1992; 85:762–763.

223. Miller HI. Acute pericarditis as a presenting feature of meningococcal speticemia. *Isr J Med Sci* 1973; 9:1570–1573.

224. Pierce HI, Cooper EB. Meningococcal pericarditis. *Arch Intern Med* 1972; 129:918–922.

225. Scott LP, Knox D, Perry LW, Pineros-Torres FJ. Meningococcal pericarditis: Report of 2 cases, 1 complicated by acute constrictive pericarditis. *Am J Cardiol* 1972; 29:104–108.

226. Symbas PN, Ware RE, DiOrio DA, Hatcher CR. purulent pericarditis: A review of diagnostic and surgical principles. *South Med J* 1974; 67:46–48.

227. Gould K, Barnett JA, Sanford JP. Purulent pericarditis in the antibiotic era. *Arch Intern Med* 1974; 134:923–927.

228. Caird R, Conway N, McMillan IKR. Purulent pericarditis followed by early constriction in young children. *Br Heart J* 1973; 35:201–203.

229. Smolar EN, Rubin JE, Avramides A, Carter AC. Cardiac tamponade in primary myxedema and review of the literature. *Am J Med Sci* 1976; 272:345–352.

230. Stanley RJ, Subramanian R, Lie JT. Cholesterol pericarditis terminating as constrictive calcific pericarditis. *Am J Cardiol* 1980; 46:511–514.

231. Brawley RK, Vasko JS, Morrow AG. Cholesterol pericarditis: Considerations of its pathogenesis and treatment. *Am J Med* 1966; 41:235–248.

232. Shojaee S, Hutchins GM. Echinococcosis complicated by purulent pericarditis. *Chest* 1978; 73:512–514.

233. Pierce RN, Walker Smith GJ. Intrathoacic manifestations of Degos' disease (malignant atrophic papulosis). *Chest* 1978; 73:79–84.

234. Mets T, Van Hove W, Louis H. Pseudomyxoma peritonei: Report of a case with extraperitoneal metastasis and invasion of the spleen. *Chest* 1977; 72:792–794.

235. Csonka GW, oates JK. Pericarditis and electrocardiographic changes in Reiter's syndrome. *Br Med J* 1957; 1:866–869.

236. Mihas AA, Dasher CA. Pericarditis associated with granulomatous colitis. *Am J Gastroenterol* 1977; 68:494–497.

237. Vlietstra RE, Lie JT, Kuhl WE, Danielson GK, Roberts MK. Whipple's disease involving the pericardium: Pathological confirmation during life. *Aust NZ J med* 1978; 8:649–651.

238. Engle MA. Cardiac involvement in Cooley's anemia. *Ann NY Acad Sci* 1964; 119:694–704.

239. Just H, Mattingly TW. Interatrial septal defect and pericardial disease. *Am Heart J* 1968; 76:157–167.

240. Westfried M, Mandel D, Alderete MN, Groopman J, Minkowitz S. Sipple's syndrome with a malignant pheochromocytoma presenting as a pericardial effusion. *Cardiology* 1978; 63:305–311.

241. Toltzis RJ, Rosenthal A, Fellows K, Castaneda AR, Nadas AS. Chylous reflux syndrome involving the pericardium and lung. *Chest* 1978; 74:457–458.

242. Rogers CI, Meredith HC. Osler revisited: An unusual cause of inversion of the diaphragm. *Radiology* 1977; 125:596.

243. Davidson ED, Horney JT, Salter PP III. Internal pancreatic fistula to the pericardium and pleura. *Surgery* 1979; 85:478–480.

244. McNicholl B, Murray JP, Egan B, McHugh P. Pneumomediastinum and diabetic hyperpnoea. *Br Med J* 1968; 4:493–494.

245. Cumming GR, Kerr D, Ferguson CC. Constrictive pericarditis with dwarfism in two siblings (mulibrey nanism). *J Pediatr* 1976; 88:569–572.

246. Scarlett JA, Kistner ML, Yang LC. Behçet's syndrome: Report of a case associated with pericardial effusion and cryoglobulinemia treated with indomethacin. *Am J Med* 1979; 66:146–148.

247. Bianchi C, DiBonito L, Fonda F, Sauli G. Pericardial perforation of a gastric ulcer secondary to phytobezoar. *Panminerva Med* 1977; 19:353–356.

248. Horowitz HW, Belkin RN. Acute myopericarditis resulting from Lyme disease. *Am Heart J* 1995; 130:176–178.

82

INFECTIVE ENDOCARDITIS

David T. Durack

Infective endocarditis is the disease caused by microbial infection of the endothelial lining of the heart. Its characteristic lesion is a *vegetation*, which usually develops on a heart valve but occasionally appears elsewhere on the endocardium. Sometimes a nidus of infection develops on the lining of a large artery, causing *infective endarteritis*; this variant can produce clinical findings that resemble those of infective endocarditis.

DEFINITIONS AND TERMINOLOGY

These abbreviations for various forms of endocarditis will be used in this chapter:

- IE: infective endocarditis
- SBE: subacute bacterial endocarditis
- ABE: acute bacterial endocarditis
- NVE: native valve endocarditis
- PVE: prosthetic valve endocarditis
- NBTE: nonbacterial thrombotic endocarditis

The terms *subacute* and *acute bacterial endocarditis* (SBE and ABE) have descriptive value when accurately applied. SBE progresses over a period of weeks to months and is usually caused by organisms of low virulence such as viridans streptococci, which possess limited ability to infect other tissues.[1–4]

In contrast, ABE evolves over a period of days to 1 or 2 weeks; the clinical progress is hectic, complications develop earlier, and the diagnosis is usually made in less than 2 weeks.[4–6] ABE is most often caused by primary pathogens such as *Staphylococcus aureus*, which are capable of causing invasive infection at many other sites in the body.

Infection engrafted upon a heart valve that was either previously normal or damaged by congenital or acquired disease is termed *native valve endocarditis* (NVE). Infection of an artificial heart valve is termed *prosthetic valve endocarditis* (PVE). This infection has been arbitrarily defined as early

PVE when onset is within the first 2 months after surgery and as late PVE thereafter.[7–9] The definition of early versus late PVE has not been standardized; some authors have defined infections occurring between 2 months and 1 year of valve replacement as intermediate PVE,[10] while others consider any prosthetic valve infection beginning before 1 year as early PVE.

Sterile vegetations sometimes develop within the heart. This condition is often termed noninfective endocarditis, but endocard*itis* is a misnomer in this context, because the lesions are primarily thrombotic rather than inflammatory.[11] This point is emphasized by use of the term *nonbacterial thrombotic endocarditis* (NBTE), which is broadly defined here to describe any sterile vegetation. This category includes a spectrum of lesions ranging from microscopic aggregates of platelets to the large vegetations of marantic endocarditis, which sometimes develop in patients with terminal malignancy or other chronic diseases.[12–14]

Infective endocarditis is designated best by naming the infecting organism, for example, "*Staph. aureus* endocarditis" or "*Candida albicans* PVE." This terminology is specific and informative, allowing useful inferences about the likely natural history, prognosis, and treatment of the case in question.

EARLY STUDIES

Riviere in 1646, Lancisi in 1706, and Morgagni in 1761 described patients who died with endocarditis in the seventeenth and eighteenth centuries.[15] Jean-Baptiste Bouillaud introduced the terms *endocardium* and *endocarditis* between 1824 and 1835. By 1846, Virchow recognized valvular vegetations at autopsy, but the microbial etiology of infective endocarditis was not fully appreciated until Virchow, Winge, and Heiberg independently demonstrated bacteria in vegetations between 1869 and 1872.[15]

William Osler studied the disease extensively, choosing infective endocarditis as the subject for his Goulstonian lectures of 1885.[16,17] Further major contributions to the knowledge of the natural history, pathogenesis, and pathology of the disease were made by Lenharz, Harbitz, and Schottmuller[15] in Germany; by Horder[18] in England; and by Blumer,[1] Thayer,[2] Allen,[19] Libman and Friedberg,[20] and Beeson[21] in the United States. The technique of blood culture was introduced in Europe and the United States between 1890 and 1910.[3] In 1955, Kerr published a classic monograph summarizing the state of knowledge on subacute bacterial endocarditis to that date.[3]

Attempts to cure endocarditis before the advent of antimicrobial drugs were unsuccessful. In 1939, one patient with infective endarteritis involving a patent ductus arteriosus was cured by surgical closure of the ductus.[22] The first successes in the treatment of endocarditis are closely linked to the history of penicillin.[23] The first patient to receive parenteral penicillin was a young man with streptococcal endocarditis who was treated in 1940 at Columbia University in New York.[24] Although the patient received far too little penicillin to effect a cure, his treatment antedated the first administration of penicillin to a patient by Florey's team in Oxford[25] by several months. After initial failures, by 1944 it had been established that penicillin,[26] unlike sulfonamides,[27] could cure most cases of streptococcal endocarditis. Subsequently, the antibiotic treatment of endocarditis was clearly established.[28–32] After antibiotics, the next great advance was cardiac valve replacement for treatment of endocarditis in 1965,[33] which provided an essential intervention to improve survival rates in selected patients.

EPIDEMIOLOGY

Incidence

The incidence of infective endocarditis is not known accurately, because it is not a notifiable disease. Various studies in developed countries have estimated the incidence to be 1.6 to 6.0 cases per 100,000 person-years.[34–38] In the United States, this would result in 4,000 to 15,000 new cases per year. In a recent study from the Delaware Valley, where the population includes a large number of intravenous drug users (IDU), the estimated rate was much higher: 11.6 cases per 100,000 per year.[39]

Evolution of the Clinical Syndrome

Infective endocarditis today is a different disease from that seen in the preantibiotic era, when its salient clinical features were exhaustively reported.[1–3] Since 1961, many authors have described the "changing face" of "modern endocarditis,"[40–45] identifying the following trends:

- Increased median age of patients
- Increased ratio of males to females
- Increased proportion of acute cases
- Reduced incidence of some of the classic physical signs of advanced SBE, such as Osler's nodes, finger clubbing, splenomegaly, or Roth's spots

- Decreased proportion of cases due to streptococci, with an increased incidence of staphylococci
- Lengthened list of etiologic organisms, with more reports of cases caused by gram-negative bacilli, fungi, and miscellaneous rare or unusual microbes
- Increased number of cases in injection drug users (IDU)
- Increased number of prosthetic valve infections
- Increased incidence of concomitant human immunodeficiency virus (HIV) infection and endocarditis

Susceptible Populations

These striking changes in the clinical features and epidemiology of infective endocarditis cannot be explained by alterations in the virulence of the infecting microorganisms. Rather, they are due to changes in susceptible populations, to earlier diagnosis and treatment of patients with subacute disease before advanced manifestations develop, and to the impact of antibiotic therapy.[44,46] The prevalence of rheumatic valvular disease, formerly the most common substrate for endocarditis, has steadily decreased in developed countries; meanwhile, the number of children with congenital heart disease surviving palliative or corrective surgery has increased. The number of individuals using illicit drugs intravenously has increased markedly in the United States and Europe since the 1960s, and more recently HIV has spread widely throughout this group.[47]

Effect of Antibiotics

Although the advent of antibiotics revolutionized treatment of endocarditis, the overall incidence of the disease has not changed strikingly during the antibiotic era. The availability of rapidly effective treatments for pneumococcal pneumonia and gonorrhea has probably been responsible for the striking decrease in the incidence of endocarditis caused by *Streptococcus pneumoniae* and *Neisseria gonorrhoeae* since 1944, while the incidence of reported cases caused by miscellaneous unusual antibiotic-resistant organisms has increased during the antibiotic era.[46,48–51] Apart from these special cases, the widespread use of antimicrobial agents seems to have exerted considerably less influence than have alterations in the populations at risk on the changing epidemiology of endocarditis.[44] Prophylactic use of antibiotics before medical procedures that cause bacteremia has not reduced the incidence of endocarditis significantly; this is not surprising, because only a small proportion of all cases can be attributed to such procedures.[52,53]

Preexisting Heart Disease

Some patients develop endocarditis even though they have no known heart disease. This is most common in cases of ABE,[54] in children less than 2 years of age,[55–61] and in IDUs.[62–67] Most patients who develop infective endocarditis, however, have a preexisting cardiac condition. Approximate figures for the frequency of the main predisposing factors in children, adults, and injection drug users are given in Table 82-1.

TABLE 82-1

APPROXIMATE FREQUENCY OF MAJOR PREEXISTING CARDIAC LESIONS IN PATIENTS
WITH INFECTIVE ENDOCARDITIS IN THE UNITED STATES

Lesion	Children under 2 years, %	Children 2–15 Years, %	Adults 15–50 Years, %	Adults >50 Years, %	Adults Who Are IV Drug Abusers, %
No known heart disease	50–70	10–15	10–20	10	50–60
Congenital heart disease[a]	30–50	70–80	25–35	15–25	10
Rheumatic heart disease	Rare	10	10–15	10–15	10
Degenerative heart disease	0	0	Rare	10–20	Rare
Previous cardiac surgery	5	10–15	10–20	10–20	10–20
Previous endocarditis	Rare	5	5–10	5–10	10–20

[a] Includes mitral valve prolapse.

Source: Adapted from Refs. 34–49, 55–67, 76, 162.

The relative propensity of various cardiac lesions to become infected can be estimated by noting their frequency in published series of cases of infective endocarditis, even though there is wide variation among individual studies. Table 82-2 ranks cardiac abnormalities according to the risk they seem to carry for development of infective endocarditis.

Mitral valve prolapse (MVP) can predispose to endocarditis.[68–74] When associated with regurgitation, this common condition increases an individual's risk for infective endocarditis five to eightfold.[69,70,74] MVP is now known to underlie 15 to 30 percent or more of cases.[34,69,71,72,75] Although MVP is common, infective endocarditis is relatively rare; thus, the risk that any individual with MVP will develop infective endocarditis during his or her lifetime remains low (see Chap. 65).[69,70]

Children

Infective endocarditis occurs at all ages but is relatively uncommon during childhood and rare during infancy.[55–61,76,77] Endocardial infection in children with no predisposing heart disease develops most often in association with infection elsewhere, often in infants and very young children.[78] Endocarditis in these settings is likely to be caused by invasive pathogens, therefore following an acute course. Infective endocarditis can occur as a rare complication of septicemia caused by staphylococci or group B streptococci or of pneumonia, other respiratory tract infections, osteomyelitis, and severe burns.[55,59] Nosocomial cases associated with intravenous catheters are important in this group.[78] Endocarditis engrafted on congenital or other preexisting heart lesions is more likely to occur in older children and more likely to present as a subacute disease without an obvious portal of entry for the organisms.[78] *Haemophilus influenzae* type b endocarditis is very rare, even though this organism was a common cause of bacteremia in children prior to introduction of conjugate vaccines.

The leading underlying cardiac lesions in children are tetralogy of Fallot and other forms of cyanotic congenital heart disease, ventricular septal defects, aortic stenosis, patent ductus arteriosus, pulmonary stenosis, and coarctation of the aorta. A high proportion of cases occur in children who have under-

TABLE 82-2

ESTIMATES OF THE RELATIVE RISK OF INFECTIVE ENDOCARDITIS POSED BY VARIOUS CARDIAC LESIONS

Relatively High Risk	Intermediate Risk	Very Low or Negligible Risk
Prosthetic heart valves	Mitral valve prolapse with regurgitation	Mitral valve prolapse without regurgitation
Previous infective endocarditis	Pure mitral stenosis	Trivial valvular regurgitation by echocardiography without structural abnormality
Cyanotic congenital heart disease	Tricuspid valve disease	
Aortic valve disease	Pulmonary valve disease	Atrial septal defects, secundum type
Mitral regurgitation	Asymmetric septal hypertrophy	Arteriosclerotic plaques
Mitral regurgitation and stenosis	Hyperalimentation or pressure-monitoring lines that reach the right atrium	Coronary artery disease
		Syphilitic aortitis
Patent ductus arteriosus	Nonvalvular intracardiac prosthetic implants	Cardiac pacemakers
Ventricular septal defect	Degenerative valvular disease in elderly patients	Surgically corrected cardiac lesions (without prosthetic implants, more than 6 months after operation)
Coarctation of the aorta		

Source: Adapted from Refs. 35, 37, 38, 42, 48, 49, 68–76, 79, 103, 295.

gone palliative or corrective surgery for congenital cardiac defects.[59,79] Atrial septal defects of the ostium secundum type very rarely become infected. In developed countries, preexisting rheumatic heart disease is now much less common than congenital disease. No underlying cardiac disease is found in about 15 percent of children with endocarditis, but the proportion is higher in those less than 2 years of age (Table 82-1).

A firm diagnosis of infective endocarditis is more difficult to make in infants and small children than in adults. Because the physician's attention is frequently focused on a serious primary bacteremic infection, endocarditis may be an unexpected finding at autopsy. Once the diagnosis is suspected, improved diagnostic criteria can help determine whether the child has definite or possible endocarditis.[78] The clinical manifestations of acute rheumatic fever may mimic endocarditis (and vice versa), but fortunately the two conditions rarely coexist.

The choice of antibiotic treatment for children should be governed by the same principles as for adults, with appropriate dose adjustment for age. As in adults, valve replacement or other potentially curative surgical treatment should not be delayed if the child has heart failure that does not respond well to medical therapy.[80]

The Elderly

The proportion of elderly people in the populations of developed countries has increased, and endocarditis in the elderly has become more common.[81–83] The median age of patients with endocarditis has risen steadily for three decades, from about 30 to about 50 years. At present, approximately one-fourth of all patients are over age 60.[34,84] The annual risk for endocarditis is strongly age-related, being about five times higher in patients over age 80.[38] Male patients now outnumber females by approximately 1.5 to 1 overall, but by as much as 8 to 1 among patients over age 60.[34,85] Elderly patients are more likely to have underlying degenerative or calcific valve lesions.[82]

Intravenous Drug Users

Illicit intravenous drug use poses a high risk for infective endocarditis.[62–67,86] Bacteremias related to parenteral drug abuse are common, either from direct intravenous injection of bacteria or arising secondarily from the skin flora and local infections at injection sites, including cellulitis, abscesses, or suppurative thrombophlebitis. Addicts seldom use sterile injection techniques, sometimes even taking water from toilet bowls to dissolve their drugs. Nevertheless, the organisms that cause drug-related endocarditis are more often derived from the addict's skin and mucosal bacterial flora than from the drug itself or its solvent.[87] Strains of *Staph. aureus* cause more than 50 percent of cases of endocarditis among parenteral drug abusers, more than all other species combined.[48,67] Infections with gram-negative bacilli, especially *Pseudomonas* species[88,89] or yeasts and other fungi,[90] are notably more common than in nonaddicts (Table 82-3). *Candida parapsilosis* and other *Candida* species are the most common fungi causing drug-related endocarditis, but occasional infections with a wide range of other fungal species have been recorded.[90,91] Polymicrobial and culture-negative cases of endocarditis occur occasionally in IDUs but together account for less than 5 percent of cases.[62,64,67,92]

TABLE 82-3

FREQUENCY OF VARIOUS ORGANISMS CAUSING INFECTIVE ENDOCARDITIS[a]

Organism	NVE, %	IV Drug Abusers, %	Early PVE, %	Late PVE, %
Streptococci	65	15–20	5	35
Viridans, alpha-hemolytic	35	5–10	<5	25
Strep. bovis (group D)	15	<5	<5	<5
Strep. faecalis (group D)	10	8	<5	<5
Other streptococci	<5	<5	<5	<5
Staphylococci	25	50	50	30
Coagulase-positive	23	50	20	10
Coagulase-negative	<5	<5	30	20
Gram-negative aerobic bacilli	<5	5	20	10
Fungi	<5	5	10	5
Miscellaneous bacteria	<5	5	5	5
Diphtheroids, propionibacteria	<1	<5	5	<5
Other anaerobes	<1	<1	<1	<1
Rickettsiae	<1	<1	<1	<1
Chlamydiae	<1	<1	<1	<1
Polymicrobial infection	<1	1–5	5	5
Culture-negative endocarditis	5–10	<5	<5	<5

[a] These are representative figures collated from the literature; wide local variations in frequency are to be expected. NVE = native valve endocarditis; PVE = prosthetic valve endocarditis.
Source: Adapted from Refs. 42, 49, 62–67, 90–97, 102, 131.

Endocarditis in addicts frequently follows an acute course,[5,62,63,91] reflecting the high frequency of *Staph. aureus* infection. This finding partly explains the overall modest increase in the proportion of acute to subacute cases that has been observed over the past 25 years.[44]

The outstanding clinical feature of endocarditis in IDUs is the high incidence of right-sided valvular infection, much higher than in any other group of patients with endocarditis. In various series, the tricuspid valve has been involved in 50 to 70 percent.[48,64,93] The aortic and/or mitral valves are involved in 30 to 48 percent.[48,93] More than one valve on either side of the heart may be infected simultaneously. Pulmonary valve infection is unusual even among injection drug users, occurring in only some 2 percent of cases.

Tricuspid vegetations commonly embolize the lungs, causing septic pulmonary infarcts, which result in multiple focal opacities on chest x-ray, sometimes with cavitation. In a drug addict with fever, this radiologic finding is a highly characteristic sign of acute right-sided endocarditis.[5,67]

Patients Infected with Human Immunodeficiency Virus

The primary risk factor for IE in HIV-infected people is the continued use of intravenous drugs. In comparison, the severe cellular immunosuppression due to HIV is not a major risk factor. Several cases of *Bartonella* endocarditis have recently been reported in patients with acquired immunodeficiency syndrome (AIDS)[94]; this appears to be a rare instance of true opportunistic infection of the endocardium. Patients in the earlier stages of HIV infection respond well to standard treatment for endocarditis, but mortality due to IE is high after the CD4+ T-cell count falls below 200/mm³ [47] (see also Chap. 79).

Post–Cardiac Surgery Patients

Intracardiac operations, especially valve replacements, have created a whole new population at risk for infective endocarditis. In the 1950s, surgeons first noted that *Staphylococcus epidermidis* endocarditis occurred fairly frequently after mitral valvotomy.[95] Probably these organisms were sometimes inoculated directly onto the endocardium through minor rents in the surgeon's gloves, made during palpation of rough, calcified valves. Subsequently, *Staph. epidermidis*, which rarely infects native valves, has become a common cause of both early and late PVE (Table 82-3).[7–10,86] Contamination of blood circulating through pump oxygenators with *Staph. epidermidis* or other organisms can initiate infection at the time of operation, resulting in early PVE. In late PVE, the causative organisms usually originate from the normal flora of the skin or gastrointestinal tract, but their portal of entry largely remains unknown. Gram-negative bacilli and fungi infect prosthetic valves much more frequently than native valves, especially in early postoperative cases.[10,86,96] The spectrum of organisms causing late PVE more nearly resembles that of subacute native valve infection (Table 82-3).

Figure 82-1 shows the curve for incidence of PVE per month after valve replacement. The peak time of onset is 3 to 9 weeks after operation, with the risk falling quickly thereafter.[8] This important time relationship emphasizes the fact that *Staph. epidermidis* and certain other organisms are often inoculated during or immediately after surgery, while streptococci infect the prosthesis during bacteremias that may occur at any time, unrelated to surgery.

The total number of cases of postsurgical endocarditis has increased along with the number of operations, even though the incidence per patient has decreased. This decrease reflects improved operative techniques and possibly the use of prophylactic antibiotics. Review of the literature indicates a rate in recent years of about 0.5 percent for early PVE, with a range of 0.3 to 1.2 percent.[7–10]

Improved survival and long-term follow-up of patients with prosthetic valves has yielded extensive experience with late PVE.[10,86,97] Patients with prosthetic valves remain at higher risk for infective endocarditis than normal people for the rest of their lives. Late PVE occurs at a rate of about 0.3 to 0.5 percent per year.[10,86,96]

Obstetric and Gynecologic Patients

Endocarditis occurring as a complication of pregnancy is most likely to develop at the time of delivery or in the puerperium.[98] Normal delivery presents a low risk of endocarditis, even in the presence of preexisting valvular disease,[99] but bacteremias associated with perinatal infective complications such as endometritis, parametritis, septic thrombophlebitis in pelvic veins, or urinary tract infection can seed the mother's endocardium.[98] Septic abortion or pelvic infection related to intrauterine contraceptive devices can also provide the portal of entry for bacteremia resulting in endocarditis.[100] The organisms most often involved are *Enterococcus faecalis*, group B streptococci, *Staph. aureus*, and occasionally gram-negative enteric bacilli or anaerobes.

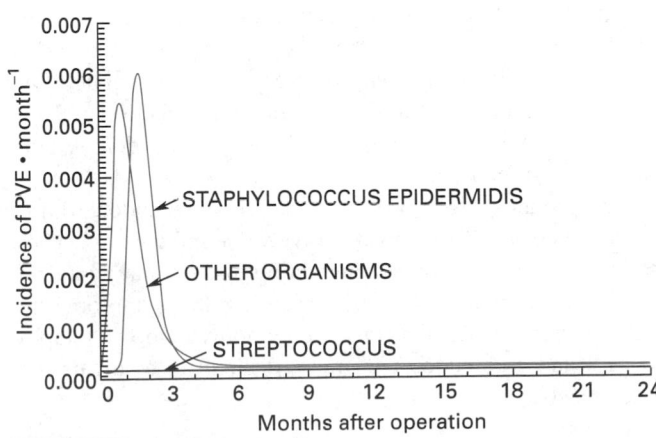

FIGURE 82-1

Incidence of prosthetic valve endocarditis (PVE) over 24 months after valve replacement. The hazard function has been stratified according to the infecting organisms. (From Ivert TSA, Dismukes WE, Cobbs CG, et al. Prosthetic valve endocarditis. *Circulation* 1984; 69:223. Reproduced with permission.)

Nosocomial Endocarditis

Hospital-acquired infective endocarditis can involve either prosthetic or native valves.[101,102] This serious complication is not rare; one study[103] reported no fewer than 35 examples of probable nosocomial endocarditis among 125 cases (28 percent), and the rate may be rising.[101] Intensive medical care can predispose to endocarditis in many ways. Endocardial damage can be produced by surgery, by intracardiac pressure-monitoring catheters, and by intravascular devices such as hyperalimentation catheters and cerebrospinal fluid shunts if they reach into the right atrium. Portals of entry for microorganisms are provided by wounds, biopsy sites, pacemakers, intravenous and arterial catheters,[104] urinary catheters, and intratracheal airways. Nosocomial bacteremias arising from local infections are common in seriously ill patients.

Many of the above-mentioned factors coexist in severely burned patients. In one study, either NBTE or infective endocarditis was found at autopsy in all of six burned patients who sustained repeated episodes of bacteremia while a pressure-monitoring catheter was maintained in the right side of the heart before death.[105] This observation has been confirmed in another autopsy study of patients with flow-directed pulmonary artery catheters.[106] Of 55 patients, 29 had one or more right-sided endocardial lesions, including 13 with thrombi and 4 with infective endocarditis. Another group at high risk are patients with prosthetic valves who develop nosocomial bacteremias, especially if the organism is a staphylococcus.[102] The portal of entry in these cases is most often an intravascular line or device, and PVE can develop later even if the patient received a course of appropriate antibiotics for the nosocomial infection. On the other hand, catheterization of the right side of the heart for brief periods in patients without bacteremia, as in a coronary care unit, presents a very low risk for infective endocarditis. Infective endocarditis is rare in patients with leukemia but has been observed in other immunocompromised patients—for example, after bone marrow transplantation[107] and heart transplantation.[108]

The leading organisms causing nosocomial endocarditis are staphylococci, enterococci, *Candida* species, and gram-negative bacilli. *Staph. aureus* is especially associated with wound infections, cellulitis, and cannula infections; *Staph. epidermidis* with ventriculoatrial shunts; and *C. albicans* with parenteral alimentation.

The prognosis for nosocomial native valve endocarditis is worse than for other forms of native valve infection.[101] These patients often have serious underlying disease that may delay diagnosis of endocarditis by obscuring the symptoms and signs, while the organisms most commonly involved (staphylococci and enterococci) are more difficult to eradicate than viridans streptococci.

Hemodialysis

Creation of arteriovenous shunts for hemodialysis predisposes patients to develop infective endocarditis by providing a ready portal of entry for bacteremias. Another possible factor is increased cardiac output. Dogs with high cardiac output due to surgically created arteriovenous fistulas are predisposed to develop not only infective endarteritis at the site of the shunt but endocarditis as well.[109] Therefore, it is not surprising that endocarditis has been reported in 2 to 6 percent of patients on long-term hemodialysis employing either arteriovenous fistulas or cannulas. *Staph. aureus* has been the most common etiologic organism, followed by viridans streptococci and *E. faecalis*.[110] The diagnosis of endocarditis is difficult in these patients, partly because coexisting intravascular infection at the shunt site often confuses the clinical picture. Mortality is high (53 percent), and early recognition and aggressive treatment of both shunt infections and endocarditis in dialysis patients are necessary to improve outcome.[110]

Infective Endarteritis

Focal intravascular infection located outside the heart itself can mimic most of the clinical manifestations of endocarditis, including vascular and immunologic phenomena.[48] In the past, about one-quarter of all patients with an uncorrected patent ductus arteriosus developed bacterial endarteritis.[3] Coarctations of the aorta also presented a significant risk, but endocarditis located on an associated bicuspid aortic valve was three times more common than endarteritis with vegetations located in the coarctation. Endarteritis occasionally complicates traumatic arteriovenous fistulas, but arteriosclerotic aneurysms rarely become infected.[48] When bacterial endarteritis does occur within an aneurysm, the organisms usually grow in a multilayered thrombus in the lumen of the aneurysm rather than in vegetations.

The spectrum of organisms causing infective endarteritis is similar to that found in endocarditis except that there is a higher frequency of infection with salmonellae in arteriosclerotic abdominal aneurysms.[48,111] The pattern of embolization observed differs according to the site of infection. Thus, petechiae may occur on the skin of the lower extremities in a patient with an infected abdominal aneurysm, and infarctions may appear in the lungs of a patient with an infected dialysis fistula in the forearm.

Because many of the congenital and acquired vascular lesions that predispose to infective endarteritis can be corrected by modern surgery, endarteritis—except in arteriovenous shunts constructed for the purpose of hemodialysis—is uncommon today in developed countries.

ETIOLOGIC ORGANISMS

The range of microbial species that can cause infective endocarditis is extraordinarily wide, yet only a few species account for the great majority of cases. On native valves, streptococci and staphylococci together cause more than 80 percent of infections.[37,42,49,103] By comparison, native valve infections caused by *Staph. epidermidis*, enteric bacilli, and fungi are uncommon. Among intravenous drug users and patients with prosthetic valves, the incidence of infection due to these organisms is higher. Table 82-3 offers representative figures from the literature on the relative frequency of the major etiologic organisms on native valves, in drug addicts, and on prosthetic valves. It should be emphasized that the relative frequency with which various organisms cause endocarditis can vary widely between countries and between medical centers.

Streptococci

Streptococci cause more cases of endocarditis than any other group of organisms.[37,49,112–114] The alpha-hemolytic or viridans streptococci account for the majority of these cases. Viridans streptococci are ubiquitous (although outnumbered by anaerobes) in the oropharyngeal and gastrointestinal flora. They are low-grade pathogens, often recovered from clinical specimens in mixed culture with other organisms but seldom themselves causing disease. Their strong association with SBE is therefore determined by the frequency with which they enter the bloodstream and by their ability to adhere to endocardium rather than by their innate virulence.

The nomenclature of these organisms is complex and has been subject to repeated revisions.[112,115,116] The following species frequently cause SBE: *Strep. sanguis*, *Strep. mitis*, *Strep. oralis*, and *Strep. gordonii*. Many other species occasionally cause SBE; for example, the *Strep. milleri* group: *Strep. anginosus*, *Strep. intermedius*, and *Strep. constellatus*.[112,114,115] A few cases are caused by strains that require media supplemented with L-cysteine or pyridoxine for growth.[117–120] These strains are more difficult to isolate from blood and seem to be more difficult to eradicate with antibiotic treatment than the other viridans streptococci.

Group D streptococci are next in frequency among the streptococci as a cause of endocarditis.[85,121,122] The nonenterococcal group D species, *Strep. bovis*, accounts for about one-fifth of streptococcal cases. Gastrointestinal lesions, especially colonic polyps and cancers, are commonly present in patients who develop *Strep. bovis* bacteremia and/or endocarditis.[123,124] Hence, recovery of this species from blood cultures should prompt investigation for colonic disease, whether or not the patient has gastrointestinal symptoms.

Strains of *E. faecalis* (enterococci) cause about 10 percent of streptococcal cases. In the past it was said that this species caused endocarditis "in young women and old men," because it was found in association with infections of the genital and urinary tract in women of childbearing age and of the urinary tract in older men with prostatic disease. Today, enterococcal endocarditis is more likely to be found in drug addicts, in patients with nosocomial endocarditis, and in those with chronic renal failure.[85] Enterococci commonly cause urinary tract, wound, and intravenous line infections, which often give rise to nosocomial bacteremias.[125,126] Fewer than 2 percent of such patients have endocarditis, but if enterococcal bacteremia is community-acquired without a primary focus of infec-

tion, about one-third will have infective endocarditis.[125] Antibiotic resistance, especially in strains of *E. faecium*, presents major difficulties in treatment of enterococcal endocarditis.[85,127–129]

Many other species and strains of streptococci occasionally cause endocarditis, but they are rare compared with the viridans and group D organisms. *Strep. pneumoniae* endocarditis has become uncommon since the advent of antibiotics. This species causes acute endocarditis.[130] In debilitated alcoholics, bacteremic pneumococcal pneumonia is occasionally complicated by development of pneumococcal endocarditis and meningitis. This triad of simultaneous pneumococcal infections carries an extremely poor prognosis.[130]

Staphylococci

Staph. aureus is the leading cause of acute bacterial endocarditis. It is the predominant etiologic organism in intravenous drug users (IDUs) with endocarditis[67] and frequently causes PVE.[86] Because it is an invasive primary pathogen, patients with staphylococcal ABE often develop disseminated disease with metastatic infections in skin and soft tissue, bone, joints, eye, or brain.[131–133]

Only a minority of all patients with *Staph. aureus* bacteremia have endocarditis, and it is often difficult to identify this subgroup. Factors that increase the probability that such a patient has endocarditis are (1) community-acquired bacteremia, (2) absence of a primary focus of infection, and (3) presence of metastatic foci of staphylococcal infection. Up to two-thirds of patients with all three of these characteristics have endocarditis.[133] *Staph. epidermidis* is a rare cause of native valve infection, usually associated with an indolent subacute or chronic course.[134] In striking contrast, it is a common cause of PVE, which may follow either an acute or subacute clinical course.[134,135]

Gram-Negative Bacteria

Although most of the species of gram-negative bacteria that colonize and/or infect humans have been reported to cause infective endocarditis, they account for only a small proportion of cases of native valve infection. A significant subgroup of cases are caused by a group of nutritionally fastidious gram-negative bacilli: *Haemophilus* species, *Actinobacillus actinomycetemcomitans*, *Cardiobacterium hominis*, *Eikenella corrodens*, and *Kingella kingae*. These are often referred to by the acronym HACEK, which is derived from their initials.[136,137] Cases caused by *Haemophilus* predominate in this group. Endocarditis caused by this genus is usually due to *Haemophilus aphrophilus*, *H. paraphrophilus*, or *H. parainfluenzae* and only rarely to *H. influenzae*, even though *H. influenzae* is more virulent and more frequently found in the blood than the other species.

The common aerobic enteric gram-negative bacilli seldom cause endocarditis. For example, cases of endocarditis caused by *Escherichia coli* and *Klebsiella* are notably rare,[89] even though these species frequently cause gram-negative bacteremia. The reasons for this striking disparity are probably multiple, including low adhesiveness of gram-negative enteric bacilli to heart valves[138] and fibrin[139] and susceptibility of many strains to complement-mediated bacteriolysis.[140] Despite these factors, two special populations are at increased risk of gram-negative endocarditis: IDUs and patients with prosthetic valves. Gram-negative bacilli account for about 5 percent of endocarditis in IDUs,[62,65–67] with *Pseudomonas* species, *Serratia*, and *Enterobacter* species predominating. Gram-negative bacilli cause 15 to 20 percent of early PVE and about 10 percent of late PVE.[10,86]

Interesting but unusual cases caused by species of *Salmonella*, *Brucella*, *Acinetobacter*, and other gram-negative bacilli have been reported.[89] *Brucella* endocarditis is well known in the Mediterranean basin[141,142] but rare in most other regions. Endocarditis caused by anaerobic bacteria is rare (1 percent or less of cases),[143,144] possibly because the oxygen tension in heart blood is too high to favor growth of these species on the endocardium.

Neisseria gonorrhoeae causes an acute form of the disease,[2] often involving the right side of the heart. Like the pneumococcus, *N. gonorrhoeae* has become uncommon as a cause of endocarditis since the introduction of penicillin.[49,50]

Yeasts and Dimorphic Fungi

Although many species of yeasts and other fungi can infect the endocardium, only two genera account for the great majority: *Candida* and *Aspergillus*.[90,91,145] *Candida* causes native valve infections in IDUs and in patients receiving parenteral alimentation, while *Aspergillus* species often involve prosthetic valves. Fungal infection of native valves in nonaddicts is rare (Table 82-3).

Miscellaneous Organisms

Many less common organisms occasionally cause endocarditis; for example, *Coxiella burnetii* (Q fever) and *Chlamydia*. Q-fever endocarditis is a chronic, febrile systemic illness with prominent hepatic as well as cardiac valvular involvement.[146–151] A recent report indicates that *Bartonella* may cause up to 3 percent of cases of IE[152]; in the past, most of these cases were listed as culture-negative, while some were misdiagnosed as chlamydial due to false-positive cross-reacting serologic tests.[152] Chlamydial endocarditis is rare; a few cases have been reported in bird fanciers.[153,154] In such cases, the etiologic diagnosis can be established only by specialized culture techniques, serologic studies, or examination of vegetations using immunofluorescent antibodies. Many unusual species occasionally infect prosthetic valves, including *Mycoplasma hominis*,[155] *Legionella* species,[51] and mycobacteria.[156] Some examples of rare or unusual organisms that have caused one or more cases of endocarditis are listed in Table 82-4.

Culture-Negative Endocarditis

This term refers to the illness of patients who have active infective endocarditis yet whose repeated blood cultures are

TABLE 82-4

SOME UNUSUAL OR RARE CAUSES OF INFECTIVE ENDOCARDITIS

Bacteria	Fungi
Bacillus cereus	*Blastoschizomyces*
Bartonella elizabethae	*capitatus*
Bartonella henselae	*Conidiobolus* sp.
Corynebacterium diphtheriae	*Curvularia lunata*
biotype *gravis*	*Engyodontium album*
Corynebacterium jeikeium	*Fusarium oxysporum*
Corynebacterium	*Histoplasma capsulatum*
pseudodiphtheriticum	*Neosartorya fischeri*
Erysipelothrix rhusiopathiae	*Phialophora richardsiae*
Haemophilus influenzae	*Pseudallescheria boydii*
type b	*Scedosporium inflatum*
Lactobacillus species	*Scedosporium apio-*
Legionella species	*spermum*
Mycoplasma hominis	*Thermomyces lanuginosus*
Rothia dentocariosa	*tsiklinsky*
Streptobacillus moniliformis	*Trichosporon beigelii*

all negative.[157–159] This syndrome was occasionally observed in the pre-antibiotic era,[160] usually in subacute cases of long duration (*endocarditis lenta*). Today, most (but not all) culture-negative cases are caused by antibiotic treatment that is sufficient to suppress the bacteremia but not to sterilize the vegetation. In most such cases, organisms will eventually reappear in the blood after antibiotics are discontinued, usually within a few days. The blood cultures from a few patients with active endocarditis remain persistently culture-negative after antibiotics are stopped.[103]

Negative blood culture results should be expected from about one-fifth of patients with NVE or PVE caused by *Candida* or other yeasts,[91] and from four-fifths of patients with endocarditis caused by *Aspergillus* or other molds.[91,145,161]

The reported incidence of culture-negative endocarditis varies widely. Among large unselected series of cases collected from several hospitals, up to 15 to 20 percent may be culture-negative.[49,157–159] Smaller series of patients studied by a single clinical and laboratory team that is experienced in evaluation of endocarditis usually show only about 5 percent culture-negative cases.[162,163] This low figure carries an important clinical implication: in a patient with suspected infective endocarditis, other diagnoses should be meticulously excluded before a diagnosis of culture-negative endocarditis is accepted. When a patient appears to have infective endocarditis but blood cultures are negative, the following checklist of possibilities should be considered:

- The patient has received some antibiotic therapy, commonly an oral drug such as ampicillin that was taken at home.
- The etiologic organism is slow-growing, requiring longer incubation of the blood culture for isolation, e.g., some

nutritionally variant streptococci, some HACEK species, or mycobacteria.

- The etiologic organism is nutritionally fastidious, requiring special procedures or supplemented media for isolation, e.g., nutritionally variant streptococci, *C. burnetii* (Q fever), *Chlamydia, Mycoplasma, Bartonella,* and *Legionella.*
- The etiologic organism is a strict anaerobe, requiring anaerobic culture conditions.
- The etiologic organism is *Aspergillus* or another mold; these are rarely recovered from blood during the course of endocarditis (although they may be recovered from an arterial embolus removed at surgery).
- The etiologic organism is nonculturable.
- The patient has an alternative diagnosis that simulates infective endocarditis—e.g., rheumatic fever, tuberculosis, brucellosis, etc.
- The patient has nonbacterial thrombotic endocarditis (NBTE) or marantic endocarditis, associated with a major underlying disease such as malignancy or tuberculosis.
- The patient has Libman-Sacks endocarditis (a variant of NBTE), associated with antiphospholipid antibody syndrome and/or systemic lupus erythematosus.

In some cases, a working diagnosis of endocarditis based on clinical manifestations can be supported by the progress of the disease and good response to empiric antibiotic treatment. If blood culture results always remain negative, a definitive etiologic diagnosis can be made only by detecting organisms in an infected embolus or in vegetations excised during surgery or at autopsy.

PATHOGENESIS AND PATHOLOGY

A general concept of the pathogenesis of NBTE and SBE is presented in Fig. 82-2.

Noninfective Endocarditis

Sterile thrombotic lesions may develop on heart valves in a variety of clinical conditions.[164] Small aggregates of platelets can occasionally be found on normal valves, but they occur frequently on the surfaces of valves damaged by congenital or rheumatic disease[165] or by infective endocarditis. These could be considered as incipient vegetations, or microvegetations.

The common factor leading to platelet deposition is endothelial damage. This exposes subendothelial connective tissue containing collagen, which in turn causes platelets to aggregate at the site. These microscopic platelet thrombi may embolize away harmlessly, or they may be stabilized and grow by deposition of fibrin and more platelets to form vegetations of NBTE. This process can be duplicated experimentally by passing a catheter into the heart of an animal; NBTE forms at sites of endothelial damage.[166] In humans, intracar-

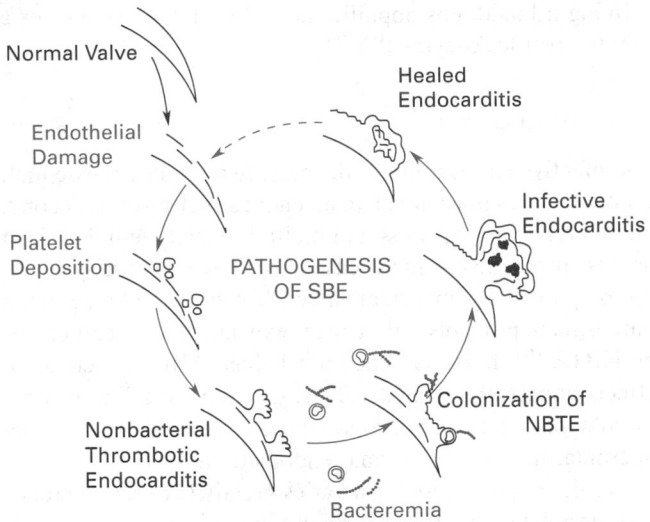

FIGURE 82-2
The main events in the pathogenesis of nonbacterial thrombotic endocarditis (NBTE) and subacute bacterial endocarditis (SBE).

diac pressure-monitoring catheters produce identical lesions.[105,106] Both experimental[167] and human[105,107,164] NBTE can be colonized by circulating bacteria, resulting in infective endocarditis.

The vegetations of marantic endocarditis occur most often in patients with advanced malignancy[12–14] but may also complicate other chronic wasting diseases, such as tuberculosis or uremia. The initiating factors for marantic endocarditis are not known. Endothelial damage caused by circulating cytokines such as tumor necrosis factor or interleukins, which can be upregulated in patients with malignancy or chronic wasting disease, might trigger focal accretions of platelets.

Sterile vegetations (termed *Libman-Sacks endocarditis—* see Chap. 85) sometimes develop in patients with systemic lupus erythematosus and/or antiphospholipid antibodies.[168] Typically, Libman-Sacks vegetations are small, sessile masses located on the ventricular surfaces of the mitral valve leaflets.

The vegetations of NBTE are friable white or tan masses, usually situated along the lines of valve closure (Fig. 82-3, Plate 63). These vary greatly in size; they are sometimes tiny but frequently rather large and exuberant, with a corresponding tendency to cause extensive infarctions when they break off and are carried to arteries supplying the myocardium, spleen, kidney, brain, mesentery, or extremities. Since there is little inflammatory reaction at the site of attachment, fresh vegetations can often be picked off easily with forceps, leaving a valve surface that may look normal to the naked eye.[164] It is not surprising that such easily dislodged vegetations embolize frequently. Histologically, the vegetations of NBTE consist of degenerating platelets interwoven with strands of fibrin,

FIGURE 82-3
See color Plate 63.

forming a bland, eosinophilic mass, featureless except for a few trapped leukocytes.[164,166]

Infective Endocarditis

For infective endocarditis to develop, two events are essential. First, microbes must attach to an endocardial surface. Second, the microbes must persist and multiply locally, eluding host defense mechanisms. In the case of SBE, which usually develops on previously abnormal valves, bacteria circulating in the bloodstream probably colonize preexisting platelet aggregates or NBTE.[164] It is not known whether ABE, which often affects apparently normal valves, develops in a like manner by colonization of microscopic sterile vegetations, or by direct microbial invasion of normal endothelium.

Ability to adhere to fibrin varies greatly between microbes and correlates with their proclivity to cause endocarditis.[48,169,170] Dextran production by oral streptococci is associated with increased adherence to fibrin, increased ability to cause endocarditis in animals, formation of larger vegetations, and relative resistance to penicillin therapy.[169] On the other hand, some streptococcal species (for example, enterococci) produce no dextran but adhere well and often cause endocarditis; thus, dextran production is not an essential virulence factor. FimA is a surface protein adhesin that mediates adherence of *Streptococcus parasanguis* in the oral cavity; deletion mutants adhere less well to fibrin and are less likely to cause endocarditis in experimental animals.[170] Binding to fibronectin appears to be an important property shared by many but not all of the bacterial species that commonly cause endocarditis.[48,169] Clumping factor produced by coagulase-positive staphylococci favors attachment to fibrinogen, adherence to platelet-fibrin clots, and ability to cause endocarditis in rats.[171]

Extracellular slime production by coagulase-negative staphylococci may favor localization in the heart, especially on prosthetic valves.[172] *Thus, microbial adherence, which can be mediated by a variety of different surface components and receptors, is a key factor for colonization of the endocardium.*[48,169]

Once lodged on NBTE, bacteria must elude local defenses, including platelet microbicidal proteins[173] and leukocytes, if they are to survive. Microbes that cannot do this may die out quickly after adhering to the endocardium.[174] Those that can survive antimicrobial defense mechanisms multiply rapidly in the vegetation, soon reaching high numbers and then entering a stationary growth phase.[167] The vegetation provides an ideal supporting stroma for the growth of microbial colonies, into which essential nutrients can diffuse from the blood. The presence of bacteria is a powerful stimulus for further thrombosis,[175,176] which may be mediated by thromboplastin generated by leukocytes when they are exposed to fibrin.[176] New layers of fibrin are deposited around growing bacteria, causing the vegetations to enlarge.[166] Inflammatory cytokines are produced by monocytes[177] (and presumably other leukocytes) in response to endocardial infection and likely cause some of the patient's symptoms.

The location of vegetations is relevant to understanding and managing endocarditis. Approximate figures for the incidence with which vegetations are found at various sites are given in Table 82-5. The frequency of involvement of each valve is directly proportional to the mean blood pressure upon it[178]; thus, the left side of the heart is involved much more often than the right. This rule is reliable for SBE but does not hold true for acute endocarditis in IDUs, in whom tricuspid infection by *Staph. aureus* predominates (Table 82-5).

Vegetations are usually located on the downstream side of anatomic abnormalities in the heart or great vessels. Rodbard[179] developed the unifying concept that vegetations usually arise at a site where blood flows from a high-pressure source (e.g., the left ventricle) through a narrow orifice (e.g., a stenotic aortic valve) into a low-pressure sink (e.g., the aorta). Illustrative examples from human disease include aortic stenosis, ventricular septal defect, coarctation, and mitral regurgitation. Experimentally, Rodbard showed that bacteria carried in an aerosol flowing through a constricted tube into an area of low pressure were deposited on the walls of the tube immediately beyond the constriction due to Venturi pressure effects and turbulence.[179] These observations fit well with the

---

TABLE 82-5

APPROXIMATE FREQUENCY OF ANATOMIC LOCATION OF VEGETATIONS
IN SBE, ABE, AND ENDOCARDITIS ASSOCIATED
WITH IV DRUG ABUSE[a]

Location	SBE, %	ABE, %	Endocarditis in IV Drug Abusers, %
Left-sided valves	85	65	40
Aortic	15–26	18–25	15–20
Mitral	38–45	30–35	15–20
Aortic and mitral	23–30	15–20	13–20
Right-sided valves	5	20	50–70
Tricuspid	1–5	15	45–65
Pulmonary	1	Rare	2
Tricuspid and pulmonary	Rare	Rare	3
Left- and right-sided sites	Rare	5–10	5–10
Other sites (patent ductus, ventricular septal defect, coarctation, jet lesions)	10	5	5

[a] SBE = subacute bacterial endocarditis; ABE = acute bacterial endocarditis.
Source: Adapted from Refs. 49, 62–67, 79, 103, 131, 178–181.

greenish-gray.[64,181] Histologically, colonies of microorganisms are found embedded in a fibrin-platelet matrix.[166,167,182,183] Although the inflammatory reaction at the site of attachment may be extensive, even progressing to form a frank abscess, the vegetations themselves characteristically contain relatively few leukocytes. Those few phagocytes present are prevented from reaching bacteria by layers of fibrin, which form protective barriers around colonies (Fig. 82-6).

Development of an abscess is one of the most important complications of valvular infection.[180,182] Abscesses often develop by direct extension of active infection into the fibrous cardiac skeleton—that is, into the rings of supporting connective tissue around the valves. From there, abscesses can extend into the adjacent myocardium. Hematogenous seeding occasionally leads to development of abscesses elsewhere in the myocardium.

Abscesses develop more often during the course of ABE, because this form of endocarditis is caused by primary pathogens adapted to invade human tissues. They are less common in SBE unless a valvular prosthesis is present. Abscesses are found in the majority of patients who die with active prosthetic valve infection, often spreading around the sewing ring of the prosthesis and causing partial dehiscence of the prosthetic valve.[10,86] Because these valve ring abscesses are located close to the cardiac conduction system, conduction disturbances commonly result.[184]

Role of Immunity

Presence of bacteria in endocardial vegetations stimulates the humoral immune system to produce nonspecific antibodies. This can result in a polyclonal increase in gamma globulins, positive rheumatoid factor, and, occasionally, false-positive serologic test results for syphilis.[185] Rheumatoid factor develops in 25 to 50 percent of patients with SBE and can provide a useful diagnostic clue; it reverts to negative after eradication of the organisms.[186–188] Antiendocardial and antisarcolemmal antibodies have been detected in 60 to 100 percent of cases[189]; they are more commonly found in SBE than in ABE.

Specific antibodies to many of the commensal organisms that cause SBE may be present in low titer before infection. Titers rise during active infection[3] and fall after treatment. Obviously, specific antibody prevents neither infection nor reinfection of the endocardium because reinfections with the same species have been reported. It has been claimed that preexisting humoral immunity actually predisposes to endocarditis[3,190] and that a "high titer of agglutinating antibody for the infecting organism" is a prime factor in pathogenesis.[190] This hypothesis, however, is based only upon theoretical considerations and uncontrolled observations in animals.[191,192] Controlled animal experiments suggest that high titers of specific antistreptococcal antibodies actually protect against streptococcal endocarditis.[193] In summary, endocardial infection stimulates an immune response, but the evidence

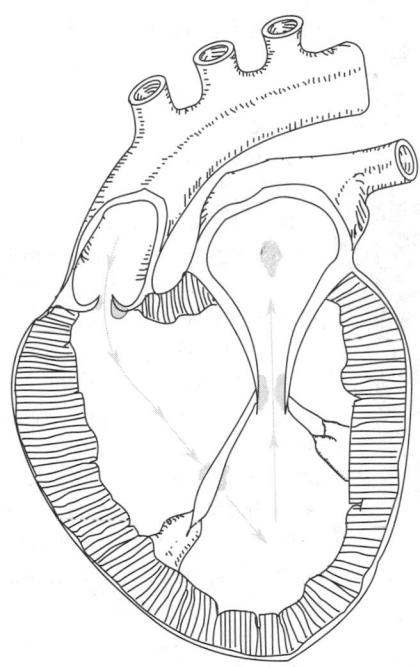

FIGURE 82-4

The sites where endocarditis occurs in aortic and mitral regurgitation. The arrows on the left indicate a high-velocity regurgitant stream passing through the orifice of an incompetent aortic valve into a low-pressure sink (left ventricle in diastole). Vegetations appear on the ventricular surface of the aortic valve. The regurgitant stream may cause a jet lesion on the chordae tendineae of the anterior leaflet of the mitral valve. The arrow on the right shows regurgitation from the high-pressure source of the left ventricle during systole into the left atrium, with vegetations developing on the atrial surface of the mitral valve. Vegetations also can occur on the jet lesion where the regurgitant stream through the mitral valve strikes the atrial endocardium, an area known as *MacCallum's patch*. (From Rodbard S. Blood velocity and endocarditis. *Circulation* 1963; 27:8. Reproduced with permission.)

actual location of vegetations found at autopsy in cases of endocarditis (Fig. 82-4). Vegetations also may develop on jet lesions, which are areas of endothelial roughening and reactive fibrosis at sites where a swift, turbulent regurgitant stream of blood strikes the endothelium.[180] *MacCallum's patch*, on the wall of the left atrium in some patients with mitral regurgitation, is an example of a jet lesion; an infected vegetation occasionally develops at this site (Fig. 82-4).

Vegetations of infective endocarditis vary greatly in morphology, from small, warty nodules to large, cauliflower-like polypoid masses (Fig. 82-5, Plate 64). Their size varies from less than a millimeter to several centimeters, which is large enough to cause functional stenosis of valve orifices. The average size of right-sided vegetations is significantly greater than that of vegetations on left-sided valves. Fungal vegetations are often larger than bacterial ones, but otherwise the etiologic species does not correlate reliably with vegetation size. Their color also varies widely, from white to tan to

FIGURE 82-5
See color Plate 64.

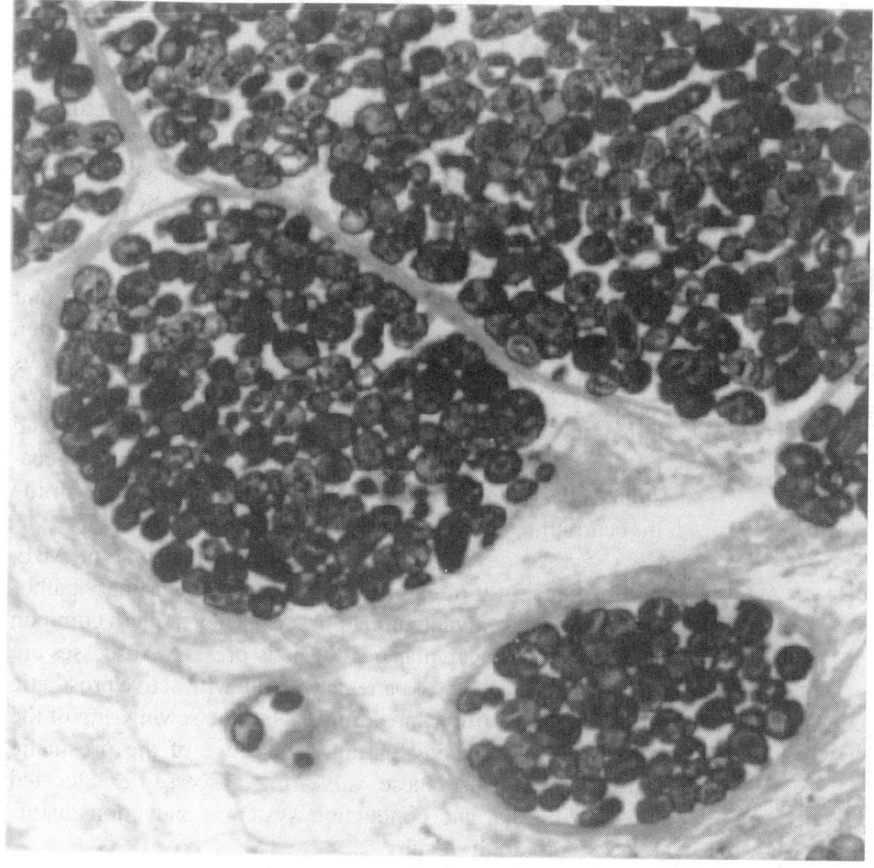

FIGURE 82-6

Electron micrograph of a vegetation of experimental streptococcal endocarditis (×7800). Note the very large number of cocci in colonies, the protective layers of fibrin, and the absence of leukocytes—all factors that may impede the efficacy of antimicrobial therapy. (From Durack DT. Experimental bacterial endocarditis: 4. Structure and evolution of very early lesions. *J Pathol* 1975; 115:81. Reproduced with permission.)

Healed Endocarditis

Even in active, untreated endocarditis, some evidence of healing can be found.[194] Histiocytes slowly advance into the base of vegetations, while endothelium begins to cover the surface from the periphery. This attempt at healing fails in untreated cases but progresses to completion during and after successful treatment. Macrophages ingest bacterial debris and fibrin, while fibroblasts organize the lesions by laying down collagen fibers. Endocardium gradually covers the surface of the shrinking vegetations. Calcium is often deposited at the site of old bacterial colonies. Dead, but still recognizable, gram-positive cocci can sometimes be found in sections of valves resected at operation or autopsy up to 3 to 6 months after infection has been eradicated by antibiotic treatment. The healed valve is often scarred and thickened by new collagen. It may also be perforated or ruptured, and the supporting structures may be damaged. Therefore, residual functional valvular abnormalities, varying from minor to severe, are common. Due to mechanical stresses, valvular function often continues to deteriorate at an unpredictable rate after infection is eradicated. Whether or not hemodynamic function is preserved, the scarred valve surface remains susceptible to reinfection.

that preexisting antibodies promote development of endocarditis remains unconvincing.[194]

Hemolytic complement levels are low in about 30 percent of patients early in the course of endocarditis, rising later and returning to normal after treatment.[195,196] The lowest levels are found in patients with immune-complex glomerulonephritis.

Circulating immune complexes have been detected in 82 to 97 percent of patients with either ABE or SBE.[195–198] Higher concentrations are correlated with the presence of extracardiac manifestations such as arthritis, splenomegaly, and glomerulonephritis; with longer duration of illness; and with hypocomplementemia. Several studies confirm that glomerulonephritis in patients with endocarditis is mediated by immune complexes.[199,200] It seems likely but unproved that arthritis and tenosynovitis—and possibly pericarditis, Osler's nodes, and Roth's spots[195,197,198]—may also represent inflammatory responses involving immune complexes. Antibodies to teichoic acids were found in the serum of 93 percent of patients with *Staph. aureus* endocarditis,[201] but this did not prove to be useful as a routine diagnostic test.

Experimental Endocarditis

Because the primary cardiac lesions are inaccessible to direct study in living patients, investigators long ago turned to animal models.[194,202,203] Bacterial infections of the endocardium in laboratory animals were successfully produced more than a century ago. The crucial importance of endothelial damage in pathogenesis was established in animals before 1890.[194,203] Later studies in animals demonstrated that arteriovenous fistulas and other high-output states predispose to endocarditis,[109] confirmed the hypothesis (derived from human autopsy observations) that the lesion of NBTE is a receptive nidus upon which circulating bacteria readily lodge,[167] and permitted study of the earliest stages of vegetation growth.[166] Experiments showing that most bacteria in vegetations are in a metabolically inactive, stationary phase helped to explain why antibiotic treatment must be continued longer to cure endocarditis than many other infections.[204] Other experiments demonstrated the reduced propensity of gram-negative bacilli and anaerobes to colonize vegetations when compared with gram-positive cocci, the role of complement in protecting against *E. coli* endocarditis,[140] and the protective effect of antibodies against oral streptococci.[193] The immune responses to endocardial infection—including demonstration of immune complexes in serum, the process of healing, the effect of anticoagulants, and the comparative efficacy of preventive and therapeutic antibiotics—have all been examined in animals with endocarditis.[11,205]

Because most of these studies could not have been performed in human beings, experimental studies have made important contributions to our understanding of this complex disease.

CLINICAL MANIFESTATIONS

Clinical and laboratory manifestations of infective endocarditis can be grouped under three headings (Table 82-6):

- Evidence of a systemic infection
- Evidence of an intravascular lesion
- Evidence of an immunologic reaction to infection

History

The symptoms of subacute endocarditis develop insidiously and with great variability.[3,42,49,103] Fevers, chills, rigors, and night sweats provide evidence of systemic infection. General malaise—with anorexia, fatigue, and weakness—is typical. Weight loss is common, along with headaches and musculoskeletal complaints, including myalgias, arthralgias, and back pains.[206] This symptom complex is often described by the patient or the physician as a "flu-like illness."

Evidence of an intravascular lesion is provided by symptoms of left- or right-sided heart failure and by manifestations of embolization, such as focal neurologic injury, chest pain, flank pain, left-upper-quadrant pain, hematuria, or ischemia of an extremity. Symptoms usually persist and worsen intermittently over 4 to 8 weeks before the diagnosis is made.[207]

In the acute form of infective endocarditis, the course is accelerated, and the symptoms are often accentuated in severity. Patients experience hectic fevers, rigors, and prostration, usually leading to admission to hospital within a few days.[5,49,93,208,209]

Symptoms of cardiac failure may develop gradually or worsen suddenly in either acute or subacute disease due to mechanical complications such as perforation of a valve leaflet, rupture of one of the chordae tendineae, rupture of a sinus of Valsalva, or development of functional stenosis from obstruction of blood flow by large vegetations.[182,210] Alternatively, heart failure may develop insidiously, or preexisting chronic heart failure may worsen due to progressive damage to the valves or associated structures. Myocarditis or myocardial

TABLE 82-6

SUMMARY OF THE MAJOR CLINICAL MANIFESTATIONS OF INFECTIVE ENDOCARDITIS

Manifestation	History	Examination	Investigations
SYSTEMIC INFECTION	Fever, chills, rigors, sweats, malaise, weakness, lethargy, delirium, headache, anorexia, weight loss, backache, arthralgia, myalgia Portal of entry: oropharynx, skin, urinary tract, drug addiction, nosocomial bacteremia	Fever, pallor, weight loss, asthenia, splenomegaly	Anemia, leukocytosis (variable), raised erythrocyte sedimentation rate, positive blood culture, abnormal cerebrospinal fluid
INTRAVASCULAR LESION	Dyspnea, chest pain, focal weakness, stroke, abdominal pain, cold and painful extremities	Murmurs, signs of cardiac failure, petechiae (skin, eye, mucosae), Roth's spots, Osler's nodes, Janeway lesions, splinter hemorrhages, stroke, mycotic aneurysm, ischemia or infarction of viscera or extremities	Blood in urine, chest roentgenogram, echocardiography, arteriography, liver-spleen scan, lung scan, brain scan, CT scan, histology, culture of emboli
IMMUNOLOGIC REACTIONS	Arthralgia, myalgia, tenosynovitis	Arthritis, signs of uremia, vascular phenomena, finger clubbing	Proteinuria, hematuria, casts, uremia, acidosis, polyclonal increases in gamma globulins, rheumatoid factor, decreased complement, immune complexes in serum, antistaphylococcal teichoic acid antibodies

Source: Adapted from Refs. 3–6, 42, 48, 49, 103.

infarction due to coronary artery embolism may contribute to heart failure.

Physical Examination

Patients with endocarditis may appear acutely or chronically ill. Intermittent chills, rigors, and sweating often provide evidence of a systemic infection. Asthenia and recent weight loss are often notable. Anemia is common,[78] especially in SBE, so many patients are pale. The skin of some patients with long-standing SBE shows the sallow hue of uremia.[3]

VASCULAR PHENOMENA

Patients with endocarditis may exhibit a variety of striking physical findings arising from vascular abnormalities. Such phenomena are diagnostically useful, even though all can sometimes occur in conditions other than endocarditis.

Petechiae

In both SBE and ABE, petechiae are common; they are rare in NBTE. In a few cases, the petechiae have a pale central spot. Most are due to microembolization to small vessels in the skin or mucous membranes. Capillary fragility, evidenced by positive tourniquet test results, accounts for the petechiae in some cases, while patients with ABE caused by a virulent bacterial pathogen may develop petechiae due to disseminated intravascular coagulation.

Splinter Hemorrhages

Linear subungual hemorrhages, resembling tiny splinters of wood under the nails but not reaching the nail margin, are found in about 20 percent of patients with SBE. They are probably caused by microembolization to linear capillaries under the nail. Because splinter hemorrhages are found in some 5 to 8 percent of patients admitted to hospital who do not have endocarditis, they are of limited diagnostic value.[211]

Osler's Nodes

These are painful, tender, erythematous nodules in the skin of the extremities, usually in the pulp of the fingers[212] (Figs. 10-17; 10-18, Plate 10). Occasionally, the center of these pea-sized, red lesions is pale, but necrosis does not occur. Osler's nodes occur in 10 to 20 percent of patients with SBE and in fewer than 10 percent of patients with ABE.[212] They are probably caused by inflammation around the site of lodgment of small, infected emboli in distal arterioles, because the etiologic organism can be recovered from some of the lesions.[213] Inflammation due to focal immunologic reactions probably contributes to formation of Osler's nodes, especially in subacute cases.[198]

Janeway Lesions

Janeway lesions are small (less than 5 mm), flat, nontender red spots, irregular in outline, found on the palms and soles of a few patients with SBE and ABE. Unlike petechiae, they are not hemorrhagic, and they blanch on pressure.[3,43]

Ocular Lesions

Conjunctival petechiae show up as small, bright-red hemorrhages that are easily seen if the upper and lower eyelids are everted. These petechiae are not specific for endocarditis, being found sometimes after cardiac surgery and occasionally in septicemia (Plate 65). Nevertheless, the discovery of conjunctival hemorrhages in a patient with unexplained fever and heart murmur makes the diagnosis of endocarditis highly likely.

Retinal hemorrhages are found in 10 to 25 percent of cases of both SBE and ABE. They are quite variable in appearance. Some simply represent petechiae in the retina; their round or flame-shaped outline is determined by the layer of the retina in which they develop. Those with a white or yellow center surrounded by a bright-red, irregular halo are known as *Roth's spots*, which probably represent cytoid bodies and associated hemorrhage caused by microinfarction of retinal vessels.

Loss of vision during the course of endocarditis can occur from embolization to the brain or to the retinal artery, from optic neuritis, or from ophthalmitis. Endophthalmitis may occur in patients with *Candida* endocarditis and/or candidemia. The typical retinal lesions are rounded, white, cotton-like exudates with extension into the vitreous and overlying vitreous haze.[214] Panophthalmitis occurs in some patients with ABE due to hematogenous spread of virulent pathogens. This phenomenon occurs most often in IDUs infected with *Staph. aureus*, *Pseudomonas*, or fungi.

CLUBBING OF THE FINGERS

Previously common in SBE, finger clubbing is now found in less than 5 percent of cases (Fig. 10-16, Plate 9), presumably because endocarditis is now diagnosed and treated earlier. The pathogenesis of this reaction, which usually resolves after eradication of the infecting organism, is not understood.

SIGNS OF EMBOLIZATION

Decreased or absent arterial pulses in an extremity may signal occlusion of a large artery by a fragment of vegetation. Focal neurologic signs may develop transiently or progress to a completed stroke due to embolization of a cerebral artery (see "Complications," below). Infarctions of the spleen, kidney, or bowel can present with pain and tenderness on palpation of the abdomen, mimicking an acute abdominal event such as bowel obstruction or peritonitis. Myocardial infarction due to obstruction of a coronary artery can cause heart failure or death and is sometimes an unexpected finding at autopsy in patients who die with active disease. These complications are illustrated in Figs. 82-8 to 82-13 (Plates 66–71).

SPLENOMEGALY

Development of splenomegaly is common, occurring in about one-quarter of patients with ABE and one-half of those with SBE. The spleen is usually soft and only slightly tender except

FIGURE 82-7
See color Plate 65.

FIGURE 82-8
See color Plate 66.

FIGURE 82-9
See color Plate 67.

FIGURE 82-10
See color Plate 68.

FIGURE 82-11
See color Plate 69.

FIGURE 82-12
See color Plate 70.

FIGURE 82-13
See color Plate 71.

in the case of recent embolic infarction, when palpation may be very painful. Radionuclide scanning may reveal infarction or, occasionally, a splenic abscess.

CARDIAC EXAMINATION

The pulse is often rapid as a result of fever or congestive failure. Irregularities of conduction may indicate the presence of an abscess near the conducting system. Underlying or newly developed aortic regurgitation associated with infective endocarditis may result in a collapsing pulse (Chaps. 10 and 63). Peripheral arteries should be palpated for evidence of occlusion by emboli or for the pulsatile swelling of a mycotic aneurysm.

One or more murmurs are present in virtually all patients at some stage of the disease. Even though some of the classic findings of infective endocarditis are less often seen today than formerly, the triad of fever, anemia, and murmur should still suggest this disease provided one remembers that these manifestations are nonspecific. They may be absent initially. *Up to 15 percent of patients do not have a murmur when first seen.* These patients are more likely to be individuals with right-sided or acute endocarditis than patients with left-sided SBE.

Murmurs present during the course of endocarditis may be due to preexisting cardiac disease, to the infection itself, or to both. Active endocarditis often causes structural damage to the valve, including deformities, tears, perforations, and rupture of chordae tendineae. Since these changes often lead to valvular insufficiency, the murmurs most often heard in association with endocarditis are those of mitral, aortic, or tricuspid regurgitation. Infective endocarditis occurs in association with pure mitral stenosis much less often than with mitral regurgitation (with or without associated stenosis) (see Chap. 64). Development of a new aortic regurgitation murmur during a febrile illness strongly suggests the diagnosis of endocarditis, because this finding is seldom associated nonspecifically with increased blood flow due to fever and anemia.

New cardiac murmurs are an important diagnostic finding in SBE and ABE. "Changing murmurs" are seldom a useful finding in SBE, however, despite a persistent misconception to the contrary. This error is partly based upon misreading of

Osler's words in which he pointed out that murmurs may not change much during SBE: "a very slight change in the character of the heart murmur in spite of the . . . most extensive vegetations and alterations in the valve."[16] Changing murmurs are more common in patients with ABE.

COMPLICATIONS

Heart Failure

Heart failure is the most important complication of infective endocarditis,[49,215–217] because it exerts a critical influence on prognosis. In 1951, Cates and Christie[215] reported a death rate of 37 percent among 314 patients with SBE who had no heart failure and 85 percent among 94 who had moderate or severe failure. In the past, congestive failure occurred in up to 55 percent of cases, being more common in patients with aortic valve disease (75 percent) than in those with mitral valve (50 percent) or tricuspid valve disease (19 percent).[216] Today, the incidence of heart failure is lower because of earlier and more effective treatment and valve replacement surgery.

Sudden onset or worsening of left ventricular failure is common during the course of ABE because of perforation or destruction of a valve leaflet or rupture of chordae tendineae, but it also occurs in some patients with SBE for the same reasons. Intractable left ventricular failure can result from rupture of a sinus of Valsalva due to infection. The right sinus of Valsalva may rupture into the right atrium or right ventricle and the left sinus into the pulmonary artery.[182] This rare condition should be suspected if the severity of heart failure seems out of proportion to the degree of valve dysfunction. Occasionally, bulky vegetations occlude the valve orifice, causing functional stenosis; this phenomenon is most likely to occur during fungal infection of prosthetic valves.[218,219]

Embolization

This important complication is recognized in 12 to 40 percent of patients during the course of SBE and in 40 to 60 percent of those with ABE, but autopsy findings indicate that many other arterial emboli go undetected. Pelletier and Petersdorf[103] reported a 50 percent incidence of major arterial emboli in 125 cases, affecting brain (25 cases), lung (17 cases), coronary artery (8 cases), spleen (8 cases), extremities (8 cases), gut (4 cases), and eye (3 cases).

Conduction Abnormalities

A conduction abnormality is detected during the course of IE in 4 to 16 percent of patients, especially in association with aortic valve infection.[184,210,220] Types of abnormalities observed include first-degree atrioventricular (AV) block (45 percent), third-degree AV block (20 percent), second-degree AV block (15 percent), and isolated bundle branch blocks (15 percent).[184] *The development of a new, unstable, or changing conduction abnormality is important because it often indicates that a focus of myocardial inflammation has extended near to or into the AV node or the bundle of His. This can be associated with or lead to formation of a valve-ring abscess, which, in turn, is associated with a worse prognosis[217] and constitutes a strong indication for surgical intervention.*

Neurologic Manifestations

Involvement of the nervous system during the course of endocarditis is both common and clinically important.[221–224] Significant neurologic abnormalities occur in 29 to 50 percent of patients with endocarditis.[221,224,225] The initial or presenting complaint involves the nervous system in 10 to 15 percent of patients with endocarditis. A wide range of syndromes occurs, including toxic confusional states, psychiatric symptoms, minor or major strokes (Fig. 82-13, Plate 71), meningoencephalitis, and cranial or peripheral nerve lesions.[224] In some recent series, neurologic complications approach or even surpass heart failure as the leading determinant of mortality[224] (see also Chap. 99).

Of 55 patients with cerebrovascular complications of endocarditis, four-fifths suffered infarction and one-fifth hemorrhage.[225] Infarction is usually due to embolism, most often to the middle cerebral arteries; hemorrhage can be a complication of either emboli or mycotic aneurysms.[103,221–223,226,227]

A meningeal reaction occurs in 7 to 15 percent of patients, especially those with staphylococcal ABE.[42,221,223–225] This reaction may be mistakenly diagnosed as acute bacterial meningitis because the cerebrospinal fluid (CSF) contains polymorphonuclear leukocytes and may have a raised protein concentration. In a minority of such cases (up to 20 percent of those with acute staphylococcal infection) CSF cultures yield the bacteria causing endocarditis. The glucose level, however, is usually normal; the results of CSF culture are usually negative; and the abnormalities usually resolve without complications during treatment of the endocarditis. Thus, these CSF abnormalities more often represent an inflammatory reaction associated with endocarditis than true bacterial meningitis. Bacterial meningitis does occur in some patients with pneumococcal endocarditis[130] and occasionally in staphylococcal ABE.

Cerebritis may develop in brain tissue surrounding small infected emboli lodged in cerebral vessels in both SBE and ABE, often with associated meningoencephalitis.[224] Computed tomography and magnetic resonance imaging often reveal multiple areas of cerebritis, especially in acute staphylococcal endocarditis, even in patients with no central nervous system (CNS) symptoms (Fig. 82-14). In patients with ABE, this inflammatory reaction in the brain may progress to form a brain abscess, but more often cerebritis will resolve uneventfully during antibiotic treatment of the underlying disease. Brain abscesses are uncommon in patients with SBE.[224]

Mycotic Aneurysm

This complication develops in only 3 to 15 percent of patients with infective endocarditis, but the local consequences of expansion and rupture can be very serious, especially in the brain (Fig. 82-13, Plate 71). In order of frequency, the sites most often involved are the proximal aorta, including the sinuses of Valsalva (25 percent of cases), arteries to the viscera (24 percent), arteries to the extremities (22 percent), and arteries to the brain (15 percent).[226–228] Unfortunately, intracerebral aneurysms are often multiple.[227,228]

Mycotic aneurysms develop when the wall of an artery is damaged by the inflammatory response to microbes.[183,194,229,230] These microbes reach the arterial wall via microemboli to the vasa vasorum or by impaction of a larger infected embolus in the lumen. The arterial wall is apparently a less favorable culture medium for bacteria than a valvular vegetation, because the organisms responsible for weakening the vessel often die out spontaneously, even if untreated. The my-

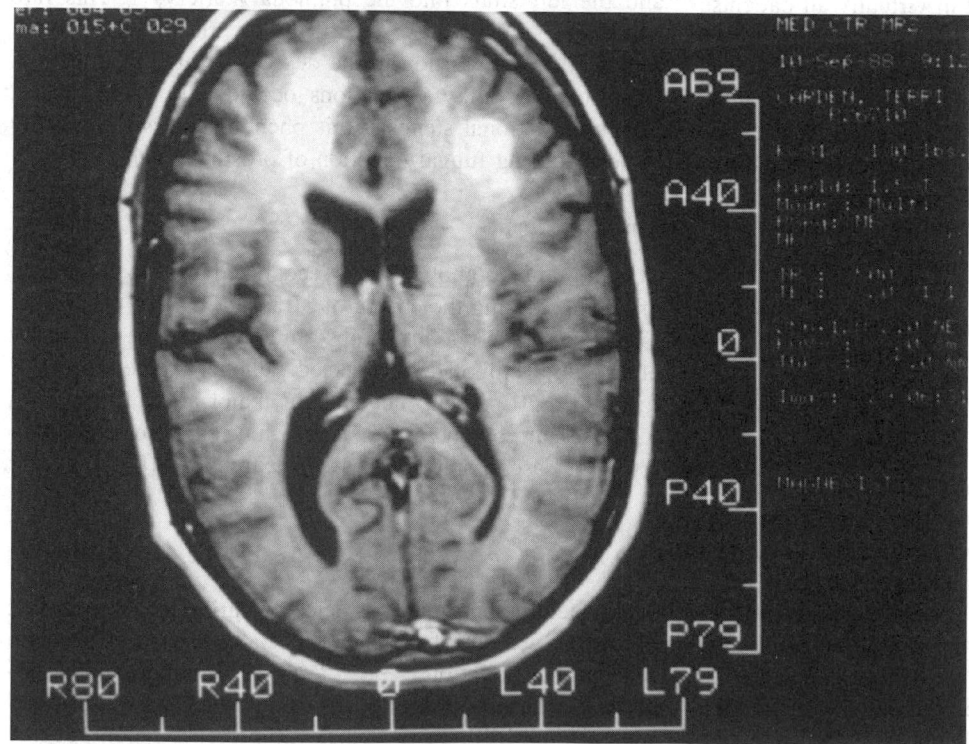

FIGURE 82-14

Magnetic resonance image of the brain in a patient with acute left-sided *Staph. aureus* endocarditis, showing multiple areas of focal cerebritis. This patient had no focal central nervous system signs and recovered fully with antimicrobial therapy. (MRI by courtesy of the Department of Radiology, Duke University, Durham, NC.)

cotic aneurysm may continue to enlarge even when living organisms are no longer present, due to the physical effects of arterial blood pressure (Fig. 82-9, Plate 67).[226–228,231]

DIFFERENTIAL DIAGNOSIS

Because the clinical manifestations of endocarditis are numerous and often nonspecific, the differential diagnosis of this disease is very wide.[3,42,103,232] Of the many conditions that may be considered, only a few leading examples are listed here.

ABE shares many clinical features with nonendocarditic septicemias due to invasive bacterial pathogens such as *Staph. aureus*, *Neisseria*, pneumococci, and gram-negative bacilli. The differential diagnosis for a case of ABE might include pneumonia, pleurisy, meningitis, brain abscess, stroke, malaria, acute pericarditis, vasculitis, and disseminated intravascular coagulation.

SBE must be considered during the workup of every patient with fever of unknown origin.[162,232,233] Its manifestations can mimic those of rheumatic fever, osteomyelitis, tuberculosis, meningitis, intra-abdominal infections, salmonellosis, brucellosis, glomerulonephritis, myocardial infarction, stroke, endocardial thrombi, atrial myxoma, connective tissue diseases, vasculitis, occult malignancies (especially lymphomas), chronic cardiac failure, pericarditis, and even psychoneurosis.

Diagnostic Criteria

Infective endocarditis can be surprisingly difficult to diagnose with certainty.[162,234] In the course of clinical practice, the diagnosis is suspected much more often than it is confirmed. This is because the presenting symptoms and signs can be highly variable and consistent with many other possible diagnoses. Furthermore, the primary lesion (an endocardial vegetation) is inaccessible to direct inspection except at surgery or autopsy. These problems can be minimized by application of carefully defined diagnostic criteria. Major and minor criteria have been defined by the Duke Endocarditis Service[162]; they are analogous to the modified Jones criteria[235] (Chap. 62) for diagnosis of acute rheumatic fever. These criteria offer improved sensitivity and specificity for diagnosis of endocarditis[79,162,163] (Tables 82-7 and 82-8).

Because the Duke criteria emphasize specificity[163,236] above sensitivity, they should not be used to guide urgent management decisions early in the course of a suspected case. To illustrate: a diagnosis of endocarditis made solely on the basis of presence of fever and a heart murmur would be very sensitive but very nonspecific. These findings might make a clinician suspect the diagnosis or even begin treatment for endocarditis, but they would not be adequate to make a final diagnosis, to decide on valve replacement, or to accept the diagnosis for the purpose of epidemiologic studies or clinical trials.

TABLE 82-7

CRITERIA FOR DIAGNOSIS OF INFECTIVE ENDOCARDITIS

Definite Infective Endocarditis

PATHOLOGIC CRITERIA
Microorganisms: demonstrated by culture or histology in a vegetation, or in a vegetation that has embolized, or in an intracardiac abscess, *or*   Pathologic lesions: vegetation or intracardiac abscess present, confirmed by histology showing active endocarditis
CLINICAL CRITERIA, USING SPECIFIC DEFINITIONS LISTED IN TABLE 82-8
Two major criteria, *or*   One major and three minor criteria, *or*   Five minor criteria

Possible Infective Endocarditis

Findings consistent with infective endocarditis that fall short of "definite," but not "rejected"

Rejected

Firm alternate diagnosis for manifestations of endocarditis, *or*   Resolution of manifestations of endocarditis, with antibiotic therapy for 4 days or less, *or*   No pathologic evidence of infective endocarditis at surgery or autopsy after antibiotic therapy for 4 days or less

Source: From Durack et al.,[162] with permission.

LABORATORY INVESTIGATIONS

Routine Laboratory Tests

Anemia usually develops during the course of SBE,[78,237] but it occurs less often in ABE. It is most often mild or moderate in degree and of the hypoproliferative type, with a normochromic, normocytic smear. Anemia may be due to hemolysis in patients with ABE. Chronic low-grade hemolysis associated with a prosthetic valve may confuse interpretation of the blood picture in a patient with PVE.

Leukocytosis is not a reliable manifestation of SBE.[78] A low-grade, variable elevation of the polymorphonuclear leukocyte count is characteristic, but in some cases the leukocyte count is normal. A high granulocyte count with an increase in band forms is commonly found in patients with ABE. These neutrophils may show toxic granulations. In a few cases of ABE, staphylococci can be identified inside neutrophils on examination of a gram-stained smear of the buffy coat of the peripheral blood,[238] and abnormal histiocytes may be found

DEFINITIONS OF TERMINOLOGY USED IN THE DIAGNOSTIC CRITERIA FOR ENDOCARDITIS

Major Criteria

POSITIVE BLOOD CULTURE FOR INFECTIVE ENDOCARDITIS

Typical microorganism for infective endocarditis from two separate blood cultures: viridans streptococci,[a] Strep. bovis, HACEK group, or community-acquired Staph. aureus or enterococci, in the absence of a primary focus, or
Persistently positive blood culture, defined as recovery of a microorganism consistent with infective endocarditis from:
1. Blood cultures drawn more than 12 h apart or
2. All of three or a majority of four or more separate blood cultures, with first and last drawn at least 1 h apart

EVIDENCE OF ENDOCARDIAL INVOLVEMENT

Positive echocardiogram for infective endocarditis
1. Oscillating intracardiac mass, on valve or supporting structures, or in the path of regurgitant jet or on implanted material, in the absence of an alternative anatomic explanation, or
2. Abscess, or
3. New partial dehiscence of prosthetic valve, or
New valvular regurgitation (increase or change in preexisting murmur not sufficient)

Minor Criteria

- Predisposition: predisposing heart condition or intravenous drug use
- Fever: ≥38.0°C (100.4°F)
- Vascular phenomena: major arterial emboli, septic pulmonary infarcts, mycotic aneurysm, intracranial hemorrhage, conjunctival hemorrhages, Janeway lesions
- Immunologic phenomena: glomerulonephritis, Osler's nodes, Roth's spots, rheumatoid factor
- Microbiologic evidence: positive blood culture but not meeting major criterion as previously defined[b] or serologic evidence of active infection with organism consistent with infective endocarditis[c]
- Echocardiogram: consistent with infective endocarditis but not meeting major criterion as previously defined

[a] Including nutritional variant strains.

[b] Excluding single positive cultures for coagulase-negative staphylococci or organisms that do not cause endocarditis.

[c] Positive serologies for Coxiella or Bartonella may be considered major criteria.[240]

HACEK = Haemophilus spp., Actinobacillus actinomycetemcomitans, Cardiobacterium hominis, Eikenella spp., and Kingella kingae
Source: Adapted from Durack et al.,[162] with permission.

in smears of peripheral blood in one-third of patients with SBE,[239] but these tests are not in routine use.

The erythrocyte sedimentation rate (ESR) is elevated in about 90 percent of cases of IE. The median ESR on admission is about 65 mm/h, but the range is wide and 10 percent are in the normal range. The median ESR rises slightly during treatment and does not fall to normal until 3 to 6 months after admission, so it is not useful as evidence of successful antibiotic therapy. The C-reactive protein is usually elevated and falls to normal more quickly than the ESR during successful treatment.

Urinalysis shows microscopic hematuria and/or slight proteinuria in about 50 percent of cases, even in the absence of specific renal complications.[3,237] Red blood cell casts and heavy proteinuria are found in those patients who develop immune-complex glomerulonephritis, often in association with decreased total serum complement.[199] Gross hematuria suggests that renal infarction has occurred.

Serologic Tests

Nonspecific serologic abnormalities are common during the course of IE. A positive rheumatoid factor is found in 35 to 50 percent of cases of SBE,[186–188] constituting a minor criterion supporting the diagnosis.[162] Rheumatoid factor is rarely positive in patients with ABE. A polyclonal increase in gamma-globulins is characteristic of active endocarditis. Occasional false-positive serologic test results for syphilis occur.[185]

Specific serologic tests are important for diagnosis of IE caused by Coxiella (Q fever) and Bartonella, both species which are difficult or slow to grow from culture. In these special cases, positive serology (1:800 anti-phase 1 IgG antibody titer for Q fever or positive microimmunofluorescence for Bartonella) or a single positive blood culture may be added as major criteria for diagnosis of IE.[152,240]

Blood Cultures

Isolation of a typical organism or detection of persistent bacteremia constitutes one of the two major criteria for diagnosis of endocarditis. Blood cultures should be drawn from all patients with undiagnosed fever and a heart murmur unless their illness is clearly due to another disease or the fever resolves within a few days without treatment. Cultures should also be taken from patients with symptoms or signs consistent with endocarditis if no other diagnosis has been made.

Bacteremia in SBE is usually continuous.[21] The number of organisms in venous blood varies widely but is usually between 1 and 200/mL in subacute cases. Because most blood cultures in untreated patients will be positive, it is seldom necessary to draw more than three separate blood specimens to isolate the organism.[241] In one study, the etiologic organism was recovered from cultures taken on the first day of admission to hospital in 93 percent of patients with culture-positive endocarditis.[242] In other studies, however, the rate of persistently positive blood cultures was lower, in the range of 62 to 68 percent.[103,162] Additional specimens obtained over a longer period may be needed to isolate the etiologic organism from patients who have received recent antibiotic therapy.

A practical approach for investigation of suspected SBE is to draw three separate samples of venous blood, each of 16 to 20 mL, on the first day, with at least 1 h between the first and last venipuncture. Half of each sample should be inoculated into aerobic broth culture medium, and the other half into another broth (usually anaerobic) medium. These media should be capable of supporting growth of fastidious, nutritionally variant bacteria[117,243] and ideally should contain a resin to remove antibiotics. As soon as a culture turns positive, Gram's stain and subculture should be performed. If all three samples (six bottles) are negative by the second or third day but the diagnosis of endocarditis still seems likely, two more samples of venous blood should be drawn for culture. If the patient had received previous antibiotic therapy, several further venous samples may be taken over the following weeks to identify a possible late recrudescence of bacteremia after partial treatment. For ABE, three venous blood samples are drawn for culture and empiric antibiotic therapy is begun at once, because in patients with acute endocarditis, treatment should not be delayed until culture results are available.

Because *Staph. epidermidis*[208] and diphtheroids[244] can cause endocarditis, special care must be taken during venipuncture to avoid contamination of the specimen with these common skin organisms, which could result in diagnostic confusion. If the diagnosis of endocarditis remains likely, cultures should be incubated for 3 weeks and Gram's stains made at 5 days, 2 weeks, and 3 weeks even if no growth is apparent on inspection. Quantitative blood cultures, although not necessary in most cases, can help to distinguish contaminants from true positive cultures.

Electrocardiography

Electrocardiographic studies should be performed initially and repeated at intervals according to progress during treatment. A disturbance of conduction that develops during the course of endocarditis suggests extension of infection into the myocardium (see above). Such extension may be due to focal myocarditis or to an abscess located close to the conduction system.[97] Thus, development of a prolonged PR interval, if due to an abscess, can have major implications: a probable need for valve replacement and a worse prognosis.[80] Electrocardiograms can reveal evidence of silent myocardial infarction due to embolization of a vegetation to a coronary artery.

Echocardiography

Echocardiographic studies are vitally important in the diagnosis of infective endocarditis.[245–249] Positive echocardiographic findings, properly defined, constitute one of the two major criteria for the clinical diagnosis of endocarditis, equaling blood cultures in practical importance.[162] Transthoracic two-dimensional echocardiography (TTE) combined with color-flow Doppler imaging (see Chap. 14) provides a wealth of information for both the diagnosis and the management of endocarditis, including the detection of vegetations, valvular perforations and other abnormalities, abscesses, pericarditis as well as the assessment of ventricular function (Fig. 82-15A–D).[246–248] Sensitivity for detection of vegetations, originally in the range of 33 to 63 percent, today is 60 to 75

percent. Sensitivity can be improved to better than 95 percent by use of transesophageal echocardiography (TEE) (see Chap. 14) in selected cases.[220,246] Transesophageal studies also detect abscesses and valve perforation with much greater sensitivity.[248] TEE is markedly better than TTE for evaluation of prosthetic valve endocarditis, especially involving mitral valves.[250]

Echocardiography has some limitations.[245] It is not cost-effective as a means of excluding IE in patients with a low pretest probability of having the disease.[251] With higher prior probability, a negative study result has useful negative predictive value, especially if transesophageal studies have been performed, but it cannot totally exclude the diagnosis of endocarditis.[137,162,251] Sensitivity for detection of vegetations is somewhat lower on the right side (about 70 percent) than on the left (better than 95 percent).[220,245] The presence of a prosthetic valve sometimes interferes with detection of vegetations, but even in these patients echocardiographic findings are usually informative. Occasionally, the specificity of echocardiography is compromised by false-positive readings for "vegetations" that do not exist. Such readings are particularly common in patients with myxomatous degeneration of valve leaflets.

Sequential echocardiograms performed during treatment can guide decisions on the need and timing for surgery by providing objective assessments of cardiac function. For example, premature mitral valve closure due to elevated end-diastolic pressure is a useful echocardiographic sign indicating severe aortic regurgitation, usually requiring urgent valve replacement (see Chap. 63).[220] Echocardiograms may detect development of an abscess, perforation of a valve, or rupture of an infected sinus of Valsalva,[182] all strong indications for surgical intervention. During successful antimicrobial treatment, vegetations may disappear, decrease in size, or even persist unchanged; therefore, serial echocardiograms should not be used as a "test of cure."[245] Significant enlargement of a vegetation during treatment, however, indicates possible treatment failure and constitutes a relative indication for surgical intervention.

Other Imaging Studies

The most important contribution of the chest x-ray in assessment of endocarditis is to provide evidence of early congestive heart failure, because this complication carries such important implications for both prognosis and management (see "Complications," above).

Various other x-ray findings can be helpful in assessment of a patient with endocarditis. The presence of multiple small, patchy infiltrates in the lungs of an IDU with fever strongly suggests the diagnosis of septic emboli arising from right-sided infective endocarditis.[62–64] Valvular calcification may identify a previously abnormal valve, thus aiding the localization of presumed intravascular infection. Widening of the aorta may be caused by a mycotic aneurysm. Fluoroscopy can demonstrate abnormal motion of a prosthetic valve, indicating

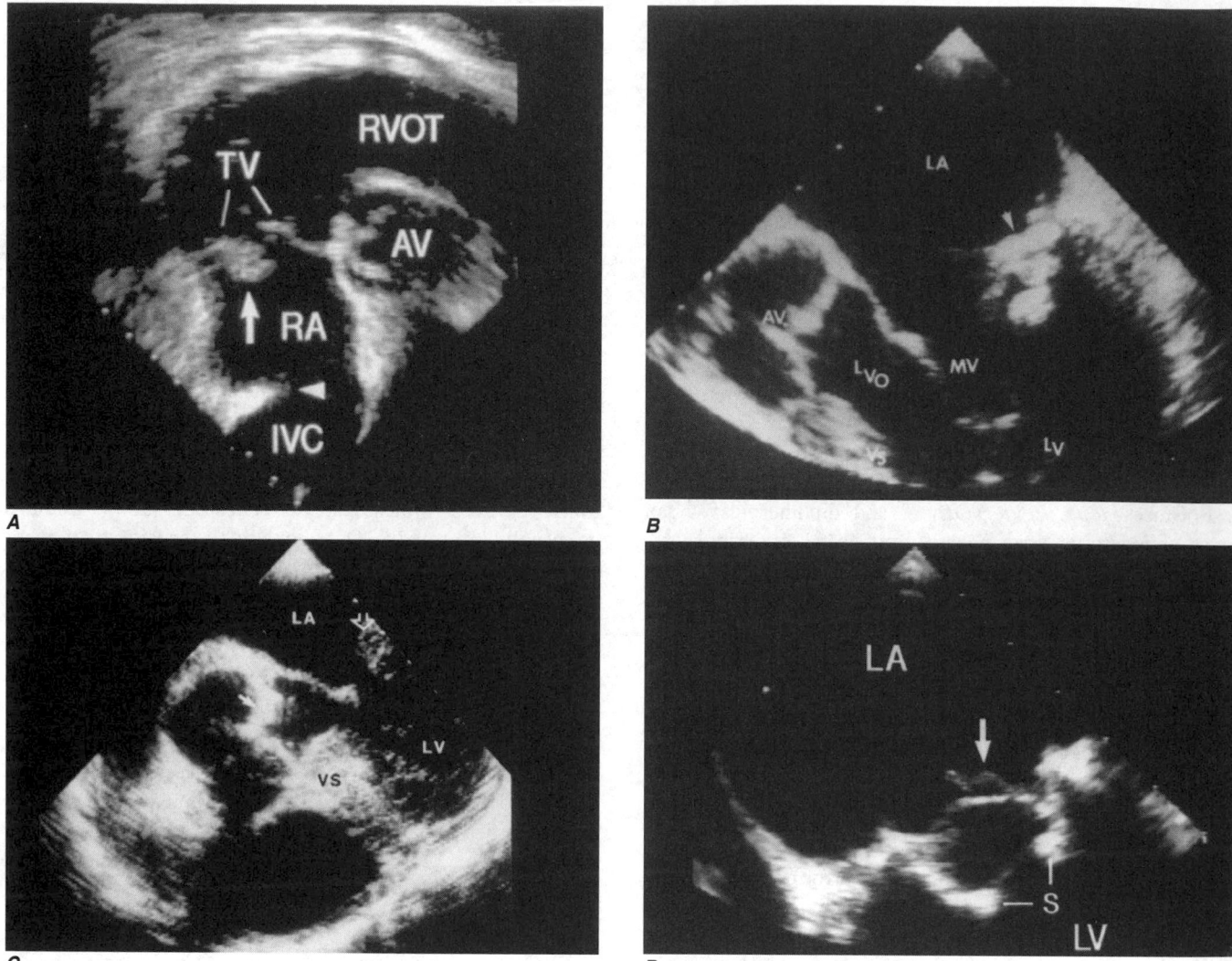

FIGURE 82-15

A–D. Echocardiograms from four patients with infective endocarditis showing vegetations located at different sites. *A.* Transesophageal echocardiogram (TEE) showing a large vegetation *(arrow)* on the tricuspid valve (TV). IVC = inferior vena cava; RA = right atrium; AV = aortic valve; RVOT = right ventricular outflow tract. *B.* Large vegetation *(arrowhead)* involving both the atrial and ventricular surfaces of the posterior mitral valve leaflet. LA = left atrium; MV = anterior leaflet of the mitral valve; LVO = left ventricular outflow tract; AV = aortic valve. *C.* TEE showing vegetations on both the mitral *(open arrow)* and aortic valve *(arrow)* in a patient with acute *Staph. aureus* endocarditis. LA = left atrium; LV = left ventricle; VS = ventricular septum. *D.* TEE showing a vegetation on the cusp of a bioprosthetic valve *(arrow).* LA = left atrium; LV = left ventricle; S = artificial valve struts. (Plates kindly provided by Dr. B. Khanderia and Dr. J. Steckelberg, Mayo Clinic.)

presence of a vegetation or partial dehiscence of the valve from the aortic root. This information often helps to decide whether or not valve replacement is needed during management of PVE.

Computed tomography (CT) (Chap. 18) and magnetic resonance imaging (MRI) (Chap. 19)[224] can be helpful in defining the cause of focal neurologic lesions in patients with endocarditis, especially infarction, hemorrhage from a mycotic aneurysm, and brain abscess. The CT scan is very effective for diagnosis of intracranial complications[252] and infected aortic aneurysms.[111] MRI adds useful information in some cases (Fig. 82-14).[253] Angiographic studies may be necessary to demonstrate mycotic aneurysms in the brain or elsewhere.[227,228]

Cardiac Catheterization and Cineangiography

This investigation is usually not necessary for patients who respond well to antimicrobial therapy without developing cardiac failure. When surgical intervention is being considered, cardiac catheterization and cineangiography (Chap. 16) can extend and add to information provided by echocardiography. The condition of the coronary arteries should be assessed before valve replacement in adults over 40 years of age, because simultaneous coronary bypass may be indicated if the patient has coronary artery disease. Other relevant anatomic abnormalities such as valvular lesions, congenital defects, asymmetric septal hypertrophy, coarctation of the aorta, or mycotic aneurysm can be better defined. Occasionally, a previously unsuspected diagnosis, such as the presence of a sinus of Valsalva aneurysm, will be made. Physiologic measurements including cardiac output, pressures in the left and right sides of the heart, and the degree of aortic regurgitation may help to decide whether or not valve replacement is indicated and may influence the timing of the operation. Among 35 patients who underwent cardiac catheterization during active endocarditis, the clinical assessment was materially modified by catheterization in 23 patients, the diagnosis of the site of valve involvement was altered in 14, and 6 valve-ring abscesses were revealed.[254] Surgery was postponed or canceled in 6 patients in whom catheterization revealed only mild hemodynamic abnormalities. There were no serious complications, indicating that catheterization should not be avoided for fear of dislodging emboli when a proper indication exists. In summary, cardiac catheterization and cineangiography should be performed in most adults with infective endocarditis who are over 40 years of age and in selected younger patients when surgery is being considered.

Radionuclide Imaging

Liver-spleen imaging may reveal defects due to splenic infarction, thus confirming embolization. This knowledge is sometimes useful diagnostically when endocarditis is suspected but unproved. In animals, experimental vegetations have been located by scanning for radiolabeled platelets deposited from the bloodstream onto a growing endocardial lesion.[255] Gallium-67 scans have shown increased uptake in the heart in some patients with endocarditis and scintigraphic studies following injection of indium-111–labeled leukocytes have detected some intracardiac abscesses,[73] but no radionuclide imaging technique has sufficient sensitivity and specificity to justify routine use for detection of vegetations in infective endocarditis. In selected cases, leukocyte scintigraphy using indium-111–labeled leukocytes can detect mycotic aneurysms and extracardiac foci of infection.[256]

TREATMENT

General Principles

Optimal management aims to eradicate the infecting organism as soon as possible, to operate with correct timing if surgical intervention should be required, and to treat complications. Because infective endocarditis carries a significant risk of death even when well managed, it is important that treatment be continued long enough to ensure that relapse will not occur. On the other hand, patients with the more easily cured forms of endocarditis should not be subjected to unnecessarily long and expensive treatment in a hospital. This can happen when physicians treat on the basis of outdated rules, such as the one stating that "endocarditis should be treated for 6 weeks." In fact, many patients can be cured in 2[257–259] or 4 weeks,[260] while some require treatment for 6 weeks or longer.

Microbiologic Tests

To choose and regulate antibiotic therapy correctly, certain basic microbiologic information about the infecting organism is required. For group A streptococcal infection, nothing more than positive identification of the organism is necessary, because these organisms, with only rare exceptions, are still sensitive to low concentrations of penicillin. For other species of streptococci, staphylococci, and most other bacteria, the minimal inhibitory concentration (MIC) of relevant antibiotics should be determined. Some of these organisms are resistant to intermediate or high concentrations of penicillin.[261,262] Many strains are tolerant—that is, inhibited but not killed by antibiotic levels achievable in serum.[263,264] Because there is no definitive evidence that tolerance determines treatment outcome in humans, however, it is not necessary to measure minimal bactericidal concentrations (MBC) in most cases.

The serum bactericidal titer (SBT, or Schlichter test) has been used frequently to monitor the treatment of endocarditis.[32,265] In this test, the infecting organism is exposed in vitro to the patient's serum, which is drawn while the patient is receiving antibiotic treatment to determine the maximal dilution of serum that will inhibit and kill the organism. On the basis of empirical clinical experience, it was said that the SBT should be 1:8 or higher at intervals during each day of treatment. For streptococcal endocarditis, this can usually be achieved without difficulty; SBTs are often high, in the range 1:128 to 1:1024. The SBT is technically difficult to perform and to standardize, however, and after years of use, its clinical utility remains unproven.[265] Therefore, SBTs are now regarded as obsolete by most experts. Rarely, measurement of the SBT might be informative: in treating unusual organisms, in using unusual antibiotics, in using unusual regimens (such as oral treatment), or when treatment appears to be failing.

Dosage regimens that result in widely fluctuating antibiotic concentrations in serum are traditionally employed for treatment of endocarditis, and they are usually effective. Whether or not the maintenance of continuous serum antibiotic concentrations offers any therapeutic benefit over intermittent dosing regimens is not known; perhaps continuous infusion of antibiotic would be desirable for treatment of some gram-negative organisms, which regrow more rapidly than most gram-positive organisms when antibiotic levels fall below the minimal inhibitory concentration.

Choice of Antibiotics

Bactericidal antibiotics are generally chosen for treatment of endocarditis whenever possible.[32,260] This is not an absolute rule; some patients have been cured with bacteriostatic drugs such as sulfonamides, tetracycline, or chloramphenicol, but the results of treatment with these agents are unreliable.[27,266,267] Bactericidal action is presumably needed because host defense mechanisms are inadequate in the vegetation; relatively few phagocytes are present, and they are hampered by protective layers of fibrin around the colonies of bacteria (Figs. 82-2 and 82-6). To effect a cure, antibiotic therapy must eradicate organisms completely, without the help of phagocytes to eliminate the subpopulation of microbes that are relatively resistant to antibiotics because they are in the resting phase. In this important respect, infective endocarditis differs strikingly from bacterial pneumonia in normal hosts, where phagocytes are plentiful and bacteriostatic antibiotics are usually effective. Nevertheless, in treating unusual organisms, it may occasionally be necessary to use a bacteriostatic antibiotic in combination with other drugs to achieve the optimal antibacterial effect. When treatment with unusual combinations of antibiotics is needed, in vitro laboratory tests can be performed to find out whether synergism, indifference, or antagonism exists between them.

For the common forms of bacterial endocarditis caused by gram-positive organisms, specific therapeutic regimens can be recommended with confidence based on extensive published experience.[257,268] Regimens for the more common forms of endocarditis are listed in Table 82-9.

Currently, increasing rates of antibiotic resistance threaten the efficacy of traditional treatment regimens. Penicillin resistance is increasing among viridans streptococci, the majority of which had previously been fully sensitive.[269,270] In 1996, 13 percent of blood culture isolates showed high-level resistance (MIC 4.0 μg/mL or greater) and 42 percent showed intermediate resistance (MIC 0.25 to 2.0 μg/mL).[270] Use of combined antibiotic regimens such as beta-lactam plus aminoglycoside or even vancomycin plus aminoglycoside should be considered for treatment of resistant strains.[269] Synergistic combinations of a beta-lactam and an aminoglycoside have been used successfully to treat enterococci for many years, but recent increasing resistance among enterococci, especially vancomycin-resistant enterococci (VRE), presents new problems for therapy. The most resistant species is *Enterococcus faecium*, which may exhibit high-level resistance to vancomycin as well as intrinsic resistance to beta-lactam antibiotics and imipenem.[85] The optimal treatment for IE

TABLE 82-9

TREATMENT REGIMENS FOR INFECTIVE ENDOCARDITIS[a,b]

Organism	Treatment Regimen: Dose and Route	Duration in Weeks	Comments
Fully penicillin-sensitive streptococci: MIC ≤ 0.1 μg/mL	1. Penicillin G 4 million units every 6 h IV *or*	4	Suitable for hospitalized patients but less convenient for outpatient therapy
viridans (α-hemolytic) streptococci; *Strep. bovis; Strep. pneumoniae; Strep. pyogenes* group A, C, etc.; *Strep. agalactiae* group B	2. Ceftriaxone 2 g IV or 1 M once daily *or*	4	For patients allergic to penicillins but not cephalosporins or for outpatient therapy in selected patients
	3. Vancomycin 15 mg/kg IV every 12 h[a,b]	4	For patients allergic to penicillins and cephalosporins
Relatively penicillin-resistant streptococci: MIC > 0.1 < 1.0 μg/mL, some viridans (α-hemolytic) streptococci; some *Strep. pneumoniae;* etc.	1. Penicillin G 4 million units IV every 4 h *plus* gentamicin 1.0 mg/kg every 12 h IV or IM (for first 2 weeks only)[a] *or*	4(2)	For outpatient therapy in selected patients, ceftriaxone 2 g IV once daily may be substituted for penicillin if ceftriaxone MIC ≤ 4 μg/mL, *plus* gentamicin 2.0 mg/kg given once daily
	2. Vancomycin 15 mg/kg IV every 12 h[b]	4	For patients allergic to penicillins
Penicillin-resistant streptococci: MIC ≥ 1.0 μg/mL, *E. faecalis, E. faecium,* other enterococci; some other streptococci	1. Penicillin G 18–30 million units/day IV continuously or in divided doses *plus* gentamicin 1 mg/kg IV or IM every 8 h *or*	4–6	Susceptibility testing needed; do not use penicillin- or ampicillin-containing regimen if strain produces β-lactamase.
	2. Ampicillin 12 g/day IV continuously or in divided doses *plus* gentamicin 1.0 mg/kg IV every 8 h, *or*	4–6	4-week regimen recommended for most cases with symptoms for <3 months, otherwise 6 weeks
	3. Vancomycin 15 mg/kg IV every 12 h *plus* gentamicin 1.0 mg/kg IV every 8 h[a,b]	4–6	For patients allergic to penicillin; 4 weeks should be adequate for most cases; serum levels should be monitored

(continued)

TABLE 82-9

TREATMENT REGIMENS FOR INFECTIVE ENDOCARDITIS[a,b] (Continued)

Organism	Treatment Regimen: Dose and Route	Duration in Weeks	Comments
Staphylococci (in the absence of prosthetic material)	Methicillin-susceptible staphylococci:		
	1. Nafcillin 2 g IV every 4 h *or*	4–6	β-lactam–containing regimens preferred over vancomycin unless patient is definitely hypersensitive to penicillins and cephalosporins; for patients with severe disseminated staphylococcal infection, antimicrobial synergy may be advantageous during early stages of treatment; therefore, gentamicin 1.0 mg/kg IV every 8 h for first 3–5 days only may be added to any of these regimens
	2. Cefazolin 2 g IV every 8 h *or*	4–6	
	3. Vancomycin 15 mg/kg IV every 12 h[b]	4–6	
	Methicillin-resistant staphylococci: Vancomycin 15 mg/kg IV every 12 h[b]	4–6	
Staphylococci (associated with prosthetic valve or other prosthetic material)	Methicillin-susceptible staphylococci: Nafcillin 2 g IV every 4 h *plus* gentamicin 1.0 mg/kg IV every 8 h[a]	≥6	Cefazolin or vancomycin may be substituted for nafcillin if necessary due to drug hypersensitivity
	Methicillin-resistant staphylococci: Vancomycin 15 mg/kg IV every 12 h *plus* gentamicin 1.0 mg/kg IV or IM every 8 h *plus* rifampin 300 mg orally every 8 h[a,b]	≥6	
HACEK group organisms: *Haemophilus* species *Actinobacillus actinomycetemcomitans* *Cardiobacterium hominis* *Eikenella* species *Kingella kingae*	1. Ceftriaxone 2 g IV or IM once daily *or*	4	Other third-generation cephalosporins may be substituted, using appropriate dose adjustment
	2. Ampicillin 12 g/day IV continuously or in divided doses *plus* gentamicin 1.0 mg/kg every 12 h IV or IM[a]	4	Less convenient for outpatient therapy
Pseudomonas aeruginosa, other gram-negative bacilli	Extended-spectrum penicillin *or* third-generation cephalosporin *or* imipenem *plus* aminoglycoside	4–6	Combination therapy recommended; final choice of antibiotic regimen to be made after sensitivity results available
Neisseria species	1. Penicillin G 2 million units IV every 6 h *or* 2. Ceftriaxone 1 g IV or IM once daily	3–4 3–4	Organisms often highly sensitive to penicillin, but must be tested for β-lactamase production; 3 weeks should be adequate for most patients without complications

[a] All gentamicin- and vancomycin-containing regimens require monitoring for potential toxicity; monitoring of serum concentrations usually will be required.

[b] Vancomycin dose not to exceed 2.0 g/24 h.

Source: Adapted from Scheld and Sande[48] and from Wilson et al.[257]

caused by these problem strains is not known. A combination of high-dose ampicillin plus imipenem (possibly with addition of a fluoroquinolone) for 6 to 12 weeks, plus valve replacement surgery, may give the best chance for cure.[85,271]

Staph. epidermidis PVE is difficult to eradicate with antibiotics alone.[135] These staphylococci are frequently resistant to semisynthetic penicillins, cephalosporins, and other antibiotics. A regimen combining vancomycin, rifampin, and an aminoglycoside chosen according to sensitivity tests is most likely to succeed. The organism may develop resistance to rifampin during treatment.

Treatment of endocarditis due to less common organisms must be chosen on the basis of more limited published experience,[48,49,137,260] together with the results of tests performed upon the infecting organism in the microbiology laboratory. Treatment must often be individualized. In general, one of the beta-lactam antibiotics should be included in the regimen whenever possible. Combinations of two or more antibiotics are often employed. The list of potentially useful regimens for these rarer forms of infective endocarditis is too long to detail here.

Empiric Therapy

When the etiologic organism is not known, the choice of empiric therapy should depend on whether the patient has acute or subacute disease. ABE requires broad-spectrum therapy that covers *Staph. aureus* as well as many species of streptococci and gram-negative bacilli. SBE requires a regimen that treats most streptococci, including *E. faecalis*. To meet these requirements, the following suggestions are offered:

- For ABE: nafcillin 2.0 g IV q 4 h plus ampicillin 2.0 g IV q 4 h plus gentamicin 1.5 mg/kg IV q 8 h. If methicillin-resistant *Staph. aureus* is considered likely (for example, in a hospital-acquired case), vancomycin 1.0 g IV q 12 h should be substituted for nafcillin in this regimen until the antibiotic sensitivity is known.
- For SBE: ampicillin 2.0 g IV q 4 h plus gentamicin 1.5 mg/kg IV q 8 h.

Treatment should be adjusted as appropriate when the etiologic organism is identified and again when antibiotic sensitivity is known. In those few cases where empiric therapy is administered as a therapeutic trial to help confirm a diagnosis, treatment should be continued without interruption or unnecessary changes for at least 2 weeks; otherwise, no useful diagnostic information will be gained.

Duration of Therapy

Extensive experience with treatment of the common forms of endocarditis provides the basis for recommendations on duration of therapy (Table 82-9). In the case of *Staph. aureus* endocarditis, the response to appropriate treatment can be variable; some patients recover swiftly without complications,

especially young IDUs, who can often be cured within 2 weeks.[67,258] In contrast, some patients remain febrile for 10 to 14 days due to complications such as abscesses or other extracardiac manifestations of disseminated staphylococcal disease. Although 4 weeks of therapy is adequate in most cases, this should not be regarded as a rigid rule, because some patients with *Staph. aureus* endocarditis require treatment for 6 weeks or longer to achieve a cure. For *E. faecalis* endocarditis, 4 weeks' treatment is usually adequate. The relapse rate, however, seems to be higher in patients with mitral valve infection and in those who have had symptoms for more than 3 months,[121] where treatment should continue for 6 weeks.

Parenteral treatment can be completed in the patient's home or in the outpatient clinic in carefully selected cases. Availability of antibiotics with long half-lives, such as vancomycin or ceftriaxone, allows once-daily administration. Supervised parenteral treatment outside the hospital should be fully effective in achieving microbiologic cure and offers obvious benefits: convenience for the patient and cost containment.[272,273] The risks posed by a possible late complication, such as an embolic stroke or the sudden onset of heart failure, must be balanced against these benefits in selecting candidates for home parenteral therapy. Further trials are needed to refine the criteria and proper applications for outpatient therapy for endocarditis, but current experience indicates that more than half of endocarditis patients could receive at least some of their treatment as outpatients.

In general, the less extensive the published experience with a particular organism and treatment regimen, the more one should lean toward prolonging treatment in order to provide a reasonable margin of safety. Guidelines for the duration of treatment of the more common etiologic organisms are listed in Table 82-9. For less common organisms, the optimal duration of treatment required may vary according to individual circumstances.

Role of Surgery

Optimal management of infective endocarditis requires operative intervention during treatment for about one-third of patients.[80,274] Correct selection of this subgroup of patients and optimal timing of surgery are both critically important.[275]

Major indications for surgery are moderate or severe heart failure not responding to medical treatment, valvular obstruction, periannular or myocardial abscess, prosthetic valve dehiscence, persistent bacteremia despite appropriate antibiotics, and fungal infection. In most such cases, surgery should proceed promptly even if the infection is still active.

Relative indications for surgery include recurrent emboli; staphylococcal and gram-negative bacillary infections, especially involving prosthetic valves; persistent fever despite treatment; and vegetations that enlarge during treatment.[10,97,217,275]

Correct timing is the essence of good surgical management of endocarditis.[274] If surgery is undertaken too soon, the risks of operative mortality and the early and late morbidity associated with valve replacement may be inflicted on the patient unnecessarily, because some patients respond well to medical therapy, allowing surgery to be postponed indefinitely. If surgery can be delayed safely, antibiotic therapy should have eradicated or at least greatly reduced the number of organisms in the vegetation and in any sites of metastatic infection, thus increasing the chance of a successful outcome if surgery becomes necessary. If time is available for the effective treatment of complications such as septicemia, renal failure, pneumonia, myocarditis, and neurologic complications[252] before surgery, the operative risk should be lower. On the other hand, if surgery is delayed too long, patients may die suddenly, or their hemodynamic status may deteriorate so seriously that surgery is no longer feasible. This would be a tragic error, because many authors have emphasized that both survival and long-term outcome can be improved by earlier operation for selected patients, even if the endocardial infection is still active.[217,276,277]

Careful, frequent reexamination of the patient, together with repeated echocardiographic studies and sometimes cardiac catheterization to confirm the clinical findings, is indicated in every case where operation might be needed. The decision to operate should also be influenced by knowledge of the natural history of the type of endocarditis being treated. For example, penicillin-sensitive streptococcal endocarditis can almost always be cured bacteriologically (Table 82-10), and the immediate prognosis is good provided that cardiac failure or other major complications do not develop. Therefore, surgery should usually be considered only for those patients with cardiac failure that does not respond well to medical treatment. Similarly, because young IDUs with acute staphylococcal endocarditis have a good prognosis,[5,258] surgery should usually be reserved for those who develop intractable heart failure or definite signs of treatment failure. In contrast, the likelihood that fungal prosthetic valve endocarditis can be eradicated with antifungal drugs alone is negligible (Table 82-10). Such patients should usually undergo valve debridement or replacement early, without waiting to test the remote possibility that antifungal treatment could eradicate the infection.[278] The development of severe aortic regurgitation, especially when accompanied by heart failure, usually requires urgent surgery. Other examples of patients who are highly likely to require operation are those with early-onset PVE, valve-ring abscesses, or gram-negative bacillary infection of prosthetic valves.[10]

TABLE 82-10

ESTIMATE OF MICROBIOLOGIC CURE RATES FOR VARIOUS FORMS OF ENDOCARDITIS[a]

Native Valve Endocarditis	Antimicrobial Therapy Alone	Antimicrobial Therapy Plus Surgery
Viridans streptococci, group A streptococci, *Strep. bovis*, pneumococci, gonococci	98	98
Enterococcus faecalis	90	>90
Staph. aureus (in young intravenous drug users)	90	>90
Staph. aureus (in elderly patients with chronic underlying diseases)	50	70
Gram-negative aerobic bacilli[b]	40	65
Fungi	<5	50

Prosthetic Valve Endocarditis	Early PVE	Late PVE	Early PVE	Late PVE
Viridans streptococci, group A streptococci, *Strep. bovis*, pneumococci, gonococci	c	80	c	90
Enterococcus faecalis	c	60	c	75
Staph. aureus	25	40	50	60
Staph. epidermidis	20	40	60	70
Gram-negative aerobic bacilli[b]	<10	20	40	50
Fungi	<1	<1	30	40

[a] Morbidity and mortality are significantly greater than these figures for microbiologic cure indicate.

[b] Excluding HACEK species.

[c] Insufficient data to estimate rates.

Source: Adapted from Refs. 8, 10, 31, 32, 97, 103, 210, 257, 258, 277, 290.

Over the past decade, surgical approaches have evolved toward increasingly radical debridement of infected tissue and more extensive use of reconstructive materials.[217,278] For example, an aortic root homograft instead of a standard prosthetic valve is now often inserted after debridement of a valve-ring abscess.[279] The Ross operation, transposing the patient's own pulmonary valve into the aortic position as an autograft after extensive debridement of infected tissue (replacing the pulmonary valve with a homograft) has recently been advocated as treatment for patients with complicated aortic root infections.[280,281]

In addition to valve replacement, several other surgical procedures may be available for the treatment of endocarditis.[275] Debridement of vegetations ("vegetectomy"), often combined with valvuloplasty, can cure the infection while sparing the native valve in selected patients.[218,219,282] This can be especially beneficial for young patients, women who wish to bear children, and patients who cannot or will not take anticoagulant therapy reliably.

Early consultation with the surgical service should be sought for most patients with endocarditis, so that an appropriate operation can be performed without delay if necessary. The sudden onset of aortic or mitral regurgitation with consequent acute left ventricular failure can occur without warning, even in the most favorable forms of endocarditis.

Anticoagulant Therapy

Even though the infected vegetation is essentially a thrombotic lesion, there is no evidence that anticoagulation has any useful therapeutic effect on the course of the endocarditis itself. On the contrary, early experience showed that simultaneous treatment with penicillin and heparin carried an increased risk of fatal intracerebral hemorrhage.[283] For this reason, anticoagulation was considered to be strongly contraindicated in patients with endocarditis until further experience showed that warfarin could be given safely during the treatment of patients with prosthetic valve infections.[284,285] Currently available information suggests the following guidelines for patients with infective endocarditis:

- Avoid use of heparin except for urgent indications such as treatment of massive pulmonary embolism.
- Discontinue or avoid oral anticoagulants if possible, especially in patients with intracranial complications.
- Anticoagulate with warfarin if there is a clear-cut indication, such as a mechanical prosthetic heart valve, taking care to regulate the prothrombin time between International Normalized Ratio (INR) 2.5 and 3.5.
- Choose an antibiotic treatment regimen that does not require intramuscular injections if anticoagulation is instituted.

Thrombolytic agents theoretically could promote lysis or resolution of vegetations. Adjunctive treatment with recombinant tissue plasminogen activator decreased vegetation size and improved the results of short-term penicillin therapy in rabbits with fresh vegetations.[11] Similarly, aspirin therapy can reduce the size of experimental vegetations and improve rate of sterilization by antibiotics.[286] The potential value of antithrombotic agents, however, has not been demonstrated in humans; thrombolytic therapy might not work on the older vegetations typical of SBE in humans and could possibly cause serious hemorrhagic complications.

Management of Complications

HEART FAILURE

The development of moderate or severe cardiac failure due to structural valvular damage indicates the need for prompt surgical intervention in most patients with endocarditis, even if the intracardiac infection is still active.[274,276] In patients with milder heart failure, the decision should be individualized, always remembering that lives may be lost unnecessarily if cardiac function suddenly worsens, so that operation becomes either hazardous or unfeasible.

EMBOLI

The occurrence of one or more significant arterial emboli during the treatment of endocarditis is a relative indication for surgery. The predictable early and long-term mortality and morbidity rates of valve replacement must be weighed against the fact that the likelihood of further emboli is highly unpredictable. For this reason, embolization is a weaker indication for valve replacement than is cardiac failure.[275,276] In the author's opinion, operative intervention during antibiotic treatment should seldom be undertaken solely to prevent further emboli unless the patient has suffered more than one or two proved major emboli. Because the frequency of emboli falls rapidly after 1 to 2 weeks of antibiotic therapy,[287] the most logical time to operate for the purpose of preventing emboli would be early, within 1 week of diagnosis.

RENAL FAILURE

In the preantibiotic era, patients with SBE frequently developed chronic renal failure before they died.[3] Subsequently, both the incidence of renal failure and its importance as a cause of death have greatly diminished. The earlier diagnosis and antibiotic treatment have forestalled the development of immune-complex glomerulonephritis in many patients. In those few (about 5 percent) who still develop this complication of SBE, timely dialysis can maintain the patient until antibiotic treatment results in disappearance of the bacterial antigens that triggered immune-complex nephritis. Renal function usually normalizes smoothly once infection has been controlled, but recovery may take weeks or months. In a few cases, creatinine clearance worsens for a time despite effective antibacterial treatment, perhaps reflecting persistence of bacterial antigen in vegetations after bacteriologic cure. Some patients with septicemia, shock, or disseminated intravascular coagulation associated with ABE develop acute renal failure and require dialysis as part of their intensive care.

MYCOTIC ANEURYSM

This complication is diagnosed in less than 5 percent of patients with infective endocarditis, but the local consequences of aneurysm expansion and rupture can be very serious, especially in the brain (see Chap. 99).[226,228,288] Small aneurysms will often thrombose or resolve spontaneously during or after antibiotic therapy. Once aneurysms exceed 0.5 to 2 cm in diameter, they are likely to enlarge and eventually rupture despite eradication of the etiologic bacteria by antibiotic therapy.[231] Surgery is indicated for accessible aneurysms before this complication occurs.

Intracranial mycotic aneurysms are especially difficult to manage. They may present with headaches, subarachnoid hemorrhage, or stroke, but many are asymptomatic. Even small aneurysms may bleed at any time; they may be multiple and/or located in inaccessible sites. This presents a therapeutic dilemma: whether to treat conservatively with antibiotics and hope for resolution (risking serious or fatal hemorrhage) or to operate (risking neurologic damage and permanent sequelae). Symptoms or signs consistent with an intracranial aneurysm indicate the need for prompt imaging, using CT and/or MRI. Cerebral angiography may be needed if the findings are inconclusive. In general, large (over 0.5 cm in diameter) or expanding aneurysms or aneurysms that have already leaked or begun to bleed should be clipped if a surgical approach is feasible. An individualized decision must be made on whether or not to operate for smaller aneurysms that have not leaked or ruptured.

PROGNOSIS

Infective endocarditis is one of the very few infectious diseases that are virtually always fatal if untreated. Spontaneous recovery was reported occasionally in the preantibiotic era,[3] but most of these patients probably had illnesses other than infective endocarditis. The interval between the onset of symptoms and death in patients with untreated subacute disease varied widely, with a median time to death of about 6 months.[3] Almost all patients with acute infective endocarditis died within less than 4 weeks.

Heart failure is the leading adverse prognostic factor.[215] Other adverse factors include central nervous system complications, renal failure, culture-negative disease, gram-negative bacillary or fungal infection, prosthetic valve infection, and development of abscesses in the valve ring or myocardium. Survival six months after PVE in a recent series was only 54 percent.[289] Six-month survival after early-onset PVE (37 percent) was significantly worse than for late-onset PVE (65 percent). Because modern treatment methods including valve replacement are effective for treatment of heart failure, central nervous system complications have replaced heart failure as the most important adverse prognostic factor in some recent case studies.[224]

Favorable prognostic factors include youth, early diagnosis and treatment, infection involving a prolapsing mitral valve, and penicillin-sensitive streptococcal infection. The prognosis is good for young IDUs with *Staph. aureus* infection of the tricuspid valve.[5,268] With earlier diagnosis and appropriate therapy including surgery, the prognosis for elderly patients can be substantially improved.[82]

Eradication of the etiologic organisms (microbiological cure) can be achieved in a high proportion of all patients with bacterial endocarditis.[6,257,272,273] Both early and long-term mortality rates remain significant, however, due to any preexisting disease and added damage caused by endocarditis before the organisms were eradicated. Survival curves after admission with infective endocarditis show a significant number of late deaths despite microbiologic cure.[8,290]

An analysis of experience over the past 25 years permits a reasonably accurate formulation of the prognosis for microbiologic cure among the various subgroups of patients with infective endocarditis. Approximate figures are listed in Table 82-10.

RECURRENT ENDOCARDITIS

Recurrent endocarditis is a general term that includes both relapses and reinfections. The term *relapse* refers to recurrence of infection with the same organism because treatment failed. The frequency of relapse can be predicted from published experience for each of the various forms of infective endocarditis (Table 82-10). Because relapses occasionally occur even after an optimal treatment regimen has been used, follow-up clinical evaluation should be meticulously performed during the first 2 months after treatment. Any clinical suspicion that relapse might have occurred indicates the need to draw blood cultures. Most relapses occur within a few weeks of ending treatment, but living organisms can persist in seemingly healed vegetations for many months and may occasionally cause late relapse.

The term *reinfection* refers to a new episode of endocarditis occurring after the cure of a previous episode.[291] Usually a different etiologic organism is involved, but if the new isolate appears similar to the initial etiologic organism, molecular typing techniques can be used to determine if the case is a relapse or a reinfection.

Patients remain permanently at risk of reinfection after cure of infective endocarditis because of residual valve damage superimposed on the original predisposing lesion (Tables 82-1 and 82-2). Recurrent episodes are fairly common, being recorded in from 2 to 31 percent of cases.[3,45,46,290,291] This wide variation in reported incidence is partly due to variable duration of follow-up. IDUs and patients with severe periodontitis are at highest risk for reinfection. Occasionally, a patient may suffer three or more separate episodes of infective endocarditis.[291] Patients who have previously had native valve endocarditis are at higher risk to develop prosthetic valve infection (often with a different organism) for reasons that are not yet understood.[8]

THE CHALLENGE OF PROPHYLAXIS

Because bacteremias occur during dental or other surgical procedures,[292–294] prophylactic antibiotics are frequently given to susceptible patients in an attempt to prevent bacterial endocarditis. Although prevention of such a serious infection is obviously desirable, many relevant questions remain unanswered. These include the following:

- Is antibiotic prophylaxis effective?
- What is the risk of developing bacterial endocarditis after an episode of bacteremia?

- Which operations and diagnostic procedures should be covered?
- Which patients should receive antibiotics?
- What antibiotic regimens will be most effective?

Although the risk of infection has not been quantitated, it is sufficiently low that most of these questions probably cannot be answered by clinical trials; the number of susceptible patients required to provide significant results would be too large.[53,276]

Less than one in five cases of SBE and even fewer cases of ABE follow identifiable medical procedures that cause transient bacteremias[52,292,293,295]; therefore, the proportion of cases that is potentially preventable by antibiotics is small. Because endocarditis causes serious morbidity and mortality, however, prevention of even a few cases could be worthwhile. For this reason, currently accepted standards of practice require that an antibiotic regimen be administered before certain dental and surgical procedures in patients with known heart lesions that pose a significant risk of endocarditis.

Because several hundred cases of streptococcal endocarditis following dental and genitourinary tract procedures have been recorded, the causative role of these procedures may be regarded as established.[292,293] A rather short "incubation period" for endocarditis is typical, in that most of these patients noticed symptoms within 2 weeks of the procedure.[207] It should be emphasized that the link between a case of endocarditis and a recent procedure causing bacteremia cannot be proved, because the infection could have been caused by one of the transient, asymptomatic, low-grade bacteremias that occur very commonly, induced by everyday events such as chewing and cleaning the teeth.[292]

In the absence of specific information, empirical recommendations[53,295,296] for prophylaxis of bacterial endocarditis must be made on the basis of indirect information. This information

TABLE 82-11

REPRESENTATIVE RATES FOR FREQUENCY OF BACTEREMIA AFTER VARIOUS DENTAL, DIAGNOSTIC, AND THERAPEUTIC PROCEDURES

Procedure	% Bacteremia	% Range (if available)
None	0	(0–3)
Oral cavity		
Extraction of teeth	60	(18–85)
Periodontal surgery	88	(60–90)
Brushing teeth or irrigation	40	(7–50)
Tonsillectomy	35	(33–38)
Respiratory tract		
Tracheal intubation	<10	(0–16)
Nasotracheal suctioning	16	
Bronchoscopy (rigid bronchoscope)	15	
Bronchoscopy (flexible bronchoscope)	0	
Genitourinary tract		
Catheter insertion and removal	3	(0–26)
Prostatectomy (sterile urine)	12	(11–13)
Prostatectomy (infected urine)	60	(58–82)
Dilatation of strictures	28	(19–86)
Normal delivery	3	(1–5)
Intrauterine device insertion or removal	0	
Gastrointestinal tract		
Upper gastrointestinal endoscopy	4	(0–8)
Transesophageal echocardiography	1	(0–17)
Endoscopic retrograde cholangiopancreatography	5	(0–6)
Barium enema	10	(5–11)
Colonoscopy	5	(0–5)
Sigmoidoscopy (rigid sigmoidoscope)	5	
Sigmoidoscopy (flexible sigmoidoscope)	0	
Proctoscopy	2	
Hemorrhoidectomy	8	
Esophageal dilatation	45	
Vascular system		
Cardiac catheterization	2	(0–5)
Insufficient data		
Insertion and removal of tympanostomy tubes		
Cesarean section		

Source: From Durack,[295] with permission.

includes the reported frequency of bacteremia after various procedures (Table 82-11); the relative risk posed by the patient's cardiac lesion (Table 82-2); case reports of prophylaxis failures[71]; in vitro susceptibility studies on the relevant organisms, especially streptococci; experimental studies in laboratory animals[205,297]; and retrospective studies in humans.[298–300]

Information from these sources indicates that experimental endocarditis in animals can definitely be prevented by antibiotics; that prevention is probably effective in humans; that only a small proportion of cases is potentially preventable by use of antibiotics[295,299]; and that the cost per prevented case would be very high.[72,299] Thus, prevention probably would not be cost-effective as a general strategy, but it might be effective for selected individuals, especially for higher-risk procedures such as tooth extractions.[295,301]

For the individual patient, the decision to administer prophylaxis should be made by assessing two main factors: the risk posed by the preexisting cardiac lesion and the risk posed by the procedure that might cause bacteremia. For example, if a patient with a prosthetic valve undergoes prostatic resection,

antibiotic prophylaxis should be given because both factors present a significant risk of endocarditis. On the other hand, if a patient with mitral valve prolapse is scheduled for gastroscopy, prophylaxis is not necessary because the risk for endocarditis in this setting is very low.[294] Such risk assessments may be difficult or inaccurate; in many situations uncertainties will remain. For these, there is no one "correct" answer; the patient's and the physician's attitudes and preferences may influence the decision to use prophylaxis. To meet a reasonable standard of care, the health care professional should know of the patient's cardiac lesion, inform the patient or his or her representative that a small risk of endocarditis exists; and then make a reasoned decision (with a written record) as to whether or not to give prophylaxis.

Attempted prophylaxis does not always succeed. Of 52 cases of apparent prophylaxis failure in one series, 42 involved patients with heart disease who received oral penicillin or erythromycin, usually to cover dental procedures.[71]

Common errors in attempted prevention of endocarditis are starting antibiotics too early, continuing too long, using low doses, covering tooth extractions but not lesser dental

---

TABLE 82-12

SUGGESTED REGIMENS FOR PROPHYLAXIS OF INFECTIVE ENDOCARDITIS[a]

Standard Regimen

For dental procedures and oral or upper respiratory tract surgery	Amoxicillin 2.0 g orally 1 h before procedure[b]

Special Regimens

Parenteral regimen for high-risk patients; also for gastrointestinal (GI) or genitourinary (GU) tract procedures	Ampicillin 2.0 g IM or IV *plus* gentamicin 1.5 mg/kg IM or IV, 0.5 h before procedure[b]; 6 h later, ampicillin 1 g IM or IV or amoxicillin 1 g orally.
Parenteral regimen for penicillin-allergic patients	Vancomycin 1.0 g IV *slowly* over 1–2 h; *plus* gentamicin 1.5 mg/kg IM or IV[b]; complete within 30 min of starting the procedure.
Oral regimen for penicillin-allergic patients (oral and respiratory tract only)	Clindamycin 600 mg orally 1 h before procedure.[b]
Oral regimen for minor GI or GU tract procedures	Amoxicillin 2.0 g orally 1 h before procedure.[b]
Parenteral regimen for cardiac surgery including valve replacement	Cefazolin 2.0 g IV on induction of anesthesia, repeated 8 and 16 h later[c] *or* Vancomycin 1.0 g IV *slowly* over 1 h starting on induction of anesthesia, then 0.5 g IV 8 and 16 h later[c]

[a] Note that (1) these regimens are empiric suggestions, no regimen has been proved effective for prevention of endocarditis, and prevention failures may occur with any regimen; (2) these regimens are not intended to cover all clinical situations, and the practitioner should use his or her own judgment on safety and cost-benefit issues in each individual case; (3) one or two additional doses may be given if the period of risk for bacteremia is prolonged.

[b] Pediatric dosages: ampicillin 50 mg/kg; gentamicin 1.5 mg/kg; amoxicillin: for children who weigh more than 60 lb, use same as for adults; for children less than 60 lb, use one-half the adult dose; vancomycin 20 mg/kg; clindamycin 20 mg/kg; cefazolin 30 mg/kg. Do not exceed 2.0 g ampicillin, 120 mg gentamycin.

[c] Vancomycin is preferred if *Staph. epidermidis* is an important cause of postoperative infection in that hospital. Gentamicin 1.5 mg/kg IV or IM may be added to each dose, only if postoperative gram-negative infections have occurred with significant frequency.

Source: Durack DT. Nine controversies in the management of infective endocarditis. In: Petersdorf RG et al, eds. *Update V: Harrison's Principles of Internal Medicine.* New York: McGraw-Hill; 1984:35; and Dajani et al. (JAMA 1997; 277:1794–1801)[296] Adapted and reproduced with permission of the publisher and author.

procedures, and confusing prevention of rheumatic fever (requiring long-term, low-dose antimicrobial drugs) with prevention of endocarditis (short-term, high-dose).[53]

On the basis of present information, prophylaxis is not necessary for minor dental procedures that do not involve the gums, such as simple fillings above the gum line, adjustment of orthodontic appliances, or root canal work. When a dentist or dental hygienist cleans and scales the teeth, however, the gums are always involved, and susceptible patients should receive a prophylactic antibiotic regimen.[296]

In the absence of pelvic infection, prophylaxis for endocarditis in patients with heart lesions is probably not required to cover normal delivery, therapeutic abortion, dilation and curettage, and insertion or removal of intrauterine contraceptive devices. Similarly, antibiotics need not be given before many common procedures, such as cardiac catheterization, insertion of temporary pacemakers, endotracheal intubation, bronchoscopy, endoscopy, or radiographic contrast studies of the upper and lower gastrointestinal tract. On the other hand, some physicians choose to cover even these low-risk procedures in patients with prosthetic valves because they are at higher risk for endocarditis than patients with native valves. Specific regimens suggested for prophylaxis of endocarditis are listed in Table 82-12.

Cardiac surgeons currently administer antibiotics to virtually all patients undergoing cardiac surgery, attempting to prevent both wound infections and endocarditis, although its efficacy in prevention of endocarditis has not been proved.[53] Current recommendations call for parenteral administration of an antistaphylococcal antibiotic just prior to operation, followed by one or two further doses (Table 82-12). The regimen may be modified if local experience shows that cases of early PVE caused by *Staph. epidermidis* or gram-negative bacilli have occurred with significant frequency (Table 82-12).

REFERENCES

1. Blumer G. Subacute bacterial endocarditis. *Medicine* 1923; 2:105–170.
2. Thayer WS. Studies on bacterial (infective) endocarditis. *Johns Hopkins Hosp Rep* 1926; 22:1–185.
3. Kerr A Jr. *Subacute Bacterial Endocarditis.* Springfield, IL: Charles C Thomas; 1955.
4. Hermans PE. The clinical manifestations of infective endocarditis. *Mayo Clin Proc* 1982; 57:15–21.
5. Chambers HF, Korzeniowski OM, Sande MA, National Collaborative Endocarditis Study Group. *Staphylococcus aureus* endocarditis: Clinical manifestations in addicts and nonaddicts. *Medicine* 1983; 170–177.
6. Korzeniowski OM, Kaye D. Infective endocarditis. In: Braunwald E, ed. *The Heart: A Textbook of Cardiovascular Medicine*, 4th ed. Philadelphia: Saunders, 1992:1078–1105.
7. Baumgartner WA, Miller DC, Reitz BA, Oyer PE, Jamieson SW, Stinson EB, et al. Surgical treatment of prosthetic valve endocarditis. *Ann Thorac Surg* 1983; 35:87–104.
8. Ivert TSA, Dismukes WE, Cobbs CG, Blackstone EH, Kirklin JW, Bergdahl LAL. Prosthetic valve endocarditis. *Circulation* 1984; 69:223–232.
9. Braimbridge MV, Eykyn SJ. Prosthetic valve endocarditis. *J Antimicrob Chemother* 1987; 20:173–180.
10. Douglas JL, Cobbs CG. Prosthetic valve endocarditis. In: Kaye D, ed. *Infective Endocarditis*, 2d ed. New York: Raven Press; 1992:375–396.
11. Meyer MW, Witt AR, Krishnan LK, Yokota M, Roszkowski MJ, Rudney JD, et al. Therapeutic advantage of recombinant human plas-

12. minogen activator in endocarditis: Evidence from experiments in rabbits. *Thromb Haemost* 1995; 73:680–682.
12. MacDonald RA, Robbins SL. The significance of nonbacterial thrombotic endocarditis: An autopsy and clinical study of 78 cases. *Ann Intern Med* 1957; 46:255–273.
13. Barry WE, Scarpelli D. Nonbacterial thrombotic endocarditis. *Arch Intern Med* 1962; 109:79–84.
14. Bryan CS. Nonbacterial thrombotic endocarditis in patients with malignant tumors. *Am J Med* 1969; 46:787–793.
15. Major RM. Notes on the history of endocarditis. *Bull Hist Med* 1945; 17:351–359.
16. Osler W. Chronic infectious endocarditis. *Q J Med* 1909; 2:219–230.
17. Osler W. The Gulstonian lectures, on malignant endocarditis. *Br Med J* 1885; 1:467–579.
18. Horder TJ. Infective endocarditis: With an analysis of 150 cases and with special reference to the chronic form of the disease. *Q J Med* 1909; 2:289–329.
19. Allen AC. Nature of vegetations of bacterial endocarditis. *Arch Pathol* 1939; 27:661–671.
20. Libman E, Friedberg CK. *Subacute Bacterial Endocarditis.* New York: Oxford University Press; 1947.
21. Beeson PB, Brannon ES, Warren JV. Observations of the sites of removal of bacteria from the blood in patients with bacterial endocarditis. *J Exp Med* 1945; 81:9–23.
22. Touroff ASW, Vesell H. Subacute streptococcus viridans endocarditis complicating patent ductus arteriosus: Recovery following surgical treatment. *JAMA* 1940; 115:1270–1272.
23. Durack DT. Review of early experience in treatment of bacterial endocarditis, 1940–1955. In: Bisno AL, ed. *Treatment of Infective Endocarditis.* New York: Grune & Stratton; 1981:1–14.
24. Dawson MH, Hunter TH. The treatment of subacute bacterial endocarditis with penicillin: Results in twenty cases. *JAMA* 1945; 127:129–137.
25. Abraham EP, Chain E, Fletcher CM, Florey HW, Gardner D, Heatley NG, et al. Further observations on penicillin. *Lancet* 1941; 2:177–189.
26. Loewe L, Rosenblatt P, Greene HJ, Russell M. Combined penicillin and heparin therapy of subacute bacterial endocarditis: Report of seven consecutive successfully treated patients. *JAMA* 1944; 124:144–149.
27. Galbreath WR, Hull E. Sulfonamide therapy of bacterial endocarditis: Results in 42 cases. *Ann Intern Med* 1943; 18:201–203.
28. Bloomfield AL, Armstrong CD, Kirby WMM. The treatment of subacute bacterial endocarditis with penicillin. *J Clin Invest* 1945; 24:251–267.
29. Hunter TH. The treatment of some bacterial infections of the heart and pericardium. *Bull NY Acad Med* 1952; 28:213–228.
30. Finland M. Treatment of bacterial endocarditis (concluded). *N Engl J Med* 1954; 250:419–428.
31. Geraci JE. The antibiotic therapy of infective endocarditis: Therapeutic data on 172 patients seen from 1951 through 1957: Additional observations on short-term therapy (two weeks) for penicillin-sensitive streptococcal endocarditis. *Med Clin North Am* 1958; 42:1101–1148.
32. Weinstein L, Schlesinger J. Treatment of infective endocarditis—1973. *Prog Cardiovasc Dis* 1973; 26:275–296.
33. Wallace AG, Young G Jr., Osterhout S. Treatment of acute bacterial endocarditis by valve excision and replacement. *Circulation* 1965; 31:450–453.
34. Harris SL. Definitions and demographic characteristics. In: Kaye D, ed. *Infective Endocarditis.* 2d ed. New York: Raven Press; 1992:1–18.
35. Steckelberg JM, Wilson WR. Risk factors for infective endocarditis. *Infect Dis Clin North Am* 1993; 7:9–19.
36. Smith RH, Radford DJ, Clark RA, Julian DG. Infective endocarditis: A survey of cases in the southeast of Scotland 1969–72. *Thorax* 1976; 31:373–379.
37. Van Der Meer JTM, Thompson J, Valkenburg HA, Michel MF. Epidemiology of bacterial endocarditis in the Netherlands: 1. Patient characteristics. *Arch Intern Med* 1992; 152:1863–1868.
38. Hogevik H, Olaison L, Andersson R, Lindberg J, Alestig K. Epidemiologic aspects of infective endocarditis in an urban population: A 5-year prospective study. *Medicine* 1995; 74:324–339.
39. Berlin JA, Abrutyn E, Strom BL, Kinman JL, Levison ME, Korzeniowski OM, et al. Incidence of infective endocarditis in the Delaware Valley, 1988–1990. *Am J Cardiol* 1995; 76:933–936.
40. Kaye D, McCormack RC, Hook EW. Bacterial endocarditis: The changing pattern since the introduction of penicillin therapy. *Antimicrob Agents Chemother* 1961; 37–46.

41. Uwaydah MM, Weinberg AN. Bacterial endocarditis—A changing pattern. *N Engl J Med* 1965; 273:1231–1235.

42. Lerner PI, Weinstein L. Infective endocarditis in the antibiotic era. *N Engl J Med* 1966; 274:199–206; 259–266; 323–331; 388–393.

43. Finland M, Barnes MW. Changing etiology of bacterial endocarditis in the antibiotic era: Experiences at the Boston City Hospital 1933–1965. *Ann Intern Med* 1970; 72:341–348.

44. Durack DT, Petersdorf RG. Changes in the epidemiology of endocarditis. In: Kaplan EL, Taranta AV, eds. *Infective Endocarditis: An American Heart Association Symposium.* Dallas: American Heart Association; 1977:3–8.

45. Baddour LM. Twelve-year review of recurrent native-valve infective endocarditis: A disease of the modern antibiotic era. *Rev Infect Dis* 1988; 10:1163–1170.

46. Garvey GJ, Neu HC. Infective endocarditis—an evolving disease: A review of endocarditis at the Columbia-Presbyterian Medical Center, 1968–1973. *Medicine* 1978; 57:105–127.

47. Pulvirenti JJ, Kerns E, Benson C, Lisowski J, Demarais P, Weinstein RA. Infective endocarditis in injection drug users: Importance of human immunodeficiency virus serostatus and degree of immunosuppression. *Clin Infect Dis* 1996; 22:40–45.

48. Scheld WM, Sande MA. Endocarditis and intravascular infections. In: Mandell GL, Douglas RG Jr, Dolin R, eds. *Principles and Practice of Infectious Diseases,* 4th ed. New York: Churchill Livingstone; 1995:740–783.

49. Weinstein L, Rubin RH. Infective endocarditis—1973. *Prog Cardiovasc Dis* 1973; 16:239–273.

50. Tunkel AR, Mandell GL. Infecting microorganisms. In: Kaye D, ed. *Infective Endocarditis,* 2d ed. New York: Raven Press; 1992:85–97.

51. Tompkins LS, Roessler BJ, Redd SC. Legionella prosthetic-valve endocarditis. *N Engl J Med* 1988; 318:530–534.

52. Bayliss R, Clarke C, Somerville W, Whitfield AGW. The teeth and infective endocarditis. *Br Heart J* 1983; 50:506–512.

53. Durack DT. Prophylaxis of infective endocarditis. In: Mandell GL, Douglas RG, Jr., Dolin R, eds. *Principles and Practice of Infectious Diseases,* 4th ed. New York: Churchill Livingstone; 1995:793–813.

54. Mansur AJ, Grinberg M, da Luz PL, Bellotti G. The complications of infective endocarditis: A reappraisal in the 1980s (see comments). *Arch Intern Med* 1992; 152:2428–2432.

55. Johnson DH, Rosenthal A, Nadas AS. A forty-year review of bacterial endocarditis in infancy and childhood. *Circulation* 1975; 51:581–588.

56. Hansen D, Schmiegelow K, Jacobsen JR. Bacterial endocarditis in children: Trends in its diagnosis, course, and prognosis. *Pediatr Cardiol* 1993; 13:198–203.

57. Saiman L, Prince A, Gersony WM. Pediatric infective endocarditis in the modern era. *J Pediatr* 1993; 122:847–853.

58. Awadallah SM, Kavey RW, Byrum CJ, Smith FC, Kveselis DA, Blackman MS. The changing pattern of infective endocarditis in childhood. *Am J Cardiol* 1991; 68:90–94.

59. Stull TL, LiPuma JJ. Endocarditis in children. In: Kaye D, ed. *Infective Endocarditis,* 2d ed. New York: Raven Press; 1992:313–327.

60. Ifere OAS, Masokano KA. Infective endocarditis in children in the Guinea savannah of Nigeria. *Ann Trop Paediatr* 1991; 11:233–240.

61. Saitoh M, Hishi T, Tamura M, Komoshita S. Forty year review of bacterial endocarditis in infants and children. *Acta Paediatr Jpn* 1991; 33:613–616.

62. El-Khatib MR, Wilson FM, Lerner AM. Characteristics of bacterial endocarditis in heroin addicts in Detroit. *Am J Med Sci* 1976; 271:197–201.

63. Reisberg BE. Infective endocarditis in the narcotic addict. *Prog Cardiovasc Dis* 1979; 22:193–204.

64. Dressler FA, Roberts WC. Infective endocarditis in opiate addicts: Analysis of 80 cases studied at necropsy. *Am J Cardiol* 1989; 63:1240–1257.

65. Weisse AB, Heller DR, Schimenti RJ, Montgomery RL, Kapila R. The febrile parenteral drug user: A prospective study in 121 patients. *Am J Med* 1993; 94:274–280.

66. Carrel T, Schaffner A, Vogt P, Laske A, Niederhauser U, Schneider J, et al. Endocarditis in intravenous drug addicts and HIV infected patients: Possibilities and limitations of surgical treatment. *J Heart Valve Dis* 1993; 2:140–147.

67. Sande MA, Lee BL, Mills J, Chambers HF III. Endocarditis in intravenous drug users. In: Kaye D, ed. *Infective Endocarditis,* 2d ed. New York: Raven Press; 1992:345–359.

68. Corrigall D, Bolen J, Hancock EW, Popp RP. Mitral valve prolapse and infective endocarditis. *Am J Med* 1977; 63:215–222.

69. Clemens JD, Horwitz RI, Jaffe CC, Feinstein AR, Stanton BF. A controlled evaluation of the risk of bacterial endocarditis in persons with mitral-valve prolapse. *N Engl J Med* 1982; 307:776–781.

70. Beton DC, Brear SG, Edwards JD, Leonard JC. Mitral valve prolapse: An assessment of clinical features, associated conditions and prognosis. *Q J Med* 1983; 52:150–164.

71. Durack DT, Kaplan EL, Bisno AL. Apparent failures of endocarditis prophylaxis: Analysis of 52 cases submitted to a national registry. *JAMA* 1983; 250:2318–2322.

72. Clemens JD, Ransohoff DF. A quantitative assessment of pre-dental antibiotic prophylaxis for patients with mitral-valve prolapse. *J Chronic Dis* 1984; 37:531–544.

73. Devereux RB, Hawkins I, Kramer-Fox R, Lutas EM, Hammond IW, Spitzer MC, et al. Complications of mitral valve prolapse: Disproportionate occurrence in men and older patients. *Am J Med* 1986; 81:751–758.

74. MacMahon SW, Hickey AJ, Wilcken DEL, Wittes JT, Feneley MP, Hickie JB. Risk of infective endocarditis in mitral valve prolapse with and without precordial systolic murmurs. *Am J Cardiol* 1986; 58:105–108.

75. MacMahon SW, Roberts K, Kramer-Fox R, Zucker DM, Roberts RB, Devereux RB. Mitral valve prolapse and infective endocarditis. *Am Heart J* 1987; 113:1291–1298.

76. Dhawan A, Grover A, Marwaha RK, Khattri HN, Anand IS, Kumar L, et al. Infective endocarditis in children: Profile in a developing country. *Ann Trop Paediatr* 1993; 13:189–194.

77. Elward K, Hruby N, Christy C. Pneumococcal endocarditis in infants and children: Report of a case and review of the literature. *Pediatr Infect Dis J* 1990; 9:652–657.

78. Del Pont JM, De Cicco LT, Vartalitis C, Ithuurralde M, Gallo JP, Vargas F, et al. Infective endocarditis in children: Clinical analyses and evaluation of two diagnostic criteria. *Pediatr Infect Dis* 1995; 14:1079–1086.

79. Kaplan EL, Rich H, Gersony W, Manning J. A collaborative study of infective endocarditis in the 1970s: Emphasis on infections in patients who have undergone cardiovascular surgery. *Circulation* 1979; 59:327–335.

80. Jung JY, Saab SB, Almond CH. The case for early surgical treatment of left sided primary infective endocarditis. *J Thorac Cardiovasc Surg* 1975; 70:509–518.

81. Bayliss R, Clarke C, Oakley CM, Somerville W, Young SEJ. Incidence, mortality and prevention of infective endocarditis. *J R Coll Phys Lond* 1986; 20:15–20.

82. Werner GS, Schulz R, Fuchs FB, Andreas S, Prange H, Ruschewski W, et al. Infective endocarditis in the elderly in the era of transesophageal echocardiography: Clinical features and prognosis compared with younger patients. *Am J Med* 1996; 100:90–97.

83. Felder RS, Nardone D, Palac R. Prevalence of predisposing factors for endocarditis among an elderly institutionalized population. *Oral Surg Oral Med Oral Pathol* 1992; 73:30–34.

84. Steckelberg JM, Melton LJ, Ilstrup DM, Rouse MS, Wilson WR. Influence of referral bias on the apparent clinical spectrum of infective endocarditis. *Am J Med* 1990; 88:582–588.

85. Eliopoulos GM. Enterococcal endocarditis. In: Kaye D, ed. *Infective Endocarditis,* 2d ed. New York: Raven Press; 1992:209–229.

86. Threlkeld MG, Cobbs CG. Infectious disorders of prosthetic valves and intravascular devices. In: Mandell GL, Bennett JE, Dolin R, eds. *Principles and Practice of Infectious Diseases,* 4th ed. New York: Churchill Livingstone; 1995:783–793.

87. Tuazon CU, Sheagren JN. Increased rate of carriage of *Staphylococcus aureus* among narcotic addicts. *J Infect Dis* 1974; 129:725–727.

88. Reyes MP, Lerner AM. Current problems in the treatment of infective endocarditis due to *Pseudomonas aeruginosa. Rev Infect Dis* 1983; 5:314–321.

89. Cohen PS, Maguire JH, Weinstein L. Infective endocarditis caused by gram-negative bacteria: A review of the literature, 1945–1977. *Prog Cardiovasc Dis* 1980; 22:205–242.

90. Rubinstein E, Noriega ER, Simberkoff MS, Holzman R, Rahal JJ. Fungal endocarditis: Analysis of 24 cases and review of the literature. *Medicine* 1975; 54:331–344.

91. Moyer DV, Edwards JE, Jr. Fungal endocarditis. In: Kaye D, ed. *Infective Endocarditis,* 2d ed. New York: Raven Press; 1992:299–312.

92. Baddour LM, Meyer J, Henry B. Polymicrobial infective endocarditis in the 1980s. *Rev Infect Dis* 1991; 13:963–970.

93. Faber M, Frimodt-Moller N, Espersen F, Skinhoj P, Rosdahl V. *Staphylococcus aureus* endocarditis in Danish intravenous drug users: High proportion of left-sided endocarditis. *Scand J Infect Dis* 1995; 27:483–487.

94. Drancourt M, Birtles R, Chaumentin G, Vandenesch F, Etienne J, Raoult D. New serotype of *Bartonella henselae* in endocarditis and cat-scratch disease. *Lancet* 1996; 347:441–443.

95. Resnekov L. Staphylococcal endocarditis following mitral valvotomy with special reference to coagulase-negative *Staphylococcus albus*. *Lancet* 1959; 2:597–600.

96. Watanakunakorn C. Prosthetic valve infective endocarditis. *Prog Cardiovasc Dis* 1979; 22:181–192.

97. Karchmer AW, Dismukes WE, Buckley MJ, Austen WG. Late prosthetic valve endocarditis: Clinical features influencing therapy. *Am J Med* 1978; 64:199–206.

98. Seaworth BJ, Durack DT. Infective endocarditis in obstetric and gynecologic practice. *Am J Obstet Gynecol* 1986; 154:180–188.

99. Sugrue D, Blake S, Troy P, MacDonald D. Antibiotic prophylaxis against infective endocarditis after normal delivery—Is it necessary? *Br Heart J* 1980; 44:499–502.

100. Cobbs CG. IUD and endocarditis. *Ann Intern Med* 1973; 78:451.

101. Fernandez-Guerrero ML, Verdejo C, Azofra J, de Gorgolas M. Hospital-acquired infectious endocarditis not associated with cardiac surgery: An emerging problem. *Clin Infect Dis* 1995; 20:16–23.

102. Fang G, Keys TF, Gentry LO, Harris AA, Rivera N, Getz K, et al. Prosthetic valve endocarditis resulting from nosocomial bacteremia: A prospective, multicenter study. *Ann Intern Med* 1993; 119:560–567.

103. Pelletier LL, Petersdorf RG. Infective endocarditis: A review of 125 cases from the University of Washington Hospitals, 1963–72. *Medicine* 1977; 56:287–313.

104. Raad II, Bodey GP. Infectious complications of indwelling vascular catheters. *Clin Infect Dis* 1992; 15:197–210.

105. Ehrie M, Morgan AP, Moore FD, O'Connor NE. Endocarditis with the indwelling balloon-tipped pulmonary artery catheter in burn patients. *J Trauma* 1978; 18:665–666.

106. Rowley KM, Clubb KS, Smith GJW, Cabin HS. Right-sided infective endocarditis as a consequence of flow-directed pulmonary artery catheterization: A clinicopathological study of 55 autopsied patients. *N Engl J Med* 1984; 311:1152–1156.

107. Martino P, Micozzi A, Venditti M, Gentile G, Girmenia C, Raccah R, et al. Catheter-related right-sided endocarditis in bone marrow transplant recipients. *Rev Infect Dis* 1990; 12:250–257.

108. Khoo DE, Zebro TJ, English TAH. Bacterial endocarditis in a transplanted heart. *Pathol Res Pract* 1989; 185:445–447.

109. Lillehei CW, Bobb JRR, Visscher MB. The occurrence of endocarditis with valvular deformities in dogs with arteriovenous fistulas. *Ann Surg* 1950; 132:577–590.

110. Cross AS, Steigbigel RT. Infective endocarditis and access site infections in patients on hemodialysis. *Medicine* 1976; 55:453–465.

111. Gomes MN, Choyke PL, Wallace RB. Infected aortic aneurysms: A changing entity. *Ann Surg* 1992; 215:435–442.

112. Brennan RO, Durack DT. The viridans streptococci in perspective. In: Remington JS, Swartz MN, eds. *Current Clinical Topics in Infectious Diseases*. New York: McGraw-Hill; 1984:253–289.

113. Sussman JI, Baron EJ, Tenenbaum MJ, Kaplan MH, Greenspan J, Facklam RR, et al. Viridans streptococcal endocarditis: Clinical, microbiological, and echocardiographic correlations. *J Infect Dis* 1986; 154:597–603.

114. Watanakunakorn C, Pantelakis J. Alpha-hemolytic streptococcal bacteremia: A review of 203 episodes during 1980–1991. *Scand J Infect Dis* 1993; 25:403–408.

115. Facklam RR. Physiological differentiation of viridans streptococci. *J Clin Microbiol* 1977; 5:184–201.

116. Douglas CWI, Heath J, Hampton KK, Preston FE. Identity of viridans streptococci isolated from cases of infective endocarditis. *J Med Microbiol* 1993; 39:179–182.

117. Carey RB, Gross KC, Roberts RB. Vitamin B6-dependent *Streptococcus mitor (mitis)* isolated from patients with systemic infections. *J Infect Dis* 1975; 131:722–726.

118. Rouff KL. Nutritionally variant streptococci. *Clin Microbiol Rev* 1991; 4:184–190.

119. Bouvet A, Grimont F, Grimont PAD. *Streptococcus defectivus* sp. nov.

120. Bouvet A. Human endocarditis due to nutritionally variant streptococci: *Streptococcus adjacens* and *Streptococcus defectivus*. *Eur Heart J* 1995; 16(suppl B):24–27.

121. Wilson WR, Wilkowske CJ, Wright AJ, Sande MA, Geraci JE. Treatment of streptomycin-susceptible and streptomycin-resistant enterococcal endocarditis. *Ann Intern Med* 1984; 100:816–823.

122. Moellering RC Jr., Watson BK, Kunz LJ. Endocarditis due to group D streptococci: Comparison of disease caused by *Streptococcus bovis* with that produced by the enterococci. *Am J Med* 1974; 57:239–250.

123. Murray HW, Roberts RB. *Streptococcus bovis* bacteremia and underlying gastrointestinal disease. *Arch Intern Med* 1978; 138:1097–1099.

124. Klein RS, Catalano MT, Edberg SC, Casey JI, Steigbigel NH. *Streptococcus bovis* septicemia and carcinoma of the colon. *Ann Intern Med* 1979; 91:560–562.

125. Maki DG, Agger WA. Enterococcal bacteremia: Clinical features, the risk of endocarditis, and management. *Medicine* 1988; 67:248–269.

126. Murray BE. The life and times of the enterococcus. *Clin Microbiol Rev* 1990; 3:46–65.

127. Megran DW. Enterococcal endocarditis. *Clin Infect Dis* 1992; 15:63–71.

128. Eliopoulos GM. Increasing problems in the therapy of enterococcal infections. *Eur J Clin Microbiol Infect Dis* 1993; 12:409–412.

129. Frieden TR, Munsiff SS, Low DE, Willey BM, Williams G, Faur Y, et al. Emergence of vancomycin-resistant enterococci in New York City. *Lancet* 1993; 342:76–79.

130. Bruyn GAW, Thompson J, Van Der Meer JWM. Pneumococcal endocarditis in adult patients. A report of five cases and review of the literature. *Q J Med* 1990; 74:33–40.

131. Pankey GA. Acute bacterial endocarditis at the University of Minnesota Hospitals, 1939–1959. *Am Heart J* 1962; 64:583–591.

132. Watanakunakorn C, Tan JS, Phair JP. Some salient features of *Staphylococcus aureus* endocarditis. *Am J Med* 1973; 54:473–481.

133. Bayer AS, Lam K, Gintzon L, Norman DC, Chiu C, Ward JI. *Staphylococcus aureus* bacteremia: Clinical, serologic, and echocardiographic findings in patients with and without endocarditis. *Arch Intern Med* 1987; 147:457–462.

134. Keys TF, Hewitt WL. Endocarditis due to micrococci and *Staphylococcus epidermidis*. *Arch Intern Med* 1973; 132:216–220.

135. Karchmer AW, Archer GL, Dismukes WE. *Staphylococcus epidermidis* causing prosthetic valve endocarditis: Microbiologic and clinical observations as guides to therapy. *Ann Intern Med* 1983; 98:447–455.

136. Chen YC, Chang SC, Luh KT, Hsieh WC. *Actinobacillus actinomycetemcomitans* endocarditis: A report of four cases and review of the literature. *Q J Med* 1992; 81:871–878.

137. Geraci JE, Wilson WR. Endocarditis due to gram-negative bacteria: Report of 56 cases. *Mayo Clin Proc* 1982; 57:145–148.

138. Gould K, Ramirez-Ronda CH, Holmes RK, Sanford JP. Adherence of bacteria to heart valves *in vitro*. *J Clin Invest* 1975; 56:1364–1370.

139. Scheld WM, Valone JA, Sande MA. Bacterial adherence in the pathogenesis of endocarditis: Interaction of bacterial dextran, platelets, and fibrin. *J Clin Invest* 1978; 61:1394–1404.

140. Durack DT, Beeson PB. Protective role of complement in experimental *E. coli* endocarditis. *Infect Immun* 1977; 16:213–217.

141. Al-Kasab S, Al-Fagih MR, Al-Yousef S, Ali Khan MA, Ribeiro PA, Nazzal S, et al. *Brucella* infective endocarditis: Successful combined medical and surgical therapy. *J Thorac Cardiovasc Surg* 1988; 95:862–867.

142. Delvecchio G, Fracassetti O, Lorenzi N. *Brucella* endocarditis. *Int J Cardiol* 1991; 33:328–329.

143. Felner JM, Dowell VR. Anaerobic bacterial endocarditis. *N Engl J Med* 1970; 283:1188–1192.

144. Nastro LJ, Finegold SM. Endocarditis due to anaerobic gram-negative bacilli. *Am J Med* 1973; 54:482–496.

145. Kammer RB, Utz JP. *Aspergillus* species endocarditis: The new face of a not so rare disease. *Am J Med* 1974; 56:506–521.

146. Turck WPG, Howitt G, Turnberg LA, Fox H, Longson M, Matthews MB, et al. Chronic Q fever. *Q J Med* 1976; 45:193–217.

147. Kimbrough RC, Ormsbee RA, Peacock M, Rogers WR, Bennetts RW, Raaf J, et al. Q fever endocarditis in the United States. *Ann Intern Med* 1979; 91:400–402.

148. Spelman DW. Q fever: A study of 111 consecutive cases. *Med J Aust* 1982; 1:547–553.

and *Streptococcus adjacens* sp. nov., nutritionally variant streptococci from human clinical specimens. *Int J Syst Bacteriol* 1989; 39:290–294.

149. Falconer H, Terry SI, Spencer H. Cryptococcosis in the West Indies. *West Indian Med J* 1980; 29:142.

150. Raoult D, Marrie T. State of the art clinical article: Q fever. *Clin Infect Dis* 1995; 20:489–496.

151. Raoult D, Brouqui P, Marchou B, Gastaut JA. Acute and chronic Q fever in patients with cancer. *Clin Infect Dis* 1992; 14:127–130.

152. Raoult D, Fournier PE, Drancourt M, Marrie TJ, Etienne J, Cosserat J, et al. Diagnosis of 22 new cases of *Bartonella* endocarditis. *Ann Intern Med* 1996; 125:646–652.

153. Ward C, Ward AM. Acquired valvular heart disease in patients who keep pet birds. *Lancet* 1974; 734–736.

154. van der Bel-Kahn J, Watanakunakorn C, Menefee MG, Long HD, Dicter R. *Chlamydia trachomatis* endocarditis. *Am Heart J* 1978; 95:627–636.

155. Cohen JI, Sloss LJ, Kundsin R, Golightly L. Prosthetic valve endocarditis caused by *Mycoplasma hominis*. *Am J Med* 1989; 86:819–821.

156. Malinverni R, Bille J, Glauser MP. Single-dose rifampin prophylaxis for experimental endocarditis induced by high bacterial inocula of *Viridans* streptococci. *J Infect Dis* 1987; 156:151–157.

157. Cannady PB Jr, Sanford JP. Negative blood cultures in infective endocarditis: A review. *South Med J* 1976; 69:1420–1424.

158. Pesanti EL, Smith IM. Infective endocarditis with negative blood cultures: An analysis of 52 cases. *Am J Med* 1979; 66:43–50.

159. Hoen B, Selton-Suty C, Lacassin F, Etienne J, Briancon S, Leport C, et al. Infective endocarditis in patients with negative blood cultures: Analysis of 88 cases from a one-year nationwide survey in France. *Clin Infect Dis* 1995; 20:501–506.

160. Libman E. The clinical features of cases of subacute bacterial endocarditis that have spontaneously become bacteria-free. *Am J Med Sci* 1913; 146:626–645.

161. Roux JP, Koussa A, Cajot MA, Marquette F, Goullard L, Gosselin B, et al. Primary *Aspergillus* endocarditis: Apropos of a case and review of the international literature. *Ann Chir* 1992; 46:110–115.

162. Durack DT, Bright DK, Lukes AS, Duke Endocarditis Service. New criteria for diagnosis of infective endocarditis: Utilization of specific echocardiographic findings. *Am J Med* 1994; 96:200–209.

163. Cecchi F, Parrini I, Chinaglia A, Pomari F, Brusasco G, Bobbio M, et al. New diagnostic criteria for infective endocarditis. A study of sensitivity and specificity. *Eur Heart J* 1997; 18:1149–1156.

164. Angrist A, Oka M, Nakao K. Vegetative endocarditis. *Pathol Annu* 1967; 2:155–212.

165. Grant RT, Wood JE Jr, Jones TD. Heart valve irregularities in relation to subacute bacterial endocarditis. *Am Heart J* 1928; 14:247–261.

166. Durack DT. Experimental bacterial endocarditis: IV. Structure and evolution of very early lesions. *J Pathol* 1975; 115:81–89.

167. Durack DT, Beeson PB. Experimental bacterial endocarditis: I. Colonization of a sterile vegetation. *Br J Exp Pathol* 1972; 53:44–49.

168. Hojnik M, George J, Ziporen L, Shoenfeld Y. Heart valve involvement (Libman-Sacks endocarditis) in the antiphospholipid syndrome. *Circulation* 1996; 93:1579–1587.

169. Livornese LL Jr, Korzeniowski O. Pathogenesis of infective endocarditis. In: Kaye D, ed. *Infective Endocarditis*, 2d ed. New York: Raven Press; 1992:19–35.

170. Burnette-Curley D, Wells V, Viscount H, Munro C, Fenno JC, Fives-Taylor P, et al. FimA, a major virulence factor associated with *Streptococcus parasanguis* endocarditis. *Infect Immun* 1995; 63:4669–4674.

171. Moreillon P, Entenza JM, Francioli P, McDevitt D, Foster TJ, Francois P, et al. Role of *Staphylococcus aureus* coagulase and clumping factor in pathogenesis of experimental endocarditis. *Infect Immun* 1995; 63:4738–4743.

172. Baddour LM, Christensen GD, Hester MG, Bisno AL. Production of experimental endocarditis by coagulase-negative staphylococci: Variability in species virulence. *J Infect Dis* 1984; 150:721–727.

173. Yeaman MR, Puentes SM, Norman DC, Bayer AS. Partial characterization and staphylocidal activity of thrombin-induced platelet microbicidal protein. *Infect Immun* 1992; 60:1202–1209.

174. Dankert J, Hess J, Durack DT. Pathogenesis of viridans streptococcal endocarditis (VSE): Disappearance of adherent streptococci from vegetations. 26th Interscience Conference on Antimicrobial Agents and Chemotherapy (abstr). 1986.

175. Drake TA, Rogers GM, Sande MA. Tissue factor is a major stimulus for vegetation formation in enterococcal endocarditis in rabbits. *J Clin Invest* 1984; 73:1750–1753.

176. van Ginkel CJW, Thorig L, Thompson J, Oh JIH, van Aken WG. Enhancement of generation of monocyte tissue thromboplastin by bacterial phagocytosis: Possible pathway for fibrin formation on infected vegetations in bacterial endocarditis. *Infect Immun* 1979; 25:388–395.

177. Capo C, Zugun F, Stein A, Tardei G, Lepidi H, Raoult D, et al. Upregulation of tumor necrosis factor alpha and interleukin-1 beta in Q fever endocarditis. *Infect Immun* 1996; 64:1638–1642.

178. Lepeschkin E. On the relation between the site of valvular involvement in endocarditis and the blood pressure resting on the valve. *Am J Med Sci* 1952; 224:318–319.

179. Rodbard S. Blood velocity and endocarditis. *Circulation* 1963; 27:18–28.

180. Edwards JE, Burchell HB. Endocardial and intimal lesions (jet impact) as possible sites of origin of murmurs. *Circulation* 1958; 18:946–960.

181. Buchbinder NA, Roberts WC. Left-sided valvular active infective endocarditis: A study of forty-five necropsy patients. *Am J Med* 1972; 53:20–35.

182. Scully RE, Mark EJ, McNeely WF, McNeely BU. Case records of the Massachusetts General Hospital. *N Engl J Med* 1996; 334:105–111.

183. McFarland MM. Pathology of infective endocarditis. In: Kaye D, ed. *Infective Endocarditis*, 2d ed. New York: Raven Press; 1992:57–83.

184. DiNubile MJ, Calderwood SB, Steinhaus DM, Karchmer AW. Cardiac conduction abnormalities complicating native valve active endocarditis. *Am J Cardiol* 1986; 58:1213–1217.

185. Phair JP, Clarke J. Immunology of infective endocarditis. *Prog Cardiovasc Dis* 1977; 22:137–144.

186. Williams RC, Kunkel HG. Rheumatoid factor, complement, and conglutinin aberrations in patients with subacute bacterial endocarditis. *J Clin Invest* 1962; 41:666–675.

187. Messner RP, Laxdal T, Quie PG, Williams RC Jr. Rheumatoid factors in subacute bacterial endocarditis—Bacterium, duration of disease or genetic predisposition? *Ann Intern Med* 1968; 68:746–754.

188. Sheagren JN, Tuazon CU, Griffin C, Padmore N. Rheumatoid factor in acute bacterial endocarditis. *Arthritis Rheum* 1976; 19:887–890.

189. Maisch B, Eichstadt H, Kochsick K. Immune reactions in infective endocarditis: I. Clinical data and diagnostic relevance of antimyocardial antibodies. *Am Heart J* 1983; 106:329–337.

190. Weinstein L, Schlesinger JJ. Pathoanatomic, pathophysiologic and clinical correlations in endocarditis. (First of two parts.) *N Engl J Med* 1974; 291:832–837.

191. Wadsworth AB. A study of the endocardial lesions developing during pneumococcus infection in horses. *J Med Res* 1919, 34:280–291.

192. Mair W. Pneumococcal endocarditis in rabbits. *J Pathol Bacteriol* 1923; 26:426–428.

193. Durack DT, Gilliland BC, Petersdorf RG. Effect of immunization on susceptibility to experimental *Streptococcus mutans* and *Streptococcus sanguis* endocarditis. *Infect Immun* 1978; 22:52–56.

194. Durack DT, Beeson PB. Pathogenesis of infective endocarditis. In: Rahimtoola SH, ed. *Infective Endocarditis*. New York: Grune & Stratton; 1978:1–53.

195. Bayer AS, Theofilopoulos AN, Eisenberg R, Dixon FJ, Guze LB. Circulating immune complexes in infective endocarditis. *N Engl J Med* 1976; 295:1500–1505.

196. Bayer AS, Theofilopoulos AN, Tillman DB, Dixon FJ, Guze LB. Use of circulating immune complex levels in the serodifferentiation of endocarditic and nonendocarditic septicemias. *Am J Med* 1979; 66:58–62.

197. Maisch B, Mayer E, Schubert U, Berg PA, Kochsiek K. Immune reactions in infective endocarditis: II. Relevance of circulating immune complexes, serum inhibition factors, lymphocytotoxic reactions, and antibody-dependent cellular cytotoxicity against cardiac target cells. *Am Heart J* 1983; 106:338–344.

198. Cabane J, Godeau P, Hereeman A, Acar J, Digeon M, Bach JF. Fate of circulating immune complexes in infective endocarditis. *Am J Med* 1979; 66:277–282.

199. Gutman RA, Striker GE, Gilliland BC, Cutler RE. The immune complex glomerulonephritis of bacterial endocarditis. *Medicine* 1972; 51:1–25.

200. Levy RL, Hong R. The immune nature of subacute bacterial endocarditis (SBE) nephritis. *Am J Med* 1973; 54:645–652.

201. Nagel JG, Tuazon CU, Cardella TA, Sheagren JN. Teichoic acid serologic diagnosis of staphylococcal endocarditis: Use of gel diffusion and counterimmunoelectrophoretic methods. *Ann Intern Med* 1975; 82:13–17.

202. Freedman LR, Valone J Jr. Experimental infective endocarditis. *Prog Cardiovasc Dis* 1979; 22:169–180.

203. Contrepois A. Notes on the history of experimental endocarditis. *Clin Infect Dis* 1995; 20:461–466.

204. Durack DT, Beeson PB. Experimental bacterial endocarditis: II. Survival of bacteria in endocardial vegetations. *Br J Exp Pathol* 1972; 53:50–53.

205. Durack DT. Experience with prevention of experimental endocarditis. In: Kaplan EL, Taranta AV, eds. *Infective Endocarditis: An American Heart Association Symposium*. American Heart Association Monograph No. 52. Dallas: American Heart Association, 1977:28–32.

206. Churchill MA, Jr, Geraci JE, Hunder GG. Musculoskeletal manifestations of bacterial endocarditis. *Ann Intern Med* 1977; 87:754–759.

207. Starkebaum MK, Durack DT, Beeson PB. The "incubation period" of subacute bacterial endocarditis. *Yale J Biol Med* 1977; 50:49–58.

208. Karchmer AW. Staphylococcal endocarditis. In: Kaye D, ed. *Infective Endocarditis*, 2d ed. New York: Raven Press; 1992:225–249.

209. Khan MY, Hall WH, Gerding DN. Infective endocarditis in narcotic addicts. *Minn Med* 1975; 83–84.

210. Steckelberg JM, Murphy JG, Wilson WR. Cure rates and long-term prognosis. In: Kaye D, ed. *Infective Endocarditis*, 2d ed. New York: Raven Press, 1992:435–453.

211. Kilpatrick ZM, Greenberg PA, Sanford JP. Splinter hemorrhages—Their clinical significance. *Arch Intern Med* 1965; 115:730–735.

212. Howard EJ. Osler's nodes. *Am Heart J* 1960; 59:633–634.

213. Alpert JS, Krous HF, Dalen JE, O'Rourke RA, Bloor CM. Pathogenesis of Osler's nodes. *Ann Intern Med* 1976; 85:471–473.

214. Edwards JE, Jr, Foos RY, Montgomerie JZ, Guze LB. Ocular manifestations of *Candida* septicemia: Review of seventy-six cases of hematogenous candida endophthalmitis. *Medicine* 1974; 53:47–75.

215. Cates JE, Christie RV. Subacute bacterial endocarditis: A review of 442 patients treated in 14 centres appointed by the Penicillin Trials Committee of Medical Research Council. *Q J Med* 1951; 20:93–130.

216. Mills J, Utley J, Abbott J. Heart failure in infective endocarditis. *Chest* 1974; 66:151–159.

217. Lytle BW, Priest BP, Taylor PC, Loop FD, Sapp SK, Stewart RW, et al. Surgical treatment of prosthetic valve endocarditis. *J Thorac Cardiovasc Surg* 1996; 111:198–207.

218. Tanaka M, Abe T, Hosokawa S, Suenaga Y, Hikosaka H. Tricuspid valve *Candida* endocarditis cured by valve-sparing debridement. *Ann Thorac Surg* 1989; 48:857–858.

219. Pruett TL, Rotstein OD, Anderson RW, Simmons RL. Tricuspid valve endocarditis: Successful treatment with valve-sparing debridement and antifungal chemotherapy in a multiorgan transplant recipient. *Am J Med* 1986; 80:116–118.

220. Sokil AB. Cardiac imaging in infective endocarditis. In: Kaye D, ed. *Infective Endocarditis*, 2d ed. New York: Raven Press; 1992:125–150.

221. Ziment I. Nervous system complications in bacterial endocarditis. *Am J Med* 1969; 47:593–607.

222. Pruitt AA, Rubin RH, Karchmer AW, Duncan GW. Neurologic complications of bacterial endocarditis. *Medicine* 1978; 57:329–343.

223. Jones HR Jr, Siekert RG. Neurological manifestations of infective endocarditis: Review of clinical and therapeutic challenges. *Brain* 1989; 112:1295–1315.

224. Francioli P. Central nervous system complications of infective endocarditis. In: Scheld WM, Whitley RJ, Durack DT, eds. *Infections of the Central Nervous System*, 2d ed. New York: Lippincott-Raven, 1997:523–553.

225. Jones HR, Siekert RG, Geraci JE. Neurologic manifestations of bacterial endocarditis. *Ann Intern Med* 1969; 71:21–28.

226. Stengel A, Wolferth CC. Mycotic (bacterial) aneurysms of intravascular origin. *Arch Intern Med* 1923; 31:527–554.

227. Brust JCM, Dickinson PCT, Hughes JEO, Holtzman RNN. The diagnosis and treatment of cerebral mycotic aneurysms. *Ann Neurol* 1990; 27:238–246.

228. Salgado AV, Furlan AJ, Keys TF. Mycotic aneurysm, subarachnoid hemorrhage, and indications for cerebral angiography in infective endocarditis. *Stroke* 1987; 18:1057–1060.

229. Nakata Y, Shionoya S, Kamiya K. Pathogenesis of mycotic aneurysm. *Angiology* 1968; 19:593–601.

230. Masuda J, Yutani C, Waki R, Ogata J, Kuriyama Y, Yamaguchi T. Histopathological analysis of the mechanisms of intracranial hemorrhage complicating infective endocarditis. *Stroke* 1992; 23:843–850.

231. Bamford J, Hodges J, Warlow C. Late rupture of a mycotic aneurysm after "cure" of bacterial endocarditis. *J Neurol* 1986; 233:51–53.

232. Bush LM, Johnson CC. Clinical syndrome and diagnosis. In: Kaye D, ed. *Infective Endocarditis*, 2d ed. New York: Raven Press; 1992:99–115.

233. Durack DT, Street AC. Fever of unknown origin—Reexamined and redefined. *Curr Clin Top Infect Dis* 1991; 11:35–51.

234. von Reyn CF, Levy BS, Arbeit RD, Friedland G, Crumpacker CS. Infective endocarditis: An analysis based on strict case definitions. *Ann Intern Med* 1981; 94:505–517.

235. Dajani AS, Ayoub E, Bierman FZ, Bisno AL, Denny FW, Durack DT, et al. Guidelines for the diagnosis of rheumatic fever: Jones criteria, 1992 update. *JAMA* 1992; 268:2069–2073.

236. Dodds GA, Sexton DJ, Durack DT, Bashore TM, Corey GR, Kisslo J. Negative predictive value of the Duke criteria for infective endocarditis. *Am J Cardiol* 1996; 77:403–407.

237. Kaye MM, Kaye D. Laboratory findings including blood cultures. In: Kaye D, ed. *Infective Endocarditis*, 2d ed. New York: Raven Press; 1992:117–124.

238. Powers DL, Mandell GL. Intraleukocytic bacteria in endocarditis patients. *JAMA* 1974; 227:312–313.

239. Engle RL, Koprowska I. The appearance of histiocytes in blood in subacute bacterial endocarditis. *Am J Med* 1959; 26:965–973.

240. Fournier PE, Casalta JP, Habib G, Messana T, Raoult D. Modification of the diagnostic criteria proposed by the Duke Endocarditis Service to permit improved diagnosis of Q fever endocarditis. *Am J Med* 1996; 100:629–633.

241. Belli J, Waisbren BA. The number of blood cultures necessary to diagnose most cases of bacterial endocarditis. *Am J Med Sci* 1956; 232:284–288.

242. Werner AS, Cobbs CG, Kaye D, Hook EW. Studies on the bacteremia of bacterial endocarditis. *JAMA* 1967; 202:127–131.

243. Ellner JJ, Rosenthal MS, Lerner PI, McHenry M. Infective endocarditis caused by slow-growing, fastidious, gram-negative bacteria. *Medicine* 1979; 58:145–158.

244. Gerry JL, Greenough WB. Diphtheroid endocarditis: Report of nine cases and review of the literature. *Johns Hopkins Med J* 1976; 139:61–68.

245. Stewart JA, Silimperi D, Harris P, Wise NK, Fraker TD Jr, Kisslo JA. Echocardiographic documentation of vegetative lesions in infective endocarditis: Clinical implications. *Circulation* 1980; 61:374–380.

246. Mugge A, Daniel WG, Frank G, Lichtlen PR. Echocardiography in infective endocarditis: Reassessment of prognostic implications of vegetation size determined by the transthoracic and transesophageal approach. *J Am Coll Cardiol* 1989; 14:631–638.

247. Pavlides GS, Hauser AM, Stewart JR, O'Neill WW, Timmis GC. Contribution of transesophageal echocardiography to patient diagnosis and treatment: A prospective analysis. *Am Heart J* 1990; 120:910–914.

248. Daniel WG, Mugge A, Martin RP, Lindert O, Hausmann D, Nonnast-Daniel B, et al. Improvement in the diagnosis of abscesses associated with endocarditis by transesophageal echocardiography. *N Engl J Med* 1991; 324:795–800.

249. Dodds GAI, Durack DT. Criteria for the diagnosis of endocarditis and the role of echocardiography. *Echocardiography* 1995; 12:663–668.

250. Morguet AJ, Werner GS, Andreas S, Kreuzer H. Diagnostic value of transesophageal compared with transthoracic echocardiography in suspected prosthetic valve endocarditis. *Herz* 1995; 20:390–398.

251. Lindner JR, Case RA, Dent JM, Abbott RD, Scheld WM, Kaul S. Diagnostic value of echocardiography in suspected endocarditis: An evaluation based on the pretest probability of disease. *Circulation* 1996; 93:730–736.

252. Gillinov AM, Shah RV, Curtis WE, Stuart RS, Cameron DE, Baumgartner WA, et al. Valve replacement in patients with endocarditis and acute neurologic deficit. *Ann Thorac Surg* 1996; 61:1125–1129.

253. Moriarty JA, Edelman RR, Tumeh SS. CT and MRI of mycotic aneurysms of the abdominal aorta. *J Comput Assist Tomogr* 1992; 16:941–943.

254. Welton DE, Young JB, Raizner AE, Ishimori T, Adyanthaya A, Mattox KL, et al. Value and safety of cardiac catheterization during active infective endocarditis. *Am J Cardiol* 1979; 44:1306–1310.

255. Riba AL, Thakur ML, Gottschalk A, Andriole VT, Zaret BL. Imaging experimental infective endocarditis with indium-111–labeled blood cellular components. *Circulation* 1979; 59:336–343.

256. Ben-Haim S, Seabold JE, Hawes DR, Rooholamini SA. Leukocyte scintigraphy in the diagnosis of mycotic aneurysm. *J Nuc Med* 1992; 33:1486–1493.

257. Wilson WR, Karchmer A, Dajani A, Taubert K, Bayer A, Kaye D, et al. Antibiotic treatment of adults with infective endocarditis due to viridans streptococci, enterococci, staphylococci and HACEK microorganisms. *JAMA* 1995; 274:1706–1713.

258. Chambers HF, Miller RT, Newman MD. Right-sided *Staphylococcus aureus* endocarditis in intravenous drug abusers: Two-week combination therapy. *Ann Intern Med* 1988; 109:619–624.

259. Wilson WR, Geraci JE, Wilkowske CJ, Washington JA. Short-term intramuscular therapy with procaine penicillin plus streptomycin for infective endocarditis due to *Viridans* streptococci. *Circulation* 1978; 57:1158–1161.

260. Baldassare JS, Kaye D. Principles and overview of antibiotic therapy. In: Kaye D, ed. *Infective Endocarditis*. 2d ed. New York: Raven Press; 1992:169–190.

261. Blount JG. Bacterial endocarditis. *Am J Med* 1965; 38:909–922.

262. Pulliam L, Inokuchi S, Hadley WK, Mills J. Penicillin tolerance in experimental streptococcal endocarditis. *Lancet* 1979; 2:957.

263. Denny AE, Peterson LR, Gerding DN, Hall WH. Serious staphylococcal infections with strains tolerant to bactericidal antibiotics. *Arch Intern Med* 1979; 139:1026–1031.

264. Brennan RO, Durack DT. Therapeutic significance of penicillin tolerance in experimental streptococcal endocarditis. *Antimicrob Agents Chemother* 1983; 23:273–277.

265. Reller LB. The serum bactericidal test. *Rev Infect Dis* 1986; 8:803–808.

266. Kane LW, Finn JJ. The treatment of subacute bacterial endocarditis with aureomycin and chloromycetin. *N Engl J Med* 1951; 244:623–628.

267. Schein J, Baehr G. Sulfonamide therapy of subacute bacterial endocarditis. *Am J Med* 1948; 4:66–72.

268. Korzeniowski O, Sande MA, National Collaborative Endocarditis Study Group. Combination antimicrobial therapy for *Staphylococcus aureus* endocarditis in patients addicted to parenteral drugs and in nonaddicts: A prospective study. *Ann Intern Med* 1982; 97:496–503.

269. Martinez F, Martin-Luengo F, Garcia A, Valdes M. Treatment with various antibiotics of experimental endocarditis caused by penicillin-resistant *Streptococcus sanguis*. *Eur Heart J* 1995; 16:687–691.

270. Doern GV, Ferraro MJ, Brueggmann AB, Ruoff KL. Emergence of high rates of antimicrobial resistance among viridans group streptococci in the United States. *Antimicrob Agents Chemother* 1996; 40:891–894.

271. Brandt CM, Rouse MS, Laue NW, Stratton CW, Wilson WR, Steckelberg JM. Effective treatment of multidrug-resistant enterococcal experimental endocarditis with combinations of cell wall-active agents. *J Infect Dis* 1996; 173:909–913.

272. Francioli P, Etienne J, Hoigne R, Thys J, Gerber A. Treatment of streptococcal endocarditis with a single daily dose of ceftriaxone sodium for 4 weeks: Efficacy and outpatient treatment feasibility. *JAMA* 1992; 267:264–267.

273. Stamboulian D, Bonvehi P, Arevalo C, Bologna R, Cassetti I, Scilingo V, et al. Antibiotic management of outpatients with endocarditis due to penicillin-susceptible streptococci. *Rev Infect Dis* 1991; 13:S160–S163.

274. Aranki SF, Adams DH, Rizzo RJ, Couper GS, Sullivan TE, Collins JJ Jr, et al. Determinants of early mortality and late survival in mitral valve endocarditis. *Circulation* 1995; 92:143–149.

275. Douglas JL, Dismukes WE. Surgical therapy of infective endocarditis on natural valves. In: Kaye D, ed. *Infective Endocarditis*, 2d ed. New York: Raven Press; 1992:397–411.

276. Durack DT. Nine controversies in the management of endocarditis. In: Petersdorf RG, ed. *Update V: Harrison's Principles of Internal Medicine*. New York: McGraw-Hill; 1984:35–45.

277. Vlessis AA, Hovaguimian H, Jaggers J, Ahmad A, Starr A. Infective endocarditis: Ten year review of medical and surgical therapy. *Ann Thorac Surg* 1996; 61:1217–1222.

278. Muehrcke D, Lytle BW, Cosgrove DM III. Surgical and long-term antifungal therapy for fungal prosthetic valve endocarditis. *Ann Thorac Surg* 1996; 60:538–543.

279. Glazier JJ, Verwilghen J, Donaldson RM, Ross DN. Treatment of complicated prosthetic aortic valve endocarditis with annular abscess formation by homograft aortic root replacement. *J Am Coll Cardiol* 1991; 17:1177–1182.

280. Joyce F, Tingleff J, Pettersson G. Expanding indications for the Ross operation. *J Heart Valve Dis* 1995; 4:352–363.

281. Joyce F, Tingleff J, Pettersson G. The Ross operation: Results of early experience including treatment for endocarditis. *Eur J Cardiothorac Surg* 1989; 9:384–392.

282. Hughes CF, Noble N. Vegetectomy: An alternative surgical treatment for infective endocarditis of the atrioventricular valves in drug addicts. *J Thorac Cardiovasc Surg* 1988; 95:857–861.

283. Katz LN, Elek SR. Combined heparin and chemotherapy in subacute bacterial endocarditis. *JAMA* 1944; 124:149–152.

284. Wilson WR, Geraci JE, Danielson GK, Thompson RL, Spittell JA Jr, Washington JA II, et al. Anticoagulant therapy and central nervous system complications in patients with prosthetic valve endocarditis. *Circulation* 1978; 57:1004–1007.

285. Kanis JA. The use of anticoagulants in bacterial endocarditis. *Postgrad Med J* 1974; 50:312–313.

286. Nicolau DP, Marangos MN, Nightingale CH, Quintiliani R. Influence of aspirin on development and treatment of experimental *Staphylococcus aureus* endocarditis. *Antimicrob Agents Chemother* 1995; 39:1748–1751.

287. Steckelberg JM, Murphy JG, Ballard D, Bailey K, Tajik AJ, Taliercio CP, et al. Emboli in infective endocarditis: The prognostic value of echocardiography. *Ann Intern Med* 1991; 114:635–640.

288. Ahern H. Cellular responses to oxidative stress: Extensively studied bacterial systems provide insights into more complex systems and, potentially, human diseases. *ASM News* 1991; 57:627–630.

289. Lu VL, Fang GD, Keys TF, Harris AA, Gentry LO, Fuchs PC, et al. Prosthetic valve endocarditis: Superiority of surgical valve replacement versus medical therapy only. *Ann Thorac Surg* 1994; 58:1073–1077.

290. Ormiston JA, Neutze JM, Agnew TM, Lowe JB, Kerr AR. Infective endocarditis: A lethal disease. *Aust NZ J Med* 1981; 11:620–629.

291. Welton DE, Young JB, Gentry WO, Raizner AE, Alexander JK, Chahine RA, et al. Recurrent infective endocarditis: Analysis of predisposing factors and clinical features. *Am J Med* 1979; 66:932–938.

292. Everett ED, Hirschmann JV. Transient bacteremia and endocarditis prophylaxis: A review. *Medicine* 1977; 56:61–77.

293. Sullivan NM, Sutter VL, Mims MM, Marsh VII, Fincgold SM. Clinical aspects of bacteremia after manipulation of the genitourinary tract. *J Infect Dis* 1973; 127:49–55.

294. Shorvon PJ, Eykyn SJ, Cotton PB. Gastrointestinal instrumentation, bacteraemia, and endocarditis. *Gut* 1983; 24:1078–1093.

295. Durack DT. Prevention of infective endocarditis. *N Engl J Med* 1995; 332:38–44.

296. Dajani AS, Taubert KA, Wilson WR, Bolger AF, Bayer A, Ferrieri P, et al. Prevention of bacterial endocarditis: Recommendations by the American Heart Association. *Circulation* 1997; 96:358–366. (JAMA 1997; 277:1794–1801)

297. Glauser MP, Francioli P. Relevance of animal models to the prophylaxis of infective endocarditis. *J Antimicrob Chemother* 1987; 20(suppl A):87–93.

298. Horstkotte D, Friedrichs W, Pippert H, Bircks W, Loogen F. Nutzen der Endokarditisprophylaxe bei Patienten mit prothetischen Herzklappen. *Z Kardiol* 1986; 75:8–11.

299. van der Meer JTM, Van Wijk W, Thompson J, Vandenbroucke JP, Valkenburg HA, Michel MF. Efficacy of antibiotic prophylaxis for prevention of native-valve endocarditis. *Lancet* 1992; 339:135–140.

300. Imperiale TF, Horwitz RI. Does prophylaxis prevent postdental infective endocarditis? A controlled evaluation of protective efficacy. *Am J Med* 1990; 88:131–136.

301. Gould IM, Buckingham JK. Cost effectiveness of prophylaxis in dental practice to prevent infective endocarditis. *Br Heart J* 1993; 70:79–83.

THIRTEEN

THE HEART, ANESTHESIA, AND SURGERY

83

PERIOPERATIVE EVALUATION AND MANAGEMENT OF PATIENTS WITH KNOWN OR SUSPECTED CARDIOVASCULAR DISEASE WHO UNDERGO NONCARDIAC SURGERY

Robert C. Schlant / Kim A. Eagle

EPIDEMIOLOGY

It is estimated that in the United States each year approximately 25 million patients have noncardiac surgery, approximately 50,000 have perioperative myocardial infarction, and more than half of 40,000 deaths are caused by cardiac events.[1–3] The number of cardiac surgeries annually exceeds 400,000, including 285,000 coronary artery bypass surgical procedures and 40,000 valve replacements.[3] As indicated in Fig. 83-1, a significant number of the 25 million patients have previously diagnosed coronary artery disease (CAD), another 2 to 3 million have two or more major risk factors for CAD (Chap. 41), and 4 million are over the age of 65. More than 25 percent of the surgical procedures are major procedures, and of patients undergoing major vascular surgery who do not have clinically evident CAD, 40 to 70 percent have been shown to have CAD at coronary arteriography.[4,5] In future years, the number of surgical patients over 65 years of age will rise, further increasing the number of noncardiac patients at risk for perioperative cardiac morbidity (PCM), which includes myocardial infarction (MI), unstable angina pectoris, congestive heart failure (CHF), serious arrhythmia, or cardiac death.[1,6–9]

PATIENTS WITH KNOWN CARDIAC DISEASE

Coronary Artery Disease

Patients with CAD have a perioperative rate of myocardial infarction after noncardiac surgery of 1.1 percent,[10] compared with a rate of 0 to 0.7 percent in the general population.[1] The reported rates of reinfarction in patients with prior MI vary overall from 5 to 8 percent: from 1 to 15 percent following vascular surgery and from 6 to 40 percent in patients with a recent MI[8] (see below). One study reported a reinfarction rate of 1.9 percent, which increased to 5.7 percent if the prior infarction occurred less than 3 months previously.[11] The risk of postoperative MI in patients with prior coronary artery revascularization has been reported to be only 0 to 1.2 percent.[8] Of significance, the mortality following a perioperative MI is higher than following a nonoperative MI (Chap. 47) and has been reported to range from 23 to 70 percent, with an average of 50 percent.[12–15] Most perioperative infarctions occur within the first 4 postoperative days and are usually clinically silent, although they are often associated with ST-segment changes in the preceding 3 to 6 h.[1,6–8] In some

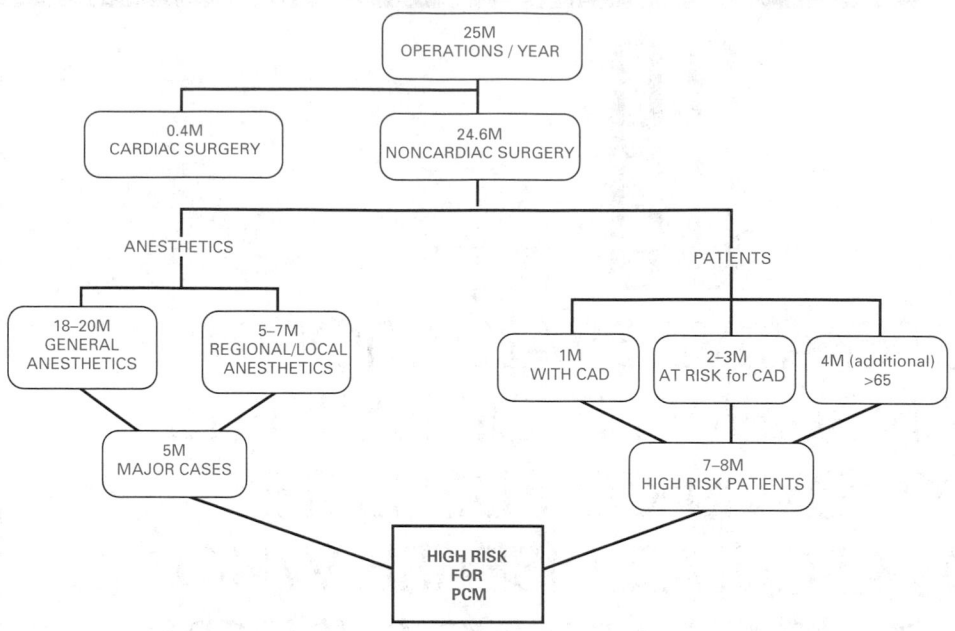

FIGURE 83-1

Estimates of the number of surgeries and anesthetics, and the patients at risk for perioperative cardiac morbidity (PCM) in the United States (1988). A total of 6 million (30 percent) surgical patients are over the age of 65. Two million of these are included in the groups with CAD and at risk for CAD, resulting in the 4 million over age 65 (and the 7 to 8 million total) shown in the figure. (Sources: National Center for Health Statistics, U.S. Public Health Service, Department of Health and Human Services; the American College of Surgeons; and the American Society of Anesthesiologists; from Mangano.[1] Reproduced with permission from the publisher and author.)

studies, non-Q-wave infarctions tended to occur in the first 2 days, whereas Q-wave infarctions tended to occur on postoperative days 2 to 4.[1,14,16–18]

Previous Myocardial Infarction

A recent (<6 months) myocardial infarction is one of two consistently proven preoperative predictors of PCM.[8] Patients with a documented history of MI have a perioperative risk of about 6 percent (range, 2.8 to 17.7 percent) of having a recurrent perioperative MI.[14] Two studies of the influence of a preceding MI on the likelihood of having a recurrent perioperative infarction during noncardiac surgery have been performed at the Mayo Clinic, covering the years 1967 to 1968[16] and the years 1974 to 1975.[19] During 1974 and 1975, the risk of perioperative reinfarction was 27 percent if the surgery was performed less than 3 months after an MI, 11 percent in patients operated upon between 3 and 6 months post-MI, and 4 to 5 percent if the surgery was more than 6 months post-MI.[17] Subsequently, Rao, et al.[11] found that reinfarction occurred in only 1.9 percent overall of patients with a history of MI, in only 5.7 percent of patients operated on less than 3 months post-MI, and in 2.3 percent of patients operated on within 4 to 6 months post-MI. They attributed this improvement to more intensive perioperative care, including use of intraarterial and pulmonary artery monitoring. Another possibility is that the early risk stratification and management of

patients following MI was improved. This may also explain why in the Coronary Artery Surgery Study (CASS) Registry, a history of MI, including MI within 6 months, did not have a statistically significant association with increased cardiac mortality or morbidity.[20]

Systemic Arterial Hypertension

Systemic arterial hypertension (SAH) is the most common cardiovascular disease in the United States, affecting more than 59 million patients.[3] It is a risk factor for CAD, CHF, stroke, and peripheral vascular disease. Some studies have indicated that untreated or poorly controlled SAH is associated with an increased incidence of perioperative myocardial ischemia, arrhythmias, and transient neurologic symptoms, although other studies have indicated that mild-to-moderate hypertension is only an intermediate risk factor for blood pressure lability and myocardial ischemia. While the influence of SAH upon perioperative risk has been poorly studied, the guidelines recently published by the American College of Cardiology/American Heart Association (ACC/AHA)[21] suggested that diastolic pressure above 110 mmHg is a reasonable cutoff to indicate a level of hypertension that should be controlled prior to embarking on elective noncardiac surgery. The availability of effective intravenous forms of beta blockers, calcium channel blockers, and angiotensin-converting enzyme (ACE) inhibitors makes rapid control of severe hypertension far less formidable than in the past. Whenever possible, SAH should be controlled prior to surgery and antihypertensive medications continued up to, during, and following surgery. Special care should be taken to avoid a rebound phenomenon with increased blood pressure and tachycardia, which can occur if therapy is not continued with clonidine or, occasionally, a beta blocker (see also Chap. 58).

Valvular Heart Disease

Patients with valvular heart disease should have antibiotic prophylaxis (Chap. 82) prior to surgery that is likely to be associated with bacteremia. Patients who are on chronic anticoagulant therapy with warfarin for a prosthetic heart valve or atrial fibrillation should have the warfarin discontinued approximately 4 to 5 days prior to elective surgery and should have a near normal international normalized ratio (INR) prior to surgery.[22] If the INR is 1.8 or higher, one may give 1 mg vitamin K_1 subcutaneously (see also Chap. 68). In patients with a prosthetic heart valve and a history of arterial embolism, intravenous heparin therapy should be begun when warfarin is discontinued and the dosage adjusted to maintain the partial thromboplastin time at 1.5 to 2.0 times the control value. The effect of heparin should be reversed by intravenous protamine sulfate immediately prior to surgery. Postoperatively, heparin and warfarin are started when there is no evidence or risk of bleeding. The heparin is discontinued when the INR is within the therapeutic range (see Chap. 52). In emergency situations, the effect of oral anticoagulants such as warfarin can be reversed by intravenous vitamin K_1 in doses of 10 to 25 mg; however, large doses of vitamin K_1 will often delay the anticoagulant effects of warfarin when it is reinstated postoperatively. In patients who do not respond to vitamin K_1, fresh frozen plasma should be given.

Patients with severe, symptomatic aortic stenosis are at substantial risk for perioperative congestive heart failure and/or death. Most such patients should have aortic valve replacement prior to elective noncardiac surgery. Rarely, either because they are not operative candidates for valve surgery or because the noncardiac operation is deemed urgent or emergent, such patients are treated with percutaneous aortic valvuloplasty prior to the noncardiac surgery (see also Chap. 63). Patients with moderately severe but asymptomatic aortic stenosis can undergo noncardiac surgery with acceptable risk; however, careful hemodynamic monitoring perioperatively is important in such patients.

Mitral stenosis involves an increased risk of perioperative congestive heart failure, particularly if rapid atrial fibrillation develops during or following surgery. Rate control, effective diuresis, and—for very fragile patients—hemodynamic monitoring are important (see also Chap. 64).

Aortic valve and mitral valve regurgitation are usually well tolerated postoperatively. Efforts to maintain proper fluid balance with diuresis and the use of afterload-reducing agents are helpful. The occasional patient with severe mitral regurgitation and borderline normal or frankly diminished left ventricular function is at substantial risk for perioperative congestive heart failure and requires special attention (see also Chap. 84).

Congestive Heart Failure

Postoperative CHF occurred in 3.6 percent of patients older than 40 years with or without CAD[14] and in 4.8 percent of patients with a history of previous MI.[11] A history of dysrhythmias or diabetes mellitus is also associated with an increased risk of postoperative CHF.[6,10,16,23,24]

Current CHF is the second consistently proven preoperative predictor of PCM.[8,10] It is important to understand the cause of CHF, particularly since diastolic dysfunction, which is the primary problem in as many as one-third of patients with heart failure, requires special attention (see also Chap. 23).

In general, patients with a moderately to severely dilated left ventricle and CHF should be treated with triple therapy, i.e., with a diuretic, an ACE inhibitor, and digoxin to optimize the symptoms and signs of CHF prior to surgery. Therapy should be given preoperatively and continued intraoperatively and postoperatively. When possible, attempts should be made to correct the hemodynamic disturbance and congestion resulting from the CHF prior to surgery. Special care should be taken to avoid hypokalemia, hypomagnesemia, excess depletion of blood volume, and excess digitalis (see also Chap. 23).

Patients without known CHF who have not been on therapy but who are found preoperatively to have moderate or marked cardiomegaly on chest film and/or decreased left ventricular function by echocardiography are more difficult to manage. In such patients, it is usually advisable to initiate therapy with an ACE inhibitor and to administer diuretics preoperatively only if there is evidence of peripheral edema on physical examination or pulmonary congestion on chest film. In this situation, digoxin is usually not given prophylactically unless the left ventricular ejection fraction is below about 40 percent, particularly if there is also evidence of edema, increased jugular venous pressure, and an S_3 gallop. If digoxin is used, it should be initiated several days prior to surgery whenever possible. In emergencies, cautious initiation of digitalis treatment can be begun preoperatively and completed postoperatively. Intra- and perioperative inotropic support can be provided in severe heart failure with intravenous dobutamine and/or milrinone (see also Chap. 84).

For patients with severe diastolic heart failure, the judicious use of diuretics to decrease congestion and beta blockers and/or calcium channel blocking agents to slow the heart rate and increase diastolic filling time are often indicated. The rare patient with hypertrophic cardiomyopathy, with or without obstruction, may have a particularly fragile hemodynamic status. Studies have shown that with careful perioperative therapy and monitoring, such patients can undergo noncardiac surgery with low risk.[25]

Congenital Heart Disease

Most patients with congenital heart disease should receive prophylactic antibiotic therapy against endocarditis when undergoing surgery that might be associated with bacteremia (see Chap. 82). Two groups of patients who may not require prophylaxis are those who have had a patent ductus arteriosus ligated and divided and those who have had an isolated ostium secundum atrial septal defect repaired more than 6 months previously. Patients with cyanotic heart disease are at increased risk of vascular thrombosis and postoperative bleeding. If their hematocrit is greater than 65 percent, such patients should undergo cautious preoperative phlebotomy with replacement of the blood volume. If possible, they should receive their own plasma back as part of the replacement fluid (see Chaps. 70 and 71).

Arrhythmia and Conduction Disorders

A history of a cardiac arrhythmia is associated with an increased likelihood of postoperative CHF.[1,10,16,23,24]

About 60 percent of all patients who have perioperative arrhythmias, most of which require no therapy. Patients who have premature atrial or junctional beats usually do not require therapy. Preoperatively, if such beats are very frequent and symptomatic and if there is adequate time, the use of a beta blocker or digoxin may be considered. Patients with frequent premature ventricular contractions (PVCs) (e.g., >5 per minute) have been shown to be at increased risk for perioperative cardiac events.[23] Much if not all of this risk is likely attributable to underlying coronary, myocardial, or valvular heart disease. Good principles in such patients are to treat maximally any known underlying heart disease, to ensure that the patient is metabolically optimized (e.g., normal K^+, Mg^{2+}), and to treat the arrhythmia itself only if symptoms or hemodynamic abnormalities occur. *Routine suppression of PVCs with lidocaine or other agents is likely not to improve outcome and, in fact, could conceivably increase the risk of more dangerous arrhythmias or asystole.*

Adults undergoing emergency surgery who have supraventricular tachyarrhythmias should be considered for either electrical conversion (Chap. 32) or rate control employing intravenous digoxin, beta blocker, verapamil, or diltiazem (see Chap. 27).

Patients with a history of Stokes-Adams attacks, complete heart block, high-degree Möbitz II atrioventricular heart block, or prolonged sinoatrial pause or block should be considered for a prophylactic temporary right heart pacemaker (see Chap. 34). Patients with asymptomatic bifascicular block (left or right bundle branch block with left anterior or posterior fascicular block) with or without prolongation of the PR interval usually do not require a prophylactic pacemaker prior to surgery, although a pacing catheter should be readily available in the operating room. If a patient with left bundle branch block requires the insertion of a pulmonary artery balloon (Swan-Ganz) catheter to monitor pressures during surgery, it is advisable to use a multipurpose catheter that permits atrial, ventricular, and atrioventricular sequential pacing (see Chap. 34).

Patients with a permanent pacemaker rarely have intraoperative pacemaker failure. When failure does occur, it may be due to electrolyte abnormalities, particularly potassium, or to myocardial ischemia and infarction. Rarely, pacemaker dysfunction may be related to use of an electrocautery. Automatic implantable cardioverter-defibrillator (ICD) units can also be temporarily or permanently inhibited by electromagnetic interference from an electrocautery. During electrocautery surgery, the electrosurgical tip and the ground plate should be as far away as possible from the pacemaker or ICD, and electrosurgery should be limited to 2- to 3-s periods if any pacemaker suppression is produced (see also Chap. 34).

Pulmonary Embolism

Patients with an increased risk of postoperative venous thromboembolism often need prophylactic measures to decrease the likelihood of such complications. Factors associated with increased risk include advanced age, prolonged immobility or paralysis, prior venous thromboembolism, malignancy, major surgery (particularly surgery involving the abdomen, pelvis, or lower extremities), obesity, varicose veins, congenital or acquired aberrations of hemostatic mechanisms (hypercoagulable states), and possibly high estrogen use.[26]

The choice of prophylactic measure or agent depends upon the type of surgery planned and the risk of venous thromboembolism. The choices include graded compression elastic stockings (ES), subcutaneous low-dose unfractionated heparin (LDUH), low molecular weight heparin (LMWH), and intermittent pneumatic compression (IPC) (see also Chap. 60 and Table 60-2).

In patients who are older than 40 years, who are undergoing major, moderate-risk general surgery, and who have no additional risk factors for thromboembolism, graded compression ES, LDUH (given 2 h before and every 12 h after operation), or IPC may be used. During operation and throughout the postoperative period, ES and IPC should be applied if possible. Patients who have additional risk factors should be given either LMWH or LDUH every 8 h. General surgery patients at very high risk should be given LDUH, LMWH, or dextran in addition to IPC. The LDUH and LMWH therapy should be started preoperatively and the dextran given intraoperatively. In selected very high risk general surgery patients, perioperative warfarin (INR, 2.0 to 3.0) may be used. Aspirin is not recommended for venous prophylaxis in general surgery patients. Patients undergoing total knee replacement should receive either LMWH subcutaneously every 12 h or IPC. Patients undergoing hip fracture surgery can be treated with either preoperative subcutaneous fixed-dose unmonitored LMWH or oral warfarin (INR, 2.0 to 3.0). In patients undergoing intracranial neurosurgery, IPC with or without ES may be used. In extremely high risk patients, one should consider the prophylactic insertion of a filter in the inferior vena cava.[26]

Diabetes Mellitus

Diabetes mellitus is a well-known risk factor for coronary atherosclerosis[27–32] (see Chaps. 41 and 78). Patients with diabetes are more likely to have asymptomatic or silent ischemia than other patients, possibly because of altered neural pain pathways in the heart. Diabetes is also associated with an increased risk of postoperative CHF.[6,16,20,23–25]

PREOPERATIVE EVALUATION OF PATIENTS WITH UNKNOWN OR SUSPECTED CARDIAC DISEASE

The two major conditions that are responsible for most perioperative cardiac morbidity and that should be especially carefully evaluated preoperatively are CAD and left ventricular dysfunction.[33–41] Several multivariate indexes of risk have been developed in an attempt to quantify the risk preoperatively. These include the factors in the Dripps–American Soci-

TABLE 83-1

THE DRIPPS-AMERICAN SOCIETY OF ANESTHESIOLOGISTS CLASSIFICATION OF PHYSICAL STATUS

1. A normal healthy patient
2. A patient with a mild systemic disease
3. A patient with a severe systemic disease that limits activity but is not incapacitating
4. A patient with an incapacitating systemic disease that is a constant threat to life
5. A moribund patient not expected to survive 24 h with or without operation

Note: In the event of emergency operation, precede the number with an E.
Source: American Society of Anesthesiologists.[42] Reproduced with permission from the publisher.

ety of Anesthesiologists (AST) classification of physical status (Table 83-1)[42] and the Goldman cardiac risk index (Table 83-2)[23,24] The clinical validity of Goldman's risk index has been confirmed by many but not all investigations.[8,34,43] Detsky et al. developed a modified risk index (Table 83-3).[44,45] At present, however, there is no consistently accurate preoperative risk index that is generally applicable and widely utilized. Such risk indexes, however, do provide useful guidelines for the identification of patients at increased risk during noncardiac surgery.

The recent ACC/AHA Guidelines for the perioperative cardiovascular evaluation for noncardiac surgery[21] provide a stepwise algorithm for clinicians that emphasizes clinical markers of risk, functional status, surgery-specific considerations, and selected use of noninvasive and invasive tests (Fig. 83-2).[21] The clinical predictors of increased perioperative cardiovascular risk are shown in Table 83-4 and the cardiac risk of various noncardiac surgical procedures is shown in Table 83-5. The greatest risk is found in patients with recent unstable coronary syndromes, advanced or poorly controlled CHF, or symptomatic arrhythmias.[40] Immediate-risk predictors include diabetes mellitus, mild stable angina, prior MI, and compensated or prior stable CHF.

The following steps and questions correspond to the algorithm in Fig. 83-2:

Step 1. What is the urgency of noncardiac surgery?
Step 2. Has the patient undergone coronary revascularization in the past 5 years?
Step 3. Has the patient had a coronary evaluation in the past 2 years?
Step 4. Does the patient have an unstable coronary syndrome or a major clinical predictor of risk?
Step 5. Does the patient have intermediate clinical predictors of risk?
Step 6. Patients without major but with intermediate predictors of clinical risk and moderate or excellent functional capacity can generally undergo intermediate-risk surgery with little likelihood of perioperative MI or death. Conversely, additional noninvasive testing is often considered for pa-

TABLE 83-2

THE GOLDMAN MULTIFACTORIAL CARDIAC RISK INDEX

Criteria	Multivariate Discriminant-Function Coefficient	Points
1. History		
Age >70 years	0.191	5
MI in previous 6 months	0.384	10
2. Physical examination		
S_3 gallop or JVD	0.451	11
Important VAS	0.119	3
3. Electrocardiogram		
Rhythm other than sinus or PACs on last preoperative ECG	0.283	7
>5 PVCs/min documented at any time before operation	0.278	7
4. General status		
P_{O_2} <60 or P_{CO_2} >50 mmHg, K<3.0 or HCO_3^- <20 meq/L, BUN >50 or Cr >3.0 mg/dL, abnormal SGOT, signs of chronic liver disease or patient bedridden from noncardiac causes	0.132	3
5. Operation		
Intraperitoneal, intrathoracic, or aortic operation	0.123	3
Emergency operation	0.167	4
Total		53

Key: MI = myocardial infarction; JVD = jugular-vein distention; VAS = valvular aortic stenosis; PAC = premature atrial contractions; ECG = electrocardiogram; PVC = premature ventricular contractions; P_{O_2} = partial pressure of oxygen; P_{CO_2} = partial pressure of carbon dioxide; K = potassium; HCO_3 = bicarbonate; BUN = blood urea nitrogen; Cr = creatinine; SGOT = serum glutamic oxaloacetic transaminase.
Source: Goldman L et al.[24] Reproduced with permission from the publisher and authors.

tients with poor functional capacity prior to moderate-risk elective and especially for patients with two or more intermediate predictors.

Step 7. Noncardiac surgery is generally safe for patients with neither major nor intermediate predictors of clinical risk and moderate or excellent functional capacity [four metabolic equivalents (METS) or greater]. Further testing may be indicated on an individual basis for patients without clinical indicators but with poor functional capacity who are facing higher-risk operations, especially patients with several minor predictors of risk who are to undergo vascular surgery.

Step 8. The results of noninvasive testing can be used to determine further perioperative management.

TABLE 83-3

THE MODIFIED MULTIFACTORIAL CARDIAC RISK INDEX

Variables	Points
CAD	
MI within 6 months	10
MI more than 6 months previously	5
Canadian Cardiovascular Society angina	
Class 3	10
Class 4	20
Unstable angina within 3 months	10
Alveolar pulmonary edema	
Within 1 week	10
Ever	5
Valvular disease	
Suspected critical aortic stenosis	20
Arrhythmias	
Sinus plus atrial premature beats or rhythm other than sinus on last preoperative ECG	5
More than 5 ventricular premature beats at any time before surgery	5
Poor general medical status[a]	5
Age over 70 years	5
Emergency operation	10

[a] Oxygen pressure <60 mmHg; carbon dioxide pressure >50 mmHg; serum potassium <3.0 meq/L (<3.0 mmol/L); serum bicarbonate < 20 meq/L (<20 mmol/L); serum urea nitrogen >50 mg/dL (>18 mmol/L); serum creatinine >3 mg/dL (>260 mmol/L); aspartate aminotransferase, abnormal; signs of chronic liver disease; and/or bedridden because of noncardiac causes.

Source: Detsky AS et al.[45] Reproduced with permission from the publisher and authors.

In most patients, preoperative risk stratification should include specific tests only if the results are likely to influence patient management. For example, most patients with lower extremity ischemic pain at rest from peripheral vascular disease and most patients with possible carcinoma in whom the chance of surgical cure would be decreased by delay do not require testing for coronary artery disease. *Preoperative testing should be limited to circumstances in which the results will affect patient treatment and results. Coronary revascularization before noncardiac surgery to enable the patient to "get through" the noncardiac procedure is appropriate for only a small subset of patients at very high risk.*

Age

Although the data supporting or refuting the predictive value of age is controversial, perioperative MI is the leading cause of postoperative death in the elderly undergoing noncardiac surgery.[1,8,14]

Twelve-Lead Electrocardiogram

A preoperative 12-lead electrocardiogram (ECG) should be obtained routinely in patients over the age of 40 and in younger patients who have increased risk factors for cardiovascular disease. While the possibility of detecting a previously undiagnosed MI is relatively low, perhaps in only 3 to 4 percent of adults,[46] the ECG may detect significant hypertrophy, conduction abnormalities, or nonspecific ST-T wave changes; in addition, it is extremely valuable for comparison postoperatively should complications occur. A preoperative ECG is also indicated in patients undergoing emergency operations; patients with conditions that can be associated with cardiac involvement; patients taking or about to receive noncardiac medications that are associated with cardiac toxicity or ECG alterations; patients at risk for major electrolyte disorders; and patients undergoing neurosurgery, intrathoracic surgery, or aortic surgery.

Chest Roentgenogram

A routine preoperative chest film in patients over the age of 40 is useful primarily as a baseline for comparison with postoperative films when the patient may have complications such as pneumonia, atelectasis, or pulmonary embolism. In addition, cardiomegaly on chest film can be the first sign of decreased left ventricular function. In patients with CAD, cardiomegaly on a 6-f (2-m) chest film indicates an ejection fraction of less than 0.40 in over 70 percent of patients.[46] The presence of a tortuous or calcified aorta may also be a predictor of increased operative risk.[47]

Exercise Stress Testing

The effectiveness of routine preoperative exercise stress testing in identifying patients at increased risk is controversial.[1,8] A poor exercise functional capacity, especially in combination with ECG evidence of myocardial ischemia (Chap. 15), is associated with a significantly increased risk during noncardiac surgery[14] (see below).

The mean sensitivity and specificity of exercise testing for obstructive coronary disease is 66 and 77 percent, respectively. The sensitivity and specificity for multivessel disease is 81 and 66 percent, and for three-vessel or left main coronary disease, 86 and 53 percent.[21] In general, individuals who are able to exercise to moderate levels [4 to 6 METS or to a maximal heart rate of 100 to 130 beats per minute (70 to 85 percent age predicted) without ischemia should be considered at low risk for perioperative ischemic events.[21]

Radionuclide Angiography

In general, the resting left ventricular ejection fraction is a relatively insensitive and nonspecific predictor of perioperative cardiac complications. Similar conclusions apply to exercise radionuclide angiography (Chap. 17), although evidence of poor functional capacity does correlate with increased cardiac risk.[14]

Radionuclide Scintigraphy

Exercise radionuclide thallium scintigraphy (Chap. 17) is very effective for identifying patients at increased risk of periopera-

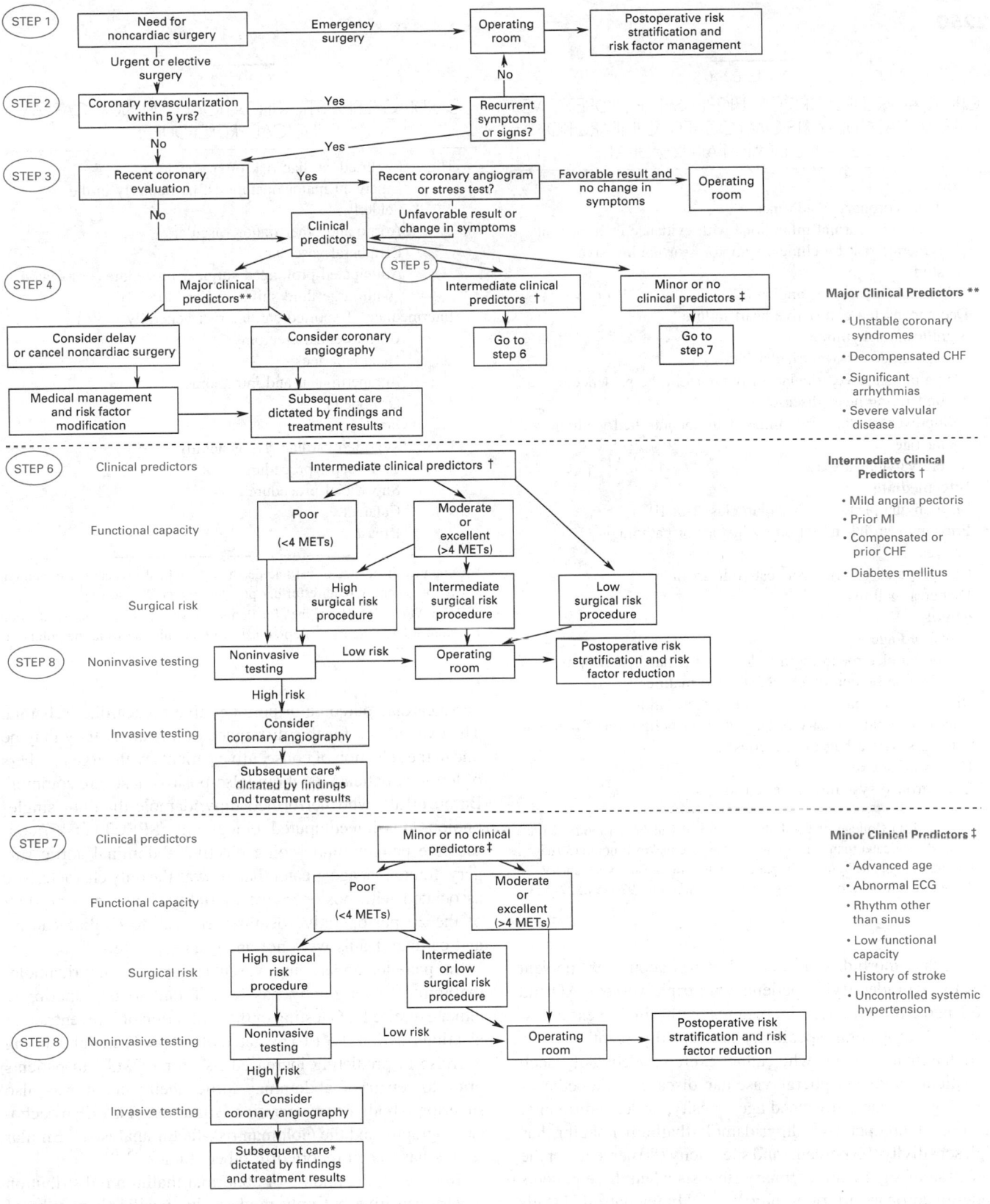

FIGURE 83-2

Stepwise approach to preoperative cardiac assessment. Steps are discussed in text.

*Subsequent care may include cancellation or delay of surgery, coronary revascularization followed by noncardiac surgery, or intensified care.

**Major clinical predictors: unstable coronary syndromes, decompensated CHF, significant arrhythmias, severe valvular disease.

† Intermediate clinical predictors: mild angina pectoris, prior MI, compensated or prior CHF, diabetes mellitus.

‡ Minor clinical predictors: advanced age, abnormal ECG, rhythm other than sinus, low functional capacity, history of stroke, uncontrolled systemic hypertension. (From the ACC/ACA Guidelines for Perioperative Cardiovascular Evaluation for Noncardiac Surgery.[21] Reproduced with permission from the publisher.)

TABLE 83-4

CLINICAL PREDICTORS OF INCREASED PERIOPERATIVE
CARDIOVASCULAR RISK (MYOCARDIAL INFARCTION,
CONGESTIVE HEART FAILURE, DEATH)

Major
Unstable coronary syndromes
Recent myocardial infarction[a] with evidence of important
ischemic risk by clinical symptoms or noninvasive
study
Unstable or severe[b] angina (Canadian class III or IV)[c]
Decompensated congestive heart failure
Significant arrhythmias
High-grade atrioventricular block
Symptomatic ventricular arrhythmias in the presence of
underlying heart disease
Supraventricular arrhythmias with uncontrolled ventricu-
lar rate
Severe valvular disease
Intermediate
Mild angina pectoris (Canadian class I or II)
Prior myocardial infarction by history or pathologic Q
waves
Compensated or prior congestive heart failure
Diabetes mellitus
Minor
Advanced age
Abnormal electrocardiogram (left ventricular hypertrophy,
left bundle branch block, ST-T abnormalities)
Rhythm other than sinus (e.g., atrial fibrillation)
Low functional capacity (e.g., inability to climb one flight
of stairs with a bag of groceries)
History of stroke
Uncontrolled systemic hypertension

[a] The American College of Cardiology National Database Library defines
recent MI as greater than 7 days but less than or equal to 1 month (30 days).
[b] May include "stable" angina in patients who are unusually sedentary.
[c] Campeau L. Grading of angina pectoris. *Circulation* 1976; 54:522–523.

TABLE 83-5

CARDIAC RISK[a] STRATIFICATION FOR NONCARDIAC
SURGICAL PROCEDURES

High (Reported cardiac risk often >5%)
Emergent major operations, particularly in the
elderly
Aortic and other major vascular
Peripheral vascular
Anticipated prolonged surgical procedures associated
with large fluid shifts and/or blood loss
Intermediate (Reported cardiac risk generally <5%)
Carotid endarterectomy
Head and neck
Intraperitoneal and intrathoracic
Orthopedic
Prostate
Low[b] (Reported cardiac risk generally <1%)
Endoscopic procedures
Superficial procedure
Cataract
Breast

[a] Combined incidence of cardiac death and nonfatal myocardial infarction.
[b] Do not generally require further preoperative cardiac testing.
Source: ACC/AHA Guidelines for Perioperative Cardiovascular Evaluation
for Noncardiac Surgery.[21] Reproduced with permission from the publisher.

tive cardiac morbidity. In general, it has about a 90 percent
sensitivity in identifying patients with triple-vessel CAD and
a 60 percent sensitivity in patients with single-vessel disease.[48–50] In general, specificity is over 90 percent.

In the many patients who cannot exercise adequately, such
as patients with peripheral vascular disease, orthopedic or
neurologic disease, advanced age, obesity, or deconditioning,
the use of preoperative dipyridamole-thallium imaging has
high sensitivity (93 percent) and specificity (80 percent) for the
detection of significant coronary stenosis when these patients
undergo coronary arteriography.[39,51–56] In uncontrolled studies of patients undergoing vascular surgery, preoperative dipyridamole-thallium or technetium-99m–sestamibi imaging
has an excellent sensitivity (89 to 100 percent) and a nearly
100 percent negative predictive value.[1,52,57–59] It is of particular value in selected patients who have stable angina pectoris,
a history of MI, or diabetes mellitus.[60,61] Mangano et al.[62]
found no association between redistribution defects and ad-

verse cardiac outcome or perioperative myocardial ischemia.
The explanation for this difference in the latter study may be
due to the selection of consecutive patients with large numbers
of low-risk patients in whom false-positive tests are common.
Baron et al., who performed dipyridamole-thallium single-
photon-emission computed tomography (SPECT) in 457 consecutive patients undergoing elective abdominal aortic surgery, found that age greater than 65 was the only characteristic
associated with postoperative mortality; however, only half
of the 20 postoperative deaths were due to cardiac causes,
and cardiac deaths were not analyzed separately.[54]

In patients undergoing vascular surgery, dipyridamole-
thallium[201] scintigraphy has been found to be superior to
either exercise ECG testing or the estimation of left ventricular
ejection fraction (LVEF) by gated blood pool scanning during
exercise in predicting increased risk for PCM.[63] In patients
prior to repair of abdominal aortic aneurysm, it was also
superior to both the preoperative estimation of LVEF by echocardiography and the Goldman risk-factor analysis.[64] Similar
results have been reported in other studies.[65–67]

In general, the finding of abnormal thallium redistribution
is very sensitive but only moderately specific. It may be of
great value in the preoperative evaluation of patients who are
scheduled for elective or semielective vascular or nonvascular
surgery and who have clinical markers of intermediate increased risk[14,60] (see Chap. 45) It also has value in predicting
long-term outcome.[68–70]

Dipyridamole-thallium testing can be associated with hypotension, which can be especially hazardous in patients with

severe carotid artery disease. Accordingly, special precautions should be taken in such patients to avoid hypotension, to correct it promptly should it occur, or to use an alternative stress test that does not severely depress blood pressure, such as dobutamine echocardiography.

It is apparent that there is a need for additional clinical trials to resolve the differences found in some studies of the predictive value and cost-effectiveness of thallium scintigraphy as a preoperative screening test, particularly in patients undergoing vascular surgery.[54,71]

Ambulatory (Continuous or Holter) Electrocardiography

Several studies have reported an increase in postoperative cardiac events in patients who have perioperative evidence of myocardial ischemia on ambulatory ECG (AECG) or Holter recordings.[6,7,72–75] On the other hand, one study found that adverse hospital outcomes were associated with evidence of myocardial ischemia on postoperative but not preoperative AECG monitoring.[76] Further studies are necessary to define better the cost-effectiveness of—and the most suitable patients for—preoperative AECG (see also Chap. 28).

Transthoracic Echocardiography

The prognostic value of preoperative transthoracic echocardiography (TTE) has not been well evaluated. It is likely to be useful to identify patients with ventricular dysfunction and/or segmental wall motion abnormalities, which have been shown to predict perioperative ventricular dysfunction when detected by radionuclide and angiographic techniques.[77,78]

Dobutamine stress echocardiography can be performed safely and with acceptable patient tolerance[59,79–84] It requires considerable operator skill, however, and the published experience is much less than that with exercise testing or intravenous dipyridamole myocardial perfusion imaging. In general, the negative predictive value has ranged from 93 to 100 percent. The predictive value of a positive test ranged from 7 to 23 percent for hard events (MI or death) and from 17 to 43 percent for all events. The degree of wall motion abnormality and/or wall motion change at low infusion rates of dobutamine appears to be especially important[21] (see also Chap. 14).

Transesophageal Echocardiography

Transesophageal echocardiography (TEE) is very useful for the early detection of intraoperative myocardial ischemia (see Chap. 14). In the future, it will likely be more widely used intraoperatively in selected high-risk patients; however, it is moderately expensive and labor-intensive.

Coronary Arteriography

Some groups had formerly recommended coronary arteriography as the routine screening test of choice for patients being considered for peripheral vascular surgery.[5,85,86] In the Cleveland Clinic experience,[4,5] severe, surgically correctable CAD

was found in 25 percent of the entire group and in 34 percent of patients clinically suspected of having CAD. Patients who have coronary artery bypass surgery for severe CAD discovered on coronary arteriography prior to vascular surgery have lower early mortality (1.5 versus 2 percent) and late mortality (12 versus 26 percent), with a higher 5-year survival rate (72 versus 43 percent). At this time, however, it is not clear whether or not preoperative coronary revascularization as a means to lower perioperative cardiac risk is justifiable.[14,18] This uncertainty relates to the significant mortality and morbidity caused by revascularization itself and the high costs associated with it.[87,88]

Such decisions are best made on an individual basis. *In patients undergoing elective aortic surgery, coronary revascularization is appropriate when the patient's symptoms and findings would themselves have been indications for coronary revascularization by either coronary angioplasty or surgery*[89] (see also Chaps. 50 and 98).

Intraoperative Use of Pulmonary Artery Catheters

The American Society of Anesthesiologists has published practice parameters for the use of pulmonary artery catheters during surgery.[90] In general, the decision is based upon three factors: the patient's condition and disease, the planned surgical procedure and anticipated intraoperative fluid shifts, and the practice setting. Catheters usually should be utilized in patients who are at risk from a major hemodynamic disturbance (for example, patients with left ventricular diastolic dysfunction, hypertrophic cardiomyopathy, severe mitral regurgitation, significant mitral or aortic stenosis) and those who are undergoing a surgical procedure likely to cause hemodynamic changes in a setting where the results would be properly interpreted. Less compelling indications exist when either the patient's condition or the procedure (but not both) is likely to place the patient at increased risk (see Chap. 84).

INTRAOPERATIVE PREDICTORS OF PERIOPERATIVE CARDIAC MORBIDITY

The classic intraoperative predictors of increased PCM include emergency surgery, vascular surgery, and prolonged (>3 h) thoracic or upper abdominal surgery[8] (see Table 83-5). Dynamic predictors of PCM include intraoperative hypotension; tachycardia; and evidence of myocardial ischemia as detected by ECG, by TEE detection of changes in wall motion and wall thickening,[91,94] by elevation of end-diastolic pulmonary artery pressure monitored by catheter[11,95,96] or by cardiokymography.[96,97] It should be noted that most of the data regarding the intraoperative detection of myocardial ischemia have been obtained during coronary artery bypass surgery rather than noncardiac surgery.

In a recent study, 300 patients over the age of 60 who were undergoing abdominal, thoracic (noncardiac), or vascular surgical procedures and who either had documented coronary artery disease or were at high risk for coronary disease were randomized to either routine thermal care or supplemental warming care during the perioperative period. The perioperative maintenance of normothermia was associated with a reduced incidence of morbid cardiac events and ventricular tachycardia.[98]

POSTOPERATIVE PREDICTION OF PERIOPERATIVE CARDIAC MORBIDITY

Postoperative Ischemia

In the past, the greatest effort has been spent in the preoperative identification and management of patients at increased risk of PCM. There is now a suggestion that the use of preoperative patient selection criteria has apparently been responsible for the observation that typical preoperative risk factors such as SAH, previous MI, or the Goldman cardiac risk factor index were found not to be predictive of ischemic events in a study of 474 men undergoing major noncardiac surgery (243 men with CAD; 231 men at high risk of CAD)[6,7] In this study, postoperative myocardial ischemia detected by two-channel AECG recording occurred in nearly all patients who subsequently had an ischemic event. The ECG evidence of postoperative ischemia, which began to become apparent in patients on the first day after surgery, occurred in most patients at least 4 h before any other clinical evidence of an event. In 13 of 15 patients who had an ischemic event, clinical symptoms occurred, the most frequent of which were dyspnea (8 patients) or chest pain (3 patients). When evidence of postoperative ischemia occurred on ECG monitoring, it was clinically silent in 97 percent, although it was associated with a ninefold increased risk of an ischemic event. On the other hand, the majority of patients who had such evidence of ischemia postoperatively did not have an ischemic event. During the first 48 h postoperatively, 41 percent (167 of 407 patients with interpretable AECG recordings) of the men had at least one episode of myocardial ischemia. This report and other recent studies emphasize the importance of giving special attention to the monitoring and management of high-risk patients during the postoperative period. A subsequent detailed analysis of the perioperative data from the same 474 men identified five major preoperative factors that were independent predictors of postoperative ischemia: ECG evidence of left ventricular hypertrophy, history of SAH, diabetes mellitus, definite CAD, and the use of digoxin.[7] The likelihood of postoperative myocardial ischemia on the continuous two-channel AECG recorded for 2 days following surgery increased progressively with the number of preoperative predictors. Thus, in this group of high-risk men, there was ECG evidence of postoperative ischemia in 22 percent of men with no preoperative predictors, in 31 percent of men with one predictor, in 46 percent of men with two predictors, in 70 percent of men with three predictors, and in 77 percent of men with four predictors. The risk of postoperative ischemia was also increased in patients who had evidence of ischemia on 12-lead ECG monitoring during surgery.

Postoperative Management

As noted above, most perioperative MIs occur in the first few days postoperatively. Most patients are asymptomatic, although they frequently have ST-segment changes in the preceding 3 to 6 h.[1,6–8] In the absence of contraindications (Chap. 54), tachycardia and hypertension should be treated with a beta blocker. Postoperative supraventricular tachycardias are most often related to noncardiac causes such as hypoxia, electrolyte abnormalities, infection, or medications. The primary treatment is to correct the cause. Atrial fibrillation with a rapid ventricular rate can be managed by intravenous diltiazem, a short-acting beta blocker (Chap. 54), or cardioversion (Chap. 32).

Surveillance for Postoperative Myocardial Infarction

In patients with known or suspected CAD who are undergoing surgical procedures with a high incidence of cardiovascular morbidity, a cost-effective strategy is to obtain ECGs at baseline, immediately after the procedure and daily for the first two postoperative days. Measurements of cardiac enzymes are best reserved for patients at high risk or those who demonstrate ECG changes or hemodynamic evidence of cardiovascular dysfunction. In patients who have no preoperative evidence of CAD, surveillance should be restricted to those who develop perioperative signs of cardiovascular dysfunction.

MYOCARDIAL REVASCULARIZATION

In a few highly selected patients, myocardial revascularization should be considered prior to elective noncardiac surgery in order to decrease perioperative cardiac morbidity and improve long-term prognosis. *In general, the indications for revascularization by coronary angioplasty or surgery are the same as they would be if the patient were not undergoing the noncardiac surgery* (see Chaps. 45, 48, and 50). Since there are no controlled trials in this area, it is necessary to extrapolate from other studies, keeping in mind the risks of the revascularization procedure in the individual patient, the added expense, and the delay in performing the noncardiac surgery.[36,50,87,99–101]

MEDICATIONS

In general, patients with known or suspected cardiac disease should have their cardiovascular medications continued before, during, and following noncardiac surgery. Preoperatively, patients who are not receiving a beta blocker should be considered for such therapy in the absence of a contraindication.[102–105] Although it is common practice, there are few data supporting the intraoperative administration of intravenous nitroglycerin in patients with CAD. One report has suggested that intraoperative intravenous diltiazem may decrease the number of ischemic episodes in patients with chronic stable angina undergoing peripheral vascular surgery.[106] This needs to be confirmed in a larger study before it can be recommended. Patients who are taking chronic low-dose aspirin should usually have this discontinued a few days prior to elective surgery in order to decrease the amount of intraoperative bleeding.

RECOMMENDED PATIENT EVALUATION AND MANAGEMENT

The evaluation of patients with known or suspected cardiac disease prior to noncardiac surgery requires an appraisal of the patient's clinical risk profile; a characterization of the type, urgency, and risks of the planned noncardiac surgery; and a knowledge of the results of coronary artery bypass surgery and coronary angioplasty at one's own institution.[14] In addition, the diagnostic accuracy of exercise treadmill testing, thallium scintigraphy, and stress echocardiography in one's institution should be known, as well as the risks and accuracy of coronary arteriography. As with most diagnostic testing, the greatest value is in patients who have an intermediate risk of having CAD on clinical grounds[14,18,43] (see also Chap. 45)

Patients who are found to be at significantly increased risk of PCM during evaluation for elective noncardiac surgery on the basis of noninvasive testing or coronary arteriography must be managed on an individual basis. Alternative recommendations include one of the following: canceling or postponing the elective surgery and instituting more intensive medical therapy; recommending an alternative lower-risk surgical procedure; proceeding with the proposed elective surgery with intensive anti-ischemic therapy and perioperative monitoring; or postponing the elective surgery until after myocardial revascularization by either coronary angioplasty or coronary artery bypass surgery.

While the overall management of cardiovascular disease in the perioperative period should closely resemble that of nonoperative patients, it is equally important to recognize that for many patients, presentation for noncardiac surgery represents the first time in years (or ever) that a careful cardiovascular assessment is performed. This may uncover coronary, valvular, electrical, and/or myocardial disease. Further, it may identify modifiable coronary risk factors that require long-term attention, such as systemic arterial hypertension, hyperlipidemia, smoking, or diabetes.

Finally, some patients will be evaluated only postoperatively, when a nonfatal cardiac event occurs. If this event is unstable angina, myocardial infarction, or ischemia-mediated CHF, the patient has a three- to fivefold increased risk of downstream MI or cardiac death as compared with patients without such complications.[21,107,108] Aggressive risk stratification, medical therapy, and risk-factor modification are important goals in such patients.

REFERENCES

1. Mangano DT. Perioperative cardiac morbidity. *Anesthesiology* 1990; 72:153–184.
2. National Center for Health Statistics. *Vital Statistics of the United States, 1980*. vol II: *Mortality*, pt A. DHHS pub no (PHS) 85-1101. Hyattsville, MD: NCHS U.S. Public Health Services; 1985.
3. National Center for Health Statistics. *Health, United States, 1988*. vol III. DHHS pub no (PHS) 89-1232. Washington, DC: U.S. Public Health Service, March 1989: 10–17, 66, 67, 100, 101.
4. Hertzer NR, Beven EG, Young JR, Ohara PJ, Ruschhaupt WF III, Graor RA. Coronary-artery disease in peripheral vascular patients: A classification of 1,000 coronary angiograms and results of surgical management. *Ann Surg* 1984; 199:223–233.
5. Hertz NR. Clinical experience with preoperative coronary angiography. *J Vasc Surg* 1985; 2:510–514.
6. Mangano DT, Browner WS, Hollenberg M, London MJ, Tubau JF, Tateo IM, et al. Association of perioperative myocardial ischemia with cardiac morbidity and mortality in men undergoing noncardiac surgery. *N Engl J Med* 1990; 323:1781–1788.
7. Hollenberg M, Mangano DT, Browner WS, London MJ, Tubau JF, Tateo IM, et al. Predictors of postoperative myocardial ischemia in patients undergoing noncardiac surgery. *JAMA* 1992; 268:205–209.
8. Mangano DT. Risk assessment for noncardiac surgery. In: Kapoor AS, Singh BN (eds). *Prognosis and Risk Assessment in Cardiovascular Diseases*. New York: Churchill Livingstone; 1993:447–467.
9. Roizen MF. Preoperative evaluation. In: Miller RD (ed). *Anesthesia*, 4th ed. New York: Churchill Livingstone, 1994:827–882.
10. Foster ED, Davis KB, Carpenter JA, Abele S, Fray D. Risk of noncardiac operation in patients with defined coronary disease: The Coronary Artery Surgery Study (CASS) Registry Experience. *Ann Thorac Surg* 1986; 41:42–50.
11. Rao TK, Jacobs KH, El-Etr AA. Reinfarction following anesthesia in patients with myocardial infarction. *Anesthesiology* 1983; 59:499–505.
12. London MJ, Mangano DT. Assessment of perioperative risk. In: Stoelting RK, Barash PG, Gallagher TJ (eds). *Advances in Anesthesia*. Vol 5. Chicago: Year Book; 1988:53–87.
13. Roberts SL, Tinker JH. Cardiovascular disease, risk and outcome. In: Brown DL (ed). *Anesthesia*. Philadelphia: Lippincott; 1988:33–49.
14. Abraham SA, Coles NA, Coley CM, Strauss HW, Boucher CA, Eagle KA. Coronary risk of noncardiac surgery. *Prog Cardiovasc Dis* 1991; 34:205–234.
15. Yeager RA, Moneta GL, Edwards JM, Taylor LM, McConnell DB, Porter JM. Late survival after perioperative myocardial infarction complicating vascular surgery. *J Vasc Surg* 1994; 20:598–606.
16. Tarham S, Moffitt EA, Taylor WF, Giuliani ER. Myocardial infarction after general anesthesia. *JAMA* 1972; 220:1451–1454.
17. Von Knooring J. Postoperative myocardial infarction: A prospective study in a risk group of surgical patients. *Surgery* 1981; 90:55–60.
18. Massie BM, Mangano DT. Assessment of preoperative risk: Have we put the cart before the horse? (editorial) *J Am Coll Cardiol* 1993; 21:1353–1356.
19. Steen PA, Tinker JH, Tarhan S. Myocardial reinfarction after anesthesia and surgery. *JAMA* 1978; 239:2566–2570.
20. Foster ED, Davis KB, Carpenter JA, Abele S, Fray D. Risk of noncardiac operation in patients with defined coronary disease: The Coronary Artery Surgery Study (CASS) Registry experience. *Ann Thorac Surg* 1986; 41:42–50.
21. Report of the American College of Cardiology/American Heart Association Task Force on Practice Guidelines (Committee on Perioperative Cardiovascular Evaluation for Noncardiac Surgery): Guidelines for perioperative cardiovascular evaluation for noncardiac surgery. *J Am Coll Cardiol* 1996; 27:910–948 and *Circulation* 1996; 93:1278–1317.
22. Kearon C, Hirsh J. Management of anticoagulation before and after elective surgery. *N Engl J Med* 1997; 336:1506–1511.
23. Goldman L, Caldera DL, Nussbaum SR, Southwick FS, Krogstad D, Murray B, et al. Multifactorial index of cardiac risk in noncardiac surgical procedures. *N Engl J Med* 1977; 297:845–850.
24. Goldman L, Caldera DL, Southwick FS, Nussbaum SR, Murray B, O'Malley TA, et al. Cardiac risk factors and complications in noncardiac surgery. *Medicine* 1978; 57:357–370.
25. Thompson RC, Liberthson RR, Lowenstein E. Perioperative anesthetic risk of noncardiac surgery in hypertrophic obstructive cardiomyopathy. *JAMA* 1985; 254:2419–2421.
26. Clagett GP, Anderson FA Jr, Heit J, Levine MN, Wheeler HB. Prevention of venous thromboembolism. *Chest* 1995; 108 (suppl):312S–334S.
27. Garcia MJ, McNamara PM, Gordon T, Kannel WB. Morbidity and

mortality in diabetics in the Framingham population: Sixteen-year follow-up study. *Diabetes* 1974; 23:105–111.

28. Dortimer AC, Shenoy PN, Shiroff RA, Leaman DM, Babb JD, Liedtke JA, et al. Diffuse coronary artery disease in diabetic patients: Fact or fiction? *Circulation* 1978; 57:133–136.

29. Kannel WB, McGee DL. Diabetes and cardiovascular risk factors: The Framingham Study. *Circulation* 1979; 59:8–13.

30. Waller BF, Palumbo PJ, Lie JT, Roberts WC. Status of the coronary arteries at necropsy in diabetes mellitus with onset after age 30 years: Analysis of 229 diabetic patients with and without clinical evidence of coronary heart disease and comparison to 183 control subjects. *Am J Med* 1980; 69:498–506.

31. Vigorita VJ, Moore GW, Hutchins GM. Absence of correlation between coronary arterial atherosclerosis and severity or duration of diabetes mellitus of adult onset. *Am J Cardiol* 1980; 46:535–542.

32. Kannel WB. Lipids, diabetes, and coronary heart disease: Insights from the Framingham Study. *Am Heart J* 1985; 110:1110–1117.

33. Mangano DT, Goldman L. Preoperative assessment of patients with known or suspected coronary disease. *N Engl J Med* 1995; 333:1750–1756.

34. Goldman L. Cardiac risk in noncardiac surgery: An update. *Anesth Analg* 1995: 80:810–820.

35. Blaustein AS. Preoperative and perioperative management of cardiac patients undergoing noncardiac surgery. *Cardiol Clin* 1995; 13:149–161.

36. Goldman L. Cardiac risk for vascular surgery (editorial). *J Am Coll Cardiol* 1996; 27:799–802.

37. Bodenheimer MM. Noncardiac surgery in the cardiac patient: What is the question? *Ann Intern Med* 1996; 124:763–766.

38. Fleisher LA, Eagle KA. Screening for cardiac disease in patients having noncardiac surgery. *Ann Intern Med* 1996; 124:767–772.

39. L'Italien GJ, Paul SD, Henel RC, Leppo JA, Cohen MC, Fleisher LA. Development and validation of a bayesian model for perioperative cardiac risk assessment in a cohort of 1,081 vascular surgical candidates. *J Am Coll Cardiol* 1996; 27:779–786.

40. Coley CM, Eagle KA. Preoperative assessment and perioperative management of cardiac ischemic risk in noncardiac surgery. *Curr Prob Cardiol* 1996; 21:291–382.

41. Eagle KA, Rihal CS, Mickel MC, Holmes DR, Foster ED, Gersh BJ. Cardiac risk of noncardiac surgery: Influence of coronary disease and type of surgery in 3,368 operations. *Circulation*, In press.

42. American Society of Anesthesiologists. New classification of physical status. *Anesthesiology* 1963; 24:111.

43. Wong T, Detsky AS. Preoperative cardiac risk assessment for patients having peripheral vascular surgery. *Ann Intern Med* 1992; 116:743–753.

44. Detsky AS, Abrams HB, McLaughlin JR, Drucker DJ, Sasson Z, Johnston N, et al. Predicting cardiac complications in patients undergoing non-cardiac surgery. *J Gen Intern Med* 1986; 1:211–219.

45. Detsky AS, Abrams HB, Forbath N, Scott JG, Hilliard JR. Cardiac assessment for patients undergoing noncardiac surgery: A multifactorial clinical risk index. *Arch Intern Med* 1986; 146:2131–2134.

46. Kannel WB, Abbott RD. Incidence and prognosis of unrecognized myocardial infarction: An update on the Framingham study. *N Engl J Med* 1984; 311:1144–1147.

47. Mangano DT. Preoperative assessment. In: Kaplan JA (ed). *Cardiac Anesthesia* 2d ed. Vol I. New York: Grune & Stratton; 1987: 341–392.

48. Dash H, Massie BM, Botvinick EH, Brundage BH. The noninvasive identification of left main and three vessel coronary artery disease by myocardial stress perfusion scintigraphy and treadmill exercise electrocardiography. *Circulation* 1979; 60:276–284.

49. Wackers FJT, Fetterman RC, Mattero JA, Clements JP. Quantitative planar thallium-201 stress scintigraphy: A critical evaluation of the method. *Semin Nucl Med* 1975; 15:46–66.

50. Seeger JM, Rosenthal GR, Self SB, Flynn TC, Limacher MC, Harward TRS. Does routine stress-thallium cardiac scanning reduce postoperative cardiac complications? *Ann Surg* 1994; 219:654–663.

51. Leppo J, Boucher CA, Okada RD, Newell JB, Strauss HW, Pohost GM. Serial thallium-201 myocardial imaging after dipyridamole infusion: Diagnostic utility in detecting coronary stenoses and relationship to regional wall motion. *Circulation* 1982; 66:649–657.

52. Leppo J, Plaja J, Gionet M, Parakos JA, Cutler BS. Noninvasive evaluation of cardiac risk before elective vascular surgery. *J Am Coll Cardiol* 1987; 9:269–276.

53. Leppo JA. Dipyridamole-thallium imaging: The lazy man's stress test. *J Nucl Med* 1989; 30:281–287.

54. Baron J-F, Mundler O, Bertrand M, Vicaut E, Barré E, Godet G, et al. Dipyridamole-thallium scintigraphy and gated radionuclide angiography to assess cardiac risk before abdominal aortic surgery. *N Engl J Med* 1994; 330:663–669.

55. Srinivas M, Roizen MF, Barnard J, Thisted RA, Ellis JE, Foss J. Relative effectiveness of four preoperative tests for predicting adverse cardiac outcomes after vascular surgery: A meta-analysis. *Anesth Analg* 1994; 79:422–323.

56. Younis L, Stratmann H, Takese B, Byers S, Chaitman BR, Miller DD. Preoperative clinical assessment and dipyridamole thallium-201 scintigraphy for prediction and prevention of cardiac events in patients having major noncardiovascular surgery and known or suspected coronary artery disease. *Am J Cardiol* 1994; 74:311–317.

57. Boucher CA, Brewster DC, Darling RC, Okada RD, Strauss HW, Pohost GM. Determination of cardiac risk by dipyridamole-thallium imaging before peripheral vascular surgery. *N Engl J Med* 1985; 312:389–394.

58. Stratmann HG, Younis LT, Wittry MD, Amato M, Mark AL, Miller DD. Dipyridamole technetium 99m sestamibi myocardial tomography for preoperative cardiac risk stratification before major or minor non-vascular surgery. *Am Heart J* 1996; 132:536–541.

59. Shaw LJ, Eagle KA, Gersh BJ, Miller DD. Meta-analysis of intravenous dipyridamole-thallium-201 imaging (1985 to 1994) and dobutamine echocardiography (1991 to 1994) for risk stratification before vascular surgery. *J Am Coll Cardiol* 1996; 27:787–798.

60. Eagle K, Singer D, Brewster D, Darling RC, Mulley AG, Boucher CA. Dipyridamole-thallium scanning in patients undergoing vascular surgery: Optimizing preoperative evaluation of cardiac risk. *JAMA* 1987; 257:2185–2189.

61. Eagle K, Coley CM, Newell JB, Brewster DC, Darling RC, Strauss HW, et al. Combining clinical and thallium data optimizes preoperative assessment of cardiac risk before major vascular surgery. *Ann Intern Med* 1989; 110:859–866.

62. Mangano D, London M, Tubau J, Browner WS, Hollenberg M, Krupski W, et al. Dipyridamole thallium-201 scintigraphy as a preoperative screening test: A reexamination of its predictive potential. *Circulation* 1991; 84:493–502.

63. Ruddy T, McPhail N, Calvin J, Sauve M, Davies R, Gulenchyn K, et al. Comparison of exercise testing, dipyridamole thallium imaging and gated blood pool scanning for the prediction of cardiac complications following vascular surgery (abstr). *J Am Coll Cardiol* 1989; 13:149A.

64. McEnroe CS, O'Donnell TF Jr, Yeager A, Konstam M, Mackey WC. Comparison of ejection fraction and Goldman risk factor analysis to dipyridamole–thallium 201 studies in the evaluation of cardiac morbidity after aortic aneurysm surgery. *J Vasc Surg* 1990; 11:497–504.

65. Lette J, Waters D, Lapointe J, Gagnon A, Picard M, Cerino M, et al. Usefulness of the severity and extent of reversible perfusion defects during thallium-dipyridamole imaging for cardiac risk assessment before noncardiac surgery. *Am J Cardiol* 1989; 64:276–281.

66. Lane SE, Lewis SM, Pippin JJ, Kosinski EJ, Campbell D, Nesto RW, et al. Predictive value of quantitative dipyridamole-thallium scintigraphy in assessing cardiovascular risk after vascular surgery in diabetes mellitus. *Am J Cardiol* 1989; 64:1275–1279.

67. Levinson JR, Boucher CA, Coley CM, Guiney TE, Strauss HW, Eagle KA. Usefulness of semiquantitative analysis of dipyridamole–thallium-201 redistribution for improving risk stratification before vascular surgery. *Am J Cardio* 1990; 66:406–410.

68. Hendel RC, Layden JJ, Leppo JA. Prognostic value of dipyridamole thallium scintigraphy for evaluation of ischemic heart disease. *J Am Coll Cardiol* 1990; 15:109–116.

69. Younis LT, Aguirre F, Byers S, Dowell S, Barth G, Walker H, et al. Perioperative and long-term prognostic value of intravenous dipyridamole thallium scintigraphy in patients with peripheral vascular disease. *Am Heart J* 1990; 119:1287–1292.

70. Daum RM, Cremisi HD, Yeager A, Udelson JE, Underhill D, Oates E, et al. Dipyridamole thallium imaging for determining perioperative and long-term prognosis in high-risk vascular disease patients (abstr). *Circulation* 1988; 77–78 (suppl 2):II–191.

71. Bry JDL, Belkin M, O'Donnell TF, Mackay WC, Udelson JE, Schmid CH, et al. An assessment of the positive predictive value and cost-

effectiveness of dipyridamole myocardial scintigraphy in patients undergoing vascular surgery. *J Vasc Surg* 1994; 19:112–124.

72. Pasternack PF, Grossi EA, Baumann FG, Riles TS, Lamparello PJ, Giangola G, et al. The value of silent myocardial ischemia monitoring in the prediction of perioperative myocardial infarction in patients undergoing peripheral vascular surgery. *J Vasc Surg* 1989; 10:617–625.

73. Ouyang P, Gerstenblith G, Furman WR, Golueke PJ, Gottlieb SO, et al. Frequency and significance of early postoperative silent myocardial ischemia in patients having peripheral vascular surgery. *Am J Cardiol* 1989; 64:1113–1116.

74. McCann RL, Clements FM. Silent myocardial ischemia in patients undergoing peripheral vascular surgery: Incidence and association with perioperative cardiac morbidity and mortality. *J Vasc Surg* 1989; 9:583–587.

75. Raby KE, Goldman L, Creager MA, Cook EF, Weisberg MC, Whittemore AD, et al. Correlation between preoperative ischemia and major cardiac events after peripheral vascular surgery. *N Engl J Med* 1989; 321:1296–1300.

76. Fegert G, Hollenberg M, Browner W, Wellington Y, Levenson L, Franks M, et al. Perioperative myocardial ischemia in the noncardiac surgical patient (abstr). *Anesthesiology* 1988; 69:A49.

77. Larsen SF, Olesen KH, Jacobsen E, Nielsen H, Nielsen AL, Pietersen A, et al. Prediction of cardiac risk in non-cardiac surgery. *Eur Heart J* 1987; 8:179–185.

78. Halm EA, Browner WS, Tubau JF, Tateo IM, Mangano DT. Echocardiography for assessing cardiac risk in patients having noncardiac surgery. *Ann Intern Med* 1996; 125:433–441.

79. Lane RT, Sawada SG, Segar DS, Ryan T, Lalka SG, Williams R, et al. Dobutamine stress echocardiography for assessment of cardiac risk before noncardiac surgery. *Am J Cardiol* 1991; 68:976–977.

80. Lalka SG, Sawada SG, Dalsing MC, Cikrit DF, Sawchuk AP, Kovacs RL, et al. Dobutamine stress echocardiography as a predictor of cardiac events associated with aortic surgery. *J Vasc Surg* 1992; 15:831–840.

81. Eichelberger JP, Schwartz KQ, Black ER, Green RM, Ouriel K. Predictive value of dobutamine echocardiography just before noncardiac vascular surgery. *Am J Cardiol* 1993; 72:602–607.

82. Langan EM III, Youkey JR, Franklin DP, Elmore JR, Costello JM, Nassef LA. Dobutamine stress echocardiography for cardiac risk assessment before aortic surgery. *J Vasc Surg* 1993; 18:905–911.

83. Davila-Roman VG, Waggoner AD, Sicard GA, Geltman EM, Schechtman KB, Perez JE. Dobutamine stress echocardiography predicts surgical outcome in patents wituh an aortic aneurysm and peripheral vascular disease. *J Am Coll Cardiol* 1993; 21:957–963.

84. Poldermans D, Fioretti PM, Forster T, Thomson IR, Boersma E, el-Said EM, et al. Dobutamine stress echocardiography for assessment of perioperative cardiac risk in patients undergoing major vascular surgery. *Circulation* 1993; 87:1506–1512.

85. Tomatis LA, Fierens EE, Verbrugge GP. Evaluation of surgical risk in peripheral vascular disease by coronary arteriography: A series of 100 cases. *Surgery* 1972; 771:429–435.

86. Hertzer NR, Young JR, Kramer JR, Phillips DF, deWolfe VG, Ruschhaupt WF III, et al. Routine coronary angiography prior to elective aortic reconstruction. *Arch Surg* 1979; 114:1336–1344.

87. Mason JJ, Owens DK, Harris RA, Cooke JP, Hlatky MA. The role of coronary angiography and coronary revascularization before noncardiac vascular surgery. *JAMA* 1995; 273:1919–1925.

88. Domanski M, Ellis S, Eagle K. Does preoperative coronary revascularization before noncardiac surgery reduce the risk of coronary events in patients with known coronary artery disease? (editorial). *Am J Cardiol* 1995; 75:829–831.

89. Anderson TJ, Meredith IT, Selwyn AP, Raby KE. Myocardial revascularization before repair of an aortic aneurysm (editorial). *Mayo Clin Proc* 1993; 68:713–715.

90. Practice guidelines for pulmonary artery catheterization: A report by the American Society of Anesthesiologists Task Force on Pulmonary Artery Catheterization. *Anesthesiology* 1993; 78:380–394.

91. Topol EJ, Weiss JL, Guzman PA, Dorsey-Lima S, Blanck TJ, Humphrey LS, et al. Immediate improvement of dysfunctional myocardial segments after coronary revascularization: Detection by intraoperative transesophageal echocardiography. *J Am Coll Cardiol* 1984; 4:1123–1134.

92. Smith JS, Cahalan MK, Benefiel DJ, Byrd BF, Lurz FW, Shapiro WA, et al. Intraoperative detection of myocardial ischemia in high-risk patients: Electrocardiography versus two-dimensional transesophageal echocardiography. *Circulation* 1985; 72:1015–1021.

93. London M, Tubau J, Wong M, Layug E, Mangano DT. The "natural history" of segmental wall motion abnormalities detected by intraoperative transesophageal echocardiography: A clinically blinded prospective approach (abstr). *Anesthesiology* 1988;69:A7.

94. Leung JM, O'Kelly B, Browner WS, Tubau J, Hollenberg M, Mangano DT. Prognostic importance of post bypass regional wall-motion abnormalities in patients undergoing coronary artery bypass graft surgery. *Anesthesiology* 1989; 71:16–25.

95. Parker J, Chiong M, West R, Case R. Sequential alterations in myocardial lactate metabolism, ST-segments and left ventricular function during angina induced by atrial pacing. *Circulation* 1969; 40:113–131.

96. Haggmark S, Hohner P, Ostman M, Friedman A, Diamond G, Lowenstein E, et al. Comparison of hemodynamic, electrocardiographic, mechanical and metabolic indicators of intraoperative myocardial ischemia in vascular surgical patients with coronary artery disease. *Anesthesiology* 1989; 70:19–25.

97. Bellows WH, Bode RH Jr, Levy JA, Foex P, Lowenstein E. Noninvasive detection of periinduction ischemic ventricular dysfunction by cardiomyography in humans: Preliminary experience. *Anesthesiology* 1984; 60:155–158.

98. Frank SM, Fleisher LA, Breslow MJ, Higgins MS, Olson KF, Kelly S, et al. Perioperative maintenance of normothermia reduces the incidence of morbid cardiac events: A randomized clinical trial. *JAMA* 1997; 277:1127–1134.

99. Fleischer LA, Skolnick ED, Holroyd KJ, Lehmann HP. Coronary artery revascularization before abdominal aortic aneurysm surgery: A decision analytic approach. *Anesth Analg* 1994; 79:661–669.

100. Elmore JR, Hallett JW Jr, Gibbons RJ, Naessens JM, Bower TC, Cherry KJ, et al. Myocardial revascularization before abdominal aortic aneurysmorrhaphy: Effect of coronary angioplasty. *Mayo Clin Proc* 1993; 68:637–641.

101. Mason JJ, Owens DK, Harris RA, Cooke JP, Hlatky MA. The role of coronary arteriography and coronary revascularization before noncardiac vascular surgery. *JAMA* 1995; 273:1919–1925.

102. Pasternack PF, Imparato AM, Baumann FG, Laub G, Riles TS, Lamparello PJ, et al. The hemodynamics of β blockade in patients undergoing abdominal aortic aneurysm repair. *Circulation* 1987; 76(suppl 3):III-1–III-7.

103. Stone JG, Foex P, Sear JW, Johnson LL, Khambatta HJ, Triner L. Myocardial ischemia in untreated hypertensive patients: Effect of a single small oral dose of a beta-adrenergic blocking agent. *Anesthesiology* 1988; 68:495–500.

104. Pasternack PF, Grossi EA, Baumann FG, Riles TS, Lamparello PH, Giangola G, et al. Beta blockade to decrease silent ischemia during peripheral vascular surgery. *Am J Surg* 1989; 158:113–116.

105. Mangano DT, Layug EL, Wallace A, Tateo I. Effect of atenolol on mortality and cardiovascular morbidity after noncardiac surgery. *N Engl J Med* 1996; 335:1713–1720.

106. Godet G, Coriat P, Baron JF, Bertrana M, Diquet B, Sebag C, et al. Prevention of intraoperative myocardial ischemia during noncardiac surgery with intravenous diltiazem: A randomized trial versus placebo. *Anesthesiology* 1987; 66:241–245.

107. Mangano DT, Browner WS, Hollenberg M, Li J, Tateo IM. Long-term cardiac prognosis following noncardiac surgery: The Study of Perioperative Ischemia Research Group. *JAMA* 1991; 268:233–239.

108. Yeager RA, Moneta GL, Edwards JM, Taylor LM Jr, McConnell DB, Porter JM. Late survival after perioperative myocardial infarction complicating vascular surgery. *J Vasc Surg* 1994; 20:598–606.

84

ANESTHESIA AND THE PATIENT WITH CARDIOVASCULAR DISEASE

David L. Reich / Joel A. Kaplan

Anesthetizing patients with cardiovascular disease is one of the most difficult challenges facing the anesthesiologist. The constellation of anesthetic drug effects, the physiologic stresses of surgery, and underlying cardiovascular diseases complicate and limit the choice of anesthetic techniques for any particular procedure. Generally speaking, the anesthesiologist's approach to the patient with cardiovascular disease is to select agents and techniques that would optimize the patient's cardiopulmonary function. The perioperative management of a patient with cardiovascular disease requires close cooperation between the cardiologist/internist and the anesthesiologist.[1] Each specialist has a unique knowledge base that complements the other's. The approach should emphasize a continuum of care from the preoperative evaluation through the extended postoperative period.

PREOPERATIVE EVALUATION

The assessment of cardiac risk and preoperative optimization of the patient's cardiovascular status are the traditional goals of the preoperative evaluation of patients with cardiovascular disease. In 1977, Goldman et al. introduced the Cardiac Risk Index Score (CRIS) to guide more quantitatively the assignment of cardiac risk in patients undergoing noncardiac surgery.[2] This study had a major impact, because clinicians concluded that improvements in factors such as congestive heart failure symptomatology and general medical condition would decrease cardiac risk. While a recent study does not support the predictive value of the CRIS or preoperative electrocardiographic (ECG) ischemic changes in patients with coronary artery disease (CAD),[3] the emphasis on preoperative optimization continues and is supported by other studies.[4] This topic is reviewed in Chap. 83. Recently, the American College of Cardiology/American Heart Association Task Force on Practice Guidelines published "Guidelines for Perioperative

Cardiovascular Evaluation for Noncardiac Surgery."[5] The algorithmic approach to preoperative evaluation described in these guidelines and that advocated by Mangano and Goldman[6] are valuable in that more consistent clinical approaches should emerge.

The information derived from the cardiac evaluation that is of particular value to the anesthesiologist can be summarized by answers to the following questions:

1. Are further diagnostic studies required prior to elective surgery?
2. Will the patient derive benefit from delaying surgery in order to optimize preoperative medical therapy?
3. Will the patient derive benefit from preoperative myocardial revascularization (angioplasty or surgical revascularization)?
4. Should there be perioperative antithrombotic therapy?
5. What is the regimen of preoperative cardiovascular medications that should be continued through the perioperative period?

The accumulation of historical, clinical, laboratory, echocardiographic, radionuclide, and cardiac catheterization data in a cogent summary form comprises the ideal "medical clearance" consultation for the anesthesiologist. With the benefit of this information, the two specialties can make intelligent decisions regarding the patient's preoperative therapy and the optimal timing of surgery.[7]

PERIOPERATIVE MONITORING

Standards for basic intraoperative monitoring were established by the American Society of Anesthesiologists in 1986.[8] Accordingly, digital pulse oximetry and capnometry have been almost universally applied in the last several years. The indications for the use of more invasive monitors, such as intraarter-

TABLE 84-1

INDICATIONS FOR INTRAARTERIAL MONITORING OF BLOOD PRESSURE

Patient characteristics
   Recent myocardial infarction, unstable angina, or severe coronary artery disease
   Decreased left ventricular function (congestive heart failure) or significant valvular heart disease
   Hypovolemic, cardiogenic, or septic shock or multiple organ failure
   Requirement for positive inotropic agents or intraaortic balloon counterpulsation
   Massive trauma
   Right heart failure, chronic obstructive pulmonary disease, pulmonary hypertension, or pulmonary embolism
   Massive ascites
   Electrolyte or metabolic disturbances requiring frequent blood samples
   Inability to measure arterial pressure noninvasively (e.g., morbid obesity)
Surgical procedures
   Major procedures involving large fluid shifts and/or blood loss
   Procedures involving the use of deliberate hypotension or deliberate hypothermia
   Cardiopulmonary bypass surgery
   Surgery of the aorta, especially that requiring cross-clamping

TABLE 84-2

INDICATIONS FOR PERIOPERATIVE PLACEMENT OF CENTRAL VENOUS LINE

Patient characteristics
   Inadequate peripheral vein access
   Major trauma
   Tricuspid stenosis
Surgical procedures
   Operations involving large fluid shifts and/or blood loss even in patients with good left ventricular function
   Procedures with a high risk of air embolism, such as sitting-position craniotomies
Access
   Intravascular volume assessment when urine output is unavailable or not reliable (renal failure, urologic surgery)
   Frequent blood sampling when an arterial line is not required
   Administration of vasoactive drugs or drugs causing thrombosis or sclerosis of peripheral veins
   Chronic drug administration
   Rapid infusion of intravenous fluids (using large cannulas)

ial, central venous, and pulmonary arterial catheters (PACs) are more controversial. Tables 84-1, 84-2, and 84-3 detail specific indications for invasive monitoring that are widely accepted.

Transesophageal echocardiography is minimally/moderately invasive and has acquired a much larger role in intraoperative management in recent years. The availability of high-frequency transducers and color-flow Doppler mapping has enhanced the ability of anesthesiologists, cardiologists, and surgeons to make intraoperative diagnoses, evaluate hemodynamic aberrations, and assess the quality of cardiac surgical interventions inter alia. Practice guidelines for transesophageal echocardiography have been published by the American Society of Anesthesiologists.[9] A list of indications for perioperative transesophageal echocardiography is presented in Table 84-4.

CHOICE OF ANESTHETIC TECHNIQUE

The choice of anesthetic technique is inherently a difficult one because multiple factors must be considered. These include the desires of the patient, the requirements of the surgical procedure, and the patient's underlying medical condition. While a specific anesthetic technique is occasionally desirable for a particular procedure (e.g., spinal anesthesia for transurethral resection of prostate), it is extremely difficult to find

scientific evidence that any particular anesthetic approach is superior to reasonable alternatives or that anesthetic technique per se influences patient outcome.[10,11]

There is controversy regarding the effects of regional anesthesia (with postoperative epidural analgesia) on cardiovascular morbidity/mortality in "high risk" patients. Five prospective randomized trials have addressed this issue. Two

TABLE 84-3

INDICATIONS FOR PULMONARY ARTERY CATHETER MONITORING

Patient characteristics
   Recent myocardial infarction or severe unstable angina
   Impaired left ventricular function (congestive heart failure) or significant mitral or aortic valvular pathology
   Pericardial tamponade
   Hypovolemic, cardiogenic, or septic shock or multiple organ failure
   Hemodynamic instability requiring positive inotropic agents or intraaortic balloon counterpulsation
   Right heart failure, chronic obstructive pulmonary disease, pulmonary hypertension, or pulmonary embolism
   Requirement for high levels of positive end-expiratory pressure
   Massive trauma
   Massive ascites
Surgical procedures
   Major procedures involving large fluid shifts and/or blood loss in patients with severe coronary artery disease
   Surgery of the aorta requiring cross-clamping
   Hepatic transplantation

TABLE 84-4

GUIDELINES FOR THE USE OF PERIOPERATIVE TRANSESOPHAGEAL ECHOCARDIOGRAPHY

Category I indications: Supported by the strongest evidence or expert opinion

Preoperative

Unstable patients with suspected thoracic aortic aneurysms, dissection, or disruption who need to be evaluated quickly

Intraoperative

Evaluation of acute, persistent, and life-threatening hemodynamic disturbances in which ventricular function and its determinants are uncertain and have not responded to treatment

Valve repair

Congenital heart surgery for most lesions requiring cardiopulmonary bypass

Repair of hypertrophic cardiomyopathy

Endocarditis when preoperative testing was inadequate or extension of infection to perivalvular tissue is suspected

Assessment of aortic valve function in repair of aortic dissections with possible aortic valve involvement

Pericardial window procedures

Postoperative/intensive care unit

Unstable patients with unexplained hemodynamic disturbances, suspected valve disease, or thromboembolic problems

Category II indications: Supported by weaker evidence and expert consensus

Preoperative

Suspected acute thoracic aortic dissections, aneurysms, or disruption

Intraoperative

Valve replacement

Repair of cardiac aneurysms

Removal of cardiac tumors

Detection of foreign bodies

Detection of air emboli during cardiotomy, heart transplant operations, and upright neurosurgical procedures

Intracardiac thrombectomy

Pulmonary embolectomy

Suspected cardiac trauma

Repair of thoracic aortic dissections without suspected aortic valve involvement

Detection of aortic atheromatous disease or other sources of aortic emboli

Evaluation of pericardiectomy or pericardial effusions or evaluation of pericardial surgery

Intraoperative evaluation of anastomotic sites during heart and/or lung transplantation

Monitoring placement and function of assist devices

Perioperative

Increased risk of myocardial ischemia or infarction

Increased risk of hemodynamic disturbances

Category III indications: Little current scientific or expert support

Intraoperative

Evaluation of myocardial perfusion, coronary artery anatomy, or graft patency

Repair of cardiomyopathies other than hypertrophic obstructive cardiomyopathy

Uncomplicated endocarditis during noncardiac surgery

Monitoring for emboli during orthopedic procedures

Assessment of repair of thoracic aortic injuries

Uncomplicated pericarditis

Evaluation of pleuropulmonary disease

Monitoring placement of intraaortic balloon pumps, automatic implantable cardiac defibrillators, or pulmonary artery catheters

Monitoring of cardioplegia administration

Source: Modified from American Society of Anesthesiologists,[9] with permission.

reported reduced cardiac morbidity with epidural anesthesia[12,13] and three studies found no difference[14–16] (Table 84-5). *While some studies suggest that regional anesthesia and epidural analgesia have salutary effects in vascular surgical patients, the issue is unresolved due to the limited and conflicting clinical evidence. In addition, there are no studies that clearly determine whether or not local anesthesia with intravenous sedation is advantageous compared with general or major regional anesthetic techniques.*[5] Therefore, it is essential that the cardiologist/internist does not specifically exclude any anesthetic technique during a preoperative consultation.

Regional anesthetics are not infrequently converted to general anesthetics intraoperatively due to unexpectedly long surgery, patient discomfort, or changes in the surgical plan. No anesthesiologist can be certain that a particular technique will be adequate for the surgical procedure, given the unpredict-

ability of the situation, and the anesthesiologist must have flexibility to alter the technique as needed.

Regional Anesthesia

The term *regional anesthesia* was coined by Cushing for operations where local anesthetics were used to operate upon localized areas of the body without loss of consciousness. The advantages of regional anesthesia include simplicity, low cost, and minimal equipment requirements. Many of the adverse effects of general anesthesia are avoided, such as myocardial and respiratory depression. The disadvantages include patients' reluctance to be awake in the operating room, anesthetic agents of insufficient duration, and local anesthetic toxicity.

There is little evidence that regional or local anesthesia with intravenous sedation offers improved cardiac morbidity in high-risk patients.

TABLE 84-5

CLINICAL TRIALS EVALUATING EFFECTS OF NEURAXIAL ANESTHESIA ON CARDIOVASCULAR MORBIDITY

Study	N	Population	Cardiac Morbidity	Vascular Graft Patency Rate
Yeager et al.,[12] 1987	53	Mixed	Reduced with epidural	Not reported
Tuman et al.,[13] 1991	80	Vascular surgery	Reduced with epidural	Improved with epidural
Baron et al.[14] 1991	173	Aortic surgery	No difference	Not reported
Christopherson et al.,[16] 1993	100	Lower extremity vascular surgery	No difference	Improved with epidural
Bode et al.,[15] 1996	423	Lower extremity vascular surgery	No difference	Not reported

Source: Modified from Christopherson R, Norris EJ: Regional versus general anesthesia. *Anesth Clin North Am* 1997; 15:37–47, with permission.

The cardiovascular side effects of regional anesthesia vary depending on the technique chosen. Spinal and epidural anesthesia, for example, may cause major decreases in cardiac preload and afterload, while local anesthetic infiltration and axillary nerve blocks have almost no cardiovascular side effects. Regional anesthetics are contraindicated in anticoagulated patients and those with coagulopathies. Regional anesthesia may also be combined with general anesthesia in adults and children in order to decrease the requirements for the general anesthetic agents and for postoperative analgesia. The institution of analgesia prior to surgical stimulation (preemptive analgesia) may have salutary effects on postoperative pain control.

LOCAL ANESTHESIC AGENTS

The local anesthetics are classified on the basis of their chemical structure as esters or amides. The esters are hydrolyzed by esterases in the plasma, and the amides are metabolized in the liver. The duration of action of local anesthetic agents is affected by the protein-binding characteristics of the molecule and the addition of vasoconstrictors to the local anesthetic solution.[17] Toxic reactions to local anesthetics are generally characterized by central nervous system excitation (seizures), which may be followed by central nervous system depression and cardiovascular collapse.

Cocaine is the original ester local anesthetic. Its clinical use is mainly restricted to topical anesthesia of the nose and airway. It is the only local anesthetic agent that is intrinsically vasoconstrictive, an effect resulting from blockade of catecholamine reuptake at sympathetic nerve terminals. Cocaine's sympathomimetic effects result in central nervous system excitation, which increases requirements for general anesthetics. Cocaine toxicity has resulted in deaths from central nervous system toxicity and dysrhythmias.[18] Cocaine can also elicit myocardial ischemia. The tachycardia associated with cocaine contraindicates its use in patients with coronary artery disease,

mitral stenosis, or obstructive cardiomyopathy (see also Chap. 80).

Tetracaine is a long-acting ester local anesthetic frequently used in spinal anesthesia. It is also used for topical anesthesia of the eye and airway but may be toxic in the larger doses required for airway topical anesthesia. Chloroprocaine is a short-acting ester local anesthetic that is often used in epidural anesthesia. This agent is very rapidly metabolized by serum cholinesterase, leading to a low incidence of toxic reactions.

Compared to the esters, the amide local anesthetics are less rapidly metabolized (in the liver), and the potential for toxic reactions is somewhat greater. Some amide compounds (e.g., lidocaine) also have potent antidysrhythmic actions (see also Chap. 30). Lidocaine and mepivacaine are agents of intermediate duration of action that are commonly used in many types of regional blocks. Etidocaine and bupivacaine are agents of higher potency and longer duration of action that also exhibit more toxicity. Bupivacaine is particularly associated with cardiovascular collapse and dysrhythmias upon inadvertent intravascular injection.

Epinephrine and phenylephrine may be added to local anesthetic solutions to prolong their duration of action by local vasoconstriction. Epinephrine is typically added in concentrations ranging from 2.5 μg/mL (1:400,000) to 10 μg/mL (1:100,000) for infiltration, nerve blocks, or epidural anesthesia. The systemic absorption of epinephrine occurs very slowly, and beta-adrenergic effects predominate, resulting in slight tachycardia and diastolic hypotension. In patients whose cardiovascular disease precludes the use of epinephrine, phenylephrine may be substituted at concentrations 10 times higher than that of epinephrine. Epinephrine may induce ventricular dysrhythmias in patients anesthetized with halothane (see below).

SPINAL ANESTHESIA

The injection into the subarachnoid space of a relatively small dose of local anesthetic that produces profound motor and sensory blockade is known as spinal anesthesia. Spinal anesthesia also produces blockade of preganglionic sympathetic fibers, which usually results in hypotension. The level of spinal anesthesia is controlled by injection of a hyperbaric or hypobaric solution into the cerebrospinal fluid. The position of the patient is then manipulated to lateralize the blockade or to move the bolus of anesthetic in a more cephalad or caudad direction. The level of sympathetic blockade is generally two dermatomal segments higher than the sensory dermatomal level.

The higher the level of sympathetic blockade, the more profound the arterial and venous vasodilation and postural hypotension. Intravenous hydration with crystalloid solutions is the primary treatment for hypotension. Intravenous ephedrine (5 to 10 mg) or phenylephrine (20 to 100 μg) are also used to temporarily increase the blood pressure during periods of relative hypovolemia. If the dermatomal level of sympathetic blockade reaches T1, then the patient is effectively sympathectomized. The loss of cardiac accelerator fiber function may lead to bradycardia. Complete sympathectomy always occurs with a "total spinal," which also produces respiratory insufficiency due to intercostal and phrenic nerve root blockade.

Spinal anesthesia must be undertaken cautiously, and with more intensive monitoring, in patients whose cardiovascular stability depends upon the maintenance of a high preload and afterload. Patients with any significant cardiac valvular disease, hypertrophic obstructive cardiomyopathy, or tetralogy of Fallot are prone to hemodynamic decompensation during spinal anesthesia. Patients with CAD usually tolerate spinal anesthesia well, so long as diastolic arterial pressure is maintained at an appropriate level to preserve coronary perfusion pressure.

EPIDURAL ANESTHESIA

The epidural space, which is filled with loose areolar tissue and a venus plexus, lies immediately external to the dura mater. An indwelling polyethylene catheter is usually placed percutaneously for intermittent bolus injections or continuous infusions of local anesthetic and/or opioids. The epidural space may be entered by thoracic, lumbar, or caudal approaches. The advantages of epidural anesthesia are similar to those of spinal anesthesia and include moderate hypotension (which tends to decrease intraoperative blood loss) and contracted bowel loops during abdominal surgery. In addition, the ability to administer dilute local anesthetics and opioids through an indwelling epidural catheter is a very effective means of postoperative analgesia.

The hemodynamic effects of epidural anesthesia are essentially similar to those of spinal anesthesia except that the onset of sympathetic blockade is more gradual. Thus, with appropriate monitoring, cautious administration of epidural anesthetics has been safely done in patients with mitral valvular disease, aortic stenosis, or hypertrophic obstructive cardiomyopathy. It should be emphasized, though, that intraarterial and PACs may be required to monitor and treat changes in preload and afterload that occur with epidural anesthesia in patients with severe cardiovascular disease.

Generally, 10 to 15 times the volume of local anesthetic is required compared to spinal anesthesia. The potential for inadvertent intravascular injection of a toxic dose of local anesthetic is present. It is also possible inadvertently to inject a large volume into the subarachnoid space and cause a "total spinal" (see above). The hemodynamic consequences of inadvertent intravenous injections of epinephrine-containing solutions may be significant for patients who cannot tolerate tachy-cardia. Opioid epidural infusions for postoperative analgesia may be complicated by pruritus, urinary retention, somnolence, and respiratory depression. Thus, appropriate monitoring and nursing care are required.

NERVE BLOCKS AND INFILTRATION OF LOCAL ANESTHETIC

Nerve blocks and local anesthetic infiltration may be performed to facilitate surgery of localized areas of the body. The brachial plexus may be blocked by interscalene, supraclavicular, or axillary approaches. The lower extremity may be anesthetized by blocking the femoral and sciatic nerves. Local anesthetic infiltration is performed in regions such as the inguinal area to facilitate herniorrhaphies. These blocks, when properly performed, have minimal cardiovascular effects. They do, however, require large volumes of local anesthetic solution, which result in toxic reactions if inadvertent intravascular injection occurs. Intercostal blocks are associated with high blood concentrations even without intravascular injection, because the neurovascular bundle enhances absorption of the local anesthetic and multiple blocks are required for clinical efficacy. Epinephrine is occasionally added to prolong the duration of block, but this may be contraindicated in certain patients with cardiovascular disease, such as those with mitral stenosis.

General Anesthesia

General anesthesia is defined as a reversible state consisting of amnesia, analgesia, immobility, and the prevention of undesirable reflexes. The general anesthetics include many drugs, almost all of which have cardiovascular side effects. Intravenous agents are nearly always used for the induction of anesthesia in adults. Anesthesia is maintained using inhalational agents, intravenous agents, or a combination of the two. Neuromuscular blocking drugs (muscle relaxants) are commonly used to facilitate tracheal intubation and to lower the requirements for anesthetic agents (i.e., the dose of anesthetic that produces adequate amnesia and analgesia may not be sufficient to prevent movement or relax the abdominal musculature). In children, the induction of anesthesia is highly individualized according to patient needs, practitioner, and institution.

The physiologic consequences of general anesthesia have changed dramatically over the last several decades with the development of modern anesthetic agents. Ether and cyclopropane have sympathomimetic properties and were often used with spontaneous ventilation. Modern, nonexplosive inhalational anesthetic agents tend to be cardiac and respiratory depressants. With the exception of brief operations, nearly all general anesthetics include tracheal intubation and mechanical ventilation. As an alternative to tracheal intubation, devices such as the laryngeal mask airway may be used to secure a patient's airway. The loss of consciousness is usually accompanied by a decrease in sympathetic tone. This, as well as the effects of positive pressure ventilation, causes a moderate decrease in cardiac output even when the anesthetic drugs are not myocardial depressants per se.

The patient with cardiovascular disease presents major concerns to the anesthesiologist. General anesthesia masks many of the symptoms of cardiovascular decompensation, such as angina, dyspnea, dizziness, and palpitations. Other signs of cardiovascular disease, such as tachycardia, are nonspecific and may be misinterpreted as hypovolemia or light anesthesia. Fluid shifts, obstructed venous return, and varying levels of noxious stimulation are other variables related to surgery that are unpredictable. It is for these reasons that appropriate monitoring and selection of anesthetic agents is vital to the intraoperative management of the patient with cardiovascular disease.

INTRAVENOUS ANESTHETICS

Intravenous anesthetic induction drugs are composed of lipophilic molecules that have an affinity for neuronal tissue or specific receptors. Their action is generally terminated by redistribution from the vessel-rich tissues (brain, heart, liver, and kidneys) to other tissues (muscle, fat, and skin). Elimination occurs via hepatic metabolism and takes place over several hours. Patients with diminished cardiac output secondary to cardiovascular disease will have prolonged effects from intravenous induction drugs.

Barbiturates

Thiopental, an ultrashort acting thiobarbiturate, is the prototype for agents of its class. It is quick, reliable, and pleasant for patients and does not have excitatory side effects. Its cardiovascular effects are marked by dose-dependent myocardial depression and dilation of venous capacitance vessels. The decrease in cardiac output is usually compensated for by arterial vasoconstriction, so that blood pressure is minimally decreased. Thiopental is a poor analgesic, however, and tachycardia and hypertension are common with tracheal intubation or any painful stimulus.

Standard doses of barbiturate for anesthetic induction are contraindicated in patients with preload-dependent cardiac lesions and/or severely impaired ventricular contractility. This includes patients with pericardial tamponade, mitral regurgitation, aortic regurgitation, mitral stenosis, and dilated cardiomyopathy. Reduced doses and slower injection of the drug will markedly decrease the cardiovascular effects.

Benzodiazepines

Benzodiazepines may be used as premedication, to induce anesthesia, or as an adjunct to regional or general anesthesia. Their most useful therapeutic effects include sedation and amnesia. They tend to be unreliable in their rapidity of induction and occasionally fail to induce unconsciousness despite high doses. When used as sole agents, the benzodiazepines have minimal cardiovascular effects. When used in combination with other drugs such as opioids and potent volatile anesthetics, benzodiazepines produce hypotension, which may be due to myocardial depression or decreased systemic vascular resistance.

Opioids

Synthetic opioids have assumed a major role in the anesthetic care of patients with cardiovascular disease. They can be used as premedication, as supplements to regional or inhalational anesthesia, as one of the main components of "nitrous-narcotic" anesthesia, or as the primary anesthetic agent (high-dose opioid anesthesia). They are often used as supplements during anesthesia induction to block the hemodynamic response to laryngoscopy and tracheal intubation. While opioids are excellent analgesics, they are unreliable amnesics, provide no muscle relaxation, and are associated with "breakthrough" hypertension and tachycardia intraoperatively.

A further problem with high doses of opioids is that they can produce truncal muscle rigidity, ocular movements, wrist flexion, and shoulder abduction—often referred to as "fentanyl seizures." These events, however, do not produce electroencephalographic changes characteristic of epileptiform activity.[19,20] The truncal rigidity does interfere with ventilation and requires the use of neuromuscular blockers. Ventilatory support is frequently continued postoperatively because the elimination half-lives of synthetic opioids are relatively long (1.5 to 4 h). Remifentanil, a new synthetic opioid that is extremely short-acting due to ester hydrolysis, has the cardiovascular advantages of the synthetic opioids without the prolonged duration of effect at high doses.[21]

Neither morphine nor meperidine is commonly used intraoperatively. Morphine is often used as premedication and for postoperative analgesia. With higher doses and rapid administration, morphine causes histamine release and is associated with hypotension and increased fluid requirements. It is also a venodilator. Meperidine produces tachycardia and histamine release, and it is a direct myocardial depressant. It has the lowest toxic:therapeutic dose ratio of the clinically relevant opioids.

Despite the disadvantages noted above, high-dose synthetic (phenylpiperidine) opioid anesthesia does not depress myocardial contractility and is devoid of histamine release. It is therefore associated with markedly stable hemodynamics during anesthetic induction and maintenance in the majority of patients with cardiovascular disease. Nevertheless, patients with high resting sympathetic tone, congestive heart failure, and severe pulmonary hypertension are prone to transient hypotension during anesthetic induction. A mild bradycardia usually occurs on anesthetic induction due to an increase in vagal tone. The bradycardia is often advantageous in patients with diseases such as CAD or mitral stenosis. The bradycardia effect is reliably antagonized by atropine or pancuronium (see below) in patients with conditions such as mitral regurgitation, which require faster heart rates. There is a recent trend to reduce the doses of opioids administered in cardiac anesthesia in order to facilitate more rapid tracheal extubation and discharge from the intensive care unit.[22]

Anesthesiologists only rarely administer naloxone or other opioid antagonists to reverse the effects of a systemic opioid in patients with cardiovascular disease. The reversal of the opioid effect results in the sudden onset of pain and surges in catecholamine levels. Naloxone administration has been complicated by pulmonary edema,[23] dysrhythmias,[24] and cardiac arrest.[25] Intravenous naloxone has been safely used to reverse the pruritus and respiratory depression associated with epidural and intrathecal opioids without reversing the analgesia.[26]

Etomidate

Etomidate is an imidazole anesthetic agent that enhances gamma-aminobutyric acid (GABA)-ergic transmission. It is associated with marked hemodynamic stability during bolus administration for anesthetic induction but does not blunt the hemodynamic response to laryngoscopy and tracheal intubation. This is one of the preferred agents for anesthetic induction in patients with valvular or ventricular dysfunction, hypovolemia, or pericardial effusion. Etomidate infusions are not used in the United States because of their association with adrenocortical insufficiency.

Propofol

Propofol is a substituted phenol (diisopropylphenol) that may be used for anesthetic induction and maintenance. It is dissolved in a soybean oil emulsion, which is mildly irritating on injection. Its main advantage is the rapid emergence and psychomotor recovery following termination of the drug infusion. Propofol causes dose-dependent hypotension that appears to be due to a combination of myocardial depression and vasodilation. It is prudent to use reduced doses of propofol in patients with aortic or mitral valvular stenosis and cardiomyopathies. Propofol is being used increasingly for sedation in intensive care units and to facilitate "fast-track" extubation following cardiac surgery.

Ketamine

Ketamine is a cyclohexanone that is chemically related to phencyclidine (PCP). Its use as a sole anesthetic is limited by its sympathomimetic effects and emergence delirium. Its sympathomimetic effects are advantageous, however, in certain groups of patients with cardiovascular disease. These include mainly those who are critically dependent on high resting sympathetic tone to maintain an adequate perfusion pressure: patients with pericardial tamponade, hypovolemia, and systemic-to-pulmonary arterial shunts. It is important to reduce the dose of ketamine in those with severe cardiac disease because ketamine is an indirect sympathomimetic and direct myocardial depressant. In patients who already have maximal sympathetic outflow, ketamine's depressant effects may be "unmasked." Ketamine is relatively contraindicated in patients who cannot tolerate tachycardia, such as those with CAD or mitral stenosis.[27]

Alpha₂-Adrenergic Agonists

Clonidine and dexmedetomidine are alpha$_2$-adrenergic agonists that are sympatholytic, sedative-anxiolytic, antidysrhythmic, analgesic, and reversible.[28,29] Clonidine has also been demonstrated to reduce anesthetic requirements and improve hemodynamic stability during the intraoperative period. Once

more convenient and specific compounds are developed, alpha$_2$-adrenergic agents may play a much larger role in the future in the perioperative management of patients with cardiovascular disease.

INHALATIONAL ANESTHETICS

Inhalational anesthetics include nitrous oxide and the potent volatile agents. The study of the uptake and distribution of inhaled drugs with cerebral and cardiovascular effects is practically unique to anesthesiology, and cardiac output is a major determinant of uptake and distribution. The alveolar concentration of a drug is generally equal to the brain concentration. Thus, anything that hastens increases in the alveolar concentration of the drug will speed the onset of anesthesia. Two factors that speed the onset of anesthesia are a diminished cardiac output and an anesthetic agent with low solubility in the blood. Thus, patients with low cardiac output secondary to cardiovascular disease will have a more rapid onset of anesthesia. Intracardiac right-to-left shunting will decrease the onset of anesthesia, whereas left-to-right shunting has negligible effects.

Nitrous Oxide

Nitrous oxide is an excellent analgesic but not a very potent anesthetic. Concentrations up to 75% may be given safely, but incomplete amnesia and movement in response to painful stimuli are likely. Thus, nitrous oxide is nearly always administered with other anesthetic agents, such as opioids or potent volatile agents, and neuromuscular blockers. It is also chosen because its relatively low solubility in the blood enhances the rapid onset and termination of its effects.

Nitrous oxide is a weak myocardial depressant, which mildly stimulates the sympathetic nervous system.[30] It does not, however, exacerbate pulmonary hypertension.[31] As a sole agent, its cardiovascular effects are minimal, but cardiac output is lowered in the presence of opioids. It also accentuates the negative inotropic effects of potent volatile agents.[32]

Nitrous oxide diffuses very rapidly into closed air spaces within the body due to its low blood solubility, high lipid solubility, and the high concentrations required. Examples of closed air spaces include bowel gas, pneumothoraces, and air emboli. Once equilibrium is reached, 75% nitrous oxide will quadruple the size of any of these spaces. For this reason, nitrous oxide must be discontinued if a pneumothorax or air embolism is suspected. It is often avoided in cardiothoracic procedures, particularly in children prone to paradoxical embolization, or after cardiopulmonary bypass.

Potent Volatile Agents

The use of inhalational anesthesia with potent volatile agents is the most common anesthetic technique because of its relatively low cost, reliable amnesia, and bronchodilation as well as the low blood solubility and overall safety record of these agents. All are myocardial depressants and vasodilators and produce some degree of hypotension. The hypotension provides some indication of the depth of anesthesia, as does monitoring of end-tidal gas concentrations.

The effect of these agents is rapidly changed when the inspiratory concentration is adjusted. The titrability of inhalational anesthesia is an advantage compared to intravenous drugs, because the duration of surgical procedures and the degree of surgical stimulation are often unpredictable. For this reason, low doses of volatile anesthetics may be added as supplements to nitrous oxide- or intravenous-based anesthetic techniques for the control of hypertension and the prevention of awareness (incomplete amnesia).

The frequent production of nodal (junctional) rhythm is also common to these agents. The loss of atrial systole may be poorly tolerated, particularly in patients with aortic stenosis, hypertrophic cardiomyopathies, or mitral stenosis. All potent volatile agents have the potential for interactions with calcium channel blockers and beta-adrenergic blockers. Negative inotropic and conduction effects of these drugs may be augmented by the volatile anesthetic agents; however, all cardiac drugs should be continued until the time of surgery.

Halothane. Halothane represented a major advance in anesthesia when it was introduced in the 1950s, but its use is restricted by its cardiovascular effects and the small incidence of hepatotoxicity. Halothane depresses the myocardium and the sinoatrial node but is not a potent vasodilator. Thus, cardiac output and heart rate are depressed in a dose-dependent fashion. Blood pressure is not severely decreased, because the decrease in systemic vascular resistance is less than with the other volatile agents at equipotent dosages. This hemodynamic profile is beneficial in situations where myocardial contractility (and oxygen consumption) should be kept low and perfusion pressure maintained high. Examples include ischemic heart disease, hypertrophic obstructive cardiomyopathy, and tetralogy of Fallot. Halothane is contraindicated in patients with dilated cardiomyopathy, congestive heart failure, aortic stenosis, aortic and mitral regurgitation, and pericardial tamponade.

Halothane lowers the threshold for epinephrine-induced ventricular dysrhythmias more than other volatile agents. As a practical matter, the initial epinephrine dose is restricted to 1.5 μg/kg during infiltration of local anesthetic solutions. If dysrhythmias occur due to an inadvertent vascular injection, the halothane should be discontinued. Approximately five times the dose of epinephrine is required to induce ventricular dysrhythmias in patients receiving enflurane and isoflurane.

Enflurane. Enflurane is almost equal to halothane in its negative inotropic effect, but it is more vasodilating and less of a negative chronotrope. Thus, cardiac output is better maintained, but blood pressure is lower than with equipotent dosages of halothane. Enflurane is often chosen as a supplement to intravenous anesthetic techniques when breakthrough hypertension occurs. Enflurane has been used less commonly in recent years for various reasons, including its cardiovascular disadvantages (compared with isoflurane).

Isoflurane. Isoflurane is somewhat less negatively inotropic than enflurane or halothane and is a potent arteriolar vasodila-

tor, which tends to maintain cardiac output. Tachycardia frequently occurs at clinical dosages because the baroreceptor reflexes are not impaired. On the basis of its hemodynamic effects, isoflurane would be beneficial in patients with mitral or aortic regurgitation with good ventricular function. It is relatively contraindicated (as a sole agent) in patients with mitral or aortic stenosis, dilated and hypertrophic cardiomyopathies, and pericardial tamponade. Isoflurane is frequently used in patients with CAD, when it is often combined with opioids or beta-adrenergic blockers to prevent tachycardia and the dose is limited to preserve coronary perfusion pressure. The use of isoflurane remains controversial in patients with coronary artery anatomy that predisposes to coronary "steal."

The coronary steal phenomenon occurs when a zone of myocardium distal to a stenotic coronary artery derives its blood supply from collateral vessels that originate in a zone of myocardium with normal coronary arterial supply. The arterioles in the normal zone are partially constricted, while those in the collateral-dependent zone are maximally dilated due to the "upstream" coronary artery occlusion. This maintains the pressure gradient across the collateral vessels and the perfusion of the collateral-dependent zone. Some arteriolar vasodilators (e.g., adenosine, dipyridamole, sodium nitroprusside) can dilate the arterioles in the normal myocardial zone, decrease the perfusion pressure across the collateral vessels, and precipitate myocardial ischemia due to coronary steal. Isoflurane has been shown to induce myocardial ischemia with collateral-dependent myocardial blood flow in canine models[33] and in humans.[34]

It remains controversial whether or not isoflurane should be used in patients with CAD, given the uncertainty regarding coronary artery anatomy in most patients. The tachycardia and hypotension associated with isoflurane, as well as evidence of maldistributed myocardial blood flow, might suggest that it should not be used. Nevertheless, a prospective clinical study in patients with "steal-prone anatomy"[35] and large outcome studies[8,9] have not found intraoperative myocardial ischemia or poorer outcome with isoflurane anesthesia. A reasonable conclusion would be that isoflurane should be used with caution and appropriate monitoring in patients suspected of having "steal-prone" coronary artery anatomy.[36]

Desflurane. Desflurane is a volatile anesthetic that was introduced into clinical practice in 1992. It is much less soluble in blood than the volatile agents described above. Its blood:gas solubility coefficient is similar to that of nitrous oxide. Thus, more rapid induction and emergence would be expected. This is particularly advantageous in ambulatory procedures. Several studies have compared emergence from anesthesia with desflurane with that from isoflurane-based anesthetics and have demonstrated that initial emergence from a given depth of anesthesia (e.g., time to eye opening or response to verbal commands) is about half as long with desflurane.[37] The coronary vascular effects of desflurane are similar to those of isoflurane, but desflurane is not associated with tachycardia at lower doses.[38] Despite desflurane's similarity to isoflurane with regard to myocardial depression and vasodilation, desflurane has a unique sympathomimetic effect. This effect is seen with rapid increases in end-tidal concentration in the absence of preanesthetic medication. The sympathomimetic effect of desflurane can be blocked by fentanyl, esmolol, and clonidine.[39]

Sevoflurane. The relatively low solubility and minimal airway irritation of sevoflurane make it a very useful anesthetic for the inhalation induction of anesthesia. Its low solubility allows rapid alterations in alveolar concentration during the maintenance period of the anesthetic, thereby improving control of the depth of anesthesia. The commercial development of sevoflurane has been slow because of concerns regarding the potential toxicity of its metabolites (e.g., fluoride-induced nephrotoxicity) and breakdown products, despite the very large clinical experience in Japan.[40]

The cardiovascular effects of sevoflurane are similar to those of isoflurane and desflurane except that sevoflurane is not associated with increases in heart rate. Sevoflurane progressively decreases blood pressure in a manner similar to the other volatile anesthetics. In animals, sevoflurane appears to be a slightly less potent coronary vasodilator than isoflurane and has not been associated with coronary steal. Myocardial contractility is depressed in a manner similar to that of equianesthetic concentrations of isoflurane and desflurane, and it does not potentiate epinephrine-induced cardiac dysrhythmias. In several prospective, randomized, multicenter studies in which patients with CAD or risk factors for CAD received either sevoflurane or isoflurane, the incidence of adverse cardiac outcomes did not differ between treatment groups.[41]

Neuromuscular Blockade

BENZYLISOQUINOLINIUM COMPOUNDS

The benzylisoquinolinium series of nondepolarizing neuromuscular blockers are all derivatives of the curare molecule. Most of these compounds have histamine-releasing properties that are dependent on the dose and rate of administration. D-Tubocurarine, metocurine, atracurium, and mivacurium are associated with clinically important histamine release following the administration of bolus doses to facilitate tracheal intubation. The newer agents, doxacurium and cisatracurium, are not associated with histamine release with large ("intubating") doses. While older agents, such as D-tubocurarine and metocurine, are mainly dependent upon renal elimination, atracurium and cisatracurium undergo a unique form of spontaneous degradation that is organ-independent (Hofmann elimination). Mivacurium undergoes enzyme-dependent ester hydrolysis.

AMINOSTEROID COMPOUNDS

Pancuronium is the classic aminosteroid nondepolarizing neuromuscular blocking drug. The atropine-like molecular structure contains two quaternary nitrogen groups. The tachycardia and hypertension associated with pancuronium have been linked to myocardial ischemia during coronary artery bypass surgery.[42] The anticholinergic effects of pancuronium, however, can be useful (e.g., in patients with mitral regurgitation) for preventing the increase in vagal tone that occurs with high-dose opioid anesthetic inductions. Vecuronium and pipecuronium have minimal cardiovascular effects at usual clinical dosages. Rocuronium is a newer aminosteroid compound with a more rapid onset of action due to its lower potency and has minimal cardiovascular side effects. While pancuronium elimination is almost entirely renal, the newer compounds are also degraded by the liver.

SUCCINYLCHOLINE

Succinylcholine, essentially di-acetylcholine molecularly, is a depolarizing short-acting neuromuscular blocker that is still used because of its low cost, rapid onset, and short duration of action. Its cardiovascular effects depend on whether nicotinic or muscarinic receptor effects predominate in a given patient. Thus, tachycardia and hypertension or bradycardia and hypotension may occur. Vagal effects tend to predominate with repeated doses or in children. In patients with various disorders (including neuromuscular diseases, recent burns, and massive trauma), hyperkalemic cardiac arrest may occur with succinylcholine administration because of exaggerated release of intracellular potassium from myocytes.

THE POSTOPERATIVE PERIOD

The emergence from anesthesia is frequently accompanied by hypertension and tachycardia, which is most often due to incomplete analgesia but may also be related to withdrawal from antihypertensive drugs, hypoxemia, delirium, or bladder distension. If an underlying modifiable cause is not identified, then intravenous drugs—such as nitroglycerin, labetalol, or esmolol—are frequently used to control hemodynamics in patients with cardiovascular disease. Shivering is another phenomenon that may occur due to hypothermia or emergence from volatile anesthetics. Shivering results in severe increases in oxygen consumption, which may be poorly tolerated by patients with cardiovascular disease. Although the mechanism is unknown, low doses of meperidine decrease or eliminate shivering.[43]

Numerous studies clearly show that the extended postoperative period entails significant cardiovascular risk. The majority of perioperative myocardial infarctions (MIs), for example, occur on postoperative days 2 through 4. Pain, high catecholamine levels, hypercoagulability, hypovolemia, anemia, intravascular volume shifts, drug effects, and a lower level of monitoring all probably contribute to this phenomenon.

Traditionally, the anesthesiologist has not played a major role in postoperative management following discharge from the recovery room/postanesthesia care unit. This situation has recently changed with the development of multidisciplinary pain services that administer epidural analgesia and patient-controlled analgesics. As noted above, it remains controversial whether or not regional anesthesia and intensive postoperative analgesia are capable of reducing morbidity and mortality. It is conceivable that more effective postoperative analgesia decreases the deleterious effects of the stress response. Future efforts to reduce perioperative risk likely will concentrate on assessing the effects of more intensive postoperative hemodynamic, analgesic, and anticoagulation management.

CONCLUSIONS

The optimal perioperative care of patients with cardiovascular disease is the joint responsibility of anesthesiologists, surgeons, and cardiologist/internists. Any anesthetic agent or technique has the potential for producing adverse effects, and the margin of safety is reduced in patients with cardiovascular disease. It is the anesthesiologist's role to acquire accurate and relevant information from the preoperative evaluation, to apply appropriate monitoring technology, to select an anesthetic technique that is suited to the planned procedure and the condition of the patient, and to manage hemodynamic alterations and analgesic requirements in the perioperative period. As cardiovascular disease continues to become more prevalent in the surgical population and preoperative testing and intraoperative monitoring become more sophisticated, the need for effective communication between the specialties of cardiology and anesthesiology will become even more important.

REFERENCES

1. Wells PH, Kaplan JA. Optimal management of patients with ischemic heart disease for non-cardiac surgery by complementary anesthesia and cardiology intervention. *Am Heart J* 1981; 102:1030–1040.
2. Goldman L, Caldera DL, Nussbaum SR, Southwick FS, Krogstad D, Murray B, et al. Multifactorial index of cardiac risk in noncardiac surgical procedures. *N Engl J Med* 1977; 297:845–850.
3. Mangano ET, Browner WS, Hollenberg M, London MJ, Tubau JF, Tateo IM, et al. Association of perioperative myocardial ischemia with cardiac morbidity and mortality in men undergoing noncardiac surgery. *N Engl J Med* 1990; 323:1781–1788.
4. Goldman L. Multifactorial index of cardiac risk in non-cardiac surgery: Ten year status report. *J Cardiothorac Anesth* 1987; 1:237–244.
5. ACC/AHA Task Force on Practice Guidelines. Guidelines for perioperative cardiovascular evaluation for noncardiac surgery. *Circulation* 1996; 93:1278–1317.
6. Mangano DT, Goldman L. Preoperative assessment of patients with known or suspected coronary disease. *N Engl J Med* 1995; 333:1750–1756.
7. Kleinman B, Czinn E, Shah K, Sobotka P, Rao TK. The value to the anesthesia-surgical care team of the preoperative cardiac consultation. *J Cardiothorac Anesth* 1989; 3:682–687.
8. American Society of Anesthesiologists. *Standards for Basic Intraoperative Monitoring* (Amended by the House of Delegates on October 18, 1989 to become effective January 1, 1990). Park Ridge, IL: ASA; 1989.
9. American Society of Anesthesiologists. Practice guidelines for perioperative transesophageal echocardiography. *Anesthesiology* 1996; 84:986–1006.
10. Slogoff S, Keats AS. Randomized trial of primary anesthetic agents on outcome of coronary artery bypass operations. *Anesthesiology* 1989; 70:179–188.
11. Tuman KJ, McCarthy RJ, Spiess BD, DaValle M, Dabir R, Ivankovich AD. Does choice of anesthetic agent significantly affect outcome after coronary artery surgery? *Anesthesiology* 1989; 70:189–198.

12. Yeager MP, Glass DD, Neff RK, Brinck-Johnsen T. Epidural anesthesia and analgesia in high-risk surgical procedures. *Anesthesiology* 1987; 66:729–736.
13. Tuman KJ, McCarthy RJ, March RJ, DeLaria GA, Patel RV, Ivankovich AD. Effects of epidural anesthesia and analgesia on coagulation and outcome after major vascular surgery. *Anesth Analg* 1991; 73:696–704.
14. Baron JF, Bertrand M, Barre E, Godet G, Mundler O, Coriat P, et al. Combined epidural and general anesthesia versus general anesthesia for abdominal aortic surgery. *Anesthesiology* 1991; 75:611–618.
15. Bode RH Jr, Lewis KP, Zarich SW, Pierce ET, Roberts M, Kowalchuk GJ, et al: Cardiac outcome after peripheral vascular surgery: Comparison of general and regional anesthesia. *Anesthesiology* 1996; 84:3–13.
16. Christopherson R, Beattie C, Frank SM, Norris EJ, Meinert CL, Gottlieb SO, et al. Perioperative morbidity in patients randomized to epidural or general anesthesia for lower extremity vascular surgery. *Anesthesiology* 1993; 79:422–434.
17. Covino BG. Pharmacology of local anaesthetic agents. *Br J Anaesth* 1986; 58:701–716.
18. Fleming JA, Byck R, Barash PG. Pharmacology and therapeutic applications of cocaine. *Anesthesiology* 1990; 73:518–531.
19. Smith NT, Benthuysen JL, Bickford RG, Sanford TJ, Blasco T, Duke PC, et al. Seizures during opioid anesthetic induction—Are they opioid-induced rigidity? *Anesthesiology* 1989; 71:852–862.
20. Murkin JM, Moldenhauer CC, Hug CC Jr, Epstein CM. Absence of seizures during induction of anesthesia with high-dose fentanyl. *Anesth Analg* 1984; 63:439–494.
21. Dershwitz M, Randel GI, Rosow CE, Fragen RJ, Connors PM, Librojo ES, et al. Initial clinical experience with remifentanil, a new opioid metabolized by esterases. *Anesth Analg* 1995; 81:619–623.
22. Glass PSA. Pharmacokinetic and pharmacodynamic principles in providing "fast-track" recovery. *J Cardiothorac Vasc Anesth* 1995; 9(5, suppl 1):16–20.
23. Prough DS, Roy R, Bumgarner J, Shannon G. Acute pulmonary edema in healthy teenagers following conservative doses of intravenous naloxone. *Anesthesiology* 1984; 60:485–486.
24. Azar I, Turndorf H. Severe hypertension and multiple atrial premature contractions following naloxone administration. *Anesth Analg* 1979; 58:524–525.
25. Andree RA. Sudden death following naloxone administration. *Anesth Analg* 1980; 59:782–784.
26. Bell SD, Seltzer JL. Postoperative pain management. In: Kaplan JA, ed. *Vascular Anesthesia*. New York: Churchill-Livingstone; 1991:565–586.
27. Reich DL, Silvay G. Ketamine: An update on the first 25 years of clinical experience. *Can J Anaesth* 1989; 36:186–197.
28. Flacke JW. Alpha$_2$-adrenergic agonists in cardiovascular anesthesia. *J Cardiothorac Vasc Anesth* 1992; 6:344–359.
29. Maze M, Tranquilli W. Alpha$_2$-agonists: Defining the role in clinical anesthesia. *Anesthesiology* 1991; 74:581–605.
30. Ebert TJ, Kampine JP. Nitrous oxide augments sympathetic outflow: Direct evidence from human peroneal nerve recordings. *Anesth Analg* 1989; 69:444–449.
31. Konstadt SN, Reich DL, Thys DM. Nitrous oxide does not exacerbate pulmonary hypertension or ventricular dysfunction in patients with mitral valvular disease. *Can J Anaesth* 1990; 37:613–617.
32. Stowe DF, Monroe SM, Marijic J, Bosnjak ZJ, Kampine JP. Comparison of halothane, enflurane, and isoflurane with nitrous oxide on contractility and oxygen supply and demand in isolated hearts. *Anesthesiology* 1991; 75:1062–1074.
33. Buffington CW, Romson JL, Levine A, Duttlinger NC, Huang AH. Isoflurane induces coronary steal in a canine model of chronic coronary occlusion. *Anesthesiology* 1987; 66:280–292.
34. Reiz S, Bälfors E, Sorensen MB, Ariola S, Friedman A, Truedsson H. Isoflurane: A powerful coronary vasodilator in patients with coronary artery disease. *Anesthesiology* 1983; 59:91–97.
35. Pulley DD, Kirvassilis GV, Kelermenos N, Kater K, Barzilai B, Genton RE, et al. Regional and global myocardial circulatory and metabolic effects of isoflurane and halothane in patients with steal-prone coronary anatomy. *Anesthesiology* 1991; 75:756–766.
36. Priebe HJ. Isoflurane and coronary hemodynamics. *Anesthesiology* 1989; 71:960–976.
37. Smiley RM, Ornstein E, Matteo RS, Pantuck EJ, Pantuck CB. Desflurane and isoflurane in surgical patients: Comparison of emergence time. *Anesthesiology* 1991; 74:425–428.

38. Saidman LJ: The role of desflurane in the practice of anesthesia. *Anesthesiology* 1991; 74:399–401.

39. Weiskopf RB, Eger EI II, Noorani M, Daniel M. Fentanyl, esmolol, and clonidine blunt the transient cardiovascular stimulation induced by desflurane in humans. *Anesthesiology* 1994; 81:1350–1355.

40. Smith I, Nathanson MH, White PF. The role of sevoflurane in outpatient anesthesia. *Anesth Analg* 1995; 81(6 suppl):S67–S72.

41. Ebert TJ, Harkin CP, Muzi M. Cardiovascular responses to sevoflurane: A review. *Anesth Analg* 1995; 81(6 suppl):S11–S22.

42. Thomson IR, Putnins CL. Adverse effects of pancuronium during high-dose fentanyl anesthesia for coronary artery bypass grafting. *Anesthesiology* 1985; 62:708–713.

43. Guffin A, Girard D, Kaplan JA. Shivering following cardiac surgery: Hemodynamic changes and reversal. *J Cardiothorac Anesth* 1987; 1:24–28.

FOURTEEN

MISCELLANEOUS DISEASES AND CONDITIONS

85

THE CONNECTIVE TISSUE DISEASES

Robert C. Schlant / Emilio B. Gonzalez / William C. Roberts

The term *connective tissue disease* includes both a group of heritable conditions and a group of nonheritable, acquired disorders. The heritable disorders of connective tissue include Marfan's syndrome (MS), the Ehlers-Danlos syndrome (EDS), pseudoxanthoma elasticum (PXE), osteogenesis imperfecta (OI), annuloaortic ectasia, and familial aneurysms.[1,2] Other heritable disorders of connective tissue that are rarely associated with cardiac defects include Stickler's syndrome, familial articular hypermobility syndrome, epidermolysis bullosa, alcaptonuria, and disorders of copper transport.[3] The nonheritable disorders of connective tissue that may have major cardiovascular involvement include systemic lupus erythematosus (SLE), polyarteritis nodosa (PN), rheumatoid arthritis (RA), ankylosing spondylitis, systemic sclerosis (SS), polymyositis/dermatomyositis, giant cell arteritis, the Churg-Strauss syndrome, the antiphospholipid syndrome, and possibly syphilis.

HERITABLE CONNECTIVE TISSUE DISORDERS

MARFAN'S SYNDROME

Epidemiology

The prevalence of the classic MS is about 5 per 100,000, without gender, racial, or ethnic predilection. Because of the great heterogeneity of the syndrome, the actual prevalence may be considerably greater, probably about 1 per 10,000.[4] MS has an autosomal dominant inheritance with high penetrance. In about 25 to 30 percent of patients, the disorder occurs without a positive family history and appears to be due to a new mutation.

Molecular Genetics

MS is associated with defects in the fibrillin-1 gene (FBN1) on chromosome 15, where more than 50 mutations have been described[5–15] (see also Chap. 69).

Clinical Features

There is considerable variation in the clinical manifestations of MS, even within one family. The ocular, skeletal, and cardiovascular systems are characteristically involved. The four major manifestations include a positive family history, ectopia lentis, aortic root dilatation or dissection, and dural ectasia.[3] Many of the other, relatively mild features of MS occur with a relatively high prevalence in the general population. These features include mitral valve prolapse, early myopia, scoliosis, and joint hypermobility. Other manifestations of MS include anterior chest deformity, especially asymmetric pectus excavatum or carinatum; long, thin extremities (dolichostenomelia) with arachnodactyly; tall stature with increased lower body height (Fig. 10-7); high, narrowly arched palate; myopia; fusiform ascending aortic aneurysm ("anuloaortic ectasia") with aortic regurgitation (Fig. 85-1); aortic dissection; mitral regurgitation, which can result from a variety of causes, including mitral valve prolapse, dilatation of the mitral annulus, mitral annular calcification, dilatation of the left ventricle, rupture of mitral chordae tendineae, papillary muscle dysfunction, or infective endocarditis; spontaneous pneumothorax; cutaneous striae; and inguinal hernia.[1–4,16–18]

In the absence of an unequivocally affected first-degree relative, requirements for the diagnosis include at least one major manifestation with involvement of the skeleton and at least two other systems. In the presence of at least one unequivocally affected first-degree relative, there should be involvement of at least two systems; the presence of a major manifestation is still preferred, but this can vary depending upon the family's phenotype.[3]

In one echocardiographic assessment of the cardiovascular abnormalities in 59 patients with MS, 57 percent had mitral

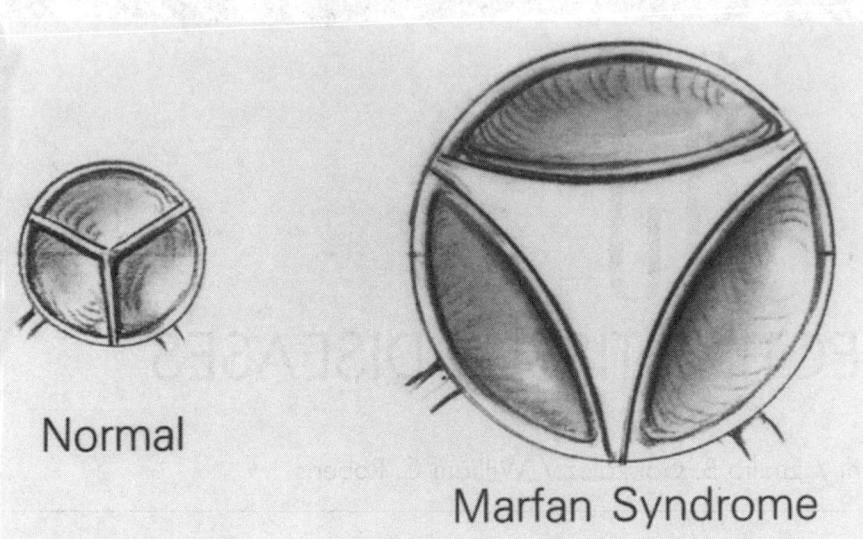

FIGURE 85-1
Mechanism of aortic regurgitation in Marfan's syndrome.

valve prolapse and 69 percent had aortic root enlargement.[19] While more than half of the patients with MS have mitral valve prolapse, primary mitral valve prolapse (Chap. 64) is not a *forme fruste* of MS,[20] although it has been suggested that the two conditions are part of a phenotypic continuum.[21]

General Evaluation

In addition to a careful personal and family history and physical examination, measurements should be made of the patient's height, arm span, and floor-to-pelvis distance. A slit-lamp ophthalmic examination and an electrocardiogram (ECG) should be obtained. Patients with MS should be seen at least yearly, and a transthoracic echocardiogram should be obtained on an annual basis. Consideration should be given to obtaining a transesophageal echocardiogram or magnetic resonance imaging (MRI). If the diagnosis is definite or probable, consideration should be given to screening first-degree relatives by echocardiography. Genetic counseling should be offered to all patients. Psychiatric counseling also is often useful. If a patient develops suggestive widening of the proximal aorta, repeat transthoracic or, in some instances, transesophageal echocardiography should be performed more frequently. Patients with possible or definite MS and evidence of mitral valve abnormality should receive antibiotic prophylaxis prior to dental procedures (see Chap. 82).

Management

Patients with MS should avoid isometric, abrupt, or strenuous exertion; contact sports; scuba diving; and trauma. Patients with aortic dilatation and aortic or mitral regurgitation should avoid competitive sports. Patients without aortic dilatation and aortic or mitral regurgitation should be allowed to perform low-to-moderate intensity static and low-intensity dynamic sports including bowling, golf, and archery.

β-Adrenergic blockade therapy should be used in all patients with MS to retard the rate of dilatation of the aortic root.[4,22–24] Although the optimal dose has not been established, some have suggested giving the largest dose that is clinically tolerated. Selective β₁-adrenergic blocking agents are preferred, although no randomized studies have been performed. Atenolol, which should be administered twice daily, appears to be the most widely used β-adrenergic blocker in this condition.

In asymptomatic patients, repair of aortic aneurysms has been recommended at different degrees of enlargement. Thus, some have advocated repair when the aortic diameter is 55 mm or greater[25,26]; at 60 mm or greater[23,27–30]; or when the aortic diameter increases to twice that of the uninvolved distal aorta.[31–34] Some patients develop aortic dissection with aortic root dimensions less than 50 to 55 mm.[12] Surgical repair is generally recommended when the diameter reaches 55 to 60 mm. Factors that encourage an earlier surgical intervention include a positive family history for aortic dissection or rupture,[35] severe aortic or mitral regurgitation, progressive dilatation of the aortic root on serial echocardiograms, the need for other major abdominal aortic or spinal surgical procedures, and planning for a pregnancy.[34,36] In most patients, the ascending aorta and aortic valve are replaced and the portion of the aorta containing the coronary ostia is reimplanted.[37] Postoperatively, annual assessment of the entire aorta by MRI is advised.[38] Patients who have aortic dissection at the time of first aortic surgery are more likely to require subsequent aortic surgery than patients who undergo prophylactic graft repair of an aortic aneurysm.

In patients who require a mitral valve procedure, valve repair is usually preferred to replacement, although repair may not be possible in patients with a large number of ruptured chordae tendineae, extensive annular calcium, or hugely dilated annuli.[12,39]

Prognosis

While earlier studies indicated that the average lifetime is decreased about 35 percent,[4,40] it is probable that beta-blocker therapy, antibiotic prophylaxis (against infective endocarditis), and aortic and valvular surgery have improved longevity. The most common causes of death of adolescents or adults with MS are rupture of a fusiform aneurysm of the ascending aorta without longitudinal dissection (Fig. 85-2), ascending aortic dissection with rupture, and congestive heart failure from aortic or mitral regurgitation[41] (Fig. 85-3). The major histologic feature in the media of the wall of an aortic aneurysm is a massive loss of elastic fibers[41] (Fig. 85-4). Factors

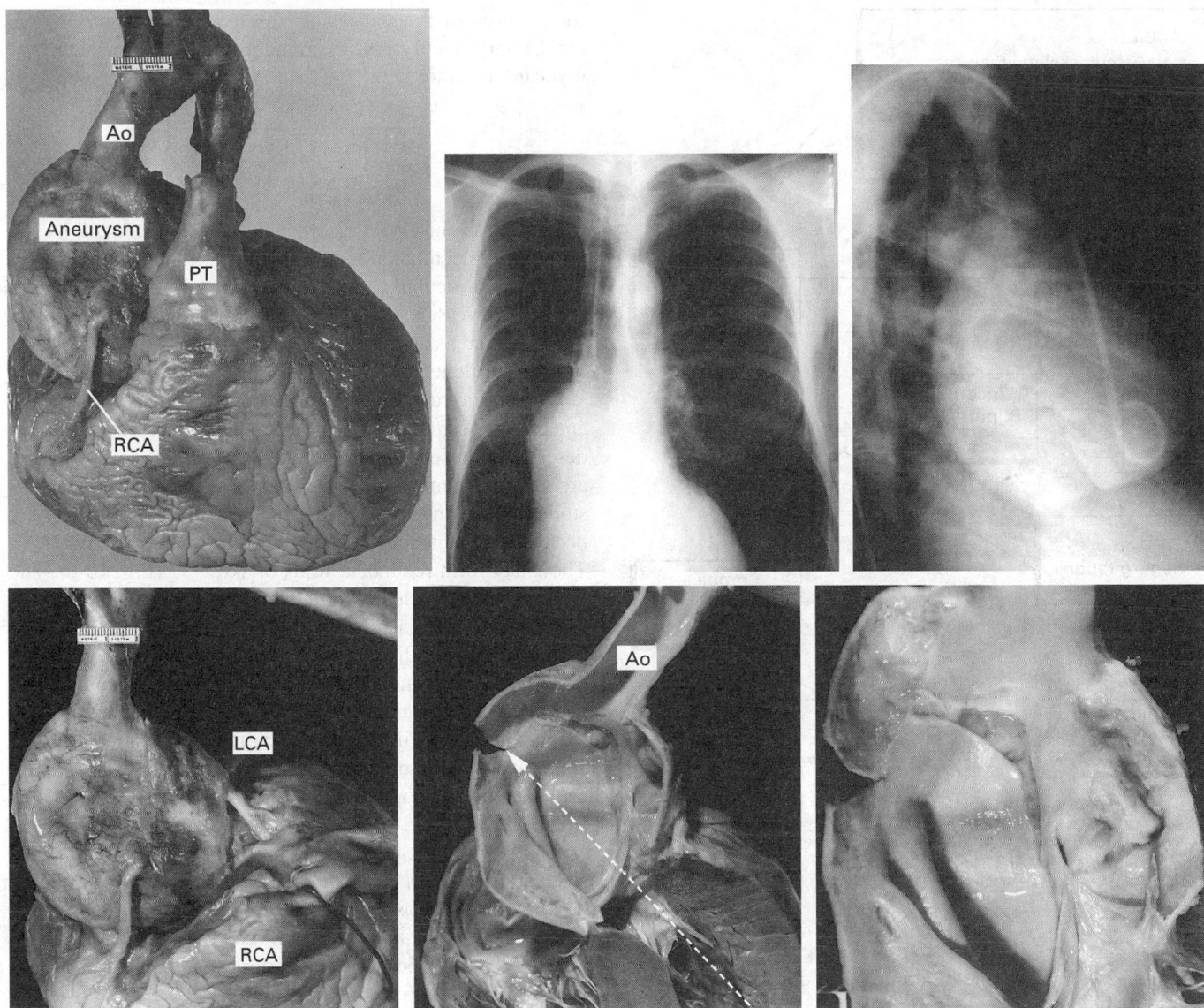

FIGURE 85-2

Heart and aorta of a 38-year-old man who was asymptomatic until exertional dyspnea appeared 5 months before death. *Upper left*. Exterior view. Ao, ascending aorta; RCA, right coronary artery; PT, pulmonary trunk. *Lower left*. Closer view of the massive aortic aneurysm after retracting the pulmonary trunk. LCA, left main coronary artery. The aneurysm does not involve the distal portion of the ascending aorta. *Lower middle*. View of heart and aorta after removing its anterior half. Death resulted from rupture of the right lateral wall of aorta at a point where blood ejected from left ventricle contacts the aortic wall (*arrow*). The aneurysmal bulge is mainly to the right. *Lower right*. Close-up view of the multiple healed tears in ascending aorta. One of the previously incomplete tears ruptured through and through. Posteroanterior chest roentgenogram (*upper middle*) and lateral aortogram (*upper right*) showing massive dilatation of the ascending aorta. (From Roberts and Honig.[41] Reproduced with permission of the publisher and authors.)

that can predispose to either aortic aneurysm or aortic dissection include systemic arterial hypertension, coarctation of the aorta, pregnancy, and trauma. In children with MS, the most common cause of death is severe mitral regurgitation (Fig. 85-5).

Pregnancy

Women with MS should be counseled regarding the approximately 50 percent risk of transmission of the condition.[42] If the woman has moderate or severe aortic regurgitation or an aortic root diameter exceeding 40 mm, she should be advised that pregnancy greatly increases her risk of premature death. Women with an aortic root diameter less than 40 mm usually tolerate pregnancy well.

β-Adrenergic blockers should be administered at least from the midtrimester onward.[43] There may be an advantage to the use of a selective β_1-adrenergic blocker.[44]

During pregnancy, transthoracic echocardiography should be performed every 6 to 10 weeks depending upon the initial findings. Using epidural anesthesia, vaginal delivery in the lateral decubitus position is preferred, and forceps or vacuum

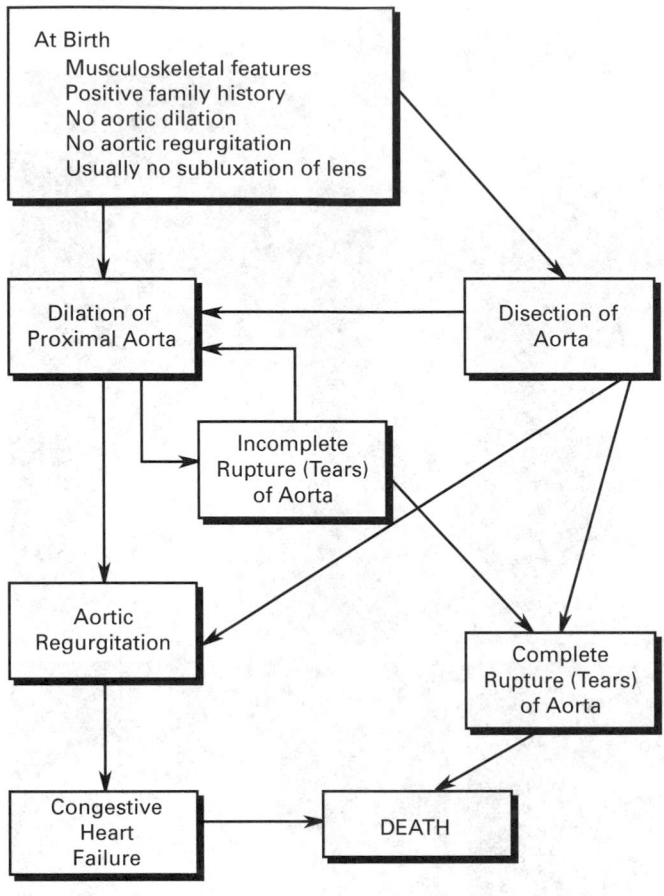

FIGURE 85-3

Scheme of development of cardiovascular complications in Marfan's syndrome. (From Roberts and Honig.[41] Reproduced with permission of the publisher and authors.)

delivery is recommended to shorten the second stage of labor. The increases in systemic blood pressure during uterine contractions should be prevented with beta-blocking agents. Postpartum hemorrhage should be anticipated. If fetal maturity can be confirmed in a patient who requires aortic surgery during pregnancy, a Cesarean section can be done before or concomitantly with thoracic surgery.[42–44]

THE EHLERS-DANLOS SYNDROME

EDS is an heterogeneous group of 14 or more disorders of connective tissue that are characterized primarily by skin fragility, easy bruising, "cigarette paper" scars, skin hyperextensibility, multiple ecchymoses, and joint hypermobility[1,45,46] (see Fig. 10-5). The numerous types of EDS have different clinical manifestations, modes of inheritance, and natural history[47] (see also Chap. 69).

In several types of EDS the heart, heart valves, great vessels, and larger conduit arteries may be involved. Some types of EDS have spontaneous rupture of the aorta or large arteries, coronary or intracranial aneurysms, and arteriovenous fistulae.[48,49] Other cardiovascular abnormalities in EDS include mitral and tricuspid valve prolapse, dilatation of the aortic

root, ectasia of the sinuses of Valsalva, aortic regurgitation, renal artery aneurysms, systemic arterial hypertension, and myocardial infarction.[50–57]

PSEUDOXANTHOMA ELASTICUM

PXE is a rare heritable disorder that is characterized by the progressive accumulation of mineral precipitants within elastic fibers, particularly those of the skin, Bruch's membrane, and blood vessels. It is transmitted both as an autosomal recessive and as an autosomal dominant trait.[1,58–60] The estimated prevalence is 1 in 160,000 (see also Chap. 69).

The elastic fiber changes cause skin, eye, gastrointestinal, and cardiovascular manifestations. The skin lesions have been described as resembling a "plucked chicken." Typically, there are yellow macules or papules that produce a rough, cobblestone texture and are maximal in the flexures of the lateral neck, axillae, antecubaital fossae, groins, and popliteal spaces. They may form redundant folds of skin[58,60] (Fig. 10-6). The retinal changes include mottled *peau d'orange* hyperpigmentation, angioid streaks, and an increased incidence of retinal hemorrhage and disk drusen. Angioid streaks, which are breaks in Bruch's membrane behind the retina and are present in 85 percent of patients with PXE, usually develop after the second decade of life. They can be found in numerous other conditions, including MS, EDS, Paget's disease, and sickle cell anemia, although PXE is most common[58,61] (see also Chap. 11).

There may be calcific deposits in the media of medium-sized arteries. Both vascular calcification similar to Mönckeberg's arteriosclerosis and intimal plaques similar to typical atherosclerotic plaques occur in the coronary, cerebral, gastrointestinal, renal, and peripheral arteries. Angina pectoris and myocardial infarction may occur.[62]

Infrequent but fairly specific lesions in PXE are calcific deposits in the mural endocardium of the ventricles, atria, and atrioventricular (AV) valves.[63–66] Restrictive cardiomyopathy has been described in PXE[65] (see also Chap. 75). Both mitral stenosis and mitral valve prolapse also have been described in PXE.[63,67,68] Surgery to remove mural endocardial calcific deposits has been performed with fair results.[69] Bleeding may occur in the gastrointestinal system, uterus, joints, and urinary bladder. It has been suggested that some bleeding complications may be prevented by avoiding aspirin and that arterial grafts not be utilized in coronary artery bypass surgery because of possible calcification of the internal elastic laminae.[60,70]

OSTEOGENESIS IMPERFECTA

OI, also known as "brittle bone disease" because of the susceptibility of affected individuals to sustain fractures from mild trauma, is a rare heritable disorder of connective tissue. It is inherited in an autosomal dominant fashion with variable penetrance. More than 80 different mutations have been identified in the genes for either of the two chains that form type I collagen, which is the major structural protein of the extracellular matrix of bone, skin, and tendon.[71] There is a wide variation in the clinical severity of OI, from some forms that are lethal in the perinatal period to other forms that may not be detected.[72–74] Most manifestations of OI are bony, ocular, otologic, cutaneous, and dental. The bony changes manifest themselves in a variety of ways including short stature, in utero fractures, severe osteoporosis, and severe bone fragility, with repeated fractures and bowing of long bones. The ocular and otologic changes include blue sclerae, angioid streaks in the retina, and hearing loss. Cutaneous and dental changes result in easy bruising and occasional dentinogenesis imperfecta. An increased risk of bleeding may also be present.[75,76]

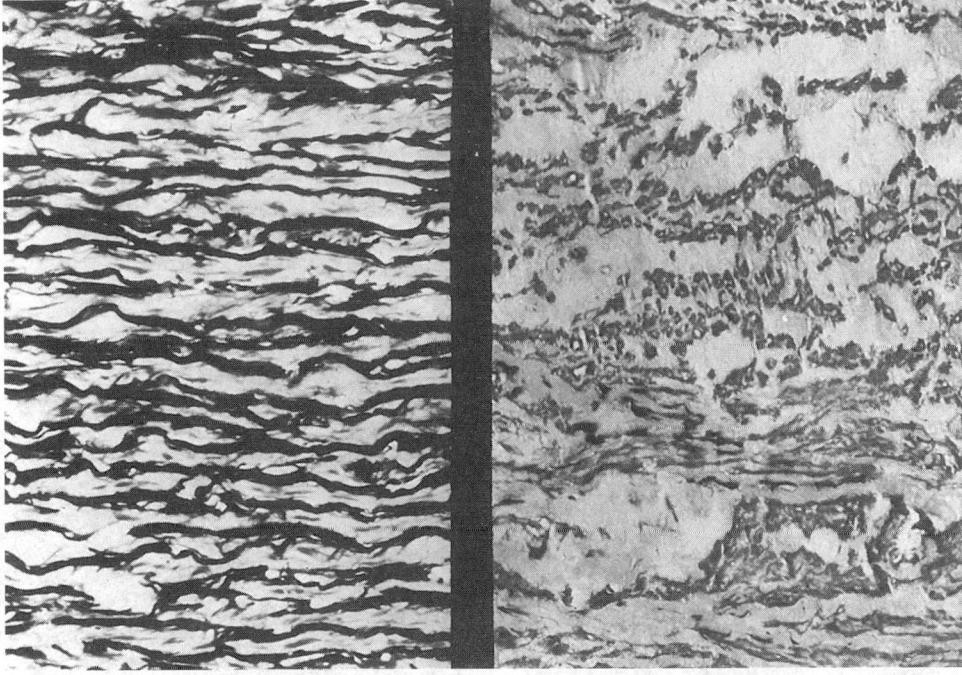

FIGURE 85-4

Left: Photomicrograph of the wall of the ascending aorta from a normal subject. *Right:* A similar histologic study (Movat stains) of the wall of an ascending aortic aneurysm in a 35-year-old woman with Marfan's syndrome. Note the virtual absence of elastic fibers. (From Roberts and Honig.[41] Reproduced with permission of the publisher and authors.)

The cardiovascular manifestations include aortic regurgitation,[76,77] aortic root dilatation,[78] aortic dissection,[79] and mitral regurgitation.[80–84] Mitral valve repair and reconstruction are occasionally feasible for patients with severe mitral regurgitation, although most patients require valve replacement. Mitral valve replacement is difficult because of weakness and friability of the tissues and poor wound healing. In addition, some patients have increased bleeding despite normal preoperative coagulation tests and bleeding times.[76]

ANNULOAORTIC ECTASIA

Annuloaortic ectasia, a pear-shaped enlargement of the sinus and the proximal tubular portions of the ascending aorta, is often part of MS, where it usually results in aortic regurgitation, partial or complete ascending aortic tears, or both. In some patients, annuloaortic ectasia is familial and no other stigmata of MS are present.[85–89] The genetic and molecular changes in these patients are not well established. Microscopically, there is severe loss of elastic fibers in the media of the ascending aorta.

FAMILIAL ANEURYSMS

Various types of familial aneurysms involving cardiovascular structures have been reported. These have included familial aortic dissection,[90] familial aneurysms of the interventricular septum,[91] familial aneurysms of the carotid arteries,[92] and familial intracranial aneurysms.[93–95] At this time, it is not established that these are heritable disorders of corrective tissue.

HOMOCYSTINURIA

See Chapter 69.

NONHERITABLE CONNECTIVE TISSUE DISEASES

The acquired or nonheritable autoimmune or connective tissue diseases represent a subset of the arthritides and rheumatic disorders. These disorders are systemic in nature; are commonly linked by a diffuse abnormality of vasculature; and are characterized by inflammatory lesions in skin, joints, muscles, and connective tissue linings such as pleura and pericardium. Involvement of the kidneys, brain, and heart is usually responsible for the fatal and most serious consequences. Specific acquired connective tissue diseases that may have major cardiac involvement include SLE, PN, giant cell arteritis, RA, ankylosing spondylitis, polymyositis/dermatomyositis, SS, and, possibly, syphilis (Table 85-1). Although certain immunogenetic factors have been identified, their etiology remains uncertain.[96,97]

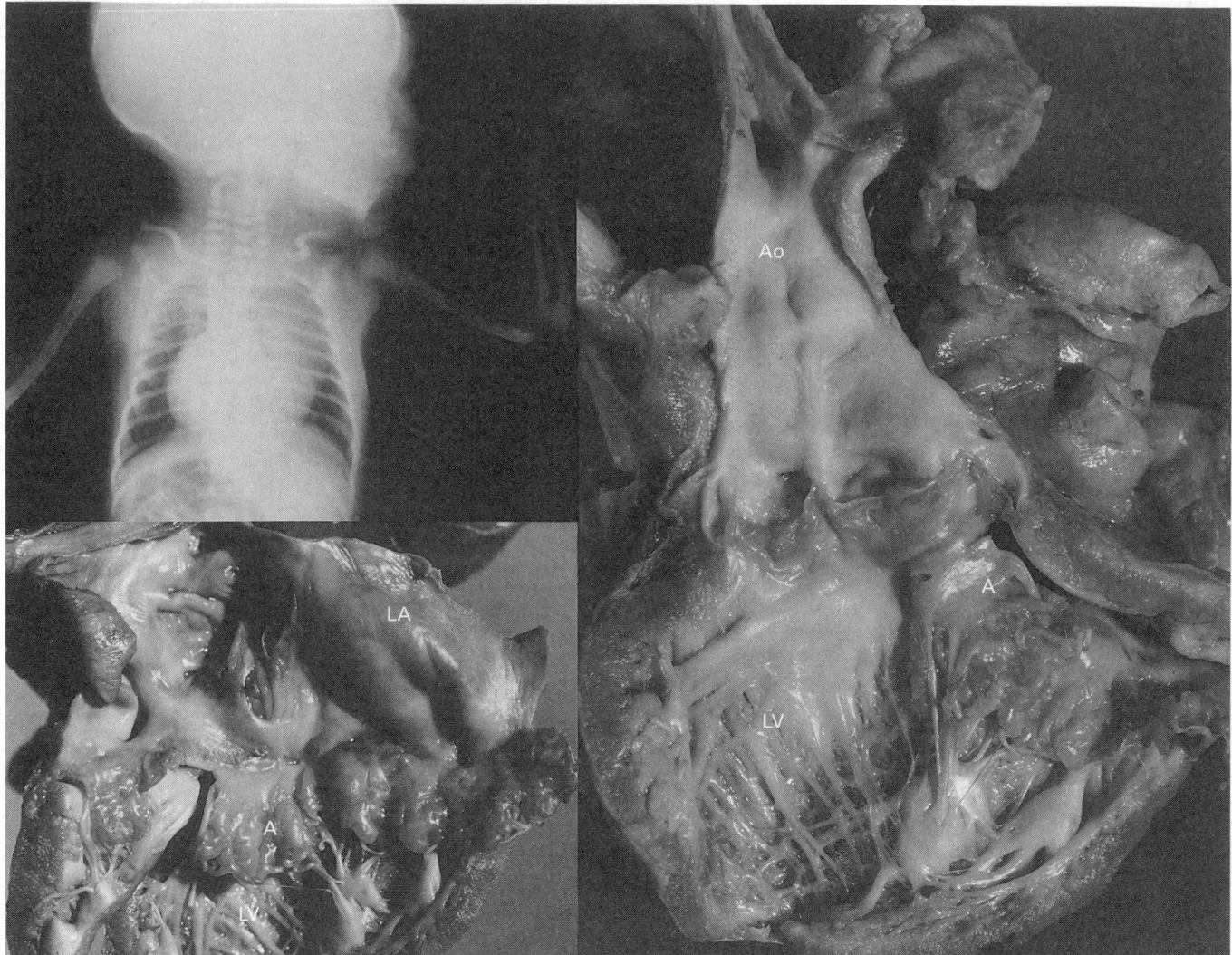

FIGURE 85-5

Congenital floppy mitral valve and floppy tricuspid valve in a 2-day-old boy who had long toes and fingers, a high-arched palate, and a grade 3/6 precordial systolic murmur typical of mitral regurgitation. The heart was enlarged (*upper left*), and he died of congestive cardiac failure. At necropsy, the intima of the ascending aorta (Ao) was wrinkled (*right*), suggesting that the underlying media was abnormal at this early stage. Shown here are the opened aorta, aortic valve, and left ventricle (LV). (A, anterior mitral leaflet.) *Lower left.* Opened left atrium (LA), mitral valve, and left ventricle (LV). The mitral leaflets are considerably elongated in both longitudinal and transverse dimensions. The left atrium is dilated. (From Roberts and Honig.[41] Reproduced with permission of the publisher and author.)

SYSTEMIC LUPUS ERYTHEMATOSUS

SLE is one of the more common autoimmune or rheumatic diseases. SLE is found worldwide and affects all races, is more common in blacks and females of child-bearing age, and is usually more severe in blacks than in whites. SLE is much more frequent in females than in males; in patients less than 40 years of age, the female:male ratio is about 8:1. In the United States, the annual incidence of SLE is about 8 per 100,000 and the prevalence rate is approximately 1 per 2000. The following genes of the human major histocompatibility locus antigens are associated with an increased risk for SLE: HLA-B8, HLA-DR2, HLA-DR3, HLA-DR5, HLA-DR7, HLA-DQ, and null alleles at the C2 and/or C4 loci. Genetic deficiencies of the complement system, i.e., deficiencies of C1q, C2, C4, and C8, predispose to SLE and SLE-like disorders.

The sterile inflammatory process of SLE involves multiple organ systems including skin, joints, kidneys, brain, heart, and virtually all serous membranes. Its clinical presentation is varied and dependent on the organ system(s) involved. Fever, arthritis and arthralgias, skin rashes (Fig. 10-24), and pleuritis are common early signs of SLE.

The immunologic abnormalities of SLE have been well characterized and enable it to be diagnosed despite the diversity of clinical presentations. Typical serologic abnormalities include the presence of antinuclear antibodies (ANA), positive serum anti-DNA antibodies, positive anti-Smith antibodies, positive anti-ribonucleoprotein (anti-RNP) antibodies, and hypocomplementemia, i.e., low serum C3 and C4. Less specific but frequently identified antibodies include anticytoplasmic antibodies, anticardiolipin (IgG-aCL) antibodies, antiphospholipid (aPL) antibodies, and rheumatoid factor. Serum complement is decreased in most patients with SLE, and, insofar as serum complement is usually normal or elevated in other connective tissue disorders (such as RA, PN, SS, and disseminated infections), this serologic test may be useful in the diagnosis of SLE.[98–100] Certain patients with SLE are more likely to have elevated levels of aPL antibodies, particularly those with recurrent venous thrombosis, thrombocytopenia, recurrent fetal loss, hemolytic anemia, livedo reticularis, leg ulcers, arterial occlusions, transverse myelitis, or pulmonary hypertension.[101] Cardiac abnormalities apparently occur more frequently in patients with increased aPL or anticardiolipin antibody titers compared to patients without increased levels, although this is controversial.[97]

Although it may have an acute, fulminating course, SLE most often is characterized by a chronic course marked with exacerbations and remissions; the 10-year survival rate exceeds 80 percent. Nephritis and seizures decrease survival approximately twofold.[102] When patients die of SLE, it is most often in the setting of acute renal failure, central nervous system disease, associated infection, infective endocarditis, or coronary artery disease (see below).

Cardiac Involvement

Probably about 25 percent of patients with SLE have cardiac involvement.[98,100,103–125] In one prospective study of 74 SLE patients, 7 (9 percent) had Libman-Sacks verrucae and 6 (8 percent) had thickened and dysfunctioning valves.[114] In addition to the valvular thickening or verrucae and mitral or aortic valvular regurgitation (or occasional stenosis), there may be pericardial thickening and/or effusion, left ventricular regional or global systolic or diastolic dysfunction, or evidence of pulmonary hypertension.[126,127] Either valvular regurgitation or stenosis due to SLE can require valve replacement.[125,128]

It is unclear whether or not cardiac abnormalities are significantly more frequent in patients with elevated titers of anticardiolipin (or aPL) antibodies.[114,125,129–135] One study of valve disease in SLE did not find an increased frequency of valve disease in patients with aPL antibodies.[136] In general, valve disease in lupus is frequent but apparently independent of the presence or absence of aPL antibodies.[125,134,135]

TABLE 85-1

PRIMARY CARDIAC MANIFESTATIONS OF THE NONHEREDITARY CONNECTIVE TISSUE DISEASES

Disease	Pericardium	Myocardium	Endocardium (Valves)	Coronary Arteries
Systemic lupus erythematosus	+ +	+	+ +	+/−
Systemic sclerosis	+	+ +	0	+ +
Polyarteritis nodosa	+/−	+	0	+ +
Ankylosing spondylitis	0	+/−	+ +	0
Rheumatoid arthritis	+ +	+	+	0
Polymyositis/ dermatomyositis	+ +	+ +	+/−	+/−

Note: + +, major site of involvement; +, may be involved, but less frequently; +/−, rarely involved; 0, not involved.

Pericarditis

SLE may cause a pancarditis with abnormalities of pericardium, endocardium, myocardium, and coronary arteries. Pericardial involvement is the most frequent, as observed clinically, by echocardiography, or at autopsy.[136,137] Pericardial effusions occur at some point in over half of the patients with active SLE. Signs of active or acute pericardial disease precede the other clinical signs of SLE in up to 4 percent of patients.[136] In most SLE patients, the pericardial involvement is clinically silent and, if manifest, runs a benign course. Pericardial tamponade may occur and should be considered in patients with unexplained signs of venous congestion.[138,139] The differential diagnosis includes infection and uremia. On rare occasions, SLE pericardial disease may lead to pericardial constriction[136,139] or to acute cardiac tamponade.[107]

Although in most instances the size of the pericardial effusion is not sufficiently large to allow aspiration, serologic studies of the pericardial fluid can be useful in diagnosing pericardial effusions due to SLE.

The most common type of pericardial disease in SLE is the presence of diffuse or focal adhesions or fibrinous deposits. The pericardial fluid usually contains mononuclear leukocytes and occasionally lupus erythematosus (LE) cells. In patients with long-standing SLE treated with anti-inflammatory agents, pericardial abnormalities appear to occur with the same frequency as in patients not receiving these agents, but at autopsy, the involvement is less extensive and more likely to be fibrous, rather than fibrinous.[137] SLE patients with fibrinous pericardial disease, particularly those with severe debilitation or renal failure, are at increased risk for purulent pericarditis, which is usually fatal.[140]

Endocarditis and Valve Disease

The cardiovascular lesion of SLE that has received the most attention is the "atypical veruccous endocarditis" first described by Libman and Sacks in 1924,[141] long before SLE was recognized as a systemic disease. The lesions, as they were first described and subsequently attributed to SLE,[142] consist almost entirely of fibrin, and although they may occur on both surfaces of any of the four cardiac valves, they are now most frequently found on the left-sided valves, particularly the ventricular surface of the posterior mitral leaflet (Fig. 85-6). These *verrucae* are similar histologically to those of nonbacterial thrombotic endocarditis or *marantic endocarditis,* the valve lesion that occurs most frequently in patients with debilitating illnesses or cancer, except that occasionally hematoxylin bodies, considered the histologic counterpart of LE cells, may be found within Libman-Sacks lesions. While valvular verrucae in SLE (Libman-Sacks lesions) are usually clinically silent, they can be dislodged and embolize and can also become infected, producing infective endocarditis.[125] It is prudent to recommend antibiotic prophylaxis against bacterial endocarditis when patients with SLE undergo procedures that may be associated with bacteremia (see Chap. 82).

Echocardiographically, SLE has a characteristic appearance, with leaflet thickening and valve masses[125,135] (see also Chap. 14). The end-stage or healed form of the verrucous endocarditis of SLE is a fibrous plaque. In some instances, if the thrombotic lesions are extensive enough, their healing may be accompanied by focal scarring and deformity of the underlying valve tissue. This healed form of SLE "endocarditis" may cause valvular dysfunction, particularly mitral and/or aortic regurgitation.[143,144]

Myocarditis

It is unclear whether or not infiltration of the myocardial interstitium with acute and/or chronic inflammatory cells and focal myocardial necrosis, i.e., myocarditis, occurs as a natural part of SLE, unassociated with anti-inflammatory drug therapy (glucocorticoid treatment). Several reports have described clinical features consistent with myocarditis, but actual visual-

ization of interstitial myocardial inflammatory cells with associated myofiber necrosis has not been demonstrated histologically. Hemodynamic and echocardiographic studies, however, have shown abnormalities in both systolic and diastolic ventricular function in some SLE patients.[139] Whether these abnormalities result from an "autoimmune attack" on the myocardium or from the effects of systemic arterial hypertension, coronary artery disease, or coexisting pericardial disease is unclear[145] (see below).

Coronary Artery Disease

Both fatal and nonfatal acute myocardial infarction from coronary artery disease may occur early in the course of SLE, particularly in young women. Studies of hearts in patients with fatal SLE have demonstrated a high incidence of coronary atherosclerosis in patients who received treatment with glucocorticoids for more than 2 years.[137,146–148] In one study of patients who had SLE for more than 2 to 3 years, death was more likely to be due to myocardial infarction than to SLE.[146] Indeed, accelerated coronary atherosclerosis is increasingly recognized as a leading cause of morbidity and mortality in young women patients with SLE who receive long-term glucocorticoid administration.[147] Although the causes of this premature coronary atherosclerosis are uncertain, glucocorticoid treatment as well as aPL antibodies have been incriminated (see "Therapy," below). It has been speculated that SLE itself may induce an underlying vasculopathy or arteritis that may facilitate premature atherogenesis from long-term glucocorticoid treatment. Coronary disease in SLE was not described before glucocorticoid therapy was introduced.[137] In one study, the presence of elevated aPL antibodies in patients with SLE correlated with left ventricular (global or segmental) dysfunction, verrucous valvular (aortic or mitral) thickening, global valvular (mitral or aortic) thickening and dysfunction,

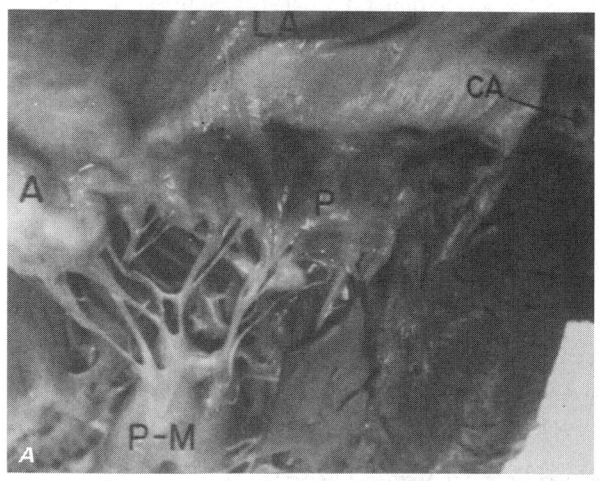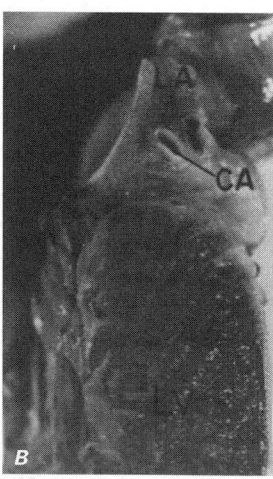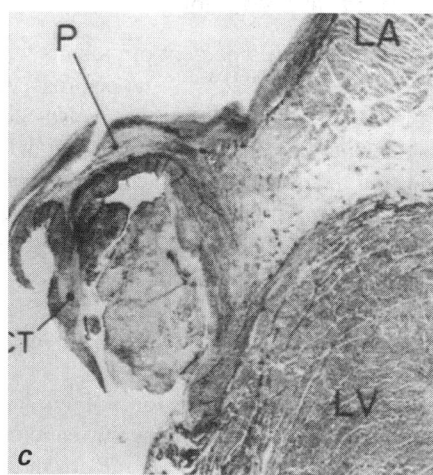

FIGURE 85-6

An example of Libman-Sacks endocarditis in systemic lupus erythematosus. *A* and *B.* The left atrium (LA) and left ventricle (LV) are open. *B* and *C.* Fibrofibrinous "verrucae," present on the undersurface of the posterior leaflet (P) of the mitral valve, are often clinically silent. A, anterior leaflet of mitral valve; CA, left circumflex coronary artery; P-M, postero-medial papillary muscle; CT, chorda tendineae. H&E, ×8. (From Bulkley and Roberts.[137] Reproduced with permission from the publisher and author.)

as well as mitral regurgitation and aortic regurgitation. Coronary thrombi may occur in patients with active lupus and an acute myocardial infarction in the presence of angiographically normal coronary arteries.[149] A fatal myocardial infarction was reported in an 8-year-old girl with SLE, Raynaud's phenomenon, and positive aPL antibodies.[150] Several case reports have described acute myocardial infarctions and the presence of coronary artery aneurysms in patients with SLE.[151,152] aPL antibodies are known to promote platelet aggregation[153] and to be associated with the presence of a clotting tendency, the so-called lupus anticoagulant syndrome.[133]

Inflammation (arteritis) of the wall of the sinus node artery in association with scarring of both sinus and AV nodes has been reported[154] and may account for some of the rhythm and conduction disturbances seen in these patients (see below).

Pregnancy and the Neonatal Lupus Syndrome

Neonatal lupus erythematosus is a rare disorder that arises when the so-called anti-Ro, or Sjögren's, (SSA) autoantibodies, mostly IgG, are formed and circulate in the pregnant patient, cross the placenta, and cause a lupus-like syndrome in the newborn with the appearance of a skin rash and transient cytopenias from passively acquired maternal autoantibodies. Since the half-life of IgG antibodies is approximately 21 to 25 days, the neonatal lupus syndrome in the newborn baby is self-limiting; it usually resolves in 3 to 6 months when all the IgG-containing anti-Ro maternal autoantibodies have been cleared from the neonate's circulation. An unfortunate exception is complete congenital heart block, which may require the implantation of a pacemaker. Once complete heart block occurs, it is usually irreversible. Second-degree heart block has also been reported as a component of the neonatal lupus syndrome. One neonate has been described with first-degree heart block at birth that resolved 6 months later. Antibodies to the Ro (SSA) ribonucleoprotein complexes are present in over 85 percent of sera from mothers of infants with complete congenital heart block. In many patients, antibodies reactive to the La (SSB) antigen as well as the U1RNP protein particle are found in association with anti-Ro (SSA) antibodies.[155]

In most cases the neonatal lupus syndrome is a benign disorder, and most babies of mothers with anti-Ro (SSA), anti-La (SSB), or anti-U1RNP antibodies do not develop neonatal lupus. *A pregnant woman with SLE with positive anti-Ro, anti-La, or anti-RNP antibodies has a risk of less than 3 percent of having a child with neonatal lupus and congenital heart block. The risk that this patient might have an infant with the neonatal lupus syndrome but without congenital heart block may be as high as 1 in 3.* The neonatal lupus syndrome mediated by the presence of maternal anti-Ro antibodies can occur in babies of mothers who do not have overt SLE, who may or may not meet criteria for a diagnosis of SLE, and who may or may not have a positive test for antinuclear antibodies.

The neonatal lupus syndrome with congenital heart block can be diagnosed by the appearance of fetal bradycardia around the 23rd week of gestation. It is thought that the cardiac damage with conduction abnormalities in the neonate results from binding of the passively transferred pathogenic anti-Ro antibodies to Ro (SSA)/La (SSB) antigens present in the fetal heart. It is not known whether these IgG anti-Ro antibodies represent "clinical markers" only or whether they are pathogenic.[155] All mothers of neonates with complete congenital heart block have been HLA-DR3 positive. If the mother is HLA-DR3 positive and has circulating IgG anti-Ro antibodies, the neonate is at risk regardless of the neonate's HLA-DR status.

Other cardiac abnormalities reported in the neonatal lupus syndrome include right bundle branch block, second-degree AV block, 2:1 AV block, patent ductus arteriosus, patent foramen ovale, coarctation of the aorta, tetralogy of Fallot, atrial septal defect, hypoplastic right ventricle, ventricular septal defect, dysplastic pulmonic valve, mitral and tricuspid regurgitation, pericarditis, and myocarditis. In one study of idiopathic congenital complete heart block, accompanying heart disease occurred in one-third of patients and only two of 35 patients reached the age of 50 years without the need for a pacemaker.[156] Most pacemakers were inserted between the ages of 10 and 49 years.

Pregnant women with SLE should have a serum anti-Ro (SSA) antibody determination as early in pregnancy as possible. Prenatal treatment of established congenital heart block has consisted of the administration of prednisone or dexamethasone and plasmapheresis from week 23 on, although heart block has persisted in most cases. One patient with SLE was successfully treated with intrauterine dexamethasone for fetal myocarditis and heart block.[157] A fetus had successful percutaneous transvenous intracardiac pacing for complete congenital heart block.[158] It is unclear whether or not aggressive anti-inflammatory therapy in an effort to diminish the generalized fetal insult and to lower the titers of circulating anti-Ro (SSA) antibodies makes a difference in fetal cardiac outcome. Fetal echocardiography is useful to follow the progression of the disease and also to help identify decreased left ventricular contractility, increased cardiac size, tricuspid regurgitation, and pericardial effusion.

Neither dexamethasone nor plasmapheresis has had much success in reversing intrauterine third-degree heart block. Glucocorticoids, however, may be helpful in suppressing an associated inflammatory response producing pleuropericardial effusions or ascites in the fetus. Close monitoring of the clinical course in the prospective mother is also essential because of the risk of exacerbation of the SLE. If fetal bradycardia is present, an "intrauterine therapeutic approach" for as long as possible is recommended to allow for fetal maturation to occur. Ultrasound images can be useful for assessing the degree of cardiac dysfunction present. Following delivery, the neonatologist should be prepared to have a cardiac pacemaker implanted. Otherwise, all the other clinical and laboratory features of the neonatal lupus syndrome (with the exception of complete heart block and/or similar severe cardiac fetal disease) should slowly and gradually disappear over the first few months of the baby's life. In one study, one-third of the children with autoantibody-associated congenital heart block died in the early neonatal period[159]; of those who survived, most required a pacemaker.

Women with SLE who are anti-Ro positive should be closely monitored during pregnancy, as should mothers of previous babies born with congenital complete heart block. Pregnant patients who are anti-Ro positive and whose babies have not had fetal bradycardia throughout most of the pregnancy should be reminded that congenital complete heart block is rare and that the neonatal cutaneous lupus syndrome is benign and transient. The long-term prognosis of the mothers of children born with congenital heart block is generally fairly good.[160] The development of subsequent valvular heart disease, possibly rheumatic, in asymptomatic mothers who have had babies born with congenital heart block, however, was common in one study.[159] In these mothers, the risk of congenital heart block in children of subsequent pregnancies was low.[159] Newborns of mothers with SLE with normal pulse rate are unlikely to have significant abnormalities in AV conduction and do not need screening ECGs at birth.[161]

A higher prevalence of clinical evidence of myocarditis and conduction defects is found in adult anti-Ro-positive patients with SLE than in patients who are anti-Ro negative or in healthy controls.[162] In general, clinical features consistent with myocarditis and conduction defects are relatively common in adults with SLE and seem associated with positive anti-Ro antibodies. Myocarditis at necropsy, however, is extremely rare.[105,137,143] In most adults with SLE, however, positive anti-Ro antibodies have uncommonly been associated with complete heart block.[162,163] The role of the anti-Ro antibody in inducing heart blocks in adult patients with SLE is disputed.[164]

Secondary Effects on the Heart

Many, if not most, of the clinically significant cardiac problems occurring in patients with SLE are secondary occurrences. Systemic arterial hypertension is common in patients with SLE, particularly those with renal disease and long-standing glucocorticoid therapy, and is a major cause of cardiac enlargement and heart failure. Pulmonary hypertension is also common,[126,127] approaching 50 percent in a 5-year follow-up study.[165] Uremic pericarditis may occur, of course, in patients with severe renal failure. Premature or accelerated atherosclerosis has been increasingly recognized in young women with SLE receiving long-term glucocorticoid treatment.

Therapy

Therapy of cardiovascular SLE is the therapy of the underlying disease and includes nonsteroidal anti-inflammatory drugs (NSAIDs), glucocorticoids, and, in severe cases, cytotoxic agents such as azathioprine and cyclophosphamide. Systemic arterial hypertension, congestive heart failure, and arrhyth-

mias should be treated with standard therapeutic measures. SLE-induced valve disease can require valve replacement[128,143,144]; pericardial tamponade may require either high-dose steroids, pericardiocentesis, or placement of a pericardial window,[139] but recurrent effusions or pericardial thickening may develop. Premature cardiovascular events from accelerated atherosclerosis may result in sudden death or myocardial infarction.[147] The antimalarial agent hydroxychloroquine lowers serum cholesterol levels in patients with SLE.[166] In addition, several earlier studies have demonstrated that antimalarials can decrease myocardial ischemic damage in dogs and other nonhuman animals.[167–169] An antimalarial such as hydroxychloroquine may be beneficial as a prophylactic agent to prevent premature or accelerated atherosclerosis in young women with SLE receiving long-term treatment with glucocorticoids. Although there are no studies documenting benefit, low-dose aspirin and hydroxychloroquine are often utilized in SLE patients receiving long-term glucocorticoid therapy.

POLYARTERITIS NODOSA

PN is characterized by segmental necrotizing inflammation of the medium- to small-sized arteries throughout the body, resulting in disease and dysfunction of multiple organ systems. The commonly involved organs are the skin, kidneys, gastrointestinal tract, spleen and lymph nodes, central nervous and musculoskeletal systems, and heart. A variety of cutaneous lesions may be seen: livedo reticularis, palpable purpura, ulcerations, infarcts of distal digits, and nodules. Evidence of glomerulonephritis ranges from low-grade proteinuria to malignant hypertension and acute renal failure.

An association between PN and hepatitis B infection has been recognized for over a decade, and recently an association with hepatitis C virus infection has also been described[170]; hairy cell leukemia has been described in a few patients with PN. Although the erythrocyte sedimentation rate and serum gamma globulins may be elevated and rheumatoid factor and antinuclear antibodies may be present, the final clinical diagnosis of PN rests on the combination of multisystem disease and biopsy evidence of active arteritis.[171,172] In PN, mesenteric vessel angiograms may show aneurysmal dilatation that mimics mycotic aneurysm in infective endocarditis. Since an inflammatory necrotizing arteritis may occur in a variety of disorders, other causes and types of arteritis must be excluded before the diagnosis of PN is made. Classed as separate entities are granulomatous or giant cell arteritis, hypersensitivity angiitis, temporal arteritis, and arteritis involving the aorta and its major branches. The designation *microscopic polyangiitis* may more appropriately describe patients who have no arteritis but who have small vessel vasculitis affecting arterioles, venules, and capillaries. Also, arteritis associated with other connective tissue disorders, for example, rheumatoid vasculitis, is not thought to represent PN when arteritis is the major clinical disease presentation.[172]

Cardiac Involvement

The heart and the coronary arteries are frequent targets of PN. Most often this involvement is a vasculitis of the distal extramural and subepicardial coronary arteries just as they penetrate the myocardium (Fig. 85-7). The lesions are characterized by inflammatory infiltrates in the media and adventitia and occasionally by necrosis of the full thickness of the vessel wall, with prominent involvement of the surrounding perivascular connective tissue (Fig. 85-7). The lumens of the involved vessels may contain thrombi, and the walls may be aneurysmal. The latter is responsible for the nodular appearance of the arteries deemed characteristic of this disorder. An even later stage of the vasculitis process is evident as the lesions heal, first showing the formation of granulation tissue and subsequently fibrous tissue replacement of the original components of the artery. In this healing phase, intimal proliferation leading to coronary artery luminal narrowing is evident.[173,174]

The coronary arterial disease of PN may lead to myocardial infarction. The myocardial necrosis and subsequent replacement fibrosis tend to be focal and patchy throughout the left ventricular wall. This is in contrast to the large areas of grossly visible, regional, subendocardial or transmural necrosis typically seen in the myocardial infarction caused by coronary atherosclerosis involving the extramural arteries (see also Chap. 42).

Conduction system abnormalities have been identified in the hearts of patients with PN.[175,176] James and Birk[175] pointed out that the size and location of the sinoatrial node and AV node arteries make them prime targets for polyarteritis. The perivascular inflammation of these vessels is more likely to lead to myocardial dysfunction, as the AV and sinoatrial node tissue closely surrounds these vessels and is included in the perivascular inflammatory reaction. Atrial and ventricular conduction disturbances may be a primary manifestation of PN, despite minimal involvement of vessels elsewhere in the heart.

Other cardiac abnormalities that may be seen in patients with PN are those that are likely secondary to the underlying systemic arterial hypertension and renal disease. Cardiomegaly and left ventricular hypertrophy most often represent secondary cardiac manifestations of this disease. Similarly, pericardial disease may develop in a patient with PN, but this is most often due to renal insufficiency.

A new autoantibody identified in the serum of patients with systemic vasculitis, especially Wegener's granulomatosis, is the so-called antineutrophil cytoplasmic antibody (ANCA).[177] The ANCA test recognizes antibodies to azurophilic granules present in the cytoplasm of neutrophils. There are two types of ANCA, c-ANCA and p-ANCA. The antigen against which c-ANCA is directed is a 29-kDa serine proteinase. Approximately 90 percent of patients with Wegener's granulomatosis have positive c-ANCA antibodies, the "c" describing the cytoplasmic staining observed under fluorescent microscopy. In contrast, other vasculitides, including PN, tend to have a positive so-called p-ANCA antibody, the "p" describing the perinuclear staining observed in the immunofluorescent assay.

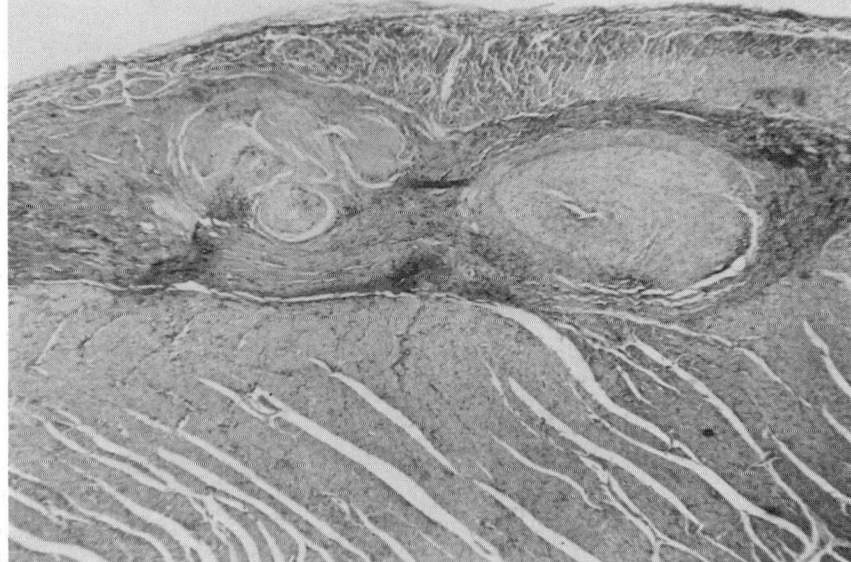

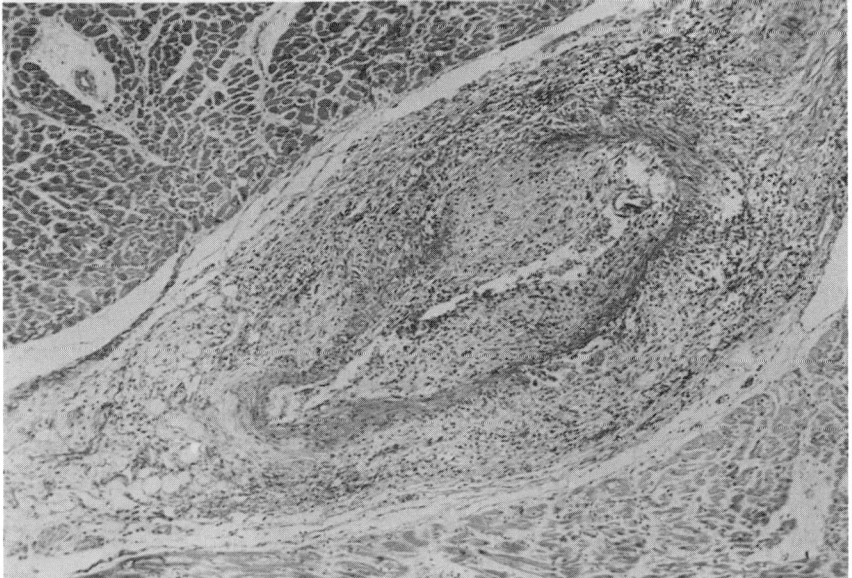

FIGURE 85-7

Polyarteritis nodosa. Examples of the necrotizing vasculitis affecting the extramural and intramural coronary arteries in polyarteritis. *Top.* Extramural coronary arteries. *Bottom.* Intramural coronary arteries. The intramural artery shows a necrotizing arteritis with inflammation involving the full thickness of the vessel. H&E, *top,* ×7; *bottom,* ×22.

The antigen responsible for the p-ANCA antibody detection appears to be a myeloperoxidase. The detection of serum ANCA levels is a useful laboratory diagnostic marker in the evaluation of the systemic vasculitides, particularly c-ANCA for Wegener's granulomatosis. Serum p-ANCA positivity seems to be nonspecific. For instance, positive p-ANCA may be seen in other chronic inflammatory disorders such as Crohn's enteritis, Felty's syndrome, Kawasaki's vasculitis, leprosy, and tuberculosis. Therefore, the detection of a positive serum p-ANCA in a patient with the clinical picture suggestive of PN should not preclude the need for a biopsy or an angiogram.

Clinical Manifestations of Cardiac Disease

Despite the dramatic involvement of coronary arteries that may accompany PN, the most frequent cardiovascular abnormalities seen in patients with PN are unrelated to the coronary arteries per se. Systemic arterial hypertension occurs in approximately 90 percent of these patients and, in combination with chronic renal failure, is the most likely cause of congestive heart failure, which may develop in up to 60 percent of patients.[171,172] Patients with PN may also develop acute myocardial infarction, which poses the diagnostic question of whether the myocardial injury is due to coronary arteritis with secondary thrombosis or to atherosclerosis, in a population that is typically middle-aged, male, steroid-treated, and susceptible to atherosclerotic coronary artery disease as well.

Therapy

Polyarteritis nodosa has a poor prognosis, especially when systemic arterial hypertension and renal disease are present. Treatment of the heart disease in PN is directed at the specific cardiac dysfunction, and glucocorticoid and other anti-inflammatory agents are administered for the underlying disease. Glucocorticoids are still the initial mainstay of therapy, although they can aggravate coexisting hypertension and even atherosclerosis. Often added to the treatment regimen are glucocorticoid-sparing agents such as cyclophosphamide, azathioprine, or methotrexate. The use of warfarin remains controversial[171]; low-dose aspirin, however, is usually recommended.

RHEUMATOID ARTHRITIS

RA, the most common of the connective tissue diseases, is characterized by its deforming erosions of the joints resulting from chronic synovial inflammation and proliferation. It tends to affect women twice as often as men and may run in families. Joint symptoms dominate its course, and symmetric involvement of the hands and wrists is most common. Other joints of the upper and lower extremities and the temporomandibular and sternoclavicular joints may also be affected. The most common systemic or extraarticular manifestations of RA include fever, weight loss, anemia, subcutaneous rheumatoid nodules, and lymphadenopathy. Less frequently, pleuritis and a diffuse, necrotizing vasculitis may occur.

Pericardial Involvement

Cardiac involvement is uncommon in RA but may take a variety of forms. A diffuse, nonspecific fibrofibrinous pericarditis occurs in about 50 percent of patients with RA; it is usually clinically silent and is overshadowed by pleuritis or joint pain.[178] The pericardial disease tends to be benign, but sizable effusions can occur and require pericardiocentesis, and pericardial constriction can rarely necessitate pericardiectomy.[179] Pericardial disease should always be considered in the differential diagnosis of patients with RA who present with right heart failure.

Constrictive pericarditis occurred in 4 of 47 patients with RA who were followed over a 10-year period.[180] The histopathologic findings in all cases after pericardiectomy were consistent with chronic fibrosing pericardial disease. The long-term outcome is good at 7- to 17-year follow-up after pericardiectomy. Another study reported on cardiac constriction from rheumatoid pericardial disease. These patients had longer disease duration, more severe disease, worse functional class, and more extraarticular features when compared with RA patients without cardiac constriction.[181] The presenting clinical features of cardiac constriction included dyspnea, edema, chest pain, and pulsus paradoxus. Chronic, symptomatic pericarditis may require glucocorticoid therapy. RA pericardial disease may shorten survival, especially in the older patients, and be associated with the presence of other cardiac disease, a greater number of extraarticular manifestations, jugular venous distenstion, and a lower mean systemic blood pressure.[182] Lymphocytic infiltrates of the CD8-positive type may occur in the pericardium of patients with rheumatoid pericardial disease, suggesting that these cells may play a role in the development of the pericardial disease[183] (see also Chap. 81).

Myocardial and Endocardial Involvement

Rarely, rheumatoid nodules may focally infiltrate the heart, including the myocardium and the four cardiac valves (Fig. 85-8).[184,185] These nodules may produce no symptoms, but, if extensive enough or strategically located, they can compromise cardiac function. A rheumatoid nodule may extend from the mural endocardium into a chamber to present as an intracausatory mass.[186] Rheumatoid nodules developing within the valve leaflets may result in mild valvular regurgitation; if the nodule becomes necrotic, perforation of the leaflet can occur and lead to severe valvular regurgitation, usually aortic.[185] The incidence of such valvular infiltration has been estimated at 1 to 2 percent in autopsy studies of patients with RA. Although distinctly uncommon, arrhythmias and conduction disturbances, including complete heart block,[184] and congestive heart failure can also result from RA involvement of the heart. One echocardiographic study of 39 patients with RA detected left ventricular abnormalities in a quarter of the patients.[187] A recent report documents catastrophic aPL syndrome in a 34-year-old woman with a 3-year history of severe seropositive RA and positive anticardiolipin antibodies; she developed a massive anterior wall acute myocardial infarction and ischemia of the lower extremities with disseminated intravascular coagulation; death ensued 7 days later from severe heart failure complicated by ventricular fibrillation.[188]

Therapy

Since most of the cardiac lesions of RA are clinically silent, it is not certain that the specific therapies used in RA, including NSAIDs, methotrexate, penicillamine, gold, and glucocorticoids, affect the cardiac involvement. Treatment of cardiac constriction from rheumatoid pericardial disease may include a trial of high-dose intravenous glucocorticoid, e.g., methylprednisolone 250 mg every 6 to 8 h, and/or surgical therapy.[180] Pericardiocentesis should be performed only as a life-saving procedure.[181]

Hydroxychloroquine and NSAIDs are often used in treating RA. Both have an anticoagulant, antiplatelet effect, which may partially explain why thrombotic events such as deep vein thrombophlebitis as well as acute myocardial infarction are relatively uncommon in patients with RA. Otherwise, conventional treatment of pericarditis, arrhythmias, and conduction disturbances is utilized when these disorders produce clinical symptoms.

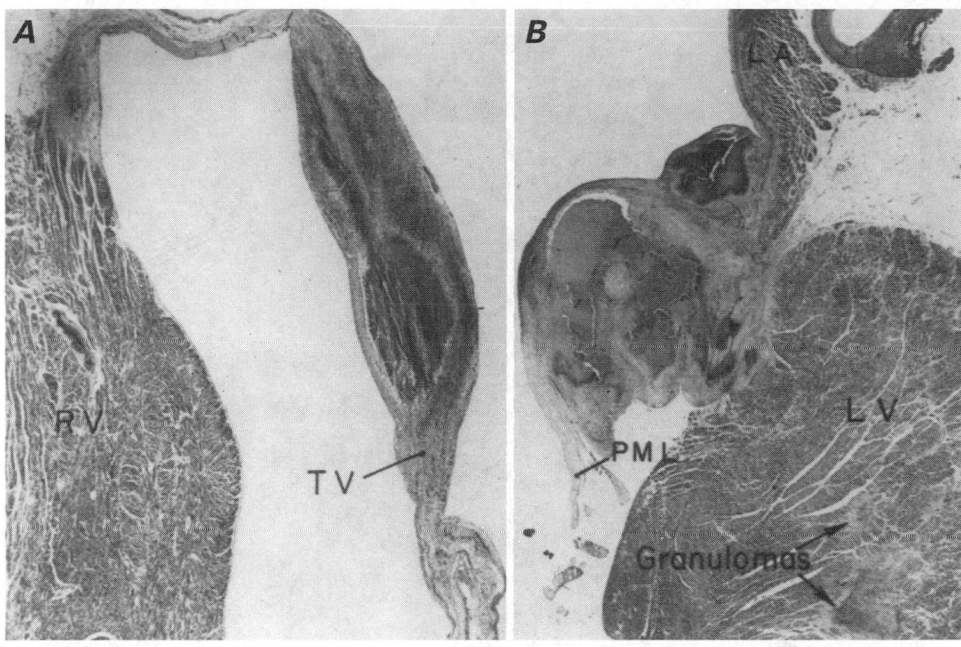

FIGURE 85-8

Rheumatoid arthritis. *A.* A tricuspid valve (TV) infiltrated by rheumatoid nodules. *B.* A mitral valve infiltrated by rheumatoid nodules. In addition, granulomas are present within the left ventricular (LV) wall. LA, left atrium; PML, posterior mitral leaflet; RV, right ventricle. (*A*) H&E, ×12. (*B*) H&E, ×65. (From Roberts et al.[185] Reproduced with permission from the publisher and authors.)

ANKYLOSING SPONDYLITIS

Ankylosing spondylitis is the prototypical example within the group of the seronegative spondyloarthropathies. It is distinctly different from RA. Ankylosing spondylitis is characterized by a progressive inflammatory lesion of the spine, leading to chronic back pain, deforming dorsal kyphosis (Fig. 10-26), and, in its advanced stage, fusion of the costovertebral and sacroiliac joints with immobilization of the spine. This condition is much more frequent in men than in women (9:1), generally first occurring early in life but with a chronic progressive course of 20 to 30 years.[189] The HLA-B27 histocompatibility antigen is found in nearly all patients with ankylosing spondylitis. Other seronegative arthritides that have a high prevalence of this antigen include Reiter's syndrome, psoriatic arthritis, and juvenile arthritis.

Cardiac Involvement

Cardiovascular disease in ankylosing spondylitis takes the form of a sclerosing inflammatory lesion that is generally limited to the aortic root area. The inflammatory process, which extends immediately above and below the aortic valve, typically causes aortic regurgitation[190,191] (Fig. 85-9). As the inflammatory process extends below the aortic valve, it can infiltrate the basal portion of the mitral valve (which is contiguous with the aortic valve) and cause mitral regurgitation.[192] Extension of the inflammatory lesion into the cephalad portion of the ventricular septum, immediately caudal to the aortic valve, accounts for the associated conduction disturbances. Ventricular diastolic dysfunction may also occur.[193]

The major clinical manifestation of ankylosing spondylitis is aortic regurgitation, which occurs in about 5 percent of patients with this condition. For example, among patients with signs of spondylitis for 10 years, only 2 percent have clinical evidence of aortic regurgitation; by 30 years, that number increases fivefold.[190] Ankylosing spondylitis may be associated with aortic root inflammatory lesions, as may other seronegative spondyloarthropathies such as Reiter's syndrome and psoriatic arthropathy.[193,194]

Therapy

Drug therapy for ankylosing spondylitis is primarily directed at relief of the pain and discomfort of back pain. This is accomplished with the use of NSAIDs, methotrexate, and sulfasalazine in addition to physical therapy; phenylbutazone

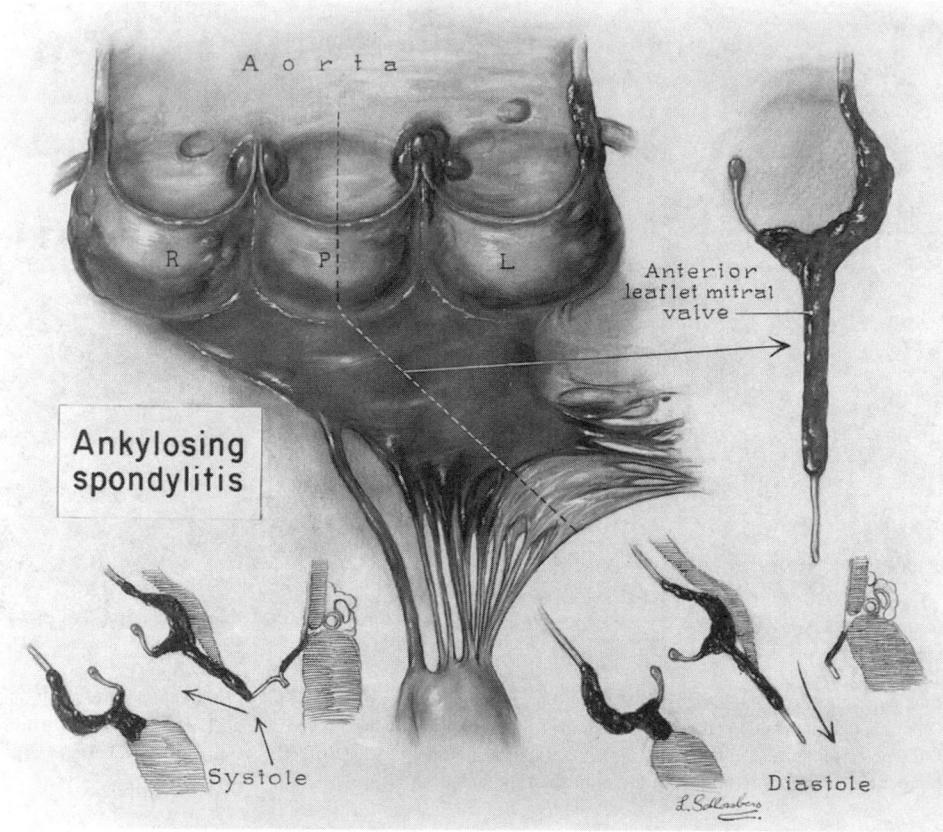

FIGURE 85-9

Diagram showing the characteristic features of ankylosing spondylitis of the heart. The aorta and aortic valve are opened, showing the thickening of the aorta in the vicinity of the aortic valve commissures and the thickening of the anterior mitral leaflet. The small diagrams at the bottom of the figure show the thickening in the wall of the aorta behind the sinuses extending below the aortic valve into the membraneous ventricular septum and anterior mitral leaflet. In the patient whose heart was portrayed by this diagram, there was also some thickening in posterior mitral leaflet.

is currently rarely used. Glucocorticoids are not used in this condition except when iritis occurs. The inflammatory lesion of the heart generally runs a clinically silent course until aortic regurgitation develops. Not infrequently, however, the aortic regurgitation of ankylosing spondylitis may become severe enough to warrant aortic valve replacement[190,191] (see also Chap. 63).

CARDIOVASCULAR SYPHILIS

Although this condition has traditionally not been considered to be a connective tissue disorder, cardiovascular syphilis has histologic features nearly identical to those of ankylosing spondylitis, and spirochetes have never been identified in the aorta of a patient with cardiovascular syphilis. The distribution of the lesions, however, is distinctly different in these two conditions. In cardiovascular syphilis, the process is usually limited to the tubular portion of ascending aorta, i.e., that portion up to the origin of the innominate artery. Because the process as a rule does not extend into the wall of aorta behind the sinuses of Valsalva, aortic regurgitation is infrequent in

syphilis. Exactly what percentage of patients with cardiovascular syphilis develop aortic regurgitation is unclear, but it is probably no more than about 15 percent and only in the patients in whom the process extends into the wall of aorta behind the sinuses of Valsalva. In syphilis, the process never involves the aortic valve cusps and never extends below (caudal to) the aortic valve. In contrast, in ankylosing spondylitis the process always involves basal portions of the aortic valve cusps and always extends into the membranous ventricular septum, the basal portion of the anterior mitral leaflet, or both. Thus, because the process in syphilis never extends below the aortic valve, bundle branch or complete heart block and mitral regurgitation never develop in cardiovascular syphilis or, if they do, they are the result of a process other than syphilis. In contrast, heart block and mitral regurgitation are common in ankylosing spondylitis.

Cardiovascular syphilis characteristically involves the entire tubular portion of the aorta, which may become either diffusely or focally dilated. In contrast, in ankylosing spondylitis, the process involves only the proximal 1 cm of the tubular portion of the ascending aorta and then usually in the areas of the aortic valve commissures. Accordingly, aneurysms of the tubular portion of the ascending aorta do not occur in ankylosing spondylitis. Syphilitic aneurysms can become so large that they burrow into the sternum or compress adjacent structures such as the right atrium, superior vena cava, or pulmonary trunk. Rupture into the adjacent structures or into the pericardial sac may also occur.

Histologically, the aortic lesions in both cardiovascular syphilis and ankylosing spondylitis are similar. Both are characterized by extensive thickening by fibrous tissue of the adventitia, with collections of plasma cells and some lymphocytes within these tissues. The vasa vasora are larger than normal, their walls are thickened, and their lumens may be severely narrowed. The inflammatory infiltrates are located primarily in the perivascular locations. The media is thinner than normal and contains scars that are generally located transversely to the long axis of the aorta. Within the scars elastic fibers may be absent. The overlying intima is thickened, and the intimal process has the "tree-bark" appearance of typical atherosclerotic plaques. The intimal thickening is greater in syphilis than in ankylosing spondylitis, probably because the patients with cardiovascular syphilis are generally much older than the patients with ankylosing spondylitis. The average age of death in patients with ankylosing spondylitis and aortic regurgitation is 48 years, whereas the typical patient with cardiovascular syphilis, with or without associated aortic regurgitations, is usually in his or her 70s or 80s.

SYSTEMIC SCLEROSIS, OR SCLERODERMA

SS, which was first identified over two centuries ago, is characterized by its striking skin manifestations; hence the name *scleroderma*. The systemic nature of this disease, and in particular its ability to affect the heart, became apparent much later. In 1943, Weiss and coworkers[195] described a pattern in the cardiac dysfunction of nine patients with scleroderma and correlated these changes with abnormalities in the heart at autopsy in two patients. Moreover, they recognized that the cardiac disease was a manifestation of an underlying primary vascular disorder.

SS is characterized by fibrous thickening of the skin (Fig. 10-22) and fibrous and degenerative alterations of the fingers and of certain target organs, particularly the esophagus, small and large bowels, kidneys, lung, and heart. Central to this degenerative process are diffuse vascular lesions. Functionally, the vascular disorder is characterized by Raynaud's phenomenon, which is a prominent feature of SS; Raynaud's disease of the digits is present in almost all patients with SS and is the first clinical symptom in most. Structurally, the vascular lesions show intimal and adventitial thickening of small- and medium-sized vessels, including arterioles. *The underlying pathophysiology of scleroderma that links structure and function is a Raynaud's-type phenomenon of visceral vasculature that leads to focal vascular lesions and parenchymal necrosis and fibrosis.* This concept is supported by findings in the heart as well as in the lungs and kidneys.[196,197] The underlying cause of the vascular disease in SS and the role of the immune system in its pathophysiology remain unclear. It has been suggested that SS may be related to increased activity of endothelial cells, mast cells, and fibroblasts, perhaps under the influence of immigrant cells, such as T cells, macrophages, or platelets.[198]

Like most connective tissue diseases, SS may have a variable clinical expression. Some patients may have skin involvement predominantly; others have minimal skin abnormalities but severe visceral disease that may therefore evade diagnosis.[199] The CREST (*c*alcinosis, *R*aynaud's phenomenon, *e*sophageal dysmotility, *s*clerodactyly, *t*elangiectasia) syndrome is an SS variant that can manifest as relatively mild skin changes limited to the face and fingers but severe lung disease with a primary pulmonary hypertension picture[200] (see Fig. 10-23).

"Overlap syndromes" are seen when a patient with typical features of SS also has features of SLE or RA. Although SS may run a long and benign course, "malignant" renal, lung, or cardiac disease can occur, with rapid deterioration and death at a young age.

The Cardiovascular System

Cardiovascular disease in patients with SS can be due to either a primary involvement of the heart by the sclerosing disease or a secondary involvement from disease of the kidney or lungs.

PRIMARY SS OF THE HEART

Myocardial involvement is a principal determinant of survival in SS. When the heart is involved directly by scleroderma, a myocardial fibrosis occurs that bears no direct relation to large- or small-vessel occlusions or other anatomic abnormalities. The fibrosis tends to be patchy, involving all levels of the myocardium unpredictably and the right ventricle as often as the left. Focal patchy myocardial cell necrosis may also be evident, and at autopsy over three-quarters of patients with myocardial SS have foci of necrosis.[197,201] The myocardial necrosis associated with patent vasculature suggests that the myocardial fibrosis of SS results de novo from repair after tissue necrosis.[197,202] The type of necrosis evident in the heart of scleroderma patients is myofibrillar degeneration, or contraction-band necrosis (Fig. 85-10). This lesion is characteristic of myocardium that is subjected to transient occlusion followed by reperfusion. This could occur with vascular spasm and may also be induced experimentally by exposing myocardium to high concentrations of catecholamine. Thus, the morphologic characteristics of the myocardial lesions of primary cardiac SS are consistent with a Raynaud's phenomenon of the heart. There is also suggestive evidence that a Raynaud's phenomenon of the pulmonary arterioles may be responsible for the "primary" pulmonary hypertension-type lesion that may occur in the CREST syndrome, and the kidneys in SS can also manifest a Raynaud's-type phenomenon. Some patients with SS have renal Raynaud's phenomenon when digital Raynaud's phenomenon is induced by cold water immersion.[203] Thus, it is likely that the major visceral manifestations of SS in the heart, lungs, and kidneys are related to the vascular spasm that is evident and readily detectable in the digits. Changes that are comparable to the necrosis and scarring of the fingertips can also develop in the viscera. Why the small vessels are hyperreactive and in spasm is not known, but a neurogenic component and defective endothelial-dependent vasodilatation are likely involved.

The cause of the myocardial necrosis and fibrosis that develops in the setting of patent extramural and intramural vessels is also unclear. That the myocardial disease relates in part to immunologic abnormalities or to primary and unrestrained fibrous tissue proliferation remains a possibility. The present evidence, however, suggests that the vascular system—and particularly the smaller arteries and arterioles—is the primary target organ of SS and that the cardiac sclerosis of scleroderma may be a consequence of focal, intermittent, and progressive ischemic injury.

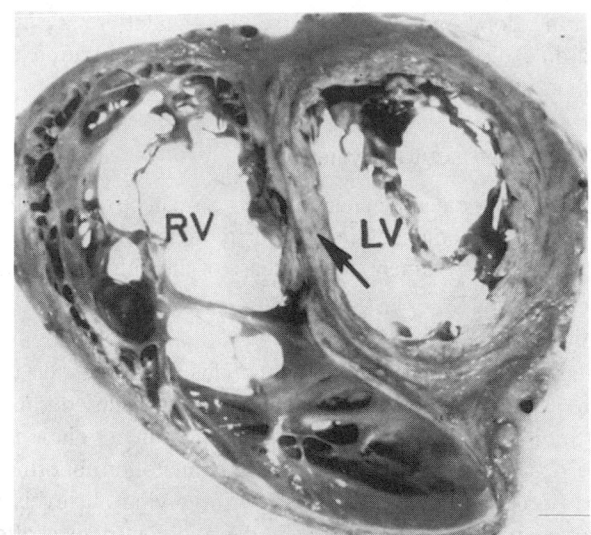

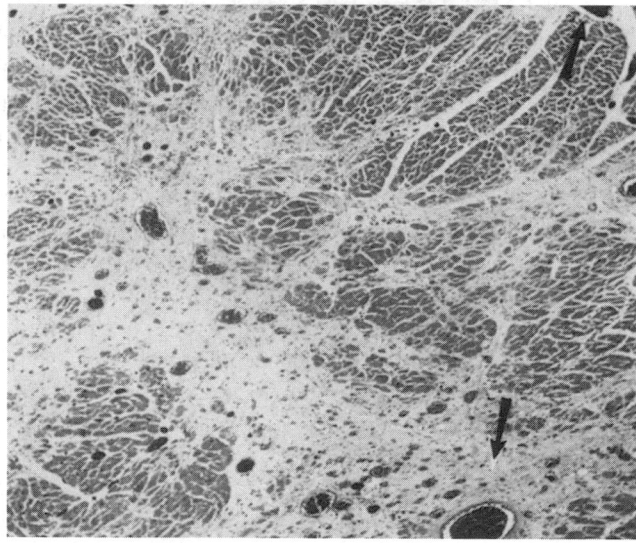 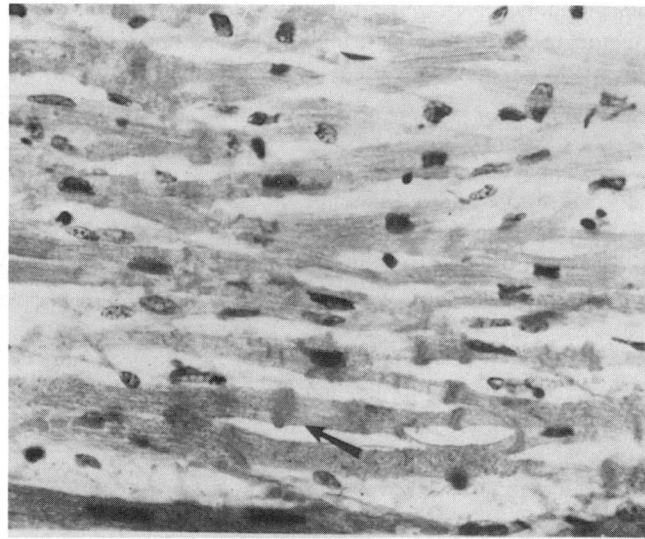

FIGURE 85-10

Systemic sclerosis. *Top.* Cross section through the dilated right (RV) and left (LV) ventricle of a patient with cardiac SS. Marked fibrous scarring of both ventricles is especially evident in the interventricular septum (arrow). *Bottom (left).* Photomicrograph of myocardium showing replacement fibrosis with patent intramural coronary arteries (arrows). *Bottom (right).* Higher-power magnification showing contraction-band necrosis of many fibers surrounding the areas of scar. H&E, ×45 and ×60. (From Bulkley.[202] Reproduced with permission from the publisher and author.)

Several functional studies have also suggested that microvascular spasm occurs in patients with cardiac scleroderma. Transient perfusion defects identified by thallium-201 radionuclide imaging in the setting of patent coronary arteries have been identified in patients with SS and symptomatic cardiac disease.[204] Some patients with SS have reversible cold-induced myocardial perfusion defects as well as cold-induced acute and reversible left ventricular dysfunction.[205,206] Decreased coronary reserve has also been reported in patients with widely patent coronary arteries.[207]

CLINICAL MANIFESTATIONS

The clinical features of myocardial SS include biventricular congestive heart failure, atrial and ventricular arrhythmias, myocardial infarction, angina pectoris, and sudden cardiac death.[202,208] These clinical manifestations reflect the underlying conditions of myocardial necrosis and fibrosis and may at times mimic ischemic heart disease due to coronary atherosclerosis. If the myocardial injury is extensive enough, leading to dilated hypodynamic ventricles, a syndrome resembling

idiopathic dilated cardiomyopathy (Chap. 73) may be simulated.

Patients with SS may have cardiac involvement but no cardiac symptoms. One study[209] examined 18 SS patients by electrocardiography, ambulatory electrocardiography, radionuclide ventriculography, myocardial scintigraphy, and echocardiography and found a high rate of cardiac abnormalities, including ventricular tachycardia in one patient, nonsustained ventricular tachycardia in five, supraventricular tachycardia in six, decreased left ventricular ejection fraction in two, decreased right ventricular ejection fraction in eight, and stress-induced reversible myocardial perfusion abnormalities in six. In other studies of patients with limited scleroderma, noninvasive cardiac techniques such as Doppler echocardiography and thallium-201 perfusion scintigraphy after a cold-stress test or radionuclide ventriculography[210] have found a number of cardiovascular abnormalities, such as mild mitral regurgitation, thickening of papillary muscles, abnormal left and right diastolic function, and systolic pulmonary arterial hypertension. A Japanese study of 13 patients with full-blown

SS concluded that patients with SS frequently have deterioration of left ventricular diastolic function, especially those with left ventricular wall thickening out of proportion to left ventricular end-diastolic dimensions.[211]

Other investigators have used electrocardiography and echocardiography to devise a simple "cardiac score" to improve the prediction of prognosis in patients with SS.[212] Skeletal muscle myositis can complicate SS, and such patients may have an increased likelihood of developing myocarditis, heart failure, symptomatic arrhythmias, and sudden death.[213,214] Accordingly, it has been suggested that serum creatine kinase with MB fractionation and studies of left ventricular function be undertaken in patients with SS who have skeletal myositis.[214] Autopsy studies have suggested that up to 50 percent of patients with SS have increased myocardial scar tissue and that up to 30 percent of patients have extensive lesions.[202,215] Some clinical cardiac abnormality, including symptoms of heart failure or abnormal rhythm with conduction disturbances, may occur in about 40 percent of patients with SS. The cardiac disorder in approximately one-half of patients has been attributed by some to a primary myocardial scleroderma. Clinically manifest cardiac disease is evident in close to 90 percent of patients with severe morphologic myocardial involvement.[202]

PERICARDIAL AND ENDOCARDIAL DISEASE

Pericardial involvement may occur in about 20 percent of patients with SS. Although the pericardial involvement is due to renal failure in as many as two-thirds of patients, some patients develop a fibrofibrinous or fibrous pericarditis for which no other apparent cause is evident. Exudative pericardial effusions may accompany scleroderma pericardial disease and can be massive.[195,216] Pericardial tamponade may occur and may precede cutaneous thickening.[217] Rarely, constrictive pericardial disease may result from the pericardial sclerosis. Mitral regurgitation is common in patients with SS.[218] Tricuspid regurgitation occurs in patients with very dilated right ventricular cavities.

SECONDARY CARDIOVASCULAR DISEASE

Since scleroderma most frequently manifests itself as renal and pulmonary parenchymal disease with pulmonary and systemic arterial hypertension, secondary cardiovascular disease is common. Left ventricular hypertrophy and congestive heart failure may be associated with long-standing systemic arterial hypertension and renal disease. Uremic pericarditis may occur. Cor pulmonale with marked right ventricular hypertrophy and right-sided heart failure may result from long-standing severe pulmonary scleroderma.

Pulmonary Hypertensive Disease

Although the pulmonary fibrosis of scleroderma had been known for years, the recognition of a "primary" pulmonary hypertensive lesion independent of parenchymal disease evolved later. Patients with this primary pulmonary vascular lesion tend to develop rapidly progressive dyspnea and right-sided congestive heart failure in the setting of clear lungs. Pulmonary pressures reach the systemic level and are refractory to treatment. Morphologically, the pulmonary arterial lesions show the range of advanced alterations (medial and intimal hyperplasia, plexiform lesions, and necrotizing arteritis) seen in Eisenmenger syndromes and idiopathic primary pulmonary hypertension. Arterial vasospasm is believed to be a major component of "primary" pulmonary hypertension, and the association is supported by angiographic studies. On occasion, vasodilators such as tolazoline may induce partial lowering of pressure, but the fixed pulmonary lesions and focal thrombotic occlusions that virtually always accompany the advanced stages of this condition make restoration of normal pressures unlikely. The fact that Raynaud's phenomenon of the digits accompanies idiopathic primary pulmonary hypertension in about one-third of patients[219] suggests that vascular hyperreactivity may be a common link between this disease and scleroderma (see also Chap. 59).

Although uncommon in scleroderma, severe pulmonary hypertension carries a grave prognosis. Sudden unexpected death occurs, and hypotension and death can occur precipitously in the setting of what would appear to be relatively benign procedures such as pericardiocentesis or cardiac catheterization.

Treatment

There is no uniformly effective therapy for the cardiovascular disease of SS. Treatment consists of standard therapy for congestive heart failure and arrhythmias. Malignant ventricular arrhythmia in SS has responded seemingly well to an implantable cardioverter defibrillator[220] (see Chap. 33). Thrombolysis may provide improvement in the Raynaud's phenomenon, cutaneous sclerosis, and digital ulcerations.[221] A pilot study of antithymocyte globulin (ATGAM) in 10 patients with scleroderma appeared ineffective in improving the skin and pulmonary features of the disease.[222] Nifedipine may improve myocardial perfusion abnormalities as well as systemic and pulmonary hemodynamics in patients with pulmonary hypertension due to SS.[223,224] Nifedipine and amlodipine may also improve Raynaud's events involving the fingers. Captopril has been shown to improve myocardial perfusion.[225,226] Potential therapeutic value for SS cardiac disease has been attributed to D-penicillamine. No therapy, however, has proved effective for either the systemic disease or its cardiac manifestations. Clinical trials with prostacyclin in the treatment of pulmonary hypertension are ongoing.

POLYMYOSITIS/DERMATOMYOSITIS

These idiopathic autoimmune inflammatory myopathies are rare in the United States, with an estimated annual incidence of about 5 to 10 new patients per million. The clinical features include a typical heliotrope rash in dermatomyositis (DM), with periorbital edema and proximal muscle weakness present in both polymyositis (PM) and DM. PM is basically the same disease except for the absence of a skin rash.[227] Typical laboratory findings include an elevated serum creatine kinase (CK) level and elevation of other muscle enzymes such as a serum aldolase, reflecting the presence of muscle breakdown from the inflammatory process. The so-called anti-Jo-1 antibody, detectable in the serum of some patients with PM/DM, has been correlated with inflammatory arthritis, Raynaud's phenomenon, interstitial lung disease, and excess mortality, mostly due to respiratory failure.

Typical changes in the electromyogram include short-wave potentials, low-amplitude polyphasic units, and increased spontaneous activity with muscle fibrillation. A positive skeletal muscle biopsy of a proximal muscle such as the deltoid is often confirmatory.[228]

In addition to skeletal muscle involvement, up to 40 percent of patients may have cardiac abnormalities, including AV conduction defects, tachyarrhythmias, pericarditis with effusion, and a dilated, poorly contracting left ventricle. A type of myocarditis leading to congestive heart failure has been found in autopsy studies.[229] Rarely, coronary arteritis has been reported in PM/DM. Accordingly, the evaluation of a middle-aged man with known PM/DM who presents with chest pain, or even classic angina with an elevated serum CK, poses a diagnostic challenge, and the differential diagnosis includes inflammatory myocarditis and coronary arteritis. It should be noted that an increase in cardiac CK-MB may be "buried" in the marked elevation of skeletal CK-MB. If coronary angiography is suggestive of coronary vasculitis rather than typical atheromatous plaques, oral high-dose prednisone, 40 to 60 mg daily, is appropriate. This is also the usual initial therapeutic approach to patients with PM/DM even when no cardiac involvement is apparent. There are no adequate large-scale, prospective, controlled clinical studies available comparing the efficacy of glucocorticoid treatment with other immunosuppressive agents such as azathioprine (Imuran), methotrexate, chlorambucil, and cyclophosphamide (Cytoxan).[229]

Most rheumatologists initially utilize a trial of glucocorticoid therapy in patients with PM/DM. If the response is suboptimal, treatment is instituted with methotrexate, azathioprine (Imuran), chlorambucil, and cyclophosphamide (Cytoxan) in that order. The response to steroids in PM/DM is unpredictable. Some patients do very well on oral prednisone therapy, while others fail to respond to all agents. A subset of patients with PM/DM who have the so-called inclusion body myositis are particularly intractable to anti-inflammatory treatment. This is also true for patients who have a rare autoantibody called the anti-signal-recognition-particle antibody, or anti-SRP antibody. Because some patients with PM/DM benefit significantly from an initial trial of high-dose oral or intravenous glucocorticoid therapy, this therapy is usually used first. Intravenous immunoglobulin appears promising in the treatment of PM/DM.[230] Finally, myopathies can arise iatrogenically from commonly used drugs such as cholesterol-lowering agents, statins, and niacin as well as from colchicine, zidovudine (AZT), and methylphenidate hydrochloride (Ritalin).

GIANT CELL (CRANIAL, TEMPORAL, GRANULOMATOUS) ARTERITIS

Temporal arteritis is a systemic inflammatory vasculitis of unknown etiology that primarily involves extracranial vessels, especially branches of the external carotid artery, but can involve almost any artery in the body as well as some veins. Giant cell arteritis occurs almost exclusively in patients over 55 years of age. Common presenting symptoms include headaches, scalp tenderness, jaw claudication, visual disturbances including blindness, diplopia, weight loss, anemia, and, in about 50 percent of patients, musculoskeletal symptoms attributable to polymyalgia rheumatica. Uncommon presentations of giant cell arteritis include fever of unknown origin, chest pain from aortitis or myocardial infarction, aortic aneurysm,[231,232] coma, peripheral gangrene, peripheral neuropathies, and large-vessel involvement with limb claudication, aortic regurgitation, or stroke. Typical physical findings include tenderness of the temporal or occipital arteries, nodulations of the artery, a pulseless artery, and a tender scalp.

Most giant cell arteritis patients have a greatly elevated erythrocyte sedimentation rate; a normal sedimentation rate is rare. The only specific diagnostic test is a temporal artery biopsy that demonstrates granulomatous arterial inflammation with disruption of the internal elastica lamina. Giant cells need not be present. Unfortunately, the positive yield for giant cell arteritis in unilateral temporal artery biopsies is no greater than 60 percent, and a contralateral biopsy may be necessary.

Since the occurrence of "skip" lesions in histologic samples is well known in giant cell arteritis, a 3- to 4-cm section of artery should be examined. Angiography is generally not helpful in diagnosis or in selecting a biopsy site. High-dose prednisone therapy, 40 to 60 mg daily, is indicated to prevent blindness or to suppress inflammation in the presence of systemic involvement. Clinical trials with methotrexate are currently ongoing.

CHURG-STRAUSS VASCULITIS

The Churg-Strauss syndrome, or allergic granulomatosis and angiitis, is a systemic vasculitis that develops in the setting of allergic rhinitis, asthma, and eosinophilia. Sinusitis and pulmonary infiltrates may cause confusion with Wegener's granulomatosis; the absence of cavitating pulmonary nodules or the presence of gastrointestinal involvement are often helpful distinguishing features. Peripheral neuropathy, cutaneous involvement, and renal disease are common clinical findings.

Pathologic studies show inflammatory lesions rich in eosinophils with intra- and extravascular granuloma formation. The major morbidity and mortality of Churg-Strauss vasculitis result from cardiac involvement. This may be associated with left ventricular dilatation and a reduced ejection fraction as well as mitral regurgitation, which may require valve replacement.[233] Left ventricular systolic function may improve significantly with glucocorticoid therapy.[234]

ANTIPHOSPHOLIPID ANTIBODY SYNDROME

The aPL antibody syndrome has been identified by the presence of aPL antibodies, usually in high titer, or the "lupus anticoagulant," and any or all of the following clinical events: recurrent arterial or venous thromboses, recurrent fetal losses, and thrombocytopenia.[235–239] Livedo reticularis is also frequently present, and nonhealing leg ulcers and Coombs'-positive hemolytic anemia may be also. Clinically, the terms *anticardiolipin syndrome, antiphospholipid syndrome,* and *lupus anticoagulant syndrome* are usually considered to be equivalent, although some individuals may have one antibody but not the other.[235] A false-positive VDRL test may also be detected in patients with aPL antibody syndrome. On the other hand, aPL antibodies may be present in asymptomatic individuals. Often, anticardiolipin antibodies cross-react with beta$_2$ glycoprotein 1 (B2GP1) antibodies. The mechanism(s) whereby anticardiolipin or aPL antibodies promote intravascular thrombosis remains uncertain. These antibodies may react with lipid antigens on endothelial cells and/or platelets. The precise nature of the antigen recognized by B2GP1-dependent anticardiolipin antibodies is under active investigation. SLE is frequently present in patients with the aPL antibody syndrome. In one study, the presence of anticardiolipin antibodies in patients with SLE was associated with prolonged activated partial thromboplastin time, thrombocytopenia, and positive Coombs' test but not with the "lupus anticoagulant" (or the aPL) syndrome[236]; the presence of a prolonged activated partial thromboplastin time was strongly associated with venous and arterial thrombosis.

Therapy depends on the clinical setting. Patients with positive aPL antibodies but without evidence of thrombosis or recurrent fetal loss should not be treated. Patients with aPL antibody syndrome who have had thrombotic events or habitual abortions should be treated. Anticoagulation and antithrombotic therapy in these patients has included heparin, warfarin, low-dose aspirin, and the antimalarial agent hydroxychloroquine.[97,237] Although there is no convincing evidence of benefit, some advocate low-dose aspirin or heparin, with or without low-dose prednisone, alone or in combination to prevent fetal loss.[238] An increased incidence of aortic or mitral regurgitation in association with the "primary" aPL antibody syndrome has been reported[239–244] as well as in patients with SLE who have aPL antibodies.[96,112,114,129–135] In one study of aPL antibody syndrome in patients with SLE and patients with primary aPL antibody syndrome, heart valve involvement was frequent but apparently unrelated to the presence or absence of aPL antibodies.[134] The aPL antibody syndrome is frequently manifest by spontaneous small- and large-vessel arterial thrombosis in the cerebral and ocular circulations.[235,245–252] In healthy men, positive anticardiolipin antibody levels were a risk factor for deep venous thrombosis or pulmonary embolus but not for ischemic stroke.[252]

Although there are no controlled trials of therapy to prevent arterial occlusion, low-dose aspirin is often used. Therapy has often included aspirin and warfarin or heparin, as well as low-dose glucocorticoids.[248,251]

REFERENCES

1. Beighton P, ed. *McKusick's Heritable Disorders of Connective Tissue,* 5th ed. St. Louis: Mosby-Year Book; 1993.
2. Prockop DJ, Kivirikko KI. Heritable diseases of collagen. *N Engl J Med* 1984; 311:376–386.
3. Beighton P, de Paepe A, Danks D, Finidori G, Gedde-Dahl T, Goodman T, et al. International nosology of heritable disorders of connective tissue, Berlin, 1986. *Am J Med Genet* 1988; 29:591–594.
4. Pyeritz PE, McKusick VA. The Marfan syndrome: Diagnosis and management. *N Engl J Med* 1979; 300:772–777.
5. Kainulainen K, Pulkkinen L, Savolainen A, Kaitila I, Peltonen L. Location of chromosome 15 of the gene defect causing Marfan syndrome. *N Engl J Med* 1990; 323:935–939.
6. Hollister DW, Godfrey M, Sakai LY, Pyeritz RE. Immunohistologic abnormalities of the microfibrillar-fiber system in the Marfan syndrome. *N Engl J Med* 1990; 323:152–159.
7. Lee B, Godfrey M, Vitale E, Hori H, Matte M-G, Sarfaraz M, et al. Linkage of Marfan syndrome and a phenotypically related disorder to two different fibrillin genes. *Nature* 1991; 352:330–334.
8. Maslen CL, Corson GM, Maddox BK, Glanville RW, Sakai LY. Partial sequence of a candidate gene for the Marfan syndrome. *Nature* 1991; 352:334–337.
9. Dietz HC, Cutting GR, Pyeritz RE, Maslen CL, Sakai LY, Corson GM, et al. Marfan syndrome caused by a *de novo* missense mutation in the fibrillin gene. *Nature* 1991; 352:337–339.
10. Dietz HC, Valle D, Francomano CA, Kendzior RJ, Pyeritz RE, Cutting GR. The skipping of constitutive exons in vivo induced by nonsense mutations. *Science* 1993; 259:680–683.
11. Dietz IIC, McIntosh I, Sakai LY, Corson GM, Chalberg SC, Pyeritz RE, et al. Four novel FBN1 mutations: Significance for mutant transcript level and EGF-like domain calcium binding in the pathogenesis of Marfan syndrome. *Genomics* 1993; 17:468–475.
12. Pyeritz RE, Francke U. The second international symposium on the Marfan syndrome. *Am J Med Genet* 1993; 47:127–135.
13. Dietz HC, Pyeritz RE. Mutations in the human gene for fibrillin-1 (FBN1) in the Marfan syndrome and related disorders. *Hum Mol Genet* 1995; 4:1799–1809.
14. Payne RM, Johnson MC, Grant JW, Strauss AW. Toward a molecular understanding of congenital heart disease. *Circulation* 1995; 91:494–504.
15. Ramirez F. Figrillin mutations in Marfan syndrome and related phenotypes. *Curr Opin Genet Develop* 1996; 6:309–315.
16. Roberts WC, Honig HS. The spectrum of cardiovascular disease in the Marfan syndrome. A clinico-morphologic study of 18 necropsy patients and comparison to 151 previously reported necropsy patients. *Am Heart J* 1982; 104:115–135.
17. Pyeritz RE, Wappel MA. Mitral valve dysfunction in the Marfan syndrome: Clinical and echocardiographic study of prevalence and natural history. *Am J Med* 1983; 74:797–807.
18. Hirata K, Triposkiadis F, Sparks E, Bowen J, Boudoulas H, Wooley CF. The Marfan syndrome: Cardiovascular physical findings and diagnostic correlates. *Am Heart J* 1992; 123:743–752.
19. Come PC, Fortuin NJ, White RI Jr, McKusick VA. Echocardiographic assessment of cardiovascular abnormalities in the Marfan syndrome. Comparison with clinical findings and with roentgenographic estimation of aortic root size. *Am J Med* 1983; 74:465–474.
20. Roman MJ, Devereux RB, Kramer-Fox R, Spitzer MC. Comparison of cardiovascular and skeletal features of primary valve prolapse and Marfan syndrome. *J Cardiol* 1989; 63:317–321.
21. Glesby MJ, Pyeritz RE. Association of mitral valve prolapse and systemic abnormalities of connective tissue: A phenotypic continuum. *JAMA* 1989; 262:523–528.

22. Child JS, Perloff JK, Kaplan S. The heart of the matter: Cardiovascular involvement in Marfan's syndrome (editorial). *J Am Coll Cardiol* 1989; 14:429–431.

23. Salim MA, Alpert BS, Ward JC, Pyeritz RE. Effect of beta-adrenergic blockade on aortic root rate of dilation in the Marfan syndrome. *Am J Cardiol* 1994; 74:629–633.

24. Shores J, Berger KR, Murphy EA, Pyeritz RE. Progression of aortic dilatation and the benefit of long-term β-adrenergic blockade in Marfan's syndrome. *N Engl J Med* 1994; 330:1335–1341.

25. Treasure T. Elective replacement of the aortic root in Marfan's syndrome. *Br Heart J* 1993; 69:101–103.

26. Gott VL, Gillinov M, Pyeritz RE, Cameron DE, Reitz BA, Greene PS, et al. Aortic root replacement: Risk factor analysis of a seventeen-year experience with 270 patients. *J Thorac Cardiovasc Surg* 1995; 109:536–545.

27. Donaldson RM, Emanuel RW, Olsen EG, Ross DN. Management of cardiovascular complications in Marfan syndrome. *Lancet* 1980; 2:1178–1181.

28. Gott VL, Pyeritz RE, McGovern GJ, Cameron DE, McKusick VA. Surgical treatment of aneurysms of the ascending aorta in the Marfan syndrome: Results of composite-graft repair in 50 patients. *N Engl J Med* 1986; 314:1070–1074.

29. Marsalese DL, Moodie DS, Vacante M, Lytle BW, Gill CC, Sterba R, et al. Marfan's syndrome: Natural history and long-term follow-up of cardiovascular involvement. *J Am Coll Cardiol* 1989; 14:422–428.

30. Gott VL, Pyeritz RE, Cameron DE, Greene PS, McKusick VA. Composite graft repair in Marfan aneurysm of the ascending aorta: Results in 100 patients. *Ann Thorac Surg* 1991; 52:38–45.

31. Svensson LG, Crawford ES, Coseli JS, Safi HJ, Hess KR. Impact of cardiovascular operation on survival in the Marfan patient. *Circulation* 1989; 80(suppl I):I233–I242.

32. Svensson LG, Crawford ES, Hess KR, Coselli JS, Safi HJ. Dissection of the aorta and dissecting aortic aneurysms: Improving early and long-term surgical results. *Circulation* 1990; 82(suppl IV):IV24–IV38.

33. Pyeritz RE. Marfan syndrome: Current and future clinical and genetic management of cardiovascular manifestations. *Semin Thorac Cardiovasc Surg* 1993; 5:11–16.

34. Smith JA, Fann JI, Miller C, Moore KA, DeAnda A, Mitchell RS, et al. Surgical management of aortic dissection in patients with the Marfan syndrome. *Circulation* 1994; 90(part 2):II235–II242.

35. Silverman DI, Gray J, Roman MJ, Bridges A, Burton K, Boxer M, et al. Family history of cardiovascular disease in the Marfan syndrome is associated with increased aortic diameter and decreased survival. *J Am Coll Cardiol* 1995; 26:1062–1067.

36. Pyeritz RE. The Marfan syndrome. In: Royce PM, Steinmann B, eds. *Connective Tissue and Its Heritable Disorders: Molecular, Genetic, and Medical Aspects.* New York: Wiley-Liss; 1993: 437–468.

37. Bachet JE, Termignon J-L, Dreyfus G, Goudot B, Martinelli L, Piquois A, et al. Aortic dissection: Prevalence, cause, and results of late operations. *J Thorac Cardiovasc Surg* 1994; 108:199–206.

38. Schaefer S, Peshock RM, Malloy CR, Katz J, Parkey RW, Willerson JT. Nuclear magnetic resonance imaging in Marfan's syndrome. *J Am Coll Cardiol* 1987; 9:70–74.

39. Gillinov AM, Hulyalkar A, Cameron DE, Cho PW, Greene PS, Reitz BA, et al. Mitral valve operation in patients with the Marfan syndrome. *J Thorac Cardiovasc Surg* 1994; 107:724–731.

40. Murdoch JL, Walker BA, Halpern BL, Kuzma JW, McKusick VA. Life expectancy and causes of death in the Marfan syndrome. *N Engl J Med* 1972; 286:804–808.

41. Roberts WC, Honig HS. The spectrum of cardiovascular disease in the Marfan syndrome: A clinico-morphologic study of 18 necropsy patients and comparison to 151 previously reported necropsy patients. *Am Heart J* 1982; 104:115–135.

42. Pyeritz RE. Maternal and fetal complications of pregnancy in the Marfan syndrome. *Am J Med* 1981; 71:784–790.

43. Rossiter JP, Repke JT, Morales AJ, Murphy EA, Pyeritz RE. A prospective longitudinal evaluation of pregnancy in the Marfan syndrome. *Am J Obstet Gynecol* 1995; 173:1599–1606.

44. Ulkayan U, Ostrzega E, Shotan A, Mehra A. Cardiovascular problems in pregnant women with Marfan syndrome. *Ann Intern Med* 1995; 123:117–122.

45. Beighton P. *The Ehlers-Danlos Syndrome*. London: Heinemann Medical; 1970.

46. Steinmann B, Royce PM, Superti-Furga A. The Ehlers Danlos syndrome. In: Royce PM, Steinmann B, eds. *Connective Tissue and Its Heritable Disorders: Molecular, Genetic, and Medical Aspects.* New York: Wiley-Liss; 1993:351–407.

47. McKusick VA, Amberger JS. The morbid anatomy of the human genome: Chromosomal location of mutations causing disease. *J Med Genet* 1994; 31:265–279.

48. Hunter GC, Malone JM, Moore WS, Misiorowski RL, Chvapil M. Vascular manifestations in patients with Ehlers-Danlos syndrome. *Arch Surg* 1982; 117:495–498.

49. Serry C, Agomuoh OS, Goldin MD. Review of Ehlers-Danlos syndrome. *J Cardiovasc Surg* 1988; 29:530–534.

50. Cabeen WR Jr, Reza MJ, Kovick RB, Stern MS. Mitral valve prolapse and conduction defects in Ehlers-Danlos syndrome. *Arch Intern Med* 1977; 137:1227–1231.

51. Leier CV, Call TD, Fulkerson PK, Wooley CF. The spectrum of cardiac defects in the Ehlers-Danlos syndrome, types I and III. *Ann Intern Med* 1980; 92(part 1):171–178.

52. Jaffe AS, Geltman EM, Rodey GE, Uitto J. Mitral valve prolapse: A consistent manifestation of type IV Ehlers-Danlos syndrome. *Circulation* 1981; 64:121–125.

53. Lüscher TF, Essandoh MD, Hollier LH. Renovascular hypertension: A rare cardiovascular manifestation of the Ehlers-Danlos syndrome. *Mayo Clin Proc* 1987; 62:223–229.

54. Kitazono T, Imaizumi T, Imayama S, Shinkai H, Takeshita A, Nakamura M. Two cases of myocardial infarction in type 4 Ehlers-Danlos syndrome. *Chest* 1989; 95:1274–1277.

55. Takahashi T, Koide T, Yamaguchi H, Nakamura N, Ohshima Y, Suzuki J, et al. Ehlers-Danlos syndrome with aortic regurgitation, dilation of the sinuses of Valsalva, and abnormal dermal collagen fibrils. *Am Heart J* 1992; 123:1709–1712.

56. Hamano K, Minami Y, Fujimura Y, Tsuboi H, Furukawa S, Oda T, et al. Emergency operation for thoracic aortic aneurysm caused by the Ehlers-Danlos syndrome. *Ann Thorac Surg* 1994; 58:1180–1182.

57. Adès LC, Waltham RD, Chiodo AA, Bateman JF. Myocardial infarction resulting from coronary dissection in an adolescent with Ehlers-Danlos syndrome type IV due to a type III collagen mutation. *Br Heart J* 1995; 74:112–116.

58. Neldner KH, Pseudoxanthoma elasticum. In: Royce P, Steinmann B, eds. *Connective Tissue and Its Heritable Disorders: Molecular, Genetic, and Medical Aspects.* New York: Wiley-Liss; 1993:425–436.

59. Contri MB, Boraldi F, Taparelli F, DePaepe A, Ronchetti IP. Matrix proteins with high affinity for calcium ions are associated with mineralization within the elastic fibers of pseudoelasticum dermis. *Am J Pathol* 1996; 148:569–577.

60. Lebwohl M, Halperin J, Phelps RG. Brief report: Occult pseudoxanthoma elasticum in patients with premature cardiovascular disease. *N Engl J Med* 1993; 329:1237–1239.

61. Coleman K, Ross MH, McCabe M, Coleman R, Mooney D. Disk drusen and angioid streaks in pseudoxanthoma elasticum. *Am J Ophthalmol* 1991; 112:166–170.

62. Slade AKB, John RM, Swanton RH. Pseudoxanthoma elasticum presenting with myocardial infarction. *Br Heart J* 1990; 63:372–373.

63. Coffman JD, Summers SC. Familial pseudoxanthoma elasticum and valvular heart disease. *Circulation* 1959; 19:242–250.

64. Mendelsohn G, Bulkley BH, Hutchins GM. Cardiovascular manifestations of pseudoxanthoma elasticum. *Arch Pathol Lab Med* 1978; 102:298–302.

65. Navarro-Lopez F, Llorian A, Ferrer-Roca O, Betriu A, Sanz G. Restrictive cardiomyopathy in pseudoxanthoma elasticum. *Chest* 1980; 78:113–115.

66. Rosenzweig BP, Guarneri E, Kronzon I. Echocardiographic manifestations in a patient with pseudoxanthoma elasticum. *Ann Intern Med* 1993; 119:487–491.

67. Lebwohl MG, Distefano D, Prioleau PG, Uram M, Yannuzzi LA, Fleischmajer R. Pseudoxanthoma elasticum and mitral valve prolapse. *N Engl J Med* 1982; 307:228–231.

68. Fukuda K, Uno K, Fujii T, Mukai M, Hauda S. Mitral stenosis in pseudoxanthoma elasticum. *Chest* 1992; 101:1706–1707.

69. Challenor VF, Conway N, Monro JL. The surgical treatment of restrictive cardiomyopathy in pseudoxanthoma elasticum. *Br Heart J* 1988; 59:266–269.

70. McKusick VA. Pseudoxanthoma elasticum. In: McKusick VA, ed. *Heritable Disorders of Connective Tissue*, 4th ed. St. Louis: Mosby; 1972:475–520.

71. Stover ML, Primorac D, Liu SC, McKinstry MB, Rowe DW. Defective splicing of mRNA from one COL1A1 allele of type I collagen in nondeforming (type I) osteogenesis imperfecta. *J Clin Invest* 1993; 92:1994–2002.

72. Sillence DO, Senn A, Danks DM. Genetic heterogeneity in osteogenesis imperfecta. *J Med Genet* 1979; 16:101–116.

73. Byers PH. Osteogenesis imperfecta. In: Royce PM, Steinmann B, eds. *Connective Tissue and Its Heritable Disorders: Molecular, Genetic and Medical Aspects,* New York: Wiley-Liss: 1993:317–350.

74. Marini JC, Gerber NL. Osteogenesis imperfecta rehabilitation and prospects for gene therapy. *JAMA* 1997; 277:746–750.

75. Hathaway WE, Solomons CC, Ott JE. Platelet function and pyrophosphates in osteogenesis imperfecta. *Blood* 1972; 39:500–509.

76. Wong RS, Follis FM, Shively BK, Wernly JA. Osteogenesis imperfecta and cardiovascular diseases. *Ann Thorac Surg* 1995; 60:1439–1443.

77. Almassi GH, Hughes GR, Bartlett J. Combined valve replacement and coronary bypass grafting in osteogenesis imperfecta. *Ann Thorac Surg* 1995; 60:1395–1397.

78. Hortop J, Tsipouras P, Hanley JA, Maron BJ, Shapiro JR. Cardiovascular involvement in osteogenesis imperfecta. *Circulation* 1986; 73:54–61.

79. Moriyama Y, Nishida T, Toyohira H, Saigenji H, Shimokawa S, Taira A, et al. Acute aortic dissection in a patient with osteogenesis imperfecta. *Ann Thorac Surg* 1995; 60:1397–1399.

80. Stein D, Kloster FE. Valvular heart disease in osteogenesis imperfecta. *Am Heart J* 1977; 94:637–641.

81. Fowler NO, Van Der Bel-Kahn JM. Indications for surgical replacement of the mitral valve with particular reference to common and uncommon causes of mitral regurgitation. *Am J Cardiol* 1979; 44:148–156.

82. White NJ, Winearls CG, Smith R. Cardiovascular abnormalities in osteogenesis imperfecta. *Am Heart J* 1983; 106:1416–1420.

83. Criscitiello MG, Ronan JA Jr, Besterman EMM, Schoenwetter W. Cardiovascular abnormalities in osteogenesis imperfecta. *Circulation* 1965; 31:255–262.

84. Wood SJ, Thomas J, Braimbridge MV. Mitral valve disease and open heart surgery in osteogenesis imperfecta tarda. *Br Heart J* 1973; 35:103–106.

85. Ellis PR, Cooley DA, DeBakey ME. Clinical consideration and surgical treatment of annulo-aortic ectasia. *J Thorac Cardiovasc Surg* 1961; 42:363–370.

86. Emanuel R, Ng RAL, Marcomichelakis J, Moores EC, Jefferson KE, Macfaul PA, et al. Formes frustes of Marfan's syndrome presenting with severe aortic regurgitation: Clinicogenetic study of 18 families. *Br Heart J* 1977; 39:190.

87. Lemon DK, White CW. Anuloaortic ectasis: Angiographic, hemodynamic and clinical comparison with aortic valve insufficiency. *Am J Cardiol* 1978; 41:482–486.

88. Savunen T. Cardiovascular abnormalities in the relatives of patients operated upon for annulo-aortic ectasia: A clinical and echocardiographic study of 40 families. *Eur J Cardiothorac Surg* 1987; 1:3.

89. Roman MJ, Devereux RB. Heritable aortic disease. In: Lindsay J, ed. *Diseases of the Aorta*. Philadelphia: Lea & Febiger; 1994:55–74.

90. Pascal N, Bloor C, Godfrey M, Hollister D, Pyeritz RE, Dittrich H, et al. Familial aortic dissecting aneurysm. *J Am Coll Cardiol* 1989; 13:811–819.

91. Chen M, Rigby ML, Redington AN. Familial aneurysms of the interventricular septum. *Br Heart J* 1991; 65:104–106.

92. Jaksche VH. Familiäre Aneurysmen: Vier Karotisaneurysmen aus einer zehnköpfigen Familie. *Zentralbl Neurochir* 1986; 47:351–353.

93. Morooka Y, Waga S. Familial intracranial aneurysms: Report of four families. *Surg Neurol* 1983; 19:260–262.

94. Verdura J, Resnikoff S, Rosenthal J, Cardenas J. Familial intracranial aneurysms, with two occurring at the distal anterior cerebral artery. *Neurosurgery* 1983; 12:214–216.

95. Elshunnar KS, Whittle IR. Familial intracranial aneurysms: Report of five families. *Br J Neurosurg* 1990; 4:181–186.

96. Steinberg AD, Gourley MF, Klinman DM, Tsokos GC, Scott DE, Krieg AM. Systemic lupus erythematosus. NIH conference. *Ann Intern Med* 1991; 115:548–559.

97. Boumpas DT, Fessler BJ, Austin HA III, Balow JE, Klippel JH, Lockshin MD. Systemic lupus erythematosus. Emerging concepts. Part 2: Dermatologic and joint disease, the antiphospholipid antibody syndrome, pregnancy and hormonal therapy, morbidity and mortality, and pathogenesis. *Ann Intern Med* 1995; 123:42–53.

98. McNeil HP, Chesterman CN, Krilis SA. Immunology and clinical importance of antiphospholipid antibodies. *Adv Immunol* 1991; 49:193–280.

99. Alarcon-Segovia D, Perez-Vasquez ME, Villa AR, Drenkard C, Cabiedes J. Preliminary classification criteria for the antiphospholipid syndrome within systemic lupus erythematosus. *Semin Arthritis Rheum* 1992; 21:275–286.

100. Wallace DJ, Hahn BH, eds. *Dubois' Lupus Erythematosus,* 4th ed. Philadelphia: Lea & Febiger; 1993.

101. Alarcon-Segovia D, Deleze M, Oria CV, Sanchez-Guerrero J, Gomez-Pacheco L, Cabiedes J, et al. Antiphospholipid antibodies and the antiphospholipid syndrome in systemic lupus erythematosus: A prospective analysis of 500 consecutive patients. *Medicine* 1989; 68:353–365.

102. Ward MM, Pyun E, Studenski S. Mortality risks associated with specific clinical manifestations of systemic lupus erythematosus. *Arch Intern Med* 1996; 156:1337–1344.

103. Brigden W, Bywaters EGL, Lessof MH, Ross IP. The heart in systemic lupus erythematosus. *Br Heart J* 1960; 22:1–16.

104. Bulkley BH, Roberts WC. Systemic lupus erythematosus as a cause of severe mitral regurgitation. *Am J Cardiol* 1975; 35:305–308.

105. Elkayam U, Weiss S, Lainado S. Pericardial effusion and mitral valve involvement in systemic lupus erythematosus: Echocardiographic study. *Ann Rheum Dis* 1977; 36:349–353.

106. Chang RW. Cardiac manifestations of systemic lupus erythematosus. *Clin Rheum Dis* 1981; 8:197–206.

107. Ansari A, Larson PH, Bates HD. Cardiovascular manifestations of systemic lupus erythematosus. *Prog Cardiovasc Dis* 1985; 27:421–434.

108. Doherty NE, Siegel RJ. Cardiovascular manifestations of systemic lupus erythematosus. *Am Heart J* 1985; 110:1257–1265.

109. Klinkhoff AV, Thompson CR, Reid GD, Tomlinson CW. M-mode and two-dimensional echocardiographic abnormalities in systemic lupus erythematosus. *JAMA* 1985; 253:3273–3277.

110. Mandell BF. Cardiovascular involvement in systemic lupus erythematosus. *Semin Arthritis Rheum* 1987; 17:126–141.

111. Doherty NE, Feldman G, Maurer G, Siegel RJ. Echocardiographic findings in systemic lupus erythematosus. *Am J Cardiol* 1988; 61:1144.

112. Galve E, Candell-Riera J, Pigrau C, Permanyer-Miralda G, Garcia-del-Castillo H, Soler-Soler J. Prevalence, morphologic types, and evolution of cardiac valvular disease in systemic lupus erythematosus. *N Engl J Med* 1988; 319:817–823.

113. Straaton KV, Chatham WW, Reveille JD, Koopman WJ, Smith SH. Clinically significant valvular heart disease in systemic lupus erythematosus. *Am J Med* 1988; 85:645–650.

114. Nihoyannopoulos P, Gomez PM, Joshi J, Loizou S, Walport MJ, Oakley CM. Cardiac abnormalities in systemic lupus erythematosus: Association with raised anticardiolipin antibodies. *Circulation* 1990; 82:369–375.

115. Leung WH, Wong KL, Lau C-P, Wong C-K, Cheng C-H, Tai Y-T. Doppler echocardiographic evaluation of left ventricular diastolic function in patients with systemic lupus erythematosus. *Am Heart J* 1990; 120:82–87.

116. Leung WH, Wong KL, Lau CP, Wong C-K, Cheng C-H. Cardiac abnormalities in systemic lupus erythematosus: A prospective M-mode, cross-sectional and Doppler echocardiographic study. *Int J Cardiol* 1990; 27:367–375.

117. Martinez-Costa X, Ordi J, Barbera J, Selva A, Bosch J, Vilardell M. High grade atrioventricular heart block in 2 adults with systemic lupus erythematosus. *J Rheumatol* 1991; 18:1926–1928.

118. Crozier IG, Li E, Milne MJ, Nicholls MG. Cardiac involvement in systemic lupus erythematosus detected by echocardiography. *Am J Cardiol* 1990; 65:1145–1148.

119. Cujec B, Sibley J, Haga M. Cardiac abnormalities in patients with systemic lupus erythematosus. *Can J Cardiol* 1991; 7:343–349.

120. Enomoto K, Kaji Y, Mayumi T, Tusda Y, Kanaya S, Nagasawa K, et al. Frequency of valvular regurgitation by color Doppler echocardiography in systemic lupus erythematosus. *Am J Cardiol* 1991; 67:209–211.

121. Cervera R, Font J, Pare C, Azqueta M, Perez-Villa F, Lopez-Soto A, et al. Cardiac disease in systemic lupus erythematosus: Prospective study of 70 patients. *Ann Rheum Dis* 1992; 51:156–159.

122. Sasson Z, Rasooly Y, Chow CW, Marshall S, Urowitz MB. Impairment of left ventricular diastolic function in systemic lupus erythematosus. *Am J Cardiol* 1992; 69:1629–1634.

123. Ong ML, Veerapen K, Chambers JB, Lim MN, Manivasagar M, Wang F. Cardiac abnormalities in systemic lupus erythematosus: Prevalence and relationship to disease activity. *Int J Cardiol* 1992; 34:69–74.

124. Sturfelt G, Eskilsson J, Nived O, Truedsson L, Valind S. Cardiovascular disease in systemic lupus erythematosus: A study of 75 patients from a defined population. *Medicine* 1992; 71:216–223.

125. Roldan CA, Shively BK, Crawford MH. An echocardiographic study of valvular heart disease associated with systemic lupus erythematosus. *N Engl J Med* 1996; 335:1424–1430.

126. Asherson RA, Oakley CM. Pulmonary hypertension in SLE. *J Rheumatol* 1986; 13:1–5.

127. Asherson RA, Hingbottam TW, Xuan ATD, Khamashta MA, Hughes GRV. Pulmonary hypertension in a lupus clinic: Experience with twenty four patients. *J Rheumatol* 1990; 17:1292–1298.

128. Alameddine AK, Schoen FJ, Yanagi H, Couper GS, Collins JJ Jr, Cohn LH. Aortic or mitral valve replacement in systemic lupus erythematosus. *Am J Cardiol* 1992; 70:955–956.

129. O'Rourke RA. Antiphospholipid antibodies. A marker of lupus carditis? *Circulation* 1990; 82:636–638.

130. Khamashta MA, Cervera R, Asherson RA, Font J, Gil A, Coltart DJ, et al. Association of antibodies against phospholipids with heart valve disease in systemic lupus erythematosus. *Lancet* 1990; 335:1541–1544.

131. Ford PM, Ford SE, Lillicrap DP. Association of lupus anticoagulant with severe valvular heart disease in systemic lupus erythematosus. *J Rheumatol* 1988; 1:597–600.

132. Chartash EK, Lans DM, Paget SA, Qamar T, Lockshin MD. Aortic insufficiency and mitral regurgitation in patients with systemic lupus erythematosus and the antiphospholipid syndrome. *Am J Med* 1989; 86:407–412.

133. Leung WH, Wong KL, Lau C-P, Wong C-K, Liu HW. Association between antiphospholipid antibodies and cardiac abnormalities in patients with systemic lupus erythematosus. *Am J Med* 1990; 89:411–419.

134. Gabrielli F, Alcini E, Di Prima MA, Mazzacurati G, Masala C. Cardiac valve involvement in systemic lupus erythematosus and primary antiphospholipid syndrome: Lack of correlation with antiphospholipid antibodies. *Int J Cardiol* 1995; 51:117–126.

135. Roldan CA, Shively BK, Lau CC, Gurule FT, Smith EA, Crawford MH. Systemic lupus erythematosus valve disease by transesophageal echocardiography and the role of antiphospholipid antibodies. *J Am Coll Cardiol* 1992; 20:1127–1134.

136. Hejtmancik MR, Wright JC, Quint R, Jennings FL. The cardiovascular manifestations of systemic lupus erythematosus. *Am Heart J* 1964; 119:119–130.

137. Bulkley BH, Roberts WC. The heart in systemic lupus erythematosus and the changes induced in it by corticosteroid therapy. A study of 36 necropsy patients. *Am J Med* 1975; 58:243–264.

138. Doherty NE, Siegel RJ. Cardiovascular manifestations of systemic lupus erythematosus. *Am Heart J* 1985; 110:1257–1265.

139. Kahl LE. The spectrum of pericardial tamponade in systemic lupus erythematosus: Report of ten patients. *Arthritis Rheum* 1992; 35:1343–1349.

140. Klacsmann PG, Bulkley BH, Hutchins GM. The changed spectrum of purulent pericarditis: An 86 year autopsy experience in 200 patients. *Am J Med* 1977; 63:666–673.

141. Libman E, Sacks B. A hitherto undescribed form of valvular and mural endocarditis. *Arch Intern Med* 1924; 33:701–737.

142. Gross L. The cardiac lesion in Libman-Sacks disease with a consideration of its relationship to acute diffuse lupus erythematosus. *Am J Pathol* 1940; 16:375–407.

143. Bulkley BH, Roberts WC. Systemic lupus erythematosus as a cause of severe mitral regurgitation: A new problem in an old disease. *Am J Cardiol* 1975; 35:305–338.

144. Paget SA, Bulkley BH, Grauer LE, Seningen R. Mitral valve disease of systemic lupus erythematosus: A cause of severe congestive heart failure reversed by valve replacement. *Am J Med* 1975; 59:134–139.

145. Winslow TM, Ossipov MA, Fazio GP, Foster E, Simonson JS, Schiller NB. The left ventricle in systemic lupus erythematosus: Initial observations and a five-year follow up in a university medical center population. *Am Heart J* 1993; 125:1117–1122.

146. Urowitz MB, Bookman AAM, Koehler BE, Gordon DA, Smythe HA, Ogryzlo MA. The bimodal mortality pattern of systemic lupus erythematosus. *Am J Med* 1976; 60:221–225.

147. Sturfelt G, Eskilsson J, Nived O, Truedsson L, Valind S. Cardiovascular disease in systemic lupus erythematosus. A study of 75 patients from a defined population. *Medicine (Baltimore)* 1992; 71:216–223.

148. Petri M, Spence D, Bone LR, Hochberg MC. Coronary artery disease risk factors in the Johns Hopkins lupus cohort: Prevalence, recognition by patients, and preventive practices. *Medicine (Baltimore)* 1992; 71:291–302.

149. Kutom AH, Gibbs HR. Myocardial infarction due to intracoronary thrombi without significant coronary artery disease in systemic lupus erythematosus. *Chest* 1991; 100:571–572.

150. Miller DJ, Maisch SA, Perez MD, Kearney DL, Feltes TF. Fatal myocardial infarction in an 8-year-old girl with systemic lupus erythematosus, Raynaud's phenomenon, and secondary antiphospholipid antibody syndrome. *J Rheumatol* 1995; 22:768–773.

151. Wilson VE, Eck SL, Bates ER. Evaluation and treatment of acute myocardial infarction complicating systemic lupus erythematosus. *Chest* 1992; 101:420–424.

152. Sumino H, Kanda T, Sasaki T, Kanazawa N, Takeuchi H. Myocardial infarction secondary to coronary aneurysm in systemic lupus erythematosus. An autopsy case. *Angiology* 1995; 46:527–530.

153. Escolar G, Font J, Reverter JC, Lopez-Soto A, Garrido M, Cervera R, et al. Plasma from systemic lupus erythematosus patients with antiphospholipid antibodies promotes platelet aggregation: Studies in a perfusion system. *Arterioscler Thromb* 1992; 12:196–200.

154. James TN, Rupe CE, Monto RW. Pathology of the cardiac conduction system in systemic lupus erythematosus. *Ann Intern Med* 1965; 63:402–410.

155. Buyon JP, Winchester R. Congenital complete heart block: A human model of passively acquired autoimmune injury. *Arthritis Rheum* 1990; 33:609–614.

156. Reid JM, Coleman EN, Doig W. Complete congenital heart block. Report of 35 cases. *Br Heart J* 1982; 48:236.

157. Carreira PE, Gutierrez-Larraya F, Gomez-Reino JJ. Successful intrauterine therapy with dexamethasone for fetal myocarditis and heart block in a woman with systemic lupus erythematosus. *J Rheum* 1993; 20:1204–1207.

158. Walkinshaw SA, Welch CR, McCormack J, Walsh K. In utero pacing for congenital heart block. *Fetal Diagn Ther* 1994; 9:183–185.

159. Waltuck J, Buyon JP. Autoantibody-associated congenital heart block: Outcome in mothers and children. *Ann Intern Med* 1994; 120:544–551.

160. Press J, Uziel Y, Laxer RM, Luy L, Hamilton RM, Silverman ED. Long-term outcome of mothers of children with complete congenital heart block. *Am J Med* 1996; 100:328–332.

161. Goble MM, Dick M 2d, McCune WJ, Ellsworth J, Sullivan DB, Stern AM. Atrioventricular conduction in children of women with systemic lupus erythematosus. *Am J Cardiol* 1993; 71:94–98.

162. Logar D, Kveder T, Rozman B, Pobovisek J. Possible association between anti-Ro antibodies and myocarditis or cardiac conduction defects in adults with systemic lupus erythematosus. *Ann Rheum Dis* 1990; 49:627–629.

163. Martinez-Costa X, Ordi J, Barbera J, Sela A, Bosch J, Vilardell M. High-grade atrioventricular heart block in 2 adults with systemic lupus erythematosus. *J Rheum* 1991; 18:1926–1928.

164. O'Neill TW, Mahmoud A, Tooke A, Thomas RD, Madison PJ. Is there an association between subclinical myocardial abnormalities, conduction defects and Ro/La antibodies in adults with systemic lupus erythematosus? *Clin Exp Rheum* 1993; 11:409–412.

165. Winslow TM, Ossipov MA, Fazio GP, Simonson JS, Redberg RF, Schiller NB. Five-year follow up study of the prevalence and progression of pulmonary hypertension in systemic lupus erythematosus. *Am Heart J* 1995; 129:510–515.

166. Petri M, Lakatta C, Madger L, Goldman D. Effect of prednisone and hydroxychloroquine on coronary artery disease risk factors in systemic lupus erythematosus: A longitudinal data analysis. *Am J Med* 1994; 96:254–259.

167. Chiariello M, Ambrosio G, Capelli-Bigazzi M, Perrone-Filardi P, Tritto I, Nevola E, et al. Reduction in infarct size by the phospholipase inhibitor quinacrine in dogs with coronary artery occlusion. *Am Heart J* 1990; 120:801–807.

168. Kimura T, Satoh S. Inhibitory effect of quinacrine on myocardial reactive hyperthermia in the dog. *J Pharmacol Exp Ther* 1985; 232:269–274.

169. Fazekas T, Szekeres L. Effect of chloroquine in experimental myocardial ischemia. *Acta Physiol Hung* 1988; 72:191–199.

170. Cacoub P, Lunel-Fabiani F, Le-Thi Huong CLT. Polyarteritis nodosa and hepatitis C virus infection. *Ann Intern Med* 1992; 116:605–606.

171. Przybojewski JZ. Polyarteritis nodosa in the adult: Report of a case with repeated myocardial infarction and a review of cardiac involvement. *S Afr Med J* 1981; 60:512–518.

172. Alarcon-Segovia D. The necrotizing vasculitides: A new pathogenetic classification. *Symp Rheum Dis* 1977; 61:241–260.

173. Holsinger DR, Osmundson PJ, Edwards JE. The heart in periarteritis nodosa. *Circulation* 1962; 25:610–618.

174. Schrader ML, Hochman JS, Bulkley BH. The heart in polyarteritis nodosa: A clinicopathologic study. *Am Heart J* 1985; 109:1353–1359.

175. James TN, Birk RE. Pathology of the cardiac conduction system in polyarteritis nodosa. *Arch Intern Med* 1966; 117:561–567.

176. Thiene G, Valente M, Rossi L. Involvement of the cardiac conducting system in panarteritis nodosa. *Am Heart J* 1978; 95:716–724.

177. Charles LA, Jennette JC, Falk RJ. The role of HLGO cells in the detection of antineutrophil cytoplasmic autoantibodies. *J Rheum* 1991; 18:491–494.

178. Bacon PA, Gibson DG. Cardiac involvement in rheumatoid arthritis: An echocardiographic study. *Ann Rheum Dis* 1974; 33:20–24.

179. Liss JP, Bachmann WT. Rheumatoid constrictive pericarditis treated by pericardiectomy: Report of a case and review of the literature. *Arthritis Rheum* 1970; 13:869–876.

180. Hakala M, Pettersson T, Tarkka M, Leirisalo-Repo M, Mattila T, Airaksinen J, et al. Rheumatoid arthritis as a cause of cardiac compression. Favourable long-term outcome of pericardiectomy. *Clin Rheum* 1993; 12:199–203.

181. Escalante A, Kaufman RL, Quismorio FP Jr, Beardmore TD. Cardiac compression in rheumatoid pericarditis. *Semin Arthritis Rheum* 1990; 148–163.

182. Hara KS, Ballard DJ, Illstrup DM, Connolly DC, Vollertsen RS. Rheumatoid pericarditis: Clinical features and survival. *Medicine (Baltimore)* 1990; 69:81–91.

183. Travaglio-Encinoza A, Anaya JM, Dupuy D'Angeac AD, Reme T, Sany J. Rheumatoid pericarditis: New immunopathological aspects. *Clin Exp Rheum* 1994; 12:313–316.

184. Ahern M, Lever JV, Cosh J. Complete heart block in rheumatoid arthritis. *Ann Rheum Dis* 1983; 42:389–397.

185. Roberts WC, Dangel JC, Bulkley BH. Nonrheumatic valvular cardiac disease: A clinicopathologic survey of 27 different conditions causing valvular dysfunction. *Cardiovasc Clin* 1973; 5:333–446.

186. Suriani RJ, Lansman S, Konstadt S. Intracardiac rheumatoid nodule presenting as a left atrial mass. *Am Heart J* 1994; 127:463–465.

187. Maione S, Valentini G, Giunta A, Tirri R, Giacummo A, Lippolis C, et al. Cardiac involvement in rheumatoid arthritis: An echocardiographic study. *Cardiology* 1993; 83:234–239.

188. Voisin L, Derumeaux G, Borg JY, Mejjad O, Vittecoq O, Tayot J, et al. Catastrophic antiphospholipid syndrome with fatal acute course in rheumatoid arthritis. *J Rheumatol* 1995; 22:1586–1588.

189. Julkunen H. Rheumatoid spondylitis—clinical and laboratory study of 149 cases compared with 182 cases of rheumatoid arthritis. *Acta Rheum Scand* 1962; 172(suppl 4):1–116.

190. Bulkley BH, Roberts WC. Ankylosing spondylitis and aortic regurgitation: Description of the characteristic cardiovascular lesion from study of eight necropsy patients. *Circulation* 1973; 48:1014–1027.

191. Kawasuji M, Hetzer R, Oelert H, Stauch G, Borst HG. Aortic valve replacement and ascending aorta replacement in ankylosing spondylitis: Report of three surgical cases and review of the literature. *J Thorac Cardiovasc Surg* 1982; 30:310–314.

192. Roberts WC, Hollingsworth JF, Bulkley BH, Jaffe RB, Epstein SE, Stinson EB. Combined mitral and aortic regurgitation in ankylosing spondylitis: Angiographic and anatomic features. *Am J Med* 1974; 56:237–243.

193. Gould BA, Turner J, Keeling DH, Hickling P, Marshall AJ. Myocardial dysfunction in ankylosing spondylitis. *Ann Rheum Dis* 1992; 51:227–232.

194. Paulus HE, Pearson CM, Pitts W. Aortic insufficiency in 5 patients with Reiter's syndrome. *Am J Med* 1972; 53:461.

195. Weiss S, Stead EA, Warren JV, Bailey OT. Scleroderma heart disease: With a consideration of certain other visceral manifestations of scleroderma. *Arch Intern Med* 1943; 71:749.

196. Sackner AM, Akgun N, Kimbel P, Lewis DH. The pathophysiology of scleroderma involving the heart and respiratory system. *Ann Intern Med* 1964; 60:611.

197. Bulkley BH, Ridolfi RL, Salyer WR, Hutchins GM. Myocardial lesions of progressive systemic sclerosis: A cause of cardiac dysfunction. *Circulation* 1976; 53:483–490.

198. Claman HN. On scleroderma: Mast cells, endothelial cells, and fibroblasts. *JAMA* 1989; 262:1206–1209.

199. Bulkley BH, Klacsmann PG, Hutchins GM. Angina pectoris, myocardial infarction and sudden death with normal coronary arteries: A clinicopathologic study of 9 patients with progressive systemic sclerosis. *Am Heart J* 1978; 95:563–569.

200. Salerni R, Rodnan GP, Leon DF, Shaver JA. Pulmonary hypertension in the CREST syndrome variant of progressive systemic sclerosis (scleroderma). *Ann Intern Med* 1977; 86:394–399.

201. Leinwand I, Duryee AW, Richter MN. Scleroderma (based on a study of over 150 cases). *Ann Intern Med* 1954; 41:1003–1041.

202. Bulkley BH. Progressive systemic sclerosis: Cardiac involvement. *Clin Rheum Dis* 1979; 5:131–149.

203. Cannon PJ, Hassar M, Case DB, Casarella WJ, Sommers SC, LeRoy EC. The relationship of hypertension and renal failure in scleroderma (progressive systemic sclerosis) to structural and functional abnormalities of the renal cortical circulation. *Medicine* 1974; 53:1–46.

204. Follansbee WP, Curtiss EI, Medsger TA Jr, Steen VD, Uretsky BF, Owens GR, et al. Physiologic abnormalities of cardiac function in progressive systemic sclerosis with diffuse scleroderma. *N Engl J Med* 1984; 310:142–148.

205. Ellis WW, Baer AN, Robertson RM, Pincus T, Kronenberg MW. Left ventricular dysfunction induced by cold exposure in patients with systemic sclerosis. *Am J Med* 1986; 80:385–392.

206. Alexander EL, Firestein GS, Weiss JL, Heuser RR, Leitl G, Wagner HN Jr, et al. Reversible cold-induced abnormalities in myocardial perfusion and function in systemic sclerosis. *Ann Intern Med* 1986; 105:661–668.

207. Kahan A, Nitenberg A, Foult JM, Amor B, Menkes CJ, Devaux JY, et al. Decreased coronary reserve in primary scleroderma myocardial disease. *Arthritis Rheum* 1985; 28:637–646.

208. Smiley JD. The many faces of scleroderma. *Am J Med Sci* 1992; 304:319–333.

209. Anvari A, Graninger W, Schneider B, Sochor H, Weber H, Schmidinger H. Cardiac involvement in systemic sclerosis. *Arthritis Rheum* 1992; 35:1356–1361.

210. Candell-Riera J, Armadans-Gil L, Simeon CP, Castell-Conesa J, Fonollosa-Pla V, Garcia-Del-Castillo H, et al. Comprehensive noninvasive assessment of cardiac involvement in limited systemic sclerosis. *Arthritis Rheum* 1996; 39:1138–1145.

211. Fujimoto S, Kagoshima T, Nakajima T, Dohi K. Doppler echocardiographic assessment of left ventricular diastolic function in patients with progressive systemic sclerosis. *Cardiology* 1993; 83:217–227.

212. Clements PJ, Lachenbruch PA, Furst DE, Paulus HE, Sterz MG. Cardiac score: A semiquantitative measure of cardiac involvement that improves prediction of prognosis in systemic sclerosis. *Arthritis Rheum* 1991; 34:1371–1380.

213. Kerry LD, Spiera H. Myocarditis as a complication in scleroderma patients with myositis. *Clin Cardiol* 1993; 16:895–899.

214. Follansbee WP, Zerbe TR, Medsger TA Jr. Cardiac and skeletal muscle disease in systemic sclerosis (scleroderma): A high-risk association. *Am Heart J* 1993; 125:194–203.

215. D'Angelo WA, Fries JF, Masi AT, Shulman LE. Pathologic observations in systemic sclerosis (scleroderma): A study of fifty-eight autopsy cases and fifty-eight matched controls. *Am J Med* 1969; 46:428–440.

216. Satoh M, Tokuhira M, Hama N, Hirakata M, Kuwana M, Akizuki M, et al. Massive pericardial effusion in scleroderma: A review of five cases. *Br J Rheumatol* 1995; 34:564–567.

217. Perez-Bocanegra C, Fonollosa V, Simeon CP, Candell J, Solans R, Gomez A, et al. Pericardial tamponade preceding cutaneous involvement in systemic sclerosis. *Ann Rheum Dis* 1995; 54:687–688.

218. Kazzam E, Caidahl K, Hallgren R, Johansson C, Waldestrom A. Mitral regurgitation and diastolic flow profile in systemic sclerosis. *Int J Cardiol* 1990; 29:357–363.

219. Walcott G, Burchell HB, Brown AL. Primary pulmonary hypertension. *Am J Med* 1970; 71:70–79.

220. Martinez-Taboada V, Olalla J, Blanco R, Armona J, Sueiro JF, Rodriguez-Valverde V. Malignant ventricular arrhythmia in systemic sclerosis controlled with an implantable cardioverter defibrillator. *J Rheumatol* 1994; 21:2166–2167.

221. Fritzler MJ, Hart DA. Prolonged improvement of Raynaud's phenomenon and scleroderma after recombinant tissue plasminogen activator therapy. *Arthritis Rheum* 1990; 33:274–276.

222. Matteson EL, Shbeeb MI, McCarthy TG, Calamia KT, Mertz LE, Goronzy JJ. Pilot study of antithymocyte globulin in systemic sclerosis. *Arthritis Rheum* 1996; 39:1132–1137.

223. Kahan A, Devaux JY, Amor B, Menkes CJ, Weber S, Nitenberg A, et al. Nifedipine and thallium-201 myocardial perfusion in progressive systemic sclerosis. *N Engl J Med* 1986; 314:1397–1402.

224. Alpert MA, Pressly TA, Mukerji V, Lambert CR, Mukerji B, Panayiotou H, et al. Acute and long-term effects of nifedipine on pulmonary and systemic hemodynamics in patients with pulmonary hypertension associated with diffuse systemic sclerosis, the CREST syndrome and mixed connective tissue disease. *Am J Cardiol* 1991; 68:1687–1690.

225. Kahan A, Devaux JY, Amor B, Menkes CJ, Weber S, Venot A, et al. The effect of captopril on thallium 201 myocardial perfusion in systemic sclerosis. *Clin Pharmacol Ther* 1990; 47:483–489.

226. Kazzam E, Caidahl K, Hällgren R, Gustafsson R, Waldenström A. Noninvasive evaluation of long-term cardiac effects of captopril in systemic sclerosis. *J Intern Med* 1991; 230:203–212.

227. Schwarz MI. Pulmonary and cardiac manifestations of polymyositis-dermatomyositis. *J Thorac Imaging* 1992; 7:46–54.

228. Plotz PH, Dalakas M, Leff RL, Love LA, Muller FW, Cronin ME. Current concepts in idiopathic inflammatory myopathies: Polymyositis, dermatomyositis, and related disorders. *Ann Intern Med* 1989; 111:143–157.

229. Dalakas MC. Polymyositis, dermatomyositis, and inclusion-body myositis. *N Engl J Med* 1991; 325:1487–1498.

230. Dalakas M, Illa I, Dambrosia JM, Soueidan SA, Stein DP, Otero C, et al. A controlled trial of high-dose intravenous immune globulin as treatment for dermatomyositis. *N Engl J Med* 1993; 329:1993–2000.

231. Gonzales EB, Varner WT, Lisse JR, Daniels JC, Hokanson JA. Giant-cell arteritis in the southern United States: An 11-year retrospective study from the Texas Gulf coast. *Arch Intern Med* 1989; 149:1561–1565.

232. Evans JM, O'Fallon M, Hunder GG. Increased incidence of aortic aneurysms and dissection in giant cell (temporal) arteritis. A population-base study. *Ann Intern Med* 1995; 122:502–507.

233. Morgan JM, Raposo L, Gibson DG. Cardiac involvement in Churg-Strauss syndrome shown by echocardiography. *Br Heart J* 1989; 62:462–466.

234. Hasley PB, Follansbee WP, Coulehan JL. Cardiac manifestations of Churg-Strauss syndrome: Report of a case and review of the literature. *Am Heart J* 1990; 120:996–999.

235. Lockshin MD. Antiphospholipid antibody syndrome. *JAMA* 1992; 268:1451–1453.

236. Abu-Shakra M, Gladman DD, Urowitz MB, Farewell V. Anticardiolipin antibodies in systemic lupus erythematosus: Clinical and laboratory correlations. *Am J Med* 1995; 99:624–628.

237. Khamashta MA, Cuadrado MJ, Mujic F, Taug NA, Hunt BJ, Hughes GRV. The management of thrombosis in the antiphospholipid-antibody syndrome. *N Engl J Med* 1995; 332:993–997.

238. Pope JM, Canny CL, Bell DA. Cerebral ischemic events associated with endocarditis, retinal vascular disease and lupus anticoagulant. *Am J Med* 1991; 90:299–309.

239. Asherson RA, Khamashta MA, Ordi-Ros J, Derksen RH, Machin SJ, Barquinero J, et al. The primary antiphospholipid syndrome: Major clinical and serological features. *Medicine* 1989; 68:366–374.

240. Harris EN. Syndrome of the black swan. *Br J Rheumatol* 1987; 26:324–326.

241. Ford SE, Charrette EJP, Knight J, Pym J, Ford P. A possible role for antiphospholipid antibodies in acquired cardiac valve deformity. *J Rheumatol* 1990; 17:1499–1503.

242. Brenner B, Blumenfeld Z, Markiewicz W, Reisner SA. Cardiac involvement in patients with primary antiphospholipid syndrome. *J Am Coll Cardiol* 1991; 18:931–936.

243. Beynon HLC, Walport MJ. Antiphospholipid antibodies and cardiovascular disease. *Br Heart J* 1992; 67:281–284.

244. Galve E, Josep O, Barquinero J, Evangelista A, Vilardell M, Soler-Soler J. Valvular heart disease in the primary antiphospholipid syndrome. *Ann Intern Med* 1992; 116:293–298.

245. Anderson D, Bell D, Lodge R, Grant E. Recurrent cerebral ischemia and mitral valve vegetation in a patient with lupus anticoagulant. *J Rheumatol* 1987; 14:839–841.

246. D'Alton JG, Preston DN, Bormanis J, Green MS, Kraag GR. Multiple transient ischemic attacks, lupus anticoagulant and verrucous endocarditis. *Stroke* 1985; 16:512–514.

247. Cronin ME, Biswas R, Van der Straeton C, Fleisher TA, Klippel JH. IgG and IgM anticardiolipin antibodies in patients with lupus with cardiolipin antibody associated clinical syndromes. *J Rheumatol* 1988; 15:795–798.

248. Brey RL. Antiphospholipid antibodies and ischemic stroke. *Heart Dis Stroke* 1992; 1:379–382.

249. Antiphospholipid Antibodies in Stroke Study Group. Clinical and laboratory findings in patients with antiphospholipid antibodies and cerebral ischemia. *Stroke* 1990; 21:1268–1273.

250. Levine SR, Brey RL, Joseph CLM, Havstad S. Risk of recurrent thromboembolic events in patients with focal cerebral ischemia and antiphospholipid antibodies. *Stroke* 1992; 23(suppl):I29–I32.

251. Rosove MH, Brewer PMC. Antiphospholipid thrombosis: Clinical course after the first thrombotic event in 70 patients. *Ann Intern Med* 1992; 117:303–308.

252. Ginsburg KS, Liang MH, Newcomer L, Goldhaber SZ, Schur PH, Hennekens CH, et al. Anticardiolipin antibodies and the risk for ischemic stroke and venous thrombosis. *Ann Intern Med* 1992; 117:997–1002.

86

NEOPLASTIC HEART DISEASE

Robert J. Hall / Denton A. Cooley / Hugh A. McAllister, Jr. / O. Howard Frazier

Tumors of the heart, while uncommon, present in protean ways and have challenged the acumen of physicians since the seventeenth century. Antemortem diagnosis, however, was rare before 1950. Intracardiac myxoma was first diagnosed with the aid of angiography in 1952, with a subsequent attempt to remove the tumor surgically. The first successful removal with the use of cardiopulmonary bypass was performed in 1954, and the patient, a 40 year-old woman, was still alive 38 years later.[1] Subsequently, increased clinical awareness, coupled with angiographic and noninvasive diagnostic techniques, has led to more frequent correct diagnoses.[2–4]

The heart may be the site of a primary tumor or may be invaded secondarily by malignancies that arise in adjacent or remote organs. Whether it is due to primary or secondary tumors, neoplastic heart disease can be expressed in only limited ways (Table 86-1). Neoplastic disease, pericardial pain, effusion, tamponade, constriction, rapid increase in heart size, new heart murmurs, electrocardiographic (ECG) changes, atrial or ventricular arrhythmias, atrioventricular (AV) block, and unexplained heart failure are all suggestive of secondary invasion of the heart. The triad of obstruction, embolization, and constitutional manifestations characterizes intracavity tumors, especially myxomas.

PRIMARY TUMORS OF THE HEART

Although they are less common than other tumors of the heart, primary tumors of the heart are far more challenging to both the physician and the surgeon. They usually present as intracavitary lesions, and more than 75 percent are benign.[5] Current surgical techniques permit removal and potential "cure" in many patients with primary tumors, necessitating an awareness of the clinical and hemodynamic presentation of these tumors.[6]

Primary tumors of the heart and pericardium are rare, occurring with a frequency of 0.001 to 0.28 percent in reported or collected postmortem series.[5] Myxomas are the most common of the primary tumors and constitute nearly 50 percent of all histologically benign tumors of the heart. The frequency and classification of 533 primary tumors and cysts of the heart and pericardium collected by the Armed Forces Institute of Pathology are listed in Table 86-2.[7]

Cardiac Myxomas

Intracardiac myxoma is the most frequent benign tumor of the heart. While most (75 percent) are located in the left atrium, myxomas are also found in the right atrium (18 percent), right ventricle (4 percent), and left ventricle (4 percent).[7]

TABLE 86-1

GENERAL MANIFESTATIONS OF NEOPLASTIC HEART DISEASE

Pericardial involvement
  Pericarditis, pain
  Pericardial effusion
  Radiographic enlargement
  Arrhythmia, predominantly atrial
  Tamponade
  Constriction
Myocardial involvement
  Arrhythmias, ventricular and atrial
  Electrocardiographic changes
  Radiographic enlargement
    Generalized
    Localized
  Conduction disturbances and heart block
  Congestive heart failure
  Coronary involvement
    Angina, infarction
Intracavitary tumor
  Cavity obliteration
  Valve obstruction and valve damage
  Embolic phenomena: systemic, neurologic, coronary
  Constitutional manifestations

TABLE 86-2

TUMORS AND CYSTS OF THE HEART AND PERICARDIUM

Type	Number	Percentage
BENIGN		
Myxoma	130	24.4
Lipoma	45	8.4
Papillary fibroelastoma	42	7.9
Rhabdomyoma	36	6.8
Fibroma	17	3.2
Hemangioma	15	2.8
Teratoma	14	2.6
Mesothelioma of the AV node	12	2.3
Granular cell tumor	3	
Neurofibroma	3	
Lymphangioma	2	
Subtotal	319	59.8
Pericardial cyst	82	15.4
Bronchogenic cyst	7	1.3
Subtotal	89	16.7
MALIGNANT		
Angiosarcoma	39	7.3
Rhabdomyosarcoma	26	4.9
Mesothelioma	19	3.6
Fibrosarcoma	14	2.6
Malignant lymphoma	7	1.3
Extraskeletal osteosarcoma	5	
Neurogenic sarcoma	4	
Malignant teratoma	4	
Thymoma	4	
Leiomyosarcoma	1	
Liposarcoma	1	
Synovial sarcoma	1	
Subtotal	125	23.5
Total	533	100.0

Source: McAllister HA Jr, Fenoglio JJ Jr. *Tumors of the Cardiovascular System.* Washington, DC: Armed Forces Institute of Pathology; 1978.

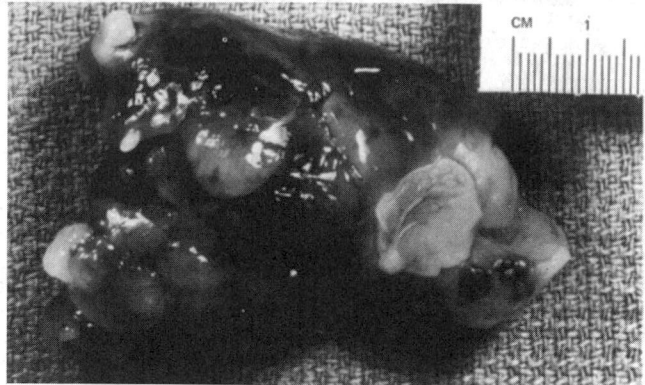

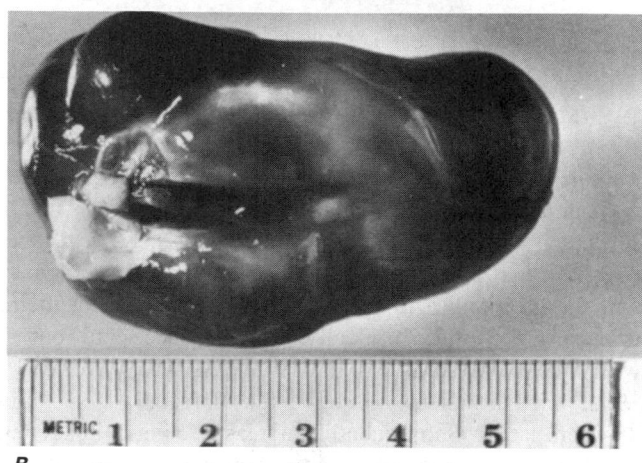

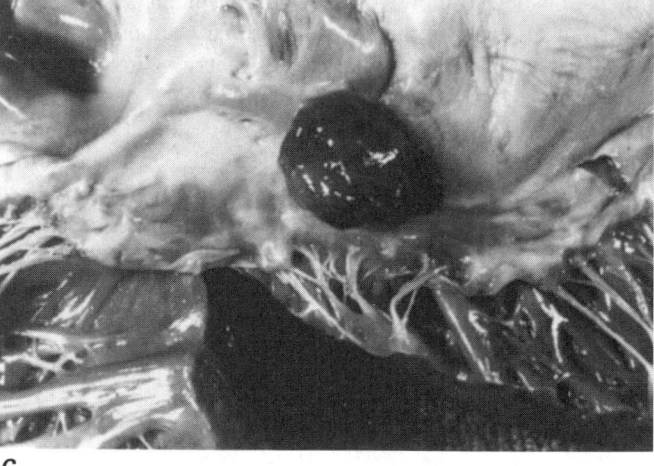

FIGURE 86-1

Left atrial myxomas. *A.* More polypoid and irregular. *B.* Smooth-surfaced and rounded. Attachment to and portion of the atrial septum is seen on each tumor. *C.* An asymptomatic sessile myxoma attached above the posterior leaflet of the mitral valve was found coincidentally at necropsy.

Cardiac myxomas usually originate from the region of the fossa ovalis but may arise from elsewhere within the atria.[7] Although myxomas have been reported as originating from the mitral annulus,[8] the mitral valve itself,[9] the aortic valve,[10] and the inferior vena cava,[11] it is likely that true myxomas arise only from the mural endocardium.[7]

PATHOLOGY

Attached to the endocardium by a broad base, myxomas are usually pedunculated, polypoid, and friable, although some may have a smooth surface and be rounded (Fig. 86-1).[12,13] Sessile myxomas are uncommon.[8] A myxoma appears as a soft, gelatinous, mucoid, usually gray-white mass, often with areas of hemorrhage or thrombosis. These lesions vary from 1 to 15 cm in diameter, with most measuring 5 to 6 cm (Fig. 86-1*A* and *B*).[7]

On microscopic examination, the myxoma is composed of an acid mucopolysaccharide myxoid matrix in which polygonal cells (lepidic cells) and occasional blood vessels are embedded. Channels, often filled with red blood cells, communicate from the surface to deep within the tumor and are lined by endothelium-like cells resembling multipurpose mesenchymal cells, from which the tumor is purported to arise. Similar endothelial cells line the surface of the tumor; however, fibrin, erythrocytes, and organized thrombi may also be present on the surface. Cystic areas, focal or gross hemorrhage, calcification, glandular elements,[14] rarely bone formation, and even hematopoietic tissue constitute the multiple although uncommon variations that may be present.[7]

A neoplastic rather than a thrombotic origin of myxomas is supported by the ultrastructural characteristics of the tumor,[15–17] the results of biochemical analyses,[18] the cultural properties of the tumor cell,[7,19,20] and DNA analysis of the tumor.[21,22] Although myxomas can recur because of their incomplete removal[23,24] and distant growth of embolic myxomatous material has been observed,[23,25,26] the existence of a true malignant cardiac myxoma remains doubtful.[5] The occurrence of multiple tumors within the left atrium, bilaterally in each atrium,[27,28] or simultaneously in the atrium and ventricle[29] raises the possibility of multicentric origin rather than metastasis of the tumor.

AGE, SEX, AND FAMILIAL OCCURRENCE

Most patients with myxomas are 30 to 60 years of age,[2] although myxomas have been discovered in children[30] and infants, neonates,[31] and the elderly.[32] Children have a higher incidence of ventricular myxoma than do adults.[30,33] A higher incidence in females characterizes most series. Familial occurrence has been reported,[34,35] more frequently in males. Tumors are divided equally on both sides of the heart, and opposite atria are usually involved in afflicted members. Familial cases are associated with a younger age at presentation and a higher recurrence rate.[34,35]

GENERAL OR CONSTITUTIONAL MANIFESTATIONS

Whereas asymptomatic patients with myxoma (Fig. 86-1C) have been reported,[29] most present with one or more features of a triad of constitutional, embolic, and obstructive manifestations.[2,8] Cardiac myxomas provoke systemic illness in 90 percent of the patients, characterized by weight loss, fatigue, fever, anemia (often hemolytic), elevated sedimentation rate, and elevated serum immunoglobulin concentration formed in response to tumor embolization, degenerative changes within the tumor (itself), or production of interleukin-6 by the tumor.[36,37] The globulin fraction most frequently elevated is immunoglobulin G (IgG); immunoglobulin A (IgA) is involved only rarely.[2,19,38] Cases involving coexisting cardiac myxoma and IgG multiple myeloma[39] and systemic AL amyloidosis have been reported.[40] Less common findings are leukocytosis, thrombocytopenia, clubbing, Raynaud's phenomenon, and breast fibroadenomas.[2] Polycythemia may result from tumor production of erythropoietin.[41]

Patients with hemolytic anemia have features of intravascular mechanical destruction, which may be accompanied by pancytopenia. Hemolytic anemia is more likely to occur in patients with calcified myxomas, more commonly in the right atrium. "Syndrome myxoma," or Carney complex, characterizes a subset of patients with cardiac myxoma associated with spotty skin pigmentation and peripheral and endocrine neoplasms. These patients, in contrast to those with "sporadic myxoma," are usually younger, have a high incidence of familial myxoma, and more frequently have multiple and recurrent tumors.[42,43] The protracted multisystemic symptoms produced by myxomas may also mimic connective tissue disease and polyarteritis nodosa.[28,44,45]

INFECTED MYXOMA

An intracavitary myxoma rarely becomes infected, and blood cultures have demonstrated a variety of organisms.[46–49] Most patients with infected myxomas experience major neurologic embolic events. Surgical resection should be carried out promptly before catastrophic embolic complications occur.[50,51]

EMBOLIZATION

Systemic tumor embolization, more commonly from myxomas with irregular, papillary frondlike surfaces,[12,13] occurs in 40 to 50 percent of patients with left atrial myxoma,[2] with tumor fragments or surface clots embolizing to arteries in the brain, kidneys, and extremities.[52,53] Rarely, a complete left atrial myxoma becomes detached and lodges in the aortic bifurcation.[48,54] The size and consistency of such an embolus may defy the usual technique of removal (using a Fogarty catheter from below) and require direct exploration of the aortic bifurcation.[55] Histologic examination of emboli recovered at operation from a peripheral artery can aid in diagnosing an otherwise unsuspected intracardiac myxoma.[5,48,56,57] Systemic embolization, especially in a young patient with normal sinus rhythm, should arouse suspicion of a myxoma once bacterial endocarditis has been ruled out.

Tumor embolization of the *central nervous system* constitutes about one-half of all embolic events caused by left atrial myxomas, may represent the first symptomatic manifestation,[19] is more common in the left hemisphere, and may be multiple and massive.[58] Embolization may be to the extracranial or intracranial cerebral vessels, with the former being amenable to surgical removal. Onset of the neurologic deficit may be gradual or sudden. Episodes of syncope can be mistaken for seizure activity and thus may delay recognition of the true cardiac cause.[59]

Intracranial arterial aneurysms secondary to myxomatous emboli have been demonstrated angiographically. Late rupture with intracranial hemorrhage has been reported. Care must be taken to avoid embolization during surgical removal of an intracardiac myxoma, not only because of the immediate consequences of an embolic phenomenon but also because viable metastatic foci may cause symptoms years later. As a consequence, the patient who has sustained cerebral emboli is not necessarily "cured" even after the primary tumor is surgically removed.[59,60]

Retinal artery embolism can occur with transient[57] or permanent[61] visual impairment, confirmed by ophthalmoscopic[57] and histopathologic[61] evidence of particulate embolic matter in the retinal artery. Only rarely has occlusion of the retinal artery occurred in the absence of multifocal neurologic manifestations, usually in the distribution of the ipsilateral middle cerebral artery.

Coronary artery embolism associated with myxoma has been documented by both angiography in living patients and histology at postmortem study.[5,62] Myocardial infarction is occasionally the first manifestation of a myxoma.[62,63]

Left Atrial Myxoma

GENERAL FEATURES

Constitutional manifestations and embolic potential are common to varying degrees in patients with myxoma in any intracavitary location. The cardiac manifestations, symptoms, and physical findings are the consequence of the intracavitary mass and are unique to the particular location of the tumor. Myxomas of the left atrium may obstruct either the mitral or pulmonary venous orifices[64] and produce symptoms and manifestations of pulmonary venous hypertension, secondary pulmonary hypertension, and right-sided heart failure. The clinical symptoms include dyspnea on exertion, orthopnea, paroxysmal nocturnal dyspnea, acute pulmonary edema, cough, and hemoptysis, along with palpitations, chest pain, fatigue, and peripheral edema. Episodes of syncope or dizziness are frequent, and sudden death may occur. If a change in the patient's position has a marked effect on the severity of any symptom, especially if recumbency relieves dyspnea,[2,65] it is suggestive of myxoma, but this occurs infrequently.

PHYSICAL EXAMINATION

On physical examination, the first heart sound is loud and frequently split, with the second component corresponding to the tumor's expulsion from the mitral orifice. The pulmonary component of the second sound is accentuated, and an early diastolic sound, the "tumor plop," is usually heard 80 to 120 ms after the aortic closure sound,[2,66] resembling an opening snap but being less sharp and of lower frequency. The tumor plop may be confused with either an opening snap of the mitral valve or a third heart sound; it follows the aortic closure sound at an interval that is intermediate between these events. Suspicion of a left atrial myxoma should be raised when one hears what is considered to be an inordinately early "third heart sound" associated with auscultatory features suggestive of mitral regurgitation or an unusually late low-pitched "opening snap" accompanying features that are consistent with severe mitral stenosis (Fig. 86-2).

An apical diastolic or systolic murmur or both are present in many patients. The auscultatory findings may vary from time to time or with a change in the patient's position.[2,65–67] Features of pulmonary hypertension are frequent and may result in a murmur of tricuspid regurgitation.[68] A shorter

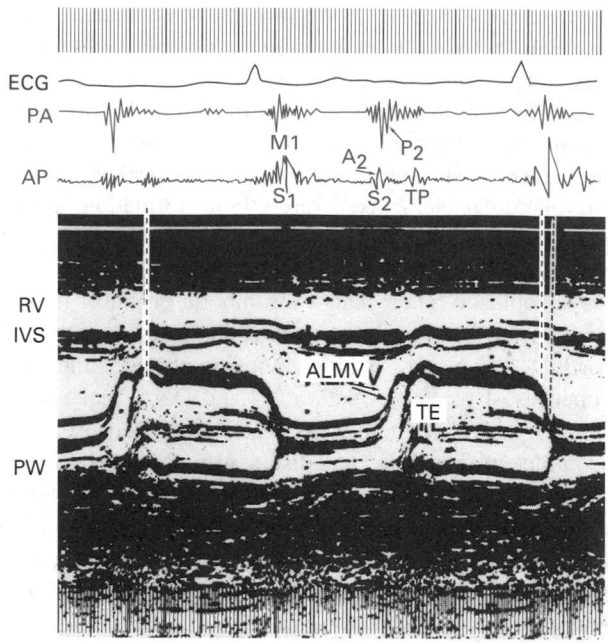

FIGURE 86-2
Recordings of a patient with a cystic left atrial myxoma including (*top*) the electrocardiogram, (*middle*) phonocardiograms from the pulmonary area (PA) at high frequency and from the apex (AP) at medium frequency, and (*bottom*) the echocardiogram at the level of the mitral valve. Time lines equal 0.01-s intervals. The right ventricle (RV), septum (IVS), and posterior wall (PW) of the left ventricle are identified. The loud component of the first sound (M_1) is delayed (Q to M_1 = 0.09 s). The pulmonic second sound (P_2) is accentuated. Multiple linear tumor echoes (TE) are seen behind the anterior leaflet to the mitral valve (ALMV), first appearing at the mitral level 0.04 s after onset of mitral opening and completing the forward movement 0.09 s after onset of mitral opening, at which point the "tumor plop" (TP) is recorded. The A_2–TP interval measures 0.010 s.

clinical history and the persistence of sinus rhythm are in contrast to features of rheumatic mitral valvular disease.

ELECTROCARDIOGRAM AND CHEST X-RAY

Results of the ECG are nonspecific, reflecting hemodynamic alterations similar to those of mitral valvular disease; however, sinus rhythm is generally the rule. The chest roentgenogram reveals left atrial enlargement and the characteristic changes of pulmonary venous congestion and pulmonary hypertension. The absence of mitral valve calcification and the presence of a smaller left atrium than might be expected in a patient with presumed severe rheumatic mitral disease are helpful clues. Calcification can be evident in the tumor even on a routine chest film,[69] but this is better visualized and motion is better appreciated on fluoroscopic examination.

The "wrecking-ball" effect of a calcified mobile myxoma may cause destruction of the mitral valve or rupture of the chordae tendineae and may produce severe mitral regurgitation.[65,70]

ECHOCARDIOGRAPHY

The value of ultrasound in the noninvasive diagnosis of intracavitary tumors has been well documented.[2,8,38] M-mode echocardiographic studies in patients with a prolapsing left atrial myxoma typically demonstrate a diminished EF slope of the anterior leaflet of the mitral valve, behind which a dense array of wavy tumor echoes is seen (see Chap. 14). These tumor echoes typically appear a short interval following the opening movement of the mitral leaflets, caused by the inertial lag in movement of the tumor after onset of diastole and opening of the mitral leaflets. The tumor plop coincides with the completion of this anterior movement of tumor echoes (Fig. 86-2). A similar array of tumor echoes may be seen in the left atrial chamber during ventricular systole. Transthoracic echocardiography (TTE) provides tomographic images of all four cardiac chambers and identifies the size, shape, point of attachment, and motion characteristics of left atrial myxomas.[3,38] Transesophageal echocardiography (TEE) permits superior imaging of the more posterior cardiac structures,[71] providing high-resolution views of both atria and the atrial septum.[72–74] Left atrial myxomas, especially their point of attachment, are better imaged by TEE (Figs. 86-3 and 86-4). (See also Chap. 14.) Visualization of all four chambers permits recognition of multiple tumors or tumors in less common locations. Doppler assessment of mitral valve and pulmonary vein flow patterns provides further information regarding the hemodynamic consequences of left atrial myxomas.[75,76]

GATED RADIONUCLIDE CARDIAC IMAGING

Gated radionuclide imaging of the isotopically tagged blood pool also has resulted in detection of left atrial myxomas.[77] This technique has also defined intracavitary tumors in other chambers[77,78] and biatrial tumors.[27]

OTHER IMAGING TECHNIQUES

Ultrafast computed tomography (CT) provides precise spatial localization of intracardiac masses[79] (Chap. 18). High resolution is similarly achieved by magnetic resonance imaging (MRI), which is demonstrating increased usefulness in the detection and characterization of intracardiac masses. The technique has been used to achieve excellent visualization of intracavitary atrial myxomas, providing information about the size, shape, attachment, and mobility of these tumors[80–82] (Chap. 19).

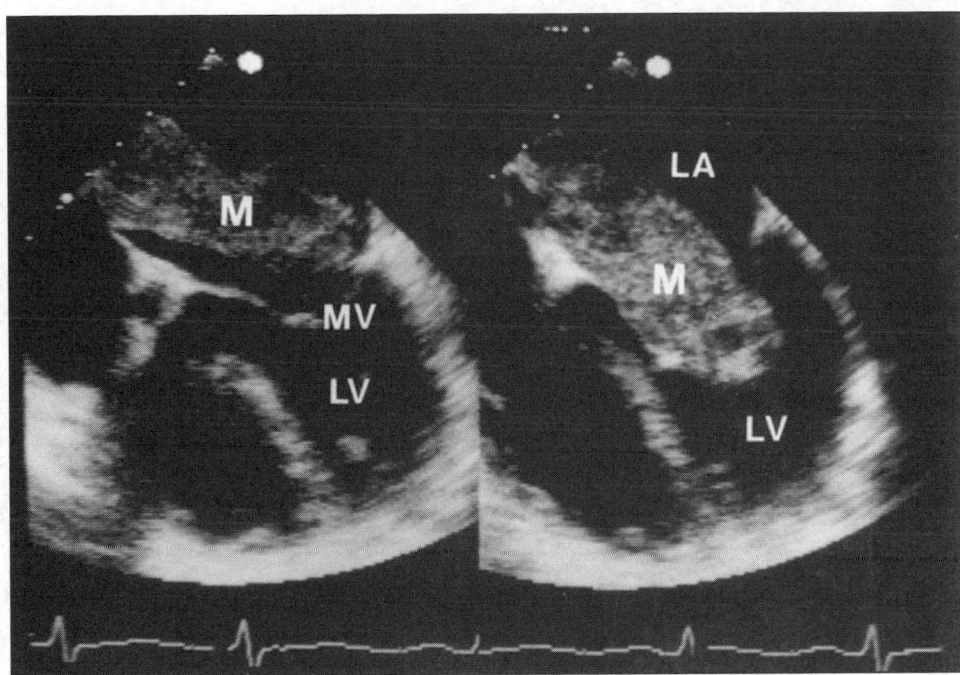

FIGURE 86-3

Transesophageal echocardiogram in the four-chamber view from a 50-year-old man who presented with exertional dyspnea and syncope. A large left atrial (LA) myxoma (M) attached to the interatrial septum is seen prolapsing across the mitral valve (MV) into the left ventricle (LV) in diastole (*right panel*). (Courtesy of Susan Wilansky, M.D., Medical Director, Noninvasive Imaging, St. Luke's Episcopal Hospital, Houston, Texas, and Bernardo Triestman, M.D.)

CATHETERIZATION

Cardiac catheterization invariably demonstrates significant pulmonary capillary wedge and pulmonary arterial hypertension.[2] A notch on the ascending limb of the left ventricular pressure curve results from expulsion of the myxoma from the left ventricle, which suddenly decreases left ventricular volume. When a large left atrial tumor or a left atrial ball thrombus obstructs the mitral orifice but does not prolapse into the left ventricular cavity, this notch is absent.[83] Similarly, a rapid *y* descent of the pulmonary wedge or left atrial pressure curve is the consequence of a sudden decrease of left atrial volume when the tumor prolapses into the left ventricle.[83] The notch, or "hold," on the rapid *y* descent appears to be caused by the slightly delayed tumor prolapse through the mitral orifice.[84] The large *v* wave, at times as high as 75 mmHg, even in the absence of significant mitral regurgitation, reflects the space-occupying effect of the tumor within the left atrium. When the clinical picture is that of mitral stenosis, these findings are highly suggestive of a space-filling defect in the atrium. Large left atrial myxomas that obstruct the mitral orifice without prolapsing into the left ventricle demonstrate a slow *y* descent.[83] Rarely, a left atrial myxoma is associated with a congenital atrial septal defect with an accompanying left-to-right shunt.[85]

ANGIOGRAPHY

Although angiography characterizes the size, location, and mobility of the tumor,[2] echocardiography and other imaging

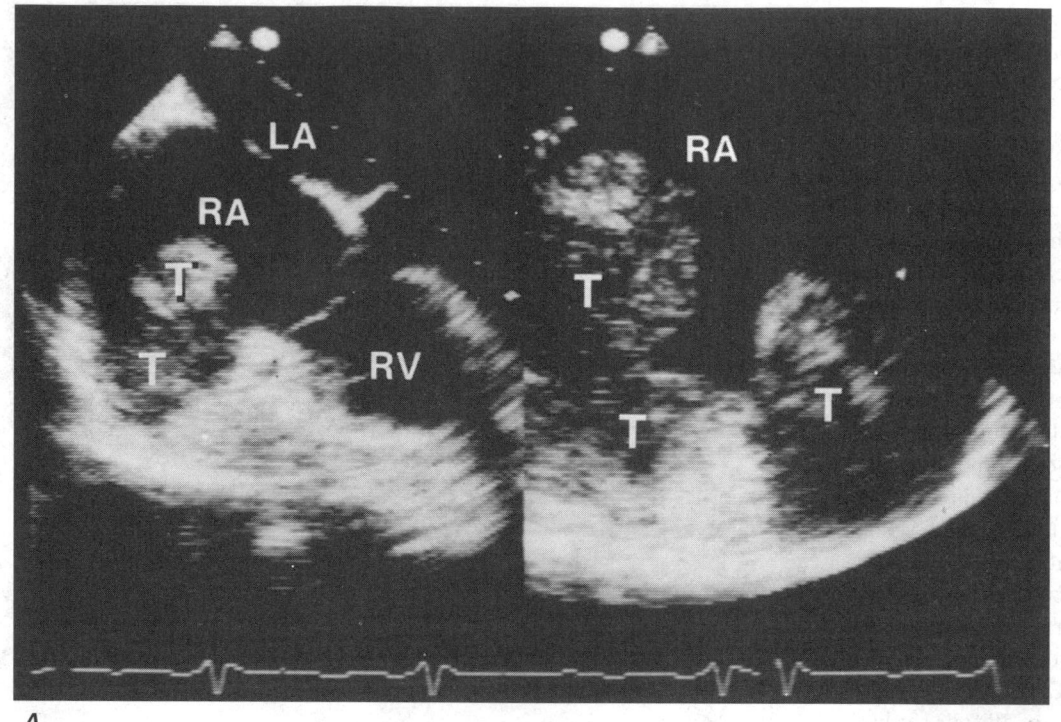

A

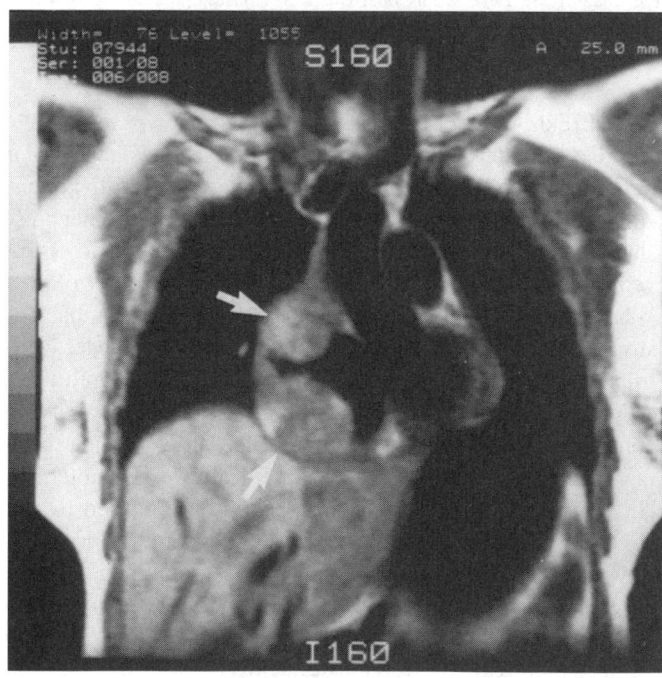

B

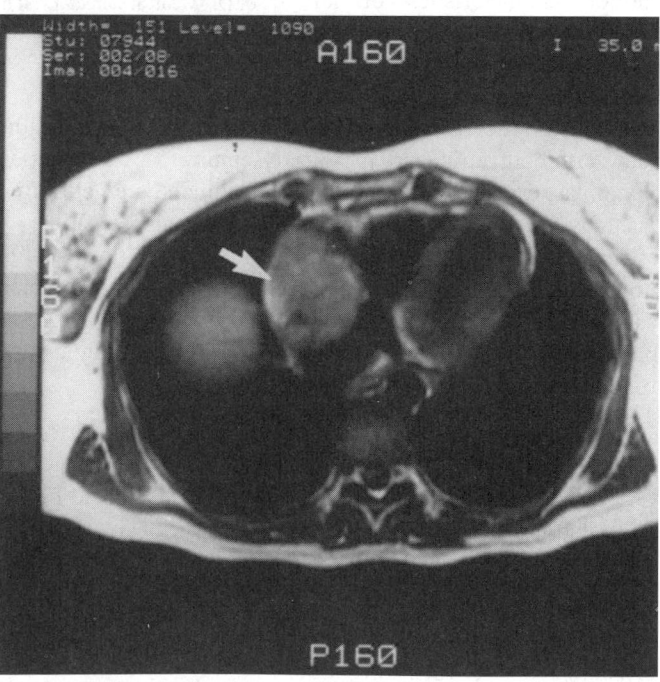

C

FIGURE 86-4

A. Biplane transesophageal echocardiogram from a 35-year-old woman who presented with shock of unknown cause. The horizontal plane seen on the left shows a tumor (T) in the right atrium (RA). The vertical plane on the right panel shows a large, bilobular tumor (T) adherent to the right atrial wall. Histology proved this to be an angiosarcoma. LA = left atrium; RV = right ventricle. (Courtesy of Susan Wilansky, M.D., Medical Director, Noninvasive Imaging, St. Luke's Episcopal Hospital, Houston, Texas.) *B* and *C.* Magnetic resonance images. Arrowheads denote a dumbbell-shaped, right atrial tumor of intermediate signal intensity, which is shown to abut the aorta in the coronal T1-weighted view, and the tricuspid valve in the axial T1-weighted view. Note the loss of the usual high-signal-intensity margin (fat) along the right lateral aspect of the aorta in the coronal plane. This raises concern for malignant invasion of the aortic wall. (Courtesy of Clark L. Carrol, M.D., St. Luke's Episcopal Hospital, Texas Children's Hospital, and Texas Heart Institute, Houston, Texas.)

techniques, because of their efficacy, have largely supplanted hemodynamic studies and contrast angiography and usually permit immediate operative intervention without additional invasive studies.[3,38,41] Catheter passage or contrast injection into the chamber containing the myxoma risks embolization of tumor fragments.[86] Injection of contrast medium into the pulmonary artery, with attention paid to the levo phase of the angiogram, is diagnostic in all patients except those with small tumors.

CORONARY ANGIOGRAPHY

Coronary angiography may demonstrate a vascular blush in the tumor from branches of both the right and/or left coronary arteries; both left and right atrial myxomas and a right ventricular myxoma have been demonstrated in this manner.[12,87,88] Neovascularization of a left atrial thrombus accompanying mitral stenosis may produce an appearance similar to that of tumor blush.[90] Aneurysms and occlusion of the coronary artery caused by tumor emboli have also been demonstrated by coronary angiography.[87] Cardiac catheterization and coronary angiography are indicated primarily for patients with additional heart disease and for those over 40 years of age to rule out concomitant coronary artery disease.[6,89]

DIFFERENTIAL DIAGNOSIS

Left atrial myxomas most often present as, and must be differentiated from, mitral valvular disease.[6] At our institution, intracavitary myxomas were discovered in approximately 1 per 100 patients presenting for mitral valve surgery.[2] Characteristically, the clinical course is relatively recent in origin, distinguishing myxoma from rheumatic mitral valvular disease; however, the course may occasionally span many years. Rarely, both conditions may coexist.[91] Fever, constitutional symptoms, and embolic phenomena mimic infective endocarditis[6]; on rare occasions the myxoma itself may be infected. Muscle pain, skin rash, and Raynaud's phenomenon may simulate peripheral vasculitis,[92] and myxomatous emboli may be found on muscle biopsy.[33] Multiple systemic arterial aneurysms secondary to myxomatous embolization to the cerebral, pulmonary, renal, and muscular arteries have mimicked polyarteritis nodosa.[28,45] Similarly, coronary ar-

tery aneurysmal dilatation and myocardial infarction have been attributed to coronary myxoma embolization.[62,87] The clinical picture has at times been suggestive of acute rheumatic fever[93] and acute myocarditis.[94] The correct diagnosis will most likely be made when the physician maintains a high index of clinical suspicion in patients with diverse and protean features, especially when cardiac, embolic, and constitutional manifestations coexist. Echocardiographic imaging of the heart has greatly facilitated the recognition of intracavitary tumors and results in detection in some patients who are asymptomatic.[46] Intracavitary thrombi may at times mimic intracardiac tumor masses (Fig. 86-5).[95]

Right Atrial Myxoma

Myxomas in the right atrial cavity constitute about one-fifth of all myxomas and tend to be more solid, have a wider attachment, and involve a greater amount of the atrial wall or septum than those in the left atrium. They originate from a variety of locations within the right atrium, including the inferior margin of the foramen ovale,[8,96] the tricuspid valve,[97] and the eustachean valve[98]; they characteristically produce tricuspid valve obstruction. A myxoma arising from the inferior vena cava has been reported.[11]

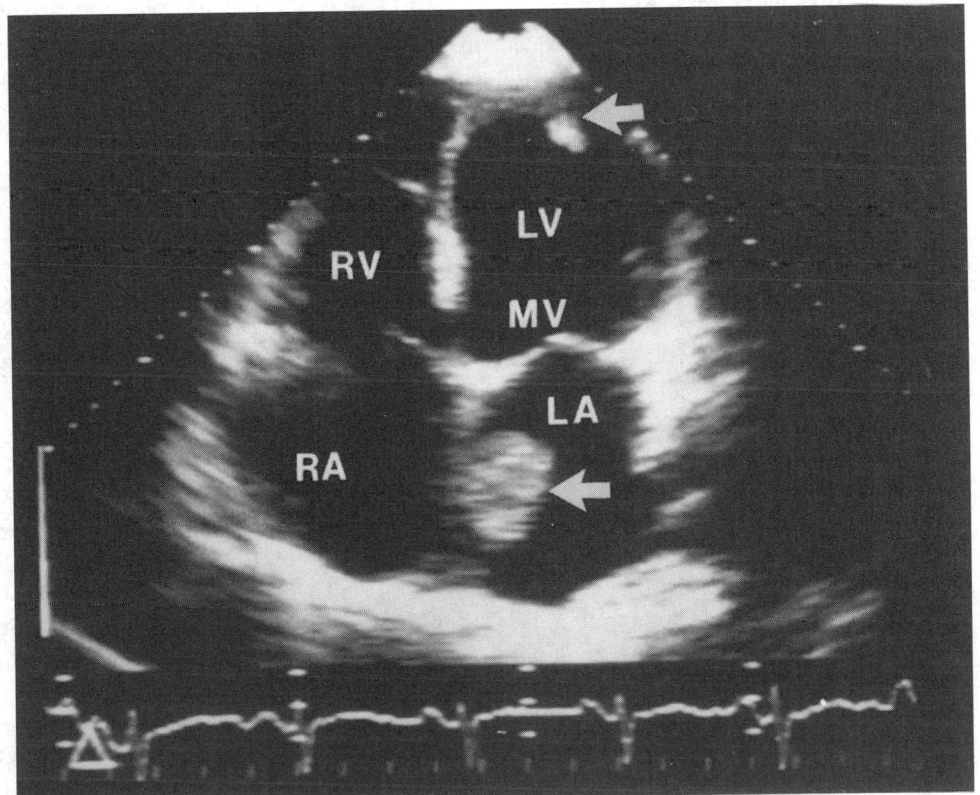

FIGURE 86-5

Two-dimensional echocardiogram, apical four-chamber view, of a patient with advanced congestive cardiomyopathy. Intracavitary masses (*arrows*), proved at autopsy to be thrombi, are present in the left atrium (LA) attached to the atrial septum (AS) and in the apex of the left ventricle (LV). The latter masses are both sessile and pedunculated. RA = right atrium; RV = right ventricle; MV = mitral valve. (Courtesy of Carlos de Castro, Department of Cardiology, St. Luke's Episcopal Hospital, Houston, Texas.)

CLINICAL MANIFESTATIONS

Clinically, symptoms of low cardiac output and manifestations of systemic venous hypertension are present with a prominent jugular venous *a* wave, hepatomegaly, ascites, edema, and cyanosis,[78] which may be episodic and may vary with the patient's position. Persistence of normal sinus rhythm is common; however, sinus rhythm is also frequent in patients with rheumatic tricuspid stenosis. Intermittent episodes of syncope and abrupt onset of dyspnea, features never seen with rheumatic tricuspid stenosis,[65] are reported in one-third of these patients.[77] The pendular action of a prolapsing right atrial myxoma ("wrecking-ball" effect),[99] especially when it is calcified, may damage or destroy the tricuspid valve and produce severe tricuspid regurgitation.[65]

PULMONARY EMBOLI

Whereas embolic tumor phenomena are reputed to occur less frequently with right than left atrial myxomas, pulmonary emboli have been reported.[96] They are sometimes extensive[99] and may produce irreversible pulmonary hypertension.[100,101] Wide dissemination of myxomatous embolization to the pulmonary arteries has been reported with active infiltration of the media[23] and formation of aneurysms.[28] Paradoxical embolization may occur if an interatrial communication exists.[50]

SYSTEMIC MANIFESTATIONS

Constitutional symptoms are less frequent in patients with a right atrial myxoma.[102] Anemia, polycythemia,[102,103] and cyanosis have been reported. Polycythemia and cyanosis may be caused by either right-to-left shunting through a patent foramen ovale or atrial septal defect,[50,104] low cardiac output and hypoxemic stimulation of the bone marrow, intravascular hemoconcentration,[103] or erythropoietin production by the tumor.[41] Mesenteric vasculitis of a nonembolic, probably autoimmune origin has been reported.[105]

AUSCULTATION

On auscultation, a loud early systolic sound may be heard. This sound occurs as late as 80 ms after the mitral component of the first sound and results from expulsion of the tumor from the right ventricle. A palpable tumor shock may coincide with this loud sound.[106] A crescendo murmur with inspiratory augmentation preceding this loud tumor expulsion sound is probably caused by early systolic tricuspid regurgitation while the valve is still held open by the tumor.[106] There may be a long diastolic murmur or, more commonly, only a late diastolic rumble, augmented by inspiration, accompanying atrial systole. If major injury to the tricuspid valve occurs, the murmur of tricuspid regurgitation will be present, and large *v* waves will be seen in the jugular venous pulse. An early diastolic sound may be heard but is less constant than the tumor plop due to a left atrial myxoma. The changing quality of the sound and murmurs, their closeness to the ear, and their friction-like quality may mimic a pericardial rub.[102] Such sounds have been said to be an endocardial friction rub (see also Chap. 10).

ELECTROCARDIOGRAM AND CHEST X-RAY

The results of the ECG are often normal, but right atrial enlargement is frequently suggested.[96] Low-voltage, right-axis deviation and varying degrees of right bundle branch block have been reported.[77] The chest roentgenogram may reveal some prominence or enlargement of the right atrial shadow and, occasionally, of the right ventricle. An important radiologic feature is the mild or moderate degree of cardiomegaly, considering the severe clinical state of the patients.[104] Calcification in the tumor may be recognized on plane film or at fluoroscopy and is more common in patients with myxomas in the right atrium.[2]

ECHOCARDIOGRAPHY

TTE and TEE provide excellent images of the right atrium.[33,71,107,108] The latter provides more detail of the tumor and defines the site of attachment with greater clarity[109–111] (see Chap. 14). A large, prolapsing atrial septal aneurysm may mimic a right atrial tumor.[112]

CATHETERIZATION AND ANGIOGRAPHY

Cardiac catheterization demonstrates elevated right atrial pressure, prominence of the *a* wave, and a diastolic gradient between the right atrium and right ventricle. Notching of the upstroke of the right ventricular pressure curve has been noted[96] and is similar to that seen in the left ventricle in patients with prolapsing left atrial myxomas. Similarly, a collapsing *y* descent has been described in the right atrium with marked inspiratory augmentation.[96] With current noninvasive imaging techniques, catheterization and angiography of the right-sided heart chambers are rarely necessary and risk embolization of tumor fragments to the pulmonary arteries.

DIFFERENTIAL DIAGNOSIS

The clinical features of right atrial myxoma resemble those of rheumatic tricuspid valvular disease, although the latter is usually accompanied by significant mitral and, frequently, aortic valve disease. There are many similarities to the manifestations of constrictive pericarditis and Ebstein's anomaly of the tricuspid valve. Episodic dyspnea, sudden syncope, and variability of symptoms and findings with position of the patient may be useful clues. Changing murmurs, along with fever and anemia, may suggest infective endocarditis. Tricuspid stenosis and regurgitation are prominent in patients with carcinoid syndrome, but involvement of the pulmonary valve and other features of a carcinoid tumor will usually distinguish it from a right atrial myxoma. Obstruction of the right ventricular outflow tract may be the dominant finding in some examples of familial obstructive myopathy and may resemble a right atrial tumor. Pulmonary embolization of other diverse etiologies, with secondary thromboembolic pulmonary hypertension and right-sided heart failure, may be mimicked by right atrial myxoma. An awareness of the protean manifestations, along with evidence from echocardiographic imaging, usually facilitates a correct diagnosis.

Bilateral Atrial Myxoma

An atrial myxoma may pass through the foramen ovale and be present in both atria. The tumor is usually shaped like a dumbbell, with the common stalk attached to the margin of the fossa ovalis. Among the cases reported, surgery was successful most often when the correct diagnosis was made preoperatively, emphasizing the importance of echocardiographic exploration of all chambers.[27] Similar echocardiographic findings have been reported in patients with discrete tumors in each atrium.[111] Multichambered cardiac myxomas occasionally involve chambers other than the usual biatrial combination and are more frequent in familial occurrences.[50]

Left Ventricular Myxoma

A myxoma originates from the left ventricle in 2.5 to 4 percent of reported myxomas.[5,113] Recorded cases are found in the younger age groups, with most patients being under age 30. Women are affected three times more often than are men, and a short duration of symptoms is also characteristic. Systemic emboli, mostly cerebral, occur in two-thirds of the patients, and constitutional symptoms are almost conspicuously absent. Emboli from left ventricular tumors may mimic multiple sclerosis.[114] Attacks of syncope occur in nearly half of the reviewed cases. Symptoms and physical findings are suggestive of aortic or subaortic obstruction. The location and movement of the tumor mass are demonstrated particularly well by TTE and TEE[115] (see Chap. 14). Echoes from an intracavitary left ventricular myxoma must be differentiated from left ventricular thrombi, which are usually apical but occasionally are pedunculated, and from ventricular septal rhabdomyomas. Left and right ventricular myxomas have been identified by MRI, which complements two-dimensional (2D) echocardiographic findings and is of higher resolution than cardiac angiography[116] (see Chap. 19). Planning for surgical excision can be based upon noninvasive imaging without resorting to cardiac catheterization unless coexistent cardiac disease is suspected.[115,116]

Right Ventricular Myxoma

Myxomas of the right ventricle are as infrequent as those occurring in the left ventricle. The patient will have symptoms and manifestations of right-sided heart failure, syncope, unexplained fever, and a murmur consistent with pulmonary stenosis. An "ejection sound" has been reported, as well as delayed closure of the pulmonary valve. A right-sided tumor plop may be heard in diastole.[117] Calcium in the tumor may be recognized on the roentgenogram. A gradient across the right ventricular outlet is characteristic,[117] and the tumor can be visualized angiographically. Pulmonary emboli may occur.[118] Echocardiographic imaging, both TTE and TEE, will detect most right ventricular myxomas.[112,119] Transvenous intracardiac biopsy may be helpful in the differential diagnosis.[120] A right ventricular myxoma has been diagnosed in a neonate and has been successfully removed surgically.[31] Other tumors, producing similar outflow tract obstruction, rarely occur within the right ventricle.[121]

Surgery for Intracavitary Myxoma

Surgical resection of a myxoma is the only acceptable therapy and, in view of the dangers of embolization and sudden death, should be performed promptly.[122] For complete removal of left atrial myxoma, we use a biatrial approach, excising a full thickness of interatrial septum if the tumor is attached to the region of the fossa ovalis (Fig. 86-6).[123,124] Right atrial myxomas are commonly attached to the fossa ovalis, and with right-sided tumors, a full thickness of atrial septum should also be resected. If a large portion of the septum is removed, a patch of knitted Dacron cloth should be used for repair to avoid distortion, arrhythmia, or possible atrial septal defect. Since fragmentation and embolization of the tumor is an ever-present threat, vigorous palpation and other manipulations of the heart should be avoided until cardiopulmonary bypass is initiated.[25] We usually induce ventricular standstill with cardioplegia solution before manipulating the heart to reduce the possibility of fragmentation of the gelatinous tumor. Left atrial myxomas have been removed successfully during pregnancy, utilizing cardiopulmonary bypass, with subsequent uncomplicated completion of a full-term pregnancy.[125,126] Surgical removal of a right ventricular myxoma in a neonate has been reported.[31]

By its movement within the heart, the tumor may traumatize either AV valve, which may require replacement or repair by annuloplasty.[2] Arrhythmias and conduction disturbances may follow surgical removal of left atrial myxomas.[127] Recurrences of atrial myxomas are rare and usually occur within a 48-month period.[24]

OTHER BENIGN PRIMARY CARDIAC TUMORS

Rhabdomyoma

The most frequent cardiac tumor in infants and children[5,128,129] is a rhabdomyoma, which is probably a hamartoma rather than a true neoplasm.[130] These tumors are usually multiple, most often involve the ventricular myocardium, and project into the cavity or move freely as a pedunculated mass.[128,131,132] Associated tuberous sclerosis is present in one-third of the patients.[133] Presenting manifestations may be caused by cardiac obstructive phenomena, arrhythmias, AV block, pericardial effusion, sudden death,[131,134,135] and ventricular preexcitation.[136] These tumors can mimic pulmonary stenosis and produce hypoxic spells like those seen with tetralogy of Fallot.[128] Ventricular outflow gradients,[137] angiographic abnormalities, echocardiography,[128,132,138,139] and MRI[140] can lead to demonstration of the tumor and successful surgical resection or heart transplantation.[141] Multiplicity of tumors does not contraindicate surgery, as these tumors appear to have little capacity for further growth. Pedunculated rhab-

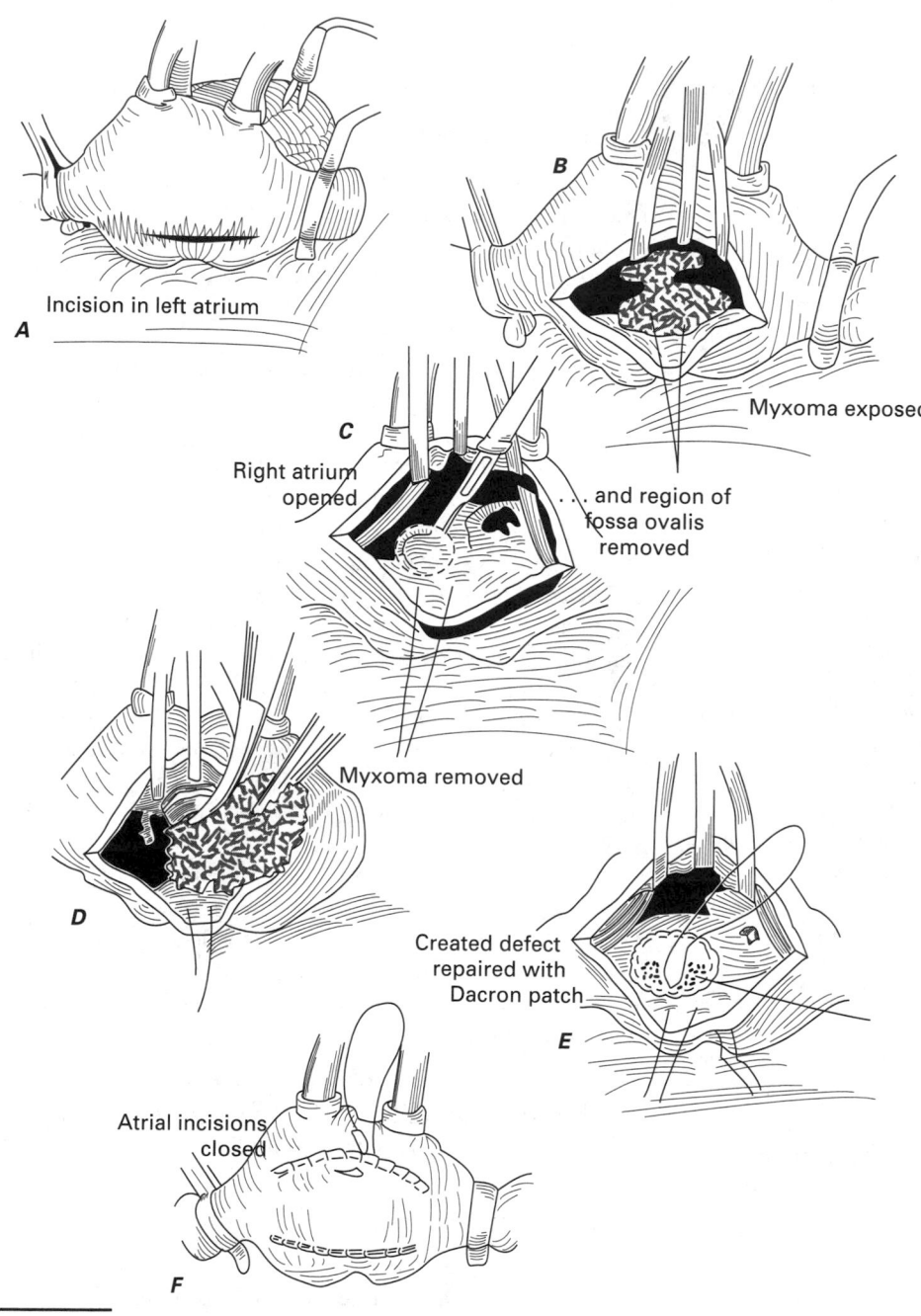

A — Incision in left atrium

B — Myxoma exposed

C — Right atrium opened ... and region of fossa ovalis removed

D — Myxoma removed

E — Created defect repaired with Dacron patch

F — Atrial incisions closed

FIGURE 86-6

Drawing illustrating resection of a typical left atrial myxoma with a broad attachment to the interatrial septum near the fossa ovalis. The ascending aorta is cross-clamped and the left atrium is opened near the interatrial groove (*A*). After the pedicle of the tumor is located (*B*), a separate incision is made in the right atrium (*C*). The interatrial septum is opened near the fossa ovalis, and a portion of the interatrial septum is excised. The tumor is removed through the left atriotomy (*D*). The resultant atrial defect is closed with a knitted Dacron patch (*E*). The atrial chambers and atrioventricular valve areas should be thoroughly inspected for additional tumor implants or fragments before the atriotomy incisions are closed (*F*). (From Cooley DA. *Techniques in Cardiac Surgery,* 2d ed. Philadelphia: Saunders; 1984:324. Reproduced with permission from the publisher and author.)

most frequent tumor found at fetal echocardiography, comprising 17 of 19 fetal tumors found in 14,000 fetal echocardiograms.[145]

Fibroma

Fibromas are usually ventricular and intramural. Although reported cases have occurred in the age range from newborn to 65 years, most occur in infants and children.[146] Calcification is common. Sudden death has been reported in nearly one-third of the patients, presumably due to involvement of the conduction system, production of arrhythmias, or obstruction of the outflow tract of the left ventricle.[147,148] 2D echocardiography accurately delineates intramural ventricular tumors.[149] Left axis deviation may occur as an interesting ECG feature. Total or partial resection of the tumor to relieve obstruction has been reported, with excellent probability of long-term survival.[123,148] Cardiac transplantation has been used in the management of a young adult with a nonresectable (1030-g) left ventricular fibroma.[150]

Papillary Fibroelastoma

Also referred to as *papillomas* or *papillary fibromas,* papillary fibroelastomas arise from the cardiac valves[151] or occasionally from the ventricular endocardium, are most commonly seen in patients over 50 years of age, and have been, in the past, seen only as a coincidental finding at surgery or postmortem examination. Grossly, these tumors resemble a sea anemone, with multiple papillary fronds attached to the endothelium by a short pedicle. There is a predilection for involvement of the aortic valve,[16,152] where angina, infarction, or sudden death may result from coronary embolization or ostial occlusion caused by the villous tumor.[5,16,153,154] Cerebral and ocular emboli from these lesions are being reported with increasing frequency.[151,155] Origin on right-sided cardiac valves is rare.[156]

domyomas that arise from the left atrium and cause mitral stenosis have been reported.[134] Discrete and multiple myocardial hamartomas and rhabdomyomas have caused incessant ventricular tachycardia in infants and have been successfully removed surgically.[123,124,142–144] Rhabdomyomas are the

Obstruction of the right ventricular outflow tract has been reported in a patient with a papillary tumor of the tricuspid valve.[157] The tumor is histologically different from Lambl's excrescences, which are degenerative in origin and usually situated on the ventricular aspect of the semilunar valve along the line of closure.[5,158,159] Papillary fibroelastomas are being discovered with increasing frequency by echocardiographic (TTE and TEE) imaging of the heart, and because of their potential for cerebral and coronary embolization, surgical excision is recommended for even small papillary fibroelastomas.[151,152,154,155,160] Papillary fibroelastomas may mimic vegetations and bacterial endocarditis.[161]

Lipoma

Lipomas may occur throughout the heart, including the pericardium. They may be massive; the largest reported cardiac tumor was an intrapericardial lipoma.[162] Intrapericardial lipomas may cause pericardial effusion, be mistaken for a pericardial cyst, or present as asymptomatic cardiac or mediastinal enlargement.[163] Intramyocardial lipomas are encapsulated and usually are small.[5] An occasional lipoma arising from the mitral or tricuspid valve may resemble an atrial myxoma on echocardiographic examination[164] and must also be differentiated from a cyst[15,103,165] or lymphangioma of the mitral valve.[102] Surgical excision of lipomas yields excellent long-term results.[123] Tissue characterization by MRI permits preoperative identification of these fatty tumors.[166]

Lipomatous hypertrophy of the atrial septum is a nonencapsulated hyperplasia of adipose tissue and may not represent a true tumor. Varying in size from 2 to 8 cm, the tumescence may bulge into the atrial cavity or superior vena cava orifice[167] and become a consideration in the differential diagnosis of intracavitary masses.[168,169] Although at times found coincidentally at postmortem study, lipomatous hypertrophy of the atrial septum can be associated with unexplained supraventricular rhythm and conduction disturbances,[170] recurrent pericardial effusion,[171] and sudden death.[5,7,172] This association has been considered fortuitous by some observers. Features of both TTE, especially from the subcostal approach, and TEE[168] are distinctive and include atrial septal thickening with a bilobed appearance due to sparing of the area of the fossa ovalis. MRI provides noninvasive tissue characterization of lipomas that echocardiography does not provide.[173] The diagnosis may be confirmed by percutaneous transvenous biopsy.[174]

Mesothelioma of the Atrioventricular Node

The smallest tumor capable of producing sudden death by causing complete heart block or ventricular fibrillation is mesothelioma of the AV node.[5,175] Patients have presented at times ranging from the newborn period to the ninth decade of life; there is a strong female preponderance. The exact origin of these cystic tumors has been disputed, but they likely arise from arrests in development[175,176]; also, other terms have been applied to them, such as *lymphangioepithelioma*[175]

and *congenital polycystic tumor of the AV node*.[177] Aside from chance intraoperative finding of this tumor,[178] in vivo recognition has not been reported, although the cystic structure may exceed 3 cm in size. The tumor is usually large enough to be recognized grossly at postmortem examination and, despite its rare occurrence, should be suspected in all cases of sudden death without apparent cause, especially in children and young adults.[5,179] Most patients with mesothelioma of the AV node have demonstrated symptomatic complete heart block. Even with complete heart block, a narrow QRS is common, and these patients may pursue a stable course for years. Electrophysiologic study discloses a block proximal to the His bundle.[179] Electronic pacing should aid in maintaining an adequate cardiac rate, but examples of electrical instability and sudden death reflect a special hazard in these patients, even during diagnostic electrophysiological studies and after initiation of effective ventricular pacing.[5,177]

Vasoformative Tumors

Hemangiomas are rare cardiac tumors usually discovered at postmortem study. Coronary angiography yields a characteristic tumor blush.[180,181] Spontaneous resolution without treatment of a large cavernous hemangioma of the right ventricle has been reported.[182] Lymphangiomas and vascular hamartomas are rare primary tumors of the heart that usually present as diffuse proliferations rather than as distinct tumors. Therefore, total excision is often not practical.[183] Cardiac transplantation may be considered as an alternative in these cases.

OTHER BENIGN TUMORS

The right side of the ventricular septum is rarely the site of congenital benign thyroid rest. Enlargement results in right ventricular outflow obstruction. Complete resection is indicated, and the condition is curable.[184] Rarely, benign teratomas occur in the ventricular myocardium and may result in sudden death.[185]

Intrapericardial Paraganglioma

Paragangliomas (pheochromocytoma, chemodectomas) may rarely be localized within the pericardium. Although these tumors may be found overlying or within any cardiac chamber, they most commonly occur over the base of the heart in the major region of vagus nerve distribution.[186] Improved detection and localization to the mediastinum have been provided by iodine-131 metaiodobenzylguanidine (^{131}I-MIBG) nuclear scanning. Magnetic resonance imaging can further localize cardiac paragangliomas without the need for contrast material and provide detailed information for guidance of surgical excision.[187] Although definitive diagnosis can only be made histologically, benign pathologic characteristics do not necessarily predict a favorable outcome. As these tumors are highly vascular, adherent, and difficult to resect, management with cardiac transplantation may be necessary.[188] Human cardiac explantation and autotransplantation have also been applied to a patient with a large cardiac pheochromocytoma.[189]

MALIGNANT PRIMARY TUMORS OF THE HEART

Angiosarcoma (Hemangiosarcoma)

Almost all primary malignant tumors are sarcomas,[190] most frequently angiosarcomas, and they usually originate in the right atrium or pericardium.[120] Intense vascularity may produce a continuous murmur.[191,192] One-fourth of all angiosarcomas will be partly intracavitary with valvular obstruction and characteristically will manifest right-sided heart failure and pericardial tamponade with hemorrhagic fluid. Cardiac rupture due to a right atrial angiosarcoma has been reported.[193] Atrial angiosarcomas exhibit highly variable histologic patterns, which may overlap those of Kaposi's sarcoma.[194] Echocardiography (Fig. 86-4A), angiography, CT, or MRI is helpful in the diagnosis.[195] Coronary angiography may demonstrate angiomatous vessels in the tumor area. The course is rapid, and widespread metastases often make surgery impractical, although tumor excision, radiation, and chemotherapy may offer some relief of symptoms and palliation.[5,124,191,194,195] An iatrogenic hemangiopericytoma of the right ventricle has been reported following intense radiotherapy to the cardiac area.[196]

Rhabdomyosarcoma

Rhabdomyosarcoma is the second most frequent primary sarcoma of the heart and, like angiosarcoma, is prevalent in males. There is no single chamber predilection; multiple sites are common, and significant obstruction of at least one valve is present in half of the patients.[197] Excision of the main tumor mass combined with radiation and chemotherapy has been advocated as the treatment for patients with primary malignant tumor of the heart, but in general the prognosis is poor and survival is short.[5,198–200]

Other Malignant Primary Tumors

Fibrosarcoma,[201] liposarcoma,[202] primary malignant lymphoma,[203,204] and occasional sarcomas of other basic cell types constitute the remaining but infrequent primary malignant cardiac tumors.[5] The fibrous histiocytoma (Fig. 86-4) has a predilection for the left atrium[205–207] and has infrequently occurred adjacent to Dacron vascular grafts and to a mitral prosthetic valve, suggesting a possible mild carcinogenic effect of these materials.[208] This tumor rarely involves right-sided cardiac chambers.[209]

Malignant primary cardiac tumors may obstruct cardiac chambers or valves[210–213] or result in peripheral embolic phenomena.

SURGERY FOR CARDIAC TUMORS

Effective palliation and local control of the disease can be achieved with extensive resection of malignant primary tumors.[124,214–216] Echocardiography (Chap. 14), MRI (Chap. 19), CT (Chap. 18), and ultrafast CT[79] are all helpful in planning operative resection of cardiac tumors, because these tests provide three-dimensional information (Fig. 86-4B and C).[82,217] Intraoperative echocardiography may be useful to guide surgical resection.[218] Adjuvant chemotherapy and radiation therapy are necessary to improve long-term prognosis,[219] and the response to therapy can be assessed by MRI.[220] Cardiac transplantation has been utilized to completely resect an "inoperable" benign tumor and an unresectable malignant primary cardiac neoplasm.[214,221,222] Cardiac explantation and autotransplantation may facilitate resection of some cardiac tumors[189] (see also Chap. 25).

TUMORS OF THE PERICARDIUM

Pericardial Cysts

Pericardial or mesothelial cysts are the most frequent benign "tumors" of the pericardium. They are usually found coincidentally on routine radiographic examination of the chest; however, 25 to 30 percent of the patients will have chest pain, dyspnea, cough, or paroxysmal tachycardia. Pericardial cysts occur most frequently in the third or fourth decade of life and are found equally among men and women.[223] The right costophrenic location is the most common, although these cysts may present in the upper mediastinum.[224] Only rarely will the cyst connect with the pericardial cavity. Clinically and radiographically, they resemble other tumors of the pericardium, such as hemangioma, lymphangioma, or lipoma, as well as retrosternal hernia, a pericardial fat pad, and eventration of the diaphragm. Echocardiography[71,225] and CT[224] are most helpful in the differential diagnosis. Surgical excision completely relieves symptoms and confirms the diagnosis[5,16]; however, percutaneous aspiration of the cystic contents is an attractive alternative to surgical resection.[224]

Teratoma

Most teratomas are extracardiac yet intrapericardial and arise and receive their blood supply from the root of the aorta or pulmonary artery through the vasa vasorum. Most are found in infants and children, with a strong female preponderance.[5] One case has been diagnosed in utero by aid of fetal echocardiography.[226] Recurrent, nonbloody pericardial effusion is common in children with this tumor; intrapericardial teratoma is the most likely diagnosis in this setting.[227] Cardiac dysfunction results from expansion of the tumor to considerable proportions, at times up to a diameter of 15 cm. Surgical excision is the only effective therapy[228] and is curative, since the tumor is rarely malignant.[228] In fact, the first successful operation for any type of cardiac tumor was done in 1938, when Beck removed an intrapericardial teratoma.[227] It is rare for a teratoma to be intracardiac and arise from the interventricular septum, but this type of tumor can be successfully excised.[229,230]

Mesothelioma

Mesothelioma ranks third in frequency among malignant tumors of the heart and pericardium.[7,231,232] The clinical manifestations resemble those of pericarditis, constrictive pericardial disease, and vena caval obstruction. Aspiration and histologic examination of the usually bloody pericardial fluid may be diagnostic. Among those affected, males outnumber females by a ratio of 2:1, with the peak incidence occurring in the third to fifth decades. The prognosis is poor, surgical excision is usually impossible, and treatment with radiation and chemotherapy generally produces only temporary improvement. Rarely, the pericardium is the site of a primary sarcoma.[233]

Primary Tumors of the Aorta

Primary tumors of the aorta are rare. Occasionally, they are benign, but most frequently they are malignant sarcomas. Presentation may mimic aortic dissection, coarctation, atherosclerotic occlusive disease, and malignancies in other organs. All portions of the aorta may be involved, and distal metastases are common. Surgical extirpation will relieve the obstructive phenomena, but distant metastases usually lead to disease progression.[234,235]

SECONDARY TUMORS OF THE HEART

General Considerations

Metastatic tumors from a primary origin in some other organ involve the heart, pericardium, or both 20 to 40 times more frequently than primary tumors of the heart.[236,237] These secondary tumors are more frequently carcinomas than sarcomas. Cardiac metastases occur most often in people above 50 years of age; the incidence is equal in both sexes. The development of otherwise unexplained cardiac symptoms or manifestations, cardiac enlargement, tachycardia, arrhythmias, or heart failure in the presence of neoplastic disease is suggestive of cardiac metastases.

Frequency and Origin of Secondary Tumors

In a report by the Harvard Cancer Commission of 4375 autopsies of patients who died of cancer, myocardial metastases were present in 146 patients (3.4 percent).[236] In a series of 2547 consecutive autopsies performed at Walter Reed General Hospital, 980 cases of malignant disease were observed. The heart was the site of metastatic tumor in 5.7 percent of the

cases and the heart, including the pericardium, in 13.9 percent.[237] In other series, cardiac metastases have been present in patients with malignant tumors in a range as wide as 1.5 to 21 percent.[238] An increased prevalence of secondary cardiac neoplasms in recent years may be related to more vigorous surgical and radiation treatment of patients with primary neoplasms.[239] The relative infrequency of cardiac metastases has been attributed to the strong kneading action of the heart, the metabolic peculiarities of striated muscle, rapid coronary blood flow, and lymphatic connections that drain afferently from the heart.[236]

Cardiac metastases occur with all types of primary tumors: carcinomas, sarcomas, leukemia, lymphomas,[240] Kaposi's sarcoma, and so on. No malignant tumor tends particularly to metastasize to the heart with the possible exception of malignant melanoma, which involves the myocardium in more than 50 percent of cases.[241] Cardiac metastases are most frequent, with bronchogenic carcinoma[242] and carcinoma of the breast occurring in one-third of the cases. Cardiac infiltration, often macroscopic, is seen in one-half the cases of leukemia and in one-sixth the cases of lymphoma.

Cardiac metastases are encountered with widespread systemic tumor dissemination; only rarely is metastatic tumor limited to the heart or pericardium. Carcinomatous metastases are generally grossly visible, multiple, discrete, small, white, firm nodules; microscopically, they resemble the primary tumor and the metastases in other organs. Diffuse infiltration is characteristic of sarcomatous metastases.

Metastatic tumors are classically thought to reach the heart by embolic hematogenous spread, lymphatic spread, or direct invasion, in descending order of frequency. Cardiac lymphatics are considered to be an important pathway of tumor metastases to the heart; lymphatic obstruction by tumor results in myocardial interstitial edema, and the secondary pressure on the myofibers may contribute to the eventual cardiac decompensation,[243] particularly in a patient with underlying atherosclerotic coronary heart disease. Lymphatic spread of tumors is particularly frequent with carcinoma of the bronchus and the breast; the proximity of the heart to major mediastinal lymphatic channels seems to explain the high incidence of cardiac metastases from mediastinal tumors.[238]

Manifestations

Secondary tumor involvement of the heart may be recognized as a pathologic finding without clinical manifestations. More often, however, such involvement is symptomatic; on rare occasions, it may be the first or only expression of a remote primary tumor. Recognition of neoplastic heart disease is dependent on the physician's awareness of the probability of its occurrence and diverse manners of presentation. At times, as with rapidly developing tamponade, recognition and appropriate therapy must be undertaken promptly. Secondary tumors of the heart may involve the pericardium, myocardium, endocardium, valves, and coronary arteries. Direct invasion of the heart through the venae cavae[244] or pulmonary veins[245]

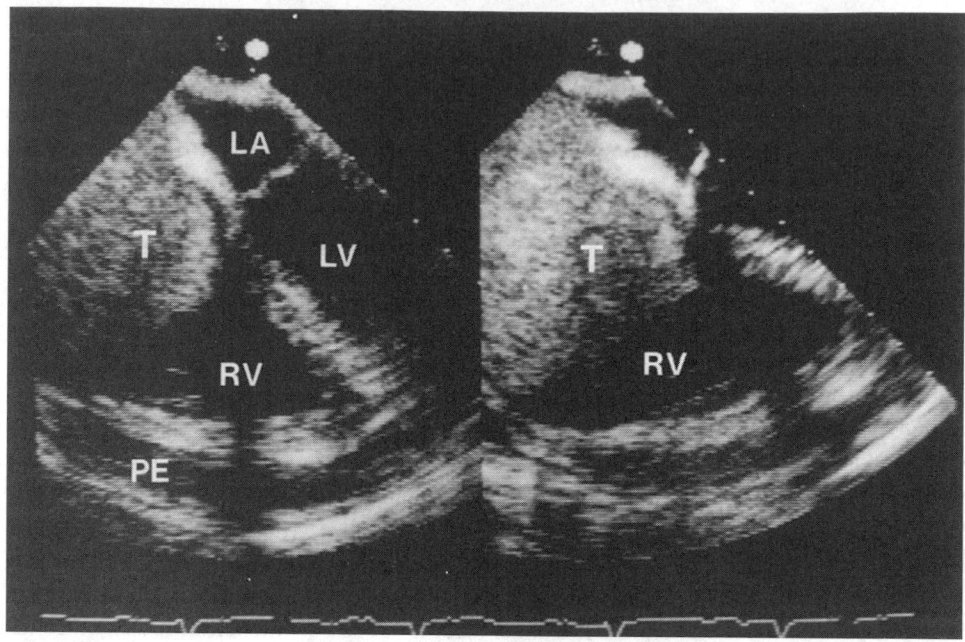

FIGURE 86-7

Transesophageal echocardiogram in a 55-year-old woman who presented with adenocarcinoma of the lung and obstructed superior vena cava syndrome. A large tumor (T) is seen in the right ventricle (RV) in systole (*left panel*) and diastole (*right panel*). Subsequent images revealed that it originated from an obstructed superior vena cava. The echo-free space anterior to the right ventricle represented pericardial effusion (PE). LA = left atrium; LV = left ventricle. (Courtesy of Susan Wilansky, M.D., Medical Director, Noninvasive Imaging, St. Luke's Episcopal Hospital, Houston, Texas.)

or through an expanding myocardial implant can produce an intracavitary tumor mass and result in obstruction to flow or cause valvular obstruction. Depending on the character and location of the cardiac lesion, a variety of manifestations may serve to identify cardiac involvement, especially in a patient with a known malignancy.

Pericardial Involvement

Pericardial involvement is often first manifest by chest pain—aggravated by inspiration—and a pericardial friction rub. Accumulation of fluid within the pericardium, often but not always bloody, may result in progressive cardiac enlargement on roentgenogram, with symptoms and signs of cardiac tamponade, and may be the first manifestation of a cardiac malignancy[246] (see also Chap. 81). Clinically, the jugular venous pressure is increased, the arterial pressure is reduced, and "pulsus paradoxus" may be present. Reduced ECG QRS voltage can be expected. Electrical alternation, which is generally seen in patients with large effusions and serious tamponade,[247] may indicate the need for prompt pericardiocentesis. The echocardiogram demonstrates pericardial fluid and may demonstrate features of hemodynamic tamponade, diastolic collapse of the right atrium and ventricle,[248,249] inferior vena cava plethora with a blunted inspiratory response,[250] and altered inspiratory intracardiac Doppler flow velocities.[251–253] Pericardial effusion and tamponade may be the first manifestation of cardiac involvement by a malignancy.[246] The associa-

tion of large quantities of pericardial fluid with tumor encasing the heart frequently results in persistent cardiac constriction, even after the fluid is withdrawn by pericardiocentesis.[238] Echocardiography and CT imaging are both useful for detecting pericardial metastases (Fig. 86-7).[238,254,255] Pericardioscopy performed during surgical drainage procedures has enabled visual diagnoses and guided biopsies of suspicious areas.[256]

Myocardial Involvement

Atrial arrhythmias are common, probably because the atrium has less mobility and hence is invaded more often. Atrial flutter and fibrillation are frequent, and a patient with either one may be unusually resistant to conventional therapy. Ventricular extrasystoles and even serious ventricular arrhythmias[257] may accompany invasion of a tumor into the myocardium. Conduction disturbances and complete heart block have been reported.[258,259] Widespread muscle involvement by tumor invasion or obstruction of the cardiac lymphatic drainage system may cause congestive failure. Rarely, a pedunculated secondary tumor mass may produce a loud murmur and palpable thrill.[260] Myocardial damage and heart failure may also result from some of the chemotherapeutic agents used in the treatment of patients with neoplastic diseases, and combined radiotherapy and chemotherapy may synergistically increase cardiac damage[261] (see Chap. 80). The most frequent ECG abnormalities seen in patients with neoplastic heart disease are nonspecific changes of the ST segment and the T wave due to myocardial or pericardial involvement by the tumor. Pronounced and prolonged ST-segment elevation in the absence of myocardial infarction may occur with tumor invasion of the heart.[262]

Coronary Artery Involvement

In patients with malignant tumor, angina or myocardial infarction may result from concomitant atherosclerosis,[261] coronary occlusion by tumor embolization,[263] or external coronary compression by the tumor, as well as from coronary fibrosis or accelerated atherogenesis in patients who have received radiation to the mediastinum.[261] The ECG pattern of myocardial infarction can also result from massive invasion of the myocardium by a tumor[261,264] or from a large pericardial effusion.[237,265]

Intracavitary Tumor

Extensions of tumors such as renal cell carcinoma,[244,266–268] hepatocellular carcinoma,[269,270] and uterine leiomyomatosis[271] along the inferior vena cava and into the right atrium can present as an intracavitary obstructive mass. Leiomyosarcoma may be primary in the vena cava, most often the inferior, and extend directly into the heart.[272,273] Intracavitary metastases or an expanding myocardial tumor may progressively obliterate a cardiac chamber or result in a valvular obstruction[274–277] and, rarely, may produce fever of unknown origin. Successful surgical resection has been reported.[91,268,270,272,278] Right atrial and tricuspid obstruction by an intracavitary mass can mimic pericardial constriction[278,279] from tumor invasion or from previous intensive radiotherapy to the mediastinum. Systemic or pulmonary emboli, so common with primary tumors of the heart, are uncommon with secondary tumors. Right-sided intracavitary thrombi may mimic primary or secondary tumors on echocardiographic imaging of the heart.[280,281]

Diagnostic Studies

Echocardiography, TTE and TEE,[71,238,254,282] CT scanning, and more recently, ultrafast CT[79] facilitate identification of pericardial effusion and intracavitary and pericardial masses (Fig. 86-7).[254,283–284] MRI provides a global view of cardiac anatomy and plays an important role in the diagnosis and evaluation of both primary and secondary tumors of the heart, providing information about the location, extent, and attachment of the tumor.[241,285] Pericardiocentesis may afford prompt symptomatic relief from pericardial tamponade and often provides a definitive cytologic diagnosis.[255] Ultrasound and fluoroscopic guidance aid in safe pericardial catheter placement[286] (see Chap. 81). The results of endomyocardial biopsy may contribute to the diagnosis in some cases.[287,288] Bone formation in metastatic osteogenic sarcoma may occasionally be visible radiographically.[289]

Treatment

Malignant pericardial effusion usually recurs rapidly after pericardiocentesis. Depending on the cytologic type and radiosensitivity of the tumor, radiation to the cardiac area, with or without systemic chemotherapy, is the treatment of choice.[255,290] The heart can tolerate 20 to 40 Gy, beyond which the risk of radiation-induced pericardial, myocardial, and valvular[291,292] damage is increased. Patients with malignant pericardial effusions have responded to systemic chemotherapy[293] and to intrapericardial administration of fluorouracil, radioactive gold (nitrogen mustard), and tetracycline.[255,294] Persistent reaccumulation of fluid may require surgical creation of a pericardial "window."[246,295–297] A pericardial-pleural "window" has also been produced with a percutaneous balloon catheter, without surgery.[298] Patients with myocardial infiltration by tumor also respond to radiation therapy and systemic chemotherapy. Heart block is treated with temporary or permanent electronic pacing, as conditions

dictate. Surgical removal of intracavitary obstructing secondary tumors may ameliorate symptoms and prolong survival,[275,283,299–303] as may chemotherapy in the occasional patient.

Documentation of tumor regression is possible with 2D echo imaging.[304,305] MRI plays an important role in characterizing the three-dimensional extent and attachment of cardiac tumors. This information is of particular importance in planning a surgical approach aimed at either complete removal or palliative debulking of a tumor mass.[241,306]

Special Considerations

LEUKEMIA

Leukemic infiltration of the heart is usually found at postmortem study and is generally not suspected before death.[238,307] Cardiac infiltrates are found in a majority of the postmortem studies of patients with acute leukemia, with most having pericardial involvement. Cardiac symptoms are unusual. Chronic lymphocytic leukemia reportedly has caused myocardial infiltration in some patients,[308] as well as mitral valve dysfunction[309] and congestive heart failure.[310] Myocardial rupture has been reported as an early manifestation of acute myeloblastic leukemia.[311] Massive pericardial effusion, often hemorrhagic,[312] and pericardial tamponade[313] have been reported, although overt pericardial effusion is not common. Management consists of pericardiocentesis and chemotherapy; occasionally, surgical decompression of the pericardium is necessitated by recurrent tamponade.[313] Infective endocarditis, commonly fungal, may complicate acute leukemia. Because of advances in treatment and improved long-term remission in patients with acute lymphoblastic leukemia, complicating infective endocarditis has been managed by valve replacement.[314]

Malignant Lymphoma

Involvement of the heart in patients with malignant lymphoma is common, although it is rarely detected before death. Cardiac or pericardial metastases occur with both Hodgkin's and non-Hodgkin's lymphoma and result from lymphatic and hematogenous spread as well as direct extension from other intrathoracic masses, resulting in predominantly epicardial and pericardial involvement.[5] Cardiac involvement may occasionally be the direct cause of death, but antemortem detection is infrequent.[315]

Acquired Immunodeficiency Syndrome and Heart Neoplasms

Two varieties of malignancies involving the heart have been described in patients with acquired immunodeficiency syndrome (AIDS): Kaposi's sarcoma[316] and, less commonly, malignant lymphoma[317,318] (see Chap. 79). Involvement of the heart by Kaposi's sarcoma may be primary or part of a widely disseminated process. The epicardium is a common location, with involvement of the underlying myocardium.

Clinical cardiac dysfunction is minimal, although fatal pericardial tamponade has been reported[319] (see also Chap. 81).

Lymphomas, usually of high-grade malignant characteristics, occur with increased frequency in patients with AIDS and other immunosuppressed states.[320] Both primary and, more commonly, secondary lymphomas involve the heart either as a diffuse infiltrative process or as focal nodules in any layer of the heart. Clinical features may be absent in approximately 50 percent of patients. When present, they include cardiomegaly, pericardial effusion and tamponade,[321] congestive failure, atrial arrhythmias,[322] and progressive heart block.[317] Echocardiography is useful and demonstrates pericardial effusion, mass lesions, and wall motion abnormalities. Transvenous biopsy can be useful in making the diagnosis.[323] There is limited experience with heart surgery in this group of patients.[324]

CARCINOID HEART DISEASE

While carcinoid tumors are never primary in the heart and only rarely metastasize to the heart and pericardium,[325–327] products of the tumor produce a distinctive endocardial and valvular pathologic pattern.[328] Tumors producing the carcinoid syndrome most commonly arise in the gastrointestinal tract, but they may also arise in the bronchus, biliary tract, pancreas, testis,[328] and ovary.[329] Appendiceal carcinoids, although common, rarely metastasize or produce the carcinoid syndrome. Ileal carcinoids, containing cytoplasmic granules that take up and reduce silver salts (argentaffinity), frequently metastasize to the liver and produce the carcinoid syndrome. These carcinoids contain a high concentration of 5-hydroxytryptamine (5-HT), which is excreted mainly as 5-hydroxyindoleacetic acid (5-HIAA) in the urine. Bronchial, pancreatic, and gastric carcinoid tumors differ morphologically and histochemically, have a worse prognosis, and metastasize more widely than do ileal tumors. They also produce 5-HT and excrete 5-HIAA in the urine; however, the clinical picture may be atypical. Carcinoid tumors of the rectum have a negative argentaffin reaction and are not associated with abnormalities of 5-HT synthesis or the carcinoid syndrome. Whereas they bear no morphologic or histochemical relation to the more typical carcinoid tumor, carcinomas of the bronchus, pancreas, or thyroid may occasionally secrete humoral substances that produce the carcinoid syndrome. In gastrointestinal carcinoid disease, the syndrome is produced by secretion of tumor products into the systemic circulation, which unfortunately delays its recognition until after liver metastases are present. The carcinoid syndrome, which results from the systemic effect of circulating vasoactive amines, consists of cutaneous flushing,[330] intestinal hypermobility, bronchial constriction, edema, and cardiac lesions.[331] Among patients with carcinoid, those with carcinoid heart disease demonstrate strikingly higher plasma serotonin and 5-HIAA levels.[332] Coronary artery spasm has also been reported in carcinoid heart disease.[333]

Cardiac Lesions

Cardiac lesions are more commonly found in the right side of the heart than in the left. Left-sided involvement[326,327] occurs with bronchial tumors, in the presence of an intraatrial communication,[334] or—in the absence of such a communication—when there is extensive right-sided heart involvement. Grossly glistening, white-yellow deposits are found on the pulmonary and tricuspid valves and, to varying degrees, on the right atrial and ventricular endocardium. Contraction of these deposits leads to tricuspid and pulmonary valve regurgitation and stenosis and occasionally may produce a restrictive type of myopathy[328] (see also Chap. 66). Mitral valve involvement may result in both stenosis and regurgitation. On microscopic examination (Fig. 86-8) the endocardial lesions consist of superficial deposits of fibrous tissue beneath a normal endothelium.[335,336] Metastatic lesions may be found in the myocardium. Serotonin, 5-HT, and bradykinin have been implicated in the pathogenesis of the cardiac lesions.[328,332] Transforming

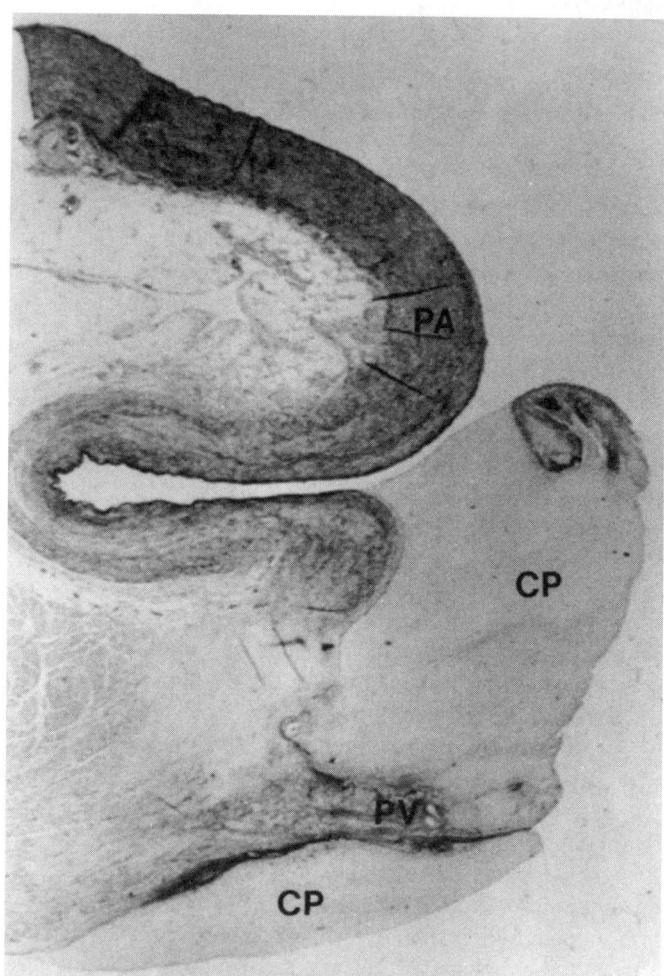

FIGURE 86-8

In carcinoid heart disease, there is either focal or diffuse plaquelike thickening of valvular and mural endocardium. When the pulmonary valve is involved, as in this patient, deposition of the fibrous tissue is almost exclusively on the arterial aspect of the valve cusps. PA = pulmonary artery; CP = carcinoid plaque; PV = pulmonary valve. (Movat Pentachrome × 10.)

growth factor-beta (TGF-β) has been shown to be produced by the fibroblasts in the carcinoid plaque and may play a critical role in progressive deposition of matrix proteins. The application of antibodies against TGF-β may potentially suppress the plaque progress.[337]

Clinical Manifestations

Carcinoid heart disease[328] cannot be recognized clinically until cardiac murmurs and signs of right-sided heart failure develop, especially elevated jugular venous pressure with inspiratory augmentation of the *v* wave, which is characteristic of tricuspid regurgitation. A harsh, holosystolic, lower sternal border murmur with inspiratory accentuation is common, frequently followed by an early diastolic filling sound and diastolic rumble (see also Chap. 66). A left upper sternal midsystolic murmur of pulmonary stenosis may or may not be identified separately. Murmurs of concomitant left-sided heart valvular involvement are rarely identified. There may be a parasternal heave and systolic pulsation of the liver, although enlargement and multinodular irregularity of the liver, ascites, and edema may be features of hepatic metastases without cardiac involvement.

Roentgenography of the chest will show the lung fields to be clear and the pulmonary trunk to be normal in size; the heart may be normal in size or show evidence of right ventricular and atrial enlargement. The ECG may show evidence of right atrial enlargement, but right ventricular hypertrophy is rare.

Echocardiographic imaging reveals right ventricular volume overload and abnormal right-sided valves. The tricuspid valve is typically thickened, retracted, and fixed in a semiopen position. Doming of the tricuspid valve may be present when the valve is predominantly stenotic. Color-flow Doppler will identify moderate to severe tricuspid valve regurgitation in the majority of patients. Pulmonary valve abnormalities are present in one-half of the patients, with pulmonary regurgitation more frequent than stenosis.[327] Left-sided valvular involvement—mitral more often than aortic—is infrequent (7 percent).[326] The echocardiographic changes are distinctive of carcinoid heart disease, are useful in following its progression, and may aid in detecting subclinical involvement.[328] TEE enhances the diagnostic accuracy and, additionally, reveals thickening of the right atrial wall.

Cardiac catheterization usually reveals predominant tricuspid regurgitation with a large right atrial systolic wave as well as some degree of tricuspid diastolic gradient. Angiography demonstrates thickening and doming of both the pulmonary and tricuspid valves. Injection of contrast medium into the pulmonary artery provides evidence of pulmonary regurgitation, which is rarely appreciated clinically from auscultation of a separate diastolic murmur. A large transpulmonary valve gradient and marked elevation of right ventricular pressure are unusual. Low cardiac output with a wide arteriovenous oxygen difference usually dominates the picture by the time cardiac catheterization is performed.

Diagnosis of carcinoid heart disease depends on clinical recognition of the characteristic right-sided heart findings in the setting of systemic features of the carcinoid syndrome. The diagnosis is sometimes made only after the tricuspid valve has been replaced.[328] In cases of ileal carcinoid disease, clinical recognition of multinodular deformity, along with radionuclide or CT imaging of the enlarged liver, serves to identify the prerequisite metastases to this organ.[328] Carcinoid tumors that originate in a location that can release metabolic products outside the portal circulation do not share the latter characteristics. Urinary excretion of 5-HIAA is markedly elevated, and heavy diversion of tryptophan to this metabolic pathway may result in profound hypoproteinemia and nicotinamide deficiency (pellagra).

Treatment

Current chemotherapeutic programs are at least partially effective in some patients with extensive liver metastases. When hepatic metastases are present, removing the primary ileal lesion is indicated only if it is large and is producing mechanical obstruction. Occasionally, large hepatic metastases are few in number and resection may afford symptomatic relief. Catheter embolization may permit segmental hepatic ablation in selected patients. In contrast, removal of an extraportal primary tumor can result in rapid resolution of cardiac failure. Some of the manifestations of the carcinoid syndrome may be blocked by alpha-adrenergic blockers, serotonin antagonists,[328,338] and somatostatin analogs.[339,340]

Valve Replacement

Because heart failure is a frequent cause of disability and death when carcinoid heart disease complicates the carcinoid syndrome, tricuspid valve replacement and pulmonary valvotomy, with outflow tract enlargement if necessary, have been recommended when hemodynamically indicated.[328] Implantation of a bioprosthetic valve[328,341,342] has generally been discouraged, although a review of reported cases of tricuspid valve replacement showed no significant difference in survival between patients with a bioprosthesis versus a mechanical valve.[328] Carcinoid plaque extending onto bioprosthetic valves as early as months after surgery has been reported.[328,342] Surgical mortality has been reported from 30 to 60 percent,[345–347] and only a small number of patients have undergone valve surgery; however, selected patients have experienced clinical improvement even in the presence of extensive hepatic metastases, reflecting the slow progression and potential for long-term survival with this tumor.[328,345–347] With proper care and planning, general anesthesia can be conducted with minimal risk.[328,348,349] Balloon valvuloplasty for tricuspid and pulmonary stenoses caused by carcinoid heart disease has been reported.[343,344]

REFERENCES

1. Chitwood WR Jr. Clarence Crafoord and the first successful resection of a cardiac myxoma. *Ann Thorac Surg* 1992; 54:997–998.

2. Peters MN, Hall RJ, Cooley DA, Leachman RD, Garcia E. The clinical syndrome of atrial myxoma. *JAMA* 1974; 230:695–701.
3. Pechacek LW, Gonzales-Camid F, Hall RJ, Garcia E, de Castro CM, Leachman RD, et al. The echocardiographic spectrum of atrial myxoma: A ten-year experience. *Texas Heart Inst J* 1986; 13:179–195.
4. Salcedo EE, Cohen GI, White RD, Davison MB. Cardiac tumors: Diagnosis and management. *Curr Probl Cardiol* 1992; 17:73–137.
5. McAllister HA Jr. Primary tumors and cysts of the heart and pericardium. In: Harvey WP, ed. *Current Problems in Cardiology*. Chicago: Year Book; 1979.
6. Reynen K. Cardiac myxomas. *N Engl J Med* 1995; 333:1610–1617.
7. McAllister HA Jr, Fenoglio JJ Jr. *Tumors of the Cardiovascular System*. Washington, DC: Armed Forces Institute of Pathology, 1978.
8. St John Sutton MG, Mercier LA, Giuliani ER, Lie JT. Atrial myxomas: A review of clinical experience in 40 patients. *Mayo Clin Proc* 1980; 55:371–376.
9. Sandrasagra FA, Oliver WA, English TAH. Myxoma of the mitral valve. *Br Heart J* 1979; 41:221–223.
10. Gorlach G, Hagel KJ, Mulch J, Scheld HH, Moosdorf R, Fitz H, et al. Myxoma of the aortic valve in a child. *J Cardiovasc Surg (Torino)* 1986; 27:679–680.
11. Devig PM, Clark TA, Aaron BL. Cardiac myxoma arising from the inferior vena cava. *Chest* 1980; 78:784–786.
12. Shimono T, Makino S, Kanamori Y, Kinoshita T, Yada I. Left atrial myxomas: Using gross anatomic tumor types to determine clinical features and coronary angiographic findings. *Chest* 1995; 107:674–679.
13. Burke AP, Virmani R. Cardiac myxoma: A clinicopathologic study. *Am J Clin Pathol* 1993; 100: 671–680.
14. Goldman BI, Frydman C, Harpaz N, Ryan SF, Loiterman D. Glandular cardiac myxomas: Histologic, immunohistochemical, and ultrastructural evidence of epithelial differentiation. *Cancer* 1987; 59:1767–1775.
15. Feldman PS, Horvath E, Kovacs K. An ultrastructural study of seven cardiac myxomas. *Cancer* 1977; 40:2216–2232.
16. Fine G. Primary tumors of the pericardium and heart. *Cardiovasc Clin* 1973; 5:207–238.
17. Wold LE, Lie JT. Scanning electron microscopy of intracardiac myxoma. *Mayo Clin Proc* 1981; 56:198–200.
18. Bashey RI, Nochumson S. Cardiac myxoma: Biochemical analyses and evidence for its neoplastic nature. *NY State J Med* 1979; 79:29–32.
19. Glasser SP, Bedynek JL, Hall RJ, Hopeman AR, Treasure RL, McAllister HA Jr, et al. Left atrial myxoma: Report of a case including hemodynamic, surgical, histologic and histochemical characteristics. *Am J Med* 1971; 50:113–122.
20. Dewald GW, Dahl R, Spurbeck JL, Carney JA, Gordon H. Chromosomally abnormal clones and nonrandom telomeric translocations in cardiac myxomas. *Mayo Clin Proc* 1987; 62:558–567.
21. Seidman JD, Berman JJ, Hitchcock CL, Becker RL, Mergner W, Moore W, et al. DNA analysis of cardiac myxomas: Flow cytometry and image analysis. *Hum Pathol* 1991; 22:494–500.
22. Kotylo PK, Kennedy JE, Waller BF, Sample RB. DNA analysis of atrial myxomas. *Chest* 1991; 99:1203–1207.
23. Read RC, White HJ, Murphy ML, Williams D, Sun CN, Flanagan WH. The malignant potentiality of left atrial myxoma. *J Thorac Cardiovasc Surg* 1974; 68:857–868.
24. Cleveland DC, Westaby S, Karp RB. Treatment of intra-atrial cardiac tumors. *JAMA* 1983; 249:2799–2802.
25. Desousa AL, Muller J, Campbell R, Batnitzky S, Rankin L. Atrial myxoma: A review of the neurological complications, metastases, and recurrences. *J Neurol Neurosurg Psychiatry* 1978; 41:1119–1124.
26. Pastakia B. Malignant atrial myxoma presenting as intercranial mass (letter). *Chest* 1979; 75:531–532.
27. Dashkoff N, Boersma RB, Nanda NC, Gramiak R, Andersen MN, Subramanian S. Bilateral atrial myxomas: Echocardiographic considerations. *Am J Med* 1978; 65:361–366.
28. Leonhardt ET, Kullenberg KP. Bilateral atrial myxomas with multiple arterial aneurysms—A syndrome mimicking polyarteritis nodosa. *Am J Med* 1977; 62:792–794.
29. Morgan DL, Palazola J, Reed W, Bell HH, Kindred LH, Beauchamp GD. Left heart myxomas. *Am J Cardiol* 1977; 40:611–614.
30. Steinke WE, Perry LW, Gold HR, McClanathan JE, Scott LP. Left atrial myxoma in a child. *Pediatrics* 1972; 49:580–589.
31. Balsara RK, Pelias AJ. Myxoma of right ventricle presenting as pulmonic stenosis in a neonate. *Chest* 1983; 83:145–146.
32. Davison ET, Mumford D, Zamah Q, Horowitz R. Left atrial myxoma in the elderly: Report of four patients over the age of 70 and review of the literature. *J Am Geriatr Soc* 1986; 34:229–233.
33. Burech DL, Teska DW, Haynes RE. Right atrial myxoma in a child. *Am J Dis Child* 1977; 131:750–752.
34. van Gelder HM, O'Brien DJ, Staples ED, Alexander JA. Familial cardiac myxoma. *Ann Thorac Surg* 1992; 53:419–424.
35. Farah MG. Familial cardiac myxoma: A study of relatives of patients with myxoma. *Chest* 1994; 105:65–68.
36. Seino Y, Ikeda U, Shimada K. Increased expression of interleukin 6 mRNA in cardiac myxomas. *Br Heart J* 1993; 69:565–567.
37. Kanda T, Umeyama S, Sasaki A, Nakazato Y, Morishita Y, Imai S, et al. Interleukin-6 and cardiac myxoma. *Am J Cardiol* 1994; 74:965–967.
38. Fyke FE III, Seward JB, Edwards WD, Miller FA, Reeder GS, Schattenberg TT, et al. Primary cardiac tumors: Experience with 30 consecutive patients since the introduction of two-dimensional echocardiography. *J Am Coll Cardiol* 1985; 5:1465–1473.
39. Graham SL, Sellers AL. Atrial myxoma with multiple myeloma. *Arch Intern Med* 1979; 139:116–117.
40. Molstad P, Smith G, Aukrust P. Left atrial myxoma and systemic AL-amyloidosis. *Eur Heart J* 1992; 13:143–144.
41. Burns ER, Schulman IC, Murphy MJ Jr. Hematologic manifestations and etiology of atrial myxoma. *Am J Med Sci* 1982; 284:17–22.
42. Carney JA. Carney complex: The complex of myxomas, spotty pigmentation, endocrine overactivity, and schwannomas. *Semin Dermatol* 1995; 14:90–98.
43. Radin R, Kempf RA. Carney complex: Report of three cases. *Radiology* 1995; 196:383–386.
44. Kaminsky ME, Ehlers K, Engle ME, Klein AA, Levin AR, Subramanian VA. Atrial myxoma mimicking a collagen disorder. *Chest* 1979; 75:93–95.
45. Boussen K, Moalla M, Blondeau P, Ayed HB, Lie JT. Embolization of cardiac myxomas masquerading as polyarteritis nodosa. *J Rheumatol* 1991; 18:283–285.
46. Markel ML, Waller BF, Armstrong WF. Cardiac myxoma: A review. *Medicine (Baltimore)* 1987; 66:114–125.
47. Joseph P, Hemmelstein DU, Mahowald JM, Stullman WS. Atrial myxoma infected with *Candida:* First survival. *Chest* 1980; 78:340–343.
48. Schweiger MJ, Hafer JG Jr, Brown R, Gianelly RE. Spontaneous cure of infected left atrial myxoma following embolization. *Am Heart J* 1980; 99:630–634.
49. ten Berg JM, Elbers HR, Defauw JJ, Plokker HW. Endocarditis on a left atrial myxoma. *Eur Heart J* 1992; 13:1592–1593.
50. Powers JC, Falkoff M, Heinle RA, Nanda NC, Ong LS, Weiner RS, et al. Familial cardiac myxoma: Emphasis on unusual clinical manifestations. *J Thorac Cardiovasc Surg* 1979; 77:782–788.
51. Flynn W, Garcia-Rinaldi R, Roehm JO Jr, Crawford ES. Surgical treatment of infected right atrial myxoma. *Ann Thorac Surg* 1979; 27:242–245.
52. Diflo T, Cantelmo NL, Haudenschild CC, Watkins MT. Atrial myxoma with remote metastasis: Case report and review of the literature. *Surgery* 1992; 111:352–356.
53. Misago N, Tanaka T, Hoshii T, Suda H, Itoh T. Erythematous papules in a patient with cardiac myxoma: A case report and review of the literature. *J Dermatol* 1995; 22:600–605.
54. McMullin GM, Lane R. A rare cause of acute aortic occlusion. *Aust NZ J Surg* 1993; 63:65–68.
55. Yeoh NTL, Clegg JF. Massive embolism from cardiac myxoma. *Angiology* 1981; 32:819–821.
56. Chadda KD, Pochaczevsky R, Gupta PK, Lichstein E, Schwartz IS. Nonprolapsing atrial myxoma: Clinical, echocardiographic, and angiographic correlations. *Angiology* 1978; 29:179–186.
57. Tipton BK, Robertson JT, Robertson JH. Embolism to the central nervous system from cardiac myxoma: Report of two cases. *J Neurosurg* 1977; 47:937–940.
58. Browne WT, Wijdicks EF, Parisi JE, Viggiano RW. Fulminant brain necrosis from atrial myxoma showers. *Stroke* 1993; 24:1090–1092.
59. Schmidley JW. Neurological presentations of atrial myxoma. *Heart Dis Stroke* 1993; 2:483–486.
60. Furuya K, Sasaki T, Yoshimoto Y, Okada Y, Fujimaki T, Kirino T. Histologically verified cerebral aneurysm formation secondary to embolism from cardiac myxoma. *J Neurosurg* 1995; 83:170–173.
61. Cogan DG, Wray SH. Vascular occlusions in the eye from cardiac myxomas. *Am J Ophthalmol* 1975; 80:396–403.

62. Tanabe J, Williams RL, Deithrich EB. Left atrial myxoma: Association with acute coronary embolization in an 11-year-old boy. *Pediatrics* 1979; 63:778–781.

63. Cheitlin MD, McAllister HA Jr, de Castro CM. Myocardial infarction without atherosclerosis. *JAMA* 1975; 231:951–959.

64. Stevens LH, Hormuth DA, Schmidt PE, Atkins S, Fehrenbacher JW. Left atrial myxoma: Pulmonary infarction caused by pulmonary venous occlusion. *Ann Thorac Surg* 1987; 43:215–217.

65. Harvey WP. Clinical aspects of cardiac tumors. *Am J Cardiol* 1968; 21:328–343.

66. Martinez-Lopez JI. Sounds of the heart in diastole. *Am J Cardiol* 1974; 34:594–601.

67. Goodwin JF. The spectrum of cardiac tumors. *Am J Cardiol* 1968; 21:307–314.

68. Cecil MP, Silverman ME. Tricuspid valve honk due to pulmonary hypertension secondary to left atrial myxoma. *Am J Cardiol* 1991; 67:321.

69. Sharratt GP, Grover ML, Monro JL. Calcified left atrial myxoma with floppy mitral valve. *Br Heart J* 1979; 42:608–610.

70. Case Records of the Massachusetts General Hospital, Weekly Clinico-pathological Exercises: Case 42-1973. *N Engl J Med* 1973; 289:853–859.

71. Reeder GS, Khandheria BK, Seward JB, Tajik AJ. Transesophageal echocardiography and cardiac masses. *Mayo Clin Proc* 1991; 66:1101–1109.

72. DeVille JB, Corley D, Jin BS, de Castro CM, Hall RJ, Wilansky S. Assessment of intracardiac masses by transesophageal echocardiography. *Tex Heart Inst J* 1995; 22:134–137.

73. Tighe DA, Rousou JA, Kenia S, Kulshrestha P. Transesophageal echocardiography in the management of mitral valve myxoma. *Am Heart J* 1995; 130:627–629.

74. Leibowitz G, Keller NM, Daniel WG, Freedberg RS, Tunick PA, Stottmeister C, et al. Transesophageal versus transthoracic echocardiography in the evaluation of right atrial tumors. *Am Heart J* 1995; 130:1224–1227.

75. Panidis IP, Mintz GS, McAllister M. Hemodynamic consequences of left atrial myxomas as assessed by Doppler ultrasound. *Am Heart J* 1986; 111:927–931.

76. Ho YL, Wu CC, Chen WJ, Chu SH, Lee YT. Flow pattern of four pulmonary veins in a case with prolapsing left atrial myxoma: A case report. *Angiology* 1995; 46:1053–1057.

77. Case Records of the Massachusetts General Hospital, Weekly Clinico-pathological Exercises: Case 14-1978. *N Engl J Med* 1978; 298:834.

78. Meyers SN, Shapiro SE, Barresi V, DeBoer AA, Pavel DI, Gracey DR, et al. Right atrial myxoma with right to left shunting and mitral valve prolapse. *Am J Med* 1977; 62:308–314.

79. Bleiweis MS, Georgiou D, Brundage BH. Detection of intracardiac masses by ultrafast computed tomography. *Am J Cardiac Imaging* 1994; 8:63–68.

80. Pflugfelder PW, Wisenberg G, Boughner DR. Detection of atrial myxoma by magnetic resonance imaging. *Am J Cardiol* 1985; 55:242–243.

81. Go RT, O'Donnell JK, Underwood DA, Feiglin DH, Salcedo EE, Pantaja M, et al. Comparison of gated cardiac MRI and 2D echocardiography of intracardiac neoplasms. *Am J Roentgenol* 1985; 145:21–25.

82. Freedberg RS, Kronzon I, Rumancik WM, Liebeskind D. The contribution of magnetic resonance imaging to the evaluation of intracardiac tumors diagnosed by echocardiography. *Circulation* 1988; 77:96–103.

83. Sung RJ, Ghahramani AR, Mallon SM, Richter SE, Sommer LS, Gottlieb S, et al. Hemodynamic features of prolapsing and nonprolapsing left atrial myxoma. *Circulation* 1975; 51:342–349.

84. Ognibene AJ, Nelson WP. Atrial myxoma: Comments on hemodynamic alterations—Report of a case. *Dis Chest* 1967; 52:699–701.

85. Hamer JPM, Nieveen J, Bergstra A, Blickman JR, Homan Van der Heide JN. Left atrial myxoma moving from right atrium to left ventricle. *Acta Med Scand* 1979; 205:527–534.

86. Pindyck F, Peirce EC II, Baron MG, Lukban SB. Embolization of left atrial myxoma after transseptal cardiac catheterization. *Am J Cardiol* 1972; 30:569–571.

87. Stewart JA, Warnica JW, Kirk ME, Winsberg F. Left atrial myxoma: False negative echocardiographic findings in a tumor demonstrated by coronary arteriography. *Am Heart J* 1979; 98:228–232.

88. Hamer AW, Weeks PA. Diagnosis of left atrial myxoma at routine coronary angiography in an asymptomatic patient. *Cathet Cardiovasc Diagn* 1993; 30:233–235.

89. Van Cleemput J, Daenen W, De Geest H. Coronary angiography in cardiac myxomas: Findings in 19 consecutive cases and review of the literature. *Cathet Cardiovasc Diagn* 1993; 29:217–220.

90. Bochna AJ, Falicov RE. Diagnosis of intracardiac thrombi in mitral stenosis and left ventricular dysfunction: Use of selective coronary arteriography. *Arch Intern Med* 1980; 140:759–762.

91. Shapiro MR, Cohen MV, Grose R, Spindola-Franco H. Diagnosis of left atrial myxoma by coronary angiography eight years following open mitral commissurotomy. *Am Heart J* 1983; 105:325–327.

92. Huston KA, Combs JJ Jr, Lie JT, Giuliani ER. Left atrial myxoma simulating peripheral vasculitis. *Mayo Clin Proc* 1978; 53:752–756.

93. Lortscher RH, Toews WH, Nora JJ, Wolfe RR, Spangler RD. Left atrial myxoma presenting as rheumatic fever. *Chest* 1974; 66:302–303.

94. Neches WH, Park SC, Lenox CC, Zuberbuhler JR, Siewers RD. Left atrial myxoma: Clinical presentation suggesting acute myocarditis. *JAMA* 1974; 229:1906–1907.

95. Warda M, Garcia J, Pechacek LW, Massumkhani A, Hall RJ. Auscultatory and echocardiographic features of mobile left atrial thrombus. *J Am Coll Cardiol* 1985; 5:379–382.

96. Roguin N, Amikam S, Riss E. Prolapsing right atrial myxoma: Clinical and haemodynamic considerations. *Br Heart J* 1977; 39:577–580.

97. Kuroda H, Nitta K, Ashida Y, Hara Y, Ishiguro S, Mori T. Right atrial myxoma originating from the tricuspid valve. *J Thorac Cardiovasc Surg* 1995; 109:1249–1250.

98. Teoh KH, Mulji A, Tomlinson CW, Lobo FV. Right atrial myxoma originating from the eustachian valve. *Can J Cardiol* 1993; 9:441–443.

99. Hickie JB, Gibson H, Windsor HM. "The wrecking ball": Right atrial myxoma. *Med J Aust* 1970; 2:82–86.

100. Miyauchi Y, Endo T, Kuroki S, Hayakawa H. Right atrial myxoma presenting with recurrent episodes of pulmonary embolism. *Cardiology* 1992; 81:178–181.

101. Heck HA Jr, Gross CM, Houghton JL. Long-term severe pulmonary hypertension associated with right atrial myxoma. *Chest* 1992; 102:301–303.

102. Vidne B, Atsmon A, Aygen M, Levy MJ. Right atrial myxoma: Case report and review of the literature. *Isr J Med Sci* 1971; 7:1196–2000.

103. Siggillino JJ, Crawley CJ, Clauss RH, Reed GE, Tice DA. Myxoma of the right atrium with polycythemia. *Arch Intern Med* 1963; 111:178–183.

104. Natarajan P, Vijayanagar RR, Eckstein PF, Bognolo DA. Right atrial myxoma with atrial septal defect: A case report and review of the literature. *Cathet Cardiovasc Diagn* 1982; 8:267–272.

105. Park JM, Garcia RR, Patrick JK, Waagner D, Anuras S. Right atrial myxoma with a nonembolic intestinal manifestation. *Pediatr Cardiol* 1990; 11:164–166.

106. Massumi R. Bedside diagnosis of right heart myxomas through detection of palpable tumor shocks and audible plops. *Am Heart J* 1983; 105:303–310.

107. Lyons SV, McCord J, Smith S. Asymptomatic giant right atrial myxoma: Role of transesophageal echocardiography in management. *Am Heart J* 1991; 121:1555–1558.

108. Smith ST, Hautamaki K, Lewis JW Jr, Serwin J, Alam M. Transthoracic and transesophageal echocardiography in the diagnosis and surgical management of right atrial myxoma. *Chest* 1991; 100:575–576.

109. Obeid AI, Marvasti M, Parker F, Rosenberg J. Comparison of transthoracic and transesophageal echocardiography in diagnosis of left atrial myxoma. *Am J Cardiol* 1989; 63:1006–1008.

110. Mugge A, Daniel WG, Haverich A, Lichtlen PR. Diagnosis of noninfective cardiac mass lesions by two-dimensional echocardiography: Comparison of the transthoracic and transesophageal approaches. *Circulation* 1991; 83:70–78.

111. Vargas-Barron J, Romero-Cardenas A, Villegas M, Keirns C, Gomez-Jaume A, Delong R, et al. Transthoracic and transesophageal echocardiographic diagnosis of myxomas in the four cardiac cavities. *Am Heart J* 1991; 121:931–933.

112. Angelini P, Wilansky S, Gaos C, Montazavi A, Boncompagni E, Cooley DA. Prolapsing large aneurysm of the atrial septum simulating a right atrial mass. *Cathet Cardiovasc Diagn* 1992; 26:122–126.

113. Meller J, Teichholz LE, Pichard AD, Matta R, Litwak R, Herman MV. Left ventricular myxoma: Echocardiographic diagnosis and review of the literature. *Am J Med* 1977; 63:816–823.

114. Albers GW, Avalos SM, Weinrich M. Left ventricular tumor masquerading as multiple sclerosis. *Arch Neurol* 1987; 44:779–780.

115. Wrisley D, Rosenberg J, Giambartolomei A, Levy I, Turiello C, Anton-

ini T. Left ventricular myxoma discovered incidentally by echocardiography. *Am Heart J* 1991; 121:1554–1555.

116. Camesas AM, Lichtstein E, Kramer J, Liebeskind D, Kronzon I, Tyras D, et al. Complementary use of two-dimensional echocardiography and magnetic resonance imaging in the diagnosis of ventricular myxoma. *Am Heart J* 1987; 114:440–442.

117. Hada Y, Wolfe C, Murray GF, Craige E. Right ventricular myxoma: Case report and review of phonocardiographic and auscultatory manifestations. *Am Heart J* 1980; 100:871–877.

118. Gonzales A, Altieri PI, Marquez E, Cox RA, Castillo M. Massive pulmonary embolism associated with a right ventricular myxoma. *Am J Med* 1980; 69:795–798.

119. Nass PC, Neimeyer MG, Brutel-de-la-Riviere A, Brune DF, Plokker HW. Left atrial and right ventricular cardiac myxoma: A case report. *Eur J Cardiothorac Surg* 1989; 3:468–470.

120. Adachi K, Tanaka H, Toshima H, Morimatsu M. Right atrial angiosarcoma diagnosed by cardiac biopsy. *Am Heart J* 1988; 115:482–485.

121. Betancourt B, Defendini EA, Johnson C, De Jesus M, Pavia-Villamil A, Cruz AD. Severe right ventricular outflow tract obstruction caused by an intracavitary cardiac neurilemoma: Successful surgical removal and postoperative diagnosis. *Chest* 1979; 75:522–524.

122. Jones DR, Warden HE, Murray GF, Hill RC, Graeber GM, Cruzzavala JL, et al. Biatrial approach to cardiac myxomas: A 30-year clinical experience. *Ann Thorac Surg* 1995; 59:851–855.

123. Cooley DA. Surgical management of cardiac tumors. In: Kapoor AS, Reynolds RD, eds: *Cancer and the Heart.* New York: Springer-Verlag; 1986:126–134.

124. Murphy MC, Sweeney MS, Putnam JB Jr, Walker WE, Frazier OH, Ott DA, et al. Surgical treatment of cardiac tumors: A 25-year experience. *Ann Thorac Surg* 1990; 49:612–618.

125. Casarotto D, Bortolotti U, Russo R, et al. Surgical removal of a left atrial myxoma during pregnancy. *Chest* 1979; 75:390–392.

126. Trimakas AP, Maxwell KD, Berkay S. Fetal monitoring during cardiopulmonary bypass for removal of a left atrial myxoma during pregnancy. *Johns Hopkins Med J* 1979; 144:156–160.

127. Bateman TM, Gray RJ, Raymond MJ, Chaux A, Czer LS, Matloff JM. Arrhythmias and conduction disturbances following cardiac operation for the removal of left atrial myxomas. *J Thorac Cardiovasc Surg* 1983; 86:601–607.

128. Mahoney L, Schieken RM, Doty D. Cardiac rhabdomyomas simulating pulmonic stenosis. *Cathet Cardiovasc Diagn* 1979; 5:385–388.

129. Abushaban L, Denham B, Duff D. 10 year review of cardiac tumors in childhood. *Br Heart J* 1993; 70:166–169.

130. Fenoglio JJ Jr, McAllister HA Jr, Ferrans VJ. Cardiac rhabdomyoma: A clinicopathologic and electron microscopic study. *Am J Cardiol* 1976; 38:241–251.

131. Howanitz EP, Teske DW, Qualman SJ, Finck S, Kilman JW. Pedunculated left ventricular rhabdomyoma. *Ann Thorac Surg* 1986; 41:443–445.

132. Spooner EW, Farina MA, Shaher RM, Foster ED. Left ventricular rhabdomyoma causing subaortic stenosis—The two-dimensional echocardiographic appearance. *Pediatr Cardiol* 1982; 2:67–71.

133. Guereta LG, Burgueros M, Elorza MD, Alix AG, Benito F, Gamallo C. Cardiac rhabdomyoma presenting as fetal hydrops. *Pediatr Cardiol* 1986; 7:171–174.

134. Kuehl KS, Perry LW, Chandra R, Scott LP III. Left ventricular rhabdomyoma: A rare cause of subaortic stenosis in the newborn infant. *Pediatrics* 1970; 46:464–468.

135. Violette EJ, Hardin NJ, McQuillen EN. Sudden unexpected death due to asymptomatic cardiac rhabdomyoma. *J Forens Sci* 1981; 26:599–604.

136. Mehta AV. Rhabdomyoma and ventricular preexcitation syndrome: A report of two cases and review of literature. *Am J Dis Child* 1993; 147:669–671.

137. Pillai R, Kharma N, Brom AG, Becker AE. Mitral valve origin of pedunculated rhabdomyomas causing subaortic stenosis. *Am J Cardiol* 1991; 67:663–664.

138. Duncan WJ, Rowe RD, Freedom RM, Izukawa T, Olley PM. Space-occupying lesions of the myocardium: Role of two-dimensional echocardiography in detection of cardiac tumors in children. *Am Heart J* 1982; 104:780–785.

139. Marx GR, Bierman FZ, Matthews E, Williams R. Two-dimensional echocardiographic diagnosis of intracardiac masses in infancy. *J Am Coll Cardiol* 1984; 3:827–832.

140. Boxer RA, LaCorte MA, Singh S, Shapiro J, Schiller M, Goldman M, et al. Diagnosis of cardiac tumors in infants by magnetic resonance imaging. *Am J Cardiol* 1985; 56:831–832.

141. Demkow M, Sorensen K, Whitehead BF, Rees PG, Sullivan ID, Elliott MJ, et al. Heart transplantation in an infant with rhabdomyoma. *Pediatr Cardiol* 1995; 16:204–206.

142. Ott DA, Garson A, Cooley DA, McNamara D. Definitive operation for refractory cardiac tachyarrhythmia in children. *J Thorac Cardiovasc Surg* 1985; 90:681–689.

143. Garson A Jr, Smith RT Jr, Moak JP, Kearney DL, Hawkins EP, Titus JL, et al. Incessant ventricular tachycardia in infants: Myocardial hamartomas and surgical cure. *J Am Coll Cardiol* 1987; 10:619–626.

144. Kearney DL, Titus JL, Hawkins EP, Ott DA, Garson A Jr. Pathologic features of myocardial hamartomas causing childhood tachyarrhythmias. *Circulation* 1987; 75:705–710.

145. Holley DG, Martin GR, Brenner JI, Fyfe DA, Huhta JC, Kleinman CS, et al. Diagnosis and management of fetal cardiac tumors: A multicenter experience and review of published reports. *J Am Coll Cardiol* 1995; 26:516–520.

146. Busch U, Kampmann C, Meyer R, Sandring KH, Hausdorf G, Konertz W. Removal of a giant cardiac fibroma from a 4-year-old child. *Tex Heart Inst J* 1995; 22:261–264.

147. Reul GJ Jr, Howell JR, Rubio PA, Petersen PK. Successful partial excision of an intramural fibroma of the left ventricle. *Am J Cardiol* 1975; 36:262–265.

148. Williams DB, Danielson GK, McGoon DC, Feldt RH, Edwards WD. Cardiac fibroma: Long-term survival after excision. *J Thorac Cardiovasc Surg* 1982; 84:230–236.

149. Biancaniello TM, Meyer RA, Gaum WE, Kaplan S. Primary benign intramural ventricular tumors in children: Pre- and postoperative electrocardiographic, echocardiographic, and angiocardiographic evaluation. *Am Heart J* 1982; 103:852–857.

150. Jamieson SW, Gaudiani VA, Reitz BA, Oyer PE, Stinson EB, Shumway NE. Operative treatment of an unresectable tumor of the left ventricle. *J Thorac Cardiovasc Surg* 1981; 81:797–799.

151. Ryan PE Jr, Obeid AI, Parker FB Jr. Primary cardiac valve tumors. *J Heart Valve Dis* 1995; 4:222–226.

152. Grote J, Mugge A, Schafers HJ, Daniel WG, Lichtlen PR. Multiplane transesophageal echocardiography detection of a papillary fibroelastoma of the aortic valve causing myocardial infarction. *Eur Heart J* 1995; 16:426–429.

153. Israel DH, Sherman W, Ambrose JA, Sharma S, Harpaz N, Robbins M. Dynamic coronary ostial obstruction due to papillary fibroelastoma leading to myocardial ischemia and infarction. *Am J Cardiol* 1991; 67:104–105.

154. Eckstein FS, Schafers HJ, Grote J, Mugge A, Borst HG. Papillary fibroelastoma of the aortic valve presenting with myocardial infarction. *Ann Thorac Surg* 1995; 60:206–208.

155. Brown RD Jr, Khanderia BK, Edwards WD. Cardiac papillary fibroelastoma: A treatable cause of transient ischemic attack and ischemic stroke detected by transesophageal echocardiography. *Mayo Clin Proc* 1995; 70:863–868.

156. Lee CC, Celik C, Lajos TZ. Excision of papillary fibroelastoma arising from the septal leaflet of the tricuspid valve. *J Cardiac Surg* 1995; 10:589–591.

157. Anderson KR, Fiddler GI, Lie JT. Congenital papillary tumor of the tricuspid valve: An unusual case of right ventricular outflow obstruction in a neonate with trisomy E. *Mayo Clin Proc* 1977; 52:665–669.

158. Cha SD, Incarvito J, Chang KS, Maranhao V, Gooch AS. Giant Lambl's excrescences of papillary muscle and aortic valve: Echocardiographic, angiographic, and pathologic findings. *Clin Cardiol* 1981; 4:51–54.

159. Fitzgerald D, Gaffney P, Dervan P, Doyle CT, Horgan J, Nelligan M. Giant Lambl's excrescence presenting as a peripheral embolus. *Chest* 1982; 81:516–517.

160. Shahian DM, Labib SB, Chang G. Cardiac papillary fibroelastoma. *Ann Thorac Surg* 1995; 59:538–541.

161. Lee KS, Topol EJ, Stewart WJ. Atypical presentation of papillary fibroelastoma mimicking multiple vegetations in suspected subacute bacterial endocarditis (review). *Am Heart J* 1993; 125:1443–1445.

162. Moulton AL, Jaretzki A III, Bowman FO Jr, Silverstein EF, Bregman D. Massive lipoma of heart. *NY State J Med* 1976; 76:1820–1825.

163. Shumacker HB Jr, Leshnower AC. Extracavitary lipoma of the heart: Operative resection. *Ann Thorac Surg* 1974; 18:411–414.

164. Barberger-Gateau P, Paquet M, Desaulniers D, Chenard J. Fibrolipoma of the mitral valve in a child: Clinical and echocardiographic features. *Circulation* 1978; 58:955–958.

165. Leatherman L, Leachman RD, Hallman GL, Colley DA. Cyst of the mitral valve. *Am J Cardiol* 1968; 21:428–430.

166. Tuna IC, Julsrud PR, Click RL, Tazelaar HD, Bresnahan DR, Danielson GK. Tissue characterization of an unusual right atrial mass by magnetic resonance imaging. *Mayo Clin Proc* 1991; 66:498–501.

167. McNamara RF, Taylor AE, Panner BJ. Superior vena caval obstruction by lipomatous hypertrophy of the right atrium. *Clin Cardiol* 1987; 10:609–610.

168. Cohen IS, Raiker K. Atrial lipomatous hypertrophy: Lipomatous atrial hypertrophy with significant involvement of the right atrial wall. *J Am Soc Echocardiogr* 1993; 6:30–34.

169. Basu S, Folliguet T, Anselmo M, Greengart A, Sabado M, Cunningham JN Jr, et al. Lipomatous hypertrophy of the interatrial septum. *Cardiovasc Surg* 1994; 2:229–231.

170. Shirani J, Roberts WC. Clinical, electrocardiographic and morphologic features of massive fatty deposits ("lipomatous hypertrophy") in the atrial septum. *J Am Coll Cardiol* 1993; 22:226–238.

171. Tschirkov A, Stegaru B. Lipomatous hypertrophy of interatrial septum presenting as recurring pericardial effusion and mistaken for constrictive pericarditis. *Thorac Cardiovasc Surg* 1979; 27:400–403.

172. Voigt J, Agdal N. Lipomatous infiltration of the heart: An uncommon cause of sudden, unexpected death in a young man. *Arch Pathol Lab Med* 1982; 106:497–498.

173. Kozelj M, Angelski R, Pavcnik D. Lipomatous hypertrophy of the interatrial septum: Diagnosis by echocardiography and magnetic resonance imaging. A case report. (review). *Angiology* 1995; 46:863–866.

174. Stone GW, O'Kell RT, Good TH, Hartzler GO. Lipomatous hypertrophy of the interatrial septum: Diagnosis by percutaneous transvenous biopsy. *Am Heart J* 1990; 119:406–408.

175. Manion WC, Nelson WP, Hall RJ, Brierty PE. Benign tumor of the heart causing complete heart block. *Am Heart J* 1972; 83:535–542.

176. Fenoglio JJ, Jacobs DW, McAllister HA Jr. Mesothelioma of the atrioventricular node. *Cancer* 1977; 40:721–727.

177. James TN, Galakhov I. De subitaneis mortibus: XXVI. Fatal electrical instability of the heart associated with benign congenital polycystic tumor of the atrioventricular node. *Circulation* 1977; 6:667–678.

178. Balasundaram S, Halees S, Duran C. Mesothelioma of the atrioventricular node: First successful follow-up after excision. *Eur Heart J* 1992; 13:718–719.

179. Hellemans IM, van Hemel NM, Kooyman CA. Atrioventricular block in childhood caused by mesothelioma. *PACE* 1981; 4:216–220.

180. Raabe DS, Fischer JC, Brandt RL. Cavernous hemangioma of the right atrium: Presumptive diagnosis by coronary angiography. *Cathet Cardiovasc Diagn* 1976; 2:389–395.

181. Boden WE, Funk EJ, Carleton RA, Benham I, Khan AH, Lasser A, et al. Left ventricular hemangioma masquerading as *Mycoplasma* pericarditis. *Am Heart J* 1983; 106:771–774.

182. Palmer TE, Tresch DD, Bonchek LI. Spontaneous resolution of a large cavernous hemangioma of the heart. *Am J Cardiol* 1986; 58:184–185.

183. Trout HH, McAllister HA Jr, Giordano JM, Rich NM. Vascular malformations. *Surgery* 1985; 97:36–41.

184. Grigg LE, Downey W, Tatoulis J, Hunt D. Benign congenital intracardiac thyroid and polycystic tumor causing right ventricular outflow tract obstruction and conduction disturbance. *J Am Coll Cardiol* 1987; 9:225–227.

185. Swalwell CI: Benign intracardiac teratoma: A case of sudden death. *Arch Pathol Lab Med* 1993; 117:739–742.

186. Hui G, McAllister HA Jr, Angelini P. Left atrial paraganglioma: Report of a case and review of the literature. *Am Heart J* 1987; 113:1230–1234.

187. Conti VR, Saydjari R, Amparo EG. Paraganglioma of the heart: The value of magnetic resonance imaging in the preoperative evaluation. *Chest* 1986; 90:604–606.

188. Jeevanandam V, Oz MC, Shapiro B, Barr ML, Marboe C, Rose EA. Surgical management of cardiac pheochromocytoma: Resection versus transplantation. *Ann Surg* 1995; 221:415–419.

189. Cooley DA, Reardon MJ, Frazier OH, Angelini P. Human cardiac explantation and autotransplantation: Application in a patient with a large cardiac pheochromocytoma. *Texas Heart Inst J* 1985; 12:171–176.

190. Raaf HN, Raaf JH. Sarcomas related to the heart and vasculature. *Semin Surg Oncol* 1994; 10:374–382.

191. Bjerregaard P, Baandrup U. Haemangioendotheliosarcoma of the heart: Diagnosis and treatment. *Br Heart J* 1979; 42:734–737.

192. Delgado Jimenez J, Tascon Perez J, Albarran Gonzalez A, Ugarte J, Gomez Pajuelo C, Carbonell Porras A, et al. Right coronary artery—Right atrium fistula in primary angiosarcoma of the heart. *Chest* 1992; 102:1629–1630.

193. Ohri SK, Nihoyannopoulos P, Taylor KM, Keogh BE. Angiosarcoma of the heart causing cardiac rupture. A rare cause of hemopericardium. *Ann Thorac Surg* 1993; 55:525–528.

194. Janigan DT, Husain A, Robinson NA. Cardiac angiosarcomas: A review and a case report. *Cancer* 1986; 57:852–859.

195. Herrmann MA, Shankerman RA, Edwards WD, Shub C, Schaff HV. Primary cardiac angiosarcoma: A clinicopathologic study of six cases. *J Thorac Cardiovasc Surg* 1992; 103:655–664.

196. Schmid KW, Thurner J Jr, Gruenewald K. Hemangiopericytoma of the heart following treatment of Hodgkin's disease: A case report. *Virchows Arch* 1987; 411:485–488.

197. Schmaltz AA, Apitz J. Primary rhabdomyosarcoma of the heart. *Pediatr Cardiol* 1982; 2:73–75.

198. Nagata K, Irie K, Morimatsu M, Nakashima T, Eriguchi N, Koga M. Rhabdomyosarcoma of the right ventricle. *Acta Pathol Jpn* 1982; 32:843–849.

199. Sholler GF, Hawker RE, Nunn GR, Bale P, Bergin M. Primary left ventricular rhabdomyosarcoma in a child: Noninvasive assessment and successful resection of a rare tumor. *J Thorac Cardiovasc Surg* 1987; 93:465–468.

200. Schwartz JE, Schwartz GP, Judson PL, Siebel JE Jr, Trumbull HR. Complete resection of a primary cardiac rhabdomyosarcoma: Case report, review of the literature, and management recommendations. *Cardiovasc Dis Bull Tex Heart Inst* 1979; 6:413–424.

201. Knobel B, Rosman P, Kishon Y, Husar M. Intracardiac primary fibrosarcoma: Case report and literature review. *Thorac Cardiovasc Surg* 1992; 40:227–230.

202. Cafferty LL, Epstein JI. Primary liposarcoma of the right atrium. *Hum Pathol* 1987; 18:408–410.

203. Cairns P, Butany J, Fulop J, Rakowski H, Hassaram S. Cardiac presentation of non-Hodgkin's lymphoma. *Arch Pathol Lab* 1987; 111:80–83.

204. Scully RE, Mark EJ, McNeely WF, McNeely BU. Case records of the Massachusetts General Hospital: Case 22-1987. *N Engl J Med* 1987; 316:1394–1404.

205. Laya MF, Mailliard JA, Bewtra C, Levin HS. Malignant fibrous histiocytoma of the heart: A case report and review of the literature. *Cancer* 1987; 59:1026–1031.

206. Stevens CW, Sears-Rogan P, Bitterman P, Torrisi J. Treatment of malignant fibrous histiocytoma of the heart. *Cancer* 1992; 69:956–961.

207. Korbmacher B, Doering C, Schulte HD, Hort W. Malignant fibrous histiocytoma of the heart—Case report of a rare left-atrial tumor. *Thorac Cardiovasc Surg* 1992; 40:303–307.

208. Holtzman E, Schiby G, Segal P, Priel I. Malignant fibrous histiocytoma complicating mitral valve replacement. *J Am Coll Cardiol* 1986; 7:956–960.

209. Teramoto N, Hayashi K, Miyatani K, Miyake K, Sarker AB, Tadashi Y, et al. Malignant fibrous histiocytoma of the right ventricle of the heart. *Pathol Int* 1995; 45:315–319.

210. Frandsen NE, Andersen L, Nielsen JR. Malignant mesenchymoma of the heart presenting as mitral stenosis. *Acta Med Scand* 1981; 209:235–237.

211. Donovan VM, Summer W, Hutchins GM. Left atrial leiomyosarcoma: Manifestation as unexplained pulmonary vascular disease. *Arch Intern Med* 1982; 142:1923–1925.

212. Terashima K, Aoyama K, Nihei K, Nito T, Imai Y, Takahashi K, et al. Malignant fibrous histiocytoma of the heart. *Cancer* 1983; 52:1919–1926.

213. Ceretto WJ, Miller ML, Shea PM, Gregory CW, Vieweg WV. Malignant mesenchymoma obstructing the right ventricular outflow tract. *Am Heart J* 1981; 101:114–115.

214. Dein JR, Frist WH, Stinson EB, Miller DC, Baldwin JC, Oyer PE, et al. Primary cardiac neoplasms: Early and late results of surgical treatment in 42 patients. *J Thorac Cardiovasc Surg* 1987; 93:502–511.

215. Putman JB Jr, Sweeney MS, Colon R, Lanza LA, Frazier OH, Cooley DA. Primary cardiac sarcomas. *Ann Thorac Surg* 1991; 51:906–910.

216. Turner A, Batrick N. Primary cardiac sarcomas: A report of three cases and a review of the current literature. *Int J Cardiol* 1993; 40:115–119.

217. Rienmüller R, Tiling R. MR and CT for detection of cardiac tumors. *Thorac Cardiovasc Surg* 1990; 38:168–172.

218. Mora F, Mindich BP, Guarino T, Goldman ME. Improved surgical approach to cardiac tumors with intraoperative two-dimensional echocardiography. *Chest* 1987; 91:142–144.

219. Burke AP, Cowan D, Virmani R. Primary sarcomas of the heart. *Cancer* 1992; 69:387–395.

220. Szucs RA, Rehr RB, Yanovich S, Tatum JL. Magnetic resonance imaging of cardiac rhabdomyosarcoma: Quantifying the response to chemotherapy. *Cancer* 1991; 67:2066–2070.

221. Goldstein DJ, Oz MC, Michler RE. Radical excisional therapy and total cardiac transplantation for recurrent atrial myxoma. *Ann Thorac Surg* 1995; 60:1105–1107.

222. Goldstein DJ, Oz MC, Rose EA, Fisher P, Michler RE. Experience with heart transplantation for cardiac tumors. *J Heart Lung Transplant* 1995; 14:382–386.

223. Feigin DS, Fenoglio JJ, McAllister HA, Madewell JR. Pericardial cysts: A radiologic-pathologic correlation and review. *Radiology* 1977; 125:15–20.

224. Stoller JK, Shaw C, Matthay RA. Enlarging, atypically located pericardial cyst. Recent experience and literature review. *Chest* 1986; 89:402–406.

225. Pezzano A, Belloni A, Faletra F, Binaghi G, Colli A, Rovelli F. Value of two-dimensional echocardiography in the diagnosis of pericardial cysts. *Eur Heart J* 1983; 4:238–246.

226. De Geeter B, Kretz JG, Nisand I, Eisenmann B, Kieny MT, Kieny R. Intrapericardial teratoma in a newborn infant: Use of fetal echocardiography. *Ann Thorac Surg* 1983; 35:664–666.

227. Reynolds JL, Donahue JK, Pearce CW. Intrapericardial teratoma: A cause of acute pericardial effusion in infancy. *Pediatrics* 1969; 43:71–78.

228. MacDonald S, Fay JE, Lynn RM. Intrapericardial teratoma: A continuing challenge. *Can J Surg* 1983; 26:81–82.

229. Maeta H, Hiyama T, Okamura K, Iriyama T, Yamaguchi T, Tamura T, et al. Successful excision of intracardiac teratoma. *J Thorac Cardiovasc Surg* 1982; 83:909–913.

230. Costas C, Williams RL, Fortune RL. Intracardiac teratoma in an infant. *Pediatr Cardiol* 1986; 7:179–181.

231. Sytman AL, MacAlpin RN. Primary pericardial mesothelioma: Report of two cases and review of the literature. *Am Heart J* 1971; 81:760–769.

232. Yilling FP, Schlant RC, Hertzler GL, Krzyaniak R. Pericardial mesothelioma. *Chest* 1982; 81:520–523.

233. Lazoglu AH, Da Silva MM, Iwahara M, Stelzer P, Marino N, Martinez A, et al. Primary pericardial sarcoma. *Am Heart J* 1994; 127:453–458.

234. Mason MS, Wheeler JR, Gregory RT, Gayle RG. Primary tumors of the aorta: Report of a case and review of the literature. *Oncology* 1982; 39:167–172.

235. Borislow DS, Floyd WL, Sane DC. Primary aortic sarcoma mimicking aortic dissection. *Am J Cardiol* 1989; 64:549–551.

236. Prichard RW. Tumors of the heart: Review of the subject and report of one hundred and fifty cases. *Arch Pathol* 1951; 51:98–128.

237. DeLoach JF, Haynes JW. Secondary tumors of heart and pericardium: Review of the subject and report of one hundred thirty-seven cases. *Arch Intern Med* 1953; 91:224–249.

238. Kutalek SP, Panidis IP, Kotler MN, Mintz GS, Carver J, Ross JJ. Metastatic tumors of the heart detected by two-dimensional echocardiography. *Am Heart J* 1985; 109:343–349.

239. Lockwood WB, Broghamer WL Jr. The changing prevalence of secondary cardiac neoplasms as related to cancer therapy. *Cancer* 1980; 45:2659–2662.

240. McDonnell PJ, Mann RB, Bulkley BH. Involvement of the heart by malignant lymphoma: A clinicopathologic study. *Cancer* 1982; 4:944–951.

241. Emmot WW, Vacek JL, Agee K, Moran J, Dunn MI. Metastatic malignant melanoma presenting clinically as obstruction of the right ventricular inflow and outflow tracts: Characterization by magnetic resonance imaging. *Chest* 1987; 92:362–364.

242. Weg IL, Mehra S, Azueta V, Rosner F. Cardiac metastasis from adenocarcinoma of the lung: Echocardiographic-pathologic correlation. *Am J Med* 1986; 80:108–112.

243. Kline IK. Cardiac lymphatic involvement by metastatic tumor. *Cancer* 1972; 29:799–808.

244. Hayashi J, Ohzeki H, Tsuchida S, Fujita Y, Tatebe S, Namura O, et al. Surgery for cavoatrial extension of malignant tumors. *Thorac Cardiovasc Surg* 1995; 43:161–164.

245. Hussain R, Neligan MC. Metastatic malignant schwannoma in the heart. *Ann Thorac Surg* 1993; 56:374–375.

246. el Allaf D, Burette R, Pierard L, Limet R. Cardiac tamponade as the first manifestation of cardiothoracic malignancy: A study of 10 cases. *Eur Heart J* 1986; 7:247–253.

247. Hernandez-Lopez E, Chahine RA. Simultaneous electrical and mechanical alternans in pericardial effusion: Echocardiographic documentation. *Arch Intern Med* 1980; 140:840–842.

248. Conrad SA, Byrnes TJ. Diastolic collapse of the left and right ventricles in cardiac tamponade. *Am Heart J* 1988; 115:475–478.

249. Levine MJ, Lorell BH, Diver DJ, Come PC. Implications of echocardiographically assisted diagnosis of pericardial tamponade in contemporary medical patients: Detection before hemodynamic embarrassment. *J Am Coll Cardiol* 1991; 17:59–65.

250. Himelman RB, Kircher B, Rockey DC, Schiller NB. Inferior vena cava plethora with blunted respiratory response: A sensitive echocardiographic sign of cardiac tamponade. *J Am Coll Cardiol* 1988; 12:1470–1477.

251. Picard MH, Sanfilippo AJ, Newell JB, Rodriguez L, Guerrero JL, Weyman AE. Quantitative relation between increased intrapericardial pressure and Doppler flow velocities during experimental cardiac tamponade. *J Am Coll Cardiol* 1991; 18:234–242.

252. Hatle LK, Appleton CP, Popp RL. Differentiation of constrictive pericarditis and restrictive cardiomyopathy by Doppler echocardiography. *Circulation* 1989; 79:357–370.

253. Burstow DJ, Oh JK, Bailey KR, Seward JB, Tajik AJ. Cardiac tamponade: Characteristic Doppler observations. *Mayo Clin Proc* 1989; 65:312–324.

254. Moncada R, Baker M, Salinas M, Demos TC, Churchill R, Love L, et al. Diagnostic role of computed tomography in pericardial heart disease: Congenital defects, thickening, neoplasms, and effusions. *Am Heart J* 1982; 103:263–282.

255. Kralstein J, Frishman W. Malignant pericardial diseases: Diagnosis and treatment. *Am Heart J* 1987; 113:785–790.

256. Millaire A, Wurtz A, de Groote P, Saudemont A, Chambon A, Ducloux G. Malignant pericardial effusions: Usefulness of pericardioscopy. *Am Heart J* 1992; 124:1030–1034.

257. Sheldon R, Isaac D. Metastatic melanoma to the heart presenting with ventricular tachycardia. *Chest* 1991; 99:1296–1298.

258. Redwine DB. Complete heart block caused by secondary tumors of the heart: Case report and review of literature. *Tex Med* 1974; 70:59–64.

259. Kubac G, Doris I, Ondro M, Davey PW. Malignant granular cell myoblastoma with metastatic cardiac involvement: Case report and echocardiogram. *Am Heart J* 1980; 100:227–229.

260. Esper RJ, Machado RA, Schapira L, de la Fuente LM, Favolaro RG. Loud systolic and diastolic murmurs originating on a right atrial metastatic tumor. *Chest* 1987; 91:926–927.

261. Kopelson G, Herwig KJU. The etiologies of coronary artery disease in cancer patients. *Int J Radiat Oncol Biol Phys* 1978; 4:895–896.

262. Hartman RB, Clarke PI, Schulman P. Pronounced and prolonged ST segment elevation: Pathognomonic sign of tumor invasion of the heart. *Arch Intern Med* 1982; 142:1917–1919.

263. Virmani R, Khedekar R, Robinowitz M, McAllister HA Jr. Tumor embolization in coronary artery causing myocardial infarction. *Arch Pathol Lab Med* 1983; 107:243–245.

264. Lubell DL, Goldfarb CR. Metastatic cardiac tumor demonstrated by 201 thallium scan. *Chest* 1980; 78:98–99.

265. Salem BI, Schnee M, Leatherman LL, de Castro CM, Benrey J. Electrocardiographic pseudo-infarction pattern: Appearance with a large posterior pericardial effusion after cardiac surgery. *Am J Cardiol* 1978; 42:681–685.

266. Nakayama DK, Norkool P, deLorimier AA, O'Neill JA Jr, D'Angio GJ. Intracardiac extension of Wilms' tumor: A report of the National Wilms' Tumor Study. *Ann Surg* 1986; 204:693–697.

267. Rothenberg DM, Brandt TD, D'Cruz I. Computed tomography of renal angiomyolipoma presenting as right atrial mass. *J Comput Assist Tomogr* 1986; 10:1054–1056.

268. Shahian DM, Libertino JA, Zinman LN, Leonardi HK, Eyre RC. Resection of cavoatrial renal cell carcinoma employing total circulatory arrest. *Arch Surg* 1990; 125:727–731.

269. Chua SO, Chiang CW, Lee YS, Lin SH, Liaw YF. Moving right atrial mass associated with hepatoma: Two cases detected by echocardiography. *Chest* 1986; 89:148–150.

270. Fujisaki M, Kurihara E, Kikuchi K, Nishikawa K, Uematsu Y. Hepatocellular carcinoma with tumor thrombus extending into the right atrium: Report of a successful resection with the use of cardiopulmonary bypass. *Surgery* 1991; 109:214–219.

271. Nakayama Y, Kitamura S, Kawachi K, Kawata T, Fukutomi M, Hasegawa J, et al. Intravenous leiomyomatosis extending into the right atrium. *Cardiovasc Surg* 1994; 2:642–645.

272. Griffin AS, Sterchi JM. Primary leiomyosarcoma of the inferior vena cava: A case report and review of the literature. *J Surg Oncol* 1987; 34:53–60.

273. Peh WC, Cheung DL, Ngan H. Smooth muscle tumors of the inferior vena cava and right heart. *Clin Imaging* 1993; 17:117–123.

274. Birmingham CL, Peretz DI. Metastatic carcinoma presenting as obstruction to the right ventricular outflow tract: Report of a case and review of the literature. *Am Heart J* 1979; 97:229–232.

275. Stark RM, Perloff JH, Glick HJ, Hirshfeld JW, Devereux RB. Clinical recognition and management of cardiac metastatic disease: Observations in a unique case of alveolar soft-part sarcoma. *Am J Med* 1977; 63:653–659.

276. Steffens TG, Mayer HS, Das SK. Echocardiographic diagnosis of a right ventricular metastatic tumor. *Arch Intern Med* 1980; 140:122–123.

277. Bartels P, O'Callaghan WG, Peyton R, Sethi G, Maley T. Metastatic liposarcoma of the right ventricle with outflow tract obstruction: Restrictive pathophysiology predicts poor surgical outcome. *Am Heart J* 1988; 115:696–698.

278. Luck SR, DeLeon S, Shkolnik A, Morgan E, Labotka R. Intracardiac Wilms' tumor: Diagnosis and management. *J Pediatr Surg* 1982; 17:551–554.

279. Kaku K, Kawashima Y, Kitamura S, Morgan E, Labotka R. Resection of leiomyosarcoma originating in internal iliac vein and extending into heart via inferior vena cava. *Surgery* 1981; 89:604–611.

280. Van Osdol KD, Hall RJ, Warda M, Massumi A, Klima T. Right ventricular thrombus: Clinical and diagnostic features. *Tex Heart Inst J* 1983; 10:359–364.

281. Heitzman M, Gibson TC, Tabakin BS. A right-sided cardiac mass. *Arch Intern Med* 1984; 144:1813–1815.

282. Schrem SS, Colvin SB, Weinreb JC, Glassman E, Kronzon I. Metastatic cardiac liposarcoma: Diagnosis by transesophageal echocardiography and magnetic resonance imaging. *J Am Soc Echocardiogr* 1990; 3:149–153.

283. Watts FB Jr, Zingas AP, Das L, Cushing BA. Computed tomographic diagnosis of an intracardiac metastasis from osteosarcoma. *J Comput Tomogr* 1983; 7:271–272.

284. Wolverson MK, Grider RD, Sundaram M, Heiberg E, Johnson F. Demonstration of unsuspected malignant disease of the pericardium by computed tomography. *J Comput Tomogr* 1980; 4:330–333.

285. Salcedo EE, Cohen GI, White RD, Davison MB. Cardiac tumors: Diagnosis and management. *Curr Probl Cardiol* 1992; 17:73–137.

286. Gatenby RA, Hartz WH, Kessler HB. Percutaneous catheter drainage for malignant pericardial effusion. *J Vasc Intervent Radiol* 1991; 2:151–155.

287. Hanley PC, Shub C, Seward JB, Wold LE. Intracavitary cardiac melanoma diagnosed by endomyocardial left ventricular biopsy. *Chest* 1983; 84:195–198.

288. Gosalakkal JA, Sugrue DD. Malignant melanoma of the right atrium: Antemortem diagnosis by transvenous biopsy. *Br Heart J* 1989; 62:159–160.

289. Seibert KA, Rettenmier CW, Waller BF, Battle WE, Levine AS, Roberts WC. Osteogenic sarcoma metastatic to the heart. *Am J Med* 1982; 73:136–141.

290. Quraishi MA, Costanzi JJ, Hokanson J. The natural history of lung cancer with pericardial metastases. *Cancer* 1983; 51:740–742.

291. Warda M, Khan A, Massumi A, Mathur V, Klima T, Hall RJ. Radiation-induced valvular dysfunction. *J Am Coll Cardiol* 1983; 2:180–185.

292. McAllister HA Jr, Hall RJ. Iatrogenic heart disease. In: Cheng TO, ed. *The International Textbook of Cardiology.* New York: Pergamon; 1986; 871–873.

293. Primrose WR, Clee MD, Johnston RN. Malignant pericardial effusion managed with vinblastine. *Clin Oncol* 1983; 9:67–70.

294. Sheppard FA, Morgan C, Evans WK, Ginsberg JF, Watt D, Murphy K. Medical management of malignant pericardial effusion by tetracycline sclerosis. *Am J Cardiol* 1987; 60:1161–1166.

295. Chan A, Rischin D, Clarke CP, Woodruff RK. Subxiphoid partial pericardiectomy with or without sclerosant instillation in the treatment of symptomatic pericardial effusions in patients with malignancy. *Cancer* 1991; 68:1021–1025.

296. Hankins JR, Satterfield JR, Aisner J, Wiernik PH, McLaughlin JS. Pericardial window for malignant pericardial effusion. *Ann Thorac Surg* 1980; 30:465–471.

297. Prager RL, Wilson CH, Bender HW Jr. The subxiphoid approach to pericardial disease. *Ann Thorac Surg* 1982; 34:6–9.

298. Palacios IF, Tuzcu EM, Ziskind AA, Younger J, Block PC. Percutaneous balloon pericardial window for patients with malignant pericardial effusion and tamponade. *Cathet Cardiovasc Diagn* 1991; 22:244–249.

299. Melvin KN, Howard RJ, Rakowski H, Goldman BS, El-Maraghi NRH. Embryonal carcinoma of the testis with metastases to the right atrium *Can J Surg* 1983; 26:86–88.

300. Poole GV Jr, Meredith JW, Breyer RH, Mills SA. Surgical implications in malignant cardiac disease. *Ann Thorac Surg* 1983; 36:484–491.

301. Lagrange JL, Despins P, Spielman M, Le Chevalier T, de Lajartre AY, Fontaine F, et al. Cardiac metastases: Case report on an isolated cardiac metastasis of a myxoid liposarcoma. *Cancer* 1986; 58:2333–2337.

302. Pillai R, Blauth C, Peckham M, Hendry W, Barrett A, Goldstraw P. Intracardiac metastases from malignant teratoma of the testis. *J Thorac Cardiovasc Surg* 1986; 92:118–120.

303. Chen RH, Gaos CM, Frazier OH. Complete resection of a right atrial intracavitary metastatic melanoma. *Ann Thorac Surg* 1996; 61:1255–1257.

304. Wiske PS, Gillam LD, Blyden G, Weyman AE. Intracardiac tumor regression documented by two-dimensional echocardiography. *Am J Cardiol* 1986; 58:186–187.

305. Atay AE, Alpert MA, Kleinsteuber WK, Freelon RL. Prolonged survival associated with spontaneous disappearance of untreated right atrial intracavitary metastasis. *Am Heart J* 1987; 114:437–440.

306. Lynch M, Balk MA, Lee RB, Martin RP. Role of transesophageal echocardiography in the management of patients with bronchogenic carcinoma invading the left atrium. *Am J Cardiol* 1995; 76:1101–1102.

307. Terry LN, Kligerman MM. Pericardial and myocardial involvement by lymphomas and leukemias. *Cancer* 1970; 25:1003–1008.

308. Schwartz JB, Shamsuddin AM. The effects of leukemic infiltrates in various organs in chronic lymphocytic leukemia. *Hum Pathol* 1981; 12:432–440.

309. Meltzer V, Korompai FL, Mathur VS, Guinn GA. Surgical treatment of leukemic involvement of the mitral valve. *Chest* 1975; 67:119–121.

310. Applefeld MM, Milner SD, Vigorito RD, Shamsuddin AM. Congestive heart failure and endocardial fibroelastosis caused by chronic lymphocytic leukemia. *Cancer* 1980; 46:1479–1484.

311. Björkholm M, Ost A, Biberfeld P. Myocardial rupture with cardiac tamponade as a lethal early manifestation of acute myeloblastic leukemia. *Cancer* 1982; 50:1867–1869.

312. Cassis N Jr, Porterfield J, Rogers JS. Massive hemopericardium as the initial manifestation of chronic myelogenous leukemia. *Arch Intern Med* 1982; 142:2193–2194.

313. Liepman MK, Goodlerner S. Surgical management of pericardial tamponade as a presenting manifestation of acute leukemia. *J Surg Oncol* 1981; 17:183–188.

314. Crofts MA, Morgan-Capner P, Sharp JC, Mcleod AA, Keates JR, Jackson G, et al. Fungal endocarditis in a patient with acute leukaemia treated by valve replacement. *Br Med J* 1982; 284:574–575.

315. Wong DWH, Guthaner DF, Gordon EP, Mitchell RS. Lymphoma of the heart. *Cathet Cardiovasc Diagn* 1984; 10:377–384.

316. Stotka JL. Cardiac Kaposi's sarcoma in a patient with acquired immunodeficiency syndrome. *N Y State J Med* 1992; 92:332–333.

317. Acierno L. Cardiac complications in acquired immunodeficiency syndrome (AIDS): A review. *J Am Coll Cardiol* 1989; 13:1144–1154.

318. Lewis W. AIDS. Cardiac findings from 115 autopsies. *Prog Cardiovasc Dis* 1989; 32:207–215.

319. Steigman CK, Anderson DW, Macher AM, Sennesh JD, Virmani R. Fatal cardiac tamponade in acquired immunodeficiency syndrome with epicardial Kaposi's sarcoma. *Am Heart J* 1988; 116:1105–1107.

320. Goldfarb A, King CL, Rosenzweig BP, Feit F, Kamat BR, Rumancik WM, et al. Cardiac lymphoma in the acquired immunodeficiency syndrome. *Am Heart J* 1989; 118:1340–1344.

321. Aboulafia DM, Bush R, Picozzi VJ. Cardiac tamponade due to primary pericardial lymphoma in a patient with AIDS. *Chest* 1994; 106:1295–1299.

322. Pousset F, Le Heuzey JY, Pialoux G, Rinaldi JP, Hernigou A, Mousseaux E, et al. Cardiac lymphoma presenting as atrial flutter in an AIDS patient. *Eur Heart J* 1994; 15:862–864.

323. Andress JD, Polish LB, Clark DM, Hossack KF. Transvenous biopsy diagnosis of cardiac lymphoma in an AIDS patient. *Am Heart J* 1989; 118:421–423.

324. Horowitz MD, Cox MM, Neibart RM, Blaker AM, Interian A Jr. Resection of right atrial lymphoma in a patient with AIDS. *Int J Cardiol* 1992; 34:139–142.

325. Schiller VL, Fishbein MC, Siegel RJ. Unusual cardiac involvement in carcinoid syndrome. *Am Heart J* 1986; 112:1322–1323.

326. Le Metayer P, Constans J, Bernard N, Roudaut R, Pellegrin JL, Lacoste D, et al. Carcinoid heart disease: Two cases of left heart involvement diagnosed by transthoracic and transoesophageal echocardiography. *Eur Heart J* 1993; 14:1721–1723.

327. Pellikka PA, Tajik AJ, Khandheria BK, Seward JB, Callahan JA, Pitot HC, et al. Carcinoid heart disease: Clinical and echocardiographic spectrum in 74 patients. *Circulation* 1993; 87:1188–1196.

328. Strickman NE, Hall RJ. Carcinoid heart disease. In: Kapoor AS, Reynolds RD, eds. *Cancer and the Heart.* New York: Springer-Verlag; 1986:135–156.

329. Artaza A, Beiner JA, Gonzalez M, Aranda I, de Teresa EG, Pulpon LA. Carcinoid heart disease: Report of a case secondary to a pure carcinoid tumour of the ovary. *Eur Heart J* 1985; 6:800–805.

330. Sane DC, Feldman JM. A blush from the heart. *Chest* 1987; 92:360–361.

331. Mattingly TW. The functioning carcinoid tumor: A serendipity in diagnosis. *Trans Am Clin Climatol Assoc* 1965; 77:190–204.

332. Robiolio PA, Rigolin VH, Wilson JS, Harrison JK, Sanders LL, Bashore TM, et al. Carcinoid heart disease: Correlation of high serotonin levels with valvular abnormalities detected by cardiac catheterization and echocardiography. *Circulation* 1995; 92:790–795.

333. Topol EJ, Fortuin NJ. Coronary artery spasm and cardiac arrest in carcinoid heart disease. *Am J Med* 1984; 77:950–952.

334. Millward MJ, Blake MP, Byrne MJ, Hung J, Gibson P. Left heart involvement with cardiac shunt complicating carcinoid heart disease. *Aust NZ J Med* 1989; 19:716–717.

335. McAllister HA Jr. Endocrine diseases and the cardiovascular system. In: Silver MD, ed. *Cardiovascular Pathology,* 2d ed. New York: Churchill Livingstone; 1991:1181–1204.

336. Lundin L, Funa K, Hansson HE, Wilander E, Oberg K. Histochemical and immunohistochemical morphology of carcinoid heart disease. *Pathol Res Pract* 1991; 187:73–77.

337. Waltenberger J, Lundin L, Oberg K, Wilander E, Miyazono K, Heldin CH, et al. Involvement of transforming growth factor-beta in the formation of fibrotic lesions in carcinoid heart disease. *Am J Pathol* 1993; 142:71–78.

338. Grahame-Smith DG. The carcinoid syndrome. In: Bondy PK, Rosenberg LE, eds. *Metabolic Control and Disease,* 8th ed. Philadelphia: Saunders; 1980:1695–1707.

339. Kvols LK, Moertel CG, O'Connell MJ, Schutt AJ, Rubin J, Hahn RG. Treatment of the malignant carcinoid syndrome: Evaluation of a long-acting somatostatin analogue. *N Engl J Med* 1986; 315:663–666.

340. Oates JA. The carcinoid syndrome. *N Engl J Med* 1986; 315:702–704.

341. Ridker PM, Chertow GM, Karlson EW, Neish AS, Schoen FJ. Bioprosthetic tricuspid valve stenosis associated with extensive plaque deposition in carcinoid heart disease. *Am Heart J* 1991; 121:1835–1838.

342. Ohri SK, Schofield JB, Hodgson H, Oakley CM, Keogh BE. Carcinoid heart disease: Early failure of an allograft valve replacement. *Ann Thorac Surg* 1994; 58:1161–1163.

343. Onate A, Alcibar J, Inguanzo R, Pena N, Gochi R. Balloon dilation of tricuspid and pulmonary valves in carcinoid heart disease. *Tex Heart Inst J* 1993; 20:115–119.

344. Hargreaves AD, Pringle SD, Boon NA. Successful balloon dilatation of the pulmonary valve in carcinoid heart disease. *Int J Cardiol* 1994; 45:150–151.

345. Knott-Craig CJ, Schaff HV, Mullany CJ, Kvols LK, Moertel CG, Edwards WD, et al. Carcinoid disease of the heart: Surgical management of ten patients. *J Thorac Cardiovasc Surg* 1992; 104:475–481.

346. Robiolio PA, Rigolin VH, Harrison JK, Lowe JE, Moore JO, Bashore TM, et al. Predictors of outcome of tricuspid valve replacement in carcinoid heart disease. *Am J Cardiol* 1995; 75:485–488.

347. Connolly HM, Nishimura RA, Smith HC, Pellikka PA, Mullany CJ, Kvols LK. Outcome of cardiac surgery for carcinoid heart disease. *J Am Coll Cardiol* 1995; 25:410–416.

348. Propst JW, Siegel LC, Stover EP. Anesthetic considerations for valve replacement surgery in a patient with carcinoid syndrome. *J Cardiothorac Vasc Anesth* 1994; 8:209–212.

349. Neustein SM, Cohen E. Anesthesia for aortic and mitral valve replacement in a patient with carcinoid heart disease. *Anesthesiology* 1995; 82:1067–1070.

87

TRAUMATIC HEART DISEASE

Panagiotis N. Symbas

Accidental or intentional trauma is the leading cause of death, hospitalization, and loss of working days in our society, particularly among young people.[1–3] Cardiac and great-vessel injuries are a major contributor to this mortality and morbidity.[4] The heart and/or great vessels may be injured from penetrating and nonpenetrating trauma. Since the diagnostic and therapeutic modalities for the management of heart diseases have become more complex and more invasive, mechanical injuries to the heart due to iatrogenic trauma have become increasingly important. These result from the complications of various diagnostic, therapeutic, and resuscitative procedures, including cardiac catheterization, percutaneous coronary angioplasty,[5,6] percutaneous aortic or mitral valvuloplasty,[7,8] insertion of pacemaker leads[9] or Swan-Ganz catheters,[10] closed- and open-chest cardiac massage, and electric defibrillation.[11,12] The increasing use of invasive catheters has also led to the more frequent migration of these catheters to the heart or pulmonary vascular beds[13–15] and to nonbacterial thrombotic endocarditis and bacterial endocarditis.

Two other types of cardiac trauma not due to mechanical injury warrant separate classification. The first type includes injury to the heart from ionizing radiation, which predominantly causes pericarditis but may also result in myocardial injury.[16–18] The second includes the group of cardiac injuries due to electric current,[19,20] which may cause asystole, ventricular fibrillation, other arrhythmias, and myocardial injury (see also Chap. 80).

Many nonpenetrating injuries and an occasional penetrating injury of the heart are well tolerated. Thus, many of these lesions are diagnosed infrequently, since their initial clinical manifestations may be none or relatively mild, and the lesion may be overlooked unless a high index of suspicion is maintained and specific studies are obtained.[21,22] Frequently, these cardiac injuries are overshadowed by the more overt manifestations of cerebral, abdominal, or musculoskeletal trauma. For these reasons and because only the more severe injuries are reflected in autopsy studies, the actual incidence of traumatic heart disease remains obscure.

PENETRATING INJURIES

Penetrating injuries are usually observed with wounds of the precordium but may also be associated with wounds elsewhere in the chest, neck, or upper abdomen. They are usually due to missile or knife wounds but are occasionally caused by a missile embolus reaching the heart through the venous system or by a needle migrating through the esophagus.

Penetrating Cardiac Trauma

Although penetrating cardiac trauma frequently involves only the free cardiac wall, injury to cardiac valves, chordae tendineae, papillary muscles, atrial or ventricular septum, coronary arteries, and conduction system may occur. The multiplicity of heart and great vessel lesions that may be produced by penetrating wounds is indicated in Table 87-1.

The relative frequency of a single, penetrating wound of the free cardiac wall is due to its area of exposure on the anterior chest wall. In decreasing order of frequency, the structures affected are the right ventricle, left ventricle, right atrium, and left atrium.[23] The cardiac wounds may be single or multiple; the latter are more commonly caused by missiles.[23,24] Over 50 percent of victims with penetrating cardiac trauma succumb shortly after injury.[25] The remaining survive for varying periods of time; many can recover completely if treated immediately.

The pathophysiologic consequences and clinical manifestations of penetrating injuries to the heart depend upon the size and site of the wound, the mode of injury, and especially the state of the pericardial wound. When the pericardial wound remains open and bleeding occurs freely into the pleural space, there are signs and symptoms of hemothorax and loss of circulating blood volume. When there is intrapericardial hemorrhage with a sealed pericardial wound, cardiac tamponade (Chap. 81) is the presenting clinical picture. The diagnosis of

TABLE 87-1

PENETRATING WOUNDS OF THE HEART

I. Pericardial damage
  A. Laceration or perforation
  B. Hemopericardium with or without cardiac tamponade
  C. Serofibrinous or suppurative pericarditis
  D. Pneumopericardium
  E. Constrictive pericarditis
II. Myocardial damage
  A. Laceration
  B. Penetration or perforation
  C. Retained foreign body
  D. Structural defects
    1. Aneurysm formation
    2. Septal defects
    3. Aorticocardiac fistula
III. Valvular injury
  A. Leaflet or cusp injury
  B. Papillary muscle or chordae tendineae laceration
IV. Coronary artery injury
  A. Laceration or thrombosis with or without myocardial infarction
  B. Arteriovenous fistula
  C. Aneurysm
V. Embolism
  A. Foreign body
  B. Thrombus (septic or sterile)
VI. Infective endocarditis
VII. Rhythm or conduction disturbances

Source: Prepared by Loren F. Parmley, MD, and Thomas W. Mattingly, and modified with permission.

cardiac injury should be suspected in a patient with chest, lower neck, epigastric, or especially precordial penetrating wounds and with symptoms and signs of cardiac tamponade and/or hemothorax and loss of circulating blood volume. The management of penetrating wounds of the heart consists of immediate thoracotomy and cardiorrhaphy.[23,25–30] When this cannot be done or while appropriate arrangements are being made for thoracotomy, the patient's blood volume should be expanded; pericardiocentesis is performed only to provide time for a safe operation.[23,31]

Although the management of the symptomatic patients with a suspected penetrating cardiac wound is clearly defined, the management of the asymptomatic patients with a penetrating precordial wound presented a considerable dilemma in the past, when the options were either exploratory surgery or observation. Currently, the use of echocardiography, either by a cardiologist or preferably by an immediately available and specially trained trauma surgeon, facilitates and makes the treatment of these patients safer by avoiding unnecessary surgery or observation, with its accompanying risk of sudden deterioration and even death.[32]

Residual or Delayed Sequelae of Penetrating Cardiac Trauma

Patients with penetrating cardiac wounds should be closely observed immediately postoperatively and after discharge for clinical manifestations of residual or delayed sequelae from the penetrating cardiac wounds. Such sequelae may include the following: (1) ventricular or atrial septal defect; (2) injury of valve cups, leaflets, or chordae tendineae; (3) aortocardiac or aortopulmonary communication, or communication from the coronary artery to the coronary vein or to the cardiac chamber; (4) ventricular aneurysms; (5) posttraumatic or postoperative pericarditis; and (6) electrocardiographic abnormalities.[33,34] When symptoms and signs of a structural defect are detected, echocardiography and/or cardiac catheterization should be performed to define the lesion and its hemodynamic significance and to determine the proper mode of therapy.[33,35]

Recurrent posttraumatic pericarditis, which is similar to the postcardiotomy syndrome seen after cardiac surgery, occurs in approximately 20 percent of all cases of penetrating heart wounds. Symptomatic management is the treatment of choice for this syndrome unless cardiac tamponade or other sequelae, such as purulent or constrictive pericarditis, require surgical intervention.

Missile wounds may also result in the presence of a projectile within the heart following either a direct injury to the heart or an injury to a systemic vein, with subsequent migration of the missile to the heart. The missile or the thrombus associated with it may embolize into the systemic or pulmonary arteries.[36–38] Bacterial endocarditis may also occur if the projectile is not completely embedded in the myocardium.[39,40] Rarely, the patient with a projectile in the heart may develop cardiac neurosis, with an almost maniacal desire for removal of the foreign body.[41] In many patients, however, the retained missile in the heart results in no ill effects over a long period of observation.[42,43] Therefore, the treatment of missiles in the heart should be individualized according to the patient's clinical course and the location, size, and shape of the missile.[42,43] Missiles that cause symptoms should be removed. Similarly, missiles that are free or partially protruding into a left cardiac chamber should be removed, because their embolization to the systemic arterial system may have serious consequences.[42,43] Missiles in the right side of the heart may either be removed or be left to embolize to the pulmonary vascular bed, from which they can easily be retrieved.[37] Intramyocardial or intrapericardial bullets or pellets are generally well tolerated and may be left in place.

A missile that has embolized to the systemic arterial bed should be surgically removed without delay unless it has resulted in a significant neurologic deficit.[38] Projectiles adjacent to or embedded within the wall of one of the great or coronary arteries should be extracted to prevent subsequent erosion and bleeding.

Coronary Artery Penetrating Trauma

Coronary artery injuries can result in cardiac tamponade and varying degrees of myocardial ischemia or myocardial infarction. The management of these wounds is dependent on the amount of myocardium at risk. Wounds of major branches of the coronary arterial system are repaired or bypassed, whereas small terminal vessels are ligated. Coronary artery aneurysms and arteriovenous fistulas are rare sequelae of injury, and their treatment should be individualized.[44]

Penetrating Trauma of the Aorta and Great Vessels

The pathophysiology of penetrating wounds to the great vessels is quite similar to that of penetrating wounds to the heart and depends on whether the site of the wound is intra- or extrapericardial.[45,46] In addition to the obvious results of either immediate or delayed hemorrhage, a penetrating wound of a great vessel may result in the formation of a false aneurysm, with possible subsequent rupture, or of an arteriovenous fistula, producing either immediate or latent signs and symptoms of congestive heart failure.[47] Traumatic arteriovenous fistulas are occasionally complicated by the development of bacterial endarteritis and endocarditis.[48] These traumatic vascular lesions should be detected and repaired as soon as possible.

NONPENETRATING INJURIES

The vast majority of blunt injuries to the heart are due to automobile accidents, although other forms of trauma from contact sports, altercations, falls, and so on may also result in such an injury. The cardiac injury is usually caused by direct compressing or decelerating forces delivered to the chest or, rarely, by an indirect force delivered to the abdomen or even to the extremities that results in a marked increase in intravascular pressures. A wide variety of injuries are produced by nonpenetrating trauma (Table 87-2).

Cardiac Contusion

Contusion of the heart usually refers to blunt injury to the heart causing identifiable histopathologic changes within the myocardium. The pathologic lesions of myocardial contusion vary considerably in extent and character, ranging from small areas of petechiae or ecchymosis, which may be either subepicardial or subendocardial, to contusion of the full thickness of the myocardial wall with or without rupture of the heart.[1]

Histologically, various degrees of subepicardial or intramyocardial hemorrhage or disruption of the myocardial fibers and leukocyte infiltration and edema may be present.[1] The forces that produce nonpenetrating lesions of the heart and great vessels are such that external evidence of chest injury may be meager or undetectable in almost one-third of the traumatized patients. This lack of evidence of chest wall injury and the frequent absence of symptoms from the cardiac or vascular injury—along with the common presence of other more obvious injuries to the body—may impede the early diagnosis of a cardiovascular injury.

TABLE 87-2
NONPENETRATING TRAUMA OF THE HEART

1. Pericardial injury
   a. Hemopericardium
   b. Rupture or laceration
   c. Serofibrinous pericarditis
   d. Constrictive pericarditis
2. Myocardial injury
   a. Contusion
   b. Rupture of free cardiac wall, early or delayed
   c. Rupture of septum
   d. Aneurysm
   e. Laceration
3. Disturbances of rhythm or conduction
4. Valve injury
   a. Rupture of valve leaflets, cusp, or chordae tendineae
   b. Contusion of papillary muscle
5. Coronary artery injury
   a. Thrombosis with or without myocardial infarction
   b. Arteriovenous fistula
   c. Laceration with or without myocardial infarction
6. Great-vessel injury
   a. Rupture
   b. Aneurysm formation
   c. Aorta–cardiac chamber fistula
   d. Thrombotic occlusion

Patients with contusion of the heart are commonly asymptomatic, but they may complain of pain that is identical in character, location, and radiation to the pain of myocardial ischemia and/or myocardial infarction.[49] The pain is usually transient unless there is concomitant coronary artery injury or occult atherosclerotic coronary heart disease.[50] Coronary thrombosis can result from nonpenetrating trauma, but this is rare and is usually associated with existing atherosclerotic coronary artery disease.[51] In 546 necropsy cases of nonpenetrating cardiac trauma, no instance of coronary thrombosis was found. Dyspnea and hypotension may also be presenting symptoms. In mild or moderate myocardial contusion, these signs may be transient and are usually absent. Cardiac failure is relatively rare; when it is present, the possibility of an associated cardiac injury, such as rupture of the ventricular septum or of one of the cardiac valves, is great. Hemopericardium, with or without signs and symptoms of cardiac tamponade, may be associated with myocardial contusion. Laceration of a coronary artery from nonpenetrating injury may also occur rarely, producing cardiac tamponade or a coronary artery fistula.[52]

The diagnosis of cardiac contusion should be suspected in all patients with significant blunt trauma, particularly to the precordium. Unfortunately, none of the currently available diagnostic tests for myocardial contusion can conclusively establish the diagnosis in all patients. The appropriate use and interpretation of the available tests, however, assist in the diagnosis of myocardial contusion with reasonable accuracy.

Electrocardiography has been the most widely used test for the diagnosis of contusion of the heart. Various electrocardiographic abnormalities have been considered indicative of cardiac contusion, such as nonspecific ST-T or Q-wave changes, supraventricular tachyarrhythmias, and ventricular arrhythmias, including fibrillation, which is usually the cause of death at the time of the traumatic impact.[53-55] On the other hand, a variety of other clinical conditions[56-59] that are frequently present in traumatized patients (i.e., pain, anxiety, hemorrhage, hypoxia, hypokalemia, head trauma, alcohol or cocaine) may cause many of these abnormalities. Therefore, the presence of these other causes must be excluded before the electrocardiographic abnormalities are attributed to contusion of the heart.[60-62]

Elevation of the serum level of the MB fraction of creatinine kinase (CK) has been extrapolated from its use in acute myocardial infarction as a diagnostic aid in patients with cardiac contusion. Other clinical conditions that cause elevation in this enzyme—i.e., tachyarrhythmias and skeletal muscle diseases, including major trauma (see Chap. 47)—must be excluded before an abnormal level is ascribed to contusion of the heart.[60-62]

Radioisotope imaging of the heart in dogs with experimentally produced cardiac contusion has identified the area of injury only in animals with full-thickness contusion.[63] Therefore, this is of diagnostic value in only a limited number of patients, since the incidence of full-thickness contusion is rare in patients surviving the initial traumatic impact.

Two-dimensional transthoracic and transesophageal echocardiography (TTE and TEE) are useful in the diagnosis of cardiac contusion and particularly of the structural lesions associated with cardiac contusion.[64-66] The sensitivity and specificity of these tests for diagnosing contusion of the heart, however, has not been clearly defined (see also Chap. 14).

The treatment of myocardial contusion is symptomatic. Appropriate limitation of activity and prevention and early treatment of arrhythmias are the most important therapeutic measures. The possible increased sensitivity of the heart to medications must also be considered when one is deciding what drugs to use in the patient with recent trauma.

Anticoagulants should not be administered because they may cause bleeding within the myocardium or pericardial space. Digitalis should be used in the presence of congestive heart failure or atrial fibrillation, and antiarrhythmic agents should be used for control of ectopic rhythms. If the myocardial contusion is severe, support with inotropic drugs (Chap. 23) may be necessary. When all these measures fail, balloon counterpulsation may be utilized.[67]

Cardiac Rupture

Although minor, insignificant myocardial contusion of the right ventricle is the most frequent blunt cardiac injury, the most fatal lesion is rupture of the heart. The rupture may occur in the free cardiac wall or the ventricular septum. Rupture of the free cardiac wall is extremely difficult to diagnose and treat in a timely manner because of the frequently rapid demise of the patient and because traumatic cardiac rupture is often only one of many other severe bodily injuries. As a result, rupture of the heart has frequently not been amenable to therapy. Readily available echocardiography in some emergency rooms, however, may increase the number of successfully treated patients. The surgical repair of interventricular septal rupture is accomplished optimally after medical therapy has stabilized the patient's hemodynamics.

Residual or Delayed Sequelae of Blunt Injury to the Heart

Contusion of the heart usually heals with little or no obvious scar or impairment of cardiac function. Large contusions, however, may cause a decrease in cardiac output, and extensive necrosis may lead to either rupture or, rarely, congestive heart failure and formation of a true or false aneurysm.[68,69] Cardiac aneurysms may cause arrhythmias, congestive heart failure, rupture, and mural thrombosis with embolism. Because of these complications, surgical repair of traumatic aneurysm is usually advisable. Localized areas of necrosis and hemorrhage involving the cardiac conduction system may produce varying degrees of atrioventricular block or any of the different types of intraventricular conduction defects.

The most commonly injured valve in surviving patients is the aortic valve, with aortic regurgitation characteristically causing the rapid development of congestive heart failure.[70] Injury of the atrioventricular valves is an infrequent result of nonpenetrating cardiac injury and usually occurs in the presence of severe cardiac trauma resulting in death. Rupture of the mitral valve leaflet can have hemodynamic consequences somewhat similar to those of aortic valve injury but is rarely encountered clinically. In contrast, tricuspid valve injury may be tolerated for years before surgical correction is required.[71]

Rupture of the papillary muscle or chordae tendineae occurs more frequently than rupture of valve leaflets. Cardiac contusion may also cause papillary muscle dysfunction with secondary mitral or tricuspid regurgitation.[72] The clinical outcome depends on whether the structures involved are on the right side of the heart, where the lesion may be well tolerated, or on the left side, where the high-pressure system can lead to more serious hemodynamic sequelae. The murmurs produced by these lesions are generally typical of valvular regurgitation, but unusual high-pitched systolic and diastolic murmurs of variable loudness may also result (see Chap. 10). Traumatic tricuspid regurgitation may be present despite the absence of any detectable murmur.[73] Prompt and correct diagnosis by echocardiographic, hemodynamic, and angiographic studies is important. Patients with hemodynamically significant valvular injury should undergo valvuloplasty or valve replacement.

Pericardial lesions are often overlooked and often heal without incident. Hemopericardium may occur but usually is due to the coexisting myocardial injury. When the hemorrhage is severe, cardiac tamponade will occur rapidly. When the oozing of blood or serum into the pericardium is slow, however, dilatation of the pericardial sac can develop over an extended period of time.

Posttraumatic pericarditis, which is similar to the post–myocardial infarction syndrome, develops less frequently with blunt than with penetrating cardiac injuries. The symptoms and signs of posttraumatic pericarditis are similar to those of pericarditis produced by a wide variety of causes (see Chap. 81). When hemopericardium or hydropericardium is suspected, echocardiography can confirm the diagnosis. Pericardial laceration is usually well tolerated, but herniation of the heart may occur, leading to more serious consequences and death.[74,75]

Aortic Rupture

Rupture of the aorta is the most common blunt injury of the great vessels. Rupture or avulsion of the innominate, carotid, or left subclavian arteries or the venae cavae has also been observed. Because of the variety of mechanical forces produced by blunt trauma (Fig. 87-1) combined with anatomic factors, the most common sites of rupture of the aorta from blunt injury are the descending aorta just distal to the origin of the left subclavian artery (aortic isthmus) and the ascending aorta just proximal to the origin of the brachycephalic artery.[76,77] Because of the high incidence of severe cardiac injury in patients with rupture of the ascending aorta, most patients who survive aortic rupture long enough to receive definitive surgical correction are those who have sustained rupture of the aortic isthmus. Occasionally, rupture at the aortic arch and at other sites of the descending and even the abdominal aorta may occur. About 20 percent of the patients with aortic rupture survive the original injury. A false aneurysm is formed in these patients at the site of rupture, the

wall of which consists of adventitia and/or parietal pleura and other mediastinal structures. The intactness of these structures maintains continuity of the circulation.

The common manifestations of traumatic rupture of the aorta are chest and/or midscapular pain, a new murmur, increased pulse amplitude, and hypertension of the upper extremities.[78] Some patients, however, are surprisingly free of any major symptoms or signs from the aortic rupture. Hoarseness, evidence of a superior vena cava syndrome, paraplegia, and anuria are rare manifestations. Although there are occasionally no obvious signs of external injury, patients with rupture of the aorta usually have associated injuries of the skeleton, abdominal viscera, or central nervous system, which can mask the signs of aortic rupture. For this reason, *any patient who has sustained severe blunt trauma or who has been exposed to major deceleration forces should be suspected of having aortic rupture if there is an increased pulse pressure, upper extremity hypertension, and especially widening of the upper mediastinal silhouette.*

Chest roentgenography is of great diagnostic value in patients with aortic rupture. Widening of the superior mediastinal shadow, depression of the left main bronchus, displacement of the trachea and esophagus to the right, and especially obliteration of the aortic knob shadow are common roentgenographic abnormalities associated with injury at the aortic isthmus (Fig. 87-2). Widening of the mediastinum has also been observed in all cases with rupture of the aortic arch and in about 79 percent with rupture of the ascending aorta (Fig. 87-3).[79] The most definitive procedure to establish the diagnosis of aortic rupture is aortography, which should be performed immediately in all patients whose history, physical examination, and particularly chest roentgenogram suggest the possibility of this injury. Aortography should include the entire aorta, since rupture may occur at sites other than the aortic segment just distal to the origin of the left subclavian artery. Computed tomography scanning is also widely used to evaluate patients with a widened mediastinum.[80] The approximately 55 percent sensitivity and 65 percent sensitivity of this test limit its contribution to the definitive management of these patients.[81] TEE appears to be a useful diagnostic test[66] (see Chap. 14), but at present there is no comprehensive study on its diagnostic value for aortic rupture. Until further experience is gained, caution should be exercised when it is used as the sole technique for establishing the diagnosis. Surgical treatment should then be undertaken as soon as possible, with particular attention to protection of the spinal cord.

A chronic false aortic aneurysm may be discovered months or years after blunt trauma to the great vessels. Rupture of the aneurysm may occur at any time after its formation. Rarely, the complications of peripheral embolization from the thrombus contained within the aneurysm or the development of bacterial endoarteritis or chronic pseudocoarctation may occur.[81] Because of the relative instability of these aneurysms and the potential complications, surgical correction is the treatment of choice.

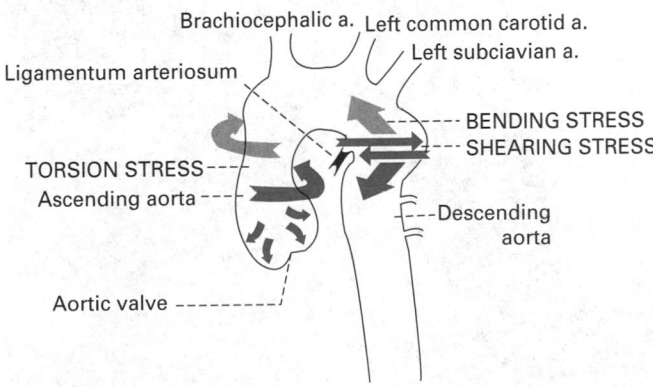

FIGURE 87-1

Diagrammatic illustration of the forces acting upon the aortic wall during rupture of the aorta from blunt trauma. (From Symbas PN. *Traumatic Injuries of the Heart and Great Vessels.* Springfield, IL: Charles C Thomas; 1971:153. Courtesy of Charles C Thomas, Publisher, Springfield, Illinois.)

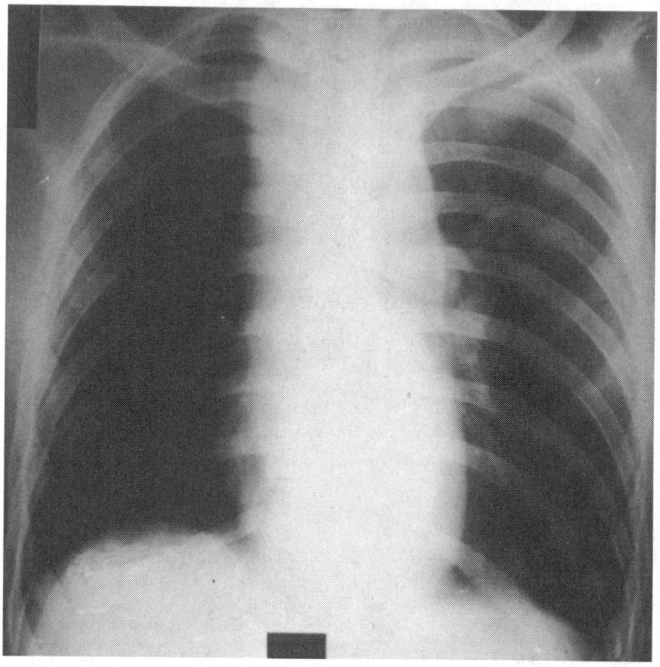

A

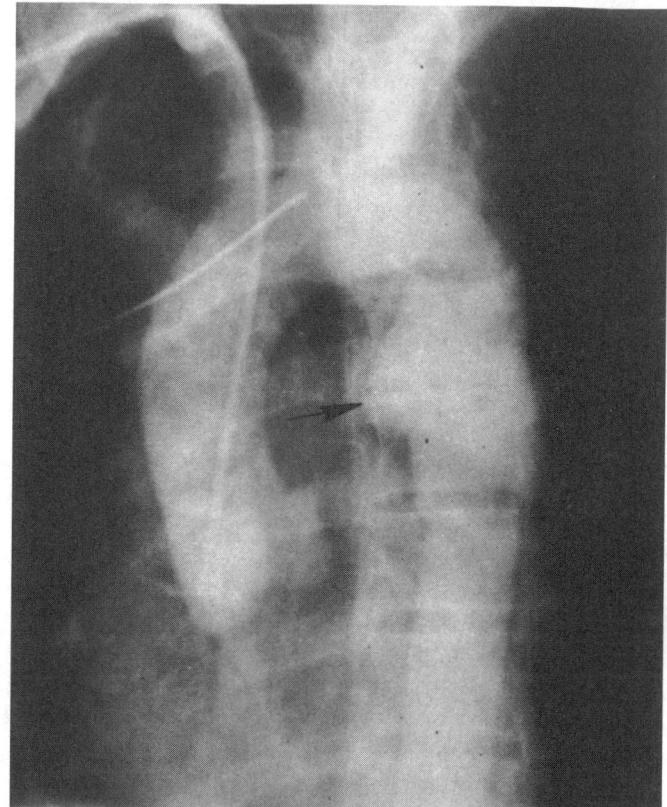

B

FIGURE 87-2

A. Chest roentgenogram of a young male who shortly before admission was involved in an automobile accident. Note the mediastinal widening. *B*. Aortogram of the same day showing a false aneurysm distal to the origin of the left subclavian artery and two filling defects, one proximal and one distal to the aneurysm.

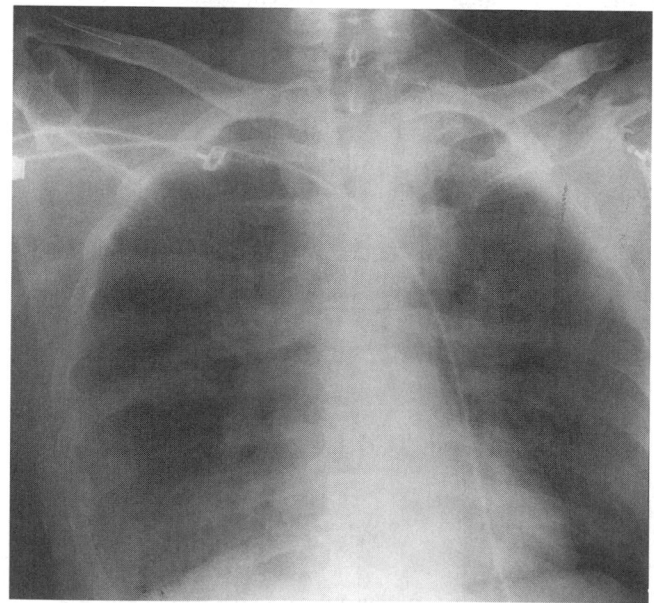

A

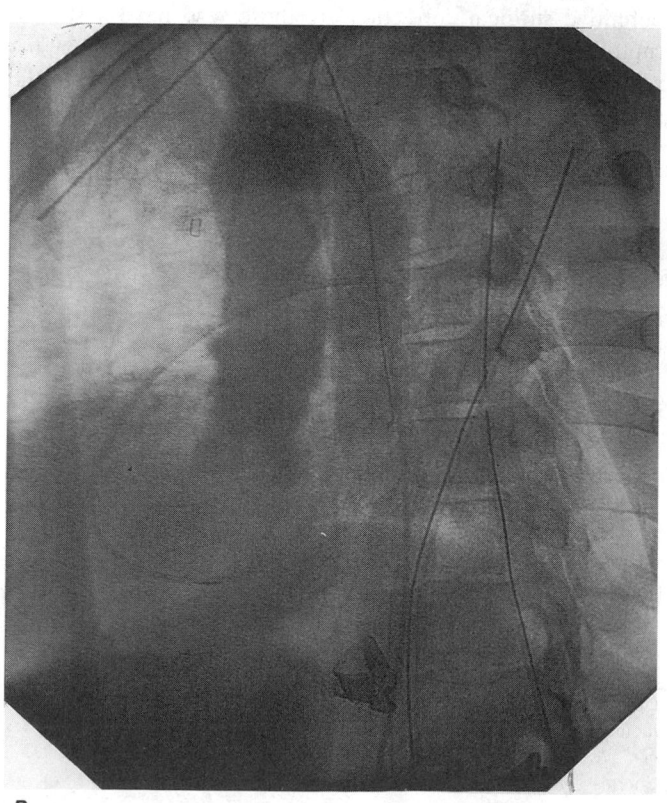

B

FIGURE 87-3

A. Chest roentgenogram of a young man shortly after a vehicular accident. *B*. Aortogram showing rupture of the ascending aorta.

REFERENCES

1. Symbas PN. *Cardiothoracic Trauma*. Philadelphia: Saunders; 1989.
2. James S. Injury mortality, *National Summary of Injury Mortality Data, 1987–1993*. Washington, DC: U.S. Department of Health and Human Services, Public Health Service Center for Disease Control and Prevention; June 1996.
3. Price PR, Mackenzie EJ. Cost of injury—United States: A report to Congress. *JAMA* 1989; 262:2803–2804.
4. Kemmerer WT, Eckert WG, Gathwright JB, Reemtsma K, Creech O Jr. Patterns of thoracic injuries in fatal traffic accidents. *J Trauma* 1961; 1:595–599.
5. Bredlau CE, Roubin GS, Leimgruber PP, Douglas JS Jr, King SB III, Gruentzig AR. In-hospital morbidity and mortality in patients undergoing elective coronary angioplasty. *Circulation* 1985; 72:1044–1052.
6. Gaul G, Hollman J, Simpendorfer C, Franco I. Acute occlusion in multiple lesion coronary angioplasty: Frequency and management. *J Am Coll Cardiol* 1989; 13:283–288.
7. Safian RD, Berman AD, Diver DJ, McKay LL, Come PC, Riley MF, et al. Balloon aortic valvuloplasty in 170 consecutive patients. *N Engl J Med* 1988; 319:125–130.
8. Nobuyoshi M, Hamasaki N, Kimura T, Nosaka H, Yokoi H, Yasumoto H, et al. Indications, complications and short-term clinical outcome of percutaneous transvenous mitral commissurotomy. *Circulation* 1989; 80:782–792.
9. Meyer JA, Millar K. Perforation of the right ventricle by electrode catheters: A review and report of nine cases. *Ann Surg* 1968; 168:1048–1060.
10. Shah KB, Rao TL, Laughlin S, El Etr AA. A review of pulmonary artery catheterization in 6,245 patients. *Anesthesiology* 1984; 61:271–275.
11. Bynum WR, Conell RM, Hawk WA. Causes of death after external cardiac massage: Analysis of observations on fifty consecutive autopsies. *Cleve Clin Q* 1963; 30:147–151.
12. Agdal N, Jorgensen TG. Penetrating laceration of the pericardium and myocardium and myocardial rupture following closed chest cardiac massage. *Acta Med Scand* 1973; 194:477–479.
13. Greene JF Jr, Fitzwater JE, Clemmer TP. Septic endocarditis and indwelling pulmonary artery catheters. *JAMA* 1975; 233:891–892.
14. Pace NL, Horton W. Indwelling pulmonary artery catheters: Their relationship to aseptic endocardial vegetation. *JAMA* 1975; 233:893–894.
15. Bloomfield DA. Techniques of nonsurgical retrieval of iatrogenic foreign bodies of the heart. *Am J Cardiol* 1971; 27:538–545.
16. Cohn KE, Stewart JR, Fajardo LF, Hancock EW. Heart disease following radiation. *Medicine* 1967; 46:281–298.
17. Morton DL, Glancy DL, Joseph WL, Adkins PC. Management of patients with radiation-induced pericarditis with effusions: A note on the development of aortic regurgitation in two of them. *Chest* 1973; 64:291–297.
18. De Silva RA, Graboys TB, Podrid PJ, Lown B. Cardioversion and defibrillation. *Am Heart J* 1980; 100:881–895.
19. Bernstein T. Effects of electricity and lightning on man and animals. *J Forens Sci* 1973; 18:3–11.
20. Jackson SH, Parry DJ. Lightning and the heart. *Br Heart J* 1980; 43:454–527.
21. Moritz AR, Atkins JP. Cardiac contusions: An experimental and pathologic study. *Arch Pathol* 1938; 25:445–462.
22. Samson PC. Battle wounds and injuries of the heart and pericardium: Experiences in forward hospitals. *Ann Surg* 1948; 127:1127–1149.
23. Symbas PN, Harlaftis N, Waldo WJ. Penetrating cardiac wounds: A comparison of different therapeutic methods. *Ann Surg* 1976; 183:377–381.
24. Symbas PN. *Cardiothoracic Trauma: Current Problems in Surgery*. St Louis: Mosby–Year Book; 1991:742–797.
25. Mattox KL, Limacher MC, Feliciano DV, Colosimo L, OMeara ME, Beall AC Jr, et al. Cardiac evaluation following heart injury. *J Trauma* 1985; 25:758–765.
26. Trinkle JK, Toon RS, Franz JL, Arom KV, Grover FL. Affairs of the wounded heart: Penetrating cardiac wounds. *J Trauma* 1979; 19:467–472.
27. Ivatury RR, Rohman M, Steichen FM, Gunduz Y, Nallathambi M, Stahl WM. Penetrating cardiac injuries: Twenty-year experience. *Am Surg* 1987; 53:310–317.
28. Attar S, Suter CM, Hankins JR, Sequeira A, McLaughlin JS. Penetrating cardiac injuries. *Ann Thorac Surg* 1991; 51:711–716.
29. Knott-Craig CJ, Dalton RP, Rossouw GJ, Barnard PM. Penetrating cardiac trauma: Management strategy based on 129 surgical emergencies over 2 years. *Ann Thorac Surg* 1992; 53:1006–1009.
30. Mitchell ME, Muakkassa FF, Poole GV, Rhodes RS, Griswold JA. Surgical approach of choice for penetrating cardiac wounds. *J Trauma* 1993; 34:17–20.
31. Cooper FW Jr, Stead EA Jr, Warren JV. The beneficial effect of intravenous infusions in acute cardiac tamponade. *Ann Surg* 1944; 120:822–825.
32. Rozycki GS, Feliciano DV, Schmidt JA, Cushman JG, Sisley AC, Ingram W, Ansley JD. The role of surgeon-performed ultrasound in patients with possible cardiac wounds. *Ann Surg* 1996; 224:1–8.
33. Symbas PN, DiOrio DA, Tyras DH, Ware RE, Hatcher CR Jr. Penetrating cardiac wounds: Significant residual and delayed sequelae. *J Thorac Cardiovasc Surg* 1973; 66:526–532.
34. Symbas PN. *Traumatic Heart Disease: Current Problems in Cardiology*. St Louis: Mosby–Year Book; 1991:539–582.
35. Whisennand HH, Van Pelt SA, Beall AC Jr, Mattox KL, Espada R. Surgical management of traumatic intracardiac injuries. *Ann Thorac Surg* 1979; 28:530–536.
36. Bland EF, Beebe GW. Missiles in the heart: A 20-year follow-up report of world war cases. *N Engl J Med* 1966; 274:1039–1046.
37. Symbas PN, Hatcher CR Jr, Mansour KA. Projectile embolus of the lung. *J Thorac Cardiovasc Surg* 1968; 56:97–103.
38. Symbas PN, Harlaftis N. Bullet emboli in the pulmonary and systemic arteries. *Ann Surg* 1977; 185:318–320.
39. Decker HR. Foreign bodies in the heart and pericardium: Should they be removed? *J Thorac Surg* 1939; 9:62.
40. Harken DE. Experiments in intracardiac surgery: I. Bacterial endocarditis. *J Thorac Surg* 1942; 11:656–670.
41. Turner GG. Bullets in the heart for 23 years. *Surgery* 1942; 9:832–852.
42. Symbas PN, Picone AL, Hatcher CR Jr, Vlasis SE. Cardiac missiles: A review of the literature and personal experience. *Ann Surg* 1990; 211:639–648.
43. Symbas PN, Vlasis SE, Picone AL, Hatcher CR Jr. Missiles in the heart. *Ann Thorac Surg* 1989; 48:192–194.
44. Konecke LL, Spitzer S, Mason D, Kasparian H, James PM Jr. Traumatic aneurysm of the left coronary artery. *Am J Cardiol* 1971; 27:221–223.
45. Symbas PN, Sehdava JS. Penetrating wounds of the thoracic aorta. *Ann Surg* 1970; 171:441–450.
46. Symbas PN, Kourias E, Tyras DH, Hatcher CR Jr. Penetrating wounds of the great vessels. *Ann Surg* 1974; 179:757–762.
47. Symbas PN, Schlant RC, Logan WD Jr, Lindsay J, MacConnell K, Zakaryia M. Traumatic aorticopulmonary fistula complicated by postoperative low cardiac output treated with dopamine. *Ann Surg* 1967; 165:614–619.
48. Parmley LF Jr, Orbison JA, Hughes CW, Mattingly TW. Acquired arteriovenous fistulas complicated by endarteritis and endocarditis lenta due to *Streptococcus faecalis*. *N Engl J Med* 1954; 250:305–309.
49. Kissane RW. Traumatic heart diseases, especially myocardial contusion. *Postgrad Med* 1954; 15:114–119.
50. Stern T, Wolf RY, Reichart B, Harrington OB, Crosby VG. Coronary artery occlusion resulting from blunt trauma. *JAMA* 1974; 230:1308–1309.
51. Levy H. Traumatic coronary thrombosis with myocardial infarction: Postmortem study. *Arch Intern Med* 1949; 84:261–276.
52. Forker AD, Morgan JR. Acquired coronary artery fistula from nonpenetrating chest injury. *JAMA* 1971; 215:289–291.
53. Louhimo I. Heart injury after blunt thoracic trauma: An experimental study on rabbits. *Acta Chir Scand Suppl* 1968; 380:1–60.
54. Dolara A, Morando P, Pampaloni M. Electrocardiographic findings in 98 consecutive nonpenetrating chest injuries. *Dis Chest* 1967; 52:50–56.
55. Jones FL Jr. Transmural myocardial necrosis after nonpenetrating cardiac trauma. *Am J Cardiol* 1970; 26:419–422.
56. Potkin RT, Werner JA, Trobaugh GB, Chestnut CH III, Carrico CJ, Hallstrom A, et al. Evaluation of noninvasive tests of cardiac damage in suspected cardiac contusion. *Circulation* 1982; 66:627–631.
57. Hoffman B. The genesis of cardiac arrhythmias. *Prog Cardiovasc Dis* 1966; 8:319–329.
58. Marriott HJ, Nizet PM. Physiologic stimuli simulating ischemic heart disease. *JAMA* 1967; 200:715.
59. Tindall GT, Iwata K, McGraw CP, Vanderveer RW. Cardiorespiratory changes associated with intracranial pressure waves: Evaluation of these changes in 27 patients with head injuries. *South Med J* 1975; 68:407–412.

60. Rapaport E. Serum enzymes and isoenzymes in the diagnosis of acute myocardial infarction. *Mod Concepts Cardiovasc Dis* 1977; 46:43–46.

61. Mamor A, Alpan G. Specificity of creatine kinase MB isoenzyme for myocardial injury. *Clin Chem* 1978; 24:2206.

62. Snow N, Richardson JD, Flynt LM Jr. Myocardial contusion: Implication for patients with multiple traumatic injuries. *Surgery* 1982; 92:744–750.

63. Gonzalez AC, Harlaftis N, Gravanis M, Symbas PN. Imaging of experimental myocardial contusion: Observations and pathologic correlations. *Am J Roentgenol* 1977; 128:1039–1040.

64. Miller FA Jr, Seward JB, Gersh BJ, Tajik AJ, Mucha P Jr. Two-dimensional echocardiographic findings in cardiac trauma. *Am J Cardiol* 1982; 50:1022–1027.

65. King RM, Mucha P Jr, Seward JB, Gersh BJ, Farnell MB. Cardiac contusion: A new diagnostic approach utilizing two-dimensional echocardiography. *J Trauma* 1983; 23:610–614.

66. Shapiro NG, Yanofsky SD, Trapp I, Purham RM, Labovitz A, Sear JE, et al. Cardiovascular evaluation in thoracic blunt trauma using transesophageal echocardiography (TEE). *J Trauma* 1991; 131:835–839.

67. Snow N, Luca AE, Richardson JD. Intra-aortic balloon counterpulsation for cardiogenic shock from cardiac contusion. *J Trauma* 1982; 22:426–429.

68. Killen DA, Gobbel WG Jr, France R, Vix VA. Post-traumatic aneurysm of the left ventricle. *Circulation* 1969; 39:101–108.

69. Singh R, Nolan SP, Schrank JP. Traumatic left ventricular aneurysm: Two cases with normal coronary angiograms. *JAMA* 1975; 234:412–414.

70. Payne DD, DeWeese JA, Mahoney EB, Murphy GW. Surgical treatment of traumatic rupture of the normal aortic valve. *Ann Thorac Surg* 1974; 17:223–229.

71. Liu S, Sako Y, Alexander CS. Traumatic tricuspid insufficiency. *Am J Cardiol* 1970; 26:200–204.

72. Schroeder JS, Stinson EB, Bieber CP, Wexler L, Shumway NE, Harrison DC. Papillary muscle dysfunction due to nonpenetrating chest trauma, recognition in a potential cardiac donor. *Br Heart J* 1972; 34:645–647.

73. Marvin RF, Schrank JP, Nolan SP. Traumatic tricuspid insufficiency. *Am J Cardiol* 1973; 32:723–726.

74. Munchow OBG, Carter R, Vannix RS, Anderson FS. Cardiac arrest due to ventricular herniation: Report of a case of two successful cardiac resuscitations. *JAMA* 1960; 173:1350–1351.

75. Anderson M, Fredens M, Olesson KH. Traumatic rupture of the pericardium. *Am J Cardiol* 1971; 27:566–569.

76. Feczko JD, Lynch L, Pless JE, Clark MA, McClain J, Hawley DA. An autopsy case review of 142 penetrating (blunt) injuries of the aorta. *J Trauma* 1992; 33:846–849.

77. Symbas PN, Tyras DH, Ware RE, DiOrio DA. Traumatic rupture of the aorta. *Ann Surg* 1973; 178:6–12.

78. Symbas PN, Tyras DH, Ware RE, Hatcher CR Jr. Rupture of the aorta: A diagnostic triad. *Ann Thorac Surg* 1973; 15:405–410.

79. Symbas PJ, Lee R, Symbas PN. Rupture of the ascending aorta and the aortic arch from blunt trauma. 1997. In press.

80. Fenner MN, Fisher KS, Sergel NL, Porter DB, Metzmoker CO. Evaluation of possible traumatic thoracic aortic injury using aortography and CT. *Am Surg* 1990; 56:497–499.

81. Miller FB, Richardson JD, Thomas HA, Cryer HM, Willing SJ. Role of CT in diagnosis of major arterial injury after blunt thoracic trauma. *Surgery* 1989; 106:596–603.

88

THE INFLUENCE OF ENVIRONMENTAL FACTORS ON THE CARDIOVASCULAR SYSTEM

Robert F. Grover / John T. Reeves / Loring B. Rowell / Claude A. Piantadosi / Herbert A. Saltzman

Cardiovascular function is regulated to preserve two vital functions, tissue oxygenation and normal body temperature. For example, during muscular exercise, the oxygen supply to the working muscles must be increased, and concurrently the increased heat generated must be dissipated. Humans are often subjected to environmental factors that stress cardiovascular regulation severely. Exposure to the atmospheric hypoxia of high altitude reduces muscular working capacity in spite of major adaptations to preserve tissue oxygenation. In hot environments, temperature regulation must compete with increased demands for oxygen during exercise, and here again, working capacity is reduced. Regrettably, our environment is now frequently contaminated with noxious substances, one of the most lethal of which is carbon monoxide. Here, artificial manipulation of the patient's environment by means of hyperbaric oxygen may assist in preserving tissue oxygenation and thereby be lifesaving. To the patient with cardiovascular disease, adaptation to such environmental stresses as heat, cold, or the hypoxia of high altitude becomes an even greater challenge. We shall examine how the body meets these challenges.

HIGH ALTITUDE

Each year millions of people visit the mountainous regions of the western United States for recreation. With modern transportation, rapid ascent to resort areas at 8000 to 9500 ft (2400 to 2900 m) in altitude is a common occurrence. Major highways cross mountain passes above 11,000 ft (3400 m) and during the summer season, half a million people drive to the summits of Pike's Peak and Mt. Evans, both exceeding 14,000 ft (4300 m). Just how severe is the stress of such altitudes?

To begin with, ascent to high altitude means exposure to a decrease in total atmospheric pressure and a parallel decrease in the partial pressure of oxygen (P_{O_2}) we breathe. At sea level, the inspired P_{O_2} is 150 mmHg; it is 125 mmHg at 5000 ft (1500 m), 100 mmHg at 10,000 ft (3000 m), and about 80 mmHg at 14,000 ft (4300 m). This is the atmospheric hypoxia to which people are exposed in the Rocky Mountains.

Circulatory Oxygen Transport

ARTERIAL OXYGENATION

Within the lung, the P_{O_2} is lowered by the presence of carbon dioxide and water vapor. Furthermore, there is imperfect matching of blood flow to regional ventilation. Consequently, the arterial P_{O_2} perfusing the body, which ranges from about 80 to 90 mmHg at sea level, is reduced to 45 to 50 mmHg at 14,000 ft (4300 m).

Although the arterial P_{O_2} on the summit of Pike's Peak is only half as great as at sea level, this does not mean that the quantity of oxygen in the blood has been reduced to one-half. That is because of the nonlinear oxygen-binding characteristics of hemoglobin. The relation between oxygen tension and oxygen saturation is defined by the hemoglobin-oxygen dissociation curve (Fig. 88-1). From this it can be seen that following adaptation to 14,000 ft (4300 m), the arterial oxygen saturation is still 85 percent compared with 95 percent at sea level. Thus, a 50 percent decrease in arterial P_{O_2} causes only a 10 percent reduction in saturation. At the more modest altitudes at which the tourist and ski resorts are situated, the fall in saturation is even less. The moderate nature of this hypoxemia should be emphasized, since many of our concepts regarding high altitude are based on much more severe hypoxic tests.

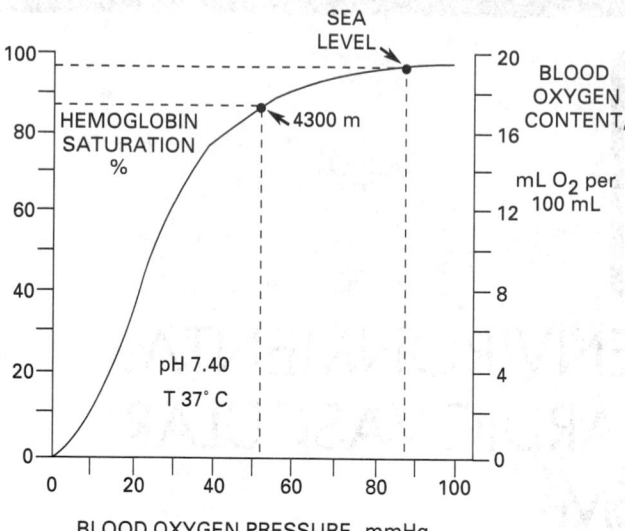

FIGURE 88-1

As a consequence of the sigmoid shape of the hemoglobin-oxygen dissociation curve, the large decrease in arterial oxygen pressure (tension) on ascent from sea level to 14,000 ft (4300 m) in altitude results in only a small decrease in hemoglobin saturation and blood oxygen content. (From Grover RF. Man living at high altitudes. In: Ives JD, Barry RG, eds. *Arctic and Alpine Environments*. London: Methuen; 1974: 822. Reproduced with permission of the publisher and author.)

The effect of a decrease in saturation on the actual amount of oxygen in the blood (arterial O_2 content) depends on the hemoglobin concentration. With a normal hemoglobin of 15 g/dL, when saturation falls to 85 percent, the arterial O_2 content is reduced from 19 to 17 mL/dL (Fig. 88-1). Within the first few hours or days at high altitude, however, plasma volume decreases while total red blood cell mass initially remains unchanged.[1] This reduction in plasma volume reflects a redistribution of body fluid[2] and is probably under control of atrial natriuretic peptide.[3,4] As a consequence, hematocrit rises, and with it hemoglobin concentration, which increases the O_2-carrying capacity of the blood. This offsets the fall in saturation and restores the arterial O_2 content to preascent values (Fig. 88-2). In other words, after a week at high altitude, even though the saturation is 85 percent, the quantity of oxygen in 100 mL of blood (milliliters of oxygen per deciliter) has been restored to normal. Even during heavy exercise at altitude, arterial O_2 content is well maintained because there is further hemoconcentration, which tends to offset the added decrease in saturation.[5] True polycythemia, reflecting an increase in total red blood cell mass resulting from bone marrow stimulation, begins to appear after about 10 days but requires many weeks of residence at altitudes high enough to cause a sustained reduction in arterial saturation before a new plateau in red cell mass is established.[6–8]

AUTONOMIC NERVOUS SYSTEM

The cardiovascular adjustments at high altitude seem to be largely under the influence of complex changes within the autonomic nervous system.[9] With regard to the adreno-sympa-

thetics, β-adrenergic stimulation, resulting in epinephrine secretion by the adrenal glands, appears to relate to the severity of the hypoxemia. Thus β activation, as determined by blood levels of epinephrine, is maximal on arrival at altitude when the hypoxemia is most severe and becomes less as the hypoxemia improves with ventilatory acclimatization. In contrast, α-adrenergic stimulation, as determined by norepinephrine levels in blood and urine, increases progressively over the first few days at 14,000 ft (4300 m) and becomes maximal in 7 to 10 days.[10] Although mechanisms are not known for α activation, it occurs in parallel with ventilatory acclimatization to high altitude and thus is increasing while β activation is decreasing. The differences between the α and β limbs in their activation sequence and in their circulatory effects contribute to complex circulatory adjustments to altitude, as diagrammed schematically in Fig. 88-3.

Heart rate increases on arrival at altitude (Fig. 88-4) and, along with epinephrine, is highest on arrival. Also, spectral analysis of heart rate suggests that early after arrival β-adrenergic tone is higher and parasympathetic tone is lower than at sea level.[11] Thus, the tachycardia on arrival is a result of β activation and concomitant parasympathetic withdrawal. As arterial oxygen saturation and content improve with ventilatory acclimatization, blood epinephrine falls and the tachycardia is ameliorated. Spectral analysis indicates that both β and parasympathetic tone are partially restored toward sea level values, with the result that heart rate is higher than at sea level but lower than on arrival.[11] Thus the directional changes in heart rate over time at altitude appear to follow changes in arterial oxygen and to result largely from complex interplay of the β-adrenergic and the parasympathetic systems.

Systemic arterial pressure, however, follows a different time course and relates to norepinephrine.[12] Pressure and norepinephrine increase progressively and together over several days at altitude. Norepinephrine levels in blood and urine

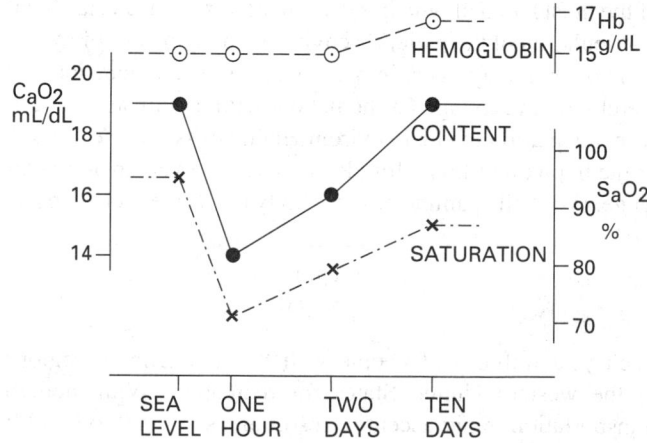

FIGURE 88-2

Arterial blood oxygenation during adaptation to high altitude. Following the initial fall, arterial saturation (SaO$_2$) improves with increasing ventilation. Concurrently, hemoconcentration increases hemoglobin (Hb) concentration and hence the O_2-carrying capacity of the blood. The net result is restoration of arterial O_2 content (CaO$_2$) to preascent values.

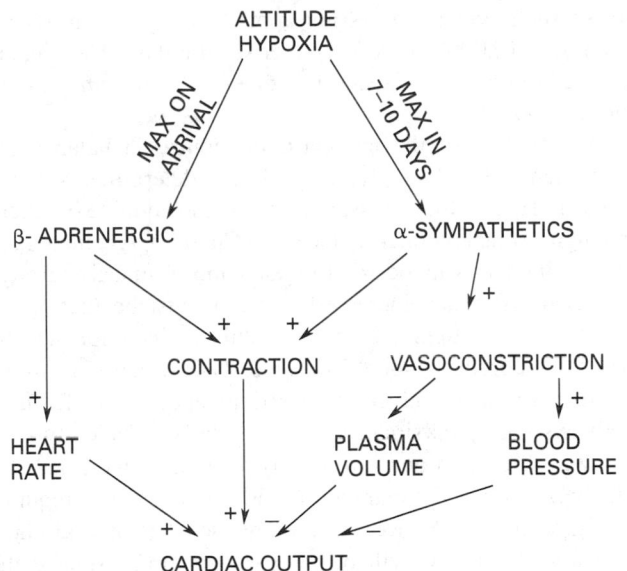

FIGURE 88-3

With ascent to high altitude, hypoxia stimulates the adreno-sympathetic system. The early β-adrenergic activation supplanted by delayed α-sympathetic activity results in a complex series of cardiovascular adjustments as indicated.

arc considered to reflect spillover from sympathetic nerve endings and, therefore, provide an index of α-neural activity.[10] Both the systemic hypertension and the norepinephrine levels return to sea level values within several months, suggesting that the activation of the α-sympathetic system at altitude may be transient in normal persons. Sympathetic activation not only increases arteriolar tone but also probably contributes to the observed increase in venous tone.[13,14] Increased venous tone likely contributes to the diuresis and the decrease in plasma volume, both of which are normal responses to altitude. Like the rise in arterial pressure, the fall in plasma volume begins soon after arrival and continues over the first days of residence.[8]

CARDIAC OUTPUT

Since the transport of oxygen by the circulation depends not only on the quantity of oxygen in each unit of blood (arterial O_2 content) but also on the number of these units of blood pumped by the heart per minute, i.e., cardiac output, let us examine the latter, including its components, heart rate (HR) and stroke volume. As stated above, HR increases with ascent to high altitude as a result of hypoxic β-sympathetic stimulation.[15] This tachycardia increases cardiac output, which offsets initial hypoxemia and preserves oxygen transport; however, this early tachycardia may not be sustained. Within a day or two, resting HR returns to preascent values, and even the tachycardia of exercise may diminish[15] (Fig. 88-4). Surprisingly, cardiac stroke volume also decreases by as much as 25 percent during the first week at high altitude.[1] As a result of these circulatory adjustments, cardiac output, both at rest and during exercise, plateaus at levels about 20 percent below the corresponding values at sea level[1] (Fig. 88-4).

Consequently, even though the quantity of O_2 in the arterial blood has been restored to normal by hemoconcentration, the amount of O_2 transported to the body is now reduced by the low cardiac output (Fig. 88-5). For the body to remain normally oxygenated, extraction of O_2 from arterial blood must be increased. Direct measurements in normal humans, both at rest and during exercise, confirm this increase in extraction (widening of the arteriovenous difference in blood O_2 content).[1]

MYOCARDIAL FUNCTION

By what mechanism does stroke volume decrease? Observations made with M-mode echocardiography in normal individuals demonstrated a progressive decrease in both end-diastolic and end-systolic diameters of the left ventricular chamber over the first week at high altitude.[16] Volumes calculated from these diameters indicated a progressive decrease in stroke volume that was highly correlated with the decrease in end-diastolic volume, while ejection fraction remained normal.

The declines in ventricular diastolic volume and stroke volume appear to reflect the reduction in blood volume from hemoconcentration induced by atrial natriuretic peptide.[3] Stroke volume remains decreased even after several weeks at high altitude. During this period of adaptation, circulating levels of norepinephrine and systemic vascular resistance rise, suggesting that ventricular afterload may now contribute to the suppression of stroke volume. However, all indices of contractility remain normal,[16] indicating that myocardial function is not compromised at moderate or even very high

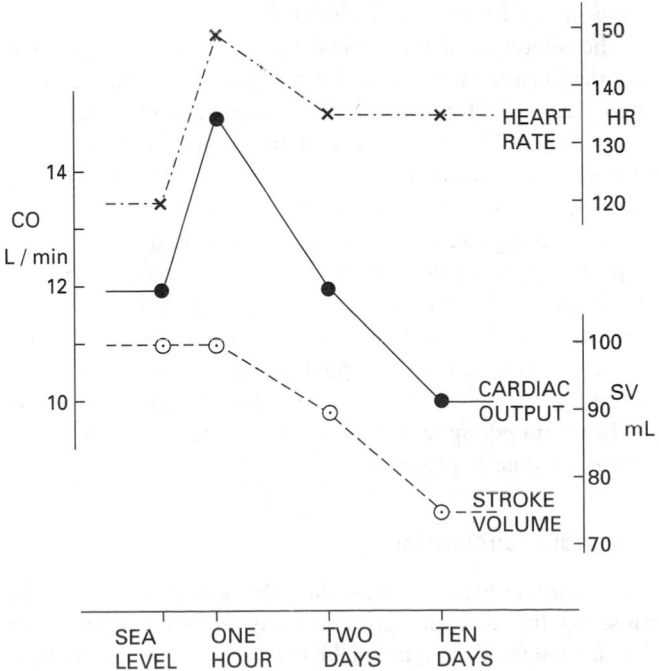

FIGURE 88-4

Time course of alterations in exercise heart rate (HR), stroke volume (SV), and cardiac output (CO) during adaptation to high altitude. After 10 days, CO is subnormal because of a significant decrease in SV.

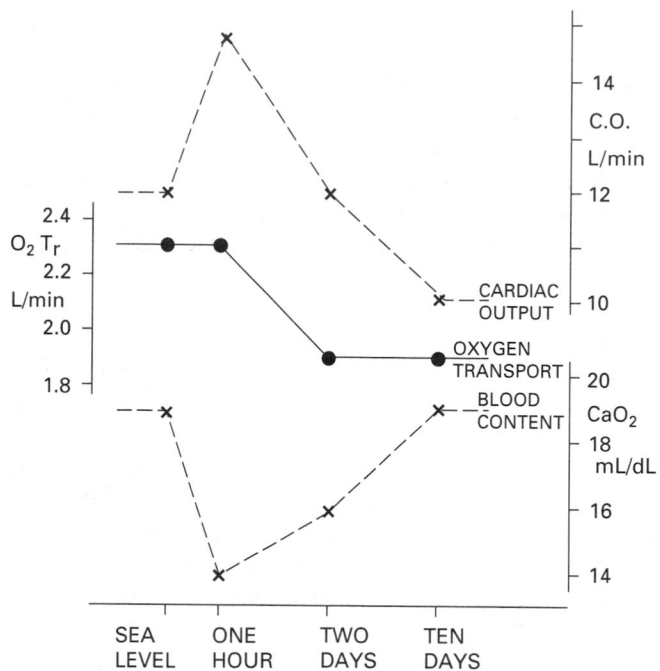

FIGURE 88-5

Oxygen transport (O_2Tr) by the systemic circulation during submaximal exercise. Upon ascent to high altitude, the fall in arterial blood O_2 content (CaO_2) is offset by an increase in cardiac output (CO). Although CaO_2 is restored within 10 days, the fall in CO to subnormal levels results in a net reduction in O_2Tr, which then requires a greater O_2 extraction from the blood to preserve O_2 delivery.

altitude. Hence, the decrease in stroke volume reflects the operation of normal physiogenic mechanisms rather than any impairment of myocardial function.

The tolerance of the normal heart to chronic hypoxemia was demonstrated dramatically in eight men during a simulated ascent of Mount Everest in a hypobaric chamber. Over a 40-day period, the pressure of the atmosphere within the chamber was reduced progressively from 760 to 240 mmHg, equivalent to an altitude in excess of 29,000 ft (8800 m). At rest and during exercise, arterial P_{O_2} was 30 and 27 mmHg, respectively, corresponding to arterial saturations of 58 and 49 percent. Pulmonary arterial wedge (left atrial) pressures were the same or less than at sea level, and the relationship between ventricular filling pressure and stroke volume remained normal.[17] Thus this index of contractile function of the heart did not appear to be adversely affected by even this severe, chronic hypoxemia.

Coronary Circulation

In considering the cardiovascular effects of high altitude, the stress on the coronary circulation is of prime importance. We are taught that hypoxia increases coronary blood flow. Evidence for this includes a study of 19 young men in whom breathing 10 percent O_2 nearly doubled coronary blood flow.[18] Breathing 10 percent O_2 at sea level, however, yields inspired O_2 tensions equivalent to sudden exposure to 18,000 ft (5500

m), so such evidence does not apply directly to tourists ascending to 10,000 ft (3000 m) over several days. Here again, the situation becomes clear when one thinks in terms of oxygen transport.

Oxygenation of the myocardium requires a balance between demand and supply. The primary determinants of demand are HR, systolic pressure (the so-called double product), and myocardial contractility (see also Chap. 3). Ascent to high altitude increases myocardial O_2 demand, primarily through increased HR. Such increased demand must be met by an increase in O_2 supply. In general, this is accomplished by increasing coronary blood flow, since O_2 extraction from the coronary arterial blood (coronary arteriovenous O_2 difference) is always nearly maximal. If the altitude is sufficiently high to lower saturation and arterial O_2 content as well, less O_2 will be available for extraction, and compensation requires even greater flow. Hence, with initial ascent to high altitude, coronary blood flow will be increased in proportion to the increase in HR and the decrease in arterial saturation.

INCREASE IN OXYGEN EXTRACTION

Within a few days at high altitude, HR will decrease and arterial O_2 content will be restored by hemoconcentration (Figs. 88-2 and 88-4). Both adjustments will tend to return coronary flow to preascent levels. In addition, a third important but subtle factor operates that permits coronary flow to decrease even further. This is a decrease in the affinity of hemoglobin for O_2, which is another aspect of adaptation to high altitude. Within the red blood cell, the concentration of 2,3-diphosphoglycerate (2,3-DPG) increases, producing a "right shift" in the hemoglobin dissociation curve,[19] lowering the saturation at any given tension. Because of the sigmoid shape of the dissociation curve, this right shift has little effect on arterial O_2 loading; however, it facilitates O_2 unloading from peripheral capillary blood.

NORMAL DECREASE IN CORONARY BLOOD FLOW

The coronary circulation is regulated to maintain the coronary sinus P_{O_2} constant at 18 mmHg. The corresponding saturation will be lowered from 34 percent at sea level to 22 percent at 10,200 ft (3100 m) as a consequence of the right shift in the dissociation curve.[20] Consequently, O_2 extraction from the coronary blood will increase significantly (wider coronary arteriovenous O_2 difference),[20] and less coronary blood flow will be needed to supply the myocardial O_2 requirements (Fig. 88-6). Literally, the right shift in the dissociation curve *permits* coronary flow to decrease. Direct measurements in normal humans studied first at sea level and again after adaptation to high altitude show a consistent decrease in coronary flow, both at rest and during exercise.[20] A decrease in coronary flow at high altitude is surprising but entirely consistent with the operation of normal physiologic mechanisms designed to preserve the constancy of myocardial tissue P_{O_2} (coronary sinus P_{O_2}). The decrease in coronary flow is required to prevent a rise in coronary sinus P_{O_2}. There is no evidence of myocardial ischemia or hypoxia; neither is there any impairment to increasing coronary flow when required to meet increased O_2 demands, as during exercise.

CORONARY ARTERY DISEASE

Does visiting high altitude pose a special risk for the patient with coronary artery disease? How do you advise the 55-year-old man from Atlanta who is contemplating a skiing vacation to Colorado? These are very practical questions, but well-controlled studies have not been conducted to provide definitive answers. All existing evidence, however, indicates that exposure to high altitude is not likely to precipitate a coronary event. For example, in almost 150,000 persons trekking in Nepal to altitudes as high as 17,700 ft (5400 m), over a 3.5-year period there were no cardiac deaths, and only 3 men required helicopter evacuation for cardiac problems.[21]

Using radiotelemetry, Grover et al.[22] recorded electrocardiograms (ECGs) from 149 men skiing at altitudes of 10,000 to 11,200 ft (3000 to 3400 m) at Vail, Colorado. Of these, 90 were age 40 or older, including 19 in their fifties and 5 in their sixties. During skiing, HRs exceeded 150 beats per minute in over half the subjects, corresponding to over 80 percent of the age-adjusted predicted maximum rate. Despite tachycardia from strenuous exercise in the cold at high altitude, the incidence of ischemic ST-segment depression was no greater than among asymptomatic older men exercising at sea level.

How do patients with known coronary artery disease respond to high altitude? In-depth studies of such patients are rare. Okin[23] conducted a study in which patients with known coronary heart disease were exercised at both low and high altitudes. Eleven men with documented previous myocardial infarction and/or angina performed a standardized step test, first at their resident altitude of 5200 ft (1600 m) and again after driving into the mountains to 8000 ft (2400 m) and then to 10,400 ft (3200 m). Although HR during exercise was greater at the higher altitudes (70 percent of predicted maximum based on age), no patient who had a normal Master's test at 5200 ft (1600 m) had a positive Master's test at higher altitude, and no patient developed symptoms at higher altitude that they did not have at 5200 ft (1600 m). Hence ischemic changes could not be produced in these patients with known coronary heart disease despite ascent from 5200 ft (1600 m) to 8000 (2400 m) and 10,400 ft (3200 m).

In another study,[24] a hypobaric chamber was employed

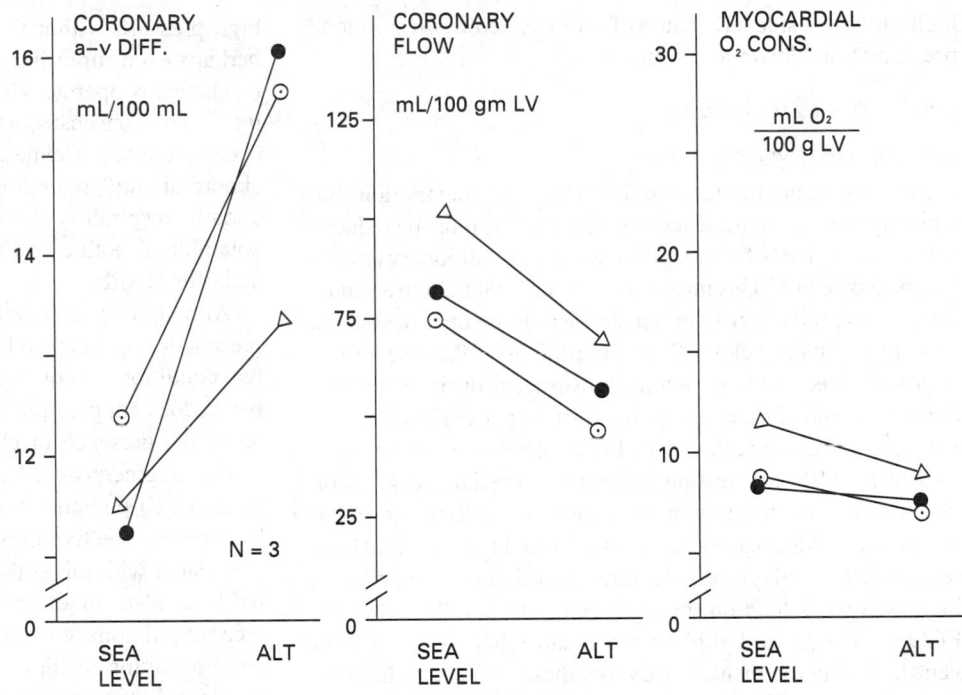

FIGURE 88-6

Alterations in the coronary circulation of the normal human heart following adaptation to 10,200 ft in altitude. Oxygen extraction from coronary blood increases, i.e., there is a significant widening of the coronary arteriovenous difference in O_2 content. This permits coronary flow to decrease while maintaining myocardial O_2 consumption unaltered. (From Grover RF. Mechanisms augmenting coronary arterial oxygen extraction. In: Vogel JHK, ed. *Myocardial Infarction—A New Look at an Old Subject. Advances in Cardiology*, Vol. 9. Basel/New York: Karger; 1973; 97. Reproduced with permission of the publisher and author.)

to simulate ascent to high altitude. Thirty men with proven stabilized ischemic heart disease performed a double Master's two-step exercise test at sea level. Within a week they entered a decompression chamber and over 10 min were taken to a simulated altitude of 15,000 ft (4600 m). After 40 min of rest, they repeated the exercise test; they were then returned to ground level. None of the subjects manifested any symptoms or arrhythmias during exercise testing at ground level or in the decompression chamber. The response to the Master's test was positive in 17 of the subjects at sea level and increased slightly to 20 at simulated altitude.

Considering the available evidence, given a patient with stable coronary artery disease and a reasonably good exercise tolerance at sea level, there is no justification for advising such a patient to avoid travel to high altitude.[25]

Paradoxically, prolonged residence at high altitude may actually reduce mortality from coronary heart disease. Mortimer et al.[26] analyzed age-adjusted mortality rates for atherosclerotic heart disease in populations living at different altitudes in New Mexico. For males, although not for females, mortality rates declined progressively from low to high altitude; the rate above 6500 ft (2000 m) was only 72 percent of the rate below 3700 ft (1100 m). This decline in rate was not explained by ethnic or socioeconomic factors and was concluded to be a true consequence of the higher altitude. The increased vascularity of the myocardium[27] in high-altitude residents may be a protective factor. In addition, left ventricular work may actually be less in high-altitude residents because of lower systemic arterial blood pressure[28] and lower heart rate.

Pulmonary Circulation

PULMONARY HYPERTENSION

Airway hypoxia stimulates pulmonary vasoconstriction, but when hypoxia is induced acutely, alvelor P_{O_2} must be reduced below 70 mmHg before a significant rise in pulmonary arterial pressure is seen.[29] This means that with ascent to high altitude, little or no pulmonary hypertension would be observed in the visitor to altitudes below 10,000 ft (3000 m). When the airway hypoxia is sustained for months, however, as during residence at high altitude, impressive pulmonary hypertension does develop.[29,30] Among residents of Leadville, Colorado, living at 10,200 ft (3100 m), resting pulmonary arterial pressures on the average are twice as high as those of individuals living at sea level. Mean pressures range from 11 to 45 mmHg at rest and frequently exceed 60 mmHg during exercise.[29] This increased work load on the right ventricle is reflected in the ECG as a rightward shift in the mean QRS axis and right ventricular enlargement.[31] Although these findings differ from those usually encountered in normal sea level residents, the pulmonary hypertension of high altitude is generally benign, nonprogressive, and reversible with descent to lower altitude. Hence, it should not be considered cardiovascular disease, and the term *cor pulmonale*, if used, is misleading.

In special circumstances, the hypoxic pulmonary hypertension of high altitude may not be entirely benign. It may delay the usual postnatal resolution of the normally high pulmonary arterial pressure in the fetus[32] and result in "persistent fetal circulation" of the newborn that may be fatal.[33] Although high-altitude pulmonary hypertension appears well tolerated by the human right ventricle, it becomes so severe in cattle that heart failure develops, and the resulting edema produces what cattle raisers call "brisket disease."[34]

HIGH-ALTITUDE PULMONARY EDEMA

Although the vast majority of people ascending to high altitude experience no pulmonary problems (apart from an awareness of the normal increase in ventilation), the occasional individual will develop acute high-altitude pulmonary edema (HAPE). The incidence is between 1 and 10 per 10,000 persons ascending rapidly to altitudes above 8000 ft (2400 m).[35,36] Symptoms almost always appear during the first 2 to 7 days at such altitudes. The patient has undue shortness of breath, cyanosis, tachycardia, moist rales, fatigue, and frequently a nonproductive cough. Untreated, HAPE tends to be progressive and fatal, whereas recovery is prompt on descent to lower altitude. During the episode of HAPE, the heart is not enlarged and heart failure is absent. This is a form of noncardiac pulmonary edema that occurs in otherwise healthy and comparatively young individuals[35,36] with no underlying cardiovascular or pulmonary disease.[37] Despite intensive research, the pathogenesis of HAPE remains uncertain. Either the lung vessel permeability has increased such that a water and protein leak overwhelm the capacity of the lymphatic drainage or

high pressure within the vessels forces fluid into the lungs, perhaps even rupturing pulmonary capillaries. Probably both mechanisms operate, since they would be mutually reinforcing.[38] The consensus is that HAPE is part of the spectrum of acute mountain sickness, with relative hypoventilation and abnormal fluid retention as underlying factors.[39,40] Consequently, respiratory stimulation, as by administration of acetazolamide, is both a rational and an effective mode of prophylaxis for HAPE.

Although acute severe pulmonary hypertension is usually present during an episode of HAPE, the relation between these two conditions is not clear. Probably pulmonary hypertension per se does not precipitate the pulmonary edema. On the other hand, the presence of elevated intravascular pressure would tend to augment fluid leakage. This may explain why nifedipine, which prevents hypoxic pulmonary vasoconstriction,[41] has proved effective in both preventing and treating HAPE.[42] Consistent with this is the observation that inhalation of nitric oxide is also an effective therapeutic modality.[43] The increased pulmonary vascular reactivity in chronically hypoxic children living at high altitude may also contribute to their predisposition to reentry HAPE[44] (see also Chaps. 21 and 59).

HEAT STRESS

Humans adjust to heat stress mainly by altering the vasomotor state of the skin to regulate heat exchange with the environment. Thermal balance is further modified by sweating and shivering. This section deals with adjustments of the systemic cutaneous and other regional circulations to regulate blood pressure and blood volume distribution along with body temperature. Reviews of this topic can be consulted for further details.[45–47]

Cutaneous Circulation

REFLEX CONTROL[48,49]

The skin receives only 5 to 10 percent of the cardiac output in normothermic individuals at rest, but it can receive 50 to 70 percent during severe heat stress. Circulatory adjustments to thermal stress can be drastically modified by cutaneous sympathetic vasoconstrictor nerve fibers releasing norepinephrine, which acts on postsynaptic α_1 and α_2 adrenoceptors.[50] These fibers are the efferent arm of (1) thermoregulatory reflexes that originate principally in cutaneous thermoreceptors, (2) cardiopulmonary and arterial baroreflexes, and (3) reflex adjustments to upright posture and exercise. The body's efforts to maintain blood pressure and support metabolic demands of other organs compete with thermoregulatory needs for skin blood flow. The temperature we maintain in conditions other than supine rest is the result of these competing nervous influences on skin blood flow.

Human skin is unique in possessing an *active vasodilator* system, the dominant effector in human cardiovascular response to rising core temperature (not skin temperature), accounting for almost all the increase in skin blood flow. The mechanism of active cutaneous vasodilation is still unknown. It requires intact sympathetic innervation and is somehow functionally linked to sweat gland function, as revealed by patients with congenital absence of sweat glands who cannot vasodilate the skin or adequately regulate body temperature.[51] Inasmuch as presynaptic blockade of sympathetic cholinergic nerves (which innervate sweat glands) with botulinum toxin selectively abolishes this active vasodilation, the response is mediated by cholinergic nerves. The vasodilation appears to be caused by a cotransmitter released from these nerves; atropine does not block the response.[52]

A rise in skin blood flow markedly increases the volume of blood within the compliant venous plexuses where it passes at reduced linear velocity just below the skin surface, increasing transcutaneous heat transfer. Cutaneous veins have a rich sympathetic nerve supply that reflexively controls the volume near the body surface in response to heat and cold. They are not responsive to baroreflexes, but they do constrict during exercise. As will be discussed, the shift in blood volume into cutaneous veins is the major regulatory problem in human cardiovascular adjustment to heat stress.[45,46]

Circulatory Adjustments to Heat Stress

AT REST IN HOT AIR ENVIRONMENTS

As long as body skin temperature (T_{sk}) is less than core temperature (T_c), body heat will be lost. The blood flow required to maintain a given T_c is proportional to the difference between T_c and T_{sk}, which is the gradient for heat transfer from body core to skin surface, where it is lost to the environment. The T_{sk} is actively controlled by the evaporation of sweat; each liter evaporated can remove 580 kcal from the body. This has permitted humans to withstand prolonged exposure to saunas at 50 to 100°C and to hot ovens reaching temperatures as high as 205°C, while meat in the same oven became well cooked.[53] Thus, even during exposure to extreme hot air environments, increments in T_c (~0.5°C) as well as in cardiac output (and thus skin blood flow) are minor as long as the water vapor pressure of ambient air is low[53]; that is, sweat evaporation is sufficient to keep T_{sk} low enough to maintain an optimal $T_c - T_{sk}$ gradient. Accordingly "heat stress" really signifies a rise in T_c that may or may not attend exposure to hot air environments, depending on the rate of sweat evaporation and the resultant gradient for heat loss.

EXPOSURE TO HOT BATHS

The current popularity of recreational hyperthermia induced by hot baths entails some risk, especially for cardiac patients. When humans are exposed to heat without the benefit of sweat evaporation, the cardiovascular response is deleterious. The ideal response to surroundings from which heat can only be gained would be the same as the response to cold. Cessation of skin blood flow by vasoconstriction would increase thermal insulation of the body and minimize the rate of heat gain from the skin circulation. The consequent retention of resting metabolic heat production would be far less serious than the rapid rate of heat gain from the hot bath.

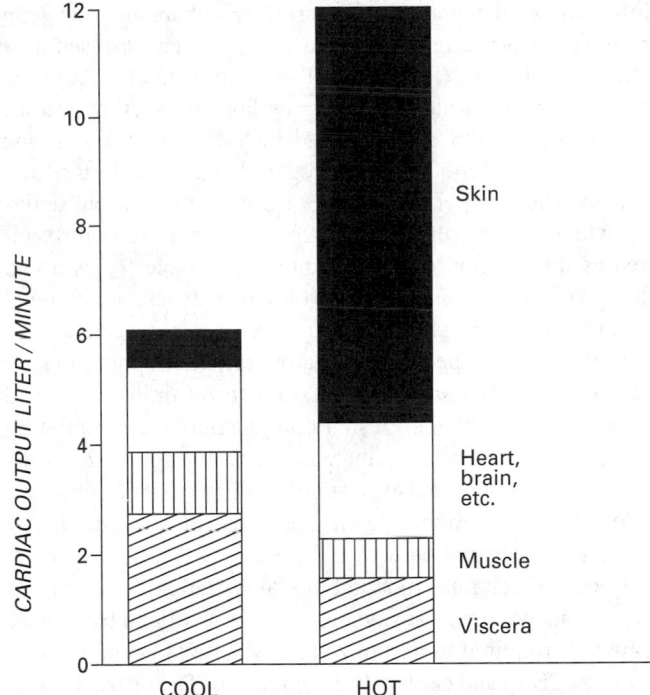

FIGURE 88-7

Bar graph showing cardiac output and its distribution among major organ systems at supine rest in normothermic (left) and hyperthermic (right) conditions. Whole body skin temperature was held at 32°C and then at 40°C for 30 to 53 min by water-perfused suits with no sweat evaporation. Rise in cardiac output plus blood flow distribution away from visceral organs and skeletal muscle went primarily to skin. (From Rowell.[46] Reproduced with permission from the American Physiological Society.)

Features unique to human skin such as its dense vascularization, capacious venous plexus, and active vasodilation system combine to accelerate the rate of heat gain. Reversal of the $T_c - T_{sk}$ gradient by hot baths generates the maximal increases in skin blood flow illustrated in Fig. 88-7. Although the marked rise in skin blood flow can reduce thermal injury to the skin, it causes hyperthermia.

Figure 88-7 shows the marked rise in cardiac output and changes in its distribution during direct heating to the limits of thermal tolerance in normal young men. Heating was achieved by holding whole body T_{sk} at 40°C by water-perfused suits that also prevented sweat evaporation. Temperature of right atrial blood (a measure of T_c) rose continuously, reaching 39.1°C in about 50 min. Cardiac output rose ~3 L/min per degree rise in T_c and reached 12 to 14 L/min.[45,46] In normal individuals, arterial blood pressure is well maintained, but right atrial and central venous pressures (CVP) decline in proportion to the rise in cardiac output. This is because the high blood flow directed to the skin vasculature raises pressure and volume* in this compliant and capacious circuit. As a consequence, blood volume as well as blood

---

* The increase in cutaneous venous volume would be most pronounced in hot humid air environments or in the water-perfused suits. In hot baths, increments in cutaneous venous volume (but not in blood flow) would be opposed by a depth-dependent counterpressure on veins from surrounding water.

flow shift to the body surface, further enhancing heat gain from the surroundings—in this case in the water-perfused suits with vapor barrier (Fig. 88-8). The main difference between exposure to hot water baths versus hot and very humid air (sweat evaporation is suppressed in both conditions) is the greater shift in blood volume to peripheral veins in the air.

Hyperthermia per se increases sympathetic nervous activity, which causes regional vasoconstriction that, in turn, increases the fraction of cardiac output available for skin and alters the distribution of blood volume. Splanchnic and renal blood flows fall in proportion to the rise in heart rate and T_c (Fig. 88-9). At the peak of the heating response approximately 60 percent of the cardiac output, or 7 to 8 L/min, is directed to the skin (Fig. 88-7). Plasma norepinephrine concentration and plasma renin activity increase in proportion to T_c; however, the renin-angiotensin system adds little to the neurogenic vasoconstriction elicited from thermoreceptors in the hypothalamus and spinal cord.[54]

Because high rates of skin blood flow can increase cutaneous venous volume, translocation of blood volume from other regions is required to minimize the reduction in central blood volume (CBV) and cardiac filling pressure. The distribution of blood volume is altered most by splanchnic vasoconstriction, which reduces the pressures throughout this capacious venous bed, which contains approximately 20 percent of total blood volume. Since splanchnic veins are normally near their maximal compliance, large decrements in intravenous volume will accompany small pressure changes. Central mobilization of blood volume is enhanced by the large pressure gradient that develops between peripheral veins and the right atrium (Fig. 88-10). We cannot say whether or not blood volume is actively expressed from visceral organs by venoconstriction, but the fall in right atrial pressure along with splanchnic vasoconstriction favors a *passive* mobilization. The *increase* in stroke volume under these conditions suggests an increase in myocardial contractile force.[45,46] Since most of the energy needed to force blood back to the heart is provided by the left ventricle [venous return to the heart is aided by the abdominothoracic pump and any suction by the right ventricle (see Chap. 3) but is not aided by compression of peripheral veins by exercising skeletal muscles at rest], an increase in myocardial contractile force would be highly advantageous during heat stress. It follows that patients in mild congestive heart failure may develop acute left ventricular failure during heat stress.[55] Also, the reduction in filling pressure caused by cutaneous vasodilation creates severe problems for patients with stenotic valvular lesions and reduced ventricular compliance.

Similar changes in blood flow are seen in patients with erythroderma; their chronically high skin blood flow leads to high-output failure with edema, venous congestion, hepatomegaly, and cardiac enlargement along with renal and gastrointestinal abnormalities.[51] Paraplegic patients show blunted responses to increased core temperature.[52] The cause is unknown; loss of thermal sensors in the spinal cord may contribute.[46] The rise in skin blood flow is also subnormal in patients with diabetic neuropathy,[53] undoubtedly because of defective neural control of skin blood vessels.

THE RISK OF HYPERTHERMIA

An issue of central importance is whether the rise in T_c during hyperthermia reflects as well the rise in brain temperature. Many mammals have specialized heat-exchange mechanisms in the head that can reduce the rate of rise of brain temperature, or portions of the brain, while at the same time body T_c reaches levels that presumably could be deleterious to cerebral function. In this "selective brain cooling,"[56,57] venous blood, which is cooled while draining the nasal cavity and skin of the head, flows into

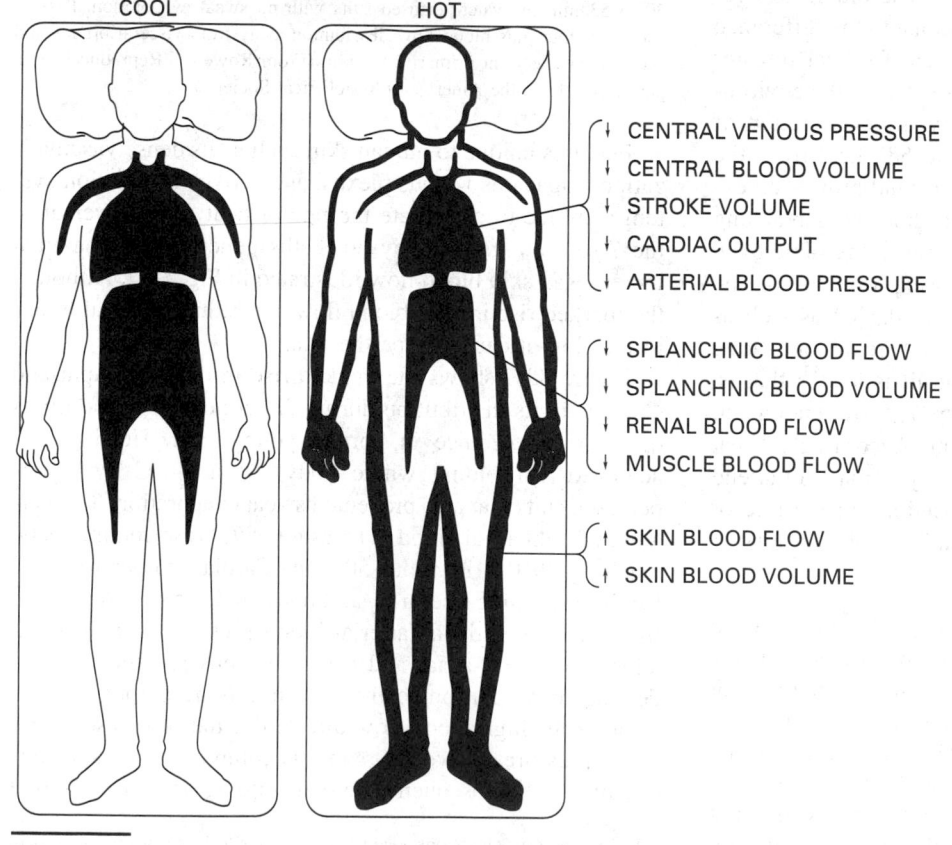

FIGURE 88-8

Hyperthermia and cutaneous vasodilation shift blood volume away from thorax and abdomen to body surface to reduce the body's thermal insulation and augment heat loss. The consequent reduction in ventricular filling reduces orthostatic tolerance. (From Rowell.[60] Reproduced with permission from Oxford University Press.)

COOL   HOT

CENTRAL VENOUS PRESSURE
CENTRAL BLOOD VOLUME
STROKE VOLUME
CARDIAC OUTPUT
ARTERIAL BLOOD PRESSURE

SPLANCHNIC BLOOD FLOW
SPLANCHNIC BLOOD VOLUME
RENAL BLOOD FLOW
MUSCLE BLOOD FLOW

SKIN BLOOD FLOW
SKIN BLOOD VOLUME

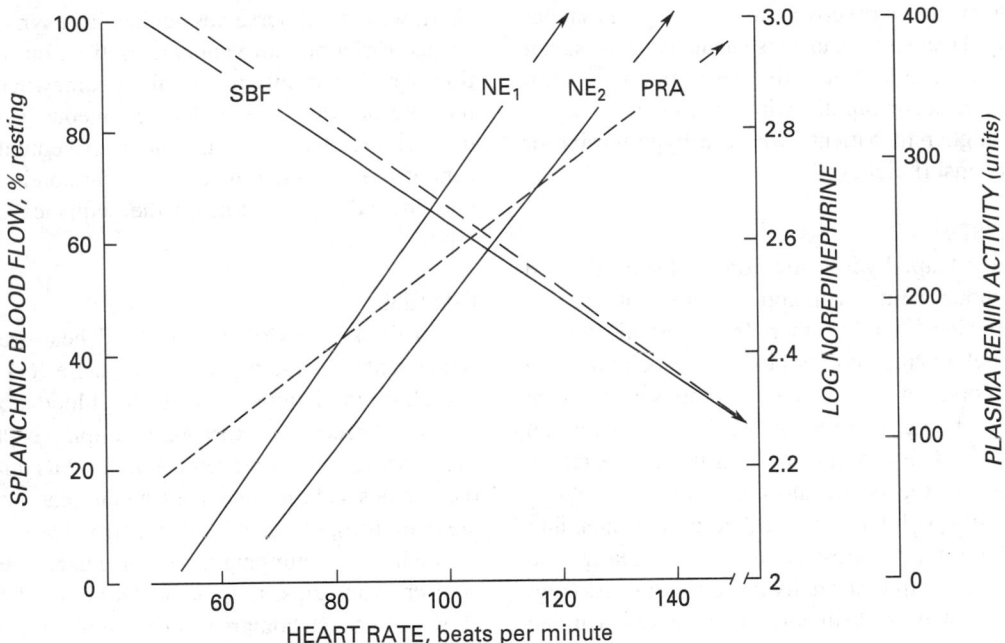

FIGURE 88-9

Relationship between splanchnic blood flow (SBF) and heart rate during heat stress. The rises in plasma norepinephrine concentration (NE_1 and NE_2 from different experiments) and plasma renin activity[54] along with the parallel declines in both SBF (and renal blood flow not shown) reflect the relative increases in sympathetic nervous activity. (From Rowell.[45] Reproduced with permission from Oxford University Press.)

venous sinuses at the base of the brain, where it removes heat from arteries supplying the circle of Willis by countercurrent exchange. Other specialized structures such as the carotid rete work similarly.

Some contend that selective brain cooling occurs in humans.[56] Others argue—more convincingly—that it does not.[57] The crux of the argument *for* selective cooling is that tympanic membrane temperature tracks brain temperature; the fall in tympanic temperature during facial cooling of hyperthermic subjects could reveal selective brain cooling. Direct measures of brain temperature in a human patient refute this claim, however.[58] Physical and anatomic arguments against selective brain cooling in humans are compelling.[57]

Accordingly in humans, the burden of guarding the central nervous system from hyperthermia falls on the entire cutaneous circulation and sweating. That is, we must control temperatures of the brain and of the whole body together as a single unit. Thus the most serious threat from hot baths stems from our lack of a significant thermal short circuit that keeps the brain—which is out of the hot bath—from experiencing the same temperatures as the remainder of the body, which is gaining heat from the bath. Although this need to cool brain and body as a single unit explains why humans require such a potent cutaneous vasodilation system and great range of skin blood flow, these same features pose a threat when the $T_c - T_{sk}$ gradient is reversed.

The strain placed on the cardiovascular system by heat stress can be severe. Patients with cardiovascular disease are

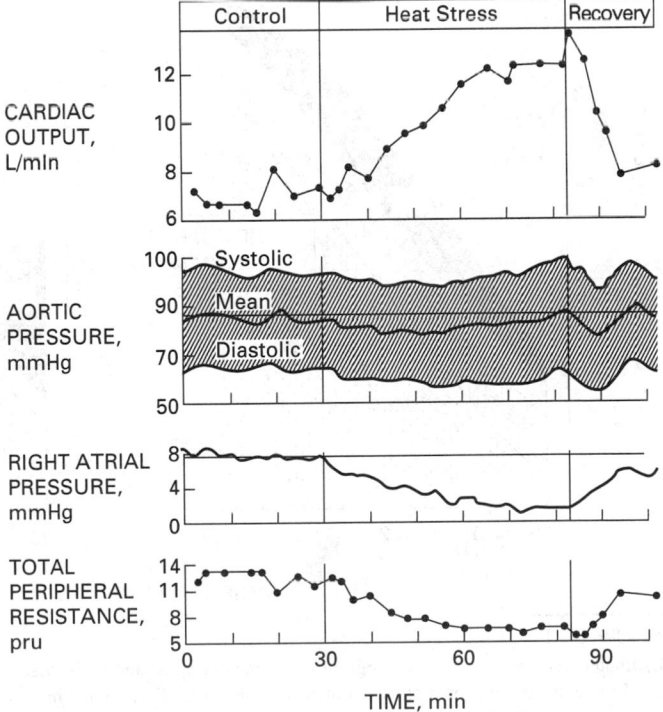

FIGURE 88-10

Responses of one normal subject to 53 min of direct whole body heating at supine rest (T_c rose to 38.7°C). The increase in cardiac output and its distribution to compliant skin lowered right atrial pressure in proportion to the rise in blood flow. (From Rowell.[60] Reproduced with permission from Oxford University Press.)

at risk, and deaths from overexposure to hot baths and saunas occur periodically. Heat stress can cause acute cardiovascular collapse in patients in mild congestive heart failure.[59] Heat injury in saunas can occur rapidly with no prodromal warnings; the risk is higher in patients who are hypertensive or prone to coronary insufficiency.[59]

STANDING AT REST

When humans stand up, hydrostatic forces displace blood volume into dependent veins, with approximately 500 to 600 mL moving into the legs[60] and another 200 to 300 mL shifting into veins of the pelvic area and buttocks. In association with increases in skin blood flow and cutaneous venous compliance during heat stress, blood volume in the legs increases an additional 200 mL.[60] This effect of heating further decreases the return of blood to the heart, and the marked reductions in CVP, CBV, stroke volume, and cardiac output attending upright posture without heat stress are now even greater. The distribution of cardiac output normally during heat stress (Fig. 88-8) provides the best example in normal humans of a cardiac output that is maldistributed to withstand orthostasis. The exaggerated fall in right and left ventricular outputs can be minimized only transiently by depletion of preventricular sumps, i.e., thoracic and splanchnic veins and the pulmonary vasculature. Without vasoconstriction in skin to supplement that occurring in other organs, syncope would occur rapidly. In short, we defend ourselves against heat syncope by cutaneous vasoconstriction, not venoconstriction; but this vasoconstriction, which can only reduce flow somewhat, merely reduces the rate at which dependent cutaneous veins fill and thus delays rather than prevents syncope. Eventually cardiac output cannot rise enough to match vascular conductance, and blood pressure falls precipitously; the sequence of events can be rapid.[61]

EXERCISE

When the stresses of exercise and heat are combined, two fundamental regulatory problems arise: (1) Skeletal muscle and skin circulations compete for blood flow because their combined needs can exceed the pumping capacity of the heart even during moderate exercise; and (2) as during rest, cutaneous venous volume increases when heat stress and exercise are combined, causing CVP and stroke volume to fall despite the maintained pumping action of muscle contraction.[45,60] In cool environments, the cutaneous veins of the legs refill so slowly after each compression by contracting muscle that their average pressure and volume remain low. In contrast, during heat stress, these veins refill so rapidly after each contraction that average venous volume is increased markedly.[45,60] Reductions in CBV, ventricular filling pressure, and stroke volume ensue. Nevertheless, during mild exercise the fall in stroke volume is well compensated by a rise in heart rate so that increased demands for skin blood flow can be met by raising cardiac output by 2 to 3 L/min.[45] During moderate to heavy exercise, however, cardiac output is maintained by increased HR but is *not* increased to meet the additional demands for skin blood flow (Fig. 88-11). Because of the decrease in stroke volume, HR approaches maximal values at submaximal levels of O_2 uptake. Eventually, because of the rapid encroachment on heart rate reserve, cardiac output is reduced below normal and combined demands for skin and muscle blood flow cannot be met. Even the most severe hyperthermia does not increase total skin blood flow to levels seen in supine individuals. Thus, cardiac output does not, as once thought, simply increase to raise skin blood flow until a maximal cardiac output is reached at submaximal levels of O_2 uptake. Again, this is prevented by the reduction in stroke volume (see also Chaps. 3 and 95).

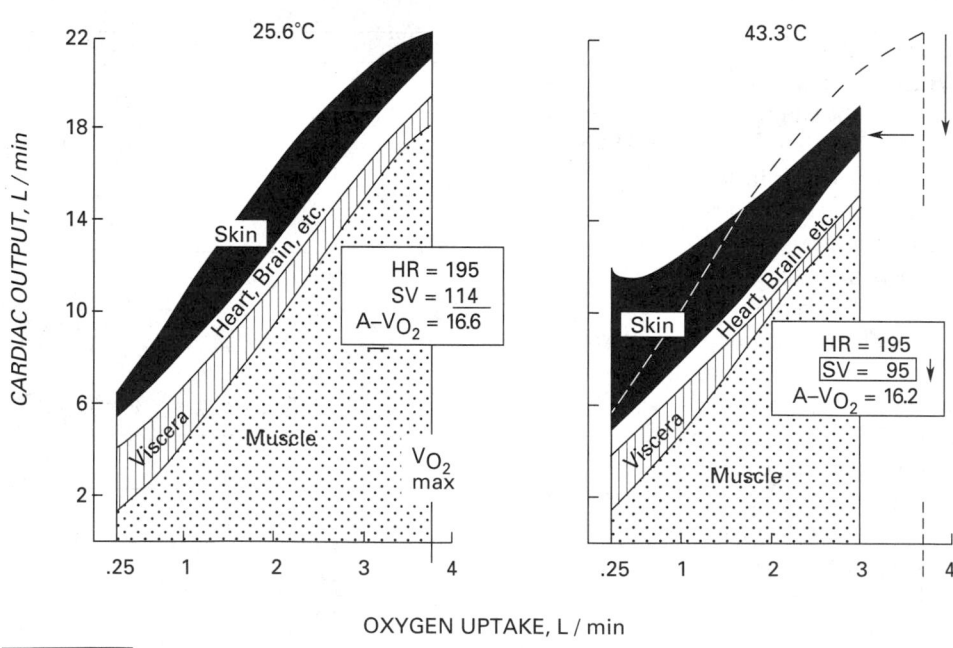

FIGURE 88-11

Estimated distribution of cardiac output between skin, heart and brain, visceral organs, and skeletal muscle over the full range of oxygen uptake from rest to maximal (V_{O_2} max) in neutral (25.6°C) and hot air (43.3°C) environments. The high skin blood flows observed by intense heating at rest cannot be achieved during exercise without compromising muscle blood flow and oxygen uptake. As oxygen uptake rises to high levels at 43.3°C, the rise in cardiac output is reduced (compare with superimposed dashed line from 25°C) owing to reduced stroke volume (SV). A reduced maximal cardiac output and a normal arteriovenous oxygen difference ($A - V_{O_2}$) are reached at a heart rate of 195 beats/min and at 3 L/min of O_2 rather than at 3.7 L/min of O_2 (V_{O_2} max). Reduction in muscle blood flow is proposed but unproven. (From Rowell.[45] Reproduced with permission of Oxford University Press.)

The limited ability of the *normal* heart to meet the combined needs of skin and muscle is partly compensated for by redistribution of blood flow away from visceral organs (Fig. 88-12). In cool environments, splanchnic and renal blood flows decrease in inverse proportion to O_2 uptake and HR during exercise while plasma norepinephrine concentration and renin activity rise. This reduction in visceral organ blood flow is increased by heat stress (along with plasma norepinephrine and renin levels), so that an additional 600 to 800 mL of blood can be redistributed from these organs to skin each minute. Inasmuch as most of the norepinephrine is derived from active muscle, vasoconstriction of these muscles (which is present during exercise in cool conditions) may also be increased.[45,60] During prolonged exercise in hot environments, splanchnic and renal blood flow decrease progressively. Reductions of 70 percent in splanchnic blood flow have been measured, and evidence indicates that function of visceral organs may be impaired.[62] The situation is analogous to that observed in cardiac patients who, being unable to raise their cardiac output adequately with exercise in cool environments, must rely instead on redistribution of cardiac output to perfuse working muscle.[63] Patients with pure mitral stenosis, for example, show marked reductions in splanchnic blood flow at low levels of work (Fig. 88-12).[64] If heat stress during exercise further reduces splanchnic blood flow in these patients (dashed line in Fig. 88-12), flow could reach critically low levels. The central lobular necrosis that can develop in such patients may result from frequent repetitions of visceral ischemia.

The cutaneous circulation does not escape the effects of altered sympathetic activity during exercise and heat stress. As core temperature rises above 38°C, the rate of rise of skin blood flow is reduced markedly and approaches an upper limit that is far below the values measured at the same core temperature in resting subjects. Surprisingly, this upper limit is caused by a withdrawal of sympathetic vasodilator activity rather than active vasoconstriction.[65] Skin blood flow, as measured in the initial stages of exercise, is reduced in patients with heart failure.[66] Cutaneous vasoconstriction can reduce or delay peripheral displacement of blood volume and help maintain blood flow, but the price is augmented heat storage. When combined skin and muscle vasodilation encroaches on cardiac pumping capacity, control of arterial pressure must demand further vasoconstriction in active muscle as well, inasmuch as it comprises 75 to 85 percent of total vascular conductance. Muscle is probably the major source of norepinephrine spillover during exercise with heat as it is with exercise alone.[60]

In the overall regulatory scheme, regulation of blood pressure during heat stress appears to have precedence unless core temperature rises beyond tolerable limits, at which point regulation fails. Such failure is most likely in patients with stenotic valvular lesions and reduced ventricular compliance because of the large reductions in cardiac filling pressure associated with heat stress. In addition, critical hepatic and renal functions are likely to be disrupted by increased diver-

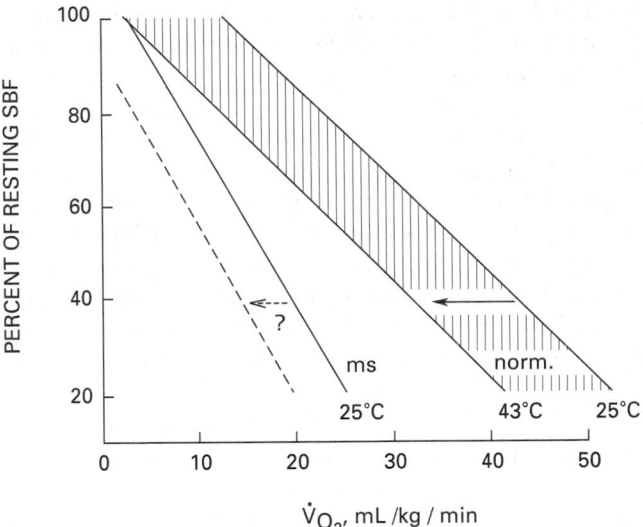

FIGURE 88-12

Summary of splanchnic vascular responses to upright exercise in normal subjects at 25 and 43°C environmental temperature. The shaded region marks the highly significant 20 percent reduction in splanchnic blood flow (SBF) at any given V_{O_2} in the heat in normal subjects. On the left is the regression line from seven patients with pure mitral stenosis (ms), who show much greater reduction in flow at any given V_{O_2}. It is not known whether these patients show further reduction in flow in the heat. (Dashed line shows result of predicted 20 percent reduction).[45,46]

sion of their blood flow. This would be most likely in patients with low output whose perfusion of visceral organs was chronically reduced at rest.

COLD STRESS

Exercise in a cold environment, as in shoveling snow, is considered particularly stressful to patients with effort angina; however, the mechanism by which cold produces angina has been elusive. In the familiar cold pressor test, intense discomfort is produced by immersion of the hand in ice water or application of ice to the forehead. Reflex sympathetic stimulation is produced, resulting in a rise in systolic blood pressure (± 12 mmHg) accompanied by a modest increase in HR that is, however, less in older men ($+4$ beats per minute) than in younger men ($+10$ beats per minute).[67] This elevation of the rate-pressure product increases cardiac work, i.e., myocardial O_2 demand, which is normally met by endothelial-dependent coronary vasodilation[68,69] mediated by nitric oxide and an increase in coronary blood flow.[68,70] In patients with coronary disease, however, there is a paradoxical decrease in coronary blood flow.[71] Apparently this results from a loss of endothelial function due to atherosclerosis, thereby leaving the constrictor influence of sympathetic stimulation unopposed.[68,72] This may explain the increase in sensitivity to catecholamines in coronary vessels with atherosclerosis.[73] Consequently, in patients with coronary artery disease, cold stress produces a discrepancy between increasing myocardial O_2 demand combined with decreasing coronary blood flow and O_2 supply that appears to be the basis for angina in this circumstance.

A less severe stimulus than the cold pressor test can also provoke angina. When coronary disease patients inhaled very cold air ($-20°$ C), some experienced typical angina chest pain even though there was only minimal change in blood pressure or HR, no increase in myocardial O_2 consumption, no change in coronary blood flow, and no angiographic evidence of coronary artery constriction. This suggests that cold air constricts minute coronary collaterals or other blood vessels specifically affecting blood flow to potentially ischemic regions of the myocardium.[74] This is at rest (see also Chap. 45).

Exercise performance in a cold environment has also been examined in men with effort angina and a history of cold intolerance.[75] During submaximal exercise on a bicycle ergometer, systolic blood pressure, HR, and the rate-pressure product were significantly higher, and angina developed at a lower work load, when the room temperature was $-10°$ C rather than $+20°$ C. Similar results could also be obtained by having the subjects inhale very cold air ($-35°$ C) during exercise in an otherwise warm room ($+20°$ C). Skin cooling, however, was considered far more important than the inhalation of only moderately cold air ($-10°$ C) in stressing the heart, presumably due to greater sympathetic stimulation.

DIVING AND HYPERBARIC MEDICINE

Diving Medicine

Underwater diving induces responses by the human cardiovascular system that have become reasonably well understood in recent years. In addition to these physiologic responses, emergencies sometimes occur that are associated with profound alterations in cardiovascular function. Divers are subject to the same cardiovascular illnesses that occur in conventional settings. In addition, the risk of an ensuing fatal consequence is infinitely greater should an acute myocardial infarction or cerebrovascular accident occur in the water.

DIVING AND IMMERSION[76–79]
Alterations in the physical environment encountered by the diver breathing air include increases in barometric pressure, density of the breathing gas, inspired P_{O_2}, and inspired pressure of nitrogen and loss of body heat to the surrounding water. The most characteristic cardiovascular effects of these physical forces, both individually and collectively, is an increase in the intrathoracic blood volume leading to increased stroke volume and increased cardiac output. These circulatory responses occur primarily in association with immersion and are modified by the effects of the temperature of the water, e.g., hypothermia.

Simple immersion in thermoneutral water produces remarkable adjustments in cardiopulmonary and renal function. These physiologic responses are attributable to the effects of increased hydrostatic pressure outside the body, which increases the pressure gradient across the diaphragm and decreases venous compliance in the lower extremities. These combined effects increase intrathoracic blood volume. This centralization of blood distends the atria and activates mechanoreceptors, initiating the immersion response. The immersion response includes both diuretic and natriuretic components, probably achieved by independent mechanisms. The primary mechanism of the diuresis is suppression of antidiuretic hormone (ADH) release by the pituitary gland (Gauer-Henry response). The natriuretic mechanism is complex and related to decrease tubular reabsorption of sodium. Natriuresis appears to be mediated by aldosterone suppression via decreased renin-angiotensin activity, increased release of atrial natriuretic peptide, and increased release of renal prostaglandins. Central hypervolemia and cardiac distension during immersion increase cardiac output by improving stroke volume through enhanced ventricular-diastolic filling (preload). Resting HR and cardiac afterload usually remain unchanged, although the HR may be increased by the Bainbridge reflex (see Chap. 3). Assessment of cardiac contractility during immersion has not provided consistent evidence of change. The cardiovascular responses to immersion have proved useful to investigators studying weightlessness in space as well as disorders of volume regulation such as congestive heart failure, chronic renal insufficiency, and chronic liver disease.

BREATH-HOLD DIVING
Cardiopulmonary alterations during breath-hold diving constitute an integrated response to the processes of immersion and apnea. Apnea and facial immersion, particularly in cold water, elicit an incomplete diving response in humans, characterized primarily by bradycardia. The diving response is more pronounced in children and may be accompanied by peripheral vasoconstriction. This response may represent an O_2-dependent function.

During a breath hold, the lungs provide a limited reservoir for exchange of O_2 and CO_2 with the blood. Aveolar P_{O_2} falls in proportion to the decline in mixed venous P_{O_2}, leading to arterial hypoxemia, decreased O_2 transport, and enhanced glycolysis. Arterial hypoxemia also elicits chemoreceptor activity, which produces peripheral vasoconstriction and helps direct a limited O_2 supply to the heart and brain. With a breath hold, the alveolar P_{O_2} rises in proportion to both pulmonary blood flow and the diffusion gradient for CO_2 between mixed venous blood and the air spaces. As CO_2 production increases, the mixed venous P_{CO_2} rises and leads to further increases in the alveolar P_{CO_2}. The point at which the high P_{CO_2} causes breathing to resume is called the *break point*. The time to the break point can be extended by maneuvers that lower the P_{CO_2}, e.g., hyperventilation. Importantly, hyperventilation does not increase the O_2 store of the body significantly because the increase in alveolar P_{O_2} produced by lowering alveolar P_{CO_2} has little effect on the O_2 content of arterial blood. Therefore, hyperventilation extends the time to the break point but may lead to severe hypoxemia before the P_{CO_2} break point is reached. These gas-exchange processes during a breath hold are affected by underwater descent when thoracic compression decreases the volume of the lungs and raises the partial pressures of the gases in the alveoli. During ascent from the breath hold dive, the lung reexpands and alveolar P_{O_2} and P_{CO_2} decline. If the dive has been unusually long, e.g., after a period of hyperventilation, the diver may experience profound hypoxemia and loss of consciousness while approaching the surface. This phenomenon, known as *shallow-water blackout*, is responsible for a significant number of drownings every year.

NEAR DROWNING

The physical environment of underwater divers and swimmers is deceptively dangerous, and relatively minor injuries or accidents may produce catastrophic results. Such catastrophes are usually the result of inhalation of water into the airways (near drowning) and subsequent asphyxia. Effective pulmonary gas exchange ceases, and the victim suffers hypoxic injuries to the brain, heart, and kidneys. Pulmonary injury is also very prominent, and the adult respiratory distress syndrome complicates near drowning in nearly half of the cases. Prolonged hypoxia leads to diffuse neuronal damage, compromise of the blood-brain barrier, and cerebral edema. As in other cases of severe cerebral hypoxia, the neurologic outcome is uncertain.

The effects of near drowning on the heart are complex. Atrial and ventricular arrhythmias, particularly ventricular fibrillation, often complicate near drowning in both fresh and salt water. These arrhythmias have been associated in animal studies with large and rapid shifts in electrolyte concentrations. Human cases generally do not provide strong evidence for such a pathophysiologic mechanism; however, pathologic studies of the human heart after either fresh or salt water drowning demonstrate changes consistent with catecholamine excess. This suggests that intense adrenergic stimulation precipitates the rhythm disturbances. Myocardial infarction may also occur in patients with coronary artery disease as either a cause or an effect of an episode of near drowning.

DECOMPRESSION SICKNESS[80-83]

Diving with compressed gases leads to increases in the partial pressures of oxygen and nitrogen in the airspaces of the lung. These gases are transported in the blood to the capillaries, where they diffuse down a concentration gradient into tissues. The oxygen is metabolized, but the inert gas, nitrogen, is taken up by the tissues of the body. Conversely, nitrogen and other inert gases are eliminated from the body after a pressure decrease during ascent from depth or to altitude. This process is known as *decompression*. Decompression sickness (DCS) occurs primarily during rapid decompression when nitrogen, dissolved in body tissues and no longer in equilibrium with a falling barometric pressure, undergoes a change in physical state. Bubbles form within tissues and venous blood, producing diverse clinical manifestations. Evolution of gas in body tissues may occur during decompression after hyperbaric exposures to more than 1.7 atmospheres absolute (ATA) or

during rapid ascent from sea level to less than 0.5 ATA [18,000 f (5500 m)]. Explosive decompression of a pressurized aircraft cabin is a familiar example of the latter circumstance. DCS is more likely to occur in association with severe exercise, after prolonged hyperbaric exposures, and with excessive body fat. These associations are related to increased uptake of nitrogen by body tissues. Other aggravating factors include increasing age, fatigue, and preexisting vascular disease, presumably related to impaired gas transport from tissues to the external environment during decompression. DCS also occurs less frequently with regular hyperbaric exposures. This acclimatization phenomenon has led to much speculation concerning mechanisms. A favored explanation is a decrease in the number of gas nuclei that act as loci for bubble formation during decompression. The pathophysiology of DCS is not explained entirely by the mechanical effects of bubbles. Gas bubbles may form in venous blood and be filtered effectively by the lungs without causing symptoms. Gas bubbles in blood and tissues, however, are also known to cause a variety of secondary manifestations related to the effects of surface activity at the gas-to-blood interface. In serious DCS, there may be loss of intravascular fluid and hemoconcentration, activation of complement, platelet aggregation, procoagulant activity, and release of vasoactive compounds such as serotonin, histamine, and bradykinin.

Overt clinical signs and symptoms of DCS are more likely to occur when bubbles lodge in regions wherein ischemia evolves with associated pain and/or perturbed function. For convenience, the clinical manifestations are classified as being either mild (type 1) or severe (type 2). Clinical manifestations of both mild and severe DCS may be present in one-third of these patients. Accordingly, a careful search for subtle manifestations of severe DCS is mandatory in every instance. The common manifestations of both mild and severe DCS are listed in Table 88-1.

The most characteristic manifestation of mild DCS is pain that is ordinarily localized within or near limb joints. After excursion dives in which compressed air is breathed, the pain is more likely to occur in the upper rather than the lower

---

TABLE 88-1

SIGNS AND SYMPTOMS OF DECOMPRESSION SICKNESS

Type 1 (mild)
  Extremities: pain (bends), paresthesia, numbness, edema
  Skin; pruritus, mottling, rash, pallor, urticaria
Type 2 (severe)
  Central nervous system: loss of consciousness, scintillating scotomata, Ménière's syndrome, vertigo, staggering gait, aphasia, paresis or paralysis, sensory loss, bladder and bowel paralysis
  Cardiorespiratory: substernal distress, paroxysmal coughing, shock, tachypnea, asphyxia (chokes), hemoconcentration, platelet–red cell aggregates
  Systemic: extreme fatigue

limbs. After prolonged exposure to compressed air, as is the case for caisson workers or after deep helium-oxygen saturation diving, pain typically occurs in the lower rather than the upper limbs. The initial symptom may be numbness. Characteristically, the discomfort becomes progressively more severe and debilitating pain may evolve, requiring potent analgesic management. At times, local edema and mottling may occur over the site of the pain. Typically, the pain subsides completely or lessens substantially during prompt recompression with oxygen breathing. Trials of recompression and oxygen breathing, singly or in combination, may be employed diagnostically as well as therapeutically. Untreated limb pain will subside gradually; however, complete resolution of pain is likely to require several days. The cutaneous manifestations of mild DCS include pruritus and patchy vasodilation, consistent with vascular stasis. Urticaria and edema may occur as well. Many patients also complain of malaise, but the etiology of this complaint is obscure.

Severe (type 2) DCS is characterized by neurologic or cardiorespiratory involvement. Manifestations are diverse, multiple, and unpredictable. The natural history is variable in the absence of recompression therapy. In fulminant cases, cardiorespiratory arrest and death may occur. Permanent serious neurologic sequelae including paralegia may also occur. In other instances, severe neurologic deficits resolve gradually over intervals of weeks and months despite the absence of appropriate treatment. Severe DCS involving the cardiorespiratory system is characterized by retrosternal discomfort, dyspnea, cough, tachypnea, and extreme fatigue. A sharp "catch" sensation during inspiration is characteristic. Divers refer to this symptom as the "chokes." Postural hypotension, oliguria, hemoconcentration, and hypovolemic shock may also occur.

Neurologic DCS involves the spinal cord relatively often. The latter manifestation reflects the consequences of ischemic injury, produced in some cases by bubble-induced stasis in the epidural venous plexus. The onset is often insidious, with initial mild symptoms of limb paresthesia and weakness. Minutes to hours later, paralysis may occur, often with impairment of bladder and bowel function. Girdle pain is a noteworthy early symptom. Visual disturbances, headaches, abnormal behavior, vertigo, nystagmus, nausea, and vomiting may develop as manifestations of upper central nervous system and labyrinthine involvement. Migraine-like symptoms may occur, particularly in patients with histories of true migraine headaches. A significant number of serious cases of DCS arise from venous gas emboli crossing a patent foramen ovale during or shortly after ascent. This cardiac anomaly, normally present in about 20 to 30 percent of the general population, is thought to be a risk factor for development of serious DCS. The associated risk is probably a function of the extent of bubble formation in the venous system during and after decompression.

Management of DCS is straightforward and very successful. Prompt recompression in a hyperbaric chamber and breathing 100 percent oxygen with short air breaks lead to relief of symptoms within a few minutes in most cases. With appropriate treatment, the recovery rate approximates 95 percent. The rationale for treatment is based on the twin principles that (1) reexposure to hyperbaric pressures facilitates the return of gas bubbles to the physically dissolved state, and (2) breathing pure oxygen lowers the concentration of inert gas in venous blood, thereby increasing the gradient for removal of nitrogen from tissue and hence from the bubbles within the tissue. Clearly, the best responses to treatment are achieved when recompression is prompt. In more severe cases of DCS, other forms of ancillary therapy may be beneficial, including volume repletion. The administration of glucocorticoids is controversial. Details of treatment schedules are outlined fully in the U.S. Navy Diving Manual.[81] These recompression tables represent treatment standards. Fortunately for the patient, even serious neurologic disability may respond to recompression therapy after a delay of several days. Furthermore, the prognosis for recovery is good even when the initial response is incomplete. Complete recovery has been observed to require as much as 2 years in some cases.

INTRAARTERIAL GAS EMBOLISM[80–83]

In compressed-air diving, arterial air (or gas) embolism may occur during ascent to the surface, particularly when the diver fails to exhale normally. Under these circumstances, as ambient hydrostatic pressure decreases during the ascent, gas within the lungs expands reciprocally according to Boyle's Law. One important consequence of this reciprocal action may not be apparent. At greater depths, a partial ascent equivalent to a barometric change of one ATA will be associated with only a small increase in gas volume, i.e., a change from 10 to 9 ATA causes only a 10 percent increase in gas volume. At shallow depths, the consequences are much greater, i.e., a change from 2 to 1 ATA will result in a 100 percent increase in gas volume. Failure to exhale under these circumstances may create a pressure gradient exceeding the compliance of lung tissue. If this positive pressure gradient between alveolar gas and the pulmonary interstitium leads to alveolar disruption and pulmonary interstitial emphysema, the diver may develop soft tissue or mediastinal emphysema, pneumothorax, or pneumopericardium. Free gas may also enter pulmonary venous blood and travel through the left heart to the arterial circulation. Air may then disperse throughout the arterial system, including the coronary and renal arteries. The most common clinical manifestations occur within the distribution of the carotid arteries, however, leading to acute profound cerebral dysfunction characterized by loss of consciousness, seizures, and paralysis. In contrast to DCS, the gas embolization does not arise from a physical change of the state of dissolved gas in tissues and, depending on the degree of pulmonary overdistension, the amount of gas disseminated into the arterial system may be very large. This severe complication of ascent can occur readily after only brief exposures or at very shallow depths in circumstances under which DCS is not a diagnostic consideration. In the absence of adequate treatment, a severe central nervous system deficit from air embolism is more likely to be permanently disabling or lethal than is DCS.

Recompression therapy should commence within minutes if a satisfactory clinical outcome is to be achieved. The principles of management are similar to those elaborated for DCS, but the magnitude, length, and number of recompression treatments are generally greater. A number of case reports describe incremental benefit from longer hyperbaric exposures configured in days rather than hours. Some observers report resolution of neurologic deficits, in some cases even after delays of treatment of more than 24 h.

Serious intraarterial gas embolism also occurs in other circumstances, for example, as a result of explosive decompression of pressurized aircraft, after accidental trauma to the great vessels, during blast injury of the thorax, and in the hospitalized patient. Arterial gas embolism in the hospital setting is not infrequent but is often unrecognized as a complication of various diagnostic and therapeutic procedures (Table 88-2). Air may enter the arterial system directly, as during cardiovascular surgery and radiodiagnostic procedures, or after venous air embolism, when acute pulmonary hypertension permits air to cross a patent foramen ovale. In the patient with serious underlying illness, the presence of a major arterial gas embolism may impose very difficult therapeutic choices for the physician. Oxygen therapy alone is not likely to produce a good functional recovery, but even when hyperbaric oxygen therapy is practical, the prognosis is relatively guarded. Whenever possible, the same principles of treatment should be employed for air embolism in the hospitalized patient as in the diver.

Hyperbaric Oxygen Therapy[84–91]

Hyperbaric oxygen therapy is defined as breathing 100 percent oxygen at greater than normal atmospheric pressures. This is achieved in special environmental chambers containing pressurized gas and at the same time providing adequate technological support for patient care. The use of hyperbaric pressure overcomes the barrier to increased oxygen transport imposed by limited solubility of oxygen in plasma. Whereas 100 mL of blood equilibrated at P_{O_2} of 100 mmHg contains only 0.3 mL of physically dissolved O_2, the latter amount can be increased to almost 6 mL by breathing 100 percent oxygen

---

TABLE 88-2

HOSPITAL PROCEDURES SOMETIMES ASSOCIATED WITH INTRAARTERIAL AIR EMBOLISM

Deep venous catheter insertion, use, and removal
Radiodiagnostic injections of contrast dye into arterial
   system
Cardiovascular surgery
Neuroradiologic and neurosurgical procedures including
   myelography
Hemodialysis
Positive pressure ventilation
Transbronchial biopsy

---

at 3 ATA. Under these circumstances, the P_{O_2} in arterial blood will approach 2000 mmHg provided pulmonary gas exchange is normal.

MECHANISMS OF ACTION OF HYPERBARIC OXYGEN

The scientific rationale for the use of hyperbaric oxygen has been based on three major principles: (1) the function of hypoxic vital organs can be maintained or restored even in the setting of decreased perfusion, (2) specific beneficial pharmacologic effects can be achieved with high oxygen pressures, and (3) removal of bubbles within tissues can be expedited greatly by the combined effects of increased hydrostatic pressure to reduce bubble size and high pressures of oxygen to accelerate washout of dissolved inert gas by providing a much larger outward diffusive gradient for elimination of inert gas molecules from the bubble. The latter principle is exploited fully in the treatment of DCS and arterial gas embolism, as outlined above. The second principle provides the rationale for use of hyperbaric oxygen in gas gangrene and other anaerobic infections. Application of the first principle, maintaining or restoring function to hypoxic or ischemic tissues, is relevant in certain cardiovascular diseases and in the management of wounded tissues with microcirculatory compromise.

The potential applicability of hyperbaric oxygen as therapy for hypoxic tissues has been constrained greatly by two biological problems: (1) ischemia is likely to prevent delivery of O_2 to the hypoxic tissue, and (2) potential toxicity to the lungs and central nervous system rules out high and continuous levels of oxygen exposure. As a practical matter, central nervous system and pulmonary oxygen toxicities are avoided by limiting hyperbaric exposures to 3 ATA or less for intervals of not more than 90 to 120 min. In practice, these intermittent, limited exposures are well tolerated, and judgments of therapeutic efficacy are based upon the success of single or repetitive treatment profiles conforming to these criteria.

INDICATIONS FOR HYPERBARIC OXYGEN THERAPY

There are only a few standard indications for hyperbaric oxygen therapy in clinical practice. Experimental and clinical evidence supporting efficacy of hyperbaric oxygen in various diseases is reviewed periodically by the Undersea and Hyperbaric Medical Society. The current approved indications are provided in Table 88-3. The applications relevant to the circulation are discussed in greater detail below, and the reader is referred to other sources for discussion of the role of adjunctive hyperbaric oxygen in the management of infectious diseases. Most observations concerning therapy of cardiovascular diseases with hyperbaric oxygen are anecdotal.

Carbon Monoxide Intoxication[88,89]

Acute carbon monoxide (CO) intoxication is the leading cause of accidental poisoning in the United States. Uptake of CO by the body impairs O_2 transport to tissues by two mechanisms. First, arterial O_2 content is decreased in a manner analogous to anemia because hemoglobin binds CO with a 200-fold greater affinity than O_2 to form carboxyhemoglobin

TABLE 88-3

APPROVED CURRENT INDICATIONS FOR HYPERBARIC OXYGEN THERAPY

Hyperbaric oxygen as a primary modality
  Decompression sickness
  Intraarterial air or gas embolism
  Serious carbon monoxide poisoning
  Exceptional blood loss with anemia
Hyperbaric oxygen as an adjunctive modality
  Clostridial myonecrosis
  Necrotizing soft tissue infections involving anaerobic
    organisms
  Enhance healing of problem wounds and compromised
    skin grafts or flaps in selected patients
Refractory chronic osteomyelitis
Radiation necrosis of bone or soft tissue

(HbCO). Second, HbCO shifts the oxyhemoglobin dissociation curve to the left, adversely affecting the release of O_2 from the remaining binding sites on the hemoglobin molecule. The net result of high circulating HbCO levels is tissue hypoxia. Despite compensatory increases in blood flow, the presence of HbCO may lead to serious functional consequences for hypoxia-sensitive organs such as the heart and the brain. Severe tissue hypoxia may set the stage for secondary mechanisms of CO toxicity related to intracellular binding of CO. When tissue P_{O_2} is low, CO may compete successfully for O_2-binding sites on intracellular hemoproteins such as myoglobin and the mitochondrial oxidase, cytochrome aa_3. This effect has potentially serious consequences for myocardial performance when myocardial O_2 demands are high, particularly in the presence of coronary artery disease.

Clinical manifestations of acute CO poisoning include headache, confusion, visual disturbances, unconsciousness, seizures, and pulmonary edema. In untreated patients, the consequences of severe intoxication may lead to death. Metabolic acidosis and rhabdomyolysis may accompany serious poisoning. Patients with mild CO poisoning are likely to recover without specific treatment other than removal from the noxious gaseous environment. With more severe forms of poisoning, the outlook is uncertain. The severity of the clinical illness often does not correlate with the measured HbCO level but corresponds more closely to the extent and duration of the exposure.

A significant number of patients will experience a delayed neurologic syndrome days to weeks after the poisoning. Patients with any form of central nervous system impairment, evidence of myocardial ischemia, or HbCO levels above 25 percent merit aggressive therapeutic intervention with hyperbaric oxygen, if it is available. The use of the modality is based primarily upon more rapid removal of the CO from hemoglobin and tissue sites. Because O_2 and CO compete for hemoglobin and tissue-binding sites, hyperbaric oxygenation greatly accelerates CO elimination. Furthermore, O_2 dissolved in plasma under hyperbaric conditions effectively bypasses

any impediment to oxygen transport imposed by HbCO. Potentially lethal cerebral hypoxia may be averted as a consequence. Twenty minutes of exposure to 100 percent oxygen at 2.5 ATA will be accompanied by release of CO from the blood equivalent to that obtained after 5 h of breathing uncontaminated air; 90 min of hyperbaric oxygen therapy at this pressure is sufficient to reduce HbCO levels to normal. Prompt recovery is the rule if treatment can be initiated before extensive and irreversible brain injury has occurred.

Although the rationale for the use of hyperbaric oxygen to treat acute CO poisoning is strong and anecdotal clinical experience positive, it has been difficult to prove the efficacy of hyperbaric oxygen in clinical trials. Part of this problem relates to the inability to identify and gather significant numbers of high-risk patients with CO poisoning, administer the therapy promptly and effectively, and obtain adequate long-term follow-up of the patients. Evidence has been accumulating, however, that prompt hyperbaric oxygen therapy will prevent the delayed neurologic syndrome.

The use of hyperbaric oxygen has also been suggested to reverse the toxic effects of other poisonous gases, such as hydrogen cyanide and hydrogen sulfide, which, like CO, interfere with cellular respiration by binding to cytochrome aa_3. Unlike CO, however, the binding process for these gases is not competitive with O_2. Consequently, reports of successful treatment of cyanide and hydrogen sulfide poisoning using hyperbaric oxygen go unexplained at present. Nevertheless, prompt O_2 administration may protect tissue viability and provide a useful adjunct to the standard antidotes.

Ischemic Heart Disease

Enthusiasm for therapeutic hyperbaric oxygen in the 1960s generated hope for benefit in ischemic heart disease. One important observation obtained largely from experimental animals was that hyperbaric oxygen exerted a predictable antiarrhythmic effect. Human observations have been sparse because available pharmacologic agents are generally successful and much easier to employ in the setting of ischemia. The implications of this antiarrhythmic effect, however, have continued to be of interest to investigators.

The concept of minimizing myocardial damage from myocardial infarction by the employment of hyperbaric oxygen has been tested experimentally with variable results. Aside from scattered anecdotal observations, only one controlled trial has been performed in human beings. In this series, overall mortality of patients treated with hyperbaric oxygen at 2 ATA was lower than that of control patients. The diversity among patients and excellent results using conventional management preclude definitive interpretation, however. The advent of fibrinolytic therapy and newer invasive techniques that improve the clinical outcome of patients with acute myocardial ischemia make it unlikely that hyperbaric oxygen will be employed widely in the management of these patients. The therapy also has limited investigational interest, particularly in view of experimental concerns that reperfusion after acute coronary occlusion may lead to tissue injury from reactive oxygen species formed as a result of cellular responses provoked by the ischemia.

Cerebrovascular Insufficiency

Very limited observations suggest that reversal of neurologic impairment associated with brief exposures to hyperbaric oxygen identifies a population of patients likely to respond well to cerebral reperfusion or revascularization after stroke. This concept has not been tested adequately using modern interventional technology; however, prompt administration of hyperbaric oxygen, combined with a therapy that restores blood flow, could allow long-term salvage of neurologic function in selected patients. The concerns about reperfusion worsening myocardial injury with hyperbaric oxygen are also valid for reperfusion after brain ischemia.

Peripheral Vascular Insufficiency

Medical management of chronic atherosclerotic peripheral vascular disease is associated with relatively limited benefit (see Chap. 100). Accordingly, there has been considerable interest in alternative therapy. Hyperbaric oxygen has yielded limited results, however, as might be expected when the fundamental problem of vascular compromise is not altered by the treatment modality. Therapeutic intervention with hyperbaric oxygen may be beneficial when superimposed acute problems occur such as infection or vascular compromise of skin grafts, provided the site of the wound is not totally ischemic.

Vasculitis, involving the skin and extremities, is more reversible than atherosclerotic vascular insufficiency. Benefit from intermittent treatment with hyperbaric oxygen has been described for forms of vasculitis causing ischemic injury, often with ulceration.

Problem Wounds

The application of hyperbaric oxygen to manage pain and ulceration caused by chronic wounds is based upon observations that tissue P_{O_2} is low and wound healing impaired in regions within the distribution of a compromised peripheral circulation. Furthermore, tissue hypoxia is a common feature of both acute and chronic wounds. Tissue P_{O_2} measurements have indicated that wound hypoxia is often sufficient to impair leukocyte function and collagen synthesis in the tissue. In selected chronic wounds, the oxygen tension can be increased with hyperbaric oxygen treatment and wound healing enhanced. Clinical treatment profiles vary, and optimal treatment schedules have not been determined for most wounds.

Another special circumstance associated with decreased capillarity and low tissue P_{O_2} is chronic radiation injury of bone and soft tissue. In this setting, chronic pain, ulceration, and tissue necrosis are common and difficult to manage. There is experimental evidence that repetitive treatments with hyperbaric oxygen increases collagen synthesis and capillary profliferation within the injured tissues. The concept has clinical support from well-controlled studies of patients with osteoradionecrosis of the mandible. Treatment with hyperbaric oxygen results in improved capillary density and P_{O_2} in the wound. This promotes more rapid healing and decreases the complications of surgery in radiated tissues.

REFERENCES

1. Alexander JK, Hartley LH, Modelski M, Grover RF. Reduction of stroke volume during exercise in man following ascent to 3,100 m altitude. *J Appl Physiol* 1967; 23:849–858.
2. Hannon JP, Chinn KSK, Shields JL. Effects of acute high-altitude exposure on body fluids. *Fed Proc* 1969; 28:1178–1184.
3. Renkin EM, Tucker VL. Atrial natriuretic peptide as a regulator of transvascular fluid balance. *News Physiol Sci* 1996; 11:138–143.
4. Albert TSE, Tucker VL, Renkin EM. Atrial natriuretic peptide levels and plasma volume contraction in acute alveolar hypoxia. *J Appl Physiol* 1996; 82:102–110.
5. Dempsey JA, Reddan WG, Birnbaum ML, Forster HV, Thoden JS, Grover RF, et al. Effects of acute though lifelong hypoxic exposure on exercise pulmonary gas exchange. *Respir Physiol* 1971; 13:62–89.
6. Weil JV, Jamieson G, Brown DW, Grover RF. The red cell mass—arterial oxygen relationship in normal man. *J Clin Invest* 1968; 47:1627–1639.
7. Grover RF, Selland MA, McCullough RG, Dahms TA, Wolfel EE, Butterfield GE, et al. β-Adrenergic blockade does not prevent polycythemia or decrease in plasma volume in men at 4,300 m altitude. *Eur J Appl Physiol* 1996; (in press).
8. Grover RF, Bṙtsch P. Blood. In: Hornbein T, Schoene R, eds. *High Altitude.* New York: Marcel Dekker; 1997: (in press).
9. Reeves JT, Moore LG, Wolfel EE, Mazzeo RS, Cymerman A, Young AJ. Activation of the sympatho-adrenal system at high altitude. In: Ueda G, Kusama S, Voelkel NF, eds. *High Altitude Medicine.* Matsumoto, Japan: Shinshu University Press; 1992; 10–23.
10. Mazzeo RS, Wolfel EE, Butterfield GE, Reeves JT. Sympathetic response during 21 days at high altitude (4,300 m) as determined by urinary and arterial catecholamines. *Metabolism* 1994; 43:1226–1232.
11. Hughson RL, Yamamoto Y, McCullough RE, Sutton JR, Reeves JT. Sympathetic and parasympathetic indicators of heart rate control at altitude studied by spectral analysis. *J Appl Physiol* 1994; 77:2537–1542.
12. Wolfel EE, Selland MA, Mazzeo RS, Reeves JT. Systemic hypertension at 4300 m is related to sympatho-adrenal activity. *J Appl Physiol* 1994; 76:1643–1650.
13. Weil JV, Battock DJ, Grover RF, Chidsey CA. Venoconstriction in man upon ascent to high altitude: Studies on potential mechanisms. *Fed Proc* 1969; 28:1160–1164.
14. Weil JV, Byrne-Quinn E, Battock DJ, Grover RF, Chidsey CA. Forearm circulation in man at high altitude. *Clin Sci* 1971; 40:235–246.
15. Grover RF, Weil JV, Reeves JT. Cardiovascular adaptation to high altitude. In: Pandolf KB, ed. *Exercise and Sport Sciences Reviews,* vol 14. New York: Macmillan; 1986:269–302.
16. Alexander JK, Grover RF. Mechanism of reduced cardiac stroke volume at high altitude. *Clin Cardiol* 1983; 6:301–303.
17. Groves BM, Reeves JT, Sutton JR, Wagner PD, Cymerman A, Malconian MK, et al. Operation Everest II: Preservation of cardiac function at great altitude. *J Appl Physiol* 1987; 63:531–539.
18. Hellems HK, Ord JW, Talmers FN, Christensen RC. Effects of hypoxia on coronary blood flow and myocardial metabolism in normal human subjects (abstr). *Circulation* 1957; 16:893.
19. Eaton JW, Brewer GJ, Grover RF. Role of red cell 2,3-diphosphoglycerate in the adaptation of man to altitude. *J Lab Clin Med* 1969; 73:603–609.
20. Grover RF, Lufschanowski R, Alexander JK. Alterations in the coronary circulation of man following ascent to 3,100 m altitude. *J Appl Physiol* 1976; 41:832–838.
21. Shlim DR, Houston R. Helicopter rescues and deaths among trekkers in Nepal. *JAMA* 1989; 261:1017–1019.
22. Grover R, Tucker C. McGroarty S, Travis R. The coronary stress of skiing at high altitude. *Arch Intern Med* 1990; 150:1205–1208.
23. Okin JT. Response of patients with coronary heart disease to exercise at varying altitudes. *Adv Cardiol* 1970; 5:92–96.
24. Khanna PK, Dham SK, Hoon RS. Exercise in an hypoxic environment as a screening test for ischaemic heart disease. *Aviat Space Environ Med* 1976; 47:1114–1117.

25. Alexander JK. Coronary heart disease at altitude. *Texas Heart Inst J* 1994; 21:261–266.

26. Mortimer E, Monson R, McMahon B. Reduction in mortality from coronary heart disease in men residing at high altitude. *N Engl J Med* 1977; 296:581.

27. Kayar SR, Banchero N. Myocardial capillarity in acclimatization to hypoxia. *Pflugers Arch* 1985; 404:319–325.

28. Marticorena E, Ruiz L, Severino J, Galvez J, Penaloza D. Systemic blood pressure in white men born at sea level: Changes after long residence at high altitudes. *Am J Cardiol* 1969; 23:364–368.

29. Grover RF. Chronic hypoxic pulmonary hypertension. In: Fishman AP, ed. *The Pulmonary Circulation. Normal and Abnormal.* Philadelphia: University of Pennsylvania Press; 1990:283–299.

30. Reeves JT, Stenmark KR. The pulmonary circulation at high altitude. In: Hornbein T, Schoene R, eds. *High Altitude.* New York: Marce Dekker; 1997.

31. Pryor R, Weaver WF, Blount SG Jr. Electrocardiographic observations of 493 residents living at high altitude (10,150 ft). *Am J Cardiol* 1965; 16:494–499.

32. Reeves JT, Grover RF. High-altitude pulmonary hypertension and pulmonary edema. In: Yu PN, Goodwin JF, eds. *Progress in Cardiology,* vol 4. Philadelphia: Lea & Febiger; 1975:99–118.

33. Sui GJ, Liu YH, Cheng XS, Anand IS, Harris E, Harris P, et al. Subacute infantile mountain sickness. *J Pathol* 1988; 155:161–170.

34. Reeves JT, Wagner WW Jr, McMurtry IF, Grover RF. Physiological effects of high altitude on the pulmonary circulation. In: Robertshaw D, ed. *Environmental Physiology III, International Review of Physiology,* vol 20. Baltimore: University Park Press; 1979:289–310.

35. Sophocles AM Jr, Bachman J. High-altitude pulmonary edema among visitors to Summit County, Colorado. *J Fam Pract* 1983; 17:1015–1017.

36. Sophocles AM Jr. High-altitude pulmonary edema in Vail, Colorado, 1975–1982. *West J Med* 1986; 144:569–573.

37. Grover RF, Hyers TM, McMurtry IF, Reeves JT. High-altitude pulmonary edema. In: Fishman AP, Renkin EM, eds. *Pulmonary Edema.* Bethesda, MD: American Physiological Society; 1979:229–240.

38. Reeves JT, Schoene RB. When lungs on mountains leak: Studying pulmonary edema at high altitudes (editorial). *N Engl J Med* 1991; 325:1306–1307.

39. Brtsch P, Shaw S, Franciolli M, Gn D, Markus P, Weidmann P. Atrial natriuretic peptide in acute mountain sickness. *J Appl Physiol* 1988; 65:1929–1937.

40. Hackett PH, Rennie D. Hofmeister SE, Grover RF, Grover EB, Reeves JT. Fluid retention and relative hypoventilation in acute mountain sickness. *Respiration* 1982; 43:321–329.

41. McMurtry IF, Davidson AB, Reeves JT, Grover RF. Inhibition of hypoxic pulmonary vasoconstriction by calcium antagonists in isolated rat lungs. *Circulation Res* 1976; 38:99–104.

42. Brtsch P, Maggiorini M, Ritter M, Noti C, Vock P, Oelz O. Prevention of high altitude pulmonary edema by nifedipine. *N Engl J Med* 1991; 325:1284–1289.

43. Scherrer U, Vollenweider L, Delabays A, Savcic M, Eichenberger U, Kleger G-R, et al. Inhaled nitric oxide for high-altitude pulmonary edema. *N Engl J Med* 1996; 334:624–629.

44. Scoggin CH, Hyers TM, Reeves JT, Grover RF. High altitude pulmonary edema in children and young adults of Leadville, Colorado. *N Engl J Med* 1977; 297:1269–1271.

45. Rowell LB. *Human Circulation. Regulation During Physical Stress.* New York: Oxford University Press; 1986.

46. Rowell LB. Cardiovascular adjustments to thermal stress. In: Shepherd JT, Abboud FM, eds. *Handbook of Physiology,* Sec 2, *The Cardiovascular System,* Vol III, *Peripheral Circulation and Organ Blood Flow.* Bethesda, MD: American Physiological Society; 1983:967–1023.

47. Brengelmann GL. Temperature regulation. In: Teitz C, ed. *Scientific Foundation of Sports Medicine.* Philadelphia: Marcel Decker; 1989:77–116.

48. Roddie IC. Circulation to skin and adipose tissue. In: Shepherd JT, Abboud FM, eds. *Handbook of Physiology,* Sec 2, *The Cardiovascular System,* Vol III, *Peripheral Circulation and Organ Blood Flow.* Bethesda, MD: American Physiological Society; 1983:285–317.

49. Rowell LB. Reflex control of the cutaneous vasculature. *J Invest Dermatol* 1977; 69:154–166.

50. Lindblad LR, Ekenvall L. Alpha-adrenoreceptors in the vessels of human finger skin. *Acta Physiol Scand* 1986; 128:219–222.

51. Brengelmann GL, Freund PR, Rowell LB, Olerud JE, Kraning KK. Absence of active cutaneous vasodilation associated with congenital absence of sweat glands in man. *Am J Physiol* 1981; 240:H571–H575.

52. Kellogg DL Jr, Pergola PE, Piest KL, Kosiba WA, Crandell CG, Grossman M, et al. Cutaneous active vasodilation in humans is mediated by cholinergic nerve cotransmission. *Circ Res* 1995; 77:1222–1228.

53. Murray RH. Cardiopulmonary effects of brief, intense thermal exposures. *J Appl Physiol* 1966; 21:1717–1724.

54. Escourro P, Freund PR, Rowell LB, Johnson DG. Splanchnic vasoconstriction in heat-stressed man—role of the renin-angiotensin system. *J Appl Physiol* 1982; 52:1438–1443.

55. Ansari A, Burch GE. Influence of hot environments on the cardiovascular system. *Arch Intern Med* 1969; 123:371–378.

56. Cabanas M. Selective brain cooling in humans: "Fancy" or fact? *FASEB J* 1993; 7:1143–1147.

57. Brengelmann GL. Selective brain cooling in humans? *FASEB J* 1993; 7:1148–1153.

58. Shiraki K, Sagawa S, Tajima F, Hashimoto M, Yokota A, Brengelmann GL. Independence of brain and tympanic temperatures in an unanesthetized human. *J Appl Physiol* 1988; 65:482–486.

59. Sohar E, Shoenfeld Y, Shapiro Y, Ohry A, Cabili S. Effects of exposure to Finnish sauna. *Isr J Med Sci* 1976; 12:1275–1282.

60. Rowell LB. *Human Cardiovascular Control.* New York: Oxford University Press; 1993.

61. Lind AR, Leethead CS, McNicol GW. Cardiovascular changes during syncope indiced by titlting men in the heat. *J Appl Physiol* 1968; 25:268–276.

62. Rowell LB, Brengelmann GL, Blackmonn JR, Twiss RD, Kusumi F. Splanchnic blood flow and metabolism in heat-stressed man. *J Appl Physiol* 1968; 24:475–484.

63. Wade OL, Bishop JM. *Cardiac Output and Regional Blood Flow.* Oxford: Blackwell Scientific; 1962.

64. Blackmon JR, Rowell LB, Kennedy JW, Twiss RD, Conn RD. Physiological significance of maximal oxygen intake in pure mitral stenosis. *Circulation* 1967; 36:497–510.

65. Rowell LB, O'Leary DS, Kellogg DL Jr. Integration of cardiovascular control systems in dynamic exercise. In: Rowell LB, Shepherd JT, eds. *Handbook of Physiology,* Sec 12, *Exercise: Regulation and Integration of Multiple Systems.* New York: Oxford University Press and American Physiological Society; 1996; 770–838.

66. Zelis R, Mason DT, Braunwald E. Partition of blood flow to the cutaneous and muscular beds of the forearm at rest and during leg exercise in normal subject and in patients with heart failure. *Circ Res* 1969; 24:799–806.

67. LeBlanc J, C_t· J, Dulac S, Dulong-Turcot F. Effects of age, sex, physical fitness on responses to local cooling. *J Appl Physiol* 1978; 44:813–817.

68. Nabel EG, Ganz P, Gordon JB, Alexander RW, Selwyn AP. Dilation of normal and constriction of atherosclerotic coronary arteries caused by the cold pressor test. *Circulation* 1988; 77:43–52.

69. Nabel EG, Selwyn AP, Ganz P. Paradoxical narrowing of atherosclerotic coronary arteries induced by increases in heart rate. *Circulation* 1990; 81:850–859.

70. Neill WA, Duncan DA, Kloster F, Mahler DJ. Response of the coronary circulation to cutaneous cold. *Am J Med* 1974; 56:471–476.

71. Mudge GH Jr, Grossman W, Mills RM, Lesch M, Braunwald E. Reflex increase in coronary vascular resistance in patients with ischemic heart disease. *N Engl J Med* 1976; 295:1333–1337.

72. Kern MJ, Horowitz JD, Ganz P, Gaspar J, Colucci WS, Lorell BH, et al. Attenuation of coronary vascular resistance by selective alpha 1-adrenergic blockade in patients with coronary artery disease. *J Am Coll Cardiol* 1985; 5:840–846.

73. Vita JA, Treasure CB, Yeung AC, Vekshtein VI, Fantasia GM, Fish RD, et al. Patients with evidence of coronary endothelial dysfunction as assessed by acetylcholine infusion demonstrate marked increase in sensitivity to constrictor effects of catecholamines. *Circulation* 1992; 85:1390–1397.

74. Hattenhauer M, Neill WA. The effect of cold air inhalation on angina pectoris and myocardial oxygen supply. *Circulation* 1975; 51:1053–1058.

75. Lassvik CT, Areskog N-H. Angina pectoris during inhalation of cold air. Reactions to exercise. *Br Heart J* 1980; 43:661–667.

76. Bert P, Hitchcock MA, trans. *La Pression Barometrique.* Columbus, OH: College Book Company; 1943.

77. Bennett PB, Elliott DH. *The Physiology and Medicine of Diving*, 3d ed. San Pedro, CA: Best Publishing; 1982.

78. Salzano J, Stolp B, Moon R, Camporesi E. Exercise at 47 and 66 ATA. In: Bachrach AJ, Matzen MM, eds. *Underwater Physiology VII, Proceedings of Seventh Symposium on Underwater Physiology*. Bethesda, MD: Undersea Med Soc; 1981; 181.

79. Lin Y. Circulatory functions during immersion and breath-hold dives in humans. *Undersea Biomed Res* 1984; 11:123–138.

80. Boycott A, Damant G, Haldane J. Prevention of compressed air illness. *J Hyg* 1908; 8:342–443.

81. *U.S. Navy Diving Manual*, NAVSEA, 0994-LP-001-9020. Washington, DC: Navy Department; 1981.

82. Bühlmann A. *Decompression-Decompression Sickness*. New York: Springer-Verlag; 1984.

83. Miller J, Fagraeus L, Elliott D, Shields T, Grimstad J, Bennett P. Nitrogen-oxygen saturation therapy in serious cases of compressed air decompression sickness. *Lancet* 1978; 2:169–171.

84. Moon RE, Camporesi EM, Kisslo JA. Patent foramen ovale and decompression sickness in divers. *Lancet* 1989; 1:513–514.

85. *Hyperbaric Oxygen Therapy: A Committee Report*. Bethesda, MD: Undersea and Hyperbaric Medical Society; 1989.

86. Holback KH, Wassman H, Banatelli A. A method to identify and treat reversible alterations of brain tissue. In: Schmiedek T, ed. *Microsurgery for Stroke*. New York: Springer-Verlag; 1977:169–176.

87. Heyman A, Saltzman HA, Whalen R. The use of hyperbaric oxygenation in the treatment of cerebral ischemia and infarction. *Circulation* 1966; 33:20–27.

88. Tsuru M, Nakagawa Y, Kitaoka K, Kwahigashi H. Treatment of cerebral ischemia by hyperbaric oxygenation. In: Shiraki K, Matsuoka S, eds. *Hyperbaric Medicine and Underwater Physiology*. Kitakyushu, Japan: Fukuoka Printing; 1983:315–327.

89. Piantadosi CA. The role of hyperbaric oxygen in carbon monoxide, cyanide and sulfide intoxication. *Respir Care* 1991; 4:215–231.

90. Davis JC, Hunt TK. *Problem Wounds. The Role of Oxygen*. New York: Elsevier; 1988.

91. Camporesi EM, Barker AC. *Hyperbaric Oxygen Therapy. A Critical Review*. Bethesda, MD: Undersea and Hyperbaric Medical Society; 1991.

89

THE HEART, EMOTIONAL STRESS, AND PSYCHIATRIC DISORDERS

Robert S. Eliot / Naresh Kumar / Hugo M. Morales-Ballejo

Numerous instances of sudden death after an emotional upset have been recorded. Evidence now documents many of the profound interrelationships of the brain and stress on human and animal physiology and confirms the link between emotions and some illnesses, including sudden death.

Stress remains ill defined. In the context of this discussion, *stress* is the body's response to real or imagined events perceived as requiring some adaptive response and/or producing strain. This definition allows differentiation between *stress*— the internally mediated adaptive response—and *stressors*— the stimuli. Stresses range from mild annoyances to death threats, from momentary scares to never-ending tension, with a corresponding spectrum of responses.

PHYSIOLOGY

The central nervous system controls cardiovascular functions through the baroreceptors and numerous afferent and efferent neuroendocrine connections of the autonomic nervous system. Animal experiments and clinical studies conclude that stress effects are mediated largely by increases in cortisol and catecholamines.[1–3] The effects are further modulated by neuropeptides, vagal stimulation, circadian influences, adaptive mechanisms, genetic susceptibilities, and the presence of disease.

In the conscious pig, stressful stimuli can increase vulnerability to ventricular fibrillation.[4] This effect is blocked by adaptation, intracerebral injection of a beta blocker, or blockade of frontocortical projections to brainstem cardiovascular nuclei. It is postulated that the pathway goes from the frontal lobes to the frontocortical brainstem, stimulating autonomic outflow (norepinephrine), increasing cyclic adenosine monophosphate (cAMP), and decreasing extracellular potassium ions.

Stress responses are divided into several patterns: those involving active coping ("fight or flight"), those associated with an aversion situation or long-term monitoring (vigilance), and those characterized by subordination, in which active coping is attempted but is not successful. In the fight-or-flight reaction, the release of catecholamines raises the blood pressure and heart rate, with increased cardiac output and decreased total peripheral resistance. The vigilance response, which seems to be mediated by the pituitary-adrenocortical system, results in elevated blood pressure with increased total peripheral resistance but decreased heart rate and cardiac output.

In studies of psychosocial effects on mice, plasma cortisol levels were highest in submissive animals, lower in subordinate animals, and lowest in dominant animals.[5] Catecholamine levels showed the opposite pattern, being highest in dominant animals. Similar patterns have been observed in other animal groups and in human beings as well. Three categories of human reactions have been described: effort without distress, effort with distress, and distress without effort.[6] In experiments with healthy subjects performing a choice-reaction task with a high degree of control or a vigilance task with no control, subjects reported that they were pleasantly challenged by the high-control task and felt some distress from the low-control task. Epinephrine increased in both, but cortisol decreased in the former and increased in the latter.

The stress of public speaking can increase platelet activation as well as serum levels of the catecholamines epinephrine and norepinephrine.[7] Propranolol treatment moderates the heart rate and systolic blood pressure during the stress period but does not block the catecholamine or platelet responses.

It has been postulated that acute (coping) response to stress is designed to provide the necessary energy for fight or flight and to protect against loss of blood and metabolites.[8] Subordinate and submissive responses are also appropriate animal behavior, generally minimizing injury while promoting survival of species. In the normal course of events, these responses are called into play for short periods and are not harmful. On the other hand, it is important to consider whether or not these reactions lead to harmful disease processes, and if so, how.

PATHOPHYSIOLOGY

Hypertension

Human primary hypertension is multifactorial, with three independent causative elements: a polygenetically transferred predisposition; environmental factors such as excitatory psychoemotional influences and habitual salt intake, which sometimes precipitate the hemodynamic expression of the genes; and structural adaptation of heart and vessels to stimulatory pressor effects, which may also be genetically reinforced.[9]

Atherosclerosis

The pathogenesis of atherosclerosis is described in detail in Chaps. 39 and 40. The general features include the development of endothelial dysfunction because of elevated cholesterol and other lipids, hypertension, smoking, diabetes, low estrogen states, and so on. Endothelial dysfunction leads to loss of endothelium-dependent vasodilator responses (because of decreased release of nitric oxide) and to the accumulation of mononuclear leukocytes and T cells in the arterial wall. Low-density lipoprotein (LDL) enters the artery wall, is modified (oxidized), and is taken up by the monocyte/macrophage to form foam cells. Macrophage/foam cells produce large amounts of the procoagulant tissue factor, which is released into the artery wall. The lipid core of an atherosclerotic lesion probably results from deposition of lipid from dying foam cells. Acute myocardial infarction generally occurs when there is localized disruption of the structural integrity of the atherosclerotic lesion, usually at a site characterized by high local concentrations of macrophages (see Chap. 40). Breakdown of the plaque results from structural weakening caused by the production of metalloproteinases, a class of proteolytic enzymes, by the macrophages; these enzymes then degrade the connective tissue framework. Plaque rupture leads to the exposure of flowing blood to tissue factors, with clot formation. If the clot occludes the arterial lumen downstream, infarction occurs.

The metabolic and physical consequences of stress can affect the process at any stage. Elevated catecholamines can increase blood pressure and hemodynamic stress on endothelium. Dysfunction can result. These hemodynamic effects can contribute to plaque rupture. Catecholamines can activate platelets, promoting thrombosis. Chronic vigilance or stress causes increased secretion of corticosteroids, leading, in turn, to increased LDL cholesterol (LDL-C) and decreased high-density lipoprotein (HDL) cholesterol.[10] This can aggravate the atherogenic process, whereas an acute stress can accelerate the thrombogenic process (Fig. 89-1).

In studies of the extent of atherosclerosis in stressed and unstressed male macaque monkeys, stress was induced by frequent disruption of social groupings.[11] Little disease was seen in unstressed monkeys on low-fat diets. On an atherogenic diet, dominant animals showed minimal lesions and subordinate animals had moderate disease. Conversely, among the stressed monkeys, lesions were more prominent in the dominant than in the subordinate animals regardless of diet; however, the extent of atherosclerosis was magnified 30-fold on the high-fat diet. In studies of female

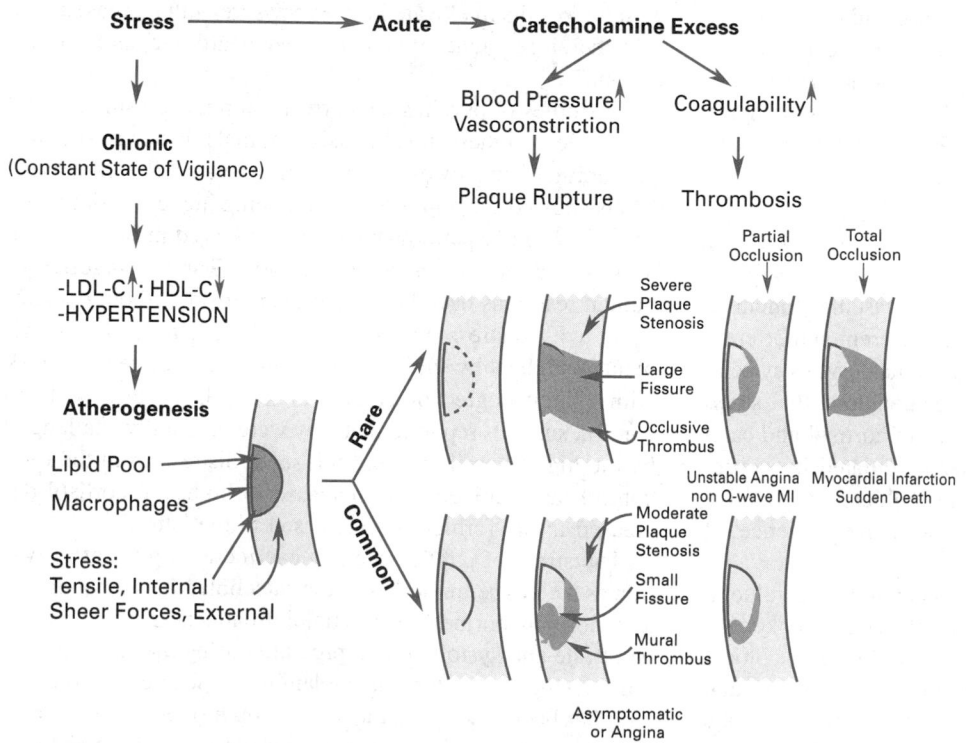

Emotional Stress & Coronary Syndrome

FIGURE 89-1

Emotional stress can precipitate cardiac events, either through a chronic state of vigilance that alters the lipids, thereby contributing to atherogenesis, or through an acute, severe emotional stress that results in catecholamine excess. The latter increases the platelet count, makes platelets more adherent, and might precipitate rupture of an atherogenic plaque. (Modified from Fuster V. Coronary artery disease: A clinical-pathological correlation. In: Fuster V, ed. *Syndromes of Atherosclerosis.* Armonk, NY: Futura; 1996:2.)

macaques,[12] dominant females seemed to be protected from atherosclerosis. Subordinate females and ovariectomized females were as affected as the males in the same groups; unstable groupings did not increase the involvement. Apparently disruption of social groupings that was very stressful to competitive males was not as stressful to the females, because they do not fight as aggressively for status as do the males.

In humans, serum cholesterol levels have been observed to rise during periods of stress, such as medical students' examination periods, soldiers' training with demolition weaponry, and anticipation of surgery.[13] Triglyceride levels are even more labile. In the course of a stressful interview, blood lipids may rise as much as 150 percent.[13]

Increased activity of the sympathetic nervous system influences lipid metabolism. Activation of alpha$_1$ receptors and possibly angiotensin II may inhibit lipoprotein lipase activity, leading to elevated very low density lipoprotein (VLDL) triglyceride and decreased HDL cholesterol levels. Sympathetic activation may also increase cholesterol by impairing LDL clearance.[14] In one study, cholesterol levels correlated positively with measures of depression, hostility, and emotional instability; they correlated negatively with motivation and happiness.[15]

Ischemia

Cardiac ischemia induced by mental stress might be produced by a combination of factors, including increased myocardial oxygen demand and reduced coronary blood flow secondary to coronary vasospasm.[16] Hemodynamic overreactivity, which can occur secondary to the mental stress often encountered in daily life situations, can induce myocardial ischemia in patients with coronary artery disease.[17] Compared with exercise testing, diastolic blood pressure increases relatively more during mental stress, and heart rate rises less. Systolic blood pressure is comparable in the two settings. Using simultaneous electrocardiographic (ECG) and blood pressure monitoring for 24 to 48 h, Deedwania and colleagues demonstrated that in two-thirds of patients with stable angina and established coronary artery disease, silent ischemia was preceded by an increase in myocardial oxygen demand secondary to an increase in systolic blood pressure and a significant increase in heart rate.[18,19]

Hemodynamic overreactivity—largely the blood pressure response—secondary to mental stress can result in increased myocardial oxygen demand, which may play a key role in the pathogenesis of ischemia observed during daily tasks associated with mental stress. The importance of increases in blood pressure is equal to or greater than that of increases in heart rate in the genesis of myocardial ischemia during daily life.[20]

Sudden Death

Ventricular fibrillation, the principal mechanism of sudden death, may be triggered by autonomic outflow from the brain, ischemia from coronary vasospasm or thrombi, or exacerba-

tion of an electrical instability caused by scar tissue from myocardial infarction or by membrane changes in myocardial hypertrophy.

THE ROLE
OF ENVIRONMENT

In modern times, the human sociocultural environment in many countries has been characterized by an increasingly hectic psychological climate and dwindling use of the somatomotor system. The ancient "emotional brain" evolved millions of years ago to cope with the comparatively infrequent but harsh physical challenges of primitive life. It now confronts stressful environmental stimuli several times each day and engages limbic-hypothalamic patterns for emotional expression. These ancient responses, designed to eliminate overt dangers by appropriate physical exertions, are frequently inadequate for dealing with the sophisticated challenges, symbolic threats, and frequent arousals typical of life in modern society.

The individual must therefore use whatever neocortical coping mechanisms he or she may have developed. When intellectual coping fails, the constraints of civilization force suppression of the more spectacular somatomotor expressions of induced emotional patterns: sudden attack or flight is seldom considered proper in polite society. When emotional tension cannot be readily diffused by physical action, it is often transmuted into sustained irritation, resentment, or frustration, thereby prolonging the associated primitive, neurohormonal adjustment of the cardiovascular system—now maladaptive in a modern context.

The cardiovascular system can be markedly and frequently engaged by environmentally induced defense reactions, with enhanced sympathetic discharge and reduced vagal tone. It is not surprising, therefore, that social status, interactions with other people, and changes in social elements can have an impact on health. When people change jobs, move their place of residence, or make other major life changes, the risk of heart disease may increase two to three times independent of such factors as age, sex, race, cigarette smoking, cholesterol, blood pressure history, physical activity, and obesity.

Hypertension was found to be less prevalent among blacks living in areas of Detroit with low ecologic stress than among their counterparts living in high-stress areas.[21] Other data suggest that there may be an interaction between stress and sodium sensitivity in black children, such that the combination of being black, on a high-salt diet, and exposed to stress produces higher than expected increases in blood pressure.[22]

A study of Japanese immigrants to the Bay Area of California found a marked increase in coronary artery disease (CAD)—up to fivefold—compared with Japanese who remained in Japan.[23] Among the Japanese immigrants in California, however, there was a group who had almost the same low incidence of CAD as those who remained in Japan. The major CAD risk factors did not appear entirely to account for the difference. This suggested that mobility per se was not a major risk factor for the immigrants. The main difference between the groups appeared to be their degree of social support.[24] The group with the highest rate of CAD had become acculturated and had adopted "Western ways." Those with a low incidence of heart disease had closer ties with other members of the Japanese ethnic group and more closely maintained their native language, diet, and customs.

A study in a more general population verified the importance of social support networks.[25] Connections were evaluated on the basis of criteria such as marital status, membership in clubs, and attendance at church or synagogue. Follow-up over the next 9 years revealed that people with fewer connections at the beginning of the study had a mortality rate two to three times higher than that of those with the greatest number of associations, even when taking into account such factors as age, race, cigarette smoking, serum cholesterol, blood pressure, family history, physical activity, obesity, socioeconomic status, and self-reported health status. Curiously, the data were for all forms of death, not just heart disease.

The protective effects of social support may help to explain two questions raised by morbidity data: (1) why certain risk factors are related not just to one disease but to a variety of diseases and (2) why the recognized risk factors—such as cigarette smoking, high blood pressure, and elevated serum cholesterol—often related imperfectly to disease incidence and outcome. It may be that some people are partially protected from the adverse effects of these factors by the positive effects of social support.

In Syme's view, life changes are important primarily when they disrupt relationships, as they do with job changes, residential moves, divorce, or the loss of loved ones.[23] Even the difference between male and female risks in CAD may be partially related to social support, as men seem to have fewer intimate ties.

The effect of social contact can also be seen in animal studies. Rabbits that were fondled and petted while on a high-cholesterol diet had a markedly lower rate of atherogenesis than a matched group that were not fondled.[26] In nonhuman primates, it was noted that affiliative behavior, such as grooming, lowers the heart rate and may have a protective effect, since increased heart rates have been correlated with increased atherosclerosis.[13]

Social Class

Socioeconomic factors influence health. The lower the socioeconomic status, the higher the rates of many diseases. The reasons for this difference are poorly understood. Hypotheses include poor nutrition, poor medical care, and heavy infectious burden, but these variables appear not to account for the entire difference.

One study compared a poor area with a more affluent area.[25] The incidence of hypertension was 50 percent higher in the poor area regardless of considerations of social interactions, medical care, smoking, and other accepted risk factors. Among the more affluent individuals living in the poor area,

however, the pattern of hypertension reflected that of the poor area as a whole rather than that of the similar income group in the affluent area. Interviews with the individuals revealed fears of robbery and violence, and there was evidence that the distribution of hypertension correlated with the number of police and fire department calls, suggesting that the increased mortality among lower socioeconomic classes might be related in part to greater levels of environmental stress.

Work

Architectural layout, danger, and excessive noise (unwanted sound) at work can have an impact on stress and health. Other stressors—such as time pressures of assembly-line workers; responsibility for others' safety, as in the case of air-traffic controllers; nonsupportive superiors; and work overload—have been alleged to be associated with an increased incidence of hypertension, myocardial infarction, and other illnesses.[27]

Much occupational stress seems to derive from feelings of lack of control. Among San Francisco bus drivers, hypertension was noted to be more prevalent among drivers than job applicants or the local population.[23] An analysis of 2000 drivers and the conditions under which they worked indicated that the bus schedules were thought to be unrealistic and rigid and that the drivers were harassed and penalized for not maintaining them.

It has been suggested that not only job demands but also the latitude of control in the job can strongly influence maintenance of health and well-being.[6] In laboratory tests of normal individuals given a timed task, those tested reported less distress when they were allowed to select their own pace than when they had no control. Physiologically, they demonstrated lower cortisol levels when they were in control. In the Framingham Study, a higher incidence of coronary heart disease was noted among women having high job demands with less supervision.[28]

The control hypothesis is the underlying explanation for how one reacts to stress. Not all stress is bad. Some types—those events that are perceived as new, interesting, and challenging, for example—are often beneficial. At the other end of the spectrum is deleterious stress associated with fear, uncertainty, and doubt that may lead to loss of control over the situation and its outcome. Lost control (or lack of it) can lead to a period of perceived struggle, with increased neurohormonal activity (cortisol, catecholamines, angiotensin) (Fig. 89-2). The so-called hemodynamic overreactor responds to these situations with marked swings in blood pressure during the day, especially during working hours (circadian pattern).[29]

Awareness of the patient's environment—cultural background, socioeconomic condition, work status, family situation—can provide the insight for effective counseling, intervention, and prevention. By identifying detrimental factors in the environment, the physician can help the patient to find areas where change is possible or to cope with unchangeable aspects. This might prevent continuing stress and adverse health consequences.

PSYCHOLOGICAL EFFECTS

Several syndromes combine anxiety and cardiovascular symptoms, including functional cardiac disorders, mitral valve prolapse, and panic disorder. There is overlap among the anxiety disorders, and their interrelationships are unclear. The presence of any of these obviously does not rule out CAD, since this can be present in addition to one of the other syndromes.

Patients with atypical chest pain and normal resting ECGs often have esophageal disease, but they may have coronary disease or both conditions. Panic disorder is also common in such patients. In one study, 43 to 61 percent of patients with chest pain and negative coronary arteriography findings had panic disorder, compared with only 5 to 23 percent of patients with pain and positive arteriography findings[30] (see Chap. 90).

In our experience, patients with high pain thresholds or denial are more apt to have or develop hypertensive and ischemic heart disease than those with high levels of anxiety.

Therapy is important for patients with chest pain even when CAD has been ruled out, since the pain can be disabling. In one study, a large percentage of patients still believed their problem was heart disease at 17-months follow-up, and more than half were unable to work because of the pain.[31]

CORONARY-PRONE BEHAVIOR

Proposed psychosocial risk factors for heart disease include type A behavior, reduced social support and isolation, lower socioeconomic status, and depression. These exert their combined influences through increased sympathetic and decreased parasympathetic nervous system function and probably also by association with an increase in risky health behaviors.

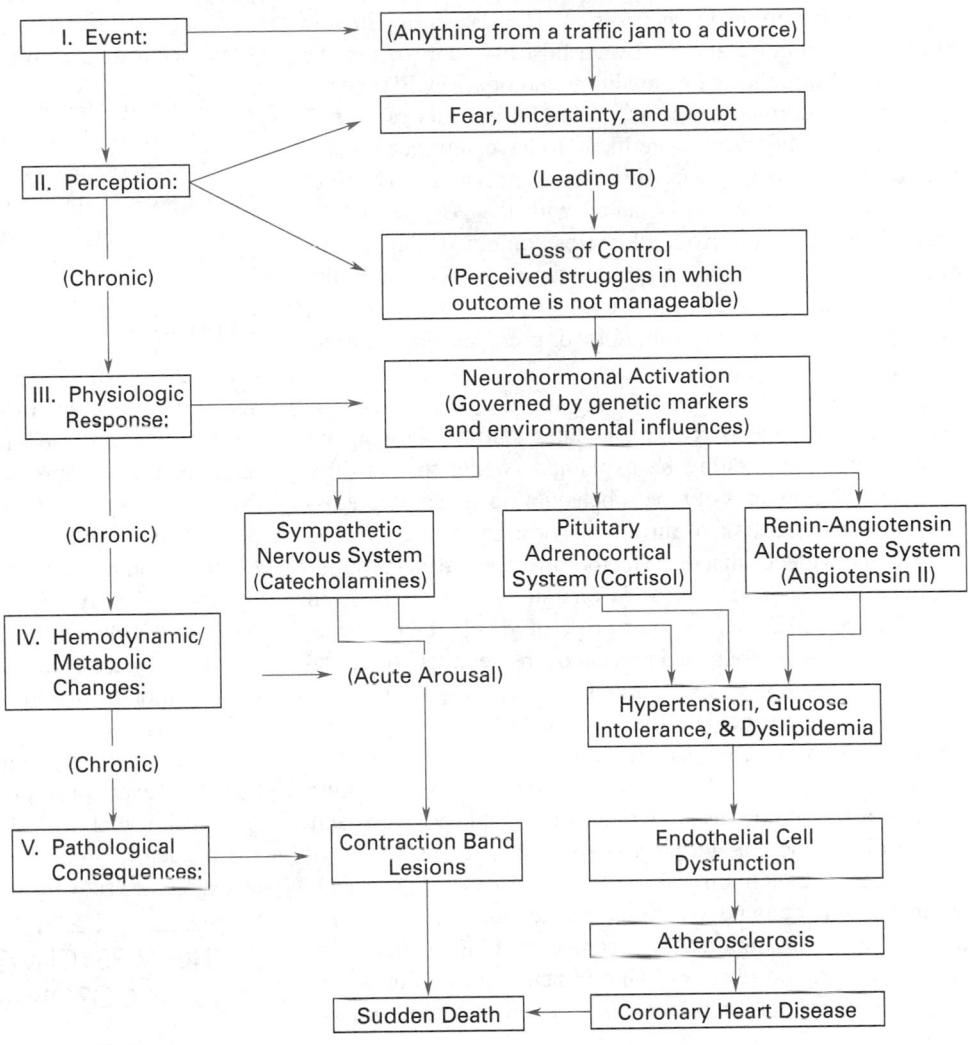

THE CONTROL HYPOTHESIS

In Hypertension, Coronary Disease, and Sudden Cardiac Death

FIGURE 89-2

Conceptual diagram of how a perceived loss of control over outcome might provoke acute and chronic neurohormonal responses. When loss of control becomes chronic, pathophysiologic consequences may ensue as diagrammed.

Type A Behavior

Of these putative psychosocial predictors of CAD, type A behavior is best known.[32] Type A individuals are characterized by a sense of urgency, explosive speech patterns, hostility, and competitiveness. In the Western Collaborative Group Study (WCGS) and other studies of middle-class American men, those with extreme type A patterns had two to four times the risk of developing CAD as individuals lacking type A characteristics (type B).[33] Later studies of different populations, however, failed to show significant differences in the risk of death.

Subsequent work addressed particular features of type A behavior, focusing on anger and hostility. Type A individuals feel a greater need to be in control. They become upset when things do not proceed according to their plans and events go beyond their control. Measures of hostility—outward-directed and inward-directed anger—correlate with CAD incidence in younger men.[33,34] Anger directed inward was also noted in high-renin hypertensive patients.[35] The Western Electric Study found a correlation between hostility scores from the Minnesota Multiphasic Personality Inventory (MMPI) and the incidence of coronary events.[36] Even individuals of type B with high hostility were more likely to have significant coronary occlusion than low-hostility type A individuals. Hostility indices were positively associated with the 20-year risk of death from CAD and from all causes combined. Suppressed anger, particularly toward a spouse, correlated with mortality in the 12-year Tecumseh follow-up.[37] The effect was strongest in combination with systolic blood pressure greater than 140 mmHg.

The inconsistency between early studies showing type A behavior predictive of CAD and later studies showing no relationship can possibly be explained. While the hostility and anger components of type A behavior do appear to predispose to increased risk of an initial coronary event, there is little if any evidence that these factors adversely affect prognosis once CAD is established. In one study, type A patients with *known* CAD had a *lower* risk of death than type B patients.[38] Ironson found a 5 percent decrease in left ventricular ejection fraction (LVEF) among a group of CAD patients asked to recall an incident that had made them angry.[39] By comparison, these same patients showed a 2 percent increase in LVEF during exercise. In another group of CAD patients, positive association was shown between hostility scores and myocardial ischemia during 24- to 48-h ambulatory ECG monitoring.[40] Our findings indicate that a lack of perceived control might activate the pituitary, adenocortical, sympathetic, and renin-angiotensin systems, leading to metabolic and hemodynamic changes. The perpetuation of this situation may contribute significantly to cardiovascular disease (Fig. 89-2).

Social Isolation

There is a twofold higher recurrence rate of myocardial infarction among patients who live alone as compared with those who live with another person.[41] Very isolated (unmarried, without a confidant) patients with angiographically documented CAD were found to have 50 percent 5-year mortality, compared with 17 percent among similar patients with a spouse, confidant, or both.[42]

Elderly persons who reported lower levels of emotional support from others were almost three times more likely to die within 6 months following a myocardial infarction than seniors with higher levels of emotional support, independent of infarction severity, comorbidity, or other risk factors for CAD.[43]

Social isolation predicted increased mortality in type A but not type B men with and without CAD.[44] The combination of type A behavior and social isolation impacted more severely on prognosis than did either psychosocial risk factor alone.

Clustering of other factors may be involved. For example, socially isolated patients are less compliant with medication and less likely to succeed in smoking cessation programs than are patients with better social supports.

Low Socioeconomic Status

The recurrence rate after myocardial infarction among patients with lower levels of education attainment is higher than it is among better educated persons.[45] Williams et al. observed an inverse dose-response effect of income on mortality among patients with angiographically documented CAD, independent of severity.[42]

Depression

Some 20 to 40 percent of CAD patients have depressive-spectrum disorders. In one study, among the 17 percent of patients who met the American Psychiatric Association's criteria for major depression in the *Diagnostic and Statistical Manual of Mental Disorders III—Revised* (DSM-IIIR), 16 percent died during the first 6 months after myocardial infarction, compared with only 3 percent among nondepressed patients.[46] Thirty percent of the same patients who had depressive symptoms (determined by a score of 10 or more on the Beck Depression Inventory) had a higher mortality rate over 18 months of follow-up than those patients without major depression.

In addition to their effect on prognosis, depressive conditions can exert profound negative effects on quality of life (physical, social, and role functioning) in patients with CAD independent of the severity of CAD, the level of disability, or degree of recovery from myocardial infarction.

HOW PSYCHOSOCIAL FACTORS AFFECT CORONARY ARTERY DISEASE

Increased sympathetic nervous system (SNS) function is the most important mechanism by which psychosocial factors may increase the risk of reinfarction or death among patients with CAD. A pharmacokinetic study documented increased SNS outflow among patients with major depression compared to nondepressed controls.[47] Fleming showed greater urinary catecholamine excretion among persons with lower levels of social support than among others with higher levels of support.[48] A similar observation has been made regarding persons with high levels of hostility versus less hostile individuals.[49] The same workers found that persons with higher hostility scores exhibited increased cardiovascular hemodynamic reactivity when angered. Chronic increase in SNS outflow as a function of low socioeconomic status was also noted by Dimsdale, reporting lower than normal lymphocyte beta-receptor density among homeless men reporting high stress during the 6 months prior to testing.[50]

Chronically increased SNS tone may increase myocardial electrical instability, platelet activation, and myocardial workload, possibly accelerating coronary atherosclerosis and acute coronary events. There is also evidence of decreased parasympathetic nervous system function in persons with the psychosocial characteristics we have cited.

As previously noted, clustering of health-damaging behaviors is also important. For example, persons with high hostility scores are more likely than those with low hostility scores to be smokers, to consume alcohol, to be overweight, and to consume caffeinated beverages. A similar pattern of health-damaging behaviors can occur in depressed persons. Hostility and depression occur more frequently in persons of low socioeconomic status. Hostility is also related to cynicism or lack of basic trust.[36]

PHYSIOLOGIC HEMODYNAMIC OVERREACTIVITY ("HOT REACTING")

The physiologic reactions that mediate the effects of personality and behavior on disease have been studied. Reactivity to laboratory-induced mental stress, however, does not necessarily follow type A-B patterns: Exaggerated cardiovascular response ("hot reacting") is often observed in individuals of type B and can be absent in type A patients. Our study found the correlation between overreactivity and type A behavior to be only 0.1 to 0.3.[51]

Reactivity patterns differ between adolescents with and without a family history of hypertension. Those with a positive family history demonstrated greater elevations of both heart rate and diastolic blood pressure after such stressors as mental arithmetic, the Stroop color test, and shock avoidance.[52]

Hypertensive patients and, perhaps, those destined to develop hypertension have a greater than expected increase in blood pressure when challenged with a simple video game or math problem.[53] The clinical value of blood pressure reactivity testing is its correlation with the working-time blood pressure, which has been found to be better than casual blood pressure measurements in predicting future target-organ damage or complications of hypertension.[54–56] Increased activity of the sympathetic nervous system may be an important component of the circadian pattern of blood pressure elevation and the increased incidence of cardiovascular events in the morning hours between 7 A.M. and noon, after awakening, and after assuming the upright position (see also Chaps. 45 and 47).

Using our standardized alpha- and beta-adrenergic low-challenge stress test with impedance cardiography monitoring, we can determine not only the elevated levels of blood pressure during stress but also the hemodynamics involved.[57,58] Using this technique during pharmacologic intervention, we can determine whether the blood pressure changes are mediated by cardiac output, total systemic resistance, or both.[59] The results before and after pharmacologic intervention can be graphically displayed to clearly identify the levels of reactivity and the hemodynamics (Fig. 89-3).

PHARMACOLOGY

Considerations in choosing drugs are their interactions with other treatment modalities, their effects on other disease conditions, and their overall effect on quality of life. Beta blockers and other cardiovascular agents can alter mood and mental acuity. Antidepressants and other psychotropic drugs can affect the heart directly and/or interact with cardiovascular agents to alter their effectiveness or to induce unwanted side effects.

Anxiety

For anxiety without depression, all benzodiazepines are about equally effective. The choice depends on the half-life desired. Even those with short half-lives should be used sparingly for the elderly, who are very susceptible to oversedation. On the other hand, if treatment with a benzodiazepine of short half-life is stopped too suddenly, the patient may experience seizures.[60] This can be avoided with proper tapering. If the patient cannot be trusted to take medication as ordered, it is best to use an agent with a long half-life, as it has a built-in tapering effect. Titrating from very low dose levels is the rule of thumb for pharmacologic management of the elderly. Minor tranquilizers do not affect blood pressure, cause cardiovascular problems, or interact with the medications commonly prescribed for hypertension or diabetes.

Short-acting tranquilizers are usually preferred for hospitalized patients; but for home use, the patient's compliance behavior determines which drug is preferable. Alprazolam has some antidepressant side effects as compared with the other minor tranquilizers.[61] Its short half-life makes it suitable for outpatient management. In general, it is safe for use in the presence of serious cardiovascular problems, including arrhythmias, post-bypass state, infarction, angina, and silent ischemia.[62]

Depression

For a patient with severe depression, electroconvulsive shock treatments (ECT) may be the safest therapy,[63] but the risks associated with the anesthesia and shock must be considered. Selective serotonin reuptake inhibitors (SSRIs) are probably the safest antidepressant drugs for cardiac patients; they have largely replaced tricyclics for outpatient management of depression.

Tricyclic antidepressants should generally not be used within 6 weeks of a myocardial infarction or in the presence of congestive heart failure, decompensation, or rhythm and conduction disturbances. Slow titration and ECG monitoring are recommended. Certain tricyclics, such as amitriptyline and imipramine, can produce postural hypotension. The hypotension effect can be minimized by using divided doses. Some tricyclics interact with other medications.

Hypertensive Patients

Many antihypertensive agents besides beta blockers can cause depression, particularly methyldopa and reserpine. With clonidine, guanethidine, and propranolol, the incidence is about 1 percent provided that doses are moderate. The patient who becomes depressed from taking an antihypertensive agent and

CARDIOVASCULAR REACTIVITY

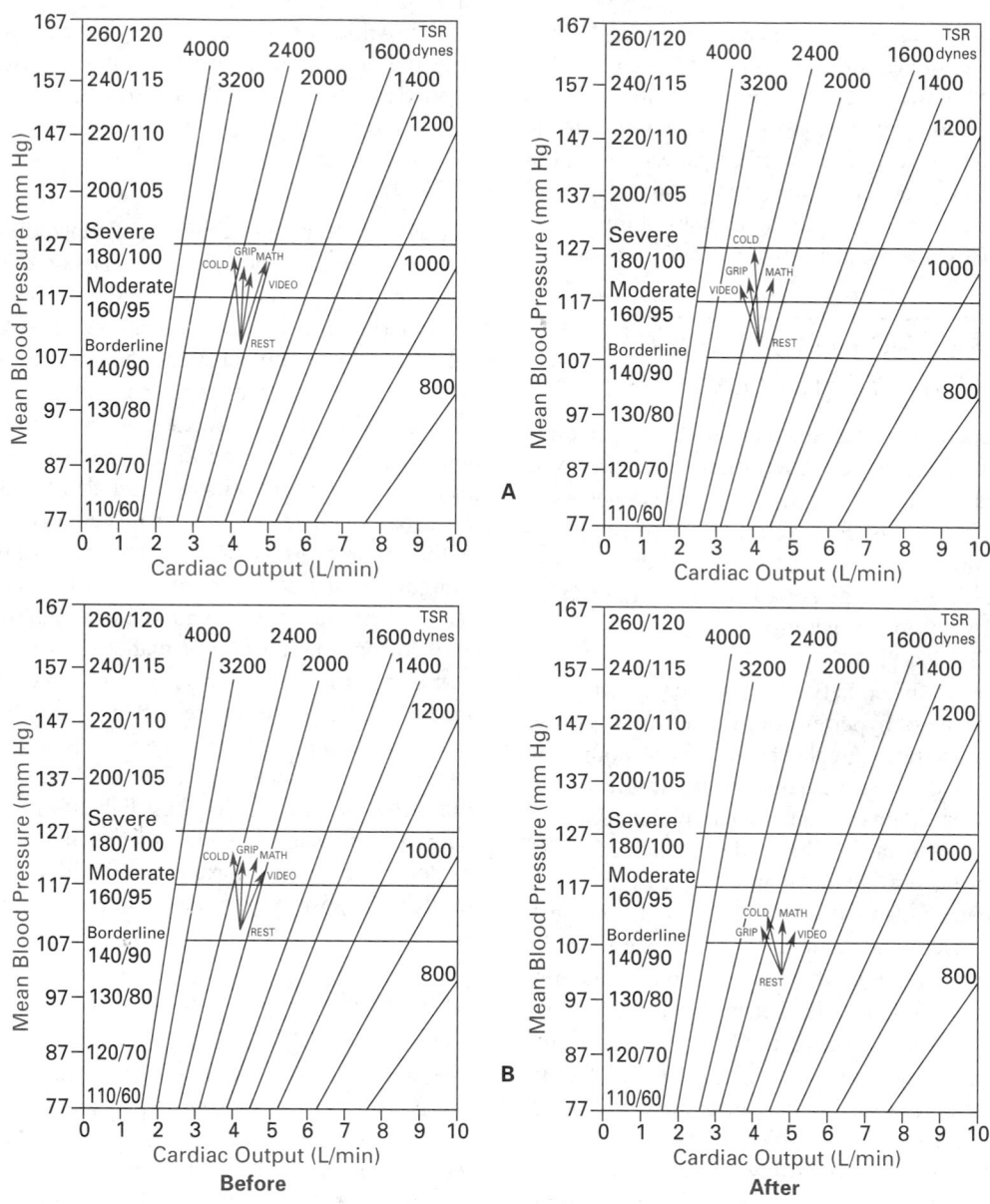

FIGURE 89-3

Cardiovascular reactivity graphs displaying levels of mean blood pressure in millimeters of mercury (*vertical axis*), cardiac output in liters per minute (*horizontal axis*), and total systemic resistance (TSR) in dynes·s·cm⁻⁵ (*radiated lines*). Blood pressure was obtained using oscillometric apparatus. Cardiac output was measured by ensemble averages of signals obtained from an impedance cardiograph. Measurements were taken during a standardized protocol at baseline (REST) and during different challenges. The arrows indicate the changes from baseline during hand grip (GRIP), cold pressor (COLD), computerized video game (VIDEO), and mental arithmetic (MATH) tests. The average hemodynamics were obtained during a double-blind, placebo-controlled study of 20 labile and mild hypertensives. *A*. Ten patients before and 2 h after oral ingestion of placebo. *B*. Ten patients before and 2 h after oral ingestion of diltiazem, 120 mg. Significant decrease in blood pressure was obtained due to reduction in total system resistance. (From Morales-Ballejo et al.,[59] with permission.)

who, for various reasons, cannot use the alternative drug can be given an antidepressant, but the patient must be cooperative, educated in the problems and limitations, and carefully monitored. SSRIs are a good choice for treating depression in hypertensive patients.

Psychosis

Neuroleptics are likely to cause disturbances in ventricular repolarization with large doses, and ventricular arrhythmias related to their use may be the cause of the occasional sudden death during long-term treatment. Major neuroleptics may also cause tardive dyskinesia (see also Chap. 80).

Cooperation between the cardiologist and the psychiatrist is necessary when severe mental conditions develop in patients with cardiovascular disorders or when mentally disturbed patients present with cardiovascular disease.

REFERENCES

1. Schneiderman N. Behaviour, autonomic function, and animal models of cardiovascular pathology. In: Dembroski TM, Schmidt TH, Blumchen G, eds. *Biobehavioral Bases of Coronary Heart Disease.* Basel: Karger; 1983:304–364.

2. Herd JA. Cardiovascular disease and hypertension. In: Gentry WD, ed. *Handbook of Behavioral Medicine.* New York: Guilford Press; 1984:222–281.

3. Corr PB, Pitt B, Natelson BH, Reis DJ, Shine KI, Skinner JE. Task Force 3: Sudden cardiac death: Neural-chemical interactions. *Circulation* 1987; 76(suppl 1):208–214.

4. Skinner JE. Psychosocial stress and sudden cardiac death: Brain mechanisms. In: Beamish RE, Singal PK, Dhalla NS, eds. *Stress and Heart Disease.* Boston: Martinus Nijhoff; 1983:44–59.

5. Henry JP. Coronary heart disease and arousal of the adrenal cortical axis. In: Dembroski TM, Schmidt TH, Blumchen G, eds. *Biobehavioral Bases of Coronary Heart Disease.* Basel: Karger; 1983:365–381.

6. Frankenhaeuser M. The sympathetic-adrenal and pituitary-adrenal response to challenge: Comparison between the sexes. In: Dembroski TM, Schmidt TH, Blumchen G, eds. *Biobehavioral Bases of Coronary Heart Disease.* Basel: Karger; 1983:91–105.

7. Levine SP, Towell BI, Suarez AM, Knierem LK, Harris MM, George JN. Platelet activation and secretion associated with emotional stress. *Circulation* 1985; 71:1129–1134.

8. Theorell T. Physiological issues in establishing links between psychosocial factors and cardiovascular illness. In: *Breakdown in Human Adaptation to "Stress."* Boston: Martinus Nijhoff; 1984:241–250.

9. Folkow B. Psychosocial and central nervous influences in primary hypertension. *Circulation* 1987; 76(suppl 1):10–19.

10. Friedman M, Rosenman RH, Carroll V. Changes in the serum cholesterol and blood clotting time in men subjected to cyclic variation of occupational stress. *Circulation* 1958; 17:852–861.

11. Clarkson TB, Weingand KW, Kaplan JR, Adams MR. Mechanisms of atherogenesis. *Circulation* 1987; 76(suppl 1):20–28.

12. Clarkson TB, Kaplan JR, Adams MR, Manuck SB. Psychosocial influences on the pathogenesis of atherosclerosis among nonhuman primates. *Circulation* 1987; 76(suppl 1):29–40.

13. Dimsdale JE, Herd JA. Variability of plasma lipids in response to emotional arousal. *Psychosom Med* 1982; 44:413–430.

14. Dzau VJ. Atherosclerosis and hypertension: Mechanisms and interrelationships. *J Cardiovasc Pharmacol* 1990; 15(suppl 5):S59–S64.

15. van Doornen LJP, Orlebeke KF. Stress, personality and serum cholesterol level. *J Hum Stress* 1982; 8:24–29.

16. Krants DS, Helmers KR, Bairey CN. Cardiovascular reactivity and mental stress induced myocardial ischemia in patients with coronary artery disease. *Psychosom Med* 1991; 53:1–12.

17. Rosanski A, Bairey C, Krantz D. Mental stress and the induction of myocardial ischemia in patients with coronary artery disease. *N Engl J Med* 1988; 318:1005–1012.

18. Deedwania PC. Increased myocardial oxygen demand and ischemia during daily life: Resurrection of age old concept. *J Am Coll Cardiol* 1992; 20:1099–1100.

19. Deedwania PC, Carbajal EV. Role of myocardial oxygen demand in the pathogenesis of silent ischemia during daily life. *Am J Cardiol* 1992; 70:19f–24f.

20. Andrews TC, Fenton T, Toyosaki N. For the Angina and Silent Ischemia Study Group (ASIS). Subsets of ambulatory myocardial ischemia based on heart rate activity: Circadian distribution and response anti-ischemic medication. *Circulation* 1993; 88:92–100.

21. Harburg E, Schull WJ, Erfurt JC, Schork MA, Rice R. A family set method for estimating heredity and stress: I. A pilot survey of blood pressure among Negroes in high and low stress areas, Detroit, 1966–1967. *J Chronic Dis* 1970; 23:83–92.

22. Faulkner B, Kushner H, Khalsa DK, Canessa M, Katz S. Sodium sensitivity, growth and family history of hypertension in young blacks. *J Hypertens* 1986; 4(suppl 5):S-381–S-383.

23. Syme SL. Socioenvironmental factors in heart disease. In: Beamish RE, Singal PK, Dhalla NS, eds. *Stress and Heart Disease.* Boston: Martinus Nijhoff; 1985:60–70.

24. Marmot MG, Syme SL. Acculturation and coronary heart disease in Japanese Americans. *Am J Epidemiol* 1976; 104:225–247.

25. Berkman LF, Syme SL. Social networks, host resistance, and mortality: A nine-year follow-up study of Alameda county residents. *Am J Epidemiol* 1979; 109:186–204.

26. Nerem RM, Levesque MJ, Cornhill JF. Social environment as a factor in diet-induced aortic atherosclerosis in rabbits. *Science* 1980; 208:1475–1476.

27. McLean AA. *Work Stress.* Reading, MA: Addison-Wesley; 1979.

28. Haynes SG, Feinleib M. Women, work and coronary heart disease: Prospective findings from the Framingham Heart Study. *Am J Public Health* 1980; 70:133–141.

29. Eliot RS. Stress and the heart. *Postgrad Med* 1992; 92:237–248.

30. Katon W. Panic disorder: Epidemiology, diagnosis and treatment in primary care. *J Clin Psychiatry* 1986; 47(suppl 10):21–27.

31. Ockene IS, Shay MY, Alpert JS, Weiner BH, Dalen JE. Unexplained chest pain in patients with normal coronary arteriograms. *N Engl J Med* 1980; 303:1249–1252.

32. Friedman M, Rosenman RH. Association of specific overt behaviour pattern with increases in blood cholesterol, blood clotting time, incidence of arcus senilis and clinical coronary heart disease. *JAMA* 1959; 169:1286–1296.

33. Rosenman RH, Brand RJ, Jenkins CD, Friedman M, Strauss R, Wurm M. Coronary heart disease in the Western Collaborative Group Study: Final follow-up experience of 8½ years. *JAMA* 1975; 233:872–877.

34. Dembroski TM, MacDougall JM. Beyond global type A: Relationships of paralinguistic attributes, hostility, and anger to coronary heart disease. In: Field T, McAbe P, Schneiderman N, eds. *Stress and Coping.* Hillsdale, NJ: Erlbaum; 1985:223–242.

35. Esler M, Julius S, Zweifler A, Randall O, Harburg E, Gardiner H, et al. Mild high-renin essential hypertension: Neurogenic human hypertension? *N Engl J Med* 1977; 296:405–411.

36. Williams RB Jr, Barefoot JC, Shekelle RB. The health consequences of hostility. In: Chesney MA, Rosenman RH, eds. *Anger and Hostility in Cardiovascular and Behavioral Disorders.* Washington, DC: Hemisphere; 1985:173–185.

37. Julius M, Harburg E, Cottingham EM, Johnson EH. Anger-coping types, blood pressure, and all-cause mortality: A follow-up in Tecumseh, Michigan (1971–1983). *Am J Epidemiol* 1986; 124:220–233.

38. Ragland DR, Brand RJ. Coronary heart disease mortality in the Western Collaborative Study Group: Follow-up experience for 22 years. *Am J Epidemiol* 1988; 127:462–475.

39. Ironson G. Effects of anger on left ventricular ejection fraction in coronary artery disease. *Am J Cardiol* 1992; 70:281–285.

40. Helmers KF. Hostility and myocardial ischemia in coronary artery disease patients: Evaluation by gender and ischemic index. *Psychosom Med* 1993; 55:29–36.

41. Case RB, Moss AJ, Case N, McDermott M, Eberly S. Living alone after myocardial infarction: Impact on prognosis. *JAMA* 1992; 267:515–519.

42. Williams RB, Barefoot JC, Califf RM, Haney TL, Saunders WB, Pryor DB, et al. Prognostic importance of social and economic resources among medically treated patients with angiographically documented coronary artery disease. *JAMA* 1992; 267:520–524.

43. Berkman LF, Leo-Summers L, Horwitz RI. Emotional support and survival following myocardial infarction: Findings from a prospective, population-based study of the elderly. *Ann Intern Med* 1992; 117:1003–1009.

44. Orth-Gomer K, Unden AL. Type A behavior, social support, and coronary risk: Interaction and significance for mortality in cardiac patients. *Psychosom Med* 1990; 52:59–72.

45. Ruberman W, Weinblatt E, Goldberg JD, Chaudhary BS. Psychosocial influences on mortality after myocardial infarction. *N Engl J Med* 1984; 311:552–559.

46. Frasure-Smith N, Lesperance F, Talajic M. Depression following myocardial infarction: Impact on 6-month survival. *JAMA* 1993; 270:1819–1825.

47. Veith RC, Lewis N, Linares OA, Barnes RF, Raskind MA, Villacres EC, et al. Sympathetic nervous system activity in major depression: Basal and desipramine-induced alternations in plasma norepinephrine kinetics. *Arch Gen Psychiatry* 1994; 51:411–422.

48. Fleming R. Mediating influences of social support on stress at Three Mile Island. *J Hum Stress* 1982; 8:14–22.

49. Suarez EC, Williams RB. Situational determinants of cardiovascular and emotional reactivity in high and low hostile men. *Psychosom Med* 1989; 51:404–418.

50. Dimsdale JE. Effects of chronic stress on beta-adrenergic receptors in the homeless. *Psychosom Med* 1994; 56:290–295.

51. Ruddel H, Langewitz W, McKinney ME, Todd GL, Buell JC, Eliot RS. Hemodynamic responses during the type A interview: A comparison with mental challenges and a clinical interview. *J Auton Nerv Syst* 1986; (suppl):685–688.

52. Jorgensen RS, Houston BK. Family history of hypertension, gender, and cardiovascular reactivity and stereotype during stress. *J Behav Med* 1981; 4:175–189.

53. Horan MJ, Lenfant C. Epidemiology of blood pressure and predictors of hypertension. *Hypertension* 1990; 15(suppl I):I-120–I-124.

54. Perloff D, Sokolow M, Cowan R. The prognostic value of ambulatory blood pressures. *JAMA* 1983; 249:2792–2798.

55. Devereux RB, Pickering TB, Harshfield GA, Kleinert HD, Denby L, Clark L, et al. Left ventricular hypertrophy in patients with hypertension: Importance of blood pressure responses to regularly recurring stress. *Circulation* 1983; 68:470–476.

56. Morales-Ballejo HM, Eliot RS, Boone JL, Hughes JS. Psychophysiological stress testing as a predictor of mean daily blood pressure. *Am Heart J* 1988; 116:673–681.

57. McKinney ME, Miner MH, Ruddel H, McIlvain HE, Witte H, Buell JC, et al. The standardized mental stress test protocol: Test-retest reliability and comparison with ambulatory blood pressure monitoring. *Psychophysiology* 1985; 22:453–463.

58. Eliot RS. The dynamics of hypertension—An overview: Present practices, new possibilities, and new approaches. *Am Heart J* 1988; 116:583–589.

59. Morales-Ballejo HM, Boone JL, Eliot RS. Influence of diltiazem-placebo on the hemodynamic changes caused by stress in mild hypertensives (abstr). *Clin Res* 1991; 39:433A.

60. Gold M, Lydiard RB, Carman J. *Advances in Psychopharmacology: Predicting and Improving Treatment Response*. Boca Raton, FL: CRC Press; 1984.

61. Feighner JP, Aden GC, Fabre LF, Rickels K, Smith WT. Comparison of alprazolam, imipramine and placebo in the treatment of depression. *JAMA* 1983; 249:3057–3064.

62. Stratton JR, Halter JB. Effect of a benzodiazepine (alprazolam) on plasma epinephrine and norepinephrine levels during exercise stress. *Am J Cardiol* 1985; 56:136–139.

63. Neshkes RE, Jarvik LF. Depression in the elderly: Current management concepts. *Geriatrics* 1986; 41:51–58.

90

PANIC ATTACKS AND THE CARDIOVASCULAR SYSTEM

David V. Sheehan / B. Ashok Raj

HISTORICAL REVIEW

Panic disorder, with its mixture of psychological and severe paroxysmal autonomic symptoms, mimics disease in varied organ systems in the body. It is chameleon-like in its presentations and has challenged the diagnostic skills of clinicians from the eighteenth century to the present time. Well-documented descriptions of this disorder are found in the literature of the mid-nineteenth century. The descriptions tend to focus on the somatic symptoms of anxiety, particularly palpitations, chest pain, shortness of breath, and choking or smothering sensations.

War stimulated many studies of this disorder in the military. In 1867, Maclean,[1] a professor of military medicine, described 252 cases of valvular disease without murmurs. He blamed the soldiers' *irritable heart* symptoms on the heavy knapsacks, chest straps, and tunics that they wore. When these accoutrements were abolished, however, the symptoms persisted. According to Skerritt,[2] in 1870, Myers, a surgeon in the Coldstream Guards, observed that functional heart disorder was more common in the army than in the navy or the Metropolitan Police. Meanwhile, Coote[3] in 1858 described a syndrome of inframammary discomfort in women that included various pains, globus hystericus, variability of temperatures, irregular pulse, palpitations, vomiting, and constipation. He felt that this was due to a local vascular problem, while others attributed its etiology to muscular disorder, uterine dysfunction, or spinal curvature. In 1871, Da Costa,[4] a Philadelphia physician, produced his classic work on the irritable heart based on his experience in treating American Civil War veterans.

By 1880, Beard and others had popularized the term *neurasthenia* to cluster a number of common symptoms like headache, pain, noise in the head, fears, and sweating, rather than just the cardiovascular symptoms or weakness. In 1894, Freud[5] separated from neurasthenia a syndrome with a smaller group of symptoms and called it *anxiety neurosis*. This disorder included free-floating anxiety and anxiety attacks, with cardiac and other symptoms that led to the development of phobias.

The medical literature from World War I includes many papers pertaining to *soldier's heart*. In 1917, Sir Thomas Lewis[6] introduced the term *effort syndrome* as a substitute for the prevailing British Army terminology *disordered action of the heart*. In 1918, Oppenheimer et al.[7] introduced the term *neurocirculatory asthenia* as a convenient way to describe a syndrome characterized by nervous and circulatory symptoms and associated with an increased predisposition to fatigue. In 1920, MacKenzie[8] suggested that the heart abnormalities were only part of a larger general condition, a *war neurosis*, with patients resembling psychoneurotic casualties. Concurrently, Culpin[9] noted the association between effort syndrome, anxiety symptoms, and phobias and suggested that treatment should be focused on the underlying nervous disorder and not on the heart.

In the post–World War I years, the term *cardiac neurosis* was used increasingly to describe a syndrome of excessive worry about heart disease, even when organic heart disease was present.[10] At this time, hyperventilation was identified either as a part of the effort syndrome or as an independent disorder.

During World War II, the focus shifted back to the effort syndrome. In 1941, Wood[11] concluded that Da Costa's syndrome and effort syndrome were the same. He advocated support and reassurance rather than physical rehabilitation as the desirable treatment. Maxwell Jones and Sir Aubrey Lewis[12] found that about 30 percent of the patients also had a psychiatric diagnosis of anxiety state. Jones[13] later noted, in 1948, that these patients would stop exercise at lower blood lactate levels than controls due to their fear of damage to their hearts—an *effort phobia*.

The irritable-heart concept continued to resurface in the descriptions of *hyperkinetic heart syndrome* by Gorlin[14] in

1962 and the *hyperdynamic beta-adrenergic circulatory state* by Frohlich et al.[15] in 1966. The cardinal feature of the latter condition was the presence of a hyperkinetic circulation with cardiac awareness, exercise intolerance, labile episodic hypertension, and high resting pulse rate. Infusion of isoproterenol induced hysterical outbursts in these individuals and propranolol blocked the symptoms. This led Frohlich to speculate that the beta-adrenergic receptors of these individuals had increased reactivity.

In 1968, Barlow et al.[16] confirmed with phonocardiography and angiography that nonejection midsystolic clicks and late systolic murmurs heard on auscultation originated from the mitral valve. In 1976 Wooley[17] suggested that Da Costa's syndrome, the effort syndrome, and neurocirculatory asthenia were all probably just earlier descriptions of the mitral valve prolapse (MVP) syndrome (see also Chap. 65).

EPIDEMIOLOGY

In the epidemiologic catchment area study, anxiety and phobic disorders were the most common disabling psychiatric disorders in the United States. Lifetime prevalence rates were estimated as 8.3 percent of the general adult population.[18] In this study, panic disorder had a lifetime prevalence of 1.5 percent of the general population (2.1 percent for females and 0.6 percent for males) and panic attack had a lifetime prevalence of 9.7 percent.[18] The criteria used to identify panic disorder were the Research Diagnostic Criteria (RDC). These criteria are more restrictive than the criteria of the *Diagnostic and Statistical Manual of Mental Disorders*, third edition, revised (DSM-III-R), which accommodates some cases that would have previously been diagnosed as generalized anxiety disorder and most cases of agoraphobia.[19] Based on DSM-III-R criteria, the more recent national comorbidity study found a lifetime prevalence of 3.5 percent for panic disorder and 15.6 percent for a panic attack in the general population.[20] The proportion of the population meeting criteria for panic disorder in any given month is about one-third the lifetime prevalence.[21] It is estimated, based on the findings of the conservative Epidemiological Catchment Area Study that 2.6 million people in the United States have panic disorder; based on the broader definition of panic disorder in the DSM-III-R, 6 million people are affected.[22] After adjustment for all other sociodemographic variables, the relative odds for having panic attacks are higher among females, for the age group 30 to 44, and for whites; they are lower in those with *higher occupational prestige*.[23]

AGE OF ONSET

The age-of-onset distribution of panic disorder is uniform and unimodal, with a peak in the twenties.[24] The mean age of onset is 23 years.[24] Panic disorder rarely starts before the age of 15 or after the age of 40. It is twice as common in the 25-to-44 age group as in the 45-to-64 age group. After the age

of 65, prevalence drops to approximately one-fifth that of the 25-to-44 age group.[21,25]

Although the unimodal age-of-onset distribution is difficult to explain in psychological terms, it is consistent with a biologic illness model of panic disorder, in which the disorder appears to afflict women preferentially in their childbearing years.

GENDER DISTRIBUTION

Approximately 70 percent of the victims of panic disorder are women.[24,26–29] There is no evidence that this gender difference is related to educational status, ethnic background, or social status. The higher risk of women for panic disorder contrasts with the equal gender distribution in some other anxiety disorders, such as obsessive-compulsive disorder.

GENETICS

Increasing data suggest that panic disorder is a genetically inherited disease. There is evidence of an increased concordance in monozygotic as compared to dyzygotic twins,[30,31] and the lifetime morbidity risk among first-degree relatives has been found to be 15 to 25 percent.[32,33] There is also evidence from the Yale Family Genetics Study that patients who are comorbid for panic disorder and major depression have *increased rates of major depression, anxiety disorders (phobia, panic disorder, and generalized anxiety disorder), and alcoholism compared with the first-degree relatives of normal controls and depressed probands without an anxiety disorder.*[34] Within families, the transmission pattern for panic disorder is consistent with inheritance for an autosomal dominant gene or with single-locus genetics.[33,35] Preliminary findings from a recent genetic linkage study suggested that panic disorder may be coded by a gene on chromosome 16, 16q22[33] but linkage was not confirmed in an interim analysis that included only 29 percent of the genome, so the issue remains to be determined.[36]

CLINICAL DESCRIPTION

The Symptom Cluster

Although *panic disorder* as a diagnostic label was first used in 1980 in the DSM-III (the American Psychiatric Association's official classification of psychiatric disorders), a similar cluster of symptoms was known in medicine for centuries under a variety of other names. The unique feature of panic disorder is the occurrence of unexpected, unprovoked panic attacks at some point in the patient's history. It is preferable to focus attention on the unexpected, unprovoked paroxysmal nature of these symptom attacks rather than on the word *panic*. A panic attack is defined as any attack with at least four of the thirteen possible symptoms listed in Table 90-1. It is not

TABLE 90-1

SYMPTOMS OF PANIC ATTACK

Shortness of breath (dyspnea) or smothering sensations
Dizziness, unsteady feelings, or faintness
Palpitations or accelerated heart rate (tachycardia)
Trembling or shaking
Sweating
Choking
Nausea or abdominal distress
Depersonalization or derealization
Numbness or tingling sensations (paresthesias)
Flushes (hot flashes) or chills
Chest pain or discomfort
Fear of dying
Fear of going crazy or of doing something uncontrolled

defined by any judgment of the intensity of the attack. The patient does not need to have an intense, cognitive feeling of panic or show signs of overt anxiety to the clinician. For example, the patient may experience skipping or racing of the heart, dizziness, a choking sensation, or pain in the left side of the chest. These symptoms may be accompanied by some cognitive anxiety, although this may not be intense. Such an attack is labeled a panic attack because the four symptoms occur suddenly and unexpectedly within a 10-min period. The important diagnostic point is to focus on the unexpected nature of the attacks and the number of symptoms in each of the patient's attacks rather than on the intensity of each attack.

The majority of patients have two to four unexpected, unprovoked anxiety attacks per week. Typically, they last about 15 to 20 min, with some lasting only 1 or 2 min and others lasting more than 1 h. There is considerable variability, many attacks having only one or two symptoms while others may have as many as 10 or 12. The typical attack usually has four to eight symptoms and is accompanied by considerable cognitive anxiety.

Mental anxiety is not a constant feature of panic attacks.[37] Approximately 20 percent of the attacks in panic disorder occur in the absence of any subjective, cognitive sense of anxiety. Certain symptoms—notably left-sided mammary chest pain, pressure, or discomfort, lightheadedness, and paresthesias—frequently arise in the absence of mental anxiety, especially when they occur as isolated somatic symptoms.

Symptom Progression over Time

The symptoms of panic disorder appear to follow an orderly progression over time and do not appear to occur in a random, haphazard fashion, as previously believed. A common sequence of stages is given in Table 90-2.

The disorder first begins in about 50 percent of cases with a full, unexpected panic attack, while in the rest it first begins with attacks limited to only one or two symptoms (limited-symptom attacks) that may occur in the absence of feeling

mentally anxious. For example, the patient may experience an episode of tachycardia or paresthesias or feel acutely short of breath for no apparent reason; several days later other symptoms from the cluster may occur, again in isolation or in pairs. Later, an attack may occur with four or more symptoms during the same attack. The patient may experience great alarm or a fear of dying, losing control, or running away.

Because the attacks often occur in an unexpected, unprovoked manner, patients may be unable to find any psychosocial reason to explain their symptoms. They interpret the events as an expression of a medical illness. Usually they first seek evaluation from an internist or a family physician rather than a psychiatrist. If one symptom dominates in their symptom cluster, they may seek the specialist who is expert in that area. For example, if they are troubled by skipping or racing of their heart, they may first consult a cardiologist. The clinician then reassures them that "there is nothing seriously wrong" and that their disorder is "just stress and nerves." They are encouraged to minimize the stress and conflict in their lives and to rest, and are reassured that the symptoms will then remit. Use of a stress and conflict model to conceptualize this disorder and the physician's reassurance that there is *nothing wrong* rarely helps. Although much was made of the value of this management strategy in the past, it can no longer be recommended as a useful strategy for managing this disorder. In choosing a treatment strategy, *clinicians can no longer rely on the stress/conflict model of panic disorder to guide them.*

Within weeks the patient usually has another unexpected panic attack and is again at a loss to explain why the attack occurred in the absence of stress or conflict. Because the physician used a stress/conflict model to identify it as an anxiety disorder and the attack occurred in the absence of stress or conflict, the patient interprets this to mean that he or she does not have an anxiety disorder. The patient often assumes that he or she has an exotic medical illness and begins to search for a specialist who has the diagnostic sophistication or the appropriate technology to make an accurate diagnosis. The patient engages in excessive health worries and goes doctor shopping in search of a solution. Reassurances that there is nothing medically wrong quickly lose all value with the next attack. Panic attacks are so terrifying that they obviate all reassurances and convince the patient that indeed there is something physically wrong and that the last physician obviously misunderstood the illness. These patients are often labeled hypochondriacs and feel embarrassed because they

TABLE 90-2

COMMON STAGES OF PANIC DISORDER

Stage 1: Limited symptom attacks
Stage 2: Panic attacks
Stage 3: Health worries
Stage 4: Limited phobias
Stage 5: Extensive phobias
Stage 6: Demoralization and depression

repeatedly call their physicians with somatic complaints in spite of no evidence of medical illness.

The majority of patients have attacks unexpectedly in a variety of situations and often begin to fear and avoid situations that they associate with their bad attacks. If the unexpected attacks continue, the phobias begin to generalize further, and patients often progress to a stage of extensive phobic avoidance behavior and some become housebound.

Approximately 24 percent of panic disorder patients have a comorbid depressive disorder.[38] Many more suffer from depressive symptoms and lose hope without fully meeting criteria for a depressive disorder.[39,40] Sixty-five percent give a history of past major depressive episodes.[40,41] Panic disorder patients with comorbid depression or a past history of depression have a worse course, more severe symptoms (of panic and phobias), longer duration of illness, and higher relapse rates.[40–42] Twenty percent of patients with panic disorder report suicide attempts, and 12 percent report suicide attempts.[43,44] In 1872, Darwin[45] put it succinctly: "If we expect to suffer, we are anxious. If we have no hope of relief, we despair."

If the unexpected attacks are very frequent and intense, the patient usually progresses through these stages (Table 90-2) very rapidly. If the unexpected attacks lessen in intensity, the disorder may abate temporarily and not progress further until the frequency and the intensity of the attacks once again increase. If the unexpected attacks stop completely, as they do in about 15 percent of all cases, the disorder moves through the stages in reverse until there is a spontaneous remission of all symptoms. In the majority of cases, however, there is a progression from unexpected attacks to progressive phobic avoidance behavior and increasing depression over time.

Life Course

Panic disorder has a chronic, fluctuating course during the middle years of life. As many as 50 percent of the victims are disabled to some degree, and 73 to 92 percent are symptomatic when they are reevaluated up to 20 years after their initial diagnosis.[2,46,47]

Patients with panic disorder also have an excess mortality from suicide and, among males, from cardiovascular disease as compared with controls matched for age and sex.[48,49]

ATYPICAL/MASKED PRESENTATIONS OF PANIC IN CARDIOLOGY

In cardiology, panic disorder is most likely to be found in patients presenting with atypical chest pain or MVP. A frequency analysis of symptoms accompanying panic attacks in the general population (Table 90-1) found that "heart pounding" was the most common symptom in the large national Epidemiologic Catchment Area study.[23]

Atypical Chest Pain and Panic Disorder

Anxiety is the most common cause of chest pain and is usually experienced as a sharp stabbing sensation in the left inframam-

mary region[50] (Chap. 10). Traditionally, this diagnosis is made by exclusion of all cardiac and other physical causes. Findings inconclusive of cardiac disease in the presence of persistent complaints of chest pain may lead to a referral for a coronary angiogram.

In cases with minimal disease or normal coronary arteries (NCAs), patients are reassured that their chest pains are not due to coronary artery disease, but they are then left with no other explanation for their symptoms. They may be told to lose weight, stop smoking, or reduce stress. They may be referred to a gastroenterologist to rule out esophageal spasm syndrome, since this disorder is reported in 17 to 100 percent of patients with chest pain and NCAs.[51,52] In one study of 25 patients with esophageal manometric abnormalities consistent with diffuse spasm syndrome, 84 percent met criteria for a psychiatric diagnosis, most frequently anxiety and depression.[53] Follow-up studies of patients with chest pain and NCAs have shown that mortality rates for these patients are no higher than those expected for the general population.[54–56] When they are evaluated from the standpoint of function, however, a different picture emerges.[57] Despite being told that they have NCAs on angiogram, a majority in one study[58] continued to complain of chest pain, 44 percent still believed they had heart disease, 51 percent were unable to work because of the chest pain, and 25 percent continued to use cardiac medications. In another study,[59] 90 percent visited the emergency room during the follow-up period complaining of chest pain, and 9 percent had a second normal coronary arteriogram.

Studies of the syndrome of chest pain with NCAs show that 33 to 48 percent of subjects meet criteria for panic disorder.[60–63] This fraction is much higher than the 2 to 5 percent rate in the community or in controls with chest pain and coronary artery disease. The pain is usually atypical; is more likely to occur in a younger female; and is accompanied by palpitations, multiple somatic complaints, multiple phobias, and depression. It is less likely to be associated with a positive stress test. This observation that chest pain secondary to panic disorder is more likely to be atypical or nonanginal in character is supported by a study of outpatients attending a cardiology clinic[64] that evaluated patients with atypical or nonanginal chest pain with or without coronary artery disease (CAD) for the presence of panic disorder. Of 74 patients with atypical or nonanginal chest pain without CAD, 59 percent had panic disorder. In this study, 50 percent of 30 subjects with atypical or nonanginal chest pain and CAD also met criteria for panic disorder. In a study of patients with acute chest pain admitted to a coronary care unit nearly one-third of the patients met criteria for panic disorder; 4 of 19 (21 percent) panic disorder patients had cardiac findings, including two myocardial infarctions. Of 27 patients with no cardiac findings 15 (55 percent) had panic disorder. These studies suggest that panic disorder and cardiac disease frequently coexist.[65] Overall, the literature supports an association between atypical or nonanginal chest pain and panic disorder. The panic disorder patients cannot be distinguished on the basis of risk factors for CAD, such as presence of diabetes, hypertension, hyperlipidemia, smoking, obesity, or a family history of CAD. In addition to the atypical nature of the chest pain, these patients can be distinguished by the fact that their symptoms are more dramatic and they show more help-seeking behaviors than do chest pain patients without panic disorder.[66] An experimental approach has suggested that by provoking panic attacks through the inhalation of 35 percent carbon dioxide, one can reliably distinguish chest pain patients with panic disorder from those without panic disorder.[67]

CLINICAL EXAMINATION

Clinical examination of the patient with panic disorder may reveal abnormalities related to the cardiovascular, respiratory, gastrointestinal, endocrine, or central nervous systems. The following discussion focuses on findings related to the cardiovascular system.

Mitral Valve Prolapse

In 1963, Barlow[16] established MVP as a separate and distinct disorder. To this day, however, there is debate about whether or not MVP and panic disorder are identical, separate and distinct, or overlapping disorders[68,69] (see Chap. 65). Clinically, both conditions are most common in women of childbearing years, and they run in families. Symptoms common to both include palpitations, tachycardia, light-headedness, dizziness, actual or near syncope, fatigue, dyspnea, and chest pain atypical of angina pectoris. The reported incidence of MVP in panic disorder ranges from 0 percent[70] to 40 to 50 percent.[71–74] Two studies[75,76] found rates of 8 and 15 percent; this was not considered significantly higher than the rates expected for the general population. The variability in results may be due to study size, diagnostic methods, and criteria for MVP. A study of 131 consecutive patients with panic disorder presenting to a psychiatric clinic rather than to cardiology used strict criteria for diagnosing MVP. The diagnosis of definite MVP was made in 34 percent of these subjects and probable MVP in another 5 percent.[77]

The prevalence of panic disorder in patients with MVP has been less extensively investigated. In a comparison of subjects with MVP, cardiac controls, and normal controls,[78] the rates of panic disorder were 12, 6, and 4.5 percent, respectively. Although the results were in the expected direction, the differences were not statistically significant. The rate of panic attacks, however, was significantly higher in patients with MVP (25 percent) than in controls (4.5 percent). The diagnosis of panic disorder was much more likely in the female subjects. In other studies, rates of 16[79] and 0 percent[80] or no increase compared to the control group have been reported.[81]

Overall, the literature supports an association between the two disorders but does not explain it. For the cardiologist in practice, MVP should serve as a marker for the possible existence of an associated panic disorder in patients who are persistently somatic and excessively disabled from their cardiovascular symptoms (see Chap. 65).

Electrocardiogram

Electrocardiographic (ECG) abnormalities, often labile, limited to T-wave inversion—mostly involving leads II, III, and aV_F but occasionally involving leads I, aV_L, and V_4, V_5, and V_6—have been reported in anxiety neurosis/panic disorder.[82–84] On the other hand, two studies found no difference in the frequency of T-wave abnormalities in anxiety neurosis and healthy controls.[85,86] Ambulatory ECG monitoring of 10 healthy women with panic disorder for 6 days did not show any ischemic changes during panic episodes, suggesting that the chest pain is not due to ischemia.[87] A number of studies have examined for cardiac rhythm changes during panic attacks.[88–92] These studies were done on small numbers of patients and used ambulatory (Holter) cardiac monitoring to detect dysrhythmias. When the panic attacks occurred during the course of cardiac monitoring, there was a mean increase in heart rate of 39 beats per minute. The most frequent pattern noted was that of a sinus tachycardia. Some subjects exhibited premature ventricular contractions, atrial tachycardia, and nonsinus atrial rhythm. A retrospective survey[93] of 107 patients referred to cardiology for treatment of paroxysmal supraventricular tachycardia (PSVT) found that the diagnosis of PSVT was initially missed in 59 (55 percent) patients. In the group where the diagnosis of PSVT was missed initially, a diagnosis of "anxiety, panic or stress" was made by physicians (nonpsychiatrists) in 32 (54 percent) of the 59 patients. The median time to diagnosis of PSVT was 3.3 years. The possibility of PSVT should be suspected if the ECG shows ventricular preexcitation in persons presenting with paroxysmal cardiac symptoms. It has been suggested that event monitoring is superior to routine Holter monitoring in making the diagnosis of PSVT.[93] The PSVT was treated in 81 percent of patients with electrophysiologically guided ablation therapy, with symptom resolution in 86 percent of those treated. Only 4 percent of subjects continued to meet criteria for panic disorder. Like MVP and panic disorder, PSVT is an illness of young adults, with a female preponderance and overlap of symptoms. A number of physical and laboratory abnormalities have been reported in panic disorder, such as MVP,[69] abnormalities of esophageal contractility,[53] decreased heart rate variability,[94] and blood pressure changes.[95,96] Whether the PSVT is a symptom of panic disorder, panic disorder is a complication of PSVT, or the two occur in the same patient independently remains unresolved. The relative merits, outcomes, and risks associated with ablation therapy versus serotonin uptake inhibitors in the treatment of this disorder merit further investigation in controlled studies.

Miscellaneous Findings

A number of physical abnormalities of interest to cardiologists have been described in panic disorder. Many of the findings reported here require further validation by replication in larger study populations. It has been reported that people with panic disorder have decreased heart rate variability, a characteristic that has been linked to a significant risk for cardiovascular disease.[94] A study of 18 frequent panickers compared them with nonanxious controls at baseline and after mild non-panic-inducing stress. At baseline, the panic patients exhibited higher forehead electromyographic activity as well as higher systolic blood pressure and heart rate. Stress led to larger increases in blood pressure and heart rate as compared with controls.[95] Others have noted higher heart rate and diastolic blood pressure in subjects with panic disorder.[96] Peripheral markers of adrenergic and serotonergic function are altered in panic disorder. It has been suggested that they may be trait markers of biogenic amine activity in panic disorder, since they do not normalize after effective treatment.[97] Clonidine pretreatment only attenuates lactate-induced panic in some

individuals. This suggests that lactate-induced panic involves more than the noradrenergic system.[98] Lactate infusions induce panic attacks; based on this, it has been generally believed that exercise will precipitate panic due to the accumulation of lactate. A study that subjected 16 panic patients and 17 controls to submaximal exercise testing did not find a difference in exercise tolerance between groups, suggesting that exercise-induced lactate increment may not cause panic attacks.[90] This issue deserves further clarification.

CONSEQUENCES OF PANIC DISORDER

There are serious and widespread medical and psychiatric consequences to missing the diagnosis or treating the disorder inadequately. The evaluation strategy outlined in Figure 90-1 should help to increase accurate diagnoses.

Medical Consequences

Significantly higher rates of hypertension and peptic ulcer have been reported in patients with panic disorder than in controls.[100,101] Increased mortality from cardiovascular disease and suicide has been reported for males with panic disorder in some studies[48,49] but not in others.[4,47,102–104] Examination of the New Haven portion of the Epidemiological Catchment Area Program suggests that the risk of stroke in persons with a lifetime diagnosis of panic disorder is twice that in persons with or without other psychiatric disorder.[105] A study[106] of patients awaiting cardiac transplant for idiopathic dilated cardiomyopathy found a high rate of panic disorder among these patients as compared with controls who had heart failure from CAD, rheumatic disease, or congenital heart disease. In the majority of cases, the panic disorder preceded the onset of heart failure. It has been suggested that some panic disorder patients may exhibit mild left ventricular hypertrophy or dilation.[107]

Another consequence of panic disorder is overutilization of medical services. Patients with panic disorder are two to three times more likely to use the

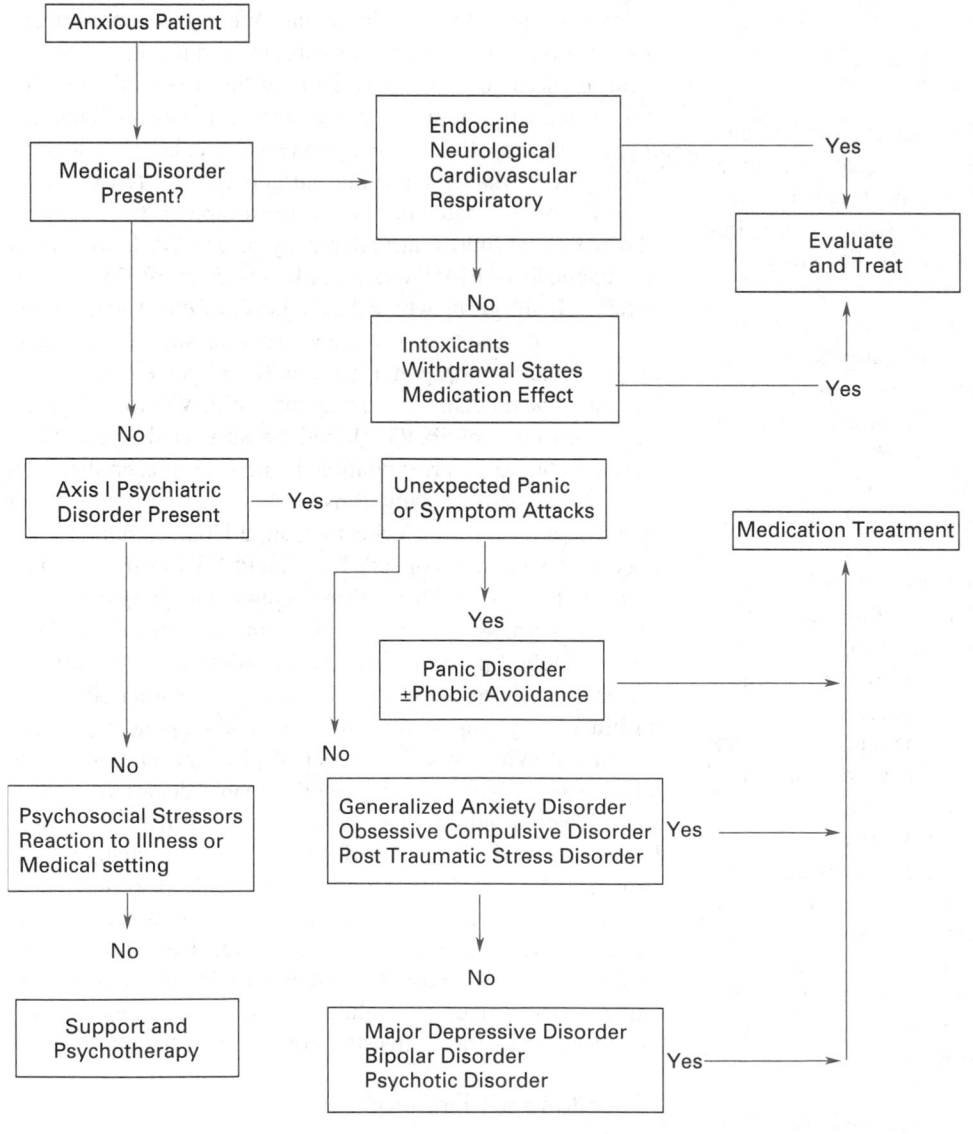

FIGURE 90-1

Evaluation strategy for the anxious patient. (Reproduced by permission. Copyright B.A. Raj, M.D., and D.V. Sheehan, M.D., 1996.)

services of an emergency room for an emotional problem than are patients with depression.[108] These patients have numerous somatic complaints, and the vast majority believe they have a physical disorder. In one study, 70 percent had 12 or more symptoms each,[109] and 70 percent of another sample had seen 10 or more physicians for somatic complaints.[110]

Some of the testing may not be inexpensive or benign. For example, subjects presenting with chest pain may end up having unnecessary coronary angiograms. Of those with normal coronary arteries and chest pain, about 33 percent will meet criteria for panic disorder.[62] A study in two primary care clinics found that 11.8 percent of the distressed high utilizers met criteria for current panic disorder and 32 percent met criteria for a lifetime diagnosis of panic disorder.[111]

Psychiatric Consequences

In a review of outcomes among patients with anxiety disorders, 6 to 60 percent of deaths during follow-up were attributed to suicide.[112] The variation in rates depends on the sample studied, with higher rates being observed in studies of panic disorder patients who had been hospitalized. In that population, 20 percent of deaths during follow-up were due to suicide.[48,49,113] Data from a community-based study of psychiatric disorders[114] showed that 7 percent of people with uncomplicated panic disorder reported a suicide attempt at some time in their lives, and the rate goes up to 20 percent if comorbid conditions coexist. These rates are similar to those observed for depression.

Criteria for the diagnosis of lifetime alcohol abuse are met among 13 percent of Americans, among 18 percent of those with depression, and among 27 perent of those with panic disorder. Some 83 percent of panic patients report that they use alcohol to mitigate their panic attacks, and 72 percent report that this is effective.[115] Studies suggest that the panic symptoms precede the alcoholism in the majority of cases.[116] Panic disorder patients are also more likely to be given symptomatic treatment and to take medications for insomnia, dizziness, and nausea. As a group, they are at high risk for unnecessary polypharmacy.[117]

TREATMENT

Panic disorder is now usually treated with a sequence of distinct approaches (Fig. 90-2). The first and most critical of

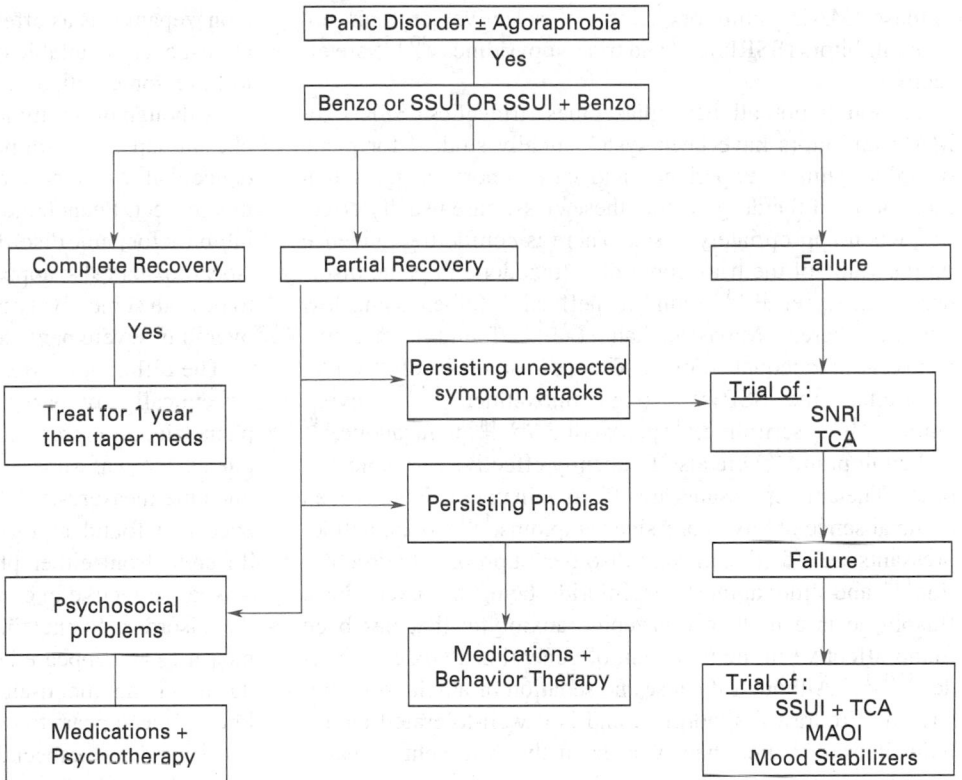

FIGURE 90-2

Management strategy in panic disorder. *Key:* Benzo = benzodiazepines; SSUI = selective serotonin uptake inhibitor; SNRI = serotonin norepinephrine uptake inhibitor; MAOI — monoamine oxidase inhibitor; TCA = tricyclic antidepressant. (Reproduced by permission. Copyright B.A. Raj, M.D., and D.V. Sheehan, M.D., 1996.)

these is the use of antipanic medication to control the unexpected attacks. *Because antipanic medications alone rarely lead to complete timely resolution of phobic avoidance behavior, in vivo exposure therapy is usually necessary to reduce phobic avoidance and anticipatory anxiety.* If there are psychosocial problems complicating recovery, psychotherapy is indicated, but it is not routinely imposed on all patients with panic disorder. Finally, to protect patients against future relapse, prepare them if they do relapse, and ensure good compliance to the other treatment steps, it is important to educate patients about their illness and the rationale for the treatments used. Relaxation treatment and exercise programs are ineffective in the treatment of panic disorder. Indeed in our experience marked exercise exacerbates the symptoms of panic disorder probably by increasing blood levels of lactic acid, to which many of them tend to be hypersensitive.

MEDICATION CHOICES

Although only two medications (alprazolam and paroxetine) have to date been formally approved by the U.S. Food and Drug Administration for the treatment of panic disorder, there is good evidence that several classes of medications may be effective. Several studies suggest that benzodiazepines,[118–120] tricyclic antidepressants,[110,121–123] monoamine oxidase (MAO) inhibitors,[110,123–128] selective serotonin uptake inhibitors (SSRIs),[129] and triazolopyridines[130,131] are effective.

Although not all benzodiazepines, tricyclics, SSRIs, or MAO inhibitors have been systematically studied for panic disorder, clinical experience and case reports suggest that most or all of the drugs within these classes are usually effective when appropriately dosed. There is conflicting evidence on the value of the triazolopyridine trazodone in panic disorder; Charney et al.[130] found it ineffective (albeit using low doses), whereas Mavissakalian et a.[131] found it effective if given in adequate doses. The newest class of "antidepressants," the SSRIs[129] (e.g., fluoxetine,[132,133] fluvoxamine,[134–141] sertraline,[142] paroxetine,[143–146] nefazadone,[147] and citalopram[148]) are also frequently effective for panic disorder. The antidepressants are effective in panic disorder even in the absence of any depressive symptoms.[110] Not all antidepressants are effective in panic disorder, bupropion hydrochloride[149] and amoxapine hydrochloride being the exceptions. Buspirone is a nonbenzodiazepine anxiolytic that has been found effective in the treatment of generalized anxiety disorder.[150–153] Although it causes no sedation or ataxia, does not have a withdrawal syndrome, and is a well-tolerated anxiolytic, it is no better than placebo in the treatment of panic disorder,[154] even when given in high doses.[155]

MEDICATION COMPARISONS

Although alprazolam is the most thoroughly studied and most widely prescribed medication for panic disorder, the preliminary evidence suggests that it may not be unique among benzodiazepines in this regard. Noyes et al.[156] have found diazepam to be effective, while Tesar et al.[157] reported that

clonazepam was as effective as alprazolam. In our experience almost every available (nonhypnotic) benzodiazepine appears to have some antipanic effects if correctly dosed.

Although imipramine is the most extensively studied tricyclic antidepressant for panic disorder, there is currently no evidence that it is superior (or inferior) to any other tricyclic in this respect. Phenelzine is the most thoroughly studied MAO inhibitor for panic disorder, although both tranylcypromine and isocarboxazid also appear effective. Tranylcypromine appears to be both subjectively better tolerated and slightly less potent overall in severe panic disorder than phenelzine.

The different classes of antipanic drugs have not all been systemically compared with each other. A study comparing phenelzine, imipramine, and placebo found evidence that phenelzine was superior to imipramine on a few but not all outcome measures.[110] A later study[123] replicated this difference and found alprazolam, overall, not to be statistically different from either phenelzine or imipramine, although it was less effective in controlling the depressive dimensions of the disorder. Phenelzine had a greater effect on disability measures and appeared to be a more potent rehabilitator, with its energizing, mood-elevating, confidence-enhancing effects. Phenelzine appears to have a margin of superiority over other antipanic drugs, especially in severe and chronic cases. Effective and safe therapy with MAO inhibitors requires a patient who will comply reliably with the required drug restrictions and low-tyramine diet.

In severe cases, phenelzine, the hydrazine MAO inhibitor, appears to be the most potent.[110,123] The SSRIs as a class, however, appear to be more effective in panic disorder than tricyclics or benzodiazepines, and the benzodiazepines seem marginally better than the tricyclics.[158] The data and the general consensus of opinion now favors SSRIs as the medications of first choice in the treatment of panic disorder (Table 90-3).

TABLE 90-3

COMPARATIVE DRUG EFFECTS ON THE DIMENSIONS OF PANIC DISORDER

Class of Drug	Panic Attacks	Anticipatory Anxiety	Phobia	Depression	Obsessions	Relative Side Effects	Overall Efficacy
Benzodiazepines							
Alprazolam, clonazepam, lorazepam	3	4	3	0–1	0–1	1–2	3
Tricyclic antidepressants (TCA)							
Clomipramine	3.5	2	2	3	3	3.5	3.5
Others	3	2	2.5	3	1	3	3
Selective serotonin uptake inhibitors							
Fluoxetine, fluvoxamine, sertraline, paroxetine, nefazodone	3.5	2	2.5	3	3	2	3.5
Monoamine oxidase inhibitors							
Phenelzine	4	3.5	3	4	3	3	4
Tranylcypromine	3	2	3	3	2.5	2	3

Key: 0 = no effect; 1 = mild; 2 = moderate; 3 = moderate plus; 4 = maximum or severe.
Source: Reproduced with permission. Copyright B.A. Raj, M.D., and D.V. Sheehan, M.D., 1996.

TABLE 90-4

RELATIVE MERITS, CONCERNS, AND DOSING OF ANTIPANIC DRUGS

	Initial Starting Dose	Final Mean Effective Dose, mg	Dose Range, mg	Advantages	Concerns
Benzodiazepines					
Alprazolam	0.5 mg t.i.d.	6	2–10	Rapid onset of action, well tolerated	Sedation, dependence, withdrawal syndrome, and no antidepressant effect
Clonazepam	0.5 mg t.i.d.	4	2–10		
Lorazepam	0.5 mg t.i.d.	6	2–10		
Cyclic agents					
Imipramine	25 mg b.i.d.	225	50–300	Effective antipanic, antidepressant and antiobsessional drugs	Anticholinergic effects; cardiotoxicity, hypotension, weight gain, poor long-term compliance, and lethality in overdose; 6–8 weeks for therapeutic benefit
Clomipramine	25 mg b.i.d.	125	75–200		
Serotonin uptake inhibitors					
Fluoxetine	10 mg q.d.	40	20–80	Well tolerated, good compliance long-term, and low lethality in overdose	Sexual dysfunction; 6–8 weeks for therapeutic benefit; potential for drug interactions due to CYP450 enzyme inhibition
Fluvoxamine	20 mg b.i.d.	200	100–300		
Sertraline	25 mg q.d.	125	50–200		
Paroxetine	10 mg q.d.	40	20–60		
Nefazodone	50 mg b.i.d.	400	300–600		
Venlafaxine	37.5 mg b.i.d.	225	150–375		
Monoamine oxidase inhibitors					
Phenelzine	15 mg q.d.	60	45–90	Very powerful antipanic, antiobsessional properties	Hypotensive; 6–8 weeks for therapeutic benefit; severe weight gain; high lethality in overdose; diet and drug restrictions
Tranylcypromine	10 mg q.d.	60	30–80		

Source: Reproduced with permission. Copyright B.A. Raj, M.D. and D.V. Sheehan, M.D., 1996.

USE OF MEDICATION

The majority of failures on antipanic drugs occur because the doses used are too low and the duration of treatment is too short (Table 90-4). Attention to these two issues is critical to good medication management. Practical guidelines for the effective use of MAO inhibitors,[128,159,160] tricyclics,[161,162] benzodiazepines,[163,164] and SSRIs[165] in panic disorder are available.

TREATMENT OF RESIDUAL PHOBIC AVOIDANCE

After the medication dosage has been correctly adjusted, some patients continue to have residual phobias that represent a learned complication of panic attacks. Behavior therapy in the form of in vivo exposure is an effective treatment for these phobias. The cardiologist should seek consultation from a behavior therapist (either a psychiatrist or psychologist) to implement this treatment.

LONG-TERM TREATMENT

If psychosocial problems complicate recovery, psychotherapy is indicated. The relapse rate is in excess of 70 percent, and many patients will require long-term medication management. The risk of relapse increases with each episode. For a first episode, most psychiatrists keep patients on antipanic medication for 1 year. If the patient suffers a recurrence, it is wise to restart the antipanic medication quickly and maintain it for at least another year. If the patient has had two or more episodes, it is now becoming the norm to keep such an individual on medication long-term.

REFERENCES

1. Maclean WC. Diseases of the heart in the British Army: The cause and the remedy. *Br Med J* 1867; 1:161–164.
2. Skerritt PW. Anxiety and the heart—A historical review. *Psychol Med* 1983; 13:17–25.
3. Coote C. Inframammary pain. *Br Med J* 1858; 1:502–503.
4. Da Costa JM. On irritable heart: A clinical study of a functional cardiac disorder and its consequences. *Am J Med Sc* 1871; 61:17–52.

5. Freud S. On the grounds for detaching a particular syndrome from neurasthenia under the description "anxiety neurosis." In: *The Standard Edition of The Complete Psychological Works of Sigmund Freud*. Vol. III (1893–1899). London: Hogarth Press; 1894.

6. Lewis T. *Report upon Soldiers Returned as Cases of "Disordered Action of the Heart" (DAH) or "Valvular Disease of the Heart" (VDH)*. Special report series no. 8, London: Medical Research Committee: 1917.

7. Oppenheimer BS, Rothschild MA. The psychoneurotic factor in the "irritable heart of soldiers." *Br Med J* 1918; 2:29–31.

8. MacKenzie J. The soldiers heart and war neurosis: A study in symptomatology. *Br Med J* 1920; 1:491–494, 530–534.

9. Culpin M. The psychological aspect of the effort syndrome. *Lancet* 1920; 2:184–186.

10. Schnur S. Cardiac neurosis associated with organic heart disease. *Am Heart J* 1939; 18:153–165.

11. Wood PW. Da Costa's syndrome (or effort syndrome). *Br Med J* 1941; 1:767–772, 805–811, 845–851.

12. Jones M, Lewis A. Effort syndrome. *Lancet* 1941; 1:813–818.

13. Jones M. Physiological and psychological responses to stress in neurotic patients. *J Ment Sci* 1948; 94:392–427.

14. Gorlin R. The hyperkinetic heart syndrome. *JAMA* 1962; 182:823–829.

15. Frohlich ED, Dustan HP, Page IH. Hyperdynamic beta-adrenergic circulatory state. *Arch Int Med* 1966; 117:614–619.

16. Barlow JB, Bosman CK, Pocock WA, Marchand P. Late systolic murmurs and non ejection ("mid-late") systolic clicks: An analysis of 90 patients. *Br Heart J* 1968; 30:203–218.

17. Wooley CF. Where are the diseases of yesteryear? Da Costa's syndrome, soldiers heart, the effort syndrome, neurocirculatory asthenia and the mitral valve prolapse syndrome. *Circulation* 1976; 53:749–751.

18. Robins LN, Helzer JE, Weissman MM, Oruaschel H, Gruenberg E, Burke JD Jr, et al. Lifetime prevalence of psychiatric disorders at three sites. *Arch Gen Psychiatry* 1984; 41:949–959.

19. American Psychiatric Association. *Diagnostic and Statistical Manual of Mental Disorders*, 3d rev ed. Washington, DC: American Psychiatric Association; 1987.

20. Eaton WW, Kessler RC, Wittcher HU, Magee WJ. Panic and panic disorder in the United States. *Am J Psychiatry* 1994; 151:413–420.

21. Raj BA, Sheehan DV. Aging issues in panic disorder. *Jpn J Psychosom Med* 1994; 34(1):33–38.

22. McGlynn TJ, Metcalf HL. *Diagnosis and Treatment of Anxiety Disorders: A Physician's Handbook*. Washington, DC. American Psychiatric Press; 1989.

23. Eaton WW, Keyl PM. The Epidemiology of panic. In: Asnis GM, van Praag HM, eds. *Panic Disorder: Clinical, Biological, and Treatment Aspects. The Einstein Psychiatry Series*. New York: Wiley; 1995:50–65.

24. Sheehan DV, Sheehan KE, Minichello WE. Age of onset of phobic disorders: A reevaluation. *Comp Psychiatry* 1981; 22:544–553.

25. Weissman MM, Myers JK, Tischler GL, Holzer CE III, Leaf PJ, Orvaschel H, et al. Psychiatric disorders (DSM-III) and cognitive impairment among elderly in a U.S. Urban community. *Acta Psychiatr Scand* 1985; 71:366–379.

26. Marks IM, Lader M. Anxiety states (anxiety neurosis): A review. *J Nerv Ment Dis* 1973; 156:3–18.

27. Weissman MM, Leaf PJ, Holzer CE III, Merikangas KR. Epidemiology of anxiety disorders. *Psychopharmacol Bull* 1985; 21:538–541.

28. Ballenger JC, Burrows GR, DuPont RL Jr, Lesser IM, Noyes R Jr, Pecknold JC, et al. Alprazolam in panic disorder and agoraphobia: Results from a multicenter trial. Efficacy in short term treatment. *Arch Gen Psychiatry* 1988; 45:413–422.

29. Eaton WW, Dryman A, Weissman MM. Panic and phobia. In: Robins L, Regier DA (eds): *Psychiatric Disorders in America*. New York: Free Press; 1991:155–179.

30. Torgersen S. Genetic factors in anxiety disorders. *Arch Gen Psychiatry* 1983; 40:1085–1089.

31. Hopper JL, Judd FK, Derrick PL, Macaskill GT, Burrows GD. A family study of panic disorder: Reanalysis using a regressive logistic model that incorporates a sibship environment. *Gen Epidemiol* 1990; 7:151–161.

32. Crowe RR, Noyes R, Pauls DL, Slymen D. A family study of panic disorder. *Arch Gen Psychiatry* 1983; 40:1065–1069.

33. Crowe RR, Noyes R, Wilson AF, Elston RC, Ward LJ. Linkage study of panic disorder. *Arch Gen Psychiatry* 1987; 44:933–937.

34. Ballenger JC, Burrows GR, DuPont RL Jr, Lesser IM, Noyes R Jr, Pecknold JC. Alprazolam in panic disorder and agoraphobia: Results from a multicenter trial. Efficacy in short term treatment. *Arch Gen Psychiatry* 1988; 45:413–422.

35. Pauls DL, Bocher KD, Crowe RR, Noyes R Jr. A genetic study of panic disorder pedigrees. *Am J Hum Genet* 1980; 32:639–644.

36. Crowe RR. The Iowa linkage study of panic disorder. In: *Genetic Approaches to Mental Disorders*. Washington, DC: American Psychiatric Press; 1994:291–309.

37. Kushner MG, Beitman BD. Panic attacks without fear: An overview. *Behav Res Ther* 1990; 28:469–479.

38. Wetzler S, Sanderson WC. Comorbidity of panic disorder. In: Asnis GM, van Praag HM, eds. *Panic Disorder: Clinical, Biological, and Treatment Aspects. The Einstein Psychiatry Series*. New York: Wiley; 1995:80–98.

39. Sanderson WC, Beck AT, Beck J. Syndrome comorbidity in patients with major depression and dysthymia: Prevalence and temporal relationships. *Am J Psychiatry* 1990; 147:1025–1028.

40. Breier A, Charney DS, Heninger GR. Major depression in patients with agoraphobia and panic disorder. *Arch Gen Psychiatry* 1984; 41:1129–1135.

41. Stein MB, Tancer ME, Uhde TW. Major depression in patients with panic disorders: Factors associated with course and recurrence. *J Affect Dis* 1990; 19:287–296.

42. Coryell W, Endicott J, Winokur G. Anxiety syndromes as epiphenomena of primary major depression: Outcome and family psychopathology. *Am J Psychiatry* 1992; 149:100–107.

43. Arnold DH, Sanderson WC, Beck AT. Panic disorder and suicidal behavior. In: Asnis GM, van Praag HM, eds. *Panic Disorder: Clinical, Biological, and Treatment Aspects. The Einstein Psychiatry Series*. New York: Wiley; 1995:99–115.

44. Weissman MM, Klerman GL, Markowitz JS, Ouellette R. Suicidal ideation and suicide attempts in panic disorder and panic attacks. *N Engl J Med* 1989; 321:1209–1214.

45. Darwin C. *The Expressions of the Emotions in Man and Animals*. London: Murray; 1872.

46. Greer S. The prognosis of anxiety states. In: Lader MH, ed. *Studies of Anxiety*. London: Royal Med Psychological Association; 1969:151–157.

47. Wheeler EO, White PD, Reed EW, Cohen ME. Neurocirculatory asthenia (anxiety neurosis, effort syndrome, neurasthenia): A twenty-year follow-up study of one hundred and seventy-three patients. *JAMA* 1950; 142:878–889.

48. Coryell W, Noyes R, Clancy J. Excess mortality in panic disorder: A comparison with primary unipolar depression. *Arch Gen Psychiatry* 1982; 39:701–703.

49. Coryell W, Noyes R, House JD. Mortality among outpatients with anxiety disorders. *Am J Psychiatry* 1986; 143:508–510.

50. Kitt TM. Recurrent atypical chest pain. *Hosp Phys* 1986; 11:57–64.

51. Dart AM, Davies AH, Dalal J, Ruttley M, Henderson AH. "Angina" and normal coronary arteriograms: A follow-up study. *Eur Heart J* 1980; 1:97–100.

52. Brand DL, Martin D, Pope CE. II. Esophageal manometrics in patients with angina like chest pain. *Dig Dis Sci* 1977; 22:300–304.

53. Clouse RE, Lustman PJ. Psychiatric illness and contraction abnormalities of the esophagus. *N Engl J Med* 1983; 309:1337–1342.

54. Bruschke AV, Proudfit WB, Sones FM. Clinical course of patients with normal and slightly or moderately abnormal coronary arteriograms: A follow-up study of 500 patients. *Circulation* 1973; 47:936–945.

55. Isner JM, Salem DN, Banas JS, Levine HJ. Long term clinical course of patients with normal coronary arteriography: Follow-up study of 121 patients with normal or nearly normal coronary arteriograms. *Am Heart J* 1981; 102:645–653.

56. Kemp HG, Vokonoas PS, Cohn PF, Gorlin R. The anginal syndrome associated with normal coronary arteriograms: Report of a six-year experience. *Am J Med* 1973; 54:735–742.

57. Beitman BD, Kushner MG, Basha I, Lamberti J, Mukerji V, Bartels K. Follow up status of patients with angiographically normal coronary arteries and panic disorder. *JAMA* 1991; 265:1545–1549.

58. Ockene IS, Shay MJ, Alpert JS, Weiner BH, Dalen JE. Unexplained chest pain in patients with normal coronary arteriograms: A follow-up study of functional status. *N Engl J Med* 1980; 303:1249–1252.

59. Lavey EB, Winkle RA. Continuing disability of patients with chest pain and normal coronary arteriograms. *J Chronic Dis* 1979; 32:191–196.

60. Bass C, Wade C. Chest pain with normal coronary arteries: A comparative study of psychiatric and social morbidity. *Psychol Med* 1984; 14:51–61.

61. Katon W, Hall ML, Russo J, Cormier L, Hollifield M, Vitaliano PP. Chest pain: Relationship of psychiatric illness to coronary arteriographic results. *Am J Med* 1988; 84:1–9.

62. Beitman BD, Lamberti JW, Mukerji V, DeRosear L, Basha I, Schmid L. Panic disorder in patients with angiographically normal coronary arteries: A pilot study. *Psychosomatics* 1987; 28:480–484.

63. Mukerji V, Beitman BD, Alpert MA, Lamberti JW, DeRosear L, Basha IM. Panic attack symptoms in patients with chest pain and angiographically normal coronary arteries. *J Anxiety Dis* 1987; 1:41–46.

64. Beitman BD, Basha I, Flaker G, DeRosear L, Mukerji V, Trombka L, et al. Atypical or nonanginal chest pain. Panic disorder or coronary artery disease? *Arch Intern Med* 1987; 147:1548–1552.

65. Carter C, Maddock R, Amsterdam E, McCormick S, Waters C, Billet J. Panic disorder and chest pain in the coronary care unit. *Psychosomatics* 1992; 33:302–309.

66. Margraf J, DeVries-Wehrhahn E, Sonnentag S. Myocardial infarct, functional heart symptoms and panic syndrome. *Psychother Psychosom Med Psychol* 1991; 41:31–34.

67. Beitman BD, Logue MB, Thomas AM, Bartels K. Response to 35% CO_2 in patients with chest pain and angiographically normal coronary arteries. *Int J Psychiatry Med* 1992; 22:197–203.

68. Gottlieb SH. Mitral valve prolapse: From syndrome to disease. *Am J Cardiol* 1987; 60:53J–58J.

69. Raj A, Sheehan DV. Mitral valve prolapse and panic disorder. *Bull Menninger Clin* 1990; 54:199–208.

70. Hickey AJ, Andrew G, Wilchen DE. Independence of mitral valve prolapse and neurosis. *Br Heart J* 1983; 50:333–336.

71. Kantor JS, Zitrin CM, Zeldis SM. Mitral valve prolapse syndrome in agoraphobic patients. *Am J Psychiatry* 1980; 137:467–470.

72. Venkatesh A, Pauls DL, Crowe R, Noyes R Jr, Van Valkenburg C, Martins JB, et al. Mitral valve prolapse in anxiety neurosis (panic disorder). *Am Heart J* 1980; 100:302–305.

73. Pariser SF, Jones BA, Pinta ER, Young ER, Fontana ME. Panic attacks: Diagnostic evaluation of 17 patients. *Am J Psychiatry* 1979; 136:105–106.

74. Gorman JM, Fyer AF, Glicklich J, King DL, Klein DF. Mitral valve prolapse and panic disorders. Effect of imipramine. In: Klein DF, Rabkin JG, eds. *Anxiety: New Research and Changing Concepts.* New York: Raven Press, 1981:317–326.

75. Mavissakalian M, Salerni R, Thompson ME, Michaelson L. Mitral valve prolapse and agoraphobia. *Am J Psychiatry* 1983; 140:1612–1614.

76. Shear MK, Devereau RB, Kramer-Fox R, Mann JJ, Frances A. Low prevalence of mitral valve prolapse in patients with panic disorder. *Am J Psychiatry* 1984; 141:302–303.

77. Liberthson R, Sheehan DV, King ME, Weyman AE. The prevalence of mitral valve prolapse in patients with panic disorders. *Am J Psychiatry* 1986; 143:511–515.

78. Kane JM, Woerner M, Zeldis S, Kramer R, Saravay S. Panic and phobic disorders in patients with mitral valve prolapse. In: Klein DF, Rabkin JG, eds. *Anxiety: New Research and Changing Concepts.* New York: Raven Press; 1981:327–340.

79. Hartman N, Kramer R, Brown WT, Devereux RB. Panic disorder in patients with mitral valve prolapse. *Am J Psychiatry* 1982; 139:669–670.

80. Mazza DL, Martin D, Spacavento L, Jacobsen J, Gibbs H. Prevalence of anxiety disorders in patients with mitral valve prolapse. *Am J Psychiatry* 1986; 143:349–352.

81. Bowen RC, D'Arcy C, Orchard RC. The prevalence of anxiety disorders among patients with mitral valve and chest pain. *Psychosomatics* 1991; 32:400–406.

82. Graybiel A, White PD. Inversion of the T waves in lead I or II of the electrocardiogram in young individuals with neurocirculatory asthenia, with thyrotoxicosis, in relation to certain infections and following paroxysmal ventricular tachycardia. *Am Heart J* 1935; 10:345.

83. Wendkos MH, Logue RB. Unstable T waves in leads II and III in persons with neurocirculatory asthenia. *Am Heart J* 1946; 31:711.

84. Levander-Lindgren M. Studies in neurocirculatory asthenia (DaCosta's syndrome): I. Variations with regard to symptoms and some pathophysiological signs. *Acta Med Scand* 1962; 172:665.

85. Kannel WB, Dawber TR, Cohen ME. The ECG neurocirculatory asthenia (anxiety neurosis or neurasthenia): A study of 203 neurocirculatory patients and 757 healthy controls in the Framingham Study. *Ann Intern Med* 1958; 49:1351.

86. Cohen ME, White PD, Johnson RE. Neurocirculatory asthenia, anxiety neurosis, or the effort syndrome. *Arch Intern Med* 1948; 81:260.

87. Lint DW, Taylor CB, Fried-Behar L, Kenardy J. Does ischemia occur with panic attacks? *Am J Psychiatry* 1995; 152:1678–1680.

88. Shear MK, Kligfield P, Hartsfield G, Devereux RB, Polan JJ, Mann JJ, et al. Cardiac rate and rhythm in panic disorders. *Am J Psychiatry* 1987; 144:633–637.

89. Jalley R, Lydiard RB, Assey ME, Usher BW, Barnwell WH, Ballenger JC. Cardiovascular status of panic disorder patients with and without prominent cardiac symptoms. *Psychosomatics* 1992; 33:81–84.

90. Taylor CB, Sheik J, Agras WS et al. Ambulatory heart rate changes in patients with panic attacks. *Am J Psychiatry* 1986; 143:478–482.

91. Lader M, Mathews A. Physiological changes during spontaneous panic attacks. *J Psychosom Res* 1970; 14:377–382.

92. Freedman RR, Lanni P, Ettedgui E, Puthezhath N. Ambulatory monitoring of panic disorder. *Arch Gen Psychiatry* 1985; 42:244–248.

93. Lessmeier TJ, Gamperling D, Johnson-Liddon V, Fromm BS, Steinman RT, Meissner MD, et al. Unrecognized paroxysmal supraventricular tachycardia: Potential for misdiagnosis as panic disorder. *Arch Int Med* 1997; 15:537–543.

94. Klein E, Cnaani E, Harel T, Braun S, Ben-Haim SA. Altered heart rate variability in panic disorder patients. *Biol Psychiatry* 1995; 1;37(1):18–24.

95. Hoehn-Saric R, McLeod DR, Zimmerli WD. Psychophysiologic response patterns in panic disorder. *Acta Psychiatr Scand* 1991; 83(1):4–11.

96. Bystritsky A, Craske M, Maidenberg E, Vapnik T, Shapiro D. Ambulatory monitoring of panic patients during regular activity: A preliminary report. *Biol Psychiatry* 1995; 38:684–689.

97. Butler J, O'Halloran A, Leonard BE. The Galway study of panic disorder II: Changes in some peripheral markers of noradrenergic and serotonergic function in DSM III-R panic disorder. *J Affect Dis* 1992; 26(2):89–99.

98. Coplan JD, Liebowitz MR, Gorman JM, Fyer AJ, Dillon DJ, Campeas RB, et al. Noradrenergic function in panic disorder: Effects of intravenous clonidine pretreatment on lactate induced panic. *Biol Psychiatry* 1992; 31(2):135–146.

99. Stein JM, Papp La, Klein DF, Cohen S, Simon J, Ross D, et al. Exercise tolerance in panic disorder patients. *Biol Psychiatry* 1992; 32:281–287.

100. Noyes R, Clancy J, Hoenk PR, Slymen DJ. The prognosis of anxiety neurosis. *Arch Gen Psychiatry* 1980; 37:173–178.

101. Katon W. Panic disorder and somatisation: A review of 55 cases. *Am J Med* 1984; 77:101–106.

102. Martin RL, Cloninger R, Guze SB, Clayton PJ. Mortality in follow up of 500 psychiatric outpatients. *Arch Gen Psychiatry* 1985; 42:47–66.

103. Black DW, Warrack G, Winokur G. The Iowa record-linkage study: III. Excess mortality among patients with "functional disorders." *Arch Gen Psychiatry* 1985; 42:82–88.

104. Winokur G, Black DW. Psychiatric and medical diagnosis as risk factors for mortality in psychiatric patients: A case controlled study. *Am J Psychiatry* 1987; 144:208–211.

105. Weissman MM, Markowitz JS, Ouellete R, Greenwald S, Kahn JP. Panic disorder and cardiovascular/cerebrovascular problems: Results from a community survey. *Am J Psychiatry* 1990; 147:1504–1508.

106. Kahn JP, Drusin RE, Klein DF. Idiopathic cardiomyopathy and panic disorder: Clinical association in cardiac transplant candidates. *Am J Psychiatry* 1987; 144:1327–1330.

107. Kahn JP, Gorman JM, King DL, Fyer AJ, Liebowitz MR, Klein DF. Cardiac left ventricular hypertrophy and chamber dilatation in panic disorder patients: Implications for idiopathic dilated cardiomyopathy. *Psychiatr Res* 1990; 32:55–61.

108. Markowitz JS, Weissman MM, Ouellette R, Lish JD, Klerman GL. Quality of life in panic disorder. *Arch Gen Psychiatry* 1989; 46:984–992.

109. Sheehan DV, Sheehan KH. The classification of anxiety and hysterical states: I. Historical review and empirical delineation. *J Clin Psychopharmacol* 1982; 1:235–244.

110. Sheehan DV, Ballenger JC, Jacobson G. Treatment of endogenous anxiety with phobic, hysterical and hypochondriacal symptoms. *Arch Gen Psychiatry* 1980; 37:51–59.

111. Katon W, Von Korf M, Lin E, Lipscomb P, Russo J, Wagner E, et al. Distressed high utilizers of medical care: DSM-III-R diagnoses and treatment needs. *Gen Hosp Psychiatry* 1990; 12:355–362.

112. Noyes R. Suicide and panic disorder: A review. *J Affect Dis* 1991; 22:1–11.

113. Allgulander C, Lavori PN. Excess mortality among 3,302 patients with pure anxiety neurosis. *Arch Gen Psychiatry* 1991; 48:599–602.

114. Weissman M, Klerman G, Markowitz J, Ouellette R. Suicidal ideation and suicide attempts in panic disorder and attacks. *N Engl J Med* 1989; 321:1209–1213.

115. Cox BJ, Norton GR, Dorward J, Ferguson PA. The relationship between panic attacks and chemical dependencies. *Addict Behav* 1989; 14:53–60.

116. Cox BJ, Norton GR, Swinson RP, Endler NS. Substance abuse and panic-related anxiety: A critical review. *Behav Res Ther* 1990; 28:385–393.

117. Ciraulo DA, Sands BF, Shader RI. Critical review of liability of benzodiazepine abuse among alcoholics. *Am J Psychiatry* 1988; 145:1501–1506.

118. Sheehan DV, Coleman JH, Greenblatt DJ, Jones KJ, Levine PH, Orsulak PJ, et al. Some biochemical correlates of panic attacks with agoraphobia and their response to a new treatment. *J Clin Psychopharmacol* 1984; 4:66–75.

119. Chouinard G, Annable L, Fontaine R, Solyom L. Alprazolam in the treatment of generalized anxiety and panic disorders: A double blind placebo controlled study. *Psychopharmacology* 1982; 77:229–233.

120. Sheehan DV, Uzogara E, Coleman JH, Greenblatt DJ, Jones KJ, Levine P, et al. The treatment of panic attacks with agoraphobia with alprazolam and ibuprofen: A controlled study (abstr). American Psychiatric Association Annual Meeting, Toronto, Canada, 1982.

121. Klein DF. Delineation of two drug-responsive anxiety syndromes. *Psychopharmacologia* 1964; 5:397–408.

122. Klein DF. Importance of psychiatric diagnosis in prediction of clinical drug effects. *Arch Gen Psychiatry* 1967; 16:118–126.

123. Sheehan DV, Claycomb JB, Surman OS, Gelles L, Gallo J, LeGros J. The relative efficacy of alprazolam, phenelzine and imipramine in treating panic attacks and phobias (abstr). In: *Scientific Proceedings of the 137th Annual Meeting of the American Psychiatric Association*, Los Angeles, 1984:83.

124. Solyom L, Heseltine GFD, McClure DJ, Solyom C, Ledwidge B, Steinberg G. Behavior therapy versus drug therapy in the treatment of phobic neurosis. *Can Psychiatr Assoc J* 1973; 18:25–31.

125. Tyrer P, Candy J, Kelly DA. A study of the clinical effects of phenelzine and placebo in the treatment of phobic anxiety. *Psychopharmacologia* 1973; 32:237–254.

126. Sheehan DV. Delineation of anxiety and phobic disorders responsive to monoamine oxidase inhibitors: Implications for Classification. *J Clin Psychiatry* 1984; 45(7, sec 2):29–36.

127. Blackwell B, Marley E, Price J, Taylor D. Hypertensive interaction between monoamine oxidase inhibitors and food stuffs. *Br J Psychiatry* 1967; 113:349–365.

128. Sheehan DV, Raj A. Monoamine oxidase inhibitors. In: Last CG, Hersen M, eds. *Handbook of Anxiety Disorders*. New York: Pergamon Press; 1988:478–503.

129. Sheehan DV, Sheehan HK. The role of SSRIs in panic disorder. *J Clin Psychiatry* 1996; 57(suppl 10):51–58.

130. Charney DS, Woods SW, Goodman WK, Rifkin B, Kinch M, Aiken B, et al. Drug treatment of panic disorder: The comparative efficacy of imipramine, alprazolam, and trazodone. *J Clin Psychiatry* 1986; 47:580–586.

131. Mavissakalian M, Perel J, Bowler K, Dealy R. Trazodone in the treatment of panic disorder and agoraphobia with panic attacks. *Am J Psychiatry* 1987; 144:785–787.

132. Gorman JM, Liebowitz MR, Fryer AJ. An open trial of fluoxetine in the treatment of panic attacks. *J Clin Psychopharmacol* 1987; 7:329–332.

133. Schneier FR, Liebowitz MR, Davies SO, Fairbanks J, Hollander E, Campeas R, et al. Fluoxetine in panic disorder. *J Clin Psychopharmacol* 1990; 10:119–121.

134. Westenberg HGM, Den Boer JA. Selective monoamine uptake inhibitors and a serotonin antagonist in the treatment of panic disorder. *Psychopharmacol Bull* 1989; 25:119–123.

135. Black DW, Wesner R, Bowers W, Gabel J. A comparison of fluvoxamine, cognitive therapy, and placebo in the treatment of panic disorder. *Arch Gen Psychiatry* 1993; 50:44–50.

136. Hoehn-Saric R, Mcleod DR, Hipsley PA. Effect of fluvoxamine on panic disorder. *J Clin Psychopharmacol* 1993; 13:321–326.

137. Sharp DM, Power KG, Simpson RJ, et al. Fluvoxamine, placebo and cognitive behavioral therapy used alone and in combination in the treatment of panic disorder and agoraphobia. *J Anxiety Dis* 1996; 10:219–242.

138. Den Boer JA, Westenberg HGM. Effect of a serotonin and noradrenalin uptake inhibitor in panic disorders: A double blind comparative study with fluvoxamine and maprotyline. *Int Clin Psychopharmacol* 1988; 3:59–74.

139. Den Boer JA, Van Viet IM, Westenberg HGM. A double blind comparative study of fluvoxamine and brofaramine. *Clin Neuropharmacol* 1992; 15(suppl 1 pt B):01B(abstr 65–96).

140. Dewulf L, Hendricks B, Lesaffre E. Epidemiological data of patients treated with fluvoxamine: Results from a 12 week non-comparative multicentre study. *Int Clin Psychopharmacol* 1995; 9(suppl 4):67–72.

141. Den Boer JA, Westenberg HG, Klamerbeek WD, Verhoeven WMA, Kahn RS. Effect of serotonin uptake inhibitors in anxiety disorders: A double-blind comparison of clomipramine and fluvoxamine. *Int Clin Psychopharmacol* 1987; 2:21–32.

142. Gorman J, Wolkow R. Sertraline as a treatment for panic disorder. *Neuropsychopharmacology* 1994; 10:35S–197S.

143. Dunbar G, Judge R, Morton N. Long-term evaluation of paroxetine, clomipramine and placebo in panic disorder. Poster, VIIth European College of Neuropsychopharmacology Venice, Italy, October 1995.

144. Steiner M, Bushnell WD, Gergel I, Wheadon D. Long-term evaluation of paroxetine, clomipramine and placebo in panic disorder. Presented at the 148th Annual Meeting of the American Psychiatric Association Miami, FL, May 20–25, 1995.

145. Oehrberg S, Christiansen PE, Behnke K, Borup AL, Severin B, Soegaard J, et al. Paroxetine in the treatment of panic disorder: A randomised, double-blind, placebo-controlled study. *Br J Psychiatry* 1995; 167:374–379.

146. Sheehan DV, Dunbar G (on behalf of the Panic Disorder Study Group). The treatment of panic disorder with paroxetine. In: Gotestam KG, Mindus P, Sheehan DV, eds. *Proceedings of the Second Novo Nordisk Symposium on Panic Disorder and OCD*. The Netherlands: Medical Forum International; 1996:29–38.

147. DeMartinis NA, Schweizer E, Rickels K. An open label trial of nefazodone in high comorbidity panic disorder. *J Clin Psychiatry* 1996; 57:245–248.

148. Humble M, Wistedt B. Serotonin, panic disorder and agoraphobia: Short-term and long-term efficacy of citalopram in panic disorders. *Int Clin Psychopharmacol* 1992; 6(suppl 5):21–39.

149. Sheehan DV, Davidson J, Manschreck TC, Van Wyck-Fleet J. Lack of efficacy of a new antidepressant (bupropion) in the treatment of panic disorder with phobias. *J Clin Psychopharmacol* 1983; 31(1):28–31.

150. Goldberg HL, Finnerty R. Comparison of buspirone in two separate studies. *J Clin Psychiatry* 1982; 43(12, sec 2):87–91.

151. Richels K, Weissman K, Norstad N, Singer M, Stoltz D, Brown A, et al. Buspirone and diazepam in anxiety: A controlled study. *J Clin Psychiatry* 1982; 43(12, sec 2):81–86.

152. Feighner JP. A double blind comparison of buspirone and diazepam in outpatients with generalized anxiety disorder. *J Clin Psychiatry* 1982; 43(12, sec 2):103–107.

153. Wheatley D. Buspirone: Multicenter efficacy study. *J Clin Psychiatry* 1982; 43(12, sec 2):92–94.

154. Sheehan DV, Raj BA, Sheehan KH, Soto S. Is buspirone effective for panic disorder? *J Clin Psychopharmacol* 1990; 10(1):3–11.

155. Sheehan DV, Raj BA, Harnett-Sheehan K, Soto S, Knapp E. The relative efficacy of high dose buspirone and alprazolam in the treatment of panic disorder: A double-blind placebo-controlled study. *Acta Psychiatr Scand* 1993; 88(1):1–11.

156. Noyes R Jr, Anderson DJ, Clancy J, Crowe RR, Slymen DJ, Ghoneim MM, et al. Diazepam and propranolol in panic disorder and agoraphobia. *Arch Gen Psychiatry* 1984; 41:287–292.

157. Tesar GE, Rosenbaum JF, Pollack MH, Otto MW, Sachs GS, Herman JB. Double-blind placebo-controlled comparison of clonazepam and alprazolam for panic disorder. *J Clin Psychiatry* 1991; 52(2):69–76.

158. Boyer W. Serotonin uptake inhibitors are superior to imipramine and alprazolam in alleviating panic attacks: A meta-analysis. *Int Clin Psychopharmacol* 1995; 10:99–121.

159. Sheehan DV, Claycomb JB. The use of MAO inhibitors in clinical practice. In: Manschreck TC, ed. *Psychiatric Medicine Update: Massachusetts General Hospital Review for Physicians*. New York: Elsevier; 1983:143–162.

160. Sheehan DV, Claycomb JB, Kouretas N. Monoamine oxidase inhibitors: prescription and patient management. *Int J Psychiatr Med* 1980; 10:99–121.

161. Sheehan DV. Traitement des troubles anxieue par les antidepresseurs. *Actualities Med Int Psychiatrie* (Suppl) 1986; 1:104–123.

162. Sheehan DV. Tricyclic antidepressants in the treatment of panic and anxiety disorders. *Psychosomatics* 1986; suppl 27(11):10–16.

163. Sheehan DV, Raj BA. Benzodiazepine treatment of panic disorder. In: Noyes R Jr, Roth M, Burrows GD, eds. *Handbook of Anxiety*. Vol. 4: *The Treatment of Anxiety*. Amsterdam: Elsevier; 1990:169–206.

164. Sheehan DV. Benzodiazepines in panic disorder and agoraphobia. *J Affect Dis* 1987; 13:169–181.

165. Sheehan DV, Raj BA. Panic disorder in primary care. *Primary Care Psychiatry* 1997. In press.

CHAPTER

91

ADVERSE CARDIOVASCULAR DRUG INTERACTIONS

Lionel H. Opie

The best-known cardiovascular drug interaction is that between quinidine and digitalis, whereby quinidine elevates digoxin levels. This interaction "caught the eye" of cardiologists because it involved two classic drugs that had been used in combination for many years. The knowledge of such an interaction alerted clinicians to the fact that apparently established properties of drugs could perhaps be explained more simply by drug interactions. For example, some arrhythmias thought to be caused by quinidine were probably evoked by the increased blood digoxin level.

Today a knowledge of cardiovascular drug interactions is regarded as basic to our understanding of the pharmacologic properties of cardiovascular drugs. Such interactions can be either *pharmacokinetic*, whereby one agent interferes with the metabolism of another, or *pharmacodynamic*, whereby the hemodynamic properties of one agent are additive or subtractive to those of another (Fig. 91-1). An example of pharmacokinetic interaction is the decreased rate of hepatic metabolism of lidocaine during cimetidine therapy, with possible risk of lidocaine toxicity. An example of a pharmacodynamic interaction arises when nifedipine is added to beta-adrenergic blockade in the therapy of severe angina, sometimes with excess hypotension as a side effect.

This chapter includes discussions of the drug interactions of the major classes of cardiovascular drugs, following an established sequence of these drugs (see Tables 91-1 to 91-7).[1]

BETA-ADRENERGIC BLOCKING DRUGS

Beta-adrenergic blockers demonstrate relatively few serious drug interactions (Table 91-1). An example of a pharmacokinetic interaction is that with cimetidine,[2] which reduces hepatic blood flow and therefore increases blood levels of propranolol and metoprolol, which are both metabolized in the liver (Fig. 91-2). However, there is no interaction of cimetidine with beta blockers such as atenolol, sotatol, and nadolol, which are not metabolized in the liver. Another pharmacokinetic interaction is when verapamil raises blood levels of metoprolol through a hepatic interaction[3]; presumably other beta blockers metabolized by the liver may be subject to a similar interaction.

Now used with increasing frequency in the acute phase of myocardial infarction, beta blockers may depress hepatic blood flow, thereby decreasing hepatic inactivation of lidocaine.[4] Thus beta blockade increases lidocaine blood levels with enhanced risk of toxicity. An example of a pharmacodynamic interaction is that with nonsteroidal antiinflammatory drugs (NSAIDs), including indomethacin, which may attenuate the antihypertensive effects of beta blockers, possibly by decreasing the formation of vasodilatory prostaglandins.[5] (For the interaction of beta blockers with disopyramide, see "Antiarrhythmic Agents," "Verapamil and Beta Blockers," and "Diltiazem," below; see also Chap. 54.)

NITRATES

The chief drug interactions of nitrates are pharmacodynamic (Table 91-2). For example, during triple therapy of angina pectoris (nitrates, beta blockers, calcium antagonists), the efficacy of the combination may be lessened, because each drug can predispose to excess hypotension.[6] Even two components of triple therapy, such as diltiazem and nitrates, may interact adversely to cause moderate hypotension.[7] Nonetheless high doses of diltiazem can improve persistent effort angina when added to maximum doses of propranolol and isosorbide dinitrate without any report of significant hypotension.[8] Therefore individual patients vary greatly in their susceptibility to the hypotension of triple therapy (see also Chap. 23). There is a newly reported beneficial interaction between nitrates and hydralazine whereby the latter helps to lessen nitrate tolerance.[9]

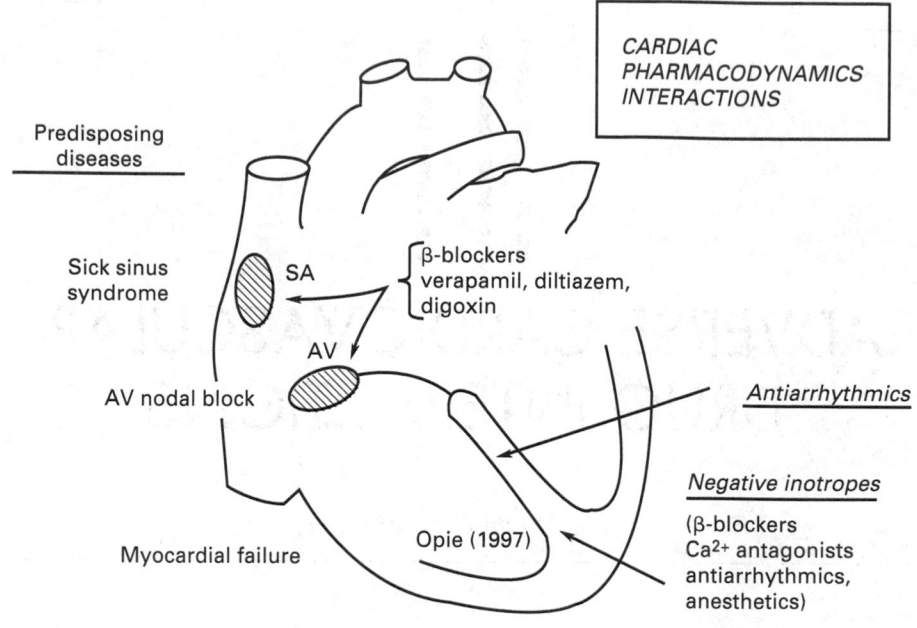

FIGURE 91-1

Cardiac pharmacodynamic interactions at the levels of the SA node, AV node, conduction system, and myocardium. The predisposing disease conditions are shown on the left. SA = sinoatrial; AV = atrioventricular. (Figure copyrighted by L. H. Opie.)

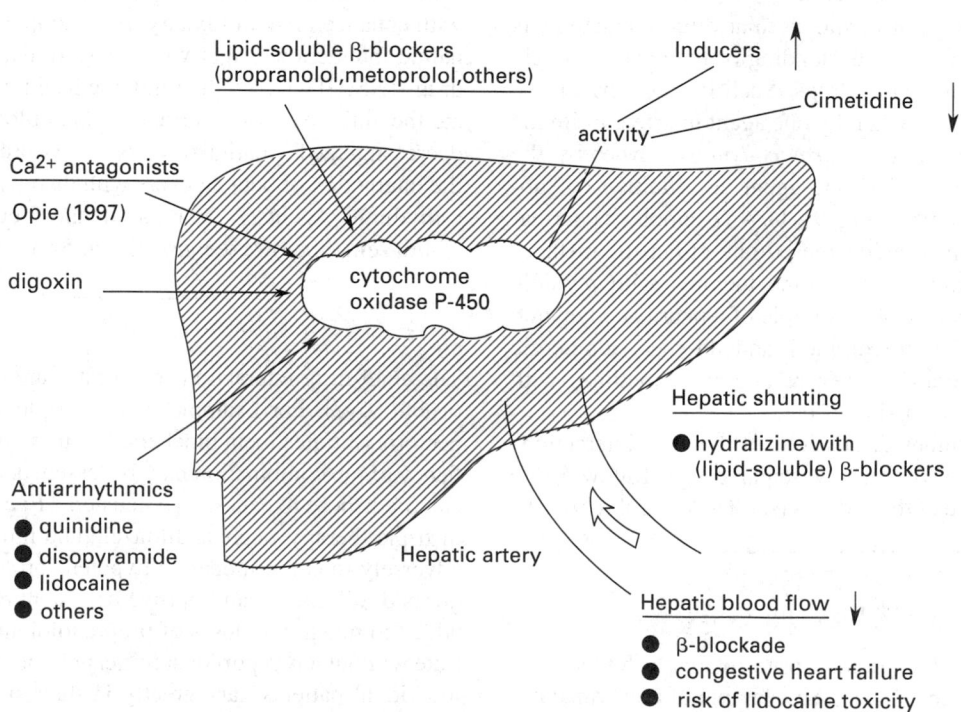

FIGURE 91-2

Potential hepatic pharmacokinetic interactions at the level of cytochrome oxidase P450 and potential pharmacodynamic interactions due to altered hepatic blood flow. (Figure copyrighted by L. H. Opie.)

TABLE 91-1

DRUG INTERACTIONS OF BETA-ADRENERGIC BLOCKING AGENTS

Cardiac Drug	Interacting Drugs	Mechanism	Consequence	Prophylaxis	Reference
HEMODYNAMIC INTERACTIONS					
All beta blockers	Calcium antagonists, especially nifedipine	Added hypotension	Risk of myocardial ischaemia	Blood pressure control, adjust doses	28
	Verapamil or diltiazem; flecainide	Added negative inotropic effect	Risk of myocardial failure Hypotension	Check for CHF, adjust doses Check LV function, flecainide levels	14
ELECTROPHYSIOLOGICAL INTERACTION					
All beta blockers	Verapamil	Added inhibition of SA, AV nodes	Bradycardia, asystole, complete heart block	Exclude "sick-sinus" syndrome, AV nodal disease, adjust dose, exclude predrug LV failure	12
	Diltiazem	Added negative inopropic effect	Excess hypotension		31
HEPATIC INTERACTION					
Propranolol (P)	Cimetidine (C)	C decreases P metabolism	Excess propranolol effects	Reduce both drug doses	3
	Lidocaine (L)	Low hepatic blood flow	Excess lidocaine effects	Reduce lidocaine dose	4
Metoprolol (M)	Verapamil (V)	V decreases M metabolism	Excess M effects	Reduce M dose	3
	Cimetidine (C)	C decreases M metabolism	Excess M effects	Reduce both drug doses	102
Labetalol (L)	Climetidine (C)	C decreases L metabolism	Excess L effects	Reduce both drug doses	103
ANTIHYPERTENSIVE INTERACTIONS					
Beta blockers	Indomethacin (I), NSAIDs	I inhibits vasodilodatory prostaglandins	Decreased antihypertensive effect	Omit indomethacin; use alternative drugs	5
IMMUNE INTERACTING DRUGS					
Acebutolol	Other drugs altering immune status: procainamide, hydralazine, captopril	Theoretical risk of additive immune effects	Theoretical risk of lupus or neutropenia	Check antinuclear factors and neutrophils; low doses during cotherapy	(-)

Abbreviations: CHF = congestive heart failure; LV = left ventricular, AV = atrioventricular; (-) = expected interaction, no reference.

CALCIUM ANTAGONISTS

Many of the interactions of calcium antagonists are pharmacodynamic (Table 91-2),[10] such as added effects on the atrioventricular (AV) or sinus nodes (verapamil or diltiazem plus beta blockers, excess digitalis, or amiodarone), or on the systemic vascular resistance (for example, nifedipine plus beta blockers causing excess hypotension). However, it is now increasingly recognized that verapamil and diltiazem (but probably not nifedipine) inhibit the hepatic oxidation of some drugs, the blood levels of which consequently increase. Such agents include cyclosporine (diltiazem), the antiepileptic carbamazepine (verapamil), prazosin (verapamil), theophylline (vera-

TABLE 91-2

DRUG INTERACTIONS OF BETA-ADRENERGIC BLOCKING AGENTS

Cardiac Drug	Interacting Drugs	Mechanism	Consequence	Prophylaxis	Reference
		HEMODYNAMIC INTERACTIONS			
All nitrates	Calcium antagonists, prazosin	Excess vasodilation	Syncope, dizziness	Monitor BP	104
	(PZ)	Excess vasodilation	Syncope, dizziness	Check BP, low initial PZ doses	
		CALCIUM ANTAGONIST DRUGS			
Verapamil (V)	Beta blockers	SA and AV nodal inhibition Myocardial failure	Added nodal and negative inotropic effects	Care during cotherapy Check ECG, BP, heart size	12
	Cimetidine	Hepatic metabolic interaction	Blood V rises	Adjust dose	64
	Digitalis poisoning	Added SA and AV nodal inhibition	Asystole; complete heart block after IV verapamil	Avoid IV verapamil in digitalis poisoning	1
	Digoxin (D)	Decreased digoxin clearance	Risk of D toxicity	Halve D dose; blood D level	21
	Disopyramide	Pharmacodynamic	Hypotension, constipation	Check BP, LV, and gut	(-)
	Flecainide (F)	Added negative inotropic effect	Hypotension	Check LV; F levels	
	Prazosin	Hepatic interaction	Excess hypotension	Check BP during cotherapy	24
	Quinidine (Q)	Added alpha-receptor inhibition; V decreases Q clearance	Hypotension; increased Q levels	Check Q levels and BP	25
	Theophylline (T)	Inhibition of hepatic metabolism	Increased blood T levels	Reduce T, check levels	27
Nifedipine (N)	Beta blockers	Added negative inotropism	Excess hypotension	Check BP, use test dose of N	28
	Cimetidine	Hepatic metabolic interaction	Increased blood N levels	Decreased N dosage by 40%	64
	Digoxin	Minor/modest changes in digoxin	Increased digoxin levels	Check D levels	105
	Prazosin (PZ)	PZ blocks alpha reflex to N	Postural hypotension	Test dose of N or PZ	30
	Propranolol (P)	N and P have opposite effects on blood liver flow	N decreases P levels; P increases N levels	Readjust P and N doses if needed	29
	Quinidine (Q)	N improves poor LV function; Q clearance faster	Decreased Q effect	Check Q levels	40
Diltiazem (D)	Beta blockers	Added SA nodal inhibition; negative inotropism	Bradycardia, hypotension	Check ECG and LV function	31
	Cimetidine	Hepatic metabolic interaction	Increased D levels	Reduce D dose by one-third	64
	Cyclosporine (C)	Hepatic metabolism of C inhibited	Increased blood C levels	Decrease C dose	32
	Digoxin (D)	Some fall in D clearance	Only in renal failure	Check D levels	64
	Flecainide (F)	Added negative inotropic effect	Hypotension	Check LV; F levels	(-)
Nicardipine (see also nifedipine)	Cyclosporine (C)	Hepatic metabolism of C inhibited	Increased blood C levels	Decrease C dose	106
	Digoxin (D)	Decreased D clearance	Blood D doubles	Decrease D, D levels	68

Abbreviations: SA = sinoatrial node; AV = atrioventricular node; LV = left ventricle; BP = blood pressure; ECG = electrocardiogram; (-) = expected interaction, no reference.

pamil), and quinidine (verapamil). In addition, nifedipine especially and also verapamil tend to increase hepatic blood flow, potentially leading to enhanced first-pass metabolism of agents such as propranolol, so that the blood levels fall (see also Chap. 54).

Verapamil (Calan, Isoptin) and Beta Blockers

Intravenous verapamil added to beta-adrenergic blockade has the additional risk of added hypotension or added nodal inhibition.[11,12] In patients with angina pectoris already receiving beta blockers, verapamil given intravenously[13] or orally[14] can reduce contractility,[14] increase heart size,[15] and cause sinus bradycardia.[16] By a hepatic pharmacokinetic interaction,[17] verapamil may raise blood levels of the beta blockers metabolized by the liver. Despite such hepatic interactions (e.g., verapamil with propranolol) in normal subjects, pharmacodynamic changes are more important.[18] The combination of verapamil and beta blockade in the therapy of angina pectoris must be used with care with preexisting depression of the sinoatrial (SA) or AV nodes and clinically detectable myocardial failure. The combination of verapamil and beta blockers improves myocardial function during exercise more than either agent alone.[19] Verapamil plus a beta blocker may have an additive therapeutic effect in hypertension, but with a small risk of excess inhibition of sinus rate, AV conduction, or left ventricular function[20] (see Chap. 58).

Other Drug Interactions with Verapamil

DIGOXIN

Verapamil can increase blood digoxin levels by over 50 percent.[21] The dose of digoxin must be cut to about half and blood levels of digoxin must then be rechecked. In digitalis toxicity, rapid intravenous verapamil is *absolutely contraindicated* because the sum of the inhibitory effects of these two agents on the AV node can be fatal. Experimentally, verapamil can inhibit the calcium-dependent delayed afterdepolarizations (DADs), which cause the ventricular automaticity found in digitalis toxicity. Oral verapamil and digitalis can, however, be combined in the absence of digitalis toxicity or AV block, because their pharmacologic sites of action are different; however, the digoxin level needs monitoring (see also Chap. 23). The combination is often used for the management of supraventricular tachycardias.

VERAPAMIL-PRAZOSIN

The combination of verapamil with prazosin for hypertension provides added and synergistic effects.[22] A hepatic pharmacokinetic interaction with enhanced bioavailability of prazosin may explain these effects.[23,24]

VERAPAMIL-QUINIDINE

Verapamil and quinidine may interact to cause excess hypotension,[25] either by combined inhibition of peripheral receptors or by increase of quinidine levels[26]; the latter may be a hepatic interaction (see Chap. 54).

VERAPAMIL-DISOPYRAMIDE

Both verapamil and disopyramide are powerful negative inotropes, so that the combination can only be given when left ventricular function is good prior to initiation of therapy and can be closely monitored.

VERAPAMIL-THEOPHYLLINE

Verapamil may inhibit the hepatic metabolism of theophylline and lead to increased blood theophylline levels.[27]

NIFEDIPINE (PROCARDIA, ADALAT)

The combination of nifedipine with beta blockade is generally well tolerated except for the risk of hypotension.[28] Nifedipine and propranolol may have a pharmacokinetic interaction whereby blood levels of propranolol are increased; it is thought that nifedipine increases the hepatic blood flow so that propranolol breakdown in the liver is lessened.[29] Although nifedipine is an afterload reducer, it also has a direct negative inotropic effect. Hence combination with beta blockers, disopyramide, or any other negative inotropic agent should be undertaken with caution. Nifedipine combined with prazosin hydrochloride may cause excess hypotension,[30] so that low initial additive doses are recommended [see "Prazosin Hydrochloride (Minipress)," below].

DILTIAZEM (CARDIZEM, TILDIEM, HERBESSER, TILAZEM)

Diltiazem, like verapamil, may increase blood digoxin levels; however, the rise is likely to be much less, and some studies report no increase at all. Diltiazem plus long-acting nitrates occasionally causes excess hypotension.[7] The combination of high-dose diltiazem with beta blockade may cause bradycardia or hypotension.[31] Relatively few life-threatening interactions have been described for diltiazem, probably because intravenous diltiazem is relatively new. However, as the application of intravenous diltiazem increases, it can be expected to produce a spectrum of drug interactions similar to that of intravenous verapamil. As diltiazem is metabolized by the liver, it interacts with cyclosporine, resulting in an increased cyclosporine blood level.[32]

ANTIARRHYTHMIC AGENTS

During antiarrhythmic therapy, numerous drug interactions are possible (Table 91-3).[33,34] Patients with serious ventricular arrhythmias frequently have associated angina (potentially necessitating calcium antagonists or beta blockers) or heart failure (requiring digitalis and diuretics). Nausea, a common symptom of patients with chronic cardiac conditions, may require cimetidine with risk of hepatic interactions (Tables 91-1, 91-3). The most frequent antiarrhythmic drug interactions are with digoxin (the levels of which increase with quinidine and verapamil), with diuretics (there is risk of QT prolongation with antiarrhythmics, such as quinidine, disopyramide, amiodarone, and sotalol, which prolong duration of the action potential), and at the level of hepatic enzyme induction (cimetidine decreases hepatic metabolism of quinidine[35]; phe-

TABLE 91-3

DRUG INTERACTIONS OF ANTIARRHYTHMIC DRUGS

Cardiac Drug	Interacting Drugs	Mechanism	Consequence	Prophylaxis	Reference
		CLASS 1A			
Quinidine (Q)	Amiodarone	Added QT effects; blood Q rises	Torsades de pointes	Check QT, potassium	43
					34
	Antibiotics (some)	Quinidine inhibits muscarinic receptors	Increased antibiotic-induced muscular weakness	Clinical care, drug levels	107
	Anticholinesterases	Quinidine inhibits muscarinic receptors	Decreased Ach efficacy in myasthenia gravis	Avoid Q if possible blood	107
	Antihypertensive agents	Added hypotensive and added SA nodal effects	Hypotension, excess bradycardia	Regulate BP Check BP, ECG	(-) 108
	Beta blockers				
	Cimetidine (C)	C inhibits oxidative metabolism of Q	Increased Q levels, risk of toxicity	Q levels, consider ranitidine	35 40
	Coumarin anticoagulants	Hepatic interaction with Q	Bleeding	Check prothrombin time	37
	Digoxin (D)	Decreased D clearance	Risk of D toxicity	Check D dose levels	36
	Diltiazem	Added inhibition of SA node	Excess bradycardia	Check ECG, heart rate	31
	Disopyramide	Added QT prolongation	Torsades de pointes	Check QT, potassium	43
	Diuretic, potassium losing	Hypokalemia and QT prolongation	Torsades de pointes	Check QT, potassium	109
	Hepatic enzyme inducers (phenytoin, barbiturates, rifampin)	Increased Q hepatic metabolism	Decreased Q levels	Q levels, doses	38
	Nifedipine	Increased Q clearance	Decreased Q levels	Q levels, doses	110 42
	Sotalol	Added QT prolongation	Torsades de pointes	Check QT, potassium	76
	Verapamil	Decreased Q clearance	Excess bradycardia	Check ECG, Q levels	25
	Warafin	Hepatic interaction with Q	Bleeding	Check prothrombin time	37
Procainamide (P)	Captopril	Combined immune effects	Theoretical risk of neutropenia	Cotherapy with care	(-)
	Cimetidine	Decreased renal P clearance	Prolonged P half-life, excess P effect	Reduce P dose; consider ranitidine	44
Disopyramide (D)	Agents prolonging APD (quinidine, amiodarone, sotalol)	Added QT prolongation especially if hypokalemia	Torsades de pointes	Check QT, potassium	1
	Beta blockers	Combined negative inotropism	Hypotension	Low doses	(-)
	Cimetidine	Hepatic D metabolism falls	Increased blood D levels		(-)
	Digitalis toxicity	Added SA, AV nodal depression	SA, AV block	Avoid D in digitalis toxicity	(-)
	Hepatic enzyme inducers (phenytoin, rifampin, barbiturates)	Enhanced D hepatic metabolism	Blood D levels fall; readjust D dose	Readjust D dose	46

(Continued)

TABLE 91-3 *(Continued)*
DRUG INTERACTIONS OF ANTIARRHYTHMIC DRUGS

Cardiac Drug	Interacting Drugs	Mechanism	Consequence	Prophylaxis	Reference
		CLASS 1A			
	Drugs inhibiting SA or AV nodes/ conduction system (quinidine, β blockers, methyldopa, digoxin)	Pharmacodynamic additive effects	SA, AV block; conduction block	Check ECG; decrease doses	(-)
	Pyridostigmine	Inhibition of cholinesterase activity	Beneficial effect of P on D; harmful effect of D on P	In myasthenia gravis, avoid D	47
		CLASS 1B			
Lidocaine (lignocaine)	Verapamil	Combined negative inotropism	Hypotension	Avoid IV D or V cotherapy	45
	Cimetidine (C)	Decreased hepatic metabolism	Increased L levels	Decrease L infusion rate	48
	Halothane	Decreased hepatic bood flow	Increased L levels	Decrease L infusion rate	49
	Propranolol	Decreased hepatic blood flow	Increased 1 levels	Decrease L infusion rate	4
	Other beta blockers	Decreased hepatic blood flow	Increased L levels	Decrease L infusion rate	111
Mexiletine	Hepatic enzyme inducers (phenytoin, barbiturates, rifampin)	Increased hepatic metabolism	Decreased plasma M levels	Increase M dose	(-)
		CLASS IC			
Flecainide (F)	Amiodarone	Unknown	Blood F rises; added effect on nodes, myocardium	Decrease F dose	58
	Digoxin (D)	Decreased D clearance	Blood D rises slightly	Check D level	57
	Drugs inhibiting SA or AV nodes, IV conduction or myocardial function	Pharmacodynamic, additive	SA, AV block; conduction block, cardiogenic shock	Avoid combinations Decrease doses	112
	Cimetidine	Decreased hepatic F loss	Blood F rises	Check F dose	59
Propafenone	Digoxin	Pharmacokinetic	Increased D level	Decrease D dose	60
		CLASS III			
Amiodarone (A)	Drugs prolonging QT interval (quinidine, disopyramide, phenothiazines, tricyclic antidepressants, thiazide diuretics, sotalol)	Pharmacodynamic additive effects	Torsades de pointes	Avoid low K^+; avoid combinations	43
	Quinidine (Q)	Pharmacokinetic	Blood O rises	Check Q levels	34
	Procainamide (P)	Pharmacokinetic	Blood P rises	Check P dose	34
Sotalol	(P) as above	Hypokalemia plus class III action	Torsades de pointes	Exclude low K^+; use K^+-retaining diuretic	76

Abbreviations: APD = action potential duration; IV = intravenous; Ach = acetylcholine; (-) = expected interaction, no reference.

nytoin and barbiturates have an opposite effect). There is also the risk of antiarrhythmic drug-drug interactions. Thus, amiodarone when added to quinidine enhances the risk of QT prolongation while quinidine levels increase, so that quinidine toxicity is also more likely[34] (see also Chap. 30). The combination of arrhythmic drugs, like amiodarone and beta blockers, can also lead to life-threatening bradycardia.

Quinidine

Because quinidine increases blood digoxin levels, the dose of quinidine must be decreased and blood digoxin levels checked.[36] Quinidine may enhance the effects of other hypotensive agents, including verapamil,[25] or of agents inhibiting the sinus node (beta blockers, verapamil, diltiazem, and methyldopa). Quinidine increases the effects of coumarin anticoagulants by a hepatic interaction.[37] When hepatic enzymes are induced by drugs such as phenytoin, phenobarbital, and rifampin (rifampicin), the hepatic metabolism of quinidine may markedly increase with decreased steady-state concentrations of quinidine.[38,39] Conversely, cimetidine can inhibit hepatic enzymes to decrease the metabolism of quinidine with opposite effects. It appears that ranitidine has no such effects.[40] Verapamil may increase quinidine levels. Conversely, nifedipine may lower plasma quinidine levels, probably by improving left ventricular systolic function.[40–42]

Hypokalemia decreases the antiarrhythmic effect of quinidine and predisposes to QT prolongation by quinidine. When quinidine is combined with other drugs that also prolong the QT interval, such as amiodarone, sotalol, or thiazide diuretics, careful monitoring of the QT interval is required.[43]

Quinidine is a vagolytic drug and reduces the effects of procedures that enhance vagal activity, such as carotid sinus massage. Quinidine also inhibits muscarinic receptors to reduce the effects of anticholinesterases in myasthenia gravis (see also Chap. 27).

Procainamide (Pronestyl)

Cimetidine inhibits the renal clearance of procainamide. The elimination half-life lengthens, so that the dose of procainamide needs reduction.[44]

Disopyramide (Norpace)

Disopyramide is negatively inotropic, so that there is a potential danger of reduction of the cardiac output in patients already receiving other negative inotropes, such as the calcium antagonists—verapamil,[45] beta blockers, or flecainide—and in patients with preexisting myocardial failure. It is also potentially dangerous to combine disopyramide with other drugs likely to depress nodal or conduction tissues, such as quinidine, digoxin, beta blockers, and methyldopa. Disopyramide is ineffective in digitalis toxicity and should be avoided. There is no interaction between disopyramide and lidocaine. The concomitant use of disopyramide with other type I antiarrhythmic agents or beta blockers should be reserved for life-threatening arrhythmias because of risk of bradycardia and hypoten-

sion. The risk of QT prolongation requires that disopyramide not be combined with other drugs prolonging the QT interval, such as the tricyclics, and certain other antiarrhythmic agents, such as amiodarone or sotalol. Phenytoin[46] and other inducers of hepatic enzymes (barbiturates, rifampin) may lower disopyramide plasma levels. Pyridostigmine bromide may interact beneficially with disopyramide by inhibiting cholinesterase activity, so that anticholinergic side effects of disopyramide are reduced.[47]

Lidocaine (Xylocaine, Lignocaine)

In patients receiving cimetidine,[48] propranolol,[4] or halothane,[49] the hepatic clearance of lidocaine is reduced, so that toxicity may occur more readily. Lidocaine may cause sinoatrial arrest, especially during coadministration of other agents potentially depressing nodal function,[50] including beta blockers.

Tocainide (Tonocard)

There are presently no known adverse drug interactions involving tocainide.

Mexiletine (Mexitil)

Narcotics delay the gastrointestinal absorption of mexiletine. Rifampin (rifampicin), barbiturates, and phenytoin all induce hepatic enzymes so that the plasma levels of mexiletine are reduced. Cimetidine should but does not increase plasma levels of mexiletine.[51] Rather, cimetidine has a beneficial side effect of decreasing the gastrointestinal symptoms associated with mexiletine. Disopyramide and mexiletine given together may predispose to a negative inotropic effect.[52] Mexiletine may, however, be combined with quinidine,[53,54] beta-adrenergic blockers,[55] and amiodarone[56] provided that the appropriate contraindications for each drug are observed and the patient is closely monitored for heart failure.

Flecainide (Tambocor)

Flecainide inhibits the sinus and AV nodal function so that its combination with beta blockers, verapamil, diltiazem, and digitalis can cause bradycardia and requires care. Flecainide also has additive negative inotropic effects that may exaggerate those of beta blockers,[57] verapamil, or disopyramide. Combined inhibitory effects on His-Purkinje conduction may arise during cotherapy with quinidine or procainamide and to a lesser extent with disopyramide. Flecainide blood levels are increased by amiodarone; when both of these drugs are used, the flecainide dose should be decreased by about one-third.[58] Studies of healthy volunteers suggest that (1) cimetidine delays the clearance of flecainide[59] and (2) flecainide increases blood digoxin levels.[57]

Propafenone (Rythmol, Arytmol, Rytmonorm)

Propafenone is a class IC antiarrhythmic drug; therefore it may interact adversely with other drugs, depressing nodal function, intraventricular conduction, or the inotropic state. Nonetheless, propafenone can be combined with quinidine or procainamide at reduced doses of both drugs.[51] Propafenone substantially increases serum digoxin levels.[60]

Amiodarone (Cordarone)

The most serious interaction of amiodarone[43] is the potential for an additive proarrhythmic effect with other drugs that prolong the QT interval, such as class IA antiarrhythmic agents, sotalol, phenothiazines, tricyclic antidepressants, and thiazide diuretics. Amiodarone does not normally depress the sinus node, yet it may do so when it is combined with calcium antagonists such as verapamil or diltiazem.[10] In patients receiving warfarin, amiodarone further prolongs the prothrombin time and if not monitored closely can lead to excessive bleeding.[61] Amiodarone may double digoxin levels (Table 91-4).

Sotalol (Sotacor), Betapace

Cotherapy with any other agents that may cause hypokalemia (such as diuretics) or prolong the action potential duration (such as quinidine, disopyramide, amiodarone, tricyclic antidepressants, or probucol) may precipitate torsades de pointes.

Bretylium (Bretylol)

Experimentally, bretylium may worsen digitalis-induced ventricular tachycardia.[62] Nonetheless, the drug may be lifesaving for patients with ventricular fibrillation thought to be induced by digitalis.[63]

POSITIVE INOTROPIC AGENTS (Table 91-4)

Digoxin

The *quinidine-digoxin* interaction is best known. Quinidine approximately doubles the blood digoxin levels, decreasing both renal and extrarenal clearance.[21,36,64] The previous dose of digoxin should be halved and the plasma digoxin rechecked. Quinine given for muscle cramps acts likewise.

The *verapamil-digoxin* interaction is equally significant; digoxin levels increase by 60 to 90 percent.[21,65] The *other calcium antagonists*, nifedipine and diltiazem, increase digoxin levels much less than verapamil.[64,66,67] Adjustment of the digoxin dose with these agents is usually not necessary except in the presence of renal failure (which decreases digoxin excretion). *Nicardipine* causes only a modest rise of digoxin levels.[68] *Nitrendipine*, however, resembles verapamil in approximately doubling the digoxin levels.[68] Thus, there are no simple rules to explain which class of calcium antagonists or which specific agent is likely to increase digoxin levels significantly.

Among other vasodilators, *prazosin* increases digoxin levels in dogs by reduction of plasma and tissue binding.[69] Among antiarrhythmics other than quinidine or verapamil,

amiodarone and *propafenone*[60] also elevate serum digoxin levels. Other antiarrhythmics, including procainamide and mexiletine, have no interaction with digoxin except for a relatively small rise of digoxin levels with flecainide.[57]

When cotherapy elevates digoxin levels, the features of digitalis toxicity may depend on the agent added. With quinidine, tachyarrhythmias becomes more likely; amiodarone and verapamil seem to repress the ventricular arrhythmias of digitalis toxicity, so that bradycardia and AV block are more likely.[70]

Diuretics may indirectly precipitate digitalis toxicity by causing hypokalemia, which, when really severe (plasma potassium below 2 to 3 meq/L), may stop the tubular secretion of digoxin. Potassium-sparing diuretics (amiloride, triamterene, and spironolactone)[71] as well as captopril decrease digoxin clearance by about 20 to 30 percent and may also elevate serum K^+ levels. When these combinations with digoxin are used in the therapy of congestive heart failure, the blood digoxin level must be watched. Unexpectedly, spironolactone and its metabolite canrenone may decrease features of digitalis toxicity,[72] probably through increased K^+ levels resulting from aldosterone inhibition. Nonetheless the combination digoxin-quinidine-spironolactone markedly elevates digoxin levels.[73]

The *gastrointestinal absorption* of digoxin may be decreased by cholestyramine, probably because of the binding of digoxin to the resin; digoxin should therefore be given several hours before the resin or else digoxin capsules may be used (Lanoxicaps; 0.2 mg = 0.25 mg of digoxin). Digoxin capsules also decrease interaction with kaolin-pectate, which reduces digoxin absorption, and with erythromycin and tetracycline, which inhibit gastrointestinal flora that inactivate digoxin and thereby increase digoxin blood levels. Cancer chemotherapeutic agents may damage intestinal mucosa to depress digoxin absorption (see Chap. 23).

SYMPATHOMIMETIC AGENTS

Dopamine (Intropin)

Dopamine is contraindicated during the use of cyclopropane or halogenated hydrocarbon anesthetics (enhanced risk of arrhythmias). Monoamine-oxidase inhibitors decrease the rate of dopamine metabolism by the tissues; the dose of dopamine should therefore be cut to one-tenth of usual.

Dobutamine (Dobutrex)

Dobutamine decreases plasma potassium and should be given with care together with diuretics, especially intravenous furosemide.

Amrinone (Inocor) and Milrinone (Primacor)

Amrinone and milrinone are phosphodiesterase inhibitors that can also provoke arrhythmias. During diuretic therapy, plasma K needs monitoring. When these drugs are combined with

TABLE 91-4

DRUG INTERACTIONS OF DIGITALIS AND OTHER POSITIVE INOTROPIC AGENTS

Cardiac Drug	Interacting Drugs	Mechanism	Consequence	Prophylaxis	Reference
POSITIVE INOTROPIC AGENTS					
Digitoxin	Verapamil	Nonrenal clearance of digitoxin falls	Digitoxin levels up by one-third	Check digitoxin levels	113
	Other drugs interacting with digoxin	? Altered digitoxin clearance	? Digitoxin levels increase	Check digitoxin levels	
Digoxin (D)	Amiodarone	Reduced renal clearance of D	D level may double	Check D level; halve dose	70
	Captopril	Reduced D clearance	Blood D increases	Check D dose	114
	Diltiazem	Variable decrease of D clearance	Variable blood D increases	Check D level	66
	Diuretics; potassium-sparing amiloride/ triamterene, spironolactone (S)	Reduced extrarenal D clearance S reduces renal D clearance	D levels up by 20% D levels increase	Check D level Complex effects; check D levels	72
	Nifedipine	Variable fall of D clearance	Variable blood D rises	Check D levels	64
	Nitrendipine	Reduced D clearance	Blood D doubles	Check D levels; halve dose	68
	Prazosin (PZ)	PZ displaces D from binding sites	Blood D rises	(Needs confirmation in humans)	69
	Propafenone	Not defined	D level increases	Check D level	60
	Quinidine, quinine	Reduced D clearance	Blood D doubles	Check D levels, halve dose	36
	Verapamil	Reduced D clearance	Blood D doubles or more	Check D levels; halve dose	21
Sympathomimetic Inotropes					
Dobutamine Amrinone Milrinone	Thiazide diuretics	Additive hypokalemic effects	Arrhythmias	Check blood potassium	(-)[a]

[a] (-) = expected interaction, no reference.

digitalis, the digoxin level does not change, but digoxin toxicity should be guarded against because of multiple mechanisms for arrhythmia development (see also Chap. 23).

DIURETICS

(Table 91-5)

Loop Diuretics

Loop diuretics given acutely and intravenously may cause hypokalemia, precipitating digitalis toxicity.[74] Furosemide decreases renal clearance of lithium. Certain NSAIDs may antagonize the action of furosemide (and other diuretics). In normal subjects, concurrent captopril therapy lessens the diuretic effect of furosemide (see also Chap. 24).

Thiazide Diuretics

Steroids, estrogens, and indomethacin and other NSAIDs lessen the antihypertensive effect of thiazide diuretics and may worsen congestive heart failure.[75] *Captopril* (Capoten) tends to be potassium-retaining and may cause hyperkalemia if combined with other potassium retainers. Diuretic-induced hypokalemia may predispose to ventricular arrhythmias including torsades de pointes; when that happens, usually an antiarrhythmic agent such as sotalol,[76] quinidine, or amiodarone (all of which may prolong the QT interval) is being used. *Probenecid* interferes with the urinary excretion of thiazide and loop diuretics, so that diuretic efficacy is reduced. Diuretics may impair the renal clearance of *lithium* so that the blood level rises with risk of lithium toxicity.[77]

TABLE 91-5

DRUG INTERACTIONS OF DIURETICS

Cardiac Drug	Interacting Drugs	Mechanism	Consequence	Prophylaxis	Reference
Diuretic loop and thiazide	Indomethacin and other NSAIDs	Pharmacodynamic	Decreased antihypertensive effect	Adjust diuretic dose or add another agent	5
	Probenecid	Decreased intratubular secretion of diuretic	Decreased diuretic effect	Increase diuretic dose	74
	ACE[a] inhibitors	Excess diuretics, high renins	Excess hypotension; prerenal uremia	Lower diuretic dose; test dose ACE inhibitor	95
Loop	Captopril	Possible interference with tubular secretion	Loss of diuretic efficacy of furoscmide	Change to another ACE inhibitor	98

[a] ACE = angiotensin-converting enzyme.

VASODILATORS

(Table 91-6)

Nitroprusside (Nipride) and Hydralazine (Apresoline)

Nitroprusside and hydralazine may decrease digoxin levels, possibly as a result of increased tubular excretion, by improving congestive heart failure, renal plasma flow, and renal excretion of digoxin[78] (see also Chap. 23). Hydralazine, by creating hepatic shunts, may substantially increase the blood levels of those beta blockers that undergo hepatic metabolism, such as propranolol and metoprolol.[79] Hydralazine interacts beneficially with nitrates, helping to lessen nitrate tolerance.[9]

Prazosin (Minipress)

DOXAZOSIN AND TERAZOSIN
There is an interaction between prazosin and the calcium antagonists verapamil and nifedipine, resulting in excessive hypotension. In the case of verapamil, part of the effect may be explained by a pharmacokinetic hepatic interaction. Both nitrates and prazosin may cause syncope, and these agents should be combined with care. Experimentally, prazosin may increase the plasma digoxin level. Similar interactions may hold for the other agents in this group.

ANGIOTENSIN-CONVERTING ENZYME INHIBITORS

In general, angiotensin-converting enzyme (ACE) inhibitors have few drug interactions.[80] The most common one is with diuretics, with risk of excess hypotension in overdiuresed patients. The K^+-retaining diuretics or K^+ supplements together with captopril can cause hyperkalemia. Indomethacin and NSAIDs may decrease the antihypertensive effects of ACE inhibitors (and almost all antihypertensives except for nifedipine, Ref. 88), and diminish the benefits of ACE inhibitors in heart failure[81] (see also Chaps. 23 and 58). Aspirin may diminish the benefit of ACE inhibitors in heart failure (Table 91-6).

Captopril (Capoten, Lopirin, Lopril)

Cotherapy of high-dose captopril with other drugs that alter or impair the immune status (such as hydralazine and procainamide) may predispose to neutropenia. Probenecid inhibits the renal tubular excretion of captopril, thereby increasing blood captopril levels[82]; doses of captopril may need downward adjustment. Captopril may decrease digoxin clearance by 20 to 30 percent.[71]

Enalapril (Vasotec, Xanef, Innovace, Renitec, Renivace)

Drug interactions are similar to those of captopril, except that the risk of neutropenia is less. It must be considered that enalapril has a longer duration of action; adverse hypotensive interactions with diuretics are therefore potentially more serious.

ANTITHROMBOTIC AND THROMBOLYTIC AGENTS (Table 91-7)

Aspirin

Blood levels of uric acid may be increased by both aspirin and thiazide diuretics, so that special care is required in patients with a history of gout.[83] Conversely, aspirin may decrease the uricosuric effects of sulfinpyrazone and probenecid. Aspirin also reduces the natriuretic effect of spironolactone. Aspirin-induced gastrointestinal bleeding may be a greater

TABLE 91-6

DRUG INTERACTIONS OF VASODILATORS AND ANGIOTENSIN CONVERTING ENZYME INHIBITORS

Cardiac Drug	Interacting Drugs	Mechanism	Consequence	Prophylaxis	Reference
VASODILATORS					
Hydralazine	Beta blockers (BB) (hepatic metabolized)	Hepatic shunting	BB metabolism ↓ Blood levels ↑	Propranolol, metoprolol dose ↓ (beneficial)	79
Hydralazine	Nitrates (N)	Renal blood flow ↑	Less N tolerance		9
Hydralazine/ nitroprusside	Digoxin (D)	Increased renal D excretion	Decreased D levels	Check D levels	78
Prazosin (P)	Nifedipine (Nif)	Pharmacodynamic	Excess hypotension	Test dose of Nif	30
	Nitrates	Pharmacodynamic	Syncope, hypotension	Decrease P dose	24
	Verapamil	Hepatic metabolism	Synergistic antihypertensive effect	Adjust doses	24
ANGIOTENSIN CONVERTING ENZYME INHIBITORS (ACEI)					
ACEI (class effect)	Diuretics	High renin levels in overdiuresed patients	"First" dose hypotension; risk of renal failure	Low test dose	95
ACEI (class effect)	Potassium-sparing diuretics	Added potassium retention	Hyperkalemia	Avoid combination	96
ACEI (class effect)	Indomethacin	Less vasodilation	Less BP↓; less antifailure effects	Avoid if possible	97 81
ACEI (class effect ?)	Aspirin	Less vasodilation	Less antifailure effects	Low dose aspirin	Unpublished SOLVD data
Captopril	Loop diuretic	Possible interference with tubular secretion	Lessened diuretic effect of furosomide	Consider alternate ACE inhibitor drug	98
Captopril (C)	Immunosuppressive drugs, procainamide, hydralazine, possibly acebutolol	Added immune effects	Increased risk of neutropenia	Avoid combination; check neutrophils	99
	Probenecid (P)	P inhibits tubular secretion of C	Small risk in C levels	Decrease dose of C	82

hazard in patients receiving other NSAIDs or corticosteroid therapy. Antacids, by altering the pH of the stomach, may decrease the efficacy of enteric-coated preparations.

Hepatic enzyme inducers (barbiturates, phenytoin, rifampicin) increase aspirin breakdown. Aspirin tends to cause hypoglycemia in patients receiving oral hypoglycemics or insulin. Aspirin, especially in high doses, may exaggerate a bleeding tendency and anticoagulant-induced bleeding.[84] The dipyridamole-warfarin combination causes less bleeding than the aspirin-warfarin combination in patients who have undergone bypass surgery.[85] All these drug interactions should be less intense if the aspirin doses are kept low, as is the current trend (see also Chap. 52).

Sulfinpyrazone (Anturane)

Sulfinpyrazone is highly bound to plasma proteins (98 to 99 percent) and may displace warfarin to precipitate bleeding.

Like aspirin, sulfinpyrazone may sensitize patients who are given sulfonylureas and insulin to hypoglycemia.

Dipyridamole (Persantine)

Dipyridamole is a potent vasodilator, so that care is required when it is used in combination with other vasodilators.

Warfarin (Coumadin)

Warfarin may be subject to many (up to 80) drug interactions.[86] A good rule is to suspect interactions unless one can be sure. The safest rule is to tell patients having oral anticoagulation not to use any new or over-the-counter drugs without consultation and for the physician to carefully check out any added compounds. More frequent measurements of the prothrombin time and dose adjustments are required when potentially interfering drugs are added.

TABLE 91-7

DRUG INTERACTIONS OF ANTITHROMBOTIC AGENTS

Cardiac Drug	Interacting Drugs	Mechanism	Consequence	Prophylaxis	Reference
Aspirin (A)	ACE inhibitors	Vasodilation ↓	Less antifailure effect	Very low A dose	Table 91-6
	Hepatic enzyme inducers (barbiturates, phenytoin, rifampin)	Increased A metabolism	Decreased A effect	Adjust A dose; check A side effects	(-)
	Sulfinpyrazone (S), probenecid (P)	A decreases urate excretion	Decreased uricosuric effect of S or P	Increase dose of S or P	83
	Thiazide diuretics	A decreases urate excretion	Hyperuricemia	Check blood urate	83
	Warfarin (W)	A is antithrombotic	Excess bleeding	Check INR or prothrombin	87
Sulfinpyrazone (S)	Warfarin	S displaces W from plasma proteins	Excess bleeding	Check INR or prothrombin	115
Warfarin (W)	Potentiating drugs				
	Allopurinol	Mechanism unknown	Excess bleeding	Check INR or prothrombin	86
	Amiodarone	Mechanism unknown	Sensitizes to W for months	Avoid combination	61
	Aspirin	Added bleeding tendency	Excess bleeding	Check INR or prothrombin	87
	Cimetidine	Decreased W degradation	Excess bleeding	Check INR or prothrombin	
	Quinidine	Hepatic interaction	Excess bleeding	Check INR or prothrombin	37
	Statins	Hepatic interaction ?	Excess bleeding	Check INR or prothrombin	116
	Sulfinpyrazone	Displaces W from plasma proteins	Excess bleeding	Check INR or prothrombin	115
	Inhibitory drugs	Decrease absorption of W	Decreased W effect	Check INR or prothrombin	86
	Cholestyramine, colestipol				
Alteplase, tPA	Nitrates	Decreased tPA effect	Less thrombolytic benefit	Avoid ?increase tPA dose	89

Abbreviations: (-) = expected interaction, no reference; INR = International Normalized Ratio; prothrombin = prothrombin time.

INTERFERING DRUGS

Interfering drugs include those that reduce absorption of vitamin K, warfarin (cholestyramine), or sulfinpyrazone and those that induce hepatic enzymes (barbiturates, phenytoin, rifampicin). The latter drugs increase the rate of warfarin metabolism in the liver (see also Chap. 52).

POTENTIATING DRUGS

Other drugs decrease warfarin degradation to increase the anticoagulant effect, including a variety of antibiotics such as metronidazole (Flagyl) and co-trimoxazole (Bactrim). Cimetidine likewise inhibits hepatic degradation; rantidine

should not. Other potentiating drugs include the cardiovascular agents allopurinol, clofibrate, quinidine,[37] and amiodarone.[61] Amiodarone is especially dangerous because of its excessively long half-life, so that this interaction can occur even after withdrawal of amiodarone. Drugs such as heparin also potentiate the risk of bleeding; there are large interindividual variations.[87] Very high doses of aspirin (six to eight tablets per day) may act differently by impairing synthesis of clotting factors. It must be restressed that sulfinpyrazone powerfully displaces warfarin from blood proteins, so that the dose of warfarin may have to be reduced to only 1 mg in some patients (see also Chap. 52).

Heparin

Physically, heparin is incompatible in a water solution with certain substances, including antibiotics, antihistamines, phenothiazines, and hydrocortisone. However, direct pharmacokinetic or pharmacodynamic drug interactions have not been described except for a controversial interaction with nitrates.[88]

Tissue-Type Plasminogen Activator

Concurrent use of intravenous nitroglycerin diminishes the efficacy of recombinant tissue-type plasminogen activator (tPA, or alteplas) possibly because of increased hepatic blood flow and enhanced catabolism of tPA.[89]

LIPID-LOWERING AGENTS (Table 91-8)

There are not many serious interactions. A number of lipid-lowering agents may interact with warfarin, either by decreased absorption (cholestyramine) or by hepatic interference (clofibrate, bezafibrate, gemfibrozil). The exact mechanism is not clear. Clofibrate, gemfibrozil, and statins all increase the effects of warfarin.

Probucol, in the presence of additional agents such as thiazide diuretics or group IA or III antiarrhythmics, may prolong the QT interval and theoretically precipitate torsades de pointes. The HMG-CoA reductase inhibitors such as lovastatin (Mevacor), simvastatin (Zocor), pravastatin (Prava-

chol), and fluvastatin should ideally not be combined with the fibrates because of the higher risk of myositis with rhabdomyolysis and possible renal failure. Likewise, concurrent therapy with niacin or cyclosporine or erythromycin may also carry a small risk of rhabdomyolysis. Adding an antifungal azole (a group that includes ketoconazole, used in transplantation) has precipitated myolysis in a patient already receiving a statin and niacin.[90] Yet in clinical practice, the advantages of better lipid control with combined therapy seems to outweigh these risks. Furthermore, a positive interaction of pravastatin with cyclosporine is reported, whereby there appears to be increased immunosuppression.[91] Serum creatine kinase levels should be checked periodically, especially after increasing doses or after starting combination therapy (see also Chap. 53).

ANTIHYPERTENSIVE DRUGS

Interactions for diuretics, beta-adrenergic blockers, calcium antagonists, ACE inhibitors, and alpha$_1$-adrenergic blockers have already been considered. In general, NSAIDs interfere severely with antihypertensive efficacy of all antihypertensives.[92] An exception is nifedipine (and, presumably, other dihydropyridines).[93] Unlike other NSAIDs, aspirin[5] and sulindac may give relative protection from the negative interaction.[92] When calcium antagonists are used as antihypertensives, part of their effect is by natriuresis, so that adding a diuretic is often relatively ineffective[94] (see also Chaps. 23 and 58).

TABLE 91-8

DRUG INTERACTIONS OF LIPID-LOWERING AGENTS

Cardiac Drug	Interacting Drugs	Mechanism	Consequence	Prophylaxis	Reference
Probucol	Thiazides, groups Ia and III, antiarrhythmics	Probucol-induced diarrhea with potassium loss?	QT prolongation	Check potassium; avoid combinations	100
Fibric acids (gemfibrozil, clofibrate, bezafibrate, fenofibrate)	Warfarin	Hepatic interference	Risk of bleeding	Check prothrombin time	86
Bile acid sequestrants (cholestyramine, colestipol)	Warfarin (W)	Decreased absorption	Decreased W effect	Check prothrombin time	86
HMG-CoA reductase inhibitors (statins) (lovastatin, simvastatin, pravastatin)	Fibrates, cyclosporine, erythromycin, nicotinic acid, antifungal azoles	Added damage to muscle with myositis	Rhabdomyolysis and risk of renal failure	Check creatine phosphokinase levels	90, 101
Statins	Warfarin	Hepatic interaction	Increased risk of bleeding	Check INR or prothrombin	(Table 91-7)
Pravastatin	Cyclosporine	?Hepatic interaction	Enhanced immunosuppression	(beneficial)	91

REFERENCES

1. Opie LH, In: Opie LH, ed. *Drugs for the Heart*. Philadelphia, Saunders. 4th ed. 1995:1–377.

2. Kirch W, Spahn H, Kohler H, Mutschler E. Influence of β-receptor antagonists on pharmacokinetics of cimetidine. *Drugs* 1983; 25(suppl 2):127–130.

3. McLean AJ, Knight R, Harrison PM, Harper RW. Clearance-based oral drug interaction between verapamil and metoprolol and comparison with atenolol. *Am J Cardiol* 1985; 55:1628–1629.

4. Ochs HR, Carstens G, Greenblatt DJ. Reduction in lidocaine clearance during continuous infusion and by coadministration of propranolol. *N Engl J Med* 1980; 303:373–377.

5. Webster J. Interactions of NSAIDs with diuretics and β-blockers: Mechanism and clinical implications. *Drugs* 1985; 30:32–41.

6. Tolins M, Weir K, Chesler E, Pierpont GL. "Maximal" drug therapy is not necessarily optimal in chronic angina pectoris. *J Am Coll Cardiol* 1984; 3:1051–1057.

7. Bruce RA, Hossack KF, Kusumi F, Day B, Kannagi T. Excessive reduction in peripheral resistance during exercise and risk of orthostatic symptoms with sustained-release nitroglycerin and diltiazem treatment of angina. *Am Heart J* 1985; 109:1020–1026.

8. Boden WE, Bough EW, Reichman MJ, Rich VB, Young PM, Korr KS. Beneficial effects of high-dose diltiazem in patients with persistent effort angina on β-blockers and nitrates: A randomized, double-blind, placebo-controlled, cross-over study. *Circulation* 1985; 71:1197–1205.

9. Gogia H, Mehra A, Parikh S, Raman M, Ajit-Uppal J, Johnson JV, et al. Prevention of tolerance to hemodynamic effects of nitrates with concomitant use of hydralazine in patients with chronic heart failure. *J Am Cardiol* 1995; 26:1575–1580.

10. Reicher-Reiss H, Neufeld HN, Ebner FX. Calcium antagonists—Adverse drug interactions. *Cardiovasc Drug Ther* 1987; 1:403–409.

11. Yeh R, Gulamhusein SS, Klein GJ. Combined verapamil and propranolol for supraventricular tachycardia. *Am J Cardiol* 1984; 53:757–763.

12. Ellrodt AG, Ault MJ, Riedinger MS, Murati GH. Efficacy and safety of sublingual nifedipine in hypertensive emergencies. *Am J Med* 1985; 79(suppl 4A):19–25.

13. Kieval J, Kirsten EB, Kessler KM, Mallon SM, Myerburg RJ. The effects of intravenous verapamil on hemodynamic status of patients with coronary artery disease receiving propranolol. *Circulation* 1982; 65:653–659.

14. Packer M, Meller J, Medina N, Yushak M, Smith H, Holt J. Hemodynamic consequences of combined beta-adrenergic and slow calcium channel blockade in man. *Circulation* 1982; 65:660–668.

15. Johnston DL, Lesoway R, Humen DP, Kostuk WJ. Clinical and hemodynamic evaluation of propranolol in combination with verapamil, nifedipine and diltiazem in exertional angina pectoris: A placebo-controlled, double-blind, randomized, cross-over study. *Am J Cardiol* 1985; 55:680–687.

16. Winniford MD, Fulton KL, Corbett JR, Croft CH, Hillis LD. Propranolol-verapamil versus propranolol-nifedipine in severe angina pectoris of effort: A randomized, double-blind, cross-over study. *Am J Cardiol* 1985; 55:281–285.

17. Hamann SR, Kaltenborn KE, Vore M, Tan TG, McAllister RG. Cardiovascular pharmacokinetic consequences of combined administration of verapamil and propranolol in dogs. *Am J Cardiol* 1985; 56:147–156.

18. Murdoch DL, Thomson GD, Thompson GG, Murray GD, Brodie MJ, McInnes GT. Evaluation of potential pharmacodynamic and pharmacokinetic interactions between verapamil and propranolol in normal subjects. *Br J Clin Pharmacol* 1991; 31:323–332.

19. Johnston DL, Gebhardt VA, Donald A, Kostuk WJ. Comparative effects of propranolol and verapamil alone and in combination on left ventricular function in patients with chronic exertional angina: A double-blind, placebo-controlled, randomized, cross-over study with radionuclide ventriculography. *Circulation* 1983; 68:1280–1289.

20. McInnes GT, Findlay IN, Murray G, Cleland JG, Dargie HJ. Cardiovascular responses to verapamil and propranolol in hypertensive patients. *J Hypertens* 1985; 3(suppl 3):S219–S221.

21. Pedersen KE. Digoxin interactions: The influence of quinidine and verapamil on the pharmacokinetics and receptor binding of digitalis glycosides. *Acta Med Scand* 1985; 697(suppl):12–40.

22. Elliott HL, Pasanisi F, Meredith PA, Reid JL. Acute hypotensive response to nifedipine added to prazosin. *Br Med J* 1984; 288:238.

23. Pasanisi F, Elliott HL, Meredith PA, McSharry DR, Reid JL. Combined alpha-adrenoceptor antagonism and calcium channel blockade in normal subjects. *Clin Pharmacol Ther* 1984; 36:716–723.

24. Reid JL, Meredith PA, Pasanisi F. Clinical pharmacological aspects of calcium antagonists and their therapeutic role in hypertension. *J Cardiovasc Pharmacol* 1985; 7(suppl 4):S18–S20.

25. Maisel AS, Motulsky HJ, Insel PA. Hypotension after quinidine plus verapamil: Possible additive competition at alpha-adrenergic receptors. *N Engl J Med* 1985; 312:167–171.

26. Trohman RG, Estes DM, Castellanos A, Palomo AR, Myerburg RJ, Kessler KM. Increased quinidine plasma concentrations during administration of verapamil: A new quinidine-verapamil interaction. *Am J Cardiol* 1986; 57:706–707.

27. Hansten PD, Horn JR. Calcium channel blocker-induced drug interactions: Evidence for metabolic inhibition. *Drug Interact Newsl* 1986; 6:35–40.

28. Opie LH, White DA. Adverse interaction between nifedipine and beta blockade. *Br Med J* 1980; 281:1462–1464.

29. Kleinbloesem CH, van Brummelen P, Sandberg TH, Danhof M, Breimer DD. Kinetic and haemodynamic interactions between nifedipine and propranolol in healthy subjects utilizing controlled rates of drug input. In: Kleinbloesem CH, ed. *Nifedipine: Clinical Pharmacokinetics and Haemodynamic Effects*. The Hague: Drukkerij JH Pasmans BV; 1985:151–165.

30. Kiss I, Farsang C. Nifedipine-prazosin interaction in patients with essential hypertension. *Cardiovasc Drugs Ther* 1989; 3:413–415.

31. Hung J, Lamb IH, Connolly SJ, Jutzky KR, Goris ML, Schroeder JS. The effect of diltiazem and propranolol, alone and in combination, on exercise performance and left ventricular function in patients with stable effort angina: A double-blind, randomized, and placebo-controlled study. *Circulation* 1983; 68:560–567.

32. Grino JM, Sabate I, Castelao AM, Alsina J. Influence of diltiazem on cyclosporin clearance. *Lancet* 1986; 2:1387.

33. Bigger JT, Giardina EG. Drug interactions in antiarrhythmic therapy. *Ann NY Acad Sci* 1984; 427:140–161.

34. Jaillon P. Antiarrhythmic drug interactions: Are they important? *Eur Heart J* 1987; 8(suppl A):127–132.

35. Hardy BG, Zador IT, Golden L, Lalka D, Schentag JJ. Effects of cimetidine on the pharmacokinetics of quinidine. *Am J Cardiol* 1983; 52:172–175.

36. Hager WD, Fenster P, Mayersohn M, Perrier D, Graves P, Marcus FI. Digoxin-quinidine interaction: Pharmacokinetic evaluation. *N Engl J Med* 1979; 300:1238–1241.

37. Koch-Weser J. Quinidine-induced hypoprothrombinemic hemorrhage in patients on chronic warfarin therapy. *Ann Intern Med* 1968; 68:511–517.

38. Dada JL, Wilkinson GR, Nies AJ. Interaction of quinidine with anticonvulsant drugs. *N Engl J Med* 1976; 294:699–702.

39. Twum-Barima Y, Carruthers SG. Quinidine-rifampicin. *N Engl J Med* 1981; 304:1466–1469.

40. Farringer JA, McWay-Hess K, Clementi WA. Cimetidine-quinidine interaction. *Clin Pharmacol* 1984; 3:81–83.

41. Green JA, Clementi WA, Porter C, Stigelman W. Nifedipine-quinidine interaction. *Clin Pharm* 1983; 2:461–465.

42. Van Lith RM, Appleby DH. Quinidine-nifedipine interaction. *Drug Intell Clin Pharm* 1985; 19:829–830.

43. Marcus FI. Drug interactions with amiodarone. *Am Heart J* 1983; 106:924–930.

44. Christian CO, Meredith CG, Speeg KV. Cimetidine inhibits procainamide clearance. *Clin Pharmacol Ther* 1984; 36:221–227.

45. Lee JT, Davy JM, Kates RE. Evaluation of combined administration of verapamil and disopyramide in dogs. *J Cardiovasc Pharmacol* 1985; 7:501–507.

46. Kapil RP, Axelson JE, Mansfield IL, Edwards DJ, McErlane B, Mason MA. Disopyramide pharmacokinetics and metabolism: Effect of inducers. *Br J Clin Pharmacol* 1987; 24:781–791.

47. Teichman SL, Fisher JD, Matos JA, Kim SG. Disopyramide-pyridostigmine: Report of a beneficial drug interaction. *J Cardiovasc Pharmacol* 1985; 7:108–113.

48. Feely J, Wilkinson GR, McAllister CB, Wood AJ. Increased toxicity and reduced clearance of lidocaine by cimetidine. *Ann Intern Med* 1982; 96:592–594.

49. Boyce JR, Cervenko FW, Wright FJ. Effects of halothane on the pharmacokinetics of lidocaine in digitalis-toxic dogs. *Can Anaesth Soc J* 1978; 25:323–328.

50. Jeresaty RM, Kahn AH, Landry AB. Sinoatrial arrest due to lidocaine in a patient receiving quinidine. *Chest* 1972; 61:683–685.

51. Klein R, Huang SK, Group Southwest Cardiology Research. Combination therapy of propafenone with quinidine or procainamide: Enhanced efficacy and reduced side-effects (abstr). *J Am Coll Cardiol* 1985; 5:423.

52. Breithardt G, Selpel L, Abendroth RR. Comparative cross-over study of the effects of disopyramide and mexiletine on stimulus-induced ventricular tachycardia (abstr). *Circulation* 1980; 62(suppl 3):153.

53. Duff HJ, Roden D, Primm RK, Oates JA, Woosley RL. Mexiletine in the treatment of resistant ventricular arrhythmias: Enhancement of efficacy and reduction of dose-related side-effects by combination with quinidine. *Circulation* 1983; 67:1124–1128.

54. Greenspan AM, Spielman SR, Webb CR, Sokoff NM, Rae AP, Horowitz LN. Efficacy of combination therapy with mexiletine and a type 1A agent for inducible ventricular tachyarrhythmias secondary to coronary artery disease. *Am J Cardiol* 1985; 56:277–284.

55. Leahey EB, Heissenbuttel RH, Giardina EG, Bigger JT. Combined mexiletine and propranolol treatment of refractory ventricular tachycardia. *Br Med J* 1980; 2:357–358.

56. Waleffe A, Mary-Rabine L, Legrand V, Demoulin JC, Kulbertus HE. Combined mexiletine and amiodarone treatment of refractory recurrent ventricular tachycardia. *Am Heart J* 1980; 100:788–793.

57. Lewis GP, Holtzman JL. Interaction of flecainide with digoxin and propranolol. *Am J Cardiol* 1984; 53:52B–57B.

58. Shea P, Lal R, Kim SS, Schechtman K, Ruffy R. Flecainide and amiodarone interaction. *J Am Coll Cardiol* 1986; 7:1127–1130.

59. Maga TB, Verbesselt R, Van Hecken A, van Melle P, De Schepper PJ. Oral flecainide elimination kinetics: Effects of cimetidine (abstr). *Circulation* 1983; 68(suppl 3):416.

60. Hodges M, Salerno D, Granrud G. Double-blind placebo-controlled evaluation of propafenone in suppressing ventricular ectropic activity. *Am J Cardiol* 1984; 54:45D–50D.

61. Martinowitz U, Rabinovich J, Goldfarb D, Many A, Bank H. Interaction between warfarin sodium and amiodarone. *N Engl J Med* 1981; 304:671–672.

62. Gillis RA, Clancy MM, Anderson RJ. Deleterious effects of bretylium in cats with digitalis-induced ventricular tachycardia. *Circulation* 1973; 47:974–983.

63. Vincent JL, Dufaye P, Berre J, Kahn RJ. Bretylium in severe ventricular arrhythmias associated with digitalis intoxication. *Am J Emerg Med* 1984; 2:504–506.

64. Peipho RW, Culbertson VL, Rhodes RS. Drug interactions with the calcium-entry blockers. *Circulation* 1987; 75:181–194.

65. Lessem J, Bellinetto A. Interaction between digoxin and the calcium antagonists nicardipine and tiapamil. *Clin Ther* 1983; 5:595–602.

66. Kirch W, Hutt HJ, Dylewicz P, Ohnhaus EE. Dose-dependence of the nifedipine-digoxin interaction. *Clin Pharmacol Ther* 1986; 39:35–39.

67. Lessem JN. Interaction between Ca^{2+} antagonists and digitalis. *Cardiovasc Drugs Ther* 1988; 1:441–446.

68. Kirch W, Hutt HJ, Heidemann H, Ramsch K, Janisch HD, Ohnhaus EE. Drug interactions with nitrendipine. *J Cardiovasc Pharmacol* 1984; 6:S982–S985.

69. Plunkett LM, Gokhale RD, Vallner JJ, Tackett RL. Prazosin alters free and total plasma digoxin levels in dogs. *Am Heart J* 1985; 109:847–851.

70. Marcus FI. Pharmacokinetic interactions between digoxin and other drugs. *J Am Cardiol* 1985; 5:82A–90A.

71. Waldorff S, Andersen JD, Heeboil-Nielsen N, Nielson OG, Moltre E, Sorensen V. Spironolactone-induced changes in digoxin kinetics. *Clin Pharmacol Ther* 1978; 24:162–167.

72. Waldorff S, Hansen PB, Egeblad H, Berning J, Buch J, Kjaergard H. Interactions between digoxin and potassium-sparing diuretics. *Clin Pharmacol Ther* 1983; 33:418–423.

73. Fenster PE, Hager WD, Goodman MM. Digoxin-quinidine-spironolactone interaction. *Clin Pharmacol Ther* 1984; 36:70–73.

74. Mudge GH. Diuretics and other agents employed in the mobilization of edema fluid. In: Gilman AG, Goodman LS, Gilman AG, eds. *The Pharmacological Basis of Therapeutics*. New York: Macmillan; 1980:892–915.

75. Dzau VJ, Packer M, Lilly LS, Swartz SL, Hollenberg NK, Williams GH. Prostaglandins in severe congestive heart failure: Relation to activation of the renin-angiotensin system and hyponatremia. *N Engl J Med* 1984; 310:347–352.

76. McKibbin JK, Pocock WA, Barlow JB, Millar RN, Obel IW. Sotalol, hypokalaemia, syncope, and torsade de pointes. *Br Heart J* 1984; 51:157–162.

77. Jefferson JW, Kalin NH. Serum lithium levels and long-term diuretic use. *JAMA* 1979; 241:1134–1136.

78. Cogan JJ, Humphreys MH, Carlson CJ, Benowitz NL, Rapaport E. Acute vasodilator therapy increases renal clearance of digoxin in patients with congestive heart failure. *Circulation* 1981; 64:973–976.

79. Schneck DW, Vary JE. Mechanism by which hydralazine increases propranolol bioavailability. *Clin Pharmacol Ther* 1984; 35:447–453.

80. Hodsman GP, Johnston CI. Angiotensin converting enzyme inhibitors: Drug interactions. *J Hypertens* 1987; 5:1–6.

81. Townend JN, Doran J, Lote CJ, Davies MK. Peripheral haemodynamic effects of inhibition of prostaglandin synthesis in congestive heart failure and interactions with captopril. *Br Heart J* 1995; 73:434–441.

82. Singhvi SM, Duchin KL, Willard DA, McKinstry DN, Migdalof BH. Renal handling of captopril: Effect of probenicid. *Clin Pharmacol Ther* 1982; 32:182–189.

83. Grayzel AI, Liddle L, Seegmiller JE. Diagnostic significance of hyperuricemia in arthritis. *N Engl J Med* 1961; 265:763–768.

84. Moroz L. Increased blood fibrinolytic activity after aspirin ingestion. *N Engl J Med* 1977; 296:525–529.

85. Chesebro JH, Fuster V, Elveback LR, McGoon DC, Pluth JR, Puga FJ. Trial of combined warfarin plus dipyridamole or aspirin therapy in prosthetic heart valve replacement: Danger of aspirin compared with dipyridamole. *Am J Cardiol* 1983; 51:1537–1541.

86. Stratton F, Chalmers DG, Flute PT, Lewis SM, MacIver J, Nelson MG. Drug interaction with coumarin derivative anticoagulants. *Br Med J* 1982; 285:274–275.

87. O'Reilly RA, Sahud MA, Aggeler PM. Impact of aspirin and chlorthalidone on the pharmacodynamics of oral anticoagulant drugs in man. *Ann NY Acad Sci* 1971; 179:173–186.

88. Koh KK, Park GS, Song JH, Moon TH. Interaction of intravenous heparin and organic nitrates in acute ischemic syndromes. *Am J Cardiol* 1995; 76:706–709.

89. Romeo F, Rosano GM, Martuscelli E, De Luca F. Concurrent nitroglycerin administration reduces the efficacy of recombinant tissue-type plasminogen activator in patients with acute anterior wall myocardial infarction. *Am Heart J* 1995; 130:692–697.

90. Lees RS, Lees AM. Rhabdomyolysis from the coadministration of lovastatin and the antifungal agent itraconazole. *N Engl J Med* 1995; 333:664–665.

91. Keogh A, Spratt P, McCosker C, MacDonald P, Mundy J, Kaan A. Ketoconazole to reduce the need for cyclosporine after cardiac transplantation. *N Engl J Med* 1995; 333:628–633.

92. Houston MC, Nonsteroidal anti-inflammatory drugs and antihypertensives. *Am J Med* 1991; 90(suppl 5A):42S–47S.

93. Salvetti A, Magagna A, Abdel-Haq B, Lenzi M, Giovannetti R. Nifedipine interactions in hypertensive patients. *Cardiovasc Drugs Ther* 1990; 4:963–968.

94. Weinberger MH. The relationship of sodium balance and concomitant diuretic therapy to blood pressure response with calcium channel entry blockers. *Am J Med* 1991; 90(suppl 5A):15S–20S.

95. Hodsman GP, Isles CG, Murray GD, Usherwood TP, Webb DJ, Robertson JI. Factors related to the first dose hypotensive effect of captopril: Prediction and treatment. *Br Med J* 1983; 286:832–834.

96. Textor SC, Bravo EL, Fouad FM, Tarazi RC. Hyperkalaemia in azotemic patients during angiotensin-converting enzyme inhibition and aldosterone reduction with captopril. *Am J Med* 1982; 73:719–725.

97. Polonia J, Boaventura I, Gama G, Camoes I. Influence of non-steroidal anti-inflammatory drugs on renal function and 24-h ambulatory blood pressure-reducing effects of enalapril and nifedipine gastrointestinal therapeutic system in hypertensive patients. *J Hypertens* 1995; 13:925–931.

98. Toussaint C, Masselink A, Gentges A, Wambach G, Bonner G. Interference of different ACE inhibitors with the diuretic action of furosemide and hydrochlorothiazide. *Klin Wochenschr* 1989; 67:1138–1146.

99. Cooper RA. Captopril associated neutropenia: Who is at risk. *Arch Intern Med* 1983; 143:659–660.

100. Browne KF, Prystowsky EN, Heger JJ, Cerimele BJ, Finebera N, Zipes DP. Prolongation of the QT-interval induced by probucol: Demonstration of a method for determining QT-interval change induced by a drug. *Am Heart J* 1984; 107:680–684.

101. Tobert JA. Rhabdomyolysis in patients receiving lovastatin after cardiac transplantation. *N Engl J Med* 1988; 318:47–48.

102. Kendall MJ, Laugher SJ, Wilkins MR. Ranitidine cimetidine and metoprolol—A pharmacokinetic interaction study (abstr). *Gastroenterology* 1986; 90:1490.

103. Daneshmend TK, Roberts CJ. Reduction in labetalol first-pass metabolism following cimetidine (abstr). *Br J Clin Pharmacol* 1983; 15:153P.

104. Kubo SH, Fox SC, Prida XE, Cody RJ. Combined hemodynamic effects of nifedipine and nitroglycerin in congestive heart failure. *Am Heart J* 1985; 110:1032–1034.

105. Kleinbloesem CH, van Brumelen P, Hilliers J, Moolenaar AJ, Breimer DD. Interaction between digoxin and nifedipine at steady-state in patients with arterial fibrillation. In: Kleinbloesem CH, ed. *Nifedipine: Clinical Pharmacokinetics and Haemodynamic Effects.* The Hague: Drukkerij JH Pasmans BV; 1985:167–173.

106. Bourbigot B, Guiserix J, Airiau J, Bressollette L, Morin JF, Cledes J. Nicardipine increases cyclosporin blood levels. *Lancet* 1986; 1:1447.

107. Aviado DM, Salem H. Drug action, reaction and interaction: I. Quinidine for cardiac arrhythmias. *J Clin Pharmacol* 1975; 15:477–485.

108. Loon NR, Wilcox CS, Folger W. Orthostatic hypotension due to quinidine and propranolol. *Am J Med* 1986; 81:1101–1104.

109. Roden DM, Woosley RL, Primm RK. Incidence and clinical features of the quinidine-associated long QT syndrome: Implications for patient care. *Am Heart J* 1986; 111:1088–1093.

110. Farringer JA, Green JA, O'Rourke RA, Linn WA, Clementi WA. Nifedipine-induced alterations in serum quinidine concentrations. *Am Heart J* 1984; 108:1570–1572.

111. Nattel S, Gagne G, Pineau M. The pharmacokinetics of lignocaine and β-adrenoceptor antagonists in patients with acute myocardial infarction. *Clin Pharmacokinet* 1987; 13:293–316.

112. Josephson MA, Kaul S, Hopkins J, Kvam D, Singh BN. Hemodynamic effects of intravenous flecainide relative to the level of ventricular function in patients with coronary artery disease. *Am Heart J* 1985; 109:41–45.

113. Kuhlmann J, Marcin S. Effects of verapamil on pharmacokinetics and pharmacodynamics of digoxin in patients. *Am Heart J* 1985; 110:1245–1250.

114. Cleland JG, Dargie HJ, Pettigrew A, Gillen G, Robertson JI. The effects of captopril on serum digoxin and urinary urea and digoxin clearances in patients with congestive heart failure. *Am Heart J* 1986; 112:130–135.

115. Bailey RR, Reddy J. Potentiation of warfarin action by sulphinpyrazone (letter). *Lancet* 1980; 1:254.

116. Trenque T, Choisy H, Germain ML. Pravastatin: Interaction with oral anticoagulant. *Br Med J* 1996; 312:886.

92

HEART DISEASE AND PREGNANCY

John H. McAnulty / James Metcalfe / Kent Ueland

This chapter is written to describe how pregnancy affects the cardiovascular system and how the heart and heart disease affect pregnancy. Even if there were no heart disease, an understanding of the cardiovascular changes of a normal pregnancy is important for optimal care. But, pregnancy in patients with heart disease is becoming more common. This is not due to a failure of health care. Rather, treatment of heart disease during childhood, usually with surgery, has resulted in an increasing number of women with treated heart disease who survive to the age of childbearing and are able to conceive. Because of this, and because failure to treat heart disease may adversely affect both the mother and the child, the person caring for a pregnant woman must recognize heart disease and direct care accordingly.

HEART DISEASE ISSUES UNIQUE TO PREGNANCY

When caring for a woman with heart disease during pregnancy, some issues are always important.

Health Priorities

Mother and child—the health of one importantly influences the other. The well-being of the fetus should be considered, but the safety of the mother is always the highest priority. Ideally, treatment of the mother with drugs, diagnostic studies, or surgery should be avoided. If required for maternal safety, however, they should be used.

Maternal Fragility

Despite the advances in recognition and management of heart disease, pregnancy puts the mother at risk. The normal hemodynamic changes of pregnancy may result in disability or death. The risk is so great with some cardiovascular abnormalities that a recommendation of avoidance or interruption of pregnancy is supportable (Table 92-1).[1] Emotional stability

is also threatened by pregnancy in the woman with heart disease. Misconceptions and apprehension are common. This previously described case provides one example of the need to keep a pregnant woman and her family informed and comfortable[2]:

A cardiac care unit nurse for 10 years, always logical and calm, and 7 months into her second pregnancy— could she be this frightened? She is, and it's about what the pregnancy will do to her heart and what her heart will do to her pregnancy. She, of course, knows too much. She has heard of a peripartum cardiomyopathy and is for some reason convinced that her labor will cause it. She is wrong about that (we believe), but she still is an appropriate representative of a prospective parent—easily worried about the effects of pregnancy on her health and worried about the baby. She knows about her ventricular ectopy. It has to be bad for the baby! She's probably wrong, but again, this is an example of how pregnancy raises issues that we ordinarily do not consider when taking care of a patient: an example of the apprehension that surrounds heart disease and pregnancy.

Fetal Vulnerability

The fetus depends on its mother for a continuous supply of oxygen and adequate nutrients. The mother must also remove the products of fetal metabolism, including heat. The maternal commitment to the fetus is exceptional, but if the mother requires a redistribution of volume for her own safety, blood is preferentially diverted away from the uterus. In the woman with a normal cardiovascular system, blood flow to the fetus seems to be adequate, even during periods of physical and emotional stress. In the woman with heart disease, however, where uterine blood flow may already be compromised, the chance of inadequate uterine perfusion increases. Treatment

TABLE 92-1

CARDIOVASCULAR ABNORMALITIES PLACING A MOTHER AND INFANT AT EXTREMELY HIGH RISK

Advise *avoidance* or *interruption of pregnancy*
  Pulmonary hypertension
  Dilated cardiomyopathy with congestive failure
  Marfan's syndrome with dilated aortic root
  Cyanotic congenital heart disease
Pregnancy counseling and close clinical follow-up required
  Prosthetic valve
  Coarctation of the aorta
  Marfan's syndrome
  Dilated cardiomyopathy in asymptomatic women
  Obstructive lesions

Source: Modified from McAnulty JH, et al.[1] Reproduced with permission from the publisher and authors.

of maternal heart disease may also jeopardize the fetus. Diagnostic studies, drugs, or surgery may increase fetal loss, result in teratogenicity, or alter fetal growth.

Newborn Infant Vulnerability

The health of a newborn infant is a concern when the mother has heart disease. This fragility may be due to a marginal uterine blood flow during pregnancy or to lingering effects of the medications used to treat the mother. Additionally, the live-born infant of a parent with congenital heart disease will have an increased incidence of congenital heart disease (see Table 92-2). Early infant nourishment may be jeopardized if maternal heart disease is severe enough to interfere with breast-feeding. Even if the mother is capable of breast-feeding, cardiovascular medications may be transmitted to the infant in breast milk. Finally, the infant is at risk of losing a parent, since life expectancy with many forms of heart disease is significantly less than normal.

Maternal Heart Disease May Not Be "Typical"

Many women with heart disease who become pregnant have a form of heart disease that is relatively new—that has existed for less than 50 years. They have mechanically "altered" heart disease. While much has been learned about hearts that have been altered by surgery (or a catheter), there is still much that is unknown. It is best not to consider a previous lesion mechanically "corrected" because there is always some residual disease. In some cases, the residual disease (a shunt, ventricular dysfunction, an arrhythmia predisposition, or persistent obstruction) may adversely affect the mother and, in turn, may harm the fetus.

CARDIOVASCULAR ADJUSTMENTS DURING A NORMAL PREGNANCY

Maternal adaptation to pregnancy includes remarkable cardiovascular changes. These explain in part why some cardiac

abnormalities are not well tolerated during pregnancy (see Table 92-1) and may result in symptoms and signs, even in a normal pregnancy, that are difficult to distinguish from those occurring with heart disease.

Hemodynamic Changes at Rest

Resting cardiac output increases by over 40 percent during pregnancy. The increase begins early, with the cardiac output reaching its highest levels by the 20th week. In the last half of pregnancy, cardiac output is significantly affected by body position (Fig. 92-1) as the enlarged uterus diminishes venous return from the lower extremities.[3–8] Compared to measurements made near term when the woman is in the left lateral position, cardiac output is lower by an average of 0.6 L/min when a woman is supine and by 1.2 L/min when she assumes the upright position.[7] In general, this results in few or no symptoms, but in some women, maintenance of the supine position may result in symptomatic hypotension, possibly in those whose collateral vessels are not well developed.[8–10] Symptoms of this "supine hypotensive syndrome of pregnancy" can be corrected by having the woman turn onto her side.

TABLE 92-2

CONGENITAL HEART DISEASE IN THE OFFSPRING OF A PARENT WITH CONGENITAL HEART DISEASE

Congenital Heart Defect in a Parent	Risk of Congenital Heart Disease in Offspring If One Parent Is Affected,[a,b] Percentage
Intracardiac shunts	
Atrial septal defect	3–11
Ventricular septal defect	4–22
Patent ductus arteriosus	4–11
Obstruction to flow	
Left-sided obstruction[c]	3–26
Right-sided obstruction	3–22
Complex abnormalities	
Tetralogy of Fallot	4–15
Ebstein's anomaly	Uncertain
Transposition of the great arteries	Uncertain
Hypertrophic cardiomyopathy with asymmetric septal hypertrophy	50
Marfan's syndrome	50

[a] The higher number in each range comes from one large series.[142,145] The incidence of congenital heart disease in the offspring tends to be closer to the lower numbers for most other reported series.[138,139]

[b] The risk in obstructive lesions is decreased by corrective surgery prior to pregnancy.[143]

[c] Includes coarctation, aortic stenosis, discrete subaortic stenosis, supravalvular stenosis.

Source: Modified from McAnulty JH, Metcalfe J, Ueland K: Cardiovascular disease. In: Burrow GN, Ferris TF, eds. *Medical Complications during Pregnancy.* Philadelphia: Saunders; 1988. Reproduced with permission from the publisher and authors.

The hemodynamic changes that are associated with or are the cause of the cardiac output variation also change dramatically (Fig. 92-2). Cardiac output is the product of heart rate times stroke volume. Its early rise is due mainly to an increase in stroke volume.[3,6] By the 20th week, stroke volume gradually begins to fall because of obstruction of the vena cava by the enlarged uterus and to increased venous bed dilation. The heart rate increases gradually throughout pregnancy, reaching a level that is approximately 25 percent above the nonpregnant levels by the time of delivery.

Cardiac output is also directly related to the mean blood pressure and inversely related to the systemic vascular resistance. There is a fall in blood pressure early in pregnancy, with a gradual return to nonpregnant levels by term. The fall in systemic vascular resistance is more marked, decreasing to one-third of resting nonpregnant values at about the 20th week of pregnancy and then gradually rising through the remainder of pregnancy, although not achieving nonpregnant levels until a few weeks after delivery.[3,6]

Finally, the cardiac output is equal to the oxygen consumption divided by the systemic arterial venous oxygen difference. The mother's oxygen consumption (which includes that of her fetus) increases by 20 percent within the first 10 weeks of pregnancy and increases steadily to a level that is approximately 30 percent above the nonpregnant levels by the time of delivery.[6] This increase is due both to the metabolic needs of the fetus and to the increased metabolic needs of the mother. The increase in cardiac output occurs earlier than the rise in oxygen consumption, and thus the arteriovenous oxygen difference narrows early in pregnancy with a gradual increase in oxygen extraction throughout pregnancy, so that by term, the systemic arteriovenous oxygen difference exceeds nonpregnant values.

At the beginning of labor, cardiac output measured in the supine position increases to over 7 L/min (Fig. 92-3). With each uterine contraction, this rises by still another 34 percent as a result of increases in heart rate as well as an increment in stroke volume resulting from extrusion of approximately 500 mL of blood into the central venous system with each contraction. Thus, at these times, the cardiac output can be as great as 9 L/min.[11] Administration of epidural anesthesia reduces this cardiac output to about 8 L/min, and the use of general anesthesia reduces it still further. Following delivery, there is a transient, marked elevation in cardiac output that

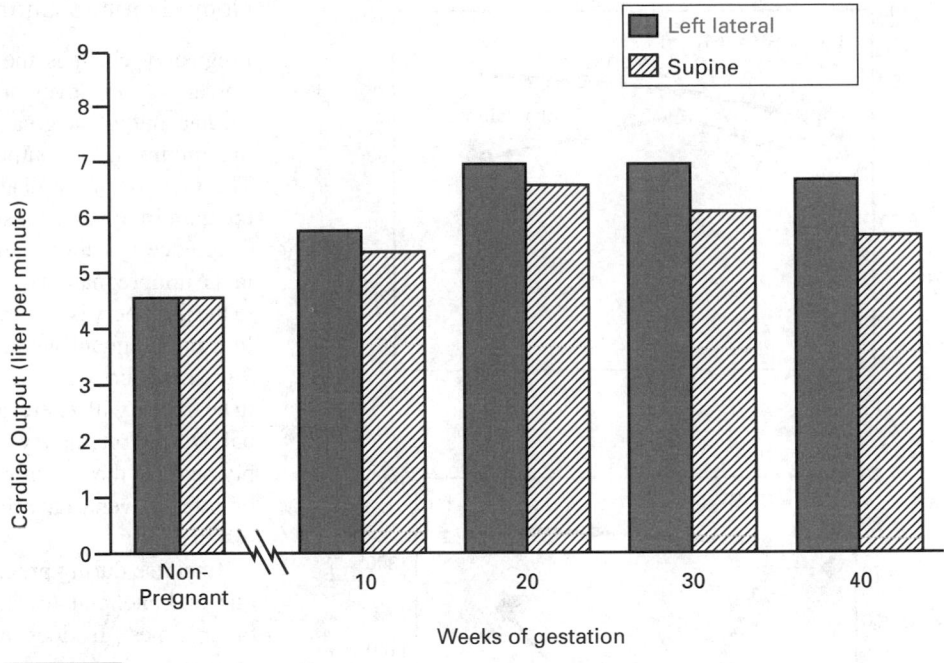

FIGURE 92-1

Normal pregnancy cardiac output values when measured in the supine and left lateral positions. The values are derived from measurements made in many studies.[3-8]

approaches 10 L/min[11] (7 to 8 L/min with cesarean section),[12] with the cardiac output falling rapidly to near-normal, nonpregnant values within a few weeks after delivery, although there is a slight elevation that can persist for as long as lactation occurs.

The increase in maternal cardiac output in women with twins or triplets is slightly greater when compared to women with single pregnancies.[13]

The distribution of blood flow is not fully understood. It is affected by changes in local vascular resistance[14] (Fig. 92-4). Renal blood flow increases by approximately 30 percent in the first trimester and stays at about that level or declines slightly throughout the pregnancy. Nonpregnant mammary blood flow is usually less than 1 percent of the cardiac output but can be approximately 2 percent of the cardiac output at term. Blood flow to the skin increases by 40 to 50 percent, a mechanism for heat dissipation.

In the nonpregnant woman, uterine blood flow is approximately 100 mL/min (2 percent of the cardiac output). This doubles by the 28th week of pregnancy and increases to approximately 1200 mL/min at term, a value approaching the mother's blood flow to her own kidneys.[15-17] During pregnancy, uterine blood vessels are maximally dilated; flow can increase, but it has to result from increased maternal arterial pressure and flow. Uterine blood flow falls if redistribution of total flow is required by the mother or if there is a fall in maternal blood pressure and cardiac output. Excitement, heat, exercise, and decrease in venous return have all been shown to decrease uterine blood flow. Vasoconstriction caused by endogenous catecholamines, vasoconstrictive drugs, maternal mechanical pulmonary ventilation, and some anesthetics, as

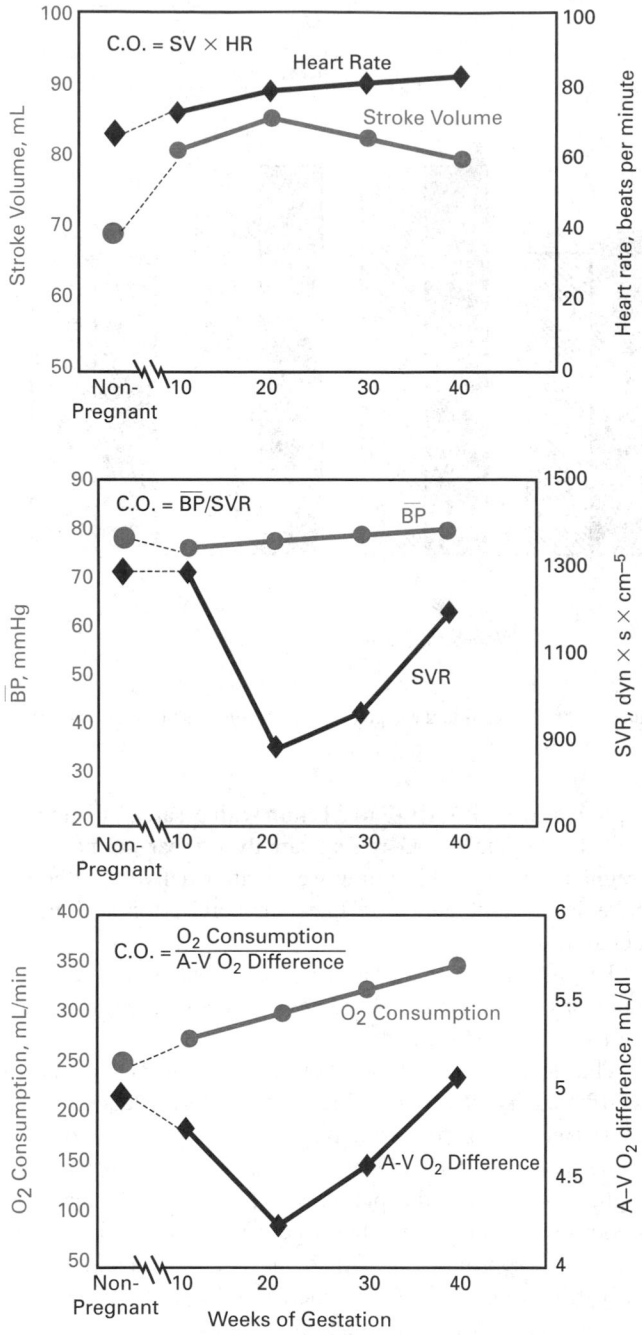

FIGURE 92-2

The cardiac output (C.O.) can be determined from other parameters in at least 3 ways: C.O. = heart rate (HR) × stroke volume (SV); C.O. = mean arterial pressure (BP) minus the RA pressure/systemic vascular resistance (SVR); C.O. = oxygen (O_2) consumption/arteriovenous (A − V) O_2 difference. The expected values for these parameters measured in the supine position during pregnancy are based on information acquired from many studies.[3–6]

well as that associated with preeclampsia and eclampsia, can decrease perfusion of the uterus. While uterine blood flow could potentially be compromised even in a healthy woman, in the mother with heart disease whose blood flow may already be compromised, the concern about diversion of flow from the uterus is greater.

Hemodynamic Changes With Exercise

Pregnancy changes the hemodynamic response to exercise. For any given level of exercise in the sitting position, the cardiac output is greater than in nonpregnant women, and maximum cardiac output is reached at lower exercise levels. The increase in cardiac output is relatively greater than the increase in oxygen consumption, so the arteriovenous oxygen difference is wider than that produced by the same exercise in the nonpregnant woman. This suggests that oxygen delivery to the periphery is somewhat less efficient during pregnancy.[18] In a nonpregnant woman, training or conditioning results in a greater increase in stroke volume and a smaller increment in heart rate with exercise as compared to an untrained individual. During pregnancy, this training effect is not seen—possibly because the increase in stroke volume is limited as a result of inferior vena cava compression or the increased venous distensibility.[19]

Exercise during pregnancy is not clearly any more dangerous or beneficial to the mother with heart disease than at other times. It does affect the fetus. In animal models, maternal exercise has been associated with a fall in uterine blood flow. In humans, it is known that the type of exercise affects maternal hemodynamics and uterine perfusion.[20,21] As an example, maximal exercise by swimming causes less fetal bradycardia (a marker of uterine blood flow) than the same level of cycling.[22] Additionally, regular aerobic endurance exercise during pregnancy has been associated with a reduction in birth weight. Since most of the reduction is due to a decrease in neonatal fat mass, it is not clear if this is detrimental.[23]

Infants born to mothers who work in a standing position may be abnormally small at birth.[24] While the long-term effects of this are not clear, the implications in relation to exercise and work in the upright position would seem to be greater for women with heart disease. This question, relating to exercise and the effect on the fetus, has become more important with an increasing enthusiasm for recreational exercise in the United States. While there is not enough evidence available to suggest that the healthy pregnant woman should avoid recreational exercise, an argument can be made for advising the woman with heart disease to keep the exercise level below that which causes symptoms.

Mechanisms for Hemodynamic Changes

The mechanisms evoking the hemodynamic adaptation to pregnancy are not fully understood. They may in part be due to volume changes. Total body water increases steadily throughout pregnancy by 6 to 8 L (most is extracellular).[25] Sodium retention results in an excess accumulation of 500 to 900 meq by the time of delivery. As early as 6 weeks after conception, plasma volume increases and approaches its maximum of 1½ times normal by the second trimester, where it stays throughout the pregnancy.[26] The red blood cell mass also increases, but not to the same degree as the increase in plasma volume. As a result, the hematocrit falls, though rarely to less than 30%. Peak hemodilation occurs at 24–26 weeks, then the hematocrit gradually increases.

Vascular alterations also contribute to the hemodynamic changes of pregnancy. Arterial compliance is increased,[27] and there is an increase in venous vascular capacitance.[28,29] These changes are advantageous in maintaining the hemodynamics of a normal pregnancy. There may be disadvantages as well. The arterial changes are associated with increased fragility; vascular accidents, when they occur in women, frequently do so during pregnancy.[30–33] The venous changes may explain, in part, the increase in thromboemboli during pregnancy.[34]

Intrinsic cardiac changes can also explain some of the hemodynamic changes.[35–37] The stroke volume increases by approximately 25 percent. The ejection fraction does not change, and thus the heart has to enlarge (since the ejection fraction is the stroke volume divided by the end-diastolic volume). Since the increases in left ventricular end-diastolic and systolic volumes are small and not adequate to explain the constant ejection fraction, the heart must become reconfigured as well. If so, this occurs with only a 10 to 15 percent increase in myocardial mass during pregnancy.[38]

The ultimate cause (or causes) for these recognized changes

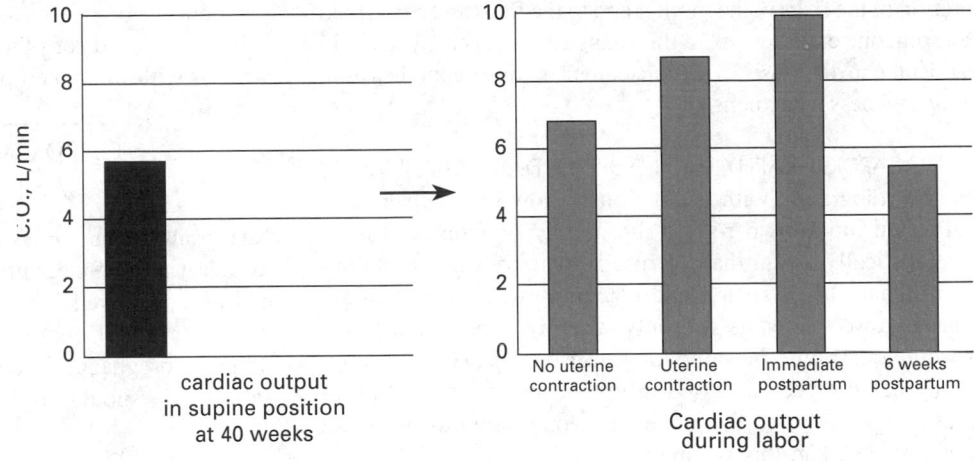

FIGURE 92-3

Cardiac output measured in the supine position is high at 40 weeks (*A*), increases during labor (*B*), particularly with contractions, and is even higher still in the minutes to hours following a vaginal delivery.[11,12]

is uncertain. Complex interactions of the renin-angiotension-aldosterone system, the reproductive hormones, prostaglandins, and atrial natriuretic factor contribute to the fluid and sodium changes.[39,40] At the present time, the effects of the increased level of circulating steroid hormones seem to explain the vascular and myocardial changes satisfactorily.

DIAGNOSIS OF HEART DISEASE

Clinical Evaluation

The recognition and definition of heart disease are difficult at any time. This is particularly true during pregnancy. Symptoms suggesting heart disease—fatigue, dyspnea, orthopnea, pedal edema, and chest discomfort—occur commonly in pregnant women with normal hearts. While they should alert a caregiver to the possibility of heart disease, the concern should increase if the dyspnea or orthopnea is progressive and limiting or if a woman develops hemoptysis, syncope with exertion, or chest pain clearly related to effort. Common examination features of a normal pregnancy include pedal edema, basilar pulmonary rales, a third heart sound, a systolic murmur, and visible neck vein pulsations. However, cyanosis or clubbing, a loud systolic murmur ($\geq$3/6), cardiomegaly, a "fixed split" second heart sound, or evidence for pulmonary hypertension (a left parasternal lift and loud P_2) do not occur as part of a normal pregnancy and deserve attention. A diastolic murmur is unusual enough during pregnancy that its presence is an indication of heart disease if care is taken to exclude the venous hum or internal mammary flow sounds (the mammary souffle), which have diastolic components and are normal.

Diagnostic Studies

It is preferable to evaluate the cardiovascular status with the history and physical examination alone. On occasion, diagnostic studies are required. They should be chosen with a consid-

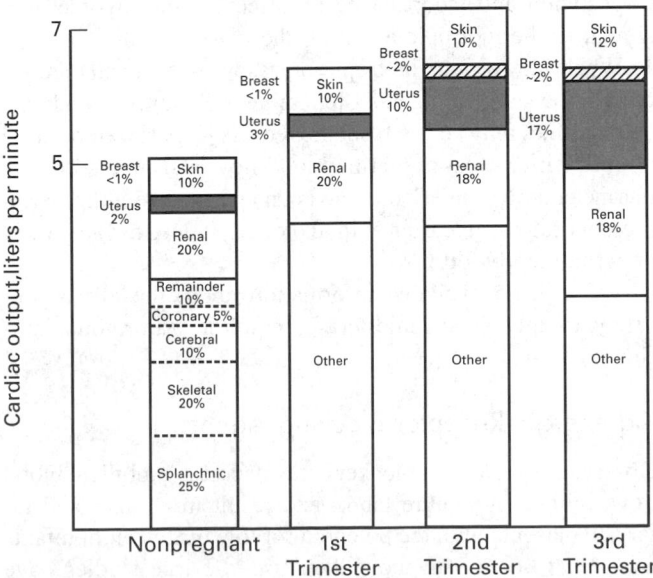

FIGURE 92-4

The changes in cardiac output and its distribution at rest in nonpregnant and pregnant women are depicted. Data used in this graph are fragmentary, especially early in pregnancy.

eration of the risks to the mother and to the fetus and performed by someone experienced in the changes of pregnancy to avoid a mistake in diagnosis, with consequent anxiety, apprehension, and unnecessary expense.

ECHOCARDIOGRAPHY WITH DOPPLER FLOW STUDIES
Echocardiography with evaluation of flow by Doppler is so safe, with no known risk to the mother or fetus, and is so diagnostically useful that overuse is the only significant concern (Chap. 14). Expense and potential misinterpretation are reasons to consider its use only when required to answer a specific question. The safety of transesophageal echocardiography has not been assessed in pregnancy. The use of anesthetic agents during the procedure would seem to create the greatest risk, and this is minor.

RADIOGRAPHIC PROCEDURES
All x-ray procedures should generally be avoided, particularly early in pregnancy. They increase the risk of abnormal fetal organogenesis or of a subsequent malignancy in the child, particularly leukemia. If a study is required, it should be delayed to as late in pregnancy as possible, the radiation dose should be kept to a minimum, and shielding of the fetus should be optimal. Interpretation should take into consideration the changes expected in a normal pregnancy. As an example, some increase in heart size and pulmonary vascular markings are common chest x-ray findings during pregnancy. Every woman of childbearing age should be questioned about the possibility of pregnancy before any x-ray procedure. Chest x-rays are performed on occasion when pregnancy is not recognized (or intentionally when it is). The exposure to a fetus is small (estimated to be 10 to 1400 μGy) and has not been associated with any recognizable increase in congenital malformations or malignancies[41]—information that can be given to worried parents if a chest x-ray was performed.

ELECTROCARDIOGRAPHY
The electrocardiogram is safe and useful for answering specific questions. Pregnancy makes interpretation of ST-T wave variations even more difficult than usual; inferior ST-segment depression is common enough to possibly be the result of a normal pregnancy. There is a leftward shift of the QRS axis during pregnancy, but true axis deviation ($-30°$) implies heart disease.

RADIONUCLIDE STUDIES
Although many radionuclides should attach to albumen and thus not reach the fetus, separation can occur and fetal exposure is possible. It is preferable to avoid these studies. On occasion, a pulmonary ventilation-perfusion scan or even a thallium myocardial-perfusion scan is required during pregnancy. Estimated exposure to the fetus is low (400 μGy).[34]

MAGNETIC RESONANCE IMAGING
While there is no available information about the safety of this procedure when used for evaluation of heart disease in

pregnancy, no adverse fetal effects have been reported when it has been used for other purposes. It should be avoided in women with implanted pacemakers or defibrillators.

CARDIOVASCULAR DRUGS AND PREGNANCY

Nearly all cardiac drugs cross the placenta and are secreted in breast milk. Since information about the use of any drug can be considered incomplete, it is best to avoid their use when possible. Definitive recommendations about the use of drugs in pregnancy is difficult, but if required for maternal safety, they should not be withheld.

Diuretics

Diuretics can and should be used for treatment of congestive heart failure that is uncontrolled by sodium restriction, and they remain frontline therapy for the treatment of hypertension. No one agent is clearly contraindicated—experience is greatest with the thiazide diuretics and with furosemide.[42] Diuretics should not be used for prophylaxis against toxemia or for treatment of pedal edema.

Inotropic Agents

The indications for the use of digitalis are not changed by pregnancy. Digoxin and digitoxin cross the placenta, and fetal serum levels approximate those in the mother. The same dose of digoxin in general will yield lower maternal serum levels during pregnancy than in the nonpregnant state.[43] If the desired clinical effect is not achieved, measuring levels may be helpful (if the assay used is not affected by an immunoreactive substance of pregnancy).[44] Digitalis may shorten the duration of gestation and labor due to an effect on the myometrium similar to the inotropic effect on the myocardium.

When intravenous inotropic or vasopressor agents are required, the standard agents (dopamine, dobutamine, and norepinephrine) may be used, but the fetus is jeopardized because all result in decreased uterine blood flow and may stimulate uterine contractions. Ephedrine is an appropriate initial vasopressor drug as, at least in animal models, it does not adversely affect uterine blood flow.

There is no available information about the efficacy or safety of the phosphodiesterase inhibitors (amrinone, milrinone).

Adrenergic Receptor Blocking Agents

Observations that beta blockers may decrease umbilical blood flow, initiate premature labor, and result in a small and infarcted placenta with the potential for low birth weight infants have led to concerns about their use.[45] Large studies have not confirmed these concerns, however, and beta-blocking drugs have been used in a large number of pregnant women without adverse effects. Their use for the usual clinical indications is reasonable.[45–47] All the available beta-blocking agents cross the placenta, are present in human breast milk, and can reach significant levels in the fetus or the newborn. If these agents are used during pregnancy, it is appropriate to monitor fetal heart rate as well as the newborn infant's heart rate, blood sugar, and respiratory status immediately after delivery.

Experience with the alpha-blocking agents phenoxybenzamine and phentolamine is sparse. Clonidine, prazosin and labetalol, with their mixed alpha- and beta-blocking effects, have been used for treatment of hypertension without clear detrimental effects.[48]

Calcium Channel Blocking Drugs

Nifedipine, verapamil, diltiazem, nicardipine, and isradipine have been used to treat hypertension and arrhythmias without an adverse effect on the fetus or newborn infant.[48–50] The drugs cause relaxation of the uterus; nifedipine has been used for this purpose.

Antiarrhythmic Agents

Atrioventricular (AV) node blockade is occasionally required during pregnancy. This can be achieved with digoxin, beta blockers, and calcium blockers. Early reports suggest adenosine can also be safely used as a node blocking agent.[51]

As a general rule, it is preferable to avoid the standard antiarrhythmic drugs in any patient. This is true during pregnancy as well. When essential for recurrent arrhythmias or for maternal safety, they should be used; however, there is insufficient accumulated information to know whether or not these drugs increase the risk to the fetus or child.[52,53] If intravenous drug therapy is required, lidocaine is reasonable first-line therapy. There has been demonstration of transient neonatal depression when the neonate's blood level exceeds 2.5 μg/L, a reason to recommend keeping maternal blood levels below 4 μg/L (since fetal levels are 60 percent of maternal levels).[54,55] Intravenous procainimide and quinidine may cause hypotension; there is no available information about intravenous amiodarone. Bretylium would seem likely to decrease uterine perfusion based on its effects on maternal blood pressure.

If oral antiarrhythmic therapy is necessary, it may still be appropriate to begin with quinidine since, given its long-term availability, it has been most frequently used without clear adverse fetal effects.[45,56] There is some information about procainamide,[57] disopyramide,[58] mexilitene,[59] flecainide,[60,61] and sotalol,[62] but it is insufficient to recommend their use unless essential for the mother. The early available information concerning amiodarone would suggest an increased likelihood of fetal loss and deformity.[63–65]

Vasodilator Agents

When needed for a hypertensive crisis or emergency afterload and preload reduction, nitroprusside is the vasodilator drug of choice. Despite a paucity of information about its use during pregnancy, this controversial recommendation is made because the drug is highly effective, works instantly, is easily tolerated, and its effects dissipate immediately when the drug is stopped. The concern about the use of this drug is that its metabolite, cyanide, can be detected in the fetus, but this has not been demonstrated to be a significant problem in humans.[66,67] This metabolite is a reason to limit the duration of use of this drug whenever possible. Intravenous hydralazine, nitroglycerin, or labetalol are options for parenteral therapy.

Chronic afterload reduction to treat hypertension, aortic or mitral regurgitation, or ventricular dysfunction during pregnancy has been achieved with the calcium blocking drugs, with hydralazine, and with methyldopa.[48,68] Adverse fetal effects have not been reported. The angiotension-converting enzyme (ACE) inhibitors are contraindicated in pregnancy.[48,68,69] They increase the risk of fetal renal development abnormalities. There are no data available on the new angiotensin II blockers, losartin and voltarin.

Antithrombotic Agents

The chronic use of warfarin is associated with a 1 to 5 percent chance per year of significant bleeding. More importantly, when considering its use during pregnancy, warfarin crosses the placenta, and fetal exposure during the first 3 months is associated with a 15 to 25 percent incidence of malformations that comprise the "warfarin embryopathy syndrome" (facial abnormalities, optic atrophy, digital abnormalities, epithelial changes, and mental impairment).[70–72] Women receiving the drug during the 7th to 12th week of gestation are particularly prone to having children with this syndrome.[73,74] Warfarin use at any time during pregnancy increases the risk of fetal bleeding or maternal uterine hemorrhage.

In women who require anticoagulation, heparin is preferable to warfarin. Self-administered subcutaneous high-dose heparin (16,000 to 24,000 units per day) has been proven feasible and efficacious.[74–78] This drug does not cross the placenta. Accumulating data suggest that low-molecular-weight heparin, while currently more expensive, is effective, is easier to use (once or twice daily without the need to follow serial blood tests), and is as safe as standard heparin therapy.

When anticoagulation is required, some have advocated using heparin for the first trimester and warfarin for the next 5 months, with a return to heparin prior to labor and delivery. While successful pregnancy has been achieved with this approach, the authors favor avoidance of warfarin during pregnancy.

Antiplatelet agents increase the chance of maternal bleeding and they cross the placenta. The most commonly used, aspirin, has some observed and theoretical disadvantages.[79] It is associated with an increased incidence of abortion and fetal growth retardation, and its inhibition of prostaglandin synthesis may result in closure of the ductus arteriosis during fetal life.[80] Still, it has been frequently used and even recommended by some for specific indications and as prophylaxis against preeclampsia.[81] These tradeoffs are difficult to evaluate, and thus aspirin should be avoided unless necessary. There are no data available on the effects of ticlopidine during pregnancy.

Obstetric Drugs and Anesthetic Agents Used During Pregnancy

Drugs used specifically for pregnancy can cause hemodynamic alterations. While there is some question as to their value,[82] beta-sympathetic amines are used to stop premature labor. All cause maternal tachycardia. Ritodrine and terbutiline have been associated with pulmonary edema, usually when glucocorticoids are being administered concurrently to promote fetal lung maturation. This pulmonary edema responds abruptly to cessation of the drugs and initiation of diuretic therapy. On other occasions, prostaglandins E_2 and F_2 are used to induce labor and have no significant hemodynamic effects.

Synthetic oxytocin (pitocin) is given to minimize blood loss after delivery. The synthetic preparation prevents vasoconstriction, but it has been associated, in turn, with transient hypotension.

Anesthesia for surgery during pregnancy and at the time of labor and delivery can adversely affect a woman with heart disease. In most cases, lumbar epidural anesthesia with a pudendal nerve block to minimize pain is effective and least likely to result in hemodynamic compromise.[83]

MANAGEMENT OF CARDIOVASCULAR SYNDROMES

Cardiovascular complications can occur with any form of heart disease. Management of each patient has to be individualized, but some recommendations are applicable in most cases.

Low Cardiac Output Syndrome

A low cardiac output is an ominous sign in any patient, and this is particularly true in pregnancy. It results in signs of poor perfusion (mental obtundation, peripheral vascular constriction, low urine output, and often a low blood pressure). While potentially treatable causes such as tamponade or severe valve stenosis should be considered, it is most often due to intravascular volume depletion. This should be prevented when possible and corrected when recognized. While it is a concern in any pregnant woman, volume depletion is particularly dangerous in those with lesions that limit blood flow such as pulmonary hypertension, aortic or pulmonic valve stenosis, hypertrophic cardiomyopathy, or mitral stenosis. Measures to prevent or treat a fall in central blood volume are outlined in Table 92-3.

Congestive Heart Failure

Management of congestive heart failure during pregnancy should not differ greatly from that at other times. Attention to reduction in salt intake and limitation of activity to a level

TABLE 92-3

MEASURES TO PROTECT AGAINST A FALL IN CENTRAL BLOOD VOLUME

Position
  45–60° left lateral
  10° Trendelenburg
Full-leg stockings
Volume preloading for surgery and delivery
  1500 mL of glucose-free normal saline
Drugs
  Avoid vasodilator drugs
  Ephedrine for hypotension unresponsive to fluid
    replacement
  Anesthetics (if required)
    Regional: serial small boluses
    General: emphasis on benzodiazepines and narcotics,
      low-dose inhalation agents

below that which causes symptoms are appropriate. In a woman with significant symptoms or pulmonary edema, standard therapy can be used with the concerns about the drugs as outlined earlier (remembering particularly that ACE inhibitors should be avoided). Congestive heart failure is one situation where maintaining a woman in the supine position may be beneficial by causing preload reduction with obstruction of return of inferior vena cava blood to the heart.

Thromboembolic Complications

The risk of venous thromboemboli increases fivefold during and immediately after pregnancy,[34,84] and there is arguably an increase in arterial emboli as well.[85,86] Both may be the result of a woman's hypercoagulable status during pregnancy, and the likelihood of venous thrombosis is increased by venous stasis. Prevention is optimal, and prophylactic full-dose heparin[87] or low-molecular-weight heparin is indicated in those at high risk of a thromboembolic complication, including women with thromboemboli during a previous pregnancy (a 4 to 15 percent risk), antithrombin III deficiency (a 70 percent risk), protein C deficiency (a 33 percent risk), protein S deficiency (17 percent), and the anticardiolipin antibody syndrome.[34] The resistance to activated protein C found in 3 to 5 percent of the population may eventually be shown to be a reason for prophylaxis as well.[88]

If a thrombus or embolus is identified, 5 to 10 days of intravenous heparin therapy followed by full-dose subcutaneous heparin is recommended.[34] If a thromboembolus is life-threatening (e.g., a massive pulmonary embolus or a thrombosed prosthetic valve), thrombolytic therapy can be used.[89]

Hypertension

Hypertension can be present before pregnancy (in 1 to 5 percent) and persist throughout pregnancy, or it can develop with pregnancy.[48,90] When normotensive women become pregnant, 5 to 7 percent will develop hypertension. Because of the marked early fall in systemic vascular resistance, this often does not occur until the second half of pregnancy. It has been called *pregnancy-induced* or *gestational hypertension* or *toxemia*. When associated with proteinuria, pedal edema, central nervous system (CNS) irritability, elevation of liver enzymes, and coagulation disturbances, the hypertension syndrome is called *preeclampsia*. If convulsions occur, the diagnosis is *eclampsia*. It is not clear that hypertension alone puts the mother or fetus at risk during pregnancy, but preeclampsia increases maternal risk (approx. 1 to 2 percent chance of CNS bleed, convulsions, or other severe systemic illness) and may cause fetal growth retardation (10 to 15 percent). Maternal and fetal morbidity and mortality increase still further with eclampsia.

Guidelines for the level of blood pressure control are not well established. Until more is known, an argument can be made for keeping the systolic pressure below 160 mmHg and the diastolic pressure below 100 mmHg. This may provide a margin of safety against severe hypertensive episodes and possibly will improve fetal survival. Nonpharmacologic therapy is preferable when possible, although it is not clearly defined. While strict bed rest may achieve blood pressure lowering, it is not generally recommended, although limitation of activity and reduction of stress is commonly advised.[68,90] Unless the patient has previously demonstrated salt-sensitive hypertension, sodium restriction is generally inadvisable, since pregnant women with hypertension have lower plasma volumes than normotensive women. If drug treatment is required, experience is greatest with methyldopa.[48] This otherwise infrequently used antihypertensive agent has been demonstrated to promote fetal survival and to result in children with normal mental and physical development. It may be that other drugs will achieve the same goal, but they have not been studied adequately. Initial therapy could also include a β-1 selective beta blocker or a diuretic. Calcium channel blockers have been proven to be effective.[49,50] As mentioned earlier, ACE inhibitors should not be used.

Pulmonary Hypertension

Whether pulmonary hypertension (Chap. 59) is primary or secondary to prolonged left-to-right shunting (Eisenmenger's syndrome), drug abuse, a primary vascular disease syndrome, or recurrent pulmonary emboli, maternal mortality ranges from 30 to 70 percent.[91-96] Even with maternal survival, fetal loss exceeds 40 percent. Maternal death can occur at any time during pregnancy, but the mother is most vulnerable during the time of labor and delivery and in the first postpartum week. If recognized early in pregnancy, interruption is advised. If this is declined, or if the pulmonary hypertension is recognized late in pregnancy, close follow-up is required. Intravascular volume depletion puts these patients at greatest risk. For this group in particular, the measures outlined in Table 92-3 are important. Systemic vascular resistance and pressure must be maintained in pulmonary hypertension patients who have a

right-to-left shunt (to minimize still further shunting), and meticulous attention to avoidance of air or thrombus emboli from intravenous catheters is essential to avoid systemic emboli in these patients. At the time of labor and delivery, a central venous line allows adequate fluid administration, and a radial artery catheter makes blood pressure and oxygen saturation determinations easier. These lines should be used for 48 to 72 h postdelivery.

Arrhythmias

In the woman with dizziness, palpitations, and lightheadedness, pregnancy offers many other explanations, but arrhythmias should be considered as a possible cause (Chap. 27). The rules for treatment should be the same as in the nonpregnant patient, with the possible exception that a rhythm causing hemodynamic instability should be treated somewhat more rapidly and aggressively because of the concern about diversion of blood flow away from the uterus. As always, if a potentially reversible cause can be identified, it should be corrected. If treatment is required, it should never be instituted without electrocardiographic documentation of the rhythm.

Tachyarrhythmias are as frequent during pregnancy as at other times. As always, the presence of *atrial* or *ventricular premature beats* or of *sinus tachycardia* are a reason to look for and to correct the cause but not a reason to institute specific treatment for arrhythmias.

Paroxysmal supraventricular tachycardia may occur somewhat more frequently than in the nonpregnant state, whether due to the mechanism of AV node reentry ("dual AV node mechanism") or to atrial ventricular reentry ("accessory pathway mechanism").[97-99] This is the most common sustained abnormal rhythm occurring with pregnancy. Initial treatment with vagal maneuvers is as appropriate as at other times. If medical treatment is required, intravenous adenosine or verapamil are effective. Cardioversion can be used if required, remembering that the rule of "never cardiovert an awake patient" is just as applicable during pregnancy as at any other time.[100] If recurrent episodes require a chronic day-to-day drug, verapamil or a beta blocker would seem optimal choices; digoxin may be effective, although it should be avoided if the patient has preexcitation. Management of *atrial fibrillation* and *flutter* should be as in the nonpregnant woman. If they occur in a woman with mitral stenosis, severe left ventricular dysfunction, or a previous thromboembolic event, antithrombotic therapy with heparin is indicated.

Ventricular tachycardia may occur during pregnancy.[101,102] If suggestive of a right ventricular outflow tract tachycardia (a left bundle branch block with vertical axis morphology), beta-blocker therapy may be effective. Emergency management of rapid ventricular tachycardia or ventricular fibrillation should be as recommended for the nonpregnant woman.[103,104] If possible, the pelvis should be rolled to the left to enhance blood return from the lower extremities.

If pregnancy has proceeded beyond 24 weeks and maternal survival is in question, emergency cesarean section could be considered.

A prolonged QT-interval syndrome can be diagnosed first during pregnancy.[105,106] If this is recognized and it is an acquired form (of course, almost always from drugs), the offending cause should be eliminated. If the syndrome is congenital, beta-blocker therapy during pregnancy is warranted. Implantable defibrillators have been used with recurrent ventricular arrhythmias, but their value remains unproven in this syndrome, even when unrelated to pregnancy. In patients with a congenital syndrome, transmission with autosomal dominance can affect the child.

Bradyarrhythmias may also occur during pregnancy. While they are a reason to look for a reversible cause, treatment is generally not required unless the patient has clear hemodynamic compromise. Complete heart block, which in this age group is most likely to be congenital in origin, is consistent with a successful pregnancy.[107] If required, a permanent pacemaker can be inserted.

Loss-of-Consciousness Spells

Pregnancy makes an assessment of a loss-of-consciousness spell even more difficult than usual. If a seizure disorder cannot be excluded as a cause, appropriate evaluation with electroencephalography is indicated. If a seizure is unlikely or excluded, the syndrome of syncope should include a consideration of the usual causes.

Endocarditis

Infective endocarditis can occur during pregnancy in women without a recognized heart abnormality, but structural abnormalities place individuals at much greater risk (Chap. 82). The clinical presentation of endocarditis is the same during pregnancy as at other times.[108,109] *Streptococcus* is the most common cause. Intravenous drug abusers are more likely to have staphylococcal infections, and women with genitourinary tract infections are more likely to have gram-negative infections, most commonly *Escherichia coli*. Optimal management includes prevention. Although it is not the recommendation of the American Heart Association committee addressing this issue,[110] most physicians caring for women with heart disease recommend antibiotic prophylaxis at the time of dental or surgical procedures or at the time of labor and delivery. If endocarditis does occur, it should be treated aggressively with medical therapy and the usual indications for surgery are appropriate during pregnancy. If open heart surgery is required late in pregnancy, simultaneous cesarean section should be considered.

Surgery

While not exactly a complication of pregnancy, pregnant women with heart disease have the same 0.5 to 2.0 percent chance of requiring surgery during pregnancy as those without heart disease. A number of rules are appropriate to consider.

Venous return must be maintained, and, when possible, surgery should be performed in the left lateral position. Unless there is severe congestive heart failure, volume loading with 1500 mL of normal saline prior to surgery or labor and delivery is important. This fluid should not include glucose at the time of labor and delivery because it can cause subsequent hypoglycemia in the newborn. In the woman who requires assisted ventilation, hyperventilation should be avoided as it decreases venous return. Pain relief should be assured to minimize the rise in catecholamine levels that would, in turn, decrease uterine blood flow. Fetal monitoring should be performed.

SPECIFIC FORMS OF HEART DISEASE

Other sections of this book discuss each of the following cardiovascular abnormalities in detail. The remainder of this chapter will relate the specific abnormalities to pregnancy and will consider the potential problems during pregnancy, the demonstrated risk to the mother and fetus, and the management of both mother and fetus during pregnancy. As discussed earlier, with each abnormality, antibiotic prophylaxis against endocarditis with dental or surgical procedures is as appropriate during pregnancy as at other times[110] and is recommended at labor and delivery.

Rheumatic Heart Disease

Worldwide, rheumatic fever remains a common and virulent disease. The resultant valve and myocardial disease is probably the most common cause of heart disease during pregnancy.[111] In the United States, clinically recognized rheumatic fever is uncommon and, when it does occur, appears to be associated with less severe heart disease.[112] Still, even in this country, there are regions where its incidence is increasing.[113] In a woman presenting with myocarditis, rheumatic fever as a cause should be considered, particularly if it is associated with fever, joint discomfort, subcutaneous nodules, erythema marginatum, or chorea, and if there is evidence of a group A streptococcal infection.[114] Rheumatic fever is the cause of almost all mitral stenosis; some isolated mitral, aortic, or tricuspid regurgitation; and of some double- and triple-valve disease. Definition of valve morphology by echocardiography can help define the etiology. Recognition of rheumatic fever as the cause of heart disease is important because it identifies those who need antibiotic prophylaxis to prevent recurrence of the disease; people at highest risk of developing rheumatic fever are those who have had it in the past. Twice-daily penicillin is the treatment regimen of choice, and this should be continued throughout pregnancy.[115]

Valve Disease

MITRAL STENOSIS
When present, mitral stenosis is caused almost exclusively by rheumatic fever, and the lesion is more common in women

than in men (Chap. 64). The increased cardiac output, tachycardia, and fluid retention of pregnancy may double the resting pressure gradient across a stenotic mitral valve.[116] Symptoms attributable to an increase in left atrial pressure with associated pulmonary vascular congestion and bronchial vein distension occur in up to 25 percent of patients with mitral stenosis during pregnancy.[117,118] They usually become apparent by the 20th week and may be aggravated still further at the time of labor and delivery with the associated increases in heart rate and cardiac output. Maternal death is rare when there is careful attention to the management of congestive heart failure. While potentially at risk from the elevated left atrial pressure, the patient with mitral stenosis also depends on this pressure to fill the left ventricle and maintain cardiac output. Because the pregnant woman is especially liable to sudden shifts in the distribution of blood volume, preservation of an adequate intravascular volume is essential to prevent a dramatic fall in cardiac output.

If a woman contemplating pregnancy has symptomatic mitral valve stenosis, balloon dilation or valve surgery is appropriate before conception. If mitral stenosis is first recognized during pregnancy and symptoms develop, standard medical therapy is appropriate. If this does not control symptoms, balloon valvuloplasty can be performed (with appropriate radiation shielding to the fetus).[119] Mitral valve surgical commissurotomy or valve replacement has been performed, but fetal loss exceeds 30 percent.[120,121] Atrial fibrillation is of particular concern during pregnancy. The usual rapid ventricular response further compromises diastolic flow time and can result in pulmonary edema. Emergency treatment should include intravenous verapamil or cardioversion. Chronic daily digoxin is recommended in patients with mitral stenosis during pregnancy to minimize the chance of a rapid ventricular response should atrial fibrillation occur.

MITRAL REGURGITATION

Mitral regurgitation may be due to rheumatic fever, but unlike mitral stenosis, the majority of cases are due to other causes. Whatever the cause, in general it is well tolerated during pregnancy. If symptoms do occur, fatigue or dyspnea is most common. Treatment for congestive heart failure should be as described earlier. Afterload reduction is an important component of this therapy, remembering that ACE inhibitors should not be used. One cause of mitral regurgitation is *mitral valve prolapse* (Chap. 65). This deserves discussion not because it carries any particular risk during pregnancy but because it is so common, occurring in 5 to 10 percent of young adults. The volume and pressure changes of pregnancy may alter examination findings in a woman with mitral valve prolapse. Possibly associated arrhythmias, endocarditis, cerebral emboli, and hemodynamically significant regurgitation are rare complications and no more likely to occur in pregnancy than at other times.[122–124] The physical examination is sufficient for diagnosis—diagnostic studies, including an echocardiogram, do little to benefit the patient. Antibiotic prophylaxis at the time of labor and delivery is recommended in those with a heart murmur.

AORTIC STENOSIS

More common in males, aortic valve stenosis is an unusual finding in pregnancy but does occur. The diagnostic criteria are the same during pregnancy as at other times. Concerns from an early review indicating high maternal and fetal mortality rates[125] should be tempered by more recent information (although still small numbers) that demonstrates that pregnancy can be carried through with little or no maternal mortality and with no clear increase in fetal loss.[126–128] The offspring can have as high as a 20 percent incidence of congenital heart disease, a value that interestingly can potentially be halved by correcting the outflow tract obstruction prior to pregnancy.[93]

If severe stenosis is recognized before pregnancy, balloon valvotomy or a surgical commissurotomy is recommended prior to conception. If pregnancy does occur in the presence of severe aortic stenosis, measures to avoid hypovolemia are particularly important (see Table 92-3). If congestive heart failure develops, it can be treated as previously described, with emphasis, again, on the need to avoid excessive diuresis. If severe symptoms persist, a balloon valvuloplasty or aortic valve surgery can be performed during pregnancy,[129,130] the latter being associated with increased fetal loss.

AORTIC REGURGITATION

Unlike aortic stenosis, which is almost always congenital in etiology, aortic regurgitation has other causes and is encountered more frequently during pregnancy. These causes include rheumatic fever, endocarditis, dilation of the aortic root, or, more ominously, aortic dissection. A dilated root or dissection should raise the consideration of Marfan's syndrome as a cause. Aortic regurgitation is generally well tolerated during pregnancy. Congestive heart failure may occur but responds to treatment, with an emphasis on afterload reduction—again with a warning to avoid ACE inhibitors. If endocarditis should occur and the infection is not rapidly controlled, mortality with medical therapy is high and surgical therapy is indicated. If this occurs late in pregnancy, consideration of associated cesarean section is appropriate.

PULMONARY VALVE DISEASE

Many women with pulmonic valve disease will have had previous valve comissurotomy or balloon valvuloplasty for valve stenosis or as part of the correction of tetralogy of Fallot. The residual stenosis and invariable regurgitation are potential concerns but in general do not adversely affect the outcome of pregnancy. The occasional patient with significant pulmonic valve stenosis who has not been treated appears to tolerate pregnancy well. Intravascular volume depletion should be avoided. If severe symptoms (recurrent syncope, uncontrolled dyspnea, and chest pain) occur, balloon valvuloplasty can be performed.

TRICUSPID VALVE DISEASE

Significant tricuspid valve disease is also uncommon during pregnancy. The incidence of regurgitation has increased because of intravenous drug use, with its resultant right-sided endocarditis. This regurgitation requires no specific therapy during pregnancy. Tricuspid stenosis is rare. If encountered, avoidance of intravascular volume depletion would seem to be important.

PROSTHETIC VALVE DISEASE

An artificial valve can perhaps be considered the ultimate form of valve disease. While many have benefitted from these valves, all are left with "prosthetic heart valve disease." Consisting of one or more of the major complications of thromboemboli, bleeding (from anticoagulation), endocarditis, valve dysfunction, reoperation, or death, this affects patients at a rate of 5 percent per year throughout their lives.[131,132] Pregnancy increases the risks of each of these complications, and the prosthetic valve and its treatment can adversely affect the fetus.[78,133–136] All these are reasons that a prosthetic valve is a relative contraindication to pregnancy. Still, women with prosthetic valves often become pregnant. Anticoagulation is required in those with a *mechanical* prosthesis. While some have suggested that warfarin is acceptable anticoagulation,[136] most would advise avoidance, particularly in the first and third trimesters.[78] Full-dose subcutaneous heparin (maintaining the partial thromboplastin time between 1.5 and 2.5 normal) is the therapy of choice. Low-molecular-weight heparin once a day may be a reasonable alternative but has not been well evaluated in patients with prosthetic valves.[87] A *heterograft* or *homograft* prosthesis is an alternative to a mechanical prosthesis. Because of their inherently lower thromboembolic rates, anticoagulation is not needed. This opportunity to avoid anticoagulation therapy is a logical argument for using these prostheses in young women who are contemplating pregnancy. However, these valves do not completely eliminate the concern about thromboemboli, and the rate of heterograft degeneration is high in young women, resulting in the need for early valve replacement[137] (see Chap. 68).

Congenital Heart Disease

Congenital heart disease is now the most common heart disease encountered in women of childbearing age in the United States. In most, it has been altered by surgery. Each abnormality is unique, but there are some issues that should be considered with all of them. First, some abnormalities significantly increase the risk of maternal morbidity and mortality during pregnancy (see Table 92-1). Second, there is an increased risk of fetal death, which increases with the severity of the maternal lesions. Third, the presence of a congenital cardiac abnormality in either parent or in a sibling increases the risk of cardiac and other congenital abnormalities in the fetus. Congenital heart disease is recognized in 0.8 percent of all live births in the United States.[138,139] Its presence in a parent increases this risk to 2 to 15 percent (see Table 92-2).[139–146] While some

have shown that the risk is two to three times greater if it is the mother rather than the father who has congenital heart disease,[144,146] this finding has not been universal.[145] Actually, the risk that a child will have heart disease can reach 50 percent when the abnormality is transmitted as an autosomal dominant trait, as in the case of Marfan's syndrome, the congenital long QT syndrome, or hypertrophic cardiomyopathy. When recognized, maternal congenital heart disease should be corrected prior to surgery. In some cases, this will make the pregnancy safer for the mother but may also provide a better intrauterine environment for fetal development. Fourth, residual or inoperable lesions require careful understanding before pregnancy is undertaken. Finally, as with valve disease, antibiotic prophylaxis against endocarditis is as appropriate during pregnancy as at other times in patients with lesions that render them susceptible to this complication.

LEFT-TO-RIGHT SHUNTS

Some women with left-to-right shunts reach adulthood and become pregnant, often without previous recognition of their disease. Although left-to-right shunting increases the chances of pulmonary hypertension, right ventricular failure, arrhythmias, and emboli, it is not clear that these complications are made more likely by a pregnancy. The degree of shunting is affected by the relative resistances of the systemic and pulmonary vascular circuits, both of which fall to a similar degree during pregnancy.[147] In general, there is no significant alteration in the degree of shunting with pregnancy. The right ventricular volume overload associated with the shunts is generally well tolerated during pregnancy.

In the United States, most patients with left-to-right shunts will have undergone surgical correction prior to pregnancy. If anything, this surgery makes pregnancy safer, and there is no clear increase in mortality in these patients with pregnancy when they are compared to women with normal hearts.[148] The surgery does not influence the incidence of congenital heart disease in the offspring.

Atrial Septal Defect

The symptoms and signs of an atrial septal defect can be subtle and the abnormality may not be recognized before pregnancy. In women with an ostium secundum defect, pregnancy is generally well tolerated by the mother and the fetus, a reason that surgical correction prior to pregnancy has no significant effect on maternal morbidity and mortality. When either parent has an atrial septal defect, 5 to 10 percent of their children will have congenital heart disease. This is not affected by corrective surgery in the mother.[144,145] Ostium primum defects are equally well tolerated during pregnancy, unless associated with other significant congenital cardiovascular abnormalities.

Ventricular Septal Defect

Over half of ventricular septal defects close in childhood, and since the murmur is usually detected in those in whom the lesion persists, an unrecognized defect at the time of pregnancy is uncommon. If present, however, pregnancy is generally well tolerated. The occasional congestive heart failure or arrhythmias developing during pregnancy can be managed as described previously. If there is no associated pulmonary hypertension, there is no increase in maternal mortality with pregnancy. Fetal loss in women with uncorrected lesions may approach 20 percent. A child has a 5 to 8 percent chance of being born with a cardiac defect; again, this incidence is not altered by previous surgical correction of the defect.[144]

Patent Ductus Arteriosus

Like the other left-to-right shunts, a patent ductus is tolerated well during pregnancy. On occasion, congestive heart failure can occur, but standard treatment is effective. Antibiotic prophylaxis against endocarditis is recommended. Fetal loss is not clearly greater than that occurring in women without heart disease.

RIGHT-TO-LEFT SHUNT ("CYANOTIC" HEART DISEASE)

Right-to-left shunting can occur through an atrial or ventricular septal defect or a patent ductus arteriosus when pulmonary vascular resistance exceeds systemic vascular resistance or when there is an obstruction to right ventricular outflow and pulmonary vascular resistance is normal. All are forms of "cyanotic" heart disease. The presence of cyanosis, especially when sufficient to result in elevated hemoglobin levels, is associated with high fetal loss, prematurity, and reduced infant birth weights (see Fig. 92-5).[93,149,150] The elevated pulmonary vascular resistance situation, Eisenmenger's syndrome, has been discussed earlier under "Pulmonary Hypertension," but it is worth repeating that with this problem it is advisable to avoid or interrupt pregnancy. When the cyanosis is not due to Eisenmenger's syndrome, maternal mortality is less, but women are at increased risk of heart failure (approximately 15 percent) from thromboemboli, arrhythmias, and endocarditis (4.5 percent).[149]

Tetralogy of Fallot

This is the most common form of right-to-left shunting resulting from obstruction to pulmonary flow when pulmonary vascular resistance is normal. If uncorrected, successful pregnancy can be achieved, but maternal mortality is high and fetal loss can exceed 50 percent. After surgical correction, maternal mortality does not clearly exceed that of a woman without heart disease[148,151]; the offspring have a 5 to 10 percent chance of having congenital heart disease.

OBSTRUCTIVE LESIONS

Two recommendations apply in women with obstructive cardiac lesions. First, volume depletion should be avoided since it can result in a significant fall in cardiac output whether the obstruction is on the left or right side of the heart. Second, surgical or catheter treatment for the obstructive lesion is recommended prior to pregnancy, not only to increase maternal safety but also to decrease the chance of congenital heart disease in the offspring.[143]

Obstruction to flow from the *right ventricle* is preferably corrected prior to pregnancy. This approach will decrease maternal morbidity and may decrease the incidence of congenital heart disease in the offspring.[143] If an obstructive lesion persists into pregnancy, prevention of intravascular volume depletion is important.

Obstructive lesions to the left side of the heart include previously described aortic valve stenosis. There is very little experience with isolated supravalvular aortic stenosis, bands, or with subvalvular bands, but the approach recommended for aortic valve stenosis would seem applicable. Two other left ventricular obstructive disease processes warrant some discussion: coarctation of the aorta and hypertrophic obstructive cardiomyopathy.

Coarctation of the Aorta

This condition is more common in men but may occur in women and, as in men, may be associated with a bicuspid aortic valve (Chaps. 70 and 71). Affected individuals may reach childbearing age and may conceive. Maternal mortality rates range from 3 to 8 percent.[152] Surgical correction prior to pregnancy reduces the risk of aortic dissection or rupture,

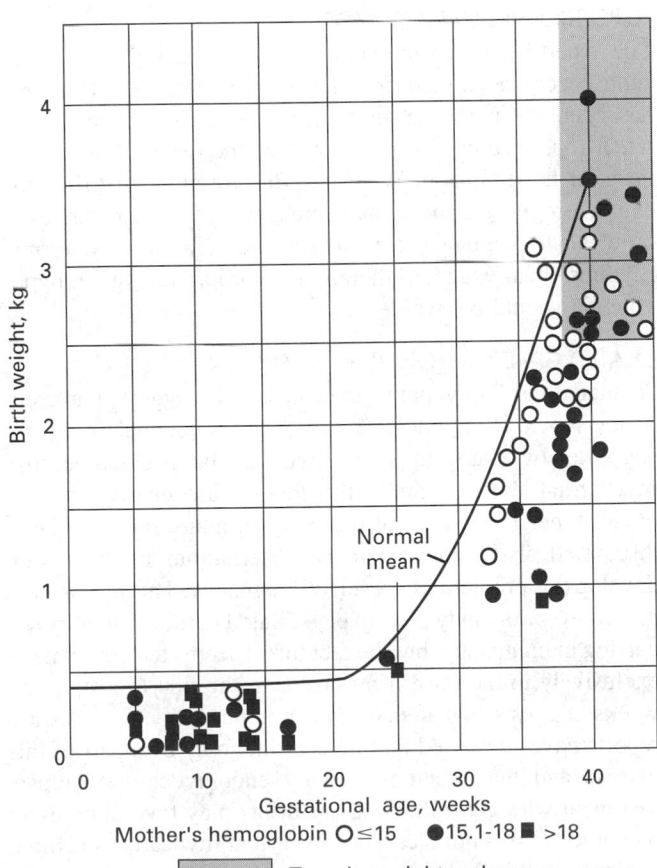

FIGURE 92-5

This figure shows that the severity of maternal cyanosis as manifest by the hemoglobin level relates directly to fetal loss (gestational age <20), to prematurity, and to infant birth weight. (From Neill and Swanson.[150] Reproduced with permission of the publisher and authors.)

and thus death, to less than 1 percent.[153,154] If pregnancy occurs in a woman with a coarctation, blood pressure control, as described previously, is appropriate. Antibiotic prophylaxis is needed because of the associated bicuspic aortic valve. The effects of catheter dilation of a coarctation on subsequent pregnancies are uncertain, but it would seem that they are as likely to decrease the risks associated with pregnancy as the surgical procedure. It is not clear if mechanical treatment decreases the rate of rupture of associated intracranial aneurisms.

Hypertrophic Obstructive Cardiomyopathy

Hypertrophic obstructive cardiomyopathy (HOCM) is inherited as an autosomal dominant trait with variable penetrance, and thus offspring have a 50 percent chance of having the same abnormality (see Chaps. 7 and 74). The fall in peripheral vascular resistance and peripheral pooling of blood can cause hypotension, and the intermittent high catecholamine state of pregnancy can increase left ventricular outflow tract obstruction. An increase in the symptoms of dyspnea, chest discomfort, and palpitations has been noted during pregnancy.[155,156] It is not clear that pregnancy increases the approximately 1 to 3 percent chance per year of sudden death, although a death has been reported with this syndrome during pregnancy.[157] This is another obstructive lesion where it is important to avoid hypovolemia. Beta-blocker therapy has been recommended at the time of labor and delivery; the concept makes sense, although it is of unproven value.

COMPLEX CONGENITAL LESIONS

The predictability of the outcome of pregnancy is more difficult as maternal abnormalities become more complex. In general, maternal and fetal morbidity and mortality are high, particularly when the abnormality results in maternal cyanosis. Still, surgery has made pregnancy a consideration, even in women with the most severe disease such as a functional single ventricle or tricuspid atresia.[158]

Transposition of the Great Vessels

Women with d-transposition of the great arteries (some with single ventricles) may become pregnant. The little available information available indicates a very poor maternal and fetal outcome.[159] Partial or complete surgical correction of the lesion prior to pregnancy improves the outcome for the mother as well as for the fetus.[159–161] If l-transposition ("corrected" transposition) is not complicated by cyanosis, ventricular dysfunction, or heart block, pregnancy should be well tolerated.

Ebstein's Anomaly of the Tricuspid Valve

This condition may be mild and unrecognized during pregnancy. Increasing problems of right ventricular dysfunction, obstruction to right-sided heart flow, and right-to-left shunting resulting in cyanosis increase the risk to the woman during pregnancy. Maternal morbidity and mortality are low if the patient does not have severe disease, and fetal loss is approximately 25 percent: significant right-to-left shunting is a reason to avoid pregnancy.[162–164]

Marfan's Syndrome

It may be difficult to make the diagnosis of Marfan's syndrome, but it is important to do so because pregnancy is particularly dangerous for affected women. First, the risk of death from aortic rupture or dissection is high during pregnancy, particularly if the aortic root is enlarged (greater than 40 mm by echocardiography has been used as one criterion).[165,166] Second, the expected life span of the woman with Marfan's syndrome is reduced to about half of normal, implying that her years of motherhood will be limited. Third, half of the offspring will be affected with the syndrome. These are reasons that women with Marfan's syndrome should be advised to avoid pregnancy.[78] The risks are sufficient to recommend interruption if pregnancy has occurred. Should the parents elect to continue the pregnancy, activity should be restricted and hypertension prevented. Beta blockade has not yet been clearly proved to be of value when used on a prophylactic basis, but its use in pregnant patients with Marfan's syndrome seems reasonable. This is the one cardiovascular syndrome where cesarean delivery is recommended to avoid the hemodynamic stresses of labor.

Myocardial Disease

HYPERTROPHIC CARDIOMYOPATHY

The hypertrophic cardiomyopathies are characterized as "concentric" or "asymmetric." The asymmetric form (HOCM) has been discussed as an obstructive lesion. A concentric hypertrophic cardiomyopathy may be the result of aortic stenosis or hypertension. When *not* due to either of these, the cause, prognosis, and management are often unclear, even unrelated to pregnancy. If congestive heart failure or abnormal rhythms occur, standard therapy is appropriate. Again, hypovolemia should be avoided.

DILATED CARDIOMYOPATHY

A dilated cardiomyopathy is a reason to suggest that pregnancy should be avoided. This strong recommendation is not supported by data from prospective trials but is given because myocardial dysfunction is the feature associated with increased maternal and fetal mortality in many forms of heart disease. It also comes from the observations of those who develop this problem as a result of pregnancy. This *peripartum cardiomyopathy* may simply be a dilated cardiomyopathy occurring in pregnancy, but the fact that it seems to occur almost exclusively in the third trimester or in the first 6 postpartum weeks suggests that it may be a unique entity.[167–169] Case reports have suggested that myocarditis may be a part of this disease and that when proven by endomyocardial biopsy, treatment with anti-inflammatory drugs may favorably affect outcome.[170] It is not clear, however, that myocarditis is more common in this form of cardiomyopathy,[171] and a large prospective trial in other myocarditis situations has failed to support the value of treatment.[172] In the woman with a dilated cardiomyopathy during pregnancy, standard treatment for heart failure, thromboemboli, and arrhythmias is appropriate.[169]

If ventricular function does not return to normal after pregnancy, subsequent pregnancies have been associated with maternal mortality rates approaching 50 percent (Chap. 73). When ventricular function returns to normal, a subsequent pregnancy is possible, but maternal mortality still approaches 10 percent.[169,170,173]

Coronary Artery Disease

Chest discomfort is common during a normal pregnancy and for the most part is due to abdominal distension or gastroesophageal reflux. Coronary artery disease is an uncommon but possible cause, and both angina and myocardial infarctions have been reported during pregnancy. Coronary artery disease in pregnancy can result from atherosclerosis, particularly in those with familial hyperlipidemia, diabetes, hypertension, or a smoking history, but this is rare. Other explanations have been dissection of the coronary artery, spasm, emboli, or vasculitis.[174–177] Vasculitis can result from Kawasaki's disease ("mucocutaneous lymph node syndrome")[178,179] or from Takayasu's disease, which is much more frequent in women than in men, causes proximal artery stenosis, and can affect the coronary arteries.[180,181] If coronary artery disease is a consideration, an electrocardiogram and exercise stress test may help with the diagnosis. If essential, thallium imaging or angiography can be performed. When suspected or demonstrated, coronary artery disease should be treated with standard medical therapy. If symptoms are not relieved, angioplasty or bypass surgery can be performed.[182,183]

Pregnancy following Cardiac Transplantation

Many cardiac transplant recipients are women of childbearing age (Chap. 25). Successful pregnancies after transplantation have been reported,[184] but the potential hazards to the mother and fetus, which include maternal heart failure, immunosuppressive therapy, maternal infections, and serial diagnostic studies, have already been recognized as causing problems in the fetus and in newborns. The potential for a shortened maternal life span must also be considered when a patient is counseled about the advisability of pregnancy.

REFERENCES

1. McAnulty JH, Morton MJ, Ueland K. The Heart and pregnancy. *Curr Probl Cardiol* 1988; 13:589–665.
2. McAnulty JH. Heart diseases in pregnancy. In: Kloner RA, ed. *Guide to Cardiology*. New York: LeJacq Communications; 1995.
3. Ueland K, Novy MJ, Peterson EN, Metcalfe J. Maternal cardiovascular dynamics: IV. The influence of gestational age on the maternal cardiovascular response to posture and exercise. *Am J Obstet Gynecol* 1969; 104:856–864.
4. Capeless EL, Clapp JF. Cardiovascular changes in early phase of pregnancy. *Am J Obstet Gynecol* 1989; 161:1449–1453.
5. Easterling TR, Benedetti TJ, Schmucher BC, Millard SP. Maternal hemodynamics in normal and preeclamptic pregnancies: A longitudinal study. *Obstet Gynecol* 1990; 76:1061–1069.
6. Robson SC, Hunter S, Boys RJ, Dunlop W. Serial study of factors influencing changes in cardiac output during human pregnancy. *Am J Physiol* 1989; 256:H1060–H1065.
7. Clark SL, Cotton DB, Pivarnik JM, Lee W, Hankins GDV, Benedetti TJ, et al. Position change and central hemodynamic profile during normal third-trimester pregnancy and post partum. *Am J Obstet Gynecol* 1991; 164:883–887.
8. Sady MA, Haydon BB, Sady SP, Carpenter MW, Thompson PD, Coustan DR. Cardiovascular response to maximal cycle exercise during pregnancy and at two and seven months post partum. *Am J Obstet Gynecol* 1990; 162:1181–1185.
9. Kerr MG. The mechanical effects of the gravid uterus in late pregnancy. *J Obstet Gynaecol Br Commonw* 1965; 72:513–529.
10. Kinsella SM, Lohmann G. Supine hypotensive syndrome, (review). *Obstet Gynecol* 1994; 83:774–788.
11. Robson S, Dunop W, Boys R, Hunter S. Cardiac output during labor. *Br Med J* 1987; 295:1169–1172.
12. James C, Banner T, Caton D. Cardiac output in women undergoing cesarean section with epidural or general anesthesia. *Am J Obstet Gynecol* 1989; 160:1178–1183.
13. Rovinsky JJ, Jaffin H. Cardiovascular hemodynamics in pregnancy. II. Cardiac output and left ventricular work in multiple pregnancy. *Am J Obstet Gynecol* 1966; 95:781–784.
14. Metcalfe J, McAnulty JH, Ueland K. *Heart Disease in Pregnancy: Physiology and Management*. Boston: Little, Brown; 1986:1–54.
15. Thoresen M, Wesche J. Doppler measurements of changes in human mammary and uterine blood flow during pregnancy and lactation. *Acta Obstet Gynecol Scand* 1988; 67:741–745.
16. Lunell NO, Nylund LE, Lewlander R, Sarby B. Uteroplacental blood flow in preeclampsia, measurement with Indium-113m and a computer-linked gamma camera. *Clin Exp Hypertens* (B) 1982; 1:105–117.
17. Thaler I, Manor D, Itskovitz J, Rottem S, Levit N, Timor-Tritsch I, et al. Changes in uterine blood flow during human pregnancy. *Am J Obstet Gynecol* 1990; 162:121–125.
18. Guzman CA, Caplan R. Cardiorespiratory response to exercise during pregnancy. *Am J Obstet Gynecol* 1970; 108:600–607.
19. Morton MJ, Paul MS, Campos GR, Hart MV, Metcalfe J. Exercise dynamics in late gestation: Effects of physical training. *Am J Obstet Gynecol* 1985; 152:91–97.
20. Veille JC, Hellerstein HK, Bacevice AE. Maternal left ventricular performance during bicycle exercise. *Am J Cardiol* 1992; 69:1506–1508.
21. Rauramo I, Forss M. Effect of exercise on maternal hemodynamics and placental blood flow in healthy women. *Acta Obstet Gynecol Scand* 1988; 67:21–25.
22. Watson WJ, Katz VL, Hackney AC, Gall MM, McMurray RG. Fetal responses to maximal swimming and cycling exercise during pregnancy. *Obstet Gynecol* 1991; 77:382–386.
23. Clapp JF III, Capeless EL. Neonatal morphometrics after endurance exercise during pregnancy. *Am J Obstet Gynecol* 1990; 163:1805–1811.
24. Naeye RL, Peters EC. Working during pregnancy: Effects on the fetus. *Pediatrics* 1982; 69:724–727.
25. Lindheimer MC, Katz AL. Sodium and diuretics in pregnancy. *N Engl J Med* 1973; 299:891–894.
26. Chesley LC. Plasma and red cell volumes during pregnancy. *Am J Obstet Gynecol* 1972; 112:440–450.
27. Hart MV, Morton MJ, Hosenpud JD, Metcalfe J. Aortic function during normal human pregnancy. *Am J Obstet Gynecol* 1986; 154:887–891.
28. Rovinsky JJ, Jaffin H. Cardiovascular hemodynamics in pregnancy. III. Cardiac rate, stroke volume, total peripheral resistance, and central blood volume in multiple pregnancy. Synthesis of results. *Am J Obstet Gynecol* 1966; 95:784–787.
29. Clark-Pearson DL, Jelovsek RD. Alterations of occlusive cuff impedance plethysmography results in the obstetric patient. *Surgery* 1981; 89:594–598.
30. Barrett JM, Vanhooydonk JD, Bochm FH. Pregnancy related rupture of arterial aneurysms. *Obstet Gynecol Surv* 1982; 37:557–566.
31. Anderson RA, Fineron PW. Aortic dissection in pregnancy: Importance of pregnancy-induced changes in the vessel wall and bicuspid aortic valve in pathogenesis. *Br J Obstet Gynaecol* 1994; 101:1085–1088.
32. Nolte JE, Rutherford RB, Nawaz S, Rosenbeger A, Speers WC, Krupsk WC. Arterial dissections associated with pregnancy (review). *J Vasc Surg* 1995; 21:515–520.
33. Elkayam U, Ostrzega E, Shotan A, Mehra A. Cardiovascular problems in pregnant women with the Marfan syndrome (review). *Ann Intern Med* 1995; 123:117–122.

34. Toglia MR, Weg JH. Venous thromboembolism during pregnancy: *N Engl J Med* 1996; 335:108–113.

35. Rubler S, Damani PM, Pinto ER. Cardiac size and performance during pregnancy estimated with echocardiography. *Am J Cardiol* 1977; 50:534–540.

36. Katz R, Karliner JS, Resnik R. Effects of a natural volume overload state (pregnancy) on left ventricular performance in normal human subjects. *Circulation* 1978; 58:434–441.

37. Sadaniantz A, Kocheril AG, Emans SP, Garber CE, Parisi AF. Cardiovascular changes in pregnancy evaluated by two-dimensional and Doppler echocardiography. *J Am Soc Echo* 1992; 5:253–258.

38. Morton MJ, Tsang H, Hohimer AR, Ross D, Thornburg K, Faber J, et al. Left ventricular size, output and structure during guinea pig pregnancy. *Am J Physiol* 1984; 246:R40–R48.

39. Milsom I, Hedner J, Hedner T. Plasma atrial natriuretic peptide (ANP) and maternal hemodynamic changes during normal pregnancy. *Acta Obstet Gynecol Scand* 1988; 67:717–722.

40. Schrier RW. Pathogenesis of sodium and water retention in high-output and low-output cardiac failure, nephrotic syndrome, cirrhosis and pregnancy. *N Engl J Med* 1988; 319:1065–1072.

41. Ginsberg JS, Hirsh J, Rainbow AG, Coastes G. Risks to the fetus of radiographic procedures used in the diagnosis of maternal venous thromboembolic disease. *Thromb Haemost* 1989; 61:189–196.

42. Collins R, Yusuf S, Peto R. Overview of randomized trials of diuretics in pregnancy. *Br Med J* 1985; 290:17–23.

43. Rogers MC, Willerson JT, Goldblatt A, Smith TW. Serum digoxin concentrations in the human fetus, neonate and infant. *N Engl J Med* 1972; 287:1010–1013.

44. Gonzalez AR, Phelps EJ, Cochran EB, Sibai BM. Digoxin-like immunoreactive substance in pregnancy. *Am J Obstet Gynecol* 1987; 157:660–664.

45. Ueland K, McAnulty JH, Ueland FR. Special considerations in the use of cardiovascular drugs. *Clin Obstet Gynecol* 1981; 24:809–823.

46. Rubin PC. Beta blockers in pregnancy. *N Engl J Med* 1982; 305:1323–1326.

47. Frishman WH, Chesner M. Beta-andrenergic blockers in pregnancy. *Am Heart J* 1988; 115:147–152.

48. Sibai BM. Treatment of hypertension in pregnant women (review). *N Engl J Med* 1996; 335:257–265.

49. Levin AC, Doering PL, Hatton RC. Use of nifedipine in the hypertensive diseases of pregnancy (review). *Ann Pharmacother* 1994; 28:1371–1378.

50. Wide-Swensson DH, Ingemarsson I, Lunell NO, Forman A, Skajaa K, Lindberg B, et al. Calcium channel blockade (isradipine) in treatment of hypertension in pregnancy: A randomized placebo-controlled study. *Am J Obstet Gynecol* 1995; 173:872–878.

51. Elkayam U, Goodwin TM. Adenosine therapy for supraventricular tachycardia during pregnancy. *Am J Cardiol* 1995; 75:521–523.

52. Cox JL, Gardner JM. Treatment of cardiac arrhythmias during pregnancy. *Prog Cardiovasc Dis* 1993; 36:137–178.

53. Page RL. Treatment of arrhythmias during pregnancy (review). *Am Heart J* 1995; 130:871–876.

54. Shnider SM, Way EL. Plasma levels of lidocaine in mother and newborn following obstetrical conduction anesthesia: Clinical applications. *Anesthesia* 1968; 29:951–955.

55. Juneja MM, Ackerman WE, Kaczorowski DM, Sollo DG, Gunzenhauser LF. Continuous epidural lidocaine infusion in the parturient with paroxysmal ventricular tachycardia. *Anesthesiology* 1989; 71:305–308.

56. Hill LM, Malkasian GD Jr. The use of quinidine sulfate throughout pregnancy. *Obstet Gynecol* 1979; 54:366.

57. Allen NM, Page RL. Procainamide administration during pregnancy. *Clin Pharm* 1993; 12:58–60.

58. Leonard RF, Braun TE, Levy AM. Initiation of uterine contractions by disopyramide during pregnancy. *N Engl J Med* 1978; 299:84.

59. Lownes HE, Ives TJ. Mexiletine use in pregnancy and lactation. *Am J Obstet Gynecol* 1987; 157:446–447.

60. Perry JC, Ayres NA, Carpenter RJ Jr. Fetal supraventricular tachycardia treated by flecainide acetate. *J Pediatr* 1991; 118:303–305.

61. Connaughton M, Jenkins BS. Successful use of flecainide to treat new onset maternal ventricular tachycardia in pregnancy. *Br Heart J* 1994; 72(3):297.

62. Wagner X, Jouglard J, Moulin M, Miller A, Petitjean J, Pisapia A. Coadministration of flecainide acetate and sotalol during pregnancy. *Am Heart J* 1990; 119:700–702.

63. Foster CJ, Love HG. Amiodarone in pregnancy. Case report and review of the literature. *Int J Cardiol* 1988; 20:307–316.

64. Ovadin M, Brito M, Hoyer GL, Marcus FI. Human experience with amiodarone in the embryonic period. *Am J Cardiol* 1994; 73:316–317.

65. Magee LA, Downar E, Sermer M, Boulton BC, Allen LC, Koren G. Pregnancy outcome after gestational exposure to amiodarone in Canada. *Am J Obstet Gynecol* 1995; 172:1307–1311.

66. Stempel JE, O'Grady JP, Morton MJ, Johnson KA. Use of sodium nitroprusside in complications of gestational hypertension. *Obstet Gynecol* 1982; 60:533–538.

67. Shoemaker CT, Meyers M. Sodium nitroprusside for control of severe hypertensive disease of pregnancy: A case report and discussion of potential toxicity. *Am J Obstet Gynecol* 1984; 149:171–173.

68. Cunningham FG, Lindheimer MD. Hypertension in pregnancy. *N Engl J Med* 1992; 326:927–932.

69. Hanssens M, Keirse MJ, Vankelecom F, Van Assche F, Van Assche FA. Fetal and neonatal effects of treatment with angiotensin converting enzyme inhibitors in pregnancy. *Obstet Gynecol* 1991; 78:128–135.

70. Fillmore SJ, McDevitt E. Effects of Coumarin compounds on the fetus. *Ann Intern Med* 1970; 73:731–735.

71. Hall JT, Pauli RM, Wilson KM. Maternal and fetal sequelae of anticoagulation during pregnancy. *Am J Med* 1980; 68:122.

72. Stevenson RE, Burton M, Frelauto GH, Taylor HA. Hazards of oral anticoagulants during pregnancy. *JAMA* 1985; 243:1549–1551.

73. Iturbe-Alessio I, Fonseca MC, Mutchinik O, Santos M, Zajarias A, Salazar E. Risks of anticoagulant therapy in pregnant women with artificial heart valves. *N Engl J Med* 1986; 315:1390–1393.

74. Ginsberg JS, Hirsh J. Use of antithrombotic agents during pregnancy: A series of eight cases. *Can J Anaesth* 1994; 41:502–512.

75. Brabeck MC. Ambulatory management of thromboembolic diseases during pregnancy with continuous infusion of heparin. *JAMA* 1987; 257:1790–1791.

76. Ginsbert JS, Kowalchuk G, Hirsh J, Brill-Edwards P, Burrows R. Heparin therapy during pregnancy. *Arch Intern Med* 1989; 149:2233–2236.

77. Anderson DR, Ginsburg JS, Brill-Edwards P, Demers C, Burrows RF, Hirsh S. The use of an indwelling teflon catheter for subcutaneous heparin administration during pregnancy. *Arch Intern Med* 1993; 153:841–844.

78. Elkayam U. Anticoagulation in pregnant women with prosthetic heart valves: A double jeopardy (editorial). *J Am Coll Cardiol* 1996; 27:1704–1706.

79. Corby DG. Aspirin in pregnancy and fetal effects. *Pediatrics* 1978; 62:930–937.

80. Werler MM, Mitchell AA, Shapiro S. The relation of aspirin use during the first trimester of pregnancy to congenital cardiac defects. *N Engl J Med* 1989; 321:1639–1642.

81. DuBard MB, Cutter GR. Low-dose aspirin therapy to prevent pre-eclampsia. *Am J Obstet Gynecol* 1993; 168:1083–1091.

82. The Canadian Preterm Labor Investigators Group. Treatment of preterm labor with the beta-adrenergic agonist ritodrine. *N Engl J Med* 1992; 327:308–312.

83. McAnulty JH. Anesthesia during pregnancy in the patient with heart disease. In: Bonica JJ, McDonald JS, eds. *Principles and Practice of Obstetric Analgesia and Anesthesia*. Philadelphia: Lea & Febiger; 1994; 1013–1039.

84. Haemostatis and Thrombosis Task Force. Guidelines on the prevention, investigation and management of thrombosis associated with pregnancy. Maternal and neonatal haemostasis working papers of the haemostasis and thrombosis task force. *J Clin Pathol* 1993; 46:489–496.

85. Kittner SJ, Stern BJ, Feeser BR, Hebel JU, Nagey DA, Buchholz DW. Pregnancy and the risk of stroke. *N Engl J Med* 1996; 335:768–774.

86. Donaldson JO, Lee NS. Arterial and venous stroke associated with pregnancy. *Neurd Clin* 1994; 12:583–599.

87. Sturridge F, de Swiet M, Letsky E. The use of low molecular weight heparin for thrombophylaxis in pregnancy. *Br J Obstet Gynaecol* 1994; 101:69–71.

88. Hellgren M, Svensson PJ, Dahlback B. Resistance to activated protein C as a basis for venous thromboembolism associated with pregnancy and oral contraceptives. *Am J Obstet Gynecol* 1995; 173:210–213.

89. Turrentine MA, Braems G, Ramirez MM. Use of thrombolytics for the treatment of thromboembolic disease during pregnancy (review). *Obstet Gynecol Surv* 1995; 50:534–541.

90. National High Blood Pressure Education Program. Working Group report on high blood pressure in pregnancy. *Am J Obstet Gynecol* 1990; 163:1691–1712.

91. Dawkins K, Burke CM, Billingham M, Jamison SW. Primary pulmonary hypertension and pregnancy. *Chest* 1986; 89:383–388.

92. Gleicher N, Midwall JJ, Hochberger D, Jaffin H. Eisenmenger's syndrome and pregnancy. *Obstet Gynecol Surv* 1979; 34:721–741.

93. Whittemore R, Hobbins JC, Engle MA. Pregnancy and its outcome in women with and without surgical treatment of congenital heart disease. *Am J Cardiol* 1982; 50:641–651.

94. Avila S, Grinberg M, Snitcowsky R, Faccioli R, Da Luz PL, Bellott G, et al. Maternal and fetal outcome in pregnant women with Eisenmenger's syndrome. *Eur Heart J* 1995; 16:460–464.

95. Smedstad KG, Cramb R, Morrison DH. Pulmonary hypertension and pregnancy: A series of eight cases. *Can J Anaesth* 1994; 41:502–512.

96. Jeyamalar R, Sivanesaratnam V, Kuppuvelumani P. Eisenmenger syndrome in pregnancy. *Aust N Z J Obstet Gynaecol* 1992; 32:275–277.

97. Widerhorn J, Woderhorn AL, Rahimtoola SH, Elkayam U. WPW syndrome during pregnancy: Increased incidence of supraventricular arrhythmias. *Am Heart J* 1992; 123:796–798.

98. Tawam M, Levine J, Mendelson M, Goldberger J, Dyer A, Kadish A. Effect of pregnancy on paroxysmal supraventricular tachycardia. *Am J Cardiol* 1993; 72:838–840.

99. Lee SH, Chan SA, Wu TJ, Chiang CE, Cheng CC, Tai CT, et al. Effects of pregnancy on first onset and symptoms of paroxysmal supraventricular tachycardia. *Am J Cardiol* 1995; 76:675–678.

100. Rosemond RL. Cardioversion during pregnancy. *JAMA* 1993; 269(24):3167.

101. Brodsky M, Doria R, Allen V, Sato D. New onset ventricular tachycardia during pregnancy. *Am Heart J* 1992; 123:933–941.

102. Varon ME, Sherer DM, Abramowicz JS, Akiyama T. Maternal ventricular tachycardia associated with hypomagnesemia. *Am J Obstet Gynecol* 1992; 167:1352–1355.

103. Lee RV, Rodgers BD, Shite LM, Harvey RC. Cardiopulmonary resuscitation of pregnant women. *Am J Med* 1986; 81:311–318.

104. Dildy GA, Clark SL. Cardiac arrest during pregnancy. *Obstet Gynecol Clin North Am* 1995; 22:303–314.

105. Nakazato Y, Nakata Y, Tokano T, Ohno Y, Fujioka H, Hisaoka T, et al. Long-term follow-up study of three patients with the long QT syndrome. *Jpn Circ J* 1992; 56:1025–1031.

106. McCurdy CM, Rutherford SE, Coddington CC. Syncope and sudden arrhythmic death complicating pregnancy. A case report of Ramano-Ward Syndrome. *J Reprod Med* 2993; 38:233–234.

107. Dalvi BV, Chaudhuri A, Kulkarni HL, Kale PA. Therapeutic guidelines for congenital complete heart block presenting in pregnancy. *Obstet Gynecol* 1994; 79:802–804.

108. Seaworth BJ, Durack DT. Infective endocarditis in obstetric and gynecologic practice. *Am J Obstet Gynecol* 1986; 154:180–188.

109. Reid CL, Elkayam U, Rahimtoola SH. Infective endocarditis. In: Gleicher N, ed. *Principles and Practice of Medical Therapy in Pregnancy*, 2d ed. Norwalk, CT: Appleton & Lange; 1992; 795–801.

110. Dajani AS, Bisno AL, Chung KJ, Durack DT, Freed M, Gerber MA, et al. Prevention of bacterial endocarditis—recommendations by the American Heart Association. *JAMA* 1990; 264:2919–2922.

111. McAnulty JH. Rheumatic heart disease. In: Gleicher N, Gall SA, Sibai BM, Elkayam U, Galbraith RM, Sarto GE, eds. *Principles and Practice of Medical Therapy in Pregnancy*, 2d ed. Norwalk, CT: Appleton & Lange; 1992; 783–788.

112. Massell BF, Chute CG, Walker AM, Kurland GS. Penicillin and the marked decrease in morbidity and mortality from rheumatic fever in the United States. *N Engl J Med* 1988; 318:280–286.

113. Veasy LG, Widemeier SE, Orsmond GS, Ruttenburg HD, Boucek MM, Roth SJ, et al. Resurgence of acute rheumatic fever in the intermountain area of the United States. *N Engl J Med* 1987; 316:421–427.

114. Special Writing Group of the Committee on Rheumatic Fever, Endocarditis, and Kawasaki Disease of the Council on Cardiovascular Disease in the Young of the American Heart Association. Guidelines for the diagnosis of rheumatic fever: Jones criteria, 1992 update. *JAMA* 1992; 268:2069–2073.

115. Dajani AS, Bisno Al, Chung KJ, Durack DT, Gerber MA, Kaplan EL, et al. Prevention of rheumatic fever. *Circulation* 1988; 78:1082–1086.

116. Bryg RJ, Gordon PR, Kudesia VS, Bhatia RK. Effect of pregnancy on pressure gradient in mitral stenosis. *Am J Cardiol* 1989; 63:384–386.

117. Ueland K, Metcalfe J. Acute rheumatic fever in pregnancy. *Am J Obstet Gynecol* 1966; 95:586–587.

118. Stephen SJ. Changing patterns of mitral stenosis is childhood and pregnancy in Sri Lanka. *J Am Coll Cardiol* 1992; 19:1276–1284.

119. Esteves CA, Auristela IOR, Braga SLN, Harrison JK, Sonsa JEMR. Effectiveness of percutaneous balloon mitral valvotomy during pregnancy. *Am J Cardiol* 1991; 68:930–934.

120. Commerford PJ, Hastie T, Beck W. Closed mitral valvotomy: Actuarial analysis of results in 654 patients over 12 years and analysis of preoperative predictors of long-term survival. *Ann Thorac Surg* 1982; 33:473–479.

121. Chambers CE, Clark SL. Cardiac surgery during pregnancy (review). *Clin Obstet Gynecol* 1994; 37:316–323.

122. Shapiro EP, Trible EL, Robinson JC, Estruch MT, Gottlieb SH. Safety of labor and delivery in women with mitral valve prolapse. *Am J Cardiol* 1985; 56:806–807.

123. Degani S, Abinader EG, Scharf M. Mitral valve prolapse and pregnancy: A review. *Obstet Gynecol Surv* 1989; 72:113–118.

124. Cowles T, Gonik B. Mitral valve prolapse in pregnancy. *Semin Perinatol* 1990; 14:34–41.

125. Arias F, Pineda J. Aortic stenosis and pregnancy. *J Reprod Med* 1978; 20:229–232.

126. Easterling TR, Chadwick IIS, Otto CM, Benedetti TJ. Aortic stenosis in pregnancy. *Obstet Gynecol* 1988; 72:113–118.

127. Lao TT, Sermer M, McGee L, Farine D, Colman JM. Congenital aortic stenosis and pregnancy—a reappraisal (review). *Am J Obstet Gynecol* 1993; 169:540–545.

128. Banning AP, Pearson JF, Hall RJ. Role of balloon dilatation of the aortic valve in pregnant patients with severe aortic stenosis. *Br Heart J* 1993; 70:544–545.

129. Lao TT, Adelman AG, Sermer M, Colman JM. Balloon valvuloplasty for congenital aortic stenosis in pregnancy. *Br J Obstet Gynaecol* 1993; 100:1141–1142.

130. Sullivan HJ. Valvular heart surgery during pregnancy (review). *Surg Clin North Am* 1995; 75:59–75.

131. Bloomfield P, Wheatley DJ, Prescott RJ, Miller HC. Twelve-year comparison of a Bjork-Shirley mechanical heart valve with porcine bioprostheses. *N Engl J Med* 1991; 324:573–579.

132. Hammermeister KE, Sethi GK, Henderson WG, Oprian C, Kim T, Rahimtoola S. A comparison of outcomes in men 11 years after heart-valve replacement with a mechanical valve or bioprosthesis. *N Engl J Med* 1993; 328:1289–1296.

133. Sareli P, England MJ, Berk MR, Marcus RH, Epstein M, Driscoll J, et al. Maternal and fetal sequelae of anticoagulation during pregnancy in patients with mechanical heart valve prostheses. *Am J Cardiol* 1989; 63:1462–1465.

134. Vitali E, Donatelli F, Quaini E, Groppelli G, Pellegrini A. Pregnancy in patients with mechanical prosthetic heart valves. Our experience regarding 98 pregnancies in 57 patients. *J Cardiovasc Surg* 1986; 27:221–227.

135. Born D, Martinez EE, Almeida PA, Santos DV, Carvalho AC, Moron AF, et al. Pregnancy in patients with prosthetic heart valves: The effects of anticoagulation on mother, fetus, and neonate. *Am Heart J* 1992; 124:413–417.

136. Salazar E, Izaguirre R, Verdejo J, Mutchinick O. Failure of adjusted doses of subcutaneous heparin to prevent thromboembolic phenomena in pregnant patients with mechanical cardiac valve prostheses. *J Am Coll Cardiol* 1996; 27:1698–1703.

137. Jamieson WR, Miller DC, Akins CW, Munro AI, Glower DD, Moore KA, et al. Pregnancy and bioprostheses: Influence on structural valve deterioration. *Ann Thoracic Surg* 1995; 60:S282–S286.

138. Mitchell SC, Korones SB, Berendes HW. Congenital heart disease in 56,109 births: Incidence and natural history. *Circulation* 1971; 43:323–332.

139. Nora JJ, Nora AH. The evolution of specific genetic and environmental counseling in congenital heart disease. *Circulation* 1978; 57:205–213.

140. Roberts N. A predictive study of congenital heart disease and need for care. *West J Med* 1978; 120:19–25.

141. McFaul PB, Dornan JC, Lamki H, Boyle D. Pregnancy complicated by maternal heart disease. A review of 519 women. *Br J Obset Gynaecol* 1988; 95:861–867.

142. Nora JJ, Nora AH. Maternal transmission of congenital heart diseases: New recurrence risk figures and the questions of cytoplasmic inheritance and vulnerability to teratogens. *Am J Cardiol* 1987; 59:459–463.

143. Whittemore R, Hobbins JC, Engle MA. Pregnancy and its outcome in women with and without surgical treatment of congenital heart disease. *Am J Cardiol* 1982; 50:641–651.

144. Morris CD, Menashe VD. Evidence for maternal transmission of congenital heart defects. *Circulation* 1993; 88(suppl):1–98.

145. Whittemore R, Wells JA, Castellsagne X. A second-generation study of 427 probands with congenital heart defects and their 837 children. *J Am Coll Cardiol* 1994; 23:1459–1467.

146. Nora J. From generational studies to a multilevel genetic-environmental interaction (editorial). *J Am Coll Cardiol* 1994; 23:1468–1471.

147. Metcalfe J, Ueland K. Maternal cardiovascular adjustments to pregnancy. *Prog Cardiovasc Dis* 1974; 16:363–374.

148. Morris CD, Manashe VD. 25-year mortality after surgical repair of congenital heart defect in childhood: A population-based cohort study. *JAMA* 1991; 266:3447–3452.

149. Presbytero P, Sommerville J, Stone S, Aruta E, Spiegelhalter D, Rabajoli F. Pregnancy and cyanotic congenital heart disease, outcome of mother and fetus. *Circulation* 1994; 89:2673–2676.

150. Neill CA, Swanson S. Outcome of pregnancy in congenital heart disease. *Circulation* 1961; 24:1003–1011.

151. Zellers TM, Driscoll DJ, Michaels VV. Prevalence of significant congenital heart defects in children of parents with Fallot's tetralogy. *Am J Cardiol* 1990; 65:523–526.

152. Deal D, Wooley CF. Coarctation of the aorta and pregnancy. *Ann Intern Med* 1973; 78:706–710.

153. Connolly HM, Ammash NM, Warnes CA. Pregnancy in women with coarctation of the aorta (abstr). *J Am Coll Cardiol* 1996; 27(suppl A):43A.

154. Pitkin RM, Perloff JK, Koos BJ, Beall MH. Pregnancy and congenital heart disease. *Ann Intern Med* 1990; 112:445–454.

155. Kolibash AJ, Ruis DE, Lewis RP. Idiopathic hypertrophic subaortic stenosis in pregnancy. *Ann Intern Med* 1975; 82:791–794.

156. Oakley GD, McGarry K, Limb DG, Oakley CM. Management of pregnancy in patients with hypertrophic cardiomyopathy. *Br Med J* 1979; 1:1749–1750.

157. Shah DM, Sunderji SG. Hypertrophic cardiomyopathy and pregnancy: Report of a maternal mortality and review of literature. *Ebstet Gynecol Surv* 1985; 40:444–448.

158. Conobbio MM, Mair DD, Velde M, Koos BJ. Pregnancy outcomes after the Fontan repair. *J Am Coll Cardiol* 1996; 28:763–767.

159. Patton DE, Lee W, Cotton DB, Miller J, Carpenter RJ Jr, Huhta J, et al. Cyanotic maternal heart disease in pregnancy. *Obstet Gynecol Surv* 1990; 45:594–600.

160. Clarkson PM, Wilson NJ, Neutze JM, North RA, Calder AL, Barratt-Boyes BG. Outcome of pregnancy after the Mustard operation for transposition of the great arteries with intact ventricular septum. *J Am Coll Cardiol* 1994; 24:190–193.

161. Perloff JK. Pregnancy and congenital heart disease. *J Am Coll Cardiol* 1991; 18:340–342.

162. Waickman LA, Skorton DJ, Varner MW, Ehmke DA, Goplerud CP. Ebstein's anomaly and pregnancy. *Am J Cardiol* 1984; 53:357–358.

163. Wooley CF, Sparks EH. Congenital heart disease, heritable cardiovascular disease, and pregnancy. *Prog Cardiovasc Dis* 1992; 35:41–60.

164. Connolly HM, Warnes CA. Ebstein's anomaly: Outcome of pregnancy. *J Am Coll Cardiol* 1994; 23:1194–1198.

165. Mor-Yosef S, Younis J, Granat M, Kedari A, Milgalter A, Schenker JG. Marfan's syndrome in pregnancy. *Obstet Gynecol Surv* 1988; 43:382–385.

166. Pyeritz RE. Maternal and fetal complications of pregnancy in the Marfan syndrome. *Am J Med* 1981; 71:784–790.

167. Damakil JG, Rahimtoola SH, Sutton GC, Meadows WR, Szanto PB, Tobin JR, et al. Natural course of peripartum cardiomyopathy. *Circulation* 1971; 44:1053–1061.

168. O'Connell JB, Costanzo-Mordin MR, Surbranian R, Robinson JA, Wallis DE, Scandon PJ. Peripartum cardiomyopathy: Clinical, hemodynamic, histologic and prognostic characteristics. *J Am Coll Cardiol* 1986; 8:52–56.

169. Lampert MB, Lang RM. Peripartum cardiomyopathy. *Am Heart J* 1995; 130:860–870.

170. Melvin KR, Richardson PJ, Olsen EG, Daly K, Jackson G. Peripartum cardiomyopathy due to myocarditis. *N Engl J Med* 1982; 308:731–734.

171. Rizeq MN, Rickenbacher PR, Fowler MB, Billingham ME. Incidence of myocarditis in peripartum cardiomyopathy. *Am J Cardiol* 1994; 74:474–477.

172. Parrilo JE, Cunnion RE, Epstein SE, Parker MM, Suffredini AF, Brenner M, et al. A prospective, randomized, controlled trial of prednisone for dilated cardiomyopathy. *N Engl J Med* 1989; 321:1061–1068.

173. Sutton MS, Cole P, Plappert M, Saltzman D, Goldhaber S. Effects of subsequent pregnancy on left ventricular function in peripartum cardiomyopathy. *Am Heart J* 1991; 121:1776–1778.

174. Ciraulo DA, Markovitz A. Myocardial infarction in pregnancy associated with a coronary artery thrombus. *Arch Intern Med* 1979; 139:1046–1047.

175. Beary JF, Summer WR, Bulkley BH. Postpartum acute myocardial infarction: A rare occurrence of uncertain etiology. *Am J Cardiol* 1979; 43:158–161.

176. Ahronheim JH. Isolated coronary periarteritis: Report of a case of unexpected death in a young pregnant woman. *Am J Cardiol* 1977; 40:287–290.

177. Jewett J. Two dissecting coronary-artery aneurysms post partum. *N Engl J Med* 1978; 298:1255–1256.

178. Nolan TE, Savage RW. Peripartum myocardial infarction from presumed Kawasaki's disease. *South Med J* 1990; 83:360–361.

179. Taubert KA, Rowley AH, Shulman ST. Nationwide survey of Kawasaki disease and acute rheumatic fever. *J Pediatr* 1991; 119:279–282.

180. Ishikawa A, Matsura S. Occlusive thromboaortopathy (Takayasu's disease) and pregnancy. *Am J Cardiol* 1982; 50:1293–1300.

181. Railton A, Allen DG. Takayasu's arteritis in pregnancy. A report of 4 cases. *S Afr Med J* 1988; 73:123–127.

182. Cowan NC, de Belder MA, Rothman MT. Coronary angioplasty in pregnancy. *Br Heart J* 1988; 59:588–592.

183. Majden JF, Walinsky P, Cowchock SF, Wagner RJ, Plzak L Jr. Coronary artery bypass surgery during pregnancy. *Am J Cardiol* 1983; 52:1145–1151.

184. Kirk EP. Organ transplantation during pregnancy. *Am J Obstet Gynecol* 1991; 164:1629–1634.

CHAPTER

93

THE HEART AND OBESITY

James K. Alexander

ADIPOSE TISSUE CIRCULATION

In adipose tissue, an extensive capillary network surrounds each adipocyte, providing morphologic evidence that the vascular bed is well dimensioned for transcapillary exchange, with passage of free fatty acids between blood and adipocyte facilitated by a high capillary filtration coefficient, almost twice that of skeletal muscle.[1] In humans, basal blood flow to adipose tissue is approximately 3 mL/min per 100 g, rising to as much as 60 mL/min per 100 g with maximal vasodilatation induced by norepinephrine infusion,[2] which is nitric oxide–dependent.[3]

Of considerable importance is the degree to which adipose tissue serves as a blood volume reservoir and to which lipocyte metabolism is flow-dependent. With hemorrhage-induced hypotension in dogs, the decrement in adipose tissue blood volume and flow is much greater than that in other organs, and adipose tissue oxygen uptake falls concomitantly.[4] In addition to metabolic demands and circulating blood volume, a variety of factors may produce profound hemodynamic alterations in the adipose tissue's vascular bed, including sympathetic nervous system influences, humoral agents, blood and tissue oxygen tension, blood pH, temperature, exercise, and mechanical compression.[1] Histologic studies have demonstrated "block devices" in the walls of small arteries and arterioles with the capacity to regulate capillary blood flow.[5]

Since the adipose tissue's blood flow is a function of both cell number and size,[6] increments in adipose depot volume secondary to either cellular hyperplasia or hypertrophy are accompanied by augmented flow. In extremely obese subjects, for example, in whom both hyperplasia and hypertrophy exist, the blood flow in adipose tissue may approximate one-half the total cardiac output at rest.[7] Weight loss in obese subjects involves a reduction in the size but not the number of adipocytes. Cardiac output falls as regression of adipocyte hypertrophy lowers the total adipose tissue weight and flow,[8] although the flow per gram of adipose tissue may actually increase.[9]

OBESITY AND HYPERTENSION

Epidemiologic studies clearly implicate obesity as a health hazard for hypertension, but the correlation between the overall incidence of hypertension and obesity is relatively low,[10] being highest in young men and black women.[11] Most obese people are not hypertensive, and even with extreme obesity, one-third are normotensive.[12] The mechanisms of obesity-induced hypertension differ from those of essential or renovascular hypertension (Chap. 56), as suggested by the observations that (1) measurements of blood volume and renin levels of obese subjects do not correlate with the presence or absence of hypertension[13] and (2) systemic vascular resistance is less while cardiac output and pulse-wave velocity are greater in obese than in lean hypertensive individuals.[13,14] A predominantly abdominal distribution of body fat appears to correlate better with the presence of hypertension than does relative weight or body mass[15] and is often associated with a triad of obesity, hypertension, and hyperinsulinemia[16] (see also Chap. 41). That insulin resistance and hyperinsulinemia may play a role in the pathogenesis of obesity-induced hypertension is suggested by a correlation of blood pressure and plasma insulin levels in obese subjects,[17,18] which also occurs with weight loss.[19] Epidemiological studies, however, suggest that hyperinsulinemia is not consistently associated with hypertension.[20] Furthermore, chronic hyperinsulinemia due to insulinoma does not cause hypertension, and blood pressure does not fall after tumor resection.[21,22] These observations and long-term laboratory studies negate hyperinsulinemia as the sole major factor in the pathogenesis of hypertension among the obese.[23] A hypertensive response to hyperinsulinemia and insulin resistance conditioned by genetic factors has been suggested, however.[24] Thus the pathophysiologic mechanism of obesity-induced hypertension is not yet defined. There is no firm supporting evidence for several other hypotheses, including elevated aldosterone levels, altered response to pressor agents, and mechanical capillary compression in adipose depots.

Direct intraarterial pressure measurements indicate that arterial hypertension is not artifactual in obese subjects.[12] When the degree of obesity is not extreme, a reasonable approximation of blood pressure level may be obtained by utilizing a cuff containing a bladder 42 cm in length.[25] In very obese individuals with unusual arm configuration, who have difficulty in wearing the cuff or whose readings are inconsistent, direct intraarterial measurement is recommended before prolonged antihypertensive therapy is initiated.

Weight reduction, an important therapeutic consideration in obesity-induced hypertension, produces a decrease in blood pressure in a large percentage of obese patients.[26,27] This decrement is poorly correlated with the amount of weight loss, often occurring early with a later plateau,[28] but it may be associated with several other potentially desirable effects, including improved glucose tolerance and less insulin resistance,[29] reduced circulating blood volume and cardiac output, regression of myocardial hypertrophy,[30] and diminution of sympathetic tone.[31] If pharmacologic therapy is required for satisfactory long-term blood pressure control, the use of thiazide diuretics and beta-adrenergic blocking agents should probably be minimized in view of their potential for lowering high-density lipoprotein (HDL) cholesterol, reducing thermogenesis, and worsening insulin sensitivity[32] (see also Chap. 58).

OBESITY AND CORONARY HEART DISEASE

Overweight greater than 30 to 40 percent above the norm is associated with excess mortality, largely due to cardiovascular disease.[33,34] Excess total fat mass, however, may have little effect on coronary heart disease (CHD) mortality in selected sex, social, ethnic, and racial groups, and physical activity may impact on coronary heart disease mortality to a greater extent than fat mass.[35] The CHD mortality rate in the United States has decreased since the 1970s despite an increase in the percentage of overweight in the population.[36]

A pattern of predominantly abdominal fat distribution, commonly identified by the ratio of waist-to-hip circumference, appears to be an independent risk factor for cardiovascular morbidity and mortality, correlating much better than total body fat with the presence of CHD.[37–39] This distribution of body fat in overweight subjects is associated with a higher incidence of coronary risk factors such as dyslipidemia, impaired glucose tolerance, insulin resistance, and hypertension.[40] The atherogenic lipid profile associated with abdominal obesity includes decreased HDL_2 levels,[41,42] preponderance of the small, dense low-density lipoprotein (LDL) subfraction, and increased concentrations of small very low density lipoprotein (VLDL).[43] In school-age children, central fat distribution is strongly related to insulin resistance independent of peripheral fat.[44] Subtle abnormalities related to carbohydrate and lipid metabolism in such children track to young adulthood, long before the clustering of risk factors and manifestation of coronary disease are found in adults.[45] This impact of obesity on clustering and tracking of multiple coronary risk factors has implications for prevention at an early age (see also Chap. 41).

Weight reduction in obese subjects to "acceptable" levels for insurance purposes over the long term is associated with a decrement in cardiovascular mortality.[46,47] The effect of weight control in relation to coronary disease appears to be mediated through favorable modification of metabolic alterations and risk factors. Weight loss in subjects with abdominal obesity may effect preferential reduction in visceral fat and waist-to-hip ratio.[48] These changes may be accompanied by significant decrements in plasma glucose and insulin as well as triglycerides, total cholesterol, and LDL cholesterol. HDL cholesterol levels may rise, while blood pressure falls to lower levels.[49] Decrements in body weight greater than 20 percent may be required for symptomatic improvement in obese subjects with stable angina pectoris.[50]

CARDIOMYOPATHY OF OBESITY

It is now well established that in morbidly obese individuals (i.e., body weight approximately 135 kg or more), there may develop a syndrome of chronic circulatory congestion associated with diastolic and sometimes systolic left ventricular dysfunction. Its pathologic, physiologic, and clinical features appear sufficiently distinctive to warrant characterization as a specific cardiomyopathy.[51] A roughly linear increment in heart weight with increasing body weight was first demonstrated at necropsy in 1933.[52] Subsequent echocardiographic studies in very obese subjects have established a similar relation for left ventricular mass with thickening of the left ventricular septum and free wall.[53] These findings are due to left ventricular hypertrophy, sometimes with accompanying right ventricular hypertrophy, and occasionally with fatty infiltration of the myocardium.[54–56] Regional blood flow in markedly obese patients is characterized by a significant increase to adipose tissue, a modest increase to the splanchnic vascular bed, and little change in flow to other organs as compared with the setting of "ideal" or "average" weight. This results in a high cardiac output at rest in absolute terms, directly related to the increment in body oxygen consumption[57] but with a quasinormal cardiac index. In markedly obese subjects with peripheral or central obesity, cardiac output, stroke volume, and left ventricular volumes are increased.[58] Circulating blood volume increases in direct proportion to cardiac output, leading to the development of a central congestive state in approximately 10 percent of morbidly obese subjects.[59] The increased left ventricular mass and altered ventricular loading conditions are accompanied by evidences of diastolic dysfunction, as indicated by Doppler interrogation of transmitral diastolic filling velocities.[60] Thus, both left ventricular diastolic dysfunction and increased pulmonary blood volume contribute to the evolution of pulmonary congestion. Elevated left ventricular diastolic pressure may cause pulmonary hypertension at rest or during exercise[60-62]; in some cases, a transpulmonary diastolic (pulmonary artery diastolic to wedge) pressure gradient is present, secondary to medial hypertrophy of small pulmonary arteries[63,64] or hypoxic pulmonary vasoconstriction (see also Chap. 59). Indices of left ventricular systolic performance such as ejection fraction and velocity of circumferential fiber shortening may be normal or depressed.[65] Increasing left ventricular cavity size and end-systolic wall tension are correlated with depression of ejection fraction[66] and tend to be more pronounced with longer duration of obesity.[67]

Thus, two mechanisms appear to operate in the pathogenesis of recurrent bouts of circulatory congestion in patients with chronic, severe exogenous obesity. In one group of patients, pulmonary and systemic vascular congestion develops as a consequence of chronic volume overload and left ventricular diastolic dysfunction. It is not unusual for patients with preserved left ventricular systolic performance to present with recurrent bouts of pulmonary and systemic congestion for many years (Fig. 93-1). In the other group, chronic volume overload and high cardiac output, with or without accompanying hypertension, appear to result in a lesser degree of myocardial hypertrophy and greater ventricular dilatation, such that ventricular end-systolic wall stress is elevated and left ventricular systolic dysfunction is superimposed. Since the clinical presentation in these two groups may be essentially the same, differentiation will usually require appraisal of left ventricular function by echocardiographic, radionuclide, or angiographic techniques.

Rapid weight gain may precipitate or exacerbate congestive symptoms. Progressively increasing dyspnea and orthopnea are characteristic, whereas acute pulmonary edema is uncommon. The terminal phase is sometimes characterized by rapid weight gain due to fluid retention, with increasing somnolence, mental confusion, and coma.[51] Sudden death is common and well documented by case reports.[68] Hypertension may or may not be present. A presystolic gallop (S_4) rhythm may be heard, but cardiac murmurs are usually absent. Frequent electrocardiograph findings include left deviation of the QRS axis in the frontal plane[69] or low-voltage, right axis deviation and P pulmonale.[70] Despite gross anatomic involvement, electrocardiographic evidence of left ventricular hypertrophy is often absent.[51] Recurrent bouts of congestion predispose to the development of atrial fibrillation or flutter, in association with left atrial enlargement[51] (Fig. 93-1). Conduction defects secondary to fatty infiltration of the conduction system may be implicated in the predisposition to sudden death.[64,71] Diuretic therapy is the most urgently indicated measure in the management of the obesity congestive state, together with judicious use of oxygen. Though cardioversion of supraventricular tachycardias may be considered in an emergency setting, the arrhythmia tends to recur, and rate control can be achieved

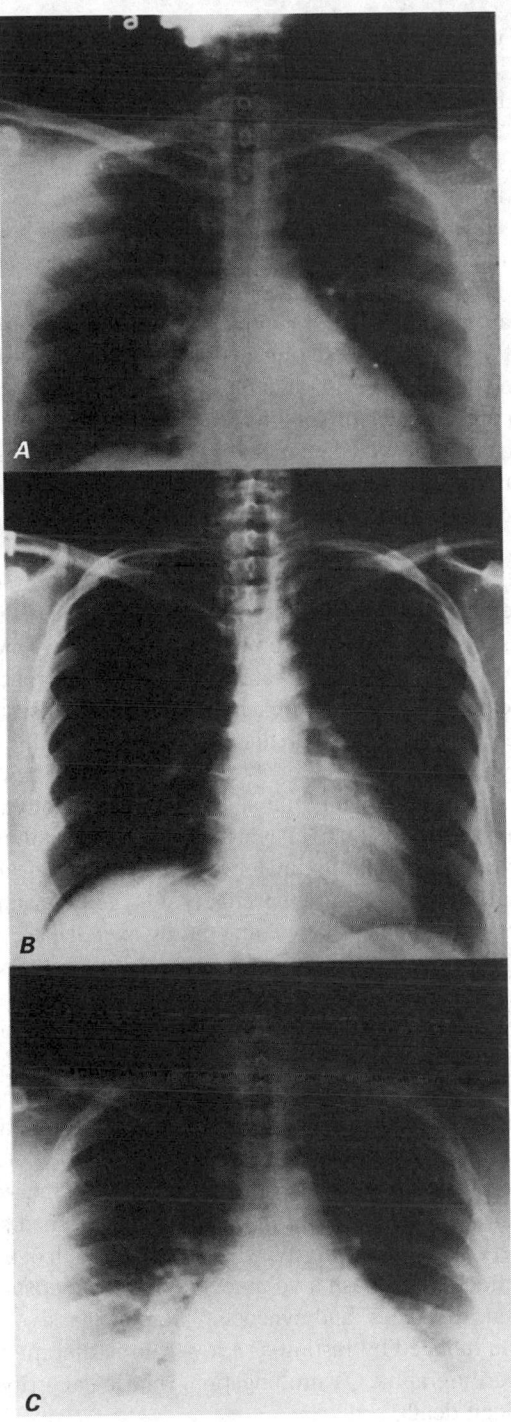

FIGURE 93-1

Chest films of a woman first presenting with severe pulmonary and systemic congestion. *A.* At age 20, weight is 184 kg. *B.* At age 31, weight reduction to 157 kg was associated with decrements in heart size as well as pulmonary congestion. *C.* Recurrence of cardiomegaly and pulmonary congestion attended regained weight at age 37. At age 43, weight 195 kg, echocardiogram demonstrated normal left ventricular systolic performance, with ejection fraction 64 percent, mean velocity of circumferential fiber shortening 1.36 cir/s. Left ventricular septal and posterior wall thickness were increased to 1.7 and 2.0 cm, respectively, and E-F slope was reduced to 30 mm/s, suggesting reduced left ventricular compliance. Left atrial dimension was enlarged to 5.2 cm. By age 48, atrial fibrillation had developed. (From Alexander JK. The cardiomyopathy of obesity. *Prog Cardiovasc Dis* 1985; 27:325–334. Reproduced with permission from Grune & Stratton, Inc., and the author.)

by the usual measures. Early appraisal of left ventricular function by echocardiographic or radionuclide study may be helpful with regard to determining the need for inotropic or angiotensin-converting enzyme (ACE) inhibitor therapy. Since there is no evidence of altered sodium, potassium, or adenosine triphosphatase (Na^+, K^+-ATPase) activity with obesity,[72] and since serum digoxin levels relate to lean body mass rather than total body weight,[73] higher digoxin dosage based on total body weight may result in toxicity. Vasodilator therapy may be indicated for control of severe hypertension and may be useful in the setting of left ventricular dysfunction (see also Chap. 23). Although there are no studies specifically examining efficacy of long-term anticoagulation therapy in very obese subjects with circulatory congestion in the absence of atrial fibrillation, consideration of such therapy would seem reasonable in view of the relatively high incidence of venous thrombophlebitis and pulmonary embolism.

The achievement of near ideal weight or long-term significant weight reduction by dietary means seldom occurs in these patients. Gastric surgery in combination with dietary measures appears to be a reasonably safe and effective approach.[74–76] Significant weight loss in subjects with marked obesity results in lowered blood pressure, reduced cardiac size, and favorable hemodynamic alterations.[8,30,61,77] Decrements in body oxygen consumption, blood volume, and cardiac output are proportional to the amount of weight loss. Blood volume and cardiac output fall approximately 30 mL and 30 mL/min per kilogram of weight loss, respectively. Oxygen consumption, cardiac output, and stroke volume during exercise are less for the same workload after weight reduction.[77] Weight loss may be accompanied by a reduction in left ventricular mass and chamber size, improvement in loading conditions and diastolic filling dynamics, and increase in ejection fraction if impaired.[78–80] Persistent elevation of left ventricular filling pressure during exercise suggests a decrement in compliance as long as 3 years after weight reduction.[8]

Experimental and clinical studies indicate that marked dietary caloric restriction or fasting leads to diminished sympathetic nervous system activity, which, together with natriuresis and contraction of plasma volume, may provoke postural hypotension, dizziness, and syncope.[81] Rapid, massive weight reduction induced by fasting or a low-calorie diet may effect electrocardiographic QT prolongation, ventricular arrhythmia, and sudden death.[82]

SLEEP APNEA AND OBESITY

Although sleep apnea occurs in a variety of clinical settings, somewhat more than 50 percent of patients so afflicted are obese.[83] The degree of obesity varies from moderate to extreme, with an incidence of sleep apnea as high as 75 percent in markedly obese subjects.[84,85] A predominance of men versus women,[86] and a higher prevalence in those with central obesity.[87] Daytime hypersomnia is frequent. Significant increases in systemic and pulmonary artery pressures occur cyclically during apnea; with a rapid succession of apneic spells there may be a progressive rise in both.[88] Apnea may be accompanied by decrements in arterial oxygen tension to 50 mmHg or less, with moderate increases in carbon dioxide tension. Cardiac arrhythmias are frequent during apnea, involving sinus arrest, asystole up to 6 s, heart block, and ventricular tachycardia.[89] All of the hemodynamic and arrhythmic effects induced by sleep apnea may be reversed in some cases by tracheostomy; when hypertension coexists, blood pressure may fall to or toward normal.[88,89]

HYPOVENTILATION SYNDROME

A syndrome of hypoventilation, cyanosis, and somnolence, with resultant chronic hypoxemia, hypercapnia, respiratory acidosis, and polycythemia, occurs in about 5 percent of extremely obese persons.[12] The sequence of physiologic events leading to the obesity hypoventilation syndrome may be initiated by the development of sleep apnea.[90] Transient bouts of hypoxia with apnea eventually cause blunting of the hypoxic ventilatory drive and, in conjunction with diminished chest wall compliance and increased respiratory work, a reduced ventilatory response to carbon dioxide as well. Obesity hypovetilation syndrome, however, may develop in the absence of sleep apnea. Chronic hypoxemia and hypercapnia stimulate pulmonary vasoconstriction, so that the effects of augmented pulmonary vascular resistance are superimposed upon the underlying hemodynamic derangements of severe obesity—namely, increased pulmonary blood volume and flow, with left atrial hypertension. Hypoventilation is reversible with weight reduction, and the attendant improvement in arterial blood gases is associated with a fall in pulmonary artery pressure and a reduction or elimination of the transpulmonary diastolic pressure gradient.[59] Several case reports document the disappearance of P pulmonale, T-wave inversion in leads V_1 to V_3, and right axis deviation in the electrocardiograms of obese subjects with the hypoventilation syndrome after weight reduction.[70,91]

REFERENCES

1. Rosell S. Microcirculation and transport in adipose tissue. In: *Handbook of Physiology*: Sec 2. Vol 4. *Microcirculation*. Bethesda, MD: American Physiological Society; 1984:949–967.
2. Kurpad A, Khan K, MacDonald I, Elia M. Haemodynamic responses in muscle and adipose tissue and whole body metabolic responses during norepinephrine infusions in man. *J Auton Nerv Syst* 1995; 54:163–170.
3. Nagashima T, Ohinata H, Kuroshima A. Involvement of nitric oxide in noradrenaline-induced increase in blood flow through brown adipose tissue. *Life Sci* 1994; 54:17–25.
4. Kovach AG, Rossell S, Sandar P, Koltay E, Kovach E, Tomka N. Blood flow, oxygen consumption and free fatty acid release in subcutaneous adipose tissue during hemorrhagic shock in control and phoenoxybenzamine-treated dogs. *Circ Res* 1970; 26:733–741.
5. Curri SB, Merlen JF. Microvascular disorders of adipose tissue. *J Mal Vasc* 1986; 11:303–309.
6. DiGirolamo M, Eposito J. Adipose tissue blood flow and cellularity in the growing rabbit. *Am J Physiol* 1975; 299:107.

7. Alexander JK, Dennis EW, Smith WG, Amad KH, Duncan WC, Austin RC. Blood volume, cardiac output and distribution of systemic blood flow in extreme obesity. *Cardiovasc Res Cent Bull* 1962; 1:39–44.

8. Alexander JK, Peterson KL. Cardiovascular effects of weight reduction. *Circulation* 1972; 45:310–318.

9. Blaak EE, Van Baak MA, Kemerink GJ, Pakbiers MT, Heidendal GA, Saris WH. Beta-adrenergic stimulation and abdominal subcutaneous fat blood flow in lean, obese, and reduced-obese subjects. *Metab Clin Exp* 1995; 44:183–187.

10. Haynes RB. Is weight loss an effective treatment for hypertension? The evidence against. *Can J Physiol Pharmacol* 1986; 64:825–830.

11. MacMahon S, Cutlar J, Brittain E, Higgins M. Obesity and hypertension: Epidemiological and clinical issues. *Eur Heart J* 1987; 8(suppl B):57–70.

12. Alexander J, Amad K, Cole VW. Observations on some clinical features of extreme obesity with particular reference to cardiorespiratory effects. *Am J Med* 1962; 32:512–524.

13. Messerli FH, Christie B, DeCarvalho J, Aristimuno GC, Suarez DH, Dreslinski GR, et al. Obesity and essential hypertension: Hemodynamics, intravascular volume, sodium excretion, and plasma renin activity. *Arch Intern Med* 1981; 141:81–85.

14. Toto MJJ, Achimastos A, Asmar RG, Hughes CJ, Safar ME. Pulse wave velocity in patients with obesity and hypertension. *Am Heart J* 1986; 112:136–140.

15. Bjorntorp P. Obesity and adipose tissue distribution as risk factors for the development of disease: A review. *Infusionsterapie* 1990; 17:24–27.

16. Black A. The coronary artery disease paradox: The role of hyperinsulinemia and insulin resistance and implications for therapy. *J Cardiovasc Pharmacol* 1990; 15:S26–S39.

17. Hall JE. Renal and cardiovascular mechanisms of hypertension in obesity. *Hypertension* 1994; 23:381–394.

18. Kaplan NM. The deadly quartet: Upper body obesity, glucose intolerance, hypertriglyceridemia, and hypertension. *Arch Intern Med* 1989; 149:1514–1520.

19. Bjorntorp P. Effects of long term physical training on body fat, metabolism, and blood pressure in obesity. *Metabolism* 1979; 28:650–658.

20. Muller DC, Elahi D, Pratley RE, Tobin JD, Andres R. An epidemiological test of the hyperinsulinemia-hypertension hypothesis. *J Clin Endocrinol Metab* 1993; 76:544–548.

21. Tsutsu N, Nunoi K, Kodama T, Nomiyama R, Iwase M, Fujishima M. Lack of association between blood pressure and insulin in patients with insulinoma. *J Hypertens* 1990; 8:479–482.

22. Pontiroli AE, Alberetto M, Pozza G. Patients with insulinoma show insulin resistance in the absence of arterial hypertension. *Diabetologia* 1992; 35:294–295.

23. Hall JE, Summers RL, Brands MW, Keen H, Alonso-Galicia M. Resistance to the metabolic action of insulin and its role in hypertension. *Am J Hypertens* 1994; 7:772–788.

24. Mark AL, Anderson EA. Genetic factors determine the blood pressure response to insulin resistance and hyperinsulinemia: A call to refocus the insulin hypothesis of hypertension. *Proc Soc Exp Biol Med* 1995; 208:330–336.

25. Nielsen PE, Larsen B, Holstein P, Poulsen HL. Accuracy of auscultatory blood pressure measurements in hypertensive and obese subjects. *Hypertension* 1983; 5:122–127.

26. Rissanen A, Pietinen P, Siljamaki-Ojansuu U, Piirainen H, Reissel P. Treatment of hypertension in obese patients: Efficacy and feasibility of weight and salt reduction programs. *Acta Med Scand* 1985; 218:149–156.

27. Reisin E. Weight reduction in the management of hypertension: Epidemiologic and mechanistic evidence. *Can J Physiol Pharmacol* 1986; 64:818–824.

28. Novi RF, Porta M, Lamberto M, Molinatti GM. Reduction of body weight and blood pressure in obese hypertensive patients treated by diet: A retrospective study. *Panminerva Med* 1989; 31:13–15.

29. Nobel F, Vangall L, Deleeuw I. Weight reduction with a high protein, low carbohydrate, calorie-restricted diet: Effects on blood pressure, glucose and insulin levels. *Neth J Med* 1989; 35:295–302.

30. Alexander JK. Cardiac effects of weight reduction in obesity hypertension. In: Messerli H ed. *The Heart and Hypertension*. New York: Yorke Medical Books; 1987:427–433.

31. Krieger DR, Landsberg L. Mechanisms in obesity-related hypertension: Role of insulin and catecholamines. *Am J Hypertens* 1988; 1:84–90.

32. Astrup AV. Obesity and diabetes as side-effects of beta-blockers. *Ugeskr Laeger* 1990; 152:2905–2908.

33. Sjostrom LV. Mortality of severely obese subjects. *Am J Clin Nutr* 1992; 55:16S–23S.

34. Troiano RP, Frongillo EA Jr, Sobol J, Levitsky DA. The relationship between body weight and mortality: A quantitative analysis of combined information from existing studies (abstr). *Int J Obesity* 1996; 20(suppl 4):109.

35. Berlin JA, Colditz GA. A meta-analysis of physical activity in the prevention of coronary heart disease. *Am J Epidemiol* 1990; 132:612–628.

36. Stern M. Epidemiology of obesity and its link to heart disease. *Metabolism* 1995; 44(suppl 3):1–3.

37. Bjorntorp P. Abdominal fat distribution and disease: An overview of epidemiological data. *Ann Med* 1992; 24:15–18.

38. Casassus P, Fontbonne A, Thibult N, Ducimetiere P, Richard JL, Claude JR, et al. Upper body fat distribution: A hyperinsulinemia-independent predictor of coronary heart disease mortality: The Paris Prospective study. *Arterioscler Thromb* 1992; 12:1387–1392.

39. Pouliot MC, Despres JP, Lemieux S, Moorjani S, Bouchard C, Tremblay A, et al. Waist circumference and abdominal sigittal diameter: Best simple anthropometric indexes for abdominal visceral adipose tissue accumulation and related cardiovascular risk in men and women. *Am J Cardiol* 1994; 73:460–468.

40. Bouchard C, Despres JP, Mauriege P. Genetic and nongenetic determinants of regional fat distribution. *Endocrinol Rev* 1993; 14:72–93.

41. Ostlund RE, Staten M, Kohrt WM, Schultz J, Malley M. The ratio of waist-to-hip circumference, plasma insulin levels, and glucose intolerance as independent predictors of the HDL_2 cholesterol level in older adults. *N Engl J Med* 1990; 322:229–234.

42. Despres JP, Moorjani S, Ferland M, Tremblay A, Lupien PJ, Nadeau A, et al. Adipose tissue distribution and plasma lipoprotein levels in obese women: Importance of intra-abdominal fat. *Arteriosclerosis* 1989; 9:203–210.

43. Terry RB, Wood PD, Haskell WL, Stefanick ML, Krauss RM. Regional adiposity patterns in relation to lipids, lipoprotein cholesterol, and lipoprotein subfraction mass in men. *J Clin Endocrinol Metab* 1989; 68:191–199.

44. Freedman DS, Srinivasan SR, Burke GL, Shear CL, Smoak CG, Harsha DW, et al. Relation of body fat distribution to hyperinsulinemia in children and adolescents: The Bogalusa Heart Study. *Am J Clin Nutr* 1987; 46:403–410.

45. Srinivasan SR, Bao W, Berenson GS. Coexistence of increased levels of adiposity, insulin, and blood pressure in a young adult cohort with elevated very-low-density lipoprotein cholesterol: The Bogalusa Heart Study. *Metabolism* 1993; 42:170–176.

46. Dublin LI. Relation of obesity to longevity. *N Engl J Med* 1953; 248:971–974.

47. Shephard WP, Marks HH. Life insurance looks at arteriosclerosis problem. *Minn Med* 1955; 38:736–741.

48. Leenen R, Van Der Kooy, Deurenberg P, Seidell JC, Weststrate JA, Schovein FJM, Hautvast JGAJ. Visceral fat accumulation in obesity subjects: Relation to energy expenditure and response to weight loss. *Am J Physiol* 1992; 263:E913–E919.

49. Dennis KE, Goldberg AP. Differential effects of body fatness and body fat distribution on risk factors for cardiovascular disease in women: Impact of weight loss. *Arterioscler Thromb* 1993; 13:1487–1494.

50. Sharma B, Thadami U, Taylor SH. Cardiovascular effects of weight reduction in obese patients with angina pectoris. *Br Heart J* 1974; 36:854–858.

51. Alexander JK. The cardiomyopathy of obesity. *Prog Cardiovasc Dis* 1985; 27:325–334.

52. Smith HL, Willius FA. Adiposity of the heart. *Arch Intern Med* 1933; 52:911–931.

53. Lauer MS, Anderson KM, Kannel WB, Levy D. The impact of obesity on left ventricular mass and geometry. *JAMA* 1991; 266:231–236.

54. Amad KH, Brennan JC, Alexander JK. The cardiac pathology of obesity. *Circulation* 1965; 32:740–745.

55. Warnes CA, Roberts WC. The heart in massive (more than 300 pounds or 136 kilograms) obesity: Analysis of 12 patients studies at necropsy. *Am J Cardiol* 1984; 54:1087–1091.

56. Duflou J, Virmani R, Rabin I, Burke A, Farb A, Smialek J. Sudden death as a result of heart disease in morbid obesity. *Am Heart J* 1995; 130:306–313.

57. White RI, Alexander JK. Body oxygen consumption and pulmonary ventilation in obese subjects. *J Appl Physiol* 1965; 20:197–201.

58. Merlino G, Scaglione R, Paterna S, Corrao S, Parinello G, Licata A, et al. Lymphocyte beta-adrenergic receptors in young subjects with peripheral or central obesity: Relationship with central hemodynamics and left ventricular function. *Eur Heart J* 1994; 15:786–792.

59. Kaltman AJ, Goldring RM. Role of circulatory congestion in the cardiorespiratory failure of obesity. *Am J Med* 1976; 60:645–653.

60. Alpert MA, Lambert CR, Terry BE, Cohen MV, Mukerji V, Massey CV, et al. Influence of left ventricular mass on left ventricular diastolic filling in normotensive obesity. *Am Heart J* 1995; 130:1068–1073.

61. Bachman L, Freyschuss U, Hallberg D, Melcher A. Cardiovascular function in extreme obesity. *Acta Med Scand* 1973; 193:437–446.

62. Alandin-Din A, Meterissian S, Lisbona R, MacLean LD, Forse RA. Assessment of cardiac function in patients who are morbidly obese. *Surgery* 1990; 108:809–818.

63. Alexander JK, Pettigrove JR. Obesity and congestive heart failure. *Geriatrics* 1967; 22:101–108.

64. James TN, Frame B, Coates EO. De subitaneis mortibus: III. Pickwickian syndrome. *Circulation* 1973; 48:1311–1320.

65. Alexander JK, Woodard CB, Quinones MA, Gaasch WH. Heart failure from obesity. In: Mancini M, Lewis B, Cantaldo F, eds. *Medical Complications of Obesity*. London: Academic Press; 1978.

66. Alpert MA, Terry BE, Lambert CR, Kelly DL, Panayiotou H, Murkevi V, et al. Factors influencing left ventricular systolic function in nonhypertensive morbidly obese patients, and effect of weight loss induced by gastroplasty. *Am J Cardiol* 1993; 71:733–737.

67. Alpert MA, Lambert CR, Panayiotou H, Terry BE, Cohen MV, Massey CV et al. Relation of duration of morbid obesity to left ventricular mass, systolic function, and diastolic filling and effect of weight loss. *Am J Cardiol* 1995; 76:1194–1197.

68. MacGregor MI, Block AJ, Ball WC Jr. Serious complications and sudden death in the Pickwickian syndrome. *Johns Hopkins Med J* 1970; 126:279–295.

69. Axelrad MA, Alexander JK. The electrocardiogram and cardiac anatomy in obesity. *Clin Res* 1965; 13:25.

70. Lillington GA, Anderson MA, Brandenburg RO. The cardiorespiratory syndrome of obesity. *Dis Chest* 1957; 32:1–20.

71. Balsaver AM, Morales AR, Whitehouse FW. Fat infiltration of myocardium as a cause of cardiac conduction defect. *Am J Cardiol* 1967; 19:261–265.

72. Beutler E, Kuhl W, Sacks P. Sodium-potassium-ATPase activity is influenced by ethnic origin and not by obesity. *N Engl J Med* 1983; 309:756–760.

73. Ewy GA, Groves BM, Ball MF, Nimmo L, Jackson B, Marcus F. Digoxin metabolism in obesity. *Circulation* 1971; 33:810–814.

74. Sugarman HJ, Baron PL, Fairman RP. Hemodynamic dysfunction in

obesity hypoventilation syndrome and the effects of treatment with surgically induced weight loss. *Ann Surg* 1988; 207:604–613.

75. Benotti PN, Hollingshead J, Mascioli EA. Gastric restrictive operations for morbid obesity. *Am J Surg* 1989; 157:150–155.

76. Kral JG. Surgical treatment of obesity. *Med Clin North Am* 1989; 73:251–264.

77. Backman L, Freyschuss U, Hallberg D, Melcher A. Reversibility of cardiovascular changes in extreme obesity. *Acta Med Scand* 1979; 205:367–373.

78. Alpert MA, Lambert CR, Terry BE, Kelly DL, Panayiotou H, Mukerji V, et al. Effect of weight loss on left ventricular mass in nonhypertensive, morbidly obese patients. *Am J Cardiol* 1994; 73:918–921.

79. Alpert MA, Lambert CR, Terry BE, Cohen MV, Mulerar M, Massey CV, et al. Effect of weight loss on left ventricular diastolic filling in morbid obesity. *Am J Cardiol* 1995; 76:1198–1201.

80. Himeno E, Nishino K, Nakashima Y, Kuriowa A, Ikeda M. Weight reduction regresses left ventricular mass regardless of blood pressure level in obese subjects. *Am Heart J* 1996; 131:313–319.

81. DeHaven J, Sherwin R, Hendler R, Felig P. Nitrogen and sodium balance and sympathetic-nervous system activity in obese subjects treated with a low calorie protein or mixed diet. *N Engl J Med* 1980; 302:477–482.

82. Van Itallie TB, Yang MU. Cardiac dysfunction in obese dieters: A potentially lethal complication of rapid, massive weight loss. *Am J Clin Nutr* 1984; 39:695–702.

83. Vgontzas AN, Tau TL, Bixler LR. Sleep apnea and sleep disruption in obese patients. *Arch Int Med* 1994; 154:1705–1711.

84. Rajala R, Partinen M, Sane T. Obstructive sleep apnea syndrome in morbidly obese patients. *J Internal Med* 1991; 230:125–129.

85. Sugarman HJ, Fairman RP, Wolfe L. Long term effects of gastric surgery for treating respiratory insufficiency of obesity. *Am J Clin Nutr* 1992; 55:597S–601S.

86. Richman RM, Elliott LM, Burns CM. The prevalence of obstructive sleep apnea in an obese female population. *Internat J Obesity* 1994; 18:173–177.

87. MIllman RP, Carlisle CC, McGarvey ST. Body fat distribution and sleep apnea severity in women. *Chest* 1995; 107:362–366.

88. Schroeder JS, Motta J, Guilleminault C. Hemodynamic studies in sleep apnea. In: Guilleminault C, Dement EC, eds. *Sleep Syndromes*. New York: Liss; 1978.

89. Tilkian A, Motta J, Guilleminault C. *Cardiac Arrhythmias in Sleep Apnea Syndromes*. New York: Liss; 1978.

90. Sharp JT, Barrocas M, Chokroverty S. The cardiorespiratory effects of obesity. *Clin Chest Med* 1980; 1:103–118.

91. Estes EH Jr, Sieker HO, McIntosh HD, Kelser GA. Reversible cardio-pulmonary syndrome with extreme obesity. *Circulation* 1957; 16:179–187.

94

THE HEART AND KIDNEY DISEASE

Stephen O. Pastan / William E. Mitch

Cardiovascular disease is a major cause of morbidity and death in patients with end-stage renal disease (ESRD) treated by chronic dialysis.[1] Forty five percent of deaths of dialysis patients in the United States are caused by cardiovascular disease; acute myocardial infarctions cause 25.8 deaths per 1000 patient-years.[2] The cardiovascular mortality rate in ESRD patients is approximately three times higher than in nonuremic, age-matched subjects without kidney disease.[3]

Specific risk factors for cardiovascular morbidity in dialysis patients include the high prevalence of hypertension and diabetes mellitus, hyperlipidemia, hypotension during hemodialysis, and abnormalities in calcium and phosphate metabolism causing hyperparathyroidism with vascular calcification. Pericardial disease, infective endocarditis, and fluid and electrolyte disturbances can contribute significantly to cardiac dysfunction in ESRD.

CARDIOVASCULAR RISK FACTORS IN CHRONICALLY UREMIC PATIENTS

Systemic Arterial Hypertension

Some 80 to 90 percent of patients with ESRD develop systemic hypertension before beginning dialysis therapy.[4] An expanded extracellular fluid volume (ECV)[5,6] and vasoconstriction mediated by the renin-angiotensin axis[6–10] probably play major roles in the pathogenesis of hypertension in patients with ESRD.

Hypertension due to sodium retention with ECV expansion in ESRD is associated with an increased cardiac output and usually an increased total peripheral vascular resistance.[11] This differs from the situation in hypertensive subjects with normal renal function, who usually have a normal cardiac output and a high peripheral resistance (see Chap. 56). The difference may be related to the anemia of ESRD, which causes a secondary increase in cardiac output. Echocardiographic evidence of left ventricular hypertrophy, which probably results from the combination of hypertension and anemia, is found in over 50 percent of patients on dialysis.

Direct evidence that ECV expansion plays a critical role in the hypertension of chronic renal failure (CRF) is found in studies demonstrating rapid resolution of hypertension in most patients after the ECV is reduced substantially by vigorous dialysis.[6,7,12] Still, there is a small group (10 to 20 percent) of ESRD patients who exhibit dialysis-resistant hypertension. These patients have high levels of plasma renin activity, and the control of their hypertension may rarely require bilateral nephrectomy. Even in this group, drugs inhibiting the renin-angiotensin axis can control hypertension, implicating the renin system in the pathogenesis of dialysis-resistant hypertension.[6,12,13]

The mechanisms for arterial vasoconstriction may be more complicated than activation of the renin system alone. A circulating inhibitor of Na^+-K^+-ATPase may mediate increased peripheral vascular resistance by causing an increase in intracellular sodium, resulting in an increase in intracellular calcium in vascular smooth muscle cells,[14] which stimulates vascular contraction. Also, overactivity of the sympathetic nervous system has been observed in CRF patients, likely due to stimulation of renal afferent nerves; this response is abolished by nephrectomy.[15] Other possible mechanisms contributing to hypertension in patients with CRF (even before the stage requiring dialysis) include a decrease in the production of vasodilator prostaglandins[16] or an increase in the levels of plasma endothelin, a vasoconstrictor.[17]

The use of recombinant human erythropoietin (EPO) to correct the anemia associated with ESRD worsens hypertension in approximately 20 to 30 percent of dialysis patients.[18] As anemia is corrected, a decline in cardiac output is accompanied by an increase in peripheral vascular resistance, in part related to increased blood viscosity; an elevation in the blood pressure may result in some patients with ESRD.[19]

The cornerstone of managing hypertension in dialysis patients is reducing the ECV effectively. This goal often requires vigorous ultrafiltration during hemodialysis to obtain a true "dry weight." The dry weight of a dialysis patient is defined as that weight at which there is no ECV expansion (e.g., edema, effusions, etc.) and a normal blood pressure. Unfortunately, antihypertensive drugs are often required, since the patients become symptomatically hypotensive before the dry weight is achieved. Regardless, the most common reason for *dialysis-resistant* hypertension is ECV expansion because of inadequate fluid removal by dialysis ultrainfiltration.

In patients who have persistent hypertension despite achieving dry weight, antihypertensive medications that inhibit the renin-angiotensin axis [beta blockers or angiotensin converting enzyme (ACE) inhibitors] appear to be the logical choice. Other antihypertensive medications, including calcium channel blockers and minoxidil, can be effective in dialysis patients but should not be used until the ECV is reduced. The dosage of antihypertensive drugs should be adjusted for the degree of renal failure; generally, the drugs are withheld on the day of hemodialysis to prevent hypotension from occurring, as ECV is reduced by ultrafiltration. Bilateral nephrectomy is rarely used to treat dialysis-resistant hypertension.

Diabetes Mellitus

Approximately 30 percent of all CRF patients who begin maintenance dialysis therapy are diabetic, and they have a significantly higher mortality rate than age-matched, nondiabetic patients. The most significant factor contributing to the high death rate in diabetic dialysis patients is coronary artery disease[20] (see also Chap. 78).

Hyperlipidemia

To measure plasma lipids, the blood sample should be obtained after a 12-h fast and before the patient is given heparin for dialysis. Approximately 50 percent of patients with ESRD have high serum levels of triglycerides and low levels of high-density-lipoprotein cholesterol.[21] Impaired degradation of very low density lipoprotein by lipoprotein lipase appears to be the major mechanism for the development of hypertriglyceridemia.[22,23] In patients treated by peritoneal dialysis, the high concentrations of glucose in the dialysate worsen the serum triglyceride level because glucose increases the production of triglycerides.

Other factors that may contribute to hyperlipidemia in ESRD include the use of diuretics and beta blockers,[24–26] the use of acetate-buffered dialysis solutions[27] or a high glucose concentration in the dialysate,[28] and possibly, carnitine deficiency.[29] Heparin given to prevent clotting in the dialyzer will cause a transient fall in serum triglycerides by increasing the activity of lipoprotein lipase.[30,31] Plasma levels of homocysteine are often elevated because of impaired renal excretion.

At present, there is no definite evidence that lowering plasma triglycerides improves survival.[32] Strategies for lowering triglycerides and low-density-lipoprotein (LDL) cholesterol include restricting dietary fat, giving fish-oil supplements, increasing exercise, and avoiding alcohol or treatment with beta blockers or diuretics[33–36] (see Chap. 53). Clofibrate or gemfibrozil, among other drugs, may be effective, but their use has been associated with an increased incidence of myositis and hepatotoxicity in dialysis patients (see Chap 53). Thus, it is particularly important to adjust the dosage for the degree of renal failure; for instance, clofibrate should be reduced to 25 to 50 percent of the usual dose. The 3-hydroxy-3-methylglutaryl coenzyme A (HMG-CoA) reductase inhibitors appear to be safe in ESRD patients and at standard doses will reduce the levels of triglycerides and LDL-cholesterol. Although definitive evidence that treatment with antihyperlipidemic drugs prevents atherosclerosis in dialysis patients is lacking, attempts at treatment seem prudent.

About 50 to 80 percent of patients undergoing renal transplantation develop hypercholesterolemia.

Hemodialysis-Associated Hypotension

Clinically significant hypotension occurs in approximately 25 percent of hemodialysis sessions.[37] Usually, the consequences are minor, but acute myocardial and cerebral ischemia have been reported. Excessive ultrafiltration is a common cause of hypotension during dialysis, leading to ECV depletion, increased venous return, and reduced cardiac output.[38] Moreover, rapid lowering of plasma osmolality during the removal or urea and other molecules causes a shift of ECV to the intracellular compartment, because these molecules do not move out of cells as rapidly as dialysis removes them from blood.[39,40] Finally, diffusion of solutes from the dialysate into the patient (e.g., acetate) can also result in vasodilatation and interfere with the hemodynamic adaptations to reduced ECV.[41]

The concentration of sodium in the dialysate is an important factor governing changes in plasma osmolality. The efficient dialyzers currently in use achieve higher rates of fluid removal (ultrafiltration), so that a higher concentration of sodium can be used in the dialysate. This practice has reduced the number of hypotensive episodes.[42]

The bioincompatibility of dialyzer membranes can activate the complement cascade and cause shunting of blood in the pulmonary vasculature, with resulting hypoxemia. This response is usually observed with cuprophane membranes and may be an important cause of hypotension during dialysis.[43] Newer dialysis membranes utilizing materials other than cuprophane cause less activation of the complement cascade.[44] Another cause of hypotension and, rarely, anaphylaxis is hypersensitivity to ethylene oxide, which is used to sterilize dialyzers.[45]

Other factors favoring hypotension during hemodialysis include (1) cardiac dysfunction from long-standing hypertension, ischemic or valvular heart disease, other causes of cardiomyopathy, or pericardial tamponade; (2) a rapid reduction in serum potassium and calcium, causing decreased contractility; (3) autonomic neuropathy (particularly in diabetic patients);

(4) sepsis; (5) occult hemorrhage (e.g., retroperitoneal hemorrhage after femoral vein catheterization); (6) ingestion of food prior to or during dialysis, resulting in splanchnic vasodilation; and (7) use of antihypertensive medications on the day of dialysis.

To reduce the incidence of hypotension, a high-sodium, bicarbonate-buffered dialysate should be used and the rate and extent of ultrafiltration monitored carefully. Antihypertensive medications should be avoided on hemodialysis days. Lowering the dialysate temperature has also been shown to reduce the incidence of hypotension.[46] Management of hypotension usually includes reducing the ultrafiltration rate, placing the patient in the Trendelenburg position, and administering saline through the arteriovenous access. Oxygen administration may be useful in patients with ischemic heart disease.

Hyperparathyroidism

Secondary hyperparathyroidism is virtually universal in dialysis patients.[47] Hyperphosphatemia due to failure to excrete dietary phosphates plays a major role in the pathogenesis of secondary hyperparathyroidism. The effects of hyperphosphatemia include a reduction in plasma-ionized calcium from direct complexing of calcium with phosphates, providing a stimulus for parathyroid hormone secretion. There is also decreased activity of 1α-hydroxylase in proximal tubule cells, leading to limited production of 1,25-dihydroxyvitamin D_3, the most active vitamin D analog.[48] All of these factors reduce the level of ionized calcium, which stimulates parathyroid hormone (PTH) secretion. The ability of ionized calcium to regulate PTH secretion is abnormal in ESRD patients. This abnormality is most likely related to a deficiency of 1,25-dihydroxyvitamin D_3,[49] a vitamin that has a direct role in suppressing PTH secretion by inhibiting transcription of the preproparathyroid gene.[50]

Unfortunately, many dialysis patients have an increased calcium × phosphate product. Morbidity in patients with a product above 60 mg^2/dL^2 includes vascular and soft tissue calcification.[51,52] Calcification can occur in coronary and peripheral arteries[53] and in the myocardium.[54] Extensive valvular calcification may result in impaired native or prosthetic valve function. Finally, it has been proposed that PTH can directly impair myocardial function,[55] but not all investigators agree.[56]

Prevention or treatment of secondary hyperparathyroidism is based on correcting hyperphosphatemia. This normalization can be accomplished only if patients will adhere to a diet containing less than 800 mg of phosphorus per day; even so, patients generally need to take phosphate binders with meals. Calcium carbonate or acetate are the preferred agents, because they avoid the risk of aluminum toxicity (including osteomalacia, anemia, and encephalopathy). If hypocalcemia persists and especially if there is evidence of secondary hyperparathyroidism, intravenous administration of 1,25-dihydroxyvitamin D_3 (calcitriol) can be used therapeutically. Vitamin D can also be given orally, but then the risk of hypercalcemia is

greater. Just as it is rarely necessary to perform bilateral nephrectomy, subtotal parathyroidectomy is also rarely needed, because severe hyperparathyroidism can usually be avoided. Prevention of hyperphosphatemia, hypocalcemia, and hyperparathyroidism are emphasized not only to avoid surgery but also because hypocalcemia after parathyroidectomy is a serious problem. These patients must take so many calcium and vitamin D tablets that compliance can be difficult.

ISCHEMIC HEART DISEASE

Acute myocardial infarctions were noted in 26 percent of autopsies of dialysis patients.[57,58] Risk factors for coronary artery disease include smoking, hypertension, insulin-dependent or non-insulin-dependent diabetes mellitus, hyperlipidemia, and hyperparathyroidism[59–61] (see also Chap. 41). In addition, factors such as hypertension, ECV overload, anemia, hypotension and hypoxia during hemodialysis, and the arteriovenous fistula can adversely affect the balance between myocardial oxygen supply and demand. In one study, electrocardiographic (ECG) changes of ischemia occurred during exercise in approximately 25 percent of dialysis patients.[62] In another study, myocardial uptake of thallium 201 during exercise was abnormal in more than 50 percent of patients, many of whom were asymptomatic during the study.[63] Of note, stress-thallium testing has been found to have a positive predictive value of only approximately 70 percent in ESRD patients.[64] Some false-positive thallium tests may relate to a decrease in the lateral-to-septal count density ratio reported in patients with renal failure and misinterpreted as a lateral wall myocardial infarction.[65] Clinically significant myocardial ischemia and angina pectoris do occur, however, in some dialysis patients who have no evidence of significant narrowing of coronary arteries on arteriography.[66]

The management of angina pectoris in uremic patients is similar to that used in patients without kidney disease except that drug dosages often have to be reduced (see Chap. 45). Nitrates, beta blockers, and calcium channel blockers are well tolerated but may need to be withheld before dialysis to avoid hypotension during the procedure. Exercise tolerance has been shown to improve in hemodialysis patients with coronary artery disease by correcting the anemia with erythropoietin.[67] Thus the hematocrit should be maintained above 30 percent by administering erythropoietin. Attention must be paid to repleting iron stores adequately; transfusion of packed red blood cells may occasionally be needed. Hypertension, ECV overload, and hyperparathyroidism should be controlled.

Treatment of angina pectoris developing during hemodialysis includes (1) stopping ultrafiltration to avoid ECV depletion, (2) reducing blood flow through the dialyzer, and (3) administering oxygen. If there is hypotension, the patient should be placed in the Trendelenburg position and saline infused through the venous line before administering sublingual nitroglycerin. If there is no hypotension, nitroglycerin can be administered immediately, with the blood pressure monitored closely. Finally, it should be emphasized that changes in serum potassium and ionized calcium during dialysis and between dialysis treatments may complicate interpretation of the ECG. Electrocardiograms obtained during angina while on dialysis will often differ from prior tracings taken between dialysis sessions.

Acute and long-term management of myocardial infarction in ESRD patients is similar to that in nonuremic patients except that changes in ECV are more critical and usually require restriction of salt and fluid intake plus judicious ultrafiltration. Rapid and/or excessive ultrafiltration should be avoided to prevent hemodynamic instability. Hypertension and anemia should be managed as discussed. Digoxin should be used in a reduced dosage and cautiously, with the plasma levels of digoxin and potassium frequently monitored. The concentration of potassium in the dialysate is commonly set at 2 meq/L, but it may be raised to 3 meq/L to prevent arrhythmias in patients receiving digoxin. When the dialysate potassium is raised, dietary potassium must be restricted to prevent hyperkalemia between treatments. The use of antiarrhythmic drugs should be carefully monitored by measuring serum levels.

The decision to perform coronary arteriography should be based upon the same criteria as for patients without kidney disease (see Chaps. 45 to 47). The dose of contrast dye should be minimized to prevent loss of residual renal function, and fluid intake (including the dose of contrast medium) should be minimized to prevent fluid overload. It is not necessary to dialyze patients immediately after arteriography unless there is concern about excess fluid or heart failure. Left ventricular function is usually determined by echocardiography or radioventriculography, which require no contrast medium.

Coronary artery bypass grafting (CABG) has been shown to have a mortality of approximately 10 percent in dialysis patients[68] as well as an increased perioperative morbidity.[69,70] Nevertheless, improved quality of life after CABG has made this a frequent operation in dialysis patients. Interestingly, *percutaneous transluminal coronary angioplasty (PTCA) has been found to have an unacceptably high rate of restenosis despite good initial angiographic success*[71]; *PTCA should therefore be reserved for dialysis patients who are not candidates for CABG.* Dialysis should be performed just before cardiac surgery to optimize ECV status and avoid hyperkalemia.

CONGESTIVE HEART FAILURE

Congestive heart failure accounts for 20 to 30 percent of the mortality in ESRD patients.[3,72] Echocardiograms reveal a high prevalence of "hypertrophic cardiomyopathy" characterized by left ventricular hypertrophy, asymmetric septal hypertrophy, and/or impaired contractility[73–76] ("uremic cardiomyopathy") as well as dilated cardiomyopathy.[77] Concentric left ventricular hypertrophy occurs in patients with current or previous systemic hypertension. Risk factors for myocardial

dysfunction in dialysis patients include hypertension, persistent ECV expansion, anemia, the arteriovenous fistula, ischemic heart disease, metabolic acidosis, electrolyte disturbances (hyperkalemia, hypocalcemia), hyperparathyroidism,[78] and possibly the uremic state itself. Hemodialysis can improve cardiac function dramatically,[79–85] presumably by controlling hypertension, correcting volume overload, removing uremic toxins, and normalizing blood pH and electrolyte levels (particularly, ionized calcium[86] and potassium[87]).

In uremic patients who develop pulmonary edema, the pulmonary capillary pressure is lower than in nonuremic patients and is less than the plasma oncotic pressure. Thus, pulmonary capillary permeability must be increased.[88,89]

The prevention of heart failure in dialysis patients requires strict control of ECV and hypertension. Salt and fluid restriction must be combined with adequate fluid removal to maintain the patient's weight as close as possible to the estimated "dry weight." Since dialysis is usually performed only three times a week, dietary salt restriction is absolutely necessary. An inappropriately high dry weight is the most common reason for persistent volume overload and hypertension in dialysis patients. Reasons for an erroneous assessment of dry weight include an unsuspected loss of muscle mass (e.g., catabolic weight loss) that is unrecognized because measured body weight does not change when fluid is retained. Finally, the influence of the arteriovenous fistula can be tested by occluding it and determining whether or not the heart rate slows (Branham's sign). When this occurs, revision of the fistula may be required to decrease excessive blood flow and oxygen demands of the heart (see Chap. 23).

Management of heart failure includes bed rest and oxygen therapy plus removal of excess fluid by ultrafiltration while excluding other causes of heart failure such as myocardial infarction, arrhythmias, or infective endocarditis. If digitalis is used, appropriate adjustment of dosage and frequent monitoring of plasma levels are necessary.

Left ventricular hypertrophy (LVH) has been found to improve after correction of anemia in dialysis patients by recombinant human erythropoietin (EPO). A recent review found that left ventricular muscle mass decreased by an average of 18 percent as the hematocrit was corrected by EPO up to 32 percent over 45 weeks.[18] Complete normalization of LVH is, however, uncommon, and it is not known whether or not a decrease in left ventricular wall thickness will result in improved patient survival.[19]

PERICARDIAL DISEASE

Before dialysis was widely available, pericarditis was regarded as a preterminal event for uremic patients. The clinical incidence of pericarditis has decreased from 50 percent to 5 to 20 percent since the predialysis era.[89–91] Although pericarditis is less common, it is still a problem.[91] Pericarditis in dialysis patients may be related to inadequate removal of uremic toxins; coincident diseases such as viral infections,[92] tuberculosis, systemic lupus erythematosus; or to drugs such as minoxidil[93] (see also Chap. 81). Pericarditis appears to occur less frequently in peritoneal dialysis patients than in hemodialysis patients. This difference has been attributed to a higher clearance of "middle molecules" by peritoneal dialysis.[94]

The primary treatment for dialysis-associated pericarditis is intensive dialysis (e.g., daily hemodialysis for 1 to 2 weeks), and heparin is eliminated to avoid pericardial hemorrhage and tamponade. Unfortunately, intensive dialysis can cause hypokalemia, hypophosphatemia, and volume depletion. An important clue to the development of cardiac tamponade is severe hypotension during dialysis, especially in the absence of volume depletion. Besides intensive dialysis, oral[95] or intrapericardial administration of corticosteroids[96] and indomethacin[97] have been used. The efficacy of indomethacin is questionable. Results from a prospective, double-blind study led to the conclusion that the predominant effect of indomethacin is to reduce fever.[98]

Pericardial effusion frequently complicates pericarditis, but cardiac tamponade is rare; the exact frequency is unknown. Small pericardial effusions are found in 15 to 20 percent of stable, asymptomatic dialysis patients.[99] It is unclear whether or not daily dialysis is beneficial in these patients, but frequent evaluation of the size and hemodynamic importance of the effusion is prudent. Treatment of a large pericardial effusion by intensification of dialysis may result in improvement[91,99]; but if there is no improvement or if hemodynamic compromise occurs, surgical drainage[91,101-104] of the pericardial effusion by subxiphoid pericardiotomy and creation of a pericardial "window" is the preferred procedure. It is usually well tolerated (see Chap. 81). Although pericardiectomy has been regarded as definitive in patients with pericarditis and clinically significant effusion, this more invasive procedure is not usually necessary.[91]

Constrictive pericarditis is rare in dialysis patients, even in patients with pericarditis.[105,106] It should be suspected when there is intractable right-sided heart failure in patients with a normal-sized or small heart. Cardiac catheterization can often verify the diagnosis, for which pericardiectomy is the definitive treatment (see Chap. 81).

INFECTIVE ENDOCARDITIS

Several factors predispose dialysis patients to infective endocarditis, the incidence of which may be as high as 3 to 5 percent.[107-109] These include a uremia-associated, immunocompromised state,[110,111] repeated puncture of the arteriovenous fistula, and infection of the arteriovenous access. In addition, calcific aortic or mitral valvular abnormalities (perhaps related to hyperparathyroidism) are present in approximately 10 percent of patients[112,113] and may serve as a nidus for infection. Bacteremia occurs in approximately 10 to 20 percent of dialysis patients.[114,115] *Staphylococcus aureus* is the most frequent organism,[109] although other microbes—

including *Staphylococcus epidermidis, Streptococcus viridans,* enterococci, and gram-negative organisms—are also reported. The diagnosis of infective endocarditis may be difficult in uremic patients because of the frequency of bacteremia and because systolic and diastolic murmurs are common (see also Chap. 82). Repeated blood cultures, physical examination, and an echocardiographic assessment are mandatory when infective endocarditis is suspected. Treatment of infective endocarditis consists of 4 to 6 weeks of parenteral antibiotics (see Chap. 82).

CARDIAC ARRHYTHMIAS

Risk factors for cardiac arrhythmias in dialysis patients include ischemic heart disease, calcification of the conduction system from secondary hyperparathyroidism and/or pericarditis, hemodialysis-associated hypotension, dialysis-induced acid-base and electrolyte disturbances (hyper- and hypokalemia, hyper- and hypocalcemia, hypermagnesemia), and hypoxemia. Fortunately, serious arrhythmias are uncommon except in patients with underlying heart disease, those receiving digitalis, or those with severe hypokalemia.[116-119] Dialysis patients receiving digitalis have an excessive risk for atrial and ventricular arrhythmias during dialysis because of rapid shifts of potassium. Therefore, digitalis should be used only when necessary and in the lowest dosage necessary. While the potassium concentration in the dialysate can be raised to decrease the risk of digitalis-toxic arrhythmias, this practice requires strict restriction of potassium intake to prevent hyperkalemia between dialyses. Hyperkalemia is believed to be responsible for a significant fraction of the 10 percent death rate from cardiac arrest in dialysis patients.[58]

RENAL FUNCTION IN HEART FAILURE

In heart failure, enhanced sympathetic activity and activation of the renin-angiotensin-aldosterone axis enhance salt reabsorption, while excess vasopressin release augments water retention.[120,121] These responses cause ECV and plasma volume expansion leading to increased end-diastolic volume plus edema. Circulating atrial natriuretic peptide (ANP) levels are increased in heart failure[20,122]; possibly, ANP modulates the antinatriuretic effects caused by sympathetic and renin system activation. Excessive vasopressin-induced water reabsorption can cause hyponatremia, which is an indicator of poor prognosis[123] (see also Chap. 21).

Renal vasoconstriction in heart failure patients can be sufficiently severe to cause prerenal azotemia, which is characterized by a blood urea nitrogen (BUN)-creatinine ratio that is greater than 10:1. The vasoconstriction causes a selective decrease in urea clearance resulting from enhanced sodium reabsorption with a secondary increase in urea reabsorption in the proximal tubule. The increased salt and water reabsorption reduces urine flow and causes a low urinary sodium excretion, as well as a high urine specific gravity and osmolality; the urinalysis is normal and there are no cellular or granular casts indicating kidney damage. Diuretic therapy can mask these characteristics by increasing urine flow and sodium excretion, thereby reducing the urine specific gravity and osmolality. Factors that can precipitate or exacerbate renal failure include excessive diuresis, use of ACE inhibitors or nonsteroidal anti-inflammatory drugs (NSAIDs), and worsening cardiac function. When renal perfusion is reduced (e.g., by heart failure), the glomerular filtration rate (GFR) becomes dependent on angiotensin II–induced efferent glomerular arteriolar constriction. Consequently, ACE inhibitors can markedly decrease the GFR.[124,125] The ACE inhibitors and other antihypertensive agents (e.g., hydralazine) can also reduce glomerular filtration by causing systemic hypotension and reducing renal perfusion pressure. NSAIDs reduce GFR by blocking the release of prostaglandins, which in turn, reduce activation of the renin-angiotensin system.

The management of renal failure in heart failure patients is aimed primarily at improving cardiac function (see Chap. 23). The NSAIDs should be avoided, and diuretics should be used judiciously because excessive diuresis can predispose to ACE inhibitor-induced renal insufficiency. Careful attention to urine flow, the BUN and serum creatinine, and potassium is mandatory to avoid these problems. It should be emphasized that ACE inhibitor therapy may sharply reduce renal clearance (i.e., cause a sharp rise in serum creatinine) by blocking angiotensin-induced glomerular efferent arteriolar vasoconstriction. Often, this is a transient problem and the serum creatinine will return to pretreatment values. If it does not, the drug should be withdrawn and a diagnosis of renal artery stenosis considered.

RENAL FAILURE FOLLOWING CARDIAC CATHETERIZATION

Contrast Nephropathy

The risk of renal damage following radiocontrast dye rises with diabetes mellitus, multiple myeloma, preexisting renal failure, volume depletion, heart failure, and with large amounts of contrast dye.[126–128] The renal failure after contrast dye is typically brief (approximately 5 to 7 days) unless there is substantial underlying renal damage. Interestingly, renal insufficiency in contrast-dye nephropathy can be associated with reduced urinary sodium excretion.[129] In high-risk patients, contrast dye studies should be avoided and noninvasive studies used to assess ventricular function and anatomy; at least the amount of contrast dye should be minimized. ECV expansion with saline prior to the studies reduces the incidence of contrast nephropathy to approximately 10 percent.[130] There is some evidence that mannitol may be protective.[130]

Atheroembolic Nephropathy

This complication usually occurs in elderly patients with erosive aortic atherosclerosis who develop cholesterol emboli to the kidneys during arterial catheterization.[126,131] Serum creatinine rises sharply and usually does not return to basal levels. At times, renal failure may worsen slowly, leading to ESRD. Hypertension due to activation of the renin-angiotensin system may be present.[132] The urinalysis typically does not reveal casts, which would suggest acute tubular damage. Atheroembolization to other locations such as the eyes (cholesterol plaques seen by fundoscopy), pancreas (pancreatitis), and skin (livedo reticularis or gangrene) may be present, suggesting the diagnosis.[133] Occasionally, immunologic activation may occur because there is an "active" urinary sediment with hematuria and cellular casts, hypocomplementemia, eosinophilia, and a high sedimentation rate.[134–136] Biopsy of an affected organ (e.g., skin, kidney) can help establish the diagnosis, but the absence of atheroemboli in a kidney biopsy does not exclude the diagnosis since affected vessels may be missed. There is no specific treatment.

Thromboembolic Renal Disease

In contrast to atheroembolic renal disease, thromboembolic renal arterial disease (e.g., in patients with atrial fibrillation or after myocardial infarction) often causes renal infarction. Such patients may present with flank pain, proteinuria, and hematuria; the serum lactate dehydrogenase (LDH) levels are increased and renal failure leads to an increased serum creatinine, particularly if both kidneys are affected.[137–139] A radioisotope scan or renal arteriography may confirm the diagnosis. Therapy includes anticoagulation, thrombolysis, and possibly surgical intervention.

CARDIAC DRUGS IN RENAL FAILURE

Many drugs used in the treatment of cardiovascular diseases undergo significant clearance by the kidneys. In order to avoid toxic side effects, the doses of these drugs must be modified depending on the level of the patient's glomerular filtration rate (see also Chap. 91). Dosing guidelines for commonly prescribed cardiovascular drugs in patients with diminished renal function are listed in Table 94-1. Specific drugs are discussed in more detail below.

Digoxin

The volume of distribution of digoxin is reduced 30 to 50 percent in ESRD patients; therefore the loading dose of digoxin should be reduced. The maintenance dosage should also be decreased because the primary route of elimination is by glomerular filtration of unmetabolized digoxin. Because of individual abnormal pharmacokinetics, only general guidelines for maintenance dosages are available: 0.0625 to 0.125 mg every other day can result in a therapeutic plasma level, but this should not be assumed, and regular monitoring of the plasma digoxin level is required. If a loading dose is not administered or if adjustments are made in the maintenance dose, the time required to attain a new steady state can be prolonged to approximately 3 weeks because of the longer half-life of digoxin in renal failure (4.4 days versus 1.6 days in normal subjects[140]). Concomitant administration of quinidine or verapamil can increase plasma digoxin levels and produce clinical toxicity (see Chaps. 23 and 91).

Procainamide

As renal function decreases, so does the ability to eliminate unmetabolized procainamide; the half-life increases from approximately 3.5 to 16 h in renal failure.[141,142] In addition, the half-life of *N*-acetylprocainamide (NAPA), an active metabolite of procainamide primarily excreted by the kidneys, is markedly prolonged in renal failure.[142] Consequently, maintenance doses should be reduced or the intervals between dosing should be prolonged; close monitoring of plasma levels of both procainamide and NAPA is necessary (see also Chaps. 30 and 91). Since both compounds are removed by dialysis, a dose of procainamide should be administered after hemodialysis.

Phenytoin

Phenytoin is bound to plasma proteins; in uremic patients, however, protein binding is reduced and hepatic elimination rises, resulting in a therapeutic concentration of free phenytoin.[143] Since most clinical laboratories measure the total phenytoin concentration (i.e., the bound plus free concentrations of the drug), attempting to maintain a "therapeutic" level of phenytoin in CRF patients by giving more drug to raise the plasma phenytoin level will cause toxicity. Fortunately, standard doses (e.g., 300 mg/day) often yield therapeutic levels of free phenytoin, so no alteration in phenytoin dosage is recommended even though the plasma level may appear to be subtherapeutic. Toxicity can be diagnosed from clinical signs (see Chap. 30).

TABLE 94-1

CARDIOVASCULAR DRUG DOSING IN RENAL FAILURE

Drug	Method of Modification	GFR >50	GFR 10–50	GFR <10	Supplemental Dose after Dialysis, mg
ADRENERGIC AGENTS					
Clonidine	D	U	U	50–75%	No
Methyldopa	I	q8h	q8–12h	q12–24h	250
Prazosin	—	U	U	U	No
ANGIOTENSIN-CONVERTING ENZYME INHIBITORS					
Benazepril	D	U	75–100%	50%	2.5
Captopril	D	U	75	50%	7.25
Enalapril	D	U	75–100%	50%	2.5–5
Fosinopril	D	U	U	75%	No
Lisinopril	D	U	50–75%	25–50%	2.5
Quinapril	D	U	75–100%	50%	2.5–5
ANTIARRHYTHMICS					
Amiodarone	—	U	U	U	No
Bretylium	D	U	25–50%	Avoid	No
Disopyramide	I	q8h	q12–24h	q24–40h	No
Flecainide	D	U	U	50–75%	No
Lidocaine	—	U	U	U	No
Procainamide	I	q4h	q6–12h	q8–24h	200
Quinidine	D	U	U	75%	100–200
Tocainide	D	U	U	50%	200
BETA BLOCKERS					
Atenolol	D	U	50%	30–50%	25–50
Esmolol	—	U	U	U	No
Labetalol	—	U	U	U	No
Metoprolol	—	U	U	U	50
Nadolol	D	U	50%	25%	40
Propranolol	—	U	U	U	No
Sotalol	D	U	30%	15–30%	80
Timolol	—	U	U	U	No
CALCIUM CHANNEL BLOCKERS—NO ADJUSTMENT NECESSARY					
CARDIAC GLYCOSIDES					
Digitoxin	D	U	U	50–75%	No
Digoxin	D	U	25–75%	10–25%	No
INOTROPIC AGENTS					
Amrinone	D	U	U	50–75%	?
Dobutamine	—	U	U	U	?
Milrinone	D	U	U	50–75%	?
VASODILATORS					
Diazoxide	—	U	U	U	No
Hydralazine	I	U	U	q8–16h	No
Minoxidil	—	U	U	U	No
Nitroprusside	—	U	U	U	No

Abbreviations: GFR = glomerular filtration rate; D = dose; U = unchanged; I = interval; ? = unknown.
Source: Adapted from Bennett WM, Aronoff GA, Golper TA, Morrison G, Brater DC, Singer I. *Drug Prescribing in Renal Failure: Dosing Guidelines for Adults,* 3d ed. Philadelphia: American College of Physicians; 1994.

Beta Blockers

Since atenolol (Tenormin) and nadolol (Corgard) are eliminated primarily by the kidneys, a dose reduction of 50 to 70 percent is necessary for CRF patients.[144] These drugs should be withheld on the morning of a hemodialysis treatment because a significant fraction is removed by the dialysis procedure. The usual dose is then given after dialysis (see also Chap. 54) (Table 94-1).

Sodium Nitroprusside

In dialysis or predialysis patients, thiocyanate will accumulate when sodium nitroprusside is infused.[145] Thiocyanate can cause neurologic toxicity such as confusion, hyperreflexia, and seizures. Consequently, the dose of nitroprusside should be minimized and the drug given for as short a period as possible. Both the cyanide and thiocyanate levels in plasma should be monitored to avoid toxicity (see also Chap. 23).

Angiotensin-Converting Enzyme Inhibitors

The doses of these drugs should be reduced by approximately 50 percent in dialysis patients because they and their metabolites are excreted by the kidney. Accumulation of converting enzyme inhibitors can cause hematologic toxicity (see also Chap. 23). These drugs have two other types of toxic effects in predialysis patients. First, in patients who are not being treated by dialysis, they can cause hyperkalemia by inhibiting angiotensin-stimulated aldosterone release, resulting in decreased potassium excretion and hyperkalemia. Second, they can cause rapid loss of renal function in patients with renal artery stenosis or other conditions associated with activation of the renin-angiotensin system, including congestive heart failure.[124,146] The mechanism for the decrease in GFR is inhibition of angiotensin-induced constriction of the efferent glomerular arterioles, which dilate and lead to a decrease in the hydrostatic pressure across the glomerular capillary wall. These drugs, like other antihypertensive agents, should be withheld on the morning of a hemodialysis treatment to avoid hypotension.

Cyclosporine

The use of cyclosporine in heart transplant recipients is often associated with loss of renal function, and some patients progress to CRF (see also Chap. 25). Cyclosporine constricts both afferent and efferent glomerular arterioles, resulting in a reduced GFR.[147] Proximal tubular injury—with vacuolar changes, inclusion bodies, and giant mitochondria—has been noted.[148] Cyclosporine usage can also cause hyperkalemia and renal tubular acidosis.[149] These effects are usually reversible if the dose is reduced or the drug is discontinued. Renal failure resembling the hemolytic uremic syndrome has been associated with cyclosporine (possibly due to endothelial damage).[148] Finally, obliterative arteriopathy with interstitial fibrosis and glomerular sclerosis can occur.[148,150]

REFERENCES

1. Rostand SG, Brunzell JD, Cannon RO, Victor RG. Cardiovascular complications in renal failure. *J Am Soc Nephrol* 1991; 2:1053–1062.
2. United States Renal Data System: 1194 Annual Report. *Am J Kidney Dis* 1994; 24(suppl 2):48–56.
3. Lazarus JM, Lowrie EG, Hampers CL, Merrill JP. Cardiovascular disease in uremic patients on hemodialysis. *Kidney Int* 1975; (suppl 2):S167–S175.
4. Ma KW, Greene El, Raji L. Cardiovascular risk factors in chronic renal failure and hemodialysis populations. *Am J Kidney Dis* 1992; 19:505–513.
5. Blumberg A, Nelp WB, Hegstrom RM, Scribner BH. Extracellular volume in patients with chronic renal disease treated for hypertension by sodium restriction. *Lancet* 1967; 2:69–73.
6. Vertes V, Cangiano JL, Berman LB, Gould A. Hypertension in end-stage renal disease. *N Engl J Med* 1991; 280:978–981.
7. Weidmann P, Maxwell MH, Lupu AN, Lewin AJ, Massry SG. Plasma renin activity and blood pressure in terminal renal failure. *N Engl J Med* 1991; 285:757–762.
8. Wilkinson R, Scott DF, Uldall PR, Kerr DNS, Swinney J. Plasma renin and exchangeable sodium in the hypertension of chronic renal failure—The effect of bilateral nephrectomy. *QJ Med* 1970; 39:377–394.
9. Kim KE, Onesti G, Schwartz AB, Chinitz JL, Swartz C. Hemodynamics of hypertension in chronic end-stage renal disease. *Circulation* 1972; 46:452–464.
10. Acosta JH. Hypertension in chronic renal disease. *Kidney Int* 1982; 22:702–712.
11. Kim KE, Onesti G, DelGuercio ET, Greco J, Fernandes M, Eidelson B, et al. Sequential hemodynamic changes in end-stage renal disease and the anephric state during volume expansion. *Hypertension* 1991; 2:102–110.
12. Lazarus JM, Hampers CL, Merrill JP. Hypertension in chronic renal failure. *Arch Intern Med* 1974; 133:1059–1066.
13. Vaughan ED, Carey RM, Ayers CR, Peach MJ. Hemodialysis-resistant hypertension: Control with an orally active inhibitor of angiotensin-converting enzyme. *J Clin Endocrinol Metab* 1991; 48:869–871.
14. Kelly RA, O'Hara DS, Mitch WE, Steinman TI, Goldszer RC, Solomon HS, et al. Endogenous digitalis-like factors in hypertension and chronic renal insufficiency. *Kidney Int* 1986; 30:723–729.
15. Converse RL, Jacobsen TN, Toto RD, Jost RD, Cosentino F, Fouad-Tarazi F, et al. Sympathetic overactivity in patients with chronic renal failure. *N Engl J Med* 1992; 327:1912–1918.
16. Cinotti GA, Pugliese F. Prostaglandins in blood pressure regulation. *Kidney Int* 1988; 35(suppl 25):57–60.
17. Shichiri M, Hirata Y, Ando K, Emori T, Ohta K, Kimoto S, et al. Plasma endothelin levels in patients with uremia. *Hypertension* 1990; 15:493–496.
18. Radermacher J, Koch KM. Treatment of renal anemia by erythropoietin substitution: The effects on the cardiovascular system. *Clin Nephrol* 1995; 44(suppl 1):S56–S60.
19. Mann JFE. Hypertension and cardiovascular effects—Long-term safety and potential long-term benefits of r-HuEPO. *Nephrol Dial Transplant* 1995; 10(suppl 2):80–84.
20. Bloembergen WE, Port FK. A comparison of cause of death between patients treated with hemodialysis and peritoneal dialysis. *Am J Kidney Dis* 1995; 6:184–191.
21. Goldberg AP, Herschel RH, Patsch W, Schechtman KB, Province M, Weerts C, et al. Racial differences in plasma high-density lipoproteins in patients receiving hemodialysis. *N Engl J Med* 1983; 308:1245–1252.
22. Goldberg AP, Applebaum-Bowden DM, Bierman EL, Hazzard WR, Haas LB, Sherrard DJ, et al. Increase in lipoprotein lipase during clofibrate treatment of hypertriglyceridemia in patients on hemodialysis. *N Engl J Med* 1979; 301:1073–1076.
23. Chan MK, Persaud J, Varghese Z, Moorhead JF. Pathogenic roles of post-heparin lipases in lipid abnormalities in hemodialysis patients. *Kidney Int* 1991; 25:812–818.
24. Ames RP, Hill P. Elevation of serum lipid levels during diuretic therapy of hypertension. *Am J Med* 1976; 61:748–757.
25. Tanaka N, Sakaguchi S, Oshige K, Niimura T, Kanehisa T. Effect of chronic administration of propranolol on lipoprotein composition. *Metabolism* 1976; 25:1071–1075.

26. Harter HR, Meltzer VN, Tindira CA, Naumovich AD, Goldberg AP. Comparison of the effects of prazosin versus propranolol on plasma lipoprotein lipids in patients receiving hemodialysis. *Am J Med* 1986; 80:82–89.

27. Rorke SJ, Shippey W, Davidson WD. Acetate delivery to hemodialysis patients (abstr). *Kidney Int* 1975; 8:433.

28. Lindholm B, Norbeck HE. Serum lipids and lipoproteins during continuous ambulatory peritoneal dialysis. *Acta Med Scand* 1986; 220:143–151.

29. Lacour B, Chanard J, Haguet M, Basile C, Assan R, Di Giulio S, et al. Carnitine improves lipid anomalies in haemodialysis patients. *Lancet* 1980; 2:763–764.

30. Teraoka J, Matsui N, Nakagawa S, Takeuchi J. The role of heparin in the changes of lipid patterns during a single hemodialysis. *Clin Nephrol* 1982; 17:96–99.

31. Wessel-Aas T, Blomhoff JP, Wideroe T-E, Wirum E, Nilsen T. The effect of systemic heparinization on plasma lipoproteins and toxicity in patients on hemodialysis and continuous ambulatory peritoneal dialysis. *Acta Med Scand* 1984; 216:85–92.

32. Ritz E, Augustin J, Bommer J, Gnasso A, Haberbosch W. Should hyperlipemia of renal failure be treated? *Kidney Int* 1985; 28:S-84–S-87.

33. Golper TA. Therapy for uremic hyperlipidemia. *Nephron* 1991; 38:217–225.

34. Goldberg AP, Hagberg JM, Delez JA, Haynes ME, Harter HR. Metabolic effects of exercise training in hemodialysis patients. *Kidney Int* 1980; 18:754–761.

35. Hamazaki T, Nakazawa R, Tateno S, Shishido H, Isoda K, Hattori Y, et al. Effects of fish oil rich in eicosapentaenoic acid on serum lipid in hyperlipidemic hemodialysis patients. *Kidney Int* 1984; 26:81–84.

36. Rylance PB, Gordge MP, Saynor R, Parsons V, Weston MJ. Fish oil modifies lipids and reduces platelet aggregability in haemodialysis patients. *Nephron* 1986; 43:196–202.

37. Degoulet P, Reach I, Di Giulio S, Devries C, Rouby JJ, Aime F, et al. Epidemiology of dialysis induced hypotension. *Proc Eur Dial Transplant Assoc* 1981; 18:133–138.

38. Kinet J-P, Soyeur D, Balland N, Saint-Remy M, Collignon P, Godon J-P. Hemodynamic study of hypotension during hemodialysis. *Kidney Int* 1982; 21:868–876.

39. Rosa AA, Shideman J, McHugh R, Duncan D, Kjellstrand CM. The importance of osmolality fall and ultrafiltration rate on hemodialysis side effects. *Nephron* 1981; 27:134–141.

40. Keshaviah P, Shapiro F. A critical examination of dialysis-induced hypotension. *Am J Kidney Dis* 1982; 2:290–301.

41. Rouby JJ, Rottembourg J, Durande J-P, Basset J-Y, Degoulet P, Glaser P, et al. Hemodynamic changes induced by regular hemodialysis and sequential ultrafiltration hemodialysis: A comparative study. *Kidney Int* 1980; 17:801–810.

42. Henrich WL, Woodard TD, McPhaul JJ Jr. The chronic efficacy and safety of high sodium dialysate: Double-blind, crossover study. *Am J Kidney Dis* 1982; 2:349–353.

43. Hakim RM, Breillatt J, Lazarus JM, Port F. Complement activation and hypersensitivity reactions to dialysis membranes. *N Engl J Med* 1984; 311:878–882.

44. Amadori A, Candi P, Sasdelli M, Massai G, Favilla S, Passaleva A, et al. Hemodialysis leukopenia and complement function with different dialyzers. *Kidney Int* 1983; 24:775–781.

45. Dolovich J, Marshall CP, Smith EKM, Shimizu A, Pearson FC, Sugona MA, et al. Allergy to ethylene oxide in chronic hemodialysis patients. *Artif Organs* 1984; 8:334–337.

46. Jost CMT, Agarwal R, Klair-el-Din T, Grayburn PA, Victor RG, Henrich WL. Effects of cooler temperature dialysate on hemodynamic stability in "problem" dialysis patients. *Kidney Int* 1993; 44:606–612.

47. Hruska KA, Teitelbaum SL. Renal osteodystrophy. *N Engl J Med* 1995; 33:166–174.

48. Portale AA, Halloran BP, Murphy MM, Morris RC Jr. Oral intake of phosphorus can determine the serum concentration of 1,25-dihydroxyvitamin D by determining its production rate in humans. *J Clin Invest* 1986; 77:7–12.

49. Delmez JA, Tindira C, Grooms P, Dusso A, Windus DW, Slatopolsky E. Parathyroid hormone suppression by intravenous 1,25-dihydroxyvitamin D. *J Clin Invest* 1991; 83:1349–1355.

50. Silver J, Russell J, Sherwood LM. Regulation by vitamin D metabolites of messenger ribonucleic acid for preproparathyroid hormone in iso-lated bovine parathyroid cells. *Proc Natl Acad Sci USA* 1985; 82:4270–4273.

51. Friedman SA, Novack S, Thomson GE. Arterial calcification and gangrene in uremia. *N Engl J Med* 1969; 280:1392–1394.

52. Ibels LS, Alfrey AC, Huffer WE, Craswell PW, Anderson JT, Weill R. Arterial calcification and pathology in uremic patients undergoing dialysis. *Am J Med* 1979; 66:790–796.

53. Lewin K, Trautman L. Ischaemic myocardial damage in chronic renal failure. *Br Med J* 1971; 4:151–152.

54. Arora KK, Lacy JP, Schacht RA, Martin DG, Gutch CF. Calcific cardiomyopathy in advanced renal failure. *Arch Intern Med* 1975; 135:603–605.

55. McGonigle RJS, Fowler MB, Timmis AB, Weston MJ, Parsons V. Uremic cardiomyopathy: Potential role of vitamin D and parathyroid hormone. *Nephron* 1984; 36:94–100.

56. Gafter U, Battler A, Eldar M, Zevin D, Neufeld HN, Levi J. Effect of hyperparathyroidism on cardiac function in patients with end-stage renal disease. *Nephron* 1985; 41:30–33.

57. Ansari A, Kaupke CJ, Vaziri ND, Miller R, Barbari A. Cardiac pathology in patients with end-stage renal disease maintained on hemodialysis. *Int J Artif Organs* 1993; 64:560–564.

58. Wing AJ, Brunner FP, Brynger H, Jacobs C, Kramer P, Selwood NH, et al. Cardiovascular-related causes of death and the fate of patients with renovascular disease. *Contrib Nephrol* 1984; 41:306–311.

59. Hahn R, Oette K, Mondorf H, Finke K, Sieberth HG. Analysis of cardiovascular risk factors in chronic hemodialysis patients with special attention to the hyperlipoproteinemias. *Atherosclerosis* 1983; 48:279–288.

60. Rostand SG, Gretes JC, Kirk KA, Rutsky EA, Andreoli TE. Ischemic heart disease in patients with uremia undergoing maintenance hemodialysis. *Kidney Int* 1979; 16:600–611.

61. Degoulet P, Legrain M, Reach I, Aime F, Devries C, Rojas P, et al. Mortality risk factors in patients treated by chronic hemodialysis. *Nephron* 1982; 31:103–110.

62. Bullock RE, Amer HA, Simpson I, Ward MK, Hall RJC. Cardiac abnormalities and exercise tolerance in patients receiving renal replacement therapy. *Br Med J* 1984; 289:1479–1484.

63. Dudczak R, Fridrich L, Derfler K, Kletter K, Frischauf H, Marosi L, et al. Myocardial studies in haemodialysis patients. *Proc Eur Dial Transplant Assoc* 1984; 21:251–261.

64. Brown JH, Vites NP, Testa HJ, Prescott MC, Hunt LP, Gokal R, et al. Value of thallium myocardial imaging in the prediction of future cardiovascular events in patients with end-stage renal failure. *Nephrol Dial Transplant* 1993; 8:433–437.

65. DePuey EG, Guertler-Krawczynska E, Perkins IV, Robbins WL, Whelchel JD, Clements SD. Alterations in myocardial thallium-201 distribution in patients with chronic systemic hypertension undergoing single-photon emission computed tomography. *Am J Cardiol* 1988; 62:234–238.

66. Roig E, Betriu A, Castaner A, Magrina J, Sanz G, Navarro-Lopez F. Disabling angina pectoris with normal coronary arteries in patients undergoing long-term hemodialysis. *Am J Med* 1981; 71:431–434.

67. Wizemann V, Kaufmann J, Kramer W. Effect of erythropoietin on ischemia tolerance in anemic hemodialysis patients with confirmed coronary artery disease. *Nephron* 1992; 62:161–165.

68. Francis GS, Sharma B, Collins AJ, Helseth HK, Comty CM. Coronary-artery surgery in patients with end-stage renal disease. *Ann Intern Med* 1980; 92:499–503.

69. Batiuk TD, Kurtz SB, Oh JK, Orszulak TA. Coronary artery bypass operation in dialysis patients. *Mayo Clin Proc* 1991; 66:45–53.

70. De Meyer M, Wyns W, Dion R, Khoury G, Pirson Y, van Ypersele De, et al. Myocardial revascularization in patients on renal replacement therapy. *Clin Nephrol* 1991; 36:147–151.

71. Cruz DN, Bia MJ. Coronary revascularization in patients on dialysis: What treatment option should we choose? *ASAIO J* 1996; 42:139–141.

72. Jacobs C, Brunner FP, Chantler C, Donckerwolcke RA, Gurland HJ, Hathaway RA, et al. Combined report on regular dialysis and transplantation in Europe, VII, 1976. *Proc Eur Dial Transplant Assoc* 1977; 14:3–69.

73. Bernardi D, Bernini L, Cini G, Ghione S, Bonechi I. Asymmetric septal hypertrophy and sympathetic overactivity in normotensive hemodialyzed patients. *Am Heart J* 1985; 109:539–545.

74. Bernardi D, Bernini L, Cini G, Geri AB, Urti DA, Bonechi I. Asymmetric septal hypertrophy in uremic-normotensive patients on regular hemodialysis. *Nephron* 1985; 39:30–35.

75. London GM, Faviani F, Marchais SJ, de Vernejoul M-C, Guerin AP, Safar ME, et al. Uremic cardiomyopathy: An inadequate left ventricular hypertrophy. *Kidney Int* 1987; 31:973–980.

76. Wizemann V, Blank S, Kramer W. Diastolic dysfunction of the left ventricle in dialysis patients. *Contrib Nephrol* 1994; 106:106–109.

77. Parfrey PS, Harnett JD, Barre PE. The natural history of myocardial disease in dialysis patients. *J Am Soc Nephrol* 1991; 2:2–12.

78. London GM, De Vernejoul M-C, Fabiani F, Marchais SJ, Guerin AP, Metivier F, et al. Secondary hyperparathyroidism and cardiac hypertrophy in hemodialysis patients. *Kidney Int* 1987; 32:900–907.

79. Pedersen T, Rasmussen K, Cleemann-Rasmussen K. Effect of hemodialysis on cardiac performance and transmural myocardial perfusion. *Clin Nephrol* 1983; 19:31–36.

80. Nixon JV, Mitchell JH, McPhaul JJ Jr, Henrich WL. Effect of hemodialysis on left ventricular function. *J Clin Invest* 1983; 71:377–384.

81. Bornstein A, Gaasch WH, Harrington J. Assessment of the cardiac effects of hemodialysis with systolic time intervals and echocardiography. *Am J Cardiol* 1983; 51:332–335.

82. Kramer W, Wizemann V, Kindler M, Thormann J, Grebe SF, Schutterle G, et al. Influence of fluid removal rate during hemodialysis on left ventricular performance and exercise tolerance in patients with coronary artery disease. *Clin Nephrol* 1984; 21:280–286.

83. Hung J, Harris PJ, Uren RF, Tiller DJ, Kelly DT. Uremic cardiomyopathy—Effect of hemodialysis on left ventricular function in end-stage renal failure. *N Engl J Med* 1980; 230:547–551.

84. Ireland MA, Mehta BR, Shiu MF. Acute effects of haemodialysis on left heart dimensions and left ventricular function: An echocardiographic study. *Nephron* 1981; 29:73–79.

85. Madsen BR, Alpert MA, Whiting RB, Stone JV, Ahmad M, Kelly DL. Effect of hemodialysis on left ventricular performance. *Am J Nephrol* 1984; 4:86–91.

86. Henrich WL, Hunt JM, Nixon JV. Increased ionized calcium and left ventricular contractility during hemodialysis. *N Engl J Med* 1984; 310:19–23.

87. Chaignon M, Chen W-T, Tarazi RC, Nakamoto S, Salcedo E. Acute effects of hemodialysis on echographic-determined cardiac performance: Improved contractility resulting from serum increased calcium with reduced potassium despite hypovolemic-reduced cardiac output. *Am Heart J* 1982; 103:374–378.

88. Rackow EC, Fein IA, Sprung C, Grodman RS. Uremic pulmonary edema. *Am J Med* 1978; 64:1084–1088.

89. Wacker J, Merrill JP. Uremic pericarditis in acute and chronic renal failure. *JAMA* 1954; 156:764.

90. Ziegler TR, Lazarus JM, Young LS, Hakim R, Wilmore DW. Effects of recombinant human growth hormone in adults receiving maintenance hemodialysis. *J Am Soc Nephrol* 1991; 2:1130–1135.

91. Rostand SG, Rutsky EA. Pericarditis in end-stage renal disease. *Cardiol Clin* 1990; 8:701–707.

92. Osanloo E, Shalhoub RJ, Cioffi RF, Parker RH. Viral pericarditis in patients receiving hemodialysis. *Arch Intern Med* 1979; 139:301–303.

93. Houston MC, McChesney JA, Chatterjee K. Pericardial effusion associated with minoxidil therapy. *Arch Intern Med* 1981; 141:69–71.

94. Silverberg S, Oreopoulos DG, Wise DJ, Uden DE, Meindok H, Jones M, et al. Pericarditis in patients undergoing long-term hemodialysis and peritoneal dialysis. *Am J Med* 1977; 63:874–880.

95. Eliasson G, Murphy JF. Steroid therapy in uremic pericarditis. *JAMA* 1974; 229:1634–1635.

96. Buselmeier TJ, Simmons RL, Najarian JS, Mauer SM, Matas AJ, Kjellstrand CM. Uremic pericardial effusion. *Nephron* 1976; 16:371–380.

97. Minuth NW, Nottebohm GA, Eknoyan G, Suki WN. Indomethacin treatment of pericarditis in chronic hemodialysis patients. *Arch Intern Med* 1975; 135:807–810.

98. Spector D, Alfred H, Siedlecki M, Briefel G. A controlled study of the effect of indomethacin in uremic pericarditis. *Kidney Int* 1983; 24:663–669.

99. Goldberg M, Lazarus JM, Gottlieb MN, Lowrie EG, Merrill JP. Treatment of uremic pericardial effusion. *Proc Clin Dial Transplant Forum* 1975; 5:20–25.

100. Singh S, Newark K, Ishikawa I, Mitra S, Berman LB. Pericardiectomy in uremia. *JAMA* 1974; 228:1132–1135.

101. Luft FC, Kleit SA, Smith RN, Glover JL, Carr JB, de Quesada AM. Management of uremic pericarditis with tamponade. *Arch Intern Med* 1974; 134:488–490.

102. Morin JE, Hollomby D, Gonda A, Long R, Dobell ARC. Management of uremic pericarditis: A report of 11 patients with cardiac tamponade and a review of the literature. *Ann Thorac Surg* 1976; 22:588–592.

103. Daugirdas JT, Leehey DJ, Popli S, McCray GM, Gandhi VS, Pifarre R, et al. Subxiphoid pericardiostomy for hemodialysis-associated pericardial effusion. *Arch Intern Med* 1986; 146:1113–1115.

104. Peraino RA. Pericardial effusion in patients treated with maintenance dialysis. *Am J Nephrol* 1983; 3:319–322.

105. Moraski RE, Bousvaros G. Constrictive pericarditis due to chronic uremia. *N Engl J Med* 1969; 281:542–543.

106. Wolfe SA, Bailey GF, Collins JJ Jr. Constrictive pericarditis following uremic effusion. *J Thorac Cardiovasc Surg* 1972; 63:540–544.

107. Dobkin JF, Miller MH, Steigbigel NH. Septicemia in patients on chronic hemodialysis. *Ann Intern Med* 1978; 88:28–33.

108. Leonard A, Raij L, Shapiro FL. Bacterial endocarditis in regularly dialyzed patients. *Kidney Int* 1973; 4:407–422.

109. Cross AS, Steigbigel RT. Infective endocarditis and access site infections in patients on hemodialysis. *Medicine* 1976; 55:453–466.

110. Goldblum SE, Reed WP. Host defenses and immunologic alterations associated with chronic hemodialysis. *Ann Intern Med* 1980; 93:597–613.

111. Ruiz P, Gomez F, Schrieber AD. Impaired function of macrophage Fc gamma receptors in end-stage renal disease. *N Engl J Med* 1990; 322:717–722.

112. Forman MB, Virmani R, Robertson RM, Stone WJ. Mitral annular calcification in chronic renal failure. *Chest* 1984; 85:367–371.

113. Maher ER, Curtis JR. Calcific aortic stenosis in chronic renal failure. *Lancet* 1985; 2:1007.

114. Keane WF, Shapiro FL, Raij L. Incidence and type of infections occurring in 445 chronic hemodialysis patients. *Trans Am Soc Artif Int Organ* 1977; 23:41–46.

115. Nsouli KA, Lazarus JM, Schoenbaum SC, Gottlieb MN, Lowrie EG, Shocair M. Bacteremic infection in hemodialysis. *Arch Intern Med* 1979; 139:1255–1258.

116. Kyriakidis M, Voudiclaris S, Kremastinos D, Robinson-Kyriakidas C, Vyssoulis G, Zervakis D, et al. Cardiac arrhythmias in chronic renal failure. *Nephron* 1984; 38:26–29.

117. Weber H, Schwarzer C, Stummvoll HK, Joskowics G, Wolf A, Steinbach K, et al. Chronic hemodialysis: High risk patients for arrhythmias? *Nephron* 1984; 37:180–185.

118. Forsstrom J, Heinonen E, Valimaki I, Antila K. Effects of hemodialysis on heart rate variability in chronic renal failure. *Scand J Clin Lab Invest* 1986; 46:665–670.

119. Wizeman V, Kramer W, Funke T, Schutterle G. Dialysis-induced cardiac arrhythmias: Fact or fiction? *Nephron* 1985; 39:356–360.

120. Dazu VJ. Renal and circulatory mechanisms in congestive heart failure. *Kidney Int* 1987; 31:1402–1415.

121. Mettauer B, Rouleau J-L, Bichet D, Juneau C, Kortas C, Barjon J-N, et al. Sodium and water excretion abnormalities in congestive heart failure. *Ann Intern Med* 1986; 105:161–167.

122. Sugawara A, Nakao K, Morii N, Yamada T, Itoh H, Shiono S, et al. Synthesis of atrial natriuretic polypeptide in human failing hearts. *J Clin Invest* 1992; 81:1962–1970.

123. Lee WH, Packer M. Prognostic importance of serum sodium concentration and its modification by converting-enzyme inhibition in patients with severe chronic heart failure. *Circulation* 1986; 73:257–267.

124. Packer M, Lee WH, Medina N, Yushak M, Kessler P. Functional renal insufficiency during long-term therapy with captopril and enalapril in severe chronic heart failure. *Ann Intern Med* 1987; 106:346–354.

125. Dzau VJ, Packer M, Lilly LS, Swartz SL, Hollenberg NK, Williams GH. Prostaglandins in severe congestive heart failure. *N Engl J Med* 1984; 310:347–352.

126. Rudnick MR. Nephrotoxic risks of renal angiography: Contrast media–associated nephrotoxicity and atheroembolism—A critical review. *Am J Kidney Dis* 1994; 24:713–727.

127. Taliercio CP, Vlietstra RE, Fisher LD, Burnett JC. Risks for renal dysfunction with cardiac angiography. *Ann Intern Med* 1986; 104:501–504.

128. Holland MD, Galla JH, Sanders PW, Luke RG. Effect of urinary pH and diatrizoate on Bence Jones protein nephrotoxicity in the rat. *Kidney Int* 1985; 27:46–50.

129. Fang LST, Sirota RA, Ebert TH, Lichtenstein NS. Low fractional excretion of sodium with contrast media–induced acute renal failure. *Arch Intern Med* 1980; 140:531–533.

130. Solomon R, Werner C, Mann D, D'Elia J, Silva P. Effects of saline, mannitol, and furosemide on acute decreases in renal function induced by radiocontrast agents. *N Engl J Med* 1994; 331:1416–1420.

131. Thadhani RI, Camargo CA Jr. Atheroembolic renal failure after invasive procedures: Natural history based on 52 histologically proven cases. *Medicine* 1995; 74:350–358.

132. Dalakos TG, Streeten DHP, Jones D, Obeid A. "Malignant" hypertension resulting from atheromatous embolization predominantly of one kidney. *Am J Med* 1974; 57:135–138.

133. McGowan JA, Greenberg A. Cholesterol atheroembolic renal disease. *Am J Nephrol* 1986; 6:135–139.

134. Richards AM, Eliot RS, Kanjuh VI, Bloemendaal RD, Edwards JE. Cholesterol embolism: A multiple-system disease masquerading as polyarteritis nodosa. *Am J Cardiol* 1965; 15:696–707.

135. Scully RE, Mark EJ, McNeely BU. Case records of the Massachusetts General Hospital. *N Engl J Med* 1986; 315:308–315.

136. Cosio FG, Zager RA, Sharma HM. Atheroembolic renal disease causes hypocomplementaemia. *Lancet* 1985; 2:118–121.

137. Lessman RK, Johnson SF, Coburn JW. Renal artery embolism. *Ann Intern Med* 1978; 89:477–482.

138. Winzelberg GG, Hull JD, Agar JWM, Rose BD, Pietka PG. Elevation of serum lactate dehydrogenase levels in renal infarction. *JAMA* 1979; 242:268–269.

139. London IL, Hoffstein P, Perkoff GT, Pennington TG. Renal infarction. *Arch Intern Med* 1968; 121:87–90.

140. Jelliffe RW. An improved method of digoxin therapy. *Ann Intern Med* 1968; 69:703–717.

141. Gibson TP, Matusik EJ, Briggs WA. *N*-acetylprocainamide levels in patients with end-stage renal failure. *Clin Pharm Ther* 1976; 19:206–212.

142. Bennett WM, Muther RS, Parker RA, Feig P, Morrison G, Golper TA, et al. Drug therapy in renal failure: Dosing guidelines for adults. *Ann Intern Med* 1980; 93:286–325.

143. Letteri JM, Mellk H, Louis S, Kutt H, Durante P, Glazko A. Diphenylhydantoin metabolism in uremia. *N Engl J Med* 1971; 285:648–652.

144. Kirch W, Gorg ER. Clinical pharmacokinetics of atenolol—A review. *Eur J Drug Metab Pharmacokinet* 1982; 7:81.

145. Cohn JN, Burke LP. Nitroprusside. *Ann Intern Med* 1979; 91:752–757.

146. Hricik DE, Browning PJ, Kopelman R, Goorno WE, Madias NE, Dzau VJ. Captopril-induced functional renal insufficiency in patients with bilateral renal-artery stenoses or renal-artery stenosis in a solitary kidney. *Med Intell* 1983; 308:373–376.

147. Barros EJG, Boim MA, Ajzen H, Ramos OL, Schor N. Glomerular hemodynamics and hormonal participation on cyclosporine nephrotoxicity. *Kidney Int* 1987; 32:19–25.

148. Myers BD. Cyclosporine nephrotoxicity. *Kidney Int* 1986; 30:964–974.

149. Bantle JP, Nath KA, Sutherland DER, Najarian JS, Ferris TF. Effects of cyclosporine on the renin-angiotensin-aldosterone system and potassium excretion in renal transplant recipients. *Arch Intern Med* 1985; 145:505–508.

150. Myers BD, Sibley R, Newton L, Tomlanovich SJ, Bashkos C, Stinson E, et al. The long-term course of cyclosporine-associated chronic nephropathy. *Kidney Int* 1988; 33:590–600.

95

EXERCISE AND THE HEART: ACUTE HEMODYNAMICS, CONDITIONING TRAINING, THE ATHLETE'S HEART, AND SUDDEN DEATH

Peter M. Buttrick / James Scheuer

In recent years considerable interest has been focused on the effects of exercise conditioning on the cardiovascular system. This is due to clinical studies that suggest that exercise increases longevity and decreases the risk and symptoms of cardiovascular disease and to animal studies that show a reduced vulnerability to ischemic insult and lethal arrhythmias in the isolated hearts of conditioned animals. Also, hypertrophy of the heart secondary to dynamic physical conditioning has intrigued cardiac physiologists because it represents a unique form of cardiac hypertrophy associated with normal or enhanced cardiac function and coronary reserve. This contrasts with hypertrophy associated with chronic systolic overload, as observed in patients with long-standing hypertension or aortic stenosis, in which impaired cardiac function and depressed coronary reserve can be seen. The current concept that exercise contributes to cardiovascular health must be contrasted with the historic view that prolonged exercise causes severe heart disease as evidenced by cardiac enlargement, significant arrhythmias, and electrocardiographic abnormalities. While this historic misconception has largely been corrected, the modern-day explosion of interest in exercise and physical fitness threatens to create a new myth of "biological arrogance" that implies that exercise can prevent or cure cardiac illness. In reality, exercise and conditioning may have broad-based, though modest, salutary effects on the heart. Exercise training, however, is not universally beneficial or even safe.

This chapter will provide physicians with an understanding of the physiologic responses that accompany acute exercise and the chronic cardiovascular adaptations that occur as a result of physical conditioning. Several excellent reviews of various aspects of exercise conditioning have been published.[1–4]

ACUTE HEMODYNAMICS

The chronic cardiac adaptations that develop as a result of conditioning reflect acute hemodynamic responses to repeated imposed loads. In this context, it is important to distinguish the acute load posed by isotonic (dynamic) exercise, which produces large increases in both cardiac output and oxygen consumption ($\dot{V}_{O_2}$) and a fall in systemic vascular resistance, from isometric (static) exercise, which acutely increases systemic vascular resistance while producing only minimal changes in cardiac output and $\dot{V}_{O_2}$.[5] Cardiovascular data illustrating these distinctions from eight normal subjects performing either isometric (in this case sustained contraction of the knee extensor muscles against a fixed load) or isotonic (two-legged exercise on a cycling ergometer) exercise are shown in Table 95-1. It should be emphasized, however, that most competitive athletes perform a combination of isotonic and isometric conditioning, and the resultant cardiac adaptations probably reflect the combined effects of these hemodynamic loads.

Isotonic, or Dynamic, Exercise

The acute cardiovascular response to isotonic, or dynamic, exercise involves complex and integrated hemodynamic and

TABLE 95-1

CARDIOVASCULAR DATA FROM EIGHT NORMAL SUBJECTS AT REST
AND WHILE PERFORMING EITHER ISOMETRIC[a] OR ISOTONIC[b] EXERCISE

	Rest	Isometric	Isotonic
Cardiac output (liters/min)	5.7 ± 0.3	6.8 ± 0.7	21.9 ± 1.0
Heart rate (beats/min)	70 ± 7	110 ± 6	164 ± 4
Stroke volume (mL)	85 ± 7	62 ± 5	131 ± 5
Mean atrial pressure (mmHg)	94 ± 3	118 ± 6	124 ± 4
Systemic vascular resistance ($dyn \cdot s/cm^5$)	1352 ± 103	1466 ± 131	461 ± 56
$\dot{V}_{O_2}$ (mL/min)	324 ± 33	556 ± 42	2758 ± 472

[a] Sustained contraction of the extensor muscles of the lower extremities at 30% of maximal effect.

[b] Two-legged cycling at 82% of $\dot{V}_{O_2}$ max.

Source: Adapted from Bezucha et al.[5] Reproduced with permission from the publisher and author.

neurohumoral functions that culminate in increased oxygen delivery to and extraction by the exercising muscles. In normal sedentary individuals, there is a 10-fold increase in oxygen consumption from rest to maximal exertion.[6] In well-trained athletes, the increase in maximal oxygen consumption can be as great as 20 to 30 times resting values, and indeed maximal oxygen consumption ($\dot{V}_{O_2max}$) is widely regarded as a measure of the training effect or the degree of fitness.[7] The various factors that contribute to oxygen consumption can be illustrated by rearranging the Fick equation:

$$\dot{V}_{O_2} = HR \times SV \times (a - \dot{V}_{O_2})$$

where $\dot{V}_{O_2}$ is oxygen consumption, HR is heart rate, SV is stroke volume, and $(a - \dot{V}_{O_2})$ is the difference between arterial and mixed venous oxygen content.

With acute dynamic exercise, heart rate, stroke volume, and $(a - \dot{V}_{O_2})$ all increase, and the net result is a marked increase in $\dot{V}_{O_2}$.

The earliest hemodynamic response to acute dynamic exercise is probably a fall in systemic vascular resistance that reflects a marked vasodilation of the resistance vessels in the exercising muscle. This is most marked at mild levels of exercise, with only minimal further decreases in vascular resistance occurring at nearly maximal work loads. The hemodynamic effects of this reflex are twofold: afterload falls and the cardiac output is redistributed. During maximal effort in human beings, more than 80 percent of cardiac output may be directed to working muscle compared with only 18 percent at rest.[8] In experimental animals a 5- to 15-fold increase in blood flow to peripheral muscle has been reported.[9] Many factors contribute, including local autoregulation that may be mediated by a fall in tissue P_{O_2} or by the release of locally acting vasodilators such as adenosine and lactic acid, and the effects of circulating catecholamines and stimulation of sympathetic vasodilatory nerve fibers. In addition, vasoconstriction of the splanchnic and renal circulation also likely occurs during acute exercise so that blood flow to these organs may actually fall, further redistributing cardiac output. A

schematic representation of the distribution of blood flow at rest and during peak exercise is shown in Fig. 95-1. Note the marked increase in flow both to the coronary arteries and to active skeletal muscles and the decrease in flow to other organs.

During sustained dynamic exercise, skeletal muscle metabolism is primarily aerobic. Therefore, it is appropriate that the increased demand for adenosine triphosphate (ATP) generation and utilization is met by a correspondingly large increase in oxygen supply. The aerobic capacity of exercising muscle is considerable and is far greater than that of the splanchnic and renal circulations, which are disproportionally perfused at rest. For this reason, oxygen extraction increases and mixed venous oxygen content decreases during acute exercise. In addition, during sustained dynamic exercise the local oxygen requirements of the *exercising* muscle are only partially met by the large increases in local flow. Therefore, at maximal exercise loads local oxygen extraction may also increase. With chronic conditioning, the aerobic capacity of skeletal muscle increases further, as evidenced by a marked increase in the activity of the enzymes of oxidative metabolism in tissue homogenates and by an increase in the size and number of mitochondria per unit of muscle.[4]

With acute dynamic exercise, the most striking cardiovascular alteration is an increase in heart rate, which is much greater in human beings than in smaller animals. Changes in heart rate correlate with both cardiac output and $\dot{V}_{O_2}$.[10] The main cause of the rise in heart rate with exercise is sympathetic stimulation. This is demonstrated by the attenuating effects of β-adrenergic blockade. Parasympathetic withdrawal also plays a definite but lesser role. During maximal effort, changes in heart rate alone cannot completely account for the improved cardiac output; in fact, clear increases in stroke volume have been shown to occur in human beings and also in experimental animals in studies in which heart rate and afterload were precisely controlled.[11] The increase in stroke volume results from a variety of factors, foremost among which are Frank-Starling effects. With acute exercise, in addition to the decrease in systemic vascular resistance mentioned above, there is an increase in venous return. This is probably mediated by sympathetic vasoconstriction of the large-capacitance veins as well as by the pumping effects of muscular contraction. It is more prominent with supine than with upright exercise. The hemodynamic effect of these volume shifts is an increase in end-diastolic volume, and the concept of diastolic or volume loading has been proposed as a feature of dynamic exercise conditioning. Studies in both dogs and human beings have shown that the increase in end-diastolic volume is most marked at maximal work loads, suggesting that both exercise type and intensity are important factors in determining the diastolic volume load to which exercised hearts are exposed. This point is quite pertinent when evaluating the prevalence and degree of cardiac hypertrophy in physically conditioned subjects. In addition, with acute exercise most researchers have reported an independent increase in inotrophy manifested by a decrease in end-systolic volume, an increase in maximum dP/dt, and an increase in fractional shortening, although given the changes in preload and afterload associated with acute exercise, this is hard to establish with certainty. The increased inotropy is probably also related to acute catecholamine effects as well as to intrinsic cardiac adaptations. The increases in cardiac output and stroke volume are paralleled by a marked increase in systolic blood pressure. Diastolic blood pressure remains unchanged and may even fall slightly, reflecting the significant decrease in peripheral vascular resistance. Therefore, mean arterial pressure increases only moderately.

Thus, the acute hemodynamic response to dynamic exercise is well adapted to provide large amounts of oxygen to exercising muscle for oxidative metabolism. This is accomplished by both central and peripheral adaptations. Heart rate, stroke volume, and $(a - \dot{V}_{O_2})$ difference increase significantly. In addition, there is a marked decrease in systemic vascular resistance and an increase in venous return. The increase in cardiac output is preferentially directed toward working muscle (see also Chap. 3).

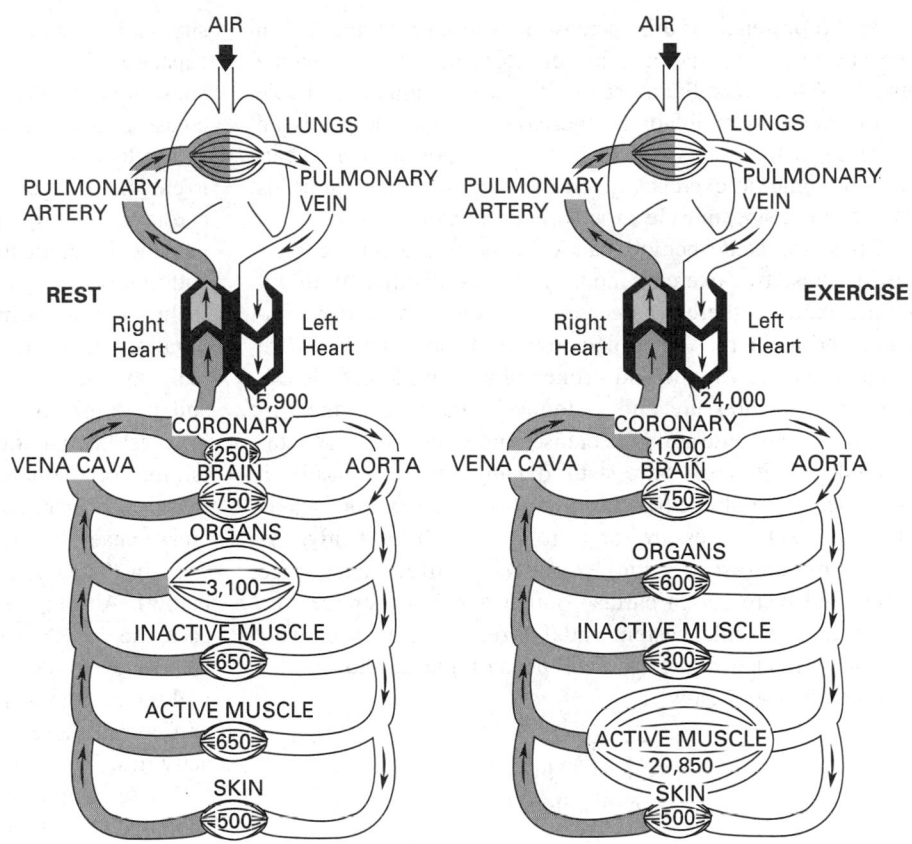

FIGURE 95-1

Schematic representation of the cardiopulmonary system at rest (*left*) and during peak isotonic upright exercise (*right*). During exercise, there are significant increases in blood flow to the exercising muscles and the coronary circulation, and flow to the organ falls. (Adapted from Mitchell JH, Blomqvist G. *N Engl J Med* 1971; 284:1018. Reproduced with permission from the publisher and authors.)

Isometric, or Static, Exercise

The acute cardiovascular responses to isometric exercise differ importantly from those to isotonic exercise. With isometric exercise a discrete muscle group is called upon to sustain a muscular contraction without performing external work. Since the muscle group involved tends to be small, the absolute oxygen requirements necessary to sustain the effort are proportionally modest. In the example shown in Table 95-1, $\dot{V}_{O_2}$ increases from 324 to only 556 mL/min with isometric exercise, compared with 2758 mL/min with an isotonic effort; however, the oxygen costs of isometric and isotonic work for a given muscular effort are similar. The increase in cardiac output required to maintain this level of oxygen consumption is also proportionally lower.

The oxygen requirements of the isometrically contracting muscle are not easily met by an increase in regional blood flow. Local vasodilatation is limited by a mechanical compression of the resistance vessels caused by sustained muscular contraction.[12] In fact, blood flow to the contracting muscle may actually fall. The combination of limited flow and increased metabolic demand appears to evoke a locally mediated pressor response that probably represents an important adaptation to maintain regional perfusion. This pressor response is at least in part mediated locally by an afferent nerve track originating in muscle, as demonstrated by studies in which an isometrically exercised muscle was maintained in an ischemic state with an occluding cuff after exercise.[13] As long as the cuff remained inflated, systemic arterial pressure was elevated; with release of the occlusion, pressure promptly normalized. The magnitude of the pressure response is proportional both to the relative tension sustained in the working muscle and the mass of the muscle groups involved, although a surprising increase in mean arterial pressure can be generated by a sustained contraction of relatively small muscle groups. For example, hand grip at 40 percent of maximal voluntary effort for 3 min can increase mean arterial pressure by 25 to 30 mmHg.

In the presence of this increase in arterial pressure and in the absence of an increase in venous return, stroke volume usually falls. Thus, the most significant mechanism available to the heart to maintain an increased cardiac output is an increase in the heart rate. In fact, the response of the heart rate to isometric exercise, given the modest metabolic needs of the exercising muscle groups, is quite exaggerated.

Thus, the acute hemodynamic loads placed on the heart during these two exercise modes are quite distinct. With dynamic exercise, there is a decrease in systemic vascular resistance and an increase in venous return leading to an increase in end-diastolic volume and stroke volume. With static loads, mean arterial pressure and systemic vascular resistance increase, venous return may decrease, and stroke volume actually falls. In its most pure state, dynamic exercise has been described as a volume (or diastolic) load, whereas static exercise represents a pressure (or systolic) load. Importantly, dynamic (in contrast to static) exercise, by virtue of the large associated increases in cardiac output and $\dot{V}_{O_2}$, stresses the entire cardiovascular system, and thus repetitive bouts of exercise may induce a spectrum of physiologic cardiovascular adaptations (see below).

CHRONIC ADAPTATIONS

With conditioning induced by chronic repetitive bouts of dynamic exercise, a number of cardiovascular adaptations develop, the effect of which is to enhance the ability of the organism to respond to exercise loads of varying type, intensity, and duration. The best single indicator of the functional capacity of the cardiovascular system is maximal oxygen consumption ($\dot{V}_{O_2max}$), and with conditioning this may increase as much as two- to threefold. About half of this increase is a reflection of adaptations that occur within the periphery to enhance oxygen extraction, and about half is due to a central cardiovascular component that serves to increase cardiac output and is characterized by changes in cardiac dimensions and indexes of systolic and diastolic performance.[14]

In addition to increasing maximal exercise intensity and duration, the trained person is also able to perform submaximal work loads with an economy of cardiovascular effort, and it is in this context that exercise conditioning has its broadest therapeutic impact. In patients with congestive heart failure, for example, the ability of the conditioned peripheral muscles to increase oxygen extraction may substantially increase anaerobic threshold and therefore functional capacity, even in the face of a fixed and limited cardiac output (see below). Alternatively, in patients with coronary artery disease, the decrease in resting heart rate and in the response of heart rate and blood pressure to a submaximal work load seen with conditioning may significantly alter patterns of angina and permit these patients to increase their meaningful daily activities.

These important points are illustrated in Fig. 95-2, which shows idealized cardiac responses to dynamic exercise in a sedentary control population and in a highly trained group of athletes. As illustrated, the trained subjects have a reduced heart rate at rest and at all submaximal workloads and are able to achieve a substantially higher level of exercise than their sedentary counterparts. Despite equivalent (or even slightly greater systolic blood pressures), the heart rate: blood pressure double product, a clinical measure of myocardial oxygen consumption, is significantly reduced at all submaximal workloads in the trained subjects.

The adaptations that occur with conditioning within skeletal muscle all serve to enhance oxygen extraction. These include changes both in structure and in metabolism. Numerous studies in experimental animals and conditioned athletes have shown an increase in capillary density and in the capillary-fiber ratio within skeletal muscle.[4,15] This, coupled with an increase in tissue myoglobin (a pigment that can serve to facilitate oxygen exchange in a fluid matrix), accounts for an increased diffusion of oxygen to the oxidative

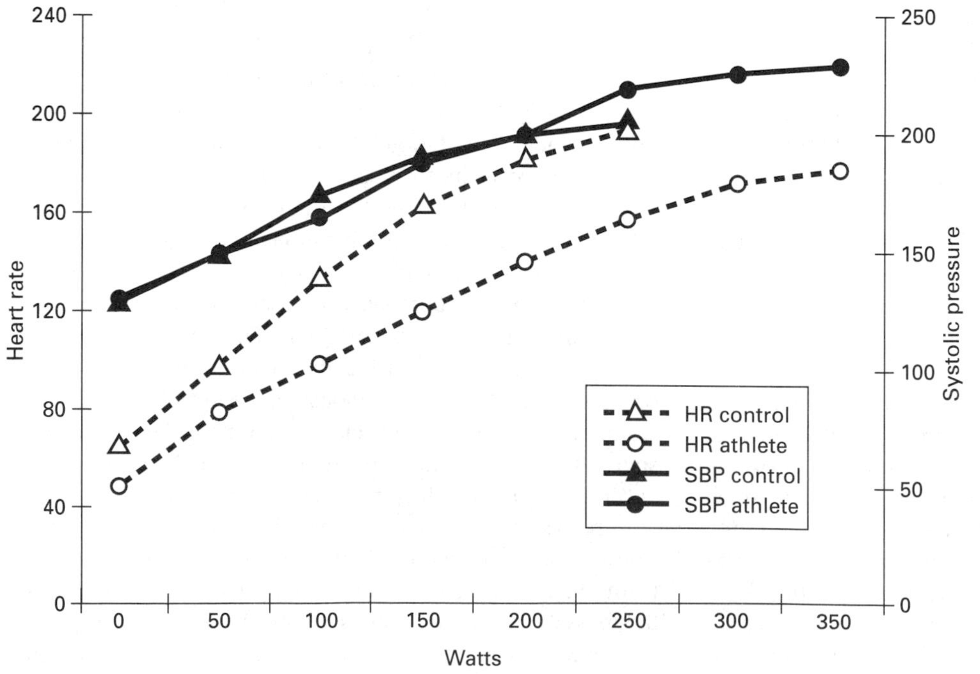

FIGURE 95-2

Cardiac responses during dynamic exercise in highly trained athletes (middle and long distance runners) and age-matched controls. The athletes have a lower double product (HR × SBP) at all workloads and are able to exercise to a higher level when compared with the controls. (Data are pooled from a number of published sources.)

machinery of the muscle cells. In addition, the muscle cells themselves have enhanced respiratory capacity. This is a reflection of the absolute increase in the size and number of mitochondria per cell and an increase in the level of respiratory enzyme capacity per mitochondrion. The myriad biochemical changes that occur within muscle cells and fibers of different types have been well reviewed.[4,14]

As mentioned above, the ability of the periphery to increase oxygen extraction accounts for approximately 50 percent of the increased $\dot{V}_{O_2 max}$ observed during exercise with training. In situations where cardiac output increases only minimally, however, the rise in oxygen extraction predominates. In fact, oxygen extraction may increase to such an extent within skeletal muscle that the increment in limb blood flow may be lower for any submaximal level of work in conditioned versus sedentary individuals. This is of practical benefit for patients with a limited cardiac reserve.

Cardiac adaptations that occur with conditioning have been more difficult to define precisely in human beings, in whom duration, mode, and intensity of conditioning protocols vary and among whom longitudinal studies are relatively rare. Therefore, much information has been derived from studies in inbred strains of animals subjected to carefully defined exercise protocols. These data can then be extrapolated to fit the available information for human beings. It is clear, however, that with conditioning in both human beings and experimental animals, significant alterations in cardiac structure and function occur that allow the heart to increase its stroke volume markedly. In athletes, during submaximal exercise a normal cardiac output is seen at a reduced heart rate compared with unconditioned controls, and at peak exercise intensity athletes have a marked increase in cardiac output at an equivalent heart rate. The mechanisms underlying this augmentation in cardiac performance reflect Frank-Starling effects (an increase in end-diastolic volume) and probably also augmented mechanisms of both myocardial contraction and relaxation.

The primary cardiac adaptation that occurs with training is an increase in heart size. In trained human beings, both longitudinal and cross-sectional echocardiographic studies have been done in trained athletes.[16,17] The left ventricular mass is increased approximately 50 percent in elite athletes compared with age-matched sedentary controls. This is predominantly due to an increase in resting end-diastolic dimension, although both posterior and septal wall thickness may slightly increase (rarely to more than 14 mm). In trained swimmers and runners, this translates into an increase in ventricular diastolic volume up to 60 to 80 percent. In longitudinal studies of swimmers, basketball players, and army recruits before and after intense conditioning programs, similar although less marked findings have been observed.[18–19] Interestingly, these changes largely regress within a few weeks following the cessation of training. A recent report in young male soldiers indicates that the hypertrophic response to training has a genetic component.[20] Subjects who had a deletion of a component of the ACE gene (DD genotype), which has

been associated with myocardial hypertrophy in other studies, had the greatest increase in myocardial mass. Representative echocardiograms (ECGs) from endurance-trained athletes and from isometrically trained athletes are shown in Fig. 95-3. In animal studies, where it is possible to control populations and the nature and degree of conditioning precisely, identical patterns of cardiac enlargement have been seen. In general, the increase in heart weight is 20 to 30 percent versus age-matched controls, and there are clear increases in diastolic dimension with preserved (or even reduced) systolic dimension. In general, the magnitude of the change in cardiac mass and dimension reflects the intensity of the trained program, and protocols that do not increase $\dot{V}_{O_2}$ to greater than 70 percent of maximum tend not to evoke this adaptation. The cardiac hypertrophy seen in response to the physiologic stress of dynamic exercise conditioning should be contrasted with the hypertrophy secondary to pathologic overload states such as hypertension and aortic stenosis, in which the increase in cardiac mass primarily reflects an increase in wall thickness with relatively preserved (at least until the late stages of illness) cavitary dimension.

The reasons cardiac dimension and mass increase with conditioning are not completely understood, but a number of factors have been identified that probably contribute. First, in a trained individual there is an increase in parasympathetic tone and a resultant bradycardia. Diastolic filling time is increased, and ventricular dilatation occurs. Also, during dynamic exercise the ventricles are exposed to an additional volume load, which in itself can lead to cardiac hypertrophy characterized by an increase in the number of mitochrondria in series and a pattern of eccentric cardiac hypertrophy.

That the mechanical properties of the physiologically hypertrophied muscle are enhanced independently of the Frank-Starling effects of increased end-diastolic volume has been suggested in studies of human beings and demonstrated in animal studies. In human beings, enhanced systolic performance during exercise has been difficult to demonstrate both because of the insensitivity of the methods employed and because of the changes in afterload that occur during exercise. In trained dogs, however, Barnard et al.[21] have shown increases in maximal dP/dt at submaximal and maximal work loads, and Stone[22] has shown that trained dogs have improved pumping ability at similar heart rates and require greater volume infusions to achieve similar left atrial pressures compared with controls. In smaller animals, several investigators have shown an increase in maximal dP/dt and in fractional shortening in hearts from conditioned rats under extreme loading conditions.[2,11,23] The diastolic properties of the physiologically hypertrophied heart have not been studied as extensively. Several studies using noninvasive imaging techniques in human beings have shown enhanced early diastolic filling and increased rates of peak myocardial lengthening during exercise in the hearts of conditioned athletes compared with controls,[24,25] and studies in isolated rat hearts have shown an increase in maximal negative dP/dt with physiologic hypertrophy.[23] All these studies are in clear contrast to work in systolic

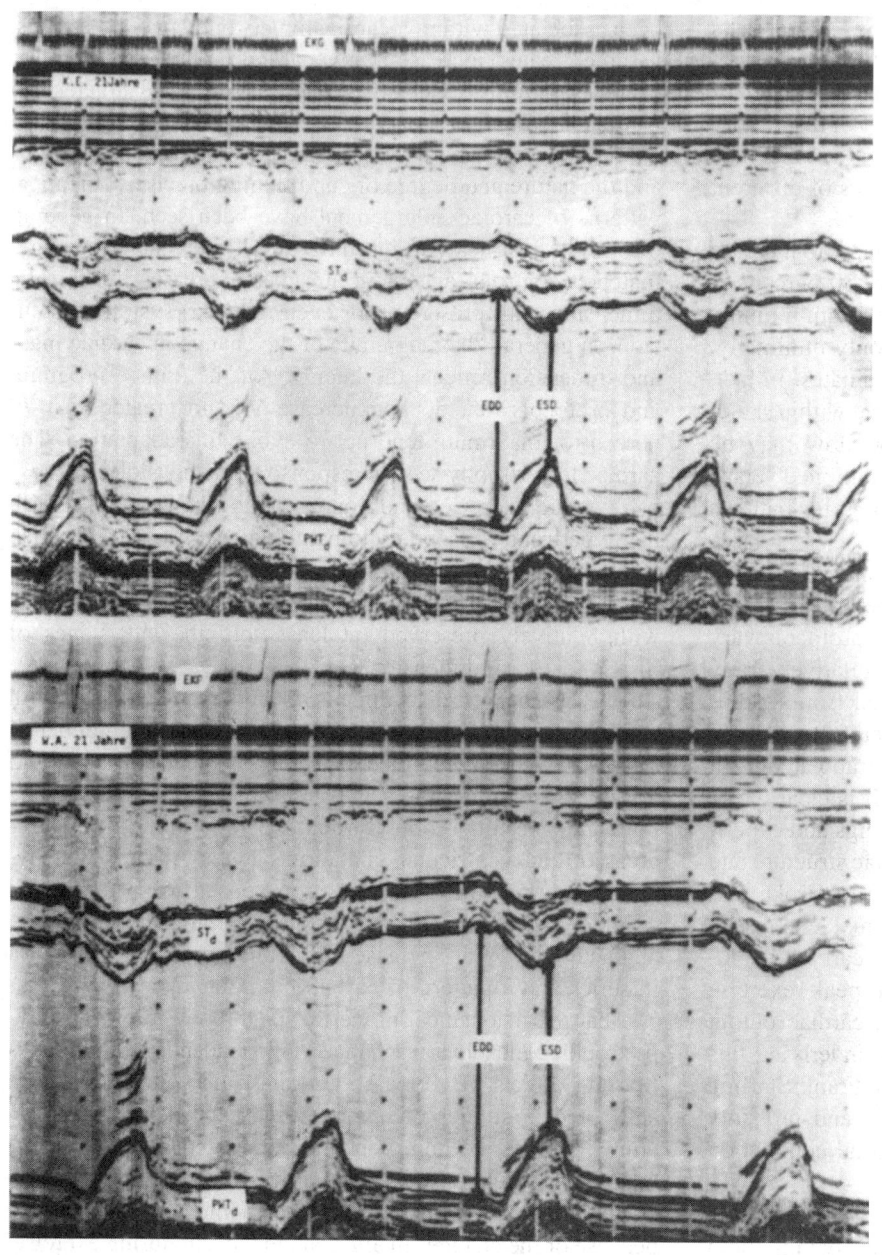

FIGURE 95-3
Representative echocardiograms from athletes trained for isometric and isotonic exercise. The left ventricle of a weight lifter (*top panel*) has an increased septal and posterior wall thickness, and that of a long-distance runner (*bottom panel*) has an increased left ventricular end-diastolic dimension. (From Keul J, Dickhuth H-H, Lehmann M. *Circ Res* 1981; 48:I-162. Reproduced with permission from the American Heart Association and authors.)

and rabbits (but not in human beings) an increase in the myosin isoenzyme of the $V_1(\alpha\alpha)$ type, which has increased adenosine triphosphatase (ATPase) activity, has been noted and correlated with the improved contractile performance seen in these hearts. In addition, alterations in sarcoplasmic reticulum and sarcolemmal function have been identified in conditioned hearts from a variety of species, suggesting alterations in calcium uptake and release that may account for the enhanced diastolic capabilities of these hearts.[26]

Adaptations also occur within the coronary circulation both at the level of the large epicardial vessels and within the microcirculation.[1,2,27] These adaptations probably help accommodate the large increases in coronary flow that occur during acute exercise. An early anecdotal report worth mentioning is the autopsy study of Clarence DeMar, who at the time of his death at age 70 had run more than 1000 long-distance races. At postmortem evaluation, his epicardial vessels were without atherosclerosis and were two to three times as large as those usually observed in septuagenarians.[28] Of course, this uncontrolled observation must be juxtaposed against examples such as that of Jim Fixx, the exercise enthusiast, who suffered a myocardial infarction while jogging and was found to have severe atherosclerotic coronary disease. Nonetheless, large necropsy studies in human beings and control studies in both dogs and rats suggest that exercise increases the cross-sectional area of the large epicardial vessels, although the functional significance of these changes is unknown. Changes that may be of more physiologic significance are observed within the microcirculation. Several animal studies have demonstrated an increase in the capillary den-

overload hypertrophied hearts, in which peak shortening and relaxation rates are consistently reduced.

A number of ultrastructural and biochemical alterations have been identified in the hearts of physically conditioned animals that underlie the physiologic adaptations outlined above.[4,14] With conditioning, the absolute myocyte size increases, as does the ratio of myofibrils and mitochondria per cell. There is an increase in the respiratory capacity of the cardiac muscle, as evidenced by an increase in lactic dehydrogenase (LDH) and pyruvate kinase activities. In rats

sity and the capillary-fiber ratio in physiologically hypertrophied hearts. Perhaps the most elegant of these studies was the careful morphometry done by Anversa et al.,[29] who studied the hearts of rats conditioned by swimming. They found a 16 percent increase in capillary density and a 41 percent increase in capillary length, which they translated into a 10 percent decrease in the diffusion distance between capillary and myocyte mitochondria. These changes in the microcirculation are small and of uncertain benefit, but they may increase the efficiency of oxygen delivery to the physiologically stressed myocardium. Also, this adaptation in physiologically hypertrophied hearts should be contrasted with systolic overload hypertrophied hearts in which capillary-fiber ratios are diminished.

In addition to defining changes in capillary number and density, several investigators have studied the effects of exercise conditioning on coronary collateral formation. The results to date have been inconclusive; however, data in both human beings[30] and experimental animals[31–33] suggest that conditioning can promote collateral growth to a potentially ischemic vascular bed. Again, the clinical significance of these changes is uncertain, especially since ischemia per se is a far more potent stimulus to collateral formation. Thus, in response to the chronic load imposed by repetitive dynamic exercise, the trained organism develops characteristic adaptations, the effect of which is to sustain large increases in oxygen delivery to the periphery. The respiratory capacity of skeletal muscles increases, and cardiac structure and function are altered to maintain an increased stroke volume without adverse metabolic cost.

EXERCISE AS THERAPY FOR CONGESTIVE HEART FAILURE

The notion that exercise might subserve an important therapeutic role in patients with congestive heart failure has recently received a good deal of attention. This follows from an appreciation of the physiology of both conditioning and of heart failure. The former is characterized by enhanced cardiac output at a reduced energy cost as well as by increased skeletal muscle flow and oxygen extraction (see above), whereas the latter has opposite effects. In particular, chronic congestive heart failure is associated with changes in skeletal muscle that are characteristic of deconditioning, including muscle fiber atrophy, reduced mitochondrial size, and respiratory capacity.[34–36] In part reflecting these peripheral abnormalities, $\dot{V}_{O_2max}$ is depressed and the anaerobic threshold is lower in patients with chronic heart failure.

A number of clinical trials have been initiated to assess the role of chronic training in the setting of heart failure, looking at skeletal muscle metabolism as one of several clinical endpoints. Several are worth comment. Sullivan et al.[37,38] evaluated a population of patients with congestive heart failure before and after 4 to 6 months of moderate level conditioning (at ~75 percent $\dot{V}_{O_2max}$). While this regimen did not affect direct measurements of cardiac function, such as ejection fraction and left and right ventricular filling pressures, in fact $\dot{V}_{O_2max}$ increased by 23 percent with training, and this reflected peripheral adaptations, including an increase in skeletal muscle blood flow and oxygen extraction and a decrease in lactate production during exercise. Hambrecht et al.[39] obtained skeletal muscle biopsies and evaluated mitochondrial respiratory capacity in a similar population of heart failure patients before and after 6 months of training. This group also showed a 20 to 30 percent increase in oxygen uptake at the ventilatory threshold and at peak exercise after training

and was able to correlate this clinical improvement with measures of oxidative capacity in the skeletal muscle, including an increase in the volume density of mitochondria and in cytochrome C oxidase activity. Finally, Piepoli et al.[40] evaluated the effects of exercise on the exaggerated neural activity of afferent fibers sensitive to skeletal muscle work (ergoreceptors) that is seen in heart failure patients. The activity of this neural axis has been proposed to disproportionately increase blood pressure and to limit blood flow to the periphery in heart failure. Six weeks of forearm training were sufficient to reduce the ergoreflex contribution to diastolic blood pressure, ventilation, and leg peripheral vascular resistance, and these reductions were disproportionate in heart failure patients versus matched controls.

In summary, there is a growing and compelling body of literature that suggests that substantial salutary effects can be derived from exercise training in patients with heart failure. These effects seem to reflect skeletal muscle and neural adaptations rather than direct cardiac effects. Unanswered at present are the nature and duration of the training program required to effect these responses, and beyond this, it is unclear if there are long-term deleterious effects associated with chronic conditioning in heart failure patients. For example, it is unknown whether chronic increases in venous return and in end-diastolic volume are potentially harmful in specific subsets of patients with heart failure.

GENDER DIFFERENCES IN CARDIOVASCULAR RESPONSE TO EXERCISE

The relative incidence of cardiovascular disease in women is increasing. Nevertheless, there is a remarkable paucity of literature describing the unique physiologic responses of women to acute and chronic exercise, although this deficiency is gradually being redressed.[41] Even large population-based epidemiologic studies describing the cardiovascular benefits of physical fitness have mainly been limited to men. Some conclusions can be drawn, however, from the literature published to date.

In general, the physiologic responses and adaptations of women to exercise are qualitatively similar to those seen in men. That is, acute dynamic exercise results in a decrease in peripheral vascular resistance and increases in venous return, stroke volume, and peripheral oxygen extraction. Acute static exercise increases peripheral vascular resistance with relatively modest changes both in stroke volume and in $(a - \dot{V}_{O_2})$. There are gender-specific differences that help identify and explain the significantly (50 percent) reduced maximal aerobic capacity seen in women relative to men when $\dot{V}_{O_2max}$ is expressed as liters per minute.[42] First, if $\dot{V}_{O_2max}$ is adjusted to lean body mass (women have a higher percentage of body fat), the difference is reduced to about 10 to 15 percent. This probably reflects a true gender-specific difference in oxygen transport and delivery, since women have a lower hemoglobin concentration and a smaller blood volume than men, although differences in fitness cannot be ruled out.

Women have a smaller cross-sectional muscle mass than men (70 to 85 percent, depending on conditioning status), although both the absolute number of muscle fibers and the fiber-type distribution in an individual muscle group appear to be similar.[43] The mechanism(s) underlying skeletal muscle hypertrophy in men relative to women is unknown. Both estrogen and androgen receptors exist in muscle, and the well-described effects of anabolic steroids on muscle mass suggest that this phenomenon may be hormonally mediated. The greater absolute (isometric) strength in men is a reflection of the increased muscle mass, since strength normalized to cross-sectional muscle area is similar.[44] Interestingly, however, the capacity to perform isotonic exercise as measured by time to muscle fatigue is probably greater in women than in men. The women's world record for the marathon is approximately 90 percent of that for men, and women generally do better than men in endurance swimming competitions despite their reduced muscle mass. This might reflect estrogen effects on muscle metabolism. Several lines of evidence both in experimental animals and humans suggest that estrogen results in preferential utilization of fatty acids as substrate during exercise, with a relative sparing of glycogen stores.[45]

The cardiac (central) response to acute dynamic exercise differs somewhat in unconditioned men and women, which may have significant clinical implications. Both genders increase stroke volume during acute isotonic exercise, although careful radionucleotide studies in humans as well as animal studies suggest that they do so through slightly different mechanisms. In general, men tend to increase their ejection fraction during moderate to marked exercise with little or no increase in end-diastolic volume, whereas women tend to increase end-diastolic volume without a significant increase in ejection fraction.[46] This may be due to differences in cardiac structure (male hearts are larger, although when adjusted for lean body mass, they are equivalent in size), differences in afterload, or real differences in inotropy (chronic testosterone administration in experimental animals has been shown to have a potent inotropic effect[47]). Regardless, the lack of a rise in ejection fraction during treadmill exercise stress testing in a woman should not be presumed to reflect cardiac pathology and may in fact be a manifestation of her normal physiology.

THE ATHLETE'S HEART

The most important distinctions that a cardiologist is called upon to make in the assessment of an athlete are (1) recognition of the distinctive physical and laboratory features that characterize the athlete's heart that themselves are manifestations of the physiologic adaptation to conditioning and (2) recognition of cardiac pathologic conditions in patients who happen to be athletic. The general physical examination of the athlete includes some characteristic but unusual features.[48,49] Notable is a resting bradycardia, generally between 40 and 60 beats per minute. In addition, the normal respiratory variation in heart rate may be exaggerated. Blood pressure and jugular venous pulsations are normal. The left ventricular enlargement discussed above may be apparent on palpation of the precordium but is usually subtle, and a widely displaced apex impulse should alert the physician to concurrent cardiac disease. The first and second heart sounds are normal; however, both S_3 and S_4 are heard in up to 50 percent of athletes. These sounds are maximal in the supine position and are without clinical significance. Short, midsystolic murmurs are quite common, presumably reflecting the large stroke volume. The presence of a thrill or a diastolic murmur warrants further investigation.

Electrocardiographic alterations are often seen.[50] Sinus bradycardia and sinus arrhythmia are extremely common and may be quite dramatic, with sinus pauses of up to 2.5 s. Therefore, it is not surprising that junctional escape beats are also frequently observed. First-degree atrioventricular (AV) block may be found in approximately 20 percent of athletes, and periods of Mobitz I second-degree AV block may also be observed.[51] These abnormalities are almost exclusively vagally mediated and disappear with exercise or atropine administration.

The clinical significance of bradycardia in athletes poses an intriguing problem for the consulting physician. This is illustrated by a recent study that contrasted 16 patients who undertook heavy exercise and developed postural syncope or Stokes-Adams attacks (group 1) with 37 elite asymptomatic athletes (group 2).[52] Ambulatory ECG recordings showed heart rates between 30 and 40 in both groups; however, electrophysiologic study revealed significant conduction abnormalities in approximately half the group 1 patients. Eight group 1 patients became asymptomatic with deconditioning, and the remainder required permanent pacemaker insertion. Group 2 patients required no specific intervention. This study highlights the distinction between the physiologic adaptations seen in the elite athletes in group 2 and the true abnormal findings in the group 1 patients that were perhaps worsened by the increased vagal tone associated with exercise conditioning.

Abnormal signal-averaged ECGs (SAECG) are seen in a relatively high percentage (8 to 10 percent) of endurance-trained athletes, but this does not appear to have any prognostic significance.[53] Supraventricular and ventricular premature contractions occur in athletes but probably no more frequently than in the general population. Certainly the development of a malignant supraventricular or ventricular tachycardia should not be ascribed to the "athlete's heart syndrome" and warrants further investigation.

Changes in P-wave and QRS morphology are commonly observed in trained athletes. Increases in P-wave voltage suggesting left or right atrial enlargement are commonly seen. An increase in QRS voltage suggesting left or right ventricular hypertrophy is seen in approximately 50 percent of athletes and is often associated with T-wave inversion in the inferior leads. Axis deviation and QRS prolongation are not commonly seen and should alert the physician to the presence of intrinsic cardiac disease. An elevated early takeoff of the T wave is common, as is T-wave inversion in the anterior leads (juvenile T-wave pattern). Downsloping ST-T changes indicating abnormal repolarization (so-called strain) are unusual, although they may occur, particularly in subjects who perform predominantly isometric exercises, such as weight lifting.

The chest x-ray in a conditioned athlete often reveals cardiomegaly. This has been recognized since the 1920s, when it was incorrectly thought to reflect significant underlying heart disease. The heart is generally globular in shape, and the cardiothoracic ratio is between 0.5 and 0.6. A disproportionate increase in the size of any one cardiac chamber is not observed.

A large number of echocardiographic studies have described the nature of the athlete's heart.[16] They are alluded to above and are illustrated in Fig. 95-3. In general, isotonically trained athletes have a slight (less than 20 percent) increase in wall thickness, a slight increase in diastolic dimension, and a normal or even slight decrease in systolic dimension reflecting preserved or augmented systolic function. In contrast, isometrically conditioned athletes may show a concentric pattern of left ventricular hypertrophy. A recent echocardiographic study of nearly 1000 elite athletes defined the limits of cardiac hypertrophy associated with exercise conditioning.[54] This study found that left ventricular wall thickness of greater than 13 mm was very uncommon in athletes (even those engaged in intense power training) and was virtually limited to athletes training in rowing sports; wall thicknesses exceeding 16 mm were not seen. The presence of asymmetric septal hypertrophy is distinctly unusual, although it can occur. In such cases it may be difficult to distinguish between physiologic hypertrophy and hypertrophic obstructive cardiomyopathy, which may pose a risk of sudden death during exercise (Chap. 74). It may therefore be necessary in these rare cases to screen first-degree relatives and/or advise a period of deconditioning during which regression of hypertrophy should be noted in athletes but not in patients with a hypertrophic myopathy.

The athlete's heart presents the clinician with a spectrum of abnormalities that reflect physiologic adaptations to the conditioned state, not intrinsic pathologic conditions. It is important for the clinician to recognize these adaptations and distinguish them from real cardiac disease, such as "sick-sinus" syndrome or hypertrophic obstructive cardiomyopathy, which are as likely to occur in athletes as in any other segment of the population.

EXERCISE AND SUDDEN DEATH

Cardiovascular death during exercise is extremely rare.[55–57] The annual incidence of sudden death in individuals under age 30 is between 2 and 7 per 100,000, of which approximately 8 percent are exercise-related. In individuals over age 30, the incidence of sudden death is between 50 and 60 per 100,000, with approximately 2 to 3 percent of these deaths occurring during exercise. Estimated mortality rates during various

modes of exercise range from 1 death per 396,000 person-hours of jogging to 1 per 13,000 to 26,000 person-hours of cross-country skiing.

Several autopsy studies of victims who died during vigorous activities indicate that most of these individuals had either recognized or occult cardiac disease.[56,58,59] As might be suspected, the epidemiologic pattern of deaths was quite different in young (below age 35) and older (above age 35) populations. The largest studies of young patients are those of Maron et al.[58,60] and Waller.[61] Structural cardiac disease was identified in 85 to 97 percent. The most common entity identified was congenital anomalies of the coronary arteries in 30 patients (35 percent). Hypertrophic obstructive cardiomyopathy was second in frequency and was found in 19 cases (22 percent). Other diagnoses included coronary artery disease (5 percent), mitral valve prolapse (4 percent), rupture or dissection of the aorta (3 percent), and dilated myopathy and myocarditis (1 percent). Another large European study[62] found a high incidence of arrhythmogenic right ventricular dysplasia. In studies of older populations,[59,61,63] up to two-thirds of patients who died during exercise had an overt history of coronary artery disease, and the majority of the remainder had recognizable coronary risk factors. Other, far less prevalent abnormalities that were reported to contribute to death during exercise in this older population included cardiomyopathies, valvular heart disease, aortic disease, abnormalities of conduction, and primary arrhythmogenic disorders.

These pathologic findings have important implications for the identification of patients at risk. In the low-risk, younger age group, the search for an individual with significant cardiac disease presents significant problems of both accuracy and expense. While it is not feasible to perform noninvasive diagnostic studies on all active young individuals prior to participation in a vigorous exercise program, the American Medical Association Committee on Medical Aspects of Sports as well as the American College of Cardiology recommend that students taking part in vigorous athletics undergo a physical examination before competing. Certainly individuals with a history of or ECG consistent with a tachyarrhythmia, a conduction abnormality, or an AV bypass tract ought to be evaluated further, and some should be excluded completely from athletics. Similarly, the appreciation of a murmur consistent with a coronary anomaly, hypertrophic obstructive cardiomyopathy, mitral valve prolapse, or aortic root disease would mandate further evaluation. Among older patients, in whom the major risk factor for sudden death is coronary artery disease, it is prudent to perform an exercise stress test in all patients with known coronary artery disease and all others with risk factors or symptoms suggesting occult coronary artery disease prior to enrollment in a program of vigorous physical activity.

A final question is whether or not exercise conditioning may actually protect against cardiovascular death, especially in patients with either overt or covert coronary artery disease who are at high risk. With conditioning, the resting heart rate is decreased and the major determinant of myocardial oxygen demand, the product of heart rate and blood pressure, is lower for any submaximal work load.[64] Coronary capillarity and capacitance may increase, and myocardial oxygen demands and coronary flow per gram of myocardium at any submaximal work load are decreased. All these factors would tend to increase the intensity level necessary to provoke coronary ischemia. In addition, blood rheology may be altered so as to diminish platelet aggregability,[65–67] and the increase in circulating high-density lipoprotein (HDL) cholesterol may actually retard the development of atherosclerotic heart disease.[68] In isolated rat hearts, physical training increases the ventricular fibrillation threshold during hypoxia and ischemia.[69] It is therefore attractive to postulate that conditioning may delay the onset of clinical coronary artery disease and actually prolong life in populations at risk.

The epidemiologic evidence necessary to support this conclusion is compelling and includes a number of large longitudinal studies compiled over the past decade. Historically, one of the first of these was a mortality study of over 6000 San Francisco stevedores.[70] Careful records of their physical activities were kept as part of their employment record, and an analysis indicated that heavy work (greater than 5.2 kcal/min) significantly decreased the relative risk of fatal myocardial infarction over the 21 years of follow-up. In a complementary study, Morris et al.[71] surveyed nearly 18,000 British civil servants with sedentary jobs about their leisure time activities and subdivided them into two groups depending on whether they exercised vigorously (greater than 7.5 kcal/min) outside of work or were sedentary. After 8 years of follow-up, the relative risk for the development of symptomatic coronary artery disease was decreased by 50 percent in the physically active group and was independent of age, smoking history, or body habitus. More recently, Paffenbarger et al.[72,73] surveyed habitual energy output and correlated it with death and the onset of symptomatic coronary artery disease in nearly 17,000 male Harvard alumni who were followed over 16 years. Rates of first coronary attack were 25 to 30 percent lower among alumni who expended 2000 kcal or more per week during exercise compared with the less active males. Mortality rates were lower among the physically active subjects and were independent of coronary risk factors. Especially noteworthy was the observation that energy expenditure at a later age was the primary determinant of risk (or benefit) and was independent of activity at a younger age. Similar data have been reported in large studies from Puerto Rico and Finland and from a retrospective analysis of the Framingham patient registry (see also Chaps. 41 and 55).

A second approach has been to evaluate the role of exercise in the secondary prevention of myocardial infarction and cardiovascular death in patients who have sustained a prior infarction. This has been attempted by several groups.[74–77] Inadequate patient numbers, inadequate control groups, and incomplete compliance with the exercise programs make these studies difficult to interpret. Nonetheless, vigorous supervised physical activity after myocardial infarction was not associated with an adverse outcome, and, in fact, a trend toward increased survival was identified in patients who complied with a long-term exercise program in several of these studies.

Thus, it is reasonable to conclude that not only is carefully prescribed physical conditioning safe but also for the majority of the population, including selected patients with coronary artery disease, it may be of benefit in preventing or at least postponing the onset of symptomatic coronary artery disease.

REFERENCES

1. Moore RL, Korzick. Cellular adaptations of the myocardium to chronic exercise. *Prog Cardiovasc Dis* 1995; 37:371–396.
2. Schaible TF, Scheuer J. Cardiac adaptations to chronic exercise. *Prog Cardiovasc Dis* 1985; 27:297–324.
3. Wagner PD. Determinants of maximal oxygen transport and utilization. *Annu Rev Physiol* 1996; 58:21–50.
4. Holloszy JO, Coyle EF. Adaptations of skeletal muscle to endurance exercise and their metabolic consequences. *J Appl Physiol* 1984; 56:831–838.
5. Bezucha GR, Lenser MC, Hanson PG, Nagle, FJ. Comparison of hemodynamic responses to static and dynamic exercise. *J Appl Physiol* 1982; 53:1589–1593.
6. Bruce RA, Kusumi F, Hosmer D. Maximal oxygen intake and normographic assessment of functional aerobic impairment in cardiovascular disease. *Am Heart J* 1973; 85:546–562.
7. Saltin B, Astrand PO. Maximal oxygen uptake in athletes. *J Appl Physiol* 1967; 23:353–358.
8. Zelis R, Flaim S. Alterations in vasomotor tone in congestive heart failure. *Prog Cardiovasc Dis* 1982; 24:437–459.
9. Vatner SF, Franklin D, Higgins CB, Patrick T, Brunwald E. Left ventricular response to severe exertion in untethered dogs. *J Clin Invest* 1972; 51:3052–3060.
10. Hellerstein HK, Ader R. Relationship between per cent maximal oxygen (% max V_{O_2}) uptake and per cent maximal heart rate (% MHR) in normals and cardiac (ASHD) (abstr). *Circulation* 1971; 43(suppl 2):76.
11. Saltin B, Blomqvist G, Michell JH. Response to exercise after bedrest and after training. *Circulation* 1968; 38(suppl V):V1–V78.
12. Asmussen E. Similarities and dissimilarities between static and dynamic exercise. *Circ Res* 1981; 48:(suppl 2):I3–10.
13. Hanson P, Nagle F. Isometric exercise: Cardiovascular responses in normal and cardiac populations. In: Hanson P, ed. *Exercise and the Heart, Cardiology Clinics*. Philadelphia: Saunders; 1987:157–170.
14. Rowell LB. Human cardiovascular adjustments to exercise and thermal stress. *Physiol Rev* 1974; 54:75–159.
15. Hermansen L, Wachtlova M. Capillary density of skeletal muscle in well trained and untrained men. *J Appl Physiol* 1971; 30:860–863.
16. Maron BJ. Structural features of the athlete's heart as defined by echocardiography. *J Am Coll Cardiol* 1986; 7:190–203.
17. Maron BJ, Pelliccia A, Spirito P. Cardiac disease in young trained athletes. *Circulation* 1995; 91:1596–1601.
18. Ehsani AA, Hagberg JM, Hickson RC. Rapid changes in ventricular dimensions and mass in response to physical conditioning and deconditioning. *Am J Cardiol* 1972; 42:52–56.
19. Crouse SF, Rohack JJ, Jacobson DJ. Cardiac structure and function in women basketball athletes: Seasonal variation and comparisons with nonathletic controls. *Res Q Exerc Sport* 1992; 63:393–401.
20. Montgomery HE, Clarkson P, Dollery CM, Prasad K, Losi M-A, Hemingway H, et al. Association of angiotensin-converting enzyme I/D polymorphism with change in left ventricular mass in response to physical training. *Circulation* 1997; 96:741–747.
21. Barnard RJ, Duncan HW, Baldwin KM, Grimditch G, Buckberg GD. Effects of intensive exercise training on myocardial performance and coronary blood flow. *J Appl Physiol* 1980; 49:444–449.
22. Stone HL. Cardiac function and exercise training in conscious dogs. *J Appl Physiol* 1977; 42:824–832.
23. Schaible TF, Scheuer J. Cardiac function in hypertrophied hearts from chronically exercised female rats. *J Appl Physiol* 1981; 50:1140–1145.
24. Matsuda M, Sugishita Y, Koseki S, Ito I, Akatsuka T, Takámatsu K. Effect of exercise on left ventricular diastolic filling in athletes and nonathletes. *J Appl Physiol* 1983; 52:323–328.

25. Granger CB, Karimeddini MK, Smith V-E, Shapiro HR, Katz AM, Riba AL. Rapid ventricular filling in left ventricular hypertrophy: Physiologic hypertrophy. *J Am Coll Cardiol* 1985; 5:862–868.
26. Scheuer J, Buttrick PM. The cardiac hypertrophic response to physiologic and pathologic overload. *Circulation* 1987; 75:I63–69.
27. Scheuer J. Effects of physical training on myocardial vascularity and perfusion. *Circulation* 1982; 66:491–495.
28. Currens JH, White PD. Half a century of running: Clinical, physiologic and autopsy findings in the case of Clarence DeMar (Mr. Marathon). *N Engl J Med* 1961; 265:988–993.
29. Anversa P, Levicky V, Beghi C, McDonald SL, Kikkawa Y. Morphometry of exercise-induced right ventricular hypertrophy in the rat. *Circ Res* 1983; 52:57–64.
30. Froelicher V, Jensen D, Atwood JE, McKirnan MD, Gerber K, Slutsky R, et al. Cardiac rehabilitation: Evidence for improvement in myocardial perfusion and function. *Arch Phys Med Rehabil* 1980; 61:517–522.
31. Eckstein RW. Effect of exercise and coronary artery narrowing on coronary collateral circulation. *Circ Res* 1957; 5:230–235.
32. Cohen MV, Yipintsoi T, Malhotra A, Penparkgal S, Scheur J. Coronary collateral stimulation by exercise in dogs with stenotic coronary arteries. *J Appl Physiol* 1978; 45:797–805.
33. Roth DM, White FC, Nichols ML, Doggs SL, Longhurst JC, Bloor CM. Effect of long-term exercise on regional myocardial function and coronary collateral development after gradual coronary artery occlusion in pigs. *Circulation* 1990; 82:1778–1789.
34. Sullivan MJ, Green HJ, Cobb FR. Skeletal muscle biochemistry and histology in ambulatory patients with long-term heart failure. *Circulation* 1990; 81:518–527.
35. Drexler H, Riede U, Munzel T, Konig H, Funke E, Just H. Alterations of skeletal muscle in chronic heart failure. *Circulation* 1992; 85:1751–1759.
36. Mancini DM, Walter G, Reichek N, Lenkinski R, McCully KK, Mullen JL, et al. Contributions of skeletal muscle atrophy to exercise intolerance and altered muscle metabolism in heart failure. *Circulation* 1992; 85:1364–1373.
37. Sullivan MJ, Higginbotham MB, Cobb FR. Exercise training in patients with severe left ventricular dysfunction. Hemodynamic and metabolic effects. *Circulation* 1988; 78:506–515.
38. Sullivan MJ, Cobb FR. The anaerobic threshold in chronic heart failure: Reaction to blood lactate, ventilatory basis reproducibility and response to exercise training. *Circulation* 1990; 81:II47–58.
39. Hambrecht R, Niebauer J, Fiehn E, Kalberer B, Offner B, Hauer K, et al. Physical training in patients with stable chronic heart failure: Effects on cardiorespiratory fitness and ultrastructural abnormalities of leg muscles. *J Am Coll Cardiol* 1995; 25:1239–1249.
40. Piepoli M, Clark AL, Volterrani M, Adamopoulos S, Sleight P, Coats AJ. Contribution of muscle afferents to the hemodynamic, autonomic, and ventilatory responses to exercise in patients with chronic heart failure: Effects of physical training. *Circulation* 1996; 93:940–952.
41. Mitchell JH, Tate C, Raven P, Cobb FR, Kraus W, Moreadith R, et al. Acute response and chronic adaptation to exercise in women. *Med Sci Sports Exerc* 1992; 24:S258–265.
42. Drinkwater BL. Women and exercise: Physiological aspects. *Exerc Sport Sci Rev* 1984; 12:21–51.
43. Costill D, Daniels J, Evans W, Fink W, Krahenbuhl G, Saltin B. Skeletal muscle enzyme and fiber type composition in male and female track athletes. *J Appl Physiol* 1976; 39:149–154.
44. Astrand PO, Rodahl K. *Textbook of Work Physiology, Physiologic Basis of Exercise.* New York: McGraw-Hill; 1986; 343–344.
45. Kendrick ZV, Steffan CA, Rumsey WL, Goldberg DI. Effect of estradiol on tissue glycogen metabolism in exercised oophorectomized rats. *J Appl Physiol* 1987; 63:492–496.
46. Higgenbotham MB, Morris KG, Coleman RD, Cobb FR. Sex-related differences in the normal cardiac responses to upright exercise. *Circulation* 1984; 70:357–366.
47. Scheuer J, Malhotra A, Schaible TF, Capasso J. Effects of gonadectomy and hormonal replacement on rat hearts. *Circ Res* 1987; 61:12–19.
48. Huston TP, Puffer JC, Rodney WM. The athletic heart syndrome. *N Engl J Med* 1985; 313:24–32.
49. Crawford MH, O'Rourke RA. The athlete's heart. *Adv Intern Med* 1979; 24:311–329.
50. Zehender P, Meinertz T, Keul J, Just H. ECG variants and cardiac arrhythmias in athletes: Clinical relevance and prognostic importance. *Am Heart J* 1990; 119:1378–1391.
51. Meytes I, Kaplinsky E, Yahini JH, Hanne-Paparo N, Neufeld HN.

Wenckebach AV block: A frequent feature following heavy physical training. *Am Heart J* 1975; 90:426–430.
52. Ector H, Verlinden M, Vanden Eynde E, Bourgois J, Herman L, Fagard R, et al. Bradycardia syncope and sports. *Lancet* 1984; 2:591–594.
53. Moroe K, Kimoto K, Inoue T, Annoura M, Oku K, Arakawa K, et al. Evaluation of signal-averaged electrocardiograms in young athletes. *Jpn Circ J* 1995; 59:247–256.
54. Pelliccia A, Maron BJ, Spataro A, Proschan MA, Spirito O. The upper limit of physiologic cardiac hypertrophy in highly trained elite athletes. *N Engl J Med* 1991; 324:295–301.
55. Mittleman MA, Siscovick DS. Physical exercise as a trigger of myocardial infarction and sudden cardiac death. *Cardiol Clin* 1996; 14:263–270.
56. Thompson PD, Mitchell JH. Exercise and sudden cardiac death: Protection or provocation. *N Engl J Med* 1984; 311:914–915.
57. McCaffrey FM, Braden DS, Strong WB. Sudden cardiac death in young athletes. A review. *Am J Dis Child* 1991; 145:177–183.
58. Maron B, Shirani J, Poliac LC, Mathenge R, Roberts WC, Mueller FO. Sudden death in young competitive athletes. Clinical demographic and pathologic profiles. *JAMA* 1996; 276:199–204.
59. Maron BJ. Triggers for sudden cardiac death in the athlete. *Cardiol Clin* 1996; 14:195–210.
60. Maron BJ, Epstein SE, Roberts WE. Causes of sudden death in competitive athletes. *J Am Coll Cardiol* 1986; 7:204–214.
61. Waller BF. Exercise-related sudden death in young (age ≤30) and old (age >30) conditioned subjects. In: Wenger NC, ed. *Exercise and the Heart*, 2d ed. Philadelphia: FA Davis; 1985.
62. Corrado D, Thiene G, Nava A, Rossi L, Pennelli N. Sudden death in young competitive athletes. Clinical pathologic correlations in 22 cases. *Am J Med* 1990; 89:588–596.
63. Waller BF, Roberts WC. Sudden death while running in conditioned runners age 40 or over. *Am J Cardiol* 1980; 45:1292–1300.
64. Amsterdam EA, Dressendorfer R, Mason DT, et al. Exercise training in coronary heart disease: Physiological rationale, clinical indications and practical application. In: Mason DT, ed. *Advances in Heart Disease*, vol 2. New York: Grune & Stratton; 1978:345–362.
65. Dix CJ, Hassall DG, Bruckdorfer KR. The increased sensitivity of platelets to prostacyclin in marathon runners. *Thromb Haemost* 1984; 51:385–387.
66. Winther K, Hillegrass W, Tofler GH. Effects on platelet aggregation and fibrinolytic activity during upright posture and exercise in healthy men. *Am J Cardiol* 1992; 70:1051–1055.
67. Williams RS, Logue EE, Lewis JL, Barton T, Stead NW, Wallace AG, et al. Physical conditioning augments the fibrinolytic response to venous occlusion in healthy adults. *N Engl J Med* 1980; 302:987–991.
68. Wood PD, Williams PT, Haskell WL. Physical activity and high density lipoproteins. In: Mill NE, Miller GJ, eds. *Clinical and Metabolic Aspects of High Density Lipoproteins.* New York: Elsevier; 1984.
69. Noakes TD, Higginson L, Opie LH. Physical training increases ventricular fibrillation thresholds of isolated rat hearts during normoxic, hypoxic and regional ischemia. *Circulation* 1983; 67:24–30.
70. Paffenbarger RS, Hale WE. Work activity and coronary heart mortality. *N Engl J Med* 1975; 292:545–550.
71. Morris JN, Everitt MG, Pollard R, Chave SP, Semmence AM. Vigorous exercise in leisure time: Protection against coronary heart disease. *Lancet* 1980; 2:1207–1210.
72. Paffenbarger RS, Hyde RT, Wing AL, Hsieh CC. Physical activity, all-cause mortality and longevity in college alumni. *N Engl J Med* 1986; 314:605–613.
73. Paffenbarger RS, Hyde RT, Wing AL, Lee I-M, Jung DL, Kampert JB. The association of changes in physical activity level and other life style characteristics with mortality in men. *N Engl J Med* 1993; 328:538–545.
74. Shaw LW. Effects of prescribed exercise program on mortality and cardiovascular morbidity in patients after a myocardial infarction. *Am J Cardiol* 1981; 48:39–46.
75. Shephard RJ, Corey P, Kavanagh T. Exercise compliance and the prevention of a recurrence of myocardial infarction. *Med Sci Sports Exerc* 1981; 13:1–5.
76. Naughton J. Role of physical activity as a secondary intervention for healed myocardial infarction. *Am J Cardiol* 1985; 55:21D–26D.
77. Lakka TA, Venalainen JM, Rauramaa R, Salonen R, Tuomilento J, Salonen JT. Relation of leisure-time physical activity and cardiorespiratory fitness to the risk of acute myocardial infarction in men. *New Engl J Med* 1994; 300:1549–1554.

96

CARDIOVASCULAR AGING AND ADAPTATION TO DISEASE

Steven P. Schulman / Myron L. Weisfeldt

DIFFICULTIES IN THE STUDY OF AGING

Many individuals have a preconception that cardiovascular function decreases substantially during later life. This bias is certainly related to the fact that cardiovascular disease is so widely prevalent in our population. Since its prevalence and severity increases with age, the perception is that nearly every older American has "heart trouble."[1–3] Therefore, it is often difficult to dissociate aging from disease. For example, for many years there had been controversy over what level of systolic blood pressure represents a normal age-associated increase and what level indicates the presence of a disease, i.e., hypertension. It is now recognized that although systolic blood pressure does gradually increase with age, an elevated systolic blood pressure is a strong risk factor for the development of future cardiovascular disease and that lowering elevated systolic blood pressure with medications reduces the risk.[4,5] In attempting to distinguish age-related changes from those of disease, one should note several important factors. In Westerners, the autopsy prevalence of ischemic disease in those over 60 years of age is approximately 50 percent.[1–3] Thus, only studies in which subjects with ischemic heart disease are eliminated can be viewed as an examination of aging separate from disease.

Furthermore, it should be recognized that the manifestations of cardiovascular disease in any given individual may be partly age-determined. The severity of the disease-induced functional decline likely depends on the aging substrate upon which the disease is superimposed. The response to treatment in the individual with cardiovascular disease may also be determined in part by aging. For example, there is some evidence of a decrease, with aging, in the potency of the inotropic response to digitalis glycosides and catecholamines.[6–11] Such an age-associated decrease in response to pharmacologic agents may well affect the response to treatment in any given older individual with severe heart disease (see also Chap. 97).

NORMAL AGING

Cardiovascular Aging as a Selective Process

Age-related cardiovascular changes appear in a selective fashion.[12] Vision is similarly affected selectively by age. Near vision decreases with age, but distant vision remains excellent unless disease appears. The ability of the cardiac muscle to develop tension is well maintained with aging,[13] as is the inotropic response of the cardiac muscle to direct stimulation of the myofibrils with calcium.[7] Such observations predict relatively normal global left ventricular function at rest.[14,15] In contrast, there is a striking decrease in the response to stimulation of beta-sympathetic receptors of cardiovascular tissues.[6,9,12] This age-associated decrease in beta-sympathetic response manifests itself in decreased inotropic response of cardiac muscle, decreased arterial vasodilating response, and decreased heart rate, or chronotropic response. When left ventricular workload is increased by exercise and other causes, there is enhanced use of the Frank-Starling mechanism to compensate for the increased workload.

Function of the Cardiac Muscle

Isolated cardiac muscle from rats, guinea pigs, and other species shows, with aging, a remarkable maintenance of abil-

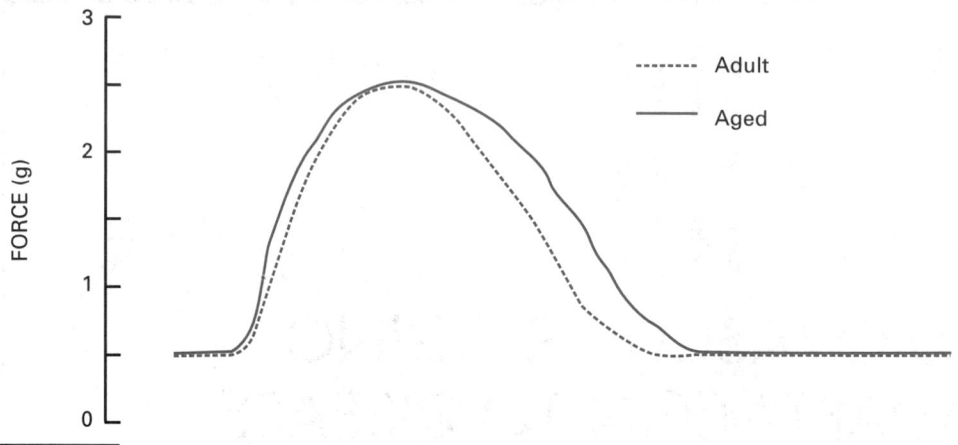

FIGURE 96-1

Typical isometric twitch in young adult (*dashed*) and in aged (*solid*) isolated cardiac muscle. Note that the rate of rise in tension and maximum tension achieved do not differ with age but that the duration of contraction is prolonged, primarily due to slowed and delayed relaxation.

In summary, in aging cardiac muscle the rate and extent of tension development are normal but there is a delayed and decreased relaxation rate. The velocity of shortening, particularly at low loads, is also decreased.

Left Ventricular Function in Human Beings at Rest

Parallel studies in humans utilizing both echocardiographic and radionuclide scintigraphy for left ventricular volume assessment have shown that resting systolic left ventricular function is well maintained with age in healthy subjects.[12,14–16] As in animal models, left ventricular mass and wall thickness increase with age in healthy individuals, probably due to the age-related increase in afterload (see below).

As in the animal models, at rest there is a slowed and delayed early diastolic left ventricular relaxation in humans.[24] As a result, noninvasive studies have shown a decrease in indices of velocity of early diastolic left ventricular filling.[15,25] This decrease in rapid filling may be consequent to several age-related changes, including a prolongation of the time constant of relaxation,[26] mild left ventricular hypertrophy,[15] an increase in afterload,[27] an increase in left ventricular chamber stiffness,[28] and an increase in regional heterogeneity in filling among left ventricular segments.[29] Unlike the animals studied, senior endurance athletes have a similar decrease in left ventricular peak filling compared to age-matched sedentary subjects in most but not all studies.[30,31] In part, the end-diastolic volume is maintained in healthy elderly subjects because of an increased atrial contribution to late left ventricular filling.[32]

In summary, in resting human beings, there is no major age-associated change in left ventricular systolic function. The characteristic prolonged relaxation of aging cardiac muscle can be identified easily in human beings. Signs include a prolonged isovolumic phase of diastole and slowed early diastolic left ventricular filling.

ity to develop tension when studied in vitro. As shown in Fig. 96-1, the rate of rise in tension and the maximum tension achieved under isometric conditions are unchanged with age. The lack of change in tension development, or the rate of tension rise, holds over the entire working range of muscle length.[13] There appears to be a small decrease in the velocity of shortening in cardiac muscle from senescent animals. This change may be related to a decrease in adenosine triphosphatase (ATPase) activity of the myofibrils, as studies show a progressive decrease in calcium-activated myosin ATPase activity with age.[17,18] It should also be noted that muscle and connective tissue stiffness increases with age, which tends to increase shortening velocity.[9]

The most striking and consistent change in mechanical performance of isolated cardiac muscle from senescent animals is prolonged duration of contraction and relaxation[19] (Fig. 96-1). The durations of contraction and relaxation are thought to be determined in part by the sarcoplasmic reticulum as well as by the duration of calcium entry during depolarization. The age-associated prolongation of relaxation can be attributed to both a decrease in the velocity of myocardial sarcoplasmic calcium uptake with increased age[20] and a prolongation of the action potential duration.[21] In younger animals, a similar prolongation of relaxation and decreased velocity of calcium uptake by sarcoplasmic reticulum is seen following hypertrophy due to pressure overload. In animals, significant myocardial cellular hypertrophy appears with aging. This hypertrophy is in part secondary to the increased impedance to left ventricular ejection as a result of stiffer arteries and to the dropout or death of some 20 to 25 percent of myocardial cells.[22] In experimental animals, the age-associated prolongation of relaxation and the decreased velocity of sarcoplasmic reticulum calcium uptake can be improved by intense exercise.[23] Thus, it is possible that the age-associated prolongation of duration of contraction is a reflection of both the age-associated myocardial hypertrophy and physical deconditioning.

CARDIOVASCULAR AGING AND ADAPTATION TO DISEASE

Although the changes in relaxation do not impact cardiovascular function significantly in healthy elderly subjects, prolonged relaxation may influence overall cardiac function in the presence of disease, particularly coronary and hypertensive heart disease, which further decrease early diastolic filling.[33,34] One would predict that in ischemic heart disease, delayed and prolonged relaxation would tend to compromise subendocardial blood flow, especially with tachycardia, since prolonged relaxation would accentuate the detrimental effect of an abbreviated diasatole by increasing diastolic pressure. Similarly, in the elderly with hypertension and left ventricular hypertrophy, dyspnea and/or fatigue may occur with the tachycardia of exercise because of an increase in left ventricular end-diastolic pressure and an inability to increase end-diastolic volume because of impaired filling of the ventricle.[35] Prolonged relaxation in the aged may contribute to the symptoms and poor tolerance of tachyarrhythmias. As discussed below, the depressed response to catecholamines and an increase in vascular load may also impair the cardiovascular adaptation to disease.

Depressed Inotropic Response to Catecholamines

Studies of isolated cardiac muscle and ventricular myocytes from older animals show a striking decrease in the inotropic response to catecholamines.[7–11,36] The inotropic response to calcium, however, is sustained, suggesting that myofibrillar contractile function and responsiveness are well maintained with aging.

The age-associated decrease in the inotropic response to catecholamines is determined partly by changes in the receptor. The number and affinity of beta-adrenergic receptors in the cardiac muscle of rats appear modestly decreased.[11] Studies in rat cardiac myocytes show a decrease in catecholamine-induced calcium release from the sarcoplasmic reticulum in senescent myocytes that correlates with reduced shortening.[37] This reduced calcium transient correlates with a reduced catecholamine-induced calcium current. The decreased catecholamine responsiveness of senescent cardiac tissue may also be contributed to by a decrease in cyclic adenosine monophosphate (cAMP) production and/or G-protein activity.[38] In contrast to the inotropic response, catecholamine-enhanced relaxation is not impaired.[12]

Thus, in senescent myocardium, the duration of contraction is shortened by catecholamines in the face of a markedly diminished inotropic effect. This age-dependent alteration results in a significantly lower peak tension developed by isolated cardiac muscle of senescent as opposed to young adult animals in the presence of beta-sympathetic stimulation (Fig. 96-2).

The inotropic response to postextrasystolic potentiation in cardiac muscle from senescent animals is well maintained and similar to the calcium response.[7] The response to digitalis glycosides in cardiac muscle of both rats and dogs, however, is markedly decreased with age. In the dog, the toxic effect of digitalis, in terms of producing ventricular tachycardia, is unchanged with age, so that the therapeutic-to-toxic ratio is much less favorable

in the senescent than in the young adult dog.[8] It is unclear, however, whether or not these observations are applicable in human beings.

Peripheral Vasculature

Several age-associated changes in arterial mechanical properties demonstrated in animal models and in humans increase the left ventricular afterload.[28,39,40] These changes consist of alterations in the composition and distribution of arterial elastin and collagen that cause a decreased elasticity or stiffening of the central arteries and changes in the distal arterioles. These changes lead to increases with age in both systemic vascular resistance, which is the nonpulsatile component of afterload, and the characteristic impedance and pulse-wave velocity, the pulsatile components of afterload.[41,42] Noninvasive measurements performed on a population of rural Chinese, who have a very low prevalence of hypertension and atherosclerosis, demonstrate a direct relationship between age and arterial stiffness as measured by pulse-wave velocity[27] (Fig. 96-3).

The increase in arterial stiffness leads to the age-associated increase in systolic blood pressure, a widening of the arterial pulse pressure, and an increase in left ventricular wall stress and metabolic demand, with a resultant increase in echocardiographically determined left ventricular mass.[9,12,15] The acute cardiac effects of directing cardiac outflow into a stiff bypass conduit have been evaluated in the canine model.[43] The marked reduction in arterial compliance results in a fall in diastolic and a rise in systolic blood pressure and an increase in left ventricular metabolic demand and systolic wall stress. Despite the fall in diastolic blood pressure, coronary blood flow was higher even at matched myocardial oxygen demand due to a marked increase in the systolic contribution to total coronary blood flow, suggesting that the pressure waveform itself may influence coronary blood flow and that systolic blood pressure may have a greater role in myocardial perfusion in the elderly than in the nonelderly. Using the same model, Kass and coworkers demonstrated that during transient

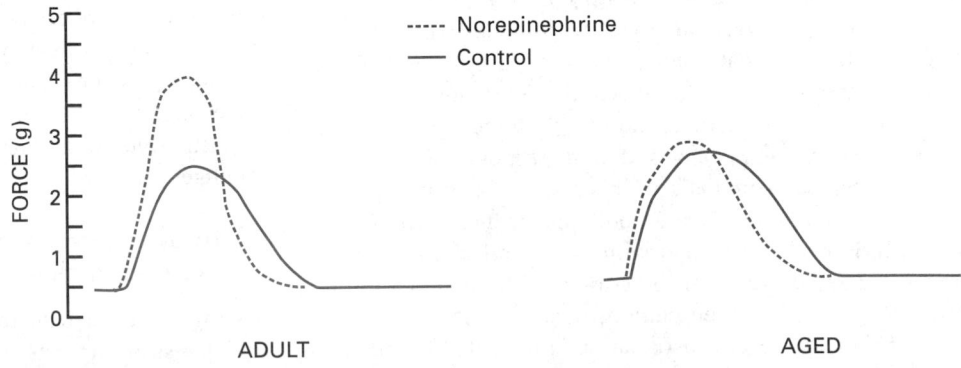

FORCE (g) — ADULT — AGED

- - - - Norepinephrine
—— Control

FIGURE 96-2

Typical isometric twitch in young adult and aged isolated cardiac muscle before (*solid*) and after (*dashed*) exposure to norepinephrine. There is no significant increase in maximum tension or rate of tension development in aged muscle, although the enhanced relaxation effect due to the catecholamines is relatively unaffected by age.

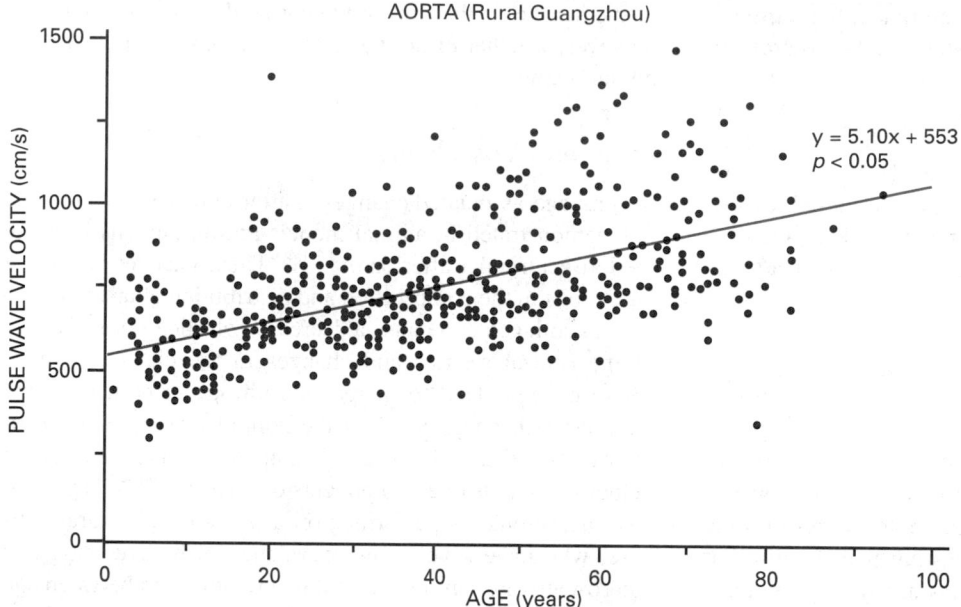

FIGURE 96-3

Relationship of pulse-wave velocity and age in males and females aged 2 months to 94 years. Pulse-wave velocity, a noninvasive measurement of aortic stiffness, increases linearly with age. *(From Avolio et al.*[27] *Reproduced with permission.)*

coronary artery occlusion, there were significantly greater increases in end-diastolic and end-systolic volumes and decreases in ejection fraction and systolic blood pressure as well as greater amounts of hypoperfused myocardium than when ejection occurred into the native aorta or during conditions of increased afterload produced by angiotensin II infusion.[44] There is relatively more coronary blood flow in systole when cardiac ejection occurs into the stiff conduit compared with the native aorta; therefore, for the same decline in mean arterial and systolic blood pressure, coronary flow is disproportionately reduced in the presence of the noncompliant conduit. These data suggest that when cardiac flow is directed into a stiffer vasculature, as occurs in the elderly, a greater degree of myocardial perfusion occurs during systole, which makes the heart more sensitive to lowering systolic and mean arterial blood pressure, potentially resulting in a greater amount of ischemia and left ventricular dysfunction. A stiffened vasculature may be a critical mechanism for the poor outcome in elderly patients with acute myocardial infarction.

As in the case of cardiac muscle,[6,45] there is distinct age-associated decrease in the vasodilating response of rat aorta to beta-sympathetic stimulation. This response appears specific, since the response to direct vasodilating agents, such as nitroglycerin, is well maintained with age. Similarly, in humans, an age-related decrease in forearm vasodilation to an isoproterenol infusion has been demonstrated.[46] Selective attenuation of beta adrenergic vasodilation is indicated by observations that elderly healthy subjects are very sensitive to direct vasodilators such as nitroprusside, which can cause a rapid fall in blood pressure and a decrease in noninvasive measurements of vascular stiffness.[47]

With exercise, systolic blood pressure reflects the net effect of the increase in cardiac output and arterial vasodilatation through beta-sympathetic stimulation and likely intrinsic endothelium-dependent vasodilatation. From the observations in isolated aorta, one can speculate that decreased arterial vasodilation during exercise is a major factor in augmenting the load on the left ventricle in older individuals. Noninvasive measurements of aortic stiffness are inversely and independently associated with maximal oxygen consumption in healthy subjects, suggesting that one factor contributing to the decline in exercise capacity in healthy elderly subjects may be the age-associated increase in central vessel stiffness.[48] Reducing arterial stiffness with nitroprusside in older, healthy individuals results in improved cardiac ejection performance during maximal exercise.[49] Similarly, exercise studies in beagles show that dynamic impedance to left ventricular ejection is greater during exercise but not at rest in 10- to 14-year-old dogs than in 1- to 4-year-old animals.[22] The lower impedance during exercise in the young dogs can be entirely eliminated by beta-sympathetic blockade. These observations, therefore, support the concept that in the young adult, sympathetic arterial vasodilation acts to decrease left ventricular load, a compensatory response lost in the aged dog.

Chronotropic Response

In addition to the decreased inotropic and vasodilator response to beta-sympathetic stimulation, there is a clear age-associated decrease in the chronotropic response to catecholamines in both animal models and humans.[10,46] The maximum heart rate response to beta-sympathetic stimulation is diminished in the senescent beagle dog both before and after vagal blockade. Older healthy subjects have a smaller increase in heart rate following an isoproterenol infusion than do younger subjects.

Cardiovascular Response to Exercise in Human Beings

The age-associated decrease in exercise capacity has long been of interest. Aging is associated with a decline in maximal aerobic capacity averaging 8 to 10 percent per decade in sedentary healthy populations.[12,28,50–52] This decline is secondary to a fall in maximal cardiac output and a decrease in arteriovenous oxygen difference, the central and peripheral components of measured oxygen consumption, respectively[53] (see also Chap. 95).

Figure 96-4 lists four factors that determine maximal cardiac output during exercise and the changes in these parameters that occur with increasing age. They are maximal heart rate, the maximal cardiac inotropic state, minimal impedance to left ventricular ejection, and the maximal use of the Frank-Starling mechanism. As discussed below, in the elderly, the Frank-Starling mechanism and increased fiber length compensate for decreases in the other three variables that might otherwise limit cardiac output capacity during exercise. There is a clear decrease in the maximum heart rate response to exercise in the elderly. There is also evidence of a decrease in cardiac inotropic response and an increase in impedance to ejection during exercise. These three age-associated alterations in cardiovascular function serve to potentially diminish maximum cardiac output capacity. There appears to be, though, a readily available and effective use of the Frank-Starling mechanism that compensates significantly in normal elderly individuals, thus maintaining cardiac output at high workload levels.

These conclusions are based on a study of 200 healthy sedentary individuals from the Baltimore Longitudinal Study on Aging of the National Institute of Aging.[54] The study population had no evidence of cardiovascular disease based on a history, physical examination, and treadmill stress test. Those subjects over the age of 40 had normal exercise thallium tests. All participants performed bicycle exercise while gated cardiac blood pool scan–derived cardiac volumes and cardiac output were obtained at each level of exercise until exhaustion. The relationship of age (22 to 86 years) and gender (121 men, 79 women) to the cardiovascular response to exercise was evaluated.

In both men and women at rest, heart rate declined and systolic blood pressure rose with increasing age. The decline in resting heart rate in men was compensated by an age-associated increase in resting end-diastolic, end-systolic, and stroke volume indices—i.e., use of the Frank-Starling mechanism (Fig. 96-5). In contrast, resting cardiac volumes in women did not vary with age. Resting ejection fraction in men and women also did not vary with age, consistent with no age-associated decline in resting systolic pump performance.

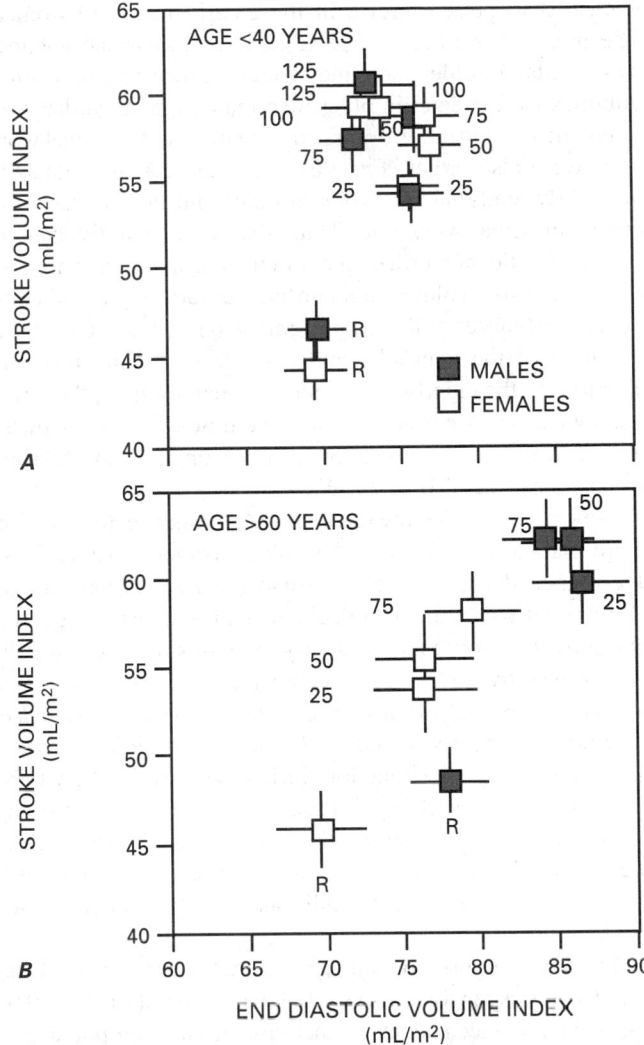

FIGURE 96-5

Relationship between rest (R) and exercise (25 through 125 watts) stroke volume and end-diastolic volume indices in younger (A) and older (B) men (*filled squares*) and women (*open squares*). Older subjects utilize the Frank-Starling mechanism to augment stroke volume with increases in end-diastolic volume index during exercise. This relationship is most evident in older men. (*From Fleg et al.*[54] *Reproduced with permission.*)

Peak exercise capacity, measured by maximal oxygen consumption and maximal work rate, declined linearly with age in men and women. With maximum exercise, there were three major age-associated changes. First, there was a lower heart rate response to maximal exercise, declining 25 percent across the age span in men and women, or a decline of about 1 beat per minute per year. Second, in the younger individuals, the end-systolic volume index diminished with exercise, reflecting the enhanced inotropic state and effective vasodilation of the arterial vasculature related to the normal beta-sympathetic response to exercise. End-systolic volume index at maximal work rate rises progressively with increasing age, reflecting both the decreased cardiac inotropic response and a decreased aortic vasodilator response or increased impedance to ejection. Third, there was an increase in the end-diastolic volume index

CONTRIBUTE TO EXERCISE CARDIAC OUTPUT	AGED	AGED AT SAME WORKLOAD
HEART RATE INCREASE	LESS	LOWER HEART RATE
AFTERLOAD DECREASE	LESS	LARGER END-SYSTOLIC VOLUME
INOTROPY INCREASE	LESS	
FRANK - STARLING USE	MORE	LARGER END-DIASTOLIC AND STROKE VOLUMES

FIGURE 96-4

Factors that contribute to increased cardiac output during stress and the influence of age on the response of these factors to exercise stress.

from rest to peak exercise in the elderly men and women. The increase from rest to peak exercise in cardiac volumes was similar in older men and women. Since resting cardiac volumes were greater in older men than women, cardiac volumes and cardiac index during submaximal and maximal work rates were also larger (Fig. 96-5). In younger individuals in this study, end-diastolic volume index did not change from rest to maximal work rate. Thus, the younger individuals in this study did not utilize the Frank-Starling mechanism to augment stroke volume and cardiac output; they relied completely and successfully on an augmented heart rate, the inotropic state of the ventricle, and a decrease in impedance to ejection. In the elderly individuals, especially men, there was a stepwise increase in end-diastolic volume with each stepwise increase in exercise, indicating a reliance on the Frank-Starling mechanism (see also Chap. 95).

Nevertheless, the lower heart rate response to exercise, more marked in older men than older women, resulted in an age-related decline in peak cardiac index. Ejection fraction at maximal work rate also declined with increasing age. Importantly, ejection fraction usually increases from rest to exercise in healthy, sedentary elderly subjects. *Thus, a decrease in ejection fraction from rest to exercise would likely reflect the presence of disease and not be due only to aging.* Furthermore, left ventricular function during exercise is likely to be affected more severely by disease in the elderly than in young individuals. Since the Frank-Starling reserve is used even in the absence of disease, there may be less reserve available for use in the presence of additional stresses superimposed by disease.

Further support for an age-related decrease in beta-adrenergic responsiveness as a key determinant of the differences in the mechanism to increase cardiac output during exercise comes from studies of 25 male participants of varying age who received intravenous propranolol prior to exercise gated blood pool scan testing.[55] The relationship of exercise hemodynamics with age in the beta-blocked subjects and 70 age-matched healthy men was evaluated and is shown in Table 96-1. Young subjects are more affected by beta blockade than older subjects, obliterating the age relationship of markedly diminished heart rate response and cardiac dilatation at maximal work and resulting in exercise hemodynamics similar to those of old, non-beta-blocked subjects. Thus, young beta-blocked subjects utilized the Frank-Starling mechanism to increase exercise cardiac output. *These data are consistent with the suggestion that the age-associated decline in maximal exercise heart rate and cardiac index, with compensation via cardiac dilatation, is due to the age-associated reduction in beta-adrenergic responsivity.*[55]

Effect of Exercise Training

The age-related changes in cardiac function—including a decline in maximal oxygen consumption, cardiac index, and ejection fraction—can be partially ameliorated by aerobic exercise training. Healthy elderly subjects who undergo aerobic conditioning have a significant increase in maximal oxygen consumption.[56–58] Recent studies utilizing serial bicycle gated blood pool scans demonstrated significant improvements in cardiac function with exercise training in elderly, previously sedentary men and deterioration in exercise cardiac function following detraining in senior master athletes.[56,57] Exercise conditioning results in an increase in left ventricular ejection fraction at peak exercise and a decrease in end-systolic volume. Maximal stroke volume index and cardiac index are also significantly greater following training. Detraining in senior master athletes results in quantitatively similar but directionally opposite changes in gated blood pool scan cardiac function. Across a broad range of cardiovascular fitness, indexed as maximal oxygen consumption, there is a linear relationship among indices of cardiac pump performance, including exercise ejection fraction and cardiac index, and an inverse relationship to end-systolic volume index. The ability of older, healthy subjects to improve cardiac pump performance with exercise training is not due to enhanced beta-adrenergic responsiveness, which does not appear to change with exercise conditioning.[59] One potential mechanism for improved systolic function is a reduced afterload following exercise training, as noninvasive indices of arterial stiffness in endurance-trained senior athletes are significantly reduced compared with those of age-matched, sedentary controls.[48]

CARDIOVASCULAR DISEASE IN AGING

Hypertension

There is a modest increase in diastolic pressure from the early portion of adulthood to age 55.[60] In contrast, systolic blood pressure increases progressively with increasing age, as does the prevalence of isolated systolic hypertension.[61] *Although systolic and diastolic blood pressure are both independent risk factors for the development of cardiovascular disease, systolic blood pressure is the stronger predictor of risk in the elderly.*[4] The prevalence of left ventricular hypertrophy, identified by electrocardiography and echocardiography, also increases with age and is an independent risk factor for the development of cardiovascular disease.[62,63] This high

TABLE 96-1

EFFECTS OF BETA-ADRENERGIC BLOCKADE ON HEMODYNAMICS COMPARED WITH AGED-MATCHED CONTROLS

	Young Beta-Blocked	Old Beta-Blocked
HR	⇓⇓	⇓
EDVI	⇑⇑⇑	=
SVI	⇑	=

Abbreviations: HR = heart rate; EDVI = end-diastolic volume index; SVI = stroke volume index.

prevalence of isolated systolic hypertension and left ventricular hypertrophy, as well as an age-specific response to different classes of antihypertensive agents, arises from age-associated hemodynamic changes. These changes include the previously mentioned increase in aortic stiffness, which is also manifest in the hypertensive population.[27] Furthermore, peripheral vascular resistance increases and cardiac output declines with increasing age in persons with hypertension.[64] This hemodynamic profile of an increase in aortic stiffness and peripheral vascular resistance, in addition to the decrease in beta-sympathetic responsiveness in the elderly, suggests that older hypertensive subjects might respond better to arteriolar vasodilators than to beta blockers[33] (see also Chap. 58).

Several large, randomized trials evaluating medical therapy for diastolic hypertension have clearly demonstrated a benefit of therapy in the elderly, with a reduction in cardiovascular mortality and stroke compared to those on placebo.[60,65] A randomized trial in elderly subjects with isolated systolic hypertension has demonstrated that treatment reduces stroke in long-term follow-up compared to placebo.[5]

Ischemic Heart Disease

In general, age is associated with increasingly severe, diffuse atherosclerosis and damage to the left ventricle. Therefore, almost all clinical manifestations of ischemic heart disease have a higher mortality rate and a worse outcome in the older as compared to the younger population. The clinical assessment of the elderly patient with coronary artery disease is often limited by the coexistence of diseases that make interpretation of symptoms difficult.[67] Thus, in the elderly, objective parameters such as stress test results are important in assessing and diagnosing ischemic heart disease. Treadmill testing is also useful to detect silent ischemia, which occurs with increasing frequency in the elderly and is a strong risk factor for the development of future symptomatic cardiac disease.[68]

Acute Ischemic Syndromes

Older patients with acute myocardial infarction are increasingly likely to be female, to have a preexisting history of angina, to have functional collateral vessels, and to have a non-Q-wave myocardial infarction.[66,69] Older patients are also more likely than are younger patients to present with atypical symptoms of acute myocardial ischemia and infarction such as shortness of breath, confusion, or failure to thrive. The acute myocardial infarction in the elderly may be completely unrecognized.[70] Age is a powerful, independent predictor of short- and long-term mortality in patients with an acute myocardial infarction.[69–72] In patients admitted with a first myocardial infarction and treated with thrombolytic therapy, in-hospital mortality increases exponentially as a function of age from 1.9 percent among patients 40 years of age or younger to 31.9 percent among patients above age 80.[71] Elderly patients with acute infarction experience an increased incidence of heart failure and cardiogenic shock in

spite of the fact that indices of infarct size, such as creatine kinase levels and QRS scores, tend to decrease with age.[69,71] The high incidence of heart failure and shock may result from age-related changes in diastolic filling, aortic compliance, and decrease in sensitivity to catecholamine stimulation, which may result in less cardiac reserve following ischemic damage. Older patients suffer less ventricular fibrillation compared to younger patients with acute myocardial infarction, but they are much more likely to have electromechanical dissociation and cardiac rupture on autopsy. The risk of death following hospital discharge also increases exponentially, by almost 6 percent per year, with increasing age.[71]

The high mortality associated with acute ischemic syndromes in the elderly dictates an aggressive approach to management. Thrombolytic therapy in acute myocardial infarction has been demonstrated to reduce mortality. In a meta-analysis of large, randomized trials of thrombolytic therapy, subjects over 75 years of age appear to benefit from thrombolysis compared to control subjects. Although the percent decrease in mortality in some studies is less in older as compared with younger patients treated with thrombolytics, the absolute benefit in terms of number of lives saved with treatment is similar or even greater.[73] In the Global Utilization of Streptokinase and Tissue Plasminogen Activator for Occluded Coronary Arteries (GUSTO) Trial,[74,75] subgroup analysis of 3655 patients over 75 years of age showed a similar absolute benefit compared with younger patients for accelerated-dosed tissue plasminogen activator compared to steptokinase for the end point of death and nonfatal disabling stroke, although this subgroup comparison was not statistically significant. The accelerated tissue plasminogen activator regimen appears to be relatively cost-effective in the elderly.[76] On the other hand, age is an important predictor of hemorrhagic stroke with thrombolytic therapy, and stroke occurs slightly more frequently with tissue plasminogen activator than with streptokinase.[74,77] Other comorbid conditions—such as cerebral vascular disease, hypertension, and body weight—must be considered in making a decision to administer thrombolytic therapy, but age alone is not a criterion for exclusion.[77]

In spite of evidence of efficacy in the elderly, the use of thrombolytic therapy decreases dramatically with increasing age. In a national registry of 350,755 patients who experienced a myocardial infarction from 1990 to 1994, thrombolytic therapy was used in nearly 51 percent of patients below age 55 years as compared with 19 and 7.4 percent of patients aged 75 to 84 years and over 85 years, respectively.[78,79] The older patients with infarction were more likely to have a nondiagnostic electrocardiogram or a non-Q-wave infarction as well as to arrive at the hospital later than younger patients. Even after adjustment for these differences, the odds of receiving thrombolytic therapy decreased progressively with increasing age.

Primary angioplasty has been compared with thrombolytic therapy in several trials and may have beneficial effects on mortality, recurrent myocardial infarction, and recurrent ischemia.[80,81] Large trials are ongoing that may delineate which modality of reperfusion most benefits the elderly patient with an acute myocardial infarction. Although elderly subjects treated with thrombolytic therapy will more often have multivessel coronary disease than will younger subjects, routine angioplasty in this clinical setting does not decrease death or recurrent myocardial infarction.[82] Angioplasty can be very effective, however, in relieving ischemia in elderly patients with postinfarction angina and unstable angina.[83,84] Although beta-blocker therapy is used less often in elderly than in younger patients with infarction, the elderly accrue similar benefits.[85] Similarly, aspirin therapy decreases mortality in elderly subjects with infarction and reduces recurrent ischemic pain in older patients with unstable angina.[85] Nevertheless, among 10,000 Medicare beneficiaries with an acute myocardial infarction with no contraindication to receiving aspirin therapy, only 61 percent of patients received it within the first 2 days in hospital.[86] Aspirin therapy in this large group of elderly patients was independently associated with a lower 30-day mortality. Furthermore, only 76 percent of elderly subjects without any contraindications are discharged home on aspirin following a myocardial infarction.[87] Aspirin use is independently associated with improved 6-month outcome in this group.

Chronic Coronary Disease

The use of percutaneous transluminal angioplasty or coronary artery bypass surgery as therapy for chronic ischemic heart disease in the elderly has increased significantly over the last decade.[88] Revascularized Medicare patients are increasingly old with an increased number of comorbid conditions. Nevertheless, 30-day and 1-year mortality have decreased significantly from 1987 to 1990 for both revascularization procedures in the elderly. The improved mortality probably represents improved technical approaches with angioplasty and with bypass surgery, including increased use of mammary grafts.

The use of bypass surgery has also increased in the very elderly, increasing 67 percent in octogenarians between 1987 and 1990. Thirty-day and 1-year mortality averaged 11.5 and 19.2 percent, respectively, both 2.5-fold greater than the corresponding operative mortality in the 65- to 70-year age group. Independent predictors of short- and long-term mortality included increasing age, female gender, admission with acute myocardial infarction, congestive heart failure, cerebral or peripheral vascular disease, and chronic renal disease. Increasing age is also a significant independent predictor of stroke, which occurs in about 8 percent of the very elderly who undergo bypass surgery.[90] In spite of the high short-term morbidity and mortality, the 3-year mortality rate of this group was similar to that in the general octogenarian population. No randomized trial of medicine compared with bypass surgery has included the elderly, although significant improvement in quality of life with relief of medically refractory angina is achieved in many elderly bypass patients.[91,92] Therefore, especially careful assessment of the risk and benefits of

bypass surgery needs be performed in the elderly, including consideration of comorbid conditions.

As with bypass surgery, angioplasty techniques and results have improved over the last several years[93] (see Chap. 48). Compared with patients in earlier data bases, elderly patients receiving the procedure recently are older, more often with a history of a myocardial infarction, prior bypass surgery, and diabetes mellitus. In spite of the increased age and comorbidities, the procedural success rate has improved significantly in the elderly to 93.5 percent, in association with a significant reduction in procedural complications, including death and myocardial infarction. The most dramatic decrease in complications was in need for emergency bypass surgery, dropping to 0.65 percent, probably because of the introduction of coronary stents.[93] Although no trial has randomized many elderly subjects with multivessel disease to angioplasty versus bypass surgery, the number of vessels with critical coronary artery disease and completeness of revascularization are powerful predictors of both short- and long-term event-free survival in elderly patients following angioplasty and should be an important factor in deciding between angioplasty and bypass surgery.[94,95]

Congestive Heart Failure

Demographic studies suggest that the prevalence of congestive heart failure is increasing in men and women of all races, with an approximate doubling in the number of hospital discharges listing this diagnosis between 1973 and 1986.[96] This increase is entirely accounted for by the steep rise in the number of elderly heart failure patients and is a consequence of at least two interacting factors. First, there is a marked age-associated increase in the prevalence of coronary artery disease and systemic arterial hypertension,[2,61] which are the two most common diseases causing myocardial damage. Improvements in therapy have led to a decrease in mortality rates of these two diseases such that many of these patients are developing heart failure as they live to older ages.[97,98] Second, there are age-related cardiovascular changes that ordinarily do not limit cardiac function; however, in the setting of myocardial damage, these may cause symptomatic heart failure to become manifest.

The age-associated factors that may affect the severity of heart failure include an increase in afterload.[40] The age-associated increase in arterial stiffness discussed previously also holds true in a heart failure population,[99] which would tend to aggravate congestive symptoms, particularly with exercise or stress. In addition, the age-associated decrease in sympathetic responsiveness limits the ability of the older person to augment heart rate and cardiac function in the presence of superimposed heart disease, particularly in the setting of acute depression of left ventricular function. Finally, the decrease in early left ventricular filling and the presumptive increase in left ventricular filling pressures during exercise may worsen heart failure symptoms, especially in association with diseases that also impair left ventricular filling, such as coronary artery disease and systemic arterial hypertension.

The treatment of congestive heart failure in the elderly is complicated by an age-associated decrease in renal function and an increase in cerebral vascular disease, both of which would increase the risks of drug side effects. Animal data suggest that digitalis glycosides may be less beneficial and potentially more toxic in the elderly than in a younger population. Vasodilator therapy for the elderly patient with heart failure is especially attractive in the setting of increased impedance to ejection. The decrease in mortality with vasodilator therapy added to therapy with digoxin and diuretics that has been demonstrated in patients generally with symptomatic heart failure holds for the subgroup of heart failure patients over 70 years old.[100] Two new agents that may eventually prove to be beneficial in the elderly include the calcium channel blocker amlodipine and the beta blocker carvedilol[101,102] (see also Chap. 54). Importantly, elderly patients with heart failure are frequently readmitted with recurrence following initial discharge from the hospital. Recently, Rich and colleagues showed that a nurse-directed, multidisciplinary approach to the treatment of the elderly patient with heart failure results in fewer hospital readmissions, reduced cost, and improved quality of life.[103]

Approximately 30 to 40 percent of elderly patients with symptomatic heart failure have normal left ventricular systolic function on echocardiography, suggesting an important role in this group for diastolic dysfunction, resulting in an abnormal diastolic pressure-volume relationship and elevated left ventricular filling pressures.[104,105] The prognosis of patients with heart failure and normal systolic function depends to a great degree on whether or not coronary artery disease is the etiology of the heart failure.[104] The clinical detection of diastolic heart failure is often difficult; therefore, determination of left ventricular function with echocardiography is an important part of the evaluation. In patients who have normal left ventricular systolic function but symptomatic heart failure from impaired left ventricular filling, beta blockers or calcium channel blockers may be beneficial[105,106] (see also Chap. 23).

Electrophysiology

Loss of pacemaker and conducting cells in otherwise normal hearts has been identified in the elderly.[107] Thus, there appears to be some age-associated predisposition in the elderly to sinus node dysfunction as well as to abnormalities of conduction in the artrioventricular (AV) node and the His-Purkinje system, including the bundle branches.

Supraventricular and ventricular arrhythmias also increase in frequency with aging,[108] but they have not been associated with specific evidence of cardiovascular disease. Arrhythmias in the elderly are to be approached in the same fashion as in younger individuals—i.e., those who are asymptomatic or who do not have evidence of cardiac disease can be viewed as less seriously ill than those with ventricular arrhythmias associated with evidence of left ventricular dysfunction and/or

ischemia. After myocardial infarction, both older and younger patients benefit from beta-blocker therapy, with a reduction in sudden death.[109] Life-threatening ventricular arrhythmias are common in the elderly patient with severe coronary disease and left ventricular dysfunction. As in the case of younger subjects, aggressive management of elderly survivors of cardiac arrest or of those with hypotensive ventricular tachycardia seems justified.[110] Antiarrhythmic therapy selected with electrophysiologic testing and/or placement of the implantable cardioverter defibrillator are well tolerated in the elderly and lead to improved mortality when compared with theoretical survival curves[111] (see also Chaps. 27 and 33).

Atrial fibrillation is common in the elderly. In five randomized trials of anticoagulation for the prevention of stroke in atrial fibrillation, the mean age of enrolled patients was 69 years, with 25 percent over the age of 75 years.[112] The population-based Cardiovascular Health Study of 5201 men and women aged ≥65 years, 4.8 percent of women and 6.2 percent of men had atrial fibrillation.[113] Atrial fibrillation in this elderly cohort correlated with increasing age and was associated with heart failure, valvular heart disease, stroke, diabetes, and hypertension.[113] In randomized trials of anticoagulation versus placebo therapy for the prevention of embolic stroke in atrial fibrillation, a significant reduction occurs with anticoagulation therapy, including patients over 75 years old.[114] This benefit of anticoagulation is greater than that of treatment with aspirin therapy in the elderly, although there is an increased rate of intracranial hemorrhage.[115] Careful monitoring of the international normalized ratio is important, as most embolic strokes in the elderly occur when the ratio is under 2 and most cerebral hemorrhages occur when the ratio is above 3[112] (see also Chaps. 27 and 99).

Valvular Heart Disease

AORTIC STENOSIS

The valvular heart disease that is relatively unique to the elderly is calcific aortic stenosis developing on a previously normal trileaflet valve[116] (see also Chap. 63). The development of clinically significant aortic stenosios may be very rapid (6 to 18 months) during clinical observation in this age group, as calcification and severe scarring can occur rather abruptly. Also, animal studies show that there is less compensatory hypertrophy to increased impedance to left ventricular ejection in the elderly, which could contribute to the appearance of heart failure.[117]

Clinical recognition of valvular aortic stenosis may be difficult in the elderly, in contrast with isolated aortic stenosis in younger subjects Table 96-2[118] (see also Chap. 63).

By far the most helpful study one can perform in screening an elderly subject for significant aortic stenosis is a Doppler echocardiogram, with which severe aortic valve calcification with decreased mobility and a significant Doppler gradient is sought (see Chap. 14). It appears that asymptomatic elderly patients with significant aortic stenosis by echocardiography can be followed carefully without surgical intervention until

TABLE 96-2
FREQUENT CHARACTERISTICS OF AORTIC STENOSIS

	Older, >65 years	Younger, <65 years
Structure	Tricuspid	Bicuspid
Origin	Degeneration	Congenital
Exam	Musical component at apex	Harsh at base, carotids delayed
	Carotids may appear normal	
Gender predominance	Women	Men

the first symptom appears.[119] Surgical therapy with aortic valve replacement often results in marked improvement in the elderly subject with symptomatic aortic stenosis. Predictors of surgical mortality with aortic valve replacement include low ejection fraction and congestive heart failure, atrial fibrillation, associated surgical procedures, and emergency operation, suggesting that aortic valve replacement for symptomatic aortic stenosis should not be delayed merely because the patient is elderly.[120–122] Percutaneous aortic valvuloplasty in the elderly is generally associated with poor outcome, including early restenosis, high mortality, and heart failure[123] (for more extensive discussion see Chap. 63).

MITRAL VALVE DISEASE

Symptomatic mitral regurgitation in the elderly is most often related to ischemic heart disease. Myxomatous degeneration of the mitral valve rather than rheumatic heart disease is probably the next leading cause of mitral regurgitation. The most common cause of mitral stenosis in the elderly is rheumatic disease, which at times may not result in symptoms until the patient reaches old age, making the diagnosis more difficult in this age group, because calcification of the valve may decrease the intensity of the first heart sound and the opening sound, and diminished cardiac output may decrease the intensity of the diastolic rumble. Doppler echocardiography is very useful in diagnosing the presence of significant disease. Balloon mitral valvuloplasty compares favorably with open surgical commissurotomy in appropriate candidates (see Chap. 64) and should be considered for elderly patients with mitral stenosis.[124,125] For elderly patients with mitral regurgitation from a myxomatous valve, mitral valve repair results in excellent long-term results.[126]

For elderly patients requiring valve replacement, the choice of a mechanical valve with the bleeding risk of lifelong anticoagulation must be balanced against a bioprosthetic valve and risk of structural deterioration. Additional factors in the choice include candidacy for anticoagulation, other requirements for anticoagulation such as atrial fibrillation, age, renal function, and valve position. In a series of elderly subjects receiving aortic or mitral mechanical valve replacements, freedom from major anticoagulant-related hemorrhage was 76 percent at 10

years.[127] A bioprosthetic valve in the mitral position deteriorates more rapidly than in the aortic position. In a large series of elderly patients receiving porcine bioprostheses, freedom from structural deterioration at 10 years for the aortic valve bioprostheses was 98 percent and 79 percent for mitral valve bioprostheses, with excellent long-term survival free of major morbidity.[128]

REFERENCES

1. White NK, Edwards JE, Dry TJ. The relationship of the degree of coronary atherosclerosis with age in men. *Circulation* 1950; 1:645–654.

2. Elveback L, Lie JT. Continued high incidence of coronary artery disease at autopsy in Olmsted County, Minnesota, 1950 to 1979. *Circulation* 1984; 70:345–349.

3. Tejada C, Strong JP, Montenegro MR, Restrepo C, Solberg LA. Distribution of coronary and aortic atherosclerosis by geographic location, race, and sex. *Lab Invest* 1968; 18:509–526.

4. Kannel WB. Blood pressure and the development of cardiovascular disease in the aged. In: Caird FI, Dall JLC, Kennedy RD, eds. *Cardiology in Old Age*. New York: Plenum Press; 1976; 143–175.

5. SHEP Cooperative Research Group. Prevention of stroke by antihypertensive drug treatment in older persons with isolated systolic hypertension: Final results of the Systolic Hypertension in the Elderly Program (SHEP). *JAMA* 1991; 265:3255–3264.

6. Fleish JH. Further studies of the effect of aging on beta-adrenoreceptor activity of rat aorta. *Br J Pharmacol* 1971; 42:311–313.

7. Gerstenblith G, Spurgeon HA, Froehlich JP, Weisfeldt ML, Lakatta EG. Diminished inotropic responsiveness to ouabain in aged rat myocardium. *Circ Res* 1979; 44:517–523.

8. Guarnieri T, Spurgeon HA, Froehlich JP, Weisfeldt ML, Lakatta ML. Diminished inotropic response but unaltered toxicity to acetylstrophanthidin in the senescent beagle. *Circulation* 1979; 60:1548–1554.

9. Lakatta EG, Yin FCP. Myocardial aging: Functional alterations and related cellular mechanisms. *Am J Physiol* 1982; 242(*Heart Circ Physiol* 11):H927–H941.

10. Yin FCP, Spurgeon HA, Greene HL, Lakatta EG, Weisfeldt ML. Age-associated decrease in heart rate response to isoproterenol in dogs. *Mech Aging Dev* 1979; 10:17–25.

11. Guarnieri T, Filburn CR, Zitnik G, Roth GS, Lakatta EG. Contractile and biochemical correlates of beta-adrenergic stimulation of the aged heart. *Am J Physiol* 1980; 239(*Heart Circ Physiol*):H501–H508.

12. Weisfeldt ML, ed. *The Aging Heart: Its Function and Response to Stress*. New York: Raven Press; 1980.

13. Weisfeldt ML, Loeven WA, Shock NW. Resting and active mechanical properties of carneae from aged male rats. *Am J Physiol* 1977; 220:1921–1927.

14. Rodeheffer RJ, Gerstenblith G, Becker LC, Fleg JL, Weisfeldt ML, Lakatta EG. Exercise cardiac output is maintained with advancing age in healthy human subjects: Cardiac dilation and increased stroke volume compensate for a diminished heart rate. *Circulation* 1984; 69:203–213.

15. Gerstenblith G, Frederiksen J, Yin FCP, Fortuin NJ, Lakatta EG, Weisfeldt ML. Echocardiographic assessment of a normal adult aging population. *Circulation* 1977; 56:273–278.

16. Yin FCP, Raizes GS, Guarnieri T, Spurgeon HA, Lakatta EG, Fortuin NJ, et al. Age-associated decrease in ventricular response to hemodynamic stress during beta-adrenergic blockade. *Br Heart J* 1978; 40:1349–1355.

17. Alpert NR, Gale HH, Taylor N. The effect of age on contractile protein ATPase activity and the velocity of shortening. In: Tanz RD, Kalaler F, Kobentz J, eds. *Factors influencing Myocardial Contractility*. New York: Academic Press; 1967:127–144.

18. Bhatnager GM, Walford GD, Beard E, Humphreys S, Lakatta EG. Dissociation of time to peak force (TPF) and myofibrillar ATPase activity (MF-ATPase) with aging of the myocardium. *J Mol Cell Cardiol* 1984; 16:203–218.

19. Lakatta EG, Gerstenblith G, Angell CS, Shock NW, Weisfeldt ML. Prolonged contraction duration in aged myocardium. *J Clin Invest* 1975; 55:61–68.

20. Froehlich JP, Lakatta EG, Beard E, Spurgeon HA, Weisfeldt ML, Gerstenblith G. Studies of sarcoplasmic reticulum function and contraction duration in young adult and aged rat myocardium. *J Mol Cell Cardiol* 1978; 10:427–438.

21. Wei JY, Spurgeon HA, Lakatta EG. Excitation-contraction coupling in rat myocardium: Alterations with adult aging. *Am J Physiol* 1984; 246:H784–H791.

22. Yin FCP, Weisfeldt ML, Milnor WR. The role of aortic input impedance in the decreased cardiovascular response to exercise with aging in the dog. *J Clin Invest* 1981; 68:28–38.

23. Spurgeon HA, Steinback MF, Lakatta EG. Prolonged contraction duration in senescent myocardium is prevented by exercise. *Physiologist* 1980; 23:56–67.

24. Harrison TR, Dixon K, Russell RO Jr, Bidwai PS, Coleman HN. The relation of age to the duration of contraction, ejection, and relaxation of the normal human heart. *Am Heart J* 1964; 67:189–199.

25. Miller TR, Grossman SJ, Schectman KB, Biello DR, Ludbrook PA, Ehsami AA. Left ventricular diastolic filling in the healthy elderly. *Am J Cardiol* 1986; 58:531–535.

26. Hirota Y. A clinical study of left ventricular relaxation. *Circulation* 1980; 62:756–763.

27. Avolio AP, Fa-Quan L, Wei-Qiang L, Yao-Fei L, Zhen-Dong H, Lian-Fen X, et al. Effects of aging on arterial distensibility in populations with high and low prevalence of hypertension: Comparison between urban and rural communities in China. *Circulation* 1985; 71:202–210.

28. Gerstenblith G, Lakatta EG, Weisfeldt ML. Age changes in myocardial function and exercise response. *Prog Cardiovasc Dis* 1976; 19:1–21.

29. Bonow RO, Vitale DR, Bacharach SL, Maron BJ, Green MV. Effects of aging on asynchronous left ventricular regional function and global ventricular filling in normal human subjects. *J Am Coll Cardiol* 1988; 11:50–58.

30. Schulman SP, Lakatta EG, Fleg JL, Lakatta L, Becker LC, Gerstenblith G. Age-related decline in left ventricular filling at rest and exercise. *Am J Physiol* 1992; 263(*Heart Circ Physiol*):H1932–H1938.

31. Douglas PS, O'Toole M. Aging and physical activity determine cardiac structure and function in the older athlete. *J Appl Physiol* 1992; 72:1969–1973.

32. Arora RR, Machac J, Goldman ME, Butler RN, Gorlin R, Horowitz SF. Atrial kinetics and left ventricular diastolic filling in the healthy elderly. *J Am Coll Cardiol* 1987; 9:1255–1260.

33. Schulman SP, Weiss JL, Becker LC, Gottlieb SO, Woodruff KM, Weisfeldt ML, et al. The effects of antihypertensive therapy on left ventricular mass in elderly patients. *N Engl J Med* 1990; 322:1350–1356.

34. Bonow RO, Bacharach SL, Green MV, Kent KM, Rosing DR, Lipson LC, et al. Impaired left ventricular diastolic filling in patients with coronary artery disease: Assessment with radionuclide angiography. *Circulation* 1981; 64:315–323.

35. Kitzman DW, Higginbotham MB, Cobb FR, Sheitch KH, Sullivan MJ. Exercise intolerance in patients with heart failure and preserved left ventricular systolic function: Failure of the Frank-Starling mechanism. *J Am Coll Cardiol* 1991; 17:1065–1072.

36. Sakai M, Danzinger RS, Xiao RP, Spurgeon HA, Lakatta EG. Contractile response of individual cardiac myocytes to norepinephrine declines with senescence. *Am J Physiol* 1992; 262:H184–H189.

37. Xiao RP, Spurgeon HA, O'Connor F, Lakatta EC. Age-associated changes in β-adrenergic modulation on rat cardiac excitation-contraction coupling. *J Clin Inves* 1994; 94:2051–2059.

38. Lakatta EG. Deficient neuroendocrine regulation of the cardiovascular system with advancing age in healthy humans. *Circulation* 1992; 87:631–636.

39. Hallock P, Benson IC. Studies of the elastic properties of human isolated aorta. *J Clin Invest* 1937; 16:595–602.

40. Yin FCP. The aging vasculature and its effect on the heart. In: Weisfeldt ML, ed. *The Aging Heart*. New York: Raven Press; 1980; 137–213.

41. Nichols WW, O'Rourke MF, Avolio AP, Yaginuma T, Murgo JP, Pepine CJ, et al. Effects of age on ventricular-vascular coupling. *Am J Cardiol* 1985; 55:1179–1184.

42. Merrillon JP, Motte G, Masquet C, Azancot Im, Buiomard A, Gourgon R. Relationship between physical properties of the arterial system and left ventricular performance in the course of aging and arterial hypertension. *Eur Heart J* 1982; 3(suppl A):95–102.

43. Saeki A, Recchia F, Kass DA. Systolic flow augmentation in hearts ejecting into a model of stiff aging vasculature. *Circ Res* 1995; 76:132–141.

44. Kass DA;, Saeki A, Tunin RS, Recchia FA. Adverse influence of systemic vascular stiffening on cardiac dysfunction and adaptation to acute coronary occlusion. *Circulation* 1996; 93:1533–1541.

45. Fleisch JH, Hooker CS. The relationship between age and relaxation of vascular smooth muscle in the rabbit and rat. *Circ Res* 1976; 38:243–249.

46. Van Brummelen P, Buhler FR, Kiowski W, Amann FW. Age-related decrease in cardiac and peripheral vascular responsiveness to isoprenaline: Studies in normal subjects. *Clin Sci* 1981; 60:571–577.

47. Nussbacher A, Fleg JL, Schulman SP, O'Connor F, Gloth ST, Lima JAC, et al. Age related mechanisms of vasodilator blood pressure reduction (abstr). *Circulation* 1994; 90:I-565.

48. Vaitkevicius PV, Fleg JL, Engel JH, O'Connor FC, Wright JG, Lakatta LE, et al. Effects of age and aerobic capacity on arterial stiffness in healthy adults. *Circulation* 1993; 88:1456–1462.

49. Nussbacher A, Schulman SP, Fleg JL, O'Connor F, Gloth ST, Townsend SN, et al. Decreasing central arterial stiffness eliminates age differences in cardiac ejection during maximal exercise (abstr). *Circulation* 1994; 90:I-15.

50. Strandell T. Circulatory studies on healthy old men. *Acta Med Scand* 1964; 175(suppl 414):1–44.

51. Dehn MM, Bruce RA. Longitudinal variations in maximal oxygen uptake with age and activity. *J Appl Physiol* 1972; 33:805–807.

52. Lakatta EG. Cardiovascular regulatory mechanisms in advanced age. *Physiol Rev* 1993; 73:413–467.

53. Ogawa T, Spina RJ, Martin WH III, Kohrt WM, Schechtman KB, Holloszy JO, et al. Effects of exercise training on cardiovascular responses to exercise. *Circulation* 1992; 86:494–503.

54. Fleg JL, O'Connor F, Gerstenblith G, Becker LC, Clulow J, Schulman SP, et al. Impact of age on the cardiovascular response to upright exercise in healthy men and women. *J Appl Physiol* 1995; 78:890–900.

55. Fleg JL, Schulman S, O'Connor F, Becker LC, Gerstenblith G, Clulow JF, et al. Effects of acute β-adrenergic receptor blockade on age-associated changes in cardiovascular performance during dynamic exercise. *Circulation* 1994; 90:2333–2341.

56. Ehsani AA, Ogawa T, Miller TR, Spina RJ, Jilka SM. Exercise training improves left ventricular systolic function in older men. *Circulation* 1991; 83:96–103.

57. Schulman SP, Fleg JL, Goldberg AP, Busby-Whitehead J, Hagberg JM, O'Connor F, et al. Continuum of cardiovascular performance across a broad range of fitness levels in healthy older men. *Circulation* 1996; 94:359–367.

58. Seals DR, Hagberg JM, Hurley BF, Ehsani AA, Holloszy JO. Endurance training in older men and women: I. Cardiovascular response to exercise. *J Appl Physiol* 1984; 57:1024–1029.

59. Stratton JR, Cerqueira MD, Schwartz RS, Levy WC, Veith RC, Kahn SE, et al. Differences in cardiovascular responses to isoproterenol in relation to age and exercise training in healthy men. *Circulation* 1992; 86:504–512.

60. Hypertension Detection Follow-up Group. Blood pressure studies in 14 communities: A two-stage screen for hypertension. *JAMA* 1977; 237:2385–2391.

61. Applegate WB: Hypertension in elderly patients. *Ann Intern Med* 1989; 110:901–915.

62. Kannel WB, Gordon T, Castelli WB, Margolis LJR. Electrocardiographic left ventricular hypertrophy and risk of coronary heart disease: The Framingham Study. *Ann Intern Med* 1970; 72:813–822.

63. Levy D, Garrison RJ, Savage DD, Kannel WB, Castelli WP. Left ventricular mass and incidence of coronary heart disease in an elderly cohort. *Ann Intern Med* 1989; 110:101–107.

64. Lund-Johansen P. Hemodynamics in essential hypertension at rest and during exercise—20-year follow-up study. *Ann Clin Res* 1988; 20(suppl 48):31–38.

65. European Working Party on High Blood Pressure in the Elderly: Mortality and morbidity results from the European Working Party on High Blood Pressure in the Elderly Trial. *Lancet* 1985; 1:1349–1354.

66. Nicod P, Gilpin E, Dittrich H, Polikar R, Hjalmarson A, Blacky R, et al. Short- and long-term clinical outcome after Q-wave and non-Q-wave myocardial infarction in a large population. *Circulation* 1989; 79:528–536.

67. Frishman WH, DeMaria AN, Ewy GA. Cardiovascular disease in the elderly: Clinical assessment. *J Am Coll Cardiol* 1987; 10:48A–51A.

68. Fleg JL, Gerstenblith G, Zonderman AB, Becker LC, Weisfeldt ML, Costa PT Jr, et al. Prevalence and prognostic significance of exercise-induced silent myocardial ischemia detected by thallium scintigraphy

and electrocardiography in asymptomatic volunteers. *Circulation* 1990; 81:428–436.

69. Goldberg RJ, Gore JM, Gurwitz JH, Alpert JS, Brady P, Strohsnitter W, et al. The impact of age on the incidence and prognosis of initial acute myocardial infarction: The Worcester Heart Attack Study. *Am Heart J* 1989; 117:543–549.

70. Nadelmann J, Frishman WH, Ooi WL, Tepper D, Greenberg S, Guzik H, et al. Prevalence, incidence and prognosis of recognized and unrecognized myocardial infarction in persons aged 75 years or older: The Bronx Aging Study. *Am J Cardiol* 1990; 66:533–537.

71. Maggioni AP, Maseri A, Fresco C, Franzosi MG, Mauri F, Santoro E, et al. Age-related increase in mortality among patients with first myocardial infarctions treated with thrombolysis. *N Engl J Med* 1993; 329:1442–1448.

72. Keller NM, Feit F. Atherosclerotic heart disease in the elderly. *Curr Opin Cardiol* 1995; 10:427–433.

73. Fibrinolytic Therapy Trialists' Collaborative Group: Indications for fibrinolytic therapy in suspected acute myocardial infarction: Collaborative overview of early mortality and major morbidity results from all randomized trials of more than 1000 patients. *Lancet* 1994; 343:311–322.

74. The GUSTO Investigators. An international randomized trial comparing four thrombolytic strategies for acute myocardial infarction. *N Engl J Med* 1993; 329:673–682.

75. White HD. Selecting a thrombolytic agent. *Cardiol Clin* 1995; 13:347–354.

76. Mark DB, Hlatky MA, Califf RM, Naylor CD, Lee KL, Armstrong PW, et al. Cost effectiveness of thrombolytic therapy with tissue plasminogen activator as compared with streptokinase for acute myocardial infarction. *N Engl J Med* 1995; 332:1418–1424.

77. Gore JM, Granger CB, Simoons ML, Sloan MA, Weaver WD, White HD, et al. Stroke after thrombolysis: Mortality and functional outcomes in the GUSTO-I Trial. *Circulation* 1995; 92:2811–2818.

78. Rogers WJ, Bowlby LJ, Chandra NC, French WJ, Gore JM, Lambrew CT, et al. Treatment of myocardial infarction in the United States (1990 to 1993): Observations from the National Registry of Myocardial Infarction. *Circulation* 1994; 90:2103–2114.

79. Gurwitz JH, Gore JM, Goldberg RJ, Rubison M, Chandra N, Rogers WJ: Recent age-related trends in the use of thrombolytic therapy in patients who have had acute myocardial infarction. *Ann Intern Med* 1996; 124:283–291.

80. Grines CL, Browne KF, Marco J, Rothbaum D, Stone GW, O'Deefe J, et al. A comparison of immediate angioplasty with thrombolytic therapy for acute myocardial infarction. *N Engl J Med* 1993; 328:672–679.

81. Jan de Boer M, Suryapranata H, Hoorntje JCA, Reiffers S, Liem Al, Miedema Km, et al. Limitation of infarct size and preservation of left ventricular function after primary coronary angioplasty compared with intravenous streptokinase in acute myocardial infarction. *Circulation* 1994; 90:753–761.

82. Aguirre FV, McMahon RP, Mueller H, Kleiman NS, Kern MJ, Desvigne-Nickens P, et al. Impact of age on clinical outcome and postlytic management strategies in patients treated with thrombolytic therapy: Results from the TIMI II Study. *Circulation* 1994; 90:78–86.

83. Iniguez A, Macaya C, Hernandez R, Alfonso F, Goicolea J, Ribera JM, et al. Long-term outcome of coronary angioplasty in elderly patients with post-infarction angina. *Eur Heart J* 1994; 15:489–494.

84. The TIMI IIIB Investigators: Effects of tissue plasminogen activator and a comparison of early invasive and conservative strategies in unstable angina and non-Q-wave myocardial infarction: Results of the TIMI IIIB Trial. *Circulation* 1994; 89:1545–1556.

85. Forman DE, Bernal JLG, Wei JY. Management of acute myocardial infarction in the very elderly. *Am J Med* 1992; 93:315–326.

86. Krumholz HM, Radford MJ, Ellerbeck EF, Hennen J, Meehan TP, Pertrillo M, et al. Aspirin in the treatment of acute myocardial infarction in elderly medicare beneficiaries. Patterns of use and outcomes. *Circulation* 1995; 92:2841–2847.

87. Krumholz HM, Radford MJ, Ellerbeck EF, Hennen J, Meehan TP, Petrillo M, et al. Aspirin for secondary prevention after acute myocardial infarction in the elderly: Prescribed use and outcomes. *Ann Intern Med* 1996; 124:292–298.

88. Peterson ED, Jollis JG, Bebchuk MS, DeLong E, Muhlbaier LH, Mark DB, et al. Changes in mortality after myocardial revascularization in the elderly: The National Medicare experience. *Ann Intern Med* 1994; 121:919–927.

89. Peterson ED, Cowper PA, Jollis JG, Bebchuk JD, DeLong ER, Muhlbaier LH, et al. Outcomes of coronary artery bypass graft surgery in 24461 patients aged 80 years or older. *Circulation* 1995; 92(suppl II):II-85–II-91.

90. Freeman WK, Schaff HV, O'Brien PC, Orszulak TA, Naessens JM, Tajik AJ. Cardiac surgery in the octogenarian: Perioperative outcome and clinical follow-up. *J Am Coll Cardiol* 1991; 18:29–35.

91. Ko W, Gold JP, Lazzaro R, Zelano JA, Lang S, Isom OW, et al. Survival analysis of octogenarian patients with coronary artery disease managed by elective coronary artery bypass surgery versus conventional medical treatent. *Circulation* 1992; 86(suppl II):II-191–II-197.

92. Glower DD, Christopher TD, Milano CA, White WD, Smith LR, Jones RH, et al. Performance status and outcome after coronary artery bypass grafting in persons aged 80 to 93 years. *Am J Cardiol* 1992; 70:567–571.

93. Thompson RC, Holmes DR, Grill DE, Mock MB, Bailey KR. Changing outcome of angioplasty in the elderly. *J Am Coll Cardiol* 1996; 27:8–14.

94. O'Keefe JH, Sutton MB, McCallister BD, Vacek JL, Piehler JM, Ligon RW, et al. Coronary angioplasty versus bypass surgery in patients >70 years old matched for ventricular function. *J Am Coll Cardiol* 1994; 24:425–430.

95. Thompson RC, Holmes DR, Gersh BJ, Bailey KR. Predicting early and intermediate-term outcome of coronary angioplasty in the elderly. *Circulation* 1993; 88:1579–1587.

96. Ghali JK, Cooper R, Ford E. Trends in hospitalization rates for heart failure in the United States, 1973–1986: Evidence for increasing population prevalence. *Arch Intern Med* 1990; 150:769–773.

97. Pomerance A. Pathology of the heart with and without cardiac failure in the aged. *Br Heart J* 1965; 27:697–710.

98. Rich MW. Epidemiology and etiology of congestive heart failure in the elderly. *Am J Geriatr Cardiol* 1996; 5:16–19.

99. Carroll JD, Shroff S, Wirth P, Halsted M, Rajfer SI. Arterial mechanical properties in dilated cardiomyopathy: Aging and the response to nitroprusside. *J Clin Invest* 1991; 87:1002–1009.

100. CONSENSUS Trial Study Group. Effects of enalapril on mortality in severe congestive heart failure: Results of the Cooperative North Scandinavian Enalapril Survival Study (CONSENSUS). *N Engl J Med* 1987; 316:1429–1435.

101. O'Connor CM, Belkin RN, Carson PE, Cropp AB, Frid DJ, Miller AB, et al. Effect of amlodipine on mode of death in severe chronic heart failure: The PRAISE Trial (abstr). *Circulation* 1995; 92:I-143.

102. Packer M, Bristow MR, Cohn JN, Colucci WS, Fowler MB, Gilbert EM, et al. The effect of Carvedilol on morbidity and mortality in patients with congestive heart failure. *N Engl J Med* 1996; 334:1349–1355.

103. Rich MW, Beckham V, Wittenberg C, Leven CL, Freedland KE, Carney RM. A multidisciplinary intervention to prevent the readmission of elderly patients with congestive heart failure. *N Engl J Med* 1995; 333:1190–1195.

104. Tresch DD, McGough MF. Heart failure with normal systolic function: A common disorder in older people. *J Am Geriatr Soc* 1995; 43:1035–1042.

105. Topol EJ, Traill TA, Fortuin NJ. Hypertensive hypertrophic cardiomyopathy in the elderly. *N Engl J Med* 1985; 312:277–283.

106. Wei JY. Age and the cardiovascular system. *N Engl J Med* 1992; 327:1735–1739.

107. Lev M. The pathology of complete atrioventricular block. *Prog Cardiovasc Dis* 1964; 6:317–326.

108. Gleg JL, Kennedy HL. Cardiac arrhythmias in a healthy elderly population: Detection by 24-hour ambulatory electrocardiography. *Chest* 1982; 81:301–307.

109. Norwegian Multicenter Study Group: Timolol-induced reduction in mortality and reinfarction in patients surviving acute myocardial infarction. *N Engl J Med* 1981; 304:801–807.

110. Tresh DD, Platia EV, Guarnieri T, Reid PR, Griffith LSC. Refractory symptomatic ventricular tachycardia and ventricular fibrillation in elderly patients. *Am J Med* 1987; 83:399–404.

111. Tresh DD, Troup PH, Thakur RK, Veseth-Rogers J, Tucker V, Wetherbee JN, et al. Comparison of efficacy of automatic implantable cardioverter defibrillator in patients older and younger than 65 years of age. *Am J Med* 1991; 90:717–724.

112. Albers GW. Atrial fibrillation and stroke. *Arch Intern Med* 1994; 154:1443–1448.

113. Furberg CD, Psaty BM, Manolio TA, Gardin JM, Smith VE, Rauta-harju PM. Prevalence of atrial fibrillation in elderly subjects (the Cardiovascular Health Study). *Am J Cardiol* 1994; 74:236–241.

114. Atrial Fibrillation Investigators: Risk factors for stroke and efficacy of antithrombotic therapy in atrial fibrillation. *Arch Intern Med* 1994; 154:1449–1457.

115. Stroke Prevention in Atrial Fibrillation Investigators. Warfarin versus aspirin for prevention of thromboembolism in atrial fibrillation: Stroke Prevention in Atrial Fibrillation II Study. *Lancet* 1994; 343:687–691.

116. Seltzer A. Changing aspects of the natural history of valvular aortic stenosis. *N Engl J Med* 1987; 317:91–98.

117. Isoyama S, Wei JY, Izumo S, Fort P, Schoen FJ, Grossman W. The effect of age on the development of cardiac hypertrophy produced by aortic constriction in the rat. *Circ Res* 1987; 61:337–342.

118. Roberts WC, Perloff JK, Costantino T. Severe valvular aortic stenosis in patients over 65 years of age. *Am J Cardiol* 1971; 27:497–506.

119. Pellikka PA, Nushimura RA, Bailey KR, Tajik AJ. The natural history of adults with asymptomatic hemodynamically significant aortic steno-sis. *J Am Coll Cardiol* 1990; 15:1012–1017.

120. Elayda MA, Hall RJ, Reul RM, Alonzo DM, Gillette N, Reul GJ, et al. Aortic valve replacement in patients 80 years and older: Operative risks and long-term results. *Circulation* 1993; 88:11–16.

121. Logeais Y, Langanay T, Roussin R, Leguerrier A, Rioux C, Chaperon J, et al. Surgery for aortic stenosis in elderly patients: A study of surgical risk and predictive factors. *Circulation* 1994; 90:2891–2898.

122. Aranki SF, Rizzo RJ, Couper GS, Adams DH, Collins JJ, Gildea JS, et al. Aortic valve replacement in the elderly: Effect of gender and coronary artery disease on operative mortality. *Circulation* 1993; 88:17–23.

123. Bernard Y, Etievent J, Mourand JL, Anguenot T, Schiele F, Guseibat M, et al. Long-term results of percutaneous aortic valvu-loplasty compared with aortic valve replacement in patients more than 75 years old. *J Am Coll Cardiol* 1992; 20:792–801.

124. Tuzcu EM, Block PC, Griffin BP, Newell JB, Palacias IF. Immediate and long-term outcome of percutaneous mitral valvotomy in patients 65 years and older. *Circulation* 1992; 85:963–971.

125. Reyes VP, Raju BS, Wynne J, Stephenson LW, Raju R, Fromm BS, et al. Percutaneous balloon valvuloplasty compared with open surgical commissurotomy for mitral stenosis. *N Engl J Med* 1994; 331:961–967.

126. Jebara VA, Dervanian P, Acar C, Grare P, Mihaileanu S, Chauvaud S, et al. Mitral valve repair using Carpentier techniques in patients more than 70 years old: Early and late results. *Circulation* 1992; 86(suppl II):II-53–II-59.

127. Holper K, Wottke M, Lewe T, Baumer L, Meisner H, Paik SU, et al. Bioprosthetic and mechanical valves in the elderly: Benefits and risks. *Ann Thorac Surg* 1995; 60:S443–S446.

128. Burr LH, Jamieson RE, Munro AI, Miyagishima RT, Germann E. Porcine bioprostheses in the elderly: Clinical performance by age groups and valve positions. *Ann Thorac Surg* 1995; 60:S264–S269.

97

GERIATRIC CONSIDERATIONS IN CARDIOVASCULAR THERAPY

Paul E. Nolan, Jr. / Frank I. Marcus

In the United States, cardiovascular disease is the leading cause of death for persons 65 years of age and older.[1] This age group accounts for about 84 percent of the deaths due to heart disease. Nevertheless, the age-adjusted death rate due to heart disease is decreasing. This decline can be attributed in part to specific medical and surgical interventions.[2] Since 13 percent of the population will be older than 65 years of age by the year 2000,[3] clinicians must understand the effects of age on cardiovascular therapy in elderly patients in order to optimize their care.

OVERVIEW OF GERIATRIC CLINICAL PHARMACOLOGY

Many physiologic functions decline with age, although considerable interindividual variability exists.[3] These changes can modify the clinical pharmacokinetics and pharmacodynamics of cardiovascular drugs. In addition, the elderly are susceptible to other chronic illnesses[3] that may further modify the disposition and response to cardiovascular drugs.

Table 97-1 provides a summary of geriatric clinical pharmacology.

Absorption

In the elderly, several physiologic alterations occur within the gastrointestinal tract, such as slower gastric emptying; elevated gastric pH; and decreased mesenteric blood flow, gastrointestinal motility, and absorptive surface area.[4] The extent of absorption of most drugs is unaltered in the elderly[4] but may be enhanced for digoxin, because of decreased gastric acid hydrolysis in hypochlorhydric or achlorhydric elderly subjects.[5] Age-related decreases in hepatic blood flow may result in enhanced oral bioavailability of highly extracted drugs (e.g., propranolol, verapamil) that undergo extensive first-pass hepatic metabolism.[4]

Distribution

BODY COMPOSITION

In the elderly, total body weight and lean body mass often decrease, but the percentage of weight due to fat increases.[4] Lean body mass is lower and the percentage of fat greater in females than in males.[6] Consequently, drugs that are relatively lipophilic (e.g., lidocaine, amiodarone) may have an increased volume of distribution in the elderly, which may prolong their elimination. Conversely, digoxin, which distributes principally to lean tissues, exhibits a reduced volume of distribution in the elderly,[7] which could result in higher serum digoxin concentrations (SDCs).

PROTEIN BINDING

The two major drug-binding proteins in the blood are albumin and alpha$_1$-acid glycoprotein (AAG). In healthy elderly, serum concentrations of albumin are minimally but significantly decreased.[8] Albumin may decrease further due to chronic malnutrition in patients with chronic disease. Concentrations of AAG are similar in the young and the elderly.[8] Conditions such as acute myocardial infarction (AMI), cardiothoracic surgical procedures, or renal failure can increase concentrations of this acute-phase reactant. The protein binding of most cardiovascular drugs should not be altered in the relatively disease-free elderly.

Hepatic Metabolism

The metabolism of drugs by the liver is determined by the intrinsic activity of phase I or II enzymes, hepatic blood flow, and hepatic volume or mass.[4] The concentration, in vitro activity, and substrate affinity of many cytochrome P450 isozymes responsible for phase I hepatic metabolism (i.e., oxidation, reduction, and hydrolysis) is unchanged in elderly

TABLE 97-1

SUMMARY OF GERIATRIC CLINICAL PHARMACOLOGY

Pharmacokinetic/ Physiologic Process	Observed Physiologic Changes	Potential Clinical Consequences
Absorption	Prolonged gastric emptying time Elevated gastric pH Decreased splanchnic blood flow Reduced gastrointestinal motility Decreased absorptive surface area	Absorption of selected drugs may be altered; increased absorption of drugs that undergo extensive first-pass metabolism
Distribution Body composition	Decreased body weight and lean body mass; increased percentage of fat weight	Increased volume of distribution and half-life of lipophilic drugs Reduced volume of distribution and elevated plasma concentrations of hydrophilic drugs
Protein binding	Decreased serum albumin, especially in chronic disease and malnutrition Possibly increased serum α_1-acid glycoprotein, especially in settings of acute myocardial infarction or cardiothoracic surgery	Possibly decreased protein binding of acidic drugs Possibly increased protein binding of basic drugs
Hepatic metabolism	Decreased hepatic blood flow and hepatic mass	Decreased excretion of drugs that are highly dependent either on hepatic blood flow or on intrinsic activity of hepatic microsomal enzymes for elimination
Renal function	Decreased renal blood flow, glomerular filtration, and renal tubular secretion	Decreased excretion of drugs that are highly dependent upon the kidney for elimination

humans.[4] Moreover, the activity and concentrations of enzymes catalyzing phase II reactions (e.g., glucuronidation, sulfation, and acetylation) are generally unaltered in the elderly.[4] However, both hepatic blood flow and liver mass decline with age.[4] These decreases may be more prominent in elderly females.[6] The reduction in hepatic blood flow may result in a decrease in clearance of drugs that are highly dependent upon hepatic blood flow for elimination (e.g., lidocaine, verapamil). For drugs with clearance principally dependent upon the intrinsic activity of phase I P450 hepatic microsomal enzymes (e.g., quinidine), the observed age-related reductions in elimination result in part from a reduced liver mass, which diminishes the absolute amount and overall functional activity of hepatic monooxygenases.

POLYMORPHIC HEPATIC METABOLISM

Several cardiovascular drugs are metabolized by hepatic enzymes that have a genetically founded polymorphic distribution. For N-acetyltransferase, a nonmicrosomal enzyme implicated in the metabolism of procainamide and hydralazine, there may be an age-related reduction in activity.[9] It is unclear whether this occurs as a consequence of a reduced functional liver mass or an actual decrease in intrinsic enzymatic activity. This may result in a phenotypically classified higher proportion of slow acetylators in the elderly. On the other hand, limited evidence suggests that cytochrome P450 2D6 (i.e., CYP2D6)—an isozyme responsible for the metabolism propa-fenone, flecainide, and the beta-adrenergic blockers propranolol and metoprolol—demonstrates no change in phenotypic distribution with age.[10]

Renal Function

The elimination of drugs that are dependent on renal excretion may diminish in the elderly, since renal blood flow, glomerular filtration, creatinine clearance, and renal tubular secretion usually decrease with age, although there is no reduction in creatinine clearance in about one-third of the elderly.[11] Serum creatinine concentration is not a reliable indicator of renal function in the elderly, since serum creatinine is determined not only by the rate of creatinine excretion but also by the rate of creatinine production, and the production of creatinine decreases due to reduced muscle mass. Therefore, creatinine clearance should be either measured or estimated by any one of several predictive equations,[12] although these equations may be inaccurate in the debilitated elderly nursing home patient.[13]

Miscellaneous Factors Affecting Drug Disposition or Response

ENVIRONMENTAL INFLUENCES

Several other factors may modify the clinical pharmacology of cardiovascular drugs in the elderly. For example, environmental influences, such as chronic cigarette smoking or alcohol ingestion, can induce specific microsomal enzymes, thereby enhancing the elimination of selected drugs.[14] In addition, cigarette smoking may antagonize the effects of antihypertensive drugs.

NUTRITIONAL FACTORS

The composition of the diet may alter the disposition of drugs. High-protein diets and cruciferous vegetables such as cabbage and brussels sprouts can enhance hepatic oxidative metabolism, whereas grapefruit juice can inhibit selected P450 isozymes.[15] Malnutrition can also affect drug metabolism.[15] Although there is a lack of data on the interaction between advanced age and diet and their effect on drug metabolism, nutritional factors may play a role in altering hepatic drug metabolism in the elderly.

ETHNIC DIFFERENCES

There is increasing evidence for interethnic variability in drug metabolism and responsiveness.[16] There is a greater prevalence of slow acetylators among Caucasians and blacks than among Chinese and Japanese.[16] Therefore, more individuals in the former groups may be at greater risk for developing drug-induced systemic erythematosus during chronic administration of procainamide or hydralazine. With respect to drug responsiveness, Chinese individuals are more sensitive to the beta-blocking and hypotensive actions of propranolol, despite a higher clearance of propranolol.[16]

GENDER DIFFERENCES

Gender differences may play an important role in the disposition of and response to cardiovascular drugs.[6] In addition, there may be greater age-related reduction in the total body clearance of lidocaine in elderly males than in elderly females.[17] The total body clearance of propranolol is greater in males than in females because of gender-related differences in selected metabolic pathways.[6] Females may be at greater risk for the development of drug-induced torsades de pointes.[18]

STEREOSPECIFIC CONSIDERATIONS

Many cardiovascular drugs are clinically available as 50/50 racemic mixtures of two enantiomers that frequently differ in their pharmacokinetic and pharmacologic properties.[19] Examples include several antiarrhythmic drugs—disopyramide, mexiletine, propafenone, flecainide, and sotalol; virtually all beta-adrenergic antagonists, including propranolol, metoprolol, and atenolol; the calcium channel antagonist verapamil; and warfarin. The disposition of the enantiomers of several of these compounds is altered as a consequence of aging.[19]

DRUG INTERACTIONS

The elderly are at an increased risk for drug interactions because of concurrent illnesses and the resultant polypharmacy.[3] In addition, specific drug interactions can be magnified in the elderly secondary to age- and disease-related changes

in physiologic functions.[3] Drug interactions may result from alterations in pharmacokinetics or pharmacodynamics.[3] An overview of cardiovascular drug interactions is beyond the scope of this chapter. The cardiovascular drugs digoxin,[20] warfarin,[21] and amiodarone[22] are frequently implicated in clinically important drug interactions (see Chaps. 23, 30, 52, and 54).

Cardiovascular, Adrenergic, and Neuroendocrine Changes

CARDIOVASCULAR CHANGES

A number of the cardiovascular, adrenergic, and neuroendocrine changes that occur during the normal aging process may modify the response to cardiovascular drugs. Resting heart rate and left ventricular systolic shortening are diminished in the healthy elderly.[23] However, ventricular performance is preserved in part by an increase in ventricular wall thickness.[23] Maximal exercise heart rate is also reduced, but cardiac output is maintained by enhanced cardiac dilatation and increased stroke volume.[23] The compliance in large arteries consistently decreases with age, but there are inconclusive data for age-related changes in the smaller-caliber resistance vessels.[23]

In addition to the age-related changes that normally occur within the cardiovascular system, the prevalence of congestive heart failure (CHF) rises progressively with increasing age for both males and females.[24] CHF may alter drug metabolism and elimination as a result of hypoperfusion of the liver and kidney.[25] Proarrhythmia, an undesirable pharmacodynamic response to antiarrhythmic drugs, is enhanced in patients with poor left ventricular function.[26]

ADRENERGIC CHANGES

Although plasma norepinephrine concentrations are generally increased in the elderly, baroreflex sensitivity to both hypertensive and hypotensive stimuli is blunted with normal human aging.[23,27] The responsiveness of cardiac beta$_1$-adrenergic receptors also declines with age, thereby diminishing the inotropic and chronotropic effects of beta$_1$-agonists.[23,27] Based upon the clinical model, vascular beta$_2$-receptor sensitivity is either diminished[27] or maintained[28] in the elderly. There is no apparent effect of age on alpha$_1$-adrenoceptor sensitivity.[27] However, both pre- and postsynaptic alpha$_2$-mediated responses seem to be attenuated with advanced age.[27]

NEUROENDOCRINE CHANGES

In the elderly, circulating levels of renin, angiotensin II, and aldosterone are decreased, and this may contribute to a diminished ability to conserve sodium.[29] Plasma concentrations of atrial natriuretic factor (ANF) increase with age and may contribute to reductions in both activity of the renin-angiotensin-aldosterone system (RAAS) and plasma concentrations of these three hormones.[30] Despite elevated ANF plasma levels, there is an increase in total body exchangeable sodium in the elderly patient with essential hypertension. The elderly may have disturbances in water balance due to a reduction in intravascular volume, diminished thirst following water deprivation, increased vasopressin secretion coupled with a diminished renal responsiveness to vasopressin, impaired sodium-conserving ability, and declining glomerular filtration.[30]

Pharmacodynamic Changes in the Elderly

There may be an increased response or enhanced sensitivity (i.e., altered pharmacodynamics) to numerous cardiovascular and noncardiovascular drugs in the elderly.[31] However, these exaggerated pharmacologic responses can often be explained by age-dependent changes in pharmacokinetics.[31] Changes in pharmacodynamics in the aged may be an indirect effect either of the normal aging process (e.g., decreased baroreflex sensitivity) or of underlying and perhaps previously undetected disease processes. Nonetheless, clinicians should be aware of the potential for exaggerated responses to cardiovascular drugs in elderly patients.

SELECTED CARDIOVASCULAR DRUGS

Antiarrhythmics

QUINIDINE

In the elderly, the total-body, renal, and nonrenal clearance of quinidine is decreased and the half-life is increased.[32] There is no change in the protein binding and volume of distribution of quinidine in healthy elderly. In addition, elderly patients may be at a potentially greater risk for accumulating the active metabolite 3-hydroxyquinidine. Elevated concentrations of this metabolite may contribute to the occurrence of quinidine-induced cardiotoxicity, such as ventricular tachycardia or excessive prolongation of the QRS interval.[33]

PROCAINAMIDE

The elimination of procainamide is diminished in elderly patients due to a reduction in the renal clearance and possibly the nonrenal clearance of procainamide.[34] These findings likely explain the longer half-life of procainamide in the aged. The clearance of n-acetylprocainamide (NAPA) is decreased,[34] the half-life is extended,[35] and the steady-state NAPA/procainamide serum concentration ratios are generally increased[34] in the elderly.

DISOPYRAMIDE

The pharmacokinetics of both total (protein-bound plus unbound) and unbound disopyramide are altered in the elderly.[36] The total body clearance is reduced; volume of distribution is increased; and half-life is prolonged for total disopyramide.[36] Although there is no change in the protein binding of disopyramide in the elderly, steady-state serum concentrations of unbound disopyramide are greater due to the reduced clearance of unbound disopyramide.[36] Serum concentrations of mono-N-dealkyldisopyramide, the active major metabolite of disopyramide, also tend to be higher in the elderly.[36] Interestingly, cigarette smoking may induce the metabolism of disopyra-

mide to a greater extent in aged individuals.[36] The elderly also appear at greater risk for the anticholingeric[36] and hypoglycemic[37] adverse effects of disopyramide.

LIDOCAINE

There is disagreement regarding age-related changes in the pharmacokinetics of lidocaine, particularly in studies following single-dose administration.[17] These studies report an increase in the half-life of lidocaine but no change in the clearance of lidocaine in elderly subjects.[17] However, another study indicates that there is a decrease in the total-body clearance of lidocaine in elderly males but not in elderly females as compared with gender-matched young control groups.[17] Following continuous infusion of lidocaine in patients with acute myocardial infarction, the total-body clearance of lidocaine decreases and serum concentrations of lidocaine rise in elderly patients with or without concomitant heart failure.[17] The protein binding of lidocaine may be increased in the elderly.[17]

MEXILETINE

The rate but not the extent of absorption of oral mexiletine is decreased in the elderly.[36] The elderly tend to have a prolonged half-life and a reduction in the oral clearance of mexiletine.

FLECAINIDE

In elderly subjects following chronic oral dosing, there is a decrease in clearance and an increase in the half-life of flecainide, perhaps because of time-dependent changes in the hepatic metabolism of this drug.[38] The Cardiac Arrhythmia Suppression Trial (CAST) study suggests that older age is an independent predictor of adverse effects in patients taking flecainide.[39]

AMIODARONE

Following single intravenous doses of amiodarone, the half-life and volume of distribution of both amiodarone and desethylamiodarone, its active metabolite, are increased, and the total-body clearance of amiodarone is decreased in older individuals.[40] Furthermore, during chronic treatment for either recurrent sustained ventricular tachycardia or fibrillation, advanced age is associated with an increased likelihood of developing amiodarone-induced adverse effects.[41] It is unknown whether this is either a direct pharmacodynamic effect of amiodarone in the aged or a secondary phenomenon due to altered pharmacokinetics.

PROPAFENONE

The metabolism and elimination of propafenone is polymorphic and stereoselective.[42] Only extensive metabolizers of propafenone (i.e., generally 90 percent or greater for most populations) form the active metabolite 5-hydroxypropafenone. Thus, for propafenone, the total-body clearance is greater and the half-life is shorter in extensive as compared with poor metabolizers. Steady-state ratios of the two enantiomers of propafenone suggest no age-related differences in the clearance of propafenone.[42]

SOTALOL

In otherwise healthy elderly hypertensive patients, the total-body and renal clearance of racemic sotalol (i.e., *dl*-sotalol) is reduced 40 to 50 percent and the half-life is increased about 60 percent relative to healthy young subjects.[43] These pharmacokinetic alterations are due to age-related decreases in renal excretion. Elderly patients may also have greater reductions in blood pressure relative to younger individuals following racemic sotalol.[43]

DIGOXIN

Both the pharmacokinetics and the pharmacodynamics of digoxin may be modified in the elderly.[7] For example, there is an age-associated reduction in the volume of distribution and total-body clearance and an increase in the half-life. In addition, the rate but not the extent of absorption of digoxin from tablets is slowed, although there may be an increase in the extent of absorption in elderly, hypochlorhydric patients.[5] Routine measurement of serum digoxin concentrations (SDCs) in elderly patients may be useful due to the difficulty in predicting digoxin dose requirements in this population.[7] There may be an increased sensitivity to the inotropic effects of digoxin in elderly patients with CHF in that an increase in resting left ventricular ejection fraction occurs at relatively low (i.e., 0.4 to 1.0 ng/mL) SDCs.[7] These data are supported by findings from the Prospective Randomized Study of Ventricular Failure and the Efficacy of Digoxin (PROVED) and Randomized Assessment of the Effect of Digoxin on Inhibitors of the Angiotensin-Converting Enzyme (RADIANCE) studies, in which the mean age exceeded 60 years. In these studies, further increases in treadmill exercise time were not observed when SDCs exceeded 1.2 ng/mL.[44] With respect to digoxin toxicity, the hospitalization rate for definite or probable digoxin toxicity for elderly patients is 0.7 percent per year (i.e., 4 percent over 6 years).[45] The coadministration of quinidine is a significant risk factor for the development of digoxin toxicity in this population.[45]

Miscellaneous Cardiovascular Agents

ANGIOTENSIN-CONVERTING ENZYME INHIBITORS

Despite lower circulating concentrations of renin, angiotensin-converting enzyme (ACE) inhibitors are frequently effective in the management of both systolic and diastolic hypertension in the aged.[46] However, some hypertensive elderly patients may have exaggerated pharmacodynamic responses to those ACE inhibitors that are principally renally eliminated (e.g., benazepril, captopril, enalapril, lisinopril, quinapril, and ramipril) because of a significant age- or disease-related decrease in glomerular filtration.[46]

The survival benefit of ACE inhibitors is clearly established in elderly patients with CHF by the results of the Cooperative North Scandinavian Enalapril Survival Study (CONSENSUS), in which the mean age for the treatment group was 71 years.[47] Other studies, in which the mean age of the patients treated with ACE inhibitors was at least 60 years, also showed favorable survival effects for ACE inhibitors.[48,49] In general, both short- and long-acting ACE inhibitors are well tolerated by older patients with CHF.[50] However, the very elderly (i.e., mean age of 83 years) with CHF may be relatively intolerant of ACE inhibitors.[51] In this age group, beginning doses of ACE inhibitors should be low (e.g., 1.25 mg of enalapril).

NITRATES

Older animals have a longer half-life and a larger volume of distribution but no change in total body clearance of nitrates.[52] Formal pharmacokinetic studies for most nitrate preparations are lacking in elderly humans.[52] An exception is isosorbide mononitrate, for which there are no age-related changes.[53]

With respect to pharmacodynamics, older patients may have a greater nitrate-induced reduction in left ventricular filling pressure, suggesting that venous smooth muscle in the aged is more sensitive to the relaxant effects of organic nitrates or that the pharmacokinetics of nitrates change with age.[52] Nitroglycerin may cause hypotension and bradycardia more commonly in elderly patients with AMI, possibly due to a dampened baroreceptor response to its hypotensive effects. Therefore, lower doses of nitrates should be used in initiating nitrate therapy in elderly patients. Interestingly, the elderly may be at a reduced risk for nitrate-induced headache.[54] There is no evidence of age-related differences in the rate or extent of development of tolerance to nitrates.[54]

HYDRALAZINE

Hydralazine undergoes phenotype-dependent, extensive first-pass metabolism that results in greater bioavailability in slow acetylators.[55] Furthermore, the first-pass metabolism is apparently saturable.[55] The total-body clearance and volume of distribution of hydralazine appear to be decreased in older hypertensive patients versus young, healthy volunteers.[55] In addition, the half-life tends to be longer in the older group. These dissimilarities may reflect differences in methodologies[55] or actual changes in rates of acetylation in the aged.[9] A q8h dosing schedule may be satisfactory in older patients, although a qid hydralazine regimen was used in the Vasodilator Heart Failure Trials (VHeFTs).[49]

CALCIUM CHANNEL BLOCKERS

Several calcium channel blocking drugs (CCBs) are used in the management of hypertension, coronary artery disease, selected supraventricular arrhythmias, and other cardiovascular disorders. The elderly have a reduced clearance and prolonged half-life relative to younger controls for a variety of CCBs, including immediate-release, first-generation CCBs (e.g., verapamil, diltiazem, nifedipine),[56] intermediate-acting CCBs (e.g., isradipine, nitrendipine),[56] long-acting CCBs (e.g., amlodipine),[56] and sustained-release CCBs (e.g., verapamil,[57] felodipine,[58] nifedipine[59] and nisoldipine[60]). In addition, CCBs may produce an increased blood pressure–lowering effect in elderly hypertensive patients generally unaccompanied by a reflex tachycardia, suggesting impaired baroreflex activity.[56] Atrioventricular conduction delay is equivalent in older and younger patients, whereas heart rate suppression may be more pronounced in older patients treated with verapamil or diltiazem.[56] Recent cohort studies in elderly hypertensive patients indicate that there may be higher rates of cancer,[61] gastrointestinal hemorrhage,[62] and mortality[63] with the use of immediate-release, first-generation CCBs as compared to beta-adrenergic antagonists and ACE inhibitors. Furthermore, the use of the intermediate-acting CCB isradipine in the treatment of hypertensive patients is associated with an increased incidence of AMI, stroke, CHF, angina, and sudden death compared to hydrochlorothiazide.[64] Prospective, controlled trials with the long-acting and sustained-release CCBs are needed to address those risks associated with the use of immediate-release and intermediate-acting CCBs.

BETA-ADRENERGIC ANTAGONISTS

Beta-adrenergic antagonists are extensively prescribed for the treatment of hypertension, arrhythmias, chronic stable angina, and to decrease mortality following AMI (see Chap. 54). For several beta blockers, there is a decreased total-body clearance, resulting in increased steady-state concentrations in elderly individuals.[65] However, the pharmacodynamic response to beta$_1$-receptor antagonism may decline with advanced age.[65] This observation suggests a diminished pharmacotherapeutic role for beta$_1$-selective and nonselective antagonists in elderly patients. However, a recent metaanalysis demonstrates the value of beta-adrenergic blockade in the treatment of diastolic or isolated systolic hypertension in the elderly.[66] In addition, beta blockers are very effective in reducing mortality in older patients following AMI.[67]

Anticoagulant and Antiplatelet Drugs

WARFARIN

The total-body clearance of warfarin is decreased in older patients.[68] In addition, elderly patients appear to have an increased sensitivity to the anticoagulant effects of warfarin.[68] A possible explanation may be that an age-related fall in functional hepatic mass results in a decrease in the absolute content of vitamin K epoxide reductase, the warfarin receptor.[68] Warfarin-related bleeding may be more common in older patients.[69]

HEPARIN

In the settings of acute coronary syndromes, recent reports suggest that advanced age significantly predicts reduced heparin dosage requirements[70] and is associated with an increased activated partial thromboplastin time.[71] As for warfarin, bleeding due to heparin may be more common in older patients.[69]

ASPIRIN

The U.S. Physicians' Aspirin Trial provides convincing evidence for the efficacy of aspirin as primary prophylaxis against AMI for males above 50 years of age.[3] The nonrandomized U.S. Nurses Study suggests similar benefit for older females.[3] Therefore, prophylactic aspirin therapy should be strongly

considered to reduce the risk for AMI in men and women above age 65, especially those at high risk for cardiovascular disease.[3,72] In addition, aspirin reduces mortality and the incidence of recurrent AMI in elderly patients after AMI.[72]

SUMMARY

The elderly are at risk for the development of cardiovascular disease frequently requiring treatment with a wide range of cardiovascular drugs. In order to optimize cardiovascular drug therapy, the clinician must (1) be aware that the disposition and response to cardiovascular drugs can be modified by the normal aging process, the presence of cardiac and extracardiac disease, and several other factors and (2) be informed of the specific alterations of these drugs in the elderly.

REFERENCES

1. *Monthly Vital Statistics Report.* Hyattsville, MD: National Center for Health Statistics; 1996; 44(7, suppl).
2. Goldman L, Cook EF. The decline in ischemic heart disease mortality rates: An analysis of the comparative effects of medical interventions and changes in lifestyle. *Ann Intern Med* 1984; 101:825–846.
3. Scheitel SM, Fleming KC, Chutka DS, Evans JM. Geriatric health maintenance. *Mayo Clin Proc* 1996; 71:289–302.
4. Iber FL, Murphy PA, Connor ES. Age-related changes in the gastrointestinal system. Effects on drug therapy. *Drugs Aging* 1994; 5:34–48.
5. Hui J, Geraets DR, Chandrasekaran A, Wang Y-MC, Caldwell JH, Robertson LW, et al. Digoxin disposition in elderly humans with hypochlorhydria. *J Clin Pharmacol* 1994; 34:734–741.
6. Harris RZ, Benet LZ, Schwartz JB. Gender effects in pharmacokinetics and pharmacodynamics. *Drugs* 1995; 50:222–239.
7. Nolan PE, Mooradian AD. Digoxin. In: Bressler R, Katz MD, eds. *Geriatric Pharmacology.* New York: McGraw-Hill; 1993:151–163.
8. Veering BT, Burm AGL, Souverijn JHM, Serree JMP, Spierdijk J. The effect of age on serum concentrations of albumin and α$_1$-acid glycoprotein. *Br J Clin Pharmacol* 1990; 29:201–206.
9. Iselius L, Evans DAP. Formal genetics of isoniazid metabolism in man. *Clin Pharmacokinet* 1983; 8:541–544.
10. Steiner E, Bertilsson L, Sawe J, Bertling I, Sjoqvist F. Polymorphic debrisoquin hydroxylation in 757 Swedish subjects. *Clin Pharmacol Ther* 1988; 44:431–435.
11. Lindeman RD. Changes in renal function with aging. *Drugs Aging* 1992; 2:423–431.
12. Luke DR, Halstenson CE, Opsahl JA, Matzke GR. Validity of creatinine clearance estimates in the assessment of renal function. *Clin Pharmacol Ther* 1990; 48:503–508.
13. Drusano GL, Muncie HL, Hoopes JM, Damron DJ, Warren JW. Commonly used methods of estimating creatinine clearance are inadequate for elderly debilitated nursing home patients. *J Am Geriatr Soc* 1988; 36:437–441.
14. Spatzenegger M, Jaeger W. Clinical importance of hepatic cytochrome P450 in drug metabolism. *Drug Metab Rev* 1995; 27:397–417.
15. Walter-Sack I, Klotz U. Influence of diet and nutritional status on drug metabolism. *Clin Pharmacokinet* 1996; 31:47–64.
16. Wood AJJ, Zhou HH. Ethnic differences in drug disposition and responsiveness. *Clin Pharmacokinet* 1991; 20:350–373.
17. Nolan PE, Otto MD. Lidocaine. In: Murphy JE, ed, *Clinical Pharmacokinetics: Pocket Reference.* Bethesda, MD: American Society of Hospital Pharmacists; 1993:115–144.
18. Makkar RR, Fromm BS, Steinman RT, Meissner MD, Lehmann MH. Female gender as a risk factor for torsades de pointes associated with cardiovascular drugs. *JAMA* 1993; 270:2590–2597.
19. Eichelbaum M, Gross AS. Stereochemical aspects of drug action and disposition. *Adv Drug Res* 1996; 28:1–64.
20. Magnani B, Malini PL. Cardiac glycosides: Drug interactions of clinical significance. *Drug Safety* 1995; 12:97–109.
21. Wells PS, Holbrook AM, Crowther NR, Hirsh J. Interactions of warfarin with drugs and food. *Ann Intern Med* 1994; 121:676–683.

22. Lesko LJ. Pharmacokinetic drug interactions with amiodarone. *Clin Pharmacokinet* 1989; 17:130–140.

23. Lakatta EG. Alterations in circulatory function. In: Hazzard WR, Bierman EL, Blass JP, Ettinger WH, Halter JB, eds. *Principles of Geriatric Medicine and Gerontology,* 3d ed. New York: McGraw-Hill; 1994:493–508.

24. Kannel WB, Belanger AJ. Epidemiology of heart failure. *Am Heart J* 1991; 121:951–957.

25. Shammas FV, Dickstein K. Clinical pharmacokinetics in heart failure. *Clin Pharmacokinet* 1988; 15:94–113.

26. Herre JM, Titus C, Oeff M. Eldar M, Franz MR, Griffin JC, et al. Inefficacy and proarrhythmic effects of flecainide and encainide for sustained ventricular tachycardia and ventricular fibrillation. *Ann Intern Med* 1990; 113:671–676.

27. Folkow B, Svanborg A. Physiology of cardiovascular aging. *Physiol Rev* 1993; 73:725–764.

28. Klein C, Hiatt WR, Gerber JG, Nies AS. Age does not alter human vascular and nonvascular β_2-adrenergic responses to isoproterenol. *Clin Pharmacol Ther* 1988; 44:573–578.

29. Belmin J, Lévy BI, Michel J-P. Changes in the renin-angiotensin-aldosterone axis later in life. *Drugs Aging* 1994; 5:391–400.

30. Miller M. Hormonal aspects of fluid and sodium balance in the elderly. *Endocrinol Metab Clin North Am* 1995; 24:233–253.

31. Feely J, Coakley D. Altered pharmacodynamics in the elderly. *Clin Geriatr Med* 1990; 6:269–283.

32. Nolan PE, Otto MD. Quinidine. In: Murphy JE, ed. *Clinical Pharmacokinetics: Pocket Reference.* Bethesda, MD: American Society of Hospital Pharmacists; 1993:225–253.

33. Bowers LD, Nelson KM, Connor R, Lais CJ, Krauss E. Evidence supporting 3(S)-3-hydroxyquinidine-associated cardiotoxicity. *Ther Drug Monit* 1985; 7:308–312.

34. Coyle JD, Lima JJ. Procainamide. In: Evans WE, Schentag JJ, Jusko WJ, eds. *Applied Pharmacokinetics: Principles of Therapeutic Drug Monitoring,* 3d ed. Vancouver, BC: Applied Therapeutics; 1992:22-1–22.33.

35. Galeazzi RL, Omar-Amberg C, Karlaganis G. N-acetyl-procainamide kinetics in the elderly. *Clin Pharmacol Ther* 1981; 29:440–446.

36. Fenster PE, Nolan PE. Antiarrhythmic drugs. In Bressler R, Katz MD, eds. *Geriatric Pharmacology.* New York: McGraw-Hill; 1993:105–149.

37. Smith RC, Sullivan M, Geller J. Inadequate adrenergic response to disopyramide-induced hypoglycemia. *Ann Pharmacother* 1992, 26:490–491.

38. McQuinn RL, Weeks CE, Kvam DC, Fredell PA, Carlson GL, Miller AM, et al. Pharmacokinetics of flecainide in elderly subjects (abstr). *Clin Pharmacol Ther* 1986; 30:210.

39. Akiyama T, Pawitan Y, Campbell WB, Papa L, Barker AH, Rubbert P, et al. Effects of advancing age on the efficacy and side effects of antiarrhythmic drugs in post–myocardial infarction patients with ventricular arrhythmias. *J Am Geriatr Soc* 1992; 40:666–672.

40. Zimmerman JJ, Klamerus KJ, Giel S, Ben-Maimon CS. Effect of age on amiodarone disposition (abstr). *Clin Pharmacol Ther* 1993; 53:201.

41. Herre JM, Sauve MJ, Malone P, Griffin JC, Helmy I, Langberg JJ, et al. Long-term results of amiodarone therapy in patients with recurrent sustained ventricular tachycardia or ventricular fibrillation. *J Am Coll Cardiol* 1989; 13:442–449.

42. Volz M, Mitrovic V, Schlepper M. Steady-state plasma concentrations of propafenone—Chirality and metabolism. *Int J Clin Pharmacol Ther* 1994; 32:370–375.

43. Ishizaki T, Hirayama H, Tawara K, Nakaya H, Sato M, Sato K. Pharmacokinetics and pharmacodynamics in young normal and elderly hypertensive subjects: A study using sotalol as a model drug. *J Pharmacol Exp Ther* 1980; 212:173–181.

44. Young JB, Gheorghiade M, Packer M, Uretsky B, Hull H. Are low serum levels of digoxin effective in chronic heart failure? Evidence challenging the accepted guidelines for a therapeutic serum level of the drug (abstr). *J Am Coll Cardiol* 1993; 21:378A.

45. Kernan WN, Castellsague J, Perlman GD. Incidence of hospitalization for digitalis toxicity among elderly Americans. *Am J Med* 1994; 96:426–431.

46. Israili ZH, Dall WD. ACE inhibitors: Differential use in elderly patients with hypertension. *Drugs Aging* 1995; 7:335–371.

47. The CONSENSUS Trial Study Group. Effects of enalapril on mortality in severe congestive heart failure: Results of the Cooperative North Scandinavian Enalapril Survival Study (CONSENSUS). *N Engl J Med* 1987; 316:1429–1435.

48. The SOLVD Investigators. Effect of enalapril on survival in patients with reduced left ventricular ejection fractions and congestive heart failure. *N Engl J Med* 1991; 325:293–302.

49. Cohn JN, Johnson G, Ziesche S, Cobb F, Francis G, Tristani F, et al. A comparison of enalapril with hydralazine-isosorbide dinitrate in the treatment of chronic congestive heart failure. *N Engl J Med* 1991; 325:303–310.

50. Giles TD, Fisher MB, Rush JE. Lisinopril and captopril in the treatment of heart failure in older patients. *Am J Med* 1988; 85(suppl 3B):44–47.

51. O'Neill CJA, Bowes SG, Sullens CM, Royston JP, Hunt WB, Denham MJ, et al. Evaluation of the safety of enalapril in the treatment of heart failure in the very old. *Eur J Clin Pharmacol* 1988; 35:143–150.

52. Alpert JS. Nitrate therapy in the elderly. *Am J Cardiol* 1990; 65:23J–27J.

53. Abshagen UWP. Pharmacokinetics of isosorbide mononitrate. *Am J Cardiol* 1992; 70:61G–66G.

54. Pahor M, Cecchi E, Fumagalli S, Manto A, Pedone C, Carosella L, et al. Association of serum creatinine and age with headache caused by nitrates. *Clin Pharmacol Ther* 1995; 58:470–481.

55. Ludden TM, McNay JL, Shepherd AMM, Lin MS. Clinical pharmacokinetics of hydralazine. *Clin Pharmacokinet* 1982; 7:185–205.

56. Schwartz JB. Calcium antagonists in the elderly: A risk-benefit analysis. *Drugs Aging* 1996; 9:24–36.

57. Gupta SK, Atkinson L, Tu T, Longstreth JA. Age and gender related changes in stereoselective pharmacokinetics and pharmacodynamics of verapamil and norverapamil. *Br J Clin Pharmacol* 1995; 40:325–331.

58. Wade JR, Sambol NC. Felodipine population dose-response and concentration-response relationships in patients with essential hypertension. *Clin Pharmacol Ther* 1995; 57:569–581.

59. Grundy JS, Foster RT. The nifedipine gastrointestinal therapeutic system (GITS): Evaluation of pharmaceutical, pharmacokinetic and pharmacological properties. *Clin Pharmacokinet* 1996; 30:28–51.

60. Plosker GL, Faulds D. Nisoldipine coat-core: A review of its pharmacology and therapeutic efficacy in hypertension. *Drugs* 1996; 52:232–253.

61. Pahor M, Guralnik JM, Salive ME, Corti M-C, Carbonin P, Havlik RJ. Do calcium channel blockers increase the risk of cancer? *Am J Hypertens* 1996; 9:695–699.

62. Pahor M, Guralnik JM, Furberg CD, Carbonin P, Havlik RJ. Risk of gastrointestinal haemorrhage with calcium antagonists in hypertensive persons over 67 years old. *Lancet* 1996; 347:1061–1065.

63. Pahor M, Guralnik JM, Corti C, et al. Long-term survival and use of antihypertensive medications in older persons. *J Am Geriatr Soc* 1995; 43:1191–1197.

64. Borhani NO, Mercuri M, Borhani PA, Buckalew VM, Canossa-Terris M, Carr AA, et al. Final outcome results of the multicenter isradipine diuretic atherosclerotic study (MIDAS): A randomized controlled trial. *JAMA* 1996; 276:785–791.

65. Abernethy DR. Altered pharmacodynamics of cardiovascular drugs and their relation to altered pharmacokinetics in elderly patients. *Clin Geriatr Med* 1990; 6:285–292.

66. Mulrow CD, Cornell JA, Herrera CR, Kadri A, Farnett L, Aguilar C. Hypertension in the elderly: Implications and generalizability of randomized trials. *JAMA* 1994; 272:1932–1938.

67. Jansen RWMM, Gurwitz JH. Controversies surrounding the use of β-blockers in older patients with cardiovascular disease. *Drugs Aging* 1994; 4:175–183.

68. Wynne H, Cope L, Kelly P, Whittingham T, Edwards C, Kamali F. The influence of age, liver size and enantiomer concentrations on warfarin requirements. *Br J Clin Pharmacol* 1995; 40:203–207.

69. Beyth RJ, Landefeld CS. Anticoagulants in older patients: A safety perspective. *Drugs Aging* 1995; 6:45–54.

70. Trujillo TC, Nolan PE, Quan RA, Slack MK, Ewy GA. Optimization of heparin therapy in patients with unstable angina or acute myocardial infarction using a multiple regression-derived dosing nomogram (abstr). *Pharmacotherapy* 1996; 16:492–493.

71. Granger CB, Hirsh J, Califf RM, Col J, White HD, Betriu A, et al. Activated partial thromboplastin time and outcome after thrombolytic therapy for acute myocardial infarction: Results from the GUSTO-1 trial. *Circulation* 1996; 93:870–878.

72. Antiplatelet Trialists' Collaboration. Collaborative overview of randomized trials of antiplatelet therapy: I. Prevention of death, myocardial infarction, and stroke by prolonged antiplatelet therapy in various categories of patients. *Br Med J* 1994; 308:81–106.

DISEASES OF THE GREAT VESSELS AND PERIPHERAL VESSELS

98

DIAGNOSIS AND TREATMENT OF DISEASES OF THE AORTA

Joseph Lindsay, Jr. / Arthur C. Beall, Jr. / Michael E. DeBakey

The aorta, structurally and functionally uncomplicated, manifests disease in a limited number of ways. Weakness of its wall may result in aneurysm, dissection, or rupture. Narrowing of the main trunk may occur but does so less frequently than does obstruction of the origin of a main branch. Finally, debris from its luminal surface may be thrown off and lodge in distal arterial beds. In contrast to this limited variety of clinical manifestations stands an array of disease processes capable of involving the aorta.

This chapter first reviews the various diseases that affect the aorta together with their pathogenetic mechanisms and characteristic pathologic features. A review of the resulting clinical problems follows.

ETIOLOGIC AND PATHOGENETIC CONSIDERATIONS IN AORTIC DISEASE

Medial Changes of Aging

With advancing age, the aortic media undergoes characteristic histologic changes. After careful and systematic study, Schlattman and Becker[1] identified these as fragmentation of elastic fibers and loss of smooth muscle cell nuclei, so-called *medionecrosis*. Collagenous tissue and basophilic ground substance replace these lost medial components. The resulting loss of compliance of the aortic wall is manifest by tortuosity and ectasia of the aorta. Although the degree to which these changes are present in any one individual varies, they appear to be an almost universal consequence of aging.

Atherosclerosis

So prevalent in the Western world is aortic atherosclerosis that its absence in middle life and beyond is noteworthy. The severity of the process varies. Diabetes, hypercholesterolemia, smoking, and hypertension are among the factors that seem to accelerate it (see Chap. 41).

The pathogenesis of aortic atherosclerosis is thought to be similar to that in the coronary arteries and elsewhere.[2,3] "Fatty streaks," the first manifestation, are recognized in childhood. These focal collections of lipid contained within macrophages ("foam cells") appear as small, yellow, circumscribed, flat or slightly raised intimal lesions. Oddly, they are common even in societies in which serum cholesterol measurements are low. By young adulthood, some but not all of these fatty streaks have evolved into "intermediate plaques" composed of layers of macrophages and smooth muscle cells. Some of these, in turn, develop into "fibrous plaques"—firm, pale gray, elevated lesions protruding into the lumen of the vessel. A dense fibrous cap in which smooth muscle cells are imbedded covers these atheromas. Contained within them are lipid-laden macrophages, smooth muscle cells, activated T lymphocytes, and a central core of amorphous yellow material consisting of extracellular lipid and cell debris. With the passage of time, many of these plaques become ulcerated and calcified. Overlying thrombus is common. The larger and more complex lesions penetrate the underlying media, producing scarring and atrophy (see Chaps. 39 and 40).

Atherosclerosis, characteristically most severe in the abdominal aorta, heavily involves the ascending segment only in a few special situations. In patients with diabetes mellitus, atherosclerosis is frequently of great severity throughout the aorta. Individuals with type II hyperlipoproteinemia represent a second exception to the rule that the ascending aorta is spared.[4] Finally, atherosclerosis can be extensive in areas overlying syphilitic aortitis involving the ascending segment. At least two explanations have been advanced for the predilection of atherosclerosis for the infrarenal aorta.[5] First, the velocity and pulsatile characteristics of blood flow in that segment differ from those found in the proximal aortic segments. Such differences may influence the interface of blood with the aortic wall so as to favor plaque development in the infrarenal segment. Second, the wall of the abdominal aorta is thinner; it has fewer elastic lamellae and more smooth muscle fibers. Moreover, it lacks the rich network of vasa vasorum found in the proximal aorta.[6]

Aortic atherosclerosis is manifest clinically in three major ways: aneurysm, obstruction of the infrarenal aorta, and embolization from atheromatous plaques to distal arterial beds.[7–9] These are addressed in that portion of this chapter dealing with the clinical manifestations of aortic disease. .

Medial Degeneration

The aortic manifestations of the Marfan syndrome (Chap. 85) are prototypical of disease processes that result from a defective aortic media. Indeed, the basis for the clinical manifestations of that syndrome has been found to be a genetically determined defect in fibrillin, a constituent of the microfibrillar component of elastin as well as other connective tissue.[10] Anuloaortic ectasia, the characteristic aortic abnormality, consists of aneurysmal dilatation of the ascending aorta that extends from the aortic sinuses to just proximal to the innominate artery.[10,11] The aorta takes on a distinctive "Florence flask" or "onion bulb" appearance. Rupture of such aneurysms or the hemodynamic effects of aortic regurgitation—a consequence of the aortic root dilatation— are responsible for most of the premature deaths from this disorder. Aortic dissection is a somewhat less common complication, although intimal tears and associated limited medial disruptions are commonly encountered within the aneurysm.

In the most complete presentation of Marfan's syndrome, skeletal, ocular, and cardiovascular anomalies are present and a family history of similar abnormalities exists.[10,11] Long extremities, particularly long, thin, hands and feet ("arachnodactyly"), and sparse muscle mass are outstanding musculoskeletal aberrations. Subluxed or frankly dislocated lenses attributable to lax supporting ligaments are characteristic. In addition to aortic aneurysm, myxomatous transformation of the aortic and mitral valves may produce valvular incompetence. Affected individuals are at risk of premature death from aortic dissection/rupture.

Annuloaortic ectasia, indistinguishable from that in Marfan's syndrome, is frequently encountered in patients who have no other detectable congenital or heritable anomaly.[11] Such patients seem to have a similar propensity to rupture and dissection. Because of the similarity of the aortic lesion to that in Marfan's patients, it is reasonable to infer that, as in Marfan's syndrome, a structural defect of the aortic media underlies this aneurysm. As yet no specific etiologic basis has been defined.

Moreover, aortic aneurysm and dissection closely mimicking the characteristic aortic lesion of Marfan's syndrome are found in a variety of other congenital or heritable disorders[12–18] (Table 98-1).

A histologic lesion, "cystic medial necrosis," was for many years considered to be the hallmark of medial degeneration.

TABLE 98-1

CONGENITAL AND HERITABLE DISEASES ASSOCIATED WITH AORTIC ANEURYSM OR DISSECTION

Bicuspid or unicuspid aortic valve[12,13]
Coarctation of the aorta[12,13]
Turner's syndrome[14]
Polycystic kidney disease[15,16]
Ehlers-Danlos sydnrome[17]
Osteogenesis imperfecta[18]

More recent observations suggest that this light-microscopic lesion is often not present in typical lesions; furthermore, it is neither specific nor accurately named.[1,19–21]

Exceptionally, medial degeneration severe enough to result in aneurysm, rupture, or dissection is found in the main pulmonary arteries or in the aorta distal to the ascending segment.

Aortitis

INFECTIVE AORTITIS

Bacteria may spread to the aortic wall directly from contiguous tissue, but more frequently invading organisms are bloodborne, entering the aortic wall from the lumen or from the vasa vasorum. Since the intact endothelium is quite resistant to bacterial invasion, a previously damaged area almost always provides the site for infection. For this reason secondarily infected aneurysms are more common than are aneurysms resulting solely from bacterial infection.[22,23]

Osler introduced the term, *mycotic aneurysm* to describe aneurysms resulting from septic emboli originating in infective endocarditis.[22,23] Typically an infected embolus lodges in a branch point of a distal artery, producing local endarteritis and a nidus for aneurysm. Because the large bore of the aorta offers few opportunities for the lodgement of small bits of infected material, embolization to the vasa vasorum has been hypothesized to explain the rare aortic aneurysm complicating endocarditis. In the antibiotic era, it is far more common to encounter bacterial aortitis attributable to contiguous spread of infection from the aortic valve to the adjacent aortic wall and adjacent tissue.[24,25] Resulting perivalvular abscesses may disrupt the junction between the aorta and the fibrous cardiac skeleton, producing aortocameral fistulas or damage to the conduction system.[24,25]

Blood-borne organisms, not related to endocarditis, may also invade the aortic wall, particularly at sites where the endothelium has been damaged. Thus, favorite sites for infectious aortitis include areas involved with atherosclerosis, sites of altered blood flow such as occur with aortic coarctation, location of aortic trauma, and areas of prosthetic replacement. A variety of organisms may be responsible, but *Staphylococcus aureus* and especially *Salmonella* species have most frequently been encountered.[22,23,26] In fact, *Salmonella* may be responsible for one-third to one-half of such infections. An unusual ability of this organism to invade endothelium has been demonstrated, and it has been suggested that this genus may produce aortic infection in areas of relatively normal endothelium.[27] The bacteremia responsible for an aortic infection need not be clinically apparent. Thus, an unexplained, persistent febrile illness, particularly in an older man in whom aortic atherosclerosis may be anticipated, may reflect an infected aortic segment.

Rupture of a secondarily infected aneurysm or of a "mycotic" aneurysm created by the aortitis is inevitable unless resection of the infected segment under cover of effective antibiotic therapy can be accomplished. Antibiotics alone are not sufficient to prevent rupture.

Unlike bacterial agents, the spirochete of syphilis produces a chronic aortitis.[22,28] During the spirochetemic phase of primary syphilis, the organisms lodge in the vasa vasorum. An obliterative endarteritis develops, resulting in destruction of the media and weakening of the aortic wall. Aneurysm—usually saccular—of the ascending aorta, arch, and proximal descending segments often complicates this process. Aortic regurgitation may result from dilatation of the proximal aorta. The frequency of syphilitic aortitis has declined dramatically in the last 25 years. As a consequence, luetic aneurysms are now quite infrequent.

Direct extension from tuberculous pulmonary or mediastinal infection to the aorta may also occur.[22] Aneurysm, rupture, or fistula may ensue.

TAKAYASU'S ARTERITIS

Narrowing of an aortic segment or of one of its branches, aneurysm formation, or aortic regurgitation may result from an aortitis associated with noninfectious inflammatory involvement of other organs, as in, for example, lupus erythematosus or rheumatoid arthritis. More often, however, it is encountered as an isolated process.

The prototype for noninfectious aortitis—whether associated with known disease or isolated—is Takayasu's arteritis. Its name is derived from the Japanese ophthalmologist who first called attention to the fundoscopic findings of the disease.[29] Because of its predilection for obstructing the brachiocephalic vessels, this arteritis has been labeled *pulseless disease* and *aortic arch syndrome*. The classic form occurs with greatest frequency in the Orient[22,29]; however, patients with nonspecific aortitis presenting a similar clinical picture are encountered worldwide.[30–32] Whether patients in widely separated geographic areas suffer from an identical disease or only a very similar one is uncertain.

Etiology

The etiology of Takayasu's arteritis remains unknown. No infectious agent has been identified. Clinical and serologic data suggest an "autoimmune" process. Support for this hypothesis is drawn from observed coincidence of the disease with rheumatoid arthritis, inflammatory bowel disease, systemic lupus, and sarcoidosis.[31] Recently, a genetic predisposition has been suggested because of clustering of the disorder in certain families and of the frequency of similar histocompatibility antigens in these kindreds.[33] Other investigators have been unable to confirm the link to the HLA antigens.[31]

Pathology

Histologic examination during active stages of the disease discloses a granulomatous arteritis resembling that of giant-cell arteritis and of the aortitis associated with seronegative spondylitis. In later stages, medial degeneration, fibrous scarring, intimal proliferation, and thrombosis result in narrowing of the affected vessel. Aneurysm formation is observed less commonly than stenosis. Aortic dissection or rupture is rare.

Detailed angiographic examination has provided a great deal of information about the distribution of the stenotic lesions.[32] The left subclavian artery, particularly in its midportion, is narrowed in about 90 percent of instances. The right subclavian, the left carotid, and the brachiocephalic trunk follow closely with regard to frequency of stenosis. Ishikawa[32] detected lesions in the thoracic aorta by angiography in two-thirds of his series. Involvement of the abdominal aorta was identified in half, but in only about 12 percent was there aortoiliac involvement. In patients studied at the Mayo Clinic,[30] involvement of the abdominal aorta, renal, and superior mesenteric arteries was even more frequent than in the Japanese series.

Evidence of pulmonary arteritis may be found in about half of these patients.[32] This may take the form of pulmonary hypertension alone or it may be combined with stenosis of a pulmonary artery.

Clinical Features

Manifestations of Takayasu's arteritis appear during the second or third decade in 70 to 80 percent of instances, but its onset has been reported in childhood and in middle life. Women are eight or nine times more often affected than are men.

During the early or "prepulseless" period of the illness, constitutional manifestations, such as fever, night sweats, malaise, nausea and vomiting, weight loss, arthralgia, and skin rash are frequently encountered. The patient may experience Raynaud's phenomenon and splenomegaly. Laboratory study may disclose an elevated erythrocyte sedimentation rate, anemia, and serum protein abnormalities.

Once the arterial disease is established, ischemic symptoms involving the extremities or central nervous system are common. Claudication and numbness of an upper extremity due to subclavian artery narrowing were encountered in about 60 percent of patients reported from the National Institutes of Health.[31] Postural dizziness, even frank syncope, usually reflecting cerebral ischemia due to narrowing of the brachiocephalic arteries—particularly a vertebral artery—is also common.

Narrowing of one or both renal arteries or of the aorta proximal to those branches accounts for nearly all of the hypertension that is observed in about half of aortitis patients. It must be remembered that difficulty may be encountered in accurately measuring arterial pressure because of arch vessel stenosis.

Cardiac manifestations may result from aortic regurgitation, coronary artery narrowing, or severe hypertension. Dilatation of the aortic root may produce aortic valve incompetence. Angina pectoris, heart failure, and myocardial infarction are reported. Pericarditis has been observed clinically, and healed pericarditis has been detected at necropsy.

The retinopathy to which Takayasu first directed attention is believed to result from ischemia of the retina. Ocular ischemia may also be manifest by transient loss of vision, cataracts, corneal opacity, and iridial atrophy. Blindness is a common complication.

Involvement of the visceral arteries occasionally results in splanchnic ischemia, and intermittent claudication due to aortoiliac obstruction may occur.

Recently attention has been directed toward the special problems that may arise during pregnancy in patients with this disorder.[31] Hypertension is a frequent and troublesome problem, but the outcome for mother and child will be acceptable when meticulous obstetric care is provided.

Diagnosis

The diagnosis of Takayasu's arteritis depends upon the recognition of the constellation of clinical findings and is supported by the presence of angiographic findings. The American College of Rheumatology identified six major criteria for the diagnosis (Table 98-2).[34] Onset of illness by age 40 years was recommended as an obligatory criterion to exclude overlap with giant-cell arteritis. The identification of two additional criteria is associated with high diagnostic accuracy.

Prognosis

During late follow-up, cerebrovascular accidents and blindness are common disabling events. Congestive heart failure and aortic rupture or dissection are less frequent. In addition, the presence of severe hypertension or of cardiac involvement predicts a shortened life expectancy.[35,36] As might be expected, patients who present with a major complication or a clinical pattern of progressively severe symptoms have a poor prognosis. In one study, one-third of patients with both succumbed within 5 years, whereas 90 percent of those with no more than one survived.[36]

TABLE 98-2

DIAGNOSTIC CRITERIA FOR TAKAYASU'S ARTERITIS

Onset by age 40 years
Claudication of an extremity (especially an arm)
Diminished brachial pulses
A difference of at least 10 mmHg in systolic blood
  pressure between arms
Subclavian or aortic bruit
Narrowing or occlusion of the aorta or its primary branches

Source: Arend et al.,[34] with permission.

Management

The benefits of any specific therapy have been difficult to assess, since the disease typically runs a chronic course. Adrenocorticoids appear to be effective in suppressing the inflamation of the active phase. Immunosuppressive therapy has also been utilized.[31,36] Operative treatment may relieve symptoms from arterial obstruction, and percutaneous angioplasty has been utilized with favorable initial results.[37,38]

GIANT-CELL ARTERITIS

Giant-cell arteritis (temporal or cranial arteritis) involves extracranial arteries, including the aorta, in at least 10 percent of cases.[39] Remarkably similar to Takayasu's aortitis in many of its clinical and pathologic characteristics, its peak incidence in late life seems to set it apart. Like that disorder, it may produce narrowing of the brachiocephalic arteries. Moreover, the frequency of aneurysm of the ascending aorta, aortic dissection/rupture, and aortic regurgitation is surprising.[40,41] Unlike Takayasu's arteritis, giant-cell arteritis rarely involves the descending thoracic or abdominal aorta (see Chap. 85).

AORTITIS IN HLA-B27–ASSOCIATED SPONDYLOARTHROPATHIES

Ankylosing spondylitis and Reiter's syndrome seem to be closely related to the histocompatibility antigen HLA-B27. More than 90 percent of individuals afflicted with one of these disorders have this marker, which is quite infrequent in the general population.[42]

A peculiar form of aortitis also seems to be associated with this antigen. It often accompanies these disorders and affects some patients with the HLA-B27 antigen who do not have spondyloarthropathy. On histologic examination, the inflammatory aortic lesion resembles that of syphilis. Focal destruction of the medial elastic tissue is seen, together with increased thickness of the intima and adventitia due to increased collagen. An obliterative arteritis of the vasa vasorum may be present.[43]

Unlike syphilis, the process is largely limited to the aortic wall behind and immediately above the sinuses of Valsalva. The thickening of the adventitia and the intimal proliferation extend below the aortic valve to involve the membranous ventricular septum and the base of the anterior leaflet of the mitral valve.[43] The aortic valve cusps are thickened and retracted, and their edges are rolled.

Such aortitis is more frequent in patients with spondylitis of long duration, in those with peripheral joint complaints in addition to spondylitis, and in patients with associated iritis.

Two clinical manifestations of this aortitis may be life-threatening. As is the case with syphilis, aortic regurgitation is the most frequent, but extension of the process onto the interventricular septum often results in atrioventricular conduction abnormalities. Further support for the association of the HLA-B27 antigen with this form of aortitis is provided by the observations that the antigen can be identified with considerable frequency among subjects with otherwise unexplained aortic regurgitation or conduction abnormalities.[42]

Congenital Anomalies of the Aorta

Patent ductus arteriosus, coarctation of the aortic isthmus, aortopulmonary window, aneurysm of the aortic sinuses, and anomalies of the aortic arch are considered in the section of this text dealing with congenital heart disease (Chaps. 70, 72).

Congenital kinking, so-called pseudocoarctation of the aorta, may be detected during the investigation of a mediastinal mass or of a systolic murmur.[44-46] An abnormally elongated thoracic aorta tethered to the ligamentum arteriosum produces a silhouette shaped like an "S" or a "3" on radiographic examination. Thus, it may resemble true coarctation; however, rib notching is not present. Exclusion of hemodynamically significant coarctation may require sophisticated imaging or the demonstration that no pressure difference exists between the upper and lower aortic segments. True coarctation may coexist and congenital cardiovascular anomalies similar to those found in true coarctation may be associated.

Some authorities believe the abnormality to be a sharp downward angulation of the aorta at the attachment of the ligamentum arteriosum as a result of elongation of the fourth aortic arch. Others consider the embryologic defect to be the same as for typical isthmic coarctation, with the difference being that in these cases the narrowing is not severe enough to result in significant obstruction.

CLINICAL MANIFESTATIONS
OF AORTIC DISEASE

Aortic Aneurysm

Aneurysms, areas of focal or diffuse dilatation of the aorta, develop at sites of congenital or acquired medial weakness. Hypertension, frequently present in patients with aneurysm, exposes weakness that might otherwise not be manifest and, in addition, probably accelerates degeneration of the aortic wall. Once begun, aneurysm formation is promoted by physical laws, particularly that of LaPlace (Chap. 3). Expansion and rupture often result unless the patient succumbs to intercurrent disease before this can occur.[47]

"Fusiform" and "saccular" aneurysms are described. In the former, circumferential dilatation, the result of a diffuse area of weakness, produces a spindle-shaped deformity. In the latter, balloon-like dilatation occurs, beginning at a relatively narrow neck. Many aneurysms are not pure examples of either. In either variety, by the time the aortic wall has been stretched to aneurysmal size, little or no recognizable medial tissue remains; the wall of the aneurysmal sac is composed of fibrous tissue.[48,49]

Whether the aneurysm is fusiform or saccular, its lumen virtually always contains laminated thrombus. Such clots may be extensive enough to fill a saccular aneurysm or to cover the circumference of a fusiform aneurysm. For this reason angiographic opacification of the aortic lumen often does not clearly delineate the size or extent of an aneurysm.

Aneurysms may result from a variety of causes. Heritable medial weakness producing aortic dilatation has been dis-

cussed previously. With the declining incidence of syphilis, aneurysms resulting from aortitis, either infectious or nonspecific, are uncommon. Saccular aneurysms are often encountered in regions of the aorta weakened by aortic dissection.[50]

Despite this variety of possibilities, the great majority of aortic aneurysms, particularly those of the descending thoracic or abdominal aorta, have been labeled "atherosclerotic."[47] A series of clinical observations support such an assumption. First, severe atherosclerosis nearly always accompanies an aneurysm. Second, aortic aneurysms are most commonly located in the infrarenal segment, the site of the most severe involvement of the aorta by atherosclerosis. Third, the usual risk factors for atherosclerosis are also risk factors for abdominal aortic aneurysm.[51] Finally, there is strong association between abdominal aortic aneurysm and coronary, cerebral, and peripheral atherosclerosis.

Challenging this assumption are a series of recent clinical and experimental observations indicating that aneurysm formation is a complex process,[48,49] and that to consider atherosclerosis to be solely responsible may be too simplistic. First, it has been suggested that atherosclerosis may an epiphenomenon inevitably accompanying the altered hemodynamics produced by aortic dilatation of any cause. In fact *atherosclerosis predictably forms on the intimal surface of any aneurysm, regardless of the etiology.* For example, atherosclerosis is characteristically seen in the false channel of a chronic aortic dissection or on the luminal surface of a luetic aneurysm. Second, the clinical features of individuals with occlusion of the infrarenal aorta by atherosclerosis differ from those of patients with infrarenal aneurysm.[48,49] Third, strong family clustering of abdominal aneurysms as well as their association with aneurysmal dilatation of other arteries provide reason to suspect that an underlying heritable medial defect may play an important role in this process.[52,53] Fourth, it has been difficult to produce abdominal aneurysms in experimental animals by feeding them an atherogenic diet.[48,49] Finally, several investigators have produced evidence of increased metabolic activity in the walls of aneurysms as compared to normal segments or those from patients with occlusive disease in the abdominal aorta. Accelerated protease activity, increased thrombolytic capacity, increased inflammatory cell presence, and increased vascularity have been demonstrated.[48,49,54]

In their recent review of this issue, Halloran and Baxter[48] concluded that "abdominal aortic aneurysms result not from passive dilatation, but from a complex remodeling process involving the synthesis and degradation of matrix proteins." Suffice it to say that the final word on the role of atherosclerosis or of a genetically determined abnormality of the media has not been heard.

THORACIC ANEURYSM

Etiology and Pathologic Anatomy

Congenital aneurysms of the aortic root and those attributable to infective endocarditis are discussed in other chapters of this text (see Chaps. 70 and 82).

Anuloaortic ectasia, the typical aortic lesion of medial degeneration, has been described as a "Florence flask" or "onion bulb" aorta. These are apt descriptors, since the dilatation is greatest in the proximal ascending aorta, including the aortic sinuses. The diameter quickly tapers, approaching a normal dimension before the takeoff of the innominate artery. Anuloaortic ectasia, the most frequent aortic manifestation of Marfan's syndrome, is often encountered in individuals with no musculoskeletal or ocular manifestations of that disorder. Limited or extensive medial dissection may complicate this lesion[10,11,55] (see Chap. 85).

Syphilitic aneurysms are still occasionally encountered. The ascending aorta and arch are most often affected, but the aortic dilatation often extends into the aortic sinuses and into the descending aortic segment. Syphilitic aneurysms are more often saccular than fusiform.

Saccular aneurysms of the aorta frequently follow aortic dissection when operative repair is not carried out. Moreover, they may develop in the descending thoracic aorta even after successful operative repair of a dissection involving the ascending aorta.[50] Such aneurysms may gradually expand over time and require operative treatment months or years after the acute dissection.

About equal in frequency to thoracic aneurysms following dissection are those that have been assumed to be atherosclerotic in origin, for the reasons noted previously. They are, however, far less common than infrarenal abdominal aneurysms. Unlike annuloaortic ectasia, these are typically located in the descending thoracic segment and are usually but not invariably fusiform. When they extend proximally into the arch or distally into the abdomen, they present a particularly difficult surgical problem. An associated abdominal aneurysm is quite frequent and should be sought whenever a thoracic aneurysm is encountered.[56,57]

Clinical Features

Aneurysms limited to the ascending aorta rarely produce symptoms directly unless they are undergoing active expansion or rupture. Findings of aortic regurgitation often draw the attention of an examiner and lead to detection of the aneurysm by one of the imaging techniques. Since the aortic root is located within the cardiac silhouette and the entire ascending aorta within the pericardial space, dilatation may not be readily appreciated on a chest radiograph.

Like aneurysms of the ascending aorta, those of the arch and descending segments are often asymptomatic and detected fortuitously in the course of an incidental chest radiograph. They are, however, more likely to produce symptoms than are those confined to the ascending aorta. These segments are fixed by the brachiocephalic arteries and lie in a position to compress a variety of mediastinal structures as well as the thoracic spine. Compression of the tracheobronchial tree may be attended by cough or dyspnea. Tracheal deviation or "tug" may be detected on physical examination. Pressure on the esophagus may result in dysphagia, rarely quite severe. Hoarseness may result from compression of the recurrent laryngeal nerve. Adjacent vascular structures may be compressed, resulting in pulmonary arterial stenosis or superior vena caval obstruction.

Chest pain, described as deep and aching or throbbing, has been the most frequent symptom reported in patients with thoracic aneurysm. Pain may also be associated with erosion of the rib cage or vertebrae. The appearance of pain clearly related to an aneurysm must be regarded as a signal of expansion and threatened rupture.[57] Rupture can be the initial manifestation of a thoracic aneurysm. Massive, usually fatal hemorrhage into the mediastinum, pleural space, esophagus, or tracheobronchial tree ensues. Rupture of an aneurysm of the ascending aorta, because of the intrapericardial location of that structure, results in acute hemopericardium and cardiac tamponade. Hemoptysis may precede, by days or weeks, fatal hemorrhage in descending thoracic aneurysms that have become adherent to adjacent lung. Rarely, aneurysms may rupture into adjacent vascular structures, producing aortovenous or aortopulmonary fistulas.

Diagnostic Studies

The aorta may now be imaged by a variety of modalities. Of these chest x-ray and transthoracic echocardiography are the most readily available and are especially useful for screening purposes. Aortography, computed tomography (Chap. 18), magnetic resonance imaging (Chap. 19), and transesophageal echocardiography (Chap. 14) all provide detailed information regarding the aorta's anatomy.[58]

Natural History and Prognosis

Most of the data concerning the natural history of thoracic aortic aneurysms come from retrospective analyses of hospital experience,[56,57] but some information from epidemiologic studies is available.[59] If anuloaortic ectasia and aortic dissection are excluded, a vast majority of cases studied have involved the descending aortic segment. Joyce's classic review[56] suggests a 50 percent 5-year and a 70 percent 10-year mortality. More recent studies have suggested that the 5-year mortality may approach 75 percent.[54,59] One-third to one-half of the deaths result from rupture of the aneurysm; most of the remainder are a consequence of other vascular diseases. The location of the aneurysm did not influence the mortality rate, but advanced age, an aneurysm more than 6 cm in size, the presence of hypertension, and the association of other cardiovascular disease all increased the risk of death. The presence of symptoms—a reflection of a large aneurysm or one threatening to rupture—was associated with a reduced rate of survival.

Insofar as the mortality data collected by Murdoch et al.[60] in patients with Marfan's syndrome apply to all patients with anuloaortic ectasia, their outlook may be even more grim than for those with aneurysm of the descending aorta. In that series, 52 of 56 patients with Marfan's syndrome died as a consequence of aortic disease at an average age of 32 years. In a more recent study, the mean age of death in Marfan's patients was 41 years.[61] This improvement may be attributable to advances in cardiovascular surgery or to improved medical therapy (including the use of beta-receptor blocking drugs), but different methods of collecting and analyzing data make the comparison debatable. It is of interest that the echocardiographic features of the aortic root (its shape,[62] size, and rate of expansion[63]) in Marfan's patients appear useful in assessing the risk of rupture (see also Chap. 85).

Management

Surgical repair constitutes the only known effective treatment for thoracic aneurysms. It is urgently indicated in patients if symptoms suggest expansion or compression of an adjacent structure. Cardiac failure from aortic regurgitation or aortocameral fistula may also necessitate early operative treatment. Available data suggest that in asymptomatic patients, the larger the aneurysm and the more rapid its increase in size, the more likely it is that rupture will occur.[64,65] Resection is less urgent in small, asymptomatic aneurysms.

Consideration of the severity of associated diseases is also important in selection of patients for surgery. Compared with the patient who has no other disease, the individual with associated coronary or cerebrovascular disease has a greater operative risk and a smaller risk of dying from rupture of the aneurysm before succumbing to the associated vascular disease.

Surgical treatment consists in replacing the resected aneurysmal segment with an albumin-coated Dacron graft attached to relatively normal aorta proximally and distally. Specific surgical procedures vary with the site of the aneurysm and the need for maintaining circulation to distal parts of the body during the necessary period of aortic occlusion (Fig. 98-1). Accordingly, thoracic aneurysms are divided into (1) those affecting the ascending aorta, (2) those affecting the arch of the aorta containing origins of the brachiocephalic vessels, (3) those affecting the descending thoracic aorta arising just distal to the origin of the left subclavian artery, and (4) thoracoabdominal aneurysms—i.e., those arising in the descending thoracic aorta and extending into the abdominal aorta.[66]

For aneurysms of the ascending aorta, total cardiopulmonary bypass is required.[67] The myocardium is protected by cold cardioplegia during the period that the coronary ostia are exposed. The aneurysm is opened, and an albumin-coated Dacron graft is sutured in place from within the aneurysm with continuous sutures, both proximally and distally. Finally, the aneurysmal sac is trimmed and sutured around the graft. If the aneurysm is associated with aortic valve incompetency, the leaflets are excised and a composite albumin-coated Dacron graft and prosthetic valve is sutured in place to the aortic annulus with interrupted sutures. Then the coronary ostia are sutured to an appropriate opening made in the composite graft or to a smaller Dacron graft which is sutured side-to-side to the composite graft. The distal anastomosis of the graft is performed as previously described.

For aneurysms of the transverse arch of the aorta, total cardiopulmonary bypass is also required. Additionally, profound hypothermia is used to protect the brain during temporary

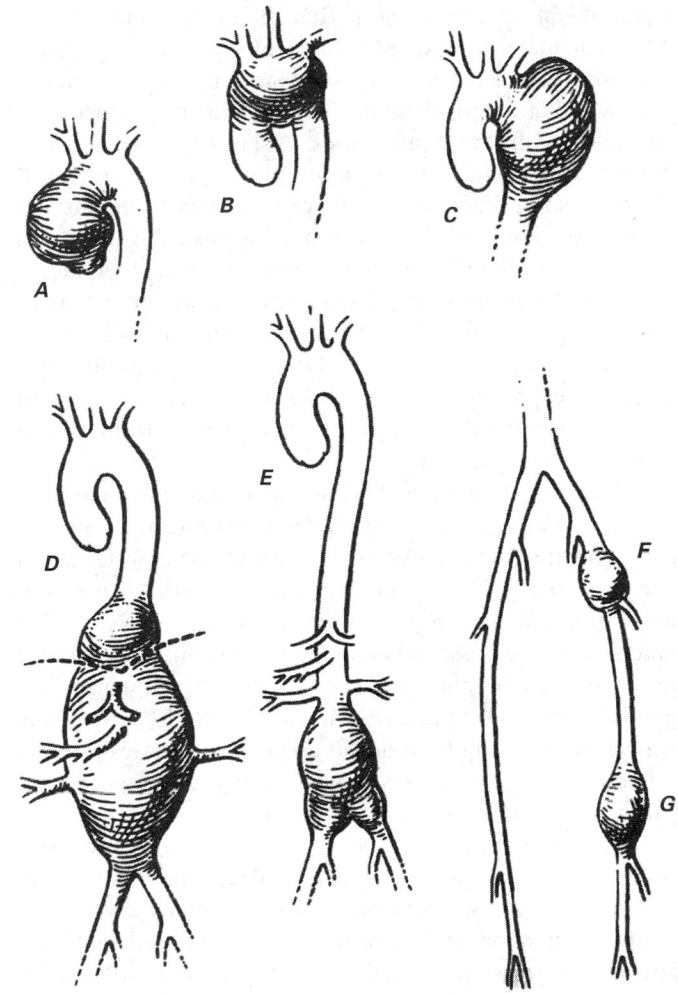

FIGURE 98-1

Most frequent sites of aneurysms of the aorta and major arteries. *A.* Fusiform aneurysm of the ascending aorta. *B.* Fusiform aneurysm of the aortic arch involving the brachiocephalic, carotid, and subclavian arteries. *C.* Fusiform aneurysm of the descending portion of the aortic arch. *D.* Large fusiform thoracoabdominal aneurysm involving the celiac, superior mesenteric, and renal arteries. *E.* Fusiform aneurysm of the abdominal aorta and iliac arteries. *F.* Fusiform aneurysm of the femoral artery. *G.* Fusiform aneurysm of the popliteal artery.

absence of circulation to the brachiocephalic vessels. Recent evidence suggests that retrograde perfusion of the brain through the superior vena cava adds further cerebral protection. An albumin-coated Dacron graft is sutured to relatively normal aorta proximally and distally from within the aneurysm, and the brachiocephalic, left common carotid, and left subclavian arteries are attached individually to appropriate openings in the graft. It is often possible to preserve the relatively normal aortic wall segment from which these vessels arise and simply anastomose this segment to an appropriate opening made in the graft for this purpose. The walls of the aneurysm are trimmed and sutured together around the grafts.

For aneurysms arising distal to the left common carotid artery, it is usually desirable to employ atrial-femoral bypass, femoral-femoral partial cardiopulmonary bypass, or various types of shunts during the period of aortic occlusion.[68,69] Although many techniques to prevent spinal cord ischemia are being studied for this purpose, there is not as yet sufficient evidence that any of them reduce the incidence of paralysis associated with these procedures. Although the evidence is not conclusive, there is reason to believe that some type of shunt is useful. The aorta is clamped proximally and distally to the aneurysm, and the aneurysm is opened. Bleeding from the orifices of the intercostal arteries is controlled within the aneurysm by figure-of-eight sutures, and a woven, albumin-coated Dacron graft is sutured to relatively normal aorta proximal and distal to the aneurysm. If one or two large intercostal arteries are present, they are attached to openings made in the graft. Finally, the walls of the aneurysm are trimmed and sutured around the graft.

Results of these methods of surgical treatment have been most encouraging. The surgical mortality rate for all aneurysms of the ascending or descending thoracic aorta ranges between 10 and 15 percent, although it is somewhat higher for those affecting the transverse arch and origins of the brachiocephalic vessels. Follow-up studies on these patients for more than 40 years provide evidence of maintenance of good results with long-term survival.[69] Deaths during this period have usually been due to associated diseases or other causes, although aneurysms occasionally develop in later years in other parts of the aorta and require surgical treatment.

The term *thoracoabdominal aneurysm,* is applied to aneurysms that arise in the descending thoracic aorta and extend distally for varying distances into the abdominal aorta as far as the bifurcation and occasionally into the common iliac arteries. They assume special significance because the arteries supplying blood to the abdominal organs arise from this portion of the aorta.

Our first successful method of surgical treatment for this type of aneurysm consisted in first applying a bypass Dacron graft from the descending thoracic aorta above the aneurysm to the normal segment of aorta below the aneurysm in the abdomen. To this Dacron graft an 8-mm Dacron tube graft was attached by end-to-side anastomosis, and the distal end of the graft was then attached to one of the abdominal visceral arteries, such as the superior mesenteric artery, by end-to-end anastomosis. Similar anastomotic grafts were then performed to the remaining arteries, including the celiac and both renal arteries, after which the aneurysm was removed.

More recently, the technical procedure has been simplified. The aneurysm is exposed through a left intercostal incision, which is extended down the midline of the abdomen, after which the diaphragm is incised and the abdominal structures are mobilized retroperitoneally to expose the entire aneurysm. The descending thoracic aorta is incised above the aneurysm, and an albumin-coated Dacron graft is attached to the proximal end of the aorta by end-to-end anastomosis. The aneurysm is opened, and bleeding vessels are controlled by oversewing. Large intercostal bleeding vessels may be attached to the Dacron graft by sewing an opening in the graft around the vessel. In most cases, it is possible to attach an opening in

the Dacron graft to the segment of the aorta from which arise the celiac, superior mesenteric, and renal arteries and thus to avoid the need to use individual grafts to each artery. Occasionally, however, because of the pathologic features of the aneurysm, it may be necessary to use a separate graft for one or more of these arteries. The terminal end of the Dacron is then anastomosed by end-to-end anastomosis to the distal end of the abdominal aorta. In the meantime, circulation can be restored to the abdominal visceral vessels by application of an occlusion clamp to the Dacron graft just distal to their attachment and releasing the proximal clamp; this reduces the period of ischemia of the abdominal organs.

Results of this operation have been highly satisfactory, with an operative mortality rate of 5 to 10 percent. Survival expectancy is reasonably good, with a survival rate of about 60 percent at 5 years. As in aneurysms of the descending thoracic aorta, paresis or paraplegia is a potential complication, occurring in about the same or perhaps somewhat higher frequency.

ABDOMINAL ANEURYSM

Responsible for nearly 15,000 deaths annually in the United States, rupture of an abdominal aortic aneurysm is the tenth leading cause of death for men 55 years of age and older. Moreover, 40,000 aneurysmectomies are undertaken each year to prevent such catastrophes. Indeed, recent evidence indicates that the incidence of abdominal aneurysms is increasing[70] despite the well-known decline in age-adjusted deaths from coronary atherosclerosis. This lesion is particularly treacherous, since it is often clinically silent until rupture occurs.

Etiology

Until recently, virtually all abdominal aneurysms have been attributed to atherosclerosis.[47,70] As discussed previously, recent evidence compels a reconsideration of this assumption.[48,48] Rarely, a traumatic, congenital, or mycotic abdominal aneurysm is encountered, and one is occasionally found as a residual of aortic dissection or in patients with Marfan's syndrome.

Pathologic Anatomy

Abdominal aneurysms are, as a rule, fusiform, but they may be saccular. Located in almost all instances distal to the renal arteries, they may extend to the aortic bifurcation and involve the iliac arteries (Fig. 98-1). Exceptionally, they extend above the renal arteries. In that case, the origins of not only the renal arteries but also the major visceral arteries may be involved. Such involvement complicates operative management.[47,70]

Some 5 to 10 percent of abdominal aneurysms are accompanied by an intense inflammatory and fibrotic reaction in the anterior and lateral periaortic tissue,[71–73] a process histologically similar to that of retroperitoneal fibrosis. It has been suggested that these "inflammatory aneurysms" result from a hypersensitivity reaction to an antigen or antigens in the atherosclerotic plaque. Systemic manifestations—such as weight loss, abdominal pain, and an elevated erythrocyte sedimentation rate—may reflect such a reaction. The difficulty of operative repair is increased.

Clinical Features

Men are three or four times more likely than women to have an abdominal aortic aneurysm. The typical patient is in the seventh or eighth decade. Most of these lesions are asymptomatic and are detected in the course of an examination directed at unrelated symptoms.[47,70]

Pain that can definitely be attributed to the aneurysm, especially when it is of recent onset, should be viewed as threatened rupture. Characteristically constant and located in the midabdomen, lumbar region, or pelvis, the pain may be severe and may be described as having a boring quality. Detection of an aneurysm that is tender to palpation carries much the same threat of rupture.[74,75] Because they present with abdominal pain and often a tender abdominal mass, inflammatory aneurysms may mimic the threat of rupture.[71–73]

Unless the patient is obese, physical examination almost always discloses an abdominal mass in the epigastrium, slightly to the left of the midline. If definite expansile movement can be detected, the diagnosis of abdominal aneurysm is reasonably secure. Bruits may be audible, and femoral pulses are reduced in some patients.

Rupture may be the initial manifestation. Rapid exsanguination may result from free rupture into the peritoneal cavity. Fortunately, more often the rupture is directed into the retroperitoneal space, where hemorrhage may be retarded. Abdominal pain and evidence of occult blood loss may persist for hours or days, allowing time for diagnosis and operative treatment. Rarely, the rupture is confined for several days to a few weeks. In such instances, the patient may present a puzzling diagnostic picture consisting of abdominal pain, fever, and slight to moderate blood loss.[74–76] Recognition of the nature of the illness can be lifesaving, since secondary rupture always ensues.

Rarely, rupture occurs into an adjacent retroperitoneal structure. When a communication develops with the vena cava or other large vein, a loud, continuous murmur in the abdomen and high-output congestive heart failure can ensue.[76] Rupture into the duodenum results in gastrointestinal bleeding,[76] but aortoduodenal fistulas are more common after graft replacement of the infrarenal aorta.

An unruptured aneurysm may also produce serious complications. Acute thrombosis may mimic saddle embolism. Furthermore, embolization of thrombus or atherosclerotic debris from aneurysms (and indeed from severely atherosclerotic but nonaneurysmal segments) to the lower extremities is far more frequent than is generally appreciated.[76,77] Secondary bacterial infection of an aortic aneurysm gives rise to fever, leukocytosis, and abdominal pain. Such infections lead to rupture of the aneurysm. As a rule, antibiotics neither eradicate the infection nor prevent the rupture.[23,26,76]

Diagnostic Studies

Anteroposterior or cross-table lateral radiographs of the abdomen often confirm the presence of aneurysm by demonstrating the characteristic "eggshell" calcification of its wall. Imaging with ultrasound (Chap. 14) provides reproducible measurements of the dimensions of the aneurysm, and computed radiographic tomography (Chap. 18) and magnetic resonance imaging (Chap. 19) provide a more definitive confirmation of the diagnosis. Aortography can be reserved for instances in which additional information regarding the extend of the aneurysm or the degree of involvement of branch arteries is required. The aortogram, a depiction of the luminal contour, may be misleading, since the aneurysm is characteristically filled or lined with thrombus.[78]

Management

Because the threat of fatal rupture looms over every patient with an abdominal aneurysm and because rupture frequently appears in a previously asymptomatic patient, screening of populations at risk by means of abdominal ultrasound has been considered. When this was undertaken in 8944 subjects at least 65 years of age, less than 5 percent were found to have abdominal aneurysms, and in less than 1 percent did such an aneurysm exceed 4 cm in diameter.[79] The cost-effectiveness of this approach has therefore been questioned.[80] The cost-effectiveness of screening could be enhanced by limiting the screening to "high-risk" populations, such as patients with a family history of aneurysmal disease or those with atherosclerotic disease in other arteries.

Abdominal aneurysms detected in asymptomatic patients during screening or the course of incidental examinations present a sometimes difficult management choice.[81] The risk of fatal rupture must be balanced against the risk of aneurysmectomy. Considerable effort has been directed to identifying the baseline characteristics of the patient and of the aneurysm that predict a high risk of rupture.[47,70,82–85] It has repeatedly been shown that the larger the aneurysm, the greater the risk of rupture. *There is, therefore, general agreement that when they are discovered in a patient who is a reasonable operative risk, aneurysms 5 cm or more in size should be resected, while those smaller than 4 cm may safely be followed pending an increase in size. Those whose diameter is more than 4 cm but less than 5 cm fall into a gray zone where there is disagreement regarding the desirability of operation.*

Cronewett et al.[82] carefully investigated other baseline factors in patients that might indicate an increased risk of rupture. They found that in addition to aneurysm size, systemic hypertension and chronic obstructive lung disease were independent predictors of increased risk.

Commonly associated with abdominal aneurysms are coronary and cerebrovascular disease.[86] Two characteristics of patients with these comorbid conditions are noteworthy. They are both less likely to die of rupture because of the lethality of their "organ-fixed" atherosclerosis, and they incur a greater operative risk for aneurysmectomy. It is important to recognize that given appropriate preoperative screening for coronary disease with noninvasive imaging or coronary arteriography and appropriate treatment of the coronary disease, the risk of aneurysmectomy is acceptable in such patients.[87–89]

Since operative repair of abdominal aneurysms can now be accomplished with a mortality rate well under 5 percent,[90] surgery can be recommended for all patients except those with advanced associated disease.

Symptomatic aneurysms require urgent surgical treatment, since early rupture can confidently be predicted. A ruptured abdominal aneurysm is a surgical emergency. Prompt surgical treatment can save most of these patients. Death is otherwise inevitable.

Surgery for an abdominal aortic aneurysm does not require maintenance of the distal circulation.[90,91] The aorta is clamped proximally between the aneurysm and the renal arteries, the iliac arteries are clamped distally, and the aneurysm is opened. Bleeding from the orifices of the lumbar arteries is controlled from within the aneurysm by figure-of-eight sutures. If the aortic bifurcation is not affected by the aneurysm, an albumin-coated Dacron tube graft may be used to restore circulation. If the bifurcation and the proximal iliac arteries are affected, an albumin-coated Dacron bifurcation graft is required. From within the aneurysm, the graft is sutured proximally to normal aorta and distally to the aortic bifurcation or individually to the iliac arteries. Finally, the aneurysmal walls are trimmed and sutured over the graft.

We have used this method of treatment in more than 10,000 patients over a period of more than 40 years. The surgical risk depends primarily on the presence or absence of rupture, associated heart disease or hypertension, and patient's age. Our experience has shown that the 5- to 10-year survival rate for patients operated on for aneurysms of the abdominal aorta closely parallels that for comparable age groups in the normal population. Surgical treatment is therefore recommended for all patients with aneurysms of the abdominal aorta unless a surgical contraindication exists.

AORTIC DISSECTION

Aortic dissection is believed to be the most common potentially fatal aortic disease, an even more frequent cause of aortic rupture than abdominal aneurysm.[92–95] Every busy general hospital will encounter several each year. Because fundamental differences exist between the pathogenesis, clinical presentation, and treatment of dissections and those of aneurysms, the confusing term *dissecting aneurysm* should be discarded.

Pathologic Anatomy

Longitudinal cleavage of the aortic media by a dissecting column of blood characterizes aortic dissection. The split in the media, not usually circumferential, typically occupies about half of the circumference of the aorta and may extend through the entire length of the vessel. The plane of dissection often follows the greater curvature of the ascending aorta and the arch. In the descending aorta, the path of the dissection is most often located lateral to the true lumen, but it may be medial and may spiral "barber pole" fashion about the long axis.[96]

In classic aortic dissection, the "false channel" created by this medial hematoma communicates with the "true lumen" through an intimal tear located near its proximal end (Fig. 98-2). Such tears are typically single and transverse in orientation, but exceptions are frequent. Multiple secondary ("reentry") tears, located more distally along the false channel, are also quite common.

Two patterns of involvement predominate. In about two-thirds of instances, the false channel originates in the ascending aorta and the intimal ("entry") tear is located a few centimeters above the aortic valve. The false channel frequently extends to the aortoiliac bifurcation. Dissections that do not involve the ascending aorta account for about one-quarter of all cases. In the latter type, the intimal tear lies in the proximal descending thoracic aorta. The medial hematoma begins in proximity to the origin of the left subclavian artery and extends distally for varying distances, often to the aortoiliac bifurcation.[92–96]

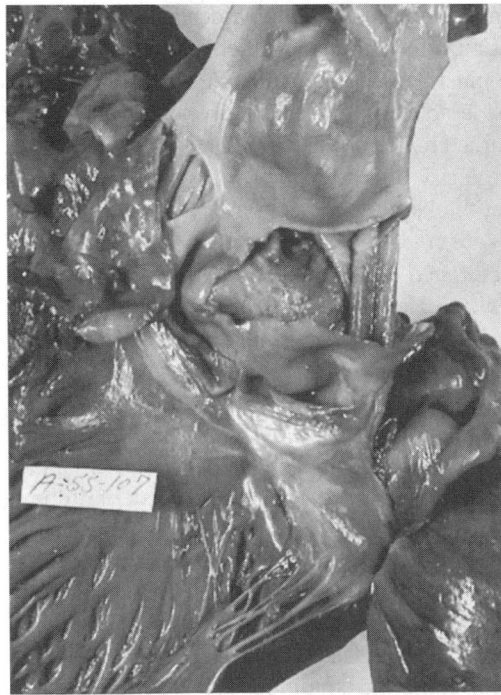
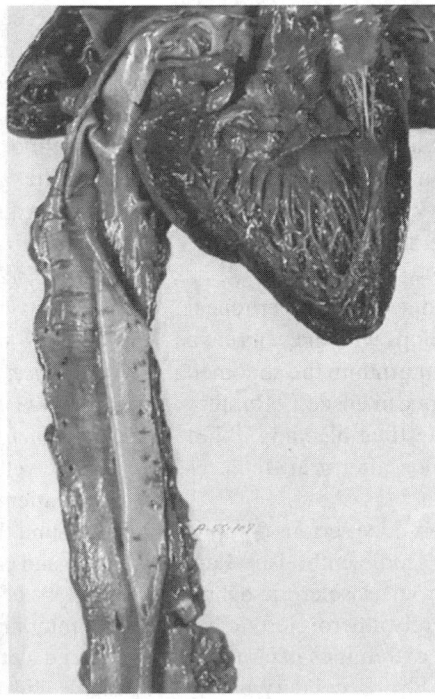

A   *B*

FIGURE 98-2

Aortic dissection. *A.* The large intimal rent may be seen a few centimeters above the aortic cusps. *B.* The false channel created by the dissecting hematoma is shown. Notice the clearly sheared layers of aortic media.

A substantial number of cases do not follow these two patterns. In some, the medial hematoma is short and limited to the arch or to the descending thoracic or abdominal segments. In another rather frequently encountered variation, an entry tear is located just beyond the left subclavian artery, but the dissection extends proximally into the ascending aorta.

The most widely applied nomenclature is that of DeBakey[92–95] (Fig. 98-3). In this classification, dissection involving the ascending aorta falls into type I, while lesions originating beyond the arch are included in type III. Type II comprises those aneurysms limited to the ascending aorta. Apart from length, many in type II are indistinguishable from type I, but others originate within chronic fusiform dilatation of the ascending aorta. In the latter, multiple intimal tears and limited medial splitting are common.

Reviews describing large numbers of patients with the clinical syndrome of aortic dissection have usually included a small number of patients with a medial hematoma but no intimal tear.[97] In recent years, imaging with computed tomography, transesophageal echocardiography, or magnetic resonance imaging has conclusively demonstrated the existence of such a subset.[98–100] These lesions are now included under the rubric *intramural hematoma*. Among 195 patients with medial hemorrhage documented with one of the tomographic imaging techniques cited, Nienaber et al.[100] found 25 with no demonstrable communicating tear. In the reported experience, the aortic segments involved with intramural hematoma and the presenting clinical picture of the process do not substantially differ from those of typical dissection.[98–100] Aortography is not ideal for the diagnosis of these abnormalities because contrast material injected into the aortic lumen does not readily enter the medial hematoma. Thus, it seems often to provide a false-negative result.[101] At present the therapeutic strategy for these lesions is the same as for typical dissection.

Imaging of the aorta with magnetic resonance, transesophageal echocardiography, or computed tomography has also allowed identification of another pathogenetic origin for medial hematoma formation, the *penetrating atherosclerotic ulcer*.[102] In these patients, a large, ulcerated atherosclerotic plaque disrupts the aortic media, creating a potential for rupture, false aneurysm formation, or dissection by hematoma. These lesions appear almost exclusively in the midthoracic and distal descending aorta. Only in exceptional instances is the medial dissection extensive enough to threaten major branch vessels or positioned to threaten the aortic valve. The initial presentation of a complication of a penetrating plaque may mimic typical aortic dissection, and surgery will be indicated in selected cases, since external rupture is a hazard.[102]

Death from aortic dissection most often occurs from disruption of the outer wall of the false channel opposite the entrance

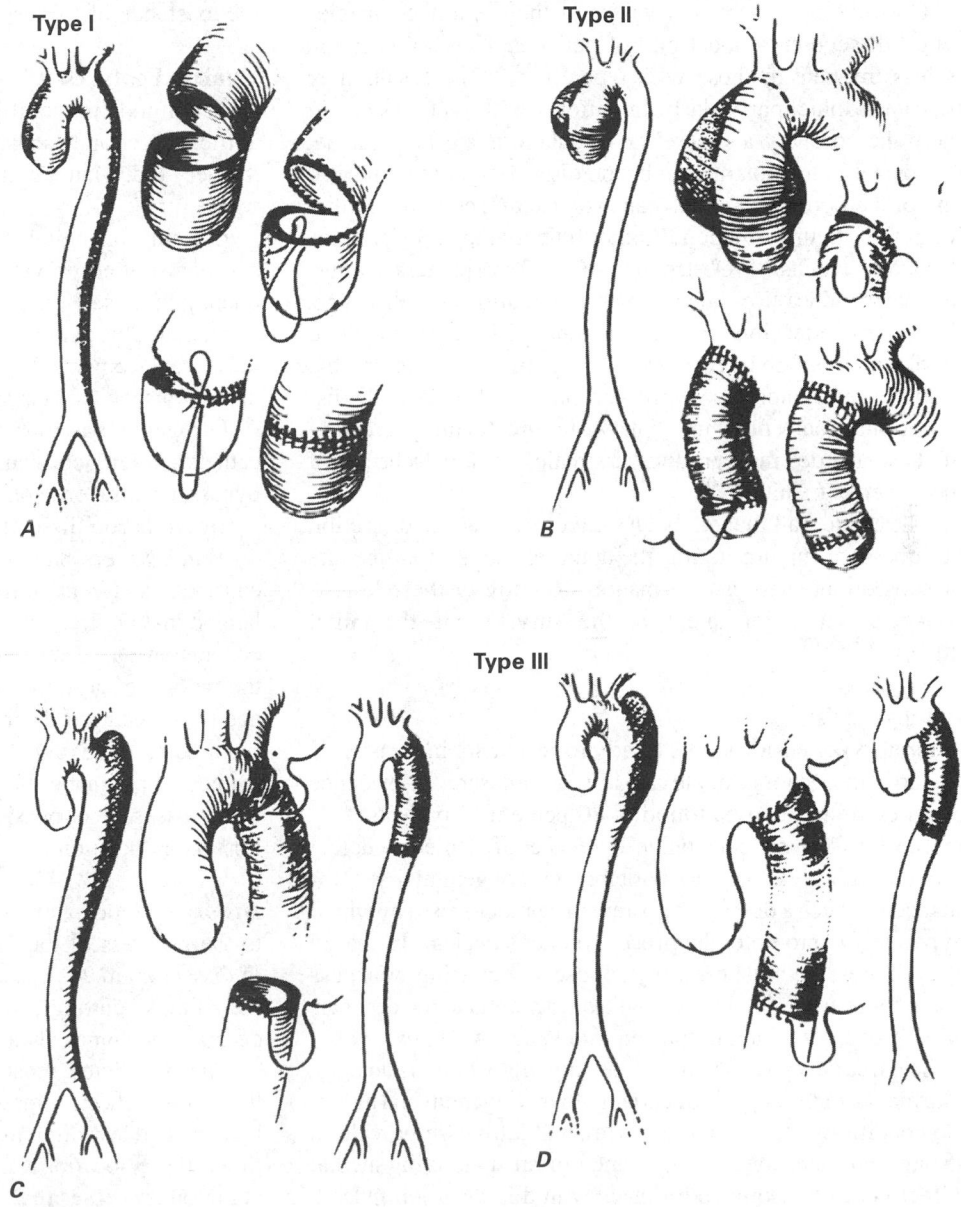

FIGURE 98-3

Surgical classification of dissecting aneurysms of the aorta based on anatomic and pathologic patterns of the lesions and their respective methods of surgical treatment.

tear.[92–97] Rupture of proximal dissection therefore produces hemopericardium and cardiac tamponade. Hemorrhage into the mediastinum or either pleural space may occur. Typically, external rupture of distal dissection results in a bloody left pleural effusion. Death from external rupture, while often abrupt, may be delayed by temporary cessation of hemorrhage attributable to falling arterial pressure and increasing tension in the periaortic tissue. Dramatic clinical syndromes result in those rare instances in which the false channel ruptures into the right heart chambers, producing a large left-to-right shunt.[103]

In approximately half of patients with proximal dissection, medial hematoma undermines the aortic valve, rendering it incompetent. Fortunately, very serious hemodynamic consequences of aortic regurgitation appear infrequently during the acute phase.[92–95]

Obstruction of a branch vessel of the aorta accompanies type I dissection in about half of patients. This complication is less frequent in those with type III.[92–95] The results may be catastrophic, particularly in patients with type I, since in them the coronary and cerebral circulations are jeopardized. Fortunately rare, obstruction by the dissection of the orifice of one of the coronary arteries can produce an acute myocardial infarction. In this situation thrombolytic therapy may produce disastrous results.[104] Obstruction of renal or splanchnic arteries may produce life-threatening complications in ether type. Severe hypertension and acute renal failure may attend involvement of the renal artery. The iliac arteries are the branch arteries most frequently compromised. Potentially disabling but usually not immediately life-threatening, narrowing of these arteries may produce dramatic, painful ischemia of the lower extremities.[105]

The aortic wall that has been weakened by aortic dissection but does not rupture during the acute phase is often the site of subsequent aneurysm formation. Rupture of these lesions constitutes a major threat to the survivor of the initial illness.[50,106,107]

Pathogenesis

Arterial hypertension seems clearly to be a factor in the genesis of aortic dissection. An elevated blood pressure, or evidence of its existence, can be found in 80 percent of patients.[92–97] In most cases, no conclusive evidence of a medial defect can be identified, and no heritable or congenital basis for suspecting such a defect is apparent. The mechanism by which hypertension promotes the process remains unclear. Increased arterial pressure must certainly expose any existing weakness of the aortic wall and may, in addition, accentuate the degenerative processes of aging that promote such weakness.

The frequency with which dissecting hematoma is noted in Marfan's syndrome,[10,11] in certain other congenital and heritable conditions,[12–18] and in experimental lathyrism provides a strong argument for the importance of an underlying medial defect in at least some individuals with this disorder. Indeed, histologic evidence of degeneration of elastin or of smooth muscle cells in the aortic media of such patients has long been noted. Recent authors, however, have thrown considerable

doubt on the specificity of the classic histologic findings. These newer studies indicate that such findings are frequently absent in patients with dissection and are remarkably similar to changes encountered in older patients without dissection.[19–21,108] It seems likely that any fundamental medial defect or defects may be unrecognizable by light microscopy.

The role of the intimal ("entry") tear in the genesis of medial dissection is debated. Many investigators feel that it exposes the media to blood under luminal pressure, and that the resulting shear forces initiate and propagate the medial cleavage. Others propose that medial weakness leads to hemorrhage from the vasa vasorum and that the resulting intramural hematoma cleaves the medial layers.[92–97] In this hypothesis the intimal tears are secondary. The instances of medial hematoma in which no intimal tear can be identified support the existence of this mechanism.[98–100]

Clinical Features

Most common in the fifth through the seventh decades of life, aortic dissection has also been reported in children as well as the very old. Men are affected at least twice as commonly as women.[92–95]

Certain congenital lesions of the aorta (e.g., coarctation and bicuspid aortic valve) are associated with increased frequency of dissection.[12] A greater-than-expected incidence is encountered in patients with aortic stenosis, even after aortic valve replacement. The same is true with certain heritable disorders such as Marfan's and Turner's syndromes.[10–18]

Iatrogenic vascular trauma—a complication of cardiac catheterization, coronary bypass surgery, cardiopulmonary bypass, or intraaortic balloon counterpulsation—may produce extensive aortic dissection.

Many writers have concluded that pregnancy, either because of its effects on the aortic wall or because of attendant hemodynamic stress, predisposes to medial dissection.[109] This conclusion has been based on the fact that half or more of the reports of aortic dissection in women below 40 years of age have occurred during pregnancy. Since the total number reported is relatively small (certainly in relation to the frequency of pregnancy) and since most reports concern one or a few cases, it is possible that selective reporting accounts for this association.[110]

History   Sudden, excruciating pain, presumably attributable to the progress of the medial cleavage, announces the onset of dissection in 90 percent of instances. Patients may describe the pain as "cutting," "ripping," or "tearing," but such vivid descriptors cannot always be elicited.[92–95]

Those afflicted most commonly locate the discomfort in the anterior chest, somewhat less frequently in the interscapular area, and less often in the epigastrium or the lumbar region. Since these locations are often the site of pain from more common processes (e.g., myocardial infarction or cholecystitis), the examiner must be alert to the possibility of aortic dissection in any patient with pain in these sites in whom the more common diagnoses are not immediately obvious.

Two features of the pain of dissection help to separate it from that of other conditions. The discomfort of dissection may not build in intensity, as is the case other disorders producing severe pain in the trunk. Rather, it is at its most intense from its inception. Moreover, it is often located either simultaneously or sequentially in more than one of the four sites mentioned above. Suspicion should be aroused particularly by pain occurring both above and below the diaphragm.[92–95]

A sudden neurologic episode accompanies the onset of most instances of "painless" aortic dissection. Syncope is the most frequent neurologic event and a particularly ominous sign. It seems always to reflect external rupture, almost always of the ascending aorta into the pericardial space. Less frequently, focal neurologic signs reflect arterial occlusion of the cerebral or spinal circulation.

When pain is not prominent, occlusion by the dissection of the femoral or the subclavian artery may be the predominant clinical feature. Arterial embolism may be simulated.[92–95]

Rarely, the acute episode goes entirely unrecognized by the patient. In such instances, diagnostic study of patients who have an abnormal chest x-ray, aortic regurgitation, or obstruction of an arterial branch of the aorta uncovers chronic dissection.

Physical Examination Although none are diagnostic of dissection, physical findings that greatly increase the probability of its presence can often be detected on examination (Table 98-3). The murmur of aortic regurgitation can be heard in about half of all patients with acute type I dissection. Loss or diminution of an arterial pulse may also be detected in half. One or both of these cardinal findings is present in all but a small minority of that subgroup. In contrast, patients with dissection limited to the descending aorta less frequently have pulse deficits and uncommonly have a murmur of aortic regurgitation. Thus, these patients often have none of these confirmatory findings.[92–95]

The frequency with which hypertension underlies aortic dissection has been mentioned, and a majority of patients presenting with dissection will have high arterial pressure. Many others will be able to provide a history of high blood pressure. Even in those with neither a history of hypertension nor a measurable blood pressure elevation, physical examination will often reveal left ventricular hypertrophy or vascular changes in the optic fundi. Blood pressure elevations may be modest during the acute process, but, particularly in those with type III dissection, extraordinarily high readings can be encountered (Table 98-3). Renal ischemia, a consequence of renal artery involvement, has been invoked to explain diastolic blood pressures that may reach 140 to 160 mmHg or more.[92–95]

Twenty percent of patients with dissection involving the ascending aorta present with hypotension. Such a presentation requires immediate consideration of operative treatment, since external rupture almost always is responsible.[92–95]

Diagnostic Studies Of the routine diagnostic studies, only the chest film provides information of much value. The aortic shadow is abnormal in 80 to 90 percent of cases but may also be abnormal in many instances in patients who do not have dissection. Dilatation of the ascending aorta, reflected by protrusion of its shadow from the right side of the mediastinum, is a characteristic finding in proximal dissection. Dilatation of the aortic knob and descending thoracic aorta is typical of distal disease (Fig. 98-4). Certain other findings—for example, progressive widening of the aortic silhouette on serial films, a lobulated or serrated margin of the aortic shadow, or a "double-lumen" effect created by a less radiopaque false channel—are less frequent but more specific. The same may be said for detection of intimal calcification more than 6 mm inside the margin of the aorta.[78]

For confirmation of the diagnosis, either computed tomography after intravenous administration of contrast material or transesophageal echocardiography may be employed with confidence. Both have high sensitivity and specificity. Some believe that magnetic resonance imaging is even more accurate; however, its value is limited in acutely ill patients because it is not available in many institutions, it requires a longer imaging time than other options, and it makes the patient relatively inaccessible during the process.[78,111,112]

An aortogram, accomplished by means of contrast injection through a catheter placed in the aorta, is occasionally required to provide details of branch vessel involvement. The findings on aortography are often quite dramatic. Two aortic channels can usually be identified because of the variation in intensity and timing of their opacification. Moreover, the aortogram may identify a linear lucency representing the aortic intima and media separating the two channels (Figs. 98-5 and 98-6). At times the false channel is not opacified because of thrombosis or because it does not communicate with the true lumen. In such cases, the true lumen may appear to be compressed and to lie at a distance from the margins of the aortic shadow. The resulting appearance of a thickened aortic wall can also be produced by thrombosis within an aneurysm, aortitis, or mediastinal hematoma or tumor. These can usually but not invariably be distinguished from dissection because in them the aortic lumen is not significantly compressed.[78,101]

TABLE 98-3

DIFFERENCES IN PHYSICAL FINDINGS BETWEEN PROXIMAL (TYPES I AND II) AND DISTAL (TYPE III) AORTIC DISSECTION

	Proximal	Distal
Aortic regurgitation	About half	Rare
Pulse deficit	About half	15–20%
Neither	15–20%	75%
Hypotension	20%	Rare
Severe hypertension	Unusual	Frequent

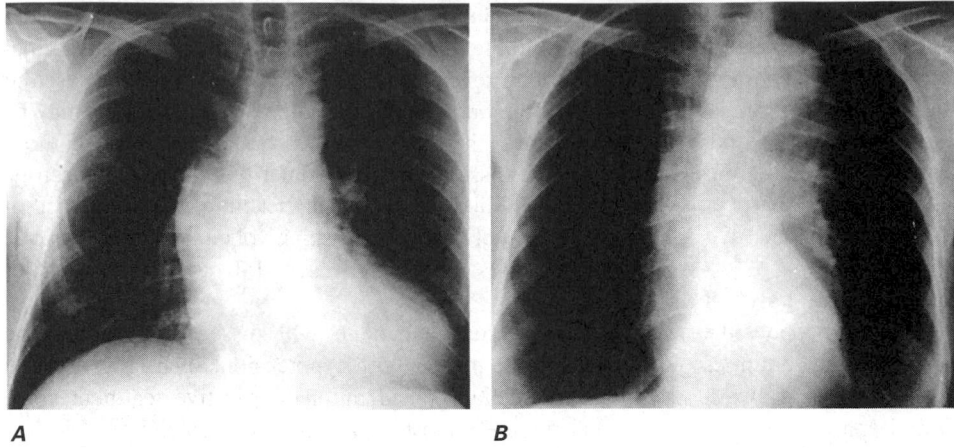

FIGURE 98-4
A. Type I aortic dissection. Characteristic appearance on chest roentgenogram. Note the marked dilation of the ascending aorta. The aorta may appear normal on the roentgenogram early in the course of aortic dissection. *B.* Type III aortic dissection. In contrast to type I, marked distortion of the aortic arch and dilation of the descending portions are typical, as seen in this radiograph of a patient with dissection beginning distal to the arch vessels.

Natural History and Prognosis

We must look to older reports of aortic dissection for information about its natural history. Since the mid 1960s, virtually all patients have received either operative intervention or aggressive antihypertensive treatment. From the classic work of Hirst and associates[97] as well as others,[113,114] it can be estimated that 35 percent of patients succumb within the initial 24 hs and that the mortality rate continues high during the first and second weeks. Fifty percent die within 48 hours, 70 percent by 1 week, and 80 percent by 2 weeks.

Certain subgroups with widely differing natural histories can be identified. Hypotension (blood pressure less than 100 mmHg) usually indicates aortic rupture and nearly certain early death. Almost all such patients have involvement of the ascending aorta; one-quarter of those with such involvement present in this way. Those with type III dissection are at the other end of the spectrum with regard to their natural history. Older reports indicate that about half survive the acute phase without aggressive treatment. Absent modern therapeutic intervention, the mortality rate of patients with type I or II dissection who are hypertensive or normotensive is intermediate between these extremes.

Patients who survive the first 2 weeks continue to experience a high mortality rate in the first year. About half of the survivors die within 3 months and an additional 10 percent within a year of the onset of their illness. The lucky few who pass the first anniversary apparently may expect reasonable longevity. Late deaths may be due to cerebrovascular complications of hypertension, heart failure from severe aortic regurgitation, or rupture of a saccular aneurysm of the residual false channel.[113–115]

Management

Sudden life-threatening complications—such as very severe hypertension, cardiac tamponade, massive hemorrhage, severe aortic regurgitation, or ischemic injury to the myocardium, the central nervous system, and kidneys—threaten the patient with aortic dissection. Optimal management requires close surveillance of vascular pressures, urine flow, mental status, and neurologic signs in an intensive care unit. Pain relief can be difficult even with potent narcotics, but it can usually be obtained with drug therapy to reduce arterial pressure.[92–95]

A successful outcome in patients with aortic dissection requires that progression of the medial cleavage be halted and that external rupture of the weakened

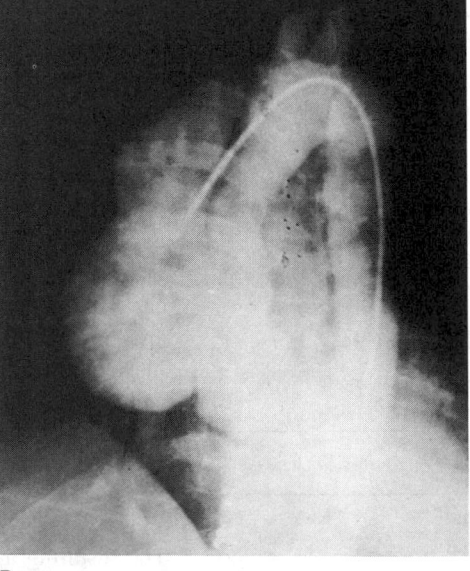

FIGURE 98-5
Serial frames from an aortogram of a patient with type I aortic dissection. Contrast material is seen to fill a tremendously dilated false channel. This accounts for the dilation of the ascending aorta noted in Fig. 98-4.

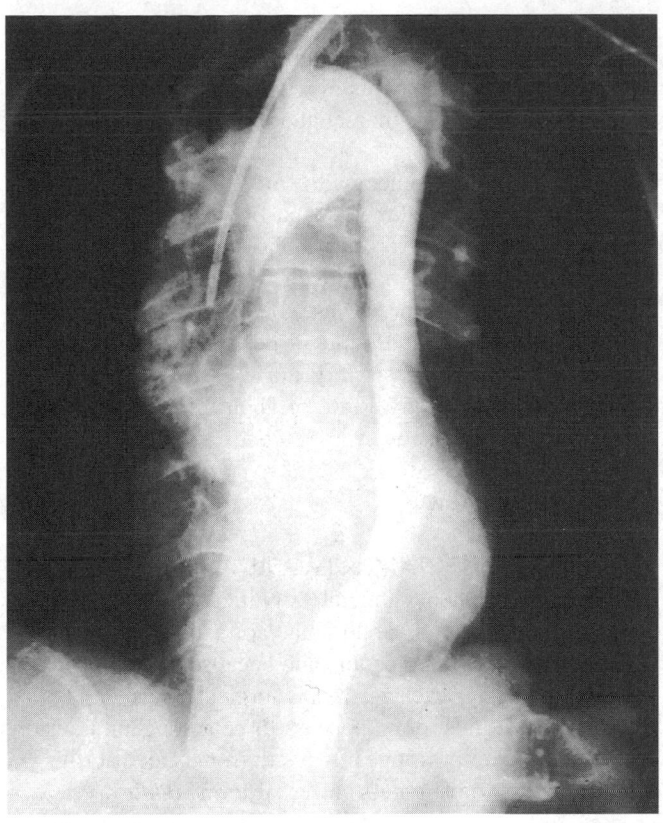

FIGURE 98-6

Aortic dissection, type III. A typical aortogram of a patient with aortic dissection beginning distal to the arch vessels. The narrowed true lumen is filled with contrast material and does not occupy the entire aortic shadow. Contrast material can be seen entering the false channel just beyond the left subclavian artery.

aortic wall be prevented. Inasmuch as the aortic defect is structural, operative treatment represents the most effective long-term remedy for many patients. Aggressive antihypertensive treatment lessens the stress on the aortic wall and thus the likelihood of progression of the dissection and of rupture of the weakened wall. Such therapy is widely employed prior to and, in selected instances, as an alternative to surgical management.[92–95]

In the acute phase, one of several drug regimens may be employed to reduce arterial pressure and its rate of rise. Aggressive use of a beta-blocking agent may be adequate in patients who present with relatively modest levels of hypertension. In others with more severe hypertension, intravenous sodium nitroprusside combined with a beta-blocking agent may be required. Drug therapy should aim to lower systolic arterial pressure to 100 to 120 mmHg. Optimal blood pressure reduction may not be possible if oliguria (less than 25 mL/h) or mental confusion appears.

At the Washington Hospital Center, intravenous esmolol is the currently preferred beta-blocking agent for acute dissection, since its effects can be readily titrated. Before infusion, this agent must be diluted to a concentration of no more than 10 mg/mL because more concentrated solutions are very

irritating to veins. An initial loading dose of 0.5 mL/kg administered over 1 min is followed by an infusion of 0.05 mg/kg per minute. The infusion rate can be increased at 4-min intervals by 0.05 mg/kg per minute. Rates beyond 0.3 mg/kg per minute have not been shown to provide added therapeutic benefit. The substantial amounts of fluid required to maintain this infusion limit the usefulness of this agent in some patients.

Alternatively, propranolol can be administered intravenously in 0.5-mg increments at 1- to 5-min intervals until the target blood pressure is achieved, the pulse rate slows, or a total dose of 1.5 mg/10 kg of body weight has been given. This scheme can be repeated at 4 to 6-h intervals. Appropriate oral doses of this agent or comparable beta-blocking agents can be given for long-term maintenance after the need for acute beta blockade has passed.

The ability of intravenous sodium nitroprusside to reduce arterial pressure promptly and consistently and the ease with which its hypotensive effects can be titrated recommend it as the current drug of choice for the patient whose blood pressure does not respond to beta blockade. As little as 0.5 μg/kg per minute may produce the desired result. Occasionally, as much as 10 μg/kg per minute is necessary. This dose, however, should not be exceeded and should be reduced as soon as practical. *A beta-blocking agent should nearly always be used in conjunction with sodium nitroprusside*, since animal data suggest that when used alone it does not reduce and may, through reflex mechanisms, enhance the rate of rise of arterial pressure.

Intravenous labetalol is another alternative to the combination of sodium nitroprusside and a beta-adrenergic blocking agent. *Hydralazine, minoxidil, and diazoxide cannot be recommended, since they produce reflex stimulation of the left ventricle and consequently an increase in the rate of rise of aortic pressure.*

Not all patients with acute aortic dissection have elevated blood pressure. Hypotension, it has been noted, reflects aortic rupture and dictates emergency operation. Some individuals have pressures only slightly higher than the target level of 100 to 120 mmHg for antihypertensive treatment. Pharmacologic treatment is of dubious value in such patients, although beta-adrenergic blockade may be tried as a means of reducing the rate of rise of aortic pressure.

As has been stated, operative treatment must be considered in all patients, but certain subgroups can be recognized whose clinical presentation dictates the timing of the surgery. At one extreme are those who are hypotensive on admission. Here, the need for emergency operation has already been noted. On the other hand, operative treatment may never be an option in those with severe comorbid illness. Further, it may not be justified in those with severe neurologic injury from the dissection. In these inoperable individuals, antihypertensive therapy is continued indefinitely by converting the drug regimen to an oral one that avoids vasodilators.

The appropriateness and urgency of surgery for aortic dissection depends upon the clinical picture presented (Table 98-4). For patients whose dissection involves the ascending

TABLE 98-4

MANAGEMENT SUBSETS IN AORTIC DISSECTION

Presentation	Management
Hypotension (rupture)	Emergency surgery
Severe comorbid disease	Antihypertensive therapy
Ascending aorta involved	Urgent surgery
Descending aorta only— uncomplicated	Antihypertensive therapy
Descending aorta only— complicated	Urgent surgery

aorta, operative repair should be undertaken as soon as the patient can be stabilized and appropriate diagnostic information compiled. Such patients are in grave danger of a fatal complication despite effective antihypertensive therapy. By contrast, *for those with uncomplicated type III dissection, it is now believed that operation during the acute phase does not improve survival beyond that achieved with drug treatment.*[92,95,116] Younger patients and those who are relatively good operative risks may benefit from operation in the subacute phase to protect them from eventual rupture of a residual saccular aneurysm.[106]

The surgical technique for aortic dissection varies with the origin of the dissecting process and its extent (Fig. 98-3).[117–119] For type I aneurysms (Figs. 98-4 and 98-5), the procedure consists in transection of the ascending aorta with use of cardiopulmonary bypass, obliteration of the false lumen by approximation of the inner and outer walls of the dissecting process with a continuous suture proximally and distally, and end-to-end anastomosis of the transected aorta. If this method of direct repair is not applicable in some patients, it may be necessary to resect the proximal segment and restore vascular continuity by means of an albumin-coated Dacron patch or tube graft. Many patients have aortic valve incompetence secondary to loss of commissural support of the valve leaflets. This condition may be corrected in some by suture approximation of the inner and outer layers of the dissecting process with resultant resuspension of the valve, although other patients may require prosthetic valve replacement.

Surgical treatment for type II aneurysms consists essentially in resection and graft replacement of the entire ascending aorta with use of cardiopulmonary bypass. Aortic valve incompetence is more common in this type than in type I and is less often amenable to reparative techniques because of the usually more chronic nature of the dissecting process. Under such circumstances, prosthetic replacement of the aortic valve is usually performed concomitantly with graft replacement of the ascending aorta.

Surgical treatment for type III aneurysms (Fig. 98-6) consists of resection of the descending thoracic aorta above the level of the origin of the dissecting process (usually at or just below the origin of the left subclavian artery), obliteration of the distal false passage by suture closure of the inner and outer layers, and replacement of the excised segment with an aortic graft. In some patients in whom the dissecting process is extensive distally, a thoracoabdominal approach may be necessary.

Analysis of experience with more than 1000 patients treated by these surgical methods at Baylor College of Medicine indicates gratifying results. The surgical mortality rate has been steadily reduced with some variation, depending on the type and stage of the disease, being about 15 percent in type I, 5 percent in type II, and 12 percent in type III. Long-term results extending over 35 years are also gratifying, with an overall 10-year survival rate of about 35 percent. In type II, this survival rate is over 50 percent.

Aortic Obstruction

ABDOMINAL COARCTATION (MIDDLE AORTIC SYNDROME)

Although rare, hemodynamically significant narrowing of the descending thoracic or abdominal aorta deserves attention because it affects young people and because it often produces life-threatening hypertension that is surgically correctable.[120–122] Although it most often appears to be a congenital lesion, at least some examples appear to result from healed aortitis.[123] For this reason, some writers prefer the term *middle aortic syndrome.*

Although the narrowed aortic segment is typically quite focal, diffuse hypoplasia of the abdominal aorta and iliac arteries may be encountered.

The renal arteries, commonly involved in this process, may be stenosed, hypoplastic, or thrombosed. As a consequence, severe hypertension is the most common presenting complaint. Involvement of the visceral arteries may result in ischemia in their distribution. Intermittent claudication from involvement of the iliac arteries is more frequent than in patients with coarctation at the aortic isthmus.

On examination, similarities to the more common postductal coarctation will be noted. Upper-extremity hypertension will be present together with feeble pulses and hypotension in the legs. Attention may be directed to the unusual location of the stenosis by a bruit in the lumbar or umbilical area.

Operative treatment is usually required, since severe hypertension significantly shortens the life expectancy of patients with this disorder.[124]

CHRONIC OBSTRUCTION OF THE TERMINAL AORTA

Etiology and Pathogenesis

The aortoiliac bifurcation is among the most common sites for atherosclerosis in the arterial tree; it therefore underlies the vast majority of instances of chronic obstruction of the infrarenal aorta.[122,125,126] Furthermore, many patients with symptomatic femoropopliteal atherosclerosis also have aortoiliac narrowing. Rarely, infrarenal coarctation, aortitis, clinically silent embolism, or in situ thrombosis produces this situation.

Rupture of atherosclerotic plaques sets the stage for mural thrombus and gradual progression on luminal narrowing and, in many instances, complete occlusion of the terminal aorta. Collateral vessels connecting the lumbar and inferior mesenteric arteries with branches of the internal iliac and common femoral arteries ameliorate the effects of the aortic narrowing. Thus, the symptoms of lower extremity ischemia typically progress over months or years. This indolent course may, however, be punctuated by abrupt acceleration of symptoms, the result of sudden increase in the size of the obstructing thrombus or its extension to a significant collateral. On the other hand, progression to complete occlusion may not be marked by a clinical event.[122,125,126]

The pathogenesis of aortoiliac atherosclerosis may differ from that of atherosclerosis in more distal segments of the arterial tree.[122,127] Patients with aortoiliac narrowing are younger and present with a shorter duration of symptoms than do those with femoropopliteal obstruction. It has been reasoned that, in the normal course of events, the narrowing in the more distal femoropopliteal arteries appears first. Only when other factors intrude, the reasoning continues, does "premature" atherosclerotic narrowing in the infrarenal aorta appear, thus the younger age.

The predilection of atherosclerosis for the terminal aorta may be enhanced in some individuals because they have anatomic variations of the aortoiliac bifurcation which produce an aortic impedance mismatch. An iliac bifurcation angle more acute than normal has been observed in some patients[128]; in others, the aorta and iliac arteries are smaller than average.[129]

Clinical Features

Men are affected far more often than women. The mean age of patients in most series falls in the sixth decade, but some are much younger. The usual "risk factors" for atherosclerosis are found with great frequency.

The original description of the clinical features of this process by René Leriche[130] still applies; however, variations on the theme are more frequent than the full-blown syndrome. Pain or tiredness in the lower back, buttocks, or thighs produced by exertion and relieved by brief periods of rest are hallmarks of aortoiliac obstruction. Claudication may occur in the calf or foot in association with the more proximal distress and can be the sole complaint. Men often complain of inability to maintain a penile erection.

Absence of or reduction in the femoral pulse is typical. More distal pulses in the legs are reduced or absent, and bruits are commonly audible over femoral arteries and in the midline of the abdomen near the umbilicus. Low skin temperature, diminished hair growth, atrophy of the skin and subcutaneous tissue, and diminished muscle bulk in the lower limbs are common but not universal signs. Frank gangrene is not common; amputation for ischemia is therefore seldom required.

The findings in patients with aortoiliac obstruction overlap those in patients with femoropopliteal narrowing. A firm identification of involvement of the aortoiliac segment may be difficult on clinical grounds. To further complicate matters, obstructing lesions are present at both levels in many patients. Fortunately, modern imaging techniques have made diagnosticians less dependent on clinical findings for the localization of the level of arterial obstruction.

Natural History and Prognosis

The survival rate for patients with the *Leriche syndrome* appears to be lower than for those in a control population matched for age and sex, but death rarely results from the aortoiliac disease. Coronary and cerebrovascular disease are largely responsible for the higher death rate. Significant morbidity or death occasionally follows occlusion of the renal arteries by proximal extension of the thrombotic process.

Management

Chronic aortoiliac occlusion may be partial or complete and may occur alone or be associated with femoropopliteal occlusive disease. For aortoiliac occlusion, the end-to-side bypass with a flexible, knitted, albumin-coated Dacron bifurcation graft is the preferable method of treatment. The trunk of the bifurcation graft is attached to a vertical incision made through the anterior wall of the uninvolved abdominal aorta above the obstruction, and the other ends are drawn through tunnels made behind the peritoneum; the ends are then attached to the sides of distal patent segments, either in the external iliac arteries or in the common femoral arteries opposite the origins of the deep femoral arteries in the groins.

In the absence of femoropopliteal occlusive disease, this method has been successful in restoring normal distal circulation in about 98 percent of patients. Even in patients with combined aortoiliac and femoropopliteal disease, bypass of the aortoiliac occlusion alone with revascularization of the deep femoral arterial system may be adequate to relieve symptoms. If symptoms are not relieved, extension of the bypass to the popliteal region can be considered. Follow-up observations in these patients for more than 40 years have provided evidence of maintenance of good long-term results with a relatively low recurrence rate of about 5 percent if only the aortoiliac region is occluded.[131]

Percutaneous transluminal angioplasty, devised by Grüntzig,[132,133] has been used in several centers in the treatment of iliac and femoropopliteal obstructive atherosclerotic disease. The early success rate appears to be satisfactory, but the long-term patency rate remains to be determined. This technique is applicable in highly selected cases of a relatively short segment of well-localized stenotic occlusion.

ACUTE OBSTRUCTION OF THE TERMINAL AORTA

Etiology

A rare event, sudden occlusion of the terminal aorta, may result from a large ("saddle") embolus, trauma, dissection, or in situ thrombosis in a severely atherosclerotic aorta or an aneurysm. When either dissection or trauma is responsible, the clinical picture usually leaves little doubt as to the reason for the aortic occlusion.[134–136]

Most emboli large enough to "saddle" and thereby occlude the terminal aorta are thrown off from the heart. Thus, embolus must be considered when acute aortoiliac occlusion occurs in patients with mitral stenosis, atrial fibrillation, or recent myocardial infarction. Rarely, embolization of a vegetation from fungal endocarditis may be large enough to occlude the aortic bifurcation.[134–136]

In situ thrombosis of an aneurysm or of a severely atherosclerotic aorta may develop when blood flow through these vessels is considerably reduced, as may be the case in shock or congestive heart failure.

Clinical Features

Unlike gradually progressive obstruction, abrupt total or near total interruption of flow through the terminal aorta or common iliac arteries produces acute, limb-threatening ischemia. Although the clinical picture will vary depending on the presence of preexisting collaterals, the full-blown syndrome is characterized by the abrupt onset of pain, typically severe and located in the lumbar area, buttocks, perineum, abdomen, and legs. Numbness, paresthesia, dysesthesia, and finally paralysis of the affected limb dominate the picture. Pulses are absent in the legs, although at times faint femoral pulsations may be detected. The legs are cold and pale. Unless circulation is promptly restored, massive muscle necrosis may produce myoglobinuria, renal failure, acidosis, and hyperkalemia.

Management

In contrast to chronic aortoiliac occlusion, acute obstruction to blood flow does not allow for the formation of collateral circulation. Immediate operation is necessary for survival. The procedure used depends on the cause of the occlusion.

Treatment for aortic dissection has been discussed above. Acute aortoiliac occlusion due to trauma with an intimal tear producing dissection may be corrected by the bypass graft technique described for chronic aortoiliac occlusion. In patients with acute aortoiliac occlusion due to a saddle embolus, consideration also must be given to treatment of the underlying disease, such as concomitant open mitral commissurotomy at the time of embolectomy, in order to prevent recurrent embolization to such vital organs as the brain.

Although aortoiliac embolectomy may be performed directly through an incision in the distal aorta or proximal iliac arteries, this approach requires laparotomy in a severely ill patient, and it does not provide the means for removing the more distally lodged embolic material often present in these patients. The preferable approach is to expose both common femoral arteries in the groins and, through transverse arteriotomies, to remove, with balloon-tipped Fogarty catheters, the embolic material lodged proximally and distally. Care must be taken to prevent further embolization in the opposite leg while these catheters are passed proximally. Even large amounts of embolic material in the distal aorta itself can be safely removed in this manner, with use of a local anesthetic when the general condition of the patient contraindicates general anesthesia.

Good circulation is usually restored after such procedures. Subsequent mortality rates, however, remain high because of the underlying disease that caused the saddle embolus in many of these patients, particularly those with myocardial infarction and a mural thrombus. Nevertheless, by the use of a local anesthetic and Fogarty catheters, surgery is possible in virtually all patients.

Obstruction of Major Aortic Branches

CHRONIC OBSTRUCTION OF AORTIC ARCH BRANCHES

Etiology and Pathology

Atherosclerosis accounts for more than 90 percent of instances of occlusion of the brachiocephalic, carotid, and subclavian arteries. Takayasu's arteritis, luetic aortitis, neoplastic obstruction, and trauma account for almost all the remainder. Lesions tend to be located at arterial bifurcations and are therefore characteristically found at the origin of the arch vessels and at the bifurcation of the common carotid arteries. The proximal left subclavian artery is the most common site of an obstructing lesion.

Clinical Features

Occlusion at the origin of one of the arch vessels often does not produce symptoms because of the many possibilities for collateral connections. Upper-extremity ischemia is particularly unusual. The occurrence of symptoms of cerebral ischemia suggests that more than one lesion is present, that there are lesions in more distal arteries, that collateral circulation is compromised, or that a "steal" syndrome is present.

The steal syndromes are of particular interest. In its classic presentation, *subclavian steal* is triggered by vigorous motion of the arm on the side of severe proximal subclavian arterial occlusion. Symptoms of cerebral ischemia result. Because of the subclavian occlusion, blood flow to the arm cannot be increased sufficiently to maintain arterial pressure in the face of exercise-induced vasodilation and blood is "stolen" from the cerebral circulation. That is, blood delivered to the brain through the carotid arteries is diverted via the circle of Willis and proceeds in a direction opposite from that of normal flow through the ipsilateral vertebral artery to the exercising arm. In brachiocephalic artery steal, a much more unusual problem, retrograde flow through the ipsilateral carotid artery, may be an additional hazard.

Meticulous assessment of the carotid, temporal, and upper extremity pulses; measurement of the blood pressure in both arms; and careful auscultation for bruits in the neck and supraclavicular areas detect brachiocephalic occlusive disease.

Diagnostic Studies

Noninvasive techniques have been developed to aid assessment of the severity of arterial obstruction in this area. These techniques are particularly pertinent to the evaluation of a patient with a carotid bruit. Duplex ultrasound examination of the carotid arteries in the neck may provide both images of the artery and with Doppler techniques identify obstructed segments and may demonstrate reversal of flow in steal syndromes. Definitive identification of the severity and location of the occlusion depends on arteriography.

Management

Occlusive diseases of the vessels arising from the aortic arch are amenable to surgical treatment when segments distally in the neck are patent. This condition is best considered as proximal or distal occlusion, although both types of occlusion may occur in the same patient. Distal occlusion usually affects the carotid bifurcations or origins of the vertebral arteries. In proximal occlusive disease, the distal segments are usually patent and therefore amenable to surgical treatment.

Proximal occlusion, usually of arch branches, occurs at or near their origins and is best corrected by the bypass procedure.[137] The proximal end of a graft is attached to the side of the ascending aorta, and the distal end or ends of the graft are attached to patent arterial segments in the neck or supraclavicular region distal to the occlusion. The ascending aorta is exposed through a second or third right anterior intercostal incision. After application of a partial occlusion clamp to the ascending aorta, a vertical incision is made in the occluded segment, and the Dacron graft is attached to this opening by end-to-side anastomosis. The patent distal arterial segments are exposed through separate incisions in the neck and supraclavicular regions. The distal end of the graft is drawn retrosternally through a tunnel made by blunt dissection and is attached to the side of the patent distal segment. In patients with multiple occlusive segments, the appropriate limbs are attached to the sides of the other patent arterial segments. Albumin-coated Dacron tubes 6 to 8 mm in diameter are used for this purpose. In some cases, the bypass may be made without opening the chest. Thus, in proximal occlusion of the left common carotid artery with a patent left subclavian artery, the bypass may be made from the latter to the former through a single incision in the neck.

Results of this form of treatment have been very gratifying. In virtually all patients with only proximal occlusion of vessels arising from the aortic arch, normal circulation has been restored. In patients with combined proximal and distal occlusion, the success rate varies with the ability to correct the distal occlusion.

ABDOMINAL ANGINA

Patients with abdominal angina may be treated by endarterectomy, excision and graft replacement, or bypass graft, the last procedure being preferable for most patients.[138] The abdominal aorta is exposed between the renal and common iliac arteries. The proximal end of the graft is attached by end-to-side anastomosis to the aorta. The distal end is carried behind the transverse mesocolon and stomach and sutured to the side of the normal hepatic or splenic artery. Since the occlusive process usually does not affect the trifurcation of the celiac artery, attachment of the graft to the hepatic or splenic arteries provides complete revascularization of the celiac distribution.

One end of a second tube is sutured to the side of the graft, and the other end is carried through a tunnel in the small-intestinal mesentery under the duodenum and attached to the side of the superior mesenteric artery distal to the site of occlusion. Albumin-coated Dacron tubes 8 mm in diameter are used in most patients.

RENOVASCULAR HYPERTENSION

Surgical treatment for renovascular hypertension is directed toward correction of renal ischemia.[139,140] Patients with well-localized disease may be treated by endarterectomy and patch-graft angioplasty. For more extensive segmental occlusion, the end-to-side bypass principle is preferred. The proximal end of an 8-mm albumin-coated Dacron graft is attached to the abdominal aorta below the origin of the renal arteries, and the distal end of the graft is attached to the side of the renal artery distal to the obstruction. The bypass-graft method has been particularly effective in restoring normal circulation to both kidneys and the lower limbs in patients with combined occlusive disease of the aorta, iliac arteries, and renal arteries.[141,142] The proximal end of the renal arterial graft is attached to the side of the aortic segment of the aortoiliac bypass graft in these patients. In a smaller number of patients, reconstructive surgery is impossible because of the site and extend of the disease. In these, total or partial nephrectomy may be required.

Results of operation are highly satisfactory, with an operative mortality rate of 1 to 2 percent. In our experience, long-term relief of hypertension was obtained in about two-thirds of the patients. Overall survival expectancy is about 50 percent at 15 to 20 years. For patients below 40 years of age, it is about 80 percent; this figure emphasizes the importance of early surgical treatment in patients whose blood pressure cannot easily be controlled with tolerable medical treatments.[143]

REFERENCES

1. Schlatmann TJM, Becker AE. Histologic changes in the normal aging aorta: Implications for dissecting aortic aneurysm. *Am J Cardiol* 1977; 39:13–20.
2. Ross R. The pathogenesis of atherosclerosis: a perspective for the 1990s. *Nature* 1993; 362:801–809.
3. Stary HC, Chandler AB, Glagov S, Guyton JR, Insull W Jr, Rosenfeld ME, et al. A definition of initial, fatty streak, and intermediate lesions of atherosclerosis: A report from the committee on vascular lesions of the Council on Arteriosclerosis, American Heart Association. *Circulation* 1994; 89:2462–2478.
4. Roberts WC, Ferrans VJ, Levy RI, Frederickson DS. Cardiovascular pathology in hyperlipoproteinemia. *Am J Cardiol* 1973; 31:557–570.
5. Zarins CK, Glagov S, Giddens DP, Ku DN. Hemodynamic factors and atherosclerotic change in the aorta. In: Bergan, JJ and Yao, JST, eds, *Aortic Surgery*, Philadelphia: Saunders; 1989:17–25.
6. Wolinsky H, Glagov S. Comparison of abdominal and thoracic aortic medial structure in mammals: Deviation of man from the usual pattern. *Circ Res* 1969; 25:677–686.
7. Tunick PA, Rosenzweig BP, Katz ES, Freedberg RS, Perez JL, Kronzon I. High risk for vascular events in patients with protruding aortic atheromas: A prospective study. *J Am Coll Cardiol* 1994; 23:1085–1090.
8. Khatibzadeh M, Mitusch R, Stierle U, Gromoll B, Sheikhzadeh A. Aortic atherosclerotic plaques as a source of systemic embolism. *J Am Coll Cardiol* 1996; 27:664–669.

9. French Study of Aortic Plaques in Stroke Group, Atherosclerotic disease of the aortic arch as a risk factor for recurrent ischemic stroke. *N Engl J Med* 1996; 334:1216–1221.

10. Roman MJ, Devereux RB. Heritable aortic disease. In: Lindsay, J Jr, ed, *Diseases of the Aorta*, Philadelphia: Lea & Febiger; 1994:55–74.

11. Savunen T. Annulo-aortic ectasia—a clinical, structural and biochemical study. *Scand J Thorac Cardiovasc Surg* 1986; (suppl 37):1–45.

12. Roberts CS, Roberts WC. Dissection of the aorta associated with congenital malformation of the aortic valve. *J Am Coll Cardiol* 1991; 17:712–716.

13. Hahn RT, Roman MJ, Mogtader AH, Devereux RB. Association of aortic dilatation with regurgitant, stenotic, and functionally normal bicuspid aortic valves. *J Am Coll Cardiol* 1992; 19:283–288.

14. Subramaniam PN. Case report: Turner's syndrome and cardiovascular abnormalities: A case report and review of the literature. *Am J Med Sci* 1989; 297:260–262.

15. Nunez L, O'Connor LF, Pinto AG, Gil-Aguado M, Gutierrez M. Annuloaortic ectasia and adult polycystic kidney—A frequent association. *Chest* 1986; 90:299–300.

16. Biagini A, Maffei S, Baroni M, Piacenti M, Terrazzi M, Paoli F, et al. Familial clustering of aortic dissection in polycystic kidney disease. *Am J Cardiol* 1993; 72:741–742.

17. Leier CV, Call TD, Fulkerson PK, Wooley CF. The spectrum of defects in the Ehlers-Danlos Syndrome, types I and III. *Ann Intern Med* 1980; 92:171–178.

18. Hortop J, Tsipouras P, Hanley JA, Maron BJ, Shapiro JR. Cardiovascular involvement in osteogenesis imperfecta. *Circulation* 1986; 73:54–61.

19. Wilson SK, Hutchins GM. Aortic dissecting aneurysms—Causative factors in 204 patients. *Arch Pathol Lab Med* 1982; 106:175–180.

20. Schlatmann TJM, Becker AE. Pathogenesis of dissecting aneurysm of the aorta—Comparative histopathologic study of significance of medial changes. *Am J Cardiol* 1977; 39:21–26.

21. Nakashima Y, Kurozumi T, Sueishi K, Tanaka K. Dissecting aneurysm: A clinicopathologic and histopathologic study of 111 autopsied cases. *Hum Pathol* 1990; 21:291–296.

22. Dollar AL. Aortitis: Inflammatory and infectious diseases of the aorta. In: Lindsay, J Jr, ed. *Diseases of the Aorta*. Philadelphia: Lea & Febiger; 1994:75–88.

23. Kearney RA, Eisen HJ, Wolf JE. Nonvalvular infections of the cardiovascular system. *Ann Intern Med* 1994; 121:219–230.

24. Daniel WG, Mugge A, Martin RP, Lindert O, Hausmann D, Nonnast-Daniel B, et al. Improvement in the diagnosis of abscesses associated with endocarditis with transesophageal echocardiography. *N Engl J Med* 1991; 324:795–800.

25. David TE, Komeda M, Brofman PR. Surgical treatment of aortic root abscess. *Circulation* 1989; 80:I-269–I-274.

26. Oskoui R, Davis WA, Gommes MN. Salmonella aortitis: A report of a successfully treated case with a comprehensive review of the literature. *Arch Intern Med* 1993; 153:517–525.

27. Cohen PS, O'Brien TF, Schoenbaum SC, Medeiros AA. The risk of endothelial infection in adults with *Salmonella* bacteremia. *Ann Intern Med* 1978; 89:931–932.

28. Jackman JD, Radolf JD. Cardiovascular syphilis. *Am J Med* 1989; 87:425–433.

29. Ito I. Aortitis syndrome (Takayasu's Arteritis)—A historical perspective. *Jpn Heart J* 1995; 36:273–281.

30. Hall S, Barr W, Lie JT, Stanson AW, Kazmier FJ, Hunder GG. Takayasu's arteritis: A study of 32 North American patients. *Medicine* 1985; 64:89–99.

31. Kerr GS, Hallahan CW, Giordano J, Leavitt RY, Fauci AS, Rottem M, et al. Takayasu arteritis. *Ann Intern Med* 1994; 120:919–929.

32. Ishikawa K. Diagnostic approach and proposed criteria for the clinical diagnosis of Takayasu's arteriopathy. *J Am Coll Cardiol* 1988; 12:964–972.

33. Takeuchi Y, Matsuki K, Saito Y, Sugimoto T, Juji T. HLA-D region genomic polymorphism associated with Takayasu's arteritis. *Angiology* 1990; 41:421–426.

34. Arend WP, Michel BA, Bloch DA, Hunder GG, Calabrese LH, Edworthy SM, et al. The American College of Rheumatology 1990 criteria for the classification of Takayasu arteritis. *Arthritis Rheum* 1990; 33:1129–1134.

35. Subramanyan R, Joy J, Balakrishnan KG. Natural history of aortoarteritis (Takayasu's disease). *Circulation* 1989; 80:429–437.

36. Ishikawa K, Maetani S. Long-term outcome for 120 Japanese patients with Takayasu's disease. *Circulation* 1994; 90:1855–1860.

37. Tyagi S, Kaul UA, Nair M, Sethi KK, Arora R, Khalilullah M. Balloon angioplasty of the aorta in Takayasu's arteritis: Initial and long-term results. *Am Heart J* 1992; 124:876–882.

38. Tyagi S, Singh B, Kaul UA, Sethi KK, Arora R, Khalilullah M. Balloon angioplasty for renovascular hypertension in Takayasu's arteritis. *Am Heart J* 1993; 125:1386–1393.

39. Klein RG, Hunder GG, Stanson AW, Sheps SG. Large artery involvement in giant cell (temporal) arteritis. *Ann Intern Med* 1975; 83:806–812.

40. Evans JM, Bowles CA, Bjornsson J, Mullany CJ, Hunder GG. Thoracic aortic aneurysm and rupture in giant cell arteritis. *Arthritis Rheum* 1994; 37:1539–1547.

41. Evans JM, O'Fallon WM, Hunder GG. Increased incidence of aortic aneurysm and dissection in giant cell (temporal) arteritis. *Ann Intern Med* 1995; 122:502–507.

42. Bergfeldt L, Insulander P, Lindblom D, Moller E, Edhag O. HLA-B27: An important genetic risk factor for lone aortic regurgitation and severe conduction system abnormalities. *Am J Med* 1988; 85:12–18.

43. Bulkley BH, Roberts WC. Ankylosing spondylitis and aortic regurgitation: Description of the characteristic cardiovascular lesion from study of eight necropsy patients. *Circulation* 1973; 48:1014–1027.

44. Hoeffel JC, Henry M, Mentre B, Louis JP, Pernot C. Pseudocoarctation or congenital kinking of the aorta: Radiologic considerations. *Am Heart J* 1975; 89:428–436.

45. Smyth PT, Edwards JE. Pseudocoarctation, kinking or buckling of the aorta. *Circulation* 1972; 46:1027–1032.

46. Grigsby JL, Galbraith T, Shurmur S, Deligonul U. Pseudocoarctation of the aorta complicated by saccular aneurysm. *Am Heart J* 1996; 131:200–202.

47. Kent KC, Boyce SW. Aneurysms of the aorta. In Lindsay, J Jr, ed, *Diseases of the Aorta*. Philadelphia: Lea & Febiger; 1994:109–125.

48. Halloran BG, Baxter BT. Pathogenesis of aneurysms. *Semin Vasc Surg* 1995; 8:85–92.

49. Patel MI, Hardman DTA, Fisher CM. Current views on the pathogenesis of abdominal aortic aneurysms. *J Am Coll Surg* 1995; 181:371–382.

50. Heinemann M, Laas J, Karck M, Borst HG. Thoracic aortic aneurysm after acute type A aortic dissection: Necessity for follow-up. *Ann Thorac Surg* 1990; 49:580–584.

51. Reed D, Reed C, Stemmermann G, Hayashi T. Are aortic aneurysms caused by atherosclerosis? *Circulation* 1992; 85:205–211.

52. Baird PA, Sadovnick AD, Yee IML, Cole CW, Cole L. Sibling risks of abdominal aortic aneurysm. *Lancet* 1995; 346:601–604.

53. Verloes A, Sakalihasan N, Koulischer L, Limet R. Aneurysms of the abdominal aorta: Familial and genetic aspects in three hundred thirteen pedigrees. *J Vasc Surg* 1995; 21:646–655.

54. Newman KM, Jean-Claude J, Li H, Ramey WG, Tilson MD. Cytokines that activate proteolysis are increased in abdominal aortic aneurysms. *Circulation* 1994; 90(part 2):II-224–II-227.

55. Smith JA, Fann JI, Miller DC, Moore KA, DeAnda A Jr, Mitchell RS, et al. Surgical management of aortic dissection in patients with the Marfan syndrome. *Circulation* 1994; 90(part 2):II-235–II-242.

56. Joyce JW, Fairbairn JF II, Kincaid OW, Juergens JL. Aneurysms of the thoracic aorta: A clinical study with special reference to prognosis. *Circulation* 1964; 29:176–181.

57. Kouchoukos NT, Dougenis D. Surgery of the thoracic aorta. *N Engl J Med* 1997; 336:1876–1888.

58. Goldstein SA, Lindsay J Jr. Thoracic aortic aneurysms: Role of echocardiography. *Echocardiography* 1996; 13:213–232.

59. Bickerstaff LK, Pairolero PC, Hollier LH, Melton LJ, Van Peenen HJ, Cherry KJ, et al. Thoracic aortic aneurysms: A population-based study. *Surgery* 1982; 92:1103–1108.

60. Murdoch JL, Walker BA, Halpern BL, Kuzma JW, McKusick VA. Life expectancy and causes of death in the Marfan syndrome. *N Engl J Med* 1972; 286:804–808.

61. Silverman DI, Burton KJ, Gray J, Bosner MS, Kouchoukos NT, Roman MJ, et al. Life expectancy in the Marfan syndrome. *Am J Cardiol* 1995; 75:157–160.

62. Roman MJ, Rosen SE, Kramer-Fox R, Devereux RB. Prognostic significance of the pattern of aortic root dilatation in the Marfan syndrome. *J Am Coll Cardiol* 1993; 22:1470–1476.

63. Legget ME, Unger TA, O'Sullivan CK, Zwink TR, Bennett RL, Byers

PH, et al. Aortic root complications in Marfan's syndrome: Identification of a lower risk group. *Heart* 1996; 75:389–395.

64. Masuda Y, Takanashi K, Takasu J, Morooka N, Inagaki Y. Expansion rate of thoracic aortic aneurysms and influencing factors. *Chest* 1992; 102:461–466.

65. Dapunt OE, Galla JD, Sadeghi AM, Lansman SL, Mezrow CK, de Asla RA, et al. The natural history of thoracic aortic aneurysms. *J Thorac Cardiovasc Surg* 1994; 107:1323–1333.

66. DeBakey ME, Noon GP. Aneurysms of the thoracic aorta. *Med Concepts Cardiovasc Dis* 1975; 44:53–58.

67. DeBakey ME, Noon GP. Aneurysms of the sinuses of valsalva. In: Sabiston DC, Spencer FC, eds, *Gibbon's Surgery of the Chest*, 3d ed. Philadelphia: Saunders; 1976:903–913.

68. Crawford ES, Rubio PA. Reappraisal of adjuncts to avoid ischemia in the treatment of aneurysms of the descending thoracic aorta. *J Thorac Cardiovasc Surg* 1973; 66:693–704.

69. DeBakey ME, McCollum CH, Graham JM. Surgical treatment of aneurysms of the descending thoracic aorta: Long-term results in 500 patients. *J Cardiovasc Surg* 1978; 19:571–576.

70. Ernst CB. Abdominal aortic aneurysm. *N Engl J Med* 1993; 328:1167–1172.

71. Pennell RC, Hollier LH, Lie JT, Bernatz PE, Joyce JW, Pairolero PC, et al. Inflammatory abdominal aortic aneurysms: A thirty-year review. *J Vasc Surg* 1985; 2:859–869.

72. Sterpetti AV, Hunter WJ, Feldhaus RJ, Chasan P, McNamara M, Cisternino S, et al. Inflammatory aneurysms of the abdominal aorta: Incidence, pathologic, and etiologic considerations. *J Vasc Surg* 1989; 9:643–650.

73. Leseche G, Schaetz A, Arrive L, Nussaume O, Andressian B. Diagnosis and management of 17 consecutive patients with inflammatory abdominal aortic aneurysms. *Am J Surg* 1992; 164:39–44.

74. Rutherford RB, McCroskey BL. Ruptured abdominal aortic aneurysms: Special considerations. *Surg Clin North Am* 1989; 69:859–868.

75. Sullivan CA, Rohrer MJ, Cutler BS. Clinical management of the symptomatic but unruptured abdominal aortic aneurysm. *J Vasc Surg* 1990; 11:799–803.

76. Bower TC, Cherry KJ Jr, Pairolero PC. Unusual manifestations of abdominal aortic aneurysms. *Surg Clin North Am* 1989; 69:745–754.

77. Keen RR, McCarthy WJ, Shireman PK, Feinglass J, Pearce WH, Durham JR, et al. Surgical management of atheroembolization. *J Vasc Surg* 1995; 21:773–781.

78. Dolmatch BL, Gray RJ, Horton KM, Rundback JH. Diagnostic imaging in the evaluation of aortic disease. In: Lindsay, J Jr, ed, *Diseases of the Aorta*. Philadelphia: Lea & Febiger; 1994:197–250.

79. Scott RAP, Wilson NM, Ashton HA, Kay DN. Is surgery necessary for abdominal aneurysm less than 6 cm in diameter? *Lancet* 1993; 342:1395–1396.

80. Frame PS, Fryback DG, Patterson C. Screening for abdominal aortic aneurysm in men ages 60 to 80 years. *Ann Intern med* 1993; 119:411–416.

81. Lederle FA. Management of small abdominal aortic aneurysms. *Ann Intern Med* 1990; 113:731–732.

82. Cronenwett JL, Murphy TF, Zelenock GB, Whitehouse WM Jr, Lindenauer SM, Graham LM, et al. Actuarial analysis of variables associated with rupture of small abdominal aneurysms. *Surgery* 1985; 98:472–483.

83. Nevitt MP, Ballard DJ, Hallett JW Jr. Prognosis of abdominal aortic aneurysm: A population-based study. *N Engl J Med* 1989; 321:1009–1014.

84. Guiruis EM, Barber GG. The natural history of abdominal aortic aneurysms. *Am J Surg* 1991; 162:481–483.

85. Nehler MR, Taylor LM Jr, Moneta GL, Porter JM. Indications for operation for infrarenal abdominal aneurysms: Current guidelines. *Semin Vasc Surg* 1995; 8:108–114.

86. Roger VL, Ballard DJ, Hallett JW Jr, Osmundson PJ, Puetz PA, Gersh BJ. Influence of coronary artery disease on morbidity and mortality after abdominal aortic aneurysmectomy: A population-based study, 1971–1987. *J Am Coll Cardiol* 1989; 14:1245–1252.

87. Graor RA. Preoperative evaluation and management of coronary and carotid artery occlusive disease in patients with abdominal aortic aneurysms. *Surg Clin North Am* 1989; 69:737–743.

88. Cambria RP, Eagle K. Cardiac screening before abdominal aortic aneurysm surgery: A reassessment. *Semin Vasc Surg* 1995; 8:93–102.

89. Bayazit M, Gol MK, Battaloglu B, Tokmakoglu H, Tasdemir O, Baya-

90. DeBakey ME, Crawford ES, Cooley DA, Morris GC Jr, Royster TS, Abbott WP. Aneurysms of the abdominal aorta: Analysis of graft replacement therapy one to eleven years after operation. *Ann Surg* 1964; 160:622–639.

91. DeBakey ME. Aneurysmectomy of the abdominal aorta. *Surg Tech Illus* 1976; 1:5–20.

92. Spittell PC, Spittell JA Jr, Joyce JW, Tajik AJ, Edwards WD, Schaff HV, et al. Clinical features and differential diagnosis of aortic dissection: Experience with 236 cases (1980–1990). *Mayo Clin Proc* 1993; 68:642–651.

93. Crawford ES. The diagnosis and management of aortic dissection. *JAMA* 1990; 264:2537–2541.

94. DeSanctis RW, Doroghazi RM, Austen WG, Buckley MJ. Aortic dissection. *N Engl J Med* 1987; 317:1060–1067.

95. Lindsay J Jr, Aortic dissection. In: Lindsay, J Jr, ed. *Diseases of the Aorta*. Philadelphia: Lea & Febiger; 1994:127–143.

96. Roberts WC. Aortic dissection: Anatomy, consequences, and causes. *Am Heart J* 1981; 101:195–214.

97. Hirst AE Jr, Johns VJ Jr, Kime SW Jr. Dissecting aneurysms of the aorta: A review of 505 cases. *Medicine* 1958; 37:217–279.

98. Robbins RC, McManus RP, Mitchell RS, Latter DR, Moon MR, Olinger GN, et al. Management of patients with intramural hematoma of the aorta. *Circulation* 1993; 88(part 2):1–10.

99. Mohr-Kahaly S, Erbel R, Kearney P, Puth M, Meyer J. Aortic intramural hemorrhage visualized by transesophageal echocardiography: Findings and prognostic implications. *J Am Coll Cardiol* 1994; 23:658–664.

100. Nienaber CA, von Kodolitsch Y, Peterson B, Loose R, Helmchen U, Haverich A, et al. Intramural hemorrhage of the thoracic aorta—Diagnostic and therapeutic implications. *Circulation* 1995; 92:1465–1472.

101. Bansal RC, Chandrasekaran K, Ayala K, Smith DC. Frequency and explanation of false negative diagnosis of aortic dissection by aortography and transesophageal echocardiography. *J Am Coll Cardiol* 1995; 25:1393–1401.

102. Movsowitz HD, Lampert C, Jacobs LE, Kotler MN. Penetrating atherosclerotic ulcers. *Am Heart J* 1994; 128:1210–1217.

103. Lindsay J Jr. Aortocameral fistula: A rare complication of aortic dissection. *Am Heart J* 1993; 126:441–443.

104. Kamp TJ, Goldschmidt Clermont PJ, Brinker JA, Resar JR. Myocardial infarction, aortic dissection, and thrombolytic therapy. *Am Heart J* 1994; 128:1234–1237.

105. Hughes JD, Bacha EA, Dodson TF, Martin T, Smith RB III, Chaikof EL. Peripheral vascular complications of aortic dissection. *Am J Surg* 1995; 170:209–212.

106. Kato M, Bai H, Sato K, Kawamoto S, Kaneko M, Ueda T, et al. Determining surgical indications for acute type B dissection based on enlargement of aortic diameter during the chronic phase. *Circulation* 1995; 92(suppl II):II-107–II-1112.

107. Moore NR, Parry AJ, Trottman-Dickenson B, Pillai R, Westaby S. Fate of the native aorta after repair of acute type A dissection: A magnetic resonance imaging study. *Heart* 1996; 75:62–66.

108. Larson EW, Edwards WD. Risk factors for aortic dissection: A necropsy study of 161 cases. *Am J Cardiol* 1984; 53:849–855.

109. Williams GM, Gott VL, Brawley RK, Schauble JF, Labs JD. Aortic disease associated with pregnancy. *J Vasc Surg* 1988; 8:470–475.

110. Oskoui R, Lindsay J Jr. Aortic dissection in women <40 years of age and the unimportance of pregnancy. *Am J Cardiol* 1994; 73:821–822.

111. Cigarroa JE, Isselbacher EM, DeSanctis RW, Eagle KA. Diagnostic imaging in the evaluation of suspected aortic dissection. *N Engl J Med* 1993; 328:35–43.

112. Erbel R, Oelert H, Meyer J, Puth M, Mohr-Katoly S, Hausmann D, et al. Effect of medical and surgical therapy on aortic dissection evaluated by transesophageal echocardiography: Implications for prognosis and therapy. *Circulation* 1993; 87:1604–1615.

113. Lindsay J Jr, Hurst JW. Clinical features and prognosis in dissecting aneurysm of the aorta: A reappraisal. *Circulation* 1967; 35:880–888.

114. Slater EE, DeSanctis RW. The clinical recognition of dissecting aortic aneurysm. *Am J Med* 1976; 60:625–633.

115. Doroghazi RM, Slater EE, DeSanctis RW, Buckley MJ, Austen WG, Rosenthal S. Long-term survival of patients with treated aortic dissection. *J Am Coll Cardiol* 1984; 3:1026–1034.

116. Glower DD, Fann JI, Speier RH, Morrison L, White WD, Smith LR,

et al. Comparison of medical and surgical therapy of uncomplicated descending aortic dissection. *Circulation* 1990; 82(suppl IV):IV-39–IV-46.

117. DeBakey ME, Beall AC Jr, Cooley DA, Crawford ES, Morris GC Jr, Garrett HE, et al. Dissecting aneurysms of the aorta. *Surg Clin North Am* 1966; 46:1045–1055.

118. DeBakey ME. The development of vascular surgery. *Am J Surg* 1979; 137:697–738.

119. DeBakey ME, McCollum DH, Crawford ES, Morris GC Jr, Howell J, Noon GP, et al. Dissection and dissecting aneurysms of the aorta: Twenty-year follow-up of five hundred twenty-seven patients treated surgically. *Surgery* 1982; 92:1118–1134.

120. Bergamini TM, Bernard JD, Mavroudis C, Backer CL, Muster AJ, Richardson JD. Coarctation of the abdominal aorta. *Ann Vasc Surg* 1995; 9:352–356.

121. Cohen JR, Birnbaum E. Coarctation of the abdominal aorta. *J Vasc Surg* 1988; 8:160–164.

122. Lindsay J Jr. Acquired obstructive disease of the aorta. In: Lindsay J Jr, ed. *Diseases of the Aorta*. Philadelphia: Lea & Febiger; 1994:145–156.

123. Lande A. Takayasu's arteritis and congenital coarctation of the descending thoracic and abdominal aorta: A critical review. *Am J Roentgenol* 1976; 127:227–233.

124. DeBakey ME, Garrett HE, Howell JF, Morris GC. Coarctation of abdominal aorta with renal artery stenosis: Surgical considerations. *Ann Surg* 1967; 165:836–843.

125. Brewster DC. Clinical and anatomical considerations for surgery in aortoiliac disease and results of surgical treatment. *Circulation* 1991; 83(suppl I):I-42–I-52.

126. Bergan JJ, Variations of the Leriche syndrome. In: Bergan, JJ and Yao, JST, eds. *Aortic Surgery*. Philadelphia: Saunders; 1989:149–159.

127. Stubbs DH, Kasulke RJ, Kapsch DN, Nichols WK, Silver D. Populations with the Leriche syndrome. *Surgery* 1981; 89:612–616.

128. Sharp WV, Donovan DL, Teague PC, Mosteller RD. Arterial occlusive disease: A function of vessel bifurcation angle. *Surgery* 1982; 91:680–685.

129. Palmaz JC, Carson SN, Hunter G, Weinshelbaum A. Male hypoplastic infrarenal aorta and premature atherosclerosis. *Surgery* 1983; 94:91–94.

130. Leriche R, Morel A. The syndrome of thrombotic obliteration of the aortic bifurcation. *Ann Surg* 1948; 127:193–204.

131. DeBakey ME. Patterns of atherosclerosis and rates of progression. In: Paoletti R, Gotto AM Jr, eds, *Atherosclerosis Reviews III*. New York: Raven Press; 1978:1–56.

132. Gruntzig A, Hopff H. Perkutane Rekanalisation chronischer arterieller Verschlusse mit einem neuen Dilatationskatheter. *Dtsch Med Wochenschr* 1974; 99:2502–2510.

133. Gruntzig A. Perkutane Dilatation von Kronarstenosen: Beschreibung eines neuen Kathetersystems. *Klin Wochenschr* 1976; 54:543–545.

134. Schatz IJ, Stanley JC. Saddle embolus of the aorta. *JAMA* 1976; 235:1262–1263.

135. Busuttil RW, Keehn G, Milliken J, Paredero VM, Baker JD, Machleder HI, et al. Aortic saddle embolus: A twenty-year experience. *Ann Surg* 1983; 197:698–706.

136. Webb KH, Jacocks MA. Acute aortic occlusion. *Am J Surg* 1988; 155:405–407.

137. DeBakey ME, Lawrie GM. Arterial occlusive disease of the major branches of the aortic arch. In: Bell PRF, Jamieson DW, Ruckley CV, eds. *Surgical Management of Vascular Disease*. London: Saunders; 1992:709–720.

138. McCollum CH, Graham JM, DeBakey ME. Chronic mesenteric arterial insufficiency: Results of revascularization in 33 cases. *South Med J* 1976; 69:1266–1268.

139. DeBakey ME, Morris GC Jr, Morgen RO, Crawford ES, Cooley DA. Lesions of the renal artery: Surgical technic and results. *Am J Surg* 1964; 107:84–96.

140. DeBakey ME, McCollum CH III. Atherosclerotic occlusive disease: V. Surgical management of atherosclerotic vascular disease. In: Gross HL, ed. *Atherosclerosis*. Kalamazoo, MI: The Upjohn Company; 1977:81–96.

141. Lawrie GM, Morris GC Jr, Soussou ID, Starr DS, Silvers A, Glaeser DH, et al. Late results of reconstructive surgery for renovascular disease. *Ann Surg* 1980; 191:528–533.

142. Lawrie GM, Morris GC Jr, DeBakey ME. Long-term results of treatment of the totally occluded renal artery in 40 patients with renovascular hypertension. *Surgery* 1980; 88:753–759.

143. Lawrie GM, Morris GC Jr, Soussou ID, Starr DS, Glaeser DH, DeBakey ME. Late results of reconstructive surgery for renovascular disease. *Ann Surg* 1980; 191:528–533.

99

CEREBROVASCULAR DISEASE AND NEUROLOGIC MANIFESTATIONS OF HEART DISEASE

Louis R. Caplan

Most vascular diseases have a tendency to affect both the heart and the brain. In addition, cardiac diseases often lead to secondary lesions and dysfunction within the brain, and central nervous system (CNS) diseases can affect the heart and its function.

BRAIN AND CEREBROVASCULAR COMPLICATIONS OF HEART DISEASE

Cerebral complications occur when (1) the heart pumps unwanted materials into the circulation that reach the brain (embolism); (2) pump function fails and the brain is hypoperfused; and (3) drugs given to treat cardiac disease have neurologic side effects.

Cardiogenic Brain Embolism

ETIOLOGY

Until recently, the diagnostic criteria of cardiogenic embolism were very restrictive. It was diagnosed when sudden focal neurologic signs, maximal at onset, developed in patients with peripheral systemic embolism and recent myocardial infarction or rheumatic mitral stenosis. By these criteria, cardiogenic embolism was diagnosed in only 3 to 8 percent of stroke patients.[1–3] None of these criteria are secure. In various stroke registries,[4–7] about 10 to 20 percent of patients did not have maximal symptoms at onset. Many other cardiac lesions are now well-accepted sources of emboli—e.g., atrial fibrillation. Only about 2 percent of patients with cardiogenic brain embolism[4] have clinically recognized peripheral emboli. In necropsy studies of patients with brain embolism, however, infarcts are commonly found in the spleen and kidneys and other organs. The symptoms of peripheral embolism are often so minor and nonspecific (transient abdominal discomfort, leg cramp, etc.) that they are seldom diagnosed correctly.

Before the advent of echocardiography, fully 30 percent of patients with stroke were believed to have cardiogenic embolism.[4] Later studies that used stricter criteria attributed 17 percent,[5] 22 percent,[8] and 14 percent[6] of strokes to cardiogenic embolism. With more advanced diagnostic techniques, more cardiac abnormalities are recognized; in the Lausanne Stroke Registry, 305 (23 percent) of 1311 patients with a first stroke had a potential cardiac source of embolism.[7,9] Because many patients have coexisting cardiac and extracranial vascular disease,[9–11] criteria for the diagnosis of cardiac embolism remain controversial.

Cardiac sources can be divided into three groups[9]: (1) *cardiac wall and chamber abnormalities*—e.g., cardiomyopathies, hypokinetic and akinetic ventricular regions after myocardial infarction, atrial septal aneurysms, ventricular aneurysms, atrial myxomas, papillary fibroelastomas and other tumors, septal defects, and patent foramen ovale; (2) *valve disorders*—e.g., rheumatic mitral and aortic disease, prosthetic valves, bacterial endocarditis, nonbacterial thrombotic endocarditis, mitral valve prolapse, and mitral annulus calcification; and (3) *arrhythmias*, especially atrial fibrillation and "sick-sinus" syndrome.

Some sources have much higher rates of initial and recurrent embolism. The Stroke Data Bank[12] divided potential sources into *strong* (valve surgery, atrial fibrillation, sick-sinus syndrome, ventricular aneurysm, akinetic segments, mural thrombi, cardiomyopathy, diffuse ventricular hypokinesia) and *weak* (myocardial infarct over 6 months old, aortic and mitral stenosis and regurgitation, congestive failure, mitral valve prolapse, mitral annulus calcification, hypokinetic ventricular segments).

Even within individual cardiac abnormalities—e.g., atrial fibrillation—there are differences in risk depending on many factors. For example, in patients with atrial fibrillation, associated heart disease, patient age, duration, chronic versus intermittent fibrillation, and atrial size influence embolic risk. A potential cardiac source of embolism does not mean that a stroke was actually caused by an embolus from the heart. Coexistent occlusive cerebrovascular disease is common. In the Lausanne registry, among patients with potential cardiac embolic sources, 11 percent of patients had severe cervicocranial vascular occlusive disease (>75 percent stenosis) and 40 percent had mild to moderate stenosis proximal to brain infarcts.[9]

Mitral valve prolapse (MVP) as a source of embolism continues to be somewhat controversial (see Chap. 65). Several clinical series indicate that MVP is associated with stroke.[13–16] Morphologic lesions, such as thrombi and fibrous lesions, clearly suggest embolism[17–19]; fibrin-platelet depositions on the surfaces of the mitral leaflets have been noted,[16–18] as well as thrombi in the angle between the posterior mitral valve leaflet and the left atrial wall.[16,19,20] Patients with MVP also have other disorders such as atrial fibrillation, syncope, and migraine. The rate of recurrence of stroke in patients with MVP as the only known cause is very low.[15,16] Given the very high incidence of MVP, the frequency of MVP-related stroke is extremely low.[16–21] Most neurologists feel that warfarin anticoagulants are ordinarily not indicated in prophylaxis of patients with MVP, even after an initial stroke. Aspirin prophylaxis (160 to 325 mg/day) is, however, advisable. Demonstration of an intracardiac thrombus by echocardiography would change that recommendation to warfarin.

Mitral annulus calcification (MAC) is an important but frequently unrecognized cause of embolism. Ulceration and extrusion of calcium through overlapping cusps have been seen at necropsy,[22] thrombi have been found on valves attached to the ulcerative process,[23] and calcific emboli have been seen in surgical embolectomies.[16,22,24] Several series show a convincing relationship between MAC and brain emboli or stroke.[5,22,25–27] Bacterial endocarditis can also develop on the MAC.

More patients have cardiogenic embolism than are presently diagnosed. Clinical features and brain investigations such as computed tomography (CT) and cerebral angiography may suggest emboli, but often a source cannot be identified. These cases, which are termed *infarcts of unknown causes* (IUC) in the Stroke Data Bank,[6,28,29] may involve 40 percent of patients.

Nonbacterial thrombotic endocarditis and Libman-Sachs endocarditis[30] are also important sources of brain embolism. Nonbacterial valve vegetations are also common in patients with the antiphospholipid antibody syndrome.[31] In infective endocarditis, embolic complications are common.[32] Mycotic aneurysms can cause fatal subarachnoid bleeding. Bleeding can also result from vascular necrosis as a result of an infected embolus.[32] Embolization usually stops when the infection is controlled.[32] Warfarin does not prevent embolization and is probably contraindicated unless there are other important lesions such as prosthetic valves or life-threatening pulmonary embolism (see also Chap. 82). In children and young adults with congenital heart defects, especially those with right-to-left shunts and polycythemia, brain abscess is an important complication (see also Chap. 70).

Emboli can arise from sources other than the heart, such as proximal arteries (intraarterial or so-called local embolism), leg veins (paradoxical emboli), fat in the liver or bones (fat embolism), and materials introduced by the patient or physician (drug particles or air).[11] The types of embolic material can also vary (Table 99-1).[11] Atheromatous plaques in the aortic arch and ascending aorta have recently been shown to be a very important and previously neglected source of embolism to the brain. Ulcerated atheromatous plaques are often found at necropsy in patients with ischemic strokes, especially in those in whom the stroke etiology was not determined during life.[33] Transesophageal echocardiography (TEE) can often show these atheromas, but technical factors limit visualization of the entire arch.[34] *Large (>4 mm), protruding, and mobile aortic atheromas are especially likely to cause embolic strokes and are associated with a high rate of recurrent strokes.*[35]

CLINICAL FINDINGS

Anterior Circulation Recipient Sites

Balloons placed into the circulation always follow the same flow patterns[36]; anterior circulation material reaches the middle cerebral arteries (MCA) and their branches.[36] The commonest sites are the mainstem MCA, the upper or lower

TABLE 99-1

EMBOLIC MATERIALS

Cardiac	Intraarterial
1. Red fibrin-dependent thrombi	1. Red fibrin-dependent thrombi
2. White platelet-fibrin nidi	2. White platelet-fibrin nidi
3. Material from marantic endocarditis	3. Combined fibrin-platelet and fibrin-dependent clots
4. Bacteria from vegetations	4. Cholesterol crystals
5. Calcium from valves and mitral annulus calcification	5. Atheromatous plaque debris
6. Myxoma cells and debris	6. Calcium from vascular calcifications
	7. Air
	8. Mucin from tumors
	9. Talc or microcrystalline cellulose from injected drugs

divisions of the MCA, or their branches. The upper division of the MCA supplies the frontal and parietal lobes above the sylvian fissure, and the inferior division supplies the convexal temporal and inferior parietal lobes. Resultant neurologic deficits include the following:

MCA Upper Division Contralateral hemiparesis, hemisensory loss; aphasia (left hemisphere); lack of awareness of deficit, neglect of the left space, motor impersistence (right hemisphere)[37]

MCA Inferior Division Wernicke-type fluent aphasia, agitation, right-upper-quadrant anopia (left hemisphere); agitation and hyperactivity, left neglect, poor drawing and copying (right hemisphere)

MCA Mainstem Infarcts—usually features of both upper and inferior division infarcts

Posterior Circulation Recipient Sites

Vertebrobasilar territory symptoms have usually been attributed to local disease within that circulation without consideration of possible cardiogenic embolism. In the major registries,[4–6,9] however, about 20 percent of emboli of cardiac origin go to the posterior circulation. Twenty percent is expected, as about one-fifth of cerebral blood flow goes to this circulation. In the posterior circulation, certain recipient sites are favored:

Posterior Cerebral Artery (PCA)[39–41] Particles and clots go to the most distal part of the system; the PCA is the terminal vessel in the vertebrobasilar circuit. The hallmark of PCA lesions is hemianopia and/or hemisensory loss contralateral to the infarct. Patients with left-PCA infarcts also commonly cannot read or name colors but retain the ability to write and spell. Amnesia is sometimes prominent and may last up to 6 months. Right-PCA infarction is often associated with left visual neglect.

Top of the Basilar Artery[40,42,43] The major clinical features are apathy and sleepiness; abnormal vertical gaze; and hallucinations, unusual reports, and other behavioral abnormalities. Bilateral PCA infarction is present, and the clinical findings include bilateral visual field loss, amnesia, and severe agitation and delirium.

Vertebral Artery (VA) Intracranially and Its Posterior Inferior Cerebellar Artery (PICA) Branch[38] Somewhat larger emboli may occlude an intracranial VA and cause cerebellar infarction involving mostly the posterior inferior surface.[40,44] Ataxia, vomiting, and occipital headache are the commonest signs.

Onset and Course

Many embolic strokes have their onset during rest or sleep. Sudden coughing or sneezing or arising at night to urinate can precipitate embolism. Although the deficit is most often maximal at outset, 11 percent of embolic stroke patients in the Harvard Stroke Registry had a stuttering or stepwise course, whereas 10 percent had fluctuations or progressive deficits. Later progression, if it occurs, is usually within the first 48 h. Progression is usually due to distal passage of emboli. "Nonsudden embolus" is explained by the embolus moving from its initial location, as demonstrated by angiography, to a more distal branch.[45] Early angiography has a very high rate of showing intracranial emboli,[4,46] but angiography after 48 h demonstrates a much lower rate of blockage. More recently, transcranial Doppler (TCD) sonography has shown a high incidence of MCA blockage acutely in patients with sudden-onset hemispheric strokes, but later, thrombolysis and normalization of the intracranial blood velocities occur.[47] As in all large infarcts, brain edema and swelling may develop during the 24 to 72 h after stroke, with headache, decreased alertness, and worsening of the neurologic signs. The edema is often cytotoxic (inside cells) and may not respond to corticosteroid treatment.

DIAGNOSTIC TESTING

Emboli usually cause occlusion of distal branches and produce surface infarcts that are roughly triangular, with the apex of the triangle pointing inward. CT and magnetic resonance imaging (MRI) can suggest the presence of embolism by the location and shape of the lesion, the presence of many superficial wedge-shaped infarcts in multiple different vascular territories, hemorrhagic infarction, and visualization of thrombi within arteries. Among 60 patients with cardiogenic sources of embolism studied by CT in whom occlusive atherosclerotic cerebrovascular disease had been excluded, 56 had superficial large or small cortical or subcortical infarcts and only 4 had deep infarcts. Emboli can block the MCA and cause solely deep infarcts because the superficial territory has good collateral flow; these infarcts are called *striatocapsular* because they involve the internal capsule and the adjacent basal ganglia, which are supplied by lenticulostriate branches of the MCA.[49] Occasionally, tiny emboli may cause small deep or superficial infarcts.

MRI is more sensitive for detection of brain infarcts than CT and is also superior in detecting hemorrhagic infarction by imaging hemosiderin. Hemorrhagic infarction has long been considered characteristic of embolism, especially when the vessel leading to the infarct is patent.[50] The mechanism of hemorrhagic infarction is reperfusion of ischemic zones, which occurs with spontaneous passage of the embolus after iatrogenic opening of an occluded artery (e.g., endarterectomy, fibrinolytic treatment) or after restoration of the circulation after a period of systemic hypoperfusion. Hemorrhage occurs into proximal reperfused regions of brain infarcts.[51] At times, it is also possible to image the acute embolus on CT.[11,52,53] In unselected series of stroke patients, transthoracic echocardiography (TTE) (Chap. 14) has been variably useful in detecting sources.[54–56] TTE is useful in patients with known cardiac disease to clarify potential embolic sources and heart function,[5] in young patients without stroke risk factors, and in stroke patients who do not have lacunar infarction or ultrasound evidence of intrinsic atherostenosis of a major extracranial and intracranial artery. TEE (Chap. 14) provides much better visualization of the aorta, atria, cardiac valves, and septal regions. Reports of TEE suggest that the diagnostic yield is 2 to 10 times that of TTE.[57–60] Aortic plaques, atrial septal aneurysms, and atrial septal defects are also much better seen with TEE. The use of an echo-enhancing agent like agitated saline helps detect intracardiac shunts.

Echocardiography has definite limitations. Particles the size of 2 mm can block major brain arteries but are probably beyond the imaging resolution of current echocardiographic technology.[11] Also, thromboembolism is a dynamic process. When a clot forms in the heart and embolizes, there may be no residual evidence until a clot reforms.[11] Cardiac thrombi may be imaged differently on sequential echocardiograms[61]; even large intracardiac thrombi seen on one echocardiogram can disappear later.[62] Platelet scintigraphy using platelets labeled with radionuclides may be helpful in localizing cardiac and intraarterial sources, but its sensitivity and specificity are undefined.[63]

Embolic signals can now also be detected by monitoring with TCD.[64–65] Embolic particles passing under the TCD probes produce transient, short-duration, high-intensity signals referred to as HITS (high-intensity transient signals). TCD monitoring of patients with atrial fibrillation,[66] cardiac surgery,[67] prosthetic valves, left ventricular assist devices,[68] carotid artery disease, and carotid endarterectomy have shown a relatively high frequency of embolic signals. In the future, monitoring of emboli with TCD may become an important diagnostic criterion to guide treatment.

PREVENTION AND TREATMENT

Early studies showed that warfarin was effective in preventing brain embolism in patients with rheumatic mitral stenosis and atrial fibrillation (AF). Previously, the intensity of anticoagulation was higher than that which is currently employed, and brain hemorrhages and other bleeding complications were more common. Trials have now shown that low-dose warfarin [International Normalized Ratio (INR) 2.0 to 3.0] is also effective in preventing brain emboli in patients with nonrheumatic AF.

In the Copenhagen Atrial Fibrillation, Aspirin, Anticoagulation (AFASAK) study, 1007 patients (median age 74.2 years) with chronic, nonrheumatic AF were assigned to warfarin (INR 2.8 to 4.2), aspirin (75 mg/day), or placebo.[69] The study was halted prematurely when analysis of effectiveness reached a predetermined level of significance in favor of warfarin treatment. The principal outcome was the composite of ischemic or hemorrhagic stroke, transient ischemic attack (TIA), and systemic embolism. The observed reduction for warfarin compared to placebo was 64 percent, an absolute risk reduction of 3.5 percent per year. An analysis by intention to treat, which excluded TIA and minor stroke, indicated a risk reduction of about 50 percent ($p < .05$) and an absolute reduction of about 1.5 percent per year.

The Stroke Prevention in Atrial Fibrillation (SPAF) study evaluated both warfarin and aspirin in patients with nonrheumatic AF.[70,74] The study evaluated two groups of patients on the basis of their eligibility for warfarin. In the first group, 627 patients judged eligible for warfarin were randomized to open-label warfarin (INR 2.8 to 4.5; prothrombin time, 1.3 to 1.8 × control) or double-blind to either aspirin (325 mg daily, enteric-coated) or matching placebo. In the second group, 703 patients ineligible for warfarin were randomized (double-blind) to aspirin (325 mg daily, enteric-coated) or placebo. The principal outcome, a composite of ischemic stroke and systemic embolism, was significantly decreased during a mean follow-up of 1.3 years. The outcome of disabling ischemic stroke or vascular death was reduced by warfarin by 54 percent ($p = .11$), an absolute reduction of 2.6 percent per year. Aspirin also decreased the principal outcome in both study groups. The risk reduction was 42 percent ($p = .02$), and the absolute reduction was 2.7 percent per year. The outcome of disabling stroke or death was reduced 22 percent by aspirin ($p = .33$), or an absolute reduction of about 1 percent per year.

In the Boston Area Anticoagulation Trial for Atrial Fibrillation (BAATAF), 420 patients with nonrheumatic AF, mean age, 68 years, were randomized unblinded to warfarin (target prothrombin time ratio, 1.2 to 1.5 × control; INR 1.5 to 2.7) or to a control group who were allowed to take aspirin.[72] The principal outcome was ischemic stroke or systemic embolism, and the mean follow-up was 2.2 years. The incidence of stroke was reduced by 86 percent in the warfarin group compared to control ($p = .002$), equivalent to an absolute risk reduction of 2.6 percent per year. There was no demonstrable benefit of aspirin, but the study was not designed to test aspirin.

In the Canadian Atrial Fibrillation Anticoagulation (CAFA) study, 187 patients were randomized to warfarin (INR target range 2.0 to 3.0) and 191 to placebo.[75] The principal outcome was the composite of nonlacunar stroke, non-CNS embolism, and fatal or intracranial hemorrhage. The relative risk reduction for warfarin was 37 percent ($p = .17$). The study was prematurely terminated when the results of the Copenhagen AFASAK and SPAF studies became known.

The Veterans Affairs Stroke Prevention in Nonrheumatic Atrial Fibrillation study was a randomized, double-blind, placebo-controlled evaluation of low-intensity anticoagulation with warfarin (prothrombin time ratio 1.2 to 1.5, corresponding to an INR of 1.4 to 2.8) in male veterans.[79] The placebo group ($n = 265$) and the warfarin group ($n = 260$) were followed for an average of 1.7 and 1.6 years, respectively. Subjects receiving warfarin had a 79 percent reduction in the risk of cerebral infarction. None of the 18 patients in this study or the 52 patients in the SPAF study who had lone AF had a cerebral infarction.

The SPAF study identified three risk factors for thromboembolism—recent congestive heart failure, history of hypertension, and previous thromboembolism—and suggested that anticoagulation with warfarin was not indicated in patients with none of the three risk factors who were at low risk for thrombo-

embolism (2.5 percent per year). In such patients the dangers of anticoagulant therapy may outweigh its benefits.[76,77] Aspirin (325 mg daily) is probably reasonable and safe therapy for patients with lone, nonrheumatic AF who are under 60 years of age and have none of the three identified risk factors.[76–79] In other patients with AF, long-term oral warfarin therapy (INR 2.0 to 3.0) should be used unless contraindicated.[78,79]

The effects of anticoagulation on embolism from other cardiac conditions have not been well studied. The rate of recurrence of stroke in patients with MVP is so low that warfarin is not recommended for prophylaxis except when a thrombus is seen on echocardiography (see also Chap. 65). Warfarin may not be effective in preventing calcific, myxomatous, bacterial, and fibrin-platelet emboli, and some researchers have suggested that warfarin may worsen cholesterol crystal embolization.[80]

The timing of the initiation of warfarin anticoagulation after embolic stroke remains controversial. Embolic brain infarcts often become hemorrhagic, and serious brain hemorrhage has occurred after anticoagulation.[81–85]

Large infarcts, hypertension, large bolus doses of heparin, and excessive anticoagulation have been associated with hemorrhage. Because most hemorrhagic transformations occur within 48 h, the recommendations of the Cerebral Embolism Task Force were to avoid early anticoagulation in patients with large infarcts or hemorrhagic transformation on repeat CT.[86,87] Studies of patients with cerebral and cerebellar hemorrhagic infarction show that, in the vast majority, the cause is embolic, that hemorrhagic infarction occurs equally with and without anticoagulation, and that the development of hemorrhagic infarction is rarely accompanied by clinical worsening.[88,89] Patients with hemorrhagic transformation who were continued on anticoagulants did not worsen.[88] The risk of reembolism must be balanced against the small but definite risk of important bleeding. If the patient has a large brain infarct, heparin should be delayed and bolus heparin infusions should be avoided. If the risk for reembolism is high, immediate heparinization is advisable, whereas if the risk seems low, it is prudent to delay anticoagulants for at least 48 h and possibly even for a period of 2 to 3 weeks.[86,87]

Brain Hypoperfusion Due to Cardiac Pump Failure

After cardiopulmonary resuscitation (CPR), the heart often recovers in individuals whose brain has been irreversibly damaged by ischemic-anoxic damage. Cardiologists must be familiar with the pathology, signs, and prognosis of brain dysfunction after periods of circulatory failure.

Different brain regions have selective vulnerability to hypoxic-ischemic damage. Those regions that are most remote and at the edges of major vascular supply are more liable to injury. These zones have usually been referred to as "border zones" or "watersheds."

The cerebral cortex is most vulnerable to injury. Damage may be diffuse or "laminar," involving layers of the cortex.

The hippocampus is one of the most vulnerable areas.[90–93] In the brain, the border zone regions are between the anterior cerebral artery (ACA) and MCA and the MCA and PCA. Damage is usually most severe in the posterior parietotemporooccipital region and in frontal areas most remote from the heart and thus called *distal fields.* A similar border zone exists in the cerebellum between the cerebellar arteries and in the brainstem between medial and lateral arteries. The basal ganglia and thalamus are most involved if hypoxia is severe but some circulation is preserved. This situation applies most to hanging, strangulation, drowning, and carbon monoxide exposure.[94] Cerebellar neurons, especially Purkinje cells, may also be selectively injured.[95]

When circulatory arrest is complete and abrupt, brainstem nuclei are especially vulnerable to necrosis, especially in young humans and experimental animals.[96] When hypoxia and ischemia are especially severe, the spinal cord may also be damaged.[97,98] When cortical damage is very severe and protracted, cytotoxic edema causes massive brain swelling, with cessation of blood flow and brain death.

CLINICAL FINDINGS

Very severe damage leads to mortal injury to the cortex and brainstem, irreversible coma, and brain death. When initially examined, such patients have no brainstem reflexes (pupillary, corneal, and oculovestibular and oculocephalic reflexes) and no response to stimuli except perhaps a decerebration response. These findings do not improve, and respiratory control is absent or lost.

When cerebral cortical damage is very severe but brainstem ischemic changes are reversible, brainstem reflexes are preserved but there is no meaningful response to the environment. Automatic facial movements such as blinking, tongue protrusion, and yawning usually persist. The eyes may rest slightly up and move from side to side. When this state does not improve, it is referred to as the *persistent vegetative state*[92,99,100] or "wakefulness without awareness." Laminar necrosis also causes seizures. These are often multifocal myoclonic twitches or jerks of the facial and limb muscles, which are very difficult to control with anticonvulsants; oversedation should be avoided.

With severe border-zone injury, there is weakness of the arms and proximal lower extremities with preservation of face, leg, and foot movement (the "man in a barrel" syndrome). With less severe ischemia, the symptoms and signs are predominantly visual. Patients describe difficulty seeing and cannot integrate the features of large objects or scenes despite retained ability to see small objects in some parts of their visual fields. Reading is impossible. There are features of Balint's syndrome,[101] including asimultagnosia (i.e., seeing things piecemeal or sequentially); optic ataxia (i.e., poor eye-hand coordination); and optic apraxia (i.e., difficulty in directing the gaze). Apathy and inertia are also common and are due to border-zone damage to the frontal lobe. Amnesia is also very common. Patients cannot make new memories and have patchy, retrograde amnesia for events during and before the hospitalization. This Korsakoff-type syndrome is due to hippocampal damage and is sometimes not reversible. Amnesia may be accompanied by visual abnormalities, apathy, and confusion, or it may be isolated.

Action myoclonus (the Lance-Adams syndrome)[95] is thought to be due to cerebellar damage. This disorder is characterized by arrhythmic fine or coarse jerking, especially on attempted movement. Reaching for an object may be accompanied by gross oscillation and tremor-like movements. Gait ataxia is also common. The findings are worsened by stress and emotion and suppressed somewhat by barbiturates and diazepam.[102]

PROGNOSIS

Shortly after resuscitation or arrest, patients with less severe cerebral injuries show some reactivity to the environment. Eye opening and restless limb movements develop. The eyes may fixate on objects. Noise, a flashlight, or a gentle pinch arouses patients to avoid or react to stimuli. Soon patients awaken fully and may begin to speak. Cognitive and behavioral abnormalities may be detected after the patient awakens, depending on the degree of injury.

Prognostic signs and variables have been extensively studied.[103,104] The initial neurologic findings and their course are helpful in predicting outcome. Among all patients who had meaningful responses to pain at 1 h, all survivors had preserved intellectual function.[103] Patients who do not respond to pain by 24 h either die or remain in a vegetative state. Being comatose predicts a poor prognosis.[105,106] *Thus, two simple observations, the presence or absence of coma and the response to pain, predict neurologic outcome very early.*[106] After hypoxic-ischemic insults, the outcome can be analyzed progressively at 3, 7, and 14 days after the event.[94]

In a study in Seattle of out-of-hospital cardiac arrests, patients who did not awaken died on average 3.5 days after arrest.[107,108] Of 459 patients, 183 never awakened (39 percent). Among those who did awaken, 91 (32 percent) had persistent neurologic deficits.[107] Prognosis could be made by analysis of pupillary light reflexes, eye movements, and motor responses.[96] Bystander initiation of CPR was not significantly related to awakening,[108] in contrast to another study that found that outcome was better if CPR was started by bystanders before the emergency team arrived.[109] Patients awake on admission were included in one study[109] but excluded in the other.[108] After in-hospital CPR, pneumonia, hypotension, renal failure, cancer, and a housebound state before hospitalization were significantly related to death in the hospital (see also Chaps. 36 and 37).[110]

DIAGNOSTIC TESTING

Neurologic imaging and other tests have proved to be relatively unhelpful, in contrast to the neurologic examination. CT is used to exclude other causes of coma such as brain hemorrhage. Electroencephalography (EEG) is helpful in studying cortical activity in unresponsive patients and in assessing brain death. Similarly, the absence of responses to visual and somatosensory stimuli is a poor prognostic sign. TCD may be helpful in the evaluation of brain death.[111–113]

TREATMENT

Other than maintaining adequate circulation and oxygenation, treatment has not been helpful in improving outcome. Increased blood sugar correlates with poor outcome,[114] and experimental animals subjected to circulatory arrest do worse if they have been fed glucose before the arrest.[115,116] Blood calcium and the presence of free radicals and excitatory neurotoxins have all been postulated to affect neuronal cell death.[116–118] A multifaceted approach to therapy has been most successful.[119]

Neurologic Effects of Cardiac Drugs

The neurologic side effects of several cardiovascular agents can mimic or cause stroke (see also Chap. 91). Digitalis can cause visual hallucinations, yellow vision, and general confusion.[120,121] Digitalis levels need not be excessively elevated, and the symptoms disappear with cessation of the drug.

Quinidine can cause confusion with delirium, seizures and coma, vertigo, tinnitus, and visual blurring.[122] Chronic cognitive and behavioral changes and "quinidine dementia" are less well known. Similar toxicity has been seen with lithium. Patients may become acutely comatose while being treated with intravenous lidocaine. This effect has been associated with the accidental administration of very large doses; more common CNS effects of less extreme toxicity include sedation, irritability, and twitching. The latter may progress to seizures accompanied by respiratory depression.

NEUROLOGIC AND CEREBROVASCULAR COMPLICATIONS OF CARDIAC SURGERY

The incidence of abnormalities of intellectual function and behavior after cardiac surgery is quite high. Fortunately, most changes are reversible with time. The reported incidence of neurologic complications after cardiac surgery varies widely from 7 to 61 percent for transient complications and from 1.6 to 23 percent for permanent complications.[123,124]

Prospectively, transient complications have been noted in 61 percent of patients.[125] In one series, 16.8 percent of patients had stroke or encephalopathy after coronary artery bypass surgery (CABS); the encephalopathies usually cleared, and only 2 percent of patients had severe strokes.[126]

Atherothrombotic, Hemodynamically Mediated Brain Infarcts

A major concern has been that the hemodynamic and circulatory stress of heart surgery will lead to underperfusion of areas supplied by already stenosed or occluded arteries, leading to brain infarcts. This concern underlies neck auscultation for bruits, ultrasound carotid artery testing, and cerebral angiography prior to CABS. Hemodynamically induced infarction, however, is a rare complication of heart surgery. Embolism is much more common and a much greater concern. *Patients with carotid bruits have a very low rate of stroke after elective surgery.*[127] *In a retrospective study of CABS patients with known carotid disease, ipsilateral strokes occurred in 1.1 percent of arteries with 50 to 90 percent stenosis, in 6.2 percent of arteries with >90 percent stenosis, and in only 2 percent of vessels with carotid occlusion.*[128,129] Stroke rates tend to be lower in those undergoing a combined as opposed to a staged procedure,[130] but definitive management of combined cerebral and coronary artery disease awaits the outcome of clinical trials. Intracranial flow and velocity do not show significant changes in patients with high-grade carotid stenosis during CABS.[131]

Most studies have relied on clinical localization of focal deficits and inference about their mechanisms. A neuroradiology study reviewed neuroimaging results from 30 patients with acute strokes in relation to CABS.[132] Only one had strong evidence of a hemodynamic atherostenotic mechanism. Thrombotic infarction may occur in the days following surgery when the cessation of anticoagulation and the activation of coagulation factors may promote hypercoagulability.

Brain Embolism

A strong point against a hemodynamic cause of many strokes is their timing. Strokes occur more frequently *after* recovery from the anesthetic. If the mechanism of stroke were hemodynamic, the major circulatory stress would be intraoperative and patients would awaken with the deficit. In two studies in which the authors record the timing of CABS-related strokes, only 16[133] and 17 percent[132] of patients had deficits noted immediately postoperatively. The distribution of infarcts and their multiplicity on neuroimaging scans were most consistent with embolism. Embolic infarcts may involve either the anterior or the posterior circulation.[126,132,133] In our own series of postoperative, posterior circulation strokes, the majority were embolic and followed cardiac surgery.[134]

Emboli may arise from preexisting cerebrovascular lesions or postoperative arrhythmias. *Mounting evidence links operative and postoperative embolism to aortic ulcerative atherosclerotic lesions. Cross-clamping of the ascending aorta and aortotomy liberate cholesterol or calcific plaque debris.*[135]

In one series in which embolic signals were monitored during CABS surgery, 34 percent of signals were detected as the aortic cross clamps were removed and another 24 percent as aortic partial occlusion clamps were removed.[135] The number of microemboli detected does correlate with abnormalities of cognitive function studied postoperatively.[136]

After cardiac surgery, severe bilateral, predominantly border-zone infarcts have been reported, and the small arteries of the brain and other viscera (heart, kidney, spleen, pancreas) may be packed with birefringent cholesterol crystal emboli.[137] TEE makes it possible to detect protruding ulcerative plaques in the aorta preoperatively and intraoperatively.[138–140] In one patient with repeated peripheral emboli, a protruding atherosclerotic plaque was removed surgically.[138] Intraaortic atherosclerotic debris identified by TEE has been found to be associated with embolic events.[139] Intraoperative B-mode ultrasonography with the probe placed on the aorta has also been used to detect severe aortic atherosclerotic plaques.[140] Ultrasonic imaging showed aortic atheromas in 58 percent of patients, whereas visual examination and palpation detected plaques in only 24 percent.[140] *Atherosclerosis of the ascending aorta is an important risk factor for post-CABS stroke.*[141]

In some patients, hypercoagulability related to surgery can precipitate occlusive thrombosis in atherostenotic arteries, and the newly formed thrombus can lead to intraarterial embolism. It is apparent that cardiac, aortic, and intraarterial embolism accounts for the vast majority of cardiac surgery–related focal neurologic deficits.

Encephalopathy

Gilman described a diffuse CNS disorder following open heart surgery—characterized by altered levels of consciousness and activity, and confusion[142]—that is now generally referred to as *encephalopathy*. Clinical and imaging studies usually do not show important focal neurologic signs or large focal infarcts. The incidence of encephalopathy varies.[124] In one series, 57 of 1669 (3.4 percent) CABS patients had postoperative mental state changes including delirium and encephalopathy.[143] In the Cleveland Clinic prospective series, 11.6 percent were "encephalopathic" on the fourth postoperative day.[126] Encephalopathy likely has multiple causes. Embolization of particulate matter has been considered to be the leading cause, and this has led to technical improvements, including the introduction of membrane rather than bubble oxygenators and on-line filtration.[129] These technical advances have led to a decrease in the risk of macroemboli (>25 mm) as a cause, but they cannot protect against microemboli of air, fat, or particles.[129]

A necropsy study of patients who died after cardiopulmonary bypass or angiography has awakened interest in this subject.[110,144] Focal, small capillary and arteriolar dilatations (SCADs) were commonly found in the brain.[144] About one-half of the SCADs show birefringent crystalline material within the dilated capillaries. SCADs could, at least in part, explain the decreased cerebral blood flow found during cardiopulmonary bypass. SCADs are iatrogenically generated microemboli, but as yet their origin is unknown. Their morphology is most consistent with air or fat.[124,144]

Other causes of encephalopathy are common. Hypoxic-ischemic insults due to hypotension and hypoperfusion do occur. *Drugs are a very common cause of encephalopathy in the postoperative period. Particularly important are haloperidol, narcotics, and sedatives.* Morphine is sometimes used heavily intraoperatively, and opiate withdrawal with restlessness and hyperactivity can result. Agitation and restlessness are often early signs of organic encephalopathy and may lead to the administration of haloperidol, barbiturates, phenothiazines, or benzodiazepines for calming and sedation. When these drugs wear off and the patient begins to awaken, agitation may occur and more sedatives may be given. Haloperidol causes rigidity, restlessness, agitation, hallucinations, and confusion. In experimental animals, haloperidol delays recovery from strokes by months and its use is not advised.[145,146] Phenothiazines and sedatives are also problematic; *in general, use of sedatives and narcotics should be minimized and they should be tapered as soon as possible.*

Intracranial Hemorrhage after Cardiac Surgery

Occasionally, intracerebral or subarachnoid hemorrhages have been reported after cardiac surgery, most commonly in children who have had repair of congenital heart disease[147] or after cardiac transplantation.[148] The postulated mechanism involves an abrupt increase in brain blood flow with rupture of small intracranial arteries unprepared for the new load. Generally, there is a prolonged period when cardiac output is low, and this output is suddenly increased by the operation. Abrupt increases in brain blood flow or pressure in other situations have also been associated with intracerebral hemorrhage.[149]

Peripheral Nerve Complications

Brachial plexus and peripheral nerve lesions frequently develop after cardiac surgery and can be confused with CNS complications.[150] In one series, new peripheral nervous system deficits occurred in 13 percent of patients.[150] The commonest deficit is a unilateral brachial plexopathy characterized by shoulder pain and usually weakness and numbness of one hand. It is probably caused by positioning of the arm during surgery, with traction on the lower trunk of the brachial plexus. Ulnar, peroneal, and saphenous nerve injuries are also common and are also related to positioning. Diaphragmatic and vocal cord paralysis are likely related to local effects of the cardiac surgery on the recurrent laryngeal and phrenic nerves.

CARDIAC EFFECTS OF BRAIN LESIONS

Information is beginning to emerge on cardiac muscle changes (myocytolysis), arrhythmias, pulmonary edema, ECG changes, and sudden death due to brain disease and sudden emotional stresses.[151]

Cardiac Lesions

The two most common lesions found in the hearts of patients dying with acute CNS lesions are patchy regions of myocardial necrosis and subendocardial hemorrhage. The changes can range from eosinophilic staining of cells with preserved striations to transformation of myocardial cells into dense eosinophilic contraction bands. These changes have been referred to as *myocytolysis*.[152] Subendocardial petechiae and frank hemorrhages are also noted. These lesions were described in

the 1950s[151–154] but were thought initially to be rare.[153,155] One study found a very high incidence of myocardial changes in patients dying of brain lesions that increase intracranial pressure rapidly.[156] Stress-related release of catecholamines and possibly corticosteroids may be responsible, at least in part, for the cardiac lesions found in patients with CNS lesions.[157–161]

Electrocardiographic and Enzyme Changes

In stroke patients, especially those with subarachnoid hemorrhage, electrocardiograms (ECGs) may show a prolonged QT interval; giant, wide, roller-coaster inverted T waves; and U waves.[162] These changes were termed *cerebral T waves*.[142] Patients with stroke who have continuous ECG monitoring have a high incidence of T-wave and ST-segment changes, various arrhythmias, and cardiac enzyme abnormalities. ECG changes may include a prolonged QT interval, depressed ST segments, flat or inverted T waves, and U waves.[162–165] Less often, tall, peaked T waves and elevated ST segments are noted (see also Chap. 12).

Cardiac and skeletal muscle enzymes, including the MB isoenzyme of creatine kinase (MB-CK), are often abnormal in stroke patients.[166–169] During the 4 to 7 days after stroke, there is usually a slow rise and later fall in serum MB-CK levels, a pattern quite different from that found in acute myocardial infarction (Chap. 47); the temporal pattern of cardiac isoenzyme release is more compatible with smoldering low-grade necrosis, such as patchy, focal myocytolysis.[153,166] The ST-segment and T-wave abnormalities and cardiac arrhythmias correlate significantly with raised levels of MB-CK in stroke patients.[153]

Arrhythmias

All types of cardiac arrhythmias have been found in stroke patients, most frequently sinus bradycardia and tachycardia and premature ventricular contractions.[163–165] Some arrhythmias are manifestations of primary cardiac problems, but others are undoubtedly secondary to the brain lesions. The incidence of sinus tachycardia and bradycardia is maximal on the first day after intracerebral hemorrhage.[170] Ventricular bigeminy, atrioventricular dissociation and block, ventricular tachycardia, atrial fibrillation, and bundle branch blocks are found less often.[170] All arrhythmias are more common with brainstem compression.

Pulmonary Edema

Acute pulmonary edema may complicate strokes, especially subarachnoid hemorrhage (SAH) and posterior circulation ischemia and hemorrhage.[153,171] Pulmonary edema has been found in 70 percent of patients with fatal SAH and correlates with the severity and suddenness of development of raised intracranial pressure.[172]

Centrally mediated sympathetic discharges such as those caused by increased intracranial pressure produce intense systemic vasoconstriction.[173] Blood shifts from the high-resistance systemic circulation to the lower-resistance pulmonary circulation. Increased pulmonary capillary pressure leads to pulmonary hypertension and rupture of pulmonary vessels, with lung hemorrhage. The pulmonary edema fluid has a high protein content and can develop despite normal cardiac function.[153,173]

Sudden Death

Sudden death associated with stressful situations, including so-called voodoo death, must involve CNS mechanisms.[174–177] Ventricular fibrillation, the presumed mechanism of sudden death, can be reliably elicited by stimulation of cardiac sympathetic nerves in both the normal and the ischemic heart.[178] Ischemia reduces the threshold for ventricular fibrillation.[153,176,179] Stress must cause CNS stimulation that triggers autonomic activation. Sudden vagotonic stimulation can cause bradycardia and cardiac standstill. The effects of vagal stimulation on the development of ventricular arrhythmias is uncertain.[178] Patients with lateral medullary and lateral pontine infarcts affecting reticular formation structures die unexpectedly; these patients have a high incidence of various types of autonomic dysregulation, such as labile blood pressure, syncope, tachycardia, and flushing.[40]

COEXISTENT VASCULAR DISEASES AFFECTING BOTH HEART AND BRAIN

Atherosclerosis

The most common and important vascular disease that affects both the brain and the heart is atherosclerosis. The most frequent cause of death in stroke patients is coronary artery disease,[180] and extra- and intracranial arterial atherosclerosis[4,181] is common in patients with coronary artery disease.

PATHOLOGY AND PREDOMINANT SITES OF DISEASE

In white men the predominant atherosclerotic lesions involve the origins of the internal carotid artery (ICA) and the VA origins in the neck.[182] Fatty streaks and flat plaques first affect the posterior wall of the common carotid artery (CCA) opposite the flow divider between the ICA and the external carotid artery (ECA), a region of low sheer stress.[183,184] Atherosclerotic plaques at this site do not differ from plaques in the aorta or coronary arteries (see Chap. 40). At first, plaques probably expand gradually and encroach on the lumen of the ICA and sometimes the CCA (Fig. 99-1). Atheromatous plaques often develop concurrently at the VA origin or spread from the parent subclavian artery to involve the VA origin.[40,185] When plaques reach a critical size, they affect turbulence, flow, and motion of the arteries, causing complications to develop within the plaques. Cracking, ulcerations, and mural thrombi develop, and the overlying endothelium is badly damaged with the development of occlusive thrombi.[186] Fresh thrombi loosely adherent to vascular walls rapidly propagate and embolize. Because the ICA has no nuchal branches, clot often propagates cranially, usually extending as far as the first branch of the ophthalmic artery, which arises from the intracranial siphon portion of the ICA. In the VA, collateral channels from the ECA and thyrocervical trunk usually provide collateral channels that reconstitute the VA in the neck and limit propagation of the thrombus. During 2 to 3 weeks after the development of an occlusive thrombus, clot gradually organizes and is much less likely to propagate or embolize. The reduction in cranial blood flow caused by severe stenosis or occlusion of the ICA or VA stimulates development of collateral circulation that usually becomes adequate.

Figure 99-2 shows diagrammatically the sites of predilection for development of atherosclerosis in the cervicocranial circulation. Note the concentration of these sites at branch points and flow dividers.

There are important race and sex differences in the distribution of cerebral atherosclerosis.[187–190] White men usually

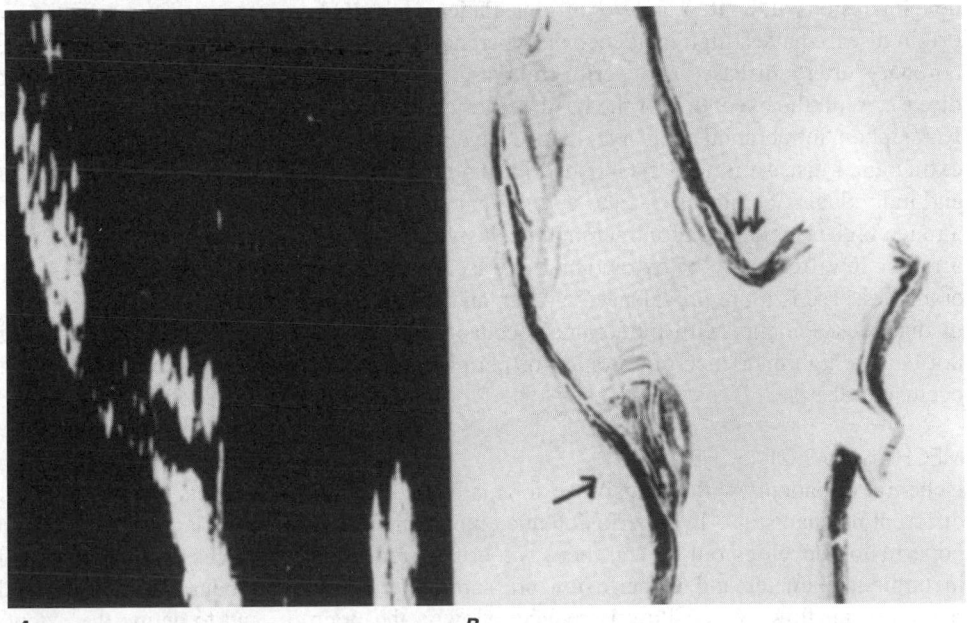

FIGURE 99-1

A. B-mode ultrasonic image showing plaque at internal carotid artery origin. *B.* A carotid specimen. The plaque (*single arrow*) is opposite the flow divider between the internal and external carotid arteries (*two arrows*). (From Hennerici M, Steinke W. Abbildende Ultraschallverfahren (B-scan) in duplex system. In: *Durchbluntungsstorungen des Gehirns—Neue Diagnostischen Möglichkeiten.* Gutersloh: Bertelsmann; 1987, with permission.)

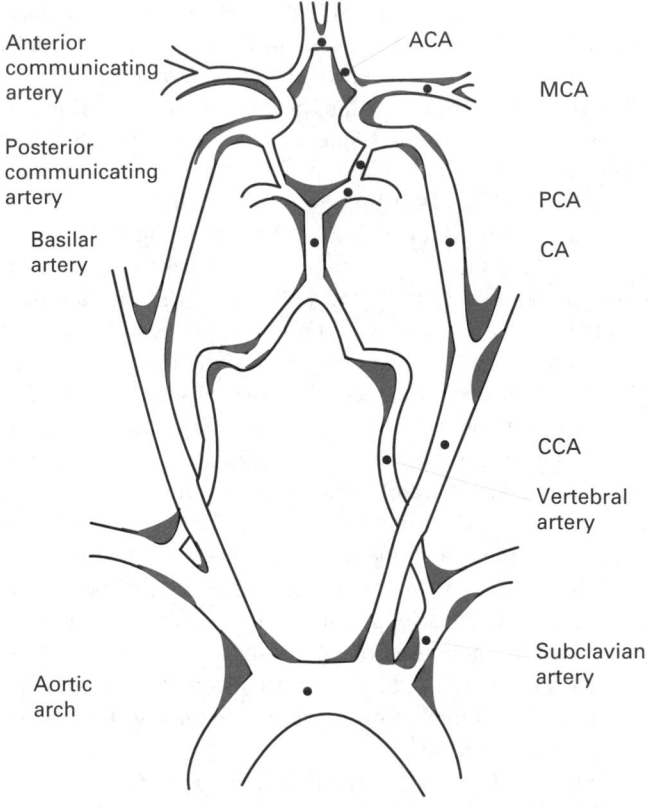

FIGURE 99-2

Sites of predilection for atherosclerotic narrowing: dark areas represent plaques. (From Caplan LR, Stein RW. *Stroke: A Clinical Approach.* Boston: Butterworth; 1986, with permission.)

develop lesions of the ICA and VA origins. Patients with ICA-origin disease have a high incidence of hypercholesterolemia, coronary artery disease, and peripheral vascular occlusive disease. With the exception of the basilar artery (BA) and the ICA siphon, intracranial occlusive disease develops only after extracranial disease is well established in this group. Blacks and individuals of Chinese, Japanese, and Thai ancestry have a much higher incidence of intracranial occlusive disease and a rather low frequency of extracranial disease.[187–191] Intracranial disease is more prevalent in women and is also found in diabetics. Patients with intracranial occlusive disease do not have a high incidence of coronary or peripheral vascular occlusive disease.

MECHANISMS OF ISCHEMIA

Ischemia in patients with occlusive lesions is caused by two different mechanisms—hypoperfusion and embolism.[192] Hypoperfusion develops only when there is a critical reduction in luminal diameter and in perfusion pressure sufficient to reduce distal flow. When flow is reduced slowly, the brain vasculature has a remarkable capacity to develop collateral circulation. Patients with severe ICA-origin occlusive disease remain asymptomatic despite marked decrease in blood flow.[179,193,194] Even when vascular occlusion is abrupt—e.g., as in tying neck arteries to treat brain aneurysms—surprisingly

few patients develop symptoms of brain ischemia. In most patients, within a few days or at most 2 weeks following an arterial occlusion, collateral circulation develops maximally and stabilizes.

Intraarterial embolism is probably a much more frequent and important cause of brain infarction than hypoperfusion. In patients with anterior circulation infarcts, angiography shows a very high incidence of intraarterial intracranial emboli distal to an ICA thrombosis.[195] These emboli most often involve the MCA and its branches. If angiography is repeated or performed later than 48 h after the stroke, the MCA occlusion is not present.[4] Intraarterial emboli often fragment and move distally. Intraarterial embolism is also very common in the posterior circulation, where the commonest donor sites are the VA origin and intracranial VA and the most frequent recipient sites for emboli are the intracranial VA, the PCA, and the distal basilar artery bifurcation.[40,196]

CLINICAL FINDINGS

Many patients with atherosclerotic occlusive disease are asymptomatic. The most frequent symptoms of hypoperfusion or embolism are headache, TIAs, and neurologic signs related to brain infarction. Headaches are due to vascular distention or brain swelling secondary to infarction. Unaccustomed headaches often precede strokes.[197] TIAs are caused by hypoperfusion or intraarterial emboli. Frequent, very brief stereotyped spells precipitated by postural changes suggest a hemodynamic mechanism. In contrast, emboli cause longer, less frequent attacks.[192,198] In many patients with clinical TIAs—i.e., with no lasting symptoms or signs—neuroimaging tests show brain infarcts.[199] Strokes may have various temporal features such as being maximal at outset, fluctuating, stepwise, or gradually progressive. The pattern is related to the adequacy of collateral circulation and the propagation and embolization of occlusive thrombi.

The neurologic signs depend on the region of brain that is ischemic. Table 99-2 outlines the most frequent clinical patterns resulting from occlusions of the major extracranial and intracranial arteries.[40,182,200]

DIAGNOSTIC TESTING

In the majority of patients, the nature and severity of the brain and vascular lesions causing the stroke can be defined. CT and MRI should localize brain lesions, distinguish between infarct and hemorrhage, and determine the location, extent, and size of the process. CT or MRI is usually the first test in patients with suspected stroke because the information allows clinicians to exclude nonvascular disease such as tumor or abscess; to differentiate hemorrhage from ischemia and show subdural hematoma; to identify the vascular territory involved; and to define the extent of brain tissue already damaged.

The vascular territory involved should be inferred by the nature of the neurologic symptoms and signs and the location of brain lesions on CT or MRI. Echocardiography, especially TEE, has dramatically improved the ability to detect potential cardiac sources of emboli (see also Chap. 14).

TABLE 99-2

COMMON SIGNS IN CEREBROVASCULAR OCCLUSIVE DISEASE AT VARIOUS SITES

ICA origin	Ipsilateral transient monocular blindness; MCA and ACA signs
ICA siphon (proximal to ophthalmic artery)	Same as ICA origin
ICA siphon (distal to ophthalmic artery)	MCA and ACA signs
ACA	Contralateral weakness of the lower limb and shoulder shrug
MCA	Contralateral motor, sensory, and visual loss
	Left: Aphasia
	Right: Neglect of left space, lack of awareness of deficit, apathy, impersistence
AChA	Contralateral motor, sensory, and visual loss, usually without cognitive changes
Subclavian artery (proximal to VA)	Lack of arm stamina, cool hand, transient dizziness, veering, diplopia
VA origin	Same as subclavian, but no ipsilateral arm or hand findings
VA intracranially	Lateral medullary syndrome; staggering and veering (cerebellar infarction)
BA	Bilateral motor weakness; ophthalmoplegia and diplopia
PCA	Contralateral hemianopia and hemisensory loss
	Left: Alexia with agraphia
	Right: Neglect of left visual space

Abbreviations: ICA = internal carotid artery; ACA = anterior cerebral artery; MCA = middle cerebral artery; AChA = anterior choroidal artery; VA = vertebral artery; BA = basilar artery; PCA = posterior cerebral artery.

Ultrasound techniques can be used to screen for obstructive lesions in the major extracranial and intracranial arteries in both anterior (carotid) and posterior (vertebrobasilar) circulation arteries. For extracranial use, the two most important are *B-mode scans* and *Doppler spectra*, both pulsed and continuous-wave (CW) Doppler. The anatomy of the carotid bifurcation (the CCA, proximal ICA, and ECA) and the proximal VAs can be imaged by high-frequency, 5- to 10-MHz, B-mode ultrasound systems, which provide images of the vessels in real time both longitudinally and in cross section (Fig. 99-3). Plaque calcifications and clot are often difficult to image. Pulsed Doppler registers frequency shifts from moving columns of blood. Doppler analysis can show the direction and velocity of blood flow. Multigated Doppler and B-mode scanning are now used together in so-called duplex systems.[200,201] The duplex system is probably more than 90 percent effective in separating three groups of vessels—those that are normal or minimally narrowed, those that have moder-

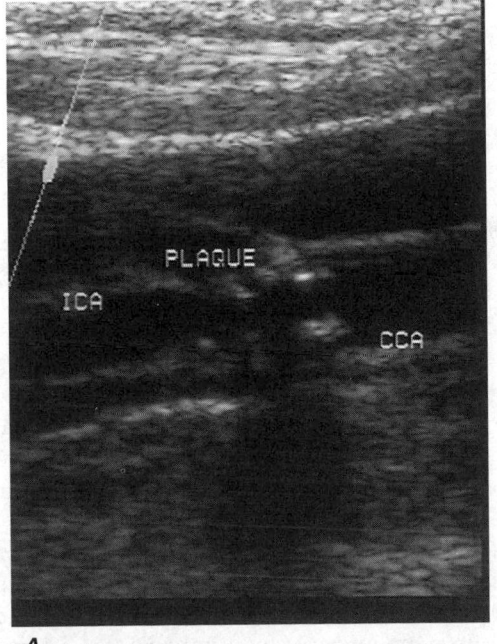

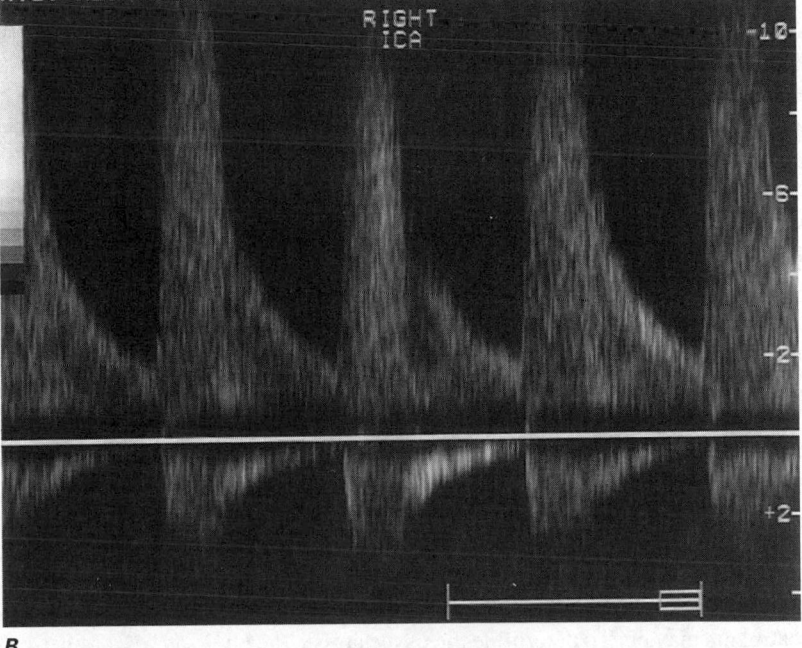

FIGURE 99-3

Duplex scan of carotid artery plaque. *A*. B-mode ultrasonic image showing plaque protruding into internal carotid artery (ICA) lumen. *B*. Doppler spectra at level of plaque showing high voltage related to stenosis.

ate disease (30 to 70 percent narrowing), and those with severe narrowing (>70 percent stenosis). B-mode scanning can sometimes suggest the presence of ulceration or hemorrhage in plaques that show heterogeneous, unusually shaped images.[202] CW Doppler also uses a movable probe to measure flow velocities along the carotid and vertebral arteries; the technique is less time-consuming and less expensive than the duplex system and in expert hands is very accurate in detecting high-grade stenosis.[201,203] Ultrasound techniques are not very accurate in separating complete occlusion from very high degrees of stenosis. Color-flow and power Doppler can often show turbulence and altered flow dynamics.

TCD ultrasound can be used to analyze the presence of intracranial arterial stenoses and to provide information about the intracranial effects of extracranial lesions. The technique takes advantage of the soft spots in the temporal bones and natural foramina (the orbit and foramen magnum) that provide windows for ultrasound recording. The depth and angle of the probe recording can be varied, allowing the recording of velocities and sound spectra from all the major intracranial arteries.[40,47,111,204] Major obstructive lesions should be detectable by the use of both extracranial ultrasound and TCD. Continuous recording of intracranial arteries with TCD is a very sensitive and accurate method of detecting emboli passing under the probes.[205,206]

Magnetic resonance angiography (MRA) provides an additional method of imaging both the extracranial and intracranial arteries for areas of stenosis and occlusion.[191,207] CT angiography (CTA), using a spiral CT machine and dye injected intravenously, can also image the major large craniocervical arteries. Standard catheter angiography is warranted when ultrasound and MRA have not sufficiently defined the vascular lesion and treatment is clinically feasible.[40,191,200]

TREATMENT

For rational treatment, the following should be known: the location, nature, and severity of the occlusive lesion; the location, extent, and reversibility of the brain lesion; and the blood constituents and coagulability.[200,208] Treatment should *not* be guided solely by the temporal pattern of the symptoms, such as TIA, progressing stroke, or so-called completed stroke.[199,200,209] These time courses do not predict the cause and mechanism of ischemia, do not tell if an infarct is present, and do not identify patients who will have further or recurrent ischemia.[209]

Physicians should first decide whether or not any specific therapy is indicated. Very severe neurologic deficits, serious intercurrent illnesses (dementia, cancer, etc.), and psychosocioeconomic considerations may make patients unsuitable for specific treatments. If treatment is feasible, the next questions to be considered are what brain tissue is at risk for further ischemia and what the benefit/risk ratio of specific treatments may be. To determine the tissue at risk, the clinician considers the cause and the deficit. For example, a man with a slight hemiplegia due to a small lacunar infarct in the anterior limb of the internal capsule may have infarcted the entire tissue supplied by an occluded small artery. In that case, treatment consists of controlling hypertension, the cause of his microvasculopathy. If, however, that same patient has a small cortical infarct in the precentral gyrus due to ICA disease, the rest of the ICA territory is at risk for further ischemia and aggressive treatment would be warranted. Suppose a patient has a moderate-sized MCA infarct. If the patient were a Chinese woman with intrinsic atherosclerotic disease of that MCA, she might have little tissue at risk for further ischemia. No aggressive treatment should be given. If that same woman's infarct were due to cardiogenic embolism, the whole remainder of the brain would be at risk for further damage from another embolus.

Patients who have little tissue at risk are not candidates for specific therapy. If there is considerable residual at-risk tissue, the guidelines in Table 99-3 are used to direct treatment, which depends upon the location and severity of the causative vascular lesions. Carotid endarterectomy (CEN) has been shown to be effective in symptomatic patients with severe ICA stenosis (>70 percent).[210,211] The Asymptomatic Carotid Artery Study (ACAS) suggested that carotid endarterectomy is slightly better than medical therapy in asymptomatic patients with severe carotid stenosis when the operation is executed by surgeons who have records of very low surgical morbidity and mortality.[212] To be effective, the operative mortality and morbidity of CEN must not be greater than 2 to 4 percent.[210–212] Surgery is also feasible on the extracranial vertebral artery in selected patients with intraarterial embolism from this site or with intractable posterior circulation hemodynamic ischemia, a rare occurrence.[40,213]

For minor and moderate degrees of stenosis in extra- and intracranial arteries, agents that alter platelet aggregation and adhesion are recommended. The most likely mechanism of ischemia in these patients is "white clot"—platelet fibrin emboli. Aspirin,[214,215] ticlopidine,[216,217] and many of the nonsteroidal anti-inflammatory drugs have antiplatelet effects, as do the omega-3 fish oils containing eicosapentaenoic acid. Aspirin is usually selected first because of the potentially serious side effects of ticlopidine (see Chap. 52).

For patients with severe stenosis of large intracranial arteries, warfarin is recommended if there are no contraindications. The anticoagulant level should be kept at an INR of 2.0 to 3.0. Anticoagulation should be continued for at least 2 months. The presence of occlusion should be detectable by duplex system, TCD, and/or MRI. The same regimen is used for patients with severe extracranial stenosis who are not operative candidates or who refuse surgery. For patients with complete occlusions when first seen, heparin and then warfarin are prescribed for 2 to 3 months.

Thrombolytic drugs, especially recombinant tissue-type plasminogen activator (rt-PA) and streptokinase, have been given intravenously and intraarterially in patients with acute brain ischemia. In a preliminary study in which the arterial lesions were not defined, intravenous therapy with rt-PA given within 90 min and 3 h of ischemia onset, in the aggregate, provided a slight statistically significant benefit.[218] Unfortu-

---

TABLE 99-3

SUGGESTED USE OF ANTICOAGULANTS AND PLATELET ANTIAGGREGANTS

HEPARIN (STANDARD DOSE)

Short term, 2–4 weeks. Usually given by intravenous infusion keeping APTT between 60 and 100 s (1.5–2 × control APTT).

1. Immediate therapy of definite cardiac-origin cerebral embolism (large cerebral infarct, hypertension, bacterial endocarditis, or sepsis would delay or contraindicate this use).
2. Patients with severe stenosis or occlusion of the ICA origin, ICA siphon, MCA, vertebral artery, or basilar artery with less than a large clinical deficit. Subsequent treatment could be warfarin or surgery.

HEPARIN (SUBCUTANEOUS MINIDOSE)

For prophylaxis of deep vein occlusion in patients immobilized by stroke (unless contraindicated). (See Chap. 60.)

WARFARIN

Usually overlapped with heparin; keeping prothrombin time around INR of 2.0–3.0 (approximately 1.3–1.5 × control).

1. Long term (>3 months)
   a. Patients with cardiogenic cerebral embolization and rheumatic heart disease, atrial fibrillation with large atria or prior cerebral embolism, prosthetic valves, and some hypercoagulable states.
   b. Patients with severe stenosis of the ICA origin, ICA siphon, MCA stem, vertebral artery, and basilar artery. Used until studies show artery has been occluded for at least 3 weeks.
2. Short term (3–6 weeks)
   a. Patients with recent occlusion of the ICA, MCA, vertebral, or basilar arteries.

PLATELET ANTIAGGREGANTS (ASPIRIN, TICLOPIDINE)

1. Patients with plaque disease of the extracranial and intracranial arteries without severe stenosis.
2. Patients with polycythemia or thrombocytosis and related ischemic attacks.

Abbreviations: APTT = activated partial thromboplastin time; ICA = internal carotid artery; MCA = middle cerebral artery; INR = International Normalized Ratio.

---

nately in this and other studies about 6 to 12 percent of patients treated with thrombolytic agents developed important intracranial bleeding. Uncontrolled studies show that patients with distal intracranial arterial embolic occlusions do well with intravenous thrombolytic therapy.[219–221] Patients with internal carotid artery occlusions in the neck and intracranially rarely reperfuse after thrombolytic therapy, especially if collateral circulation is poor. Patients with in situ thrombosis superimposed upon preexistent severe atherostenosis do less well than patients with embolism. The dose, timing, mode of delivery, and target group for therapy remain unsettled.

Because all patients with atherosclerosis are at risk of developing more lesions, control of risk factors is very important and generally should be begun in the hospital. Risk factors include smoking, hyperlipidemia, obesity, inactivity, and hypertension (see also Chap. 41). Blood pressure should not be excessively lowered during the acute ischemic period as this may decrease flow in collateral arteries. Blood pressure therapy and control can be instituted 3 to 4 weeks after the stroke. Rehabilitation must also begin early.

MANAGEMENT OF COEXISTENT CORONARY AND CEREBROVASCULAR DISEASE

Many patients have both coronary and cerebrovascular occlusive disease. In candidates for both CABS and CEN, there is controversy regarding which surgery should be done first or whether or not both procedures should be done together under the same anesthetic. *In general, the most symptomatic system should be operated on first.* Thus, if the patient has severe coronary disease with active cardiac ischemia but asymptomatic severe extracranial occlusive disease, he or she should have a CABS procedure and CEN could be considered later. On the other hand, if the patient has active cerebrovascular symptoms (recent TIAs or nondisabling stroke within 3 months) and minor or stable coronary symptoms, a CEN would be in order without a CABS. If the patient has both active coronary and cerebrovascular symptoms, the CEN and CABS should be performed together.[222–224] The reasons for this view are as follows: (1) The morbidity and mortality of the two procedures done together are considerably higher than those of either alone. The stroke risk is especially high.[231] (2) Patients with asymptomatic bruits and even severe stenosis have a very low rate of stroke due to hemodynamic changes during CABS or other surgery. Most operative and postoperative strokes are embolic. (3) With good medical care, the risk of myocardial infarction during CEN in patients with stable coronary disease is relatively low (see also Chap. 101).

It is important to define the extent of cerebrovascular disease preoperatively by noninvasive means (ultrasound and/or MRA) as well as to define cardiac and coronary artery anatomy and function when indicated. Staged surgical procedures are sometimes warranted. In some patients with excessive surgical risks, anticoagulation represents an alternative treatment. Clearly, optimal medical therapy should be instituted preoperatively unless symptoms are emergent.

Systemic Arterial Hypertension

High blood pressure, both acute and chronic, damages deep, penetrating, small intracranial arteries; accelerates the development of atherosclerosis in the extracranial and large intracranial arteries; and results in ischemic syndromes of lacunar infarction,[225,226] diffuse ischemic changes in white matter and basal gray structures (Binswanger's disease[227]), and intracerebral hemorrhage. Hypertension is also frequent in patients with aneurysmal SAH and may contribute to enlargement and rupture of congenital and acquired aneurysms.

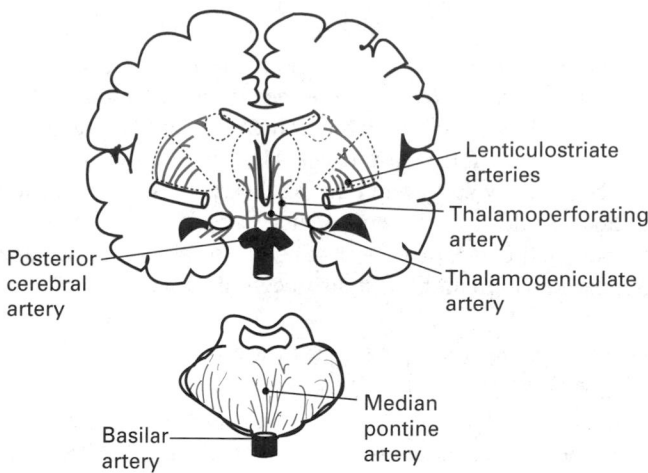

FIGURE 99-4

Deep penetrating arteries prone to the development of lipohyalinosis and microaneurysms (dark blue). Occlusion of these arteries causes lacunar infarcts, and rupture of these arteries causes intracerebral hemorrhage. (From Caplan LR, Stein RW. *Stroke: A Clinical Approach.* Boston: Butterworth; 1986, with permission.)

Hypertension especially damages the deep arteries that penetrate perpendicularly from the major intracranial arteries (Fig. 99-4) (see also Chap. 57). Serial sections of these arteries in patients with hypertension show characteristic abnormalities consisting of focal microaneurysmal enlargements and small hemorrhagic extravasations through the arterial walls. Subintimal foam cells may obliterate the lumen, and pink-staining amorphous fibrinoid material is found within the walls of the small arteries. The media are often considerably thickened. In places, the vessels are often replaced by whorls, tangles, and wisps of connective tissue that completely obliterate the usual vascular layers, causing segmental arterial disorganization as a consequence of *lipohyalinosis* and *fibrinoid degeneration*.[228,229] Microaneurysms are particularly common in patients with hypertensive intracerebral hemorrhages and in hypertensive older patients.[149,230–234]

The two major patterns of brain ischemia in patients with hypertension are *discrete lacunar infarcts* and a more *diffuse patchy white and gray matter degeneration with gliosis*. Both are thought to be caused by sclerotic changes in deep intracerebral arteries and arterioles. The term *lacune* (hole) refers to small, deep infarcts caused by lipohyalinosis of the penetrating artery feeding the ischemic brain.[228] Other vascular pathologic processes such as microdissections and tiny emboli also cause lacunes.[228,229] Some patients are normotensive and have miniature atherosclerotic lesions (so-called microatheromas) at the orifices of the branches or within the parent arteries blocking or extending into the branches.[40,225,235,236] Amyloid angiopathy can cause small, deep infarcts in normotensive and hypertensive patients. Single lacunes cause discrete clinical syndromes.[237,238] The most common are pure motor hemiparesis,[239] pure sensory stroke,[240] ataxic hemiparesis,[241] and the dysarthria–clumsy hand syndrome[242] (see Chap. 57).

Since the advent of CT and MRI, it has become widely appreciated that hypertensive patients with lacunes often have more diffuse changes in the white matter of the brain, referred to as *leukoariosis*.[227,243] The clinical picture consists of acute strokes; subacute progression of neurologic signs; dementia, especially the frontal lobe apathetic type; gait disorder; and parkinsonian, pyramidal, and pseudobulbar signs.[227,244,245] The clinical signs and gross pathology are identical to those partially described by Otto Binswanger in 1894 and 1895[233] and by his students Alzheimer and Nissl.[229,233,234] The deep arteries are thickened and hyalinized and show lipohyalinosis and sometimes amyloid angiopathy in regions of white matter atrophy and gliosis. Invariably, lacunar infarcts are also found. The pathogenesis most likely is related to diffuse vascular narrowing in deep arteries and altered microvascular flow and perfusion. Some studies suggest altered hemorheology and increased blood viscosity, and some patients have had polycythemia vera. The diagnosis is made on the basis of the clinical findings, the CT and MRI findings, and the absence of cortical infarcts, larger artery occlusive disease, or cardioembolic sources.

HYPERTENSIVE INTRACEREBRAL HEMORRHAGE

Intracerebral hemorrhage (ICH) accounts for about 10 percent of all strokes.[4,6] Head trauma, vascular malformations, bleeding diatheses, drugs (especially amphetamines and cocaine), amyloid angiopathy, and intracranial aneurysms account for some cases.[230,246] The majority of patients without these conditions have a spontaneous ICH. Traditionally, spontaneous ICH has usually been equated with hypertensive hemorrhage. Many of these patients, however, have no history of hypertension and no associated changes of hypertensive vasculopathy at necropsy.[149,230,247,248] Acute elevations of blood pressure and/or blood flow to the brain (Table 99-4) can cause ICH by the sudden increase in blood pressure, causing breakage of capillaries and arterioles.[149,230]

TABLE 99-4

CAUSES OF ACUTE CHANGES IN BLOOD PRESSURE OR BLOOD FLOW THAT CAN RESULT IN INTRACEREBRAL HEMORRHAGE

Drugs, especially cocaine and amphetamines
Recent onset of arterial hypertension
Pheochromocytoma
Cold hemorrhages (exposure to freezing ambient temperatures)
Dental chair hemorrhages
Intracranial operations on the fifth cranial nerve
Stereotactic treatment of the fifth cranial nerve for trigeminal neuralgia
Carotid endarterectomy (reflex hypertension and reperfusion)
Cardiac transplantation, especially in children
Surgical repair of congenital heart disease in children
Migraine

Hypertensive ICH issues from the deep penetrating arteries, so the location parallels the distribution of these arteries. Hematomas develop in the same sites as lacunes, the most frequent being the putamen/internal capsule (30 to 40 percent), caudate nucleus (8 percent), lobar white matter (20 percent), thalamus (15 percent), pons (10 percent), and cerebellum (10 percent).[230] In fatal hematomas, microaneurysms and lipohyalinosis are prevalent in penetrating arteries, but the hematomas obscure findings in the middle of the lesions.[249] Along the outside, circumferentially, fibrin globules represent rupture sites.[249] Arterioles or capillaries rupture in the center of the lesion, suddenly increasing local tissue pressure and leading to pressure on adjacent capillaries, which then rupture. As the hematoma gradually grows on its periphery (Fig. 99-5), local tissue pressure and finally intracranial pressure increase until the hematoma is contained. Alternatively, the pressure is decompressed by the lesion emptying into the ventricular system or into the subarachnoid space on the brain surface.

Clinical Findings

Contrary to popular belief, patients with ICH have a gradual evolution of neurologic signs; symptoms do not begin abruptly, as in SAH.[230] The first neurologic signs are related to the bleeding site; e.g., left putaminal hematoma patients might first notice right arm weakness or numbness, whereas cerebellar hematoma patients stagger and feel off balance. As the hematoma grows, focal signs worsen. When and if the hematoma increases sufficiently in size to increase intracranial pressure, headache, vomiting, and decreased levels of alertness develop.[230] In the presence of small, restricted hemorrhages, headache is absent and the patient remains alert. The course and findings mimic so-called progressing ischemic stroke. Headache is absent or not a very prominent symptom in more than half of the patients with ICH. Loss of consciousness is also not invariable but is a bad prognostic sign when present. Clinical localization of the hematoma rests on an analysis of pupillary responses, eye movements, and the presence and distribution of motor signs.

Diagnosis

CT accurately shows the location, size, shape, and extent of hematomas. Also shown is the presence of ventricular and surface drainage, surrounding edema, and pressure shifts in surrounding tissues. MRI in the patient with an acute hematoma is more difficult to interpret, but old hematomas are more readily shown by imaging hemosiderin-containing cavities. MRI is superior to CT in suggesting arteriovenous malformations and cavernous angiomas. Lumbar puncture is seldom warranted. Atypical location, absence of hypertension, and abnormal vascular echoes on MRI are indications for angiography.

Prognosis and Treatment[230,250]

Coma, increased intracranial pressure, and large hematoma size (>3 cm in one dimension on CT) all indicate a poor prognosis.[250] Ordinarily, severe systemic hypertension should be reduced, but not excessively. The hematoma causes increased intracranial pressure, and the spinal fluid pressure and pressure in the dural sinuses increase pari passu. Patients with ICH can die from raised pressure. In order to perfuse the brain and to maintain the arteriovenous pressure gradient, the systemic arterial pressure must rise. Overzealous reduction of systemic blood pressure may make the patient worse. The patient's state of alertness and neurologic signs should be carefully monitored, together with the blood pressure.

Recent hematomas in the brain lobes, cerebellum, and right putamen are sometimes drained surgically without leaving a major deficit, at times using stereotactic equipment with CT guidance. The indications for drainage are increased pressure and the presence of lesions that require removal (tumor, arteriovenous malformations, aneurysm). When hematomas resolve, they leave a hole disconnecting but not destroying the overlying cortex.

In general, small hematomas resolve well without specific therapy except blood pressure control, whereas massive hematomas usually kill or maim patients before they can be treated. Medium-sized hematomas (2 to 4 cm), which increase pressure and cause worsening signs or decreased consciousness while patients are under observation, are indications for drainage if the hematoma is favorably located.

SUBARACHNOID HEMORRHAGE

SAH is not directly caused by hypertension in most cases, although an abrupt increase in blood pressure (e.g., due to cocaine or amphetamines) can sometimes lead to SAH, as can a bleeding diathesis, trauma, and amyloid angiopathy. The most frequent lesions causing SAH are abnormal vessels such as aneurysms and vascular malformations on or near the surface of the brain. SAH describes bleeding directly into the subarachnoid space with rapid dissemination into the cerebrospinal fluid (CSF) pathways. Usually blood is suddenly released under systemic arterial pressure, causing an abrupt rise in intracranial pressure and producing headache, vomiting, and interruption of conscious behavior and memory, at least temporarily.[251] In some patients, the jet and spread of blood cause neckache, backache, or sciatica instead of headache. Patients are usually agitated and restless or sleepy and have a stiff neck.

The most frequent cause of SAH is leakage from a berry aneurysm. Often there has been a past history of a "warning leak"—that is, a sudden-onset headache unusual for the patient

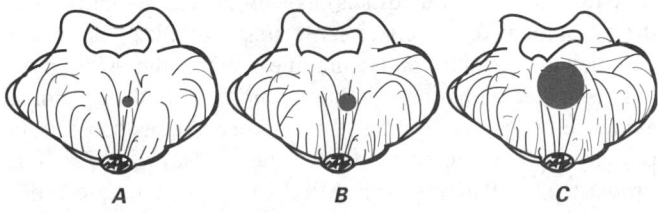

FIGURE 99-5

Gradual evolution of a hypertensive pontine intracerebral hematoma. *A.* The earliest leakage of blood from a paramedian penetrating artery. *B* and *C.* The hematoma has grown. (From Caplan LR, Stein RW. *Stroke: A Clinical Approach.* Boston: Butterworth; 1986, with permission.)

that lasts days and usually prevents normal daily activities.[251,252] Aneurysms are most often located at bifurcations of major intracranial arteries. The commonest sites are the ICA–posterior communicating artery junction, the ACA–anterior communicating artery junction, and the MCA bifurcation. CT can often suggest the site of rupture if blood is pooled locally near a typical site.[253] Large aneurysms are occasionally visible on contrast-enhanced CT or MRI. Lumbar puncture is very important in the diagnosis of SAH.[254] The absence of blood in the CSF effectively excludes the diagnosis of SAH if the fluid is examined within 24 h of the onset of the headache, although bleeds that are very small in volume or older than 72 h can be missed. The CSF pressure, presence of xanthochromia, and quantification of the hemoglobin and bilirubin content of the CSF by spectrophotometry can help establish and date the bleeding and document increased intracranial pressure.[254]

The two most important complications of aneurysmal SAH are rebleeding and brain ischemia due to vasoconstriction (so-called vasospasm). Once an aneurysm has ruptured, either a tiny cap of platelets and fibrin seals the point of rupture or continued bleeding leads to death. Lysis of the fibrin cap initiates rebleeding. Surgical clipping of the aneurysmal sac or obliteration of the aneurysm by endovascular use of balloons or other devices should be attempted before rebleeding occurs.

Vasoconstriction of arteries is thought to be due to blood or blood products that bathe the adventitia of arteries.[255–258] In the presence of a large accumulation of blood, there is a much higher incidence of arterial vasoconstriction and resultant brain ischemia and infarction. Delayed ischemia can also develop postoperatively, as manipulation of vessels can precipitate or potentiate vasoconstriction. The clinical findings in patients with vasoconstriction confirmed by angiography are often those of diffuse brain swelling, such as headache, decreased alertness, and confusion. When vasoconstriction is focal or multifocal, the clinical findings are those of focal ischemia, such as hemiparesis, aphasia, hemianopia, and so on. Vasoconstriction usually has its onset 3 to 5 days after hemorrhage, and the peak time for constriction is days 5 to 9; vasoconstriction usually improves after the second week unless there is rebleeding.[259]

Vasoconstriction has been detected by angiography in 30 to 70 percent of patients with SAH, depending on the timing of the study.[259,260] Severe vasoconstriction is manifested by a lumen size of <0.5 mm, delayed anterograde flow, and evidence of collateral filling distal to the vasoconstricted vessel. TCD is effective in monitoring for the presence of vasoconstriction, which increases blood flow velocities.[261] Single-photon emission computed tomography (SPECT) can also show regions of poor perfusion and document the presence of delayed ischemia.[256]

Many treatments have been tried to prevent or treat vasoconstriction after SAH.[263] These include removal of blood by lumbar puncture or at the time of early surgery; pharmacologic agents such as calcium channel blockers to minimize contraction of the arterial wall; and hypervolemia to prevent ischemia

by maintaining perfusion. At present, the most popular approaches are early surgery, nimodipine (a calcium channel blocker), and hypervolemic therapy, especially after aneurysmal clipping. Hypovolemia is common after SAH, as is hyponatremia. Hypervolemia does not reverse the vasoconstriction but helps maintain brain perfusion.

Coagulopathies

Hypercoagulability and bleeding due to decreased coagulability affect most body organs, including the brain and heart. An increased tendency for clotting can be caused by abnormalities of the formed blood elements or serologic factors.[264–266] Increased numbers of red blood cells and platelets and qualitative abnormalities such as sickle cell disease can cause excess intravascular clotting, especially in the presence of dehydration and reduced plasma volume. Excessive platelet activation, or so-called sticky platelets, can also explain increased coagulability but has proved hard to measure reliably in vitro.[267,268] The level of β-thromboglobulin is a good marker for platelet activation (see also Chap. 52). Serologic abnormalities may be congenital or acquired. Decreased amounts of natural anticoagulants (antithrombin III, protein C, and protein S) and resistance to activated protein C can cause hypercoagulability.[264–266,269] These proteins may be decreased in patients with hypoproteinemia, especially that due to the nephrotic syndrome and urinary protein loss.[261] Fibrinogen levels and the levels of the various coagulation factors such as factors VIII and XI may also be high in patients with a prothrombotic state (see also Chap. 52). In many of these patients—e.g., those on high-dose estrogen birth control pills, pregnant women, and patients with cancer—serologic and standard coagulation tests (in vitro) do not clarify the mechanism of the excessive clotting in vivo. Stroke patients may have serologic evidence of platelet activation and increased fibrin formation but decreased natural fibrinolytic and anticoagulant activity.[266,269]

Recently, measurement of various serum antiphospholipid antibodies has elicited considerable interest. The usually measured substances are the so-called lupus anticoagulant[270–272] and anticardiolipin antibodies. Increased activity of antiphospholipid antibodies (APLA) is found in patients with systemic lupus erythematosus, acquired immunodeficiency syndrome (AIDS), giant cell arteritis, and Sneddon's syndrome[276] (livedo reticularis and strokes) as well as in association with the use of many drugs (e.g., phenytoin, phenothiazines, procainamide, hydralazine, and quinidine). When the APLAs are not associated with other conditions and the patient has clinical evidence of excess clotting, the disorder is considered to be primary and is referred to as the *primary APLA syndrome*.[277–279] Patients with APLAs have an increased incidence of spontaneous abortions, venous occlusive disease of the legs and pulmonary embolism, brain infarcts (often multiple), thrombocytopenia, and false-positive syphilis serologic tests. Some older patients with APLAs also have important risk factors for stroke.[276–279]

Patients with systemic illnesses often have elevated erythrocyte sedimentation rates, and strokes and pulmonary emboli often follow and complicate myocardial infarction (see Chap. 47). Customarily, such brain infarcts have been attributed to cardiogenic embolism, but some undoubtedly are secondary thromboses precipitated by increased levels of acute-phase reactant coagulation proteins. Cancer, especially mucinous adenocarcinoma, has been associated with multiple vascular occlusions, large and tiny brain infarcts, and venous and arterial occlusions.[280]

Deficient coagulability can lead to serious intracranial bleeding. The hemorrhage can be into the brain (ICH), CSF (SAH), or the subdural and epidural compartments. Thrombocytopenia, hemophilia, and leukemia are common conditions leading to intracranial hemorrhage. The most common iatrogenic cause of bleeding is anticoagulation with heparin or warfarin.[230,281] Brain hemorrhage has also been described after fibrinolytic treatment of patients with coronary artery disease[282,283] and after rt-PA infusion to treat cerebrovascular occlusive disease (see also Chaps. 47 and 52).

Anticoagulant-related ICH, which is often a catastrophic complication with high morbidity and mortality, is relatively rare considering the frequency of anticoagulant use. Anticoagulant-related hemorrhages develop more insidiously and evolve more slowly and more often than do other causes of ICH.[281] Many are erroneously attributed to brain ischemia, especially if anticoagulants had been prescribed to treat TIAs. Any patient taking anticoagulants who develops CNS symptoms should be considered to have anticoagulant-related ICH until CT or MRI excludes the diagnosis. The hematoma grows slowly and insidiously increases intracranial pressure. Many patients require surgical drainage of their hematomas to ensure survival. Anticoagulants should be stopped immediately and their effect reversed by fresh frozen plasma or vitamin K. It is probably safe to resume anticoagulation 10 days to 2 weeks after the ICH if indicated—e.g., for prophylaxis in patients with artificial heart valves.[284] In patients treated with fibrinolytic agents, hemorrhages are most often lobar or cerebellar and may be multiple. ICH may be more common when there is a past stroke, when heparin or other agents that affect coagulation are given with or after fibrinolytic agents, and when there is a hemostatic defect secondary to treatment.[230,282,283]

Arterial Dissections

Aortic dissections involving the innominate or carotid arteries (Chap. 98) are a well-known cause of stroke or other manifestations of cerebral ischemia. Less well known are the syndromes produced by dissections of the extracranial and intracranial arteries, which are especially likely to occur in young, active individuals without risk factors for atherosclerosis or stroke but after trauma or chiropractic or other neck manipulations. They are also associated with fibromuscular dysplasia, Marfan's syndrome, pseudoxanthoma elasticum, and migraine.

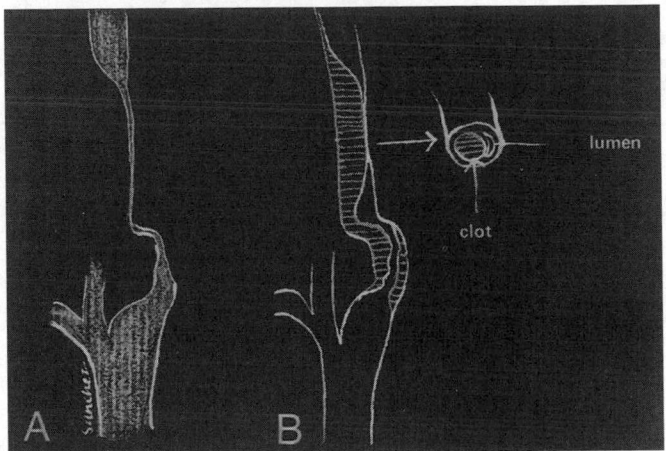

FIGURE 99-6

Diagrams of a carotid artery dissection. *A.* The lumen encroached upon by the intramural clot. *B.* The dissection (*cross-hatched*). (From Caplan LR, Stein RW. *Stroke: A Clinical Approach.* Boston: Butterworth; 1986, with permission.)

Dissection starts with a tear in the media and spread longitudinally (Fig. 99-6), often disrupting adventitial fibers or even rupturing through the adventitia to produce an extravascular hematoma and a false or pseudoaneurysm within muscle and connective tissue. Intracranially, such a rupture can produce SAH. Other dissections cause arterial obstruction and secondary thrombosis of the narrowed vascular lumen. Most recognized cerebrovascular dissections occur in the extracranial vessels, particularly the pharyngeal portion of the internal carotid artery or the nuchal vertebral arteries.[285-289]

Extracranial dissections produce sharp pain and throbbing headache; brain and retinal ischemic episodes, which may occur in rapid-fire attacks ("carotid allegro"[290]); and pressure on adjacent structures. Strokes, usually from embolization of clots, are common but often have a benign course. Intracranial dissections have a poorer prognosis, often with vascular rupture and SAH.

The diagnosis is confirmed by angiography, CT, or MRI. Ultrasound studies can be helpful in suggesting the diagnosis of dissection in the neck.[291]

Treatment consists of the use of heparin acutely, followed by warfarin for 6 to 12 weeks to prevent intraarterial thrombus and peripheral embolism. Intracranial dissections with SAH have been treated surgically.[286,292,293] Surgery on extracranial dissections has also been performed, but the results are not better than medical management.

REFERENCES

1. Aring C, Merritt H. Differential diagnosis between cerebral hemorrhage and cerebral thrombosis. *Arch Intern Med* 1935; 56:435–456.
2. Whisnant J, Fitzgibbons J, Kurland L, Sayre GP. Natural history of stroke in Rochester, Minnesota 1945–1954. *Stroke* 1971; 2:11–22.
3. Matsumoto N, Whisnant J, Kurland L, Okazaki H. Natural history of stroke in Rochester, Minnesota 1955–1969. *Stroke* 1973; 4:2–29.
4. Mohr J, Caplan LR, Melski J, Duncan G, Goldstein R, Kistler JP, et

al. The Harvard Cooperative Stroke registry: A prospective study. *Neurology* 1978; 28:754–762.

5. Caplan LR, Hier D, D'Cruz I. Cerebral embolism in the Michael Reese Stroke Registry. *Stroke* 1983; 14:530–536.

6. Foulkes MA, Wolf PA, Price TR, Mohr JP, Hier DB. The Stroke Data Bank: Design, methods, and baseline characteristics. *Stroke* 1988; 19:547–554.

7. Bogousslavsky J, Van Melle G, Regli F. The Lausanne Stroke Registry: Analysis of 1000 consecutive patients with first strokes. *Stroke* 1988; 19:1083–1092.

8. Kunitz S, Gross C, Heyman A, Kase C, Mohr JP, Price TP, et al. The Pilot Stroke Data Bank: Definition, design and data. *Stroke* 1984; 15:740–746.

9. Bogousslavsky J, Cachin C, Regli F, Despland PA, Van Melle G, Kappenberger L. Cardiac sources of embolism and cerebral infarction—clinical consequences and vascular concomitants: The Lausanne Stroke Registry. *Neurology* 1991; 41:855–859.

10. Halperin J, Hart RG. Atrial fibrillation and strokes: New ideas, persisting dilemmas. *Stroke* 1988; 19:937–941.

11. Caplan LR. Of birds and nests and brain emboli. *Rev Neurol (Paris)* 1991; 147:265–273.

12. Kittner SJ, Sharkness CM, Sloan M, Price TR, Dambrosia JM, Tuhrim S, et al. Infarcts with a cardiac source of embolism in the NINDS Stroke Data Bank: Neurologic examination. *Neurology* 1992; 42:299–302.

13. Barnett HJM, Jones MW, Boughner DR, Kostuk WJ. Cerebral ischemic events associated with prolapsing mitral valve. *Arch Neurol* 1976; 33:777–782.

14. Barnett HJM, Boughner DR, Taylor DW, Cooper PE, Kostuk WJ, Nichol PM. Further evidence relating mitral valve prolapse to cerebral ischemic events. *N Engl J Med* 1980; 302:139–144.

15. Sandok BA, Giuliani ER. Cerebral ischemic events in patients with mitral valve prolapse. *Stroke* 1982; 13:448–450.

16. Lauzier S, Barnett HJM. Cerebral ischemia with mitral valve prolapse and mitral annulus calcification. In: Furlan AJ, ed. *The Heart and Stroke*. London: Springer-Verlag; 1987:63–100.

17. Pomerance A. Ballooning deformity (mucoid degeneration) of atrioventricular valves. *Br Heart J* 1969; 31:343–351.

18. Pomerance A, Davies MJ. Strokes: A complication of mitral leaflet prolapse. *Lancet* 1977; 2:1186.

19. Kostuk WJ, Boughner DR, Barnett HJM, Silver MD. Strokes: A complication of mitral-leaflet prolapse. *Lancet* 1977; 2:313–316.

20. Hanson MR, Conomy JP, Hodgman JR. Brain events associated with mitral valve prolapse. *Stroke* 1980; 11:499–506.

21. Jones HR, Naggar CZ, Selyan MP, Downing ZZ. Mitral valve prolapse and cerebral ischemic events: A comparison between a neurology population with stroke and a cardiology population with mitral valve prolapse observed for 5 years. *Stroke* 1982; 13:451–453.

22. Pomerance A. Pathological and clinical study of calcification in the mitral valve ring. *J Clin Pathol* 1970; 23:354–361.

23. Stein JH, Soble JS. Thrombus associated with mitral valve calcification. *Stroke* 1995; 26:1697–1699.

24. Fulkerson PK, Beaver BM, Auseon JC, Graven HL. Calcification of the mitral annulus—etiology, clinical associations, complications and therapy. *Am J Med* 1979; 66:967–977.

25. deBono DP, Warlow CP. Mitral-annulus calcification and cerebral or retinal ischemia. *Lancet* 1979; 2:383–385.

26. Korn D, DeSanctis RW, Sell S. Massive calcification of the mitral annulus. A clinicopathological study of fourteen cases. *N Engl J Med* 1962; 267:900–909.

27. Benjamin EJ, Plehn JF, D'Agostino RB, Belanger AJ, Comai K, Fuller DL, et al. Mitral annular calcification and the risk of stroke in an elderly cohort. *N Engl J Med* 1992; 327:374–379.

28. Sacco RL, Ellenberg JH, Mohr JP, Tatemichi T, Hier DB, Price TR, et al. Infarcts of undetermined cause: The NINCDS Stroke Data Bank. *Ann Neurol* 1989; 25:382–390.

29. Mohr JP. Infarct of unclear cause. In: Furlan AJ, ed. *The Heart and Stroke*. London: Springer-Verlag; 1987:101–116.

30. Galve E, Candell-Riera J, Pigrau C, Permanyu-Miralda G, Garcia del Castillo H, Soler-Soler J. Prevalence, morphology, types and evaluation of cardiac valvular disease in systemic lupus erythematosus. *N Engl J Med* 1988; 319:817–823.

31. Barbut D, Borer JS, Wallerson D, Ameisen O, Lockshin M. Anticardiolipin antibody and stroke: Possible relation of valvular heart disease and embolic events. *Cardiology* 1991; 79:99–109.

32. Kanter MC, Hart RG. Neurologic complications of infective endocarditis. *Neurology* 1991; 41:1015–1020.

33. Amarenco P, Duyckaerts C, Tzourio C, Henin D, Bousser M-G, Hauw JJ. The prevalence of ulcerated plaques in the aortic arch in patients with stroke. *N Engl J Med* 1992; 326:221–225.

34. Amarenco P, Cohan A, Baudrimont M, Bousser M-G. Transesophageal echocardiographic detection of aortic arch disease in patients with cerebral infarction. *Stroke* 1992; 23:1056–1061.

35. The French Study of Aortic Plaques in Stroke Group. Atherosclerotic disease of the aortic arch as a risk factor for recurrent ischemic stroke. *N Engl J Med* 1996; 334:1216–1221.

36. Gacs G, Merel MD, Bodosi M. Balloon catheter as a model of cerebral emboli in humans. *Stroke* 1982; 13:39–42.

37. Fisher CM. Left hemiplegia and motor impersistence. *J Nerv Ment Dis* 1956; 123:201–218.

38. Caplan LR, Kelly M, Kase CS, Hier DB, White JL, Tatemichi T, et al. Infarcts of the inferior division of the right middle cerebral artery: Mirror image of Wernicke's aphasia. *Neurology* 1986; 36:1015–1020.

39. Caplan LR. Posterior cerebral artery. In: Bogousslavsky J, Caplan LR. *Stroke Syndromes*. New York: Cambridge University Press; 1995:290–299.

40. Caplan LR. *Posterior Circulation Vascular Disease: Clinical Findings, Diagnosis, and Management*. Boston: Blackwell Science; 1996.

41. Pessin MS, Lathi E, Cohen MB, Kwan E, Hedges TR, Caplan LR. Clinical features and mechanisms of occipital infarction in the posterior cerebral artery territory. *Ann Neurol* 1987; 21:290–299.

42. Caplan LR. Top of the basilar syndrome: Selected clinical aspects. *Neurology* 1980; 30:72–79.

43. Mehler MF. The rostral basilar artery syndrome: Diagnosis, etiology, prognosis. *Neurology* 1989; 39:9–16.

44. Amarenco P. The spectrum of cerebellar infarctions. *Neurology* 1991; 41:973–979.

45. Fisher CM, Perlman A. The nonsudden onset of a cerebral embolism. *Neurology* 1967; 17:1025–1032.

46. Fieschi C, Argentino C, Lenzi GL, Sacchetti ML, Toni D, Bozzao L. Clinical and instrumental evaluation of patients with ischemic stroke within the first six hours. *J Neurol Sci* 1989; 91:311–322.

47. Kushner MJ, Zanotte EM, Bastianiello S, Mancini G, Sachetti M, Carolei A, et al. Transcranial Doppler in acute hemispheric brain infarction. *Neurology* 1991; 41:109–113.

48. Ringlestein EB, Koschorke S, Holling A, Thron A, Lambertz H, Minale C. Computed tomographic patterns of proven embolic brain infarcts. *Ann Neurol* 1989; 26:759–765.

49. Bladin PF, Berkovic SF. Striatocapsular infarction. *Neurology* 1984; 34:1423–1430.

50. Fisher CM, Adams RD. Observations on brain embolism. *J Neuropathol Exp Neurol* 1951; 10:92–94.

51. Fisher CM, Adams RD. Observations on brain embolism with special reference to hemorrhagic infarction. In: Furlan AJ, ed. *The Heart and Stroke*. London: Springer-Verlag; 1987:17–36.

52. Gacs G, Fox AJ, Barnett HJ, Vinuela F. CT visualization of intracranial arterial thromboembolism. *Stroke* 1983; 14:756–763.

53. Tomsick T, Brott T, Barsan W, Broderick J, Haley C, Levy D, et al. Thrombus localization with emergency cerebral computed tomography. *Stroke* 1990; 21:180.

54. Bergeron GA, Shah PM. Echocardiography unwarranted in patients with cerebral ischemic events. *N Engl J Med* 1981; 304:489.

55. Greenland P, Knopman D, Mikell F, Asinger R, Anderson D, Good D. Echocardiography in diagnostic assessment of stroke. *Ann Intern Med* 1981; 95:51–54.

56. Donaldson R, Emmanuel R, Earl C. The role of two-dimensional echocardiography in the detection of potentially embolic intracardiac masses in patients with cerebral ischemia. *J Neurol Neurosurg Psychiatry* 1981; 44:803–809.

57. Tegeler CH, Downes TR. Cardiac imaging in stroke. *Stroke* 1991; 22:1206–1211.

58. Pop G, Sutherland GR, Koudstaal PJ, Sit TW, de Jong G, Roelandt JR. Transesophageal echocardiography in the detection of intracardiac embolic sources in patients with transient ischemic attacks. *Stroke* 1990; 21:560–565.

59. Zenker G, Ecbel R, Kramer G, Mohr-Kahaly S, Drexler M, Harnoncourt K, et al. Transesophageal echocardiography in young patients with cerebral ischemic events. *Stroke* 1988; 19:345–348.

60. Cohen A, Chauvel C. Transesophageal echocardiography in the man-

agement of transient ischemic attack and ischemic stroke. *Cerebrovasc Dis* 1996; 6(suppl 1):15–25.

61. Yasaka M, Yamaguchi T, Miyashita T, Park YO, Sawada T, Omae T. Predisposing factors of recurrent embolization in cardiogenic cerebral embolism. *Stroke* 1990; 21:1000–1007.

62. DeWitt LD, Pessin MS, Pandian NG, Pauker SG, Sonnenberg FA, Caplan LR. Benign disappearance of ventricular thrombus after embolic stroke: A case report. *Stroke* 1988; 19:393–396.

63. Ezekowitz MD, Wilson DA, Smith EO, Burow RD, Harrison L, Parker D, et al. Comparison of indium-III platelet scintigraphy and two-dimensional echocardiography in the diagnosis of left ventricular thrombi. *N Engl J Med* 1982; 306:1509–1513.

64. Markus HS, Droste DW, Brown MM. Detection of symptomatic cerebral embolic signals with Doppler ultrasound. *Lancet* 1994; 343:1011–1012.

65. Markus HS, Harrison MJ. Microembolic signal detection using ultrasound. *Stroke* 1995; 26:1517–1519.

66. Tong DC, Bolger A, Albers GW. Incidence of transcranial Doppler-detected cerebral microemboli in patients referred for echocardiography. *Stroke* 1994; 25:2138–2141.

67. Barbut D, Hinton RB, Szatrowski TP, Hartman GS, Bruefach M, Williams-Russo P, et al. Cerebral emboli detected during bypass surgery are associated with clamp removal. *Stroke* 1994; 25:2398–2402.

68. Nabavi DG, Georgiadis D, Mumme T, Schmid C, Mackay TG, Scheld HH, et al. Clinical relevance of intracranial microembolic signals in patients with left ventricular assist devices: A prospective study. *Stroke* 1996; 27:891–896.

69. Petersen P, Boyscn G, Godtfredsen J, Andersen ED, Andersen B. Placebo-controlled, randomized trial of warfarin and aspirin for prevention of thromboembolic complications in chronic atrial fibrillation: The Copenhagen AFASAK Study. *Lancet* 1989; 1:175–179.

70. Stroke Prevention in Atrial Fibrillation Study Group Investigators. Preliminary report of the Stroke Prevention in Atrial Fibrillation Study. *N Engl J Med* 1990; 322:863–868.

71. Chesebro JH, Fuster V, Halperin J. Atrial fibrillation—risk marker for stroke. *N Engl J Med* 1990; 323:1556–1558.

72. The Boston Area Anticoagulation Trial for Atrial Fibrillation Investigators. The effect of low-dose warfarin on the risk of stroke in patients with nonrheumatic atrial fibrillation. *N Engl J Med* 1990; 323:1505–1511.

73. Cairns JA, Connolly SJ. Nonrheumatic atrial fibrillation: Risk of stroke and role of antithrombotic therapy. *Circulation* 1991; 84:469–481.

74. Stroke Prevention in Atrial Fibrillation Investigators: The stroke prevention in atrial fibrillation trial: Final results. *Circulation* 1991; 84:527–539.

75. Connolly SJ, Laupacis A, Gent M, Roberts RS, Cairns JA, Joyner C. Canadian Atrial Fibrillation Anticoagulation (CAFA) study. *J Am Coll Cardiol* 1991; 18:349–355.

76. The Stroke Prevention in Atrial Fibrillation Investigators. Predictors of thromboembolism in atrial fibrillation: I. Clinical features of patients at risk. *Ann Intern Med* 1992; 116:1–5.

77. The Stroke Prevention in Atrial Fibrillation Investigators. Predictors of thromboembolism in atrial fibrillation: II. Echocardiographic features of patients at risk. *Ann Intern Med* 1992; 116:6–12.

78. Pritchett ELC. Management of atrial fibrillation. *N Engl J Med* 1992; 326:1264–1271.

79. Ezekowitz MD, Bridgers SL, James KE, Carliner NH, Colling CL, Gornick CC, et al. Randomized trials of warfarin for atrial fibrillation. *N Engl J Med* 1992; 327:1451–1453.

80. Moldveen-Geronimus M, Merriam JC. Cholesterol embolization: From pathologic curiosity to clinical entity. *Circulation* 1967; 35:946–953.

81. Shields RW Jr, Laureno R, Lachman T, Victor M. Anticoagulant-related hemorrhage in acute cerebral embolism. *Stroke* 1984; 15:426–437.

82. Lieberman A, Hass WK, Pinto R, Isom W, Kupersmith M, Bear G, et al. Intracranial hemorrhage and infarction in anticoagulated patients with prosthetic heart valves. *Stroke* 1978; 9:18–24.

83. Drake ME, Shin C. Conversion of ischemic to hemorrhagic infarction by anticoagulant administration: Report of two cases with evidence from serial computed tomographic brain scans. *Arch Neurol* 1983; 40:44–46.

84. Cerebral Embolism Study Group. Immediate anticoagulation of embolic stroke: A randomized trial. *Stroke* 1983; 13:668–676.

85. Toni D, Fiorelli M, Bastianello S, Sacchetti ML, Sette G, Argentino C, et al. Hemorrhagic transformation of brain infarct. *Neurology* 1996; 46:341–345.

86. Cerebral Embolism Task Force. Cardiogenic brain embolism. *Arch Neurol* 1986; 43:71–84.

87. Cerebral Embolism Task Force. Cardiogenic brain embolism: The second report of the Cerebral Embolism Task Force. *Arch Neurol* 1989; 46:727–743.

88. Pessin MS, Estol CJ, Lafranchise F, Caplan LR. Safety of anticoagulation after hemorrhagic infarction. *Neurology* 1993; 43:1298–1303.

89. Chaves CJ, Pessin MS, Caplan LR, Chung C-S, Amarenco P, Breen J, et al. Cerebellar hemorrhagic infarction. *Neurology* 1996; 46:346–349.

90. Brierley J, Meldrum B, Brown A. The threshold and neuropathology of cerebral "anoxic-ischemic" cell change. *Arch Neurol* 1973; 29:367–373.

91. Brierley JB, Adams JH, Graham DI, Simpson JA. Neurocortical death after cardiac arrest: A clinical, neurophysiological report of two cases. *Lancet* 1971; 2:560–565.

92. Dougherty JH, Rawlinson DG, Levy DE, Plum F. Hypoxic-ischemic brain injury and the vegetative state: Clinical and neuropathologic correlation. *Neurology* 1981; 31:991–997.

93. Cummings JL, Tomiyasu U, Read S, Benson DF. Amnesia with hippocampal lesions after cardiopulmonary arrest. *Neurology* 1984; 34:679–681.

94. Dooling E, Richardson EP. Delayed encephalopathy after strangling. *Arch Neurol* 1976; 33:196–199.

95. Lance J, Adams RD. The syndrome of intention and action myoclonus as a sequel to hypoxic encephalopathy. *Brain* 1963; 86:111–133.

96. Gilles F. Hypotensive brainstem necrosis. *Arch Pathol* 1969; 88:32–41.

97. Silver JR, Buxton PH. Spinal stroke. *Brain* 1974; 97:539–550.

98. Caronna JJ, Finkelstein S. Neurological syndromes after cardiac arrest. *Stroke* 1978; 9:517–520.

99. Jennett B, Plum F. Persistent vegetative state after brain damage: A syndrome in search of a name. *Lancet* 1972; 1:734–737.

100. Levy DE, Knill-Jones RP, Plum F. The vegetative state and its prognosis following non-traumatic coma. *Ann NY Acad Sci* 1978; 315:293–306.

101. Hecaen H, Ajuriaguerra J. Balint's syndrome and its minor forms. *Brain* 1954; 77:373–400.

102. Sherwin I, Redman W. Successful treatment in action myoclonus. *Neurology* 1969; 19:846–850.

103. Willoughby J, Leach B. Relation of neurological findings after cardiac arrest to outcome. *Br Med J* 1974; 3:437–439.

104. Plum F, Caronna J. Can one predict outcome of medical coma? In: *Outcome of Severe Damage to the Central Nervous System. A CIBA Foundation Symposium.* New York: Elsevier; 1975:121–139.

105. Bell JA, Hodgson HJ. Coma after cardiac arrest. *Brain* 1974; 97:361–372.

106. Levy D, Carrona JJ, Singer BH, Lapinski RH, Frydman H, Plum F. Predicting outcome from hypoxic-ischemic coma. *JAMA* 1985; 253:1420–1426.

107. Longstreth WT, Inui TS, Cobb LA, Copass MK. Neurologic recovery after out-of-hospital cardiac arrest. *Ann Intern Med* 1983; 38:588–592.

108. Longstreth WT, Diehr P, Inui TS. Prediction of awakening after out-of-hospital cardiac arrest. *N Engl J Med* 1983; 308:1378–1382.

109. Thompson RG, Hallstrom AP, Cobb LA. Bystander-initiated cardiopulmonary resuscitation in the management of ventricular fibrillation. *Ann Intern Med* 1979; 90:737–740.

110. Bedell SE, Delbanco TG, Cook EF, Epstein FH. Survival after cardiopulmonary resuscitation in the hospital. *N Engl J Med* 1983; 309:569–576.

111. Caplan LR, Brass LM, DeWitt LD, Adams RJ, Gomez C, Otis S, et al. Transcranial Doppler ultrasound: Present status. *Neurology* 1990; 40:696–700.

112. Kirkham F, Levin S, Padayachee T, Kyme M, Neville B, Gosling R. Transcranial pulsed Doppler ultrasound findings in brainstem death. *J Neurol Neurosurg Psychiatry* 1987; 50:1504–1513.

113. Ropper A, Kehne S, Wechsler L. Transcranial Doppler in brain death. *Neurology* 1987; 37:1733–1735.

114. Longstreth WT, Inui TS. High blood glucose level on hospital admission and poor neurological recovery after cardiac arrest. *Ann Neurol* 1984; 15:59–63.

115. Myers C, Yamaguchi S. Nervous system effects of cardiac arrest in monkeys. *Arch Neurol* 1977; 34:65–74.

116. Plum F. What causes infarction in ischemic brain. *Neurology* 1983; 33:222–233.

117. Collins RC, Dobkin BH, Choi DW. Selective vulnerability of the brain: New insights into the pathophysiology of stroke. *Ann Intern Med* 1989; 110:992–1000.

118. Albers G, Goldberg M, Choi D. N-methyl-D-aspartate antagonists: Ready for clinical trial in brain ischemia? *Ann Neurol* 1989; 25:398–403.

119. Giswold S, Safar P, Rao G, Moosy J, Kelsey S, Alexander H. Multifaceted therapy after global brain ischemia in monkeys. *Stroke* 1984; 15:803–812.

120. Volpe BT, Soave R. Formal visual hallucinations as digitalis toxicity. *Ann Intern Med* 1979; 91:868–869.

121. Closson RG. Visual hallucinations as the earliest symptom of digoxin intoxication. *Arch Neurol* 1983; 40:386.

122. Gilbert GJ. Quinidine dementia. *JAMA* 1977; 237:2093–2094.

123. Slogoff S, Girgis KZ, Keats AS. Etiologic factors in neuropsychiatric complications associated with cardiopulmonary bypass. *Anesth Analg* 1982; 61:903–911.

124. Gilman S. Neurological complications of open heart surgery. *Ann Neurol* 1990; 28:475–476.

125. Shaw PJ, Bates D, Cartlidge NEF, Heaviside D, Julian DG, Shaw DA. Early neurological complications of coronary artery bypass surgery. *Br Med J* 1985; 291:1384–1387.

126. Breuer AC, Furlan AJ, Hanson MR, Lederman RJ, Loop FD, Cosgrove DM. Central nervous system complications of coronary artery bypass graft surgery: Prospective analysis of 421 patients. *Stroke* 1983: 14:682–687.

127. Ropper AH, Wechsler LR, Wilson LS. Carotid bruit and the risk of stroke in elective surgery. *N Engl J Med* 1982; 307:1388–1390.

128. Furlan AJ, Craciun AR. Risk of stroke during coronary artery bypass graft surgery in patients with internal carotid artery disease documented by angiography. *Stroke* 1985; 16:797–799.

129. Sila C. Neuroimaging of cerebral infarction associated with coronary revascularization. *AJNR* 1991; 12:817–818.

130. Hertzer NR, Loop FD, Beven EG, O'Hara PJ, Krajewski LP. Surgical staging for simultaneous coronary and carotid disease: A study including prospective randomization. *Vasc Surg* 1989; 9:455–463.

131. VonReutern G-M, Hetzel A, Birnbaum D, Schlosser V. Transcranial Doppler ultrasound during cardiopulmonary bypass in patients with internal carotid artery disease documented by angiography. *Stroke* 1988; 19:674–680.

132. Hise JH, Nippu ML, Schnitker JC. Stroke associated with coronary artery bypass surgery. *AJNR* 1991; 12:811–814.

133. Wijdicks EFM, Jack CR. Coronary artery bypass grafting-associated stroke. *J Neuroimag* 1996; 6:20–22.

134. Tettenborn B, Caplan LR, Sloan MA, et al. Postoperative brainstem cerebellar infarcts. *Neurology* 1993; 43:471–477.

135. Barbut D, Hinton RB, Szatrowski TP, Hartman GS, Bruefach M, Williams-Russo P, et al. Cerebral emboli detected during bypass surgery are associated with clamp removal. *Stroke* 1994; 25:2398–2402.

136. Pugsley W, Paschalis C, Treasure T, Harrison M, Newman S. The impact of microemboli during cardiopulmonary bypass on neuropsychological functioning. *Stroke* 1994; 25:1393–1399.

137. Price DL, Harris J. Cholesterol emboli in cerebral arteries are a complication of retrograde aortic perfusion during cardiac surgery. *Neurology* 1970; 20:1207–1214.

138. Tunick PA, Culliford AT, Lamparello PJ, Kronzon I. Atheromatosis of the aortic arch as an occult source of multiple systemic emboli. *Ann Intern Med* 1991; 114:391–392.

139. Karalis DG, Chandrasekaran K, Victor MF, Ross JJ, Mintz GS. Recognition and embolic potential of intraaortic atherosclerotic debris. *J Am Coll Cardiol* 1991; 17:73–78.

140. Marshall JNG, Barzilai B, Kouchoukos N, Saffitz J. Intraoperative ultrasonic imaging of the ascending aorta. *Ann Thorac Surg* 1989; 48:339–344.

141. Gardner TJ, Horneffer PJ, Manolio TA, Pearson TA, Gott VL, Baumgartner WA, et al. Stroke following coronary artery bypass grafting: A ten-year study. *Ann Thorac Surg* 1985; 40:574–581.

142. Gilman S. Cerebral disorders after open-heart operations. *N Engl J Med* 1965; 272:489–498.

143. Coffey CE, Massey EW, Roberts KB, Curtis S, Jones RH, Pryor DB. Natural history of cerebral complications of coronary artery bypass graft surgery. *Neurology* 1983; 33:1416–1421.

144. Moody DM, Bell MA, Challa VR, Johnston WE, Prough DS. Brain microemboli during cardiac surgery or aortography. *Ann Neurol* 1990; 28:477–486.

145. Feeney DM, Gonzalez A, Law WA. Amphetamine, haloperidol and experience interact to affect the rate of recovery after motor cortex injury. *Science* 1982; 217:855–857.

146. Houda DA, Feeney DM. Haloperidol blocks amphetamine induced recovery of binocular depth perception after bilateral visual cortex lesions in the cat. *Proc West Pharmacol Soc* 1985; 28:209–211.

147. Humphreys RP, Hoffman JH, Mustard WT, Trusler GA. Cerebral hemorrhage following heart surgery. *J Neurosurg* 1975; 43:671–675.

148. Sila CA. Spectrum of neurologic events following cardiac transplantation. *Stroke* 1989; 20:1586–1589.

149. Caplan LR. Intracerebral hemorrhage revisited. *Neurology* 1988; 38:624–627.

150. Lederman RJ, Breuer AC, Hanson MR, Furlan AJ, Loop FD, Cosgrove D, et al. Peripheral nervous system complications of coronary artery bypass graft surgery. *Ann Neurol* 1982; 12:297–301.

151. Natelson BH. Neurocardiology: An interdisciplinary area for the 80's. *Arch Neurol* 1985; 42:178–184.

152. Schlesinger MJ, Reiner L. Focal myocytolysis of heart. *Am J Pathol* 1955; 31:443–459.

153. Norris JW, Hachinski V. Cardiac dysfunction following stroke. In: Furlan AJ, ed. *The Heart and Stroke*. London: Springer-Verlag; 1987: 171–183.

154. Smith RP, Tomlinson BE. Subendocardial hemorrhages associated with intracranial lesions. *J Pathol Bacteriol* 1954; 68:327–334.

155. Cropp GJ, Manning GW. Electrocardiographic changes stimulating myocardial ischemia and infarction associated with spontaneous intracranial hemorrhage. *Circulation* 1960; 22:25–38.

156. Kolin A, Norris JW. Myocardial damage from acute cerebral lesions. *Stroke* 1984; 15:990–993.

157. Samuels MA. Electrocardiographic manifestations of neurologic disease. *Semin Neurol* 1984; 4:453–459.

158. Myers MG, Norris JW, Hachinski V, Sole MJ. Plasma norepinephrine in stroke. *Stroke* 1981; 12:200–204.

159. Marion DW, Segal R, Thompson ME. Subarachnoid hemorrhage and the heart. *Rev Neurosurg* 1986; 18:101–106.

160. Haggendal J, Johansson G, Jonsson L, Thoren-Tolling K. Effect of propranolol on myocardial cell necrosis and blood levels of catecholamines in pigs subjected to stress. *Acta Pharmacol Toxicol* 1982; 50:58–66.

161. Hunt D, Gore J. Myocardial lesions following experimental intracranial hemorrhage. *Am Heart J* 1972; 83:232–236.

162. Burch GE, Myers R, Abildskov JA. A new electrocardiographic pattern observed in cerebrovascular accidents. *Circulation* 1954; 9:719–723.

163. Dimant J, Grob D. Electrocardiographic changes and myocardial damage in patients with acute cerebrovascular accidents. *Stroke* 1977; 8:448–455.

164. Rolak LA, Rokey R. Electrocardiographic features: In: Rolak LA, Rokey R, eds. *Coronary and Cerebral Vascular Disease*. Mt. Kisco, NY: Futura; 1990:139–197.

165. Goldstein DS. The electrocardiogram in stroke: Relationship to pathophysiological type and comparison with prior tracings. *Stroke* 1979; 10:253–259.

166. Puleo P. Cardiac enzyme assessment. In: Rolak L, Rokey R, eds. *Coronary and Cerebral Vascular Disease*. Mt. Kisco, NY: Futura; 1990;199–216.

167. Fabinyi G, Hunt D, McKinley L. Myocardial creatine kinase isoenzyme in serum after subarachnoid hemorrhage. *J Neurol Neurosurg Psychiatry* 1977; 40:818–820.

168. Neil-Dwyer G, Cruickshank J, Stratton C. Beta-blockers, plasma total creatine kinase and creatine kinase myocardial isoenzyme, and the prognosis of subarachnoid hemorrhage. *Surg Neurol* 1986; 25:163–168.

169. Myers MG, Norris JW, Hachinsky VC, Weingert ME, Sole MJ. Cardiac sequelae of acute strokes. *Stroke* 1982; 13:838–842.

170. Stober T, Sen S, Anstatt T, Bette L. Correlation of cardiac arrhythmias with brainstem compression in patients with intracerebral hemorrhage. *Stroke* 1988; 19:688–692.

171. Hoff JT, Nishimura M. Experimental neurogenic pulmonary edema in cats. *J Neurosurg* 1978; 18:383–389.

172. Wier BK. Pulmonary edema following fatal aneurysmal rupture. *J Neurosurg* 1978; 49:502–507.

173. Theodore J, Robin ED. Pathogenesis of neurogenic pulmonary edema. *Lancet* 1975; 2:749–751.

174. Engel GL. Psychologic factors in instantaneous cardiac death. *N Engl J Med* 1976; 294:664–665.

175. Engel GL. Psychologic stress, vasodepressor (vasovagal) syncope and sudden death. *Ann Intern Med* 1978; 89:403–412.

176. Lown B. Sudden cardiac death: The major challenge confronting contemporary cardiology. *Am J Cardiol* 1979; 43:313–328.

177. Lown B, Temte JV, Reich P, Gaughan C, Registeen Q, Hai H. Basis for recurring ventricular fibrillation in the absence of coronary heart disease and its management. *N Engl J Med* 1976; 294:623–629.

178. Talman WT. Cardiovascular regulation and lesions of the central nervous system. *Ann Neurol* 1985; 18:1–12.

179. Schwartz PJ, Stone HL, Brown AM. Effects of unilateral stellate ganglion blockage on the arrhythmias associated with coronary occlusion. *Am Heart J* 1976; 92:589–599.

180. Adams H, Kassell N, Mazuz H. The patients with transient ischemic attacks. Is this the time for a new therapeutic approach? *Stroke* 1984; 15:371–375.

181. Hennerici M, Aulich A, Sandmann W, Freund HJ. Incidence of asymptomatic extracranial arterial disease. *Stroke* 1981; 12:750–758.

182. Caplan LR. Cerebrovascular disease: Large artery occlusive disease. In: Appel S, ed. *Current Neurology*: vol 87. Chicago: Year Book; 1988:179–226.

183. McMillan DE. Blood flow and the localization of atherosclerotic plaques. *Stroke* 1985; 16:582–587.

184. Zarins CK, Giddins DP, Bharadvaj BK, Sottivrai VS, Mabon R. Carotid bifurcation atherosclerosis. *Circ Res* 1983; 53:502–514.

185. Hutchinson EC, Yates DO. The cervical portion of the vertebral artery: A clinicopathologic study. *Brain* 1956; 79:319–331.

186. Fisher CM, Ojemann RG. A clinico-pathologic study of carotid endarterectomy plaques. *Rev Neurol (Paris)* 1986; 142:573–589.

187. Caplan LR, Gorelick PB, Hier DB. Race, sex, and occlusive vascular disease: A review. *Stroke* 1986; 17:648–655.

188. Gorelick PB, Caplan LR, Hier DB, Patel D, Langenberg P, Pessin MS, et al. Racial differences in the distribution of posterior circulation occlusive disease. *Stroke* 1985; 16:785–790.

189. Gorelick PB, Caplan LR, Hier DB, Patel D, Parker S. Racial differences in the distribution of anterior circulation occlusive cerebrovascular disease. *Neurology* 1984; 34:54–59.

190. Feldmann E, Daneault N, Kwan E, Ho K, Pessin MS, Langenberg P, et al. Chinese-white differences in the distribution of occlusive cerebrovascular disease. *Neurology* 1990; 40:1541–1545.

191. Caplan LR, Wolpert SM. Angiography in patients with occlusive cerebrovascular disease: Views of a stroke neurologist and neuroradiologist. *AJNR* 1991; 12:593–601.

192. Pessin MS, Duncan GW, Mohr JP, Poskanzer DC. Clinical and angiographic features of carotid transient ischemic attacks. *N Engl J Med* 1977; 296:358–362.

193. Chambers BR, Norris JW. Outcome in patients with asymptomatic neck bruits. *N Engl J Med* 1986; 315:860–865.

194. Hennerici M, Hulsbomer HB, Rautenberg W, Hefter H. Spontaneous history of asymptomatic internal carotid occlusion. *Stroke* 1986; 17:718–722.

195. Ringelstein EB, Zeumer H, Angelou D. The pathogenesis of strokes from internal carotid artery occlusion: Diagnostic and therapeutical implications. *Stroke* 1983; 14:867–875.

196. Caplan LR, Tettenborn B. Embolism in the posterior circulation. In: Berguer R, Caplan L, eds. *Vertebrobasilar Arterial Disease*. St Louis: Quality Medical Publishers; 1991; 52–65.

197. Gorelick PB, Hier DB, Caplan LR, Langenberg P. Headache in acute cerebrovascular disease. *Neurology* 1986; 36:1445–1450.

198. Pessin MS, Hinton RC, Davis KR, Duncan G, Roberson G, Ackerman R, et al. Mechanism of acute carotid stroke. *Ann Neurol* 1979; 6:245–252.

199. Caplan LR. TIAs—we need to return to the question, what is wrong with Mr. Jones? *Neurology* 1988; 791–793.

200. Caplan LR. *Stroke: A Clinical Approach*, 2d ed. Boston: Butterworth; 1992:195–271.

201. Hennerici M, Freund H. Efficacy of C-W Doppler and duplex system examinations for the evaluation of extracranial carotid disease. *J Clin Ultrasound* 1984; 12:155–161.

202. O'Donnell TF, Erdoes L, Mackey WC, McCullough J, Shepard A, Heggerick P. Correlation of B-mode ultrasound imaging and arteriography with pathologic findings at carotid endarterectomy. *Arch Surg* 1985; 120:443–449.

203. Zwiebel WJ, Zagzebski JA, Crummy AB, Hirscher M. Correlation of peak Doppler frequency with lumen narrowing in carotid stenosis. *Stroke* 1982; 13:386–391.

204. Hennerici M, Rautenberg W, Sitzer G, Schwartz A. Transcranial Doppler ultrasound for the assessment of intracranial arterial flow velocity: I. Examination technique and normal values. *Surg Neurol* 1986; 315:860–865.

205. Russell D, Madden KP, Clark WM, Sandset PM, Zivin JA. Detection of arterial emboli using Doppler ultrasound in rabbits. *Stroke* 1991; 22:253–258.

206. Spencer MP, Thomas GI, Nicholls SC, Sauvage LR. Detection of middle cerebral artery emboli during carotid endarterectomy using transcranial Doppler ultrasonography. *Stroke* 1990; 21:415–423.

207. Edelman RR, Mattle HP, Atkinson DJ, Hoogewoud HM. MR angiography. *AJR* 1990; 154:937–946.

208. Caplan LR. Treatment of cerebral ischemia: Where are we headed? *Stroke* 1984; 15:571–574.

209. Caplan LR. Are terms such as completed stroke or RIND of continued usefulness? *Stroke* 1983; 14:431–433.

210. North American Symptomatic Carotid Endarterectomy Trial (NASCET) Collaborators. Beneficial effect of carotid endarterectomy in symptomatic patients with high-grade carotid stenosis. *N Engl J Med* 1991; 325:445–453.

211. European Carotid Surgery Trialist's Collaborative Group. MRC European Carotid Surgery Trial: Interim results for symptomatic patients with severe (70–99 percent) or with mild (0–29 percent) carotid stenosis. *Lancet* 1991; 1:1235–1243.

212. Executive Committee for the Asymptomatic Carotid Atherosclerosis Study. Endarterectomy for asymptomatic carotid artery stenosis. *JAMA* 1995; 273:1421–1428.

213. Berguer R, Caplan LR, eds. *Vertebrobasilar Arterial Disease*. St Louis: Quality Medical Publishers; 1991:201–261.

214. Fields WS, Lemak NA, Frankowski RF, Hardy RJ. Controlled trial of aspirin in cerebral ischemia. *Stroke* 1977; 8:301–314.

215. Canadian Cooperative Study Group. A randomized trial of aspirin and sulfinpyrazone in threatened stroke. *N Engl J Med* 1978; 299:53–59.

216. Hass WK, Easton JD, Adams HP, Pryse-Phillips W, Molony BA, Anderson S, et al. A randomized trial comparing ticlopidine hydrochloride with aspirin for the prevention of stroke in high risk patients. *N Engl J Med* 1989; 321:501–507.

217. Warlow CP. Ticlopidine, a new antithrombotic drug: But is it better than aspirin for long term use? *J Neurol Neurosurg Psychiatry* 1990; 53:185–187.

218. The National Institute of Neurological Disorders and Stroke rt-PA Study Group. Tissue plasminogen activator for acute ischemic stroke. *N Engl J Med* 1995; 333:1581–1587.

219. del Zoppo GJ, Poeck K, Pessin MS, Wolpert SM, Furlan AJ, Ferbert A, et al. Recombinant tissue plasminogen activator in acute thrombotic and embolic stroke. *Ann Neurol* 1992; 32:78–86.

220. Wolpert SM, Bruckmann H, Greenlee R, Wechsler L, Pessin MS, del Zoppo GJ, et al. Neuroradiologic evaluation of patients with acute stroke treated with recombinant tissue plasminogen activator. *AJNR* 1993; 14:3–13.

221. Pessin MS, del Zoppo GJ, Furlan AJ. Thrombolytic treatment in acute stroke: Review and update of selected topics. In: Moskowitz MA, Caplan LR, eds. *Cerebrovascular Diseases: Nineteenth Princeton Stroke Conference*. Boston: Butterworth-Heinemann; 1995:409–418.

222. Pettigrew LC. Surgical considerations. In: Rolak L, Rokey R, eds. *Coronary and Cerebral Vascular Disease*. Mt Kisco, NY: Futura; 1990:349–377.

223. Hertzer NR, Loop FD, Beven EG. Management of coexistent carotid and coronary artery disease: A surgical viewpoint. In: Furlan A, ed. *The Heart and Stroke*. London: Springer-Verlag; 1987:305–318.

224. Easton JD, Hart RG. Asymptomatic carotid artery disease in patients undergoing open heart surgery: A neurologic viewpoint. In: Furlan A, ed. *The Heart and Stroke*. London: Springer-Verlag; 1987:319–327.

225. Caplan LR. Intracranial branch atheromatous disease. *Neurology* 1989; 39:1246–1250.

226. Caplan LR. Lacunar infarction: A neglected concept. *Geriatrics* 1976; 31:71–75.

227. Caplan LR. Binswanger's disease revisited. *Neurology* 1995; 45:626–633.

228. Fisher CM. The arterial lesions underlying lacunes. *Acta Neuropathol* 1969; 12:1–15.

229. Fisher CM. Lacunes, small deep cerebral infarcts. *Neurology* 1965; 15:774–784.

230. Kase CS, Caplan LR. *Intracerebral Hemorrhage.* Boston: Butterworth-Heinemann, 1994.

231. Rosenblum WI. Miliary aneurysms and "fibrinoid" degeneration of cerebral blood vessels. *Hum Pathol* 1977; 8:133–139.

232. Cole F, Yates P. Intracerebral microaneurysms and small cerebrovascular lesions. *Brain* 1966; 90:759–767.

233. Fisher CM. Pathological observations in hypertensive cerebral hemorrhage. *J Neuropathol Exp Neurol* 1971; 30:536–550.

234. Fisher CM. Cerebral miliary aneurysms in hypertension. *Am J Pathol* 1972; 66:314–324.

235. Fisher CM, Caplan LR. Basilar artery branch occlusion: A cause of pontine infarction. *Neurology* 1971; 21:900–905.

236. Fisher CM. Bilateral occlusion of basilar artery branches. *J Neurol Neurosurg Psychiatry* 1977; 40:1182–1189.

237. Mohr JP. Lacunes. *Stroke* 1982; 13:3–11.

238. Fisher CM. Lacunar strokes and infarcts: A review. *Neurology* 1982; 32:871–876.

239. Fisher CM. Pure motor hemiplegia of vascular origin. *Arch Neurol* 1965; 13:30–44.

240. Fisher CM. Pure sensory stroke and allied conditions. *Stroke* 1982; 13:434–447.

241. Fisher CW. Ataxic hemiparesis. *Arch Neurol* 1978; 35:126–128.

242. Fisher CM. A lacunar stroke, the dysarthric-clumsy hand syndrome. *Neurology* 1967; 17:614–617.

243. Hachinski VC, Potter P, Merskey H. Leukoaraiosis. *Arch Neurol* 1987; 44:21–23.

244. Caplan LR, Schoene W. Subcortical arteriosclerotic encephalopathy (Binswanger disease): Clinical features. *Neurology* 1978; 28:1206–1219.

245. Babikian V, Ropper AH. Binswanger's disease: A review. *Stroke* 1987; 18:2–12.

246. Kase CS. Intracerebral hemorrhage: Non-hypertensive causes. *Stroke* 1986; 17:590–594.

247. Bahemuka M. Primary intracerebral hemorrhage and heart weight: A clinicopathological case-control review of 218 patients. *Stroke* 1987; 18:531–536.

248. Brott T, Thalinger K, Hertzberg V. Hypertension as a risk factor for spontaneous intracerebral hemorrhage. *Stroke* 1986; 17:1078–1083.

249. Fisher CM. Pathological observations in hypertensive cerebral hemorrhages. *J Neuropathol Exp Neurol* 1971; 30:536–550.

250. Tuhrim S, Dambrosia JM, Price TR, Mohr JP, Wolf PA, Heyman A, et al. Prediction of intracerebral hemorrhage survival. *Ann Neurol* 1988; 24:258–263.

251. Adams HP, Jergenson DD, Kassell NF, Sahs AL. Pitfalls in the recognition of subarachnoid hemorrhage. *JAMA* 1980; 244:794–796.

252. Ostergaard JR. Warning leaks in subarachnoid hemorrhage. *Br Med J* 1990; 301:190–191.

253. Weisberg L. Computed tomography in aneurysmal subarachnoid hemorrhage. *Neurology* 1979; 29:802–808.

254. Caplan LR, Flamm ES, Mohr JP, Toole J, Plum F, Fisher CM, et al. Lumbar puncture and stroke. *Stroke* 1987; 18:540A–544A.

255. Heros R, Zervas NT, Varsos V. Cerebral vasospasm after subarachnoid hemorrhage: An update. *Ann Neurol* 1983; 14:599–608.

256. Kassell N, Sasaki T, Colohan A, Nazar G. Cerebral vasospasm following aneurysmal subarachnoid hemorrhage. *Stroke* 1985; 16:562–572.

257. MacDonald RL, Weir BK. A review of hemoglobin and the pathogenesis of cerebral vasospasm. *Stroke* 1991; 22:971–982.

258. Wilkins RH. Attempts at prevention or treatment of intracranial arterial spasm: An update. *Neurosurgery* 1986; 18:808–825.

259. Weir B, Grace M, Hansen J, Rothberg C. Time course of vasospasm in man. *J Neurosurg* 1978; 48:173–178.

260. Kwak R, Niizuma H, Ohi T, Suzuki J. Angiographic study of cerebral vasospasm following rupture of intracranial aneurysms: I. Time of the appearance. *Surg Neurol* 1979; 11:257–262.

261. Sloan MA, Haley EC, Kassell NF, Henry ML, Stewart SR, Beskin RR, et al. Sensitivity and specificity of transcranial Doppler ultrasonography in the diagnosis of vasospasm following subarachnoid hemorrhage. *Neurology* 1989; 39:1514–1518.

262. Davis S, Andrews J, Lichtenstein M, Kagi A, Tress B, Rossiter S, et al. A single-photon emission computed tomography study of hypoperfusion after subarachnoid hemorrhage. *Stroke* 1990; 21:252–259.

263. Wilkins RH. Attempted prevention or treatment of intracranial arterial spasm: A survey. *Neurosurgery* 1980; 6:198–210.

264. Hart RG, Kanter MC. Hematologic disorders and ischemic stroke: A selective review. *Stroke* 1990; 20:1111–1121.

265. Coull BM, Goodnight SH. Current concepts of cerebrovascular disease and stroke: Antiphospholipid antibodies, prothrombotic states and stroke. *Stroke* 1990; 21:1370–1374.

266. Feinberg WM, Bruck DC, Ring ME. Hemostatic markers in acute stroke. *Stroke* 1989; 20:592–597.

267. Holliday P, Mammen E, Buday J, Gilroy J, Barnhart M. "Sticky platelet" syndrome and cerebral infarction. *Neurology* 1983; 33(suppl 2):145.

268. Wu K, Hoak J. Increased platelet aggregation in patients with transient ischemic attacks. *Stroke* 1975; 6:521–524.

269. Feinberg WM. Coagulation. In: Caplan LR, ed. *Brain Ischemia: Basic Concepts and Clinical Relevance.* London: Springer-Verlag; 1995:85–96.

270. Hart R, Miller V, Coull B, Bril V. Cerebral infarction associated with lupus anticoagulants: Preliminary report. *Stroke* 1984; 15:114–118.

271. Levine SR, Welch KMA. The spectrum of neurologic disease associated with antiphospholipid antibodies, lupus anticoagulants, and anticardiolipin antibodies. *Arch Neurol* 1987; 44:876–883.

272. Kushner M, Simonian N. Lupus anticoagulant, anticardiolipin antibodies and cerebral ischemia. *Stroke* 1989; 20:225–229.

273. Levine SR, Langer SL, Albers JW, Welch KMA. Sneddon's syndrome: An antiphospholipid antibody syndrome. *Neurology* 1988; 38:798–800.

274. Rebollo M, Vol JF, Garijil F, Quintana F, Bercinao J. Livedo reticularis and cerebrovascular lesions (Sneddon's syndrome): Clinical, radiologic, and pathologic features in eight cases. *Brain* 1983; 106:965–979.

275. Bruyn RP, VanderVeen JP, Donker AJ, Valk J, Wolters EC. Sneddon's syndrome: Case report and literature review. *J Neurol Sci* 1987; 79:243–253.

276. Antiphospholipid Antibodies in Stroke Study Group (APASS). Clinical and laboratory findings in patients with antiphospholipid antibodies and cerebral ischemia. *Stroke* 1990; 21:1268–1273.

277. DeWitt LD, Caplan LR. Antiphospholipid antibodies and stroke. *AJNR* 1991; 12:454–456.

278. Asherson RA. A "primary antiphospholipid syndrome"? (editorial). *J Rheumatol* 1988; 15:1742–1746.

279. Coull BM, Boudette DN, Goodnight SH, Briley DP, Hart R. Multiple cerebral infarction and dementia associated with anticardiolipin antibodies. *Stroke* 1987; 18:1107–1112.

280. Amico L, Caplan LR, Thomas C. Cerebrovascular complications of mucinous cancers. *Neurology* 1989; 39:522–526.

281. Kase C, Robinson R, Stein R, DeWitt LD, Hier D, Harp D, et al. Anticoagulant-related intracerebral hemorrhage. *Neurology* 1985; 35:943–948.

282. Bovill EG, Terrin ML, Stump DC, Berke AD, Frederick M, Collen D, et al. Hemorrhagic events during therapy with recombinant tissue-type plasminogen activator, heparin, and aspirin for acute myocardial infarction. *Ann Intern Med* 1991; 115:256–265.

283. Kase CS, Pessin MS, Zivin JA, Del Zoppo GJ, Furlan AJ, Buckley JW, et al. Intracranial hemorrhages following coronary thrombolysis with tissue plasminogen activator. *Am J Med* 1992; 92:384–390.

284. Babikian V, Kase C, Pessin M, Caplan L, Gorelick P. Resumption of anticoagulation after intracranial bleeding in patients with prosthetic valves. *Stroke* 1988; 19:407–408.

285. Hart RG, Easton JD. Dissections of cervical and cerebral arteries. *Neurol Clin North Am* 1983; 1:255–282.

286. Anson J, Crowell RM. Cervicocranial arterial dissection. *Neurosurgery* 1991; 29:89–96.

287. Caplan LR, Zarins CK, Hemmati M. Spontaneous dissection of the extracranial vertebral arteries. *Stroke* 1985; 16:1030–1036.

288. Mas JL, Bousser MG, Hasboun D, Laplane D. Extracranial vertebral artery dissections. *Stroke* 1987; 18:1037–1047.

289. Mokri B, Houser W, Sandok B, Piepgras D. Spontaneous dissections of the vertebral arteries. *Neurology* 1988; 38:880–885.

290. Ojemann RG, Fisher CM, Rich JC. Spontaneous dissecting aneurysms of the internal carotid artery. *Stroke* 1972; 3:434–440.

291. Hennerici M, Steinke W, Rautenberg W. High-resistance Doppler flow pattern in extracranial carotid dissection. *Arch Neurol* 1989; 46:670–672.

292. Berger MS, Wilson CB. Intracranial dissecting aneurysms of the posterior circulation. *J Neurosurg* 1984; 61:882–894.

293. Friedman AH, Drake CG. Subarachnoid hemorrhage from intracranial dissecting aneurysm. *J Neurosurg* 1984; 60:325–334.

100

DIAGNOSIS AND MANAGEMENT OF DISEASES OF THE PERIPHERAL ARTERIES AND VEINS

John W. Joyce / Thom W. Rooke

Diseases of the arteries and veins are common, recurrent events in many active medical practices. The vascular system parallels the heart in that its many structural and hydraulic disorders cause major symptoms and findings that are often accessible to the eye, ear, and hand. Clinical syndromes are clearly defined, and the diagnosis is usually established through knowledge of the natural history of each entity and by a competent historical and physical examination. Both invasive and indirect testing modalities are well developed and can provide confirmation, quantitation, and in some instances clarification of the diagnosis. Assessment of the vascular system is an intrinsic component of a general examination and an essential extension of the cardiac evaluation for three reasons: heart disease extends to the vascular tree through macro- and microembolic events, endocarditis, congestive failure, tricuspid and aortic regurgitation, and complicating venous thromboembolism. In turn, arterial and venous diseases may produce many cardinal cardiac manifestations including dyspnea, syncope, edema, chest pain, hypertension, aortic valve disease, and congestive failure (Fig. 100-1). Several congenital or heritable disorders have both valvular and aortic components. Finally, of fundamental importance is an appreciation of the comorbidity of atherosclerosis in the aorta, carotid, renal, visceral, and peripheral arteries in the diagnosis and management of coronary artery disease (CAD). This chapter represents a synopsis and overview of peripheral vascular disorders.

CLINICAL ASSESSMENT OF ARTERIAL DISEASE

The History

Certain general information is always pertinent in the assessment of arterial disease and includes the patient's age, sex, and associated problems; the presence of risk factors for atherosclerosis; and knowledge of prior trauma, procedures, and drug use. Specific symptoms are evaluated for tempo, progression, factors that aggravate or alleviate, and their relationship to other medical events. Interrogation of other individuals and prior records are often essential when the patient is impaired. *Claudication and ischemic distress are the major symptoms of occlusive arterial disease.*

CLAUDICATION

Claudication (literally, "limping") is a stereotyped, reproducible distress in muscle groups brought on by sustained exercise and relieved by 3 to 6 min of rest. The distress may be described as numbness, weakness, giving way, aching, cramping, or pain. It may change character and location with progression of the causative lesion. Claudication occurs at shorter distances when the workload is increased by a rapid pace, carrying of a burden, or walking uphill or over rough terrain. When the claudication distance is abruptly decreased, there may be thrombosis in situ of occlusive or aneurysmal disease or, on occasion, embolization from these sources, the heart, or proximal vessels. Claudication limits often decrease after a period of inactivity but can usually improve to prior levels with reconditioning. Claudication as defined is a most reliable symptom.

It is essential to establish that the distress occurs in muscle groups, that relief is timely, and that it does not occur at rest. When these criteria are not met, musculoskeletal or neurologic disorders should be suspected. Quantitation by history alone, however, is quite variable because of differences in pace, workload, and estimates of distance. Standardized treadmill testing utilizing ankle/brachial indices at rest and after the reproduction of symptoms confirms the diagnosis, can identify

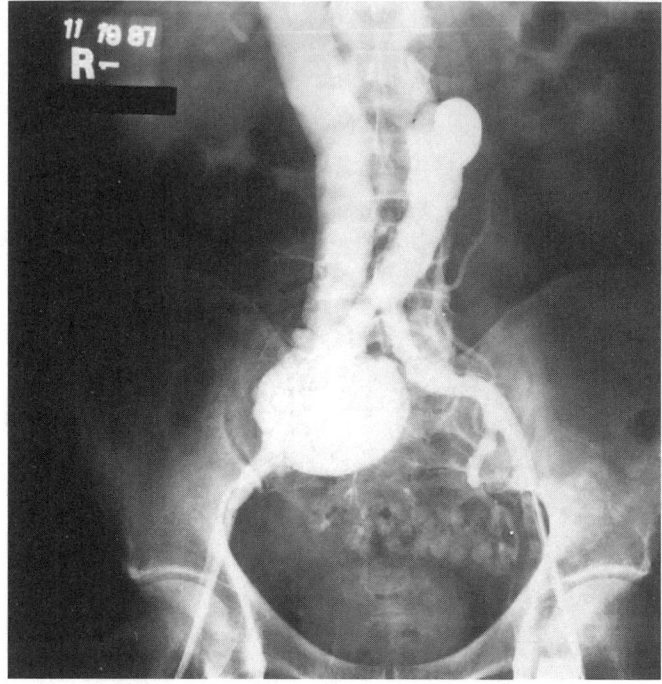

FIGURE 100-1
This 72-year-old man led a vigorous life until he was hospitalized twice in a single month for progressive fatigue, dyspnea, orthopnea, and paroxysmal nocturnal dyspnea. A continuous bruit in the right lower quadrant, noted during his second hospital stay, defined the cause of his high-output cardiac failure. Rupture of an iliac artery aneurysm into the adjacent iliac vein, shown in this aortogram, was repaired and he regained his prior vitality.

TABLE 100-1
VARIANTS OF CLAUDICATION

"Vasospastic" claudication
Pseudoclaudication
   Neurogenic claudication
   Myogenic claudication
Venous claudication

various pain syndromes not of arterial origin, and documents the claudication distance for follow-ups.

The site of claudication localizes the occlusive process when it is a single, focal lesion. Foot claudication results from pedal and low calf occlusive disease; calf and pedal distress, from tibioperoneal trunk lesions; and low calf discomfort, from popliteal disease. Superficial femoral disease causes claudication of the entire calf, and both thigh and calf symptoms occur with common femoral and external iliac lesions. Depending upon its distribution, aortoiliac occlusive disease may produce unilateral or bilateral claudication of the calf, thigh, buttocks, and occasionally the low back. The symptoms usually progress from caudad to cephalad but may be limited to the calf or buttocks and thighs. This distribution may reflect a given individual patient's particular gait or associated involvement of the internal iliac arteries. When the occlusive process is at multiple levels, the initial site of claudication usually reflects the most distal significant lesion or the area with the least collateral flow. Many patients with bilateral disease on examination will report only unilateral symptoms, since a more critical lesion induces claudication before a lesser lesion in the contralateral limb.

VARIANTS OF CLAUDICATION

Three causes of leg distress induced by exercise can be perplexing (Table 100-1). In the first, a classic claudication history is obtained, but on examination pulses are normal and

no bruits are noted. This apparent contradiction is clarified by exercising the patient on the examining table step or treadmill until the symptoms are reproduced, then promptly repeating the examination. Pedal pulses will now be absent, the feet pale, and proximal bruits noted, and the ankle/brachial indices will drop. The symptoms and findings will normalize within minutes with rest. Vasospasm was thought to explain this quandary,[1] but arteriography shows early occlusive disease in proximal vessels, usually of atherosclerotic origin.[2] Entrapment or adventitial cystic disease of the popliteal artery can also cause the syndrome.[3] The phenomenon of *vasospastic claudication* is explained by a stenosis, subcritical at rest, that causes blood to be shunted into collateral arterial muscular beds dilated by exercise, depriving downstream arteries of flow.[2] Of note, arterial spasm induced by ergot toxicity causes a fixed lesion and abnormal examination findings.

A second variant is *pseudoclaudication*, which may be of neurogenic or muscular origin. The patient with neurogenic claudication will describe exercise-induced distress. It often has a dysesthetic quality; however, it clears slowly or may require a specific posture for relief; clumsiness may develop as walking progresses; and the distress also occurs with prolonged standing or in given fixed positions. A history of current or prior back distress should be sought. Compression of the distal spinal cord by hypertrophic bone, disk protrusion, or tumor causes the syndrome.[4] The arterial examination is normal at rest. Arterial and neurogenic disease coexist, and in this situation, the dominant lesion may be identified by observing the symptoms and measuring the arterial indices with exercise.[5]

Muscular distress induced by exercise is common in amyotrophic lateral sclerosis, muscular dystrophy, and McArdle's syndrome. The muscular deficits are apparent by history and examination, and exercise testing will clarify the status of the arterial system.

Venous claudication is described as a congestive, often "bursting" distress of thighs and calves induced by running and sometimes walking. Relief with rest is slow and notably accelerated when the patient reclines and elevates the legs. It occurs with significant iliocaval obstruction. Signs of venous hypertension of the legs and sometimes lower abdomen are noted.

ISCHEMIC DISTRESS

With severe perfusion deficits the patient can experience persistent distress of two types: rest pain and ischemic neuropathy. *Rest pain* is constant, agonizing, and confined to the digits, foot, or hand. It may localize to focal sites of infarction, ulceration, or infection. Such small lesions can occur with vasculitis, microembolization, or thrombosis but more often represent trauma to an area of poor perfusion from chronic occlusive disease. The patient may be unaware of injury, but it is important to inquire of new shoes, ingrown nails, or recent trimming of callus or nails. Rest pain is first noted at night, interrupting sleep, and may be partially relieved by hanging the limb dependently, sleeping in a chair, or walking about. It later becomes constant, can suppress appetite and weight, and requires large doses of analgesics. The patient may become depressed. The area is tender and sensitive to touch by clothing and bedding. Muscular atrophy and contractures of ankle, knee, and hip joints can result when the limb is protected by fixed postures and immobility.

Ischemic neuropathy is constant distress described as aching, throbbing, burning, pulling, or tearing. It is diffuse, often affecting the entire lower leg or forearm, and may shift its focus of intensity. Momentary jabs or lancinating pain are often experienced. Paroxysms of exacerbation lasting hours may occur, and these may be accompanied by a diffuse cyanosis and coolness of the skin.

THE ARTERIAL EXAMINATION

Arteries routinely palpated are the radial, ulnar, subclavian, carotid, aortic, femoral, popliteal, posterior tibial, and dorsalis pedis. When a pulse is abnormal or absent, its course should be traced as far as muscle or bony anatomy allows. Collateral arteries are sought under several circumstances: scapular and rib with thoracic coarctation, superficial epigastric and hypogastric with abdominal coarctation, and geniculates with chronic popliteal occlusion. The temporal and occipital arteries are palpated when temporal arteritis is suspected.

The following techniques will serve the examiner well:

1. Both patient and examiner should be in a relaxed position.
2. Use the surface area of three or more fingers when possible.
3. Control and relax any nearby joint with the other hand.
4. Begin with light pressure, increasing and varying it for difficult examinations.
5. Avoid use of the thumb, as the examiner's pulse can be transmitted.

The most challenging pulse is the pulse not found. The history and ancillary findings may support that it should be absent. When in doubt, Doppler signals and pressures can establish whether the pulse is absent or just obscured.

Individual arteries are palpated sequentially as the arm, neck, trunk, and legs are examined. Paired vessels are compared. Blood pressure is taken bilaterally, and a difference of 10 mmHg or more is significant if duplicated after several readings. The following pulses are easily identified. The radial pulse is quite accessible, particularly when the examiner uses his or her other hand to relax the wrist tendons into flexion.

The posterior tibial is identified by controlling the ankle with one hand and cupping three to four fingers of the other about the posteroinferior surface of the medial malleolus. The subclavian pulse is best felt with the patient sitting and by curling two to three fingers into the supraclavicular space and slowly increasing pressure. The common femoral artery is easily felt just below the inguinal ligament. The limb should be uncrossed and rotated laterally to relieve muscle tension. Firm pressure may be required for the obese patient. Examination of the carotid is done with gentle pressure of two or three fingers, palpating the artery from the clavicle to the mandibular angle. It is prudent to examine each carotid individually and with the patient semirecumbent. Of note, what seems to be a normal internal carotid may actually be the external carotid, which is often prominent when the internal carotid is highly stenotic.

The dorsalis pedis is commonly felt between the tendons of the first and second toes, 5 to 7.5 cm below the joint crevice. It may, however, be more lateral and is sometimes congenitally absent. The abdominal aorta is best examined with the patient supine on a firm surface, knees flexed and arms at the side. Examination is initiated with the gentle pressure of eight fingers spread across the epigastrium to appreciate any diffuse pulsation. Then two or three fingers of each hand are gradually brought deeper on either side of the aorta until its pulsation and dimensions are defined. It is helpful to coach the patient to breathe and relax, warning that modest discomfort may be felt, and penetrating deeper with each expiration.

The popliteal artery can be challenging to examine when musculoskeletal structures are prominent or relaxation is poor. It is best approached with the patient supine and the knee relaxed into the cradle of eight examining fingers, varying the pressure according to the resistance felt. When a pulse is not found, it may sometimes be located by palpating lower between the heads of the gastrocnemius muscle. Popliteal examination should routinely include both of these sites and is not completed until the adductor muscle mass distal to the adductor hiatus is compressed between both hands. Aneurysms can occur at any of these three locations (Fig. 100-2).

The ulnar artery, a particularly important parallel vessel because of the impact of wrist punctures, is subject to variation and not infrequently is obscured by tendons. The *Allen test* can ascertain its patency. This test depends upon the integrity of the radial, ulnar, and palmar arch arteries. It is performed by occluding the radial or ulnar artery with firm digital pressure, having the patient exsanguinate the hand by making a fist and then relaxing both the hand and wrist. When the noncompressed artery is patent, flushing will occur within 3 s. Delayed refilling is diagnostic of occlusive disease in the noncompressed vessel and may also define digital or microcirculatory deficits when focal refilling is slow in the digits.[6] It is imperative that the wrist be relaxed to avoid false-positive results caused by ligamentous compression.[7] Thus, the Allen test is valuable in assessing occlusive disease of the radial, ulnar, palmar, and digital arteries.

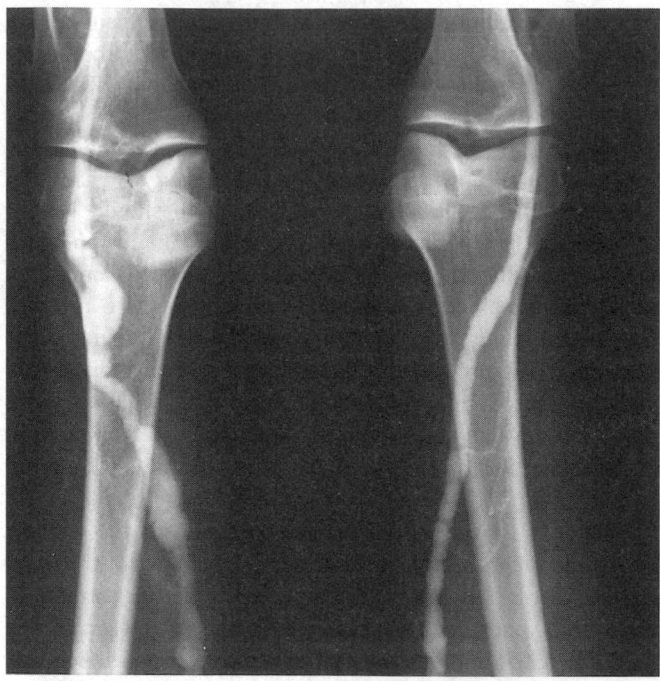

FIGURE 100-2
Popliteal artery aneurysmal disease located at the adductor hiatus. This is a common site for aneurysms and is easily overlooked unless the area is routinely examined. The popliteal arteries are normal at the joint crevice. Typical arteriomegaly is seen in both superficial femoral arteries.

ANEURYSMS

Arterial aneurysms are a major cause of death and disability. Early detection allows definitive repair. The three most common aneurysms are accessible to examination; 40 to 60 percent of abdominal aortic and almost all popliteal and femoral aneurysms are detected by examination.[8–11]

The size and pulsatility of paired arteries are normally of similar magnitude, and ectasia is suspected when a pulse is larger or more forceful than others in a given patient. *Aneurysm* is defined as a focal enlargement 1½ or more times larger than the usual diameter of the artery; diagnosis is established when a palpable, often visible pulsation is transmitted to the fingers on each side of an enlarged vessel. A mass pulsating on only part of its surface is a mass with a transmitted pulse. Lesions adjacent to the abdominal aorta that produce this phenomenon include mesenteric and pancreatic cysts, horseshoe kidney, and retroperitoneal tumors. Tortuosity of the right carotid, abdominal aorta, or wrist arteries can mimic an aneurysm. Ultrasound or angiographic studies may be needed to clarify this question when the examination is uncertain.

Many abdominal aortic aneurysms may be detected by palpation, which reveals a pulsating mass below the xiphoid and above the umbilicus, often filling the epigastrium. Most aneurysms are centered to the left of the midline, but tortuosity may occasionally result in placing the mass more to the right. Slight patient discomfort is usual during examination, but significant tenderness suggests an inflammatory aneurysm,

recent expansion, or a contained rupture. When the mass extends below the umbilicus, it may represent either extension into the iliac arteries or a large, overlapping aortic aneurysm. Isolated iliac aneurysms are usually hidden in the pelvis, and less than a fifth are detected by abdominal or digital examination of the rectum or pelvis. Most are found incidental to imaging or symptoms.[12] Femoral aneurysms are often first noted by the patient, but popliteal lesions are easily overlooked unless the popliteal space is routinely examined at all three sites described (Fig. 100-2). Femoral and popliteal aneurysms are often first detected when the patient presents with acute thrombosis, distal micro- or macroembolization, or edema from venous compression or thrombosis.[10,11]

Most thoracic and thoracoabdominal aneurysms are diagnosed incidentally by imaging procedures. Both may also be found during investigation of pain, cough, dysphagia, hemoptysis, or dysphonia. Physical signs are late manifestations of thoracic aneurysms and include those of aortic valve incompetence, unilateral or bilateral jugular venous distention, and pulsatility in the upper intercostal spaces or of the precordium. Carotid and axillosubclavian aneurysms are easily diagnosed by palpation, and some present with local pain, thrombosis, or distal embolic complications.[13,14] Visceral aneurysms are rarely large enough to be palpated, 3 to 5 percent present as rupture, and the majority are found incidental to surgery or imaging.[15,16]

BRUITS

Bruits ("noise") represent turbulent flow in arteries or veins and can be caused by stenosis, extrinsic compression, aneurysm, or hyperdynamic flow; they can be palpable as a thrill. The proximal limit of a bruit defines the site of the lesion. Bruits usually transmit an additional 4 to 6 cm or further downstream in vessels with high-velocity flow. Coarse, low-pitched bruits are generated in larger vessels such as the proximal limb arteries, carotid, or aorta, while bruits of a higher pitch occur in smaller arteries or mark a high-grade stenosis in any vessel. The duration and pitch increase as stenosis progresses. A bruit may disappear when a critical narrowing is reached. Conversely, a mild stenosis may be silent until flow is increased by exercise, emotion, or drugs.

A continuous bruit throughout systole and diastole and repeated without pause in the next cardiac cycle is nearly pathognomonic of arteriovenous fistula at the site of its greatest intensity. Continuous bruits occur at acquired fistula of named arteries and veins (Fig. 100-1); over multiple congenital fistulas of the liver, lung, soft tissue, or skull; and over areas of tumor necrosis or prior biopsies. There are three innocent bruits. The first is the classic jugular venous hum of the youthful, which is heard with the patient upright and clears with the Valsalva maneuver, with head rotation, or upon reclining. The innocent supraclavicular bruit of young patients disapears with shoulder hyperabduction.[17] An epigastric bruit may represent celiac compression or organic visceral or renal artery stenosis but may be heard, especially in the young, in the absence of vascular disease.[18]

EXTENSIONS OF THE ARTERIAL EXAMINATION

The value of the Allen test in establishing patency of the radial, ulnar, and digital arteries has been discussed. The exercise test was described for the patient having a positive claudication history but a negative exam ("vasospastic" claudication). It is just as useful for the patient with a positive examination but negative history. The workload imposed exceeds the patient's usual activity level, and claudication is experienced, confirming the examination. In a third application, observation and interrogation during exercise may clarify an unclear history or separate claudication from other symptoms.

Pedal perfusion has traditionally been tested by timing elevation pallor and venous refilling. With the patient supine, both feet are elevated to 60° for 1 min. If no pallor is seen, perfusion is judged normal. The appearance of pallor before 15 s suggests poor healing capacity, and pallor without elevation is indicative of severe ischemia. The patient then sits upright and refilling of the pedal veins is timed. Normal filling occurs in less than 15 s, filling between 30 and 45 s suggests slow healing, and values beyond 60 s confirm severe ischemia. Venous incompetence invalidates venous filling times, and the test is not practical with significant edema or obesity. Grossly abnormal tests correlate well with the presence of rest pain or ulceration.

Several maneuvers are used to screen for arterial, venous, and neurogenic compression syndromes of the thoracic outlet. Because these tests are frequently abnormal in the normal population, and because of the complexity of the syndromes, the reader is referred to detailed reviews.[19,20]

THE SKIN

Occlusive arterial disease can alter skin temperature, color, and nutrition. Skin temperature is reduced in the zone of reduced perfusion caused by acute or chronic occlusive disease. Differences are best felt with the dorsum of the fingers, and comparisons to the contralateral or proximal limb should be made. Profound coolness indicates severe ischemia. Generalized body coolness may denote shock, hemorrhage, or poor cardiac output. Chronically cool hands and feet reflect the basic vasomotor tone of some patients. Limbs with neurologic damage, immobility, and reflex sympathetic dystrophy are often cool. Edema can accompany these states, obscuring pulses. Doppler systolic indices will differentiate occlusive disease from these vasomotor changes.

Skin color varies with blood flow and therefore with temperature, activity, and emotional stimuli. A red or purplish color of the forefoot is common with chronic ischemia and increases with dependency. It represents chronic arteriolar dilation in response to inadequate flow. Pallor can be seen with acute ischemia or on elevation with chronic ischemia. Skin that is chronically deprived of blood can become thin, translucent, and shiny. Thick calluses and nails may develop. Age and various dermatologic disorders can also cause these findings, and a circulatory deficit should be established before a causal role is presumed.

Additional skin lesions and color changes are described in the subsequent discussion of vasomotor and microcirculatory syndromes.

Clinical Syndromes

CHRONIC OCCLUSIVE ARTERIAL DISEASE

Atherosclerosis obliterans is the usual cause of chronic occlusive disease of the legs, including patients under age 35.[21] Coexistent CAD is clinically apparent in 40 percent or more, and additional occult disease is found by screening patients whose exercise is limited by claudication.[22,23] CAD is the major cause of operative death and subsequent shortened life span.[22,24] In addition, there is at least a 15 percent prevalence of coexisting carotid occlusive disease and abdominal aortic aneurysms in males beyond 65 years of age.[22,25,26] Sound management requires a careful analysis of the entire cardiovascular system. *The limb lesion often serves as the initial marker of these comorbid conditions and of the risk factors of smoking, hypertension, diabetes, and hyperlipidemia that accelerate the atherosclerotic process.*

Natural History

Occlusive disease can manifest as asymptomatic pulse reductions or bruits, claudication, ischemic syndromes, and microcirculatory embolic events. Common sites of focal lesions are the aortoiliac, superficial femoral (often at the adductor hiatus), and popliteal arteries. Patients present with claudication when collateral vessels are patent, and their limitation can be stable or progress slowly over several years when risk factors are controlled. Over 80 percent of such patients avoid ischemic complications or amputation for 5 or more years.[27,28] Up to 15 percent of those who continue smoking undergo amputation within 5 years, however, and diabetics have an amputation rate of 25 percent within 9 years.[27,29] Ischemic complications are more frequent when two or three levels (aortoiliac, femoropopliteal, tibioperoneal) are diseased or significant collaterals are impaired. Such diffuse disease usually reflects significant risk factors. As previously noted, rest pain, infarcts, and ulcers often result from local trauma to a limb with borderline perfusion. Further, thrombosis in situ superimposed on chronic stenosis may initiate distal ischemic lesions.

Clinical Strategy

Ideally, all patients would be returned to normal by a procedure. The majority, however, are not limited enough to warrant repair and are managed with medical measures and control of risk factors. In some, repair is precluded by coexistent disease or by technical limitations. The usual logic is to establish a diagnosis clinically, to confirm and quantify by the vascular laboratory, and to reserve angiography for those patients needing repair. *Surgical indications are limiting claudication, ischemic complications, and requirement of removal of proximal sites causing microembolization* (see Chap. 101). The indications for angiography are extended in three circumstances: to define etiology in young patients, when an uncommon lesion is suspected, and when juxtarenal occlusion of the aorta with azotemia or hypertension is suspected (Fig. 100-3). If the renal arteries are stenotic in this latter syndrome, surgery can prevent premature death from renal failure.[30] Percutaneous angioplasty is an effective alternative or adjunct to surgery when the location, extent, and configuration are carefully selected by an experienced operator. Morbidity and mortality are low, but durability is less than with conventional repair; this may improve as stenting techniques evolve (see Chap. 102 for a detailed discussion).

Medical Therapy

Vasodilating drugs do not improve claudication.[31] These agents increase only cutaneous flow and may accelerate healing of minor wounds when ischemia is mild. Anticoagulants are utilized only when a clotting disorder or a cardiac source of embolism is identified. Pentoxifylline, 400 mg orally three times daily, can improve claudication distance 30 to 60 percent in some patients.[32,33] More significant help for most patients is a walking program of 30 to 45 min (with interruptions for claudication) performed on four or more days weekly. This approach frequently increases walking distance by 200 percent or more.[34] *Patients with occlusive disease should receive careful instruction in good foot care.* Regular follow-up is required to monitor disease management, detect other atherosclerotic manifestations, and control risk factors.

Unusual Causes

Leg claudication and ischemia can result from numerous disorders, most of which are listed in Table 100-2. Many are suggested by the history or clinical constellation (acute arterial

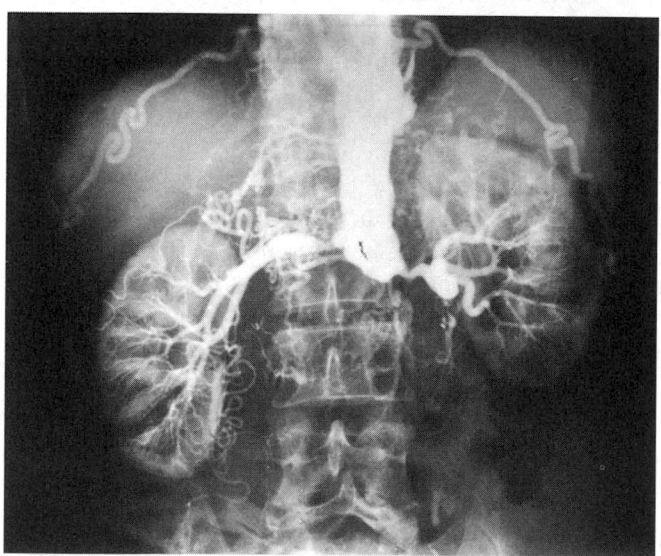

FIGURE 100-3
Classic juxtarenal aortic occlusion. These lesions start as significant plaque at the aortic bifurcation, and thrombus propagates proximally until the high flow into the renal arteries limits its progression. Subsequent renal artery occlusion leads to premature death unless repair is accomplished. This 42-year-old male smoker presented with uncontrolled hypertension and claudication. Note the hypertrophied intercostal arteries serving as collaterals to the legs.

TABLE 100-2

CAUSES OF LEG CLAUDICATION

Atherosclerosis obliterans	Temporal arteritis
Acute arterial occlusion	Takayasu arteritis
Occluded aneurysms	Popliteal entrapment
Thromboangiitis obliterans	Adventital cystic disease
Fibromuscular dysplasia	Aortic coarctation (thoracic, abdominal)
Aortic dissection	Pseudoxanthoma elasticum
Radiation fibrosis	Primary arterial tumor
Retroperitoneal fibrosis	Iliac endofibrosis (cyclists)
Ergot toxicity	

occlusion, aortic dissection, temporal and Takayasu's arteritis, radiation therapy, ergot use, and competitive cycling), some by physical findings (coarctation, pseudoxanthoma elasticum, occluded aneurysms), and others only through imaging. The distinctive features of several warrant a brief profile.

Thromboangiitis obliterans (TAO) is the most frequent of these random occlusive disorders. Buerger described an inflammatory vasculopathy, with a characteristic, highly cellular intraluminal thrombus affecting small and medium-sized arteries and veins. TAO is always associated with, and may be an autoimmune response to, tobacco use. Buerger's disease is seen in most races predominantly in males in the second through fifth decades, although the incidence in women is rising. Clinically, TAO differs from atherosclerosis: upper extremity involvement is usual; initial involvement is distal in digital, pedal, and hand vessels; and progression to calf, thigh, and forearm is brisk over a few months or years. Rare manifestations are due to coronary, cerebral, or visceral artery lesions. Bilateral leg and often arm involvement is noted at presentation. One-third of patients will also report Raynaud's phenomenon and/or episodes of superficial phlebitis of calves or forearms. Biopsy of acute lesions, particularly accessible veins, is diagnostic, and angiographic features are characteristic. Progressive tissue loss is inevitable until tobacco is stopped, when stability or improvement will be seen. Surgical sympathectomy and intravenous prostacyclin analogs can accelerate healing of ischemic lesions, but amputation of damaged digits and limbs is often needed.[35–38]

Two congenital lesions peculiar to youthful claudicants are noteworthy. The popliteal artery can be entrapped by the medial gastrocnemius or various muscular and ligamentous bands, causing claudication and later occlusion. Second, adventitial cystic disease is a slowly enlarging growth in the popliteal or occasionally common femoral artery, analogous in structure and content to a ganglion. It also causes claudication and subsequent occlusion. Both warrant surgical repair upon diagnosis but often are discovered only after occlusion or distal embolization.[39,40] Takayasu's arteritis involves the aorta and iliofemoral system, and temporal arteritis involves the profunda femoral, superficial femoral, and distal vessels in 5 to 10 percent of cases. This involvement is usually bilateral and results in claudication that progresses briskly over a few months. Ischemia is rare. Both have characteristic clinical and laboratory findings. Arteriographic features are typical. These arteritides are unique among all arteriopathies in that stenotic lesions are significantly improved in their acute phase by steroid therapy. Adjunctive cytotoxic drugs are also useful.[41–43]

Ergot toxicity can induce Raynaud's phenomenon, claudication, acute ischemia, or tissue infarction depending on the dose taken. It is usually seen with overuse of rectal suppositories for migraine. Intravenous nitroprusside drip is advised for acute ischemic events. Lesser syndromes will clear over several days after stopping ergot.[44]

ACUTE ARTERIAL OCCLUSION

The mechanisms causing acute arterial occlusion may place both life and limb in jeopardy. Significant acute or chronic cardiac disease coexists with most thrombotic or embolic occlusions. It is the major determinant of immediate and long-term survival, and death exceeds limb loss in all major reports. Acute arterial occlusion is an event of high priority that requires prompt evaluation of the limb, heart, and other problems common to these patients.[45–47]

Etiology

The etiology of acute arterial occlusions is classified into three groups—trauma, thrombosis in situ, and embolism—each with a subset of specific mechanisms. Attention to arterial integrity is of prime importance in all penetrating (including medical interventions), crushing, and deceleration injuries and fractures. In situ thrombosis occurs with both occlusive and aneurysmal disease. Any of the lesions listed in Table 100-2—aneurysms, clotting disorders, but predominantly atherosclerosis with its multiple manifestations and risk factors—can be the substrate of thrombosis.

A small percentage of acute emboli come from proximal occlusive or aneurysmal arterial lesions, but the majority originate in the heart. Both the left ventricle and atrium may harbor thrombus, and ischemic heart disease now exceeds valvular problems as a cause of emboli.[48] Atrial fibrillation is common to both. Emboli tend to be multiple and recurrent and to distribute randomly, mostly to the legs but with a significant incidence of cerebral, renal, visceral, and arm events.[49] Venous thrombi from the right heart or limbs can pass across septal defects or patent foramen ovali and cause arterial events, often cerebral. Such paradoxical embolism can be both a diagnostic and a therapeutic challenge.[50]

There are two exceptions to the diagnostic triad. First are the branch vessel deficits of aortic dissection that may be subtle on examination, attributed to other causes, or confusing because no history of chest pain is given. The second is ergot toxicity, which is usually diagnosed only when the question of drug use is asked.[44]

Manifestations

The site and spectrum of manifestations are dependent on the location of the occlusion and the status of collateral and distal arteries. The presentation may be the silent loss of a pulse, a sudden reduction in walking distance, or a major clinical event. Acute occlusion is abrupt, evolving over moments or a few hours: the tempo of onset does not differentiate embolic from thrombotic events.[51] Examination reveals absent pulses and distal ischemia of varying degrees manifest by skin pallor and coolness, muscle tenderness or hardness, and reduced motor and sensory power. Coolness begins several inches distal to the occlusion and helps localize its site, similar to claudication in chronic disease. When collateral vessels are also obstructed, the coolness approximates the obstructed site. All findings can be increased by clot propagation or, on occasion, decreased by clot fragmentation.

Management

Immediate measures are directed to urgent care of all associated problems (usually cardiac) and protection of the limb from trauma by a bulky dressing. Heparin is given to prevent clot propagation and venous thromboembolism and to control embolic sources when present.[45,52] It can be reversed quickly if surgery follows. The etiology is established at the original assessment. Angiography is required to plan repair when there is preexisting occlusive or aneurysmal disease or when the etiology is uncertain. Many surgeons will perform balloon embolectomy without angiography when an embolic source is certain and the vessel was previously normal.

Ideally, all acute occlusions warrant repair, the urgency of which is governed by the degree of ischemia. Severe ischemia is manifest by pallor at rest, profound coolness, tender or hard muscles, and loss of motor and sensory power; repair must occur within hours of onset to salvage the limb. Additional days for care of ancillary problems can be taken with lesser degrees of ischemia, and sometimes no repair is elected when the occlusion has minimal impact on the patient's lifestyle. When acute, unstable cardiac events create prohibitive risks for surgery on concomitant severe limb ischemia, the heart may be stabilized over a few hours and the limb then improved by interventional embolectomy under local anesthesia, with minimal risk.[53,54] When not contraindicated, lysis of acute occlusion not requiring immediate relief can be effective.[55,56]

Prevention

Acute arterial occlusion is often preventable. The need for meticulous technique during interventional procedures is apparent. Conditions known to cause occlusion warrant definitive treatment. Surgical treatment is recommended for aneurysms, thoracic outlet arteriopathy, adventitial cystic disease and popliteal entrapment syndromes, and atrial myxoma. Treatable medical disorders include vasculitis, hematologic disorders, and thyrotoxicosis. Cardiac disease prone to atrial or ventricular thrombi, atrial fibrillation, acute myocardial infarction, profound congestive failure, cardiomyopathy, and prosthetic valves all warrant antithrombotic therapy (see Chap. 52).

MICROCIRCULATORY DISORDERS

Digital and microcirculatory ischemia may present as focal digital cyanosis, petechiae, splinter hemorrhages, ulcer, infarction, or gangrene and may be accompanied by livedo reticularis and Raynaud's phenomenon. Lesions may be single or multiple and usually are acute. Most initial lesions heal spontaneously with little or no tissue loss, but recurrences are common, compound the ischemia, and can result in loss of phalanges, digits, or large areas of skin (Fig. 100-4).

Etiologic mechanisms include (1) trauma in an area of preexistent occlusive disease, (2) atherothrombotic emboli, and (3) humoral and systemic disease (Table 100-3). Microemboli almost always originate from a proximal ulcerative plaque or aneurysm and only rarely from the heart, in contrast to macroembolic events. Solitary lesions showering atheroemboli are readily treated surgically.[57] When lesions are found at several levels, surgical choices are more difficult. Suprarenal and thoracoabdominal ulcerative or aneurysmal sources can cause progressive azotemia or intestinal ischemia and require a formidable repair.[58] Thromboulcerative disease of the entire aorta can shower randomly to the brain, viscera, kidneys, skin, and muscle; anemia, leukocytosis, elevated sedimentation rate, azotemia, and abnormal urinary sediment are usually noted, and the syndrome is differentiated from vasculitis by biopsy.[59] Microembolic events may be spontaneous or precipitated by surgery, instrumentation, or anticoagulant therapy.[58] Antiplatelet agents have been advised to pre-

TABLE 100-3

MICROCIRCULATORY DISEASE: ETIOLOGY

I. Occlusive disease
    Trauma
II. Microembolism
    Spontaneous
    Instrumentation
    Surgery
    Anticoagulants
III. Specific diseases
    Vasculitis
    Endocarditis
    Ergot toxicity
    Cold injury
    Malignancy
    Hepatitis antigenemia
    Hematologic disorders
        Polycythemia vera
        Thrombocytosis
        Intravascular coagulopathy
        Dysproteinemia
        Cryoglobulinemia
        Cold agglutinins
        Circulating anticoagulants
        Antiphopholipid antibodies
        Thrombotic thrombocytopenic purpura
        Heparin-induced thrombocytopenia

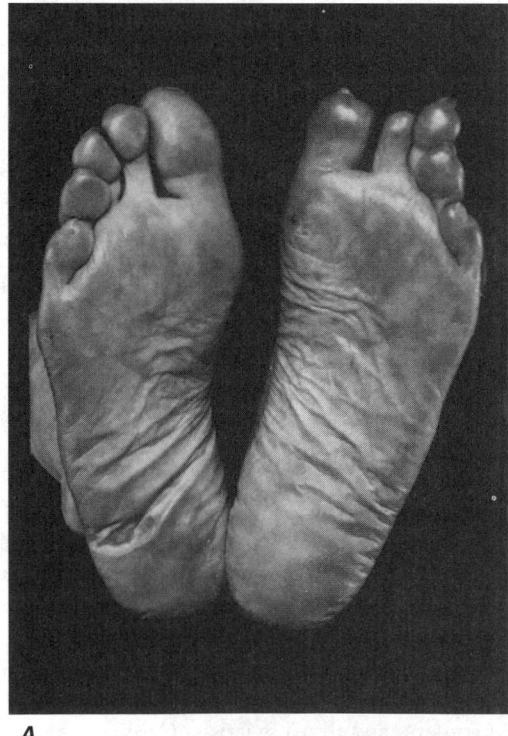

A

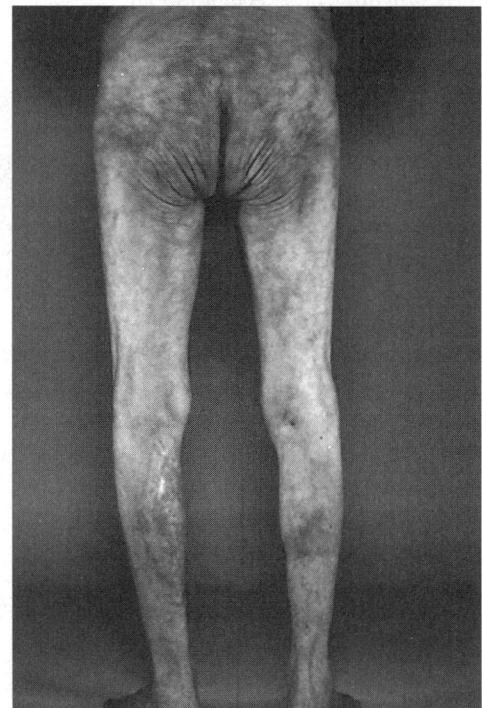

B

FIGURE 100-4

A. Cyanotic toe pads, livoid plantar skin, and prior tissue loss typical of recurrent showers of atherothrombotic microemboli. This 73-year-old man presented because of ischemic rest pain of the left great toe. *B.* In the same patient, extensive secondary livedo reticularis was seen only from the waist down. These microcirculatory phenomena led to the diagnosis and successful repair of a 7-cm abdominal aortic aneurysm.

vent recurrences when surgery is not feasible; their efficacy is poorly documented.[60]

The systemic disorders listed are diagnosed by clinical features and selective tests. Most are treatable. Vasculitic syndromes respond to steroids and/or cytotoxic agents. Anticoagulants are given for associated circulating anticoagulant[61] or antiphospholipid syndromes. Myeloproliferative disease and dysproteinemias are treated with chemotherapy, sometimes enhanced by plasmaphoresis. Clotting syndromes are controlled by anticoagulants, and may also involve large arteries and veins. Culture-sensitive antibiotics are essential for endocarditis and infected prosthetic valves must usually be removed (Chap. 82). Digital ischemia with advanced malignancy is rare and may be idiopathic or explained by a coagulopathy, dysproteinemia, or marantic endocarditis.

VASOSPASTIC DISORDERS

The color and warmth of the acral parts vary considerably from person to person in a normal population, reflecting individual vasomotor tone. Livedo reticularis, acrocyanosis, and Raynaud's phenomenon are distinctive clinical syndromes manifest by abnormal color and temperature changes of the skin. These are induced or intensified as a result of stimuli from cold, emotion, or drugs and cause spasm in digital arteries, arterioles, and perhaps venules. These syndromes are usually benign, lifelong, primary processes; the features of each may combine in a given patient, but all three syndromes can have important secondary causes. Careful clinical examination and selective testing will usually confirm the specific etiology and define prognosis and the direction of therapy.

Livedo Reticularis

Livedo reticularis is characterized by a persistent, symmetric, bluish, meshlike pattern on the extremities and sometimes the trunk that is variable in its extent and intensity. It is most apparent after stimulation by cold or emotion and fades with warmth and exercise. It is first seen in childhood or at puberty and is more common in women and fair-skinned individuals. It is so frequent in its milder form that it is overlooked or considered a variant of normal skin, which it is. The skin overall is often somewhat cool. It is postulated that spasm of cutaneous arterioles with secondary dilation of the capillaries and venules causes slow flow, increased oxygen uptake, and more reduced oxyhemoglobin, producing the color changes. Primary livedo reticularis is often seen with acrocyanosis and primary Raynaud's disease. Treatment is rarely needed.

Secondary livedo reticularis is patchy, focal, or asymmetric in distribution, of late onset, and may be complicated by local infarction or ulceration. The lesions may be elevated or tender when caused by vasculitis. Causes of the secondary syndrome include atherothrombotic emboli (Fig. 100-4), systemic and cutaneous vasculitis, amantadine and beta-blocker therapy, and limbs with neurogenic disuse, including reflex sympathetic dystrophy. Therapy is directed at the underlying cause (Table 100-4). Vasodilators and sympathectomy are of unpredictable, anecdotal value for healing painful ulcers.

TABLE 100-4
LIVEDO RETICULARIS: SECONDARY CAUSES

Atherothrombotic emboli
Collagen-vascular disease
Cutaneous vasculitis
Thrombocytosis
Dysproteinemia
Amantadine therapy
Neurogenic disuse
Erythema ab igne

Hemosiderin deposition can occur in secondary and, on occasion, primary livedo reticularis. *Erythema ab igne* can be confused with livedo reticularis. This is a focal, well-defined livoid lesion with broader bands of fixed red color, often with a hemosiderin stain. It is a reaction to chronic, local heat exposure, such as a heating pad or fireplace.

Acrocyanosis

This finding is a benign, persistent cyanotic discoloration and coolness of the hands and fingers, sometimes the feet, seen predominantly in women. Mild local edema is not uncommon; on occasion, an associated hyperhidrosis can be most bothersome and may require treatment. It is painless and does not ulcerate. Cold and emotion will intensify whereas warmth and exercise ameliorate the findings. It is a bothersome cosmetic defect for some. Calcium entry blockers or alpha$_1$ antagonists will often reduce the symptoms. A modest degree of acrocyanosis is sometimes seen in limbs immobilized by neurogenic deficits. Rarely, beta blockade will induce the syndrome.

Raynaud's Phenomenon

The diagnosis of Raynaud's phenomenon is made from a reliable history alone. It is difficult to demonstrate, even with ice immersion, as generalized cooling is usually needed to bring out the findings. The syndrome is defined as episodes of blue or white color changes of the digits, often followed by reactive hyperemia during recovery; it is induced by cold or emotional stimuli. Most patients describe the white phase, some blue to white, a few blue only, and most note the subsequent hyperemia. A dead, numb feeling but rarely pain accompanies the ischemic phase, and dysesthetic, throbbing, or painful sensations are common in recovery. Fingers are involved more often than toes—initially the distal phalanges and later all, but rarely the palm. Thumbs are often spared. The recovery time is 3 to 10 min but can exceed 1 h in advanced cases, usually of secondary origin.

The prime question is whether the phenomenon will remain a benign, lifelong vasospastic event, or whether it is secondary to systemic disease or obstructive arteriopathy. *Allen and Brown*[62] *defined primary Raynaud's as episodes of bilateral color changes, induced by cold or emotion, and without evidence of ischemia or other disease for 2 years.* The later development of secondary disease was noted in 2 to 5 percent of patients.[63–65] A recent prospective study confirms that patients without laboratory evidence of digital occlusive, clotting, or serologic abnormalities have a benign course, with only 2 percent showing secondary causes in the subsequent decade.[66]

Disorders causing secondary Raynaud's phenomenon are extensive and diverse (Table 100-5). Most can be defined by a sound history and examination, knowledge of their natural behavior, vascular laboratory measurements of digital obstruction, and screening clotting and serologic tests. Arteriography (from the arch through the digits) is reserved for unusual problems or for planning surgery when needed. Trophic skin changes and ischemic lesions usually reflect occlusive etiologies, while unilateral Raynaud's suggests a secondary process.[65,67]

Most patients with primary Raynaud's phenomenon require no therapy and quickly learn to keep not only hands but the whole body warm. Treatment of secondary forms is directed to their cause when feasible. Calcium channel blockers and non-beta-adrenergic blocking sympatholytics alone or in combination can suppress the episodes in some patients, but drugs and sympathectomy have little impact on ischemic complications: these are best treated with local debridement and control of infection and pain.

ANEURYSMAL DISEASE

Effective repair of aneurysms has been defined for several decades. (The indications and risks of surgery are discussed in Chap. 101.) For this large group of patients to benefit from repair, it is essential that the lesion be identified and that the ancillary disease that is so often present be fully assessed.

TABLE 100-5

RAYNAUD'S PHENOMENON: SECONDARY CAUSES

Collagen-vascular	Drugs
Scleroderma	Beta blockers
Mixed connective	Ergot
tissue disease	Methysergide
Rheumatoid arthritis	Vinblastine, ? bleomycin
Polymyositis,	Estrogens
dermatomyositis	Imipramine
Sjögren's syndrome	Occlusive diseases
Necrotizing vasculitis	Microcirculatory (see Table
Hematologic (see Table	100-3)
100-3)	Buerger's disease
Neurogenic	Hypothenar hammer
Outlet irritation	Environmental
Carpal tunnel	Prior cold injury
Neuropathy	Vibration syndrome
Miscellaneous	Vinyl chloride disease
Myxedema	
Acromegaly	
Pulmonary	
hypertension	

Examination techniques and the role of imaging have been presented. An appreciation of three general characteristics of aneurysms adds to the logic of approach. *First, most aneurysms progressively enlarge; the tempo for degenerative etiologies extends over years, whereas infectious or traumatic lesions progress in days or months. Second, aneurysms tend to be multiple. Some 5 to 10 percent of patients with an aortic aneurysm and 50 percent or more with peripheral aneurysms will have additional lesions.*[68,69] *A final generalization reviews aneurysm behavior. Rupture is the dominant threat of thoracic and abdominal aortic, iliac, and visceral artery aneurysms, while thrombosis, microembolism, and macroembolism are rare. In contrast, the latter complications are typical of carotid and limb aneurysms and rupture is rare.* Any aneurysm can cause dysfunction of adjacent structures by compression or can form a fistula with contiguous viscera or veins (Fig. 100-1). Ascending thoracic aorta aneurysms may cause aortic valve regurgitation or dissect, particularly when caused by cystic medial disease or congenital defects of the arterial wall (see also Chap. 98).

Patients should be screened for aneurysmal disease by examination or various imaging techniques in two sets of circumstances: (1) certain clinical problems and (2) specific settings. Aneurysms should be considered with discovery of an aneurysm elsewhere, unexplained occlusion of a distal artery, microembolic syndromes, limb edema possibly caused by aneurysm compression or fistula, and any continuous bruit. Aneurysms should be sought with given diseases known to cause them, including syphilis, the heritable disorders of connective tissue, several of the vasculitides, and atherosclerosis. Hypertension, smoking, and age predispose to aneurysm formation; abdominal aneurysms were found in 15 percent of males over age 65 screened by ultrasound,[70] and a familial tendency for aneurysms in both males and females has been identified.[71]

The current mortality and morbidity of aneurysm repair result more from chronic, concurrent medical problems than from surgical complications. The remarkable success of contemporary surgery is dependent upon the recognition and perioperative care of the multiple problems common to these patients. The patient should be free of infection to minimize the chance of graft infection. A simple hematologic screen will exclude bleeding disorders, intravascular coagulopathy, and platelet deficits. A history of prior venous thromboembolic disease warrants postoperative prophylaxis. The kidneys should be screened for renal artery stenosis, obstructive uropathy, and horseshoe kidney. Surgery can be performed with serum creatinine values below 4 mg/dL. Values above this level do not preclude surgery, but the need for dialysis increases.[72,73] Spirometry and blood gas values predict the need for pulmonary preparation and later ventilatory support. Death from respiratory failure is rare, even in patients with a P_{O_2} of less than 50 torr, mean forced expiratory flow (FEF_{x-y}) less than 26 percent of predicted normal, and those on oxygen.[74]

Carotid screening by duplex ultrasound is logical for those patients with bruits or a prior history of stroke or transient ischemic attacks. Angiography and possible prophylactic repair is warranted with significant bilateral stenosis found on scanning and those with recent ischemic events.[75] Significant hypertension, congestive failure, and hazardous rhythm problems should be identified and treated before repair. Critical aortic stenosis should not be overlooked. Coronary artery disease is the major determinant of both operative and long-term survival of the patient with atherosclerotic aneurysmal disease. A logical screening protocol is essential for all patients.

UPPER EXTREMITY ARTERIAL DISEASE

The diagnosis of these lesions can be demanding for three reasons: they are relatively rare, the etiology is very varied, and the combinations of associated vasospastic and microcirculatory disorders are common. The principles of diagnosis and treatment learned from the leg provide a reliable background logic; *upper extremity lesions are also categorized as acute and chronic occlusive disease, microcirculatory and vasospastic disorders, and aneurysmal disease*, Most problems are seen in one or more of three anatomic zones: at or near the origins of the brachiocephalic arteries in the chest, the axillosubclavian area, or the hand. Lesions in the muscular portion of the arm are infrequent. Causes include embolic occlusion, direct or iatrogenic trauma, and, on occasion, vasculitis, fibromuscular dysplasia, or embolic infections. When required, noninvasive testing should survey the entire limb, and angiography should include the aortic arch and extend through the hand, with adequate vasodilation for the delineation of the digital arteries.

Chronic atherosclerotic occlusive disease is seen predominantly at the origin of the innominate or, more commonly, the left subclavian artery. Claudication is infrequent or modest because of the intermittent use of the arm and because of its excellent collateral circulation. Radiologic or ultrasound evidence of "steal" from the vertebral artery is not uncommon, but any neurologic symptoms are most often explained by associated carotid disease rather than the subclavian lesion.[76] Acute macroemboli to the arm come predominantly from the heart and only occasionally from proximal aneurysmal or occlusive lesions. Most acute in situ occlusions reflect direct or iatrogenic trauma, aneurysm thrombosis, and the occasional clotting disorder. Acute or chronic microcirculatory disease of the hands may be generated by any of the numerous mechanisms listed in Table 100-3. Most are caused by connective tissue or hematologic disorders, emboli from proximal occlusive and aneurysmal disease, or occupational trauma. Raynaud's phenomenon may accompany any acute or chronic occlusive process. It may also reflect neural irritation at the thoracic outlet. Aneurysms are rare, usually located in the proximal brachiocephalic or axillosubclavian arteries; atherosclerosis, trauma, or the outlet syndrome are the usual etiologies. Thrombosis, distal micro- and macroemboli, and a painful mass are expected presentations. Rupture is rare except with infected lesions.[77]

Several specific entities should be remembered. Thromboangiitis obliterans may present initially with Raynaud's phenomenon or hand ischemia. It is bilateral, leg involvement is usual, and its clinical features, selective testing, and angiography separate it from other causes of hand ischemia.[78] The arteriopathic variant of the thoracic outlet syndrome usually reflects an osseous lesion (most commonly a cervical rib) that causes an aneurysm, or, less frequently, a stenosis. As noted, these produce complications by thrombosis, distal micro- or macroembolization, and Raynaud's phenomenon, alone or in combination (Fig. 100-5). Treatment is surgical.[79] Many patients with Takayasu's syndrome and one-tenth of those with temporal arteritis have lesions of the proximal arm arteries. Limiting arm claudication develops rapidly over a few months, but the process can be halted or improved by steroid therapy.[42,43] Repetitive trauma to the hypothenar area from using the hand as a hammer on wrenches, levers, or other devices causes occlusion or aneurysm formation of the ulnar artery at the hammate bone. Digital ischemia and Raynaud's phenomenon of one or more digits can result from distal emboli. Improvement follows if the trauma is stopped, but continued manifestations require surgical treatment.[80] Vibratory tools such as chain saws, grinders, and jackhammers can induce hand dysesthesias and Raynaud's phenomenon after several years. Symptoms initially occur during use, later becoming chronic; but ischemia is a rare and late occurrence.[81]

LABORATORY ASSESSMENT: ARTERIAL DISEASE

Indications

DIAGNOSIS OF VASCULAR DISEASE

Vascular disease cannot always be diagnosed by history and physical examination alone. When doubt exists, vascular testing may help to define an underlying problem or establish a specific diagnosis.

ASSESSMENT OF DISEASE SEVERITY

In many cases the diagnosis of vascular disease has been made, but the exact severity of the disease is uncertain. Specific testing may help to quantify disease severity in these situations.

MONITORING THE PROGRESSION/REGRESSION OF VASCULAR DISEASE

People with peripheral vascular disease may not be aware that their condition is slowly worsening over time, even when the symptoms become relatively severe and/or disabling. Objective testing enables the physician to identify and follow these changes. After medical, radiologic, or surgical intervention has been performed, serial noninvasive vascular testing enables the caregiver to determine the efficacy of therapy over time.

DOCUMENTATION OF VASCULAR DISEASE

Insurance companies and other third-party payers often require definitive documentation of vascular disease before au-

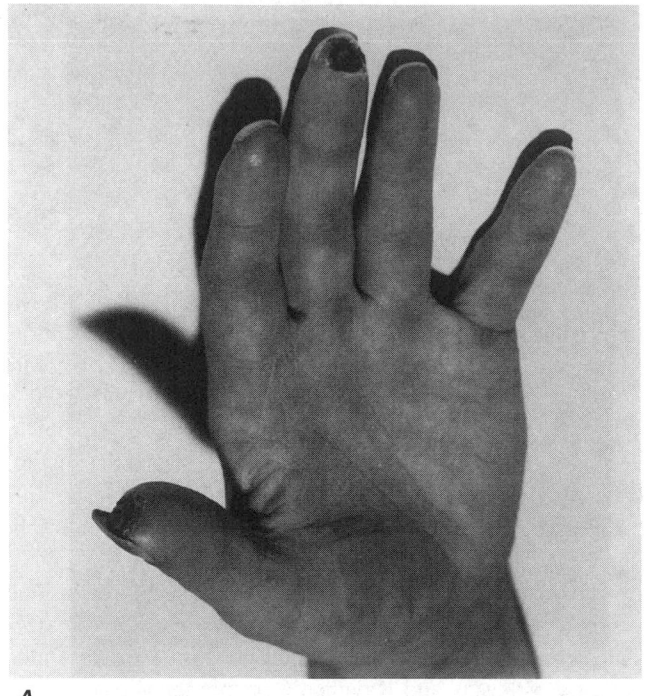

A

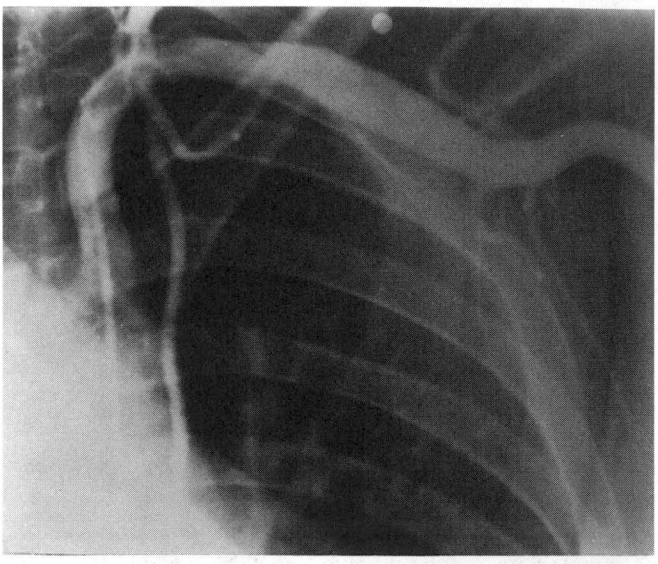

B

FIGURE 100-5

A. This 24-year-old house painter presented with rest pain and ischemic ulcers of digits 1 and 3. He had experienced bilateral arm claudication for 2 years and Raynaud's phenomenon for 9 months before admission. Steroids had been given for a diagnosis of vasculitis. *B.* In the same patient, radial and ulnar pulses were normal. Hyperabduction and costoclavicular maneuvers were abnormal bilaterally. Cervical ribs were noted on cervical spine roent-genograms. Note the subtle shadow suggesting thrombus in the mid-upper portion of the poststenotic aneurysm. The digital lesions healed slowly following resection of the cervical and first rib, aneurysmorrhaphy, and cervical sympathectomy. A similar, asymptomatic lesion on the right was subsequently repaired.

thorizing treatment. In some cases, objective vascular testing may be necessary to meet these increasing requirements for documentation.

Types of Tests

Vascular tests are generally classified as *invasive* (such as angiography) or *noninvasive*, although some tests such as computed tomography may be considered *minimally invasive* because they require the administration of intravenous contrast. This section focuses on noninvasive testing.

Vascular tests can be divided into three broad categories, depending upon the type of information they generate. These include the following.

ANATOMIC STUDIES

Imaging techniques—including two-dimensional (2D) real-time ultrasound, magnetic resonance imaging, computed tomography, and angiography—provide *anatomic* information about blood vessels. The presence or absence of aneurysms, dissections, stenotic lesions, arterial occlusions, etc., can be determined by these tests.

HEMODYNAMIC STUDIES

These techniques provide information about the *hemodynamic* importance of a given vascular lesion. For example, angiog-raphy may demonstrate an *anatomically* significant 60 percent stenosis in a vessel, but it does little to assess the lesion's *hemodynamic* significance. In contrast, tests that measure the pressure drop across the stenosis or that evaluate the increase in blood-flow velocity across the lesion provide information about the *hemodynamic* impact of the narrowed segment.

FUNCTIONAL STUDIES

In some cases the information obtained by anatomic or hemodynamic testing is insufficient to explain the symptoms or impairment described by the patient. In this case a *functional* vascular test may be helpful. Functional tests assess the impact of vascular disease on the limb, and often involve some form of "stress." Consider a hypothetical example in which two patients each present with comparable degrees of arterial obstruction. Despite having similar anatomy and resting hemodynamics, one of the subjects is physically well conditioned and has excellent collateral vessels, while the other is poorly conditioned and has minimal collateral development. In this situation, an exercise study will clarify the difference between the two subjects and allow the clinician to implement appropriate treatment.

Specific Arterial Tests

Table 100-6 lists some of the more commonly used noninvasive arterial tests and characterizes each in terms of the anatomic, hemodynamic, or functional information it provides.

CONTINUOUS-WAVE DOPPLER

The most widely used continuous-wave (CW) Doppler devices are simple hand-held units, which can be purchased for a few hundred dollars and are easily carried on a belt or in a coat pocket. Most modern 2D ultrasound imaging devices also have CW Doppler capabilities (*duplex scanning*). The Doppler detects blood motion and may be used by itself as a means of screening for vascular disease,[82,83] or it may be an integral part of other tests such as segmental pressure determination (described below).

In a normal artery, the pulsatile waveform is usually *triphasic*; during cardiac systole, there is forward flow in the arteries; during early diastole, the flow reverses direction (because of the elastic recoil of the peripheral arteries); and during mid- to late diastole, there is a return to forward flow as arterial blood runs off through the small distal vessels.[84] When a blood vessel is interrogated by Doppler at a site distal to a hemodynamically significant stenosis, this normal triphasic signal becomes altered. If the degree of stenosis is minimal, subtle changes such as dampening of the signal and/or loss of the middiastolic forward flow component may be noted. As the severity of the stenosis worsens, the signal will eventually become *monophasic*. By assessing the Doppler signal at multiple sites along the limb, the evaluator can determine whether or not hemodynamically significant lesions are present and roughly localize them to a particular area of the limb.

The CW Doppler is inexpensive, and testing with it can be performed at the bedside as an extension of the vascular examination by those who are skilled in its usage. It requires training and practice to use the Doppler effectively, however, and the information obtained may be limited by the fact that it is a "blind" technique; duplicated vessels, anatomic variations, and obesity may lessen its accuracy. It is therefore primarily used as a screening tool.

TABLE 100-6

TYPES OF INFORMATION PROVIDED BY NONINVASIVE ARTERIAL TESTS

Tests	Anatomic	Hemodynamic	Functional
Continuous-wave Doppler	+	+ +	0
Segmental pressure (with exercise)	+	+ +	+ + +
Pulse volume recorder	+	+	+
Transcutaneous oximetry	0/ +	0	+ + +
Imaging studies (ultrasound/CT/MRI)	+ + +	0/ + [a]	0

[a] Poor for CT/MRI; better for ultrasound with Doppler or magnetic resonance angiography.

Key: 0 to + + + indicates a range from "not useful" to "very useful."

SEGMENTAL PRESSURES

Segmental pressures are measured by placing inflatable cuffs at multiple levels around the limb or digit and then sequentially inflating and deflating each to determine the arterial pressure at each cuff site.[85] Pneumatic cuffs are typically placed around the thigh, calf, ankle, upper or lower arm, or digits (Fig. 100-6). A CW Doppler (see above) is positioned over an artery at a site *distal* to the pressure cuff(s) and is used to determine the systolic pressure at which arterial flow resumes during cuff deflation. The limb pressures are typically divided by a reference arterial pressure (usually the brachial artery systolic pressure) to create an *index*. The most commonly reported segmental pressure is the *ankle-brachial index* (ABI).

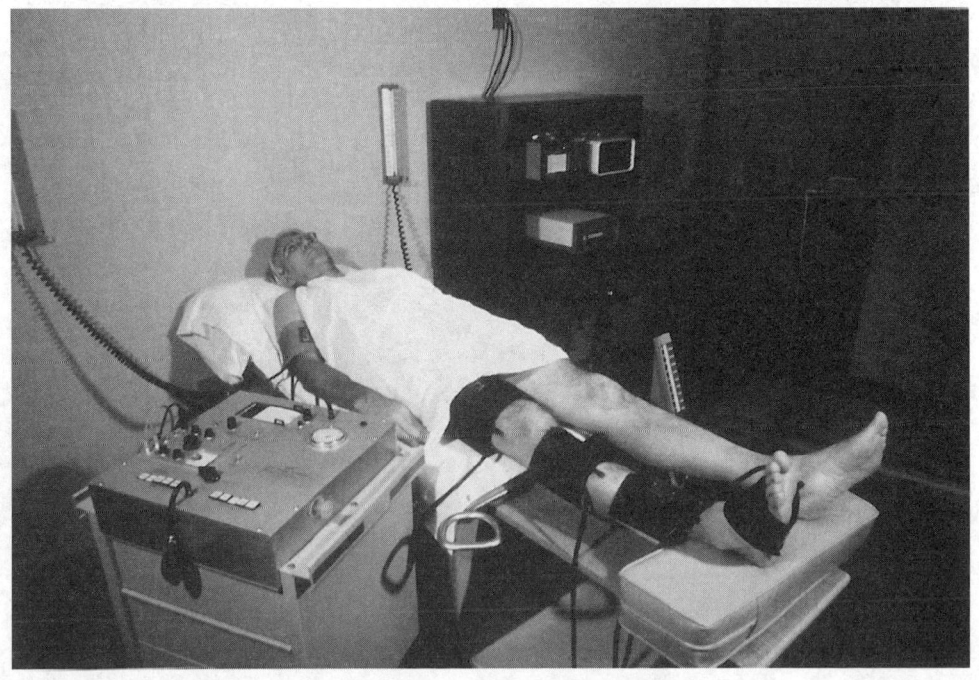

FIGURE 100-6

Segmental pressures. Pressure cuffs are placed at multiple levels along the limb and are used to determine the systolic blood pressure at each cuff site. An arm pressure is also obtained for comparison.

Segmental pressures provide a simple, reproducible, inexpensive, and accurate method of determining whether or not arterial obstruction is present, the severity of the obstruction, and the approximate location of the obstructed region(s). For example, if pressure is normal at the thigh cuff and is attenuated at the calf cuff, a hemodynamically significant blockage is likely to be present somewhere between the thigh and the calf. In most vascular laboratories, an ABI greater than 1.0 is considered normal, 1.0 to 0.8 is considered to represent *mild* disease, 0.8 to 0.5 reflects *moderate* disease, and less than 0.5 is a manifestation of *severe* disease.

Arterial lesions that are too minor to produce pressure drops at rest can be identified by exercising the patient. The subject is placed on a treadmill and ambulated according to a specific protocol; these protocols may be "fixed" (for example, 2 mi/h up a 12 percent incline for a maximum of 5 min) or may utilize "graded" exercise similar to those used in cardiac exercise studies.[86] Elements of the lower extremity study (i.e., as ABIs or CW Doppler analysis) are performed before and after exercise to determine the magnitude of change produced by walking. Exercise studies can be used to identify parameters such as the minimum walking distance that will produce claudication, the walking distance at which a patient would normally stop, the maximum walking distance, and so on.

The biggest disadvantage of segmental pressure measurement is that it cannot be used in patients whose blood vessels are noncompressible due to calcification of the arterial wall,[87] as occurs most commonly in diabetics. When vessels are stiff, the cuff cannot produce sufficient pressure to obliterate blood flow and the arterial pressure cannot be determined. Even when the large vessels of the limb are noncompressible, however, the digital vessels in the toes and fingers often remain uncalcified and can be used to estimate pressure if an appropriately small cuff is available.

PULSE VOLUME RECORDING

Pulse volume recording (PVR) is used to assess the arterial pulsatility of the limb.[88] It is measured by placing a pneumatic pressure cuff around the limb at a given level; the cuff is filled with air to a low pressure (typically 40 to 60 mmHg) and is connected by a flexible hose to a pressure transducer. The blood ejected from the left ventricle during cardiac systole causes a transient distention of the limb, which, in turn, produces a transient rise in cuff pressure. The cyclic changes in cuff pressure with each heartbeat provide an index of arterial "pulsatility." Measurements are typically made at multiple levels along the limb, as is done with segmental pressures, and the tracings are analyzed to determine whether or not there is a particular level at which the waveform changes shape or pulse dampening occurs.[89] When an altered pulse is found, it can be inferred that there is a hemodynamically signficant lesion proximal to the site of the cuff.

PVR is simple to perform and provides quick information about the presence and location of arterial occlusive disease. It has, however, a number of limitations, including *poor reproducibility* and the fact that pulsatility is a *qualitative* rather than *quantitative* measurement. Any situation that reduces pulsatility (such as aortic stenosis, rerouting of blood through collateral vessels, etc.) will attenuate the PVRs even when the actual blood flow is normal. Conversely, conditions that accentuate pulsatility (such as aortic regurgitation) or an arteriovenous fistula may produce large, abnormal PVR excursions even when overall forward arterial blood flow is reduced. PVR appears to be most useful for determining large-vessel patency and is often used by vascular surgeons to demonstrate the improvement in vascular patency after surgical revascularization or to monitor grafts for restenosis.

TRANSCUTANEOUS OXIMETRY

Transcutaneous oxygen (TcP_{O_2}) measurement is used to evaluate skin blood flow.[90] Oxygen-sensing Clark-type electrodes are attached to the skin by means of adhesive rings (Fig. 100-7), which create an airtight seal and ensure that the only oxygen reaching the electrode is that which diffuses into it from the skin. The surface temperature of the electrode is maintained at a

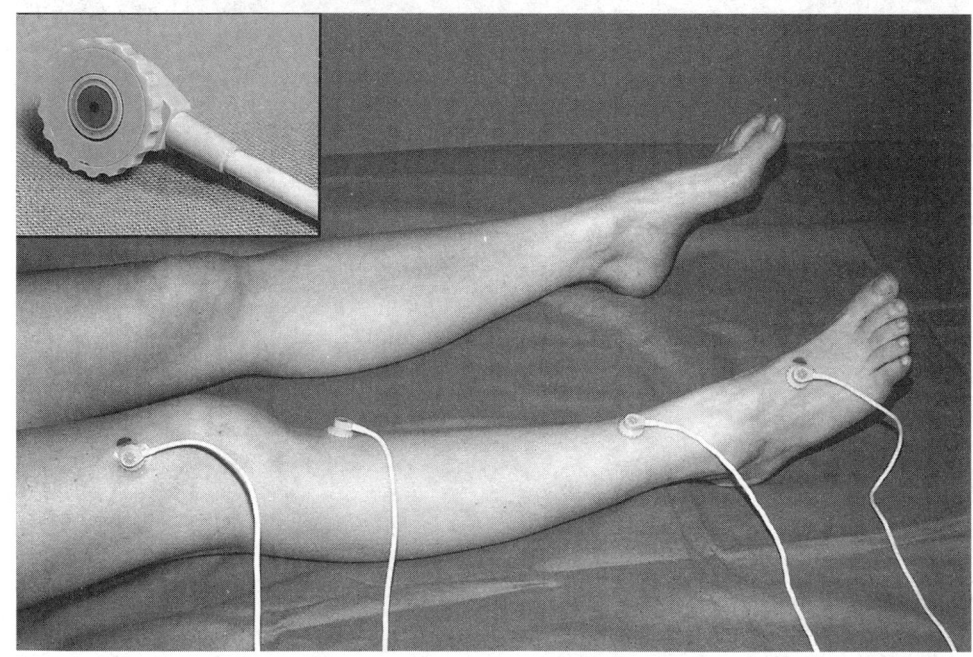

FIGURE 100-7
Transcutaneous oxygen can be measured at multiple sites along the limb. An airtight attachment is formed between the electrodes (*insert*) and the skin using a sticky adhesive.

relatively high temperature (43 to 45°C) so that the small vessels underlying the electrode become maximally dilated and the cutaneous blood flow is therefore determined primarily by the patency of the proximal arteries.[91] The amount of oxygen that diffuses out of the skin depends upon numerous factors including the arterial P_{O_2}, the cutaneous blood flow, and the rate of oxygen consumption by the skin. When the cutaneous blood flow is high (relative to the metabolic rate of the skin), the TcP_{O_2} may approach the arterial O_2; in contrast, when the cutaneous blood flow is low, the TcP_{O_2} is reduced. TcP_{O_2} is not so much a measurement of skin blood flow as it is a measurement of the *adequacy* of skin blood flow.

Transcutaneous oximetry has been shown to be useful in a number of situations, including *evaluation of critical ischemia*. It may be difficult to determine the functional severity of arterial occlusive disease solely on the basis of historical or clinical findings, even when basic noninvasive testing is available. This difficulty is especially relevant when the clinician is attempting to determine whether or not limb revascularization will be essential for pain relief, ulcer healing, or limb salvage.

Transcutaneous oximetry can be used to predict whether or not the cutaneous perfusion is adequate for healing at a given amputation site. Values above 40 mmHg are typically sufficient for healing, while those below 20 mmHg are not.[92]

Certain disease states may affect the small vessels or microcirculation without involving larger arteries; when this occurs, techniques such as CW Doppler, segmental pressures, PVR, and so on will not detect a significant abnormality. In contrast, TcP_{O_2} measurement usually demonstrates the inadequacy of circulation when it is due to small-vessel occlusive disease.

ASSESSMENT OF DIABETICS

TcP_{O_2} determination is often valuable in the assessment of patients with diabetes because they may have noncompressible vessels, small-vessel disease, and so on and are therefore not easily studied by other noninvasive functional tests.[93]

Although TcP_{O_2} measurement is an accurate way to assess the severity of cutaneous ischemia, it has several limitations. These include its inability to localize the occlusive disease to a particular segment or vessel and the fact that each laboratory must standardize and validate the technique before the results can be relied upon for diagnostic/therapeutic decisions.[94,95]

IMAGING TECHNIQUES

Imaging modalities such as 2D real-time ultrasound, computed tomography (CT) (Chap. 18), and magnetic resonance imaging (MR) (Chap. 19) are increasingly used as substitutes for the invasive technique of angiography, especially for the evaluation of structural abnormalities such as aneurysm, dissection, and arterial rupture. In addition, new acquisition and processing techniques are enabling CT scanning and *MR angiography* (MRA) (Fig. 100-8) to replace conventional angiography as a means of identifying arterial stenoses and occlusions. Continued technological advances in these noninvasive

modalities may allow them to eventually replace conventional arteriography in all but a few selected circumstances.

CLINICAL ASSESSMENT: VENOUS DISEASE

Diseases of the venous system are often a challenge. They require careful, skillful examination, selective testing, and prudent treatment. Skin lesions that appear as common superficial phlebitis, stasis change, or isolated varicosity may distract the physician from appropriately diagnosing vasculitis or lymphatic or cardiac disease. Deep venous thrombosis may

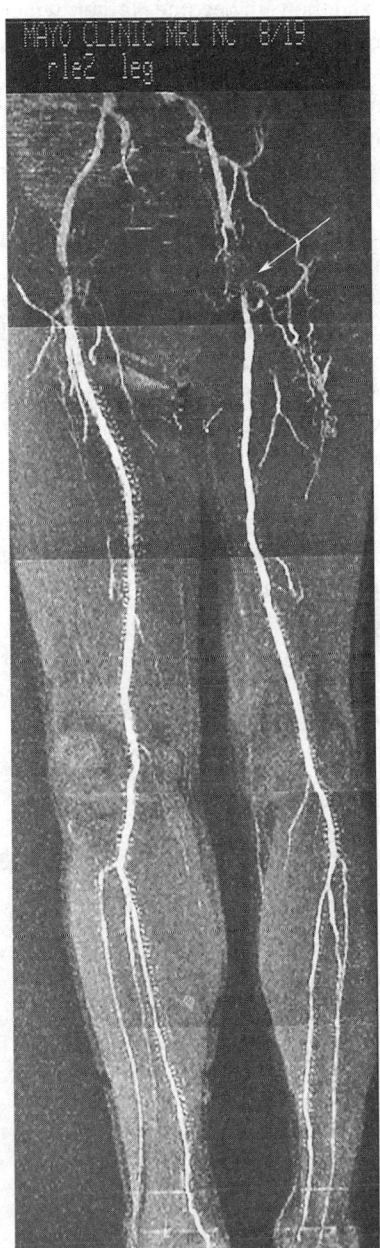

FIGURE 100-8
Magnetic resonance angiogram. This study shows an occlusion (*arrow*) of the left common femoral artery with collateral vessel development around it.

be subtle and easily overlooked, exposing the patient to risk of thromboembolism. In turn, what appears as classic deep vein thrombosis is often explained by venous compression or other disorders causing edema and limb pain (Table 100-7). Antithrombotic therapy is constantly being refined, surgical management of deep venous obstruction and incompetence is evolving, and new imaging techniques are enhancing diagnosis.[96,97]

Varicose Veins

Varicosities begin with the leakage of one or more valves. Local venous pressure is increased, additional valves become incompetent, and the vein becomes larger, wider, and tortuous over time. Primary varicosities are often a familial trait and are accelerated by lifestyles requiring prolonged standing, by obesity, and by pregnancy. Secondary varicosities reflect underlying perforator and deep venous obstruction and/or incompetence; the deep venous disease may result from venous compression, prior deep vein thrombosis of any cause and, on occasion, congenital lesions, arteriovenous fistulas, or right heart disease. Edema and stasis changes are rare with primary varicosities and usually signal an underlying secondary process. Bidirectional Doppler or color duplex ultrasound can usually differentiate primary from secondary varicosities. Primary varicosities are not often symptomatic, but they may ache or burn with chronic, recurrent standing. Both symptoms and progression can be ameliorated by light compression hose or a procedure. Sclerotherapy is effective for short primary varicosities and cutaneous "spiders." Surgical removal is indicated for longer segments of symptomatic or undesirable varicosities, for complications of subcutaneous or external hemorrhage, or for recurrent thrombosis in a varix (see Chap. 101).

TABLE 100-7

THE SWOLLEN LEG: DIFFERENTIAL DIAGNOSIS OF LOCAL CAUSES

Deep venous thrombosis	Acute arthritis with edema
Chronic venous insufficiency	Neurogenic pain with orthostatic edema
Congestive episodes	Tendonitis with orthostatic edema
Lymphedema	Achilles
Lipedema	Adductor
Muscle hemorrhage	Anserine
Trauma	Venous compression
Blood dyscrasia	Baker's cyst
Anticoagulants	Aneurysm
Muscle tear	Bone, muscle tumor
Ruptured Baker's cyst	Femoral bursitis
Sustained cramp	Heterotopic bone
Orthopedic vascular surgery	May-Thurner syndrome
Factitial	

Superficial Thrombophlebitis

The presence of a warm, tender, erythematous, and indurated linear lesion in the anatomic course of a superficial vein is diagnostic. Ultrasound can differentiate an atypical presentation from lymphangitic streaks, erythema nodosum, and other nodose lesions. The process most often occurs in a varix or at sites of indwelling catheters or needles. Active infection may be associated with the latter or with use of illicit street drugs; septic lesions are treated with culture-sensitive antibiotics and may require drainage. It may also be seen after direct trauma or in zones of severe acute arterial ischemia. Lesions occurring in a previously normal vein, whether single or migratory, can be idiopathic but more often are associated with malignancy, thromboangiitis obliterans, or vasculitis. The lesions of the latter two conditions may be nodular rather than linear and require diagnostic biopsy.[98] Superficial thrombophlebitis is usually self-limited, but healing can be accelerated by rest, intermittent warmth, and anti-inflammatory agents. Systemic anticoagulation is appropriate for lesions that progress despite conservative care and those located where the lesser or greater saphenous veins enter the deep system.[99]

Deep Venous Thrombosis

The diagnosis of deep venous thrombosis should be objectively documented, when feasible, for three reasons. First, this establishes the need for treatment to accelerate healing, to prevent clot propagation, and to prevent the sequelae of chronic venous insufficiency and pulmonary embolism. A firm diagnosis facilitates treatment choices when anticoagulation is relatively or absolutely contraindicated. Second, if the diagnosis is disproved, the cost of treatment and the risks of hemorrhage, heparin-induced thrombocytopenia, and warfarin necrosis are avoided.[100,101] Third, other diagnoses are sought when thrombosis is not found. The cardinal manifestations of deep vein thrombosis are a prominent superficial venous pattern, edema, and muscle turgidity and discomfort. These findings, however, may be absent or subtle. Very importantly, a broad spectrum of mechanisms can mimic deep venous thrombosis. These are diagnosed by their clinical findings and confirmed by appropriate testing (Table 100-7). *Less than half of patients considered to have deep venous thrombosis have the diagnosis confirmed when tested objectively.*[102–104]

Contemporary tests for venous disease are discussed below. Tests chosen for diagnosing deep venous thrombosis can be selected either for accuracy of definitive diagnosis or for clinical outcome. The various forms of isotope venography, plethysmography, and CW Doppler may be 95 percent sensitive to thigh obstructions, but are less accurate below and above this level. They do not exclude external compression and all are operator-dependent to some degree. When the need to know a definitive diagnosis is high, because of contraindications to therapy or for prognostic requirements, direct visualization by color ultrasound or venography is advisable. Venography remains very definitive, but attention must be paid to inadequate filling or defects in the lumen caused by inflow from collaterals without contrast.[105]

Treatment with heparin and subsequently warfarin for 12 to 16 weeks is highly effective in preventing clot propagation and pulmonary embolism (see Chaps. 52 and 60). Heparin-induced thrombocytopenia is minimized by monitoring platelets at 2- to 3-day intervals, and warfarin necrosis is avoided by overlapping heparin with warfarin for 4 to 5 days.[100,101] The risk of major hemorrhage from anticoagulation is 1 to 2 percent when laboratory control is precise and attention is paid to drugs enhancing warfarin effects.[106] Thrombus isolated to the calf rather than the thigh is less threatening, but upward of 20 percent of such thrombi extend proximally and 10 percent embolize; laboratory surveillance of the lesion is required if anticoagulants are not used.[107] Caval occlusive procedures, particularly filters causing minimal obstruction, are used when anticoagulants are contraindicated or have failed. Thrombolytic therapy,[108] given early, accelerates recovery and may reduce the postphlebitic syndrome.

Phlegmasia cerulea dolens is a rare, extensive iliofemoral and distal thrombosis characterized by rapid, massive edema, severe pain, and cyanosis of the limb. A third of patients succumb to pulmonary embolism and a half develop distal gangrene, often with cutaneous blebs. It is seen most commonly with advanced malignancy or severe infections but can follow surgery, fractures, and other common precipitants of thrombosis.[109] Urgent treatment is essential to minimize loss of life or limb and may include placing a caval filter, heparinization, and, often, debulking of the clot by thrombectomy and sometimes thrombolysis.

There are numerous local causes of repetitive episodes of limb pain and swelling that suggest acute recurrent deep venous thrombosis and that may warrant objective testing (Table 100-7). Fibrinogen uptake, D-dimer, duplex ultrasound, or venography confirms a new thrombus in only about one-third of such episodes.[110] Patients who have chronic deep venous insufficiency are especially likely to be symptomatic with these other conditions. Such patients may have acute episodes of pain and swelling that mimic new thrombosis, especially if they are not managed with adequate elastic support or if the limb is stressed by increased dependency, travel, hot weather, increased sodium intake, or sodium retention from drugs.

Prophylactic anticoagulation by various protocols is warranted in many patients with prior venous thromboembolism or known clotting disorders who are stressed by trauma or by medical or surgical illness or who are at bed rest for major skeletal trauma or surgery, congestive failure or debility, particularly when aged or obese.[97,108,111] When thromboembolic events occur without a recognized stimulus of venous stasis or injury, a search for venous compression, clotting defects, or systemic disease is appropriate. Such screening is valuable, even when the results are negative, in planning the duration of therapy and establishing prognosis (see also Chap. 60).

Central Venous Thrombosis

Occlusion of the superior (SVC) or inferior vena cava (IVC) may be an acute thrombotic event or may occur gradually, reflecting slow compression with subsequent thrombosis. The acute syndromes produce massive regional swelling and discomfort. Venous collaterals are prominent in chronic occlusion; the collaterals of the IVC syndrome are best appreciated with the patient upright. Malignancy is the cause of over 80 percent of SVC and about half of IVC obstruction. Relatively benign causes of the SVC syndrome include a growing incidence caused by indwelling catheters and fibrosing mediastinitis.[112] Inferior vena caval obstruction is often an extension from leg thrombosis, and both syndromes may be the initial manifestation of a clotting problem. Lytic therapy may clear thrombosis if given early. Bypass surgery is effective and durable in select instances of both syndromes.[113] Acute and chronic hepatic vein thrombosis presents with varying degrees of hepatic failure and ascites. Clotting disorders, tumors, and congenital venous anomalies are the usual causes.[114] Acute axillosubclavian thrombosis is often attributed to unusual effort; in these cases there is often an associated outlet lesion. Compression by tumor or aneurysm, indwelling catheters, and clotting defects arc other causes. Lytic therapy can be effective when given early and should be followed by anticoagulation. Patients with local outlet lesions can be further improved by subsequent balloon dilatation or surgery.[115]

Chronic Venous Insufficiency

Chronic deep venous incompetence or obstruction causing venous hypertension in the upright position may produce chronic venous insufficiency. This is characterized by leg edema, venous dilation, and intradermal deposition of proteins and hemosiderin. Cutaneous changes of fibrosis, lichenification, cellulitis, and ulceration follow. Edema of the foot and toes characteristically distinguishes lymphedema from the edema of chronic venous insufficiency (Fig. 100-9). Symptoms include heavy, congested limbs, venous claudication, pruritus, and skin ulceration that is often painful. Prior deep venous thrombosis, chronic right-sided heart disease, or arteriovenous fistula produce the syndrome. Increased ambulatory pressure can be confirmed by direct measurement or plethysmography. Both incompetence and obstruction can be documented by bidirectional Doppler, ultrasound, or color duplex scanning and venography.[116] Successful management has two stages: the initial healing of the skin, including ulcer grafting when required, and then lifelong control of venous hypertension utilizing rigid or elastic support generating 30 to 40 mmHg of compression. Repair or replacement of incompetent proximal valves and bypass of iliocaval obstruction are promising in a select subset of patients. The initial durability of these operations is encouraging.[117,118]

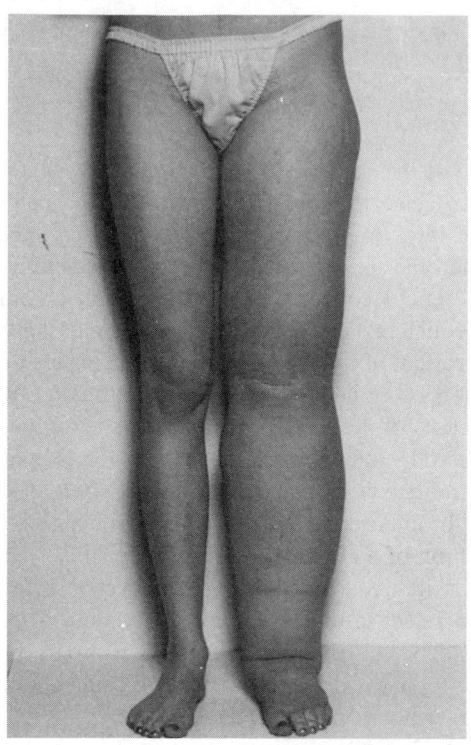

FIGURE 100-9
Massive painless edema and skin thickening in a 19-year-old woman that had evolved in less than 2 years. This constellation of historical and physical events is diagnostic of lymphedema praecox.

LABORATORY ASSESSMENT: VENOUS DISEASE

As with arterial testing, the indications for peripheral venous testing include the diagnosis of venous disease, assessment of disease severity, monitoring of disease progression/regression, and objective documentation of the presence of venous disease. Venous tests may be *invasive* (like venography) or *noninvasive*, and the information they provide may be *anatomic*, *hemodynamic*, or *functional*.

Specific Venous Tests

Table 100-8 lists the more commonly used venous tests and characterizes each in terms of the anatomic, hemodynamic, or functional information provided.

TABLE 100-8

TYPES OF INFORMATION PROVIDED
BY NONINVASIVE VENOUS TESTING

Test	Anatomic	Hemodynamic	Functional
Continuous-wave Doppler	+	+ +	0
Plethysmography (exercise or outflow)	0/ +	+ +	+ + +
Imaging studies (ultrasound/CT)	+ + +	0/ + [a]	0

[a] Poor for CT; better for ultrasound with Doppler.
Key: 0 to + + + indicates a range from "not useful" to "very useful."

CONTINUOUS-WAVE DOPPLER

As described previously, CW Doppler acts primarily by detecting the movement of blood. In contrast to the normal arterial signal, which is usually triphasic and synchronous with the cardiac cycle, the normal venous signal is much more complex. The components of venous flow that can be evaluated by CW Doppler include the following.

Spontaneity

When the Doppler is placed over a large vein, a spontaneous venous flow signal should be heard. Minor repositioning should be all that is necessary to obtain a detectable flow signal in most veins. If more extraordinary measures are needed—such as elevating, compressing, or otherwise manipulating the limb—it suggests a possible abnormality in venous flow.

Phasicity

Venous return Doppler signals vary with the respiratory cycle. Above the diaphragm there is an *increase* in venous return during *inspiration*. Below the diaphragm there is a *decrease* in venous return during *inspiration*, which occurs because the increased intraabdominal pressure during inspiration opposes venous return. A loss of phasicity with respiration suggests possible venous obstruction.

Augmentation

If a Doppler is placed over a vein in the proximal limb (for example, the femoral vein) and a distal portion of the limb (for example, the calf) is compressed, there should be a sudden increase in venous return. This phenomenon, called *augmentation*, will occur only if the vein is patent between the site of compression and the site of Doppler interrogation.

Competency

If a normal limb is compressed proximally (for example, over the thigh) or if a Valsalva maneuver is performed, the Doppler flow signal obtained distally (for example, over the popliteal vein) should temporarily cease as retrograde flow is stopped by the closure of venous valves. If the valves are incompetent, a retrograde flow signal will be noted.

Pulsatility

Unlike arterial flow, venous flow is not necessarily pulsatile. When significant pulsatility is noted, it raises the possibility of tricuspid regurgitation, right heart failure, pulmonary hypertension, volume overload, arteriovenous fistula, or some other disorder.

The CW Doppler provides qualitative (but not quantitative) information about the presence of hemodynamically significant reflux or obstruction; by interrogating the limb at multiple levels, it can be used to roughly localize the abnormality. Wheeler and Anderson[119] have analyzed multiple reports in which venography was used to confirm a proximal deep venous thrombosis and have demonstrated an overall accuracy rate of 87 percent for CW Doppler (specificity 88 percent, sensitivity 85 percent). It is a poor technique for evaluating partially obstructing thrombus or calf deep venous thrombosis. Although it is relatively sensitive for detecting areas of hemodynamically significant valvular incompetence, it is also a poor test for determining the functional significance of venous incompetence.

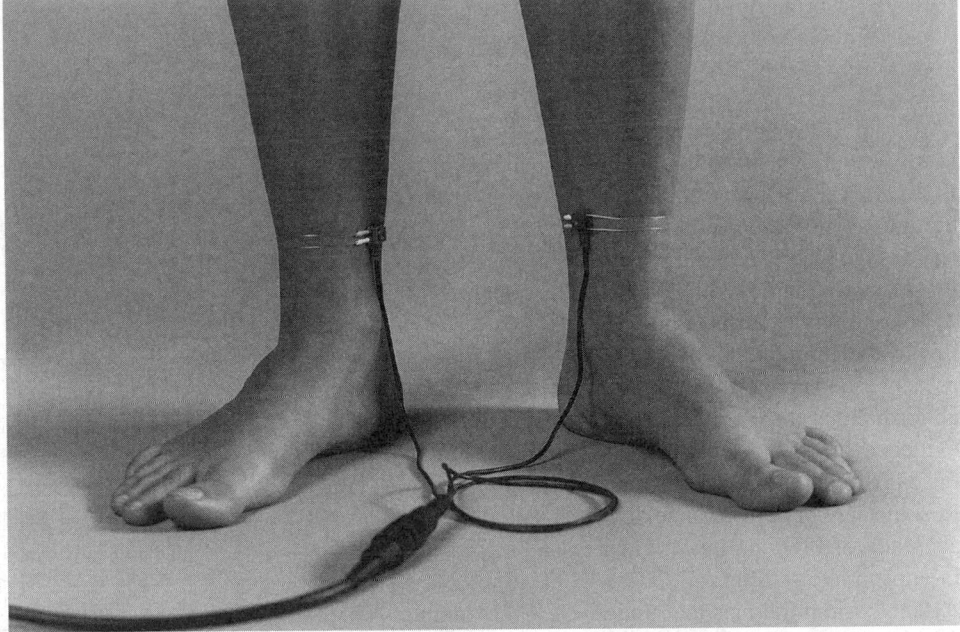

A

VENOUS PLETHYSMOGRAPHY

Various plethysmographic techniques can be used to measure the changes in limb volume that occur when venous return is enhanced or impeded. A variety of plethysmographic approaches have been developed, the most popular of which are *strain gauge* plethysmography, *air* plethysmography, and *impedance* plethysmography. A fourth modality, *photo* plethysmography,[120] is not a true plethysmographic technique but instead estimates the amount of blood in the limb by reflecting infrared light off blood cells flowing through the cutaneous vasculature.

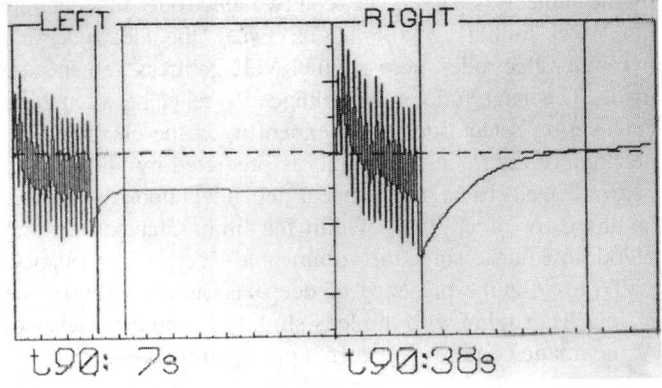

B

Plethysmography for Reflux

Venous reflux can be diagnosed and quantified using plethysmographic measures.[121,122] The patient is placed in an upright position (sitting or standing) and an air cuff or strain gauge is positioned around the lower portion of the limb. Once a steady volume measurement is obtained, the patient is tipped back and the legs are elevated to drain them of blood. The plethysmographic reading falls as blood drains from the veins and the limb becomes smaller. Once the blood has been emptied, the patient returns to the upright position and the veins begin to refill. If the valves are competent, refilling must occur in an antegrade fashion through the arteries and capillaries. In normal individuals, this may take a minute or more. If there is venous incompetence, the veins refill quickly and the leg volume likewise returns to baseline more rapidly than normal. If the incompetence is primarily *superficial* in location, the rapid refill rate can be normalized by placing tourniquets around the leg and/or directly compressing the incompetent superficial vein with the fingers.

Exercise Venous Plethysmography

This approach is used to assess the function of the "muscle pump" that normally compresses the veins and ejects blood

FIGURE 100-10

Exercise venous plethysmography. *A.* Mercury electrodes (or air cuffs) are placed around the lower extremities of the patient. *B.* Volume tracings of the right and left limb are obtained during and after exercise. In this example, the right limb falls during exercise and slowly refills during the recovery period. The T-90 (time to reach 90% refilling) is 38 s. Volume in the left limb does not fall nearly as much during exercise and recovers more quickly (T-90 of 7 s). This is consistent with hemodynamically significant venous insufficiency of the left leg.

out of the limb whenever muscular contraction occurs.[121,122] As above, the plethysmograph is usually placed around the lower limb or ankle while the patient is in an upright (sitting or standing) position (Fig. 100-10A). Once a stable baseline volume measurement is achieved, the patient is instructed to exercise the lower limb; this may consist of a series of toe or heel raises or deep knee bends. If a treadmill is available, the patient may be instructed to walk on it. In patients with normal venous pump function, the leg volume decreases during exercise. At the end of exercise, the volume returns to baseline as the veins refill. Legs with impaired venous pump function (caused by either venous obstruction, valvular incompetence, or primary pump failure) cannot decrease their plethysmographic volume during exercise to the same extent as normal limbs (Fig. 100-10*B*).

Outflow Plethysmography

Plethysmographic techniques can also be used to evaluate limbs for venous obstruction or deep venous thrombosis. Although any of the plethysmographic techniques are valid, impedance plethysmography (IPG) is the best studied and the most widely employed.[123–125] Unlike "anatomic" tests such as venography or ultrasound scanning (i.e., tests that directly image the thrombus), functional tests like IPG identify the presence of venous thrombi by detecting the hemodynamic abnormalities they produce. Because IPG relies on indirect evidence of venous obstruction, it may be subject to more false positives and negatives than the imaging tests; nevertheless, the ease of performance, low cost, and reasonable overall accuracy of IPG continue to make it a useful screening tool in appropriate settings.

The basic principles that underlie IPG are simple. A high-frequency, low-intensity electrical current (too weak to be felt by the subject) is passed between two electrodes that encircle the lower limb (Fig. 100-11). Between the electrodes are two other electrodes, across which voltage measurements are made. The magnitude of the voltage difference between these "measuring" electrodes is dependent upon the electrical impedance of the underlying limb as predicted by Ohm's law; in turn, the electrical impedance is dependent upon the volume of blood (or other fluid) within the limb. Changes in limb blood flow thus change the volume and electrical impedance.

To test for the presence of deep venous thrombosis, the patient lies supine with the legs slightly flexed and elevated. A pneumatic compression cuff is placed around the thigh and

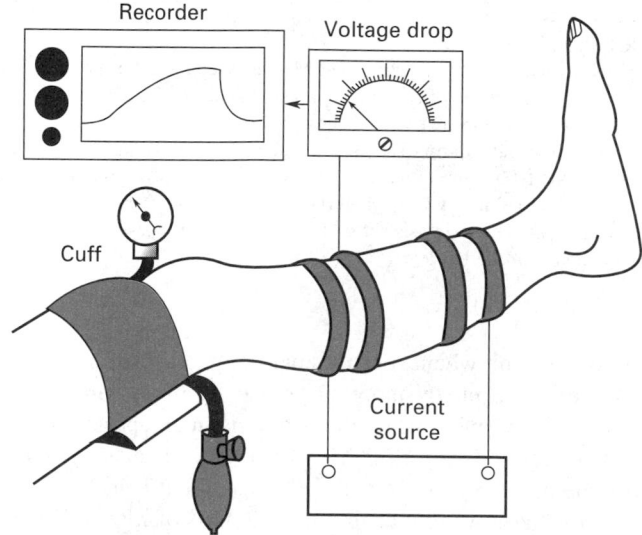

FIGURE 100-11

Schematic representation of impedance plethysmography (IPG). A high-frequency, low-intensity electrical current is passed between the two outer electrodes, and the voltage change is measured between the two inner electrodes. An inflatable thigh cuff is used to produce venous occlusion.

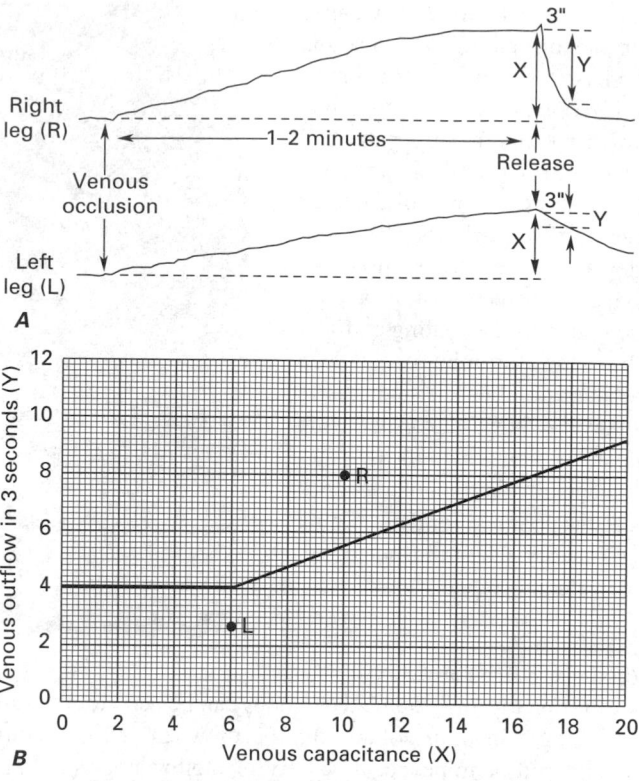

FIGURE 100-12

A. An IPG tracing from a normal right limb (*above*) and an obstructed left limb (*below*). When venous obstruction is present, IPG is typically affected in two ways: (1) the rise in leg volume occurring during venous occlusion is decreased (because the deep venous thrombosis has already occluded venous outflow and thus causes limb distention and a reduction in limb compliance); (2) the decrease in leg volume occurring during the first 3 s following cuff deflation is reduced (i.e., the rate of venous outflow is reduced). *B.* The changes in volume produced by cuff inflation and deflation can be plotted on a standard diagram. The line separating normal (*above*) from abnormal (*below*) has been empirically derived by comparing IPG results from limbs with and without deep venous thrombosis, as determined using a "gold standard" such as venography for the diagnosis.

inflated to a pressure above venous pressure but below arterial pressure (typically 40 to 50 mmHg); this produces venous occlusion, during which blood flows into the leg but not out. As blood becomes trapped beyond the cuff, the volume of the lower leg increases and the electrical impedance and voltage change (Fig. 100-12*A*). After an inflation period of typically 1 to 2 min, the cuff is rapidly deflated and venous flow is allowed to resume. As blood drains from the limb, the volume and voltage rapidly change. Values for the increase in leg volume produced by cuff inflation and the decrease in leg volume 3 s after cuff deflation are plotted on a standard diagram (Fig. 100-12*B*) and the presence or absence of deep venous thrombosis is determined.

CLINICAL APPLICATION

The accuracy of IPG as a means of detecting proximal deep venous thrombosis has been studied extensively with generally impressive results. One analysis that compared IPG with

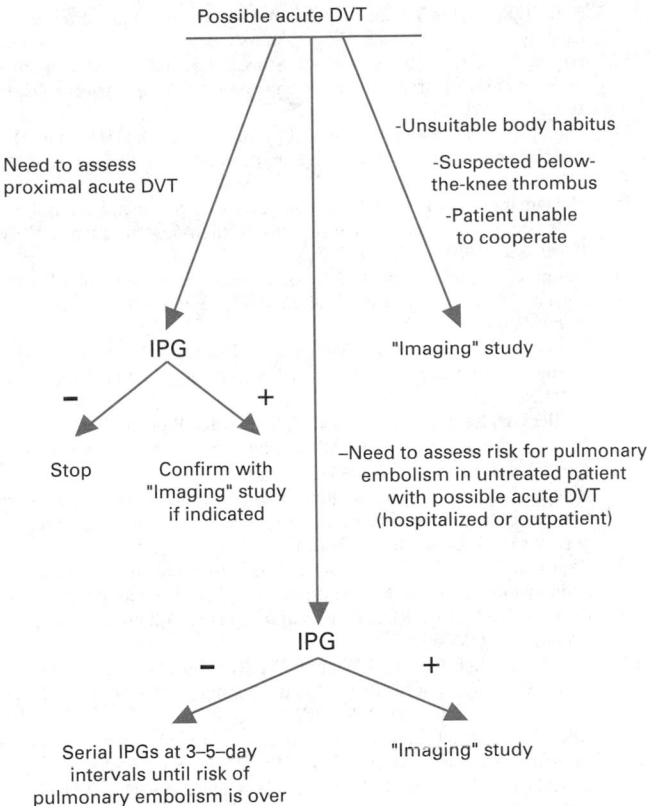

FIGURE 100-13
Algorithm for the use of IPG in the diagnosis of acute deep venous thrombosis (DVT).

venography in 2561 limbs demonstrated a sensitivity of 93 percent, a specificity of 94 percent, and an overall accuracy of 94 percent.[119] False positives occur when conditions other than acute deep venous thrombosis cause and mimic venous obstruction; the most common examples of these include elevated venous pressure from congestive heart failure, extrinsic vein compression, or "old" nonrecanalized venous thrombi. In contrast, false-negative tests are usually due to below-the-knee thrombi or nonoccluding proximal thrombi. As one would predict, the accuracy of IPG is variable and depends upon the subgroup of patients being studied. For example, although there is ample documentation that the test is useful when applied to symptomatic patients, concern has been raised about its reliability as a tool for screening high-risk, asymptomatic patients. Other pitfalls of testing include unsuitable body habitus (such as morbid obesity or severe limb edema) and inability on the part of the patient to cooperate during the examination (as may occur with patients who are comatose or in those with severely reduced limb mobility due to recent limb fracture, joint replacement, or other cause).

Despite potential pitfalls with its sensitivity and specificity, IPG appears to offer considerable prognostic information about the likelihood of a subsequent pulmonary embolism in patients suspected of having deep venous thrombosis. In one report involving short-term follow-up on 1074 patients with bilaterally negative IPG, there were no fatal pulmonary em-

boli; there was only a 1 percent incidence of clinical suspicion for nonfatal pulmonary emboli.[126] Other plethysmographic techniques have demonstrated similar good results.

The IPG remains best suited for use with cooperative, anatomically suitable patients in whom there is either a clinical suspicion of acute proximal deep venous thrombosis or a need to demonstrate that the patient is not at high risk for pulmonary embolism if anticoagulation therapy is withheld. The algorithm in Fig. 100-13 has proved to be a useful guideline for the clinical application of the test (see also Chap. 60).

REFERENCES

1. Leary WV, Allen EV. Intermittent claudication as a result of arterial spasm induced by walking. *Am Heart J* 1941; 22:719–725.
2. DeWeese JA. Pedal pulses disappearing with exercise. *N Engl J Med* 1960; 262:1214–1217.
3. Barnett AJ, Dugdale L, Ferguson I. Disappearing pulse syndrome due to myxomatous degeneration of the popliteal artery. *Med J Austr* 1966; 2:355–358.
4. Kavanaugh GJ, Svein HJ, Holman CB, Johnson RM. "Pseudoclaudication" syndrome produced by compression of the cauda equina. *JAMA* 1968; 206:2477–2481.
5. Goodreau JJ, Creasy JK, Flanigan DP, Burnham SJ, Kudrna JC, Schafter MF, et al. Rational approach to the differentiation of vascular and neurogenic claudication. *Surgery* 1978; 84:749–757.
6. Allen EV. Thromboangiitis obliterans: Methods of diagnosis of chronic occlusive arterial lesions distal to the wrist with illustrative cases. *Am J Med Sci* 1929; 178:237–244.
7. Kamienski RW, Barnes RW. Critique of the Allen test for continuity of the palmar arch assessment by Doppler ultrasound. *Surg Gynecol Obstet* 1976; 142:861–864.
8. Lederle FA, Walker JM, Reinke DB. Selective screening for abdominal aortic aneurysms with physical examination and ultrasound. *Arch Intern Med* 1988; 148:1753–1756.
9. Littooy FN, Stefan G, Greisler HP, White TL, Barker WH. Use of sequential B-mode ultrasonography to manage abdominal aortic aneurysms. *Arch Surg* 1989, 124:419–421.
10. Wychulis AR, Spittell JA Jr, Wallace RB. Popliteal aneurysms. *Surgery* 1970; 68:942–951.
11. Pappas CK, James JM, Bernatz PE, Schirger A. Femoral aneurysms: Review of surgical management. *JAMA* 1964; 190:489–493.
12. McCready RA, Pairolero PC, Gilmore JC, Kazmier FJ, Cherry KJ Jr, Hollier LH. Isolated iliac artery aneurysms. *Surgery* 1983; 688–693.
13. Zwolak RM, Whitehouse WM, Knake JE, Bernfeld BD, Zelenock GB, Cronenwett JL, et al. Atherosclerotic extracranial carotid artery aneurysms. *J Vasc Surg* 1984; 1:415–422.
14. Pairolero PC, Walls JT, Payne WS, Hollier LH, Fairbairn JF II. Subclavian-axillary artery aneurysms. *Surgery* 1981; 90:757–763.
15. Stanley JC, Thompson NW, Fry WJ. Splanchnic artery aneurysms. *Arch Surg* 1970; 101:689–697.
16. Trastek VF, Pairolero PC, Joyce JW, Hollier LH, Bernatz PE. Splenic artery aneurysms. *Surgery* 1982; 91:649–699.
17. Perloff JK: *Physical Examination of the Heart and Circulation*. Philadelphia: Saunders; 1982:215.
18. McLaughlin MJ, Colapinto RF, Hobbs BB. Abdominal bruits: Clinical and angiographic correlation. *JAMA* 1975; 232:1238–1242.
19. Beven EG. Thoracic outlet syndromes: In: Young JR, Graor RA, Olin JW, Bartholomew JR, eds. *Peripheral Vascular Diseases*. St. Louis: Mosby–Year Book; 1991:497–509.
20. Stoney RJ, Cheng SWK. Neurogenic thoracic outlet syndrome. In: Rutherford RD, ed. *Vascular Surgery*, 4th ed. Philadelphia: Saunders; 1995:976–992.
21. Pairolero PC, Joyce JW, Skinner CR, Hollier LH, Cherry KJ. Lower limb ischemia in young adults: Prognostic implications. *J Vasc Surg* 1984; 1:459–464.
22. Szilagyi ED, Elliott JP Jr, Smith RF, Reddy DJ, McPharlin M. A thirty-year survey of the reconstructive surgical treatment of aortoiliac occlusive disease. *J Vasc Surg* 1986; 3:421–436.

23. Hertzer NR, Beven EG, Young JR, O'Hara PJ, Ruschhaupt WF III, Graor RA, et al. Coronary artery disease in peripheral vascular patients: A classification of 1000 coronary angiograms and results of surgical management. *Ann Surg* 1984; 199:223–233.

24. Criqui MH, Langer RD, Fronek A, Feigelson HS, Klauber MR, McCann TJ, et al. Mortality over a period of 10 years in patients with peripheral arterial disease. *N Engl J Med* 1992; 326:381–386.

25. Turnipseed WD, Berkoff MA, Belzer FO. Postoperative stroke in cardiac and peripheral vascular disease. *Ann Surg* 1980; 192:365–368.

26. Collin J, Araujo L, Walton J, Lindsell D. Oxford screening programme for abdominal aortic aneurysm in men ages 65 to 74 years. *Lancet* 1988; 2:613–615.

27. Juergens JL, Barker NW, Hines EA Jr: Arteriosclerosis obliterans: Review of 520 cases with special reference to pathogenic and prognostic factors. *Circulation* 1960; 21:188–195.

28. Imperato AM, Kim GE, Davidson T, Crowley JG. Intermittent claudication: Its natural course. *Surgery* 1975; 78:795–799.

29. Schadt DC, Hines EA Jr, Juergens JL, Barker NW. Chronic atherosclerotic occlusion of the femoral artery. *JAMA* 1961; 175:937–940.

30. Starrett RW, Stoney RJ. Juxtarenal aortic occlusion. *Surgery* 1974; 76:890–897.

31. Coffman JD: Principles of conservative treatment of occlusive arterial disease. In: Spittel JA Jr, ed. *Clinical Vascular Disease.* Philadelphia: Davis; 1983:1–13.

32. Porter JM, Cutler BS, Lee BY, Reich T, Reichle FA, Scogin JT, et al. Pentoxifylline efficacy in the treatment of intermittent claudication: Multicenter controlled double-blind trial with objective assessment of chronic occlusive arterial disease patients. *Am Heart J* 1982; 104:66–72.

33. Porter JM, Baur GM. Pharmacologic treatment of intermittent claudication. *Surgery* 1982; 92:966–971.

34. Ekroth R, Dahllof AG, Gundevall B, Holm J, Scherstein T. Physical training of patients with intermittent claudication: Indications, methods, and results. *Surgery* 1978; 84:640–643.

35. Lie JT. The rise and fall and resurgence of thromboangiitis obliterans (Buerger's disease). *Acta Pathol Jpn* 1989; 39:153–158.

36. Mills JL, Taylor LM Jr, Porter JM. Buerger's disease in the modern era. *Am J Surg* 1987; 154:123–129.

37. Olin JW, Young JR, Graor RA, Ruschhaupt WF, Bartholomew JR. The changing clinical spectrum of thromboangiitis obliterans (Buerger's disease). *Circulation* 1990; 82:(suppl IV):IV-3–IV-8.

38. Fiessinger JN, Schafter M. Trial of iloprost versus aspirin treatment for critical limb ischaemia of thromboangiitis obliterans. *Lancet* 1990; 335:555–557.

39. Collins PS, McDonald PT, Lim RC. Popliteal artery entrapment: An evolving syndrome. *J Vasc Surg* 1989; 10:484–490.

40. Ishikawa K. Cystic adventitial disease of the popliteal artery and of other stem vessels in the extremities. *Jpn J Surg* 1987; 17:221–229.

41. Klein RG, Hunder GG, Stanson AW, Sheps SG. Large artery involvement in giant cell (temporal) arteritis. *Ann Intern Med* 1975; 83:806–812.

42. Hall S, Barr W, Lie JT, Stanson AW, Kazmier FJ, Hunder GG. Takayasu arteritis: A study of 32 North American patients. *Medicine* 1985; 64:89–99.

43. Kerr GS, Hallahan CW, Giordano J, Leavitt RY, Fauci AS, Rottem M, et al. Takayasu arteritis. *Ann Intern Med* 1994; 120:919–929.

44. Shepherd RFJ. Ergotism. In: White RA, Hollier LH, eds. *Vascular Surgery: Basic Science and Clinical Correlations.* Philadelphia: Lippincott; 1994:177–191.

45. Green RM, DeWeese JA, Rob CG. Arterial embolectomy before and after the Fogarty catheter. *Surgery* 1975; 77:24–33.

46. Blaisdell FW, Steele M, Allen RE. Management of acute lower extremity arterial ischemia due to embolism and thrombosis. *Surgery* 1978; 84:822–834.

47. Abbott WM, Maloney RD, McCabe CC, Lee CE, Wirthlin LS. Arterial embolism: A 44 year perspective. *Am J Surg* 1982; 143:460–464.

48. Hight DW, Tilney NL, Couch NP. Changing clinical trends in patients with peripheral arterial emboli. *Surgery* 1976; 79:171–176.

49. Darling RC, Austen WG, Linton RR. Arterial embolism. *Surg Gynecol Obstet* 1967; 124:106–114.

50. Meister SG, Grossman W, Dexter L, Dalen JE. Paradoxical embolism: Diagnosis during life. *Am J Med* 1972; 53:292–298.

51. McKechnie RE, Allen V. Sudden occlusion of the arteries of the extremities: A study of 100 cases of embolism and thrombosis. *Surg Gynecol Obstet* 1936; 63:231–240.

52. Holm J, Schersten T. Anticoagulant treatment during and after embolectomy. *Acta Chir Scand* 1972; 138:683–687.

53. Fogarty TJ, Cranley JJ, Krause RJ, Strasser ES, Hafner CD. A method for extraction of arterial emboli and thrombi. *Surg Gynecol Obstet* 1963; 116:241–244.

54. Thompson JE, Weston AS, Sigler L, Raut PS, Austin DJ, Patman RD. Arterial embolectomy after acute myocardial infarction: A study of 31 patients. *Ann Surg* 1970; 171:979–986.

55. McNamara TO, Fischer JR. Thrombolysis of peripheral arterial and graft occlusions: Improved results using high-dose urokinase. *Am J Roentgenol* 1985; 144:769–775.

56. Ouriel K, Veith FJ, Sasahara AA. for the TOPAS Investigators. Thrombolysis or peripheral arterial surgery: Phase I results. *J Vasc Surg* 1996; 23:64–75.

57. Karmody AM, Powers SR, Monaco VJ, Leather RP. "Blue toe" syndrome: An indication for limb salvage surgery. *Arch Surg* 1976; 111:1263–1268.

58. Hollier LH, Kazmier FJ, Ochsner J, Bowen JC, Procter CD. "Shaggy" aorta syndrome with atheromatous embolization to visceral vessels. *Ann Vasc Surg* 1991; 5:439–444.

59. Richards AM, Eliot RS, Kanjuh VI, Bloemendaal RD, Edwards JE. Cholesterol embolism: A multiple-system disease masquerading as polyarteritis nodosa. *Am J Cardiol* 1965; 15:696–707.

60. Kaufman JL, Shah DM, Leather RP. Atheroembolism and microembolic syndromes (blue toe syndrome and disseminated atheroembolism). In: Rutherford RB, ed. *Vascular Surgery,* 4th ed, Philadelphia: Saunders; 1995:669–677.

61. Gastineau DA, Kazmier FJ, Nichols WL, Bowie EJW. Lupus anticoagulant: An analysis of the clinical and laboratory features of 219 cases. *Am J Hematol* 1985; 19:265–275.

62. Allen EV, Brown GE. Raynaud's disease: A critical review of minimal requisites for diagnosis. *Am J Med Sci* 1932; 183:187–200.

63. DeTakats G, Fowler EF. Raynaud's phenomenon. *JAMA* 1962; 179:99–106.

64. Priollet P, Vayssairat M, Housset E. How to classify Raynaud's phenomenon: Long-term follow-up study of 73 cases. *Am J Med* 1987; 87:494–498.

65. Gifford RW Jr, Hines EA Jr. Raynaud's disease among women and girls. *Circulation* 1957; 16:1012–1021.

66. Landry GJ, Edwards JM, McLafferty RB, Taylor LM Jr, Porter JM. Long-term outcome of Raynaud's syndrome in a prospectively analyzed patient cohort. *J Vasc Surg* 1996; 23:76–86.

67. Coffman JD. *Raynaud's Phenomenon.* New York: Oxford; 1989.

68. Dent TL, Lindenauer M, Ernst CB, Fry WJ. Multiple arteriosclerotic aneurysms. *Arch Surg* 1972; 105:338–344.

69. Joyce JW, Fairbairn JR II, Kincaid OW, Juergens JL. Aneurysms of the thoracic aorta: A clinical study with special reference to prognosis. *Circulation* 1964; 29:176–181.

70. Bergqvist D, Bengtsson J, Sternby NH. Associated atherosclerotic manifestations. In: Greenhalgh RM, Mannick JA, eds. *The Cause and Management of Aneurysms.* London: Saunders; 1990:47.

71. Johansen K, Koepsell T. Familial tendency for abdominal aortic aneurysms. *JAMA* 1986; 256:1934–1936.

72. Johnson KW, Scobie TK. Multicenter prospective study of nonruptured abdominal aortic aneurysms: Population and operative management. *J Vasc Surg* 1988; 7:69–81.

73. Cohen JR, Mannick JA, Couch NP, Whittemore AD. Abdominal aortic aneurysm repair in patients with preoperative renal failure. *J Vasc Surg* 1986; 3:867–870.

74. Hollier LJ, Reigel MM, Kazmier FJ, Pairolero PC, Cherry KJ, Hallett JW Jr. Conventional repair of abdominal aortic aneurysm in the high risk patient: A plea for abandonment of nonresective therapy. *J Vasc Surg* 1986; 3:712–717.

75. Hart RG, Easton JD. Management of cervical bruits and carotid stenosis in preoperative patients. *Stroke* 1983; 14:290–297.

76. Walker PM, Paley D, Harris KA. What determines the symptoms associated with subclavian artery occlusive disease. *J Vasc Surg* 1985; 2:154–157.

77. Bower TC, Pairolero PC, Hallett JW Jr, Cherry KJ. Brachiocephalic aneurysms: The case for early recognition and repair. *Ann Vasc Surg* 1991; 5:125–132.

78. Hirai M, Shionaya S. Arterial obstruction of the upper limb in Buerger's disease: Its incidence and primary lesion. *Br J Surg* 1979; 66:124–128.

79. Kieffer E, Ruotolo C. Arterial complications of thoracic outlet com-

pression. In: Rutherford RB, ed. *Vascular Surgery*, 4th ed. Philadelphia: Saunders; 1995:992–999.

80. Conn J Jr, Bergan JJ, Bell JL. Hypothenar hammer syndrome: Posttraumatic digital ischemia. *Surgery* 1970; 68:1122–1127.

81. *Vibration Syndrome: Current Intelligence Bulletin 38.* Washington DC: National Institute of Occupational Safety and Health; 1982.

82. Strandness DE Jr, McCutcheon EP, Rushmer RF. Application of transcutaneous Doppler flowmeter in evaluation of occlusive arterial disease. *Surg Gynecol Obstet* 1966; 122:1039–1045.

83. Strandness DR Jr, Schultz RD, Sumner DS, Rushmer RF. Ultrasound flow detection: A useful technic in the evaluation of peripheral vascular disease. *Am J Surg* 1967; 113:311–320.

84. Johnston KW. Processing continuous wave Doppler signals and analysis of peripheral arterial waveforms: Problems and solutions. In: Bernstein EF, ed. *Vascular Diagnosis*, 4th ed. St. Louis: Mosby; 1993:149–159.

85. Yao JST. Pressure measurement in the extremity. In: Bernstein EF, ed. *Vascular Diagnosis,* 4th ed. St. Louis: Mosby; 1993:169–175.

86. Regensteiner JG. Exercise rehabilitation for patients with peripheral arterial disease. *Exerc Sport Sci Rev* 1995; 23:1–24.

87. Hobbs JT, Yao JST, Lewis JD, Needham TN. A limitation of the Doppler ultrasound method of measuring ankle systolic pressure. *Vasa* 1974; 3:160–164.

88. Darling RC, Raines JK, Brener BJ, Austen WG. Quantitative segmental pulse volume recorder: A clinical tool. *Surgery* 1973; 72:873–877.

89. Symes JF, Graham AM, Mousseau M. Doppler waveform analysis versus segmental pressure and pulse-volume recording: Assessment of occlusive disease in the lower extremity. *Can J Surg* 1984; 27:345–347.

90. Rooke TW. The use of transcutaneous oximetry in the noninvasive vascular laboratory. *Int Angiol* 1992; 11:36–40.

91. Rooke TW, Hollier LH, Osmundson PJ. The influence of sympathetic nerves on transcutaneous oxygen tension in normal and ischemic lower extremities. *Angiology* 1987; 38:400–410.

92. Bacharach JM, Rooke TW, Osmundson PJ, Gloviczki P. Predictive value of transcutaneous oxygen pressure and amputation success by use of supine and elevation measurements. *J Vasc Surg* 1992; 15:558–563.

93. Rooke TW, Osmundson PJ. The influence of age, sex, smoking, and diabetes on lower limb transcutaneous oxygen tension in patients with arterial occlusive disease. *Arch Intern Med* 1990; 150:129–132.

94. Rooke TW, Osmundson PJ. Variability and reproducibility of transcutaneous oxygen tension measurements in the assessment of peripheral vascular disease. *Angiology* 1989; 40:695–699.

95. Rooke TW, Heser JL, Hallett JW, Gloviczki P, Johnson CM. Hemodynamic changes following the surgical revascularization of lower limbs in patients with arterial occlusive disease: A comparison of six methods. *J Vasc Technol* 1993; 17:27–31.

96. Hirsh J, Hull RD. *Venous Thromboembolism: Natural History, Diagnosis and Management.* Boca Raton, FL: CRC Press; 1987.

97. LeClerc JR. *Venous Thromboembolic Disorders.* Philadelphia: Lea & Febiger; 1991.

98. Zimran A, Shilo S, Dallberg L, Herskro C. Chronic cutaneous polyarteritis nodosa simulating recurrent thrombophlebitis. *Isr J Med Sci* 1985; 21:154–156.

99. Plate G, Eklof B, Jensen R, Oblin P. Deep vein thrombosis, pulmonary embolism, and acute surgery in thrombophlebitis of the long saphenous vein. *Acta Chir Scand* 1985; 151:242–246.

100. Ansell J, Deykin D. Heparin-induced thrombocytopenia and recurrent thromboembolism. *Am J Hematol* 1980; 8:325–333.

101. Colp MS, Minifee PK, Wolma FS. Coumadin necrosis: A review of the literature. *Surgery* 1988; 103:271–277.

102. Haeger K. Problems of acute deep vein thrombosis: The interpretation of signs and symptoms. *Angiology* 1969; 20:219–223.

103. Barnes RW, Wu KK, Hoak JC. Fallibility of the clinical diagnosis of venous thrombosis. *JAMA* 1975; 234:605–607.

104. Ouriel K, Whitehouse WM Jr, Zarins CK. Combined use of Doppler ultrasound and phlebography in suspected deep venous thrombosis. *Surg Gynecol Obstet* 1984; 159:242–246.

105. LeClerc JR, Illegcas F, Jarzem P. Diagnosis of deep vein thrombosis. In: LeClerc J, ed. *Venous Thromboembolic Disorders.* Philadelphia: Lea & Febiger: 1991:176–228.

106. Robitaille P, LeClerc JR, Brave G. Treatment of venous thromboembolism. In: LeClerc J, ed. *Venous Thromboembolic Disorders.* Philadelphia: Lea & Febiger; 1991:267–302.

107. Kakkar VV, Howe CT, Nicholdes AN, Rennen JG, Clark MB. Deep vein thrombosis of the leg: Is there a higher risk group? *Am J Surg* 1970; 120:527–530.

108. Comerota AJ. Venous thromboembolism. In: Rutherford RB, ed. *Vascular Surgery*, 4th ed. Philadelphia: Saunders; 1995:1785–1814.

109. Brockman SK, Vasko JS. Phlegmasia cerulea dolens. *Surg Gynecol Obstet* 1965; 121:1347–1356.

110. LeClerc JR, Jay RM, Hull RD. Recurrent leg symptoms following deep vein thrombosis: A diagnostic challenge. *Arch Intern Med* 1985; 145:1867–1869.

111. Hyers TM, Hull RD, Weg JG. Antithrombosis therapy for venous thromboembolic disease. *Chest* 1989; 95(suppl):375–515.

112. Parish BM, Marschke RF Jr, Dines DE, Lee RE. Etiologic considerations in superior vena cava syndromes. *Mayo Clin Proc* 1981; 56:407–413.

113. Lochridge SK, Kibbe WP, Doty DB. Obstruction of the superior vena cava. *Surgery* 1979; 85:14–19.

114. Lillimoe KD, Cameron JL. The Budd-Chiari syndrome. In: Rutherford RB, ed. *Vascular Surgery.* Philadelphia: Saunders; 1989:1195–1202.

115. Machleder HI. Evaluation of a new treatment strategy for Paget-Schroetter syndrome: Spontaneous thrombosis of the axillary-subclavian vein. *J Vasc Surg* 1993; 17:305–317.

116. Nicholaides A, Christopoulos D, Vasdekis S. Progress in the investigation of chronic venous insufficiency. *Ann Vasc Surg* 1989; 3:278–292.

117. Kistner RL, Ferris EB. Technique of surgical reconstruction of femoral vein valve. In: Bergan JJ, Yao JST, eds. *Operative Techniques of Vascular Surgery.* New York: Grune & Stratton; 1980.

118. Lalka SG. Management of chronic obstructive venous disease of the lower extremity. In: Rutherford RB, ed. *Vascular Surgery*, 4th ed. Philadelphia: Saunders; 1995:1862–1882.

119. Wheeler HB, Anderson FA Jr. Use of noninvasive tests as the basis for treatment of deep vein thrombosis. In: Rutherford RB, ed. *Vascular Diagnosis*, 4th ed. St. Louis: Mosby; 1993:862–874.

120. Abramowitz HB, Queral LA, Flinn WR, Nora PF Jr, Peterson LK, Bergan JJ, et al. The use of photoplethysmography in the assessment of venous insufficiency: A comparison to venous pressure measurements. *Surgery* 1979; 86:434–441.

121. Katz ML, Comerota AJ, Kerr R. Air Plethysmography (APG): A new technique to evaluate patients with chronic venous insufficiency. *J Vasc Tech* 1991; 15:23–27.

122. Rooke TW, Heser JL, Osmundson PJ. Exercise strain-gauge venous plethysmography: Evaluation of a "new" device for assessing lower limb venous incompetence. *Angiology* 1992; 43:219–228.

123. Brown JG, Ward PE, Wilkinson AJ, Mollan RAB. Impedance plethysmography: A screening procedure to detect deep-vein thrombosis. *J Bone Joint Surg* 1987; 69B:264–267.

124. Huisman MV, Buller HR, TenCate JW, Vreeken J. Serial impedance plethysmography for suspected deep venous thrombosis in outpatients: The Amsterdam General Practitioner Study. *N Engl J Med* 1986; 314:823–828.

125. Patterson RB, Fowl RJ, Keller JD, Schomaker W, Kempczinski RF. The limitations of impedance plethysmography in the diagnosis of acute deep venous thrombosis. *J Vasc Surg* 1989; 9:725–730.

126. Wheeler HB, Anderson FA Jr, Cardullo PA, Patwardhan NA, Ming LJ, Culter BS. Suspected deep vein thrombosis: Management by impedance plethysmography. *Arch Surg* 1982; 117:1206–1209.

101

SURGICAL TREATMENT
OF PERIPHERAL VASCULAR DISEASE

Thomas F. Dodson / Robert B. Smith III

THE SURGICAL TREATMENT
OF PERIPHERAL VASCULAR DISEASE

Vascular surgery, generally slow to change and conservative in nature, is undergoing an evolutionary upheaval due to two ongoing forces in medicine today: (1) the emergence of managed care and for-profit hospital businesses in this decade[1] and (2) the advent of minimally invasive procedures readily adopted by general surgeons and accepted by the public.[2] For the first time, doctors and hospitals are being forced to confront the possible limitation of expensive specialty care as well as monetary incentives in order to provide "cost-effective care." Endovascular procedures[3] and laparoscopic techniques[4] are being utilized in vascular surgery in ever-increasing numbers and with limits bounded only by the imagination of the surgical investigator. Additionally, on the horizon is the potential utilization of gene therapy and molecular biology to manage the problems of restenosis and neointimal hyperplasia after endovascular procedures.[5,6]

Amid these technologic innovations, a few voices have been raised in dissent.[7,8] Expressed concerns have ranged from a "paucity of publications" in support of laparoscopic methods to a lack of "objective proof of efficacy" in patients undergoing endovascular procedures. As surgeons, we realize that randomized, controlled trials are necessary to solve many of the questions that remain in vascular surgery. It has been noted that lack of this methodology continues to be a stumbling block in the assessment of surgical therapies.[9] The recent publication of the Bypass Angioplasty Revascularization Investigation (BARI) shows that such studies *can* be carried out and comparisons made between interventional and surgical techniques[10] (see also Chaps. 48 and 102).

This chapter is divided into three sections: (1) carotid endarterectomy, (2) upper and lower extremity revascularization; and (3) upper and lower extremity venous thrombosis. As we acknowledged in an earlier edition, vascular surgery is directed toward the "palliative management" of patients with atherosclerotic and venous disease, but we recognize that "cure" clearly resides in the province of the gene rather than the scalpel.

CAROTID
ENDARTERECTOMY

Stroke continues to be the third leading cause of death in the United States, outranked only by heart disease and cancer. There are nearly 500,000 cases of stroke each year in this country, with approximately one-third of patients dying as a result.[11] Yet, encouragingly, there has been a decline over the past four decades in both the incidence of stroke as well as the mortality resulting from it. In the past several years, however, evidence has suggested that this long decline in stroke mortality and morbidity may have plateaued in the Minneapolis–St. Paul area.[12] Ironically, recent data from the Mayo Clinic in Rochester, Minnesota, noted that, in the period 1985 to 1989, there was a continuance of an earlier "leveling off" of incidence rates and a suggestion that stroke rates have actually increased over the past 10 years.[13,14] While it has been suggested that "environmental factors" influence the risk of stroke, certainly better control of hypertension, a gradual reduction in the percentage of individuals who smoke cigarettes, an increased awareness of the benefits of a physically active lifestyle, greater attention to cholesterol reduction and dietary modification, and greater use of anticoagulants in patients with atrial fibrillation have probably all contributed to the decline in stroke deaths in the United States.

Interestingly, "new" etiologies of stroke have been identified in the past decade, giving both medical and surgical investigators better insight into the underlying problems of stroke victims. The increased importance of a patent foramen ovale and associated paradoxical embolism was brought to light by Lechat and colleagues in France.[15] The subsequent development of transesophageal echocardiography has enhanced our ability not only to see the patent foramen ovale but also to identify the approximately 15 percent of patients who suffer ischemic strokes as a result of cardiogenic emboli.[16] Investigators from both the United States and England have identified a relationship between homocysteine concentrations and carotid artery disease.[17,18] While the former group noted an association between plasma homocysteine concentrations and extracranial carotid artery stenoses, the group from England found an association between serum total homocysteine concentrations and stroke in a sample of middle-aged men. They confirmed, in a prospective manner, a "strong independent association" between total homocysteine concentration and stroke in this population. In a metaanalysis of the literature on this topic, Boushey et al. concluded that there was an increased risk of arteriosclerotic vascular disease in patients with elevated total homocysteine levels, and they recommended clinical trials utilizing increased folic acid intake, since folic acid appears to be effective in reducing elevated total homocysteine.[19] An important addition to the understanding of various etiologies of stroke has been provided by The French Study of Aortic Plaques in Stroke Group. While their first paper in 1994 indicated a definite association between atherosclerotic disease of the aortic arch and the risk of ischemic stroke, a recent paper showed that the presence of plaques in the aortic arch ≥ 4 mm in thickness gave rise to a "high risk" recurrence of strokes and other vascular events.[20,21] It probably will be no surprise to physicians treating patients with vascular disease to learn that 26 of the 45 patients with plaques ≥ 4 mm thickness in the aortic arch were smokers.

In terms of who should undergo operation for carotid artery disease, we are finally on relatively firm ground. There have been six prospective randomized trials published on this topic since 1991, five of which have shown a benefit for surgery in preventing cerebral ischemia (Table 101-1).[22–27] At present, patients who present with transient ischemic attack or recent minor strokes without an obvious cardiac source are evaluated by duplex scanning of their carotid arteries. If patients are found to have significant stenosis, it is currently recommended that they have a four-vessel angiographic study of the cerebral circulation. If the arteriogram confirms the ultrasound evaluation (Fig. 101-1) and the patient is an otherwise acceptable operative candidate, a carotid endarterectomy is recommended. With respect to patients who have asymptomatic carotid lesions, we have not adopted entirely the recommendations of the Asymptomatic Carotid Atherosclerosis Study (ACAS) group.[24] While ACAS has suggested that patients with asymptomatic carotid artery stenosis causing a 60 percent or greater reduction in diameter and who are in generally good health were candidates for operation, we have somewhat arbitrarily adhered to a higher degree of stenosis of 70 to 80 percent as the criterion for surgical intervention in these individuals.

The generally accepted policy of requiring a preoperative

angiogram before every carotid endarterectomy is currently undergoing reevaluation. This reassessment is based on two factors: (1) there is a small but substantial morbidity related to angiography, documented in both the ACAS (1.2 percent)[24] and the North American Symptomatic Carotid Endarterectomy (NASCET) (0.7 percent) studies[27]; and (2) the use of the combination of duplex imaging and magnetic resonance angiography (MRA) when both document severe disease (greater than 70 percent stenosis) has been shown to reduce both morbidity and cost by avoiding angiography.[28,29] Others have noted that MRA adds little to the information provided by duplex ultrasonography, and they have recommended duplex scanning as the only preoperative imaging test before carotid endarterectomy.[30–32]

The great majority of our patients have their carotid endarterectomies done under local anesthesia with light sedation given by the anesthesiologist.[33] Others have utilized cervical block anesthesia with similarly good results.[34,35] We feel that these techniques are safer than a general anesthetic and provide moment-to-moment assessment of the patient's neurologic condition, avoiding the necessity of concern at the end of the case as the patient awakens from general anesthetic. We also shunt the patient routinely (Fig. 101-2), realizing, however, that approximately 80 percent of patients can undergo operation safely without the use of a shunt.

A carotid endarterectomy performed under local anesthesia with intraoperative sedation imposes a low degree of surgical stress on the patient with only a rare need for blood transfusion. The risk of operation rises with increases in the patient's symptomatology: the asymptomatic patient has the lowest risk, about 1 percent perioperative morbidity and mortality; the patient with transient ischemic attacks has a perioperative risk of about 3 percent, with a doubling of the yearly stroke risk from 1 percent (in the asymptomatic patient) to 2 percent; the patient who has had a completed stroke has a perioperative risk of about 5 percent, with a yearly stroke risk of 4 percent.[36]

For the past 2 years, we have adopted a clinical pathway for patients undergoing carotid endarterectomy that utilizes the postanesthesia care unit (PACU) for several hours after operation, with subsequent transfer to the vascular surgery ward rather than to the intensive care unit (ICU). Only patients with complications, with coexistent carotid and coronary disease awaiting cardiac surgery, or with instability are admitted to the ICU. While the majority of our patients are discharged on the second postoperative day, other groups have demonstrated the safety and cost reductions possible with discharge within 24 h of operation.[31,37,38]

A recent addition to the treatment of carotid artery disease has been the utilization of carotid angioplasty. This technique has been popularized by Dietrich and others,[39] but concerns have been raised by prominent vascular surgeons.[40,41] The current state of the dispute between radiologists and vascular surgeons is well illustrated in two recently published letters showing distrust on both sides.[42] Such controversy can be settled only by large, randomized, controlled trials to evaluate the efficacy of radiologic versus surgical techniques.

TABLE 101-1

CAROTID ENDARTERECTOMY: RANDOMIZED STUDIES

Symptomatic	Size of Study	Study Methods	Outcome
Mayberg et al.,[25] 1991	193 patients	92 patients treated surgically 101 patients treated medically	Significant reduction in stroke or TIAs in patients who received carotid endarterectomy (7.7%) compared with patients treated medically (19.4%)
European Carotid Surgery Trial,[26] 1991	2200 patients	219 patients treated surgically with mild stenoses (0–29%) 155 patients treated medically with mild stenoses 455 patients treated surgically with severe stenoses (70–99%) 323 patients treated medically with severe stenoses	Sixfold reduction in ipsilateral ischemic stroke for those patients who underwent carotid endarterectomy and had severe stenoses
NASCET,[27] 1991	659 patients	328 patients treated surgically 331 patients treated medically	Risk for reduction of 17 ± 3.5% for those patients who underwent carotid endarterectomy with high-grade stenoses (70–99%)

Asymptomatic	Size of Study	Study Methods	Outcome
CASANOVA Group,[22] 1991	410 patients	206 patients had surgery unilaterally or bilaterally 160 patients had no initial surgery (if bilateral, more affected side operated upon)	No significant difference in number of neurologic deficits and deaths between the two groups
Hobson et al.,[23] 1993	444 patients	211 patients treated surgically 233 patients treated medically	Endarterectomy reduced the overall incidence of ipsilateral neurologic events by 4.7%; no difference between combined incidence of stroke and death
ACAS Study,[24] 1995	1662 patients	825 patients treated surgically 834 patients treated medically	Carotid stenosis patients with 60% or greater reduction in lumen diameter had reduced 5-year risk of ipsilateral stroke if endarterectomy was performed with <3% perioperative morbidity and mortality

The treatment of carotid artery disease represents a benchmark for many other common vascular problems. Large randomized studies were performed to answer difficult questions. The economic milieu made a search for more cost-effective and efficient care a necessity, and we have responded by diminishing invasive preoperative testing and markedly shortening hospital stay, both of which were accomplished without sacrifice of quality of care.[43] Other questions remain to be answered, in a similar fashion.

UPPER EXTREMITY REVASCULARIZATION

Chronic arterial insufficiency of the upper extremity is most often due to occlusive disease of the aortic arch branches near their origin, either the subclavian artery or the brachiocephalic trunk. Symptoms may either be limited to ischemic manifestations of the arm and hand or may include posterior circulation insufficiency of the brain due to subclavian steal syndrome. Patient selection for surgical intervention is extremely important in this group of disorders, as many patients have few or no symptoms and should not be subjected to an operative procedure simply for the correction of an anatomic or radiologic finding.[44,45] Individuals who are significantly limited by arm claudication or those who have symptomatic subclavian steal syndrome should be thoroughly evaluated by vascular examination and complete angiography. Since the patterns of occlusive lesions are extremely variable, any surgical procedure must be carefully planned. Generally, extrathoracic bypass procedures are preferred if a normal donor artery is available; otherwise, a transthoracic procedure may be required to originate a prosthetic bypass from the aortic arch itself. If an extrathoracic bypass is feasible, the operation imposes a low degree of surgical stress, and there is little likelihood of a need for blood transfusions. General anesthesia

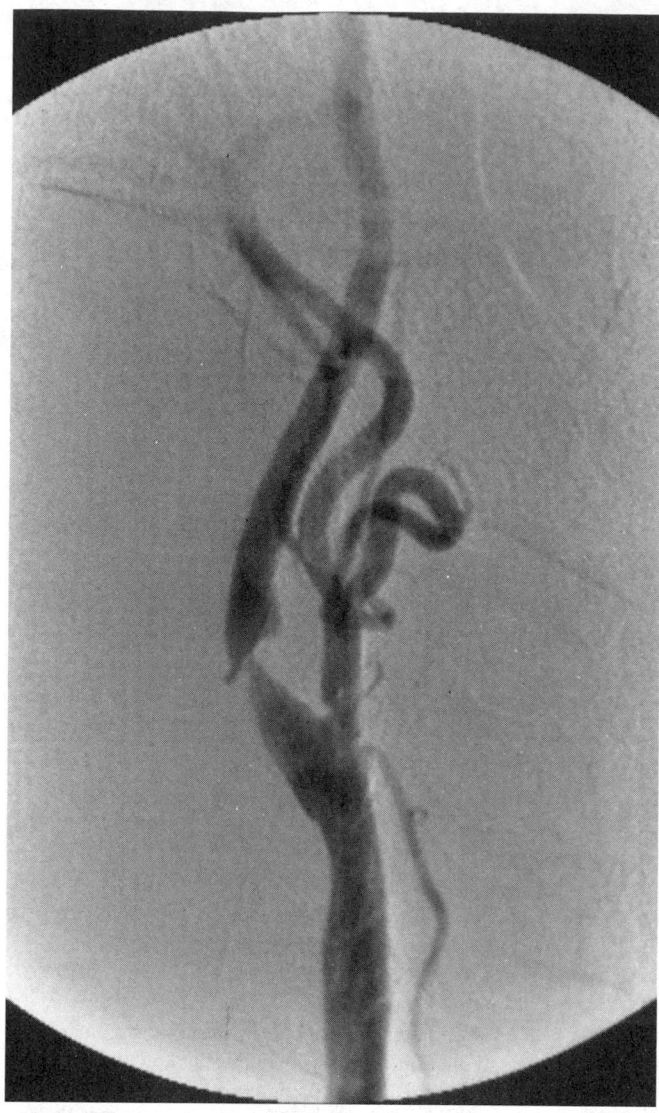

FIGURE 101-1
Carotid arteriogram in a 70-year-old man with asymptomatic, high-grade carotid stenosis.

is preferred, but selected operations for poor-risk patients can be performed with local anesthesia, if necessary.

Atheromatous occlusive disease of the subclavian artery is the most common lesion involving the proximal branches of the aortic arch. Extrathoracic revascularization of this vessel can be achieved by one of several techniques, depending on the pattern of obstruction and the relationship of the artery in question to a patent donor vessel. When the ipsilateral common carotid is patent and has minimal or no disease, it is frequently chosen as the site of arterial inflow. Perler and colleagues performed carotid-subclavian bypasses or transposition procedures on 31 individuals for a variety of conditions between 1979 and 1989. They achieved relief of symptoms in 30 patients (97 percent), with symptom-free survival of 89 percent at 1 year and 84 percent at 2 years.[46]

Vein grafts are often utilized to improve flow to the upper arm or forearm. Since the demonstration of this technique in

1965 by Garrett et al.,[47] others have published their series of bypass grafts for upper limb ischemia.[48,49] In the largest such series, comprising 74 patients who underwent 95 separate operations over a 15-year period, there were no operative mortalities and only a single major amputation. The survival rate was 86 percent at 5 years, with an overall patency rate of 61 percent at that time. Vein grafts were superior at all sites as compared with prostheses.[50]

A third alternative (after transthoracic or transsternal operations and extraanatomic bypasses) to improve perfusion to the upper extremity is the utilization of endovascular techniques for aortic arch lesions. In a recent review of 30 patients treated in this manner, success (defined as the ability to cross the lesion with a guidewire and to stent or angioplasty the lesion, leaving no residual pressure gradient or stenosis) was achieved in 27 of 30 lesions. The remaining three patients underwent extrathoracic bypasses. There were no procedure-related deaths and no strokes. The authors stated that "long-term arterial patency" was achieved in 24 of 30 instances, giving a success rate of 80 percent.[51] In view of the remarkably low incidence of stroke in this small series, it will be interesting to see if similar results are found in larger trials with longer follow-up.

LOWER EXTREMITY REVASCULARIZATION

Just as patients with asymptomatic carotid bruits have a higher risk of a cardiac ischemic event than of a stroke,[52] patients with peripheral vascular disease have an increased risk of death from cardiovascular causes. In a study of 565 men and

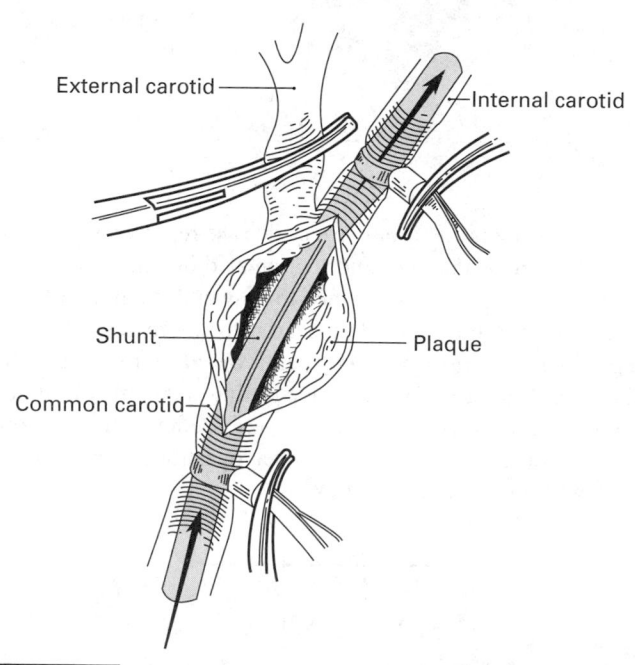

FIGURE 101-2
Indwelling shunt in place to preserve internal carotid flow during the endarterectomy.

women who were evaluated for the presence of large-vessel peripheral arterial disease (abnormal segment-to-arm blood pressure ratios or abnormal flow velocities) (see Chap 111) 67 subjects with peripheral arterial disease were identified. During a follow-up of 10 years, 21 of 34 men (61.8 percent) and 11 of the 33 women (33.3 percent) died. In patients without evidence of arterial disease, the death rates were 16.9 percent for the men and 11.6 percent for the women.[53] The same conclusion was found by Vogt and colleagues, who demonstrated that patients with a diminished ankle–arm blood pressure index of 0.9 or less had a crude overall mortality rate about fivefold greater than that of patients with a higher value of this index.[54]

PATIENTS WITH CLAUDICATION

A conservative approach to patients with claudication is generally appropriate. This conservatism is based on the relatively benign prognosis of the disorder itself, with a low risk of limb loss (approximately 1 percent per year) but a significant mortality rate (approximately 5 percent per year).[55] Furthermore, smoking cessation and structured exercise programs influenced the outcome of patients with claudication favorably.[56] A recent metaanalysis of exercise rehabilitation programs noted that the greatest improvement occurred with a duration of walking greater than 30 min per session, the use of near maximal pain during training as the end point, a frequency of at least three sessions per week, and a program length of greater than 6 months.[57]

On the other hand, an aggressive surgical approach to claudication involving femorotibial bypass has been advocated.[58] Over a 16-year period, a total of 57 tibial reconstructions were performed in 53 patients, which represented, however, only 5 percent of all the group's infrainguinal reconstructions. Autogenous vein was the conduit in all cases. There were no perioperative deaths, but there was a major complication rate of 9 percent (five patients total, with two cerebrovascular events and single episodes of pulmonary embolism, renal failure, and myocardial infarction). The overall survival at 5 years was 54 ± 15 percent.[58] We do not favor this aggressive approach to patients with claudication and would consider such distal bypasses only in patients whose claudication severely affected their lifestyles, such as inability to work or to perform the activities of daily living.

PATIENTS WITH REST PAIN

Ischemic rest pain is frequently an intolerable symptom and implies potential loss of the foot or limb. Whereas patients with claudication are generally managed in a conservative or nonoperative manner, patients with rest pain or a nonhealing lesion are evaluated, frequently as outpatients in the increasingly cost-conscious environment, for a potential operation.

The question of amputation versus revascularization for rest pain or a nonhealing lesion arises, especially in the elderly. A partial answer was provided by Veith and colleagues, who detailed a fall in the primary amputation rates from 41 to 5 percent during 1974 to 1989. These results were achieved with limb salvage in 90 percent of patients operated upon, with only a 3.3 percent mean procedural mortality.[59] Four studies that addressed this issue in the past decade are listed in Table 101-2.[60–63] While the numbers vary somewhat, revascularization seems to be appropriate in the great majority of patients (approximately 95 percent), while approximately 5 percent of patients should have amputation due to their moribund condition, little chance of functional recovery, or irretrievable limb ischemia.

We are in a period of transition in terms of the imaging of carotid artery disease, and approaches to imaging of the vasculature of the extremities are also evolving. We continue to order arteriograms to assess the vasculature of the arms and legs (Fig. 101-3), but MRA may ultimately supplant contrast arteriography.[64–67] MRA has also been utilized in graft surveillance, with an accuracy of 95 percent when combined with color-flow duplex imaging.[68] We currently utilize MRA to identify runoff vessels in patients who are otherwise candidates for revascularization but in whom contrast angiography has been of poor quality or has failed to demonstrate patent runoff vessels. The utility of MRA in this setting has recently been confirmed by investigators who noted a limb-salvage rate of 78 percent in patients with angiographically occult runoff vessels that were detectable by MRA.[69]

In our institution, the majority of patients who are being evaluated for potential vascular procedures are seen by cardiology consultants and undergo noninvasive cardiac testing to better define their cardiac risk. The utility of this approach remains controversial, with no clear answer despite several recent attempts to resolve the issue.[70–75] Chapter 83 addresses this question in greater detail.

Although we prefer to utilize the greater saphenous vein as a conduit in almost all infrainguinal bypasses, there are a number of alternatives,.[76,77] Most investigators acknowledge the relatively poor long-term results with polytetrafluoroethylene (PTFE) bypasses to infrapopliteal arteries, but some authors still recommend its utilization in the above-knee position.[78,79] In 1992, Taylor and colleagues described improved long-term results using PTFE and an anastomotic vein patch (now known as the "Taylor patch").[80] They documented a 5-year patency rate of 54 percent using this technique in infrapopliteal grafts. In a recent report of 63 patients in whom an autologous vein was not available and who underwent 66 PTFE bypasses to a tibial or peroneal artery *without* a distal anastomotic vein cuff, the results were described as "not significantly different" from those reported by Taylor.[81] Umbilical vein grafts are utilized by our group infrequently, although other authors have found them "an acceptable alternative."[82] Cryopreserved saphenous vein allografts have also been utilized as conduits for revascularization, but concerns remain about their thrombogenicity, antigenic nature, and consider-

TABLE 101-2

LOWER EXTREMITY AMPUTATION VERSUS REVASCULARIZATION

Author	Size of Study	Study Methods	Results
Ouriel et al.,[60] 1988	362 patients	158 patients, below-knee amputation 204 patients, revascularization	Patients who underwent revascularization had a lower perioperative mortality rate, a shorter length of stay, and an increased long-term survival rate.
Taylor et al.,[61] 1991	498 patients	498 patients with 627 critically ischemic legs treated with revascularization regardless of operative risk or operative difficulty.	Mortality for revascularization was 2.3% and median hospital stay was 11 days. In patients with gangrene and no distal vein, 14 primary amputations were performed. Renal failure had an adverse influence on limb salvage. Life-table survival at 5 years was only 38%.
Bunt and Malone,[64] 1994	767 patients	302 patients, revascularization 465 patients, primary major amputation	Revascularization patients had an 8% mortality at 30 days. In the 253 patients >70 years old, mortality of amputation was also 8%. Of all survivors of amputation, 50% died within 1 year.
Schina et al.,[63] 1994	266 patients	211 patients, revascularization 55 patients, amputation	Procedure-specific mortality was 2% for primary revascularization and 4% for amputation. Of the 12 deaths in the entire series, 9 were of cardiac etiology.

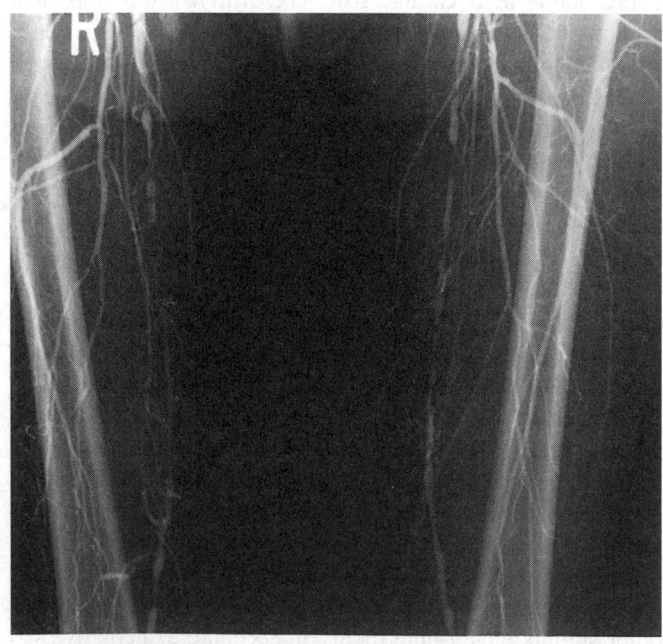

FIGURE 101-3

Arteriogram of the legs in a 75-year-old man with rest pain and bilateral superficial femoral artery occlusions.

able expense.[83–86] We do not currently utilize this vascular conduit.

In the largest series on long-term results of in situ saphenous vein bypass grafts, Shah et al. documented a cumulative secondary patency rate of 91 and 81 percent at 1 and 5 years, respectively, and a limb salvage rate of 97 and 95 percent at 1 and 5 years, respectively.[87] These results set the standard for infrainguinal reconstruction performed today. It has also been shown in a prospective, randomized, multicenter study that a comparison of in situ (Fig. 101-4) and reversed saphenous vein bypasses revealed "no significant differences" in overall patency rates.[88] The authors concluded that surgeons should therefore be adept at both procedures. We are increasingly utilizing "vein mapping" to help locate acceptable venous conduits preoperatively; these veins include the accessory ipsilateral greater saphenous vein, the contralateral greater saphenous vein, the lesser saphenous vein, and arm veins. Again, Shah et al. have shown that utilization of "spliced" excised vein segments will yield a primary patency rate of 72 percent at 1 year and 45 percent at 4 years.[89] There presently seem to be few fundamental impediments to the ability of vascular surgeons to operate on distal extremity vasculature. Current innovations include bypasses to the lat-

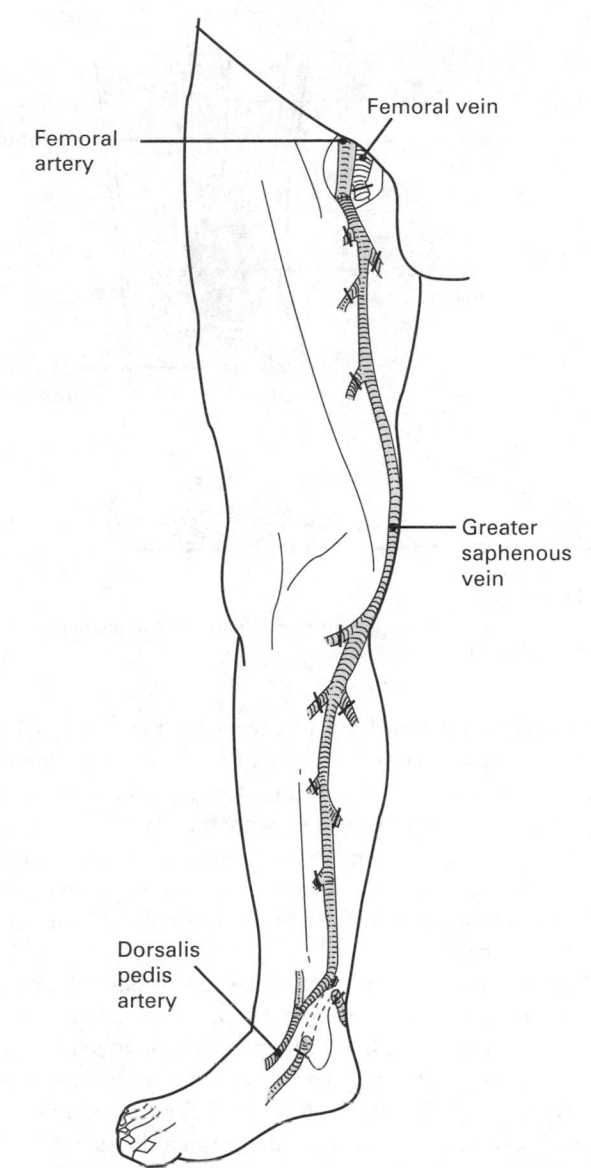

Femoral
artery

Femoral vein

Greater
saphenous
vein

Dorsalis
pedis
artery

FIGURE 101-4
In-situ bypass from femoral artery to dorsalis pedis artery.

eral plantar artery[90] and utilization of the operating micro-scope by teams at the Mayo Clinic[91] and The University of California—Los Angeles (UCLA).[92] Intensive surveillance, involving utilization of duplex scanning of vein grafts at 1 month, 3 months, 6 months, and every 6 months thereafter, seems to aid in detecting graft-threatening lesions, although it also adds to cost.[93]

Angioplasty of the femoral, popliteal, and even tibio-peroneal vessels has been recommended by some investiga-tors,[94–99] and some individuals have even recommended angioplasty for mild intermittent claudication.[100] Random-ized controlled trials are needed to determine the efficacy of these approaches.[101] Endovascular techniques such as stent placement[102] and percutaneous femoropopliteal graft place-ment[103,104] are also being evaluated in patients with femoral and popliteal artery disease. Cost-effective analyses of femor-

opopliteal revascularization procedures are just becoming available, and more are to follow.[105,106] (see Chap. 102).

UPPER EXTREMITY VENOUS THROMBOSIS

Deep venous thrombosis of the upper extremity is a relatively rare occurrence and represents only 2 to 3 percent of all diagnosed deep venous thromboses.[107] There are generally three etiologies of this uncommon problem: (1) central venous lines or devices; (2) cancer (pulmonary carcinoma, Hodgkin's disease, or lymphoma), especially in patients undergoing oper-ation or radiation; and (3) idiopathic causes including thoracic outlet syndrome and effort thrombosis.[108,109] In one report of 40 patients, who were found to have subclavian vein throm-bosis, 45 percent had anatomic abnormalities, 32 percent had intravenous catheters, and 23 percent had carcinoma. Pulmo-nary emboli have been thought to be less common as a conse-quence of upper extremity venous thrombosis than with thrombosis in the lower extremity. A recent report, however, has documented a 36 percent incidence of pulmonary emboli in 27 patients with venography-confirmed upper extremity deep vein thrombosis.[110] Compression ultrasonography and color-flow Doppler imaging were effective diagnostic modali-ties. Recurrences were observed and several patients had post-thrombotic sequelae. Venous gangrene is a rare but devasta-ting complication of upper extremity venous thrombosis; if it occurs, over half of the patients may need amputation and over one-third may die.[107] Patients with upper extremity thrombosis caused by a central line or device should have the line or device removed (if possible) and then should be treated by heparin, followed by warfarin sodium. Often the edema goes away with removal of the line, suggesting that the pa-tient's own fibrinolytic system deals effectively with the thrombus. Patients with cancer are the most difficult to treat, but elevation of the extremity and heparin followed by warfa-rin sodium are the mainstays of therapy. Effort thrombosis of the subclavian vein has received renewed attention in the past several years. The general tenets of therapy are as follows: (1) phlebogram to diagnose the abnormality; (2) lytic therapy in the acute phase; and (3) operation to decompress the tho-racic outlet. In patients with more chronic venous obstruction, vein patch angioplasty may also be required.[109,111–113]

LOWER EXTREMITY VENOUS THROMBOSIS

Deep venous thrombosis (DVT) of the lower extremities is an insidious and potentially lethal problem in hospitalized patients. It has been estimated that there are approximately 600,000 cases of venous thromboembolism in the United States each year.[114] Risk factors have been detailed in multiple publications and include age above 40, past history of DVT, general anesthesia, operations, pregnancy, malignant disease, hypercoagulable states, and trauma.[114] Hypercoagulable states (Fig. 101-5) have received renewed attention in recent

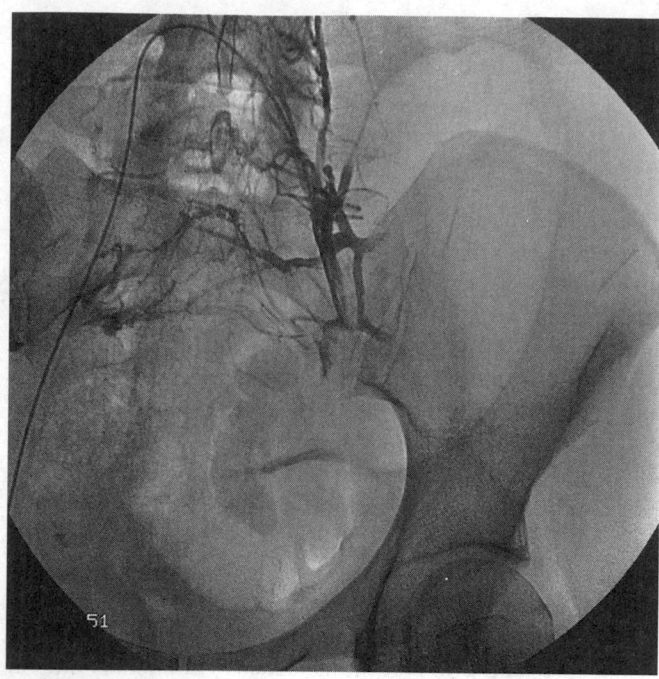

FIGURE 101-5
Venogram in a 31-year-old woman with a swollen leg, hypercoagulable state, and left iliac vein occlusion.

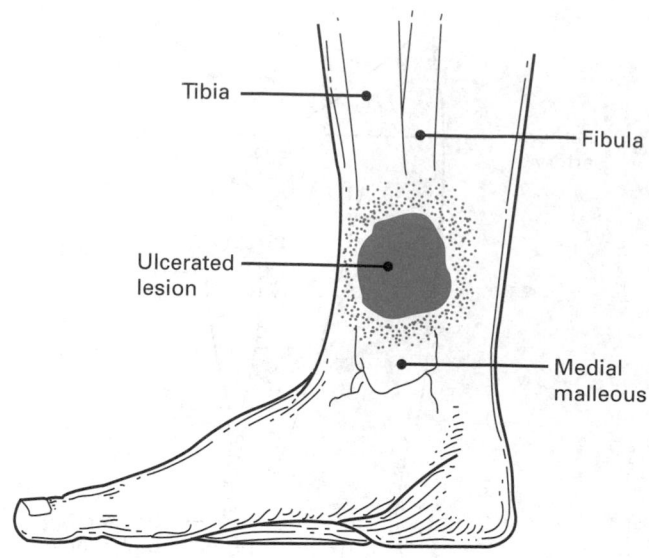

FIGURE 101-6
Venous stasis ulceration of the lower extremity after an episode of deep venous thrombosis.

years.[114–119] Studies have documented DVT in 58 percent of trauma patients,[120] 11 percent of patients undergoing lower extremity amputation,[121] and 33 percent of patients in a medical ICU.[122]

Patients with DVT are effectively treated by heparin given either by continuous intravenous infusion or by subcutaneous injection. The past decade has brought a number of changes in the therapeutic approach to patients with clot in major lower extremity veins: (1) a 5-day course of heparin has been shown to be as effective as a 10-day course[123]; 6 months of oral anticoagulant therapy has been shown to have a lower recurrence rate than the same dose given for 6 weeks[124]; and low-molecular-weight heparin has been found effective in treating patients at home with proximal DVT.[125,126] This last discovery was said to be "a major contribution to the treatment of deep vein thrombosis" in an editorial commenting on the findings.[127]

In recent years there has been some enthusiasm for lytic therapy in patients with DVT. The reasoning has been that lytic therapy could lyse the clot, restore normalcy to the leg and, more importantly perhaps, to the valves of the affected leg, thereby reducing the long-term sequelae of DVT (primarily the postphlebitic syndrome, which manifests as edema, hyperpigmentation, and ulceration and occurs in up to one-third of patients) (Fig. 101-6).[128] The obvious issue is weighing the risks of lytic therapy versus the chronic problems of the postphlebitic syndrome.

This issue was addressed by O'Meara et al., who used decision analysis after estimating the probabilities of various adverse outcomes of treatment and found that all 36 patients

interviewed were unwilling to accept an increased risk of death from lytic therapy in order to avoid the postphlebitic syndrome. In other words, in this study, all the patients selected heparin when presented with the data.[129] A recent report describing a spontaneous spinal epidural hematoma with subsequent paraplegia in an 18-year-old female after heparin and urokinase therapy for deep vein thrombosis lends credence to their decision.[130]

Patients with extensive clot in the lower extremities may go on to *phlegmasia curulea dolens* or acute iliofemora venous thrombosis. This condition, which is characterized by near total venous occlusion, may lead to total venous occlusion and venous gangrene. Venous thrombectomy for this condition has received renewed enthusiasm in the surgical literature,[131,132] but lytic therapy[133,134] and nonoperative therapy[135] also have their proponents.

While heparin and warfarin sodium are excellent therapy for the majority of patients with deep vein thrombosis, not all patients can tolerate the complications of these agents. Such patients include individuals with recent trauma, active bleeding or hemolysis, those with complications of heparin therapy, and patients with inferior vena caval clot or iliofemoral venous thrombosis.

A 20-year review of the clinical experience with Greenfield caval filters documented a caval patency rate of 96 percent, with a rate of recurrent emboli of 4 percent. There was no procedural mortality, and morbidity was minimal.[136] Interestingly, with the advent of percutaneous placement of prophylactic filters, concern has been raised about the possibility of overuse of these devices.[137] Lending another note of caution to the issue was the documentation of four patients who developed phlegmasia cerulea dolens after percutaneous placement of filters and cessation of anticoagulation.[138] A careful review of this topic was recently written by Greenfield and Proctor.[139]

REFERENCES

1. Kuttner R. Columbia/HCA and the resurgence of the for-profit hospital business. *N Engl J Med* 1996; 335:362–367.

2. Soper NJ, Brunt LM, Kerbl K. Medical progress: Laparoscopic general surgery. *N Engl J Med* 1994; 330:409–419.

3. Marin ML, Veith FJ, Cynamon J, Sanchez LA, Lyon RT, Levine BA, et al. Initial experience with transluminally placed endovascular grafts for the treatment of complex vascular lesions. *Ann Surg* 1995; 222:449–469.

4. Ahn SS, Clem MF, Braithwait BD, Concepcion B, Pavel BS, Petrik PV, et al. Laparoscopic aortofemoral bypass: Initial experience in an animal model. *Ann Surg* 1995; 222:677–683.

5. Lafont A. Guerot C, Lemarchand P. Which gene for which restenosis? *Lancet* 1995; 346:1442–1443.

6. McCarthy M. Reason for optimism over vascular gene therapy. *Lancet* 1996; 347:752.

7. Porter JM. Endovascular arterial intervention: Expression of concern. *J Vasc Surg* 1995; 21:995–997.

8. Treacy PJ, Johnson AG. Is the laparoscopic bubble bursting? *Lancet* 1995; 346:23.

9. McLeod RS, Wright JG, Solomon MJ, Hu X, Walters BC, Lossing A. Randomized controlled trials in surgery: Issues and problems. *Surgery* 1996; 119:483–486.

10. The Bypass Angioplasty Revascularization Investigation (BARI) Investigators. Comparison of coronary bypass surgery with angioplasty in patients with multivessel disease. *N Engl J Med* 1996; 335:217–225.

11. Bronner LL, Kanter DS, Manson JE. Primary prevention of stroke. *N Engl J Med* 1995; 333:1392–1400.

12. McGovern PG, Burke GL, Sprafka JM, Xue S, Folsom AR, Blackburn H. Trends in mortality, morbidity, and risk factor levels for stroke from 1960 through 1990: The Minnesota Heart Survey. *JAMA* 1992; 268:753–759.

13. Brown RD, Whisnant JP, Sicks JD, O'Fallon WM, Wiebers DO. Stroke incidence, prevalence, and survival: Secular trends in Rochester, Minnesota, through 1989. *Stroke* 1996; 27:373–380.

14. Bonita R, Beaglehole R. The enigma of the decline in stroke deaths in the United States: The search for an explanation. *Stroke* 1996; 27:370–372.

15. Lechat PH, Mas JL, Lascault G, Loron PH, Theard M, Klimczac M, et al. Prevalence of patent foramen ovale in patients with stroke. *N Engl J Med* 1988; 318:1148–1152.

16. Daniel WG, Mugge A. Transesophageal echocardiography. *N Engl J Med* 1988; 332:1268–1279.

17. Selhub J, Jacques PF, Bostom AG, D'Agostino RB, Wilson PWF, Belanger AJ, et al. Association between plasma homocysteine concentrations and extracranial carotid-artery stenosis. *N Engl J Med* 1995; 332:286–329.

18. Perry IJ, Refsum H, Morris RW, Ebrahim SB, Uelane PM, Shaper AG. Prospective study of serum total homocysteine concentration and risk of stroke in middle-aged British men. *Lancet* 1995; 346:1395–1398.

19. Boushey CJ, Bereford SAA, Omenn GS, Motulsky AG. A quantitative assessment of plasma homocysteine as a risk factor for vascular disease: Probable benefits of increasing folic acid intakes. *JAMA* 1995; 274:1049–1057.

20. Amarenco P, Cohen A, Tzourio C, Bertrand B, Hommel M, Besson G. Atherosclerotic disease of the aortic arch and the risk of ischemic stroke. *N Engl J Med* 1994; 331:1474–1519.

21. The French Study of Aortic Plaques in Stroke Group. Atherosclerotic disease of the aortic arch as a risk factor for recurrent ischemic stroke. *N Engl J Med* 1996; 334:1216–1221.

22. The CASANOVA Study Group. Carotid surgery versus medical therapy in asymptomatic carotid stenosis. *Stroke* 1991; 22:1229–1235.

23. Hobson RB II, Weiss DG, Fields WS, Goldstone J, Moore WS, Towne JB. Efficacy of carotid endarterectomy for asymptomatic carotid stenosis. *N Engl J Med* 1993; 328:221–279.

24. Executive Committee for the Asymptomatic Carotid Atherosclerosis Study: Endarterectomy for asymptomatic carotid artery stenosis. *JAMA* 1995; 273:1421–1428.

25. Mayberg MR, Wilson SE, Yatsu F, Weiss DG, Messina L, Hershey LA, et al. Carotid endarterectomy and prevention of cerebral ischemia in symptomatic carotid stenosis. *JAMA* 1991; 266:3289–3294.

26. European Carotid Surgery Trialists' Collaborative Group: MRC European carotid surgery trial: Interim results for symptomatic patients with severe (70–99%) or with mild (0–29%) carotid stenosis. *Lancet* 1991; 337:1235–1243.

27. North American Symptomatic Carotid Endarterectomy Trial Collaborators: Beneficial effect of carotid endarterectomy in symptomatic patients with high-grade carotid stenosis. *N Engl J Med* 1991; 325:445–453.

28. Turnipseed WD, Kennell TW, Turski PA, Archer CW, Hoch JR. Magnetic resonance angiography and duplex imaging: Noninvasive tests for selecting symptomatic carotid endarterectomy candidates. *Surgery* 1993; 114:643–649.

29. Kent KC, Kuntz KM, Patel MR, Kim D, Klufas RA, Whittemore AD, et al. Perioperative imaging strategies for carotid endarterectomy: An analysis of morbidity and cost effectiveness in symptomatic patients. *JAMA* 1995; 274:888–893.

30. Moneta GL, Saxn RR, Taylor LM, Porter JM. Carotid imaging before carotid endarterectomy. *Semin Vasc Surg* 1995; 8:21–28.

31. Kraiss LW, Kilberg L, Critch S, Johansen KH. Short-stay carotid endarterectomy is safe and cost-effective. *Am J Surg* 1995; 169:512–518.

32. Muto PM, Welch HJ, Mackey WC, O'Donnell TF. Evaluation of carotid artery stenosis: Is duplex ultrasonography sufficient? *J Vasc Surg* 1996; 24:17–24.

33. Chaikof EL, Dodson TF, Thomas BL, Smith RB III. Four steps to local anesthesia for endarterectomy of the carotid artery. *Surg Gynecol Obstet* 1993; 177:308–310.

34. Allen BT, Anderson CB, Rubin VG, Thompson RW, Gyle MW, Young-Beyer P, et al. The influence of anesthetic technique on perioperative complications after carotid endarterectomy. *J Vasc Surg* 1994; 19:834–843.

35. Shah DM, Darling RC, Chang BB, Bock DEM, Paty PSK, Leather RP. Carotid endarterectomy in awake patients: Its safety, acceptability, and outcome. *J Vasc Surg* 1994; 19:1015–1019.

36. Moore WS, Quinones-Baldrich WJ. Extracranial Cerebrovascular disease—The carotid artery. In: Moore WS, ed: *Vascular Surgery: A Comprehensive Review*, 3d ed. Philadelphia: Saunders; 1991: 434–472.

37. Collier PE. Are one-day admissions for carotid endarterectomy feasible? *Am J Surg* 1995; 170:140–143.

38. Katz SG, Kohl RD. Carotid endarterectomy with shortened hospital stay. *Arch Surg* 1995; 130:887–891.

39. Diethrich EB, Ndiaye M, Reid DB. Stenting in the carotid artery: Initial experience in 110 patients. *J Endovasc Surg* 1996; 3:42–62.

40. Beebe HG, Archie JP, Baker WH, Barnes RW, Becker GH, Bernstein EF, et al. Concern about safety of carotid angioplasty. *Stroke* 1996; 27:197–198.

41. Beebe HG. The carotid angioplasty premise. *Vasc Surg* 1996; 30:269–273.

42. Roubin GS, Yadav J, Iyer S, King P, Vitek J. Concern about safety of carotid angioplasty with response by Beebe HG. *Stroke* 1996; 27:1130–1131.

43. Hirko MK, Morasch MD, Burke K. Greisler HP, Litooy FN, Baker WH. The changing face of carotid endarterectomy. *J Vasc Surg* 1996; 23:622–627.

44. Fields WS, Lemak NA. Joint study of extracranial arterial occlusion. *JAMA* 1972; 222:1139–1143.

45. Hafner CD. Subclavian steal syndrome. *Arch Surg* 1976; 111:1074–1080.

46. Perler BA, Wiliams GM. Carotid-subclavian bypass: A decade of experience. *J Vasc Surg* 1990; 12:716–723.

47. Garrett ED, Morris GC, Howell JF, DeBakey ME. Revascularization of upper extremity with autogenous vein bypass graft. *Arch Surg* 1965; 91:751–757.

48. McCarthy WJ, Flinn WR, Yao JST, Williams LR, Bergan JJ. Result of bypass grafting for upper limb ischemia. *J Vasc Surg* 1986; 3:741–746.

49. Katz SG, Kohl RD. Direct revascularization for the treatment of forearm and hand ischemia. *Am J Surg* 1993; 165:313–316.

50. Mesh CL, McCarthy WJ, Pearce WH, Flinn WR, Shireman PK, Yao JST. Upper extremity bypass grafting: A 15-year experience. *Arch Surg* 1993; 128:795–802.

51. Queral LA, Criado FJ. Endovascular treatment of aortic arch occlusive disease. *Semin Vasc Surg* 1996; 9:156–163.

52. Chambers BR, Norris JW. Outcome in patients with asymptomatic neck bruits. *N Engl J Med* 1986; 9:860–865.

53. Criqui MH, Langer RD, Fronek A, Feigelson HS, Klauber MR, McCann TJ, et al. Mortality over a period of 10 years in patients with peripheral arterial disease. *N Engl J Med* 1992; 326:381–386.

54. Vogt MT, Cauley JA, Newman AB, Kuller LH, Hulley SB. Decreased ankle/arm blood pressure index and mortality in elderly women. *JAMA* 1993; 270:465–469.

55. Imparato AM, Kim GE, Davidson T, Crowley JG. Intermittent claudication: Its natural course. *Surgery* 1975; 78:795–799.

56. Radack K, Wydersky RJ. Conservative management of intermittent claudication. *Ann Intern Med* 1990; 113:135–145.

57. Gardner AW, Poehlman ET. Exercise rehabilitation programs for the treatment of claudication pain: A meta-analysis. *JAMA* 1995; 274:975–980.

58. Conte MS, Belkin M, Donaldson MC, Baum P, Mannick JA, Whittemore AD. Femorotibial bypass for claudication: Do results justify an aggressive approach? *J Vasc Surg* 1995; 21:873–881.

59. Veith FJ, Gupta SK, Wengerter KR, Goldsmith J, Rivers SP, Bakal CW, et al. Changing arteriosclerotic disease patterns and management strategies in lower-limb-threatening ischemia. *Ann Surg* 1990; 212:402–414.

60. Ouriel K, Fiore WM, Geary JE. Limb-threatening ischemia in the medically compromised patient: Amputation or revascularization? *Surgery* 1988; 104:667–672.

61. Taylor LM, Hamre D, Dalman RL, Porter JM. Limb salvage vs amputation for critical ischemia. *Arch Surg* 1991; 126:1251–1258.

62. Bunt TJ, Malone JM. Amputation for revascularization in the 70 year old. *Am Surg* 1994; 60:349–352.

63. Schina MJ, Atnip RG, Healy DA, Thiele BL. Relative risks of limb revascularization and amputation in the modern era. *Cardiovasc Surg* 1994; 2:754–759.

64. Owen RS, Carpenter JP, Baum RA, Perloff LJ, Cope C. Magnetic resonance imaging of angiographically occult runoff vessels in peripheral arterial occlusive disease. *N Engl J Med* 1992; 326:1577–1581.

65. Carpenter JP, Baum RA, Holland GA, Barker CF. Peripheral vascular surgery with magnetic resonance angiography as the sole preoperative imaging modality. *J Vasc Surg* 1994; 20:861–871.

66. Carpenter JP, Owen RS, Holland GA, Baum RA, Barker CF, Perloff LJ, et al. Magnetic resonance angiography of the aorta, iliac, and femoral arteries. *Surgery* 1994; 116:17–23.

67. Baum RA, Rutler CM, Sunshine JH, Blebea JS, Blebea J, Carpenter JP, et al. Multicenter trial to evaluate vascular magnetic resonance angiography of the lower extremity. *JAMA* 1995; 274:875–880.

68. Turnipseed WD, Sproat IA. A preliminary experience with use of magnetic resonance angiography in assessment of failing lower extremity bypass grafts. *Surgery* 1992; 112:664–669.

69. Carpenter JP, Golden MA, Barker CF, Holland GA, Baum RA. The fate of bypass grafts to angiographically occult runoff vessels detected by magnetic resonance angiography. *J Vasc Surg* 1996; 23:483–489.

70. Wong T, Detsky AS. Preoperative cardiac risk assessment for patients having peripheral vascular surgery. *Ann Intern Med* 1992; 116:743–753.

71. Ashton CM, Petersen NJ, Wray NP, Kief CI, Dunn JK, Wu L, et al. The incidence of perioperative myocardial infarction in men undergoing noncardiac surgery. *Ann Intern Med* 1993; 118:504–510.

72. Mason JJ, Owens DK, Harris RA, Cooke JP, Hlatky MA. The role of coronary angiography and coronary revascularization before noncardiac vascular surgery. *JAMA* 1995; 273:1919–1925.

73. Mangano DT, Goldman L. Preoperative assessment of patients with known or suspected coronary disease. *N Engl J Med* 1995; 333:1750–1756.

74. Fleisher LA, Eagle KA. Screening for cardiac disease in patients having noncardiac surgery. *Ann Intern Med* 1996; 124:767–772.

75. Bodenheimer MM. Noncardiac surgery in cardiac patient: What is the question? *Ann Intern Med* 1996; 124:763–766.

76. Bergan JJ, Veith FJ, Bernhard VM, Yao JST, Flinn WR, Gupta SK, et al. Randomization of autogenous vein and polytetrafluoroethylene grafts in femoral-distal reconstruction. *Surgery* 1982; 92:921–930.

77. Veith FJ, Gupta SK, Ascer E, White-Flores S, Samson RH, Scher LA, et al. Six-year prospective multicenter randomized comparison of autologous saphenous vein and expanded polytetrafluoroethylene grafts in infrainguinal arterial reconstructions. *J Vasc Surg* 1986; 3:104–114.

78. Prendiville EJ, Yeager AN, O'Donnell TF, Coleman JC, Jaworek A, Callow AD, et al. Long-term results with the above-knee popliteal

79. O'Riordain DS, Buckley DJ, O'Donnell JA. Polytetrafluoroethylene in above-knee arterial bypass surgery for critical ischemia. *Am J Surg* 1992; 164:129–131.

80. Taylor RS, Loh A, McFarland RJ, Cox M, Chester JF. Improved technique for polytetrafluoroethylene bypass grafting: Long-term results using anastomotic vein patches,. *Br J Surg* 1992; 79:348–354.

81. Parsons RE, Suggs WD, Veith FJ, Sanchez LA, Lyon RT, Marin ML, et al. Polytetrafluoroethylene bypasses to infrapopliteal arteries without cuffs or patches: A better option than amputation in patients without autologous vein. *J Vasc Surg* 1996; 23:347–356.

82. Dardik H, Miller N, Dardik A, Ibrahim IM, Sussman B, Berry SM, et al. A decade of experience with the glutaraldehyde-tanned human umbilical cord vein graft for revascularization of the lower limb. *J Vasc Surg* 1988; 7:336–346.

83. Walker PJ, Mitchell RS, McFadden PM, James DR, Mehigan JT. Early experience with cryopreserved saphenous vein allografts as a conduit for complex limb-salvage procedures. *J Vasc Surg* 1993; 18:561–569.

84. Shah RM, Faggioli GL, Mangione S, Harris LM, Kane J, Taheri SA, et al. Early results with cryopreserved saphenous vein allografts for infrainguinal bypass. *J Vasc Surg* 1993; 18:965–971.

85. Harris RW, Schneider PA, Andros G, Oblath RW, Salles-Cunha S, Dulawa L. Allograft vein bypass: Is it an acceptable alternative for infrapopliteal revascularization: *J Vasc Surg* 1993; 18:553–560.

86. Mastroroberto P, Chello M, Zofrea S, Cirillo F, Marchese AR. Preliminary experience with cryopreserved saphenous vein allografts as a conduit for femoropopliteal revascularization. *Vasc Surg* 1996; 30:103–107.

87. Shah DM, Darling RC, Chang BB, Fitzgerald KM, Philip BS, Paty SK, et al. Long-term results of in situ saphenous vein bypass: Analysis of 2058 cases. *Ann Surg* 1995; 222:438–448.

88. Wengerter KR, Veith FJ, Gupta SK, Goldsmith J, Farrell E, Harris PL, et al. Prospective randomized multicenter comparison of in situ and reversed vein infrapopliteal bypasses. *J Vasc Surg* 1991; 13:189–199.

89. Chang BB, Darling RC, Bock DEM, Shah DM, Leather RP. The use of spliced vein bypasses for infrainguinal arterial reconstruction. *J Vasc Surg* 1995; 21:403–412.

90. Andros G, Harris RW, Salles-Cunha SX, Dulawa LB, Oblath RW. Lateral plantar artery bypass grafting: Defining the limits of foot revascularization. *J Vasc Surg* 1989; 10:511–521.

91. Gloviczki P, Morris SM, Bower TC, Naessens JM, Stanson AW. Microvascular pedal bypass for salvage of the severely ischemic limb. *Mayo Clin Proc* 1991; 66:243–253.

92. Quinones-Baldrich WJ, Colburn MD, Ahn SS, Gelabert HA, Moore WS. Very distal bypass for salvage of the severely ischemic extremity. *Am J Surg* 1993; 166:117–123.

93. Bergamini TM, George SM, Massey HT, Henke PK, Klamer TW, Lambert GE, et al. Intensive surveillance of femoropopliteal-tibial autogenous vein bypasses improves long-term graft patency and limb salvage. *Ann Surg* 1995; 221:507–516.

94. Polak JF. Femoropopliteal angioplasty with US guidance: An example of a niche market. *Radiology* 1996; 199:317–318.

95. Bakal CW, Cynamon J, Sprayregen S. Infrapopliteal percutaneous transluminal angioplasty: What we know. *Radiology* 1996; 200:36–43.

96. Fraser SCA, Al-Kutoubi MA, Wolfe JHN. Percutaneous transluminal angioplasty of the infrapopliteal vessels: The evidence. *Radiology* 1996; 200:33–36.

97. Kalman PG, Johnston KW, Sniderman KW. Indications and results of balloon angioplasty for arterial occlusive lesions. *World J Surg* 1996; 20:630–634.

98. Treiman GS, Treiman RL, Ichikawa L, Allan RV. Should percutaneous transluminal angioplasty be recommended for treatment of infragenic-ulate popliteal artery or tibioperoneal trunk stenosis? *J Vasc Surg* 1995; 22:457–463.

99. Stanley B, Teague B, Raptis S, Taylor DJ, Berce M. Efficacy of balloon angioplasty of the superficial femoral artery and popliteal artery in the relief of leg ischemia. *J Vasc Surg* 1996; 23:679–685.

100. Whyman MR, Ruckley CV, Fowkes FGR. Angioplasty for mild intermittent claudication. *Br J Surg* 1991; 78:643–645.

101. Bradbury AW, Ruckley CV. Angioplasty for lower-limb ischemia: Time for randomized controlled trials. *Lancet* 1996; 347:277–278.

102. White GH, Liew SCC, Waugh RC, Stephen MS, Harris JP, Kidd J, et al. Early outcome and intermediate follow-up of vascular stents in

the femoral and popliteal arteries without long-term anticoagulation. *J Vasc Surg* 1995; 21:270–281.

103. Cragg AH, Dake MD. Percutaneous femoropopliteal graft placement. *Radiology* 1993; 187:643–648.

104. Shapiro MJ, Levin DC. Percutaneous femoropopliteal graft placement: Is this the next step? *Radiology* 1993; 187:618–619.

105. Hunink MGM, Cullen KA, Donaldson MC. Hospital costs of revascularization procedures for femoropopliteal arterial disease. *J Vasc Surg* 1994; 19:632–641.

106. Hunink MGM, Wong JB, Donaldson MC, Meyerovitz MF, de Vries J, Harrington DP. Revascularization for femoropopliteal disease: A decision and cost-effectiveness analysis. *JAMA* 1995; 274:165–171.

107. Smith BM, Shield GW, Riddell DH, Snell JD. Venous gangrene of the upper extremity. *Ann Surg* 1985; 201:511–519.

108. Kunkel JM, Machleder HI. Treatment of Paget-Schroetter syndrome. *Arch Surg* 1989; 124:1153–1158.

109. Hill SL, Berry RE. Subclavian vein thrombosis: A continuing challenge. *Surgery* 1990; 108:1–8.

110. Prandoni P, Polistena P, Bernardi E, Cogo A, Casara D, Verlato F, et al. Upper-extremity deep vein thrombosis: Risk factors, diagnosis, and complications. *Arch Intern Med* 1997; 157:57–62.

111. Thompson RW, Schneider PA, Nelken NA, Skioldebrand CG, Stoney RJ. Circumferential venolysis and paraclavicular thoracic outlet decompression for "effort thrombosis" of the subclavian vein. *J Vasc Surg* 1992; 16:723–732.

112. Molina JE. Need for emergency treatment and surgery in subclavian vein effort thrombosis. *J Am Coll Surg* 1995; 181:414–420.

113. Machleder HI. Thrombolytic therapy and surgery for primary axillo-subclavian vein thrombosis: Current approach. *Semin Vasc Surg* 1996; 9:46–49.

114. Weinmann EE, Salzman EW. Deep-vein thrombosis. *N Engl J Med* 1994; 331:1630–1641.

115. Svensson PJ, Dahlback B. Resistance to activated protein C as a basis for venous thrombosis. *N Engl J Med* 1994; 330:517–522.

116. Ridker PM, Hennekens CH, Lindpaintner K, Stampfer MJ, Eisenberg PR, Milltich JP. Mutation in the gene coding for coagulation factor V and the risk of myocardiac infarction, stroke, and venous thrombosis in apparently healthy men. *N Engl J Med* 1995; 332:912–917.

117. Khamashta MA, Cuadrado MJ, Mujic F, Taub NA, Hunt BJ, Hughes GR. The management of thrombosis in the antiphospholipid-antibody syndrome. *N Engl J Med* 1995; 332:993–997.

118. Mandel H, Brenner B, Berant M, Rosenberg N, Lanir N, Jakobs C, et al. Coexistence of hereditary homocystinuria and factor V Leiden—Effect on thrombosis. *N Engl J Med* 1996; 334:763–768.

119. Den Heijer M, Koster T, Blom HJ, Bos GMJ, Briet E, Reitsma PH, et al. Hyperhomocysteincmia as a risk factor for deep-vein thrombosis. *N Engl J Med* 1996; 334:759–762.

120. Geerts WH, Code KI, Jay RM, Chen E, Szalai JP. A prospective study of venous thromboembolism after major trauma. *N Engl J Med* 1994; 331:1601–1606.

121. Yeager RA, Moneta GL, Edwards JM, Taylor LM, McConnell DB, Porter JM. Deep vein thrombosis associated with lower extremity amputation. *J Vasc Surg* 1995; 22:612–615.

122. Hirsch DR, Ingenito EP, Goldhaber SZ. Prevalence of deep venous thrombosis among patients in medical intensive care. *JAMA* 1995; 274:335–337.

123. Hull RD, Raskob GE, Rosenblood D, Panju AA, Brill-Edwards P, Ginsberg JS, et al. Heparin for 5 days as compared with 10 days in the initial treatment of proximal venous thrombosis. *N Engl J Med* 1990; 332:1260–1264.

124. Schulman S, Rhedin AS, Lindmarker P, Carlsson A, Larfars G, Nicol P, et al. A comparison of six weeks with six months of oral anticoagulant therapy after a first episode of venous thromboembolism. *N Engl J Med* 1995; 332:1661–1665.

125. Levine M, Gent M, Hirsh J, Leclerc J, Anderson D, Weitz J, et al. A comparison of low-molecular-weight heparin administered primarily at home with unfractionated heparin administered in the hospital for proximal deep-vein thrombosis. *N Engl J Med* 1996; 334:677–681.

126. Koopman MMW, Prandoni P, Piovella F, Ockelford PA, Brandjes DPM, van der Meer J, et al. Treatment of venous thrombosis with intravenous unfractionated heparin administered in the hospital as compared with subcutaneous low-molecular-weight heparin administered at home. *N Engl J Med* 1996; 334:682–687.

127. Schafer AI. Low-molecular-weight heparin—An opportunity for home treatment of venous thrombosis. *N Engl J Med* 1996; 334:724–726.

128. Prandoni P, Lensing AWA, Cogo A, Cupini S, Villalta S, Carta M, et al. The long-term clinical course of acute deep venous thrombosis. *Ann Intern Med* 1996; 125:1–7.

129. O'Meara JJ, McNutt RA, Evans AT, Moore SW, Downs SM. A decision analysis of streptokinase plus heparin as compared with heparin alone for deep-vein thrombosis. *N Engl J Med* 1994; 330:1864–1869.

130. Krieger NR, Mehigan JT. Spontaneous spinal epidural hematoma after combined urokinase and heparin thrombolytic therapy for deep venous thrombosis. *Vasc Surg* 1996; 30:67–70.

131. Plate G, Einarsson E, Ohlin P, Jensen R, Qvarfordt P, Eklof B. Thrombectomy with temporary arteriovenous fistula: The treatment of choice in acute iliofemoral venous thrombosis. *J Vasc Surg* 1984; 1:867–876.

132. Solis MM, Ranval TJ, Thompson BW, Eidt JF. Results of venous thrombectomy in the treatment of deep vein thrombosis. *Surg Gynecol Obstet* 1993; 177:633–639.

133. Elliot MS, Immelman EJ, Jeffrey P, Benatar SR, Funston MR, Smith JA, et al. The role of thrombolytic therapy in the management of phlegmasia caerulea dolens. *Br J Surg* 1979; 66:422–424.

134. Hood DB, Weaver FA, Modrall JG, Yellin AE. Advances in the treatment of phlegmasia cerulea dolens. *Am J Surg* 1993; 166:206–210.

135. Patel KR, Paidas CN. Phlegmasia cerulea dolens: The role of nonoperative therapy. *Cardiovasc Surg* 1993; 1:518–523.

136. Greenfield LJ, Proctor MC. Twenty-year clinical experience with the Greenfield Filter. *Cardiovasc Surg* 1995; 3:199–205.

137. Arnold TE, Karabinis VD, Mehta V, Dupont EL, Matsumoto T, Kerstein MD. Potential of overuse of the inferior vena cava filter. *Surg Gynecol Obstet* 1993; 177:463–467.

138. Harris EJ, Kinney EV, Harris EJ, Olcott C, Zarins CK. Phlegmasia complicating prophylactic percutaneous inferior vena caval interruption: A word of caution. *J Vasc Surg* 1995; 22:606–611.

139. Greenfield LJ, Proctor MC. Current indications for caval interruption: Should they be liberalized in view of improving technology? *Semin Vasc Surg* 1996; 9:50–58.

102

ANGIOPLASTY OF PERIPHERAL BLOOD VESSELS

Kenneth Rosenfield / Robert M. Schainfeld / Jeffrey M. Isner

The pioneering work of Dotter, Judkins, Gruentzig, and others opened the door for percutaneous, "less-invasive" strategies to treat peripheral artery disease (PAD). In the early years of percutaneous transluminal angioplasty (PTA), the availability of only large-profile balloons, nonyielding guide wires, and imaging equipment that dictated the need for large volumes of contrast sometimes meant that the hazards of percutaneous therapy were comparable to that of surgical revascularization. Recent innovations, however, have resolved many of these early limitations. Catheter profiles have been reduced, limiting complications related to vascular access. The use of novel materials for balloon and guide wire construction has facilitated passage through occluded vessels and permitted routine access to more remote vascular sites with less risk and greater efficacy. Directional and rotational atherectomy now enable "debulking" of atheroma that are eccentric and/or heavily calcified. Endovascular stents have dramatically improved both short- and long-term outcomes of aortoiliac, renal, and coronary PTA (see Chap. 48).[1-4] Improvements in imaging techniques have also enabled better appreciation of the results of catheter-based interventions. On-line intraprocedural imaging using intravascular ultrasound (IVUS), which provides a cross-sectional view of the vessel similar to a histologic section,[5,6] along with digital enhancement of conventional contrast images have led to better comprehension of the mechanisms responsible for successful angioplasty[7,8] (see Chap. 49).

Market forces have also made percutaneous revascularization increasingly attractive. Providers and insurers realize that PTA is a potentially cost-saving approach for treating vascular disease. Moreover, many patients favor the potential for reduced morbidity afforded by using less-invasive techniques, even in those instances where symptomatic improvement may not be as durable or the degree of revascularization as complete as in higher-risk surgical revascularization. Nowhere

has the wisdom of this philosophy become more evident than in the treatment of infrapopliteal disease in high-risk patients with limb-threatening ischemic ulceration. *Recognition that even short-term restoration of antegrade flow by PTA can result in ulcer healing and—barring any trauma to the limb—long-term limb salvage has provided a viable alternative to surgery in these patients.*[9] Lastly, as the population in the United States ages, the prevalence of PAD is increasing, thus compelling health care providers to optimize treatment strategies. People over 65 years of age now constitute nearly 15 percent of the population, a figure expected to double in the next 35 years. Judicious treatment of older patients disabled by PAD may enable them to experience the well-documented benefits of exercise and physical activity. In consideration of these goals, the availability of effective, "less invasive" percutaneous options for revascularization in this group of patients with a high risk profile due to comorbid conditions had led to a reevaluation of the threshold for intervention. For example, a patient whose claudication is not severe enough to warrant major surgical bypass may nonetheless be appropriate for PTA. The increasing popularity of percutaneous intervention as first-line therapy for patients with PAD underscores the need for vascular specialists and interventionalists to have a comprehensive understanding of the mechanisms of angioplasty, indications for intervention, expected outcomes, and potential complications.

MECHANISMS OF SUCCESSFUL PERCUTANEOUS ANGIOPLASTY

Pathologic evaluation of dilated vessels typically discloses plaque fractures and stretching of the arterial wall; the exact contribution of these, versus plaque compression and other factors, remains controversial. Most in vivo attempts to identify the mechanisms responsible for successful PTA have been limited by the lack of ability—using standard angiographic imaging methods—to assess the morphology and geometry of a lesion adequately before and after treatment and at the time of restenosis. Conventional contrast angiography, the time-honored approach for lesion characterization, remains limited by the fact that it depicts the vessel lumen only; plaque and vessel wall are viewed as a "negative imprint" upon the contrast-filled lumen.[10–13] While this allows for characterization of lumen topography, irregularities within the vessel wall may only be inferred from the negative imprint. Furthermore, contrast angiography is limited to a single planar view per injection; as such, information regarding the circumferential nature of the plaque is not provided.

Intravascular Ultrasound

IVUS has become a potent adjunctive imaging technique to contrast angiography, addressing many of the limitations of the latter (see Chap. 49). IVUS is unequivocally superior to contrast angiography in its ability to demonstrate detailed characteristics at the interface of the lumen and vessel wall. IVUS also depicts structures below that interface, within the plaque and vessel wall. Indeed, experimental and clinical experience to date indicate that IVUS images correlate remarkably well with histologic examination. IVUS is exquisitely sensitive in detecting plaque and other details that are angiographically "silent."[5,14–16] For instance, angiographically normal sites that are adjacent to target lesions almost always demonstrate disease when imaged by IVUS; indeed, it is not uncommon that an angiographically normal-appearing vessel will be found by IVUS to have diffuse, ubiquitous distribution of plaque throughout, indicating a much more advanced stage of atherosclerosis than would have been presumed otherwise. This revelation has obvious implications regarding assessment and selection of device size and in determination of relative luminal narrowing. Similarly, calcified plaque, characterized by "acoustic shadowing," is detected by IVUS in a majority of vessels undergoing angioplasty. This important feature is grossly underappreciated by angiography.

IVUS AND MECHANISMS OF ANGIOPLASTY

IVUS, because it consistently demonstrates exquisite detail regarding morphologic alterations in the arterial wall similar in perspective to that achieved by histologic examination, has provided new insight into the effects of angioplasty.[17,18] This unique feature of IVUS has been used to good advantage to study the mechanisms by which balloon angioplasty, directional atherectomy, stent deployment, and laser angioplasty enhance luminal area. Observations from IVUS suggest that plaque fracture and/or dissection are associated with balloon dilation in the majority of angiographically and hemodynamically successful procedures.[5,19] Vessels in which directional atherectomy is performed demonstrate less prominent plaque–arterial wall disruption; instead, the perimeter of the neolumen is typically smooth and uninterrupted, with discrete "bites"

corresponding to individual passes of the cutting blade. Signs of arterial wall trauma—including severe disruption—are most commonly ameliorated on IVUS images recorded following delivery of an endovascular stent.[20,21]

REGIONS OF INTEREST

The enhanced imaging capability and the evolution in catheter technology over the past two decades have permitted improved procedural results in certain sites, e.g., infrapopliteal arteries, previously considered to be inaccessible by the percutaneous approach. Likelihood of success and chances for clinical improvement, however, vary in degree according to the vascular region of interest and extent of disease within the peripheral circulation. Weighted consideration of these issues is required to determine, for any given combination of lesions, the appropriateness of nonsurgical revascularization.

Aortoiliac Disease

PTA remains the treatment of choice for aortoiliac stenoses. The application of endovascular prostheses (stents) to aortoiliac lesions has dramatically altered both the short- and long-term results. Palmaz[22] and others have documented the extent to which stents may be used expertly to rescue flow-limiting complications of iliac PTA (Fig. 102-1). Preliminary findings reported by Richter and colleagues[23] have suggested that significant improvements in long-term patency may be achieved in patients randomized to PTA-and-stent versus PTA alone: the *angiographic* patency (93 percent) in patients studied at 5-year follow-up rivals the best *clinical* patency reported at a similar time interval in patients undergoing operative revascularization. These excellent procedural and long-term results of percutaneous revascularization in patients with iliac lesions thus make the physical finding of a diminished femoral pulse a useful sign for identifying patients who are likely to benefit from percutaneous revascularization.

Iliac occlusions may also be treated percutaneously with a high degree of success. There are two specific considerations in this regard. The first is the ability to traverse the segment of occluded artery. This issue has been addressed by the use of novel technical approaches, such as the so-called pull-through technique and hydrophilic guide wires.[24] The combination of these has yielded an extremely high procedural success rate. The second issue concerns distal embolization, previously reported to occur with alarming frequency.[25] While the specter of acute limb-threatening ischemia resulting from embolization may serve as a deterrent to direct (nonlytic) recanalization of occluded iliac arteries, the current incidence of embolization in this setting is exceedingly low. Such is particularly the case if one employs a strategy of initial underdilation followed by stent deployment; the stent provides a scaffold that, in theory, affixes the thrombus/plaque to the vessel wall, thus reducing the likelihood of distal embolization. Given the low incidence of embolization with this strategy, primary recanalization and stenting—without lytic therapy—provide excellent results and avoid the potential hazards of thrombolytic therapy. The exception to this is in the case of documented recent thrombosis, where lysis is undoubtedly indicated (Fig. 102-1).

Clearly, the most common indication for iliac angioplasty is claudication. In many patients with claudication, and in some patients with limb ischemia, the iliac lesion coexists with more distal disease involving the superficial femoral artery (SFA) and/or infrapopliteal vessels; in such cases, initial treatment of the iliac obstruction is based on the premise that improving inflow will secondarily improve outflow, either via the profunda in the case of an occluded SFA or by increasing the head of perfusion pressure to the infrapopliteal circulation. Implicit in this strategy is the lesser degree of technical difficulty, high rate of procedural success, and low incidence of restenosis associated with iliac PTA. A similar strategy underlies the preparatory role of iliac angioplasty in patients undergoing surgical revascularization, such as femoral-femoral or femoral-popliteal bypass, for treatment of distal disease.[26] Such a strategy may lower the anatomic site or complexity of bypass and thereby reduce the risk of operative revascularization.

Two additional issues regarding percutaneous treatment of aneurysmal or stenotic aortoiliac disease deserve specific comment. The first concerns the role of percutaneous revascularization in modifying the treatment in such patients with coexisting cardiac disease, who heretofore would have required high-risk abdominal surgery.[27,28] Recent work from several groups[29,30] has demonstrated the feasibility of intraluminal insertion of a stent graft prosthesis for the treatment of abdominal aortic aneurysms. Although much less common than aneurysmal dilation, stenoses of the aorta are routinely and effectively treated by PTA and stents.[31] The second issue involves angiographic assessment of aortic and iliac stenoses. Clinical

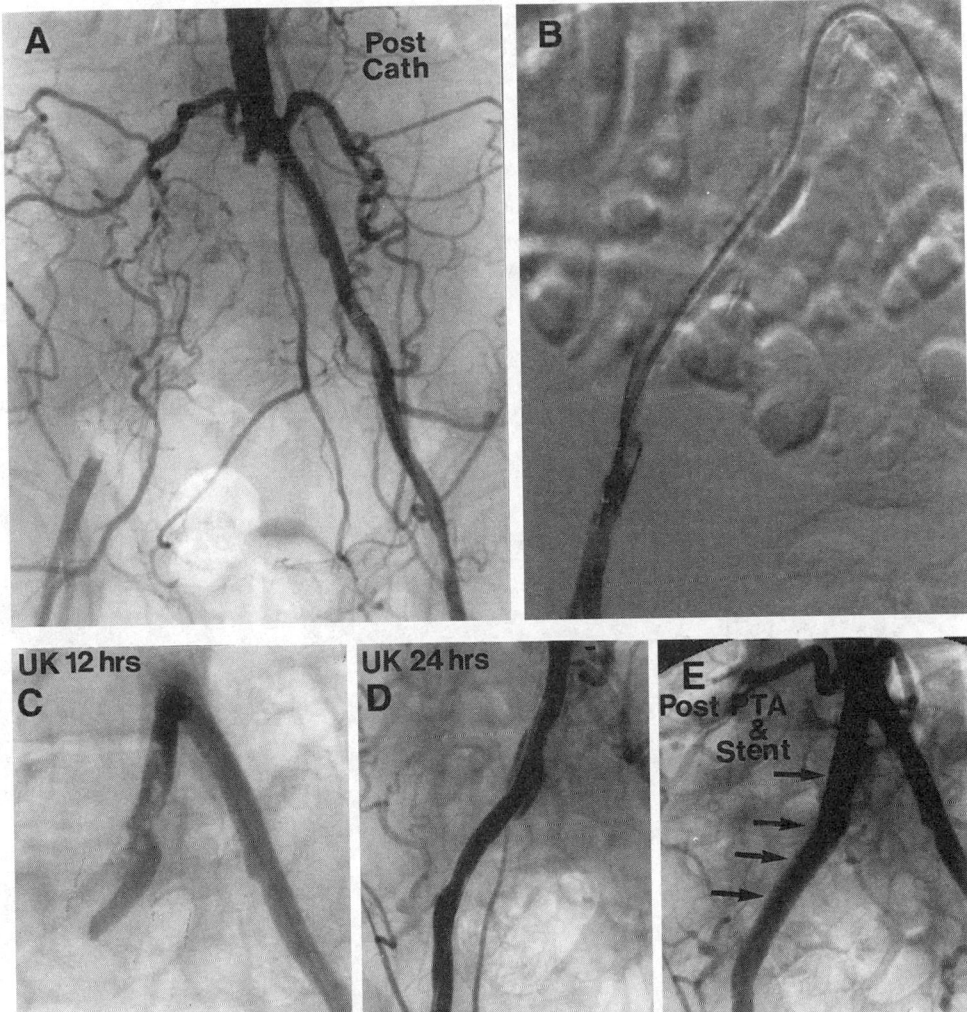

FIGURE 102-1

Thrombolysis, percutaneous transluminal angioplasty, and stent deployment in a patient who developed cold right leg following diagnostic cardiac catheterization. *A.* Baseline arteriogram demonstrates lengthy fresh occlusion of right common iliac artery, with reconstruction of common femoral artery by collaterals. *B.* Occlusion crossed in antegrade fashion from contralateral side, and infusion of urokinase begun. *C.* Following 12 h of urokinase (UK), common and external iliac arteries now partially patent but have extensive dissection, residual thrombus, and blind cul-de-sac. Thrombolytic therapy therefore continued. *D.* Following 24 h of UK, vessel now patent and thrombus resolved, but extensive dissection remains. *E.* Following deployment of two Palmaz stents, iliac artery widely patent, with amelioration of dissection/cul-de-sac. Patient remains asymptomatic 30 months later.

experience with IVUS has documented the extent to which conventional diagnostic angiography may underestimate hemodynamically significant luminal narrowing in the aorta and in tortuous iliac arteries. IVUS permits direct planimetry of luminal cross-sectional narrowing at these sites, obviating the multiple, angulated angiographic views required to eliminate sites of vessel overlap, which may obscure important luminal obstruction. The use of IVUS is particularly imperative during complex revascularization of the aorta, where the difficulty obtaining an angulated view and presence of multiple important side branches can obscure the outcome of revascularization. IVUS in such cases may greatly facilitate the safe and effective execution of percutaneous procedures (Fig. 102-2).

Femoral and Popliteal Arteries

The acute procedural success that may be currently achieved using conventional guide wires and standard PTA in SFA stenoses is similar to that reported for iliac stenoses, approaching 100 percent. Long-term patency in the SFA, however, is clearly inferior to that which may be expected in iliac stenoses. Five-year primary patency rates varying from 43 to 70 percent[32–35] have been reported for SFA revascularization; the variability in long-term follow-up results is due in part to

the multiple lengths and morphologies of SFA lesions selected for treatment, including a mixture of stenoses with occlusions. These factors, however, pale by comparison to the variable manner in which vessel patency has been defined and/or evaluated, whether initial failures are or are not excluded from long-term analyses, and the statistical measures employed to analyze long-term follow-up.[36,37]

A variety of novel technologies, including directional atherectomy, laser angioplasty, rotational atherectomy, and stents, have been investigated as potential means of improving long-term patency and reducing restenosis following SFA revascularization. Directional atherectomy has the unique capability of resecting intact atherosclerotic plaque, which can

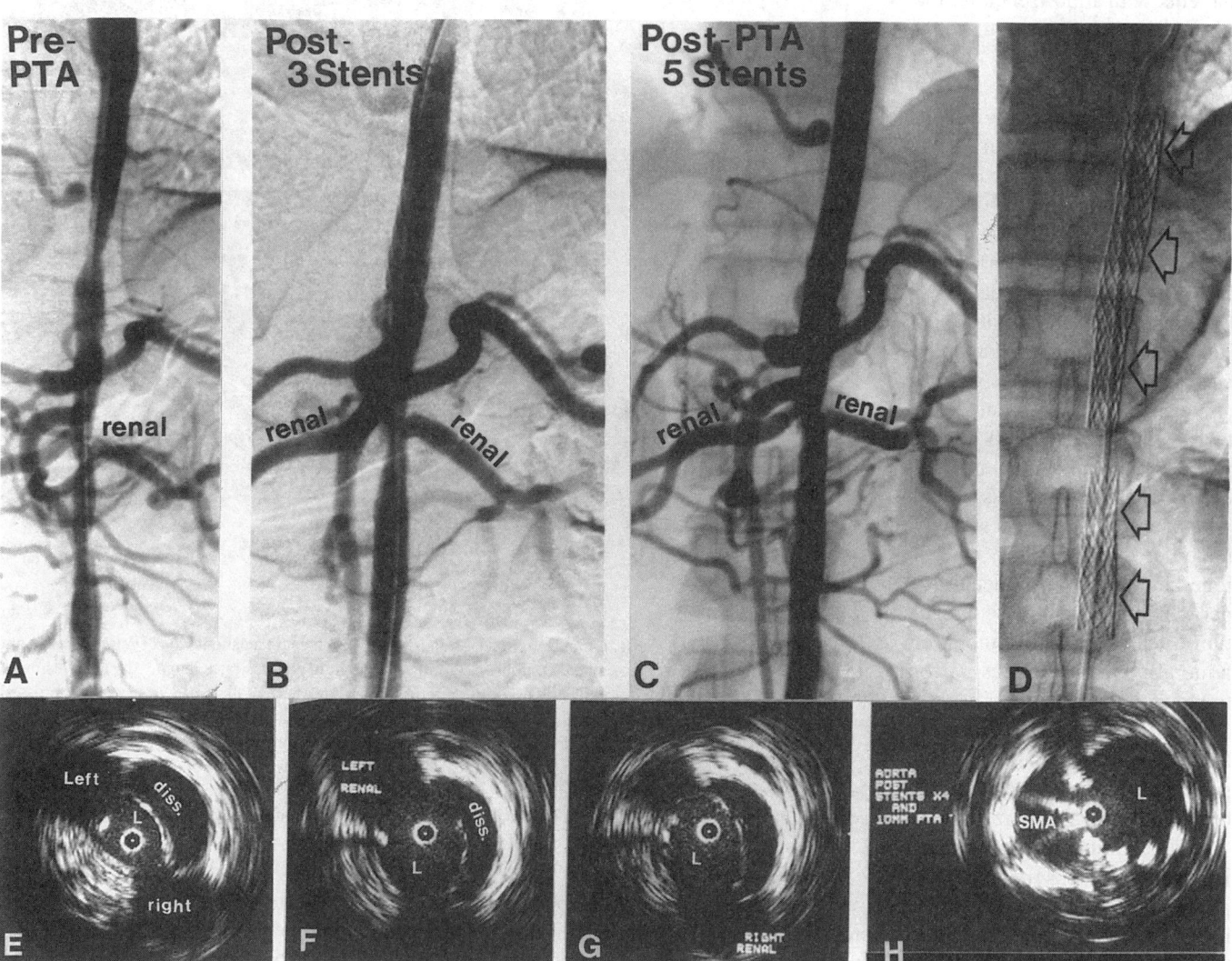

FIGURE 102-2

Revascularization of abdominal aortic stenosis with percutaneous transluminal angioplasty (PTA)/multiple stents under intravascular ultrasound (IVUS) guidance. This 30-year-old woman presented with malignant hypertension and nonpalpable femoral pulses due to abdominal aortic coarctation, thought to be secondary to Takayasu's disease, now quiescent. *A*. Angiogram pre-PTA demonstrates extensive disease in aorta, both above and below the renal arteries. *B*. Following PTA above and below the renal arteries and placement of three stents; result appears reasonable by angiography, although moderate stenosis remains below/at level of renal arteries. IVUS image (*E*) at origins of renals ("left" and "right") demonstrates large dissection (diss.) extending from proximal aorta PTA site, encroaching upon renal artery ostia and narrowing aortic lumen (L). *C*. Redilated aorta, with two additional stents, now has less encroachment at level of renal arteries; IVUS frames (*F*) and (*G*) show persistence of dissection (diss.), but concurrent enlargement of aortic lumen (L) and elimination of obstruction leading into renal arteries ("left renal," "right renal"). *D*. Stents (*arrows*) in aorta. *H*. IVUS of stent in midaorta depicts struts overlying origin of superior mesenteric artery (SMA); struts cast "shadows" into SMA but do not compromise blood flow (*C*).

be preserved in a form that is suitable for a variety of laboratory analyses. Studies of atherectomy specimens performed using light microscopy[38] as well as more contemporary molecular biologic techniques[39–41] suggest that this technique may play an important role in providing human tissues to develop novel biopharmaceutical agents to prevent restenosis.[42] The superiority of directional atherectomy from a therapeutic standpoint remains less clear. In patients with short, eccentric lesions, directional atherectomy appears to offer satisfactory acute procedural results similar to PTA.[43,44] The impact of directional atherectomy upon subsequent restenosis, however, remains controversial; unlike the recently completed CAVEAT investigation,[45] no randomized trial of PTA versus directional atherectomy has yet to be reported. Most nonrandomized studies have so far failed to demonstrate significant reduction in restenosis.

Rotational atherectomy[46] has not yet been demonstrated to have an advantage for SFA revascularization, save for those rare patients in whom the extent of calcific deposits renders the lesions refractory to alternative techniques. In the smaller popliteal artery, it is possible that the debulking effect of rotational atherectomy may ultimately prove to offer some benefit over balloon angioplasty alone.

In contrast to the documented benefits achieved by the use of endovascular stents for iliac PTA, experience with stents in the SFA has been less favorable. Stents can dramatically enhance acute outcome, especially where they are used to rescue a flow-limiting dissection resulting from PTA. Early results with a variety of stent designs,[47,48] however, failed to demonstrate a significant reduction in restenosis following SFA revascularization. More recent uncontrolled studies employing the Palmaz stent[49] and the Wallstent[50] demonstrated modest improvement in intermediate-term patency when compared to historic controls using balloon angioplasty alone. These nonrandomized studies indicate that, much as with balloon angioplasty alone, the most favorable long-term results from stents are seen in the proximal SFA. The fate of stents placed at or caudal to the adductor canal is more sobering. The description of deformation or compression of stents placed within the adductor canal, a finding that led to the premature termination of a randomized trial between SFA stent implantation versus PTA alone, suggests that the design of stents currently available in the United States may be suboptimal for use in the SFA.[51]

OCCLUSION OF THE SFA AND POPLITEAL ARTERY

Among patients studied angiographically for consideration of revascularization, occlusions are more prevalent than stenoses. Two technical advances have facilitated treatment of SFA occlusions, including lengthy (>10 cm) segments. The first is the use of hydrophilic (so-called Glide) wires. Among 109 consecutive patients at the authors' institution in whom the Glidewire was used to attempt percutaneous revascularization of SFA total occlusions, the Glidewire was successfully advanced across the occluded segment in 107 (98 percent); PTA alone or in combination with directional atherectomy and/

or laser angioplasty was then used to complete percutaneous revascularization in all 107 patients.[24] Ankle-brachial index improved from 0.48 ± 0.02 before to 0.82 ± 0.02 after revascularization. Improvement in Rutherford class by one or more grades was observed in 96 (94.1 percent) of 102 patients seen at 1-month follow-up. This experience was noteworthy for two reasons in particular: first, among the 107 SFA occlusions, 50 measured 5 to 10 cm in length and 21 were >20 cm long; consequently, mean occlusion length (9.8 cm) exceeded that reported in most previous series. Second, IVUS examination during these procedures demonstrated, in approximately one-third of patients, a subintimal route of recanalization.[52]

The second advance that has contributed to improved procedural success in recanalizing SFA occlusions is the use of thrombolytic therapy. Lytic therapy has in fact been proven effective even for *chronic* total occlusions; this is because occlusion of the lower extremity arteries is typically characterized by a lengthy, metastable, gelatin-like thrombus superimposed upon a less lengthy, high-grade atherosclerotic lesion. In such cases, lytic therapy can be effective in converting a long occlusion to one that is either shorter or no longer occlusive and is thereby more amenable to mechanical revascularization. The efficacy of this approach recently underwent systematic, multicenter investigation in patients with lower extremity occlusions who were randomized to lytic versus operative therapy within the Surgery and Thrombolysis for Ischemia of the Lower Extremity (STILE) Trial.[53] Data from the STILE trial suggest that successful recanalization of *chronic* SFA occlusions using thrombolytic agents (tissue plasminogen activator or urokinase) is technically feasible and, in many instances, associated with an excellent outcome. Reestablishing patency by this approach, however, is less reliable for lengthy and/or "flush" total occlusions than surgical bypass, and for these lesions the outcomes of surgery are more durable. The use of thrombolytic therapy for *acute* occlusions (≤14 days' duration) appears to be more favorable. Both the STILE trial and a similar randomized investigation executed by Ouriel and associates[54] demonstrated that, for acute or subacute occlusions, thrombolysis and surgery were equivalent in terms of restoration of patency and limb salvage. An unexpected finding in Ouriel's study, with a similar trend in the STILE trial, was a significant reduction in the frequency of both in-hospital complications and 12-month mortality in patients receiving thrombolysis versus those treated surgically. *Thus, there is compelling evidence to support a strategy of primary thrombolysis for acute occlusions of the SFA.*

The extent to which favorable acute procedural results in patients with chronic total occlusion will ultimately extend the role of percutaneous revascularization remains to be defined. Certainly for patients with nonhealing lesions and/or threatened limb loss in whom the risks of surgery are considered prohibitive or in whom veins are unavailable for distal bypass, percutaneous revascularization of lengthy, occluded segments may facilitate healing. In similar types of patients with rest pain or severe claudication, PTA may be employed to achieve pain relief at a lower risk than conventional surgical reconstruction. For patients with less severe symptoms, improved ability to revascularize does not in and of itself constitute a sufficient basis for routine invasive therapy.

Two anatomic issues concerning femoral arterial revascularization deserve additional, specific comment. The first involves lesions of the common femoral artery. Such lesions may be accessed without great difficulty, and results of PTA (Fig. 102-3) or directional atherectomy can be quite favorable. However, the concern that PTA-induced plaque fractures could propagate into the common femoral bifurcation, leading to compromise of both the SFA and profunda, implicitly suggests that PTA of the common femoral artery must be undertaken with caution, especially given the ease of surgical access in this location. The second anatomic consideration is the combination of a stenotic profunda with a proximal occlusion of the SFA. Technically satisfactory results of profunda PTA have been described previously[55] and in this particular situation might well be more easily accomplished than revascularization of a coexisting, proximal, long SFA occlusion. Should revascularization of the profunda—a site not currently favored for stent deployment—be complicated by acute occlusion, however, complete interruption of antegrade flow via both femoral arteries may result in an acutely ischemic limb. For this reason, the authors advocate caution when considering a percutaneous approach to this combination of lesions.

Infrapopliteal Arteries

Published clinical experience involving percutaneous revascularization of the anterior tibial, tibioperoneal trunk, posterior tibial, and peroneal arteries, while dating to the time of Dotter's original work,[56] has nevertheless been far more limited than that described for aortoiliac and SFA sites. This is related to several issues: (1) claudication is rarely due to isolated disease of the infrapopliteal arteries, (2) knee-to-foot patency of one of the three major branches is generally regarded as sufficient to prevent critical lower limb ischemia, (3) restenosis rates in these vessels have typically been the highest of any of the lower extremity sites, and (4) obstructive disease in these arteries is often occlusive or diffuse and complicated by heavy calcific deposits. There is little question that the application of techniques employed for coronary arterial revascularization has resulted in more widespread use of percutaneous therapy for infrapopliteal disease.[57] Several reports[58,59] have now documented that stenotic and even short occlusions of one or more infrapopliteal arteries can be revascularized percutaneously with a very high degree of efficacy and at extraordinarily low risk.

It must be emphasized that the goals of infrapopliteal revascularization often differ from those of above-the-knee therapy. *Claudication is rarely the result of infrapopliteal obstruction alone.* Thus, when infrapopliteal disease coexists with above-knee lesion(s), the requirement for below-knee angioplasty is not automatic; often, treatment of the proximal disease alone is sufficient for symptomatic relief. *In patients with rest pain or ischemic ulceration, restoring patency of at least one of the three major infrapopliteal arteries is generally sufficient to obviate symptoms and/or heal a distal ischemic lesion.* In this group of patients, aggressive application of percutaneous revascularization may achieve extremely gratifying results, even in patients with calcified or lengthy occlusions.

One point concerning percutaneous infrapopliteal revascularization requires special emphasis: the incidence of restenosis, which remains high in these patients, should not be a factor in the decision to employ a percutaneous approach for what is, in many of these patients, a short-term problem. If uninterrupted patency of even one vessel can be achieved, the improvement in antegrade nutrient flow is typically adequate to facilitate limb salvage. Once healed, most patients will do satisfactorily, even in the face of documented restenosis, if they can avoid subsequent foot trauma. This strategy is further supported by the fact that both the short- and long-term outcomes of distal surgical reconstruction for infrapopliteal disease are likewise imperfect.

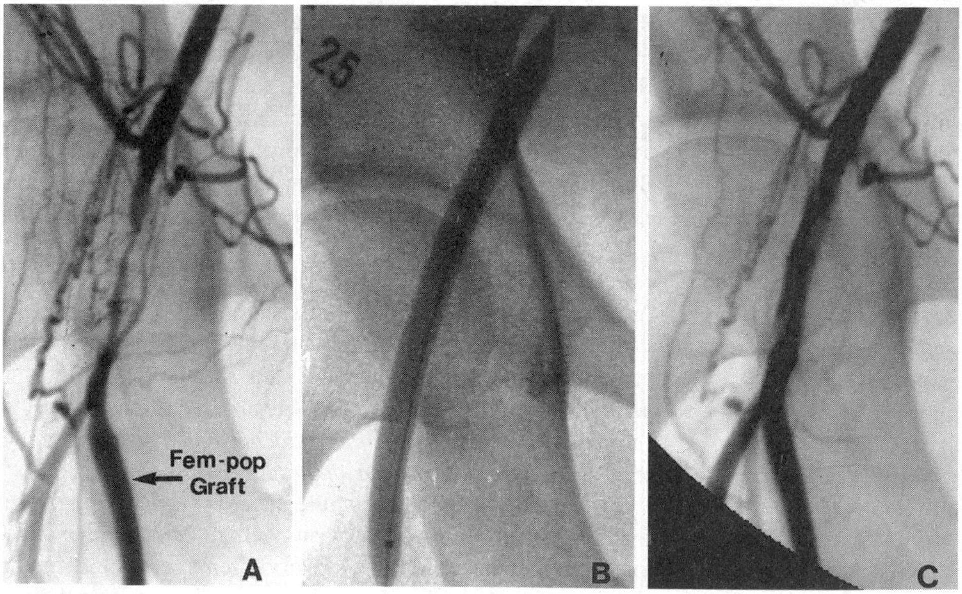

FIGURE 102-3
Balloon angioplasty (percutaneous transluminal angioplasty—PTA) of common femoral artery in patient with severe scarring from multiple previous surgical interventions of right groin. *A.* High-grade, diffuse stenosis in right common femoral artery, with extensive collateral flow, supplying profunda and femoropopliteal (fem-pop) graft. *B.* PTA via contralateral approach. Balloon inflated to 15 ATM. *C.* Post-PTA angiogram demonstrates mild plaque fracture, with excellent patency. Patient's claudication symptoms resolved, and he continues to be minimally symptomatic 2 years later.

Bypass Grafts

Percutaneous revascularization represents an alternative to operative reconstruction for achieving so-called secondary patency[36] of failing or failed native or prosthetic conduits. Nonsurgical revascularization has several obvious advantages: it saves the patient the morbidity and additional hospitalization associated with a repeat surgical procedure; it does not require the availability or utilization of additional native veins; and in certain cases it may obviate the need to employ prosthetic materials for distal reconstruction, an application for which such materials have been shown to confer lower patency rates.[60] The published results of PTA of *stenotic* lower-extremity bypass grafts is extremely variable. Series in the surgical literature suggest that, while PTA can be acutely successful, the long-term patency is inferior to that associated with surgical revision.[61,62] Employment of a strategy of regular surveillance, with appropriately timed intervention—even repeated—for impending graft failure, can optimize the results of percutaneous therapy.[63] The authors' approach to stenotic grafts is to make at least one attempt at percutaneous revascularization. This approach is derived from consideration of several issues. First, percutaneous revascularization of stenotic grafts is most often technically straightforward. Second, the risk of serious complications is low. Third, the contribution of adjunctive diagnostic and therapeutic techniques, including intravascular ultrasound, directional atherectomy, and endovascular stents, to preservation of graft patency remains essentially untested. Fourth, surgical revision itself is complicated by imperfect long-term patency.[64–66]

Subclavian and Innominate Arteries

Angioplasty of the subclavian and innominate arteries produces results comparable to those in iliac vessels. Confounding the results of studies is the fact that there is a learning curve associated with this procedure, that equipment used in earlier years was less advanced, and that most reports are limited to small (≤50) numbers of patients. In spite of these mitigating factors, reported technical success and complication rates are >90 percent and <10 percent, respectively.[67] The application of stents to this site may further improve the results, which already compare favorably to surgical alternatives, including common carotid to subclavian bypass. Clinical indications for subclavian PTA include symptomatic ischemia of the posterior fossa and/or upper extremity, with or without subclavian steal syndrome, and for preservation of flow, where thrombosis or progressive stenosis could have devastating consequences. While no randomized trials exist comparing surgery and PTA for subclavian disease, PTA is now considered first-line therapy for focal subclavian stenoses. *Occlusive* disease is more controversial because of the potential to embolize thrombus or atheroma into the intracerebral circulation. PTA has potential advantages over surgery, namely, obviating the need for general anesthesia, shortening hospital stay, and reducing morbidity. Moreover, the carotid artery is often stenotic and, consequently, may be unsuitable as a donor artery.

Percutaneous recanalization of subclavian occlusions has been shown to be technically feasible,[68] but safety and efficacy compared to surgery have not been evaluated. Nonetheless, based on the favorable results of several investigators,[69,70] PTA appears to be an appropriate strategy for symptomatic patients.

A special category of patients with subclavian obstruction—those with so-called coronary-subclavian steal syndrome—respond quite well to PTA and stent deployment. In such patients, restoration of antegrade flow into the carotid and internal mammary artery can be life-saving (Fig. 102-4).[71]

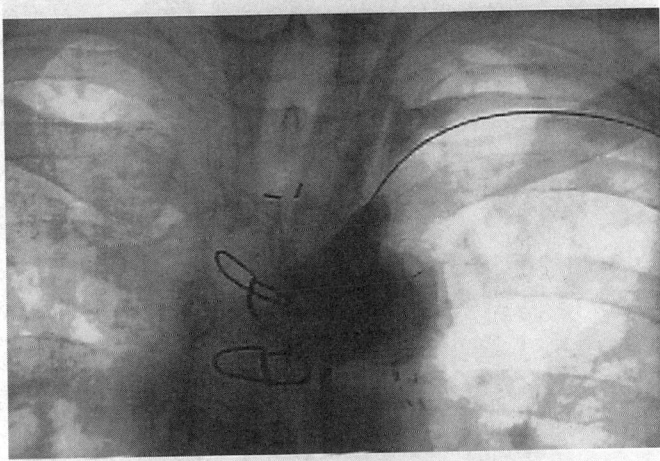

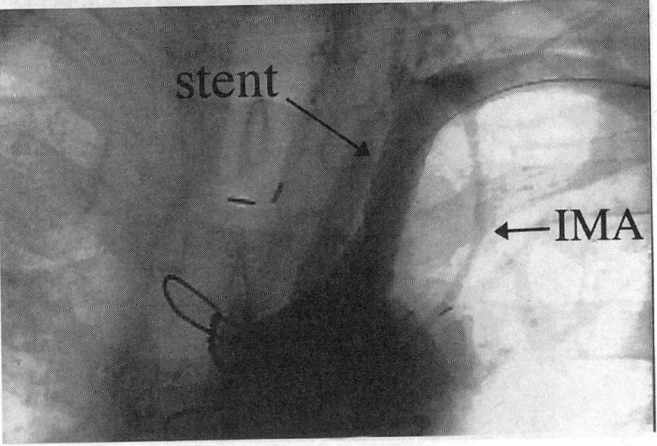

FIGURE 102-4

Coronary-subclavian steal syndrome following coronary artery bypass grafting—treatment with percutaneous transluminal angioplasty (PTA)/stent. *Top:* Angiogram of left subclavian artery pre-PTA shows near occlusion, with no antegrade flow into internal mammary (IMA) bypass graft to LAD. Left main coronary injection in same patient demonstrates retrograde flow up IMA into subclavian artery, indicating coronary steal syndrome. Patient had severe angina as a result. *Bottom:* Following PTA and stent, antegrade flow restored in IMA and angina resolved.

Carotid Arteries

Revascularization of carotid arteries has, until recently, been considered to be exclusively within the purview of vascular surgery. Indeed, since the first surgical carotid endarterectomy over 30 years ago, the morbidity, mortality, cost, and patient inconvenience associated with this procedure have been reduced considerably. Carotid endarterectomy performed by experienced vascular surgeons on appropriately selected patients can be accomplished with a very favorable risk-benefit ratio. To date, percutaneous treatment of carotid arteries has been reserved for those circumstances wherein the surgical risk is excessive, such as patients with either a high cervical lesion or stenosis in the proximal common carotid artery, which would require an intrathoracic surgical approach. In addition, patients with prior neck irradiation, previous radical neck dissection, or restenosis at a previous endarterectomy site have been considered reasonable PTA candidates, due to the increased risk of surgery in these subsets. Successful PTA in these high-risk patients, especially with the adjunctive use of endovascular stents, has led to consideration that a less-invasive, percutaneous approach might be applied more widely for carotid artery disease (Fig. 102-5). Recent reports from several groups have indicated that carotid PTA and stent deployment are feasible in most cases and may be associated with an acceptable risk of neurologic events, comparable to that of carotid endarterectomy.[72–75] Notably, many of the patients treated in these series would have been considered high risk for carotid endarterectomy, by virtue of their lesion site or comorbid conditions (e.g., unstable angina). Furthermore, the percutaneous procedures were performed using technology and stents that were not devised specifically for application in carotid arteries. When one considers these facts, the initial results of PTA with stenting appear even more promising. Further study will be required to define the role for this novel procedure, vis-à-vis carotid endarterectomy.

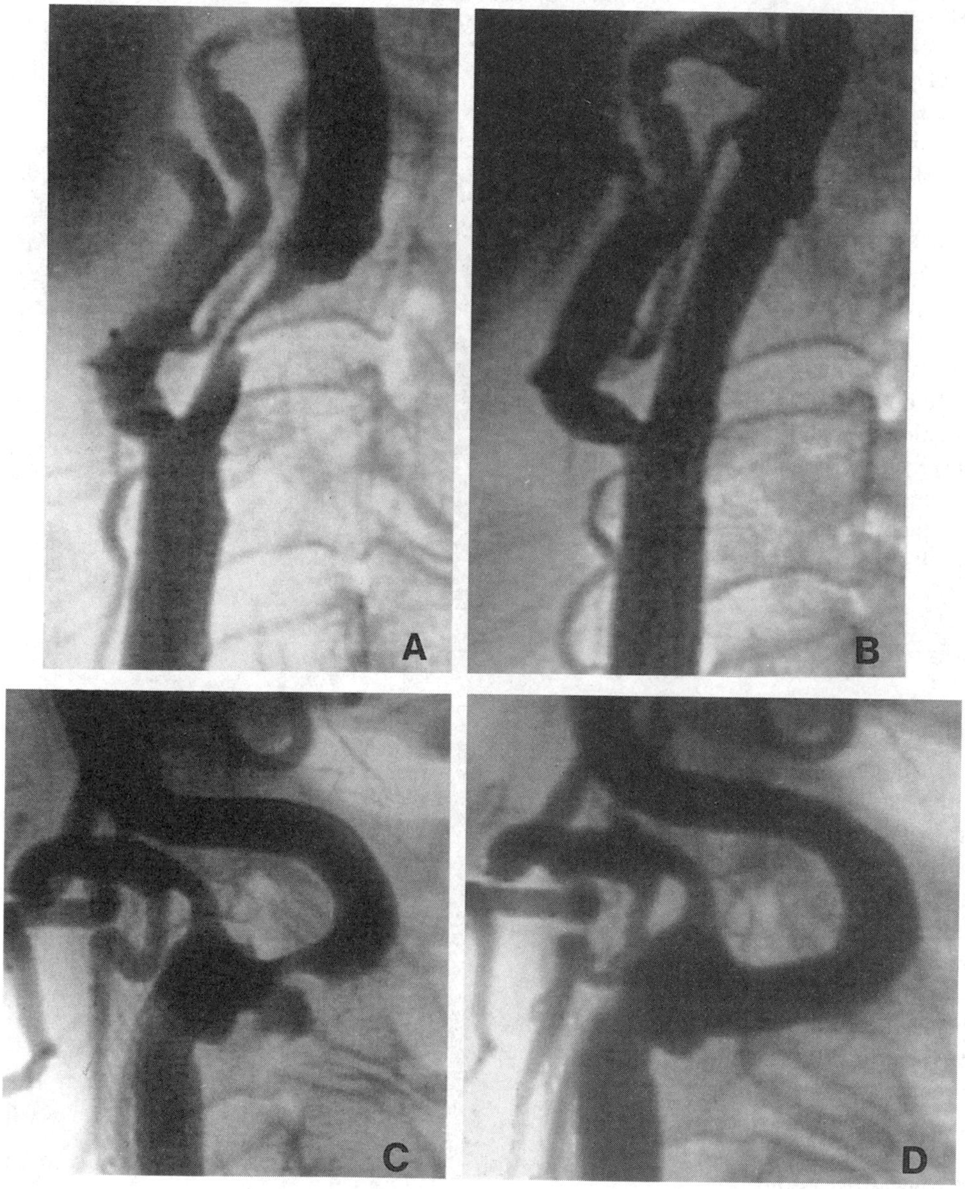

FIGURE 102-5

Bilateral carotid artery revascularization with balloon angioplasty and stent deployment in an 82-year-old asymptomatic male with "isolated hemispheres." *A*. High-grade stenosis of right internal carotid artery. *B*. Status after percutaneous transluminal angioplasty (PTA) and Wallstent deployment, with marked improvement and only mild residual narrowing. Wallstent extends into common carotid artery. No significant compromise in external carotid artery. *C*. High-grade, ulcerated stenosis in proximal left internal carotid artery. Patient brought back for revascularization of this side 4 weeks after PTA of contralateral side. *D*. Status after PTA and Palmaz stent deployment in proximal left internal carotid artery. Both procedures were uneventful, and patient remains asymptomatic at 1 year.

Renal Arteries

The primary goals of renal artery revascularization are to preserve or restore renal function, improve control of hypertension, and eliminate congestive heart failure. Associated secondary benefits can include reduction in antihypertensive medications and, occasionally, elimination of the need for dialysis (Fig. 102-6). For patients with chronic congestive heart failure and/or cardiomy-

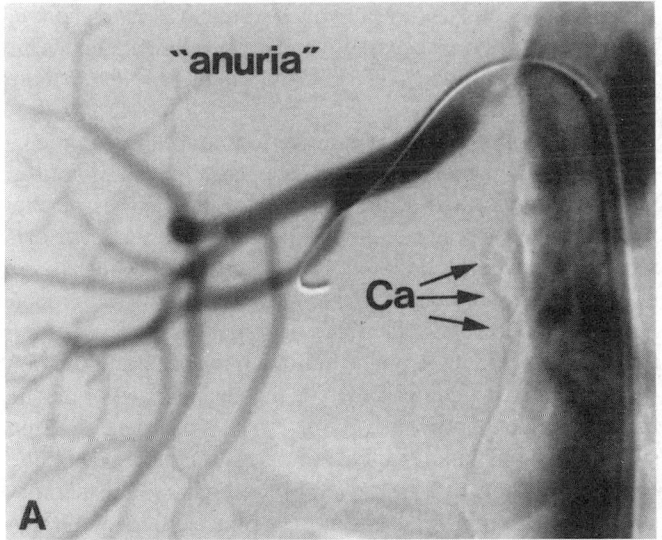

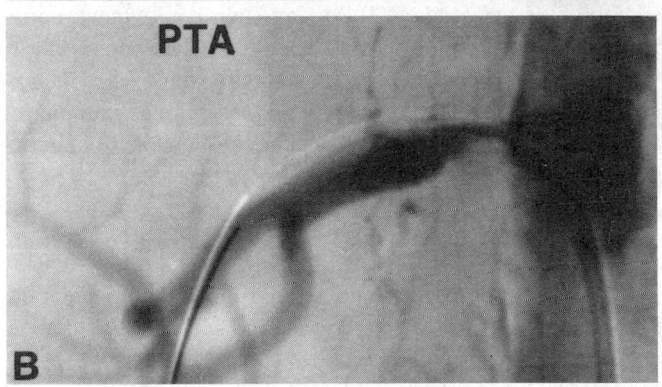

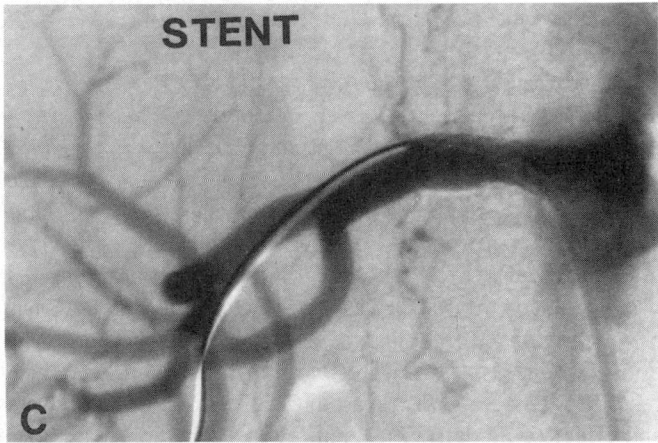

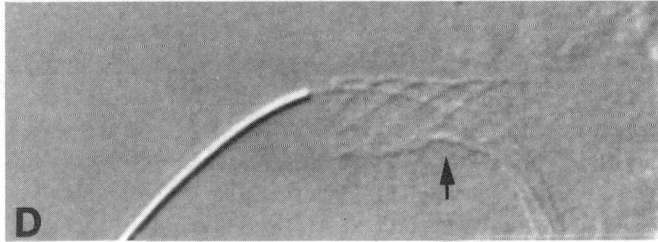

FIGURE 102-6

"Salvage" renal angioplasty and stent deployment in a woman with recent onset of renal failure, anuria, and severe, refractory congestive heart failure requiring intubation and dialysis. *A.* Baseline angiogram obtained after traversing subtotal occlusion of right renal artery with guidewire. Aorta is very heavily calcified (Ca), and left renal artery is occluded, left kidney nonfunctional. *B.* Status after balloon angioplasty alone (percutaneous transluminal angioplasty) for this heavily calcified ostial stenosis: extensive recoil is evident. *C.* Vessel widely patent following stent deployment; not significantly obstructive. *D.* Stent configuration without contrast demonstrates minor dimple along inferior border, caused by resistant aortic plaque. Patient began making urine immediately while on the angiographic table. Dialysis was discontinued immediately, and patient left the hospital with a creatinine of 1.2 off dialysis 4 days after stent deployment. She remains off dialysis 2 years later.

opathy, correction of renal artery stenosis (RAS) may enable safe institution of angiotensin-converting enzyme inhibitor therapy. Percutaneous revascularization offers an attractive alternative to surgical bypass or endarterectomy, which are more invasive and associated with higher morbidity.

Since Gruntzig first reported successful application of balloon catheters for renal angioplasty, controversy has persisted regarding which lesions to treat by percutaneous revascularization versus surgery and at what threshold revascularization should be recommended. The paucity of controlled trials comparing medical therapy, surgery, and percutaneous revascularization or even of standardized definitions as to what constitutes a successful therapeutic outcome precludes formulation of conclusions regarding the relative merits of each strategy. Notwithstanding this lack of standardized data, certain lesions are now deemed appropriate for percutaneous revascularization; others may be more definitively treated by surgical means or are best treated medically. The distinction between these anatomic substrates is based upon lesion etiology (fibromuscular versus atherosclerotic) and lesion location (ostial, midvessel, or branch). Additional considerations include the condition of the adjacent aorta and the presence of comorbid conditions such as coronary artery disease. Finally, *preliminary experience suggests that the use of stents for adjunct therapy in percutaneous revascularization promises to greatly enhance the success of percutaneous renal revascularization.*

FIBROMUSCULAR DISEASE

Results of surgical revascularization for severe hypertension due to fibromuscular disease can be exemplary in the hands of surgeons with extensive experience.[76] Nonetheless, the role of surgery in fibromuscular disease has declined significantly, a reflection of the fact that this entity is treated quite effectively with percutaneous revascularization. When the disease is primarily localized in the main renal artery, initial technical success exceeds 90 percent.[77] Initial clinical success (elimination or significant reduction in hypertension at 6 months) occurs in >80 percent of patients undergoing percutaneous revascularization. Recurrence is infrequent (<20 percent). Experience with this technique for branch stenosis due to fibromuscular disease is limited. The approach advocated thus far for these lesions has been surgical; however, recent reports suggest that fibromuscular branch stenoses may be treated effectively with percutaneous revascularization.[78]

ATHEROSCLEROTIC RENAL ARTERY STENOSIS

Percutaneous treatment of atherosclerotic RAS has been less gratifying than that of fibromuscular disease. In a pooled analysis of multiple studies, Rimmer and Gennari describe improvement in renal function in 43 percent of patients, stabilization in 35 percent, and no beneficial effect of percutaneous revascularization in 22 percent.[79] Interpretation of the results of percutaneous revascularization in atherosclerotic RAS has been complicated by a lack of consistency regarding definitions of success and failure. Despite this inconsistency in reporting, percutaneous revascularization can provide a safe and effective modality for renal revascularization, with a favorable risk-benefit ratio. The mortality rate in most series is <1 percent, contrast-related and atheroembolic events are surprisingly infrequent, and the majority of reported complications are related to vascular access. Surgical revascularization in appropriately selected cases has also been shown to be quite effective, with regard to both restoring or preserving renal function and reducing hypertension.[79,80] The mortality associated with surgical revascularization can be significant, however, between 2 and 17 percent.[79,81,82] Novick and colleagues correctly point out that surgical experience and technique have progressed over the past 20 years and complications have decreased.[76]

A balanced assessment regarding the role of percutaneous revascularization versus surgery has recently been provided by Weibell et al.,[83] who carried out one of the only randomized prospective trials comparing percutaneous revascularization (without stents) to surgical reconstruction in atherosclerotic RAS. Among the 58 patients randomized to percutaneous revascularization or surgery, there was no statistically significant difference in acute outcome. At 24 months, the primary patency in the percutaneous revascularization group was only 62 percent, but secondary patency (90 percent), achieved by repeat revascularization or surgery, was comparable to that of patients initially randomized to surgery (97 percent). Results with regard to improvement in hypertension and frequency of complications were also similar. *The conclusion of Weibell et al. was that a strategy of initial percutaneous revascularization is indicated for RAS, with close follow-up and additional percutaneous surgical revascularization for cases of initial failure or restenosis.* Employing this strategy, one can expect that approximately 60 percent of patients will not require additional treatment after initial percutaneous revascularization; of those with recurrent symptoms, 50 percent will require repeat percutaneous revascularization, the other 50 percent surgery. Interestingly, over the 2-year study period,

14 percent of patients developed a new stenosis in the contralateral renal artery, necessitating additional treatment. This makes the case for less-invasive initial therapy even more compelling.

The factor that is most predictive of initial failure or recurrence following percutaneous revascularization is lesion location: stenoses located at the ostium are generally associated with an acute success rate of ≤50 percent and high restenosis rates.[77,84,85] While modifications in angioplasty technique, such as use of guiding catheters,[86] and enhancement in imaging using IVUS[87] may facilitate percutaneous revascularization, it is likely that the major limitation to successful dilation of ostial lesions will continue to be the elastic recoil of plaque that is partially aortic in origin. Recent experiences using stents during percutaneous revascularization have been quite encouraging (Fig. 102-6). Several investigators have demonstrated more complete amelioration of the stenosis and transstenotic pressure gradient following stent deployment, compared to balloon angioplasty alone.[88–90] These preliminary results support the routine use of stents for renal ostial stenoses. This hypothesis is currently being tested in a randomized trial between percutaneous revascularization alone or in combination with stents.

CURRENT RECOMMENDATIONS FOR THE TREATMENT OF RAS

Patients with progressive renovascular disease in association with steady decline in renal function, hypertension that is accelerated or difficult to control, and/or congestive heart failure will generally benefit from renal revascularization. Patients who have recently developed end-stage renal disease, partly or wholly due to RAS, may also benefit from revascularization[82,91,92]; percutaneous revascularization may enable such patients to discontinue or avoid imminent dialysis (Fig. 102-6). The role of stents, which may ultimately revolutionize treatment of RAS, is currently being evaluated.

Hemodialysis Conduits

Patients dependent on hemodialysis number in excess of 120,000. Recent evidence shows this number to be increasing at a rate of 10 percent per year.[93] As the population of patients on dialysis expands and life expectancy on dialysis increases, preservation of vascular access sites has become increasingly important. Repeated large-gauge needle punctures three times per week, increased sheer forces and intraluminal pressure during dialysis, and postdialysis compression of puncture sites are all factors that may contribute to the high incidence of stenosis and thrombosis that occur in dialysis conduits, be they arteriovenous (AV) fistulas or Gore-tex grafts. AV fistulas tend to develop fibrous strictures at, and proximal to, sites of repeated puncture. Gore-tex grafts develop stenoses principally localized to the venous and arterial anastomoses; accumulation of pseudointima within the body of the graft may also predispose to graft failure. Surgical revision typically involves several days of hospitalization and placement of temporary access. A more important consequence of surgical revision, however, is the use of proximal vein, which may limit options for future surgical management. *PTA has played an increasingly important role in maintaining the functional status of hemodialysis access conduits.* The use of PTA for dialysis conduits requires a different perspective from PTA at other sites: because the patency of dialysis conduits is problematic, regardless of whether surgery or other approaches are utilized, restenosis is tolerated at a higher frequency than under nearly all other circumstances.

Percutaneous treatment of stenotic or occluded grafts or fistulae is usually technically straightforward. Acute success rates of 70 to 95 percent have been reported.[93–95] Primary restenosis rates are higher than for PTA in most other vascular beds, however, up to 60 percent and 80 percent at 1 and 2 years, respectively.[95,96] *Secondary* patency, however, has been quite acceptable (>70 percent at 2 years) in series where the investigators closely monitored graft function and performed early angiography and repeat PTA in cases of recurrent stenosis.[95] Thus, while the average graft may only remain functional for 4 to 6 months after a single PTA, as opposed to 14 to 18 months after surgical revision,[93] close monitoring of graft function and appropriately timed intervention can enhance the results of the percutaneous strategy and delay the need for graft revision.

Angioplasty of offending lesions in dialysis conduits often requires use of high pressure (up to 20 ATM) inflation, due to the fibrotic nature of the strictures within the venous system and at the graft anastomosis. IVUS is particularly useful for determining the reference diameter and quantifying the extent of recoil.[7] Even aggressive angioplasty using oversized balloons, however, is often insufficient, in which case adjunctive treatment with directional atherectomy may be useful to "cut" the fibrous band. Endovascular stents have also been investigated, but their role remains to be determined.

Management of dialysis conduits requires the cooperative efforts of a team consisting of nephrologists, vascular surgeons, and interventionalists.[93,94,97] The nephrologists and dialysis nursing staff must pay close attention to the hemodynamic function of access sites during dialysis. Increase in venous pressure, decrease in arterial flow, increase in recirculation, and poor dialysis efficiency are all factors that should trigger the request for a diagnostic angiogram. Focal stenoses can be treated initially using PTA and, for resistant lesions, directional atherectomy. Thereafter, patients should be monitored particularly closely, as one can expect a high incidence of restenosis. Repeated percutaneous interventions, in the interest of preserving the access site and avoiding the need to sacrifice additional vein, are appropriate. In cases of recurrent early failure and/or extensive graft degeneration, however, surgical revision becomes necessary.

CURRENT TREATMENT OF PERIPHERAL ARTERY DISEASE

The therapeutic armamentarium for, and clinical experience with, percutaneous revascularization described above has markedly improved the prospects of patients with PAD (see Chap. 101). In the bygone era when vascular surgery was the only effective option available to patients with claudication or threatened limb loss, there was little reason to perform diagnostic angiography unless surgery was indicated. And there were justifiable reasons, given the risks of major reconstructive surgery in a population of patients riddled with coronary and cerebrovascular disease, to restrict surgery to patients with altogether disabling claudication or threatened limb loss.

In the current era, intervention at an earlier stage of symptomatic disability is possible due to the lower risks and lower costs of nonsurgical revascularization. As has been pointed out by Kumpe and Rutherford,[98] ". . . the advantages to the patient able to undergo angioplasty rather than surgery . . . are lower initial morbidity and mortality, no need for general anesthesia, shorter hospital stay, [and] less trauma." Complications of PTA are, for the most part, minor and typically do not require surgical treatment. Access-related events account for most complications (2 percent to 8 percent in most series[98,99]); these range from the less serious and more common (e.g., groin hematoma) to the serious but rare (e.g., retroperitoneal hematoma).[100] The incidence of complications at the angioplasty site—1 to 7 percent in most series[98,99]—is similar to percutaneous transluminal coronary angioplasty, the main one being acute occlusion; as with coronary angioplasty, many of these complications can be managed with lytic or adjunctive mechanical therapy, including stents, so that the need for emergent surgery due to a jeopardized limb is rare. Distal embolization has been reported in up to 5 percent of cases; most, however, are clinically silent,[99] and even those that might be potentially problematic can often be obviated before PTA or treated successfully afterwards by judicious use of lytic therapy.

It is nevertheless true that both the risks and cost of percutaneous revascularization increase with the complexity and extent of anatomic involvement. The decision to revascularize the patient with claudication in the current era must therefore take into account two principal considerations. The first is the patient's symptoms and physical findings. Noninvasive testing[101–104] remains an indispensable initial step in the evaluation of PAD; but, importantly, failure to detect an abnormal ankle-brachial index at rest does not exclude the presence of severe obstruction, particularly in diabetic or other patients with noncompressible arteries. Exercise stress testing may be required to elicit hemodynamic evidence of vascular obstructions. Duplex,[101] including color-flow,[103] examinations may help to clarify such discrepancies. Angiographic examination, however, is still required to define the second consideration, namely, the full extent and complexity of the anatomic basis for symptomatic disability.

Once having clarified the anatomic basis for claudication, the recommendation to advise percutaneous revascularization is then individualized. Two patients, for example, may be similarly limited, and in both the degree of limitation may be inadequate to justify the risks of vascular surgical reconstruction. Angiography may suggest that percutaneous revascularization has a high likelihood of technical success in one patient, who may thus be a suitable candidate for PTA. In the second patient, anatomic factors suggesting a low likelihood of acute and/or long-term success may dictate that only surgical revascularization would constitute effective therapy, in which case it may be appropriate to defer the risk of surgery until the patient is more critically disabled. Angiography may thus critically raise or lower the threshold for recommending that an intervention be performed. In previous days, when surgery represented the sole option to medical and exercise therapy, it could be reasonably argued that the decision to proceed with angiography could come down to consideration of severe disability only. The option of performing lower-risk and lower-cost PTA, however, implies that the threshold for responding to a given level of symptomatic disability may be lowered, depending upon the complexity of anatomic findings.

Should the patient treated by percutaneous revascularization return with clinical evidence of restenosis, repeat percutaneous intervention is probably indicated for the same reasons that led to the recommendation for the original procedure. A certain proportion of these patients—as has been clearly documented in certain patients undergoing one or more repeat coronary angioplasty procedures[105]—will achieve a satisfactory long-term result following the second intervention (see Chap. 48). In those who fail repeated percutaneous attempts to achieve long-term patency, the decision to undergo surgical revascularization may involve a reassessment of the patient's anatomy and clinical status.

To adopt this approach with maximum concern for safety and efficacy clearly requires *coordinated* input from enlightened experts in cardiology, radiology, and vascular surgery. The cost of underutilizing such enlightened and coordinated input will be reflected in loss of both dollars and patient years that might have been otherwise fulfilling and useful.

Acknowledgment

The expert assistance of Ms. Susan Panzica in the preparation of this chapter is greatly appreciated. The collaboration of Dr. Syed Razvi and our surgical colleagues as well as Dr. Eugene Langevin and our radiology colleagues in the care of patients discussed in this chapter is gratefully acknowledged.

REFERENCES

1. Fischman DL, Leon MB, Baim DS, Schatz RA, Savage MP, Penn I, et al. A randomized comparison of coronary-stent placement and balloon angioplasty in the treatment of coronary artery disease. *N Engl J Med* 1994; 331:196–501.
2. Dorros G, Jaff M, Jain A, Dufek C, Mathiak L. Follow-up of primary Palmaz-Schatz stent placement for atherosclerotic renal artery stenosis. *Am J Cardiol* 1995; 75:1051–1055.
3. Isner JM, Rosenfield K. Redefining the treatment of peripheral artery disease. Role of percutaneous revascularization. *Circulation* 1993; 88:1534–1557.
4. Long AL, Page PE, Raynaud AC, Beyssen BM, Fiessinger JN, Ducimetiere P, et al. Percutaneous iliac artery stent: Angiographic long-term follow-up. *Radiology* 1991; 180:771–778.
5. Isner JM, Rosenfield K, Kelly K, Losordo DW, DeJesus ST, Palefsky P, et al. Percutaneous intravascular ultrasound examination as an ad-

6. Rosenfield K, Isner JM. Intravascular ultrasound in patients undergoing coronary and peripheral arterial revascularization. In: Topol EJ, ed. *Textbook of Interventional Cardiology*, 2d ed. Philadelphia: Saunders; 1994:1153–1185.
7. Isner JM, Rosenfield K, Losordo DW, Rose L, Langerin RE, Razvi S, et al. Combination balloon-ultrasound imaging catheter for percutaneous transluminal angioplasty. *Circulation* 1991; 84:739–754.
8. Losordo DW, Rosenfield K, Pieczek A, Baker K, Harding M, Isner JM. How does angioplasty work? Serial analysis of human iliac arteries using intravascular ultrasound. *Circulation* 1992; 86:1845–1858.
9. Isner JM, Pieczek A, Rosenfield K. Untreated gangrene in patients with peripheral artery disease. *Circulation* 1994; 89:482–483.
10. Pepine CJ, Feldman RL, Nichols WW. Coronary arteriography: Potentially serious sources of error in interpretation. *Cardiovasc Med* 1977; 2:747–752.
11. Isner JM, Kishel J, Kent KM, Ronan JA Jr, Ross AM, Roberts WC. Accuracy of angiographic determination of left main coronary arterial narrowing: Angiographic-histologic correlative analysis in 28 patients. *Circulation* 1981; 63:1056–1064.
12. White CW, Wright CB, Doty DB. Does visual interpretation of the coronary arteriogram predict the physiologic importance of a coronary stenosis? *N Engl J Med* 1984; 310:819–824.
13. Isner JM, Donaldson RF. Coronary angiographic and morphologic correlation. *Cardiol Clin* 1984; 2:571–592.
14. Nissen SE, Gurley JC, Grines CL, Booth DC, McClure R, Berk M, et al. Intravascular ultrasound assessment of lumen size and wall morphology in normal subjects and patients with coronary artery disease. *Circulation* 1991; 84:1087–1099.
15. Davidson CJ, Sheikh KH, Harrison JK, Himmelstein SI, Leithe ME, Kisslo KB, et al. Intravascular ultrasonography versus digital subtraction angiography: A human in vivo comparison of vessel size and morphology. *J Am Coll Cardiol* 1990; 16:633–636.
16. Mecley M, Rosenfield K, Kaufman J, Langevin RE, Razvi S, Isner JM. Atherosclerotic plaque hemorrhage and rupture associated with crescendo claudication. *Ann Intern Med* 1992; 117:663–666.
17. Tobis JM, Mallery JA, Gessert JM, Griffith JM, Mahon DJ, Bessen M, et al. Intravascular ultrasound cross-sectional arterial imaging before and after balloon angioplasty in vitro. *Circulation* 1989; 80:873–882.
18. Nishimura RA, Edwards WD, Warness CA, Reeder GS, Holmes DRJ, Tajik AJ, et al. Intravascular ultrasound imaging: In vitro validation and pathologic correlation. *J Am Coll Cardiol* 1990; 16:145–154.
19. Honye J, Mahon DJ, Jain A, White CJ, Ramee SR, Wallis JB, et al. Morphologic effects of coronary balloon angioplasty in vivo assessed by intravascular ultrasound imaging. *Circulation* 1992; 85:1012–1025.
20. Nakamura S, Colombo A, Gaglione A, Almagor Y, Goldberg SL, Maiello L, et al. Intracoronary ultrasound observations during stent implantation. *Circulation* 1994; 89:2026–2034.
21. Rosenfield K, Losordo DW, Ramaswamy K, Pastore JO, Langevin RE, Razvi S, et al. Three-dimensional reconstruction of human coronary and peripheral arteries from images recorded during two-dimensional intravascular ultrasound examination. *Circulation* 1991; 84:1938–1956.
22. Palmaz JC, Richter GM, Noeldge G. Intraluminal stents in atherosclerotic iliac artery stenosis: Preliminary report of multicenter study. *Radiology* 1988; 168:727–731.
23. Richter GM, Roeren T, Brado M. Further update of the randomized trial: Iliac stent placement versus PTA-morphology, clinical success rates, and failure analysis. *J Vasc Interv Radiol* 1993; 4:30.
24. Pieczek AM, Langevin RE Jr, Razvi S, Rosenfield K. Successful percutaneous revascularization of 180/190 (95%) consecutive peripheral arterial total occlusions using hydrophilic ("Glide") wire (abstr). *Circulation* 1992; 86:I-704.
25. Ring E, Freiman D, McLean G, Schwartz W. Percutaneous recanalization of common iliac artery occlusions: An unacceptable complication rate? *Am J Roentgenol* 1982; 139:587–589.
26. Brewster DC, Cambria RP, Darling RC, Athanasoulis CA, Waltman AC, Geller SCM, et al. Long-term results of combined iliac balloon angioplasty and distal surgical revascularization. *Ann Surg* 1989; 210:324–331.
27. Isner JM, Rosenfield K. Reducing the cardiac risk associated with vascular surgical procedures: Balloons as prophylactics. *Mayo Clin Proc* 1992; 67:95–98.

28. Eagle KA, Coley CM, Newell JB, Brewster DC, Darling RC, Strauss HW, et al. Combining clinical and thallium data optimizes preoperative assessment of cardiac risk before major vascular surgery. *Ann Intern Med* 1989; 110:859–866.

29. Laborde JC, Parodi JC, Clem MF, Tio FO, Barone HD, Rivera FJ, et al. Intraluminal bypass of abdominal aortic aneurysm: Feasibility study. *Radiology* 1992; 184:185–190.

30. Razavi MK, Dake MD, Semba CP, Nyman UR, Liddell RP. Percutaneous endoluminal placement of stent-grafts for the treatment of isolated iliac artery aneursysms. *Radiology* 1995; 197:801–804.

31. Isner JM, Kaufman J, Rosenfield K, Pieczek A, Schainfeld R, Ramaswamy K, et al. Combined physiologic and anatomic assessment of percutaneous revascularization using a Doppler guidewire and ultrasound catheter. *Am J Cardiol* 1993; 71:70D–86D.

32. Krepel VM, vanAndel HJ, vanErp WFM, Breslau BJ. Percutaneous transluminal angioplasty of the femoropopliteal artery: Initial and long-term results. *Radiology* 1985; 165:325–328.

33. Hewes RC, White RI, Murray RR. Long-term results of superficial femoral artery angioplasty. *Am J Roentgenol* 1986; 146:1025–1029.

34. Johnston KW. Femoral and popliteal arteries: Reanalysis of results of balloon angioplasty. *Radiology* 1992; 183:767–771.

35. Hunink MG, Donaldson MC, Meyerovitz MF, Polak JF, Whittemore AD, Kandarpa K, et al. Risks and benefits of femoropopliteal percutaneous balloon angioplasty. *J Vasc Surg* 1993; 17:183–184.

36. Rutherford RB, Becker GJ. Standards for evaluating and reporting the results of surgical and percutaneous therapy for peripheral arterial disease. *Radiology* 1991; 181:277–281.

37. Matsi PJ, Manninen JI, Vanninen RL, Suhonen MT, Oksala I, Laakso M, et al. Femoropopliteal angioplasty in patients with claudication: Primary and secondary patency in 140 limbs with 1- to 2-year follow-up. *Radiology* 1994; 191:727–733.

38. Johnson DE, Hinohara T, Selmon MR, Braden LJ, Simpson JB. Primary peripheral arterial stenoses and restenoses excised by transluminal atherectomy: A histopathologic study. *J Am Coll Cardiol* 1990; 15:419–425.

39. Leclerc G, Isner JM, Kearney M, Simons M, Safian RD, Baim DS, et al. Evidence implicating nonmuscle myosin in restenosis: Use of in situ hybridization to analyze human vascular lesions obtained by directional atherectomy. *Circulation* 1992; 85:543–553.

40. Nikol S, Isner JM, Pickering JG, Kearney M, Leclerc G, Weir L. Expression of transforming growth factor-β_1 is increased in human vascular restenosis lesions. *J Clin Invest* 1992; 90:1582–1592.

41. Pickering JG, Weir L, Jekanowski J, Kearney M, Isner JM. Proliferative activity in peripheral and coronary atherosclerotic plaque among patients undergoing percutaneous revascularization. *J Clin Invest* 1993; 91:1469–1480.

42. Simons M, Leclerc G, Safian RD, Isner JM, Weir L, Baim DS. Relation between activated smooth muscle cells in coronary artery lesions and restenosis after atherectomy. *N Engl J Med* 1993; 328:608–613.

43. vonPolnitz A, Nerlich A, Berger H, Hofling B. Percutaneous peripheral atherectomy: Angiographic and follow-up of 60 patients. *J Am Coll Cardiol* 1990; 15:682–688.

44. Gordon IL, Conroy RM, Tobis JM, Kohl C, Wilson SE. Determinants of patency after percutaneous angioplasty and atherectomy of occluded superficial femoral arteries. *Am J Surg* 1994; 167:115–119.

45. Topol EJ, Leya F, Pinkerton CS, Shitlow PL, Hofling B, Simonton CA, for the CAVEAT study group. A comparison of directional atherectomy with coronary angioplasty in patients with coronary artery disease. *N Engl J Med* 1993; 329:221–227.

46. Dorros G, Lyer S, Zaitoun R, Lewin R, Cooley R, Olson K. Acute angiographic and clinical outcome of high speed percutaneous rotational atherectomy (Rotablator). *Cathet Cardiovasc Diagn* 1991; 22:157–166.

47. Rousseau HP, Raillat CR, Joffre FG, Knight CJ, Ginested MC. Treatment of femoropopliteal stenoses by means of self-expandable endoprostheses: Midterm results. *Radiology* 1989; 172:961–964.

48. Sapoval MR, Long AL, Raynaud AC, Beyssen BM, Fiessinger J-N, JeGaux J-C. Femoropopliteal stent placement: Long-term results. *Radiology* 1992; 184:833–839.

49. Henry M, Amor M, Ethevenot G, Henry I, Amicabile C, Beron R, et al. Palmaz stent placement in iliac and femoropopliteal arteries: Primary and secondary patency in 310 patients with 2–4 year follow-up. *Radiology* 1995; 197:167–174.

50. Do DD, Triller J, Walpoth BH, Stirnemann P, Mahler F. A comparison study of self-expandable stents vs balloon angioplasty alone in femoropopliteal artery occlusions. *Cardiovasc Intervent Radiol* 1992; 15:306–312.

51. Rosenfield K, Schainfeld R, Pieczek A, Haley L, Isner JM. Restenosis of endovascular stents due to stent compression. *J Am Coll Cardiol* 1997; 29:328–338.

52. Rosenfield K, Losordo DW, Ramaswamy K, Langevin RE Jr, Razvi S, Kosowsky BD. Three-dimensional reconstruction of intravascular ultrasound images recorded in 68 consecutive patients following percutaneous revascularization of totally occluded arteries: In vivo evidence that the neolumen frequently includes subintimal component (abstr). *Circulation* 1991; 84:II-686.

53. Comerota AJ, Weaver FA, Graor RA, Hosking JD, Froelich J, Sussman B, et al. Surgery versus thrombolysis for occluded lower extremity bypass grafts: Results of a prospective randomized trial. *Ann Surg* 1994; 220:251–268.

54. Ouriel K, Shortell CK, DeWeese JA, Green RM, Francis CW, Azodo MV, et al. A comparison of thrombolytic therapy with operative revascularization in the initial treatment of acute peripheral arterial ischemia. *J Vasc Surg* 1994; 19:1021–1030.

55. Motarjeme A, Keifer J, Ziska A. A percutaneous transluminal angioplasty case selection. *Radiology* 1980; 135:573–581.

56. Dotter CT, Judkins MP. Transluminal treatment of arteriosclerotic obstruction. Description of a new technic and a preliminary report of its application. *Circulation* 1964; 30:654–670.

57. Bakal CW, Sprayregen S, Scheinbaum K, Cynamon J, Veith FJ. Percutaneous transluminal angioplasty of the infrapopliteal arteries: Results in 53 patients. *Am J Roentgenol* 1990; 154:171–174.

58. Schwarten DE, Cutclif WB. Arterial occlusive disease below the knee: Treatment with percutaneous transluminal angioplasty performed with low-profile catheters and steerable guide wires. *Radiology* 1988; 169:71–74.

59. Dorros G, Lewin RF, Jamnadas P, Mathiak LM. Below-the-knee angioplasty: Tibioperoneal vessels, the acute outcome. *Cathet Cardiovasc Diagn* 1990; 19:170–178.

60. Veith FJ, Gupta SK, Ascer E, White-Flores S, Samson RH, Scher LA, et al. Six-year prospective multicenter randomized comparison of autologous saphenous vein and expanded polytetrafluoroethylene grafts in infrainguinal arterial reconstructions. *J Vasc Surg* 1986; 3:104–114.

61. Perler BA, Osterman FA, Mitchell SE, Burdick JF, Williams GM. Balloon dilatation versus surgical revision of infra-inguinal autogenous vein graft stenoses: Long-term follow-up. *J Cardiovasc Surg* 1990; 31:656–661.

62. Whittemore AD, Donaldson MC, Polak JF, Mannick JA. Limitations of balloon angioplasty for vein graft stenosis. *J Vasc Surg* 1991; 14:340–345.

63. Berkowitz HD, Fox AD, Deaton DH. Reversed vein graft stenosis: Early diagnosis and management. *J Vasc Surg* 1992; 15:130–142.

64. Veith FJ, Gupta SK, Wengerter KR, Goldsmith J, Rivers SP, Bakal CW, et al. Changing arteriosclerotic disease patterns and management strategies in lower-limb-threatening ischemia. *Ann Surg* 1990; 212:402–414.

65. Brewster DC, LaSalle AJ, Robison JG. Factors directing patency of femoropopliteal bypass grafts. *Surg Gynecol Obstet* 1983; 157:437–442.

66. Whittemore AD, Clowes AW, Couch NP. Secondary femoropopliteal reconstruction. *Ann Surg* 1981; 193:35–42.

67. Millaire A, Trinca ZM, Marache P, de Groote P, Jabinet JL, Ducloux G. Subclavian angioplasty: Immediate and late results in 50 patients. *Cathet Cardiovasc Diagn* 1993; 29:8–17.

68. Burke DR, Gordon RL, Mishkin JD, McLean GK, Meranze SG. Percutaneous transluminal angioplasty of subclavian arteries. *Radiology* 1987; 164:699–704.

69. Hebrang A, Maskovic J, Tomac B. Percutaneous transluminal angioplasty of the subclavian arteries: Long-term results in 52 patients. *Am J Roentgenol* 1991; 156:1091–1096.

70. Dorros G, Lewin RF, Jamnadas P, Mathiak LM. Peripheral transluminal angioplasty of the subclavian and innominate arteries utilizing the brachial approach: Acute outcome and follow-up. *Cathet Cardiovasc Diagn* 1990; 19:71–76.

71. Mufti SI, Young KR, Schulthesis T. Restenosis following subclavian artery angioplasty for treatment of coronary-subclavian steal syndrome: Definitive treatment with Palmaz-stent placement. *Cathet Cardiovasc Diagn* 1994; 33:172–174.

72. Satler LF, Hoffmann R, Lansky A, Mintz GS, Popma JJ, Pichard AD, et al. Carotid stent-assisted angioplasty: Preliminary technique, angiography, and intravascular ultrasound observations. *J Invas Cardiol* 1996; 8:23–30.

73. NACPTAR (North American Cerebral Percutaneous Transluminal Angioplasty Registry). Update of the immediate angiographic results and in-hospital central nervous system complications of cerebral percutaneous transluminal angioplasty (abstr). *Circulation* 1995; 92:I-383.

74. Diethrich EB, Ndiaye M, Reid DB. Stenting in the carotid artery: Initial experience in 110 patients. *J Endovasc Surg* 1996; 3:42–62.

75. Yadav JS, Roubin GS, Iyer S, Vitek J, King P, Jordan WD, et al. Elective stenting of the extracranial carotid arteries. *Circulation* 1997; 95:376–381.

76. Novick AC, Ziegelbaum M, Vidt DG, Gifford RW, Pohl MA, Goormastic M. Trends in surgical revascularization for renal artery disease: Ten years experience. *JAMA* 1987; 257:498–501.

77. Sos TA, Pickering TG, Phil D. Percutaneous transluminal renal angiography in renovascular hypertension due to atheroma or fibromuscular dysplasia. *N Engl J Med* 1983; 309:274–279.

78. Cluzel P, Raynaud A, Beyssen B, Pagny JY, Gaux JC. Stenoses of renal branch arteries in fibromuscular dysplasia: Results of percutaneous transluminal angioplasty. *Radiology* 1994; 193:227–232.

79. Rimmer JM, Gennari FJ. Atherosclerotic renovascular disease and progressive renal failure. *Ann Intern Med* 1993; 118:712–719.

80. Libertino JA, Flam TA, Zinman LN, Ying CY, Breslin DJ, Swinton NW, et al. Changing concepts in surgical management of renovascular hypertension. *Arch Intern Med* 1988; 148:357–359.

81. Hansen KJ, Ditesheim JA, Metropol SH, Canzanello VJ, Graves J, Plonk GW. Management of renovascular hypertension in the elderly population. *J Vasc Surg* 1989; 10:266–273.

82. Libertino JA, Bosco PJ, Ying CY, Breslin DJ, Woods BO, Tsapatsaris NP. Renal revascularization to preserve and restore renal function. *J Urol* 1992; 147:1485–1487.

83. Weibell H, Bergqvist D, Bergentz SE, Jonsson K, Hulthen L, Manhem P. Percutaneous transluminal renal angioplasty versus surgical reconstruction of atherosclerotic renal artery stenosis: A prospective randomized study. *J Vasc Surg* 1993; 18:841–852.

84. Tegtmeyer CJ, Dyer R, Teates CD, Ayers CR, Carey RM, Wellons HA, et al. Percutaneous transluminal dilatation of the renal arteries. *Radiology* 1980; 135:589–599.

85. Sos TA. Angioplasty for the treatment of azotemia and renovascular hypertension in atherosclerotic renal artery disease. *Circulation* 1991; 83(suppl I):I162–I166.

86. White CJ, Ramee SR, Collins TJ, Dearing B, Rees AP, Granke K, et al. Guiding catheter-assisted renal artery angioplasty. *Cathet Cardiovasc Diagn* 1991; 23:10–13.

87. Rosenfield K, Losordo DW, Harding M, Pieczek A, Waters J, Isner JM. Intravascular ultrasound of renal arteries in patients undergoing percutaneous transluminal angioplasty: Feasibility, safety, and initial findings, including 3-dimensional reconstruction of renal arteries (abstr). *J Am Coll Cardiol* 1991; 17:204A.

88. Rees CR, Palmaz JC, Becker GJ, Ehrman KO, Richter GM, Noeldge G, et al. Palmaz stent in atherosclerotic stenoses involving the ostia of the renal arteries: Preliminary report of a multicenter study. *Radiology* 1991; 181:507–514.

89. Dorros G, Prince C, Mathiak L. Stenting of a renal artery stenosis achieves better relief of the obstructive lesion than balloon angioplasty. *Cathet Cardiovasc Diagn* 1993; 29:191–198.

90. Hennequin LM, Joffre FG, Rousseau HP, Aziza R, Tregant P, Bernadet P, et al. Renal artery stent placement: Long-term results with the Wallstent endoprosthesis. *Radiology* 1994; 191:713–719.

91. Jamieson GG, Clarkson AR, Woodroff AJ, Faris I. Reconstructive renal vascular surgery for chronic renal failure. *Br J Surg* 1984; 71:338–340.

92. Morris GC, DeBakey ME, Cooley DA. Surgical treatment of renal failure of renovascular origin. *JAMA* 1962; 182:609–612.

93. Gaylord GM, Taber TE. Long-term hemodialysis access salvage: Problems and challenges for nephrologists and interventional radiologists. *J Vasc Interv Radiol* 1993; 4:103–107.

94. Kumpe DA, Cohen MA, Durham JD. Treatment of failing and failed hemodialysis access sites: Comparison of surgical treatment with thrombolysis/angioplasty. *Semin Vasc Surg* 1992; 5:118–127.

95. Turmel-Rodrigues L, Pengloan J, Blanchier D, Abaza M, Birmele B, Haillot O, et al. Insufficient dialysis shunts: Improved long-term patency rates with close hemodynamic monitoring, repeated percutaneous balloon angioplasty, and stent placement. *Radiology* 1993; 187:273–278.

96. Glantz S, Gordon DH, Lipkowitz GS, Butt K, Hong J, Sclafani SJ. Axillary and subclavian vein stenosis: Percutaneous angioplasty. *Radiology* 1988; 168:371–373.

97. Sullivan KL, Besarab A, Bonn J, Shapiro MJ, Gardiner GA, Moritz MJ. Hemodynamics of failing dialysis grafts. *Radiology* 1993; 186:867–872.

98. Kumpe DA, Rutherford RB. Percutaneous transluminal angioplasty for lower extremity ischemia. In: Rutherford RB, ed. *Vascular Surgery*, 3d ed. Philadelphia: Saunders; 1992:759–761.

99. O'Keeffe ST, Woods BO, Beckmann CF. Percutaneous transluminal angioplasty of the peripheral arteries: In: Breslin DJ, ed. *Cardiology Clinics. Peripheral Vascular Disease in the Elderly*. Philadelphia: Saunders; 1991:519–521.

100. Trerotola SO, Kuhlman JE, Fishman EK. Bleeding complications of femoral catheterization: CT evaluation. *Radiology* 1990; 174:37–40.

101. Kohler TR, Nance DR, Cramer MM, Vandenburghe N, Strandness DE Jr. Duplex scanning for diagnosis of aortoiliac and femoropopliteal disease: A prospective study. *Circulation* 1987; 76:1074–1080.

102. Johnston KW, Hosang MY, Andrews DF. Reproducibility of noninvasive vascular laboratory measurements of the peripheral circulation. *J Vasc Surg* 1987; 6:147–152.

103. Rosenfield K, Kelly SM, Fields CD, Pastore JO, Weinstein R, Palefski P, et al. Non-invasive assessment of peripheral vascular disease by color flow Doppler/two-dimensional ultrasound. *Am J Cardiol* 1989; 64:247–251.

104. Bandyk DF. Postoperative surveillance of infrainguinal bypass. *Surg Clin North Am* 1990; 70:71–85.

105. Teirstein PS, Hoover C, Ligon B, Girogi LV, Rutherford BD, McConahay DR, et al. Repeat restenosis: Efficacy of the third and fourth coronary angioplasty (abstr). *J Am Coll Cardiol* 1987; 9:63A.

COST-EFFECTIVE STRATEGIES, INSURANCE, AND LEGAL PROBLEMS

103

COST-EFFECTIVE STRATEGIES
IN CARDIOLOGY

Joel Kupersmith

In the United States, cardiovascular diseases cost over $128 billion in treatments and lost productivity.[1] For this reason, they are a major topic in the continuing public discussion of health care expense and an important target for cost containment. This chapter will briefly review concepts necessary to understand cost-effective strategies, and then discuss approaches in specific disease categories. Outcomes of therapies will not be specifically considered; for these the reader is referred to other sections of this textbook.

COST, VALUE, AND COST EFFECTIVENESS

Cost Effectiveness

GENERAL

The term *cost effective* is often loosely applied in the absence of data to measures or approaches that save, or appear to save, dollars. However, *cost effectiveness*, in its proper use, is a specific term that describes the cost of an intervention in relation to its medical benefit or effectiveness, i.e., not only cost but, more broadly, value.

In formal "cost-effective analysis," economic and clinical information are combined in one formula in which cost in currency is in the numerator and effectiveness in the denominator. Effectiveness may be expressed in several ways: (1) years of life saved (YLS) or prolonged—*cost-effectiveness analysis*, (2) quality of life—*cost-utility analysis*, or (3) health benefit translated into dollars (i.e., monetized)—*cost-benefit analysis*. (Note the term *cost-effectiveness analysis* has also been used as an overall rubric to describe all of these approaches.) A cost-only study is called *cost-minimization analysis*, where it is assumed, though frequently not proven, that effectiveness is approximately equal between alternatives.[2,3]

In their usual method of use, cost-effectiveness analyses are incremental, i.e., they compare two competing strategies. Here, the total cost and life expectancy of the strategy to be analyzed is determined and then the cost and life expectancy of a competing strategy is subtracted. For example, in the case of coronary artery bypass graft (CABG) surgery versus drug therapy, one determines the entire costs (including those of follow-up and future events) and life expectancy of the surgical strategy and subtracts the costs and life expectancy of drug therapy as follows:

$$Cost\ effectiveness = \frac{\Delta Cost}{\Delta LE} = \frac{Cost_{CABG} - Cost_{Drug\ Rx}}{LE_{CABG} \quad LE_{Drug\ Rx}}$$

$$= Cost/YLS$$

where *LE* is life expectancy and Drug Rx is drug therapy. In cost-utility analysis, the denominator would be the difference in quality-adjusted life years (QALYs), a unit that combines life expectancy and quality of life.[2,3]

EVALUATING ANALYSES

To assure that analyses are rigorous and relevant, one should carefully evaluate the source of cost and effectiveness data, whether the data are from randomized trials, and other aspects of their quality, as well as their applicability to one's local situation, and whether an adequate sensitivity analysis was performed.[2] It should be noted that while randomized trials are considered a "gold standard," the fact that they compare a careful and limited selection of patients and providers may influence their applicability to the routine clinical situation. In addition, even if effectiveness data are from trials, costs used in the analyses are often derived from other sources.[2] Database analyses may represent effectiveness in routine clinical practice but may be associated with selection bias.

COST-EFFECTIVE RANGES

It has been considered that approximately $20,000 to $40,000 or $50,000 per year of life saved (depending on the dollar year) is the cost-effective range; borderline to expensive is defined as >$60,000/YLS and "highly expensive" as >$100,000/YLS.[4,5] Although it is uncommon, treatment strategies sometimes actually save money by substantially reducing future medical events and costs; in these cases they are termed *dominant*.

Cost Determination

COST COMPONENTS OF A STRATEGY

There are usually many components of cost and a variety of resources consumed in a medical strategy. For example, CABG surgery includes not only the cost of surgery but also the cost of various medications, complications, testing, and possibly screening for coronary artery disease (CAD) in certain individuals. Compared to medical therapy, CABG surgery may lead to savings in myocardial infarctions (MIs) averted, which include their own set of testing and therapy costs as well as those for emergency room visits, ambulances, etc. Some of these costs are obvious and some, such as ambulance and screening costs, may be more subtle and overlooked in the usual analysis. Initiation of programs with new technologies also involves start-up and learning-curve costs, which decline with a variable time course. Other costs also may not be static, e.g. drug costs, such as those for ACE inhibitors and statins, may decline due to loss of patent protection and increased competition, thereby improving cost effectiveness.

COST PERSPECTIVE

Perspective refers to who pays the bill or may receive benefits from efficiencies. Entities include insurance companies, health maintenance organizations, hospitals, providers, patients, or society as a whole. At times perspectives of these entities may clash. For example, shortened length of stay (LOS) benefits the hospital because payment from insurance companies is prospective (diagnosis-related group: DRG) and irrespective of LOS. On the other hand, for the patient, it may be economical to stay in the hospital since there are many out-of-pocket costs at home. From the societal perspective, both the hospital and the long-term outpatient costs would be considered. Managed care creates a physician's perspective on hospital payments since there is a designated "hospital pool" available to the physician if unused. All cost-reduction strategies must be considered in relation to whose perspective they benefit.

TYPES OF COSTS

In analyses, the term *cost* may refer to actual cost, i.e., resources spent, of a service or to charges (fees) or payments (reimbursements) for them. Costs themselves can be categorized in several ways, some of which are relevant to the text of this chapter. Direct costs of illness in one context refer to both medical and nonmedical expenditures involved in delivering medical care, e.g., hospitalization and physician services, while indirect costs (or "indirects") would be those that occur from a loss of income and productivity because of illness or death. In another context, e.g., in hospitals, direct costs may refer to those directly related to medical care, while indirects refer to nonmedical costs such as building maintenance.[2,6–8]

Variable costs differ according to the quantity of services provided (e.g., supplies or personnel working flexible hours), while fixed costs remain the same (e.g., regular staff). Average (or unit) costs refer to total costs divided by total units, while marginal (or "incremental" or "differential") costs are those of adding an additional unit of service and are dependent on the infrastructure in place and its prior utilization. For example, the cost to hospitals of 1000 cardiac catheterizations may be $200,000, or $200 per catheterization. If the schedule is not full and there is nonutilized capacity, however, the cost of adding 50 catheterizations would be much less, perhaps $50 per catheterization; when capacity is fully utilized, the cost, which now includes overtime wages, etc., is greater.

Cost-Reduction Methods

Interventions to control costs[9] may be applied locally or globally; aimed at patients or providers; directed at administrative or overhead costs, clinical decision-making (e.g., reduced cardiac procedures), or a combination of these (e.g., chest pain clinics); and mildly or severely coercive.[6,9] In these, it is important to remember that the denominator of the cost-effectiveness formula is effectiveness. Cost reduction that also reduces quality is not cost effective. The other issue is affordability, however; no matter how cost effective a Rolls Royce is, it may not be affordable.

Some knowledge of cost determination and cost allocation is also necessary since cost shifting and other issues influence the consequences of cost-cutting measures.[2,6–8] Goals of cost cutting may not be achieved if administrative fixed and other costs remain flat or if cost allocations disfavor them. For these reasons, one should always judge cost-reduction measures by actual dollars saved, including the costs of the measure itself, and not merely by tests, procedures, or hospital days reduced.

Relevant Specific Topics

CASE MANAGEMENT AND CRITICAL PATHWAYS

Case management and critical pathways have quickly emerged in the health care world as cost-reduction and quality-improvement measures. Case management refers to a coordinated, patient-oriented process to standardize and increase the efficiency of care and discharge planning. Continuous quality improvement and total quality management are vehicles for quality improvement in industry[10] from which derive critical pathways. Continuous quality improvement in particular is designed to rule out random and assignable variations in process, most commonly systems problems as well as those related to physicians' practice patterns and employee factors. In a critical (also called "clinical") pathway, steps in care are reviewed and fine-tuned to achieve cost-effectiveness goals (at present usually in ideal or uncomplicated cases).[11–15]

TABLE 103-1

COST EFFECTIVENESS OF PREVENTIVE INTERVENTION IN HIGH- VERSUS LOW-RISK PATIENTS[a]

	High Risk Untreated	High Risk Treated	Low Risk Untreated	Low Risk Treated
Annual death rate	10%	5%	1%	0.5%
Years of life saved (YLS)[b]	0	5209	0	614
Cost of intervention ($ millions) at $2000/year	0	90.5	0	99.0
Annual CABG rate	6%	3%	0.6%	0.3%
Cost CABG	$20,000	$20,000	$20,000	$20,000
Annual AMI rate	4%	2%	0.4%	0.2%
Cost/AMI	$10,000	$10,000	$10,000	$10,000
Annual rate of other events	4%	2%	0.4%	0.2%
Cost per other event	$5000	$5000	$5000	$5000
Medical costs ($ millions)[c]	70.0	39.7	8.8	4.4
Total cost ($ millions)	70.0	130.2	8.8	103.4
Total cost difference[d] ($ millions)		60.2		94.8
Approximate $/YLS		$11,500		$155,000

[a] Hypothetical intervention in 10,000 patients for 5 years; simplified so that the intervention reduces all risks by 50%, neither costs nor health effects discounted, all patients are assumed to die at midyear, and the analysis considers only the first 5 years.

[b] By life table analysis. Considers CABG but not PTCA.

[c] Total costs of CABG, AMI, and other events in the 10,000 patients.

[d] Costs of treated less costs of untreated patients.

Note: In the example, an intervention reduces risk by 50% in high-risk (10% mortality, 6% annual CABG rate, and 4% annual rate of AMI) and low-risk (1%, 0.6%, 0.4%, respectively) patients. Note that the dollar savings in prevention of events ("medical costs") and effectiveness in years of life saved are greater in the high-risk patients.

Abbreviations: CABG, coronary artery bypass graft surgery; AMI, acute myocardial infarction; YLS, year of life saved, PTCA, percutaneous transluminal coronary angioplasty.

Source: From Goldman et al.[16] Reproduced with permission of the publisher and authors.

RISK AND COST EFFECTIVENESS

Patient targeting is an important determinant of cost effectiveness, and a prominent patient characteristic is the pretreatment risk situation. Table 103-1 shows a hypothetical preventive intervention.[16] Here, for the same proportional benefit (50 percent reduction in mortality), cost effectiveness is more favorable for the individual at high risk ($11,500/YLS) than for the one at low risk ($155,000/YLS). Although the details and reasons vary, this principle applies to many situations. Exceptions would pertain to patients with very shortened life expectancy, particularly those undergoing procedural therapy, where there is insufficient time to gain the benefits of high initial costs. Age and cost effectiveness have a complex interaction. In the elderly, there is an interplay between higher risk, shorter life expectancy, and a tendency toward lower efficacy coefficients.

DIAGNOSTIC TESTING

The cost effectiveness of diagnostic testing is important in many cardiovascular diseases. Table 103-2 lists factors (Baysian and otherwise) in the cost effectiveness of these tests (see also Chap. 15). Evaluation of the cost effectiveness of diagnostic testing tends to be complex, as it involves not only the test itself but also the treatment strategies that follow.

Inflation Adjustments

Inflation of medical costs has been somewhat variable between categories and locations, and no overall measure is exact, especially as more recent marketplace forces have come into play. For purposes of comparison among strategies in this chapter, earlier costs will be adjusted to 1993 dollars using the medical consumer price index,[17] as this is the latest dollar year used in the majority of the analyses to date.

TABLE 103-2

FACTORS IN COST EFFECTIVENESS OF DIAGNOSTIC TESTING

Use of test results
  Test is involved in clinical decision-making
  Test leads to choice of a cost-effective treatment strategy
Pretest probability of disease
  Clinical evaluation of patient
Predictive accuracy of test
Posttest probability of disease
  Pretest vs. posttest probability
Cost of test
Morbidity of test

PREVENTIVE THERAPIES

At a superficial glance, preventive strategies in CAD would seem to be cost effective. There are wide variations, however, depending upon patient targeting, level of risk, and appropriate choice of screening and treatment.[18] As in other situations, identification and treatment of high-risk patients, including those with manifestations of target organ disease, multiple risk factors, or intense alterations of a single risk factor, are associated with the most favorable cost effectiveness (Table 103-1).[16]

Costs of preventive programs include the following: (1) screening, an important factor in primary but generally less in secondary prevention where patients are already in the health care system; (2) medical treatments; and (3) lifestyle changes, which are individually variable depending on motivation. Cost savings from prevention programs are derived from avoidance of acute myocardial infarction (AMI) and other morbid events.

Hyperlipidemia

In analyses based on the Lipid Research Clinics Coronary Primary Prevention Trial (see Chap. 53), the cost effectiveness of lipid-lowering therapy in general was not terribly favorable and was in the $100,000 to $200,000 per YLS range.[19,20] Cost effectiveness was somewhat improved when indirect costs (i.e., forgone earnings) were taken into account and much improved when oat bran (which was not part of the Lipid Research Clinics trial) was modeled in place of cholestyramine ($31,600/YLS or $16,300/YLS with indirects included).[19]

When targeted to specific patient groups, however, lipid-lowering therapy can be highly cost effective. Figure 103-1 shows the cost effectiveness of lovastatin therapy in primary prevention related to age, sex, and risk.[21] Data for this figure were derived from an analysis based on drug trials, with low-density lipoprotein levels as end points and Framingham data for outcomes at each level of low-density lipoprotein. *Note that as risk factors accumulate and become more severe, cost effectiveness improves; it is also better in males.* Variations with age tend to be in a U-shaped curve, with more expense in the younger (lower risk, more years of therapy until events occur, and thus more cost) and the oldest patients (shortest life expectancy and, therefore, less gain). When the lovastatin-induced increase in high-density lipoprotein was added to the model, there was about a 40 to 50 percent improvement in cost effectiveness, somewhat less at younger ages.[22] In a similar analysis, treatment of the highly risky heterozygous familial hypercholesterolemia with lovastatin also tends to be cost effective,[23] but less so as the dose rises above 20 mg/day.

Secondary prevention tends to be highly cost effective. Figure 103-2 shows results of a recent analysis (using Swedish costs) based on the "4S" study of simvastatin post-AMI. Here, the intervention was highly cost effective in all subjects and

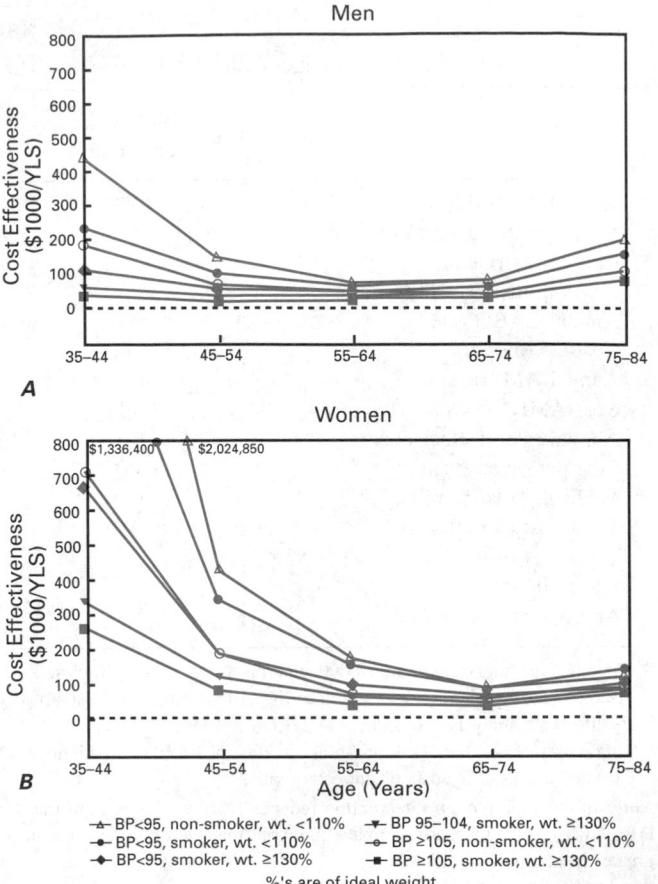

FIGURE 103-1

Cost effectiveness of lovastatin (20 mg/day) used for primary prevention in men (*A*) and in women (*B*) at varying accompanying risk. Pretreatment cholesterol level was >300 mg/dL. Age is on the horizontal and cost effectiveness on the vertical axis. Accompanying risk is shown by the symbols. Note that therapy was more cost effective in men and at greater risk and that it varied with age. (From Kupersmith et al.,[18] based on data from Goldman et al.[21] Reproduced with permission of the publishers and authors.)

more so in males, at higher cholesterol levels, and when indirect costs were added (i.e., those related to lost work). With direct costs only (Fig. 103-2*A*), cost effectiveness of simvastatin was more advantageous at older ages, but when indirects were included (Fig. 103-2*B*), it became much more favorable at younger ages because of the value of a lifetime of work in these individuals. Numbers were somewhat higher substituting U.S. drug costs, but since U.S. procedure rates are also higher, there may be more long-term savings via prevention.[24] In the analysis using the same methodology as in Fig. 103-1, lovastatin was also cost effective in secondary prevention but not in all situations and less so overall.[23]

In summary, lipid-lowering drug therapy is a cost-effective strategy for secondary prevention and in high-risk individuals for primary prevention.[18] It is not cost effective for those at low risk.

Adequate cost data are not yet available on lifestyle interventions in broad populations, nor have screening and other less obvious costs been considered sufficiently in analyses.

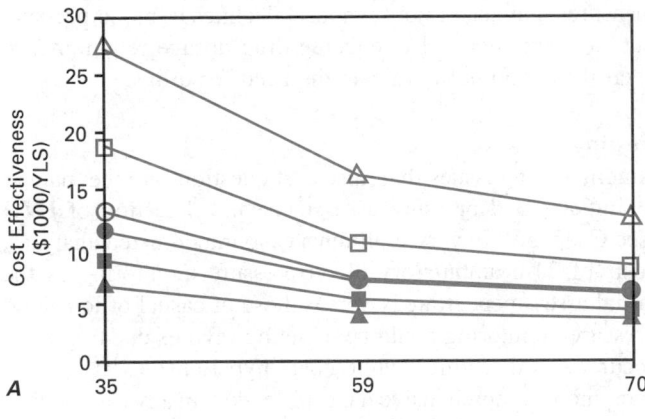

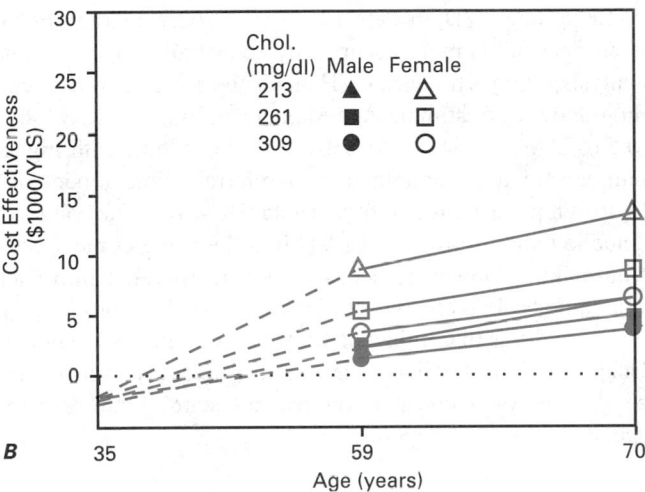

One analysis modeled in Australian men found that a media campaign based on the Stanford Three Cities Study was less than one-tenth the cost per event saved of screening strategies aimed at moderate- to high-risk individuals in general practitioners' offices ($26,578, $368,943, and $294,739 per event saved, respectively).[25]

Smoking Cessation

Since cigarette smoking is a substantial risk factor and its effect on CAD completely reversible, efforts at cessation are highly cost effective.[26–30] In primary prevention, cigarette cessation programs including physician counseling, nicotine gum, and nicotine patch are all highly cost effective at <$10,000 per YLS or QALY, assuming 1-year quit rates of about 1.5 to 2.7 percent. They are somewhat more expensive

but still cost effective as quit rates drop to 1 percent and recidivism after 1 year rises.[26,27,29] In the Stanford Five Cities Preventive Program, various public campaigns were also highly cost effective at <$1000 per quitter.[30] In secondary prevention post-AMI, where quitting may be more likely, cost effectiveness was $250/YLS in a model with a 26 percent quit rate and remained very favorable even when only 1 percent of patients quit ($6800/YLS).[28]

Thus, smoking cessation programs are highly cost-effective strategies, though it should be noted that long-term recidivism rates are not known. Also, the above programs were focused on highly motivated individuals and they may be less cost effective when extended to the general public unless there are motivational inputs.

Hormone-Replacement Therapy

Based on epidemiologic data, with an assumed 50 percent decrease in CAD mortality and also considering effects on hip fracture and breast cancer, estrogen alone was cost effective in 50-year-old women with no uterus ($11,300 to $15,600 per YLS over 15 and 10 years). However, combined therapy with progesterone (assumed, perhaps erroneously, to completely reverse estrogen effects on CAD) was not cost effective in women with an intact uterus ($106,500/YLS to $109,500/ YLS).[31]

Thus, hormone-replacement therapy seems to be cost effective, but this will be clarified when clinical data from randomized trials become available. In translating these results to routine care, it should be noted that the commercially available preparations of estrogen and progesterone vary widely in cost and content.

Exercise

For the most part, exercise programs appear to be cost effective. For example, in primary prevention, a 2000 kcal/week jogging program predicted to decrease CAD incidence by 50 percent in 35-year-old men[32] was analyzed using nonrandomized data. When both direct and indirect costs were considered, cost utility was $22,400/QALY. In a subgroup who loved exercise and did not consider it work, e.g., health club devotees, cost utility was highly favorable at $2500/QALY. For those who hated exercise, it jumped to $86,500/QALY.

Hypertension

OVERALL COST EFFECTIVENESS

Hypertension affects over 60 million individuals in the United States and costs over $15 billion/year. Antihypertensive measures have been highly successful in reducing morbidity and mortality from stroke, heart disease, and renal disease, with modest adverse effects.

Strategies to manage hypertension are clearly cost effective,[18,33–35] as shown in a landmark analysis on screening and treatment of hypertension by Weinstein and Stason in 1976.[33,34] Assuming stepped care (see Chap. 58) and then available drugs and that given levels of blood pressure had the same consequences whether spontaneous or arrived at by treatment, cost utility in patients with mild hypertension (diastolic pressure of 90 to 104 mmHg) was $41,900/QALY and with severe hypertension (≥105 mmHg), was $20,600/QALY. Overall, about 22 percent of drug costs were recovered over a lifetime in prevention of stroke and MI in treating severe hypertension and 15 percent in mild hypertension. Treatment was more cost effective in men (greater risk) and probably in the elderly.[35–37]

SPECIFIC ISSUES

Screening

Screening, drugs, testing, and follow-up visits are the major cost issues that arise in hypertension. Regarding screening, costs of a community program in severe hypertension increased cost utility only from $20,600 to $29,700 per QALY overall, to $25,900/QALY if targeted to blacks, and to $24,600/QALY if performed along with routine office visits.[33,34] Thus, treatment of hypertension including these programs appears to be cost effective, especially when screening is performed in physicians' offices where it is part of a multifaceted approach targeting lipids and other risk factors.

Drugs

Drug costs account for up to half of the costs of antihypertensive treatment strategies,[35,38,39] and, in analyses, cost effectiveness among drugs has varied mainly with drug cost (even when additional blood tests required with certain drugs are included). For example, in one analysis, the two least expensive categories of agents, beta blockers (propranolol) and diuretics, had the most favorable cost effectiveness, $16,900 and $25,400 per YLS, respectively, and the currently expensive angiotensin-converting enzyme (ACE) inhibitors the least favorable (captopril, $111,600/YLS, subject to change of course with any price reduction).[39] Analyses, however, have been based on level of blood pressure attained, with derived morbid outcomes. The hierarchy of cost effectiveness may change if the effectiveness of certain drugs in avoiding end-organ effects differs for the same blood pressure number attained, as data on left ventricular hypertrophy (LVH) may suggest.[40] In addition, certain drugs, such as ACE inhibitors, appear to have the advantage in quality of life, though major adverse effects occur in only a small number of hypertensive patients with modest proportional cost impact.

Cost-reduction measures for hypertension include substitution of cheaper drugs in the same class or, in selected instances, in other classes and use of half of a scored tablet as the prescribed dose.[41] Compliance with drug regimens also enhances cost effectiveness. In one analysis, the same dollars applied to measures to enhance compliance led to blood pressure control in about one-third more patients than when applied to screening.[34]

The cost effectiveness of nonpharmacologic measures to control hypertension has not been analyzed adequately. These measures may lead to only modest declines in blood pressure but can save money by reducing drug dosage requirements, even if they do not eliminate the need for drugs.

Testing

Among testing issues that raise cost questions are the manner of initial blood pressure assessment and detection of LVH (see Chap. 56). In very preliminary, nonrandomized analyses, costs of 24-h ambulatory blood pressure monitoring as the initial assessment strategy versus those of casual office blood pressure monitoring could be offset by savings due to greater accuracy in detecting "white coat" hypertensives[42,43]; however, more comprehensive data are needed. In any case, ambulatory blood pressure monitoring does not seem appropriate for all patients and is often not covered by insurance.[43]

Regarding LVH, its detection by electrocardiogram (ECG) is cheaper but is more accurate by echocardiography. In one analysis, charges for each LVH incidence detected by echocardiography were estimated to be about half those of ECG ($644 to $1672 versus $1320 to $3019 per detection), with higher numbers in a general than in a referral clinic model due to lower pretest probability (Table 103-2).[44] The value of detection and follow-up of LVH in influencing clinical decision-making, however, needs to be incorporated into such calculations. If there is little influence on decisions, e.g., if the same drugs that influence LVH are used in any event (see Chap. 58),[40] test value is less. An efficient approach may be the use of a cheaper, limited echocardiogram directed specifically to the detection of LVH.

Follow-up

Follow-up office visit costs in hypertension are in general amenable to steps toward managerial efficiency, i.e., diminished lengths of visits, increased patient turnover, decreased number of visits per year, and less costly personnel to monitor blood pressure. But in one study performed almost 20 years ago, creation of a specific hypertension clinic appeared to be more costly and less cost effective than usual care, even though it included nurse practitioners.[45]

Anticoagulation

Data are available on anticoagulation for atrial fibrillation, a treatment that is, for the most part, highly cost effective. In a model of mitral stenosis with atrial fibrillation, anticoagulation was valued at $4200/QALY (for a 35-year-old woman), while with normal sinus rhythm it was $174,100/YLS.[46]

In an analysis of nonvalvular atrial fibrillation using randomized trials data for event rates, cost effectiveness of warfarin and aspirin[47] varied with risk for thromboembolism. In 65-year-old patients, warfarin dominated over no therapy in the high- and medium-risk groups and was cost effective in those at low risk (about $14,000/QALY). Warfarin was also highly cost effective versus aspirin in all but the low-risk group, where it was >$350,000/QALY. It was also generally less cost effective at the younger ages of patients in the trial, i.e., 50 years. In this analysis, data were considered insufficient to compare aspirin to no therapy.

Assumed rates of stroke and hemorrhage strongly influenced results. At >4.6 percent stroke rates, warfarin dominated aspirin, and at 1.1 percent, aspirin dominated warfarin. At higher rates of hemorrhage, the cost effectiveness of anticoagulant therapy declined. It has been estimated that rates of hemorrhage are twofold higher in routine use than in clinical trials,[47] at which level aspirin dominates over warfarin in low-risk patients. *In this regard, precise use of INRs is cost effective,[48] and specialized anticoagulation clinics seem to reduce costs resulting from hemorrhage.[49]*

ACUTE MYOCARDIAL INFARCTION

Coronary Care Units and Triage of Chest Pain Patients

COST EFFECTIVENESS AND TRIAGE

Evaluation and treatment of AMI are expensive, effective, and epitomize modern "high-tech" care. Their elaboration has been through the coronary care unit (CCU), which, since its inception, has changed from a predominantly passive monitoring unit to an active unit that deals with expensive drugs and intense technologies.

For AMI patients, CCUs are highly cost effective (<$15,000 per life saved in the author's community-based study).[50] On the other hand, for patients requiring low intensity of care, CCUs are costly and inefficient.[51] A recent analysis based on the Multicenter Chest Pain Study (a prethrombolytic database) assumed that the survival benefit for AMI in the CCU versus intermediate care was 15 percent. Cost effectiveness varied with AMI probability, age, and risk from <$15,000/YLS to >$1.5 million/YLS. In patients aged 55 to 64 years, cost per YLS was <$100,000 if the probability of AMI was >.15, <$75,000/YLS if p > .20, and <$50,000/YLS if p > .29. Figure 103-3 shows results at various ages and AMI probabilities. Thus, in its classic form, the CCU is clearly not cost effective for those at low probability of AMI, making triage of chest pain patients a most important issue.[52,53] In sensitivity analysis, when the mortality benefit of CCU versus intermediate care was modeled to be less than 15 percent, which may be likely, the CCU was much less cost effective.[52]

Unfortunately, persons with nonischemic or low-level ischemic chest pain syndromes ("rule out MIs") rather than AMIs have constituted the majority of patients admitted to CCUs at a cost of $3.5 to $4 billion per year in the United States.[54] To address this problem, chest pain observation units [also called short-stay units, chest pain clinics, or coronary observation units (COUs)] evolved for low-risk chest pain syndromes. These units, generally tied to emergency room staff,[55] monitor and observe patients for 12 to 24 h (or "overnight"), following which, in the absence of events or diagnosis of AMI, stress tests are usually performed for further triage. One nonrandom-

ized study compared patients eligible for such a COU with those sent to ward care, stepdown units (SDUs), CCUs, or discharged. Outcomes were similar, and median 6-month costs along with mean initial LOS were $2800 and 2.3 days in COU, $6847 and 6.3 days in wards, $5857 and 5.1 days in SDU, $13,079 and 6.9 days in CCU, and $586 for patients discharged (all p < .0001 versus COU).[55]

Chest pain observation units thus appear to be cost effective. Also of interest is the fact that when CCU beds are scarce and patients are sent elsewhere, there is little effect on outcome.[56] As CCU bed capacity increases in an institution, the proportion of patients with AMI on it decreases,[57] an example of cost expanding with resource availability. For these reasons, it is also a cost-effective strategy to maintain an optimal number of CCU beds, as determined by case-mix analysis.

COST REDUCTION

At present, CCUs account for a substantial proportion of total AMI charges, though these are variable depending on case mix and local administrative and practice pattern factors. Given its complexity and the need for integration of many hospital services, the CCU offers an excellent venue to use practice guidelines, critical pathways, and systems approaches.[13,58,59] Critical pathways should address the following: (1) staffing (e.g., adjusted personnel hours for high-load time, which decreases cost and converts fixed to variable costs); (2) other

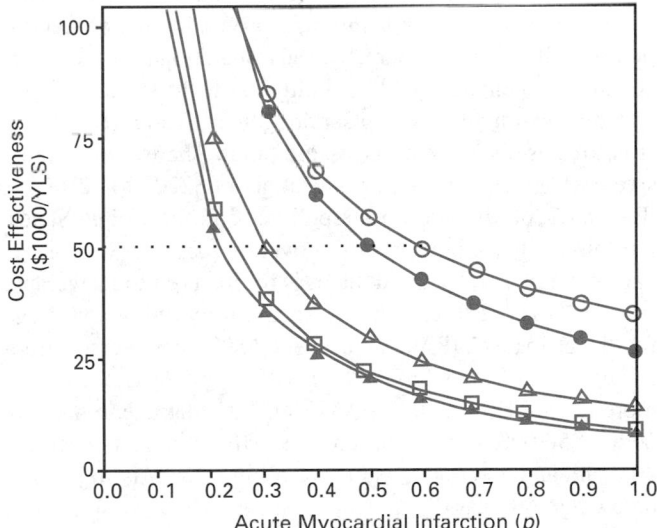

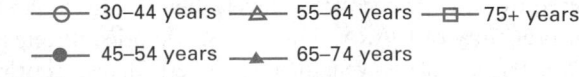

FIGURE 103-3

Cost effectiveness of coronary care unit (CCU) versus intermediate care for patients at various age groups as the probability (p) of acute myocardial infarction (AMI) varied. Also shown are threshold probabilities at $50,000 per year of life saved (YLS). CCU was assumed to confer a 15 percent mortality benefit. (From Tosteson et al.[52] Reproduced with permission of the publisher and authors.)

flexibilities so as to give an appropriate and not excessive intensity of care to individual patients; (3) efficient purchasing and tracking of supplies; (4) coordination of physician and staff activity centered around patient needs; and (5) good coordination between the CCU and other sites, including appropriate timing of physician rounds for efficient procedure and CCU discharge orders. Information systems are most helpful for the evaluation and tracking of these measures, since administrative (billing) data may be insufficient for these particular purposes.[13,60]

Reperfusion

THROMBOLYSIS

Thrombolytic therapy is undoubtedly a cost-effective strategy when applied to all appropriate patients and with all reasonable assumptions in sensitivity analysis, as shown in both overseas and U.S. analyses[61] (though some analyses are presented in cost per life saved, which is difficult to compare with costs per YLS).[62,63] In one U.S. analysis of the elderly using effectiveness data from large randomized trials, streptokinase was valued at $27,700/YLS[64] (effectiveness of thrombolytics is somewhat lower in the elderly, but the AMI risk is higher).

In models targeting subgroups, cost effectiveness of thrombolysis generally becomes more favorable in the higher-risk group, e.g., in anterior versus inferior AMIs[63,65]; with more accurate diagnosis of AMI; and with fewer complications (though the last two have less impact with clinically reasonable alternative assumptions).[62] It also improves with earlier and efficient drug administration,[65] prompting the concept of prehospital treatment; here, various operational costs versus actual time benefit would be additional factors to consider.

Comparison of tissue plasminogen activator (tPA) with streptokinase is a major discussion point. There is an impressive cost spread between agents, at about $2200 to $2700 for tPA and $200 to $400 for streptokinase in the United States, but this is only a portion of the overall cost of AMI, a large part of which in the United States is for interventional therapy. In the GUSTO-I trial, there was a slight mortality advantage for "front-loaded" tPA, and its cost effectiveness versus streptokinase was about $32,700/YLS ($36,400/QALY). It was more favorable for anterior AMIs and at older age, remaining below $50,000/YLS for all anterior MIs in patients over age 40 years and above this value for all inferior MIs in patients below age 60 years.[66]

Thus, tPA appears to be a cost-effective strategy versus streptokinase in more high-risk situations and when administered by strict protocols; however, there is also a question of affordability of tPA. Assuming a $2000 price difference and 750,000 AMIs per year in the United States, of which 40 percent receive thrombolysis,[50] the total additional cost of tPA would be $600 million for 18,361 life-years. In Europe, the price of tPA is less, with about a $800 rather than a $2000 difference from streptokinase,[67] leading to greater affordability and a very favorable cost effectiveness of $13,900/YLS.[66] It is to be hoped that future competition or other factors will

lower the price of tPA in the United States. One controversial suggestion is a copayment for those who prefer tPA.

PRIMARY PERCUTANEOUS TRANSLUMINAL CORONARY ANGIOPLASTY (PTCA)

In randomized trials, primary PTCA achieved higher reperfusion rates and reduced mortality versus thrombolysis, with a greater mortality difference in higher-risk patients (see Chap. 47). The approach has a higher procedural cost than thrombolysis, but there is a reduction in recurrent ischemia, hemorrhagic complications, and LOS. In randomized trials, costs of initial hospitalizations in the United States have been lower with primary PTCA ($23,330 and 7.6 days LOS versus $26,744 and 8.4 days for tPA, excluding physician fees, which would have narrowed the gap somewhat; $p = .04$ for both), as were costs over the first year.[68] These data suggest that the strategy is dominant. Estimated charges per 1 percent of myocardial salvage were similar with both strategies ($2321 for tPA versus $1770 for primary PTCA).[69]

Recently, an even more daring approach of very early discharge after primary PTCA was studied—possible because of a shorter time window for recurrent ischemia than with thrombolysis. In the PAMI-2 study, low-risk patients undergoing emergency catheterization (42.8 percent of the total) with the intent of subsequent PTCA (carried out in 89 percent) were randomized to traditional versus accelerated care (heparin for 60 h, no noninvasive testing, and discharge planned in 3 days, with intructions to return to work in 2 weeks). Average length of stay declined from 7.1 to 4.2 days ($p < .001$), and hospital charges from $20,197 to $16,193 ($p < .0001$). There was no difference in outcome over 6 months, and a very low mortality of 0.4 percent in both groups.[70]

However, in contradistinction to the above studies, an AMI registry in Seattle hospitals[71] showed no difference in 3-year mortality between primary PTCA and thrombolytic treatment patients (74 percent of whom received angiography and 32 percent PTCA). While hospital stay in the primary PTCA group was 1.1 days less (mean 6.8 versus 7.9 days) ($p < .001$), both initial and 3-year hospital costs were about $3000 more and with a higher rate of procedures subsequent to hospitalization.

Thus, while primary PTCA appears to be a cost-effective strategy in randomized trials, at least one outcomes analysis casts doubt on this in routine clinical practice. At present, 18 percent of hospitals have a PTCA capacity with surgical backup,[72] but many can undertake primary PTCA only if the patient arrives during routine laboratory hours. Also, while surgical backup was not required to perform PTCA in the PAMI-2 study, it has been noted that 5 percent of study patients randomly assigned to PTCA had to have emergency CABG.[72] If primary PTCA is, in fact, the preferred strategy overall or in certain subgroups, the cost and affordability of creating an infrastructure for widespread capability, which was not included in the above analyses, should be considered.

LENGTH OF STAY FOR AMI

Until the late 1950s, 6 weeks was the rule for LOS in patients with AMI, then 3 weeks, and, by the 1980s, 7 to 10 days[73] (median 8.1, mean 10.1 days in the author's community-based study).[50] Advances in interventional and pharmacologic therapy have been such that patients can now return home earlier and with patent coronary arteries. This change has increased the ratio of direct to indirect medical costs, with proportionally more money spent on medical care than on "hotel" and other indirect costs, and thus has made management of AMI more cost effective. On the other hand, some caveats have been expressed about the consequences of early discharge in that patient education may be insufficient,[73] anxiety may be high, and some cost shifting to patients or other (albeit less expensive) provider entities such as home care or nursing homes may occur.

LATER TRIAGE AND THE INVASIVE APPROACH

A crucial time in AMI is the triage made after the initial phase, when identification of jeopardized myocardium is an important issue. Approaches include angiography only in those who have had either spontaneous or stress-induced ischemia (demonstrated by ECG and/or thallium; the so-called TIMI-IIB conservative approach)[74] or direct angiography, either immediately after thrombolysis or deferred.

Factors involved in cost effectiveness of these diagnostic tests are similar to those in other situations (Table 103-2). While ECG and the more costly thallium stress tests are initially cheaper than angiography and appear safe in appropriate patients at 3 to 4 days,[75] their predictive value in post-thrombolysis patients has been questioned.[76] Also, if a high proportion of patients go on to angiography in any event, the overall expense of the strategy will be higher than for direct angiography.[77] In addition, after thrombolysis, earlier discharge may be feasible when coronary arteries are made more patent by PTCA, possibly avoiding the continuing incidence of recurrent ischemia and infarction (6 to 7 percent and 1 to 2 percent, respectively after day 4).[78] Immediate angiography post-thrombolysis is favorable for those in whom thrombolysis has failed and may also avoid reocclusions.

Unfortunately, cost data are incomplete. Analyses have shown a slight cost advantage for the conservative versus the deferred invasive strategy and modest[79] or no[80] advantage for deferred versus immediate angiography, all with similar outcomes.[73,81] However, these studies cannot be considered conclusive, their costs are very influenced by study protocols, and in any case they do not generally apply to patients not receiving thrombolytic agents, presently about 60 to 70 percent of AMI patients.[50] Practice patterns in the United States are highly variable in these situations, with a tendency to favor interventional approaches.

Recently, an analysis of angiography after AMI using comprehensive data inputs found that clinical predictors were most helpful in decision-making. Specifically, the following points emerged, among others: (1) With angiography, almost all subgroups had a QALY (i.e., a clinical) benefit; (2) cost effec-

tiveness varied from about $17,000/QALY to >$1,000,000/QALY, depending on age and clinical factors; (3) for the most part, angiography had a more favorable cost effectiveness in those at higher risk except for certain subgroups aged >75 years, where survival was very poor in any case; (4) *prior AMI and inducible myocardial ischemia (strongly positive ECG exercise test or severe post-AMI angina pectoris) were the most influential factors in determining cost effectiveness, and age and left ventricular ejection fraction were also important*; and (5) with inducible ischemia, cost effectiveness was <$50,000/QALY in almost all categories (exceptions tended to be certain older patients with short life expectancies). Without inducible ischemia the converse was also true, though men aged 45 to 74 years with prior MI and ejection fraction >0.50 were exceptions. Here, cost effectiveness was still <$50,000/QALY with direct angiography, whether or not an exercise test was performed.[82]

Thus, clinical factors are useful in determining cost-effective strategies related to post-MI angiography, and, for certain subgroups, direct angiography without preceding stress test is cost effective. It is also important to note that if angiography is performed under any triage scheme, the decision for intervention must be made judiciously and not automatically.

Long-Term Post-MI Strategies

Randomized trials have identified a number of beneficial cost-effective pharmacologic strategies after AMI, including aspirin, beta blockers, ACE inhibitors, and, as indicated above, lipid-lowering therapy.

Long-term beta blockade is highly cost effective. In a U.S. analysis, cost effectiveness of propranolol was <$10,000/YLS in medium- and high-risk situations and $20,200/YLS in those at low risk (assuming gradual decline of effectiveness after the 6-year run of available beta-blocker data; results were similar assuming abrupt decline).[83] In another analysis, over the 3 years of a randomized trial in Sweden, metoprolol was cost-saving and more so when indirects were included.[37]

ACE inhibitors used prophylactically in patients with ejection fraction <40% post-MI are also highly cost effective. Using effectiveness and resource use data from the SAVE trial (see Chap. 47), cost effectiveness of captopril was valued at <$12,000/QALY if a persistent benefit after the 4-year duration of this study was assumed. With a limited poststudy benefit, the drug remained similarly cost effective in all but the youngest (50 year) age group.[84]

The cost effectiveness of aspirin after MI was modeled based on pooled outcome data. It was found to be <$600/YLS in men and cost-saving in women.[85] There are overseas data showing that anticoagulation with coumadin may also be cost effective,[86] but comparison studies with aspirin are needed and are underway. It has been estimated that if an aspirin strategy attained ≥41 percent of the effectiveness of anticoagulants in this situation, its cost effectiveness would still be more favorable.[87]

Rehabilitation after MI

A number of studies have suggested benefits of post-MI rehabilitation programs, but a problem in determining cost effectiveness is that their components are so variable and may be designed for either medical or marketing purposes. Services include not only exercise but also expert advice regarding lifestyle and medications.

A Canadian[88] and a Swedish study[89] suggested that rehabilitation in their health care settings could be cost effective. Of particular interest was the high return to work rate (58.1 percent versus 27.4 percent at 5 years in the Swedish study) ($p < .01$).[89] Because of their components and style, rehabilitation programs in the United States tend to be expensive. Development of "essentials-only" low-cost programs would be of considerable use, probably cost effective, and especially relevant as transition programs after early discharge of AMI patients from hospital.

DIAGNOSTIC STRATEGIES IN CORONARY ARTERY DISEASE

General

Since CAD is so prevalent in the United States and the Western world, its detection is a most important enterprise and consumes considerable resources. Strategies for specific diagnosis of this condition include coronary angiography, considered the "gold standard" test, and a variety of stress tests (see Chap. 45) for which the substantial relevant data are nonrandomized and still only on exercise ECG and thallium.

The cost effectiveness of diagnostic testing depends on its added value in establishing the diagnosis of CAD,[4,90,91] according to the factors listed in Table 103-2. Where CAD is unlikely (e.g., young woman, atypical chest pain, no risk factors), many tests have to be performed to detect one CAD patient, and this patient will benefit only slightly from treatment. Costs are high and ultimately effectiveness is low. Where CAD is highly likely (e.g., 60-year-old man, typical chest pain, three risk factors), the stress test offers little added value and direct angiography is more cost effective. Between these extremes, stress testing has value.

The above principles are demonstrated in two published analyses of stress testing. In one, stress testing as screening for asymptomatic individuals without risk factors was decidedly not cost effective, except possibly in 60-year-old men. Here, cost effectiveness was $38,100/YLS and was more favorable with a strategy beginning with an ECG and followed by thallium testing. It also improved somewhat if the test was confined to individuals with at least one risk factor (increased pretest probability of CAD), or if a 2-mm cutoff was used (more specificity).[92]

Figure 103-4 shows another intensive analysis. It was based on a literature review of nonrandomized data and, though some of its inputs are unclear, offers a framework for thinking. Four strategies were analyzed, and in ascending order of their predictive accuracy and cost (see legend for Fig. 103-4) they

are: exercise ECG, thallium single-photon emission tomography, positron emission tomography (each leading to angiography next if positive), and direct angiography. Figure 103-4A shows that as pretest probability of CAD rises, more patients will go on to further testing and there will be more expense, except in the case of angiography, which is the "final" test. On the other hand, as pretest probability of CAD rises, cost per CAD diagnosis and cost per QALY fall (Figs. 103-4B and C), i.e., there is more detection of CAD and thus more appropriate therapy. Note also that the cost utility of primary angiography crosses over to a more favorable zone versus the other tests beginning with the least predictively accurate: about 20 percent pretest probability of CAD for ECG alone, 35 percent for exercise thallium, and 55 percent for positron emission tomography. Also, at least in this analysis, thallium remains more cost effective than ECG testing over the range of probability of CAD.[91] Other data on this issue are various,[91-93] and ECG testing may be more favorable as the initial step at low probability of CAD (possibly when leading to thallium next).[92] Positron emission tomography was the most favorable noninvasive test, but more data here would be helpful as this test is not in widespread use. Another factor is the consequences of misdiagnosis. At less test sensitivity and higher pretest probability of CAD, more patients with CAD will be missed and mortality greater (Fig. 103-4D).

Thus, based on clinical models, stress testing to diagnose CAD is cost effective in appropriate patients, and choice of test versus direct angiography depends on clinical evaluation of risk. Models incorporating both risk and niceties of interpretation may be helpful here. One should also note that the cost effectiveness of other stress test uses, such as for evaluation of prognosis in established CAD or of significance of an angiographically detected coronary artery lesion, has not been determined.

Preoperative Testing

One focused use of CAD testing is in preoperative evaluation of asymptomatic patients for noncardiac surgery. Approaches vary considerably and can be expensive.[94] Neither direct angiography[95] nor dipyridamole stress testing[96] prior to vascular surgery was cost effective when used broadly (nonrandomized data), nor is it clear whether they would be in patients with increased clinical risk. The unfavorable cost effectiveness of these strategies is in part due to the mortality and morbidity of PTCA and CABG relative to that of the vascular surgery,[95] for which mortality has decreased.[97]

INTERVENTIONAL CARDIOLOGY AND SURGERY

Cardiac Catheterization

Over the years, cardiac catheterization in the uncomplicated patient has become an efficient procedure requiring only a short outpatient stay.[98,99] One cost issue is the use of nonionic, low-osmolarity contrast material at 10 to 20 times the price of the ionic alternative used in catheterization laboratories for many years. Estimates are that nonionic agents cost about $2196 per avoidance of (generally mild) adverse effects if given to all patients, $1444 if given only to patients >60 years old or with unstable angina, and $7557 if given to the others.[100] It has been suggested that these agents be used only in high-risk patients.[100]

Percutaneous Transluminal Coronary Angioplasty

CONVENTIONAL PTCA

Cost Effectiveness
At the time of this writing, the only formal cost-effectiveness analysis on PTCA was based on a literature review of nonrandomized studies. Here, PTCA was generally cost effective in

patients with severe angina pectoris and one- to three-vessel disease, at <$20,000/QALY compared to medical therapy (in 55-year-old men with type A lesions). In mild angina pectoris, because impact on quality of life was less, cost per QALY was usually >$100,000, though it improved with a positive prescreening stress test. As lesions became technically more difficult (type C), cost effectiveness also became less favorable.[101] In the next few years, further cost-effectiveness data should emerge from some of the large randomized trials (see Chap. 48).

Cost Reduction
Costs of PTCA include not only those related to the initial procedure, such as catheters and surgical standby, but also those due to failures, complications, and, most importantly, obligatory repeat procedures for restenosis. Substantial variation exists in these costs, attributed to clinical markers,

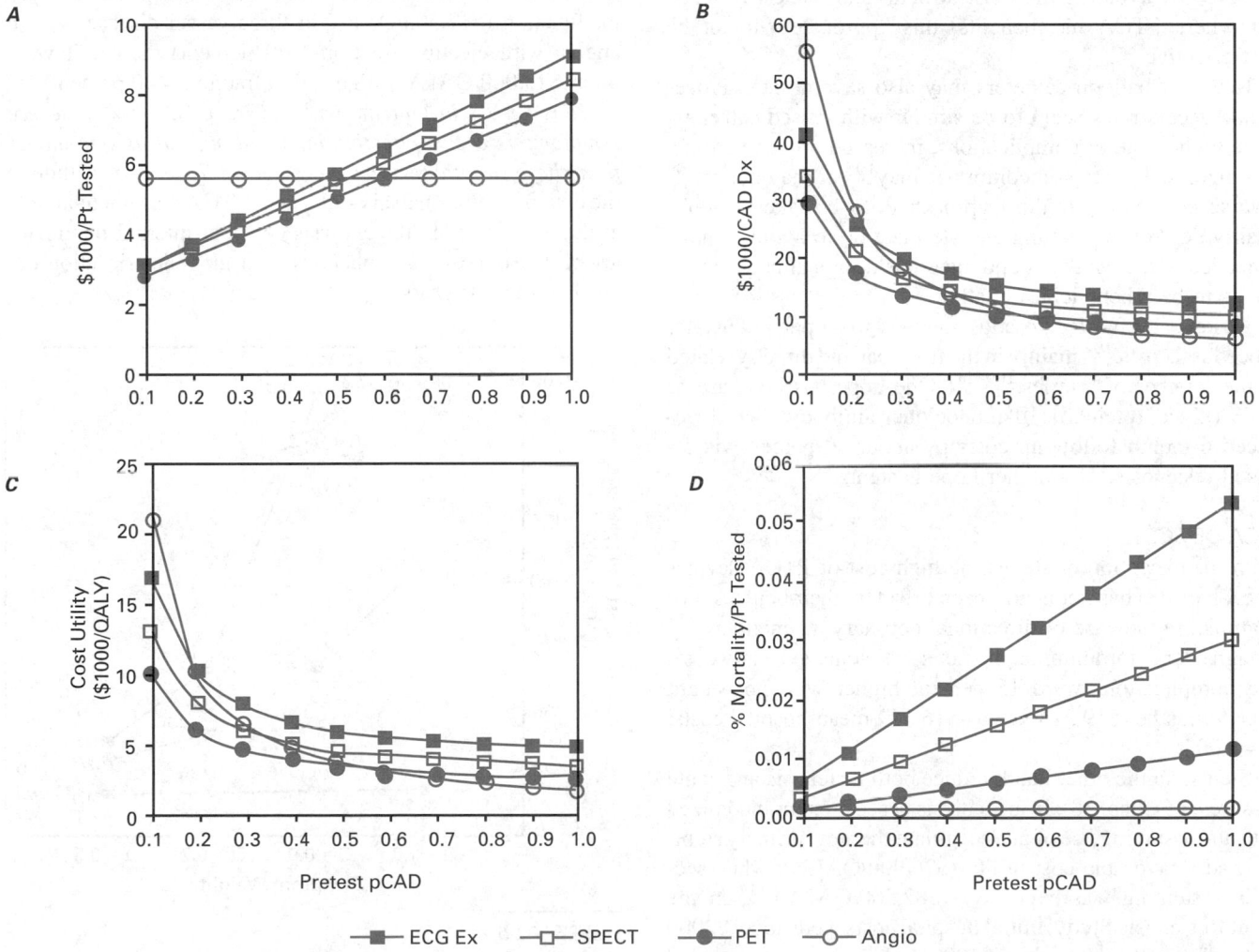

FIGURE 103-4

Costs, cost effectiveness, and mortality for potential coronary artery disease (CAD) patients examined by exercise ECG (assumed cost $330, sensitivity 0.68, specificity, 0.77), thallium single-photon emission tomography (SPECT) ($1,200, 0.84, 0.87), positron emission tomography (PET) ($1,800, 0.95, 0.95), and coronary angiography ($4,800, 1.0, 1.0). Clinical algorithm to approach diagnostic testing was stress test first, followed by angiography if positive. *A.* Cost per patient tested. *B.* Costs per CAD diagnosis. *C.* Cost per quality-adjusted life years (QALY). *D.* Mortality per patient tested. See text for further discussion. pCAD, pretest probability of CAD. (From Patterson et al.[91] Reproduced with permission of the publisher and authors.)

complications, hospital factors, and, at times, physician operator.[11,15,102] Also, private insurance charges were found to be lower in the northeast, in hospitals with training programs, and when preceding exercise tests were performed.[103]

These variations suggest that guidelines, case management, and operational efficiencies are likely to be useful cost-reduction methods.[14] For the most part, hospitals are now efficient, with <2 h of total laboratory time for PTCA and overnight stays in uncomplicated patients. Due to revised scheduling, the cost of surgical standby has fallen from over $1700 in the early 1980s[104] to less than $100. Moving from a two- to a one-stage angiogram/PTCA procedure saves fluoroscopy time, contrast media dose, and total procedure time (94 versus 150 min) ($p < .001$); LOS (8.0 to 5.6 days); and about 18 percent in total charges.[105] Perhaps 5 to 10 percent of patients are not candidates, however, because of the need to review complex anatomy or contrast media limits. Dollars might also be saved by avoiding the most difficult and riskiest patients, but where PTCA has benefits, this approach will not be cost effective.

Reuse of balloon catheters may also save dollars. Procedural success rates seem to be similar with reused catheters, but a higher rate of complications, increased procedure time, and increased contrast medium use may[106] or may not[107,108] reverse cost gains. If this approach is to be taken, careful quality control in cleaning and sterilization to avoid damage is needed. Future catheter and materials design aimed at reuse seems to be a beneficial initiative.

Restenosis after PTCA adds about 35 to 45 percent in later procedural costs,[102] mainly in the first year and directly related to the number of arteries.[109–111] One hope has been use of c7E3 (glycoprotein IIb/III monoclonal antibody), which reduced 6-month follow-up costs by about 30 percent via reduced restenosis.[112] Another hope is stents.

PTCA DEVICES

With the exception of stents, the high cost of PTCA devices (see Chap. 48) has not nearly been offset by their benefits. For example, in the case of directional coronary atherectomy,[113] though a large intraluminal diameter was achieved, early costs and complications were 15 percent higher with no benefit over 6 months ($19,214 versus $16,769 mean hospital costs; $p = .004$).

Stents, on the other hand, reduce both restenosis and acute closure (see Chap. 48). In an analysis based on nonrandomized data and assuming use of anticoagulant therapy, primary stenting had a favorable cost utility ($26,900/QALY), while secondary stenting was expensive ($82,500/QALY).[114] In the Stent Restenosis Study, initial hospital costs were about $2000 higher but fell to less than $1000 at 1 year due to reduced subsequent procedures and hospitalization.[115]

Beyond this, however, cost effectiveness of stents is enhanced by the fact that antiplatelet therapy with ticlopidine plus aspirin, rather than coumadin anticoagulation, will suffice. This capability reduces initial complication cost and LOS

(by >$4000 in procedural and nonprocedural costs and by 2.3 days in LOS in one retrospective analysis)[116] and perhaps will allow next-day discharge.[117]

Coronary Artery Bypass Graft Surgery

COST EFFECTIVENESS

In an early formal analysis based on both randomized and nonrandomized effectiveness data, cost utility depended on the severity of both angina pectoris and CAD (Fig. 103-5). The procedure was cost effective in all instances of left main and three-vessel coronary artery disease (<$20,000/QALY; male, age 55 years; ejection fraction $\geq$ 40 percent) and at all levels of CAD severity when symptoms were very severe (<$45,000/QALY when Q (quality adjustment factor) = 0.5; see Fig. 103-5). It was not cost effective in one- or two-vessel disease with a lesser severity of angina pectoris, where numbers could rise above $1 million/QALY. Cost utility was also somewhat more favorable with good ventricular function ($17,500/QALY in three-vessel disease, severe angina with ejection fraction >40 percent) than if it were poor ($25,000/QALY with ejection fraction <40 percent).[118]

Thus CABG in patients with severe CAD or with severe symptoms is a cost-effective intervention, but as one moves from these situations, it becomes decidedly less so. Although the data from this analysis still stand, PTCA was not available at that time, nor did the analysis consider internal mammary artery anastamosis or saphenous vein graft deterioration occurring after 10 years.

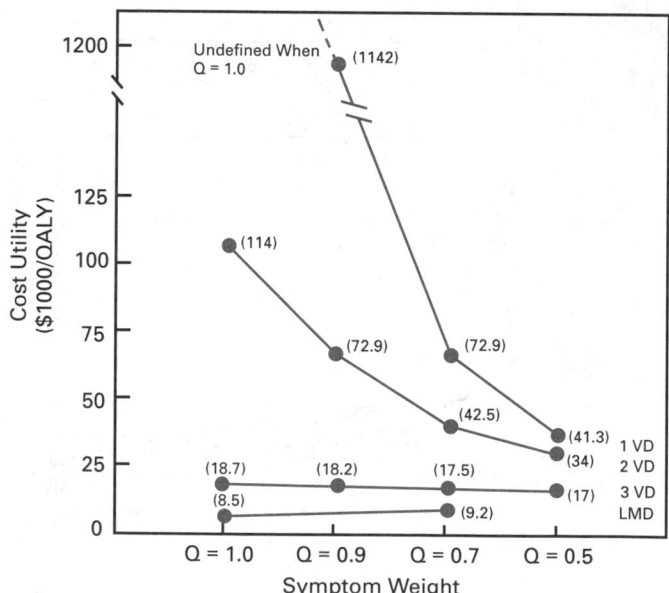

FIGURE 103-5

Cost utility of coronary artery bypass graft surgery in 1-, 2-, and 3-vessel disease (VD) and left main disease (LMD). Q (quality adjustment factor) = 1.0, no angina or concern over pain; Q = 0.9, mild angina, sedentary life style; Q = 0.7, severe angina, active life style; Q = 0.5, very severe angina or serious psychological effect. Numbers in parentheses show cost utilities ($1000/QALY). (From Kupersmith et al.[4]; adapted from Weinstein and Stason.[118] Reproduced with permission of the publishers and authors.)

COST REDUCTION

As with PTCA, considerable variation in hospital costs and charges for CABG occurs within[12] and between institutions, e.g., almost threefold among six Illinois hospitals.[119] These variations are in part explicable by complications, case mix,[12,119,120] and individual surgeons' practice styles, even when surgical outcomes were similar.[12]

Cost savings can be achieved by case management approaches to address different patterns of care[121] (e.g., reduction of LOS from 7.4 to 5.8 days in one retrospective analysis; $p < .05$).[122] Minimizing complications, in part based on good case selection, is also an obvious goal and will be helped by guidelines if they are adhered to. Minimally invasive CABG (see Chap. 50) is also expected to be less expensive, but at the time of this writing, cost data are not yet available for the procedure in routine use. One increasingly popular procedure, autologous donation of blood, while rather inexpensive, is also not terribly cost effective (over $500,000/QALY depending on number of units,[123] somewhat less at centers with high numbers of transfusions).

PTCA versus CABG

The initial PTCA procedure is about two-thirds the cost of CABG (including physician fees),[102] but the gap narrows to about 80 to 90 percent over the next 1 to 3 years, due mainly to post-PTCA restenosis in the first year.[4,71,102,124–126] (Disparity is greater using charges because of CABG's higher charge/cost ratio.) The number of vessels treated is important. For PTCA, follow-up costs rise stepwise with the number of vessels reperfused, due to greater likelihood of restenosis, while they remain similar for CABG. Thus, the long-term cost gap between procedures is virtually abolished in three-vessel disease.[109,127,128] Studies extending beyond 10 years, however, may be less favorable to CABG because of saphenous vein graft deterioration.

Return to work following interventions is an important economic factor, which in the past was disappointing after CABG and variable after PTCA. Work status appears to be related more to preceding functional status and disability benefits than to clinical or angiographic findings. In a recent cohort analysis of patients following cardiac catheterization and adjusted for baseline factors, 84 percent of PTCA patients, 80 percent of CABG patients, and 79 percent of medical therapy patients returned to work after 1 year. Because of a 1- to 2-month earlier return of PTCA patients, however, estimated dollar value of the lost work was $3024 for PTCA, $7509 for CABG, and $5064 for medical therapy.[129]

Conclusions

Based on data available now, both CABG and PTCA appear to be cost-effective interventions when, and only when, used narrowly and efficiently for currently accepted indications. Further refinements of our knowledge on precise case selection, costs, and outcomes will be of value in selecting these interventions versus what at least nonrandomized comparisons have shown to be less-expensive medical strategies.[109,130]

CONGESTIVE HEART FAILURE

Scope

Congestive heart failure (CHF) is a very costly condition. In 1991, Medicare DRGs related to CHF cost $5.45 billion, or 4.8 percent of the total DRG budget (as against $2.2 billion for cancer and $3.2 billion for AMI). In the private sector, an estimated $38.1 billion, or 5.4 percent of all private health care expenditures, was spent on CHF, with hospitalizations ($23.1 billion) the major cost.[131] Efforts to reduce hospital costs using drug therapy and case management strategies are therefore highly worthwhile.

Pharmacotherapy

Digoxin, ACE inhibitors, and the hydralazine-isosorbide combination are all highly cost effective in CHF.[132–134] In data modeled from the RADIANCE and PROVED withdrawal trials, digoxin, which is inexpensive, reduced hospitalization in mild to moderate CHF and was cost-saving. It remained so in patients taking ACE inhibitors and even with very generous assumptions regarding the incidence of digitalis toxicity.[133]

Based on data from the SOLVD and VHeFT trials (see Chap. 23), with U.S. costs modeled, hydralazine-isosorbide versus standard treatment (digoxin and diuretics) cost $5900/YLS for patients with class II to IV CHF, while enalapril at 20 mg/day versus hydralazine-isosorbide was $10,300/YLS.[132] Regarding patient targeting, in the Munich Mild Heart Failure trial, ACE inhibition with captopril was much more cost effective in the more risky and expensive progressive CHF patients than in the stable group.[135] ACE inhibitors also reduce hospitalizations in patients with asymptomatic left ventricular dysfunction,[136] but analyses here would also have to consider detection costs.

Among other drugs, prazosin and milrinone do not reduce hospitalizations; prazosin, in fact, increases them. Home intravenous therapy with amrinone[137] or dobutamine may save hospital days, but there are no reliable data on their overall cost effectiveness.

Case Management

CHF patients are prone to repeat emergency room visits and long stays, often related to medication noncompliance and lack of programs designed to increase activity capabilities. Case management strategies are, therefore, useful. One program consisting of comprehensive, nurse-directed education of patient and family, a prescribed diet, social service consultations, planning for early discharge, review of medicines, and intensive follow-up for 90 days in hospitalized CHF patients ≥70 years old at high risk for readmission was the subject of a randomized outcomes and cost trial. Patients selected were considered to be at high risk for readmission. Reduction in CHF readmissions was as great as that achieved in ACE inhibitor studies (Fig. 103-6), and the savings over 90 days were $460 out of total costs of $5275. Quality-of-life measures and patient knowledge of CHF also improved, and there was a trend toward decreasing non-CHF admissions. Benefit appeared to hold over 1 year.[138] Thus, highly favorable results can be gained by such a program, although its application beyond this high readmission risk and presumably cooperative group would be more expensive.

Cardiac Transplantation

Although the cost of individual heart transplants is high, it represents a rather small proportion of total CHF cost, about $270 million.[131] Transplant costs are about $10,000 to $25,000, preadmission; $100,000 to $150,000 for hospital admission (but can exceed $1 million in outliers, especially in inefficient centers); and $7000 to $15,000 per year subsequently.[139] In a very preliminary analysis, overall cost effectiveness of heart transplant was estimated at $44,300/YLS.[140] One-third to one-half of the 60 percent of patients who can return to work do so.[141]

Cost-saving strategies for heart transplant include good case selection so that hearts will not be wasted and disastrous expensive cases avoided; intensive case management; avoidance of "gaming," to position patients better on lists; use of ketoconazole[142] or, to a lesser extent, diltiazem to decrease the dose and costs of cyclosporine; echocardiographic rather than fluoroscopically guided biopsies,[141] and management by experienced cardiologists.

ARRHYTHMIAS

Diagnostic Testing

Effective arrhythmia diagnosis and management can be expensive, and third party payers have raised questions as to the extent to which sophisticated testing and devices should

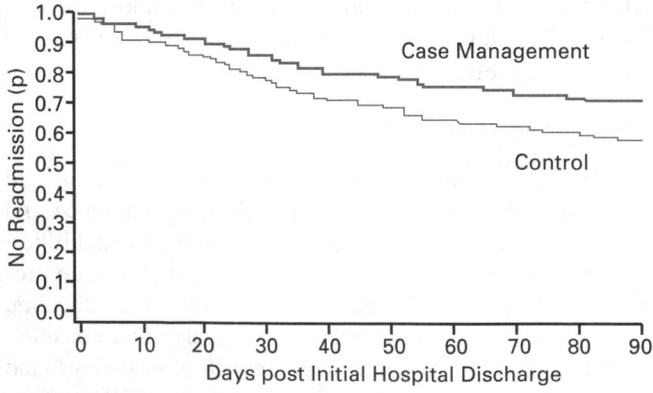

FIGURE 103-6

Effect of case management strategy on hospital readmission in congestive heart failure patients at high risk for readmission ($p = .035$ versus control). (From Rich et al.[138] Reproduced with permission of the publisher and authors.)

be reimbursed. Initial evaluation of patients with arrhythmias has been by hospital or ambulatory ECG monitoring or electrophysiologic testing as a prelude to antiarrhythmic drugs or interventional therapy, including radiofrequency ablation (RFA), implantable cardioverter-defibrillators (ICDs), or arrhythmia surgery (see Chap. 27). These diagnostic technologies are costly and in the past have been used inefficiently, with long hospital stays especially for drug testing, followed by numerous outpatient ambulatory ECGs. One must also consider, however, that a delicate balance exists between efficiency and safety in high-risk situations where there is a need for careful in-hospital observation, especially since antiarrhythmic drugs have proarrhythmic potential.

In the case of electrophysiologic testing, cost-conscious streamlining has considerably reduced LOS (see also Chap. 29). Measures include limits on the number of drug trials; close coordination with planned subsequent interventions, e.g., RFA (see Chap. 31); and general case management. In addition, outpatient electrophysiologic testing saves as much as 23 percent of charges ($8493 versus $3081; $p <$ .001),[143,144] but it should be reserved for low-risk patients, i.e., generally those with atrial arrhythmias, and since patients destined for certain procedures will also be excluded, this approach has less applicability.

To determine the need for electrophysiologic testing in selecting drug therapy, the ESVEM study compared it to ambulatory ECG monitoring in patients with frequent ventricular premature complexes plus ventricular tachycardia. Hospital charges and LOS were significantly higher in the electrophysiologic testing group (means, $47,794 versus $34,103, $p = .0015$, and 19.6 versus 13.9 days, respectively, $p = .0007$). A large factor in this difference was the greater efficiency of ambulatory ECG monitoring in finding an effective antiarrhythmic drug. Charges were more clustered around patients achieving (mean about $24,000) or not achieving (about $59,100) an efficacy prediction, whether randomized to electrophysiologic or ambulatory ECG monitoring. Charges were also higher in CHF (26 percent) and cardiac arrest screening (28 percent) patients.[145] In a previous trial, initial results were similar to ESVEM, but hospital costs equilibrated over 2 years.[146] Although ESVEM patients represent a small proportion of those with ventricular arrhythmias, the most useful observation is perhaps that efficiency in finding a treatment is the important cost-effectiveness issue.

Regarding ambulatory ECG monitoring, one analysis of relatively high-risk patients has shown that 24-h monitoring is relatively inefficient for detection and management of arrhythmias.[147] Here, management decisions were made in only 18 percent of patients, at $3384 per decision, with 5.4 ambulatory ECGs required per decision. Specifically, numbers were reasonable in two categories: (1) for dizziness/lightheadedness plus cardiac symptoms, $1925 per decision and 3.5 ambulatory ECGs per resulting clinical decision, and (2) for palpitations, $2816 and 4.5, respectively. The numbers were worse in others as follows: For detection of arrhythmias in patients with any suggestive symptoms, $9638 and 15.4, in patients with cerebrovascular accidents to detect previously unknown atrial fibrillation, $15,803 and 25.0, for determination that the patient has symptoms without arrhythmia, $15,357 and 24.5, and for detection of potentially significant arrhythmia, $17,361 and 27.7, where the numbers are cost per decision and number of ambulatory ECGs per decision, respectively. Another use, evaluation of established antiarrhythmic therapy, is clouded by this questionable value of a negative 24- or 48-h monitor in the situation (see Chap. 28). A similar low yield for ambulatory ECG was found earlier[148] although results will depend on the case mix of the population tested (Table 103-2).

Patient- or arrhythmia-activated event monitors, worn for several weeks, appear to be a more cost-effective approach and in one crossover study dominated over 48-h ambulatory ECGs (cost savings of $169 per additional diagnostic ECG detected during symptoms and $296 for clinically significant arrhythmias detected). Many patients, however, were not eligible for such a device.[149]

Implantable Cardioverter-Defibrillators

The ICD is an expensive (about $27,000) but also cost-effective device.[4] In three separate analyses using nonrandomized data, the epicardial (epi) ICD was cost effective at <$50,000/YLS when compared to electrophysiologically guided drug therapy or empirical amiodarone.[150–152] Cost effectiveness improved with longer battery life ($29,400/YLS assuming 3 years versus $18,700/YLS assuming 8 years).[152] It was, however, less favorable in patients when ejection fraction was lower ($44,000/YLS for ejection fractions <.25 versus $27,200/YLS for those ≥.25) due to a very high nonarrhythmic mortality.[150]

The endocardial (endo) ICD is more economical and is associated with a postimplant LOS of 3.1 days (including very little intensive care unit time) versus 7.2 days with the epi ICD. Initial hospital charges are about 25 to 30 percent less than with the epi device[153] but can probably decline further with case management strategies. In one model, cost effectiveness with efficient ICD implantation was $15,000/YLS.[150]

An interesting randomized trial of 60 patients compared the strategy of directly implanting (mainly epi) ICDs without performing a preceding electrophysiologic test to that of electrophysiologically guided therapy in post-AMI cardiac arrest survivors. Median cost effectiveness

in the ICD group was $66/patient per day alive versus $99/patient per day alive in the latter group. Costs in the latter group were initially lower but were overtaken at 2 to 3 months by frequent crossovers to ICD and arrhythmia surgery because of drug treatment failures (Fig. 103-7). Overall, the ICD was dominant, saving an estimated $12,000/YLS.[154] In an analysis at the author's institution, the model of direct ICD implant without preceding electrophysiologic testing was also a favored approach.[150]

It is important to note that ICD cost effectiveness is very much influenced by the presumed effectiveness coefficient, i.e., YLS gained using the device.[155] Thus, the ICD appears to be cost-effective[150–152] especially with primary implantation.[154] It is important to note that the device's cost effectiveness is very much influenced by the presumed effectiveness coefficient, i.e., YLS using the device,[155] and a number of studies have been and are under way to address this issue. Thus far, AVID, comparing the ICD with sotalol or amiodarone and MADIT, a prophylactic study in post-MI patients, had favorable results.

Radiofrequency Ablation

Since RFA can effect a cure for supraventricular arrhythmias, it is a desirable form of therapy and, *in the long run*, cost effective. Compared to surgery for either accessory pathways or AV nodal reentrant tachycardia, RFA is effective, less expensive,[156] and less bothersome, has fewer complications, and is therefore now preferred. Compared with medical therapy, the situation is more complex. In the Wolff-Parkinson-White syndrome, a formal cost utility analysis using nonrandomized data found that RFA dominated over other strategies

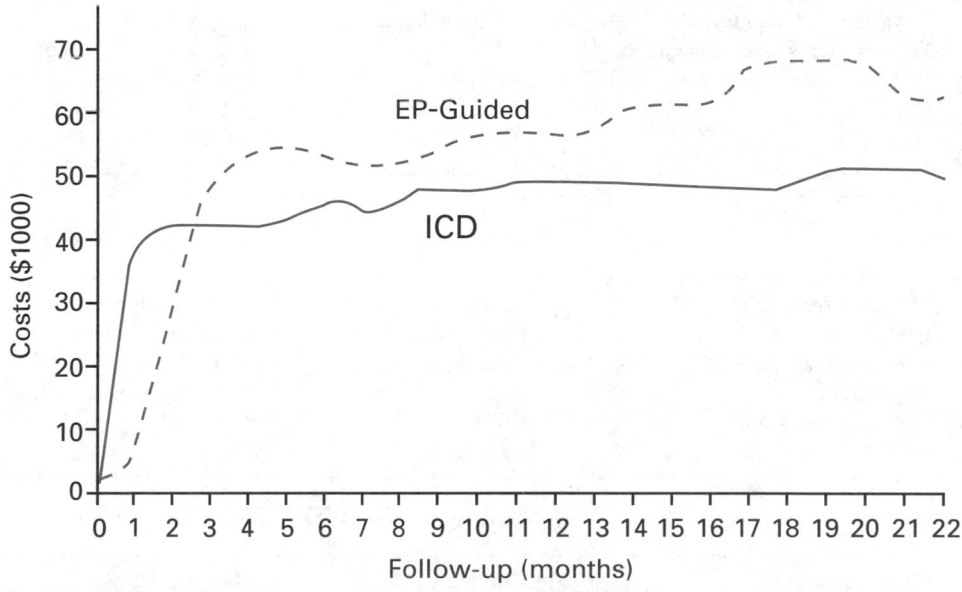

FIGURE 103-7

Medians of total cost per patient at monthly intervals for survivors of the direct implantable cardioverter-defibrillator (ICD) (solid line) and electrophysiologically (EP) guided (dashed line) strategies. Dips in the curves are due to deaths of patients with high costs. Costs of EP-guided therapy overtake those of direct ICD at 2 to 3 months. (From Wever et al.[154] Reproduced with permission of the publisher and authors.)

TABLE 103-3

COST EFFECTIVENESS OF HEART DISEASE STRATEGIES[a]

Strategy	Condition	Patient Targeting	$/YLS $/QALY
Highly Cost Effective (<$20,000/YLS or QALY)			
Anticoagulant[47]	AF	Nonvalvular disease, high/moderate risk, age 65	Dominant[b]
Digoxin[133]	CHF	Mild to moderate	Dominant[b]
ICD, no EP[154c]	VT/VF		Dominant[b]
Aspirin[85]	Post-MI	♀	Dominant[b]
Lovastatin, 20 mg/day[21d]	Hyperlipidemia	2°, chol ≥ 250 mg/dL, ♂, ages 45–54	Dominant[b]
Radiofrequency ablation[157]	WPW	PSVT/AF, hemodynamic compromise	Dominant[b]
Physician advice/nicotine gum[26]	Smoking	♂, age 50–54	1300
Beta blocker[83]	Post-MI	High risk	3600
Anticoagulant[46]	Mitral stenosis	AF, ♀, age 35	4200
Lovastatin, 20 mg/day[21d]	Hyperlipidemia	2°, chol ≥ 250 mg/dL, ♀, ages 45–54	4700
CABG surgery[118]	Chronic CAD	Severe angina, left main disease[e]	9200
Captopril[84]	Post-MI	EF ≤ .40, age 60	10,200
Enalapril, 20 mg/day[132f]	CHF		10,300
Anticoagulant[47g]	AF	Nonvalvular disease, low risk, age 65	14,000
Endocardial ICD with EP[150c]	VT/VF		15,000
Estrogen (10 years)[31]	Postmenopausal, ♀	Age 50 years, no uterus	15,600
CABG surgery[118]	Chronic CAD	Mild angina, 3 VD[e]	18,200
Angiogram[82]	AMI	♀, age 55–64 ET⁺, EF ≥ .50, prior MI[h]	18,500
Cost Effective ($20,000–$40,000/YLS or QALY)			
Beta blocker[83]	Post-MI	Low risk	20,200
CCU[52]	Possible AMI	pAMI = .77, age 55–64	20,200
Lovastatin, 20 mg/day[21d]	Hyperlipidemia	1°, chol ≥ 300 mg/dL, 3 RF, ♀, ages 55–64	20,200
Common regimen[33]	Hypertension	Diast ≥ 105 mmHg	20,600
Exercise[32]	Prophylaxis	♂, 35 year old	22,400
Lovastatin, 20 mg/day[21d]	Hyperlipidemia	2°, chol < 250 mg/dL, ♂, ages 55–64	22,900
Primary stents w/anticoagulation[114]	CAD	Angina, 1 VD, ♂, age 55	26,800
Streptokinase[64]	AMI	Age ≥ 75	27,700
Oat bran[20]	Hyperlipidemia	LRC-CPPT Pt[h], Chol ≥ 265 mg/dL	31,600
Angiogram[82]	AMI	♂, age 55–64, ET⁻, EF ≥ .50, prior MI	35,400
ECG exercise testing[92]	Asymptomatic	♂, age 60, ≥ 1 RF	37,700
Borderline (>$40,000–$60,000/YLS or QALY)			
Common regimen[33]	Hypertension	Diast 95–104 mmHg	41,900
CABG surgery[118]	Chronic CAD	Severe angina, 2 VD[e]	42,500
Lovastatin, 20 mg/day[21]	Hyperlipidemia	2°, chol < 250 mg/dL, ♀, ages 55–64	48,600
Angiogram[82]	AMI	♀, ages 55–64, ET⁻, EF ≥ .50, prior MI	52,500
Radiofrequency ablation[157]	WPW	Asymptomatic, age 40	57,100
CCU[52]	Possible AMI	pAMI = .28, age 55–64	58,700
Expensive (>$60,000–$100,000/YLS or QALY)			
CABG surgery[118]	Chronic CAD	Mild angina, 2 VD[e]	72,900
Angiogram[82]	AMI	♂, age 55–64, ET⁻, EF ≥ .50, no prior MI	78,300
Lovastatin, 20 mg/day[21]	Hyperlipidemia	1°, chol ≥ 300 mg/dL, no RF, ♂, ages 55–64	78,300

(Continued)

TABLE 103-3

COST EFFECTIVENESS OF HEART DISEASE STRATEGIES[a] (Continued)

Strategy	Condition	Patient Targeting	$/YLS $/QALY
		Very Expensive (>$100,000/YLS or QALY)	
Cholestyramine—bulk drug[20]	Hyperlipidemia	LRC-CPPT Pt[i], chol ≥ 265 mg/dL	115,500
ECG exercise testing[92]	Asymptomatic	♂, age 40	124,400
Lovastatin, 20 mg/day[21]	Hyperlipidemia	1°, chol ≥ 300 mg/dL, no RF, ♂, ages 45–54	148,500
Anticoagulant[46]	Mitral stenosis	NSR, ♀, age 35	174,100
CABG surgery[118]	Chronic CAD	Mild angina, 1 VD[e]	1,142,000
CCU[52]	Possible AMI	pAMI = .02, age 45–54	1,147,400
Lovastatin, 20 mg/day[21]	Hyperlipidemia	1°, chol ≥ 300 mg/dL, no RF, ♀, ages 35–44	2,024,800
Drug therapy[157]	WPW	Asymptomatic, age 60	6,042,000

[a] Representative list of formal analyses. Note certain qualifications in evaluating comparisons made in this table: analyses are expressed in both $/YLS and $/QALY, and these may not be strictly comparable; omitted are those in $/LS or other units. Analyses are from societal perspective and make use of varied types of assumptions and of data (randomized, nonrandomized, literature reviews, costs, charges, use of physician fees, etc.) as indicated in the text. Data inputs may not be applicable to one's local situation. Cost effectiveness is dependent on competing strategy selected. All earlier values updated to 1993$, but inflation corrections may be oversimplifications.[4,16] Categorization of values as "cost effective" or otherwise depends on dollar year.

[b] Saves both money and lives or QALYs.

[c] Versus EP-guided therapy. ICD without EP findings are from different analyses[150,154] with the former modeling a streamlined admission. See text.

[d] See also Fig. 103-2 for recent randomized data on simvastatin in 2° prevention.[24]

[e] Analysis was versus medical therapy of 55-year-old, EF ≥ .40.

[f] Versus hydralazine-isosorbide.

[g] However, versus aspirin cost effectiveness is >$350,000/QALY. See text.

[h] Plus mild post-AMI angina pectoris. For (♂) in the category 17,600.

[i] LRC-CPPT patients were men (avg. age 48 years), 38% smokers, cholesterol ≥ 265 mg/dL, LDL ≥ 190 mg/dL.

Abbreviations: 1°, primary prevention; 2°, secondary prevention; AF, atrial fibrillation; CABG, coronary artery bypass graft; CAD, coronary artery disease; CCU, coronary care unit; CHF, congestive heart failure; chol, pretreatment cholesterol; Diast, diastolic blood pressure; ECG, electrocardiogram; EF, ejection fraction; EP, electrophysiologic testing; ET⁺/ET⁻, strongly positive/negative ECG exercise test (>2 mm ST↓); ICD, implantable cardioverter-defibrillator; LAD, left anterior descending coronary artery; LRC-CPPT, Lipid Research Clinics Coronary Primary Prevention Trial; MI, myocardial infarction; NSR, normal sinus rhythm; NYHA, New York Heart Association; p, probability; PSVT, tachycardia; RF, other risk factors; VD, vessel disease; VT/VF, ventricular tachycardia/fibrillation; WPW, Wolff-Parkinson-White syndrome.

Source: Adapted from Kupersmith, et al.[4] Reproduced with permission of the publisher and authors.

for patients with cardiac arrest or those with hemodynamic compromise. In patients with arrhythmias but without hemodynamic compromise, it was still highly cost effective ($7,300, $10,900, and $20,900 per QALY at 20, 40, and 60 years of age, respectively). It was generally not cost effective in asymptomatic individuals, however, except perhaps, in the young (aged 20 years).[157]

In the case of AV nodal reentrant tachycardia, which rarely causes mortality, the trade-off in RFA is a high up-front cost to effect a cure, with little or no subsequent expense. Thus, continuing drug therapy will eventually catch up and overtake the cost of RFA.[156,158,159] In one retrospective review of patients with a successful RFA and high resource use (4.5 episodes of tachycardia/month), catch-up was in 2 years, i.e., $18,085 initial and no subsequent charges versus $8706/year on drugs. Absenteeism from work also declined from 13 days/ year to zero. Catch-up in hypothetical patients with low resource utilization (one emergency room visit per year) was at about 10 years.[158] Missing from this analysis, however, were RFA failures (up to 11 percent)[159,160] and AV block (about 4.7 percent in early use),[160,161] both of which would be responsible for continuing post-RFA costs for some patients.

Thus, in patients with AV nodal tachycardia and frequent resource use, RFA is associated with lower costs than drugs and, by reversing tachycardia episodes, probably a better quality of life, the important effectiveness measure in the absence of mortality improvement. On the other hand, for patients with infrequent episodes of tachycardia and low resource utilization, the procedure is costly. For all indications, minimizing complications and performing the procedure close to the electrophysiologic study to reduce hospital costs and improve efficiency are helpful.

Pacemakers

Since their inception in the late 1950s, pacemakers have become highly technologically sophisticated and extended their use from the original indication of complete heart block to sick sinus syndrome and tachycardias. Cost-effectiveness data are scant, but overuse in general and use of excessive technological sophistication in particular[162] are important cost issues. For example, dual-chamber pacemakers are more expensive and shorter lived.

Scrutiny and peer review of pacemaker implants to reduce

cost is a long-standing tradition. The workings of these programs have been questioned, however, and they may have had little impact.[163,164] There are also guidelines with staged indications promulgated by major societies,[165] but, at least in the U.K., they did not reduce (and may have increased) the implant of expensive sophisticated devices.[166] More efficient hospital stays and moving implantation from the operating room to the cardiac catheterization laboratory[167] have reduced costs. Same-day implantation and recycling of devices have also been advised[168] but are not now in common practice.

Overall, although there are currently no data, pacemakers are undoubtedly cost effective in complete heart block but probably less so in other indications. Regarding technological sophistication, there is evidence from Medicare databases that dual-chamber pacemakers are an independent predictor of survival,[169] although trials are needed. In any case, if either the device or specific aspects of its expensive technological accoutrements provide a better quality of life for certain patients, cost effectiveness of focused, appropriate use will be favorable.

COST-EFFECTIVENESS COMPARISONS

Table 103-3 is a "league table" comparing the cost effectiveness of a number of cardiac treatment strategies grouped by expense ranges in 1993 dollars (issues related to league tables are discussed in reference 4). Included are only those where a formal cost-effectiveness analysis in cost per YLS or cost per QALY was performed. The table makes several instructive points. First, no type of strategy is favored. Preventive, pharmacologic, and interventional treatment strategies are interspersed along the entire scale, and the cost effectiveness of any intervention would be difficult to predict without data.[4] There are important differences in timing: interventional treatments have high up-front costs and immediate benefits, while preventive treatments have continuous costs and later benefits. *Note also that patient targeting, based in large part on identification of risk, is highly important for any intervention, as especially exemplified by lipid-lowering therapy, which appears at both the most and least favorable cost effectiveness ends.*

On the other hand, neither the relative position on the list nor the absolute cost effectiveness number is fixed; all are potentially mobile. Many strategies can be made more cost effective by the physician- and administrator-driven efficiencies noted in this chapter. In addition, a more competitive marketplace will be a major factor. For example, it is hoped that drug pricing will be influenced by cost-effectiveness data as well as by the competitive factors noted earlier. Programs for prevention have and will continue to become more refined, efficient, and effective. High-tech interventions are helped by diminished hospital LOS and greater hospital efficiency. Also, as time goes by, new technologies, such as ICD, tend to become less expensive due to the learning curve and further technological advance. Many economic forces are at work to favor these beneficial movements and to drive the research programs that will fill in the numerous gaps still present in Table 103-3.

REFERENCES

1. American Heart Association publication no. 44-1027 (OPA) 1993.
2. Kupersmith J, Holmes-Rovner M, Hogan A, Rovner D, Gardiner J. Cost-effectiveness analysis in heart disease, I: General principles. *Prog Cardiovasc Dis* 1994; 37:161–184.
3. Eisenberg JM. Clinical economics: A guide to the economic analysis of clinical practices. *JAMA* 1989; 262:2879–2886.
4. Kupersmith J, Holmes-Rovner M, Hogan A, Rovner D, Gardiner J. Cost-effectiveness analysis in heart disease, III: Failure, and arrhythmias. *Prog Cardiovasc Dis* 1995; 37:307–346.
5. Goldman L, Gordon DJ, Rifkind BM, Hulley SB, Detsky AS, Goodman DW, et al. Cost and health implications of cholesterol lowering. *Circulation* 1992; 85:1960–1968.
6. Mark DB. Medical economics and health policy issues for interventional cardiology. In: Topol EJ, ed. *Interventional Cardiology*, 2d ed. Philadelphia: Saunders; 1994:1323–1353.
7. Rice DP, Hodgson TA, Kopstein AN. The economic costs of illness: A replication and update. *Health Care Finance Rev* 1985; 7:61–80.
8. Finkler SA. The distinction between cost and charges. *Ann Intern Med* 1982; 96:102–109.
9. Rice T. Containing health care costs in the United States. *Med Care Rev* 1992; 49:19–65.
10. Deming WE. *Out of the Crisis*. Cambridge, MA: Massachusetts Institute of Technology Center for Advanced Engineering Study; 1982.
11. Heidenreich PA, Chou TM, Amidon TM, Ports TA, Browner WS. Impact of the operating physician on costs of percutaneous transluminal coronary angioplasty. *Am J Cardiol* 1996; 77:1169–1173.
12. Smith LR, Milano CA, Molter BS, Elbeery JR, Sabiston DC, Smith PK. Preoperative determinants of postoperative costs associated with coronary artery bypass graft surgery. *Circulation* 1994; 90:II124–II128.
13. Califf RM, Bartrug B, Rogers MC, Roth D, Bride W, Fitzpatrick K, et al. Developing a rational system to contain costs on the cardiac care unit. In: Califf RM, Mark DB, Wagner GS, eds. *Acute Coronary Care*, 2d ed. St. Louis: Mosby-Year Book; 1995:895–912.
14. Paul SD, DiSalvo TG, Mahjoub ZA, O'Gara PT, Eagle KA. Care of patients with acute myocardial infarction: Patients characteristics and therapeutic options that influence direct costs (abstr). *Circulation* 1995; 92(suppl 1):I510–I511.
15. Ellis SG, Miller DP, Brown KJ, Omoigui N, Howell GL, Kutner M, et al. In-hospital cost of percutaneous coronary revascularization. *Circulation* 1995; 92:741–747.
16. Goldman L, Garber AM, Grover SA, Hlatky MA. Task Force 6. Cost effectiveness of assessment and management of risk factors. *J Am Coll Cardiol* 1996; 27:964–1047.
17. *Consumer Price Index, US City Average*. Chicago, IL: US Department of Labor, Bureau of Labor Statistics; 1994.
18. Kupersmith J, Holmes-Rovner M, Hogan A, Rovner D, Gardiner J. Cost-effectiveness analysis in heart disease, II: Preventive therapies. *Prog Cardiovasc Dis* 1995; 37:243–271.
19. Oster G, Epstein AM. Cost-effectiveness of antihyperlipemic therapy in the prevention of coronary heart disease: The case of cholestyramine. *JAMA* 1987; 258:2381–2387.
20. Kinosian BP, Eisenberg JM. Cutting into cholesterol: Cost-effective alternatives for treating hypercholesterolemia. *JAMA* 1988; 259:2249–2254.
21. Goldman L, Weinstein MC, Goldman PA, Williams LW. Cost-effectiveness of HMG-CoA reductase inhibition for primary and secondary prevention of coronary heart disease. *JAMA* 1991; 265:1145–1151.
22. Hamilton VH, Raciciot FE, Zowall H, Coupal L, Grover SA. The cost-effectiveness of HMG-CoA reductase inhibitors to prevent coronary heart disease. *JAMA* 1995; 273:1032–1038.
23. Goldman L, Goldman PA, Williams LW, Weinstein MC. Cost-effectiveness considerations in the treatment of heterozygous familial hypercholesterolemia with medications. *Am J Cardiol* 1993; 72:75D–79D.

24. Johannesson M, Johnsson B, Kjekshus J, Olsson A, Pedersen T, Hans W. Cost effectiveness of simvastatin treatment to lower cholesterol levels in patients with coronary heart disease. *N Engl J Med* 1997; 336:332–336.

25. Kinlay S, O'Connell D, Evans D, Halliday J. The cost-effectiveness of different blood-cholesterol-lowering strategies in the prevention of coronary heart disease. *Aust J Public Health* 1994; 18:105–110.

26. Cummings SR, Rubin SM, Oster G. The cost-effectiveness of counseling smokers to quit. *JAMA* 1989; 261:75–79.

27. Oster G, Huse DM, Delea TE, Colditz GA. Cost-effectiveness of nicotine gum as an adjunct to physician's advice against cigarette smoking. *JAMA* 1986; 256:1315–1318.

28. Krumholz HM, Cohen BJ, Tsevat J, Pasternak RC, Weinstein MC. Cost-effectiveness of a smoking cessation program after myocardial infarction. *J Am Coll Cardiol* 1993; 22:1697–1702.

29. Fiscella K, Franks P. Cost-effectiveness of the transdermal nicotine patch as an adjunct to physicians' smoking cessation counseling. *JAMA* 1996; 275:1247–1251.

30. Altman DG, Flora JA, Fortmann SP, Farquhar JW. The cost-effectiveness of three smoking cessation programs. *Am J Public Health* 1987; 77:162–165.

31. Tosteson ANA, Weinstein MC. Cost-effectiveness of hormone replacement therapy after the menopause. *Baillieres Clin Obstet Gynaecol* 1991; 5:943–959.

32. Hatziandreu EI, Koplan JP, Weinstein MC, Caspersen CJ, Warner KE. A cost-effectiveness analysis of exercise as a health promotion activity. *Am J Public Health* 1988; 78:1417–1421.

33. Weinstein MC, Stason WB. *Hypertension—A Policy Perspective.* Cambridge, MA: Harvard University; 1976.

34. Stason WB, Weinstein MC. Allocation of resources to manage hypotension. *N Engl J Med* 1977; 296:732–739.

35. Littenberg B, Garber AM, Sox HC. Screening for hypertension. *Ann Intern Med* 1990; 112:192–202.

36. Johannesson M, Dahlof B, Lindholm LH, Ekbom T, Hansson L, Oden A, et al. The cost-effectiveness of treating hypertension in elderly people: An analysis of the Swedish Trial in Old Patients with Hypertension (STOP Hypertension). *J Intern Med* 1993; 234:317–323.

37. Jonsson B. Improving patient care: Consequences for resource allocation. *Cardiology* 1994; 84:420–426.

38. Stason WB. Opportunities to improve the cost-effectiveness of treatment for hypertension. *Hypertension* 1991; 18(suppl I):I161–I166.

39. Edelson JT, Weinstein MC, Tosteson AN, Williams L, Lee TH, Goldman L. Long-term cost-effectiveness of various initial monotherapies for mild to moderate hypertension. *JAMA* 1990; 263:407–413.

40. Eagle KA, Blank DJ, Aguiar F, Firth LM. Economic impact of regression of left ventricular hypertrophy by antihypertensive drugs. *J Hum Hypertens* 1992; 7:341–351.

41. Joint National Committee on Detection, Evaluation, and Treatment of High Blood Pressure. The fifth report of the joint national committee on detection, evaluation, and treatment of high blood pressure (JNC V). *Arch Intern Med* 1993; 153:154–183.

42. Krakoff LR, Eison H, Phillips RH, Leiman SJ, Lev S. Effect of ambulatory blood pressure monitoring on the diagnosis and cost of treatment for mild hypertension. *Am Heart J* 1988; 116:1152–1154.

43. Yarows SA, Khoury S, Sower JR. Cost effectiveness of 24-hour ambulatory blood pressure monitoring in evaluation and treatment of essential hypertension. *Am J Hypertens* 1994; 7:464–468.

44. Devereux RB, Casale PN, Wallerson DC, Kligfield P, Hammond IW, Liebson PR, et al. Cost-effectiveness of echocardiography and electrocardiography for detection of left ventricular hypertrophy in patients with systemic hypertension. *Hypertension* 1987; 9(suppl II):II69–II76.

45. Christianson JB, Krishan I, Nobrega FT, Davis CS, Smoldt RK, Harris AM. The Mayo three-community hypertension control program v. cost-effectiveness of intervention. *Mayo Clin Proc* 1981; 56:11–16.

46. Eckman MH, Levine HJ, Pauker SG. Decision analytic and cost-effectiveness issues concerning anticoagulant prophylaxis in heart disease. *Chest* 1992; 102(suppl):538S–549S.

47. Gage BF, Cardianalli AB, Albers GW, Owens DK. Cost-effectiveness of warfarin and aspirin for prophylaxis of stroke in patients with nonvalvular atrial fibrillation. *JAMA* 1995; 274:1839–1845.

48. Eckman MH, Levine HJ, Pauker SG. Effect of laboratory variation in the prothrombin-time ratio on the results of oral anticoagulant therapy. *N Engl J Med* 1993; 329:696–702.

49. Chiquette I, Amato MG, Bussey HI. Comparison of an anticoagulation clinic with routine medical care (abstr). *Circulation* 1995; 92(suppl 1):I686.

50. MICH Investigators. Michigan State University Inter-Institutional Collaborative Heart Study, unpublished observations.

51. Lee TH, Cook EF, Fendrick AM, Shammash JB, Wolfe EP, Weisberg MC, et al. Impact of initial triage decisions on nursing intensity for patients with acute chest pain. *Med Care* 1990; 28:737–745.

52. Tosteson ANA, Goldman L, Udvarhelyi S, Lee TH. Cost-effectiveness of a coronary care unit versus an intermediate care unit for emergency department patients with chest pain. *Circulation* 1996; 94:143–150.

53. Fineberg HV, Scadden D, Goldman L. Care of patients with a low probability of acute myocardial infarction: Cost-effectiveness of alternatives to coronary-care-unit admission. *N Engl J Med* 1984; 310:1301–1307.

54. Madias JE. Shifting paradigms of diagnosis and care in a cost-conscious environment. *Chest* 1995; 108:1483–1484.

55. Gaspoz JM, Lee TH, Weinstein MC, Cook EF, Goldman P, Komaroff AL, et al. Cost-effectiveness of a new short-stay unit to "rule out" acute myocardial infarction in low risk patients. *J Am Coll Cardiol* 1994; 24:1249–1259.

56. Strauss MJ, LoGerfo JP, Yeltatzie JA, Temkin N, Hudson LD. Rationing of intensive care unit services: An everyday occurrence. *JAMA* 1986; 255:1143–1146.

57. Thibault GE. Making the coronary care unit cost-effective. *Am J Cardiol* 1985; 56:35C–39C.

58. Weingarten S, Ellrodt AG. The case for intensive dissemination: Adoption of practice guidelines in the coronary care unit. *QRB Qual Rev Bull* 1992; 18:449–455.

59. Eagle KA, Mulley AG, Skates SJ, Reder VA, Nicholson BW, Sexton JO, et al. Length-of-stay in the intensive care unit: Effects of practice guidelines and feedback. *JAMA* 1990; 264:992–997.

60. Iezzoni LI, Burnside S, Sickles L, Moskowitz MA, Sawitz E, Levine PA. Coding of acute myocardial infarction. *Ann Intern Med* 1988; 109:745–751.

61. Levin LA, Jonsson B. Cost-effectiveness of thrombolysis: A randomized study of intravenous rt-PA in suspected myocardial infarction. *Eur Heart J* 1992; 13:2–8.

62. Midgette AS, Wong JB, Beshansky JR, Porath A, Fleming C, Pauker SG. Cost-effectiveness of streptokinase for acute myocardial infarction. *Med Decis Making* 1994; 14:108–117.

63. Naylor CD, Bronskill S, Goel V. Cost-effectiveness of intravenous thrombolytic drugs for acute myocardial infarction. *Can J Cardiol* 1993; 9:553–558.

64. Krumholz HM, Pasternak RC, Weinstein MC, Friesinger GC, Ridker PM, Tosteson AN, et al. Cost effectiveness of thrombolytic therapy with streptokinase in elderly patients with suspected acute myocardial infarction. *N Engl J Med* 1992; 327:7–13.

65. Vermeer F, Simoons ML, de Zwaan C, van Es GA, Verheugt FWA, van der Laarse A, et al. Cost benefit analysis of early thrombolytic treatment with intracoronary streptokinase. *Br Heart J* 59:527–534.

66. Mark DB, Hlatky MA, Califf RM, Naylor CD, Lee KL, Armstrong PW, et al. Cost effectiveness of thrombolytic therapy with tissue plasminogen activator as compared with streptokinase for acute myocardial infarction. *N Engl J Med* 1995; 332:1418–1424.

67. de Boer MJ, van Hout BA, Liem AL, Suryapranata H, Hoorntje JCA, Zijlstra F. A cost-effectiveness analysis of primary coronary angioplasty versus thrombolysis for acute myocardial infarction. *Am J Cardiol* 1995; 76:830–833.

68. Stone GW, Grines CL, Rothbaum D, Catlin T, O'Neill WW. Primary angioplasty reduces hospital costs while improving outcomes in AMI comprehensive cost efficacy analysis from the PAMI study. (Personal communication.)

69. Reeder GS, Bailey KR, Gersh BJ, Holmes DR, Christianson J, Gibbons RJ, et al. Cost comparison of immediate angioplasty versus thrombolysis followed by conservative therapy for acute myocardial infarction: A randomized prospective trial. *Mayo Clin Proc* 1994; 69:5–12.

70. Grines C, Marsalese D, Brodie B, Griffin J, Donohue B, Costantini C, et al. Emergency cardiac catheterization and angioplasty allows risk stratification and early discharge of patients with acute myocardial infarction. PAMI-2. (Personal communication.)

71. Every NR, Parsons LS, Hlatky M, Martin JS, Weaver WD. A comparison of the thrombolytic therapy with primary coronary angioplasty for acute myocardial infarction. *N Engl J Med* 1996; 335:1253–1260.

72. Lange RA, Hillis LD. Immediate angioplasty for acute myocardial infarction. *N Engl J Med* 1993; 328:726–728.

73. Conti CR. Early discharge after acute myocardial infarction. *Clin Cardiol* 1992; 15:229–230.

74. TIMI Study Group. Comparison of invasive and conservative strategies after treatment with intravenous tissue plasminogen activator in acute myocardial infarction. Results of the Thrombolysis in Myocardial Infarction (TIMI) Phase II Trial. *N Engl J Med* 1989; 320:618–627.

75. Topol EJ, Burek K, O'Neill WW, Kewman DJ, Cander NH, Shea MJ, et al. A randomized controlled trial of hospital discharge three days after myocardial infarction in the era of reperfusion. *N Engl J Med* 1988; 318:1083–1088.

76. Topol EJ, Holmes DR, Rogers WJ. Coronary angiography after thrombolytic therapy for acute myocardial infarction. *Ann Intern Med* 1991; 114:877–885.

77. Udvarhelyi IS, Goldman L, Komaroff AL, Lee TH. Determinants of resource utilization for patients admitted for evaluation of acute chest pain. *J Gen Intern Med* 1992; 7:1–10.

78. Newby LK, Califf RM, Guerci A, Weaver WD, Col J, Horgan JH, et al. Early discharge in the thrombolytic era: An analysis for criteria for uncomplicated infarction from the global utilization of streptokinase and t-PA for occluded coronary arteries (GUSTO) trial. *J Am Coll Cardiol* 1996; 27:625–632.

79. Mark DB, Lam LC, Hlatky MA, Melton JR, Davidson-Ray L, Woodlief L, et al. Effects of three thrombolytic regimens and two interventional strategies on acute MI costs: Results from a prospective randomized trial (abstr). *Circulation* 1991; 84:221.

80. Charles ED, Rogers WJ, Reeder GS, Chesebro JH, Papapietro SE, Maske L, et al. Economic advantages of a conservative strategy for AMI management: rt-PA without obligatory PTCA (abstr). *J Am Coll Cardiol* 1989; 13:152A.

81. SWIFT Trial Study Group. SWIFT trial of delayed elective intervention v conservative treatment after thrombolysis with anistreplase in acute myocardial infarction. *BMJ* 1991; 302:555–560.

82. Kuntz KM, Tsevat J, Goldman L, Weinstein MC. Cost-effectiveness of routine coronary angiography after acute myocardial infarction. *Circulation* 1996; 94:957–965.

83. Goldman L, Sia STB, Cook EF, Rutherford JD, Weinstein MC. Costs and effectiveness of routine therapy with long-term beta-adrenergic antagonists after acute myocardial infarction. *N Engl J Med* 1988; 319:152–157.

84. Tsevat J, Duke D, Goldman L, Pfeffer MA, Lamas GA, Soukup JR, et al. Cost-effectiveness of captopril therapy after myocardial infarction. *J Am Coll Cardiol* 1995; 26:914–919.

85. Gaspoz JM, Goldman P, Williams L, Weinstein M, Goldman L. Cost-effectiveness of aspirin in secondary prevention of coronary heart disease (abstr). *Circulation* 1995; 92(suppl I):I47.

86. van Bergen PFMM, Jonker JJC, van Hout BA, van Domburg RT, Deckers JW, Azar AJ, et al. Costs and effects of long-term oral anticoagulant treatment after myocardial infarction. *JAMA* 1995; 273:925–928.

87. Cairns JA, Markham BA. Economics and efficacy in choosing oral anticoagulants or aspirin after myocardial infarction. *JAMA* 1995; 273:965–967.

88. Oldridge N, Furlong W, Feeny D, Torrance G, Guyatt G, Crowe J, et al. Economic evaluation of cardiac rehabilitation soon after acute myocardial infarction. *Am J Cardiol* 1993; 72:154–161.

89. Levin LA, Perk J, Hedback B. Cardiac rehabilitation: A cost analysis. *J Intern Med* 1991; 230:427–434.

90. Kotler TS, Diamond GA. Exercise thallium-201 scintigraphy in the diagnosis and prognosis of coronary artery disease. *Ann Intern Med* 1990; 113:684–702.

91. Patterson RE, Eisner RL, Horowitz SF. Comparison of cost-effectiveness and utility of exercise ECG, single photon emission computed tomography, positron emission tomography, and coronary angiography for diagnosis of coronary artery disease. *Circulation* 1995; 91:54–65.

92. Sox HC, Littenberg B, Garber AM. The role of exercise testing in screening for coronary artery disease. *Ann Intern Med* 1989; 110:456–469.

93. Christain TF, Miller TD, Bailey KR, Gibbons RJ. Exercise tomographic thallium-201 imaging in patients with severe coronary artery disease and normal electrocardiograms. *Ann Intern Med* 1994; 121:825–832.

94. Brenner S, Cohen M, Talley JD, Eagle K, Gershony G, Chaitman B, et al. Striking hospital to hospital variation in pre-operative cardiac work-up for patients referred for major non-cardiac surgery (abstr). *Circulation* 1995; 92(suppl 1):I679.

95. Mason JJ, Owens DK, Harris RA, Cooke JP, Hlatky MA. The role of coronary angiography and coronary revascularization before noncardiac vascular surgery. *JAMA* 1995; 273:1919–1925.

96. Bry FDL, Belkin M, O'Donnell TF, Mackey WC, Udelson JE, Schmid CH, et al. An assessment of the positive predictive value and cost-effectiveness of dipyridamole myocardial scintigraphy in patients undergoing vascular surgery. *J Vasc Surg* 1994; 19:112–124.

97. Shaw LJ, Miller DD. Cost-effectiveness analysis of preoperative pharmacologic stress myocardial imaging in 3,623 vascular surgery candidates (abstr). *Circulation* 1995; 92(suppl 1):I521–I522.

98. Lee JC, Bengtson JR, Lipscomb J, Bashore TM, Mark DB, Califf RM, et al. Feasibility and cost-saving potential of outpatient cardiac catheterization. *J Am Coll Cardiol* 1990; 15:378–384.

99. Block PC, Ockene I, Goldberg RJ, Butterly J, Block EH, Degon C, et al. A prospective randomized trial of outpatient versus inpatient cardiac catheterization. *N Engl J Med* 1988; 319:1251–1255.

100. Steinberg EP, Moore RD, Powe NR, Gopalan R, Davidoff AJ, Litt M, et al. Safety and cost effectiveness of high-osmolality as compared with low-osmolality contrast material in patients undergoing cardiac angiography. *N Engl J Med* 1992; 326:425–430.

101. Wong JB, Sonnenberg FA, Salem DN, Pauker SG. Myocardial revascularization for chronic stable angina: Analysis of the role of percutaneous transluminal coronary angioplasty based on data available in 1989. *Ann Intern Med* 1990; 113:852–871.

102. Weintraub WS, Mauldin PD, Becker E, Kosinski AS, King SB. A comparison of the costs of and quality of life after coronary angioplasty or coronary surgery for multivessel coronary artery disease. *Circulation* 1995; 92:2831–2840.

103. Topol EJ, Ellis SG, Cosgrove DM, Bates ER, Muller DWM, Schork NJ, et al. Analysis of coronary angioplasty practice in the United States with an insurance-claims data base. *Circulation* 1993; 87:1489–1497.

104. Wilson JM, Dunn EJ, Wright CB, Bailey WW, Callard GM, Melvin DB, et al. The cost of simultaneous surgical standby for percutaneous transluminal coronary angioplasty. *J Thorac Cardiovasc Surg* 1986; 91:362–370.

105. O'Keefe JH, Gernon C, McCallister BD, Ligon RW, Hartzler GO. Safety and cost effectiveness of combined coronary angiography and angioplasty. *Am Heart J* 1991; 122:50.

106. Burton J, Tymchak W, Dzavik V, Lucas A, Muzyka T, Hogg N, et al. Randomized controlled trial of reuse of PTCA balloon catheters (abstr). *Circulation* 1996; 92 (suppl I):I662.

107. Mak KH, Eisenberg MJ, Eccleston DS, Brown KJ, Ellis SG, Topol EJ. Cost-efficacy modeling of catheter reuse for percutaneous transluminal coronary angioplasty. *J Am Coll Cardiol* 1996; 28:106–111.

108. Plante S, Strauss BH, Goulet G, Watson RK, Chisholm RJ. Reuse of balloon catheters for coronary angioplasty: A potential cost-saving strategy? *J Am Coll Cardiol* 1994; 24:1475–1481.

109. Mark DB. Implications of cost in treatment selection for patients with coronary heart disease. *Ann Thorac Surg* 1996; 61:512–515.

110. Califf RM. Restenosis: The cost to society. *Am Heart J* 1995; 130:680–684.

111. Reeder GS, Krishan I, Nobrega FT, Naessens J, Kelly M, Christianson JB, et al. Is percutaneous coronary angioplasty less expensive than bypass surgery? *N Engl J Med* 1984; 311:1157–1162.

112. Mark DB, Talley JD, Lam LC, Davison-Ray L, Bowman L. Reduced restenosis from aggressive platelet inhibition reduces costs of high risk angioplasty: Results from the EPIC randomized trial (abstr). *Circulation* 1994; 90(suppl IV):IV44.

113. Topol EJ, Leya F, Pinkerton CA, Whitlow PL, Hofling B, Simonton CA, et al. A comparison of directional atherectomy with coronary angioplasty in patients with coronary artery disease. The CAVEAT Study Group. *N Engl J Med* 1993; 329:221–227.

114. Cohen DJ, Breall JA, Ho KKL, Kuntz RE, Goldman L, Baim DS, et al. Evaluating the potential cost-effectiveness of stenting as a treatment for symptomatic single-vessel coronary disease. *Circulation* 1994; 89:1859–1874.

115. Cohen DJ, Krumholz HM, Sukin C, Ho KKL, Siegrist RB, Cleman M, et al. In-hospital and one-year economic outcomes after coronary stenting or balloon angioplasty: Results from a randomized clinical trial. *Circulation* 1995; 92:2480–2487.

116. Goods CM, Liu MW, Iyer SS, Yadav SS, Al-Shaibi KF, Negus BH, et al. A cost analysis of coronary stenting without anticoagulation versus stenting with anticoagulation using warfarin (abstr). *Circulation* 1995; 92(suppl I):I796–I797.

117. Kiemeneij F, Laarman GJ. Next-day discharge after transradial Palmaz-Schatz coronary stenting: A first step towards outpatient coronary stent implantation (abstr). *Circulation* 1994; 90(suppl I):I620.

118. Weinstein MC, Stason WB. Cost-effectiveness of coronary artery bypass surgery. *Circulation* 1982; 66(suppl III):56–66.

119. Taylor GJ, Mikell FL, Moses HW, Dove JT, Katholi RE, Malik SA, et al. Determinants of hospital charges for coronary artery bypass surgery: The economic consequences of postoperative complications. *Am J Cardiol* 1990; 65:309–313.

120. Mauldin PD, Weintraub WS, Becker ER. Predicting hospital costs for first-time coronary artery bypass grafting from preoperative and postoperative variables. *Am J Cardiol* 1994; 74:772–775.

121. Strong AG, Sneed NV. Clinical evaluation of a critical path for coronary artery bypass surgery patients. *Prog Cardiovasc Nurs* 1991; 6:29–37.

122. Bolling SF, Walters J, Monaghan H, Watts J, Schlafer J, Deeb GM. Case management, critical pathways and patient outcome after coronary artery bypass (abstr). *Circulation* 1995; 92(suppl 1):I47.

123. Birkmeyer JD, AuBuchon JP, Littenberg B, O'Connor GT, Nease RF, Nugent WC, et al. Cost-effectiveness of preoperative autologous donation in coronary artery bypass grafting. *Ann Thorac Surg* 1994; 57:161–169.

124. Cohen DJ, Breall JA, Ho KKL, Weintraub RM, Kuntz RE, Weinstein MC, et al. Economics of elective coronary revascularization: Comparison of costs and charges for conventional angioplasty, directional atherectomy, stenting and bypass surgery. *J Am Coll Cardiol* 1993; 22:1052–1059.

125. Rodriguez A, Boullon F, Perez-Balino N, Paviotti C, Liprandi MIS, Palacios IF. Argentine randomized trial of percutaneous transluminal coronary angioplasty versus coronary artery bypass surgery in multivessel disease (ERACI): In-hospital results and 1 year follow-up. *J Am Coll Cardiol* 1993; 22:1060–1067.

126. Hlatky MA, Lipscomb J, Nelson C, Califf RM, Pryor D, Wallace AG, et al. Resource use and cost of initial coronary revascularization: Coronary angioplasty versus coronary bypass surgery. *Circulation* 1990; 82(suppl IV):IV208–IV213.

127. Kelly ME, Taylor GJ, Moses HW, Mikell FL, Dove JT, Batchelder JE, et al. Comparative cost of myocardial revascularization: Percutaneous transluminal angioplasty and coronary artery bypass surgery *J Am Coll Cardiol* 1985; 5:16–20.

128. Hlatky M, William R, Iain J, Boothroyd D, Brooks M, Bertram P, et al. Medical care costs and quality of life after randomization to coronary angioplasty or coronary bypass surgery. *N Engl J Med* 1997; 336:92–99.

129. Mark DB, Lam LC, Lee KL, Jones RH, Pryor DB, Stack RS, et al. Effects of coronary angioplasty, coronary bypass surgery, and medical therapy on employment in patients with coronary artery disease. *Ann Intern Med* 1994; 120:111–117.

130. van den Brand M, van Halem C, van den Brink F, de Feyter P, Serruys P, Suryapranata H. Comparison of costs of percutaneous transluminal coronary angioplasty and coronary bypass surgery for patients with angina pectoris. *Eur Heart J* 1991; 11:765–771.

131. O'Connell JB, Bristow MR. Economic impact of heart failure in the United States: Time for a different approach. *J Heart Lung Transplant* 1993; 13:S107–S112.

132. Paul SD, Kuntz KM, Eagle KA, Weinstein MC. Costs and effectiveness of angiotensin converting enzyme inhibition in patients with congestive heart failure. *Arch Intern Med* 1994; 154:1143–1149.

133. Ward RE, Gheorghiade M. The economic outcomes of withdrawal of digoxin therapy in adult patients with stable heart failure: A decision analysis. *J Amer Coll Cardiol* 1995; 93–101.

134. Hart W, Rhodes G. The cost effectiveness of enalapril in the treatment of chronic heart failure. *Br J Med Econ* 1993; 6:91–98.

135. Kleber FX, Niemöller L, Doering W. Impact of converting enzyme inhibition on progression of chronic heart failure. Results of the Munich Mild Heart Failure Trial. *Br Heart J* 1992; 67:289–296.

136. SOLVD Investigators. Effect of enalapril on mortality and the development of heart failure in asymptomatic patients with reduced left ventricular ejection fractions. *N Engl J Med* 1992; 327:685–691.

137. Levinoff Roth SN, Moe G. Intermittent intravenous amrinone infusion: A potentially cost effective mode of treatment of patients with refractory heart failure. *Can J Cardiol* 1993; 9:231–237.

138. Rich MW, Beckham V, Wittenberg C, Leven CL, Freedland KE, Carney RM. A multidisciplinary intervention to prevent the readmission of elderly patients with congestive heart failure. *N Engl J Med* 1995; 333:1190–1195.

139. Mills A, Drummond MF. Economic evaluation of health programmes: Glossary of terms. *World Health Stat Q* 1985; 38:432–434.

140. Evans RW. Cost-effectiveness analysis of transplantation. *Surg Clin North Am* 1986; 66:603–616.

141. Evans RW. Organ procurement expenditures and the role of financial incentives. *JAMA* 1993; 269:3113–3118.

142. Eggers PW, Kucken LE. Cost issues in transplantation. *Surg Clin North Am* 1994; 74:1259–1267.

143. Kadish A, Calkins H, de Buitler M, Morady F. Feasibility and cost savings and outpatient electrophysiologic testing. *J Am Coll Cardiol* 1990; 16:1415–1419.

144. May CD, Davis MJE. The safety and economic advantages of day case electrophysiologic studies. *Aust NZ J Med* 1992; 22:240–242.

145. Omoigui NA, Marcus FI, Mason JW, Hahn EA, Hartz VL, Hlatky MA. Cost of initial therapy in the electrophysiological study versus ECG monitoring trial (ESVM). *Circulation* 1995; 91:1070–1076.

146. Mitchell LB, Duff HJ, Manyari DE, Wyse DG. Drug therapy of ventricular tachycardia: A cost-comparison of randomized noninvasive and invasive approaches. *Can J Cardiol* 1992; 8:487–494.

147. Kessler DK, Kessler KM, Myerburg RJ. Ambulatory electrocardiology: A cost per management decision analysis. *Arch Intern Med* 1995; 155:165–169.

148. DiMarco JP, Philbrick JT. Use of ambulatory electrocardiographic (Holter) monitoring. *Ann Intern Med* 1990; 113:56–68.

149. Kinlay S, Leitch JW, Neil A, Chapman BL, Hardy DB, Fletcher PJ. Cardiac event recorders yield more diagnoses and are more cost-effective than 48-hour Holter monitoring in patients with palpitations. *Ann Intern Med* 1996; 124:16–20.

150. Kupersmith J, Hogan A, Guerrero P, Gardiner J, Mellits ED, Baumgardner R, et al. Evaluating and improving the cost-effectiveness of the implantable cardioverter-defibrillator. *Am Heart J* 1995; 130:507–515.

151. Kupperman M, Luce BR, McGovern B, Podrid PJ, Bigger JT, Rushkin JN. An analysis of the cost effectiveness of the implantable defibrillator. *Circulation* 1990; 81:91–100.

152. Larsen GC, Manolis AS, Sonnenberg FA, Beshansky JR, Estes NAM, Pauker SG. Cost-effectiveness of the implantable cardioverter defibrillator: Effect of improved battery life and comparison with amiodarone therapy. *J Am Coll Cardiol* 1992; 19:1323–1334.

153. Williamson BD, Man KC, Neibauer M, Daoud E, Strickberger SA, Hummel JD, et al. The economic impact of transvenous defibrillation lead systems. *Pacing Clin Electrophysiol* 1994; 17:2297–2303.

154. Wever EFD, Hauer RNW, Schrijvers G, van Capelle FJL, Tijssen JGP, Crijns HJGM. Cost-effectiveness of implantable defibrillator as first-choice therapy versus electrophysiologically guided, tiered strategy in postinfarct sudden death survivors. *Circulation* 1996; 93:489–496.

155. Owens D, Sanders G, Harris R, McDonald K, Heidenreich P, Dembitzer A, et al. Cost-effectiveness of implantable cardioverter defibrillators relative to amiodarone for prevention of sudden cardiac death. *Ann Intern Med* 1997; 126:1–12.

156. Weerasooriya HR, Murdock CJ, Harris AH, Davis MJE. The cost-effectiveness of treatment of supraventricular arrhythmias related to an accessory atrioventricular pathway: Comparison of catheter ablation, surgical division and medical treatment. *Aust NZ J Med* 1994; 24:161–167.

157. Hogenhuis W, Stevens SK, Wang P, Wong JB, Manolis AS, Estes NA 3d, et al. Cost-effectiveness of radiofrequency ablation compared with other strategies in Wolff-Parkinson-White syndrome. *Circulation* 1993 88(suppl II):II437–II446.

158. Kalbfleisch SJ, Calkins H, Langberg JJ, El-Atassi R, Leon A, Borganelli M, et al. Comparison of the cost of radiofrequency catheter modification of the atrioventricular node and medical therapy for drug-refractory atrioventricular node reentrant tachycardia. *J Am Coll Cardiol* 1992; 19:1583–1587.

159. Kertes PJ, Kalman JM, Tonkin AM. Cost effectiveness of radiofrequency catheter ablation in the treatment of symptomatic supraventricular tachyarrhythmias. *Aust NZ J Med* 1993; 23:433–436.

160. Lee MA, Morady F, Kadish A, Schamp DJ, Chin MC, Scheinman MM, et al. Catheter modification of the atrioventricular junction with radiofrequency energy for control of atrioventricular nodal reentry tachycardia. *Circulation* 1991; 83:827–835.

161. Calkins H, Sousa J, El-Atassi R, Rosenheck S, de Buitleir M, Kou WH, et al. Diagnosis and cure of the Wolff-Parkinson-White syndrome or paroxysmal supraventricular tachycardias during a single electrophysiologic test. *N Engl J Med* 1991; 324:1612–1618.

162. Bush DE, Finucane TE. Permanent cardiac pacemakers in the elderly. *J Am Geriatr Soc* 1994; 42:326–334.

163. Falk RH. Impact of prospective peer review on pacemaker implantation rates in Massachusetts. *J Am Coll Cardiol* 1990; 15:1087–1092.

164. Parsonnet V. Role of peer review of pacemaker implantations. *J Am Coll Cardiol* 1990; 15:1093–1094.

165. Dreifus LS, Fisch C, Griffin JC, Gillette PC, Mason JW, Parsonnet V. Guidelines for implantation of cardiac pacemakers and antiarrhythmia devices. *Circulation* 1991; 84:455–467.

166. Ray SG, Griffith MJ, Jamieson S, Bexton RS, Gold RG. Impact of the recommendations of the British Pacing and Electrophysiology Group on pacemaker prescription and on the immediate costs of pacing in the Northern Region. *Br Heart J* 1992; 68:531–534.

167. Stamato NJ, O'Toole MF, Enger EL. Permanent pacemaker implantation in the cardiac catheterization laboratory versus the operating room: An analysis of hospital charges and complications. *Pacing Clin Electrophysiol* 1992; 15:2236–2239.

168. Tyers GFO. Recycling and 'transplantation' of implantable electronic devices. *Can J Cardiol* 1992; 8:683–684.

169. Lamas GA, Pashos CL, Normand ST, McNeil BJ. Permanent pacemaker selection and subsequent survival in elderly Medicare pacemaker recipients. *Circulation* 1995; 91:1063–1069.

GENERAL READING

Detsky AS, Naglie IG. A clinician's guide to cost-effectiveness analysis. *Ann Intern Med* 1990; 113:147–154.

Drummond MF, Stoddart GL, Torrance GW. *Methods for the Economic Evaluation of Health Care Programmes.* Oxford, UK: Oxford University; 1987.

Finkler SA. The distinction between cost and charges. *Ann Intern Med* 1982; 96:102–109.

Kamlet MS. *A Framework for Cost-Utility Analysis of Government Health Care Programs.* Washington, DC: US Government Printing Office; 1992: publication no. 617-025/68280.

Kupersmith J, Holmes-Rovner M, Hogan A, Rovner D, Gardiner J. Cost-effectiveness analysis in heart disease, I: General principles. *Prog Cardiovasc Dis* 1994; 37:161–184.

Rice DP, Hodgson TA, Kopstein AN. The economic costs of illness: A replication and update. *Health Care Finance Rev* 1985; 7:61–80.

Russell LB, Gold MR, Siegel JE, Daniels N, Weinstein MC. The role of cost-effectiveness analysis in health and medicine. *JAMA* 1996; 276:1172–1177.

Siegel JE, Weinstein MC, Russell LB, Gold MR. Recommendations for reporting cost-effectiveness analyses. *JAMA* 1996; 276:1339–1341.

Sox HC, Blatt MA, Higgins MC, Martin KI. *Medical Decision Making.* Stoneham, MA: Butterworth, 1988.

Warner KE, Hutton RC. Cost-benefit and cost effectiveness analysis in health care: Growth and composition of the literature. *Med Care* 1980; 18:1069–1084.

Weinstein MC, Fineberg HV, Elstein AS, Frazier HS, Neuhauser D, Neutra RR, et al. *Clinical Decision Analysis.* Philadelphia: Saunders, 1980.

Weinstein MC, Siegel JE, Gold MR, Kamlet MS, Russell LB. Recommendations of the panel on cost-effectiveness in health and medicine. *JAMA* 1996; 276:1253–1258.

104

INSURANCE ISSUES IN PATIENTS WITH HEART DISEASE

Michael B. Clark / William T. Friedewald

INSURANCE MEDICINE AND CARDIOLOGY

The purpose of insurance is to provide for financial relief in the event of significant economic loss. Insurance usually takes the form of a contract—a legal agreement between insurer and insured—specifying those losses that are to be covered and the insurance benefit agreed upon. Under specific conditions, including definable losses that occur by chance within large populations at risk, the laws of probability can be applied using actuarial methods to predict the total amount of loss for a group of individuals over some defined period of time.[1] For life and health insurance, an evaluation process described as *insurance underwriting* serves to identify the potential risk of loss for each individual. When a premium proportional to that risk is assessed, the result is an insurance system that allows for economic risk to be spread over large groups of people, with contributions from each insured proportional to the risk assumed by the insurer for that individual.

These concepts of insurance and insurance underwriting are not new; insurance for commercial ventures existed in some form by the Middle Ages, and life insurance had appeared by the seventeenth century. Private medical insurance, usually for catastrophic illnesses, was available in the 1800s.[2] Within the past 100 years, there has been an explosion in the amount of life and health insurance available and in the diversity of insurance products. This includes group employee-sponsored health and life insurance, insurance options offered by health maintenance and managed care organizations, and government-sponsored health insurance plans for indigent, disabled, and elderly populations. Within the medical community, the impact of this changing insurance climate has been enormous.[3,4] Nevertheless, as medical care providers and as consultants, cardiologists continue to play an important role in insurance underwriting evaluation.

MEDICAL UNDERWRITING FOR LIFE INSURANCE

Medical Risk Assessment

As a first step in the risk assessment process for an insurance applicant with a cardiac impairment, the patient's physician submits medical information to the insurance company in the form of the Attending Physician Statement (APS). This may include an outline of recent medical history and will often contain office and hospital records for review. Clinical problems identified in the APS are analyzed for severity of disease, extent of clinical evaluation, and thoroughness of clinical follow-up to provide data for risk assessment.

After the development of any additional information provided by authorized query to one of the national insurance company data-base exchanges, the next step in the medical underwriting evaluation involves, in most cases, the insurance medical examination. Comprehensive history taking and physical examination are routine in these examinations. Noninvasive cardiac testing may also be required by the insurance company, particularly if large amounts of insurance are requested or if additional information is required to permit a proper assessment of cardiac risk. A cardiology consultant may serve as a member of the medical underwriting team itself at this stage, reviewing all of the cardiac information obtained as part of the evaluation, including electrocardiograms and stress test tracings.

To complete the risk assessment process, each medical condition identified during the medical underwriting evaluation must be correlated with long-term survival data relevant to that disease process. From these data, a mortality ratio is derived (observed deaths in a population of individuals affected by the condition divided by the expected deaths for a comparable standard population).[5,6] This quantitative prognostic index serves as a standard, which is useful for comparing mortality projections among the various medical conditions. In general, the higher the mortality ratio calculated for a particular impairment, the greater the mortality and, thus, the greater the relative risk assumed by the company to provide insurance for individuals affected by that impairment. The mortality ratios calculated for various medical conditions are integrated into a table of risk classes or "ratings"; applicants within a rating class are grouped together to be assessed similar insurance premiums. The relationship of risk class to premium is complex and often varies by company and by insurance product, but the final result is coverage for financial loss, with the contribution to the total insurance pool proportional to the medical risk assumed by the insurance company. This equitable arrangement has the additional benefit of making insurance coverage possible for many people with cardiac disease who would otherwise be uninsurable.[7,8]

Published data relevant to mortality assessment derive from several sources. Excellent long-term follow-up data are available for insured populations based on medical conditions, demographic characteristics, and personal habits identified at the time of original insurance application (Table 104-1). Results are usually expressed as mortality ratios to address directly the prognostic, as opposed to diagnostic, significance of examination and laboratory abnormalities such as "heart murmur on exam" or "low serum albumin." This information, while particularly relevant to insurance underwriting, may not be directly comparable to standard mortality data derived from the general population, as the insured population data more precisely relate to large groups of *selected* individuals (those people willing and able to purchase life insurance). A further limitation of such data is that they typically involve follow-up intervals as long as 20 to 30 years. Significant medical advances, as well as changes in demographics or personal lifestyles that occur during the period of study,

may significantly limit the applicability of the information developed.

Long-term clinical and epidemiologic studies published in the medical literature are also useful for mortality assessment and are generally more readily available for most medical impairments. In such studies, the survival data as reported can be extrapolated to provide actuarial information useful to the calculation of mortality risk. A common shortcoming in such clinical studies, however, is the single reporting of the observed mortality for the population recruited into the study without sufficient information to allow one to extrapolate the findings to the larger population from which they were selected.[9] This actuarial problem for many of the studies reported in the clinical literature was recently identified in a review[10] of a reported study of survivors of asymptomatic myocardial infarction.[11] *Good* long-term prognosis was the conclusion of the clinical investigation, which followed 48 patients with a mean age of 36 years for approximately 6 years; the observed mortality in this population was 10 percent for the entire period. However, reference to the U.S. Standard Life Tables (1979–1981) reveals a much lower expected mortality (approximately 1.46 percent) at this age for the same length of follow-up. The estimated mortality ratio of 685 percent (10 percent/1.46 percent $\times$ 100), represents a high substandard risk level for life insurance purposes, even though it may represent good clinical results in young patients with severe cardiac disease.

CORONARY HEART DISEASE: ANGINA PECTORIS AND MYOCARDIAL INFARCTION

One long-term follow-up study in the insured population[12] has shown initial and short-term mortality following the diagnosis of coronary disease to be relatively high (estimated at up to 1150 percent of standard mortality depending on the presenting manifestations of disease) and quite variable for clinical subpopulations. This initial period of unstable risk is followed by a plateau phase during which the mortality rate (found to be close to 390 percent of standard) is relatively stable and thus more predictable. Other studies in insured individuals have confirmed this pattern,[13,14] which has led to the common practice of postponing consideration for life insurance for periods of up to one year following the initial presentation of coronary heart disease (CHD). Over the next several years, the excess *short-term* mortality demon-

TABLE 104-1

MORTALITY RATIOS IN CARDIAC IMPAIRMENTS: SELECTED DATA

Medical Finding or Condition	Age Interval, Years	Number of patients	Mortality Ratio, Percent
ECG findings in males	40–64	21,415	
Axis deviation (symptomatic)			225
Axis deviation (asymptomatic)			139
ST depression (symptomatic)			420
ST depression (asymptomatic)			220
Heart murmurs	50–59	21,295	
Apical systolic (not transmitted to neck; presumed functional)			114
Apical systolic (transmitted)			178
Basal systolic			276
Acute myocardial infarction	30–59	1,608	145
Coronary bypass reoperation	50–59	1,608	145

Source: Adapted from Refs. 14, 29, 32, and 33.

strated for this disease is reflected in a series of short-term extra premium charges. Upon reaching the more predictable plateau phase, a permanent, somewhat substandard rating is usually applied to correspond to the more stable, but still greater than expected, mortality rate seen in individuals with CHD.

To facilitate appropriate risk assessment, special attention is directed to the presence of known CHD risk factors such as high blood pressure, diabetes mellitus, hyperlipidemia, smoking history, and obesity. In addition, a strong family history of cardiovascular disease has been confirmed in studies in insured as well as in other broader-based epidemiologic populations to be an independent risk factor for coronary heart disease with mortality ratios in insureds of 189 and 121 percent for men and women, respectively.[14]

Long-term prognosis in patients with CHD may be influenced by intercurrent clinical interventions, such as the use of thrombolytic drugs or the performance of coronary angioplasty and coronary bypass surgery. Commonly, life insurance consideration for patients having undergone these procedures is initially postponed to allow for review of the clinical course soon after the intervention. Underwriting risk assessment after this initial period is quite similar to that for the coronary syndromes as described above, with particular consideration given to the status of left ventricular function before and after intervention, the number and extent of coronary artery lesions seen on coronary angiography, and the results of electrocardiographic, echocardiographic, and radionuclide stress testing. In addition, the presence or absence of coronary artery risk factors, and in particular smoking, will influence the level of the final medical rating. The frequency and thoroughness of follow-up care may also influence the medical underwriter in otherwise borderline cases.

Mortality risk assessment is considerably more difficult when only limited information is available. For example, the record from the patient's physician may include, in its assessment of an individual presenting with chest pain, a simple statement such as "possible angina, trial of nitroglycerin initiated" with no further cardiac testing indicated at the time of insurance review. For purposes of risk assessment, this information would commonly be rated as "definite angina" until further clinical follow-up or noninvasive cardiac testing results were made available. Exercise electrocardiograms are, in general, routinely required for applicants requesting large amounts of insurance, although some insurance companies have recently discontinued this requirement. Even for such companies, however, these tests continue to be ordered when indicated by the presence of strong risk factors for CHD or by suggestive clinical presentations documented in the attending physician's medical summary forwarded to the insurance company. An abnormal stress test will, in most cases, result in a recommendation for a less than standard insurance rating. These judgments can be revised, however, based on supplementary evidence provided by the applicant's personal physician, including the results of stress testing with cardiac imaging or the findings on coronary angiography.

HIGH BLOOD PRESSURE

Since 1925, the life insurance industry has published several major comprehensive studies demonstrating increased mortality among insured populations with high blood pressure.[15-17] All of these show a direct, nearly linear relation between systolic and diastolic blood pressure and mortality. The latest such study, the 1979 Blood Pressure Study,[17] dealt in the main with the mortality experience between 1954 and 1972 of 4,350,000 men and women aged 15 to 60. An estimated 530,000 of these men and women had borderline or definite high blood pressure, obviously an unusually large population of people with this diagnosis. During this study's follow-up phase, the first effective (and later routinely) used treatment for high blood pressure was introduced in the United States, and thus the 1979 study, unlike previous studies, was influenced by the increasing use of antihypertensive medication. Mortality ratios for mildly or moderately hypertensive individuals were approximately 20 percent lower than for those with more severe elevations of blood pressure. In a subgroup of applicants who were taking antihypertensive medication at the time of entry and whose blood pressure was well controlled, mortality was closer to normal (mortality ratio in males under 50 years of age at the time of insurance review, 175 percent; in males over 50 years old, 95 percent). Thus, consideration of less than standard or declined insurance applications would generally apply only to patients with untreated hypertension, for noncompliance with prescribed medical regimens, or with hypertension complicated by end-organ damage (ventricular hypertrophy or cerebrovascular or renal disease). Although such developments are often identified in the clinical record, at times additional testing is performed by the insurance company and may include electrocardiography and qualitative urinary protein measurement. On rare occasions, echocardiography may be ordered to assess the degree of cardiac impairment as a result of long-standing hypertension where other clues are ambiguous or contradictory.

VALVULAR HEART DISEASE

The Medical Impairment Study of 1983 provided long-term survival data in the insured population with heart murmurs.[14] Information extracted from that study has been used to provide mortality projections in people with valvular heart disease (Table 104-1). Advances in cardiac diagnostic technology since publication of that study, particularly the development of echocardiographic and Doppler imaging systems, have allowed better definition of valvular pathology. With these and other advances in medical and surgical intervention, it has become more difficult to accumulate data concerning the natural history of unoperated cardiac valvular impairments.[18,19]

Mitral Valve Prolapse

This is, at present, the most common valve condition reported to insurance companies. Although most such patients are offered standard insurance rates, a small subset of patients with frequent chest pain, cardiac arrhythmias, and significant mitral regurgitation may be rated below standard.[20]

Congenital Valvular Heart Disease

Most companies postpone consideration of life insurance for an infant with known or suspected congenital heart disease until the child reaches 1 or 2 years of age. Even then, the history must include a definitively proven diagnosis as well as successful repair of all surgically correctable lesions before the applicant can be considered for life insurance. After successful restoration of normal cardiac hemodynamics, most applicants with congenital defects—including those with atrial and ventricular septal defects, corrected pulmonic stenosis, patent ductus, or coarctation of the aorta (once blood pressure has returned to normal)—can be considered as standard risks.[21] Uninsurable applicants would include most cases of transposition of the great vessels, Ebstein's anomaly, anomalous venous return, and Eisenmenger's syndrome.

Congenital bicuspid aortic valve remains a difficult clinical and underwriting problem.[8] Estimation of prognosis in this impairment when applicants present in the second and third decades of life is often problematic. In the absence of associated echocardiographic left ventricular enlargement, most companies are willing to assess this risk as only mildly substandard. Left ventricular dilatation or hypertrophy seen on echocardiography, or the presence by Doppler analysis of any significant degree of aortic stenosis or regurgitation, will usually require a more substantial rating assessment.

Acquired Valvular Heart Disease

To perform risk assessment in applicants known to have acquired valvular disease, the underwriter will usually first consider the clinical and electrocardiographic findings on the insurance examination. The degree of cardiac enlargement and severity of left ventricular dysfunction will also be considered and will commonly be outlined in the APS. The medical underwriter will also give consideration to the attendant risk of anticipated surgical valve repair or replacement as well as to the risk of lifelong anticoagulation following such surgery. Applicants with valvular disease who show evidence of marked cardiomegaly, especially with prior history or physical examination findings consistent with left-sided or right-sided heart failure, cannot usually be offered life insurance. Other significant complications, such as new-onset atrial fibrillation or systemic embolization, will usually result in a postponement for up to 1 year prior to reconsideration. In most other cases, life insurance can be offered, albeit at rates significantly below standard.[8,19,22] Early follow-up studies of patients undergoing surgical procedures that preserve the native cardiac valve have demonstrated an improvement in perioperative and short-term postoperative survival.[20] As more complete long-term data in patients undergoing these procedures become available, further liberalization of risk penalties may be possible.

OTHER CARDIAC DISEASES OR ABNORMAL LABORATORY FINDINGS

Cardiomyopathy

Insurance risk assessment of the applicant with cardiomyopathy is based on the initial clinical presentation of the patient and the subsequent clinical and physiologic evaluation. Life insurance cannot usually be offered to those diagnosed with dilated (congestive) cardiomyopathy or amyloid heart disease. Systemic diseases with cardiac involvement, such as scleroderma and sarcoidosis, are most often assessed on the basis of overall disease activity and response to therapy. Insurance, however, may be available to many in this latter group of patients, albeit at rates below standard.[8]

Evaluation of the asymptomatic individual with a strong family history of inheritable heart disease or in whom a heart murmur has been discovered may at times produce findings consistent with the obstructive or nonobstructive cardiomyopathies. Complete information concerning the natural history of these impairments is not yet available, particularly in the mild, asymptomatic cases.[23] As a result, most clinical reports are of severe and fatal outcomes, leading many insurance companies currently to decline or rate highly any applicant with an established diagnosis of hypertrophic cardiomyopathy.[8]

Arrhythmias

Most insurance companies will consider applicants who give a history of paroxysmal or chronic atrial arrhythmias in the context of the presence and severity of coexisting cardiac disease. One series in an insured population with paroxysmal atrial tachycardia noted mortality rates quite similar to those of the standard population; the mortality ratio for this condition was estimated to be 73 percent.[14] This can be contrasted with mortality ratios of 700 percent or greater in the presence of atrial fibrillation.[24] In the apparently asymptomatic young individual with new-onset atrial arrhythmias, particular attention is paid to social history and habits such as smoking or excessive alcohol use. In the middle-aged or older applicant, the possibility of asymptomatic coronary heart disease must also be assessed.

Ventricular arrhythmias have remained a difficult risk assessment problem. In many cases, isolated ventricular ectopy can be rated in the context of the underlying cardiac impairment, such as coronary artery or valvular heart disease. Particular attention is directed during the review of the medical record to the results of clinical cardiac evaluation, including stress testing and noninvasive analysis of cardiac function.[25] Survivors of sudden death will, in most cases, be declined—

a situation that may change as long-term data on the benefits of automatic implantable defibrillator (AID) become available. This change would probably apply to those patients in whom AID implantation has been performed as prophylaxis in the setting of high clinical risk for sudden death[26] (see also Chap 33).

Heart Transplantation

Heart transplantation techniques and immunosuppressive strategies have continued to evolve and have been associated with significant improvement in 5- to 10-year survival (see also Chap 25). Most insurance companies would continue to decline such patients, however, until additional long-term survival data became available.

Insurance Laboratory Evaluation Abnormalities

Life insurance underwriting protocols generally include a clinical laboratory panel with a full lipid profile and a resting electrocardiogram. Depending on the age of the applicant and the amount of life insurance requested, additional testing, including stress testing and echocardiography, may be required. In most cases, abnormalities revealed during this laboratory evaluation are fully consistent with the clinical history as reported in the APS. In a minority of applicants, however, medical history is scanty or medical records are unavailable. In such patients, medical underwriting risk assessment is then based primarily on the findings from the insurance physical and laboratory examination. Studies in insured as well as in general populations provide the necessary mortality projections for underwriting risk assessment using these parameters (Table 104-1). The Medical Impairment Study (1983), for example, confirmed the benign prognosis of incidental bradycardia found on insurance examination, with mortality ratios of 73 to 80 percent reported.[14] On the other hand, a relative mortality of 250 percent was found for the finding of tachycardia.[14] Additional information is available to perform risk assessment for findings such as overweight and underweight,[12,27] low serum albumin,[28] and an abnormal electrocardiogram.[29,30]

HEALTH AND DISABILITY INSURANCE

Health insurance continues to evolve in terms of overall cost, quality, and availability within the current environment of health care reform. Further, the delivery of health care under managed care plans by both governmental and employer insurance plans has begun to redefine many aspects of the traditional patient–doctor, doctor–doctor, and doctor–insurer relationship.[3,4]

Within this environment, cardiologists remain vitally important, functioning both as clinical consultants to primary care providers as well as professional consultants to managed care organizations and indemnity insurance plans. This latter role deserves special emphasis. Cardiologists will often be called upon to provide the expertise essential to the determination of the medical necessity and appropriateness of care for health insurance case management and claim review. Assessment of new technology in its evolution from experimental procedure to accepted standard of care is a particularly important responsibility of the insurance consultant in the managed care environment.[31]

The role of the physician in disability determination is more complex, often requiring legal interpretation of disability based on the results of medical data available. The expertise of medical specialists—including physiatrists, physical and occupational therapists, and social workers—may be required for complete evaluation and recommendations. In general, thorough analysis coupled with appropriate goal-directed therapy often allows for return to work in a supportive environment accommodated to individual needs.

For practical purposes, the patient with known heart disease of any kind is going to have difficulty in obtaining standard individual health or disability insurance. As in patients with high blood pressure, however, effective subclassification of patients and effective new therapies may allow insurance to become available to more and more patients who were considered unacceptable insurance risks in the past.

ACKNOWLEDGMENTS

We gratefully acknowledge the work of Dr. M. Irene Ferrer and Dr. Joseph A. Wilber in previous editions of this textbook, from which we drew for this current chapter.

REFERENCES

1. Morton GA. *Principles of Life and Health Insurance.* Atlanta: Life Office Management Association; 1984.
2. Brackenridge RDC, Brown AE. A historical survey of the development of life assurance. In: Brackenridge RDC, Elder WJ, eds. *Medical Selection of Life Risks,* 3d ed. New York: Stockton Press; 1992:3–17.
3. Billi JE, Wise CG, Bills EA, Mitchell RL. Potential effects of managed care on specialty practice at a university medical center. *N Engl J Med;* 1995; 333:979–983.
4. Weisbuch JB, Roberts NK. Without the denominator, where is the quality improvement paradigm in the nation's health care reform? *J Ins Med* 1995; 27:12–14.
5. Pokorski RJ. Mortality methodology and analysis seminar test. *J Ins Med* 1995; 20:20–45.
6. Seltzer F. Choosing a standard for adjusted mortality rates. *Stat Bull* 1996; 77:13–19.
7. Cumming GR, Croxson R. Cardiovascular disorders: Part I. Coronary heart disease. In: Brackenridge RDC, Elder WJ, eds. *Medical Selection of Life Risks,* 3d ed. New York: Stockton Press; 1992:251–323.
8. Croxson RS. Cardiovascular disorders: Part II. Other cardiovascular disorders. In: Brackenridge RDC, Elder WJ, eds. *Medical Selection of Life Risks,* 3d ed. New York: Stockton Press; 1992:324–431.
9. Singer RB. Pitfalls of inferring annual mortality from inspection of published survival curves. *J Ins Med* 1994; 26:333–338.
10. Iacovino JR. A "quick hit" method to assess insurance mortality from a clinical article. *J Ins Med* 1994; 26:317–318.
11. Negus BH. Coronary anatomy and prognosis of young, asymptomatic survivors of myocardial infarction. *Am J Med* 1994; 96:354–358.
12. Clarke RD. Mortality of impaired lives 1964–73 (abstr). *J Inst Act* 1979; 100(part 1). In: Lew EA, Gajewski J, eds. *Medical Risks: Trends in Mortality by Age and Time Elapsed.* New York: Praeger; 1990: 7–119, 120.

13. Jarvis HJ. Development of the diabetic, coronary, and blood pressure pools (abstr). *Cooperation Internationale pour les Assurances des Risques Aggraves,* 1986. In: Lew EA, Gajewski J, eds. *Medical Risks: Trends in Mortality by Age and Time Elapsed.* New York: Praeger; 1990:7–121, 122.

14. Medical Impairment Study 1983 (abstr) I. Boston: Society of Actuaries and Association of Life Insurance Medical Directors of America, 1986. In: Lew EA, Gajewski J, eds. *Medical Risks: Trends in Mortality by Age and Time Elapsed.* New York: Praeger; 1990:6–77, 6–78.

15. *Build and Blood Pressure Study 1959.* Chicago: Society of Actuaries, 1959.

16. *Mortality Investigation of Declined Lives in Japan.* Tokyo: The Life Insurance Association of Japan; 1979.

17. *Blood Pressure Study 1979.* Boston: Society of Actuaries and Association of Life Insurance Medical Directors of America; 1980.

18. Borer JS, Kligfield P. Aortic regurgitation: Making management decision. *ACC Curr J Rev* 1995; 4:30–32.

19. MacKenzie BR. Long-term mortality and complications of Bjork-Shiley spherical-disc valves—A life table analysis. *J Ins Med* 1992; 24:128–132.

20. Jeresaty RM. Mitral valve prolapse: An update. In: Arnold CB, ed. *Transactions of The American Academy of Insurance Medicine: One Hundred and First Annual Meeting.* Tampa, FL: Klay Printing, 1993:24–33.

21. Singer RB, Gajewski J. Cardiovascular diseases I. In: Lew EA, Gajewski J. *Medical Risks: Trends in Mortality by Age and Time Elapsed, 1.* New York: Praeger; 1990:6-30–6-38.

22. Cumming GR. Survival after valve replacement. In: Arnold CB, ed. *Transactions of The America Academy of Insurance Medicine: One Hundred and First Annual Meeting.* Tampa, FL: Klay Printing, 1993:40–55.

23. Elliott PM, Saumarez RC, McKenna WJ. Recent clinical advances in hypertrophic cardiomyopathy. *Heart Failure* 1995; 11:15–25.

24. Gajewski J, Singer RB. Mortality in an insured population with atrial fibrillation. *JAMA* 1981; 245:1540–1544.

25. Chait L. Electrocardiography. In: Brackenridge RDC, Elder WJ, eds. *Medical Selection of Life Risks,* 3d ed. New York: Stockton Press; 1992:433–472.

26. Gorlin R. Cost-effectiveness of ICD therapy for ventricular arrhythmias. *Prim Cardiol* 1995; 21:32–38.

27. *Build Study 1979.* Boston: Society of Actuaries and Association of Life Insurance Medical Directors of America; 1980.

28. Segel L. Serum albumin: "Phoenix" of the blood profile. *On The Risk* 1995; 11:81–83.

29. Rose G, Baxter PJ, Reid DD, McCartney P. Prevalence and prognosis of electrocardiographic findings in middle-aged men (abstr). *Br Heart J* 1978; 40:636–643. In: Lew EA, Gajewski J, eds. *Medical Risks: Trends in Mortality by Age and Time Elapsed.* New York: Praeger; 1990.

30. Ferrer MI: A survey of 19,734 electrocardiograms obtained in insurance applicants. *J Ins Med* 1985; 16:6–13.

31. Privette M, ed. Court overrules HCFA 1986 investigational devices payment policy. *Cardiology* (American College of Cardiology newsletter) 1996; 25:4.

32. Singer RB. Comparative mortality by sex and age in residents of Rochester, Minnesota, with acute myocardial infarction during 1960–1979 (sudden deaths included). *J Ins Med* 1995–96; 27:235–240.

33. Hutchinson R. Additional follow-up of patients with coronary bypass reoperation at Cleveland Clinic. *J Ins Med* 1994; 26:324–328.

105

CARDIAC EVALUATIONS FOR LEGAL PURPOSES

Elliot L. Sagall

SUMMARY

This chapter describes for the physician the scope of the legal areas where issues concerning heart disorder are key elements of the litigation. The following will be discussed: (1) the essential components of a medicolegal cardiac evaluation; (2) the legal and medical concepts, definitions, and criteria for determinations of diagnosis, the time of occurrence of specific cardiac lesions, causality, disability, medical malpractice, prognosis, life expectancy, and other medicolegal assessments; and (3) the formulation of a report of the physician's findings and opinions that will be meaningful and helpful to the legal forum assigned to resolve the disputed medical problems of the case in hand.

The socioeconomic ramifications of heart disease have long been a source of vexing legal as well as medical problems with no easy resolution as yet forthcoming. Nationwide, claims instituted by heart patients and/or their beneficiaries alleging heart disorder, disability, and cardiac death as a workplace or accidental injury or as due to the negligent action of a health care provider are burgeoning in number and scope. The existence of a heart disorder may also be the key issue in the legal determination of an individual's physical capacity to participate as a defendant or witness in a legal proceeding, to drive a motor vehicle, to pilot an airplane, to engage in "substantial" gainful activity, to write a legally valid will or contract, to enable an insurer to recover some of the moneys paid to a worker as compensation for a work-related injury, or to invalidate a life insurance policy. It may be the basis for suit by a handicapped employee against the employer for illegal job discrimination.

The rapidly expanding interrelationships of heart disorders and the law necessarily will involve physicians who examine and treat cardiac patients more and more frequently in the legal processes concerned with resolution of disputed medical aspects of these claims in one or combinations of several roles, as follows: (1) as a *factual* witness called upon to present the history personally received and the findings of physical and other examinations performed and treatment rendered, (2) as an *expert* witness called by one side or the other in the legal dispute to present opinions on the issues under consideration, (3) as an *impartial* witness called by the presiding judicial arbiter for opinion testimony, or (4) as a *defendant* in a suit for medical malpractice.

The question of a cardiac patient's eligibility for certain statutory or common law benefits is basically a legal rather than a medical problem. Accordingly, the ultimate determination is assigned to a court, jury, administrative agency, commissioner, referee, or some other duly appointed person or persons referred to as a "fact finder." The legal resolution of disputed issues of a medical nature, however, almost invariably necessitates consideration of expert medical opinion testimony by the legal fact finder. Crucial areas such as diagnosis, extent, degree, and causation of disability, the existence and time frame of "conscious" pain and suffering, the necessity and reasonableness of past and projected medical and surgical treatment, the charges rendered, the role of preexisting conditions, losses of bodily functions, scarring and disfigurement, reduction of life expectancy, prognosis, whether an "end result" has been reached, and the many other items that determine damages to be awarded to the victim of a cardiac injury or benefits available under covering workers' compensation or other legislative acts, and the causal relationship of each to the alleged injury, generally require medical substantiation or refutation.

LEGAL ACTIONS REQUIRING CARDIAC MEDICAL EVALUATIONS

The spectrum of legal actions where medical evaluations relating to cardiology become key issues is vast, varied, and limited only by the ingenuity and imagination of the claimants' attorneys involved in the case.[1–3] The most common areas include the following:

1. Claims brought under various state workers' compensation statutes and similar federal legislation (e.g., the Federal Longshoremen's and Harbor Workers' Compensation Act and the Federal Employees' Compensation Act), where cardiac disorder disability, treatment, or death is alleged a consequence of a work-related heart "injury" or as an "occupational disease."

2. Tort claims under common law seeking damages for alleged cardiac "injury" due to negligence on the part of another person or persons, including suits for medical malpractice.

3. Claims against insurers, including the Social Security Disability Insurance program, for pensions, covered medical expenses, losses of income, or accidental death benefits resulting from heart disease.

4. Questions as to the fitness of a person with a heart disorder to return to a specific job, to drive a motor vehicle, to operate machinery or other equipment, to pilot an airplane, to participate in a legal proceeding, to serve a prison sentence, or to prepare a will.

5. Claims instituted by insurers alleging preexistent heart disease as a basis for qualifying under "second injury funds" for reimbursement of workers' compensation benefits, the voiding of an insurance contract by reason of the applicant's fraudulent concealment of a preexisting heart disorder, or the nonpayment of special benefits provided in the insurance contract for death or injury due to an accident because of the contribution thereto by a preexistent cardiac disorder.

6. Claims under the newly enabled Americans with Disabilities Act.

Of these, the most commonly encountered are claims that a cardiac disorder is a workplace injury covered by the applicable workers' compensation statute.

Although individual state and federal workers' compensation acts differ somewhat in requirements for eligibility and benefits provided to injured workers and their dependents, with frequent legislative changes as well,[4] the fundamental social principle common to all compensation statutes is that the financial costs of work-related injuries should be assumed to a large extent by the employer as an expense of production and not by the injured worker or the public dole. Without exception, all compensation acts embrace the basic concept that the right to compensation for work-incurred injury is afforded to the injured employee without regard to fault or to demonstrable negligence of the employer. Legal defenses available under common law to employers to avoid or to mitigate liability such as *assumption of the risk* of the job by the employee's acceptance of the employment or *contributory negligence* by the employee or fellow employees (the *fellow servant rule*) are specifically excluded from workers' compensation. In turn, the benefits potentially accruing to an injured employee are generally limited to a portion of the lost wages plus allowances for dependents and reasonable and necessary medical expenses. Items such as pain and suffering and loss of consortium, which may play a large role in the determination of an award to an injured person in actions for tort (negligence) under common law, are excluded.

In workers' compensation, legal liability attaches to the employer (or insurance carrier) for the consequences of an injury, including heart disorder, disability, or death,[1,4–8] demonstrated to have occurred during "the course of" *and* to have arisen "out of" employment—a formula that has aptly been characterized as "deceptively simple and litigiously prolific."

Under some compensation statutes, the basic formula of compensable injury has been modified by specific legislative restrictive definitions that require that the alleged work injury be suffered "by accident" or be due to "unusual stress" or to "stress greater than normal nonwork life" or to have been contributed "substantially" to by the work. In most jurisdictions, an identified time and place of injury must be demonstrated for coverage to apply. And in one compensation act (Wyoming's), further restriction has been placed for legal acceptance of an alleged work-related cardiac injury in that no more than 4 h must elapse between the claimed time of injury and the first clinical manifestations of same.[9]

The imposition of these restrictions indicates a legislative attempt to distinguish alleged work-related heart injuries and consequences thereof from those that occur as a result of the natural progression of the underlying disease—an effort not often successful. Along these lines, one state (Nevada) even went so far as to exclude "coronary thrombosis, coronary occlusion, or any other ailment or disorder of the heart, and any death or disability ensuing therefrom" as an injury by accident arising out of and in the course of employment, except under certain circumstances for firemen, police officers, prison guards, and several other favored categories of public employees.[10]

In many states the concept of "accidental" disability* for purposes of workers' compensation or retirement has been extended for certain named occupational groups, particularly uniformed police and firefighters, by legislative inclusion in the covering statutes of a presumption of job causation for disabling heart disease or hypertension. Although theoretically rebuttable, such presumptions, from a practical viewpoint, generally cannot be overcome, particularly in the absence of generally recognized risk factors for coronary artery disease. The result is that applicants under these laws (commonly referred to as "Heart Laws") often need only establish the existence of a disabling heart disorder or hypertension and

---

* *Accidental disability* retirement applies to a permanent work incapacity as a result of a work-related injury or a hazard experienced in the performance of job duties. *Ordinary disability* retirement applies to permanent work incapacity due to sickness or injury that is not job-related.

Since the financial benefits of an accidental disability retirement generally are significantly greater than those of an ordinary disability retirement in that the awards usually are free from federal and state income tax, applicants for disability understandably seek the greater "take-home" pay of an "accidental disability."

not the causal connection to the employment, although in some jurisdictions, e.g., Massachusetts, the existence of significant nonemployment risk factors such as tobacco abuse may overcome the presumption of job-related causation.

The Massachusetts statute[11] is a typical example:

> Notwithstanding the provisions of any general or special law to the contrary . . . any condition of impairment of health caused by hypertension and heart disease resulting in total or partial disability or death to a uniformed member of a paid fire department or permanent member of a police department . . . shall, if he successfully passed a physical examination on entry into such service which examination failed to reveal any evidence of such condition, be presumed to have been suffered in line of duty, unless the contrary be shown by competent evidence.

The first step in the process of determining eligibility of an applicant for the benefits provided under this statute usually is an examination by a medical panel appointed for the purpose of determining the existence of heart disease or hypertension, the resulting job disability, the permanency thereof, and job causation. The medical panel's findings, however, are only advisory and are not binding on the designated retirement board. Inasmuch as the etiology of most forms of heart disease and hypertension is not currently known, the medical panel, most often, cannot provide "competent evidence" to offset the legislative presumption of job causation embodied in the covering statute, and an accidental disability can be awarded if the medical panel has found the existence of a disabling cardiac or hypertensive condition.

The applicant's probative task under many of these statutes is further eased by the definition of *job disability* as an incapability of the applicant to perform the full range or "all" of the duties, including response to emergency situations inherent in the course of police or firefighting activities.

The legal dependents of deceased Heart Law retirees do not automatically receive death benefits. They usually have the burden of establishing by medical evidence that the death was causally related to the condition for which retirement was awarded. Thus, a statement on a death certificate that the immediate cause of death was "cardiac arrest" is not sufficient to establish legal causation since cardiac arrest is frequently only a terminal event, not necessarily related to a condition of preexistent heart disease or hypertension. However, medical opinion that the death was hastened to some degree, even by as short a period as seconds to minutes, by reason of reduced cardiac and/or coronary reserve related to the underlying heart disorder, although not a direct consequence thereof, may be sufficient to satisfy the legal issue of causality.

Particularly important in adjudication of claims for cardiac injury, disability, or death under workers' compensation and in actions in tort for injury due to negligence is the universal legal acceptance of the common law precept that prior infirmity is no bar to benefits even though the injured person would not have suffered injury, as is the case in most cardiac claims, had there not been underlying heart disease, whether previously known or unknown. Legally, the injured person may be entitled to benefits if it can be shown that the employment or an act of negligence in some way aggravated a preexisting condition to lead to injury, disability, or death *sooner* than would otherwise have been expected during the natural history of the underlying disorder.

Under many state compensation acts, the burden of proving job causation generally assigned to the claimant is eliminated when the worker is found deceased or otherwise medically unable to testify at the place of employment, e.g., as from a stroke. By the statutory adoption of presumption or even *prima facie* evidence of work relationship in such situations, the burden of disproving causation is placed upon the employer. Under the Federal Longshoremen's and Harbor Workers' Compensation Act, a set of presumptions effectively requires that the employer establish noncausation to the job for almost all medical conditions that may render an employee permanently or partially disabled from work.[12]

Under actions in tort in common law, recovery of "damages" may be obtained when the plaintiff or those claiming through the plaintiff can show that the disorder and its consequences arose from or were aggravated by the negligent activity of another (commonly referred to as a *tortfeasor*). Unlike the doctrine of workers' compensation, liability in actions of tort is predicated on fault. To be awarded "damages," the injured party must show (1) that the defendant owed the plaintiff a duty, i.e., the duty to adhere to an accepted standard of medical or other care and the duty to refrain from negligence; (2) that the defendant's conduct breached that duty; (3) that the plaintiff suffered injuries or "harms"; (4) that the defendant's negligent conduct was the proximate cause of the damage (harms) allegedly suffered by the plaintiff; and, generally, (5) that the victim's own negligence did not contribute to his or her harms (the *doctrine of contributory negligence*). Again, susceptibility to injury by reason of preexisting infirmity does not bar recovery.

Actions in tort alleging cardiac injury most commonly arise from motor vehicle accidents where it is claimed that a myocardial contusion, an acute coronary artery occlusion, an acute myocardial infarction, a cardiac death, or some other acute cardiac episode resulted from, or was hastened in occurrence by, mechanical or physical trauma or the psychological consequences of the accident. Most difficult in both medical determinations and legal handling are those situations where it is alleged that a preexisting condition of stable angina pectoris has been aggravated, as evidenced by a change in a preexisting symptom complex, or by an increase in the frequency and severity of attacks after an accident, or when new-onset or unstable angina allegedly occurs after an accident, but with no objective evidence to support the claimed aggravation.

Another commonly encountered vexing medicolegal problem is whether a fatal cardiac episode was "the result of" or "the cause of" an accident—a determination also of import when insurance contracts provide double indemnity or other specified benefits for "accidental" death or injury.

Other frequently encountered actions in tort involving cardiac patients are those in which it is alleged that heart problems have stemmed from trauma or stress subsequent to negligent conduct, such as from falling objects, slipping, and other accidentally induced falls; from exposure to food poisonings; from toxic fumes; from menacing animals; and from long-term psychological "stress" claimed as a consequence of a chronic pain syndrome or from an anxiety-producing situation of an injury, such as the need for repeated hospitalizations or surgery and/or from resulting financial hardships attributable to an original noncardiac injury.

In addition, the Americans with Disabilities Act, initially phased in on July 26, 1992, promises new areas of litigation by prohibiting employment discrimination against an employee "who meets the skill, experience, education and other job-related requirements of a position held or desired, and who, with or without reasonable accommodation, can perform the essential functions of a job."[13]

Medical malpractice suits, often referred to as "professional negligence" suits to lessen the sting, fall within the province of actions in tort and are subject to the same legal considerations affecting all claims for "damages" due to "negligence." In malpractice cases, as with other actions in tort, the aggrieved patient or those acting for the plaintiff have the burden of demonstrating by factual and opinion evidence: (1) that the defendant doctor or other health care provider named in the legal action breached a standard of care owed in an established physician-patient relationship, and (2) that this breach did in fact cause the plaintiff "harm." In evidentiary proof, the plaintiff must define by expert medical opinion the standard of care alleged to have been breached. The plaintiff must further establish the existence of alleged "harms" or "damage" and also must then show, again by expert medical opinion, that the alleged deviation from the acceptable standard of care was the cause of the claimed "damages." Finally, in many jurisdictions it must further be demonstrated that the plaintiff's conduct did not negligently contribute to the claimed harms. Again, unless all these criteria are satisfied, the burden of proof legally assigned to the plaintiff will not be considered to have been met and a directed verdict for the defendant may be ordered by the judge, thereby effectively dismissing the plaintiff's legal action unless later reversed on appeal to a higher court.

In some legal actions, the known existence of a prior cardiac disorder is of importance in the assessment of financial awards. Under the *Second Injury Funds* of the Federal Longshoremen's and Harbor Workers' Compensation Act and of many state workers' compensation acts, some financial relief is afforded the employer or insurer for disability payments to an injured worker if it can be demonstrated that the work incapacity following an accepted or assigned work injury was made substantially greater than would otherwise have been the case because of a known preexistent medical condition or that death would not have occurred absent the preexisting physical impairment.

In other instances, the demonstration of a heart disorder may be of key importance in a legal decision as to whether a worker can return to a prior job that an employer claims involves physical or psychological stress potentially harmful to a person with known heart disease or where the operation of machinery by a person subject to sudden incapacity, as from an acute cardiac dysrhythmia, would endanger others; whether a person should be rejected from driving a motor vehicle, particularly one used in public transportation, or from piloting an airplane; whether a heart patient can participate in a court trial as a defendant or witness or serve a prison term, write a valid will, or be forced to pay alimony or other financial assessment; whether certain items claimed as income tax–deductible medical expenses are medically justified as treatment; whether an insurance contract can be voided because of the applicant's fraudulent concealment of a known cardiac disorder in the original application for the policy; and in other situations where the question of preexistent heart disorder may be of importance for legal and insurance determinations of eligibility for "accidental death" benefits.

A large area of litigation involving heart disorder concerns the many applicants for disability benefits under the Social Security Disability Insurance Program, public welfare programs, the Veterans Administration service- and non-service-related pensions, and privately purchased disability, accident, and health insurance contracts. In most of these situations, the legal issue to be decided is the work capacity of the individual, as defined in the covering statute or insurance contract, based on a demonstrated medical condition, not the question of causation.

Miscellaneous legal actions that may require expert medical opinions on heart disorders and their consequences include determination of the existence and extent of "conscious pain and suffering" as an element of tort "damages," losses of bodily functions under certain workers' compensation statutes, reduction of life and/or work-year expectancy due to a cardiac disorder or worsening thereof, projected reasonable medical expenses of future treatment in a cardiac patient, relationship of a coronary artery bypass grafting or other treatments to a compensable myocardial infarction, prognosis, projected life span, and many other medicolegal issues too numerous to list.

THE CARDIOLOGIST IN THE COURTROOM

It is in the role of an expert witness that cardiologists most often find themselves involved with the legal profession. Any duly licensed physician, however, whether a general practitioner or a specialist, is considered legally qualified to present opinion testimony when the medical issues of the matter in hand are not patently discernible as a matter of common knowledge or are not within the recognized ken of a layperson, as in most cardiac cases. The appropriateness of a particular physician's competency to testify as an expert, however, can be raised by either side to the dispute and put before the court or other legal body involved for its evaluation and acceptance or rejection on the basis of the physician's training and experience as well as demonstrated bias. Once a physician has been accepted as an expert witness, the weight to be attached to the medical conclusions presented is determined by a legally appointed fact-finding body. Since the current state of scientific knowledge in cardiology does not provide, in many instances, clear-cut definitive answers to many of the courtroom medical questions raised in individual cases, there not infrequently is a difference between the conclusions reached by the expert witnesses called by the disputants in the litigation. In such instances, the legal fact finder can adopt as "factual" that opinion believed most likely to conform to the facts in the case and reach a decision on that basis. In some legal actions the fact finder may elect to call on an outside court-appointed physician for an "impartial" opinion, usually subject to cross-examination if requested by either side, but is not bound to accept the opinions so proferred. Thus, almost every legal decision in medical matters has to be supported by the testimony of a physician "expert witness." It is imperative, therefore, that legal decisions should be in accord with the main current of medical thinking and the testimony of the "experts" should be within the boundaries of presently acceptable scientific beliefs and concepts.

The physician who testifies as an expert witness need not have personally examined the claimant nor even have any personal knowledge of the claimant's medical condition prior to or following an alleged incident. The medical expert may reach conclusions solely from a review of the medical records of the claimant and other factual data that have been admitted into evidence. Alternatively, the expert may be presented by either counsel with a hypothetical question, or questions, that contains a set of facts he or she is obliged to accept as true and that are then to be utilized as the factual basis for the conclusions reached and the opinions expressed. The law, however, does require that those facts put forth in hypothetical questions be supported by the evidence presented in the case. Thus, the fact finder cannot adopt the opinion expressed by an expert in answer to a hypothetical question unless the evidence on hand is sufficient to establish legally the truth of the evidence to be assumed as factual. When the factual evidence is conflicting, as is frequently the case, it is within the province of the fact finder to determine which evidence is to be believed and adopted as "factual." The hypothetical question posed to a medical expert in courtroom proceedings need not include all the evidence previously presented in the case. It may be limited to a partisan recital of that evidence most favorable to the proponent's side. However, the adversary party, in cross-examination of the expert, can propose a counter-hypothetical recital of alleged facts to provide data omitted or now added to the original hypothetical question posed in direct examination. The medical expert can then be queried as to whether the newly assumed factual changes or additions alter or modify the opinions previously expressed. In this manner, both parties in the legal dispute have full opportunity to pose to medical experts respective versions of what they believe is factual. Again, however, the ultimate determination of medical issues for legal purposes

rests with the duly appointed fact finder, not with the medical experts.

Generally, it is not sufficient for an expert witness to present conclusions alone without supporting reasoning. The basis on which the opinion rendered rests also may be subject to attack in cross-examination so that the testimony presented can be weighed by the fact finder in reaching a decision as to which of conflicting medical opinions to adopt.

In formulating an opinion, the medical expert must appreciate the degree of certainty required in reaching medical conclusions when such opinions are to be expressed in the courtroom and not in a medical forum per se. The legal system recognizes the current inability of medical science to answer definitively and with absolute certainty many of the medical questions raised in individual cases. Yet the legal body before which the claimant's case ultimately (often after long delay) has been placed for final legal resolution must answer as best it can all the issues raised at the time of trial. The law does not have the luxury of being able to defer resolution of controverted medical issues until medical science has advanced to the point of providing clear-cut answers to the questions on hand. Legal proof, therefore, cannot be equated with scientific proof. Although pure science seeks absolute certainty or positive proof before reaching a determination, legal decisions necessarily are far less exacting in their demands. In civil cases, decisions are based primarily upon such standards as a *preponderance of the evidence* and *clear and convincing evidence,* whereas in criminal matters, the requirements are more stringent, usually *beyond a reasonable doubt.*

For answers to medical questions, the law generally requires that these be expressed in terms of *reasonable medical certainty* or *probability* rather than mere *possibility.* In essence, this means that the conclusions reached by an expert are believed to be *more likely than not* true with a tilting of the balance scale to as little as 50.1 percent versus 49.9 percent sufficient to determine the courtroom outcome, although such a difference would not be acceptable to a body of scientists. In accord with this legal philosophy, *reasonable medical certainty* generally means reasonable *legal* certainty—a far less exacting criterion of proof than that required for rigid medical *scientific* certainty.

In cases involving cardiac claims, as in most civil cases, the burden of proof generally is placed on the claimant, who must show by a preponderance of supporting evidence, including expert opinion when necessary, that the allegations are true. For example, in a claim alleging a cardiac disorder and its consequences as a workplace injury, the claimant must provide the fact finder with sufficient supporting medical expert testimony attesting not only to the existence of a cardiac disorder but also to its causal relationship to some element of the employment; otherwise the claim will fail. A claimant's burden of proof generally is not met when a medical expert merely acknowledges the *possibility* of the truth of the allegations rather than asserting their *probability.* Phraseology frequently employed by physicians in medical reports and testimony such as "may," "could," or "might have" serves no useful purpose in the courtroom. Additionally, the burden of proof is not met, nor is it sustained, when the medical supportive conclusions are shown to be based on speculation, surmise, or conjecture rather than on *reasonable medical certainty* or *probability,* or when the medical expert admits that acceptance and denial of the allegations are *equal* possibilities that cannot be differentiated. As pointed out earlier in this chapter, under many workers' compensation acts, when a worker is found dead or unable to testify (e.g., poststroke) at the place of employment, the burden of disproving causation by the job is placed on the employer. The Federal Longshoremen's and Harbor Workers' Compensation Act even goes a step further by stating that "In any proceeding for the enforcement of a claim for compensation under this Act it shall be presumed, in the absence of substantial evidence to the contrary. . . . That the claim comes within the provisions of this Act. . . ."[12] And in actions for medical malpractice the burden of proof of lack of causation by negligence may be shifted to the defendant health care provider when the doctrines of *res ipsa loquitur* ("the thing speaks for itself") and *the captain of the ship,* i.e., the operating room surgeon, become applicable.

When expert medical opinions presented by the respective litigants contradict or conflict, the fact finder must choose between them with the choice subject to reversal on appeal to a higher court only when contrary to the weight of the evidence or the result of an error in legal procedure, as with acceptance of evidence inadmissible under the law. Since reached by a lay fact finder, often without adequate scientific background, legal decisions in many instances appear contrary to the main current of medical/scientific thinking.

THE MEDICOLEGAL CARDIAC EVALUATION

Medical examinations and evaluations performed specifically for legal and insurance reasons necessarily emphasize aspects of the medical situation not customarily addressed by physicians, since the primary purpose of such evaluations is the answering of legal questions and not the providing of medical care.

The scope of potential medicolegal questions where heart disorder is germane to the litigation is too vast and varied for detailed discussion within the constraints of this chapter. Certain inquiries, however, are fundamental to most claims alleging cardiac injury, disorder, dysfunction, or death and warrant further consideration and elaboration. These are (1) the cardiac diagnosis that is to be accepted legally as established in a given claimant; (2) the time of onset of each specific cardiac lesion or dysfunction, particularly those with legal import; (3) the causal relationship, if any, between the factor or factors under legal examination and the cardiac disorder found or some aspect thereof; (4) the medical determination of the impairment to be assessed on the basis of the claimant's overall cardiovascular status and, more specifically, to each component of the cardiac condition that has legal significance in its derivation; and (5) the medical consid-

erations in allegations of professional negligence in the physicians' and/or other health care providers' handling of a cardiac patient as the basis of a claim for resulting harm. Additionally, in some legal actions arising under workers' compensation and some insurance policies, questions as to the role of preexisting disease or infirmity in contributing to the covered impairment or death may be of paramount import in determining eligibility for benefits as well as the amount of benefits to be paid by the employer or insurer.

Defining the Cardiac Diagnosis

From the medical viewpoint, the diagnosis is the foundation on which the treatment of the patient is constructed. From the legal viewpoint, the diagnosis is the foundation upon which many decisions and rulings concerning issues of causation, eligibility for disability and retirement pensions, awards for damages, and many other matters arising in the litigation on hand are made.

Although the diagnosis, in actuality, has to be made by a physician based upon medical data, legally it is considered to be but one of the various factual determinations within the province of the fact-finding body assigned to adjudicate the case.

The diagnosis reached by a physician after the gathering, reviewing, and studying of the medical data is, in essence, merely an opinion based on the individual examiner's specialized training, study, experience, and interpretation of the medical findings. As such, it is open to question both medically and legally as to reasonableness, accuracy, and completeness. Since the diagnostic conclusions in individual instances reached by a medical examiner may not be concurred in by other physicians evaluating the same data, opinions expressed in court concerning the diagnosis, as with all medical conclusions, are subject to interrogation by counsel during cross-examination.

The cardiac diagnosis should be established in each instance as fully as possible in terms of (1) an *etiologic* diagnosis that describes the underlying disease processes basically responsible for the structural and functional disorders found in the patient/claimant, (2) an *anatomic* diagnosis that describes the specific structural abnormalities (lesions) found in the cardiovascular examination, and (3) a *physiologic* diagnosis that describes the resulting disturbances of cardiovascular action and function. These should be delineated in generally accepted terminology, such as recommended by the Criteria Committee of the New York Heart Association in that committee's publication, "Nomenclature and Criteria for Diagnosis of the Heart and Great Vessels."[14]

Because of varying connotations and implications, nonspecific terms, such as *heart attack, coronary, mild or massive heart attack,* and *heart disease,* without adequate qualification as to specific meaning, should not be employed in the cardiac evaluator's written report or testimony. Similarly, umbrella terms, such as *unstable angina, preinfarction angina, acute coronary deficiency,* and *acute coronary insufficiency,* at times popular in medical jargon to designate certain symptom complexes encountered during the course of ischemic heart disease, should be avoided unless they are precisely defined (see Chap. 46).

The *etiologic diagnosis* should be reached after consideration of both the structural and functional disturbances found. If two or more etiologic bases for a person's heart disorder are present, each should be listed. Legally, the identification of the etiologic basis of a cardiac disorder or disorders becomes important in a causality assessment where an aggravation or worsening of a preexistent cardiac condition is claimed as a "personal injury" and must be differentiated from the expected natural progression of an underlying cardiac disorder and in legal actions where an estimation of life expectancy is of importance in determining awards for "damages" or in settlement proceedings.

The *anatomic diagnosis* comprises that component of the total cardiac diagnosis that describes the specific structural lesions present in the heart and great vessels. A complete description of the anatomic alterations often constitutes an important aspect of the legal determinations of a cardiac "personal injury" and of disability. Thus, for example, there may be considerable differences in the benefits or awards available legally for the sustaining of an episode of prolonged ischemic cardiac pain when diagnosed as an intermediate coronary syndrome attack with no documented new myocardial damage or when diagnosed as acute myocardial necrosis with resulting permanent new or added heart damage and a change in the preexistent condition.

Anatomic lesions of the heart and great vessels frequently can be delineated clinically on the basis of the history, the findings of physical examination, and the results of specialized cardiac diagnostic studies. Certain anatomic lesions, e.g., a coronary artery thrombotic occlusion, however, cannot be diagnosed with reasonable certainty unless established by coronary angiography or other reliable objective means. Thus, diagnoses of *coronary thrombosis* and *microscopic myocardial necrosis,* terms not infrequently encountered in cardiac medicolegal reports and expert testimony, should usually be reserved for the radiologist or pathologist. When more than one anatomic abnormality is found, each should be included in the final diagnosis.

The *physiologic diagnosis* specifies the alterations in cardiovascular dynamics and function that have resulted from the cardiac pathology. The physiologic diagnosis includes a description of the cardiac rhythm and whether of normal or abnormal mechanism; disturbances in cardiac impulse conduction; disturbances in supravalvular, valvular, or subvalvular function; malfunctions of prostheses, homografts, and cardiac pacemakers; disturbances in myocardial pump action; disturbances in intravascular pressures; abnormal communications (shunts) in the heart or great vessels; and the anginal syndromes.

A cardiac diagnosis presented in the courtroom should be supported, wherever possible, by objective measures of cardiac structure and function, where indicated and within limitations of practicality and risk. A diagnosis based solely on a claimant's history, although in many cases the only diagnostic tool available to the medical expert, is not on secure grounds and, accordingly, is subject to strong attack on cross-examination. Many symptoms common to cardiac disorders, in particular, chest pain, shortness of breath on exertion, palpitations, and fatigue, are not pathognomonic for heart disorder since they are commonly found in a variety of noncardiac conditions. Symptoms alone are difficult to evaluate, since they may be exaggerated by self-serving or other purposes. Symptoms, per se, also defy quantifying. On the other hand, the severity of symptoms in cardiac patients often does not correlate with the degree and severity of the found impairment of heart structure and function, and some cardiac disorders, e.g., a "silent" myocardial infarction, may result in no, minimal, or nonspecific symptoms.

The physician performing a cardiac evaluation for legal purposes must determine whether the patient-claimant had heart disease prior to the alleged potentially harmful exposure under legal consideration and, if so, whether there was a change in the preexistent cardiac status after the exposure. If a change is found, the physician must then define its nature, degree, and extent, whether permanent or temporary. In this regard it is important to distinguish between a demonstrated structural change in a preexisting heart disorder, e.g., a coronary artery occlusion by thrombosis or a rupture of a heart valve or other part of the heart, and an alleged hastening of an expected consequence, e.g., an acute myocardial infarction, by reason of the progression of an underlying process of atherogenesis in the coronary artery tree.

Diagnoses, as with other medical opinions, presented to a legal forum must be established in terms of reasonable medical certainty, which means in terms of *probability. Possible, potential, or suspected* heart disorder has no place in the courtroom or in other legal determinations.

Timing the Onset of Cardiac Lesions and Dysfunctions

Determining the time of onset of a specific cardiac pathology or dysfunction is an essential part of many cardiac medicolegal evaluations, often the crux of an issue of causation or of eligibility for the benefits of an insurance contract. Because of the vagaries of clinical presentations, individual differences in response to and manifestations of illness, and the frequent initial "silent" development of many cardiac pathologies with no symptoms or abnormal signs evident until the process has progressed to an advanced state, the current methodology frequently prevents timing the onset of cardiac pathologies and/or dysfunctions within the precise framework sought by the law. Additionally, the sequence of development of the pathophysiologic process underlying various pathologies cannot be delineated. Yet, though difficult, the time of onset of cardiac lesions and dysfunctions must be defined by the cardiac examiner as best as it can be within frameworks of reasonable medical certainty and probability.

The time of occurrence of a single episode of angina pectoris is fairly easy to pinpoint since, in most cases, the symptoms of the attack are clear-cut and abrupt in onset, thereby allowing a reasonably accurate timing of the commencement of the individual attack. Similarly, the end of the attack is evidenced by the disappearance of symptoms, although some degree of subsiding silent myocardial ischemia may be present for a short time thereafter.

Delineating the time of onset of an episode of myocardial infarction is more difficult because of variable clinical presentations. The classic textbook presentation of sudden crushing anterior chest pain associated with profuse diaphoresis, dyspnea, weakness, and other cardinal symptomatology is a generally acceptable index of the occurrence at that time of significant discrete acute myocardial tissue necrosis, although the possibility that some degree of myocardial necrosis has occurred previously (silently or with atypical manifestations) cannot be excluded. In some patients, the process of acute myocardial infarction is an ongoing ischemic/necrotic process that may start minutes to hours to several days prior to the initial appearance of recognizable symptoms, signs, and laboratory or electrocardiographic abnormalities. In some patients, an acute myocardial infarction, although evident at a later date on an electrocardiogram or at postmortem examination, is clinically silent at the time of occurrence. In other patients, the clinical picture is one of waxing and waning ischemic symptoms or signs over the course of one or more days (a state currently popularly referred to as *unstable angina* or *preinfarction angina*), with or without culmination in a bout of classic, prolonged chest discomfort that heralds the infarction of a larger discrete mass of myocardium. In still other patients, the first anginal attack (*new-onset angina*) may actually represent an acute myocardial infarction. And in patients with previous angina pectoris, an acute myocardial infarction may be manifested by an anginal attack of greater severity and duration or of radiation and location different from that previously experienced. And in some 15 to 25 percent of cases, the occurrence of an acute myocardial infarction is clinically silent and cannot be pinpointed as to time of happening (see Chap. 47).

Thus, the time of occurrence of an acute myocardial infarction, if determinable, does not necessarily reflect the time of onset of underlying atherosclerotic coronary heart disease or the time of initiation of a culprit thrombotic coronary artery occlusion or of other pathophysiologic processes that may result in infarction of the myocardium.

Indexes, sometimes of help in the attempt to time the onset of an acute myocardial infarction, may be provided by the time of appearance of certain signs, laboratory findings, and the time sequence of development of electrocardiographic changes during the acute phases of the illness. Thus, a retrospective correlation of the time of enzyme results with the clinical picture may permit a rough extrapolated determination of the time of occurrence of infarction. Additional guides for such temporal extrapolations, but not as useful or as precise as serial cardiac enzyme and isoenzyme determinations, include the times of initial and peak leukocytosis, the development of postmyocardial infarction fever, the occurrence of a pericardial friction rub or of a rupture of infarcted myocardium, and other potential concomitants of an acute myocardial infarction. From the viewpoint of the pathologist, the time of onset of a process of myocardial infarction can be roughly estimated by correlation of the gross and microscopic postmortem appearance of the involved tissue with that generally expected (on the basis of accumulated experience and knowledge) at different time periods after the beginning of the attack.

Unless otherwise determinable, the time of onset of a cardiac arrhythmia generally is accepted as the time of occurrence of identifying symptoms such as palpitation or initial awareness of heartbeat irregularity or of a sudden collapse, as with a cardiac arrest due to ventricular tachycardia or fibrillation.

The time of onset of coronary atherosclerotic, valvular, hypertensive, and most other heart disorders generally cannot be determined medically with any greater accuracy other than that the underlying etiologic condition must have been present for some time (usually only measurable in months or years) prior to the initial clinical manifestations or abnormality that led to its detection.

The occurrence of sudden collapse, acute pulmonary edema, cardiogenic shock, or severe pain provides an index of the time of rupture of an aortic aneurysm or of a cardiac valve, papillary muscle, chordae tendineae, or infarcted myocardium. However, the commencement of the pathophysiologic processes underlying such rupture most often cannot be pinpointed with accuracy because of subtle or silent initial clinical manifestations for a variable period of time preceding the end-stage catastrophic event.

Assessment of Causality

The determination of causation is vital to legal actions in which a heart disorder or its consequences is claimed as a compensable "work injury," as an injury due to "negligence," or as an "accident" under an insurance contract in which benefits are specifically provided for injury, disability, or death due to an "accident" rather than the result of "illness."

In general, legal claims and medical acceptance of cardiac injury or sudden cardiac death generally allege as *a* or *the* cause (1) an isolated, specifically identified incident, event, accident, trauma, or exposure; (2) a complication of medical or surgical treatment or other alleged so-called triggers[5,6] or (as in a malpractice action) a negligent treatment or negligent failure to institute indicated treatment; (3) a set of repetitive, cumulative factors[7] that, although subliminal individually, have combined in additive effect to produce cardiovascular harm, such as repeated subthreshold inhalation of carbon monoxide or a recent period of days, weeks, or months of mounting physical or psychological stress as might be associated with unduly long work hours, an impending deadline or quota, trying business conditions, a forthcoming surgical procedure, or some other presumed stressful happenings; (4) long-term "overall" job or situational physical or psychological "stress"; or (5) a combination of one or more of the preceding.[6,7]

In such actions, the claimant must first establish the existence of a cardiac disorder that can be accepted as an "injury" and the causal connection thereof to an item with attached legal liability and then establish a causal connection between such injury and the alleged harmful consequences (disability, medical and surgical treatment and diagnostic expenses, pain and suffering, death, and other items of "harms") for which benefits are claimed. The claimant usually has the further burden of disproving any contributions to the alleged harms from intervening causes or from personal negligence should such charges be raised by the defendant.

In disputed issues involving causality questions in medical disorders, the fact finder in reaching the legal decision must rely on the evidence put forth by the respective litigants, particularly expert medical opinion testimony. Physicians presenting such testimony in cause-and-effect assessments must appreciate the different weights assigned by the legal profession to the various elements that comprise a legal causality determination from those assigned by the medical profession to a pure medical assessment of causality (see Table 105-1). Because of differences in training and orientation backgrounds, causation often means one thing to a physician and quite another to an attorney, judge, or administrative hearing official. On occasions, medical opinion testimony based on traditional medical concepts of causality differs dramatically from answers based primarily on legal concepts utilized by a fact finder in reaching courtroom decisions.

The differences between the medical and legal approaches to solving causality problems are many.[15–20] The physician, for example, in viewing a patient's medical problems, instinctively searches for the basic cause or causes underlying the overall disorder, whereas legal and judiciary professionals generally limit their concern to the one or more items under legal scrutiny as an "injury," independent of other causes. The physician generally defines *cause* as the production of a new condition or a new pathology or dysfunction, whereas the law in its definition accepts the aggravation of an underlying disorder by the worsening, hastening, or acceleration of its progression to lead to impairment, bodily harm, or death sooner than otherwise would have occurred during the natural history of the preexisting condition without the claimed noxious exposure. The law thus includes in its framework of causation not only the production of a *de novo* condition but also the "triggering" or "proximate precipitation" of a new stage of pathology or of a new dysfunction in an underlying disorder and the worsening of an ongoing pathologic process.

Physicians are reluctant to assign causal responsibility when the degree of aggravation of a preexisting condition is small in overall relationship to the extent of the underlying abnormality or when the degree of hastening of an inevitable end result is minor in relation to the entire clinical condition. The law, on the other hand, emphasizes the fact of hastening

TABLE 105-1

MEDICAL VERSUS LEGAL EMPHASIS IN CAUSALITY ASSESSMENT

Medical Emphasis	Legal Emphasis
The etiologic bases of a disease or disorder	The proximate ("triggering") cause of an injury, disability, or death
The causes of disease	A cause of injury, disability, or death
The producing cause of the entire disorder	An aggravation of a preexisting condition
The key role of preexisting disease	"The victim is taken as found," not as a normal, healthy person, but subject to whatever existing medical disorders were present at the time of exposure
The end result was inevitable because of the expected progression of the preexisting disease	A determination of whether the end result was hastened, not the time amount of hastening
The degree of aggravation was small in the light of the entire clinical picture	The crux is aggravation, not degree
The alleged causative element(s) not unique or unusual	The key element is the causative element(s), not the characteristics
The multiplicity of causes and their interrelationships	The key is the causative element(s) under legal scrutiny, independent of other coexisting or interrelating causes
Scientific proof of causation required	Establishment of causation generally is defined in terms of *reasonable medical certainty,* i.e., *probable vs. possible, more likely than not,* a 50.1% chance of relationship
Equally consistent theories of causation acceptable in differential diagnosis and choice of therapies	Equally consistent theories of causation do not satisfy standards for legal proof
The ultimate answer to causations can be deferred, pending new scientific advances	The issue of causation must be decided legally when presented
In assessment of damages (harms), there should be an apportionment of the role of each causative element	Generally, a total responsibility is assigned for the end result, if such is deemed due to a legally indicated exposure

Source: Adapted from Sagall and Reed,[3] Sagall,[18] and Danner and Sagall.[19]

or aggravation, not the quantitative aspects. The crux of legal causation thus is the occurrence of an aggravation of an underlying disorder, not the degree to which it was aggravated, or the hastening of an end result to cause it to occur sooner than otherwise would have been the case, not the extent to which it was hastened.

Physicians in their assessments of causation are particularly impressed that the alleged injurious results, as is true in most cardiac cases, would not have occurred in the absence of a preexisting disorder that rendered the patient susceptible to harm from the alleged exposure. Legal fact finders, however, see it as immaterial that the event in question would not have caused injurious consequences had the victim been in good or average health. In all *personal injury* legal actions, the victim is "taken as he is found." Preexisting infirmity does not bar legal recovery, nor is it an acceptable excuse to relieve a defendant from legal responsibility or to mitigate the damages to be assessed. An illustration is the case of the proverbial "straw that broke the camel's back." To the physician, the proverb emphasizes the obvious predisposition to break down because of existing overload. The physician thus assigns the cause of the camel's collapse to the prior strain on his back, not to the added straw. The law, on the other hand, asserts that although loaded to the breaking point, the back had held up without breaking. Accordingly, the added straw must be viewed as the cause of the collapse and the person who placed the straw on that loaded back as legally responsible for the consequences. Most often, the assignment of legal liability in such situations is made without attempt to apportion a percentage of harm between the triggering straw and the preload.

Unfortunately, the many current deficiencies in medical knowledge concerning the etiology and pathogenesis of most cardiac disorders and the limitations of presently available cardiac diagnostic testing procedures often prevent medical science from defining precisely the complete cardiac diagnosis, the nature and extent of the underlying pathology, the pathophysiologic mechanisms that have led to the end result, the sequence in which pathologic lesions have developed, the time of onset of certain lesions, and the answers to the many medical questions that may be of key importance in the legal matter on hand. The medical determination of causation is further made difficult because the very nature of most cardiac disorders categorized legally as *personal injuries* does not, in contrast to lesions such as burns or lacerations, present clinical or pathologic features pathognomonic of trauma or of an external cause. Thus, the question of whether some identified external element or stress played a contributory or precipitating role in their development or whether the disorder found stemmed from the natural, expected progression of an underlying cardiac disease unrelated to and unaffected by the item under legal scrutiny quite frequently is not amenable to clearcut, noncontroversial answers or to overall causality guidelines or criteria.

Similarly, differences in the provisions of the individual state and territorial workers' compensation acts under which most cardiac claims arise, differences in legal philosophy among the many persons assigned fact-finding roles in disputed litigation, subtle differences in fact situations of claims that are seemingly identical, and the often diametrically opposed medical conclusions presented in a given case by equally competent medical experts preclude the formulation of legal standards of causality that can be applied uniformly to cover all instances. Accordingly, each case must be decided, both medically and legally, on its own set of facts and medical testimony.

Certain precepts, however, should govern medical assessments of causality in cardiac claims. For an alleged causal connection to be accepted in a cardiac case as *probable* or with *reasonable medical certainty,* the following criteria should be satisfied:

- The cardiac diagnosis should be delineated completely and established, as far as reasonably possible, by objective means, and those portions of the cardiac condition under consideration as potential "injuries" specified.
- The alleged causative element presented for legal consideration should be one that is currently recognized medically and scientifically as capable, under appropriate circumstances, of producing the heart disorder or injury found.
- Conversely, the cardiac condition or dysfunction diagnosed must be one generally recognized medically as a possible resultant of the alleged harmful exposure.
- The time interval elapsing between the alleged noxious exposure and the medically manifest evidence of heart damage or dysfunction must be consistent with currently accepted scientific concepts of pathogenesis.
- The proposed cause-and-effect relation, although not always fully explainable in terms of present-day scientific knowledge, must still be consistent with current scientific concepts.

As an aid to medical assessment of causality in coronary artery heart disease and its ischemic sequelae, which is the cardiac disorder that is by far the most frequent basis of heart claims, the reader is referred to "Report of the American Heart Association's Committee on Stress, Strain, and Heart Disease."[20] Although originally published in 1977, the conclusions of this committee, supported by more recent studies,[21–32] are currently valid with only minor modification, have not been supplanted by any other formal set of medical causality guidelines, and are generally accepted by the medical profession.

The conclusions currently pertinent to a medical assessment of causality in cardiac claims are summarized below:

- Long-term repetitive physical effort, such as is inherent in many occupations, cannot currently be regarded medically as a causative element in the development of atherosclerotic coronary heart disease. Such activity, if playing any role in this disease process, is believed beneficial by preventing or slowing the rate of atherosclerotic progression.[20]

- Long-term repeated physical effort of work and/or non-work activities in persons with underlying heart disease theoretically may hasten the development of congestive heart failure by reason of the additional work load imposed upon an already weakened heart. It is not possible within the present state of medical knowledge, however, to determine in any given heart patient when congestive heart failure would have occurred as the result of the expected natural progression of the underlying cardiac disorder in the absence of such exertional efforts; hence in these situations a causative or aggravating role to such stress most often cannot be assigned with "reasonable medical certainty."[20]

- Continued, psychological emotional stress and job demands to which an individual may have been subjected over a protracted period of time, though commonly accepted by the public and many physicians, have not been established scientifically as a causative or worsening agent in the genesis or acceleration of atherosclerotic disease,[20–36] although the possibility of some contribution cannot be excluded in individual cases.

- A single, isolated, identified physical or emotional stress in individuals rendered susceptible to harm therefrom by reason of preexistent heart disease, whether or not previously known or symptomatic, if of sufficient intensity and duration, is capable of eliciting adverse cardiac responses that, in turn, can "trigger" or hasten certain cardiac lesions and dysfunctions such as an attack of angina pectoris, a myocardial infarction, a sudden cardiac dysrhythmia, sudden cardiac death, rupture of a diseased cardiac structure, coronary artery vasospasm, an acute coronary artery occlusion, flash pulmonary edema, and a bout of congestive heart failure.[20–32]

- The shorter the time interval between the exposure of an individual to a potentially noxious stimulus and the appearance of clinical or pathologic evidence of new heart disease or dysfunction, the more likely there is a causal relationship between the two. Conversely, the farther apart in time, the less likely is a cause-and-effect relation.[20]

- The exposure of a person with underlying heart disease to a stimulus potentially capable of eliciting harmful cardiovascular responses does not necessarily mean that such will be elicited, even when the exposure would be advised against medically because of the possibility of ensuing harm[20].

The elements most often accepted by workers' compensation adjudicators in cardiac cases as work-related *competent-producing* causes of injury, disability, or death are identified incidents of physical work effort (usual, unusual, or of a degree greater than accustomed nonwork exertion, depending on the covering compensation act requirements); adverse work environments, e.g., excessive heat or cold, noxious fumes; an acute psychological trauma such as a heated argument or a sudden fright; an accidental electric shock; a severe nonpenetrating blow or other mechanical injury to the chest cage; and adverse cardiac reactions to medical, surgical, corrective, and rehabilitative therapy of an industrial injury not originally involving the cardiovascular system.

Nationwide, burgeoning claims under workers' compensation alleging illnesses such as coronary heart disease, hypertension, stroke, gastrointestinal disorders, and neuropsychiatric states as initiated or worsened by overall job-related "stress" are straining the workers' compensation system.[36] Frequently cited as "harmful" to the cardiovascular system are adverse mental reactions stemming from harassments from superiors, frustrations from dealing with the public, tensions created by imposed deadlines and quotas, boredom or excessive responsibility in job duties, threats of job termination or changes, insufficient vacations and time off, changing work shifts, long work hours, ongoing business financial problems, and others too numerous to list.

In the cardiac "stress" cases that have reached state supreme court levels on appeals, the decisions have been mixed and have not established uniform case law precedents. For example:

- In New Hampshire, medical opinion that the continuing "stress" of a failing business over a 2-year period did *not* cause the fatal myocardial infarction suffered by the owner on a Sunday morning at home was upheld and compensation to his widow denied.[37]

- On the other side of the coin, a Rhode Island trial commissioner's denial of compensation to the widow of a newspaper sports editor who suffered a fatal cerebral hemorrhage at home was reversed. The court concluded that medical testimony that the deceased was suffering from high blood pressure of the type that would rise whenever he was under stress plus evidence that the decedent attended a professional football game earlier in the day of his death that placed him "under pressure" to meet a reporting deadline were sufficient to support the claim that his death that night was due to a cerebral hemorrhage resulting from aggravation of his preexisting hypertension.[38]

- In Colorado, the denial of compensation by the Industrial Commission to the widow of a fire department lieutenant with preexisting mitral valve prolapse and hypertension who died at home on the tenth day of a vacation absence from work was vacated. As grounds for the reversal and for an award of compensation, the court concluded that uncontroverted testimony from the fire chief, coworkers, and widow that the decedent had suffered a great deal of cumulative tension and frustration relating to his being overlooked in favor of junior firefighters for promotion and to his differing from superiors in department training and communication policies with no other significant sources of mental stress in his life qualified this "stress" legally as an injury or occupational disease arising out of and in the course of employment. On this basis, the court remanded the claim to the referee to make specific findings whether the job-related stress was the proximate cause of the death as was testified to by the decedent's doctor, who opined that the likely cause of death was an irregular heart rhythm that, when combined with a preexisting mitral valve prolapse and job-related stress, resulted in a fatal arrhythmia. The doctor further testified that the imminence of the decedent's return to work may have exacerbated his stress level, thereby increasing his hypertension just prior to his scheduled return to work, and was a contributory cause of his death.[39]

- In Connecticut, the court affirmed a commissioner's decision that unjust criticism of a bank employee on a number of occasions by superiors so aggravated her condition of obstructive coronary disease as to lead to a continued work disability from angina pectoris from intermittent coronary artery spasm still unrelieved by a coronary artery bypass surgery some 2 years later, despite the ruling out of an acute myocardial infarction during hospitalization shortly after the harassments and the presence of multiple coronary atherosclerosis risk factors of long-standing, including extensive cigarette smoking, obesity, and a positive family history of premature coronary disease.[40]

So-called major risk factors, such as cigarette smoking, elevated blood cholesterol, diabetes mellitus, hypertension, and positive family history of coronary disease, are often put forth by defense counsels as mitigating or alternative, not of legal liability, elements arguing against the claim's validity in regard to questions of causality assessments in coronary heart disease. Conversely, in a New Hampshire Supreme Court decision, the absence of identified risk factors in a firefighter with catheter-documented coronary atherosclerotic disease was deemed to support the *prima facie* presumption in the state's Workers' Compensation Act that heart disease in firefighters is occupationally related.[41]

In evaluating the role of risk factors in cardiac claims, it should be recognized that risk factors are of importance primarily in epidemiologic studies applicable to groups, not to an individual. For any given person, the presence or absence of medical background risk factors does not necessarily indicate the premature development of this condition or an escape therefrom. Thus, although statistically related to the presence of coronary heart disease, generally accepted risk factors for coronary atherosclerosis cannot be viewed medically as legally causative elements in the production of the disease. In any consideration of so-called personality types A and B as risk factors, it should further be recognized that, in addition to the practical impossibility of definitively separating human beings categorically into type A or type B personalities, the role of personality type, if any, in the pathogenesis of coronary atherosclerosis has not been scientifically established and, therefore, should not be presented to a court of law as within the realm of medical probability or reasonable medical certainty.

Additionally, in medical causality assessments in atherosclerotic coronary heart disease, although physical stress may be definable quantitatively to some degree, emotional stress defies quantitative measurement. Nor can presumed long-term

effects of an occupational endeavor or a presumed unpleasant life situation incident be separated from similar effects inherent in day-to-day life and interpersonal contacts. Finally, the effects of so-called psychological stress are primarily, as with beauty, in the eyes of the beholder. A psychological situation that may be upsetting and possibly harmful to one person may be but an exhilarating, stimulating challenge to another.

Not all cardiac claims require legal causality determinations. For example, in claims instituted under the Social Security Disability Insurance Program, the primary issue is whether the applicant is unable to engage in substantial gainful employment as defined in the covering statute, not the medical or legal relationship of the disability to a particular causative element. Similarly, eligibility for benefits in most privately acquired insurance contracts is based on the fact of disability, generally independent of cause unless the applicant must demonstrate that disability stems from an "accident" rather than an illness, in which case the issue of causation has to be established.

Evaluation of Disability

Evaluation of disability for legal and insurance purposes is a complex process necessarily involving more than one professional discipline. The evaluation generally requires interrelating the fields of medicine, law, insurance, judiciary, vocational counseling, and rehabilitation. As a minimum, a cardiac disability evaluation is twofold: first, a medical assessment must be made of the extent of the patient-claimant's impairment in terms of what the patient can and cannot do and what the patient should not do by reason of the cardiac disorder and, second, there must be a legal translation of the medically determined impairments into the specific definition of disability incorporated in the applicable statute or insurance contract, the latter often involving questions of total versus partial disability, permanent disability, house-confining, and other qualifying or restrictive adjectives that may affect benefits.

As with most medicolegal evaluations, contested claims for disability benefits are decided by legal or administrative fact finders, with the physician's role limited to providing the fact finder with medical data and opinion testimony that can be utilized in reaching a conclusion.

As a minimum, the physician examining a patient-claimant for disability evaluation purposes should attempt to determine the following:

- The full cardiac diagnosis, including etiology when known, and all anatomic and functional derangements found, together with the supporting clinical evidence.
- The clinical manifestations of the disorder revealed by the medical examination, including all subjective complaints and, more important, all objective confirmatory findings that support the presence of a heart disease or disorder medically recognized as capable of producing the symptoms alleged as the basis for disability.
- The restrictions in the patient's physical activities and mental capacity that have resulted from the disorders found

in terms of limitations of walking, stair climbing, standing, sitting, reaching, lifting, bending, pushing, pulling, gripping, running, work hours, work pace, ability to concentrate, and capacity to work under conditions of tension, heat, cold, etc.

• Those restrictions of nonwork and work activities medically imposed to prevent an aggravation of the underlying heart disorder or to prevent further heart damage, such as advice to postmyocardial infarction patients not to subject themselves to sudden bursts of strenuous physical effort.

In those instances where the law requires that causation be apportioned between the parties (e.g., work-related versus non-work-related disabilities), the physician may be asked to furnish an opinion as to the causation of each of the impairments found. For example, in claims based on myocardial infarction, the physician may be asked what aspects of the impairments found are related to the underlying coronary atherosclerotic disease for which there may not be legal liability and what are related to the myocardial infarction itself for which there may exist legal responsibility.

In those situations where a patient-claimant has impairments coexisting from cardiac as well as noncardiac disorders, the physician may be asked to separate the impairments due to each disorder and, in assessing the overall combined impairments, whether noncardiac impairments, if present, magnify the impairment attributable to the heart disorder.

Where workers' compensation acts provide *second injury funds,* the examining or treating physician may be asked whether the disability from a cardiac injury in an employee with a known physical impairment from a congenital or acquired heart condition was made substantially greater by reason of the combined effects of such impairment and subsequent personal injury than that disability that would have resulted from the subsequent personal injury alone or if the death of the claimant would not have occurred except for the contribution of the preexisting physical impairment.

In reaching the conclusions expressed in the medical assessment of disability, all currently available objective means of diagnosis and measurement of cardiac function should be used within practical limits of risk to the patient and cost of the testing and in terms of the information to be obtained relative to the assessment. Wherever feasible, medical evaluations of disability should be based on objective findings to obviate depending only on subjective complaints, which are often unreliable because they are self-serving.

Medical assessments of cardiac impairment are significantly hampered by the following:

1. Reliance in most cases on subjective complaints.
2. Individual variations in symptoms, motivation, adjustment, and return-to-work desires among persons with similar cardiac abnormalities.
3. Paucity and limitations of currently available means for quantitative measurement of cardiac functional reserves.
4. Frequent discrepancy between objective findings and subjective complaints.

5. Practical difficulties in transferring the results of objective test measurements, such as those of exercise stress testing, under controlled environmental conditions, into the uncontrolled, variable environment of the workplace or other real-life settings in which hostile environments, often immeasurable, may significantly affect the demands placed on the heart.
6. The fact that most cardiac impairments are rarely static and cannot be considered to have reached an end result but are subject, because of the progressive nature of the underlying disorder and variations in therapeutic responses, to sudden change so that an impairment assessment or disability evaluation at a given date may be unpredictably rendered invalid for a later time.

The definition of disability from cardiovascular and/or other conditions for adults to qualify for benefits under the Social Security Insurance program requires an "inability to engage in any substantial gainful employment by reason of any medically determinable physical or mental impairment which can be expected to result in death or has lasted or is expected to last for a continuous period of not less than 12 months." The listing of impairment for each major body system, the applicable medical criteria, and the key concepts of medical evaluations are outlined and defined in the agency's handbook *Disability Evaluation under Social Security*[42] and on its web site on the internet.[43]

In workers' compensation, for both cardiac and noncardiac conditions, administrators in more and more states have turned to the American Medical Association's *Guides to the Evaluation of Permanent Impairment*[44] for determinations of qualifying disability as well as for rating the impairment in terms of percentage degree of functional loss that may qualify the injured worker for additional benefits in addition to lost wages.

The New York Heart Association's[14] grading system of cardiac functional capacity provides an easily understood, readily applicable guide to the medical description of cardiovascular impairment:

Class I. Patients with cardiac disease, but without resulting limitation of physical activity. Ordinary physical activity does not cause undue fatigue, palpitation, dyspnea, or anginal pain.

Class II. Patients with cardiac disease resulting in slight limitations of physical activity. They are comfortable at rest. Ordinary physical activity results in fatigue, palpitation, dyspnea, or anginal pain.

Class III. Patients with marked limitation of physical activity. They are comfortable at rest. Less than ordinary physical activity causes fatigue, palpitation, dyspnea, and anginal pain.

Class IV. Patients with cardiac disease resulting in inability to carry on any physical activity without discomfort. Symptoms of heart failure or of the anginal syndrome may be present even at rest. If any physical activity is undertaken, discomfort is increased.

For further discussion of medical evaluations and legal definitions of disability under a variety of situations plus extensive legal and medical references to disability assessments the reader is referred to the *Disability Handbook* of Balsam and Zabin[45] and its updated supplements.[46]

The legal aspects of commonly sought medical assessments of physical impairment by third-party physicians and the legal relationship of the third-party physician and the person being examined are discussed by Rothstein.[47]

As with causality assessments, medical and legal assessments of disability may vary considerably because of the difference in emphasis necessarily placed by each profession on individual aspects of the impairment in the disability rating process. Although a physician might consider a patient not disabled and, therefore, employable, the fact finder may declare the same person disabled from work activity under the terms of the applicable law or insurance contract. Here the physician must appreciate that in reaching the legal decision as to work capacity, the fact finder frequently has to include nonmedical elements such as age, sex, educational background, motivation, and prior work training and experience. Additionally, the fact finder's decision may be influenced by the availability of certain types of employment in the local or national labor market, the problems imposed by transportation to and from work sites, language or other communication problems, and other factors that, as a practical matter, so restrict a given person's opportunity for gainful employment as to make that individual practically disabled from gainful employment although medically cleared for work.

It is also important to recognize that because of differing statutory and contractual definitions, a person declared disabled and awarded benefits under one disability program may not be deemed eligible for benefits under another program. Thus, an award for disability by one agency or insurer does not, by itself, bind another agency or insurer. Each insurance contract or other disability benefit program or statute must be considered individually and separately for each claim raised, although the claim in each instance is based on the same medical disorders and impairments.

Prognosis and Life Expectancy Assessments

When considering a lump sum settlement of a disputed cardiac claim or when setting up a dollar reserve to cover future benefits, defendant attorneys and insurers often ask their cardiology expert for an opinion as to a claimant's future course, anticipated future treatment, and/or life expectancy based upon the medical findings and records. Estimates of the number of years a claimant with heart disease can reasonably be expected to live not only are utilized legally to establish economic and other losses in the consideration of awards for "damages" in tort cases of cardiac injury, but also may be significant in limiting potential "damages" by reason of the heart condition's expected reduction of life span in cases where the legal liability is for a noncardiac injury.[48]

Prognostic and life expectancy determinations realistically have to be based to a large extent upon statistical considera-

tions and parameters in reported series involving large numbers of patients. While statistical conclusions do not necessarily apply to a given individual patient, a medical assessment of a cardiac patient's expected need for and extent of future treatment and of life expectancy, formulated after thorough medical examination and based on valid scientific guidelines, can be relatively accurate within certain ranges, barring events unpredictable as to time of occurrence and, accordingly, of practical usefulness to the legal resolution of cardiac claims of persons with heart disease.

Determination of Malpractice

The risk of a physician being sued for professional negligence should a patient suffer an untoward result during the course of diagnosis and treatment is an inescapable fact of today's professional life. Choosing cardiology as a specialty increases this risk[49] because of a variety of reasons, particularly (1) the ever-present threat of sudden, unpredicted death due to the relentless progressive nature of most heart diseases independent of treatment or lack of treatment; (2) the adverse reactions often attributable to the narrow overlap between therapeutic and toxic ranges of commonly employed cardiac medications; (3) the inherent hazards and complications of exercise stress testing, invasive diagnostic procedures, and cardiac surgery; (4) the often-encountered lack of clear-cut diagnostic evidence or an atypical clinical presentation in the early stages of an acute myocardial infarction, thereby leading to the *emergency room turnaway* of patients in the throes of an attack, possibly resulting in late dire consequences; (5) the unavoidable mortality and morbidity associated with "last-ditch" heroic medical and surgical treatment of desperately ill patients in the end stages of heart disease; and (6) the many problems involved in obtaining *informed consent* for procedures beyond the understanding of most lay persons, particularly when frightened by the threats of a cardiac illness.

In medical malpractice cases, the aggrieved patient or those instituting the claim have the legal burden of demonstrating by factual and opinion evidence (1) that the defendant doctor or other health care provider named in the suit owed a duty to the plaintiff as is legally and morally implied in the physician-patient relationship; (2) that the defendant violated that duty by breaching the standard of care owed; (3) that the patient suffered injury or harm; (4) that the physician or other health care provider's negligence was the proximate cause of that harm; and (5) in some jurisdictions, that the patient's conduct did not negligently contribute to the alleged harm (the doctrine of contributory negligence). Unless all these elements are established in the courtroom by the plaintiff, the legal action will fail.

The evidentiary proof required of the plaintiff in establishing the bases of his or her action generally necessitates that expert medical opinion be provided that (1) defines the standard of care due the plaintiff by the defendant(s), (2) establishes the breach or failure to conform to that standard of care, (3) defines the injuries or "harms" claimed, and (4) causally relates the harms found to the claimed negligent action or failure to act on the part of the defendant(s).

Should a patient suffer harm during the course of medical diagnosis and treatment, the physician and/or other health care providers may be liable, separately or additionally, to two other legal actions besides that in tort. The first constitutes charges that the patient or those acting for him or her were not given sufficient information by the responsible professional persons to allow a legally valid "informed" consent to be made to a medically prescribed diagnostic test or treatment that resulted in injury and that, therefore, performance of the procedure or treatment was legally an "assault," subject to evidentiary requirements less stringent than those required in actions in tort as well as protected by a differing statute of limitations. The second possible legal action is one based on alleged *breach of contract* should a particular result or cure allegedly promised and thereby "guaranteed" not be achieved. In both of these actions, supportive expert medical opinions may not be necessary to substantiate the claim since the legal issue in dispute often hinges on the factual determination of whether the defendant physician did or did not say what the patient alleges was actually said or not said in information imparted or in guarantee of results and may not therefore require a separate demonstration of professional negligence.

Medical evaluation of a malpractice claim requires a careful review of all the claimant's medical records with particular attention, first, to whether the defendant's professional actions were in accord with generally accepted and proper standards of professional conduct and, second, to whether the alleged "harms" were causally related to the defendant's professional actions or failure to act.

In a medical evaluation of alleged professional negligence, the fact that a patient suffered injurious effects during or after a prescribed treatment or procedure does not by itself raise a legal presumption of negligence as a causative factor. A physician is not legally responsible for want of success in professional endeavors unless it is proved that the want of success followed from want of professional care and diligence ordinarily possessed by others in the profession. The determination, however, must give due regard to the state of advancement of medical science at the time of the treatment or procedure performance. Nor is a physician legally responsible for untoward results from errors in judgment in areas where reasonable doubt and uncertainty exist as to the course of action to be taken and no negligent act has been performed. As long as the professional judgment exercised does not represent a departure from the requirements of accepted medical practice or does not result in a failure to do something that accepted medical practice obligates or in a procedure that accepted medical practice precludes, the physician is not guilty of malpractice.

THE MEDICOLEGAL CARDIAC EXAMINATION

The techniques employed in medicolegal cardiac examinations are essentially the same as in medical examinations performed for treatment purposes. Generally, the basic components of history taking, physical examination, resting electrocardiogram, and chest roentgenogram plus review and study of the available medical records suffice. In claims where the patient-claimant is not available for examination, the evaluation may have to be made entirely on the basis of medical records provided. Rarely do the legal questions require the employment of one or more of the specialized cardiac diagnostic techniques. In such cases, the recommending physician must keep in mind the principles that govern the use of each diagnostic testing to be considered, the information it can be expected to provide, the limitations of results, the pitfalls in interpretation, the availability and cost of the procedure, and the inherent risks and hazards to the patient. All must be weighed carefully against the legal need for the information to be obtained.

Because of the key role of the medical history in legal issues of liability and disability rating, and because the special components of such history taking are not generally appreciated or utilized by physicians primarily interested in treating the patient, specific discussion of history taking for medicolegal evaluations and its implications is warranted.

When cardiac disorders have legal consequences, the content of the medical history ultimately accepted by the legal arbiter of the claim frequently makes or breaks the action instituted by the plaintiff-claimant. For example, in many workers' compensation cases there is often no dispute legally concerning insurance coverage and the presence of a disabling cardiac disorder for which benefits might be available under the law; rather, the key issue is whether a work-connected factor played a role in precipitating, triggering, hastening, aggravating, or otherwise "causing" the disorder or disability for which benefits are claimed. The crucial element in such causality assessments frequently is the medical history ultimately accepted by the fact finder as depicting the sequence of events and circumstances surrounding the occurrence of cardiac symptoms and the findings claimed to represent an injury.

In those situations where it is alleged or where it can be anticipated that it will later be alleged that the patient's heart disorder arose in some part out of employment, thereby entitling the person to workers' compensation benefits for disability, loss of earning capacity, and medical expenses, the examining physician should inquire about and include in the written history the sequence of events preceding and leading to the onset of symptoms for which the patient sought medical attention. Inquiry should also be made as to the specific work activities engaged in before, during, and after an alleged cardiac incident; whether these were customary and usual for the employee or comprised unaccustomed, unusual activities; and whether there were associated hostile environmental conditions that could have intensified the potential physiologic demands and thereby the cardiostressful attributes of the work effort, e.g., excessive heat or cold, humidity, dust or other respirator irritants, or undue associated psychological stress.

Similarly, in situations where mechanical trauma is alleged to be a cause of heart injury, as in tort cases involving motor vehicle accidents, inquiry should be directed to the exact type of mechanical forces involved, particularly the point or points of bodily contact; the effect on the patient's body such as jarring, whiplash, and dislodgment; the development and objective evidence of trauma such as cuts, lacerations, external bleeding, bruises, and ecchymoses; and the precise time and sequence of occurrence of symptoms and signs consistent with cardiac injury.

The list of potential questions that may be pertinent in the medicolegal history thus is virtually endless. In each case, therefore, the examiner's questioning must be tailored to provide the information needed to reach a reasonable medical conclusion for the facts on hand.

Hospital records generally contain more than one written history, depending on the number of persons who may be involved in the treatment of the patient. Significant historic facts, often of key legal significance, may be found in the admitting histories and progress notes of physicians, interns, residents, nurses, and medical students and in reports of consultants and occupational and physical therapists as well as in less obvious places, such as in requests for x-rays, laboratory determinations, and various diagnostic tests and reports. Accordingly, the physician asked to make a medical evaluation for legal purposes should request from the referring party, when deemed appropriate, the complete hospital records rather than only the discharge summary, so as to have the benefits of all the histories contained therein.

Because the medical history is derived by a question-and-answer interview between a physician and a patient-claimant, simultaneously or later transposed into a written narrative record, it is subject to many limitations of content, distortion, and error that may affect its legal value. Many of these limitations stem from a failure of the interviewer to ask pertinent questions, a failure of the interviewed patient to understand the questions asked or to respond appropriately, a bias of the interviewer, and self-serving motives of the interviewed patient. Typically, histories contained in hospital records are devoid of those items that later are of key importance in legal resolution of the claim. This is quite common in the history recorded at the time the patient is first seen with an actual or suspected acute myocardial infarction. In such situations, brevity in history taking is essential because of the urgent need to establish a diagnosis and institute lifesaving therapy rapidly. Characteristically, such histories make no mention of details relevant to causation that are crucial in later legal actions. In many instances, the attending physician, not aware of the potential legal actions that may stem from the patient's cardiac disorder, fails to record the detailed history necessary to resolve the legal aspects of the patient's illness, making it necessary that a detailed history be obtained at a later date at a time when the patient has become suspect as to reliability because of elements of financial or other gain associated with the institution of a claim for benefits.

THE MEDICOLEGAL
REPORT

The report prepared by the physician of the cardiac evaluation is an important document with far-reaching practical conse-

quences.[50] For the attorney or insurer to whom it is addressed, the report forms the basis for determining the pretrial acceptance or denial of the claim, the consideration of settlement negotiations, the pretrial preparation, and the courtroom presentation of the medical aspects of the case. For the physician, the time put forth in compiling a comprehensive medical report of the examination findings, summary of medical records, and conclusions drawn therefrom will later provide a useful refresher for the marshaling of the pertinent medical findings and the bases for the conclusions reached should the matter come to trial at some later date when details of the original examination have been forgotten or have dimmed with the passage of time. Carelessly composed, poorly prepared, or obviously biased medical reports frequently prove damaging and embarrassing to the physician called upon to testify at trial if they contain inaccuracies, inconsistencies, unwarranted medical conclusions, or omissions.

The composition of a medical report for legal and insurance purposes differs from that of the usual medical report in that it often requires inclusion of information not directly related to the treatment of a patient but essential for answering the various medical questions posed by the impending litigation. In most situations, the medicolegal report of a cardiac examination and findings is best presented in narrative form. As a minimum such a report should cover the following topics, preferably in the order listed:

- A recounting of the history personally related to the examining physician by the patient-claimant or outlined in the medical records reviewed should the evaluation have to be made without opportunity to examine the claimant, with particular emphasis on the sequence of events leading to the seeking of medical attention. In a workers' compensation claim, adequate facts must be recorded in the medical history as to the overall job duties and requirements, including consideration of possible noxious occupational exposures and psychological "stress," "pressures," and "tensions." There should also be detailed recounting of the work activity before, during, and after an alleged cardiac event. In an automobile accident or other situation where trauma is alleged as a cause of a cardiac "personal injury," there should be a description of the mechanical aspects of the contact or psychological sequelae that are important in an evaluation of the competency of the alleged trauma or stress to precipitate cardiac lesions and/or dysfunctions. The significant past medical history should be detailed, with particular reference to recognized background medical risk factors favoring premature development of atherosclerotic coronary heart disease and the existence of prior heart disorder or of other conditions that might affect the patient's susceptibility to cardiac injury and/or current medical status.

- A chronologic listing, with summary of the contents deemed important, of the various hospital and medical reports and other data reviewed by the physician and utilized in the formulation of the opinions reached. If death has occurred, the pertinent findings of autopsy.

- A detailing of the physical examination findings with description of all the abnormalities detected as well as the important negatives.
- The results of the various diagnostic studies performed or utilized by the examining physician in reaching conclusions of the evaluation.
- A statement of the complete cardiac diagnosis with substantiating reasons if the diagnosis is questionable or not firmly established.
- The examiner's opinion concerning each of the various medicolegal questions posed in the individual case with substantiating reasons that support the conclusions expressed.

The medicolegal report should conclude with the physician's signature in black ink for photocopy purposes and a certification—a simple maneuver that in many cases suffices for the report to be accepted into evidence without need for the personal appearance of the author to verify its authenticity. The following is an example that has been successfully employed:

CERTIFICATION: I hereby swear that I am a physician duly licensed in the state of _____ and further state that this written report of _____ pages dated _____ represents my report concerning _____ and is signed under the pains and penalties of perjury pursuant to the laws of this state, as cited in Chapter _____, Section _____.

Signed _____
Board certified in Internal Medicine
and Cardiovascular Diseases

Finally, it is imperative that the physician submitting a medicolegal report recognize that the report, in most cases, will be made available to opposing counsel in sufficient time for detailed close study and conference with his or her medical expert in preparation for a potential intensive cross-examination.

REFERENCES

1. McNiece HF. *Heart Disease and the Law*. Englewood Cliffs, NJ: Prentice-Hall; 1961.
2. Sagall EL, Reed BC. *The Heart and the Law—A Practical Guide to Medicolegal Cardiology*. New York: Macmillan; 1968.
3. Sagall EL, Reed BC. *The Law and Clinical Medicine*. Philadelphia: Lippincott; 1970.
4. "Analysis of Workers' Compensation Laws," prepared and published annually by the Chamber of Commerce of the United States, 1615 H Street, NW, Washington, DC 20062.
5. Sagall EL. Heart disease, workmen's compensation and the practicing physician. *N Engl J Med* 1961; 264:699–705.
6. Sagall EL. Compensable heart disease. *Trial* 1969; 5:29–31.
7. LaDou J, Mulryan LE, McCarthy KJ. Cumulative injury or disease claims: An attempt to define employers' liability for workers' compensation. *Am J Law Med* 1980; 6:1–28.
8. Sullivan RT. Heart injuries under workers' compensation: Medical and legal considerations. *Suffolk Univ Law Rev* 1980; 14:1365–1401.
9. Wyo Stat § 27-12-603(b) (1977).
10. (a) Nev Rev Stat Ann, Title 53, Ch 616.110 (1985). (b) Nev Rev Stat Ann, Title 53, Ch 617.457 (1973).
11. Mass. Gen. Laws Ch 32 § 94 (1956).
12. Longshoremen's and Harbor Workers' Compensation Act, Amendments of 1972, Sec. 20.
13. The Americans with Disabilities Act 42 U.S.C. 12101, *et seq.*
14. Criteria Committee of the New York Heart Association. *Nomenclature and Criteria for Diagnosis of Diseases of the Heart and Great Vessels*, 9th ed. Boston: Little, Brown;1994.
15. Small B. Gaffing at a thing called cause: Medico-legal conflicts in the concept of causation. *Texas Law Rev* 1953; 31:630–659.
16. Sagall EL. Heart disease and the law—medico-legal considerations of causality. *Tenn Law Rev* 1963; 30:517–535.
17. Sagall EL, Reed BC. The legal assessment of causality. *Med Science* 1967; 18(July):51–54.
18. Sagall EL. Causality assessment—medical vs. legal. *Trial* 1969; 5(June/July):59–60.
19. Danner D, Sagall EL. Medicolegal causation: A source of professional misunderstanding. *Am J Law Med* 1977; 3:303–308.
20. American Heart Association. Report of the Committee on Stress, Strain, and Heart Disease. *Circulation* 1977; 55:825A–835A.
21. Muller JE, Toffler GH, Stone PH. Circadian variation and triggers of onset of acute cardiovascular disease. *Circulation* 1989; 79:733–743.
22. Brodsky MA, Allen BJ. Stress, cardiac arrhythmias, and sudden cardiac death. *Practical Cardiol* 1989; 15:49A–55A.
23. Muller JE, Toffler GH, eds. A symposium: Triggering and circadian variation of acute cardiovascular disease. *Am J Cardiol* 1990; 66:1G–70G.
24. Johnson RJ. Sudden death during exercise. A cruel turn of events.*Postgrad Med* 1992; 92:195–206.
25. Mittleman MA, Maclure M, Toffler GH, Sherwood JB, Goldberg RJ, Muller JE. Triggering of acute myocardial infarction by heavy physical exertion. Protection against triggering by regular exertion. *N Engl J Med* 1993; 329:1677–1690.
26. Muller JE, Abela GS, Nesto RW, Toffler GH. Triggers, acute risk factors and vulnerable plaques: The lexicon of a new frontier. *J Am Coll Cardiol* 1994; 23:809–813.
27. Taylor CB. Anger, angina, and ischemia. *J Myocard Ischemia* 1994; 6:11–17.
28. Gottdiener JS, Krantz DS, Howell RH, Hecht GM, Klein J, Falconer JJ, et al. Induction of silent myocardial ischemia with mental stress testing: Relation to triggers of ischemia during daily life activities and to ischemic functional severity. *J Am Coll Cardiol* 1994; 24:1645–1651.
29. Maron BJ, Poliac LC, Kaplan JA, Myeller FO. Blunt impact to the chest leading to sudden death from cardiac arrest during sports activities. *N Engl J Med* 1995; 333:337–342.
30. Mittleman MA, Maclure M, Sherwood JB, Mulry RP, Toffler GH, Jacobs SC, et al. Triggering of acute myocardial onset by episodes of anger. *Circulation* 1995; 92:1720–1725.
31. Gabbay FH, Krantz DS, Kop WJ, Hedges SM, Klein J, Gottdiener JS, et al. Triggers of myocardial ischemia during daily life in patients with coronary artery disease: Physical and mental activities, anger and smoking. *J Am Coll Cardiol* 1996; 27:585–592.
32. Krantz DS, Kop WJ, Gabbay FH, Rozanski A, Barnard M, Klein J, et al. Circadian variation of ambulatory myocardial ischemia. Triggering by daily activities and evidence of an endogenous circadian component. *Circulation* 1996; 93:1364–1371.
33. Sagall EL, Reed BC. Heart disorder due to emotional stress: Medical and legal aspects. *Med Counterpoint* 1969; 1(April):15–43.
34. *Proceedings of the Conference on Stress, Strain, Heart Disease and the Law,* Boston, Jan. 26–28, 1978. US Government Printing Office, Publication 790-281-412/107, 1979.
35. *Stress in the Workplace: Costs, Liability and Prevention.* Rockville, MD: The Bureau of National Affairs; 1987.
36. Hlatky MA, Lam LC, Lee KL, Clapp-Channing NE, Williams RB, Pryor DB, et al. Job strain and the prevalence and outcome of coronary artery disease. *Circulation* 1995; 92:327–333.
37. *New Hampshire Supply Company, Inc. et al.* v. *Edith Steinberg et al.* 121 N.H. 506, 433 A.2d 1247 (1981).
38. *Helen F. Mulcahey* v. *New England Newspapers, Inc.* 488 A.2d 681 (R.I. 1985).
39. *City of Boulder* v. *Barbara E. Streeb et al.* 706 P.2d 786 (Colo. 1985).
40. *Rosalie McDonough* v. *Connecticut Bank and Trust Company et al.* 204 Conn. 104 527 A. 2d 664 (1987).
41. *Cunningham* v. *City of Manchester Fire Department.* 129 N.H. 232.

42. *Disability Evaluation under Social Security.* DHEW Publication No. 05-10089, Washington, DC, US Government Printing Office, February 1986.

43. http://www.ohsu.edu/disability/adult.html.

44. Committee on Rating of Mental and Physical Impairment, American Medical Association. *Guides to the Evaluation of Permanent Impairment,* 4th ed. Chicago: American Medical Association; 1993.

45. Balsam A, Zabin AP. *Disability Handbook.* Colorado Springs: Shepard's/McGraw-Hill; 1990.

46. Balsam A, Zabin AP. *Disability Handbook. 1995 cumulative supplement. Current through December, 1994.* Colorado Springs: Shepard's/McGraw-Hill; 1995.

47. Rothstein MA. Legal issues in the medical assessment of physical impairment by third-party physicians. *J Leg Med* 1984; 5:503–548.

48. Sagall EL. Life expectancy determination. *Trial* 1969; 5(Aug/Sep):59–62.

49. Sagall EL, Lucas I, eds. *Malpractice Hazards in Cardiology* (proceedings, symposium, Boston, May 12, 1971). Boston: Massachusetts Heart Association; 1973.

50. Sagall EL. Physician's medical report. *Trial* 1972; 8(Jan/Feb):59–62.

NOTES

NOTES

NOTES

NOTES

NOTES

NOTES

INDEX

Numbers followed by an "f" or a "t" refer to figures or tables.

INDEX